Forfar and Arneil's
Textbook of Pediatrics

For Churchill Livingstone

Commissioning Editors: Timothy Horne, Inta Ozols
Project Editor: Antonia Seymour
. *Project Controller:* Kay Hunston
Project Assistant: Isobel Black
Copy Editors: Susan Beasley, Stephanie Pickering, Holly Regan-Jones
Design Direction: Judith Wright
Designer: Keith Kail
Indexer: John Sampson

Forfar and Arneil's
Textbook of Pediatrics

Edited by

A. G. M. Campbell
MB FRCP(Edin) HonFRCPCH DCH
Emeritus Professor of Child Health, University of Aberdeen,
Aberdeen, UK

Neil McIntosh
DSc(Med) FRCP(Edin) FRCP(Lond) FRCPCH
Professor of Child Life and Health, University of Edinburgh,
Edinburgh, UK

FIFTH EDITION

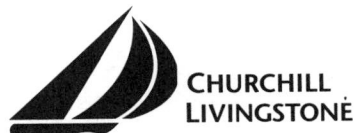
CHURCHILL
LIVINGSTONE

NEW YORK EDINBURGH LONDON MADRID MELBOURNE SAN FRANCISCO AND TOKYO 1998

CHURCHILL LIVINGSTONE
Medical Division of Pearson Professional Limited

Distributed in the United States of America by Churchill Livingstone Inc., 650 Avenue of the Americas, New York, N.Y. 10011, and by associated companies, branches and representatives throughout the world.

First edition 1973
Second edition 1978
Third edition 1984
Fourth edition 1992
Fifth edition 1998

ISBN 0 443 053936

British Library Cataloguing in Publication Data
A catalogue record for this book is available from the British Library.

Library of Congress Cataloging in Publication Data
A catalog record for this book is available from the Library of Congress.

Note
Medical knowledge is constantly changing. As new information becomes available, changes in treatment, procedures, equipment and the use of drugs become necessary. The authors and the publishers have, as far as it is possible, taken care to ensure that the information given in this text is accurate and up to date. However, readers are strongly advised to confirm that the information, especially with regard to drug usage, complies with latest legislation and standards of practice.

The publisher's policy is to use paper manufactured from sustainable forests

Printed in Great Britain by BPC Wheatons Ltd, Exeter

Contents

Preface   vii
Acknowledgments   viii
Contributors   ix
Color plates   xv–xxvi

1   Demography, vital statistics and the pattern of disease in childhood   1
2   History taking and physical examination   16
3   Genetics   45
4   Obstetric aspects of perinatal care   79
5   The newborn   93
6   Infant feeding   326
7   Preventive pediatrics   337
8   Physical growth and development   349
9   Psychomotor and intellectual development   381
10   Fluid, electrolyte and acid-base disturbances   402
11   Disorders of the alimentary tract and liver   423
12   Respiratory disorders   489
13   Cardiovascular disease   584
14   Disorders of the central nervous system   641
15   Disorders of the blood and reticuloendothelial system   847
16   Oncology and terminal care   884
17   Disorders of the urinary system   934
18   Gynecological diseases   985
19   Endocrine gland disorders and disorders of growth and puberty   996
20   Inborn errors of metabolism   1099
21   Nutrition   1179
22   Immunodeficiency   1231
23   Infections   1273
24   Disorders of bone, joints and connective tissue   1544
25   Diseases of the skin   1616
26   Disorders of the eye   1649
27   Disorders of the ear, nose and throat   1679
28   Allergic disorders   1689
29   Poisoning, accidents and sudden infant death syndrome   1705
30   Psychiatric disorders   1727
31   Surgical pediatrics   1768
32   Emergency care   1802
33   Practical procedures   1829
34   Social and legal aspects of pediatrics   1848
35   Child care in developing countries   1882
36   Practical aspects of diagnostic imaging   1894
37   Biochemical and physiological tables and reference ranges for laboratory tests   1921
38   Pediatric prescribing   1953
Index   1981

Preface

To the Editors, and no doubt the contributors, it seems only a short time since the publication of the 4th edition. However, it soon became obvious that a new edition was necessary by 1998 if we were to keep pace with current progress in pediatrics and child health. This 5th edition also gives us an opportunity to respond to some of the helpful suggestions made by those readers who kindly took the time to comment on the 4th edition.

Most chapters and sections have been revised by the original authors but the introduction of some new contributors has meant that some chapters have been extensively rewritten with the advantage of a fresh approach. Two new chapters have been added: one dealing with Accident and Emergency Pediatrics and Intensive Care; and one on Disorders of the Ear, Nose and Throat. Pediatric Gynecology is no longer embedded within the Urogenital System but appears as a separate chapter. Considering how much time most of our contributors need to spend on the increasing demands and responsibilities of their employment, some delay from the originally planned publication date was probably inevitable but, like all editors, we are particularly grateful to the authors who kept to their deadlines.

We welcome all new contributors and, at the same time, wish to express our gratitude and thanks to those who have departed. Their efforts contributed greatly to the success of previous editions and much of their work is still apparent in these pages.

Our thanks are also due to the many secretaries in the UK and elsewhere without whose efforts no books of this size would be possible. Particular thanks are due to Elaine Forbes and Lisa M. Horsburgh in Edinburgh.

We are also grateful to Lucy Gardiner, Inta Ozols, Antonia Seymour and Graham Birnie of Churchill Livingstone for their help and advice at various stages of the project.

Aberdeen and Edinburgh 1998

A.G.M.C.
N.McI.

Acknowledgments

We gratefully acknowledge the following material that has been borrowed from the copyright holders listed below. We have sought permission wherever possible but if we have inadvertently missed any, we should like to be informed so that we can make changes at the first possible opportunity.

Fig. 3.29: Oxford University Press, Oxford
Fig. 4.2: British Medical Journal 285 (1982) – BMJ Publishing Group, London
Fig. 5.2: Journal of Pediatrics 81 (1972) – Mosby-Year Book, St Louis
Fig. 5.6: Charles C. Thomas Publisher, Springfield
Fig. 5.13: Blackwell Science, Oxford
Fig. 5.15, 5.19: Archives of Disease in Childhood 48 (1973) – BMJ Publishing Group, London
Fig. 5.44: Academic Press, New York
Fig. 5.45: Gastroenterology 74 (1978) – W B Saunders, Orlando
Fig. 5.47: Journal of the American Chemical Society 104 (1982) – American Chemical Society, Washington
Fig. 5.59: Developmental Medicine and Child Neurology 30 (1988) – MacKeith Press, London
Fig. 6.2: Early Human Development 9 (1984) – Elsevier Science Ireland, Co. Clare
Figs 8.1, 8.6, 8.8: Blackwell Science, Oxford
Figs 8.3, 8.11: Archives of Disease in Childhood 41 (1966) – BMJ Publishing Group, London
Figs 8.7, 8.10: Dr J M Tanner
Fig. 8.9: Archives of Disease in Childhood 45 (1970) – BMJ Publishing Group, London
Fig. 8.13: University of Minnesota Press, Minneapolis
Fig. 8.14: Clinical Endocrinology 27 (1987) – Blackwell Science, Oxford
Fig. 11.1: John Wiley, Chichester

Fig. 11.18: Butterworth-Heinemann, Oxford
Table 13.2: British Heart Journal 46 (1981) – BMJ Publishing Group, London
Table 13.6: Journal of Clinical Pharmacology 4 (1984) – Lippincott-Raven, Philadelphia
Figs 14.23, 14.24: Developmental Medicine and Child Neurology 35 (1993) – MacKeith Press, London
Figs 15.1, 15.2, 15.14: Butterworth-Heinemann, Oxford
Fig. 15.6: Pediatric Clinics of North America 19 (1972) – W B Saunders, Philadelphia
Figs 15.7, 15.8, 15.11: Blackwell Science, Oxford
Fig. 19.19: Journal of Clinical Endocrinology and Metabolism 70 (1990) – The Endocrine Society, Bethesda
Fig. 22.7: W B Saunders, Philadelphia
Table 23.23: Archives of Disease in Childhood 70 (1994) – BMJ Publishing Group, London; and Dr J Darbyshire
Figs 23.9, 23.10, 23.14, 23.15, 23.16, 23.17, 23.20, 23.21, 23.22: Mosby-Year Book, St Louis
Table 23.10: Oxford University Press, Oxford
Fig. 23.47: Nature 212 (1966) – Macmillan Magazines, London
Table 24.2: Professor Robert J Gorlin
Table 24.3: Journal of Pediatrics 71 (1967) – Mosby-Year Book, St Louis
Figs 24.5, 24.8, 24.9, 24.18: Blackwell Science, Oxford
Figs 24.10, 24.22: Journal of Bone and Joint Surgery 50B (1968) and 72B (1990), London
Fig. 24.46: Georg Thieme, Stuttgart
Table 30.3: John Wiley, Chichester
Tables 37.2 and 37.3: Pediatrics 98 (1966) – American Academy of Pediatrics, Illinois

Contributors

N. Archer MA FRCP DCH
Consultant Paediatric Cardiologist, John Radcliffe Hospital, Oxford; Honorary Clinical Senior Lecturer, Department of Paediatrics, University of Oxford, Oxford, UK

Alastair James Baker MBChB MRCP(UK)
Consultant Paediatric Hepatologist, The Variety Club Children's Hospital, Kings College Hospital, London, UK

A. P. Ball BSc MBChB FRCP(Edin)
Honarary Senior Lecturer, Department of Medical Sciences, University of St Andrews, St Andrews, UK

Frank N. Bamford MD FFPHM FRCP HonFRCPCH
Retired. Reader and Honorary Consultant in Developmental Paediatrics, University Department of Child Health, St Mary's Hospital, Manchester, UK

Donald Barltrop MD BSc FRCP DCH
Professor of Child Health, Charing Cross and Westminster Medical School, Academic Department of Child Health, Chelsea and Westminster Hospital, London, UK

Ross St C. Barnetson MD FRCP FRACP FACD
Professor of Dermatology, University of Sydney, New South Wales, Australia

D. G. D. Barr MBChB FRCP(Edin) DCH
Consultant Paediatrician, Royal Hospital for Sick Children, Edinburgh; Senior Lecturer, Department of Child Life and Health, University of Edinburgh, Edinburgh, UK

Thomas F. Beattie MB FRCS(Edin) FFAEM DCH
Consultant, Paediatric Accident and Emergency Care, Royal Hospital for Sick Children, Edinburgh, UK

Neville R. Belton BSc PhD CChem MRSC FRCPCH
Senior Lecturer, Department of Child Life and Health, University of Edinburgh, Edinburgh, UK

Guy T. N. Besley PhD
Head of Laboratory, Willink Biochemical Genetics Unit, Royal Manchester Children's Hospital, Manchester, UK

W. Michael Bisset BSc MBChB DCH MSc MD FRCP
Consultant in Paediatrics and Paediatric Gastroenterology, Royal Aberdeen Children's Hospital, Aberdeen, UK

Bernard John Brabin MBChB MSc PhD FRCPC FRCPCH
Senior Lecturer in Tropical Paediatrics, Liverpool School of Tropical Medicine; Honorary Consultant Community Paediatrics, Royal Liverpool Children's Hospital NHS Trust, Alder Hey, Liverpool, UK

John Keith Brown MBChB FRCP DCH
Consultant Paediatric Neurologist, Royal Hospital for Sick Children, Edinburgh, UK

Elaine Buchanan BSc SRD
Senior I Dietitian, Yorkhill NHS Trust, Glasgow, UK

Neil R. M. Buist MBChB FRCPE DCH
Professor, Paediatrics and Medical Genetics, Oregon Health Sciences University, Portland, Oregon, USA

A. G. M. Campbell MB FRCP(Edin) HonFRCPCH DCH
Emeritus Professor of Child Health, University of Aberdeen, Aberdeen, UK

Harry Campbell MD FRCP MFPHM
Senior Lecturer, Department of Public Health Sciences, University of Edinburgh, Edinburgh, UK

James Stanley Cant MBChB FRCS(Edin) FRCS(Glas) FRCOphth DO(Eng)
Visiting Ophthalmic Surgeon (retd), Royal Hospital for Sick Children, Glasgow, UK

Brenda J. Clark BSc(Hons) SRD
Chief Dietitian, Yorkhill NHS Trust, Glasgow, UK

G. J. Connett MBChB DCH MRCP MD
Paediatric Respiratory Consultant, Southampton University Hospital, Southampton, UK

G. C. Cook MD DSc FRCP FRACP FLS
Physician, Hospital for Tropical Diseases and University College London Hospitals, London; Lecturer, London School of Hygeine and Tropical Medicine, London, UK

J. Brian S. Coulter MD FRCPI DCH
Senior Lecturer in Tropical Child Health, Liverpool School of Tropical Medicine; Honorary Consultant, Royal Liverpool Children's NHS Trust, Alder Hey, Liverpool, UK

David L. Cowan MBChB FRCSE
Consultant Otolaryngologist, Royal Hospital for Sick Children, Edinburgh and Honorary Senior Lecturer, University of Edinburgh Medical School, Edinburgh, UK

Patricia M. Crofton MA PhD
Principal Grade Biochemist, Department of Paediatric
Biochemistry, Royal Hospital for Sick Children, Edinburgh, UK

William A. M. Cutting MBChB FRCPE DCH
Reader in Child Health, University of Edinburgh; Honorary
Consultant Paediatrician, Royal Hospital for Sick Children,
Edinburgh, UK

Mohul Dattani MBBS DCH MRCP MD
Lecturer in Paediatric Endocrinology, Institute of Child Health,
London, UK

Timothy J. David PhD MD FRCP DCH
Professor of Child Health and Paediatrics, University of
Manchester and Honorary Consultant Paediatrician, Booth Hall
Children's Hospital, Royal Manchester Children's Hospital and
St Mary's Hospital, Manchester, UK

E. Graham Davies MA FRCP
Consultant and Senior Lecturer in Child Health, St George's
Hospital Medical School, London

Ruth E. Day MBChB FRCP
Consultant Paediatrician, Department of Neurology and Child
Development, Royal Hospital for Sick Children, Glasgow, UK

P. R. F. Dear MD FRCP DCH
Consultant and Senior Lecturer in Neonatal Medicine, St
James's University Hospital, Leeds, UK

Edward Doyle MD FRCA
Consultant Anaesthetist, Royal Hospital for Sick Children,
Edinburgh; Part-time Senior Lecturer, University of Edinburgh,
Edinburgh, UK

Tim O. B. Eden MBBS DRCOG FRCP(Edin) FRCP FRCPath MRCPCH
Cancer Research Campaign Professor of Paediatric Oncology,
University of Manchester and Honorary Consultant, Christie
Hospital NHS Trust and Manchester Children's Hospitals Trust,
Manchester, UK

Christine A. Edwards BSc PhD
Senior Lecturer, Department of Human Nutrition, Glasgow
University, Yorkhill Hospitals, Glasgow, UK

T. Eldridge SCM NNEB ENB 401 Course
Senior Midwife, Neonatal Unit, St George's Hospital, London,
UK

T. J. Evans FRCP
Consultant Paediatrician, Royal Hospital for Sick Children,
Yorkhill, Glasgow, UK

T. R. Fenton MD FRCP MSc
Consultant Paediatrician, Department of Paediatrics, Greenwich
District Hospital, London, UK

John Fernandes MD
Emeritus Professor of Paediatrics, Beatrix Children's Hospital,
University Hospital Groningen, Groningen, The Netherlands

Alistair R. Fielder FRCP FRCS FRCOphth
Kennerley Bankes Professor of Ophthalmology, Academic Unit
of Ophthalmology, Imperial College School of Medicine at St
Mary's Western Eye Hospital, London, UK

Peter J. Fleming MBChB PhD FRCP FRCP(C) MRCPCH
Professor of Infant Health and Developmental Physiology;
Consultant Paediatrician, Institute of Child Health, Royal
Hospital for Children, Bristol, UK

John O. Forfar MC FRSE BSc MD FRCP(Edin) FRCP(Lond)
FRCP(Glas) DCH FACN FRCPCH(Honorary)
Professor Emeritus of Child Life and Health, University of
Edinburgh; Former Consultant Physician, Royal Hospital for
Sick Children, Edinburgh and Consultant Paediatrician, Simpson
Memorial Maternity Pavilion, Royal Infirmary, Edinburgh, UK

Anne S. Garden MBChB FRCOG
Senior Lecturer, Obstetrics and Gynaecology and Lecturer in
Child Health (Gynaecology), University of Liverpool; Honorary
Consultant Obstetrician and Gynaecologist, Liverpool Women's
Hospital Trust, Liverpool, UK

Alasdair M. Geddes CBE MBChB FRCP FRCPath
Professor of Infection, Department of Infection, University of
Birmingham, Birmingham, UK

M. J. Godman MBChB FRCP(Edin)
Consultant Paediatric Cardiologist, Royal Hospital for Sick
Children; Senior Lecturer, Department of Child Life and Health,
University of Edinburgh, Edinburgh, UK

Krishna Goel MD FRCP(Lond, Edin and Glas)
Consultant Paediatrician and Honorary Clinical Senior Lecturer,
Royal Hospital for Sick Children, Glasgow, UK

John M. Goldsmid MSc PhD FRCPath FACTM FASM FIBiol FAIBiol
Professor in Medical Microbiology, Division of Pathology,
University of Tasmania, Hobart, Tasmania

I. Gordon FRCR
Consultant Radiologist, Great Ormond Street Hospital for
Children, London, UK

Diab Farhan Haddad MD MRCP
Lecturer in Child Health, Ninewells Hospital and Medical
School, University of Dundee, Dundee, UK

Henry L. Halliday MD FRCPE FRCP MCPCH DCH D(Obst)RCOG
Consultant Neonatologist, Royal Maternity Hospital, Belfast,
Royal Belfast Hospital for Sick Children, Jubilee Maternity
Hospital, Belfast and Mater Hospital, Belfast; Honorary
Professor of Child Health, The Queen's University of Belfast,
Belfast, UK

Ian M. Hann MD FRCP FRCP(Glas) FRCPCH FRCPath
Consultant Haematologist, Department of Haematology, Great
Ormond Street Children's Hospital, London, UK

Khalid N. Haque FRCP(Lond, Edin, Ire) FAAP FPAMS(Pak) FICP
MRCPCH MBA DCH(Lond) DTM&H
Senior Lecturer and Consultant Neonatologist, St Helier
Hospital, Carshalton, UK

Paul T. Heath MBBS FRACP
Paediatric Research Fellow, Department of Paediatrics, John
Radcliffe Hospital, Oxford, UK

John Henderson MD FRCP
Consultant Paediatrician, Bristol Royal Hospital for Sick
Children; Senior Lecturer, University of Bristol, Bristol, UK

George Michael A. Hendry MBBS DMRD FRCR
Consultant Paediatric Radiologist, Royal Hospital for Sick
Children, Edinburgh, UK

Peter Hoare DM FRCPsych
Senior Lecturer, University of Edinburgh; Honorary Consultant
Psychiatrist, Royal Hospital for Sick Children, Edinburgh, UK

Alan B. Houston MD MBChB FRCP(Glas) DCH
Consultant Paediatric Cardiologist, Royal Hospital for Sick
Children, Glasgow, UK

Robert Hume BSc MBChB PhD FRCP(Edin)
Reader, Department of Child Health, University of Dundee;
Consultant Paediatrician, Ninewells Hospital and Medical
School, Dundee, UK

David Isaacs MBBChir MD MRCP FRACP
Clinical Associate Professor and Head, Department of
Immunology and Infectious Diseases, New Children's Hospital,
Westmead, Sydney, Australia

Huw R. Jenkins MA MD FRCP MCPH
Consultant Paediatric Gastroenterologist, University Hospital of
Wales, Cardiff, UK

Alison M. Johnston BSc SRD
Senior 1 Paediatric Dietitian (Diabetes), Diabetes Service, Royal
Hospital for Sick Children, Yorkhill, Glasgow, UK

Frank D. Johnstone MD FRCOG
Senior Lecturer, Department of Obstetrics and Gynaecology,
University of Edinburgh; Consultant Obstetrician and
Gynaecologist, Simpson Memorial Maternity Pavilion,
Edinburgh, UK

Christopher J. H. Kelnar MA MD FRCP FRCPCH DCH
Consultant Paediatric Endocrinologist, Royal Hospital for Sick
Children, Edinburgh; Senior Lecturer, Department of Child Life
and Health, University of Edinburgh, Edinburgh, UK

Nancy G. Kennaway DPhil
Professor of Molecular and Medical Genetics and Director of the
Biochemical Genetics Laboratory, Oregon Health Sciences
University, Portland, USA

Alastair I. G. Kerr MB FRCS(Edin and Glas)
Consultant Otolaryngologist, Edinburgh Royal Infirmary and
Royal Hospital for Sick Children, Edinburgh; Honorary Senior
Lecturer, University of Edinburgh, Edinburgh, UK

M. A. Kibel MBBCh(Wits) FRCP(Edin) DCH(Lon)
Emeritus Professor of Child Health, University of Cape Town,
Cape Town, South Africa

Derek J. King MBChB FRCP(Edin) FRCPath
Consultant Haematologist, Royal Aberdeen Children's Hospital;
Clinical Senior Lecturer, University of Aberdeen, Aberdeen, UK

Ian A. Laing MA MD FRCPE
Clinical Director, Neonatal Unit, Simpson Memorial Maternity
Pavilion, Edinburgh; Senior Lecturer, Department of Child Life
and Health, University of Edinburgh, Edinburgh, UK

David P. Lessels LLB BPhil
Senior Lecturer in Law, University of Aberdeen, Aberdeen, UK

Malcolm I. Levene MD FRCP
Professor of Paediatrics and Child Health, University of Leeds,
The General Infirmary at Leeds, Leeds, UK

Jean-Pierre Lin BSc(MedSci) MBChB MRCP(UK)
Consultant Paediatric Neurologist, Newcomen Centre and One
Small Step Gait and Movement Laboratory, Guy's Hospital,
Guy's and St Thomas' Hospital Trust, London, UK

Roxy N. S. Lo MBBS DCH(Ire) MRCP(UK) FRCP(Glas)
Honorary Consultant Paediatric Cardiologist, Department of
Paediatric Cardiology, Grantham Hospital, Hong Kong

Robert W. Logan TD MBChB BSc(Hons) FRCP(Glas) FRCPath
Senior Lecturer in Clinical Biochemistry, University of Glasgow;
Honorary Consultant Medical Biochemist, Royal Hospital for
Sick Children and Queen Mother's Hospital, Glasgow, UK

A. M. MacConnachie BSc(Hons) MSc MRPS MCPP
Principal Pharmacist and Honorary Lecturer, Ninewells Hospital
and Medical School, University of Dundee, Dundee, UK

Mary E. McGraw MBChB FRCP DCH
Consultant Paediatric Nephrologist, Children's Renal Unit,
Southmead Hospital, Bristol, UK

Neil McIntosh DSc(Med) FRCP(Edin) FRCP(Lond) FRCPCH
Professor of Child Life and Health, University of Edinburgh,
Edinburgh, UK

Sheila McKenzie MD FRCP
Consultant Paediatrician and Honorary Senior Lecturer, Queen
Elizabeth Hospital for Children, London, UK

Gordon A. MacKinlay MBBS LRCP FRCS(Edin) FRCS
Senior Lecturer, Department of Clinical Surgery, University of
Edinburgh; Consultant Paediatric Surgeon, Royal Hospital for
Sick Children, Edinburgh, UK

A. McMillan MD FRCP(Lond) FRCP(Edin)
Consultant Physician, Department of Genito-urinary Medicine,
Royal Infirmary, Edinburgh; Part-time Senior Lecturer and Head
of Genito-urinary Medicine Unit, Department of Medicine,
University of Edinburgh, Edinburgh, UK

Janice Main MBChB FRCP(Edin & Lond)
Senior Lecturer, Department of Medicine, St Mary's Hospital,
London, UK

Duncan J. Matthew MBChB FRCP DCH
Clinical Director of Paediatrics, King Fahd Armed Forces
Hospital, Jeddah, Saudi Arabia; Honorary Consultant, Great
Ormond Street Hospital for Children, London, UK

A. E. Mills MA MB DCP DPath FRCPA FFPath RCPI FACTM
Pathologist, Bendigo, Victoria, Australia; Formerly Senior
Specialist and Senior Lecturer, Red Cross Children's Hospital
and University of Cape Town, Cape Town, South Africa

Robert A. Minns PhD FRCP(Edin) FRCPCH
Senior Lecturer, Department of Child Life and Health,
University of Edinburgh; Consultant Paediatric Neurologist,
Department of Paediatric Neurology, Royal Hospital for Sick
Children, Edinburgh, UK

Jacqueline Y. Q. Mok MD FRCP(Edin) DCH(Glas) MBChB
Consultant Paediatrician, Edinburgh Sick Children's NHS Health
Trust; Part-time Senior Lecturer, Department of Child Life and
Health, University of Edinburgh, Edinburgh, UK

Malcolm E. Molyneux MD FRCP
Professor of Tropical Medicine, Wellcome Trust Centre, College
of Medicine, University of Malawi, Malawi

The late A. P. Mowat MBChB FRCP DObst&RCOG DCH
Consultant Paediatrician and Paediatric Hepatologist; Professor
in Child Health, Kings College Hospital School of Medicine and
Dentistry, London, UK

E. Richard Moxon MB BChir FRCP
Professor (Action Research) of Paediatrics, University of
Oxford, Oxford, UK

Miranda Mugford BA(Hons) DPhil
Senior Lecturer (Health Services Research), School of Health
Policy and Practice, University of East Anglia, Norwich, UK

Dilip Nathwani FRCP(Edin) DTM&H
Consultant Physician and Honorary Senior Lecturer in Medicine
and Infectious Diseases, Dundee Teaching Hospital NHS Trust,
Dundee, UK

Simon J. Newell MD MRCPCH FRCP
Consultant in Neonatal Medicine and Paediatrics, St James's
University Hospital, Leeds; Honorary Senior Clinical Lecturer,
University of Leeds, Leeds, UK

Angus Nicoll MA MSc FRCP FFPHM
Consultant Epidemiologist, PHLS Communicable Disease
Surveillance Centre and Medical Adviser (Infectious Diseases),
British Paediatric Surveillance Unit (Royal College of
Paediatrics and Child Health), London, UK

Vas Novelli FRCP FRACP
Consultant in Paediatric Infectious Diseases, Great Ormond
Street Children's Hospital, London, UK

Anne E. O'Hare MD FRCP
Consultant Paediatrician, Department of Community Child
Health, Edinburgh; Senior Lecturer, Department of Child Life
and Health, University of Edinburgh, Edinburgh, UK

Richard E. Olver BSc MBBS FRCP FRCPE
Professor and Head of Department of Child Health, University
of Dundee, Ninewells Hospital and Medical School, Dundee, UK

Mary E. O'Regan MB MRCP(UK) DCH
Research Fellow, Department of Paediatric Neurology, Royal
Hospital for Sick Children, Edinburgh, UK

Clodagh O' Reilly FRCP(Ire)
Consultant Paediatrician, Cavan General Hospital, Cavan,
Republic of Ireland

Michael A. Patton MB MA MSc FRCP
Reader in Medical Genetics, St George's Hospital Medical
School, London; Consultant Clinical Geneticist, S. W. Thames
Regional Genetic Service, London, UK

M. A. Preece MD MSc FRCP
Professor of Child Health and Growth, Institute of Child Health,
University College London Medical School, London, UK

John W. L. Puntis DM FRCP MRCPCH
Senior Lecturer, Division of Paediatrics and Child Health,
University of Leeds; Consultant Paediatric Gastroenterologist,
The Children's Centre, The General Infirmary at Leeds, Leeds,
UK

T. M. S. Reid BMedBiol MBChB FRCPath FRCP(Edin)
Consultant Microbiologist, Aberdeen Royal Infirmary, Aberdeen,
UK

John Reilly BSc PhD
Lecturer, Department of Human Nutrition, University of
Glasgow, Yorkhill Hospitals, Glasgow, UK

Janet M. Rennie MA MD FRCP DCH
Consultant in Neonatal Medicine, King's College Hospital,
London, UK

Peter H. Robinson BSc MRCP
Consultant Paediatrician, Royal Hospital for Sick Children,
Glasgow, UK

Maureen Rogers MBBS FACD
Head, Department of Dermatology, Royal Alexandra Hospital
for Children, Westmead, New South Wales, Australia

Peter Rudd MD FRCP
Consultant Paediatrician, Royal United Hospital Bath Trust;
Honorary Senior Lecturer, University of Bath, Bath, UK

George Russell MB FRCP FRCPE FRCPCH
Reader in Child Health, University of Aberdeen; Consultant in
Medical Paediatrics, Royal Aberdeen Children's Hospital,
Aberdeen, UK

Nicholas Rutter MD FRCP
Professor of Paediatric Medicine, Nottingham University and
Honorary Consultant Paediatrician, Nottingham City and
University Hospitals, Nottingham, UK

R. B. H. Schutgens Prof dr
Department of Clinical Chemistry, University Hospital of the
Vrije Universiteit, Amsterdam, The Netherlands

Jo Sibert MA MD FRCP MRCPCH DCH
Professor of Community Child Health, University of Wales
College of Medicine, Academic Centre, Llandough Hospital,
Penarth, UK

Michael Silverman MD FRCP
Professor in Child Health, University of Leicester; Honorary
Consultant Paediatrician, Leicester Children's Hospital, Leicester
Royal Infirmary, Leicester, UK

Peter J. Smail MA BM FRCP FRCPCH
Clinical Director of Child Health, Aberdeen Royal Hospitals
Trust; Clinical Senior Lecturer, University of Aberdeen,
Aberdeen, UK

David H. Smith MBBS FRCP DTM&H
Senior Clinical Lecturer and Head of Division of Tropical
Medicine; Honorary Consultant Physician in Tropical Medicine,
Liverpool School of Tropical Medicine, Liverpool, UK

A. J. W. Steers MBBS FRCS
Consultant Neurosurgeon, Western General Hospital and Royal
Hospital for Sick Children, Edinburgh, UK

Robert D. Steiner MD
Assistant Professor, Pediatrics and Molecular and Medical Genetics, Oregon Health Sciences University, Portland, USA

Ben J. Stenson MD MRCP
Lecturer in Paediatrics, Department of Child Life and Health, University of Edinburgh, Edinburgh, UK

Terence Stephenson BSc DM FRCP
Professor of Child Health, Nottingham University; Honorary Consultant Paediatrician, University Hospital, Nottingham, UK

James Syme MBChB FRCP FRCPE FRCP(Glas) HonFRCPCH
Formerly Consultant Paediatrician and Honorary Senior Lecturer, Royal Hospital for Sick Children, Edinburgh, UK

William O. Tarnow-Mordi BA MBChB DCH MRCP(UK)
Honorary Consultant Neonatologist, Department of Child Health; Reader in Neonatal Medicine and Perinatal Epidemiology, University of Dundee, Ninewells Hospital and Medical School, Dundee, UK

Christopher Mark Taylor FRCP DCH
Consultant Paediatric Nephrologist, The Birmingham Children's Hospital; Honorary Senior Clinical Lecturer, University of Birmingham, The Birmingham Children's Hospital, Birmingham, UK

Carolyn Thompson MBChB FRCP(Edin)
Consultant in Genitourinary Medicine, Kirkcaldy Acute Hospitals NHS Trust, Kirkcaldy, UK

Thomas L. Turner MB FRCP(Edin and Glas)
Consultant Paediatrician and Senior Clinical Lecturer, Queen Mother's Hospital, Royal Hospital for Sick Children and Department of Child Health, University of Glasgow, Glasgow, UK

William S. Uttley MB FRCP DCH
Consultant Children's Physician, Royal Hospital for Sick Children, Edinburgh; Honorary Senior Lecturer, University of Edinburgh, Edinburgh, UK

Kerry Walker BSc SRD
Senior 1 Dietitian, Royal Hospital for Sick Children, Yorkhill NHS Trust, Glasgow, UK

Euan M. Wallace MBChB MRCOG
Senior Lecturer, Monash University; Specialist Obstetrician, Monash Medical Centre, Victoria, Australia

John O. Warner MD MRCPCH FRCP DCH
Professor of Child Health, University of Southampton; Honorary Consultant Paediatrician, Southampton General Hospital, Southampton, UK

A. C. H. Watson FRCS(Edin)
Formerly Consultant Plastic Surgeon, Royal Hospital for Sick Children, Edinburgh, UK

Alan R. Watson BSc(Hons) MBChB FRCP(Edin)
Consultant Paediatric Nephrologist, City Hospital; Clinical Teacher, University of Nottingham, Nottingham, UK

Lawrence T. Weaver MA MD FRCP DCH
Professor of Child Health, University of Glasgow, Royal Hospital for Sick Children, Glasgow, UK

Philip D. Welsby FRCP(Edin)
Consultant Physician in Infectious Diseases, City Hospital, Edinburgh, UK

Richard J. West MD FRCP FRCPCH
Honorary Consultant, Royal Hospital for Sick Children, Bristol; Regional Postgraduate Dean, Academic Centre, Frenchay Hospital, Bristol, UK

Brian A. Wharton BA MBA MD DSc FRCP FRCPH
Director-General, British Nutrition Foundation, London

A. Graham Wilkinson MB BS MA MRCP FRCP
Consultant Paediatric Radiologist, Royal Hospital for Sick Children, Glasgow, UK

David Will BSc MBChB FRCPsych
Consultant in Adolescent Psychiatry, Young People's Unit, Royal Edinburgh Hospital, Edinburgh, UK

Anthony F. Williams DPhil FRCP
Senior Lecturer in Paediatrics, Department of Child Health, St George's Hospital Medical School, London, UK

Louise E. Wilson MD FRCP
Consultant Intensivist, Royal Hospital for Sick Children, Edinburgh; Senior Lecturer (Part-time), University of Edinburgh, Edinburgh, UK

Dieter Wolke PhD DiplPsych
Professor of Psychology (Research), Department of Psychology, University of Hertfordshire; Honorary Director of Psychology of Bavarian Longitudinal Study, University of Munich Children's Hospital, Germany

Hock-Boon Wong MBBS FRCP(Lond) FRCP(Edin) FRCP(Glas) FRACP DCH(Lond)
Consultant Pediatrician, Pediatric Clinic, Thomson Medical Centre, Singapore; Professorial Fellow and Emeritus Professor, Department of Pediatrics, National University of Singapore, Singapore

Robert M. Wrate MBBS FRCPsych
Consultant in Adolescent Psychiatry, The Young People's Unit, Royal Edinburgh Hospital; Honorary Senior Lecturer, Department of Psychiatry, Royal Edinburgh Hospital, University of Edinburgh, Edinburgh, UK

Hugh Young PhD FRCPath
Clinical Lecturer, Department of Medical Microbiology, University of Edinburgh Medical School; Honorary Consultant Clinical Scientist, Edinburgh Royal Infirmary NHS Trust, Edinburgh, UK

D. A. Zideman QHP(C) BSc MBBS FRCA DipIMC
Consultant Anaesthetist, Hammersmith Hospital Trust; Honorary Senior Lecturer, Royal Postgraduate Medical School, London, UK

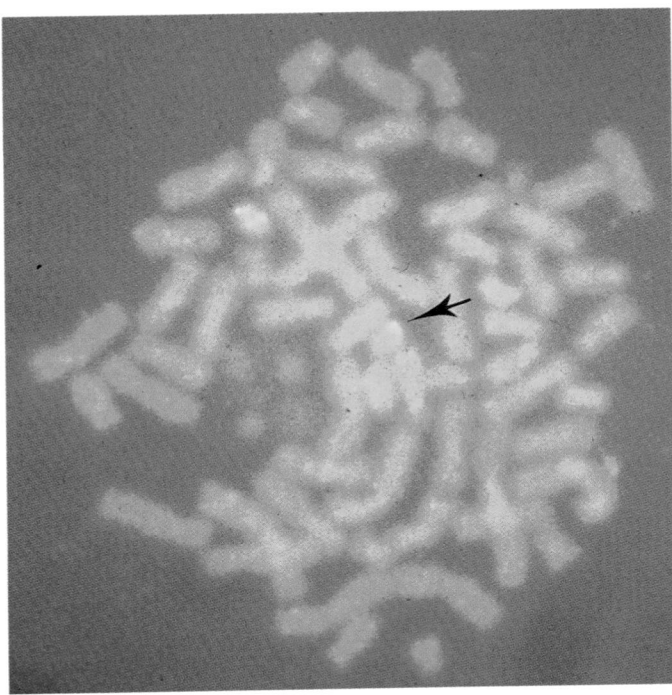

Plate 3.1   Fluorescent in situ hybridisation (FISH) using probes on
chromosome 22. The normal chromosome 22 has two pairs of signals
indicating the control probe and the critical region, while the deleted
chromosome 22 (marked with the arrow) shows only the control probe. This
indicates the patient has Di George Syndrome (see p. 50).

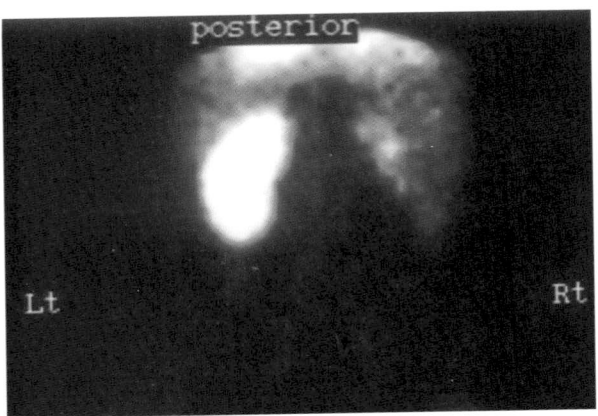

Plate 17.13a   MAG 3 scan in 6-year-old boy with history of UTI and small
right kidney on ultrasound (see p. 955).

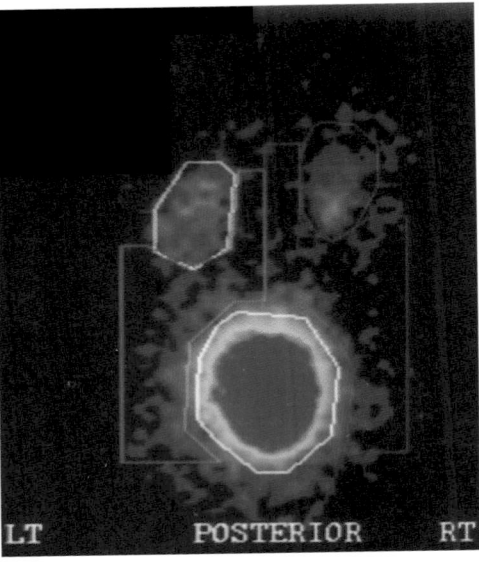

Plate 17.13b   Indirect micturating cystogram showing gross reflux right
side reflected in increased counts in right ureter and kidney (see p. 955).

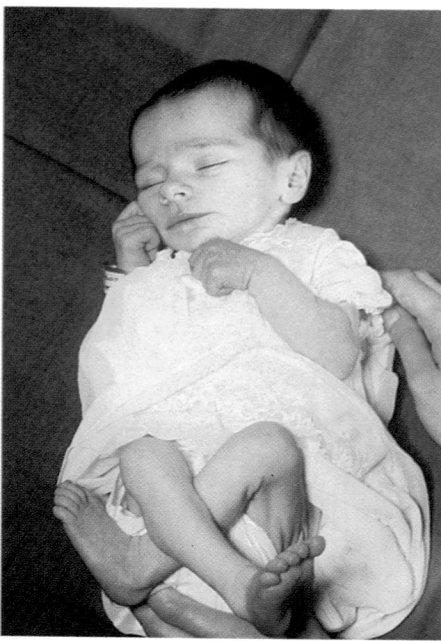

Plate 21.1   Infant with failure-to-thrive secondary to insufficient breast milk intake (see p. 1191).

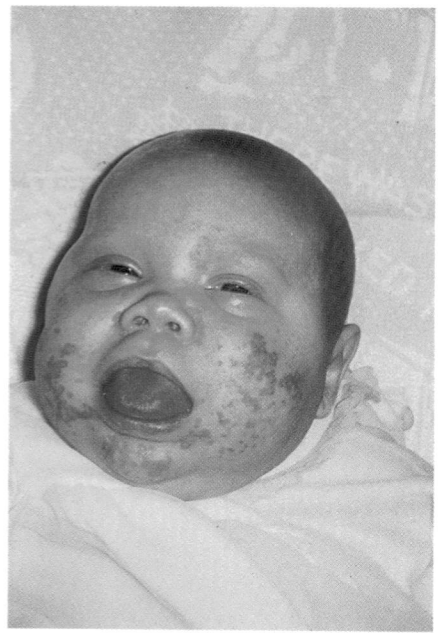

Plate 21.2   Skin changes in zinc deficiency (see p. 1201).

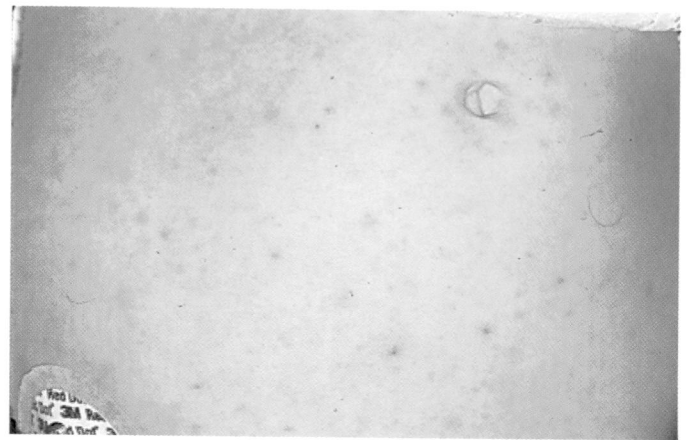

Plate 23.1   Maculopapular/morbilliform rash of early meningococcemia (see pp. 1285, 1314). (Courtesy of Department of Medical Illustration, University of Aberdeen.)

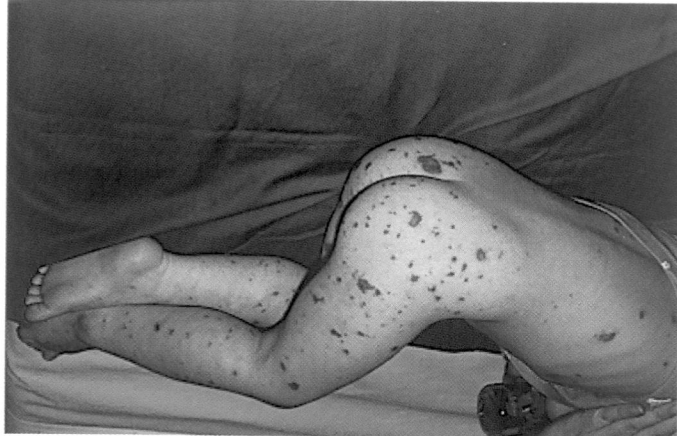

Plate 23.2   Purpuric rash of meningococcemia (see pp. 1285, 1290, 1314). (Courtesy of Department of Medical Illustration, University of Aberdeen.)

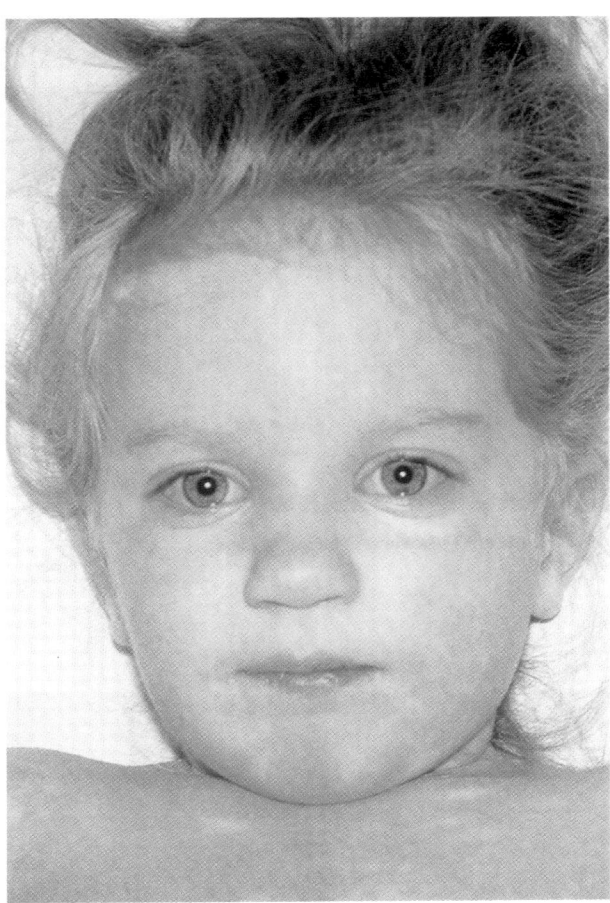

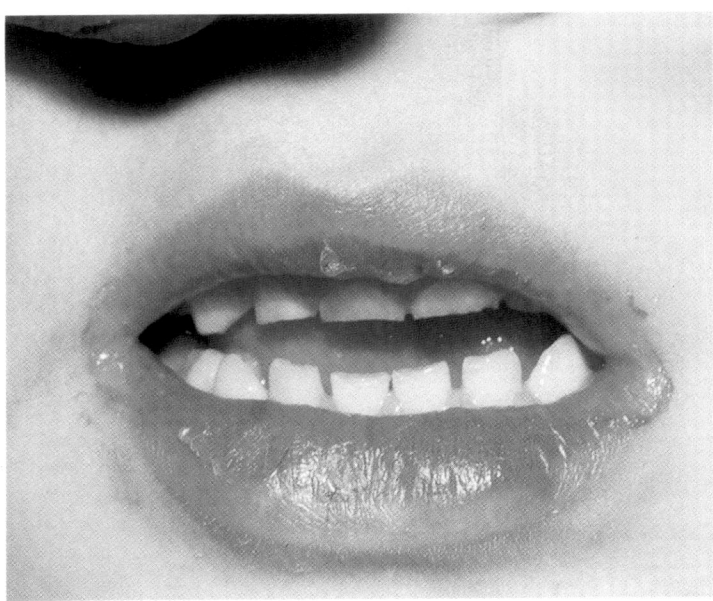

Plate 23.4   Reddened, cracked lips (see p. 1479).

Plate 23.3   Facial appearance in Kawasaki disease (see p. 1479) (reproduced with permission of the family).

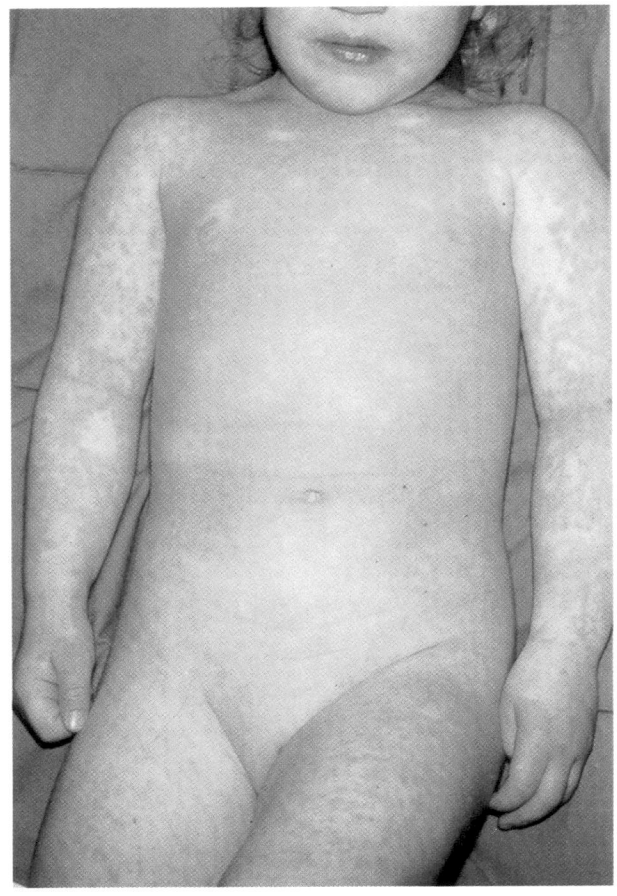

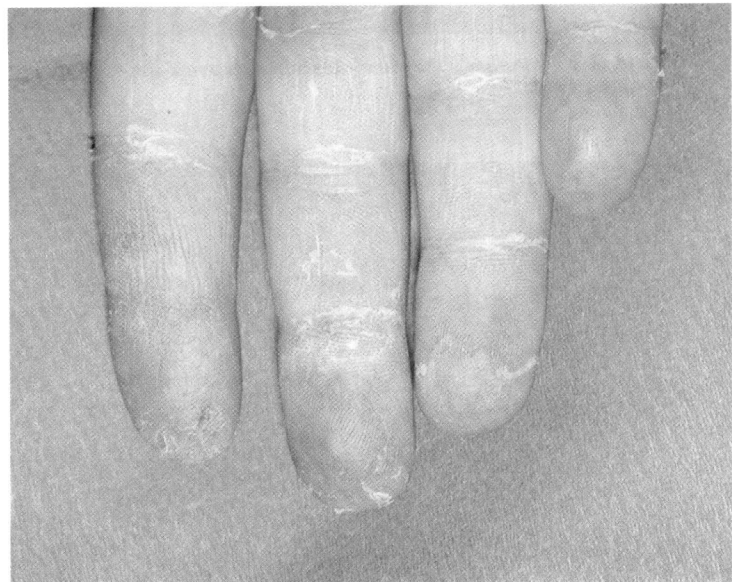

Plate 23.5   Finger desquamation starting at the tips (see p. 1479).

Plate 23.6   Generalized rash (see p. 1479).

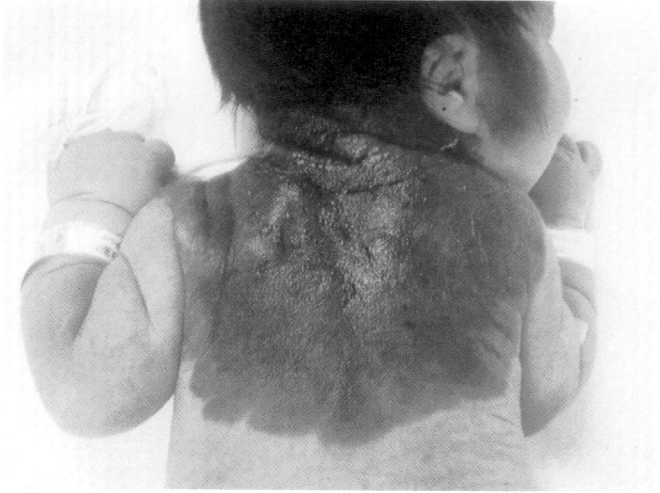

Plate 25.1   Congenital melanocytic nevus (see p. 1617).

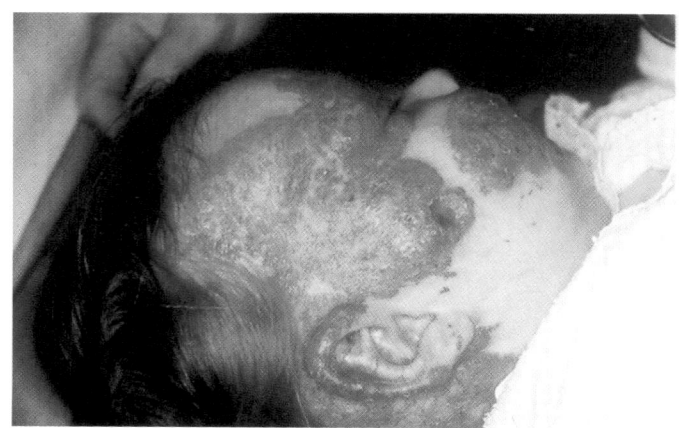

Plate 25.2   Capillary (stawberry) hemangioma (see p. 1619).

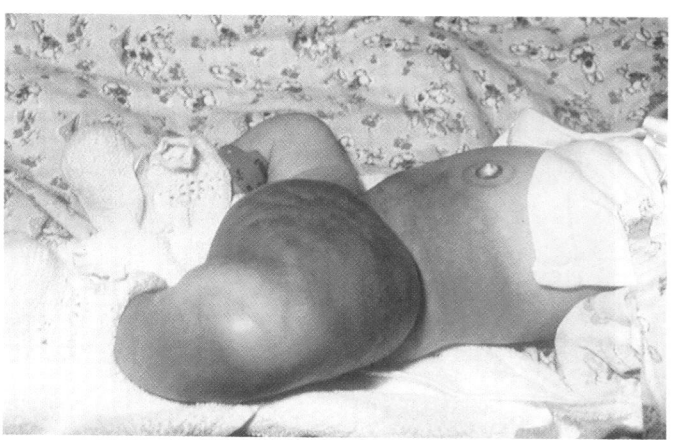

Plate 25.3   Kasabach–Merritt syndrome (see p. 1619).

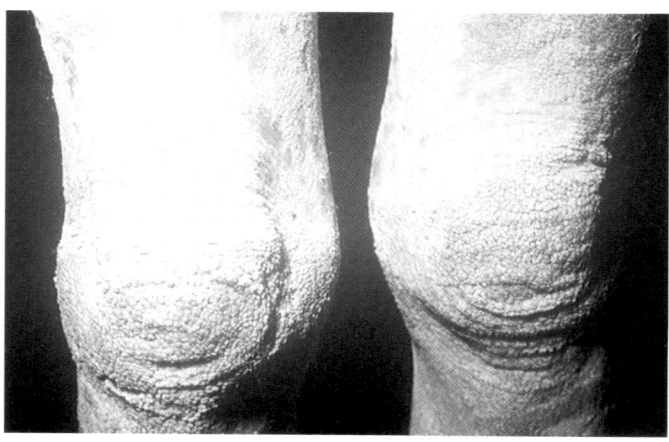

Plate 25.4   Lamellar ichthyosis (congenital ichthyosiform erythroderma) (see p. 1620).

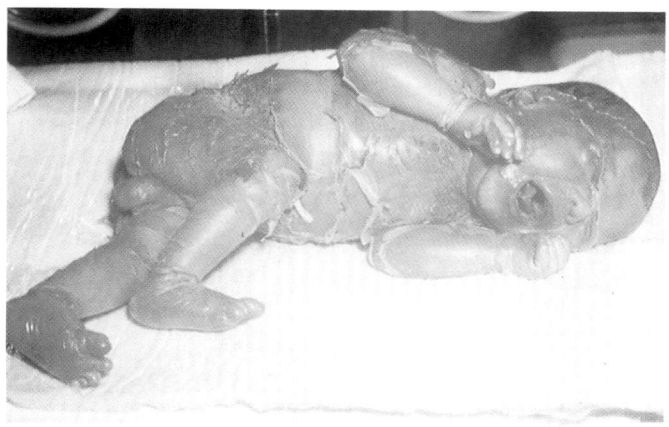

Plate 25.5   Collodion baby (see p. 1621).

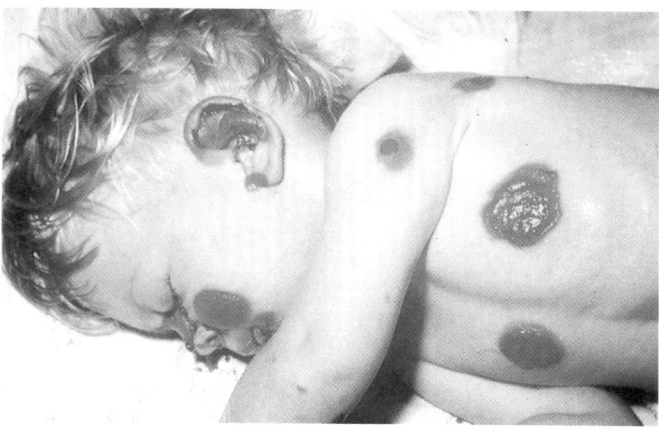

Plate 25.6   Junctional epidermolysis bullosa (see p. 1622).

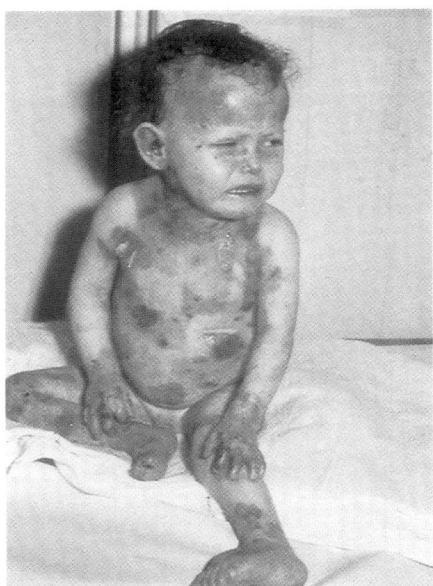

Plate 25.7 Dystrophic epidermolysis bullosa (see p. 1622).

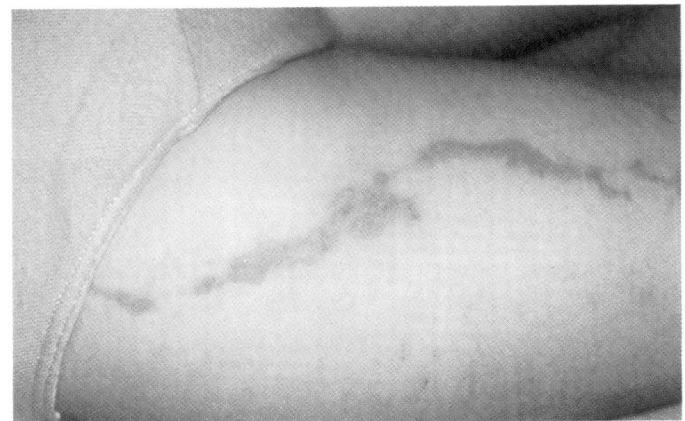

Plate 25.8 Incontinentia pigmenti: pigmented stage (see p. 1626).

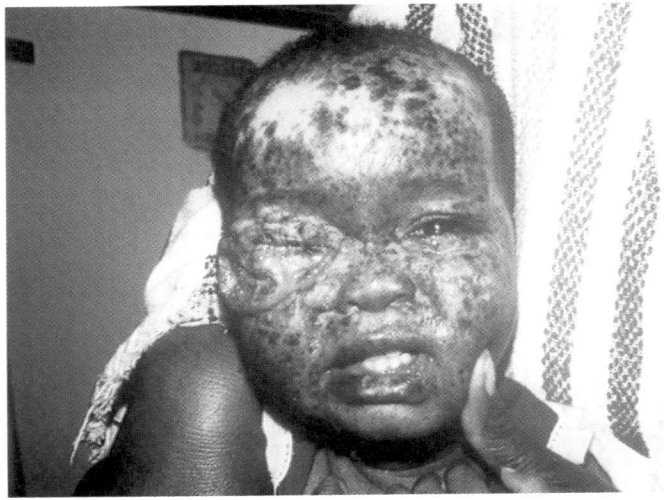

Plate 25.9 Xeroderma pigmentosum (see p. 1630).

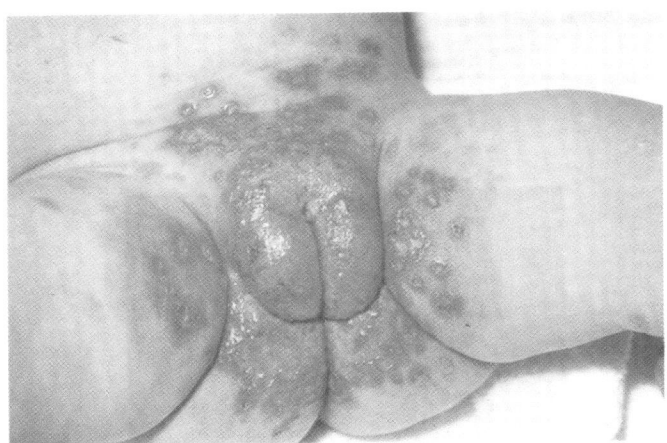

Plate 25.10 Perineal herpes simplex (see p. 1631).

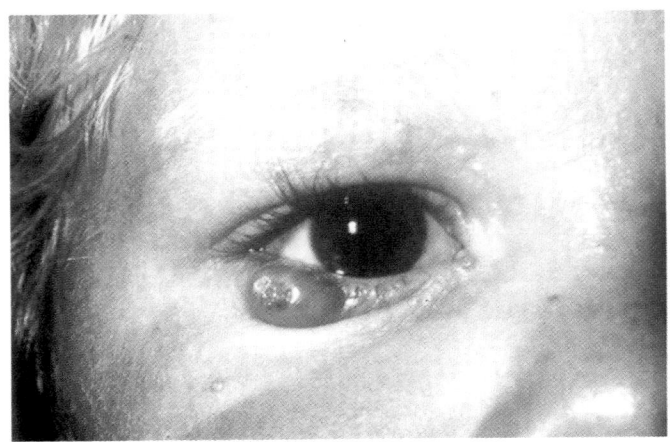

Plate 25.11 Molluscum contagiosum (see pp. 1388, 1633).

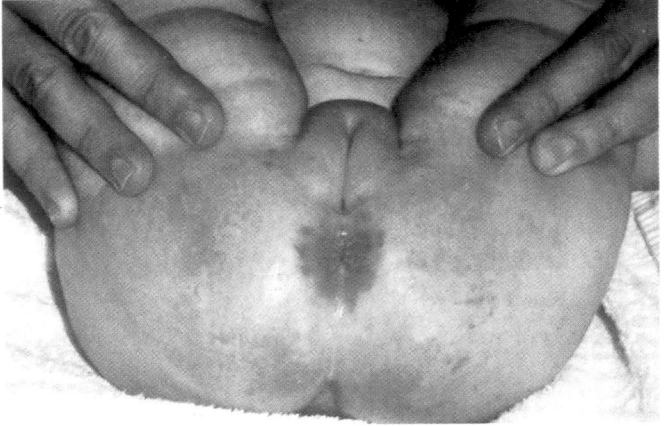

Plate 25.12 Streptococcal perianal cellulitis (see p. 1635).

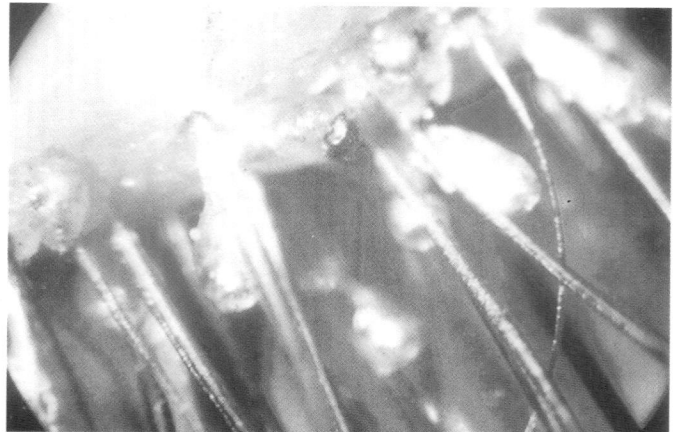

Plate 25.13   Pediculosis of eyelid (see p. 1638).

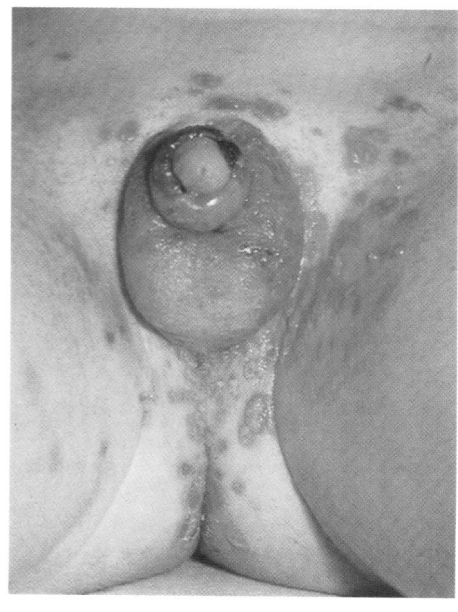

Plate 25.14   Chronic bullous disease of childhood (see p. 1640).

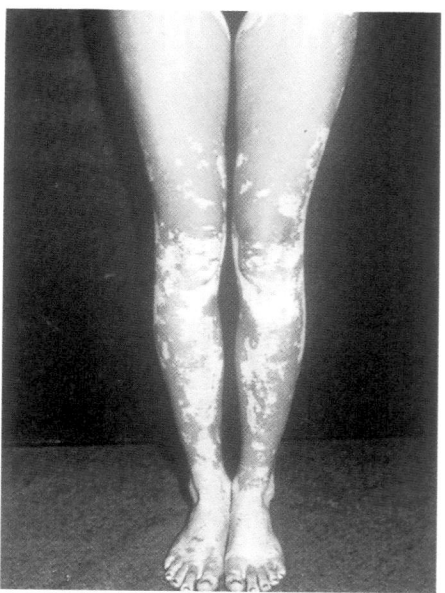

Plate 25.15   Vitiligo (see p. 1640).

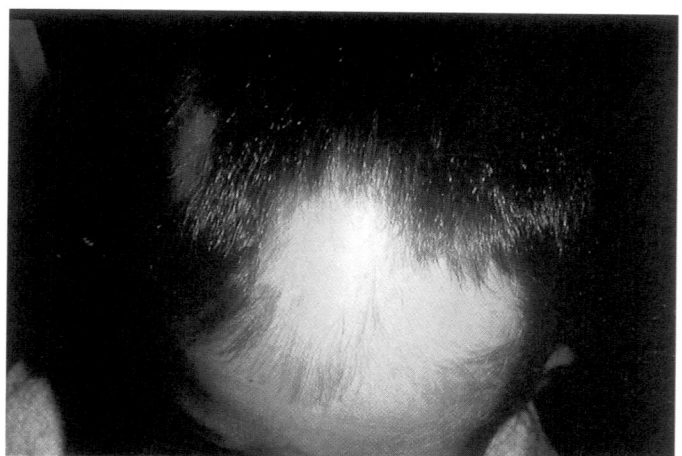

Plate 25.16   Alopecia areata (see p. 1640).

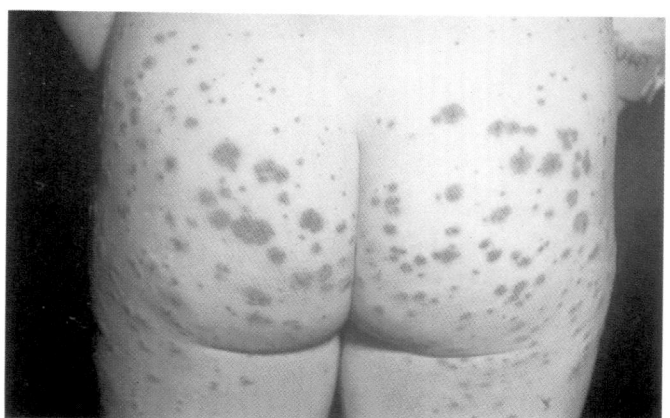

Plate 25.17   Henoch–Schönlein purpura (see p. 1640).

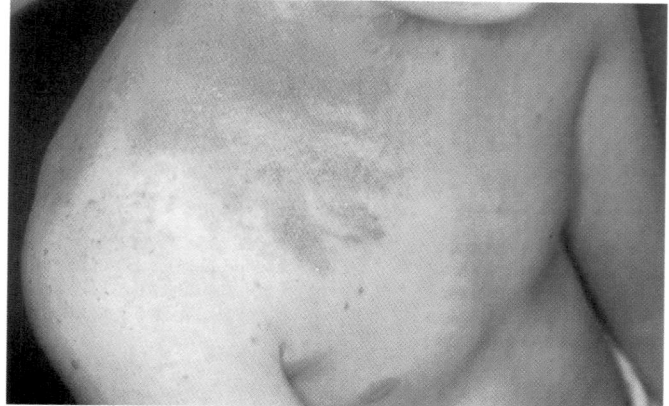

Plate 25.18   Plant (*Rhus*) dermatitis (see p. 1641).

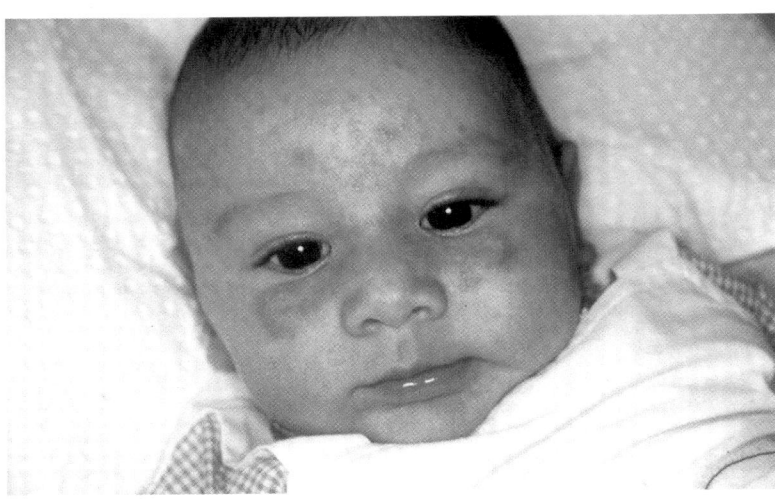

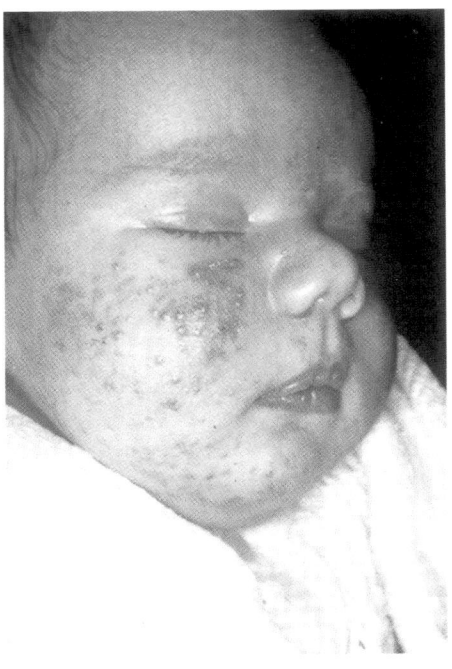

Plate 25.19 Neonatal lupus erythematosus (see p. 1644).

Plate 25.20 Pustular miliaria (prickly heat) (see p. 1646).

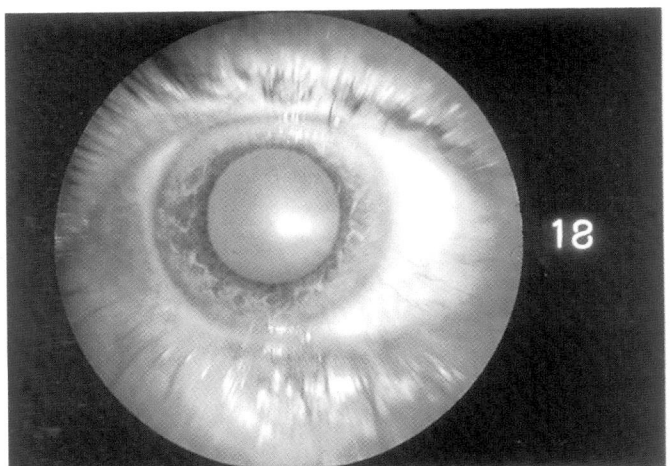

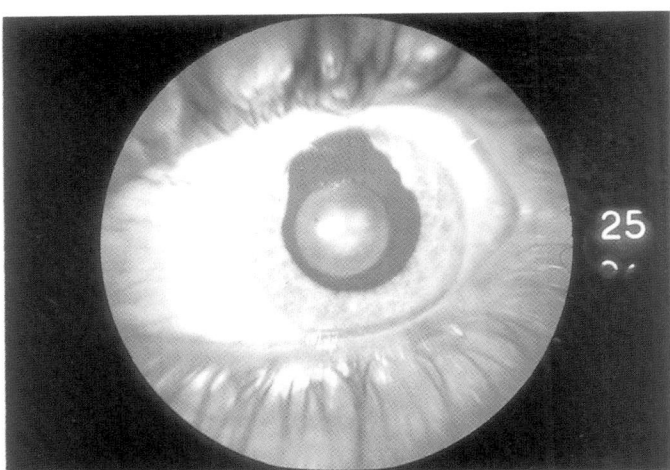

Plate 26.1 The normal red reflex. This is the view when the red reflex is examined with a direct ophthalmoscope held at arm's length and close to the observer's eye. The pupil is fully dilated. A clear red reflex of the fundus is seen indicating clear media. A small light reflex from the ophthalmoscope is seen in the pupil. (See p. 1651.)

Plate 26.2 An abnormal red reflex. The patient has an upper iridectomy and there is a cataract situated centrally in the pupil (see p. 1651).

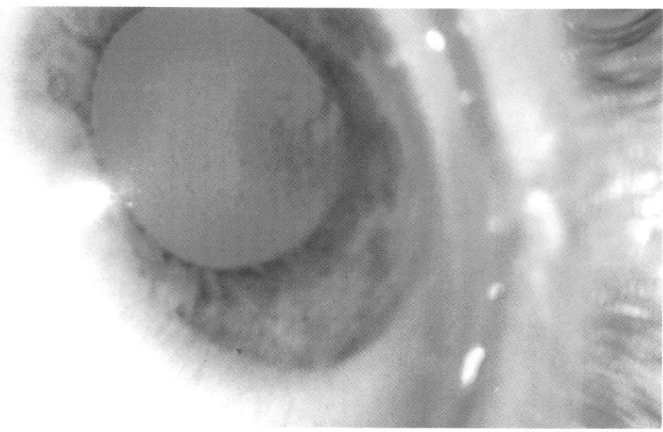

Plate 26.3   The red reflex interrupted by discrete lens opacities due to partial cataract (see p. 1651).

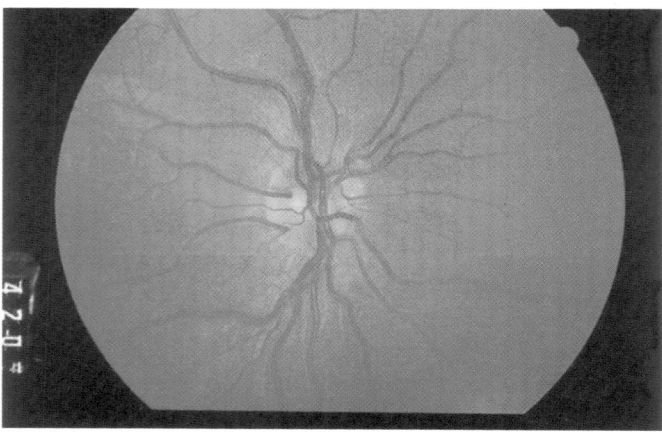

Plate 26.4   The normal fundus of the eye seen with a direct ophthalmoscope held close to the observer's eye and also close to the patient's eye with the pupil fully dilated. The normal background color and normal color of the optic disk and blood vessels can be seen. (See p. 1651.)

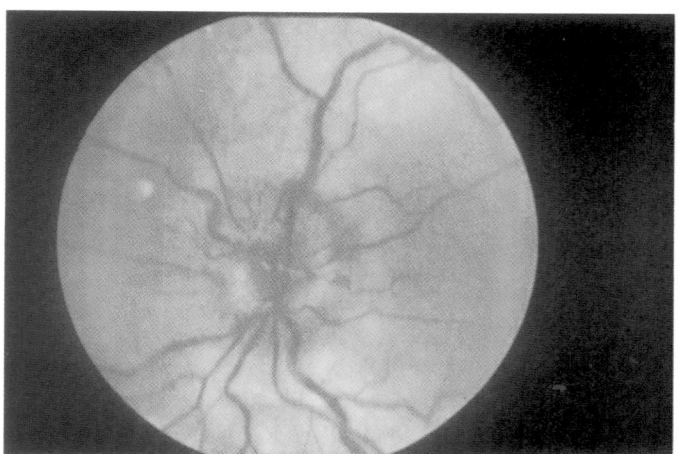

Plate 26.5   The optic disk in early papilledema showing apparent enlargement of the disk with blurred disk outlines and tortuous blood vessels (see p. 1652).

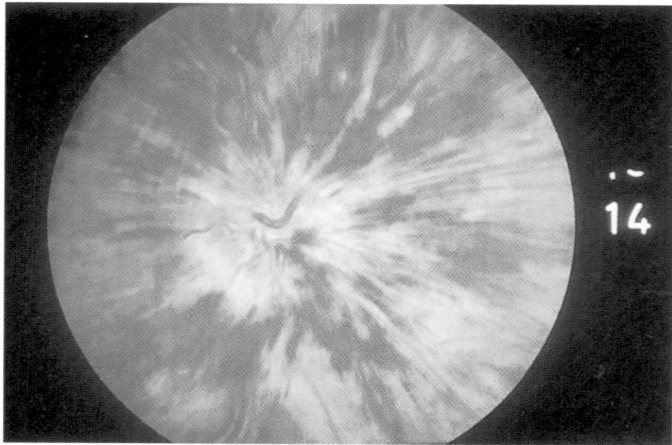

Plate 26.6   Established papilledema. The optic disk margins are blurred and the disk is elevated. The retinal vessels are engorged and the optic disk is surrounded by hemorrhage. (See p. 1652.)

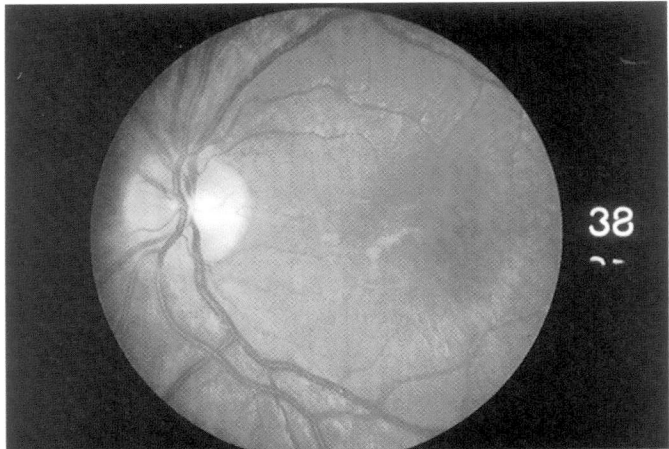

Plate 26.7 Conmotio retinae – traumatic edema at the posterior pole of the eye. This can be difficult to detect but explains reduced central visual acuity following undisclosed trauma. (See p. 1652.)

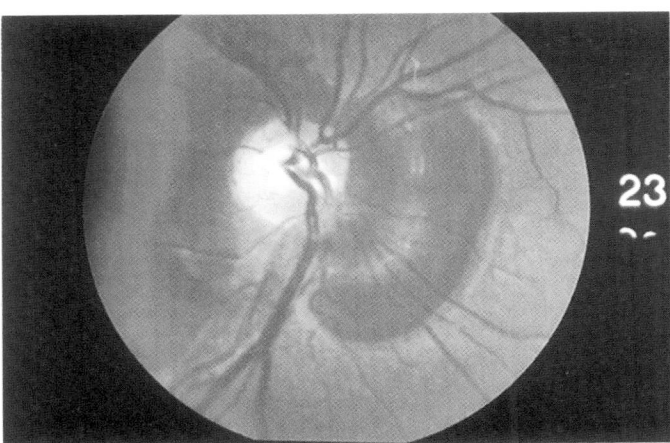

Plate 26.8 Traumatic rupture of the choroid (see p. 1652).

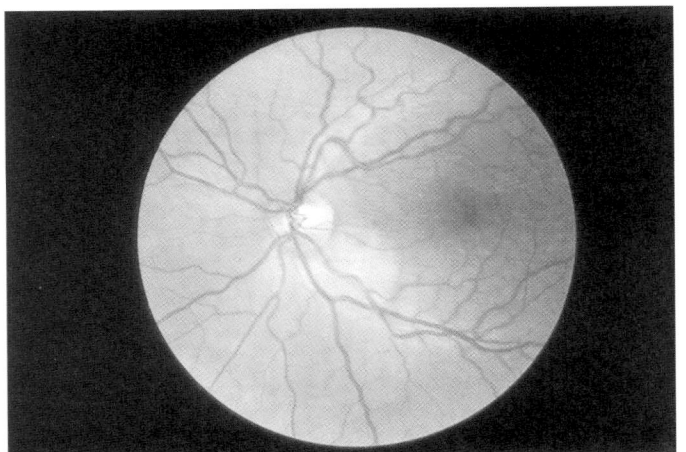

Plate 26.9 Choroidal folds. Choroidal or 'chorioretinal' folds are occasionally seen in the fundi typically in disthyroid conditions. In this patient there was a reduction in vision due to increased orbital pressure caused by an orbital tumor (Fig. 25.1). When the tumor was removed vision returned to normal. (See p. 1652.)

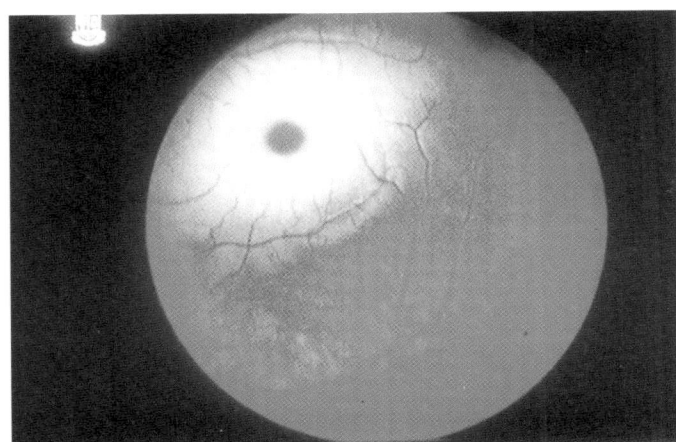

Plate 26.10 Tay–Sachs disease. A cherry-red spot is seen at the posterior pole due to the presence of ganglioside in the ganglian cells of the macula. There are no ganglian cells at the fovea which presents as a red spot but the surrounding area appears white or milky in color. (See p. 1655.)

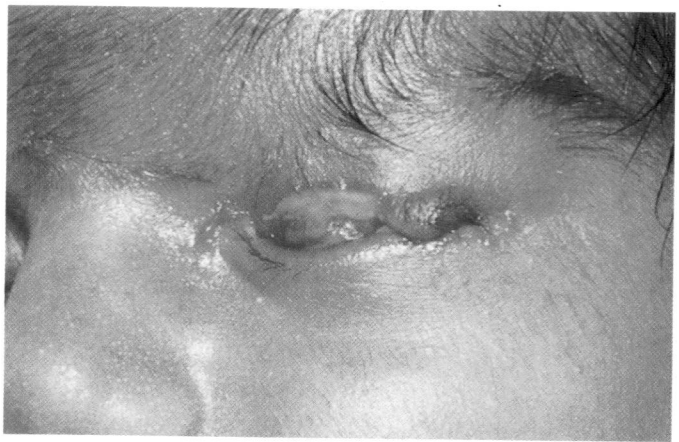

Plate 26.11 Coloboma of the eyelid. This child was born with a totally exposed left eye due to a large coloboma of the left upper eyelid in the superomedial position. An attempt at temporary repair was made on the day following birth and subsequent lid plastic surgery was carried out but even 1 day's total exposure resulted in drying of the eye and subsequent loss of the eye. (See p. 1662.)

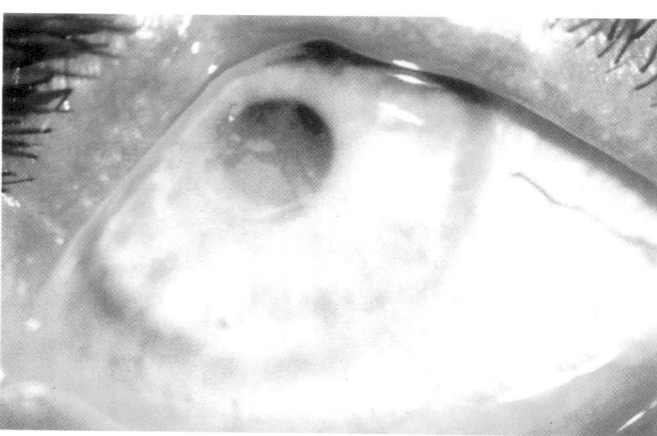

Plate 26.12 Vaccinia keratoconjunctivitis. Fluorescein has been instilled in the conjunctival sac and shows ulcerated areas on the cornea. This child has touched a vaccination lesion on another child's arm and subsequently rubbed his own eye. (See p. 1663.)

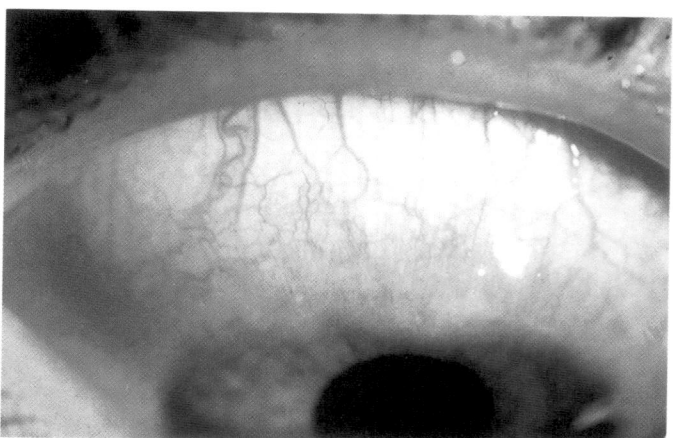

Plate 26.13 Allergic conjunctivitis showing the typically hyperemic conjunctiva (see p. 1664).

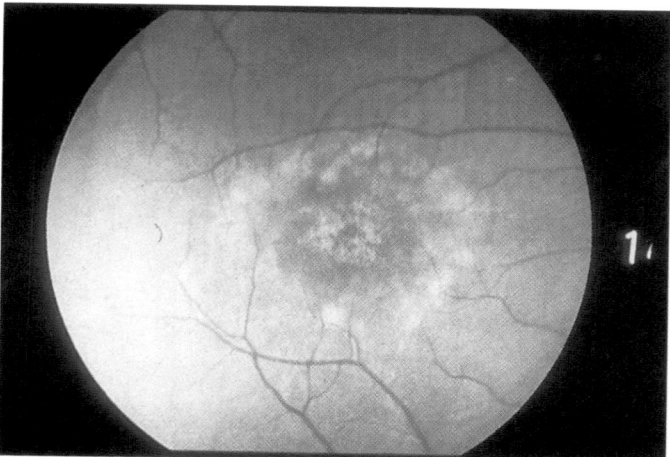

Plate 26.14 Stargardt's disease. This is the commonest form of macular degeneration in childhood. Initially there is pigment stippling at the macula and eventually the typical circular area of depigmentation and atrophy develops at the posterior pole. Total blindness does not occur. (See p. 1666.)

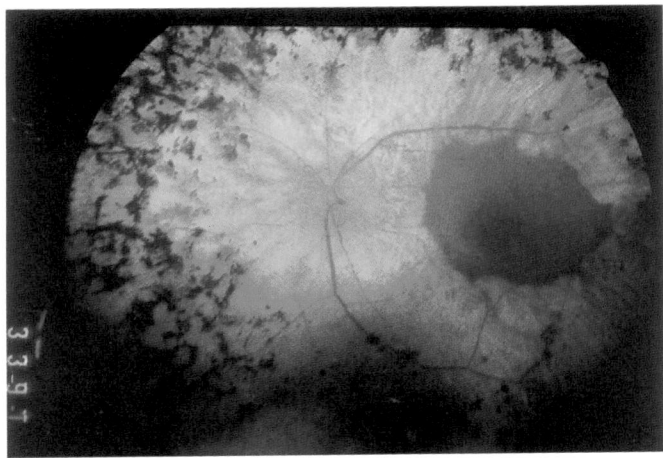

Plate 26.15 Retinitis pigmentosa. This is an advanced case of retinitis pigmentosa showing attenuation of the retinal vessels and irregular pigmentary distribution in the mid-periphery. (See p. 1667.)

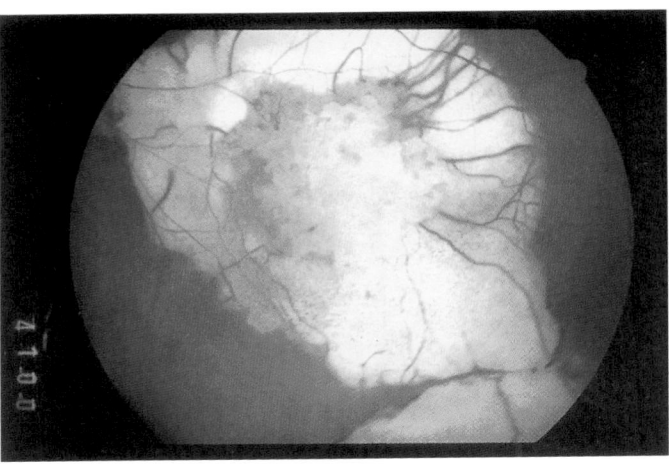

Plate 26.16 Retinoblastoma. An extensive light-colored tumor is seen in the fundus (see pp. 1667, 1670).

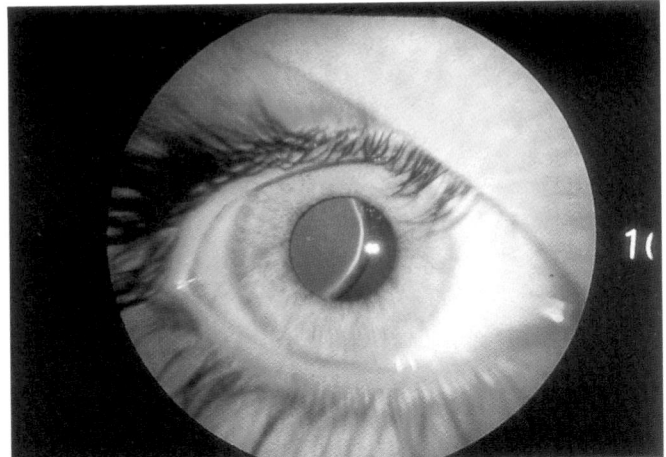

Plate 26.17 Dislocation of the lens seen in the red reflex. The lens is dislocated laterally and slightly upward. When it moves toward the pupil the child will be myopic but when there is no lens in the pupillary area the child will be hypermetropic (aphakic). In the photograph the edge of the lens is cutting the axial area with the result that there will be an irregular refractive error with an irregular astigmatism. (See p. 1670.)

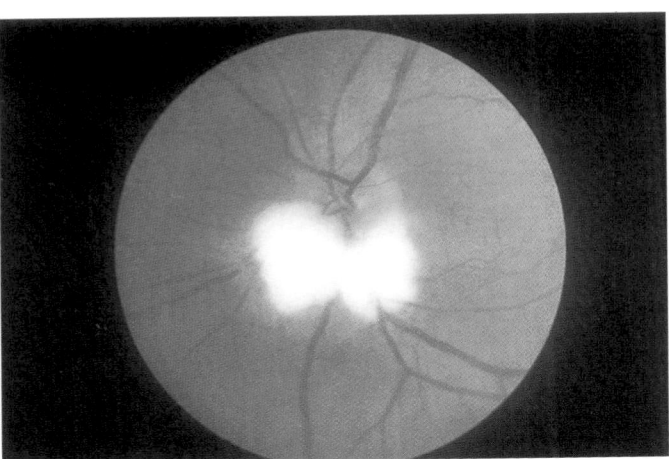

Plate 26.18 Myelinated nerve fibers. Myelin which is white can be seen extending from the optic disk onto the retina. This is a developmental abnormality of no significance and should not be confused with papilledema. (See p. 1671.)

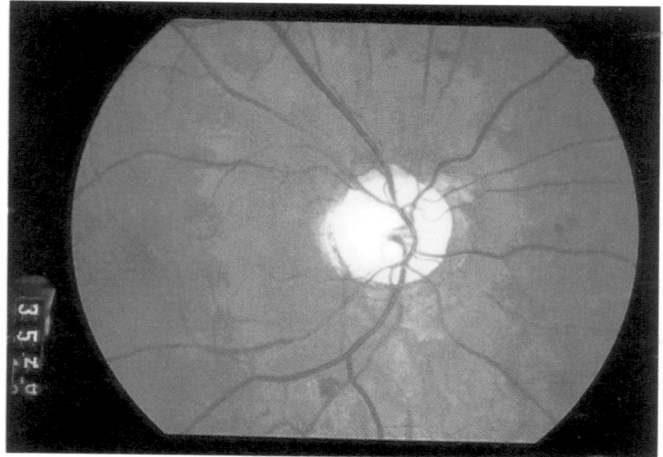

Plate 26.19 Primary optic atrophy. The optic disk is pale with sharply cut margins and appears to be avascular. (See p. 1671.)

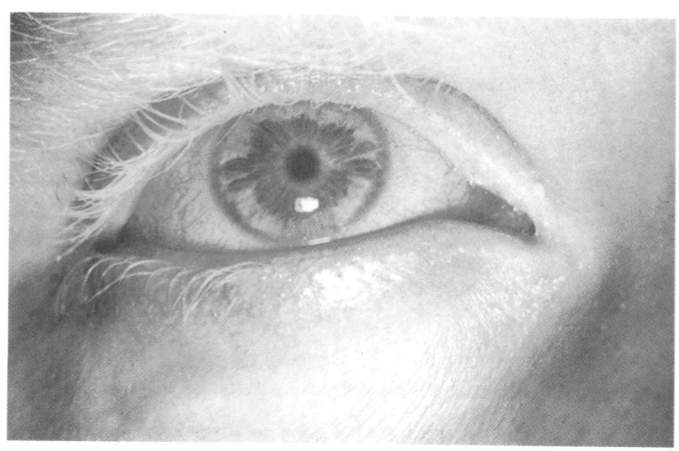

Plate 26.20 Albinism. The eye appears to be pink in direct illumination and the iris is atrophic and light gray in color. (See p. 1673.)

1 Demography, vital statistics and the pattern of disease in childhood

J.O. Forfar

Child population   1
United Nations convention on the rights of the child
  (1989)   1
Birth   1
Population density   2
Life expectancy   2
Childhood mortality   2
  Definitions   3
  Stillbirths (late fetal mortality)   3
  Perinatal mortality   3
  Early neonatal mortality   4
  Late neonatal mortality   4
  Neonatal mortality   4
  Postneonatal mortality   5
  Infant mortality   5
  Age-specific deaths   5
  Mortality in the developing world   7
  Trends in mortality from individual diseases   7

Childhood morbidity   8
  Childhood morbidity: general practice   8
  Notifiable infectious disease   9
Hospital services   9
  Outpatients   9
  Inpatients   9
Age incidence of disease in childhood   9
  Fetal   11
  Birth   13
  Neonatal   13
  Early infancy (1–6 months)   13
  Later infancy (6 months to 1 year)   13
  Early childhood (preschool 1–5 years)   13
  Later childhood (school 5–15 years)   13
Combined mortality and morbidity   13
Chronic and handicapping illness in childhood   13
Child health indicators, social and environmental influences   13
References and bibliography   14

CHILD POPULATION

The present world population is 5600 million, one-third being children under the age of 15 years. The child population has doubled since 1950 with large increases in the developing countries and small in the developed (Fig. 1.1). 14% of children live in developed and 86% in developing countries. Population statistics for world regions are shown in Table 1.1 and British age-group populations in Table 1.6.

UNITED NATIONS CONVENTION ON THE RIGHTS OF THE CHILD (1989)

This embodies the right of every child to:

Equality regardless of race, religion, nationality or sex
Special protection for full physical, intellectual, moral, spiritual and social development in a healthy and normal manner
A name and nationality
Adequate nutrition, housing and medical services
Special care if handicapped
Love, understanding and protection
Free education, play and recreation
Priority for relief in times of disaster
Protection against all forms of neglect, cruelty and exploitation
Protection from any form of discrimination, and the right to be brought up in a spirit of universal brotherhood, peace and tolerance.

These rights were amplified at the World Summit for Children (1990) but in some countries are largely ignored and in most are moral principles rather than legal requirements. Expanding world population is an important factor in frustrating the achievement of these rights.

BIRTH

Live birth is the complete expulsion or extraction from its mother of a product of conception, irrespective of the duration of pregnancy, which after such separation breathes or shows any evidence of life such as beating of the heart or pulsation of the umbilical vessels whether or not the umbilical cord has been cut or the placenta is attached. Each product of such birth is considered liveborn.

Crude birth rate is the number of live births per annum per 1000 population. The falling birth rate in Scotland over the past century is shown in Figure 1.3. The UK rate (1992–94) is 13.4, nearly one-third of live births being conceived outside marriage.

Standardized birth rate is an arbitrary population standardized for age structure and allows comparisons to be made between different countries, or different epochs in the same country.

Birth rate may also be expressed as a *fertility index*, the number of births per 1000 women in the child-bearing period 15 to 44 years or, sometimes, 15 to 49 years.

The highest rates are found in Africa, Asia and South America, the lowest in Europe, North America and developed Far-Eastern countries such as Japan and Hong Kong (Table 1.1). In countries with both white and nonwhite ethnic groups the birth rate in the latter may be 50% higher than in the former.

Table 1.2 shows the distribution of births among social classes, birthweights, parities and maternal ages.

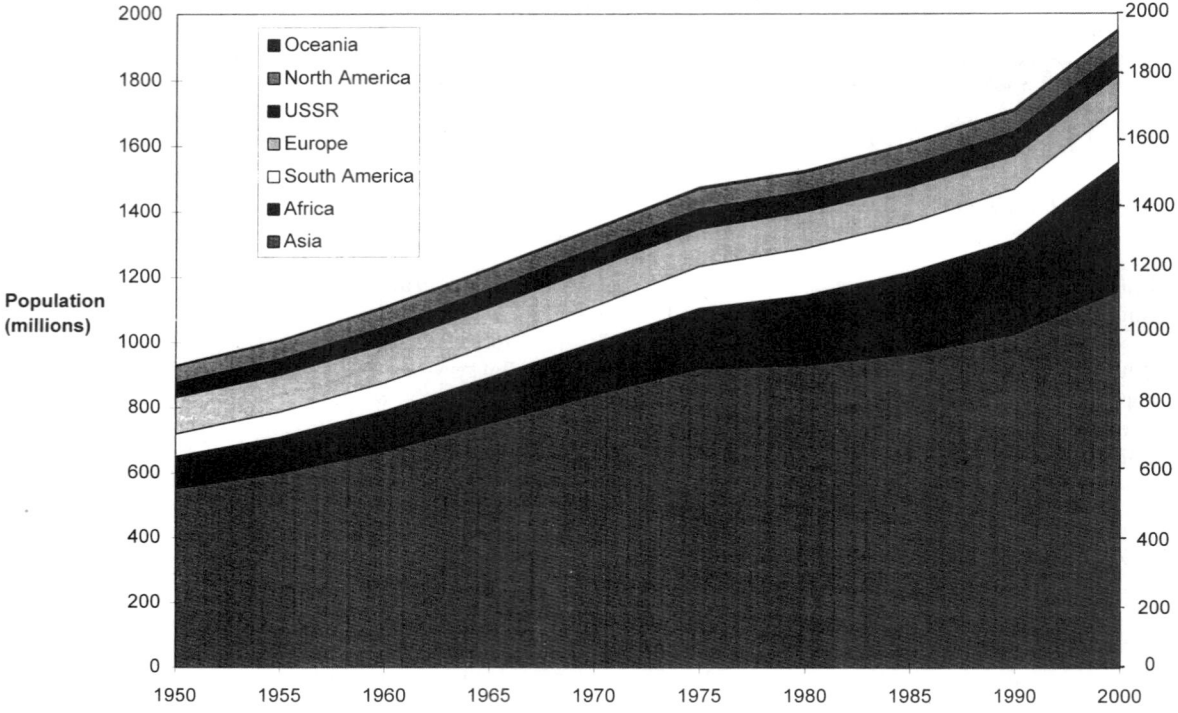

Fig. 1.1   World population of children 0–14 years, 1950–2000.

POPULATION DENSITY

Worldwide population densities are shown in Table 1.1.

LIFE EXPECTANCY

Table 1.1 indicates life expectancy at birth in various parts of the world and Figure 1.3 the changes in Britain over the past century. Worldwide, life expectancy at birth is increasing. In India it increased from 27 to 61 years between 1946 and 1993. There are significant correlations between birth rate and both life expectancy at birth and the under-5 mortality rate – among the world's 20 most populous countries the correlation is negative (– 0.5; $P = 0.005$) in the former relationship, and positive (0.9; $P < 0.001$) in the latter.

The life expectancy of children as a group is one-third of the total life expectancy of the nation (UK).

CHILDHOOD MORTALITY

Although widely used, mortality statistics (Fig. 1.2) are limited indicators of disease and health. Morbidity, rather than mortality,

Table 1.1   The world's children

	Population* (%)	Child population* (0–14 years) (%)	Birth† rate	Life expectancy (years)	Annual population increase (%)	Area (1000 sq. km)	Population density (per sq. km)	Infant‡ mortality	Early childhood (0–5 years) mortality§
WORLD	5600 (100)	1828 (100)	28	64	1.8	136 255	41	64	90
The developed countries	1230 (22)	260 (14)	14	76	0.6	58 205	22	16	19
Europe	510 (9)	95 (5)	13	76	0.5	5108	101	8	8
North America	277 (5)	62 (3)	16	75	1.2	21 962	13	9	9
Former USSR	292 (5)	75 (4)	16	69	0.8	22 227	13	35	42
Japan	125 (2)	23 (1.5)	11	79	0.7	372	336	5	6
Oceania	26 (0.5)	5 (0.3)	16	70	1.3	8536	3	7	8
The developing countries	4370 (78)	1568 (86)	30	61	2.1	78 050	56	78	100
Asia	3000 (54)	1020 (56)	27	63	1.9	27 210	118	64	89
Africa	900 (16)	390 (21)	41	55	3.0	30 305	24	91	141
Latin America	470 (8)	158 (9)	26	68	2.1	20 535	23	38	48
United Kingdom	58 (1)	11 (0.6)	14	76	0.2	244	238	7	8
Hong Kong	6 (0.1)	1 (0.06)	13	77	1.4	1	5400	6	7
China	1205 (26)	327 (18)	21	71	1.6	9536	125	35	43

* Millions; †per 1000 population; ‡per 1000 live births; §per 1000 in age group.

Table 1.2 Factors influencing childhood mortalities

	Proportion %	SBR	PMR	NMR	PNMR	IMR
Social class						
All	100	4.3	7.5	4.2	2.2	6.4
I	9.2	3.4	6.3	3.6	1.5	5.0
II	28.7	3.5	6.1	3.4	1.2	4.6
IIIN	11.0	3.4	6.8	4.2	1.3	5.5
IIIM	34.1	4.1	7.0	3.7	1.8	5.6
IV	12.7	4.6	7.3	3.5	2.4	5.8
V	4.5	5.2	8.8	5.2	2.7	7.8
Birthweight						
All	100	4.3	7.5	4.2	2.2	6.4
< 1500 g	1.0	100.5	250.4	203.4	36.4	239.8
1500–1999 g	1.3	46.5	61.6	21.2	11.2	32.3
2000–2499 g	4.4	14.5	19.1	6.3	6.0	12.3
2500–2999 g	16.7	3.9	5.3	2.2	2.6	4.8
3000–3499 g	36.5	1.8	2.5	1.1	1.5	2.6
3500 g and over	40.1	1.2	1.8	0.8	1.0	1.8
Parity (within marriage)						
All	100	4.0	7.0	3.8	1.8	5.6
0	39.3	4.4	7.7	4.3	1.6	6.0
1	36.5	3.2	5.7	3.2	1.5	4.7
2	15.8	3.9	6.9	3.7	2.2	5.9
3 and over	8.5	5.8	9.4	4.7	3.0	7.6
Maternal age						
All	100	4.3	7.5	4.2	2.2	6.4
< 20	6.9	4.4	8.3	5.3	4.2	9.6
20–24	23.7	4.5	8.2	4.9	3.1	8.0
25–29	35.5	3.6	6.4	3.6	1.8	5.4
30–34	24.2	4.1	7.1	3.8	1.5	5.3
35 and over	9.7	6.2	10.2	5.0	1.9	6.9
Multiple birth						
All	3	14.4	39.5	29.1	6.6	35.7

SBR = stillbirth rate; PMR = perinatal mortality rate; NMR = neonatal mortality rate; PNMR = postneonatal mortality rate; IMR = infant mortality rate.

should be the main determinant of the needs and character of the child health services. Mortality at different ages is shown in Figure 1.2.

Definitions

Childhood is taken as the first 15 years of life.

Stillbirth (or late fetal mortality) rate (SBR). The number of infants born after the 28th week of gestation who do not breathe or show any other sign of life per 1000 total births (sometimes, e.g. United Nations statistics, expressed as per 1000 live births). In the UK the period of gestation defining stillbirth was reduced in 1992 to 24 or more completed weeks of gestation.

Perinatal mortality rate (PMR). The number of stillbirths plus first week deaths per 1000 total births. (WHO has suggested that national perinatal statistics should include delivered fetuses and infants weighing at least 500 g or, when birthweight is unavailable, of gestational age of 22 weeks or crown–heel length of 25 cm, whether alive or dead.)

Early neonatal mortality rate (ENMR). The number of deaths in the first 6 days of life per 1000 live births.

Late neonatal mortality rate. The number of deaths occurring from the 7th to the 27th days of life per 1000 live births.

Neonatal mortality rate (NMR). The number of deaths in the first 27 days of life per 1000 live births.

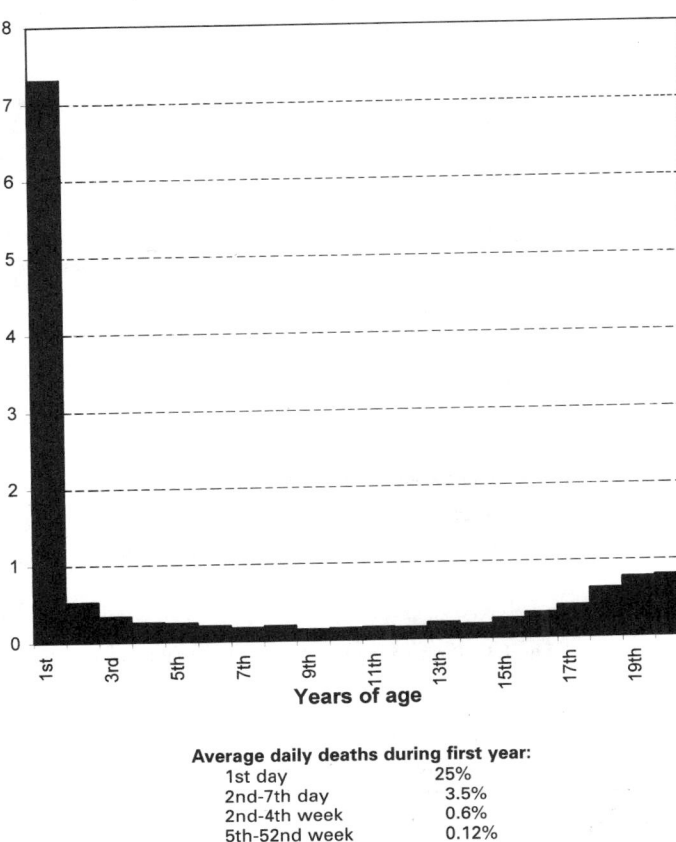

Average daily deaths during first year:

1st day	25%
2nd-7th day	3.5%
2nd-4th week	0.6%
5th-52nd week	0.12%

Fig. 1.2 Mortality rate/1000 in age group; England and Wales 1993.

Postneonatal mortality rate (PNMR). The number of deaths at age 28 days and over to the end of the first year of life per 1000 live births.

Infant mortality rate (IMR). The number of deaths in the first year of life per 1000 live births.

Under-5 mortality rate. Annual number of deaths of children under 5 years of age per 1000 live births.

Age-specific death rates. Number of deaths in an age group per specified population in the group.

Births outside marriage involve mortality rates 12–40% higher than those within marriage.

Stillbirths (late fetal mortality)

In Britain the rate has fallen from 42 to 4.3 during the past half century (Fig. 1.3). There are 175 live births for every stillbirth (1992). The influence of social class, maternal age, parity, birthweight and multiparity on the stillbirth rate is indicated in Table 1.2 and the pathology in Table 1.3.

Perinatal mortality

The UK rate (1992–94) is 7.5. The falling rate over the past half century is shown in Figure 1.3. Influencing factors are indicated in Table 1.2. Under least favorable circumstances the PMR can be three or more times that under the most favorable.

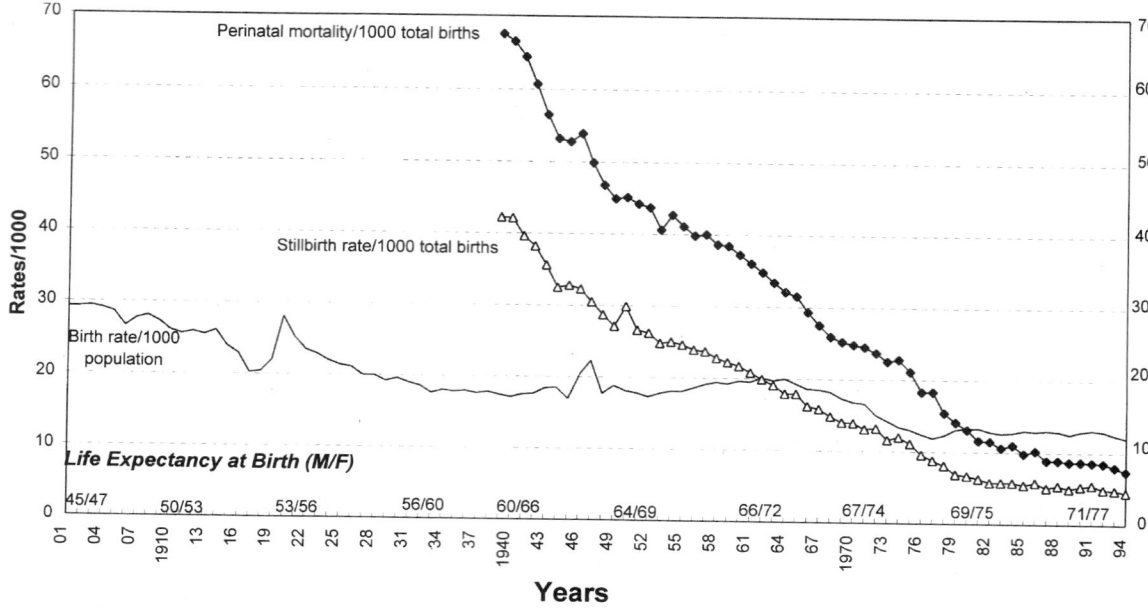

Fig. 1.3   Birth, stillbirth and perinatal mortality rates, and life expectancy; Scotland 1900–1994.

Table 1.3   Causes of stillbirth

	%	%
Congenital abnormalities		7.0
CNS	2.3	
Congenital heart disease	0.7	
Genitourinary	0.5	
Musculoskeletal	0.7	
Chromosomal	1.4	
Prematurity (IUGR, short gestation, low birthweight)		5.0
Birth trauma		0.3
Intrauterine hypoxia and birth asphyxia		20.0
Infection		0.7
Other perinatal causes		10.0
Maternal causes		14.0
No fetal abnormality		43.0
Total		100.0

Early neonatal mortality

The UK rate (1992–94) is 3.5. 80% of neonatal, 49% of infant and 32% of childhood deaths occur in the first week of life. The fall in ENMR over the past six decades is shown in Figure 1.4.

Late neonatal mortality

The UK rate (1992–94) is 1.

Neonatal mortality

Neonatal deaths account for 40% of childhood deaths. The fall in neonatal mortality rate throughout the 20th century is indicated in Figure 1.4 and influencing factors in Table 1.2. Causes are shown in Table 1.4.

Table 1.4   Causes of neonatal death

	%	%
Congenital abnormalities		24.8
Anencephalus	0.6	
Spina bifida	0.3	
Other CNS	1.7	
Congenital heart disease	10.4	
Respiratory system	4.1	
Cleft lip and palate	0.7	
Genitourinary	1.0	
Musculoskeletal	2.3	
Chromosomal	2.3	
Other	1.1	
Prematurity (short gestation and low birthweight)		28.4
Birth trauma		3.8
Intracranial hemorrhage	3.7	
Fetal and neonatal asphyxia		5.3
Noninfectious respiratory disorders		20.1
RDS	10.0	
Other	10.1	
Infections		5.0
Meningitis	0.5	
Pneumonia	0.8	
Other	3.3	
Fetal and neonatal hemorrhage		3.7
Perinatal digestive disorders		1.5
Disordered temperature regulation		0.9
Sudden infant death syndrome		1.7
Other fetal and perinatal		4.9
Total		100.0

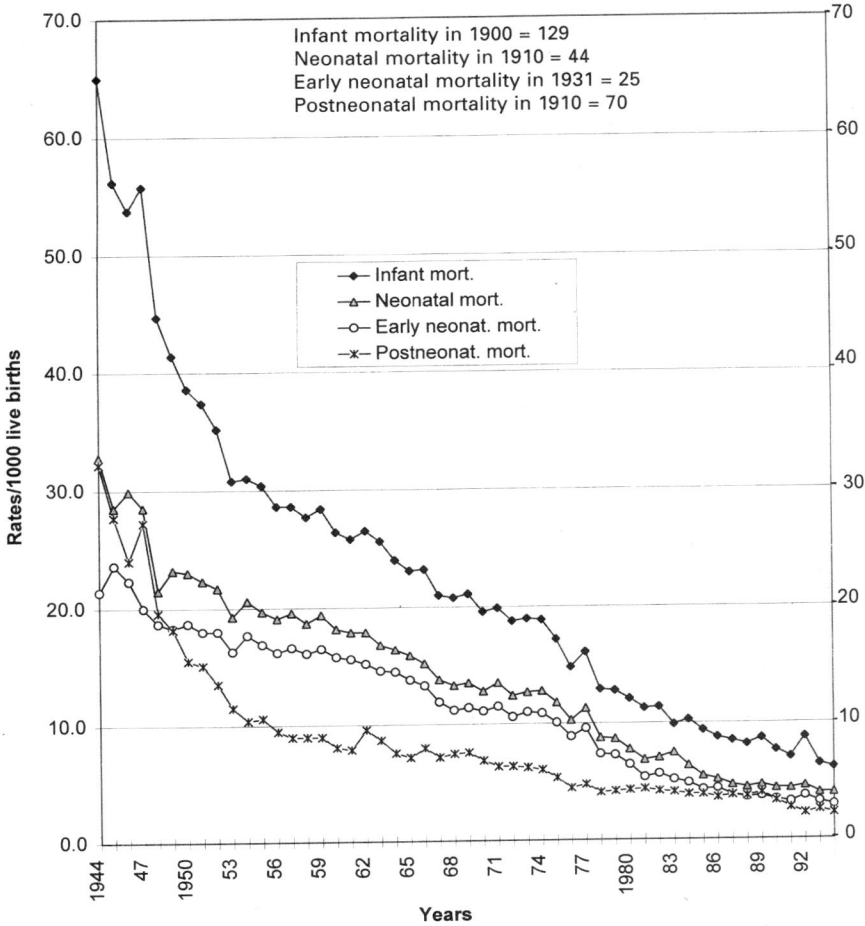

Infant mortality in 1900 = 129
Neonatal mortality in 1910 = 44
Early neonatal mortality in 1931 = 25
Postneonatal mortality in 1910 = 70

Fig. 1.4 Infant, neonatal, early neonatal and postneonatal mortality; Scotland 1944–1994.

Postneonatal mortality

Worldwide, postneonatal mortality rates show enormous variation – from 2 in some developed to over 80 in certain developing countries. The UK rate (1992–94) is 2.2. Figure 1.4 illustrates the fall during the last 50 years, Table 1.2 influencing factors and Table 1.5 causes. The recent fall from 4.1 to 3.0 per 1000 live births is due almost entirely to the fall in sudden infant deaths.

Table 1.5 Causes of postneonatal deaths

	%	%
Infection and parasitic disorders (excluding respiratory tract)		5.8
Disorders of respiratory tract		9.5
Upper respiratory	0.6	
Acute bronchitis	1.4	
Pneumonia	4.4	
Congenital anomalies		27.2
CNS	4.0	
Congenital heart disease	14.6	
Other disorders originating in perinatal period		17.4
Sudden infant death syndrome		34.1
External causes of injury and poisoning		6.0
Total		100.0

Infant mortality

World IMRs are listed in Table 1.1. Rates for individual countries (1993) range from nearly 200 in Niger to 4 in Finland. The UK rate (1992–94) is 6.4. The change over the past century is shown in Figure 1.4, influencing factors in Table 1.2 and causes in Table 1.6. Infant deaths account for approximately 65% of all childhood deaths.

Age-specific deaths

Figure 1.5 compares the change in the 0–14 age group mortality over the past 65 years with the 15–54 group.

UK age-specific death rates per 100 000 are shown in Table 1.6 which gives the main causes of death by age group and the percentages of deaths attributable to different causes. In the *first year of life* the major toll is taken by neonatal disorders such as congenital abnormalities, prematurity, asphyxia, the respiratory distress syndrome, sudden infant death, infections, birth trauma, CNS disorders and accidents; in the *1–4 years age period* by accidents, congenital abnormalities, infections (especially meningitis and respiratory infection), CNS disorders and malignant neoplasms; in the *5–9 years age group* by malignant neoplasms, accidents, infections and congenital abnormalities; and in the *10–14 years age group* by accidents, malignant

Table 1.6 Causes of death in childhood (age group populations: numbers by age group: rates)

International Detailed List numbers	Cause of death	Number of deaths					%
	Age group	< 1	1–4	5–9	10–14	0–14	
	Population (thousands)	732.7	3025.2	3643.0	3511.7	10 915.7	
	All causes of death (rates/100 000 in age group)	4740 (647)	940 (31)	499 (14)	641 (18)	6820 (62)	100*
001–139, 320–326, 380–384, 460–489, 513, 540–543, 590, 680–686, 771	I. Infective and parasitic diseases	350	159	57	55	621	9.1
001–009	Enteritis	22	2	1	28	53	0.8
036, 320–323	Meningitis and encephalitis	58	65	14	5	142	2.1
045–049	Viral and chlamydial infection	10	10	6	6	32	0.5
464–465	Acute laryngotracheitis and upper respiratory tract infection	5	3	3	2	13	0.2
466	Acute bronchitis and bronchiolitis	27	13	1	1	42	0.6
480–487	Pneumonia	71	49	20	13	153	2.2
771	Neonatal infection	106	–	–	–	106	1.6
140–239	II. Malignant neoplasms	29	95	135	130	389	5.7
170–171	Bone and connective tissue	–	10	4	19	33	0.5
191–192	Brain and spinal cord	7	19	42	38	106	1.6
204–208	Leukemia	3	18	44	46	111	1.6
240–279	III. Endocrine, metabolic and immunological disorders	48	35	22	28	131	1.9
280–289, 773–776	IV. Disorders of blood-forming organs (including hemolytic and aplastic anemia and coagulation defects)	38	9	6	17	70	1.0
776	Hematological disorders of newborn	22	–	–	–	22	0.3
290–319	V. Mental disorders	–	3	–	7	10	0.1
330–379, 430–438	VI. Nervous system (excluding congenital abnormalities and infective disorders of the CNS)	96	107	61	68	332	4.9
335	Anterior horn disease	20	15	1	3	39	0.6
342–344	Cerebral palsy	19	32	20	22	93	1.4
345	Epilepsy	7	13	15	16	51	0.7
430–438	Cerebrovascular disease	14	4	2	4	24	0.4
390–414, 420–424, 429, 440–459	VII. Circulatory system (excluding congenital heart disease)	31	21	12	11	75	1.1
490–512, 514–519	VIII. Respiratory system (excluding newborn and infection)	49	23	13	19	104	1.5
490–493	Asthma and emphysema	5	10	7	11	33	0.5
520–537, 550–579, 777	IX. Digestive system (excluding congenital abnormalities)	83	27	5	5	120	1.8
777	Neonatal disorders of the digestive system	53	–	–	–	53	0.8
580–589, 591–629	X. Genitourinary system (excluding congenital abnormalities)	6	5	4	3	18	0.3
690–709	XII. Skin and subcutaneous tissue	1	–	–	–	1	.01
359, 710–739	XIII. Musculoskeletal system	10	5	5	19	39	0.6
359	Muscular dystrophy	9	2	1	16	28	0.4
415–417, 425–428, 740–759	XIV. Congenital abnormalities	1127	191	48	67	1433	21.0
415–417	Pulmonary circulation disorders	12	9	4	1	26	0.4
425	Cardiomyopathy	19	12	4	10	45	0.7
740	Anencephalus	29	–	–	–	29	0.4
741	Spina bifida	13	–	2	5	20	0.3
742	Other CNS anomalies	89	36	11	13	149	2.2
745–747	Congenital morbus cordis including TGA, VSD, Fallot's tetralogy and others	473	101	22	28	624	9.1
748	Respiratory system	156	6	–	1	163	2.4
749–751	Cleft lip and palate	37	7	3	1	48	0.7
753	Genitourinary system	36	3	–	–	39	0.6
754–756	Limb and skeletal abnormalities	96	6	2	2	106	1.6
758	Chromosomal abnormalities	112	10	–	3	125	1.8
760–770, 772, 778–779	XV. Certain neonatal conditions	2190	36	4	–	2230	32.7
760–763	Complications of pregnancy and labor	57	–	–	–	57	0.8
764, 765	Short gestation, low birthweight, intrauterine growth retardation	1001	–	–	–	1001	14.7
768	Birth trauma	151	1	–	2	154	2.3
769	Asphyxia	364	–	–	–	364	5.3
770	RDS	419	–	–	–	419	6.1
772	Other respiratory disorders	121	–	–	–	121	1.8
778	Disordered temperature regulation	27	–	–	–	27	0.4
780–799	XVI. Symptoms and ill-defined disorders	615	31	1	3	650	9.5
798	Sudden infant death	484	17	–	–	501	7.3
E800–E999	XVII. Injury and poisoning	69	193	126	209	597	8.8
E810–E829	Road accidents	7	55	69	100	231	3.4
E850–E869	Poisoning	1	15	4	9	29	0.4
E880–E888	Falls	3	13	11	11	38	0.6
E890–E899	Burns and scalds	4	31	10	2	47	0.7
E910	Drowning	3	25	9	7	44	0.6

* Percentage of childhood deaths attributed to the diagnosis. Based on the Annual Report of the Registrar General, Scotland 1994 (HMSO) and OPCS Surveys, Mortality Statistics, Cause, 1993 and Mortality Statistics, Perinatal and Infant: Social and Biological Factors 1992 (HMSO).

0-14 years
15-54 years
Mortality rate/1000
Years
1930
1995
0
1
2
3
4
5
6
7
8
9
10

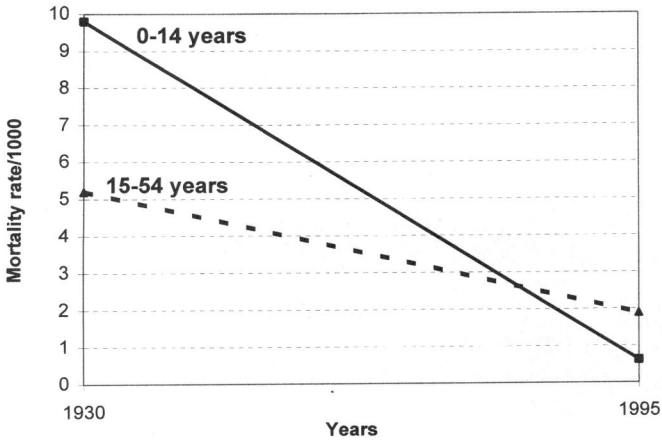

Fig. 1.5 Relative child/adult mortalities 1930 to 1995.

neoplasms, CNS disorders, congenital abnormalities and infections.

Thus, after the first year, accidents are the main cause of childhood deaths followed by neoplasms, congenital abnormalities, infections, CNS disorders and endocrine disorders.

Table 1.6 shows the age-related incidence of different accident mortalities.

Figure 1.6 shows, in broad categories, the causes of death throughout childhood.

Mortality in the developing world

In many developing countries, mostly Africa, Asia and South America, the mortality rate is 10 or more times that in Britain (Table 1.1). Figure 1.7 illustrates the main causes of death among 12.9 million children under 5 in the world's least developed countries (1990).

Trends in mortality from individual diseases

The mortality rate per million children 50 years ago was 20 times greater than it is now. Reduction has not occurred uniformly. The incidence of *tuberculosis* and *acute rheumatism* and certain infectious fevers such as *whooping cough* and *measles* has fallen significantly. *Diphtheria* and *poliomyelitis* have been virtually eliminated. Death from *neonatal asphyxia/birth injury* (Fig. 1.8) showed a stepwise fall during the periods 1941–50 and 1965–80. 60 years ago the mortality from *pneumonia/bronchitis* (Fig. 1.8) was 100 times greater than it is today. Deaths from *nontuberculous meningitis* had fallen from 300 to 6 per million by 1977 but have recently shown a slight rise. The fall in *congenital*

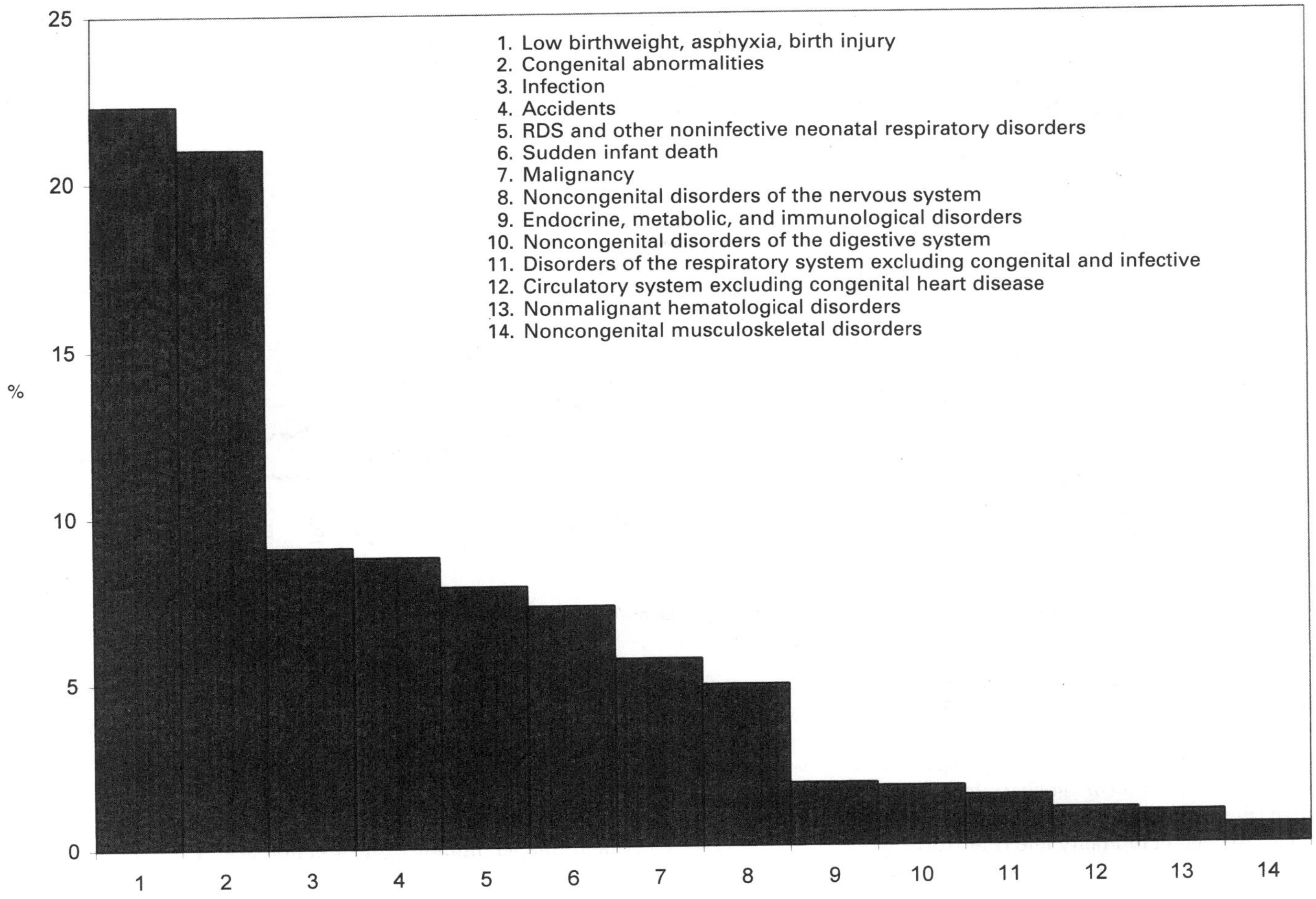

%
0
5
10
15
20
25
1. Low birthweight, asphyxia, birth injury
2. Congenital abnormalities
3. Infection
4. Accidents
5. RDS and other noninfective neonatal respiratory disorders
6. Sudden infant death
7. Malignancy
8. Noncongenital disorders of the nervous system
9. Endocrine, metabolic, and immunological disorders
10. Noncongenital disorders of the digestive system
11. Disorders of the respiratory system excluding congenital and infective
12. Circulatory system excluding congenital heart disease
13. Nonmalignant hematological disorders
14. Noncongenital musculoskeletal disorders
1
2
3
4
5
6
7
8
9
10
11
12
13
14

Fig. 1.6 Causes of death throughout the period of childhood (0–14 years); Scotland (1994), England and Wales (1992–93) combined.

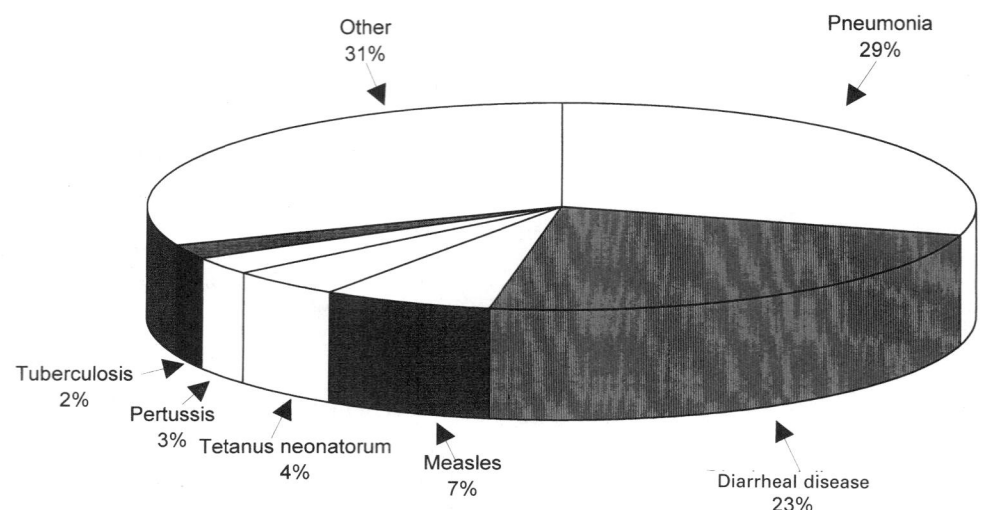

Fig. 1.7   Main causes of death in children (0–5 years) in developing countries.

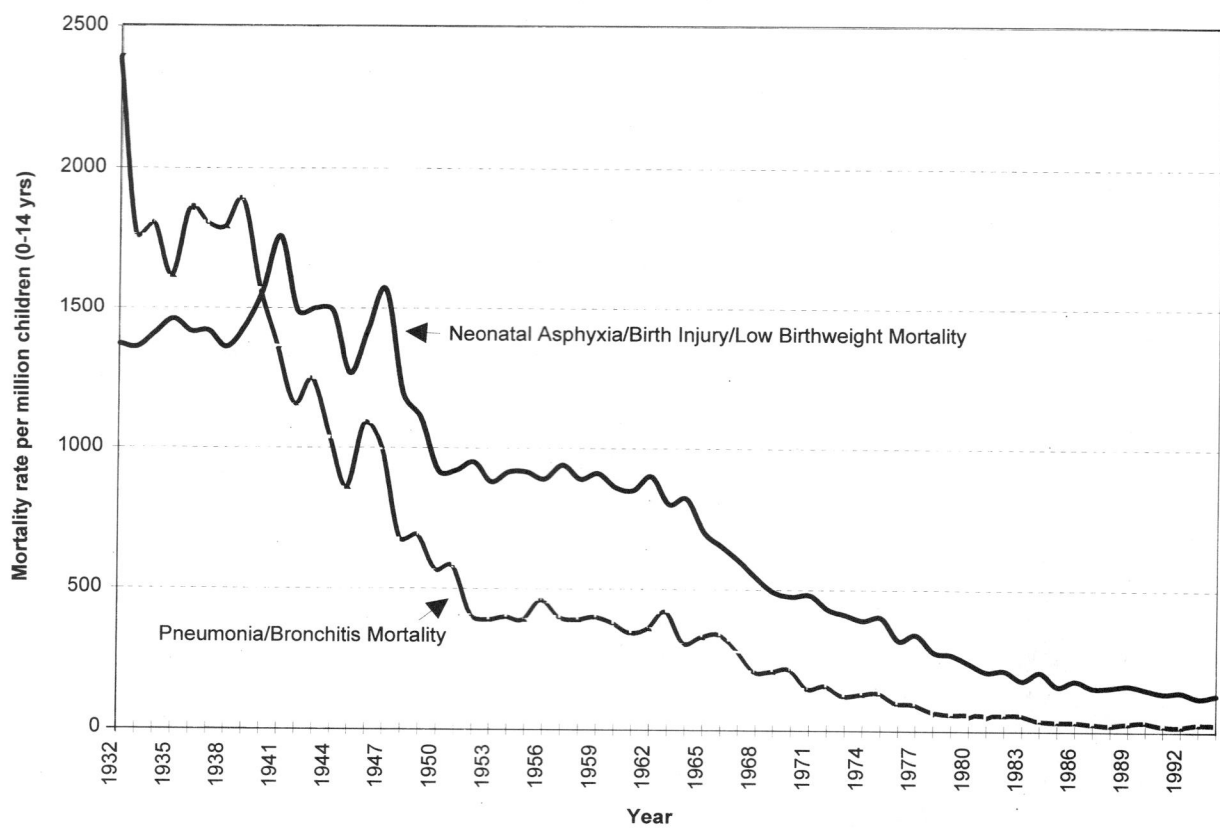

Fig. 1.8   Neonatal asphyxia/birth injury/low birthweight and pneumonia/bronchitis mortalities; Scotland 1932–1994.

abnormalities (Fig. 1.9) can be related to improved treatment for some, genetic counseling, prenatal diagnosis and termination of abnormal pregnancies, rather than to removal of primary causes. Less improvement is evident with *congenital heart disease* (Fig. 1.9). Although *accident numbers* have increased mortality has fallen (Fig. 1.9). Improving prognosis in *malignancy* has yet to be better reflected in mortality rate (Fig. 1.9).

CHILDHOOD MORBIDITY

More and more children recover from disease. Lower mortalities and surviving children require more child health services, not less.

Childhood morbidity: general practice

Among the 11 million British children in 1991–92 there were

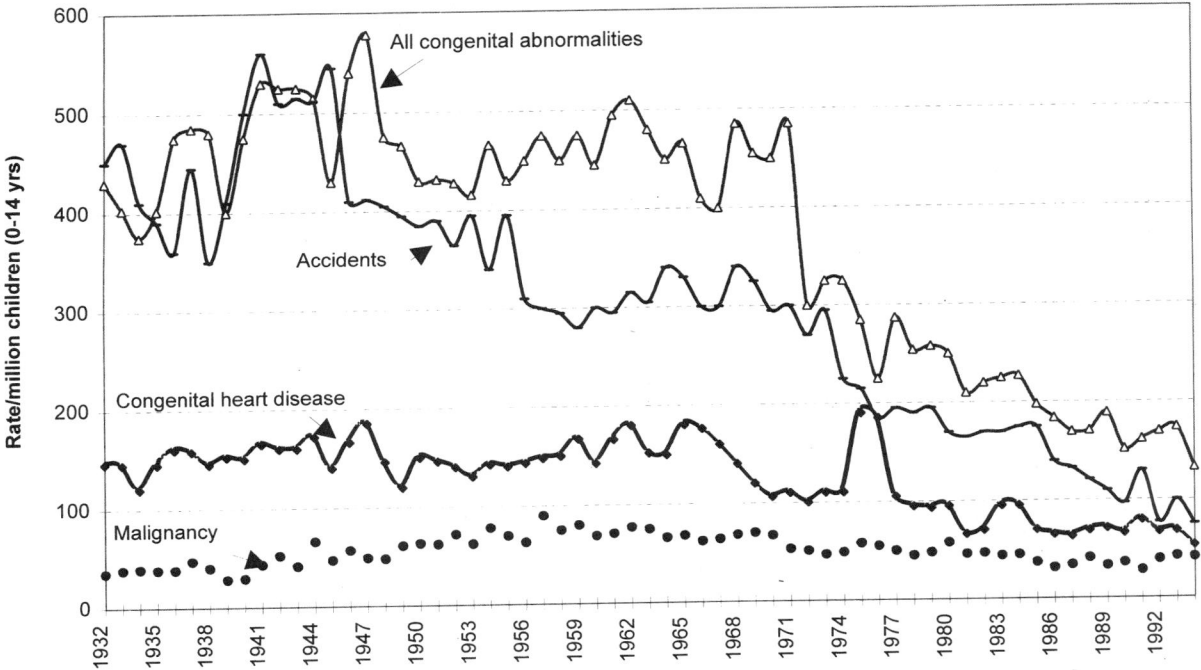

Fig. 1.9   Childhood (0–14 years) mortalities: congenital abnormalities, malignancy, accidents 1936–1994.

approximately 25 million general practitioner (GP) *consultations* per year, 14 million in the 0–4 year group and 11 in the 5–14 group. Children consulting their GP averaged 6 consultations per year in the 0–4 age group and 2.5 in the 5–14 group. The male/female ratio was 1.1. In the 0–4 group illness was considered serious in 7%, intermediate in 44% and minor in 49%. In the 5–14 year group the percentages were 10, 40 and 50. Only 10% of visits were home visits.

Table 1.7 shows, by age groups, the common childhood disorders seen in the community. Infections predominate, particularly in the early years of life.

GPs (1991–92) referred annually: for *hospital admission* 1 in 40 of their patients in the 0–4 year group and 1 in 135 of those aged 5–14; for *outpatient consultation* 1 in 10 and 1 in 14; and for *treatment in accident and emergency departments* 1 in 23 and 1 in 57.

Notifiable infectious disease

Table 1.8 presents the 1993 notifications for infectious disease in England and Wales. These imply that each year 1 child in 200 suffered from an infectious disease which is notified. Notifications may under-represent true incidence.

HOSPITAL SERVICES

Outpatients

On average, 1 child in 5 attends a hospital each year, either at an A&E department (2 million attendances; Table 1.9) or consultative clinic, and visits two to three times. Accidents,

respiratory disorders, neonatal problems, problems of development and behavior and handicapping disorders preponderate. 1 child in 300 attends a child psychiatry unit.

Inpatients

1 in 8 children aged 0–4 years and 1 in 16 aged 5–14 was admitted into hospital in 1993–94. 56% were boys. Duration of stay averaged 3.0 days in the 0–4 group and 2.7 days in the 5–14 group. For all causes there were annually 1.7 million finished consultant episodes (FCE = the period a patient using a hospital bed spends in the continuous care of one consultant, or in the care of two or more consultants with equal responsibility). Less than 1% of FCEs in the 0–4 group but nearly 25% in the 5–14 group were devoted to day cases. Table 1.10 shows FCE-based diagnoses in age groups, sorted for descending frequency in the 0–14 group.

Over the past half century the number of children admitted into hospital has increased, accompanied by a compensating reduction in length of stay (Fig. 1.10). This exemplifies the changing role of the pediatric unit from a last ditch refuge for the seriously ill to a service based on specialization and appropriate investigative procedures effecting early diagnosis, early institution of appropriate therapy and early return to parental and GP care.

AGE INCIDENCE OF DISEASE IN CHILDHOOD

Pediatrics involves medical care from intrauterine to adolescent life conducted against a range of biological change in its patients far wider than that encountered in any other branch of medicine. Particular diseases tend to reveal themselves at particular times in the biological calendar.

Table 1.7 General practice

Patient consulting rates per 10 000 persons at risk	Age (years) 0–4	Age (years) 5–15	Age (years) 0–14
All diseases	10 221	7234	8322
Acute respiratory disorders excluding pneumonia and influenza	6082	2861	3971
Potential health hazards related to communicable disease	4546	790	2084
Disorders of the ear mostly otitis media	2933	1350	1896
Ill-defined symptoms and nonspecific abnormalities	2821	1289	1814
Skin infections	2393	1115	1555
Disorders of the eye	1980	522	1024
Chronic obstructive respiratory disease and allied conditions	938	771	829
Other viral disease and chlamydia	633	783	731
Intestinal infections	338	771	622
Related to development	1838	81	607
Other disorders of the respiratory tract	328	641	533
Viral exanthematous disease	841	313	495
Helminthiasis	659	278	409
Superficial injuries, contusions and crushing	357	393	381
Open wounds	242	195	211
Other infections and parasitic diseases	226	199	208
Disorders of the intestine and peritoneum and noninfective enteritis and colitis	383	114	207
Arthropathies and dorsopathies	77	276	207
Pneumonia and influenza	239	187	205
Mental disorders – nonpsychiatric	228	191	204
Disease of oral cavity and salivary glands	344	121	198
Rheumatism	52	159	122
Congenital abnormalities	217	59	113
Sprains	94	107	103
CNS disorders	35	135	101
Fractures and dislocations	54	117	95
Osteopathies and acquired musculoskeletal deformities	37	82	66
Disease of esophagus, stomach and duodenum	80	53	62
Certain conditions in the neonatal period	173	0	60
Intracranial injuries and fractures	78	48	58
Metabolic disorders	60	43	57
Hematological disorders	58	56	57
Benign neoplasms	40	64	56
Burns	68	20	37
Foreign body entering an orifice	43	24	31
Hernia – abdominal	70	9	30
Total	29 585	14 217	19 513

The cumulative totals exceed the number of patients as the same patient may have suffered from several disorders and have made multiple visits.

Table 1.8 Infectious disease notifications (numbers), 0–14 years, England and Wales, 1993

Age (years)	Measles	Rubella	Pertussis	Meningitis All	Meningitis Meningo-coccal	Meningitis Pneumo-coccal	Meningitis H. influenzae	Meningitis Viral	Dysentery	Scarlet fever	Mumps	Viral hepatitis	Food poisoning
< 1	1920	1408	537	473	125	62	44	22	159	99	39	13	
1	1660	1002	353	216	113	22	39	4	362	190	106	11	
2	728	463	349	150	81	8	31	3	359	473	169		1350*
3	531	412	377	107	66	5	17	5	359	607	174	73†	
4	492	432	407	64	45	1	9	0	346	811	211		
5	408	490	418							808	204		
6	397	426	328							531	149		
7	332	337	270	30‡	19‡	16‡	1‡	3‡	305‡	358	115	188‡	
8	283	311	219							235	91		807§
9	275	344	187							188	85		
10–14	1982¶	203¶	75¶	23¶	14¶	1.2¶	0.6¶	1.8¶	76¶	102¶	52¶	140¶	

Annual averages: *0–4 years; †2–4 years; ‡5–9 years; §5–14 years; ¶10–14 years.

Table 1.9 Childhood accidental injuries treated in accident and emergency departments annually in England and Wales

Type of injury	Number	%
Cuts and bruises	800 000	40
Sprains and fractures	500 000	25
Head injuries	400 000	20
Foreign body in orifice	60 000	3
Eye injuries	60 000	3
Burns and scalds	40 000	2
Poisonings	40 000	2
Inhalations and ingestions	40 000	2
Bites and stings	40 000	2

From: Basic Principles of Child Accident Prevention (Child Accident Prevention Trust 1989).

Fetal

The fetus tends to be involved in diseases in which heredity and/or disturbed intrauterine environment play a part. The former include dominantly inherited disorders (e.g. achondroplasia), recessive disorders (e.g. autosomal such as cystic fibrosis or X-linked such as hemophilia), or polygenic disorders (e.g. spina bifida); the latter maternal infections (e.g. rubella, syphilis, toxoplasmosis, cytomegalic inclusion disease and AIDS) and drugs which may have a teratogenic effect (e.g. warfarin and sodium valproate).

Premature birth may have a profound effect on subsequent development, particularly neurological and intellectual (Forfar et al 1994).

Table 1.10 Annual hospital and day case admissions (finished consultant episodes*) (England and Wales) 1993–4 in descending order of diagnoses frequency, with distribution of age frequency and gender ratio (M/F)

	0–4 years	5–14 years	0–14 years	%	M/F
All causes	**1 181 142**	**500 546**	**1 681 688**		
All diagnoses	**738 477**	**478 202**	**1 216 679**	**100**	**1.41**
Certain perinatal conditions	**195 954**	**320**	**196 274**	**17**	**1.53**
Hypoxia, asphyxia, RDS	77 667	4	77 671		1.21
Obstetric complications affecting fetus	16 779	0	16 779		1.11
Birth trauma	5620	41	5661		1.49
Hemorrhagic disease of newborn	1206	0	1206		1.08
Diseases of the respiratory system	**124 108**	**41 964**	**168 072**	**14**	**1.41**
Upper respiratory tract infection	53 290	19 202	72 492		1.49
Asthma and asthmatic bronchitis	33 537	17 508	51 045		1.01
Other respiratory disorders	27 616	2789	30 405		1.45
Pneumonia	7665	2395	10 060		1.08
Disorders of the ear	**45 869**	**84 289**	**130 158**	**11**	**1.49**
Otitis media	26 033	31 423	57 456		1.31
Chronic disease of tonsils and adenoids	15 081	41 785	56 866		0.82
Deafness	2649	4000	6649		1.17
Injuries and poisoning	**51 974**	**76 586**	**128 560**	**11**	**1.42**
Fractures	9122	32 905	42 027		0.94
Intracranial injury and concussion	10 904	15 901	26 805		1.59
Poisoning	11 337	5879	17 216		0.97
Open wounds	6538	7695	14 233		1.69
Complications of trauma and other injuries	3953	5937	9890		1.20
Complications of medical and surgical care	2393	3652	6045		1.05
Foreign body entering an orifice	3843	2199	6042		1.29
Burns	3843	1044	4927		2.04
Sprains and dislocations	248	1612	1860		2.18
Ill-defined symptoms	**71 035**	**42 656**	**113 691**	**10**	**1.02**
Abdominal pain	3631	21 389	25 020		0.48
Pyrexia of unknown origin	4926	1411	6337		1.28
Symptoms involving the heart	2239	91	2330		0.73
Digestive system	**47 934**	**61 198**	**109 132**	**9**	**1.13**
Oral cavity, salivary glands, teeth	9455	33 293	42 748		0.85
Abdominal hernia	11 290	4793	16 083		2.55
Appendicitis	481	10 885	11 366		1.20
Intestinal obstruction	1021	220	1241		0.82
Other disorders of alimentary tract	25 687	12 007	37 694		0.68
Congenital abnormalities	**62 190**	**23 824**	**86 014**	**7**	**1.89**
Undescended testicles	5730	6476	12 206		–
Congenital heart disease	9410	2239	11 649		1.07
Digestive system	7317	1539	8856		1.78
Congenital dislocation of hip	6251	253	6504		0.40
Talipes	3499	353	3852		0.92
Cleft lip and palate	2478	698	3176		1.38
Spina bifida and hydrocephalus	975	772	1747		1.07
Disorders of genitourinary system	**26 271**	**27 318**	**53 589**	**5**	**–**
Redundant prepuce and phimosis	10 619	11 444	22 063		–
Other urinary disorders	9133	5424	14 557		–
Hydrocele	2316	1412	3728		–
Nephritis and nephrosis	1067	1540	2607		1.59
Infections of kidney including cystitis	126	360	486		0.34

Table 1.10 *Cont'd*

	0–4 years	5–14 years	0–14 years	%	M/F
Neoplasms	**13 604**	**19 368**	**32 972**	**3**	**1.11**
Malignant neoplasms	9841	12 608	22 449		1.39
Leukemia and other lymphatic tissue	5383	8911	14 294		1.39
Benign neoplasms	3763	6760	10 523		0.67
Musculoskeletal system	**7509**	**19 023**	**26 532**	**2**	**0.96**
Arthropathies excluding rheumatoid arthritis	3722	8395	12 117		0.63
Rheumatism excluding rheumatoid arthritis	2291	4474	6765		0.85
Rheumatoid arthritis	253	652	905		0.33
Dorsopathies	222	688	910		0.80
Osteomyelitis	282	357	639		1.41
Other disorders of joints	3113	7443	10 556		1.39
Disorders of the eye	**11 839**	**10 803**	**22 642**	**2**	**0.86**
Strabismus	5827	7068	12 895		0.95
Disorders of the lachrymal system	2659	392	3051		0.68
Conjunctivitis	599	49	648		1.02
Cataract	187	237	424		0.57
Skin and subcutaneous tissue	**10 195**	**10 640**	**20 835**	**2**	**1.22**
Infection of skin and subcutaneous tissue	4927	2781	6708		1.17
Mental disorders	**4353**	**14 170**	**18 523**	**2**	**1.14**
Mental retardation	1457	9128	10 585		1.24
Diseases of the blood-forming organs	**6294**	**11 663**	**17 957**	**2**	**1.11**
Anemia	2673	4975	7648		0.75
Disorders of the central nervous system	**7983**	**9877**	**17 860**	**1**	**0.95**
Epilepsy	3831	4490	8321		1.14
Cerebral palsy	1062	1888	2950		1.51
Degenerative and hereditary disorders	1216	753	1969		0.91
Cerebrovascular disorders	747	1132	1879		0.89
Meningitis	793	241	1034		0.94
Intracranial hemorrhage	150	198	348		1.12
Endocrine, metabolic and immunological disorders	**4974**	**9498**	**14 472**	**1**	**1.00**
Diabetes	557	2987	3544		1.03
Disorders of the circulatory system	**1633**	**2206**	**4550**	**< 1**	**1.19**
Heart disease (excluding congenital heart disease)	1593	1077	2605		1.03
Dysrhythmias	550	525	1075		1.06
Other reasons for contact with the health service	**442 665**	**22 339**	**465 004**		**1.03**
Housing, household and economic circumstances	2765	7736	10 501		0.90
Holiday relief care	1123	4979	6102		0.89

* See text.

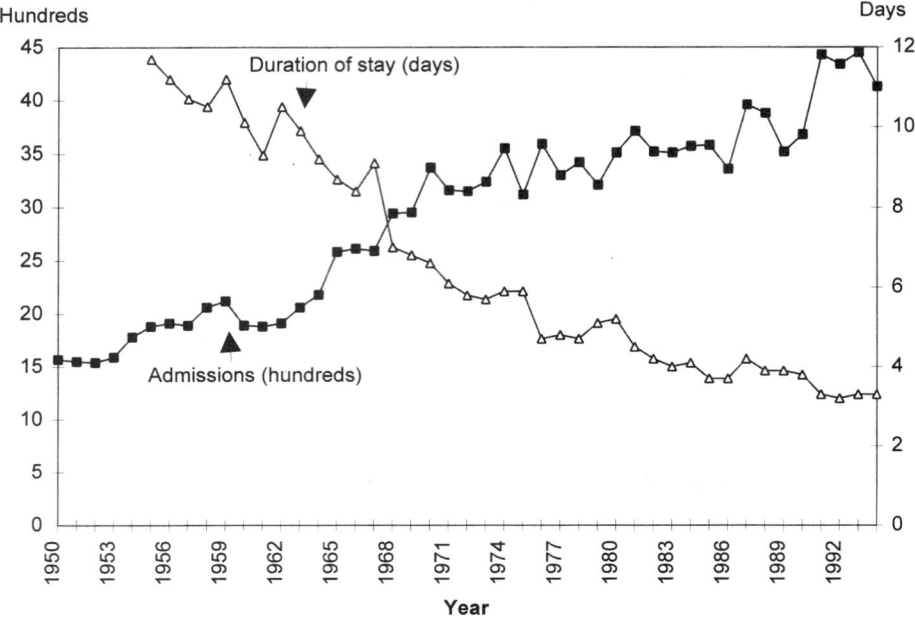

Fig. 1.10 Medical admissions and duration of stay; RHSC Edinburgh 1950–1994.

Birth

Disturbance of the physiological adaptations occurring before and after birth involving particularly placental function and the cardiorespiratory system (e.g. hypoxia, ischemia, RDS), mechanical stresses induced by abnormal presentation and/or instrumentation (e.g. intracranial bleeding) and the revelation of previously undetected congenital abnormalities (e.g. diaphragmatic hernia) may create immediate problems.

Neonatal

During the first month the pathological agenda includes congenital disorders, prematurity, the aftermath of fetal asphyxia and/or the development of postnatal asphyxia, infection, disseminated intravascular coagulation, anemia from blood loss or hemolysis and periventricular hemorrhage.

Early infancy (1–6 months)

Feeding problems may occur. Resistance to infection is poor with the intestinal and respiratory tracts particularly vulnerable. Cot death is a serious but enigmatic problem. Surgical treatment for developmental defects may be required.

Later infancy (6 months to 1 year)

The child is nearing the end of very rapid growth (at no other time in extrauterine life is growth of this order) and this predisposes to nutritional deficiencies such as rickets and iron deficiency anemia. Cerebral development is now such that convulsions are prone to occur. Liability to infection remains.

Early childhood (preschool 1–5 years)

The child, more mobile, mixes with other children and is liable to contact infection (e.g. the exanthemata). Mobility, curiosity and lack of judgment and experience mean more accidents. Consciousness of his/her identity and peer jealousies may promote behavior disorders.

Later childhood (school 5–15 years)

Schooling may reveal deficiencies of intellect (with learning problems) and/or of sensory organ function, and create psychological problems. With adolescence sexual problems and problems of identity may develop. The exuberance of youth predisposes to accidents.

COMBINED MORTALITY AND MORBIDITY

On average in the UK 18 British children die every day, 2500 are admitted to hospital, 3600 attend hospital outpatient departments,

Table 1.11 Daily mortality and morbidity rates per million children aged 0–14 years, UK 1993

Deaths	1.6
Admitted to hospital	230
Seen at hospital outpatient departments	330
Seen at accident and emergency departments	400
Seen by general practitioner	10 000

4400 attend accident and emergency departments and 110 000 consult general practitioners (Table 1.11).

CHRONIC AND HANDICAPPING ILLNESS IN CHILDHOOD

Impairment implies a pathological process such as spina bifida, *disability* a consequence of an impairment, and *handicap* ('a disability of body or mind which interferes with the ability to lead a normal life or to benefit from a normal education') the social consequence of impairment or disability. The assessed frequency of handicap varies according to the criteria used for diagnosis and the timing of the assessment. At birth 16 per 1000 liveborn infants exhibit major congenital abnormalities whereas 1 week later, due to early deaths, the incidence is 13 per 1000.

Minor impairments such as limited limb deformity, skin abnormalities, congenital dislocation of the hip, hydrocele, penile abnormalities and accessory auricles occur at a frequency of 33 per 1000 births (Nelson & Forfar 1969). Table 1.12 indicates the prevalence of impairment among school pupils and Table 1.13 that of severe childhood handicap (7.2 per 1000). Many of the latter (half affected physically and half intellectually, with considerable overlap) are unable to achieve independence. In keeping with the tendency for multiplicity in severe handicap, one-third have a single handicap, one-third have two, and one-third have three to five. Broad etiologic categories can be identified as genetic in 55%, acquired in 20% and chromosomal in 10%.

CHILD HEALTH INDICATORS, SOCIAL AND ENVIRONMENTAL INFLUENCES

The health and welfare of children are significantly influenced by social and environmental factors. Some of these are indicated in Table 1.14.

Table 1.12 Prevalence of impairment: school pupils

Learning disability	3.1
Speech impairment	1.8
Mentally retarded	1.0
Emotionally disturbed	0.6
Multiple handicap	0.2
Hearing impairment	0.1
Orthopedically impaired	0.1
Other health impaired	0.05
Deaf/blind	0.03
Total	6.98

After Vanderheiden (1990).

Table 1.13 Severe handicapping disorders: 10 077 severely handicapped children* aged 0–15 years

Disorder	Main subgroups within each major diagnostic group (with percentage frequency within the group)	Percentages of disorders (primary) among handicapped children	Percentages of handicapped children affected
Mental retardation	Down syndrome 18%, diseases causing neurological effects 18%, perinatal disorders 14%, unknown etiology 20%	38	67
Neurological disorders		22	39
Epilepsy	Grand mal 86%, myoclonic epilepsy 7%, petit mal 6%, mental retardation 1%	8	
Cerebral palsy	Perinatal 52%, developmental 27%, postinfective 11%, post-traumatic 4%	8	
Spina bifida and hydrocephalus	Meningomyelocele with hydrocephalus 37%, meningomyelocele 21%, hydrocephalus 39%	4	
Hereditary and familial CNS disorders	Microcephaly 65%	2	
Special sense and speech disorders		15	26
Deafness	(Needing special education 82%), (mentally defective 32%), congenital rubella 25%, cerebral palsy 7%	7	
Visual defects	Blind 34%, strabismus 23%, cataract 14%, congenital nystagmus 11%, retroplental fibroplasia 4%	6	
Speech and learning disorders	Speech disorders 83%, learning disorders 17%	3	
Psychiatric disorders	Hyperactivity 39%, behavior disorders 35%, autism 13%	6	11
Skeletal, joint and muscular disorders	Muscular dystrophies 25%, scoliosis 11%, congenital dislocation of hip 8%, talipes equinovarus and calcaneovalgus 7%	6	11
Alimentary disorders	Cystic fibrosis 46%, congenital abnormalities of alimentary tract 31%, celiac disease 16%	4	7
Cardiovascular disorders	Congenital heart disease 83%	3	5
Metabolic and endocrine disorders		2	4
Inborn errors of metabolism	Phenylketonuria 52%	1	
Other	Diabetes mellitus 32%, dwarfism 32%, thyroid disorders 16%	1	
Neoplastic disease	Leukemia 52%	2	3
Respiratory disorders	Asthma 72%	1	2
Genitourinary disorders	Chronic nephritis/pyelonephritis 20%	1	2
Disorders of the blood	Hemophilia 48%	< 1	1
Disorders of the skin, hair and nails		≤ 1	< 1
Total		100	

After Dykes (1978). *Boys 58%, girls 42%.

REFERENCES AND BIBLIOGRAPHY

Bone M, Meltzer H 1989 The prevalence of disability among children. OPCS survey. HMSO, London
Botting B (ed) 1995 The health of our children. OPCS survey. HMSO, London
British Paediatric Association 1991 Towards a combined health service. BPA, London
British Paediatric Association 1995 Child health rights. BPA, London
British Paediatric Association 1995 Health needs of school age children. BPA, London
Central Statistical Office 1992 Social trends 22. HMSO, London
Child Accident Prevention Trust 1989 Basic principles of child accident prevention. Child Accident Prevention Trust, London
Dykes J 1978 Ten thousand severely handicapped children. Australian Publishing Service, Canberra
Forfar J O (ed) 1988 Child health in a changing society. British Paediatric Association. Oxford University Press, Oxford
Forfar J O, Hume R, McPhail F et al 1994 Low birth weight: a 10-year outcome study of the continuum of reproductive casualty. Developmental Medicine and Child Neurology 36: 1037–1048
Government Statistical Service 1995 Hospital episode statistics vol 1. Finished consultant episodes by diagnosis, operation and specialty 1993–94. Department of Health, HMSO, London
Nelson M M, Forfar J O 1969 Congenital abnormalities at birth; their association in the same patient. Developmental Medicine and Child Neurology 11: 3–16
Office of Health Economics 1995 Compendium of health statistics. OHE, London
Office of Population Censuses and Surveys (England and Wales): 1992 Series DH2 No. 20 Mortality statistics, cause: 1992 Series DH6 No. 6 Mortality statistics, childhood: 1992 Series DH3 No. 26 Mortality statistics, perinatal and infant; social and biological factors: 1993 Series DH2 No. 20 Mortality statistics: 1993 Series MB2 No. 2 Communicable disease statistics. HMSO, London
Registrar General for Scotland, Annual Reports 1992, 1993, 1994. General Registrar Office, Edinburgh. HMSO, Edinburgh
Royal College of General Practitioners, OPCS, Department of Health 1995 Morbidity statistics from general practice, fourth national survey, 1991–92. HMSO, London
UNICEF 1992, 1993, 1994 The state of the world's children. Oxford University Press, Oxford
United Nations convention on the rights of the child 1989 UN, New York
United Nations 1992 Demographic year book. UN, New York
Vanderheiden G C 1990 30 something millions; should they be exceptions? Human Factors 32: 383–396
Wenlock R W, Disselduff M M, Skinner R K et al 1986 The diets of British schoolchildren. Department of Health and Office of Population Censuses and Surveys, London
World Health Organization 1994 WHO statistics. WHO, Geneva

Table 1.14   Child health indicators, social and environmental influences (UK)

Population and births:

The relative proportions of boys and girls (0–14 years) are boys 51.2% and girls 48.8%

The average number of births per female is 1.8 (1990)

Over the past 25 years the number of children born to women over the age of 30 years has increased but for other age groups has changed little or has fallen. Thus the proportion of births to women over the age of 30 has increased

Between 1983 and 1991 the proportion of liveborn babies weighing less than 1500 g increased from 0.84 to 0.93%

In 1992, 1 in 40 liveborn infants was a twin and 1 in 1000 a triplet. In singletons the risk of cerebral palsy is 2 per 1000. It is six times that rate in twins and 38 times in triplets

In 1991 there were 9.9 conceptions per 1000 women aged under 16 and 51% ended in abortion

Mothers:

About 12% of mothers work full time and 30% part time

70% of mothers in social class I are breast-feeding their babies at 6 weeks but there is a steady downward incidence by social class to 20% in class V. Overall only 1 in 4 mothers breast-feeds for 4 months after birth

Children:

1 in 5 children lives in lone parent families: 18% of families with dependent children are headed by lone mothers and 1.5% by lone fathers

Daily food intake by social class 10/11-year-old children per two parent family:*

Social class	I/II (m/f)	IIIN (m/f)	IIIM (m/f)	IV/V (m/f)	Unemployed (m/f)
Energy (kJ)	8990/7610	8060/7630	8710/7790	8440/7710	8820/7640
Protein (g)	63.5/64.1	60.8/53.2	60.4/52.9	57.9/53.1	60.5/51.3
Fat (g)	90.8/77.6	81.0/78.1	88.0/79.5	84.0/79.8	90.1/77.8
Carbohydrate (g)	277/238	252/239	276/247	271/240	278/243
Vitamin C	60.7/60.7	45.6/60.7	46.4/45.5	40.2/40.6	39.5/36.7
Height (cm)	144.4/143.1	144.7/144.0	141.9/143.6	141.9/142.8	140.8/140.0

The number of children in care in England, Wales and Northern Ireland fell from over 100 000 in 1980 to 65 000 in 1990

For both boys and girls the amount of exercise which they take declines across the 11 to 15 year period

Among children aged 11–15 (1990) 15% in Wales, 16% in England, and 20% in Scotland were regular or occasional smokers

Approximately 9% of 13-year-old children and 29% of 15-year-old children are weekly drinkers of alcohol

About 30% of 15-year-old boys and 4% of girls abuse volatile substances

Approximately 10% of children belong to ethnic minority groups. In these, congenital abnormalities, iron deficiency anemia, tuberculosis, vitamin D deficiency and inherited diseases such as thalassemia and sickle cell disease are more common but sudden infant death is less common

Among children fires are the main cause of accidental deaths in the home

Between 1981 and 1991 notified rates for babies born with central nervous system malformations fell from 19 per 10 000 births to 4.6

By 1991 92% of children aged less than 2 years had been immunized against measles, mumps, rubella, diphtheria, tetanus, whooping cough and poliomyelitis

Between 1983 and 1993 the number of children free from dental caries had risen from 7 to 37%

* After Wenlock et al (1986). (m/f) = male/female.

2 History taking and physical examination

J. O. Forfar

History 16
History of present illness 16
Previous history 18
    Birth history 18
    Feeding 18
    Previous illnesses 18
    Contact with infectious disease 18
    Residence abroad 18
    Prophylactic inoculations 18
Family history 18
Developmental history 18
Social and environmental history 18
Physical examination 18
Relationship of examiner to child and parents 19
General inspection 19
Physical measurements 19
    Weight 19
    Length 19
    Head circumference 20
    Temperature 20
    Blood pressure 20
Examination of individual systems and regions 20
Head and neck 20
    Cranium 20
    Ears 20
    Facies 21
    Eyes 21
    Nose 27
    Mouth 27
    Neck 29
    Lymph nodes 30
Chest and lungs 30
Cardiovascular system 30

Abdomen 32
    Examination of stools 33
Perineum and genitalia 33
    Anus 33
    Rectal examination 33
    Genitalia 34
Nervous system 34
    Inspection 34
    Cranial nerves 34
    Muscle tone 35
    Motor power 35
    Coordination 35
    Sensation 35
    Reflexes 35
    Other neurological signs 38
Higher nervous activities 38
Locomotor system 38
    Fractures 38
    Deformities of the trunk and neck 38
    Deformities of limbs 38
    Muscles 39
    Joints 39
Examination of the newborn 41
Medical history of parents, siblings and other relatives 41
Birth history 41
Gestational age 41
The transition period 42
Routine examination 42
    Measurements 42
    Excreta 43
    Instrumental procedures 43
Neurological assessment 43
References 44

HISTORY

Clinical examination in pediatrics relies on the classic principles of history taking and physical examination, applied appropriately in the circumstances of childhood and supplemented by such supplementary investigations as are necessary. The history has often to be obtained from parents or attendants so that the examiner has to be alert to the possibility that they may introduce secondary bias and make preconceived judgments based on limited knowledge or folklore.

Firstly, parents should be encouraged to give a spontaneous account of a child's illness subject to such curbs on irrelevance or verbosity as the examiner deems expedient and secondly the examiner can ask specific questions to amplify and clarify the parents' description. Older children can provide much history, usually give an accurate account of their symptoms and answer questions directly without bias. The examiner has to decide before or during the history taking whether it is desirable for the child to be present.

Children can be divided into age groups:

Neonatal	1st 4 weeks of life
Infant	1st year
Preschool	2 to 4+ years
School	5 to 15 years
Childhood	1 to 15 years
Adolescent	13 to 19 years

HISTORY OF PRESENT ILLNESS

Specific points for inquiry or amplification are:
Age and sex. Note date of birth.

Symptoms of abnormalities complained of and their duration.

The precise order of symptoms including any repeated episodes (e.g. asthma or epilepsy).

Changes noted since the onset of illness contrasting present with previous condition.

Activity or apathy may be gauged by the child's movements in pram or cot, performance in normal household activities, interest in people and things, willingness to walk to school or shops, tiring easily or returning early from play.

Feeding and appetite. Temporarily or persistently impaired (this may lead to an assessment of daily caloric intake which with babies can usually be assessed in terms of intake of milk, amount of sugar and other elements, and with older children by analyzing a recorded daily diet), food fads or dislikes; unusual parental ideas regarding diet; daily intake of vitamin supplements?

Difficulty in swallowing is commonly functional rather than organic and related to attempts to persuade the child to eat against his will with resultant choking and gagging. The child with organic dysphagia may swallow food but will regurgitate it shortly thereafter.

Thirst. If present, assess the total daily intake of fluid and output of urine.

Vomiting. Amount; frequency; duration; effortless or projectile; nature of vomitus (e.g. stained with bile or blood); an isolated symptom or associated with abdominal pain (e.g. constipation), pyrexia or impairment of consciousness? In a baby the possibility of rumination necessitates questions regarding observed movements of the mouth and glottis prior to vomiting.

Abdominal pain is probably thought to occur much more frequently than it actually does in babies due to their propensity for drawing up their legs and crying as a result of pain wherever it occurs. Toddlers, asked frequently if they have a 'sore tummy' in the presence of any upset, may come to use this term for pain at any site. With abdominal pain ascertain its nature; timing; duration; constancy or intermittence; site; aggravation by breathing or movement; relationship to food, bowel movement or micturition; association with anorexia, diarrhea, melena, constipation, vomiting, sore throat, cough or purpura.

Abdominal distention. Generalized or localized; distended abdominal veins; past or present only; duration; associated pain?

State of bowels and character of the stools. Normally infants pass several semisolid mustard-colored stools per day. Ascertain the frequency of bowel movement, character of the stools (hard or soft, watery, accompanied by mucus, blood-streaked or mixed with blood, bulky, dark or pale, floating on water, malodorous), presence of involuntary fecal soiling (encopresis), pain or crying on defecation (e.g. anal fissure)?

Loss of, or gain in, weight. Has the child become thinner or fatter judged by general appearance, recent looseness or tightness of clothing, wasting, swelling or puffiness?

Discharge from eyes, ears, nose or other sites. Purulent, watery or bloodstained, profuse or scanty, continuous or intermittent?

Sore throat. Babies and toddlers do not complain of sore throat although parents often assume this to be present (e.g. when there is refusal of food). Older children can localize pain.

Cough. Ascertain duration; character; dry or moist; paroxysmal; more severe by day or night; disturbing of sleep; associated with pain, whoop, vomiting, chest pain, wheeze, nasal discharge; accompanied by sputum (swallowed or expectorated, watery, mucoid, mucopurulent or bloodstained).

Breathlessness. Present only on activity (exercise tolerance) or at rest; persistent or intermittent; of gradual or sudden onset; exercise induced; nocturnal or diurnal; associated with cough, cyanosis or breath holding?

Cry or voice. Any change noted?

Mouth breathing. Mouth habitually open or shut, snores?

Stridor. Continuous or intermittent, inspiratory or expiratory, duration?

Wheeze. Inspiratory or expiratory; continuous or intermittent; precipitating factors; duration?

Abnormalities of the breath. Sweet smell (acetone) or fetor?

Other localized pain. Extent, nature, degree of severity, intermittent or continuous, duration and direction of radiation?

Localized swellings. Site, size, color, consistency, presence or absence of local pain, tenderness, duration?

Rashes or other skin lesions. Site, color, number and size of lesions; vesicles, ulcers, papules, macules, petechiae, itch?

Jaundice. Time of onset, duration, any abnormality in the stools or urine, vomiting?

Cyanosis. Peripheral or central, persistent or intermittent, affected by environmental temperature?

Pallor. Intermittent or persistent (many children are naturally pale but pallor tends to cause anxiety in parents)?

State of the musculature. Normal active movements or not? Does the mother feel the limbs to be stiff (hypertonicity or spasticity), or 'floppy', slipping through her hands on lifting (hypotonicity)?

Changes in posture or in walk. Of long duration or recently developed; holding the body in any unusual way (e.g. torticollis or scoliosis); abnormality in gait (examine wear in shoes); falling frequently?

Coordination. Dropping things, spilling from a cup, impairment of fine movement (e.g. writing or buttoning clothing)?

Involuntary movements. Nature of these; the same movement repeated or different movements; any injury suffered as a result of the movements; aggravated by emotional stress?

States of reduced consciousness. Degree; premonitory symptoms or aura; duration; subsequent awareness of events; injury sustained; response to stimuli?

Convulsions and fits. State of the child prior to the convulsion, any precipitating factor (e.g. pyrexia), any premonitory symptoms, type of movement observed (e.g. tonic or clonic); duration of various stages, state of consciousness, loss of posture, incontinence; uprolling of the eyes, biting of the tongue or other injury; sleep or headache afterwards?

Speech. Delay in onset or loss of speech, nature of speech (e.g. gruff, aphonic, slurred), change in character, difficulty in comprehension or expression?

Defects in vision. Able to follow a moving object with eyes, difficulty in reading or in distance vision, colliding with objects, color blindness?

Headache. Site, manner of onset, severity, and accompanying symptoms (e.g. vomiting), aura (e.g. migraine)? Younger children seldom complain of headache.

Hearing. Parental or teacher appreciation of hearing loss; unresponsiveness or inattentiveness; any evidence of mental retardation, behavior disorder or circumstance suggesting organic or functional deafness?

Dysuria. Pain, burning or cry related to micturition?

Frequency of micturition. How frequent, any recent change in pattern?

Bed wetting and incontinence. Always present or recently developed; any polyuria, dysuria, frequency of micturition, or thirst; do particular circumstances produce the symptoms and what is the parental reaction to them (e.g. punishment or ridicule); unhappiness or bullying at school?

Volume of urine. Evidence of actual volume passed (parents tend to overestimate the amount of urine passed per day).

Character of the urine. Color (e.g. amber, red, smoky, like tea or cola drink), abnormal odor?

Manipulative ability. Ability to handle objects, use spoon, knife and fork, dress and undress himself, tie shoe laces (c. 6 years), write.

Behavior and mood (best discussed in the absence of the child). Active or hyperactive; quiet or lethargic; loquacious or silent; given to 'cocktail party' chatter (common in hydrocephalus); disobedient; aggressive; negative; reluctant to go to school; refusing food; withdrawn; averse to social activities; resistance to bedding; reluctant to sleep; fearful of the dark; frequent awakening during the night; subject to nightmares or night terrors, temper tantrums, nail biting and thumbsucking; carefree or anxious; whining, nagging, demanding attention; fastidious or careless; 'highly strung' or placid; crying too readily; jealous; volatile or stolid; speech disturbed? Relationship with parents, siblings, schoolmates and teachers?

Treatment already given must be ascertained.

Selectivity of questioning. Not all of the questions indicated above will be asked in every instance; some will be secondary questions dependent on positive answers to primary questions. Better to ask too many rather than too few questions: the more extensive the questioning the more likely are forgotten points of history to be uncovered.

PREVIOUS HISTORY

Mostly a history about past illness in a child has to be obtained from parents, guardians or others. Baby books, photographs, health visitor and infant clinic records may help.

Birth history

An account of the mother's pregnancy and the birth is a necessary part of history taking in the case of an infant or young child. Ascertain illnesses which the mother had before or during pregnancy, exposure to drugs or radiation, hydramnios, hypertension, edema, albuminuria, threatened abortion or antepartum hemorrhage, length of gestation, duration of labor (prolonged or precipitate), type of delivery (high forceps and breech carry particular risk). Note the infant's birthweight, state at delivery (e.g. Apgar score), and postnatal history regarding events such as convulsions, breathing difficulties, cyanosis, jaundice, vomiting, infection, special or intensive care.

Feeding

Nature of the feed, its composition, volume, frequency, any additional supplements and the state of the appetite?

Previous illnesses

Diagnosis, dates of occurrence, duration and severity?

Contact with infectious disease

Include contact with animals.

Residence abroad

Country and any particular hazards it holds?

Prophylactic inoculations

Inoculations received and any reaction to them?

FAMILY HISTORY

Parents' ages, present state of health, past health and possible consanguinity? Previous stillbirths or miscarriages (mothers who have had difficulty in conceiving and have had abortions, stillbirths, infant deaths or abnormal children are more likely to have children who suffer from congenital abnormalities and cerebral palsy)? Past or present illnesses or deaths (with cause of death) of siblings? Illnesses of other relatives or occupants of the house? Hereditary traits require inquiry regarding a much wider circle of relatives.

DEVELOPMENTAL HISTORY (see Chs 8 and 9)

This involves the time of achievement of milestones of motor, vision/fine motor, social/adaptive and hearing/language progress. Note any evidence of dissociated development (e.g. delay in reaching linguistic compared with motor milestones would raise the question of hearing impairment or speech disorder; standing holding on to furniture before sitting, cerebral diplegia; normal manipulative ability combined with retarded postural milestones, ataxic cerebral palsy). Approximately 15% of mentally retarded children reach normal motor milestones during infancy.

SOCIAL AND ENVIRONMENTAL HISTORY

With most disorders it is necessary to build up a picture of the child's social and cultural environment; to appreciate fears and stresses both at home (e.g. parental attitudes, separation and divorce, absence of a parent, illness or chronic disability in the family, jealousy at the arrival of a new baby, the possible death of a near relative) and at school (e.g. a change of school, difficulty in meeting educational standards, overrigid discipline or bullying); to judge intelligence and ability as they affect capacity to meet the demands of communal living and education; to ascertain the occupation of the father, the size and condition of the child's home. Inadequately explained injuries or neglected appearance may raise the possibility of child abuse.

PHYSICAL EXAMINATION

The examination of infants and children is an art demanding qualities of understanding, sympathy, patience and at times finesse and subtlety. The pediatric patient who enters the consulting room or is ill in bed may be a bawling infant whom nothing will pacify, a toddler clinging to his mother and burying his tearful face in her lap at the slightest movement of the examiner towards him, a more robust young man of early school age who stoutly and persistently resists all attempts to remove his clothing, particularly his trousers, an uninhibited hyperactive child who moves rapidly round the room deploying his destructive interest against toys, instruments or the examiner's papers, or an apprehensive schoolgirl who just retains her self-control during questioning but recoils in terror at the production of a sphygmomanometer or ophthalmoscope.

RELATIONSHIP OF EXAMINER TO CHILD AND PARENTS

The child should be placed where he wishes, be it on the parent's knee or on a chair by himself. Removal of clothing or a visit to the examination couch may come later. The examiner must remain patient and confident even if provoked and not be too conscious of his own dignity.

Impatience and irrascibility will deprive him of information which might be available. His demeanor should be friendly, sociable, tolerant, good-natured and restrained as he listens, observes, notes and judges. He should encourage the mother and child no matter how the latter behaves. Loud noise tends to alarm children, a soft persuasive voice is more likely to be effective than stentorian exhortation. Conversation should be attuned to the intellectual and social level of the child. Talk to him/her and explain what is being done. Disturbing or painful procedures should be kept to the end.

GENERAL INSPECTION

Clinical examination of a child begins from the moment of first meeting. A glance will reveal the state of consciousness. Much may be learned from first impressions of the child's appearance, demeanor, state of nutrition, reaction to the environment, relationship with parents (Fig. 2.1), conversation, speech, cry, size relative to age, state of nutrition, state of activity, posture, overt deformity, injury or hemorrhage. The facies may indicate pain or anxiety, the blankness of mental retardation, wasting (Fig. 2.4n) or the spasmodic movement of the tic. Weight loss or dehydration may be revealed by hollow cheeks and sunken eyes, edema by periorbital swelling (Fig. 2.4q). Mouth breathing, jaundice or cyanosis may be present. Some disorders, e.g. mongolism, cretinism (Fig. 2.4c), gargoylism (Fig. 2.4f), de Lange syndrome (Fig. 2.4e) and sometimes tetanus (Fig. 2.4o) may be diagnosed immediately by the characteristic facies which they exhibit. Rashes call for appreciation of color, size, distribution and nature. The skin may be dry and loose in dehydration with loss of elasticity on lifting up skin folds, loose but not inelastic in weight loss, ulcerated, infected, dry, ichthyotic, angiomatous, abnormally pigmented, sweating abnormally, shiny and tense, edematous pitting on pressure (Fig. 2.6i), showing localized swellings (Fig. 2.4d) or striae.

The nails may be bitten and show abnormalities including deficient formation, ridging, abnormal curving, infection. Finger clubbing may be present.

Disturbance of rate or pattern of breathing or dyspnea may be visible. Abnormal sounds such as high pitched cry, cough,

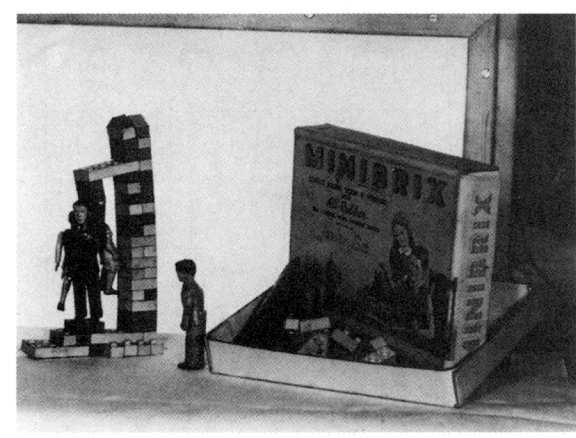

Fig. 2.1 Symbolic play in disturbed boy aged 8 years – he is hanging his father. (Courtesy of Dr T. S. Ingram.)

wheeze, stridor or whoop may be heard. Abnormal smells such as acetone (usually in a child who is refusing food) or the mousy odor of phenylketonuria may be detected.

Posture may be abnormal as in opisthotonus, kyphosis or torticollis (Fig. 2.4n).

A few moments may tell much of a child's psychological make-up and intelligence. Is he nervous, excitable, distractible, withdrawn, intelligent or stupid? What is his emotional relationship with his parents?

PHYSICAL MEASUREMENTS

Weight (pp. 354, 355)

Over the first few days of life physiological weight loss of up to 15% of bodyweight with return to birthweight (BW) by 7 to 10 days is common followed by weight gain of approximately 25 g per day up to 3 months. Expected weight in kilograms can be calculated as follows:

First year: during 1st 4 months: BW + (age in months × 0.8)
during 2nd 4 months: BW + (age in months × 0.7)
during 3rd 4 months: BW + (age in months × 0.6)
(Infants normally double their birthweight by 5 months and treble it by 1 year)

Between 1 and 9 years add 4 to the age in years and multiply by 2.
Between 9 and 12 years treble the age in years.
One standard deviation from these figures = $12\frac{1}{2}\%$ of their value.

Length (pp. 354, 355)

At birth, length is approximately 50 cm (20 in), at 6 months 68 cm (27 in), at 1 year 75 cm (30 in), at 2 years 85 cm (34 in), at 3 years 95 cm (37 in) and at 4 years 100 cm (39 in). Over the next 8 years there is an annual increase of approximately 5.5 cm (2 in). One standard deviation from these figures = 4% of their value.

In infancy, because of the difficulty of measuring crown–heel length accurately (see Fig. 8.1), crown–rump length is the most

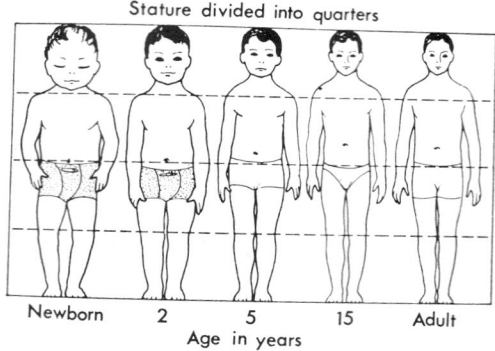

Fig. 2.2 Body proportions at different ages.

representative measurement of length (see p. 363). The mean crown–rump length at birth is 34 cm (13 in), at 2 weeks 34.5 cm ($13\frac{1}{2}$in) and at 6 months 43.5 cm (17 in).

Body proportions and shape change with age (Fig. 2.2).

Measurement of the arms should be from the tip of the acromium to the tip of the middle finger and of the legs from the anterior superior iliac spine to the internal malleolus.

Coincidental measurements of length and weight can be used to calculate 'weight for length' which may be of value in the diagnosis of certain diseases, e.g. hypothyroidism (Fig. 2.4c), Marfan's syndrome or, as nutrition indices. Length for age, weight for age or weight for length below the 5th centile would indicate undernutrition in the absence of any disease process.

Head circumference (p. 363)

At birth 35 cm (14 in), 6 months 43.5 cm (17 in), 1 year 46.5 cm (18 in), 2 years 49 cm (19 in): increases annually by approximately half a centimeter from 2 to 7 years and by one-third of a centimeter from 8 to 12 years. One standard deviation from these figures = $2\frac{1}{2}$% of their value.

A cranial hemicircumference less on one side than the other may indicate hemiplegia on the contralateral side.

Temperature

Pyrexia is a common concomitant of disease in the child but hypothermia may also be so, particularly in the newborn. The infant's temperature can be taken in the groin with the thigh flexed on the abdomen (normal = 37°C or 98.4°F) or in the rectum (normal = 37.5°C or 99.5°F). In older children the axilla is more suitable. Low reading thermometers covering the range 29–43°C (85–109°F) are necessary in assessing hypothermia and should be used routinely in pediatric practice. Premature infants have temperatures 1°F or so lower than full-term infants.

Blood pressure

The normal *auscultatory method* can be carried out over the age of 3 years but is more difficult in younger children in whom sedation may be necessary. The cuff width should be two-thirds of the upper arm (cuffs of 5 cm (2 in) and 7.5 cm (3 in) are available). Auscultatory blood pressure determination in the legs is difficult. The palpatory method (systolic pressure) may be

employed with babies and toddlers and where neither of these methods is possible the *flush method* may be used. A suitably sized cuff is applied loosely round the upper arm or thigh, the limb below the elbow or knee is blanched either by manual compression or an elastic bandage and the cuff inflated above 200 mmHg. The compression is then released and the cuff pressure lowered slowly, the point at which the blanched area flushes being noted. This flush pressure is midway between systolic and diastolic pressures.

Noninvasive automatic methods of measuring blood pressure utilize the Doppler principle and oscillometry and are valuable for monitoring (e.g. in intensive care).

Average blood pressures (mmHg) are:

Newborn (range of flush method)	35–85
Infancy (systolic/diastolic)	80/55
Preschool child (systolic diastolic)	85/60
School child (systolic diastolic)	90/60

EXAMINATION OF INDIVIDUAL SYSTEMS AND REGIONS

Individual systems can be examined in a standard sequence but in practice this is seldom appropriate. It is better to begin with the system which is likely to reveal the most information and to leave to the last disturbing procedures and systems likely to yield least information.

HEAD AND NECK

Cranium

Pathological *cranial shapes* are illustrated in Figure 2.3.

Note color, quantity and character of the hair and level of the hair line.

The *anterior fontanel* measures approximately 2.5 cm (1 in) × 2.5 cm at birth and does not close until 18 months (delay may be seen in rickets, increased intracranial tension or abnormal development of cranial bones). Assess tension (bulging or sunken) visually and by palpation. The *posterior fontanel* measures 0.5 cm ($\frac{1}{4}$ in) in diameter at birth and closes shortly thereafter.

Cranial sutures such as the sagittal and coronal are easily palpable at birth but the edges are not widely separated (e.g. as in raised intracranial pressure). Sutures may be prematurely closed and the edges heaped up in cranial synostosis. *Scalp veins* may be distended (Fig. 2.4t).

Craniotabes (seen in prematurity and rickets) is a reduction in the rigidity of the cranial bones which can be indented by finger pressure over the parieto-occipital region. Structural defects such as lacunae or areas of thickening may be detected by palpation. *Cranial bruits* may be audible on auscultation over the vertex, occipital or temporal regions. After the fontanel has closed a 'cracked pot' sign (raised intracranial pressure) may be elicited by a sharp tap over the cranium.

Ears

The external auricle may be deformed, the meatus narrowed or absent or the ears low set (one-third of the external auricle should be above a horizontal line at eye level. Low-set ears are often associated with other congenital abnormalities (Figs 2.3a and 2.3e).

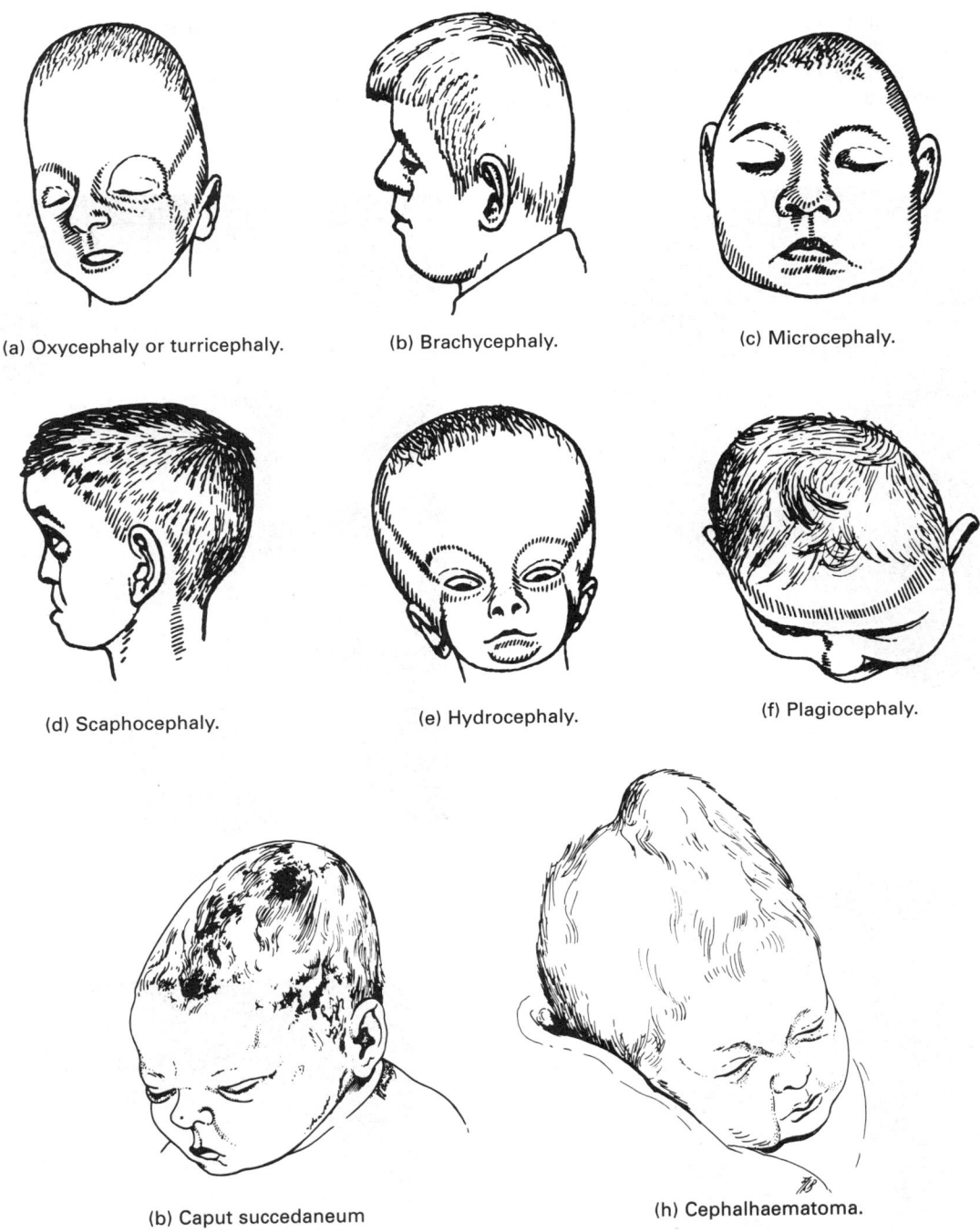

(a) Oxycephaly or turricephaly.

(b) Brachycephaly.

(c) Microcephaly.

(d) Scaphocephaly.

(e) Hydrocephaly.

(f) Plagiocephaly.

(b) Caput succedaneum

(h) Cephalhaematoma.

Fig. 2.3 Head shapes.

Auroscopic examination (the speculum should be appropriate to the size of the infant) may reveal wax or purulent discharge (if necessary clear with a metal loop or cotton wool on an orange stick), a tympanic membrane (eardrum) which is dusky, bulging, retracted or perforated. Distortion of the cone of light which normally extends forward from the tip of the handle of the malleus usually indicates infection, undue prominence of the malleus retraction of the drum. Perforations are most likely in the upper part of the drum.

Facies

Apart from the general aspects of facial appearance mentioned above the face may indicate specific disease as exemplified in Figures 2.4a–2.4w.

Eyes

Distance apart may be measured in terms of inner canthal distance, mid-pupillary distance or outer canthal distance. Age and racial differences can be offset by using the canthal index (100 × inner canthal distance divided by the outer canthal distance) which is 38 (SD 2.4) for boys and 38.5 (SD 2.4) for girls. The eyes are wide apart (*telecanthus*) (Fig. 2.4k) in acrocephalosyndactyly (Apert), hypertelorism, Waardenburg syndrome and craniofacial dysostoses such as Crouzon's. They may be close spaced (e.g. Down syndrome) or displaced downwards (the 'sunset sign') in hydrocephalus.

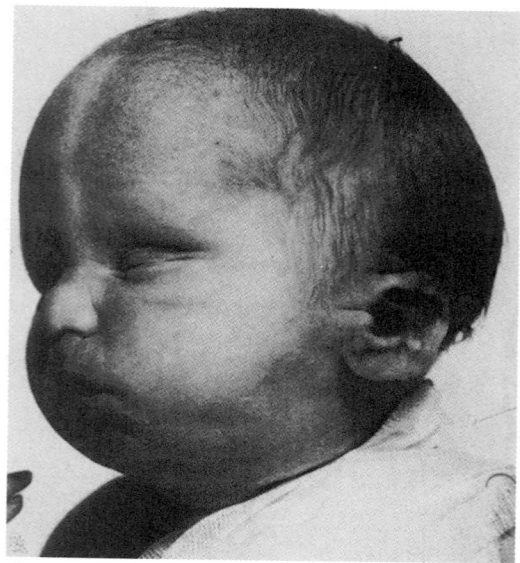

Fig. 2.4a   Renal agenesis – low-set ears, rounding of nose, marked nasolabial line.

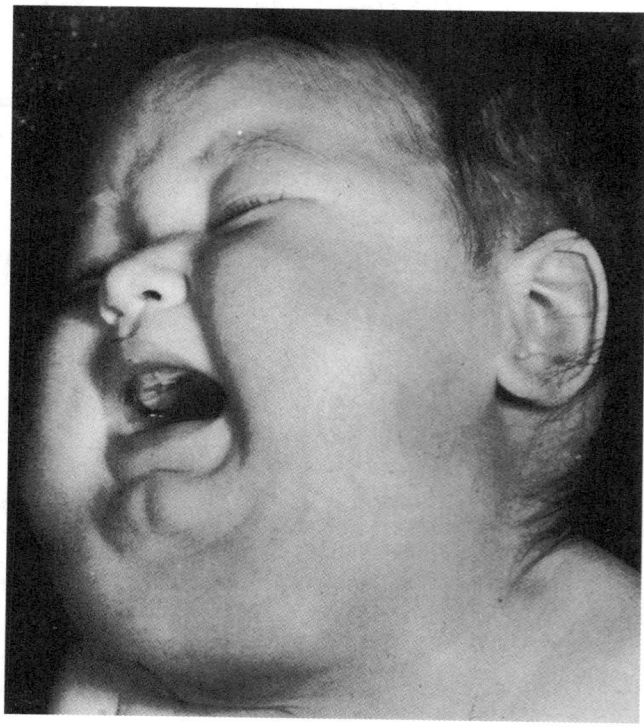

Fig. 2.4b   Cystic hygroma in submental region.

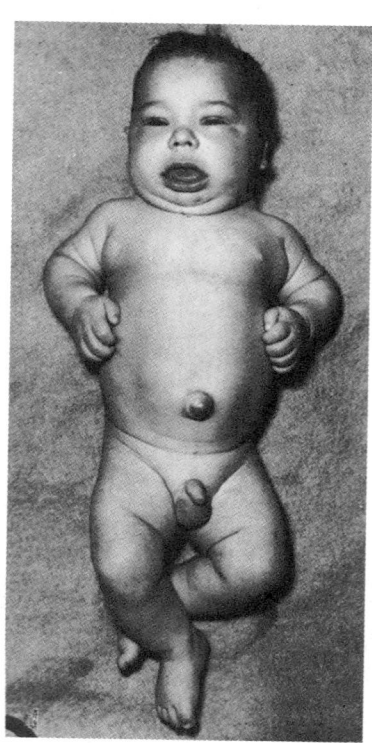

Fig. 2.4c   Cretinism – large tongue, expressionless face, umbilical hernia.

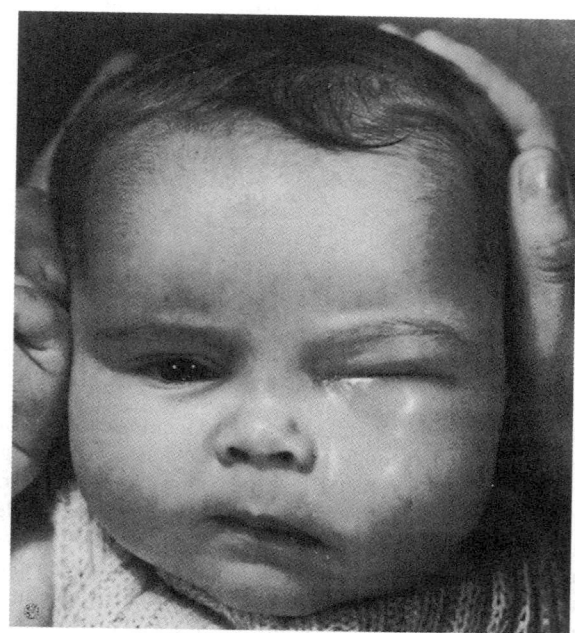

Fig. 2.4d   Osteomyelitis of the left maxilla.

Ptosis (Figs 2.4g and 2.4h) is drooping of the eyelids. The color of the mucous membrane of the lower eyelid may give some indication of anemia. The *eyeballs* may be prominent (exophthalmos), sunken (enophthalmos), enlarged (buphthalmos) (Fig. 2.4u) and may exhibit nystagmus, squint (strabismus),

conjunctivitis, icterus, hemorrhage, congenital defects (e.g. colobomata (Fig. 2.4l) or aniridia), abnormal iris pigmentation, Brushfield's spots (small whitish inclusions in the iris (Fig. 2.4v) – often present in Down syndrome), opacities of the cornea, lens (Fig. 2.4i) or intraocular chambers. The *pupils* may be different in

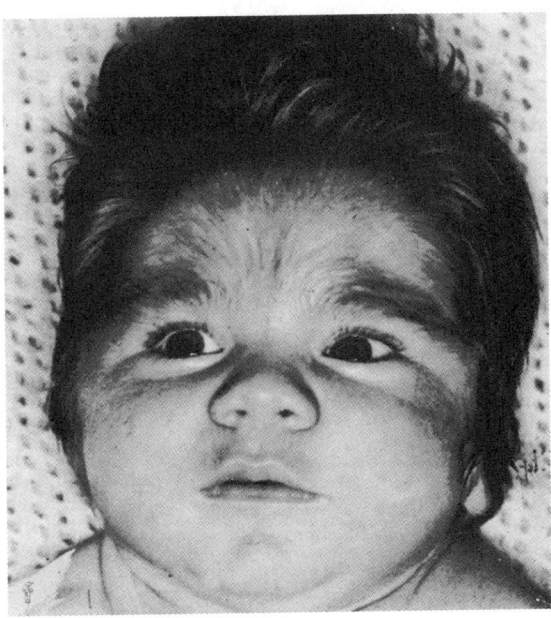

Fig. 2.4e de Lange syndrome (Amsterdam dwarf) – snub nose, low hairline, hairy forehead.

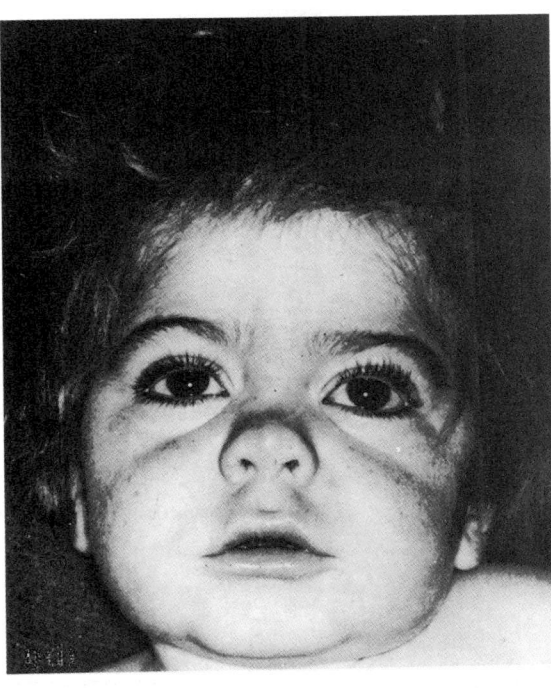

Fig. 2.4f Gargoylism (Hurler's syndrome) – sunken nasal bridge, tow-like hair, corneal opacities.

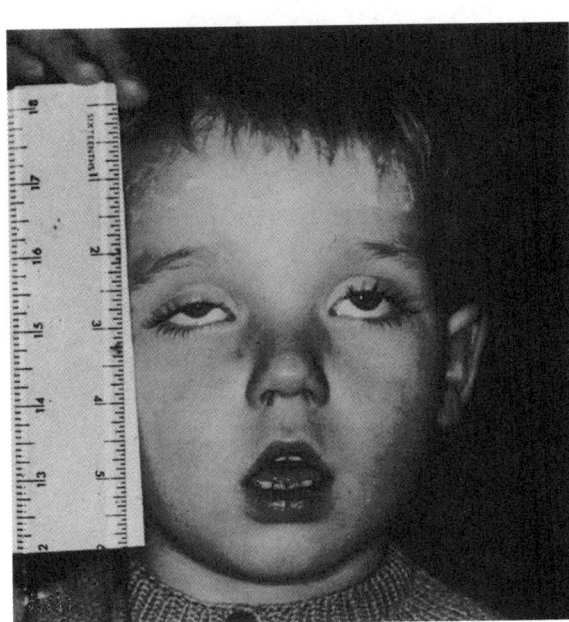

Fig. 2.4g Myasthenia gravis – attempting to look up.

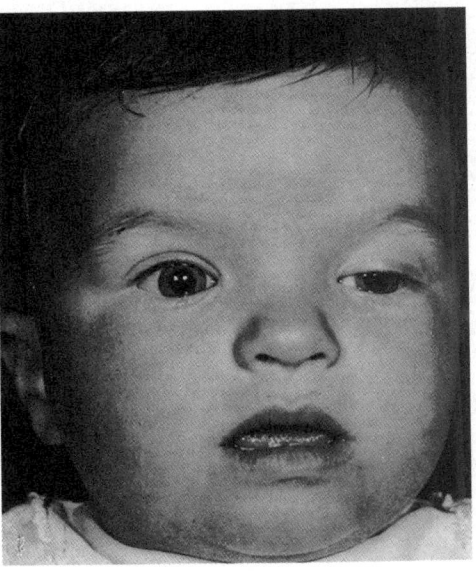

Fig. 2.4h Congenital ptosis – left eye.

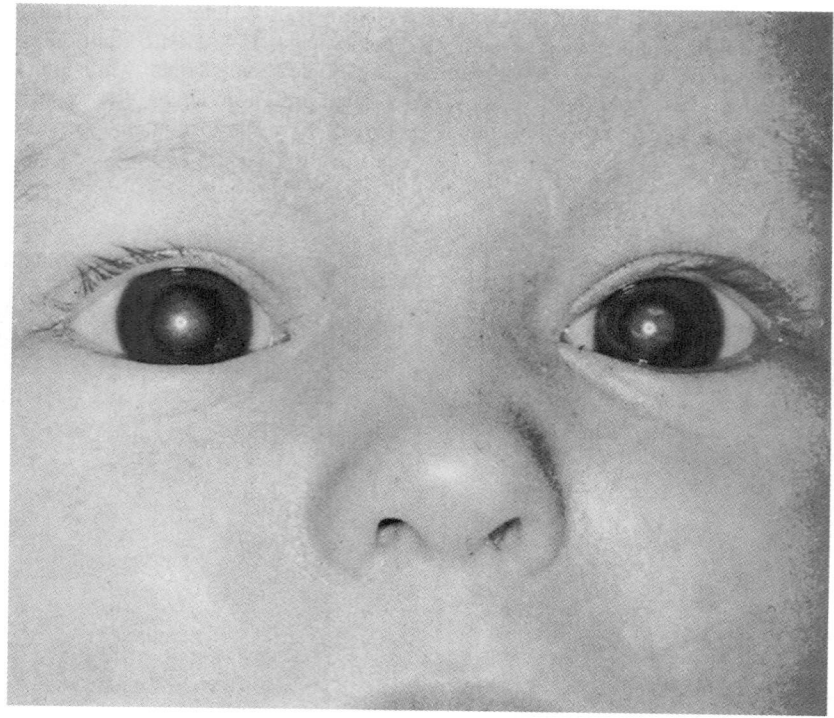

Fig. 2.4i Cataract associated with the rubella syndrome.

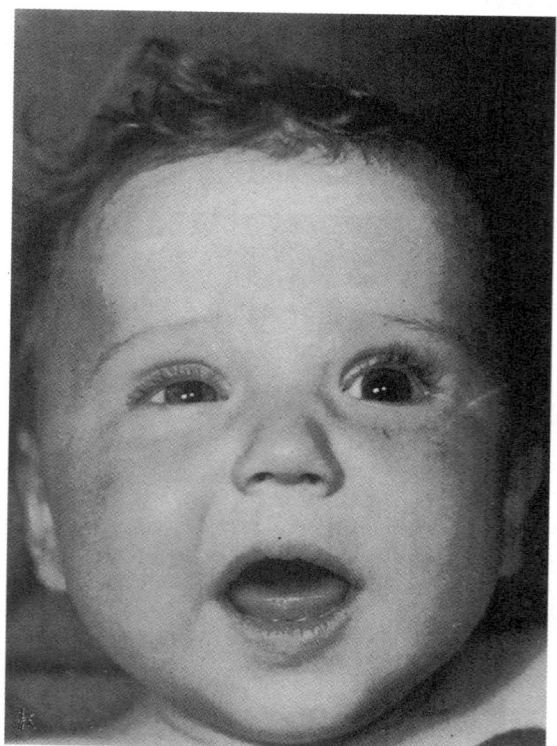

Fig. 2.4j Horner's syndrome (right) enophthalmos and meiosis on affected side.

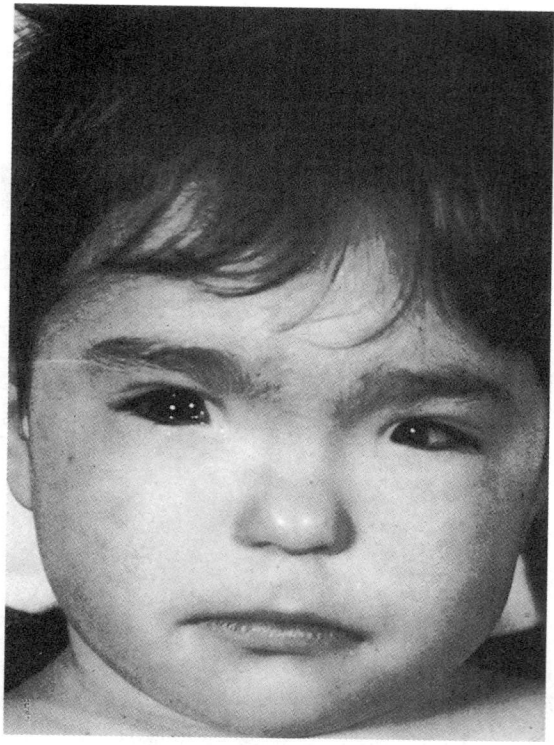

Fig. 2.4k Telecanthus (hypertelorism).

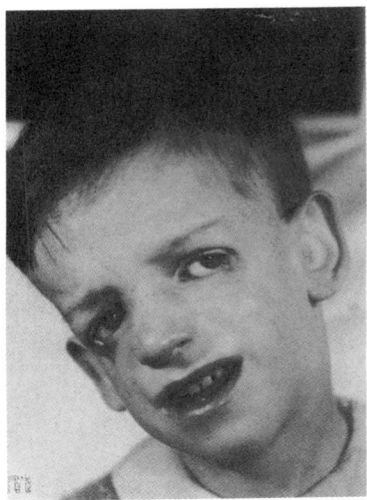

Fig. 2.4l Treacher Collins' syndrome – downward sloping palpebral fissure, coloboma of lower eyelids, sunken cheek bones.

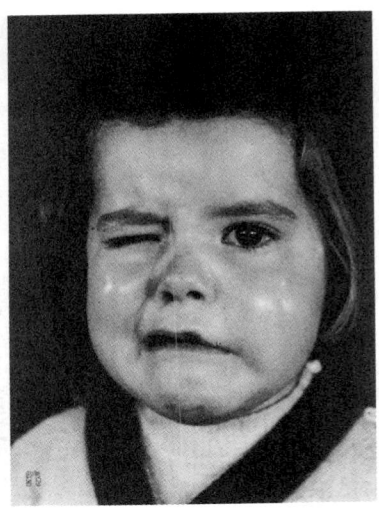

Fig. 2.4m Left facial palsy – child crying.

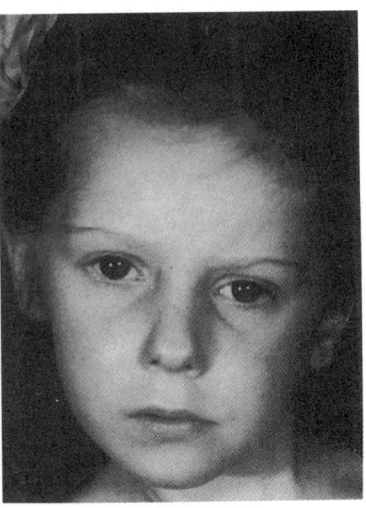

Fig. 2.4n Torticollis with facial wasting (asymmetry) on left side.

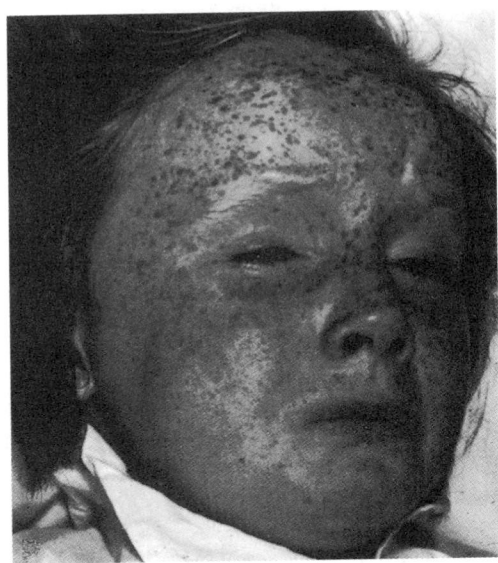

Fig. 2.4o Tetanus – risus sardonicus (normal freckling).

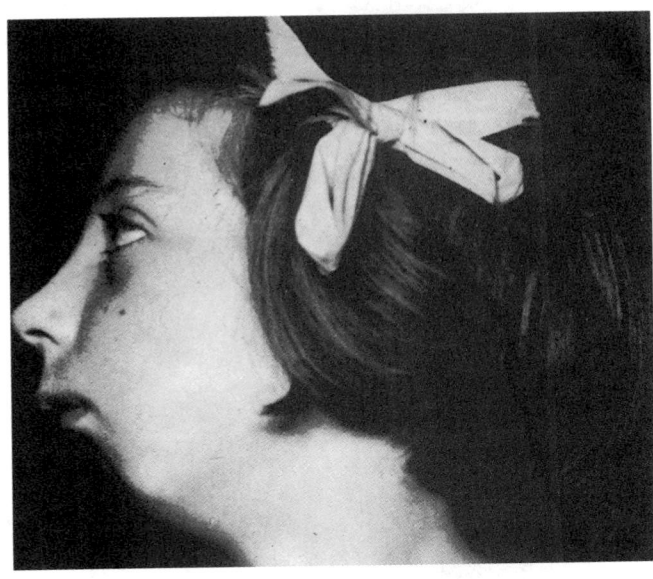

Fig. 2.4p Micrognathia.

size (e.g. contracted (myosis) due to unopposed action of the 3rd nerve in Horner's syndrome (Fig. 2.4j), or larger than normal in an amblyopic eye); they should react to light and accommodation. *Vision* in babies can be tested crudely by observing whether they follow an object held 46 cm (18 in) in front of the face and moved from side to side through an arc of 30°.

Ophthalmoscopic examination is best carried out in a dim room. The examiner's eye should be as near as possible to the ophthalmoscope and his head placed so that it does not obstruct the gaze of the child's other eye. If observer and patient each have normal vision no lens ('O') is necessary. The need to use a plus (+) lens indicates hypermetropia, a minus (–) lens myopia. An examiner with a refractive error should correct this with a lens of the ophthalmoscope. To get the young child to look in a fixed direction get him to look with some expectancy in the required direction and periodically fulfill his expectations, e.g. 'tell me when the torch flashes' – a helper being prepared to flash the torch at the appropriate moment. Babies looking backwards over the mother's shoulder tend to open their eyes. Dilatation of the pupils is not usually necessary routinely but for full examination 1%

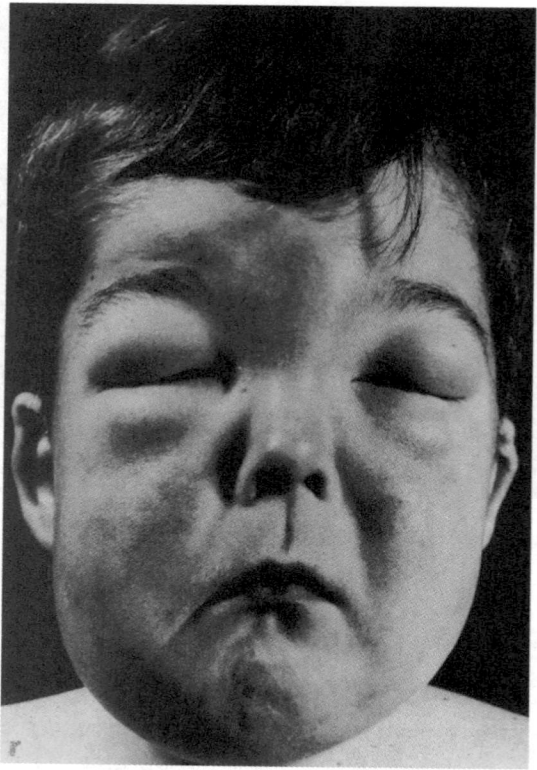

Fig. 2.4q Facial edema in nephrosis.

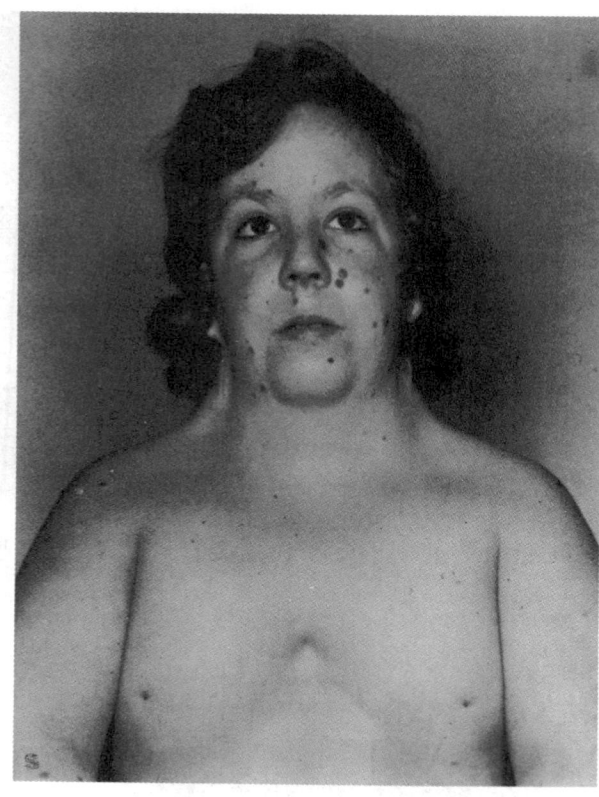

Fig. 2.4r Turner's syndrome – webbing of neck, multiple pigmented moles.

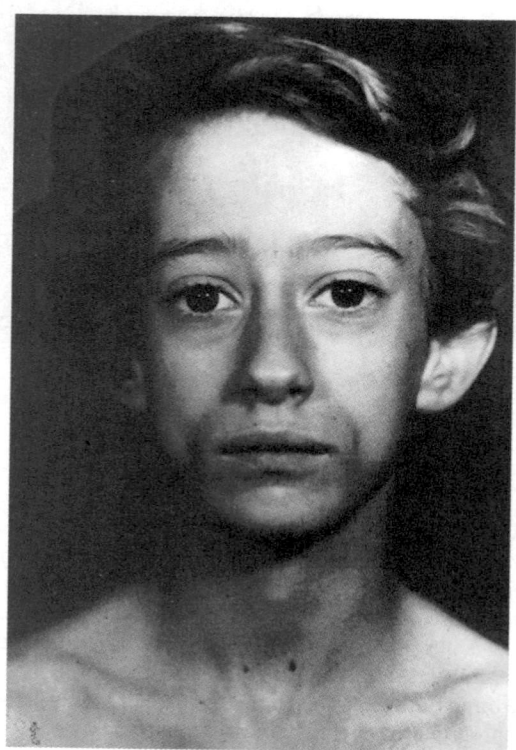

Fig. 2.4s Lipodystrophy.

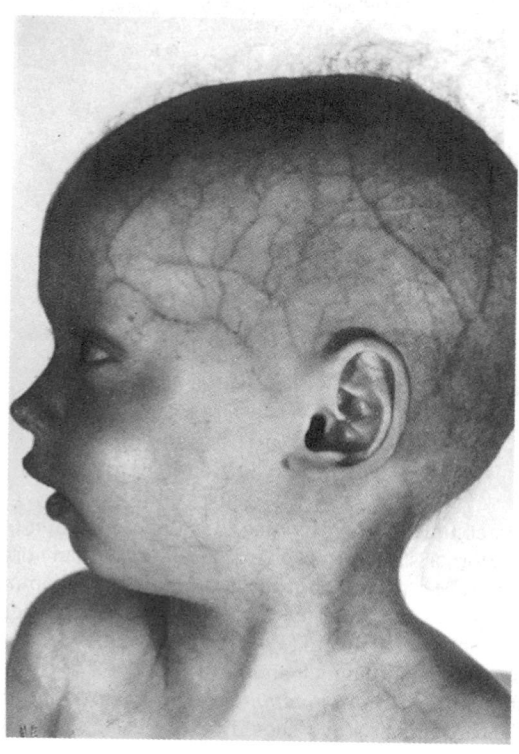

Fig. 2.4t Progeria – sparse hair, distended scalp veins, peaked nose.

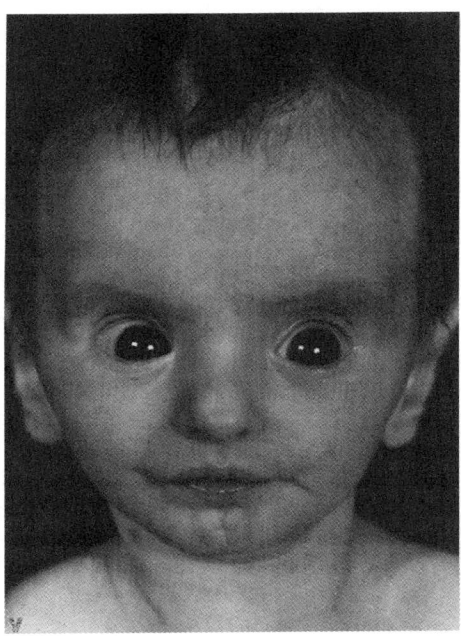

Fig. 2.4u Congenital glaucoma (buphthalmos).

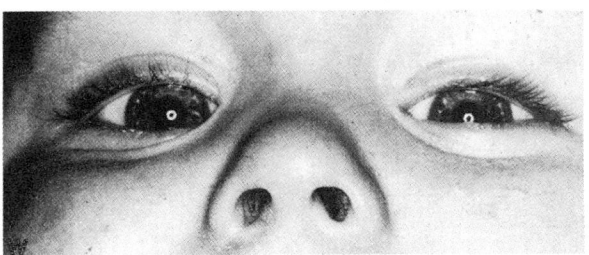

Fig. 2.4v Brushfield's spots in iris.

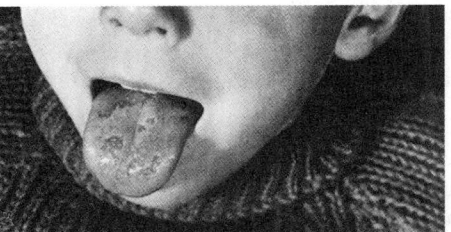

Fig. 2.4w Geographic tongue.

homatropine may be used. Ophthalmoscopy may reveal opacities of the media, refractive errors, retinal hemorrhage, venous engorgement, papilledema with blurring of the disc edges or filling of the optic cup with vessels coming into focus in front of the disc, pallor of the disc, exudate, choreoretinitis, abnormal pigmentation, cherry-red spots or choroidal tubercles.

In older children it is usually possible to map *visual* fields against the examiner's fields, each looking straight at the other's pupil 46 cm (18 in) apart, the examiner frequently moving a cotton wool pledget on the end of an orange stick midway between himself and the patient who indicates each time when the cotton wool enters his visual field.

Nose

The nose may show evidence of infection or allergy in the form of a purulent or watery discharge. Movement of the alae nasi may indicate respiratory difficulty. The nasal mucosa may be pale, congested, watery or dry; the septum may be deflected; polyps may be present. By closing off the mouth, blockage of the nasal passages may be demonstrated.

Mouth

The *lips* may show edema, pallor, cyanosis or ulceration. The mouth may be examined with the cooperation of the child or without it (Fig. 2.5). *Mucosae* may be moist, dry, well colored or pale, ulcerated, blistered, bleeding or purpuric, exhibiting the white curd-like plaques of thrush which will not easily scrape off, or Koplik's spots (measles) on the buccal mucosa. The *gums* may be ulcerated or hypertrophied (e.g. phenytoin). The *teeth* can be observed for number, whether primary or secondary, size and

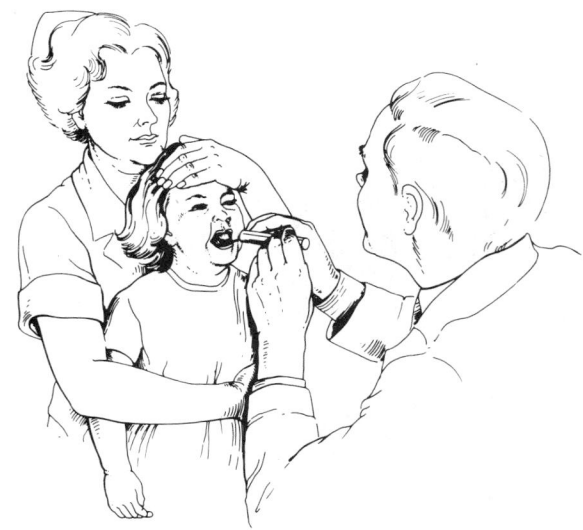

Fig. 2.5 Examining the mouth – uncooperative child.

shape, pigmentation, caries and enamel defect (Fig. 2.6a). The average times of eruption of the teeth are as follows:

Deciduous (primary) teeth		Eruption	Shedding
central incisors	lower	} 7th month	75 months
	upper		
lateral incisors	upper	} 9th month	86 months
	lower		
first molars		12th month	100 months
canines		18th month	122 months
second molars		24th month	109 months

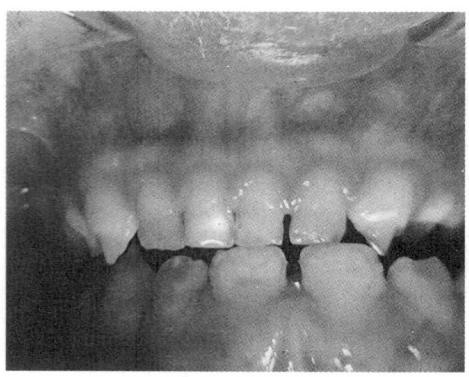

Fig. 2.6a   Enamel defect of the primary dentition following neonatal hypocalcemia.

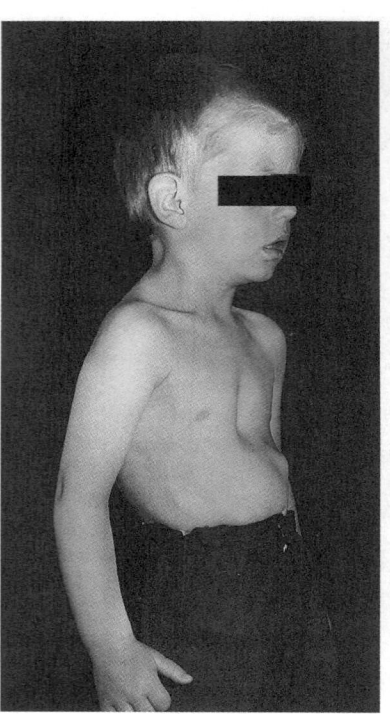

Fig. 2.6b   Pectus excavatum.

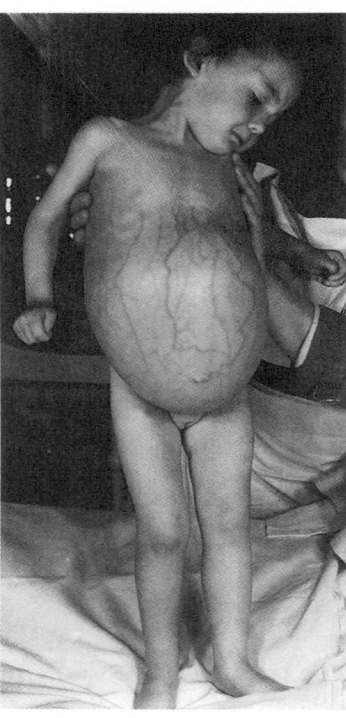

Fig. 2.6c   Ascites with distended abdominal wall veins following hepatic vein thrombosis.

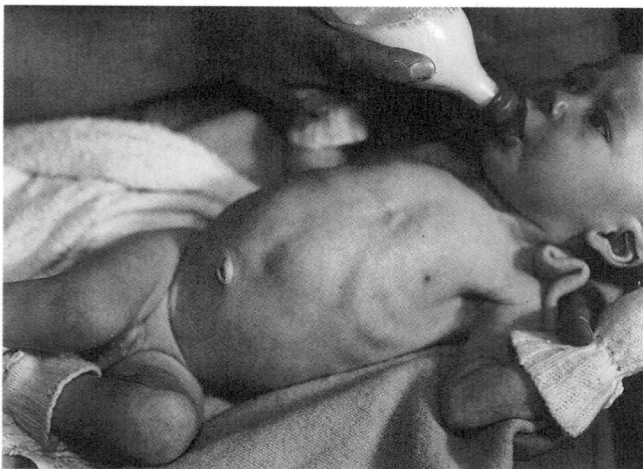

Fig. 2.6d   Peristaltic wave during feeding in pyloric stenosis.

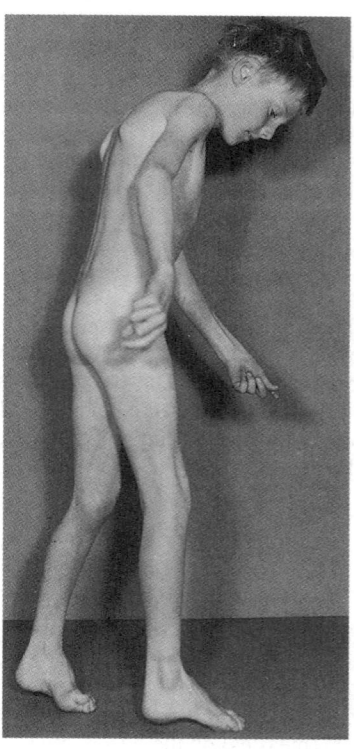

Fig. 2.6e   Gait, posture, plantar flexion of foot and pes cavus in Friedreich's ataxia.

The teeth in the lower jaw are shed earlier than those in the upper and girls' teeth earlier than boys' teeth.

Permanent dentition		Eruption
first molars	lower upper }	6th year
central incisors	lower	6th year
	upper	6th to 7th year
lateral incisors	lower	7th year
	upper	8th year
canines	lower	10th year
	upper	10th to 11th year
first premolars	upper	10th year
	lower	10th to 11th year
second premolars	upper	11th year
	lower	11th to 12th year
second molars	lower	11th to 12th year
	upper	12th year
third molars		20th year

Tongue: size, shape, 'geographic' appearance (Fig. 2.4w)? *Palate*: cleft or high arched, any abnormality of the uvula? If the child is willing to say 'ah' examination of the posterior *pharynx* is easy; otherwise induce the gag reflex by touching the posterior pharyngeal wall with a spatula and take advantage of the few brief moments during which the posterior pharynx is revealed on gagging (Fig. 2.5). *Tonsils*: size, presence of infection, exudate, pitting, peritonsillar swelling? *Posterior phalangeal wall*: inflammation, postnasal discharge, presence of lymphoid tissue?

Neck

Examine from front and back noting any shortening, webbing (Fig. 2.4r), torticollis (Fig. 2.4n), head retraction or neck stiffness (by passive flexion), limitation of flexion (ask child to put nose on knees while sitting with knees drawn up), abnormal swellings (e.g. lymph glands, thyroid, cystic hygroma (Fig. 2.4b) – transilluminable). A sternomastoid tumor (early infancy) is a hard visible nodule within the body of the sternomastoid muscle.

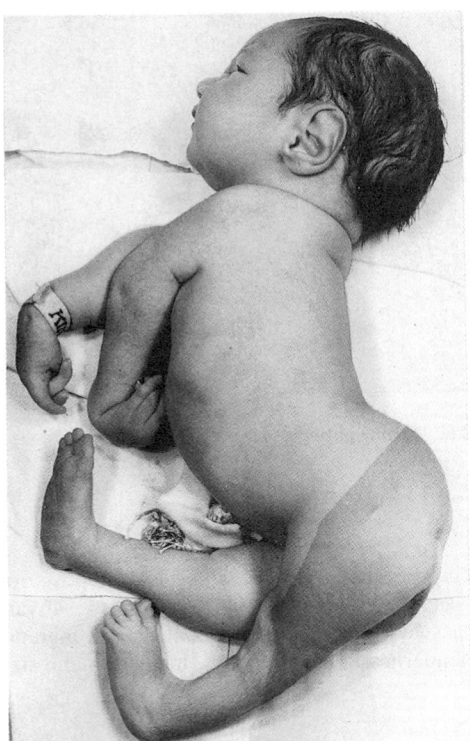

Fig. 2.6g Arthrogryposis multiplex congenita.

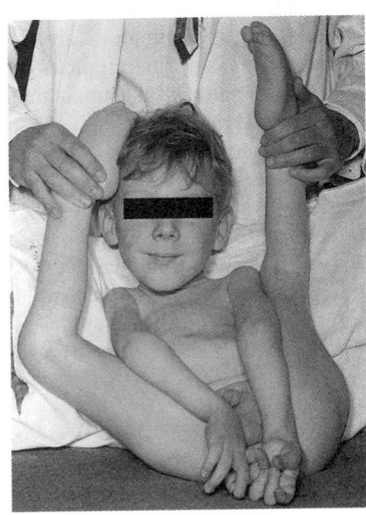

Fig. 2.6f Gross hypotonia.

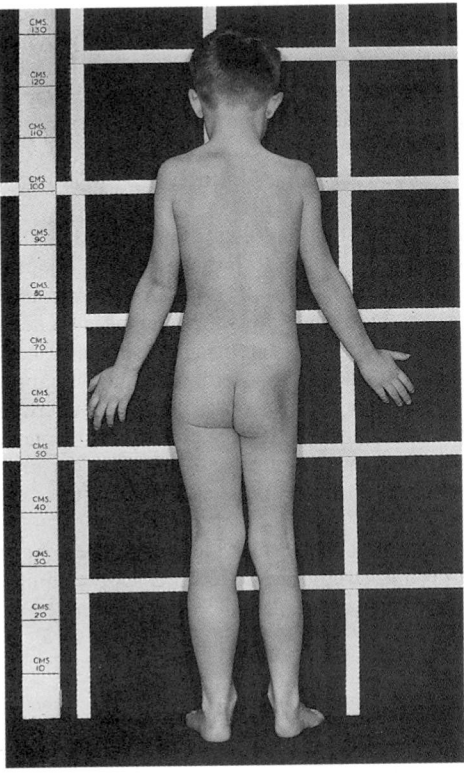

Fig. 2.6h Pseudohypertrophic muscular dystrophy involving predominantly the left leg and buttock.

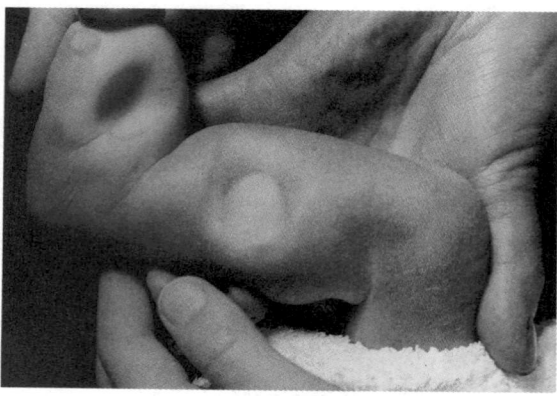

Fig. 2.6i   Edema pitting under pressure.

Lymph nodes

Enlargement may occur in the anterior and posterior cervical triangles, occipital and submental (lateral to salivary glands) regions – as well as axillary, epitrochlear and inguinal regions. Ascertain tenderness, inflammation, fluctuation and size.

CHEST AND LUNGS

Inspection

The cross-section of the infant's chest is circular compared with elliptical for the older child or adult. This imposes limitations on expansion so that respiration is diaphragmatic and abdominal and dyspnea is reflected in both respiratory and abdominal movements. In infancy overinflation of the chest (e.g. in bronchiolitis) is most evident in the upper half of the chest anteriorly. Chronic emphysema can cause an increase in the anteroposterior diameter of the chest (pigeon chest) which is normally less than the lateral diameter.

Chest circumference ranges from 32 ± 5 cm at birth to 75 ± 16 cm at 14 years.

Chest expansion measured at the nipple line between full inspiration and expiration can be measured in cooperative older children. It should be 4 cm ($1\frac{1}{2}$ in) or more. Asymmetry is best detected by watching chest movement on taking a deep breath.

Visible deformities of the chest include pectus excavatum (Fig. 2.6b), Harrison's sulcus (at insertion of diaphragm), precordial bulging, thickening of the costochondral junctions (rickety rosary), the dinner fork deformity of the costochondral junction (scurvy) and anterior prominence of the ribs on one side with frontal skull prominence on the same side (the 'squint baby' syndrome).

The *respiratory rate* must be measured when the infant is at peace, not crying, struggling or feeding. Upper limits of normal for various ages are as follows:

0 to 2 years	40 per minute
2 to 6 years	30 per minute
6 to 10 years	25 per minute
over 10 years	20 per minute

Respiratory rhythm may be disturbed in time and amplitude particularly in premature and asphyxiated babies. Infection can cause *respiratory inversion* – the respiratory cycle changing from inspiration/expiration/pause to expiration/inspiration/pause, often described by the mother as a 'catch' in the infant's breathing. The normally longer inspiratory phase of respiration may be exceeded by a lengthened expiratory phase (e.g. in asthma).

The pliable chest wall of the infant readily reflects changes in intrathoracic pressure, increased inspiratory effort or obstruction of air flow resulting in *intercostal indrawing and costal margin recession*.

Abnormal *respiratory noises* include inspiratory and expiratory stridor, wheeze, cough and grunting respiration.

Palpation

The chief *landmarks* of the child's chest are shown in Figure 2.7. Palpation with the palm of the hand may reveal a cardiac thrill, palpable rhonchi, the crepitant sensation of subcutaneous emphysema, local tenderness or swelling. Due to the mobility of the trachea in infancy and childhood tracheal displacement is not a reliable sign. *Axillary lymph* nodes should be examined by abducting the arm from the trunk, inserting the fingers into the axilla and palpating, with the arm replaced beside the trunk.

Percussion

Percussion landmarks are shown in Figure 2.7. The percussion note is more resonant in the child than in the adult and percussion should be lighter: significant impairment usually means extensive consolidation or fluid in the chest. Hyperresonance occurs in overinflation, emphysema or pneumothorax; reduced cardiac dullness is a valuable concomitant sign of these.

Auscultation

The *breath sounds* in infants and children are harsh (bronchovesicular). The inspiratory sound is normally two to three times longer than the expiratory and followed by a pause. Breath sound intensity may be reduced in conditions such as bronchiolitis, emphysema, pneumothorax and pleural effusion and increased with consolidation or collapse where an affected lobe or segment collapses against a bronchus giving rise to bronchial breathing (sounds similar to those heard on auscultation over the trachea). Rhonchi and coarse crepitations are usually associated with infection or bronchospasm, fine crepitations with infection. The wheezing sounds associated with asthma are high pitched and musical. Pleural friction is a creaky leathery sound giving the impression of being close to the ear.

Vocal resonance, heard on auscultation of the chest when the patient speaks (e.g. says 'one two three'), may be diminished (e.g. pleural effusion) or increased (e.g. consolidation). If whispering is easily audible on auscultation *whispering pectoriloquy* (associated with lung consolidation) is present.

Abnormal signs in the cardiovascular system such as displacement of the apex beat may be due to respiratory disease.

CARDIOVASCULAR SYSTEM

Inspection

Cardiovascular disease may be accompanied by a range of general signs such as poor physical development, squatting, dyspnea,

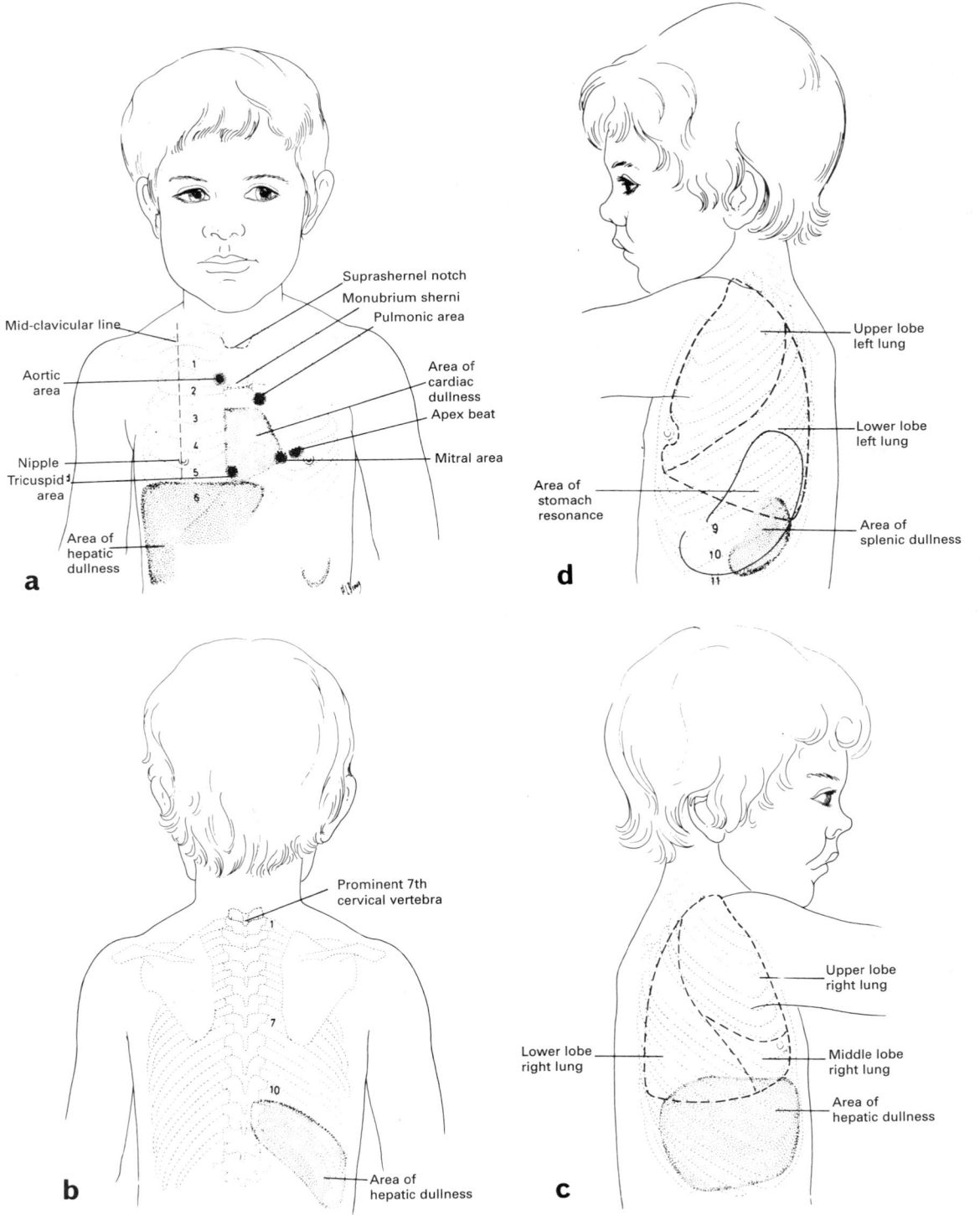

Fig. 2.7   Landmarks in a child's chest: (**a**) anterior, (**b**) posterior, (**c**) right lateral, (**d**) left lateral.

tachypnea, central cyanosis, edema, finger clubbing and distention of superficial veins. *Cardiac enlargement* may be associated with precordial bulging and abnormal pulsation – right ventricular hypertrophy causing increased pulsation in the central and superior parts of the precordium, left ventricular hypertrophy increased pulsation and visible lifting of the apical precordium.

The position of the *apex beat* is an important landmark (Fig. 2.7). *Jugular venous pressure* (increased if above the level of the manubrium sterni) can be assessed in older children but this is rarely practicable in infants due to their shortness of the neck, mobility and lack of cooperation.

Palpation

Applying the palm of the hand to the chest, thrills, increased precordial pulsation (apical in left ventricular hypertrophy and basal and right sided in right ventricular hypertrophy) and diastolic shock (in the pulmonary area in pulmonary hypertension) may be felt. The *apex beat*, normally in the fourth or fifth intercostal space within the mid-clavicular line, can be identified at the point of maximum impulse.

The *pulse* can be examined at the wrist (radial) or inguinal region (femoral). Sinus arrhythmia (increase in rate on inspiration with decrease on expiration) is common in most children. A bounding pulse is usually associated with lesions causing shunting (e.g. VSD or PDA), a weak pulse with restriction of left-sided cardiac outflow (e.g. aortic stenosis), a collapsing (water hammer) pulse with wide pulse pressure – difference between systolic and diastolic pressures – (e.g. aortic regurgitation). The latter is best felt with four fingers laid across the pulse with the patient's arm elevated. In coarctation of the aorta the femoral pulses may be absent, or delayed compared with the radial, and in older children pulsating collateral vessels may be detected in the scapular region.

Percussion

The thin chest wall of the child makes cardiac percussion of more value than in the adult. The right cardiac border does not normally extend beyond the right sternal edge: the upper border is at the level of the second intercostal space (Fig. 2.7). In conjunction with the position of the apex beat (and the character of precordial pulsation) these assessments are of some value in determining cardiac size and/or displacement. Diminished or absent cardiac dullness is found in emphysema and pneumothorax.

Auscultation

The ranges for *heart rate* in infancy and childhood are:

Newborn	Infant	Preschool child	School child
70/120	80/160	75/120	70/110

Auscultation should be carried out over the areas shown in Figure 2.7. Auscultatory assessment concerns cardiac *rhythm*, *heart sounds*, and *murmurs*. Sinus arrhythmia (see above) is normal in children: triple or gallop rhythm is usually associated with cardiac failure: irregular irregularity (e.g. due to extra systoles or, rarely in childhood, atrial fibrillation) may occur. Close splitting of the second heart sound in the pulmonic area (often present on inspiration and absent on expiration) is common in normal children: pathological splitting is wider and does not vary with respiration. The commonly heard and often physiological third heart sound is differentiated from a split second sound by being heard best at the apex, widely separated from the second heart sound and of lesser intensity. An ejection click may be associated with stenosis of a valve. There is diminished intensity of heart sounds in cardiac failure or pleural effusion; and of the pulmonic second sound in pulmonary stenosis and aortic second sound in aortic stenosis. Cardiac hypertrophy accentuates heart sounds. Description of murmurs should include *site* (Fig. 2.7), *intensity* (graded 0–6) with point of maximum intensity, *timing* (systolic: pan, early or late; or diastolic: early diastolic, mid-diastolic or presystolic) (Fig. 2.8), *propagation* (mitral systolic murmurs radiate to the left axilla, aortic systolic to

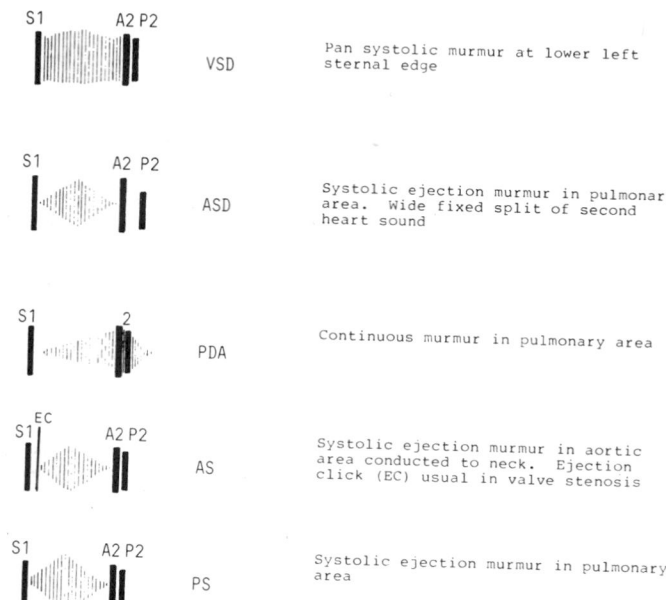

Fig. 2.8 Symbolic depiction of cardiac sounds and murmurs.

the neck, aortic regurgitant down the left sternal edge) and *variation with position*. Coarctation of the aorta may produce a murmur audible over the back. A *venous hum* is a continuous loud murmur at the root of the neck abolished by pressure over the jugular vein or placing the child in the head-down position. A pericardial *friction rub* is a to and fro leathery sound heard by the examiner, on auscultation, as if close to his ear.

Cardiovascular disorder may also be revealed in other systems, e.g. by hepatic enlargement in cardiac failure.

ABDOMEN

Inspection

Disease may reveal itself by *distention* with shiny tense abdominal skin and distended abdominal veins (Fig. 2.6c), or a *scaphoid* abdomen with lax wrinkled skin. Absent abdominal wall movement on respiration may indicate a disorder such as peritonitis. *Visible peristalsis* may be seen in obstruction (e.g. in the epigastrium in pyloric stenosis (Fig. 2.6d)): obstruction low down in the gut may cause a *ladder pattern*. A distended *bladder* may show as a rounded swelling in the suprapubic region. *Umbilical abnormalities* include hernia, omphalocele, infection or discharge. Other *herniae* may be present and *inguinal lymph glands* may be enlarged.

Palpation

Should be carried out with warm hands usually with the examiner seated beside the child lying recumbent or held on the mother's knee, head supported, knees and hips flexed. Crying children relax the abdominal muscles during inspiration allowing the examiner a brief moment when palpation is possible. *Tenderness* should be sought using gentle palpation followed by deeper palpation, while simultaneously looking for evidence of pain in the form of facial grimacing. Rebound tenderness (sudden withdrawal of the hand on deep palpation) may confirm doubtful tenderness. *Guarding* of the abdominal wall may be localized or generalized and in severe degrees may amount to boarding. Palpation of a pyloric *tumor* (start with the stomach empty and give a feed) is carried out as in Fig. 2.9: the tumor may harden and relax intermittently and be impalpable when relaxed.

The lower border of the *liver* is normally 1 cm below the costal margin in infants and children and can be felt rolling under the finger as it descends during inspiration (Fig. 2.10). *Liver span*, measured in the mid-clavicular line, is the distance between the upper border of the liver (Fig. 2.7) determined by percussion and the lower edge. At a body weight of 20 kg the mean span (± 2 SD) is 8 cm (± 1.8 cm), and at 60 kg 10.2 cm (± 2.0 cm).

An enlarged *spleen* is felt in the left hypochondrium possibly extending into the left iliac fossa in infancy and the right in older children. In lesser degrees of splenic enlargement the tip can be felt descending superficially below the costal margin on deep inspiration (Fig. 2.11). The *kidneys* can be palpated bimanually at the end of forced expiration (Fig. 2.12). A distended bladder may reach the umbilicus. *Tumors* (e.g. Wilms' or neuroblastoma) may be felt, and the soft sausage-shaped tumor of intussusception be found in the right upper quadrant during relaxation. A strangulated *hernia* (e.g. inguinal) may be hard, irreducible and very tender. With *ascites* a fluid thrill may be detected, the wave caused by flicking the abdominal wall on one side being transmitted to a hand-held flat on the other side, with the hand (hypothenar edge) of a second person placed on the abdomen in the longitudinal axis of the patient to suppress any transmission of shock waves through the fat of the abdominal wall. Enlarged *inguinal lymph glands* may be palpable.

Percussion

When supine, dullness due to free fluid may be present in both flanks but on turning the patient on to one side disappears from the upper side while the level of dullness rises over the lower side (*shifting dullness* – allow half a minute for change to take place). A distended *bladder* will cause increased dullness in the suprapubic area. Intra-abdominal *masses* may impair percussion.

Auscultation

Tinkling, crackling bowel sounds are normally audible intermittently over the abdomen, are accentuated with increased peristalsis (e.g. obstruction) and absent with ileus (e.g. peritonitis).

Examination of stools

Note color, consistency and the presence of abnormalities such as blood, mucus or pus. Bright red blood suggests bleeding from the lower alimentary tract, melena from the upper while streaking suggests local bleeding (e.g. anal fissure). Threadworms may be noted on the stool.

PERINEUM AND GENITALIA

Anus

Examine for normality of position and abnormalities such as

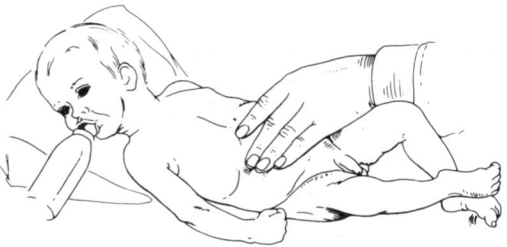

Fig. 2.9   Palpation of pyloric tumor in pyloric stenosis.

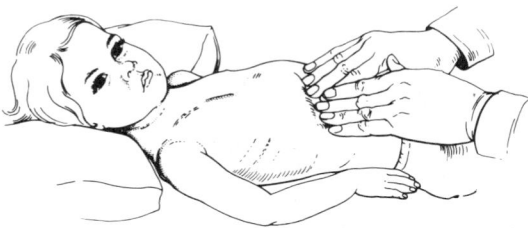

Fig. 2.10   Palpation of liver.

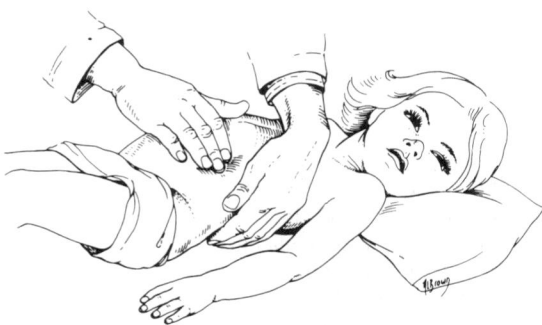

Fig. 2.11   Palpation of spleen.

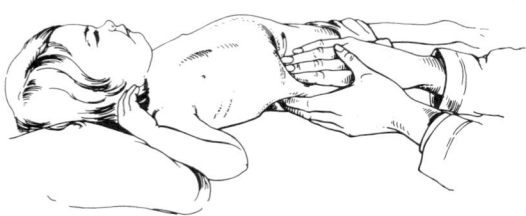

Fig. 2.12   Palpation of kidney.

stenosis, paralysis, fissure, prolapse or evidence of trauma – as may occur in sexual abuse.

Rectal examination

Use a finger appropriate to the size of the patient to detect the tone of the anal sphincter; fecal masses, including their character; gripping of the finger (e.g. anal stenosis, or narrowed segment in Hirschsprung's disease), intrapelvic masses or undue pain. Note material on the withdrawn finger (e.g. blood).

Genitalia

Female genitalia may show labial adhesions, clitoral enlargement, abnormal discharge, abnormality of the vaginal introitus (e.g. sexual abuse) or urethra. In the male note the size of the penis and any developmental abnormality such as hypospadias, phimosis or prepucial infection (balanitis). The testes should be examined for presence in the scrotum (in a warm room with warm hands as cold will cause retraction), abnormality in size and shape: if palpable in the inguinal canal see if they can be maneuvered gently into the scrotum. *Transillumination* may reveal the nature of a scrotal swelling (e.g. hydrocele is transilluminable, solid tumor is not). The assessment of secondary sexual characteristics is described in Chapter 8.

NERVOUS SYSTEM

The nervous system can be examined in the older child with the same exactitude as in the adult but in the infant and young child has not achieved the functional precision with which it operates later; intelligent cooperation is also likely to be lacking. Neurological deficits are often more easily observed in the course of everyday activities than on formal examination: they may reveal neglect of a limb (e.g. hemiplegia), strabismus, clumsiness, incoordination, intention tremor, ataxia and neglect of sound.

Developmental assessment is largely the assessment of the maturation of the nervous system (Ch. 9).

Inspection

After infancy it is usually possible to test specific aspects of neurological function and intelligence separately but during infancy neurological and intellectual disorders tend to express themselves in terms of disturbed motor function. A neurological lesion may be appreciated as impaired intelligence and vice versa.

Note *state of consciousness*, such as degree of alertness, interest, memory for events, hyperexcitability, hyperirritability, unresponsiveness, drowsiness, semiconsciousness or unconsciousness.

Disorders of *posture and movement* may result from neurological disease. In recumbency is he too inactive and is posture unduly affected by gravity (hypotonia)? Are there normal limb, trunk and head movements or abnormal movements (e.g. the writhing movements of choreoathetosis, intention tremor or the repetitive involuntary movement of tics) or purposeless roving movements of the eyes (blindness)? Can he/she sit and stand? Are there any convulsive movements, generalized, localized, or the 'salaam' attacks of myoclonic epilepsy (in which the sitting infant suddenly falls forward or drops his head)? Is there any *incoordination*, clumsiness, abnormality of *gait* (e.g. the broad-based groping walk of ataxia; stiff-legged scissoring gait of spasticity with difficulty in putting the heel to the ground; the outward flinging and stiffness of one leg with adduction, elbow flexion and limited swinging of the arm on the same side seen in hemiplegia; the awkward gait and pes cavus of Friedreich's ataxia (Fig. 2.6e) or the staggering gait of cerebellar disturbance)? Are there any *palsies* (e.g. facial (Fig. 2.4m) or Erb's, or wrist drop). Cry and *speech* may be affected (e.g. the high-pitched cry of cerebral injury, the peculiarly specific cry of the cri-du-chat syndrome, delayed speech with mental retardation and autism, lack of speech intelligibility in mental retardation or cerebral palsy, aphonia in chorea, stammering, monotony and lack of expression in deafness and certain types of cerebral damage). Range of vocabulary, language and ideas give some indication of intelligence.

Cranial nerves

With younger children lack of cooperation will diminish ability to test the cranial nerves although with practice observation of the child's movements may enable a limited examination to be made.

1st (olfactory) nerve. Only older children have the experience and ability to distinguish smells such as orange, lemon or chocolate.

2nd (optic) nerve. Can the infant and toddler see and follow (later name) objects? For older children use Snellen types. Test visual fields (p. 27). Ophthalmoscopic examination (pp. 25 and 1649).

3rd (oculomotor), 4th (trochlear) and 6th (abducens) nerves. Test eye movements in all directions (the common abnormalities are inability to deviate the eyes fully upward or abduct the eyes fully). 3rd nerve paralysis causes ptosis, lateral deviation of the eye (unopposed action of 6th nerve) and pupillary dilation; 4th nerve paralysis (often along with 3rd nerve paralysis) diplopia on looking downwards and medially (e.g. going down stairs), 6th nerve paralysis (of lateral rectus muscle) loss of abduction of the eyes (paralytic squint) on looking to the affected side. Paralysis of the sympathetic innervation of the pupil (usually damage to the cervical sympathetic chain) results in a contracted pupil (myosis) still reacting to light and accommodation, along with ptosis, enophthalmos and loss of sweating (anhidrosis) on the affected side of the face (*Horner's syndrome* – Fig. 2.4j).

The assessment of *squint* is discussed in Chapter 26.

5th (trigeminal) nerve. Test sensation over the area supplied by the sensory branch – forehead, cheek and lower jaw – and by the corneal and jaw reflexes; motor function by palpating contraction in the masseter muscle when the patient clenches the teeth.

7th (facial) nerve. Upper motor neuron lesions affect the lower part only of one side of the face so that the teeth cannot be shown effectively and the lips formed for whistling; lower motor neuron lesions affect the whole of one side of the face so that, in addition to the above, eye closure, forehead wrinkling and smiling are affected (Fig. 2.4m).

8th (auditory) nerve. Damage to the auditory branch impairs hearing (see Ch. 9 for testing): damage to the vestibular branch may result in impaired balance and positional nystagmus (following sudden rotating movement of the head).

9th (glossopharyngeal) and 10th (vagus) nerves. Test their motor function by asking the patient to say 'ah' – paralysis on the affected side results in the palate being drawn to the healthy side or merely lack of movement. X-ray palatography may help. For diagnosis of paralysis of the recurrent laryngeal branch of the vagus see Chapter 14. Enlarged adenoids may also limit palatal movement.

11th (spinal accessory) nerve. Demonstrate trapezius weakness by exerting downward pressure on the patient's shoulders as he tries to shrug them.

12th (hypoglossal) nerve. Paralysis affects the same side of the tongue which deviates to the affected side on protrusion, or waggling shows limited movement towards one side.

Muscle tone

Handling of the child and passive movements of limbs indicate muscle tone (Fig. 2.6f). Muscle softness, floppiness, excessive laxity of joints (with hyperextensibility of the digits, elbows and knees) are the features of *hypotonia*; excessive firmness of muscles, stiffness and limited mobility on passive movement indicate *hypertonia*. Spasticity in the upper limbs can be tested by extending the arm fully at the elbow, supinating the forearm and seeing if there is a pronator flick when the limb is released. Hypertonia may be 'clasp knife' (stretching the muscle beyond a certain range results in sudden relaxation of tone), generalized or regionalized (e.g. adduction of the thighs and shortening of the tendo-Achillis with plantar flexion of the foot – spastic diplegia (Little's disease)).

Motor power

Assessed by observing capacity for muscular activity and ability to overcome resistance (by examiner) to various movements.

Coordination

Specific tests such as the finger–nose test or the picking up of small objects (see Fig. 9.2) may examine this. *Dysdiadochokinesis* (inability to carry out rapid repetitive movements such as patting the back of the hand or asymmetry of footsteps heard on running) is a feature of ataxic cerebral palsy. A tendency to run on the toes suggests cerebral diplegia. A hemiplegic posturing of the limb on one side may be most obvious on running.

Sensation

Pin prick, normally causing a withdrawal response, can be used to test sensory loss. In older children sensation can be tested by light touch (cotton wool), two-point discrimination (compass points normally recognized 2–3 cm apart), temperature appreciation (hot or cold water in test tubes), positional sense (ask the child to state the position of a joint passively moved and screened from him, e.g. 'is the toe pointing up or down'?), rombergism (ability to maintain balance with eyes shut), vibration sense (detection of vibration of a tuning fork applied to a bony point) and astereognosis (inability to tell by touch the nature of a familiar object such as a coin placed in the hand).

Cutaneous nerve segments (Fig. 2.13) can be used to judge levels of cord damage in respect of sensory loss.

Reflexes

In early infancy there are a number of *primitive reflexes* peculiar to this period of life (Table 2.1) whose absence or persistence beyond the time of normal disappearance often has pathological significance (Fig. 2.18).

After infancy the main *superficial and deep reflexes* used in neurological examination, and their segmental innervations, are:

Jaw jerk	pons
Biceps jerk	C5
Supinator jerk	C6
Triceps jerk	C6, C7
Abdominal reflex	Th8–12
Cremaster reflex	L1
Knee jerk	L3, L4
Ankle jerk	L5, S1
Plantar response	S1

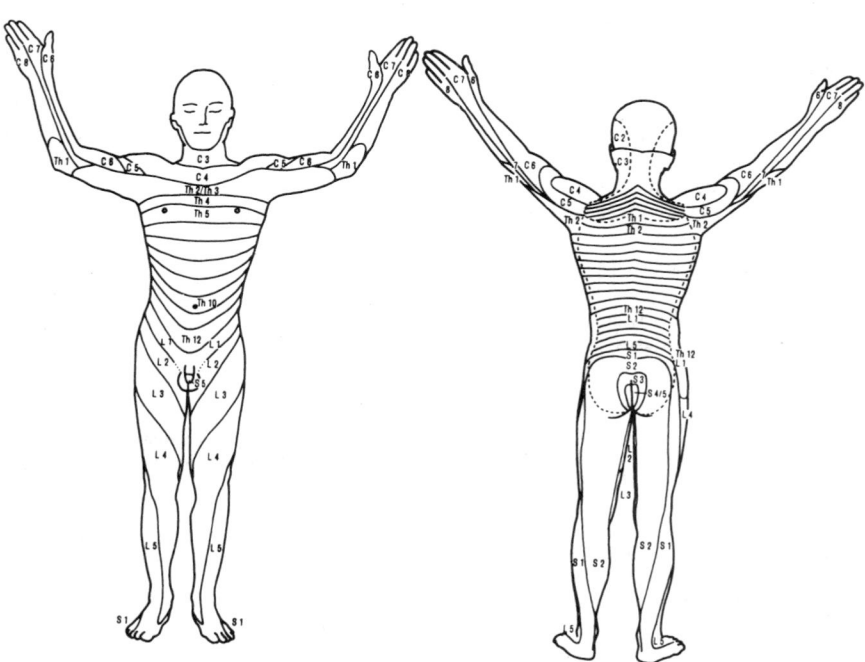

Fig. 2.13 Sensory nerve segments (reproduced from *Folia Medica, Geigy Scientific Table* by permission of Geigy J.R. Basle, S.A., Switzerland).

Table 2.1   Neonatal reflexes

	How elicited	Time of appearance	Usual time of disappearance of those reflexes which are time limited	Possible significance if abnormal
Primitive reflexes				
Cranial nerve reflexes (relevant cranial nerves)				
Sucking (IX, X, XII)	On feeding	Birth	When voluntary control of feeding achieved at 6–9 months	General neurological depression, hypotonia, immaturity or bulbar palsy
Swallowing (IX, X, XII)	On feeding	Birth	When voluntary control of feeding achieved at 6–9 months	General neurological depression, hypotonia, immaturity or bulbar palsy
Rooting (V)	On light contact with infant's cheek the infant turns towards the point of contact	Birth	9 months	General neurological depression, hypotonia, immaturity or bulbar palsy
Glabella (V, VII)	A sharp tap on the glabella produces momentary tight closure of the eyes	Birth	Variable persistence	Apathy or facial palsy if absent; accentuated in hyperexcitability
Head turn to light (II)	With infant supine light from a diffuse source is allowed to fall on one side and then on the other side of the infant's face and he turns his head to the light (the infant must be in a quiet relaxed state)	Several weeks	–	General neurological depression, hypotonia, ? impaired vision
Pupillary (II, also III and V)	Shade one eye with the hand for a moment or two and then withdraw it	Birth	–	General neurological depression, ? impaired vision
Optic blink (II)	Shine a bright light suddenly at the eyes	Birth	–	General neurological depression, ? impaired vision
Doll's eye (III, IV, VI)	Turn head slowly to right or left watching position of eyes (normally eyes do not move with head)	Birth	2 weeks	Ophthalmic muscle palsies (ophthalmoplegia)
Acoustic blink (VIII)	Clap the hands about 30 cm from the infant's head. Avoid producing an air stream across the face. Rapid habituation – no response to test – normally achieved	After a few days	–	? Impaired hearing
Labyrinthine (rotation) (VIII, also III, IV, VII) (see also Fig. 2.14)	(a) Hold baby upright with examiner's hands under infant's arms. Spin round so that baby turns with examiner, first one direction then other (the head should turn towards direction in which baby is being turned)	Birth	–	Disturbed vestibular function or ophthalmoplegia
	(b) Baby similarly held but head held firmly by examiner's forefinger and middle finger which, on each side, are extended upwards against the side of the baby's head. Similar rotation (the baby's eyes should turn towards the turning direction)			Disturbed vestibular function or ophthalmoplegia
Gag (IX, X, XII)	Touch posterior pharynx, e.g. with spatula	Birth	–	General neurological depression or bulbar palsy
Cough (IX, X, XII)	Generated spontaneously on irritation of the respiratory passages	Weak for several weeks after birth	–	General neurological depression
Cutaneous reflexes				
Palmar/foot grasp (Fig. 2.18a)	Place the examiner's forefinger in the palm/sole of the infant's hand/foot which then closes round the examiner's finger maintaining a grip	Birth	2–3 months (palmar), 7–8 months (foot)	General neurological depression, hypotonia: hemisyndromes, Erb palsy or clavicular fracture. May persist beyond normal time in spastic cerebral palsy
Abdominal	Stroke a pin or thumbnail from the side to the center of the abdomen (a response is only possible if muscles are fully relaxed)	7 days	–	Absence does not necessarily imply abnormality
Anal	Contraction of the external anal sphincter when the skin round it is stroked with a pin	Birth	–	Damage to sacral cord (e.g. spina bifida)

Table 2.1 *Cont'd*

	How elicited	Time of appearance	Usual time of disappearance of those reflexes which are time limited	Possible significance if abnormal
Cremaster	Stroking the medial side of the thigh with a pin or thumbnail results in pulling up of the testes	10 days	–	Absent in spinal cord lesion
Withdrawal	On pricking the sole of the foot with a pin there is rapid flexion of the hip, knee and foot	Birth	–	Hemisyndromes; absent or weak in spina bifida and after breech delivery with extended legs
Plantar (Babinski)	Stroking the foot along the lateral side with pin or thumbnail produces dorsal flexion of the big toe and spreading of the other toes in infancy (and plantar flexion of the other toes in older children who are walking). Do not mistake a grasp reflex of the foot for a flexor plantar response	Birth	–	Defects of lower spinal cord, Hemisyndromes
Extensor reflexes Asymmetrical tonic neck (Fig. 2.18b)	With baby in supine position rotate the head to one side. This produces increased tone in, and partial extension of, the arm and leg on the side to which the head is rotated, and there may be flexion of the arm and leg on the contralateral side	1 month	3–5 months	Medullary or spinal cord damage. Readily elicited in immature infant. May persist beyond normal time in cerebral palsy
Crossed extensor reflex	Passively extend one lower limb pressing the knee down, and with a pin stimulate the sole of the foot of this fixated leg. Flexion and slight adduction of the unstimulated lower limb normally occurs	A few days after birth	1 month	Absent in lesions of spinal cord and weak in peripheral nerve damage
Trunk incurvation (Galant)	Stroke a pin or thumbnail along the paravertebral line about 3 cm from the midline from the shoulder to the buttock (the back should curve with the concavity to the stimulated side)	5–6 days	7–8 days	Hemisyndromes; spinal cord damage – with indication of segmental level
Perez	Elicited as for Galant but by stroking over central vertebral spines (the infant arches backwards, the buttocks rise and the anus dilates)	5–6 days	–	As for trunk incurvation reflex
Moro	Hold baby in supine position with shoulders and back supported on left hand and arm of the examiner and head (occiput) on the right hand. Allow the head to fall back suddenly (catching it again with the right hand after it has fallen a short distance) while the rest of the body remains supported. The arms rapidly abduct and come together again with an embracing movement and the legs flex	Birth	2–3 months	General neurological depression, hypotonia. Prolongation of tonic phase of response in immaturity. Hemisyndromes, fractured clavicle or humerus. May persist beyond normal time in cerebral palsy
Hand opening	Stroke the dorsum of the hand	Birth	2–3 months	General neurological depression. Hemisyndrome
Progression Walking/stepping (Fig. 2.19)	Hold infant in standing position and place foot on a flat surface. The leg extends to take the infant's weight (supporting reaction), the opposite leg flexes then extends, and as it takes weight the original leg flexes	4 days	2 months	General neurological depression, hypotonia: paresis of lower limbs
Placing	With the baby held upright between the hands of the examiner the dorsal part of the foot is brought lightly in contact with the edge of the table. Normally the baby flexes knee and hip and places foot on the table	4 days	5–9 months	General neurological depression, hypotonia: paresis of lower limbs

Table 2.1 *Cont'd*

	How elicited	Time of appearance	Usual time of disappearance of those reflexes which are time limited	Possible significance if abnormal
Crawling	Infant prone. Crawling movements may occur spontaneously but can be reinforced by the examiner pressing his thumb gently into the sole of the infant's foot (the crawling reflex is more easily elicited in the immature infant than the walking reflex)	4 days	4 months	General neurological depression, hypotonia: paresis of lower limbs
Tendon reflexes				
Jaw jerk	Sharp tap on examiner's index finger placed on patient's chin below the lip	2 days	–	Absent in brainstem lesions or 5th cranial nerve damage; exaggerated in hyperexcitability, e.g. hypocalcemia
Biceps	A tap on the examiner's finger placed on the biceps muscle causes contraction of the muscle	2 days	–	Absent in general neurological depression and hypotonia; exaggerated in hyperexcitability
Knee jerk	A tap on the patellar tendon with the knee in the flexed position produces quadriceps contraction	2 days	–	Absent in general neurological depression and hypotonia; exaggerated in hyperexcitability
Ankle	With infant prone, knee slightly flexed and the fore part of the foot held lightly in the examiner's hand a tap over the tendo-Achillis produces plantar flexion of the foot (response better felt than seen)	Birth	–	Absent in general neurological depression and hypotonia; exaggerated in hyperexcitability
Ankle clonus	Rapid dorsiflexion of the foot with the examiner's hand on the distal part of the sole produces a succession of rapid contractions of the calf muscle (only briefly sustained in normal infant)	Birth	–	Absent in general neurological depression and hypotonia; exaggerated in hyperexcitability

Other neurological signs

In *Kernig's sign* extension of the flexed knee with the child supine and hips at a right angle is resisted or impossible. In *Brudzinski's sign* flexion of the head produces flexion of the knees and thighs. In impairment of *straight leg raising*, the leg, with the knee fully extended, cannot be raised to a right angle with the patient supine. 'Balancing' movements reflect labyrinthine function (Fig. 2.14).

HIGHER NERVOUS ACTIVITIES

Past history, place in school, relationship with peers and routine clinical examination may reveal much about higher nervous function; accurate assessment will involve psychometric testing and formal speech and language analysis.

LOCOMOTOR SYSTEM

Examination of the nervous system and of the locomotor system may be closely interrelated.

Fractures

Fractures may be visible or suspected because of deformity, crepitus (which should not be actively elicited), pain on movement and local tenderness – which could be due to other conditions such as bruising or osteomyelitis.

Deformities of the trunk and neck

These may be spinal such as *scoliosis* (best recognized when the child bends forward to touch his toes (Fig. 24.22) or suspected if skin creases in the flanks are asymmetrical and fail to disappear when the spine is passively flexed to the opposite side), *kyphosis* (anterior bowing) or *lordosis* (posterior bowing). Ribs may be absent. With *torticollis* (Fig. 2.4n) the head is tilted towards the affected side, the chin points in the opposite direction and rotation of the head away from the affected side may be limited.

Deformities of limbs

Normally children are mildly bow-legged before the age of 2 years and knock-kneed between the ages of 2 and 12 years: thereafter the legs straighten spontaneously (Fig. 24.16). Deformities may consist of absence of bones (e.g. radius with severe flexion and lateral twisting of the hand and wrist, or phocomelia), shortening or deformity of bones, increased carrying angle at the elbow (Turner's syndrome – Fig. 2.4r), incurving of the little finger (Down syndrome), the 'dinner fork' deformity of the wrists with the hands outstretched (chorea) and flexion deformities (e.g. arthrogryposis multiplex congenita Fig. 2.6g).

Lower limb deformities include genu valgum and genu varum, talipes equinovarus (club foot), talipes calaneovalgus, metatarsus varus, absence of part of a limb, shortening or unequal development (e.g. hemiatrophy or hemihypertrophy). Excessive

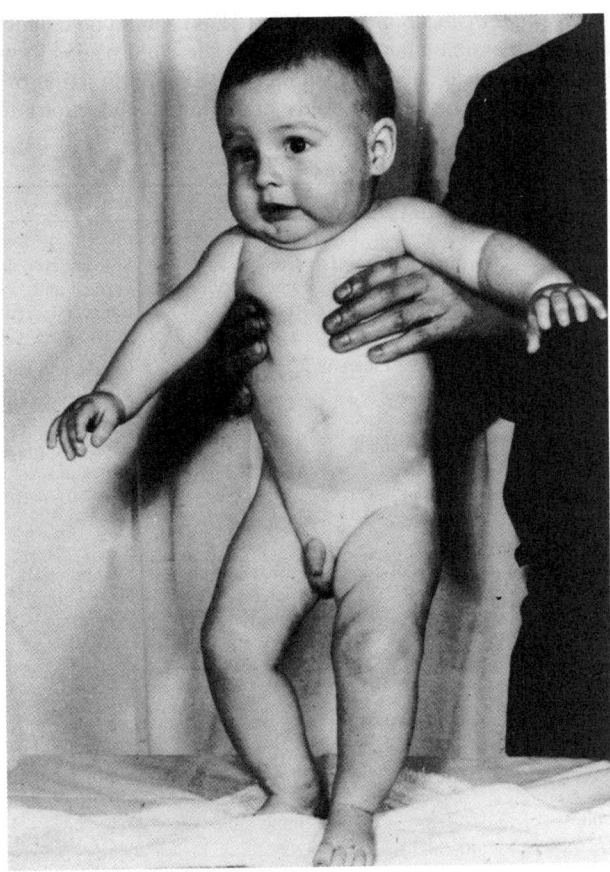

Fig. 2.14 Normal labyrinthine reflexes at the age of 7 months. The infant makes reflex 'balancing' movements with the arms as he is tilted from side to side.

joint mobility is seen in hypotonia, Ehlers–Danlos syndrome and diastrophic dwarfism.

Measurement of limb length is discussed on page 20. Finger shortening (brachydactyly; e.g. Down and the Ellis–van Creveld syndrome) or lengthening (arachnodactyly; e.g. Marfan's syndrome) may be expressed in terms of finger length relative to palm length – the middle finger length (tip to proximal crease) is 43% of the total hand length (tip of the middle finger to the distal palmar crease).

Muscles

May be wasted, hypertrophied (e.g. pseudohypertrophic muscular dystrophy Fig. 2.6h) or absent (e.g. Poland's syndrome). Fasciculation or fibrillary movements may be noted in the tongue, thenar eminence or elsewhere. Muscle tone – see page 35.

Joints

Examination will include assessment of joint temperature relative to other body areas, range of movement, swelling, local tenderness or pain on active or passive movement. Dislocation may cause gross deformity. In the knee, synovial effusion is likely

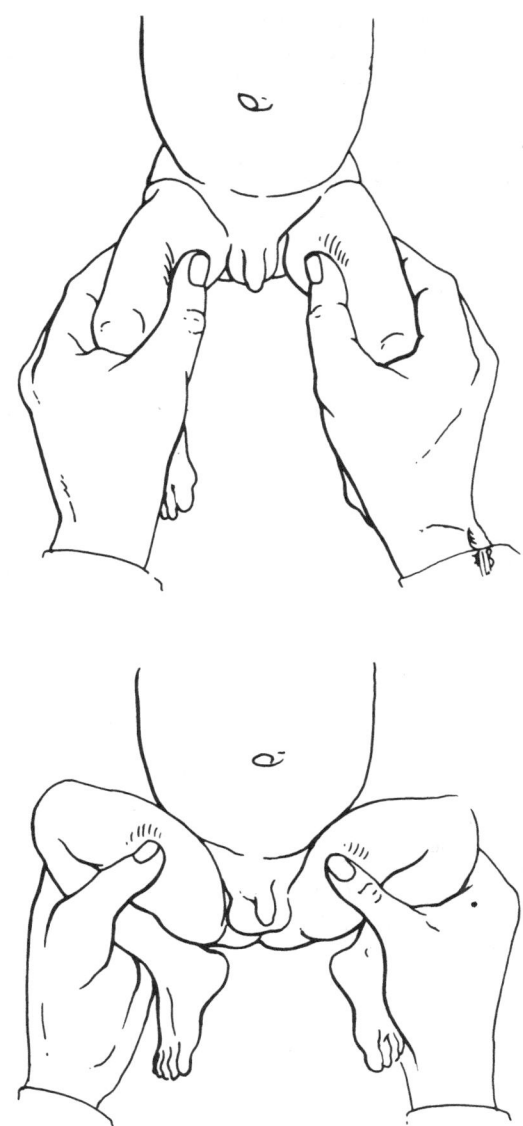

Fig. 2.15 Examination for congenital dislocation of the hip.

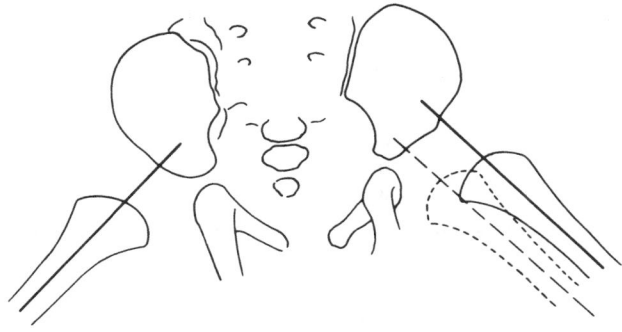

Fig. 2.16 X-ray – congenital dislocation of the hip. Hips abducted 45° from the midline. Line drawn through the center of the shaft of the femur lies outside the upper edge of the acetabulum.

to give rise to *patellar tap* – with the knee joint extended and the thigh gripped just above the patella, the patella, on being sharply depressed, is felt to tap against the underlying bone. Dislocation may cause gross deformity.

Congenital dislocation of the hips (CDH) should be diagnosed as soon as possible after birth, not after the child begins to walk when the classical late signs (shortening, external rotation of the limb, asymmetry of thigh folds and limited abduction) have

Table 2.2 Clinical assessment of gestation age in the newborn infant

	28 weeks	30 weeks	32 weeks	34 weeks	36 weeks	38 weeks	40 weeks
External characteristics							
Sole creases					Anterior transverse crease only	Creases on anterior two-thirds	Sole covered with vertical and transverse creases
Breast nodule diameter					2 mm	4–5 mm	7–10 mm
Scalp hair					Fine and fuzzy		Coarse and silky
Ear lobes					Pliable, no cartilage	Some cartilage	Stiffened by thick cartilage
Testes and scrotum					Scrotum small, few rugae Testes in lower canal	Intermediate	Extensive rugae Testes in scrotum
Muscle tone							
Posture	Completely hypotonic Total extension	Beginning of flexion of thigh and hip	Stronger flexion of hips and knees	Frog-like attitude – lower limbs flexed, upper limbs extended	Flexion of all four limbs	Flexion of all four limbs – hypertonic	Flexion of all four limbs – very hypertonic
Arm and leg recoil on sudden extension	Nil – arms and legs in extension		Slight – legs	Good – legs	Slight – arms	Good – arms	
Head rotation	Chin well past acromion				Chin still passes acromion	Chin to acromion	
Scarf sign	No resistance		Slight resistance		Elbow slightly past midline		Elbow almost reaches midline
Heel to ear maneuver	No resistance		Some resistance	Difficult		Impossible	
Dorsiflexion – angle between dorsum of foot and tibia			40–50°	40–50°	40–50°	20°	0°
Popliteal angle – with thigh in knee–chest position	180°	160°	150°	120°	100°	90°	90°
Head lag – on pulling to sitting position from supine	Head pendulant		Contraction of muscles visible but no movement of head	Head beginning to right itself but still hanging back at end of movement	Head hangs back at first then goes forward on to chest with sudden movement	Head begins to follow trunk, keeps in line for a few seconds in upright position	Keeps head in line with trunk for more than a few seconds
Reflexes							
Pupillary reaction	Appears (29–31 weeks), thereafter present						
Head turning in prone position	Appears, thereafter present						
Head turning to light			Appears (32–36 weeks), thereafter present				
Glabellar tap response			Appears (32–34 weeks), thereafter present				
Neck-righting reflex				Appears (34–37 weeks), thereafter present			
Trunk incurvation on stroking paravertebral area	Present	Present	Present	Active	Present	Present	Weak
Asymmetrical tonic neck reflex	+	+	++	++	+	+	–
Grasp reflex	Finger grip good, reaction spreads up whole upper limb		Stronger		Infant can be lifted up off bed		
Moro reflex	Weak and easily exhaustible		Good	Complete			
Crossed extension reflex	Flexion and extension in a random pattern		Extension but no adduction	Extension and some fanning of toes	Extension, adduction and fanning of the toes		
Rooting	Latency and slow response		More rapid	Full			
Sucking	Weak		Stronger and synchronous with deglutition	Fully developed			
Automatic walking	Nil		Minimal		On toes		Flat foot

developed. Ortolani's test is used in diagnosis: the thighs are abducted while the middle finger of each hand presses the greater trochanter forward (Fig. 2.15); if the hip is dislocated the femoral head during abduction can be felt to slip forward with a 'clunk' (similar to the sensation of changing gear in a car and to be differentiated from the common nonsignificant minor muscular clicks). An extension of the test (Barlow maneuver) consists in applying pressure backwards and outwards with the thumb on the inner side of the thigh as abduction is commenced. If the femoral head slips out over the posterior lip of the acetabulum and returns when pressure is released and abduction continues the hip is unstable. These tests should not be repeated more than necessary. Dislocation may be confirmed by radiology or ultrasound. In anteroposterior radiographs, with the hips and knees extended, thighs medially rotated and abducted 45° from the midline, a line along the center of the femoral shaft lies outside the upper lip of the acetabulum (Fig. 2.16).

EXAMINATION OF THE NEWBORN

Gross physical abnormalities are obvious at birth but other manifestations of disease tend to be less specific. Examination has a threefold purpose – recognizing (1) physical defects, (2) disease and (3) establishing a baseline to which later clinical assessments can relate.

MEDICAL HISTORY OF PARENTS, SIBLINGS AND OTHER RELATIVES

The mother's previous pregnancies may indicate factors such as prolonged involuntary infertility, habitual abortion or frequent fetal loss implying higher risk of congenital abnormality. Parents, siblings or other relatives may suffer, or have suffered, from disorders which carry hereditary risks. Certain maternal diseases may have profound influence on the fetus. The social history may imply disadvantage.

BIRTH HISTORY

Note birth rank and maturity, evidence of fetal distress, early rupture of the membranes, induction of labor, prolonged or rapid labor, type of delivery, obstetric estimate of gestation, birthweight, Apgar score, apnea, need for resuscitation, special or intensive care.

GESTATIONAL AGE

Important in making judgments concerning diagnosis and management, this may be assessed by (1) mother's 'dates' (p. 79), (2) obstetric examination (p. 80), (3) ultrasound measurements of fetal growth (p. 80), (4) clinical examination of the infant. Gestation age may be assessed using external characteristics, muscle tone and primitive reflexes (Table 2.2). Dubowitz & Dubowitz (1977) have derived a score based on (a) neurological criteria and (b) external criteria convertible into gestation age (Fig. 2.17). A more rapid method relies on skin color and texture, breast development and ear firmness (Parkin et al 1976).

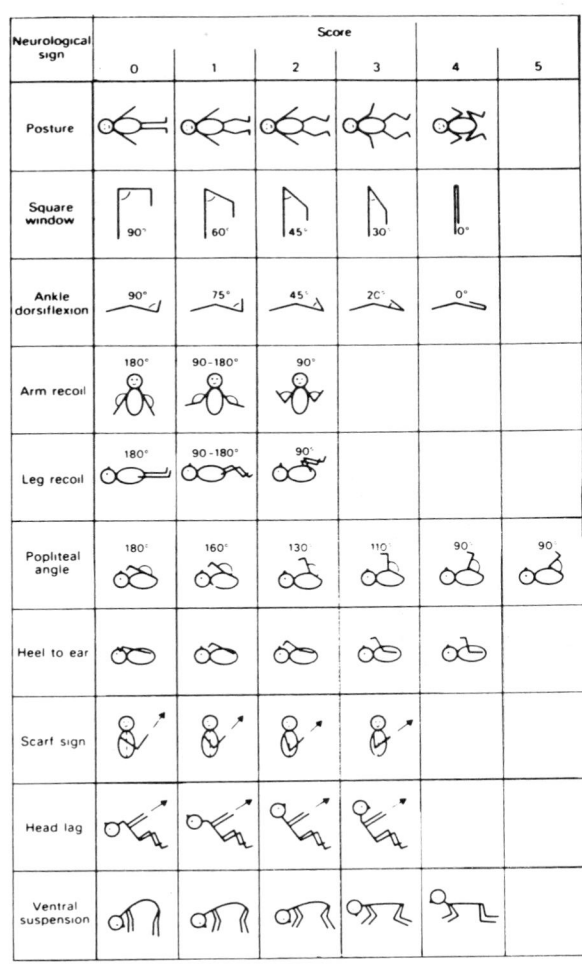

POSTURE. Observed with infant quiet and in supine position. Score 0: Arms and legs extended; 1: beginning of flexion of hips and knees, arms extended; 2: stronger flexion of legs, arms extended; 3: arms slightly flexed, legs flexed and abducted; 4: full flexion of arms and legs.

SQUARE WINDOW. The hand is flexed on the forearm between the thumb and index finger of the examiner. Enough pressure is applied to get as full a flexion as possible, and the angle between the hypothenar eminence and the ventral aspect of the forearm is measured and graded according to diagram. (Care is taken not to rotate the infant's wrist while doing this manoeuvre.)

ANKLE DORSIFLEXION. The foot is dorsiflexed onto the anterior aspect of the leg, with the examiner's thumb on the sole of the foot and other fingers behind the leg. Enough pressure is applied to get as full flexion as possible, and the angle between the dorsum of the foot and the anterior aspect of the leg is measured.

ARM RECOIL. With the infant in the supine position the forearms are first flexed for 5 seconds, then fully extended by pulling on the hands, and then released. The sign is fully positive if the arms return briskly to full flexion (Score 2). If the arms return to incomplete flexion or the response is sluggish it is graded as Score 1. If they remain extended or are only followed by random movements the score is 0.

LEG RECOIL. With the infant supine, the hips and knees are fully flexed for 5 seconds, then extended by traction on the feet, and released. A maximal response is one of full flexion of the hips and knees (Score 2). A partial flexion scores 1, and minimal or no movement scores 0.

POPLITEAL ANGLE. With the infant supine and his pelvis flat on the examining couch, the thigh is held in the knee-chest position by the examiner's left index finger and thumb supporting the knee. The leg is then extended by gentle pressure from the examiner's right index finger behind the ankle and the popliteal angle is measured.

HEEL TO EAR MANOEUVRE. With the baby supine, draw the baby's foot as near to the head as it will go without forcing it. Observe the distance between the foot and the head as well as the degree of extension at the knee. Grade according to illustrations. Score 0: Elbow reaches the knee. Note that the knee is left free and may draw down alongside the abdomen.

SCARF SIGN. With the baby supine, take the infant's hand and try to put it around the neck and as far posteriorly as possible around the opposite shoulder. Assist this manoeuvre by lifting the elbow across the body. See how far the elbow will go across and grade according to diagram. Score 0: Elbow reaches opposite axillary line; 1: Elbow between midline and opposite axillary line; 2: Elbow reaches midline; 3: Elbow will not reach midline.

HEAD LAG. With the baby lying supine, grasp the hands (or the arms if a very small infant) and pull him slowly towards the sitting position. Observe the position of the head in relation to the trunk and grade accordingly. In a small infant the head may initially be supported by one hand. Score 0: Complete lag; 1: Partial head control; 2: Able to maintain head in line with body; 3: Brings head anterior to body.

VENTRAL SUSPENSION. The infant is suspended in the prone position, with examiner's hand under the infant's chest (one hand in a small infant, two in a large infant). Observe the degree of extension of the back and the amount of flexion of the arms and legs. Also note the relation of the head to the trunk. Grade according to diagrams.

If the score for an individual criterion differs on the two sides of the baby, take the mean.

Fig. 2.17a Dubowitz score: neurological criteria.

External (superficial) Criteria

EXTERNAL SIGN	SCORE				
	0	1	2	3	4
OEDEMA	Obvious oedema hands and feet; pitting over tibia	No obvious oedema hands and feet; pitting over tibia	No oedema		
SKIN TEXTURE	Very thin, gelatinous	Thin and smooth	Smooth; medium thickness. Rash or superficial peeling	Slight thickening. Superficial cracking and peeling esp ' hands and feet	Thick and parchment-like; superficial or deep cracking
SKIN COLOUR (Infant not crying)	Dark red	Uniformly pink	Pale pink variable over body	Pale. Only pink over ears, lips, palms or soles	
SKIN OPACITY (trunk)	Numerous veins and venules clearly seen, especially over abdomen	Veins and tributaries seen	A few large vessels clearly seen over abdomen	A few large vessels seen indistinctly over abdomen	No blood vessels seen
LANUGO (over back)	No lanugo	Abundant; long and thick over whole back	Hair thinning especially over lower back	Small amount of lanugo and bald areas	At least half of back devoid of lanugo
PLANTAR CREASES	No skin creases	Faint red marks over anterior half of sole	Definite red marks over more than anterior half; indentations over less than anterior third	Indentations over more than anterior third	Definite deep indentations over more than anterior third
NIPPLE FORMA-TION	Nipple barely visible; no areola	Nipple well defined; areola smooth and flat diameter <0.75 cm.	Areola stippled, edge not raised; diameter <0.75 cm.	Areola stippled, edge raised diameter >0.75 cm.	
BREAST SIZE	No breast tissue palpable	Breast tissue on one or both sides < 0.5 cm. diameter	Breast tissue both sides; one or both 0.5-1.0 cm	Breast tissue both sides; one or both > 1 cm	
EAR FORM	Pinna flat and shapeless, little or no incurving of edge	Incurving of part of edge of pinna	Partial incurving whole of upper pinna	Well-defined incurving whole of upper pinna	
EAR FIRMNESS	Pinna soft, easily folded, no recoil	Pinna soft, easily folded, slow recoil	Cartilage to edge of pinna, but soft in places, ready recoil	Pinna firm, cartilage to edge, instant recoil	
GENITALIA MALE	Neither testis in scrotum	At least one testis high in scrotum	At least one testis right down		
FEMALES (With hips half abducted)	Labia majora widely separated, labia minora protruding	Labia majora almost cover labia minora	Labia majora completely cover labia minora		

Fig. 2.17b Dubowitz score: external (superficial) criteria.

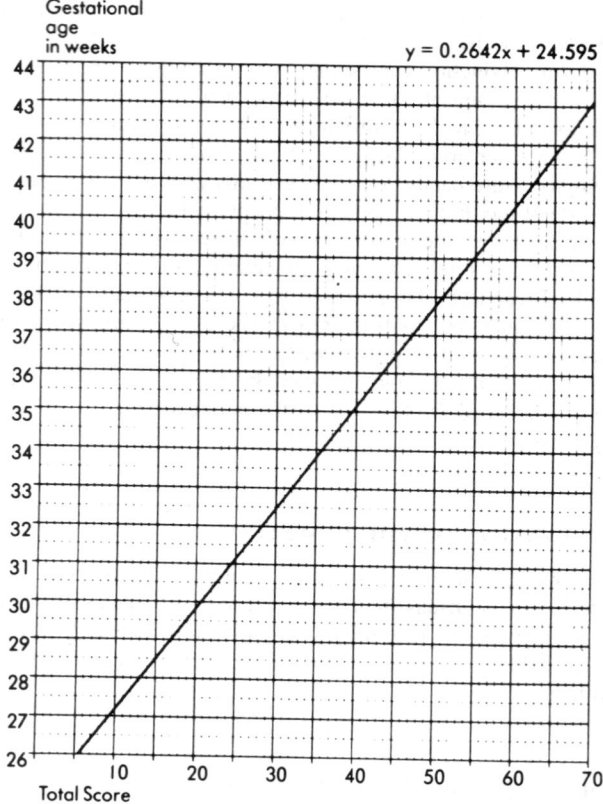

Fig. 2.17c Dubowitz score: graph for converting score into gestational age. (Forms available from Spastics International Medical Publications, 5A Netherhall Gardens, London)

THE TRANSITION PERIOD

Respiration, which may be irregular in rate and depth in the immediate neonatal period, should be established within half a minute of delivery. Diffuse motor activity at birth peaks at half to 1 hour then diminishes and the infant often passes into sleep.

ROUTINE EXAMINATION

Usually carried out on the first day of life and again on discharge when signs not evident on the first day may be evident (e.g. the murmur of ventricular septal defect).

Measurements

Weight, length (crown–heel or crown–rump), skull circumference, respiration rate and temperature are standard.

Inspection

Gross *deformities* such as excessive cranial molding, caput succedaneum, cephalhematoma, abnormal facies (e.g. Down syndrome or renal agenesis (Fig. 2.4a)), spina bifida, absent or deformed limbs, tumor masses (e.g. sacrococcygeal teratoma), herniae (e.g. umbilical) may be evident.

Posture and *movement* (see below).

Healthy *skin* will be pink and elastic; unhealthy may be cracked and parchment-like (placental insufficiency), abnormally pallid (fetal exsanguination), cyanosed (asphyxia or severe congenital heart disease), shiny (edema), jaundiced, desquamating (e.g. Ritter's disease), loose and inelastic (prematurity), dry and turgorless (dehydration), blemished (angiomata, nevi or milia) or pustular (infection). Neonatal urticaria (erythema toxicum), petechiae or ecchymosis (consumption coagulopathy), Mongolian blue spots (patchy accumulations of pigment over the lumbar region and buttocks) and rarer disorders such as Harlequin color change (the body pale on one side and deep red on the other with a clear line of demarcation between) or the 'collodion baby' may occur. Dermal sinuses may be present in the region of the coccyx. Cyanosis or pallor may be evident.

The *umbilical cord* and stump may show an omphalocele, bleeding, infection or other discharges. A single umbilical artery (1% of singletons, higher in twins) is sometimes associated with severe congenital abnormalities. Note the shape of the *head* and character and size of the anterior *fontanel*. Prematurely born infants tend to develop side-to-side flattening due to their readily moldable skulls.

The *eyes* are usually closed but pupillary shape and size can be examined. Nystagmus (if transitory unimportant, but if persistent probably pathological), microphthalmia, eyeball enlargement (buphthalmos – Fig. 2.4u), corneal clouding, cataract (Fig. 2.4i), defects of the iris (coloboma or aniridia) may be present. Eye movements may be absent (ophthalmoplegia).

The *mouth* may reveal deformities such as cleft palate. The mucous membranes may be moist, dry, ulcerated or infected. The jaw may be small and retracted (micrognathia – Fig. 2.4p). Epstein's pearls (nodules just lateral to the midline on the hard palate) are normal. Facial asymmetry may be noted (in the neonate the corner of the mouth is actively depressed on crying so that in facial palsy the depressed side is the normal).

Inspect the *chest* for asymmetry, the pattern and rate of respiration, evidence of respiratory distress (tachypnea, grunting, intercostal and costal margin recession), respiratory depression (slowness and shallowness of respiration), precordial bulging or abnormal precordial pulsation, breast enlargement or secretion of milk.

Note any abnormal shape of the *abdomen* (e.g. scaphoid, distended, showing peristaltic waves) and any impairment of normal abdominal respiration.

Watch *feeding* for vigor and coordination of sucking, swallowing and possible vomiting.

Note any imperforation, malposition or abnormal structure (e.g. lax and patulous) of the *anus* or structural abnormality of the *urethra* (e.g. hypospadias) or *genitalia* (e.g. scrotal swelling or testicular abnormality). In the newborn female, particularly the premature, the clitoris and labia minora are usually prominent.

The *cry* may be abnormal (e.g. stridulous or high pitched as in cerebral irritation). *Hiccup* is common in normal newborn infants.

Palpation

Handling will reveal *muscle tone*.

Note the size and tension of the anterior *fontanel*, degree of closure of the posterior fontanel, state of the sutures (widening or overriding).

Edema pits on pressure (Fig. 2.6i); *sclerema* neonatorum presents as lardlike hardening of subcutaneous tissue, *subcutaneous fat necrosis* as areas of rubbery consistency usually on the neck posteriorly and outer aspect of the thighs, *surgical emphysema* as a crepitant sensation over the root of neck and thorax.

Palpation and handling will reveal abnormal *precordial pulsation*, position of the apex beat, enlarged viscera and other *masses*, mobility and range of movements of *joints* (cf. Ortolani maneuver), position of the *testes*, possibly *fractures*.

Percussion

May reveal lung *hyperresonance* (e.g. lobar emphysema), lung *consolidation*, *cardiac displacement* and possibly size, *fluid* in the abdomen.

Auscultation

Reveals *breath sounds* and associated adventitious sounds,

cardiac murmurs (often transitory in the first few days of life), *bowel sounds* (bowel sounds in the chest are unique in diaphragmatic hernia), *cranial bruits*.

Excreta

The nature and manner of passage of *meconium*; the frequency, consistency, color, odor and possible blood staining of the stools; the visual, chemical and bacteriological examination of the *urine* may be important.

Instrumental procedures

Laryngoscopy (frequently used for intubation); ophthalmoscopy (detection of early retinopathy of prematurity; retinal bleeding, exudate or defect; cataract and corneal opacity); *auriscopic examination*; *transillumination* (e.g. hydranencephaly or hydrocele); *lumbar puncture*; *subdural tapping*; *suprapubic aspiration of the bladder*; blood *culture* and culture of various other discharges.

NEUROLOGICAL ASSESSMENT

Neurological assessment of the newborn infant gives an indication of the presence or likely development of disorders such as cerebral palsy, microcephaly, hydrocephaly, the 'clumsy child' and intellectual impairment.

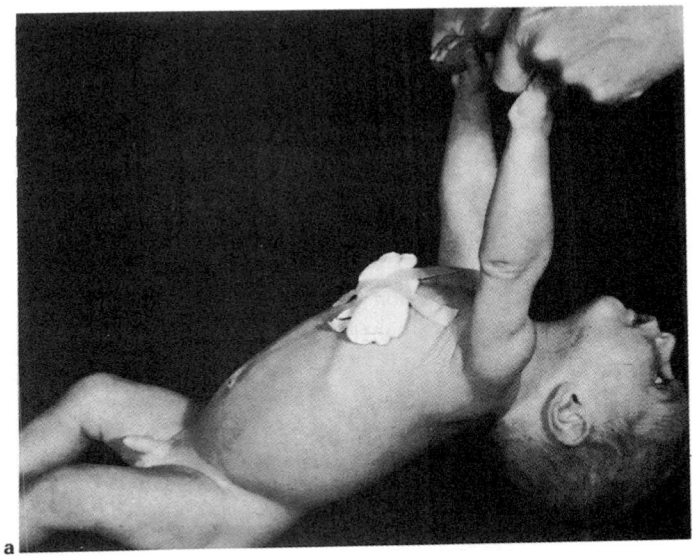

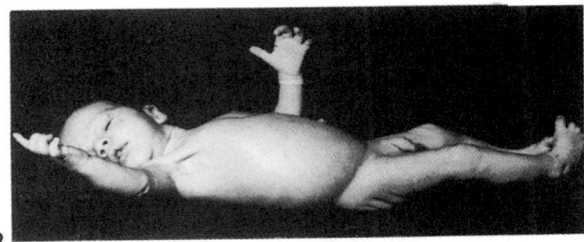

Fig. 2.18 (a) Hand grasp (note poor head control). (b) Marked asymmetrical tonic reflex in infant aged 4 months suffering from diplegic cerebral palsy.

Behavioral characteristics: was breathing established spontaneously at birth or intubation required? What is the *state of consciousness*, response to stimuli, amount of spontaneous movement (or lack of it)? Have there been *convulsions* (localized or generalized). Are *sucking* and *swallowing* impaired (e.g. in bulbar palsy) necessitating tube feeding? Are there normal *crying* responses to hunger and pain? Is there a normal state of alertness, or *apathy*? Does sleep occupy the normal 20 out of 24 hours?

Posture in the newborn is one of flexion; the arm will remain flexed at the elbow on 'pulling to sit', the popliteal angle remains at 90° on straight leg raising (in contrast dorsiflexion of the foot against the tibia reveals the diminished extensor tone – Table 9.1), sudden passive extension (stretch) and then release of the elbow will result in forearm recoil; in the prone position the lower limbs are flexed under the abdomen, the arms flexed at the elbows and adducted beside the trunk (Fig. 9.1); on ventral suspension the dangling limbs remain flexed (Table 9.1). Disturbance of the normal postural flexion is likely to indicate neurological dysfunction. In generalized *hypotonia* the infant is 'floppy' with a 'flat' posture in recumbency. Regional hypotonia is seen for instance in the bilateral lower limb paresis of spina bifida or in Erb's palsy. In generalized *hypertonia* (extensor hypertonus) the legs are usually more affected than the arms, the trunk tends to be opisthotonic and the extensor tone in the neck results in seemingly good head control in ventral suspension but poor head control on 'pulling to sit' (Fig. 2.18a). In more severe cases, the arms are also involved, the position being one of decerebrate rigidity. In hypertonia static postures may be interrupted by 'cycling' movements of the lower limbs, 'doggy paddling' of the upper and generalized 'jitteriness': tendon reflexes are usually exaggerated. Transient or persistent *hemisyndromes* may occur in which one side of the body may show increased or diminished tone relative to the other (tonic hemisyndrome); reflexes, particularly the extensor reflexes, such as the asymmetrical tonic neck reflex (Fig. 2.18b), may be accentuated unilaterally (reflex hemisyndrome) or one side may be paralyzed (paralytic hemisyndrome).

Spontaneous movements exhibited by the newborn infant include rotation of the head, movement of the arms, sucking the thumb, movement of the lower limbs (more than the arms).

The *primitive and tendon reflexes* which can be used in neurological assessment are described in Tables 2.1 and 2.2.

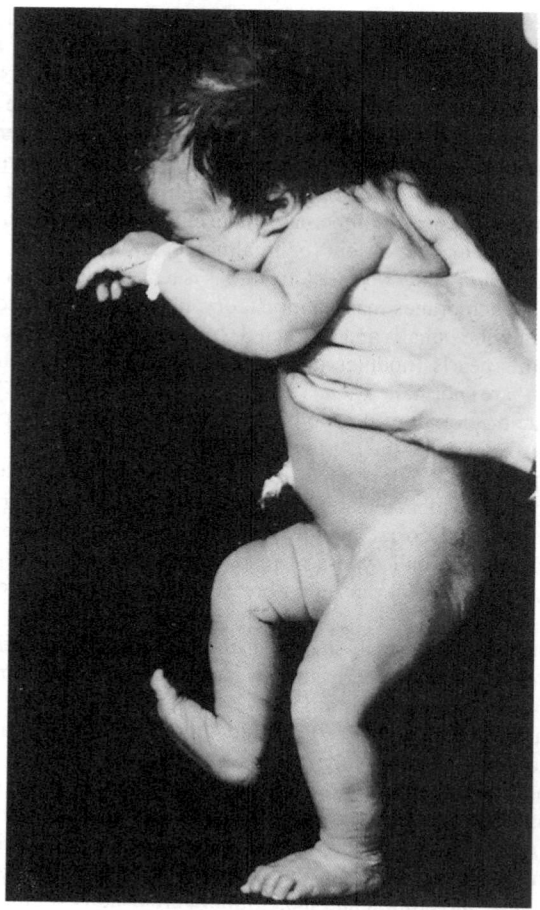

Fig. 2.19   Normal stepping reflex.

REFERENCES

Dubowitz L M S, Dubowitz V 1977 Gestational age of the newborn. Addison-Wesley, London
Parkin J M, Hey E N, Cloews J S 1976 Rapid assessment of gestational age at birth. Archives of Disease in Childhood 67: 444–447

3 Genetics

Michael A. Patton

Introduction **45**
Epidemiology **45**
Mitosis and meiosis **47**
Mitosis: cell division **47**
Meiosis: production of gametes **47**
 Spermatogenesis and oogenesis **48**
Chromosomes **48**
Preparation of chromosomes **48**
 Standard preparations from blood **48**
 Staining techniques **48**
 Preparation of chromosomes from other tissues **49**
 Fluorescent in situ hybridization (FISH) **50**
 Indications for chromosome studies **50**
Types of chromosome abnormality **51**
 Numerical abnormalities **51**
 Structural abnormalities in chromosomes **51**
Nomenclature **53**
Chromosomal syndromes **54**
Down syndrome (trisomy 21) **54**
 Incidence **54**
 Clinical features **54**
 Cytogenetics **55**
 Genetic counseling and screening **56**
Trisomy 18 (Edwards' syndrome) **57**
 Clinical features **57**
 Cytogenetics **57**
Trisomy 13 (Patau's syndrome) **57**
 Clinical features **57**
 Cytogenetics **58**
4p⁻ (Wolf–Hirschhorn) syndrome **58**
5p⁻ (cri du chat) syndrome **58**
18q⁻ syndrome **58**
Deletions of 13q **59**
Newer chromosomal syndromes **59**
Other autosomal abnormalities **60**
Sex chromosome abnormalities **60**
Turner's syndrome **60**

Clinical features **60**
Cytogenetics **61**
47XXX **62**
Klinefelter's syndrome (47XXY) **62**
 Cytogenetics **62**
48XXXY and 49XXXXY **62**
XX males **62**
XYY syndrome **62**
Fragile X mental retardation **62**
 Clinical features **63**
 Molecular genetics **63**
Single gene disorders: inheritance **64**
Drawing the pedigree **65**
Autosomal dominant inheritance **65**
Autosomal recessive inheritance **66**
Codominance **66**
X-linked recessive inheritance **66**
X-linked dominant inheritance **67**
Mitochondrial inheritance **68**
DNA and gene action **68**
Structure and function of genes **68**
 Mutations at a molecular level **69**
Techniques used in molecular genetics **70**
 The preparation of gene probes and gene library **70**
 DNA extraction **70**
 Southern blotting **70**
 Polymerase chain reaction **70**
 Gene sequencing **72**
Gene mapping **72**
The use of molecular genetics in diagnosis **73**
Multifactorial inheritance **74**
Malformation syndromes **75**
The clinical approach to the diagnosis of a dysmorphic syndrome **76**
Counseling and genetic services **76**
Organization of services **76**
Approaches to genetic counseling **77**
References **78**

INTRODUCTION

There have been many advances in the understanding of human genetics in the last 10–15 years and the purpose of this chapter is to present some of the basic concepts of genetics in relation to pediatric practice. Rather than becoming polarized in an argument about which disorders are due to 'nature' and which are due to 'nurture', it is more fruitful to consider human disease as a spectrum from those conditions like Duchenne muscular dystrophy and Down syndrome, which are purely genetic, through to those which are purely environmental such as scurvy and tuberculosis (Fig. 3.1). Between the two extremes are many common diseases like diabetes mellitus, ischemic heart disease and congenital malformations in which both genetic and environmental factors are involved. Such conditions may be referred to as multifactorial. Disorders which are at the genetic end of the spectrum are either due to changes in a single gene or to visible changes in the chromosomes.

EPIDEMIOLOGY

The frequency of genetic disorders has not increased, but they

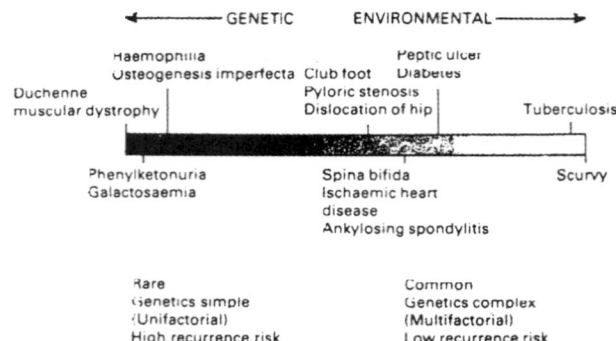

Fig. 3.1 Human disease may be seen as being on a spectrum from those diseases which are exclusively genetic to those which are exclusively environmental (reproduced from Emery & Mueller 1988).

have become relatively more important with the decline in mortality from infectious diseases that has resulted from vaccination, improved living standards and antibiotic therapy. The relative importance of genetic disease is also increasing for other reasons. There is rapidly increasing knowledge in the field of medical genetics. The number of human chromosomes was only established in 1956 and since then many forms of mental handicap, malformation and intersex have been attributed to chromosome abnormality. Prenatal diagnosis has offered the opportunity of preventing an increasing number of serious handicaps, and the developments in DNA technology have meant that many of the genes that predispose to common adult disorders such as heart disease and cancer are now being identified and may play a major role in identifying the predisposition in these disorders, and developing strategies for their prevention.

Genetic disorders are a major component in childhood mortality (Table 3.1) with up to half of childhood deaths in hospital having a genetic or partly genetic cause. In addition to mortality, genetic disorders produce a substantial morbidity. They often require frequent hospital admissions or complex surgery and this is reflected in a number of studies on the incidence of genetic disorders amongst pediatric inpatients; the incidence of genetic or partially genetic disease amongst pediatric inpatients in New York in 1974 was 12.5% of admissions. Other similar studies have found incidences of between 11 and 27% (Emery & Rimoin 1990). It should also be noted that many chronic genetic disorders may place a considerable financial strain on health resources, e.g. the average annual cost of a patient with cystic fibrosis in 1990 was £8000 (Cuckle et al 1995) and the lifetime cost of continual nursing care for a severely handicapped individual may be in the region of £1 000 000.

In the field of mental handicap the genetic contribution is even greater. With the recognition of chromosomal disease it has been found that around one-third of mental handicap is due to chromosomal abnormality and future studies which include analysis for fragile X are likely to find an even greater contribution from chromosomal abnormality. Overall more than 50% of mental handicap is due to genetic factors, and many of these could be prevented by genetic counseling and prenatal diagnosis (Table 3.2).

The same situation applies in visual handicap and profound childhood deafness. In previous generations retrolental fibroplasia and ophthalmia neonatorum contributed significantly to childhood blindness but the frequency of these disorders is declining with improved medical care. One survey (Philips et al 1987) conducted in a national school for children who are registered blind has shown that about 50% of childhood blindness has a genetic basis and that this is largely due to single gene disorders (Table 3.3). In studies on congenital deafness around 30% has been attributed to genetic factors and once again many of these are due to single gene disorders (Table 3.4).

Even before birth chromosome abnormalities are a major cause of fetal wastage with between 15 and 30% of all human conceptions having an abnormal karyotype and being spontaneously aborted or failing to implant (Epstein 1986).

The incidence of genetic disorders is roughly comparable in different parts of the world, but the frequency of specific disorders may vary for reasons such as inbreeding, selective advantage and genetic isolation (Mueller & Young 1995). The frequency of

Table 3.2 Causes of severe mental retardation

Etiology	Frequency (%)
Chromosomal	33
Single gene disorder	15
Malformation syndrome	13
CNS malformation	7
Perinatal factors	15
Infections, trauma	3
Unknown	14

(Based on a regional study of mentally handicapped children in Hertfordshire, Laxova et al 1977.)

Table 3.3 99 Children in blind school, Edinburgh (1988)

Genetic = 50%	Nongenetic = 50%
Congenital cataract	Birth asphyxia
Anophthalmos	Optic nerve hypoplasia
Leber's amaurosis	Cortical blindness
Laurence–Moon–Biedl	Retrolental fibroplasia
Retinitis pigmentosa	Hydrocephalus
Retinal dystrophy	Nonaccidental injury

(Modified from Philips et al 1987.)

Table 3.1 Genetic and nongenetic causes of childhood deaths in United Kingdom Hospitals 1914–1976

	Nongenetic	Genetic		
		M	C	MF
London (1914)	83.5%	2%	–	14.5%
Edinburgh (1976)	50.0%	8.9%	2.9%	38.2%

M = monogenic; C = chromosomal; MF = multifactorial. (Modified from Carter 1956, and Emery & Rimoin 1983.)

Table 3.4 Causes of severe childhood deafness

Etiology	Frequency (%)
Genetic	30
Acquired	40
Unknown	30

Table 3.5 Racial and geographic differences in the frequency of genetic disease

Disease	Racial/geographic group	Birth incidence
Sickle cell disease	African	1 in 50
Thalassemia	Mediterranean	1 in 100
Oculocutaneous albinism }	Hopi Indians	1 in 250
	N. Europeans	1 in 40 000
Congenital adrenal hyperplasia }	Yupik Eskimos	1 in 500
	N. Europeans	1 in 10 000
Cystic fibrosis	N. Europeans	1 in 2000
	Orientals	Very rare
Tay–Sachs disease	Ashkenazi Jews	1 in 3600
Neural tube defects	N. Ireland	1 in 300
Ellis–van Creveld syndrome }	Amish	1 in 200
	N. European	1 in 60 000

sickle cell disease mirrors the frequency of malaria since carriers of sickle cell trait have a greater resistance to *Plasmodium falciparum* malaria. This frequency has taken many generations to develop from a relatively small selective advantage and will remain in those racial groups for a very considerable number of generations even after they have moved to countries without malaria. Cystic fibrosis is one of the most frequent single gene disorders in Western Europe, and although this may be attributable to a selective advantage in gene carriers this has yet to be demonstrated. For other recessive disorders in small isolated communities the frequency of affected children may be increased by inbreeding, e.g. oculocutaneous albinism in the Hopi Indians, congenital adrenal hyperplasia in the Yupik Eskimos and Ellis–van Creveld syndrome in the Amish community (Table 3.5). It should be noted that genetic disease may pose a major health problem even in underdeveloped countries where infections are still a major cause of childhood deaths, e.g. in Thailand up to 500 000 children suffer from variable degrees of chronic ill health due to the interaction of different thalassemia genes.

MITOSIS AND MEIOSIS

Chromosomes are the means whereby the units of genetic information (or genes) are transmitted from one cell generation to the next. This transmission of genetic information must be precise and accurate and is achieved via one of the two mechanisms of cell division, either mitosis (division of somatic or body cells) which results in the growth of specific organs or the overall body, or meiosis, the specialized cell division which results in gamete formation, and may be referred to as 'reduction division' since it involves the reduction of the original *diploid* (2n) complement of 46 chromosomes to the *haploid* (n) complement of 23 chromosomes.

MITOSIS: CELL DIVISION

Somatic cell division is a cyclical procedure, the length of the total cycle varying from organism to organism and between cell types. Essentially the cycle can be divided into the *interphase* stage during which DNA synthesis (and hence chromosome replication) occurs, and the mitotic stage during which the actual division process takes place. During interphase the chromosomes are not condensed and are invisible other than as a mass of chromatin, but the mitotic phase is characterized by the gradual condensation of the chromatin through *prophase* into recognizable chromosomes,

each comprising two sister chromatids held together at the centromere and aligned on the equatorial plate of the cell. This stage of the cell division is known as *metaphase* and is the stage at which the chromosomes are usually visualized. The centromere divides longitudinally and under the influence of the 'spindle apparatus' homologous daughter chromatids move to opposite cell poles (*anaphase*), where they are included in separate daughter nuclei (*telophase*). The products of mitotic division, therefore, are two daughter cells identical in all respects with the parent cell from which they have arisen.

MEIOSIS: PRODUCTION OF GAMETES

Meiosis comprises a single replication of the genetic material in interphase followed by two successive nuclear divisions.

As chromosomes begin to condense into the prolonged prophase characteristic of this type of division, homologous chromosomes pair closely with one another (*synapsis*) to form bivalents, and exchange segments of genetic material in a process known as *meiotic recombination* (Fig. 3.2). This recombination ensures the individuality of the offspring in much the same way as shuffling a pack of cards ensures that in each game the players will receive a different combination of cards. As condensation of chromatin continues the centromeres of the paired chromosomes repel one another, and eventually two daughter chromosomes of differing genetic constitution are formed from each bivalent (*metaphase I*). These daughter chromosomes each contain a mixture of genetic material from both parents of the individual concerned and they segregate at random (but in equal numbers) into the daughter nuclei formed at this stage in the cycle (*anaphase I*), thus completing the first stage of the process. The

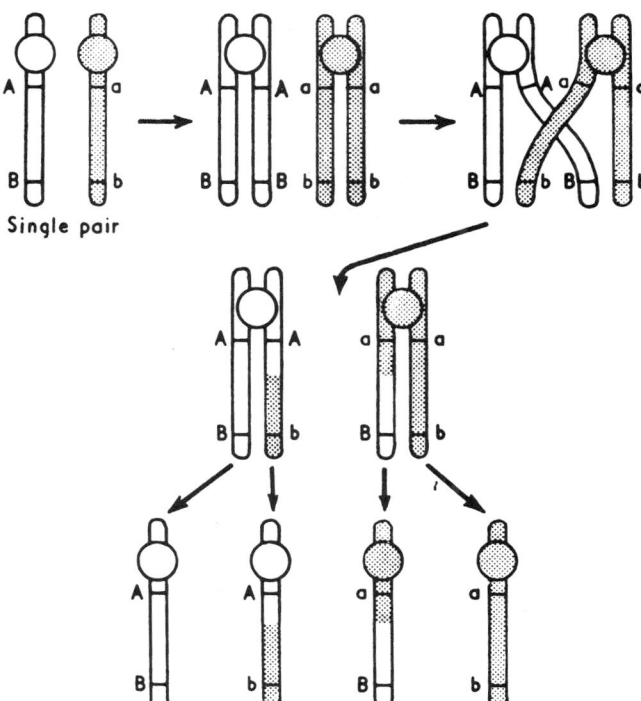

Fig. 3.2 'Crossing over' – the exchange of genetic material between homologous chromosomes.

second stage is a straightforward mitotic division in which the centromeres of the daughter chromosomes divide and homologous centromeres with their attached chromatids travel to opposite cell poles.

The outcome of this two-stage division process is a quartet of nuclei, each with half (n) the original number (2n) of chromosomes, and with new combinations of parental genes.

Spermatogenesis and oogenesis

The basic pattern of chromosome behavior is the same during meiosis in both male and female gametogenesis, but there are differences in timing of the various stages. Spermatogenesis begins around puberty, and continues throughout life, with spermatozoa produced by continuing meiotic division of primary spermatocytes.

On the other hand, oogenesis commences in intrauterine life but is arrested at a very early stage in meiosis I, with completion of the cycle only when ovulation occurs, anything up to 50 years later (Fig. 3.3).

Spermatogenesis and oogenesis also differ in that, while the former gives rise ultimately to four functional sperm, the latter normally yields only a single functional ovum, with the other three products of the division process forming what are known as 'polar bodies', each with its haploid chromosome constitution, but with only a relatively small amount of cytoplasm. The first polar body arises from the eccentric division of the cytoplasm at the end of meiosis I. This polar body divides further in parallel with the oocyte. The oocyte undergoes further division to form the functional ovum and a residual polar body.

The polar bodies are generally nonfunctional but in exceptional circumstances may be fertilized simultaneously with the ovum, subsequent development resulting in an individual derived from fusion of two distinct zygotes. One example of this unusual situation may be the XX/XY patient with ambiguous sexual development.

CHROMOSOMES

PREPARATION OF CHROMOSOMES

Standard preparations from blood

The original demonstration that there are 46 chromosomes in the human cell was made using fibroblast cultures from fetal lung (Tijo & Levan 1956). In routine clinical practice, however, it is

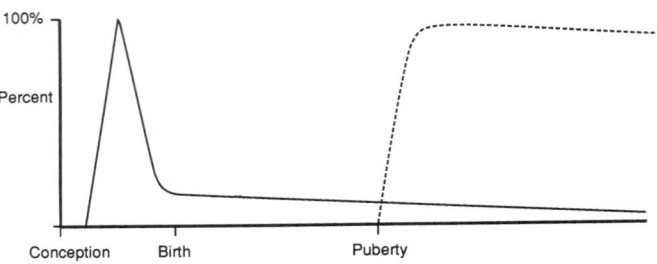

Fig. 3.3 Relative populations of germ cells in males (.....) and females (——) by age. In the female the maximum number of germ cells is reached before birth, whereas in the male sperm are not produced until puberty and the production continues throughout adult life.

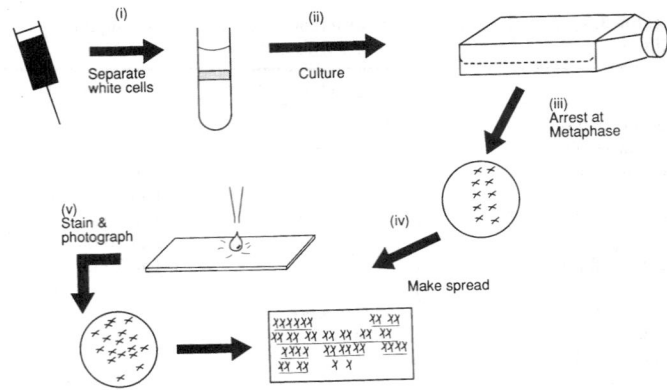

Fig. 3.4 Preparation of a chromosome karyotype from a blood sample.

human lymphocytes that are used for the standard chromosome analysis since a blood sample is convenient to obtain and relatively easy to prepare.

The standard preparation of chromosomes from a blood sample is illustrated in Figure 3.4 (see Rooney & Czepulskowski 1992 for further details). The first stage of the process (i) is to separate the white cells from the rest of the blood sample. This is done by centrifugation using a medium such as Ficoll, which leaves the lymphocytes in a buffy coat at the top of the tube. The second stage (ii) is to cultivate the lymphocytes in vitro. The lymphocyte rarely divides in circulation but when a *mitogen* (a chemical which stimulates mitosis or cell division) such as phytohemagglutinin is added the lymphocytes undergo a cell division in about 48 h and a further cell division at 72 h. The third stage (iii) is to arrest the cell division in metaphase when the chromosomes are at their most contracted and are best visualized. This is done by adding colchicine to the culture at 69–70 h. The fourth stage (iv) is to release the chromosomes from the nucleus and spread them on a microscope slide. This is carried out by placing the cultured cells in hypotonic saline and dropping the solution carefully onto a microscope slide from a sufficient height to give a reasonable spread of chromosomes. The fifth stage (v) is to fix and stain the spread for microscopic analysis (Fig. 3.5). Most of the analysis is carried out under the microscope, but a photograph of the spread may be taken and a mounted karyotype prepared as a permanent record or for further analysis.

Staining techniques

When stained and viewed under the microscope, chromosomes are visualized as a continuous series of light and dark *bands*. These bands are numbered using a standard nomenclature (see below).

The types of banding most commonly used are:

G-banding uses a Giemsa dye mixture as the staining agent, following treatment of the chromosome preparations by one of a variety of methods, among which are included incubation at various temperatures, denaturation of the chromosomal DNA or treatment with various proteolytic enzymes, e.g. trypsin (Fig. 3.5). Such techniques result in the production of a large number of dark- and pale-staining bands comparable in general distribution with the Q-bands (see below) but allowing rather better resolution and greater permanence than the Q-bands. This is the most widely used technique.

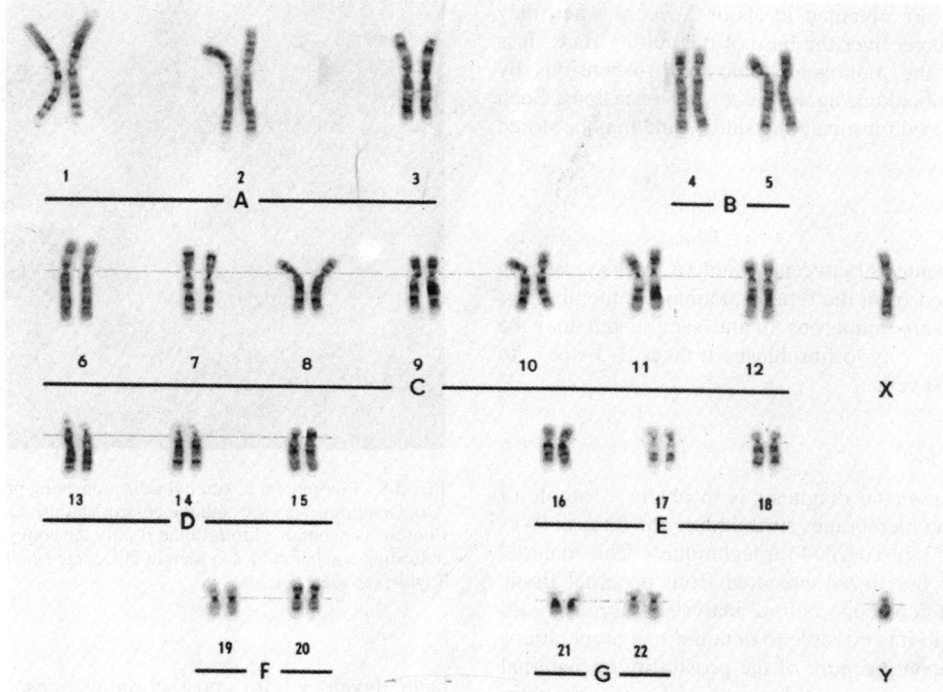

Fig. 3.5 Normal human chromosomes: after being cut out and arranged as a karyotype.

Q-banding in which the chromosome preparation is stained with a quinacrine compound and subsequently examined using fluorescence microscopy. This was the first banding method to be brought into regular use, and is of major significance in the investigation of the human Y chromosome, which exhibits particularly brilliant fluorescence. In metaphase spreads, the fluorescent segment of the Y chromosome can be identified in the distal portion of the long arm while in interphase nuclei, the presence of a Y chromosome can be inferred by detection of a brilliantly fluorescent Y chromatin body.

C-banding (centromeric banding) stains the centromeres of the chromosomes (Fig. 3.6). There are occasions when an extra fragment of a chromosome or marker chromosome is identified in a metaphase spread. It may be difficult to determine the significance of this finding but if there is a centromere present on C-banding then it is more likely to segregate at mitosis and to be of greater clinical significance. In the absence of a centromere such fragments are more likely to get lost in cell division and therefore to be of less significance.

Preparation of chromosomes from other tissues

Bone marrow

Bone marrow contains many rapidly dividing cells and thus it is possible to locate cells which are already in metaphase. When the marrow preparation is appropriately spread it is possible to obtain a direct preparation in this way for analysis. However, short-term culture is generally used. Marrow analysis is used in leukemias where chromosome abnormalities may be present in the marrow but not in the peripheral blood. It is of value both for diagnosis and prognosis (Ch. 15).

Fibroblasts

Culture of connective tissue in vitro will result in the growth of fibroblasts, which may be used for chromosome culture. In the live patient the most common source of fibroblasts is in the skin. At postmortem connective tissue may be obtained from many different sources, but usually it is adequate to take a sample of skin under sterile conditions for culture.

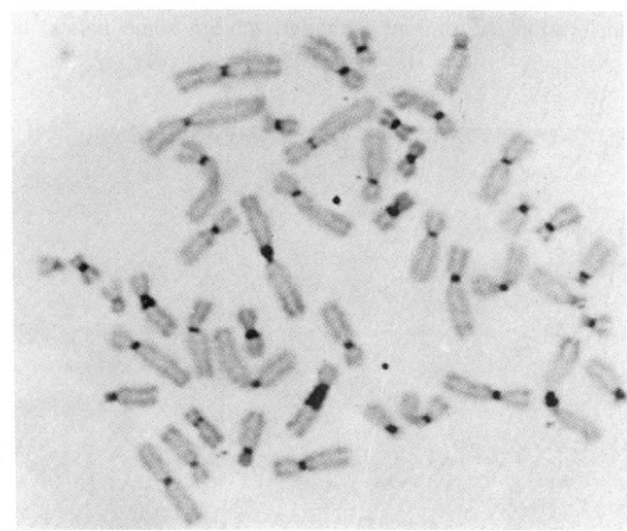

Fig. 3.6 Chromosomes stained by the C-banding technique to show the centromeres.

Fibroblast cultures are obtained in about 2 weeks when they have formed a monolayer over the base of the culture flask. It is possible to disperse the monolayers into cell suspensions by adding trypsin and subculture again on several occasions. Such cultures may also be used for metabolic studies and may be stored long term at –70°C.

Amniocentesis

Fluid taken at amniocentesis between 12 and 16 weeks' gestation contains skin cells shed from the fetus and amniotic membranes. These cells are not very numerous in the sample but may be cultured up in a similar way to fibroblasts. It takes 2–3 weeks to culture and analyze the cells.

Chorionic villus samples

Another approach to prenatal diagnosis is to obtain a sample of chorionic villi from the membranes surrounding the fetus at 9–11 weeks' gestation (Fig. 3.7; see Ch. 4 for techniques). This material is fetal in origin, but has to be separated from maternal tissue under the dissecting microscope before analysis. Chorionic villi are rapidly dividing and it is possible to obtain direct preparations without culture. However, because of the possibility of maternal contamination and mosaicism most diagnostic laboratories prefer to wait until culture is also available at 1–2 weeks before giving a definitive result.

Fluorescent in situ hybridization (FISH) (Fig. 3.8)

There has been a considerable gap between cytogenetic analysis at the microscopic level and molecular genetics at the gene level, but the development of combining the use of gene probes with fluorescent dyes has bridged that gap. It is now possible to combine a gene specific probe with a fluorescent dye and to demonstrate the location of that gene on the chromosome spread.

Instead of using a probe specific to one gene, probes which are specific and unique to one chromosome have been developed and these can act as a 'chromosome paint' to identify the origin of a chromosome fragment or for further analysis of a chromosome translocation. At present, although 'chromosome paints' have

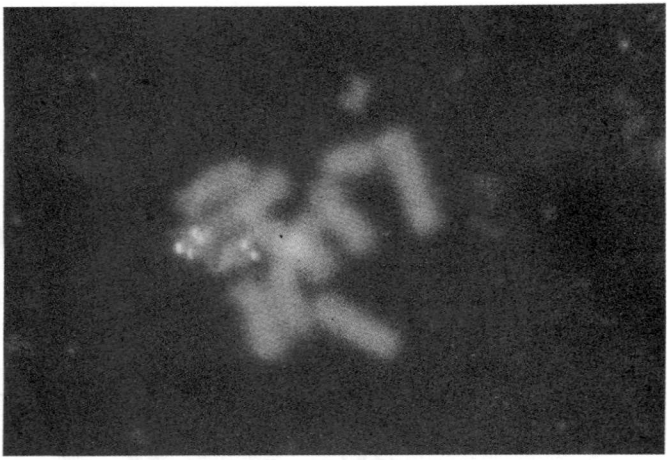

Fig. 3.8   Fluorescent in situ hybridization using probes for chromosome 22q. On chromosome A both the control and the 22q probe show fluorescence, but on chromosome B only the control probe shows up indicating a deletion of 22q seen in DiGeorge syndrome. (Courtesy of Dr J. Taylor; see Plate 3.1.)

been developed for most chromosomes, there are insufficient fluorescent dyes to allow one color for each chromosome, but it is likely that this will be a short-term problem in this rapidly developing field.

It is not necessary to culture the cells and prepare a metaphase spread in order to use FISH probes. They can be applied to the interphase cell and as such could provide a rapid process for diagnosing abnormalities of chromosome number. It might also be possible to semiautomate some of the routine cytogenetic analysis. A review of the techniques used in the laboratory is provided by Rooney & Czepulskowski (1992).

Indications for chromosome studies

Chromosome analysis can be a most valuable diagnostic test, allowing precise clinical diagnosis and offering the opportunity for prevention of serious handicap by prenatal diagnosis. However, as cytogenetic investigations require highly skilled scientific staff and are very time consuming, the clinician will have to exercise some discretion in requesting these investigations. It will often be helpful to discuss the need for genetic testing with the clinical geneticist or laboratory concerned.

The indications for chromosome studies in pediatric practice include:

1. Mental retardation especially if there is a family history of mental retardation or when associated with physical abnormalities. It should be borne in mind that there are specific tests now for some forms of mental handicap, e.g. fragile X, Prader–Willi syndrome, Williams syndrome, and these will need to be requested separately with appropriate samples.

2. Multiple congenital abnormalities. It should be remembered that even if the diagnosis of Down syndrome is obvious clinically, it is still important to determine whether it is a standard trisomy 21 or not.

3. Intersex conditions manifesting as the presence of ambiguous genitalia in the newborn, inguinal herniae in a girl or

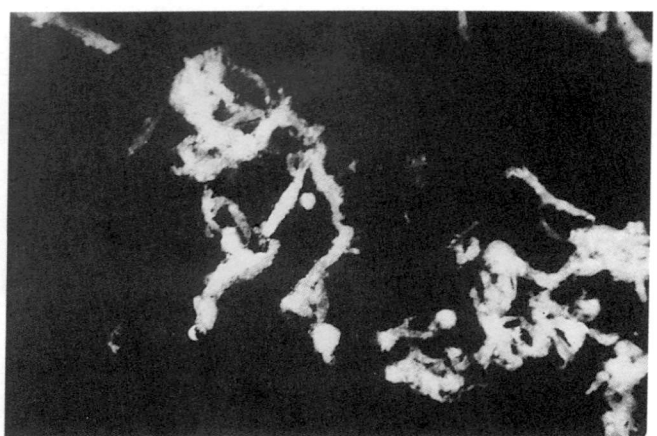

Fig. 3.7   Chorionic villi under dark ground low power magnification.

the failure of development of secondary sexual characteristics at adolescence. Cryptorchidism or minor degrees of hypospadias alone are unlikely to be manifestations of a chromosome abnormality.

4. Congenital lymphedema may be a manifestation of Turner's syndrome and Noonan's syndrome, and part of the investigation should include chromosome analysis.

5. Gross failure to thrive which is prenatal in origin may be due to a chromosome abnormality especially when accompanied by minor physical abnormalities or mental handicap.

6. Childhood leukemias and malignancies will often reveal major chromosomal rearrangements in the cancerous cells and these may be an indicator of the prognosis.

TYPES OF CHROMOSOME ABNORMALITY

The chromosome abnormalities fall into two categories: (a) abnormalities of number and (b) abnormalities of structure.

Numerical abnormalities

Numerical abnormalities may be euploid or aneuploid and arise from errors in cell division.

Euploidy describes chromosome constitutions which are multiples of the haploid (n) number (23 in man), thus diploid, 2n = 46, triploid, 3n = 69, or tetraploid, 4n = 92. Multiples greater than 2n are designated by the general term *polyploid*.

Aneuploidy refers to those karyotypes in which the chromosome complement is not an exact multiple of the haploid number and includes both the trisomic and monosomic states.

Polyploids (other than triploids) usually result from the occurrence of nuclear division without simultaneous cell division, so that the chromosome complement of a single cell is doubled. Triploidy usually arises from the fertilization of a single ovum by two spermatozoa (*dispermy*).

Nondisjunction is the term used to describe the failure of homologous chromosomes or sister chromatids to separate and migrate to opposite poles of the nucleus during cell division and is the major mechanism by which monosomic and trisomic states originate. The consequences of nondisjunction vary depending on whether the event occurs during meiosis, or mitosis. Nondisjunction occurring in meiosis will give rise to trisomy or monosomy, but nondisjunction taking place in mitosis in the early embryo will give rise to mosaicism.

There seems no doubt that in some families there is a predisposition towards nondisjunctional events. The number of families in which aneuploidy recurs and the occurrence of individuals who possess two different aneuploidy states, e.g. both Down and Klinefelter's syndromes, are suggestive evidence of this predisposition.

Structural abnormalities in chromosomes

Structural chromosome abnormalities can be subdivided into those involving a definite loss or gain of genetic material, and those in which the existing genetic material is rearranged in some way. Obviously all structural abnormalities involve at least one chromosomal breakage but in fact it is generally accepted that two breakages are probably obligatory in the etiology of virtually all rearrangements.

Figure 3.9 presents in diagrammatic form the mechanisms of origin of the common structural abnormalities.

Deletions

Deletions (Fig. 3.9a) result when one or more breakages occur along the chromosome with subsequent loss of the resulting fragment, and may be either terminal or interstitial.

Ring chromosomes

Ring chromosomes (Fig. 3.9b) result from simultaneous breakage in both long and short arms of a chromosome with subsequent fusion of the ends of the remaining centric fragment and loss of the acentric terminal segments. Ring chromosomes are notoriously unstable during cell division and break down readily so that the proportion of cells with a clear ring may vary considerably in cultures from the same individual, as also may the actual form and number of the rings observed.

Inversions

Inversions (Fig. 3.9c), as their name suggests, result from a reversal of the sequence of genes in a segment of chromosome lying between two points of breakage. Inversions may be either *paracentric* involving double breakage in only one arm of a chromosome without any alteration in arm ratio, or *pericentric* involving breakage on either side of the centromere. While paracentric inversions can be identified only by the use of banding techniques, pericentric inversions frequently result in an alteration in arm ratio such that the abnormality is easily identifiable in mitotic chromosomes even without banding.

The clinical significance of inversions is a subject for debate. If there is no loss of genetic material then the significance may be minimal, provided only that the rearrangement in sequence of the genes on the inverted segment does not, per se, result in abnormal expression of those genes. The vast majority of paracentric inversions are likely to be harmless; however, the risk of having an unbalanced rearrangement in offspring would be increased if there is a family history of recurrent miscarriage of congenital malformations. Small pericentric inversions, including the relatively common pericentric inversions of chromosome 2 and 9, also seem to be associated with a relatively small risk of unbalanced chromosome arrangements in offspring, and in some cases might be regarded as normal variants. However, the effects of inversions can be unpredictable and the risks in the individual case should be assessed in the light of the family history and cumulative experience from the medical literature.

Isochromosomes

An isochromosome is a chromosome in which the two arms are genetically and structurally identical, e.g. two short arms from the same chromosome. Such chromosomes are thought to arise as a direct result of misdivision of the centromere in the transverse rather than the longitudinal plane, with subsequent reunion of the centric elements of sister chromatids (Fig. 3.9d). Individuals carrying an isochromosome are therefore effectively trisomic for one part of the genetic material and monosomic for another.

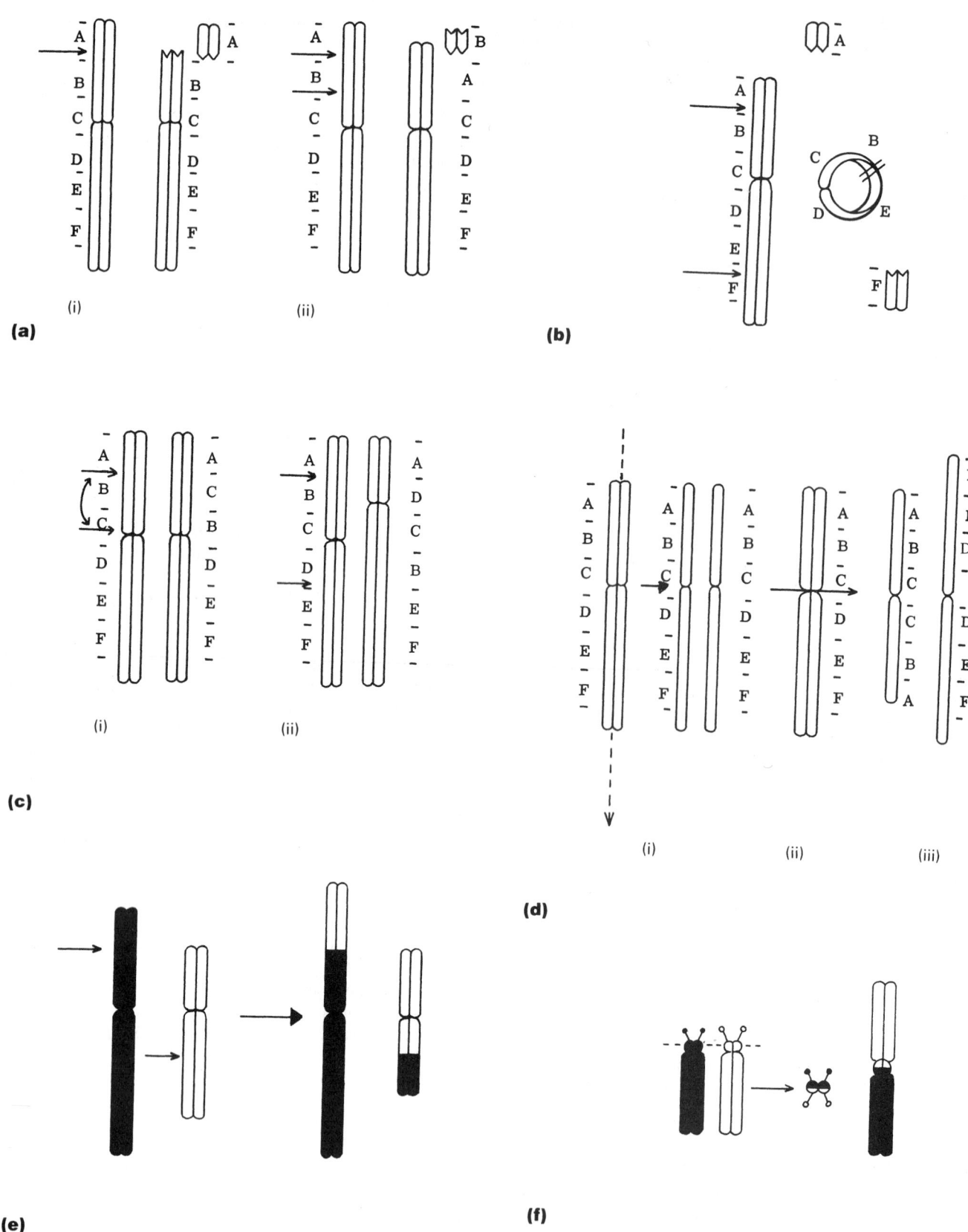

Fig. 3.9 Structural rearrangements in chromosomes. (**a**) Deletions may be (i) terminal or (ii) interstitial. (**b**) Ring chromosome. (**c**) Inversions may be (i) paracentric or (ii) pericentric. (**d**) Isochromosome formation: (i) normal mitosis with longitudinal division of the centromere; (ii) misdivision of the centromere in the transverse plane leading to the products (iii) of either isochromosome of the short arm or of the long arm. (**e**) Balanced reciprocal translocation. (**f**) Robertsonian or centric fusion translocation.

Translocations

In a translocation there is a transfer of genetic material from one chromosome to another. When there is a mutual exchange of segments with no associated loss of genetic material this is termed a *balanced reciprocal translocation*. Such translocations may involve either homologous or nonhomologous chromosomes and can be the result of no more than two breaks, one in each of the chromosomes involved (Fig. 3.9e).

Provided that the translocation does not result in the loss or gain of genetic material there will be no harm to the carrier, although the potential effect for the offspring of carriers may be considerable. Many carriers are first identified following the detection of one or other product of a reciprocal rearrangement in an abnormal infant, in a stillbirth, or in an early abortus. Family studies following such observations frequently uncover a history of previously unexplained abortion in phenotypically normal individuals, who are found subsequently to be carriers of the rearrangement. Such translocations can often be traced through many generations of a large pedigree. Translocations involving chromosome 9 and those between chromosome 11 and 22 appear to carry a particularly high risk of an unbalanced defect.

One of the most commonly occurring structural rearrangements in man is the centric fusion or Robertsonian translocation, involving, by definition, only acrocentric chromosomes. The break points occur close to the centromere, either one in the short arm and one in the long arm, in which case the metacentric chromosome formed has a single centromere, or in both short arms with a resultant dicentric chromosome (Fig. 3.9f). The deleted short arm material is generally lost without any apparent effect on phenotype, presumably because it is heterochromatin without structural genes. Robertsonian translocations may occur between homologous chromosomes or between nonhomologous chromosomes.

A Robertsonian translocation between chromosomes 13 and 14 is thought to be one of the most common structural rearrangements in man, with a frequency of 0.05–0.08% in the newborn population. This rearrangement appears to function more or less normally during meiosis, as large pedigrees are recorded in which abnormal offspring are not reported, and in which there is little or no history of early spontaneous abortion.

Of considerable clinical significance are the translocations t(14q,21q) and t(21q,22q). The birth of a second child with Down syndrome in a sibship may be related to such translocations, especially in younger couples, where one or other partner is a carrier of such a rearrangement. There are differences in the risk of recurrence of affected offspring, dependent on the sex of the carrier parent, with a level of 10–15% if the mother is the carrier, and probably less than 5% if the father is the carrier.

Mosaicism

Significant levels of mosaicism are reasonably easy to demonstrate. The examination of 30 metaphases will be sufficient to demonstrate mosaicism at the 10–15% level, but many more metaphases would be needed to exclude lower levels of mosaicism. It may be difficult to exclude mosaicism as a diagnosis, and failure to demonstrate mosaicism in blood need not necessarily exclude the diagnosis as a possibility in other less available tissues. Inevitably the question must arise of how many cases of maldevelopment with an apparently normal karyotype are due to the genetic effects of a second, abnormal cell line which has become extinct. However, changes in frequencies of cell lines of congenital origin with the complete elimination of one cell line have only rarely been documented.

The phenotypic effects of chromosomal mosaicism vary widely, ranging from the full syndrome as determined by the aneuploid cell line to virtually no abnormality whatsoever.

NOMENCLATURE

In the normal human somatic cell nucleus there is a complement of 46 chromosomes (the diploid, or 2n complement) comprising 22 pairs of homologous autosomes, and one pair of *sex chromosomes*, represented as XX in females and XY in males.

Chromosomes can be arranged in pairs on the basis of certain morphological features. Such morphological features include size, centromere position, and the presence of satellites or secondary constrictions.

The *centromere* is the point of union of the two chromatids which constitute a single chromosome. The position of the centromere in relation to the *telomeres* (or chromosome ends) determines the actual shape of the chromosome and divides it into two segments or *arms* which vary in length, being either short (p), or long (q) (Fig. 3.10). Where the centromere is median in position and the arms are of approximately equal length, the chromosome is described as *metacentric*. Where the arms are of unequal length, the chromosome is described as *submetacentric*. Where the centromere is more nearly terminal so that the short arms are minute, the chromosome is described as *acrocentric*. Small condensations of heterochromatin or satellites may occur on the short arms of acrocentric chromosomes.

The Paris Conference on Standardization in Human Cytogenetics 1971 devised a system of chromosome nomenclature and symbols (Table 3.6). The conventions which apply in use of this nomenclature are as follows. The number of chromosomes is given first followed by the sex chromosome constitution, e.g. 45X in Turner's syndrome and 47XXY in Klinefelter's syndrome. Autosomal aneuploidies are indicated by a numerical alteration, the extra or deficient chromosome being designated by a + or − before the chromosome involved, e.g. 47XX,+21, a female with Down syndrome, or 45XX, −21, a female missing a 21

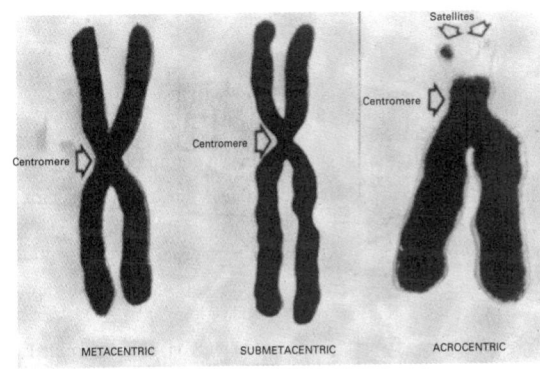

Fig. 3.10 One of the main features of the human chromosomes which can be seen with the light microscope is the centromere. The centromere is the point at which the two strands (chromatids) are joined down the longitudinal axis. The shorter arm is referred to as p (= petit) and the longer arm as q. Chromosomes are classified by the position of the centromere: metacentric, submetacentric and acrocentric.

Table 3.6 Table of nomenclature symbols (Chicago Conference 1966; Paris Conference 1971)

A–G	The chromosome groups
1–22	The autosome numbers (Denver system)
X, Y	The sex chromosomes
Diagonal (/)	Separates cell lines in describing mosaicism
Plus sign (+) or minus sign (–)	When placed immediately before the autosome number or group letter designation indicates that the particular chromosome is extra or missing; when placed immediately after a symbol it means an increase or decrease in length of the chromosome
Question mark (?)	Indicates questionable identification of chromosome or chromosome structure
Asterisk (*)	Designates a chromosome or chromosome structure explained in text or footnote
ace	Acentric (absence of centromere)
cen	Centromere
dic	Dicentric (presence of 2 centromeres)
tri	Tricentric (presence of 3 centromeres)
end	Endoreduplication
h	Secondary constriction or negatively staining region
i	Isochromosome
inv	Inversion
inv (p+ q–) or inv (p– q+)	Pericentric inversion
mar	Marker chromosome
mat	Maternal origin
p	Short arm of chromosome
pat	Paternal origin
q	Long arm of chromosome
r	Ring chromosome
s	Satellite
t	Translocation
repeated symbols	Duplication of chromosome structure
del	Deletion
der	Derivative chromosome
dup	Duplication
ins	Insertion
inv ins	Inverted insertion
rep	Reciprocal translocation
rec	Recombinant chromosome
rob	Robertsonian translocation ('centric fusion')
tan	Tandem translocation
ter	Terminal or end (pter = end of short arm; qter = end of long arm)
:	Break (no reunion, as in a terminal deletion)
::	Break and join
–	From – to

All symbols for rearrangements are placed before the designation of the chromosome or chromosomes involved and the rearranged chromosome or chromosomes should always be placed in parentheses.

chromosome. When placed after a symbol a + or – means an increase or decrease in the length of a chromosome, e.g. 18p – represents deletion of the short arm of chromosome 18. Diagonals are used in the description of mosaicism, e.g. 45XO/46XX represents a Turner mosaic and 45XX/47XX,+21 a female with mosaic Down syndrome. Translocation is designated by the letter t followed in brackets by an indication of the nature of the translocated chromosome. An isochromosome is indicated by the letter i before the chromosome arm involved, e.g. 45X,i(Xq) represents an isochromosome for the long arm of one X chromosome. Ring chromosomes are designated by the letter r placed before the chromosome involved, e.g. 46X,r(X). Bands on chromosomes are numbered outwards from the centromere and are represented by a number written after p or q representing the short or long arms, e.g. 8q24 represents a region on the long arm of chromosome 8 and t(8;14)(q24;q32) a translocation between chromosome 8 and 14 involving region 24 on the long arm of chromosome 8 and region 32 on the long arm of chromosome 14.

CHROMOSOMAL SYNDROMES

DOWN SYNDROME (TRISOMY 21)

Incidence

Since the original description of the condition by Langdon Down in 1866, this disorder has been recognized to be the commonest single cause of mental handicap occurring in approximately 1 in 700 of all live births. A comparable birth incidence has been found in most populations. However, the incidence varies with the age of the mother: the incidence for mothers aged 25 years is 1 in 1400 and increases to reach an incidence of 1 in 46 for mothers aged 45 years (see Fig. 3.11).

Clinical features (Fig. 3.12)

In most instances Down syndrome is recognizable at birth by the craniofacial features. The head circumference is small with a

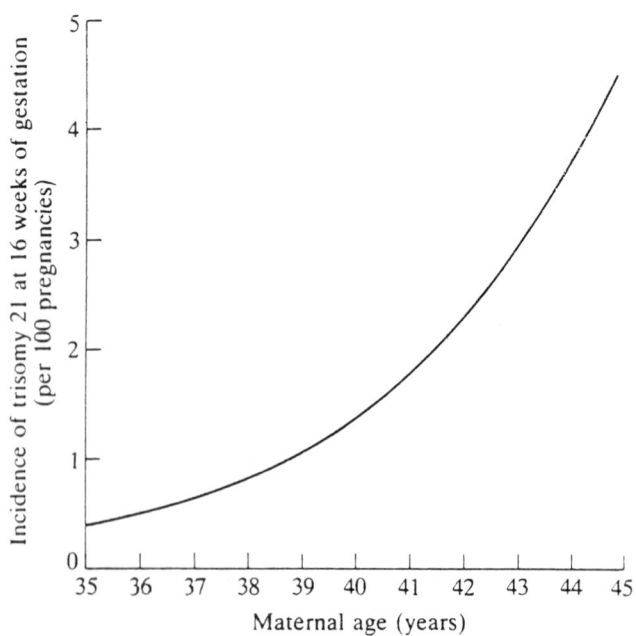

Fig. 3.11 The frequency of Down syndrome increases with maternal age.

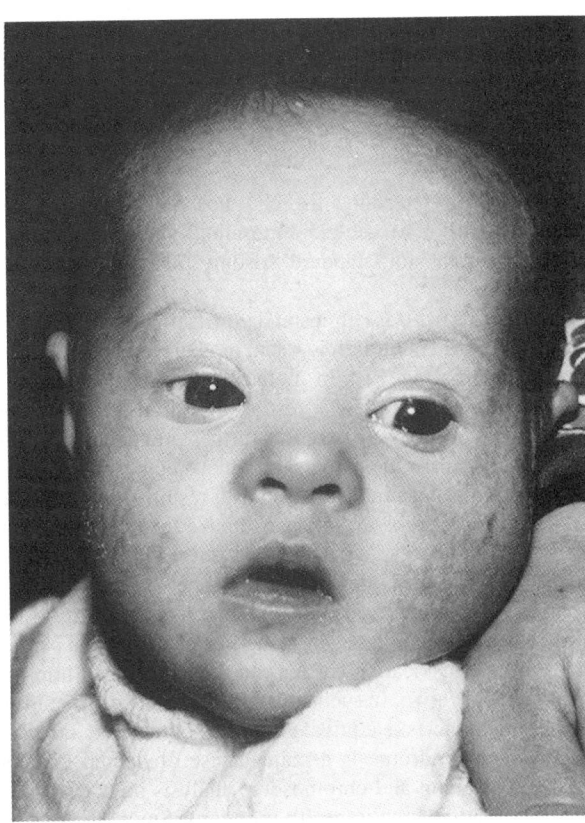

Fig. 3.12 Facial features of Down syndrome.

brachycephalic skull and there is often a third fontanel. The neck is short and thick. The palpebral fissures slope upwards (i.e. the outer canthus is higher than the inner canthus) and there may be marked epicanthic folds. Brushfield's spots (whitish spots scattered round the periphery of the iris) are found more frequently in Down syndrome than in the general population. There is an increased incidence of lens opacities. The ears are small with an overfolding helix. The nasal bridge is flat. The tongue appears large and may protrude because the mouth is relatively small. Eruption of the teeth is frequently delayed with abnormalities in positioning. The hair may be fine and sparse.

The hands are short and broad. The fifth finger is short and incurved (clinodactyly). Radiologically this feature is accompanied by shortening of the shaft of the middle phalanx. A single transverse palmar crease (or simian crease) is seen in both hands in at least 50% of children with Down syndrome. A unilateral transverse palmar crease may be demonstrated in 2–5% of chromosomally normal infants. A deep plantar crease between the first and second toe may also be a helpful diagnostic sign. The other dermatoglyphic features noted in Down syndrome include an increase in ulnar loops, a single flexion crease on the fifth finger and a distal axial triradius.

Congenital heart disease occurs in between 40 and 60% of infants with Down syndrome. Atrioventricular canal and ventricular septal defects are the commonest types of cardiac lesion seen. Intestinal atresia, in particular duodenal atresia, is also considerably more common in Down syndrome. One-third of cases of congenital duodenal atresia occur in Down syndrome.

Initially a child with Down syndrome may be hypotonic, but the early developmental milestones are eventually reached. The ultimate IQ ranges from 20 to 75 with a mean around 50. The earlier assessment of development tends to be more favorable than the formal measurement of IQ in later childhood. Children with Down syndrome are often affectionate and good humored but like all stereotypes this tends to underestimate the range of personality and behavioral traits seen in a defined group.

Intellectual function shows a decline with age in adults with Down syndrome and this has been attributed to a presenile dementia. It is, therefore, particularly interesting to note the relationship between Down syndrome and Alzheimer's disease (Oliver & Holland 1986). The neuropathology of both conditions is very similar with senile plaques and neurofibrillary tangles; however, while there is a generalized depletion of all neurotransmitters in Down syndrome, in Alzheimer's disease it is more specifically a depletion of the cholinergic neurotransmitters. Gene mapping studies have found mutations in the amyloid precursor protein gene on chromosome 21 in some early onset familial cases of Alzheimer's disease (Goate et al 1989).

The development of secondary sexual characteristics is delayed in Down syndrome. In males infertility is the rule and there are no proven cases of a fully affected male fathering a child. In females, although puberty is delayed they are usually fertile.

The incidence of leukemia, but not other malignancies, is greater in Down's children. A transient leukemoid reaction may occur in newborns with Down syndrome. In the first year of life acute nonlymphoblastic leukemia predominates, but in older children it is predominantly acute lymphoblastic leukemia. Overall the incidence is 10–18 times greater than that in the general childhood population.

A generation ago two-thirds of children with Down syndrome died in early childhood usually from the associated congenital abnormalities. Now only about 20% die in the first year and 45% of individuals with Down syndrome will survive to 60 years of age (Baird & Sadovnick 1988). This is less than the general population where 86% can be expected to live to 60 years of age.

Cytogenetics

Standard trisomy 21

Approximately 95% of children with Down syndrome have 47XX,+21 or 47XY,+21. Trisomy 21 arises as a result of meiotic nondisjunction usually from the maternal side.

Translocation as a cause of Down syndrome

A number of different translocations may give rise to Down syndrome. They account for 2–3% of Down's individuals.

The most frequent is a Robertsonian 14,21 translocation (Fig. 3.13). In this form the carrier would have one 14 chromosome, one 21 chromosome and one fused 14,21 chromosome giving a total of 45 chromosomes, e.g. 45XX, −14, −21 complement, and is phenotypically normal. However, when a carrier produces offspring there is a risk of producing an unbalanced karyotype.

In Figure 3.13, when an individual with a 14,21 translocation produces offspring with an individual with a normal karyotype then three viable chromosome arrangements may be produced: (i) a normal karyotype, (ii) a balanced translocation and (iii) an unbalanced translocation giving 46 chromosomes with trisomy

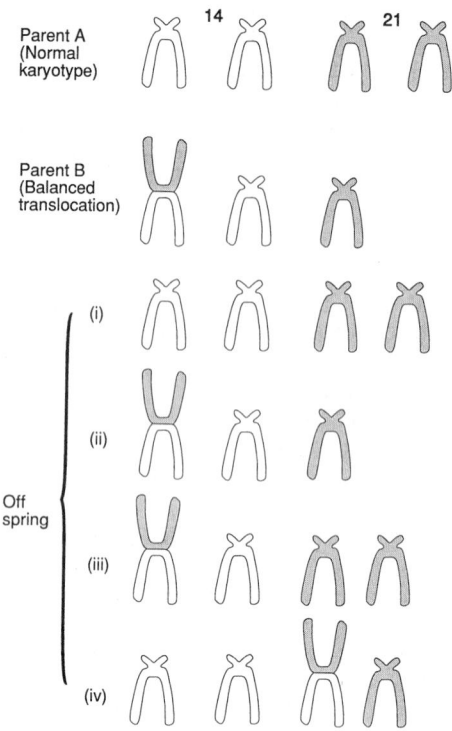

Fig. 3.13 Segregation of a 14,21 translocation. Four combinations may be produced: (i) normal karyotype; (ii) balanced translocation; (iii) unbalanced trisomy 21; (iv) unbalanced trisomy 14 (lethal).

21. Other arrangements can be produced, but these will be nonviable or lead to early miscarriage, e.g. monosomy 21, monosomy 14 or trisomy 14. While in theory it may appear that one-third of pregnancies would produce an unbalanced translocation with trisomy 21, this does not take into account the selective disadvantage that acts on gametogenesis, fertilization or the early zygote. From analysis of pooled family data the likelihood of a female carrier producing an unbalanced trisomic child is 15%, and the likelihood of a male carrier producing an unbalanced trisomic child is 2.5%. The different risks may be explained by selective disadvantage in the sperm carrying the extra 21 chromosome.

The second commonest translocation to give rise to Down syndrome is a 21,22 Robertsonian translocation. It may give rise to trisomy 21 due to unbalanced translocation karyotypes in a similar manner to those described for the t(14,21) carrier. Translocations between chromosome 13 or chromosome 15 and chromosome 21 have been reported but are rare.

Very rarely a t(21q,21q) may arise. Carriers of this translocation can only produce zygotes which are monosomic or trisomic for chromosome 21, and since monosomy 21 would almost always be lethal the risk of producing a child with trisomy 21 is virtually 100%.

Mosaic trisomy 21

In about 2.5% of individuals with Down syndrome there is a mosaic combination of cells with a normal karyotype and cells with trisomy 21. The phenotypic variation produced may range from apparently normal individuals to those with typical Down syndrome. Occasionally unsuspected low grade maternal mosaicism (at the level of 2–3% trisomic cells) may be uncovered when more than one child with trisomy 21 is born into a family.

Genetic counseling and screening

It is essential to determine the chromosome karyotype in the affected child prior to genetic counseling, since the recurrence risks are different for standard trisomy 21 and translocation trisomy 21.

In the case of a child with a standard trisomy 21 the chance of recurrence in further children is 1% in mothers under 35 years and twice the maternal age risk in mothers over 35 years. Since the trisomy has not arisen as a result of a translocation and a chromosome test will be offered in further pregnancies, it is not necessary to examine the parents' chromosome karyotype.

When Down syndrome has arisen as a result of an unbalanced translocation, it is necessary to check both parents' chromosomes and if one is found to be a carrier, then further family studies are necessary to determine which other members of the family are also carriers. The recurrence risks for carriers of a 14,21 translocation carrier are given above. In some instances neither parent is found to be a translocation carrier and the unbalanced translocation has arisen de novo. In such situations the chance of recurrence in further pregnancies is equivalent to the population risk.

Since Down syndrome is a major cause of mental handicap, pregnancy screening and chromosome analysis have been incorporated into various public health programs. Since the incidence of Down syndrome increases with increasing maternal age, amniocentesis has been offered to mothers of 35 and above. This approach, if fully taken up by all mothers, would diagnose 30% of all pregnancies with Down syndrome, and the remaining 70% would occur in younger mothers. It should be remembered that the vast majority of pregnancies occur in mothers under 35 years, and to offer amniocentesis to all mothers irrespective of age would be unacceptable because of the small but significant risk of miscarriage.

Another approach to screening in pregnancy is to look at the level of α-fetoprotein in maternal serum (MSAFP) from blood samples taken around 12 weeks' gestation. Higher levels of MSAFP are associated with an increased risk of neural tube defects because of the leakage of α-fetoprotein across the defect into the amniotic fluid and hence into the maternal serum. A fortuitous observation was made that the level of MSAFP tends to be *lower* in pregnancies with trisomy 21. The physiological basis for this observation is not clear, but it has been possible to combine the levels of MSAFP with maternal age in screening for Down syndrome. By using the combined parameters the percentage of pregnancies with Down syndrome detected in pregnancy could be increased from 30% to 35% without in theory increasing the amniocentesis rate.

This work has been expanded to look not simply at one parameter in maternal serum but three. Wald and his colleagues (1988) have suggested that by combining the levels of MSAFP, estriol and human chorionic gonadotrophin with maternal age, it is possible to predict those pregnancies at greater risk of having trisomy 21 in all ages and to diagnose 60% of pregnancies with Down syndrome without increasing the amniocentesis rate (Harris & Andrews 1988). Another approach to screening is to use ultrasound scanning in the first trimester and to measure the amount of thickening over the back of the neck, i.e. nuchal translucency. Increased nuchal translucency has been associated with a greater risk of chromosome abnormalities. It is estimated from preliminary studies that this approach could diagnose up to 80% of Down syndrome in the early stages of pregnancy (Nicolaides et al 1994)

TRISOMY 18 (EDWARDS' SYNDROME)

First described in 1960 (Edwards et al 1960). Although much rarer than Down syndrome, it is the second commonest autosomal trisomy with an incidence between 1 in 3500 and 1 in 7000. It is associated with increased maternal age, the mean being about 32 years. There is a slight preponderance of females.

Of the affected infants some 80–90% die within the first week usually from cardiopulmonary failure. A few cases have been reported surviving into the teens, but they have all been profoundly retarded (Mehta et al 1986).

Clinical features

There is often polyhydramnios and intrauterine growth retardation. The cranium is long and narrow with a prominent occiput. The ears are low set and frequently underdeveloped. The facies characteristically shows micrognathia and narrow sloping palpebral fissures. The hands are clenched with the second and fifth fingers overlapping the third and fourth fingers (Fig. 3.14a). There may be other flexion deformities. The nails are hypoplastic. The feet show a 'rocker bottom' appearance like the appearance of the runners of a rocking chair (Fig. 3.14b).

A variety of congenital malformations are present. Anomalies of the gastrointestinal tract are particularly common, e.g. intestinal atresias, malabsorption and exomphalos. Around one-third of cases of exomphalos detected prenatally on ultrasound have trisomy 18. Renal abnormalities are also frequent with renal hypoplasia or cystic dysplasia being one of the commoner and more serious abnormalities. Congenital heart defects, ocular abnormalities and neural tube defects can also occur.

In the past a number of conditions which clinically appeared similar to trisomy 18 but showed normal karyotypes were

described as pseudotrisomy 18. Some of these cases were probably Pena-Shokier syndrome (Smith 1988) which is autosomal recessive. It presents with a combination of microcephaly, joint contractures, pulmonary hypoplasia and cataracts, and should be considered in the differential diagnosis when the karyotype is normal.

Cytogenetics

The vast majority of cases arise as a result of primary nondisjunction and have a regular trisomy 18. Like trisomy 21, it is associated with increased maternal age and thus may be diagnosed on screening prenatally. After the birth of one affected child, the chance of recurrence is 1% in younger mothers.

A partial trisomy 18 may arise in the offspring of carriers of reciprocal translocations involving chromosome 18. Available data suggest it is the proximal region of the long arm (pter to q21) that primarily determines the phenotypic features of Edwards' syndrome.

TRISOMY 13 (PATAU'S SYNDROME)

This syndrome has an incidence around 1 in 6000 (Patau et al 1960). The majority of affected children have multiple malformations and succumb in the first few months. The few cases reported with longer survival have all been severely retarded. There is some maternal age effect, but probably not as significant as that seen in trisomy 21 or trisomy 18.

Clinical features

The affected children show intrauterine growth retardation. There may be marked microcephaly. Structural malformations of the brain are common and this may alter facial development. Instead of two cerebral hemispheres with lateral ventricles, a single forebrain with a single ventricle may form. This malformation sequence is known as holoprosencephaly (Fig. 3.15). The process alters the development and separation of optic vesicles from the forebrain and the migration of the median process from the

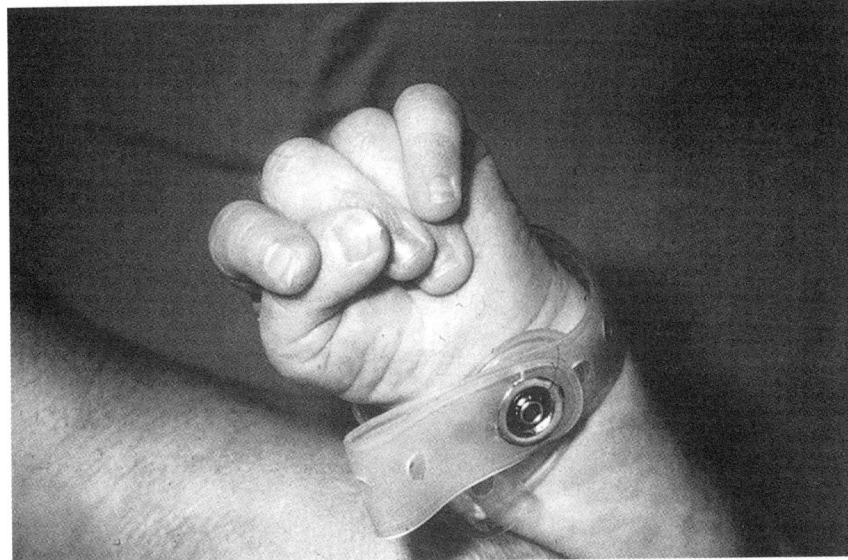

a

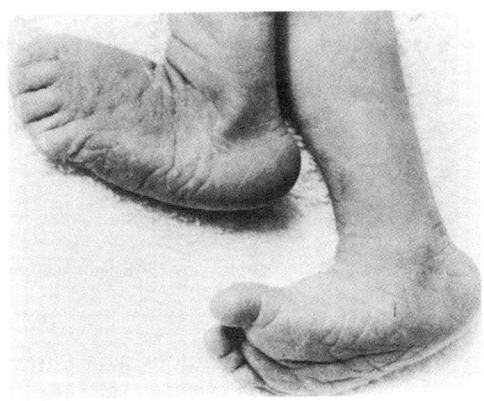

b

Fig. 3.14 The typical appearance of the hands (**a**) and feet (**b**) in trisomy 18 (Edwards' syndrome).

NORMAL DEVELOPMENT

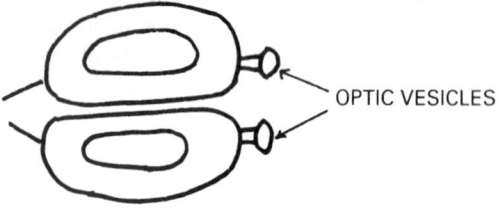

OPTIC VESICLES

HOLOPROSENCEPHALY

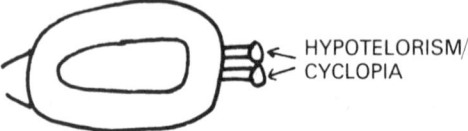

HYPOTELORISM/
CYCLOPIA

Fig. 3.15 Holoprosencephaly sequence. The forebrain divides into two hemispheres and the optic vesicles develop from these to form the eyes. In holoprosencephaly the forebrain divides incompletely and the optic vesicles develop in close proximity, leading to hypotelorism or cyclopia.

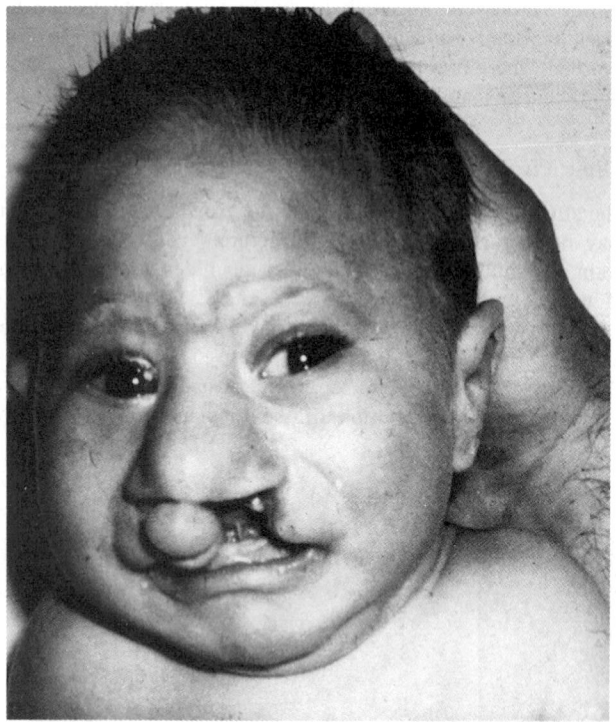

Fig. 3.16 Facial features of trisomy 13 (Patau's syndrome).

forehead to form the nose. In its most extreme form the optic vesicles may fuse to give cyclopia. More usually (Fig. 3.16) there is marked hypotelorism with a small nose and cleft lip and palate. Ocular abnormalities such as microphthalmos are common, often reflecting the underlying cerebral abnormality.

In the hands, postaxial polydactyly is frequent. Flexion contractures and 'rocker bottom' feet may also be present. Scalp defects may be helpful diagnostically as they rarely appear in

other abnormalities. Internally, in addition to cerebral malformations, renal and cardiac abnormalities are also frequent.

Cytogenetics

The majority of cases of trisomy 13 arise as a result of primary nondisjunction.

It may occasionally arise from an unbalanced chromosome translocation t(13q,14q). In the vast majority of cases carriers of a t(13q,14q) do not produce unbalanced progeny. In 230 pregnancies to carriers of a t(13q,14q) studied in a European collaborative study there were no cases of unbalanced progeny, but in practice it is appropriate to counsel such carriers with a small recurrence risk and offer amniocentesis.

4p⁻ (WOLF–HIRSCHHORN) SYNDROME

This syndrome gives a clearly recognizable phenotype. The features include microcephaly, hypertelorism, low set simple ears, coloboma (25%), cleft palate (30%), renal abnormalities, heart defects (50%) and intrauterine growth retardation. The facial features (Fig. 3.17) are described as resembling a Greek helmet since the flat nasal bridge appears to run in continuity from the glabella in much the same way that the protective nose piece is incorporated into a helmet.

Death usually occurs in early childhood (at least one-third die in the first year of life) and survivors invariably show profound mental retardation with seizures. Two-thirds of cases are female. As 10% arise from balanced translocations it is important to examine the parents' chromosomes.

The deletion required to produce this syndrome may be very small and may require specific tests with fluorescent probes in situ to identify it.

5p⁻ (CRI DU CHAT) SYNDROME

This is one of the commoner autosomal deletion syndromes with an estimated incidence of 1 in 50 000. About 70% of affected newborns are female, but the survival rate appears to be better for males than females. Survival into adult life with severe mental retardation has frequently been described.

The syndrome derives its name from the striking cat-like cry that is heard in infancy. This cry is related to the hypoplastic larynx and tends to lessen with increasing age and growth of the larynx. In the newborn the face is round with microcephaly, micrognathia and down-slanting palpebral fissures. With further growth the microcephaly remains but the face becomes long and narrow.

The deletion may involve a variable amount of the short arm of chromosome 5 but band 5p15 is invariably involved. About 15% of cases arise from a balanced reciprocal translocation.

18q⁻ SYNDROME

The cardinal features of this syndrome are intra-uterine growth retardation, profound mental retardation and a 'carp-shaped mouth'. Cleft palate, heart defects and ocular defects are also common. Genital hypoplasia may occur. Serum IgA is decreased in about half the affected individuals.

Survival to adult life has been reported although with severe mental handicap. The majority of cases arise de novo.

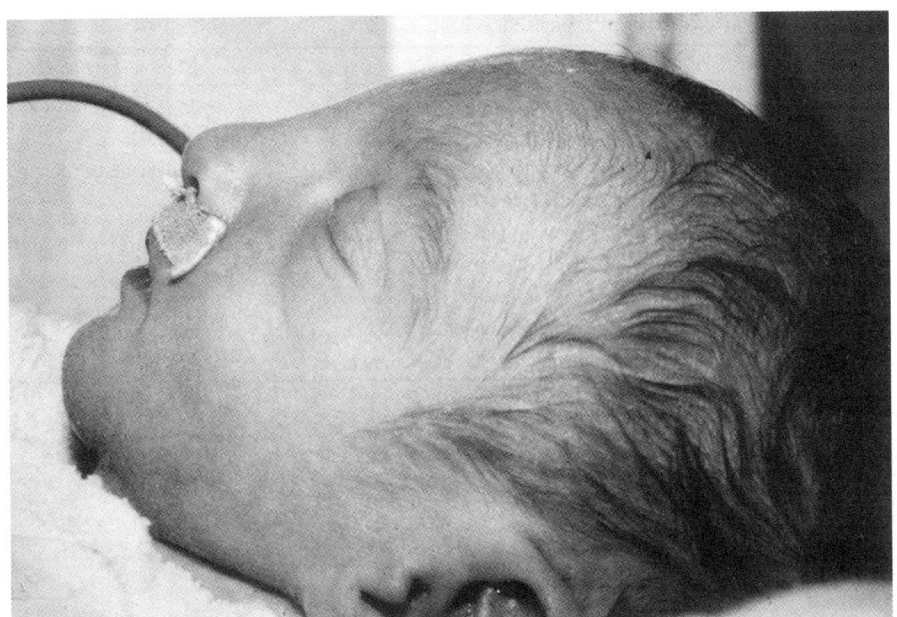

Fig. 3.17 Facial features of 4p⁻ (Wolf–Hirschhorn) syndrome.

DELETIONS OF 13q (Fig. 3.18)

Deletions of 13q14 and terminal deletions of 13 produce different recognizable phenotypes, and have been helpful in gene mapping.

Deletions of 13q14 are associated with retinoblastoma. The dysmorphic features associated with this deletion are variable. Further genetic analysis of the interstitial 13q14 deletions has led to a recognition that this chromosomal region contains an anti-oncogene responsible for inhibiting the proliferation of embryonic retinal cells. In the presence of a homozygous deletion or a deletion in one allele with a mutation in the other allele, retinal cells continue to proliferate in a malignant fashion producing a retinoblastoma which is usually bilateral. Isolated cases of retinoblastoma which are usually unilateral are the result of somatic mutation in the same region of the chromosome.

Terminal deletions of 13 may also produce eye abnormalities but not retinoblastoma. They also characteristically have hypoplastic thumbs and anal atresia. Most die in the neonatal period.

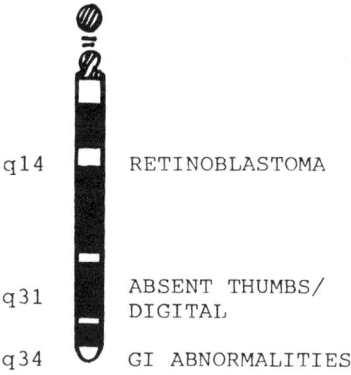

q14   RETINOBLASTOMA

q31   ABSENT THUMBS/ DIGITAL

q34   GI ABNORMALITIES

Fig. 3.18 Deletions of the long arm of chromosome 13.

NEWER CHROMOSOMAL SYNDROMES

With the introduction of extended banding techniques a number of disorders which were not previously recognized to be chromosomal have been demonstrated to have chromosomal microdeletions. One of these is the aniridia–Wilms' tumor syndrome. In this condition bilateral aniridia, Wilms' tumor, hypogonadism occur with retardation of growth and development. This particular combination is due to the deletion of a small number of adjacent or contiguous genes in band 11p13. This concept may well have wider application in explaining the occurrence of apparently unrelated clinical features in other malformation syndromes.

In other syndromes which have been thought of as single gene disorders, small chromosomal deletions have been found in a proportion of cases. For example in the Prader–Willi syndrome a small interstitial deletion at 15q12 has been found in some cases and molecular analysis showed that a deletion was present in the majority of cases even if it was not microscopically visible (Butler et al 1986). More surprising was the discovery that the deletion always arose in the chromosome 15 that was paternally inherited. Subsequently work on Angelman syndrome, which has very different clinical features, found that in this syndrome there was also a deletion present in 15q12. The difference is explained by the fact that the deletion in Angelman syndrome arises from the maternally inherited chromosome 15 and that in early fetal development genes from both chromosome 15s are required. The phenomenon of different phenotypes arising depending whether the gene is maternally or paternally derived is referred to as *imprinting* (Malcolm et al 1991).

Other new syndromes with deletions which can be visualized by fluorescent gene probes include Williams syndrome (Lowery et al 1995), DiGeorge syndrome (Fig. 3.8) and Miller Dieker syndrome (see Table 3.7).

Another characteristic chromosomal syndrome is the Killian–Pallister syndrome (Reynolds et al 1987). It is unusual in

Table 3.7 Chromosomal microdeletion syndromes

Syndrome	Features	Chromosome defect
Angelman	Mental retardation, ataxia, seizures	15q12 del
Aniridia–Wilms'	Aniridia, Wilms' tumor, mental retardation	11p13 del
Beckwith–Wiedemann	Macroglossia, exomphalos	11p dup/del
DiGeorge	Cardiac and immunological defects	22q del
Langer–Giedion	Sparse hair, bulbous nose, digital abnormalities	8q del
Miller Dieker	Lissencephaly, fits	17p del
Prader–Willi	Obesity, hypogonadism, mental retardation	15q12 del
Rubenstein–Taybi	Broad thumb, mental retardation, characteristic facies	16p del
Smith–Magennis	Severe self-mutilation, mental retardation	17q del

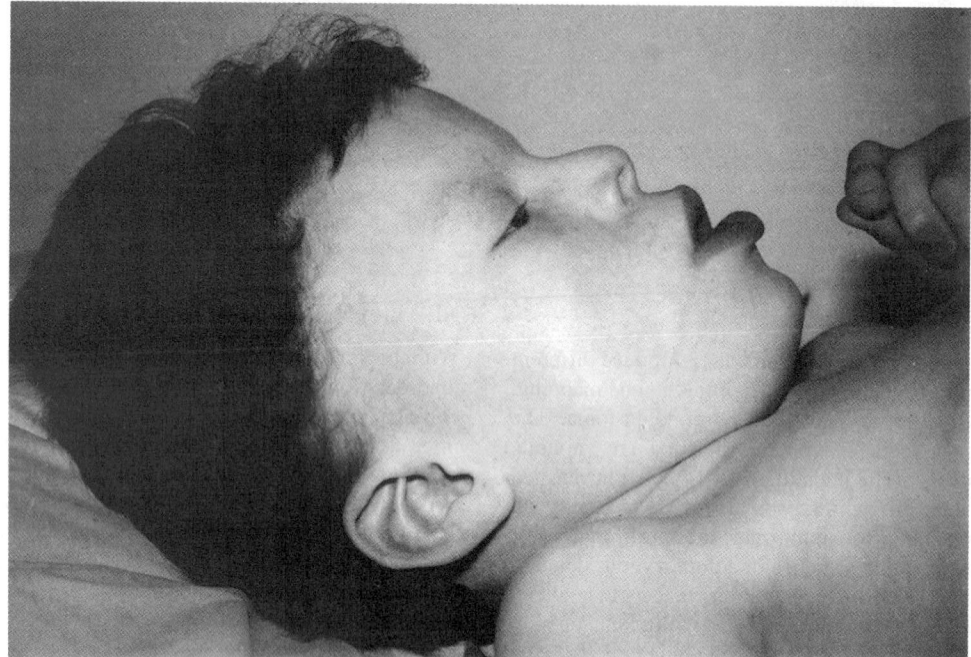

Fig. 3.19 The Killian–Pallister syndrome is caused by a mosaic isochromosome 12p, which is present in skin culture but not in blood culture. The syndrome has a characteristic coarse facies.

that a mosaic cell line containing tetrasomy 12p is found in the skin fibroblasts but not in the blood. Although the mosaicism is relatively tissue specific the effects are generalized. There is severe mental retardation with coarse facial features and a characteristic bitemporal loss of hair growth (see Fig. 3.19).

OTHER AUTOSOMAL ABNORMALITIES

Many other aberrations involving the autosomes have been described. As a general rule they are associated with low birthweight, mental retardation and physical malformations. In many instances a specific phenotype cannot be delineated because gene dosage will depend on the exact breakpoints and in the case of unbalanced translocations, which other chromosome is involved.

It is recommended that the reader refers to a chromosomal atlas such as de Grouchy & Turleau (1984) or Schnizel (1984) for details of other autosomal abnormalities.

SEX CHROMOSOME ABNORMALITIES

TURNER'S SYNDROME (see also p. 370)

The syndrome was first described in 1938 and subsequently became the first disorder recognized to have a chromosomal basis.

It is a frequent finding in first trimester abortions, but, as many 45X conceptuses are nonviable, the frequency at birth is 1 in 3000 liveborn females.

Clinical features

At birth there is lymphedema (Fig. 3.20) especially in the dorsum of the hand and there may be redundant skin over the back of the neck. Hydrops and cystic hygroma are seen in utero and may occasionally be present in the neonate.

In childhood, Turner's syndrome may present with short stature (Fig. 3.21). There is a short webbed neck with low posterior hairline. The chest is shield shaped with widely spaced nipples.

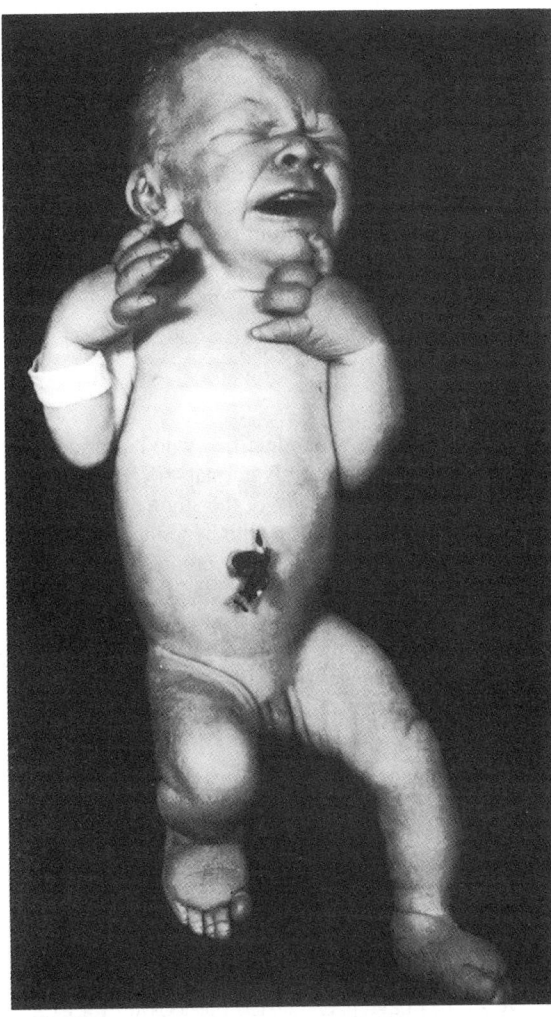

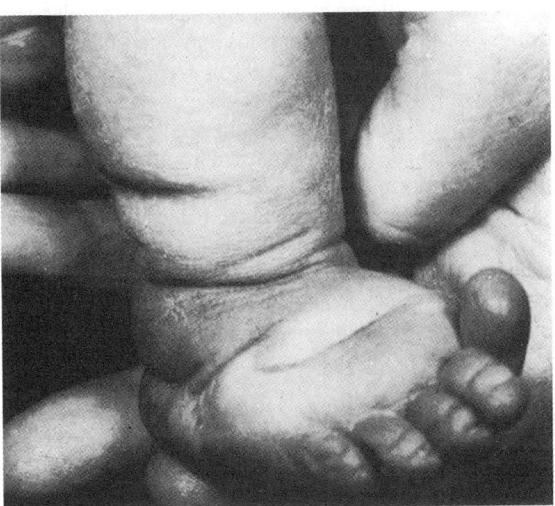

Fig. 3.20 Turner's syndrome in the neonate may present with edema of the hands and feet.

The carrying angle at the elbow is increased (cubitus valgus). Pigmented nevi and a tendency to keloid scarring are frequently found. Coarctation of the aorta may also be present. Around 60% will have renal tract abnormalities, which include horseshoe

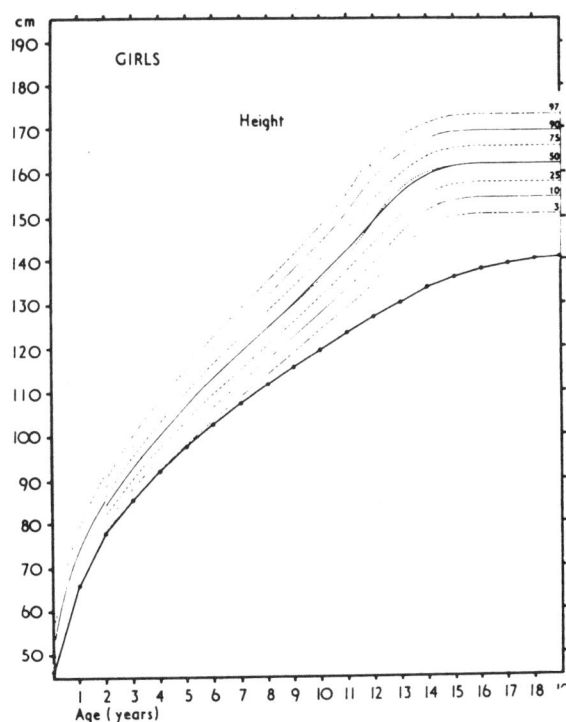

Fig. 3.21 Growth chart for Turner's syndrome (reproduced with permission).

kidneys and duplex ureters, but do not usually compromise renal function. Mental development is normal although detailed psychometric testing may demonstrate a minor defect in spatial perception.

At puberty Turner's syndrome may present for the first time with primary amenorrhea and failure of secondary sexual development. Streak gonads are found with ultrasound and at laparotomy. The patients are almost invariably sterile, but menstruation and secondary sexual development may be induced by estrogen replacement (see Ch. 19).

Girls with Turner's syndrome have a normal life span. It is now recognized that hypertension may be a complication in adult life, and in the absence of hormone replacement osteoporosis may also develop.

Cytogenetics

Although 60% of patients with Turner's syndrome have a 45X karyotype, a variety of chromosome abnormalities are seen with the syndrome (Table 3.8).

Table 3.8 Chromosome abnormalities in Turner's syndrome

45XO	60%
Mosaic XX/XO	15%
Isochromosome Xq or Xp	10%
46X del (X)	5%
46X ring (X)	5%
With Y chromosome	5%

Mosaic cell lines arise from mitotic nondisjunction in early embryogenesis. On the whole the phenotype with mosaicism is similar to the classical features of Turner's syndrome. When the mosaicism involves an XY cell line there is an increased risk of gonadoblastoma, and the streak ovaries should be removed. In the rare situation of an unbalanced X:autosome translocation and in some cases of ring X, mental retardation may occur.

Turner's syndrome is not associated with increased maternal age and as it usually arises from mitotic rather than meiotic error is not associated with an increase of recurrence in further pregnancies.

47XXX

When triple X (47XXX) was first identified the majority of patients were thought to be mentally retarded and infertile, but with prospective ascertainment a truer picture has emerged. Their height tends to be greater than average. The majority of girls with triple X attend normal schools although special educational assistance and possibly speech therapy may be required. Prospective studies have shown on average there is a slight lowering of mean IQ, but no specific abnormal behavioral patterns. Fertility is normal. In theory there should be an increased risk of sex chromosome aneuploidy in the offspring of these girls, but in practice the risk may be very small and should be more accurately known with long-term follow-up of the prospectively ascertained individuals.

The presence of further extra X chromosomes in 48XXXX and 49XXXXX is associated with microcephaly, mental retardation and dysmorphic facial features.

KLINEFELTER'S SYNDROME (47XXY) (see p. 1036)

The syndrome of gynecomastia, small atrophic testes and absent spermatogenesis (azoospermia) in phenotypic males was first described in 1942 and associated with an abnormal karyotype (47XXY) in 1959. The incidence is around 1 in 1000 liveborn males.

The clinical features are not usually evident in the first few years of life although it may be discovered incidentally in apparently normal male infants. At puberty, however, the secondary sexual characteristics develop poorly and body fat tends to take on a feminine distribution with gynecomastia in 50% of cases. Beard growth is minimal and in adult life patients will rarely need to shave more than twice a week. The testes remain small and infertility may be the presenting feature in adult males. Sexual function is normal although the libido is reduced. The testosterone levels are low and the gonadotrophin levels elevated. Testicular histology shows an increase in Leydig cells and interstitial fibrosis. Height is usually increased with relatively long limbs. The mean intelligence is on average slightly reduced in Klinefelter's syndrome, but this rarely poses a problem. In adult life risk of breast cancer is the same as in 46XX females.

Cytogenetics

About two-thirds of XXY males are the result of disjunctional errors either during oogenesis or in the early zygote cleavage having two copies of the maternal X chromosome as detected by chromosomal markers. As would be predicted from this the incidence of Klinefelter's syndrome increases with maternal age.

In about 15% of patients with Klinefelter's there is a mosaic XY/XXY form. If the XY cell line exerts a predominant genetic effect then the individual may be fertile but up to half of XY/XXY males have azoospermia and gynecomastia.

48XXXY AND 49XXXXY

These karyotypes produce more clinical disturbance than 47XXY. Mental retardation is more frequent and there may be skeletal abnormalities, especially radioulnar synostosis (leading to inability to supinate the forearm). The facies may also be dysmorphic with hypertelorism, epicanthic folds, broad nose and large open mouth.

XX MALES

A group of patients have been identified who have an essentially male phenotype with an apparently normal 46XX karyotype. They are very rare. They exhibit many of the stigmata of Klinefelter's syndrome, including small testes, with hypoplastic genitalia prior to puberty, gynecomastia in a large proportion of cases, and infertility. Skeletal proportions and intelligence are generally normal.

On molecular analysis these males will almost invariably be found to have the SRY gene which is the major gene determining male development (Ferguson-Smith et al 1990)

XYY SYNDROME

The initial reports of males with 49XYY came from studies of males in institutions for mentally ill criminals and this biased ascertainment has distorted the clinical picture of this chromosomal disorder.

It is relatively common with an incidence of 1 in 1000 males. In order to obtain a truer picture of the syndrome a number of prospective studies have been carried out looking for example at the karyotypes of all newborn children in a particular area and following those with sex chromosome abnormalities through childhood (Ratcliffe & Paul 1985). The XYY karyotype is associated with a normal birthweight but increased growth in early to mid-childhood. About a third are in the 90th centile for height. Intelligence is not significantly different from their chromosomally normal siblings. Detailed psychological testing does reveal a tendency to compulsive behavior, which in certain settings may lead to socially deviant behavior, but in the presence of a stable family background this can be more appropriately channeled. It should be remembered that the vast majority of males with 47XYY remain undetected in the community.

FRAGILE X MENTAL RETARDATION

Although it has long been recognized that there is a considerable excess of males in the mentally handicapped population, it has only recently been realized that this is due to a number of X-linked forms of mental retardation. The most significant of these is mental retardation associated with the Xq27 folate-sensitive fragile site.

In 1969 Lubs demonstrated a fragile site on the X chromosome in a family with mental retardation, but it was initially regarded as an isolated curiosity. Around the same time Turner et al studied a number of X-linked mental retardation families in a mental handicap institution and described their relatively 'normal looking' appearance together with large testes. Lubs had described the cytogenetic finding and Turner the phenotypic appearance of fragile X mental retardation. Several years later connection between the clinical and laboratory findings was firmly established (Sutherland & Hecht 1985) and the condition is now recognized as the second commonest cause of mental handicap in males after Down syndrome. The incidence of fragile X mental retardation is 1 per 1000 males. In a study of autism 5% of the male patients were found to have fragile X mental retardation.

Clinical features

The phenotype of fragile X mental retardation is not as striking as that of Down syndrome, but with experience can be recognized (Fig. 3.22). Fragile X males have a large forehead, large head, long nose, prominent chin and long ears. The facial phenotype, however, becomes more obvious with age and is not easily recognizable in younger children.

Fragile X males tend to be larger at birth and taller than other children, but do not achieve the full growth predicted by the centile chart. In adult life fragile X males tend to be short. The head circumference is increased with many having a head circumference greater than the 97th centile. Similarly the ear length is increased. This is an extremely useful clinical sign and may be measured and compared with a centile chart prepared from a normal population (Smith 1988).

Macro-orchidism is present in 80% of adult fragile X males and 15% of prepubertal fragile X boys. The size of the testes may be

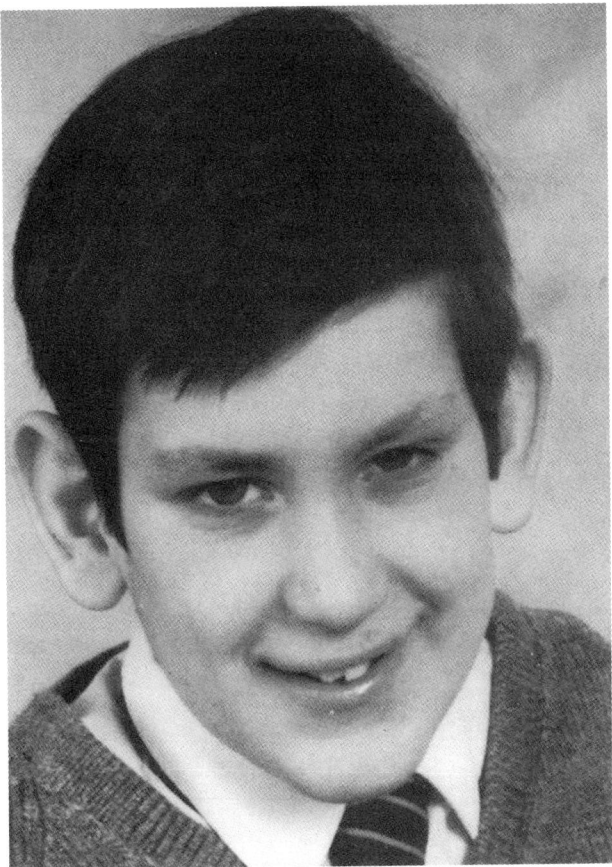

Fig. 3.22 Facial features of fragile X mental retardation (reproduced with permission).

considerably enlarged. In one series (Sutherland 1983) the range was 15–127 ml (the Prader orchidometer can only be used for testicular volumes up to 25 ml!). The large testes are functionally normal and the increased size may be due to an increase in interstitial edema or connective tissue. Large testes are a relatively rare feature in other syndromes with mental handicap.

It has been suggested that there may be a connective tissue abnormality in fragile X. There is a slight, but clinically insignificant, increase in the frequency of mitral valve prolapse, aortic root dilation and hernias. More striking clinically is the soft skin and joint hypermobility, which may be helpful diagnostically.

The range of intellectual handicap in fragile X males varies but most are moderately to severely retarded. Females tend to be more mildly affected. There is also a suggestion that intelligence may decline with age. Speech development is particularly affected in fragile X males and behavioral changes and seizures may occur. The level of intellectual deficit can, to some extent, be determined by the molecular testing. Medical treatment with folate therapy has been suggested to improve behavior and improve IQ, but it does not appear to be effective in properly controlled trials (Neri et al 1988).

Molecular genetics

The fragile site in the X chromosome was initially used to diagnose this disorder but in affected males only 5–20% of cells will demonstrate the fragile site and in female carriers only half of the carriers could be detected by the cytogenetic test. It is now recognized that the fragile site is a marker for the disease rather than its cause.

The diagnostic difficulties were resolved by the identification of the FMR 1 gene at Xq27 (Verkerk et al 1991, Hirst et al 1992). This gene has within it a repeating sequence of three nucleotides CGG. Normal individuals have up to 50 copies of the nucleotide repeat. If the number of repeats is greater than 50 it becomes unstable in meiosis and can then increase in repeat number. The initial increase to between 50 and 150 repeats is referred to as the *premutation*. It may be found in intellectually normal males and female carriers. However, after passing through meiosis in the female the size of the repeats increases to the *full mutation* of greater than 150 repeats and can then produce learning difficulties in both males and females. In a male with the premutation the repeat length is not significantly increased in spermatogenesis. Repeat number may increase or decrease in the full mutation during somatic cell division and therefore somatic mosaicism can be detected in some affected individuals. The full mutation affects the methylation of the DNA and this in turn switches off the FMR 1 gene and will affect both intellectual function and the cytogenetic fragility. At present the exact function of the gene is not clear but the gene product has been identified (Willemsen et al 1995) and a transgenic mouse model is available for further research (Hergersberg et al 1995).

In terms of inheritance therefore it appears very similar to X linked recessive inheritance as the condition is passed through females and will affect males, but daughters may also be affected with a degree of learning difficulties and the mutation can arise from unaffected males.

The discovery of the FMR-1 gene has meant that accurate follow up and counseling of families is possible (Fig. 3.23). Prenatal diagnosis using CVS and molecular analysis is possible in the first trimester of pregnancy.

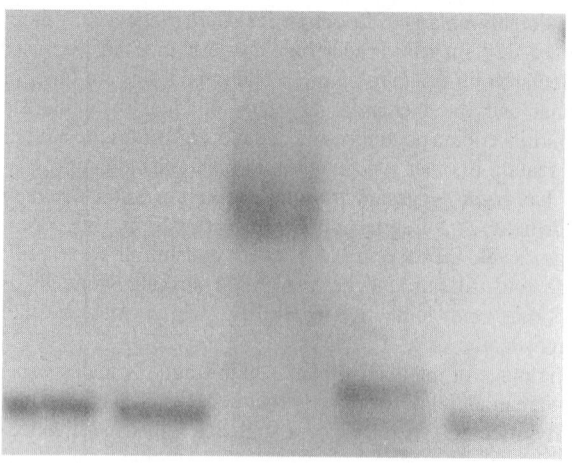

Fig. 3.23 Autoradiograph of Southern blot looking for fragile X. The DNA has been digested by the restriction enzyme Eco R1 and probed with FMR-1 probe OX1.9. The normal fragment size is seen in lanes 1, 2 and 5. In lane 3 there is an expanded fragment (< 500 repeats) indicating an affected boy. In lane 4 there is a female with a normal band and a slightly larger band above, indicating a carrier of a premutation. (Courtesy of R. Taylor).

SINGLE GENE DISORDERS: INHERITANCE

Distributed amongst the 46 chromosomes, there are approximately 100 000 structural genes which code for specific proteins. The position at which the structural gene lies on the chromosome is referred to as the *locus*. At the locus there is a pair of alleles. If an individual possesses two alleles which are the same, the individual is said to be *homozygous* for that particular trait. If the two alleles are different, the individual is said to be *heterozygous*. A gene which is manifest in the heterozygote is *dominant*, whereas a gene which is only manifest in the homozygote is *recessive*. These terms do not refer to the characteristics of the genes, but only to their manifestations. It is, therefore, more correct to refer to a 'dominant disorder' rather than a 'dominant gene'.

A trait or disorder which is determined by a gene on an *autosome* is said to be inherited as an autosomal trait and may be dominant or recessive. A trait or disorder which is determined by a gene on one of the *sex chromosomes* is said to be sex linked and may also be either dominant or recessive. A variety of single gene disorders are listed in Table 3.9.

Table 3.9 Modes of inheritance in some genetic disorders

Autosomal dominant	Autosomal recessive	X-linked recessive
Achondroplasia	Adrenal hyperplasia	Aldrich syndrome
Congenital spherocytosis	Albinism	Anhidrotic ectodermal dysplasia
Diaphyseal aclasis	Alkaptonuria	Choroideremia
Ehlers–Danlos syndrome	Amaurotic idiocy	Color blindness
Epidermolysis bullosa – simplex types	Ataxia telangiectasia	Deutan and protan color blindness
Hemoglobin variants	Crigler–Najjar syndrome	Diabetes insipidus (nephrogenic)
Holt–Oram syndrome	Cystic fibrosis	G-6-PD deficiency
Huntington's chorea	Cystinosis	Fabry's disease
Hypercholesterolemia	Dubin–Johnson disease	Chronic granulomatous disease
Marfan's syndrome	Dysautonomia	Hemophilia A and B
Myotonic dystrophy	Ellis–van Creveld syndrome	Hunter's syndrome
Muscular dystrophy – facioscapulohumeral type	Epidermolysis bullosa – dystrophic and lethal types	Lesch–Nyhan syndrome
Neurofibromatosis	Friedreich's ataxia	Lowe's syndrome
Osteogenesis imperfecta	Galactosemia	Muscular dystrophy – Duchenne type, Becker type
Periodic paralyses	Hartnup disease	Nephrogenic diabetes insipidus
Polycystic kidney disease	Homocystinuria	Ocular albinism
Polyposis coli	Hurler's syndrome	Oculocerebrorenal syndrome
Porphyria variegata	Laurence–Moon–Biedl syndrome	Retinitis pigmentosa
Retinoblastoma (bilat.)	Maple syrup urine disease	Retinoschisis
Tuberous sclerosis	Morquio's syndrome	Vit. D-resistant rickets (X-linked dominant)
Waardenburg syndrome	Muscular dystrophy – limb girdle type Niemann–Pick disease	
	Phenylketonuria	
	Pendred's syndrome	
	Pseudoxanthoma elasticum	
	Refsum's syndrome	
	Sickle cell anemia	
	Werdnig–Hoffmann disease	
	Wilson's disease	

DRAWING THE PEDIGREE

The first stage in analyzing the pattern of inheritance in a family is to draw up a pedigree. This is a shorthand method of putting all the relevant family information together in a systematic way. The symbols used in drawing up a pedigree are illustrated in Table 3.10. Each individual in a pedigree is identified from his generation (Roman numerals) and his location in the generation (Arabic numerals). Thus the index case or proband in Figure 3.24 is IV.4. It is usually necessary to ask specifically about consanguinity and miscarriages as most patients will not realize details are relevant.

AUTOSOMAL DOMINANT INHERITANCE

In an autosomal dominant disorder an affected individual possesses the abnormal (mutant) gene and its normal allele. When an affected individual marries a normal person, on average half their children will be affected. This is because an affected person produces gametes that have either the mutant allele for the

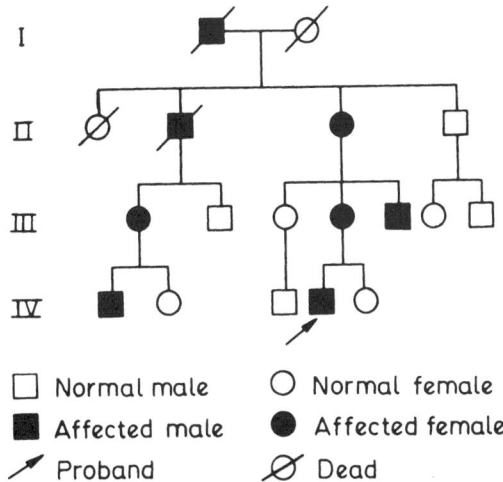

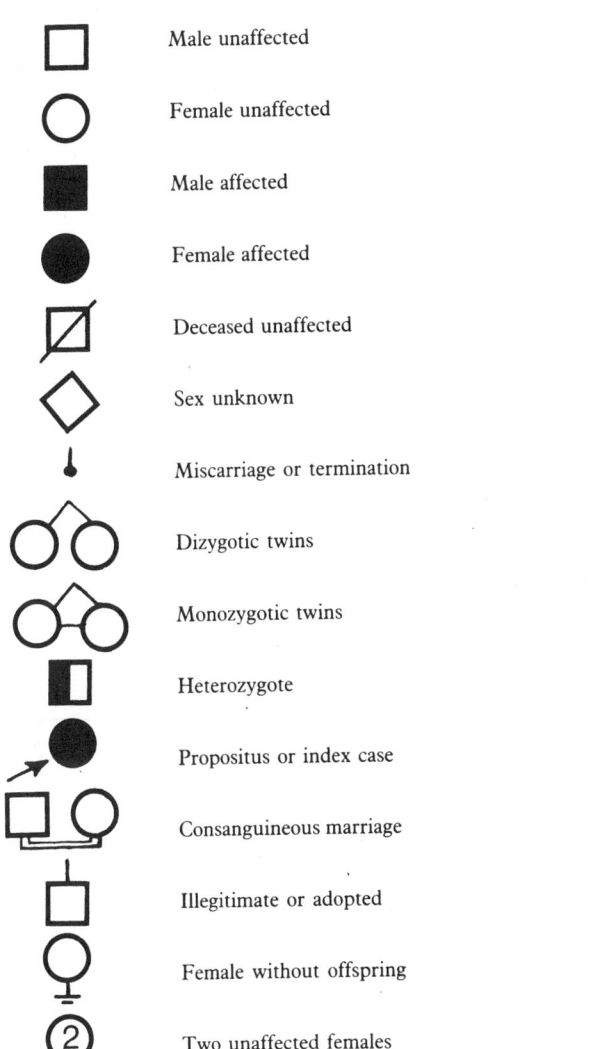

Fig. 3.24 Pedigree pattern of an autosomal dominant trait.

disorder or the normal allele. If the normal allele is represented as 'a' and the abnormal allele as 'A' then the various combinations are illustrated in Table 3.11.

Classically an autosomal dominant disorder can be traced back through several generations, but if the condition is severe, affected individuals may not survive to have children and transmit the disease to subsequent generations. In such cases the affected individual is 'sporadic', as the condition in the individual has arisen as a new mutation and they will not live to reproduce. The frequency of new mutations arising varies from condition to condition, e.g. about 50% of cases of neurofibromatosis arise from new mutations whereas new mutations are extremely rare in Huntington's disease.

Autosomal dominant traits affect both males and females (Fig. 3.24). They may show great variation in severity (= *expressivity*) as in neurofibromatosis, which may range from being a relatively mild pigmentary skin disorder to a cause of severe deformity. Sometimes the gene may not express itself at all in which case it is said to be nonpenetrant. This phenomenon explains apparent skipped generations in certain pedigrees. The *penetrance* of the trait is the proportion of heterozygotes who express a trait even if mildly.

Some autosomal genes are expressed more frequently in one sex than the other. This is referred to as sex-influenced inheritance or, in the extreme case in which only one sex is affected, as *sex-limited inheritance*. Possible examples of sex influenced autosomal dominant traits include hemochromatosis, gout and male pattern baldness.

Table 3.10 Pedigree symbols

□	Male unaffected
○	Female unaffected
■	Male affected
●	Female affected
⊘	Deceased unaffected
◇	Sex unknown
↓	Miscarriage or termination
○○	Dizygotic twins
○△○	Monozygotic twins
▣	Heterozygote
●	Propositus or index case
□○	Consanguineous marriage
□	Illegitimate or adopted
○	Female without offspring
②	Two unaffected females

Table 3.11 Autosomal dominant inheritance

			Affected parent (Aa) ↓ gametes	
			A	a
Normal parent (aa)	→ gametes	a	Aa affected	aa normal
		a	Aa affected	aa normal

In myotonic dystrophy it was suggested that the severity of the condition tended to increase with each generation, e.g. the grandparent could have had cataracts only, while the mother had myotonia and muscle weakness and the affected child had the disorder in its congenital form with developmental delay. This was referred to as *anticipation*. It was initially thought that the cause of this was a bias in ascertainment but it is clear now that the mutation which is a triplet repeat in the myotonin gene can increase with each meiotic transmission.

AUTOSOMAL RECESSIVE INHERITANCE

Autosomal recessive traits affect both sexes and only homozygotes are affected. The affected individuals in a family are all in one sibship, i.e. they are brothers and sisters (Fig. 3.25). The parents of an affected child or children are both heterozygotes, and are perfectly healthy. It is, therefore, not possible to trace the disease through several generations unless there is complex inbreeding. With rare recessive traits the parents of affected individuals are often related, the reason being that cousins are more likely to carry the same genes because they inherited them from a common ancestor.

When parents have a child affected by an autosomal recessive disorder the likelihood of the next pregnancy being similarly affected is 1 in 4. The risk remains 1 in 4 for each successive pregnancy no matter how many children may be affected in the family. If the normal allele is represented as 'A', and the abnormal allele as 'a', then the possible combinations are illustrated in Table 3.12.

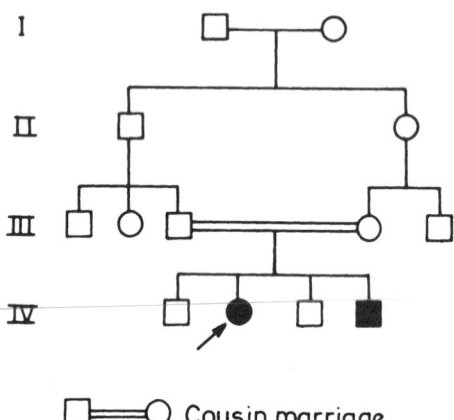

Cousin marriage

Fig. 3.25 Pedigree pattern of an autosomal recessive trait.

Table 3.12 Autosomal recessive inheritance

		Normal heterozygous parent (Aa) ↓ gametes	
		A	a
Normal heterozygous parent (Aa) → gametes	A	AA normal	Aa unaffected heterozygote
	a	Aa unaffected heterozygote	aa affected

Nowadays, since families tend to be small, it frequently happens that an autosomal recessive condition appears sporadic with only one affected person in the family.

The majority of inborn errors of metabolism are due to deficiencies of specific enzymes and are inherited as autosomal recessive traits. In some instances it may be possible to demonstrate that individuals are heterozygotes in these disorders by finding an intermediate level of enzyme activity.

Where a number of different mutant alleles exist it is occasionally possible to find an individual who is heterozygous for two different mutant alleles. An example of this is seen in the hemoglobinopathies. An individual may be heterozygous for both HbS and HbC. Such double heterozygotes or 'genetic compounds' have a disease intermediate in severity between sickle cell disease and HbC disease.

CODOMINANCE

Codominance is the term used for two traits which are both expressed in the heterozygote. An example of codominance is the inheritance for the blood groups A and B. An individual with both alleles will have the blood group AB. When it is possible to demonstrate by appropriate biochemical tests the presence of the mutant gene in heterozygotes the terms dominant and recessive become less meaningful.

X-LINKED RECESSIVE INHERITANCE

In theory sex-linked inheritance could be either X linked or Y linked, but as there are no structural genes other than those determining sexual development on the Y chromosome, sex linkage is effectively the same as X linkage.

An X-linked recessive trait is one which is due to a mutant gene on the X chromosome, and is carried by females to affect males (Figs 3.26 and 3.27). The affected males are *hemizygous* (with the mutant gene on their single X chromosome) while the carrier females are heterozygous and are usually perfectly healthy. X-linked disorders may also be transmitted by affected males through their daughters unless the disorder is so severe that affected males do not survive to have children (e.g. Duchenne muscular dystrophy). Hemophilia is an X-linked recessive disorder where improvements in medical treatment and surgical techniques have led to affected males often surviving into adult

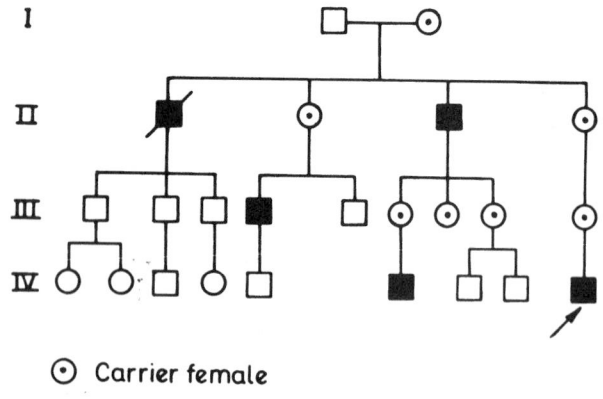

⊙ Carrier female

Fig. 3.26 Pedigree pattern of an X-linked recessive trait in which affected males reproduce.

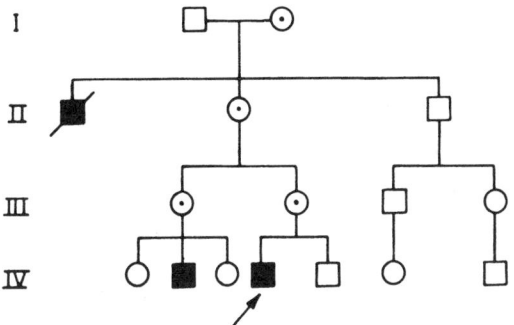

Fig. 3.27 Pedigree pattern of a severe X-linked recessive trait in which affected males do not survive to have children.

life. If an affected male marries a normal female and if the hemophilia gene is represented as X^h and the normal gene as X, then the various gametic combinations that can occur are represented in Table 3.13.

Thus, all daughters of an affected male are carriers and all his sons are normal.

In the case of a woman who is a carrier (XX^h) and marries a normal male then half her sons will be affected and half her daughters will be heterozygote carriers (Table 3.14).

Quite often in serious X-linked conditions there is only one affected boy in a family. Such a sporadic case may be the result of a new mutation in the affected boy's X chromosome and in such cases recurrence would not occur in the family. It is also possible that the mother might be a carrier, and by chance the mutant gene has not been transmitted to any of her other male offspring. In families with predominantly female offspring an X-linked

mutation may be inherited through the female line for a few generations without affected males. In one-third of isolated cases of Duchenne muscular dystrophy the mutation occurs in the affected boy, and in two-thirds of cases the mother is a carrier. It is obviously of vital importance to determine if the mother is a carrier in order to provide accurate information about recurrence risks. The probability of the mother being a carrier can be calculated using knowledge of the numbers of unaffected males in the family (the more unaffected males the less chance the mother is a carrier), the level of creatine kinase (female heterozygotes have slightly higher levels than female controls from the general population) and using information from DNA studies. This analysis is well reviewed in Emery (1987).

In a number of special circumstances a female may exhibit manifestations of an X-linked recessive trait. It may occur as a result of random inactivation or lyonization of the X chromosome. In early embryogenesis in the female zygote one of the X chromosomes is inactivated in each cell. This process is random so that on average half the cells in a female will have one X chromosome inactivated and half will have the other X chromosome inactivated. However, occasionally by chance the majority of cells will have the X chromosome with the normal allele inactivated and the mutant allele will be partially expressed. This situation is seen in female carriers of Duchenne muscular dystrophy where about 5% of female carriers may show some muscle weakness. It may also occur in the rare situation when a female is both a carrier of an X-linked mutation and has an XO karyotype (Turner's syndrome). Finally it can also occur in common X-linked disorders such as red–green color blindness where an affected male marries a female heterozygote and produces a daughter in whom both X chromosomes possess the mutant allele.

Table 3.13 X-linked inheritance: the offspring of affected males

		Affected male (X^hY) ↓ gametes	
		X^h	Y
Normal female (XX) → gametes	X	XX^h carrier daughter	XY normal son
	X	XX^h carrier daughter	XY normal son

Table 3.14 X-linked inheritance: the offspring of affected carrier females

		Normal male (XY) ↓ gametes	
		X	Y
Carrier female (XX^h) → gametes	X	XX normal daughter	XY normal son
	X^h	XX^h carrier daughter	X^hY hemophiliac son

X-LINKED DOMINANT INHERITANCE

An X-linked dominant disorder is one which is manifest in the heterozygous female as well as in the hemizygous male. The pedigree pattern superficially resembles that of autosomal dominant inheritance, but in an X-linked dominant disorder an affected male transmits the disease to all his daughters and to none of his sons. Affected females transmit the disease equally to sons and daughters half of whom, on average, will be affected (Fig. 3.28).

There are relatively few X-linked dominant disorders. One example is vitamin D-resistant rickets (hypophosphatemia). In some X-linked dominant disorders the condition is lethal in males and so only females are affected (e.g. incontinentia pigmenti).

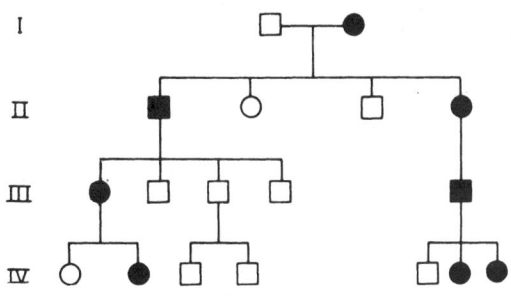

Fig. 3.28 Pedigree pattern of an X-linked dominant trait.

MITOCHONDRIAL INHERITANCE

While the vast majority of genes are located on the chromosomes in the nucleus of the cell and segregate according to Mendelian principles, a relatively small number of genes are located in the mitochondria. The segregation of mitochondrial genes follows a very different and unpredictable pattern. Mitochondrial genes are not transmitted paternally, because the sperm has very little cytoplasm and thus few mitochondria. The ovum, on the other hand, has a large volume of cytoplasm and many mitochondrial genes are transmitted maternally. The exact proportion of maternal offspring affected will depend on the proportion of mitochondria containing the mutation in the particular ovum fertilized. It is thus difficult to give specific recurrence risks for mitochondrial disorders and it is best to rely on statistical data from family studies.

Examples of mitochondrial disorders include mitochondrial cytopathy and Leber's optic atrophy (Riordan-Eva & Harding 1995, Harding 1993).

DNA AND GENE ACTION

STRUCTURE AND FUNCTION OF GENES

The genetic material that is capable of providing a perfect replica in cell division is in the form of a molecule of DNA (deoxyribonucleic acid). While it is possible to study chromosomes at a microscopic level, the genes are well below the resolution of the microscope. Looking at the chromosomes under the microscope is rather like looking at the wrapping around the genes. In rough terms a 5-cm length of DNA is compressed into a chromosome 10 000 times smaller by tight coiling and packing with proteins called histones.

DNA consists of long chains of molecules called *nucleotides*. Each nucleotide consists of a nitrogenous base (*adenine, thymine, guanine* or *cytosine*), a pentose sugar and a phosphate group. The pentose sugar in DNA is deoxyribose. The DNA (unless denatured) is in the form of two polynucleotide chains arranged in a double helix (Fig. 3.29). The arrangement of the bases in the double helix is not random since adenine in one chain always pairs with thymine, and in the other cytosine always pairs with guanine. Thus the arrangement of nucleotides in the two chains is *complementary*, and in cell division using one chain a complementary chain may be synthesized, thus preserving the sequence of bases in each daughter cell.

The sequence of bases is important, because the arrangement of the bases provides the genetic code from which proteins may be made (Fig. 3.30). The genetic information in the DNA is first *transcribed* with messenger ribonucleic acid (mRNA) and this in turn is *translated* into the synthesis of a polypeptide chain. RNA is very similar to DNA in structure except (i) the thymidine is replaced by uracil, (ii) the deoxyribose is replaced by ribose and (iii) it is a single-stranded rather than double-stranded polynucleotide chain.

The DNA, which is responsible for the synthesis of specific proteins, forms the structural genes. The information is in the form of a *triplet code*, a sequence of three bases or a *codon* determines one amino acid. Since there are four bases involved the possible combination that could be provided is $4^3 = 64$. Since there are only 20 amino acids this code is said to be degenerate and most amino acids can be coded for by more than one triplet

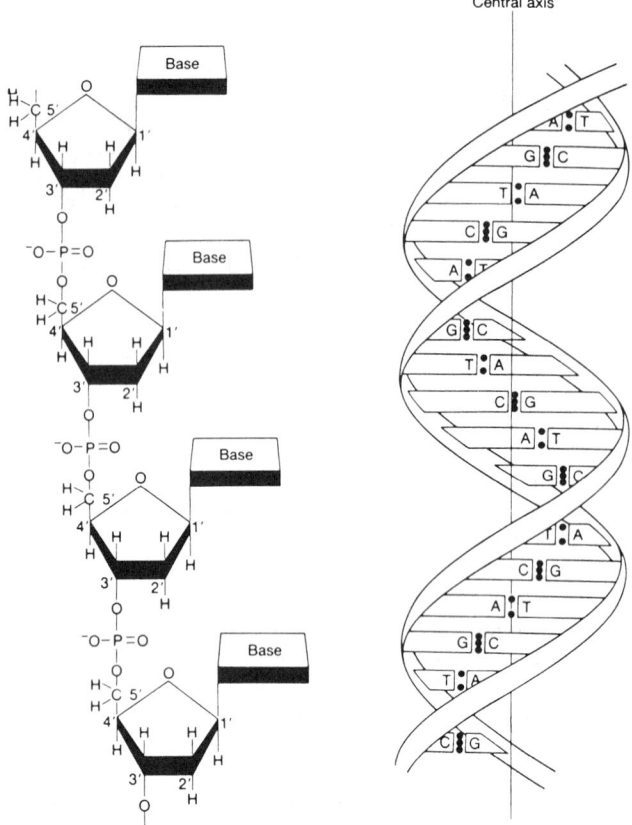

Fig. 3.29 The structure of DNA (reproduced with permission from Weatherall 1986).

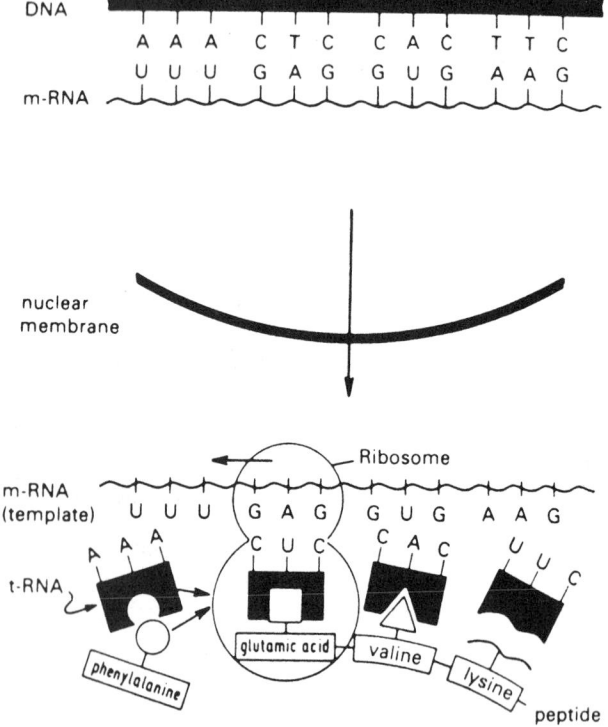

Fig. 3.30 The production of proteins from DNA (modified from Emery with permission).

Table 3.15 Base sequences (coding triplets) in RNA for certain amino acids

	Code			Amino acid
	UGG			Tryptophan
	AUG			Methionine
GAA	GAG			Glutamic acid
UUU	UUC			Phenylalanine
AUU	AUC	AUA		Isoleucine
GUU	GUC	GUA	GUG	Valine
CGU	CGC	CGA	CGG	Arginine
AGA	AGG			

U = uracil, C = cytosine, A = adenine, G = guanine.

sequence (see Table 3.15). The code also provides codons to initiate and terminate synthesis.

In the first stage of protein synthesis the DNA sequence between the initiation codon and the stop codon is transcribed into mRNA. The mRNA then moves from the nucleus to the ribosomes in the cytoplasm. Here the second stage takes place, viz. the translation of mRNA into a polypeptide chain. The ribosome binds to the initiation site on the mRNA and for each codon an amino acid is added on using transfer RNA. Transfer RNA (tRNA) is another form of RNA, which because of its molecular configuration is able to carry an amino acid and match it to the appropriate codon.

It has become apparent that the majority of DNA does not code for proteins and is not transcribed at all. The total amount of human DNA is 3 billion bases and if each gene were around 2000 bases in length this would allow for 1.5 million genes. Instead it is estimated that there are around 100 000 structural genes and 90% of the genome is DNA which does not code for proteins. Much of this is highly repetitive in its sequences and may have some as yet undefined function in the control of gene action.

The structural gene has an ordered sequence that is illustrated in Figure 3.31. Upstream of the structural gene there is highly repetitive DNA and within this there are two promoter regions, which regulate gene transcription. The beginning of the structural gene is marked by an initiation codon AUG which indicates where transcription begins. Within the region that is transcribed, the DNA may be divided into *exons* and *introns*. The exons mark the regions of DNA that code for the amino acids in the translated protein, whereas the introns or intervening sequences are spliced out of the processed RNA before it migrates to the cytoplasm as mRNA. The introns probably have a role in gene regulation. The complexity of genes varies, e.g. insulin has two introns, whereas some collagen genes may have as many as 50 introns. At the end of the transcribed gene there is a stop codon and further downstream an AATAA sequence that allows the release of the RNA.

Mutations at a molecular level

A *mutation* represents a change in the genomic material. Mutations may occur in somatic cells or germinal cells. Somatic cell mutation may predispose to malignancy, but will not be inherited. Mutations to the germinal cells, on the other hand, may be transmitted in the form of genetic disease. Mutations may be in the form of large chromosomal rearrangements as described in the earlier part of the chapter or may occur at molecular level in a single gene.

At a molecular level the following types of mutation have been described.

1. *Point mutations* – these involve the substitution of one base for another. A classical example of such a mutation is sickle cell disease in which an A to T substitution in the 6th codon of the globin gene changes GAG to GTG and hence leads to the substitution of valine for glutamic acid and the subsequent physiological effects on the hemoglobin molecule.

2. *Frameshift mutations* – if a single base is omitted or inserted this will alter the reading frame for all subsequent codons in the gene since the nucleotides are read in 'threes'.

3. *Termination mutations* – a base change may alter a codon to one of the stop codons (UAA or UAG or UGA) and produce premature termination of the transcription. Alternatively a mutation in the stop codon may convert it to code for an amino acid and the transcription carries on producing an abnormally long polypeptide.

4. *Deletions* – deletions may arise which involve variable lengths of the DNA in the structural gene. Many examples of these are known, e.g. at least 60% of mutations in Duchenne muscular dystrophy are gene deletions.

5. *Deletions in promoter sequences or introns* – deletions of this type have been reported in β thalassemia and affect the rate of β globin synthesis rather than its structure.

6. *Triplet repeats* – when a sequence of three nucleotides increases within a gene beyond a certain point the repeat sequence becomes genetically unstable and may increase further affecting the function of the gene. Examples of this are increasingly being recognized, e.g. fragile X mental retardation, myotonic dystrophy, Huntington's disease.

It should be noted that a number of different mutations can produce the same clinical phenotype. This phenomenon is often referred to as molecular heterogeneity.

While most mutations produce either no change or a decreasing function in a gene and may lead to disease, it should be remembered that mutations also provide the basis of genetic individuality and in some cases may produce beneficial results leading to evolutionary advance. Unfortunately medical research is orientated to disease and beneficial mutations are almost certainly overlooked.

Mutations usually produce a permanent change in the gene, but DNA has some ability to repair itself. This has largely been

Fig. 3.31 The structural gene consists of promoter and terminator sequences that are located at either end of the gene. The coding sequence of the gene is made up of exons and introns (the mRNA of which will eventually be spliced out before translation into a protein).

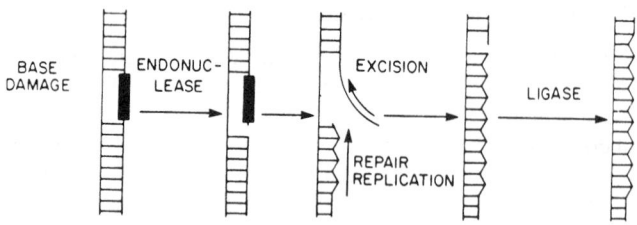

Fig. 3.32 DNA may be damaged but has a capacity to repair itself (reproduced with permission from Bundey 1985).

studied from disorders where DNA damage leads to malignancy. Ultraviolet exposure leads to the formation of pyrimidine dimers binding the nucleotide bases. In the rare skin disorder xeroderma pigmentosa such abnormal dimers cannot be repaired because of an enzyme deficiency and ultimately skin tumors develop. The stages in the normal repair are illustrated in Figure 3.32. Firstly, the single strand of DNA with the dimer formation is excised and removed, then using a DNA replicase a new strand is synthesized using the complementary strand as a template; finally the new strand is fixed into strands of the original using a DNA ligase.

TECHNIQUES USED IN MOLECULAR GENETICS

The recent rapid advances in medical genetics have come about largely because of the development of DNA technology. Some knowledge of the technology is helpful in understanding its practical application in the diagnosis of genetic disease. A more detailed review of the laboratory techniques may be found in Davies (1986) and Emery & Malcolm (1995).

The preparation of gene probes and gene library

A *gene probe* is a single-stranded segment of DNA which can be used to determine whether a particular DNA sequence is present or absent in an individual's genome. Gene probes may be prepared in three ways:

1. If the DNA sequence is fully known, then a small oligonucleotide probe may be synthesized in vitro.
2. If there is a ready source of mRNA such as the mRNA for α and 1β globin in reticulocytes then complementary DNA (cDNA) may be made using reverse transcription.
3. If the DNA sequence is not known, then an isolated segment of DNA which is known to be situated very close to the same region of the chromosome may be selected and used to track the inheritance of a specific structural gene within a family.

In practice most gene probes used in clinical work have been isolated from individual chromosomes sorted by their differential fluorescence, and prepared as a gene library by cloning the smaller fragments into bacterial plasmids. Once in this form the probes can be multiplied up by growing the bacteria and will be available for repeated use.

To illustrate how a gene probe could be used in diagnosis the example in Figure 3.33 is given. If it is necessary to determine whether a blood sample is from a male or female, DNA is extracted from the sample and denatured to make it single stranded. This DNA is then put on a filter and a Y-specific probe with an isotope (32P) attached is added to the filter. The Y-specific

probe is a DNA sequence derived from the Y chromosome and only found on the Y chromosome. If the individual is male, the Y-specific probe will bind on to the individual's DNA and when this is exposed to a radiological plate, it shows up as a hot dot. If the individual is female then the Y-specific probe will not find a complementary sequence to bind to and is washed off the filter, so that when the filter is exposed to radiographic plate, no dot shows up.

DNA extraction

DNA may be extracted from many different tissues. In practice extraction from blood or chorionic villi is the most widely used. The DNA is obtained by lysing the cells, digesting the proteins by a proteinase and purifying the DNA by serial extractions with phenol and chloroform. The purity of the DNA obtained is then determined by spectroscopy and running an electrophoretic gel. Full details of the technique may be found in Davies (1988).

Southern blotting

This technique has been widely used in both research and diagnosis. The DNA is extracted and cut into small fragments with a *restriction enzyme* which will recognize specific DNA sequences and cleave the DNA at these points. The DNA may then be electrophoresed so that the smallest fragments move fastest through the gel. If this is compared to a control sample the specific size of the DNA fragment may be estimated. Throughout the genome there will be variations or polymorphisms in the cutting sites for the restriction enzymes (*restriction fragment length polymorphisms* (RFLPs)) and therefore it will be possible to study the pattern of inheritance of these RFLPs within a family. If a particular RFLP is located close to a disease gene locus, it will be possible to follow the segregation through the family and make use of this in predicting whether or not a disease has been passed on in prenatal diagnosis. The main disadvantages of using Southern blotting are that it involves the use of radioisotopes and may require some days to develop the X-ray plate.

It should be noted that this technique is named after its originator (Southern 1975), but rather confusingly a geographical nomenclature has been applied to other techniques, e.g. a DNA–RNA blot is known as a Northern blot, and a protein–monoclonal antibody analysis is known as a Western blot!

Polymerase chain reaction

The polymerase chain reaction (PCR) is now the most frequently used technique in molecular biology. It basically is used to study a specific area of DNA using short complementary sequences of DNA (*oligonucleotides*) from both the 3′ and the 5′ ends of the DNA to be studied. These oligonucleotides build copies of the DNA using a *heat stable polymerase* (Taq 1). It is then possible to heat the mixture and the DNA strands will separate. On cooling, the DNA can once more be duplicated and the process repeated again and again leading to an exponential increase in the copies of the two fragments. The main advantages of this technique are that it is very quick, and it can be used to study mRNA as well as DNA. It can also be used to study very small amounts of almost any tissue, e.g. the blood spots on a Guthrie card or the cells found in a mouth wash sample (Lancet 1988, Lench et al 1988). The

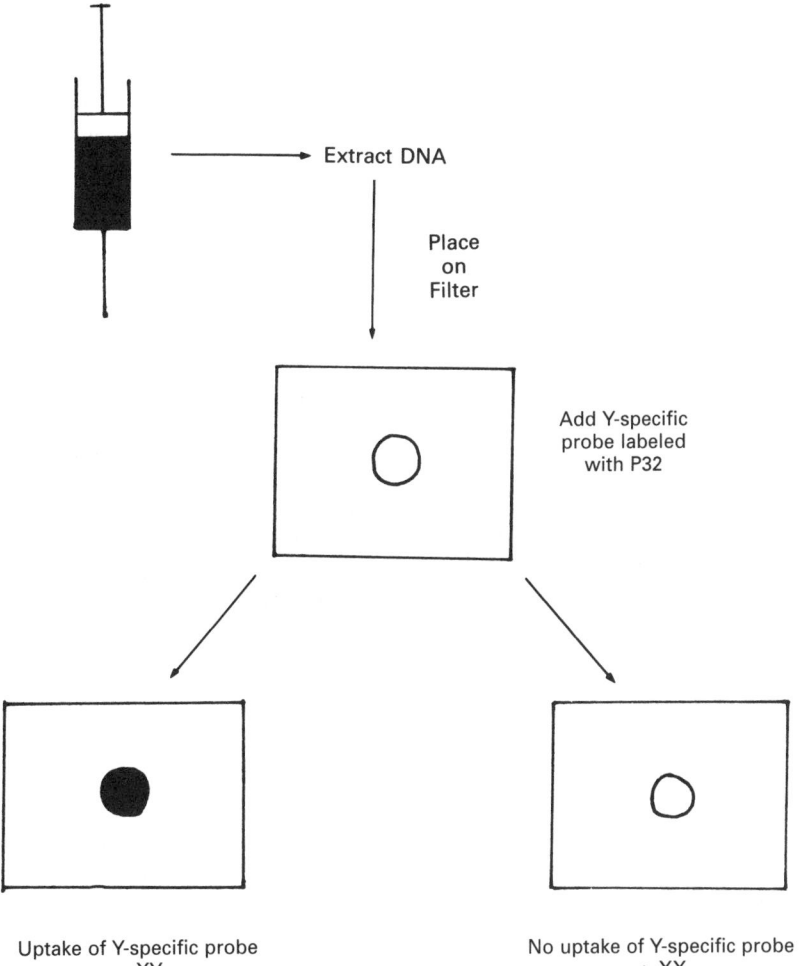

Extract DNA

Place
on
Filter

Add Y-specific
probe labeled
with P32

Uptake of Y-specific probe
∴ XY

No uptake of Y-specific probe
∴ XX

Fig. 3.33 Dot blotting using a Y-specific probe.

technique is widely used in molecular diagnosis of genetic disease (Figs 3.34 and 3.35). It is also being used in infectious disease to confirm the presence of infectious agents and in immunology to identify the HLA haplotype.

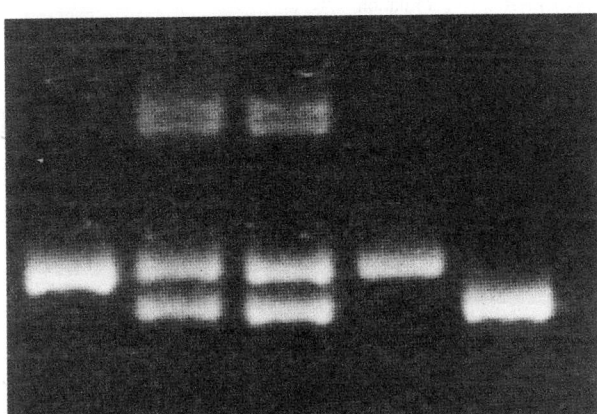

Fig. 3.34 PCR of exon of CFTR gene. Lanes 1 and 4 show homozygous normal individuals. Lanes 2 and 3 show heterozygous carriers of the ΔF508 mutation and lane 5 shows an affected homozygous ΔF508 individual. (Courtesy of R. Taylor)

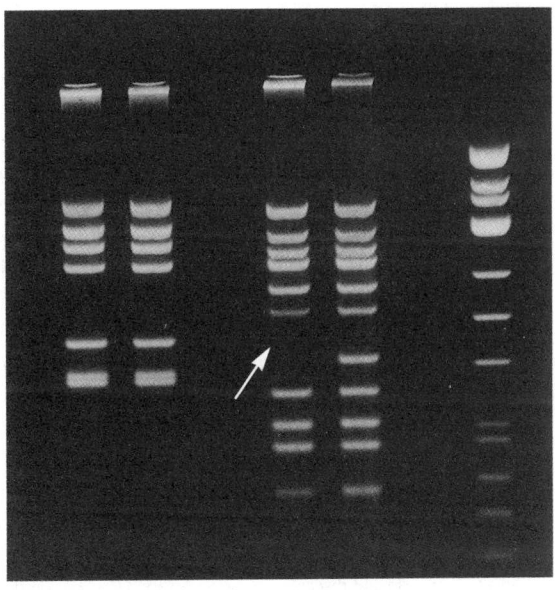

Fig. 3.35 Multiplex PCR testing for deletions in the dystrophin gene. The third lane from the left shows a band missing in amplifying exons from the 3′ end of the gene, indicating a patient affected with Duchenne muscular dystrophy. (Courtesy of R. Taylor)

Gene sequencing

There are now a number of techniques available to decode or sequence a gene with its component nucleotide bases. This is likely to be important in the future as in many diseases there is no one single mutation to look for but could be many hundreds of different mutations; short of sequencing most of the gene the confirmation or exclusion of the disease may be difficult. At the present time the process is very time consuming, but with the development of semiautomatic gene sequencers there is now a possibility that it will become more widely used in clinical diagnosis.

GENE MAPPING

When two genetic loci are close together on the same chromosome they are said to be *linked*. If two loci are at different ends of the chromosome then it is very likely that they will be separated during meiosis since there are two or three crossovers for each chromosome (see Fig. 3.2). The closer together they are the less likely that they will be separated during meiosis. Thus a measure of how close gene loci are to each other is the frequency of recombination. This is measured in *map units* or *centiMorgans* where 1 centiMorgan is equivalent to a 1% chance of recombination.

Locating the position of genes on the chromosomes (*gene mapping*) has become a major area of research in human genetics. There are in the region of 4000 genes or genetic disorders mapped to specific chromosome sites. This represents about 4% of the total, but the number of new gene localizations is increasing weekly. Some of the important gene localizations are illustrated in Table 3.16.

Gene mapping has been of considerable practical value in medical genetics. There are a large number of single gene disorders in which the underlying biochemical abnormality and gene mutation are unknown, but because the location of the disorder on the gene map is known, it is possible to track the disease through a family using linked polymorphic markers and offer prenatal diagnosis or, in the case of adult disorders, presymptomatic diagnosis. It has also been possible to progress from gene localization to sequencing the gene and to identifying the gene product. A good example of this was the research that led to the discovery of dystrophin as altered gene product in Duchenne muscular dystrophy (Witkowski 1988). This approach is known as *reverse genetics*, since it reverses the usual approach of identifying the gene mutation from the enzyme or protein abnormality.

Genes may be mapped in a number of ways:

1. *Pedigree analysis*: if the pattern of inheritance conforms with X-linked inheritance, then the gene in question is on the X

Table 3.16 Single gene disorders with their chromosome locations and approaches to diagnostic testing

Disease	Location(s)	Molecular tests
Adrenoleukodystrophy	Xq27	Linkage or biochemical
Adult polycystic kidney disease	16p13, 4q13	Linkage
Alpha-thalassemia	16p13	Mutation
Beta-thalassemia	11p15	Mutation
Charcot-Marie-Tooth disease	17p11, 1q21, Xq13	Linkage, mutation
Color blindness	Xq27	Research
Congenital adrenal hyperplasia	6p21	Mutation
Cystic fibrosis	7q31	Mutation
Duchenne muscular dystrophy	Xp21	Mutation or linkage
Emery-Dreifus muscular dystrophy	Xq27	Linkage
Facioscapulohumeral MD	4q34	Linkage
Fragile X mental retardation	Xq27	Mutation
Friedreich's ataxia	9q13	Mutation
Galactosemia	9p13	Linkage or biochemical
Hemophilia A & B	Xq28	Mutation/hematological
Hypertrophic cardiomyopathy	14q12	Linkage
Marfan's syndrome	15q21	Linkage
Myotonic dystrophy	19q13	Mutation
Neurofibromatosis type 1	17q11	Linkage
Neurofibromatosis type 2	22q11	Mutation
Noonan's syndrome	12q23	Research
Oculocutaneous albinism	11q14	Research
Osteogenesis imperfecta	7q21, 17q21	Linkage
Phenylketonuria	12q24	Mutation
Polyposis coli	5q21	Mutation or linkage
Sickle cell disease	11p15	Mutation
Tuberous sclerosis	9q33, 11q23, 12q23	Linkage
Von Hippel-Lindau syndrome	3p25	Mutation
Werdnig-Hoffman disease	5q	Mutation & linkage

chromosome. This simple approach has made the X chromosome the most fully mapped chromosome.

2. *Chromosome rearrangement*: if an association is found between a disorder and a specific chromosome rearrangement, then the gene for that disorder may be located at the chromosome breakpoints, e.g. patients were found with retinoblastoma and deletions of 13q14 and further research has identified the gene responsible for retinoblastoma to be located in this region.

3. *In situ hybridization*: if the amino acid structure of a protein is known then it is possible to predict which codons would code for it and therefore to synthesize a short oligonucleotide gene probe from it and label that probe with an isotope. The gene probe is then added to a chromosome spread and will hybridize to the complementary DNA in the chromosome. The localization of the gene is thus identified by an increased uptake of isotope at a specific site on the karyotype.

4. *Somatic cell hybridization*: using a virus it is possible to fuse human and mouse cells into a single hybrid cell. With subsequent cell divisions the human chromosomes are gradually lost, until there are cell lines with just one or two human chromosomes. By comparing the biochemical activity of a specific enzyme with the chromosome complement in each hybrid cell line, it is possible to deduce which chromosome the gene for the specific enzyme is on.

5. *Linkage analysis*: if a specific genetic marker such as a blood group or RFLP segregates in a family with a single gene disorder, then the gene for that disorder will be located on the same chromosome as the marker and the position of two genes can be estimated from the frequency of crossovers. For example, in Figure 3.36, a large family with an autosomal dominant disorder is studied with a DNA polymorphism which gives four alleles, A, B, C and D. In the first generation the disease is inherited with the B allele from the grandfather (I.1) to his son (II.1). In other words the DNA polymorphism B and the disease allele are on the same particular chromosome and the linkage phase is established. In the third generation it is possible to see if any recombination takes place. In all but one of the eight children the B polymorphism segregates with the disease and the D polymorphism segregates with the normal allele. The exception is III.7 in whom there has been a recombination. Thus there has been one recombination out of eight meioses and the recombination rate is 12.5% or 0.125. Obviously not all families are so obligingly large and informative, but it is still possible to carry out linkage analysis with smaller families because the number of meioses may be added together.

The usual way of expressing linkage is as the log of the odds of linkage or the *lod score* and this is expressed in terms of genetic distance by the recombination fraction θ. A recombination fraction of 0.05 represents a 5% chance of recombination. A lod score of 3 or over, for a recombination fraction of 0.05 or less, is significantly close linkage for prenatal diagnosis.

THE USE OF MOLECULAR GENETICS IN DIAGNOSIS

The techniques of molecular genetics have moved out of the research laboratory into the diagnostic genetic laboratory. There are now many diseases in which gene analysis may help in diagnosis. A summary of these is given in Table 3.16. The tests roughly fall into three groups:

1. *Fully diagnostic* – in these diseases there is only one mutation and analysis of this will give a clear and conclusive result. Examples of these are sickle cell disease where the only mutation is the point mutation in position 6 of the β globin chain and in myotonic dystrophy and fragile X where there is an expansion of a triplet repeat sequence.

2. *Partially diagnostic* – in these disorders there is more than one mutation that may cause the disorder and while it may be possible to make a clear positive diagnosis it is more difficult to exclude the diagnosis without fully sequencing the whole gene. There are many examples of this, but two will illustrate the point.

In cystic fibrosis around 70–80% of patients have a deletion of the codon for phenylalanine at position 508 (ΔF508) and if a patient is found to be homozygous for this mutation the diagnosis is confirmed (Fig. 3.34). If, however, the patient without a family history of cystic fibrosis is tested for ΔF508 and is found not to have it, the diagnosis is not completely excluded as it is possible to have any one of 200 other mutations. Rather than trying to test for such a large number of mutations it is possible to test for the commonest four to five mutations and this will give a 95% exclusion which is sufficient in most cases. The problem also exists if the patient is found to be heterozygous for ΔF508. The patient might be an unaffected heterozygote carrier or could be an affected homozygote with another rarer mutation on the other chromosome 7.

The other example is Duchenne muscular dystrophy. By using a combination of gene probes it is possible to look for several possible deletions in the dystrophin gene. If a deletion is found the diagnosis is confirmed (Fig. 3.35). However, the absence of the deletion only provides a 60% exclusion of the diagnosis.

In both these examples the molecular test has to be used in conjunction with the other clinical information and the accuracy and limitations of the tests must be appreciated.

3. *Genetic linkage tests* – in these cases the location of the gene is known but not the specific mutation. By using linked genetic polymorphisms it is possible to follow the inheritance of the disease through the family and make a prediction of whether other members of the family may be carriers or become affected. These tests will have a small chance of error (usually about 3–5%) due to the possible recombination between the disease gene and the genetic polymorphism. As these are indirect tests it is also important to be certain of the diagnosis and whether there is more than one gene locus causing the disorder.

The family structure and the ability to collect sufficient samples from the relevant members of the family may limit the use of this approach.

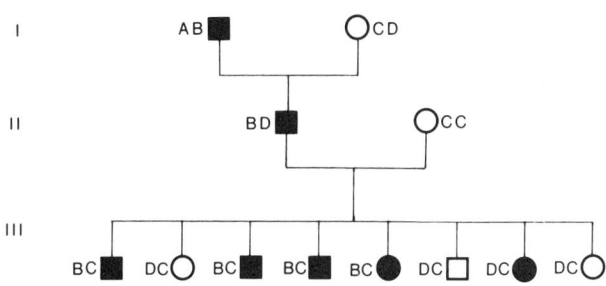

Fig. 3.36 Gene mapping by linkage analysis. In this pedigree the polymorphic marker B is segregating with the disease, with the exception of III.7 where a meiotic recombination between the polymorphic marker and the disease has occurred.

MULTIFACTORIAL INHERITANCE

Many common disorders including congenital malformations show some increase in frequency within families, but follow no simple Mendelian pattern of inheritance. In these disorders the condition becomes manifest when there is a sufficient combination of genetic predisposition and environmental factors. These disorders are, thus, referred to as multifactorial.

One way of understanding multifactorial inheritance is to consider an individual's *liability* to a particular disorder to be a combination of genetic and environmental factors. The distribution of liability in the general population will have a normal distribution and it is only those whose liability goes beyond a certain threshold who will show the disease or malformation (Fig. 3.37). This would be a relatively small proportion of the general population. First degree relatives of those who manifest the disorder will have half the genes in common with their affected relatives and therefore have a greater proportion of the genetic predisposition than the general population. If one then looked at the distribution of liability in first degree relatives it would be shifted away from the distribution in the general population, so that a greater proportion of first degree relatives would be affected than that in the general population (Fig. 3.37).

While the mathematical model of liability may be helpful in understanding the principles of multifactorial inheritance it is not of practical value in providing information on recurrence risks for genetic counseling. These are best provided by the statistical analysis of family studies. For example the recurrence of neural tube defects in those families who had already had an affected child is around 5% or 15 times the risk for the general population. Similar studies looking at the offspring of those affected by spina

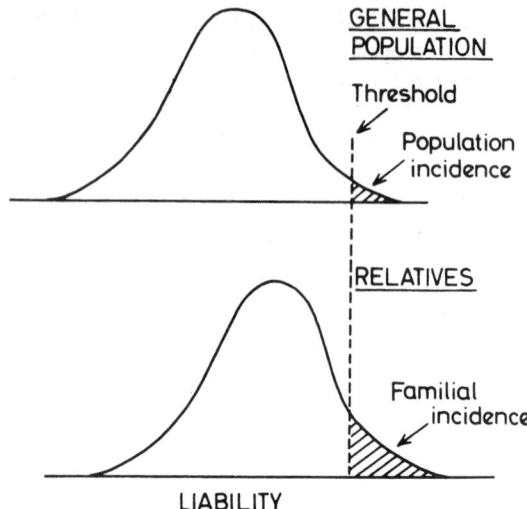

Fig. 3.37 Hypothetical curve of liability in the general population and in relatives for a hereditary disorder in which the genetic predisposition is multifactorial.

bifida have shown a 5% risk for their offspring. Table 3.17 gives some of the empiric risks for common disorders calculated from family studies. With new techniques in molecular biology it may become possible to identify the genetic factors in multifactorial disorders. This has to some extent already been achieved in ischemic heart disease where many of the genes involved in lipoprotein metabolism have been identified.

Table 3.17 Recurrence risks (%) for some common disorders (from Emery 1983)

Disorder	Incidence	Sex ratio M:F	Normal parents having a second affected child	Affected parent having an affected child	Affected parent having a second affected child
Anencephaly	0.20	1:2	5*	–	–
Asthma	3–4	1:1	10	26	–
Cleft palate only	0.04	2:3	2	7	15
Cleft lip ± cleft palate	0.10	3:2	4	4	10
Club foot	0.10	2:1	3	3	10
Congenital heart disease (all types)	0.50	–	1–4	1–4	–
Diabetes mellitus (early onset)	0.20	1:1	8	8	10
Dislocation of hip	0.07	1:6	4	4	10
Epilepsy ('idiopathic')	0.50	1:1	5	5	10
Hirschsprung's disease	0.02	4:1	–	–	–
Male index			2	–	–
Female index			8	–	–
Mental retardation ('idiopathic')	0.30–0.50	1:1	3–5	–	–
Profound childhood deafness	0.10	1:1	10	8	–
Pyloric stenosis	0.30	5:1			
Male index			2	4	13
Female index			10	17	38
Renal agenesis (bilat.)	0.01	3:1			
Male index			3	–	–
Female index			7	–	–
Schizophrenia	1–2	1:1	10	16	–
Scoliosis (idiopathic, adolescent)	0.22	1:6	7	5	–
Spina bifida	0.30	2:3	5*	3*	–

*Anencephaly *or* spina bifida.

With multifactorial inheritance there are some general rules which are helpful.

1. The risk for sibs is approximately equal to the risk for offspring. On the whole the risks are lower than those for Mendelian inheritance.

2. The risks for second degree relatives (uncles, aunts, nephews and nieces) is considerably smaller than those for first degree relatives. The risks for third degree relatives (cousins) are for practical purposes more or less the same as those for the general population.

3. If the frequency of a multifactorial disorder is q, then the risk for first degree relatives is approximately the square root of q, e.g. esophageal atresia occurs in 1 in 10 000 births; the risk for further offspring is the square root of 0.0001 = 1/100.

4. If there is a sex difference in the frequency of the disorder, then the risks are greater for further relatives of the rarer sex. For example, with pyloric stenosis males are affected five times as frequently as females. After an affected male the risk of further affected children is 2%, but after an affected female the risk is 9%.

5. The risks increase with the number of affected individuals in the family. The risk after a second affected child is more than twice the risk after a single affected child. For example after one child with a cleft lip and palate the risk is 4%, but after two affected children it is 10%.

6. In theory the recurrence data collected from family studies are only relevant for the same racial group and geographical area. If there are differences in the incidence of a disorder in different racial groups and countries, then care must be taken in applying the data, e.g. the recurrence risk for anencephaly and spina bifida is less in blacks than whites.

MALFORMATION SYNDROMES

The majority of single congenital malformations have a multifactorial inheritance and a relatively low risk of recurrence. In the case of multiple malformations or the combination of mental handicap and congenital abnormalities, then considerable care needs to be exercised, since a proportion of such cases are caused by single gene mutations and consequently have a high risk of recurrence.

Another reason why it is important to recognize when a malformation is part of a syndrome is that it may give a better indication of the ultimate prognosis or likelihood of subsequent complications. For example, the Stickler syndrome is an autosomal dominant disorder with variable expression. It may present in the newborn with a cleft palate and micrognathia and a characteristic facial appearance with a flat nasal bridge (Fig. 3.38). There is often severe myopia and possibly retinal detachment; by anticipatory follow-up the retinal detachment can be prevented by early treatment.

The clinical approach to the diagnosis and study of malformations and birth defects is known as *dysmorphology* (Smith 1988). There are a number of concepts that are useful in delineating patterns of malformation.

1. A *syndrome* is a recognized pattern of clinical abnormalities that have a single cause, e.g. the Meckel syndrome is an autosomal recessive disorder in which postaxial polydactyly, encephalocele, cystic dysplastic kidneys and hepatic fibrosis occur together.

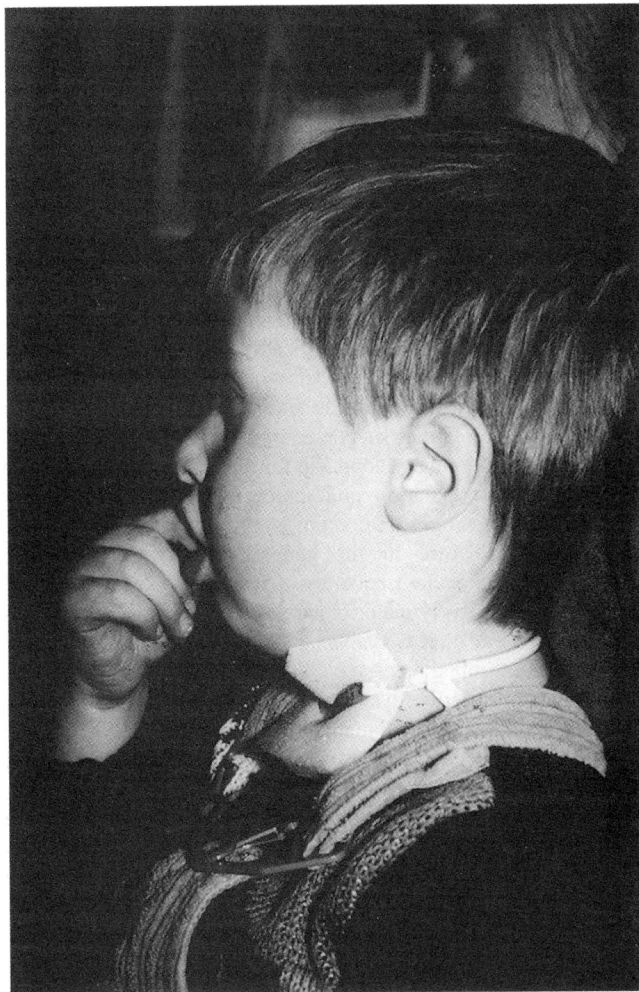

Fig. 3.38 Stickler's syndrome.

2. An *anomalad* is a recognized pattern of congenital abnormalities that may have several different causes, e.g. the Robin anomalad of micrognathia, cleft palate and posteriorly displaced tongue may be a feature of Stickler's syndrome, fetal compression, cerebrocostal syndrome and others.

3. An *association* is a combination of congenital abnormalities that occur together at a frequency greater than by chance alone, but do not appear to recur in families, e.g. the VATER association is a combination of Vertebral abnormalities, Anal atresia, TracheoEsophageal fistula, Radial and Renal abnormalities. The combination of abnormalities might represent an insult at a specific point in embryonic development which affects all systems developing at that particular time in embryogenesis.

4. A *sequence* is a series of malformations that arise secondary to one specific developmental incident, e.g. in the prune belly sequence urethral or bladder neck obstruction leads to bladder distention which in turn leads to abdominal distention, hydronephrosis and possibly interference with testicular descent and the iliac blood supply. When the pressure is sufficient to overcome the obstruction the bladder may deflate leaving the characteristic wrinkled prune belly appearance.

5. A *deformation* arises not from an error in embryological development but because normal fetal growth is restricted, e.g. the

low-set ears, micrognathia and joint contractures seen with oligohydramnios in utero.

THE CLINICAL APPROACH TO THE DIAGNOSIS OF A DYSMORPHIC SYNDROME

With the exception of radiological and cytogenetic investigations the diagnosis of a dysmorphic syndrome rarely depends on laboratory investigations. It is primarily a clinical diagnosis based on the assessment of the clinical signs and knowledge of the pattern of abnormalities seen in the dysmorphic syndromes.

In trying to weigh up the significance of specific dysmorphic features it is helpful to consider whether they are relatively common or rarely seen outside the context of a dysmorphic syndrome. Abnormalities such as a single palmar crease or partial syndactyly between the second and third toes are commonly seen in the general population and therefore are relatively minor clinical signs. Features like retinitis pigmentosa, cleft lip and polydactyly are rare in the general population as single abnormalities, and are frequently a feature of syndromes and therefore are relatively major clinical signs. Occasionally there is a specific feature that is diagnostic like the 'hitchhiker thumb' seen in the autosomal recessive diastrophic dwarfism (Fig. 3.39).

In trying to describe dysmorphic features, in particular facial characteristics, everyday language may be very unprecise and subjective so it is helpful to use defined terms (Table 3.18) as far as possible and to keep photographic records. The objectivity may be improved also by anthropometric measurements. There is a considerable literature on the use of anthropometric measurements in dysmorphology but some of the more useful measurements are listed in Smith (1988).

The diagnosis of a dysmorphic syndrome depends primarily on pattern recognition and knowledge. The task has been helped by the publication of some excellent photographic atlases, e.g. Smith (1988), Baraitser & Winter (1983). As there are now some 1700 malformation syndromes described, a computerized database is a great asset in the recognition of rare syndromes which may have been described on only a few occasions (Winter et al 1984, Patton 1987).

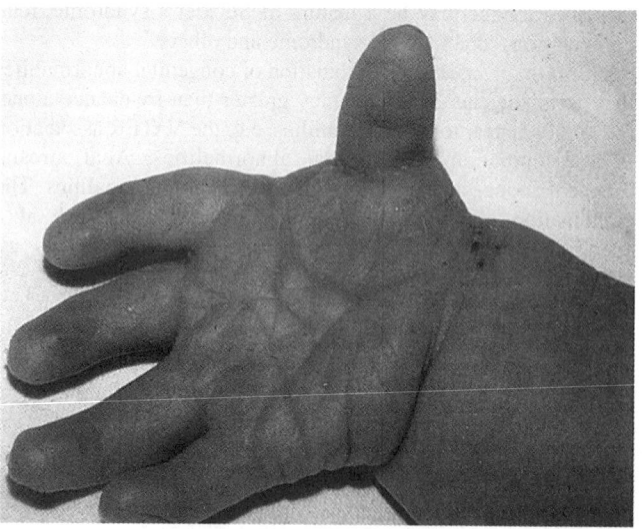

Fig. 3.39 'Hitchhiker thumb' in diastrophic dwarfism.

Table 3.18 Descriptive terms used in dysmorphology

Hypertelorism	Increased distance between the eyes
Hypotelorism	Decreased distance between the eyes
Blepharophimosis	Narrowed palpebral fissures
Synophyris	Medial fusion of the eyebrows
Nasal bridge	Upper part of nose between eyes
Alae nasi	Lateral border of nostril
Columella	Medial part or septum of nostril
Philtrum	Vertical folds on upper lip
Pterygium	Webbing, e.g. webbing of neck = pterygium colli
Syndactyly	Fusion of digits
Preaxial polydactyly	Extra digit(s) on lateral border of limb
Postaxial polydactyly	Extra digit(s) on medial border of limb
Clinodactyly	Incurving usually of 5th digit
Brachydactyly	Short fingers or toes
Camptodactyly	Bent and contracted digits
Ectrodactyly	Cleft hand or foot
Symphalangism	Fusion of phalanges
Phocomelia	Absence of limb
Rhizomelia	Shortening of proximal segment of limb
Mesomelia	Shortening of middle segment of limb
Acromelia	Shortening of distal segment of limb
Dysplasia	Generalized abnormality of development, e.g. skeletal dysplasia

The subject of dysmorphology has proven itself in identifying the genes that control normal development. Genetic studies in Waardenburg syndrome which is deafness, heterochromia and depigmentation has lead to the identification of a developmental gene responsible for the migration of cells from the neural crest (Tassabehji et al 1992). Studies on craniosynostosis syndromes such as Pfieffer's and Apert's syndrome have identified a group of genes such as fibroblast growth factor or fibroblast growth factor receptor genes which play a very significant part in skeletal development (Park et al 1995).

COUNSELING AND GENETIC SERVICES

ORGANIZATION OF SERVICES

While all pediatricians and other doctors will be involved in providing some genetic information and counseling to their patients, the increasing complexity of medical genetics has led to the development of a new specialty which links the clinical and laboratory aspects. In England each regional health authority (population 1.5–4.5 million) has a regional genetic service, which combines clinical and laboratory skills. One of the important aspects of such a service is that it is orientated towards the extended family rather than the individual, and as such can provide the follow-up required for chromosome translocations or single gene disorders. Separate family records are kept on a long-term basis as opposed to the relatively short periods individual records are kept in most general hospitals. In addition to this, DNA may be 'banked' from family blood samples and be available for family studies in the future. Coordinating this may require a computerized follow-up or genetic register. The philosophy of family orientated screening can provide a highly personalized service which is very cost effective in terms of preventing handicap.

APPROACHES TO GENETIC COUNSELING

As in all areas of medicine the first stage of genetic counseling is to establish an accurate diagnosis. Without accurate diagnosis the counseling may be erroneous. There are a number of problems in establishing a diagnosis which are unique to medical genetics. The first is the enormous number of genetic disorders which have now been described. McKusick lists 5710 single gene traits or disorders (McKusick 1992). In addition to this, there are many chromosomal abnormalities and malformation syndromes, and the number of disorders described is increasing exponentially (Fig. 3.40). The second problem is that the disorders are often very rare and thus even a specialist covering a relatively large population cannot rely solely on his own personal experience, but must be familiar with the medical literature. A third problem is heterogeneity. *Heterogeneity* may be at the clinical or molecular level. At the clinical level it means that two or more disorders may have the same phenotype, e.g. both Marfan's syndrome and homocystinuria have dislocation of the lenses with a similar physical habitus, but Marfan's syndrome is autosomal dominant, whereas homocystinuria is autosomal recessive. At a molecular level it means that a number of different allelic mutations can cause the same disease. This point is of considerable practical significance if a specific DNA diagnosis is to be made. Fourthly, the individuals who come to the genetic clinic may not themselves have any clinical features of the genetic disorder in question and so clinical examination will not necessarily provide the appropriate diagnosis. It is essential before seeing the individual in the clinic to obtain as much background medical information about the family as possible. This may mean a careful search of hospital records and considerable ingenuity in tracking the results of autopsies or laboratory investigations.

Having established the correct diagnosis it is then necessary to discuss the prognosis and likelihood of recurrence. It is particularly important to discuss the prognosis in the case of parents whose experience of a disorder may be limited because, for example, the disease has not yet progressed to any significant extent in their affected child. It should also be remembered that some conditions, such as neurofibromatosis, may show a considerable range of expression and this should be taken into account in giving advice. The risk of passing on the gene for neurofibromatosis is 1 in 2, but as only about one-third of patients have severe medical complications from the disease the risk of severe complications in offspring is $1/2 \times 1/3$ or 1 in 6.

Having diagnosed the disorder and given guidance about recurrence and prognosis, the next stage is to discuss the options that may be available to the couple (Table 3.19). It must be stressed that these reproductive discussions are personal choices rather than medical decisions and the counselor should remain nondirective in his approach. The immediate aim of genetic counseling is to inform and support families faced with genetic disease rather than reduce the frequency of genetic handicap per se.

Choosing the right time for genetic counseling is very important. The couple whose child has just died from a major congenital malformation will usually want to come to terms with their loss before considering the recurrence in further pregnancies. On the other hand, leaving genetic counseling until pregnancy is advanced may produce an emotional crisis which could have been avoided by anticipation. It is to the advantage of the family and the geneticist if the initial referral is made before pregnancy.

While the above description outlines one approach to genetic counseling, it is important that the counselor should be flexible in his approach. It is important to allocate sufficient time for the counseling session and to be able to elucidate the couple's feelings with open ended questions. It should be noted that a report from a working party of the Clinical Genetics Society in the UK (endorsed by Royal College of Paediatrics and Child Health) regarded genetic screening of children for late-onset disorders when there is no treatment for the disorder screened (e.g. Huntington's disease) to be completely unethical (Clarke 1994).

It has been shown that a patient's comprehension of the genetic information is limited by anxiety and the counselor must ensure that the patient is given every opportunity to express his or her feelings and be put at ease as far as possible. It is often helpful to follow the session with a letter to the family outlining the important pieces of information and give them the opportunity of a further session or sessions to discuss the matter further. The consequences of genetic counseling can be profound and far reaching and so such advice should not be given lightly. Further information on genetic counseling is given elsewhere (Harper 1993).

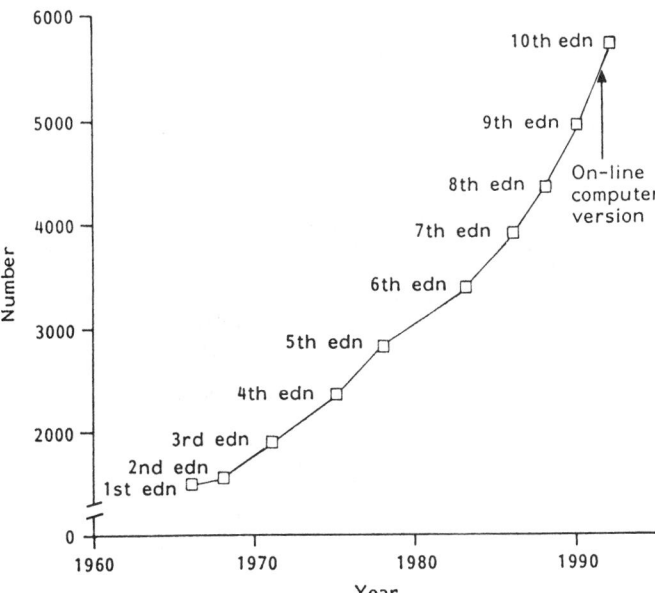

Fig. 3.40 Numbers of confirmed gene loci given in McKusick's catalogs from 1966 to 1992. Including unconfirmed loci the total number of disorders listed by 1992 was 5710 (reproduced with permission from Emery & Malcolm 1995).

Table 3.19 Options which may be available for couples receiving genetic counseling

No further action
Restrict family size
Adoption
Artificial insemination by donor
Ovum donation
Prenatal diagnosis and selective termination

REFERENCES

Baird P A, Sadovnick A D 1988 Life expectancy in Down syndrome adults. Lancet ii: 1354–1356

Baraitser M, Winter R M 1983 A colour atlas of clinical genetics. Wolfe Medical Publications, London

Bundey 1985 Genetics and neurology. Churchill Livingstone, Edinburgh

Butler M G, Meaney F J, Palmer C G 1986 Clinical and cytogenetic survey of 39 individuals with the Prader–Labhart–Willi syndrome. American Journal of Medical Genetics 23: 793–809

Carter C 1956 Changing patterns in the cause of death at the Hospital for Sick Children. Great Ormond Street Journal 11: 65–68

Chicago Conference 1966 Standardization in human genetics. Birth Defects ii, no. 2

Clarke A 1995 The genetic testing of children – Report of a working group of the Clinical Genetics Society – Chairman, Dr Angus Clarke. March 1994. Journal of Medical Genetics 1994; 34: 785–797

Cuckle H S, Richardson G A, Sheldon T A, Quirke P 1995 Cost effectiveness of antenatal screening for cystic fibrosis. British Medical Journal 311: 1460–1463

Davies K E 1986 Human genetic disease. IRL Press, Oxford

Davies K E 1988 Genomic analysis: a practical approach. IRL Press, Oxford

Edwards J H, Harnden D G, Cameron A H et al 1960 A new trisomic syndrome. Lancet i: 787–790

Emery A E H (ed) 1983 Principles and practice of medical genetics. Churchill Livingstone, Edinburgh

Emery A E H 1987 Duchenne muscular dystrophy (revised edn). Oxford University Press, Oxford

Emery A E H, Malcolm S 1995 An introduction to recombinant DNA in medicine, 2nd edn. John Wiley, Chichester

Emery A E H, Mueller R F 1988 Elements of medical genetics, 7th edn. Churchill Livingstone, Edinburgh

Emery A E H, Rimoin D L (eds) 1990 Principles and practice of medical genetics, 2nd edn. Churchill Livingstone, Edinburgh

Epstein C J 1986 The consequences of chromosome imbalance. Cambridge University Press, Cambridge

Ferguson-Smith M A, Cooke A, Affara N A, Boyd E, Tolmie J L 1990 Genotype–phenotype correlations in XX males and their bearing on current theories of sex determination. Human Genetics 84: 198–202

Goate A M, Haynes A R, Owen M J et al 1989 Predisposing locus for Alzheimer's disease on chromosome 21. Lancet i: 352–355

Grouchy J, Turleau C 1984 Clinical atlas of human chromosomes, 2nd edn. John Wiley, Chichester

Harding A E 1993 Mitochondrial genes and neurological disease. Clinical and Experimental Neurology 30: 1–16

Harper P S 1993 Practical genetic counselling, 4th edn. John Wright, Bristol

Harris R, Andrews T 1988 Prenatal screening for Down's syndrome. Archives of Disease in Childhood 63: 705–706

Hergersberg M, Matuso K, Gassmann M et al 1995 Tissue specific expression of a FMR-1/beta galactosidase gene in transgenic mice. Human Molecular Genetics 4: 359–366

Hirst M C, Suthers G K, Davies K E 1992 X-linked mental retardation: the fragile X syndrome. Hospital Update 18: 736–742

Lancet Editorial 1988 DNA diagnosis and the polymerase chain reaction. Lancet i: 1372–1373

Laxova R, Ridler M A C, Bowen-Bravery M 1977 An etiological survey of the severely retarded Hertfordshire children who were born between January 1 1965 and December 31 1967. American Journal of Medical Genetics 1: 75–86

Lench N, Stanier P, Williamson R 1988 Simple non-invasive method to obtain DNA for gene analysis. Lancet i: 1356–1358

Lowery M C, Morris C A, Ewart A et al 1995 Strong correlation of elastin deletions detected by FISH with William's syndrome: evaluation of 235 patients. American Journal of Human Genetics 57: 49–54

McKusick V A 1992 Mendelian inheritance in man. Catalogs of autosomal dominant, autosomal recessive and X linked phenotypes, 10th edn. Johns Hopkins University Press, Baltimore

Malcolm S, Clayton-Smith J, Nichols M et al 1991 Uniparental paternal disomy in Angelman's syndrome. Lancet 337: 694–697

Mehta L, Shannon R S, Duckett D P et al 1986 Trisomy 18 in a 13 year old girl. Journal of Medical Genetics 23: 256–278

Mueller R F, Young I D 1995 Emery's elements of medical genetics. Churchill Livingstone, Edinburgh

Neri G, Opitz J M, Mikkelsen M et al 1988 Conference report: third international workshop on the fragile X and X-linked mental retardation. American Journal of Medical Genetics 30: 1–29

Nicolaides K, Brizot M L, Snijders R J M et al 1994 Fetal nuchal translucency: ultrasound screening for fetal trisomy in the first trimester of pregnancy. British Journal of Obstetrics and Gynaecology 101: 782–786

Oliver C, Holland A J 1986 Downs syndrome and Alzheimer's disease: a review. Psychological Medicine 16: 307–322

Paris Conference 1971 Standardization in human cytogenetics. Birth defects: original articles series, viii, 1972 & Supplement 1975 xi, 9. New York

Park W J, Bellus G A, Jabs E W 1995 Mutations in the fibroblast growth factor receptors: phenotypic consequences during eukaryotic development. American Journal of Human Genetics 57: 748–754

Patau K, Smith D W, Therman E et al 1960 Multiple congenital anomaly caused by an extra autosome. Lancet i: 790–793

Patton M A 1987 A computerized approach to dysmorphology. MD Computing 4: 33–39

Philips C I, Levy A M, Newton M et al 1987 Blindness in schoolchildren: importance of heredity, congenital cataract and prematurity. British Journal of Ophthalmology 71: 578–584

Ratcliffe S G, Paul N 1985 Prospective studies on children with sex chromosome aneuploidy. Birth defects: original articles series Vol 22, No 3. Alan Liss, New York

Reynolds J F, Daniel A, Kelly T et al 1987 Isochromosome 12p mosaicism (Pallister mosaic aneuploidy of Pallister–Killian syndrome): report of 11 cases. American Journal of Medical Genetics 27: 257–274

Riordan-Eva P, Harding A E 1995 Leber's hereditary optic neuropathy: the clinical relevance of different mitochondrial DNA mutations. Journal of Medical Genetics 32: 81–87

Rooney D E, Czepulskowski B H (eds) 1992 Human cytogenetics: a practical approach, 2nd edn. IRL Press, Oxford, vols I, II

Schnizel A 1984 Catalogue of unbalanced chromosome aberrations in man. Walter de Gruyter, Berlin

Smith D W 1988 Recognisable patterns of human malformation, 4th edn. W B Saunders, Philadelphia

Southern E M 1975 Detection of specific sequences among DNA fragments separated by gel electrophoresis. Journal of Molecular Biology 98: 503–517

Sutherland G R 1983 The fragile X chromosome. International Review of Cytology 81: 107–143

Sutherland G R, Hecht F 1985 Fragile sites on human chromosomes. Oxford University Press, Oxford

Tassabehji M, Read A P, Newton V E et al 1992 Waardenburg's syndrome patients have mutations in the human homologue of the Pax 3 paired box gene. Nature 355: 635–636

Tijo J H, Levan A 1956 Chromosome number in man. Hereditas 42: 1–6

Verkerk A J M H, Pieretti M, Sutcliffe J S et al 1991 Identification of a gene (FMR-1) containing a CGG repeat coincident with a breakpoint cluster region exhibiting length variation in a fragile X syndrome. Cell 65: 905–914

Wald N J, Cuckle H S, Densem J W et al 1988 Maternal serum screening for Downs syndrome in early pregnancy. British Medical Journal 297: 883–887

Weatherall D J 1986 The new genetics and clinical practice, 2nd edn. Oxford University Press, Oxford

Willemsen R, Mohkamsing S, de Vries B et al 1995 Rapid antibody screening test for fragile X syndrome. Lancet 345: 1147–1148

Winter R M, Baraitser M, Douglas J M 1984 A computerized database for the diagnosis of rare dysmorphic syndromes. Journal of Medical Genetics 21: 121–124

Witkowski J A 1988 The molecular genetics of Duchenne muscular dystrophy: the beginning of the end. Trends in Genetics 4: 27–30

4 Obstetric aspects of perinatal care

I. A. Laing   E. M. Wallace

Introduction   79
Pregnancy   79
Preconceptional care   79
Antenatal care   80
    Booking/early pregnancy   80
    Mid-pregnancy   81
    Late pregnancy   81
    Postterm pregnancy   83
Intrapartum care   83
    Place of delivery   83
    Onset of parturition   84
    Progress in labor   84
    Induction of labor   87
    Breech delivery   87
Postpartum care   88

Obstetric complications   88
Antepartum hemorrhage   88
    Placental abruption   88
    Placenta previa   88
Multiple pregnancy   90
Hypertensive disorders   90
Effects of maternal drugs on fetus and newborn   90
References   91

INTRODUCTION

All obstetricians and midwives should have some knowledge of neonatology, to be able to provide all routine and some emergency care for the infants they have delivered, to be aware of the eventual outcome of the children for audit of their practice, and to be able to discuss with parents the infant's future. More recently it has become equally important for both neonatologist and general pediatrician to have a sound basic knowledge of obstetrics. Only then can they contribute to the team providing counseling for parents before and during a high-risk pregnancy. Discussions may include the effects of maternal disease or drugs on the fetus, the implications of labor and delivery, and the planning of future pregnancies in the light of past medical and obstetric history. Improved knowledge of each other's disciplines allows the obstetrician and neonatologist to discuss together the implications of a high-risk pregnancy, and in consultation with the parents select a time and mode of delivery which may be safest for mother and child.

Confronted with a difficult pregnancy with increased risk of mortality or morbidity to mother or fetus, the obstetrician may need to coordinate many different hospital specialties (e.g. diabetic, renal, cardiac, ultrasonographic, anesthetic and respiratory) in addition to maintaining liaison with the neonatology department. This chapter describes the assessment and management of a normal pregnancy and delivery, introducing aspects of decision-making about problems that are either commonly encountered in pregnancy or that are relatively uncommon but are nonetheless important because of the associated risks to the mother and/or her fetus.

PREGNANCY

The process of having a baby, while a continuum, may be viewed as a number of discrete stages in terms of the care provided: preconceptual care, antenatal care, intrapartum care and postpartum care. While there is much debate about who should deliver this care and where it should be delivered (Calder 1994), it is generally accepted that women who receive no care have much poorer outcomes (Chamberlain 1978).

PRECONCEPTIONAL CARE

Preconceptional or prepregnancy care is not an established feature of care for a prospective mother in the same way as antenatal care clearly is. However, care delivered before pregnancy, often only in the form of advice, may be of considerable benefit in preventing problems during pregnancy. Most women first seek confirmation of pregnancy from their family doctor when they are already 6–8 weeks pregnant and the first hospital antenatal booking visit is usually scheduled for 12–14 weeks' gestation. Embryogenesis therefore largely occurs without any medical input but it is the time when teratogenic influences exert their effects. Thus any modification of risk must be initiated prior to pregnancy. In women with pre-existing medical conditions optimization of their current therapies in preparation for pregnancy is often necessary. In women with diabetes mellitus for example, improved glycemic control is important to reduce the risks of fetal abnormality, while in women with epilepsy trying a reduction in drug therapy is often worthwhile for the same reasons. Indeed, if there has been a 2- or 3-year seizure-free period then gradual total withdrawal of medication should be considered. Women who have hypertension managed by angiotensin-converting enzyme inhibitors (ACE inhibitors) should have their medication changed prior to pregnancy as these drugs are associated with fetal loss in animals (Broughton Pipkin et al 1980) and growth retardation in humans (Greer 1992).

Even in women with no pre-existing health problems prepregnancy advice can be beneficial. All women considering pregnancy should take folate supplementation to reduce the risk of neural tube defects (Expert Advisory Group 1992) and general advice may be given about diet, smoking and alcohol and work. It is clear that smoking has many detrimental effects on pregnancy, including increasing the risks of miscarriage, preterm labor and growth retardation (Poswillo & Alberman 1992). While many women will stop smoking of their own accord once pregnant, a measure of the public awareness that smoking is unhealthy, reaffirmation of this by health professionals is worthwhile. Likewise, excessive alcohol consumption is harmful to the fetus and it is generally considered that women should not drink alcohol during pregnancy (Royal College of Obstetricians and Gynaecologists 1985). There is no good evidence, however, that moderate or social levels of consumption are harmful. Type of work may also affect pregnancy outcome. Heavy manual work or work involving standing is associated with a significantly increased risk of preterm labor (Papiernik 1993, Henriksen et al 1995). Empowered with this knowledge, it may be possible for a woman to identify such risks and organize ways to reduce them. Indeed, in France a national program aimed at improving perinatal outcome reduced the number of deliveries before 34 weeks by 50% with just such strategies (Papiernik 1993).

ANTENATAL CARE

The aims of antenatal care are to provide advice, education and support to the woman and her family during pregnancy, to assess risks of harm to the mother and her baby, to screen for various disorders and to treat any problems that arise during pregnancy. As the pregnancy proceeds the style of care provided will change to reflect risks or problems that are common to the different gestations. Likewise, care should be tailored to the individual women, with women at low risk receiving different care from women with pre-existing indicators of high risk (House of Commons Health Committee 1992). While this might seem self-evident a recent survey showed that this was not reflected in practice, with low-risk and high-risk women receiving similar care (Tucker et al 1994). It is generally accepted, however, that a woman should be seen during pregnancy monthly until 28 weeks, 2-weekly until 36 weeks and thereafter weekly until delivery (American College of Obstetricians and Gynecologists 1988). The care offered during this time can be divided into four parts:

10–16 weeks	Booking/early pregnancy
16–28 weeks	Mid-pregnancy
28–41 weeks	Late pregnancy
Over 41 weeks	Postterm

Booking/early pregnancy

At the first (booking) visit to the antenatal clinic a record will be drawn up as a basis for all future maternal visits to the clinic. The format of these records is similar throughout the UK and it is accepted that a women will carry her records herself so that information can be extracted quickly in an emergency wherever the woman is during her pregnancy. Information should include age, parity, personal medical history, family history, and details of past obstetric experience. Smoking and drinking habits, drugs taken, and contacts with infectious diseases (including hepatitis B

and human immunodeficiency virus (HIV)) are all recorded. Accurate dating of the pregnancy is assisted by detailing length and regularity of previous menstrual cycles, previous contraceptive methods, and whether the last period was normal in time, duration and character. Dating is usually confirmed by an ultrasound examination. Measurement of the crown–rump length by ultrasound in the first trimester is accurate to within 1 week; biparietal diameter between 14 and 20 weeks is accurate to within 2 weeks. Thereafter ultrasonography is less reliable as a tool for the assessment of gestational age because of the variation in fetal growth rates. Accurate gestational dating is important to time interventions in later pregnancy, such as screening for Down syndrome or neural tube defects and the offer of labor induction for post-dates pregnancies.

A full medical examination is carried out during the first visit, including recordings of maternal height, weight and blood pressure. The cardiovascular and respiratory systems are carefully examined, and the breasts and nipples inspected and palpated. A cervical smear is taken if required. A specimen of blood is taken for full blood count, blood group and blood group antibodies, syphilitic serology and rubella status. Different ethnic or geographical groups require additional testing, such as hemoglobin electrophoresis for α and β trait-thalassemia (North Africa, East Mediterranean, Middle East), Sickledex test for sickle cell trait (sub-Saharan Africa, Caribbean) and hepatitis serology (Far East). Urine is tested for the presence of protein and glucose and a mid-stream specimen sent for bacteriological culture. Many centers also offer screening for cystic fibrosis, performed by analyzing DNA collected from a mouthwash for the major known mutations. If both partners have a mutation they would be offered a diagnostic test such as amniocentesis or chorion villus sampling (see below). Diet during pregnancy is discussed as well as social aspects such as housing, pets, work, etc. and advice given as appropriate. Further, breast-feeding is discussed and the mother is offered access to parenting classes which help prepare her for labor and the arrival of her baby. These classes run throughout her pregnancy and the attendance of her partner is encouraged.

At 16 weeks, gestation screening for neural tube defects and Down syndrome is offered. This is by the estimation of risk calculated from the mother's age and the measurement of α-fetoprotein (AFP) and human chorionic gonadotropin (hCG) in maternal blood (Wald 1995). In pregnancies complicated by a neural tube defect maternal serum AFP is elevated and in pregnancies complicated by Down syndrome AFP is reduced while hCG is elevated. If a woman is given a high risk of a neural tube defect then she would be offered a detailed fetal anomaly ultrasound scan for diagnostic purposes. Detection rates of approximately 90% (5% false positive rate) can be achieved by such an approach. A number of conditions are associated with an elevated maternal serum AFP (Table 4.1) but all of them can potentially be diagnosed by detailed ultrasound scanning – even threatened abortion which may be associated with an intrauterine hematoma can be directly imaged. If a woman has an increased risk of having a fetus affected by Down syndrome then she would be offered an amniocentesis or chorion villus sampling (CVS) giving detection rates of approximately 70% for a 5% false positive rate (Royal College of Obstetricians and Gynaecologists 1993). Both amniocentesis and CVS examine of the fetal karyotype but CVS is particularly useful for DNA analysis and the diagnosis of inborn errors of metabolism since the enzyme deficiency underlying these can be detected in the trophoblastic

Table 4.1 Causes of elevated maternal serum α-fetoprotein

Threatened abortion

Multiple pregnancy

Intrauterine death

Myelomeningocele

Anencephaly

Exomphalos

Gastroschisis

Turner's syndrome

Meckel–Gruber syndrome

Hemangioma of placenta/cord

Teratoma

villi. Table 4.2 lists the indications for amniocentesis and CVS. Initial studies suggested that CVS carried a higher risk of pregnancy loss than amniocentesis but this is no longer thought to be the case. However, CVS can be performed earlier in pregnancy than amniocentesis (from 10 weeks compared to 14 weeks) and a result thus obtained sooner. Thus CVS offers a diagnosis much earlier in pregnancy than amniocentesis. Some centers perform early amniocentesis (10–14 weeks) but no data from randomized trials exist to assess critically pregnancy outcome following this procedure and the pregnancy loss rates do appear to be higher (Byrne 1994). Few centers now perform CVS before 10 weeks following reports of fetal limb reduction defects at gestations earlier than this (Firth et al 1991).

It is also recognized that in pregnancies in which there are unexplained high maternal serum AFP and/or hCG levels there is an increased risk of preterm delivery, intrauterine growth retardation, antepartum hemorrhage and pregnancy-induced hypertension. The primary defect is thought to be an abnormality in placentation and subsequent close monitoring of maternal blood pressure and fetal growth is mandatory in these pregnancies.

The future management of a woman during her pregnancy depends on the problems already identified and further difficulties which may present during subsequent surveillance. Full hospital care, shared care with a local general practice, total general practitioner care, and community care by a midwife are all options which should be available to and discussed with the woman. While women with high-risk features such as a significant pre-existing medical disorder or a previous poor obstetric performance should receive obstetrician-led care, the majority of women should be able to receive their care in the community from midwives and/or general practitioners with few visits to hospital specialists. Formalized assessment of risk, however, has not been

Table 4.2 Indications for amniocentesis and chorion villus sampling

Chromosomal abnormality

Fetal sexing

DNA analysis

Inborn errors of metabolism

Neural tube defects*

Bilirubin estimation (suspected red cell hemolysis)*

* Amniocentesis only

found to be specific or sensitive enough to be of practical use. High risk status is more often than not a retrospective assessment.

Mid-pregnancy

At 18–20 weeks' gestation some centers offer routine fetal anomaly screening using ultrasound scanning and although detection rates differ, depending on the population and the expertise of the center, detection rates of 75% with a false positive rate of 0.02% have been reported (Chitty & Campbell 1992). Further, it has been shown that the perinatal mortality rate can be reduced with the use of routine fetal assessment by ultrasound (Saari-Kemppainen et al 1990).

At each routine visit blood pressure is checked, maternal weight taken and the urine is examined for protein and glucose. If a mother is rhesus negative and antibody negative at booking then blood is taken for repeat antibody screening at approximately 24 weeks. If she has antibodies present at booking then more frequent assessment of the titer is required with the sampling interval indicated by the previous result. Abdominal palpation allows measurement of the symphysis fundal height (SFH) which is a crude measurement of fetal growth: this value in centimeters should approximate to the gestational age in weeks. However, the value of the SFH in detecting babies that are small for gestational age (SGA) is disputed with sensitivities varying between 27% and 86% (Pearce & Robinson 1995). Nonetheless the routine measurement of the SFH is accepted practice and as such is an established component of antenatal surveillance.

In mothers assessed as high risk for the development of hypertension or fetal growth problems, either from a past history or from the results of screening tests, Doppler ultrasound examination of uterine artery blood flow may be useful. Women who have a persistent notch in the uterine artery waveform, indicative of impaired trophoblastic invasion of the spiral arterioles, have an almost 70-fold increase in the risk of developing pre-eclampsia (Bower et al 1993). Such women would thereafter have more intensive assessment of blood pressure and fetal growth/well-being. Despite previous small studies showing aspirin improved the outcome of high risk pregnancies (e.g. McParland et al 1989), a recent large trial and subsequent meta-analysis showed that this drug was not useful in the prevention of pre-eclampsia and IUGR (CLASP 1994).

Late pregnancy

From 28 weeks' gestation onwards the practitioner's attention focuses more on the maternal blood pressure and urinalysis, fetal growth and movements and latterly on fetal lie and presentation. Should an abnormality in any of these be detected then referral to an obstetrician would be expected. Measurement of the SFH has been discussed above and any pregnancy suspected to be SGA by this method would then be examined ultrasonographically. However, the most sensitive approach to the detection of SGA babies is to offer all women two ultrasound measurements rather than scanning only those thought to be at risk clinically. Indeed, many centers will routinely offer 'growth' scans to all pregnancies. While a number of different ultrasound measurements of the fetus can be taken the abdominal (trunk) circumference is the most sensitive and specific (Neilson et al 1980) largely because the biparietal diameter (BPD) is often difficult to measure in late pregnancy consequent upon the head being low in the pelvis and also because 'head-sparing' may occur in growth retardation.

If growth retardation is detected (less than the 5th percentile for gestation) then further investigation of the pregnancy is merited. The importance of being SGA is highlighted by a study from Dobson and co-workers (1981) who demonstrated that the perinatal mortality rates for babies with birthweights below the 5th percentile was 15 times that of babies with a birthweight above the 10th percentile. In the same study almost 17% of babies with a birthweight below the 5th percentile were found to have a major abnormality and ultrasound assessment for abnormality is an important investigation in such pregnancies. Indeed, the earlier the growth retardation the more likely it is that there will be an abnormality, particularly a chromosomal abnormality. Thus, the attending obstetrician will often consider cordocentesis or chorion villus biopsy if a fetus is shown to be severely growth retarded very early in pregnancy, particularly before 28 weeks of gestation. However, being SGA does not necessarily equate with growth retardation. Rather intrauterine growth retardation (IUGR) describes babies that are not fulfilling their growth potential. Thus many SGA babies will not have IUGR and as such will have a normal perinatal mortality rate. Similarly some babies with IUGR will have normal birthweights but still have a high perinatal mortality rate as a population. The challenge to the obstetrician is to discern IUGR babies from the rest of the population, whether SGA or not.

The most common cause of growth retardation is uteroplacental insufficiency, often in association with pre-eclampsia – the maternal expression of the same underlying process. Further investigation of SGA babies involves Doppler assessment of the uteroplacental and fetal circulations. In early pregnancy (before 28 weeks' gestation) if IUGR is suspected then assessment of the uterine arteries is worthwhile. Most likely these will be abnormal and low-dose aspirin might be considered as discussed above. Assessment of the fetal middle cerebral artery is also helpful and predictive of fetal compromise. In fetuses with IUGR the pulsatility index (PI = (systolic velocity × diastolic velocity)/mean velocity) of the Doppler waveform from the cerebral arteries decreases secondary to vasodilation. This arises as a result of centralization of the circulation, where there is decreased flow in the splanchnic circulation and increased flow in the cerebral circulation brought about as a protective mechanism by a fetus that is becoming hypoxic and acidemic. There is a correlation between the PI of the middle cerebral artery and umbilical PO_2 and pH in SGA babies (Vyas et al 1990) and a relationship between reduced cerebral vascular resistance and subsequent neurological abnormality (Rizzo et al 1989). Figure 4.1 demonstrates a suggested course of events at the most extreme end of the spectrum of the processes described above.

In pregnancies where IUGR is suspected at a more advanced gestation the umbilical artery Doppler flow velocity waveform (FVW) is the most useful investigation. Small fetuses with a

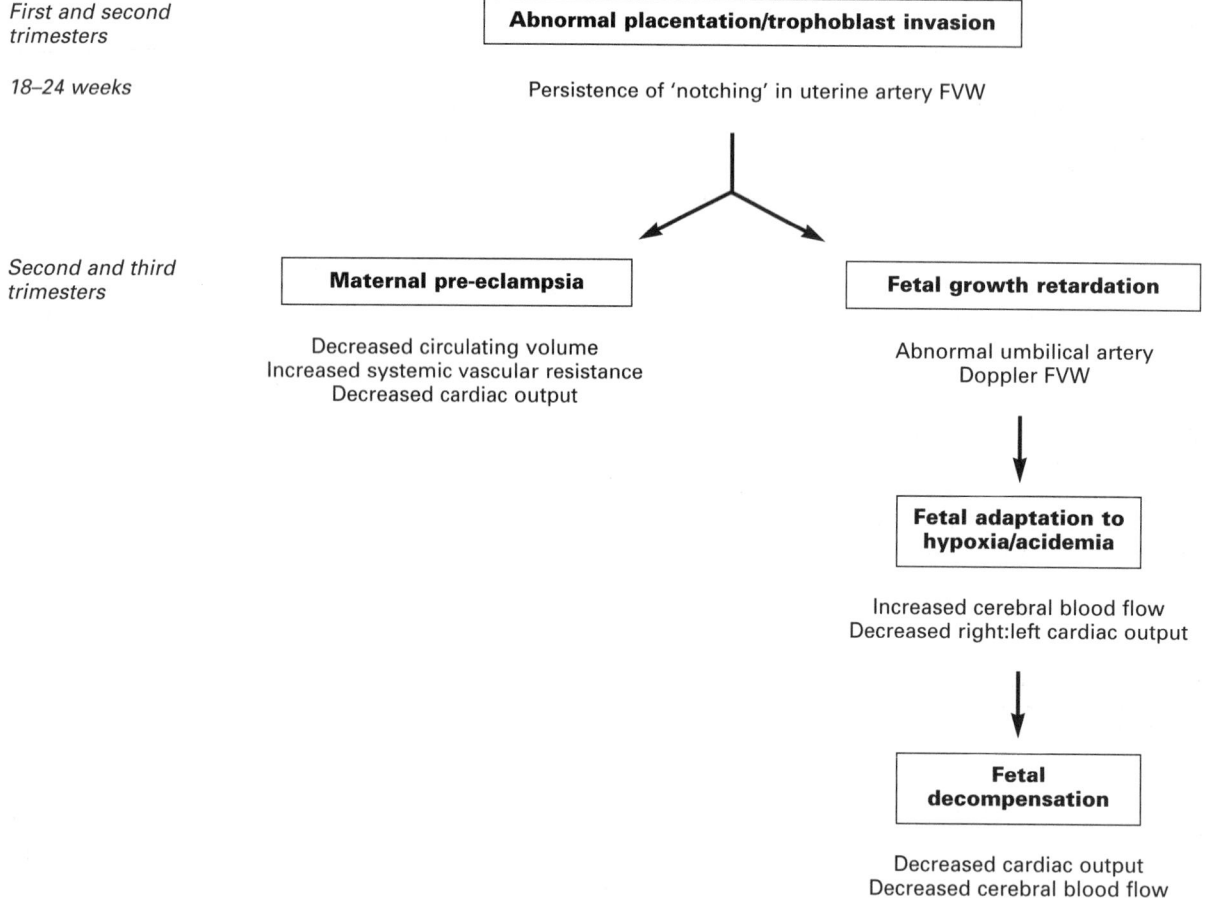

Fig. 4.1 Progression of fetal and maternal disease and Doppler flow velocity waveforms (FVWs) in pregnancies complicated by placental dysfunction.

normal umbilical artery Doppler FVW are not at increased risk antenatally and therefore discriminate those that are normal and constitutionally small from those SGA from IUGR. Unfortunately, when applied to the whole population Doppler assessment of the umbilical artery has not been shown to be as discriminating and has no screening role in unselected women. Interestingly, while absence of end-diastolic flow in the umbilical artery is associated with fetal hypoxia and an increased perinatal mortality, routine fetal monitoring of these pregnancies has not been shown to improve outcome (Mohide & Kierse 1989).

Near term assessment of the fetal lie and presentation becomes important. Although this is regularly assessed by abdominal-palpation throughout pregnancy it is of no particular significance until 36 weeks or later since no further action is usually required if an abnormal lie or presentation is found before this. Prior to discussing this further, some basic definitions are given below to aid understanding.

Lie: the relationship of the long axis of the fetus to that of the uterus – usually longitudinal, but occasionally transverse or oblique.

Presentation: the part of the fetus occupying the lowermost pole of the uterus – at term 96% are cephalic, 3% breech, and the remaining 1% include brow, face and shoulder.

Position: relationship of presenting part to the maternal bony pelvis – thus for vertex presentation the position may be occipitoanterior, occipitoposterior or occipitolateral. The position is not usually noted before labor and is of little significance until then.

Station: the height of the presenting part during labor, related to the ischial spines on vaginal examination. Before labor, and with vertex presentation, the station is assessed by abdominal examination and classified as 0/5 to 5/5 depending on the amount of head palpable above the pelvic brim: 5/5 head free; 0/5 head deeply engaged and impalpable.

Table 4.3 details causes of an abnormal lie or a high head at term. These should be considered particularly in primigravidae in whom it is expected that the head will be fixed in the pelvis by term. Further investigation, usually by ultrasound, will exclude these causes. If no cause can be found and the head is presenting but high there is no cause for concern. However, if there is an abnormal lie (oblique or transverse) then admission to hospital is usually recommended. If labor were to start and the membranes rupture in such cases then there is a high risk of cord prolapse and subsequent fetal demise. Should the lie remain abnormal but mobile then a stabilizing induction can be considered or delivery by Cesarean section performed by 41 weeks.

Table 4.3 Causes of malpresentation at term

Fetal abnormality
Placenta previa
Fibroid uterus
Multiple pregnancy
Multiparity
Polyhydramnios
Pelvic tumor
Contracted pelvic inlet
No abnormality

The diagnosis of a breech presentation is also important antenatally because it has significant implications for delivery. If suspected it is useful to confirm by ultrasound to exclude fetal abnormality, which is more common in pregnancies with a persistent breech presentation, or an abnormal placental site and to estimate fetal size which may be helpful in deciding further management. The dilemmas presented by a breech pregnancy at term relate to mode of delivery (see below) and can be avoided if the baby can be turned to a cephalic presentation. Instructing the mother to adopt a knee–elbow position encourages the breech to fall away from the pelvis and allows the baby to kick its own way round. In an uncontrolled trial such treatment when practiced for 15 minutes every 2 hours was shown to be beneficial but controlled trials have been less convincing (Chenia & Crowther 1987). However, there have been six randomized controlled trials of external cephalic version (ECV) at term and meta-analysis of these reveals a typical odds ratio of a noncephalic birth of 0.15 (95% confidence intervals 0.11–0.21) (Hofmeyer 1993). Thus ECV should be offered if there are no contraindications but only performed at term; ECV before term is not beneficial – most babies turn back spontaneously.

Postterm pregnancy

42 weeks of gestation (294 days from the last menstrual period) is traditionally accepted as postterm but it is now believed by many that pregnancies extending beyond 41 weeks are at an increased risk of perinatal problems including fetal death associated with asphyxia and meconium aspiration. Approximately a quarter of pregnancies will complete 41 weeks and 10% will complete 42 weeks. Postterm pregnancy is a considerable clinical problem. The clinician has essentially two management options: expectant management with close fetal surveillance or induction of labor. Of the various tests available for fetal surveillance, assessment of amniotic fluid volume is believed to be one of the most sensitive and now the most well established (Johnson et al 1986) although Doppler assessment of umbilical blood flow is also helpful (Pearce & McParland 1991). However, meta-analysis of trials comparing surveillance with induction reveals that induction of labor results in less fetal distress, fewer macrosomic babies, fewer meconium-stained liquor and fewer perinatal losses. Perhaps surprisingly, induction of labor is also associated with a reduced risk of Cesarean section or instrumental delivery, largely because of a reduction in the incidence of intrapartum fetal distress (Hannah 1993). Thus the evidence for encouraging women in whom pregnancy extends beyond 41 weeks to undergo induction of labor is compelling, although the final decision should of course remain with the mother.

INTRAPARTUM CARE

Place of delivery

The birth attendant constantly strives to deliver an infant in the best possible condition, avoiding asphyxia, trauma and infection. However, while most obstetricians might believe that this is optimally obtainable only in a hospital environment, this is not universally accepted and there are no controlled data to support this view. Nonetheless, the number of babies born in hospital in the UK has increased from 15% in the 1920s to 99% in the 1980s. Recognizing that there is some variation in parental wishes as to the site of delivery, particularly in the vocal middle classes, the UK government has recently called for increased choice in childbirth and, in particular, more home confinements (DoH 1993). The debate about the implications of the Government's wishes rage on and are well discussed elsewhere (Chamberlain & Patel 1994) but it is clear that while some mothers may feel reassured by delivering in a large referral center where complex modern technology is available, others desire the comfort of smaller midwife/GP units while others still prefer to deliver at home. The 'Domino' scheme is designed to allow a midwife to provide antenatal care in the community, and then to deliver the infant in hospital, returning the family to home a few hours later. The parents and their advisors have the extra responsibility of knowing that 'choice' for the parents must be compatible with the eventual well-being of the infant who has no vote. Recently the relative merits of midwife-run units and traditional consultant-led units for women assessed as low risk have been assessed by randomized trials. Essentially, while these have shown that in midwife units there is less intrapartum intervention with no increase in neonatal morbidity compared to consultant-led units, 40–50% of women will require transfer to a consultant unit, with approximately half of these transferred in labor (McVicar et al 1993, Hundley et al 1994). It would seem sensible therefore that if midwife/GP units are to be developed and encouraged they should be located within a consultant facility to ease transition of care.

Onset of parturition

In the human it is not yet clear what initiates the process of labor. In the sheep, which has been used extensively as an experimental model, there is a clear endocrine sequence, with activation of the fetal hypothalamopituitary–adrenal axis, resulting in alteration in the balance of placental production of estrogen (more) and progesterone (less), and this in turn stimulates the release of prostaglandins to initiate parturition. Similar systemic endocrine changes cannot be demonstrated in human pregnancies prior to labor although similar local changes within the uterus have been demonstrated. It is likely therefore that in human pregnancy the controlling mechanisms are paracrine and not endocrine.

Prior to labor, changes in the human cervix and myometrium occur that facilitate labor onset. To understand these changes the cervix and the corpus (myometrium) should be considered as separate organs, both anatomically and functionally. The uterine cervix is largely a connective tissue organ composed of collagen fibrils within a glycoprotein matrix, with a small component of elastin and smooth muscle. During normal pregnancy the ordered collagen fibrils responsible for the integrity and rigidity of the cervix in nonpregnancy and early pregnancy, become progressively less ordered, possibly resulting from exposure to collagenases and other proteases. Indeed, it has been shown that as pregnancy continues, protease activity within the cervix increases, a phenomenon associated with a decrease in total collagen content (Uldbjerg et al 1983). To explain this effect, the cervical leukocytes responsible for collagenase and other protease release may increase in both number and activity towards term (Junqueira et al 1980, Osmers et al 1992). This influx of activated neutrophils may be mediated by a combined effect of endogenous prostaglandins (e.g. PGE_2) and chemokines, such as interleukin-8 (IL-8) (Kelly 1994). In the corpus, towards term there is an increase in the production of gap junctions, allowing the uterus to contract as a syncytium and prostaglandins also upregulate the expression of oxytocin receptors in the myometrium, although increased secretion of oxytocin does not appear to occur. Prostaglandins, particularly PGF_2, also cause the myometrium to contract directly.

Progress in labor

The labor which progresses normally should involve gradual dilation of the cervix and descent of the presenting part, while uterine contractions become more frequent, more prolonged and usually more forceful and painful – eventually occurring every 3 min lasting 1–2 min with only 1–2 min in between. The muscle fibers of the uterus contract, relax, and retract, i.e. the resting length becomes less than when the contraction began. In many centers labor is displayed on a partogram, which usually describes cervical dilation in centimeters against time (Fig. 4.2).

Since the 1970s intervention in the form of routine amniotomy and early intravenous oxytocin to stimulate uterine activity has been widely practiced in primigravidae in the belief that it shortened labor, reduced fetal distress and lowered both Cesarean section and instrumental delivery rates. These and other measures were introduced by the National Maternity Hospital, Dublin as 'the active management of labor' (O'Driscoll et al 1967) and continue to form an essential component of routine labor management in many units around the world.

However, while active management certainly shortens labor and reduces operative intervention, the routine practice of amniotomy and the use of oxytocin probably have a limited role in these effects. Early amniotomy does modestly shorten labor but the most significant component of active management is the presence of a companion in labor (Klaus et al 1986, Thornton & Lilford 1994). This has been shown to afford all the effects that active management does and meta-analysis of trials assessing separately the components of active management show minimal effects of all except support. Indeed, the beneficial effects of support extend beyond the labor with more women breast-feeding for longer durations if they had a supporter in labor.

During labor the fetus undergoes a number of maneuvers, guided by the shape of the pelvis and the pelvic floor, ensuring that the narrowest part of the presenting part negotiates the widest part of the birth canal. Usually the fetal head enters the pelvic brim well flexed with the occiput directed laterally (left occipitolateral, right occipitolateral) and as descent progresses there is further neck flexion induced by pressure exerted from above. The fetal head then rotates (internal rotation) through the pelvis so that the occiput turns anteriorly. The fetal shoulders undergo the same rotation. The head on emergence should then be occipitoanterior, and it then 'restitutes' to take up the same alignment as the shoulders. The shoulders then descend into the lower pelvis, occupy an anteroposterior position, and the anterior shoulder emerges first from under the symphysis pubis, closely followed by the posterior shoulder. The second stage of labor is of mean duration 39 min in primigravid women and 15 min in parous women.

The labor partogram (Fig. 4.2) contains all observations made on mother during routine labor. Pulse, blood pressure, temperature, urine volume and urine content of ketones, protein and glucose, may be recorded. A careful assessment of pelvic size should be made on initial examination to determine the risk of cephalopelvic disproportion. Time zero on the partogram refers to the time of the mother's admission to the labor ward. Cervical

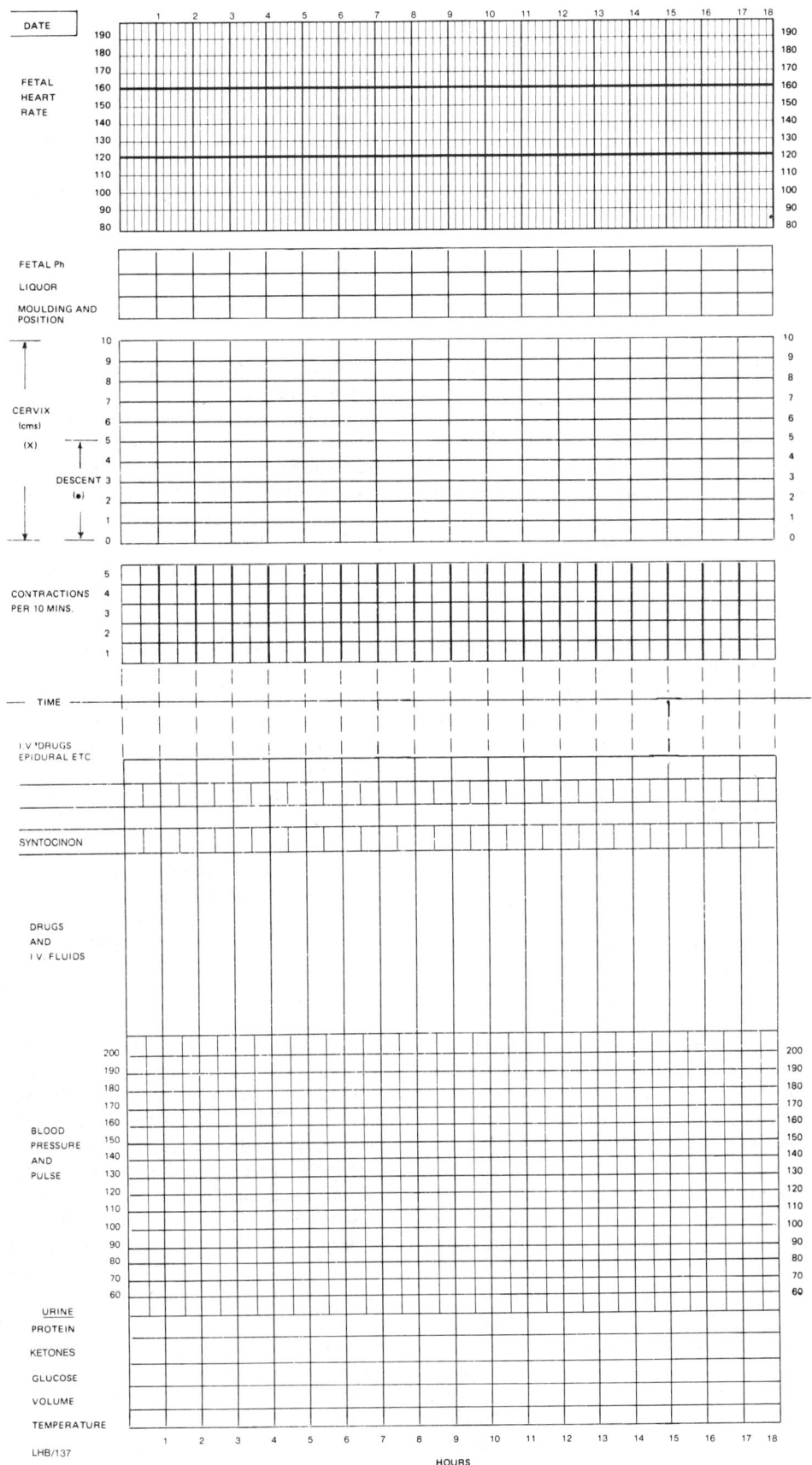

Fig. 4.2   Partogram in current use in the Simpson Memorial Maternity Pavilion, Edinburgh.

dilation, station of presenting part relative to the ischial spines measured in centimeters, fetal head position, degree of caput and molding, and the color of the liquor may all be recorded. Further, as labor progresses the use of analgesia and other interventions (amniotomy/oxytocin) are also noted. In this way the current maternal condition and changes in it over time are pictorially represented and readily interpreted, facilitating the recognition of problems.

It is also important to monitor the fetus during labor and record the findings on the partogram. Traditionally fetal monitoring was done by auscultation with a Pinard stethoscope. In the 1970s, however, electronic fetal monitoring (cardiotocography) was introduced to reduce the incidence of intrapartum stillbirth. Since then the routine use of CTGs has become widespread in modern labor wards with the added expectation of reducing neonatal morbidity. However, this hope has not been realized and prospective evaluation of electronic fetal monitoring versus intermittent auscultation in labor has revealed that electronic monitoring (EFM) does not decrease neonatal morbidity or mortality but instead increases the Cesarean section rate. This effect can be neutralized if EFM is supplemented by fetal blood sampling, assessing fetal acid–base balance (Neilson 1995), although using this approach the odds ratio of a Cesarean section for fetal distress compared to intermittent auscultation is still almost 2.0 with no improvement in neonatal outcome. Cardiotocography therefore, should not be used routinely in labor but instead reserved for when there are abnormalities on intermittent auscultation, the presence of antenatal risk factors or meconium-stained liquor (Neilson 1993).

Abnormalities of fetal heart rate during labor can be described in three categories:

1. changes in baseline heart rate
2. lack of baseline variability of heart rate
3. periodic changes with uterine contractions.

1. Changes in baseline heart rate. The normal baseline fetal heart rate is between 110 and 150 beats per minute. The very preterm infant may have a baseline heart rate greater than 160 per min, but fetal tachycardia also occurs with maternal or fetal infection, maternal anxiety, maternal hyperthyroidism, fetal anemia, and maternal exhaustion and dehydration. Similarly the postterm fetus may have a baseline heart rate below 110 per min, but constant bradycardia may also be a feature of congenital heart block, associated with maternal systemic lupus erythematosus. Profound maternal hypotension following an epidural insertion may also cause an acute onset of bradycardia, usually responding to correction of the maternal blood pressure.

2. Variability of heart rate. The length of time between successive heart beats varies from beat to beat in the normal fetus, reflecting the balance between the sympathetic and parasympathetic drives to the heart. This variation is usually 5–15 beats per min in amplitude and may be best observed on a cardiotocographic tracing. It is normal for baseline variation to be less in the preterm infant which may make interpretation more difficult. Variation is also diminished by maternal opiates, sedatives and local anesthetic agents but it is an important indicator of fetal hypoxia. Indeed, of the three elements baseline variability is the most useful in determining the well-being of a fetus

3. Periodic changes with uterine contractions. While accelerations in fetal heart rate are normal during uterine contractions and fetal movements, decelerations may be of pathological significance and should be examined carefully. They are generally classified as (a) early, (b) variable, (c) late. Early decelerations are relatively rare and are coincident with the uterine contraction, mirroring the contraction with the trough of the heart rate coinciding with the peak of the contraction and a return to the previous baseline by the time the contraction has ceased. This is a normal phenomenon due to pressure on the fetal head as it descends in the pelvis causing increased intracranial pressure and thus vagal slowing of the heart. Indeed, the commencement of deep early decelerations often heralds the second stage of labor. Variable decelerations are inconsistent in time of onset and in their shape on the cardiotocograph. They are commonly due to umbilical cord compression. Cord compression causes first occlusion in the umbilical vein, thus reducing venous return to the fetal heart, lowering blood pressure and so inducing a transient acceleration in the fetal heart rate. Then the umbilical arteries are occluded, inducing hypertension and thus a transient bradycardia or deceleration. As the contraction eases, the effects reverse, again with a transient acceleration at the end. These accelerations are often known as shouldering. On their own variable decelerations are not sinister and a healthy fetus can withstand the cord compressions without difficulty. However, if recurrent and persistent the fetus will become hypoxic and the baseline rate will rise and the variability decrease. The resulting complicated fetal tachycardia is sinister. Nursing the mother on her side, tilting the head end of the bed downwards, and giving her enriched facial oxygen to breathe may improve the fetal cardiotocograph tracing and if oxytocin is being administered it should be reduced. Late-onset decelerations are commonly due to fetal hypoxia or acidosis. Uterine contractions exacerbate the problems of the already compromised fetus, increasing the hypoxia, and causing fetal bradycardia which does not recover until after the contraction is over. The deceleration typically is most pronounced after the peak of the contraction when retroplacental oxygen reserves have been exhausted.

As described above the use of EFM without fetal scalp sampling cannot be sustained in modern obstetric practice. Capillary blood sampling from the fetal scalp is a logical and necessary sequel to the identification of an abnormal fetal heart rate either on cardiotocography or clinical auscultation. During the first stage of labor the mean fetal scalp blood pH is 7.33 and a value above 7.25 is widely regarded as normal. If a well-taken sample shows a pH less than 7.20, acidosis is present and delivery should be either anticipated or effected. Capillary pH values of between 7.20 and 7.25 merit careful clinical decisions to be taken on the basis of all information available, but, if no new factors occur, it may prove reasonable to wait and repeat the sample 1 hour later.

Despite the use of these monitoring techniques significant benefit in terms of improved fetal outcome has not been demonstrated when compared to simple intermittent auscultation. A possible reason for this was suggested by Murphy and co-workers (1990) who demonstrated that while gross CTG abnormalities were present in 87% of asphyxiated babies, but only in 29% of normal babies, labor staff were apparently unable to distinguish between severe and moderate CTG changes. Thus while the technology is able to detect fetal compromise arising in labor the attendants are failing to recognize it and take appropriate action. Further Nielson et al (1987) showed that even among experts there is very little agreement about the degree of severity of CTG abnormalities. These problems could be addressed by improved training for midwifery and junior medical staff, and the widespread introduction of computerized CTG analysis.

Induction of labor

The incidence of labor induction varies from unit to unit, depending on both the population and the attending obstetricians. Approximately 1 in 5 of all pregnancies will be induced in a modern maternity hospital but this rate can be reduced with accurate gestational dating, avoiding the induction of pregnancies erroneously thought to be postterm. The major indications for induction are: prolonged pregnancy, hypertensive disorders, fetal growth retardation or other concern for fetal well-being, maternal diabetes, and antepartum hemorrhage. Induction is most likely to succeed if the process mimics that of normal labor and in this regard it is important to achieve the changes described above prior to the commencement of uterine activity.

Throughout history a number of different, usually mechanical, methods of labor induction have found favor for periods of time. However, in modern obstetric practice the principal method of labor induction over the past 25 years, until fairly recently, was the stimulation of uterine activity using amniotomy and oxytocin (Turnbull & Anderson 1968). This was certainly used to good effect, which was probably due in part to the stimulated release of endogenous prostaglandins, but it became clear that such an approach was less efficient in women with an unripe cervix denoted by a low Bishop's score, particularly primigravidae (Calder 1977). In these women, while uterine activity was easily achievable, the duration of labor was often very prolonged and there was an unacceptably high incidence of complications necessitating Cesarean section. From such studies where induction of labor was undertaken in women with a low Bishop's score, it became clear that the uterine cervix, rather than the corpus, held the key to a successful outcome of labor induction. This understanding has led to the concept of artificial cervical ripening. Prostaglandins, particularly PGE$_2$, have been shown to have a role in bringing about the structural changes that constitute cervical ripening and it is now well established through considerable clinical research that the pharmacological use of prostaglandins is highly effective in achieving this ripening artificially (Kierse 1992). Indeed, meta-analysis of 35 trials, where prostaglandins have been evaluated against either placebo or no treatment, have shown that, disregarding the dose or route of prostaglandin administered, prostaglandins will confer a number of beneficial outcomes when used to ripen the cervix (Table 4.4). Overall therefore, it can be appreciated that the use of prostaglandins for cervical ripening is associated with significant

Table 4.4 Effects of prostaglandin vs placebo for cervical ripening on induction and labor

Improved cervical score
Earlier onset of labor
Shorter labor
Less epidural uptake
Fewer induction failures
Fewer Cesarean sections
Fewer instrumental vaginal deliveries

changes in the cervix, with a 60% reduction in induction failures and with a less complicated labor once induced (Kierse 1992). As with cervical ripening, there is now a large body of evidence from clinical research showing that prostaglandins are highly effective in labor induction even when the cervix is already ripe (Kierse 1993). Indeed when used to induce labor, compared to oxytocin, prostaglandins will confer a significantly shorter duration of labor, a lower rate of instrumental vaginal delivery, less uptake of analgesia and higher rates of maternal satisfaction (Kennedy et al 1982). It has also been shown that postpartum hemorrhage is significantly decreased in women receiving a prostaglandin induction compared to those undergoing amniotomy and oxytocin labor induction (Calder & Embrey 1975).

A number of PG preparations and routes of PG administration are available to the clinician for cervical priming and labor induction but in the UK the intravaginal administration of either prostaglandin gel, or more recently of retrievable slow-release preparations, has found most favor largely because of the ease of administration and established efficacy. In mainland Europe however, intracervical administration remains popular. While oral prostaglandin preparations exist, they have not been found to be particularly useful because of unpleasant systemic side effects.

Breech delivery

The management of a persistent breech presentation at term continues to arouse considerable debate in both obstetric and pediatric circles. There are no randomized controlled trials to guide practice, explaining the continued and significant differences of opinion. In a recent review of mature breech deliveries in London, UK (Thorpe-Beeston et al 1992) it was reported that the risk of intrapartum and neonatal death in association with vaginal delivery was almost 30 times that of Cesarean section (0.83% vs 0.03%). While this was an uncontrolled study and no data were given to judge whether the losses were attributable to the mode of delivery, such are the perceived risks to the fetus of a vaginal breech delivery that in the US over a 15-year period from 1970, the Cesarean section rate for breeches rose from almost 12% to almost 80% (Croughan-Minihane et al 1990). There is now a real risk that a generation of obstetricians is being trained which has little or no experience of vaginal breech delivery. If current trends continue therefore they will be almost irreversible, removing real choice from the population. Despite these increased rates of operative delivery there is no evidence that there has been an associated improvement in either immediate or long-term neonatal well-being (Green et al 1982). Such findings, the uncontrolled nature of existing trials, the maternal risks of Cesarean section and personal clinical experience have encouraged many clinicians to continue offering vaginal delivery in well-selected cases. It is this selection along with clinical experience that is the key to successful management of the term breech.

The management of preterm breech is no less confusing with numerous, uncontrolled trials showing that Cesarean section is safer than vaginal delivery and an equal number of equally uncontrolled trials showing that the mode of delivery does not significantly affect neonatal outcome. The problem peculiar to the preterm breech is that the head is large in proportion to the breech. Thus the breech may readily move through the pelvis leaving the unmolded head to become trapped in a partially dilated cervix. In one series 25% of deaths in preterm breeches delivered vaginally were due to head entrapment (Westergren et al 1985) although overall the outcomes for vaginal delivery were not significantly poorer than those for Cesarean births. While it is likely that the most important predictor of outcome is gestation, rather than mode of delivery, preterm infants, particularly those of gestation less than 34 weeks, are vulnerable to intraventricular hemorrhages which are commoner if the infant is delivered vaginally. It is therefore accepted practice to deliver abdominally babies presenting by the breech and weighing between 1000 and 1500 g while allowing the remainder to deliver vaginally if the expertise is available. Such a management strategy, however, is not evidence based (Myers & Gleicher 1987).

POSTPARTUM CARE

It should be clear that the quality of care that a woman receives during her pregnancy and labor may have important sequelae in the postpartum period. This is important not only for herself but also for her new baby and for the rest of the family. Many psychosocial problems encountered in the postnatal period can be prevented or helped by antenatal education, intrapartum support and postnatal support. For the baby one of the most important benefits of this care is the increased likelihood of breast-feeding and its longer maintenance once commenced.

OBSTETRIC COMPLICATIONS

The topics selected here are those relevant to pediatricians in their management of infants and in discussions with obstetricians and parents. The effects on the fetus and newborn of rarer maternal diseases are presented in Table 4.5.

ANTEPARTUM HEMORRHAGE

Before 24 weeks gestation significant vaginal bleeding is traditionally referred to as a threatened abortion while after 24 weeks gestation such bleeding is termed antepartum hemorrhage (APH). Bleeding at any stage of pregnancy occurs in approximately 10% of pregnancies and is associated with an increased perinatal mortality rate. Most commonly no cause is found, but it is essential to exclude placental abruption and placenta previa which are associated with considerable maternal and perinatal morbidity and mortality.

Placental abruption

Placental abruption (or accidental hemorrhage) is when there is hemorrhage from the decidual attachment of the placenta to the uterine wall. It occurs in approximately 1% of pregnancies, with a slightly increasing risk associated with increasing parity and maternal age. The exact etiology remains unknown but pregnancies associated with increased maternal serum markers in the second trimester are at increased risk (see above). Table 4.6 also shows other associated conditions. Classically, placental abruption will present with continuous, sometimes severe abdominal pain associated with vaginal bleeding. A posteriorly lying placenta may cause backache rather than abdominal pain. Because much or even all of the blood loss is hidden between decidua and chorionic membrane the degree of maternal shock

can be out of all proportion to the apparent blood loss. Abdominal palpation reveals a tense, hard and tender uterus and it may be difficult to identify the fetal heart by auscultation, whether or not fetal death has occurred. Placental abruption must be treated as a continuing emergency, since the placental separation can extend, threatening the life of both fetus and mother.

The continued management of a women with a placental abruption depends on the extent of the abruption, maternal well-being, fetal well-being and gestation. Clearly, at 38 weeks gestation delivery of a woman who has had only a minor abruption is often sensible while at 24 weeks gestation conservative management may be required even in the face of considerable blood loss. In any event the first priority is resuscitation of the mother with adequate intravenous access and the use of plasma expanders or whole blood as indicated. As the apparent blood loss may be significantly less than actual loss, a common mistake is to undertransfuse. The mother's coagulation status is ascertained and deficiencies are corrected; coagulation abnormalities are common consequent on the systemic release of placental thromboplastins.

Management thereafter, if the mother is stable, is dependent upon fetal well-being. If fetal demise has occurred then delivery is effected as soon as practicable to minimize further coagulation disturbance and potential DIC with other organ failure. Delivery is usually vaginal. If the fetal heart beat is still audible the senior obstetrician managing the emergency will take a clinical decision regarding the most appropriate course. Many women with an abruption will progress into labor, often laboring quickly, and with satisfactory fetal monitoring a vaginal delivery can be anticipated. The risk of profound asphyxia, however, is ever-present, since abruption may extend during the second stage of labor and in the face of fetal distress, or a labor progressing poorly, or a labor which may last several further hours, Cesarean section may be the safest course provided mother's coagulation status is under control. Fetal death and significant neonatal asphyxia are two significant complications of this acute obstetrical emergency. An expert pediatric presence at the delivery is essential.

Placenta previa

Placenta previa, when the placenta encroaches on the lower uterine segment, complicates approximately 0.5% of all pregnancies. Table 4.7 shows known associations. It is associated with significant maternal and neonatal morbidity and mortality (McShane et al 1985). Placenta previa usually presents as small quantities of painless bleeding, but in early labor hemorrhage may be torrential. The diagnosis may be suspected from an abnormal or unstable lie, especially a persistent transverse lie, but in many cases routine ultrasound scanning of fetus and placenta may reveal the problem. Unlike placental abruption, the maternal condition is usually good unless major hemorrhage has already occurred. Nevertheless an intravenous infusion should be started and cross-matched blood made available. The mother and fetus are carefully monitored.

There are many different classifications of placenta previa in the literature, each attempting to reflect the degree of previa and the implications for further management. It is now clear that the extent of the previa (i.e. how low it is and whether it partially or totally covers the internal cervical os) is not predictive of outcome with regard to likelihood of bleeding or the requirement for an emergency delivery (Love & Wallace 1996). Antenatal

Table 4.5 Maternal conditions and their effects on fetus and neonate

Maternal condition	Effects on fetus and pregnancy	Effects on infant	Maternal condition	Effects on fetus and pregnancy	Effects on infant
Diabetes mellitus	Macrosomia Microsomia Unexpected death Preterm delivery Polyhydramnios Fetal distress	RDS Hypoglycemia Hypocalcemia Polycythemia Poor feeding Sacral agenesis, other congenital anomalies	Congenital spherocytosis	Usually nil	50% chance of inheritance, jaundice
Hyperthyroidism (Graves' disease)	Transient goiter and hypothyroidism if mother treated with propylthiouracil or iodides	Thyrotoxicosis due to thyroid-stimulating immunoglobulins	Glucose-6-phosphate dehydrogenase deficiency	Nil	Jaundice, anemia
			Appendicitis	Abortion, preterm labor	Problems of prematurity
Hypothyroidism Acquired	Usually nil	Small decrease in IQ if mother's treatment inadequate	Intrahepatic cholestasis	Hypoxia, preterm labor	Prematurity, asphyxia
Familial thyroiditis	Usually nil	Usually nil	Rhesus sensitization	Hydrops fetalis, pleural effusions	Anemia, jaundice, hydrops
Hyperparathyroidism	Increased fetal loss	Tetany	Dystrophia myotonica	Decreased fetal activity, may be polyhydramnios	50% chance of inheritance, respiratory distress
Polycystic disease (adult type)	50% have polycystic disease	Usually nil in childhood	Rubella	Growth retardation	Nerve deafness, cataract, microphthalmos, congenital heart disease, mental retardation
Cushing's syndrome	Death in utero Growth retardation Preterm delivery	Problems of low birthweight			
Epilepsy	Intermittent hypoxia with maternal seizures, teratogenic effects of anticonvulsants	Maternal phenytoin may cause cleft lip and palate, heart defects, anemia	Sickle cell disease (homozygous HbSS)	Growth retardation, preterm delivery, hemorrhage, death	Asphyxia
Myasthenia gravis	Nil	10% have transient myasthenia and some need treatment with anticholinesterase	Sickle cell trait (heterozygous HbAS)	Nil	No clinical problem
			α-thalassemia	Anemia, hydrops	Anemia
Viral hepatitis	Abortion, stillbirth, preterm delivery	Problems of prematurity, viremia, hepatitis, later cirrhosis and hepatocellular carcinoma	β-thalassemia	Anemia	Jaundice, anemia
			Disseminated intravascular coagulation	Death, asphyxia, preterm delivery	Asphyxia, prematurity
Acyanotic heart disease	Premature labor, growth retardation	Problems of low birthweight	Idiopathic thrombocytopenic purpura	Thrombocytopenia	Thrombocytopenia, hemorrhage
Cyanotic heart disease	Premature labor, growth retardation, asphyxia, death	Problems of low birthweight	Urinary tract infection	Preterm delivery	Prematurity, congenital infection
Thromboembolism	Warfarin causes teratogenesis and fetal hemorrhage		Systemic lupus erythematosus	Heart block	Thrombocytopenia, lupus syndrome, heart block

Table 4.6 Conditions associated with placental abruption

Hypertensive disorders

Trauma

Uterine abnormalities

Placental abnormalities

Smoking

Poverty

Table 4.7 Conditions associated with placental previa

Increasing maternal age

Increased parity

Previous uterine surgery

Placental abnormalities

Smoking

Multiple pregnancy

management should therefore not be based on the degree of previa. Rather, it is the management at delivery that depends on this. Thus a simple but useful classification is:

Major previa: a previa requiring delivery by Cesarean section
Minor previa: a previa consistent with a vaginal delivery.

Since the 1940s management of this condition has been conservative and supportive, delivering only when the fetus is mature or when there is persistent bleeding compromising either mother or fetus. Once bleeding has stopped it has been traditional that mothers are maintained in hospital until delivery but this approach has recently been questioned (Silver et al 1984, Rosen & Peek 1994) and outpatient care would appear safe for most women. Rather than the antenatal period, it is delivery that is associated with significant risk. Cesarean section for placenta previa may be hazardous, particularly if the placenta is anterior, since the obstetrician may be compelled to cut through it despite the risks of major fetal blood loss. Such are the risks of maternal death that successive reports, e.g. Confidential Enquiries into Maternal Deaths in the United Kingdom (HMSO 1994) have recommended that a senior obstetrician is present at delivery.

MULTIPLE PREGNANCY

The incidence of multiple pregnancy in the UK is approximately 1 in 80, although the incidence is increasing in the West secondary to assisted reproductive technologies. Monozygotic twins occur with an incidence of 1 in 250. Dizygotic twins are commoner if there is a family history (on mother's side) and also may vary with race, age, parity, and response to drug-induced ovulation. The perinatal mortality rate of twin pregnancies is approximately six times that for singleton pregnancies (Neilson & Crowther 1993) primarily because of the increased chance of preterm delivery, growth abnormalities, congenital anomaly, and asphyxia of the second twin. Early identification of multiple pregnancy by ultrasound affords the opportunity to organize specialist care aimed at minimizing risk factors for the most significant of these complications – preterm labor – and the early identification and management of growth problems. Ultrasound also allows assessment of zygosity which is important because monozygotic pregnancies, particularly monochorionic, monoamniotic, are at very high risk of perinatal loss.

Antenatal visits should be at 2-weekly intervals after 20 weeks and some authorities recommend cervical assessment to predict preterm labor (Neilson & Crowther 1993). While labor cannot be effectively prevented, knowledge of a likely delivery allows the administration of corticosteroids to the mother, a strategy that will significantly improve neonatal outcome should delivery occur preterm. Further, from 28 weeks gestation 2-weekly assessment of fetal growth by ultrasound is helpful in the detection of growth retardation. Discrepancy in growth between the fetuses of over 20% is suggestive of twin–twin transfusion, a complication that is associated with significant perinatal loss. Hypertension, anemia and placenta previa are associated with multiple pregnancies, and should be sought and treated.

Labor is also a time of particular risk for twin pregnancies. Satisfactory monitoring of both fetuses is often difficult and usually requires a fetal scalp electrode for the first twin and external monitoring of the second. Vaginal delivery can be anticipated if the first twin is cephalic, irrespective of the presentation of the second (Adam et al 1991) but most authorities would recommend Cesarean section if the lead twin is breech. During labor epidural anesthesia is the pain relief of choice as it allows internal manipulation of the second twin should a malpresentation arise (Jarvis & Whitfield 1981). The mean interval between delivery of twins is approximately 20 minutes but as long as the fetal heart rate of the second twin is satisfactory there is no evidence that a delay is harmful and so delivery should

not be expedited. After delivery zygosity should be determined by careful examination of the placenta.

HYPERTENSIVE DISORDERS

Hypertensive disorders complicate 10% of all pregnancies, and are the leading cause of maternal mortality in the UK and a leading cause of perinatal morbidity and mortality. There are a number of different classifications of the disorders (Roberts & Redman 1993, Chari et al 1995), used by different authorities. However, essentially all classifications attempt to discern chronic hypertension existing before pregnancy from new-onset hypertension during pregnancy. For the latter, it is also worthwhile differentiating between those women without proteinuria (pregnancy-induced hypertension) and those with proteinuria (pre-eclampsia).

The underlying pathophysiology of pre-eclampsia/pregnancy-induced hypertension (PIH) is not fully understood but involves a primary placental abnormality resulting in the release of unknown factors which exert the well-described features of the disease. Thus the disease can be predominantly expressed in the mother (hypertension, platelet activation, proteinuria, etc.), in the fetus (growth retardation, hypoxia) or in both. The course of the disease is unpredictable, sometimes remaining stable for weeks and occasionally progressing rapidly, requiring emergency delivery. However, in general the earlier the disease onset the more severe it will be.

Management of PIH or pre-eclampsia depends on the predominant expression. If hypertension is the most significant problem then the risks are to the mother. The most significant risk is of cerebral hemorrhage or edema and so the hypertension requires correction. This can be achieved by either delivering the fetus (and therefore placenta) if mature, or, if preterm, by using antihypertensive medication to allow improved fetal maturity. Throughout treatment close observation of the fetus should be made and assessment of umbilical artery FVWs is useful in directing management. In addition to the hypertension, maternal urinary protein should be measured over a 24-hour period, plasma urea, electrolytes, creatinine and urate assessed and maternal platelet count measured. These will assist in the assessment of risk to both mother and fetus (Redman et al 1976).

If fetal expression predominates, then assessment of fetal well-being will allow continuation of the pregnancy until a desirable maturity or until it becomes obvious that the fetus would be better delivered. Close observation of the mother is still required to detect any developing abnormalities. In essence then management of pre-eclampsia/PIH is dependent on the gestation of the pregnancy, how the disease is expressed and the severity of the abnormalities. For more complete discussion of this important condition the interested reader is referred to specialist texts (Greer 1992, Redman & Roberts 1993, Chari et al 1995).

EFFECTS OF MATERNAL DRUGS ON FETUS AND NEWBORN

Since the thalidomide disaster there has been increased awareness of drug teratogenicity. Agents administered in the early days after fertilization may cause abortion. Teratogens later in the first trimester may result in severe malformations. Late in pregnancy toxic effects are much less likely and usually cause only minor disturbances. The effects of some maternal drugs on the fetus and neonate are shown in Table 4.8.

Table 4.8 Effects of maternal drugs on fetus and neonate

Maternal drug taken during pregnancy	Effects on fetus/newborn
Alcohol	Low birthweight, microcephaly, congenital heart disease, mental retardation
Androgens	Teratogenesis in first trimester, virilization of female fetus
Atropine	Tachycardia
Beta-blockers	Decreased physiological response to asphyxia
Busulfan	Uncertain
Cyclophosphamide	Teratogenesis in first trimester
Diuretics	? decreased birthweight
Diazepam	Respiratory depression
Diethylstilbestrol	Genital anomalies, females may develop clear cell carcinoma of the vagina many years later; males, infertility
Hydralazine	Hypotension and hypothermia
Magnesium sulfate	Hypotonia, lethargy, ileus
Methotrexate	Cranial and digital malformations
Phenobarbitone	Dysmorphic facies, hypocalcemia and coagulation defects
Phenytoin	Embryopathy includes dysmorphic facial features, microcephaly and motor and intellectual retardation
Ritodrine	Hypoglycemia
Tetracycline	Tooth enamel hypoplasia and cataracts
Thalidomide	Phocomelia
Valproate	? spina bifida
Warfarin	Embryopathy including central nervous system anomalies

REFERENCES

Adam C, Allen A C, Baskett T F 1991 Twin delivery: influence of the presentation and method of delivery on the second twin. American Journal of Obstetrics and Gynecology 165: 23–27

American College of Obstetricians and Gynecologists 1988 Guidelines for prenatal care. American Academy of Pediatricians and American College of Obstetricians and Gynecologists, Washington DC, pp 54–55

Bower S, Bewley S, Campbell S 1993 Improved prediction of preeclampsia by two-stage screening of uterine arteries using the early diastolic notch and color Doppler imaging. Obstetrics and Gynecology 82: 78–83

Broughton Pipkin F, Turner S R, Symonds E M 1980 Possible risks with captropril in pregnancy: some animal data. Lancet i: 1256

Byrne D L 1994 Early amniocentesis. Fetal and Maternal Medicine Review 6: 203–218

Calder A A 1977 The unripe cervix. 57th William Blair Bell Memorial Lecture, June 1977. Royal College of Obstetricians and Gynaecologists, London

Calder A A 1994 Contributions of the professions. In: Chamberlain G, Patel N (eds) The future of the maternity services. RCOG Press, London

Calder A A, Embrey M P 1975 Comparison of intravenous oxytocin and prostaglandin E2 for induction of labour using automatic and non-automatic infusion techniques. British Journal of Obstetrics and Gynaecology 82: 728–733

Chamberlain G 1978 A re-examination of antenatal care. Journal of the Royal Society of Medicine 71: 662–668

Chamberlain G, Patel N (eds) 1994 The future of the maternity services. RCOG Press, London

Chari R S, Friedman S A, Sibai B M 1995 Antihypertensive therapy during pregnancy. Maternal and Fetal Medicine Reviews 7: 61–75

Chenia F, Crowther C 1987 Does advice to assume the knee-chest position reduce the incidence of breech presentation at delivery? A randomised clinical trial. Birth 14: 75–78

Chitty L, Campbell S 1992 Ultrasound screening for fetal abnormalities. In: Brock D J H, Rodeck C H, Ferguson-Smith M A (eds) Prenatal diagnosis and screening. Churchill Livingstone, Edinburgh, pp 595–610

CLASP Collaborative Group 1994 CLASP: a randomised trial of low-dose aspirin for the prevention and treatment of pre-eclampsia among 9364 pregnant women. Lancet 343: 619–628

Croughan-Minihane M, Petitti D, Gordis L, Golditch I 1990 Morbidity among breech infants according to method of delivery. Obstetrics and Gynecology 75: 821–825

Department of Health 1993 Changing childbirth. HMSO, London

Dobson P C, Abell D A, Beischer N A 1981 Mortality and morbidity of fetal growth retardation. Australian and New Zealand Journal of Obstetrics and Gynaecology 21: 69–72

Expert Advisory Group Report 1992 Folic acid and the prevention of neural tube defects. Department of Health, London

Firth H V, Boyd P A, Chamberlain P, MacKenzie I Z, Lindenbaum R H, Huson S M 1991 Severe limb abnormalities after chorion villus sampling at 55–66 days gestation. Lancet 337: 762–763

Green J F, McLean F, Smith L P, Usher R 1982 Has an increased cesarean section rate for term breech delivery reduced the incidence of birth asphyxia, trauma, and death? American Journal of Obstetrics and Gynecology 142: 643–648

Greer I A 1992 Hypertension. In: Calder A A, Dunlop W (eds) High risk pregnancy. Butterworth Heinemann, Oxford, pp 30–93

Hannah M E 1993 Postterm pregnancy: should all women have labour induced? Maternal and Fetal Medicine Reviews 5: 3–18

Henriksen TB, Hedegaard M, Secher N J, Wilcox A J 1995 Standing at work and preterm delivery. British Journal of Obstetrics and Gynaecology 102: 198–206

HMSO 1994 Confidential enquiries into maternal deaths in the United Kingdom 1988–1990. HMSO, London

Hofmeyer G 1993 External cephalic version at term. Maternal and Fetal Medicine Reviews 5: 213–222

House of Commons Health Committee 1992 Second report on the maternity services. HMSO, London

Hundley V A, Cruickshank F M, Lang G D, Glazener C M A, Milne J M, Turner J M, Blyth D, Mollison J, Donaldson C 1994 Midwife managed delivery unit: a randomised controlled comparison with consultant led care. British Medical Journal 309: 1400–1404

Jarvis G T, Whitfield M F 1981 Epidural analgesia and the delivery of twins. Journal of Obstetrics and Gynaecology 2: 90–92

Johnson J M, Harman C R, Lange I R, Manning F A 1986 Biophysical profile scoring in the management of the postterm pregnancy: an analysis of 307 patients. American Journal of Obstetrics and Gynecology 154: 269–273

Junqueira L C U, Zugaig M, Montes G S, Toledo O M S, Kriszian R M, Shigihara K M 1980 Morphologic and histochemical evidence for the occurrence of collagenolysis and for the role of neutrophilic polymorphonuclear leukocytes during cervical dilation. American Journal of Obstetrics and Gynecology 138: 273–281

Kelly R W 1994 Pregnancy maintenance and parturition; the role of prostaglandin in manipulating the immune and inflammatory response. Endocrine Reviews 15: 684–706

Kennedy J H, Stewart P, Barlow D H, Calder A A 1982 Induction of labour: a comparison of a single prostaglandin E2 vaginal tablet with amniotomy and intravenous oxytocin. British Journal of Obstetrics and Gynaecology 89: 704–707

Kierse M J N C 1992 Any prostaglandin/any route for cervical ripening. In: Enkin M W, Kierse M J N C, Renfrew M J, Nielson J P (eds) Pregnancy and childbirth module, Cochrane database of systematic reviews: review no: 04534. Update Software, Oxford

Kierse M J N C 1993 Any prostaglandin (by any route) vs oxytocin (any route) for induction of labour. In: Enkin M W, Kierse M J N C, Renfrew M J, Nielson J P (eds) Pregnancy and childbirth module, Cochrane database of systematic reviews: review no: 04536. Update Software, Oxford

Klaus M H, Kennel J H, Robertson S S, Sosa R 1986 Effects of social support during parturition on maternal and infant morbidity. British Medical Journal 293: 585–587

Love C D B, Wallace E M 1996 Pregnancies complicated by placenta praevia; what is appropriate management? British Journal of Obstetrics and Gynaecology 103: 864–867

McParland P, Pearce J M, Chamberlain G V P 1989 Doppler ultrasound and aspirin in recognition and prevention of pregnancy-induced hypertension. Lancet 335: 1552–1555

McShane P M, Heyl P S, Epstein M F 1985 Maternal and perinatal morbidity resulting from placenta previa. Obstetrics and Gynecology 65: 176–182

McVicar J, Dobbie G, Owen-Johnstone L, Jagger C, Hopkins M, Kennedy J 1993 Simulated home delivery in hospital: a randomised controlled trial. British Journal of Obstetrics and Gynaecology 100: 316–323

Mohide P, Kierse M J N C 1989 Biophysical assessment of fetal wellbeing. In: Enkin M, Kierse M J N C, Chalmers I (eds) Effective care in pregnancy and childbirth. Oxford University Press, Oxford

Murphy K W, Johnson P, Moorcraft J, Pattison R, Russell V, Turnbull A 1990 Birth asphyxia and the intrapartum cardiotocograph. British Journal of Obstetrics and Gynecology 97: 470–479

Myers S A, Gleicher N 1987 Breech delivery: why the dilemma? American Journal of Obstetrics and Gynaecology 154: 900–903

Neilson J P 1993 Cardiotocography during labour. British Medical Journal 306: 347–348

Neilson J P 1995 EFM + scalp sampling vs intermittent auscultation in labour. In: Enkin M W, Kierse M J N C, Renfrew M J, Neilson J P (eds) Pregnancy and childbirth module of the Cochrane database of systematic reviews, 1995 [updated 24 February 1995]

Neilson J P, Crowther C A 1993 Preterm labour in multiple pregnancies. Maternal and Fetal Medicine Reviews 5: 105–119

Neilson J P, Whitfield C R, Aitchison T C 1980 Screening for the small-for-dates fetus: a two stage ultrasound examination schedule. British Medical Journal 2280: 1203–1206

Nielson P, Stigsby B, Nickelson C, Nim J 1987 Intra- and inter-observer variability in the assessment of intrapartum cardiotocograms. Acta Obstretrica et Gynaecologica Scandinavica 66: 421–424

O'Driscoll K, Jackson J A, Gallagher J T 1967 Prevention of prolonged labour. British Medical Journal ii: 477–480

Osmers R, Rath W, Adelmann-Grill B C, Fittkow C, Kuloczik M, Szeverenyi M, Tschesche H, Kuhn W 1992 Origin of cervical collagenase during parturition. American Journal of Obstetrics and Gynecology 166: 1455–1460

Papiernik E 1993 Prevention of preterm labour and delivery. Bailliere's Clinical Obstetrics and Gynaecology 7: 499–522

Pearce J M, McParland P J 1991 A comparison of Doppler flow velocity waveforms, amniotic fluid columns, and the non-stress test as a means of monitoring post-dates pregnancies. Obstetrics and Gynecology 77: 204–208

Pearce J M, Robinson G 1995 Fetal growth and intrauterine growth retardation. In: Chamberlain G (ed) Obstetrics. Churchill Livingstone, Edinburgh, pp 299–312

Poswillo D, Alberman E 1992 Effects of smoking on the fetus, neonate and child. Oxford University Press, Oxford

Redman C W G, Roberts J M 1993 Management of pre-eclampsia. Lancet 341: 1451–1454

Redman C W G, Beilin L J, Bonnar J et al 1976 Plasma urate measurement in predicting fetal death in hypertensive pregnancy. Lancet i: 1370–1373

Rizzo G, Luciano R, Arduini D, Rizzo C, Tortorolo G, Romanini C, Mancuso S 1989 Prenatal cerebral Doppler ultrasonography and neonatal neurologic outcome. Journal of Ultrasound in Medicine 8: 237–240

Roberts J M, Redman C W G 1993 Pre-eclampsia: more than pregnancy-induced hypertension. Lancet 341: 1447–1451

Rosen D M B, Peek M J 1994 Do women with placenta praevia without ante-partum haemorrhage require hospitalisation? Australian and New Zealand Journal of Obstetrics and Gynaecology 342: 130–134

Royal College of Obstetricians and Gynaecologists 1985 Statement of Scientific Advisory Committee on alcohol consumption in pregnancy. RCOG, London

Royal College of Obstetricians and Gynaecologists 1993 Report of the RCOG working party on biochemical markers and the detection of Down's syndrome. RCOG Press, London

Saari-Kemppainen A, Karjalainen O, Ylostalo P, Heinonen O P 1990 Ultrasound screening and perinatal mortality: a controlled trial of systematic one-stage screening in pregnancy. Lancet 336: 387–391

Silver R, Depp R, Sabbagha R E, Dooley S L, Socol M I, Tamura R K 1984 Placenta previa: aggressive expectant management. American Journal of Obstetrics and Gynecology 150: 15–22

Thornton J G, Lilford R J 1994 Active management of labour: current knowledge and research issues. British Medical Journal 309: 366–369

Thorpe-Beeston J G, Banfield P J, Saunders N J St G 1992 Outcome of breech delivery at term. British Medical Journal 305: 746–747

Tucker J S, Howie P W, Florey C D U V, McIlwaine G, Hall M H 1994 Is antenatal care apportioned according to risk? Journal of Public Health Medicine 16: 60–70

Turnbull A C, Anderson A B M 1968 Induction of labour; results with amniotomy and oxytocin titration. Journal of Obstetrics and Gynaecology of the British Commonwealth 75: 32–41

Uldbjerg N, Ekman G, Malmstrom A 1983 Ripening of the human uterine cervix related to changes in collagen, glycosaminoglycans and collagenolytic activity. American Journal of Obstetrics and Gynecology 147: 662–666

Vyas S, Campbell S, Bower S, Nicolaides K H 1990 Middle cerebral artery flow velocity waveforms in fetal hypoxaemia. British Journal of Obstetrics and Gynaecology 97: 797–803

Wald N J 1995 Biochemical detection of neural tube defects and Down's syndrome. In: Chamberlain G (ed) Obstetrics. Churchill Livingstone, Edinburgh, pp 195–209

Westergren L M R, Songster G, Paul R H 1985 Preterm breech delivery: another retrospective study. Obstetrics and Gynecology 66: 481–484

5 The newborn

Chapter editor: N. McIntosh

Introduction
Definitions – World Health Organization (WHO) 94
N. McIntosh
Epidemiology, birthweight standards, perinatal
    mortality and morbidity 94
N. McIntosh
The environment of care 96
D. Wolke T. Eldridge
The ethics of newborn care 100
A. G. M. Campbell
The economics of newborn care 104
M. Mugford
The normal fetal–neonatal transition 106
N. McIntosh
Routine care of the full-term infant
Examination of the neonate 109
N. McIntosh
Labor ward routines 111
N. McIntosh
Postnatal ward routines 111
N. McIntosh
Feeding the full-term newborn 112
N. McIntosh
The high-risk fetus and infant
High-risk pregnancy 113
F. D. Johnstone
High-risk delivery 116
F. D. Johnstone
Birth trauma 120
N. McIntosh
Birth asphyxia 123
M. I. Levene
Hypoxic-ischemic encephalopathy (HIE) 125
M. I. Levene
Resuscitation of the newborn 132
M. I. Levene
The small for gestational age infant 136
N. McIntosh
The large for gestational age infant 138
N. McIntosh
Care of the preterm infant
Delivery room care 138
N. McIntosh

Special care 139
    Fluid balance 139
    T. Stephenson N. Rutter
    Sodium and potassium 143
    T. Stephenson N. Rutter
    Thermoregulation 145
    N. Rutter
    Enteral nutrition 150
    P. R. F. Dear S. J. Newell
Intensive care 155
    Organization of neonatal intensive care services 155
    N. McIntosh
    Practical parenteral nutrition 157
    N. McIntosh
    Blood gases and respiratory support 159
    W. Tarnow-Mordi B. Stenson
    Neurodevelopmental outcome 165
    J. M. Rennie
    Neonatal death 172
    N. McIntosh
Problems of the newborn
Pulmonary disorders and apnea 175
H. L. Halliday
Neonatal cardiovascular disease 198
L. N. J. Archer
Gastrointestinal problems and jaundice of the neonate 206
T. R. Fenton
Hematological problems of the newborn 221
T. L. Turner
Neonatal neurology 235
J. M. Rennie
Renal disease in the neonate 253
W. S Uttley
Eye problems and the newborn 262
A. R. Fielder
Infection and immunity in the newborn 273
K. H. Haque
Neonatal neoplasia 289
N. McIntosh
Neonatal metabolic disorders 290
R. Hume
References 309

INTRODUCTION

DEFINITIONS – WORLD HEALTH ORGANIZATION (WHO)

GESTATION (INDEPENDENT OF BIRTHWEIGHT)

1. Preterm = less than 37 completed weeks of gestation (258 days).
2. Full term = between 37 weeks and 42 completed weeks of gestation (259–293 days).
3. Post-term or postmature = more than 42 completed weeks (294 days).

Dates are taken from the first day of the last menstrual period. Conception is presumed to be approximately 2 weeks after this date. Ultrasound dates are based on conception and have to be altered to fit with the dates estimated from the last menstrual period.

BIRTHWEIGHT (INDEPENDENT OF GESTATION)

1. Low birthweight = less than 2500 g.
2. Very low birthweight = less than 1500 g (accepted by convention).
3. Extremely low birthweight (USA – very, very low birthweight) = less than 1000 g (accepted by convention).
4. Impossibly or incredibly low birthweight = (less than 750 g).

SIZE FOR GESTATION (Fig. 5.1)

1. Small for gestation (SGA) = less than 10th centile in weight expected for gestation (small for dates).
2. Appropriate for gestation (AGA) = between 10th and 90th centiles of weight expected for gestation.
3. Large for gestation (LGA) = more than 90th centile in weight expected for gestation.

NB: The expected weight centiles will vary with the population. The terms immature, premature and dysmature should no longer be used.

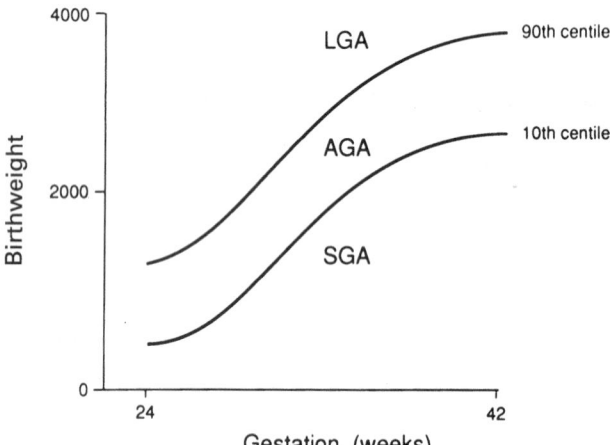

Fig. 5.1 Size for gestation based on population centiles for birthweight with gestation: LGA – large for gestational age; AGA – appropriate for gestational age; SGA – small for gestational age (less than the 10th centile expected weight for gestation).

AGE

In utero

1. Less than 1 week = fertilized egg to the formation of the blastocyst.
2. 1–12 weeks = embryo.
3. 12 weeks–delivery = fetus.
4. 24 weeks or more = current period of 'legal' viability in the UK.

In the UK it is uncommon to terminate a pregnancy after 20 weeks of gestation, though it is legal through to term for major fetal anomaly or maternal life-threatening problem (Human Embryo and Fertilization Act 1990).

Abortion is the expulsion of the dead fetus prior to 24 weeks' gestation (168 days). A dead fetus expelled after this time is a **stillbirth**. Note that a liveborn baby is a baby of *any gestation* that has signs of life (e.g. only a heart beat) at delivery. Many miscarriages before 20 weeks' gestation will show signs of life.

The neonate

1. Perinatal period = the period from 24 weeks' gestation or the time of the live birth if less than 24 weeks' gestation, to 7 days of postnatal age.
2. Early neonatal period = the first 7 days of life of a liveborn infant of *any* gestation.
3. Late neonatal period = 8–28 days after birth.
4. Neonatal period = the first 28 days of life of a liveborn infant of *any* gestation.
5. Infancy = the first year of life.

MORTALITY RATES

1. Stillbirth rate = number of stillbirths per 1000 total births.
2. Perinatal mortality rate (PMR) = number of stillbirths + early (up to 7 days) neonatal deaths per 1000 total births.
3. Neonatal mortality rate (NNMR) = number of deaths in the first 28 days per 1000 live births.
4. Infant mortality rate (IMR) = number of deaths in the first 365 days per 1000 live births.

Maternity units should collect the figures for PMR, NNMR and also neonatal deaths before discharge from hospital. Reduction of NNMR simply by postponing the deaths out of the neonatal period is not the ideal of neonatal care. Bronchopulmonary dysplasia, infection and necrotizing enterocolitis are the current problems that lead to late deaths after 28 days. The 'corrected' WHO neonatal mortality rate is the number of deaths in the first 28 days of life (birthweight greater than 1000 g) per 1000 live births.

EPIDEMIOLOGY, BIRTHWEIGHT STANDARDS, PERINATAL MORTALITY AND MORBIDITY

Neonatal mortality will vary with the health of the population and the expertise and facilities provided by the medical system. The western world perinatal mortality rates (PMR) are now less than 15/1000 total births and the neonatal mortality rate (NNMR) is less than 5/1000 live births (Ch. 2). Some populations are prejudiced against, thus the PMR of black Americans is still almost double that of white Americans.

Risk of death varies with size and gestation (Fig. 5.2) as does incidence of congenital abnormalities and infection (Fig. 5.3).

Morbidity is also clearly related to both gestational age and size. However, some population studies would indicate that if congenital abnormalities are excluded there may not be a significant increase in morbidity with reducing size when neonatal intensive care is offered (Van Zeben et al 1989).

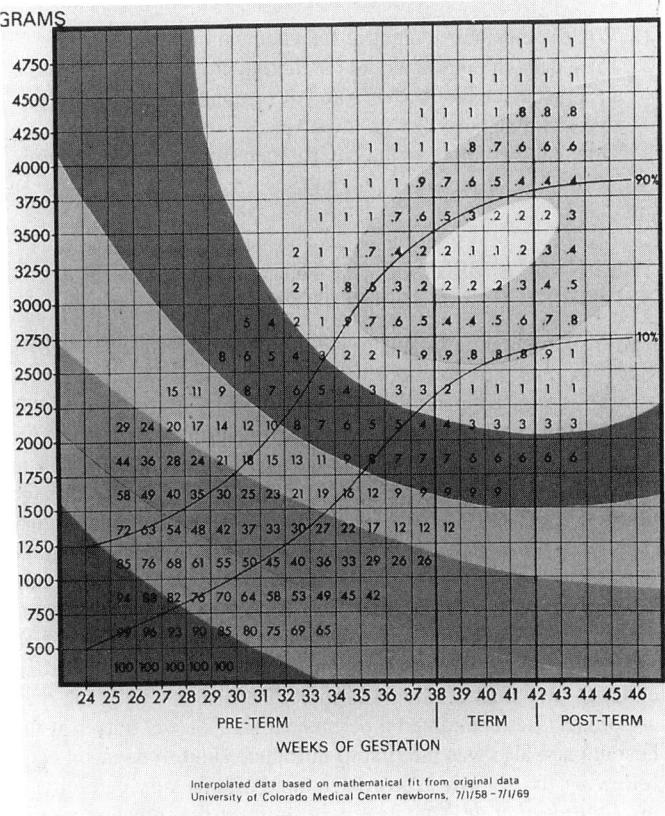

Fig. 5.2 Newborn classification and neonatal mortality risk by birthweight and gestational age (from Lubchenko et al 1972, with permission).

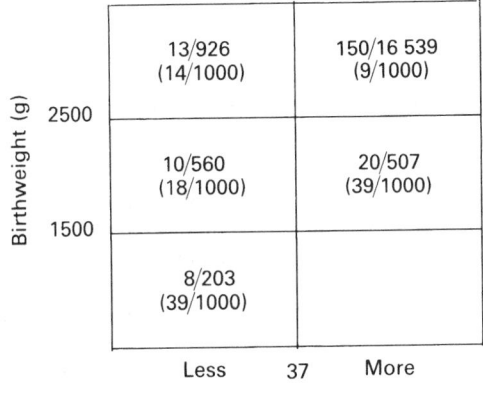

Fig. 5.3 Incidence of congenital heart disease by birthweight and gestational age (Yerushalmy 1969).

CARE

All newborn infants should receive special care as all babies are special. Babies with minor deviations of normality should if at all possible be nursed with their mothers after birth. A baby should be admitted to a neonatal unit *only* if special treatment is required which cannot be given on a postnatal ward or when sophisticated observation is required which cannot be carried out on the postnatal ward with the mother. *All* babies should receive independent casenotes whether or not they receive any extra care – they are independent beings.

Different degrees of care may be required in the neonatal unit. These have been defined by the British Paediatric Association (BPA) and British Association of Perinatal Medicine (BAPM).

Definitions of care (BPA and BAPM)

1. Intensive care = care given in a special or intensive care nursery which provides continuous skilled supervision by nursing and medical staff.
2. Special care = care given in the special care nursery or on a postnatal ward which provides observation and treatment falling short of intensive care but exceeding normal care.
3. Normal care = care given usually by the mother in a postnatal ward, supervised by a midwife and doctor but requiring minimal medical or nursing advice.

The clinical categories of care (BPA and BAPM)

Intensive care

1. Babies receiving assisted ventilation or continuous positive airways pressure, and in the first 24 h following its withdrawal.
2. Babies receiving total parenteral nutrition.
3. Babies who have cardiorespiratory disease which is unstable, including recurrent apnea requiring constant attention.
4. Babies who have had major surgery, particularly in the first 24 postoperative hours.
5. Babies of less than 30 weeks' gestation during the first 48 h after birth.
6. Babies who are having convulsions.
7. Babies transported by the staff of the unit concerned between hospitals or for special investigations or treatment.
8. Babies undergoing major medical procedures, such as arterial catheterization, peritoneal dialysis or exchange transfusion.

Special care

1. Babies who require continuous monitoring of respiration or heart rate or oxygen by transcutaneous transducers.
2. Babies who are receiving additional oxygen.
3. Babies who are receiving intravenous glucose and electrolyte solutions.
4. Babies who are being tube fed.
5. Babies who have had minor surgery in the previous 4 h.
6. Babies with a tracheostomy.
7. Dying babies.
8. Babies who are being barrier nursed.
9. Babies receiving phototherapy.
10. Babies who receive special monitoring (e.g. glucose or bilirubin estimations).

11. Other babies receiving constant supervision (e.g. the babies of drug-addicted mothers).
12. Babies receiving antibiotics.
13. Babies with conditions requiring radiological examination or other methods of care.

Resources required for neonatal care (BPA and BAPM)

Intensive care

1. Medical staff: the minimum medical staff should be an experienced pediatric registrar and SHO on duty and available in the intensive care area at all times with an appropriately trained consultant in charge.
2. Nursing staff: there should be a minimum establishment to allow a ratio of four *trained* nurses (with neonatal intensive care experience) to each cot. This ratio allows for 24-h cover and leave. The optimum ratio is 5.5 : 1.
3. Equipment: the following should be available for any baby receiving intensive care:

   Intensive care incubator or unit with overhead heater
   Respiratory or apnea monitor
   Heart rate monitor
   Blood pressure transducer (either intravascular or surface)
   Transcutaneous PO_2 or intravascular oxygen transducer
   Transcutaneous PCO_2 monitor
   Two syringe pumps
   Two infusion pumps
   Ventilator
   Continuous temperature monitor
   Phototherapy unit
   Ambient oxygen monitor.

   There should be facilities for frequent blood gas analysis using micromethods. There should be access to ultrasound equipment and radiological equipment.

Special care

1. Medical staff: minimum medical staff for 24-h cover are an experienced SHO with a more senior member of staff on call with a consultant pediatrician in charge.
2. Nursing staff: there should be a minimum establishment to allow a ratio of 1.25 nurses (with neonatal experience) to each cot. This ratio allows for 24-h cover and leave. The optimum ratio is 1.5 : 1.
3. Equipment: the following equipment must be available for each baby in special care:

   Incubator or cot for adequate temperature control
   Ambient oxygen analyzer
   Apnea alarm
   Heart rate monitor
   Infusion pump
   Phototherapy unit.

   There should be access to ventilators for short-term ventilation, access for biochemical analysis by micromethods and radiology.

THE ENVIRONMENT OF CARE

INTRODUCTION

Improved diagnosis and treatment both as a result of technological advances and increased pediatric and nursing specialization in neonatal intensive care have led, over the last decade, to impressive falls in neonatal mortality. Concern has been expressed, however, that the development and application of new medical technology has outpaced considerations for the psychological well-being of the very young patient in hospital. Current neonatal environments and invasive treatment may exert adverse iatrogenic effects on preterm and sick newborn which may hamper their recovery and healthy development.

It is important that certain questions be asked:

1. What is the environment of the neonatal unit like today?
2. How does the physical and caretaking environment of such a unit influence the recovery and development of the preterm and sick newborn that go there?
3. How can we improve the environment for the biobehavioral well-being of the small patient?

THE ENVIRONMENT OF THE PRETERM NEONATE: A BRIEF HISTORICAL REFLECTION

The term 'premature infant' entered the English language in 1870. Prior to this infants born before term were referred to as 'weaklings' or 'congenitally debilitated' babies. Before the middle of the 19th century infants, whether full term or preterm, were rarely weighed at birth and preterm infants were often allowed to 'pine away' and die and no special care was provided. Although the first children's hospitals were established in the 18th century (i.e. Halle, Germany, in 1701; Children's Hospital in Lamb's Conduit Street by Thomas Coram in 1741), the first premature baby unit was not established until 1895 by Pierre Budin at the Hôpital Port Royale in Paris. He stated: 'with weaklings we shall have to consider three points, one, their temperature and their chilling, two, their feeding and three, the diseases to which they are prone.' He maintained a permanent staff of wet nurses at the hospital and also was the first to introduce audit to neonatal care, following the growth of his discharged infants very carefully in his *Consultation de Nourissons*. Because of the infection rate in the premature infants at his hospital, he designed a special unit for premature infants, allowing separation of healthy from sick infants with daily disinfection of incubators and the staff gowned and scrubbing before handling the infants. Although Budin himself encouraged the visiting of parents, a pupil, Martin Couney who introduced Budin's principles throughout the US in the first half of the 20th century, separated the parents from their infants, discouraging them from visiting and certainly prohibiting their sharing of care. This complete separation and more recently the separation of parents from their infants through gowning, sterile procedures and the physical restrictions of incubators and heat shields continued until the 1970s. Both Budin and Couney recognized that on many occasions when the infants were ready to go home, it was difficult to get the mothers to accept the children back and later, separation of parents and their infants was identified as a possible cause (Klein & Stern 1971, Klaus & Kennel 1976). Thus from the 1970s the opening of nurseries to parents, with visiting and social contact with their preterm infants, became the predominant theme of change in the social environment of the preterm newborn. While technological and medical advances are continuing, the adverse side effects of more vigorous treatment have only recently become a focus of systematic research. Changes in the physical and caretaking environment have continued to be determined by accommodating equipment and staff needs rather than the needs of the patient, the small newborn infant.

PHYSICAL AND CARE ENVIRONMENT: DEFINITION

In theory two types of environment can be distinguished. First, the physical environment consisting of the nursery design and factors such as noise and light levels, the placing of infant (e.g. cot versus incubator, the bedding, the distance between cots and incubators, etc.) and the objects which are close to the infants (e.g. monitors and mobiles etc.). Second, the social environment which relates to the opportunities for social experience by the preterm infant: this includes handling by staff and parents and the provision of auditory, visual, tactile and vestibular stimulation. In practice such a distinction is blurred and not particularly useful because factors in the physical environment partly determine social encounters with the infant.

There are two pathways by which the environment can exert effects on the newborn. *Direct* influences are those characteristics of the physical, care or social environment which lead to immediate responses detectable in the physiological, motor and state organization of the infant. Alternatively, if better care is provided for parents and staff then they are able to provide better care for the infant. This is an *indirect* effect promoting the infants' development (Kennel & Klaus 1971).

ADVERSE EFFECTS OF THE NEONATAL INTENSIVE CARE UNIT ENVIRONMENT

Noise pollution

Preterm infants are exposed to moderate noise levels for weeks and months without having any control over the noise exposure. The mean noise levels outside the incubator are in the range 55–75 dB(A). This resembles the noise pollution found in a busy office environment. Incubators of the 1990s comply with British safety standards which require that the mean noise level inside an incubator should not exceed 60 dB(A). Protection from continuous background noise is not given in open cots.

Frequencies of less than 500 Hz easily penetrate the incubator but human voices which are in the 100–5000 Hz range are masked. Tape recordings from inside an incubator pick up only muffled and indistinct human speech. It is difficult to make sense of the sound source and type. The background noise in the incubator is often rhythmic due to the ventilators; other prominent sounds are metallic and high frequency from squeaking door hinges, bowls being placed on the top or equipment knocking the incubator. Impulse sound pressures of 114 dB(SPL) occur when incubator portholes are opened and shut in older incubators. Noise levels are generally higher in intensive compared to special care nurseries.

Adverse effects of noise

The risk of hearing loss due to SCBU noise levels in the absence of other severe complications is negligible (Abramovich et al 1979) but sudden loud noises often lead to adverse physiological and behavioral effects, including sleep disturbance, motor arousals such as startles and crying, hypoxemia, tachycardia and increased intracranial pressure (Wolke 1987). The latter might contribute to the development of intraventricular hemorrhage when associated with poor autoregulation of cerebral blood flow in the preterm infant's brain. Conversely the masking of meaningful sounds makes it unlikely that the infant will acquire recognition and integration of, for example, a voice with a particular visual stimulus (i.e. face). This cross-integration is acquired by full-term infants in the first month of life. Bushnell & Slater (1986) suggested that preterm infants have problems in concept learning and recognition and this may be related to poor cross-integration after birth.

Light exposure

The intensity of light in hospital neonatal intensive care units has increased five to tenfold in the past two decades. A randomized trial indicated that normal neonatal intensive care unit light levels may contribute to retinopathy of prematurity in vulnerable extremely low birthweight infants (Glass et al 1985). The effects were more severe when extremely low birthweight infants were nursed near the nursery window allowing long-term exposure to sunlight.

Handling and social contacts

The amount of handling received by the preterm infant has increased drastically from about 32 episodes/day in the early 1970s to a mean of 132–234 handling procedures/day in current intensive care units in the mid-80s (Murdoch & Darlow 1984). Very preterm infants in intensive care are handled, on average, every 5–10 min and handling accounts for 4 h in a 24-h period. The main disturbers are nursing and support staff, then the pediatricians and only lastly the parents. The sickest and most fragile infants are handled most frequently. Less aversive and less frequent handling by staff occurs as the infant's condition improves. Most handling is with nursing and medical routine procedures and social contact such as talking, gentle touching or rocking occur infrequently. Social activities account for no more than a quarter of the contact of the infant in the intensive care and only up to one-third in the postintensive care nurseries. Handling by nursing and medical staff disrupts the young infant's sleep pattern and is associated with a significantly higher incidence of hypoxemia, bradycardia, apnea and behavioral distress (Gorski et al 1990). The most uncomfortable and adverse procedures leading to a marked increase in cerebral blood flow and intracranial pressure are endotracheal suctioning and chest physiotherapy. Lagercrantz et al (1986) showed that the handling also leads to increased release of catecholamines which in the reported levels are only found in the stressed human organism.

Handling and high impulse sounds are also likely to increase the time the infant is spending in REM sleep and apnea is more common during REM compared to deep non-REM sleep.

In contrast to staff handling, parental handling is mostly benign and parents often intuitively talk to and gently stroke their infants (Wolke 1987).

The indiscriminate encouragement of parents by nursing staff and pediatricians to hold even the very sick and ventilated preterm infant has arisen from false interpretations of the concept of bonding and it is possible that a 'too pushy' approach may interfere with intuitive parenting, i.e. gentle stroking and minimal handling of the sick infant with the natural acquisition of a close relationship. Offering close contact (i.e. kangarooing) in a selective manner, depending on infant and parent state, has no adverse and usually beneficial effects (Anderson 1991).

Daily rhythms

Diurnal rhythms are characteristic features of human behavior and day/night rhythms in sleeping and waking are acquired in the early months of human life. In many intensive care units there is still no pronounced diurnal rhythm for noise, light levels or staff activities. While the lack of day/night cycle before 35 weeks' gestation has little influence on the acquisition of post-term sleeping behavior (Wolke et al 1995), the introduction of reduced noise, light and handling at night in intensive care units reduces staff interventions, supports longer periods of deep sleep and fewer state changes in vulnerable preterm infants (Fajardo et al 1990). Longer-term positive influences such as more rapid post-discharge weight gain have also been reported (Mann et al 1986).

PAIN IN THE NEONATE

Pain is an unpleasant sensation with strong emotional connotations. Early studies and theoretical views led to the pervasive view that newborns do not perceive pain. Strictly speaking nociceptive activity rather than pain should be discussed with regard to the neonate (Anand & Hickey 1987). Recent research indicates that the anatomical, neurochemical and functional requirements for nociception and the ability to respond to such inputs in an organized way are present in the infant at 22–26 weeks' gestation (Anand & Hickey 1987, Fitzgerald et al 1988a,b). Although the preterm infant cannot verbally express pain and discomfort, physiological and behavioral changes in response to insults provide a window into the preterm infant's nociceptive reception. Cardiorespiratory, hormonal and metabolic changes, simple motor responses, facial expressions, crying and complex behavioral responses such as state changes all indicate that the preterm infant can respond to noxious stimuli in all these areas of functioning. Similar adverse responses have been reported to handling and noise which indicates that certain aspects of the caretaking and the physical environment in current special care units may be stressful for the preterm or sick newborn.

OPPORTUNITIES FOR EARLY LEARNING

The term 'infancy' derives from the Latin *infans* which means speechless. Young infants have no verbal language apart from crying and they acquire concepts about the world through sensorimotor experiences and by making associations between stimuli. Sensorimotor experiences are exposures to tactile, kinesthetic, vestibular, motor, auditory and visual experiences. Basic processes of learning are habituation, classical and instrumental conditioning and more advanced processes such as complex learning, concept learning and language acquisition. During the early stages of development the function and structure of the brain are particularly dependent on interaction with the environment (Greenough W T et al 1987); motor skills and perceptual and intellectual performances consolidate and are consolidated by learning in early infancy (Slater 1989) and the resilience and plasticity of the central nervous system allow recovery from moderately adverse early influences. The current intensive and special care baby unit environments give little opportunity or support for early constructive learning (Wolke

1991). Many sensory and motor experiences are unpleasant and during incubator nursing there are few opportunities for cross-modal integration and concept learning. Most of the handling and human sounds are noncontingent on the infant's state and the preterm infant can exert little control over stimuli in the environment. Furthermore, although the preterm infant's capacities for social interaction increase as he recovers and graduates to the postintensive care nursery, the staff to patient ratio changes equally dramatically. There are fewer nurses to look after the more alert infant who is now potentially more often able to invite and cope with increased social action.

A number of follow-up studies have noted that preterm infants have qualitatively poorer and quantitatively different interactions with their caretaker. Poor attention span, irritability and restlessness may interfere with structured learning though cognitive capacities may be in the normal range (Riegel et al 1995). This has been noted in the neonatal nursery and in infancy and early childhood (Buka et al 1992). These observed problems in healthy, very and extremely low birthweight infants after discharge are likely to result from complex interactions of neonatal medical problems, the neonatal unit and the home environment. However, some current evidence suggests that being housed in the neonatal unit may contribute to subsequent development in ways not directly related to the reasons for being on such a unit (Lawson et al 1985, Als et al 1994).

IMPROVING THE ENVIRONMENT

Principles of care

Preterm infants are not, as previously proposed, either understimulated or overstimulated: rather the preterm infant receives stimulation which is ignorant and not adapted to his developmental level. The premature neonate is neither similar to the fetus nor a deficient full-term infant but is a unique organism, a medical artifact with special needs. It is therefore inappropriate to supply supplemental stimulation mimicking the environment of the womb or the outside world of the full-term infant (Wolke 1991). There is no easy recipe for optimal psychological development. The care needs of the infant should be adapted to the developmental level of the individual infant while in hospital care (Wolke 1987) and adhere to three principles:

1. Observe the baby. How does he react to noises, light, handling and attempts at social interaction? How does he show his distress? Infants who are reacting to minimal stimuli with physiological changes are the most fragile and need reduced stimulation while those coping with moderate stimulation should be provided with meaningful social stimulation.

2. Design an individual care plan. All involved in the care of the preterm infant (nurses, neonatologists, parents, physiotherapist and psychologist) should design an individual care plan on the basis of the detailed observations. Developmental support is a significant corollary of medical care: it is defined as the provision of a nursery environment which reinforces the emerging abilities of the maturing infant.

3. Grow up with the patient. The preterm infant develops during his time in the hospital. He will become more alert, robust and available to higher social interaction. It is important that the care adapts adequately to these changes (Wolke 1987, 1991).

Recent controlled studies have evaluated the introduction of these principles into neonatal intensive care practices (Als et al 1994, Becker et al 1991, Meyer et al 1994). Very preterm infants cared for by individualized behavioral and environmental care had briefer stay on the respirator and more optimal respirator status. They graduated earlier to oral feeding and had lower morbidity, shorter hospitalization and improved behavioral organization. Many aspects of such care can be introduced without great cost (and even with savings) and are outlined below.

Prevention of invasive treatment

Antenatal referral patterns and the routine application of invasive medical procedures for VLBW infants in the first 24 h often determine the environmental experiences of vulnerable infants in the SCBU. Both regionalization of intensive care in perinatal centers with efficient antenatal screening and in utero referral (i.e. delivery of inborns) and abandoning routine use of intubation for VLBW or ELBW infants are beneficial in reducing the need for invasive and disturbing treatments. The need for transport to a NICU increases intubation rates and the subsequent need for invasive and disturbing interventions (Riegel et al 1995).

Great differences in rates of intubation exist between different NICUs without apparent differences in populations (Avery et al 1987, Hack et al 1991). Wolke (1997), comparing neonatal treatment approaches in South Germany and South Finland for infants of < 32 weeks gestation, found a much decreased use of intubation and subsequent use of parenteral feeding and reduced hospitalization length in Finland; the lower rates of intubation and less invasive treatment had no detrimental effects on developmental outcome in the first 5 years of life. Individualized and restrained decisions to intubate based on observations of respiratory progress in the first 2 h of life (i.e. using CPAP as an alternative) have been shown to reduce intubation rates to below 35% (Jacobson et al 1993) for VLBW infants, without adverse effects on medium-term outcome.

Reduction of noise

Reduction of noise pollution can be achieved by changing staff behavior. Radio playing should be reduced in the unit, talking should be at a considerate low level and loud laughter should be discouraged. Cot-side ward rounds should be abandoned if no patient contact is necessary and only X-rays or medical records are reviewed. No bowls or other equipment should be placed on the incubator and incubator portholes should be opened and shut gently. The telephone should not be placed in or immediately adjacent to the unit. Sounds from monitoring equipment should be muffled or be replaced by light signal systems. Ideally, new nursery design should include sound-proofing for ceilings, walls and floors, and manufacturers of medical equipment and incubators should be encouraged to reduce noise levels in their products. A no-noise policy should be applied at nighttime. Indistinct background noise should be replaced by meaningful sounds such as gentle music or recordings of one of the parents reading stories. These should be played at a low sound level from a tape recorder from within the incubator and only when the infant is awake.

Light reduction

Flexible point lighting sources should be introduced. It is unnecessary that a whole room is brightly lit if only one infant is to be examined. The smallest and most fragile infants should not be placed in sunlight. The incubators of very ill infants could be covered with light density filter sheets. Unit lighting should be controllable by a dimmer switch and there should be a positive policy to induce day/night rhythms.

Handling

Procedures such as suction or chest physiotherapy should not be used routinely but only if absolutely necessary. Handling by different staff should be sequenced more sensibly (Gorski et al 1990). Routine monitoring and investigations should be carried out only when the infant is awake. Access for staff (but not parents) may be restricted by a primary nurse assigned to a specific infant. Infants should be contained and gently stroked during painful procedures and calmed down before being left after the intervention. Analgesia and anesthesia should, if possible, be used to reduce suffering. A minimal handling policy should apply for the smallest and most fragile infants.

Appropriate stimulation

A whole range of different hospital-based stimulation programs targeted at taste and sucking stimulation, tactile, auditory, vestibular, multimodal and social stimulation of the preterm infants have been proposed and evaluated (from sucking to waterbeds to kangarooing). Most of these rather specific methods have shown some limited positive effects on the growth and development of the preterm infant in the short term but not improved long-term development (Helders 1989). No single stimulation program has been found beneficial for all preterm infants (Lacy & Ohlsson 1993). Instead, environmental care must be individualized and finely attuned to the developmental status of the preterm infant, his family and their special needs (Wolke 1991, Als et al 1994, Meyer et al 1994).

THE ROLE OF THE PARENTS

The aim of neonatal intensive care is to discharge a healthy infant into the gentle loving care of his parents. In supporting this process the following should always be kept in mind:

1. The *infant is the patient* requiring special care by professionals for a limited period of time but the *parents are the caregivers*.
2. The parents have *rights* to make informed choices and are competent agents in early care.
3. Society represented by the neonatal carers *expects* from parents certain levels of involvement.

Professionals have pointed out factors in certain parents ('difficult parents', 'disturbed', etc.) that mitigate against joint care involvement.

Parents have also identified issues in neonatal care which make it difficult for them to be more involved (Lucey 1993). The most important issue raised by parents is that they often feel that *open and honest communication* between parents and professionals on medical and ethical issues is lacking. Neonatologists often feel they need to protect the parents by communicating with vague statements to shield parents from being overwhelmed, because it may disrupt the 'bonding' process or because the treatment outcome is uncertain. Such well-intentioned shielding has proved to be fallacious in dealing with stillbirth and is wrong, as perceived by parents, when discussing their critically ill newborn (Harrison 1993).

Furthermore, neonatologists have allowed the media to widely publicize their successes ('miracle babies'), but have minimized their failures to the public (Stahlman 1990). This has raised parents' expectations. Parents wish a more sober and realistic appraisal of what neonatal medicine can and cannot do from the medical community and media. They wish for honest communication, to be informed about treatment choices and to be involved in making decisions in medical situations involving very high mortality and morbidity and regarding further highly invasive treatments for their infant (Harrison 1993). The situation should be explained in plain and common language adapted to the parents.

Instead of assuming that parents do not want to be involved, neonatal carers should consider parents as wanting but not always able to be involved. The high-tech, noisy and busy environment of the neonatal unit, and the anxieties regarding the intact survival of the small preterm infant, can lead to the perception that only the experts (medical and nursing staff) can provide the right care. Parents thus withdraw, particularly in the early acute stages, from more involvement (Affleck et al 1991). Anxieties, shock and emotional turmoil and sometimes financial restraints and the attention demanded by siblings of the preterm infant make it difficult for parents to do what the neonatal carers expect.

Simple changes can help to make parents more welcome:

1. Unrestricted access to neonatal units by parents, grandparents, siblings and close friends. Late visits should not interfere with the policy of reduced, noise, light and handling levels at night.

2. Practical help in the form of financial support for traveling and caretaking arrangements (e.g. play areas for siblings) are important to enable parents to visit the unit, as well as a direct telephone line for contact with parents.

3. The surroundings of the unit should be attractive and comfortable (i.e. wallpaper, pictures, etc.) and ideally should also allow for some privacy for parents. The setting should be baby centered (e.g. mobiles, toys, etc.). Parents should have comfortable seating such as rocking chairs which also facilitate nursing in the postintensive care nursery.

4. The small infant and his microenvironment (incubator or cot) can be made attractive by clothing and toys.

5. Encouragement by neonatal unit staff should not end with providing parents with a booklet about the unit and explaining the equipment and medical condition of the infant. Nursing and medical staff should work with the parents to explore areas where the parents themselves can provide an important part of the care within a warm and trusting atmosphere (e.g. the provision of soothing techniques for the agitated infant during and after painful procedures). Parents can be encouraged to keep records of their infant's behavior, which are valuable for the medical and nursing team in designing an individual care plan for the patient. Parents can carry out tube feeding and hygiene care and in the transitional and special care nurseries, if given the information, can stimulate their infant at appropriate times and learn how to read the infant cues for sensitive interaction and care. Breast-feeding should be encouraged and facilities for rooming in should be available.

6. Self-help groups or educational classes for parents should be established and have been shown to be beneficial. Psychological support has been shown to reduce anxiety and depression (Meyer et al 1994).

7. Medical and nursing staff can only provide emotional support to parents if they themselves are emotionally available and coping. Support for the staff can be by various means including team work, staff support groups, and regular formal and informal meetings between the different professions to enhance the work ethos and atmosphere. Occasionally individual counseling may be warranted.

Parents are individuals with their own characteristics and needs. There is no easy recipe or approach which is right for all parents to help them in coping. An individual care approach should be adopted for all members of each family to promote the contact necessary to encourage the development of the infant in the best way possible.

Finally, NICU professionals need to acknowledge that critically ill newborns can be harmed not only by undertreatment but also by overtreatment, a feature now reflected in some legal proceedings (Silverman 1992). Treatment policies for the infant and family need to be based on compassion.

THE ETHICS OF NEWBORN CARE

This review addresses two ethical issues that trouble pediatricians working in neonatal intensive care units where, perhaps more than anywhere else, doctors and nurses are aware of the impact of new knowledge, new skills and new technology. Difficult ethical decisions in medical practice result from our increased ability to sustain life in patients who, in years past, would not have survived. When little or nothing could be done, death was accepted as inevitable and perhaps 'for the best'. Developments in medical technology, the creation of newborn intensive care units (NICU) and the emergence of specialists in perinatology/neonatology – accompanied by improved health, nutrition and socioeconomic circumstances for mothers – have led to an impressive reduction in perinatal mortality since the Second World War. For the tiniest infants this improved survival is particularly noteworthy. First noted in the US, which pioneered intensive care for the smallest infants, equally encouraging results have been reported from other countries. Extremely low birthweight (ELBW) infants (< 1000 g) seem a constant preoccupation in neonatal units; they occupy a very considerable portion of the time, skills, energies and emotions of the staff, and take up a major part of the resources allocated for neonatal care. Fortunately, the majority who survive are healthy and free from major neurological disability but recent statistics suggest that, although the proportion of infants who survive in good health has increased, the absolute number left with some physical or mental disability also may have increased. 'The future continues to lie in the development of the methodology to prolong the sojourn in utero, rather than in dramatic biophysical biochemical and technologic advances' (Hack & Fanaroff 1988).

WITHHOLDING OR WITHDRAWING INTENSIVE CARE

The technical details of caring for premature infants or for those born with disabling congenital abnormalities are described elsewhere. This review focuses on the moral uncertainties that are inseparable from some medical decisions, decisions with profound implications for the infant and family. For most families recent advances in obstetric and neonatal care have brought blessings beyond measure. For some, the consequences of modern neonatal intensive care have been devastating and tragic (Stinson & Stinson 1983). Questions continue to be asked about the wisdom of using modern medical technology to save or sustain life in all circumstances; about what some view as the unnecessary and cruel prolongation of dying; and about the medical, moral and legal justification of continuing 'futile' treatment in patients who are not dying. Arguments about the relative roles and responsibilities for making such decisions continue to occupy not only those directly involved, but lawyers, philosophers, theologians and others.

In withholding or withdrawing certain intensive life-prolonging treatments, not care, five questions are considered here:

1. For an infant who lacks decision-making capacity, who should decide?
2. What is the basis for such a fundamental decision? What criteria should be used?
3. Which infants are involved?
4. If treatments are withheld or withdrawn, what alternative care is appropriate?
5. Are there implications for others? What about 'society' or 'the law'?

Who should decide?

Doctors, with or without parental knowledge or consent, have made such decisions for generations. They based them on the medical realities of diagnosis and prognosis and on what they (and the parents when consulted) believed to be the child's best interests. In the ethical climate of today such paternalism is unfashionable, even unacceptable. Since many of the issues raised by life and death dilemmas are moral and not medical, some commentators, notably philosophers and lawyers, believe that doctors and parents are no longer competent to make such decisions on their own. Legislative actions to limit the discretion traditionally granted to doctors and parents in these essentially private family tragedies were particularly evident in the US during the 1980s and the interested reader is directed to the extensive literature on this debate (Angell 1983, Annas 1984, Caplan et al 1992).

In the UK and in most other countries, doctors are still granted considerable discretion in deciding what forms of intensive treatment should or should not be used, but there are a growing number of cases where court help has been sought in resolving such dilemmas. In this author's view such decisions should continue to be made primarily by the doctors and parents but the burden of decision making, if not the final responsibility, should be shared with others closely involved. The vast majority of such decisions are made in this way. On occasions, especially if there is disagreement, it will be necessary and prudent to seek court help. At all costs a 'rush to judgment' must be avoided. Extensive consideration of all the options and implications and adequate time for reflection are important safeguards. Nowadays it must be rare for such decisions to be made paternalistically by one doctor. They are made by exhaustive consultation and consensus in an intensive care unit staffed by nurses, junior doctors and others whose views are all relevant to moral decision making. In establishing the facts of diagnosis and prognosis, the unit doctors will consult with specialist colleagues. The family doctor may provide important insights to the parents' understanding of the issues and their ability to cope with the implications of the various treatment options. The parents may seek the views of grandparents, relatives, clergymen, friends and perhaps many others. This pattern of decision making has been described as 'family centered' because families are most familiar with their own strengths, weaknesses and resources and must live with the consequences of any decision.

American pediatricians responded to federal intervention by broadening the decision-making process through the establishment of hospital infant bioethical committees. They contain both professional and lay membership, advise on policy; review decisions for critically ill infants, and provide 'ethical comfort' for the staff (Fleischman 1986). In such a role they can be helpful to the staff of neonatal units, but unfortunately a few committees became too involved in the actual medical decisions. This led to accusations that an occasional decision was being made in the legal and fiscal interests of the institution rather than in the personal, medical and social interests of the infant and family. Ethics committees of this type are still not common in the UK. Many British neonatologists use a multidisciplinary group informally to discuss difficult cases at length, and there is encouraging evidence from America that the traditional primacy of the responsible doctor and the parents in making such decisions is once again being recognized and respected (American Academy of Pediatrics 1995).

Criteria for withholding or withdrawing intensive care

When doctors and parents consider withholding or withdrawing treatment, the infant's 'best interests' are paramount. If an individual method of treatment will not benefit the infant it may justifiably be withheld. If it is likely to be beneficial it should be used and should not be withdrawn. Doctors are not required, nor should they be forced, to overtreat patients when, in their best medical judgment, the treatment is inappropriate. Acceptance of the 'best interests' principle in this way means that we believe that some infants are better off dead, a view supported by the US President's Commission of 1983, which considered that there are some disabilities and impairments so severe 'that continued existence would not be a net benefit to the infant.' A competent autonomous adult may reach such a conclusion for himself or herself and refuse life-saving treatment but it is indeed an awesome decision for a parent or doctor to make on behalf of an infant. It requires assessment of what would be a 'life worth living' from the infant's point of view.

In choosing options for treatment in these always difficult and often tragic situations, doctors are sometimes accused of occupying polarized positions, either obsessively adhering to a 'sanctity of life' principle or allowing infants to die on vague 'quality of life' criteria that, to some, are unacceptable and unethical. This is unfortunate, because they are both important elements in making these decisions. It is possible to respect life yet recognize that an 'infant's best interests' standard must include quality of life considerations. Quality of life judgments, far from being discriminatory as has been alleged, are a necessary component of a patient-centered approach to decision making, particularly at the beginning of life (Campbell 1995a).

It is axiomatic that before any decision is made to withhold or withdraw intensive treatment every effort is made to ensure that the diagnosis and prognosis are accurate. Only then can treatment be decided at the appropriate level based on the expected outcome – an 'individualized prognostic strategy' (Rhoden 1986). The most important criterion is whether the abnormality or combination of abnormalities, especially if involving the brain, are likely to prevent the infant from 'having a life' as an integrated and interrelating human being, instead of merely 'being alive' in the biological sense. Recent developments in medical imaging and neurophysiological measurement have improved the ability to recognize brain damage but it must be emphasized that there are considerable limitations in our understanding of neurological integrity in the early newborn period (Coulter 1987).

Which infants are involved?

There are two particular groups of infants where such decisions may be appropriate:

1. The very immature infant. With more and more tiny infants surviving at the limits of viability it is difficult to know where to 'draw the line' at intensive care or indeed if it is ever justifiable to draw such a line. Any 'cutoff' must be flexible enough to recognize individual viability and circumstances. The decision to withhold or withdraw treatment must be carefully considered, not the result of a 'snap judgment' made in the delivery room or elsewhere. This means that the vast majority of infants who are born with signs of life, whatever the gestation age or weight, should be resuscitated and given a 'trial of life'. Recommendations about continuing or withdrawing treatment will depend on frequent re-evaluations of the infant's condition and prognosis.

2. The severely damaged or malformed infant. More than anything else, parents worry about the consequences of brain damage for their child's future health, happiness and independence. There are a number of conditions where the prognosis can be estimated with a reasonable degree of accuracy, and where doctors and parents together may decide to allow an infant to die. Specific examples include infants brain damaged by severe birth asphyxia or virus infection, infants with major and often multiple congenital abnormalities such as neural tube defects, and certain chromosomal disorders, for example trisomy 13 or 18.

In deciding for or against treatment we all tend to 'draw lines'. Some doctors who would not hesitate to withhold intensive care from an infant with anencephaly will insist on aggressive treatment for severe forms of spina bifida or for an infant of 650 g with intracranial hemorrhage. There will be considerable differences in individual moral reasoning which make such decisions acceptable or unacceptable. Above all, doctors and nurses must be sensitive to the parents' concerns and opinions. Parents may have cultural, religious and ethnic backgrounds that are very different from those of the doctors and nurses concerned.

All decisions and the actions taken must be accurately recorded in a manner that facilitates objective review of the decision-making process. The record should include notes of discussions held with the infant's parents. Full explanation of the circumstances and the reasons for any decision to withdraw life-sustaining treatment will do much to demonstrate trustworthiness, which must be a key component of medical decisions if public acceptability is to be retained. Although there will be times when

wider family and social interests must also be considered, doctors should keep the decision firmly focused on the best interests of the child. There will be times when doctors must steer a difficult course between forcing unwelcome choices on families through a sense of moral superiority and yielding to family demands in violation of their own principles. They may need to guide parents towards a decision that is not only acceptable medically and morally but is compatible with the law of the land.

After the decision – alternative care

Withholding or withdrawing life-sustaining treatment in these circumstances does not mean withdrawal of care. All that we associate with good medical and nursing practice must continue – cherishing, warmth, relief of hunger and thirst, toileting, and treatment aimed to relieve any distress or pain. Withdrawing parenteral feeding on the basis that it is a medical treatment is controversial, highly emotional and becoming subject to review in the courts. It is this author's view that oral feeds should be offered as tolerated but that once the decision is taken to allow an infant to die it is illogical and pointlessly cruel to prolong dying unnecessarily by introducing or continuing i.v. infusions or tube feedings. Each case must receive careful individual consideration and particular attention should be paid to the views of the parents. It is also illogical to treat infections with antibiotics. The important question that should always be asked is, 'Will this treatment benefit my patient?' If not, it should not be used.

According to the family wishes, arrangements may be made for the infant to die at home with the appropriate support provided. Circumstances will vary from family to family and unit to unit but when an infant is dying in hospital, time should be allowed for family members to interact with the infant as they wish. Baptism and photographs may be important to them. When death is imminent, the staff should inquire if the parents wish to leave, wish to remain beside their baby's incubator or cot as much as possible, or would prefer to cradle their dying infant with all tubes and apparatus removed in a private room. 'Immediately they chose the last. In the company of the doctor they held their infant for 55 minutes while he died. ... They came to think of this experience as a fitting funeral from which they found greater strength for living' (Duff & Campbell 1976).

Legal and social implications

By studying the cases that have come to court in recent years, it is possible to gain some idea of how the courts might respond to the facts of an individual case (Campbell 1995b). However, considerable areas of uncertainty remain and are unavoidable, e.g. the way judges will view 'intolerable quality of life' or 'demonstrably awful abnormalities' will be variable and unpredictable.

The law confers protection on all infants born alive at any gestational age but it does not insist that all available treatments be used to maintain life in all circumstances. Thus while strongly protective of life, it recognizes the need for discretion in using life-sustaining treatment. Experience suggests that most legislators are reluctant to see formal regulations directing British pediatricians as to how they should care for impaired newborn infants. The 'Baby Doe' experience in the US demonstrated that legislation is simply too blunt an instrument to resolve these highly individual and tragic problems. Legislators are responsive to a consensus of social interests and expectations and at present, as far as can be judged, the general public prefers that these decisions remain the responsibility of parents and doctors.

It should not be necessary to defend carefully considered decisions to withdraw intensive treatment against warnings of the 'slippery slope'. If, through the application of rigid laws, a state or committees made these decisions, the dangers would be great, but not if decisions are made only by those who care most for the patient and who must bear the consequences. If the process of decision making is conducted openly and properly documented, 'bad' decisions should be rare and easy to detect.

RESEARCH IN THE NURSERY

The importance of good research to infant care hardly needs emphasis here yet history contains examples of useless or unsafe treatments adopted without adequate research or any proper regard to safety (Silverman 1985). If public trust is to be maintained, research on such vulnerable subjects as infants and children must be of high quality and be able to withstand intense scrutiny as to its scientific validity and ethical acceptability.

Authoritative guidelines are available for those wishing to carry out research using child subjects (British Paediatric Association 1992).

They incorporate several basic principles:

1. Research involving children is important for the benefit of all children and should be supported and encouraged, and conducted in an ethical manner.
2. Research should never be done on children if the same investigation can be done using adult subjects.
3. Research which involves a child but is of no benefit to that child (nontherapeutic research) is not necessarily either unethical or illegal.
4. The degree of benefit resulting from research should be assessed in relation to the risk of disturbance, discomfort or pain – the 'risk/benefit ratio'.

Although often blurred in practice, there is an important distinction between therapeutic research conducted as part of necessary treatment and nontherapeutic research which, though it may result in important advances in medical care, is not of direct value to the participant. Nontherapeutic research is acceptable only if associated with negligible risk. Before any study can proceed, the investigator must have the written permission of the parents or legal guardian, and it is now essential to have the approval of a research ethics advisory committee.

Parental consent

Though 'informed consent' is perhaps an ideal rarely achieved in practice, neonatal investigators should provide parents with sufficient information in an understandable form to allow an informed choice. Understanding can be facilitated by including a written explanation provided prior to obtaining consent. (Ideally this documentation should also be submitted with the application for ethical approval.) Particular problems arise immediately after birth when the mother may not be in a fit state to give consent and the father may not be available. It may be desirable to include infants in studies of various treatment alternatives starting from birth. Without such research the benefits and risks of new

treatments may never be properly evaluated, yet, to parents at this anxious time, any suggestion that their infant be part of an 'experiment' to determine the better or best treatment may cause considerable anxiety and distress. However, there is likely to be equal, if not greater, distress with loss of confidence and trust if parents later discover that their infants have been involved without their knowledge. Provisional permission obtained prenatally with more formal consent after birth is usually possible. Parents are often aware of the benefits to be derived from the skills and technical facilities available in major hospitals where most research is conducted. In most cases they will cooperate willingly if given the appropriate information and approached with the right attitude.

Advisory committee approval

In preparing a protocol for submission to an ethics advisory committee the investigators should pay particular attention to the following:

Justification

Why is the study necessary on newborn infants instead of older children or adults? Are animal data available? If already done elsewhere, why is the research being repeated? A review of past work should be included.

Feasibility

Is it possible to achieve the aims of the study with the proposed design? Will the result be interpretable? Is the study to be randomized and controlled? Can nonrandomization be justified? Has expert statistical advice been obtained? Would a large-scale multicenter study not be more appropriate?

Conduct

What are the practical implications for the infants and parents? Will efforts be made to minimize expense, disruption of normal routines and separation of infant from parents? Are risks being minimized using the safest procedures consistent with research design? Have arrangements been made for early data analysis so that possible harm or lack of benefit might be identified quickly and the study terminated prematurely if necessary? How will privacy and confidentiality be protected? Have others directly or indirectly involved been consulted, e.g. nurses and laboratory workers?

Consent

How will informed consent be obtained? What information will be provided for the parents? (A copy of information for parents should be included.) As well as the potential benefits, have the possible risks been discussed? Will there be opportunities for parents to withdraw consent? Will they be assured that refusal or withdrawal of consent will in no way prejudice their infant's care?

If neonatal research is seen by the public as essential to progress and neonatologists are seen to be worthy of trust in their conduct of research, it may become an accepted component of high quality infant care.

THE ECONOMICS OF NEWBORN CARE

Choices will always have to be made between different and competing ways of using medical resources. The development of expensive technologies and the corresponding increase in the costs of caring for some babies at a time of increasing demands for funds for health care has added urgency to questions about the relationship between the costs and the benefits. Optimization of the benefit to be gained from limited resources is the central theme of economics, and this chapter outlines the methods used in economic evaluation of health care, with examples taken from studies of neonatal care.

COMPARING ALTERNATIVES

The value of a particular health program depends on whether more could be gained by using the resources in a different way. Therefore, all economic evaluations start with the question: what are the alternatives being compared? This might be a comparison of the relative costs and benefits of caring for different risk groups in a neonatal unit, a comparison of the care given in different settings (e.g. district and referral), or a comparison of different treatment strategies.

MEASURING RESOURCES

Once the alternatives are specified, the next stage is to identify how resource use and outcomes differ between the strategies compared. Costs and benefits are then estimated, comparing the alternatives with respect to the difference in the value of resources used as a result of the practices compared, and the difference in the health outcomes.

The resources used in health care include human skills and time, buildings, equipment, drugs, consumables, laboratory and radiology services, heat, light and power.

Costs also arise beyond the health sector. Parents forego other productive activities (paid or unpaid work) in order to be with their sick newborn babies, and incur costs of transport and care for other children. Other agencies may also be involved: for example parents of babies discharged from hospital early may require more support from community health and family practice staff, when compared to low weight babies who are kept in hospital for longer.

MEASURING OUTCOMES

The most efficient allocation of resources is one which maximizes the benefit to be gained. Any ineffective or harmful treatment is inefficient, because benefits could be increased by stopping such practices and using the resources for more effective practices. This might seem obvious, but there are many aspects of perinatal care that are still routine in some places for which there is inadequate evidence of effectiveness or which have been shown to be ineffective in comparison with alternative practices (Chalmers et al 1989). The importance of basing practice on good evidence from controlled research designed to minimize observer bias is illustrated in the example of the use of oxygen for preterm infants. It was initially assumed that little harm could result from high doses, at the cost of increased occurrences of retinopathy of prematurity (Silverman 1980).

The least biased evidence comes from randomized controlled trials, and much useful evidence about effectiveness of different aspects of care can be derived from analyses synthesizing data from trials of the same procedure (Cochrane Database of Systematic Reviews 1997). Examples (Enkin et al 1995) of some practices which have been shown in randomized controlled trials not to be of clinical benefit include: sodium bicarbonate administration to asphyxiated neonates; performing gastric suctioning on all infants routinely; separating healthy mothers and babies routinely; routine nursery care for all newborn infants; routine use of gowns and masks in normal newborn nurseries; giving free formula samples to breast-feeding mothers; and test weighing breast-fed infants. Care that the same authors recommend for further evaluation includes: routine pharyngeal suctioning of all neonates at birth; tracheal suction for meconium-stained neonates at birth; and antiseptic dressings for the umbilical cord. A similar review of neonatal care has been conducted and extends this list to aspects of neonatal care beyond the immediate care of the newborn (Sinclair & Bracken 1992). Recent evidence of effective forms of care to prevent or treat neonatal respiratory distress syndrome includes antenatal administration of corticosteroids to the mother where preterm delivery is anticipated (Crowley 1995), and administration of surfactant to babies at high risk of RDS (Soll 1991).

Outcomes used in trials include changes in mortality rates and differences in specific aspects of morbidity. Occasionally, trials are designed to include measures both of parents' views and of costs arising from the alternative treatments compared.

Relatively few well-designed clinical comparisons of perinatal care have included enough long-term follow-up data to assess the longer-term implications of treatment for outcomes and resources. Evaluation of neonatal care is hampered by lack of good population-based observational data about long-term outcomes. Mortality and other outcome data for neonatal unit babies can be affected by definitions of viability, or by admission criteria: differences in outcomes between centers cannot be assumed to reflect differences in the effectiveness of neonatal care.

VALUING RESOURCES AND OUTCOMES: COSTS AND BENEFITS

The economic cost of using staff or equipment in one particular way is the lost value of the best alternative use of those resources. For example, increasing staff in the neonatal unit may reduce the number of staff available for routine postnatal support in the maternity unit. This could possibly affect outcomes such as breast-feeding success or postnatal infection rates. Such forgone benefit is known as the *opportunity cost* of the resources, and it is this concept that economists have in mind when they measure costs.

Once the differences in the physical amounts of resource use and outcome are known, they must be expressed in comparable units which are weighted to convey their relative values. Monetary values are used in most economic studies, but arriving at the correct value raises questions about what is the best indicator of the opportunity cost. Should drug costs include the overheads of running the hospital pharmacy? Should the cost of caring for a disabled child be based on institutional costs, or loss of parents' earning power? Does the current market value of a product used in neonatal care reflect its opportunity cost? Published economic analyses make different assumptions, and it is important to be clear what these assumptions are before comparing results from different studies. For example, costs of neonatal care in the US are frequently quoted as very much higher than they are in British studies, even after converting dollars to sterling values. Apart from the higher salary bill in the US, one reason for this may be that hospital billing systems are used as the basis for the costs in US studies, and these accounting systems are designed to recoup from the payers the overheads of running the hospital (and sometimes include an element of profit). Costing data from studies of NHS neonatal care do not necessarily include the full overhead and administrative costs of the hospital.

If valuation of physical resources is difficult, there is even more controversy about attempts to express outcomes of care in monetary or other comparable units. The extent to which such valuation of benefits is required depends on the nature of the question being asked. A simple approach is to ask what are the relative costs of achieving a particular outcome in different ways. Resource effects are summarized by a monetary value, outcomes in units such as life years gained or morbidity averted. This approach is known as *cost-effectiveness analysis*.

If the question is whether the extra resources used by the program are justified by the benefits, an attempt is sometimes made to value the outcomes explicitly in the same monetary units that are used for resources. Known as *cost-benefit analysis*, this approach has attracted much criticism for the valuing of life or disability in monetary terms (Sugden & Williams 1978).

An alternative approach, *cost utility analysis*, is to construct a single index of outcome which reflects people's valuation of each possible outcome. The technique uses data about how people choose between different health outcomes to estimate the effect of different treatments on quality adjusted life years (QALYs). There is debate about how this should be done, and how it can contribute to the final decision between health care options. However, where the concept has been used, it emphasizes how including considerations about long-term disability may affect conclusions about life-saving procedures. In a study comparing the costs and outcomes before and after introduction of regional neonatal intensive care in Hamilton County, Ontario, in the early 1970s, Boyle et al (1983) estimated that the additional cost of intensive care per life year gained for babies weighing less than 1000 g was eight times more than for those weighing between 1000 and 1499 g, but that this difference increases to a 17-fold increase in cost per QALY for babies less than 1000 g when quality of life is taken into account (see Table 5.1).

The weight of value put on different outcomes depends on prevailing ethical and moral standards about life, death and disability. In some cases this rules out consideration of certain options, such as some forms of prenatal screening in a country where abortion is illegal. Where there are differences within a society, economic evaluation should be explicit about whose values are being considered. For example, in the case of neonatal intensive care, Boyle and colleagues based assessments on a survey of the views of parents of school age children. In that study, some parents ranked severe disability as worse than death. It is possible that other groups would place different weights on the possible outcomes of neonatal intensive care. It is not the place of the economist to judge the 'correct' values, but to show decision makers how different values will affect choices about the best way to use resources.

CHOOSING BETWEEN OPTIONS

Choices about the benefit from different uses of resources are

Table 5.1 Measures of economic evaluation of neonatal intensive care, according to birthweight class

Period	Birthweight class	
	1000–1499 g ($)	500–999 g ($)
To hospital discharge Cost/survivor* at hospital discharge	59 500	102 500
To age 15 (projected)† Cost/life-year gained Cost/QALY gained	6100 7700	12 200 40 100
To death (projected)† Cost/life-year gained Cost/QALY gained Net economic benefit (loss)/live birth	2900 3200 (2600)	9300 22 400 (16 100)
Net economic cost/life-year gained	900	7300
Net economic cost/QALY gained	1000	17 500

Based on a comparison of births in 1964–1969, without regional neonatal intensive care, and 1973–1977, with a regional neonatal intensive care service (see Boyle et al 1983). Values are expressed in 1978 Canadian dollars, a discount rate of 5% per annum has been used for valuation of long-term costs and benefits (see Drummond et al 1986).
* Costs and benefits are marginal. They are measured as those which are *additional* to those resulting from care without a regional neonatal intensive care service.
† Projections of life expectancy and lifetime earning capacity and needs are based on pediatric assessments at upwards of 18 months.

seldom 'all or nothing' decisions. Care that is clearly good for some may be of less benefit for others. Cost–benefit analysis seeks to find the point, known as the *margin*, at which the additional benefit to be gained by the treatment is outweighed by the additional costs. For example, Boyle et al (1983) found that, for babies born weighing less that 1500 g between 1973 and 1977, the added benefit of neonatal intensive care was outweighed by the additional costs, but that this additional cost was significantly higher per unit of benefit for the babies of extremely low weight (under 1000 g) than for those weighing between 1000 and 1499 g. There is considerable variability of cost per case within these birthweight groups, so the results do not provide a decision rule for allocation of resources at the level of individual patient care. Changes in neonatal care over the last decade have altered the equation, but more recent research suggests that there is still, on average, a decreasing ratio of benefits to costs with decreasing birthweights (Mugford 1995).

RESULTS OF ECONOMIC RESEARCH

There is an increasing number of published studies of the economics of neonatal care, mostly on the narrower subject of the hospital costs of neonatal care. In general these show that: costs per patient day are high initially for individual babies but fall over the length of time they are in hospital; costs of intensive care constitute the largest part of the overall neonatal care cost; nursing costs are the largest single category of cost for a neonatal unit; and the costs of neonatal care, on average, increase with decreasing birthweight and gestation. Comparisons of data about cost-utility of different programs are complicated by differences in methodology between studies (Mason et al 1993), but suggest that neonatal intensive care for babies weighing 500–999 g costs less per QALY than continuous ambulatory peritoneal dialysis or hospital hemodialysis, both of which are widely accepted health care technologies in many countries. There are, however, many programs that have been shown to be more cost-effective, and many more that are still unevaluated. Current practices in neonatal care which are demonstrated not to be effective are an inefficient use of resources.

THE NORMAL FETAL–NEONATAL TRANSITION

The most vital change immediately after birth is for the lungs to expand to take in air. If lung expansion fails, death will occur quite rapidly and shortly after the umbilical cord is clamped. Almost as important as lung expansion is the change from the fetal type circulation, with the cardiac output bypassing the lungs, to the postnatal pattern where the cardiac output from the right side of the heart will perfuse the lungs and be oxygenated (Fig. 5.4). Less-urgent changes in the other organ systems must take place over the next days and weeks in order to ensure a viable postnatal existence.

THE LUNGS (Fig. 5.5)

The lungs of the fetus in utero are filled with a unique fluid which near term is being produced at a rate of about 3 ml/kg/h. Clearance of this fluid is crucial for successful air breathing and begins during labor. Each uterine contraction has been shown to generate surges of fetal catecholamines which reduce the rate of lung liquid secretion and, as labor progresses, lead to active resorption. Elective delivery of the baby before labor will lead to babies being born with wet lungs which result in transient tachypnea of the newborn (p. 182). Additional lung fluid is dispersed during the second stage of labor by a compression force of up to 160 cm of

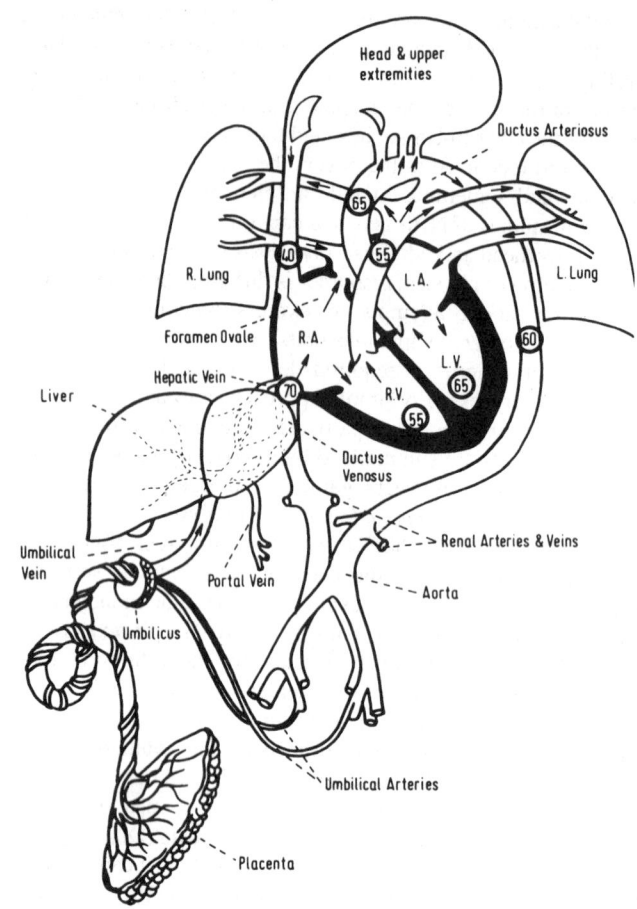

Fig. 5.4 Fetal circulation. The circled figures indicate oxygen saturation at various points, e.g. blood 70% saturated at point where inferior vena cava enters right atrium.

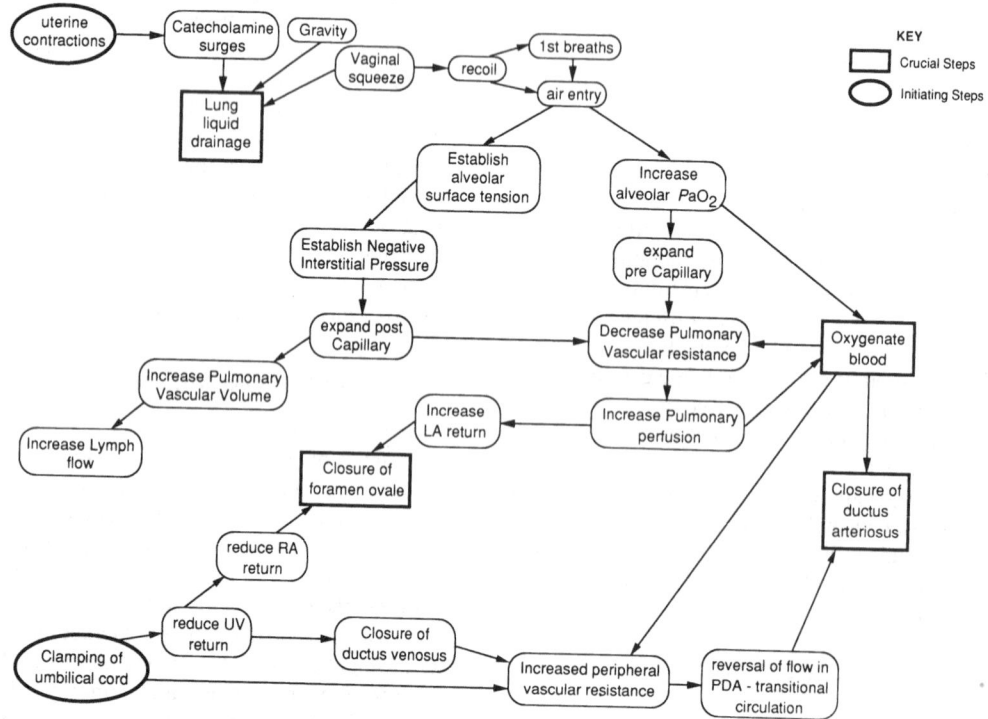

Fig. 5.5 The steps involved in lung expansion and the change in circulation after birth.

water and the elastic recoil from this vaginal squeeze may draw up to 50 ml of air into the chest. Where a mother delivers her infant from a squatting position, further fluid drains by gravity in the vertex delivery. Cesarean section can reduce the effectiveness of all these mechanisms to give an increased incidence of respiratory problems from wet lungs, but even the normal vaginally delivered infant will have a quantity of fluid in his lungs at the moment of birth.

The first gasps or cries of the baby achieve a transthoracic pressure of 70–90 cm of water and a tidal wave of air passes into the upper respiratory passages and larynx. This air initiates Head's paradoxical reflex which potentiates the first gasp. The Valsalva maneuver achieved by the infant crying against a partially closed glottis pushes further fluid from the airway through to the lymphatics. The first breath may generate a pressure as high as 70–120 cm water and may achieve a volume of 80 ml of air in the lungs. The gasps occurring immediately after birth are crucial for the success of air breathing. It is not clear which of the many stimuli that occur after birth are most important in initiating breathing. It may be the deluge of sensory information as the baby delivers – tactile (midwife's hands), thermal (air temperature in the delivery room and evaporation of liquor from the skin), noise, position, light, gravity, pain, etc. It is likely that chemoreceptor input caused by hypoxia and hypercarbia in the last moments before delivery (physiological asphyxia) are also important; however, severe hypoxia and acidemia may depress the respiratory center.

There are two major reasons for the failure of the lungs to expand at birth:

1. The lungs may be unable, physically, to expand either because they have failed to develop properly in utero (e.g. Potter's syndrome, prolonged liquor leakage, diaphragmatic hernia) or because the airway is obstructed (congenital laryngeal web, acquired meconium aspiration).

2. The brain may fail to initiate the expansion of the lungs (e.g. extreme immaturity, oversedation with obstetric prescribed narcotics or brain damage occurring during either the pregnancy or the delivery).

Effective means of resuscitation at birth are crucial in these situations (p. 132) and in developed countries should be available to all infants born.

HEART AND CARDIOVASCULAR SYSTEM

The left and right ventricles of the fetus both receive blood returning from the body (cf. after birth). Partly oxygenated blood ($PaO_2 = 3.7–4.7$ kPa (25–35 mmHg)) returning from the placenta via the ductus venosus and inferior vena cava is returned to the right atrium but is deflected by the 'valve' of the inferior vena cava through the patent foramen ovale into the left atrium. In utero only 5–10% of the cardiac output goes to and returns from the lungs; therefore the blood passing from the left atrium to the left ventricle is largely the oxygenated supply from the placenta. Left ventricular contraction powers blood to the aortic arch with its major vessels; thus the coronary and carotid arteries of the fetus, the priority areas, receive blood with the best possible oxygen content. Blood returning from the coronary sinus and the superior vena cava to the right atrium passes to the right ventricle and the pulmonary trunk. The high pulmonary vascular resistance of the fetus and the presence of the patent ductus arteriosus ensure that the right ventricular output predominantly (90%) supplies the

descending and abdominal aorta and the viscera. 50% of the abdominal flow goes via the two umbilical arteries to the placental bed where exchange of blood gases and other nutritional and excretory substances occurs (Fig. 5.5). The distribution of blood flow in utero is primarily dependent on the high vascular resistance of the unexpanded fetal lung and the low vascular resistance of the placenta. Fetal pulmonary arterioles have a thick medial muscle layer. The low fetal PaO_2 is thought to keep the vessels constricted. With the first gasps there is a rapid rise in the oxygen tension within the alveoli, and the arteriolar musculature relaxes and pulmonary perfusion occurs. The sudden increase in pulmonary venous return of well-oxygenated blood to the left atrium functionally closes the foramen ovale within minutes or hours of birth and this now well-oxygenated blood (PaO_2 greater than 7 kPa (50 mmHg)) is ejected up the aortic arch from the left ventricle. The closure of the ductus arteriosus is thought to be a result of the increased oxygen content. The ductal muscle in utero is maintained in a relaxed state by the combination of the relative hypoxia and the presence of high circulating levels of prostaglandins produced by the placenta.

The clamping of the umbilical cord raises the systemic vascular resistance and, as a consequence, blood may pass in the reverse direction through the patent ductus. This 'transitional circulation' may revert back to the fetal situation (right to left) if satisfactory oxygenation is not achieved (PPHM, p. 204). Functional closure of the ductus usually takes place within the first 24 h (and usually much earlier) after birth but before this, a systolic murmur may be present at the base of the heart from transient left to right ductal flow. After birth the pulmonary artery pressure falls from about 3.3–5.3 kPa (25–40 mmHg) on the first day to 2 kPa (15 mmHg) after 6 weeks. During this time there is a rise in the systemic blood pressure from 45–55 mmHg (6–7.3 kPa) to approximately 70 mmHg (9.3 kPa).

BRAIN AND CENTRAL NERVOUS SYSTEM

The brain and central nervous system develop steadily through fetal life, infancy and childhood. There are no dramatic changes that occur with or because of birth itself although sensory experience following birth is obviously different. At birth the cerebellum is more maturely developed than the cerebrum. Neuronal development and dendritic connections are more evident and myelination is already occurring from the oligodendroglia. Cerebral myelination and dendritic connections are predominantly postnatal events.

Brainstem and higher reflexes develop in late fetal life in an orderly fashion and can be used to estimate gestation (Ch. 2). Interruption at any stage will cause damage. The seriousness of ensuing problems will depend on the maturity of the brain at the time the damage occurs.

Some recognition patterns seem innate in the newborn. Immediately after birth many newborns will follow a simple stylized face through 180° though if the features are scrambled this will not occur. Other experiments show rapid learning ability; for example by the fifth day of life the breast-fed infant will be able to detect his own mother by his sense of smell.

THE GUT AND DIGESTION

Swallowing is well developed by the fourth month of in utero life. The inability to swallow in utero leads to hydramnios. Sucking develops rapidly after birth; usually the baby increases the number of sucks in a burst from 5–6 on the first day to 30 or more by day 3. Babies born at 28 weeks' gestation may also suck but the coordination of sucking, swallowing and breathing does not occur until 34–35 weeks' gestation. The importance of sucking and swallowing after birth is obvious but these have to be matched by the ability of the rest of the gastrointestinal tract to digest and absorb the food. Intestinal motor activity and the migrating motor complex are developed by 34 weeks' gestation but it is possible that feeding facilitates this development in a baby born earlier (Bisset et al 1989). Radiological investigation will show that air usually passes to the large bowel by 2 h of postnatal age, even in the very preterm infant. Most of the intestinal enzymes are present at birth but their full activity and that of the various gastrointestinal hormones are further induced by feeding. Breast milk is undoubtedly and not surprisingly better tolerated than other food and no additional nutritional supplements are required for at least 4–5 months of life in the full-term infant.

Meconium should be passed within 24 h of birth (95%). Should the baby fail to pass meconium, medical staff should be notified as an intestinal atresia, Hirschsprung's disease or meconium ileus may be the cause.

THE KIDNEYS AND RENAL FUNCTION

Dynamic measurements of bladder volume by ultrasound show that the fetus at full term will be producing 7 ml of urine/kg/h; thus glomerular filtration from the full complement of nephrons (present by 35 weeks' gestation) is considerable. Fine control of water balance in utero has been the concern of the placenta and after birth both glomerular and tubular immaturity mean that fluid and electrolyte insults on the newborn are poorly tolerated. The GFR of the term infant is only 10 ml/min/m², increasing to 15 ml/min/m² by the end of the first week. Renal blood flow is low at birth and the juxtaglomerular nephrons are preferentially perfused. Sodium resorption is well developed in the full-term infant (though not in the preterm) as the tubules are comparatively mature and the circulating aldosterone levels are high. The maximum urine osmolality is relatively low, not because of the baby's inability to secrete the antidiuretic hormone, arginine vasopressin (AVP), from the posterior pituitary but because the low solute and nitrogen content of breast milk result in a low solute concentration of the interstitial compartment of the medulla. Increasing the protein intake of the infant increases the maximum urine osmolality that is possible.

The renal bicarbonate threshold is low and there may be limited hydrogen ion excretion due to reduced phosphate availability. Both of these may lead to acidosis. The tubular cells are also less able to produce ammonia. This is more marked in preterm infants particularly with high protein and acid loads and leads to the late metabolic acidosis of prematurity.

The breast-fed infant receives low solute food with adequate nitrogen and calories: there is little stress on the kidneys. Unmodified cow's milk or solids contain too much solute and nitrogen and can rapidly lead to metabolic difficulties such as cow's milk tetany (p. 299) and hypernatremia (p. 144).

Congenital abnormalities of the kidney and renal excretory systems lead to metabolic upset developing over the first days or weeks of life depending on their severity. The common coexistence of pulmonary hypoplasia with complete renal agenesis (Potter's syndrome) ensures this abnormality presents as an acute respiratory difficulty, usually with rapid death.

LIVER FUNCTION

Immaturity of liver function leads to jaundice (p. 216) and also to the newborn's inability to tolerate drugs which are usually excreted via the biliary tree. The 'gray baby' syndrome is due to increased free and conjugated chloramphenicol levels in the serum leading to vomiting, poor sucking, respiratory distress, abdominal distention, diarrhea and eventually collapse. Liver immaturity may be a factor in the development of hemorrhagic disease of the newborn (p. 229) though damage to the liver from hypoxia and an inadequate supply of vitamin K are likely to be more important components.

BLOOD

The fetal hemoglobin predominant in the full-term newborn (80%) is ideal for oxygen uptake across the placenta at the low oxygen tensions that are present in utero. After birth this fetal hemoglobin is less able to unload oxygen at the tissues. Red cell 2,3-diphosphoglycerate levels increase rapidly in the newborn period to improve oxygen delivery and release, and the oxygen dissociation curve shows a shift to the right.

The blood volume of the newborn depends on the age at which the umbilical cord is clamped. Clamping within the first 15 s after delivery leads to a blood volume of around 75 ml/kg but delayed clamping increases this, the contracting uterus expelling blood from the sinuses of the placenta to the baby (Fig. 5.6). If the cord is not clamped for 3 min after delivery, the blood volume may be 95–100 ml/kg. In the term baby this is associated with a higher incidence of respiratory problems and jaundice but in the preterm infant, where the hemoglobin and red cell volume at birth tend to be lower, a 30-s delay in cord clamping with the newborn infant lower than the placenta may reduce the respiratory problems and the subsequent requirement for top-up blood transfusions.

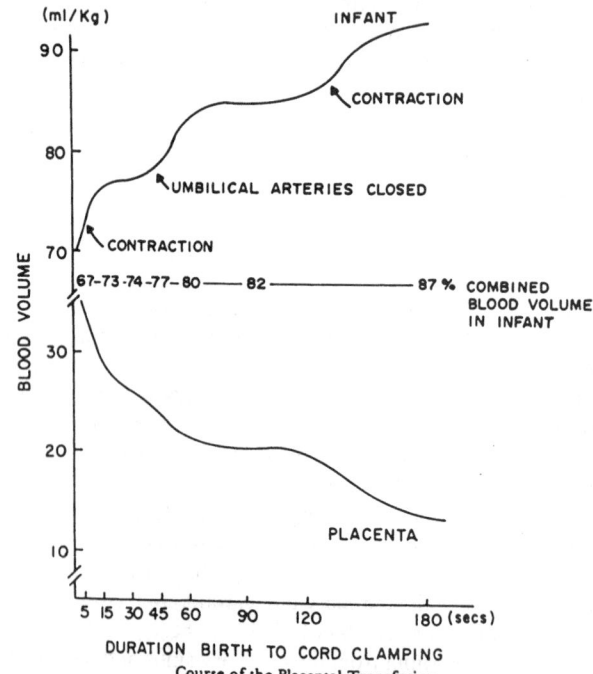

Fig. 5.6 Variation in infants' blood volume with time of clamping of the umbilical cord (from Smith & Nelson 1976 with permission).

ENDOCRINE SYSTEM

Numerous hormonal changes take place during labor and immediately after birth which allow the infant to adjust to the change in the environment and the loss of the placental supply of nutrients and minerals. There is a rapid surge in thyroid hormones, thought to be a response to cold exposure. Cortisol and ACTH rise with labor and peak a few hours after delivery in response to stress. Intact pituitary, thyroid, parathyroid, adrenal and pancreatic function are required to maintain glucose, calcium and electrolyte homeostasis. Babies with disorders of pituitary function may present with hypoglycemia or prolonged jaundice, and this may be associated with midline structural abnormalities of the brain (septo-optic dysplasia). Inborn errors of adrenocortical steroid synthesis (congenital adrenal hyperplasia) can present with ambiguous genitalia and/or salt loss.

THE IMMUNE RESPONSE AND INFECTION

Once delivered from the protected environment of the uterus, the baby is subjected to many potentially infectious agents. IgG transferred actively across the placenta in the last trimester of pregnancy will last for only a short time (up to 6 months). During this time the infant must develop his own antibodies. Although both B and T cells are potentially functional in utero the virginal experience (in relation to foreign antigen) in the uterus leads to a gap of cell-mediated immunity in the neonatal period. It is sensible for people overtly suffering with viral or bacterial infections not to be intimately involved with the management of newborn infants. Exposure to a pathogen leads to a response at a rate similar in the baby to that seen in older age groups. Absence of either B or T cell functions after birth leads to severe infections and if the diagnosis is not considered, the infant may die (Ch. 22).

ROUTINE CARE OF THE FULL-TERM INFANT

EXAMINATION OF THE NEONATE

Every doctor should develop a systematic and thorough routine for examining the neonate. The routine examination immediately after birth is a screening test and may be performed by midwife, general practitioner or hospital doctor. It ensures that the transition from fetal to postnatal life has been effected smoothly and reveals congenital abnormality that may impair normal development. At a later stage examination should in addition elicit minor blemishes in the baby that may cause the parents much worry and necessitate considerable reassurance. With each contact it should be ensured that the mother is providing appropriate care for her baby.

HISTORY

It is always essential to discuss details of the pregnancy and delivery with the mother. A systematic and thorough approach to the history taking is outlined in Table 5.2. This approach may appear rather complex and time consuming but in most cases can be significantly abbreviated.

Table 5.2 Outline of a suitable approach to history taking

Mother	Father
Age	Age
Race	Race

Past medical history of mother
Illnesses such as diabetes, hypertension, heart disease, kidney disease, or sickle cell disease

Family history of hereditary diseases
Hereditary disorders on either side of the family, such as cystic fibrosis, adrenogenital syndrome and hemophilia

Past obstetric history
Have all previous pregnancies, deliveries and babies been normal?
If not, why not?
Full details of all abnormalities

History of pregnancy
Date of last menstrual period
Results of ultrasound scans and, if performed, amniocentesis
Illnesses during pregnancy (e.g. rubella)
Complications (e.g. pre-eclampsia, antepartum hemorrhage, intrauterine growth retardation, polyhydramnios)

History of labor
Gestation at onset
Length of time membranes ruptured
Length of labor
Drugs used
Fetal heart irregularities
Fetal distress

History of delivery
Spontaneous, assisted (forceps), vertex, breech or Cesarean section (elective or emergency)

Resuscitation of baby
Oxygen, bag and mask intubation
Drugs given (e.g. naloxone, bicarbonate, other)
Condition of infant as assessed by Apgar score

EXAMINATION

Each doctor should develop a systematic routine for the examination of the neonate in order that the examination is thorough. Potentially painful maneuvers, such as checking for a cleft palate and testing for congenital dislocation of the hip, are best left until last. A possible regimen is outlined in Table 5.3.

Table 5.3 A systematic approach to examination of the neonate

General appearance
Lanugo or evidence of postmaturity
Pallor, jaundice or cyanosis
Features of Down syndrome, Turner's syndrome or Marfan's syndrome, etc.
Is the baby of appropriate weight for the period of gestation, or small or large for gestational age?

Skin
Birthmarks, meconium staining, traumatic cyanosis, purpura

Head
Size and tension of anterior and posterior fontanels
Cephalhematoma or depressed fracture
Head circumference
Sternomastoid swelling

Face
Potter's facies
Pierre Robin jaw (the combination of a receding jaw with cleft palate), harelip, accessory auricles, ptosis or cataract (red reflex), subconjunctival hemorrhage

Arms and hands
Proportions of arms and fingers, number of fingers, normal movements, Erb palsy, palmar creases, edema

Chest
Distortion, recession, distress, respiratory rate (<60 breaths/min), air entry, additional sounds, breast enlargement

Cardiovascular system
Apex precordial impulse, quality of pulses (brachial and femoral), heart sounds and murmurs

Abdomen
Palpate carefully for renal, bladder and other masses. Liver is normally palpable, but the spleen is never palpable. Lower poles of kidneys are commonly palpable

Genitalia
Male: testes (normal, undescended or maldescended), hernia or hydrocele, penis size, position of urethral orifice
Female: posterior vaginal skin tag is common, clitoromegaly, vaginal bleeding

Legs and feet
Proportions of legs and feet, club foot, femoral pulses

Back
Scoliosis, spina bifida, sacral pit

CNS
Are all four limbs moving normally?
Is the baby alert and vigorous when awake or quiet?
Is the cry normal?
Are the Moro and grasp reflexes symmetrical?

Mouth
Is there a cleft soft palate (or worse)?
Is saliva profuse (? esophageal atresia)?
Are Epstein's pearls present (nodules on the hard palate)?

Test for congenital dislocation of the hip
With the hips and knees flexed at right angles the thighs are abducted. During this maneuver, a dislocated femoral head will 'clunk' back into the acetabulum

TRANSITIONAL PROBLEMS

Respiratory problems Premature babies and babies with some congenital malformations may have difficulty in achieving satisfactory pulmonary gas exchange after birth. A rapid respiratory rate, intercostal recession or cyanosis may be seen. It is most important to have good lighting where a baby is delivered or cyanosis may be missed.

Liver. Serological jaundice is invariably present between days 2 and 6 though it may not be clinically evident. If jaundice is seen in the first 36 h or lasts longer than 10 days or rises to high levels, further investigation is indicated.

Gut. Failure to pass meconium within 24 h may indicate Hirschsprung's disease or meconium ileus.

Micturition. Urine is normally passed within 24 h. If it is not, it was probably passed during the delivery but it is important to check for the characteristic low-set ears of Potter's facies (which is associated with abnormalities of the renal tract) or a palpable bladder.

Genital bleeding. Vaginal bleeding may occur at about 5–7 days following the rapid excretion of maternal and placental estrogens transmitted to the fetus before birth. Considerable reassurance may be required for the parents when this happens.

Breast enlargement and production of milk (witch's milk). This may occur in either male or female. Milk production is due to the placental transfer of estrogens from the mother. Considerable reassurance may be required.

Birth trauma. See page 120.

CONGENITAL ABNORMALITIES

Congenital abnormalities may be extremely obvious as in the case of talipes, meningomyelocele or Down syndrome. Furthermore a complete physical examination should reveal most immediately life-threatening internal abnormalities (e.g. cyanosis or heart murmur are indicative of congenital heart lesion, enlarged kidneys suggestive of bilateral hydronephrosis or palpable bladder secondary to urethral valves). Many very minor abnormalities or even deviations from the 'norm' can cause parents to panic and considerable reassurance may be required.

Birthmarks, e.g. nevus flammeus, strawberry marks, blue spots, port-wine stains, pigmented nevi, see Chapter 25.

Other skin problems such as erythema toxicum, milia, see Chapter 25.

Minor toe webbing. This is a minor deviation of no clinical significance. It may be familial.

Sacral pit. If the bottom of the pit is visible, there need be no anxiety. If the bottom cannot be seen or there is an associated hemangioma the infant should be referred to a pediatrician for X-ray and probably MRI.

Umbilical hernia. This is more common in the Afro-Caribbean infant than in other races. Treatment need never be given during the first year of life since such hernias do not obstruct. Even large hernias almost invariably disappear with time.

Other abnormalities. Parents should be reassured if possible but should always be given simple clear and full information. A second opinion is often appropriate and does not reflect any inadequacy in the first doctor.

SATISFACTORY CARE

The mother's handling of her baby while the history is taken and her behavior during the examination will usually alert the doctor to any problem in the developing relationship between mother and baby. The doctor should also consider the following points: Is the baby satisfactorily nourished? Has the weight gain been satisfactory since birth? If not, is the artificial feed being made up incorrectly, or is the mother persevering with breast-feeding when she is not actually producing any milk? The progress of weight, length and head circumference should always be plotted on a centile chart.

LABOR WARD ROUTINES

ENSURE AIRWAYS ARE CLEAR

As the head and airways deliver through the mother's perineum the nasal passages and mouth should be gently cleared of liquor, vaginal secretions and other matter. In the past this has been done by an orally controlled mucus extractor. Worries about possible HIV transmission from mother to attendant now make it more appropriately done by a gently applied suction catheter. Note that vigorous pharyngeal suction causes reflex vagal bradycardia and sometimes apnea. Once the airway is cleared suction is *not* the way to stimulate a baby to breathe.

TEMPERATURE CONSIDERATIONS

The most potent cause of heat loss in the newborn infant is evaporation. This can be reduced by wiping the baby dry with a warm towel immediately after delivery. It takes less than 10 s and is also a very good stimulus for the baby to breathe. Warm towels should always be available.

THE CORD

The cord should be clamped by a disposable cord clamp or tied firmly twice with cord ligature. Cord clamps are unlikely to slip. Two cord ties with ligature are unlikely both to work loose. The cord separates by an inflammatory reaction later.

MOTHER'S PROPERTY AND SUCKLING

After respiration is achieved and the cord clamped the baby should be given to the mother. If she has elected to breast-feed, the baby should be suckled there and then, nude baby on the mother's bare chest. Although babies are supposed at this stage only to lick the nipple, they have not read the textbooks and some try to suck very maturely. Suckling in the labor ward/delivery room is associated with a much higher rate of successful breast-feeding.

APGAR SCORES

The 1-min score will probably need to be calculated as the cord clamp is being secured. The 5-min Apgar score will often be while the baby is being suckled by the mother. In the uncomplicated delivery the baby can frequently be at the breast by 2 min of age.

OTHER RITUALS

The baby should be weighed at a convenient point: this does not have to be immediately after birth, though sometimes the parents like to know the weight early on. Labels should be put on the infant after the parents have made physical and emotional welcome to their baby and before they leave the delivery room so that there is no possibility of losing or confusing babies later. At this stage vitamin K may be given if it is the hospital routine (p. 230). A nasogastric tube may be passed to rule out esophageal atresia and choanal atresia but in an otherwise apparently normal baby we believe this routine is unnecessary. If meconium has not been passed the temperature may be taken rectally to ensure the anus is patent. The baby is then clothed as the parents wish and a nappy is put on.

We believe that all babies should be delivered in hospital *in case* there is a rapidly developing problem. When the delivery and baby are obviously normal the parents should be allowed to be with their new family member from then on.

POSTNATAL WARD ROUTINES

On the postnatal ward the baby should be kept with the mother. A baby should only go to a ward nursery at night if it is the mother's *spontaneous* request: staff should then ensure that they know whether the mother would like the infant brought to her for feeding and changing in the middle of the night.

On first admission it is traditional to take the temperature (rectally) and count the pulse rate and respiratory rate. There may be a practical reason for the last of these (early detection of intrapartum pneumonia or respiratory distress syndrome) but the taking of rectal temperatures is an unnecessarily invasive ritual if the baby is otherwise normal. Repeated measurements of pulse and respiration and particularly temperature should be discouraged if the baby is clinically well.

VITAL FUNCTIONS

Urine should be passed in the first 24 h of life (95%). Most of the remainder have micturated at the time of delivery without it being observed. 99% of babies pass urine in 48 h. Urine flow is 24–48 ml/kg in the first 36 h of life and at least double this thereafter. Isolated oliguria or anuria is very uncommon.

Meconium is frequently passed soon after delivery. Failure of passage by 24 h may indicate Hirschsprung's disease or meconium ileus and investigations should proceed for these conditions if there is clinical suspicion. After 2–3 days of milk feeding the dark green meconium (bile-stained intestinal secretions, intestinal debris and cells) becomes mixed with a milk stool and after a further 2–3 days the yellow milk stool is present. Over the first week the baby usually opens his bowels many times a day. If breast-fed this is usually with every feed and the stool is loose in consistency. Mothers need to be warned that this is not diarrhea. The bottle-fed infant opens his bowels less frequently and the stool is usually the consistency of pale yellow toothpaste.

All babies lose weight after birth. A 10% weight loss over the first 4 days is not unusual and reflects the edematous state of the baby at birth. After the fourth or fifth day the fluid shifts (extracellular water is both excreted and to a lesser extent shifted intracellularly) are complete and the baby should begin to put on weight at a rate of approximately 25 g/day until discharge. Test weighing breast-fed babies is both highly inaccurate and also demeaning to both mother and baby. It is rarely if ever required.

Vomiting is common in the normal newborn but can occasionally be an early warning sign of abnormality. Mucus or milk vomiting can be accepted if occasional. Bile- or bloodstained vomit should always be promptly investigated (p. 209).

Bloodstained vomit may be the result of swallowing maternal blood during delivery.

BABY CARE

Mothering does not often come naturally and the postnatal period can be used by mother and staff as an education period, consolidating the antenatal classes.

The cord should be cleaned with spirit daily. It is common and not necessarily bad to then dust the base with antistaphylococcal powder (chlorhexidine). If the cord becomes sticky or purulent or the periumbilical area becomes inflamed a medical opinion should be sought.

Bathing is unnecessary on the first day but on the second day and subsequently the mother can be instructed on how to bath the baby. Particular attention should be paid to the groin and buttocks and creases of the neck. Ordinary baby soap should be used.

Mothers are sometimes worried about the baby's temperature control. If the surroundings (postnatal ward or bedroom) are suitable in temperature for a mother clothed only in a nightdress then a baby in a gown or babygrow and under two blankets should be quite warm enough. Do not supply extra heat either by nearby radiators or hot water bottles. Epidemiological data show it is safer for an infant to sleep supine.

GENITALIA

Foreskins, like vaginas, should be left severely alone by both parents and doctors. Circumcision of either sex is a nonmedical ritual.

FEEDING THE FULL-TERM NEWBORN (Ch. 6)

BREAST MILK

The milk of the mother has been uniquely developed to be appropriate in composition for the human newborn infant (Table 5.4). The rise in prolactin from the anterior pituitary during pregnancy is inhibited from producing milk by the high pregnancy levels of progesterone but with the delivery of the baby, further prolactin secretion and the withdrawal of other circulating hormones (progesterone, estrogens and placental lactogen) leads to lactogenesis. Nipple stimulation (suckling) exaggerates prolactin production; thus after birth the baby is literally switching on the mother's milk production. Nipple stimulation also causes secretion of oxytocin from the posterior pituitary which leads to contraction of the myoepithelial cells surrounding the milk-filled lactiferous sinuses to cause milk ejection (the let-down reflex). Oxytocin release (and let-down) may also come from visual, auditory and other stimuli.

Over the first 48–72 h the secretions from the breast (colostrum) are high in protein, hormones, immunoglobulins and white cells but are low in volume. After this time the milk 'comes in' sometimes causing extreme tenseness and tenderness of the breasts. Continued suckling by the infant empties the breast and stimulates further milk production. Once the baby is feeding well the breast will be emptied in about 5 min and further time is for emotional and physical satisfaction of mother and baby as much as for nutrition.

Breast milk is variable in composition both with the stage of lactation and as the feed progresses (towards the end of the feed, it is high in fat and calories). The latter may be important for appetite development. The data in the literature are variable as to whether the mother who has had a preterm infant has more concentrated milk than the mother of the full-term infant and, because the composition is anyway variable, it is probably only of academic interest.

BREAST MILK SUBSTITUTES (Table 5.4)

Formula feeds are derived from cow's milk. Although the overall calorie density of unmodified cow's milk (65 cal/100 ml) is similar to human breast milk, the composition is very different. Modification involves reducing the high protein and particularly casein concentration and substituting lactalbumin (whey protein). The high sodium and phosphate concentrations are reduced, iron and vitamin D are added and the fatty acid composition is made more like breast milk. Despite all these modifications and accepting that modified formulae are generally safe when made up as recommended with a sterile water supply, they are all *very second rate* compared to breast milk. In the western world where water supplies are well prepared there is usually no problem using a powdered milk formula but in the developing world where water

Table 5.4 Composition of milks

Per 100 ml	Colostrum	Mature breast milk	Drip breast milk (foremilk)	Unmodified cow's milk	Ostermilk*	Aptamil*
Energy calories	67	70	45	65	68	67
Protein (g)	2.3	1.34	1.0	3.2	1.45	1.5
Fat (g)	2.95	4.2	2.2	3.8	3.82	3.6
Carbohydrate (g)	5.7	7.1	6.5	4.7	7.0	7.3
Sodium (mg)	50	19		77	19	18
Calcium (mg)	48	27		137	35	59
Phosphorus (mg)	16	14		91	29	35
Iron (µg)	100	50		45	650	700
Vitamin A (µg)	161	60		23	100	61
Vitamin C (µg)	7.2	5.2		1.1	6.9	6.0
Vitamin D (µg)	0.04	0.1		0.02	1.0	1.0
Vitamin E (mg)	1.5	0.24		0.06	0.48	0.7
Vitamin B$_6$ (mg)	–	0.018		0.05	0.035	0.03
Folic acid (µg)	0.05	2.4		3.8	3.4	10

* Ostermilk and Aptamil are two commercial full-term baby formulae available in Europe from Farley Health Products Ltd (The Boots Company PLC, UK) and Milupa Ltd (Altana AG, West Germany), respectively.

supplies are frequently contaminated their use may lead to disastrous gastroenteritis, other infections and death.

Milk derived from soya or other sources, for instance goats, have *no place* in the feeding of normal newborn infants and may be very dangerous.

PRACTICAL BREAST-FEEDING

Successful breast-feeding depends on both the mother and infant being relaxed. It is more difficult for the mother to relax in a hospital environment and this is definitely on the negative side with regard to hospital delivery. There has been a great tendency for hospital routines developed pseudoscientifically to dominate both midwifery and medical staff (4-hourly feeds, timed at the breast) and the power of the bottle of formula left at the end of the bed 'just in case' to erode maternal confidence cannot be minimized. It has now been clearly shown that breast-feeding early in the delivery room, rooming in, demand feeding and untimed suckling all increase the chances of successful breast-feeding for the mother. An empathetic midwife or other counselor with previous experience can be extremely helpful in showing the mother useful tips.

Over the first 24 h the baby will probably only wish to feed three to four times and may be quite sleepy between feeds. By the fifth day the baby at the breast will be demanding feeds nearly 2-hourly. He is switching on his mother's supply at this stage but not because she has not the potential to produce enough milk. After the milk has come in the baby will settle down by 10–12 days to $3\frac{1}{2}$- to 4-hourly feeds in most instances. Breast-feeding mothers should be taught this antenatally so they do not become unnecessarily despondent (Fig. 5.7).

PRACTICAL BOTTLE-FEEDING

The practice of using ready-to-feed milk in hospitals is convenient but means that the mother who has chosen to bottle-feed may not have seen or made up a bottle of milk when she returns home. Midwives should ensure that the mother who is choosing to bottle-feed sees how to prepare such a bottle. Powdered milk must

be reconstituted in the way stated on the packet with water that has boiled and cooled a few minutes previously. The practice of adding extra scoops is still not uncommon in western cultures and may be dangerous if the baby has a free water loss from any cause, though hypernatremia is uncommon with modern commercial milks. (In the developing world the high cost of milk formulae leads to overdilution on economic grounds so that infants fail to thrive for lack of sufficient calories and nutrition; Ch. 6).

Bottles and teats should be carefully cleaned soon after use and should be kept in a 1% hypochlorite solution to ensure sterility.

After the first few days of life the bottle-fed baby usually demands food about 4-hourly. If the baby is demanding food more often and is irritable it may be that thirst rather than hunger is the problem and clear fluid (pure water is best) may be needed.

THE HIGH-RISK FETUS AND INFANT

HIGH-RISK PREGNANCY

'High-risk' pregnancy is a concept which has evolved over the last two decades, and is now an integral part of obstetric thinking. It defines a pregnancy where mother or fetus has a disorder which puts one or other at increased risk of morbidity or mortality. Risk assessment is important not only in identifying the pregnancy at high risk, so that the appropriate expertise and resources can be directed towards that woman and fetus, but also in defining low-risk pregnancy, so that the majority of women with normal pregnancies can be spared overinvestigation, overattendance at clinics and medicalization of their pregnancy. However, it is clear that many pregnancies not initially recognized as high risk become so (for example with unexpected preterm labor) and conversely many 'high-risk' pregnancies proceed to uncomplicated delivery of a mature healthy baby. Although the concept of 'risk' is important in planning care, and some genuinely high-risk conditions can be easily defined, the prediction of risk at a population level is very imprecise.

PREDICTION OF 'HIGH RISK'

The initial and important step in antenatal care is to obtain a comprehensive history. Risk features can then be highlighted, and a strategy for antenatal management developed. The traditional type of history taking has faults, and various attempts at a more structured and formalized approach have been made. The most powerful predictors of 'high risk' in the history are certain medical conditions and previous obstetric history; but there are cumulative risks of maternal age, parity, social class, smoking, attitude to pregnancy and acceptance of medical care which may increase the risk of any pregnancy complication which does develop.

Several schematic approaches to objective assessment of risk, both at booking and throughout pregnancy, have been devised. However Alexander & Keirse (1989) reviewing formal risk scoring systems, concluded that current evidence did not support their use outside the context of a well-defined trial.

When a particular high-risk feature is identified, appropriate strategy for management has to be followed. The highest risk of perinatal death usually occurs amongst those mothers who suffer from multiple problems of social, biological and pathological

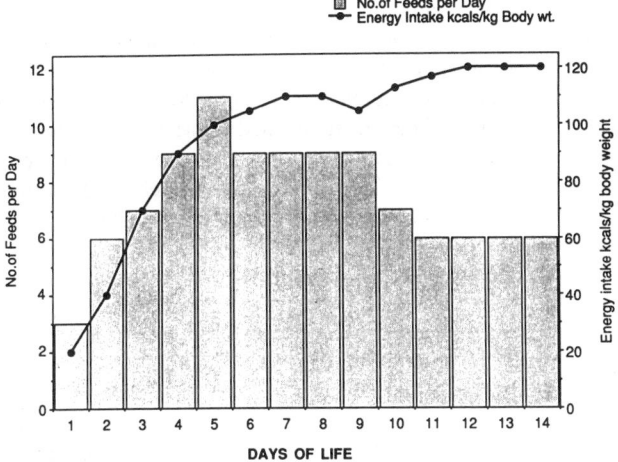

Fig. 5.7 Line graph – daily spontaneous energy intake of bottle-fed babies offered as much as they would take (Faber 1922). Histogram – the number of feeds chosen each day during the first 14 days of life by an infant on self-regulation (Simsarian & McLendon 1942).

origin. At the same time, those women who have the highest cumulative risk can sometimes be those who have the poorest medical care. 'High-risk' labeling should focus attention on that pregnancy to ensure that appropriate specialized care is delivered in a way that is acceptable, and increasingly this involves close liaison with community services.

PREPREGNANCY CARE

Many fetal anomalies have their origin early in pregnancy before a woman is likely to present for antenatal care. One of the major remaining problems in the management of a diabetic pregnancy, for example, is the high incidence of serious structural congenital anomalies. The incidence of congenital anomaly in the offspring of diabetic mothers is increased two- to fourfold over that in nondiabetic pregnancies, ranging from 4 to 11% in published series. In addition, the abnormalities are more likely to be severe and more often multiple and fatal. There is evidence that inadequate diabetic control is a teratogenic factor as several workers have shown an association between high glycosylated hemoglobin levels in early pregnancy and congenital anomalies. Because the defects typically occur before the seventh week, the problem cannot be prevented by improving diabetic control after the woman has attended for routine antenatal care. Thus attention has focused on prepregnancy counseling, with explanation of risks and advice about diabetic control as a way of preventing anomalies (Drury & Dodridge 1992). There is much circumstantial evidence that such an approach does reduce the risk of fetal malformation and this justifies the attempt to achieve good metabolic control around the time of conception (Fuhrmann et al 1989, Steel et al 1990).

Genetic counseling is well established as part of prepregnancy care. This should include not only those at risk because of family history or a previously affected baby, but also those at risk from hemoglobinopathies where screening should ideally occur before pregnancy. This allows testing of the partner, discussion of the issues, and explanation of the available methods of prenatal diagnosis.

Women with epilepsy should have their medication reviewed. There is a general belief that all anticonvulsant drugs are mildly teratogenic. The most common malformations are NTDs and facial clefts and congenital heart defects. Some women may be able to stop therapy before pregnancy if they no longer need their anticonvulsants. For the remainder, the aim should be monotherapy, in the lowest dose that effectively controls seizures. Of the four well-established front line antiepileptic drugs (valproate, carbamazepine, phenytoin, phenobarbitone) valproate may have the highest teratogenic risk but studies have produced conflicting results. Since no definite agreement has been reached, consensus opinion is to continue the one of these drugs which successfully controls seizures in a given patient (Delgado-Escueta & Janz 1992). A diet containing adequate folate should be advised, but in addition 5 mg folic acid is recommended.

There are a number of other medical conditions where special investigations can be performed before pregnancy, and management during pregnancy usefully discussed. These include systemic lupus erythematosus, hypertension, hemoglobinopathies and renal disease.

Finally, prepregnancy care has enormous potential for all pregnancies if it can concentrate attention on changing harmful aspects of lifestyles such as smoking, alcohol use and poor nutrition. The question of whether folate helps prevent recurrence of neural tube defects was finally settled by a randomized control trial (MRC Vitamin Study Research Group 1991). This study showed a reduction of 72% in recurrence of neural tube defect with folate supplementation. Based on this, the current recommendations for women with a *history* of neural tube defect is to take 5 mg folic acid daily before pregnancy and for the first 12 weeks. If there is *no* previous history, women are advised to take 400 μg folic acid daily.

PRENATAL THERAPY

There are still few ways of improving the intrauterine environment for the fetus. One of the most promising was the use of low-dose aspirin as prophylaxis of uteroplacental insufficiency and pre-eclampsia. This drug, in a dose of 60–75 mg daily, has been shown to inhibit thromboxane production by fetal platelets without affecting prostacyclin production in umbilical vessels. This has considerable potential benefit in certain high-risk pregnancies, particularly with hypertension where platelet aggregation, alterations in the prostacyclin–thromboxane ratio and uterine and placental vasoconstriction are important in the pathophysiology. Five small randomized controlled trials provided evidence for the value of low-dose aspirin. Despite the high hopes, large randomized controlled trials have failed to confirm benefit. The largest trial (Farrell 1994) involved 9364 pregnant women selected on risk, and randomized to receive either aspirin (60 mg) or placebo. No overall benefit was identified, and only small differences were found in subsequent subgroup analysis. However, there were no adverse effects. A further trial in 1009 women selected on risk similarly showed no difference in pre-eclampsia, premature delivery, growth retardation or complications (ECPPA 1996). It remains possible that small subgroups of very high-risk women may benefit, but aspirin has not fulfilled its early promise.

An area which may assume greater importance in future is the manipulation and early maturation of fetal enzyme systems. A most important development has been the consensus on the benefit of antenatal steroids for the prevention of hyaline membrane disease. Reduction in respiratory distress syndrome and neonatal death in preterm delivery were shown in a meta-analysis of 15 randomized controlled trials including 3560 neonates (Crowley 1995) and with observational evidence of effectiveness in more than 35 000 infants (Wright et al 1995). There is theoretical potential for harmful long-term effects but none have so far been demonstrated. Currently therefore this seems to be a major advance in perinatal care. Unfortunately, a possible potentiating effect of thyrotropin-releasing hormone (TRH) has been disproved, and indeed, this drug showed adverse effects (ACTOBAT 1995).

Other examples of nonsurgical interventions in prenatal therapy include the use of aspirin and steroids or aspirin and heparin in women with antiphospholipid antibody syndrome (Rai et al 1996) and the occasional use of digoxin and verapamil in persistent fetal tachycardias.

Of surgical interventions, the diagnostic techniques of chorionic villus sampling and fetal blood sampling are well established. Direct intravascular fetal transfusion has proved a very effective approach in treating very severe rhesus disease. A similar technique has been used in alloimmune thrombocytopenia though this probably has a limited place (Mueller-Eckhart et al

1989). Traditional surgery for congenital diaphragmatic hernia has been performed in utero, but with mixed results (Harrison et al 1993). New, and preliminary developments include operative fetoscopy, possible applications being umbilical cord ligation of acardiac twins (Quintero et al 1994) and laser photocoagulation of communicating vessels in twin–twin transfusion (Ville et al 1995).

Further examples of invasive surgical techniques include in utero shunting of obstructive uropathies. This is limited to the small group of fetuses with normal chromosomes, no associated fetal anomaly, bilateral urinary obstruction accompanied by oligohydramnios with reasonable residual renal function at a gestation of less than 32 weeks. The place of in utero shunting in congenital hydrocephalus is uncertain and clinical experience has so far been disappointing.

FETAL SURVEILLANCE

Assessment of growth has always been an important determinant of fetal well-being, with the most accurate measurement being that of serial abdominal circumference with ultrasound (Bucher & Schmidt 1993, Ewighman et al 1993). Much more attention needs to be paid to growth velocity, rather than size, and charts for this purpose have been produced (Owen et al 1995). However, clinical examination is important, and measurement of symphysis–fundal height with a tape measure may be as effective as ultrasound in screening for growth retardation (Pearce & Campbell 1987).

The only investigation which has been shown on meta-analysis of randomized controlled trials to reduce fetal mortality is Doppler assessment of flow velocity waveform in the umbilical artery (Alfirevic & Neilson 1995). This measures downstream vascular resistance, dependent on placental tertiary villous arterioles, and hence gives prognostic information of uteroplacental problems. Absent end-diastolic frequency in high-risk pregnancies is associated with poor clinical outcome and a high chance of fetal acidosis. Normal Doppler in a stable clinical situation is highly predictive of fetal well-being. The test is helpful in segregating pregnancies into those requiring intensive surveillance and those where more relaxed clinical or biophysical monitoring is adequate. In meta-analysis the odds ratio for reduction in fetal death was 0.62 with 95% confidence interval 0.45 to 0.85. More sophisticated assessment of the fetal vascular system is targeted at the detection of centralization of blood flow (increased in the middle cerebral artery) in comparison to decreased abdominal aortic flow.

Short-term well-being of the fetus can be assessed by fetal movement counting by the woman herself. The baby in the third trimester makes an average of approximately 800 body movements per 24 h and reduction in movement, and then cessation, will usually precede intrauterine death by at least 12 h. One randomized controlled trial in high-risk patients did show a significant reduction in perinatal death in the group asked to count fetal movement. A large, multicenter trial showed no benefit (Grant et al 1989) but this study included all hospital pregnant women and clear management protocols were not defined.

Nonstressed fetal heart testing (cardiotocography) is still widely used. The critical sign of well-being is the presence of accelerations above baseline (greater than 15 beats/min in amplitude and lasting longer than 15 s) in association with fetal movement or uterine contractions. A persistently nonreactive tracing in the absence of maternal sedation, fasting or a fetal cardiac anomaly, is very likely to be due to serious fetal compromise. However, despite the huge amount of evidence that nonstressed testing (NST) does accurately reflect short-term well-being, evidence that the use of cardiotocography improves perinatal outcome is lacking.

Measurement of amniotic fluid volume by ultrasound gives further indication of fetal response to chronic hypoxic stress. Oligohydramnios, with no renal abnormality and an intact sac may reflect decreased renal blood flow and where this is 'absolute' (no cord-free pool greater than 2 cm) this usually mandates delivery. Amniotic fluid volume is of particular value in post-term pregnancies, where oligohydramnios may occur quite quickly and where fetal hypoxia can result from cord compression.

A combination of ultrasound, visualization of fetal movement, fetal breathing, fetal tone and amniotic fluid volume, together with a nonstress test was developed by Manning et al (1987) as a 'biophysical profile'. The application of this test has been well described (Harman et al 1994). Although there are no randomized controlled trials showing reduction in perinatal death with use of biophysical profile, the corrected stillbirth rate in the pregnancies monitored because of risk, was significantly lower than for the untested, apparently normal pregnancies. The technique requires experience, but is quick and appears to have advantages over NST alone.

A problem with the above tests is that they rely on fairly gross signs of cerebrocardiac response. Abnormality therefore occurs late in the course of the evolution of chronic hypoxia, and an abnormal test may mean that already some damage is done. In addition, a central problem of monitoring is that clinical criteria for monitoring are not very discriminatory, and many monitored pregnancies are not at risk, and are monitored unnecessarily. Generally speaking, current testing works well in conditions involving uteroplacental supply problems and growth retardation. The tests appear to be less predictive in normal-size babies and in other conditions (Soothill et al 1993).

PRETERM LABOR

Preterm labor is the major obstetric factor determining perinatal mortality and long-term handicap. Spontaneous labor is only one reason for early delivery but is a very significant one. Several different prediction scores have been developed, the best known being that of Creasy et al (1980). Patients classified as high risk by this score at the initial clinic visit comprised 9% of the population but accounted for 44% of the preterm births. However, the efficacy of the scoring system relies heavily on a previous history of preterm delivery. Only 31% of primigravid preterm deliveries were predicted. On the other hand approximately 15% of women with one previous preterm delivery and 40% of those with two previous preterm deliveries will deliver preterm in a subsequent pregnancy.

General advice about daily work activity, avoidance of stress, support at home and smoking seems reasonable, but is of unproven value. The same applies to explanation of the possibility of very early preterm delivery, early recognition and early hospital admission. However, patient education may result in women attending earlier in the course of labor and this may allow tocolysis to be successful, give enough time for antenatal steroids to be effective, or allow the baby to be delivered in optimal conditions with ideal circumstances for initial resuscitation and stabilization. Detection of fetal fibronectin in the vagina may predict preterm delivery in high-risk asymptomatic pregnancies (Leeson et al 1996) but the place of this test is not yet established.

There is sufficient evidence to justify antibiotic treatment of asymptomatic bacteriuria, and also to justify aggressive treatment of vaginal infection in high-risk cases, though the relationship between infection and preterm birth is still under discussion.

In particular, recent interest surrounds the association of bacterial vaginosis with preterm delivery, odds ratios of 2–4 typically being found (Hillier et al 1995, Hay et al 1994). Two randomized placebo-controlled studies have shown modest reductions in the rate of preterm delivery in high-risk groups given antibiotic treatment for bacterial vaginosis (Morales et al 1994, Hauth et al 1995). The role of antibiotics in established preterm labor or preterm premature rupture of the membranes is still undefined. Benefits seem to outweigh harms but this is currently the subject of a large multicenter RCT (ORACLE).

Unequivocal evidence of cervical incompetence is found uncommonly, but cervical suture transforms the outlook for these few cases. Cervical suture does seem to have some place in less classical cases of previous loss (MRC/RCOG 1993) and assessment of cases may be helped by measurement of the cervix in the nonpregnant state.

The role of home uterine monitoring with tocography has not been established (Colton et al 1995). There is no indication that prophylactic beta-sympathomimetic drugs decrease the incidence of preterm labor (Keirse et al 1989). The use of prophylactic maternal corticosteroids to enhance fetal lung maturity in women at very high risk has not been examined in detail. Hospitalization has not been shown to be effective in twin pregnancy (Maclennan et al 1990).

There is a persistent belief that a comprehensive program of care can decrease the incidence of preterm labor, but although this has been claimed for a total population, the effect did not seem to extend to those women at highest risk (Papiernik et al 1985).

The diagnosis of ongoing preterm labor is difficult and in most series around 60% of untreated cases do not progress to delivery. The presence of fetal breathing movements makes it less likely that premature labor will become established (Agustsson & Patel 1987). A number of drugs have been used in an attempt to suppress preterm labor. The most widely used have been sympathomimetic amines. These are potentially dangerous drugs and they cause unpleasant symptoms of tachycardia, tremor, restlessness and anxiety. Pulmonary edema is a particular concern, often but not always associated with fluid overload or synergistic effects of other drugs, and maternal deaths have been reported. Although they clearly do inhibit contraction in the short term, tachyphylaxis is a problem and there is continuing doubt about their effectiveness in reducing perinatal mortality and morbidity. There are no trials which are ideally designed and large enough to provide convincing evidence of their benefit. The largest (Merkatz et al 1980) took 7 years and involved 11 institutions and although it did show apparent benefit there are several features of design which are not optimal.

Other drugs are largely experimental. Prostaglandin inhibitors are effective in suppressing uterine activity, but again there are no studies demonstrating effectiveness in reducing mortality or morbidity, and there are concerns about premature closure or constriction of the fetal ductus arteriosus, persistent pulmonary hypertension in the newborn, decreased urine production, oligohydramnios and animal work showing decreased placental blood flow. Calcium channel antagonists have not been

adequately evaluated, and there are concerns about maternal and fetal safety. Oxytocin antagonists (Atosiban) are being intensively studied but their role is not yet clear.

Preterm labor remains a major obstetric concern, with the etiology poorly understood and treatments of uncertain value. In many cases, the role of the obstetrician remains in ensuring that the mother gets antenatal corticosteroids, that there is enough time for these to be effective, and that the baby is delivered in optimal condition.

HIGH-RISK DELIVERY

Much obstetric attention centers around judging the optimal time and mode of delivery and ensuring that the neonatologist receives the baby in as good a condition as possible, free from the effects of asphyxia, infection, trauma and hypothermia. This often involves balancing risks of quite different natures, for example a very small risk of very serious abnormal outcome (fetal death) against a high risk of relatively minor abnormal outcome (minor neonatal morbidity, maternal morbidity from Cesarean section). In high-risk pregnancy there is an inherent risk of intrauterine death in continuing pregnancy but this is kept at a minimum with careful surveillance and this remote risk may be run in order to improve neonatal and maternal morbidity. This has been well demonstrated in diabetic pregnancy where the tendency to allow uncomplicated pregnancies to reach term has greatly improved neonatal well-being. Cesarean section, which must often seem the simple way out of a high-risk situation, carries a sixfold increase in maternal mortality compared with vaginal delivery, is associated with postnatal depression, delays postpartum recovery and can sometimes mean repeat Cesarean section in another pregnancy. Obstetrics has become more invasive and more technological, and while this has brought undoubted benefits, it has also brought public disquiet. Cesarean section rates of around 15% in the UK and 21% in the US, as they now are, have been the target of particular criticism. It is against this background that the neonatologist should view the obstetrician's attempts to balance competing risks and make the correct judgment in an individual high-risk pregnancy.

MONITORING IN LABOR

Much information can be obtained clinically about the likely fetal state in labor. Antenatal risk factors and monitoring are important while abnormal progress of labor, particularly prolonged delay in the active phase, or obstetric intervention in the form of induction of labor, epidural analgesia or oxytocin infusion, are all much more likely to be associated with fetal acidosis. Finally, clinical monitoring should include intermittent auscultation of the fetal heart rate with either a Pinard stethoscope or with Doppler. Fetal heart rate should be recorded at least every 15 min in the first stage of labor and after every contraction in the second stage of labor.

The importance of meconium staining has been emphasized by O'Driscoll & Meagher (1986). These authors recognize three grades of meconium which they describe as follows: Grade I – a good volume of liquor, lightly stained with meconium; Grade 2 – a reasonable volume of liquor, with a heavy suspension of meconium; Grade 3 – thick meconium, which is undiluted, and resembles sieved spinach. They recommend Cesarean section in Grade 3 unless easy vaginal delivery is imminent, because of the risk of hypoxia and meconium aspiration. Fetal blood sampling is considered mandatory in Grade 2 meconium with continuous electronic monitoring if this is satisfactory.

Continuous electronic monitoring of the fetal heart rate (EFM) has become the norm in high-risk deliveries and there are good descriptions of interpretation (e.g. Gibb & Arulkumaran 1992). The key features are rate, short-term variability and deceleration. A useful terminology used in the Dublin monitoring trial

Table 5.5 Fetal heart rate pattern: terminology I*

Baseline rate	
Normal	120–160 beats/min
Tachycardia	Moderate (160–180 beats/min)
	Severe (>180 beats/min)
Bradycardia	Moderate (100–120 beats/min)
	Severe (100 beats/min)
Variability	
Normal	> 5 beats/min
Reduced	3–5 beats/min
Absent	< 3 beats/min
Periodic changes	Duration at least 10 min
Acceleration	Repetitive increase in rate coincident with contraction
Deceleration	Early: repetitive deceleration coincident with contraction with return to baseline before end of contraction
	Late: repetitive deceleration with lag time between peak of contraction and trough of deceleration
	Variable: repetitive decelerations with variable waveform time of onset or relation to contractions

* As used in Dublin fetal heart rate monitoring trial (MacDonald et al 1985), adapted from Boylan (1987) with permission.
The more usually accepted baseline rate is 110–150 beats/min.

Table 5.6 Fetal heart rate pattern: terminology II*

Variable decelerations	
Mild	Amplitude < 50 beats/min, regardless of duration
	Amplitude > 50 beats/min, duration < 30 s
Moderate	Amplitude > 50 beats/min, duration 30–60 s
Severe	Amplitude > 50 beats/min, duration > 60 s

* As used in the Dublin fetal heart rate monitoring trial (MacDonald et al 1985), adapted from Boylan (1987) with permission.

Table 5.7 Classification of fetal heart rate patterns*

Ominous	Marked tachycardia with reduced variability
	Prolonged, > 10 min, marked bradycardia
	Late deceleration pattern
	Severe variable deceleration pattern
Suspicious	Marked tachycardia
	Moderate tachycardia with reduced variability
	Moderate bradycardia with reduced variability
	Minimal variability, normal rate
Nonreassuring	Moderate tachycardia, normal variability
	Mild variable deceleration pattern
	Early deceleration pattern
	Reduced variability
Reassuring	Normal baseline
	Normal variability
	Acceleration pattern
	Moderate bradycardia, normal variability

* As used in the Dublin fetal heart rate monitoring trial (MacDonald et al 1985), adapted from Boylan (1987) with permission.

(MacDonald et al 1985) is shown in Tables 5.5–5.7 as presented by Boylan (1987). Examples are shown in Figures 5.8a–d. Although much information can be obtained from fetal heart tracings alone there is a tendency to overdiagnose fetal compromise and EFM tends to be associated with an increased rate of Cesarean section and forceps delivery. For this reason it is important to combine EFM with fetal blood sampling as the final arbiter of fetal distress. When this is done, Cesarean section rates for the population can be as low as found with intermittent auscultation although with a doubling of the rate of Cesarean section specifically for fetal distress.

The definitive study on the value of EFM compared with intermittent auscultation was the randomized controlled trial of MacDonald et al (1985) in the National Maternity Hospital in Dublin. This trial excluded only those 6% of labors where there was Grade 2 meconium or absent liquor. The authors studied 13 084 babies delivered and found no difference in perinatal mortality, or frequency of Cesarean section. However, EFM significantly reduced the incidence of seizures in surviving neonates and this was particularly pronounced in those labors which lasted for longer than 5 h. Despite this, a 4-year follow-up

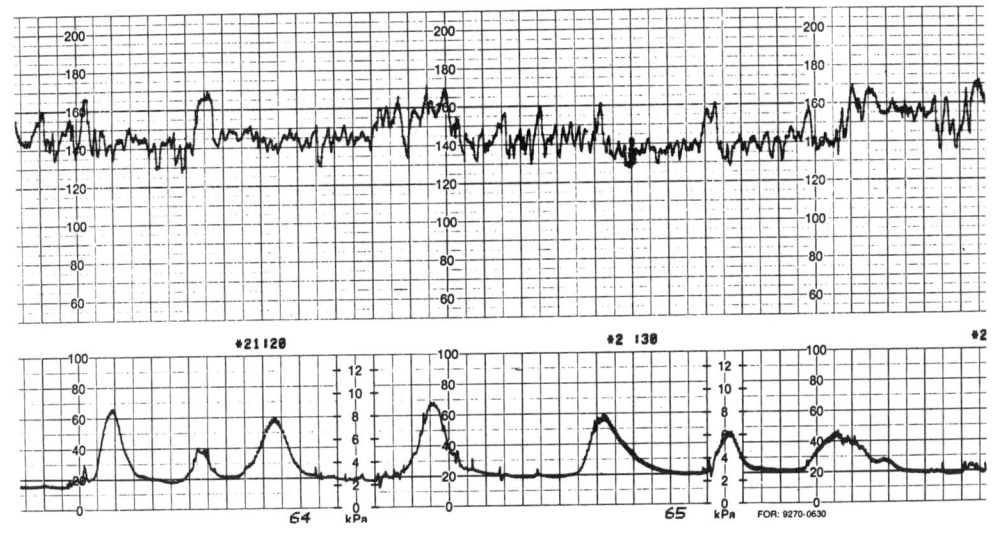

a

Fig. 5.8a

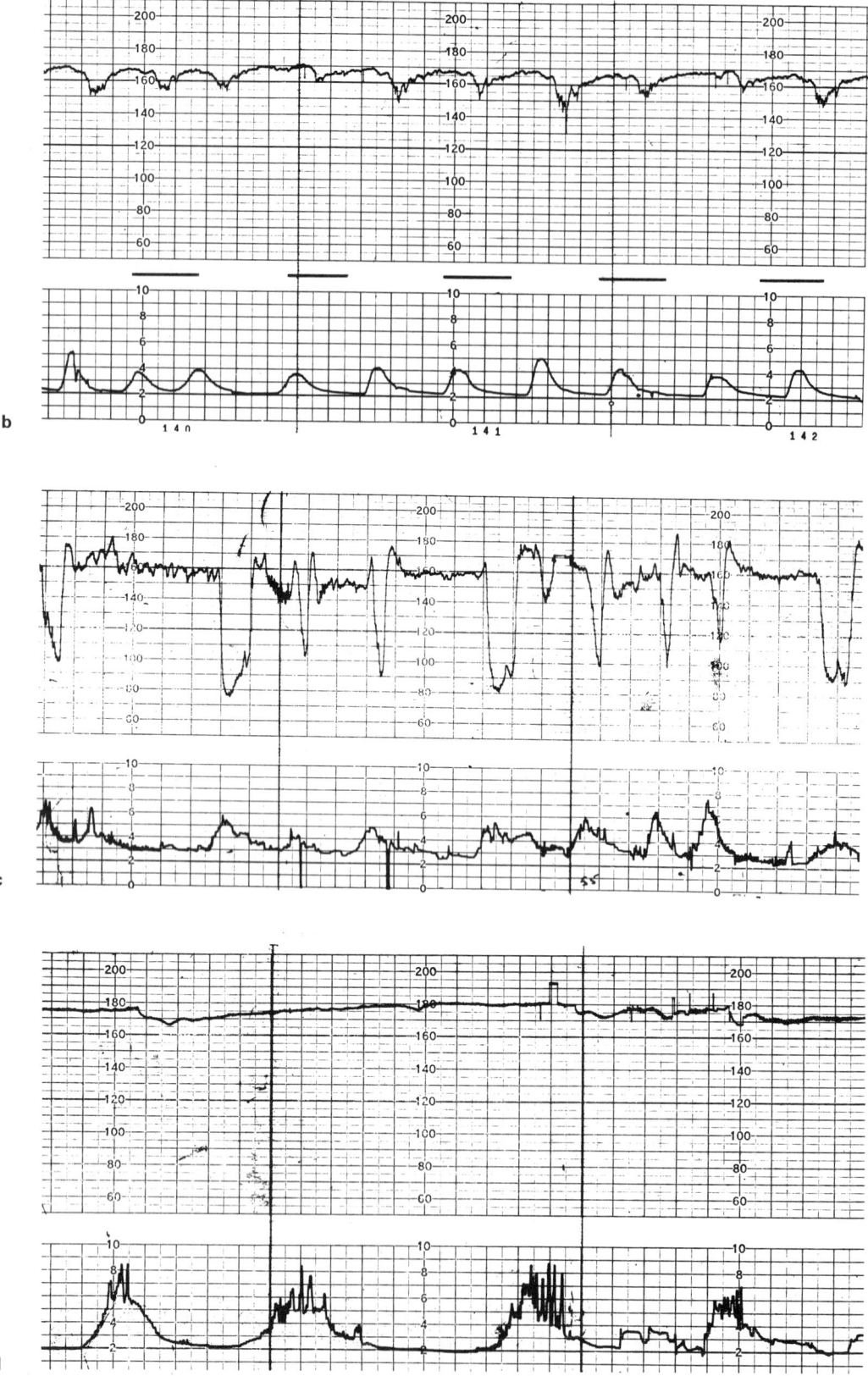

Fig. 5.8   Cardiotocograms. Graphs on scale 60–200 are the heart rate (beat to beat) and on scale 0–10 the uterine contractions. (**a**) Normal; (**b**) late decelerations – fetal tachycardia; (**c**) variable decelerations; (**d**) loss of variability, fetal tachycardia, late decelerations.

Table 5.8 Limits of normal values

pH	Down to 7.25
Base deficit	Down to − 8 mmol/l
Lactate	Up to 3.0 nmol/l
Δ pH (maternal–fetal)	Up to 0.15
Δ Lactate (fetal–maternal)	Up to 2.0 nmol/l

* Adapted from Smith (1987) with permission.

(Grant et al 1989) has shown no difference between the two groups in the incidence of cerebral palsy. This has fueled the debate about the relationship between asphyxia in labor and subsequent cerebral palsy. Current opinion is that cerebral palsy is associated with (though not necessarily caused by) obvious problems with labor, delivery and birth asphyxia in only approximately 10% of cases.

Scalp sampling is a simple technique which should be carried out with the mother in the left lateral position to avoid fetal hypoxia due to caval and aortic compression. It is indicated where the fetal heart trace is suspicious but not so ominous that immediate delivery is required. Normal values quoted by Smith (1987) are shown in Table 5.8. Using Apgar score as a criterion, scalp blood pH has a high false positive and false negative rate. This is partly because of deficiencies in the Apgar scoring system. Nevertheless, duration of acidosis, tissue perfusion, coexisting head compression, respiratory drive and perhaps most important, vulnerability of the baby will all influence neonatal condition. It is therefore essential to see EFM and scalp pH as only part of the overall assessment of the case.

Continuous tissue pH monitoring is likely to become clinically available in the near future and this may remove some current uncertainties. Earlier equipment had technical problems which limited use but more robust and reliable equipment is now being tested in clinical trials. Similarly, continuous fetal monitoring with pulse oximetry may add to information from heart rate monitoring although the available sensor generates only a limited amount of signal time (Luttkus et al 1995).

THE MANAGEMENT OF PRETERM LABOR

If suppression of preterm labor is unsuccessful or inadvisable the baby must be delivered in optimum condition avoiding as far as possible hypoxia, infection and precipitate or traumatic delivery. Initial assessment should include estimation of fetal weight and gestation, exclusion of multiple pregnancy and obvious fetal abnormality and confirmation of presentation. Ultrasound is helpful and many units now have a machine on labor wards for this purpose. A decision is then made about mode of delivery as Cesarean section may be indicated in some cases. Consultation with the neonatologist is essential at this point.

Pain relief is an important part of the management of a vaginal delivery. The woman will not be prepared for her unexpected preterm labor and will have all the anxieties about the outcome for her baby. The previous tendency to avoid opiates is unnecessary, providing the neonatologist in charge of resuscitation is informed. Epidural anesthesia is, however, the preferred method of pain relief having the important advantage that precipitate delivery is less likely. This also allows a gradual controlled second stage employing the techniques of passive pushing to minimize expulsive forces.

At the first vaginal examination a high vaginal swab should be sent for bacteriology. In general it is better not to rupture the membranes early in the labor as this increases cephalic compression and may in turn stress cerebral vasculature. Cord compression and infection may also be more common. It is essential to monitor the fetal heart rate carefully to detect early signs of fetal distress but in most cases this can be done satisfactorily by continuous external recording. Although there are differences in fetal heart recordings in the very preterm fetus (a tendency to baseline tachycardia and reduced variability), such recordings still accurately reflect fetal status. Thus a normal pattern predicts satisfactory outcome at birth and ominous patterns correlate with acidosis, abnormal neurological behavior in the neonatal period and long-term neurodevelopmental delay. Because of the particular vulnerability of the very preterm fetus to hypoxia, evidence of fetal distress should be managed very aggressively with Cesarean section when necessary.

The progress of the labor should be carefully assessed in order to prevent rapid unattended delivery and this may need frequent vaginal examination. Great care should be taken with delivery. This should often involve routine generous episiotomy and controlled delivery of the head without forceps but outlet forceps should be applied readily if there is delay or fetal distress. The routine use of forceps 'to protect the head' is no longer advocated, and indeed the use of elective episiotomy is not supported by convincing evidence.

A further important point about preterm delivery is the question of viability and the appropriateness of Cesarean section at very early gestations. These are questions that each unit should examine in relation to its own data on survival and follow-up. At the time of writing the chances of survival at gestations of less than 26 weeks or birthweights less than 750 g mean that Cesarean section is generally inappropriate, though there will be exceptions. However, this does not mean that an attitude of fatalism should be adopted or that the baby should be 'written off'. Indeed, estimates of weight and gestation may be misleading and it is essential that fetuses of 22–25 weeks are offered the best possible care short of performing Cesarean section. In our opinion this may include fetal heart rate monitoring and should certainly include careful supervision of labor progress and delivery by experienced staff and assessment at birth by a neonatologist.

CESAREAN SECTION

The place of Cesarean section in preterm delivery

There are several reasons why Cesarean section might be the optimal method of delivery for the very preterm infant. Compared with vaginal delivery Cesarean section probably reduces the risk of trauma, may have less potential for asphyxia and ensures that skilled neonatal care will be present at delivery. However, it should be made clear that there have been no adequate randomized controlled trials examining this question and information from retrospective studies is subject to several sources of bias. This whole subject has been authoritatively discussed by Westgren & Paul (1985). To summarize a large literature, there is no convincing evidence that abdominal delivery is the optimal method where the low birthweight fetus presents by the vertex. There is, however, a consensus of obstetric opinion that prognosis for very preterm breech infants may be better after Cesarean section than after vaginal delivery. The results of 14 retrospective reviews published since 1977 have been summarized by Westgren & Paul (1985). These all indicate reduced mortality in the preterm breech delivered abdominally though the authors of this review point out the inherent sources of bias. In addition in very low birthweight breech infants, Cesarean section may be associated with a reduced incidence of intraventricular hemorrhage and neurological abnormalities on long-term follow-up. A UK multicenter randomized controlled trial addressing this issue could not be completed due to inadequate recruitment.

Thus there are inadequate data on which to base definitive statements about the ideal mode of very preterm delivery. However, a reasonable approach in line with present thinking might be as follows: where there is any suggestion of asphyxia or where this might reasonably be expected to follow (a primigravida with severe pre-eclampsia and a closed cervix, for example) delivery should be by Cesarean section. Where labor is spontaneous, the presentation vertex and other factors are favorable, the aim should be vaginal delivery. Where presentation is breech with spontaneous labor, then an individual case assessment must be made, with a decision towards Cesarean section where problems are anticipated.

Type of incision

The lower segment operation is the procedure used in nearly all term deliveries, occasional exceptions being made for fibroids occupying the lower segment, transverse lie with ruptured membranes, occasional cases of placenta previa and other unusual situations. The operation is associated with less short-term morbidity than classical Cesarean section and is much safer in subsequent pregnancies. It is mandatory to deliver by repeat Cesarean section after classical Cesarean section and such scars can rupture before labor. This is virtually unknown after lower segment incision.

In very preterm delivery the lower segment may not have formed and delivery through an inappropriately small and poorly placed incision in the lower segment may result in serious trauma to the fetus. In addition, malpresentation at this gestation is common with 25% of babies at 28 weeks presenting by the breech. Where possible a low transverse uterine incision should still be used, with scissors used to make an upward or J-shaped curve which will give ample space in most cases. However, in some cases where there is a poorly formed lower segment and a malpresentation, classical Cesarean section is preferred. This decision can only be made intraoperatively.

Operative vaginal delivery

'Outlet' forceps delivery can be described as occurring where the scalp has been visible at the introitus without separation of the labia, the skull has reached the pelvic floor and the sagittal suture is in the anteroposterior diameter of the pelvis. This is a safe procedure and there is no evidence that this type of forceps delivery is harmful to the mature baby. 'Midcavity' forceps delivery is where the above conditions are not met and may involve delivery as occipitoposterior or rotation from an oblique posterior or transverse position. These procedures have the potential to cause trauma. However, comparison with Cesarean section in this situation has given conflicting results. Where possible, it is better for the baby to be delivered by propulsion rather than traction, by giving oxytocin in second stage if necessary (O'Driscoll & Meagher 1986). Where delivery is necessary before the fetal head has reached the pelvic floor, a careful assessment is required by an experienced obstetrician to decide whether delivery can safely be achieved by midcavity forceps or whether Cesarean section is preferable.

In many centers the vacuum extractor is preferred to forceps for operative vaginal delivery. A number of randomized comparisons of the use of the vacuum extractor compared with forceps have been completed (e.g. Johanson et al 1989) and have suggested that selection of the vacuum extractor as the instrument of first choice results in considerable reduction in maternal morbidity with no differences in neonatal morbidity. Chalmers & Chalmers (1989) suggest that use of the vacuum extractor should be the first choice for operative vaginal delivery in most assisted vaginal deliveries, and this is the trend worldwide. Vacuum delivery is though associated with a higher incidence of cephalhematoma, and forceps are still preferred for the preterm delivery.

BIRTH TRAUMA

A birth injury is a potentially avoidable mechanical injury occurring during labor or delivery (thus excluding damage from amniocentesis or intrauterine transfusion). Asphyxia and injury may occur together as the identification of a fetus in suboptimal condition inevitably leads to a rushed delivery. Even competent obstetric intervention in this situation may lead to injury but it is often possible that more serious damage such as severe asphyxia or death may have been prevented. Improvements in antenatal care and obstetric practice have reduced the incidence of birth trauma but where obstetric provision is poor, injuries are both common and severe. In the western world, possibly because of the low incidence, obstetric anxiety and guilt may be an inevitable sequel to each case. It is important that information is given to the parents immediately problems are identified in order to avoid misunderstandings and recrimination. Sensitive counseling is a most important aspect of management. Estimates of incidence are meaningless as the frequency varies with the quality of obstetric practice but the more difficult or prolonged the labor and delivery, the more likely it is that trauma will occur. Conditions predisposing to injury are listed in Table 5.9.

SOFT TISSUE INJURIES

Abrasions and *blisters* from forceps or vacuum deliveries, *punctures* from scalp electrodes or blood samples and *incisions* from hurried Cesarean sections lead to potential infection sites. *Bruises* from trauma may be severe in preterm deliveries and extensive into the buttocks following breech deliveries leading later to jaundice and anemia and occasionally disseminated

Table 5.9 Conditions predisposing to birth injury

Poor maternal health	Cephalopelvic disproportion
Maternal age (very young and old)	Hydrocephalus
Grand multiparity	Macrosomia
Twins (particularly the second)	Dystocia
Prematurity/low birthweight	Contracted pelvis
Malpresentation	Instrumental delivery

Table 5.10   Fractures

	Specific cause	Potential problem	Treatment	Comment
Skull				
Linear	1. Forceps pressure 2. Pubic pressure 3. Sacral pressure 4. Ischial spine pressure	Usually none, rarely subdural or extradural hemorrhage		
Depressed	Forceps	Underlying brain injury	1. If asymptomatic, none 2. If symptomatic, elevate	Prevent sustained cortical pressure
Occipital subluxation	Traction on spine in breech deliveries with head fixed in the pelvis	Rupture of underlying venous sinus		Usually fatal from subdural hemorrhage or tentorial tear
Clavicle (common)	1. Breech – extended arms 2. Difficult shoulder in vertex delivery	Associated brachial plexus injury	1. None – or if pain: 2. Bandage arm to chest with pad in axilla for 10 days	Prognosis excellent
Humerus	Breech – bringing down a displaced arm	Nerve damage	As for clavicle	Prognosis excellent
Femur	Extended breech	Sciatic nerve damage	1. Immobilize leg onto abdomen for 2–4 weeks (the in utero position) 2. Gallows traction	Position unimportant, molding will repair
Epiphyseal separation		Callus interferes with joint mobility and bone growth		1. On the upper femur, pain on external rotation 2. Outlook good
Nose	Dislocation of nasal cartilage	Difficulty feeding	1. Insert oral airway 2. Straighten surgically	Nares asymmetrical and nose flat

intravascular coagulation. Vitamin K should be given and phototherapy considered early. The *sternomastoid tumor* is originally a hemorrhage (p. 1784). Do *not* call it a tumor in front of parents. It may require passive physiotherapy. *Petechiae* are common over the head and neck following shoulder dystocia, face presentation or a nuchal cord. *Subconjunctival hemorrhages* are common in spontaneous deliveries (the mother may be worried about the baby's vision – reassure). *Subcutaneous fat necrosis* may be from obvious pressure from forceps or mother's pelvis, the thickened rubbery skin sometimes softening with resolution. This necrosis may occur over the back of head, cheek, outside of upper arm or greater trochanter of the femur. No treatment is required. *Fractures* (Table 5.10), deformity or pseudoparalysis may be observed and crepitations or later callus may be palpable. Pain relief is important.

INTRA-ABDOMINAL INJURIES

Hepatosplenomegaly (e.g. rhesus hemolytic disease), coagulation disorders and hypoxia, breech deliveries and cardiac massage all predispose to *subcapsular hematomas of the liver and spleen*. Anemia, pallor, tachycardia and tachypnea may be the presenting features or rupture may occur (immediately or days later) to give hypovolemic shock and death. *Adrenal hemorrhages* may follow severe infection, severe asphyxia or coagulation disorder. Hypovolemic shock with a flank mass and overlying skin discoloration may be evident. Adrenal failure may require treatment (p. 1067) and later calcification may occur. All hemorrhages predispose to jaundice. Ultrasound assists in diagnosis.

EXTRACRANIAL INJURIES

The *caput succedaneum* (present at birth) is a serosanguineous subcutaneous effusion over the presenting part in a vaginal delivery. It crosses the suture lines and disappears rapidly. *Subaponeurotic hemorrhages* are rare. They may follow vacuum deliveries or less commonly other instrumental deliveries. The hemorrhage is between the scalp aponeurosis and the periosteum and if it is massive it may present with hypovolemic shock and be fatal. Vitamin K (1 mg) intramuscularly should be given to all vacuum deliveries. Once diagnosed full clotting tests should be performed and 10 ml/kg of fresh frozen plasma should be given followed by cross-matched blood. Later there may be jaundice and anemia. The *chignon* is usual from a vacuum delivery and requires no treatment. A *cephalhematoma* may follow an instrumental or less commonly a spontaneous delivery. This subperiosteal hematoma is limited by each cranial bone and is probably always associated with a hairline fracture. There is no scalp discoloration and it appears *after* birth. Jaundice may develop and phototherapy may be required. The hematoma usually resolves over 2–8 weeks with hardening of the edge and at this stage may mimic a depressed fracture. Thickening of the diploë on skull X-ray may be apparent for years. The commonest site is parietal (sometimes bilateral) followed by frontal and then occipital. No treatment is required. Do *not* drain as this allows infection into the hematoma.

INTRACRANIAL INJURIES

Asphyxia and intracranial birth injury show similar clinical features and frequently coexist. Prenatal asphyxia or congenital abnormality may have initiated an instrumental delivery so it may be impossible to attribute abnormal features neonatally or later neurodevelopmental problems to one cause rather than the other. It is also possible that prenatal asphyxia may make a baby more vulnerable to birth injury by causing a high venous pressure, acidosis or disordered coagulation.

Intraventricular hemorrhage (p. 249)

This hemorrhage usually found in preterm infants is not now thought to be related to birth injury. In the asphyxiated full-term infant the choroid plexus may bleed into the ventricle.

COMPRESSION HEAD INJURIES

Cephalopelvic disproportion and instrumental delivery will predispose to intracranial injury. In many cases there will be obvious extracranial injury. Hypoxic-ischemic encephalopathy and cerebral edema (p. 126) may contribute to the clinical signs. If intracranial hemorrhage is massive, resuscitation may prove impossible or when initially successful the infant may survive only a few hours with generalized hypotonia progressing later to rigidity with convulsions and deep gasping respirations. Supratentorial bleeds lead to a tense fontanel but posterior fossa bleeds do not. Head retraction may be marked, retinal hemorrhages may occur rapidly and the infant may have a high-pitched cry or may moan continuously. If unconscious the infant may make no sound.

Less severe hemorrhage leads to apathetic periods interspersed with periods of extreme irritability. The hemisyndrome may be evident with eyes and head turned to one side and paucity of movement on the other. Up to 50% of such infants convulse and tonic fits have a worse prognosis.

Subarachnoid hemorrhage

This may occur in preterm and term infants following perinatal hypoxia. The baby may be pale and irritable with a high-pitched cry, neck retraction and sometimes a full fontanel. Diagnosis is difficult by ultrasound but the presumptive diagnosis by lumbar puncture may be confirmed by CT scan.

Subdural hemorrhage (hematoma)

Tears of the tentorium cerebelli or less often the falx cerebri are rare nowadays. If the hemorrhage is not rapidly fatal and if it is supratentorial, localization leads to hematoma. Signs of cerebral irritation settle after 48–72 h but later in the first week the head circumference begins to increase fast and there is clinical deterioration. Vomiting is common. Diagnosis is by CT scan and treatment by subdural taps at the lateral edge of the anterior fontanel. Ultrasound may show midline shift but it is frequently difficult to see the subdural region to visualize the hemorrhage itself.

Management of intracranial injury

Any baby suspected of having an intracranial injury should be closely observed in an incubator with monitoring of PaO_2 and $PaCO_2$. Temperature, blood pressure, fluid balance, and metabolic problems of blood sugar, calcium and coagulation should be corrected.

Phenobarbitone 4 mg/kg/12 h may help prevent convulsions but if these occur a loading dose of 20 mg/kg intravenously followed by the sedative dose should be used. Breakthrough convulsions may require diazepam, paraldehyde or phenytoin or other anticonvulsant (p. 246). Careful fluid balance is needed and it is wise to restrict intake initially to intravenous 10% dextrose at 50 ml/kg/24 h (to reduce edema secondary to inappropriate vasopressin secretion). Manual expression of the bladder may be needed.

The sedation is reduced from 48–72 h of age but is reintroduced if convulsions recur. Treatment may be required for cerebral edema (p. 126).

Prognosis

Prediction of late effects from brain damage is notoriously difficult. A recent Edinburgh study showed 9% died, 29% were handicapped (12% severely) and 62% were normal. The bad outcome is usually due to diskinetic or hemiplegic cerebral palsy with some degree of mental retardation and sometimes epilepsy.

PERIPHERAL NERVE INJURIES

Sixth nerve palsy seen for a few days after birth is probably associated with cerebral edema and trapping of the nerve on the tentorium. *Facial nerve damage (VII)* is usually peripheral from forceps pressure or from pressure on the maternal pelvis (spontaneous deliveries). No facial movement or forehead movement is seen when the infant cries. The corner of the mouth droops with dribbling at feeds and the eye fails to close (this requires protection). Recovery usually occurs over weeks but if after months there has been no recovery surgical neuroplasty should be considered. Rarely a central nuclear agenesis leads, if one sided, to paralysis of the lower half of the face.

Neck retraction in breech deliveries or shoulder dystocia damages the upper brachial plexus roots to give *Erb palsy (C5, C6)* or *phrenic palsy (C3, C4, C5)*. The arm is limp with forearm pronated and wrist flexed (waiter's tip position) from paralysis of deltoid, biceps, brachioradialis and long wrist extensors. Finger movements and therefore grasp reflex are normal. The biceps and Moro reflexes are absent on the affected side. Initial splinting of the arm to the side of the head probably makes little difference to the rate of recovery which is usually within 3 weeks (if severe it may take up to 2 years). Phrenic involvement presents as acute cyanosis and irregular labored breathing. There are reduced breath sounds and an absent abdominal bulge on inspiration because of paradoxical diaphragmatic movement. Diagnosis is by ultrasound or fluoroscopy. Treatment is with oxygen and intravenous fluids and then the gradual introduction of enteral feeds. If there is no improvement in 2 months (on ultrasound), diaphragmatic plication is indicated to prevent recurrent infection and bronchiectasis. *Klumpke palsy (C8, T1)* may occur with a breech delivery when the arms are extended up beside the head and the lower roots are stretched. The hand and forearm are paralyzed and there may be an ipsilateral Horner's syndrome. Edema and hemorrhage cause temporary problems but avulsion leads to permanent disability. Traditional treatment strapping the upper limb to the trunk probably makes little difference to the rate of recovery. *Radial nerve* damage is temporary and leads to wrist drop. It may be due to fat necrosis involving the nerve but frequently no predisposing factor can be found. Treat with a cock up splint.

In general peripheral nerve injuries need gentle passive exercise of the limb several times a day with splinting to avoid contractures. If paralysis continues for more than 3 months, recovery is unlikely. Neuroplasty and tendon transplant have usually been considered at 3–4 years of age but there has been a recent move in brachial plexus injuries to explore and attempt repair at 3–6 months if there has been no improvement since birth.

SPINAL CORD INJURIES

The lower cervical or upper thoracic cord may be bruised or rarely transected by forceful longitudinal or lateral traction on the spine. Subluxation or fractures of the vertebrae may occur with breech deliveries where the head is hyperextended or in a vertex delivery with shoulder dystocia. Coincident brachial plexus injury is common. The infant may be normal at birth or shocked but paralysis with flaccidity below the lesion quickly occurs with accompanying constipation and urinary retention. Intercostal paralysis leads to respiratory recession (Fig. 5.9). Spinal reflex activity returns after a short time. The initial flaccidity and immobility are replaced after several weeks by rigid flexion at hip, knee and ankle with increased tone and spasms. Absent sensation and automatic bladder function necessitate treatment similar to that of the baby with a meningomyelocele (p. 653). Diagnosis may be confined by MRI or myelography. There is no reparative treatment but multidisciplinary involvement inclusive of physiotherapy may prevent or reduce contractural difficulties in the future.

BIRTH ASPHYXIA

Birth asphyxia is the most common and important cause of preventable cerebral injury occurring in the neonatal period, but although asphyxia at birth is a commonly made diagnosis, there is no accepted definition for it. The term is used to imply an abnormal process and one that, if untreated, may cause permanent injury. Asphyxia, at a pathophysiological level, is the simultaneous combination of both hypoxia and hypoperfusion which impairs tissue gas exchange leading to tissue acidosis. Almost any organ can be affected, but the brain, myocardium, kidneys and bowel appear to be most sensitive to severe damage. Cerebral complications are the most devastating as full recovery may not occur and the child may be left with lifelong neurological impairment and in some cases devastating disability.

THE FETAL RESPONSE TO HYPOXIC STRESS

Hypoxia, and to a lesser extent placental underperfusion, both hallmarks of asphyxia, are relatively common events during labor and ones to which the fetus is well adapted. These adaptations are summarized in Table 5.11 and each is discussed briefly below. It is most important to realize that these are physiological responses to perturbations in the fetal environment which are common enough during labor to be considered 'normal'.

Reflex activity

Certain diving marine mammals have the ability to redistribute their cardiac output to vital organs and to slow their heart rate to extraordinarily low levels in order to remain under water for up to an hour in some cases. The fetus has been shown to have adaptive mechanisms during periods of normal hypoxic stress of labor in some ways similar to those of the diving seal. There is a reduction of blood flow through the descending aorta, together with reflex bradycardia. This reflex is mediated through a number of mechanisms discussed below.

Redistribution of blood flow

Episodes of hypoxemia cause a reduction in the fetal heart rate and an increase in blood pressure. This results in a net fall in cardiac output during the hypoxemic event. The overall reduction in cardiac output is more than compensated by a simultaneous

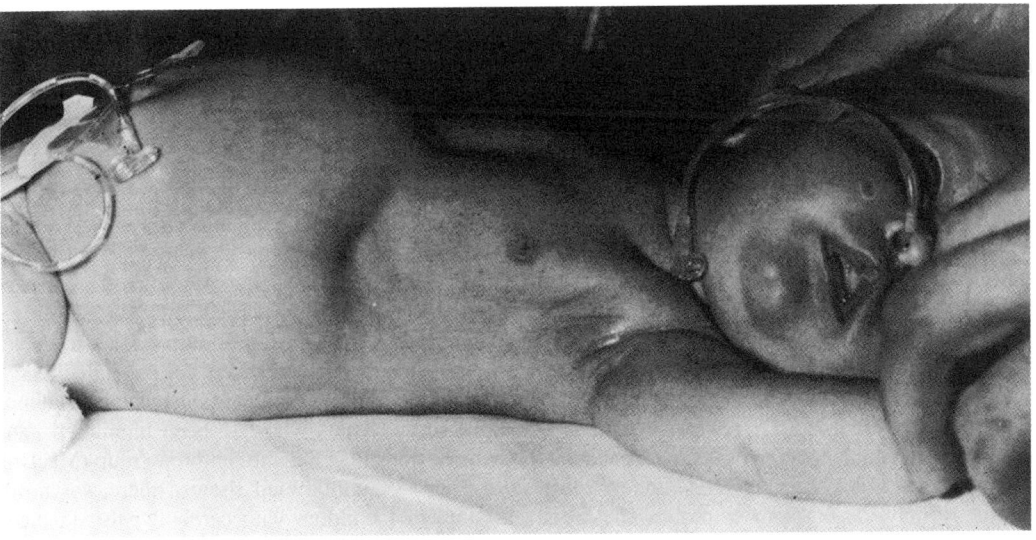

Fig. 5.9 Thoracic indrawing in newborn infant with broken neck.

Table 5.11 Important physiological adaptations to short episodes of fetal hypoxic stress

---

Cardiovascular responses
  'Diving seal' reflex
    – bradycardia
    – increase in blood pressure
  Redistribution of blood flow
    – towards brain, myocardium and adrenals
    – away from gut, lungs and carcass
  Regional cerebral blood flow changes
    – relative increase to brainstem
    – relative decrease to cerebral cortex

Autonomic responses
  In premature animals:
    – net parasympathetic response
  In full-term animals:
    – net sympathetic response
  Catecholamine surge

Biochemical response
  Glycolysis
    – switch from aerobic to anaerobic metabolism

---

redistribution of blood flow to vital organs with marked increase to the fetal brain, heart and adrenals. These increases occur at the expense of a redistribution of flow away from the placental circulation, lungs, gut and carcass. Although there is an increase of up to 100% in the total cerebral blood flow (CBF) during episodes of fetal hypoxia, regional CBF also shows consistent adaptive changes. Blood flow to the brain is distributed towards the phylogenetically more primitive regions, particularly the brainstem, at the expense of the cerebral cortices, thus protecting function in the most basic and 'vital' centers. During fetal stress, high levels of circulating cortisol are produced (Procianoy et al 1988), which may mediate some of the vascular effects seen in the normal fetus during periods of hypoxia. The autonomic nervous system is also closely involved with the fetal responses to stress.

Glycolytic activity

Glucose and oxygen are the metabolic fuels of the developing brain. Metabolism can switch to anaerobic glycolysis during periods of hypoxia with the production of lactic acid. This is a normal metabolic adaptation. It has been known for three centuries that the immature animal is more resistant to asphyxia than more mature animals of the same species. This resistance is in part due to the increased resilience of the immature cardiovascular system, but the brain also appears to have greater resistance and this may be due to either augmented glycolytic ability (production of more fuel) or lower utilization of glucose by the brain.

Stress vs distress

It is clear from the above that the fetus is a beautifully adapted organism with a number of interrelated mechanisms to protect him or her from the rigors of labor, both hypoxic and ischemic. Stress is an invariable accompaniment of the birth process and one which the fetus is well able to withstand under most circumstances. Distress may result from a prolonged stress response and the two may merge as an imperceptible continuum. It may be extremely difficult to separate fetal stress from distress using currently available clinical methods. Fetal distress may occur as the result of a single period of hypoxia which is too long, or periods which occur too frequently.

Currently, methods used to detect 'fetal distress' such as cardiotocography and fetal scalp pH assessments are really detecting degrees of fetal stress. These tests may be misinterpreted by the obstetrician as fetal distress, but an understanding of the fetal responses to the stress of uncompromised labor might encourage the fetus' medical attendants that s/he requires no assistance.

What is asphyxia?

There is no clinically accepted definition for asphyxia, although many suggested definitions have been put forward. The suggestion that asphyxia occurs when there is hypoxia together with accumulation of carbon dioxide and if prolonged this leads to an eventual state of respiratory and then metabolic acidosis ignores the fact that this may be an entirely normal sequence of physiological events. The clinical detection of acidosis as an indicator of asphyxia is discussed in more detail below. A recent statement recommended that the term 'birth asphyxia' should not be used (Bax & Nelson 1993). The concept that 'birth asphyxia' is a syndrome, or collection of features, with the exclusion of alternative conditions (Levene 1995) is becoming more widely accepted.

Clinical methods which have been suggested to be diagnostic for intrapartum asphyxia are described here.

Meconium staining of the amniotic fluid

Heavy or thick meconium staining is considered to be a marker of more prolonged or severe asphyxial episodes. Meconium staining is seen in up to 18% of all labors and is present during labor in 11% of full-term pregnancies where there is no evidence, other than the meconium, of asphyxia (Curtis et al 1988).

This sign is poorly predictive of adverse outcome and, in one study, more than half of infants who had early neonatal seizures (a possible indicator of intrapartum asphyxia) showed no evidence of meconium staining. Furthermore, if cerebral palsy is taken as the end point of a major asphyxial event in the perinatal period, then 99.6% of normal birthweight infants with meconium staining had no evidence of this condition (Nelson & Ellenberg 1984).

The cardiotocograph (CTG)

A normal CTG trace appears to be a good indicator that metabolic acidosis is not developing, but a severely abnormal trace with late decelerations in the fetal heart rate is associated with significant fetal acidosis in only about 50% of cases. The use of routine CTG monitoring in low-risk pregnancies certainly causes a two- to threefold increase in the number of forceps deliveries and Cesarean sections undertaken for presumed fetal distress.

A large controlled study of intrapartum fetal monitoring showed that those infants who had been monitored had fewer neonatal convulsions than the unmonitored group (MacDonald et al 1985), but at 4-year follow-up showed there was no difference in the number of children with cerebral palsy in the two groups. No studies have ever shown that CTG monitoring actually prevents impairment resulting from intrapartum asphyxia.

It must, however, be stressed that in high-risk labors, CTG monitoring is likely to detect those fetuses who become severely compromised, although there are a significant number of false positive results. The prolonged and severely compromised fetus will probably show a pattern of abnormality in the heart rate described as the terminal trace and the longer the trace is abnormal, the more likely the child is to be abnormal if he survives.

Acidosis

Acidosis is a marker of CO_2 accumulation (respiratory acidosis) and/or metabolic acidosis as the result of anaerobic metabolism. Severe fetal or cord blood acidosis is a marker of impaired tissue gas exchange, but there is no evidence that acidosis *per se* is a cause of further tissue damage. There is poor correlation between cord blood acidosis and depression of Apgar scores. A pH level < 7.00 or 7.05 represents a figure at which intrapartum compromise may have been severe enough to be associated with organ dysfunction (Carter et al 1993).

Apgar score

Depression of the Apgar score is the most widely used criterion for diagnosing birth asphyxia. The Apgar score assesses five variables easily elicitable at birth (Table 5.12) and is a useful method for describing the condition of any infant at varying times from birth. Depression of the score, however, may be due to factors such as gestational age, maternal medication, cardiovascular disease of the infant and a variety of congenital neuromuscular problems quite apart from asphyxia. It has been shown that the more immature the infant, the more the respiratory effort, muscle tone and reflex irritability will be reduced, irrespective of any degree of depression due to other causes (Catlin et al 1986). Premature infants born in optimal condition normally have a lower Apgar score than full-term infants also born in good condition.

In full-term infants there is a direct relationship between severe depression of the Apgar score (0–3) and risk of death but generally the Apgar score is poorly predictive of adverse outcome and as such is not a very useful method of defining significant asphyxia. As well as being an insensitive predictive method, it is also poorly specific: 50% of children with cerebral palsy evident at 7 years of age had an optimal Apgar score of 7–10 at 1 min (Nelson & Ellenberg 1981).

Delay in establishing spontaneous respiration

Asphyxia has been defined as delay in establishing spontaneous respiration or the need for more than 1 min of positive pressure ventilation. Unfortunately, this is very unreliable in premature infants who commonly have apnea at birth for reasons related to their prematurity. Other infants may fail to breathe because of maternal anesthesia or opiate administration. In many hospitals, very premature infants are electively intubated as this is believed to improve outcome, thereby further reducing the value of defining asphyxia on the basis of respiratory activity at birth.

HYPOXIC-ISCHEMIC ENCEPHALOPATHY (HIE)

If the full-term brain has been compromised during delivery, it is likely that the infant will show clinically evident disturbance in neurological behavior, a state referred to as hypoxic-ischemic encephalopathy. HIE cannot be reliably diagnosed in premature babies. Infants show a continuum of encephalopathic behavior depending on the severity and duration of the asphyxial event and grading systems have been published to define the degree of encephalopathy (Sarnat & Sarnat 1976, Levene et al 1985). Table 5.13 describes the major clinical features. Early neonatal seizures are also considered to be a good marker of intrapartum asphyxia (Curtis et al 1988).

The severity of postasphyxial encephalopathy (PAE) is the best clinical method currently available to predict subsequent outcome following asphyxia (see section on outcome), but it has a number of disadvantages. Firstly, the severity of PAE can only be determined retrospectively as the clinical neurological features of asphyxia take some time to evolve. Secondly, other organs such as the kidneys and heart may be compromised due to asphyxia, but the fetus preserves blood flow to his brain thereby sparing cerebral function. The lack of encephalopathy does not necessarily indicate that the infant has not suffered from significant intrapartum asphyxia. Thirdly, other neurological lesions can cause encephalopathy including cerebral hemorrhage and hypoglycemia. These must be excluded before a diagnosis of postasphyxial encephalopathy can be made.

The American Academy of Pediatrics (1986a) have considered that for the diagnosis of substantial cerebral hypoxia (asphyxia) which may cause neurological impairment to be made, three clinical criteria must be present:

1. Apgar score 0–3 at 10 min (other causes of depression having been excluded)
2. the infant remains hypotonic for at least several hours
3. the presence of neonatal seizures.

Table 5.12 The Apgar score

Sign	0	1	2
Heart rate	Absent	< 100/min	> 100/min
Respiratory effort	Absent	Weak cry	Strong cry
Muscle tone	Limp	Some flexion	Good flexion
Reflex irritability on suctioning pharynx	No response	Some motion	Cry
Color	Pale with general cyanosis	Centrally pink, peripheral cyanosis	Pink

Table 5.13 The major clinical features for grading the severity of postasphyxial encephalopathy

Mild	Moderate	Severe
Irritability	Lethargy	Coma
Hyperalert	Seizures	Prolonged seizures
Normal tone	Differential tone (legs > arms) (neck extensors > flexors)	Severe hypotonia
Weak suck	Poor suck, requires tube feeds	No sucking reflex
Sympathetic dominance	Parasympathetic dominance	Coma, requires respiratory support

INCIDENCE

The incidence of birth asphyxia depends largely on the definition used to diagnose the condition as well as the gestational age of the infant. As discussed above the diagnosis of asphyxia in immature infants is extremely difficult as all the available methods have considerable practical problems when used in premature infants. The incidence of low Apgar scores in babies with birthweights < 1500 g is 15-fold higher than in infants weighing > 3000 g (Palme-Kilander 1992).

The incidence of birth asphyxia ranges from 3.7 to 9.0 per 1000 infants based on different definitions of birth asphyxia. There appears to have been a significant reduction in the incidence of birth asphyxia in recent years, but only in mature newborn infants. In a study from Leicester, the overall incidence of postasphyxial encephalopathy was reported to be 6 per 1000 full-term liveborn infants, of whom 1.1 per 1000 and 1.0 per 1000 had moderate and severe encephalopathy, respectively (Levene et al 1985). Two cohorts of full-term infants born in England in 1976–80 and 1984–88 showed that there had been a decline in incidence of HIE from 7.7 per 1000 to 4.6 per 1000 in the intervening 4 years (Hull & Dodd 1992).

PATHOLOGY

The type of brain pathology seen in infants depends on the duration and intensity of the asphyxial event and the gestational age of the baby at the time the insult occurred. The type of pathology expected with insults at different stages of development is summarized in Figure 5.10. An asphyxial insult occurring very early in development (< 20 weeks) may cause a disorder in neuronal migration, but once neuronal migration is complete by 20 weeks an asphyxial insult cannot damage the brain in the same way since all the neurons have completed their migration by then. A severe insult at 24–34 weeks of gestation is likely to cause periventricular leukomalacia (p. 250), but by 35 weeks of gestation brain maturation no longer predisposes to this type of pathology. By 35 weeks onwards a new watershed vulnerability is exposed and subcortical leukomalacia (p. 250) may occur. In the term brain and for a number of weeks after term an asphyxial insult may lead to damage primarily in the parasagittal area or in the basal ganglia.

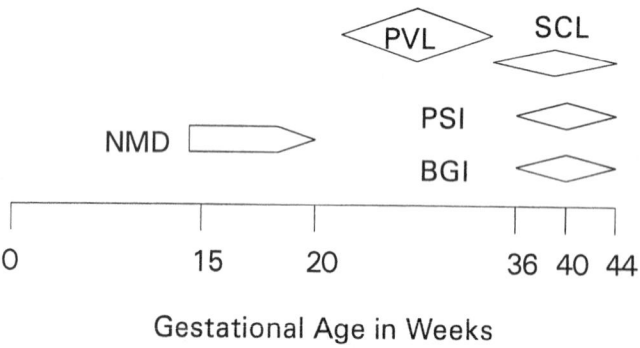

Fig. 5.10 Vulnerable periods for the development of different forms of pathology as the result of an hypoxic ischemic insult: NMD – neuronal migration disorder; PVL – periventricular leukomalacia; SCL – subcortical leukomalacia; PSI – parasagittal injury; BSI – basal ganglia injury.

As mentioned above the brain has the ability to redistribute regional cerebral blood flow away from the cortical areas to the more primitive brainstem, basal ganglia and cerebellum. The classical studies of Windle (1966) and Myers (1972) distinguished two forms of neuropathology dependent on the pattern of asphyxiating insult; the partial or intermittent model and the sudden and complete form. In partial fetal asphyxia (the clinically more common form) the cortical mantle is more likely to be affected in the parasagittal distribution whereas in the acute and total form of asphyxia, the lesions affect mainly the basal nuclei and brainstem. These patterns of damage are only seen in the term baby's brain as described above and can be recognized on brain imaging (see below).

Hemorrhage

Although intracranial hemorrhage is a common condition in premature infants, its incidence in more mature asphyxiated babies is much less. Subdural hemorrhage is the best-described hemorrhagic lesion associated with birth asphyxia in full-term infants, but it probably occurs in only 5% of such infants. Some subarachnoid hemorrhage is commonly found at autopsy examination, but this is not usually severe and its frequency is not known in surviving infants. Hemorrhage may occur into the choroid plexus, cerebellum and thalamus in asphyxiated infants, but these are all relatively uncommon.

Cerebral edema

Two forms of cerebral edema have been described: cytotoxic and vasogenic edema, and both occur in the neonatal brain following asphyxia. Injury to the cellular pump mechanism causes sodium and water to enter the cell causing it to swell (cytotoxic edema). Injury to the blood–brain barrier causes it to become leaky and fluid enters the cerebral extracellular compartment with consequent brain swelling. This is known as vasogenic edema.

Cerebral edema does not become apparent clinically until 24–48 h after the asphyxial event, by which time progressive swelling is obvious on macroscopic examination with flattening of the gyri and obliteration of sulci. Rarely, herniation of the uncus through the tentorium or cerebellar displacement through the foramen magnum is found. Cerebral edema may be detected either clinically or by imaging.

The causes of neuronal death

It is often not appreciated that the neuron is a cell which is particularly resistant to asphyxia. In experimental studies on the isolated neuron, cellular and electrical activity may recover after 1 h of total asphyxia. In many cases, neuronal death eventually occurs due to a cascade of events which occurs following asphyxia, associated with deranged cellular biochemistry or vascular injury. The concept of delayed neuronal injury is now well accepted. It is not known how long it takes for the neuron to die and the time has been estimated to vary between hours and days. Wyatt et al (1989) have used magnetic resonance spectroscopy to show a delayed deterioration in the brain energy state, suggestive of a slowly progressive disruption of oxidative phosphorylation in brain tissue over 48 h. The cellular mechanisms for neuronal death are discussed below.

Apoptosis has been suggested as an alternative or second mechanism for delayed neuronal death. Apoptosis refers to programmed cell death. It appears that cells require constant signaling from adjacent cells to continue to function. Withdrawal of this signaling stimulus causes cell death. In asphyxia disruption of cellular mechanisms may cause the cell to enter a death cycle.

Calcium and cell death

Intraneuronal calcium concentration is carefully regulated to ensure that the gradient of Ca^{2+} within the cell is of the order of 10^4 less than the extraneuronal concentration. Calcium enters through a number of different sites in the cell wall. These can be divided into either receptor-operated channels (ROCs) or voltage-dependent channels (VDCs). The main entry site is through excitatory amino acid-sensitive ROCs, of which glutamate is the most commonly expressed in the developing brain. Glutamate is an excitatory neurotransmitter which causes sensitive receptors to open with entry of calcium into the neuron. Asphyxia causes excessive glutamate release with sustained stimulation of ROCs and excessive entry of Ca^{2+}. There are at least three glutamate-like receptor ligands, which are named from the agents that individually excite them and can be divided into either NMDA receptors or non-NMDA receptors. Mg^{2+} operates a voltage-dependent block deep within the NMDA calcium channel which is relieved when the membranes depolarizes. Ca^{2+} also enters through VDCs of which there are a number of types, some of which are predominantly expressed in the neuron. The VDCs are situated on both pre- and postsynaptic dendritic terminals, but do not appear to control the major flux of calcium into the neuron. Excessive intraneuronal calcium sets up a cascade of destructive biochemical processes including activation of lipases, proteases and endonucleases which lead to disruption of the neuronal cytoskeleton with eventual neuronal necrosis. This process may take many hours to complete. A number of substances act as NMDA-receptor antagonists, and these may protect the immature brain when used following an asphyxial insult (see below).

Free radicals are particularly likely to occur as the result of asphyxial insults and are thought to play a major role in the pathophysiology of postasphyxial damage. They are highly aggressive substances which damage cell membranes by lipid peroxidation. The mitochondrion is particularly sensitive to free radical attack. During hypoxia, ATP is degraded with the production of adenosine, inosine and hypoxanthine. During resuscitation and reperfusion the enzyme xanthine oxidase uses any available oxygen to convert hypoxanthine or xanthine to uric acid with the production of large quantities of free radicals. This may cause progressive mitochondrial compromise. Nitric oxide (NO) has a neurotransmitter role which is closely related to the NMDA receptor. Intraneuronal Ca^{2+} binds with calmodulin and activates nitric oxide synthase which releases NO. NO itself acts as a free radical and under some circumstances may be neurotoxic in the presence of excessive calcium entry.

CLINICAL FEATURES

There is a characteristic sequence of abnormal clinical neurological signs associated with birth asphyxia. These have been well described and Table 5.13 lists the major clinical features. In the majority of cases the clinical pattern of postasphyxial encephalopathy is only consistent for relatively mature newborn infants with a gestational age of 35 weeks or above. The very premature infant has a less well-developed nervous system and similar clinical signs may not be evident. In addition, other neuropathological conditions such as hemorrhage or periventricular leukomalacia are much more common in these infants, and any clinical signs are more likely to be related to these conditions. Nevertheless, very immature infants have been reported to develop the typical features of severe postasphyxial encephalopathy, but this is rare. The description that follows is most relevant to the more mature infant.

Mild encephalopathy

Babies with mild encephalopathy exhibit relatively subtle abnormalities which last no longer than 2 days. They show no depression in conscious level, but are described as being 'hyperalert'. This refers to the appearance of hunger, yet not feeding well together with a wide-eyed gaze, but failure to fixate. They are overly responsive to external stimuli and show exaggerated and excessive numbers of spontaneous Moro reflexes. These babies often do not feed well and may need occasional gavage feeding. There is a net sympathetic effect with mydriasis and tachycardia. Clinically evident seizures are not a feature of mild encephalopathy.

Moderate encephalopathy

These children are more severely neurologically abnormal and show evidence of seizures. These may be relatively subtle including lip smacking, excessive sucking-type movements as well as the more typical tonic or clonic convulsive activity. The infants also show differential tone. This refers to increased lower limb tone compared with that in the upper limbs as well as increased neck extensor tone compared with that of the neck flexors. This is best elicited by placing the baby in a sitting position with the head first extended and then flexed on the trunk. The baby's spontaneous movements are observed and if the infant holds his head in the extended position with little effort to flex it, then this confirms neck extensor muscle hypertonus. Lethargy is the other constant feature of moderate encephalopathy with reduction in spontaneous movements. The baby requires a higher sensory input to elicit a response. The Moro and other primitive reflexes are usually lost in the early stages, but the tendon jerks are often exaggerated. The infants show predominantly parasympathetic activity with relative bradycardia and constricted pupils. Recovery begins within the first week after birth and full recovery (if it occurs) may be delayed for a number of weeks.

Severe encephalopathy

These infants develop coma, although it may take several hours before the infants show severe respiratory depression and require mechanical ventilation. Seizures are also a prominent feature and these may be prolonged and very frequent. In the most severely asphyxiated infants, there may be no seizure activity either clinically or evident on EEG monitoring as the brain's energy supply has been completely exhausted. Babies with severe encephalopathy are severely hypotonic and show little spontaneous movement other than that due to seizures. Reflex activity is usually lost. These infants may die in the acute phase of their illness, but if they recover, their abnormal neurological signs may progress from hypotonia through to excessive hypertonia. Complete recovery may occur, but may take up to 6 weeks. Persistently abnormal neurological signs beyond this time are ominous predictors of subsequent cerebral palsy.

MONITORING TECHNIQUES

Biochemical markers of asphyxia

Biochemical markers of asphyxial insult can be considered to be either brain-specific or derived from many tissues within the body. Some studies have attempted to measure CSF levels of these substances in order to more accurately assess brain-derived biochemical markers of asphyxial injury, but this clearly limits the use of the test. In particular, CSF levels of neuron-specific enolase correlated with outcome (Thornberg et al 1995). In general, studies have failed to show a major role for biochemical or hormonal markers of significant birth asphyxia (Ruth 1989, Ruth et al 1988).

Spectroscopy

Magnetic resonance spectroscopy (MRS) has been used in vivo to evaluate ATP energy states within the immature human brain following perinatal hypoxic-ischemic brain injury (Wyatt 1994). These studies have shown that during the first 24 h after delivery the phosphorus spectra remain normal, but show increasing deterioration after this time with falling phosphocreatine (PCr) and a reciprocally increased proportion of inorganic phosphorus (Pi) indicating degradation of ATP which they have suggested is evidence of 'delayed' or 'secondary' energy failure. The ratio of PCr : Pi appears to accurately predict those babies who will show major neurological impairment at 1 year and those who die of their asphyxial injury. Proton MRS allows identification of choline, creatine, N-acetyl aspartate (NAA) and lactate within different brain regions (Hashimoto et al 1995) and preliminary data suggest that severe perinatal asphyxia causes marked elevation of brain lactate with reduced intraneuronal NAA (Wyatt 1994).

Imaging

Ultrasound imaging is of particular value in the immature infant as hemorrhagic and ischemic lesions can be readily identified. Ultrasound imaging is of less value in the full-term infant as these lesions occur less frequently. The main role of ultrasound in the term baby who has suffered severe birth asphyxia is as a screening test to identify shift of the midline structures associated with subdural hemorrhage. This is an uncommon lesion (see above) and, if suspected, a CT scan should be performed as it may require surgical evacuation.

CT scanning is of value in the accurate prediction of outcome, but only when the scan is performed in the second week of life. Extensive areas of low attenuation are associated with a high risk of adverse outcome (Lipper et al 1986). More recently magnetic resonance imaging (MRI) has been used to observe the evolution of hypoxic-ischemic injury in the immature brain (Fig. 5.11), but to date the number of reports have been few (Martin & Barkovich 1995). There appears to be a consistent pattern of abnormalities seen in full-term asphyxiated infants which first become apparent 2–3 days after the injury and persist for many weeks. Martin &

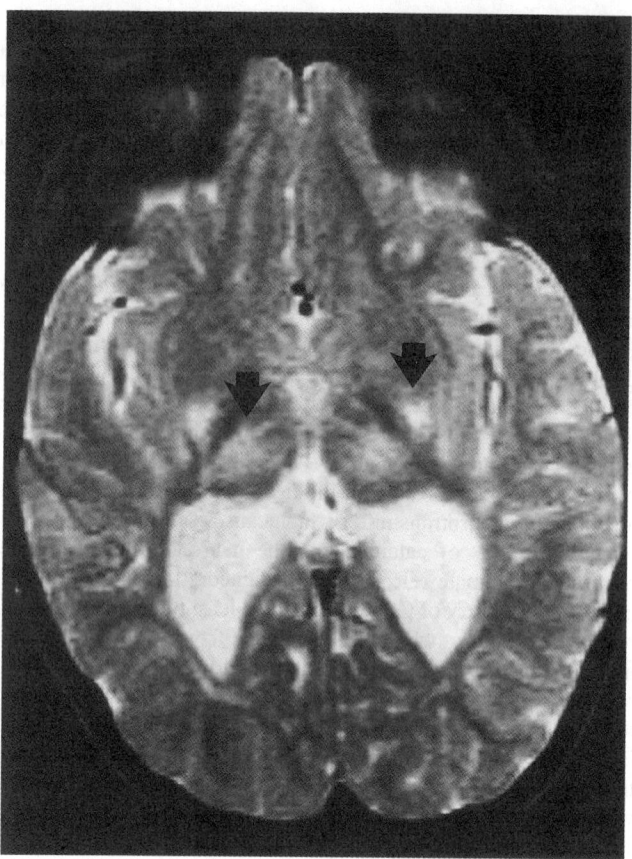

Fig. 5.11 MR scan (T2 weighted image) in axial plane from a 2-year-old showing abnormal signal (arrows) in the basal ganglia. The baby had sustained a severe asphyxial injury due to acute cord prolapse in the neonatal period.

Barkovich (1995) report that a normal MRI scan in the first 24–72 h of life always predicts favorable outcome even after severe asphyxia and, conversely, evidence of extensive cerebral edema at this time carries a poor prognosis.

Intracranial pressure monitoring

Intracranial hypertension due to cerebral edema is a commonly anticipated complication in asphyxiated infants, but in fact probably occurs in less than 50% of such infants and a sustained rise in pressure exceeding 15 mmHg is rare (Levene & Evans 1983). In those infants who develop intracranial hypertension, the marked increase does not occur for 24 h after the initial asphyxial event; the determining factor in whether a child survives to be normal is the severity of the underlying asphyxia. Monitoring ICP does not appear to be of significant benefit to the asphyxiated child (Levene et al 1987).

Assessment of cerebral hemodynamics

Doppler ultrasound has been used to assess cerebral hemodynamics following birth asphyxia and there are a number of reports of a consistent abnormality seen on the Doppler sonogram in severely asphyxiated infants. In some such babies, the difference between the maximum systolic and minimum diastolic frequencies is reduced and this is reflected in a falling Pourcelot resistance index (PRI). It has been shown that in some asphyxiated infants the appearance of a low PRI (< 0.55) correlates well with adverse outcome – either handicap or death (Archer et al 1986). In addition a high mean flow velocity above 3 standard deviations has also been shown to correlate very well with adverse outcome (see section on prognosis). Unfortunately these abnormalities do not reliably occur within 24 h of the asphyxial event which tends to limit their clinical utility. Near Infrared Spectroscopy (NIRS) has shown that both cerebral blood volume and flow were significantly greater in acutely asphyxiated infants than in controls, but the cerebral vascular resistance was reduced (Wyatt 1994). The Doppler and NIRS data suggest a progressive vasoparalysis following a severe asphyxial event in full-term babies.

Electroencephalography

EEG has been widely used for many years to assess the severity of cerebral insults. In the asphyxiated newborn, EEG monitoring has two main indications. First, to assess whether there is subclinical seizure activity which may require treatment and second, to evaluate the background trace which may aid prognosis.

EEG may be monitored either continuously using one or two electrodes or by short intermittent studies using a six or twelve electrode array. Persistently low-amplitude, discontinuous, or unreactive traces are particularly associated with poor outcome and may be particularly valuable in predicting outcome (see Prognosis, p. 131).

COMPLICATIONS

The fetus copes with an asphyxial event by a number of protective reflexes to preserve function to vital organs. Less well-perfused tissues may be particularly vulnerable to hypoxic-ischemic injury. In one study, a third of full-term asphyxiated infants developed asphyxia-related complications in two different organ systems (Perlman et al 1989). The kidney appears to be most vulnerable, followed by the brain and then the heart. Gastrointestinal complications of asphyxia were uncommon. This section reviews organ damage at sites other than the brain.

Lungs

During intrapartum asphyxia, the fetus commonly passes meconium and gasping may occur due to brainstem compromise. The gasp causes meconium to be aspirated deep into the bronchial tree and this may cause a chemical pneumonitis with severe pulmonary hypertension and a high risk of air leak. The management of meconium aspiration is discussed on page 185. Those infants who are pharmacologically paralyzed in order to facilitate mechanical ventilation for this condition will not show the clinical signs of postasphyxial encephalopathy and coincidental cerebral injury may not be recognized. These infants should have continuous EEG monitoring to assess cerebral function.

Cardiovascular system

Blood flow to the myocardium is preserved during asphyxial episodes, but cardiac compromise is a relatively common complication of hypoxic-ischemic injury. Myocardial dysfunction detected by Doppler ultrasound studies has been reported in 28–40% of asphyxiated infants (Perlman et al 1989, Van Bel & Walthor 1990). Recognized complications include cardiogenic shock and hypotension, functional tricuspid incompetence secondary to acute cardiac dilation, arrhythmias and myocardial ischemia which may be diagnosed from the electrocardiogram.

Renal impairment

Acute tubular necrosis and oliguria occurs commonly following episodes of asphyxia. This usually recovers with supportive treatment alone. Acute renal failure was reported in 19% of asphyxiated infants (Roberts et al 1990). Acute retention of urine is also a relatively common complication following birth asphyxia and usually indicates very severe compromise, often associated with severe cerebral injury. Renal failure following asphyxia has also been reported to be due to myoglobinuria.

Gastrointestinal tract

Necrotizing enterocolitis (see p. 210) is associated with hypoxic-ischemic events, but in mature infants this is rarely seen in conjunction with hypoxic-ischemic encephalopathy.

Metabolic disorders

One of the commonest metabolic complications of birth asphyxia is inappropriate ADH secretion with concentrated urine, dilute plasma and hyponatremia (p. 1040). Transient hyperammonemia has been reported with asphyxia but the precise cause of this metabolic compromise is not known.

Hematological disorders

Disseminated intravascular coagulation (DIC) is a well-recognized complication of birth asphyxia and usually presents with excessive bleeding from puncture sites together with petechial hemorrhages. Secondary complications such as intracranial hemorrhages may occur as the result of the DIC.

MANAGEMENT

The management of birth asphyxia can be considered under a number of headings including diagnosis during the intrapartum period with rescue by expeditious delivery, effective resuscitation, general support of the infant, management of complications, brain-orientated intensive care and more speculative and novel treatments directed towards the early pharmacological management of the basic pathophysiology which leads to neuronal injury.

Intrapartum care

Modern obstetrics is directed towards the recognition of the high-risk fetus together with careful monitoring and early delivery if fetal distress is suspected. As discussed above, although there has been a marked increase in the proportion of pregnancies terminated by operative delivery, it is by no means certain that routine CTG monitoring has reduced the prevalence of hypoxic-ischemic cerebral injury and subsequent handicap.

Resuscitation

It is vital to ensure that the newborn infant is effectively resuscitated following intrapartum compromise and this may reduce the risk of subsequent complications. Neonatal resuscitation is discussed in detail on page 132.

General support

The asphyxiated infant may develop complications in almost any organ system and the infant who is recognized to have suffered from hypoxic-ischemic injury should be carefully monitored. Table 5.14 lists the categories of general support which should be considered. Any infant with major complications involving any organ system should be given the benefit of modern intensive care with very careful monitoring undertaken by experienced nursing and medical staff. The specific management of noncerebral asphyxial injury is discussed elsewhere in this book. A particularly important and common complication of birth asphyxia is systemic hypotension and this should be detected by careful blood pressure monitoring. Undetected or inadequately treated hypotension will cause the already compromised brain to be further underperfused.

Brain-oriented care

The practical management of moderate and severe HIE is listed in Table 5.15. More detailed discussion of some of these points is warranted.

Table 5.14 General methods for managing the asphyxiated infant and organ-related complications

General support	
Nurse in thermoneutral environment	
Avoid hypo- and hyperglycemia	
Measure blood gases:	
treat hypoxia with oxygen	
treat hypercarbia with IPPV	
Review infection risk and treat with antibiotics if appropriate	
Adequate hydration, do not dehydrate	
Treat hyperbilirubinemia	
Cardiovascular	
Hypotension	Plasma, inotrope support
Myocardial failure	Digoxin, inotrope support
Renal	
Oliguria	Careful assessment of fluid status
Acute tubular necrosis	Renal failure regimen
	Peritoneal dialysis if necessary
Pulmonary	
Meconium aspiration	Respiratory support
Metabolic	
Inappropriate ADHS	Restrict fluids
Hypoglycemia	Give glucose, but avoid inducing hyperglycemia
Hematological	
DIC	No specific therapy
Gastrointestinal	Antibiotics, avoid enteral feeds
NEC	

Table 5.15 Brain-oriented management. The dosages of the anticonvulsants are discussed in the text

Cerebral perfusion
Carefully monitor blood pressure and maintain a mean arterial blood pressure > 40 mmHg in full-term infants
Seizures
Treat seizures with phenobarbitone
If intermittent seizures, give paraldehyde
If persistent seizures, consider:
clonazepam
lignocaine
phenytoin best avoided for maintenance therapy
Intracranial hypertension
Give 20% less than daily fluid requirements
If full fontanel and seizures, give mannitol 20% (1 g/kg), avoid if the baby is oliguric

Seizures

These are very common following intrapartum asphyxia and may be clinically evident or only detected on EEG monitoring. Treatment is often relatively unsuccessful and not infrequently multiple anticonvulsant medication may be necessary. It is not known whether seizures cause additional neuronal injury above that generated by the acute hypoxic-ischemic event. Seizures probably only represent underlying neuronal compromise and as such abolition of all convulsions is both illogical and potentially dangerous. Exposing the infant to the minimum number of anticonvulsants is obviously important. It is not necessary to abolish all convulsions, but treatment should be started for frequent (> 3 per h) or prolonged (≥ 3 min) convulsions. The following drugs are used to treat postasphyxial convulsions.

Phenobarbitone. This is the first-line anticonvulsant for neonatal seizures. The loading dose is 20 mg/kg followed 12 h later by 6 mg/kg/24 h given twice daily. High-dose phenobarbitone monotherapy has been suggested to be a useful method for treating seizures resistant to standard phenobarbitone treatment (Gilman et al 1989). They suggest that if seizures continue, a further infusion of 5–10 mg/kg of phenobarbitone is given over a 10- to 15-min period and repeated every 20–30 min until seizures stop or the serum level of drug exceeds 40 μg/ml. Two-thirds of convulsing neonates responded to this form of management.

Clonazepam. This is my preferred second-line anticonvulsant in mature infants, but its effect is not well documented in the baby born prematurely. The loading dose is 0.25 mg with 0.05 mg 12-hourly. With severe seizures a continuous infusion may be used.

Phenytoin. This drug has also been widely used to treat neonatal convulsions but has two disadvantages compared with phenobarbitone. Firstly, it is potentially cardiotoxic and secondly it is an unpredictable drug in terms of maintenance dosage. There is a progressive fall in half-life over the early postnatal months, and particularly in the first week. It is best used intravenously in a loading dose only (20 mg/kg) to control convulsions in a baby who has already received other anticonvulsants, but not given as maintenance therapy once convulsions have been controlled.

Brain swelling

Treatment is commonly directed towards the prevention and reduction of raised intracranial pressure. It is traditional to keep asphyxiated infants relatively dehydrated. It is most appropriate to carefully monitor serum electrolytes and urinary specific gravity and give just enough fluid to keep the infant on the dry side of normal hydration. Fluid restriction (20% less than daily requirements) is only necessary for the first 48 h of life.

There is no evidence that the treatment of cerebral edema or raised intracranial pressure improves outcome (see above). Mannitol has been shown to significantly reduce brain water in an animal model when given immediately after an asphyxial event (Mujsce et al 1988), but it did not reduce the severity or distribution of brain damage. Although 20% mannitol infusion reduced intracranial pressure, we found no improvement in outcome in babies given intravenous mannitol (Levene & Evans 1985). The routine measurement of intracranial pressure is not indicated, but if the infant is neurologically abnormal and has a bulging fontanel, 20% mannitol may reduce intracranial hypertension and should be given as a 20% solution, 1 g/kg by continuous infusion over 20 min. Mannitol is contraindicated in the presence of oliguria or severe renal compromise as this may cause a rebound effect with increased swelling of the brain and an increase in pressure due to failure of the infant to excrete the drug.

In older children and adults with presumed or actual cerebral edema the $PaCO_2$ is usually adjusted to between 3.5 and 4 kPa. This reduces intracranial pressure by reducing intracranial blood volume but there is no evidence that this actually improves outlook. It is now apparent that hyperventilation with reduction in $PaCO_2$ increases neuropathology in immature experimental animals (Vannucci et al 1995) and human premature infants (Fujimoto et al 1994). Limited data in mature newborn animals do not suggest a similar adverse effect (Rosenberg 1992). In the human infant there is no evidence that maintaining a $PaCO_2$ lower than the normal range is of any benefit and it is potentially dangerous in immature babies as cerebral ischemia may be induced.

Steroids have no effect on experimental global cerebral edema when given following birth asphyxia. Corticosteroid treatment may be associated with adverse outcome and should not be used.

Early prevention of neuronal injury

The neuron may be particularly resistant to asphyxial injury and neuronal death results from a cascade of biochemical and vascular complications during the stage of reperfusion as discussed above. There is some evidence from animal experiments that early treatment immediately after the immature animal is resuscitated may limit cerebral injury, but it must be stressed that at the present time no such treatment is available in the neonatal unit and this section should be read as a possible signpost towards future management.

Free radical scavengers

The majority of free radicals are produced during resuscitation following an asphyxial insult (Pourcyrous et al 1993). Xanthine oxidase inhibition with either allopurinol or oxypurinol reduces both free radical production (Pourcyrous et al 1993) and neuropathological lesions if given prior to the asphyxial event (Palmer et al 1990). Recently, it has been shown that allopurinol given after a hypoxic-ischemic insult results in a significant reduction in cerebral edema and neuronal destruction (Palmer et al 1993). Prevention of intraneuronal NO production by a nitric oxide synthase inhibitor reduced neuronal damage only when this agent was given prior to the asphyxial event and not after it (Hamada et al 1994). This probably has an effect by reducing free radical damage.

Calcium channel blockers

Flunarizine when given prior to a hypoxic-ischemic insult protects against neuronal injury in the immature rat brain (Gunn et al 1989), but there are no studies showing calcium channel blockers to have a protective effect when given after the asphyxial insult. In four severely asphyxiated human infants the calcium channel blocker, nicardipine, was associated with severe hypotension in two cases. These drugs have a general vasodilating action on the systemic vascular bed and inadvertent hypotension may be a side effect which renders these drugs of little value in the newborn infant.

Excitatory neurotransmitter antagonists

A variety of drugs have been shown to act as NMDA receptor antagonists and reduce the severity and extent of neuronal necrosis in neonatal animal models (Levene 1992). The best-studied antagonist is MK-801 which when given 120 min after insult gives 70% neuroprotective effect (McDonald et al 1990a). Unfortunately, MK-801 is toxic and cannot be used in neonates. Mg^{2+} may have a neuroprotective role following neonatal asphyxial insult by preventing Ca^{2+} entry into the neuron and a number of studies have shown that treatment with $MgSO_4$ after the insult significantly reduces neuropathology (McDonald et al 1990b, Marret et al 1995). This is now the subject of a large international multicenter trial in human birth asphyxia.

Hypothermia

Adult studies have shown that even a small reduction in brain temperature ameliorates cerebral injury following hypoxic-ischemic insult. A recent study in newborn piglets has confirmed that depression of core temperature to 35°C for 12 h significantly reduced the secondary energy failure and this effect persisted after rewarming the animals (Thorensen et al 1995).

PROGNOSIS

The outcome for birth asphyxia depends upon the criteria used to make the diagnosis. As discussed above, the diagnosis of birth asphyxia in premature infants is more difficult than in the full-term infant and obvious neuropathology evident on imaging is much more commonly detected in the premature group. The prognosis in premature infants is usually more accurately made on the basis of whether the infant has parenchymal hemorrhage or periventricular leukomalacia than how low the Apgar score was or the need for intubation or resuscitation. The prognosis related to these specific neuropathological events is discussed on pages 167 and following.

There is a close relationship between depression of Apgar score and mortality (Table 5.16). This is almost linear for full-term babies (Nelson & Ellenberg 1981) but in premature infants there is a 84% mortality rate with Apgar scores of 0–3 at 15 min. The mortality has also been reported to be very high in babies who have not established regular spontaneous respiration by 30 min

Table 5.16 Risk of death or cerebral palsy (CP) in infants with Apgar scores of 0–3 at varying times from birth (data from Nelson & Ellenberg 1981)

Age (min)	Death in first year < 2500 g (%)	CP < 2500 g (%)	Death in first year > 2500 g (%)	CP > 2500 g (%)
1	26	2	3	0.7
5	55	7	8	0.7
10	67	7	18	5
15	84	0	48	9
20	96	0	59	57

after birth. Failure to breathe spontaneously is, however, related to many different factors and these should be carefully considered during resuscitation before a decision to abandon resuscitative efforts is made.

Depression of Apgar scores is an insensitive method for predicting handicap in newborn infants. The risk of death or handicap (cerebral palsy) in infants with severely depressed Apgar scores is shown in Table 5.16. It is not until the Apgar score remains at 0–3 by 20 min that there is a relatively high risk of cerebral palsy. Such a small proportion of newborn infants have depression of the Apgar score to this degree as to make its predictive ability of little relevance. Thomson et al (1977) reported that 93% of infants with an Apgar score of 0 at 1 min and/or 0–3 at 5 min were entirely normal at follow-up. Levene et al (1986) graded the severity of Apgar score depression according to different criteria in an effort to establish how predictive these scores were for serious impairment at a median age of 2.5 years. They found that an Apgar score of 5 or less at 10 min was the most sensitive for adverse outcome, but that this was far less good than a prediction based on encephalopathy.

A number of studies have reported outcome related to the severity of postasphyxial encephalopathy (Levene 1988, Peliowski & Finer 1992). There was a remarkable consensus in prediction, although many of the grading systems had slight variations in detail. All referred to three grades of encephalopathy considered to be mild, moderate or severe. No infant with mild encephalopathy alone developed significant impairment. The median risk of impairment from five follow-up studies in full-term infants with moderate encephalopathy (seizures, but not coma) was 25% (range 17–27%) and for severe encephalopathy (seizures and coma) 92% died or were severely handicapped (range 75–100%) (Levene 1988). Mortality in the group of infants with moderate HIE is 4.5%, compared with 62% mortality in those with severe HIE (Peliowski & Finer 1992). Of the surviving infants with severe HIE, 71% were severely handicapped. The accuracy of prognosis based on postasphyxial encephalopathy is far better than Apgar scores or delay in establishing respiration.

Imaging with CT and MR both give good prognostic information, but these techniques are of limited value in the early prognosis of severe asphyxia because abnormalities may not be apparent in the first 24 h (see above).

Doppler assessment is also an accurate predictor of adverse outcome in asphyxiated full-term infants (Levene et al 1989, Eken et al 1995). A low PRI (see above) or a high mean flow velocity above 3 SD from the mean has a positive predictive value for adverse outcome of 94% (Levene et al 1989). These Doppler abnormalities do not occur within the first 24 h of life and repeated Doppler estimates must be performed.

Assessment of cerebral function by EEG is a very useful prognostic tool. An overview of four studies (Peliowski & Finer 1992) found that a normal or mildly abnormal EEG had an excellent prognosis (likelihood ratio of adverse outcome 0.03 CI 0.01–0.11) compared with a likelihood ratio of 1.56 (CI 0.82–2.96) for moderate EEG abnormality (slow wave activity). A severely abnormal EEG (burst suppression, low voltage or isoelectric EEG) gave a very poor prognosis with a likelihood ratio for adverse outcome of 18.60 (CI 6.88–50.00). A recent study using early modified EEG assessment (Cerebral Function Monitor – CFM) found that major abnormality at 6 h or later was associated with a poor prognosis (Eken et al 1995). At 6 h of age the CFM was the best predictor of any test of outcome in asphyxiated full-term infants with a positive and negative predictive value of 84.2% and 91.7% respectively.

Practical approach to prognosis

At the present time there is no proven effective treatment in asphyxiated infants. It may be appropriate to recognize a group of infants with very poor prognosis so that an informed discussion about withdrawal of intensive care can be conducted with the parents. I suggest that two separate assessments with both EEG (or CFM) and Doppler should be carried out at 6 h and 24 h. If the EEG (CFM) is severely abnormal at 6 and 24 h and the Doppler is abnormal at 24 h then the prognosis is extremely poor and the parents should be made aware of this.

RESUSCITATION OF THE NEWBORN

Approximately 1% of all newborn infants will need vigorous resuscitation involving artificial respiration. Although only 0.5% of full-term infants will need intubation, 50% of infants born at or below 28 weeks will require vigorous resuscitation with the need for intubation. Dawes (1968) has described the sequence of events that occur during experimental asphyxia of fetal rhesus monkeys. Initially there is an episode of small-volume but regular breaths, followed by apnea and a fall in heart rate with the animal becoming cyanosed. This period of primary apnea lasts for up to a minute and is followed by spontaneous gasping which is maintained for a further 4–5 min before a second period of apnea develops. If resuscitation is not undertaken at the stage of secondary or terminal apnea, then the animal will die. These events are represented in Figure 5.12, and are applicable to the human situation.

Many, but by no means all, infants who are born in a depressed state can be anticipated and Table 5.17 lists the indications for calling a pediatrician or other person competent to resuscitate the newborn infant. Some of these indications require some qualification.

Prematurity It is not necessary for a pediatrician to be present at the delivery of every premature infant. Approximately 5% of infants born at 35 weeks' gestation require active resuscitation and this should be the gestational age cutoff at which a pediatrician is routinely called assuming there are no other risk factors.

Fetal distress As discussed above the term 'fetal distress' usually refers to the detection of fetal stress, which the fetus is often able to cope with. Meconium staining of the liquor is seen in 18% of deliveries (Nelson & Ellenberg 1984) and if the

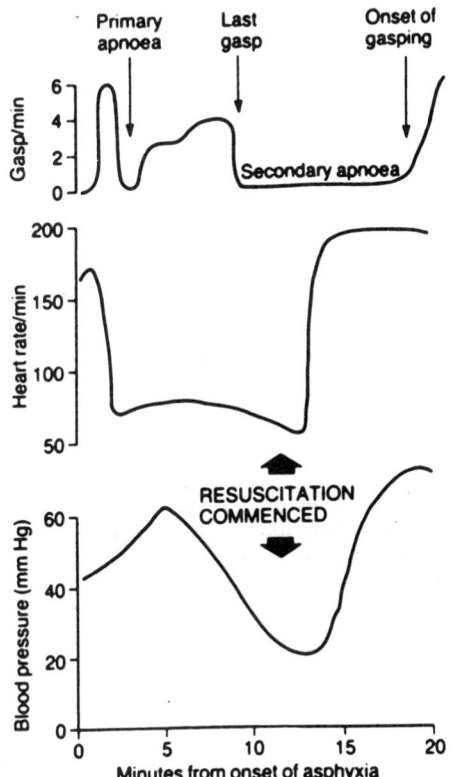

Fig. 5.12 The effects of asphyxia on a newborn animal showing primary and secondary apnea. (Redrawn from Dawes (1968) with permission of Blackwell Scientific Publications.)

Table 5.17 Indications for calling a pediatrician to be present at a delivery

Prematurity
  Gestation < 36 weeks

Fetal distress
  Thick meconium staining
  Severely abnormal CTG
  Fetal scalp acidosis (pH < 7.2)

Operative delivery
  Any delivery under general anesthesia
  Mid-cavity or rotational forceps

Multiple pregnancy

Significant antepartum hemorrhage

Fetal disease
  Known major congenital abnormality
  Rhesus disease

meconium staining is light, then there is only a very small risk that this reflects fetal distress. Thick meconium in the amniotic fluid indicates the need for a pediatrician to be in attendance at the delivery. Type II decelerations, fetal scalp blood acidosis (pH < 7.2) and fetal bradycardia indicate possibly significant distress and a pediatrician should be alerted.

Operative delivery. A pediatrician should be present for the delivery of all babies born to a mother who is having a general anesthetic. Cesarean section under epidural anesthesia does not necessitate a pediatric presence providing the delivery is not considered high risk for any other reason. Lift out forceps deliveries should be treated as low risk, but a pediatrician should be present for all complicated or rotational forceps deliveries.

PREPARATION PRIOR TO DELIVERY

The pediatrician called for a high-risk delivery should spend some time prior to delivery acquainting him- or herself with the mother's medical and antenatal history. It is important that s/he checks all the equipment that may be required prior to delivery and not rely on the fact that this should have been done by others.

Resuscitation trolley. The infant should be laid on a flat surface which is inclined so that the head is about 15° below the feet and facing towards the pediatrician. This facilitates drainage of secretions. A stop clock should be permanently fixed to the trolley and is started at delivery, giving the operator a reference point for the duration of resuscitation. Another important component of the resuscitation trolley is an integral overhead heater. This should be of fixed height above the infant with a dial to give variable temperature settings.

Medical gases. It is most important that both air and oxygen are readily available, together with appropriate reduction valves so that a variable and measurable flow of gas can be given to the infant. One gas line must be available for face mask oxygen and another that can be attached to an endotracheal tube via a Y-piece connector. The arm of the Y-piece not connected to the ET tube can be occluded by the pediatrician's thumb which will direct the gas mixture into the baby's lungs at regular intervals for predetermined periods of time. As well as controlling the flow of gas a blow-off valve must be fitted so that the baby's lungs are not overdistended by unacceptably high pressures. On many resuscitation trolleys a water manometer valve is used, set to blow off at a maximum of 30 cm of water.

Ideally there should be a mixing valve to allow a variable concentration of oxygen to be given to the baby. It is not generally appreciated that air is probably a more valuable gas than 100% oxygen in the immediate resuscitation of the newborn infant as the nitrogen will not be absorbed thereby maintaining expansion of the lungs. Oxygen is rapidly absorbed and atelectasis may ensue if mucous plugs are present which cause the oxygen to be trapped. The potential hazardous effects of oxygen are discussed below.

Suction. The presence of suction apparatus on the resuscitation trolley is essential. This must also be fitted with an accurate valve device with a display of negative pressure as too high a suction pressure may damage the infant's respiratory tract. A variety of electric suction devices are manufactured for use in neonatal resuscitation and are perfectly acceptable. Mouth suction must no longer be used. A number of suction catheters of different sizes (FG 4, 6 and 8) must also be at hand with appropriate connectors to attach to the suction device.

Bag and mask. Bag and mask resuscitation equipment is essential in every hospital where babies are delivered or cared for and all staff must be familiar with their effective use. The method for appropriate bag and mask ventilation is described below.

A number of different bags exist, the best being the Laerdal type. These are fitted with blow-off valves which can be adjusted to give a maximum inflation pressure. Tubing can be fitted to these devices so that the baby can be ventilated with additional oxygen. As well as the bag, a tight-fitting face mask is essential. These should be of variable sizes (Bennett 2 and 3) to fit the faces of the smallest and the biggest babies likely to be encountered.

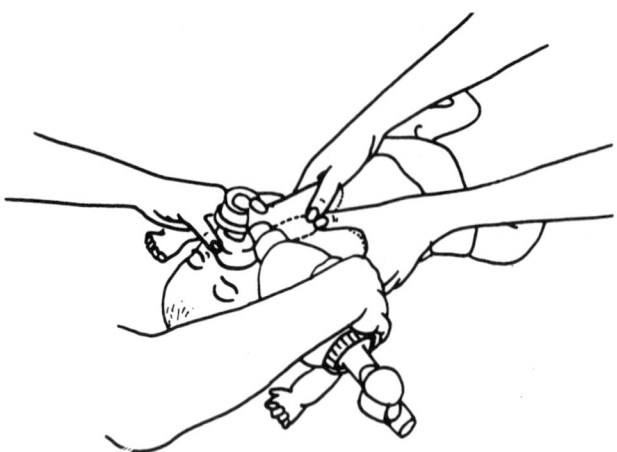

Fig. 5.13 Cardiorespiratory resuscitation. One operator inflates the baby's lungs with the bag and mask. The head is slightly extended and the chin pulled forward. The other operator gives external cardiac massage with hands encircling the chest. (Reproduced from Levene et al (1987) with permission of Blackwell Scientific Publications.)

Table 5.18 Drugs that should be immediately available to the pediatrician at delivery

Glucose 25% solution
Sodium bicarbonate 8.4%
Adrenaline 1: 1000 (0.5–1 ml i.v.)
Naloxone (10 μg/kg i.m. or i.v.)
Calcium gluconate 10% (1 ml i.v.)
Normal saline
Plasma
Atropine (0.1 mg i.v.)
Isoprenaline

The technique is shown in Figure 5.13. The baby's head is slightly extended and one hand elevates the mandible. The tightly fitting Silastic face mask covers the mouth and nose and is pressed down to form an airtight seal. The bag is then squeezed using two or three fingers just hard enough to produce good symmetrical chest expansion. More forceful inflation is unnecessary and dangerous.

Intubation equipment. Two laryngoscopes should be available with fresh batteries and these should be checked prior to delivery of the baby. A variety of laryngoscope blades should also be available of varying sizes and shapes. One kind should be curved and the other flat to suit the preferences of different staff. A selection of endotracheal tubes should be present varying in size from 2.5 to 4.0 mm. The correct connector must also be available together with a malleable metal introducer. Reliable means of securing the tube to the baby's face should also be present and the assisting nurse must be skilled in the fixation of the tube. A stethoscope should be worn by the resuscitator prior to delivery of the baby.

Drugs. Table 5.18 lists the drugs that should be available to the pediatrician in the labor ward. They should always be kept in a box by the side of the resuscitation trolley and not locked in the main drug cupboard.

ASSESSMENT AT BIRTH

At birth, the newborn infant's condition should be rapidly assessed. If the baby is breathing regularly and is pink, s/he should be dried, wrapped in a warm towel and given to the mother. The baby with impaired breathing may remain cyanosed, have bradycardia or develop hypopnea. Such infants should be dried rapidly and observed naked under a radiant heater. The baby's mouth and nose should be gently suctioned with a soft catheter and oxygen blown onto his face from a funnel. Most babies improve with such stimulation. If the baby fails to improve, then further management is discussed in the next section.

The Apgar score is the best method of recording the infant's condition at birth and in the ensuing minutes after birth. The Apgar score has five components, each of which can be graded as 0, 1 or 2. Table 5.12 lists the components of the Apgar score. Although it is a useful device for recording the condition of the baby at one moment in time it has a number of deficiencies which are discussed on page 125.

The baby may present to the pediatrician in a variety of degrees of depression and the resuscitative efforts depend on the degree of apnea or shock.

THE BABY WHO DOES NOT BREATHE

As discussed above, apnea following birth can be either primary or secondary. In the primary form the baby is blue due to hypoxia but has an adequate circulation. In secondary apnea the baby is white due to impaired circulation and poor cardiac output. In practice it may be difficult to distinguish the two and infants with apnea must always be carefully assessed. The medical attendant's response to apnea may also vary depending on whether the infant is immature or full term.

The mature infant

The apneic newborn infant should initially be stimulated by flicking the heels or gently sucking out the nares. This in most cases is enough to produce gasping which should rapidly give way to regular respiration. A flow of oxygen directed towards the infant's nose and mouth may be a further stimulus to breathe. If regular respiration is not established by 1 min, or if the cardiovascular system is depressed (poor cardiac output or bradycardia), artificial ventilation should be started. This is done either with a bag and mask or by intubation. An infant laryngoscope is used to visualize the glottis and a soft suction catheter should be introduced into the trachea which is gently sucked out. An appropriately sized endotracheal tube is then inserted. Once the baby has established regular respirations and the cardiac output is good, the baby can be extubated. If the birth attendant cannot intubate the apneic infant, then a bag and mask should be used to inflate the baby's lungs (Fig. 5.13).

Naloxone. Some babies may be apneic because their mothers have recently been given an opiate for pain relief. Naloxone is a specific antagonist to opiates and should be given to the baby if the mother has had pethidine or a similar opiate-like drug within 4 h of delivery. The dose of naloxone is 10 μg/kg by deep intramuscular injection.

The immature infant

Birth of the immature infant should always be anticipated and a pediatrician should be present. If the infant has not achieved regular respiration and good color within 20 s of delivery the child should be intubated. In some centers, elective intubation is undertaken in all very premature infants as soon as they are born, but there is little evidence that this is of benefit. There is, however, no point in delaying intubation in depressed premature infants if they clearly have not established spontaneous respiratory effort shortly after birth. They should then be transferred to the neonatal unit with an endotracheal tube in situ and not extubated until they can be appropriately monitored in an incubator.

THE INFANT WITH LITTLE OR NO CARDIAC OUTPUT

These infants have bradycardia and are pale and shocked. This represents a severe form of terminal apnea and unless they are resuscitated rapidly they will surely die. They should be intubated immediately and ventilated in high concentrations of oxygen at a rate of 30–40 breaths/min at the lowest inflating pressure necessary to obtain good chest movements. In some cases bradycardia will improve with effective ventilation alone and the baby will become pink. If the pulse rate is still slow and the baby pale, then support of the cardiovascular system should be undertaken in the following sequence.

1. *External cardiac massage.* This is performed by placing both hands around the infant's chest and back to encircle the chest with the two thumbs on either side of the midsternal area (Fig. 5.13). The sternum is then depressed 1–3 cm according to the size of the baby 80–100 times a minute. This approach produces a better cardiac output than is obtained with two fingers over the sternum. A peripheral pulse (femoral or carotid) should be monitored by an assistant to ensure that the cardiac massage produces effective cardiac output.

2. *Cardiac stimulants.* A variety of drugs can be considered once effective ventilation and cardiac output have been established. These drugs should only be used in the presence of a working cardiorater which shows the electrocardiogram (ECG) signal. Adrenaline is a powerful cardiac stimulant and is used for asystole or severe bradycardia where there is little cardiac output. The dose is 0.5–1 ml of 1 : 1000 adrenaline. This is best given into a central vein, but if venous access is not available this can be given directly into the heart or down the endotracheal tube (see below). It can be repeated after 5 min if there is no response.

Calcium gluconate is a useful cardiac stimulant, particularly in babies with persistent bradycardia and low cardiac output. The dose is 1 ml of 10% solution intravenously. This should not be given directly into the heart, because inadvertent injection into the myocardium causes severe and extensive muscle fibrosis.

The following drugs may be used in infants who have a persistent bradycardia unresponsive to the above measures: atropine (0.1 mg i.v.); isoprenaline (bolus dose of 1–2 ml and continuous infusion of 0.1–0.4 µg/kg/min).

3. *Other agents.* Metabolic acidosis inevitably accompanies asphyxia and some authorities recommend the routine use of sodium bicarbonate solution. The majority of severely asphyxiated babies do not require this substance during the course of resuscitation, particularly if the infant improves rapidly. If the baby has a good cardiac output and effective ventilation then he will correct his own acidosis. It is only those babies who require prolonged cardiorespiratory support for more than 5 min who will require an intravenous infusion of 8.4% sodium bicarbonate solution (10 ml/kg).

The role of routine glucose infusion during resuscitation is the subject of some controversy and is discussed below. Glucose must be given if the baby is found to be hypoglycemic.

Intracardiac injection

This should only be used if all other methods have failed to resuscitate the infant. The skin in the epigastric region is cleaned with an alcohol swab and a 21 G needle, attached to a syringe containing the drug to be given, is introduced just below the xiphisternum and angled up towards the left shoulder. Following insertion to 2–3 cm, the syringe is aspirated and if blood is obtained the drug is injected. The needle is then withdrawn.

THE INFANT WHO DOES NOT RESPOND TO RESUSCITATION

The majority of infants respond rapidly to intubation, but if there is failure to respond then there are a number of conditions which must be considered and rapidly eliminated by appropriate tests.

1. *Poor technique.* The baby may not be ventilating because the bag and mask is being used inappropriately, or the endotracheal tube is not sited appropriately in the trachea.

2. *Iatrogenic disease.* Pneumothorax may occur due to overvigorous resuscitation (p. 187).

3. *Underlying disease.* Consider anatomical abnormalities such as diaphragmatic hernia (p. 1769), tracheo-esophageal fistula (p. 1770), congenital cyanotic cardiac abnormality (p. 613) or hypoplastic lungs (p. 191).

Current controversies in neonatal resuscitation

The routine use of additional oxygen. During resuscitation after asphyxia, free radicals are produced which may be an important factor in subsequent neuronal necrosis (see above). Routine use of 21% oxygen (air) during the course of resuscitating asphyxiated infants has been shown to be as effective as 100% oxygen (Ramji et al 1993). In another study, premature infants (< 33 weeks) were shown to have a significantly lower cerebral blood flow at 2 h if they had been resuscitated in 80% oxygen compared with air (Lundstrom et al 1995). These data suggest that neonates requiring resuscitation should be initially ventilated in air, and oxygen given only if they are subsequently shown to remain hypoxic.

The routine administration of glucose. In a series of elegant experiments on immature rat pups, Vannucci & Mujsce (1992) have shown that hyperglycemia *prior* to a hypoxic-ischemic insult had a dramatic effect on protecting the brain from infarction. Controversy remains as to whether glucose given immediately *after* the hypoxic-ischemic event is of benefit. Recent reports on the use of glucose in immature animal models have given conflicting results. One study has shown evidence of brain protection (Hattori & Wasterlain 1990) and the other showed severe neuronal damage in the hyperglycemic group (Sheldon et al 1992). This issue requires further investigation but it is clear that hypoglycemia during and after resuscitation must be vigorously treated. At the present time the routine use of glucose during resuscitation cannot be recommended.

When to stop resuscitation

All babies deserve to be considered for active resuscitation, unless they are macerated or show an obvious lethal congenital abnormality. In those infants with no cardiac output after 10 min active resuscitation should be abandoned.

A more difficult question is how long to pursue resuscitation if the infant fails to breathe? Other causes of respiratory failure must first be considered such as maternal drug effect and neuromuscular disorders. If the baby is not breathing by 40 min and particularly if he remains extremely depressed with severe hypotonia, then further active resuscitation should be considered to be inappropriate. It is best for the most senior doctor available to make this decision. If there is any doubt it is best to take the baby to the neonatal unit for intensive care until such time as a full assessment can be made. It is much easier for the parents to mourn the loss of their baby if they are convinced that a full resuscitation was attempted and they will come to terms with it better if they have time to understand the severe problems that are present. Parents should be encouraged to hold their baby at whatever stage resuscitative efforts are abandoned.

THE SMALL FOR GESTATIONAL AGE INFANT (Fig. 5.14)

The World Health Organization in 1950 defined a baby as small for gestational age (SGA) when it was below the 10th weight centile for gestation. At that time perinatal mortality of this group even in the western world was very high. Obstetric deaths due to placental failure in utero and acute intrapartum asphyxia were relatively common. Neonatal problems such as pulmonary hemorrhage and hypoglycemia were inadequately treated and the mortality and morbidity from congenital rubella was commoner (immunization schedules were not introduced until 1966 in the UK). Times have now changed but the definition has not. With modern antenatal and intrapartum care it is unusual for the pediatrician to be confronted by an unexpectedly small baby. Intrauterine and peripartum asphyxia and death are rarities. Rubella embryopathy is much less common and ultrasound policies for infants early diagnosed as small may allow termination of pregnancy for a lethal congenital abnormality. Better feeding policies postnatally have made all but the smallest of light for dates babies (SGA) manageable with care on the postnatal wards. It is unlikely that the baby more than 1800 g birthweight will need to be transferred to the neonatal unit if delivery care and care on the postnatal wards are appropriate (Jones & Roberton 1986).

ETIOLOGY

Maternal causes

In utero starvation and placental insufficiency (essential hypertension, pregnancy associated hypertension (PET), chronic renal disease, longstanding diabetes, heart disease in pregnancy, multiple pregnancy, poor socioeconomic circumstances with severe malnutrition, excess smoking, excess alcohol, living at high altitude). Classically, placental insufficiency leads to

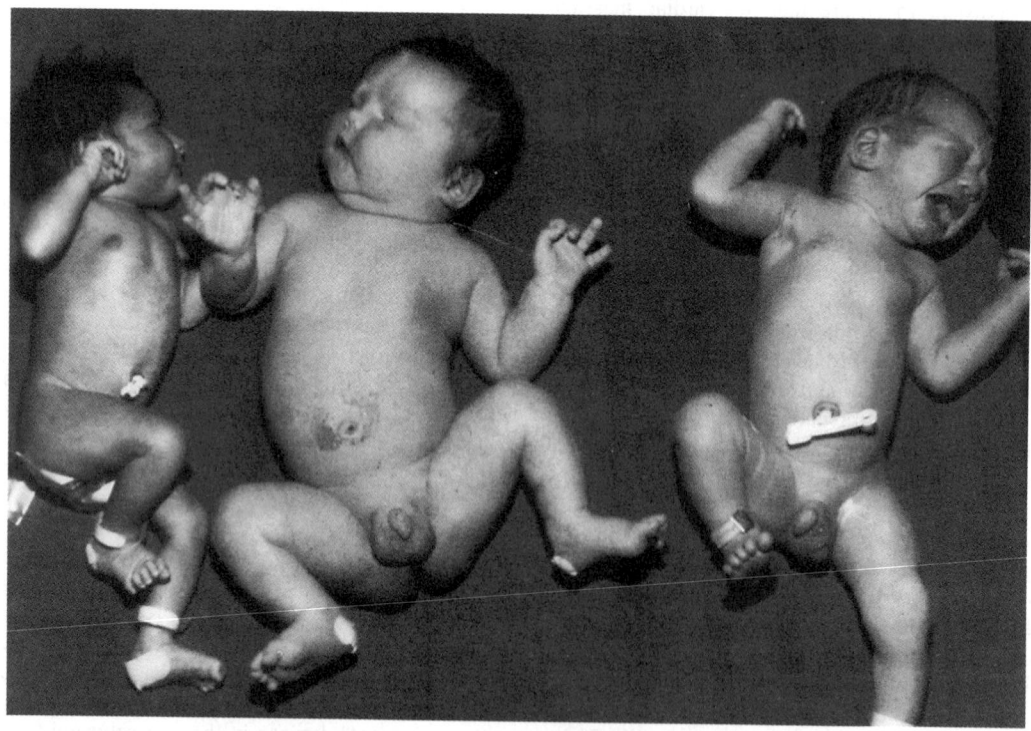

Fig. 5.14 Size with gestation. The baby on the left at 1.7 kg and 39 weeks is small for gestational age. The baby on the right is 1.9 kg and 34 weeks' gestation and is both appropriate for gestation and preterm. The center baby at 4.4 kg and 39 weeks' gestation is large for gestational age.

asymmetric growth retardation, the weight being more affected than the length or particularly the head circumference. The obstetrician may identify this problem in utero, ultrasound showing a small abdominal and thoracic circumference and a relatively spared head circumference. Small mothers and elderly primigravidae tend to have smaller than average babies.

Fetal causes

Congenital abnormality (chromosomal and many syndromes, e.g. Potter's) and congenital infection (rubella, toxoplasmosis, cytomegalovirus, herpes simplex and syphilis). Early fetal toxins such as alcohol, phenytoin and warfarin. Such infants usually display symmetrical growth retardation, the head size being as retarded as the weight and length.

PROBLEMS OF THE SGA BABY

Hypoglycemia

Before modern neonatal treatment developed, 60% of preterm babies who were also SGA and 30% of full-term SGA babies developed hypoglycemia. Hypoglycemia may be present before birth. The etiology after birth is complex.

1. Reduced glycogen deposits (in liver, muscle and heart).
2. The brain and heart (but not the liver, spleen, thymus and adrenals) are large in proportion to the rest of the body and have high energy substrate demands.
3. A reduced catecholamine response to a falling blood sugar suggests that the adrenal medulla is failing with consequent reduced glycogenolysis.
4. Rapid glucose disappearance may in some cases be due to high insulin levels. However many infants show a reduced insulin response to a glucose load which suggests either a defect in peripheral glucose utilization or reduced insulin sensitivity.
5. Defective lipolysis is suggested by reduced levels of β-hydroxybutyrate and lack of the normal inverse relationship between free fatty acids and blood sugar.
6. Hepatic gluconeogenesis is reduced. Frequently there are elevated levels of alanine, lactate and pyruvate and an alanine load does not provoke an appropriate increase in blood sugar. There may be a delay in the postnatal development of hepatic gluconeogenic enzymes.

Hypoglycemia may lead to neuroglycopenia. Clinical signs of apnea and convulsions do not occur until a blood sugar of less than 1 mmol/l has been present for several hours, probably because alternative substrates are available (glycerol, lactate, β-hydroxybutyrate, acetoacetate). Nevertheless, Koh et al (1988) have shown that auditory evoked potentials are compromised at much higher blood sugar levels so it is important to be obsessional in blood sugar management in these small infants.

Practically, in all except the very small for gestational age (less than 3rd centile), management can and should be on the postnatal ward.

Breast-feeding mothers are encouraged to breast-feed 3-hourly, and prefeed dextrostix or BM stix are done after 6 h for 48 h. If hypoglycemia less than 2.6 mmol/l is detected, 8 ml/kg of formula are given after each breast-feed on day 1 and 12 ml/kg after each feed on day 2, if necessary by nasogastric tube. After 48 h, if there has been no hypoglycemia the bottle feeds after the breast can be withdrawn gradually as the mother's milk comes in.

Bottle-fed babies should be given 90, 120, 150 ml/kg/day respectively on each of the first 3 days of life. Prefeed dextrostix or BM stix should be done at 6, 9, 12, 18, 24, 30, 36 and 48 h. If the blood sugar is low, < 2.6 mmol/l, or the baby is asymptomatic add 2 ml/kg/feed of 50% dextrose. If the dextrostix is still low or the baby is vomiting or the hypoglycemia is symptomatic a drip of at least 90 ml/kg/24 h of 10% dextrose is required.

Hypoglycemia is unlikely to be problematic after 48 h of age if it has not been so beforehand.

A baby both small for gestational age and less than 1800 g should probably be admitted to the neonatal unit for observation and treatment.

Infants with transient diabetes mellitus are usually small for gestational age.

Hypothermia

SGA infants may be born with a temperature above mother's as the inefficient placenta will not exchange heat. The scraggy baby with large surface area : bodyweight ratio may cool fast after delivery if appropriate steps are not taken to prevent this (p. 147).

Polycythemia

The high altitude effect associated with poor placental oxygen transfer leads to increased packed cell volume, red cell mass and high erythropoietin levels. This may lead to viscosity problems. Sheer stresses may reduce the platelet count and on rare occasions liberated platelet thromboplastins may set off disseminated intravascular coagulation (DIC). It is appropriate if the baby looks plethoric to do a venous packed cell volume (PCV) and also platelet count and clotting tests. Treatment with partial exchange transfusion may be required on occasions and vitamin K should be given (p. 230).

Neutropenia and thrombocytopenia

Severely SGA infants particularly those less than 1000 g birthweight may show neutropenia and thrombocytopenia (McIntosh et al 1988) Platelets may be reduced in number partly by the mechanisms mentioned above but it may be that the marrow in utero is more committed to manufacture of red cell series (high normoblasts) because of hypoxia and there is a temporary reduction in the ability to produce other cells after birth.

Hypocalcemia

This is less commonly seen now that babies are delivered in good condition by the obstetric team. It was probably related to perinatal asphyxia but the pathophysiology is not clear.

Infection

With modern management it is rare for SGA infants to develop a postnatal infection unless they are in addition very preterm.

Congenital abnormality

3–6% of SGA babies have congenital abnormalities; these are usually obvious and lethal such as the chromosome abnormalities,

Potter's syndrome and the baby with disseminated congenital infection.

Meconium aspiration

Rare with modern obstetric management.

Pulmonary hemorrhage

This was probably related to intrapartum asphyxia and polycythemia. Modern obstetric and pediatric practice should identify and rectify these problems before hemorrhage results.

Other humoral and metabolic abnormalities

High ammonia, urea and uric acid levels after birth may reflect the reduced calorie reserve of these infants or a protein catabolic state. High circulating cortisol, corticosterone and growth hormone levels have also been demonstrated at birth.

CLINICAL FEATURES OF SGA BABIES

A minority of infants will have obvious congenital abnormalities, chromosome defects or intrauterine infection. Most infants will be scraggy individuals with wasting, particularly of the thighs. The fingernails are mature and long and cracks and desquamation of the skin begin rapidly after birth. The infant is usually active and vigorous and apparently anxious lest his starved state in utero may continue after birth. Sucking is usually strong and the weight loss after birth is less than for an appropriately sized baby.

MANAGEMENT

Early obstetric diagnosis should be followed by a planned delivery in the presence of pediatric staff capable of skilled resuscitation. Labor and birth are asphyxial stresses so labor should be carefully monitored. The baby may be hypoglycemic at birth so a dextrostix should be performed immediately. If there are no signs of anomaly or infection the major pediatric concerns are to prevent hypothermia and hypoglycemia hopefully on the normal postnatal ward.

OUTCOME

Babies with asymmetric growth retardation usually catch up to within the normal centiles after birth whereas many symmetrically growth retarded infants do not. Unless they suffer symptomatic hypoglycemia, they will in all probability develop with a normal DQ and later IQ. Babies SGA because of syndromes, chromosome abnormalities and intrauterine infections will have a high neonatal mortality and later morbidity.

THE LARGE FOR GESTATIONAL AGE INFANT (Fig. 5.14)

By definition heavier than the 90th weight centile for gestation.

ETIOLOGY

1. Constitutionally large baby from heavy large mother.
2. Maternal diabetes or prediabetes – the infant of the diabetic mother (IDM) or the infant of the gestational diabetic mother (IGDM).
3. Severe erythroblastosis.
4. Other causes of hydrops fetalis and ascites.
5. Transposition of the great arteries (sometimes).
6. Syndromes:
   a. Beckwith–Wiedemann (BW) syndrome (p. 295)
   b. Sotos' syndrome (p. 1043)
   c. Marshall syndrome
   d. Weaver syndrome.

PROBLEMS OF LARGE FOR GESTATIONAL AGE (LGA) BABIES

Birth asphyxia and trauma

Shoulder dystocia may delay delivery leading to low Apgars, acidosis, meconium aspiration and hypoxic-ischemic encephalopathy and the consequent interventions may lead to fractured clavicle or long bones, brachical plexus injury (Erb ± phrenic palsy), subdural or cephalhematoma and skin bruising (later resulting in jaundice).

Hypoglycemia

The IDM, IGDM, baby with erythroblastosis and BW syndrome baby all have hyperinsulinism leading to reactive hypoglycemia after birth.

Polycythemia

Unusual.

Apparent large postnatal weight loss

A 5-kg baby may naturally lose more than 0.5 kg in weight over a few days (10% bodyweight being 500 g) even if supplied with adequate milk.

CARE OF THE PRETERM INFANT

DELIVERY ROOM CARE

A pediatrician or person trained in resuscitation should be present at the delivery of any preterm infant to ensure that air breathing is established rapidly and effectively and that the circulation changes appropriately from that of the fetus to that of the newborn infant (p. 106). If the infant is very immature (less than 32 weeks' gestation) two such people are better than one. Many preterm and particularly growth-retarded infants withstand a normal vaginal delivery poorly and the more gentle delivery by 'protective forceps' or Cesarean section may be very traumatic for the infant.

32–36 WEEKS' GESTATION

At this gestation the infant is usually quite robust. He should be dried thoroughly and the oro- and nasopharynx should be cleared of foreign material. If his Apgar scores (Table 5.12) are good he should be wrapped warmly and given to his mother. If less good, resuscitation may be required – page 132.

32 WEEKS' GESTATION OR LESS

Use gentle suction to clear oro- and nasopharynx and then rapidly and completely dry the infant with a warm towel to prevent evaporative heat loss (p. 146). Late clamping of the umbilical cord after the pulsation has ceased reduces the necessity for subsequent top-up transfusions and also reduces the incidence of respiratory distress (Kinmond et al 1990) – this is in contrast to cord clamping in the full-term infant which is probably best done early.

Many then advocate endotracheal intubation as a routine for all infants unless they are so vigorous that it will obviously be a traumatic procedure. Once intubated the infant is ventilated until pink and making good attempts to breathe spontaneously with an adequate cardiac output (assessed by feeling the femoral and brachial pulses). If the infant is large and robust and has responded vigorously to such care, extubation may be carried out at this stage. If the baby is small or feeble or the resuscitation has been prolonged, extubation would invite trouble which would not be optimally handled during the transfer between wards!

If there is a persistent bradycardia or a poor cardiac output it may be appropriate for the second resuscitator to insert an umbilical venous or arterial catheter to give volume support or drugs while the other maintains ventilation. Management is helped considerably by an early estimation of arterial blood gas. An early blood sugar measurement is vital in small infants as they may be hypoglycemic from birth and require 10% dextrose infusion immediately. The maintenance of warmth is best done by a continuous supply of warm towels to put over the baby.

Once the baby is stabilized it is important that the parents know what has happened and what will go on in the future. If at all possible the parents should see and touch their infant in the delivery room. If the baby is large the mother may be able to cuddle her infant. If the baby is small and supported on a ventilator the parents can usually still make contact with their newborn in the portable incubator. This important early contact should only be curtailed if the mother is anesthetized and without a partner; otherwise the father at least should be involved.

SPECIAL CARE

FLUID BALANCE

Even the anephric fetus enjoys biochemical homeostasis but immediately following birth, the kidney is crucial for chemical and fluid balance. The preterm infant is particularly vulnerable and dehydration and hyponatremia are the commonest problems (Simpson & Stephenson 1993).

Body water content and distribution

Perinatal changes

The ratio of intracellular fluid (ICF) to extracellular fluid (ECF) increases in the immediate postnatal period owing to water loss from the ECF space. A postnatal weight loss of 5–8% is common in term infants, the nadir occurring around the fifth day with birthweight usually regained by the 10th day. An even greater percentage loss of 12–21% may occur in premature infants (Gill et al 1986).

Some of this weight loss is meconium, vernix and umbilical stump but most is water derived from the ECF space. The ECF is comprised of interstitial fluid and circulating blood and much of the early postnatal weight loss is due to a reduction in interstitial fluid volume since plasma volume is well maintained over the first week of postnatal life. The interstitial fluid is lost from the body as urine which is virtually isotonic (Hamilton & Shaw 1984) and the negative sodium and water balance and weight loss which result from this appear to be obligatory as they are not prevented by administration of water, sodium or both (Rees et al 1984). The magnitude of this postnatal weight loss does not appear to alter short-term prognosis, at least up to 15% of birthweight.

Changes in body fluid related to delivery

At the time of delivery, stress hormones such as glucocorticoids, aldosterone, antidiuretic hormone and angiotensin (Stephenson et al 1991) are all elevated in the newborn and may contribute to salt and/or water retention. Moreover, crystalloid fluids administered to laboring mothers equilibrate across the placenta and increase fetal ECF volume, and plasma sodium concentration in the newborn correlates closely with maternal plasma sodium concentration at delivery (Tarnow-Mordi et al 1981).

Water balance

To maintain a stable water balance:

Water intake = water for growth
     + respiratory losses
     + transepidermal losses } insensible losses
     + sweat
     + urine } sensible losses
     + fecal losses

In addition, to achieve a 'normal' water balance, rather than maintaining the status quo, pre-existing deficits or overload must also be corrected.

Water for growth

Approximately 75% of increase in weight in utero is water. If this growth velocity of approximately 16 g/kg/24 h (Keen & Pearse 1985) is to be sustained in infants born prematurely, 12 ml/kg/24 h of water intake will be diverted towards growth, mostly into the ICF space. This is equivalent to the water of oxidation generated from infant feeds (13.5 ml/kg/24 h for an infant fed on a regime of 120 kcal/kg/24 h) (Shaw 1988). If the infant is not being fed enterally or parenterally, this consideration of water for growth is irrelevant as intravenous crystalloid solutions contain no nitrogen for anabolism.

Respiratory water losses

Inspired air is humidified and warmed by the respiratory tract so that expired air leaves the nose and mouth almost fully saturated at a temperature of 35–36°C. The amount of water lost from the respiratory tract is inversely proportional to the humidity of the inspired air, highest when the inspired air is dry and nonexistent when it is fully saturated. It will also depend on the minute volume, the product of tidal volume and respiratory rate. The amount is 7 ml/kg/24 h at an ambient humidity of 50% in term infants (Riesenfeld et al 1987) and will be similar in preterm infants in the absence of respiratory disease.

Transepidermal water loss

Transepidermal water loss (TEWL) is the passive diffusion of water through the epidermis and is dependent on the ambient humidity and temperature. TEWL is low in the full-term newborn (6–10 ml/kg/24 h), lower than the child or adult. Values are higher in preterm infants and very high before 30 weeks' gestation in the early newborn period. This is a result of a poorly developed horny layer of the epidermis – as the stratum corneum rapidly matures in the first 2 weeks of life, TEWL falls towards term values (Hammarlund et al 1983). There is an inverse correlation of TEWL with ambient relative humidity, so that TEWL is much higher if the surrounding air is dry and is abolished when it is fully saturated. The management of the fluid balance of a tiny, very immature infant is therefore simplified if a high ambient humidity is provided. TEWL is also increased by phototherapy and radiant heat.

Respiratory and transepidermal water loss together make up insensible water loss. This has been measured as insensible weight loss and is about 15 ml/kg/24 h for a term infant. Values in preterm infants are higher (especially in the very immature infant in the early neonatal period, because TEWL is so high), ranging from 15 to 120 ml/kg/24 h depending on the gestational age, postnatal age and the ambient conditions (Costarino & Baumgart 1986). Since published values of insensible weight loss are based on such a wide range of infants in differing environments, they are not useful for practical management of fluid balance. Insensible water loss is best derived by adding 7 ml/kg/24 h (respiratory water loss) to the values of TEWL shown in Table 5.19.

Sweating

The ability to sweat is impaired in the term newborn compared with children or adults. If the heat stress is sufficient to raise the body temperature above 37.5°C, evaporative water loss increases by a factor of 2–4. This means an increase from 15 to 30–60 ml/kg/24 h. Below 36 weeks' gestation sweating does not appear until a few days after birth and is limited compared with a term infant. Before 30 weeks' gestation, sweating is absent in the first 2 weeks and can be ignored in fluid balance consideration.

Fecal water loss

An allowance of 5–10 ml/kg/24 h is reasonable unless the infant has diarrhea or an enterostomy.

Urinary losses

In the immediate period after birth, urine production falls and the urine becomes more concentrated. Failure to pass urine

Table 5.19 Average values of transepidermal water loss (in ml/kg/24 h) at an ambient relative humidity of 50%. There is wide individual variation in the higher values. Data from Hammarlund et al (1983)

Gestation (weeks)	Postnatal age (days)						
	1	3	5	7	14	21	28
25–27	110	71	51	43	32	28	24
28–30	39	32	27	24	18	15	15
31–36	11	12	12	12	9	8	7
37–41	6	6	6	6	6	6	7

Table 5.20 Normal renal function in newborn infants in the first week of life

Glomerular filtration rate	0.35–0.85 ml/kg/min
Urine flow rate	1.0–3.0 ml/kg/h
Urine osmolality	45–800 mOsm/kg

postnatally is not significant until 24 h have elapsed, unless there are other pointers to a urogenital abnormality.

This oliguric period may be due to the high levels of antidiuretic hormone in the newborn following birth as there is no evidence of a fall in glomerular filtration rate (GFR). Indeed, over the first week of postnatal life, both GFR (Wilkins 1992a) and blood pressure increase in term and premature infants and the initial period of oliguria and relatively concentrated urine is followed by a diuresis of isotonic or even hypotonic urine (Hamilton & Shaw 1984) and contraction of the ECF volume.

During early postnatal life, the kidney of even a full-term infant has a limited capacity to produce concentrated urine and fractional sodium excretion is high. In the VLBW infant, GFR varies from 0.4 to 1.0 ml/min/kg with a mean of 0.7 ml/min/kg at 26 weeks' gestation and 0.84 ml/min/kg at 33 weeks (Wilkins 1992a). Given the reported maximum concentrating capacity (Table 5.20) and average renal solute load, fluid intake should be such as to maintain a minimum urine output of 1 ml/kg/h.

Water requirements

The aims of fluid management are to maintain satisfactory volumes of TBW, ICF and ECF, and a normal plasma sodium concentration. Changes in plasma sodium during the first week of life are usually due to changes in water balance rather than sodium balance (Rees et al 1984). Therefore, if water requirements are given according to Table 5.21, and provided there is no water retention due to inappropriate secretion of ADH or excessive water loss due to transepidermal evaporation, plasma sodium should remain constant as urinary losses are initially isotonic.

Fluid requirements depend on gestational age. The premature infant has a greater surface area to volume ratio, a thinner epidermis and more limited renal water conservation than a term infant. The premature infant is also more likely to require ventilation and phototherapy, and be nursed under a radiant heater.

Fluid requirements also vary with postnatal age, increasing during the first week of life to cope with the transition from oliguria to diuresis and reaching a plateau as water balance is restored and birthweight is regained. Fluid requirements do not fall again until after the first 6 months of life.

If the infant is fed enterally, all or part of the water requirement is delivered in breast or formula milk. If the infant is not fed, all the water must be administered intravenously, as 10% dextrose solution on the first day and 10% dextrose/0.18% saline thereafter (see section on sodium balance). Alternatively, the water requirement can be incorporated into a total parenteral nutrition regime.

The fluid regime recommended in Table 5.21 may need to be

Table 5.21 Recommended daily fluid requirements (ml/kg/24 h)

	Day 1	Day 2	Day 3	Day 4	Day 5
Premature infants	60	90	120	150	150–180
Term infants	40	60	80	110	150

Table 5.22 Fluid intake alterations

Conditions in which fluid restriction should be considered
Patent ductus arteriosus, especially if indomethacin given
Hypoxic-ischemic encephalopathy
Severe respiratory distress
Oliguric renal failure
Inappropriate release of ADH

Conditions in which fluid requirements are increased
Very low birthweight infant with excessive insensible water loss
Use of a radiant warmer
Phototherapy
Vomiting
Diarrhea
Polyuria (e.g. due to glycosuria or following relief of obstructive uropathy)

modified in the light of continuing assessment of fluid balance or the presence of the conditions in Table 5.22.

Assessment of water balance

Water balance cannot be assessed independently of sodium balance. Together, they constitute the major solute and solvent of the ECF and most clinical and laboratory observations give information about the ECF volume rather than ICF volume.

Clinical examination

Heart rate, systemic arterial blood pressure, central venous pressure and skin–core temperature gradient are all variables which are related to intravascular volume and cardiac output. However, these signs are crude monitors of fluid balance and tachycardia, hypotension and poor perfusion are features of decompensation following significant hypovolemia. Moreover, many factors other than fluid balance modulate cardiovascular responses.

Classical signs of decreased interstitial fluid volume are sunken eyes, a depressed fontanel and reduced skin turgor but only semiquantitative interpretation is possible and this is much more difficult in premature infants in whom these skin changes may be less apparent. Nor is edema a reliable sign of fluid overload in the premature infant (Cartlidge & Rutter 1986).

Fluid balance charts

If obsessionally maintained, these are a helpful guide to monitoring fluid balance. Obviously they give no information about insensible losses and the cumulative arithmetic balance may become very misleading if this is overlooked. Sources of error in recording fluids administered are the omission of drug vehicle volumes and omission of the volumes of heparinized saline used to flush vascular cannulae. A common error in the 'out' column of the chart is the omission of blood sample volumes which may cause significant cumulative losses leading to anemia (Obladen et al 1988) and even hypovolemia.

Bodyweight

This is the best cotside guide to TBW. Where fluid balance is important, the infant should be weighed daily, on the same scales and at the same time, particularly in relation to feeds. Serial bodyweights are of great help in distinguishing hyponatremia due to water overload from that due to sodium depletion.

A stable or increasing bodyweight may be falsely reassuring under circumstances in which TBW and intravascular volume do not move in parallel, e.g. concealed losses from the intravascular compartment into the so-called 'third space' in peritonitis, ileus, hydrops and congestive cardiac failure.

Urine flow rates

The normal range is given in Table 5.20. Catheterization should be avoided wherever possible but urine output must be assessed in all infants when fluid balance is considered critical, particularly if there is evidence of renal disease. Bag collections are more reliable in male infants but the adhesive used may damage the skin of a very immature infant. Alternatively, the infant may be nursed on a dimple plastic sheet and the urine collected with a syringe, or nursed on cotton wool which is weighed before and after micturition. All three methods also allow the collection of samples for urine chemistry (see below), urine pH, glucose testing, specific gravity and osmolality (Fig. 5.15). A urine specific gravity of between 1.005 and 1.012 is desirable as the newborn kidney is not then at the limits of its concentrating or

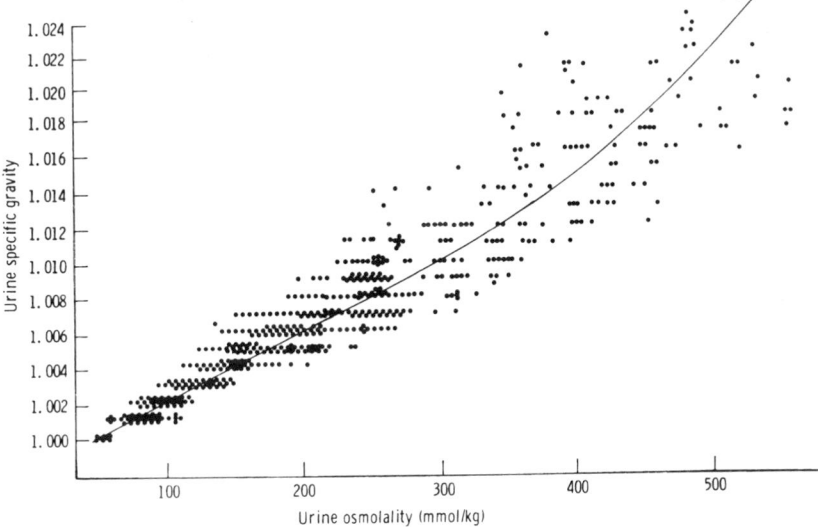

Fig. 5.15 Comparison of urinary specific gravity and urinary osmolality in 1000 urine samples. Third order regression line is shown: $r = 0.97$. (Reproduced with permission from Jones et al 1976.)

diluting capacity. Specific gravity and osmolality are unreliable in the presence of glycosuria or significant proteinuria.

Urine and plasma biochemistry

Plasma creatinine concentration is of limited value as an index of glomerular filtration in the newborn because:

1. initially the neonatal concentration mirrors the maternal concentration before birth
2. noncreatinine cromogens interfere with measurement
3. the normal range is wide (Wilkins 1992a, 1992b).

The interpretation of urinary electrolytes is difficult as the ranges encountered are so wide (Table 5.23). Interpretation should always be made in the light of simultaneous plasma electrolytes and a clinical assessment. Moreover, fractional sodium excretion declines with increasing gestation and increasing postnatal age so that fluid intake is best adjusted to maintain a normal plasma sodium concentration rather than relying on urinary measurements.

Nevertheless, urinary chemistry is obviously of value in distinguishing oliguria due to hypovolemia when fluid intake should be increased from established renal failure when fluid intake should be restricted. Another cause of oliguria is inappropriate ADH secretion, and urinary electrolytes and osmolality are necessary for the definitive diagnosis before initiating fluid restriction. In VLBW infants, random urine creatinine concentration is related to instantaneous urine flow rate by the formula: urine flow rate (ml/kg/24 h) = 90/urine creatinine concentration (μmol/l). However, the 95% confidence limits are wide (± 40%; Wilkins 1992b).

Plasma albumin and colloid osmotic pressure

Albumin concentration accounts for 70% of colloid osmotic pressures (COP). The two measurements are closely correlated in the premature newborn and both increase postnatally, in a similar fashion to the increase in fetal albumin concentration in utero. However, low albumin concentrations correlate poorly with clinical edema (Cartlidge & Rutter 1986) and although high albumin concentrations may reflect reduction in plasma volume ('hemoconcentration'), this relationship has not been demonstrated directly.

Packed cell volume

Packed cell volume (PCV) falls with decreasing gestation and increasing postnatal age, but with great variability between individuals, so that single measurements are a poor guide to fluid balance. However, if serial measurements of PCV (a simple and reproducible task using a microhematocrit meter) show a rising trend in a sick infant, in whom erythropoiesis is usually depressed, then fluid intake is probably insufficient. Falling levels of PCV may be due to blood loss or hemodilution and are therefore difficult to interpret.

Consequences of water overload and deficiency

Poor control of water balance leads to both volume and osmolar changes within body fluid compartments. The consequences of pure water overload and deficiency are discussed in the section on sodium under the headings hyponatremia and hypernatremia. Perhaps more common in the neonatal period is overload of water *and* sodium, which if it is isotonic expands only the ECF, and this has been implicated in the pathogenesis of a number of neonatal disorders.

Respiratory distress syndrome (RDS)

In infants with RDS, the oliguric phase following birth persists for longer and there is correlation between the degree of oliguria and the minimum PaO_2 (Tuck 1986). There is also correlation between the duration of oliguria, the duration of oxygen therapy and the risk of bronchopulmonary dysplasia (BPD). Partly, the sodium and water retention accompanying RDS is due to prerenal factors rather than lung disease per se and ventilation may also be contributory as increased positive pressure used in the absence of lung pathology for recurrent apneas is also associated with a decrease in GFR and urine flow rate. The use of paralysis in RDS exacerbates this fluid retention as pancuronium is associated with passage of concentrated urine, peripheral edema and weight gain (Greenough et al 1986).

The orthodox view is that the onset of the diuretic phase precedes improvement in respiratory function but this has been questioned (Modi 1988, Wilkins 1992c). In either case, high levels of ADH (Tuck 1987) and angiotensin II have been reported in RDS, which would contribute to salt and water retention, and increased levels of ANP (Stephenson et al 1994), which would antagonize these hormones, have been reported during the diuretic phase of RDS (Kojima et al 1987). The use of frusemide in the treatment of RDS has given differing results and its role remains unclear.

Patent ductus arteriosus (PDA)

PDA is extremely common in premature infants and this is associated with high fluid intake (Bell et al 1980). The persistence of the duct may be due to failure of the usual postnatal contraction in ECF and this in turn may be responsible for the elevated levels of ANP found with PDA (Rascher & Seyberth 1987, Andersson et al 1987). Moreover, PGE_2, which is the most potent dilator of the

Table 5.23 Normal reference values for urinary excretion

Term infants		
	Mean	SD
Sodium*	1.63	(0.78) mmol/kg/24 h
Potassium*	0.68	(0.31) mmol/kg/24 h
Creatinine†	0.45	(0.23) mmol/24 h
Urea‡	3.34	mmol/24 h
Preterm infants		
	Median	Range
Sodium§	2.23	(0.18–4.12) mmol/kg/24 h
Potassium§	0.75	(0.06–3.50) mmol/kg/24 h
Creatinine§	0.06	(0.03–0.36) mmol/kg/24 h
Urea§	2.44	(0.67–7.04) mmol/kg/24 h

* Full-term, appropriate weight, breast-fed babies during the first and second weeks of life (Slater 1961).
† Normal full-term infants during the first month of life (Flood & Pinelli 1949).
‡ Normal full-term infants during the first week of life (Barlow & McCance 1948).
§ Male infants, 24–36 weeks' gestation, during the first week of life (Stephenson & Broughton Pipkin, unpublished observations).

duct (Wilkinson 1988), is also involved in regulation of sodium balance, causing natriuresis. Elevated levels of PGE_2 may therefore be provoked by salt and water retention.

There has been no systematic trial of the place of fluid restriction in the treatment of PDA and, as in cardiac failure, it may be more rational to restrict sodium intake and maintain fluid and hence calorie intake, using diuretics to reduce fluid overload. Diuretics could also be used with indomethacin in the treatment of PDA since PGE_2 synthesis is inhibited and fluid retention may result.

Higher fluid intakes have also been reported in association with bronchopulmonary dysplasia (BPD) and necrotizing enterocolitis but the evidence is less compelling than for RDS and PDA and the relationship with BPD was not confirmed by a prospective study (Bell et al 1980).

In a number of other conditions, such as cardiac failure, renal failure or ascites, salt and water overload occurs as a consequence of organ dysfunction rather than as an etiologic factor.

SODIUM AND POTASSIUM

Body sodium content and distribution

Sodium is the major extracellular cation. As the percentage of body weight which is ECF falls during fetal life, so the sodium content in the fetus falls from 94 mmol/kg at 25 weeks' gestation to 74 mmol/kg at term. Despite this, there is a daily accretion of sodium in utero of about 1 mmol/kg/24 h.

Because of the isotonic contraction of the ECF following birth, there is an inevitable loss of sodium during the first week which averages 14 (range 6–22) mmol/kg. This loss cannot be prevented but may be excessive if sodium intake is inadequate. Negative sodium balance is maximal on day 4 and becomes positive by day 6 or 7 (Rees et al 1984) provided sodium intake is maintained at 6–8 mmol/kg/24 h.

Regulation of sodium homeostasis

The control of sodium and water balance is regulated by a number of homeostatic mechanisms to maintain a normal plasma sodium concentration (132–142 mmol/l) and normal circulating volume. Moreover, there must be a net stimulus to conserve sodium throughout childhood as this is essential for growth. The regulating mechanisms are:

1. sodium and water intake under the influence of thirst
2. glomerular filtration rate which determines the amount of sodium and water delivered to the renal tubules
3. reabsorption of sodium and water by the renal tubules and collecting ducts.

The healthy term infant can respond to thirst by demand feeding but an infant of less than 34 weeks' gestation has no control over intake. Moreover, as the rise in GFR over the first week outstrips the more gradual improvement in renal tubular sodium reabsorption, transient glomerulotubular imbalance develops and a high fractional sodium excretion results. Sodium sensors in the macula densa are stimulated by this high delivery of sodium to the distal tubule, as shown by correlation between urinary sodium and plasma renin even in very premature infants (Broughton Pipkin & Stephenson 1989), but the immature nephron appears to be unresponsive to the high circulating concentrations of angiotensin

II and aldosterone generated by this system. Atrial natriuretic peptide (ANP) levels are high in the immediate newborn period (Ito et al 1988) and ANP inhibits the sodium-retaining actions of both angiotensin and aldosterone (Stephenson & Broughton Pipkin 1990).

This initial sodium-losing state continues until the end of the first week following which positive sodium balance ensues to ensure growth. Maturation of the aldosterone-dependent distal tubular reabsorption, which is gestation dependent but accelerated by birth, appears to be responsible for the transition to net sodium gain, since proximal tubular reabsorption is unchanged.

During the initial period of glomerulotubular imbalance, urine flow rates do not increase significantly (Modi 1988) although GFR is increasing. This suggests that the collecting ducts are sensitive to ADH, the levels of which are high in the immediate newborn period (Rees et al 1984). The feedback control of ADH secretion is operative from 26 weeks' gestation, although inappropriate secretion of ADH also occurs commonly in this group (Rees et al 1984), and plasma osmolality is normally maintained within a narrow range of 282–298 mOsm/kg despite variable water intake.

Sodium balance

To maintain a stable plasma sodium and allow growth:

sodium intake = sodium for growth (mostly increase in ECF)
+ sodium lost in urine
+ sodium lost in sweat (only after 36 weeks' gestation)
+ sodium lost in feces

In a healthy term infant, urinary sodium losses (1–2 mmol/kg/24 h) far exceed the other terms in this equation. In VLBW infants, urinary sodium losses up to 20 mmol/kg/24 h are seen (Wilkins 1992c). Sodium for growth is roughly 1–2 mmol per week over the first year of life and fecal sodium losses are trivial (0.23 mmol/kg/24 h) in the absence of diarrhea.

Therefore, for the first 24 h of life no sodium is required as there is oliguria; during the succeeding week, 4–8 mmol/kg/24 h should be adequate; thereafter, term infants require as little as 1 mmol/kg/24 h whereas immature infants may require 8–12 mmol/kg/24 h if 'late' hyponatremia is to be avoided (see below). The needs of a term infant are ideally supplied by human breast milk which, on a nominal intake of 150 ml/kg/24 h provides 4 mmol/kg/24 h on day 3 but only 1.2 mmol/kg/24 h after a month, the sodium concentration of breast milk naturally falling with time. Human milk obviously provides insufficient sodium for premature infants. Either preterm formulae should be used (14–26 mmol/l) or sodium supplements given with expressed breast milk.

If parenteral fluids are given, the same sodium intakes as above can be achieved by giving 10% dextrose on day 1 and 10% dextrose and 0.18% saline thereafter at the rates recommended in Table 5.21, thus delivering 4.5 mmol/kg/24 h of sodium by day 5. Changes in plasma sodium concentration during the first week of life are more often due to changes in water balance than sodium balance (Rees et al 1984) so the volumes of water suggested in Table 5.21 may need to be adjusted on the basis of frequent plasma sodium estimations.

In premature infants, a high incidence of 'late' hyponatremia is well recognized and, in contrast to the first postnatal week, this is due to total body sodium depletion (accompanied to a lesser extent by water depletion) and there is poor weight gain or even weight loss. The sodium depletion is due to prolongation of the period of obligate renal sodium loss, possibly due to a delay in endocrine maturation, so that plasma sodium concentration is dependent on sodium intake which must be increased accordingly, usually by oral supplements of 30% NaCl (5 mmol/ml).

Hyponatremia

The causes of hyponatremia (plasma sodium < 130 mmol/l) are listed in Table 5.24. Water overload is the major cause during the first week of life but thereafter sodium depletion becomes more important. Under conditions of sodium depletion, initially the kidney loses water to maintain a normal plasma osmolality but eventually the need to conserve plasma volume becomes the overriding stimulus, there is appropriate release of ADH and hyponatremia occurs.

The clinical features have three origins:

1. Hypotonia, lethargy and convulsions due to the hyponatremia, irrespective of the cause. These symptoms are not usually seen until plasma sodium falls below 125 mmol/l and are partly related to the acuteness of the fall.

2. Inappropriate weight gain with water overload or weight loss with sodium depletion.

3. Features associated with the underlying disease. The underlying cause should be treated but in the interim symptomatic treatment may be necessary to achieve a safe plasma sodium concentration. It is critical that a definitive diagnosis is made as the appropriate treatment may be either fluid restriction or sodium supplementation.

If there is a sodium deficit, the number of millimoles required is given by the formula:

$$(135 - \text{plasma sodium concentration}) \times \text{bodyweight (kg)} \times 2/3$$

Table 5.24 Causes of hyponatremia in the newborn

A. Water overload
  1. Maternal water overload prior to birth
  2. Iatrogenic water overload following birth
  3. Decreased free water clearance in a sick preterm infant
  4. Inappropriate release of antidiuretic hormone
    Cerebral disease (birth asphyxia, meningitis)
    Respiratory disease (pneumonia, collapse, pneumothorax)

B. Sodium depletion
  This is usually accompanied by a lesser degree of water depletion
  1. Excessive gastrointestinal losses (vomiting, diarrhea, nasogastric aspirate, enterostomy loss)
  2. Excessive removal (repeated drainage of ascites, pleural fluid or cerebrospinal fluid)
  3. Excessive renal losses
    a. Primary renal tubular disease
      (i) 'late' hyponatremia of prematurity
      (ii) following relief of obstructive uropathy
      (iii) Fanconi's syndrome
      (iv) Bartter's syndrome
    b. Hypoadrenalism
      (i) congenital adrenal hyperplasia
      (ii) congenital adrenal hypoplasia
      (iii) hypoaldosteronism
      (iv) pseudohypoaldosteronism

Hypernatremia

This is almost invariably the result of water depletion (Table 5.25). There is usually failure to thrive or weight loss and irritability, hypertonicity and convulsions may occur when plasma sodium exceeds 150 mmol/l. A 'doughy' quality of the skin and a paradoxically full fontanel may also suggest hypernatremic dehydration. The osmotic gradient favors maintenance of the ECF at the expense of the ICF and the diagnosis may be delayed as signs of hypovolemia and decreased skin turgor occur late.

Treatment is difficult as persistence of hypernatremia is associated with cerebral hemorrhage and renal vein thrombosis in the newborn but overaggressive correction may cause cellular overhydration in the brain. A solution of 0.18% saline and 10% dextrose should be used judiciously to correct the deficit over 48 h.

Body potassium content and distribution

Potassium is the major intracellular cation, 'of the soil and not the sea, of the cell and not the sap'. It is not surprising then that whilst fetal growth must be accompanied by a more than commensurate increase in total body potassium (as the ICF fraction of TBW increases), the potassium concentration in blood throughout life is virtually unchanged from 15 weeks' gestation (Moniz et al 1985). Likewise, as only 2% of total body potassium is found in ECF, large changes may occur in total body potassium without significantly altering plasma potassium concentration. For example, in ventilated premature infants a negative potassium balance of 10% of total body potassium occurs over the first 4 postnatal days, but hypokalemia is a rare problem. Subsequently, positive potassium balance is restored and net potassium accumulation then continues at an average of 1 mmol/24 h over the first year of life (approximately 0.3 mmol/kg/24 h initially and 0.05 mmol/kg/24 h at 1 year). Nevertheless, plasma potassium concentration is a major determinant of the cell membrane potential and if significant changes do occur, they must be corrected quickly.

Potassium balance

Intake = potassium for growth
        + potassium lost in urine
        + potassium losses from the gastrointestinal tract

As with sodium balance, urinary losses far exceed the other terms, particularly during early newborn life when prostaglandin E_2 levels are high. As these levels decline, the distal tubule is

Table 5.25 Causes of hypernatremia in the newborn

A. Water depletion
  1. Inadequate intake
  2. Excessive transepidermal water loss
  3. Excessive renal losses
    a. Glycosuria
    b. Diabetes insipidus

B. Sodium overload
  Isolated sodium overload is rare as water is usually retained with sodium. It is caused by the administration of hypertonic solutions, such as sodium bicarbonate

becoming more aldosterone responsive so that urinary potassium to sodium ratio continues to increase with postconceptional age. Urinary potassium excretion in VLBW infants is 1–5 mmol/kg/24 h (Guignard & John 1986, Wilkins 1992c). Gastrointestinal losses are normally less than 0.5 mmol/kg/24 h but very significant cumulative losses of potassium can occur if there is prolonged nasogastric suction, diarrhea or ileus.

A daily potassium intake of 3 mmol/kg/24 h should be more than adequate. Human breast milk provides 2.25 mmol/kg/24 h (assuming 150 ml/kg/24 h intake). The sodium : potassium ratio in mature human breast milk is about one, the same as the ratio in the urine of healthy term infants (Wilkins 1992c).

Hypokalemia

Symptoms rarely occur until the plasma potassium concentration is more than 0.5 mmol/l below the lower limit of the normal range (3.0–6.6 mmol/l up to 1 month of age). A concomitant increase in plasma bicarbonate is common. The clinical features (weakness, hypotonia, hyporeflexia, lethargy) are extremely difficult to recognize in the newborn and therefore plasma potassium should be measured frequently in sick infants. Such infants should receive continuous cardiac monitoring (ECG features of hypokalemia are small T waves, depression of the ST sequence, and the appearance of U waves) because cardiac arrhythmias may occur. Loop diuretics and aminophylline (Wilkins 1986) predispose to hypokalemia in the newborn and hypokalemia sensitizes the heart to digoxin.

Causes of hypokalemia are listed in Table 5.26. Treatment is by oral or intravenous (5 ml of 20% solution contains 1 g or 13 mmol) potassium chloride administration, depending on the infant's condition and the severity of the hypokalemia, and by reversal of the underlying cause if possible. Intravenous potassium supplements should not exceed a concentration of 40 mmol/l. ECG monitoring is mandatory, infusion through a central venous catheter is preferable (provided the tip is not in the right atrium), and potassium added to fluid in plastic containers must be well mixed to prevent adherence. Potassium should not be added to blood products as it may cause red cell lysis. Oral potassium supplements should be avoided in gastrointestinal disorders because they may cause vomiting, ulceration and stricture. Diuretics should be stopped if possible or the potassium-sparing aldosterone antagonist spironolactone added.

Hyperkalemia

Plasma potassium concentrations above the 'normal' range occur in 3.5% of infants under 1500 g and there is an association with cerebral lesions (Shortland et al 1987) and gestation less than 28 weeks (Wilkins 1992c). Acute rises in plasma potassium can occur with intravenous administration but apart from this hyperkalemia due to excessive intake is rare because the kidney has a large reserve for potassium excretion. Hyperkalemia is more commonly due to a failure of excretion by the distal tubule, and this is supported by the finding of impaired renal function in 50% of cases of hyperkalemia in VLBW infants (Shortland et al 1987). The causes of hyperkalemia are listed in Table 5.27.

As with hypokalemia there may be apathy, weakness, hypotonia and hyporeflexia and also ileus. The ECG shows tall peaked T waves and arrhythmias occur in 60% of premature infants with serum potassium above 7.5 mmol/l, the commonest being supraventricular tachycardia (Shortland et al 1987).

Hyperkalemia > 7.5 mmol/l requires urgent treatment (or 6.5–7.5 mmol/l if associated ECG abnormalities) to redistribute potassium into cells as measures to improve renal excretion are too slow. The myocardium is stabilized by intravenous calcium whilst the other measures in Table 5.28 take effect. Exchange transfusion with washed red cells has also been used effectively but needs further evaluation.

THERMOREGULATION

Children and adults maintain a constant deep body temperature over a wide range of ambient thermal conditions. This is achieved by physiological and behavioral responses which control the rate at which heat is produced or lost. The newborn infant is also homeothermic but control of body temperature can only be

Table 5.27 Causes of hyperkalemia in the newborn

Excessive intake
Iatrogenic supplementation of i.v. fluids or parenteral nutrition

Inadequate excretion
Acute renal failure
Hypoadrenalism (especially congenital adrenal hyperplasia and hypoplasia)
Hypoaldosteronism

Table 5.26 Causes of hypokalemia in the newborn

Gastrointestinal losses
Vomiting or excessive nasogastric aspirate
Diarrhea
Enterostomy losses
Ileus

Renal losses
Bartter's syndrome
Fanconi's syndrome
Following relief of obstructive uropathy
Diuretic therapy
Alkalosis from any cause

Inadequate intake
Inadequate enteral or intravenous supplements

Table 5.28 Management of hyperkalemia in the newborn

1. Intravenous 10% calcium gluconate 1 ml/kg slowly

2. Intravenous 4.2% sodium bicarbonate 4 ml/kg slowly. This should be given via a different vein or after flush to prevent precipitation

3. Calcium resonium enema 0.5 g/kg, retained for at least 30 min. This can be repeated 8-hourly

All potassium administration, potassium-conserving diuretics and potentially nephrotoxic drugs should be stopped. Any prerenal failure due to hypovolemia should be corrected, sepsis should be treated (avoiding potassium-containing penicillin salts), and nutrition should be provided to minimize catabolism. The ECG should be monitored continuously

If hyperkalemia persists, 5 ml/kg 20% dextrose and 0.3 units/kg of soluble insulin should be given intravenously over 2 h. These should be mixed in the same syringe. The venous blood sugar and plasma potassium concentrations should be measured hourly and dialysis considered achieved over a narrower range of ambient conditions. The preterm infant has even greater difficulty in body temperature control, and the most immature infants behave at times as if they are poikilothermic – their body temperature tending to drift up and down with the ambient temperature. The aim in neonatal care is to provide a thermal environment which keeps body temperature in the normal range, and which does not stress the infant to produce or lose large amounts of heat. This is not just instinctive common sense. Several studies have shown that if sick or preterm infants are allowed to become cold their chances of becoming ill are higher, they do not grow as well and they are more likely to die.

Heat balance

By the law of conservation of energy:

heat production = heat lost by convection + radiation
+ evaporation + conduction

Heat production

Heat is produced as a byproduct of cell metabolism. The lowest obligatory rate of heat production occurs when an individual is starved, quiet and resting (basal metabolic rate) but a newborn infant is rarely in this state. It is usual therefore to measure resting metabolic rate as the minimal rate of oxygen consumption in an infant who is lying still and asleep at least 1 h after a feed in a neutral thermal environment. Values depend on gestation and postnatal age. Heat production per unit area is lower in preterm infants, particularly below 28 weeks' gestation. In all infants there is a progressive rise over the first weeks of life so that by about 6 months of age adult values are reached.

Heat loss

Convection. Heat is lost from the skin surface to the surrounding air by convection. Loss is high if the air is cold, the skin surface is exposed and there is rapid movement of air over the skin. A naked baby in a cold drafty room has a high convective heat loss.

Radiation. Heat is lost from the skin surface to the nearest surface which faces the skin by means of radiation. It varies with the temperature of that surface and its distance from the skin but is independent of the temperature of the intervening air. A naked infant can radiate large amounts of heat to the cool inner walls of an incubator even if the air is warm. An overhead warmer provides heat by radiation.

Evaporation. Heat is lost as water evaporates from the surface of the skin (560 cal/ml of water). Evaporative heat loss is low in mature infants unless they are sweating in response to heat stress. Losses are high in preterm infants who have a high transepidermal water loss (TEWL) due to passive diffusion of water vapor through the thin, poorly keratinized immature epidermis. A newly born infant wet with amniotic fluid loses heat as the skin dries.

Conduction. Newborn infants are not usually in direct contact with a structure of high thermal capacity, so conductive losses are small.

Response to thermal stress

There is a range of environmental temperatures over which an infant has a minimum rate of heat production and is not sweating

– small adjustments to thermal control can be made by alterations in posture, activity and skin blood flow, and deep body temperature remains constant within the normal range defined for children and adults. This is the thermoneutral range. The range widens and falls if the infant is well insulated by clothes and bedding but is narrow and high if the infant is small and naked. As environmental temperature falls below the lower end of the thermoneutral range, metabolic heat production increases (Fig. 5.16). This may be partly due to increased activity but is mainly the result of oxidation of brown adipose tissue. This is distributed in the neck, between the scapulae and along the aorta. As the environmental temperature falls, nerve endings in the skin are stimulated, catecholamines are released and the brown adipose tissue is metabolized to produce heat. This is nonshivering thermogenesis. A term newborn infant can double his resting heat production in this way without any increase in activity. As environmental temperature continues to fall, heat production reaches a maximum (summit metabolism) and below this point the body temperature starts to fall. As environmental temperature rises above the upper end of the thermoneutral range, sweating occurs until a point is reached when the heat lost by sweating is not enough and body temperature starts to rise.

Nonshivering thermogenesis is impaired in preterm infants and there is doubt that it occurs at all in very immature infants. It is impaired in all newborn infants in the first 12 h after delivery, especially if there is asphyxia, hypoxia or maternal sedative

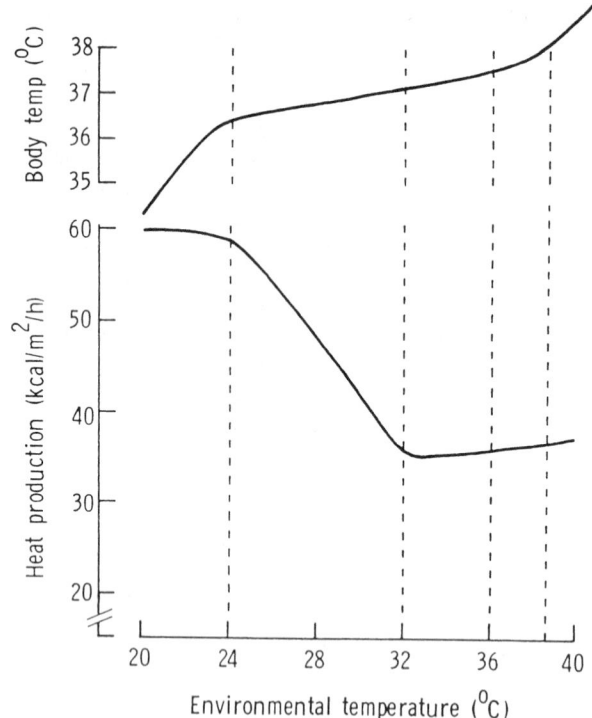

Fig. 5.16 The effects of environmental temperature on heat production and body temperature of a 1.9-kg infant of 34 weeks' gestation, nursed naked in surroundings of uniform temperature and moderate humidity. Between 32 and 36°C, heat production is minimal, there is no sweating, and the body temperature is normal (neutral thermal range). When the environmental temperature exceeds 36°C the infant sweats and above 38°C the body temperature rises rapidly. Below 32°C heat production increases by nonshivering thermogenesis, but below 24°C heat production has reached its maximum and body temperature rapidly falls (Rutter 1986).

administration. Sweating in response to heat stress occurs from birth in most infants beyond 36 weeks' gestation but takes 2 or 3 weeks to appear in the most immature infants. This is a result of neurological rather than glandular immaturity. Sweating is a relatively poor defense against overheating in the newborn because the production of sweat per unit area of skin is low compared with a child or adult. Alteration of skin blood flow by vasoconstriction and vasodilation results in an increase or decrease in the amount of heat lost by convection and radiation, particularly if the infant is unclothed. The term newborn can alter skin blood flow effectively but this is impaired in the very immature infant. Alteration of posture to increase or decrease the surface area available for heat loss by convection and radiation is important in thermoregulation. It occurs in the healthy term infant and to some extent in the preterm infant but not in the presence of illness.

Body temperature and its measurement

Measurement of body temperature in the newborn is a crude way of assuring the effectiveness of the thermal environment, although it is clear from the heat production diagram that an infant has to be considerably heat or cold stressed for the body temperature to rise or fall outside the normal range. An infant can have a normal body temperature but still be too hot or too cold. The most immature and smallest infants who are nursed naked for observation have a very narrow neutral thermal range and a limited ability to respond to heat or cold. Their body temperature tends to rise and fall according to environmental conditions and therefore a normal temperature suggests a suitable environment. It is essential to record body temperature in infants nursed under radiant warmers as a check against overheating. Instability of body temperature, particularly a mild pyrexia, may be an early sign of infection.

Deep body temperature is usually measured as rectal temperature. Colonic temperature can be recorded with a soft flexible probe inserted several centimeters past the anal margin but such probes are easily extruded. Esophageal and tympanic membrane temperatures are only useful in research. Rectal temperature under-records deep body temperature especially if the bulb of the mercury in glass thermometer is only just inserted into the anal canal – 3 cm in term and 2 cm in the preterm are recommended depths of insertion and at least half a minute is required to obtain a stable reading. The normal range is 36.6–37.1°C. Hemorrhage or bowel perforation are rare but well-described complications, and rectal temperature should not be measured in infants with colitis.

Axillary temperature is a reasonable guide to deep body temperature and is less invasive. The bulb of the thermometer should be held in the roof of the axilla with the infant's arm pressed against the side of the chest until a stable reading is obtained, usually by 3 min. The normal range is 36.3–37.0°C. Skin temperature reflects tissue insulation and environmental conditions as well as deep body temperature and is therefore less useful. However, if an infant lies on a skin temperature probe which is insulated on the outside, the recorded temperature is close to rectal temperature.

Problems of temperature control in the preterm infant

The smaller and more immature the infant, the greater the difficulties in temperature control. The major problem is hypothermia and there are physical and physiological reasons for this. Size alone places the small infant at a thermal disadvantage. Heat production is related to mass which is low – heat loss is related to surface area which is relatively high. Lack of subcutaneous tissue means poor insulation of the heated core from the cool surroundings. A poorly developed stratum corneum results in a very high evaporative water and therefore heat loss. The ability to conserve heat by vasoconstriction and increase heat production by metabolism is reduced. Overheating is rarely a problem unless the infant is warmed by a very powerful heating device where output is uncontrolled.

Management of the thermal environment

At delivery

The delivery room and operating theater are usually kept at a temperature considered suitable for adults but which is cold for the newborn. The naked infant loses heat by convection and radiation, and by evaporation of amniotic fluid from the wet skin. The body temperature of a small preterm infant can easily fall by 1°C every 5 min and this is particularly likely to occur if delivery takes place unexpectedly at home. The healthy term infant does not appear to suffer from this transient cold exposure at birth but in the preterm infant a fall in body temperature is associated with an increased risk of acidosis, hypoxia and respiratory distress. The newborn infant should be dried at delivery, wrapped in a warm dry blanket and given to the mother – skin to skin contact with the mother is an effective way of maintaining body warmth. Exposure for weighing, cord care and fixing of namebands should be minimized and bathing avoided. The small preterm infant should be dried, wrapped and removed to a warm environment as soon as possible. If an infant requires resuscitation, a supplementary heat source such as a radiant warmer is necessary.

Nursing

Most healthy term and preterm infants can be nursed clothed and wrapped in a blanket in a cot in a warm room. This is both comfortable and thermally safe. Very small infants may need to be nursed clothed in an incubator to provide a sufficiently warm ambient temperature.

Over 2 kg: nurse clothed, with bedding in a cot, in a room temperature of about 24°C.

1.5–2 kg: nurse clothed with a bonnet and bedding in a cot, in a room temperature of about 26°C.

Below 1.5 kg: nurse clothed with a bonnet, in an incubator temperature of 30–32°C.

Heated cot

A heated water-filled mattress can be used to provide conductive heat to a preterm infant nursed in a cot in the usual way. The mattress is a polyvinyl chloride bag filled with 10 l of water which is heated electrically by a foil pad and controlled to provide a set temperature between 35 and 38°C. It has been shown that the heated cot is just as effective as the incubator in keeping small babies warm and results in similar rates of resting metabolism and growth (Sarman & Tunell 1989). Its advantages are that it is cheap, simple and does not depend on a constant unbroken supply of electricity (because of its stored heat), so that it is particularly useful in developing countries. It is also more comfortable for the infants and appealing to their mothers, but is only of use if the infants are healthy and do not need to be nursed naked for observation and access. It has been effectively used as a method of rewarming cold preterm infants (Sarman et al 1989).

Incubator

The incubator provides a warm environment suitable for nursing small or sick infants, particularly if they need to be naked for observation and access. Air within the Perspex canopy is warmed by a heater and circulated by a fan. The heater output can be controlled in two ways. In air mode the incubator air temperature is set to a point between 30 and 37°C and the heater is thermostatically controlled to reach and maintain this temperature. In servo mode a thermister probe is taped to the infant's abdominal skin and the desired skin temperature is set – the heater output varies to provide an air temperature which maintains the set skin temperature. In practice, air mode control is simpler to use, safer and results in a very constant ambient air temperature regardless of the condition of the infant and the amount of care he is receiving. Servo control results in wide fluctuations in air temperature during periods of handling, the probe can become detached or wet, and the infant's own attempts at thermoregulation are overridden so that a fever is disguised.

Suggested air temperature (Table 5.29) and skin temperature settings (Table 5.30) for the two modes of control are shown. In a single-walled incubator the inner wall is cooler than the air in the canopy and the naked infant therefore loses heat by radiation as well as convection. This can be reduced by raising the temperature of the nursery, raising the incubator air temperature, using a radiant heat shield within the incubator which warms to the air temperature and shields the infant from the inner wall of the canopy, or by using a double-walled incubator.

In most infants it is not necessary to humidify the incubator air. In infants below 30 weeks' gestation, weighing less than 1 kg, evaporative water loss and therefore heat loss is high during the first few days of life and may exceed the infant's own heat production. Thus a very immature infant may have a subnormal deep body temperature although the incubator air temperature is on the maximum setting. Raising the humidity of the air around the body will reduce evaporative losses so that a normal body temperature can be achieved. Some (but not all) incubators have humidifiers which will produce an ambient relative humidity within the canopy of 90% or more (compared with 30–40% relative humidity without use of the humidifier). At such high humidity the infant's evaporative water and heat losses are very low, it is easy to control body temperature and fluid balance is simplified. Beyond 1 week of age the immature infant's skin has matured to such an extent that evaporative water and heat losses are less important and added humidity is no longer required. There is always the concern that use of humidity predisposes the infant to bacterial infection, particularly by *Pseudomonas* or *Klebsiella* species, although in practice this does not seem to be a major problem. The humidifier water should be drained and replaced with sterile water each day, with a brief period in between where the incubator is run dry. An alternative to humidifying the incubator air is the use of a waterproof covering over the infant. This raises the humidity close to the skin surface and therefore reduces evaporation – it reduces visibility though and when the covering is removed the evaporative losses are high.

The incubator provides a constant, bland thermal environment which keeps the infant's heat losses by radiation and convection to levels which are balanced by his own heat production. It is difficult to get at the infant for examination and practical procedures (not always a disadvantage) and parents sometimes find the physical barrier distressing.

Radiant warmer

The infant lies naked on a platform exposed to a radiant heat source suspended horizontally above him. The output of the heater is controlled by a temperature sensor in contact with the infant's skin which is set to the desired temperature. The sensor should be taped to the abdomen or chest rather than a limb and should be shielded from the heat source. The normal range of abdominal skin temperature under neutral thermal conditions for infants of different size is shown in Table 5.30 – this is a good guide to the set temperature which should be chosen.

Since the infant is exposed to the cool drafty nursery air and walls, heat losses by convection and radiation are high when radiant warmers are used. Evaporative water loss is also increased as a result of the drafts and a direct effect of radiant heat on the infant's skin. These losses are all balanced by a large radiant heat gain from the powerful heater. Wide fluctuations in heater output

Table 5.29   Average incubator air temperatures needed to provide a suitable thermal environment for naked, healthy infants (from Hey 1975 and Sauer et al 1984)

Birthweight (kg)	Environmental temperature					
	37°C	36°C	35°C	34°C	33°C	32°C
Less than 1.0	For 1 day	After 1 day	After 2 weeks	After 3 weeks	After 4 weeks	After 6 weeks
1.0–1.5			For 10 days	After 10 days	After 3 weeks	After 5 weeks
1.5–2.0				For 10 days	After 10 days	After 4 weeks
2.0–2.5				For 2 days	After 2 days	After 3 weeks
More than 2.5					For 2 days	After 2 days

Note: 1. In a single-walled incubator the environmental temperature needs to be increased by 1°C for every 7°C difference between room and incubator temperature.
2. Infants below 1.0 kg and below 30 weeks' gestation need a humidified incubator in the first week of life.
3. Clothed infants need lower incubator temperatures.
4. Values are average ones but there is considerable variation in individual requirements.

Table 5.30 Suggested abdominal skin temperature settings for infants nursed in servo mode incubators or under radiant warmers (Rutter 1986)

Weight (kg)	Abdominal skin temperature (°C)
Less than 1.0	36.9
1.0–1.5	36.7
1.5–2.0	36.5
2.0–2.5	36.3
More than 2.5	36.0

occur, producing a very uneven, asymmetrical thermal environment compared with an incubator. In the more immature infants, evaporative water loss may lead to hypernatremia and dehydration. The wide fluctuations in thermal environment and high evaporative water losses can be conveniently reduced by placing a small clear plastic canopy over the infant – radiant heat can still reach the infant but heat losses by convection, radiation and evaporation are greatly reduced.

Radiant warmers are powerful devices and therefore inherently more hazardous than incubators. Overheating can occur and regular measurement of the infant's body temperature by an independent method is essential. If the heater is switched off, moved to one side or if something is interposed between the infant and the heat source, the infant's heat losses are very great and rapid cooling occurs. Their advantage is that they allow access to the infant for practical procedures whilst keeping the infant warm. They are ideally suited to the care of a small or large sick infant in the early neonatal period when the illness is evolving, but less suitable for the care of the stable or improving infant.

Both devices have been in use in neonatal intensive care for over 20 years and there is no evidence that either is superior. Several studies have shown that infants nursed under radiant warmers have slightly higher metabolic rates (10–20%) compared to infants nursed in incubators but this has not been shown to have any adverse effect.

Transport

A small sick infant who is transferred from one hospital to another for intensive care is thermally vulnerable. The body temperature is often low before the journey, the ability to produce and conserve heat is limited, the outside temperature may be very low indeed and the transport incubator is less sophisticated than the usual nursing incubator. It is important to cover the infant to reduce radiant heat losses which may be very high – a waterproof covering is useful if evaporative water loss is likely to be high. The infant therefore has to be monitored indirectly rather than by direct observation. In spite of the risk of cold stress during transport, studies have shown that body temperature does not usually fall during the journey but may actually increase.

Surgery

A newborn infant who needs surgery is at risk of cold stress. He is usually starved and drugged, thus reducing the normal metabolic response to cold. The operating theater may be a journey away, it is drafty and has cool walls and often cool air. The infant needs to be exposed for the operation and exposed moist organs lose heat by evaporation. To minimize cold stress and hypothermia, the infant should be well insulated before the journey to theater and the minimum area exposed for surgery in theater. The theater air temperature should be raised to 28–30°C and a supplementary source of heat such as an electric warming pad or radiant warmer should be provided.

Disorders of body temperature in the newborn

A low body temperature (below 36°C)

Acute hypothermia in the newborn is not uncommon – it is usually mild (rectal temperature 34–36°C) but may be moderate (30–34°C) or severe (below 30°C). Of the several causes, accidental hypothermia due to cold exposure is the commonest, particularly in the moderate or severe cases. Accidental hypothermia is likely to occur in hospital when low birthweight infants require resuscitation or when infants are exposed to a cool delivery room or operating theater. If careful attention is paid to keeping infants warm after delivery it should happen infrequently. It commonly occurs when infants are born outside hospital, either unexpectedly or after a concealed delivery – if the infant is small, born into a toilet, abandoned, or inadvertently exposed to cold, severe hypothermia may result. Accidental hypothermia also occurs later on in the newborn period or early infancy because of inadvertent cold exposure due to inadequate clothing or cold thermal environments – it may occur chronically. Infants with bacterial sepsis or with respiratory syncytial virus infection are prone to mild hypothermia – so too are infants in severe heart failure or with marked cyanosis. Malnutrition predisposes to hypothermia because of poor tissue insulation and an impaired metabolic response to cold. Hypothyroidism also results in an impaired metabolic response to cold too. Drugs given to the mother which cross the placenta have a similar effect on the newborn infant, particularly the long-acting sedatives such as diazepam. Finally intentional hypothermia is used as an adjunct to cardiopulmonary bypass when newborn infants have major heart surgery – body temperature is lowered to about 28°C by surface cooling with ice. The infants tolerate this brief, acute severe hypothermia well but it has not been successful as a method of preventing brain damage in severe birth asphyxia.

Hypothermic infants develop symptoms when their deep body temperature falls below 34°C. They become lethargic, feed poorly, have a weak cry and reduced movements. If exposure to cold has been persistent there may be peripheral edema, sclerema, and marked facial erythema in the presence of a strikingly cold skin – these are the features of neonatal cold injury. In very severe hypothermia there is profound bradycardia with slow, shallow respiration and the infant may appear to be dead. There are anecdotal reports of such infants being left for dead yet eventually making a full recovery. The diagnosis of hypothermia is made by recording a low rectal temperature – it is important that a low reading thermometer is used, not the standard clinical thermometer with a minimum reading of 35°C.

The treatment of accidental hypothermia is rewarming – if there is an underlying cause, this obviously needs to be treated too. There is limited information about the speed of rewarming cold infants. In cases of mild hypothermia rewarming can take place rapidly. In moderate or severe cases there is concern that rapid rewarming of the infant's surface causes peripheral vasodilation, diversion of blood from the core and therefore hypotension. Use of a plasma expander during rewarming has been advocated. Very slow rewarming over a period of several days has been used in infants with cold injury but after acute accidental hypothermia it appears to be safe to restore deep body temperature to normal over a few hours. This can be achieved using a radiant warmer, an incubator or a heated cot (Sarman et al 1989).

Hypoglycemia may occur during rewarming – it should be anticipated and treated or better still prevented by a slow intravenous infusion of 10% dextrose. Care should be taken in interpreting blood gas results – a metabolic acidosis at 37°C is less severe at 30°C and should not be overenthusiastically treated. Abdominal distention is common as a result of ileus and feeding should not be started until a normal body temperature is achieved. Necrotizing enterocolitis and hemorrhagic pulmonary edema have been described and are sinister complications. The reported mortality rate in severe hypothermia is 25–50% but this includes infants with overwhelming sepsis or congenital abnormalities which predisposed them to cold. Most survivors develop normally.

A high body temperature (above 38°C)

An infant with a high body temperature may be febrile or overheated. A febrile infant has a high set point temperature and behaves as if cold. He makes physiological and behavioral responses which reduce heat loss, increase heat production and therefore raise body temperature. An overheated infant makes physiological and behavioral responses in an effort to increase heat loss and therefore lower body temperature. The distinction is an important one which can be made clinically (Table 5.31). Overheated infants simply need a cooler environment, not a series of painful investigations to find an infective cause for the 'fever'. In a large study of term infants with a high body temperature, 90% were found to be overheated and only 10% had infection.

The newborn infant may develop a raised body temperature in the presence of infection but this is usually not marked. It may be masked if the infant is being nursed in a servo control incubator or radiant warmer. It is not known why serious infection in a newborn seems to elicit such a mild febrile response when mild infection in a toddler is often associated with a very high body temperature. Infection is not the only cause of a raised set point temperature in the newborn; it is also caused by a severe cerebral abnormality, either congenital (holoprosencephaly, hydranencephaly, encephalocele) or acquired (birth asphyxia). Such infants have hypothalamic dysfunction leading to poor temperature control.

Table 5.31 Differences between a healthy infant who is overheated and a febrile infant with a raised set point (Rutter 1986)

Overheated infant	Febrile infant
High rectal temperature	High rectal temperature
Warm hands and feet	Cool hands and feet
Abdominal exceeds hand skin temperature by less than 2°C	Abdominal exceeds hand skin temperature by more than 3°C
Pink skin	Pale skin
Extended posture	Lethargic
Healthy appearance	Looks unwell

Overheating is less common than accidental hypothermia in the newborn. It is invariably the cause of hyperpyrexia (rectal temperature above 41°C). Mild degrees occur when active, large infants are overwrapped and left in a warm room, or when small infants are overheated by an incubator or radiant warmer. Severe overheating occurs when there is electrical or mechanical failure of a warming device, or when an incubator is exposed to direct sunlight (this turns it into a greenhouse). It can also occur if infants are left in closed cars exposed to direct sunlight.

Mild overheating has been suggested as a predisposing factor in apnea of prematurity but is otherwise not dangerous. Severe overheating leading to hyperpyrexia has caused sudden death in the newborn without prior symptoms. In this context it is interesting that sudden death in infancy has been linked to overheating, and is described in families with a history of malignant hyperpyrexia and anhidrotic ectodermal dysplasia.

ENTERAL NUTRITION

The preterm baby has very little stored energy and urgently needs an adequate supply of food in order to survive beyond a few days. Subsequently, good nutrition is essential to promote the rapid growth which characterizes this period of life, and is important for long-term outcome (Lucas et al 1994). Nutrients can be provided either parenterally or enterally but the aim in all infants is to use full enteral feeding as soon as it is safe to do so. The section that follows reviews the balance of benefits and risks of enteral feeding and recommends suitable intakes, aimed at promoting growth and avoiding deficiencies.

Development of gut function

The motility, digestive and absorptive functions of the gut, and hence its ability to deal with food, develop in utero. Gut development continues postnatally and enteral feeding has an important influence on this. An understanding of gut development is essential to the discussion of benefits and risks of enteral feeding.

Sucking, swallowing, gastric emptying and small gut peristalsis are inefficient in the preterm baby (Kelly & Newell 1994). The fetus begins to swallow at 16 weeks but in babies born before 34 weeks' gestation feeding behavior is characterized by short bursts of sucking, a small intake of milk, uncoordinated swallowing, and nonpropagative, disorganized esophageal motor activity. Lower esophageal sphincter pressure is low (Newell et al 1986), predisposing to gastroesophageal reflux. Gastric emptying time is prolonged to about twice that of the term infant, and is even longer in the presence of illness or when feeds are of high energy density, fat or carbohydrate content (Kelly & Newell 1994). In the fetus small intestinal transit is seen from 30 weeks, but the normal pattern of migrating motor complexes and peristalsis is not observed until a few weeks later (Bisset et al 1988). The coincidence of nutritive sucking, swallowing and gut motor activity at about 34 weeks is a good example of developmental coordination.

Gastric acid production has been shown from 24 weeks' gestation (Kelly et al 1993). Pepsin production is low, but this does not appear to inhibit utilization of dietary protein. In fact, low gastric proteolytic activity may enhance the passage of intact IgG and IgA into the small bowel. Pancreatic enzyme secretion is reduced in the term infant, and in the preterm infant levels of trypsin, lipase, amylase, and bicarbonate secretion are further reduced (McClean & Weaver 1993). In the preterm baby, studies using test meals have demonstrated inadequate intraluminal digestion of fat, protein and carbohydrate, but clinical malabsorption is rare. Fat absorption, for example, limited by low pancreatic lipase and low intraluminal bile salt concentration, may be improved by the high contribution of lingual and gastric lipase. α-glucosidase (sucrase, maltase and isomaltase) activities are about 70–80% of normal at 32 weeks' gestation. Lactase is at 25% of adult levels at 26 weeks and increases markedly towards term (Schmitz 1991).

Intestinal permeability is increased in the preterm baby and results in increased macromolecular transport across the epithelium (Jakobsson et al 1986). This may be relevant to the development of necrotizing enterocolitis (NEC) by allowing bacteria and their antigens to penetrate the gut wall.

The effect of enteral nutrition on the gut

Enteral feeding promotes both structural and functional changes in the gut and its associated organs, which occur less well, or not at all, during enteral starvation. In animals, enteral feeds enhance digestive capacity, with increase in gastric lipase, intestinal lactase activity, and pancreatic responsiveness to glucose. In the human infant, the use of nutritionally inconsequential amounts of milk, as trophic feeding, may improve lactase activity (Mayne et al 1986), and pancreatic function (Kolacek et al 1990), but has its principal advantage in inducing maturation of motor function (Berseth & Nordyke 1993). Preterm infants receiving small volume milk feeds, more rapidly tolerate full enteral feeding, achieve full feeds from breast or bottle earlier, need less phototherapy and show better weight gain (Dunn et al 1988, Slagle & Gross 1988). These effects may be mediated through feed-related release of gut hormones (Lucas et al 1986) or nonnutritional components of breast milk. If prolonged total parenteral nutrition is required, however, most preterm babies make the transition to milk feeds with relatively little difficulty.

Introduction of enteral feeds

The healthy preterm baby should be fed within 1 or 2 h of birth, in order to prevent hypoglycemia and to maintain hydration. Deciding when to enterally feed the sick baby in intensive care is a more contentious matter about which many strong views are held, and practice varies widely (Newell et al 1989b). Most would not attempt feeds in the ill preterm infant, unstable in intensive care. The small for gestational age (SGA) infant also merits particular care. In intrauterine growth retardation with abnormal fetal Doppler studies, fetal gut perfusion is reduced, predisposing the infant to NEC (Malcolm et al 1991) and poor tolerance of milk (Ewer et al 1993). Delay in the introduction of milk feeds in the infant who is SGA is therefore advised (Newell 1996).

In the preterm infant, stable on intensive care and receiving ventilatory assistance, should milk feeds be given? The main arguments for not feeding are the fear of milk aspiration into the lungs, respiratory embarrassment through gastric distention, and NEC (see Complications of feeding). With a cautious approach, however, many neonatal units successfully milk feed babies on ventilators. When full enteral feeding is not thought wise, trophic feeding should be considered with the benefit of stimulating gut growth and development. Milk feeds should always be stopped

for at least 12 h following extubation, to allow recovery of laryngeal protective reflexes, and are generally not given to babies receiving CPAP.

Nutritional requirements of the preterm infant

Table 5.32 compares some aspects of size and body composition between a baby of 26 weeks' gestation and a term baby. Clearly, the metabolic demands of fetal life are quite different from those which pertain after birth, and nutrient requirements based on prenatal growth may not be appropriate for the preterm baby. Current consensus, however, is that the fetal growth curve seems a reasonable 'gold standard' by which to judge the effectiveness of nutritional intake, and a growth rate falling far below it should be regarded as a potential risk factor for poor long-term outcome. Intrauterine growth rates are high, 15–18 g/kg/day, and allowance must be made for the composition of growth during late fetal life. For example, in the term infant, during the first weeks after birth over 40% of weight gain is fat and about 12% protein, whereas in late fetal life only 15–20% of the weight gain is fat, and protein accretion rates are higher (Widdowson 1980).

The nutritional requirements of the preterm baby for the major nutrients, electrolytes, minerals, vitamins and trace elements remain a subject of debate and disagreement. European consensus was reached by ESPGAN, and these figures have been used widely (ESPGAN 1987). A recent attempt to achieve transatlantic agreement is now gaining acceptance (Tsang et al 1993). Differences between the two recommendations are small in relation to the major nutrients. Assuming a growth rate approaching the intrauterine rate of 15 g/kg/day, and allowing for incomplete absorption, the requirements of the preterm baby for the major nutrients are shown in Table 5.33. Table 5.34 completes the picture with details of the requirements for electrolytes, minerals, vitamins and trace elements. The stated values and ranges are culled from many sources and there is still debate and disagreement about some of them.

Table 5.32 Some aspects of body size and composition at 26 weeks' gestation and at term

	26 weeks	40 weeks
Weight	850 g	3500 g
Length	34 cm	51 cm
Brain weight	260 g	490 g
Body water	730 ml	2400 ml
Body sodium	70 mmol	280 mmol
Total nitrogen	10 g	60 g
Fat	6 g	540 g
Calcium	6 g	35 g
Phosphate	3 g	18 g

Table 5.33 Requirements of the preterm baby for the major nutrients

Calories	130 kcal/kg/day
Water	150–180 ml/kg/day
Carbohydrate	16 g/kg/day
Fat	7 g/kg/day
Protein	3.5 g/kg/day

Table 5.34 Requirements of the preterm baby for electrolytes, minerals, trace elements and major vitamins

Sodium	2.5–5 mmol/kg/day
Potassium	2.5–3.5 mmol/kg/day
Chloride	2.5–3.5 mmol/kg/day
Calcium	150 mg/kg/day
Phosphate	100 mg/kg/day
Magnesium	15 mg/kg/day
Iron	2 mg/kg/day
Copper	120 µg/kg/day
Zinc	1 mg/kg/day
Vitamin A	500 µg/day
Vitamin D	25–30 µg/day
Vitamin C	40 mg/day
Vitamin E	5 mg/day
Vitamin B_{12}	0.5 µg/day
Folic acid	100 µg/day

The choice of milk for the preterm infant

The choice of milk has effects upon neurodevelopmental outcome and intelligence. All mothers of preterm infants should be encouraged to express their milk, which is the feed of choice for the preterm infant (Lucas et al 1992b). Long-term results with preterm formula are almost as good (Lucas et al 1994). In the intensive care unit the immediate concern is that the composition of a milk should meet the nutritional requirements for growth and prevention of deficiencies, while being well tolerated, digested and absorbed. Breast milk is better tolerated and absorbed, but is of variable composition and contains inadequate quantities of some nutrients.

Human milk

In the preterm infant, human milk is better tolerated than any currently available formula, gastric emptying is quicker (Ewer et al 1994) and stool frequency greater (Weaver & Lucas 1993). These are especially important considerations during the introduction of enteral feeds.

The advantages of human milk are now well established: NEC is many times less likely if expressed breast milk is given (Lucas & Cole 1990); protection against gastrointestinal and respiratory tract infection in the first years of life (Howie et al 1990); reduction in atopic symptoms in infants with a family history of atopy (Lucas et al 1990a); and, most importantly, its association with optimal neurodevelopmental and intellectual outcome (Lucas et al 1992b, Lucas et al 1994). The mechanism behind this intellectual benefit is not known, but may relate to long chain polyunsaturated fatty acids. These semi-essential fats are structurally important, and subtle differences between those found in human and cow's milk are important in the developing, immature nervous system (Desci & Koletzko 1994). Breast milk may also protect against adult disease, like diabetes mellitus and Crohn's disease through nutritional programming, whereby early nutritional experience exerts a later effect upon health, independent of other influential factors during life (Standing Committee on Nutrition of the British Paediatric Association 1994, Barker 1988). Human milk also contains hormones, such as calcitonin and insulin, and growth factors, such as epidermal

growth factor, in higher concentration than in maternal plasma, and these may have a role in the growth and development of the gut (Kelly & Newell 1994), as well as possible systemic effects.

There are two main problems with human milk: it is not always available, and its energy, protein, calcium, phosphate and sodium content do not meet theoretical nutrient requirements, based on fetal accretion rates. This is in spite of the fact that absorption of nutrients from human milk is more complete, and its composition results in a lower energy cost of growth.

Breast milk varies in composition, and is particularly affected by gestation, postnatal age and method of collection. The mothers of term and preterm infants produce milk which is different in important respects during the first 2–3 weeks after birth. Preterm milk has about a three times higher concentration of sodium, protein and IgA, and a lower water content producing a variable but general increase in the concentration of most constituents, but not calcium or phosphate. Method of collection is important, and drip milk is of lower energy content than expressed milk (Table 5.4). Banked donor milk from term mothers produces less good weight gain than either expressed preterm milk or preterm formula.

When the preterm mother's own milk is available, it is the feed of choice and can be given in larger volumes than formula milk, at around 180 ml/kg/day. It is necessary, however, to compensate for its nutritional deficiencies, and fortification of breast milk is now used in 85% of regional neonatal units in the UK (McClure 1996 in press). Two breast milk fortifiers are currently available in the UK, and both increase energy, protein, carbohydrate, sodium, calcium and phosphate contents of the milk. There is some concern that they might alter tolerance of feeds (Metcalf et al 1994) but we have not found this, and gastric emptying during introduction of milk feeds is the same whether breast milk is fortified or not (McClure 1996). The optimal use of breast milk fortifier is not established. Our practice is routinely to add it, once maternal breast milk is being produced and given in a volume exceeding 90 ml/kg/day.

If donated milk is used, great care must be taken to prevent transmission of HIV (Zeigler et al 1985), through screening of donors once before the donation and again 3 months later. Donated milk should be pasteurized and records kept on all donors and recipients. This disincentive to the use of donor milk, has led to a reduction of milk banking. The use of bank breast milk may again become more prevalent with improved methods of viral screening.

Preterm formula milks

The preterm formulae are based upon human milk. The principal differences are: more protein (approx. 1.8–2.5 g/100 ml); more energy (approx. 75–90 kcal/100 ml); higher sodium, calcium and phosphorus content; and the addition of iron and vitamins, especially D, E and the B complex. Some lactose is replaced with glucose or its polymers, and a small proportion of fat may be given as medium chain triglyceride to improve fat absorption. The recent addition of long chain polyunsaturates (see above), similar to those found in breast milk, has been shown to produce more rapid maturation of the visual pathway, and may confer neurodevelopmental advantage (Desci & Koletzko 1994). New, purified sources of these fats will allow their routine addition to formula milk. Preterm formulae work well, growth rates are good, nutritional deficiencies are rare, and long-term outcome almost matches that seen with breast milk (Lucas et al 1994).

Other milks

Term formula is not adequate for the preterm infant (Lucas et al 1990b). Preterm formula is given until an infant weighs 2.0–2.5 kg. Most, who are not breast-fed, then go on to a whey-dominant term formula. Better weight gain may be seen after discharge home if a formula of composition between preterm and term formula is given (Lucas et al 1992a), but whether this confers benefit upon the infant is currently unknown. At no time during the first year of life is unprocessed cow's milk a suitable food for the preterm baby.

Special milks are occasionally required to treat cow's milk protein or lactose intolerance in the postoperative neonate and in inborn errors of metabolism. This should be done in collaboration with a pediatric dietitian. Soya milks have not been properly evaluated in the preterm baby and should probably be avoided. Goat's milk is suitable for goats.

Feeding in practice

Enteral feeding should be introduced gradually and increased with care. Tolerance should be assessed at each stage so that complications can be averted as far as possible, and, whenever possible, infants should be weighed and measured regularly to assess growth. It is reasonable to begin with as little as 0.5–1 ml/h in a baby of less than 28 weeks' gestation, increasing by 0.5–1 ml every 6 h. In more mature babies, larger starting volumes and a faster rate of progress may be indicated. In a healthy baby, enteral feeds may be given at 75 ml/kg on day 1, 90 ml/kg on day 2, 120 ml/kg on day 3, 135 ml/kg on day 4 and 150 ml/kg on day 5, with subsequent increases up to a maximum of 200 ml/kg/day according to tolerance and growth rate. We routinely increase preterm formula feeds to 165 ml/kg/day, and fortified breast milk to 165–180 ml/kg/day. If the enteral route is chosen during intensive care, the amount given should be monitored closely and parenteral nutrition added if necessary.

Full nipple feeding from breast or bottle depends upon maturity and health. In most it is achieved at a postmenstrual age of 34–37 weeks. The extra respiratory reserve required to successfully feed directly means that babies recovering from RDS or those with BPD will reach feeding independence later.

Continuous or intermittent feeds?

The main argument in favor of continuous feeding is that there should be less gastric distention, with its attendant risks of respiratory embarrassment and pulmonary aspiration, unless the tube becomes misplaced. Randomized studies of these two techniques show little difference, although there is a suggestion of slightly better weight gain with continuous feeds in infants of birthweight 1000–1249 g (Toce et al 1987). Others have shown loss of energy due to adhesion of fat to the tubing and syringe during continuous infusion. A number of potentially adverse effects of continuous feeding have been reported: increased bacterial growth in the milk after 5 h; delay in the development of circadian rhythms; and attenuation of the gut hormone response to feeding (Lucas et al 1986). On balance, there seems more to recommend intermittent than continuous feeding.

Feeding tube placement

The other major differences in tube feeding practice which exist between neonatal units concern preferences for locating the tip of the tube in the stomach or the upper small bowel (transpyloric), and for passing the tube via the nose or the mouth.

Transpyloric feeding had its vogue, but is demanding of staff time and skill, and is associated with excess loss of nitrogen and fat in the stools. Meta-analysis of seven studies has now shown, compared with gastric feeding, a 15% (95% CI 5–23%) increase in mortality in association with transpyloric feeding which can no longer be recommended (Steer et al 1992).

The choice between nasal and oral tube passage is more a matter of aesthetics than of clinical importance. Nasal tubes are commoner because they are easier to fix than oral tubes, which babies have a remarkable ability to dislodge and regurgitate. However, a nasal tube increases resistance to air flow through the nose and this may increase the work of breathing. The use of a palatal appliance (Fig. 5.17) enables secure fixation of an orally

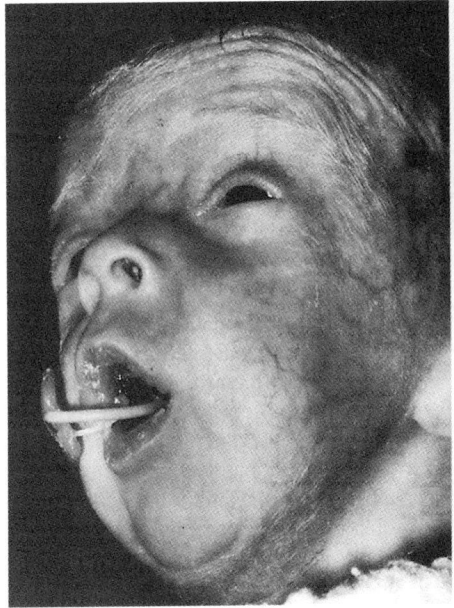
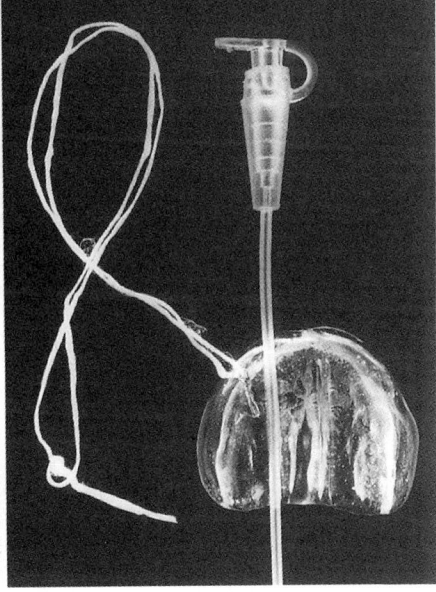

Fig. 5.17 Palatal appliance.

placed tube. This technique leads to a slight reduction in the frequency of apnea and episodes of periodic breathing. In our experience, the mothers' preference for the palatal appliance over the passage of tubes through the nose is a good recommendation for the technique, although it does require the help of an orthodontist or orthodontic technician. In 12 years of using 'feeding plates' routinely in babies of less than 1500 g, we have encountered no adverse effects other than the very occasional area of soreness in the mouth, easily remedied by slight reshaping of the plate.

Nonnutritive sucking (use of a dummy during gastric tube feeds) accelerates maturation of sucking, measured by pressure and pattern of sucking, and leads to more rapid transition to full nipple feeding. Nonnutritive sucking has no effect upon gastric emptying or nutrient absorption, but meta-analysis shows a small, associated increase in weight gain, and a mean reduction of hospital stay of 6 days (95% CI 2–10) (Steer et al 1992).

Weaning from tube to bottle or breast feeds is usually a gradual process and most experienced neonatal nurses say that if rushed, it will take longer. There is no doubt that sucking a whole feed can be a tiring experience for an immature baby especially if there is residual lung dysfunction. The ability to feed independently often determines when babies are discharged, and there may be parental pressure to accomplish the task as soon as possible. Special soft teats are available for preterm babies and do seem to have some advantages over conventional teats.

Nutritional supplements

Protein and energy

There is no need to supplement routinely preterm formulae that are specifically designed to meet the requirements of the preterm infant. Increasingly, as discussed above, expressed breast milk is routinely fortified with a commercial breast milk fortifier once enteral feeding is established. Occasionally the use of an energy supplement, in the form of glucose polymers or a mixture of glucose polymers and fat, is worth considering in a baby who is not growing satisfactorily on its mother's milk or a preterm formula and who cannot cope with larger volumes, say because of incipient heart failure. These supplements are usually well tolerated when added to milk at a rate of 5 g/100 ml. It is important to ensure that the ratio of energy to protein is not increased too much as this may result in relative protein deficiency. A maximum of 100 kcal/2 g of protein should not be exceeded.

Vitamins

Preterm formulae contain vitamins, but, because of instability, do not provide for all the preterm infant's anticipated needs. The following additions to breast milk are recommended by the Committee on Nutrition of the Preterm Infant of the European Society of Pediatric Gastroenterology and Nutrition (ESPGAN 1987):

vitamin A – 500 μg/day
vitamin D – 25 μg/day
vitamin B$_6$ – 100 μg/day
vitamin C – 20 mg/day
folic acid – 100 μg/day.

Routine use of a multivitamin preparation is therefore common practice in breast- and formula-fed infants. The widely used Abidec (Warner Lambert), 0.6 ml/day, will provide enough vitamins A, B$_6$ and C, but additional vitamin D (about 15 μg/day) and folic acid (100 μg/day) are needed to meet the full recommended intakes. The dose of Abidec may be doubled to meet the vitamin D requirement without providing toxic amounts of vitamin A. Several other multivitamin preparations are available, some compounded by hospital pharmacies.

Multivitamin supplements are maintained until full mixed feeding is established, although the extra vitamin D may be reduced to 10 μg (400 IU) per day (equivalent to Abidec 0.6 ml daily) when a weight of about 2250 g is reached.

All infants of all gestations should receive vitamin K prophylaxis against hemorrhagic disease of the newborn (HDN) very soon after birth. In most very low birthweight infants, oral prophylaxis is inappropriate, and a single intramuscular dose of 0.5 mg should be given. Recent controversy about the route of administration should not lead to infants being left without protection against HDN (Newell 1995). If oral vitamin K is given, and the infant breast-fed, further doses should be given at 1 and 4 weeks of age. After intramuscular prophylaxis, additional vitamin K is rarely given after the initial labor ward dose and later bleeding problems from vitamin K deficiency are rare. Extra vitamin K should be given intramuscularly if the preterm baby needs to undergo surgery, has clinical liver disease, or severe diarrheal illness during the first 4 months of life.

Sodium

The preterm infant requires 2.5–4 mmol/kg/day of sodium, usually as chloride. When intake is poor, urinary excretion may well exceed the intake, leading to poor growth and hyponatremia. Routine supplementation of preterm formula or fortified breast milk is not necessary. One reason, as suggested above, to fortify breast milk only when lactation is established is because preterm milk may contain as much as 20 mmol/l of sodium. This is, however, not sustained and falls to levels seen in mature human milk, at about 7 mmol/l. Thus, when feeding with unfortified breast milk is maintained, or donor milk is used, a sodium supplement should be considered. Certainly, if a preterm baby is not growing well, it is always worth checking the serum and urinary sodium concentrations, as the response to an additional 2–4 mmol/kg/day of sodium (as chloride) can be dramatic. The serum concentrations should be monitored during therapy.

Calcium and phosphorus

Osteopenia (also known as metabolic bone disease of prematurity and, previously, neonatal rickets) is now believed to be caused by calcium and phosphate deficiency which is the almost inevitable consequence of preterm delivery. In fetal life, active transport of these minerals across the placenta, during the final trimester, results in fetal accretion rates which cannot be matched by enteral or parenteral supplementation after birth because when sufficient calcium and phosphate is added to feeds, precipitation of insoluble salts occurs. It is, however, known that addition of calcium and phosphate to enteral feeds will result in improved bone mineral density and lower levels of alkaline phosphatase (Bishop et al 1993, Steer et al 1992).

Addition of calcium and phosphate to preterm formulae or fortified breast milk is probably unnecessary. If unsupplemented breast milk is used, on the basis of current knowledge, the addition of calcium (as gluconate) to provide about 100 mg/100 kcal and phosphorus (as buffered sodium phosphate) to provide about 50 mg/100 kcal is recommended.

Iron

Iron absorption from human milk is very efficient, but its iron content is low. Larger amounts of iron are contained in some of the preterm formulae. Late iron deficiency anemia is a regular occurrence among nonsupplemented preterm infants from about 2 months of age. It can largely be prevented by giving 2 mg/kg/day of iron from 4–8 weeks of age until about 12 months. The relative indications for delaying supplemental iron until around 6 weeks are:

1. It is not well absorbed before 4 weeks of age
2. It predisposes to gastrointestinal infection by saturating lactoferrin
3. It predisposes to vitamin E-deficient hemolysis, which is otherwise very rare among breast-fed preterm babies.

Complications of feeding

Milk aspiration

Regurgitation of milk into the esophagus, as shown by esophageal pH monitoring, is common among preterm babies (Newell et al 1989a) and the presence of an endotracheal tube does not prevent pulmonary aspiration (Goodwin et al 1985). Gastroesophageal reflux, however, is reduced during ventilation compared with normal breathing (Newell et al 1989b), and significant aspiration is uncommon in infants receiving milk feeds during intensive care. In a few infants, definite episodes of milk aspiration can be diagnosed by history, resulting in temporary respiratory difficulty and chest X-ray changes. The extent to which milk aspiration contributes to chronic lung disease (Hrabovsky & Mullett 1986) or recurrent apneic attacks (Newell et al 1989a) remains uncertain, but in the infant who has atypical disease, with unexplained deterioration, or failure to respond to standard therapy, gastroesophageal reflux and aspiration should be considered. Prone positioning, thickening agents and smaller, more frequent, feeds may help. Xanthines may be withdrawn or feeds stopped. Cisapride (Janssen Pharmaceutical Ltd.) has now an established place in the management of reflux in infants and children, and may be used in preterm infants at 0.1–0.3 mg/kg/dose, given orally t.d.s.

Respiratory embarrassment resulting from gastric distention

When the lungs are normal, tube feeding has little or no effect on lung function, but when the lungs are abnormal a tube feed of only 5 ml of milk has been shown to produce a small reduction in arterial PO_2 for about 30 min. During suckling, a fall in arterial PO_2 and a small rise in arterial PCO_2 has been shown in preterm infants. It is important to be aware of this effect in babies recovering from respiratory distress syndrome and those with bronchopulmonary dysplasia.

Necrotizing enterocolitis (NEC)

There is a definite association between enteral feeding and NEC, in that it is unusual in babies who have not received milk feeds. It is speculated that the introduction of milk provides a food substrate for bacterial multiplication, and that these bacteria subsequently invade the bowel wall, which has been rendered susceptible by hypoxia or ischemia. A causal effect for feeding in the generation of NEC has not been established but the epidemiology of the disease is complex. For example, some neonatal units with a policy of introducing milk feeds to all babies in the first few days of life hardly ever see a case of NEC, whereas a unit with a more conservative feeding policy may see quite a lot. Breast milk protects against NEC (Lucas & Cole 1990). Other trials of feeding practice on the incidence of NEC have failed to provide clear guidance, although occasional studies have suggested that delaying the introduction of milk feeds, or at least increasing them very slowly, may reduce the incidence (Ng et al 1988). There is clear evidence for caution in infants with intrauterine growth retardation (see above).

Food intolerance

Intolerance of cow's milk protein seems uncommon among preterm babies, perhaps reflecting the relative unresponsiveness of their immune system. It may present as colitis with fresh bleeding per rectum. Lactose intolerance is commoner, especially after NEC or gut surgery. Treatment by exclusion diet is appropriate as long as the substitute food is carefully chosen with the nutritional needs of the preterm baby in mind. The advice of the pediatric dietitian is helpful in this situation.

Nutritional assessment

The final validation of any nutritional regime is that it supports a satisfactory rate and quality of growth, and prevents deficiency states. Careful and frequent assessments of the growth of the preterm baby should be made. Weight, length and occipitofrontal circumference are measured at least weekly, and related to centile charts. In addition to the routine measurements, reference data are now available for skinfold thickness, mid-upper arm circumference (MUAC) and MUAC : head circumference ratio (Sasanow et al 1986) which can be used as indicators of fat deposition and lean body mass.

Hematological and biochemical assessments should be undertaken to look for signs of nutritional deficiency such as: anemia due to vitamin E or iron deficiency; pancytopenia due to folate deficiency; raised alkaline phosphatase and low serum phosphate related to osteopenia; hypoalbuminemia suggesting absolute or relative protein deficiency; hyponatremia; hypocalcemia; metabolic acidosis due to excessive protein intake, etc.

Finally, growth monitoring and dietary advice, are an important part of follow-up for the very low birthweight infant after discharge, and throughout the first year.

INTENSIVE CARE

ORGANIZATION OF NEONATAL INTENSIVE CARE SERVICES

In 1983 it was suggested that one intensive care cot and five special care cots are needed to manage the problems resulting from each 1000 yearly deliveries (BPA/RCOG 1983). The Royal College of Physicians in 1988 adjusted the cot number required for intensive care to 1.5/1000 deliveries recognizing that intensive care was both more frequently possible and could be more prolonged (Royal College of Physicians of London 1988). Each unit providing for anything other than anticipated normal deliveries should have special care back-up facilities. The belief by many obstetricians and pediatricians in the UK that a normal delivery is only diagnosable in retrospect has encouraged moves to ensure that all deliveries occur in hospital.

Intensive care equipment is reasonably centralized to a few centers where 24-h support for its use can be guaranteed. Nursing and medical staff have to be properly trained to use 'high-tech' sophisticated machinery or the baby may be at risk from the equipment itself. Continuous back-up maintenance and service support is needed for machines that are themselves in use all day every day. Without a certain critical level of expertise neonatal care becomes a very dangerous provision.

Hierarchy of care

Each and every hospital concerned with the delivery of babies should at all times provide expertise for the resuscitation of the newborn. The functioning equipment – mucus aspirators, bag and mask, oxygen, endotracheal tubes and laryngoscope – and a person who is familiar with their correct use (not necessarily a doctor) should be available at all times.

In addition, all district hospital maternity services should have a neonatal unit that can provide special care. This care can be given by midwives under the supervision of staff trained in neonatal care but the skill mix must be adequate. There should be medical personnel on site at all times with pediatric experience. The special care unit (level 1 care – USA) must be capable of providing safe oxygen therapy, intravenous access and therapy, and treatment for hypoglycemia, hypocalcemia, hyperbilirubinemia and infection. Though not intended to carry out sophisticated intensive care, the special care unit must still provide expertise for the safe resuscitation and stabilization of the unexpected critically ill child with respiratory failure while help arrives.

The subregional center (level 2 – USA) will usually be sited in a larger hospital and will be able to offer short-term neonatal intensive care to their own deliveries. Infants likely to require long periods of intensive care (e.g. the extremely low birthweight infant or infant requiring surgical treatment) would reasonably be diverted to the perinatal intensive care unit (PICU) which when busy could itself refer shorter-term problems and high-dependency cases back. The subregional center should be capable of intensive care with the exception of surgery; its specialist staffing will be less broad.

Each region should have one or more PICUs (level 3 – USA) (Table 5.35) dealing with the very high-risk mother and infant. These centers not only provide care for all the most difficult medical and surgical problems of the region but also are intimately concerned with the improvements of standards in the region by specialist education and research.

Categories of neonatal care

In 1984 the categories of care required for babies were more

Table 5.35 The perinatal intensive care unit (PICU) (at least one in every health region)

Facilities
1. Obstetric ICU facilities
2. Neonatal ICU facilities
   a. Minimum medical provision
      SHO (experience in pediatrics) always on duty
      Registrar (experience in neonates) always on duty
      Consultant (experienced in neonatal intensive care) always on call
   b. Nursing provision
      One neonatal intensive care nurse per intensive care baby per shift*
   c. 24-hour back-up provisions
      Radiology service to the unit
      Biochemistry with blood gases and electrolytes
      Hematology service for diagnosis and transfusion
      Microbiological service
      Medical physics and electronics

Responsibilities
1. Provision of medical neonatal intensive care
2. Provision of surgical neonatal intensive care
   THE BUCK STOPS HERE!
3. Administrative liaison within the region
4. Neonatal education for the region
   a. Ward rounds and seminars for nursing and medical visitors to the PICU
   b. Medical and nursing outreach by staff to the district and subregional centers
5. Regional audit
6. Training base for medical and neonatal nursing
7. Research
   Epidemiological
   Applied
   Basic

* Although recommended and ideal, the provision of one NNIC trained nurse per IC baby per shift is not available anywhere in the UK at this stage. One is forced back to stipulating that there be adequate overall numbers of trained nurses and a reasonable skill mix of trainers to trainees. This in fact means that most units are unable to take all the sick infants that they are asked to because of insufficient nursing staff.

clearly defined – see Definitions (p. 94). Despite these and other sensible recommendations made by the Short Report (1980), the House of Commons Social Services Committee (1984) and the Maternity Services Advisory Committee (1985) few recommendations have been implemented. Although it is true that such organization is expensive, there is little doubt that it is extremely cost effective (see Economics of care, p. 104). Most expensive is the trained neonatal nurse staffing – the latest recommendations are that there should be 5.5 trained nurses per intensive care cot and 1.5 per special care cot. Medical, laboratory and paramedical back-up services add in lesser costs.

Transport of sick or high-risk neonates

Introduction

Except in the remoter areas of Scotland or under extreme weather conditions, road transfer is the usual means of transporting babies from one center to another in the UK. It is also the rule to use ambulances provided by the health service as these are available at all times. They have the added advantage that the crew have expert knowledge of the hospitals and the major and minor routes between them, thus enabling the use of alternative routes if traffic conditions are problematic and there is no police escort. It is usual for the PICU to provide the transport team to pick up the sick infant: the ambulance traveling with the emergency siren will get the expert team to the baby with the greatest possible speed. Returning the sick infant to the PICU should be done at a steady pace rather than a rush and, if there is a problem in transit, it is wise to stop and sort it out, not run for the home base. When the infant no longer requires intensive care, the local hospital sends a team to collect the infant, again using the local ambulance service.

Equipment

The equipment needed for transferring sick newborn infants is almost identical to that required in the PICU. The infant is stabilized in a portable transport incubator which enables management of the infant in the optimal thermal environment with good visibility and access. Full respiratory support must be possible using ventilator or CPAP and adjustable oxygen concentration. All the supporting equipment such as laryngoscope, endotracheal tubes, chest drains etc. and drugs must be available in a compact and portable travel case. Except for diagnostic services (e.g. radiology and blood gases) the transport team should be independent of the district hospital.

Indications

The indication for postnatal transfer is the perceived inability by the district hospital to provide a satisfactory level of diagnosis or care on that site, either at that moment or in the immediate future. This may be a result of lack of equipment or adequately trained staff. One important job of the PICU is to ensure that staff at district hospitals are given training, both in-service by outreach and by clinical meetings. A level of expertise is then always available for the management of stable but high-dependency problems on site. In this way the district hospital can take infants back before they are 'low risk' thus allowing a greater turnover of patients at the center.

Antenatal (in utero) transfer (Table 5.36)

With few exceptions the best portable incubator for the high-risk problem is the uterus, with delivery of the infant where support and expertise are readily available. Such transfers should be with agreement between district and central obstetric consultants and should also involve the neonatal staff of the PICU. Mothers in advanced stages of preterm labor should be delivered peripherally to avoid the danger of a delivery in the ambulance. The mother with severe pregnancy-associated hypertension or antepartum hemorrhage should be stable before transfer and an obstetric doctor should accompany her.

Table 5.36 Indicators for antenatal (in utero) transfer

1. Obstetric assessment of the high-risk fetus where urgent delivery is likely (e.g. IUGR)
2. The severely ill mother (e.g. with pregnancy-associated hypertension) at an early stage of pregnancy with a potentially viable fetus
3. Early preterm labor where the referring hospital has inadequate facilities
4. Hemolytic disease with a severely affected fetus
5. Fetal malformation needing postnatal surgery
6. Prolonged and preterm rupture of the fetal membranes with resulting oligohydramnios

PRACTICAL PARENTERAL NUTRITION (see also Ch. 21)

All tertiary neonatal services and many secondary units should be able to provide optimal parenteral nutrition for sick, full-term and preterm infants. All regimens should provide full and adequate nutrition with minimal adverse nutritional or other consequences. The variations used to reduce complications are numerous.

Indications in the neonatal unit

Parenteral nutrition may provide for all the nutritional requirements of the infant (total parenteral nutrition, TPN) or may supplement inadequate enteral nutrition.

There are three major indications for parenteral nutrition in the neonatal unit:

1. Surgical lesions such as omphalocele or gastroschisis, or following extensive bowel resections and anastomoses (usually TPN, occasionally supplemental).
2. The medical (and surgical) treatment of necrotizing enterocolitis (NEC) (usually TPN).
3. In immature and usually very premature infants where enteral feeds cannot be fully established and the provision of good nutrition is essential. Here the provision may be TPN or supplemental. It may be prudent to supply parenteral nutrition in other postoperative situations and acute disease but it is advisable that systemic infection is under control before these highly nutritious solutions are used.

Nutritional requirements

Protein

Although milks provide between 2 and 4 g of protein per kg daily most preterm infants require only 2.5 g/kg/day of parenteral amino acids and they may develop a metabolic acidosis if given more (Adamkin 1986). The biological availability of amino acids is variable but the use of crystalline L-amino acids maximizes effect. Ideally the proportions of essential to nonessential amino acids should be approximately equal and the branched-chain amino acids should form about 25% of the total (Adamkin 1986). There are additional amino acids essential in the preterm infant, e.g. cysteine, histidine, arginine and tyrosine. Provision of amino acids to achieve a plasma aminogram similar to that of the fetus in the last trimester seems logical (McIntosh et al 1984, Soltesz et al 1985). For optimal nitrogen utilization adequate calories must also be provided, the ideal calorie to nitrogen ratio being between 150 and 250.

Table 5.37 shows the amino acid solution profile of three commonly used European preparations. The addition of cysteine is necessary as it is an essential amino acid in the newborn and there is evidence to suggest that retinal damage may occur if taurine is not provided. The balance of amino acids is probably very important and the reports of hyperphenylalaninemia and hypertyrosinemia using some amino acid solutions may reflect the fact that these solutions are not originally designed for newborn or preterm infants (Puntis et al 1986, Mitton et al 1988). Aminograms of preterm infants given Primene R 10% (Cernep Synthelabo) fall consistently within the reference range of the fetus in the last trimester in utero (Rigo et al 1987, McIntosh & Mitchell 1990).

Table 5.37 Amino acid profile of solutions available in UK (each amino acid expressed as percentage of total)

	Vamin-9-Glucose*	Vamin Infant*	Primene R 10%†
Essential			
Isoleucine	5.5	4.8	6.7
Leucine	7.5	10.7	10.0
Valine	6.1	5.5	7.6
Lysine	5.5	8.6	11.0
Methionine	2.7	2.0	2.4
Phenylalanine	7.8	4.1	4.2
Threonine	4.3	5.5	3.7
Tryptophan	1.4	2.1	2.0
Nonessential			
Alanine	4.3	9.7	8.0
Arginine‡	4.7	6.3	8.4
Histidine‡	3.4	3.2	3.8
Proline	11.5	8.6	3.0
Serine	10.7	5.8	4.0
Tyrosine‡	0.7	0.8	0.5
Glycine	3.0	3.2	4.0
Aspartic acid	5.8	6.3	6.0
Glutamic acid	12.8	10.9	10.0
Taurine	–	–	0.6
Cysteine‡	2.0	1.5	2.5
Ornithine	–	–	2.5

* KabiVitrum, Stockholm, Sweden.
† Cernep Synthelabo, Paris, France.
‡ Probably essential in the preterm newborn.

Fat

The absence of an intravenous fat emulsion in early parenteral nutrition regimens led to a syndrome of essential fatty acid deficiency with inadequate growth and a scaly dermatitis. In the UK and Europe Intralipid (KabiVitrum) can be obtained as a 10% or 20% solution with 1.1 or 2.2 calories per ml respectively. This soya bean oil : egg yolk phospholipid emulsion is both a good calorie source and a source of essential fatty acids and phosphatides and with gradual increase preterm infants can tolerate up to 4 g/kg/day (36 calories/kg/day as lipid). Heparin increases the clearance of lipid from the circulation probably by promoting the release of lipoprotein lipase from hepatic and extrahepatic tissues. There is a belief, though not weighty evidence, that addition of 1 IU/ml to parenteral nutrition solutions preserves i.v. line patency and promotes lipolysis.

Carbohydrate

Glucose is the usual carbohydrate used for the neonate although galactose, fructose and ethanol have been tried in the past. It is usual to start with a 10% dextrose solution at approximately 4 mg/kg/min and to increase this if there is no hyperglycemia and particularly glycosuria.

Vitamins and minerals

The vitamin requirements are shown in Table 5.38. These are conveniently given as:

1. 2 ml Vitlipid N infant (Kabi Pharmacia Ltd.) in each 100 ml of Intralipid for the fat-soluble vitamins retinol, ergocalciferol, tocopherol and vitamin K.

Table 5.38 A typical parenteral nutrition prescription for a 16-day-old infant of 1600 g with necrotizing enterocolitis

Solution 1		Solution 2	
Primene 10%*	17.05 ml	Intralipid 10%‡	60 ml
Dextrose 20% w/v	47.75 ml	Vitlipid Infant‡	6 ml
Multibionta†	0.3 ml		
Sodium chloride 30% w/v	0.67 ml		66 ml
Potassium chloride 29% w/v	0.81 ml		
Pedel‡	3.4 ml		
Calcium gluconate 10% w/v	0.3 ml		
Water for injections	30.23 ml		
	100 ml		

The final solution has the following composition:

Amino acids	1.7 g		Retinol	410 mg
Carbohydrate	9.51 g		Ergocalciferol	6 mg
Sodium	3.4 mmol		Tocopherol	3.84 mg
Potassium	2.1 mmol		Phytomenadione	120 mg
Calcium	0.57 mmol		Lipid	6 g
Phosphate	0.26 mmol			
Magnesium	0.13 mmol			
Chloride	6.29 mmol			
Vitamin A palmitate	0.18 mg			
Vitamin B HCl	1.5 mg			
Vitamin B$_2$	0.3 mg			
Nicotinamide	3.0 mg			
Pantothenyl alcohol	0.75 mg			
Vitamin B$_6$ HCl	0.45 mg			
Vitamin C	0.15 mg			
Vitamin E acetate	0.15 mg			
Iron	1.7 µg			
Zinc	0.5 µg			
Manganese	0.85 µg			
Copper	0.26 µg			
Fluoride	0.6 µg			
Iodine	0.03 µg			
Phosphorus	2.25 µg			

The final solution has the following composition shown in the right column above.

Start at 130 ml/kg/day and increase to 145 ml/kg/day after 24 h

Start at 15 ml/kg/day and increase if tolerated to 30 ml/kg/day

Weekly supplements intramuscularly: (1) vitamin B$_{12}$ 5 mg; (2) folic acid 0.5 mg.
* Cernep Synthelabo, Paris, France.
† Merck Ltd, Alton, Hants GU34 5HG, UK.
‡ KabiVitrum Ltd, Bourne End, Bucks SL8 5XF, UK.

2. 2 ml of Solivito (Kabi Pharmacia Ltd.) (vitamins B$_1$, B$_2$, nicotinamide, B$_6$, pantothenic acid, biotin, folic acid, B$_{12}$ and vitamin C) in 100 ml of dextrose.

3. 1 ml of Peditrace (Kabi Pharmacia Ltd.)/kg/day containing calcium, magnesium, iron, zinc, manganese, copper, chloride, phosphate, fluorine and iodine – also added to the dextrose. In addition, sodium, potassium and extra calcium, magnesium and phosphate may be required (see Table 5.38).

Technique of administration

Whether the final solution is infused by central or by peripheral vein, it should be made up by pharmacy under laminar flow conditions to prevent contamination. It should be run through from the bag to the giving set delivery point so that all that is required on the neonatal unit is the linking of the sterile connection of the set to the intravenous line on the baby. The lipid should join the main set by a Y-connector just prior to this connection. The use of millipore filters does little to reduce infection and introduces a further junction into the system which potentially increases the risk. Orange bags and giving sets reduce the photodegradation of vitamins but are expensive and covering the bags with colored polyethylene is almost as effective.

Since Wilmore & Dudrick's original description in 1968 central lines have frequently been used to give parenteral nutrition. They can often last for weeks but line colonization and systemic infection is common even when they are placed surgically under strict aseptic conditions and maintained in the best possible way. The placement of a fine Silastic catheter percutaneously reduces the need for surgical help and has been widely used in the UK (Shaw 1973) with practiced units showing infection rates of less than 10%. If the infant with a central line behaves in any way as if infected the line should be removed immediately.

Many units use peripheral infusions to give parenteral nutrition. Although this reduces the incidence of systemic infection the amount of extra handling that the infants receive is very significant and the medical staff time involved in maintenance of the infusions to provide the nutrition is considerable.

Complications

1. Catheter related:
   a. Sepsis – common and not wholly confined to central lines. It may be bacterial or fungal.
   b. Thrombosis/obstruction – more common with peripheral lines but more serious with possible embolus and infection if on a central line.
   c. Hemorrhage – more related to central lines.
   d. Extravasation of fluid from peripheral lines with chemical burns, skin sloughing and infection.
2. Metabolic related:
   a. Cholestasis – total parenteral nutrition for more than 2–3 weeks is commonly associated with cholestatic jaundice and mild hepatocellular damage. Many factors have been postulated as important in the pathogenesis but the actual cause is uncertain. The liver biopsy shows fatty infiltration and a little hepatocellular injury without significant inflammation. The condition is completely reversible (Adamkin 1986) and reduced by minimal enteral feeding.
   b. Fat embolism – this has not been convincingly associated with 10% Intralipid given throughout the 24 h. Some recommend a check for clear serum by eye (unreliable) or nephelometry when using 20% Intralipid. If large amounts of lipid are given, serum triglycerides should be checked periodically.
   c. Hyperglycemia and glycosuria – reduce the infusion rate.
   d. Hypocalcemia, hypophosphatemia, hypokalemia – from inadequate intake.
   e. Hyperammonemia and acidosis – these may result from either too fast an infusion of amino acids or inadequate clearance in a sick infant.
   f. Hyperaminoacidemia – related to rate of infusion, the maturity of the infant and probably the balance of the intravenous solution.

Despite the large possible numbers of complications, good catheter insertion and management in tertiary centers ensures that the benefits far outweigh the risks. Where less adequate supervision of infants is possible, parenteral nutrition may be extremely hazardous. A typical parenteral nutrition prescription is seen in Table 5.38.

BLOOD GASES AND RESPIRATORY SUPPORT

The physiological basis of neonatal gas exchange and respiratory control has been reviewed by Carlo & Chatburn (1988) and Henderson-Smart (1992). Successful management demands obsessional recording of blood gases, ventilator settings, blood pressure and other variables, and careful interpretation of their physiological significance. To achieve adequate gas exchange with minimal complications requires a knowledge of:

1. lung mechanics
2. the principles of gas exchange
3. measurement of blood gases
4. probable mechanisms of lung injury from ventilation
5. recommended blood gas values.

Lung mechanics

To inflate the lungs, work must be done against their elastic recoil and resistance. Even with adequate surfactant most of this elastic recoil is attributable to surface tension. The higher the elastic recoil the lower the compliance. Compliance depends on the number of recruited alveoli. Resistance reflects airway caliber and is increased at lower lung volumes or in airway obstruction.

The pressure–volume curve of the lungs

When a lung is inflated from complete collapse (atelectasis) the relationship between increasing pressure and volume follows three phases. First, as alveoli are opened, large increases in pressure achieve only small increases in volume. Second, once alveoli are recruited inflation is easier and small increases in pressure achieve larger changes in volume. Third, as the lungs become overinflated and stiff, increases in volume per unit pressure become progressively smaller. During deflation lung volume remains higher at all pressures than during the three phases of inflation. In health, the alveoli do not collapse and about 30 ml/kg bodyweight of gas remains at the end of expiration. This volume is the functional residual capacity (FRC). If the alveoli are unstable and collapse, the 'pressure-inefficient' process of alveolar recruitment must be repeated. Surfactant deficiency leads to instability during deflation with low expiratory lung volume and impaired gas exchange.

The time required to inflate or deflate the lungs depends on the volume moved, the pressure applied and the resistance to flow. Where resistance is high as in chronic lung disease or obstruction of the endotracheal tube the same volume takes longer to be exchanged. Where compliance is low, as in hyaline membrane disease, the lungs are stiffer and empty more rapidly. Strategies for respiratory support should achieve adequate alveolar recruitment, appropriate inflation and deflation times and avoid overinflation.

Principles of gas exchange

In pulmonary gas exchange the gas tensions in the blood equilibrate by diffusion with those in the air spaces, if both ventilation and perfusion are adequate. Mechanisms that lead to ventilation/perfusion mismatching are illustrated in Figure 5.18.

Intrapulmonary right-to-left shunting

Right-to-left shunting of blood in alveoli occurs when they collapse or are filled with blood, edema or exudate. Alveolar ventilation with fresh gases is inversely related to the respiratory dead space and is proportional to minute ventilation, which is the tidal volume multiplied by the number of breaths per minute. Minute ventilation may be inadequate with poor respiratory drive, airway obstruction, increased dead space or widespread atelectasis.

Extrapulmonary right-to-left shunting

Pulmonary vascular resistance is increased by acidosis, hypoxia and hypercapnia. It may be increased in lung disease, or after asphyxia, causing blood to bypass the lungs through fetal channels, the foramen ovale or ductus arteriosus. This is called persistent fetal circulation or pulmonary hypertension. This right-to-left shunting is exacerbated by low systemic arterial blood pressure. When cardiac output is low the blood entering the alveoli has lower oxygen tension and higher carbon dioxide tension than normal and equilibration with alveolar gas may be incomplete. If blood volume is low the increased rate of circulation may also reduce the time for equilibration.

Mild degrees of right-to-left shunt can be corrected by increasing the inspired oxygen concentration and hence alveolar PO_2. In severe lung disease causing intrapulmonary shunt or in severe cyanotic heart disease or asphyxia causing extrapulmonary shunt, total right-to-left shunt is substantial. If the hemoglobin in pulmonary capillaries is already saturated, systemic arterial oxygen tension (PaO_2) cannot be restored to normal simply by raising the alveolar PO_2. While this raises the oxygen tension of pulmonary capillary blood it does not significantly increase its total oxygen content, as oxygen is relatively insoluble. Severely inadequate oxygenation can only be improved by increasing the number of ventilated lung units when there is intrapulmonary right-to-left shunting or by improving pulmonary perfusion when there is extrapulmonary right-to-left shunting. Correction of hypotension by volume expansion or pressors may improve gas exchange without altering ventilator settings, by improving pulmonary perfusion.

Because carbon dioxide is highly soluble in plasma and its pulmonary diffusion capacity greater than that of oxygen, carbon dioxide is more easily exchanged. The relationship between blood carbon dioxide content and $PaCO_2$ is linear. In mild respiratory failure the carbon dioxide tension in alveoli with good ventilation/perfusion matching is lowered by hyperventilation. This leads to normal or even reduced $PaCO_2$, despite the elevated carbon dioxide content of blood leaving lung units with poor matching. Only when total alveolar ventilation or perfusion is severely reduced does $PaCO_2$ rise.

Measurement of blood gases

All neonatal units should have immediate 24-h access to an automated blood gas analyzer. Blood samples are usually obtained from an umbilical arterial catheter, or by indwelling catheter or needle puncture from the radial or posterior tibial arteries after confirming that the collateral circulation is adequate. Use of end arteries (temporal, brachial or femoral) is not advisable because of the risk of irreversible ischemia.

Measurements of oxygen tension (PO_2) in capillary or venous blood underestimate arterial oxygen tension (PaO_2) and cannot be relied on, even if the skin is warmed to 40°C. Capillary blood obtained by heel prick provides an acceptable estimate of arterial PCO_2, pH and base excess, but warming the heel to 40°C does not significantly improve accuracy of PO_2 (McLain et al 1989).

Continuous monitoring of blood gas tensions or oxygen saturation is a useful supplement to, but not a substitute for, intermittent sampling. Changes in oxygenation following procedures such as endotracheal suction or surfactant administration can be detected and quickly corrected. Continuous information on PaO_2 can be obtained from an indwelling oxygen electrode in the umbilical artery. A less invasive method is transcutaneous measurement of oxygen tension (tcPO_2) with a heated electrode. TcPO_2 underestimates PaO_2 when the skin is (a) poorly perfused in hypovolemic shock, (b) compressed over a bone, or (c) thicker after the first 8 weeks of life (Hamilton et al 1985). In very immature infants repeated reattachment of electrodes damages the skin. This can be prevented by a layer of plastic spray-on film (Op-Site) without loss of accuracy of tcPO_2 (Evans & Rutter 1986).

Continuous transcutaneous monitoring of hemoglobin saturation (tcSaO$_2$) by pulse oximetry has some advantages over tcPO_2 monitoring (Southall et al 1987). A nonadhesive, unheated probe wrapped around a hand or foot measures the light absorption characteristics of arterial oxygenated hemoglobin. A pulse oximeter requires no calibration and is not affected by changes in skin thickness or perfusion. It is easily applied without injury to immature infants, but is more sensitive to movement artifact than tcPO_2 monitoring. In the steep portion of the oxygen–hemoglobin dissociation curve small changes in PO_2 cause large changes in O$_2$ saturation, so the pulse oximeter reflects hypoxia and oxygen availability to tissues better than tcPO_2 measurements in this range. In the flat portion of the oxygen–hemoglobin dissociation curve large changes in PO_2 cause small changes in O$_2$ saturation, so hyperoxia cannot safely be excluded when tcSaO$_2$ is 95–100% and tcPO_2 monitoring is more reliable in this range.

Probable mechanisms of lung injury from ventilation

Lung injury from ventilation is often referred to as barotrauma. Many now prefer the term volutrauma, since overdistention caused by inappropriate pressure may be harmful, rather than

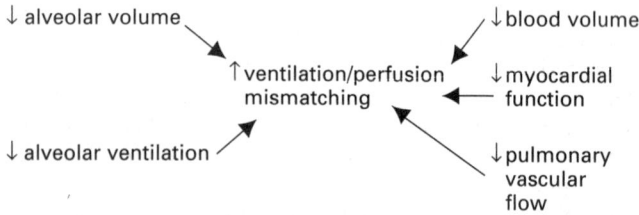

Fig. 5.18 Mechanisms leading to ventilation/perfusion mismatching.

pressure itself (Parker et al 1993). Oxygen in high concentration generates free oxygen radicals, which are toxic. The preterm infant has poorly developed antioxidant lung defenses and may therefore be at greater risk.

Recommended blood gas values

Ideally, recommendations should be based on prospective studies which compare outcomes among infants randomly allocated to specific ranges of blood gas values. Until this is done, recommendations must depend on physiological reasoning and clinical observations.

Oxygenation (PaO₂, tcPO₂ and tcSaO₂)

Values for $tcPO_2$ and $tcSaO_2$ in the first weeks of life for healthy term and preterm infants (Mok et al 1986, 1988) are shown in Table 5.39. Prolonged, severe hypoxia causes brain damage. Hyperoxia can predispose to retinopathy of prematurity, particularly in infants below 31 weeks' gestation (Prendiville & Schulenberg 1988). A reasonable policy in newborn infants receiving respiratory support is *to aim for PaO₂ or tcPO₂ between 6.7 and 10.7 kPa (50–80 mmHg) or tcSaO₂ between 87 and 94%.* Factors contributing to poor oxygenation are shown in Table 5.40.

Table 5.39 Normal range of $tcPO_2$ and $tcSaO_2$ in healthy infants in air* (adapted from Mok et al 1986, 1988)

	Awake	Quiet sleep	Active sleep
Term infants (*n* = 55)			
$TcPO_2$ (kPa†)			
Postnatal age			
<1 week	8.5–13.0	7.8–12.1	6.7–12.8
6 weeks	9.1–12.2	7.1–12.3	7.1–12.4
$TcSaO_2$ (%)			
Postnatal age			
<1 week	91.8–100	87.4–98.3	86.1–98.4
6 weeks	95.0–99.0	89.4–98.1	87.5–98.5
Preterm infants (*n* = 28)			
$TcPO_2$ (kPa†)			
Postconceptional age			
29–34 weeks	4.7–11.0	6.4–11.7	4.7–11.1
36–38 weeks	6.8–12.5	7.0–12.9	6.7–12.0
$TcSaO_2$ (%)			
Postconceptional age			
29–34 weeks	86.6–96.3	86.0–96.1	86.6–96.5
35–38 weeks	86.8–96.8	87.6–97.9	88.6–96.8

* No infant appeared cyanosed or had signs of respiratory distress during any of the studies.
† To convert oxygen tension in kPa to mmHg, multiply by 7.5.

Table 5.40 Factors contributing to poor oxygenation

1. Intrapulmonary right-to-left shunt caused by alveolar hypoventilation or collapse

2. Extrapulmonary right-to-left shunt through ductus arteriosus, foramen ovale or both

3. Low cardiac output or hypovolemia

Carbon dioxide tension

Hypercapnia produces pulmonary vasoconstriction, but cerebral vasodilation. In a prospective study of 200 very low birthweight infants, $PaCO_2 > 7$ kPa (52.5 mmHg) was associated with both periventricular hemorrhage and periventricular leukomalacia (Trounce et al 1988), an important predictor of later disability (Graham et al 1987). Severe hypocapnia profoundly reduces cerebral blood flow, and is associated with periventricular leukomalacia and cerebral palsy (Calvert et al 1987, Ikonen et al 1992, Graziani et al 1992b).

Broad consensus in current practice is to keep $PaCO_2$ between 4.7 and 8 kPa (35–60 mmHg) (HIFI Study Group 1989). However, in severe respiratory failure some authors keep $PaCO_2$ between 6.7 and 8 kPa (50–60 mmHg) or higher, provided arterial pH remains above 7.25. By allowing lower ventilator pressures this, it is suggested, may increase survival without chronic lung disease (Rhodes et al 1983, Wung et al 1985, Avery et al 1987, Kraybill et al 1989). Whether it may also increase the risk of cerebral insult and disability in preterm infants must be resolved by controlled trials. A reasonable compromise is to aim for $PaCO_2$ between 5.3 and 7.0 kPa (40–52.5 mmHg) in preterm infants below 33 weeks' gestation in their first 3 days.

pH

Acidosis causes cerebral vasodilation, while alkalosis reduces cerebral blood flow. In preterm infants, values of pH < 7.20 have been associated with periventricular hemorrhage (Skoutelli et al 1985) and values of pH < 7.1 with periventricular leukomalacia (Trounce et al 1988). In 140 very low birthweight infants, pH < 7.20 appeared to be more strongly associated with subsequent retinopathy of prematurity than either hyperoxia or prematurity (Prendiville & Schulenberg 1988). A reasonable policy for infants receiving respiratory support is to keep pH between 7.25 and 7.45.

Respiratory support

Reducing the need for respiratory support by antenatal steroids

Use of antenatal steroids in mothers at risk of preterm delivery reduces infants' risks of hyaline membrane disease, death and brain damage by around 50% (Crowley et al 1990) and should be a standard of care subjected to routine audit (Scottish Neonatal Consultants Collaborative Study Group and International Neonatal Network 1996).

Continuous positive airway pressure (CPAP)

Continuous positive airway pressure (CPAP) is currently given by facemask, nasal prongs or endotracheal tube. Early application of continuous distending pressure in hyaline membrane disease appears to preserve an adequate alveolar air–liquid interface, conserving surfactant and promoting its release (Wyszogrodski et al 1975). This may reduce disease severity, further respiratory support and subsequent complications. The need for clinical trials to test this hypothesis is reemphasized by an observational study of chronic lung disease among 1625 infants of 700–1500 g birthweight in eight centers (Avery et al 1987). Fewer were dependent on oxygen at 28 days in Columbia University.

One policy unique to that center was use of nasal CPAP within minutes after birth for infants with respiratory distress after resuscitation.

Nasal CPAP has been combined with surfactant to treat hyaline membrane disease (Verder et al 1994). Infants with worsening respiratory failure are sedated, intubated, surfactant is administered and the infants are extubated and returned to CPAP. This may reduce the number of infants that require ventilation but further trials of its impact on death, chronic lung disease and brain damage and costs would be valuable. Continuous negative extrathoracic pressure (CNEP) may supplement or replace mechanical ventilation in infants with hyaline membrane disease or bronchopulmonary dysplasia (Samuels & Southall 1989) but in small preterm infants an adequate neck seal might lead to raised intracranial pressure with cerebral hemorrhage. Nasal CPAP and CNEP have been used as an adjunct to early extubation. It is unclear whether the elective use of CPAP following extubation decreases the need for reintubation (So et al 1995, Annibale et al 1994, Chan & Greenough 1993).

Indications for respiratory support by endotracheal tube

An endotracheal tube poses several hazards. In babies with hyaline membrane disease who are 'grunting' (forced expiration against partly closed vocal cords), endotracheal intubation without adequate end expiratory pressure leads to loss of lung volume and rapid hypoxia. Other complications include blockage or malplacement of the tube, inadequate humidification, airway injury, depression of mucociliary clearance, tracheal injury, secondary infection and aspiration, which all may lead to chronic lung disease.

No consensus exists about indications for intermittent positive pressure ventilation (IPPV) by endotracheal tube. Wung initiated nasal continuous positive airway pressure at 5 cmH$_2$O immediately after birth if any chest wall retractions or other signs of respiratory distress were seen, and only started intermittent positive pressure ventilation when $PaCO_2 > 8$ kPa (60 mmHg) (Avery et al 1987). Others adopt earlier intubation with CPAP or IPPV by endotracheal tube.

Controlling gas exchange by mechanical ventilation

Despite the enormous variation in type and severity of neonatal respiratory disorders, specific alterations in ventilator settings often have predictable effects on oxygenation and $PaCO_2$. These are summarized in Tables 5.41 and 5.42.

Table 5.41 Ventilator settings and gas exchange: methods of increasing oxygenation

Maneuver	Probable underlying mechanisms
1. ↗ FiO$_2$	a. ↑ Saturation of alveolar capillary blood b. Relieving hypoxia can decrease pulmonary vascular resistance, reducing extrapulmonary right-to-left shunt through fetal channels
2. Adding CPAP	Maintains lung volume in spontaneously breathing infants with reduced lung compliance

Table 5.41 *Cont'd*

Maneuver	Probable underlying mechanisms
3. ↑ PIP 4. ↑ PEEP 5. ↑ I:E ratio	These maneuvers increase mean airway pressure (MAP), hence lung volume and oxygenation The stiffer the lungs, the greater the MAP needed for optimum lung expansion NB: In mild or improving disease, excessive MAP may cause hypoxia by obstructing the pulmonary circulation (causing right-to-left shunt) and it may also decrease cardiac output
6. Achieving synchronous ventilation	a. Maximizes efficiency of baby's contribution to gas exchange b. ?Minimizes compression of pulmonary circulation during ventilator inflation and consequently reduces right-to-left shunting
7. Correcting hypotension	If there is evidence of hypovolemia (systemic hypotension ± peripheral vasoconstriction), correcting it with an infusion of blood, plasma or an inotrope may reduce extrapulmonary right-to-left shunt, improving pulmonary perfusion and oxygenation without a change in ventilator settings
8. Percutaneous oxygenation	Direct absorption of ambient oxygen by the immature skin (infants < 30 weeks' gestation)
9. Exogenous surfactant	?Decreases alveolar surface tension

Table 5.42 Ventilator settings and gas exchange: methods of decreasing $PaCO_2$

Maneuver	Probable underlying mechanisms
1. Reduce excess CPAP	In a spontaneously breathing baby, excess CPAP a. Decreases compliance and tidal volume b. Obstructs the pulmonary circulation c. Increases the work of breathing
2. ↑ Ventilator rate	Increases minute volume
3. ↑ PIP 4. ↓ PEEP	Increases tidal volume and therefore minute volume
In severe disease, with stiff lungs: 5. ↑ Inspiratory time	If expansion of the chest wall is poor and $PaCO_2$ is elevated, increasing the inspiratory time may improve alveolar ventilation and decrease $PaCO_2$. *Increasing the expiratory time may have the opposite effect*
In mild or improving disease, with compliant lungs: 6. ↑ Expiratory time	Compliant lungs need longer to deflate. If expiratory time is too short, inadvertent PEEP is produced and alveolar ventilation is decreased. Inadvertent PEEP can be reduced by increasing expiratory time.

Mean airway pressure and oxygenation

Herman & Reynolds (1973) showed in infants with severe hyaline membrane disease a linear relationship between mean airway pressure and oxygenation, expressed as the alveolar–arterial oxygen difference (A-adO$_2$) (Fig. 5.19). Improved oxygenation was mainly attributed to improved alveolar inflation with reduced intrapulmonary right-to-left shunt. Increases in (1) peak pressure, (2) inspiratory : expiratory ratio and (3) positive end expiratory pressure were thought to (a) expand collapsed lung units, (b) hold them open longer and (c) prevent their collapse during expiration, respectively. The use of positive end expiratory pressure and high inspiratory : expiratory ratios above 1 : 1 enabled peak pressures to be decreased, which may have reduced mortality from bronchopulmonary dysplasia (Reynolds & Taghizadeh 1974). With stiff lungs in severe hyaline membrane disease, high mean airway pressures had no effect on cardiac output or arterial blood pressure. In milder or improving hyaline membrane disease, lower inspiratory : expiratory ratios and ventilator pressures were recommended, to prevent impaired gas exchange from obstruction of the pulmonary and systemic circulation. Nowadays with improved antenatal and early neonatal care hyaline membrane disease is usually less severe and inspiratory times of 0.75–1.0 s at rates of 20–40/min may increase the risk of pneumothorax in comparison with high frequency positive pressure ventilation using inspiratory times of 0.33–0.5 s at 60 breaths per min (OCTAVE Study Group 1991). Inspiratory times shorter than 0.75–1.0 s therefore seem preferable when compliance is not severely impaired. However, extremely short inspiratory times may achieve insufficient lung inflation. Field et al (1985) found a significant fall in tidal volume at inspiration times under 0.3 s.

Stewart et al (1981) achieved the greatest increase in oxygenation per unit increase in mean airway pressure in hyaline membrane disease by raising positive end expiratory pressure (PEEP). Increases in inspiratory: expiratory ratio and peak inspiratory pressure (PIP) produced smaller increments in oxygenation per unit increase in mean airway pressure. PEEP may prevent alveolar collapse, maintaining the lung on the deflation limb of the pressure–volume curve. In mild disease, it may minimize compression of the pulmonary circulation and extrapulmonary right-to-left shunting.

Minute ventilation, carbon dioxide exchange and inadvertent PEEP

Herman & Reynolds (1973) showed that $PaCO_2$ (a) falls with increasing ventilator rate (increased minute volume), and (b) rises with increases in PEEP (i.e. decreased minute volume). Bartholomew et al (1994) showed that the average effect on tidal volume of a 1 cmH$_2$O change in PEEP was comparable to that of a 2 cmH$_2$O change in PIP in infants with hyaline membrane disease. This probably reflects the triphasic, or sigmoid, shape of the pulmonary pressure–volume curve.

Inadvertent PEEP may cause hypercapnia (Simbruner 1986). It occurs when the ventilator expiration time is too short for adequate deflation before the next inflation is imposed. The pressure within the lungs does not fall as far as the PEEP set on the ventilator, causing unseen or inadvertently elevated PEEP within the lungs. This trapped gas can increase respiratory dead space and compress the pulmonary circulation, occasionally with dangerous consequences (Stenson et al 1995). Inadvertent PEEP is most likely when lung compliance is improving, particularly with elevated airway resistance as in chronic lung disease. Paradoxically, reducing the ventilator rate by lengthening the expiration time may improve gas exchange by allowing more complete expiration. This is not recommended in *severe* hyaline membrane disease as increasing the ventilator expiratory time may reduce the already low lung volume, causing further hypoxia, alveolar hypoventilation and an *increase* in $PaCO_2$.

Humidification and tracheal lavage

Bypassing the upper airway with an endotracheal tube renders a baby dependent on an external source of humidification. Excess humidification causes fluid overload, increases respiratory system resistance and may inactivate surfactant. Inadequate humidification slows mucociliary clearance causing viscid respiratory secretions and may also predispose to pneumothorax and chronic lung disease (Tarnow-Mordi et al 1989). Condensate in the ventilator tubing indicates that gas relative humidity is close to 100% at that point but does not guarantee that the absolute humidity of the gas is well above the minimum International Standard, unless the temperature of the gas at that point exceeds 30.5°C (equivalent to 31 mgH$_2$O/l at 100% relative humidity). Inspired gas temperature or humidity may vary considerably (Tarnow-Mordi et al 1986, O'Hagan et al 1991) and should be measured continuously, as close as possible to the patient's airway.

Endotracheal lavage, suction and physiotherapy

Clearance of secretions by intermittent endotracheal tube lavage and suction reduces respiratory system resistance (Prendiville et al 1986). However, endotracheal suction is associated with hypoxia, bradycardia, and increased blood pressure. The need for routine endotracheal suction has been questioned, particularly in the first 48 h of life when secretions are scant. Randomized trials would be informative (Tarnow-Mordi 1991).

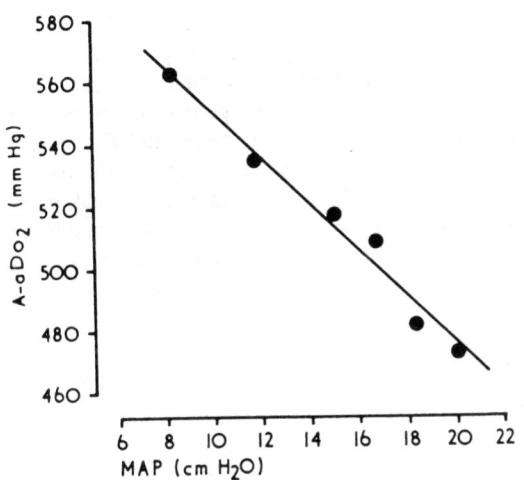

Fig. 5.19 Inverse relationship between mean airway pressure (MAP) and A-adO$_2$ in severe hyaline membrane disease, indicating that MAP is directly proportional to oxygenation. (Reproduced with permission from Herman & Reynolds 1973.)

Additional techniques

Synchronous ventilation

Greenough et al (1987a) investigated the effects of ventilator rates of 30, 60 and 120/min on oxygenation in 32 babies of 25–33 weeks' gestation with hyaline membrane disease, half of whom were paralyzed with pancuronium. Inspiratory : expiratory ratios of 1 : 1 or 1 : 1.2 were used. There was a significant *increase* in oxygenation when the ventilator rate was increased to 120/min compared with rates of 30 and 60/min, but only in the nonparalyzed babies. This increased oxygenation was attributed to the babies' *synchronous respiration* with the ventilator, which could usually be achieved by setting the ventilator at a rate slightly faster than the babies' own spontaneous respiratory rate (Greenough et al 1987b). Similar improvements in oxygenation were seen in synchronous ventilation by South & Morley (1986) and in patient triggered ventilation by Mehta et al (1986) and Greenough & Greenall (1988). Synchronous ventilation may prevent potentially harmful fluctuations in cerebral blood flow velocity (Rennie et al 1987).

Synchronized ventilation is conveniently divided into synchronized intermittent mandatory ventilation (SIMV) and patient triggered ventilation (PTV). Another term for PTV is assist control ventilation. In SIMV, the ventilator rate, inspiratory time and pressures are set by the clinician. The ventilator then divides the minute up into equal blocks of time. In the first part of each time block (trigger window) the ventilator can sense an inspiratory effort and deliver a triggered breath. If it does not, a mandatory breath is delivered later in the time block. There is then a brief refractory phase. Weaning is accomplished as the clinician chooses. The need for a trigger window, a preset inspiratory time and a refractory phase in each time block limits effective SIMV to slower respiratory rates. In PTV all respiratory efforts made by the infant of greater than trigger threshold are rewarded by a ventilator breath. The infant therefore determines the ventilator rate and the clinician the inspiratory time and pressures. A mandatory back-up rate is also set to be delivered in the event of apnea or failure to trigger. Weaning is accomplished by diminishing the pressures. Neither SIMV or PTV has been proved superior for weaning infants from the ventilator (Chan & Greenough 1994a).

Bernstein et al (1994a) and Cleary et al (1995) demonstrated improved tidal volume and gas exchange with synchronized versus conventional ventilation. Govindaswami et al (1993) demonstrated a decrease in the variability of cerebral blood flow velocity on SIMV versus conventional ventilation. Bernstein et al (1994b) demonstrated no advantage to SIMV versus conventional ventilation in terms of mortality or intraventricular hemorrhage in a multicenter randomized study enrolling 306 infants. Fewer infants under 1000 g who received SIMV required supplemental oxygen at 35 weeks postconceptional age. Further trials are needed.

Paralysis

In randomized trials, Greenough et al (1984) demonstrated that infants breathing asynchronously sustained fewer pneumothoraces if paralyzed with pancuronium, and Shaw et al (1993) showed that routine paralysis of all ventilated infants offered no advantage over selective paralysis of those breathing asynchronously. When pancuronium is administered rapid hypoxia can result if ventilation is inadequate. Hypotension has

also been observed. Prolonged neuromuscular blockade is associated with decreased lung compliance (Bhutani et al 1988) and edema.

High frequency ventilation

High frequency ventilation describes any technique of respiratory assistance using ventilator rates of 60/min or more. It can be divided into three major types: high frequency positive pressure ventilation (HFPPV 60–150/min – see OCTAVE Study Group (1991) and previous discussion on synchronous ventilation); high frequency oscillatory ventilation (HFOV 180–3000/min); and high frequency jet ventilation (HFJV 200–600/min).

High frequency oscillatory ventilation. HFOV exploits the remarkable observation that when the airways are subjected to rapidly oscillating pressure at 3–50 Hz with appropriate mean airway pressure, spontaneous respiration stops but respiratory gases diffuse along their concentration gradients sufficiently rapidly to achieve adequate gas exchange. As with conventional ventilation, oxygenation is determined by the mean airway pressure. If lung recruitment is adequate (Froese & Bryan 1987), the FIO_2 is often substantially reduced. The mechanism of carbon dioxide exchange is uncertain and likely to be multifactorial. The tidal volumes are less than the respiratory dead space and carbon dioxide elimination is proportional to the square of the tidal volume rather than directly proportional (Boynton et al 1989). Only about 10% of the pressure oscillation measurable in the ventilator circuit is transmitted to the airspaces. Increases in frequency reduce the volume delivered for a given pressure amplitude (Chan et al 1993). Carbon dioxide elimination is optimal at frequencies around 10 Hz (Chan & Greenough 1994b). In a multicenter randomized controlled trial to compare HFOV with conventional ventilation in 673 preterm infants, HFOV did not reduce mortality or chronic lung disease and was associated with an increase in intracranial hemorrhage and periventricular leukomalacia (HIFI Study Group 1989). The trial has been criticized for failing to ensure adequate lung volume recruitment in the HFOV group (Bryan & Froese 1991) or to stratify infants in both groups by severity of disease (Tarnow-Mordi et al 1994). Further evaluation is needed.

High frequency jet ventilation. The principles of ventilation strategy with HFJV are similar to those with HFOV (Gerstmann et al 1991). With this technique high frequency positive pressure pulses of gas are introduced into the endotracheal tube through a cannula within its lumen. These pulses entrain additional gas through the endotracheal tube. In contrast to HFOV, expiration in HFJV is passively dependent on lung elastic recoil and is promoted by the use of low I : E ratios. Rate, peak pressure and inspiratory time are controlled and tidal volume and mean airway pressure depend on them. The optimum rate for carbon dioxide elimination tends to be lower than with HFOV. Although HFJV has been associated with improved gas exchange in hyaline membrane disease (Carlo et al 1987), adverse outcome was not reduced in a small trial of HFJV versus conventional ventilation (Carlo et al 1990).

Extracorporeal membranous oxygenation (ECMO)

This technique uses cardiopulmonary bypass to allow gas exchange to occur outside the body in an artificial membrane oxygenator. It is used where there is severe respiratory failure as in persistent pulmonary hypertension of the newborn, severe lung disease, or diaphragmatic hernia. Although survival rates after ECMO in severe respiratory failure are high (Glass et al 1989), similar results are reported after conventional ventilation without hyperventilation (Wung et al 1985, Dworetz et al 1989). A trial of ECMO versus conventional ventilation which allocated treatment by a controversial 'play the winner' technique (Bartlett et al 1985) was inconclusive. However, among 190 infants in severe respiratory failure the risk of death or disability at 1 year was reduced by 50% among those randomly allocated to be transferred to an ECMO facility versus those allocated to remain in their local referral center (UK Collaborative ECMO Trial Group 1996).

Pulmonary vasodilators

Pulmonary vasodilators may improve oxygenation where there is extrapulmonary right-to-left shunt secondary to increased pulmonary vascular resistance. *Tolazoline*, the most widely used agent, may also produce systemic vasodilation and hypotension, and should be used while continuously monitoring blood pressure with colloid ready for infusion. Other agents include prostacyclin (PGI_2), glyceryl trinitrate, nitroprusside and magnesium sulfate. No pulmonary vasodilator has ever been shown in controlled trials to reduce mortality or major morbidity.

Inhaled nitric oxide

Vascular smooth muscle relaxation is induced by an endogenous vasodilator previously known as endothelium-derived relaxing factor, now known to be nitric oxide (Ignarro 1989). Inhaled nitric oxide is inactivated by combining with hemoglobin to form methemoglobin in pulmonary capillaries, so its effects can be confined to the lungs. Nitric oxide also reacts with oxygen to form nitrogen dioxide, nitric and nitrous acid raising the issue of toxicity. As US safety regulations recommend that nitrogen dioxide exposure should not exceed 5 p.p.m. in an 8-h period, it is of interest that Miller et al (1994) found that in an infant ventilator circuit, nitric oxide concentrations greater than 80 p.p.m. resulted in nitrogen dioxide levels greater than 5 p.p.m. in the presence of 90% oxygen. Nitric oxide concentrations of less than 70 p.p.m. did not result in excess nitrogen dioxide. In newborn infants with persistent pulmonary hypertension, oxygenation improved with concentrations of inhaled nitric oxide between 5 and 100 p.p.m. (Kinsella et al 1993, Finer et al 1994) but no large randomized studies have assessed its effects on outcome.

Hyperventilation

Hyperventilation to highly unphysiological levels of pH > 7.6 can reverse extrapulmonary right-to-left shunt in severe pulmonary hypertension, but its clinical value is uncertain (Wung et al 1985, Dworetz et al 1989). A similar effect is achieved through infusion of alkali to high pH (Schreiber et al 1986). Both maneuvers may cause cerebral ischemia.

Percutaneous oxygenation

In infants of less than 30 weeks' gestation, the immature skin can absorb therapeutic quantities of oxygen during the first week of life (Cartlidge & Rutter 1988). Management in 95% ambient oxygen can usefully supplement PaO_2 and may allow ventilator pressures to be reduced. However, it is recommended that SaO_2 or intra-arterial oxygen tension is monitored continuously during this treatment because percutaneous oxygenation masks cyanosis and makes transcutaneous PO_2 monitoring unreliable.

Liquid ventilation

Despite advances in treatment a significant number of infants die of respiratory failure. The high surface tension at the air–liquid interface in immature lungs is virtually eliminated if they are filled with liquid. Perfluorocarbon liquid is biologically inert, will not mix with water, has low surface tension and a high solubility for oxygen and carbon dioxide. After filling the lungs completely with perfluorocarbon, compliance and gas exchange improved in lambs (Shaffer et al 1983) and infants with severe hyaline membrane disease (Greenspan et al 1990). Liquid ventilation requires specialized ventilation equipment and the high flow resistance of the liquid in the airways prevents effective spontaneous breathing. An alternative approach, called partial liquid ventilation or perfluorocarbon associated gas exchange (PAGE), is to fill the lungs with perfluorocarbon liquid to FRC only. Conventional tidal gaseous ventilation is then undertaken with standard equipment. Seven infants with severe hyaline membrane disease showed improved oxygenation, carbon dioxide elimination and lung compliance with PAGE (Leach et al 1995). Animal studies suggest that PAGE is compatible with concurrent nitric oxide treatment (Leach et al 1995). This technique must be further evaluated in randomized controlled trials.

The need for more and better controlled trials

Most infants receiving respiratory support still have hyaline membrane disease, which varies considerably in its severity. Other common diagnoses include transient tachypnea of the newborn, apnea of prematurity, pneumonia, birth asphyxia and pulmonary hypertension with persistent fetal circulation, which is often associated with severe meconium aspiration. Very few methods of respiratory support have been tested by controlled trials of adequate size and design which compare mortality and complications among infants specifically stratified by diagnosis, stage and severity of respiratory disease. Because of this, vigorous debate persists about the precise indications and optimum use of even long-established techniques, such as continuous positive airway pressure (CPAP) and intermittent positive pressure ventilation (IPPV) (Ramsden et al 1987). These questions require resolution because, with the rapid introduction of new technologies, there is a danger that relatively simple treatments like these may be replaced by much more expensive and potentially more hazardous ones, for want of proper evaluation.

NEURODEVELOPMENTAL OUTCOME

Apart from death, severe neurodevelopmental disability is the worst outcome associated with prematurity. Since Little's original description of cerebral palsy a link has been established between certain types of spasticity and prematurity. The types of disability seen amongst preterm survivors include spastic diplegia, spastic hemiplegia and quadriplegia with and without intellectual impairment. Other problems include blindness, deafness and severe epilepsy. Minor motor problems, specific learning disorders and attention deficits are commonly recognized amongst

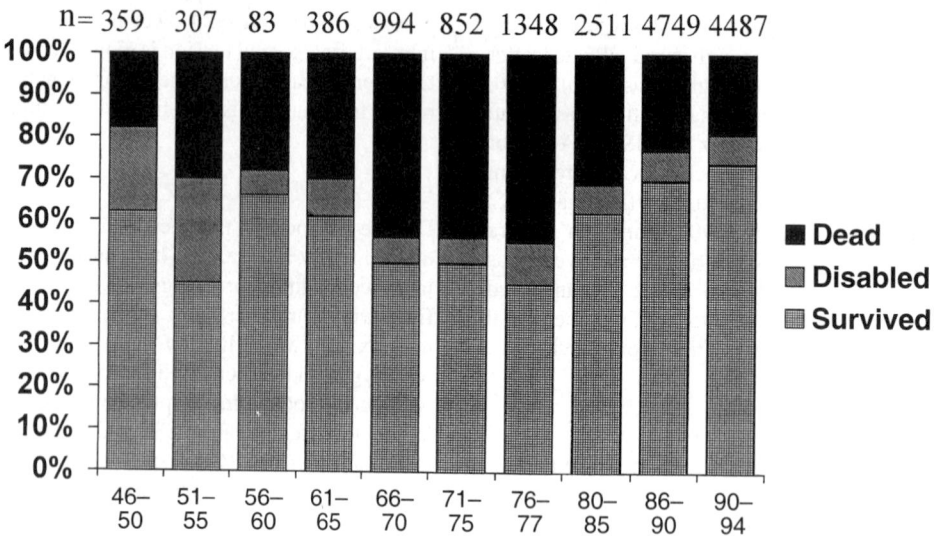

Fig. 5.20 Trends in outcome for VLBW between 1946 and 1994.

school-age survivors. The median prevalence of cerebral palsy in a meta-analysis of 111 studies reporting outcome for very low birthweight (VLBW) survivors was 7.7% (Escobar et al 1991). The median incidence of any disability in VLBW survivors was high at 25% with a positive correlation between the reported incidence of disability and length of follow-up. Follow-up studies from the US report better survival and worse neurodevelopmental outcome than current European studies; the lower incidence of disability and higher mortality in Dutch preterm survivors when compared to those in Oxford, England was thought to reflect the more aggressive Dutch approach to the withdrawal of intensive care (Ens-Dokkum et al 1994). Time trends show that the prevalence of cerebral palsy is increasing, particularly amongst the very low birthweight population. The prevalence of cerebral palsy amongst babies born in the Mersey region between 1966 and 1977 was 1.5 per 1000 live births overall but 15.5 per 1000 live births amongst those born weighing less than 1500 g (Pharoah et al 1987). Subsequently the same group have shown a threefold increase in all types of cerebral palsy for infants of birthweight below 1500 g with a rate of 50 : 1000 (Pharoah et al 1990). This figure is in remarkable agreement with those from the Western Australia register of cerebral palsy, the Scottish low birthweight study and a large geographical study in California (Stanley & Watson 1992, Scottish Low Birthweight Study Group 1992a,b, Cummins et al 1993). Whilst increasing survival means that there has been a net gain of normal survivors amongst the VLBW group over time, these trends and the fact that disabilities are more often multiple in preterm infants can leave no room for complacency. Figure 5.20 updates the summary published by Stewart et al (1981), giving a general overview of VLBW outcome by 5-year time cohorts since 1946. Further information is contained in this chapter reviewing the literature reporting neurodevelopmental outcome by gestational age, 250 g weight groups and the prediction of outcome from neonatal cranial ultrasound studies.

Evaluating the outcome studies

The vast literature reporting the outcome of preterm babies can be a minefield for the unwary reader. The results of outcome studies show a huge variation and there has been little improvement in methodology over time (Aylward et al 1989, Escobar et al 1991). In order to evaluate the studies and to plan better research in future the following guidelines should prove helpful. Further detail is contained in the article by Mutch et al (1989).

Population

Most reports of preterm morbidity are hospital based making it difficult to compare results as referral practices vary widely between units. Birthweight cutoffs are extensively used, perhaps the most frequent being the reporting of the outcome for babies less than 1500 g. Small for dates infants of around 30 weeks' gestation are thus over-represented. Resuscitation of infants who are at the borderline of viability varies so that the number of recorded live births and stillbirths at 23–24 weeks of gestation differs. This affects the denominator used to calculate prevalence rates per number of live births. The ideal study would report results from an entire geographical region and contain information about the outcome of all pregnancies ending between 22 and 32 weeks' gestation.

Missing cases

Tracing the movements of babies is never easy. Frequent changes of surname and address are common and some leave the country of their birth altogether. Work from Newcastle has shown that the last few babies remaining to be found in a follow-up study contain a disproportionate number of handicapped infants (Wariyar & Richmond 1989). The reasons for this discrepancy include the fact that the parents of the handicapped infants are already busy with hospital attendances or that they do not wish to confront the adverse outcome. Studies reporting less than 95% follow-up are likely to be underestimating handicap and an ideal study would have 100% ascertainment. Parental consent for inclusion may become more of a problem in future studies in the UK: refusal often accounts for a large proportion of missing data in current North American studies.

Duration and timing of follow-up

The diagnosis of cerebral palsy cannot be made with any degree of confidence before 2 years, and may not be stable until 5 years or more (Victorian Infant Collaborative Study Group 1995). Late deaths will alter the denominator if the handicap rates are to be reported for survivors rather than for live births, another potential source of difficulty when trying to compare studies. Some report neonatal survival, some survival to discharge, and some survival to the time of late follow-up. There is a tendency to use cranial ultrasound results as a proxy for the more expensive and time-consuming neurodevelopmental assessments; this will underestimate the number of cases and is becoming less accurate as the incidence of large hemorrhages and periventricular leukomalacia continues to reduce.

Definition of disability

This is perhaps the most variable of the many problems with outcome studies. The international classification of impairment, disabilities and handicap contains useful definitions which are listed in Table 5.43. Usually major handicap includes cerebral palsy, severe developmental delay (more than two or three standard deviations below the mean on the particular test used), blindness and deafness. There are differences of opinion regarding inclusion of conditions such as epilepsy and shunted hydrocephalus. The latter can cause impairment without disability, as can a mild hemiplegia. Types of cerebral palsy include spastic, ataxic, dyskinetic (athetoid and dystonic) and hypotonic and can involve a single limb through to quadriplegia. Evans & Alberman (1985) have designed a form for recording details of cerebral palsy which incorporates a scoring system from 0 to 4 where 4 means that no useful function of the limb is possible, and 1 means no significant functional impairment but that there are abnormal neurological signs in the limb. Few groups have enough subjects to allow analysis of outcome according to type of cerebral palsy: Powell et al (1988a,b) have shown different associated antecedent variables for spastic diplegia and hemiplegia in their large cohort, and this group have made the point that important associations may be missed by 'lumping' adverse outcome.

Minor disability, clumsiness, language disorder, school failure and behavior disorder are even more difficult to define and the wide range in the reported incidence between studies reflects this.

Table 5.43   WHO definitions

Impairment
Any loss or abnormality of psychological, physiological or anatomical structure or function: in principle impairments represent disturbances at organ level.

Disability
Any restriction or lack (resulting from an impairment) of ability to perform an activity in the manner or within the range considered normal for a human being. A disability thus reflects the consequence of an impairment in terms of functional performance and activity by an individual.

Handicap
A disadvantage for a given individual resulting from an impairment or disability that limits or prevents the fulfillment of a role that is normal (depending on age, sex and social and cultural factors). Handicap thus reflects interaction with the surroundings and is a difficult outcome to use for comparison as it depends on attitudes within the family and society to disability.

Diagnosis of disability

The tests used to diagnose disability should be reproducible and have been previously evaluated in an appropriate population in order to minimize problems such as interobserver variability. At present there are a large number of tests applied at different ages by people of varying levels of experience and this can severely bias results. Well validated in this respect are the Bayley and Griffiths scales of infant development. Amiel-Tison & Stewart (1989) have tackled the difficulties of uniformity in recording neurological impairment, together with the problems of children who are too disabled to be tested conventionally and those in whom cooperation cannot be obtained. The latter may refuse to be tested because they know they cannot perform the task (Stewart et al 1987) and this in itself may therefore be an important observation.

Control groups

In a cohort descriptive follow-up study of all children below a certain weight there can be no control group. Consideration needs to be given to the inclusion of control subjects such as term infants, however, particularly in view of the known effects of socioeconomic deprivation on the incidence of prematurity. As studies of preterm outcome begin to report school performance, variables such as birth order and social class will become relatively more important factors than they are in the current descriptions of the prevalence of major handicap. There is always an excess of twins and higher multiple births in VLBW cohorts and although some say that the outlook is not different in preterms (Leonard et al 1994) there is increasing evidence that twinning is associated with an increased risk of cerebral palsy.

Outcome related to birthweight, sex and gestational age

That the incidence of handicap increases with decreasing birthweight and gestational age was shown as early as 1956. Most large regional studies reporting the outcome of very low birthweight babies born during the last 50 years record serious disability in less than 10% of the survivors, increasing to 13–25% of affected children when moderate disability is included. The interaction of birthweight and gestational age on survival and disability can be studied by those who have access to large datasets. One approach is to calculate the birthweight ratio, which is the actual birthweight divided by the mean birthweight for the same gestational age (Morley et al 1990). A birthweight ratio of 0.8 corresponds to the 10th centile. This is a statistically useful tool because the number generated is a normally distributed continuous variable. In a cohort of 429 very low birthweight infants Morley and her colleagues were unable to show any association between birthweight ratio and neurodevelopmental outcome at 18 months, but Cooke (1994) reported that his population was skewed to the right, suggesting a higher mortality for very preterm growth retarded infants. Synnes et al (1994) showed either a U-shaped curve or a negative correlation between mortality and weight at each gestational age between 23 and 26 weeks. A collaborative network in the USA has presented very valuable information based on a large recent cohort (1991–92) which allow the calculation of mortality risk by sex, birthweight and gestational age (Fanaroff et al 1995). Male sex has been associated with a doubling of the risk of death and/or handicap in almost every study which has included sex as a factor in logistic regression analysis (Brothwood et al 1986, Cooke 1993, Rennie et al 1996).

Outcome related to gestational age

22–23 weeks. Survival at 22 weeks' gestation has been claimed (Nishida 1993). At 23 weeks the chance of a handicapped survivor outweighs that of a normal survivor, and many would argue that this means the parents should be fully informed of the experimental nature of intensive care at these low gestations (Rennie 1996).

24 weeks. Since the last edition of this book the survival rate for 24-week gestation infants has improved from virtually zero to 25% (Fig. 5.21, Table 5.44). All the infants born at 24 weeks' gestation in Holland during 1983 died (Van Zeben et al 1989), and only one baby survived in the same year in the Northern region of England (Wariyar et al 1989a). Hack & Fanaroff (1989) report a 15% survival between 1982 and 1988 but give no information about the quality of life for the survivors. Cooke (1988) reporting the outcome for 31 infants admitted to the Mersey Regional Intensive Care Unit between 1980 and 1985 found three intact survivors from a total of 31. From his own unit he now reports over 30% survival (Cooke 1993). Recent North American studies claim survival of around 50% for this group, and we found a

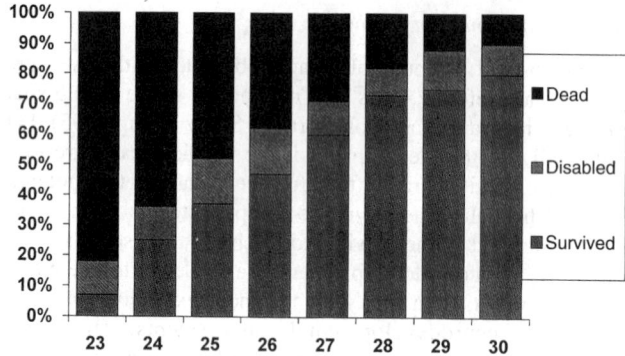

Fig. 5.21   Outcome by gestational age.

similar survival rate in Cambridge during the late 1980s (Synnes et al 1994, Fanaroff et al 1995, Table 5.44). At least 30% of the survivors have a significant disability (Table 5.45), and in addition many more children have school failure. The confidence intervals for prediction of outcome at this gestation are wide because the numbers followed are still small. The disabled and nondisabled survivors are just about in balance at 24 weeks, with the trend shifting in favor of intact survival.

Table 5.44   Summary of published literature reporting survival by gestational age: babies born 1977–1993

Place	Year of birth	23 weeks	24 weeks	25 weeks	26 weeks	27 weeks	28 weeks	29 weeks	30 weeks	Reference
Royal Women's, Melbourne, Australia	1977–1982		2/27	11/54	36/80	47/67	76/98			Kitchen et al 1985
Victoria, Australia	1977–1986	2/31	13/40	19/61	44/78	71/106	86/119	90/99	83/91	Yu et al 1986, 1992
Ontario, Canada	1979–1982	1/7	9/23	28/44	34/45	45/60	71/88			Milligan et al 1984
Nova Scotia, Canada	1980–1982	0/7	1/10	5/13	6/13	13/17				Nwaesi et al 1987
Liverpool, UK	1982–1993				80/180	122/191	205/277			Cooke 1994
		7/27	30/84	62/134						Cooke 1996
Ontario, Canada	1982–1987	12/55	49/114	109/175	152/223					Whyte et al 1993
Cleveland, USA	1982–1988	3/37	8/51	42/80	52/82	59/82				Hack & Fanaroff 1989
Maine, USA	1982–1992	31/114*		57/100	62/96	48/60	38/44	15/15		Philip 1995
Haifa, Israel	1982–1986		5/40	2/27	8/19	23/33	37/50			Weissman et al 1989
Northern Region, UK	1983		2/19	7/22	13/27	15/30	28/30	38/46	63/76	Wariyar et al 1989a,b
Holland	1983	0/19*		7/48	29/77	37/67	57/85	86/124	107/130	Verloove-Vanhorick et al 1986, Veen et al 1991
Vancouver, Canada	1983–1989	9/32	46/87	88/143	111/170	144/188	192/222			Synnes et al 1994
Oxford, UK	1984–1986	5/60*		10/45	32/66	44/69	84/102			Johnson et al 1993
Copenhagen, Denmark	1984–1987		0/3	7/8	18/40					Eg-Andersen 1989
Tokyo, Japan	1984–1990	3/7	14/15	17/20	21/25					Nishida 1993
Scotland, UK	1985	0/6	1/21	6/32	29/61	31/64	62/78			Working Group on the VLBW Infant 1990
Leiden, Holland	1985–1987		3/4	7/14	6/10					Ruys et al 1989
Dusseldorf, Germany	1986	0/2	0/3	2/5	3/17	11/22	20/31			Working Group on the VLBW Infant 1990
North Carolina, USA	1986–1988		1/10	9/25	24/30					Wood et al 1989

Table 5.44 *Cont'd*

Place	Year of birth	23 weeks	24 weeks	25 weeks	26 weeks	27 weeks	28 weeks	29 weeks	30 weeks	Reference
Minneapolis, USA	1986–1990	12/32	28/75	54/90	72/113					Ferrara et al 1994
Cambridge, UK	1985–1992	2/9	13/28	26/55	43/80	72/116	95/110	124/140		Unpublished
Baltimore, USA	1988–1991	6/40	19/34	31/39						Allen et al 1993
Detroit, USA	1988–1991	2/28	13/40	11/44	35/62					Holtrop et al 1994
North Carolina, USA	1989–1991	0/21	5/11	14/22	18/25					Katz & Bose 1993
NICHD†, USA	1991–1992	58/292	134/280	252/361	363/438	400/488	490/545	495/538	440/473	Fanaroff et al 1995
Trent Region, UK	1991–1993	1/37	27/95	38/104	73/132					Bohin et al 1995
TOTALS		118/670	428/1174	921/1765	1364/2189	1182/1660	1541/1879	848/962	693/770	
%		18%	36%	52%	62%	71%	82%	88%	90%	
95% CI		(15–20)	(34–39)	(50–54)	(60–64)	(69–73)	(80–84)	(86–90)	(88–92)	

* Not included in totals.
† National Institute of Child Health and Development.

Table 5.45 Summary of the number of handicapped children/total survivors by gestational age: babies born late 1970s to early 1990s

Place	Year of birth	23 weeks	24 weeks	25 weeks	26 weeks	27 weeks	28 weeks	29 weeks	30 weeks	Reference
Queen's, Melbourne	1977–1986	1/2	2/13	5/11	9/35					Yu et al 1986, 1992
Royal Women's, Melbourne	1977–1982		1/2	3/6	3/21					Kitchen et al 1985
Ontario, Canada	1979–1982	0/1	3/8	4/27	3/27					Milligan et al 1984
Nova Scotia, Canada			0/1	3/5	0/6					Nwaesi et al 1987
Liverpool, UK	1980–1993		3/8	12/46	16/73	10/122	10/205			Cooke 1994
Haifa, Israel	1982–1986		2/5	1/2	2/8	1/20	2/30			Weissman et al 1989
Northern Region, UK	1983		0/1	2/6	2/12	3/15	2/28	2/38	3/63	Wariyar et al 1989a,b
Holland	1983					3/37	5/57	15/86	14/107	Veen et al 1991
Vancouver, Canada	1983–1989	6/9	16/43	25/77						Synnes et al 1994
Oxford, UK	1984–1986		4/5*	6/9	12/31	13/44	20/84			Johnson et al 1993
Copenhagen, Denmark	1984–1987			2/7	2/18					Eg-Andersen 1989
Minneapolis, USA	1986–1990	7/12	8/28	16/54	23/72					Ferrara et al 1994
Cambridge, UK	1985–1992	2/2	3/13	8/27	10/43	17/72	10/71	20/83		Unpublished
Leiden, Holland	1985–1987		2/3	0/7	2/6					Ruys et al 1989
TOTALS		16/26	39/125	82/278	79/331	62/408	68/604	42/288	25/228	
%		62%	31%	30%	24%	15%	11%	15%	11%	
95% CI		(41–80)	(23–39)	(24–35)	(20–29)	(12–19)	(9–14)	(11–19)	(7–15)	

* Not included in totals.

25–28 weeks. For the baby born between 25 and 28 weeks' gestation the risk of severe disability in survivors falls from about 25% to about 13% (Table 5.45). Perhaps surprisingly the risk of disability does not decrease markedly with increasing gestational age. The risk of dying correlates better with the degree of immaturity. Figure 5.21 expresses the information from the studies which report outcome related to gestational age. From this it can be seen that the chance of taking home a normal survivor (providing the infant survives long enough to be admitted to an intensive care unit) increases from 8% at 23 weeks through 45% at 26 weeks to 72% at 28 weeks. This chance increases to about 80% at 30 weeks and above.

Very few studies have addressed the problem of predicting outcome prior to delivery. This is important as a significant number of very preterm babies will die during delivery or cannot be resuscitated. More information about the mother's chance of taking home a normal baby, which can be used to counsel her and to advise her obstetrician so that he or she can make an informed choice about the timing and mode of delivery is essential. Unfortunately at present such decisions have to be taken using very little information as there was no legal requirement to register stillborn deliveries below 28 weeks' gestation until 1992. Wariyar et al (1989b) have shown that neonatal death represents only a small portion of fetal loss at low gestational ages, and that overall between 24 and 31 weeks' gestation 25% of deaths occurred antepartum or intrapartum. Intrapartum deaths accounted for only 5% of loss, meaning that the risks presented above can be helpful once the mother is established in labor with a live fetus.

Summary

In summary, whilst it is generally true that survival increases and the percentage risk of handicap remains the same as pregnancy advances the accruing data shows some gradation of risk (Table 5.45). There are still insufficient good quality national studies on which to base important decisions. These data provide no justification for failure to offer intensive care at 25 or 26 weeks, and the contrast with the figures presented in the last edition show that this is still a moving target.

Outcome related to birthweight

Figure 5.22 and Table 5.46 shows the results from 13 large studies

Percentage survival

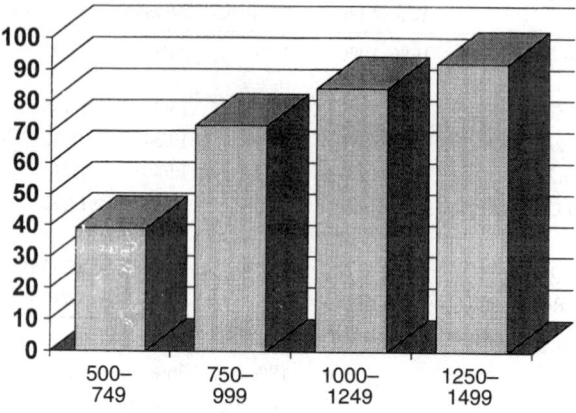

Fig. 5.22   Outcome by 250-g birthweight groups.

reporting the current mortality for babies by 250 g birthweight groups. Not all these studies followed all the children; preterm babies born in The Netherlands during 1983 have been extensively studied (Van Zeben et al 1989, Verloove-Vanhorick et

Table 5.46   Survivors by 250 g weight cohort, VLBW babies born in the 1980s and 1990s

Place	Year of birth	500–749 g	750–999 g	1000–1249 g	1250–1499 g	Reference
Newfoundland, Canada	1980–1981	2/23	13/32	33/46	34/40	Johnson et al 1987
Cambridge, UK	1985–1992	29/69	122/185	199/249	262/292	Personal observation
Toronto, Canada	1980–1987	91/223	239/339	240/398	356/397	Wojtulewicz et al 1993
Maine, USA	1982–1985	25/70	60/97	87/99	98/106	Philip 1995
Maine, USA	1986–1989	24/71	53/80	106/121	106/113	Philip 1995
NIH* Centers, USA	1987–1988	108/349	252/382	419/480	514/554	Hack et al 1991
Maine, USA	1990–1991	21/35	51/57	58/62	53/54	Philip 1995
Neonatal Network, USA	1989–1990	128/329	325/423	447/498	515/554	Hack et al 1995
Neonatal Network, USA	1991–1992	382/869	785/982	1060/1153	1211/1275	Fanaroff et al 1995
Alberta, Canada	1990	24/63	61/72	87/106		Robertson et al 1994
Holland	1983	16/42	80/151	173/227	188/221	Verloove-Vanhorick et al 1988
Alberta, Canada	1988–1989	27/66	70/109	100/116		Robertson et al 1992
Victoria, Australia	1985–1987	212/560†				VICS 1991
Ontario, Canada	1981–1984	122/266†				Saigal et al 1989
Scotland, UK	1984	78/204†		327/398†		Scottish LBW Study Group 1992a,b
TOTAL		877/2209	2111/2909	3009/3555	3337/3606	
%		39%	72%	84%	92%	
CI%		(37–41)	(70–74)	(83–85)	(91–93)	
Handicapped infants by survivors						
Newfoundland, Canada	1980–1981	1/2	2/13	1/33	4/34	Johnson et al 1987
Cambridge, UK	1985–1992	7/29	25/95	24/149	35/181	Personal observation
Toronto, Canada	1980–1987	16/87	28/226	25/306	18/297	Wojtulewicz et al 1993
Alberta, Canada	1990	3/20	6/57	5/84		Robertson et al 1994
Alberta, Canada	1988–1989	7/27	9/70	14/100		Robertson et al 1992
Victoria, Australia	1985–1987	64/212				VICS 1991
Ontario, Canada	1981–1984	21/122				Saigal et al 1989
Scotland, UK	1984	8/60		14/298		Scottish LBW Study Group 1992a,b

* National Institute of Health
† Not included in the totals.

al 1988, Ruys et al 1989, Veen et al 1991). A 97.4% follow-up was achieved at 2 and 5 years. Major handicap was diagnosed when severe retardation or a severe neurological disorder was present, and the definition included children with sensory defects and psychosocial problems which seemed likely to prevent the child from attending normal school. 82% of the surviving preterm children had no handicap, 11% had minor handicap and 6% a major handicap. Increasingly studies report outcome by gestational age rather than birthweight and more emphasis has been given to these data than in the previous edition in view of the need for antenatal counseling.

Sensory handicap

In addition to the cerebral palsy rate of about 7% in very low birthweight infant survivors there are a significant number of visually impaired children as a consequence of retinopathy of prematurity. Table 5.47 gives the number of blind children diagnosed in several follow-up studies. In addition many more have severe myopia: a quarter of the children followed by Saigal et al (1990) were wearing prescription glasses. Deafness afflicts slightly fewer children but is still a problem in about 1%. Early diagnosis by screening can help limit the handicap resulting from this latter disability.

Minor handicaps and school failure

Follow-up to school age and beyond has been reported for several cohorts of ex-preterm children. More of the children are left-handed, which has been suggested as a possible risk factor for a later risk of schizophrenia. More are hyperactive with a short attention span and thus require special help at school (Robertson et al 1990, Pharoah et al 1994). Calame et al (1986), in a population-based controlled study, found 22% of VLBW babies were failing at school. The meta-analysis of Aylward et al (1989) showed a mean reduction of 6 points in IQ when disabled survivors were excluded. These results are similar to those of Saigal et al (1991), who found that two-thirds of a < 1 kg cohort were performing adequately at school but very few children were performing in the high range. There is a considerable overlap between behavioral disorders, neurodevelopmental abnormalities and school problems – 'clumsiness' may be a marker for this type of dysfunction. More (14%) Finnish low birthweight children born in 1966 than controls (6%) were educationally subnormal at the age of 14, but when the disabled survivors were excluded similar numbers succeeded in higher education (Olsen et al 1994).

Table 5.47 Visual handicap in survivors

Number blind	Number followed	Cohort defined as	Reference
7	611	< 1500 g	Scottish LBW Study 1992a
5	122	< 1000 g	Saigal et al 1989
8	113	< 1000 g	Saigal et al 1991
6	197	< 1250 g	Robertson et al 1992
2	143	< 1250 g	Robertson et al 1994
9	212	< 1000 g	VICS 1991

Outcome related to cranial ultrasound appearance

Cohort screening of asymptomatic VLBW infants with cranial ultrasound has uncovered a high incidence of lesions involving the periventricular zone. Although damage to premyelin cells abundant in this region provides a convenient explanation for the high prevalence of cerebral palsy, a causal relationship remains to be proven. Cysts in the parenchyma and cerebral atrophy indicate loss of white matter and are the strongest predictors yet found for cerebral palsy (Paneth et al 1994, Pinto-Martin et al 1995). Delayed myelination has been confirmed with later MRI studies, suggesting that the cysts are markers of even more diffuse injury to oligodendroglia (van de Bor et al 1989, 1992, Guit et al 1990, De Vries et al 1993). Most studies are in remarkable agreement, showing a fivefold increase in the risk of cerebral palsy following ultrasound diagnosis of any parenchymal lesion, and a 15-fold increase in the presence of bilateral occipital periventricular leukomalacia. Accumulated experience is still relatively meager, however, and the predictions have wide confidence intervals due to the small numbers of cases. Prediction of learning difficulties, which in some cases may be due to lesser degrees of white matter damage, is still imprecise (Levene et al 1992). Visual handicap can be accurately predicted from ultrasound abnormalities (Hungerford et al 1986, Scher et al 1989, Weisglas-Kuperus et al 1993, Eken et al 1994, Pike et al 1994).

White matter damage carries a high probability of cerebral palsy but by no means all cases in VLBW survivors have early ultrasound abnormalities. All but 7 of 45 children with cerebral palsy had periventricular cysts or echodensity detected in the neonatal period, as did 16 of 18 preterm cerebral palsied children in Oxford (Graziani et al 1992a,b, Murphy et al 1996). Prolonged artificial ventilation for bronchopulmonary dysplasia may be a factor in those without obvious intracranial pathology (Wheater & Rennie 1994, Pinto-Martin et al 1995). Inadequate or incorrect nutrition at a critical period may be another (Lucas et al 1990). A normal scan is not therefore a guarantee of a normal outcome, although the chances are about 90% (Ng & Dear 1990).

Normal ultrasound scan

The outcome of over 3500 preterm infants enrolled in 18 studies has now been reported: over 2000 of these infants had a normal scan and of these 89% were normal at follow-up (Rennie 1997). The risk of a significant disability is very small for a preterm infant who has a normal cranial ultrasound scan in the neonatal period, particularly if this is repeated before discharge. Only 128 of these children had a major handicap (6% : 95% confidence intervals from 5 to 7).

Germinal matrix hemorrhage, subependymal hemorrhage

There is consistent agreement that the appearance of increased echodensity in the region of the germinal matrix capillary bed carries no increased risk of adverse outcome (Levene 1990). This is also true for intraventricular hemorrhage which is not associated with ventricular enlargement.

Ventricular dilation and progressive hydrocephalus

The natural history of ventriculomegaly secondary to the presence of blood in the ventricular cavity in VLBW infants is that about 50% will progress to require a ventriculoperitoneal (VP) shunt insertion and the remainder will arrest or regress. Attempts at preventing the progression by early cerebrospinal fluid drainage have proved unsuccessful (Ventriculomegaly Trial Group 1990). Many of these infants have associated parenchymal lesions of the brain making the assessment of risk due to persistent dilation alone very difficult. Most of the 127 infants with ventriculomegaly followed in the aforementioned large collaborative study had a poor outcome: only 11 of 112 were normal at 30 months (Ventriculomegaly Trial Group 1994).

The outcome for 54 babies requiring VP shunt insertion was reported by Cooke (1987b). 50% had an adverse outcome, the major determinants of which were the presence of a parenchymal lesion or the occurrence of fits in the neonatal period.

Noncavitating transient parenchymal echodensity

This is perhaps the most variable of the ultrasound diagnoses discussed. The incidence with which a 'flare' or 'blush' is seen in the parenchyma surrounding the ventricle varies widely with the observer and the frequency of scanning. Graham et al (1987) described a slightly increased risk related to a flare which persisted for 2 weeks compared to a normal ultrasound scan (8%). Appleton et al (1990) found handicap in 4 of 15 (26%) survivors who had 'isolated and transient' intracerebral flares seen with ultrasound during the neonatal period. This lesion may not be completely benign but at the time of writing too few studies have accurately recorded this appearance to enable assessment of risk.

Persistent parenchymal echodensities and porencephalic cysts

A single large echodense area in the parenchyma of the brain may be the end result of one or several pathological events including venous infarction, secondary hemorrhage into an ischemic area or a primary hemorrhagic event due to transmission of a hypertensive peak or release of vasoactive substances. Large hemorrhages into the brain often cause death in VLBW infants so the number of survivors with this diagnosis is small. However, the overall risk of major neurodevelopmental handicap of 75% is the best estimate that can be given until more consensus regarding definition of diagnosis is reached.

Large parenchymal lesions often cavitate to form parenchymal cysts: these are associated with a similar risk of handicap of about 83%. As expected this abnormality is usually correlated with a hemiplegia rather than spastic diplegia. Parenchymal lesions predict motor outcome better than cognitive outcome and from the studies completed so far periventricular leukomalacia is more likely to be associated with a cognitive and motor defect than a parenchymal hemorrhagic lesion or porencephalic cyst (Costello et al 1988).

Periventricular leukomalacia

There is no doubt that cystic periventricular leukomalacia is the most powerful predictor of cerebral palsy amongst the neonatal cranial ultrasound lesions so far described. In many cohort follow-up studies almost all the cases of cerebral palsy had bilateral occipital leukomalacia in the neonatal period (Graham et al 1987, Pidcock et al 1990). Cysts involving more than one zone have a particularly poor prognosis (Shortland et al 1988). Earlier studies, reporting an association between ventricular dilation and adverse outcome probably included some undiagnosed cases of periventricular leukomalacia owing to poor resolution of the older, 5 MHz scanheads. Single cysts and cysts confined to the frontal region have a better outcome than multiple bilateral occipital cysts, where the outlook is universally dismal. Too few studies have reported the outcome of anterior or central cysts to make it possible to give a confident prediction of a good outcome, although most of the reported survivors with single unilateral cysts or cysts confined to the frontal zone are normal at follow-up (Graham et al 1987, Shortland et al 1988, Fazzi et al 1992, Fawer & Calame 1991).

NEONATAL DEATH

Although neonatal deaths have become steadily less common, they are still frequent enough both on the labor ward and on the neonatal unit for consideration of best management to be important. PICUs have developed to rescue preterm and sick infants but there is still a steady trickle of deaths in a neonatal unit from congenital abnormality and the problems occurring in the very immature baby. With all formal nursing and medical training geared to rescue, the death of the patient is often regarded as failure. If it is an occasional event, a neonatal death may be rapidly 'set aside', but in a referral unit the frequency and regularity means that such events cannot be easily avoided. The emotional load of guilt and depression occurring with frequent deaths on a unit almost certainly plays a part in the high turnover of nursing staff and the incidence of 'burn out' in physicians. In the arena of neonatal intensive care, perinatal mortality meetings and more universally perinatal mortality statistics, highlight the unsatisfactory nature of death, yet many will be inevitable.

Parental grief

The grief of the parents after a neonatal death seems independent of the size of the offspring. Such grief is present even when the infant is nonviable or lives for only a very short time. It has also been shown that parents go through an identical reaction after a stillbirth. Cullberg in 1972 showed that the failure of a mother to come to terms with a perinatal death could lead to a very high incidence of emotional problems. Over 30% of mothers in his study had overt psychiatric problems in the 2 years after such an event. It was the recognition that psychiatric sequelae could be considerably reduced by parents touching their infants before and after death that led to an acknowledgment that the management of death is as important as the rescue of life.

The death

The death of a baby in the neonatal unit is a very undignified event for the baby and the family, especially when 'rescue therapy' is applied until the last moment. It is difficult for the parents to express their true emotions in the intensive care unit where staff are busy with other critically ill patients. It is difficult for staff to cope on the one hand with the rescue care for some patients and still provide sensitivity for grieving parents in the same nursery, and it is particularly difficult for parents of other babies in a unit with an open visiting policy. The emphasis in neonatal death must be changed from a medical failure which must be rapidly forgotten to an event, tragic indeed, but in which the parents are if at all possible closely involved. Deaths in a neonatal unit should occur, if possible, with the parents present and life support can often be withdrawn with the baby in the mother's or father's arms. Thus in many instances the time of death is itself organized for the benefit of the parents. Death then becomes a reality and with this involvement parents may feel, in retrospect, that they have done their best for their infants by allowing death to occur in a dignified way in the presence of love and company. In an attempt to dissociate death from the urgency of the intensive care unit it is helpful to set aside for the parents a room in the unit which can be used for terminal care. This room should be less clinical than the main nurseries with wallpaper, curtains, a rug and easy chairs. Full supportive care may still be given but in this setting the parents will be more able to supply care of the hospice type for their infant's last hours or sometimes days and will more easily be able to come to terms with the impending death. The availability of a special room allows extended families to be involved in culturally important ritual. During the terminal period a senior member of the nursing and medical staff must be available to provide continuity and it must be made clear to the parents that someone will always be present unless they wish otherwise. The cultural and religious background of the families must be acknowledged so that a flexible and individual approach can be developed. Discussions early on with the parents should elaborate their religious beliefs and standpoints and outside support from a priest, mullah, rabbi, etc. should be encouraged if indicated. The introduction of this support at an early stage in a critically ill infant is important as it allows more constructive relationships to develop than when the meeting is for the baptism of a terminally ill infant. In Christian families hospital chaplains and social workers can be actively involved with the family. The presence of young siblings can enrich the feeling of family togetherness at this time of grief and is unlikely to damage the siblings. Ritual is important. If an emergency baptism is required this should be memorable with a proper silver christening bowl (rather than a plastic galley pot) to facilitate baptism with meaning and dignity. I believe it is important to *suggest* to parents that they might like to hold or groom their dead infant. This is usually met with agitation and a certain degree of horror, particularly by European parents, but after a short time many mothers will request such involvement. In some instances parents have left the hospital to obtain their own baby clothes in which to dress their infant in the laying out process. Photographs of the infant will usually have been taken during life but if the life span has been short it is suggested that pictures of the dead infant are taken, often in the parents' arms. Frequently the baby can be specially clothed to enable a better photograph for remembrance to be taken than the ones in life, with evidence of intensive care support. The neonatal unit can provide the parents with a bereavement folder which combines advice and information (to help them at this time) with mementos of their baby (lock of hair, name band, hand and foot prints, etc.).

The immediate aftermath of death (SANDS 1986)

Their baby's death is an intensely private and personal experience for all parents. Many will wish to follow the customs of their own culture or the rights of their own particular religion and these wishes should be respected. It is important that no assumptions are made. It may be helpful to ask parents as sensitively and gently as possible to explain their needs. If language problems make this or any other discussion with parents difficult every effort should be made to find an appropriate and skilled interpreter. Parents who do have a specific religious commitment may want to make contact with their minister, priest or other religious leader and he or she will probably advise them about their baby's funeral as well as provide support and help. Some parents who do not hold any particular religious belief will still find comfort in holding a simple ceremony in the hospital, perhaps in the hospital chapel with their families and the nursing and medical staff involved in the care of their infant taking part. This may be suggested bearing in mind that it is not appropriate for all parents. Parents will inevitably be bewildered by a neonatal death. It may be their first experience of losing a close relative and sensitivity is required by staff at all stages.

Autopsy in the UK

The parents themselves may request an autopsy. If they make such a request it should always be fulfilled. The autopsy may be necessary because the cause of death is unclear. In this case a coroner (or in Scotland, a procurator fiscal) will be involved because the medical practitioner is unable to issue a death certificate of the medical cause of death. In this situation it is not open to the parents to withhold their consent but parents can withhold their consent if the medical practitioner is prepared to put a cause of death on the death certificate. I believe that all babies should have an autopsy independent of whether the cause of death is apparently known. I believe this because:

1. In 25% of autopsies further information is discovered which has a direct bearing on the counseling of the parents for the future (Porter & Keeling 1987).
2. It is important for the medical staff to know that their diagnosis has been accurate. It is only in this way that medical science can progress.
3. At some stage in the future it is not uncommon that parents will have anxieties that something went undiscovered in their baby and that this led to the death.

Where the parents consent is necessary, it is highly desirable that they can give their consent freely. An honest and unhurried approach to parents by consultant or senior resident (not a junior staff member), explaining the reasons for an autopsy and what it involves, will help them to reach a decision. Parents will also feel more comfortable if the request is made as a normal rather than an exceptional procedure. Although the consent of only one parent is required by law, it is advisable that whenever possible parents should be asked to sign the consent form together. A duplicate copy of the consent form should be given to the parents to keep. It will help parents to make their decision if they are given clear information about the following:

1. Why it is thought an autopsy is necessary and why therefore their consent is being sought. Although many parents wish to be given the reason for their baby's death, many also find the thought of an autopsy very distressing. It is important that they can feel their baby is still theirs and not becoming a hospital specimen.
2. The possible outcome of the examination. While it should be explained that an autopsy can provide a definite cause of death, parents should also be warned that an indecisive result is possible.
3. Where, when and by whom the autopsy will be performed. Parents are also likely to want information and reassurance about the whereabouts of and their access to their baby and, if the

autopsy is to be performed at another hospital, the body should not be removed to that hospital until the day of the autopsy and should be returned as quickly as possible after the examination.

4. When, to whom and how the results of the autopsy will be made available. If you are not prepared to transmit the full information to the parents you should not be doing an autopsy.

Most parents feel anxious about giving their consent to an autopsy and need reassurance. A particular fear is the damage which will be done to their baby. With good practice, by the pathologist (who can be introduced to the parents), it is possible for the baby to be restored and carefully dressed so as to be acceptable for the parents to see again before the funeral. If the parents are to hold their infant following the autopsy, they should be warned that he or she will be lightweight as in most cases the brain will be removed for later processing. It may also be suggested that the parents might like to provide clothes including a bonnet for the baby to be dressed in after the autopsy or the parents may prefer a funeral director to prepare the baby for them.

The results of an autopsy are anxiously awaited by most parents and there should be a minimum of delay in providing parents not only with the results but also with the opportunity to discuss them fully. I believe that the full autopsy report should be sent to the parents with an appointment shortly after so that they can bring it and discuss it fully with the pediatrician involved. In this way they have both written information and the access to a pediatrician to discuss all the implications. If necessary the results can be discussed also with an obstetrician. If an autopsy shows the baby's death to be the result of a genetic disorder, parents should be offered the opportunity for later genetic counseling.

Certification and registration procedures in the UK

When a baby is born alive and subsequently dies, irrespective of the gestation or the duration of life, the medical practitioner who attended the baby is required by law to issue a medical certificate giving the cause of death. This certificate is required to enable the death to be registered. If the cause of death is not immediately apparent the medical practitioner may have to report the death to the coroner (or in Scotland, a procurator fiscal). The law requires that all births and deaths be notified to the registrar of births and deaths. It is best if parents can deal with registration themselves and *both together* and this is necessary where the couple are unmarried and wish both parents' names entered on the certificate. The medical practitioner who attended the baby during his or her last illness will issue a medical certificate giving the cause of death. This certificate must be produced to the registrar of births and deaths within 5 days of the baby's death (8 days in Scotland). The registrar will issue a green certificate after registration (the certificate for disposal) to permit burial or cremation. This certificate is required before the funeral can take place. It is free of charge. The registrar will also issue, on request, a copy of a certified entry (a death certificate) currently priced at £7.00. It is helpful if parents are told in advance that this certificate is available since to many parents it is a valuable memento of their baby. Parents should be told in advance when registering a baby's death that the registrar can enter the baby's forename as well as the surname if they so wish. This may be particularly important for those parents where the baby died soon after birth, as they can then give some thought to the naming of the child, before registering the death.

'Death grants' have now been abolished in the UK, but parents can apply to the Department of Social Security for a grant or loan to cover the funeral expenses. In Scotland, the health board will meet the funeral costs for stillborn babies and terminations.

The funeral in the UK

It is the parents' choice whether they wish to arrange a funeral privately or to accept a health authority's offer to arrange a funeral on their behalf, though the latter will only happen if the infant is stillborn or lives for only a very short time after birth. Ceremonies can take many different forms and may be religious or nonreligious. The certificate of disposal (Form 14) issued after registration is needed by the undertaker before a cremation can take place but is not needed for a burial. It should be handed to the funeral director or if the parents have asked the hospital to take responsibility for the funeral, to the hospital. The funeral director involved will complete all necessary documentation according to the kind of funeral requested. It is also the parents' choice whether their baby is buried or cremated. The cremation of a baby leaves no remains whatsoever (ashes) and the parents should be aware of this. A baby cannot be cremated without the parents' formal consent. If the funeral is privately arranged the funeral director will organize all steps in conjunction with the parents. If on the other hand the parents wish for a hospital contract funeral, they must be aware that there may be some emotional risks in accepting this option. If there is any anxiety about this the parents can always contact the British Institute of Funeral Directors or the Stillbirth and Neonatal Death Society (SANDS).

Graves, memorials and remembrance

Depending on the funeral that the parents opt for, the baby may be buried with other babies in a common grave though this practice is becoming less common. Many parents find it comforting to know that their baby is buried with other babies but for others this is distressing and sometimes it takes a while before the grave is full (usually no more than 10 babies should be buried in one grave). Most parents accept a multiple grave so long as they are told about it in advance and do not find out about it when it is too late to consider alternatives. The common grave should be located in a special children's area of a cemetery with a general memorial stone. Parents should be warned that unless they purchase exclusive right to burial, they do not have the right to erect any kind of memorial of their own. If the parents buy exclusive right of burial they can mark their baby's grave with a memorial provided that it complies with local regulations. All crematoria and some cemeteries have a book of remembrance for individual entries. Many specialist neonatal units also have a book of remembrance for infants dying in their units. This book may be located on the neonatal unit or in the hospital chapel. A full page can be allocated to each baby with a personal inscription designed by the parents. This can be made in copperplate writing. The parents can then see the book at any time by arrangement with the hospital chaplain or neonatal unit staff.

Late bereavement counseling and support

It is now accepted that the aftercare of the parents and siblings is important for subsequent emotional well-being. The parents should be seen several times after the death of their infant. On the first occasion, usually on the day of death, sympathy is shown for the parents' situation. Explanation, I believe, is inappropriate at this stage and intrudes into the grief. Over the next few days necessary formalities have to be completed and this can be a bewildering time. The parents need to be seen on the day after the death to explain what has to be done. If the mother is mobile (that is, not just postoperative after a Cesarean section) it is appropriate to encourage both parents to complete the formalities together rather than the man take on an organizational role. A social worker or member of the clergy if indicated can frequently be involved in shepherding through these routines. It is also at this second interview that permission is asked for the autopsy (by a senior pediatrician). We do not pressurize parents for this permission but find it is exceptional for them to be unwilling when the reasons are explained unless there are cultural or religious differences and these can usually be resolved by contact with the local mosque or temple. The final task on this second visit is to guide the parents through a few of the reactions and emotions that they will suffer in the ensuing period. At between 1 and 2 weeks after the death the parents are seen a third time. They will have received a copy of the autopsy report and this interview will explain the findings of the autopsy. If possible, the senior nurse who has been involved in the terminal events will also be present. The interview will last between half and 1 h. It is important not to see the parents in the neonatal unit or in the middle of the busy outpatient session where other babies and infants intrude too easily into their consciousness. The distress and anxieties of the ensuing weeks are again raised and suggestions are made as to how best to deal with them. Finally at this time an appointment is given for an optional visit at about 3 months at which outstanding questions may be clarified and at which pathological grief, if present, should be evident. At all stages hospital social workers and chaplains should be informed (not necessarily to be active) of what is proceeding. The GP should have a full letter with regard to each interview. Genetic counseling should be arranged for the future if this is appropriate from the results of the autopsy.

Voluntary support organizations

The Stillbirth and Neonatal Death Society (SANDS), 28 Portland Place, London WIN 4DE (Tel. 0171 436 5881).
The British Institute of Funeral Directors, 11 Regent Street, Kingswood, Bristol (Tel. 01272 614 737).

Booklets

The Loss of Your Baby produced by the Health Education Council in conjunction with the Stillbirth and Neonatal Death Society and the National Association for Mental Health.
Saying Goodbye to Your Baby by Priscilla Alderson. Available from SANDS and the National Childbirth Trust, 9 Queensborough Terrace, London W2 3TB.
Miscarriage, Stillbirth and Neonatal Death: Guidelines for Professionals. Available from SANDS.

Staff support

With the realization that the support and understanding of health professionals can play a vital role in the eventual recovery of the parents, there has also come the realization that this involvement can itself cause depression and emotional tension in the staff.

After a death I believe that it is important not only to analyze in detail traditional physiological and pathological events but also the stress aspects for the parents and the nursing and medical staff. Some units may feel it is important to involve formal psychiatric help in this process but regular discussion on a less formal basis (and at particular times of need) are as important (our regular involvement of chaplaincy staff with parents in a neonatal unit pays dividends for the staff themselves at 'crisis times'). In this way we hope that the people involved in a neonatal death and who will inevitably be under considerable stress will not reach the point of physical and emotional exhaustion.

PROBLEMS OF THE NEWBORN

PULMONARY DISORDERS AND APNEA

DEVELOPMENT OF THE LUNG

The viability of the preterm baby is limited by lung development; it is not until 26–28 weeks that potential airway development and capillary proliferation around the airway are sufficient for gas exchange.

The airways begin as an outpouching from the primitive gut at 24 days and by 26 days two primary branches, which will go to form the major bronchi, can be discerned. For the next 3 months growth consists of branching of the endodermal tube into the surrounding mesenchyme (glandular phase). By 10 weeks cartilage is deposited in the bronchi and by 16 weeks formation of new bronchi is almost complete. Canalization of the airways begins at about 20 weeks with the development of a cuboidal cell lining (canalicular phase). The terminal air sacs or alveoli appear as outpouchings of the bronchioles after 28 weeks and increase in number to form multiple pouches of a common chamber called the alveolar duct. Also, at 26 weeks the capillary network, which arises at about 20 weeks from vascular structures in the mesenchyme, proliferates close to the developing airway (alveolar phase). Before 26 weeks gas exchange must take place across terminal bronchioles into the developing capillary network.

Growth of the lung

Mechanical and humoral factors influence growth of the fetal lung and the former are more important (Liggins & Kitterman 1981). Lung growth is regulated by distention in the fluid-filled lung with tracheal fluid acting as an internal template or splint (Alcorn et al 1977). There are also external forces which include the phasic negative pressure of fetal breathing and the tonic negative pressure of diaphragmatic tone. Normal lung growth is dependent upon fetal breathing movements but the mechanism is unclear. It is unlikely to be due to increased lung distention as only 1 ml of tracheal fluid is displaced during fetal breathing movements. Lung hypoplasia may be caused by oligohydramnios from renal agenesis, bladder neck obstruction or rupture of the membranes before 20 weeks. These lungs, although structurally immature with persistent cuboidal epithelium and lack of elastic tissue, are also biochemically immature containing low levels of phospholipids. Hypoplastic lungs may also result from absence of fetal breathing movements in babies with central nervous system anomalies, congenital muscle disorders, absent diaphragm or exomphalos. These lungs, although small, appear to be appropriately developed and have normal content of phospholipids. Pulmonary hypoplasia may also be caused by thoracic space-occupying lesions such as diaphragmatic hernia, lung cysts, or pleural effusions which may be associated with severe erythroblastosis.

Maturation of the lung

After birth alveolar stability is dependent upon the release of pulmonary surfactant into the lumen. Synthesis and release of surfactant rely more on humoral control mechanisms than mechanical factors (Liggins & Kitterman 1981). Alveolar type II cells, which synthesize surfactant, have microvilli on the luminal surface and contain lamellar bodies. They constitute 16% of alveolar cells but only 7% of the alveolar surface area and can differentiate to form the larger, thinner type I cell which covers the remaining 93% of the alveolar surface. The lamellar bodies (storage sites for surfactant) are first recognized at about 22 weeks and contain about 80% phosphatidylcholine (much as dipalmitoylphosphatidylcholine (DPPC) but also unsaturated phosphatidylglycerol (PG)). PG is used as a marker of lung maturity and levels rise as phosphatidylinositol levels decrease towards term. Lamellar bodies also contain many enzymes and two protein groups, a glycoprotein of 28–36 kDa (SP-A) and two very hydrophobic low molecular weight proteins (SP-B and SP-C). The major pathway for surfactant synthesis uses choline incorporation (Fig. 5.23). The mechanisms controlling surfactant synthesis and secretion are not fully understood but humoral factors are important.

Humoral factors

Glucocorticoids

These induce both structural and biochemical changes in alveolar type II and type I cells. Glucocorticoids act on lung fibroblasts to produce fibroblast pneumocyte factor which in turn stimulates surfactant synthesis by alveolar type II cells. They also increase the numbers of lamellar bodies, the rate of choline incorporation into phosphatidylcholine, the amount of DPPC in tracheal fluid and the lung content of SP-A. The induction of fibroblast pneumocyte factor is relatively slow, which may account for the delayed clinical effect of maternal corticosteroid treatment (Halliday 1993).

Thyroid hormones

Thyroid hormones increase the synthesis of surfactant lipids in type II cells, probably by making the cells more responsive to fibroblast pneumocyte factor. They act earlier in the phospholipid

biosynthetic pathway and are synergistic when used with glucocorticoids (Ballard & Gonzales 1984). Synthetic analogues of T_3 and thyrotropin releasing hormone (TRH) cross the placenta (Ballard 1984).

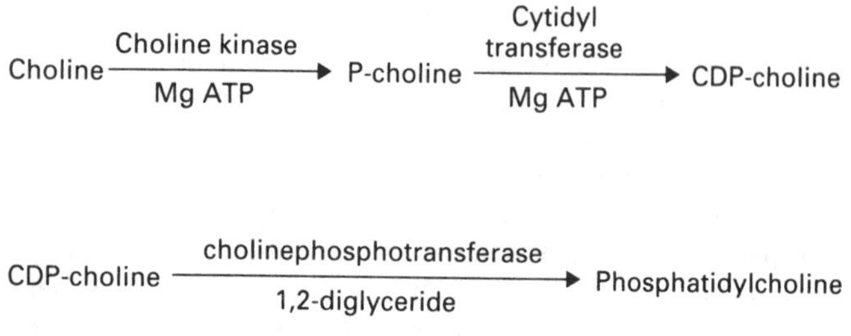

Catecholamines

Adrenaline but not noradrenaline decreases tracheal fluid secretion (Walters & Olver 1978) and increases surfactant release (Lawson et al 1978). The concentration of β-adrenergic receptors in the lung increases at term and in response to glucocorticoids. β-adrenergic agents delay preterm labor; if used in association with betamethasone, they have a synergistic effect in preventing respiratory distress syndrome (Faxelius et al 1983).

Other hormones and agents

Prolactin levels are lower in babies with respiratory distress syndrome. Estrogen, testosterone, epidermal growth factor, prostaglandins, cholinergic agonists and leukotrienes have all been postulated as having roles in fetal lung development. These roles remain to be defined but it is possible that many aspects of lung development are regulated by various hormones acting in concert (Hawgood 1987).

Role of surfactant and fetal lung fluid

The fetal lung is filled with liquid secreted by the epithelium of potential air spaces. Absorption across the epithelium is initiated by increased circulating catecholamines associated with the contractions of labor. The air-filled lung after birth retains a thin fluid layer in the alveolus. Surface tension at this air–fluid interface tends to decrease its area and this must be overcome by the transpulmonary pressure, if alveolar collapse is to be avoided. Pulmonary surfactant forms an insoluble film at the alveolar air–liquid interface replacing water molecules in the surface layer and lowering surface tension. Alveolar stability during expiration is due to low surface tension from surfactant during surface compression. At functional residual capacity surface tension is close to zero, but without surfactant it would be 70 mN/m at 37°C.

Surfactant allows very low transpulmonary pressures to be used during normal respiration and may also have a role in the host defense mechanisms of the lung. The mechanisms controlling surfactant secretion are unclear.

Although β-adrenergic agents have been shown to initially increase secretion, prolonged use could deplete surfactant stores if rate of synthesis is low. Lung inflation also stimulates surfactant secretion but this may be mediated by humoral mechanisms. The apoprotein SP-A has a role in the feedback control of surfactant secretion. When surfactant is released the contents of the lamellar bodies are extruded into the alveoli. After secretion the tightly packed lamellae of the lamellar bodies are left as tubular myelin which may also have an active role in lowering surface tension.

The surface film needs to be constantly replenished from freshly secreted surfactant and recycling occurs within the type II cells. As much as 85–90% of surfactant is recycled (Goerke & Clements 1986). The clearance of surfactant is rapid and may be increased in the newborn period or after hyperventilation. Specific proteins may regulate the clearance of surfactant back to type II cells and small amounts are also phagocytosed by alveolar macrophages and cleared up the airways.

Choline $\xrightarrow[\text{Mg ATP}]{\text{Choline kinase}}$ P-choline $\xrightarrow[\text{Mg ATP}]{\text{Cytidyl transferase}}$ CDP-choline

CDP-choline $\xrightarrow[\text{1,2-diglyceride}]{\text{cholinephosphotransferase}}$ Phosphatidylcholine

Fig. 5.23 Synthesis of phosphatidylcholine by choline incorporation.

Postnatal lung growth

The terminal air sacs are shallow and wide mouthed in the newborn baby; several months later they assume a cup shape. Growth of the lung occurs by increasing the number of bronchiolar divisions, alveoli, alveolar diameters and surface area for gas exchange. Fortunately, alveoli may continue to form as long as body length increases. The numbers of alveoli and airways increase approximately 10-fold from infancy to adulthood (30 million to 300 million) and lung surface area increases 20-fold. This capacity for growth and repair is of benefit to babies recovering from bronchopulmonary dysplasia.

Interalveolar communications (pores of Kohn) are few in number in the neonate and become prominent only after the age of 7 years. The absence of this 'collateral ventilation' probably increases the risk of pulmonary atelectasis in the neonate and young child.

RESPIRATORY DISTRESS SYNDROME (HYALINE MEMBRANE DISEASE)

Respiratory distress syndrome (RDS), also known as hyaline membrane disease because of the histological features at autopsy, is caused by surfactant deficiency and affects mainly preterm infants. The incidence is 1–3% of all births but it is important as it is responsible for the deaths of many preterm infants throughout the world each year. The incidence of RDS is inversely proportional to gestational age (Taeusch & Boncuk-Dayahikli 1995). Apart from prematurity certain other factors are known to affect the incidence of RDS (Table 5.48).

Pathogenesis

Deficiency of surfactant leads to alveolar collapse, reduced lung volume, decreased lung compliance and ventilation–perfusion abnormalities. Right-to-left shunting of up to 70% or more occurs through collapsed lung (intrapulmonary) or across the ductus arteriosus and the foramen ovale (extrapulmonary) if pulmonary hypertension is severe. Persistent hypoxemia (< 4 kPa) causes metabolic acidosis and respiratory acidosis will also be present because of alveolar hypoventilation. This further reduces surfactant production and affects pulmonary vascular resistance, myocardial contractility, cardiac output and arterial blood pressure. Perfusion of the kidneys, gastrointestinal tract, muscles and skin is reduced leading to edema and electrolyte disorders.

Table 5.48 Factors affecting the incidence of RDS

Decrease	Increase
Intrauterine growth retardation	Asphyxia
Prolonged rupture of membranes	Erythroblastosis
Maternal steroid therapy	Maternal diabetes
Sickle cell disease	Antepartum hemorrhage
Heroin	Elective Cesarean section
Alcohol	Second twin
Black infants	Family history
Girls	Boys

Oxygen delivery is affected by arterial oxygen tension, oxygen-carrying capacity, oxygen affinity, peripheral blood flow, temperature and pH. Fetal hemoglobin allows more oxygen to be carried in the blood at any oxygen tension (greater affinity) but less oxygen will be released to the tissues. The newborn and especially the preterm infant has a reduced level of 2,3-DPG and this may be improved by giving transfusions of adult blood or exchange transfusion.

Pathology

Macroscopically the lungs appear collapsed and liver-like and sink in water. Microscopic examination shows generalized collapse of alveoli with eosinophilic membranes in infants surviving more than a few hours. The membranes begin to break up by the third day and are removed by macrophages. Sometimes there is frank pulmonary hemorrhage and interstitial emphysema. The muscle layer of the walls of the pulmonary arterioles is thickened and pulmonary lymphatics are dilated.

Clinical features

The disease has a wide spectrum of severity from mild respiratory distress lasting 2 or 3 days to a rapidly fatal illness causing death within a few hours. The early clinical signs are shown in Table 5.49. When at least two of these signs are present after the first hour of life and the chest radiograph is typical (see below) diagnostic criteria are fulfilled. Each of these clinical signs may be explained by disturbed lung function. Increased respiratory rate is caused by the demand of increased alveolar ventilation and is related to blood gas changes of hypercarbia and hypoxemia. Later slow or decreasing respiratory rate which may progress to apnea may be related to diaphragmatic muscle fatigue.

The sternal and intercostal recession or retractions are due to reduced lung compliance as a result of surfactant deficiency. Expiratory grunting results from expiration against a partially closed glottis in an attempt to prevent alveolar collapse. It may be absent in the very immature or seriously ill baby. Cyanosis is due to decreased arterial oxygen tension caused by right-to-left interatrial and ductus shunts and to increasing intrapulmonary shunting after the first 12 h of life due to perfusion of collapsed or poorly ventilated parts of the lungs. These right-to-left shunts contribute to total venous admixtures of up to 75% of the cardiac output.

In severe disease, immature babies or those with asphyxia may need positive pressure ventilation from birth. In more mature babies grunting and retractions are prominent and cyanosis may be apparent from soon after birth. Oxygen concentrations of greater than 60% are often needed to abolish cyanosis and respiratory failure with hypercarbia and acidosis frequently

Table 5.49 Early clinical signs of respiratory distress syndrome

Tachypnea (> 60/min)
Expiratory grunting
Sternal and intercostal recession
Cyanosis in room air
Delayed onset of respiration in very immature babies

Table 5.50 Nonrespiratory clinical signs in severe respiratory distress syndrome

Hypotonia	Jaundice
Decreased movements	Hypothermia
Edema	Abdominal distention
Loss of heart rate variability	Decreased urinary output

supervene, so that mechanical ventilation becomes necessary. Clinical signs outside the respiratory system also occur (Table 5.50).

Investigations

The initial radiographic signs are a diffuse reticulogranular pattern of mottling of the lung fields and an 'air bronchogram' appearance due to air in the major bronchi being highlighted against the white opacified lung (Fig. 5.24). With increasing severity the granular areas increase and become confluent so that the lung has a homogeneous ground glass appearance and the heart borders are obscured. Grading of the severity of respiratory distress syndrome using radiological criteria (Table 5.51) is useful although certain methods of treatment such as application of continuous positive airway pressure (CPAP) or surfactant replacement may improve the radiographic appearances considerably. Many other

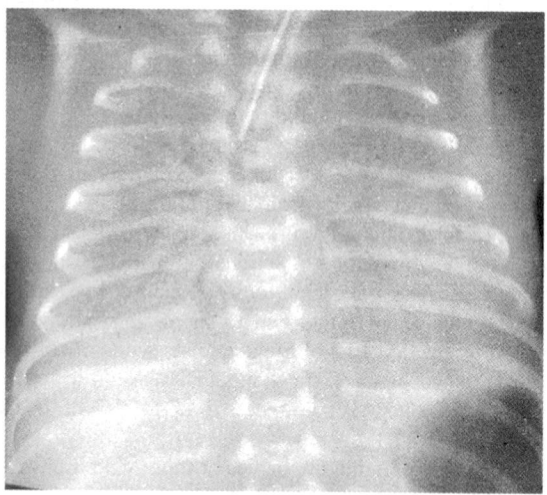

Fig. 5.24 Severe respiratory distress syndrome with widespread reticulogranular mottling and air bronchograms amounting to grade IV disease (see Table 5.51).

Table 5.51 Radiological grading of severity of respiratory distress syndrome

Grade I	Fine reticulogranular mottling, good lung expansion
Grade II	Mottling with air bronchograms
Grade III	Diffuse mottling, heart borders just discernible, prominent air bronchograms
Grade IV	Bilateral confluent opacification of lungs ('whiteout')

Table 5.52 Differential diagnosis of respiratory distress syndrome

Congenital pneumonia
Aspiration pneumonia
Meconium aspiration syndrome
Air leak – pneumothorax, pulmonary interstitial emphysema and pneumomediastinum
Transient tachypnea of the newborn
Lobar emphysema
Pulmonary hypoplasia
Diaphragmatic hernia
Heart failure
Persistent pulmonary hypertension
Asphyxia and raised intracranial pressure
Metabolic acidosis
Congenital neuromuscular disorders
Anemia and hypovolemia

pulmonary and some nonpulmonary disorders present with signs of respiratory distress (Table 5.52). History of pregnancy, labor and delivery are sometimes helpful to distinguish these disorders but often a chest radiograph is needed to make an accurate diagnosis. Serial analyses of pH and arterial blood gases are also essential for clinical evaluation. These measurements may be made from indwelling arterial catheters or by intermittent arterial puncture. Continuous measurements of oxygen and carbon dioxide tensions may be made transcutaneously, and oxygen saturation can be assessed noninvasively by means of pulse oximetry. These measurements are necessary to follow the clinical course of a baby with RDS and to detect impending respiratory failure so that assisted ventilation may be used before irreversible clinical deterioration has occurred. Direct measurements of surfactant activity by estimation of lecithin : sphingomyelin ratio of amniotic fluid, hypopharyngeal aspirate, tracheal aspirate or gastric aspirate help to confirm the diagnosis of surfactant deficiency but are less useful in monitoring the course of RDS in an individual baby. Rapid tests of pulmonary maturity can be used to guide the neonatologist in the need for surfactant treatment.

Natural history

The clinical course of classical RDS is that of increasing severity during the first 24–48 h of life, followed by a period of stability lasting another 48 h before improvement occurs. The severity of the disease may be expressed in terms of oxygen requirements and need for assisted ventilation. In the 24 h prior to recovery a diuresis usually occurs but diuretic therapy does not alter the course of RDS.

Prevention

Antenatal glucocorticoid administration reduces the incidence and the severity of RDS provided 48 h of treatment is possible. Improved survival and reduced risk of complications such as pneumothorax, intraventricular hemorrhage, patent ductus arteriosus and bronchopulmonary dysplasia have also been demonstrated (Crowley et al 1990, Halliday 1993). Combination treatment with glucocorticoids and thyrotropin-releasing hormone is currently under investigation and holds promise as an improvement on steroids alone (see p. 114). Ambroxol, if given intravenously for 5 days to women in preterm labor, appears to reduce the incidence of RDS (Wauer et al 1982). This drug is popular in some European countries but, because of the long treatment period it is not used widely in the UK.

RDS may also be prevented or at least ameliorated if care is taken to prevent hypoxemia, acidosis and hypothermia in preterm babies. Good resuscitation at birth with early expansion of the alveoli or terminal airways in the preterm baby is very important and for babies of less than 30 weeks' gestation endotracheal intubation may lead to improved outcome (Drew 1982).

Surfactant replacement will also modify the course of RDS and in general the earlier it is given the greater the benefit (Jobe 1993). Babies that might benefit most from prophylactic treatment at birth are those of less than 30 weeks' gestation, those needing endotracheal intubation for resuscitation or those who were not treated with prenatal corticosteroids.

Treatment

The objectives of treatment are to maintain normal blood gases, pH, biochemistry and physiology (blood pressure, temperature and renal function) and in addition to prevent complications of both the disease and the treatments. Surfactant replacement therapy is an effective way of accomplishing these objectives (Halliday & Speer 1995). There are two basic types of surfactant, synthetic and natural.

A synthetic surfactant (ALEC), pioneered in Cambridge, is a mixture of DPPC and PG (7 : 3) and this has been shown, in a large randomized controlled trial, to reduce the severity of RDS and mortality from 27 to 14% in babies treated prophylactically at birth (Ten Centre Study Group 1987). Another synthetic surfactant, Exosurf, has been extensively studied and reduces neonatal mortality and incidence of pneumothorax in babies with RDS (Dechant & Faulds 1991). This surfactant is also protein-free, containing DPPC, tyloxapol and hexadecanol. There are also a number of studies of natural surfactants (prepared from calf, pig and cow lungs) showing them to be effective when used either prophylactically or to treat established severe RDS (Halliday 1989, Jobe 1993). Meta-analyses of over 30 randomized controlled trials (over 3500 babies) show a consistent 40% reduction in the risk of death and between 30 and 70% decrease in the risk of pneumothorax with the use of surfactant treatment (Soll & McQueen 1992). Examples of natural surfactants are Survanta (bovine) and Curosurf (porcine). The optimal dose of surfactant is about 100 mg/kg and repeated doses may be needed for babies who show relapse (Halliday & Speer 1995). Natural surfactants have a more rapid onset of action than artificial preparations and there is now some evidence that they may be more effective (Halliday 1996). Synthetic surfactants may have a role in the prevention of RDS whilst natural surfactants should probably be given to babies with moderate to severe RDS as soon after birth as possible.

Maintenance of temperature (p. 147)

Preterm infants should be nursed in an incubator or under a radiant warmer.

Maintenance of normoxemia (p. 161)

The aim is to keep arterial oxygen tension in the range of 6–10 kPa (45–75 mmHg). For babies with spontaneous respiration, humidified oxygen should be given into a Perspex headbox. Excessive handling should be avoided as this causes hypoxemia and leads to deterioration. Monitoring of oxygenation is essential (Dear 1987) as too little oxygen will cause hypoxemia, metabolic acidosis and tissue damage and too much oxygen has been associated with the development of retinopathy of prematurity. Measurement of arterial oxygen tension is the best method of assessing adequate oxygenation. An initial right radial artery blood sample is helpful to assess oxygen requirements and to determine the need for an indwelling arterial catheter. For all babies needing greater than 40% oxygen after the first hour, an arterial catheter should be inserted. For babies of less than 1200 g birthweight more than 30% oxygen should be taken as a guide for insertion of an arterial catheter. Continuous methods of assessing oxygenation such as the intravascular oxygen electrode, transcutaneous oxygen monitor and pulse oximeter also have their place, but these devices do not remove the need for intermittent arterial blood sampling to check calibration and measure pH, arterial carbon dioxide tensions and base deficit. In severe RDS, peripheral perfusion and tissue oxygen delivery may be improved by transfusion of fresh blood which will increase the circulating blood volume and 2,3-DPG levels allowing additional release of oxygen to the tissues.

When respiratory failure supervenes, some form of assisted ventilation becomes necessary (see below).

Correction of acid–base abnormalities (p. 421)

Respiratory acidosis due to raised arterial carbon dioxide tensions is common in severe RDS. Hypercarbia can only be treated adequately by improving ventilation. Metabolic acidosis may arise from hypoxemia, hypotension, infection, renal failure, persistent ductus arteriosus or intraventricular hemorrhage. Treatment of the underlying cause, for example by increasing oxygen concentrations or giving blood or plasma transfusions, may be more appropriate than infusion of sodium bicarbonate. The aim should be to keep the pH above 7.25 and if the base deficit becomes greater than 10 mmol/l then sodium bicarbonate should be given. The dose may be calculated as follows:

$$\text{dose (mmol)} = \text{base deficit (mmol/l)} \times \text{weight (kg)} \times 0.3$$

Molar sodium bicarbonate 8.4% (1 mmol/ml) is the most frequently used alkali in clinical practice but it has some disadvantages (Table 5.53).

In practice molar sodium bicarbonate should be diluted and given slowly (not faster than 1 mmol/min) by peripheral venous infusion. The total amount of bicarbonate should be restricted to 10 mmol/kg/day to lessen risks of hypernatremia and intraventricular hemorrhage.

Table 5.53 Disadvantages of sodium bicarbonate therapy

1. May raise $PaCO_2$ unless ventilation is adequate (Eidelman & Hobbs 1978)

2. Hyperosmolar – associated with intraventricular hemorrhage

3. High sodium content

Energy, fluid and electrolyte requirements

The preterm baby with RDS has reduced stores of carbohydrate (as glycogen), fat and protein (as skeletal muscle), and at the same time has increased metabolic requirements as a result of the extra work of breathing. Providing adequate exogenous sources of energy as parenteral nutrition for these sick babies is technically difficult, if not impossible. For the first 24–48 h protein and fat requirements are not met and in practice only an infusion of 10% dextrose in water at 60–90 ml/kg is given on the first day. Fluid requirements may be monitored by looking at urine output and specific gravity, osmolality and by regular weighing.

Excessive fluid intake is associated with an increased incidence of persistent ductus arteriosus, necrotizing enterocolitis and bronchopulmonary dysplasia.

Oliguria in severe RDS is not unusual for the first 48 h due to the effects of asphyxia, hypotension and possibly inappropriate ADH secretion. Care must be taken to avoid fluid and electrolyte overload. Subsequently, when the diuretic phase occurs, the large urinary losses mean that extra fluid, sodium and potassium intake will be necessary to prevent hyponatremia or hypokalemia (see pp. 144–145).

Once the baby shows signs of recovery, extra energy should be provided in the form of either small oral milk feeds or parenteral amino acid and fat solutions.

Assisted ventilation

CPAP is a distending pressure which prevents alveolar collapse during expiration and thus improves oxygenation. The indications for using CPAP in RDS are not absolute and may depend upon the maturity of the baby (Table 5.54).

Large babies tolerate CPAP better than very immature ones, and its application may prevent progression to IPPV. Methods of

Table 5.54 Indications for CPAP in RDS

1. Oxygen concentrations > 60% to keep PaO_2 > 8 kPa (60 mmHg)
2. Recurrent apneic attacks
3. Weaning from IPPV

applying CPAP include facemask, face chamber, nasal prongs, nasopharyngeal tube and Gregory box. For small babies endotracheal intubation is often necessary. This allows for easy changeover to IPPV if this becomes necessary. A CPAP circuit is shown in Figure 5.25 but use of existing ventilator circuits or driving systems is more common.

Mechanical ventilation is used to treat respiratory failure and intractable apnea (Table 5.55 and p. 196). The smaller the baby the more likely it is that IPPV will be needed. For babies less than 30 weeks' gestation, $PaCO_2$ of > 8 kPa (60 torr) is usually accepted as an indication for IPPV. Use of mechanical ventilation requires considerable expertise and meticulous attention to detail by both medical and nursing staff. The quality of the intensive care team may determine outcome to a greater degree than the type of ventilator used. Suitable ventilators are pressure limited and time cycled, and allow variation of inspired oxygen concentration, flow rate, peak airway pressure, positive end expiratory pressure (PEEP), ventilation rate and inspiratory and expiratory times. IPPV is performed through an endotracheal tube (2.5–3.5 mm) inserted through either the nose or mouth into the mid-trachea. The initial ventilator settings employed will depend upon the maturity of the baby and the severity of the lung disease. For the baby weighing less than 1200 g, which corresponds to a gestational age of less than 30 weeks, with severe lung disease the aim of IPPV should be to expand the lungs as early as possible with the lowest peak airway pressure possible. The effect of

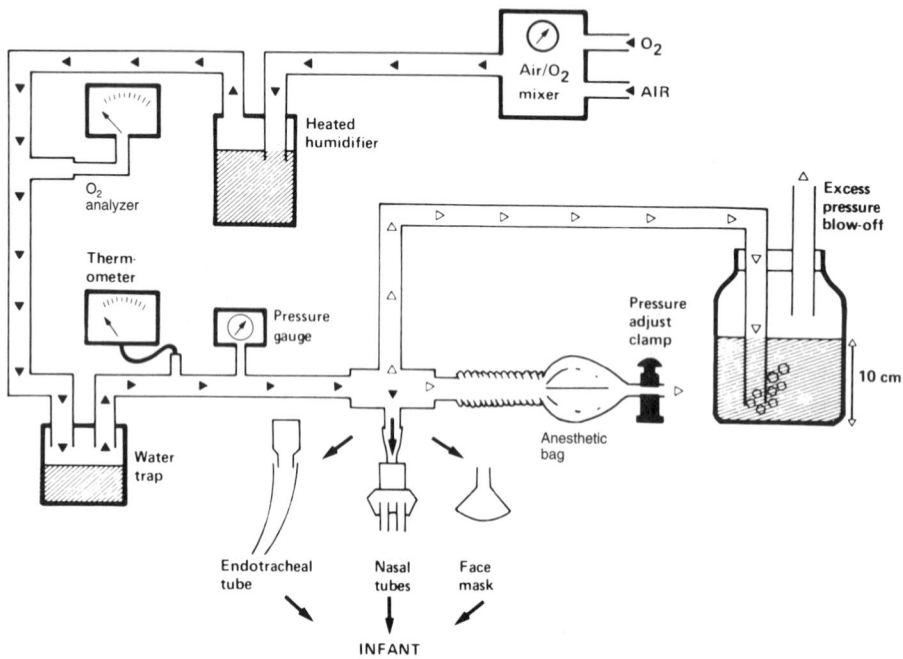

Fig. 5.25 Arrangement of the gas flow circuit used in application of CPAP.

Table 5.55 Indications for IPPV in RDS

1. Failure to establish respiration at birth
2. Intractable apneic attacks
3. Incipient or actual collapse
4. Respiratory failure
    pH < 7.20
    $PaCO_2$ > 9 kPa (68 mmHg)
    PaO_2 < 7 kPa (53 mmHg) in 90% oxygen

Table 5.56 Complications of RDS

1. Persistent ductus arteriosus
2. Intraventricular hemorrhage
3. Pulmonary
    a. Air leaks
        Pneumothorax
        Pneumomediastinum
        Pulmonary interstitial emphysema
        Pneumopericardium
        Pneumoperitoneum
        Air embolism
        Subcutaneous emphysema
    b. Bronchopulmonary dysplasia
    c. Pneumonia
        – Aspiration
        – Bacterial
4. Complications of mechanical ventilation (see above)
5. Long-term neurological sequelae

ventilation may be checked by observing chest wall movement and measuring arterial blood gases and pH. Peak airway pressures of 15–25 cmH$_2$O are often needed initially, with PEEP of 3–5 cmH$_2$O and ventilator rate of 60–120/min. These faster rates are preferred by smaller babies who may often be induced to breathe synchronously with the ventilator without resort to muscle relaxants. (South & Morley 1986, Greenough et al 1987b). Inspiratory times of 0.3–0.5 s are used so that the inspiratory to expiratory time (I : E) ratio is about 1 : 1. Inspired oxygen concentration should be adjusted to keep PaO_2 levels and oxygen saturation in the normal range.

Mechanical ventilation of the more mature baby with severe RDS can often be adequately performed using lower ventilator rates (30–40/min) and longer inspiratory times (0.8–1.0 s) with reversed I : E ratios (1.5 or 2 : 1) (Ramsden et al 1987). Sometimes muscle relaxants are needed to prevent these babies 'fighting' the ventilator which will increase the risk of pneumothorax. To improve oxygenation one may increase either the inspired oxygen concentration or the mean airway pressure (MAP). MAP is dependent upon peak airway pressure, PEEP and inspiratory time and increases in any of these parameters should increase PaO_2. If oxygenation remains poor PaO_2 < 4 kPa, the alternatives include muscle relaxation with pancuronium (0.03 mg/kg) to allow further increase in peak pressures, or use of a pulmonary vasodilating drug such as tolazoline (1–2 mg/kg) (McIntosh & Walters 1979). Inhaled nitric oxide is an experimental therapy for pulmonary hypertension.

As the baby's condition improves the ventilator settings can be reduced. Peak airway pressure should be lowered first, along with inspired oxygen concentration as guided by blood gas analysis. Later, ventilator rates can be lowered keeping inspiratory time constant at about 0.4–0.5 s to prevent air trapping. Intermittent mandatory ventilation (IMV) is possible with all of the newer pressure-limited ventilators and this allows ventilator rates to be lowered with the baby breathing as he or she wishes between each ventilator breath. A period of CPAP is sometimes tried before extubation but in the immature baby, longer periods of IMV (rates 10/min) may be necessary. Theophylline has been used to successfully wean very low birthweight infants from mechanical ventilation. Patient triggered ventilation may also have a role to play in weaning.

Complications of RDS (Table 5.56)

Persistent ductus arteriosus (PDA)

The ductus arteriosus is likely to remain open in babies with severe RDS for a number of reasons: prematurity with poorly developed ductus musculature, reduced arterial oxygen tensions and inadequate metabolism of prostaglandins in the lungs

(Halliday 1988). Fluid overload and surfactant replacement may also increase the risk of PDA. The management is discussed on page 204.

Intraventricular hemorrhage (IVH) (p. 249)

IVH can both cause acute deterioration in a baby having mechanical ventilation for RDS, and be predisposed to by other causes of collapse such as pneumothorax (Lipscomb et al 1981). Maintenance of physiological stability and prevention of air leak by manipulation of ventilator settings or surfactant replacement (McCord et al 1988) should reduce the incidence of IVH.

Pulmonary air leaks (p. 187)

The incidence of these depends upon the severity of the RDS and the need for assisted ventilation. For babies with RDS not needing assisted ventilation the incidence is 5–10%. In the decades of the 1970s and 1980s, if CPAP was needed the incidence was about 10–15% and with IPPV 10–30% (Ogata et al 1975). Since that time high rate ventilation, muscle relaxation and surfactant replacement (McCord et al 1988) together with better ventilators have been shown to reduce the incidence of pneumothorax (Halliday 1992).

Bronchopulmonary dysplasia (p. 193)

This condition was not described until after the introduction of mechanical ventilation to treat RDS. Positive pressure ventilation with an endotracheal tube is necessary for its development, but other factors such as oxygen toxicity, infection and fluid overload probably have a significant role in pathogenesis. About 20% of babies needing mechanical ventilation for RDS will develop this complication (Corcoran et al 1993).

Pneumonia (p. 183)

This may be a secondary bacterial pneumonia due to the presence of an endotracheal tube. Cultures of tracheal aspirates are of limited use in diagnosing this complication but may guide the choice of antibiotics should the infant develop pulmonary or systemic signs. The presence of both pus cells and organisms in tracheal aspirates, development of patchy opacity on chest radiograph and general deterioration often with positive blood cultures help to make the diagnosis (Giacoia et al 1981). Appropriate antibiotic treatment is then necessary in conjunction with careful tracheal toilet. The role of chest physiotherapy is probably limited. Aspiration pneumonia may be common. In one study it occurred in up to 80% of mechanically ventilated neonates (Goodwin et al 1985) and it may be responsible for acute deterioration. Chest radiograph may show areas of collapse and consolidation especially in the right upper or right lower lobes. The presence of gastroesophageal reflux increases the risk of this complication and transpyloric feeding may reduce the risk. Antibiotic therapy and possibly gentle chest physiotherapy may be helpful.

Long-term neurological sequelae (p. 171)

There is recent evidence that modern neonatal intensive care has not only reduced neonatal mortality very considerably, but has also improved the quality of survival. A major contributing factor is the improved understanding of the pathogenesis of RDS as well as improved methods of prevention and treatment. For babies of more than 30 weeks' gestation, ventilatory techniques are now well standardized and technical difficulties are minimal. Babies in whom RDS is the primary indication for mechanical ventilation are unlikely to develop permanent brain injury unless there is severe asphyxia or extensive intraventricular hemorrhage.

TRANSIENT TACHYPNEA OF THE NEWBORN

This occurs in both term and preterm babies. First described in 1966 (Avery et al 1966), it has also been called type II RDS and wet lung disease.

Incidence

Tachypnea after normal vaginal delivery is relatively common occurring in about 5% of full-term babies. After Cesarean section the incidence is about 9% although only about 6 per 1000 babies need treatment with oxygen. The timing of elective Cesarean section is important with the risk decreasing from 25% to 15% from 37 to 40 weeks' gestation (Krantz et al 1986).

Etiology and pathogenesis

Transient tachypnea has been attributed to delayed resorption of fetal lung fluid and predisposing factors include elective Cesarean section, perinatal asphyxia, excessive maternal analgesia or hypothermia, maternal diabetes and male sex. Many of these factors are associated with increased production or decreased resorption of lung fluid. Catecholamine levels after elective Cesarean section are lower than those following vaginal delivery with the result that fetal lung fluid production continues after birth (Walters & Olver 1978). The time of cord clamping is related to tachypnea after birth with delayed clamping being associated with an increased incidence of respiratory distress in both term and preterm babies. Late cord clamping leads to increased placental transfusion to the baby and may cause left ventricular dysfunction which has been found in echocardiographic studies of babies with transient tachypnea of the newborn. Asphyxia exacerbates this left

ventricular failure in some babies who resemble those with persistent fetal circulation.

Clinical presentation

Most affected babies are either large preterm or term infants with a male preponderance of 3 to 1. Tachypnea is apparent from about 1 h after birth, with respiratory rates of up to 120/min. Subcostal recession, grunting and cyanosis may be present but are not prominent features of the syndrome. Affected babies have barrel chests with increase in anteroposterior diameter. Babies with a picture of persistent fetal circulation are uncommon, but present with marked cyanosis and often need mechanical ventilation (Tudehope & Smyth 1979).

Diagnosis

The chest radiograph shows hyperinflated lung fields, perihilar opacities, increased vascular markings, fluid in the transverse fissure and small pleural effusions (Fig. 5.26). The presence of biochemically mature lungs, e.g. normal shake test, helps to confirm the diagnosis. Two important differential diagnoses should be considered in atypical infants. Early onset group B β-hemolytic streptococcal sepsis can mimic transient tachypnea of the newborn initially but if unrecognized and untreated will be fatal. Blood culture, examination of gastric aspirate and full blood picture will help to make this diagnosis. Some forms of congenital heart disease, for example anomalous pulmonary venous drainage, can also mimic TTN. Chest radiograph and echocardiography are helpful if a cardiac anomaly is suspected.

Management

Oxygen is often needed for 2 or 3 days but respiratory failure is very uncommon. Pulse oximetry may be useful in monitoring the oxygen needs of affected term babies. Only rarely are oxygen concentrations above 40% necessary. Penicillin should be given if any doubt about congenital pneumonia exists. There is no evidence that frusemide treatment hastens recovery (Wiswell et al 1985).

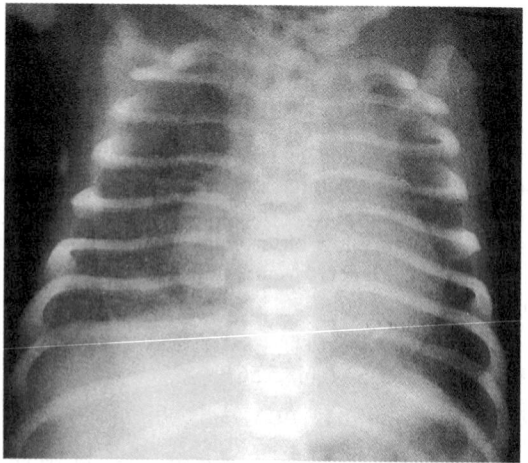

Fig. 5.26 Transient tachypnea of the newborn with overinflated lungs, fluid in the right costophrenic angle and horizontal fissure. The skinfold line seen at the right base may be mistaken for a pneumothorax.

Outcome

Most infants recover within 2–3 days and there are no long-term sequelae. Up to 10% of babies develop pneumothoraces and a few may need mechanical ventilation. The mortality rate should approach zero and survivors should have normal neurodevelopment (Halahakoon & Halliday 1995).

PNEUMONIA

Pneumonia is probably the most common serious infection of the newborn baby. It may be either congenital or acquired, although intrapartum infection can occur and may not fit easily into either category (Table 5.57).

Incidence

Preterm babies are more commonly infected for at least three reasons. Firstly congenital infection may stimulate preterm labor, secondly preterm babies have problems with host defense mechanisms and thirdly they are more likely to need intensive care and thus be exposed to the risks of acquired infections. Early-onset pneumonia has been estimated to occur in 1.79 per 1000 live births (Webber et al 1990). Nosocomial infection causing pneumonia was found in about 8% of babies in a neonatal intensive care unit (Hemming et al 1976). Pneumonia as a complication of endotracheal intubation for mechanical ventilation has an incidence of about 30% (Giacoia et al 1981).

Pathogenesis

Pneumonia that is acquired congenitally or intrapartum (Table 5.57) will usually present within the first 4–6 h and may then be described as early onset. Nosocomial infections are usually late onset although colonization with organisms acquired intrapartum can lead to subsequent infection occurring after 7 days.

Transplacentally acquired pneumonia may be due to viruses (cytomegalovirus, coxsackie, Herpes simplex and rubella), bacteria (*Listeria monocytogenes*, coliforms, pneumococci and streptococci) or toxoplasmosis (Halahakoon & Halliday 1995). The ascending route of infection is the most important in early-onset infection and the organisms found in the maternal genital tract and in the baby's lungs are very similar. Prolonged rupture of the membranes is commonly found in cases of ascending infection and as the duration of membrane rupture increases up to 3 days the incidence of chorioamnionitis increases to about 50% and neonatal infection to about 8%. Ascending infection can occur through intact membranes and cause illness or perinatal death (Naeye & Peters 1978) although this is less common. Organisms involved in ascending infection are coliforms, streptococci,

Haemophilus influenzae, pneumococci, staphylococci and Herpes simplex virus.

Intrapartum aspiration of infected secretions can cause infection with *Listeria monocytogenes*, streptococci, Herpes simplex and varicella. Nosocomial or environmentally acquired infection can be transmitted by hospital staff usually from poor handwashing. The organisms involved are staphylococci, streptococci and respiratory syncytial virus. Sometimes infection is acquired from nursery equipment and the organisms involved are pseudomonas, serratia, klebsiella and listeria. Late-onset infection may also be due to delayed invasion of organisms acquired at birth. This typically occurs with certain serotypes of streptococci and listeria.

Early-onset pneumonia

Clinical features

Intrapartum stillbirth may occur, but often the baby is born alive with signs of asphyxia and needs resuscitation. The onset of respiratory symptoms may be more gradual with a clinical picture very similar to that of RDS (Table 5.49). Helpful distinguishing features include temperature instability, hypotension, apneic spells and acidosis. Sometimes a skin rash or hepatosplenomegaly (listeriosis) will be present or the baby may be foul smelling (coliforms or bacteroides). The severity of respiratory distress is variable and some babies may have profound shock and metabolic upsets with right-to-left shunting and a clinical course resembling severe persistent fetal circulation.

A chest radiograph is necessary to exclude other causes of respiratory distress. With transplacentally acquired infection there are diffuse, interstitial opacities giving a ground glass, reticular pattern which may be indistinguishable from RDS or there may be extensive consolidation (Fig. 5.27). With ascending infection there may be alveolar involvement which produces bilateral coarse opacities which are much less uniform (Fig. 5.28). Air

Table 5.57 Pathogenesis of neonatal pneumonia

Congenital (transplacental acquisition)

Intrapartum
  a. Ascending infection and chorioamnionitis
  b. Aspiration of infected secretions at delivery

Acquired
  Nosocomial – often during mechanical ventilation or late infection
  after colonization at birth

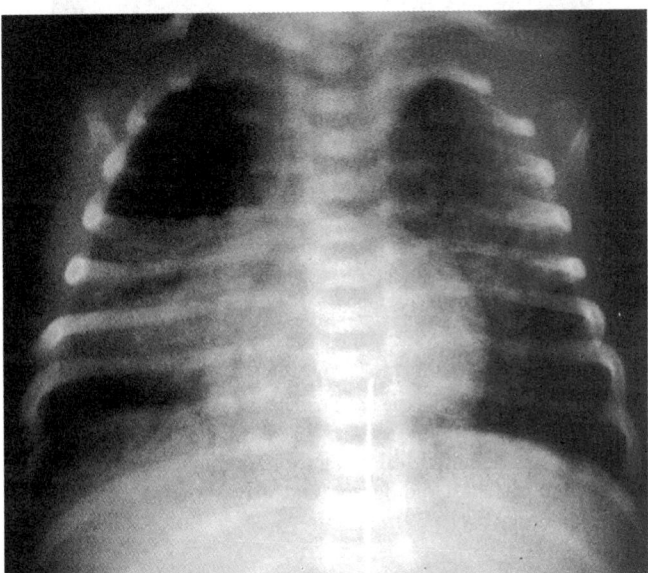

Fig. 5.27 Congenital listeriosis showing extensive consolidation in both midzones but more marked on the right. An arterial catheter is seen with its tip at T7 and T8.

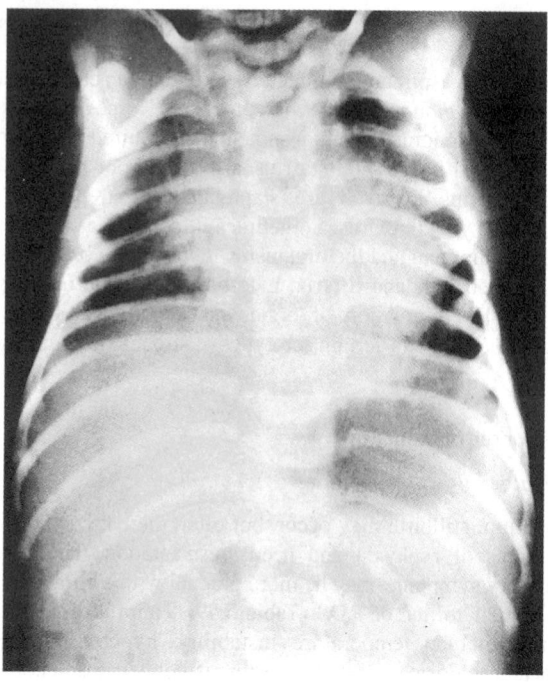

Fig. 5.28 Intrauterine pneumonia from ascending infection showing patchy bronchopneumonic consolidation.

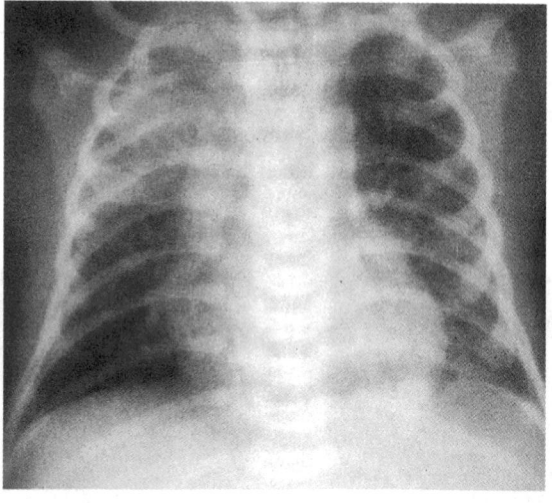

Fig. 5.29 Chest radiograph showing aspiration pneumonia with collapse and consolidation in right upper lobe.

bronchograms may also be seen especially if the opacities become confluent.

Pneumonia acquired following aspiration is usually less evenly distributed on chest radiograph and may show as segmental or lobar collapse (Fig. 5.29).

Diagnosis

The clinical diagnosis is confirmed by culturing organisms from tracheal fluid, blood or gastric aspirate, although the last is less reliable. There is not time to wait for culture results before starting treatment and hematological and biochemical tests are not sensitive enough to be relied upon if negative. If in doubt, it is best to start antibiotics after cultures have been taken. Direct examination of gastric aspirate has been used to guide antibiotic therapy but any polymorphonuclear leukocytes present are probably of maternal origin and any organisms seen on Gram stain may be contaminants rather than the pathogens causing the pneumonia. If tracheal aspirate can be obtained and examined within 8 h of birth there is a good correlation between organisms seen and those subsequently cultured.

Differential diagnosis

This includes respiratory distress syndrome, transient tachypnea of the newborn and meconium aspiration syndrome in addition to causes of severe asphyxia at birth including pulmonary hypoplasia. Sometimes these conditions can coexist so that if any doubt exists antibiotic cover especially for group B β-hemolytic streptococcal (GBS) infection should be given. Severe pneumonia may also be difficult to distinguish from cyanotic heart disease and persistent fetal circulation.

Management

Prevention. Early-onset GBS infection can be predicted from maternal risk factors such as prolonged rupture of the membranes, spontaneous preterm labor and maternal pyrexia in labor. When women with these risk factors who are known to be colonized with GBS are treated with intravenous ampicillin in large doses during labor there is a significant reduction in neonatal infection (Boyer & Gotoff 1986). Ampicillin may also be effective in pregnancies complicated by infection with listeria, haemophilus and pneumococci but other Gram-negative organisms and anaerobes will not usually be sensitive. A combination of ampicillin and metronidazole would improve the spectrum of cover in these high-risk cases.

Treatment. Babies born to mothers with the risk factors mentioned above should have cultures taken and be given antibiotic prophylaxis. There is no evidence that routine penicillin prophylaxis for all preterm babies is effective and this approach might increase the risk of Gram-negative infections. Routine monitoring of the respiratory rate for 24 h on the postnatal ward has been shown to be effective in shortening the time to diagnosis and treatment of the occasional late-presenting case (Mifsud et al 1988).

For symptomatic infants with respiratory distress, penicillin therapy should be started after appropriate cultures have been taken; the antibiotic can be stopped after 48 h if the cultures are negative and the baby's condition improved or a clear diagnosis of noninfective illness has been made. If infection is strongly suspected, cultures become positive or the infant deteriorates, an aminoglycoside such as gentamicin should be added to the antibiotic regimen.

Treatment of the ill baby requires good resuscitation, stabilization and respiratory support, in addition to antibiotics given after cultures have been taken. Blood or plasma transfusion, inotropic drugs and correction of acidosis are all important. Penicillin or ampicillin and gentamicin or netilmicin in combination provide the best cover for early-onset pneumonia.

Late-onset pneumonia

This may be associated with mechanical ventilation, aspiration, bacteremia or occur secondary to late invasion with an organism acquired during birth, e.g. GBS or *Listeria monocytogenes*. Occasionally unusual organisms such as chlamydia, candida, cytomegalovirus, Herpes simplex, respiratory syncytial virus or mycoplasma are implicated although staphylococci and coliforms are much more commonly found.

Clinical features

Late-onset pneumonia occurs after 24 h and presents with signs of respiratory distress although preterm babies may develop apnea. There may be systemic signs with pyrexia in term babies and hypothermia in preterm ones. Bacteremia and meningitis can be present at the same time.

A chest radiograph is necessary for diagnosis, and culture of blood, tracheal aspirate and CSF should also be performed. The differential diagnosis includes persistent ductus arteriosus and heart failure, aspiration pneumonia, Wilson–Mikity syndrome or an inborn error of metabolism.

Management

General supportive measures, antibiotics and perhaps gentle chest physiotherapy form the basis of management. Antibiotic selection must cover staphylococci and Gram-negative organisms and if meningitis is suspected be capable of penetrating the CSF. A combination of flucloxacillin and netilmicin or one of the third generation cephalosporins, e.g. cefotaxime, is usually satisfactory. For pseudomonas infections ceftazidime is used.

Outcome

Early-onset pneumonia has a high mortality of about 50% especially when due to GBS which often affects very immature babies who have septicemia with pneumonia. Late-onset pneumonia has a mortality rate of less than 15% despite its association with bacteremia and meningitis.

MECONIUM ASPIRATION SYNDROME

This is a serious and potentially preventable condition occurring usually in term and post-term babies.

Incidence

Meconium staining of the amniotic fluid is found in about 9% of deliveries at term, and at birth 56% of these babies have meconium in their tracheas. However, only 20% of babies born through meconium-stained liquor develop pulmonary disease requiring oxygen supplementation or have a pulmonary air leak (Gregory et al 1974). The incidence may be lower in the UK where obstetricians manage prolonged pregnancy more aggressively (Cardozo et al 1986).

Etiology and pathogenesis

In the term or post-term infant asphyxia prior to birth stimulates intestinal peristalsis and relaxation of the anal sphincter. Meconium passage is most likely to occur in the post-term baby, the term baby after asphyxia or the baby with intrauterine growth retardation. It rarely happens in the preterm baby of less than 34 weeks' gestation as even with severe asphyxia the anal sphincter does not usually relax.

If meconium staining does occur in preterm labor one should consider an alternative cause such as congenital infection, especially that due to listeriosis (Halliday & Hirata 1979). Once meconium reaches the major airways, respiration after birth ensures distal migration into the smaller airways. This may lead to obstruction with air trapping and atelectasis and pneumothorax is a common complication.

Other factors producing lung disease are chemical pneumonitis and secondary bacterial infection. There may be abnormal pulmonary vascular spasm with arteriolar thickening causing pulmonary hypertension.

Clinical features

Affected babies are usually post-term or growth retarded. There may be meconium staining of the skin, umbilical cord and nails. The baby may present with respiratory distress from birth but more usually the respiratory symptoms develop over 12 h with tachypnea, cyanosis, indrawing and a hyperinflated chest. There may be profound hypoxemia although hypercarbia is less common. Metabolic acidosis and hypoglycemia are common and postasphyxial signs may be found in the central nervous system, kidneys and heart. Pneumothorax complicates about 30% of cases of severe meconium aspiration syndrome.

Diagnosis

The diagnosis is made on the basis of meconium-stained amniotic fluid, presence of meconium in the trachea and radiological changes. On chest radiograph there is overinflation of the lungs with widespread coarse, fluffy opacities (Fig. 5.30). Sometimes the appearances are confined to the right lung or right upper lobe. Pneumothorax, pneumomediastinum and cardiomegaly may be

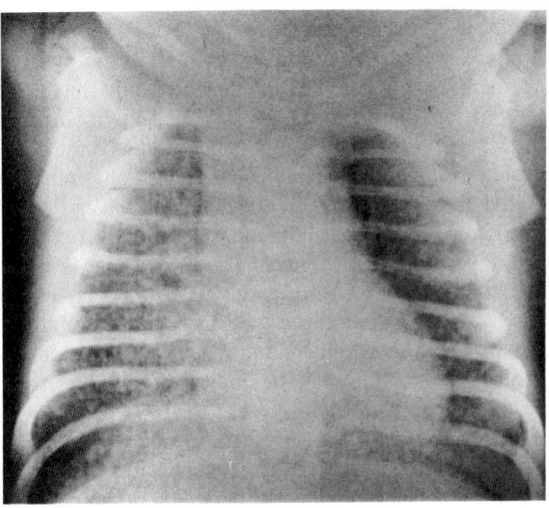

Fig. 5.30 Meconium aspiration syndrome with overinflated lungs, depressed diaphragm and coarse modular opacities alternating with areas of focal overinflation.

present. There is usually slow radiological clearing over 10 days but in some babies the meconium disappears within 2–3 days possibly by ciliary action, phagocytosis or enzymatic lysis (Halahakoon & Halliday 1995).

Management

This comprises prevention by intervention in pregnancy or labor, and the treatment of established aspiration.

Prevention

Meconium aspiration syndrome should be largely preventable by careful antenatal monitoring, rapid delivery for fetal distress and rapid resuscitation and tracheal suctioning at birth. A pediatrician skilled at neonatal resuscitation should attend all deliveries complicated by meconium staining of the amniotic fluid. If the meconium staining is thick and particulate ('pea soup'), an attempt to clear the mouth and pharynx should be made as soon as the head has been delivered. After birth the larynx should be inspected directly and, if meconium is found, the trachea should be carefully intubated and meconium aspirated from the airway.

Intubation of all meconium-stained babies and careful tracheal toilet has been advocated as a method of reducing mortality and severity of subsequent respiratory distress. A large randomized study, however, showed no benefit of routine endotracheal intubation in these circumstances and indeed the babies whose airways were aspirated had more respiratory problems than the control infants (Linder et al 1988). Intubation is best reserved for babies with signs of respiratory depression and asphyxia or those born through thick, particulate meconium-stained liquor. Tracheal aspiration using an endotracheal tube adaptor should be repeated until the trachea is cleared and saline lavage should be avoided as this may help to liquefy the meconium allowing it to pass distally (Halahakoon & Halliday 1995). Positive pressure ventilation with oxygen to achieve oxygenation must be balanced with tracheal aspiration during the resuscitation.

Treatment

All babies with meconium below the vocal cords should be admitted to the neonatal unit for observation and further management. All symptomatic babies should have a chest radiograph performed and oxygen supplements as indicated by blood gas analyses. Babies with mild disease may need only humidified oxygen in a headbox. Gentle chest physiotherapy and postural drainage may be helpful but lung lavage should be avoided. Broad spectrum antibiotics should be given to treat a coexistent pneumonia or congenital sepsis. There is no benefit from the use of hydrocortisone and it may even delay recovery.

Severely asphyxiated babies with meconium aspiration often have multisystem involvement and require careful management. Mechanical ventilation may be indicated to treat respiratory failure and severe hypoxemia.

Rapid ventilator rates with low PEEP are advised because of the risk of pneumothorax and cardiovascular side effects. Muscle relaxation or sedation with morphine is often necessary. If hypoxemia due to right-to-left shunting persists the PEEP may be increased up to 6 cmH$_2$O and a tolazoline infusion may be helpful. The use of inhaled nitric oxide remains experimental but treatment with surfactant might be beneficial (Davis et al 1992).

Outcome

Infants with mild disease who do not require assisted ventilation recover within a few days. Recent reports suggest lower mortality rates of about 10% (Wiswell et al 1990, Halahakoon & Halliday 1995). Both mortality and long-term neurodevelopmental sequelae are related to the severity of the underlying perinatal asphyxia. There is an increased risk of asthma among survivors of meconium aspiration syndrome compared with the general childhood population (Macfarlane & Heaf 1989).

OTHER ASPIRATION PNEUMONIAS

Aspiration may occur before, during or after birth. Apart from meconium the substances aspirated may be amniotic fluid, blood, secretions or milk.

Incidence

This is unknown but early contrast radiography studies showed that 10–15% of newborn babies aspirate fluid into their lungs during the first few days after birth. It is likely that the incidence of milk aspiration in preterm babies has substantially decreased as a result of more widespread use of intravenous fluids which allows the volume of feeds to be gradually increased. Preterm babies with endotracheal tubes for mechanical ventilation probably aspirate secretions frequently; one study suggested that this occurred in 80% of such babies (Goodwin et al 1985).

Etiology

Aspiration can occur before birth and amniotic debris including squamous cells have been found in the lungs of stillborn babies. Aspiration of small amounts of fetal and maternal blood do not appear to cause major problems and are rapidly removed from the lungs. If purulent secretions are aspirated during birth there is an increased risk of subsequent bacterial pneumonia. Aspiration of milk may occur in the very preterm infant, those with swallowing disorders, and those with esophageal atresia and tracheoesophageal fistula. Before 34 weeks, sucking and swallowing are uncoordinated and most babies need gastric tube feeds. Aspiration of liquids may cause apnea as part of a protective laryngeal reflex.

Clinical features

Aspiration before or during birth may cause signs of asphyxia and immediate respiratory distress in the same way as meconium aspiration syndrome. Aspiration after birth presents with apneic or cyanotic attacks and there may be choking or signs of airway obstruction. After such an episode there may be tachypnea and indrawing.

Apart from immaturity, babies at risk of aspiration are those who have suffered asphyxia or those with neuromuscular disorders who may also have drooling, poor suck and myopathic facies. If there are recurrent episodes of aspiration, an underlying disorder such as H-type tracheoesophageal fistula or posterior laryngeal cleft should be excluded. In supine infants aspiration is most likely to occur into the right upper lobe and crepitations may be heard there. Occasionally there may be complete collapse of a lobe with shift of the mediastinum towards the affected side.

Diagnosis

The chest radiograph may be clear or show localized or diffuse opacities and areas of atelectasis. These changes are most frequently seen in the right upper lobe (Fig. 5.29). Aspirate from the lung may show fat-laden macrophages in babies who have aspirated milk or medium chain triglycerides. If gastroesophageal reflux is suspected, barium swallow, esophageal manometry or pH studies and endoscopy may be necessary.

Management

Direct laryngoscopy and careful suction of the airways should be performed to resuscitate babies who have aspirated. Supportive care includes oxygen to correct hypoxemia, intravenous fluids and the treatment of acidosis. Broad spectrum antibiotics should be given if the extent of the aspiration is large or the secretions aspirated appear to be infected. Careful nursing is important, gastric emptying is most rapid with the baby lying either prone or on the right side.

PULMONARY AIR LEAKS

These comprise pneumothorax, pulmonary interstitial emphysema, pneumomediastinum, pneumopericardium, pneumoperitoneum, subcutaneous emphysema and air embolism. They are related conditions of varying severity which have a common etiology and pathogenesis (Halahakoon & Halliday 1995).

Etiology and pathogenesis

Alveolar rupture occurs more commonly in the neonate than any other time of life. It is more likely to occur in states of hyperinflation of the chest and the risk is increased because of lack of pores of Kohn which are communications between alveoli.

Air leak occurs at the base of a group of alveoli and tracks into the perivascular sheath at the center of the pulmonary lobule (Plenat et al 1978). Air later tracks along the bronchovascular spaces to the hilum where it dissects into the mediastinum and pleural space. Air may also form subpleural blebs which can later rupture to cause a pneumothorax. Extension of air into the subcutaneous tissues of the neck will cause surgical emphysema, and down along perivascular or periesophageal tissue sheaths to form a pneumoperitoneum. A pneumothorax may result from high transpulmonary pressures generated by the first breath but it more usually arises later because of some underlying lung pathology such as respiratory distress syndrome, aspiration syndromes, pulmonary hypoplasia and positive pressure ventilation. Traumatic pneumothorax may occur from perforation of the lung by a suction catheter or a chest drain. Although the more mature lung ruptures at lower transpulmonary pressures than the immature lung, pneumothorax is commoner in the preterm baby who is more likely to have respiratory distress.

Pneumothorax

This is accumulation of air within the pleural cavity and usually occurs following a pneumomediastinum, although the latter may not be obvious clinically or radiologically.

Incidence

About 1% of term babies have an asymptomatic pneumothorax.

Symptomatic pneumothorax is less common occurring in about 1 in 1000 live births. With mild RDS the incidence of pneumothorax is about 5% increasing to 10–20% when continuous positive airways pressure is used, and to 20–40% for babies having mechanical ventilation. About 10% of babies with transient tachypnea of the newborn and 40% of those with meconium aspiration syndrome develop pneumothoraces (Halliday 1992).

Clinical presentation

Most babies with spontaneously occurring pneumothoraces who have no underlying lung pathology have minimal signs of respiratory distress and the pneumothorax is seen as an incidental finding on a chest radiograph taken for another reason. However, most significant pneumothoraces occur in babies with underlying pulmonary disease and the diagnosis should be suspected in any such baby whose condition suddenly deteriorates. If the baby is breathing spontaneously, tachypnea, grunting and cyanosis are often the presenting signs. In a unilateral pneumothorax there may be shift of the mediastinum (apex beat) away from the side of the pneumothorax and breath sounds may be reduced on the affected side. The affected hemithorax or the abdomen may appear distended because of increased tension within the pleural space. There may be hyper-resonance to percussion on the affected side and hypotension may occur because of venous compression and reduced cardiac output. In the baby with a small pneumothorax there may be an increase in cardiac output, heart rate and blood pressure so that continuous monitoring of blood pressure can help to make the diagnosis (Goldberg 1981).

In about 10% of babies pneumothoraces will be bilateral and this causes a major hemodynamic upset which for the very preterm baby may prove fatal. In survivors there is an increased likelihood of intraventricular hemorrhage (Lipscomb et al 1981).

Diagnosis

The chest radiograph is the usual method of confirming the diagnosis and anterior-posterior (Fig. 5.31) and lateral views should be taken (Swischuk 1976). The lateral will show air in the

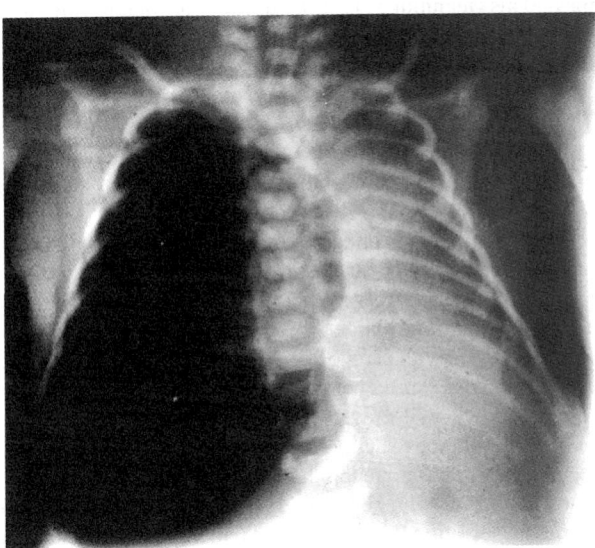

Fig. 5.31 Right tension pneumothorax with depression of the diaphragm and shift of the mediastinum to the left. There is also mediastinal herniation.

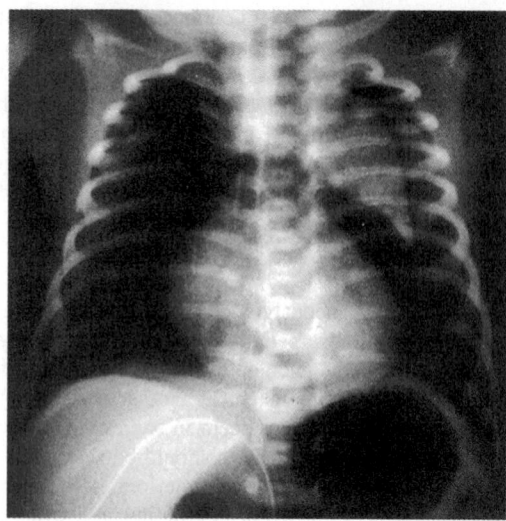

Fig. 5.32 Bilateral pneumothoraces and large pneumomediastinum with elevation of the lobes of the thymus clear of the cardiac shadow (the sail sign). The endotracheal tube is shown with its tip in the right mainstem bronchus.

anterior mediastinum and the thymus may be lifted up, which may also be evident on the AP film (Fig. 5.32). If the pneumothorax is extensive there will be collapse of the lung and shift of the mediastinum away from the affected side (Fig. 5.31). Sometimes a pneumothorax may only be seen medially and may be mistaken for a pneumomediastinum. Ultrasound scanning may be helpful in distinguishing these (Van Gelderen 1992). For the baby who deteriorates suddenly, there may not be time to wait for a chest radiograph, and two alternative methods of confirming the diagnosis of pneumothorax have been used. For the baby in extremis diagnostic pleural aspiration using a needle, syringe and three-way tap can be performed without delay. The second or third intercostal space in the mid-clavicular line should be used for this procedure which is both diagnostic and therapeutic. Transillumination of the chest with a fiberoptic bright light can be used to rapidly diagnose large pneumothoraces in less severely ill babies. This technique is less useful for diagnosing small pneumothoraces or those occurring in term babies.

Treatment

No treatment is necessary if the infant is asymptomatic. For term babies with mild symptoms, nitrogen washout by breathing high oxygen concentrations may be used to accelerate resorption of gas loculated within the pneumothorax. The only satisfactory treatment of a tension pneumothorax is insertion of a pleural drain connected to a nonreturn valve such as an underwater seal drain. The drain should be large bore and placed in the anterior mediastinal space with care to avoid perforation of the lung. Local anesthetic should be used before making a small skin incision and an artery forceps will prevent overpenetration of the trocar into the chest. Continuous suction of 10–20 cmH$_2$O helps to prevent reaccumulation of the pneumothorax.

Careful fluid balance should be observed as increased vasopressin secretion, leading to fluid retention, may occur after a pneumothorax although this is not common (McIntosh et al 1990). Fibrin glue pleurodesis has been used to treat persistent

pneumothorax with bronchopleural fistula (Berger & Gilhooly 1993).

Prevention

The incidence of pneumothorax may be reduced by muscle relaxation for babies with severe RDS having mechanical ventilation (Greenough et al 1984), rapid rate conventional ventilators with reduced inspiratory time (Heicher et al 1981) and natural surfactant replacement used either prophylactically at birth in babies of less than 30 weeks' gestation or to treat babies with severe RDS (Collaborative European Multicenter Study Group 1988, Soll & McQueen 1992, Halliday 1992).

Prognosis

Pneumothorax is associated with a high morbidity and mortality which depends upon the nature of the underlying lung disease and the gestational age of the baby. Both mortality rate and intraventricular hemorrhage rate are doubled following pneumothorax.

Pulmonary interstitial emphysema

This is the presence of air in the interstitium or perivascular tissues of the lung and it is probably a prerequisite of all other forms of air leak.

Incidence

The true incidence is uncertain but interstitial emphysema has been described in about 10% of neonatal autopsies. The incidence in control groups of the randomized surfactant trials varies from 25–50% (Halliday 1992).

Pathogenesis

After alveolar rupture, air escapes into the pulmonary interstitium to form regular air-filled cysts varying from 0.1 to 1.0 cm in diameter. These are localized to the interlobular septa and extend radially from the hila of each lung to form a diffuse or a localized pattern. Lung function is impaired by compression of normal lung tissue, decreased compliance and obstruction of pulmonary blood flow. Interstitial emphysema is associated with raised leukocyte elastase levels in tracheal aspirates suggesting that intrauterine infection may predispose (Fujimura et al 1993).

Clinical presentation

When interstitial emphysema is localized there may be no symptoms or the baby may gradually deteriorate. If the condition becomes diffuse there is progressive hypoxemia and ventilation–perfusion imbalance necessitating an increase in ventilator settings. There is usually decreased chest wall movement with hyperinflation of the chest and muffling of the heart sounds.

Diagnosis

The chest radiograph may show areas of translucency and collapse scattered throughout the lung fields rather like a

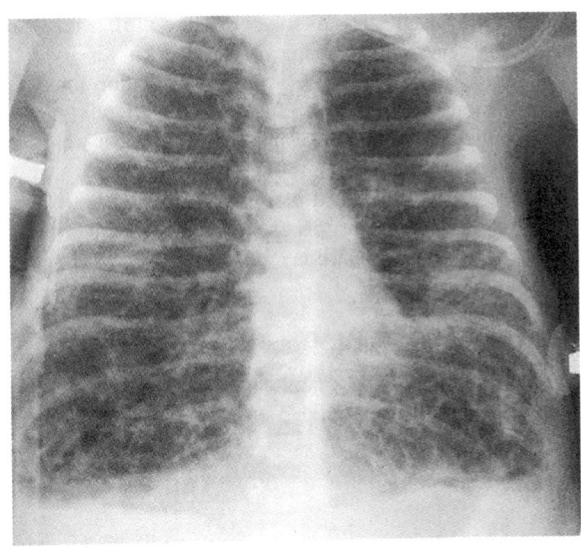

Fig. 5.33 Bilateral diffuse pulmonary interstitial emphysema with marked overinflation of the chest, lowered diaphragm and narrowed heart shadow.

snowstorm (Fig. 5.33). If the changes are localized to one lung there may be marked overinflation and shift of the mediastinum as in a tension pneumothorax. Pseudocysts may form within the pulmonary parenchyma beneath the visceral pleura or along fissure lines.

Treatment

For diffuse interstitial emphysema, fast rate mechanical ventilation using low pressures has been advocated and periods of fast rate hand bagging up to 140 breaths/min may also be of benefit. A more conservative approach has been suggested with postural drainage and chest physiotherapy especially in cases of unilateral interstitial emphysema under tension. More aggressive treatment has also been used to manage the severe unilateral form of interstitial emphysema and includes selective intubation of the normal lung to allow the emphysematous lung to collapse, (Rettwitz-Volk et al 1993), selective bronchial obstruction of the affected side, artificial creation of a pneumothorax by probing (Dear & Conway 1984) or some form of surgical procedure.

Prognosis

Severe diffuse interstitial emphysema occurring soon after birth has a very high mortality rate. For babies weighing less than 1000 g, mortality at 67% is more than twice that of babies without interstitial emphysema (Hart et al 1983). Complications such as pneumothorax and intraventricular hemorrhage are common and affected babies need prolonged ventilator support. Surviving infants have an increased risk of developing bronchopulmonary dysplasia.

Pneumomediastinum

Incidence

Pneumomediastinum probably occurs prior to all cases of pneumothorax but it often goes unrecognized.

Clinical presentation

Pneumomediastinum may occur with other air leaks or in isolation, when it is asymptomatic in over 90% of cases, being noticed incidentally on a routine chest radiograph. If there are symptoms the baby may have tachypnea, cyanosis and an overinflated chest which is hyper-resonant to percussion. Occasionally a large pneumomediastinum causes severe symptoms by compressing the heart and lungs.

Diagnosis

Confirmed by chest radiograph. The lateral view is most helpful to demonstrate air lying anteriorly. The thymus may be lifted off the mediastinum in the anteroposterior view giving rise to the 'sail sign' or 'spinnaker sign' (Fig. 5.32).

Treatment

In pneumomediastinum the air is loculated so that drainage is impracticable. The rate of absorption can be accelerated by breathing high oxygen concentrations provided that the infant is full term.

Pneumopericardium

This occurs in about 1.6% of babies with respiratory distress syndrome (Madansky et al 1979).

Clinical presentation

Occasionally asymptomatic but more usually presents with pallor, shock and hypotension due to cardiac tamponade. In most cases other forms of air leak are associated.

Diagnosis

Chest radiograph shows a complete ring of air around the heart. The transverse diameter of the heart is reduced if tamponade is present and substernal transillumination may be used to make a rapid diagnosis in the baby who suddenly deteriorates during mechanical ventilation.

Treatment

The only effective treatment for pneumopericardium with tamponade is immediate drainage of air from the pericardial sac using a needle and syringe directed anteriorly and superiorly from below the xiphisternum. Recurrence of tamponade is common and permanent drainage is often needed.

Prognosis

The mortality is high despite early drainage with more than half of affected babies dying.

Pneumoperitoneum

Air in the peritoneal cavity may be the result of a pulmonary air leak or a ruptured abdominal viscus.

Incidence

The incidence of pneumoperitoneum as a complication of mechanical ventilation is about 2% (Madansky et al 1979).

Clinical presentation

This may be asymptomatic or present as abdominal distention. There are usually other signs of air leak (Fig. 5.34).

Treatment

Aspiration is only necessary if abdominal distention is severe enough to compromise ventilation.

Subcutaneous emphysema

This is rare in the neonate and when it does occur it is usually associated with pneumomediastinum. Air from the superior mediastinum passes along the perivascular fascia to the subclavicular area before spreading subcutaneously. Apart from swelling and a typically crackling feel to the affected skin there are few other signs and the air usually absorbs in a few days.

Air embolism (pneumatosis arterialis)

This is an uncommon and almost universally fatal condition which may present as air being withdrawn from an umbilical arterial catheter in an infant who has collapsed (Fenton et al 1988). Air embolism results from rupture of pulmonary veins associated with raised intra-alveolar pressure during mechanical ventilation of very preterm babies. Affected babies have other forms of air leak and deteriorate acutely with pallor, bradycardia and hypotension. Chest and abdominal radiographs show gas shadows in the heart chambers and major arteries. Massive air embolism is usually fatal but one surviving baby has been reported where the embolism was minor (Kogutt 1978). There is no effective treatment but prevention involves avoidance of unnecessary barotrauma (Halliday 1992).

PULMONARY HEMORRHAGE

Sometimes called massive pulmonary hemorrhage, this poorly understood condition has a sudden onset and a high mortality.

Incidence

Isolated pulmonary hemorrhage is a rare condition occurring in approximately 1 per 1000 live births. Between 2 and 5% of babies with RDS develop pulmonary hemorrhage (Raju & Langenberg 1993).

Etiology and pathogenesis

Pulmonary hemorrhage can occur in small for gestational age babies with no underlying lung disease but more usually there has been a history of severe perinatal asphyxia, hypothermia, rhesus isoimmunization, pneumonia, hypoglycemia, coagulation disorder or fluid overload, particularly when a patent ductus arteriosus is present. It is likely that pulmonary hemorrhage is a form of hemorrhagic pulmonary edema which occurs secondary to left ventricular failure and damage to pulmonary capillaries. The edema fluid usually has an hematocrit of less than 10% and is probably a filtrate from pulmonary capillaries. Pulmonary hemorrhage may sometimes be secondary to aspiration, hypoproteinemia and lung tissue damage from pneumonia, RDS, oxygen toxicity or mechanical ventilation. There is an association with surfactant treatment especially in the very immature infant (Stevenson et al 1992, Raju & Langenberg 1993).

Clinical presentation

The onset is frequently between the second and fourth day after birth when an infant with respiratory distress shows sudden deterioration with shock, cyanosis, bradycardia and apnea. Pink or red frothy fluid is aspirated from the mouth and lungs and the baby needs urgent resuscitation to prevent death. In ventilated babies, bloodstained fluid appears in the endotracheal tube during suctioning. Auscultation of the chest will reveal widespread crepitations.

Diagnosis

Chest radiograph shows large areas of consolidation with areas of diffuse opacification. In its worst form the lungs may appear completely white and there may be cardiomegaly. Sometimes the diagnosis is only confirmed at autopsy when widespread intra-alveolar and interstitial hemorrhage is found (van Houten et al 1992).

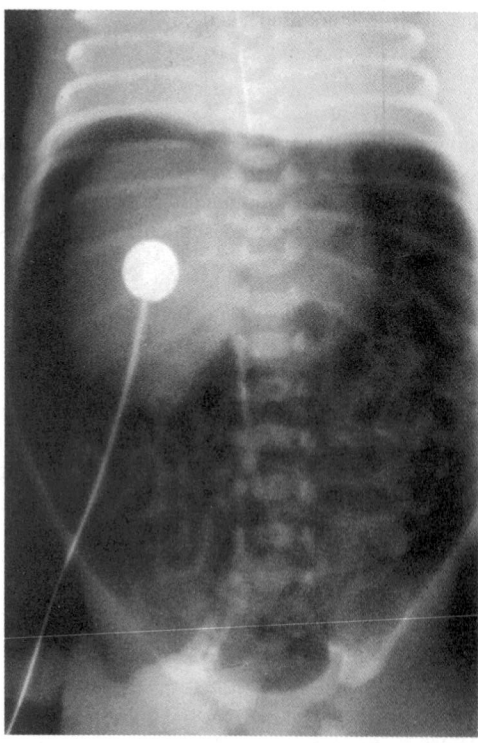

Fig. 5.34 Large pneumoperitoneum with the liver clearly outlined by the air in the peritoneal cavity. The lungs appear collapsed and airless.

Treatment

Immediate resuscitation of the collapsed baby is important with endotracheal intubation for mechanical ventilation and volume expansion with blood or plasma. High positive end expiratory pressures (PEEP) may help to reduce bleeding by tamponade, and a diuretic such as frusemide may reduce pulmonary edema. Correction of acidosis and underlying coagulation disorder is beneficial and antibiotics should be given if infection is suspected. Repeated doses of surfactant may be beneficial (Pandit et al 1995a).

Prognosis

Until recently massive pulmonary hemorrhage was invariably fatal but prompt use of mechanical ventilation and transfusions of fresh whole blood have improved the outlook (Halahakoon & Halliday 1995).

Prevention

Prevention is most important because of the poor outlook once pulmonary hemorrhage has occurred. Small for gestational age babies should not be allowed to develop asphyxia, hypothermia, hypoglycemia or acidosis. Coagulation defects in these babies should be corrected early.

DEVELOPMENTAL ANOMALIES OF THE LUNG

Pulmonary hypoplasia

In this condition, which is frequently bilateral, the lungs are smaller than normal. Unilateral hypoplasia may be primary but is more often associated with other congenital malformations such as diaphragmatic hernia.

Incidence

Pulmonary hypoplasia is present in 15 to 20% of early neonatal deaths and is now the commonest single abnormality at autopsy (Wigglesworth & Desai 1982).

Etiology and pathogenesis

Pulmonary hypoplasia occurs as a primary lesion in about 10% of cases but is most often associated with other malformations that restrict lung growth (Table 5.58). Pulmonary hypoplasia, as a result of oligohydramnios, is caused by the combined effects of reduced lung volume and impaired fetal breathing.

Table 5.58 Pathogenesis of pulmonary hypoplasia

1. Oligohydramnios: renal agenesis, urinary tract obstruction, prolonged rupture of the membranes

2. Lung compression: diaphragmatic hernia, lung cysts, pleural effusions, erythroblastosis, chondrodystrophies

3. Absent fetal breathing movements: anencephaly, neuromuscular disorders

Clinical presentation

The diagnosis may be suspected prenatally if there has been prolonged rupture of the membranes or an ultrasound scan has demonstrated congenital diaphragmatic hernia or a chondrodystrophy. Babies with pulmonary hypoplasia may present at birth with signs of asphyxia and difficulties in resuscitation. Some of these babies have Potter's syndrome and do not survive; pneumothoraces readily develop during resuscitation. With less severe degrees of hypoplasia the presentation is less acute with mild but prolonged respiratory distress and oxygen dependency. Congenital diaphragmatic hernia must be excluded by chest radiograph (Fig. 5.35). Such a hernia is usually left sided, in 80% of cases occurring through the foramen of Bochdalek and there is displacement of the mediastinum to the right by stomach and bowel. About 25% of cases have associated congenital heart lesions which increase mortality.

Diagnosis

In life it is difficult to confirm the diagnosis unless an associated abnormality such as Potter's syndrome, diaphragmatic hernia, Jeune's syndrome or prolonged oligohydramnios is present. Sometimes chest radiograph shows small lungs with a bell-shaped thorax. At autopsy lung : bodyweight ratio may be helpful in making the diagnosis provided that there is no postnatal complication such as pneumonia or pulmonary hemorrhage. A lung : bodyweight ratio of less than 0.012 for babies over 28 weeks' gestation and less than 0.015 for lower gestations is used to define pulmonary hypoplasia (Wigglesworth & Desai 1981). Strict confirmation of the diagnosis requires more sophisticated autopsy analysis such as radial alveolar counts or DNA estimation.

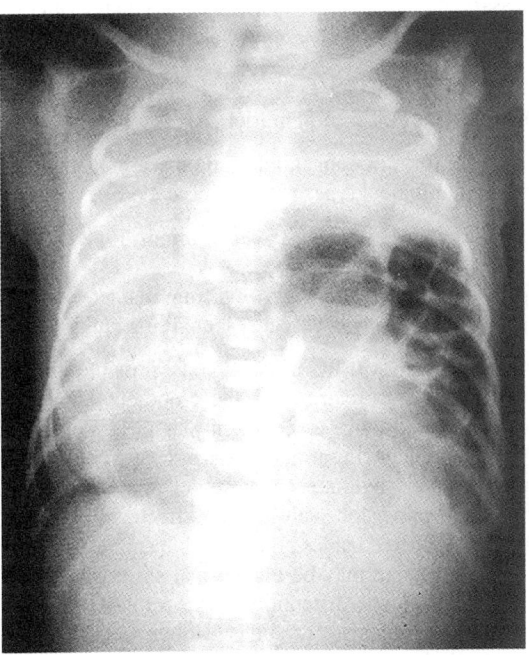

Fig. 5.35 Large left-sided diaphragmatic hernia with mediastinal shift to the right. Air in the stomach and intestine is due to resuscitation with bag and mask.

Management

The outlook depends upon the severity of the respiratory signs and the associated congenital anomalies. Severe pulmonary hypoplasia occurring with oligohydramnios is usually fatal but on occasions mechanical ventilation with high pressures has been successful in 'opening up' the lungs (McIntosh 1988). Although surfactant deficiency is present in some cases surfactant replacement therapy is not successful (Tubman & Halliday 1990). Babies with diaphragmatic hernia need surgical correction, but even with this, severe unilateral pulmonary hypoplasia can be associated with marked pulmonary hypertension which does not respond to mechanical ventilation or vasodilators such as tolazoline. Extracorporeal membrane oxygenation (ECMO) and inhaled nitric oxide remain as experimental treatments (Milner & Fox 1995). For babies who survive the neonatal period, lung growth occurs and their prognosis improves.

Congenital lobar emphysema

This is an uncommon condition where overinflation of one or more lobes occurs secondary to bronchial obstruction or deficiency of bronchial cartilage. The left upper lobe and the right middle lobe are most commonly affected and the babies present with signs of respiratory distress and occasionally wheezing. Boys are affected twice as commonly as girls (Milner & Fox 1995). The chest radiograph may initially show lobar opacification due to fluid trapped beyond the obstruction but later the affected lobe becomes overdistended and there may be shift of the mediastinum (Fig. 5.36).

Bronchoscopy is often needed to make the diagnosis and to remove any cause of bronchial obstruction. If symptoms are slight, conservative management is preferred and continuous positive airway pressure may be beneficial. For babies with persistent respiratory failure, surgical excision of the affected lobe is necessary. In about 30% of affected babies there is an associated congenital heart defect.

Cystic adenomatoid malformation

This is a rare form of congenital cystic disease of the lung which has three pathological types (Stocker et al 1978):

Type I   multiple large cysts which mimic Type III lobar
          emphysema (70%)
Type II   medium-sized cysts (< 12 mm diameter) (20%)
Type III small cysts evenly distributed in a bulky lung (10%).

Antenatal diagnosis by ultrasound is possible. Half of the affected babies are preterm and about one-quarter are stillborn with boys affected twice as commonly as girls. Polyhydramnios and hydrops occur in about one-third of cases. Associated anomalies include hydranencephaly and prune-belly syndrome. The middle or upper lobes are usually affected and the condition is unilateral. Affected babies present with respiratory distress soon after birth, and there may be mediastinal shift. Chest radiograph shows the cystic overdistention of the affected lung and the differential diagnosis includes lobar emphysema and diaphragmatic hernia. Treatment is by lobectomy which gives a generally good prognosis in Type I but survival is reduced in Types II and III largely because of the severity of associated anomalies.

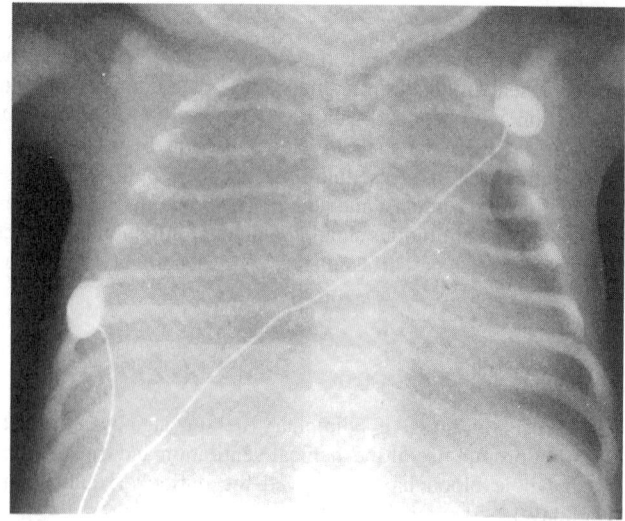

a

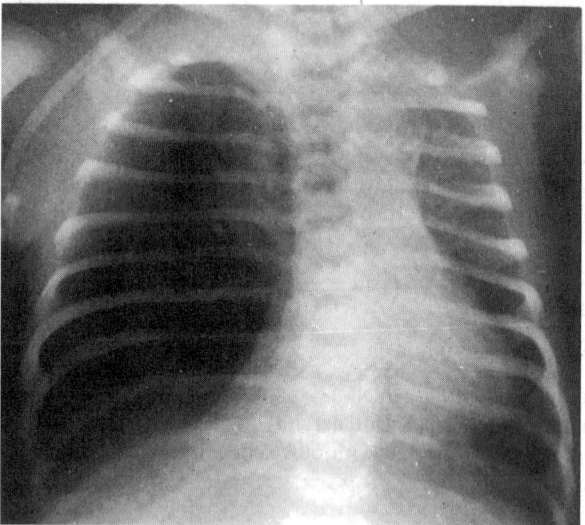

b

Fig. 5.36 (a) Congenital lobar emphysema showing retained lung fluid on the right as a result of bronchial obstruction, and displacement of the heart shadow to the left. (b) After 24 h with clearance of the lung fluid the right lung shows gross overinflation and the mediastinal displacement is more clearly demonstrated.

Other lung cysts

Neurenteric cysts present as a mediastinal mass on chest radiograph in association with vertebral anomalies. Gastrogenic cysts, containing gastric mucosa, may ulcerate and cause hemoptysis. Duplication cysts of the duodenum may extend through the diaphragm and, if associated with a vertebral anomaly, can cause meningitis.

Bronchogenic cysts

These may present as episodes of wheezing or stridor. They are found near the carina but may be radiolucent on chest radiograph. If bronchial obstruction occurs there may be retained lung fluid giving rise to confluent opacity of one lung or lobe on radiography. Antenatal diagnosis by ultrasound scan is possible.

Sequestration of the lung

This is a mass of embryonic lung tissue that does not communicate with the bronchial tree, and has a systemic rather than a pulmonary arterial supply. It may be intra- or extralobar and in the latter communication with the foregut, and other congenital anomalies including congenital heart disease are common. Males are more commonly affected and in about three-quarters of cases the sequestration is on the left side. Ultrasound can be used to make the diagnosis prenatally. Extralobar lesions are more likely to be symptomatic but abnormality on chest radiograph is the most usual presentation. A triangular density at the left lung base extending to the mediastinum gives rise to the 'scimitar sign'. Bronchoscopy, radionuclide scanning or aortography may be needed to confirm the diagnosis. In 65% of cases there are associated anomalies (Stocker 1986). Surgery for intralobar sequestrations prevents repeated respiratory infections and may also be needed for extralobar lesions that are symptomatic.

Chylothorax

This is a form of pleural effusion in which chyle or lymphatic fluid appears in the pleural cavity. The condition may be spontaneous or acquired, both being more common in males and typically unilateral with 60% occurring on the right side. In spontaneous chylothorax there is usually an anomaly of lymphatic drainage and chylous ascites and lymphedema may be associated. Acquired chylothorax may follow birth trauma or thoracotomy. About half of affected babies present with respiratory distress soon after birth and a further one-quarter have symptoms by the end of the first week. Breath sounds are reduced on the affected side and there is mediastinal shift away from this side. Chest radiography shows diffuse opacity with depressed diaphragm and mediastinal shift. A pleural tap will show clear yellow fluid soon after birth and only after feeding does the effusion appear chylous. The fluid is sterile and contains large numbers of lymphocytes and fat globules. Treatment is initially by thoracocentesis and most babies recover after one or two drainage procedures. Occasionally several drainage attempts are necessary and there is a risk of protein and lymphocyte depletion in these babies. If reaccumulation becomes a problem, use of a milk formula containing medium chain triglycerides will reduce the production of chyle. Pleural effusion can also occur in cases of hydrops, Turner's syndrome, pneumonia and congestive heart failure.

Pulmonary lymphangiectasis

In this rare condition there is bilateral cystic dilation of pulmonary lymphatics with obstruction of lymph drainage. Three types have been described: a primary isolated developmental defect accounting for 70% of cases; a generalized type which presents with generalized edema, malabsorption, hemihypertrophy and other anomalies; and thirdly a type associated with congenital heart disease and obstruction of pulmonary venous return (total anomalous pulmonary venous drainage, closure of atrial septum in hypoplastic left heart syndrome or pulmonary vein atresia).

There may be polyhydramnios and antenatal diagnosis by ultrasound scan is possible. Babies with primary lymphangiectasis are often born at term and have progressive respiratory distress which is usually fatal. Clinical and radiological features mimic respiratory distress syndrome so that there is underdiagnosis of this condition. Chest radiograph may show reticulogranular mottling with hyperaeration, and dilated lymphatics may sometimes be seen. Confirmation of the diagnosis is by lung biopsy or at autopsy.

Choanal atresia

This obstruction to the nasal airway may be unilateral or bilateral, membranous or bony. The incidence is about 0.3 per 1000 births with girls affected twice as commonly as boys. About two-thirds of cases are unilateral and in about half there are associated anomalies such as coloboma, heart defects, micrognathia and tracheoesophageal fistula. If the obstruction is bilateral, babies often present with great distress at birth, although when crying they may remain pink. Babies with unilateral choanal atresia may be asymptomatic or present later with a purulent nasal discharge. The diagnosis may be confirmed by attempting to pass a fine feeding tube or suction catheter, although use of a radiopaque dye and radiograph is sometimes necessary. The infant with bilateral choanal atresia needs an oral airway or oral endotracheal intubation followed by a surgical procedure. A transnasal or transpalatal approach may be used to open the posterior choanae and patency is maintained by inserting Silastic tubes for up to 2 months. Operative correction of unilateral choanal atresia may be postponed until the child is several years old.

Laryngomalacia

This is a condition where the larynx appears soft and flexible, associated with an elongated, floppy epiglottis and loose aryepiglottic folds which tend to be drawn over the glottis during inspiration. Also known as congenital laryngeal stridor, it needs to be distinguished from other causes of stridor such as vocal cord paralysis, vascular rings, laryngeal webs and cysts, and papillomata. The onset of stridor is usually on the second day of life but delay of up to 4 months is possible. Usually the stridor persists for less than 1 year. The diagnosis is confirmed by direct laryngoscopy which will help to exclude other causes of stridor. No specific treatment is required apart from reassurance of the parents although occasionally long-term feeding problems and speech difficulties occur.

CHRONIC LUNG DISEASES

The prevalence of chronic pulmonary disorders has increased because of more intensive respiratory support and improved survival of small preterm babies.

Bronchopulmonary dysplasia (BPD)

This form of chronic lung disease occurs in babies who have needed mechanical ventilation. It was first described in large babies who had been ventilated at high pressures and with high oxygen concentrations (Northway et al 1967). More recently it has become common in small preterm babies who, although ventilator dependent for long periods, have not needed high pressures or oxygen concentrations (Corcoran et al 1993).

Incidence

The incidence varies according to the definition used with rates between 5 and 40% of babies following mechanical ventilation being reported. The presence of oxygen dependency at 28 days is not sufficient to make the diagnosis and the chest radiograph should show cystic areas and strands of opacity corresponding to the Northway grades of III and IV (Northway et al 1967). With this definition about 10% of babies weighing less than 1500 g at birth and about 20% of those weighing less than 1000 g develop bronchopulmonary dysplasia. To simplify the definition of chronic lung disease, it has recently been suggested that oxygen dependency and other signs of respiratory distress at a postconceptional age of 36 weeks be used (Shennan et al 1988). With this stricter definition the incidence of BPD is reduced by about 50%.

Etiology and pathogenesis

Factors associated with the development of BPD are listed in Table 5.59. The single most important factor is the need for mechanical ventilation through an endotracheal tube. The role of barotrauma in the pathogenesis of lung damage is supported by the finding of increased airways resistance in the survivors of RDS who were treated with mechanical ventilation and low oxygen concentrations. Respiratory distress syndrome is not an absolute prerequisite for BPD as babies treated with mechanical ventilation for apnea or meconium aspiration syndrome also develop this complication. Oxygen concentrations in excess of 60% are toxic to the lungs of newborn mice causing proliferative changes in the alveoli rather than the smaller airways. Perhaps the combination of 'oxygen plus pressure plus time' is important. The role of pulmonary infection has probably been underestimated and the presence of an endotracheal tube with retention of secretions and recurrent infection is probably an important cause of lung damage. Other factors suggested as important in the pathogenesis of BPD include pulmonary interstitial emphysema, patent ductus arteriosus and fluid overload, and deficiency of vitamins A and E (Yu & Ng 1995).

Pathology

BPD is a disease of scarring and repair which affects lung growth. Histological abnormalities may be found in babies dying before the development of the clinical disease (Thurlbeck 1979). Babies dying of severe BPD have hyperinflated lungs with extensive destruction of alveoli causing widespread emphysema and fibrosis. There is also bronchial necrosis, peribronchial fibrosis and squamous metaplasia giving an obliterative bronchiolitis. Active epithelial regeneration is not uniform and there may be marked thickening of the intima of pulmonary arterioles which causes progressive pulmonary hypertension.

Table 5.59 Factors associated with BPD

Respiratory distress syndrome

Mechanical ventilation

Oxygen therapy

Pulmonary infection

Pulmonary interstitial emphysema

Patent ductus arteriosus

Fluid overload

Vitamin A or E deficiency

Clinical presentation

The diagnosis is rarely made clinically before the age of 3 weeks. The usual history is of a preterm baby treated with mechanical ventilation for RDS whose condition improves and then deteriorates so that he becomes ventilator or oxygen dependent.

Mild cases need increased inspired oxygen concentrations for a few weeks but in severe cases there may be progressive respiratory failure with tachypnea, indrawing, wheezing and recurrent apnea with cyanotic spells. Cor pulmonale may develop secondary to pulmonary hypertension, and these babies show hepatomegaly, increased weight gain and edema which is often found in the face and neck region (Halahakoon & Halliday 1995).

Diagnosis

BPD must be distinguished from Wilson–Mikity syndrome, chronic pneumonia, recurrent aspiration and heart failure due to patent ductus arteriosus. Chest radiographs show hyperinflation, coarse streaking and cystic changes most marked at the lung bases (Fig. 5.37, Table 5.60) (Northway et al 1967). Cytological examination of tracheal aspirate shows epithelial cell necrosis, squamous metaplasia and later regeneration which may be used to help in making the diagnosis and excluding chronic infection.

Management

In general babies should be ventilated and in oxygen for the shortest possible time; however, the arterial oxygen tension

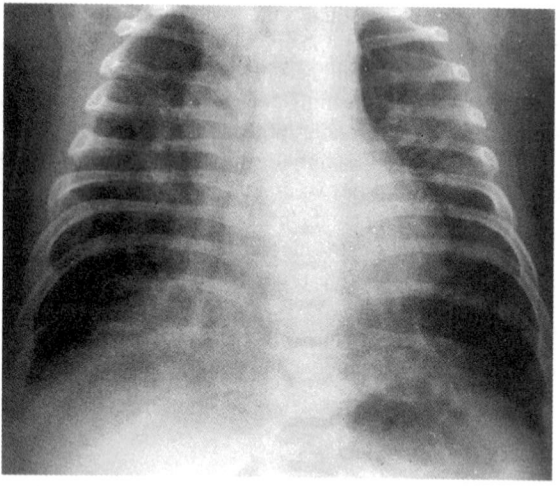

Fig. 5.37 Established bronchopulmonary dysplasia with basilar emphysema, coarse stranding and cystic changes amounting to stage 4 (see Table 5.60).

Table 5.60 Radiological stages in BPD

Stage 1: indistinguishable from respiratory distress syndrome (first week)

Stage 2: generalized opacity and pulmonary plethora (second week)

Stage 3: cystic changes with stranding (third week)

Stage 4: hyperinflation, widespread stranding, cardiomegaly (after fourth week)

should be maintained above 7 kPa as below this level there is an increase in pulmonary vascular resistance and a risk of cor pulmonale. Transcutaneous oxygen monitoring may under-estimate PaO_2 beyond the age of 10 weeks so that pulse oximetry may be preferable.

Weaning from the ventilator may be helped by allowing $PaCO_2$ levels to rise to 7–9 kPa so that peak inspiratory pressures can be lowered. Reduced fluid intake, diuretic therapy and closure of the ductus arteriosus may all assist in weaning. Theophylline has also been shown to improve lung function and shorten the duration of ventilation. Dexamethasone improves BPD in the short term sometimes allowing rapid weaning from the ventilator but the long-term efficacy of steroids have not been proven (Collaborative Dexamethasone Trial Group 1991). There are concerns about side effects (Ng 1993) so their use should be limited to babies who are ventilator-dependent. The role of steroids in the prevention of BPD is promising (Yeh et al 1990, Sanders et al 1994) and is currently being evaluated using both systemic and inhaled drug in a large international trial. Adequate nutrition is important and supplemental calories may be given in the form of long chain glucose polymers so that fluid restriction is possible without reducing energy intake. Blood transfusions should be given to keep the hematocrit above 40% and chest infections should be promptly treated with antibiotics and chest physiotherapy. In later infancy respiratory syncytial virus infections may cause acute deterioration and ribavirin has been advocated in these babies. Experimental treatments include inhaled nitric oxide and surfactant replacement (Pandit et al 1995b).

Prognosis

Many babies with BPD require prolonged oxygen therapy which may conveniently be given via a nasal catheter. For babies needing low flow rates home oxygen therapy significantly shortens the period in hospital.

Mortality in babies with severe BPD is about 25–30%. Surviving babies have frequent lower respiratory tract infections and often require hospital admission with persistent tachypnea, intermittent wheezing and subcostal retractions. Growth and development depend upon the severity of the lung disease and adverse perinatal events. Growth retardation is present in about one-third of survivors and major developmental defects in about 25%.

Wilson–Mikity syndrome

Wilson–Mikity syndrome is a form of chronic lung disease in very low birthweight babies who usually have not been treated with mechanical ventilation (Wilson & Mikity 1960).

Incidence

About 2% of babies with a birth weight less than 1500 g develop this condition (Lupton et al 1987).

Etiology and pathogenesis

This is uncertain. Air trapping due to compliant and collapsible airways was originally proposed and lung damage from pulmonary edema secondary to excessive fluid administration or chronic patent ductus arteriosus, rickets, recurrent aspiration, chronic surfactant deficiency and infection all have their advocates.

Clinical presentation

Very small preterm babies are affected with onset of symptoms after the first week of life. Affected babies have not had RDS and the onset is insidious with cyanosis, tachypnea, indrawing and recurrent apnea. Respiratory distress usually progresses to reach a peak at 4–8 weeks of age. Some infants die during this phase but most recover slowly without developing cor pulmonale.

Diagnosis

The chest radiograph is usually clear during the first week, with gradual appearance of a diffuse streaky infiltrate with small cystic areas throughout both lungs beginning after this time. Later, there is hyperinflation of the chest with large cystic areas which are often basal (Fig. 5.38). Radiological resolution lags behind clinical improvement and may take from 3 months to 2 years.

Treatment

Supportive care includes supplemental oxygen and mechanical ventilation if respiratory failure supervenes. Fluid restriction and diuretic therapy may help prevent cor pulmonale. Antibiotics, digoxin and steroids are ineffective.

Prognosis

The overall survival is about 80% and most survivors are asymptomatic by age 2 years. Persisting small airway damage is found on pulmonary function testing of some children at age 8 years.

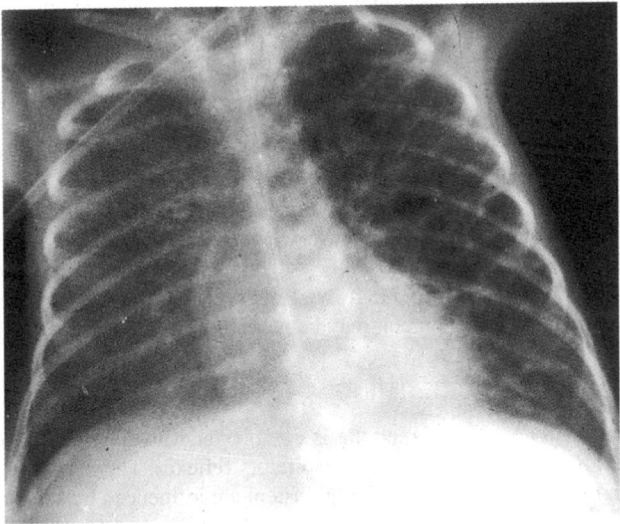

Fig. 5.38 Wilson–Mikity syndrome with overinflation and an irregular pattern of stranding and cystic changes most marked in the left lung.

Chronic pulmonary insufficiency of prematurity

This condition clinically resembles the Wilson–Mikity syndrome and similarly occurs in very preterm babies. Radiologically, however, this condition is different and the lungs show a characteristic, hazy appearance suggestive of reduced lung volume or pulmonary edema. Proposed mechanisms include chronic surfactant deficiency, persistent lung fluid secretion and respiratory muscle fatigue. Continuous positive airways pressure is helpful to reduce oxygen requirements and treat apnea. Most babies improve within 6 weeks of birth.

Chronic pulmonary infection

This may account for a small proportion of cases of chronic lung disease in the newborn. Infection with cytomegalovirus may be congenital or acquired although pneumonitis is uncommon in congenitally infected babies (Whitley et al 1976). Interstitial pneumonitis can also occur with congenital toxoplasmosis, rubella, varicella and Herpes simplex virus. Acquired infections with enteroviruses, adenovirus, respiratory syncytial virus and rhinovirus can cause acute pneumonitis.

Chlamydia may cause a late pneumonitis with tachypnea, cough and a chest radiograph showing disproportionately severe infiltrates and hyperinflation. Erythromycin treatment for 14 days is effective. Pneumocystis pneumonia has also been reported in preterm infants and should be treated with co-trimoxazole. One prospective study found chlamydia in 25%, ureaplasma in 21%, cytomegalovirus in 20% and pneumocystis in 18% of preterm babies with pneumonitis (Stagno et al 1981). How relevant this study of infants from the southern states of the USA is to a UK population of babies is unknown.

Subglottic stenosis

Subglottic stenosis may be congenital or acquired. Acquired subglottic stenosis is due to prolonged endotracheal intubation and occurs in a severe form in about 1% of ventilated babies. Use of endotracheal tubes that are too big, oral rather than nasal intubation and repeated intubations may increase the risk of subglottic stenosis. Presentation is with stridor and respiratory distress after extubation although there may be a delayed onset of symptoms for several months with difficulty apparently precipitated by an upper respiratory tract infection.

In mild cases treatment with high humidity and supplemental oxygen is sufficient, but use of dexamethasone or inhaled adrenaline has been advocated in more severe cases prior to a trial of extubation. Sometimes tracheostomy is needed but cryosurgery (Strome & Donahoe 1982) or minor surgery to split the cricoid cartilage anteriorly (Cotton & Seid 1980) have been successful as an alternative to tracheostomy which often proves difficult to close. Dilation of the narrowed segment at intervals by an experienced ENT surgeon may be necessary.

CONTROL OF BREATHING

Postnatal control of breathing is complex and involves chemical and nonchemical stimuli and respiratory reflexes. The inspiratory and expiratory centers in the brainstem are influenced by sensors (central and peripheral chemoreceptors) monitoring arterial blood and they maintain normal oxygen tensions and pH despite wide variations in oxygen demand and carbon dioxide production.

Chemical stimuli

Hypoxemia and hypercapnia are the most important chemical stimuli to respiration. For the first week after birth there are three phases of the respiratory response to hypoxemia: (1) stimulation of peripheral chemoreceptors causing transient hyperventilation in a warm environment; (2) central depression; (3) central stimulation by severe hypoxemia causing gasps.

Hypoxemia depresses ventilation and blunts the ventilatory response to hypercapnia. In the preterm baby these responses may persist for up to 6 weeks after birth. Breathing oxygen reduces ventilation by an effect on carotid body chemoreceptors but after several minutes hyperventilation occurs secondary to carbon dioxide retention.

The response to hypercapnia, mediated by hydrogen ion receptors in the medulla, increases with gestational and also with postnatal age.

Sleep state

In rapid eye movement (REM) sleep respiration is intrinsically driven with little chemical control. There is inhibition of intercostal muscles which results in distortion of the rib cage and this can lead to diaphragmatic fatigue with apnea. In nonrapid eye movement (NREM) sleep control of respiration is chemical rather than intrinsic and apnea is less common.

Respiratory reflexes

The Head and Hering–Breuer reflexes, arising from lung stretch receptors and mediated through the vagus nerve, are important in the modulation of respiratory center output in the newborn. Head's paradoxical reflex, which is present for the first few days after birth, causes an extra inspiratory effort when the upper airways are distended. Its importance is in aeration of lungs soon after birth. In the Hering–Breuer reflex sustained lung inflation inhibits respiration causing apnea in inspiration. This inflation reflex is stronger in preterm infants than term babies. The Hering–Breuer deflation reflex consists of an increase in respiratory rate in response to reduced lung volume and may also be important in the preterm baby. There are irritant receptors in the hypopharynx and larynx which, if stimulated by vigorous suctioning or cow's milk, cause apnea.

Apneic attacks

Apnea in the newborn is cessation of breathing for more than 20 s and this is significant if it is associated with bradycardia and/or cyanosis. Periodic breathing is a series of respiratory pauses of about 10 s duration alternating with periods of hyperventilation of up to 15 s and occurring at least three times per min. It is not associated with cyanosis and bradycardia and may be a physiologic response in the preterm baby (Henderson-Smart 1995).

Incidence

Apneic attacks occur in most infants of less than 30 weeks' gestation and in about half of babies of 30–32 weeks decreasing to less than 10% of babies at 34 weeks' gestation. Periodic breathing is also common, occurring in nearly all low birthweight babies and about one-third of term babies.

Etiology and pathogenesis

There are many clinical conditions that are associated with apnea (Table 5.61). Only after exclusion of the disorders listed from 1 to 6 can a confident diagnosis of apnea of prematurity be made. Immaturity of the brainstem respiratory neurons is probably a major underlying factor and apnea may also occur if the medullary centers are immature or depressed by hypoxia.

Pathophysiology

During a significant apneic attack the preterm baby has bradycardia, peripheral vasoconstriction and a variable alteration of blood pressure which may increase or decrease slightly. The interval between the onset of apnea and bradycardia varies between 2 and 30 s. There are three types of apnea based upon polygraphic recordings (Table 5.62). In preterm babies central apnea and mixed apnea occur with about equal frequencies (Henderson-Smart 1995). The use of apnea monitors which detect chest wall movement and bradycardia will underestimate the incidence of apnea and suggest that isolated bradycardia is occurring.

Diagnosis

The infant should be examined carefully to look for signs of infection, airway obstruction, seizures or patent ductus arteriosus. Laboratory investigations might include full blood picture, blood culture, blood glucose, electrolytes and calcium.

Chest radiography, blood gas analysis and pH and examination of CSF might also be indicated. Only after exclusion of infection, biochemical or drug causes of apnea can an infant be confidently labeled as having apnea of prematurity.

Table 5.61 Clinical conditions associated with apnea

1. Hypoxemia: respiratory distress syndrome, pneumonia, chronic lung disease, recurrent aspiration, airway obstruction
2. Infection: septicemia or bacteremia, meningitis, necrotizing enterocolitis
3. Metabolic disorder: hypoglycemia, hypocalcemia, hypomagnesemia, hypernatremia, hyponatremia, acidosis
4. CNS disorder: seizures, intracranial hemorrhage, drugs and drug withdrawal, kernicterus, cerebral malformation
5. Circulatory disorder: hypotension, congestive heart failure, patent ductus arteriosus, anemia, polycythemia
6. Temperature instability: hyperthermia, hypothermia
7. Apnea of prematurity: diagnosis by exclusion

Table 5.62 Polygraphic classification of type of apnea

1. Central apnea: simultaneous cessation of respiratory effort and air flow at the end of expiration. Probably due to cessation of motor output from the respiratory center in the brainstem
2. Obstructive apnea: cessation of airflow while respiratory effort continues. Seen in babies with the Pierre Robin syndrome for example
3. Mixed apnea: cessation of airflow with continued respiratory effort on some occasions and not on others. Both central and obstructive apneas occur during the same episode (Milner et al 1980)

Treatment (Table 5.63)

All preterm babies < 34 weeks' gestation should have continuous monitoring of heart and respiratory rate until 5 days have elapsed without apnea. Pulse oximetry or transcutaneous oxygen monitoring is also desirable in less mature babies. Monitors which respond to chest wall movement (the apnea mattress, pressure sensor pad or pressure-sensitive capsule) will fail to detect obstructive apnea as long as respiratory movement continues. In order to detect obstructive or mixed types of apnea, the heart rate must also be monitored. Sometimes a simple adjustment of environmental temperature or feed frequency will prevent apneic attacks. During resuscitation, overzealous suctioning must be avoided as this stimulates irritant receptors in the pharynx and perpetuates the apnea and bradycardia. Many apneic attacks are self-resolving and provided bradycardia and hypoxemia (oxygen desaturation) do not occur these are probably not harmful to the baby.

Repeated stimulation

Stimulation by stroking, gentle rubbing or rocking, e.g. rocking water beds, often prevents or shortens apneic attacks by increasing the input to the immature respiratory center by cutaneous, vestibular or proprioceptive pathways.

Intermittent bag and mask ventilation

When peripheral stimulation fails, bag and mask ventilation, using the same oxygen concentration as the baby is breathing, will stimulate spontaneous respiration without increasing the risk of retinopathy of prematurity.

Continuous positive airway pressure (CPAP)

CPAP reduces apnea by improving oxygenation and increasing functional residual capacity. It may also stabilize the chest wall and eliminate the Hering–Breuer deflation reflex. CPAP decreases the incidence of both mixed and obstructive apneas but does not affect central apneas so that it might work by helping to relieve upper airway obstruction. A nasopharyngeal tube or nasal prongs may be used to deliver the CPAP at 3–4 cmH$_2$O.

Drug therapy

Theophylline is useful in central as well as obstructive apnea and works by increasing the sensitivity of the respiratory center to

Table 5.63 Management of apnea

1. Immediate resuscitation
2. Exclude underlying cause (Table 5.61)
3. Lower environmental temperature 0.5°C
4. Correct mild hypoxemia and anemia
5. Repeated stimulation
6. Intermittent bag and mask ventilation
7. Continuous positive airway pressure
8. Drug therapy – aminophylline, theophylline, caffeine, doxapram
9. Mechanical ventilation

Table 5.64 Drug therapy of apnea

Drug	Route	Loading dose (mg/kg)	Maintenance dose (mg/kg)	Frequency	Therapeutic range
Aminophylline	Oral, rectal, i.v.	6	1–2	8- to 12-hourly	5–20 mg/l
Theophylline	Oral, i.v.	5–6	1–2	8- to 12-hourly	5–15 mg/l (28–84 μmol/l)
Caffeine	Oral, i.v.	10	2.5	24-hourly	5–20 mg/l
Doxapram	i.v.	–	1–2.5	1-hourly	< 5mg/l

hypercapnia, increasing minute ventilation and oxygen consumption. Other effects are stimulation of the diaphragm, positive inotropic and chronotropic effects, mild diuresis and increased heat production through utilization of brown fat. Unwelcome effects include decreased cerebral blood flow and some uncertainty about long-term outcome (Howell et al 1981). Dosage schedule and therapeutic range are shown in Table 5.64. Caffeine is also effective in treating apnea, and has a wider margin of safety than theophylline (Scanlon et al 1992). Doxapram is a direct respiratory stimulant which has undergone limited study in the treatment of neonatal apnea and has the side effect of jitteriness and raised blood pressure (Barrington et al 1986).

Mechanical ventilation

This is reserved for babies whose apnea is resistant to other measures. Very immature infants and those with bacteremia often need mechanical ventilation and low inflating pressures should be used as lung compliance is normal.

Prognosis

Recurrent apnea has been associated with spastic diplegia and delayed development, especially if associated with an underlying cause but more recently uncomplicated recurrent apnea has been associated with a poor neurological outcome (Koons et al 1993). Overall mortality of babies with apnea less than 33 weeks' gestation is one-third though this reflects the illness of the baby rather than the apnea per se. The relationship between apneic spells in the neonatal period and subsequent SIDS is uncertain. Apnea can recur within 2 months of discharge from hospital if there is a respiratory infection or if general anesthesia is needed for surgery (Liu et al 1983).

NEONATAL CARDIOVASCULAR DISEASE

A logical approach to suspected cardiac disease in the newborn is important for correct management, and must be based on awareness of the changes occurring in the circulation in the perinatal period (see Fig. 5.5). This section first considers how these processes or disturbance of them affects clinical presentation of cardiac problems in the newborn period. Certain situations characteristically associated with the newborn period are then covered in detail. Congenital and acquired cardiac diseases are considered in Chapter 13.

PERINATAL CARDIOVASCULAR PHYSIOLOGY

Figure 5.4 illustrates fetal circulatory pathways. Labor and delivery trigger a number of cardiovascular events (Fig. 5.5), the occurrence or failure of which have clinical implications.

Pulmonary vascular resistance

In healthy term babies the postnatal fall in pulmonary vascular resistance results in a rapid fall in right heart pressures over a few days with adult pulmonary to systemic pressure ratios being established by 2–3 weeks of age. Many factors can inhibit, delay or reverse pulmonary vasodilation in the newborn and these are listed with clinical examples in Table 5.65. The fall in resistance may occur more slowly in certain congenital cardiac abnormalities, such as a large ventricular septal defect (VSD). This delayed fall has implications for the time at which heart murmurs, clinical left-to-right shunting and heart failure develop. Thus, a very small VSD is more likely to produce a murmur in the first few days after birth than a large one, and a large VSD rarely causes heart failure in the first few weeks of life. In some congenital heart lesions, pulmonary vascular resistance never falls to normal and pulmonary vascular disease develops without clinical evidence of a large shunt ever having been present. This happens not infrequently in complete atrioventricular septal defect (AVSD), but can also happen with large VSD, in both cases particularly if the child has Down syndrome.

Ductus arteriosus

As gestation progresses, ductal smooth muscle becomes less sensitive to dilating circulating prostaglandins and more sensitive to oxygen, which causes it to constrict. At term, increasing arterial oxygen tension causes functional closure of a normal ductus within the first 2–3 days in virtually all babies. In preterm babies without respiratory distress the time of ductal closure is similar (Evans & Archer 1990). Babies with structural abnormalities of the cardiovascular system may maintain ductal patency longer than normal before spontaneous closure occurs. There are two groups of congenital heart lesions which are critically dependent on ductal patency for the baby to remain alive (Table 5.66). The

Table 5.65 Situations associated with delay in or reversal of postnatal fall in pulmonary vascular resistance

Factor	Comment
Acidosis, hypoglycemia, hypoxemia, hypercapnia, polycythemia	Wide range of neonatal diseases
High altitude	Mediated via lower oxygen tension
Cardiac disease	See Table 5.73
Respiratory disease	Any cause
Ductal closure in utero	Maternal prostaglandin synthetase inhibitor ingestion
Obstructed middle or upper airway	Any cause

Table 5.66 Duct-dependent congenital heart lesions

Obstruction to flow through right heart
    Pulmonary atresia with intact ventricular septum
    Critical pulmonary stenosis
    Severe tetralogy of Fallot
    Pulmonary atresia with VSD
    Tricuspid atresia

Obstruction to flow through left heart
    Aortic atresia
    Critical aortic stenosis
    Hypoplastic left heart syndrome
    Interrupted aortic arch
    Severe coarctation

first group, those with duct-dependent pulmonary circulation, show appearance of or worsening in cyanosis on ductal closure. The second group are those conditions in which the systemic circulation is dependent on the ductus and collapse with gross heart failure occurs when the ductus closes. An important part of resuscitation in both these groups of infants is the use of prostaglandin E$_1$ or E$_2$ to reopen and maintain ductal patency. Patent ductus arteriosus, either isolated or in association with other cardiac abnormalities, may also be a structural abnormality which will never close. If a normal ductus arteriosus is subject to abnormal conditions, its closure may be delayed. This situation is frequently seen in preterm babies with lung disease and may respond to prostaglandin synthetase inhibitor administration.

Foramen ovale

Increased pulmonary venous return after birth results in closure of the flap-like structure of the foramen ovale as left atrial pressure rises. With abnormal hemodynamics shunting can occur through the foramen ovale, in either direction. Thus, left-to-right shunting at atrial level may occur in babies with an overloaded left atrium (owing to left-to-right shunting through a patent ductus or to obstruction to forward flow of blood through the left heart) and right-to-left shunting at atrial level with arterial desaturation can occur in persistent pulmonary hypertension or mechanical obstruction to blood flow through the right heart.

Ductus venosus

Blood flow through the ductus venosus falls dramatically when umbilical venous return ceases. Functional closure of the ductus venosus occurs in the first few days but an umbilical venous catheter can be passed through it into the inferior vena cava and right atrium for over a week after birth. Clinical relevance of patency of the ductus venosus relates to its usefulness as a route to the heart for central venous pressure monitoring or cardiac catheterization (Ashfaq et al 1991) and also to the fact that when it closes, obstruction to pulmonary venous drainage becomes severe in total anomalous pulmonary venous return to the portal vein, causing marked cyanosis and respiratory distress.

CARDIOVASCULAR EXAMINATION OF THE NEWBORN

The present history, perinatal and family histories may all give valuable clues to a diagnosis. Routine examination of well babies should include an assessment of the presence or absence of central cyanosis, an evaluation for evidence of heart failure and observations about pulse rate, regularity and character with special reference to the nature of the femoral pulses when compared simultaneously to the right brachial pulse. If the femoral pulses cannot be satisfactorily palpated or are markedly different from right arm pulses, a more thorough cardiovascular assessment including four-limb blood pressure reading, ECG and chest X-ray should be performed. Auscultation of the heart should be performed with an attempt to ensure that heart sounds are louder in the left chest than the right. Then attention should be given to whether the second sound is single or fixedly split and then to murmurs. The presence or absence of murmurs is only part of the neonatal cardiovascular examination. Some murmurs are innocent and many severe lesions have unimpressive murmurs or even none.

If cardiac disease is suspected, the precordium, suprasternal notch and subxiphoid region should be palpated for thrills or abnormal impulses, the skull auscultated for bruits, and a more detailed cardiac auscultation for added sounds and full murmur characterization carried out. Reliable blood pressure measurement in newborn infants requires a quiet and relaxed infant and a cuff of appropriate size (a cuff which covers two-thirds of the length of the upper arm and in which the bladder either encompasses the entire circumference of the arm or is positioned in such a way as to have the center of the bladder over the brachial artery). Detection of pulse reappearance can be by palpation but a Doppler probe is more sensitive. Auscultation is very difficult and the flush technique is rarely used. Oscillometric devices are not suitable for definitive diagnostic readings and are also second best to direct invasive continuous monitoring in immobile ill patients (Diprose et al 1986). The same cuff can be used on the calf with detection of posterior tibial or dorsalis pedis pulses for lower limb systolic pressures. Normal values for systolic pressures in term babies measured noninvasively are given in Table 5.67. Acceptable values in ill preterm babies are different and less clearly defined (Table 5.68). A difference of up to 20 mmHg systolic between arm

Table 5.67 Systolic blood pressure: term infants, neonatal period (noninvasive measurements) (from Wilkinson & Cooke 1986)

	Mean (95% confidence limits)			
	Day 1	Day 4	Day 30	Day 42
Systolic	70 (56–81)	74 (63–96)	99 (77–111)	95 (76–112)
Diastolic	40 (30–50)	–	57 (40–74)	–
Mean	50 (43–62)	–	–	–

Table 5.68 Systemic blood pressure in the neonatal period. Day 1: direct aortic measurement (from Wilkinson & Cooke 1986)

		Mean	(95% confidence limits)
1000 g	Systolic	47	(35–57)
	Diastolic	26	(17–35)
	Mean	35	(25–45)
2000 g	Systolic	53	(44–65)
	Diastolic	30	(22–41)
	Mean	41	(30–50)
3000 g	Systolic	62	(50–72)
	Diastolic	35	(27–47)
	Mean	47	(36–55)
4000 g	Systolic	70	(56–81)
	Diastolic	40	(30–50)
	Mean	52	(43–62)

and leg pressures can be normal; discrepancies between arm pressures may give clues as to the site of an aortic arch obstruction or interruption. Significant coarctation may occasionally be associated with an aberrant right subclavian artery arising distal to the left subclavian, in which case upper to lower limb pulse discrepancy will not exist. Upper limb pressures may be raised in coarctation but in sick infants poor left ventricular function may prevent hypertension.

CARDIOVASCULAR INVESTIGATION OF THE NEWBORN

Chest X-ray

A systematic approach to the chest X-ray allows maximum information to be obtained; the particular points of relevance to cardiovascular diagnosis are listed in Table 5.69. Immediate management of a baby with a cardiac lesion may be greatly influenced by deciding whether lung blood flow is increased (plethoric lung fields, Fig. 5.39) or decreased (oligemic lung fields, Fig. 5.40). Pulmonary venous obstruction produces X-ray appearances often hard to distinguish from respiratory pathology. Clinical conditions associated with each of these abnormalities are given in Table 5.70.

Table 5.69   Chest X-ray: points to look for with reference to the cardiovascular system

Bronchial situs	
Lung fields	Oligemia
	Plethora
	Venous engorgement
	Lung pathology
Heart	Position, apex side
	Size
	Contour
	Aortic arch side
Abdomen	Visceral situs
Skeleton	Abnormalities

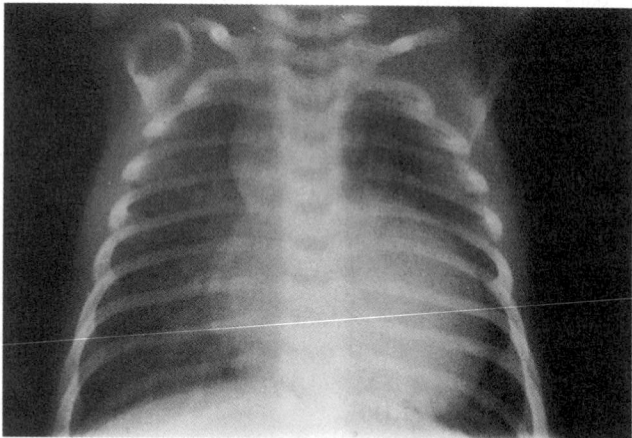

Fig. 5.39   Chest X-ray on cyanotic newborn infant. Lung fields are plethoric (double inlet left ventricle).

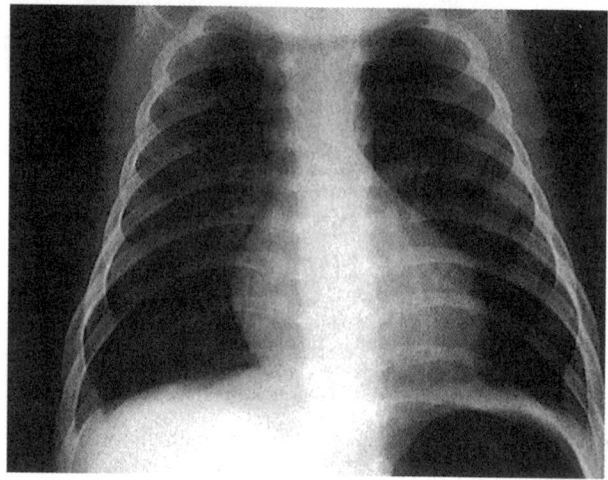

Fig. 5.40   Chest X-ray on cyanotic newborn infant. Lung fields are oligemic (tetralogy of Fallot).

Table 5.70   Lung vascularity on chest X-ray

Oligemia	Tricuspid atresia (unless large VSD)
	Ebstein's anomaly
	Pulmonary atresia or critical stenosis
Plethora	Any left-to-right shunt
	Common mixing without pulmonary stenosis
	Transposition of great arteries
Venous congestion	Obstruction to flow into or through left heart

Electrocardiography

This can provide important diagnostic information when significant heart disease is suspected. A detailed consideration of the subject will be found in Chapter 13. It is important to recognize the normal evolution of the ECG in the newborn and to have access to reference information. (Davignon et al 1979) (Table 5.71).

Hyperoxia (nitrogen washout) test

If cyanosis is due to a cardiac cause, high concentrations of inspired oxygen rarely relieve it significantly, although there are exceptions, for example some common mixing conditions. If respiratory disease is the cause there is often relief from increasing inspired oxygen, although there are exceptions such as severe respiratory disease or persistent pulmonary hypertension. This is the basis for the hyperoxia test. If a baby is put in 85%+ inspired oxygen for 15–20 min, a right radial arterial blood or right upper trunk transcutaneous oxygen tension should rise to well above 20 kPa. Failure to do so supports a desaturating cardiac abnormality. Transcutaneous oxygen tension monitors placed on the right upper thorax can give similar information to right radial artery samples but pulse oximetry can be misleading in that elevation of saturation to normal, even to 100%, would not necessarily mean that arterial oxygen tension had risen above 20 kPa. Theoretical fears about precipitating ductal closure mean that the baby should be closely observed during the test; however, the risk of precipitating a problem is extremely small. Marked

Table 5.71   Selected ECG measurements in normal pediatric patients

	0–3 days	3–30 days	1–6 months	6–12 months	1–3 years	3–5 years	5–8 years	8–12 years	12–16 years
Heart rate (per minute)	90 → 160	90 → 180	105 → 185	110 → 170	90 → 150	70 → 140	65 → 135	60 → 130	60 → 120
PR (msec) lead II	80 → 160	70 → 140	70 → 160	70 → 160	80 → 150	80 → 160	90 → 160	90 → 170	90 → 180
QRS (msec) lead V_s	25 → 75	25 → 80	25 → 80	25 → 75	30 → 75	30 → 75	30 → 80	30 → 85	35 → 90
QRS axis (degrees)	60 → 195	65 → 185	10 → 120	10 → 100	10 → 100	10 → 105	10 → 135	10 → 120	10 → 130
QRS V_1									
Q (mV)	0	0	0	0	0	0	0	0	0
R (mV)	0.5 → 2.6	0.3 → 2.3	0.3 → 2.0	0.2 → 2.0	0.2 → 1.8	0.1 → 1.8	0.1 → 1.5	0.1 → 1.2	0.1 → 1.0
S (mV)	0 → 2.3	0 → 1.5	0 → 1.5	0 → 1.8	0.1 → 2.1	0.2 → 2.1	0.3 → 2.4	0.3 → 2.5	0.3 → 2.2
QRS V_6									
Q (mV)	0 → 0.2	0 → 0.3	0 → 0.25	0 → 0.3	0 → 0.3	0.02 → 0.35	0.02 → 0.45	0.01 → 0.3	0 → 0.3
R (mV)	0 → 1.1	0.1 → 1.3	0.5 → 2.2	0.5 → 2.3	0.6 → 2.3	0.8 → 2.5	0.8 → 2.6	0.9 → 2.5	0.7 → 2.4
S (mV)	0 → 1.0	0 → 1.0	0 → 1.0	0 → 0.8	0 → 0.6	0 → 0.5	0 → 0.4	0 → 0.4	0 → 0.4
TV_1 (mV)	− 0.4 → 0.4	− 0.5 → − 0.1	− 0.6 → 0.1	− 0.6 → − 0.1	− 0.6 → − 0.1	− 0.6 → 0	− 0.5 → 0.2	− 0.4 → 0.3	− 0.4 → 0.3

Reproduced from Emmanouilides et al 1995, as adapted from Davignon A, Rautaharju P, Barselle E, Soumis F, Megelas M 1979/80 Normal ECG standards for infants and children. Pediatric Cardiology 1: 123–124.
Values reported as 2% → 98% (approximate).

prematurity is a contraindication because of the possible consequence of retinopathy.

Echocardiography

Clinical evaluation should always precede echocardiography. Resuscitation and stabilization must always be achieved before transfer to another unit for evaluation. Ultrasound imaging and Doppler ultrasound allow a precise anatomical and functional diagnosis in the majority of symptomatic neonates with cardiac disease, so that surgery, be it palliative or definitive, is frequently not preceded by cardiac catheterization.

Cardiac catheterization

Although echocardiography has made neonatal diagnostic cardiac catheterization uncommon, there has been an increase in the number and scope of interventional therapeutic catheterizations in neonates. Good neonatal care is required throughout the procedure. The heart can be approached via umbilical vessels, femoral vessels percutaneously or by cut-down, or rarely by axillary vessel cut-down. The procedure has mortality and morbidity, though these have been greatly reduced by good general neonatal care and by anatomical information obtained from prior echocardiography.

PATTERNS OF CARDIOVASCULAR DISEASE IN THE NEWBORN

Congenital disease accounts for most cardiac disease in the newborn but acquired disease can occur as a result of birth asphyxia, viral infections and other severe postnatal illnesses. Congenital heart disease presents in the newborn period in

approximately 4 per 1000 live births. Congenital heart disease may be structural or functional, the latter group being conditions such as conduction disturbances and dysrhythmias where a structural defect as an underlying cause or associated problem usually needs to be carefully excluded.

PRESENTATION AND MANAGEMENT OF CARDIOVASCULAR DISEASE IN THE NEWBORN

Fetal diagnosis (Wyllie et al 1994, Allan 1995)

Detailed fetal echocardiography may show cardiac abnormalities from 16 to 18 weeks' gestation onwards. Investigation is performed when a factor increasing the risk of heart disease is identified. When a baby is born in whom a fetal diagnosis has been made, this must be confirmed by postnatal echocardiography. A normal fetal cardiac scan should not prevent postnatal echocardiography being performed if clinical features point to the possibility of cardiac disease in the newborn.

Cyanosis

To be certain of clinical cyanosis in a newborn infant is not always easy. Factors which complicate the assessment include a high hematocrit, traumatic petechiae on the face, racial pigmentation and acrocyanosis. A plethoric newborn infant may be normally saturated but still have enough deoxygenated hemoglobin to look centrally cyanosed. Occasionally noninvasive monitoring or blood gas sampling will be needed for confirmation. Some 'cyanotic' congenital heart disease may not produce recognizable cyanosis in a newborn baby (unobstructed total anomalous pulmonary venous drainage, double inlet and double outlet ventricles with high lung blood flow and good mixing, and tetralogy of Fallot in which right ventricular outflow obstruction progresses through infancy and is often only mild in the newborn period). Once central cyanosis is identified the immediate priority is to assess that respiration is adequate, regardless of suspected cause. A careful review of history, a complete physical examination and measurement of four-limb blood pressure are then important. Features of the different groups of causes and management pathways for a suspected cardiac cause are given in Tables 5.72 and 5.73, respectively. In an ill infant with cyanosis

Table 5.72 Clinical features and investigations which help rapid differentiation of causes for central cyanosis

Causes of cyanosis	Clinical features	Investigations
Respiratory	Marked respiratory distress (unless PPHN in addition) Color improves in oxygen usually	Abnormal lung fields on X-ray Hypercapnia Hyperoxia test (pass)
Cardiac	May have other cardiac signs May have little or no respiratory distress	X-ray may help, lung pathology absent Normo- or hypocapnia Hyperoxia test (fail) ECG abnormal
Neurological (respiratory depression)	Slow respiration Color improves on stimulation and in oxygen. May have other neurological or syndrome features	X-ray normal Hypercapnia Hyperoxia test (pass)
Hematological (methemoglobinemia)	Black mucous membranes, not typical cyanosis, usually very well	Blood gas normal Hyperoxia test (pass)

In all groups history may provide valuable clues.

Table 5.73 Management approach to cyanosis due to a suspected cardiac cause

1. General measures	Temperature control, avoid hypoglycemia ensure ventilation adequate
2. Arterial blood gas	Treat respiratory acidosis Treat metabolic acidosis Ventilate if necessary (hypoxemia alone not indication to ventilate) Consider value of hyperoxia test

3. Chest X-ray	Diagnostic clues may be present
	Management
	  Oligemia – trial of prostaglandin
	  Plethora – trial of prostaglandin if very hypoxemic or metabolic acidosis

4. ECG	May help with specific diagnosis
5. Drugs	Prostaglandin Alkali } see above Diuretics if heart failure/pulmonary congestion Antibiotics if significant risk of serious infection
6. Echocardiography	Precise diagnosis often possible (transfer if necessary when stable)

Table 5.74 Drug dosage table

Drug	Route	Dose	Frequency
Prostaglandin			
E_1	i.v.	0.005–0.1 mcg/kg/min	—
E_2	i.v.	0.005–0.05 mcg/kg/min	—
E_2	Nasogastric	25 mcg/kg/h	Hourly initially
Indomethacin	i.v.	0.2 mg/kg over 30 min	8- to 12-hourly × 3
Tolazoline	i.v.	0.5 mg/kg over 5 min then 0.5 mg/kg/h	—
Prostacyclin	i.v.	2–20 ng/kg/min	—
Dopamine	i.v.	2–20 mcg/kg/min	—
Dobutamine	i.v.	2–20 mcg/kg/min	—
Captopril	Oral/nasogastric	0.1–0.5 mg/kg/dose Start with lowest dose	8-hourly

from cardiac disease, the most important specific issue is whether or not ductal patency needs to be secured with prostaglandin; if in doubt, a trial of the drug is appropriate. Prostaglandin E_1 or E_2 may be given intravenously; prostaglandin E_2 may be given orally or nasogastrically, hourly in the first instance. Doses are given in Table 5.74.

Oxygenation is improved by prostaglandin in conditions with obstructed right heart flow (oligemic lungs on X-ray) and in many cases of transposition of the great arteries. Short-term side effects of prostaglandin include pyrexia, apnea, jitteriness, convulsions, flushing and diarrhea. These often respond to dosage reduction without loss of therapeutic effect. The drug should be stopped if no benefit is seen after 1–2 h. Persistent pulmonary hypertension in the newborn (PPHN, see below) can at times be difficult to distinguish from cardiac disease even with echocardiography and the two may coexist (Table 5.75).

Heart failure

Features of heart failure include respiratory distress, sweating, hepatomegaly and in severe cases, particularly where failure has been present antenatally, ascites, generalized edema, pleural and pericardial effusions. Tachycardia, gallop rhythm and clinical features of the cause should also be looked for. Structural heart disease (particularly severe left ventricular outflow obstruction),

Table 5.75 Structural cardiac lesions which may be associated with persistent pulmonary hypertension in the newborn infant

Pulmonary venous hypertension	Pulmonary vein stenosis Obstructed total anomalous pulmonary venous drainage Absent left atrioventricular connection with restrictive foramen ovale Left ventricular dysfunction (any cause) Left ventricular outflow obstruction (any cause)
Left-to-right shunts independent of pulmonary vascular resistance	Atrioventricular septal defect Cerebral arteriovenous malformation Coronary arteriovenous fistula
Severe tricuspid regurgitation	Ebstein's anomaly

rhythm disturbances, myocardial ischemia, myocarditis and noncardiac diseases may all cause heart failure. Intracerebral and more rarely other arteriovenous malformations, viral and bacterial infections, storage diseases, noncardiac hypoxemia, severe anemia, marked polycythemia and excessive fluid administration may need to be considered as possible causes.

Cyanosis and heart failure

Cyanosis is only a feature of very severe heart failure and heart failure does not develop in many conditions which cause severe cyanosis. Thus, if both cyanosis and heart failure are present, this may be a useful diagnostic aid (Table 5.76).

Collapse

This may be caused by closure of the ductus arteriosus when the systemic circulation is dependent upon its patency, for example in hypoplastic left heart syndrome, interrupted aortic arch or severe coarctation. Such diagnoses are supported by respiratory distress, massive hepatomegaly, cardiomegaly with congested lung fields on X-ray, right ventricular dominance on ECG, and metabolic acidosis. Differential diagnosis includes septicemia and metabolic disorders but if any doubt exists, resuscitation should include prostaglandin, which will almost invariably produce rapid improvement if the diagnosis is cardiac.

Arrhythmia

Tachyarrhythmia may produce collapse, although supraventricular tachycardia (SVT) may produce no symptoms or may cause heart failure severe enough to produce hydrops fetalis. Ventricular tachycardia may be life threatening or asymptomatic. It is an indication for urgent cardiological referral. Complete heart block may be well tolerated especially if the ventricular rate is above 55 per min and rises on activity. Although Stokes–Adams attacks may occur, cardiac failure is the more usual problem in the neonate with complete heart block and both are indications for pacemaker insertion. Chronotropic drugs rarely have much effect on ventricular rate in symptomatic cases. The association of rhythm disturbance with structural heart disease must be remembered and in complete heart block without structural heart disease at least 50% have mothers with positive serology suggesting lupus erythematosus or other collagen vascular disease (McCue et al 1977). Supraventricular ectopics are not rare in normal newborns; they are not always conducted to the ventricles. All other arrhythmias except those clearly related to a metabolic disturbance in an ill baby are indications to have structural cardiac lesions excluded by ultrasound.

Cardiac murmur

Murmurs are often heard at routine examination of newborn infants. Symptoms or any other sign of cardiac disease must be carefully sought. Asymptomatic murmurs with no other abnormal features may be innocent; Table 5.77 lists features of innocent neonatal murmurs. If doubt exists, blood pressure measurements, ECG and chest X-ray may still allow early discharge and outpatient follow-up. Tricuspid regurgitation and ventricular septal defect (VSD) may produce similar pansystolic murmurs at the lower left sternal edge in the first few days of life (Kelly & Guntheroth 1988). Tricuspid regurgitation producing a murmur in an otherwise well baby is of no long-term significance; a VSD heard in the early neonatal period may never cause symptoms. Aortic and pulmonary valve stenosis will produce a murmur at birth or shortly after; careful evaluation including ECG and chest X-ray and possibly echocardiography is necessary before allowing a baby home. The normal murmur from pulmonary artery branches in the newborn is not as loud or as harsh as that from semilunar valve stenosis. Babies with critical aortic or pulmonary stenosis will have symptoms, other signs and ECG abnormalities.

Hypertension

Neonatal hypertension is usually only identified in infants with other cardiovascular signs or in those known to be at increased risk such as survivors of severe respiratory illness or the infants of cocaine-using mothers. Treatment of neonatal hypertension is

Table 5.76 Structural cardiac lesions characteristically showing both heart failure and arterial desaturation in the newborn period. Such lesions with pulmonary stenosis in addition are unlikely to have heart failure

Transposition	(i) with large VSD and PDA
	(ii) with coarctation
Truncus arteriosus	
Tricuspid atresia	(i) with large VSD
	(ii) with TGA and coarctation
Double inlet ventricle	
Total anomalous pulmonary venous drainage with obstructed pulmonary veins	
Hypoplastic left heart syndrome	
Cerebral arteriovenous malformation (vein of Galen aneurysm)	

Table 5.77 Features of innocent neonatal murmurs: in all groups the remainder of the examination is normal

Source/type	Features of murmur	Other points
Pulmonary arteries	Bilateral, base of heart, also over scapulae and lateral chest High pitched mid-systolic	Gone by 6 months
Ductus arteriosus	Pulmonary area rarely diastolic	Gone by 2–3 days
Tricuspid regurgitation	Same as VSD, heard day 1	May be perinatal asphyxia Goes in a few days–weeks
Still's innocent murmur	Vibratory Mid-systolic Between LLSE and apex	Rarely heard in newborn May last years

LLSE = lower left sternal edge.

Table 5.78 Causes of hypertension in the newborn

Renal	Renal vein thrombosis
	Renal arterial emboli/thrombosis
	Dysplastic renal disease
	Polycystic renal disease
	Urinary tract obstruction
	Renal infection
	Renal failure (any cause)
Cardiovascular	Coarctation
Endocrine	Congenital adrenal hyperplasia
	Hyperaldosteronism
	Hyperthyroidism
	Pheochromocytoma
	Neuroblastoma
Respiratory disease	Bronchopulmonary dysplasia (mechanism unknown)
Neurological disease	Raised intracranial pressure (any cause)
Drugs	Corticosteroids
	Methylxanthines
	Phenylephrine (in eyedrops)

only occasionally necessary, but attention to the underlying cause is always appropriate (Table 5.78).

Association with other abnormalities

Many syndromes include cardiac abnormalities; in some the cardiac malformation may be a major determinant of length or quality of life. Any infant with a congenital abnormality should at very least have a full physical examination of the cardiovascular system. Babies undergoing major surgery on congenital abnormalities which may be associated with cardiac problems should have a full cardiovascular evaluation to identify possible management problems, as well as to allow comprehensive information to be passed to the family (Tulloh et al 1994).

CARDIOVASCULAR ASPECTS OF NEONATAL DISEASES

Respiratory distress syndrome (RDS)

Patent ductus arteriosus (Archer 1993)

Patency of the ductus arteriosus is associated with worse RDS and delayed closure of the ductus can result in the need for continuing ventilation. The typical clinical features of a patent ductus arteriosus (PDA) may be hard to detect in a baby with respiratory disease and a PDA may cause no murmur or more usually just a systolic one. Other features of PDA in the context of the preterm include apnea, hypotension, heart failure, necrotizing enterocolitis and metabolic acidosis. When ventilator requirements are increasing after apparently passing the peak of RDS, and a continuous murmur is present, the diagnosis is easy; when features are less obvious, the possibility of left-to-right shunting through a PDA must be remembered. The ECG is not usually helpful, and chest X-ray is often noncontributory. If there is clinical doubt, echocardiography imaging and Doppler examination are required (Evans 1993). Careful fluid management reduces the incidence of symptomatic PDA in preterm infants. Prophylactic duct closure with indomethacin reduces but does not abolish the occurrence of later symptoms (Cotton et al 1991) but is not widely utilized as early prediction of

which babies are at great risk of symptomatic PDA is unreliable and indomethacin is not without side effects. Symptomatic PDA should be vigorously treated with fluid restriction and correction of anemia. Digoxin is not widely used and regular frusemide has disadvantages including electrolyte imbalance and possible antagonism of ductal closure. If conservative measures do not rapidly control the situation, indomethacin has long been known to be effective in closing the ductus in approximately 70% of premature infants (Gersony et al 1983). Intravenous indomethacin (0.2 mg/kg) for three doses 8–12 h apart should be used; an infusion over at least 30 min is preferable to a bolus injection because of effects on blood pressure and cerebral circulation (Evans et al 1987, Colditz et al 1989), although even slow infusions reduce cerebral oxygen delivery (Edwards et al 1990). It has been suggested that ibuprofen may be less active on the cerebral circulation and just as effective at closing the ductus, although this needs to be confirmed (Patel et al 1995). Fluid retention and elevation of creatinine are temporary adverse effects of indomethacin; thrombocytopenia is usually considered a contraindication to its use, as are renal failure and necrotizing enterocolitis. A repeat course may be used if the beneficial effect is transient. A 5-day course of indomethacin (Hammerman & Aramburo 1990) or a 6-day low dose course (Rennie & Cooke 1991) are effective at closing the ductus with a lower relapse rate. Biochemical evidence of renal dysfunction is less on the low dose regime. The effect on cerebral hemodynamics of prolonged indomethacin treatment has not been studied. Two unsuccessful short courses, unacceptable side effects or a definite contraindication, mean that surgical ligation or clipping of the ductus should be carried out. This can be done in the neonatal nursery with very low mortality and morbidity.

Persistent pulmonary hypertension of the newborn (PPHN)

Pulmonary hypertension may complicate a variety of neonatal respiratory illnesses (Table 5.65). Diagnosis is based on knowing a risk situation exists, and excluding structural heart disease. Lower saturations in the feet than the right hand are characteristic and specific echocardiographic features are reported but are not always distinct. If hypercapnia exists this should be treated; if it cannot be controlled the problem is probably chiefly one of intrapulmonary shunting producing hypoxemia and not of pulmonary arteriolar constriction with associated extrapulmonary right-to-left shunting.

Management in general consists of treating predisposing and aggravating factors aggressively, ensuring normal or slightly alkalotic acid–base balance with a carbon dioxide tension of 3–4 kPa. Consideration can then be given to the use of vasodilators. Oxygen and inhaled nitric oxide (Roberts et al 1992, Kinsella et al 1992) are the only specific pulmonary vasodilators, although endotracheal tolazoline has been used (Welch et al 1995). Magnesium sulfate (Abu-Osba et al 1992), prostacyclin (Bush et al 1988) and tolazoline are all effective. All infused drugs will lower systemic as well as pulmonary vascular resistance, so blood pressure must be invasively and continuously monitored when they are used. Plasma expansion and inotropes may both be needed. Extracorporeal membrane oxygenation (ECMO) is effective in PPHN but exact indications for its use are unclear, as newer treatment protocols are more effective than those used when ECMO was first introduced. In many countries, including the UK, ECMO is available in only a small number of centers

(O'Rourke et al 1989, Dworetz et al 1989, Stolar et al 1991, Schumacher 1993).

Asphyxia

Persistent pulmonary hypertension

This may also be a feature of perinatal asphyxia, with or without meconium aspiration pneumonitis (see above).

Myocardial ischemia

Electrocardiographic (Jedeikin et al 1983) and pathological studies indicate that myocardial ischemia is common in neonates stressed by asphyxia. Even in mild cases there may be the murmur of tricuspid regurgitation which may be associated with ischemic ECG changes. In severely asphyxiated infants, hypotension from myocardial dysfunction may need inotrope support, and atrial and ventricular arrhythmias can also occur.

Infection

Bacterial and viral infections in the newborn may cause PPHN. Myocarditis is a feature of disseminated viral infections and heart failure, shock and arrhythmias may all result. Shock may also be caused by peripheral vasodilation and capillary leakage in severe bacterial sepsis. Endocarditis is increasingly being recognized in already sick newborn infants. Clinical features are nonspecific. There may be unrecognized underlying heart disease. Diagnosis is often at autopsy but certain clinical features such as multiple septic lesions appearing over time or recurrent septicemia, particularly in the presence of intravenous long lines, should alert one to the possibility. Ultrasound scanning can make, but not exclude, the diagnosis. Prolonged appropriate multiple antimicrobial therapy is indicated (Millard & Shulman 1988).

Metabolic diseases

There are many inborn errors of metabolism and storage diseases which may be associated with cardiomyopathy. Hypertrophic cardiomyopathy seen in the newborn infants of diabetic mothers is worth specific mention because although it is frequently asymptomatic it may cause severe heart failure with gross cardiomegaly and ECG changes. The role of cardiac dysfunction in the respiratory problems encountered in some infants of diabetic mothers needs careful individual assessment, as in some it will be a major contributory factor. This cardiomyopathy is however self-limiting, resolving completely in 6–12 months (Way et al 1979). Digoxin, other inotropes and vasodilators should be avoided in this condition because they may aggravate left ventricular outflow obstruction. Dilated cardiomyopathy may present symptomatically in the newborn period and a vigorous search for infective and metabolic causes is indicated.

GENERAL MANAGEMENT OF NEONATAL HEART DISEASE

All the principles for care of the newborn infant apply to the baby with definite or suspected cardiac disease. These principles should not be neglected because of a desire to get the correct diagnosis.

Ductal manipulation

The major resuscitative decision with respect specifically to heart disease is whether or not to use prostaglandin. Pharmacological duct closure with indomethacin is never as urgent and if any doubt exists about the diagnosis, echocardiography is essential, as indeed it is before surgical intervention.

Heart failure

Fluid restriction, optimal oxygenation and the treatment of anemia are important. Digoxin use is time honored but controversial in the treatment of heart failure when associated with left-to-right shunt. It is probably not necessary in PDA in the preterm, but in some other conditions it is still widely used. Diuretics, usually frusemide with or without spironolactone, are particularly effective. Vasodilators in neonatal heart failure are relatively untried, although angiotensin-converting enzyme inhibitors are widely used in infants (Shaw et al 1988, Leversha et al 1994). Aggressive drug therapy for heart failure is appropriate in order to allow adequate nutrition.

Low output states

It is not clear to what extent newborn infants can increase cardiac output by increasing myocardial contractility rather than heart rate. An inappropriately low heart rate resulting in circulatory compromise should be treated by identifying and removing the cause, by drugs such as atropine and isoprenaline or by pacing. Most babies with shock or heart failure have tachycardia. Attention to obtaining optimal circulating volume should precede or accompany inotrope support with dopamine or dobutamine (Keeley & Bohn 1988). Repeated boluses of colloid for hypotension in preterm infants are inadvisable, cardiac function may well need support (Gill & Weindling 1993). Echocardiography is helpful if doubt about the need for inotrope support exists, central venous pressure measurements may help (Skinner et al 1992) and clinical assessment of end organ perfusion is just as important as aiming at a particular blood pressure.

Arrhythmias

Management of these in newborn babies is governed by the same principles as throughout infancy and is discussed in Chapter 13.

Drug therapy

Recommended drugs and dosages for the treatment of neonatal cardiovascular disease are given in Table 5.74.

Interventional cardiac catheterization

Rashkind balloon atrial septostomy still forms part of the emergency management of a number of conditions, particularly transposition of the great arteries (TGA). If diagnostic catheterization is not needed, a balloon atrial septostomy can be performed by an experienced operator under ultrasound control in the neonatal nursery (Ashfaq et al 1991). Balloon valvuloplasty is used in some centers for both critical aortic and critical pulmonary valve stenosis (Hanley et al 1993). Balloon dilation of neonatal coarctation is generally not as effective as surgery. The role of ductal stenting in duct-dependent lesions is being explored (Salmon et al 1993). Transcatheter ductal closure is not yet feasible in premature newborns.

Surgery

Cardiac surgery in the newborn can be palliative or corrective, closed or open. Surgical treatment for particular conditions is discussed in Chapter 13 and it must be remembered that local practices vary a great deal. In general there is a trend towards performing corrective open procedures at increasingly younger ages. Whatever approach is taken results are better when infants come to operation well resuscitated and stable.

STRUCTURAL HEART DISEASE IN THE PRETERM INFANT

Respiratory pathology and infective processes are so common in the preterm infant that cardiac disease can be forgotten or masked. It is extremely important to bear in mind the possibility of structural and functional cardiac disease as the cause of or a contributory factor to symptoms and signs in the premature infant. In many cases pharmacological or surgical management is possible with ultimate good outcome. Preterm babies may go into heart failure at an earlier postnatal age with a given condition, such as VSD, than a term baby for reasons that are not entirely clear.

CARDIOVASCULAR ASPECTS OF CHRONIC PULMONARY DISEASE IN THE NEWBORN

The role of PDA in prolonging acute respiratory failure in RDS has been discussed above. Chronic lung disease will make clinical features of a left-to-right shunt of any sort very hard to recognize but treatment of the cardiac abnormality may help the respiratory condition. Chronic respiratory failure may cause right heart failure; it is important to avoid hypoxemia in such infants and to treat intercurrent infections and secretion retention vigorously.

GASTROINTESTINAL PROBLEMS AND JAUNDICE OF THE NEONATE

EMBRYOLOGY

The gut is derived from the embryonic yolk sac which differentiates in early life into the fore-, mid- and hindgut. The foregut gives rise to the pharynx, thyroid, thymus, parathyroid glands, respiratory tract, esophagus, stomach, upper duodenum, liver and pancreas. The midgut gives rise to the lower half of the duodenum, small intestine and large intestine as far as the distal third of the transverse colon. The rest of the large bowel arises from the hindgut.

Between 4 and 6 weeks of fetal life the cranial portion of the foregut differentiates into a complicated branchial arch system which is transitory and obliterated by 7 weeks. Failure of obliteration may result in a persistent sinus, fistula or epithelial lined cyst (e.g. neurenteric cyst). The partitioning of the foregut into the pharynx and trachea may also be incomplete and various types of tracheoesophageal fistula with or without esophageal atresia will result. Abnormal development of the lower end of the foregut may result in a diaphragmatic hernia whilst failure of

esophageal differentiation causes achalasia of the cardia or more rarely an esophageal web.

The stomach is relatively immune to disorders of embryogenesis. However, the terminal portion of the foregut and cranial end of the midgut undergo major growth in length with consequent herniation from the umbilical cavity (Fig. 5.41). As it returns to the abdomen there is a complex counterclockwise rotation (ultimately 270°) resulting in the fixation of the cecum in the right iliac fossa and the passage of the transverse colon and mesentery over the second and third parts of the duodenum. The first possible failure is that of the endoderm of the yolk sac to separate from the notochord during the third week which results in a variety of reduplications of the intestine. Failure of the vitellointestinal duct to regress in the fifth week results in a Meckel's diverticulum and other vestigial abnormalities. Finally failure in herniation return and fixation of the intestine between the fifth and twelfth weeks may cause major defects such as exomphalos and malrotation.

The cloaca is divided by a membrane at 6 weeks into the sagittally oriented rectum posteriorly and the urogenital sinus anteriorly. Anomalies in rectal differentiation cause a variety of defects ranging from imperforate anus and rectovaginal fistulae to sacral sinus formation. Because rectal differentiation is cotemporaneous with that of esophageal differentiation, defects in both structures are often found in the same patient.

The liver is derived from an outpouching of the ventral portion of the duodenum at 4 weeks and defects in its development are rare (Fig. 5.42). Defects in the development of the biliary tree from the cystic duct are more common with either cystic dilation (choledochal cyst) or failure of canalization (biliary atresia) being

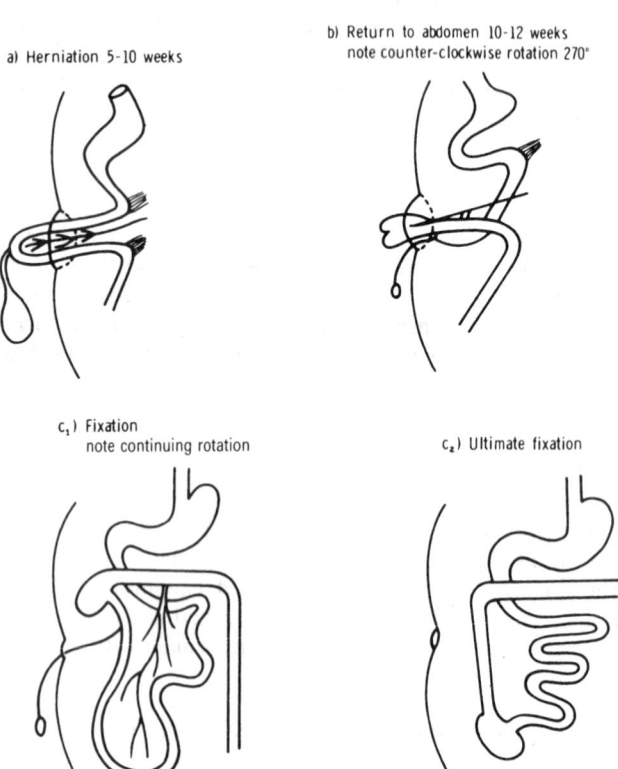

a) Herniation 5-10 weeks

b) Return to abdomen 10-12 weeks note counter-clockwise rotation 270°

c₁) Fixation note continuing rotation

c₂) Ultimate fixation

Fig. 5.41 The course of events leading to fixation and final position of the gut within the abdomen. (From Lebenthal et al 1988.)

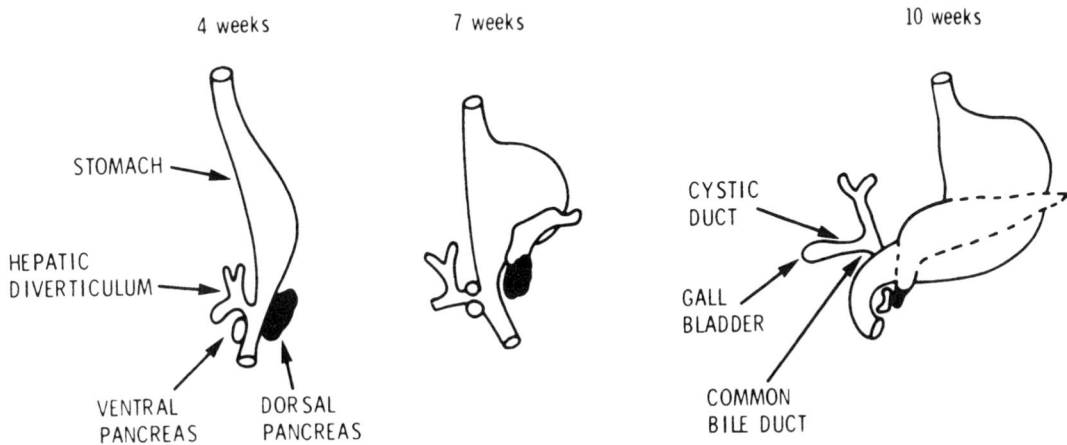

Fig. 5.42   The development of the liver/pancreas from an outpouching of the ventral portion of the duodenum. (From Lebenthal et al 1988.)

the commonest disorders. Defects in pancreatic development are also rare but because the final gland is produced by the fusion of a dorsal pancreas from an outpouching of the duodenum just cranial to the hepatic diverticulum and a ventral pancreas from an outpouching in the caudal angle between the gut and hepatic diverticulum (Fig. 5.42) failure of this fusion process may result in an annular pancreas. Cellular differentiation of all the organs of the gut occurs early and is complete in most cases by the end of the first trimester. Intestinal epithelial cells of the first trimester human fetus resemble immature crypt cells of the adult intestine. Morphogenesis of the intestinal epithelium (including differentiation of crypts and villi as well as the intracellular organelles) is completed by about 22 weeks' gestation. Thus, the anatomical development of the gut is complete by the birth of even the 24-week infant and the limiting factor in feeding is the maturation of functional activity.

ONTOGENY OF GUT FUNCTION

Carbohydrate absorption

The absorption of carbohydrates seems to pose no problem even for premature neonates. Human milk and most formula milks usually contain only lactose, thus pancreatic digestion is relatively unimportant and the low levels of amylase detected in the duodenal juice of premature and term infants do not matter. More modified milks, however, contain such elements as corn syrup, amylose or maltodextrins in order to reduce their osmolality and it is possible that intolerance to these moieties sometimes occurs, although glucoamylase and sucrose isomaltase activity should be adequate for their digestion. The disaccharidases develop in close association with the enterocyte itself and disaccharidase activity first appears with the villus formation. Lactase, however, develops later in comparison with sucrase isomaltase activity (8–10 months' gestation) but lactose intolerance is very rarely seen in the very low birthweight infant, presumably because of enzyme induction.

Intestinal absorption of nutrients and electrolytes is dependent on the development of appropriate cellular transport processes. Studies of everted fetal intestinal sacs have shown that sodium-dependent cotransport of glucose/galactose is present as early as 10 weeks and there is a threefold increase in the uptake by 18

weeks. Studies of glucose-evoked potential difference across the duodenum in neonates have confirmed the presence of active glucose transfer in premature neonates, although the number of transporting sites (carriers) is reduced in the premature compared with the term infant. Thus carbohydrate digestion/absorption is adequate in the premature infant.

Protein absorption

Protein digestion is initiated in the stomach and gastric peptic activity increases rapidly after birth (from 2 to 50% adult reference levels by 2 months in term infants). Gastric acid secretion (which is necessary for full peptic activity, the pH optima of pepsin being 4–5) does not occur at maximal activity in the preterm infant for about 1 month. It is, however, rapidly buffered by milk because of the overall decreased secretory mass in these infants.

Although tryptic activity is low at birth, pancreatic enzyme induction results in high levels by the first week of life in term preterm/infants. Brush border oligopeptidase activity is similar to that found in adults by the early part of the second trimester and protein digestion appears adequate. Active absorption of L-alanine and L-leucine has also been demonstrated in everted sacs from both 10- and 18-week fetuses. Peptides as well as amino acids can be absorbed by the enterocyte which further enhances the efficiency of protein absorption. The diminished tryptic activity seen initially in premature infants may result in pathological intestinal colonization (see below under Necrotizing enterocolitis).

Fat absorption

Lipid digestion is more complex and requires more adaptive mechanisms to ensure maximal absorption of this major source of energy by preterm infants. Three major lipases exist: (1) lingual lipase – this is often bypassed by nasogastric tubes although nonnutritive sucking may increase the contribution of this enzyme; (2) gastric lipase (first demonstrated as having a role in the gastric aspirates of infants with esophageal atresia); (3) pancreatic lipase (this shows rapid substrate induction). These contribute more than sufficient lipolytic activity even in the preterm infant. Unfortunately, bile salt production in such infants barely reaches the critical micellar concentration and this becomes the rate-limiting factor in fat digestion. However, the palmitic acid of human milk fat is predominantly esterified at the triglyceride 2 position which matches the stereospecificity of pancreatic lipase reducing the need for bile salts. Furthermore, the packaging epithelial lining of fat globules in the milk contains a highly active breast milk lipase. Milk manufacturers lacking these resources have tended to compensate for the inefficient fat absorption of their milks by supplementing them with medium chain triglycerides (at the expense of increasing osmolality). The transport of fats by diffusion and the re-esterification within the enterocyte has not been studied but is presumed adequate.

Salt and water absorption

Salt and water absorption by the enterocyte is present in the early stages of cellular differentiation. It has been shown that adenylate cyclase and Na/K ATPase activities, both closely related to the electrolyte transport processes, develop concomitantly with the brush border translocation mechanisms. Equilibrium dialysis studies of colonic transport mechanisms in the premature infant have demonstrated that the sodium chloride exchange mechanisms are highly active (presumably under the influence of the high levels of aldosterone seen in these infants). Basic transport processes clearly function in early life.

Intestinal motility

The limiting factor in feeding premature infants is the intestinal motility. The ability to suck is not present until about 34 weeks' gestation (although it can occur earlier) but this can be bypassed by tube feeding. Gastric emptying although poor at birth, is fully functional by 24 h postnatally. It is controlled by duodenal receptors in similar fashion in both premature and mature infants by nutrient density and specific constituents of the meal and is inhibited by pathological processes (e.g. RDS and asphyxia). Small intestinal motor activity is divided into fasting and postprandial motor patterns. The fasting migrating motor complex does not fully develop until about 34 weeks' gestation (in association with the onset of the sucking) (Bisset et al 1988, 1989). Postprandial activity does not occur until later and seems to be a learned phenomenon increasing with the increasing nutritional density of the feeds. Before 34 weeks a highly propulsive activity, the fetal motor complex, is seen which allows the intestine to function and feeding to be effective. Before 26 weeks, only small nonpropagated contractions are seen and so enteral feeds may not be tolerated initially. More mature motor function may be induced by feeding, allowing many infants of lower gestation to tolerate enteral feeding. The development of colonic motility has not been studied but appears to be adequate although regular glycerin suppositories may be needed initially. It is also clear that the gut motor function is critically dependent upon the well-being of the infant. Thus, sick infants will show delayed maturation (or regression) of gut motor activity and it is this which causes the functional ileus or pseudo-obstruction seen in such infants. More rarely disorders of the nervous system of the gut may present with a true pseudo-obstruction and disordered distal migration of the myenteric nerves can give rise to aganglionic segments as in Hirschsprung's disease.

Table 5.79 Feeding disorders

Etiology	Investigations
a. 'Not tolerating feeds'	
Prematurity	History and examination
Pseudo-obstruction	Nursing observation
Sepsis	Abdominal distention
Major clinical deterioration	Septic screen
Necrotizing enterocolitis (NEC)	Distention – abdominal wall crepitus, tenderness
	Abdominal X-ray
	Proctoscopy
Asphyxia	
Drugs	
All causes of vomiting	
b. 'Feeding difficulties'	
Maternal factors	History and examination
Poor milk supply	Nursing observation
Cracked nipples/breast abscess	
Tension/anxiety	
Poor ability to suck	
Tachypnea/RDS	
Anatomical abnormality	
Micrognathia	
Macroglossia	
Cleft palate	
Asphyxia	
Bulbar/suprabulbar palsy	Jaw jerk positive
Moebius' syndrome	
Myopathies	Absent reflexes
	EMG nerve conduction studies
Familial dysautonomia	Jewish race
	Histamine prick test
	Pupillary response to metacholine

PROBLEMS

'Not tolerating feeds' (Table 5.79)

This is a common problem in the neonatal nursery becoming manifest as increasingly large aspirates and failure to tolerate milk in the tube-fed infant. Care must be taken to check for blood or bile in the aspirate. The former suggests a gastritis and the latter functional or surgical obstruction. Prematurity is the usual cause for failure to tolerate feeds although most infants after the age of 28 weeks will tolerate continuous tube feeds which are started gradually at 1 ml/h and increased, as tolerated, to full requirements over the course of the first week. Hourly intermittent bolus feeds are then introduced and by about 34 weeks' gestation, with the onset of suckling, the infant will tolerate 3- to 4-hourly feeds and is ready for the introduction of orogastric feeding. Attempts to introduce these steps too quickly will result in an increase in the volume of stomach contents aspirated before the next feed (or hourly if continuously fed). Experienced nurses are normally able to distinguish such an increase in aspirate from that occurring unexpectedly and indicating pathology in the gastrointestinal tract. Most of the causes of vomiting in the neonatal period could present in this manner but most commonly such an increase in aspirate heralds the onset of pseudo-obstruction secondary either to sepsis, a major deterioration in the child's general condition or necrotizing enterocolitis. Asphyxia may be complicated by gastric stasis and is the commonest organic cause of poor feeding postnatally in the term infant. Failure to start oral feeding for more than 1 week indicates a poor prognosis. Drugs used postnatally, especially phenobarbitone and diazepam, can delay gastric emptying and enteral feeding is often not possible in the ventilated and paralyzed infant.

Feeding difficulties (Table 5.79)

It may be difficult to establish feeding even in the term infant. Breast disorders such as cracked nipples or a breast abscess prevent breast-feeding but the baby will quickly accept bottle-feeding. Maternal anxiety, however, may prevent the establishment of breast-feeding and can also lead to clumsy or inappropriate methods of bottle-feeding (resulting usually in overfeeding and vomiting but occasionally in inadequate feeding and failure to thrive).

Disorders of sucking and swallowing can occur. Anatomical abnormalities such as micrognathia, macroglossia and cleft palate often result in poor sucking and slow feeding. Neurological conditions other than asphyxia tend to present with uncoordinated sucking and swallowing causing oral or nasal regurgitation, sometimes accompanied by the signs of a suprabulbar palsy with tongue thrust and a positive jaw jerk. The rare congenital Moebius' syndrome with bilateral facial palsy (and other cranial nerve palsies) due to congenital agenesis of the cranial nerves also results in a poor suck and uncoordinated swallowing. Unilateral nerve lesions do not usually cause problems and where present should be distinguished from myopathies such as mitochondrial cytopathy which may cause dysphagia in the neonatal period. The Riley–Day syndrome (familial dysautonomia) may also present in the neonatal period with disorders of swallowing but usually dysphagia occurs later in childhood. Where there is excessive drooling of saliva in association with swallowing difficulties a tracheoesophageal fistula should be considered although the usual clinical picture (coughing, excessive saliva, cyanotic and apneic spells) is quite distinctive and is rapidly diagnosed within a few hours of birth by a plain X-ray with a 'nasogastric' tube inserted.

Vomiting

Posseting

Posseting (the regurgitation of small amounts of milk after feeds) is common in the neonatal period and is easily distinguished from pathological vomiting by experienced mothers and midwives. Regurgitation and vomiting both indicate underlying disorders in the newborn period (vomiting is a more serious problem). Rumination is a rare disorder, possibly familial. The baby regurgitates small amounts of food into the mouth which is then chewed with apparent self-gratification. It usually presents after the neonatal period.

Feeding disorders

Feeding disorders are the commonest cause of vomiting in the first month of life after leaving hospital. Greedy babies swallow air. This leads to excessive posseting or vomiting and can usually be recognized by experienced health visitors. Overfeeding or the improper preparation of the bottles is more difficult to spot and commonly presents as vomiting to casualty departments. A careful history of type, amount and constitution of feed is vital in every case of vomiting. With correction of mother's mistakes the symptoms rapidly resolve. However, maternal anxiety or depression is often a coexistent factor in such cases and contributes to the fussy eating and vomiting in these babies. Evidence of affective disorder or postnatal depression in the

mother should be sought during history taking and a full family history often reveals predictable stressors such as death of a sibling or other close relative, or a previous stillbirth or neonatal death.

Organic causes of vomiting

Vomiting in the first week of life. Vomiting at this time may be due to difficulties in establishing appropriate feeding. However, more specific organic causes must be excluded by appropriate means. All causes of vomiting (Table 5.80) may

Table 5.80 Vomiting

Etiology	Investigations
Feeding disorders	
Overfeeding	Feeding history and observation
Air swallowing	
Maternal stress	Family history
Esophageal disorders	
Tracheoesophageal fistula/frothy vomit day 1	CXR/AXR with large nasogastric tube
Hiatus hernia	Barium swallow/pH study
Gastric disorders	
(Gastritis)	
Maternal debris	Stomach washout
Blood – hemorrhagic disease of the newborn	Clotting screen
Maternal stress illness	History
Pyloric stenosis	Test feed
	Ultrasound/barium meal
Small intestinal disorders	
Congenital	
Duodenal atresia	AXR
Extrinsic duodenal obstruction	AXR
Malrotation	AXR
Volvulus	AXR
Meconium ileus	AXR (calcification)
Intestinal duplication	AXR
Acquired	
Pseudo-obstruction/sepsis	Full blood count, septic screen
Necrotizing enterocolitis	AXR – free or intramural gas
Proctocolitis	Stool cultures
Dietary protein intolerance	Dietary manipulation
Incarceration/strangulation	Inspection
Inguinal herniae	AXR
Extraintestinal disorders	
Intracranial lesions	
Asphyxia, meningitis	
Intracranial hemorrhage	
Hydrocephalus/SOL	
Renal disorders	
UTI	MSU/bag urine
Obstructive uropathy	Renal ultrasound
Metabolic disorders	
Galactosemia	Urine sugar
Hyperammonemias	Urine amino acids
Phenylketonuria	Urine amino acids
Hereditary protein intolerance	
Organic acidemias	pH urine
Congenital adrenal hyperplasia	Electrolytes
Drugs	Theophylline

CXR = chest X-ray; AXR = abdominal X-ray.

present at any time, but in this early period, consideration of the vomitus and baby together with an abdominal X-ray can narrow the differential diagnosis. For example:

1. Vomitus
   - Frothy
     – tracheoesophageal fistula
   - Blood
     – maternal – swallowed
     – hemorrhagic disease
     – gastric erosions/stress ulcers
   - Bile
     – intestinal obstruction
     – intestinal perforation/peritonitis
     – intestinal pseudo-obstruction
   - Milk only
     – feeding disorder
     – gastroesophageal reflux
     – milk allergy/intolerance
2. Baby well: abdomen normal
   - AXR – fluid level
     – duodenal/intestinal atresia
     – meconium ileus
     – large bowel obstruction/Hirschsprung's disease
   - AXR – no fluid levels
     – gastroesophageal reflux
     – milk allergy/intolerance
3. Baby sick
   - Abdomen normal: AXR – no or occasional fluid levels + watery diarrhea
     – sepsis/UTI
     – increased intracranial pressure/meningitis
     – renal tract disorders
     – metabolic disorders
   - Abdomen distended/tender: AXR – fluid levels ± watery diarrhea or bloody diarrhea
     – necrotizing enterocolitis
     – obstruction/perforation
     – volvulus
     – intussusception

The commonest cause for vomiting in the first 2 days of life is undoubtedly a neonatal gastritis due to irritation from swallowed liquor and debris from the birth canal. One or two stomach washouts usually suffice to identify the debris (and the altered maternal blood) and to cure the problem. The baby remains well throughout. If the baby is sick, other signs are present or the vomiting persists, then fuller investigations are required. Clearly a septic screen (comprising FBC, clotting studies, blood cultures, MSSU and probably LP) is indicated in a baby who is unwell and all vomiting babies need urea and electrolytes checked. Hematemasis may require transfusion and treatment with vitamin K or FFP as indicated. Stress ulceration is rare but usually settles with i.v. ranitidine and aggressive neutralization of the gastric acid with sodium bicarbonate washouts. In extremis intravenous prostaglandins may arrest the bleeding.

Bile-stained vomiting is a more sinister sign and usually indicates necrotizing enterocolitis, obstruction or some other surgical condition. The higher the obstruction, the earlier the presentation; thus duodenal atresia, jejunal atresia, malrotation and volvulus and high duplications all present in the first 2 days of life with marked vomiting and intolerance of feeds. Low obstructions due to Hirschsprung's disease, milk plug, functional obstruction and anal atresia may present more insidiously with a period of obstipation or constipation before the vomiting starts towards the end of the first week. Meconium ileus due to cystic fibrosis presents at any time in the first week (usually in the first few days). Acquired obstruction obviously tends to present later but one should always examined the abdomen carefully for signs of strangulated herniae and intussusception and the presence of anal atresia. These conditions are discussed in more detail elsewhere.

The abdominal X-ray is pivotal in making the initial diagnosis. Fluid levels indicate both the obstruction and the level of obstruction. Duodenal atresia causes a classic double bubble whilst high obstructions reveal small bowel fluid levels with no gas in the rectum. Colonic disorders may have many fluid levels but often require contrast enemas to distinguish between long segment Hirschsprung's disease, meconium ileus of cystic fibrosis (although abdominal calcification may be seen following intrauterine perforation) and the even more rare true pseudo-obstruction (visceral myopathy or neuropathy). Free abdominal gas indicates an intestinal perforation (usually due to NEC but occasionally spontaneous or associated with an atretic segment). Volvulus secondary to malrotation is dramatic with large dilated loops (the American football sign) or may be inferred from the abnormal distribution of the bowel gas in malrotation (although this usually requires upper gut contrast studies for accurate delineation). When fluid levels are less marked and the infant is sick or jaundiced, pseudo-obstruction due to sepsis is likely.

Surgical disorders when identified will require prompt transfer to a unit specializing in neonatal surgery. An intravenous infusion of 10% dextrose should be started and the infant kept warm in the incubator. The stomach should be aspirated hourly and the aspirate replaced as normal saline intravenously. If the infant is shocked, resuscitation with 10–20 ml/kg of plasma is required. If the infant is sick, parenteral antibiotics must be started whilst awaiting the result of the septic screen. In cases of tracheoesophageal fistula, a large bore double lumen tube (replogle tube) is passed into the proximal pouch. Air is passed into one lumen and aspirated with any secretions from the other. Continuous drainage in this way prevents apnea and aspiration episodes. The infant is nursed prone with a slight head tilt.

Necrotizing enterocolitis. Necrotizing enterocolitis (NEC) is a much feared condition in every neonatal unit (having a much higher incidence in the very low birthweight baby). The etiology is unknown but is likely to be multifactorial with superinfection by gas-forming bacteria and failure of the mucosal barrier in the immature gut, playing important roles. Precipitating factors include hyperosmolar feeds, perinatal asphyxia, polycythemia and umbilical vessel catheterization. More recently a clear association has emerged between the presence of reversed end-diastolic flow in the umbilical artery in utero in the severely growth retarded infant and the development of NEC in the first weeks of life (Hackett et al 1987). It has also been postulated that left-to-right shunt through a patent ductus and retrograde flow in the aorta during diastole may contribute to the pathogenesis. Breast milk is partly protective (Lucas & Cole 1990).

The disease presents with increasing aspirates (usually bile stained) or vomiting (usually bilious but occasionally bloodstained). Diarrhea follows (or occasionally precedes) the failure to tolerate feeds and may be watery or contain mucus and visible blood and pus. The baby is often unwell, lethargic and having apneic episodes. Examination reveals a tense distended tender abdomen which is quiet (or silent if perforation has taken place). Tenderness and/or guarding suggest peritonitis has supervened and in the later stages there may be edema and inflammation of the abdominal wall (producing a 'peau d'orange' appearance in the skin) or an underlying abdominal mass. Blood cultures are positive in 18–60% of cases and septic or hypovolemic shock may be a complication and the infant may collapse and die. Diagnosis is classically made on the plain abdominal X-ray. This initially shows separation of the bowel loops due to ascites with fluid levels. Then the periluminal tramlines indicating intramural gas appear (Fig. 5.43a) especially in the cecum, ascending and descending colon and sigmoid. Later signs include gas in the portal tree (Fig. 5.43b) and gas under the diaphragm following perforation. In the early stages the diagnosis may also be suggested by the presence of a proctocolitis using an auroscope as a proctoscope.

A pancolitis is usually found at postmortem. The histology reveals a characteristic hemorrhagic inflammatory infiltration. The differential diagnoses include generalized sepsis, meconium ileus, malrotation and volvulus, hemorrhagic disease of the newborn, cow's milk colitis and intussusception and the even rarer neonatal appendicitis. The other causes of abdominal distention (Table 5.81) must also be considered especially spontaneous perforation of the gut and other causes of ascites.

Management is initially medical and conservative (Walshe &

Table 5.81 Cause of abdominal distention

1. Intestinal obstruction
2. Intestinal pseudo-obstruction
3. Intestinal perforation – Congenital/spontaneous
   Acquired
4. Ascites – Congestive cardiac failure/hydrops fetalis
   Peritonitis/necrotizing enterocolitis
   Hypoalbuminemia/nephrotic syndrome
   Urinary/ruptured urinary tract with urethral valves
   Biliary/spontaneous rupture of bile duct
   Chylous/disordered lymphatic drainage
5. Mass – Hydronephrosis
   Congenital malignancy, Wilms'/neuroblastoma
   Reduplication
   Ovarian

Klugman 1986). Oral feeds should be stopped and the stomach placed on free drainage. A septic screen is performed and it is customary to give intravenous antibiotics (e.g. penicillin, gentamicin and metronidazole) to cover the bacteremia. Oral vancomycin has a role in prophylaxis and may be a valuable adjunct to treatment. Blood counts, clotting screen, urea and electrolytes and albumen are checked and appropriate supportive management given as indicated. Most surgeons insist that

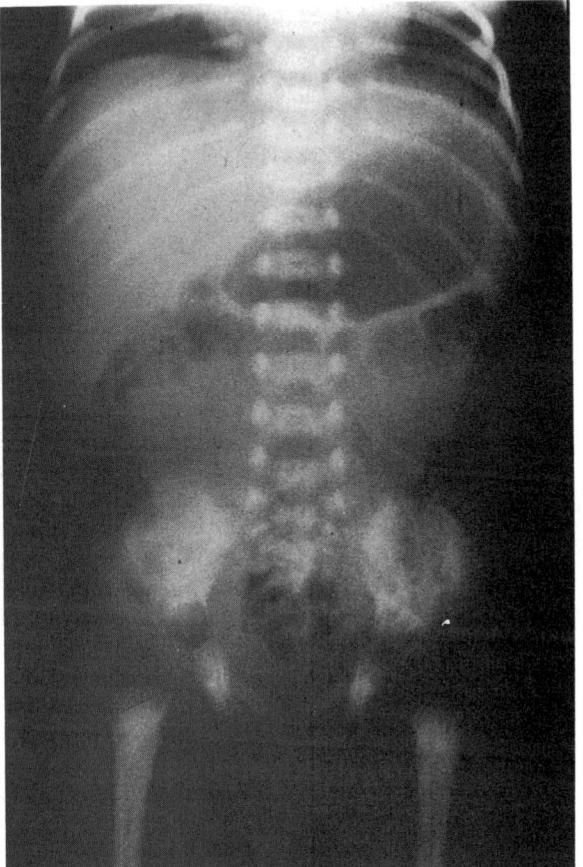 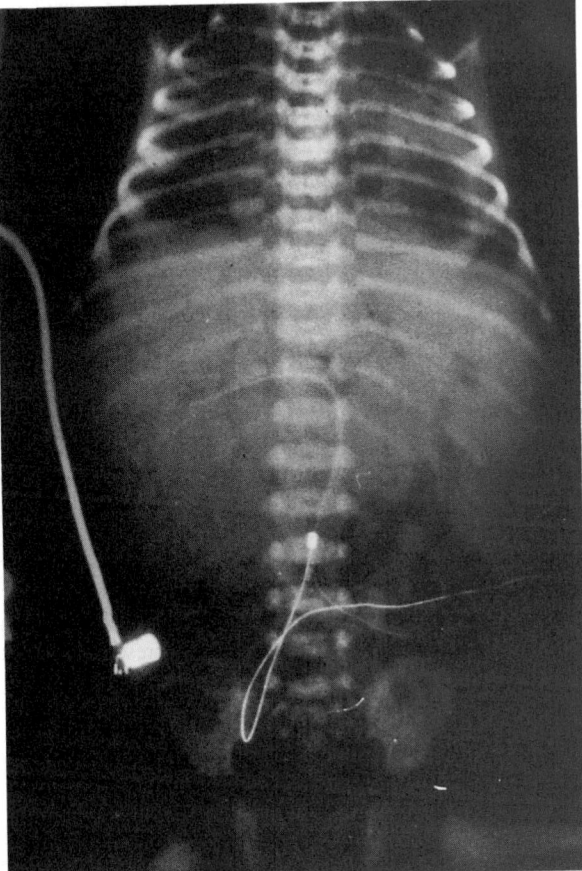

Fig. 5.43 (a) Necrotizing enterocolitis. Double lumen to the colon can be seen clearly at the hepatic flexure and triple lumen in the descending colon – both effects caused by intramural gas. (b) Gas tracts ramifying throughout the liver in portal vessels and periportal tissue. Arterial catheter is adequately sited. The venous catheter passes into the right hepatic vein.

intravenous feeding through a central line should be instituted for 10 days and the bowel rested. Afterwards feeds should be introduced slowly. Expressed breast milk or a hypoallergenic milk such as Pregestimil must be used as lactose and cow's milk protein intolerance are often seen in the recovery phase in these infants. Surgery is required for the acute complications of perforation and sometimes bleeding or if there is failure to improve with medical therapy. Later complications (stricture formations with subacute small bowel obstruction, obstipation, blind loop syndrome and rectal bleeding) may also require surgery as may a recurrence which occurs in 10% of patients.

General disorders. Nongastrointestinal causes for vomiting must always be borne in mind. Sepsis will cause pseudo-obstruction as already described. Urinary tract infection without bacteremia, however, has long been recognized to present with gastrointestinal symptoms, most commonly with vomiting. (Obstructive renal disease, e.g. ureteral valves, may also present in this way in the absence of infection.) Urine culture microscopy must always be performed. Plasma urea and electrolytes are also important to identify acidosis (renal and metabolic disease) and alkalosis (pyloric stenosis occasionally presents early in the neonatal period). Intracerebral asphyxial insults may cause vomiting acutely due to raised intracranial pressure, and meningitis may present as vomiting at any age. Other cerebral causes of vomiting such as hydrocephalus, space-occupying lesions and the diencephalic syndrome rarely present in this fashion in the neonatal period. Metabolic disorders are a cause of vomiting in the neonatal period and should always be considered if metabolic acidosis (and/or hypoglycemia) is present. Galactosemia may present as early as the first day and the urine must always be tested for reducing substances. Usually the infants with metabolic disorders start vomiting after milk feeding has been established and they have been exposed to a reasonable protein load (e.g. the hyperammonemias, disorders of amino metabolism and the nonketotic hypoglycemias). The presence of constipation as well as vomiting in a dysmorphic infant may alert one to the presence of idiopathic hypercalcemia and vomiting with dehydration and electrolyte disturbance to congenital adrenal hyperplasia which may also present with diarrhea. The organic acidemias must be excluded by specific assays (dicarboxylic aciduria) on acute phase urines collected when the patient is symptomatic and, where possible, acidotic. After the first week of life acquired metabolic disorders such as Reye's syndrome, diabetic ketoacidosis and Munchausen syndrome by proxy may rarely have to be considered.

Persisting vomiting/vomiting after the first week of life. Babies presenting after the first week of life tend to have acquired problems although lower intestinal obstructions, malrotation and in the very low birthweight baby, necrotizing enterocolitis may present later. Vomiting is one of the commonest presentations to a pediatric unit and consideration of the baby's clinical state again allows a fairly rapid differentiation.

- Baby well: abdomen normal
  - posseting
  - feeding disorder
  - gastroesophageal reflux
  - cow's milk protein intolerance
  - pyloric stenosis
  - urinary tract infection.
- Baby unwell: abdomen distended

  - late obstruction
  - peritonitis/appendicitis
  - intussusception.

Persistent vomiting even in a relatively well baby, especially if accompanied by failure to thrive may indicate a more serious underlying disorder. If investigations are normal, a feeding disorder is excluded and the vomiting still persists then the differential diagnosis usually rests between a dietary food intolerance and gastroesophageal reflux.

Gastroesophageal reflux (GOR). GOR may present with vomiting in the first month of life. In the term baby this is investigated with pH meter or radiolabel milk scan and treated in the normal way. In the premature infant recurrent consolidation due to aspiration from GOR may lead to a disorder indistinguishable from bronchopulmonary dysplasia. GOR may also be a major cause of apneic spells resistant to methylxanthine therapy. pH studies will confirm this although they undoubtedly underestimate postprandial reflux in the preterm baby where the decreased acid production of the stomach is readily buffered for prolonged periods by the milk feed. Sometimes it is more practicable to treat such infants empirically with thickening agents or cisapride and ranitidine. A milk scan when available may give a more definitive diagnosis in these patients.

Dietary intolerance. Dietary intolerance can present as vomiting in the first few weeks of life in its own right. Cow's milk protein intolerance, due either to allergy or enteropathy, often presents this way although lactose intolerance more commonly presents as diarrhea (see below). Midwives often find that changing the formula milks from whey-based formulae to casein-based formulae leads to a more contented baby and less posseting but there is no obvious rationale for this. Gastric emptying may be slower but it is more likely that the taste or the texture suits the baby better.

Neonatal diarrhea (Table 5.82)

Diarrhea is a relatively uncommon symptom in the neonatal period although most breast-fed children will have loose yellow seedy stools. Mothers and midwives are very clear when the stools are pathological, usually because they are watery with little or no solid matter, are increased in frequency or contain blood and mucus. The commonest cause of loose stools is phototherapy but this causes no harm as long as the fluids are increased appropriately. The loose stools due to nasojejunal tube feeding are similarly of little importance and usually pass unnoticed by nursing staff. The commonest serious causes of diarrhea are gastroenteritis and necrotizing enterocolitis and the latter should always be considered in infants with diarrhea. Usually, however, the characteristic bloody/mucusy stool together with the abdominal extension and X-ray signs give the diagnosis.

Outbreaks of viral gastroenteritis are not unknown in the neonatal unit and the infants respond to the normal management of such infections. Stools should be sent for cultures and electron microscopy for viruses. A full infection screen should be performed to exclude systemic causes of diarrhea. If formula fed the feeds should be stopped and i.v. fluids instituted. When the diarrhea has stopped in the neonatal period it is probably wise to regrade the infant on to full strength feeds slowly. Babies who are breast-fed should continue with breast milk but the stool, as in all infants with diarrhea, should be tested for reducing substances

Table 5.82 Neonatal diarrhea

Etiology	Investigations
Iatrogenic	
Phototherapy	
Nasojejunal tube feeding	
Infective	
Gastroenteritis	
Viral	Stool electron microscopy
Bacterial	Culture
Parenteral diarrhea	Infection screen
Thrush	Culture
Surgical	
Necrotizing enterocolitis	Abdominal X-ray
Appendicitis	
Hirschsprung's disease	Rectal examination, biopsy
Congenital enteropathy	
Lactose intolerance	Stool sugars – Clinitest, Chromatography
Sucrase isomaltase deficiency	Biopsy
Glucose galactose malabsorption	
Congenital Na/H exchange deficiency	
Congenital chlorodiarrhea	Stool electrolytes/osmolality
Congenital microvillus atrophy	
Abetalipoproteinemia	Fasting cholesterol/lipids + biopsy
Acrodermatitis enteropathica	Plasma zinc
Acquired enteropathy	
Cow's milk colitis	Family history, eosinophilia on biopsy
Immunodeficiency (SCID)	Immunoglobulins, lymphopenia
Metabolic disorders	
Congenital adrenal hyperplasia	Electrolytes
Dicarboxylic aciduria	Venous pH, urine organic acids
Iatrogenic	
Narcotic withdrawal	Drug history – maternal, neonatal
Drugs	
Antibiotics	
Prostaglandins	
Theophylline	
Pancreatic insufficiency	
Cystic fibrosis	
Schwachman's syndrome	

since lactose intolerance secondary to gastroenteritis is not uncommon at this age. Other complications of diarrhea include electrolyte disturbance with acidosis, nosocomial spread of the disease (the infants should be isolated) and secondary cow's milk protein intolerance.

Other causes of diarrhea are all rare (Muller & Milla 1988). Primary lactose intolerance is more common among infants of African origin but is still rare compared to a secondary intolerance. Congenital disorders of the enterocyte usually cause loose stools in the neonatal period although they may present later with intractable diarrhea since the pathological nature of the stools is not always appreciated initially. An antenatal ultrasound may have shown distended fluid-filled bowel loops. Cow's milk protein intolerance may present as diarrhea or vomiting. The more specific entity of cow's milk colitis, however, presents with bloody diarrhea and must be differentiated from NEC and other conditions (CF, intussusception, Meckel's diverticulitis and volvulus). Diagnosis rests on the resolution of the symptoms after appropriate substitution of the feed. Where the infant's size and condition permit, a rectal biopsy may show eosinophils in the inflammatory infiltrate. Immunodeficiency, especially severe

combined immunodeficiency, may present with diarrhea and often a protein-losing enteropathy in the neonatal period. Lymphopenia on the blood film and other coexistent signs of infection (such as an interstitial pneumonia on chest X-ray) should alert one to this diagnosis. Similarly, abnormalities of the urea and electrolytes or acidosis should suggest the possibility of a metabolic disorder and one should always inquire jointly of the mother's and baby's drug history.

Neonatal constipation

The failure to pass meconium in the first 24 h in a term baby is a significant symptom and should prompt a search for the underlying cause. In a preterm baby, however, failure to open the bowels is not uncommon and many neonatal units use glycerin suppositories (chips) from day 1 to encourage bowel actions and facilitate tolerance of enteral feeds. After prematurity the most common organic cause of constipation in the first weeks of life is Hirschsprung's disease and this must be excluded by rectal examination followed by suction biopsy in all term infants when constipation follows on failure to pass meconium within the first 48 h. Neonatal constipation should always be taken seriously; failure to open the bowels at least every other day is outside the range of normality. Clinical findings and simple investigations as outlined in Table 5.83 should allow one to identify most organic causes.

Overfeeding is a common cause of constipation in older neonates. In this situation either the baby is very greedy or mother mistakes thirst for hunger and the baby is offered, and takes, more and more milk. (It is almost unknown as a cause of constipation in the breast-fed infant when autoregulation of the maternal milk

Table 5.83 Neonatal constipation

Etiology	Investigation
1. Pseudo-obstruction	
Prematurity	
Major insult – sepsis	
asphyxia	
Neuropathy	Abdominal X-ray, barium meal and follow through
Myopathy	Rectal biopsy
2. Meconium plug	
3. Low bowel obstruction	
Meconium ileus/cystic fibrosis	Immunoreactive trypsin
Hirschsprung's disease	Rectal examination, barium enema
Colonic atresia	
4. Anorectal anomalies	
Imperforate anus – anal atresia	Rectal examination
anorectal	
atresia	
Rectal atresia	
Anal stenosis/stricture	
Rectal stenosis/stricture	
5. Metabolic disorder	
Hypothyroidism	Thyroxin, TSH
Hypercalcemia	Calcium
Salt- and water-losing states	Urea and electrolytes
Renal tubular acidosis	Urine pH
6. Overfeeding	

allows a more diluted milk to be provided for the baby as the volume of milk taken increases.) An accurate feeding history soon identifies this problem. It is, however, rare in the early neonatal period.

The management of simple constipation in the neonatal period is similar to that at an older age. Correction of a feeding disorder and provision of an adequate amount of extra water to slake thirst (especially in hot weather) will correct most cases. If this proves insufficient, intermittent suppositories are occasionally successful but more usually infants will need a stool softener (lactulose 2.5 ml b.d.) for a period of time to regularize the bowel habit. Rarely a bowel stimulant such as Senokot is needed.

BILIRUBIN METABOLISM (Weinberg 1986)

Bilirubin is one of the end products of heme catabolism and in normal circumstances has to be processed by the liver for its excretion. In early neonatal life there is a much greater production of bilirubin. The hemoglobin mass at birth is high (and further increased by such factors as delayed clamping of the cord) and contains approximately 80% fetal hemoglobin. This is replaced within 4 months by adult hemoglobin. This obligatory red cell turnover is the major factor in the excess bilirubin production (each 1 g Hb produces 600 μmol of bilirubin). To this must be added the bilirubin produced by bruising, cephalhematoma and shunt bilirubin (bilirubin produced by heme pigments in the reticuloendothelial system that are never incorporated into

hemoglobin: approximately 20% of the total bilirubin production).

Heme is metabolized to biliverdin by heme oxygenase (Fig. 5.44) which is found in the liver, spleen and macrophages and whose activity is increased manyfold in the face of such an increased substrate load. The biliverdin is rapidly reduced to bilirubin by biliverdin reductase using NADPH as a proton donor. The end product, bilirubin XIIa, is insoluble because of the hydrogen bonding between the two pyrrole rings (a process facilitated by the ionization of the molecule that occurs below pH 7.4) (Fig. 5.45). The insoluble bilirubin is bound to albumin (binding capacity 0.5–1.0 mmol bilirubin per mol albumin). At a bilirubin concentration of 340 mmol/l the molar ratio exceeds 1 : 1 and dissociation of the bilirubin occurs readily. Because of its fat solubility (increased at low pH) this bilirubin is readily deposited in the tissues.

Bilirubin is transported through the hepatocyte membrane by a carrier-mediated process (Fig. 5.46) and is then carried to the smooth endoplasmic reticulum by ligandin or Y protein. This has a low concentration at birth but increases to adult levels by 5–10 days of age. In the smooth endoplasmic reticulum the bilirubin is conjugated with a uridine moiety to bilirubin monoglucuronide by the enzyme glucuronyltransferase. This too has a low activity at birth but following induction by the high bilirubin load, adult levels are reached by 14 days of age irrespective of gestation (a birth-related event). The activity of this enzyme can be induced by phenobarbitone or other microsomal enzyme-inducing drugs. The

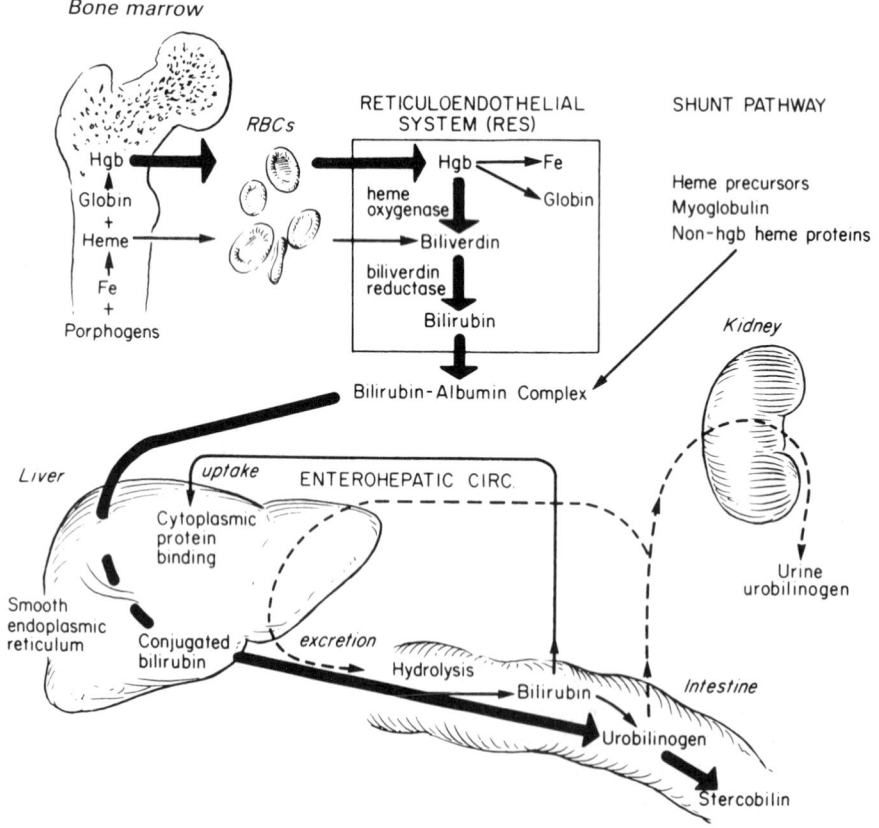

Fig. 5.44 The pathway of bilirubin production, transport and metabolism. (From Garcia 1972, reprinted with permission.)

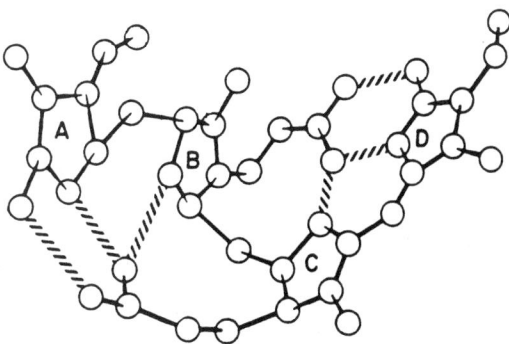

Fig. 5.45 Primary structure of bilirubin above, and below tertiary structure with hydrogen bonds shown as shaded lines. This folded structure serves to mask the polar carboxyl residues and renders the bilirubin molecule water insoluble/fat soluble. (From Schmidt 1978.)

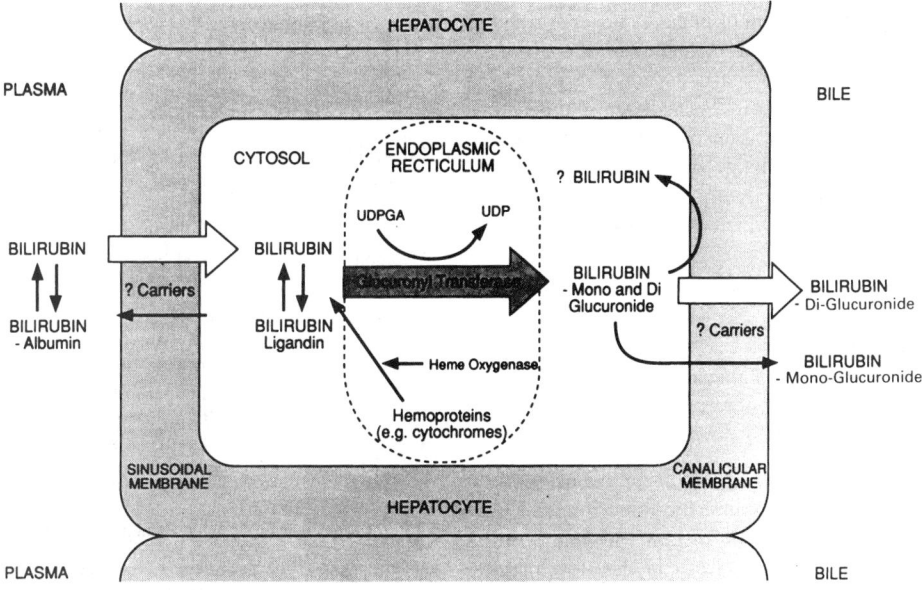

Fig. 5.46 Bilirubin handling by the liver. For explanation see text. (Modified from Schmidt 1978.)

bilirubin monoglucuronide is converted to bilirubin diglucuronide by glucuronyltransferase (requiring UDP glucuronic acid) and then transported across the canalicular membrane by an energy-dependent carrier-mediated system.

The excretory mechanisms described above result in a high concentration of bilirubin in the bile. In the adult this consists mostly of bilirubin IXa, a pigment which cannot be excreted without conjugation which alters its involuted hydrogen-bonded conformation. However, the other bilirubin isomers can be excreted directly in the bile since they are naturally water soluble. The major photochemical effect of phototherapy makes use of this fact. Under blue light (420–480 nm) bilirubin IXa is converted by

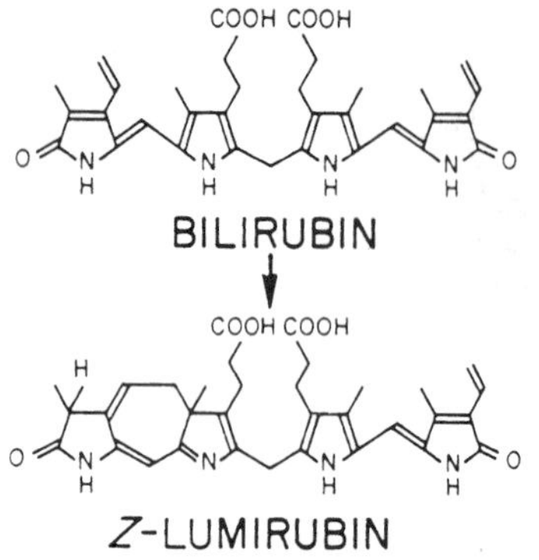

BILIRUBIN

↓

Z-LUMIRUBIN

Fig. 5.47 Photoisomerization by light converts the stable isomer of bilirubin to the thermodynamically unstable Z-lumirubin. (From McDonagh et al 1982, reprinted with permission.)

photoisomerization to Z-lumirubin (Fig. 5.47). There is a 180° rotation of a terminal pyrrole which prohibits intramolecular hydrogen bonding, thus disrupting the tertiary structure of the bilirubin IXa isomer, and exposes the carboxyl radical, thus creating a polar water-soluble pigment which can be excreted in the bile.

It is clear from the above that the neonate arrives in the world unable to cope with the normal bilirubin load and thus a degree of jaundice is to be expected. This is recognized by the term physiological jaundice of the newborn. Postnatally there is a rapid rise in the bilirubin due to a combination of high bilirubin load and decreased hepatic excretion. Following the initial rise there is a slow fall due to the slow development of hepatic carrier proteins (induction of ribosomal enzyme complexes). The maximum allowable level of physiological jaundice is not clear. A level as low as 210 μmol/l by the third day of life has been claimed to indicate the need for further investigation but, in practice, most clinicians probably would not investigate the cause of jaundice unless the patient required phototherapy or other clinical features were present, the most important of which is the postnatal age of patient.

NEONATAL JAUNDICE (Table 5.84)

Early jaundice (< 10 days)

First 24 hours (hemolytic disease of the newborn, HDN)

This is by far the most dangerous form of jaundice in the newborn as the bilirubin levels can rise rapidly into the toxic range. The most common cause is rhesus hemolytic disease although with current obstetric management it is now rare in the developed world. Sensitization of the mother (usually by small fetomaternal transfusions in previous pregnancies and particularly deliveries) will result in the production of anti-D IgM and IgG. The latter is responsible for rhesus disease in the neonate which is characterized by a (often highly) positive Coombs' test and extravascular hemolysis in the spleen. ABO incompatibility, now the most common cause for HDN (mother usually blood group O, infant blood group A or B) in the UK occurs in 15% of pregnancies. It is particularly common in Negros. Again the IgG antibody is the important hemolysin but in this case the Coombs' test is often negative (possibly due to the decreased number of A

Table 5.84 Neonatal jaundice

Mechanism	Cause	Investigation
1. Early jaundice (<10 days)		
a. *First 24 hours*		
Immune hemolysis	Rhesus disease	Direct Coombs' test Maternal/infant blood group
	ABO incompatibility Rare blood group antibodies	
Nonimmune hemolysis	Glucose-6-phosphate dehydrogenase (G6PD) deficiency	Family history G6PD assay
	Pyruvate kinase (PK) deficiency	PK assay
	Congenital spherocytosis	Blood film
Sepsis		Full blood count Septic screen
b. *After 24 hours*		
Physiological jaundice	Prematurity Hypoglycemia Hypoxia Dehydration Intestinal stasis	
Excess bilirubin production	Bruising cephalhematoma Disseminated Intravascular coagulation/ Intraventricular hemorrhage	
	Polycythemia Ingestion maternal blood (Melena)	Full blood count
Infection	Sepsis Intrauterine infection	Septic screen IgM, torch screen
Congenital hemolytic anemia	Crigler–Najjar syndrome	
	Gilbert's syndrome	
Metabolic	Galactosemia	Urine-reducing substances
2. Prolonged jaundice (>10 days)		
a. *Prolonged unconjugated hyperbilirubinemia*		
Breast milk	Breast milk jaundice Inhibitor of glucuronyl transferase Lucey–Driscoll syndrome	Trial of formula milk Navajo Indians
Sepsis	New/persisting i.v. alimentation	Full blood count, septic screen
Metabolic	Hypothyroidism Aminoacidemias	Thyroxine, TSH Plasma/urine amino acids
	Galactosemia	Urine-reducing substances
	Fructosemia Cystic fibrosis	Liver function tests Immunoreactive trypsin
Increased enterohepatic circulation	Intestinal obstruction Pyloric stenosis Atresia Hirschsprung's disease Meconium ileus Meconium plug	Abdominal X-ray

Table 5.84 *Cont'd*

Mechanism	Cause	Investigation
	Pseudo-obstruction	
	Fasting	
	Underfeeding	
	Drugs	
Persisting hemolysis	Rhesus incompatibility (inspissated bile syndrome) Hemoglobinopathy G6PD deficiency, PK deficiency Vitamin E deficiency	
Congenital nonhemolytic hyperbilirubinemia	Crigler–Najjar syndrome Gilbert's syndrome	
Decreased hepatic uptake	Persisting shunt through ductus venosus	

b. *Prolonged conjugated hyperbilirubinemia*
Intrahepatic cholestasis
  Infections

Mechanism	Cause	Investigation
Acquired	Septicemia/bacteremia	Septic screen, chest X-ray
	Urinary tract infection	MSU
	Listeriosis	
	Tuberculosis	
Congenital	Syphilis	
	Malaria	
	Toxoplasmosis	Torch screen
	Hepatitis	Hepatitis B antigen, hepatitis A IgM
	Epstein–Barr virus	Viral titers
	Rubella	Viral titers
	Coxsackie B, A9	Viral titers
	Cytomegalovirus	Viral titers
	Varicella-zoster.	Viral titers
	Herpes simplex	Viral titers
	Echovirus, adenovirus	Viral titers
	Aids HIV infection	Maternal HIV titers
Metabolic disorders	α_1-antitrypsin deficiency	α_1-antitrypsin
	Cystic fibrosis	Immunoreactive trypsin Sweat test
	Galactosemia	Urine reducing substances
	Fructosemia	WBC enzyme assay
	Tyrosinosis	Plasma/urine amino acids
	G_{M1} gangliosidosis	Storage vacuoles Lymphocytes
	Gaucher's syndrome	WBC enzyme assays
	Nieman–Pick disease	Urine oligosaccharides
	Mucopolysaccharidosis	Urine mucopolysaccharides
	Sialosis	
	Wolman's disease	
	Zellweger syndrome	Serum catalase/VLC fatty acids
	Dubin–Johnson syndrome	
	Rotor's syndrome	
	Glutaric aciduria Type II	Urine organic acids
Endocrine	Hypothyroidism	Thyroxine, TSH
	Hypoadrenalism	Urea and electrolytes, 17-OH-progesterone, cortisol, aldosterone

Table 5.84 *Cont'd*

Mechanism	Cause	Investigation
	Hypopituitarism	ACTH
	Diabetes insipidus	Plasma/urine osmolality
	Hypoparathyroidism	
Vascular	Veno-occlusive disease	Ultrasound liver
	Poor perfusion syndromes	
	Hemangioendothelioma	
	Lymphatic defects, familial	
	Cholestasis with lymphedema	
Miscellaneous	Infantile polycystic disease	Ultrasound kidney and liver
	Toxins	
	Parenteral nutrition	
	Drugs	
	Halothane	
	Chromosomal disorders–trisomies 21, 18, 13	Chromosomes
	Biliary hypoplasia (Alagille's syndrome)	
	Familial neonatal steatosis (Byler's syndrome)	
	Posthemolytic hepatic dysfunction	
Idiopathic neonatal hepatitis		
Extrahepatic cholestasis	Extrahepatic biliary atresia	
	Choledochal cyst	Ultrasound liver
	Bile duct stenosis	
	Spontaneous perforation of bile duct	Abdominal X-ray ascites
	Gallstones	
	Ascending cholangitis	

and B sites on the fetal erythrocyte). Laboratory investigation is notoriously unreliable at predicting infants at risk from ABO hemolytic disease but microspherocytosis on the blood film is a useful diagnostic pointer to the condition (Brouwers et al 1988). Red blood cell destruction occurs primarily by extravascular mechanisms and is more rapid in ABO incompatibility with the antibody disappearing within 2–3 days. Occasionally minor blood group antibodies (anti-Kell, anti-Duffy) cause hemolytic disease and these are usually Coombs' positive.

Hemolysis also occurs in the absence of blood group incompatibility. Sepsis is said to cause jaundice at this age and should always be excluded. In fact, it rarely turns out to be responsible for such early jaundice but congenital infections, e.g. rubella, syphilis and toxoplasmosis, can present this way. The most common nonimmunological cause of hemolytic jaundice within 24 h is congenital hemolytic anemia due to a red cell metabolic defect (e.g. glucose-6-phosphate dehydrogenase (G6PD) deficiency or pyruvic kinase (PK) deficiency) or structural defect (congenital spherocytosis, elliptocytosis and pyknocytosis). In these cases there is often a family history. G6PD deficiency occurs more commonly in patients of Mediterranean, African or Oriental origin. Appropriate hematological investigations and enzyme assays usually provide a rapid diagnosis.

After 24 hours

65% of normal neonates exhibit clinical jaundice (85 μmol/l or 5 mg/dl). In most patients excessive jaundice at this stage is due to exacerbation of the normal physiological jaundice of the newborn. The 95th percentile for term infants is 190 μmol/l (11.5 mg/dl) for bottle-fed and 240 μmol/l (14.5 mg/dl) for breast-fed infants. The more premature the infant the more immature the liver although this may be balanced by decreased bilirubin production since exchange transfusion is rarely required despite the almost obligatory use of phototherapy in infants of less than 30 weeks' gestation. Excessive production of bilirubin from severe bruising or cephalhematomata, polycythemia or ingestion of maternal blood commonly causes jaundice in this period.

The most important cause to consider is acquired bacterial infection or rarely congenitally transmitted infections (CMV, rubella, toxoplasmosis, syphilis). Direct involvement of the liver by the infective process is one reason for the jaundice, as is increased bilirubin breakdown with disseminated intravascular coagulation. However, it is likely that the nature of the hyperbilirubinemia is multifactorial.

Inadequate calorie intake and decreased glucose production will lead to a reduction in glycogen and energy available for the production and conversion of the uridine diphosphoglucuronic acid required for the conjugation of the bilirubin glucuronyltransferase. Acidosis may increase bilirubin levels but, more importantly, increases bilirubin toxicity due to the alteration of the equilibrium between free bilirubin and its acid salt, thus decreasing the maximum tolerable level of bilirubin. Dehydration probably increases the bilirubin levels by prolonging gut transit and therefore increasing the enterohepatic circulation. In such conditions as failure to pass meconium, pyloric stenosis and cystic fibrosis with meconium ileus, there will be an increase in the hydrolysis of the conjugated bilirubin by the alkaline duodenal juices and the mucosal β-glucuronidases of the small intestine, thus increasing the bilirubin returned to the blood via the enterohepatic circulation.

In most cases of neonatal jaundice, the bilirubin levels will fall below the phototherapy range before the end of the second week of life. However, in the premature infant phototherapy may be required for longer. One group of patients that presents with severe early neonatal jaundice that continues beyond the first 10 days (and may also present later) is the rare patient with congenital nonhemolytic hyperbilirubinemias. The most important of these, Crigler–Najjar syndrome, presents as two variants:

1. the autosomal recessive Type I with absence of uridine diphosphoglucuronyltransferase (UDPGT) in the liver, characterized by persistent severe unconjugated hyperbilirubinemia
2. the autosomal dominant Type II with defective rather than absent UDPGT activity in which the bilirubin levels are lower (< 340 μmol/l).

This latter variant (known also as Arias syndrome) may present much later in life and for this reason is said to merge diagnostically into the commonest of the unconjugated hyperbilirubinemias, Gilbert's syndrome, which is more common in men and usually presents after puberty. The other familial conjugated hyperbilirubinemias (Dubin–Johnson and Rotor's syndrome) hardly ever present at birth.

Management of early jaundice

Investigation and treatment of cause. It is important that the etiology of the hyperbilirubinemia should be established. A careful obstetric and family history (e.g. spherocytosis) is important. A full blood count, direct Coombs' test, grouping of mother and baby and testing the urine for reducing substances are the usual minimum of investigations required. If infection is suspected a septic and TORCH (congenital infection) screen can be added. Where the hemolysis remains unexplained further hematological investigation (e.g. enzyme assays for G6PD deficiency and PK deficiency) will be needed. In most cases no treatment for the cause of the hemolysis will be available though it behoves the pediatrician to ensure that the mother is given anti-D globulin where indicated. Advice on drugs to be avoided in the future must be made available to the patients with G6PD deficiency. Infection should be treated as indicated.

Treatment of jaundice. *Phototherapy.* The aim of therapy is to keep the level of bilirubin below the toxic level. Phototherapy must be started early enough to prevent the expected rise in bilirubin but not at a level which causes unnecessary work for the nursing staff and, more importantly, an unnecessary separation of mother and baby. Most units have their own chart for plotting bilirubin levels and action lines to indicate the levels at which phototherapy (and exchange transfusion) are indicated. Where a rapidly rising bilirubin is expected such as hemolytic disease and jaundice at less than 24 h, phototherapy should be started straight away and the sequential bilirubin results should be graphed. At a later stage the need for phototherapy is more debatable. As a general rule the more premature the infant the lower the levels of bilirubin that are tolerated and thus a good guiding figure is that phototherapy is indicated when the bilirubin rises above a level given by the formula: birthweight in kg × 100. In term babies phototherapy should be given when the bilirubin rises above 300 μmol/l.

There are many potential complications to phototherapy:

1. Equipment failure/design drawbacks: the lamps must produce radiation in the blue range of 450–460 nm with a minimum irradiance of flux of 4 μW/m²/nm. The new generation of phototherapy units are much more efficient than the old (although the blue light is off-putting for the parents). It seems prudent to protect the eyes since changes of premature aging have been induced by phototherapy in newborn monkeys but no detrimental effect is recorded in the human infant.
2. Dehydration: this is by far the most important complication and is the result of increased insensible water loss through the skin and increased stool water content. Increasing the fluid intake of infants under phototherapy by 15 ml/kg/day will correct this.
3. Loose stools: Z-lumirubin excreted in the bile is a highly polar, nonphysiological substance which has a direct secretory effect on intestinal mucosa leading, inevitably, to loose stools. These are not troublesome and frank diarrhea never results. The increased fluid intake is the only therapeutic manipulation required. (Lactose intolerance, however, may also occur.)
4. Parental anxiety: the separation of mother and baby and the terrible color given to the infant by the effective blue lamps are naturally upsetting to parents and a sympathetic explanation of

what is happening is mandatory. The best way of minimizing this anxiety is to pay scrupulous attention to the need for phototherapy and to minimize the duration of such therapy.

5. Other effects have been noted experimentally (copper retention, abnormal porphyrin metabolism and damage to DNA in cell cultures) but they do not seem relevant in clinical practice. Bronzing or discoloration of the skin can also occur when phototherapy is used in patients with a cholestatic element to their jaundice.

Exchange transfusion. The exchange transfusion of blood via an umbilical artery or vein is the most efficient way of removing bilirubin (and other noxious substances). It is employed when bilirubin levels reach the toxic range determined both by the gestational age and the clinical state of the baby. Sicker babies with their attendant metabolic derangements such as acidosis are transfused at lower levels. Acceptable criteria for exchange transfusion would be a serum bilirubin of 340 μmol/l (term babies), 300 μmol/l (infants < 2500 g), 250 μmol/l (infants < 1500 g) and 170 μmol/l (infants < 1000 g). In practice, however, most exchange transfusions in the smaller infants (< 1500 g) are performed for reasons other than jaundice (usually a septic child in extremis or DIC). Most physicians would not immediately exchange an asymptomatic term baby even with severe physiological jaundice greater than 340 μmol/l assuming there was a fairly prompt response to phototherapy (usually given with double lamps in such situations). The commonest indication for exchange transfusion is a rapidly rising bilirubin in the first 24 h of life in babies with hemolytic disease of the newborn (p. 232). The technique is described on page 1838. The complications are listed in Table 5.85 together with suitable avoiding action.

Other methods. Attention to clinical detail (for example the correction of acidosis, treatment of infection and maintenance of hemodynamic stability) is valuable. In the small premature infant judicious use of 20% albumen (4–5 ml/kg) will buy time under

phototherapy and often obviate the need for a formal exchange transfusion. In the rarer congenital nonhemolytic disorders (Crigler–Najjar Type II and Rotor's syndrome) hepatic enzyme inducers such as phenobarbitone (1–8 mg/kg/24 h) are used in addition to prolonged daily phototherapy to control the bilirubin levels.

Prolonged jaundice

Any jaundice beyond 10 days in a term infant is pathological but preterm infants (especially very low birthweight infants) often have jaundice that persists beyond this time for which no cause is found. It is probably wise, however, to investigate all these patients in the same way so that rarer conditions presenting in premature infants are not missed. The basic investigation is the estimation of the percentage of conjugated bilirubin by the Van den Bergh method. The majority of patients will have an unconjugated hyperbilirubinemia (conjugated bilirubin < 30% of total). Conjugated hyperbilirubinemia (> 80% of total) is an indication of intra- or extrahepatic cholestasis and is accompanied by bilirubinuria and dark urine (conjugated bilirubin > 25 μmol/l). Although there would appear to be a large gray area between 30 and 80%, in practice this is not often a problem. Such patients will probably have intrahepatic cholestasis and should be investigated accordingly.

Prolonged unconjugated hyperbilirubinemia

Breast milk jaundice. The usual cause of such prolonged jaundice is breast milk jaundice but to diagnose this without estimating the percentage of conjugated bilirubin would be negligent. The bilirubin rises to values of between 255 and 360 μmol/l (usually less than 20% conjugated); the patient, however, is well and no treatment is necessary. The jaundice usually settles by about 6 weeks although it may occasionally continue up to 4 months. Discontinuation of breast-feeding leads to a rapid fall in the bilirubin. The etiology of this condition long remained obscure and was thought to be due to various constituents of the milk. Breast milk consists of milk constituents which are parceled in maternal breast milk membrane prior to their secretion from the acini of the gland. This membrane is a protein structure and has a functional activity in its own right, e.g. enzymatic (breast milk lipase) and transport (membrane-bound iron). Both of these greatly increase the nutritional efficiency of milk. In patients with breast milk jaundice a β-glucuronidase has been shown to be present in mother's milk and in the infant's feces (the activity in the stool disappearing with the cessation of breast-feeding coincident with a fall in unconjugated hyperbilirubinemia). It seems likely, therefore, that breast milk jaundice is due to the breast milk β-glucuronidase causing deconjugation of the bilirubin diglucuronide and intestinal absorption of the fat-soluble bilirubin through the intestinal mucosa, increasing the enterohepatic circulation of bilirubin (Fig. 5.44) and thus increasing the level of unconjugated bilirubin in the blood (Gourley & Arend 1986). It is relevant at this point to contrast this with the mechanism seen in the very rare Lucey–Driscoll syndrome in which there is a definite inhibitor of bilirubin glucuronide in mother's milk (recoverable in the infant's serum) and which results in the development of jaundice in all of the mother's offspring (despite her apparent good health). This entity may present in the first few days of life and is occasionally severe

Table 5.85 Complications of exchange transfusion

Infection	Sepsis	Strict aseptic technique Fresh blood
	CMV	Appropriate screening donors
	Hepatitis	
Hypothermia		Warm blood/baby
Cardiovascular instability	Transient hypovolemia Hypervolemia	Small aliquots (10–20 ml) Meticulous recording of exchanges
	Cardiac dysrhythmia	Cardiac monitoring
Electrolyte disorders	Hyperkalemia	Monitor electrolytes and blood sugar before and after exchange
	Hypoglycemia Hypocalcemia	Check citrate concentration of donor blood
	Acidosis	
Complications of catheter	Embolic	Minimize duration of catheterization
	Hemorrhage (late portal vein thrombosis)	
Inadequate exchange		Use 170–200 ml/kg over 100 min for full exchange

enough to require exchange transfusion. (A true inhibitor of glucuronyltransferase has also been found in the Navajo American Indians.)

Hypothyroidism. It is mandatory to exclude hypothyroidism as a cause of persistent unconjugated hyperbilirubinemia although in countries with a neonatal screening program for hypothyroidism this is hardly ever a presenting symptom.

Intestinal stasis. The second most common cause now for persistent unconjugated jaundice is an increased enterohepatic circulation of bilirubin. In the normal situation 25% of the conjugated bilirubin reaching the duodenum is deconjugated and reabsorbed. This may be increased in situations of stasis where the alkaline intestinal juices and the mucosal bilirubin diglucuronidases (together with bacterial organisms in conditions of overgrowth) have longer to act on this substrate. Thus surgical conditions such as Hirschsprung's disease, intestinal atresia, pyloric stenosis and the meconium ileus of cystic fibrosis are often complicated by jaundice. Cystic fibrosis may also cause unconjugated jaundice due to hepatic involvement, and such involvement may explain why other conditions can present in this fashion (i.e. sepsis, galactosemia and fructosemia).

Hemolytic causes. Finally, the hemolytic anemias, especially rhesus hemolytic disease and more consistently the rare hemolytic congenital hyperbilirubinemias, will be a cause of prolonged unconjugated jaundice. The management of all such jaundice is the identification and treatment of the underlying disorder as indicated in Table 5.84.

Prolonged conjugated hyperbilirubinemia

This discussion will center on the presentation of the child with prolonged conjugated jaundice to the general pediatrician. The more complicated perspective of the specialist referral center will be dealt with in the section on liver disease (p. 470). The main aim of the general pediatrician is to recognize that a cholestatic syndrome is present. The signs listed in Table 5.86a, should alert the physician to the presence of such a syndrome. Whilst jaundice is the usual presenting symptom other complications, especially bruising and other evidence of defective hemostasis, hypoalbuminemia or hypoglycemia may also be presenting features. (One should never diagnose hemorrhagic disease of the newborn, especially in a jaundiced child, without checking the liver function tests and percentage conjugated bilirubin.) Clues that suggest an underlying disorder are shown in Table 5.86b.

The management of prolonged cholestatic jaundice is aimed at identifying conditions requiring immediate treatment and supportive therapy and then distinguishing between intra- and extrahepatic cholestasis. Blood cultures and a septic screen together with a screen for intrauterine infections (TORCH, VDRL) should be sent in all infants. Parenteral antibiotics should be started if the infant appears unwell. Urine should be tested for reducing substances and sent for sugar chromatography to exclude galactosemia and fructosemia. It is also sensible to exclude galactose and fructose from the diet until the results of this are known. It should be remembered that all infants less than 2 weeks of age (and babies with renal tubular disorders, e.g. Lowe's syndrome) can have reducing substances in the urine. Furthermore, infants with liver disease can both have sugar in the urine and present with septicemia. Initial investigations should include urine for amino acid chromatography to identify particularly tyrosinemia and to send blood for α_1-antitrypsin

Table 5.86 Clinical features that alert one to the presence of conjugated hyperbilirubinemia

a. Evidence of hepatic disease

Jaundice	Urine – yellow, not colorless from birth. Dark later with bilirubin ++ on Clinistix
	Stools – Pale yellow to white (may be green)
Hepatomegaly	
Pruritus	
Splenomegaly, ascites, edema	
Evidence of bleeding tendency – Bruising	
	Bleeding
Failure to thrive	
Investigations – Increased bilirubin, conjugated bilirubin >80%	
	Increased alanine aminotransferase
	Increased aspartate transaminase
	Increased γ-glutamyltransferase
	Increased α-fetoprotein
	Prolonged prothrombin time
	Low albumin
	Low blood sugar

b. Features of underlying etiology

Maternal history, skin lesions	– Congenital infections
Purpura, choroidoretinitis	– Congenital infections
Cataracts	Galactosemia (urine positive for reducing substances)
	Lowe's syndrome (aminoaciduria)
Multiple congenital abnormalities	– Trisomy 13, 18, 21
Ascites, bile-stained hernia	– Spontaneous perforation of bile ducts
Cystic mass below the liver	– Choledochal cyst
Situs inversus, midline liver, malposition of the viscera	– Extrahepatic biliary atresia
	– Biliary hypoplasia
Systolic murmur, dysmorphic facies	
Cutaneous hemangioma	– Hepatic/biliary hemangiomata
Marked splenomegaly	– Lysosomal storage disorder
Hypoglycemia	– Pituitary deficiency

c. Features indicating the nature of the cholestasis

Incomplete stool pallor	– Intrahepatic cholestasis plus low birthweight, moderate hepatomegaly
Complete stool pallor: <10 days transient	– Intrahepatic cholestasis
>10 days permanent	– Extrahepatic cholestasis plus normal birthweight, firm hard hepatomegaly

phenotyping (PiZZ; PiNul,Nul; PiZ,Nul) and serum immunoreactive trypsin. Endocrinological disorders and other rare metabolic disorders should be considered and investigated as seems appropriate to the infant. Liver function tests are not discriminatory but serum α-fetoprotein is particularly raised in tyrosinemia and bile duct hypoplasia. A hemorrhagic diathesis should be treated with vitamin K (1 mg i.v.) and fresh frozen plasma if bleeding continues. Other supportive measures for liver failure may be needed.

The next step is to distinguish between intra- and extrahepatic cholestasis. The color of the stool is a useful guide (Table 5.86c). Incomplete stool pallor together with evidence of intrauterine growth retardation suggests a prenatal hepatitis causing intrahepatic cholestasis. Complete stool pallor lasting longer than 2 weeks, especially if accompanied by a large hard liver or a conjugated bilirubin level of > 80%, suggests extrahepatic biliary obstruction and referral to a specialist to exclude biliary atresia is required without delay. Where the diagnosis is less clear cut or delay in referral is experienced a hepatic ultrasound (to exclude a

Table 5.87 Laboratory investigations of suspected extrahepatic cholestasis (EHC)

1. Conjugated bilirubin	>80% – EHC
2. Liver function/clotting disorders	γ-glutamyltransferase : aspartate transaminase = 2 : 1 – EHC
3. Ultrasound scan liver/gallbladder	Cystic dilation – choledochal cyst
4. ¹³¹I Rose Bengal excretion test	<10% in stool in 72 h – EHC
5. ⁹⁹ᵐTc DIDA scan	
6. Liver biopsy – Neonatal hepatitis	Hepatocellular necrosis, giant cell transformation, disorganized/inflammatory infiltrate of portal tracts, cholestasis, bile duct proliferation
Extrahepatic biliary atresia	Widened portal tracts with prominent distorted angulated bile ducts. Increased fibrosis with inflammatory cell infiltrate. Cholestasis with bile lakes. Giant cell transformation
Alagille's syndrome biliary hypoplasia	Paucity of interlobular ducts compared with portal areas. Mild fibrosis
Nonsyndromic biliary hypoplasia	Paucity of interlobular ducts with variable portal fibrosis

choledochal cyst) and I-131 rose bengal fecal excretion test (> 10% of i.v. dose excreted over 72 h excludes biliary atresia) or technetium-99m HIDA cholescintography (to demonstrate hepatic uptake and functional bile flow) may all be considered. The gold standard for the diagnosis of intra- and extrahepatic cholestasis remains, however, the percutaneous liver biopsy (see Table 5.87). This will also provide for the differentiation between neonatal hepatitis syndrome and interlobular biliary hypoplasia. Biliary hypoplasia may be further differentiated into Alagille's syndrome (characteristic facies, butterfly wing vertebra, peripheral pulmonary artery stenosis and retinopathy) and secondary biliary hypoplasia, by the degree of portal fibrosis (although such fibrosis may result from a variety of infective or metabolic insults). Neonatal hepatitis is the end result of many hepatic insults. In the majority of cases, however, no cause can be found and the final diagnosis is idiopathic neonatal hepatitis. These entities are discussed further in Chapter 11.

HEMATOLOGICAL PROBLEMS OF THE NEWBORN

DEVELOPMENTAL HEMOPOIESIS

Unlike in the older child and adult, fetal hemopoiesis is principally extramedullary and develops over three main overlapping phases: mesoblastic (yolk sac), hepatic and myeloid (bone marrow) (Fig. 5.48).

A few days after implantation solid masses of cells called blood islands form within the yolk sac and by 14 days of gestation they have differentiated into either peripheral cells which form the vascular endothelium or central cells which become the primitive blood cells. These pluripotent stem cells are remarkable for their ability to both replicate themselves and to produce daughter cells which are committed to differentiation along one or more hemopoietic lines. Pluripotent cells are almost certainly responsible for seeding the later developing sites of hemopoiesis (liver, spleen and bone marrow). The progenitor stem cells (CFU-GEMM: colony-forming unit, granulocyte erythrocyte megakaryocytic macrophage cells) (Fig. 5.49) are able to produce either red cells, platelets or white cells except lymphocytes (Hann

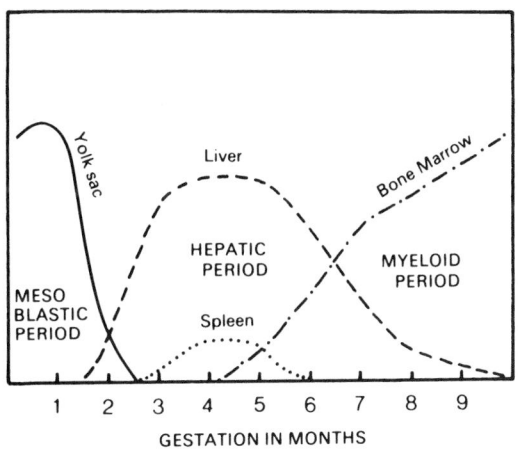

Fig. 5.48 Stages of hemopoiesis in the developing embryo and fetus. (From Roberton 1986.)

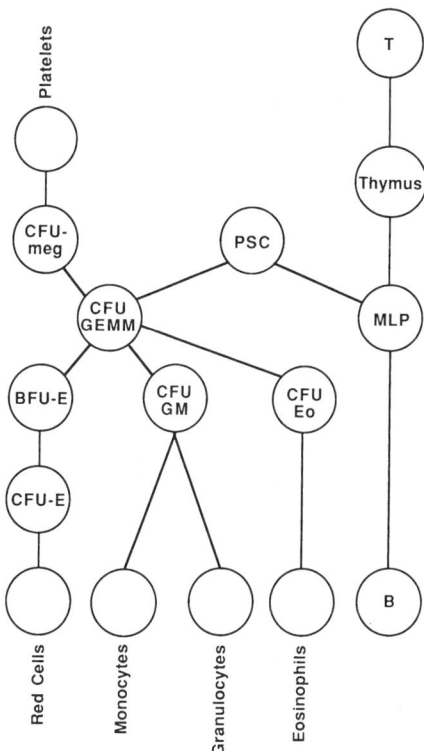

Fig. 5.49 Schematic outline of hematopoietic stages: PSC = pluripotent stem cell; CFU = colony-forming unit; BFU = burst-forming unit; MLP = mixed lymphoid progenitor; T = T lymphocyte; B = B lymphocyte; GEMM = granulocyte erythrocyte megakaryocyte monocyte; Eo = eosinophil. (Adapted from Hann et al 1983.)

et al 1983). Such early cells are morphologically similar to small lymphocytes. Hepatic hemopoiesis develops between 6 and 10 weeks gestation and diminishes towards term. Bone marrow hemopoiesis begins about 10 weeks' gestation and increases steadily towards term when it is almost entirely responsible for hemopoietic function. Extramedullary hemopoiesis may persist into the neonatal period if there has been excessive intrauterine hemolysis (e.g. rhesus disease). It can also reactivate in later life when the marrow is stressed by increased demand. During the second trimester there is a period when hemopoietic activity can be found in the kidney and spleen but in normal circumstances neither site retains function beyond term.

Erythropoiesis

In the mesoblastic phase the red cell is megaloblastic, nucleated and identical to other cell lines. By 6 weeks the red cell series are more readily identified and the first red cells observed are large (normoblastic) and well filled with hemoglobin. As gestation progresses the red cell becomes smaller, contains less hemoglobin and more mature forms evolve. Thus the hemoglobin concentration of the fetus steadily rises, as does the packed cell volume (PCV) and red blood cell (RBC) count. The percentage of nucleated cells and reticulocytes falls steadily towards term (Table 5.88). The control of erythropoiesis is primarily by erythropoietin (EPO) but this appears to operate only during the hepatic and myeloid phases (Zanjani et al 1977). Other growth factors are important, the major being the degree of oxygen delivery to the fetal tissues. This is reflected in the higher cord hemoglobin concentrations in growth-retarded infants, infants of smoking mothers, infants of diabetic mothers and those infants delivered at high altitudes. It is likely that the principal source of erythropoietin production in the human fetus is the liver and that this switches to the adult renal site some time after birth. The plasma concentration of erythropoietin at birth is similar to that in the adult but falls rapidly over the next few days to increase following a hiatus of 6–8 weeks of postnatal life.

Hemoglobin changes

The primitive hemoglobins Hb Gower 1 and 2 and Hb Portland disappear by the end of the first trimester and are replaced by fetal hemoglobin (HbF; α_2,γ_2). This remains the predominant hemoglobin of the fetus but HbA (α_2,β) can be detected by 10–12 weeks and rises to 10% by 32 weeks. Towards term the HbA production increases rapidly to 20–30%. The proportion of HbF continues to fall over the next 6 months by which stage it comprises barely 1% of the total. Small quantities of HbA_2 (α_2, δ_2) appear during the third trimester (approx. 1%).

Leukopoiesis

Granulocytes can be detected in small numbers during the first few months of gestation but increase in number during the fifth month in the connective tissue of the portal spaces. During the last trimester there is a rapid increase in number so that at term the white cell count exceeds the normal adult value. Eosinophils and basophils appear between 14 and 16 weeks and monocytes can be found by 8–10 weeks' gestation. About this time large and small lymphocytes also appear. Production of granulocytes is under the control of granulocyte colony-stimulating factor (GCSF) which has been used therapeutically in severe neutropenia.

Thrombopoiesis

Megakaryocytes appear in the mesoblastic period and continue to be produced in the bone marrow and liver until term. From 30 weeks the platelet count is similar to that of the adult. Platelet production is regulated by thrombopoietin which is in significantly lower concentrations at birth than in older children. It rises over the next 4 months and is closely linked to interleukins.

BLOOD VOLUME CHANGES

The blood volume and hemoglobin concentration at birth are significantly affected by the degree of transplacental transfusion which in turn is dependent on the timing of cord clamping after birth and the relative positioning of the infant to the placenta. The volume of transplacental transfusion may be as high as 125 ml and this volume could clearly affect the infant's clinical condition at birth by posing either the risks of anemia and polycythemia or the benefits of improved tissue perfusion. In normal circumstances in preterm infants it is probably wise to delay clamping of the cord for at least 30 s after birth with the infant at or lower than the level of the placenta. In term infants this is not necessary. Kinmond et al (1993) have demonstrated the value of placental transfusion in reducing the oxygen requirements of preterm infants.

Table 5.88   Red cell parameters in the fetus (adapted from Oski & Naiman 1982)

Age (weeks)	Hb (g/dl)	PCV	RBC ($\times 10^{12}$/l)	MCV (fl)	MCH (pg)	MCHC (g/dl)	Nucleated RBC (% of WBC)	Reticulocytes (%)
12	8.0–10.0	0.33	1.5	180	60	34	5.0–8.0	40
16	10.0	0.35	2.0	140	45	33	2.0–4.0	10–25
20	11.0	0.37	2.5	135	44	33	1.0	10–20
24	14.0	0.40	3.5	123	38	31	1.0	5–10
28	14.5	0.45	4.0	120	40	31	0.5	5–20
34	15.0	0.47	4.4	118	38	32	0.2	3–10
Term 40 cord	16.8	0.53	5.25	107	34	31.7	0.01	3–7

PCV = packed cell volume, MCV = mean cell volume, MCH = mean corpuscular hemoglobin, MCHC = mean corpuscular hemoglobin concentration.
(From Roberton 1986.)

During the first few hours of life, plasma leaves the circulation and the blood volume stabilizes with an increase in the PCV and hemoglobin concentration. The normal blood volume in a term infant is 80–90 ml/kg and nearer 100 ml/kg with decreasing maturity.

RED CELL MASS (RCM)

Ultimately the oxygen carrying capacity of the blood is controlled by the total circulating red cell mass (ml/kg bodyweight). The normal red cell mass of infants can vary from 30 to 50 ml/kg depending on whether the cord is clamped immediately at birth. Hemoglobin concentration and hematocrit bear a very variable relationship to total RCM. The poor correlation between hemoglobin concentration and red cell mass is a particular problem in preterm infants. By contracting the plasma volume the infant may be able to mask the fall in hemoglobin concentration and hematocrit for some time (Phillips et al 1986). For example, the hematocrit of 0.3 is frequently seen to correspond to RCM values ranging between 12 and 24 ml/kg in infants who have 'compensated' by reducing their plasma volume to this essential hematocrit level which seems to be optimal for oxygen transport at rest to vital organs such as the brain and heart (Ersley & Caro 1984).

BLOOD PARAMETERS AT BIRTH

Table 5.89 demonstrates the usual findings at birth and the changes which occur in the subsequent weeks. Because of the shortened life span of neonatal red cells (40–70 days) the hemoglobin concentration falls to around 11 g by 10 weeks. Red cell filterability is significantly poorer than in adults. Prematurity, hypothermia, acidosis and nutritional status exaggerate these differences. Blood group antigens only develop to adult levels by the age of 2. The blood film shows marked variations in the size and shape of red cells, the presence of spherocytes, target cells and fragments. The neutrophil count rises initially after birth to 60%

of the total white cell count and falls between the fourth and seventh day. At this time there is a reversal of the granulocyte/lymphocyte ratio with a steady rise in the latter. Band (immature) forms and myelocytes are commonly observed. The proportion of T and B lymphocytes in cord blood mimics that found in adult blood. The functional capacity of granulocytes and lymphocytes is reduced relative to older child values. The eosinophil counts rise after birth from 2% to 4–6% by the age of 1 month, but may become markedly raised in incontinentia pigmentii. Small for gestational age infants (SGA) often have a pronounced leukopenia at birth and an excess of normoblasts associated with an above normal hemoglobin concentration (McIntosh et al 1988).

ANEMIA IN THE NEWBORN INFANT

Capillary blood samples can give hemoglobin concentrations 1–2 g/dl higher than simultaneous venous samples. In the first week of life it is usual to diagnose anemia when the venous hemoglobin concentration is less than 14 g/dl.

Physiological anemia

There are progressive changes in the newborn infant's hemoglobin concentration after birth which are related to the initial degree of placental transfusion at birth and the speed at which erythropoiesis commences after birth. Whilst the average cord blood hemoglobin concentration is 16 g/dl this may vary between 14 and 20 g/dl. The subsequent fall in hemoglobin concentration is due to the physiological absence of erythropoietin, the shortened red cell life span and the increasing blood volume due to growth. The hemoglobin concentration usually reaches its nadir at 8–10 weeks (9.5–11 g/dl). Although erythropoietin cannot readily be detected until 8–12 weeks after birth, erythroid activity commences a few weeks after birth when the hemoglobin concentration falls to 10–11 g/dl.

Table 5.89 Blood parameters at birth and over the subsequent 4 weeks

	Cord blood	24 h	1 week	1 month
Hemoglobin (g/dl)	16.8	18.4	17.0	13.7
Packed cell volume (PCV)	0.53	0.58	0.54	0.43
Red cell count (× 10¹²/l)	5.25	5.8	5.2	4.2
Mean corpuscular volume (MCV, fl)	107	108	98	101
Mean corpuscular hemoglobin concentration (MCHC, g/dl)	31.7	32	33	32.1
Mean corpuscular hemoglobin (MCH, pg)	34	35	32.5	32.5
Reticulocytes (% of red cells)	3–7	3–7	0–1	1–10
Nucleated red cell count (/mm³)	500	200	0	0
Total leukocytes (range × 10⁹/l)	9.1–30	9.4–34	5.0–21	5.0–19.5
Neutrophils (range × 10⁹/l)	6.0–26.0	5.0–21.0	1.5–10.0	1.0–9.0
Lymphocytes (range × 10⁹/l)	2.0–11.0	2.0–11.5	2.0–17.0	2.5–16.5
Monocytes (% leukocytes)	6	6	9	7
Eosinophils (% leukocytes)	2	2	4	3

(From Roberton 1986.)

Hemorrhagic anemia

Fetomaternal hemorrhage

Infants may lose blood from one or more of the causes shown in Table 5.90. Before delivery fetomaternal hemorrhage is the most common cause. The mechanism is not clear in most instances but a Kleihauer test, which relies on the resistance of fetal cells to acid elution, can readily detect as little as 0.5 ml of fetal blood in the maternal circulation. Blood loss commonly occurs in the second and third stages of labor and is responsible for rhesus immunization in susceptible pairings. Iatrogenic causes of fetomaternal bleeding include attempts at amniocentesis, fetal blood sampling and external cephalic version. At the time of the episode the mother may experience mild shivering or discomfort if a considerable degree of fetomaternal hemorrhage has occurred. A 40 ml fetomaternal transfusion or more occurs in at least 1% of all pregnancies. Depending on the timing and degree of blood loss, the infant may be stillborn, hydropic, shocked at birth or merely anemic.

Fetofetal transfusion

This condition is not uncommon and may occur in up to 15% of twin pregnancies. Bleeding occurs through a communicating vessel between the placentae. If this is from the artery of one twin to the vein of the other, blood transfer will occur, the donor twin becoming progressively more anemic and intrauterine death may occur. The recipient twin will become plethoric and is generally the larger of the two at birth. A difference in hemoglobin concentration of 5 g or more at birth indicates a probable twin-to-twin transfusion. Estimations of every twin infant's hemoglobin concentration (4–6 h after birth) should be routine practice. If both twins are born alive, either may require treatment; replacement transfusion for the anemic twin or treatment of polycythemia for the plethoric.

Table 5.90 Causes of acute blood loss

Before or during delivery
Fetomaternal transfusion
Fetofetal transfusion
Rupture of placental vessels
Placenta previa; vasa previa
Placental abruption
Surgical incision of fetus or placenta
Rupture of cord vessels

After delivery
External blood loss
Cord stump
Gastrointestinal tract
  Hemorrhagic disease
  Acute gastric/duodenal erosion
  Meckel's diverticulum
Skin injury
Menstruation in females

Internal blood loss
Cephalhematoma
Subaponeurotic hemorrhage
Intracranial hemorrhage
Liver or splenic rupture
Adrenal and intrarenal hemorrhage
Retroperitoneal hemorrhage
Gluteal hemorrhage (breech)
Pulmonary hemorrhage

Iatrogenic blood loss (sampling)

Blood loss from placental or cord vessels, vasa previa or cord rupture generally occurs as a result of trauma but abnormal vessels may rupture with minimal injury. Fetal blood loss can be recognized in the presence of maternal vaginal blood loss by the Apt test (see below).

Postnatal hemorrhage

After delivery blood loss may be recognized easily if it is external as from a cord stump hemorrhage or the gastrointestinal tract. Swallowed maternal blood can be excluded by the Apt test (fetal blood resists denaturation by 1% sodium hydroxide solution and remains pink whilst adult (maternal blood) is denatured to a brownish-yellow color). Internal hemorrhage can lead to a serious and rapidly fatal deterioration in condition and this is more likely to occur where cerebral hemorrhage has occurred. Subaponeurotic hemorrhage can produce a substantial blood loss and clinical shock. Rupture of the liver or spleen is usually associated with breech delivery and is often subcapsular initially. This produces abdominal swelling. If a subcapsular hematoma ruptures death may be very rapid. Intrarenal and splenic hemorrhages are also features of breech delivery and can cause major blood loss. Adrenal hemorrhages are more likely to occur as a result of severe birth asphyxia and its secondary hemorrhagic problems. Pulmonary hemorrhage is most often secondary to right heart failure but can occur in the presence of hypothermia, severe birth asphyxia and respiratory distress syndrome.

Diagnosis and treatment of acute blood loss. Since the hemoglobin concentration and hematocrit may not fall for some time after acute blood loss, the diagnosis may be difficult to confirm immediately. However, the infant will be pale, vasoconstricted and hypotensive with a tachycardia, tachypnea and a large peripheral core temperature differential. The central venous pressure (CVP) will be low or negative. It is an undoubted neonatal emergency when the infant shows acute symptoms and the immediate treatment is to infuse 20 ml/kg of group O negative blood over 5–10 min. Uncrossmatched whole blood is always available in a maternity unit and should be used in this circumstance. The infant will also need oxygen therapy and correction of acid–base status. If the infant responds rapidly, repeat the hemoglobin concentration or PCV and reassess the infant. If the infant remains shocked a further 20–30 ml/kg transfusion should be given over 20–30 min. The aim of therapy is to achieve a normal blood pressure and CVP. When prenatal blood loss has been less acute, e.g. fetofetal transfusion, it may be more appropriate to perform a single blood volume (80–90 ml/kg) exchange transfusion with semipacked red blood cells. Where the blood loss has been more chronic, transfusion may be unnecessary but oral iron and folate supplements may be required to replenish stores and raise the hemoglobin level.

ANEMIA OF PRETERM INFANTS

Since the major function of hemoglobin is to maintain adequate tissue oxygenation, anemia especially in the vulnerable preterm infant can prove a critical factor in the healthy survival or otherwise of such infants. The main determinants of adequate tissue oxygenation are hemoglobin concentration, oxygen affinity of red blood cells and the circulating red cell mass (RCM). The causes of low hemoglobin concentrations are discussed later; hemoglobin–oxygen affinity is largely a factor of the hemoglobin

F concentration of neonatal red cells. Hemoglobin F has high oxygen affinity designed for the low oxygen tensions of in utero life, but unfortunately it releases oxygen only poorly at the higher oxygen values encountered after birth. Thus after birth the availability of oxygen to tissues per gram of hemoglobin F is 20–30% less than per gram of hemoglobin A. Combining this with the lower red cell mass of preterm infants, the inability to bring forward the rate of hemoglobin A production after preterm birth, and the already high cardiac output of even healthy preterm infants there is little wonder that the infant has little reserves during illness. Available oxygen (AO) calculated from the hemoglobin concentration, PaO_2 and the oxygen dissociation property of the red cells (i.e. the p_{50} upon which depends the ability of the blood to release oxygen) gives a realistic assessment of the need for the transfusion. In term infants the AO is usually between 12.5 and 10.5 ml oxygen/dl for the first month of life. Many preterm infants have AO significantly below this value and this oxygen lack gives symptoms and signs of anemia in preterm infants even at rest and with hemoglobin concentrations as high as 10.5 g/dl. Brown (1988) offers an excellent review of the subject.

Hematinic and nutrient deficiencies

Iron (3 mg/kg/day) from the end of the first month of life until mixed feeding is established is necessary because of the low iron stores in preterm infants. Folic acid (15 μg daily) is also required. It should be commenced from the age of 7 days and continued until the age of 3 months, especially in very low birthweight infants. Vitamin B_{12} is largely acquired during the last trimester and the daily requirement is thought to be 3–5 μg daily. It is unusual for supplementation to be required routinely.

The role of vitamin E is still unclear despite its known antioxidant properties. Some centers give 25 mg/day in a water-soluble form (tocopherol succinate) until the age of 6 weeks to infants under 1500 g at birth at risk of oxygen toxicity. Deficiency of vitamin E produces a hemolytic anemia by shortening the red cell life span. The dietary requirement of vitamin E increases if there is an excessive intake of polyunsaturated fatty acid (PUFA) and this can occur in artificially fed infants. It is also exacerbated by the poorer intestinal absorption of fat-soluble vitamins. Vitamin E deficiency presents clinically with a low hemoglobin concentration, facial puffiness due to periorbital edema and edema of the lower limbs. There is usually an associated tachypnea and poor feeding. The hematological changes include red cell fragments (pyknocytes) and an increased sensitivity of red cells to hydrogen peroxide. The platelet count is also elevated. Large doses of iron magnify the effects of vitamin E deficiency.

Deficiency of protein will also lead to anemia in preterm infants and deficiency of the trace element copper has been linked to anemia. Ceruloplasmin is important for the absorption of iron, and copper is necessary for iron metabolism within the erythroid precursors. Clinical features of copper deficiency include hypochromic microcytic anemia, neutropenia, peripheral edema and facial swelling. Low birthweight formulae for preterm infants have had their copper/zinc ratios adjusted to improve the bioavailability of copper.

Blood losses

In addition to the causes of blood loss described previously, preterm infants are vulnerable to spontaneous intracranial bleeds (periventricular and intraventricular hemorrhage). Sampling losses can prove colossal relative to the preterm infant's blood volume. It is important to keep a careful record of blood sampling volumes and to minimize them whenever possible. Early clamping of the umbilical cord at birth may also lead to inadequate placental transfusions and hence effective blood loss for the preterm infant.

Refractory early anemia of prematurity (REAP)

This anemia of prematurity is probably due to a combination of erythropoietin deficiency and the shortened life span of the fetal red cell. Shannon et al (1987) have demonstrated that erythroid progenitor cells in the blood of infants with REAP have normal responsiveness to EPO. The production of erythropoietin in preterm infants seems to be less responsive to anoxic stimuli than that found in term infants. In utero this may well be important to prevent excessive degrees of hyperviscosity but following preterm delivery this certainly has disadvantages for the sick, preterm infant. The balance between fetal and adult erythropoiesis depends on postconceptional age and conditions such as placental insufficiency. Maternal diabetes may delay the switchover from fetal to adult cell formation. Recent work in several centers (Maier et al 1994, Shannon et al 1995) has suggested that recombinant human EPO, 600–750 u/kg per week, by the subcutaneous route may have an important role in reducing REAP if supported by adequate intakes of protein and iron.

Fetal red cells have rheological problems which compromise the microcirculation because of their large cell volumes. This is worsened by acidosis. The life span of the fetal red cell post-delivery is half that of adult cells. Fetal RBCs have reduced enzyme complement and membrane properties for survival in the circulation. Figure 5.50 presents a suggested protocol for red cell transfusion in preterm infants relevant to their clinical status and hemoglobin concentration.

Anemia due to hemolysis

The commonest presentation of hemolysis in the newborn infant is jaundice. Anemia may not be a major finding nor may

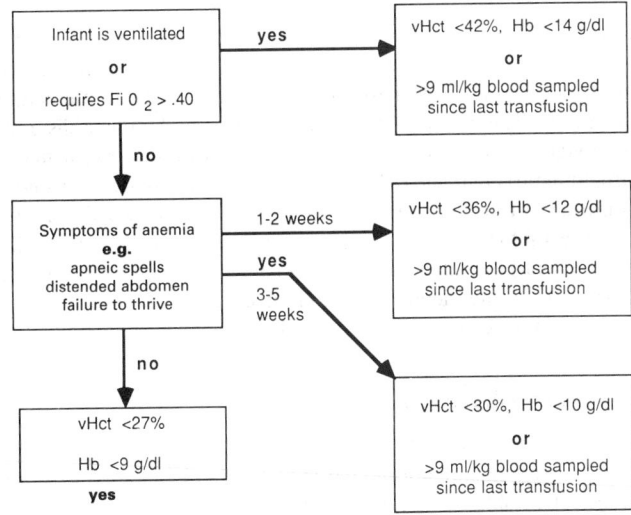

Fig. 5.50 Criteria for red cell transfusion: FiO_2 = inspired oxygen; vHct = venous hematocrit.

reticulocytosis be present. The commonest cause of hemolysis is blood group incompatibility (p. 231). It should not be forgotten that infection, acidosis, oxidizing agents (e.g. naphthalene) and disseminated intravascular coagulation can all cause rapid hemolysis in the newborn. Rarely transplacental autoimmune hemolytic anemia in the mother or maternal disseminated lupus erythematosis may be the cause of neonatal hemolytic anemia. Red cell enzyme abnormalities, red cell membrane disorders and disorders of hemoglobin synthesis are the main congenital causes responsible for abnormalities in the newborn period.

RED CELL ENZYME ABNORMALITIES

While there are several varieties of this disorder only two cause significant clinical problems.

Glucose-6-phosphate dehydrogenase (G6PD) deficiency

G6PD deficiency has a worldwide distribution but is particularly prevalent in the Middle East, China and West Africa. The gene for G6PD is located on the X chromosome so that clinical problem occurs much more frequently in males than in females. G6PD is the first enzyme in the hexose monophosphate shunt and is important in generating NADHP for red cell protection against oxidative damage. There are many varieties of the disorder which usually produce only a mild chronic hemolysis. Acute hemolysis is usually triggered by infection or drug administration and it is important when the condition is recognized that the parents and their family practitioners are given information on drugs which might be of relevance to this condition (Table 5.91).

Pyruvate kinase (PK) deficiency

PK deficiency is an autosomal recessive disorder which is rare but it may be important because of neonatal jaundice or chronic low grade anemia. The enzyme is at the lower end of the Embden–Myerhof pathway and normally prevents hemolysis.

RED CELL MEMBRANE DISORDERS

Hereditary spherocytosis

Instead of the normal biconcave disc, the red cell shape becomes biconvex and the resultant larger cell is unable to traverse the microcirculation (especially of the spleen) without premature disruption. The cause of this usually autosomal dominant disorder is thought to be a defect in the production of spectrin, a major structural protein in the red cell membrane. The diagnosis is usually confirmed from the family history and the increased osmotic fragility of the red cells, although the in vitro tests are usually delayed until the infant is several months old. There is no specific treatment in the neonatal period other than the treatment of jaundice and the provision of folic acid supplements (0.5 mg daily).

Hereditary elliptocytosis

This condition is usually dominantly inherited and seldom causes clinical problems. In normal individuals up to 15% of red cells are elliptical in shape but this percentage rises to 25% or more in affected infants. This is due to abnormal structural membrane proteins. Treatment of the resultant jaundice is the only necessary treatment.

Table 5.91 Some agents reported to produce hemolysis in patients with G6PD deficiency

Antimalarials	Others
Primaquine	Dimercaprol (BAL)
Pamaquine	Methylene blue
Pentaquine	Naphthalene
Plasmoquine	Phenylhydrazine
Quinocide	Acetylphenhydrazine
Quinacrine (Atabrine)	Probenecid
Quinine*	Vitamin K (large doses of water-
	soluble analogues)
	Chloramphenicol*
Sulfonamides	Quinidine*
Sulfanilamide	Fava beans*
N^2-acetylsulfanilamide	Chloroquine
Sulfacetamide (Sulamyd)	Nalidixic acid (Negram)
Sulfamethoxypyridazine	Orinase
(Kynex, Midicel)	
Salicylazosulfapyridine	Infections
(Azulfidine)	Respiratory viruses
Sulfafurazole (Gantrisin)	Infectious hepatitis
Sulfapyridine	Infectious mononucleosis
	Bacterial pneumonias
Nitrofurans	
Nitrofurantoin (Furadantin)	Diabetic acidosis
Furazolidone (Furoxone)	
Furaltadone (Altafur)	
Nitrofurazone (Furacin)	
Antipyretics and analgesics	
Acetylsalicylic acid (in large doses)	
Acetanilide	
Acetophenetidin (Phenacetin)	
Antipyrine*	
Aminopyrine*	
p-aminosalicylic acid	

* To date, only in white races.

Sickle cell anemia

This condition only rarely presents before 3 months of age when the proportion of HbF falls below 35%.

Hemoglobin synthesis disorders

Apart from the rare homozygous state of α-o thalassemia (hemoglobin Barts) which usually produces hydrops or death within the first hour of life, neither α- or β- thalassemia produces neonatal problems. The importance lies in the possibility of prenatal diagnosis and in the early recognition and appropriate treatment in later infancy.

POLYCYTHEMIA IN THE NEWBORN INFANT

This is still a somewhat controversial condition and no clear definition of what constitutes polycythemia has yet evolved. It does appear, however, that a central venous hematocrit of greater than 0.65 is accompanied by a greater than proportional increase in blood viscosity. However, if peripheral venous blood is used, a hematocrit of 0.7 is probably more representative of the condition. Infants who have experienced intrauterine hypoxia such as that due to maternal diabetes, pre-eclampsia, maternal heart disease and maternal smoking, as well as postmature and growth-retarded infants, may all show polycythemia. The increased production of erythropoietin found in Down syndrome infants has led to the association of polycythemia with this condition and it is also seen in the other trisomies. The other main group of infants who experience polycythemia are those in whom there has been either intrauterine transfusion (either maternofetal or twin to twin) or very delayed cord clamping. The hyperviscosity of polycythemia leads to sludging and microthrombi in the peripheral circulation. There is in addition reduced deformability of red cells and resultant tissue hypoxia. Features such as renal vein thrombosis, necrotizing enterocolitis and seizures have been described and the affected infant is usually lethargic and hypotonic but irritable when aroused. Feeding is usually poor and hyperbilirubinemia may become a management problem. Because of local aggregation of platelets in the peripheral circulation there may be thrombocytopenia. It is still unclear whether treatment of asymptomatic infants is required but studies (Black & Lubchenco 1982) have suggested that any complications may be minor. Symptomatic infants require urgent treatment with partial exchange transfusion to remove whole blood and replace it with an equal volume of fresh frozen plasma to achieve a hematocrit of 50–55% as below.

$$\text{Plasma volume required} = \text{estimated blood volume} \times \frac{\text{observed Hct} - \text{desired Hct}}{\text{observed Hct}}$$

COAGULATION DISORDERS IN NEWBORN

With the exception of the inherited disorders the frequency of coagulation problems increases with decreasing gestational age. Term infants seldom have bleeding disorders apart from the congenital variety unless there is associated hypoxia or sepsis which leads to disseminated intravascular coagulation (DIC). Hemorrhagic disease of the newborn (see below) is preventable. The various complications of prematurity lead to significant increased risks of coagulation disorders.

Any approach to the investigation and management of coagulation problems in the newborn must be based on knowledge of the physiological processes involved and the related gestational variations. There must also be an appreciation of the normal values obtained in each investigating laboratory. Sampling methods present an important variable in infants and a major challenge to interpretation of the resultant investigations. Most laboratories still require a 'clean' venepuncture sample, although capillary methods are available. Laboratory cooperation is necessary so that appropriate anticoagulants and inhibitors can be provided for samples and full use can be made of the limited sample size. Heparin must be avoided because of its adverse effect on coagulation testing. Table 5.92 gives appropriate blood volumes required to produce standard anticoagulant/blood ratios with 0.1 ml citrate anticoagulant.

An essential element in the investigation of any infant with coagulation disorder is a full family history.

Physiology of hemostasis

The aim of the normal hemostatic process is to produce a stable, established repair at the site of blood vessel injury. The coagulation process and its counterpart (fibrinolysis) should therefore remain in balance in health. There are three main components of hemostasis: platelets, vascular factors and the coagulation system.

Platelets

Platelets contain granules which have a variety of functions ultimately directed towards platelet adherence. The plasma component, the Von Willebrand factor, and platelet membrane released factors, lead to binding of platelets to vessel collagen. Adenosine diphosphate (ADP) derived from the granules, serotonin and thrombin generated by release of tissue thromboplastin stimulate platelet aggregation. Subsequently there is conversion of platelet membrane arachidonic acid by cyclooxygenase to the endoperoxides PGG_2 and PGH_2 and ultimately to thromboxane A_2 which produces further platelet aggregation. Release of platelet factor 3 (PF3) and platelet factor 4 (PF4) activates the coagulation factor cascade.

Vascular

In normal circumstances prostacyclin (PGI_2) synthesized in the vessel wall acts as a powerful inhibitor of platelet aggregation and thrombus formation. Damage and exposure of the vascular lining reduces PGI_2 availability and also exposes collagen and myofibrils which encourage platelet aggregation. Tissue factor III (tissue thromboplastin) and factor VIII released from vessel walls along with high molecular weight kininogen and prekallikrein all act to stimulate coagulation (Mann 1984).

Coagulation system

All clotting factors (procoagulants) are high molecular weight proteins which as zymogens (inactive forms) do not cross the placenta. Most are liver produced. Inherited deficiencies of all except factors VIII and IX, which are sex linked, follow the autosomal recessive pattern.

Following activation, these zymogens behave as serine proteases with narrow substrate specificity and depend on a cascade process in which the intrinsic and extrinsic pathways combine and overlap to produce activated factor X which activates thrombin. This in turn converts fibrinogen to fibrin monomer which is incorporated in the platelet clot under the influence of factor XIII (Fig. 5.51).

Procoagulant inhibitors

Protein C, a vitamin K-dependent inhibitor and its cofactor protein S (produced in the liver and endothelium respectively) on activation by thrombin rapidly inactivates factors Va and VIIIa in the presence of thrombomodulin. Deficiency of proteins C and S leads to excessive intravascular thrombosis. Antithrombin III is the main inhibitor of coagulation and its action is accelerated by heparin. It also acts on factors IXa, XIa and XIIa. At birth it is thought to have concentrations of 50% of adult values. α_1-antitrypsin and α_2-macroglobulin also have inhibitor effects.

Table 5.92 Blood volumes required to produce standard anticoagulant/blood ratios with 0.1 ml citrate anticoagulant

Hct	0.30	0.35	0.40	0.45	0.50	0.55	0.60	0.65	0.70	0.75
Specimen vol. (ml)	0.8	0.85	0.9	1.0	1.1	1.2	1.3	1.5	1.8	2.15

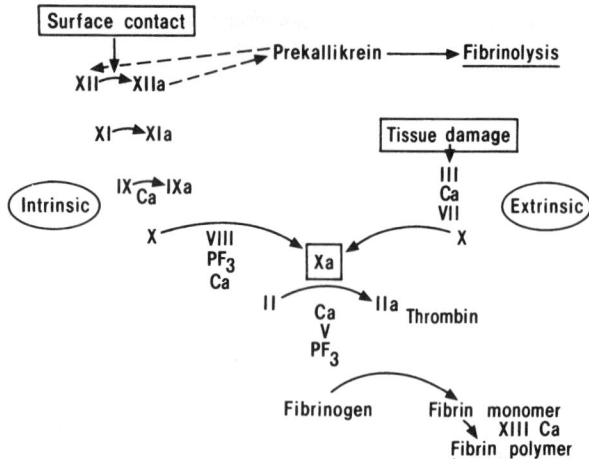

Fig. 5.51 Schematic representation of the coagulation cascade. (From Roberton 1986.)

Fibrinolysis

With the inhibitors, fibrinolytic compounds help maintain the normal balance between the hypercoagulable and bleeding states. Plasmin, the end product of plasminogen activation, is responsible for fibrin lysis. The result of this fibrin degradation is the production of products (FDPs) which can be identified in the serum as D dimers and other split products. Plasmin itself is usually inhibited by α_2-antiplasmin, α_2-macroglobulin and α_2-antitrypsin. Exogenous compounds such as streptokinase and labile endogenous activators (prekallikrein and urokinase) also have powerful fibrinolytic properties. It is imperative that fibrinolysis be inhibited in any sample collected for assay. Epsilonaminocaproic acid (EACA) and aprotinin (Trasylol) are antiplasmins used in this role.

Screening test of hemostasis

A full blood count including a film for fragments and platelet number is an essential element in any hemostatic investigation. The bleeding time (BT) by standardized methods reflects platelet number and function and whilst normally between 2 and 6 min in older children it is frequently around 90 s in normal newborn infants. It is not often used for diagnostic purposes. The prothrombin time (PT) measures factors I, II, V, VII and X (extrinsic pathway) whilst variations of the partial thromboplastin time (PTT) activated by cephalin or kaolin measure the intrinsic path (factors I, II, V, VIII, IX, XI, XII). Heparin severely prolongs this assay. Thrombotest gives a rapid assay of factors II, VII, IX and X. The thrombin time (TT) and fibrinogen concentrations evaluate fibrinogen function and concentration and are sensitive to the effects of heparin and FDPs, respectively. The reptilase time (RT) also reflects fibrinogen status but is not heparin sensitive. FDPs such as D dimers can also be assayed. It is not usually necessary to assay individual procoagulants but a well-documented history and family history may indicate a specific need to do so.

Normal hemostatic values

Table 5.93 reflects commonly used laboratory values for the standard screening tests. There is of necessity a variability due to

Table 5.93 Commonly used hemostatic screening tests with normal values in first 72 h

Screening test	Preterm (30–36 weeks)	Term	Adult
Prothrombin (PT, s) (I, II, V, VII, X)	13–23	13–17	13–16
Thrombotest (TT)%	15–50	15–60	80–100
Partial thromboplastin time (PTT, s)	35–100	35–70	35–45
Thrombin time (s)	12–24	12–18	10–14
Reptilase time (s)	18–30	18–24	18–22
Platelet count ($\times 10^9$/l)	100–350	150–400	150–400
Fibrinogen concentration (g/l)	1.2–3.8	1.5–3.5	1.5–3.5

Table 5.94 Commonly tested hemostatic factors with 'normal' values (venous) used in the first 72 h

Factor		Preterm (30–36 weeks)	Term
II	(% of normal adult values)	30–65	40–65
V	(% of normal adult values)	50–100	50–100
VII	(% of normal adult values)	20–50	40–70
VIII	(% of normal adult values)	60–120	70–150
IX	(% of normal adult values)	10–30	15–55
X	(% of normal adult values)	10–45	20–55
XI	(% of normal adult values)	10–50	15–70
XII	(% of normal adult values)	20–50	25–70
XIII	(% of normal adult values)	50–100	50–100

laboratory methods and each laboratory should attempt to establish its own standards. Table 5.94 indicates the usually accepted variations caused by gestation in the individual factor levels.

Thrombocytopenia

Thrombocytopenia occurs when the platelet count is less than 100 $\times 10^9$/l. 15–20% of preterm infants and 1% of term infants have thrombocytopenia. The nadir is usually around day 2 and resolves by day 8 in most. Spontaneous bleeding seldom occurs if the count is above 40×10^9/l. The clinical features include purpura, bleeding from injection sites and occasionally from the gastrointestinal tract or into the central nervous system. Thrombocytopenia usually results from either excessive platelet consumption or abnormally low production, whilst on occasions a combination of both may be found. Occasionally, thrombocytopenia may be due to platelet loss during exchange transfusion or hemorrhage.

Alloimmune (isoimmune) neonatal thrombocytopenic purpura (INP)

This condition results from the transplacental passage of maternal specific IgG platelet antibody in a mother who has a normal platelet count. The platelet antigen-negative mother is sensitized by transplacental passage of fetal platelets which carry one of the common platelet antigens, usually PLA1 (85% of cases) (Deaver et al 1986). 98% of the population are PLA1 antigen positive and the remainder PLA2 or other antigen positive. Maternal serological testing will confirm the presence of the isoantibody. The diagnosis is usually made on observing that washed maternal platelets lead to a rapid rise in the thrombocytopenic infant's platelet count, whereas random washed platelet transfusions (since they are likely also to be PLA1 positive) produce only a very short-lived increase in the platelet count. Most infants demonstrate a mild degree of thrombocytopenia although up to a third in some series (Deaver et al 1986) have been suspected of having intracranial hemorrhage. Treatment is usually reserved for those infants with either evidence of clinical bleeding or a platelet count below $20 \times 10^9/l$. Washed maternal platelets or platelets from known specific platelet antigen-negative donors are indicated. Derycke et al (1985) have used intravenous IgG for affected infants with some success and we now use it. As in other forms of thrombocytopenia, the use of steroids (2 mg/kg/day) is controversial although their ability to reduce capillary fragility may be of value. Intramuscular drugs should be avoided. It is important to investigate the antigen status of other family members especially women of child-bearing age when the condition is suspected or confirmed, as elective Cesarean section may be a safer mode of delivery in the presence of isoantibodies. Family members also provide a worthwhile source of platelet antigen-negative donors. There is still controversy over maternal management in pregnancy but where a previous infant has been severely affected some centers now perform antenatal cordocentesis from 20 to 34 weeks of pregnancy to identify fetal thrombocytopenia, transfuse the fetus with washed irradiated compatible platelets regularly and treat the mother with weekly intravenous IgG (Bussel et al 1988, Kroll et al 1994).

Autoimmune neonatal thrombocytopenia (ANT)

Passive transfer of maternal lymphocyte-produced IgG antiplatelet antibodies (PAIgG) causes this form of thrombocytopenia. There is a significant risk of thrombocytopenia in the infants of mothers with idiopathic thrombocytopenic purpura (ITP) but less so with systemic, i.e. lupus erythematosus (SLE). Although the perinatal mortality is low (less than 2%) morbidity is more significant. Up to 4% of infants will be severely thrombocytopenic at birth and almost 50% of those with platelet counts close to $100 \times 10^9/l$ at birth will show a further drop in the platelet count during the first week of life. Mothers who have had splenectomy for ITP may still produce antibodies and the infants may be affected. It is possible to attempt to identify fetal thrombocytopenia by direct measurement of platelets from fetal scalp samples during labor and the risk of intrapartum damage due to intracranial bleeding may be reduced if fetuses with platelet counts less than $50 \times 10^9/l$ are delivered by Cesarean section. Cordocentesis for fetal sampling is probably not justified in ITP. There is no evidence that antenatal use of maternal steroids has a role to play in the management. Prenatal maternal high dose IgG immunoglobulin has also been used (Sidiropoulos 1986) and may reduce the risks of fetal thrombocytopenia. It is a routine form of therapy at present in some centers when maternal platelet count falls below $50 \times 10^9/l$. When there is either clinical bleeding or the platelet count is below $10 \times 10^9/l$ in the infant, most still use steroids to reduce capillary fragility and random platelet transfusions although their effect is of very short duration. Exchange transfusion may help to remove unbound PAIgG and intravenous IgG also improves platelet life span and is usually used.

Infection

Thrombocytopenia is a frequent early marker of neonatal infection and is usually caused by either megakaryocyte or platelet damage due to endotoxin or disseminated intravascular coagulation (DIC). Both congenital and acquired infections are important causes of thrombocytopenia although congenital virus infection usually results in thrombocytopenia at birth. Gram-negative septicemia is a particularly important cause of rapid onset thrombocytopenia in preterm infants.

Drugs

Tolbutamide is probably the only drug with a substantial literature to support the association between its maternal use and neonatal thrombocytopenia. Platelet function, however, is clearly disturbed by salicylates, thiazide diuretics and intravenous fat solutions.

Bone marrow defects

Any condition which leads to bone marrow replacement may ultimately produce neonatal thrombocytopenia. Letterer–Siwe disease, neuroblastoma and neonatal leukemia all produce thrombocytopenia. The congenital syndromes of Fanconi's pancytopenia, pure congenital amegakaryocyte thrombocytopenia, Wiskott–Aldrich syndrome and the association of absent radii with thrombocytopenia complex (TAR) are all rare causes.

Platelet function disorders

These disorders seldom cause significant symptoms in the newborn period. The commonest hereditary disorders are Glanzmann's disease, an autosomal recessive disorder where there is probable deficiency of the platelet membrane components and ADP storage pool disease, both of which cause mild clinical features (due to defective formation of the platelet granules which store ADP). Bernard–Soulier syndrome, another autosomal recessive disorder, produces a moderate bleeding disorder in the presence of giant platelets and decreased platelet adhesiveness. The condition is probably due to lack of receptor sites for factor VIII-related antigen on the platelets. As previously noted, drugs are the commonest cause of platelet function disorders. Aspirin and indomethacin probably produce their effects by inhibiting cyclooxygenase which ultimately reduces thromboxane A_2 production.

Coagulation factor deficiencies

In infants who otherwise appear healthy, vitamin K_1 deficiency or an inherited specific coagulation factor disorder are the likeliest cause, whereas in preterm and ill infants most coagulation deficiencies are secondary in origin, associated with either hypoxia, infection, necrotizing enterocolitis, liver damage or rhesus isoimmunization.

Hemorrhagic disease of the newborn (HDN)

It is now over a century since Townsend described gastrointestinal bleeding in a group of breast-fed infants during their first week of life (Townsend 1894). He also noted that survivors appeared to have normal hemostasis thereafter. These observations were later linked with hypoprothrombinemia and prolongation of the prothrombin time. Townsend also recognized that infants who received cow's milk formula did not develop HDN. Once the link with vitamin K_1 was established the main controversy has been whether or not this fat-soluble vitamin should be given routinely to all infants. As well as having low hepatic levels of vitamin K_1, plasma vitamin K levels in infants at term are almost undetectable. The maternal : cord plasma vitamin K ratio is 30 : 1. To achieve adequate neonatal vitamin K_1 levels at birth it is necessary for mothers to be given prolonged vitamin K prophylaxis (20 mg daily for 2 weeks for mothers on anticonvulsants). The type of feed is probably the most important determinant of the development of HDN. Breast milk contains only a twelfth of the vitamin K_1 of most artificial feeds (2 μg compared with 30 μg). In addition, the bacterial flora of breast-fed infants may delay full maturation of vitamin K_1 levels. Other factors which may contribute to a lower vitamin K_1 level in infants include abnormal fat absorption and hepatic function. Substances which might interfere with vitamin K function such as some cephalosporins, high levels of vitamin E and maternal anticonvulsant therapy should be avoided.

Early hemorrhagic disease of the newborn. This variety of HDN presents within the first 48 hours of life. It is usually associated with maternal anticonvulsant therapy.

Classical hemorrhagic disease of the newborn. This variety of HDN is almost always associated with breast-feeding; it occurs between the third and seventh days of life and has an incidence of 1–1.6 per thousand infants in the UK. There is usually gastrointestinal hemorrhage, which needs to be distinguished by the Apt test from swallowed maternal blood (breast origin), or less frequently but catastrophically bleeding into the central nervous system. There may also be epistaxis, unexplained bruising, or oozing from the umbilicus or the Guthrie test site. The diagnosis is confirmed by finding a prolonged prothrombin time and/or a reduced thrombotest. Immediate treatment with parenteral vitamin K_1 (1 mg) is necessary and in some circumstances blood transfusion or fresh frozen plasma (FFP) may be necessary.

Late-onset HDN. In this variety of vitamin K_1 deficiency, which occurs between the age of 8 days and 6 months, bleeding is often into the central nervous system. The most frequent association has been with breast-feeding although many infants have had associated gastrointestinal or hepatic disorders or have been administered broad spectrum antibiotics. Treatment is also with vitamin K_1 intravenously, fresh frozen plasma or blood transfusion. Neurological handicap is likely among those infants who have suffered substantial intracranial hemorrhage.

Vitamin K prophylaxis

A substantial body of opinion now considers that vitamin K prophylaxis is warranted for all infants. How the vitamin K should be given is still unresolved. There is no doubt that intramuscular vitamin K_1 (1 mg) provides satisfactory prophylaxis and 1 mg orally at birth or with the first feed provides adequate protection against early and classical hemorrhagic disease. The peak levels reached by a single dose orally do not have sufficient effect on stores to prevent the late-onset disorder in breast-fed infants. Some centers give several doses of vitamin K_1 orally during the first 6 weeks of life but compliance is a problem. A new formulation of vitamin K_1 (mixed micellar) may improve absorption and plasma levels thus increasing the interval between doses and still give adequate protection. Intramuscular vitamin K_1 prevents late hemorrhagic disease and the author's practice is to give vitamin K_1 0.5 mg intramuscularly to term infants at birth (0.25 mg <34 weeks) with parental consent.

Vitamin K and cancer controversy

Golding and her coworkers in 1990 and 1992 reported an association with childhood cancers and the neonatal administration of intramuscular but not oral vitamin K_1 (odds ratio 2 : 1). This observation has not been borne out by subsequent studies of much larger populations in the USA and Scandinavia (Klebanoff 1993, Ekeland 1993). Currently most authorities recommend continuing with the intramuscular route until a satisfactory oral preparation has been evaluated.

Maternal anticonvulsant therapy

There is an increased risk of HDN in infants whose mothers have taken phenytoin or phenobarbitone during pregnancy. It is preventable by maternal supplementation (20 mg daily for 2 weeks prior to delivery) or by routine administration of vitamin K_1 at birth.

Maternal anticoagulant therapy

Oral anticoagulants in late pregnancy can increase the risk of fetal bleeding during labor and should be avoided. There is little risk of similar problems with the use of maternal heparin. Fetal anomaly is associated with warfarin use in the first trimester. Prophylactic vitamin K_1 should be given at birth to all infants of mothers who have had anticoagulant therapy in pregnancy. It is not advisable to use coumarin anticoagulants in lactating mothers but both warfarin and heparin are safe.

Parenteral nutrition

Infants of very low birthweight who require prolonged parenteral nutrition require regular vitamin K_1 supplementation as do infants with significant malabsorption disorders or chronic hepatic disease who are at the risk of late hemorrhagic disease.

Inherited procoagulant deficiencies

Afibrinogenemia and hypofibrinogenemia occur rarely but may present as cord hemorrhage, hematoma or bleeding after neonatal surgery. There is often a family history. Defective biological activity of fibrinogen (dysfibrinogenemia) can also occur. Treatment involves the use of cryoprecipitate or fresh frozen plasma (FFP). Other equally rare procoagulant factor deficiencies include hypoprothrombinemia and factor X deficiency, both of which respond to FFP replacement.

The commonest procoagulant deficiencies are hemophilia A and Christmas disease. Either may present with bleeding from the cord, injection sites or occasionally from a scalp electrode site. Factor assay will define the disorder and factor VIII or IX replacement is indicated. Cryoprecipitate also provides factor VIII whilst factor IX is available in FFP.

Von Willebrand's disease (factor VIII-related antigen) produces platelet function disorders and bleeding from mucous membranes. This condition responds well to factor VIII replacement.

Factor XIII deficiency usually presents with cord oozing or intracranial hemorrhage (Kitchens & Newcombe 1979). Treatment is with FFP.

Disseminated intravascular coagulation (DIC) (secondary hemorrhagic disease, consumption coagulopathy)

Most disorders of the coagulation system in newborn infants are secondary to varying degrees of disseminated intravascular coagulation (DIC). DIC is a 'process characterized by widespread activation of the coagulation system with formation of soluble or insoluble fibrin and in which clotting factors and platelets are commonly consumed with secondary activation of fibrinolysis'. The result is widespread intravascular thrombosis with associated disturbance of organ function. The level of ATIII in newborn infants increases the risk of intravascular thrombosis and poor hepatic function delays the rate of factor replacement. Sepsis is the most common cause of DIC in infants and is frequently seen in the low birthweight infant. Hypoxia is another effective trigger and there is a close association with conditions such as necrotizing enterocolitis and intracranial hemorrhage. Any condition leading to hypoxia and/or acidosis may also act as a trigger to DIC and there is a close association with respiratory distress syndrome. Rivers et al (1975) demonstrated that neonatal monocytes release tissue factor on exposure to Gram-negative endotoxin. Similar mechanisms occur with the IgG anti-D erythrocyte immune complexes of rhesus isoimmunization.

Occasionally, chronic DIC can occur in untreated polycythemia or low grade sepsis.

Localized DIC can occur where there is consumption of platelets and coagulation factors within large cavernous hemangiomas (Kasabach–Merritt syndrome) and this in turn may lead to generalized DIC. The diagnosis is usually made in an at-risk infant when bleeding occurs from injection sites or from the gastrointestinal tract.

Investigation reveals thrombocytopenia of varying severity associated with prolongation of screening tests (APTT) and low plasma fibrinogen concentration (less than 1 g/l). D dimers are elevated as are other FDPs. The hemoglobin concentration usually falls and red cell fragments are observed on a peripheral blood film. It is clear that the main bulwarks of management are adequate treatment of the precipitating factor, e.g. infection, hypoxia, hypotension and acidosis. Replacement component therapy is indicated when there is bleeding or extensively prolonged screening test abnormalities. Von Kreis et al (1985) have demonstrated that the intravenous use of ATIII may be of value whilst platelet transfusions and FFP may be adequate to control bleeding tendencies. Exchange transfusion has been used in some circumstances, particularly where there has been poor response to other methods, but the use of heparin has not been shown to offer any substantial advantage.

Major vessel thrombosis

These conditions usually occur in the presence of indwelling umbilical venous or arterial catheters or when there is polycythemia. Treatment involves the removal of the provoking cannula and the use of heparinization (15–25 units/kg/h as continuous infusion following priming with heparin 100 units/kg). Renal vein thrombosis also occurs, often in association with polycythemia or hypoxia, and requires heparinization. Laboratory control of heparinization is usually established by monitoring the PTT and maintaining it at approximately twice the normal level. The use of thrombolytic agents in the newborn remains controversial but both streptokinase and urokinase have been employed. Congenital ATIII and proteins C and S deficiency can also produce major blood vessel thrombosis and when diagnosed require specific replacement treatment.

BLOOD GROUP INCOMPATIBILITIES

Pathogenesis

Blood group incompatibility between fetus and mother occurs where the fetus possesses an antigen on the red blood cells derived from the father which is not present on the maternal red cells. Transplacental passage of fetal red cells can be recognized by examining the maternal blood by the Kleihauer acid elution technique and is found to occur more frequently and in greater volumes about the time of delivery. The 'Kleihauer test' involves the immersion of a blood smear from the mother in a citrate phosphate buffer of acid pH. Under these conditions, HbA is eluted from the maternal red cells but cells containing HbF are not affected. After staining, the cells containing HbF take up the stain but cells which had contained HbA appear as ghosts. The relative proportions of cells containing HbF and HbA can, therefore, be determined. In the normal adult, the film will show a vast majority of ghost cells with only a rare, faintly stained cell. Obstetric complications such as toxemia of pregnancy, Cesarean section and breech delivery increase the risk of fetomaternal transfusion. The foreign antigen on the transfused cells may stimulate antibody formation by the mother. Should such antibodies pass back into the fetus, either during that current pregnancy or during a later pregnancy, they may become attached to the fetal red cells which are then removed from the circulation and destroyed by cells of the reticuloendothelial system. As a result the fetus becomes anemic and were it not for the clearing action of the placenta, would also become jaundiced. In the most severely affected, the anemia may be sufficiently severe to cause cardiac failure or death. An affected liveborn infant suffers hemolytic disease of the newborn. As the anemia stimulates additional hemopoiesis, the condition is also called erythroblastosis fetalis.

Incidence

The proportions of the different blood groups vary in different racial groups and hemolytic disease of the newborn in any population will depend upon its ethnic composition. In populations of European origin, ABO accounts for the majority of hemolytic disease of the newborn. About 9% of fetuses are Rh (D)-positive with a Rh (D)-negative mother. Before preventive measures were instituted the incidence of rhesus hemolytic disease in those of European origin was 6–7 per 1000 live births (this is about 1 in 12 of those where Rh (D) incompatibility is present – this difference being due to the 'protection' of a coincident ABO incompatibility which causes fetal cells entering the maternal circulation to be destroyed before sensitization to the Rh (D) antigen takes place). Rhesus hemolytic disease now affects about 2.5 per 1000 live births as against an expected figure of 1.5 per 1000 were all susceptible mothers treated with anti-D Ig. The minor blood groups are now responsible for about 10% of cases of hemolytic disease of the newborn. Overall about 1 in 500 Rh-positive mothers develop red cell antibodies, mostly anti-E and anti-C or non-Rh antibodies such as anti-Kell. These may have resulted from earlier blood transfusions.

Rhesus incompatibility

Rh genotypes, phenotypes and zygosity

There are six antigens in the Rh system: C, D, E, c, d, and e. Specific sera are available to detect five of these antigens but the existence of d is hypothetical. Any gene complex containing D is classified as Rh positive. In any individual, the genes are carried as a pair of gene complexes and the frequency of such pairs in a white population is shown in Table 5.95.

Hemolytic disease of the newborn is most commonly associated with a Rh-negative (cde) mother with a Rh-positive (D) infant and further discussion will use this situation as a model. Rarely, other factors represented in the Fisher nomenclature, such as C, E, c, e, act antigenically. Where the father of the child is heterozygous Rh (D) positive, there is a one in two chance that his infant will be Rh (D) positive, whereas if the father is homozygous Rh (D) positive, all his children will be Rh (D) positive. It is not possible to tell with certainty whether an individual is homozygous or heterozygous for the D antigen unless a previous baby is Rh negative, showing that both parents possess a gene complex containing 'd'.

Factors in sensitization

ABO incompatibility between mother and fetus protects against Rh immunization as naturally occurring anti-A and anti-B antibodies in the A, B or AB mother destroy incompatible fetal red cells immediately on entering to the maternal circulation.

The volume of fetal blood required to produce sensitization of the mother after a fetomaternal transfusion has been estimated to be 0.25 ml or more. Complications of pregnancy or operative manipulations at delivery will all lead to greater fetomaternal transfusions. Destruction of such red blood cells before they can produce immunity in the mother is the basis for the prophylactic treatment of Rh incompatibility using anti-D immunoglobulin. Management depends on the detection of antibodies in the mother by the indirect Coombs' test and, if present, assessment of the likely severity of the hemolytic disease in the fetus by maternal antibody quantitation and studies of the bilirubin content of amniotic fluid.

Clinical types and features

Anti-Rh (D) antibody derived from the mother will result in hemolysis of fetal Rh (D)-positive cells. The degree of hemolysis will vary with the degree of antibody passage from mother to fetus. Destruction of fetal red cells probably takes place mainly in the spleen. The fetus responds by increasing its output of red cells (erythroblastosis) but if the fetus cannot compensate for the hemolysis, anemia will result. The resultant hemolytic anemia may be slight, when there will be no interference with the progress of pregnancy with normal growth of the infant and a relatively normal appearance at birth. In more severe cases hemolysis outstrips hemopoiesis and the fetus becomes progressively more anemic in utero. With severe degrees of anemia there is heart failure and this, in combination with hypoproteinemia, may lead such infants to be delivered in a grossly edematous, anemic state – hydrops fetalis. Between the mild and the hydropic cases many infants will be born anemic to become later severely jaundiced – these suffer from icterus gravis neonatorum.

Rhesus hemolytic anemia. In Rh (D) incompatibility the danger of early death from anemia is confined to those infants whose cord hemoglobins are below 7 g/dl. These may die from heart failure before jaundice has had time to develop. If the hemolytic anemia is clinically evident at birth it should be treated by exchange transfusions (see below) but even after such treatment anemia may develop after jaundice has faded, usually maximal at the end of the third week. Treatment at any stage is by a simple top-up transfusion.

Icterus gravis neonatorum. The affected Rh (D) infant who is neither hydropic at birth nor severely anemic will develop jaundice after birth which may quickly deepen. The anemia will also worsen over the first few hours or days but it is the urgency to treat increasing jaundice before danger levels are reached which is paramount. Hyperbilirubinemia constitutes a second major risk requiring (further) exchange transfusion for its control. After the bilirubin is lowered by exchange transfusion, the level may rise again requiring subsequent further exchange transfusions. Initially, the hyperbilirubinemia is due predominantly to unconjugated bilirubin but an obstructive element may develop with the presence of bile in the urine though the stools are seldom pale. Thrombocytopenia is not uncommon in severe Rh (D) disease and may be clinically manifest as skin petechiae.

If the hyperbilirubinemia of icterus gravis neonatorum is untreated or inadequately treated, bilirubin encephalopathy with irritability, apnea, convulsions and opisthotonus may develop and if the infant dies the typical yellow staining of the basal ganglia and other cerebral nuclei may be evident (kernicterus; see p. 753).

Hydrops fetalis. The very severely affected Rh (D) fetus may develop gross subcutaneous edema, pleural effusions and ascites in utero – hydrops fetalis. The liver and spleen are usually greatly enlarged and there are frequently skin hemorrhages from thrombocytopenia on such infants. The visceromegaly and generalized edema may severely compromise lung expansion and diaphragmatic movement (see below). The hemoglobin is generally below 5 g/dl and may be below 3 g/dl. Good obstetric management should prevent the fetus reaching this stage by monitoring and intrauterine transfusion (see Ch. 4).

Diagnosis

The antenatal diagnosis of Rh (D) incompatibility and the management of the affected pregnancy are discussed in Chapter 4.

Diagnosis of hemolytic disease of the newborn at birth will depend upon foreknowledge of the likelihood of a baby being affected, the possible presence of the appropriate clinical features and examination of the cord blood for hemoglobin and for antibody using the direct Coombs' test. A positive direct Coombs' test with a lowered hemoglobin in the infant of a sensitized

Table 5.95 Distribution of Rh genotypes in a white population (bracketed figures indicate Wiener designations)

Rh positive 83% (D or Rh$_0$)	Heterozygous D.d 49%	CDe.cde (R$_1$r)	32%
		cDE.cde (R$_2$r)	11%
		Other D.d (Rh$_0$r)	6%
	Homozygous D.D. 34%	CDe.CDe (R$_1$R$_1$)	16%
		CDe.cDE (R$_1$R$_2$)	11%
		cDE.cDE (R$_2$R$_2$)	2%
		Other D.D. (Rh$_0$ Rh$_0$)	5%
Rh negative 17% (d or r)	Homozygous d.d.	cde.cde (rr)	15%
		Other d.d. (rr)	2%

mother indicates hemolytic disease of the newborn. Additional information can be gained from the reticulocyte count, high levels of which indicate active erythropoiesis and a severe hemolytic disorder even though the hemoglobin may not be greatly reduced. High nucleated red cell counts and a low platelet count are generally found in severely affected infants who may show skin and other hemorrhages at or shortly after delivery. Edema is an index of cardiac failure and sometimes of associated hypoproteinemia. With the severe anemia it demands immediate treatment. Although the cord and skin may be yellow (vernix), jaundice is not a diagnostic feature at delivery though it may develop very rapidly in severe cases.

Conditions entering into the differential diagnosis of Rh (D) incompatibility are infections such as syphilis, cytomegalic inclusion disease, rubella, septicemia and toxoplasmosis and hemolytic disease due to other causes (p. 234).

Treatment

General organization. Regional centers where antenatal management and postnatal management proceed with continuity provide the best results. The pediatrician should work in close collaboration with obstetrician, hematologist and blood transfusion service and should meet the expectant mother so that she can know who will be dealing with her infant after birth and be informed of the action which may have to be taken.

The obstetrician and pediatrician should jointly decide when the baby should be delivered. It is best to avoid delivery of the severely affected infant on a Friday afternoon with a Bank Holiday weekend ahead. The dangers of preterm delivery must be balanced against the risk of increasing severity of hemolytic disease of the newborn with prolongation of the pregnancy. In general, induction before 30 weeks' gestation is not justifiable (Ch. 4).

Management after birth. Any infant anticipated to have Rh (D) hemolytic disease should be admitted to a neonatal unit. Cord blood should be sent for urgent hemoglobin, bilirubin and Coombs' testing and the blood group of the baby should be determined. Urgent exchange transfusion may be required but in the less severely affected infant, it is important to perform regular and frequent serial estimations of serum bilirubin, plotting the values on a time-based graph. It is only with a knowledge of the rate of rise that exchange transfusion can be carried out at the appropriate time. Phototherapy should be given to all Rh (D)-sensitized infants from birth.

Exchange transfusion. After delivery, immediate exchange transfusion is urgently required for those infants who are in danger of death from anemia or cardiac failure. This will include all infants showing evidence of edema and any infant with a cord hemoglobin below 7 g/dl. Severely edematous infants with ascites and hydrothorax may have difficulty with respiration until fluid has been removed from chest and abdomen by aspiration. Such infants almost invariably need respiratory support and may need moderately high pressure ventilation because of pulmonary edema and pulmonary hypoplasia.

When it is expected that an infant may be severely affected, preparations for an immediate exchange transfusion at birth should have been made before delivery. This will involve the provision of group O Rh (D)-negative blood crossmatched against the mother which should be available at body temperature when the infant is born. Such urgency is only necessary for a small minority of very severely affected and usually hydropic infants.

In less seriously anemic infants, exchange transfusion may be required because of anemia or jaundice. Opinions differ as to the degree of anemia which should be used as an indication for exchange transfusion in the first few hours of life. Most pediatricians would carry out an early exchange (in the first few hours of life) if the cord hemoglobin were equal to or less than 10 g/dl or the cord bilirubin greater than 70 μmol/l or if there were a very strongly positive Coombs' test – all these indicating that the hemolytic process is already quite rampant. After the immediate urgency at birth the main indication for exchange transfusion is the level of serum bilirubin. In general, the policy is to prevent the serum bilirubin level exceeding 340 μmol/l but in the presence of adverse factors such as low pH, hypoxia, hypoglycemia and particularly prematurity or in the presence of a rapidly rising serum bilirubin, exchange transfusion should be carried out at lower bilirubin levels.

The technique of exchange transfusion is discussed in Chapter 33, p. 1838. The donor blood should be compatible with mother and infant, but Rh (D) negative. When the infant is severely anemic and in early failure, packed cells should be used and the blood volume should first be reduced by replacing less blood than has been removed until the venous pressure has been reduced to less than 10 cmH$_2$O. In the presence of moderate to severe heart failure, a venous catheter should be used to measure the central venous pressure regularly as the exchange proceeds. If there is hypoproteinemia, the donor exchange blood (with a normal protein content) will 'suck' edema fluid back into the vascular compartment as the exchange progresses. The circulating blood volume will therefore steadily rise and serial steps may be necessary to reduce this.

Full correction of the hemoglobin after an exchange transfusion is not always achieved and is very much dependent on the hematocrit of the donor blood being used in the second half of the exchange. If later anemia develops, this should be treated by simple transfusion.

Continuous phototherapy may reduce the degree of hyperbilirubinemia without reducing the hemolytic antibody concentration. This may reduce the number of exchange transfusions required but increase the likelihood of an anemia that will later require top-up transfusion.

Other Rh incompatibility

Although Rh disease is most usually caused by anti-D incompatibility, anti-c, anti-E or anti-C has also been described.

ABO hemolytic disease

Although 20% of mothers have incompatibility of their blood groups with their fetus, hemolytic disease due to ABO incompatibility is uncommon, mild disease affecting 1 : 150 deliveries and severe 1 : 3000 deliveries. This is because most naturally occurring anti-A or anti-B in the mother is IgM and therefore does not cross the placenta. Although there are small quantities of anti-A or anti-B IgG these are rapidly tissue-bound by the fetus and the binding sites on the fetal red cells seem poorly developed; thus sensitization is uncommon. ABO incompatibility rarely presents with an anemic infant but usually with jaundice in the first 24 h; the infants are never hydropic. ABO incompatibility may affect a first pregnancy as frequently as a subsequent one. It is not possible to predict ABO hemolytic disease antenatally, even if the blood group set-up is correct.

The diagnosis in the newborn infant is usually made on investigation of an infant for jaundice presenting in the first 24 h. The ABO incompatibility set-up must be correct (usually mother O, baby A or B); the demonstration of a weakly positive Coombs' antiglobulin test in the newborn together with large numbers of spherocytes in the newborn infant's blood film makes the diagnosis likely and the demonstration (in the mother) of anti-A or anti-B IgG hemolysins makes the diagnosis almost certain.

Although it is uncommon for ABO incompatibility to require more than phototherapy for management, exchange transfusion may occasionally be necessary and in the UK this indication for exchange transfusion is more frequent now than rhesus hemolytic disease. The blood needed for the exchange is either group O with the Rh (D) group of the baby, or better, O cells resuspended in AB plasma.

Atypical isoimmunization

Severe isoimmunization can be due to anti-Kell or anti-Fyᵃ

antibodies. Whereas the antibodies directed against c, C, e and E are usually generated during pregnancy, the anti-Kell and anti-Fyᵃ antibodies are usually a result of previous maternal transfusion. If the Coombs' test demonstrates atypical antibodies in early pregnancy, the zygosity of the father should be investigated and serial antibody levels monitored during pregnancy. The treatment of the fetus and infant are similar to that in rhesus disease.

HYDROPS FETALIS

Although originally fetal hydrops was defined as universal edema of the fetus unassociated with erythroblastosis, the term now includes erythroblastosis as a cause. Hydropic infants are then subdivided to immune hydrops associated with erythroblastosis and nonimmune hydrops. The mechanism for the hydropic state is disputed and may differ with different causes. It is likely that there are three main mechanisms: firstly severe anemia, secondly congestive heart failure with hypervolemia and thirdly hypoproteinemia. Experimentally and clinically, none of these

Table 5.96 Causes and association of hydrops fetalis

a. *Fetal conditions*	
1. *Hematological*	Isoimmune – rhesus, ABO, minor blood factors
	Nonisoimmune – homozygous α-thalassemia, chronic fetomaternal hemorrhage, chronic twin-to-twin transfusion, glucose-6-phosphate dehydrogenase deficiency
2. *Cardiovascular*	Congenital heart disease – hypoplastic left heart, aortic stenosis, pulmonary valvular incompetence, prenatal closure of ductus arteriosus, prenatal closure of foramen ovale, atrial septal defect, ventricular septal defect, endocardial cushion defect, hypoplastic aorta, subaortic stenosis, anomalous pulmonary venous drainage, transposition of the great arteries, tricuspid atresia, pulmonary atresia, tetralogy of Fallot, Ebstein's malformation, mitral insufficiency, endocardial fibroelastosis, Uhl's anomaly
	Arrhythmias – congenital heart block, atrial flutter, paroxysmal supraventricular tachycardia
	Myocarditis – Coxsackie B virus, nonspecific
	Miscellaneous – hemangiomata, arteriovenous malformations, arterial calcification, cardiac tumors, thrombosis of the vena cavae, embolism of the coronary arteries
3. *Pulmonary*	Congenital cystic adenomatoid malformation, pulmonary lymphangiectasia, pulmonary sequestration, pulmonary hypoplasia, diaphragmatic hernia
4. *Renal*	Urinary obstruction, congenital nephrosis, cystic malformations, renal dysplasia, renal hypoplasia, renal vein thrombosis
5. *Gastrointestinal*	Tracheoesophageal fistula, duodenal stenosis and atresia, jejunal atresia, intestinal volvulus, congenital meconium peritonitis, cystic meconium peritonitis
6. *Hepatic*	Congenital hepatitis, cirrhosis, intrauterine infections, vascular tumors
7. *Intrauterine infections*	Syphilis, rubella, cytomegalovirus, toxoplasmosis, leptospirosis, Chagas' disease
8. *Neoplasms*	Hemangiomata, cardiac tumors, congenital neuroblastoma, sacrococcygeal teratoma, intrapericardial teratoma
9. *Chromosomal*	Turner's syndrome (45X), Down syndrome (trisomy 21), Edwards' syndrome (trisomy 18), triploidy, minor chromosomal defects
10. *Congenital anomalies*	Achondroplasia, thanatophoric dwarfism, asphyxiating thoracic dystrophy, osteogenesis imperfecta, sacral agenesis, multiple anomalies
11. *Miscellaneous*	Tuberous sclerosis, cystic fibrosis, theca lutein cysts in the mother, Gaucher's disease, gangliosidosis G_{M1}, Hurler's syndrome, mucopolysaccharidosis VII, retroperitoneal fibrosis, intracranial hemorrhage, cystic hygroma
b. *Placental and cord conditions*	
1. *Chorioangioma*	Associated hemagiomas may be found in the fetus and disseminated intravascular coagulation may be a complication
2. *Chorionic vein thrombosis*	
3. *Umbilical vein thrombosis*	
4. *Placental insufficiency*	
c. *Maternal conditions*	
1. *Diabetes mellitus*	
2. *Toxemia*	
3. *Anemia*	
d. *Idiopathic*	About half the cases of nonimmunological hydrops

mechanisms is wholly convincing; thus the sheep fetus can be chronically bled to be extremely anemic without the hydropic state developing and in the erythroblastotic fetus there is considerable overlap between the degree of anemia and the degree of hydrops. Similarly, in the erythroblastotic hydropic fetus, hypervolemia is uncommon though experimental atrial pacing of the fetal sheep will lead to hydrops possibly by this mechanism. Hypoproteinemia is common in severe erythroblastosis but the hydropic situation is unusual in the congenital nephrotic syndrome. The many associated causes of hydrops fetalis are indicated in Table 5.96. The investigation and management of the baby with hydrops depends on the time of diagnosis. More and more commonly, infants are being identified in utero and the investigations appropriate are outlined in Table 5.97. Investigation in utero may not lead to a diagnosis and when this happens or when such a baby is not diagnosed until delivery, the postnatal investigations outlined in Table 5.98 are appropriate. The outlook for the condition depends on the diagnosis, being much better in recent years for erythroblastosis but still poor for the nonimmune hydrops where 50–95% succumb (Castillo et al 1986).

Where a clear diagnosis is not established in utero or postnatally and the fetus or infant dies, it is extremely important to have a complete pathological investigation including the placenta (Keeling et al 1983) as a definitive diagnosis can be established in a proportion of cases by autopsy and these may have a significant genetic component.

NEONATAL NEUROLOGY

NEUROLOGICAL ASSESSMENT

Introduction

Clinical examination of the neonatal nervous system is, of

Table 5.97 Investigation of fetal hydrops

Maternal
Full blood count
Blood group
Hemoglobin electrophoresis
Kleihauer stain of peripheral blood
IgG and IgM antibody titers for congenital infections, e.g. syphilis, TORCH, parvovirus
Anti-R_o antibodies
Oral glucose tolerance test
Glucose-6-phosphate dehydrogenase assay

Fetal
Cardiac assessment and full ultrasound assessment
Limb length, fetal movement

Amniocentesis
Karyotype
α-fetoprotein
Viral cultures
Establish culture for appropriate metabolic or DNA testing
Lecithin : sphingomyelin ratio

Fetal blood sampling
Karyotype
Hemoglobin analysis
Blood groups
IgM; specific cultures
Albumin and total protein
Placental biopsy for karyotype

Table 5.98 Diagnostic evaluation of newborn babies with nonimmune hydrops

Cardiovascular	Echocardiogram Electrocardiogram
Pulmonary	Chest radiograph Pleural fluid examination
Hematologic	Complete blood cell count Blood reticulocytes and Coombs' test Hemoglobin electrophoresis Glucose-6-phosphate dehydrogenase assay
Gastrointestinal	Abdominal radiograph Abdominal ultrasound Liver enzymes Peritoneal fluid examination Total protein, albumin
Renal	Urinalysis BUN, creatinine
Genetic	Chromosomal analysis Skeletal radiographs Genetic consultation
Congenital infections	Viral cultures or serology (including TORCH agents and parvovirus)
Pathology	Complete autopsy Placental examination – histology or culture

necessity, dominated by assessment of motor function. The following description is based on the work of pediatric neurologists such as Saint-Anne Dargassies (1977), Amiel-Tison & Grenier (1986), Prechtl & Bientema (1964), Prechtl (1977), Brazelton (1973) and Dubowitz & Dubowitz (1981). Gestational age and drugs can affect tone and reflex response so that an accurate maternal and neonatal history is essential. In term infants the best time to perform a neurological examination is when the infant is quiet and alert having awakened spontaneously after a feed.

State

Normal babies show different states of alertness (Table 5.99). The fetus exhibits similar states, apart from crying (Prechtl 1985).

Table 5.99 Normal neonatal states of Prechtl and Brazelton

Prechtl & Bientema (1964)		
	State 1	Eyes closed, regular respiration, no movements
	State 2	Eyes closed, irregular respiration, no movements
	State 3	Eyes open, no gross movements
	State 4	Eyes open, gross movements, no crying
	State 5	Crying
Brazelton (1973)		
	State 1	Deep sleep, regular breathing, no movements
	State 2	Light sleep, irregular respiration, rapid eye movements, eyes closed
	State 3	Drowsy, eyes open or closed, some activity – smooth
	State 4	Alert, minimal motor activity
	State 5	Eyes open, considerable motor activity
	State 6	Crying

Babies born before 36 weeks' gestation spend a great deal of time asleep and fall asleep easily when awakened. Preterm sleep states are less easily characterized than at term. Term babies spend about 50 min of each hour asleep, 50% of the time in quiet sleep. Babies who are continually in one state may be abnormal. One example is a baby who is 'hyperalert' due to withdrawal symptoms after maternal drug abuse, who spends little time asleep and more time crying than is usual. Inability to rouse a baby from sleep is pathological and a baby who is persistently in state 1 is in a coma.

Crying and consolability

During an examination most infants will cry but are consolable. Soundless or hoarse crying results from damage to the larynx from intubation or a congenitally abnormal larynx. High pitched crying is more than just a subjective phenomenon: spectral analysis of the sound frequencies contained in cries reveals patterns which can predict outcome (Lester 1987). Asymmetrical crying facies is often due to facial palsy.

Posture, spontaneous movement and tone

Normal muscle offers a resistance to stretch felt by the examiner as tone. Tone increases with gestational age and is very high in term babies. Their limbs lie flexed and adducted, unlike preterm infants who adopt an extended posture (Fig. 5.52). Asymmetrical tone does not always indicate asymmetrical pathology in the newborn period. A pattern of mixed change in tone with hypertonia in the limbs and hypotonia in the trunk is abnormal. Tone can alter considerably in relation to feeds and sleep state, and repeated examinations are required to confirm physical signs. Passive tone matures from below upwards, and this forms the basis of several methods of assessing gestational age. This type of assessment is not suitable for ill babies.

A term newborn makes smooth, spontaneous symmetrical limb movements which stop when the infant's attention is diverted (Prechtl 1990). Finger movements are elegant and varied, involving the thumb which can be abducted away from the palm by term (Ferrari et al 1990). A persistently adducted thumb (cortical thumb) is abnormal, and brain-damaged infants often have fisted hands and a paucity of fine finger movements.

Jitteriness

The normal term newborn is in a state of hypertonicity, with brisk reflexes tending to clonus. This 'transient spasticity' gradually relaxes over the first 8–10 months in a caudocephalad direction. The high tone can lead to the clinical sign of jittering. Jittering is a high frequency, generalized, symmetrical tremor of the limbs which is stilled by flexion or by inducing the infant to suck on a finger. Jittering is common in the first 2 or 3 days in term babies but if it is excessive or persistent deserves investigation. Repetitive chewing movements or tongue thrusting are not part of jitteriness and imply seizures. Jitteriness is stimulus-sensitive whereas seizures are not. In seizure the movement has a fast and slow component whereas in jittering the tremor is symmetrical.

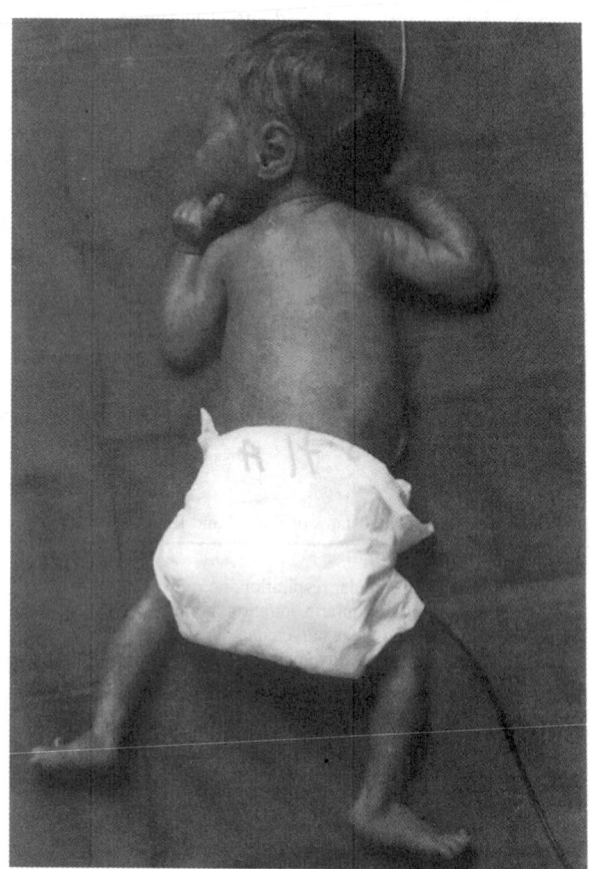 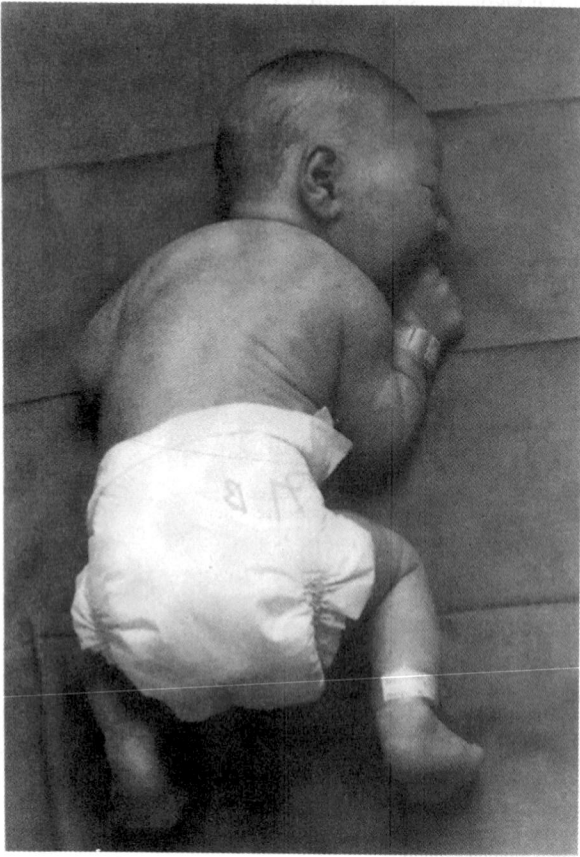

Fig. 5.52 Comparison between low tone in preterm infant (normal) (left) and the high flexor tone of a healthy term baby (right).

Jittering is never accompanied by physiological changes due to the autonomic nervous system such as tachycardia, hypertension or apnea.

Limb tone and power

Before passive movements are used to assess tone it may be possible to observe spontaneous movements of the limbs against gravity. Failure to move part or whole of a limb may be due to pain or paralysis. Limb tone is influenced by the tonic neck reflex in newborns which means it is important to have the head in the midline before beginning to elicit passive movements. These involve gentle flexion of the upper and lower limbs, then rapid extension and observation of recoil. A summary is contained within the protocol suggested by Dubowitz & Dubowitz (1981) (Fig. 5.53). This examination system, like that of Amiel-Tison (1995), involves assessing angles made by bending and manipulating the limbs. These include the popliteal angle, the foot

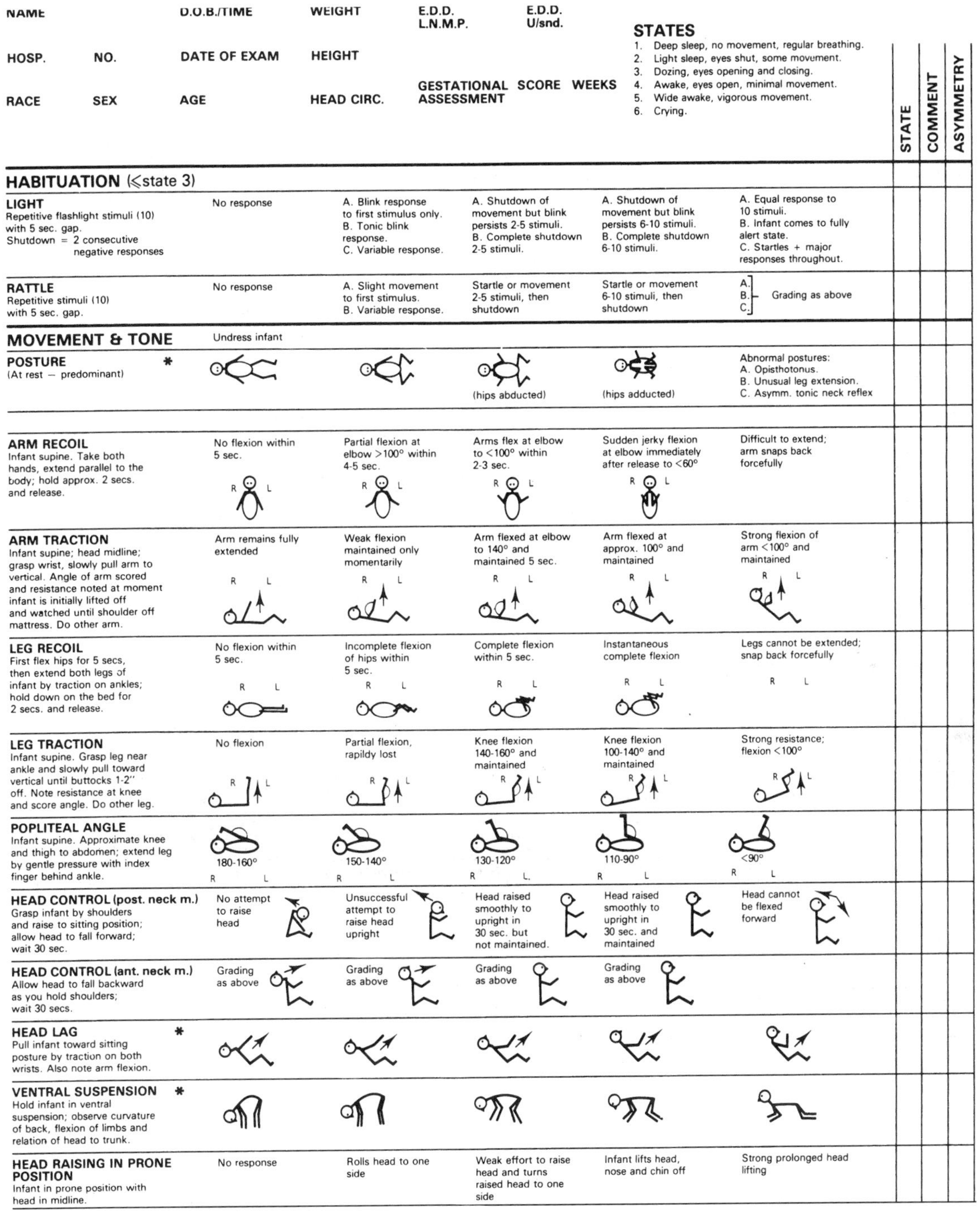

						STATE	COMMENT	ASYMMETRY
NAME	D.O.B./TIME	WEIGHT	E.D.D. L.N.M.P.	E.D.D. U/snd.	**STATES** 1. Deep sleep, no movement, regular breathing. 2. Light sleep, eyes shut, some movement. 3. Dozing, eyes opening and closing. 4. Awake, eyes open, minimal movement. 5. Wide awake, vigorous movement. 6. Crying.			
HOSP. NO.	DATE OF EXAM	HEIGHT						
RACE SEX	AGE	HEAD CIRC.	GESTATIONAL SCORE WEEKS ASSESSMENT					

HABITUATION (≤state 3)

LIGHT Repetitive flashlight stimuli (10) with 5 sec. gap. Shutdown = 2 consecutive negative responses	No response	A. Blink response to first stimulus only. B. Tonic blink response. C. Variable response.	A. Shutdown of movement but blink persists 2·5 stimuli. B. Complete shutdown 2·5 stimuli.	A. Shutdown of movement but blink persists 6-10 stimuli. B. Complete shutdown 6-10 stimuli.	A. Equal response to 10 stimuli. B. Infant comes to fully alert state. C. Startles + major responses throughout.			
RATTLE Repetitive stimuli (10) with 5 sec. gap.	No response	A. Slight movement to first stimulus. B. Variable response.	Startle or movement 2·5 stimuli, then shutdown	Startle or movement 6-10 stimuli, then shutdown	A. B. Grading as above C.			

MOVEMENT & TONE — Undress infant

POSTURE (At rest — predominant) *			(hips abducted)	(hips adducted)	Abnormal postures: A. Opisthotonus. B. Unusual leg extension. C. Asymm. tonic neck reflex			
ARM RECOIL Infant supine. Take both hands, extend parallel to the body; hold approx. 2 secs. and release.	No flexion within 5 sec.	Partial flexion at elbow >100° within 4-5 sec.	Arms flex at elbow to <100° within 2-3 sec.	Sudden jerky flexion at elbow immediately after release to <60°	Difficult to extend; arm snaps back forcefully			
ARM TRACTION Infant supine; head midline; grasp wrist, slowly pull arm to vertical. Angle of arm scored and resistance noted at moment infant is initially lifted off and watched until shoulder off mattress. Do other arm.	Arm remains fully extended	Weak flexion maintained only momentarily	Arm flexed at elbow to 140° and maintained 5 sec.	Arm flexed at approx. 100° and maintained	Strong flexion of arm <100° and maintained			
LEG RECOIL First flex hips for 5 secs, then extend both legs of infant by traction on ankles; hold down on the bed for 2 secs. and release.	No flexion within 5 sec.	Incomplete flexion of hips within 5 sec.	Complete flexion within 5 sec.	Instantaneous complete flexion	Legs cannot be extended; snap back forcefully			
LEG TRACTION Infant supine. Grasp leg near ankle and slowly pull toward vertical until buttocks 1-2" off. Note resistance at knee and score angle. Do other leg.	No flexion	Partial flexion, rapidly lost	Knee flexion 140-160° and maintained	Knee flexion 100-140° and maintained	Strong resistance; flexion <100°			
POPLITEAL ANGLE Infant supine. Approximate knee and thigh to abdomen; extend leg by gentle pressure with index finger behind ankle.	180-160°	150-140°	130-120°	110-90°	<90°			
HEAD CONTROL (post. neck m.) Grasp infant by shoulders and raise to sitting position; allow head to fall forward; wait 30 sec.	No attempt to raise head	Unsuccessful attempt to raise head upright	Head raised smoothly to upright in 30 sec. but not maintained	Head raised smoothly to upright in 30 sec. and maintained	Head cannot be flexed forward			
HEAD CONTROL (ant. neck m.) Allow head to fall backward as you hold shoulders; wait 30 secs.	Grading as above	Grading as above	Grading as above	Grading as above				
HEAD LAG Pull infant toward sitting posture by traction on both wrists. Also note arm flexion. *								
VENTRAL SUSPENSION Hold infant in ventral suspension; observe curvature of back, flexion of limbs and relation of head to trunk. *								
HEAD RAISING IN PRONE POSITION Infant in prone position with head in midline.	No response	Rolls head to one side	Weak effort to raise head and turns raised head to one side	Infant lifts head, nose and chin off	Strong prolonged head lifting			

Fig. 5.53 The Dubowitz score.

ARM RELEASE IN PRONE POSITION Head in midline. Infant in prone position; arms extended alongside body with palms up.	No effort	Some effort and wriggling	Flexion effort but neither wrist brought to nipple level	One or both wrists brought at least to nipple level without excessive body movement	Strong body movement with both wrists brought to face, or 'press-ups'			
SPONTANEOUS BODY MOVEMENT during examination (supine). If no spont. movement try to induce by cutaneous stimulation.	None or minimal Induced	A. Sluggish. B. Random, incoordinated. C. Mainly stretching.	Smooth movements alternating with random, stretching, athetoid or jerky	Smooth alternating movements of arms and legs with medium speed and intensity	Mainly: A. Jerky movement. B. Athetoid movement. C. Other abnormal movement.		1 2	
TREMORS Mark: Fast (>6/sec.) or Slow (<6/sec.)	No tremor	Tremors only in state 5-6	Tremors only in sleep or after Moro and startles	Some tremors in state 4	Tremulousness in all states			
STARTLES	No startles	Startles to sudden noise, Moro, bang on table only	Occasional spontaneous startle	2-5 spontaneous startles	6 + spontaneous startles			
ABNORMAL MOVEMENT OR POSTURE	No abnormal movement	A. Hands clenched but open intermittently. B. Hands do not open with Moro.	A. Some mouthing movement. B. Intermittent adducted thumb	A. Persistently adducted thumb. B. Hands clenched all the time.	A. Continuous mouthing movement. B. Convulsive movements.			

REFLEXES

TENDON REFLEXES Biceps jerk Knee jerk Ankle jerk	Absent		Present	Exaggerated	Clonus			
PALMAR GRASP Head in midline. Put index finger from ulnar side into hand and gently press palmar surface. Never touch dorsal side of hand.	Absent	Short, weak flexion	Medium strength and sustained flexion for several secs.	Strong flexion; contraction spreads to forearm	Very strong grasp. Infant easily lifts off couch			
ROOTING Infant supine, head midline. Touch each corner of the mouth in turn (stroke laterally).	No response	A. Partial weak head turn but no mouth opening. B. Mouth opening, no head turn.	Mouth opening on stimulated side with partial head turning	Full head turning, with or without mouth opening	Mouth opening with very jerky head turning			
SUCKING Infant supine; place index finger (pad towards palate) in infant's mouth; judge power of sucking movement after 5 sec.	No attempt	Weak sucking movement: A. Regular. B. Irregular.	Strong sucking movement, poor stripping: A. Regular. B. Irregular.	Strong regular sucking movement with continuing sequence of 5 movements. Good stripping.	Clenching but no regular sucking.			
WALKING (state 4, 5) Hold infant upright, feet touching bed, neck held straight with fingers.	Absent		Some effort but not continuous with both legs	At least 2 steps with both legs	A. Stork posture; no movement. B. Automatic walking.			
MORO One hand supports infant's head in midline, the other his back. Raise infant to 45° and when infant is relaxed let his head fall through 10°. Note if jerky. Repeat 3 times.	No response, or opening of hands only	Full abduction at the shoulder and extension of the arm 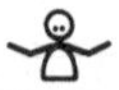	Full abduction but only delayed or partial adduction 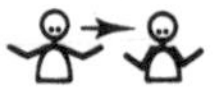	Partial abduction at shoulder and extension of arms followed by smooth adduction 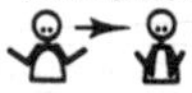 A. Abd>Add B. Abd=Add C. Abd<Add	A. No abduction or adduction; extension only. B. Marked adduction only. 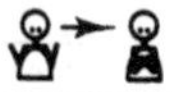		J S	

NEUROBEHAVIOURAL ITEMS

EYE APPEARANCES	Sunset sign Nerve palsy	Transient nystagmus. Strabismus. Some roving eye movement.	Does not open eyes	Normal conjugate eye movement	A. Persistent nystagmus. B. Frequent roving movement. C. Frequent rapid blinks.			
AUDITORY ORIENTATION (state 3, 4) To rattle. (Note presence of startle.)	A. No reaction. B. Auditory startle but no true orientation.	Brightens and stills; may turn toward stimuli with eyes closed	Alerting and shifting of eyes; head may or may not turn to source	Alerting; prolonged head turns to stimulus; search with eyes	Turning and alerting to stimulus each time on both sides		S	
VISUAL ORIENTATION (state 4) To red woollen ball	Does not focus or follow stimulus	Stills; focuses on stimulus; may follow 30° jerkily; does not find stimulus again spontaneously	Follows 30-60° horizontally; may lose stimulus but finds it again. Brief vertical glance	Follows with eyes and head horizontally and to some extent vertically, with frowning	Sustained fixation; follows vertically, horizontally, and in circle			
ALERTNESS (state 4)	Inattentive; rarely or never responds to direct stimulation	When alert, periods rather brief; rather variable response to orientation	When alert, alertness moderately sustained; may use stimulus to come to alert state	Sustained alertness; orientation frequent, reliable to visual but not auditory stimuli	Continuous alertness, which does not seem to tire, to both auditory and visual stimuli			
DEFENSIVE REACTION A cloth or hand is placed over the infant's face to partially occlude the nasal airway.	No response	A. General quietening. B. Non-specific activity with long latency.	Rooting; lateral neck turning; possibly neck stretching.	Swipes with arm	Swipes with arm with rather violent body movement			
PEAK OF EXCITEMENT	Low level arousal to all stimuli; never > state 3	Infant reaches state 4-5 briefly but predominantly in lower states	Infant predominantly state 4 or 5; may reach state 6 after stimulation but returns spontaneously to lower state	Infant reaches state 6 but can be consoled relatively easily	A. Mainly state 6. Difficult to console, if at all. B. Mainly state 4-5 but if reaches state 6 cannot be consoled.			
IRRITABILITY (states 3, 4, 5) Aversive stimuli: Uncover Ventral susp. Undress Moro Pull to sit Walking reflex Prone	No irritable crying to any of the stimuli	Cries to 1-2 stimuli	Cries to 3-4 stimuli	Cries to 5-6 stimuli	Cries to all stimuli			
CONSOLABILITY (state 6)	Never above state 5 during examination, therefore not needed	Consoling not needed. Consoles spontaneously	Consoled by talking, hand on belly or wrapping up	Consoled by picking up and holding; may need finger in mouth	Not consolable			
CRY	No cry at all	Only whimpering cry	Cries to stimuli but normal pitch	Lusty cry to offensive stimuli; normal pitch	High-pitched cry, often continuous			

NOTES ✱ If asymmetrical or atypical, draw in on nearest figure

Record any abnormal signs (e.g. facial palsy, contractures, etc.).

Record time after feed:

Fig. 5.53 The Dubowitz score (contd). Scheme for the neurological examination of the newborn infant at term. (From Dubowitz & Dubowitz 1981, courtesy of Spastics International Publishers Ltd.)

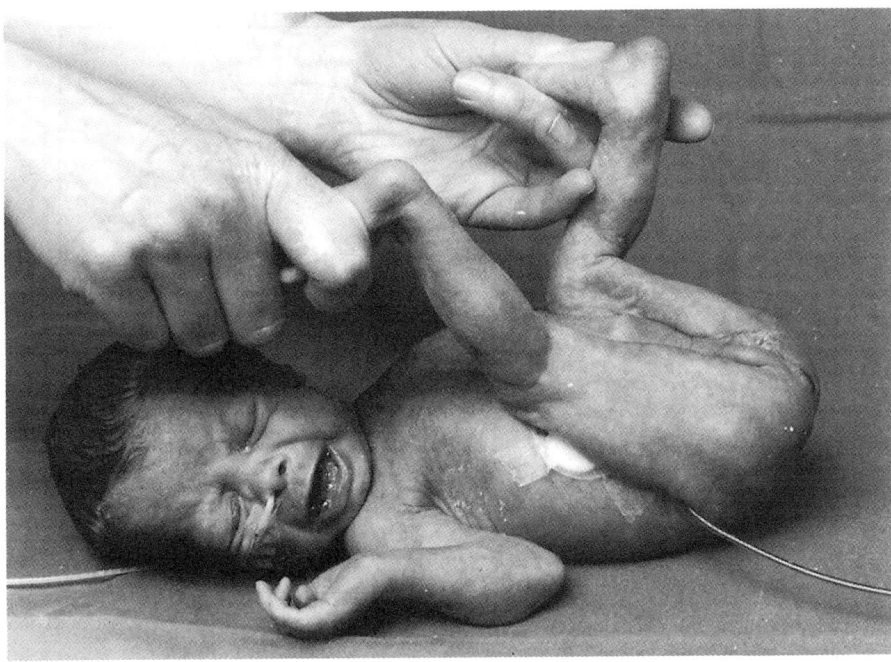

Fig. 5.54 Asymmetrical popliteal angle in a preterm baby with a unilateral cerebral lesion.

dorsiflexion angle, the square window and the scarf sign. A reduced popliteal angle (Fig. 5.54) and clusters of abnormal signs have been shown to be a sensitive indicator of later outcome.

Trunk and neck tone and power

Normal term infants have sufficient power in their neck muscles to lift their heads slightly when prone or supine. Preterm babies can manage to turn their heads from side to side but have much less power with complete head lag when pulled to sit. In order to judge tone in the neck and trunk, babies should be pulled to sit by holding them at the shoulders (Fig. 5.55) and then allowed to fall back again to the couch. If the head is unsupported it will gradually fall forwards or backwards: normal term infants will be able to raise their heads to the vertical again from either direction. There is balance between the neck flexors and extensors during pull-to-sit and back-to-lying maneuvers at term so that the head is held in line with the body during both phases. Immature infants usually have better control in back-to-lying. To assess truncal tone, lie the child on his back and try to push his bottom towards his head using his thighs (Fig. 5.56). With the infant lying on his side, hold the lumbar region and pull both legs backwards with the other hand grasping the ankles. Trunk flexion should always exceed extension. Arching of the trunk is abnormal; backwards arching of the whole back and neck is called opisthotonos.

Reflexes

Tendon and Babinski reflexes

Eliciting tendon reflexes is of less value in the newborn period than later in childhood. Knee and biceps jerks can usually be obtained. Reflexes at term are very brisk due to the high tone, and a few beats of clonus at the ankle are usual. The plantar reflex of

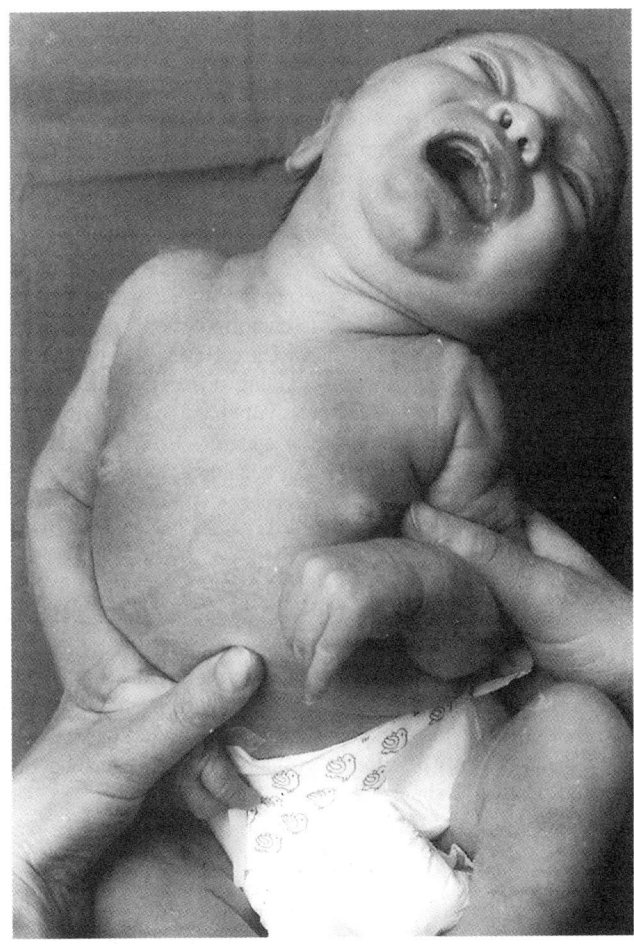

Fig. 5.55 Poor tone in the neck muscles in a baby with birth asphyxia.

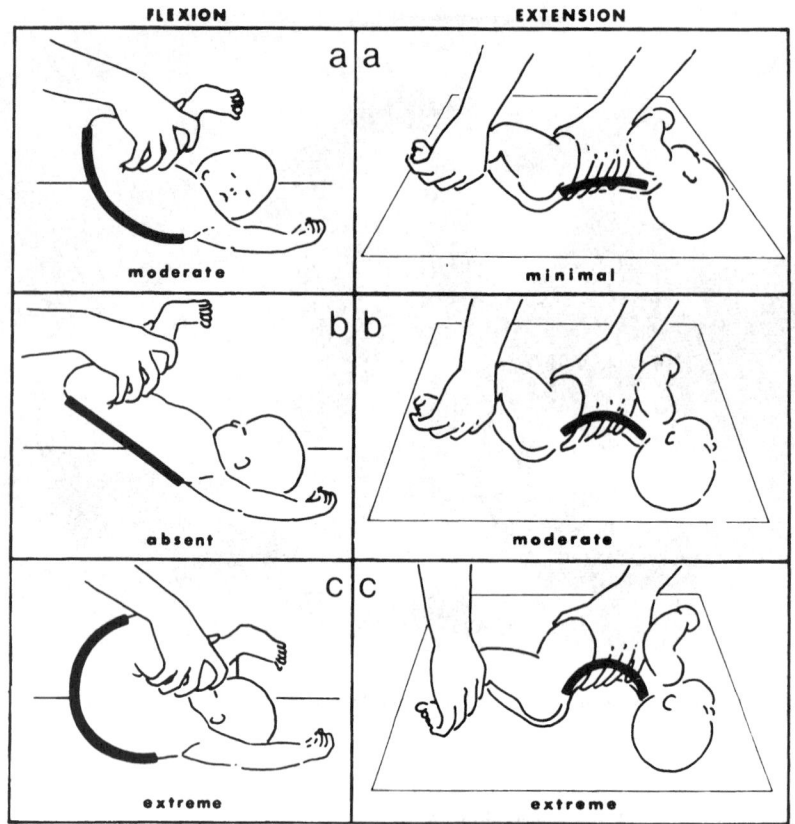

Fig. 5.56 Amiel-Tison system for assessing truncal tone. (Reproduced with permission from Amiel-Tison 1995.)

Babinski is always extensor and is best omitted as the stimulus often results in a withdrawal response.

Primary neonatal reflexes

Whilst the multiplicity of these responses and the timing of their appearance and disappearance is fascinating it is only necessary to have a working knowledge of a few. The reflexes have parallels in animals; the Moro reflex enables young primates to hold on to their mothers. Primitive reflexes normally habituate after repeated performance: this 'conditioning' is apparent even in fetal life. Persistence of neonatal reflexes can considerably inhibit normal movement in children with cerebral palsy.

Moro

This reflex is elicited by allowing the previously supported head of a baby to fall backwards slightly, whereupon the baby extends and adducts both upper limbs, opening the hands (Fig. 5.57). Babies of greater than 33 weeks' gestation subsequently adduct their arms. The Moro response is present from 28 weeks of gestation and usually disappears by 4 months. Persistence beyond 6 months is always abnormal.

Asymmetric tonic neck reflex

Starting with the infant supine and the head in the midline the head is slowly turned to one side. This results in increased extensor tone in the arm on the side to which the head is turned and increased flexor tone in the arm on the opposite side (fencing posture).

Symmetric tonic neck reflex

This reflex helps the child to push up on his arms later; when the head is extended on the neck tone increases in the upper limbs and when it is flexed tone reduces.

Crossed extension (adduction) reflex

One leg is held in extension and the sole of the foot is rubbed. The other leg first withdraws and then extends with fanning of the toes. Finally adduction brings the foot towards the foot which was stimulated. Eliciting the knee jerk produces this reflex in the neonatal period, which should not persist after 8 months of age.

Placing and stepping

By stimulating the dorsum of the foot, usually by bringing it into contact with the edge of the couch, a mature baby can be induced to 'step' over the edge. With the feet in contact with a solid surface the baby will 'walk'.

Rooting, sucking and swallowing

Stroking the upper lip of a baby of 28 weeks' gestation and above

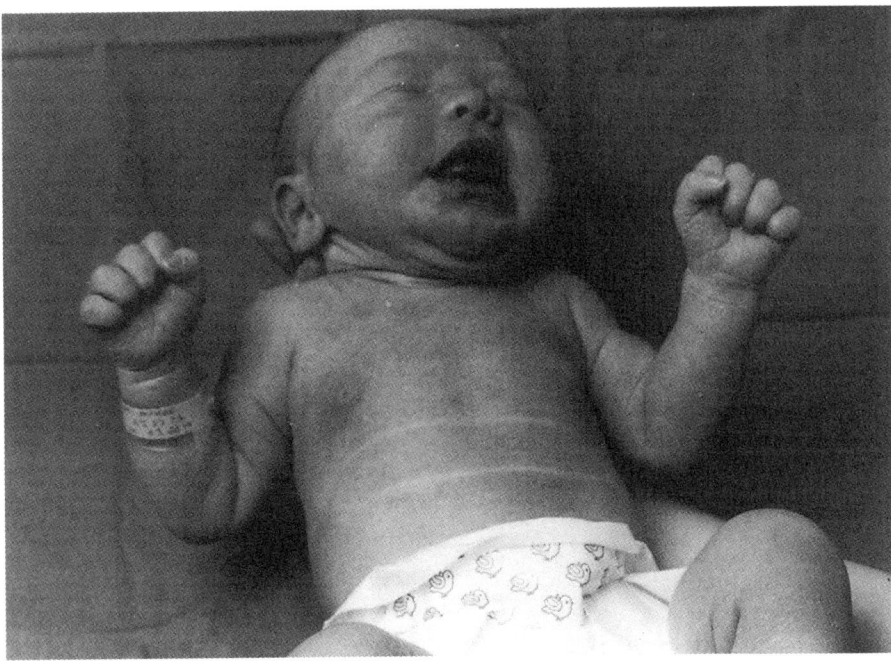

Fig. 5.57 The fully developed Moro reflex, abduction phase.

results in the baby searching for the nipple and tests the sensation in the distribution of the 5th cranial nerve. Sucking involves the motor activity of cranial nerves V, VII, XII; swallowing involves IX and X. The sensory input for the sucking reflex comes from the hard palate, not the tongue or cheek. Coordination between sucking and swallowing exists from 28 weeks' gestation but the strength to sustain it and to synchronize breathing is only adequate after 32–34 weeks' gestation. Sucking gradually builds up from bursts of three at a time to eight or more, with a reduction in the interburst interval. If sucking is absent test the gag reflex by gently stroking the soft palate with a cotton bud.

Palmar and plantar

The palmar reflex results from stroking the palmar surface of the hand, eliciting a grasp that is often strong enough to lift the baby from the crib. It is present from 26 weeks' gestation and persists up to 4 months. Stroking the ball of the foot results in curling of the toes in a similar manner to the palmar response.

Special senses

Examination of the eyes and vision

Infants can usually be induced to open their eyes by holding them face to face and spinning them round, or they often open their eyes when sucking. The eyes are in alignment, although a slightly dysconjugate horizontal position is not abnormal in the first 6 weeks. Vertical or skew deviation is always abnormal and has been seen in association with periventricular hemorrhage (Volpe 1995). Sunsetting (Fig. 5.58) should be noted although it is not as reliable a sign of raised intracranial pressure as later in childhood. The 'doll's eye' maneuver induced by rotating the head from side to side results in reflex deviation of the eyes to the opposite side.

It is normally present even in preterm babies, and absence of this reflex indicates severe brainstem damage. Pupil reactions to light are present after 31 weeks' gestation. Visual fixation of a suitable target such as a red woolen ball or a target of broad concentric rings is present from 32 weeks' gestation, and by 34 weeks infants track briefly. By term babies can reliably fix and track an object held 20–30 cm away from the face, and persistent failure to follow a suitable object should give rise to concern. Blinking in response to a bright light is a subcortical response and has been recorded in anencephalic and holoprosencephalic infants. Tracking in infancy is not a guarantee of later intact visual function and may be subcortically mediated (Dubowitz et al 1986). Optokinetic nystagmus is present from 36 weeks and preferential looking towards gratings of varying thickness can be used to assess acuity. Visual cortical function is achieved by 6 weeks (Braddick et al 1986). Visual evoked potentials are discussed below in the investigation section.

Hearing

Infants from 28 weeks' gestation onwards can be shown to respond to noise, usually by turning the head or increased body movements. For electrophysiological methods of assessing the auditory pathway, see investigation section below.

Sensory testing

Withdrawal

Babies respond to pinprick stimuli with gross body movements or grimacing and there is no doubt that very preterm babies feel pain (Anand & Hickey 1987) and indeed may be exquisitely sensitive to it (Fitzgerald et al 1988a). The classical withdrawal response of flexion of the lower limb and extension of the opposite leg in

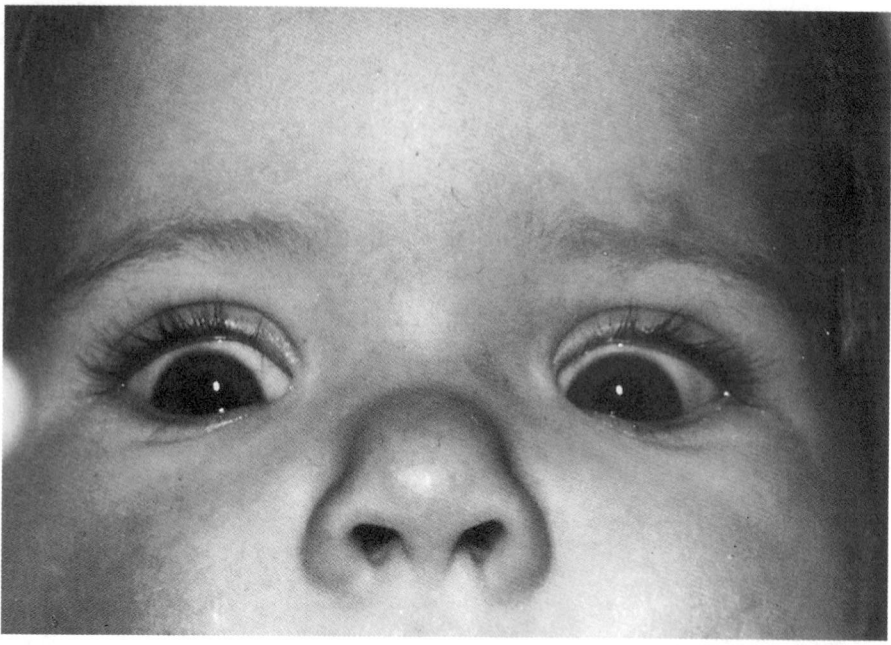

Fig. 5.58   Sunsetting in a baby with raised intracranial pressure.

response to pricking the sole of the foot requires motor integrity also, and habituates easily.

Occipitofrontal head circumference and fontanels

Examination is not complete without measuring and charting the occipitofrontal circumference and noting the presence and tension of the fontanels. An extremely large anterior fontanel can indicate hypothyroidism, a nonexistent fontanel can mean craniosynostosis. Useful information can be obtained by palpation of the sutures which can be widely spaced (diastasis) or overlapping. During the first 3 months of life the head grows at least half a centimeter a week, and insufficient head growth is an ominous sign.

INVESTIGATION OF THE NEWBORN NERVOUS SYSTEM

Imaging

Ultrasound is the imaging procedure of first choice in the newborn. The method is relatively cheap, portable and safe enabling repeated examination even of infants in an incubator. Periventricular and other forms of hemorrhage can be identified fairly reliably (Trounce et al 1986). The cystic lesions of periventricular leukomalacia can be imaged down to a resolution of 1–2 mm. The method is insensitive for the detection of cerebral edema, lesions of the extracerebral space and in the posterior fossa. Several excellent atlases of cranial ultrasound pictures exist (De Vries et al 1990, Rennie 1997).

CT scanning provides better information about the posterior fossa and the subdural space than ultrasound, with the disadvantages of X-ray exposure and the need for the infant to travel. Magnetic resonance imaging (MRI) appears entirely safe but brings its own problems relating to ferrous metals in life-support and monitoring devices. The improved detail, the ability to distinguish gray and white matter and to combine imaging with spectroscopic information means that MRI is preferred where there is access to the equipment. For those who wish to learn more about MRI images the book edited by Faerber (1995) is a useful resource.

Examination of cerebrospinal fluid

Lumbar puncture is often easier with the baby sitting up in the newborn period, and this position results in a more stable oxygen level. The spinal cord of the newborn extends to L3 so that the L3/L4 space is the best one to choose. A blood sample for plasma glucose estimation should be collected before performing the lumbar puncture as the stress response raises the blood sugar level. The cerebrospinal fluid glucose value is usually 70–80% of the plasma glucose and should be at least 50% of it. A proper styleted lumbar puncture needle should be used as there have been cases of epidermoid tumors resulting from the implantation of a tiny core of skin during neonatal lumbar puncture with an unstyleted needle. In the neonatal period cerebrospinal fluid may be xanthochromic because of jaundice or old intraventricular hemorrhage. The cell count is higher than later in childhood. In preterm neonates the red and white cell counts can each be up to 30/mm^3 (Table 5.100). In term infants after the first week of life more than 10 cells of each type per cubic millimeter is abnormal. A white cell count of more than 30/mm^3 with neutrophils more than 66% of the total is suspicious, although in cases of meningitis the white cell count is usually more than 100/mm^3. Seizures do not influence the results. Red cell counts of more than 1000/mm^3 make the interpretation of cerebrospinal fluid results impossible: applying correction factors using the ratio of white cells to red cells has been shown to be inaccurate. The only course of action is to repeat the lumbar puncture after 12 h.

Table 5.100 Normal values for CSF in neonates (adapted from Rennie 1995)

Type of infant	Red cell count (per cubic mm)	White cell count (per cubic mm)	Protein (g/l)	Glucose (mmol/l)
Preterm < 7 days	30 (0–333)	9 (0–30)	1 (0.5–2.9)	3 (1.5–5.5)
Preterm > 7 days	30	12 (2–70)	0.9 (0.5–2.6)	3 (1.5–5.5)
Term < 7 days	9 (0–50)	5 (0–30)	0.6 (0.3–2.5)	3 (1.5–5.5)
Term > 7 days	< 10	3 (0–10)	0.5 (0.2–0.8)	3 (1.5–5.5)

Estimation of intracranial pressure (ICP)

ICP usually refers to pressure within the cerebrospinal fluid space, and when subtracted from the arterial pressure gives the cerebral perfusion pressure. Rising ICP results in a reduction in cerebral perfusion unless the usual reflex elevation in systemic blood pressure occurs (the Cushing response). The Cushing response may be inadequate in the newborn (Kaiser & Whitelaw 1988).

Normal value of ICP in the newborn

Measured directly with accurate pressure transducers at lumbar puncture the pressure is 0–5.5 mmHg (Kaiser & Whitelaw 1985). Noninvasive devices designed to be stuck to the fontanel are numerous: the Ladd monitor works using light and a mirror and pneumatic devices working within a plastic blister (Rochefort et al 1987) can give good correlations when used with care, but are not accurate enough for clinical decision making.

Electroencephalography (EEG)

Conventional multichannel EEG recordings are difficult to obtain in newborn infants. The montage of electrodes is hard to apply and maintain and many babies requiring investigation are in intensive care units which are electrically noisy. Short recordings are of less value than prolonged ones as the EEG shows wide variability and changes not only with sleep state but also with the length of the preceding sleep epoch (Eyre et al 1988). Continuous monitoring is possible with either a cerebral function monitor, which displays the amplitude of one or two channels of processed EEG, or the Oxford Medilog system which records two channels of EEG on audio tape requiring later analysis. The output can be displayed on a laptop computer at the cot side.

Maturation of EEG

The EEG of very preterm babies is markedly discontinuous (Fig. 5.59, Eyre et al 1988) with a pattern of high voltage slow activity with suppressed EEG activity termed 'trace alternant'. This pattern can still be seen during normal sleep in mature babies, but with increasing gestation there is a reduction in amount and duration of trace alternant activity. There is also a pattern, called 'delta brush' of fast waves superimposed on delta waves which can be misinterpreted as convulsive activity. Abnormal background EEG activity correlates well with later adverse outcome in both preterm and asphyxiated term babies (Hellstrom-Westas et al 1995, Eken et al 1995).

Investigation of the visual pathway

Visual evoked potentials (VEP) are produced within the occipital cortex as a result of repeatedly applying an appropriate visual stimulus so that the minute electrical response to it, which will be identical each time, can be extracted from the random background electrical noise (EEG) by computerized averaging. Stroboscopic or flashing red lights are used which can penetrate closed eyelids. The electrical response 'matures' with advancing gestation and can be detected from 25 weeks. Study of VEPs has been found to be of value in predicting outcome after birth asphyxia (Taylor et al 1992), and is a sensitive test for the integrity of the visual pathway. Absent VEPs predicted cortical blindness in preterm infants with extensive cystic leukomalacia (de Vries et al 1987).

Investigation of the auditory pathway

Neural pathways for hearing are established and can be tested within hours of birth. The fetus responds to low frequency sounds applied to the maternal abdomen from 19 weeks of gestation, with a gradual increase in the range of frequency response and sensitivity (Hepper & Shahidullah 1994). Young children who are fitted with hearing aids early have an excellent chance of developing normal speech, but the current average age for the acquisition of hearing aids is often almost 2 years (Robertson et al 1995). Bilateral sensorineural deafness occurs in about 1.5 per 1000 children. This has led to the suggestion that all newborns,

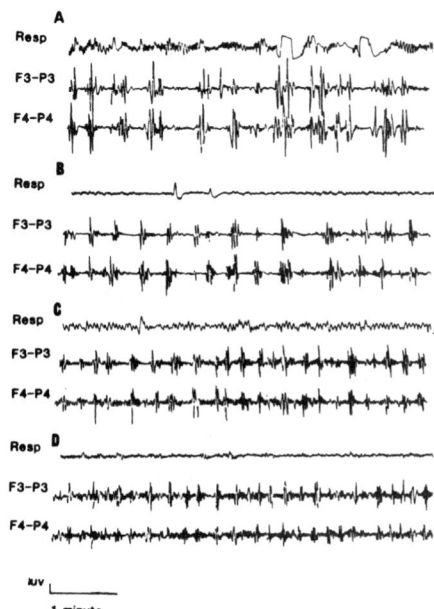

Fig. 5.59 Maturation of the normal EEG in preterm babies: (A) 26 weeks; (B) 32 weeks; (C) 35 weeks; (D) 42 weeks. (From Eyre et al 1988, with permission.)

and certainly those at high risk of deafness by virtue of a positive family history, neonatal illness, cleft palate or low birthweight should be screened for hearing loss (Stapells & Kurtzberg 1991, Kennedy et al 1991). The latter approach will identify 40% of the hearing-impaired children for the work of screening about 10% of the whole population. A successful universal neonatal screening program has been established in north London (Watkin 1996), and is being developed in the US but is not supported by all (Bess & Paradise 1994). Neonatal screening programs will never eliminate the need to monitor hearing with distraction testing at 7–9 months because many cases of infant hearing loss are conductive and acquired later due to secretory otitis media. The poor performance of the current distraction testing program is providing a stimulus for discussion regarding a different approach to hearing screening in the UK (Haggard 1990). A combination approach using screening for high-risk newborns, dissemination of information for parents derived from McCormick (1988), and training of health visitors led to a reduction in the median age at which hearing aids were fitted in one district (Scanlon & Bamford 1990). There are three main ways in which hearing can be assessed in the neonatal period. These are the auditory response cradle, automated auditory evoked brainstem potentials and otoacoustic emissions.

Auditory response cradle

This test involves placing the infant in a special crib which monitors body movement, respiration and head turning via a pressure-sensitive mattress. The infant is exposed to sounds with a threshold of 90 dB. 1.7% of 6000 children failed this test in one west London hospital; 20% of these were subsequently confirmed to have significant hearing loss (Tucker & Battacharya 1992). Seven children who passed the test in the neonatal period were found to be deaf subsequently; five had a progressive hereditary condition or definite postnatal factors. The test also had a high false positive rate in a group of babies tested in Nottingham, and has not been widely adopted. The US equivalent, the Crib-O-Gram, has not proved a success either.

Brainstem auditory evoked potential

These indicate electrical events generated in the brainstem auditory pathway in response to sound (usually a click) presented at the ear. The electrical signals are recorded with EEG electrodes on the scalp. The results of many click stimulations are summed by a computer which uses coherent averaging to eliminate the background noise generated by the local EEG signal. The mature pattern consists of seven waves, but these are poorly developed with increased latency and require a larger stimulus in order to elicit them in babies, in whom the response is present from 24 weeks. Prolongation of brainstem auditory evoked potentials have been described with hyperbilirubinemia and gentamicin toxicity. Automated brainstem response equipment eliminates the need for extensive operator training and is the most widely used method of hearing screening. Ex-preterm infants are tested as near to term as possible in order to reduce the false positive failure rate to a minimum.

Otoacoustic emissions

Otoacoustic emissions were discovered in 1978. They are low amplitude sound waves which are produced by the inner ear; they occur spontaneously as well as in response to a click stimulus. The automated method depends on the fact that a click stimulus, when presented to an intact hearing ear, evokes an otoacoustic emission which can be detected by a probe lying in the ear canal. Programmable software for measuring otoacoustic emissions has been developed (POEMS) and the system evaluated as a screening method in high-risk newborn babies in Sheffield and Southampton (Stevens et al 1989, Kennedy et al 1991). POEMS was quicker to administer than the automated evoked brainstem response method (no scalp electrodes) but there were more false positive results. It has been proposed that POEMS should be used for the first screen with automated brainstem evoked potentials available for those who fail.

CONVULSIONS IN THE NEWBORN

Diagnosis and incidence

Convulsions are more frequent on the first day of life than at any other time, although the diagnosis is easily missed because their manifestations can be extremely subtle. Subtle seizures were the most common type seen in several surveys, occurring in 75% of the cases described by Scher et al (1993). Repetitive lip smacking, cycling or swimming movements, deviation of the eyes and apnea can all be convulsive in origin but are sometimes difficult to distinguish from normal movements or jittering (see Table 5.101).

Continuous monitoring has shown that electrical seizures occur more frequently in the newborn than clinically suspected seizures, and conversely that stereotyped repetitive activity which looks like a seizure is not always associated with EEG change (Connell et al 1989a, Weiner et al 1991). There is as yet no evidence that treating clinical and electrically manifest seizures to electrical silence improves the outcome. There is also controversy about whether the lack of surface EEG activity truly confirms that a suspicious clinical event is not a seizure. There may be EEG change in 'hidden' electrical sites in the hippocampus or brainstem with poor transmission to the scalp because of the reduced myelin content of the neonatal brain. Recognition of seizure activity may be particularly important in babies who are paralyzed as prolonged seizures (> 30 min in animals) are accompanied by an increase in cerebral metabolic rate which outstrips the available energy supply and leads to cerebral damage. Changes in cerebral energy metabolites have been seen

Table 5.101 Types of seizure in the newborn (adapted from Volpe 1989)

Type	Clinical manifestation
Subtle	Eye signs – eyelid fluttering, eye deviation, fixed open stare, blinking
	Apnea. Cycling, boxing, stepping, swimming movements of limbs
	Mouthing, chewing, lip smacking, smiling. Often no EEG changes – most likely with ocular manifestations
Tonic	Stiffening. Decerebrate posturing. EEG variable
Clonic	Repetitive jerking, distinct from jittering. Usually EEG change
Myoclonic	Rare, but sleep myoclonus is benign. EEG often normal, although background EEG can be abnormal

even in the brief seizures characteristic of the human neonate (Young et al 1986).

The incidence of seizures in term babies is reported at between 1.6 and 14 per 1000 deliveries. Higher incidences were reported prior to the introduction of low-phosphate milks and half the babies in early series were hypocalcemic. More recent series give an estimate of around 5 per 1000; in most a quarter of the cases are amongst infants of less than 30 weeks' gestation and a half are less than 37 weeks (Lanska et al 1995). The incidence of clinically diagnosed seizures in very low birthweight infants varies from 50–60 per 1000 (Lanska et al 1995, Van Zeben et al 1990) and 90–130 per 1000 (personal observations, Watkins et al 1988).

Etiology

Intracranial injury

The majority of cases of seizures in term infants are associated with hypoxic-ischemic encephalopathy (Table 5.102). Newer imaging methods reveal middle cerebral artery infarction (stroke) to be more common than previously suspected (Koelfen et al 1995). This condition often accompanies perinatal asphyxia but also occurs in association with hypertension and polycythemia. Focal seizures are particularly likely to be caused by arterial infarction and MR imaging should be requested in these cases, with a repeat scan at 2 weeks if an early result is negative. Intracranial hemorrhage was diagnosed in 17% of Levene & Trounce's series (1986) which included cranial ultrasound but not MRI amongst the investigations. These workers were unable to assign a cause in only 8% of cases.

Maternal drug withdrawal

In some inner city neonatal units this is fast taking over from hypoxic-ischemic encephalopathy as the most common cause of seizure in term infants. Methadone withdrawal is more likely to produce seizures than heroin. The mean time of seizure onset in one series was 10 days but there was a wide range from 3–34 days. Urine testing can fail to reveal the metabolites which may be detected in hair or nails from the infant.

Metabolic causes

The metabolic causes of hypocalcemia, hypoglycemia, hyponatremia and hypomagnesemia now account for less than 10% of cases of neonatal seizure but remain important because they are readily treatable. Hypomagnesemia coexists with hypocalcemia about half the time, and recognition is important because administration of calcium can cause the serum magnesium to drop further. Recently a new congenital disorder involving an abnormality of glucose transport across the blood–brain barrier has been recognized (Fishman 1991). The cerebrospinal fluid glucose is low whereas the blood glucose is normal, and the condition is treatable. Pyridoxine dependency can be a difficult diagnosis to make; the disorder is autosomal recessive and the fits are intractable until an infusion of 100 mg pyridoxine is given, ideally under EEG monitoring. The response may take up to half an hour. Pyridoxine is necessary for the manufacture of γ-aminobutyric acid, which is the major inhibitory neurotransmitter, and hence in the familial form of the disease replacement needs to be lifelong. Temporary deficiency has also arisen following vomiting and incorrectly designed formula baby milks. Inborn errors of metabolism such as nonketotic hyperglycinemia can cause seizure and these should be suspected if the onset is late and related to milk feeds. Preterm infants can develop transient hyperammonemia and hyperlactemia causing seizures. 'Fifth day fits' were commonly reported in the 1970s and 1980s, but recent reports have failed to identify any cases.

Infection

Infection accounts for about 8% of neonatal fits and evidence of bacterial or viral infection should always be sought, including congenital infections such as cytomegalovirus.

Inherited and congenital disorders

Benign familial convulsions are dominantly inherited, and occur in the first 3 weeks of life. The fits can be very frequent but they are usually brief and the prognosis is excellent. The diagnosis rests on excluding other causes and the presence of a positive family history. The chromosomal defect has recently been mapped to the long arm of chromosome 20. Benign neonatal sleep myoclonus may give rise to dramatic manifestations in otherwise entirely healthy newborns who have a normal prognosis.

Sometimes neonatal seizures are the first manifestation of a congenital neurological disorder and these are more likely if the fits are intractable. The condition called 'early infantile epileptic encephalopathy' presents as severe tonic spasms and many of these babies have cerebral malformations. Cases of Aicardi's syndrome (female children with infantile spasms, agenesis of the corpus callosum and a characteristic EEG) would also fall into this group. The phakomatoses occasionally present in the neonatal period, and syndromes like Zellweger's or Smith–Lemli–Opitz can cause neonatal seizures.

Table 5.102 Causes of neonatal convulsions in order of current importance; percentage incidences included where available

Cause	1*	2†	3‡	4§
Hypoxic-ischemic encephalopathy	53%	16%	53%	30%
Intracranial hemorrhage	17%			
Cerebral infarction (stroke)				
Meningitis	8%	3%	8%	7%
Maternal drug withdrawal				
Hypoglycemia	3%	2%	3%	5%
Hypocalcemia, hypomagnesemia				22%
Rapidly changing serum sodium				
Congenitally abnormal brain		8%		4%
Fifth day fits		52%		
Benign familial neonatal seizures				
Pyridoxine-dependent seizures				
Hypertension				
Inborn errors of metabolism				

* Data from Levene & Trounce (1986).
† Data from Goldberg (1983).
‡ Data from Watanabe et al (1980).
§ Data from Bergman et al (1983).

Investigations

These follow from the possible causes listed above. Information regarding the delivery is vital to exclude hypoxic-ischemic encephalopathy. Essential laboratory investigations include estimation of calcium, magnesium, glucose, acid–base balance and sodium in the blood together with a full infection screen including a lumbar puncture, specimens for virology and a congenital infection screen. A cranial ultrasound scan should be included. If the cause is not revealed second line investigations include magnetic resonance imaging, samples to look for maternal 'street' drugs, urinary and blood amino acid estimation, chromosomal analysis, blood ammonia, measurement of organic acids and consideration of a trial of pyridoxine. The value of an EEG examination has already been discussed. A normal background interictal EEG is useful in prognosis (Connell et al 1989a).

Treatment

General guidelines

Treatment is best given intravenously as intramuscular absorption is erratic and the neonate has little muscle mass. Facilities to site and maintain intravenous lines and to institute artificial ventilation are necessary as many of the available drugs depress respiration and ventilation can become inadequate due to frequent convulsions. The high total body water of the neonate means a large volume of distribution hence the relatively large loading doses suggested in Table 5.103. Many of the drugs are protein bound and can interact with other drugs and bilirubin. Probably the best advice is to use phenobarbitone in an adequate dose with an early blood level, and to follow with intravenous phenytoin, then sodium valproate or rectal paraldehyde. Thiopentone coma did not improve the outcome in a controlled clinical trial (Goldberg et al 1986) and in resistant cases I would currently consider lignocaine (Hellstrom-Westas et al 1988).

Phenobarbitone

Note the large loading dose, and it is reasonable to give 30 mg/kg if the patient is already ventilated, otherwise use 15–20 mg/kg. Gilman et al (1989) achieved seizure control with phenobarbitone alone in 77% of cases using a rapid sequential method in which they gave 15–20 mg/kg initially then further doses of 5–10 mg/kg every 30 min up to a maximum of 40 mg/kg and serum level of over 40 mg/l. The half-life is very long and there have been concerns about toxic effects on the developing brain. Nevertheless the drug has other actions, reducing cerebral metabolic rate and acting as a free radical scavenger, which make it a good choice as the first line anticonvulsant. EEG response to anticonvulsant treatment is variable (Connell et al 1989b).

Phenytoin

There is some suggestion that more rapid control of seizures can be achieved with this agent, although its usefulness is limited by the myocardial depressant effect in some babies. Long-term treatment is not suggested because of the side effects and unpredictable metabolism.

Paraldehyde

Rectal administration of paraldehyde has been used for many years with safety and the drug is a useful second line anticonvulsant. There is some experience with intravenous infusions which can be inconvenient as the drug must be light-protected. Concern has been raised regarding pulmonary edema and hepatic necrosis. Intramuscular administration often leads to sterile abscess formation and should be abandoned.

Sodium valproate

Concern about the hepatotoxic effects, hyperammonemia and hyperglycinemia may limit its use in the newborn. Valproate proved effective in six intractable cases of neonatal seizure (Gal et al 1988). The oral solution is apparently absorbed from the rectum (Steinberg et al 1986).

Table 5.103 Anticonvulsant drugs in the newborn

Drug	Initial dose	Route	Maintenance dose	Route	Therapeutic level	Half-life	Mode of excretion
Phenobarbitone	15–30 mg/kg	i.v.	5 mg/kg/24 h – single dose	i.v./oral	14–40 mg/l 60–180 μmol/l	100–200 h	Hepatic P_{450} cytochrome oxidase
Phenytoin	20 mg/kg in two doses 1 h apart	i.v.	8 mg/kg/24 h in two doses	i.v./oral	10–20 mg/l 40–80 μmol/l	20 h (75 prems)	Liver glucuronidation
Paraldehyde	0.1 mg/kg	p.r.	150 mg/kg/h as dilute 5% solution	i.v.		10 h	Lungs and liver
Diazepam	0.2 mg/kg	i.v.	0.2 mg/kg/h	i.v.		20–60 h	Liver glucuronidation
Clonazepam	0.2 mg/kg	i.v.	0.01 mg/kg/h	i.v.		30 h	Liver glucuronidation
Valproate	20–25 mg/kg	i.v.	5–10 mg/kg/day	Oral	40–50 mg/l 275–350 μmol/l	26–47 h	Hepatic
Lignocaine	1–2 mg/kg	i.v.	2 mg/kg/h	i.v.	2.4–6 mg/l in adults	200 min	Liver and kidney

Duration of treatment

Concern about the effects of anticonvulsant treatment on the developing brain means that most neonatologists would only discharge a baby on maintenance phenobarbitone if the neurological examination was abnormal, discontinuing treatment before discharge in those who were neurologically normal (Volpe 1995). As many as 56% of infants developed subsequent epilepsy in one series (Ledigo et al 1991) although 20–30% is probably a more realistic figure (Scher et al 1993). For infants who are discharged on anticonvulsants consider discontinuation of treatment if the baby is seizure-free at 9 months.

Prognosis

This is related to the cause of the seizures. Following hypoxic-ischemic encephalopathy at term about 25% of those who fit will have sequelae (p. 125). Of 70 cases of clinical seizure in very low birthweight infants followed in Cambridge, 43 (59%) died, 16 (22%) had a major handicap and 11 (15%) were normal at 18 months. These data are remarkably similar to those of Watkins et al (n = 65, 1988), Van Zeben et al (n = 72, 1990), and Scher et al (n = 62, 1993) although in earlier series as many as 90% of the preterm infants died. The prognosis after hypocalcemic seizure and in familial neonatal seizure is excellent. Symptomatic hypoglycemia and meningitis have a 50% chance of sequelae in the survivors. A normal background interictal EEG at term is a good prognostic factor, with fewer than 10% of such infants experiencing sequelae. The value of a normal neurological examination at discharge in providing early reassurance should not be underestimated either; in one series 11 of 14 infants with seizures who were normal at 4 years were assessed as normal at this stage. However, this apparently normal group of Oxford children then had problems with spelling and memory in adolescence (Temple et al 1995).

INFECTION OF THE NERVOUS SYSTEM IN THE NEWBORN

Neonatal meningitis

Incidence and cause

Meningitis is more common during the first month of life than at any other time: the incidence has been estimated as 0.25–0.5 per 1000 in normal weight babies and 1–2 per 1000 in those below 2.5 kg at birth. Gram-negative organisms are more often implicated than later in childhood. The commonest causative organisms are *Escherichia coli* and group B streptococcus, the latter reflecting the association with septicemia. *Listeria monocytogenes* is becoming less frequent in the UK since the Government issued advice to pregnant women about avoiding soft cheese and carefully reheating cook–chill food. A wide variety of different organisms have been reported, particularly in the low birthweight baby. Staphylococci have a predilection for ventriculoperitoneal shunts. Table 5.104 lists 10 important causative bacteria.

Clinical signs and diagnosis

The diagnosis can be difficult and if infection is considered as a cause for a newborn's symptoms then a lumbar puncture must be performed. Examples include babies who are shocked and with

Table 5.104 Bacterial causes of neonatal meningitis (adapted from Rennie 1995)

Organism	Incidence
Escherichia coli	34%
Group B streptococci	30%
Other Gram-negative bacilli	8%
Listeria monocytogenes	6%
Staphylococci	4.5%
Other streptococci	4%
Pneumococcus	3%
Pseudomonas	3%
Haemophilus	2%
Meningococcus	2%

respiratory distress early in life in whom group B streptococcal infection or hyaline membrane disease (or both) could be the cause, and babies presenting later with subtle signs such as apnea, lethargy or regurgitation of milk. Babies developing hydrocephalus deserve one lumbar puncture even if the etiology is thought to be posthemorrhagic as ventriculomegaly can result from low-grade staphylococcal infection. Cerebral ultrasound scans may reveal intraventricular strands. The difficulty in distinguishing group B streptococcal infection from RDS at birth has led to the practice of performing a routine lumbar puncture in all such babies who require artificial ventilation. The yield of positive cultures in this situation is low, and the practice should be abandoned. The white blood cell count and the C reactive protein are raised and the platelet count may be low.

Treatment

Antibiotics alone do not treat meningitis, and the importance of supportive treatment must not be underestimated. Babies are often shocked requiring measures such as artificial ventilation, inotropic support, frequent monitoring of their acid–base state, careful fluid balance and maintenance of nutrition. There is no convincing evidence that adjunctive therapy such as steroid or immunoglobulin administration, exchange transfusion or monoclonal antibody treatment helps in neonatal meningitis.

Most treatment is started without knowledge of the infecting organism. Third generation cephalosporins offer excellent penetration into CSF with wide spectrum of activity including Gram-negative organisms. Of those available cefotaxime is probably the best choice with 100% survival reported in one small study though treatment failures and rapid development of resistance have occurred with cefuroxime. Ampicillin or penicillin should also be used to cover *Listeria*. Combination therapy of cefotaxime and ampicillin or triple therapy of penicillin, gentamicin and cefotaxime should be used until the infecting organism is identified and then rationalized. Antibiotics should be continued for 3 weeks after the CSF is sterilized. A repeat lumbar puncture should be carried out if there is a failure of clinical response and/or a failure of the laboratory indices of infection to return to normal. An intraventricular tap may be required if the ventricles are seen to enlarge on serial ultrasound scans, and intraventricular therapy should be considered via a surgically implanted reservoir in this situation.

Prognosis

The probability of survival relates mainly to the infecting organism and the gestational age of the baby. Gram-negative meningitis now has a 70% survival rate, a considerable improvement on the previous figures of 40–75% mortality. Neurodevelopmental sequelae in the survivors continues to be a problem with approximately one-third of the survivors sustaining an impairment of which deafness is the most frequent.

Viral and protozoal infections

These may be acquired in utero or postnatally and can cause severe neurological impairment. The acronym TORCH has been used to summarize the infections *Toxoplasma*, rubella, cytomegalovirus and herpes to which should be added human immunodeficiency virus and varicella-zoster.

Rubella infection in the first 16 weeks of pregnancy can result in a severely damaged baby with cataracts, sensorineural deafness, congenital heart disease, microcephaly, hepatospleno-megaly and thrombocytopenia. The condition is preventable by achieving high immunization coverage.

Cytomegalovirus can present in a dramatic form with jaundice and petechiae, the 'blueberry muffin' baby. Most infants who are symptomatic at birth will be handicapped. Only 1% of infants born with congenital cytomegalovirus infection are symptomatic, however, most infants being clinically unaffected by the infection. Perhaps 6% have significant hearing loss at follow-up (Peckham et al 1987).

Varicella-zoster can result in severe damage with cicatricial skin scarring, cataracts and seizures. Sequelae are more likely following infection in the first trimester when the risk was 1/11 in one study (Paryani & Arvin 1986). Transmission later in pregnancy can result in zoster or chickenpox in the newborn. If the maternal infection occurs within − 5 to + 5 days of delivery, the fetus will be unprotected by maternal antibody and should be treated with acyclovir and zoster immune globulin.

Herpes simplex virus can result in severe illness in newborns. There is a high incidence of meningitis and encephalitis. The infection should be treated with acyclovir. Herpes can be difficult to diagnose but the virus can be identified on electron microscopy. There have been case reports of congenitally infected neonates presenting like congenital varicella.

Human immunodeficiency virus: this retrovirus can cause meningitis and encephalopathy. Vertical transmission occurs in 13–45% of cases: a risk which can be reduced by zidovudine (Editorial 1994) and possibly by Cesarean section delivery. About one-third of infected children will present in the first year of life. Neurological manifestations include encephalopathy and microcephaly. Calcification of the basal ganglia has been seen with CT scanning (Epstein et al 1987).

Toxoplasma gondii: this protozoan can cause neurological sequelae when acquired in uterine life and the diagnosis is important because the condition is treatable. The organism is mainly acquired from cat litter or consumption of undercooked meat, and the infection may produce only mild symptoms in the mother. Birth prevalence is about 0.5 per 1000 in the UK. The classic triad of hydrocephalus, chorioretinitis and intracranial calcification is extremely rare, with four such cases in the UK between 1975 and 1980. Specific IgM antibody can be demonstrated in the baby who should be treated with pyrimethamine + sulfadiazine followed by spiramycin. The prognosis of symptomatic congenital toxoplasmosis is poor, with 50% suffering impaired vision and 85% mental retardation.

Spirochetal and fungal infections

The incidence of congenital syphilis is rising commensurate with the rise in the use of crack cocaine. All infants with suspicion of congenital syphilis should receive penicillin, and this is also the drug of choice for neonatal Lyme disease. Fungal meningitis and abscess formation is mainly a problem of the very low birthweight infant requiring intensive care, in whom the mortality from this complication is high.

DEVELOPMENTAL ABNORMALITIES

See Chapter 14 for further information about these conditions.

METABOLIC AND ENDOCRINE DISORDERS

Introduction

Whilst adequate energy is essential to sustain adequate growth of the brain, nutrients also need to be in the appropriate concentrations and supported by the correct hormonal milieu. Inborn errors of metabolism can alter the relative concentrations of amino acids and many of these conditions present in the newborn period with neurological symptoms. High ammonia levels are toxic to the nervous system so that disorders of the urea cycle also present with severe derangement of neurological function. Lack of thyroid hormone causes failure of neurological maturation which rapidly results in permanent damage; the prevention of cretinism by early identification of such individuals with screening and replacement therapy has been a significant advance. Preterm babies have low thyroxine in early postnatal life; two studies suggest a correlation between low levels of thyroid hormones and adverse neurodevelopmental outcome (Lucas et al 1988a, Den Ouden et al 1996).

Urea cycle defects

Hyperammonemia may present with severe neurological disturbance in the newborn period. Recognition is important because many of the conditions are inherited and the babies often succumb without the correct diagnosis being made. There may be lethargy, vomiting and convulsions. Plasma ammonia concentrations above 200 mg/l are toxic and can result from liver failure, enzyme defects of the urea cycle or other disorders of amino acid metabolism such as propionic acidemia and lysine intolerance. Further investigation consists of enzyme assay using leukocytes or liver cells.

Hyperbilirubinemia

Unconjugated bilirubin is lipid soluble and hence able to cross the blood–brain barrier. The classical neurological syndrome of kernicterus presented with opisthotonic posturing and fits is now rare. Such babies were subsequently severely damaged. Damage to the auditory pathways can be demonstrated with prolongation of auditory evoked potentials which return to normal with exchange transfusion, and a reduced incidence of hearing loss in preterm survivors has been claimed to be due to adoption of a policy attempting to prevent high bilirubin levels (above 200 µmol/l).

Hypoglycemia

Prolonged low glucose levels damage the newborn nervous system which is unable to utilize alternative energy sources. There has been some debate recently regarding the degree of hypoglycemia which is required to inflict permanent damage with the suggestion that for preterm babies below 2.6 mmol/l was associated with a reduction in Bayley motor and mental development scores at 18 months (Lucas et al 1988b). Much more evidence is needed before definite guidelines can be formulated regarding moderate hypoglycemia. The damage which can result from severe reduction in glucose levels is not in doubt, however, and is highlighted by the incidence of impairment in survivors of nesidioblastosis of the pancreas who often have intractable hypoglycemia. Symptomatic hypoglycemia has at least a 50% chance of sequelae in the survivors.

NEONATAL CEREBRAL INJURY

Perinatal stress such as hypotension or trauma can result in cerebral injury. The preterm brain is particularly vulnerable, as are the brains of more mature infants who have been subjected to in utero insults. Neonatal brain injury is best considered as a spectrum with the end result depending on the type and degree of insult, the gestational age of the baby and any underlying factors. The problem is an important one because there is a relationship with later handicap (Stewart et al 1987, de Vries et al 1985, Cooke 1987a).

Periventricular hemorrhage (PVH)

The preterm brain contains a unique structure, the germinal matrix, containing actively dividing neuroblasts and glioblasts.

The blood supply is via a capillary bed supplied by Heubner's artery, which is a branch of the anterior cerebral artery. The region of the germinal matrix which is situated at the head of the caudate nucleus is prone to bleeding, and this is the most common form of intracranial hemorrhage in preterm babies. The incidence of intracranial hemorrhage diagnosed with ultrasound in very low birthweight infants has reduced from around 40% to 15–20% since the widespread introduction of antenatal steroids and postnatal surfactant (Szymonowicz et al 1986, Strand et al 1990). The trend seen in inborn very low birthweight infants in Cambridge is shown in Figure 5.60. A falling incidence has not been reported from all centers (Cooke 1991).

The term PVH is often used as a generic one, encompassing several different types of hemorrhage in preterm infants. The mildest form is germinal matrix or subependymal bleeding alone. This is often abbreviated to GLH or SEH and is equivalent to Grade 1 PVH in the classification of Levene & De Crespigny (1983) and Grade 1 in the classification of Papile et al (1978). Bleeding into the ventricular system, or intraventricular hemorrhage (IVH) was classified by Levene in 1983 as Grade 2 PVH and was subdivided by Papile into Grade 2 when the ventricle is not distended and Grade 3 where it is. Finally, bleeding into the parenchyma of the brain (ParH) was Levene Grade 3 PVH in 1983 and Grade 4 in the Papile classification. A parenchymal hemorrhagic lesion is illustrated with the ultrasound scan appearance in Figure 5.61. Because few now believe that parenchymal hemorrhage represents direct extension of intraventricular bleeding, and because it is now clear that all echodense lesions diagnosed with ultrasound are not certain to be hemorrhagic a new classification has been proposed by Levene & de Vries (1995). They suggest that the term GMH-IVH is used to describe bleeding into the germinal matrix and the ventricle, and that all other intracranial hemorrhage should be described as carefully as possible with ultrasound, and photographic records kept. Parenchymal echodense lesions visualized with ultrasound can represent various forms of pathological lesion including hemorrhagic lesions. Some parenchymal lesions represent

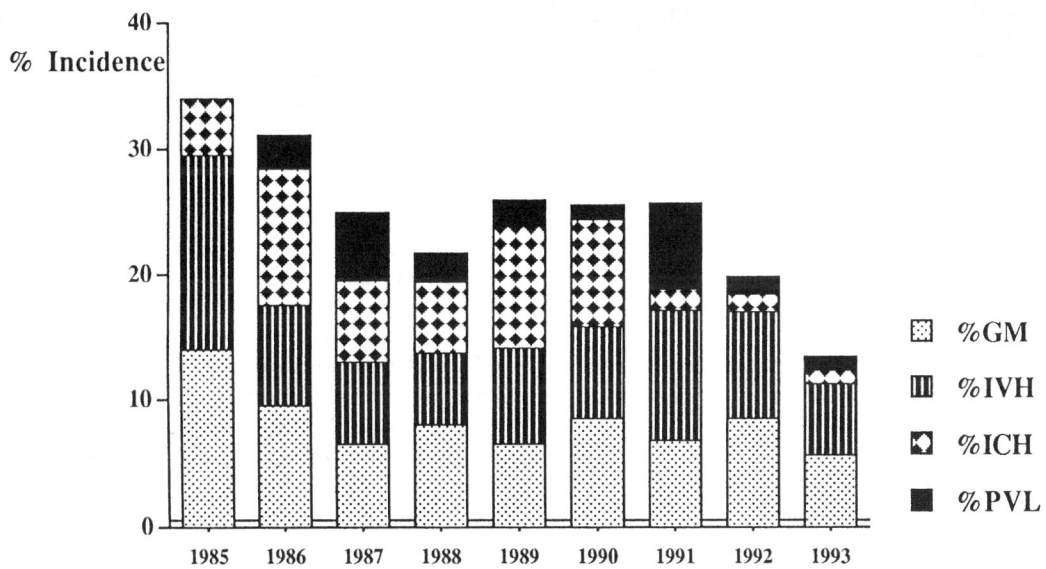

Fig. 5.60 Incidence of brain injury in VLBW infants born in hospital 1985–1993: GM = germinal matrix; IVH = intraventricular hemorrhage; ICH = intracranial hemorrhage; PVL = periventricular leukomalacia.

bleeding into areas of brain that were previously ischemic. One explanation for the frequent association of unilateral hemorrhagic parenchymal lesions with the presence of a germinal matrix hemorrhage is that the latter reduces the perfusion to the adjacent white matter by obstructing venous drainage, causing an infarction (Gould et al 1987). The ultrasound scan appearance of

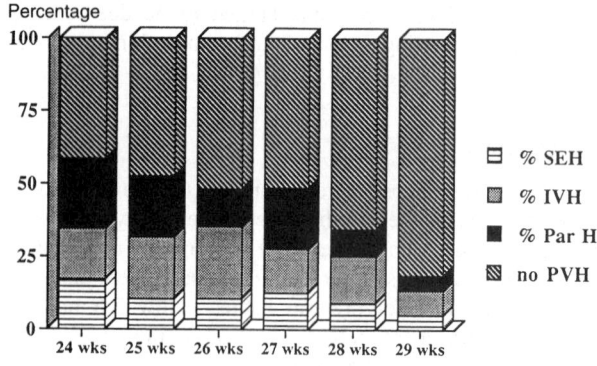

Fig. 5.62 Relationship of gestational age to brain injury: SEH = subependymal hemorrhage; IVH = intraventricular hemorrhage; Par H = parenchymal hemorrhage; PVH = periventricular hemorrhage.

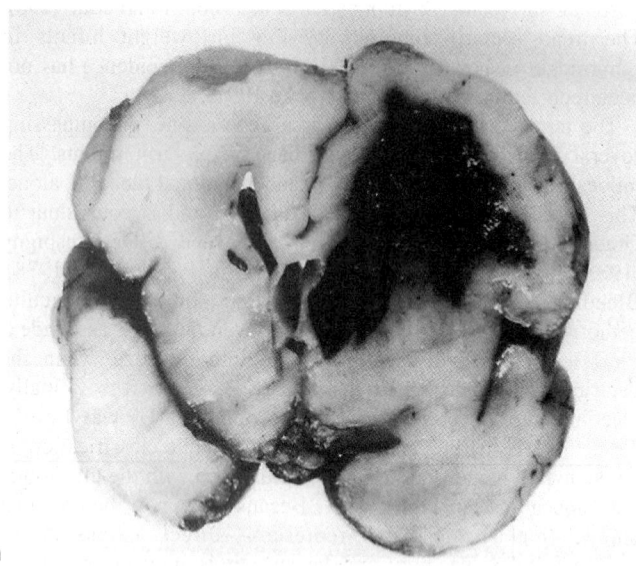

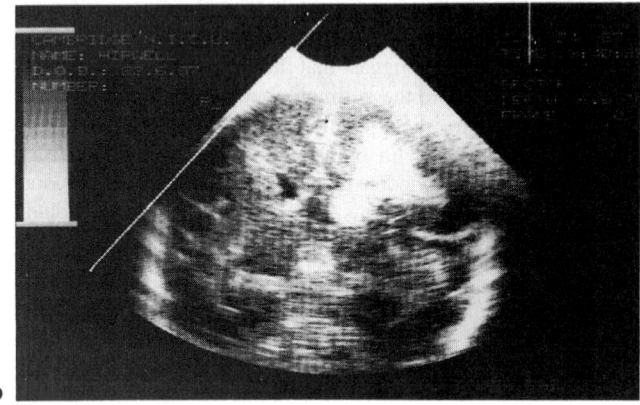

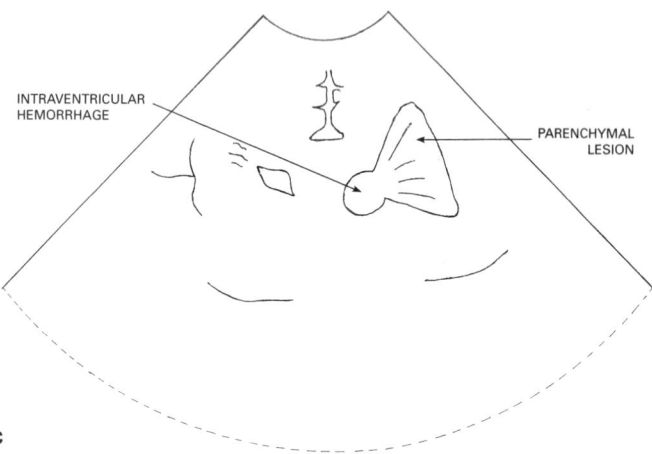

Fig. 5.61 Periventricular hemorrhage, at postmortem (**a**) and imaged with ultrasound in life ((**b**), with diagrammatic representation (**c**)).

this lesion is that the shape is triangular with the apex at the lateral border of the lateral ventricle (Fig. 5.61). The lesion is often preceded by an ipsilateral GMH-IVH. Distinction is important as the prognosis is different from hemorrhagic periventricular leukomalacia.

Repeated ultrasound scanning of cohorts of VLBW infants has revealed that the incidence and degree of hemorrhage relates to the birthweight and gestational age (Fig. 5.62). The complication develops in early postnatal life, with as many as 36/47 (77%) of lesions present by 6 h in one study and all by 72 h in another. There are several undisputed risk factors. These are:

- gestational age
- birthweight
- respiratory distress syndrome
- artificial ventilation
- hypercarbia
- pneumothorax.

Less conclusive evidence exists for variables such as the mode and place of delivery, use of β-sympathomimetics during labor, presence of coagulopathy, acidosis, bicarbonate administration, low blood pressure and fluctuating cerebral blood flow velocity (Miall-Allen et al 1987) and the administration of vasodilators such tolazoline. The main problem is in distinguishing antecedent from associate. The best 'unifying hypothesis' (Levene 1987) is that GMH-IVH results from a disturbance of cerebral blood flow in babies who are poor at cerebral autoregulation, and in whom there is often a bleeding tendency.

Attempts to prevent PVH have included administration of agents such as fresh frozen plasma, phenobarbitone in nine trials, indomethacin six trials (Ment et al 1994), tranexamic acid, ethamsylate (EEC Working Group 1994), vitamin E, and pancuronium. A useful reduction was also obtained with surfactant in the British multicenter trial (Ten Centre Study Group 1987). At the present time there is insufficient evidence to recommend wholesale prophylaxis in the nursery.

Periventricular leukomalacia

Periventricular leukomalacia (PVL) was first recognized by pathologists. The 'white spots' appear at the boundary zone of the cerebral circulation in the immature brain and it seems likely that a period of low cerebral blood flow is often exacerbated by flow–metabolism uncoupling. Small cysts can now be diagnosed during life with ultrasound (Fig. 5.63) (Trounce et al 1986). Cysts can be imaged in between 8 and 17% of babies less than 1500 g. Some series include parenchymal echodense lesions persisting for more than 2 weeks but not evolving into cysts, with a higher incidence of 25% (Trounce et al 1986). There can be some difficulty in distinguishing this type of 'flare' from the peritrigonal

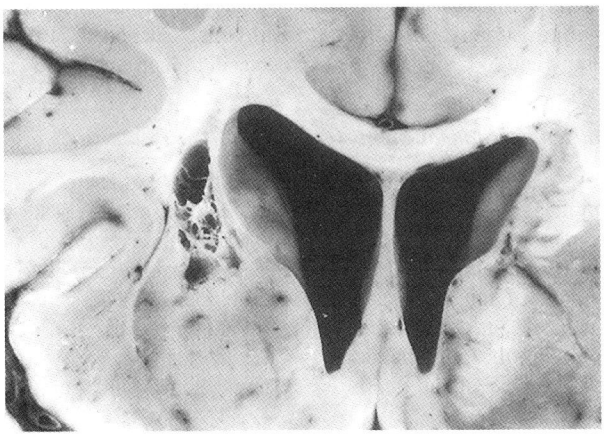

a

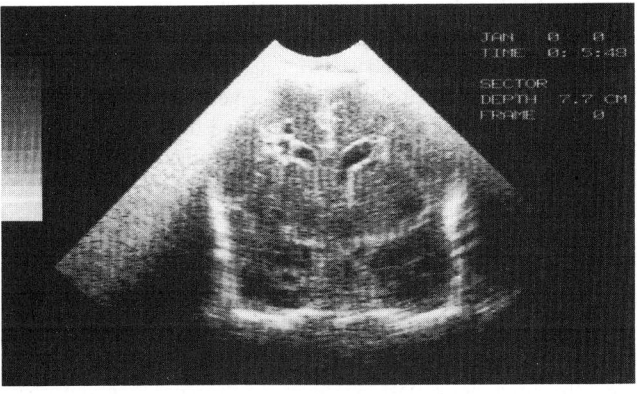

b

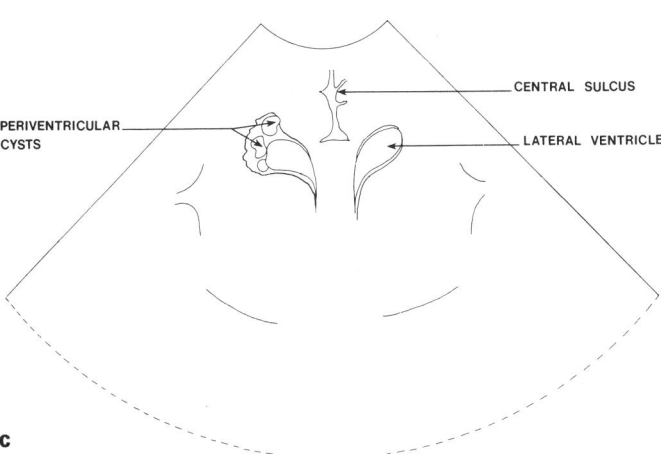

c

Fig. 5.63 Periventricular leukomalacia at postmortem (**a**) and imaged with ultrasound in life ((**b**), with diagrammatic representation (**c**)).

'blush' described by Di Pietro et al (1986) which is normal. It is very important to describe the ultrasound appearances in detail; an echodense lesion in a 1-day-old preterm baby is a long way from the pathological identification of cystic change in the white matter and should not be confidently diagnosed as PVL. Paneth et al (1994) found white matter damage at postmortem in preterm infants with cerebral echodensity during life, but in very few were the lesions typical of classical periventricular leukomalacia. In many the white matter damage, with liquefactive necrosis and perivascular hemorrhage, was not restricted to the periventricular region. They suggest that the lesion seen in today's very preterm population differs from that originally described. Cysts disappear after a few months and are replaced by a thinning of the myelin layer. Magnetic resonance imaging confirms reduction in myelin content of the brain.

No agreement has yet been reached on the precise definition of the ultrasound appearances of a 'flare' but follow-up suggests that they are predictive of outcome and hence represent injury (Graham et al 1987, Appleton et al 1990). These early echodense lesions appear 24–48 h after an insult and are often followed in 2–4 weeks by appearance of cystic change. Studies are still emerging regarding the antecedents: antepartum hemorrhage, asphyxia and surgery particularly for necrotizing enterocolitis have been suggested (Calvert et al 1987, Trounce et al 1988). Hypocarbia and hyperbilirubinemia are others (Calvert et al 1987, Ikonen et al 1988, 1992, Fujimoto et al 1994). The outlook for the survivors has so far proved extremely poor: of 82 babies reported in several series almost all have severe cerebral palsy. Bilateral cysts greater than 1 cm diameter in the occipital cortex have the worst prognosis.

Intracerebellar hemorrhage

Cerebellar blood can occur as an extension from intraventricular or subarachnoid bleeding or as an isolated event in premature babies. It has been described in association with tight bands around the head. Management is usually conservative and a good outcome has been described at term although preterm babies often succumb as the condition forms part of more extensive PVH.

Thalamic hemorrhage

This type of intracranial bleeding may be primary or secondary to extension from germinal matrix bleeding. Term babies with this condition may present aged about 10 days of age with eye signs (deviation and sunsetting) and fits. 18-month follow-up has revealed no abnormality, in contrast to the babies with 'bright thalamus' described by Shen et al (1986) who were all suffering from severe birth asphyxia and subsequently developed cerebral palsy.

Subdural hemorrhage

The incidence of this complication has fallen with more careful obstetric practice, and usually results from tearing of the bridging veins. Babies may present with shock, bradycardia and are frequently asphyxiated. Ultrasound is poor at detecting subdural hemorrhage and suspicion of the diagnosis is an indication for CT scan.

Subarachnoid hemorrhage

Like cerebellar and thalamic bleeding blood in the subarachnoid space is often secondary to PVH, but primary subarachnoid hemorrhage has been described in cases of vitamin K deficiency. Convexity subarachnoid hemorrhage has been diagnosed with ultrasound in a group of babies who had undergone exchange transfusion for rhesus disease.

HYDROCEPHALUS AND VENTRICULOMEGALY

For more information on these conditions see Chapter 14. The following discussion is limited to preterm posthemorrhagic hydrocephalus and the outcome after an in utero diagnosis of ventriculomegaly.

Etiology

Important causes to consider in the newborn period include:

1. Cerebral malformations: Arnold–Chiari malformation, Dandy–Walker cysts, aqueduct stenosis, arachnoid cysts
2. Craniosynostosis, e.g. Apert's syndrome
3. Obstruction by a mass: vein of Galen aneurysm, tumors
4. Posthemorrhagic hydrocephalus, particularly in preterm babies
5. Postmeningitic hydrocephalus
6. X-linked congenital hydrocephalus.

Posthemorrhagic hydrocephalus in preterm infants

This is now the most frequent cause of acquired hydrocephalus in infants and occurs secondary to periventricular hemorrhage. The distance from the midline to the lateral border of the ventricle in a coronal ultrasound view should be measured and plotted on a centile chart – the ventricular index. A ventricular size greater than the 97th centile occurred in 15 of 68 survivors with periventricular hemorrhage from a cohort of 202 VLBW babies. The risk relates to the degree of hemorrhage.

The natural history of ventricular dilation secondary to PVH is that at least half the cases will not progress to require shunting, an important consideration when assessing uncontrolled studies claiming effective 'cures' (Whitelaw et al 1992). The percentage of babies of birthweight less than 1500 g who required ventriculoperitoneal shunt insertion was 1.8% in Liverpool (Cooke 1987a).

Treatment

There is now no place for compressive head wrapping, glycerol or isosorbide in the treatment of hydrocephalus in infants. The definitive treatment is surgical placement of a ventriculo-peritoneal shunt and this will be required in most cases of congenital hydrocephalus. The difficulty usually occurs in the cases of posthemorrhagic dilation as some will spontaneously arrest and in some cases the babies are too ill to permit surgery. Suggestions that shunt placement could be avoided by early intervention have not been borne out by a multicenter study in England, Eire and Switzerland enrolling 157 infants with posthemorrhagic hydrocephalus (Ventriculomegaly Trial Group 1990). Repeated percutaneous drainage of CSF did not reduce the

eventual requirement for shunt surgery nor improve the neurodevelopmental status at 18 months except in the subgroup with parenchymal lesions. Management of this condition should therefore include a single diagnostic lumbar puncture in order to establish the intracranial pressure, whether the ventriculomegaly is of the communicating type and to exclude infection, and then a wait-and-see policy should be adopted with intervention planned if the head growth is more than twice the usual rate or the infant develops symptoms of raised intracranial pressure. Intervention should be surgical if the baby is fit enough, but acetazolamide (25–100 mg/kg/day) may allow delay and reduce the number of lumbar/ventricular taps which have to be done in babies who are awaiting surgery. Electrolyte disturbance secondary to drug therapy and to CSF drainage can occur in this group.

Ventriculoperitoneal shunts

These can be inserted in babies as small as 1500 g. There is a high complication rate in such infants, 30% in some series, with frequent episodes of blockage. Many surgeons like to wait until the CSF protein is below 1.5 g/l before insertion, particularly in posthemorrhagic hydrocephalus when blood in the CSF makes it viscous. Ventriculoatrial shunting is no longer the method of choice, as the complications specific to this route are serious; these include shunt nephritis, systemic sepsis and pulmonary hypertension.

Prenatally diagnosed ventriculomegaly

Pediatricians are increasingly asked for help in counseling parents whose fetus has enlarged ventricles diagnosed on an antenatal ultrasound scan. The usual basis is a ventricle/hemisphere ratio more than 0.5. More than 50% will have other problems, and a search should be made for intrauterine infection, chromosomal abnormality and spina bifida. Even in the best hands some important associated cerebral malformations can be missed antenatally. The outlook for this group is generally poor and many couples choose termination of pregnancy after counseling if the diagnosis is made early enough. Of those diagnosed later, the differentiation between progressive and nonprogressive enlargement needs to be made. If the hydrocephalus is progressive and the pregnancy past 32 weeks' gestation then delivery is probably the best option. Fetuses with nonprogressive enlargement without associated abnormality have the best chance of a normal outcome although most were eventually shunt dependent in one series (Hudgins 1988). This selected subgroup also did well in a series from London (Nicolaides et al 1990) but these formed only 7% of the total of 267 cases. The chance of chromosomal malformation was 3% if the ventriculomegaly was isolated and 36% when another abnormality, such as syndactyly, was present.

Prognosis

This depends on the underlying condition, and is worse for posthemorrhagic hydrocephalus than the congenital syndromes. Surgery has radically improved the outlook for some children with hydrocephalus, who can now expect to survive and attend normal school. Overall about 86% now survive and two-thirds will have normal intelligence. For preterm babies the prognosis relates to the severity of the associated periventricular hemorrhage and the presence of fits in the neonatal period (Cooke 1987b). About half of these children will have significant neurodevelopmental delay.

RENAL DISEASE IN THE NEONATE

INTRAUTERINE DEVELOPMENT

Embryology

Three distinct pairs of primitive kidneys are induced successively from the third week of gestation in mesenchyme lying at the lateral edges of the high thoracic somites. Only the third pair, the metanephros, persist and secrete urine from 10 weeks onwards. Nephrogenesis is induced by a cephalic extension of the Wolffian duct which comes to lie anterior to mesenchyme. A succession of dichotomous branchings by this duct or ureter leads firstly to the formation of renal pelvis and calyces (five branchings) and secondly to the induction of nephrons. Continuity between collecting ducts derived from ureteric branchings and the distal convoluted tubules of induced nephrons is established by assimilation of the cells between them.

Early changes in position of the kidneys comprise migration from fetal pelvis to a subdiaphragmatic position and a concomitant external rotation to bring the ureters into a medial relationship.

Older nephrons induced by branchings 6 to 12 lie deeply in a juxtamedullary position and have long loops of Henle and a blood supply suitable for urinary concentration/dilution and the reabsorption of solute. Younger nephrons from branchings 13 to 15 are cortical in site, comprise 75% of mature nephrons and have short tubules with a capacity for solute excretion.

Each kidney has 10^6 nephrons when nephrogenesis is complete at 36 weeks. Thereafter renal growth reflects an increase in nephron size.

Development of renal function in utero

Urine production increases throughout fetal life until an abrupt decline which occurs just before term. Urine is initially an ultrafiltrate of plasma. The volume varies from 4.5 ml/kg/h at 20 weeks to 6 ml/kg/h at 32 weeks and to 8 ml/kg/h at 39 weeks. Up to 600 ml of amniotic fluid is swallowed daily, 10% of which is derived from nonrenal sources including gut, skin, lungs and amniotic membrane. An adequate volume of amniotic fluid is necessary for the normal development of the lungs, facial morphology and limbs.

The kidney is in a state of water diuresis. Sodium is resorbed increasingly with maturation. Its content in amniotic fluid decreases from 120 mmol/l at 20 weeks to 50 mmol/l at term. Glomerular tubular imbalance is present due to the reabsorptive capacity of the relatively smaller and more immature tubules being exceeded by the glomerular filtrate delivered to them. This is a developmental feature and the absence of glucose, phosphate and amino acid in amniotic fluid by term is indicative of tubular maturation.

CONGENITAL ABNORMALITIES OF THE KIDNEY AND URINARY TRACT

The overall frequency of major and minor congenital abnormality of the kidneys and urinary tract is of the order of 10% and a small

Table 5.105   Causes of an upper abdominal mass in the newborn

1. Multicystic kidney
2. Polycystic kidneys
3. Adrenal hemorrhage
4. Hydronephrosis
5. Renal vein thrombosis
6. Renal tumor
7. Left lobe of liver
8. Splenomegaly
9. Gastric reduplication
10. Ovarian cysts and tumors

increase in this figure is seen where a single umbilical artery is present. Many will be palpable and detected during routine clinical examination of the newborn (Table 5.105). Three-quarters of major renal malformations have major malformations in other systems. Likewise approximately one-third of anorectal, one-quarter of cardiac and one-fifth of spinal malformations have an accompanying urinary tract or renal anomaly.

Renal abnormalities may be classified as those of size and position or as abnormalities of differentiation.

Urinary tract abnormalities involve obstruction or embryological malformation of ureters, bladder or urethra. Obstruction of any part of the urinary tract during nephrogenesis will lead to an associated renal abnormality, usually of differentiation. The earliest obstructions have the most severe effect.

Renal abnormalities of size and position

Bilateral renal agenesis

This has a frequency of 1 per 5000 births and is usually sporadic. The postulated cause is a failure of renal induction by the ureteric branchings. The diagnosis may be made antenatally by ultrasound following the detection of oligohydramnios.

The condition is a major cause of the Potter syndrome of facial dysmorphism, pulmonary hypoplasia and abnormality of the limbs which results from a lack of amniotic fluid during the second and third trimesters of pregnancy. The facial characteristics include deformed and low-set ears, squashed beaked nose, epicanthic folds, hypomandibulosis and a rounded head.

Although biochemistry of the infant is normal at birth owing to the function of the placenta, death generally occurs shortly after birth from pulmonary insufficiency.

Unilateral renal agenesis

With a frequency of 1 per 1000, this is not associated with symptoms and is mostly found by accident.

Renal hypoplasia

This is defined when only five-eighths or less of a kidney is present and has a unilateral frequency of 1 per 500. Although rare in a bilateral form it may account for up to 20% of cases of renal failure in infants and children. The Ask-Upmark kidney is a particular example where hypoplasia of segmental type is found in association with a deep transverse scar. This may cause hypertension in later childhood.

Oligomeganephronia

This is a very rare form of bilateral hypoplasia which presents with renal insufficiency, polyuria and dehydration in the first weeks of life. It is characterized by a paucity of nephrons which are seen to be greatly enlarged at histology. The etiology is thought to be a failure of development of the later generations of nephrons.

Horseshoe kidney

This anomaly results from early fusion of the two kidneys which thus remain pelvic in position and palpable as a firm mass. The ureters are in an anterior relationship which may lead to obstruction and urinary infection.

Ectopic kidney

An ectopic kidney may be pelvic on its normal side, crossed to its opposite side or even fused to the contralateral kidney. The organ is often discoid in shape and may also present as a mass or with infection.

Renal abnormalities of differentiation

Polycystic kidney disease (PCK)

These conditions are genetic and affect both kidneys equally and diffusely. The liver is also commonly affected by cyst formation. Two distinct patterns are recognized.

Autosomal recessive polycystic kidney disease (ARPKD), formerly described as infantile polycystic kidney disease is well developed by birth and has a frequency of 1 in 6000 to 1 in 40 000. There may be renal enlargement sufficient to obstruct normal labor whilst poor production of urine may have led to Potter's syndrome. Cases can be detected in utero by ultrasonography.

The kidneys are easily felt on abdominal palpation. Confirmation of diagnosis is by renal and liver ultrasound. Intravenous urography should demonstrate the characteristic dilated collecting ducts radiating laterally from the renal pelves but films may be of poor quality due to impaired function.

The immediate prognosis at birth will depend on the pulmonary status but thereafter the degree of renal function available must be assessed and the management of chronic renal failure and its complications instituted as appropriate. In a proportion of cases early progress may be reasonably satisfactory only for esophageal bleeding to occur secondary to hepatic fibrosis and portal hypertension and it is not yet clear whether or not this is a separate diagnostic category. Renal size may diminish with age due to fibrosis. Half the affected children are alive at 10 years but of those surviving the first year, three-quarters attain the age of 15 (Kaplan et al 1989).

Autosomal dominant polycystic kidney disease (ADPKD), or adult polycystic kidney disease is more common with a frequency of 1 in 200 to 1 in 1000. The abnormal gene is found on chromosome 6. Small cysts are occasionally detectable at birth by ultrasonography. Signs and symptoms typically found later in life such as abdominal mass, urinary infection, hematuria or hypertension are uncommon but have been described (Cole et al 1987). Pediatricians specifically asked for a diagnosis in affected families should refer to a geneticist for application of a genetic probe rather than depend on ultrasound alone. Investigation is best deferred to 18 years of age in members of affected families and proven cases followed up for the development of hypertension.

Renal dysplasia

This term implies the presence within the renal substance of abnormal tissue and includes cysts lined with columnar epithelium, fibrous tissue, cartilage and other embryonic rests. The condition results from obstruction to the urinary tract during early renal development. The kidneys may be totally nonfunctioning or show severe impairment, and may be associated with posterior urethral valves, prune belly or other forms of obstructive uropathy.

The large multicystic kidney is one manifestation of this type of dysplasia and may be detected in utero by ultrasonography and postnatally by palpation of the abdominal mass. The cysts are large, smooth and variable in size. The kidney is nonfunctional. If there is no doubt as to the diagnosis and the kidney is not too large, it may be left to atrophy in situ. Otherwise surgical removal is undertaken.

The small button kidney as the name suggests is a tiny nonfunctional nub of dense cystic tissue, sometimes classified as aplasia. The condition when unilateral is usually discovered fortuitously as for example during investigation for urinary infection when an associated gross and longstanding intrauterine vesicoureteric reflux may also be found. Indeed the prenatal determination of renal dysplasia by vesicoureteric reflux may account for many of the scars found on cortical scanning after urinary tract infection and hitherto ascribed to infection (Risdon 1987).

Syndromic cystic disease

An increasing number of recognizable syndromes feature cortical or medullary cysts (Table 5.106). In only a few of these are renal symptoms of early significance. These include the survivors of Jeune's asphyxiating thoracic dystrophy and tuberous sclerosis.

Table 5.106 Recognized syndromes involving renal cystic disease

1. Trisomies 13 and 18
2. Triploidy
3. Meckel–Gruber
4. Zellweger
5. Laurence–Moon–Biedl
6. Jeune
7. Roberts
8. Tuberous sclerosis
9. Nail–patella
10. Orofacial–digital
11. Beckwith

Medullary cystic disease (familial juvenile nephronophthisis)

This may be inherited as either autosomal dominant or recessive and is an important cause of chronic renal failure early in childhood. Its particular characteristics are hyposthenuria and profound anemia. Retinal changes may be present and the diagnosis must be confirmed on renal biopsy when ectasia of the collecting ducts and fibrosis of the interstitium are seen. This condition should not be confused with the relatively harmless medullary sponge kidneys of later life.

Microcystic disease

Microcystic disease is so named on the basis of its ultrasonographic and pathological findings and causes a congenital nephrotic syndrome (see below).

Congenital mesoblastic nephroma

This tumor of the neonate is formed from fibroblasts or myofibroblasts with entrapped nephrons and presents as a firm solid infiltrative mass within the kidney. It is usually single and not malignant and is therefore best treated by simple removal. Exceptionally a particularly cellular growth should receive chemotherapy as for Wilms' tumor.

Renal abnormalities due to obstruction

Hydronephrosis

Dilation of the renal pelvis may be due to any anatomical or functional obstruction within the urinary tract. The diagnosis is most easily confirmed by ultrasonography both before and after birth. In each instance it is important to identify and assess the function of the contralateral kidney as bilateral involvement is common. The site of obstruction must be identified.

Pelviureteric junction (PUJ) obstruction may be due to a fibrous band or to an aberrant renal artery supplying the lower pole. The degree of obstruction may be assessed postnatally by ultrasonography following a water load. If immediate release of obstruction is felt to be necessary to preserve function, nephrostomy or insertion of a pigtail drain will allow pyeloplasty to be delayed beyond early infancy.

Vesicoureteric junction (VUJ) obstruction may occur at the ureteric insertion into the bladder or be due to a ureterocele perhaps in association with a duplex drainage system.

Vesicoureteric reflux may be secondary to urethral or neurogenic obstruction as defined below. Raised intravesical pressure can lead to major upper urinary tract dilation. Primary reflux may also cause hydronephrosis.

Megacystis–megaureter is the result of longstanding intrauterine vesicoureteric reflux without obstruction. Gross dilation of the bladder, ureters and renal pelves is found and there is a generalized flaccidity within the urinary tract.

Whatever the type of obstruction it should be remembered that there may be associated renal dysplasia, interference with urinary concentrating ability and a vulnerability to urinary infection.

Posterior urethral valves

This problem occurs only in males and although of varying severity it is usually detectable at birth or even during prenatal ultrasonography. The valves comprise an incomplete membrane across the proximal urethra with resultant proximal urethral dilation, thickening, hypertrophy and palpable enlargement of the bladder. There is a variable degree of ureteral dilation and renal dysplasia dependent on the presence and severity of vesicoureteric reflux.

Presentation is by the observation of a poor stream on micturition, the palpation of persistent bladder enlargement or urinary infection. In particularly severe examples a Potter facies may be apparent. Diagnosis should be apparent with ultrasound examination but it is normally confirmed by micturating cystourethrography with lateral views. Transurethral fulguration is the usual treatment but drainage of the upper urinary tract by nephrostomy may also be required. The long-term outcome depends on the remaining renal function and the early initiation of treatment for chronic renal failure.

Triad (prune belly) syndrome

This is an association of dilation of the urinary tract with hypoplasia of the abdominal musculature and ectopic testes. Antenatal findings with ultrasound now strongly support the theory that severe urethral obstruction in early embryogenesis is the cause. Gross fusiform dilation of the penile urethra has been described and presumed to be due to a delay in the joining of the penile portion of the urethra with the glandular portion which has a separate embryological origin. The severe abdominal distention with muscular hypoplasia and failure of testicular descent are secondary to massive dilation of the renal pelves, ureters and bladder. After the urethra has canalized the penis assumes a more regular appearance but in many cases is abnormally small at birth.

Diagnosis is straightforward on the basis of the wrinkled and flaccid appearance of the abdomen with visceroptosis and impalpable testes. Gross urinary tract dilation is shown on ultrasound. The long-term outcome again depends on the degree of renal dysplasia and the remaining renal function together with the early initiation of treatment for chronic renal failure as appropriate.

Other abnormalities of the urinary tract

Double ureters

These have a frequency as high as 2%, may be bilateral and are best classified as either bifid or duplex.

Bifid ureters have twin pelves at a renal level but meet at a variable point in the manner of a 'Y' prior to insertion in the bladder. There is a tendency for a yo-yo movement of urine between the two upper arms and this leads to infection and renal scar formation.

Duplex ureters remain separate until their insertion into the bladder but cross each other along their course. The lower-pole ureter is inserted at the usual site but may be associated with vesicoureteric reflux which tends not to undergo spontaneous resolution. The upper-pole ureter terminates ectopically and variably in the trigone, lower bladder or into the urethra either above or below the internal sphincter. Obstruction of the ectopic ureter may lead to hydronephrosis affecting the upper pole alone. Infection produces a pyonephrosis. Tight obstruction causes a cyst-like swelling palpable on abdominal examination. In the event of insertion distal to the sphincter a ureterocele is formed which may lead to total urethral obstruction.

Ureterocele

This is a dilation of the terminal part of the ureter.

Simple ureterocele. Simple ureterocele is caused by obstruction at the vesicoureteric junction of a normally situated ureteric orifice.

Ectopic ureterocele. Ectopic ureteroceles are formed as described above. Diagnosis is best by ultrasonography but a double shadow in the bladder is typical both on IVU and MCU. Ectopic ureteroceles are likely to be the most troublesome causing bladder outlet obstruction. If they are of long standing, obstructive nephropathy will be present. Surgical treatment is required.

Hypospadias

This is an abnormal emergence of the urethra onto the ventral surface of the penis resulting from a deficiency in anterior urethral development. The frequency in boys is of the order of 0.5% and there is a familial tendency. The majority involve the distal or medial shaft and the ectopic urethral meatus is not associated with other anomalies in these cases.

Parents are exceedingly upset by the condition and need reassurance particularly with regard to eventual sexual function.

Treatment is surgical with the MAGPI (meatal advancement, glanduloplasty) procedure being performed later in the first year in these uncomplicated cases.

Approximately 20% have a posterior outlet and should be investigated for upper urinary tract anomaly, inguinal hernia, undescended testes and intersex. Chromosomes should be analyzed. This group with proximal outlets and associated chordee (fibrosis and ventral concavity) require a more specialized surgical approach (Sheldon & Duckett 1987).

Exstrophy of the bladder and epispadias

These comprise a spectrum due to abnormal development of the cloacal membrane. They are rare anomalies with incidences of 1 per 30 000 and 1 per 120 000 respectively and a male : female sex ratio of 2.5 : 1. These are reviewed by Jeffs (1987).

Exstrophy. Exstrophy of the bladder is obvious on inspection with defects of the abdominal wall and penile epispadias being found. Separation of the pubic rami is visible on X-ray. The neonatologist must arrange immediate transfer to a specialist center. Meanwhile the bladder mucosa is protected by soaks of normal saline. The best results are obtained when closure is achieved within the first 24 h.

Sexual assignment can be difficult. Only minute amounts of phallic tissue may be present in some males and it would be preferable to assign a female gender.

Epispadias. This is found in both sexes as an isolated lesion. In the male the urethral outlet is proximal and dorsal, in the female it is anterior to the clitoris and causes constant dribbling.

Cloacal exstrophy. Cloacal exstrophy is the most severe example of this spectrum comprising anal and rectal anomalies as well as the bladder and urethral defects. There is also a higher incidence of upper urinary tract maldevelopment.

Antenatal diagnosis of urinary tract abnormality

Antenatal ultrasonography of the mother is now widely practiced and has lead to the diagnosis in utero of a wide variety of congenital defects of which urinary tract anomalies comprise a large part and have a frequency of about 0.2% (Colodny 1987).

The kidneys and bladder may be visualized from the 15th week onwards. A positive family history, oligo- and polyhydramnios are indications for a close examination. Hydronephrosis and other obstructive lesions are most common, one-third of the former being due to PUJ.

The severity of obstructive nephropathy may be reflected by amniotic fluid concentrations of sodium above the normal for the period of gestation. The temptation to treat such obstructions by the insertion of drains from the viscus into the amniotic fluid has lead to disappointing results with frequent fetal loss, chorioamnionitis and intestinal perforation. Misdiagnosis has also been surprisingly common. The results of early treatment of obstructions associated with the Potter syndrome have been particularly disappointing and the failure of pulmonary development after treatment has given rise to speculation that the fetal kidney may secrete substances which promote pulmonary development. Poor prognostic features include early detection, high grade obstruction, bilateral disease, hyperechoic characteristics of dysplasia on ultrasound and oligohydramnios.

Thus the decision to treat is difficult on medical as well as ethical grounds. If treatment is to be attempted then only bilateral progressive and destructive cases with oligohydramnios ought to be considered. However, it is noted that 80% of obstructive anomalies suspected antenatally are asymptomatic at birth. (Estes & Harrison 1993). Infants shown to have vesicoureteric reflux are particularly at risk in view of the relationship with dysplasia and the risks of subsequent infection. (Anderson & Rickwood 1991).

All cases require postnatal follow-up with urinalysis, culture, ultrasound and functional assessment. Prophylactic antibiotics, e.g. trimethoprim 1–2 mg/kg nocte, may be required until the problem is resolved.

DEVELOPMENT OF RENAL FUNCTION AFTER BIRTH

Glomerular filtration rate (GFR)

The GFR at birth is directly proportional to gestation. There is an immediate increase in the first few days after birth depending on factors which include renal plasma flow and its distribution, perfusion pressure and basement membrane permeability. The rate of postnatal increase in GFR is linear but is less rapid in the preterm. Even after correction for surface area, values comparable to the adult may not be reached until 1 year. Limited delivery of water, sodium, phosphate and acid radicals to the tubules also restricts the excretory capacity of the kidneys for these substances. These principles are important when drugs eliminated by the kidneys are prescribed. Values are shown in Table 5.107.

Renal tubular function

Sodium reabsorption

Prior to birth urinary sodium content is high for all fetuses but declines logarithmically with gestation. Fractional excretion of sodium, FE_{Na}, at birth varies from 3% at term to between 5 and 15% in extremely low birthweight infants (ELBW).

In all infants FE_{Na} falls after delivery due to increasing activity

Table 5.107   Glomerular filtration rates and plasma creatinine (P^{Cr}) values

Weeks		After 1 week	1 month	After 2 months
25–28	GFR (ml/min/1.73 m^2)	11	15	50
	GFR (ml/min)	0.6	0.9	6
	P^{Cr} (μmol/l)	123	80	35
29–34	GFR (ml/min/1.73 m^2)	15	30	50
	GFR (ml/min)	1.2	2.5	11
	P^{Cr} (μmol/l)	80	62	35
38+	GFR (ml/min/1.73 m^2)	41	66	96
	GFR (ml/min)	5	11	21
	P^{Cr} (μmol/l)	44	35	35

Figures for GFR derive from creatinine clearance. For routine clinical purposes a reasonable guide to GFR is available from the formula:

$$\text{GFR (ml/min/1.73 m}^2\text{)} = k \times \text{length (cm)}/P^{\text{creatinine}}\ (\mu mol/l)$$

Values for k of 30 for infants of 25–34 weeks' gestation and 40 for term infants are applicable for the rest of the first year. (Data from Schwartz et al 1987). Average surface areas are 0.1 m^2 at 1.0 kg body weight and 0.2 m^2 in a 3.5 kg infant at term.

of the renin–angiotensin–aldosterone system (RAAS) which facilitates distal tubular sodium reabsorption. Soon there is a net retention of sodium which is needed for growth.

The degree and rate of fall of FE^{Na} also varies with gestational age. In term infants it drops to below 0.3% in 3 days. In preterm low birthweight (LBW) infants it may remain between 1 and 5% over the first week of life despite negative sodium balance and ELBW infants' FE^{Na} of 5–15% may be sustained for several weeks with consequent severe sodium loss. These features are due to tubular immaturity related to the development of Na/K ATPase-dependent reabsorptive pathways and to distal tubular unresponsiveness to RAAS.

Conversely the natriuretic response to a sodium load is sluggish and care is required not to overload infants of any gestation with saline drips or sodium supplements.

Urinary dilution and concentration

The capacity to dilute the urine is well developed both in term and preterm infants with urinary concentration as low as 40 mosmol/kg being achieved. However, free water excretion in response to a water load is blunted.

Urinary concentrating ability is also well developed at birth in term babies, a response to arginine-vasopressin of 400–500 mosmol/kg being rapidly achieved. Thereafter the limiting factor appears to be the availability of solute for the countercurrent multiplier and the establishment of medullary hypertonicity.

Urinary concentrating ability is much less well established in LBW and ELBW infants where maximum values of under 350 mosmol/kg only are obtained and represent a threat to water balance should a dehydration stress occur.

Syndrome of inappropriate antidiuretic hormone secretion (SIADH). This results in water retention and cerebral swelling and can occur in the newborn as a response to cerebral injury, meningitis or asphyxia. The diagnosis is made by the finding of urinary concentration greater than plasma whilst there is plasma hypotonicity. Treatment is by fluid restriction to 50–75% of requirements for hyponatremia and by i.v. mannitol for cerebral edema.

Sodium, water and the diuresis

Urine concentration increases and volume decreases immediately after birth because of the release of antidiuretic hormone (ADH) triggered by the stress of delivery.

The initial oliguria for 24–36 h is followed by a diuresis as the extracellular fluid (ECF) compartment diminishes by a total of 3% and 5% or more in term and LBW infants, respectively. This loss may be mediated by atrial natriuretic polypeptide (ANP) and is accompanied by continuing sodium excretion and a temporary increase in FE^{Na} (Kojima et al 1987).

In term infants the diuresis may be imperceptible and then FE^{Na} falls rapidly. In preterms the diuresis is proportionately larger and longer. The reduction in body water and the ECF may be a necessary stimulus for the kidney to assume its final role in the net conservation of sodium which is a feature of both renal maturity and growth of the infant.

In preterm infants with respiratory distress syndrome sodium retention persists and the diuresis is delayed. Respiratory improvement is accompanied by the onset of diuresis and Modi (1988) has suggested that changes in pulmonary function and dynamics initiate the diuresis by a mechanism involving ANP. Infants with RDS and a delay in diuresis beyond 72 h are more likely to develop bronchopulmonary dysplasia.

Bicarbonate reabsorption

There is a reduced bicarbonate threshold in the newborn which is more marked in the preterm. Plasma bicarbonate is 18–20 mmol/l, some 4–6 mmol/l lower than adults. Maximum net acid excretion is limited in preterms during the first weeks as there is a direct relationship between ammonia synthesis and gestational age. However, the ability to generate an acid urine in response to an acid load is well developed and acid–base homeostasis is well maintained in the absence of hypoxia or high protein feeds.

Glucose reabsorption

Normal term babies have no glycosuria when normoglycemic. Significant glycosuria was seen in the majority of preterms at plasma concentrations of 8.3 mmol/l in a study by Stonestreet et al (1980) and renal thresholds as low as 5.5 mmol/l have been shown in tiny preterms presumably due to nephron heterogeneity and splay. After birth the increase in maximal tubular reabsorption of glucose corresponds to GFR.

Phosphate reabsorption

Fractional excretion of phosphate is higher in the first week in preterm as compared to full-term infants but is low in both thereafter as would be appropriate for growth. Subsequent development is also related to increases in GFR.

DISORDERS OF FUNCTION

Acute renal failure

93% of infants pass urine in the first day and 99.5% by 2 days. A diagnosis of acute renal failure (ARF) is made when electrolyte and water homeostasis cannot be sustained. In practice a rise in plasma creatinine greater than 2 SD above normal for age will be diagnostic. Normal values at 1 week are shown in Table 5.107. Renal failure might also be assumed where urine volume fails to exceed 1 ml/kg/h but up to 25% of neonatal ARF may be polyuric.

Etiology

Recognized causes are indicated in Table 5.108. Up to 6–7% of admissions to neonatal units may have ARF.

Prerenal failure. 75% of cases of ARF in neonates are prerenal. Usually hypovolemia has led to oliguria and a rise in plasma urea but an immediate return to normal function can be anticipated following rehydration.

Intrinsic renal failure. This is excluded by the finding of FE^{Na} less than 2.5% or urine/plasma osmolality ratio greater than 1, i.e. features of prerenal failure. In practice all infants can be given an i.v. fluid load of 10–20 ml/kg 5% dextrose together with 2 mg/kg frusemide. The patients are catheterized and a continuing lack of urine will confirm a diagnosis of intrinsic renal failure as discussed below.

Postrenal or obstructive failure. Total anuria suggests a diagnosis of postrenal or obstructive failure and this is confirmed by ultrasonography which should be carried out in all cases of ARF.

Table 5.108 Renal failure in the neonate

1. Prerenal
   a. Hypotension, poor perfusion
      (i) Respiratory distress syndrome
      (ii) Antepartum hemorrhage
      (iii) Fetomaternal transfusion
      (iv) Twin-to-twin transfusion
   b. Cardiac surgery
   c. Heart failure
   d. Asphyxia
   e. Dehydration

2. Intrinsic renal failure
   a. Congenital abnormalities
      (i) Polycystic kidneys
      (ii) Dysplasia
      (iii) Hypoplasia
   b. Vascular
      (i) Renal cortical necrosis
      (ii) Renal venous thrombosis
      (iii) Renal arterial thrombosis
      (iv) Disseminated intravascular coagulation
   c. Acute tubular necrosis
      (i) Respiratory distress syndrome
      (ii) Asphyxia
      (iii) Dehydration
      (iv) Poor perfusion
      (v) Cardiac surgery
   d. Interstitial nephritis
   e. Infections
      (i) Urinary tract infection
      (ii) Congenital infections

3. Postrenal
   a. Hydronephrosis
   b. Neurogenic bladder
   c. Posterior urethral valves
   d. Ureterocele
   e. Urethral obstruction
   f. Meatal/foreskin obstruction
   g. External pressure
      (i) Sacrococcygeal tumor

Clinical features of intrinsic renal failure

These are dominated by the causative illness but hypertension, blood pressure > 90/65 at term and > 80/45 preterm, edema and abdominal masses should be sought. Abdominal ascites is a feature in obstructive uropathy.

Acute tubular necrosis (ATN). This is the most common example of intrinsic failure to result from poor perfusion in the neonate. Ultrasonography shows mild bilateral renal enlargement and hyperechoic medullary pyramids. Histological findings vary from a few breaks in tubular epithelium to the absolutely normal! The period of oliguria is variable but full recovery of function can be anticipated.

Renal cortical necrosis. Renal cortical necrosis may occur alone or as a result of arterial and venous occlusion. Histologically there are diffuse or patchy ischemic changes in the nephron. Calcification in the cortex may be seen in survivors on ultrasonography or X-ray.

Renal vein thrombosis. Renal vein thrombosis is the more common form of the two renovascular problems and is often associated with the hypercoagulability which accompanies asphyxia, hyperosmolar dehydration, polycythemia and the nephrotic syndrome at all ages. It is more common in infants of diabetic mothers. Clinically there is an enlarged kidney, hematuria and proteinuria, and often hematological evidence of intravascular coagulation such as consumption coagulopathy and raised FDPs.

Renal arterial thrombosis. This may be a sequel to sepsis, umbilical arterial catheterization and traumatic interventional procedures on the kidneys such as transcutaneous nephrostomy. Hypercoagulable states may also be present.

In the renovascular disorders lack of renal perfusion is best shown by Doppler ultrasonography or isotope renograms which will also reveal congenital renal artery stenoses where present. Hypertension is frequent and ultimately may only respond to nephrectomy.

Management of intrinsic renal failure

A catheter is inserted initially to allow assessment of urine flow rates but is removed as soon as practicable. Urine is sent for qualitative analysis, electrolytes and culture. Blood is taken for creatinine, urea and electrolytes, acid/base, hematology including coagulation studies and culture. Chest X-ray and ECG are obtained and heart rate, respiratory rate, blood pressure and fluid balance are monitored carefully. A CVP line should be considered.

Particular problems which may be met relate to the following.

Hydration. Many infants have substantial edema by the time diagnosis is made yet treatment for associated conditions may lead to continued fluid administration. These infants may require hypertonic peritoneal dialysis (PD) or extracorporeal hemofiltration to remove water. If dialysis is not required, fluids are administered as saline of similar sodium concentration to urine to replace urinary losses and as 10% dextrose to replace insensible water losses. Insensible water losses are increased by prematurity, fever, radiant heaters, phototherapy and diarrhea but decreased by ventilation.

Hyperkalemia. Coexisting multisystem failure exacerbates hyperkalemia in many cases of ARF. The newborn is more resistant to hyperkalemia than older age groups but there is a clear threat to life through cardiac toxicity when high peaked T-waves and widening of the QRS complex are present. All potassium-containing fluids and drugs should be discontinued. Cardiotoxicity is minimized by correction of acid–base balance and any calcium abnormality. Moderate hyperkalemia of 6.5–7.5 mmol/l with mild ECG changes such as peaked T-waves may be treated by i.v. 8.4% sodium bicarbonate 2 ml (2 mmol)/kg given slowly over 10–15 min and a small but temporary reduction of concentration achieved. Extreme hyperkalemia with potassium levels in excess of 7.5–8.0 mmol/l may cause more ominous cardiotoxicity with a widened QRS complex. This may be alleviated by i.v. 10% calcium gluconate, 0.5 ml (0.1125 mmol)/kg given slowly over 10–15 min. Potassium concentration is temporarily reduced by administration of insulin 0.1 unit/kg together with glucose 1 g/kg. Neither method removes potassium from the body. Calcium resonium 1 g/kg inserted rectally for 3–4 h effects a modest removal but is a messy procedure and PD or hemofiltration should be considered dependent on further progress of the infant.

Acidosis. This is treated by i.v. infusion over 12 h of 8.4% sodium bicarbonate calculated as base deficit × 0.3 × kg bodyweight.

Hypertension. In this age group hypertension is most commonly caused by volume overload which may therefore become an indication for dialysis. Extremes of pressure can be treated with labetalol 1–3 mg/kg/h i.v. or diazoxide 5 mg/kg given rapidly i.v. Otherwise drugs referred to under chronic renal failure should be utilized.

Other problems. Infection, hypocalcemia, hyperphosphatemia and anemia may be anticipated and are treated symptomatically.

Dialysis and hemofiltration

Peritoneal dialysis is the treatment of choice in small infants. Recommended catheters include the short soft Pendlebury inserted under local anesthetic using a Seldinger technique and if prolonged anuria is anticipated a conventional Silastic Tenchoff placed surgically. Edema is removed by hypertonic (2.2% glucose or greater) dialysate and, with decreasing efficiency, potassium, hydrogen ion, urea and phosphate. The method is safe and efficient but is unsuitable where necrotizing enterocolitis or transperitoneal abdominal operations may have occurred. The technique in very small infants is discussed by Steele et al (1987).

Extracorporeal hemofiltration has been utilized for neonates in a number of centers but although helpful, mortality has been high because of the severity of the conditions or disease underlying the renal failure. Vascular access is established from any artery including the umbilical and a bloodline led to a low volume hemoperfusion membrane. Ultrafiltration of plasma takes place and the procedure is particularly efficient with regard to fluid removal. Hemofiltration is discussed by Pascual et al (1987).

Prognosis

When ATN has occurred oliguria may be as short as 24 h but periods of up to 2–3 weeks have been described before diuresis and its attendant electrolyte losses ensue.

When cortical necrosis has occurred whether due to shock, toxemia or renal vascular disease only partial recovery of function may be expected. This diagnosis is suggested by prolonged oliguria and the appearance of calcification on ultrasonography or X-ray, and should eventually be confirmed by biopsy. Chronic renal failure is the most likely outcome.

A relationship has been shown in the asphyxiated newborn infant between the severity of the renal injury and the neurological outcome (Perlman & Tack 1988). Whatever the renal classification, however, mortality in the acute phase is high from the associated conditions.

Chronic renal failure

Chronic renal failure (CRF) will not be apparent in the first few days of life owing to placental clearance of the waste products of metabolism. Maternally derived high plasma creatinine values normally clear after the first 48–72 h and a persistent elevation beyond this time above the normal 30–40 μmol/l for term infants will become diagnostic.

The major etiologies of chronic renal failure in the neonatal period include the obstructive uropathies, recessive PCK and renal hypoplasia. These conditions often display an obligatory water-losing state accompanied by salt loss and hypertension is rare as a consequence of this. The provision of extra water and electrolyte is essential in many cases.

Conversely where CRF is due to cortical necrosis, for instance after hemorrhagic or septic shock, then oliguria, raised circulating volumes and hypertension are to be expected.

Whilst general supportive measures may preserve life, delay in the provision of adequate energy or of renal replacement therapy may irreversibly impair the potential for both physical and intellectual growth even by the end of the first year. Decisions about feeding routines and/or dialysis require the full awareness, agreement, education and cooperation of parents and community services as well as the hospital staff.

The major problems which will be encountered in management include nutrition, hydration, acidosis, hyponatremia and hypokalemia, bone disease, hypertension and anemia. These issues along with the indications and techniques for dialysis and transplantation are discussed in Chapter 17, pp. 980–1.

Renal tubular disorders

The proximal tubule is responsible for the isotonic reabsorption of 80% of the filtrate content of chloride, sodium and water, and also of phosphate, glucose and amino acids. It contributes to acid–base homeostasis by the regeneration and reabsorption of bicarbonate with the aid of brush border carbonic anhydrase, and by the secretion of hydrogen ion.

The loop of Henle is concerned with the establishment of renal medullary hypertonicity and the dilution of urine.

The distal tubule reabsorbs sodium in an exchange for potassium and/or hydrogen ion and is stimulated by aldosterone and the renin–angiotensin system (RAAS). Further water is reabsorbed.

The collecting duct and antidiuretic hormone (ADH) determine the final concentration of urine and therefore of the amount of urine passed in health.

As the absorptive pathways are genetically determined a variety of congenital disorders of isolated tubular functions occur in addition to those problems caused by more widespread congenital or acquired renal damage (Table 5.109). Only those likely to be found in the neonate are discussed here.

Renal tubular acidosis. This is by definition only found in children with normal glomerular function and is typified by a hypokalemic hyperchloremic metabolic acidosis. Thus the anion

Table 5.109 Examples of renal tubular dysfunction

	Genetics
1. Specific	
a. Primary proximal renal tubular acidosis	Various
b. Primary distal renal tubular acidosis	Various
c. Congenital nephrogenic diabetes insipidus	X-linked recessive
d. Familial hypophosphatemia	X-linked dominant
e. Cystinuria	Autosomal recessive
f. Hartnup disease	Autosomal recessive
g. Renal glucosuria	Autosomal dominant
h. Bartter's syndrome	Sporadic
2. Generalized	
a. Cystinosis	Autosomal recessive
b. Galactosemia	Autosomal recessive
c. Tyrosinemia	Autosomal recessive
d. Hereditary fructose intolerance	Autosomal recessive
e. Lowe's syndrome	X-linked recessive
f. Interstitial nephritis	Acquired
g. Medullary cystic disease	Autosomal recessive
h. Heavy metal poisons	Acquired
i. Heavy proteinuria	Acquired
j. Hyperparathyroidism	Acquired

gap is normal ($[Na] - [Cl] - [HCO_3] < 12$ mmol/l). Most cases are sporadic but both autosomal dominant and recessive families have been described in each of the two major types. Symptoms may begin from a few weeks to a few years of age. Diagnosis is reviewed by Chan (1983).

Proximal renal tubular acidosis (RTA type 2) results from a defect in the reabsorption of sodium bicarbonate and there is in effect a reduced bicarbonate threshold. Clinically the infants fail to gain weight and exhibit signs of muscle weakness. Glycosuria and generalized aminoaciduria may also be present. Hypercalciuria is not a feature and thus nephrocalcinosis is rare. The bicarbonate leak is confirmed by an assessment of the fractional excretion of bicarbonate which exceeds 15% (normal < 5%). Urine pH may fall below 5.5 in response to an acid load, e.g. NH_4Cl 0.1 g/kg orally stat. Treatment is by generous supplements of sodium bicarbonate 2–15 mmol/kg/24 h which also causes a requirement for additional potassium supplementation.

Secondary proximal renal tubular acidosis is also seen in infancy as a developmental problem in some babies fed on high protein formulae, i.e. late metabolic acidosis of infancy, and when tubular damage has occurred in Lowe's syndrome, cystinosis, tyrosinosis and galactosemia.

Distal renal tubular acidosis (RTA type 1) results from a defect in hydrogen ion secretion in the distal convoluted tubule and a failure to maintain a pH gradient between the tubular cells and the filtrate. Failure to thrive and weakness are marked. Glycosuria and generalized aminoaciduria are not seen but nephrocalcinosis may ensue later and is the limiting factor to prognosis. The fractional excretion of bicarbonate is normal, less than 5%, but urine pH does not fall below 5.5 in response to an acid load. Treatment is by bicarbonate supplements 2–10 mmol/kg/24 h sufficient to correct systemic acidosis.

Secondary distal renal tubular acidosis is seen in later life.

Renal tubular acidosis type 3 is a mixed form of types 1 and 2. And is often seen as a transient defect. The proximal tubular disorder tends to predominate.

Renal tubular acidosis type 4 is misnamed and due to congenital hypoaldosteronism (both true and pseudo), i.e. end-

organ failure. Thus it is characterized by hyperkalemia as well as hyperchloremia and acidosis. Some cases are associated with obstructive uropathy. Treatment is with dietary potassium restriction and a potassium-losing diuretic such as frusemide. Sodium bicarbonate may also be indicated.

Bartter's syndrome. This appears to be due to a failure of proximal tubular reabsorption of chloride and therefore also of sodium. The physiological outcome is profound hypokalemia with metabolic alkalosis, polyuria with dehydration, activation of RAAS and prostaglandin synthesis, and hyponatremia. The clinical outcome is a constipated, weak and dry infant with marked growth failure. The condition may be mimicked by magnesium- or calcium-losing tubulopathies and the differential diagnosis is from other potassium-losing tubulopathies and from chloride-losing diarrhea (Linshaw 1987). Treatment is with heavy potassium supplementation, the need for which may be reduced by prostaglandin-synthetase inhibitors.

Congenital nephrogenic diabetes insipidus. This is an X-linked failure of the distal nephron to respond to antidiuretic hormone. There is a failure to produce or release cyclic adenosine monophosphate following desmopressin (DDAVP) administration. Male infants present with severe hypernatremic dehydration and shock and will rapidly succumb unless given substantial fluid replacement. Diagnosis of diabetes insipidus is first made by the demonstration of a failure to concentrate the urine up to plasma in the face of a supervised weight loss of 5% achieved by thirsting, i.e. to 300 mmol/kg. The nephrogenic nature is confirmed by a failure to respond to intranasal desmopressin 2 μg. Differential diagnosis is from central diabetes insipidus, other tubulopathies and any congenital or acquired pathology affecting the renal medulla, the countercurrent multiplier and the establishment of medullary hypertonicity. Female infants and carriers are rarely symptomatic but commonly show an impaired concentrating ability on testing. Management comprises the addition of water as 5% dextrose, not milk, to the feeding regimen and can be given by nasogastric tube. The quantity of fluid required may paradoxically be reduced by the administration of a proximal tubular diuretic such as hydrochlorothiazide although this causes potassium loss. Long-term problems include hypocaloric growth failure, mental retardation unless repeated episodes of hypernatremia are avoided and dilation of the urinary tract.

Familial hypophosphatemia. Familial hypophosphatemia (vitamin D-resistant rickets, X-linked hypophosphatemia, phosphate diabetes) is the commonest of the inherited forms of rickets and the only one likely to be picked up in the neonatal period on account of the hypophosphatemia. There is a dual defect involving a reduction in the renal tubular reabsorption of phosphate and of the l-alpha hydroxylation of vitamin D. Clinical manifestations of rickets and shortness of stature are not seen at this age but their development may be minimized by the use of a vitamin D analogue and phosphate supplements.

HEMATURIA, PROTEINURIA AND URINARY INFECTION

Neonatal hematuria

Hematuria is a nonspecific but important sign of renal and urinary tract disorder (Table 5.110). Clinical examination should be directed towards the detection of other evidence of bleeding, palpation of abdominal masses (Table 5.105), ascertainment of edema and measurement of blood pressure. Investigations should

Table 5.110 Neonatal hematuria

1. Coagulation disorders
   a. Hemorrhagic disease of the newborn
   b. Thrombocytopenia
   c. Disseminated intravascular coagulation

2. Urinary tract infection

3. Acute tubular necrosis

4. Renal vascular disease

5. Neonatal glomerulopathy
   a. Syphilis
   b. Toxoplasmosis
   c. Cytomegalovirus
   d. Nail–patella syndrome

6. Interstitial nephritis
   Drugs (i) aminoglycosides
          (ii) penicillins

7. Obstructive uropathies
   a. Hydronephrosis
   b. Posterior urethral valves

8. Cystic diseases

9. Renal tumors

10. Urethral and meatal abnormality

be performed to exclude disorders of coagulation, urinary infection, congenital abnormality, obstructive nephropathy, renal failure (Table 5.108) and renal damage due to drugs or glomerulonephritis. These will include in the first place urinalysis and culture, estimation of plasma creatinine, urea and electrolytes, immunoglobulin and complement assay coagulation screen, and ultrasonography.

Neonatal proteinuria

The presence of protein is physiological in neonatal urine averaging 500 mg/l at 1 day and falling to an average of 175 mg/l at 5 days. It is found in at least small quantities in all cases of hematuria as shown in Table 5.110. Heavy isolated proteinuria is rare.

The nephrotic syndrome ensues whenever proteinuria (any etiology) is sufficiently heavy to lead to the development of hypoproteinemia and thus to edema and hypercholesterolemia. Protein loss is greater than 40 mg/m^2/h and plasma albumin falls below 25 g/l.

Congenital Nephrotic Syndrome, Finnish type (CNF) is an autosomal recessive condition and can be detected in utero by the finding of raised levels of α-fetoprotein in maternal plasma or in amniotic fluid due to prenatal proteinuria. The first postnatal clue to diagnosis may be the large placenta which exceeds 25% of the infant's typically low birthweight. Edema develops in half the infants by 1 week and in the rest by 3 months. The proteinuria is highly selective in character but steroid resistant. Other aspects of renal function are not initially abnormal, rather the main problems are recurrent infection due to antibody deficiency and failure to thrive due to heavy protein losses. Pathology shows a diffuse cystic dilation of the proximal tubules on microscopy and there is a virtually diagnostic pattern of cortical bright-up on ultrasonography. The condition is due to a fundamental disorder of glomerular basement membrane. Diagnosis is from other causes of nephrotic syndrome or of edema such as congestive heart failure or injudicious fluid and electrolyte management. Symptomatic management is ineffective and the only prospect for survival is dialysis and eventual transplantation. Unilateral or even bilateral nephrectomy may be the only way of effectively controlling the proteinuria, growth failure and recurrent infection.

Other causes of nephrotic syndrome in the neonate include early-onset minimal lesion glomerulopathy, glomerulopathy due to focal glomerulosclerosis or diffuse mesangial sclerosis, glomerulonephritis due to syphilis, toxoplasmosis or cytomegalovirus, nail–patella syndrome (hereditary onycho-osteo dysplasia – HOOD) and severe infantile sialosis. The topic is reviewed by Hoyer & Anderson (1981) and by Mahan et al (1984).

Urinary tract infection

Urinary tract infection (UTI) is found in the neonate with a frequency of 1–2% and a M : F ratio of 2 : 1. The infecting organism is most commonly *E. coli* but other Gram-negative bacteria can be found. The bacteria may be hematogenously acquired unlike in other age groups where ascending infection is the norm. Thus bacteremia is present in more than 60% of cases, and many babies are extremely ill and toxic.

Vulnerability to UTI is often the result of inadequate drainage of urine and the obstructive uropathies and vesicoureteric reflux are therefore important risk factors. UTI is said to be more common in uncircumcised infants (Ginsburg & McCracken 1982). In other cases, however, bacteriuria is asymptomatic and may be due only to pre-foreskin organisms.

Clinical features

Infants can be irritable, febrile, reluctant to feed and liable to vomit in the early stages but then proceed to generalized toxicity and even shock. They are often septicemic and may have infection at other sites including the meninges. Less severe cases present with vomiting, failure to thrive, exacerbation of unconjugated hyperbilirubinemia or more rarely with the well-recognized conjugated hyperbilirubinemia. The nappies may be reported as having a fishy odor.

Diagnosis

This must rest on the finding of more than 10^2 organisms/ml in urine obtained by suprapubic aspiration, or less reliably and particularly in boys on more than 10^5 organisms/ml in clean catch (or, even worse, bag) urine. The finding of pus cells or of protein in the urine is of interest but not of diagnostic value. Hematuria may be present. UTI must be considered in the differential diagnosis of vomiting, failure to thrive, PUO, toxicity and shock and of the various types of jaundice.

Treatment

This must be initiated immediately with a nonnephrotoxic antibiotic i.v. in any but the mildest case. Co-amoxyclav (Augmentin) 25 mg/kg 12-hourly or ceftazidime 12–30 mg/kg 12-hourly would be appropriate. Antibiotics are continued until the results of imaging are known.

Investigation

Immediate investigation once the diagnosis is suspected bacteriologically includes estimation of hemoglobin, white cell and platelet counts and a blood culture. An assessment of overall renal function is best shown by plasma creatinine concentration and urea and electrolytes including bicarbonate.

Imaging in neonatal UTI is mandatory in view of the particular risks associated with vesicoureteric reflux at this age. Ultrasonography will reveal obstruction and significant renal anomaly. Doppler ultrasound will show renal blood flow.

A micturating cystourethrogram is necessary to establish the presence of reflux, but must be delayed until the urine is sterile. Other forms of imaging, e.g. excretory urogram, isotope scan and renogram, may be difficult to interpret in the neonate and can usefully be deferred for several months.

Outcome

Even in the absence of underlying abnormalities recurrence of infection is common so that follow-up of all cases is advised. Cases where vesicoureteric reflux is present should be placed on chemoprophylaxis at least for the first year and then reassessed.

VESICOURETERIC REFLUX AND REFLUX NEPHROPATHY

Introduction

Vesicoureteric reflux is the abnormal retrograde passage of urine from bladder to kidneys due to incompetence of the vesicoureteric junction. It may be primary or secondary to obstruction. The mechanism has long been held to be a shortening of the intramural ureteric segment and a reduction in the ratio between this and its diameter. Primary nonobstructive reflux is a congenital abnormality with a familial element as shown by its finding in around 20% of first degree relatives. The natural history of reflux is of probable spontaneous resolution over 2–5 years in the great majority of milder cases but only in 40% of severe cases with urinary tract dilation. Reflux may be sustained by infection (Roberts et al 1988). Prior to resolution the main associated features are recurrent urinary infection, renal growth failure and most importantly reflux nephropathy.

Diagnosis

Reflux is best demonstrated by a micturating cystourethrogram, usually performed for investigation after UTI. Intrarenal reflux should be carefully sought. Over one-third of children with UTI under 1 year show reflux. Ultrasonography and indirect voiding isotope renograms are less secure means of detection.

Reflux nephropathy

Segmental scars are found in up to a half of the cases of vesicoureteric reflux in the first year and in the long term may cause hypertension, or end-stage renal failure if bilateral.

The majority of scars are formed as a result of urinary infection involving the pyramids and distal nephrons. The 'big bang' theory (Ransley & Risdon 1979) proposes that only one episode of infection is required to create a scar. High pressure sterile reflux is also accepted as a cause in obstruction and in these cases scarring may have been established in utero and indeed there may also be dysplasia. The role of sterile low pressure reflux is controversial but the long-term water hammer effect of repeated bladder contractions and emptyings may be proved important.

The importance of age cannot be overstressed. Whatever the mechanism the younger the patient the more likely it is that scarring will result. This is explained by the pivotal role of intrarenal reflux in the genesis of scarring (Rolleston et al 1970) which is facilitated by the presence of immature compound papillae found only in the first 1–2 years of life or by the distortions due to pre-existing scars. Thus new scars tend not to appear after 5 years of age in previously normal kidneys.

Management

The most important aspect of treatment in the newborn is the maintenance of sterility within the urinary tract. Usually the drugs used to prevent further UTI are the same but in half the dose required for the acute infection. At least monthly follow-up is required. Meanwhile renal function, extent of the nephropathy, blood pressure and growth can also be supervised. This approach protects the kidneys, whilst allowing the reflux to improve spontaneously and the child to grow. Thus if surgery does become indicated on the grounds of failure of medical treatment then the operation of ureteric reimplantation ought to be technically easier. The Birmingham Reflux Study Group (1983) showed no difference of outcome in a prospective trial of operative versus nonoperative treatment even in severe vesicoureteric reflux. Cystoscopic periureteric injection is now undertaken in many centers in this age group (the sting procedure – p. 1794).

EYE PROBLEMS AND THE NEWBORN

A normal visual input is important for a child's development. This section will be concerned with the immature visual system, and the various problems which may befall it in the neonatal period, and for the first 6 months of life.

THE IMMATURE VISUAL SYSTEM

Ocular growth

The eye of the infant born at term is at a relatively advanced stage of development as it grows only three times in volume, to reach adult size, compared to the rest of the body's 20 times. While the length of the globe does not reach its adult value of 24 mm until the second decade, the anterior segment of the eye is further advanced, and the cornea is fully grown within a month or so after birth. Thus, most of the postnatal growth of the eye takes place in its posterior segment, particularly in the peripheral regions of the retina.

Between 6 months gestational age (GA) and term, at a time when many preterm babies are already born, ocular growth is particularly active, as retinal surface area doubles during this period. Over the ensuing 2 years it increases by a further 50%.

Vascular development

Transient vascular systems. In fetal life there are two transient vascular systems – the hyaloid vascular complex which fills the vitreous cavity and extends forwards and also contributes to the second system, the tunica vasculosa lentis, a vascular structure which surrounds the lens. The hyaloid artery has disappeared by 7 months and the tunica vasculosa lentis regresses between 28 and 34 weeks GA. As the latter can easily be visualized by direct ophthalmoscopy the degree of regression can be used as a crude estimate of gestational age.

Retinal vasculature. Until the fourth month of gestation the retina is avascular, relying entirely on the underlying choroidal circulation for its nutrients. From this time the mesenchymal precursors of the retinal vessels grow out from the optic disc and reach the periphery of the nasal retina around 8 months GA, whilst in the temporal retina, which is the last area to be vascularized, this process is not complete until after term.

Visual pathway development

The retina has its full complement of cells by the sixth month GA, but retinal maturational changes continue, particularly in the fovea, for another 4 years. Myelination between the globe and the lateral geniculate nucleus commences at about 6 months GA and is complete by 2 years. In the posterior visual pathway dendrite formation and synaptogenesis both lead to an increase in volume of the lateral geniculate nucleus and the visual cortex over the first 6 or so months of postnatal life.

Ocular growth, the maturational changes within the eye and the posterior sections of the visual system, are all dovetailed so that they proceed at a predetermined and relatively unimpeded rate to a successful functional outcome in most infants and children. This is even more remarkable for the baby born before term, who is reared in a hostile, brightly lit environment.

THE NEONATAL PERIOD

Ophthalmia neonatorum

This is defined as conjunctivitis developing within the first 4 weeks of life (Fig. 5.64). It is a notifiable condition as in the past ophthalmia neonatorum was one of the most important causes of childhood handicap. Fortunately the situation has now changed, but even today permanent ocular damage can result and treatment must be prompt and appropriate. Although the clinical features of the various types of ophthalmia neonatorum are suggestive of a particular diagnosis they are not sufficiently characteristic to make a definitive diagnosis. A large number of organisms have been implicated and in order of frequency these are *Chlamydia trachomatis, Staphylococcus aureus, Neisseria gonorrhoeae, Streptococcus viridans, Haemophilus* group, *Escherichia coli,* and less frequently a number of other organisms including *Pseudomonas aeruginosa* and the herpes simplex virus.

Chlamydia trachomatis. This is the commonest cause of ophthalmia neonatorum (developing in 18–50% of those infants exposed) and although the clinical picture may be mild, subclinical infections are unusual. The incubation period is 7–28 days with a peak incidence in the second week. The condition can be unilateral or bilateral and may range from a mild erythematous response to a severe pseudomembranous conjunctivitis (streptococci are another cause of a pseudomembranous reaction). Only in the most severe infection is the discharge copious and purulent. Even mild disease can cause corneal scarring (pannus), but the risk of this complication is lessened by prompt treatment.

Neisseria gonorrhoeae. This infection is acquired during passage down the birth canal in the mother who has either untreated or partially treated gonorrhoea. The incubation period is 4–7 days. Characteristically it causes a marked inflammatory reaction with lid and conjunctival edema, and there is a copious purulent, greenish, sometimes bloodstained, discharge held under pressure by the swollen eyelids. This organism is particularly virulent as it alone can penetrate the intact cornea, hence its propensity to cause blindness.

Herpes simplex virus. When ophthalmia neonatorum is caused by this virus it is usually as part of a generalized infection. In addition to the conjunctivitis, corneal clouding and dendritic ulceration occur. In contrast to herpes simplex infections developing at other times of life, neonatal herpes has a propensity to affect both eyes.

Other organisms. These do not individually give rise to distinctive clinical features, although in general a purulent discharge indicates bacterial origin or secondary involvement.

Chemical conjunctivitis. In those countries where prophylaxis against ophthalmia neonatorum is still practiced a chemical conjunctivitis with 1% silver nitrate drops is the rule, occurring 24 h after treatment. This subsides spontaneously within 2–3 days.

Diagnosis and treatment

As the clinical features are at best suggestive but not pathognomonic, accurate diagnosis rests with laboratory tests. No topical antibiotic should be administered until swabs have been taken. Culture media (blood and chocolate agar) should be inoculated at the cot side. A further specimen which must contain epithelial cells is applied directly to microscope slides and stained by Gram and Giemsa stains, looking in the latter for the cytoplasmic inclusions of chlamydia and multinucleated giant cells and intranuclear inclusions of herpes simplex. Impression cytology of conjunctival cells is a rapid technique for diagnosing chlamydia.

In several countries, but not the British Isles, prophylaxis is routinely performed using either silver nitrate 1%, tetracycline ointment 1%, or erythromycin ointment 0.5%. Whichever preparation is used it is applied once to both eyes soon after birth.

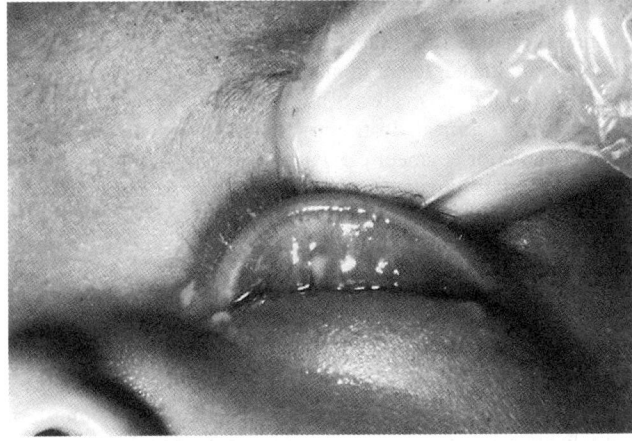
Fig. 5.64 Ophthalmia neonatorum.

All cases of ophthalmia neonatorum should be managed as though they are contagious. Treatment must be started immediately, guided by clinical findings and the results of the histological stains. If there is any evidence of systemic involvement topical and systemic therapy are necessary and all cases of gonococcal and chlamydial infections are so treated. Gonococcal infections are treated with systemic and topical penicillin; the eyedrops are instilled intensively, initially at 15-min intervals decreasing to 3- to 4-hourly after about 6 h. The copious purulent discharge should be washed away by saline irrigation before instilling topical antibiotics. For chlamydial infection systemic erythromycin is administered for 2 weeks. Topical tetracycline or sulfacetamide ointment is also used.

Birth trauma

Eyelids and orbit

Ecchymosis of the eyelids is common but is of no long-term consequence. Dislocation of the globe from the orbit has been reported rarely and is particularly prone to occur in certain of the craniofacial anomalies such as Apert's syndrome. Although alarming to all, replacement can be achieved by gentle pressure on the globe. Orbital hemorrhage causing proptosis occurs occasionally and is usually the consequence of a prolonged and difficult labor.

Ocular hemorrhages

Hemorrhages into various ocular tissues are frequent with all types of delivery. Conjunctival hemorrhages resolve rapidly and without sequelae. It is not uncommon for the iris blood vessels to be markedly engorged following birth and on occasion bleeding occurs causing a hyphema which also settles spontaneously.

The retina is the most frequent site of hemorrhage (up to 50% of all births). Frequently, but not invariably bilateral, most resolve spontaneously without trace over the ensuing days and weeks, although if the hemorrhage is large and has a preretinal or vitreous extension this process may take up to 2–3 months. Neonatal retinal hemorrhages do not cause amblyopia. Sometimes it can be difficult to differentiate between retinal hemorrhages due to the birth process or a later acquired nonaccidental injury. The distinction, which can be extremely difficult, rests on the history, and whether the features of the hemorrhage are compatible with the history.

Cornea

The cornea may be damaged by forceps injury. This is usually unilateral and causes a cloudy cornea. Although this clears over the ensuing few weeks, in the long term astigmatism, amblyopia and strabismus are likely sequelae. It is important but not always simple to distinguish corneal cloudiness due to injury and infantile glaucoma (buphthalmos – Fig. 5.65). Although in glaucoma the corneae are characteristically enlarged, in the neonatal period this may be yet to develop and it is essential to measure the intraocular pressure, which can usually be done at this age without sedation. The following features may also help: history and signs of trauma and the direction of fine lines in the deeper corneal layers. These are breaks in Descemet's membrane and are vertically directed in injury whilst in glaucoma are almost horizontal.

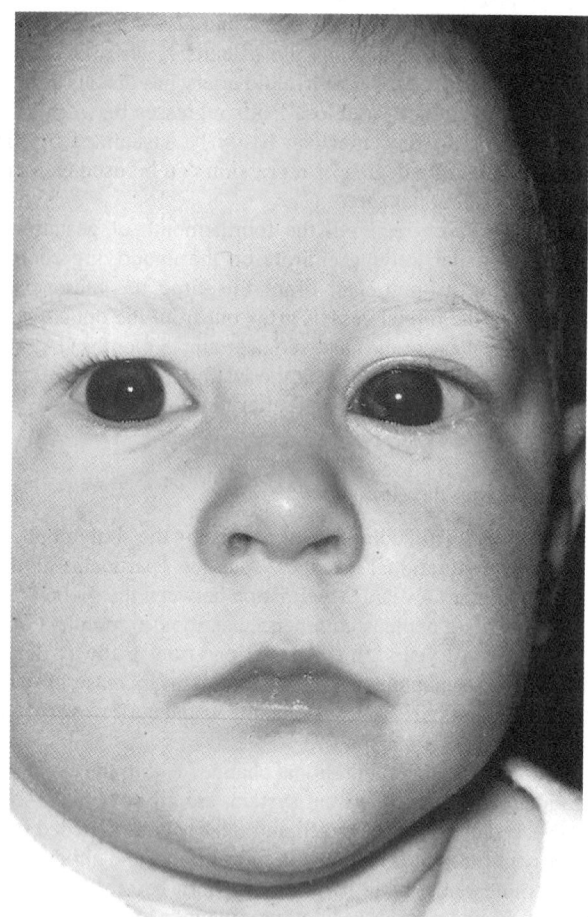

Fig. 5.65 Congenital glaucoma in the left eye. This eye is larger than its fellow, and the cornea is also slightly hazy (dulled corneal light reflex).

Cranial nerve palsies

Palsy of one of the ocular motor nerves is not rare, and has in the past often been attributed to birth trauma – almost certainly incorrectly.

Cornea

The normal cornea is hazy until about 27 weeks GA. Slight haze in preterm and term infants is not rare and clears rapidly, depending on the degree of immaturity. The following causes of a cloudy cornea must also always be considered: infantile glaucoma (see above), a corneal dystrophy, malformation of the anterior segment (anterior segment cleavage syndrome – Fig. 5.66), and rarely congenital rubella causes a self-limiting cloudy cornea due to keratitis.

Lens

Subtle lens opacities are quite common in preterm neonates. These are in the form of vacuoles and are best seen using the direct ophthalmoscope. They are transient, of no long-term significance and their etiology is unknown. Congenital cataract is considered elsewhere (p. 1667).

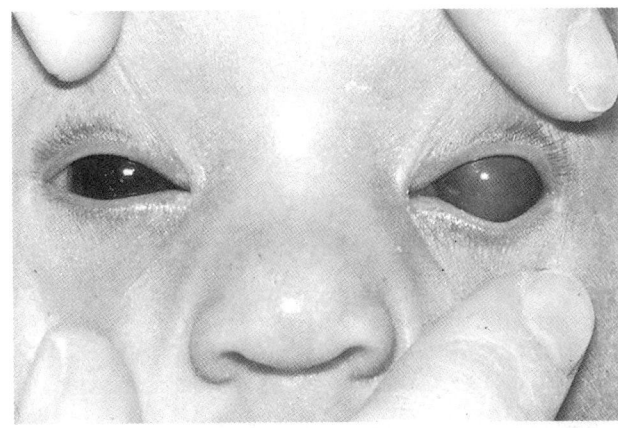

Fig. 5.66 Left cloudy cornea due to malformation of the anterior segment, the so-called anterior cleavage syndrome.

Eye movements

Strabismus and amblyopia are discussed elsewhere (Ch. 26); see also Leigh & Zee (1991). Here it is only necessary to discuss those aspects of eye movements relevant to the neonatal period. Certain eye movements which would be considered abnormal later in infancy and childhood and warrant urgent neurological investigation are commonly seen in the neonatal period with usually less serious connotations. The eyes of healthy neonates frequently appear to be divergent but this is largely due to the shape of the neonatal eye. 'Congenital' esotropia (convergent strabismus) is rarely, if ever, present at birth and is therefore more appropriately named infantile esotropia. Rarely a sixth nerve palsy producing a convergent strabismus can be present at birth. It is usually an isolated abnormality which resolves over a few weeks. In general, congenital cranial nerve palsies are rare, and the role of birth trauma in their pathogenesis has been overemphasized. However, maldevelopment of, or in utero damage to, the ocular motor nuclei or nerves causes the well-known syndromes including Duane's and Moebius' syndromes. Although a third or sixth nerve palsy is simple to diagnose, this is not so for the fourth nerve and a palsy of this nerve may remain undetected for years until the compensatory head posture is noticed. It is important to recall that a squint may be the first sign of a serious neurological or ophthalmic abnormality and therefore any deviation, be it divergent or convergent, persisting beyond the neonatal period must be taken seriously.

During the neonatal period a few beats of up- or downbeat nystagmus are commonly seen, and sometimes abnormalities of other conjugate movements such as ocular flutter, opsoclonus (bursts of rapid eye movements) or skew deviation. The significance of these movements is unknown. Sustained nystagmus is rarely if ever seen at this time but roving eye movements have been reported in association with intraventricular hemorrhage. A variety of supranuclear eye movement disorders including saccadic and gaze palsies can result from neurological insults.

Retinopathy of prematurity

Retinopathy of prematurity (ROP) is a potentially blinding disorder affecting infants born prematurely. Described first in the 1940s there was an epidemic of retrolental fibroplasia (RLF) as it was then known which was brought to an end in the early 1950s by the discovery that the high concentrations of oxygen being given at that time were important in its production. Concomitant with the increased survival of the extremely immature neonate in recent years the incidence of ROP has again risen.

Pathogenesis

ROP is a condition of the immature retinal vasculature and does not develop after the retina is fully vascularized. Retinopathy develops at the junction of the vascularized and yet to be vascularized retina. There are three theories. According to the first classic theory (Ashton 1980, Patz 1980) the retinal vessels constrict and their endothelial cells are damaged due to raised (i.e. above normal for the fetus) PaO_2 levels. This leads to ischemia and the production of angiogenic factors and subsequent vasoproliferation. The second theory (Kretzer & Hittner 1988) also postulates the production of angiogenic factors but proposes that this is not induced by vasoconstriction but by direct oxidative insult to the mesenchymal precursors (spindle cells) which then synthesize and secrete angiogenic factors generating the vasoproliferative response by the retinal vessels.

Both theories invoke an oxidative insult which might be due to a direct cytotoxic action of oxygen itself (Ashton 1980), indirectly due to ischemia consequent upon the vasoconstriction (Patz 1980), or indirectly by oxygen-generated free radicals (Kretzer & Hittner 1988). The most recent, third, theory invokes growth factors and apoptosis (Alon et al 1995). The maintenance of the retinal vascular tree depends on a continuous supply of survival factors which can be downregulated by oxygen. Thus hyperoxia induces a shutdown of vascular endothelial growth factor (VEGF) which induces endothelial apoptosis and excessive capillary regression. The ischemia which follows generates an upregulation of VEGF which induces angiogenesis and the vasoproliferative response of ROP.

All theories concur that oxygen is implicated directly or indirectly in the initiation of ROP. However, once ROP has developed the retina is rendered ischemic and it is this ischemia which contributes to the vasoproliferative response of severe disease.

Risk factors

ROP is not a totally preventable condition. By far the most powerful risk factor is the degree of immaturity and recently clinicians have tended to regard severe ROP as an inevitable, albeit unpredictable, consequence of extreme prematurity. Numerous risk factors have been implicated of which the best known is supplemental oxygen administration. Interest in the role of oxygen in its pathogenesis has reawakened with the finding that oxygen administration in the first few weeks of life is a risk factor for ROP incidence and severity. Fluctuations, even within the normal range, can increase the risk of severe ROP, and PaO_2 monitoring – being intermittent – may mask important variations (Cunningham et al 1995). These findings have major implications for neonatal care. Nevertheless, it has not been possible to define a concentration, or duration, of oxygen which is, or is not, associated with ROP. The current consensus is that hyperoxia can be important in ROP initiation. Hypoxia on the other hand may increase the severity of established ROP, which is known to be ischemic. Other possible risk factors include blood transfusions, apneic episodes, hypercarbia, low pH, intraventricular hemorrhage and periventricular leukomalacia. The role of early exposure to light as an etiologic agent has yet to be determined.

Classification

Clinically, ROP is classified by the International Classification of Retinopathy of Prematurity (CCRoP 1984, 1987). The severity of acute ROP is classified by stage, but its location within the retina is also important (Fielder & Levene 1992).

Acute ROP (Fig. 5.67):

Stage 1 – demarcation line, lying within the plane of the retina at the junction of the vascularized and avascular retina. The demarcation line is the accumulation of the mesenchymal precursors of the retinal vessels.

Stage 2 – ridge; the demarcation line extends out of the plane of the retina.

Stage 3 – ridge with extraretinal fibrovascular proliferation. This is the stage of frank neovascularization, i.e. definitive new vessels are formed.

Stage 4 – subtotal retinal detachment.

Stage 5 – total retinal detachment.

'Plus' disease – signs of activity, which in order of severity include: congestion of the retinal vessel of the posterior pole, congestion of the iris vessels so that the pupil does not dilate readily with mydriatics (iris rigidity), and vitreous haze.

Regressed ROP. Not all ROP undergoes complete resolution. Signs in the fundus which signify previous acute ROP are

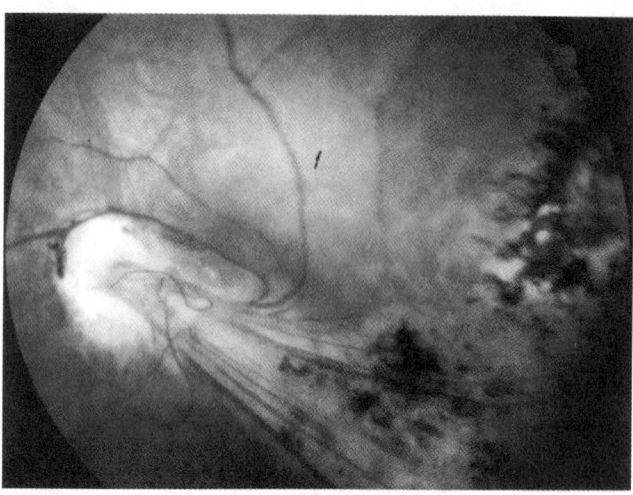

Fig. 5.68 Signs of regressed ROP. Retinal fold extending from the 'dragged' optic disc. Peripheral pigmentation corresponds to the site of the acute lesion. (Reproduced with permission, Editor of the Practitioner.)

described according to their location – posterior or peripheral – and according to the structures involved, thus:

Vascular – tortuosity, abnormal branching and arcades, and the straightening ('dragging') of the vessels around the disc (Fig. 5.68).

Retinal – pigmentation, folding, stretching, detachment and vitreoretinal membranes.

Incidence. The incidence and severity of acute ROP rises with decreasing birthweight and gestational age. Quoted figures vary widely, probably due more to examination technique and frequency than neonatal factors. About 30–60% of babies weighing less than 1500 g develop some ROP. Severe disease is virtually confined to those infants < 1500 g birthweight and affects about 6% infants < 1250 g birthweight.

Natural history

As the temporal retina is the last area to be vascularized, most acute ROP develops in that region, although in extremely immature babies it often starts in the nasal retina. The age at onset of acute ROP is governed by the postconceptual age (PCA) of the baby rather than neonatal events. Thus contrary to expectation, ROP develops later postnatally in the smaller, very immature baby who is ill, compared to his larger, usually fitter more mature counterpart. Retinopathy of prematurity infrequently starts before 31 weeks PCA, and never after complete retinal vascularization. Stage 3 acute ROP affects almost exclusively infants < 32 weeks GA, and < 1500 g and develops between about 33 and 41 weeks PCA.

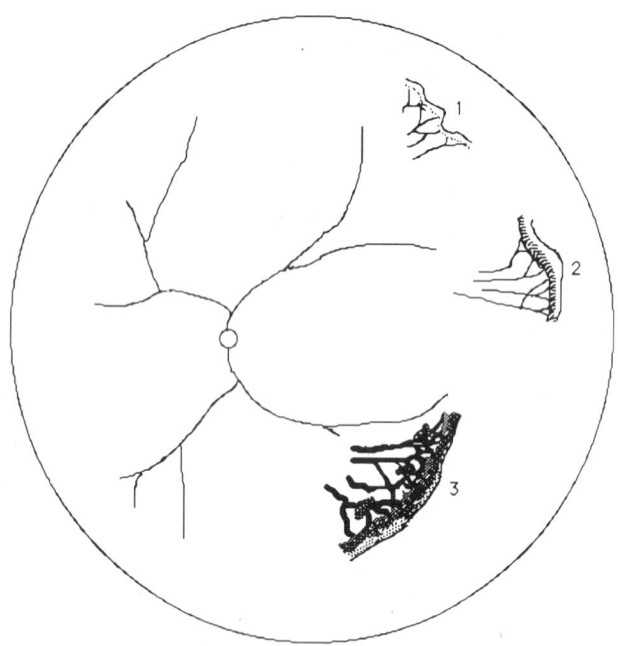

Fig. 5.67 Acute ROP: the first three stages of acute ROP presented for diagrammatic purposes on one retina. Each is shown as a short segment, but can extend over 360°. Stage 1, demarcation line; stage 2, ridge; and stage 3, ridge with extraretinal fibrovascular proliferation. Note abnormal peripheral vascular arborization in all stages, but in stage 3 the vessels are engorged and the lesion is more posteriorly located. Note also that the retina is not fully vascularized.

Outcome

Spontaneous and complete regression is the rule for all stage 1 and 2 acute ROP. Some babies with stage 3 also undergo resolution, but at this stage the likelihood of significant sequelae is very high and some babies become blind – hence the use of the term severe to describe stage 3 and above. All stage 4 and 5 ROP has a poor visual outcome.

Treatment

As mild ROP spontaneously resolves and the outcome for stages 4 and 5 is dismal, therapeutic intervention can only be considered at stage 3. The current indication for intervention is 'threshold' at which stage the untreated risk of blindness is 50% (CRPCG 1988). 'Threshold' is defined as stage 3 ROP which extends over five or more continuous, or eight or more cumulative, clock hours of the retinal circumference, in the presence of 'plus' disease. It is important to emphasize that the time available for treatment once 'threshold' ROP has been reached is short, and ideally treatment should be undertaken within 2–3 days (Royal College of Ophthalmologists and British Association of Perinatal Medicine Joint Working Party 1995).

Cryotherapy and laser. Until recently ROP could neither be prevented nor treated. This changed in 1988 when the US-based Multicenter Trial of Cryotherapy for ROP demonstrated that cryotherapy reduced the unfavorable outcome of 'threshold' stage 3 ROP by about 50% (CRPCG 1988). This single study has changed clinical practice worldwide and now cryotherapy is recommended for babies reaching this stage.

More recently laser, delivered via an indirect ophthalmoscope, has been used to treat severe ROP. Both modalities have their indication, but laser is increasingly the method of choice. Either cryotherapy or laser is applied to the peripheral retina anterior to the ridge – over the full circumference of the globe. The procedure can be performed either under general anesthesia or sedation. Not all babies respond to treatment and it is likely that treatment criteria will change in the future.

ROP screening

Screening is now recommended (Fielder & Levene 1992, Royal College of Ophthalmologists and British Association of Perinatal Medicine Joint Working Party 1995) and has the aim of identifying babies at risk of developing stage 3 ROP – these babies require either treatment or, because of sequelae, continued ophthalmic surveillance. UK guidelines specify that all babies of birthweight < 1500 g and < 32 weeks GA are screened at least fortnightly, commencing at 6–7 weeks postnatal age and continuing until retinal vascularization is into zone 3 (i.e. peripheral).

Treatment for end-stage disease

Not all ROP responds to treatment and retinal detachment surgery and vitrectomy have been used for end-stage ROP. Vitrectomy is technically well within the scope of many surgeons but to date the visual results have been so poor that it is not recommended. Acute glaucoma sometimes develops in advanced disease. Removal of the lens may be helpful although there is a risk of globe shrinkage.

Differential diagnosis

For the preterm neonate this question hardly ever arises but there are a number of conditions simulating ROP which may present in the full-term baby or in later life. These include autosomal dominant familial exudative vitreoretinopathy, fetal ischemia (porencephaly, anencephaly), Coats' disease. The distinction may be impossible on ophthalmological criteria alone, and the family history and systemic aspects must be taken into account.

Ophthalmic sequelae of preterm birth

Sequelae of ROP

All mild ROP (stages 1 and 2) regresses without significantly affecting eye growth and visual function. Severe disease, even after treatment, generates sequelae which include refractive errors (myopia, astigmatism), strabismus, and visual deficits ranging from the very mild to complete blindness. A serious late complication of ROP is retinal detachment which can develop at any age, even in adulthood.

Sequelae of prematurity

Visual development proceeds according to postconceptional age rather than postnatal age and failure to appreciate this can result in unnecessary concern about visual functions. Infants and children who were born prematurely, even after ROP has been accounted for, are more prone to suffer visual pathway defects – although in reality the effects of ROP and neurological insults cannot be differentiated as the proportional effect of neurological damage suffered in the perinatal period compared to that due to prematurity per se is unknown. Neurological insults can vary in location and severity and not surprisingly result in a range of neuro-ophthalmic defects including; reduced vision, eye movement disorders, refractive errors and optic atrophy. The causes of reduced vision depend on the nature of the insult (see elsewhere in this chapter), and the severity of the deficit can range from minimal to severe (cortical visual impairment). Eye movement disorders include strabismus, gaze and saccadic palsies, and nystagmus and are commonly associated with neurological insult; indeed the last three mentioned are almost certainly its direct consequence. The incidence of squint ranges from 11% to over 20% and is particularly high in those with neurological damage such as cystic periventricular leukomalacia, especially if this is posteriorly located. Myopia can be due to ROP, but the ex-prematurely born teenager who did not have ROP is more likely to be myopic than his ex-full-term counterpart.

Routine neonatal eye examination

Every baby should have an eye examination in the very early neonatal period before discharge from hospital or equivalent. The following aspects need to be included and although the list looks formidable at first glance each examination need not take more than a minute or so.

Look for conditions affecting both eyes, but be especially suspicious of asymmetry between the eyes.

Signs of significant birth trauma

These have already been covered, and the word significant is included so that the pediatric resident performing this examination does not feel obliged to dilate pupils in order to look for retinal hemorrhage. Using the direct ophthalmoscope as a torch light, the anterior segment of the eye can be examined for corneal cloudiness, hyphema, etc.

Ocular malformation

With the ophthalmoscope the following are examined:

- *Lids* – ptosis, hemangioma, dermoids
- *Globe size*
  - microphthalmos
  - macrophthalmos, most important as this could be infantile glaucoma, but in the neonatal period the eyes may still be of normal size as the process is at an early stage
- *Conjunctiva* – dermoid
- *Cornea* – cloudiness, consider infantile glaucoma (Fig. 5.65). Opacities may be part of a malformation (Fig. 5.66)
- *Iris* – coloboma.

Leukocoria (white pupil)

An important clinical sign, which may signify a condition that is potentially lethal or may have severe consequences for vision. The red reflex is looked for by viewing the undilated pupil, viewing through an ophthalmoscope which is held at 33 cm from the eye (without a correction dialed in), or with + 10 dialed in and held close to the infant's eye. This writer prefers the former as it provides a better 'feel', and the location of an opacity can be better determined. The absence of a red reflex must always be taken seriously and it requires *urgent* specialist referral.

Causes of leukocoria (Fig. 5.69) include: cataract, malformations (persistent hyperplastic primary vitreous, coloboma, retinal dysplasia as in Norrie's disease and lissencephaly), tumors (retinoblastoma), myelinated nerve fibers, and inflammations (endophthalmitis). Conditions such as end-stage ROP, Coats' disease and toxocariasis also can give a white pupil but usually after the neonatal period.

Ophthalmic family history

It is important to examine the eyes if there is a family history of a serious ophthalmic problem. In some conditions, for example dominantly inherited retinitis pigmentosa, the eyes at this time will be normal and it is not possible to determine whether or not the baby will be affected later. Certain fears can only be eliminated by a detailed examination and the diplomatic effect of this early examination is considerable and provides a good start to any subsequent involvement. A positive family history of infantile

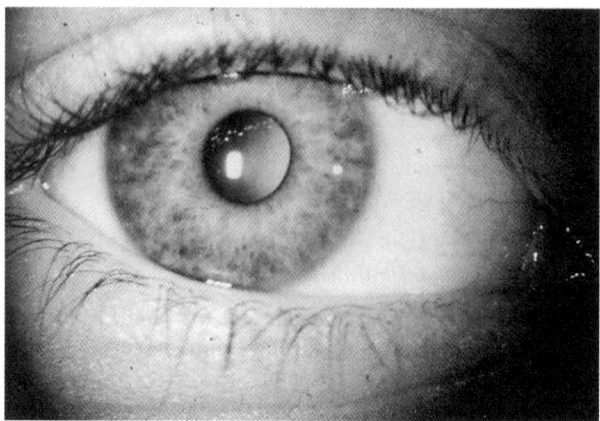

Fig. 5.69 Leukocoria, a frequent presenting sign of retinoblastoma.

glaucoma and retinoblastoma even in the presence of a *normal* neonatal eye examination requires urgent referral and continued ophthalmological review.

NORMAL DEVELOPMENT OF VISION

The visual responsiveness of a baby never fails to delight, and is one of the great rewards of infancy. Vision can be demonstrated in the infant even before term, and reaches about 6/60 and 6/18 at 3 and 12 months of age respectively. As mentioned, for the infant born prematurely development is governed by postconceptional age. Adult acuity levels of 6/6 are not reached until the third or fourth year of life. Attempting to measure the visual responses of an infant or lively preschool child even up to the age of 5 years, remains one of the major challenges of pediatric ophthalmology.

Visibility and resolution

Before considering individual tests of visual acuity, or even the value of a history, the distinction between visibility and resolution must be understood.

- *Visibility* is the ability to identify a single object such as a sweet, thread on a carpet, airplane in the sky. Clinical tests based on this principle use white balls of varying size, e.g. Stycar balls, or black spots on a white background, i.e. the Catford drum.
- *Resolution* is the ability to distinguish between two points or lines. Tests of resolution include black and white stripes (gratings) of varying widths, and the standard Snellen test, which also contains a recognition element (recognition of letter shape).

Visibility and resolution are not comparable and measure different neurological substrates. While tests of visibility clearly indicate that a baby has vision, they significantly overestimate the result obtained by resolution tests – to the extent that results so obtained can be seriously misleading.

Qualitative assessment

Most assessments of infant vision are qualitative. The eyelids are fused until about 25 weeks GA and the blink reflex to a bright light is present from about this time. From 30 weeks GA visual fixation can be observed during periods of alertness, and these naturally increase in frequency and length with development. After about 32 weeks GA head turning to a light can be observed and just over half babies at term will follow a target such as a red woollen ball. During early infancy following eye movements are slow and jerky so it is important not to move the target too quickly. Visually elicited smiling commences around 6 weeks, and as this response often has such an important visual component, its absence within about a week or so of this age, is useful in alerting carers to the possibility of a significant visual deficit. Visually directed reaching commences around 2–3 months of age.

History

A parent's concern for her infant's vision must always be taken seriously, as it is exceptionally rare for such concern to be unfounded. The converse is of course less reliable and the parent of an infant with a serious visual problem may not express concern for the following reasons: first, expectancy for early vision may be low, particularly for the firstborn when parental experience is naturally limited. Second, parents cannot differentiate visibility and resolution, and the clinician should be aware that when using the word vision, a parent (in this context) is referring to her infant's visibility, whereas to the clinician the same word denotes resolution ability. Third, the parent may await the opinion of the professional before volunteering his or her own view.

Quantitative tests

It has been argued that quantifying the vision of infants and young children is clinically irrelevant. This view is no longer tenable for the following reasons. Both qualitative assessments and ophthalmic findings are poor guides to the level of vision. In addition objective assessment can influence medical and surgical management. Finally, the finding of normal acuity can prevent unnecessary anxiety and although many causes of reduced vision are untreatable, detailed knowledge of the level of vision can help parents understand the severity of the defect and other helpers in the care of the child with a visual problem.

Behavioral tests of vision

Preferential looking. This technique is based on the observation known to mothers' since time immemorial – that a face is a powerful visual stimulus to an infant. In the 1970s these observations led to the development of more formal testing procedures with the mother's face being replaced by a patterned stimulus, namely black and white stripes (gratings). In preferential looking (PL) the infant is presented with two stimuli, one patterned, the other blank, and if the pattern is seen the infant will prefer to look towards it. The infant is held in front of a screen containing the gratings, with the tester behind observing the infant's looking responses through a peephole in the screen. Successively finer gratings are presented until no looking response is elicited. Threshold, i.e. the visual acuity of the baby, is the finest grating to induce a looking response. The term 'forced-choice' is often used to describe this technique because the tester is unaware of the grating location and is 'forced' to determine this 'choice' based on the looking response. Although forced-choice PL is a powerful investigative tool which has provided much information about normal and abnormal visual development, the technique is lengthy and tedious, and consequently has not found favor in routine clinical practice.

Acuity card procedure. A clinical adaptation of PL has been introduced – the acuity card procedure (ACP). In contrast to formal PL procedures in which the gratings are TV generated, in ACP both grating and blank are contained on a single hand-held card presented through a large aperture in a gray cardboard screen placed in front of the infant (Figs 5.70 and 5.71). The tester views the infant through a central peephole in the card and proceeds approximately as in PL. Ideally cards are stacked in order before commencing the test and selected in such a way that the tester is ignorant of grating location and consequently able to make an unbiased judgment. Toys can be introduced through the aperture to maintain interest and fixation can be confirmed by a sideways movement of the card. Older children may point rather than look at the grating. ACP has considerable advantages over any other test currently available in that it allows the rapid quantitative estimation of acuity in infants and young children. ACP can be used from birth, even if preterm, and the success rate of ACP testing binocular acuity up to around 30 months is between 80% and almost 100%. Between 18 and 24 months of age this is reduced to about 75%. The success rate for testing monocular vision is lower in the routine clinical setting. The test is relatively simple to use, especially in early infancy, and is now finding clinical favor.

There are problems: looking responses can be difficult to judge especially in the older infant, in the presence of a squint, field

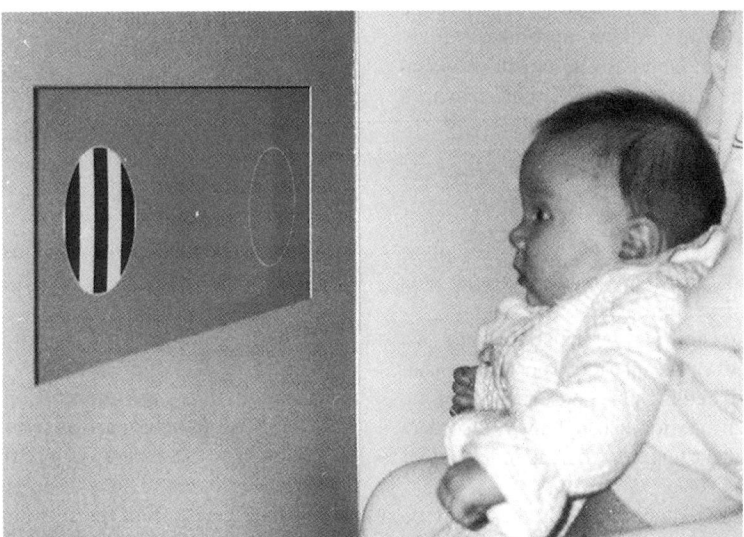

Fig. 5.70 Acuity card procedure: infant looking at the grating. The observer judges the infant's looking response through the peephole in the center of the card.

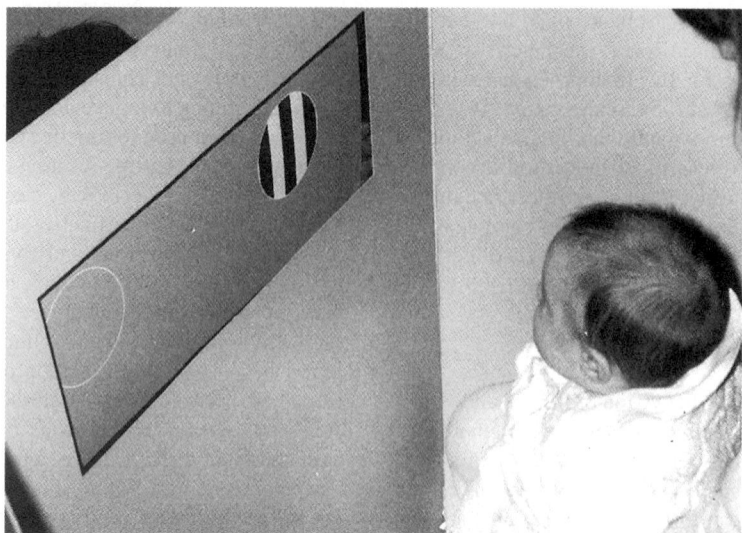

Fig. 5.71 The card is hand-held, and can be moved sideways by a small amount to confirm fixation. The introduction of toys through the aperture rekindles flagging interest.

defect or nystagmus. In addition grating (ACP) and Snellen acuities do not always correlate, particularly in amblyopia. Despite these problems PL-based tests offer the clinician the first opportunity to quantify the vision of infants and young children.

Electrophysiological tests of vision

Visually evoked potentials. (see also pp. 1655 and 1656). The visually evoked potential (VEP) in response to a flash stimulus (flash VEP) cannot measure acuity, or necessarily even the presence of vision, but does give a valuable indication of visual pathway maturation. To obtain a measure of acuity, a pattern VEP must be obtained employing white and black gratings or checkerboards. The stimulus can be presented using either a pattern reversal or pattern-onset paradigm. A recent modification includes a high stimulation rate with rapid sweep through a range of stimuli – the sweep VEP. Although the equipment is widely available, the expertise is not, and the VEP assessment of visual acuity remains within the domain of the research electrophysiologist.

THE INFANT WITH REDUCED VISION

The infant thought to have severely reduced vision presents a difficult clinical problem. The causes are numerous and it is appropriate to take a broad clinical approach to this topic.

Conditions causing reduced vision can be separated into two major groups; those involving either the anterior or posterior visual pathways. There is clinical sense to this as the consequences of the visual defect are different; thus in anterior visual pathway disorders sustained nystagmus is a prominent feature, whereas in lesions of the posterior visual pathway it is not.

Multiple pathology is not rare, and consequently there may be involvement of more than one part of the visual pathway. Only those conditions affecting the vision of both eyes will be discussed.

Anterior visual pathway disorders

Conditions included under this heading involve the eye, optic nerve or chiasm. Despite the anterior location there is not always an ophthalmoscopically visible explanation. In addition to the visual deficit the characteristics of this group are the presence of nystagmus – a nonspecific response to a visual deficit involving the *anterior* visual pathway in early life. Although nystagmus is rarely, if ever, present at birth, it is usually seen by the time concern is expressed, between 2 and 6 months of age.

Corneal disorders

Corneal opacities are relatively infrequent as a cause of blindness in the developed world. The most commonly seen are the neural crest malformations of the ocular anterior segment the so-called anterior cleavage syndromes, including sclerocornea and Peters' anomalies. These can occur as isolated anomalies or as part of a syndrome, in which latter case developmental delay is often a feature. Other causes include certain corneal dystrophies and buphthalmos (infantile glaucoma).

Disorders of the lens

Cataract is considered elsewhere as is the differential diagnosis of the white pupil.

Retinal disorders

With obvious ophthalmoscopic signs. Several disorders produce obvious signs such as retinal folds, coloboma, retinopathy of prematurity (see below) or scarring from chorioretinitis.

Cherry-red spot. This classic sign, which is subtle and fades with time, results from the accumulation of abnormal substances in the retinal ganglion cells in conditions such as Tay–Sachs, Sandhoff's, Niemann-Pick and Farber's diseases, metachromatic leukodystrophy and the mucolipidoses.

Without obvious ophthalmoscopic signs. Ophthalmoscopic abnormalities are present in many of the conditions included here, but they are often extremely subtle, particularly in the early stages.

Leber's amaurosis. This autosomal recessively inherited retinal dystrophy is characterized by blindness or severely reduced vision from birth, an absent or markedly reduced electroretinogram in the presence of a normal or near normal retina. Leber's amaurosis is one of the more common causes of blindness in early life and has many possible ocular and systemic associations. The latter include a variety of neurodevelopmental disorders, renal disorders, including nephronophthisis, and skeletal abnormalities. Leber's amaurosis is not a single entity but a group of conditions associated with a retinal dystrophy in early infancy. In Zellweger syndrome (cerebrohepatorenal syndrome) a retinal dystrophy develops as a consequence of the underlying peroxisomal disorder, but whether this is really Leber's amaurosis is less pertinent than appreciating that some retinal dystrophies can be progressive and indicate an underlying metabolic disorder.

Achromatopsia. Congenital absence of retinal cones is inherited as an autosomal recessive trait. Affected infants have poor vision which worsens dramatically when the illumination is bright. They also exhibit nystagmus and when old enough to be tested are found to be completely color blind. Ophthalmoscopic examination is normal and before reaching the age at which color vision can be tested, the diagnosis can only be made electrophysiologically (absent electroretinogram at 30 Hz).

Retinal dysplasia. In this group of conditions the retina is poorly differentiated and presents clinically as a white pupil (leukocoria) and is mentioned above.

Pigmentary retinopathies. A large heterogeneous group of tapetoretinal degenerations, including such conditions as retinitis pigmentosa and the Laurence–Moon–Biedl (Bardet–Biedl) syndrome; all usually present later on in childhood.

Optic nerve disorders

Optic atrophy. This is frequently a subtle sign. The degree or extent of pallor is not a guide to the level of vision. Optic atrophy can indicate pathology from the retina to the lateral geniculate nucleus and, in the infant only, as far back as the visual cortex.

Intrauterine disease. Infections, asphyxia and cerebral malformations.

Perinatal damage. The precise mechanism(s) by which damage occurs is often lacking.

Inflammatory. From meningoencephalitis.

Compression. Stretching or compression of the optic nerves can be caused by hydrocephalus or tumor, such as craniopharyngioma or glioma.

Metabolic. Rare causes of optic atrophy including the lipid storage disorders (e.g. Tay–Sachs disease), osteopetrosis, etc.

Retinal disease. Severe retinal disease may lead to optic atrophy, as in the tapetoretinal degenerations or retinal dystrophies such as Leber's amaurosis, retinitis pigmentosa, Laurence–Moon–Biedl and Zellweger syndromes.

Hereditary optic atrophy. Rare in infancy, but Behr's autosomal recessive optic atrophy, associated with mental retardation, ataxia and hypertonia, has its onset within the first year of life.

Optic nerve hypoplasia. In its severe form optic nerve hypoplasia (ONH) is relatively easy to diagnose, but none of the following features is pathognomonic – small disc, peripapillary

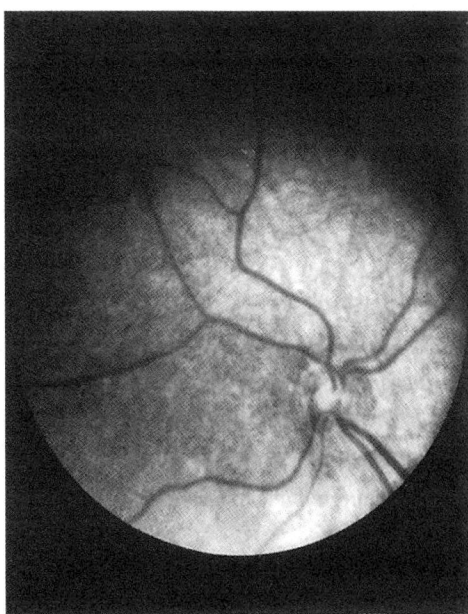

Fig. 5.72 Optic nerve hypoplasia. The pigmented double-ring sign. The remaining optic nerve is the small central white area, which as frequently occurs is atrophic.

pigmented ring (Fig. 5.72), slightly tortuous retinal vessels or thinned nerve fiber layer. ONH is a relatively common malformation and visual function may range from near normal to total blindness.

ONH is not inherited and its pathogenesis is unknown, but is thought to represent a nonspecific response by the developing visual system to an early insult; consequently a degree of optic atrophy is a common accompaniment (see above). ONH, particularly if bilateral, can be associated with a large variety of ocular and/or systemic malformations and abnormalities. The former include microphthalmos and aniridia, whilst systemic associations include absence of the septum pellucidum, hydranencephaly, porencephaly, cerebral atrophy, leukomalacia, etc.

Neuroendocrine dysfunction occurs in 20–30% of patients with ONH, with or without a structural CNS anomaly, and as it may not become apparent for years; surveillance throughout early childhood is required. Growth, thyroid and gonadotrophic hormones can all be affected. In the neonatal period transient cholestatic jaundice and hypoglycemia have been reported.

Other optic nerve malformations. These include colobomas of the optic disc, the morning glory syndrome, optic nerve pit, etc.

Nystagmus

Defined as a rhythmic oscillation of the eyes, its classification and pathophysiology are so bewildering that only a few clinical aspects relevant to early life will be mentioned here. The reader keen to delve further into this perplexing topic is advised to consult specialized texts (e.g. Leigh & Zee 1991).

Nystagmus is a sign, not a diagnosis, and excepting for certain occasions in the neonatal period, an explanation for its presence must be sought. It is described by the direction of its fast phase, rate and amplitude, and the terms pendular and jerk are not useful.

Physiological nystagmus

This includes, caloric and optokinetic and nystagmus induced by rotation.

Nystagmus due to central nervous system conditions

Nystagmus is seen in many CNS conditions due to pathology in a variety of locations, including the cerebellum, brainstem and vestibular apparatus. In infancy its features do not have much specific diagnostic value. CNS-generated nystagmus can be present at any age, even in the neonatal period (a roving nystagmus has been seen with intraventricular hemorrhage), at which time it does not have major connotations for future vision. Certain specific patterns of nystagmus do have important neurological connotations and can have localizing value. These include, see-saw, downbeat, upbeat, retraction, dissociated nystagmus and ocular bobbing (Leigh & Zee 1991).

Nystagmus due to reduced vision

Reduced vision in early life causes nystagmus, but only if the pathology lies in the anterior visual pathway, such as an ocular disorder. It develops at about 2 to 3 months of age and in general the lower the vision the slower the speed of the nystagmus – the totally blind patient exhibits a slow, roving oscillation.

Certain conditions are associated with a pattern of nystagmus which is clinically indistinguishable from congenital nystagmus. These include albinism, achromatopsia, aniridia and milder forms of optic nerve defects, and the link between them is probably the relatively mild deficit.

Infantile (congenital) nystagmus

This is rarely, if ever, present at birth; thus the term infantile is preferred. The oscillation is characteristically binocular, symmetrical, and uniplanar – beating horizontally in all positions of gaze. It can be inherited by dominant, recessive or X-linked traits. Head nodding is sometimes present.

Spasmus nutans

A syndrome consisting of nystagmus, head nodding and torticollis, it commences in infancy and resolves within a year or so. Not all features are obvious and nystagmus may be the only sign. It can be unilateral or asymmetric – the other cause being monocular blindness. Spasmus nutans is also a diagnosis of exclusion as the infant may harbor an intracranial tumor.

The investigation of nystagmus

Take care to differentiate neurological, ocular and congenital types – this is not always possible by clinical examination. Thus every patient should have a detailed and appropriate ophthalmological *and* pediatric assessment. In many cases it is appropriate to include neuroradiology and ophthalmic electrodiagnosis (especially the electroretinogram).

Posterior visual pathway disorders

The two major conditions in this group are delayed visual maturation (DVM; Fielder 1995, Fielder & Mayer 1991) and cortical visual impairment (CVI; Good et al 1994). In contrast to disorders of the anterior visual pathway the overall ophthalmic clinical picture is one of reduced vision in the absence of both ocular signs and nystagmus.

Delayed visual maturation

This is a clinical term describing the infant with reduced visual responsiveness from birth in whom the vision subsequently improves. Known for over a century, it has become increasingly appreciated that delayed visual maturation (DVM) is not a single clinical entity, but represents a spectrum. Four types are recognized.

Clinical features – all types. DVM is a diagnosis of exclusion, and can only be made retrospectively. Certain features are common to all types during the period of blindness. The onset of visually directed smiling is delayed – a useful historical point. Because the infants are blind the eyes often diverge slightly, but apart from this there are no abnormal ocular signs. Thus pupillary responses are normal and there is no sustained nystagmus at this stage, even for type 3 infants. Except for a few type 3 infants there is no ophthalmoscopic abnormality.

Type 1: DVM as an isolated anomaly. Apart from the finding of reduced vision there are no abnormal findings and the baby is otherwise normal. The onset of visual improvement is usually between 10 and 20 weeks of age and once begun the change is rapid (over a few days) and complete. Some of these infants have experienced perinatal problems or been born prematurely. Nevertheless, the outlook for vision and development is excellent although a few develop mild neurodevelopmental sequelae.

Type 2: DVM with severe and permanent neurodevelopmental problems. In contrast to type 1 DVM, the neurodevelopmental aspects dominate the clinical picture and the visual deficit is often identified only during assessment. The age at which vision improvement commences is variable, ranging from about 6 to 18 months, the rate of change is slow, and the eventual level of vision achieved is limited and determined by the extent of CNS damage. This type of DVM and pre- and perinatal causes of cortical visual impairment (see below) are indistinguishable.

Type 3: DVM associated with infantile nystagmus or albinism. One of the striking features of DVM is the absence of nystagmus – *during the period of blindness*. Infants with type 3 DVM do not have nystagmus during the period of blindness but this hallmark sign develops around the time of visual improvement. As with type 1, improvement commences between about 10 and 25 weeks, but the eventual level of vision is governed by the nystagmus, and other ocular anomalies, if present. The nystagmus, when it develops is characteristic of the so-called infantile (congenital), horizontal, uniplanar type. The commonest causes are infantile nystagmus and albinism.

Clearly DVM must be a diagnosis of exclusion and can only be made in retrospect following the improvement of vision. Although clinical features may point to this diagnosis, during the phase of blindness, it is essential that the improvement is not openly anticipated to the parents, for early falsely optimistic advice causes far more distress than the subsequent delight of unexpected improvement, however limited.

Type 4: DVM with severe congenital, structural ocular abnormalities (excluding albinism). Surprisingly, some infants – but not all – who are blind in infancy with severe ocular abnormalities exhibit a limited but useful degree of improvement.

Examples include ONH, coloboma and Leber's amaurosis. Although this clinical picture fits uncomfortably within the DVM spectrum, by definition it requires to be included. Because the ocular disorder dominates the clinical picture, the clinician should experience no difficulty in differentiating this entity from DVM types 1–3.

Cortical blindness or cortical visual impairment

This term describes the blind infant or child with a normal ophthalmic examination, including preservation of the pupillary responses. Although a few beats of poorly sustained nystagmus may be seen, the absence of *sustained* nystagmus is an important diagnostic feature. The VEP is not always abnormal in cortical blindness. Although the visual defect may be total initially, some improvement is common and the term cortical visual impairment (CVI) is now often preferred to cortical blindness. There is clearly some overlap between this condition and DVM, which has yet to be delineated. The degree of improvement in CVI is often incomplete and influenced by the etiology and severity of the insult. Most children achieve at least navigational vision and sometimes much more. Recovery may take from a few hours to more than 2 years. Full recovery has been reported after head injury and cardiac arrest, but is less likely after bacterial meningitis and is not expected in children with neurodegenerative disorders.

The causes of cortical blindness include:

1. *Prenatal*: malformations, intrauterine infections and toxemia
2. *Perinatal*: neonatal asphyxia, intracerebral hemorrhage, hypoglycemia, meningitis and encephalitis
3. *Acquired*: trauma, cardiac arrest, meningitis, encephalitis, neurodegenerative disorders, cortical vein thrombosis and shunt failure.

Investigation of the infant who appears to be blind

Assessment must be systematic taking care not to 'destroy' the evidence, for instance by dilating the pupil before its reactions have been tested.

Investigation should include the following:

1. *Vision assessment*. Ideally a quantitative behavioral PL-based test such as ACP. Always repeat a low reading.
2. *Full ophthalmic examination*. Look for:
   a. *Pupillary reflexes* – normal in disorders of the posterior visual pathway but abnormal in conditions involving the retina, optic nerve, or chiasm – especially the last two
   b. *Nystagmus* – presence of sustained nystagmus indicates involvement of the anterior, rather than posterior, visual pathway
   c. *Fundus* – to include the optic disc and retina.
3. *Full pediatric examination*. Many conditions causing reduced vision in infancy have important systemic associations.
4. *Electrophysiology*. Some conditions exhibit few clinical signs, and a diagnosis cannot be made without electrophysiological tests. The electroretinogram (ERG) and the visually evoked potential (VEP), can be performed simply and without sedation. It is important to recognize that obtained this way, they should be regarded as qualitative rather than quantitative. In practice this is of minor importance as the finding of a good ERG excludes a retinal dystrophy; however, a reduced response must be repeated, and if still abnormal, an ERG under general anesthetic should be considered. The ERG is the most important of these tests, and is the only method of identifying, or eliminating a retinal dystrophy. The ERG should be performed at 2 Hz (rod and cone response) and 30 Hz (cone response).

The VEP is useful as its presence may indicate a favorable prognosis, but it may be normal in DVM and some cases of CVI.

5. *Other special tests*. The need for neuroradiological, ocular or cranial ultrasound, etc. are indicated by the results of the clinical examination. Ophthalmic examination under anesthesia, should only rarely be necessary, with one important indication being equivocal results on electrophysiological testing.

INFECTION AND IMMUNITY IN THE NEWBORN

Despite the advances in perinatal care and improved survival rates of smaller babies, mortality from neonatal sepsis remains around 20% (Gerdes 1991). There are three main reasons for this:

1. deficient host defense mechanisms in the newborn, particularly when preterm
2. lack of a specific and sensitive test to diagnose sepsis early
3. little use of host defense modulating therapies in neonatal sepsis.

The ability to defend oneself against infection requires a very large number of responses working in unison. The front line of defense is the physical barrier of intact skin and mucus membrane. Once the bacterium enters through these barriers, it is attached and lysed by the cellular component (see below) of the defense system. During lysis Gram-positive bacteria release peptiglycans whilst Gram-negative bacteria release lipopolysaccharide-A (LPS-A) or endotoxin. These initiate a cascade of events that lead to the sepsis syndrome, septic shock, multiple organ failure and death (Fig. 5.73).

Bacterial fragments and endo- or exotoxins stimulate monocytes and neutrophils to produce a variety of inflammatory mediators. They also activate complement, coagulation and fibrinolytic cascades leading to the formulation of vasoactive and proinflammatory fragments.

Proinflammatory mediators produced by macrophages include arachidonic acid and its metabolites, e.g. prostaglandin E_2, along with free radicals, e.g. nitric oxide and PAF (platelet activating factor). Macrophages and other cells also produce a multitude of cytokines of which tumor necrosis factor α (TNF-α), interleukin-1β (IL-1β), IL-6, IL-8 and IL-10 have been identified as important in sepsis. Most of these mediators can inhibit or stimulate the release of themselves or other mediators.

These mediators either singly, or sequentially, or in concert, lead to chemical and electrical change in the microvascular environment of the endothelium (in one or many organs) leading to adhesion and diapedesis of polymorphoneutrophils into the tissue. This results in the clinical features seen in sepsis syndrome and septic shock.

CELLS IN HOST DEFENSE

Of the many cells involved in response to infection perhaps the macrophage is the most important. When stimulated

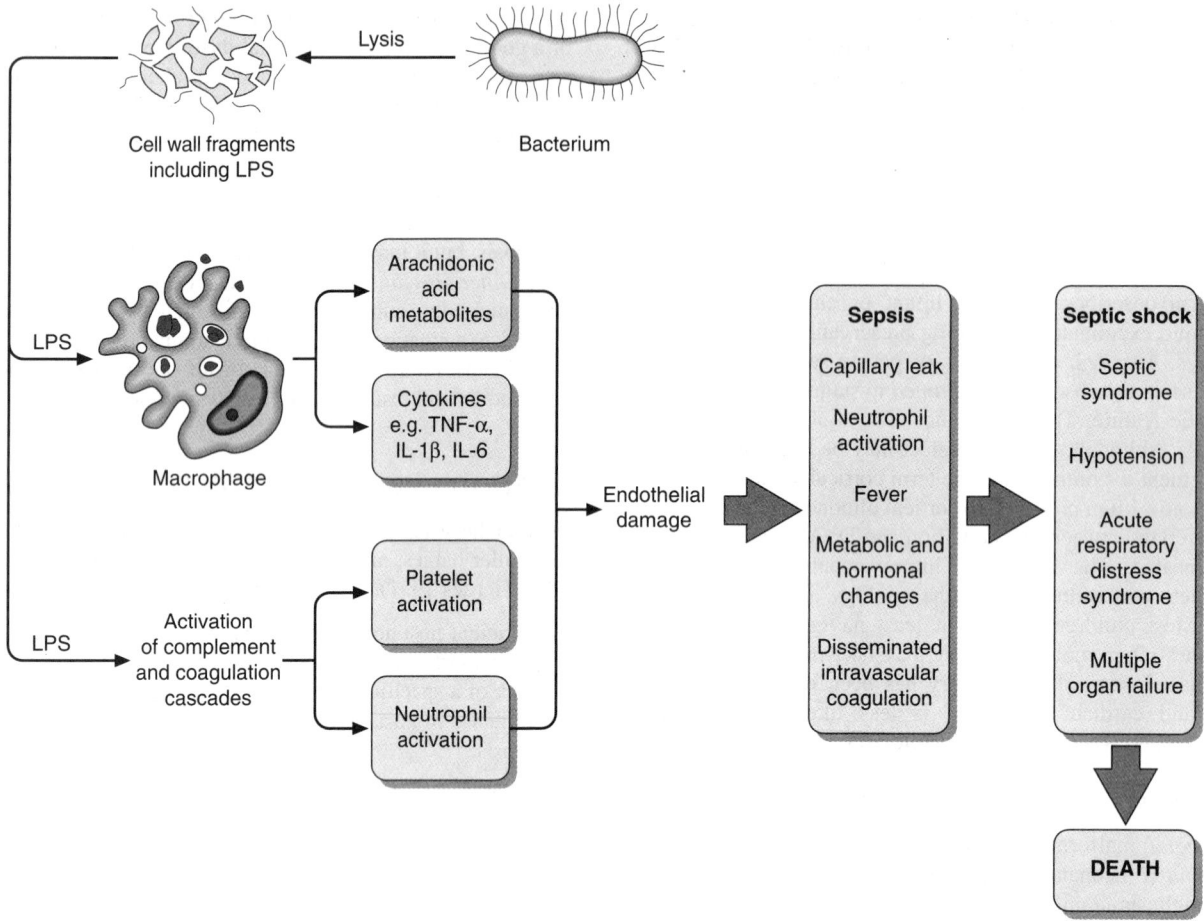

Fig. 5.73 The 'sepsis cascade': LPS – lipopolysaccharide; TNF – tumor necrosis factor; IL – interleukin. (Published with permission and courtesy of Dr S. K. Jackson and Bayer plc UK from their publication *Endotoxin and Septic Shock – the Antibiotic Connection* 1994.)

the macrophage produces three groups of powerful mediators (Fig. 5.74).

These mediators in general produce beneficial effects but when they are overproduced, as in sepsis, they lead to harmful effects like hypotension and DIC.

Phagocytes

To adequately combat the invading microorganism, the polymorphonuclear leukocytes (PMNs) must arrive at the site of infection within a critical period (2–4 h). This chemotaxis is in response to factors released by the bacteria or from the complement system (C5a). In the newborn, PMNs exhibit less chemotactic activity than they do in adults. This may be due to marked decrease in membrane deformability of the newborn PMN and the deficiency of C3 and C5 in the newborn. Other factors like Ca^{2+}, zinc and cyclic AMP may also be involved. PMNs in the newborn are also deficient in their phagocytic capacity compared to adults (Miller 1969). This may be due to decreased expression of the complement receptor CR3 in the newborn (about 60% of adult values – Berger 1990).

Prior to killing the microbe, the PMN or macrophage must attach and opsonize it, (with the help of many factors, such as immunoglobulins (mainly IgM) and complement (C3, C5 and

C3PA)). The attachment is poor in the newborn. Following opsonization, the organism can be ingested in preparation for killing.

For killing (digestion), a number of toxic oxygen products are generated including the superoxide and hydroxyl radicals and hydrogen peroxide. The cationic proteins, lactoferrin and a lysosomal enzyme (myeloperoxidase) interact with hydrogen peroxide to form the hypochlorite ion which is bactericidal. PMNs of newborns are poor in opsonization because of their inability to generate Ca^{++} ions and killing is depressed owing to poor production of hydroxyl radicals. All these essential functions are further depressed when the infant is stressed by infection.

Lymphopoietic system (T and B cells)

These form the basis of the adaptive or specific host defense system:

1. thymus-dependent cell-mediated immunity – T cell
2. bursal-dependent antibody (humoral) mediated immunity – B cell.

T lymphocytes. 70% of these cells are CD4 (helper/inducer) and only 30% form the CD8 (suppresser/cytotoxic) population. These cells are capable of producing the lymphokines which are

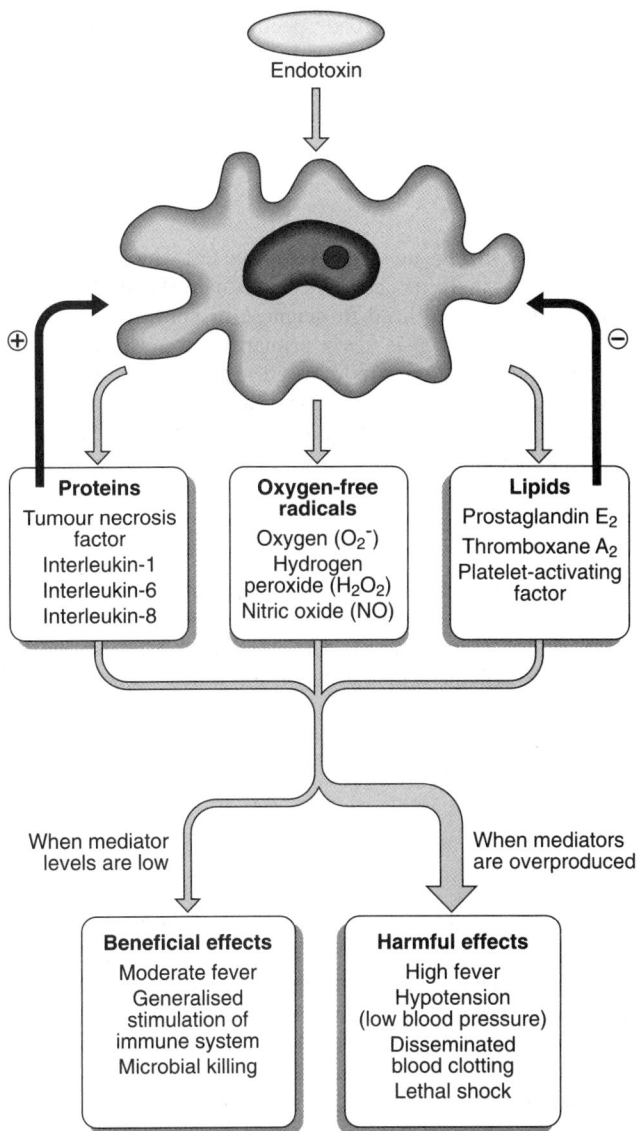

Endotoxin

$\oplus$ $\ominus$

Proteins
Tumour necrosis factor
Interleukin-1
Interleukin-6
Interleukin-8

Oxygen-free radicals
Oxygen (O_2^-)
Hydrogen peroxide (H_2O_2)
Nitric oxide (NO)

Lipids
Prostaglandin E_2
Thromboxane A_2
Platelet-activating factor

When mediator levels are low

When mediators are overproduced

Beneficial effects
Moderate fever
Generalised stimulation of immune system
Microbial killing

Harmful effects
High fever
Hypotension (low blood pressure)
Disseminated blood clotting
Lethal shock

Fig. 5.74 Endotoxins stimulate macrophages to produce three groups of powerful mediators – proteins, oxygen free radicals and lipids. These mediators may act independently, together or in sequence to engender various effects. In addition to its other functions tumor necrosis factor amplifies mediator synthesis; prostaglandin E_2 inhibits such synthesis. (Published with permission from Scientific American, August 1992, 267(2): 54–61, *Bacterial Endotoxins* by E T Rietschel and Helmut Brade.)

critical for the immune response against infection. They also retain memory.

B lymphocytes. These are concerned with humoral immunity or antibody synthesis.

HUMORAL FACTORS IN HOST DEFENSE

Antibodies

Antibodies are produced by B lymphocytes and plasma cells. In addition to their direct effect in reacting with antigens, antibodies appear to play a significant role in chemotaxis, phagocytosis and the release of mediators.

The production of immunoglobulins by the fetus is limited.

Only minute amounts of IgM are produced from 8 weeks' gestation. IgM and IgA do not cross the placenta and thus do not appear in the infant to any significant extent. IgG, however, is actively transported through the placenta from 32 weeks' gestation onwards so that the term infant has an IgG level equal to or slightly greater than the maternal level. Unfortunately, not all subclasses of IgG are transferred equally across the placenta, IgG_2 and IgG_4 being transferred in very small amounts. Preterm infants born prior to 30 weeks' gestation are deficient in all classes of IgG.

Secretory IgA inhibits the adherence of bacteria to mucosal surfaces and is present in large amounts in the colostrum and breast milk. IgE and IgD have no known role in host defense.

Complement

The circulating proteins of this system play a major role in the body's defense against bacterial, viral and fungal infections. The classical pathway is activated mainly by antigen–antibody complexes or aggregated immunoglobulins. The alternative (properdin) pathway is activated by endotoxins or complex polysaccharides in the absence of antibodies.

C_3, C_4 and C_5 are the most important functional components of the complement system and are approximately 50% of adult level in term infants. Much lower levels are seen in preterm infants. The receptor for C3b1 component on neonatal PMN, is decreased leading to depressed cell adherence, phagocytosis, mobility and activation of adhesion reactions (Berger 1990).

Cytokines

These are glycoproteins secreted by a variety of cells particularly the macrophage, to act as self-regulating proinflammatory mediators. Cytokines also play a role in modulating immune responses by acting as molecular messengers between cells.

The production of interferon-α (IFN-α) in newborn T cells is 10-fold less than in the adult (Wilson & Lewis 1990). TNF-α production is also around 50% of adult levels. These deficiencies, plus the reduced capacity to produce interleukins, lead to reduced expression of adhesion molecules on both endothelial and phagocytic cells.

Fibronectin

This glycoprotein, which is present in and around most cells in the body has a scavenging role, promoting the removal of immune complexes, fibrin and other collagenous debris by phagocytes. In the newborn, levels are 30–50% of adult values.

Adhesion molecules

Glycoproteins which mediate cell to basement membrane and cell to cell attachment are being increasingly recognized (intracellular adhesion molecules (ICAM), endothelium–leukocyte adhesion molecule (ELAM), etc.). Activated phagocytic cells induce expression of these adhesion molecules.

EPIDEMIOLOGY

The exact incidence of serious sepsis in the newborn is uncertain and underreporting is common (de Louvois & Harvey 1988).

Estimates range from 1 to 14 per 1000 live births. Gram-positive organisms were more than twice as common as Gram-negative until 1943, but between 1958 and 1965 Gram-negative organisms were responsible for three-quarters of the isolates. Since then, Gram-positive organisms have once again gained ascendancy due to the increasing importance of *Staphylococcus epidermidis*, previously not considered as a pathogen. The concept that certain bacteria are 'nonpathogenic' is not safe in neonatology and constant vigilance is required. Though mortality from sepsis has fallen considerably (over 60% since 1930) rates between 3.3 and 45% are still being reported.

Newborns are colonized with both Gram-negative and Gram-positive organisms within a few days after birth and with candida within the first 5 days of life. Other vaginal organisms, e.g. *Ureaplasma urealyticum* and *Mycoplasma hominis* may also play a role in chronic lung disease and congenital pneumonia.

In the UK the common organisms causing infection in the newborn are shown in Table 5.111.

A significant proportion of neonatal infections are due to organisms which can be cultured readily from the cervix and vaginal canal of normal pregnant women and prolonged rupture of membranes (more than 24 h), amnionitis and maternal urinary tract infection are all associated with a higher risk of neonatal infection. Maternal socioeconomic status, race and the mother's own susceptibility towards certain pathogens (e.g. rubella, cytomegalovirus) may increase the risk of transmission of microorganisms transplacentally to the fetus. Undoubtedly, the greatest hazard predisposing to infection is prematurity and low birthweight. These babies have a 3- to 10-fold greater chance of sepsis and/or meningitis compared with term infants. Male babies are twice as likely to have infection as female babies. Fetal growth retardation is also associated with higher rates of infection. Similarly, excessive manipulation during birth, resuscitation with endotracheal intubation, umbilical catheterization, insertion of long lines, hyperbilirubinemia, iron therapy, total parenteral nutrition, bottle-feeding and poor handwashing practice all predispose the newborn baby to infection.

In neonatal units, babies may be infected directly by contact with infected parents or staff or indirectly by contaminated equipment. The best and perhaps the only method to prevent nosocomial infection is to reduce these two factors. Handwashing is the single most important measure in decreasing the incidence of nosocomial infection (Haque & Chagla 1989). Though surveillance of the pattern of infection in individual units is important, routine superficial swabbing of all babies admitted to the neonatal unit or special care unit is unwarranted, as is the use of prophylactic antibiotics or antifungal creams for preterm babies. Repeated use of broad spectrum antibiotics should be curtailed as it encourages the growth of multiresistant bacteria and fungi.

DIAGNOSTIC TESTS

Microbiological test

Unfortunately, there is no single diagnostic test which can reliably diagnose sepsis in the newborn, therefore many diagnostic tests or groups of tests are utilized to diagnose or confirm sepsis. The ultimate proof of sepsis rests primarily on recovery of the infecting organism from a body fluid, e.g. blood, cerebrospinal fluid (CSF), urine, pus or other exudate aspirated from an infected lesion or tissue. The list of diagnostic tests is ever increasing. An important combination of tests is given in Table 5.112.

Blood culture

Although essential for diagnosis and appropriate management, positive blood culture results are not immediately available and their yield is poor (6–42%). The yield is dependent on skin disinfection, volume and the site from which blood is taken. Ideally 3 ml of blood is inoculated for both aerobic and anaerobic cultures. A Gram stain on buffy coat smear may give early help, and it may be helpful to repeat the blood culture on two or three occasions.

CSF culture

Meningitis may accompany neonatal sepsis in up to one-third of infants so a lumbar puncture should rarely be omitted from 'septic screen' in a stable infant. Although some have questioned the wisdom of doing routine lumbar puncture in every septic screen (McMahon et al 1990), we would recommend doing it. If CSF examination is omitted as part of the early neonatal sepsis evaluation, the diagnosis of bacterial meningitis will occasionally be delayed or completely missed (Wiswell et al 1995). Interpretation of the values in the newborn requires care as they differ from older children (Sarff et al 1976) (Table 5.113).

Urine culture

Urine is difficult to obtain; the best method is a suprapubic aspiration. Infection should be considered present if there are

Table 5.111 Common organisms causing neonatal infection

	Organism	%
Early-onset sepsis (0–4 days)	GBS	55
	Escherichia coli	14
	Other streptococci	10
	Haemophilus influenzae	8
Late-onset sepsis (5–30 days)	*Staphylococcus epidermidis*	30
	Escherichia coli	21
Late, late-onset sepsis (> 30 days)	*Staphylococcus epidermidis*	66
	Candida	9

Source: Glaxo Microdata Base 1994.

Table 5.112 Important combination of investigations for neonatal sepsis

Tests	Sensitivity %	Specificity %
1. Total white cell count < 5000/mm^3	29	81
2. Immature/total neutrophil ratio > 0.2	90–100	50–78
3. C-reactive protein > 10 mg/dl	47–100	83–94
4. Micro-ESR > 15 mm/h	27–50	83–97
5. Increased platelet size	42–52	79–95
6. Blood culture	11–60	90–100
7. Seven point hematological score ≥ 3*	93	82
8. ICAM-1 (> 300 ng/ml)	88	86

* Rodwell et al 1995.

Table 5.113 CSF values in high-risk infants without meningitis*

	Term	Preterm
Protein Mean (range)	0.9 g/l (0.2–1.7)	1.15 g/l (0.65–1.5)
Cells† Mean (range)	8.2/ml (0–32)	9.0/ml (0–29)
Glucose As percentage of blood glucose level	81%	74%

* Adapted from Sarff et al (1976) by Davies & Gothefors (1984).
† Approximately 60% were polymorphonuclear leukocytes; there was no obvious association between red and white cell counts.

more than 10 leukocytes/mm³ in an uncentrifuged and well-shaken specimen or when there are more than 105 colony-forming units/ml of freshly passed urine (or suprapubic aspiration) on two consecutive samples. Urine examination becomes more sensitive when illness occurs after the third day of life (Polin & St Gene 1992).

Superficial and other cultures

Routine cultures from the umbilicus, skin, nose, rectum, etc. frequently show colonization and positive culture does not imply invasive disease. Positive culture from trachea, joint, abscess and gastric aspirates may be more relevant. Tips of catheters, long lines and endotracheal tubes should be sent routinely for culture.

Hematological tests

White blood cells

Though total white cell counts are unhelpful profound neutropenia or neutrophilia is frequently found in sepsis. More important is the absolute early 'band' (metamyelocyte and myelocyte) count and its ratio with total neutrophils (I : T ratio). An I : T ratio greater than 0.2 is very suggestive of infection. Other characteristics, e.g. toxic granulation, vacuolation, Dohle bodies, decreased leukocyte alkaline phosphatase activity, are not invariably present. There is now some evidence that decrease in the proliferative pool in the bone marrow may be the earliest sign of sepsis (Cairo 1989).

There are usually some coagulation factor abnormalities but these are not specific, though a platelet count of less than 50 × 10⁹/l and increase in platelet size, carries a poor prognosis.

Erythrocyte sedimentation rate (ESR)

This is a sensitive but nonspecific index of infection. It is usually very low in the first days of life and inversely related to the hematocrit. A micro-ESR (done using a hematocrit tube) greater than 15 mm in the first hour is suggestive of sepsis.

Acute phase reactants

C-reactive protein (CRP), an acute phase reactant, is often raised nonspecifically in infection. CRP determination alone lacks the necessary sensitivity and specificity for the diagnosis of neonatal sepsis. Haque et al (1986) found that latex agglutination was not helpful but quantitative values of greater than 10 mg/l are considered significant by some. CRP levels are perhaps more important in monitoring sepsis than in its early diagnosis allowing the earlier discontinuation of antibiotic treatment.

Fibrinogen, haptoglobin and orosomucoid are other acute phase reactants which are nonspecifically raised in infection. The nitroblue tetrazolium (NBT) test, a test of white cell phagocytosis, is abnormal in infection but has a high rate of false positives in the newborn.

Tests for rapid diagnosis

New tests for early diagnosis largely lack the required specificity and sensitivity so cannot be recommended for routine septic screening. Counterimmunoelectrophoresis (CIE) is useful but due to lack of suitable antisera, is not routinely applicable in newborn infections. Latex agglutination tests are useful in the diagnosis of group B streptococcal and *Haemophilus influenzae* type B infections. Considerable differences in sensitivity have been found amongst different commercially available kits. False positive rates are high.

Blood, CSF and urine specimens along with cord blood IgM levels should be taken for virology and serology whenever intrauterine TORCH infections or syphilis are considered. A bone marrow aspirate may be done to confirm the diagnosis of tuberculosis. Placental histology is also very useful in the diagnosis of congenital infections (especially syphilis and listeria).

A chest X-ray is often included in a septic screen but X-rays are probably of greater help in the follow-up of infection rather than in making an early diagnosis.

Candida can be rapidly diagnosed by detection of its circulating cell wall or cytoplasmic antigens. Candida fragments may also be seen in urine and fungal balls may be detected on renal ultrasound examination.

Newer tests like the polymerase chain reactions (PCR) are not universally available and there is also a great deal of cross-sensitivity thus reducing specificity. ICAM-I is an important new tool in the early diagnosis of neonatal sepsis.

NEONATAL SEPSIS

Incidence of neonatal sepsis varies from 2.7/1000 live births in developed countries to 10–50/1000 live births in developing countries though underreporting is common in both. Incidence in preterm infant rises to 1/250 live premature births.

Predisposing factors for infection may be maternal, perinatal or environmental. Maternal factors like chorioamnionitis and urinary tract infection increase the risk of infection in the baby three- to fourfold. Prematurity increases the risk of infection 20-fold but there is considerable debate about the risk of infection following prolonged rupture of membranes. Our own experience (Haque 1993) is that factors which predispose a baby to infection after PROM are any one or more of the following: chorioamnionitis, birth at or before 32 weeks of gestation and PROM for 72 h or longer.

Even today, mortality from neonatal sepsis is around 20% and has not fallen for the last decade or so. Moreover, most babies who die from sepsis, die within the first 14 days of life. This may be due to the increasing number of very premature or low birth-weight babies being delivered.

Clinical manifestations

The signs and symptoms of sepsis in the newborn are often nonspecific (Table 5.114) and may evolve differently in each baby. Sepsis may be fulminant leading to death in several hours or may be more protracted. The most frequent symptoms are lethargy, poor feeding and abdominal distention, and the most frequent signs are prolonged capillary filling time, glucose intolerance with or without glucosuria and unexplained persistent acidosis.

Microbiology

Organisms responsible for infections in the newborn constantly change and every unit should constantly monitor its pattern of sepsis. *Escherichia coli* (Table 5.115) has continued to be the most important Gram-negative organism while group B streptococcus (GBS) and *Staphylococcus epidermidis* are the two most frequent Gram-positive organisms. GBS presents most frequently early and with signs and symptoms mimicking respiratory distress syndrome. The high incidence may be due to lack of maternal GBSIII serotype antibody. *Staph. epidermidis* is more frequent in very tiny babies with indwelling catheters or long lines and usually presents after the first 48 h.

Diagnosis

Whenever the diagnosis of sepsis is entertained, a septic screen should be performed (Table 5.112).

Treatment

Prompt initiation of supportive and antimicrobial therapy may be the most important factor in the outcome. Supportive therapy like the maintenance of blood pressure, fluid, electrolyte and acid–base balance, temperature and nutrition are dealt with

Table 5.114 Most frequent signs and symptoms in neonatal sepsis

Symptoms	Signs
Lethargy	Temperature instability
Poor feeding	Prolonged capillary filling time (hypotension)
'Does not look well'	
Apnea	Widening toe–core temperature difference
Respiratory distress	Hepatomegaly
Pallor	Splenomegaly
Mottling	Full fontanel
Cyanosis	Abnormal neurological reflexes
Abdominal distention	Glucose intolerance
Vomiting/increasing gastric residue	a. Hyper/hypoglycemia b. Glucosuria
Jaundice	Persistent acidosis
Petechiae, purpura, bleeding from prick sites	Painful bones/joints
Irritability	
Seizures	
Sclerema	

Table 5.115 Most frequently infecting organisms

From the mother (pre/perinatal)	From the environment (postnatal)
1. *Escherichia coli*	1. *Staphylococcus aureus*
2. Group B streptococci	2. *Staphylococcus epidermidis*
3. *Staphylococcus aureus*	3. *Pseudomonas aeruginosa*
4. *Streptococcus pneumoniae*	4. *Serratia* species
5. *Haemophilus influenzae*	5. Hemolytic streptococci
6. *Neisseria gonorrhoeae*	6. *Citrobacter* species
7. *Proteus* species	7. *Enterobacter* species
8. *Ureaplasma ureolyticum*	8. *Salmonella*
9. *Listeria monocytogenes*	9. Enterococci
10. *Mycoplasma hominis*	10. *Proteus* species
11. *Clostridium perfringens*	11. *Clostridium* species
12. *Mycobacterium tuberculosis*	
13. Other streptococcal species	
14. *Chlamydia trachomatis*	
15. *Treponema pallidum*	
16. *Candida albicans*	
17. TORCH organisms	
18. Malaria	
19. Viruses: vaccinia, Coxsackie, echovirus, varicella, herpes, adenovirus, respiratory syncytial, hepatitis, polio, rota and Western equine encephalitis	

TORCH = *Toxoplasma gondii*, rubella, cytomegalovirus and herpes/hepatitis.

elsewhere. Broad spectrum and bactericidal antimicrobial therapy should be started as soon as cultures have been taken.

Prognosis

With conventional therapy, the mortality from neonatal sepsis ranges from 10–40%. The most frequent complications are meningitis, jaundice and toxic effects of the antimicrobials used.

Prevention

Identification of high-risk pregnancies and where possible, e.g. GBS carrier mothers, interruption of vertical transmission is ideal, but rarely achievable. The most successful strategy is to deliver the baby under hygienic conditions and to diagnose and treat sepsis promptly. Obsession with handwashing is the key.

ANTIMICROBIAL THERAPY

The newborn is unique in its handling of drugs because of the evolving physiology. Thus most antimicrobial drugs in the newborn require modification of dose, dose intervals and duration. For detailed information about absorption, metabolism, distribution and excretion of each antimicrobial the reader is referred to specialized texts on the subject (McCracken & Nelson 1983).

The most important limiting factor in the pharmacokinetics of an antimicrobial in the newborn is the slow metabolism and the delayed excretion of the drug, which prolong the half-life. This makes it necessary to adjust the dose interval. Other factors which need to be considered are the large volume of extracellular fluid, the amount of serum protein available for binding and drug competition with bilirubin at protein binding sites. The specific antimicrobial agent(s) chosen to treat infection are determined by knowledge of local pathogens and their susceptibilities, the nature of the infectious illness and the policy employed within a neonatal unit. Since initial blind treatment in suspected neonatal sepsis cannot provide cover for all possible pathogens; value judgments have to be made.

Antibiotics for neonatal sepsis may be divided into: those that are used for initial blind therapy, e.g. ampicillin plus an aminoglycoside or a third generation cephalosporin, and those that are used for specific infection, e.g. erythromycin or vancomycin.

Most antibiotics can be administered either intravenously or intramuscularly (painful) with perhaps the exception of chloramphenicol which is poorly absorbed after intramuscular administration. Absorption after oral therapy is erratic and cannot be relied on but transdermal applications are being tried in preterm infants.

Drug levels of some antibiotics should be carefully monitored, and dosage and dose interval adjusted. There is no consensus on the duration of therapy. If the cultures are negative and the baby is well, antibiotic therapy should be stopped after 48 h. However, if the cultures were positive or the clinical suspicion of sepsis remained strong in face of negative cultures we would give antibiotic therapy for 5–7 days. Bacterial meningitis requires 2–3 weeks of parenteral therapy while osteomyelitis should be treated for 4–6 weeks, the initial 2 weeks being given by the parenteral route.

HOST DEFENSE MODULATION

The antibiotics commonly used in neonatal sepsis are given in Table 5.116. Additional modalities of therapy (Table 5.117) which have been tried and shown to be useful are granulocyte transfusion (Christensen et al 1982), exchange transfusion which has shown promise but lacks controlled studies (Hall et al 1983), and immunotherapy (Baley 1988).

Granulocyte and granulocyte–macrophage colony-stimulating factors (G-CSF, GM-CSF) have been used as adjuvant to antimicrobial therapy in neonatal sepsis with equivocal success (Cairo et al 1990, Roberts et al 1991).

IMMUNOTHERAPY

Recently pooled human immunoglobulins have been used intravenously both for prevention and treatment of neonatal sepsis. Intravenous immunoglobulins are known to stimulate release of PMNs into the tissues so increasing the number of antigen-presenting cells and potentiating the action of complement. Intravenous immunoglobulins have reduced the mortality from neonatal sepsis when used in conjunction with antibiotics; however, the best duration and dosage remain unclear. Currently, we use a pooled human IgG preparation intravenously for the prevention of sepsis. 100–250 mg/kg are infused over 2–3 h within the first hours of birth to infants weighing 1200 g or less. For the treatment of proven sepsis we either use an IgG preparation or an IgM-enriched preparation in conjunction with antibiotics. The preparation is infused over 2–3 h in a dosage of 250 mg/kg/day given once every 24 h for 4 days. No major side effects of this therapy have been noted so far (Chirico et al 1987, Weisman et al 1992, Haque et al 1995).

Table 5.116   Antibiotics commonly used in the newborn (in alphabetical order)

Drug	First week of life or preterm			Term infant, more than 7 days old			Comment
	Dosage (mg/kg/day)	Route	Frequency (h)	Dosage (mg/kg/day)	Route	Frequency (h)	
1. Amikacin	10–15	i.v./i.m.	8–12	22.5	i.v./i.m.	8	Infuse over 30 min
2. Ampicillin	100	i.v./i.m.	8–12	150–300	i.v./i.m.	6–8	Use higher dose for meningitis
3. Cefotaxime	100–150	i.v./i.m.	12	150–200	i.v.	6–8	Use higher dose for meningitis
4. Ceftazidime	50–100	i.v./i.m.	12	50–100	i.v.	12	
5. Ceftriaxone	50–100	i.v.	12–24	50–100	i.v.	12–24	
6. Chloramphenicol*	25	i.v.	8–12	50	i.v.	6–8	
7. Erythromycin	40–60	i.v.	6	40–60	i.v./p.o.	6–8	Infuse over 60 min
8. Gentamicin*	5	i.v./i.m.	12–18	7.5	i.v./i.m.	8–12	Infuse over 30 min
9. Kanamycin*	15	i.v./i.m.	12–18	25	i.v./i.m.	8–12	
10. Methicillin	100	i.v./i.m.	8	200	i.v./i.m.	6–12	
11. Metronidazole	20	i.v.	8	20	i.v.	8	
12. Moxalactam	100	i.v./i.m.	12	100–200	i.v./i.m.	8–12	Do not use as a single drug in neonatal sepsis
13. Netilmicin*	5	i.v./i.m.	12	5	i.v./i.m.	12	
14. Nystatin	200 000–400 000	p.o. or local	6	200 000–400 000	p.o. or local	12	
15. Penicillin	30–50	i.v./i.m.	12	40–60	i.v./i.m.	8	
16. Tobramycin*	4.5	i.v./i.m.	12	5–7.5	i.v./i.m.	6–8	Infuse over 30 min
17. Vancomycin*	20–40	i.v.	12	30–60	i.v.	6–8	Infuse over 60 min

* Monitor concentration levels.

Table 5.117 Therapeutic strategies to boost host defenses in neonatal sepsis

Target	Strategies
1. Leukocyte depletion	Leukocyte transfusion G-CSF/GM-CSF Intravenous immunoglobulin Exchange transfusion
2. Bacterial products	Plasma Antiserum Intravenous immunoglobulin (standard or hyperimmune) Monoclonal antibody
3. Endorphin blockade	Corticosteroids Naloxone Pentoxifylline
4. Cytokine blockade	Cytokine receptor antagonist Corticosteroids Monoclonal antibodies
5. Leukocyte activation	Nitric oxide Free radical scavengers Pentoxifylline
6. Eicosanoid blockade	Indomethacin Ibuprofen
7. Endothelium–leukocyte interaction	Intravenous immunoglobulin Pentoxifylline

Recently this mode of therapy has been questioned (Lacy & Ohlsson 1995), but we continue to believe that intravenous immunoglobulin has a significant role to play in the treatment of neonatal sepsis (Haque et al 1995).

TYPES OF INFECTIONS

Pneumonia (p. 183)

In spite of the recent advances in neonatal care, 35% of newborns at autopsy are found to have significant pneumonia.

Transplacental (or truly congenital) pneumonia

This may be part of the TORCH group of infections, or due to chorioamnionitis. Organisms like *Treponema pallidum*, *Mycoplasma hominis* and *Listeria monocytogenes* most frequently cause congenital pneumonia.

Aspiration pneumonia

The majority of infants swallow material during passage through the birth canal but pneumonia is seen in very few. It usually presents within the first 24–48 h of life. The most common organisms are *Staph. aureus*, group B streptococci, *E. coli*, *Haemophilus influenzae*, *Klebsiella* spp. and *Streptococcus pneumoniae*. The role of *Chlamydia trachomatis* and *Ureaplasma urealyticum* remains controversial, but should be actively looked for in babies who do not improve on conventional therapy (Wang et al 1995).

Acquired pneumonia

This is acquired usually in the immediate postpartum period or during the first week of life in preterm infants and usually after the first week in term infants. Common organisms involved are *Staph. aureus*, and *Staph. epidermidis*, and rarely *Pseudomonas aeruginosa*.

Clinical manifestations

Clinical features are similar in all the three categories, i.e. tachypnea, tachycardia, cyanosis and expiratory grunt. Symptoms and signs are nonspecific except for *Chlamydia trachomatis* infection where there may be a classical staccato cough. Babies may show signs of cerebral irritation or be hypotonic and lethargic. They do not feed well and may go into heart failure.

Diagnosis

This is based on the history, blood culture, microscopy and culture and Gram stain of the tracheal aspirate. An early chest radiograph may not be helpful but may be confirmatory if taken 48–72 h after onset of symptoms. Serology may also be helpful.

Treatment

The treatment depends on the etiologic agent. The initial therapy should be with ampicillin/penicillin and an aminoglycoside. Erythromycin should be reserved for ureaplasma and chlamydial infections. Flucloxacillin should be used for *Staph. aureus*. Vancomycin is preferred for *Staph. epidermidis* and methicillin-resistant *Staphylococcus*. Acyclovir and ribavirin are effective in pneumonia due to herpes simplex and respiratory syncytial virus but their routine use is not well substantiated.

Supportive therapy with oxygen, i.v. fluids, suction and physiotherapy should also be given. Drainage of a pleural effusion or empyema may be necessary but the overall prognosis is good.

Group B streptococcal infection

In Europe and North America, GBS is the most common Gram-positive bacterium causing neonatal septicemia. This, however, is not the case in most Afro-Asian countries (Haque et al 1989). The reason is unclear. About 35–40% of female genital tracts are colonized by GBS and although the vertical transmission rate is approximately 50–70% the attack rate for neonatal infection is less than 0.3%.

Clinical manifestations

Serotypes Bla and III are the most frequent offenders, the latter predominantly causing meningitis. Though classically two distinct clinical syndromes, early-onset disease (within the first 72 h) and late-onset disease (from 7 days to 6 weeks) are seen, about a quarter of GBS infections do not fit into this division.

The early-onset disease is characterized by signs and symptoms of severe sepsis, and may be indistinguishable from respiratory distress syndrome due to surfactant deficiency. It is usually a rapidly progressive disease and death may occur within hours or days.

Late-onset disease has a wider spectrum of presentation with meningitis being the most common but conditions like cellulitis, abscesses, otitis media, arthritis, osteomyelitis, ethmoiditis, fasciitis and conjunctivitis also occurring. Cultures are diagnostic;

rapid diagnosis may be made using either latex agglutination, complement fixation or countercurrent immunoelectrophoresis.

Treatment

Penicillin G is the drug of choice and should be given in large doses parenterally. Improved results have been shown by using GBS-specific (hyperimmune) gammaglobulins intravenously. Monoclonal antibody therapy may be another beneficial technique but is currently only experimental. Mortality from GBS infection remains high – 20–70% in early-onset disease and 15–50% in late-onset disease.

Staphylococcus infection

Most infants are colonized with *Staphylococcus* by the fifth day of life. The infection rate is less than 0.3%. Coagulase-positive *Staph. aureus* infections were common in the late 1950s and early 1960s but with improved recognition of hygiene and handwashing, *Staph. aureus* is not a major cause of infection in neonatal units now, though conditions like conjunctivitis and Ritter's disease still occur.

Systemic staphylococcal infections are uncommon (less than 1%). They usually take the form of osteomyelitis, septicemia or pneumonia. Staphylococcal pneumonia is characterized by the formation of pneumatoceles and/or pyopneumothoraces, or empyema.

Superficial infections include conjunctivitis which usually occurs after the first 48 h, characterized by scanty but thick, sticky yellow discharge which is more obvious in the mornings. The usual skin lesions are crops of 'pustules' with golden centers surrounded by erythema, which may be seen on any part of the body. The more sinister skin infection is the 'scalded' skin syndrome or Ritter's disease due to coagulase-positive, phage group II (3A, 3C, 55, 71). Paronychia are also seen with *Staph. aureus* infection.

It is important to recognize early osteitis due to *Staph. aureus*. The head of the femur is often involved but any bone may be affected. The infant is usually pyrexial, lethargic and may have a pseudoparalysis of the involved limb. There is usually localized swelling with or without discoloration of the overlying skin.

Coagulase negative staphylococcal infection is the disease of the 1990s. Of the 21 recognized species, *Staph. epidermidis* is the most significant in the newborn unit. Mortality from *Staph. epidermidis* infection is low but morbidity is high. This infection is associated mostly with long lines and central catheters along which it grows and forms a biofilm over itself, secreting an exopolysaccharide called 'slime'. This prevents it being attacked by antibiotics (Fleer et al 1985). Like others (Scheifele 1990) we have also seen cases of necrotizing enterocolitis due to the delta-like toxin produced by *Staph. epidermidis*.

Treatment

Most skin and nailbed lesions can be treated by local cleaning and the application of 1% aqueous gentian violet solution or 3% hexachlorophene solution. Conjunctivitis is best treated by application of 0.5% ointment of chloramphenicol after cleaning the eye with either saline or warm water. For systemic therapy, vancomycin is our first choice followed by teicoplanin as 25% of strains are resistant to flucloxacillin.

Prevention

There is no evidence that masking and wearing of gowns or isolation of the baby is effective against *Staphylococcus* crossinfection (Haque & Chagla 1989). The use of topical antiseptic and antibiotic creams is not recommended as routine, nor is the use of subtherapeutic infusion of vancomycin through a long line to prevent *Staph. epidermidis* infection (Harins et al 1995).

Overcrowding in the nursery should be avoided. Handwashing should be mandatory and meticulous and the use of chlorhexidine (Hibiscrub) for handwashing is recommended.

Neonatal meningitis (see also p. 247)

Incidence

Although meningitis is more common in the neonatal period than any other period of life, its incidence is much lower than the widely quoted figure of one-third of all septicemias. The exact incidence is not known but lies somewhere between 0.2 and 1.36 per 1000 live births.

Microbiology

Any of the organisms tabulated in Table 5.115 may cause meningitis. The most frequent organisms are *E. coli* carrying the K1 capsular antigen, group B streptococci type III and the serotype IVb of *Listeria monocytogenes*. More recently, *Staph. aureus* and *Staph. epidermidis* have become common organisms causing ventriculitis in infants with ventricular shunt placement for posthemorrhagic hydrocephalus.

Aseptic or viral meningitis is rare in the newborn, though Coxsackie B, adeno- and herpes viruses have been implicated.

Pathogenesis and pathology

Babies with myelomeningocele, congenital dermal sinus, infected cephalhematoma, osteomyelitis of the skull and otitis media have increased risk of meningitis.

At autopsy subarachnoid inflammatory exudate is more prominent at the base of the brain than over the cortex. Ventriculitis may lead to encephalopathy and blockage of the foramina and aqueduct result in hydrocephalus. Vasculitis is common, and both thrombosis and infarction may occur. Hemorrhagic cerebral necrosis is most characteristic of *Proteus* infection.

Clinical manifestation

Any of the clinical signs and symptoms listed in Table 5.114 may be present in meningitis. Pyrexia, lethargy and food intolerance are more frequent. A bulging or full fontanel and neck stiffness are late manifestations and occur in only 28 and 15% of cases, respectively (Siegel 1985).

Diagnosis

Diagnosis requires careful evaluation of the CSF with isolation of the infecting organism. A Gram stain of CSF must always be made. The cell count and the protein content are raised while glucose may be reduced. However, these results should be interpreted in the light of normal values for the newborn (Table 5.113). Countercurrent immunoelectrophoresis or latex agglutination tests may permit an etiologic diagnosis within minutes. A blood culture may grow the organism, though as many as 15% with positive CSF culture have negative blood culture.

Treatment

Treatment consists of antibiotic therapy and full supportive care. It is essential to maintain normal blood pressure because this affects cerebral blood flow. Fluctuations in the latter may predispose to cerebral ischemia or hemorrhage. Convulsions should be controlled with phenobarbitone and in the face of hyponatremia due to inappropriate secretion of antidiuretic hormone secretion fluid restriction may be necessary.

Antibiotic therapy should be aimed at sterilizing the CSF by achieving adequate levels of the drug in the CSF. Until a definitive diagnosis has been made, a combination of ampicillin and an aminoglycoside (gentamicin) or a third generation cephalosporin should be started intravenously immediately after cultures have been drawn. There is no benefit in giving the drugs intrathecally or into the ventricles. Indeed they may be harmful (Mustafa et al 1989). Once a specific pathogen has been isolated and its susceptibilities identified, the best drug or combination of drugs should be employed.

Benzyl penicillin is the drug of choice for group B streptococcal infection. A combination of ampicillin and gentamicin which have synergistic action is preferred in infections with *Listeria monocytogenes*, *P. mirabilis* and enterococci. A combination of an aminoglycoside with either an ureidopencillin (azlocillin or piperacillin) or a cephalosporin such as ceftazidime should be chosen for meningitis due to *Pseudomonas aeruginosa* or *Serratia marcescens*. Cefotaxime is preferred by us to other third generation cephalosporins because it is not excreted in the bile and there is more clinical experience with this drug in the newborn. Chloramphenicol until recently was the antibiotic of choice in neonatal meningitis due to its superior penetration into CSF. Despite its well-known toxicity, if serum concentrations are kept between 15 and 25 mg/l, toxicity from this drug is extremely rare. However, with the advent of third generation cephalosporins, chloramphenicol is now not recommended for routine use in neonatal meningitis.

Whatever drugs are used, careful monitoring of levels in both the serum and perhaps the CSF is essential for effective treatment. Antimicrobial therapy should be continued for a minimum of 14 days for Gram-positive organisms and 21 days for Gram-negative organisms (Volpe 1995). The question about repeating the lumbar puncture remains debatable (Schwersenki et al 1991). We do not recommend a repeat lumbar puncture unless in the rare case with totally normal CSF findings but continuing suspicion of meningitis.

Prognosis and complications

Mortality ranges between 20 and 40% dependent on gestational age, causative organism and the duration between the onset of the disease and initiation of therapy. Hydrocephalus occurs in about 30% whilst conditions like blindness, deafness, epilepsy and spastic cerebral palsy occur in another 30%. Brain abscesses are common in *Citrobacter* infections. Currently there is no evidence

that adjuvant dexamethasone therapy reduces morbidity in infants under 6 weeks of age with meningitis.

Gastroenteritis

This condition is uncommon in the neonatal period and is seen usually as a result of epidemics. Serotypes of *E. coli*, *Salmonella*, *Shigella*, *Campylobacter* and *Yersinia* are the usual bacterial agents. More frequent, however, are the viral agents, rota-, echo- and adenovirus.

The infant may be symptomatic with vomiting, diarrhea, feed intolerance, dehydration and may become febrile. The basis of management is correction of dehydration and if the organism is considered to be invasive, then antibiotics should be considered.

Necrotizing enterocolitis (NEC) (see also p. 210)

This is a major disease in the newborn period particularly in small preterm infants. It occurs both in endemic and epidemic forms. It is an illness of many predisposing causes. The precise role played by bacteria remains uncertain.

NEC occurs when the intestinal mucosal integrity has been disturbed. Many predisposing factors have been enumerated, e.g. low birthweight, hypoxia, patent ductus arteriosus, umbilical catheterization, early onset of feeding, particularly with hyperosmolar milk, Hirschsprung's disease, hyperviscosity syndromes and infective diarrheas. Antenatal Doppler studies showing reduced placental perfusion (absent/reversed end-diastolic flow) may be another risk factor.

In the majority of cases (60% in our series), no organism is isolated. Organisms which have been reported in the literature include *E. coli*, *Klebsiella pneumoniae*, *Clostridium butyricum*, *C. perfringens*, *C. difficile*, *Salmonella*, *Proteus mirabilis* and *Pseudomonas aeruginosa*. Viruses like adeno type 19, Coxsackie, corona and unspecified enterovirus have also been implicated.

Clinical manifestations

NEC is commonly seen in the first 10 days after birth and in babies weighing 1500 g or less. There is no sex predisposition. The most commonly encountered presentations are abdominal distention, increasing gastric residue which soon becomes bile stained, absent bowel sounds, vomiting and passage of blood in the stools. X-ray of the abdomen may show bowel wall edema in the early stages followed by pneumatosis, perforation and gas in the portal tract, the latter being a very sinister sign.

Treatment

Medical management consists of withdrawal of oral feeds, gastric suction and administration of i.v. fluids. We use parenteral ampicillin, gentamicin and metronidazole for at least 7–10 days and do not favor the use of aminoglycosides orally. Indications for surgery are debatable and are discussed on page 1782. Mortality varies from 0 to 25% and morbidity from 12 to 37%.

Osteomyelitis and septic arthritis

During the first year of life, capillaries perforating the epiphysial plate of the long bone provide communication between the joint space and the metaphysis. Thus, septic arthritis and osteomyelitis often occur together.

The source of infection is usually hematogenous but direct trauma during arterial or venous puncture has also been implicated as a cause. Organisms vary but the most predominant are *Staph. aureus* followed by group B streptococcus and Gram-negative organisms like *Klebsiella* and *E. coli*. In underdeveloped countries, *Salmonella* osteitis is frequent. In the extremely preterm, low birthweight babies who are cared for in tertiary care units, *Staph. epidermidis*, and *Candida albicans* are emerging as important agents.

Clinical manifestations

The majority of the cases present very insidiously in a 'benign' manner. There may be the nonspecific symptoms of sepsis such as poor feeding, lethargy and decreased activity. We have also found slight unexplained acidosis as an important presentation. Local signs are swelling over the affected area or joint, irritability on handling that part of the body and a low grade fever.

Diagnosis

Diagnosis is based on radiological confirmation. Technetium-99m scan is highly sensitive while conventional radiographs may miss an early lesion. Whole body scanning is preferable as there may be more than one focus of infection. Repeated cultures should be taken.

Treatment

We favor the use of flucloxacillin and cefotaxime but these should be changed according to culture and sensitivity results. Therapy should be continued for at least 6 weeks (at least 3 weeks parenterally). There is evidence that surgical aspiration and instillation of antibiotic at the site of the lesion is superior to parenteral therapy alone. Orthopedic consultation should always be sought. Mortality is low; however, reports have indicated a 25% morbidity particularly if hip or knee joints are involved.

Urinary tract infection (see also p. 261)

With improved techniques of collecting urine and radiology, the incidence is considered to be 3% in preterm and 1% in term infants. It is more common in males and in infants with kidney or renal tract abnormalities, e.g. obstructive uropathy. It is also seen more frequently in babies whose renal parenchyma may have been damaged, e.g. from asphyxia or dehydration.

The most frequent infecting organism is *E. coli* but *Klebsiella* spp. may account for 7–11% of infections. In very preterm low birthweight babies who have received long courses of antibiotics, *Candida albicans* is also an important etiologic agent.

Clinical manifestations

The clinical signs and symptoms are nonspecific but may include poor weight gain, unusual jaundice, hepatomegaly, palpable kidneys and rarely be part of generalized septicemia. Diagnosis is confirmed by a positive urine report (greater than 100 000 colony-forming units/ml and > 10 white cells/ml in a freshly voided or aspirated urine.

Treatment

Usually, a 5- to 10-day course of ampicillin plus gentamicin is sufficient; however, there is a recurrence rate of up to 10%, so follow-up is essential. We favor doing at least an ultrasound examination of the kidneys as in up to 45% of cases, radiological abnormalities have been found. With current therapy, the prognosis is excellent where there has been no renal parenchymal damage or where there are no congenital abnormalities.

Conjunctivitis (see p. 263)

The exact incidence is not known but varies between 0.5 and 3%. The higher figure comes mainly from premature infants nursed on neonatal intensive care units.

Clinical manifestations

Gonococcal conjunctivitis usually presents within the first week while *Chlamydia* infection, though it can present within the first 24 h, more usually presents after the first week. Gonococcal infection if untreated may lead to corneal ulceration and perforation, iridocyclitis, anterior synechiae and panophthalmitis. Chlamydial infection producing a similar clinical picture does not involve the cornea but involves the tarsal aspect of the conjunctiva.

Diagnosis

This is based on the clinical history, timing, site of the lesion and cultures of the discharge. Chlamydial infection may be diagnosed by obtaining scrapings from the tarsal conjunctiva and staining these with Giemsa stain for intracytoplasmic inclusions.

Treatment

For gonococcus the eye should be cleaned with frequent eye washes of normal saline or water (every 15–30 min at first) followed by instillation of penicillin drops; 100 000–150 000 units/kg/day of penicillin G are also given parenterally for 5–7 days.

For chlamydial infection, 0.5% erythromycin ophthalmic ointment is used with systemic erythromycin therapy for 7–14 days.

Chloramphenicol and sulfacetamide ophthalmic preparations may be useful for staphylococcal colonization.

The instillation of 1% silver nitrate drops to newborns led to the decline in gonococcal conjunctivitis, but this treatment has generally been abandoned as it leads to more chemical conjunctivitis.

Otitis media

Examination of the eardrum, particularly of the preterm infant, should be a mandatory part of routine examination when sepsis is suspected.

The exact incidence of otitis media is not known but it is likely to be appreciable (0.6–2.4%) due to the shorter, widely patent and horizontally placed eustachian tube. Predisposing factors are chorioamnionitis, asphyxia, prematurity, ventilatory support and infants with cleft palate or Down syndrome. *Streptococcus pneumoniae* and *Haemophilus influenzae* are by far the commonest organisms involved though *Staphylococcus epidermidis*, *Branhamella catarrhalis* and *Mycobacterium tuberculosis* have also been recorded. Presentation is nonspecific like any other infection. Otoscopic examination reveals a dull tympanic membrane which is bulging and has reduced or absent mobility on pneumatic otoscopy. Treatment includes tympanocentesis and appropriate antibiotics. Outcome is usually favorable but the recurrence rate is high and up to 33% develop chronic otitis media.

SPECIFIC INFECTIONS

The possible clinical involvement and the infecting organisms are shown in Table 5.118. Only a few specific infections will be discussed in detail.

Listeriosis

Listeria monocytogenes, a short Gram-positive bacillus, causes either an early- or late-onset disease. Early-onset disease is predominantly due to serotypes Ia and Ib. It is frequently associated with signs of maternal infection, which results in abortion, stillbirth or preterm delivery and the infant is likely to have pneumonia. Late-onset disease due to serotype IVb is likely to present with meningitis or with signs and symptoms of septicemia.

Microabscess, skin granulomas, hepatosplenomegaly and passage of meconium by preterm infants should arouse the suspicion of *L. monocytogenes* infection.

Diagnosis is based on culture and ELISA (enzyme-linked immunosorbent assay). Ampicillin is very effective and gentamicin acts synergistically but mortality from early-onset infection still remains high.

Syphilis

Congenital syphilis is now uncommon in the developed world with only eight confirmed cases in the UK between 1993 and 1995 (BPASU 1995). *Treponema pallidum* is the etiologic agent. Transplacental infection rarely occurs before 18 weeks' gestation as the Langhans layer of the chorion prevents the passage of the *Treponema*. It is possible that infection does occur prior to 18 weeks but the fetus is only able to respond to it by 20–25 weeks' gestation when the fetus becomes immunocompetent.

Treatment of the mother before the 18th week of gestation will almost always completely protect the fetus while the chances of the fetus being uninfected are negligible if the mother is not treated. If the mother has early or latent syphilis then the fetus has 20–70% chance of being infected.

Clinical manifestations

Hematogenous spread in prenatal life dictates the number of organs and tissues involved in the fetus. Abortion, stillbirth and hydrops occur in 40% of pregnancies. There may be severe anemia, hepatosplenomegaly or pneumonia soon after birth. 1–3 weeks later the stigmata of congenital syphilis become evident, e.g. nasal obstruction with serosanguineous discharge, copper-

Table 5.118 Lesions that may be caused by prenatally acquired nonviral infections

Possible clinical involvement	Infecting organisms
Central nervous system	
Meningitis, meningoencephalitis (manifestations may include microcephaly, hydrocephaly, and hydranencephaly, abnormal CNS signs, convulsions, and cerebral calcification)	*Candida albicans, Cryptococcus neoformans, Escherichia coli,* Group B streptococcus, *Listeria monocytogenes, Staphylococcus aureus, Streptococcus pneumoniae, Toxoplasma gondii, Treponema pallidum*
Special sensory organs	
Eye	
Cataracts	*Cryptococcus neoformans, Toxoplasma gondii, Treponema pallidum*
Choroidoretinitis*	*Cryptococcus neoformans, Toxoplasma gondii, Treponema pallidum*
Acute iritis, chronic iridocyclitis, vitritis, glaucoma	*Treponema pallidum*
Optic atrophy	*Toxoplasma gondii, Treponema pallidum*
Uveitis	*Toxoplasma gondii*
Endophthalmitis	*Cryptococcus neoformans*
Conjunctivitis	*Chlamydia trachomatis, Neisseria gonorrhoeae*, and other bacteria
Ear	
Eighth nerve damage	*Toxoplasma gondii, Treponema pallidum*
Otitis media	*Mycobacterium tuberculosis* and other bacteria
Cardiovascular system	
Pericarditis	*Mycoplasma hominis* and other bacteria
Myocarditis	*Toxoplasma gondii, Trypanosoma cruzi*
Respiratory system	
Pneumonia/pneumonitis	*Candida albicans, Chlamydia trachomatis, Cryptococcus neoformans, Mycobacterium tuberculosis, Toxoplasma gondii, Treponema pallidum*, and many other bacteria
Pleural effusion	*Coccidioides immitis*, Group B streptococcus
Skeletal system	
Periostitis and/or defective mineralization and growth disturbances	*Toxoplasma gondii, Treponema pallidum*
Septic arthritis	*Viridans* streptococci and other bacteria
Gastrointestinal system	
Hepatosplenomegaly with or without jaundice	*Cryptococcus neoformans*, Group B streptococcus, *Escherichia coli, Mycobacterium tuberculosis, Plasmodium, Toxoplasma gondii, Treponema pallidum*
Enteritis	Enteropathogenic *Escherichia coli, Listeria monocytogenes, Salmonella, Shigella*
Genitourinary system,	
Nephritis, nephrotic syndrome	*Plasmodium, Toxoplasma gondii, Treponema pallidum*
Miliary abscesses	*Coccidioides immitis, Cryptococcus neoformans, Listeria monocytogenes*
Vulvovaginitis	*Neisseria gonorrhoeae, Trichomonas vaginalis*
Balanitis	*Chlamydia trachomatis*

Table 5.118 *Cont'd*

Possible clinical involvement	Infecting organisms
Hematopoietic system	
Anemia, sometimes hemolytic, with jaundice	*Toxoplasma gondii, Treponema pallidum*
Petechiae or purpura, with or without disseminated intravascular coagulation. (Some hemorrhagic skin nodules are erythropoietic in nature)	*Toxoplasma gondii, Treponema pallidum*, and other bacteria
Lymphatic system	
Enlarged lymph glands	*Coccidioides immitis, Mycobacterium tuberculosis, Toxoplasma gondii, Treponema pallidum*
Skin and mucous membranes	
Vesicular lesions, single, grouped or scattered, sometimes unilateral	*Treponema pallidum*
Macular or maculopapular lesions	*Listeria monocytogenes, Toxoplasma gondii, Treponema pallidum*, and other bacteria
Maculopapular, vesicular, or scaling lesions	*Candida albicans*
Pustules, abscesses	*Staphylococcus aureus*
Ecthyma gangrenosum	*Pseudomonas aeruginosa*
Intrauterine growth retardation	*Plasmodium, Treponema pallidum*

Adapted from Davies et al (1972).
Infecting organisms are listed alphabetically and not in order of likelihood.
* The choroidoretinitis caused by *Toxoplasma gondii* and *Treponema pallidum* has been confused with the Aicardi syndrome, in which the lesions are always bilateral, rarely peripheral, and lack pigments, in contrast to that due to these two organisms.

colored maculopapular rash, perianal condylomata, rhagades and there may be loss of hair, exfoliation of the nails, iritis and choroiditis. Poor feeding and fever may be accompanied by jaundice, generalized lymphadenopathy and signs of pancreatitis or hepatitis. Bone lesions are seen in nearly all the infants beyond the neonatal period.

Diagnosis

This is based on either the complement fixation (Wasserman) or flocculation tests (Kahn, VDRL). The *Treponema pallidum* immobilization (TPI) test and the fluorescent *Treponema* antibody absorption IgM test (FTAABS IgM) are more specific. These are positive in the blood and CSF. PCR is highly sensitive.

Treatment

Symptomatic or CNS syphilis should be treated with aqueous crystalline penicillin G 50 to 100 000 units/kg/day parenterally in two divided doses for at least 10 days. For asymptomatic syphilis, we favor benzathine penicillin G 50 to 100 000 units/kg given as a single intramuscular injection. We would recommend treatment of any infant if maternal treatment was unknown, inadequate or given during the last 4 weeks of pregnancy or if the treatment was by any drug other than penicillin. Penicillin-allergic patients can be given cephalosporins.

Tetanus

This is very unusual in developed countries but neonatal tetanus

in some parts of the world is responsible for 30–40% of all neonatal deaths. The causative organism is *Clostridium tetani*, a Gram-positive anaerobic spore-forming bacillus which produces a toxin, tetanospasmin, which is responsible for muscle spasms and convulsions. The toxin once fixed to the nervous tissue cannot be neutralized by antitoxins. Mothers who are immunized protect the fetus by actively transporting antitoxins across the placenta.

Clinical manifestations

Though the incubation period is between 3 days and 3 weeks, most neonatal disease occurs between 3 and 10 days after birth. The umbilicus is the main route of entry. The infant usually presents with difficulty in sucking (due to upper lip spasm), excessive irritability and trismus. This is followed very soon by generalized muscle spasms, convulsions, rigidity and fever. There may also be cardiorespiratory difficulties.

Diagnosis

This is usually easy but meningitis, metabolic disorders and ingestion of phenothiazines must be considered in countries where tetanus is unusual.

Treatment

This is based on the provision of an adequate airway and ventilation, neutralization and elimination of toxins, prevention of spasms and convulsions and maintaining the infant's hydration and nutrition. Diazepam, either as a bolus (0.1–2 mg) or as a continuous infusion (10–140 mg/kg/day) is useful. Paraldehyde or barbiturates may also be used. Human tetanus immune globulin (500–3000 units) should be given if possible as a single dose but equine tetanus antitoxin may also be used (50 000–80 000 units). Parenteral penicillin 100 000–150 000 units should be given for at least 10 days. Fluid, electrolytes and nutrition should be maintained. Where facilities are available, mechanical ventilation and neuromuscular blockade has improved the outcome which generally, in developing countries, remains gloomy.

Tuberculosis

It is rare to see tuberculosis during the first month of life. The mother may transmit the disease either through the placenta or the baby may acquire it by aspiration of infected amniotic fluid or vaginal secretions. The signs and symptoms are nonspecific and the diagnosis is made on the basis of maternal history, placental histology and culture of gastric washings or bone marrow aspiration from the infant.

If the mother does not have an active lesion, the infant should be given INH (10 mg/kg/day) for 4–6 weeks after which a Mantoux test should be done. If this is negative BCG should be given. If the mother has active lesions, the infant should be separated from the mother and should remain separated from the mother until a BCG-induced tuberculin (Mantoux) response has been demonstrated. In situations where it is difficult to separate the infant from the mother, the infant is given INH-resistant BCG and started on INH. The infant remains with the mother and it is ensured that the mother is receiving adequate antituberculous therapy.

VIRAL INFECTIONS

Viral infections of the fetus and the newborn other than CMV are infrequent. Viral infections may cause abortion, stillbirth, congenital malformations, intrauterine infection, acute disease during the neonatal period or infancy or manifest only after a prolonged period (Fig. 5.75). Most virus infections of the neonate are transmitted from the mother and their manifestations are given in Table 5.119. Rubella and varicella-zoster are truly teratogenic but CMV and herpes zoster lead to an inflammatory destruction of organs.

Rubella

Rubella infection inhibits fetal cell multiplication. The risk of a congenitally infected infant varies with the gestation when maternal infection occurs. Though 68% of infected infants do not show any signs or symptoms at birth, between 50 and 80% are infected if the maternal infection occurs prior to the eighth week of gestation, 20–60% are infected if the maternal infection occurs during the second trimester, but fetal infection is uncommon if maternal infection is in the third trimester. Between 1990 and 1994, BPASU have reported 32 confirmed cases of congenital rubella in the UK.

Clinical manifestation

The common manifestations of congenital rubella infection are shown in Table 5.120. Important clinical manifestations are intrauterine growth retardation, microcephaly, microphthalmia, cataract, thrombocytopenia, congenital heart disease (PDA, peripheral pulmonary artery stenoses), linear bone lesions, retinitis and convulsions. The majority of manifestations, however, present much later in life. These include hearing loss 87%, congenital heart disease 46–60%, mental or psychomotor retardation 30–50%, and cataract or glaucoma 30–40%. Up to 20% may die in infancy. Progressive rubella encephalitis, diabetes mellitus, thyroid dysfunction and infantile autism have been reported as late sequelae of rubella infection.

Diagnosis

Virus isolation, either from nasopharyngeal washing, urine or CSF is the most direct method of diagnosis. A positive rubella-specific

Table 5.119 Lesions that may be caused by prenatally acquired viral infections

Pathogen	Clinical sequelae
1. Coxsackie virus	Abortion, mild febrile disease, rash, meningitis, hepatitis, gastroenteritis, myocarditis, congenital heart disease and neurological deficits
2. Cytomegalovirus	Microcephaly, hydrocephaly, microphthalmia, retinopathy, cerebral calcification, deafness, psychomotor retardation, anemia, thrombocytopenia, hepatosplenomegaly, jaundice and encephalopathy
3. Echovirus	Same as Coxsackie virus
4. Hepatitis B virus	Low birthweight, asymptomatic hepatitis carrier, acute hepatitis, chronic hepatitis
5. Herpes simplex virus	Abortion, microcephaly, cerebral calcification, retinopathy, encephalitis, multiple organ involvement
6. Human immune deficiency virus	Abortion, hydro/microcephaly, limb deformities intrauterine growth retardation, failure to thrive, rash, hepatosplenomegaly, pneumonia
7. Influenza virus	Abortion
8. Measles virus	Abortion, congenital measles
9. Polio virus	Abortion, congenital poliomyelitis with paralysis
10. Rubella virus	Abortion, microcephaly, cataract, microphthalmia, congenital heart disease, deafness, low birthweight, hepatosplenomegaly, petechiae, osteitis
11. Vaccinia virus	Abortion, congenital vaccinia
12. Varicella-zoster virus	Abortion, limb, cerebral and skin malformation Stillbirth, low birthweight, chorioretinitis, congenital chickenpox, or disseminated neonatal varicella or zoster
13. Variola virus	Abortion, congenital variola

In alphabetical order and not in order of frequency or seriousness.

IgM would suggest recent infection, a positive hemagglutination inhibition (HAI) test would suggest infection in the past and a positive complement fixation test indicates infection within the past 2 years. Newer tests include avidity-ELISA and PCR. The latter has crossreactivity with parvovirus B19.

Management

There is no specific treatment for rubella infection. In countries where routine rubella vaccination has been used, the infection rate has been considerably reduced. Seronegative women of childbearing age should be offered vaccination either after a pregnancy test or immediately postpartum. Rubella immunization to 13-year-old girls, which started in 1970 reduced the incidence

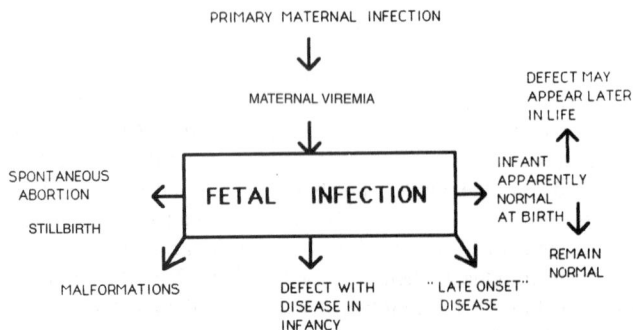

Fig. 5.75 Consequences of intrauterine virus infection.

Table 5.120 Clinical features of rubella, cytomegalovirus and toxoplasmosis

	Cytomegalovirus	Rubella	Toxoplasmosis
CNS			
Hydrocephaly	+	−	+++
Microcephaly	+	+++	−
Calcification	+++	+	++
Deafness	++	+++	++
Encephalitis	−	−	+
Eyes			
Microphthalmia	+	+	+++
Cataracts	−	++	+
Chorioretinitis	+	+	+++
Intrauterine growth retardation	+	+++	+
Cardiac lesion	−	++	+
Purpuric rash	++	+++	−
Pneumonia	+++	++	++
Hepatosplenomegaly	++	+++	++++
Lymphadenopathy	−	−	+
Bony lesion	+	+++	−

considerably and the use of MMR vaccine in the UK from 1988, will make congenital rubella rare. Most new reports of congenital rubella in the UK are of infants born to mothers who were themselves born abroad and came to the UK after the age of schoolgirl immunization.

Cytomegalovirus (CMV)

This is the most common congenital infection in Europe with a prevalence of 3–4 per 1000 births. It is a member of the herpes group of viruses and may be transmitted transplacentally or through genital secretions, breast milk or blood transfusion.

About 50% of women of childbearing age in the UK remain susceptible to CMV infection and 1% of those susceptible at the beginning of pregnancy will have a primary infection during pregnancy. Unlike rubella, fetal damage may follow primary infection or recurrent infection at any stage of pregnancy.

Clinical manifestations

In about 40% of primary infections of the mother the fetus will be infected but will nearly always be asymptomatic. When symptomatic, the main clinical features are as shown in Table 5.119. Intrauterine growth retardation, hyperbilirubinemia, chorioretinitis and intracerebral periventricular calcification are frequent. Those infants who have symptoms in the newborn period nearly always have subsequent handicap. Of the infected infants 10% will have CMV-related problems by 3 years of age, the most common problem being sensorineural hearing loss (Peckham & Logan 1989).

Diagnosis

Diagnosis is based on isolation of the virus in the throat washings or urine. Demonstration of CMV-specific IgM antibody in neonatal serum can be diagnostic. ELISA and PCR are newer sensitive methods of diagnosis.

Treatment and prevention

Antiviral drugs have not proved effective but CMV-specific hyperimmune immunoglobulin plus ganciclovir therapy holds prospect. Infected infants should be isolated. Work is in progress towards production of a vaccine.

Varicella-zoster (chickenpox)

Primary infection early in pregnancy usually leads to miscarriage, but occasionally the pregnancy survives and there may be limb hypoplasia and malformation of the eye. Later there is no problem until term. If the mother then develops chickenpox within 5 days either side of delivery, the infant may be infected. Such a mother and her infant should be isolated and given hyperimmune gammaglobulin (ZIG).

Herpes simplex virus (HSV)

Neonatal HSV infection is invariably symptomatic and carries a high mortality. Neonatal infection is due to HSV type 2 in nearly three-quarters of the cases and the rest are due to type 1. In most the infection is acquired from the maternal genital tract or oral lesions. Transmission from a primary lesion is about 50%, while from recurrent lesions it may be less than 5%.

Clinical manifestations

These may be divided into two groups. The disseminated form commences about 1 week of age with constitutional signs and symptoms of sepsis, encephalitis, seizures and a shock-like syndrome. Skin lesions, e.g. vesicles, appear in 50% of the cases. In this group, the mortality may be as high as 80%. The second group presents later (up to 3 weeks) and shows predominantly herpetic skin vesicles. 30–50% of these infants will also develop eye, skin and oral lesions and CNS symptoms without visceral involvement. A unique feature of the skin, oral and possibly the corneal infection is its tendency for recurrence.

Diagnosis

This is based on cytologic examination or direct viral culture of skin, mouth or eye lesions. Complement fixation, passive hemagglutination, neutralization, inhibition and immunofluorescence tests are available but analysis of infants' IgM-specific antibody response and PCR are the most rapid diagnostic test.

Treatment and prevention

Mothers with primary lesion should be delivered electively by Cesarean section while mothers with recurrent lesions, if they have a negative culture and do not have lesions or prodrome of infection, may be delivered vaginally. The infant should be screened for infection.

Acyclovir (Zorivax), 30 mg/kg/day in three divided doses given intravenously for 14–21 days, has reduced the mortality appreciably. The same drugs can also be used locally on skin lesions.

Hepatitis

Hepatitis A infection is rarely transmitted transplacentally. Hepatitis B transmission, however, is common. The rate of vertical transmission varies between different races being very high in Orientals. The rate of transmission is greatest with the presence of the e antigen (HBeAg). Only a small percentage of infants are likely to get infected if maternal hepatitis occurs during the first two trimesters of pregnancy, but up to 80% of infants are likely to get infected when maternal hepatitis occurs during the third trimester. If the mother is an asymptomatic HBsAg and HBeAg-positive HBsAb-negative carrier the vertical transmission rate is also very high. Transmission of hepatitis C is nearly always through contaminated blood or blood products.

Clinical manifestation

Though congenital malformations have not been implicated with hepatitis infection, growth retardation and premature delivery are frequent. Infants may either remain asymptomatic or develop hepatitis and jaundice, or go on to develop chronic aggressive hepatitis and cirrhosis.

Prevention and treatment

All infants born to HBsAg-, HBeAg-positive mothers should be given as soon as possible 0.5 ml of hepatitis immunoglobulin (HBIG) and three doses of hepatitis vaccine (10 μg). The first dose of vaccine is given along with HBIG on the first day of life but with a separate syringe at a different site. The second and third doses of the vaccine are given 1 and 6 months after the first (American Academy of Pediatrics 1986b). These infants should be tested at 9 months and if negative given a fourth dose and retested 1 month later (Stevens 1991).

Parvovirus B19

B19 is a small, nonenveloped single-stranded DNA virus. Though associated with many conditions, it primarily effects the fetus and the newborn by lytic infection of the human erythroid progenitor cell. B19 infection is the most important cause of nonimmune hydrops in the fetus and the newborn. Treatment is symptomatic but commercial IVIG preparations have been used with benefit (Schwarz et al 1990).

Human immune deficiency virus (HIV) (see pp. 1392–1398)

Between June 1986 and December 1994 over 850 children with HIV infection had been reported in the UK (BPASU 1995), 523 have been born to HIV-infected mothers. The vertical transmission rate varies from 14.4% in Europe, 30% in USA to 50% in Africa (European Collaborative Study 1992, Hutto et al 1991, Van de Perre et al 1991). It is generally considered that HIV infection is transmitted either peripartum or postpartum, but there is increasing evidence that HIV transmission may be intrapartum (Douglas & King 1992). It is interesting that if the firstborn twin is infected, only 42% of the second-born siblings are infected and, if the firstborn escapes HIV infection, then only 13% of second-born twins are infected (De Martino et al 1991). Most perinatally infected infants develop AIDS within 12 months. With new

laboratory tests, (P24 antigen, PCR) HIV infection can usually be diagnosed by 3–4 months of age.

Clinical manifestation

Signs and symptoms are nonspecific but may include a runny nose, chronic otitis media, rash, poor weight gain and lymphadenopathy.

Treatment

Treatment of the infant is symptomatic along with Septrin prophylaxis for *Pneumocystis carinii* infection. Breast-feeding is contraindicated in Europe but may be less dangerous than formula-feeding in the developing world. A careful watch should be kept for fungal and atypical mycobacterium infection.

In the BPASU database of the 523 children born to HIV-infected women (June 1986 to January 1995), 26 of the infected children have died.

PARASITIC INFECTIONS

Toxoplasmosis

Toxoplasmosis is a worldwide disease. In the UK between 20 and 40% of the population have been infected with this protozoan by adult life. Human to human transmission only occurs from mother to fetus. The rate of transmission varies from 5 per 1000 in Paris where the disease is particularly common to 1 per 5000. Overall the rate of transmission is about 40% of which 6% abort, 4% are stillborn and 30% are born alive but only a few with severe disease. The rate of fetal transmission is about 60% of third trimester maternal infections and 20–30% during the first two trimesters. Despite such high transmission rates, BPASU have recorded an incidence of 14 cases/year in the UK.

Clinical manifestations

Severe disease may be seen in 80% and 50% of infants delivered to mothers who acquired the infection in the first and second trimesters, respectively.

The classical triad of hydrocephalus, chorioretinitis and cerebral calcification is seen in more than two-thirds of infected infants. Other important clinical features are given in Table 5.120. The prognosis for patients with CNS involvement must be extremely guarded.

Diagnosis

This is usually based on toxoplasma dye test, immunofluorescent IgG toxoplasma antibody test or toxoplasma IgM antibody test. Sensitivity of IgM-ISAGA test is probably the highest.

Treatment

Two synergistic antimicrobials are used. Sulfadimidine or sulfadiazine 100–150 mg/kg/day in divided doses given every 6 h, and pyrimethamine 2 mg/kg/day in two divided doses per day for first 72 h, then 1 mg/kg/day. Therapy should be continued for 30 days. Corticosteroids should be used in presence of chorioretinitis or raised CSF protein. Clindamycin and photocoagulation have been used for ocular toxoplasmosis in older children.

Malaria

Placental transmission of malaria is extremely rare but transfusion-induced malaria is being increasingly recognized. Clinical presentation may be indistinguishable from sepsis, or the infant may present with jaundice due to hemolysis.

Diagnosis is made on seeing malarial parasites in the blood film. Treatment should be with chloroquine 5–10 mg/kg/day in divided doses for 3–5 days.

FUNGAL INFECTIONS

Candida

Disseminated candidiasis is occurring with increasing frequency, 3–4% in very low birthweight infants. Cutaneous and oral thrush lesions are common. The infant may acquire the infection from the mother's vagina, nipples, hands or from contaminated bottles. Lesions appear between the seventh and tenth day and are usually seen initially as a small papular rash which soon coalesces to form cheesy white patches in the mouth, nappy area, groin or axillae. Occasionally oral thrush may extend to cause esophagitis.

Systemic candidiasis is increasingly recognized in very low birthweight infants who receive intensive care, prolonged antibiotic therapy and parenteral nutrition, particularly with intralipid. The signs and symptoms are indistinguishable from bacterial sepsis. Renal disease, joint effusions, endophthalmitis and involvement of the CNS in the form of brain abscesses or meningitis are recognized features. Gradual respiratory deterioration with increasing infiltration of the chest on X-ray is highly suggestive.

Diagnosis

The diagnosis of local lesions is easy and can be confirmed by taking scrapings from the margins of the lesions. Urine may show yeasts or hyphae in systemic candidiasis. Candida antigen or antibody detection is useful but not immediately available. Ultrasound of the kidneys may reveal fungal balls.

Treatment

Local lesions may be treated by nystatin, 100 000 units four times a day for 5 days, or with miconazole gel (orally) and cream (to the perineum and buttocks). Nystatin with corticosteroid ointment may be used in severe cases of candida dermatitis.

Systemic candidiasis is best treated by removing all central long lines and indwelling catheters and starting the infant on intravenous amphotericin B, initially 0.25 mg/kg/day diluted in 5% D/W to 1.0 mg/10 ml. The daily dose is increased by 0.25 mg/kg/day every other day until a maximum of 1 mg/kg/day is reached. Treatment should be given for 4–6 weeks, with a total dose of 25–35 mg/kg. The infusion must be given slowly and to prevent detoxification of the drug, the infusion bottle and tubing should be covered with foil. Renal and hematological parameters should be closely monitored. The best results are obtained when amphotericin B is combined with 5-flucytosine intravenously 4.5

mg/m^2/day in two divided doses. Miconazole 20–40 mg/kg 6- to 8-hourly intravenously may also be added. There is little experience in the newborn with fluconazole or liposomal amphotericin B.

A mortality of 54% and morbidity of 25% have been reported following systemic candida infection in very low birthweight infants.

Malassezia furfur and *M. pachydermatis* which are associated with parenteral nutrition have a much better prognosis.

NEONATAL NEOPLASIA

Neoplasia presenting at birth or in the neonatal period are rare and less than half will be malignant. Knowledge of the natural history is important as even huge tumor masses or apparently disseminated disease may regress completely and spontaneously. As survival from childhood cancer has improved, death certificate data have become progressively less accurate as an indicator of frequency. Estimates of incidence vary because most reports are referral center based rather than population based and some exclude benign tumors. In the USA the best estimate of different malignancies is based on an analysis of 10% of the total population over a 3-year period. This suggests an overall incidence of 1 per 27 000 live births (Table 5.121, column 5 for proportions of different tumors). In the UK a prevalence of 1 per 12 500 to 1 per 17 500 has been found but this was inclusive of benign neoplasia (Table 5.121, column 1). Overall approximately 1.9% of childhood malignancy will present in the first 28 days of life: 43% of these will present on the first day; 66% by the end of 1 week (Campbell et al 1987); and 0.6% of pediatric malignant deaths will occur during this period.

ETIOLOGY

1. Transplacental metastases of maternal choriocarcinoma, melanoma and leukemia are well described but very rare.
2. Transplacental carcinogenesis. This is definite for maternal stilbestrol usage which leads to vaginal adenocarcinoma – the latent period is 10–15 years and it has not been reported neonatally. It is also probable for infantile neuroblastoma in the fetal phenytoin syndrome and it is possible for hepatoblastoma when the mother has been taking estrogens in the first trimester.
3. Genetic
   a. Chromosomal
      (i) Down syndrome 21X3 – acute myelogenous and occasionally acute lymphoblastic leukemia presents neonatally. Leukemoid reactions are comparatively common in the neonatal period; they are difficult to distinguish and 15% will go on to develop leukemia later.
      (ii) Kleinfelter's syndrome XXY – breast cancer (not reported neonatally), and recent reports of a higher incidence of leukemia.
      (iii) Gonadal dysgenesis 46XY, 45X/46XY, other mosaics – dysgerminomas (not reported neonatally).
      (iv) 13q$^-$ retinoblastoma – may present neonatally, the only known inheritable malignancy.
      (v) Fanconi's anemia – leukemia (not reported neonatally).
      (vi) Bloom's syndrome – leukemia (not reported neonatally).

Table 5.121 Comparative frequencies of neonatal neoplasms in different series

	Barson (1978)[1] UK (dates variable)	Davis et al (1988) Glasgow, UK (1955–1988)	Broadbent (1986) Oxford, UK (1970–1977)	Campbell et al (1987) Toronto (1922–1982)	Bader & Miller (1979) USA (1969–1971)[2]	Bader & Miller (1979) Deaths, USA (1960–1969)	Fraumeni & Miller (1969) Deaths, USA (1960–1964)
Leukemia	17	Not surveyed	17	8[3]	5	101	44
Teratoma	67	19	16 (malig.)	Not surveyed (regarded benign)	Not surveyed (regarded benign)	11	9
Neuroblastoma	64	7	27	48 (44%)	21	70	27
Soft tissue sarcoma (rhabdo-, leio-, fibro-)	22	8	13	12 (17%)	4	29	12
Wilms' and mesoblastic nephroma	20	9	8	4 (75%)	5	21	9
CNS	17		12	9 (11%)	1	12	7
Hepatoblastoma		3	3	1	0	15	10
Retinoblastoma		4		7 (76%)	0	1	
Others	78[4]	1	5	3 (100%)	3	35	12
Total	285	51	101	102[5] (42%)	39	295	130[6]
Sex incidence	–	–	1:1	1.7:1	–	–	–

[1] Benign and malignant.
[2] Third National Cancer Study (10% US population surveyed); overall incidence neonatal malignancy USA = 130 cases/year.
[3] Long-term survival.
[4] Unclear from report.
[5] Represents 1.9% of all childhood malignancy.
[6] Represents 0.6% childhood deaths from malignancy.

(vii) Ataxia telangiectasia – lymphoma and gastric carcinoma (not reported neonatally).
b. Malformation syndromes
  (i) Aniridia – nephroblastoma (possible neonatally).
  (ii) Hemihypertrophy syndrome – nephroblastoma and hepatoblastoma (not recorded neonatally).
  (iii) Beckwith–Wiedemann syndrome – nephroblastoma and hepatoblastoma (not recorded neonatally).
  (iv) Cryptorchidism – testicular tumors (not recorded neonatally).
  (v) Other syndromes – chondrosarcoma (not recorded neonatally).

GENERAL MANAGEMENT

The variety of neonatal neoplasia makes it extremely important that all should be referred to recognized specialist centers with facilities for diagnostic imaging, expert pathology and prediction, surgery, radiotherapy, chemotherapy and hematology. Tumor markers have an increasingly important role in both diagnosis and monitoring the response to treatment (Table 5.122). Large tumors may be problematic more from their size interfering with organ function rather than because of tumor load. Surgery can frequently be more conservative than is generally appreciated but may often be curative. Postoperative intensive care back-up is essential. Neonatal tissue (especially brain, bone, lungs, liver and kidneys) is very sensitive to radiotherapy and the anxieties of infection secondary to immune suppression, or the development of second malignancies means that this form of therapy should be avoided if possible. Cytotoxic chemotherapy may reduce the infant's

effective immune response so that there is a higher incidence of complications and particularly infection. Chemotherapy can potentially affect a child's subsequent development but will often reduce tumor size very significantly even when used at 50% of the dose recommended in older children. Centralization of referral also allows more realistic parental and family support.

SPECIFIC DIAGNOSIS AND MANAGEMENT

See Table 5.122.

NEONATAL METABOLIC DISORDERS

HYPOGLYCEMIA

Glucose homeostasis in the fetus and newborn

The fetus receives a constant supply of glucose across the placenta and this largely determines fetal blood glucose concentrations. Fetal metabolism is directed towards the synthesis of protein, fat and glycogen with insulin acting as the principal anabolic hormone. Hepatic glycogen accumulates during gestation and mobilization of this reserve is the principal source of glucose for the first hours of postnatal life. At delivery, the constant transplacental glucose supply is interrupted, blood glucose falls and the processes of glycogenolysis and gluconeogenesis are activated mainly by a rise in glucagon, catecholamines and cortisol and a concomitant decrease in insulin levels. Active gluconeogenesis is required for the first few postnatal days to maintain glucose homeostasis until milk feed intakes increase to levels where this is the main source of glucose precursors.

Table 5.122 Features of tumors presenting in the neonatal period

Tumor	Presentation	Investigations	Markers	Treatment	Incidence per 100 000 live births in UK	Notes

Teratoma
a. Sacrococcygeal
b. Head and neck
	1. Prenatal ultrasound
	2. Obvious mass
	  a. On buttocks: may be so large as to obstruct delivery
	  b. On neck: may lead to airway obstruction
		1. Lateral abdominal X-ray for anterior displacement of rectum ± calcification
		2. Neck X-ray
		3. Chest X-ray – pulmonary metastases
			1. α-fetoprotein: raised malignant; normal benign
			2. Beta human chorionic gonadotropin often raised
				1. Benign – surgery (remove coccyx or local recurrence common)
				2. Malignant – surgery then chemotherapy, radiotherapy
					0.27	1. At birth 90% benign, 10% malignant (if present after 2 years 90% malignant)
						2. 4:1 females:males
						3. 20% of those with intra-abdominal extension are malignant (Altman et al 1974)
						4. α-fetoprotein raised in 70% of malignant variety
						5. Solid tumors are more likely to have malignant elements
						6. Teratoma rarely present as retroperitoneal (abdominal) mass

Leukemia a. Acute myelogenous (nonlymphocytic)	1. Hepatosplenomegaly 2. Petechiae + bruising 3. Skin infiltration (nodules) 4. Respiratory distress (infiltration) 5. Bone pain 6. Meningeal involvement	1. WBC variable blasts ++ platelets reduced 2. Bone marrow ± biopsy 3. Biopsy skin plaque	1. Enzymes 2. Monoclonal membrane markers 3. Chromosomes (Greaves 1979)	Invariably fatal despite modern chemotherapy ± intrathecal methotrexate	0.29	1. 25% of cases are Down syndrome 2. Differential = hemolytic disease, congenital infection, disseminated neuroblastoma 3. Skin lesions may suggest monocytic leukemia 4. Null acute lymphoblastic leukemia may rarely present neonatally
b. (Leukemoid reactions)	1. Down syndrome child with leukemoid blood reaction	1. WBC 2. Marrow		Spontaneous remission, support with platelets, blood, ± antibiotic	—	1. Down syndrome frequent but may be normal karyotype + phenotype 2. Indistinguishable from leukemia but regresses over 1–3 months
Neuroblastoma	1. Abdominal mass 2. SVC obstruction 3. Respiratory obstruction 4. Leukoerythroblastic anemia 5. Bluish s.c. nodules 6. Spinal cord compression with pain and paraplegia 7. Horner's syndrome from cervical chain involvement	Stage i confined to structure of origin ii, local unilateral spread iii, bilateral spread iv, remote disease ivs i or ii, with remote disease 1. 24 h catecholamines VMA-HVA excretion 2. Calcification on X-ray 3. US 4. IVP 5. bone marrow 6. skel. survey or bone scan	1. VMA ⎱ in up 2. HVA ⎰ to 95% 3. Vasointestinal peptide (serum) 4. Neuron specific enolase (serum)	Stage i, total excision ii, maximal excision ± chemotherapy iii, chemotherapy plus excision iv, chemotherapy ivs, spontaneous regression usual	0.45	1. 1:40 neonatal autopsies (Guin et al 1969) 2. Spontaneous regression common (Bolande 1971) 3. 60% occur in the abdomen or pelvis 4. Prognosis excellent (cf. later in childhood, p.910) 5. Accounts for 30–50% neonatal malignancy 6. Mostly stage ivs 7. Associated congenital abnormalities are common (Isaacs 1985)

Table 5.122 *Cont'd*

Tumor	Presentation	Investigations	Markers	Treatment	Incidence per 100 000 live births in UK	Notes
Soft tissue sarcomas Fibro-, spindle cell leio-, myo-, rhabdomyo-, hemangiopericytomas	1. Mass – particularly in head, neck, extremities	1. Biopsy		1. Excision if possible 2. ± cytotoxics at a reduced dose	0.3	1. If benign soft tissue sarcomas (fibromatosis and myofibromatosis) are included, the incidence is greater than either leukemia or neuroblastomas 2. Locally aggressive 3. Metastases rare (compare older age groups, p. 915)
Renal a. Nephroblastoma (Wilms') (rare)	1. Prenatal US 2. Postnatal abdominal mass 3. Hematuria – rare	1. US 2. Chest X-ray (pulmonary metastases) 3. Staging – almost always local I or II (see p. 914)	1. ↑ Inactive renin (Carachi et al 1987)	a. Stage I, surgery + vincristine. II, surgery + vincristine + actinomycin (chemotherapy at 50% dose)	0.13	1. A neonatal renal mass is not likely to be malignant 2. True Wilms' tumors are associated with hemihypertrophy, aniridia, Beckwith's, UG abnormalities 3. Nephroblastomatosis is present in 1:400 autopsies (Machin 1980)
b. Congenital mesoblastic nephroma (more common) (Bolande 1974)	1. Prenatal (US) 2. Postnatal abdominal mass 3. Hematuria – rare	1. US 2. CXR (pulmonary metastases) 3. Staging – almost always local I or II (see p. 915)	1. ↑ Inactive renin (Carachi et al 1987)	b. Stage I, surgery II, surgery		1. Commoner than Wilms' and do not metastasize 2. Outlook extremely good
CNS Astrocytomas, teratomas, ependymomas oligodendrogliomas, craniopharyngiomas medulloblastomas	1. Prenatal US 2. Hydrocephalus cephalopelvic disproportion bulging fontanel suture separation 3. Increased intracranial pressure with vomiting 4. Convulsions	1. US 2. CT 3. NMR		1. Surgery 2. Probably not radiotherapy 3. ± shunt 4. Chemotherapy	0.2	1. High incidence of teratomas 2. Predominantly supratentorial (astrocytomas) 3. Often large at diagnosis with high incidence of hemorrhage 4. Prognosis poor 5. Best to avoid RT until ≥ 2 years
Hepatoblastoma + hemangio- endotheliomas (rare)	1. Hepatomegaly 2. ± Respiratory distress 3. ± GI symptoms	1. US	1. αFP	1. Surgery 2. ± Prepo. chemotherapy 3. ± Low dose radiotherapy preoperative 4. Postop. chemotherapy in low dose	0.05	1. A neonatal liver mass is not likely to be malignant, it is more likely to be a hemangioma or mesenchymal hamartoma and may present with cardiac failure or DIC 2. Secondary neuroblastoma or leukemia is a commoner cause of hepatomegaly than is hepatoblastoma 3. Associated with hemihypertrophy and Beckwith's syndrome

Table 5.122 *Cont'd*

Tumor	Presentation	Investigations	Markers	Treatment	Incidence per 100 000 live births in UK	Notes
Retinoblastoma	1. White eye and squint 2. Heterochromia iridis 3. Abdominal mass	1. CT 2. Chest X-ray 3. Abdominal US	1. Operation – enucleation 2. If bilateral – laser photocoagulation ± RT			1. Family history in 25% and this usually bilateral 2. Abnormality of chromosome 13 common 3. Orbital mass may be an orbital teratoma
Langerhans cell histiocytosis (no longer considered a neoplastic process Chu et al 1987)	1. Skin rash, particularly groins, axillae, neck and behind ears. Occasionally trunk. Usually brown-red raised macules which may coalesce or even ulcerate in skinfolds 2. A 'cradle cap' like skin lesion on the scalp 3. Respiratory distress from infiltration 4. Hepatosplenomegaly 5. Lymphadenopathy 6. Usually little systemic upset	1. Skin biopsy 2. Chest X-ray 3. Skeletal survey for punched-out bone lesions 4. Osmolality of urine for diabetes insipidus		1. Spontaneous remissions 2. If systemic upset/ progression steroids ± vincristine or vinblastine ± VP16		1. Proliferation of tissue macrophages. T-suppressor lymphocytes normally control the macrophages – these are deficient tissue macrophages: liver histiocytes, Kupffer cells lung alveolar histiocytes skin Langhans cells pleura + peritoneum lymph nodes gut microglia osteoclasts

VMA = vanilyl mandelic acid; HVA = homovanilic acid; US = ultrasound; IVP = intravenous pyelogram; CT = computerized tomography; NMR = nuclear magnetic resonance; RT = radiotherapy.

The maintenance of normoglycemia during the newborn period is dependent on adequate fetal glycogen reserves, effective glycogenolysis and gluconeogenesis, an appropriate balance of insulin : glucagon and the need for increasing postnatal nutritional intake to maintain homeostasis. Hypoglycemia will result if any of these processes are inadequate.

Neuropathology

Glucose is an essential primary fuel for the brain and as this is large in relation to total mass, cerebral glucose consumption is proportionately high. It seems likely that the brain of the newborn infant can utilize ketones, lactate or amino acids as an alternative to glucose. This may explain the apparent vulnerability of infants with nonketotic hypoglycemia to cerebral damage. Neurons and glial cells are susceptible to hypoglycemia and vulnerable areas are the cerebral cortex, particularly posteriorly in the parieto-occipital region. Less commonly involved are neurons of the hippocampus, caudate nucleus and putamen but any level of the central nervous system may be involved including anterior horn cells of the spinal cord. Glial injury may relate to subsequent disturbances of myelination.

Definitions of hypoglycemia

In the past, hypoglycemia was defined as a glucose concentration less than one standard deviation below the mean for a particular population; for example, hypoglycemia in the preterm or low birthweight infant was defined as < 1.1 mmol/l during the first week of life. In full-term infants the corresponding value was < 1.7 mmol/l for the first 72 h of life with a value of < 2.2 mmol/l after 72 h of age. These criteria imply that preterm infants compared to term are less prone to neurological impairment secondary to hypoglycemia and that resistance to hypoglycemia is greatest in the immediate postpartum period. A more satisfactory approach is to define significant biochemical hypoglycemia in the context of acute or chronic neurological dysfunction. This approach has shown that moderate hypoglycemia, < 2.6 mmol/l, in preterm infants is associated with reduced mental and motor developmental scores as well as a higher incidence of neurodevelopmental pathology (Lucas et al 1988b).

The *symptomatic* response of the neonate to low blood glucose is variable with clinical features which are in general nonspecific and include pallor, feeding difficulties, hypotonia, tachypnea, abnormal cry, jitteriness, apnea, irritability, coma and convulsions. This lack of symptomatic specificity can make the interpretation of biochemical hypoglycemia difficult. This is particularly so in the intensively cared for infant where concurrent pathologies cause the same pattern of clinical features or where symptomatic responses may be depressed with therapeutic muscle paralysis, severe birth asphyxia or extreme prematurity. Hypoglycemia may be intermittent and it is important to check blood glucose at times of vague but suspicious symptoms.

Some otherwise well infants with low blood glucoses are *asymptomatic* suggesting that alternative metabolic substrates are available for brain metabolism. Such infants in general have a favorable prognosis. However, acute cerebral dysfunction, as measured by auditory and somatosensory evoked potentials, occurred in the majority of neonates when blood glucose levels fell below 2.6 mmol/l even though 50% of them were still asymptomatic (Koh et al 1988).

As a consequence of these relationships between blood glucose levels and acute and chronic neurological dysfunction, *blood glucose levels < 2.6 mmol/l are accepted as indicating hypoglycemia* which requires treatment regardless of gestation or postnatal age

A classification of neonatal hypoglycemia with practical clinical value is to divide the cause or exacerbating factors into two main groups: *transient* and *persistent* hypoglycemia (Aynsley-Green & Soltesz 1985) as in Table 5.123.

Transient neonatal hypoglycemia

Intrauterine growth retardation

Fetal growth retardation can result from many causes. Infants with asymmetric growth retardation with disproportionate preservation of head size in relation to body mass are particularly prone to both in-utero and postnatal hypoglycemia. The etiology of the hypoglycemia can be multifactorial with metabolic demands of a relatively large brain, depleted glycogen, fat and protein reserves as well as limited gluconeogenic and ketogenic responses which in some are secondary to poorly coordinated counterregulatory mechanisms (Hawdon et al 1993a,b). The presence of prematurity, birth asphyxia or polycythemia can compound the problem.

Table 5.123   Causes of neonatal hypoglycemia

Transient hypoglycemia	Persistent hypoglycemia
Intrauterine growth retardation	Hyperinsulinism
	Nesidioblastosis
	Insulinoma
Prematurity	
	Inborn errors of metabolism
Birth asphyxia	Glycogen storage disease
	GSD types I, III, IV
Neonatal sepsis	Galactosemia
	Hepatic gluconeogenic deficiencies
Neonatal cold injury	Fructose-1,6-diphosphatase
	Pyruvate carboxylase
Starvation	Phosphoenolpyruvate carboxylase
	Defects in amino acid metabolism
Congenital heart disease	Maple syrup urine disease
	Methylmalonic acidemia
Hyperinsulinism	HMG-CoA lyase deficiency
Infant of diabetic mother	Beckwith–Wiedemann syndrome
Erythroblastosis fetalis	Proprionic acidemia
Maternal drugs	Tyrosinemia type I
Maternal glucose infusions	Mitochondrial fatty acid oxidation defects
Idiopathic hyperinsulinism	MCAD deficiency
	LCAD deficiency
	Electron transport defects
	MAD-S deficiency
	MAD-M deficiency
	RR-MAD deficiency
	Hormonal deficiencies
	Congenital hypopituitarism
	Cortisol deficiency
	Congenital glucagon deficiency

Birth asphyxia should be avoided by monitoring and intervention in labor (p. 84) and neonatal polycythemia if present should be corrected (p. 226). Enteral feeds should start early, usually within an hour of birth. Blood glucose should be monitored frequently, usually hourly, until normoglycemia is attained when the interval can be extended to 2- then 4-hourly. If normoglycemia is not attained, then a background intravenous infusion of dextrose is required, starting around 5 mg/kg/min but increasing this if necessary, usually by increasing the dextrose concentration rather than the volume per kg. Enteral feeds are gradually increased in volume with reciprocal decreases in intravenous dextrose if normoglycemia is maintained. With the discontinuation of intravenous dextrose, the frequency of enteral feeds can be sequentially reduced to 2-, 3- and 4-hourly if normoglycemia is established. In a minority of infants where attaining normoglycemia is problematic and i.v. glucose requirements are high or prolonged, in spite of established enteral nutrition, concurrent pathology should be considered.

Prematurity

The immaturity of gluconeogenesis and glycogenolysis as well as limited glycogen and fat reserves make this group vulnerable to hypoglycemia. The problem is greater with decreasing gestational age. Early hypoglycemia, < 1 h, occurs in up to 70% of infants < 30 weeks' gestation before intravenous dextrose infusions are established and thereafter glucose homeostasis can be unstable in sick premature infants and may require frequent monitoring (Lyall et al 1994). Hypoglycemia is usually transient and correctable with a dextrose infusion of 5 mg/kg/min but a higher caloric intake to meet energy demands, either parenterally or enterally, should be established early. In addition, preterm infants will only partially suppress endogenous glucose production with glucose infusions (van-Goudoever et al 1993, Tyrala et al 1994) but also fail to inhibit proteolysis (Hertz et al 1993) and early introduction of complete parenteral nutrition (day 1) improves not only energy–nitrogen balance but reduces hypoglycemic episodes (Murdock et al 1995). Hypoglycemia in preterm infants is common and this may impair the early detection of underlying metabolic abnormalities whether developmental delay or genetic disorders affecting glucose homeostasis (Hume et al 1992, Hume & Burchell 1993)

Birth asphyxia

Perinatal stress will deplete glycogen reserves and mitochondrial damage may uncouple oxidative phosphorylation with subsequent anaerobic glycolysis and generation of lactate. Hypoglycemia is usually transient and correctable with an intravenous infusion of dextrose at around 5 mg/kg/min. Glucose homeostasis may be unstable. Hyperglycemia should be avoided as it may exacerbate existing metabolic acidosis and compound the hyperosmolar state. Prematurity, intrauterine growth retardation, adrenal hemorrhage and transient hyperinsulinism are common associations.

Neonatal sepsis

Hypoglycemia and sepsis are commonly associated. Pyrexia may increase the metabolic rate, caloric intake may be decreased and insulin sensitivity may be increased.

Neonatal hypothermia

Hypoglycemia is a common feature and glucose homeostasis should be established as part of the resuscitative measures.

Starvation

Failure to establish adequate enteral intake in full-term infants can result in hypoglycemia and this effect is exaggerated by intrauterine growth retardation, prematurity or birth asphyxia.

Congenital heart disease

Hypoglycemia per se can result in transient cardiomegaly. An association exists between hypoglycemia and acute congestive cardiac failure; the etiology of this may be multifactorial with decreased caloric intake, increased metabolic rate, decreased hepatic perfusion or even focal hepatic necrosis. Hypoglycemia has also been observed in children with severe congenital heart disease but without cardiac failure. Management consists of restoration of normoglycemia with intravenous glucose and in the longer term adequate caloric intake.

Transient hyperinsulinemia

Infant of diabetic mother

Fetal blood glucose uptake is directly related to maternal blood glucose levels and fetal hyperglycemia results in hyperplasia of the islets of Langerhans, increased peripheral insulin receptors, a decreased glucagon response to postnatal hypoglycemia and delayed evocation of hepatic gluconeogenic pathways. Meticulous control of maternal diabetes in pregnancy and labor can prevent or reduce the severity of neonatal hypoglycemia and in parallel the incidence of macrosomia, respiratory distress syndrome, hyperbilirubinemia, polycythemia and hypocalcemia. The incidence of congenital malformations is higher in this population and includes congenital heart disease, abnormalities of the central nervous system, vertebral anomalies and the caudal regression syndrome which may present in various forms including sacral agenesis, femoral hypoplasia or sirenomelia. Careful control of maternal diabetes preconceptually and in the early weeks of pregnancy may reduce the incidence of malformations.

In the majority of infants, postnatal hypoglycemia is transient, < 6 h, and asymptomatic. Blood glucose is usually monitored at birth, 1, 2, 4 and 6 h. Enteral feeds are established within the first hour and thereafter 2-hourly until normoglycemia is established. In the minority of infants hypoglycemia may be more prolonged, up to 3 days, and if normoglycemia is not maintained the infants may become symptomatic. In asymptomatic infants who fail to establish normoglycemia with enteral feeds, a single dose of glucagon (0.03–0.1 mg/kg) may prevent recurrence. In the sick infant, or those intolerant of enteral feeds or where hypoglycemia is prolonged, normoglycemia should be maintained by i.v. infusions of dextrose (4–8 mg/kg/min). Symptomatic hypoglycemia requires an initial bolus of i.v. dextrose (0.25–0.5 g/kg and thereafter a constant i.v. infusion. Enteral feeds are introduced when appropriate with reciprocal reduction in i.v. infusion rates maintaining normoglycemia and avoiding abrupt changes which can result in reactive hypoglycemia. Rarely, in prolonged hypoglycemia unresponsive to the above measures, hydrocortisone 5 mg/kg 12-hourly has been used.

Erythroblastosis fetalis

An association exists between moderate to severe erythroblastosis fetalis and neonatal hypoglycemia secondary to hyperinsulinism. It is estimated that around 20% of infants with cord hemoglobins < 10 g/dl will have significant hypoglycemia. It is important to monitor blood glucose, not only in the early neonatal period, but during and after exchange transfusions.

Beckwith—Wiedemann syndrome

Affected infants may have exomphalos, macroglossia, visceromegaly, giantism, parallel creases on the ear lobes, hyperinsulinemic hypoglycemia and an increased risk of Wilms' tumor and other malignancies (Elliot et al 1994). All features may not be present and infants with only giantism or exomphalos should have blood glucose levels monitored.

The etiology of this syndrome is unknown with no obvious maternal risk factors but abnormalities of growth hormone, somatomedin and of the adrenal glands may indicate a disturbance of fetal growth factors. The majority of cases are sporadic with a female predominance but in familial forms possible patterns include autosomal dominant, multifactorial and autosomal dominant sex-dependent inheritance. Genomic imprinting has been implicated. Chromosomal abnormalities are present at 11p15.3 with close associations to IGF-II and tumor suppresser genes (Mannens et al 1994).

Hypoglycemia is usually transient but may be prolonged and severe and occasionally persists into adulthood. Symptomatic hypoglycemia is estimated to occur in around 50% of individuals and may contribute to the mental deficiency recognized as part of this syndrome. The management of persistent hyperinsulinemia is discussed below.

Maternal drugs

β-mimetic agents used in the management of premature labor stimulate the fetal pancreas to produce insulin and also reduce fetal hepatic glycogen deposition. Hyperinsulinemia is usually transient and related to cord levels of the β-mimetic agent but may go undiagnosed since the majority of infants are preterm and at risk of hypoglycemia for other reasons. Maternal administration of β-mimetics is usually discontinued when preterm delivery is planned or is inevitable as these agents can also have profound effects on neonatal cardiorespiratory function.

Neonatal hyperinsulinemic hypoglycemia has been reported after maternal administration of *chlorpropamide* and mothers should not be managed on this agent in pregnancy. Thiazide diuretics were at one time prescribed to control pregnancy-associated edemas and were postulated to stimulate β-cell function. The evidence was not conclusive and their use in pregnancy is now rare.

Intrapartum glucose infusion

Fetal insulin secretion can be induced by intrapartum maternal glucose infusions. The incidence of resultant neonatal hypoglycemia is related to maternal blood glucose levels particularly when above 6.6 mmol/l or when maternal glucose infusions are greater than 20 g/h.

Idiopathic transient neonatal hyperinsulinism

The etiology of hypoglycemia in growth-retarded infants is multifactorial but in some infants where normoglycemia is not established by 72 h, in spite of adequate nutrition, the possibility of hyperinsulinism should be considered and investigated. This syndrome also occurs in full-term, appropriate for gestational age infants after normal pregnancies and deliveries, without histories of maternal diabetes or drug ingestion. The resolution of transient hyperinsulinemia may take days, weeks or in some instances months, and on occasions diazoxide is required to control hypoglycemia. The etiology of transient hyperinsulinism is unknown and is regarded as a temporary imbalance in the regulatory development of insulin secretion.

Persistent hypoglycemia

Organic or persistent hyperinsulinemia

This is characterized by recurrent or persistent hyperinsulinemia and is the commonest cause of prolonged severe hypoglycemia during the first year of life. In the neonatal group, the underlying pathology is usually nesidioblastosis whereas in older children solitary islet cell adenomas predominate. However, congenital islet cell adenomas are described in neonates and hyperinsulinemic hypoglycemia, with the features of nesidioblastosis, has been described in adults.

Histological features of nesidioblastosis vary widely. In most instances there is an increase in pancreatic (β) cells either organized in groups or as individuals. Somatostatin (δ) cells are usually decreased. Some individuals show no obvious histological abnormality. In functional terms, all have an uncontrolled release of insulin.

The majority of organic hyperinsulinisms present with early neonatal hypoglycemia and are recognized causes of neonatal death and sudden infant death syndrome. Fetal hyperinsulinism results in a phenotype similar to that of the infant of the diabetic mother. The majority of cases of nesidioblastosis are sporadic but familial cases suggest an autosomal recessive inheritance and it may also occur in familial endocrine adenomatosis.

Diagnosis of hyperinsulinism

Normoglycemia, > 2.6 mmol/l, may only be attained in infants with hyperinsulinism with increased glucose infusion rates (> 8 mg glucose/kg/min and in individual cases sometimes > 20 mg glucose/kg/min). Insulin secretion is inappropriately high in comparison to simultaneously measured blood glucose. In normal, fasted individuals, insulin levels are low or undetectable, but in organic hyperinsulinism they remain elevated even in the presence of hypoglycemia. Insulin prevents ketogenesis by inhibiting lipolysis and in hyperinsulinism there is no increase in blood ketones with decreasing glucose concentrations in comparison to healthy normals or patients with ketotic hypoglycemia. Plasma levels of branched chain amino acids are sensitive indicators of circulating plasma insulin concentrations and are decreased in hyperinsulinemia. Insulin increases hepatic glycogen reserves and liver size may increase due to glycogen deposition.

Management

Immediate management is to maintain normoglycemia by intravenous infusion of dextrose and this may require rates > 15 mg/kg/min. Glucagon may be useful as a temporary measure, e.g. resiting i.v. sites, as it provokes an exaggerated glycemic response compared with normals and those with ketotic hypoglycemia but paradoxically may also increase insulin secretion. Somatostatin has been used as a short-term measure as it decreases endogenous insulin production and increases blood glucose but may inhibit other endocrine responses with long-term use. Diazoxide inhibits insulin release, increases adrenaline secretion and activates glycogenolysis. The therapeutic effects are variable and unpredictable, some infants showing initial benefit with a subsequent return to hypoglycemia. Diazoxide in oral dosage up to 25 mg/kg/day is usually combined with a thiazide diuretic, which potentiates its effects and reduces water retention. Complications of diazoxide therapy include fluid retention, edema, nonketotic–hyperosmolar coma and blood dyscrasias. In many cases, however, long-term treatment with diazoxide is successful. Surgery may have to be considered in infants who are already prescribed diazoxide–thiazide, and whose glucose requirements are still > 25 mg/kg/min and where hypoglycemia is still problematic. There is no diagnostic metabolic or endocrine test to distinguish a diffuse pancreatic disorder from an adenoma. Localization of an adenoma by angiography, ultrasonography or palpation at laparotomy allows resection which is curative. Where no tumor is localized pre- or perioperatively, subtotal or total pancreatectomy may have to be considered, balancing the detrimental effects of hypoglycemia against postpancreatectomy diabetes.

Leucine-sensitive hypoglycemia may be a reflection of an individual tendency to hyperinsulinism rather than a specific and distinct pathological entity. A decrease in plasma glucose and an increase in insulin after administration of leucine has been used as a test of excessive insulin secretion. Not all patients respond in this manner and leucine can stimulate insulin secretion in normal individuals. In hyperinsulinemic states, short clinical trials of low leucine diets may be tried but the mainstay of treatment remains diazoxide–surgery.

Inborn errors of metabolism

Glycogen storage disease (p. 1135)

Type I glycogen storage disease, glucose-6-phosphatase deficiency and the associated transporter defects, may present in its severest form in the neonatal period with hepatomegaly, profound hypoglycemia and lactic acidosis (Chen & Burchell 1995).

Hepatic gluconeogenic enzyme deficiencies

Fructose-1,6-diphosphatase (p. 1135) is a key hepatic gluconeogenic enzyme and deficiency causes a similar biochemical profile to glucose-6-phosphatase deficiency with fasting hypoglycemia, lactic acidosis, ketosis, hyperuricemia and hyperlipidemia. Hepatomegaly in this condition is secondary to lipid accumulation. Around half the cases present in the newborn period and require frequent feeding of a high carbohydrate diet.

Phosphoenolpyruvate carboxykinase (p. 1131) converts oxaloacetic acid to phosphoenolpyruvate. Defects of the enzyme restrict the utilization of lactate and gluconeogenic amino acids and this results in hypoglycemia, lactic acidosis and hyperalaninemia.

Pyruvate carboxylase converts pyruvate to oxaloacetic acid and deficiency will limit gluconeogenesis from lactate and alanine. Hypoglycemia may not be a prominent feature as other gluconeogenic amino acids can enter the tricarboxylic acid cycle and be converted through oxaloacetic acid to glucose.

Galactosemia (p. 1132)

Galactosemia commonly presents in the neonatal period with vomiting, diarrhea, failure to thrive, cataracts, hyperbilirubinemia and hypoglycemia.

Defects in amino acid metabolism

Maple syrup urine disease (p. 1116) in neonates may present with vomiting, failure to thrive, a characteristic odor and hypoglycemia with a rapid progression to severe neurological symptoms. Early recognition is important to prevent long-term neurological damage.

3-hydroxy-3-methylglutaryl-CoA lyase deficiency (HMG-CoA lyase deficiency) (p. 1118) is usually classified as a disorder of leucine metabolism with biochemical features of hypoglycemia, hyperammonemia and metabolic acidosis without ketonuria. Initial presentation may be in infancy, early childhood or the neonatal period (Gibson et al 1988).

Methylmalonic acidemia (p. 1117) and proprionic acidemia (p. 1117) can present in the neonatal period with hypoglycemia and metabolic ketoacidosis.

Mitochondrial defects of fatty acid oxidation

Medium chain or general acyl-CoA dehydrogenase (MCAD) deficiency (p. 1129). This is the commonest of the inborn errors of mitochondrial fatty acid catabolism and crises are commonly precipitated by infectious episodes with fever, diarrhea, vomiting, poor feeding, lethargy and coma. Hepatomegaly is inconsistently found but if biopsy is performed shows fatty infiltration. Hypoglycemia is always present. Plasma ammonia may be normal or slightly elevated. Ketonuria is classically absent or inappropriately low. MCAD deficiency has been reported as a cause of sudden and unexpected death in infants. The diagnosis of MCAD deficiency can be made by DNA molecular analysis (90% have a common allelic variant) and/or plasma acylcarnitines (Roe & Coates 1995). The severity of clinical symptoms can be prevented by frequent meals, additional carbohydrate intake during stress and supplements of carnitine if required.

Long chain acyl-CoA dehydrogenase (LCAD) deficiency (p. 1129). Attacks of hypoglycemia and hypotonia occur with hepatocardiomegaly during episodes of exacerbation. In a few infants a sensorimotor neuropathy or pigmentary retinopathy has been described (Roe & Coates 1995). The earliest presentation of LCAD deficiency was thought to be 2 months until the case report of Chalmers et al (1987) who described a sudden neonatal death at 31 h in a full-term infant who was appropriately grown and without dysmorphic features. Initially the infant appeared healthy but fed poorly and was lethargic at 27 h. Liver, kidneys and muscle showed fatty infiltration.

Hormone deficiencies

Congenital hypopituitarism (p. 1039). Early hypoglycemia may be a presenting feature. Infants are usually at term, normally grown and without other central nervous system defects but there may be a conjugated or unconjugated hyperbilirubinemia. In affected males external genitalia may be small with micropenis. A few infants have associated midline defects including cleft lip and palate or septo-optic dysplasia. Pituitary hormone deficiencies may be partial or complete and are usually multiple. Cortisol and thyroid replacement may be required from the newborn period.

Cortisol deficiency states. Hypoglycemia may be seen in congenital adrenal hyperplasia (p. 1061), bilateral adrenal hemorrhage (p. 121) and congenital adrenal hypoplasia (p. 1067).

Congenital glucagon deficiency. This is rare with two cases reported and where deficiency contributed to the hypoglycemia.

Investigation of hypoglycemia

The majority of infants will have transient hypoglycemia associated with a clinical risk factor (Table 5.123) and do not require extensive investigation. If hypoglycemia persists or is recurrent the infant should be investigated. The priority of investigations may be determined by clinical features or a family history of inborn errors of metabolism or sudden infant death syndrome.

Hypoglycemia should always be confirmed by formal laboratory analysis using a method specific for glucose. Fluoride oxalate tubes should be used to inhibit glycolysis. Glucose requirements of the infant should be calculated in mg/kg/min.

Investigations include a full blood count to exclude polycythemia, a blood gas to determine the presence of a metabolic acidosis and plasma electrolytes, essential if adrenal dysfunction is suspected.

Plasma should be collected at the time of hypoglycemia for insulin, ketone bodies (usually β-hydroxybutyrate), amino acids, lactate, growth hormone, cortisol and ACTH levels. Blood for insulin and ACTH should be collected into lithium heparin tubes, immediately stored on ice and plasma separated within 20 min. Blood for lactate should be collected into a fluoride oxalate tube. The total blood volume required need not be large, 2.5–3 ml. Prior discussion with the investigating laboratory is essential.

Urine should be collected at around the time of hypoglycemia and screened for pH, reducing compounds (Clinitest) (p. 137), ketones and keto acid with 2,4-dinitrophenylhydrazine and for the variety of compounds that react with ferric chloride. Urine should also be analyzed for amino acid and organic acids.

These investigations may give the definitive diagnosis or guide to further more specific investigation or analysis. Complete characterization of a metabolic defect may require provocation or loading tests or enzyme studies on fibroblasts, leukocytes or tissue biopsies or molecular analysis of DNA.

HYPERGLYCEMIA

Hyperglycemia in the newborn is defined as a blood glucose > 7 mmol/l after a 4-h fast and this value may be used in the diagnosis and subsequent management of the rare phenomenon of transient neonatal diabetes mellitus.

Hyperglycemia in preterm infants

Hyperglycemia is seen in nonfasting preterm infants where blood glucose concentrations > 10 mmol/l are not uncommon, may occasionally exceed 20 mmol/l and are most frequently associated with either dextrose infusions or parenteral nutrition. The pathogenesis of this hyperglycemia is uncertain and may include failure to suppress endogenous glucose production, an attenuated insulin release or a decrease in end-organ sensitivity to insulin (Hawdon et al 1993c). Some regimens for parenteral nutrition include insulin to control not only the hyperglycemia but to improve anabolism and activate lipid clearance.

The adverse effects of hyperglycemia include osmotic diuresis and dehydration, an increase in plasma osmolality and generation of a metabolic acidosis through lactate production.

Blood glucose values which constitute hyperglycemia in preterm infants are not well defined. Most clinicians would consider it desirable to maintain blood glucose < 10 mmol/l either by decreasing the amount of dextrose infused or prescribing insulin 0.05–0.1 IU/kg. Careful monitoring of blood glucose at least hourly is essential and intermittent doses of insulin are often preferred to a continuous infusion. Whether to control moderate hyperglycemia, 5–10 mmol/l, depends on clinical circumstances. Glucose renal thresholds can be as low as 5 mmol/l in extremely preterm infants and a glucose-induced osmotic diuresis might be an indication to treat with insulin.

Hyperglycemia is also associated with infection, intracranial hemorrhage, severe respiratory distress syndrome or necrotizing enterocolitis. Aminophylline and dexamethasone may exacerbate hyperglycemic tendencies.

Hyperglycemia in full-term infants

Early postnatal hyperglycemia has been described in association with compensatory responses to birth asphyxia. The mechanism is thought to involve rapid mobilization of hepatic glycogen by a combination of glucagon and adrenaline secretion and suppression of insulin release. Early hypoglycemia is much more common in this group although late hyperglycemia and instability of glucose homeostasis is seen in severely birth asphyxiated infants who often have associated hepatic damage.

Transient diabetes mellitus

The onset of permanent diabetes mellitus is rare in infants less than 6 months of age. A transient form of diabetes mellitus may present as early as the first postnatal day or as late as 6 weeks of age. The infants are usually small for gestational age and present, in spite of adequate nutrition, as failure to thrive with wasting and dehydration but with a characteristic 'alert appearance'. Blood glucose levels are variable and may be as low as 13 mmol/l or as high as 110 mmol/l. Glycosuria leads to dehydration which may be rapid in onset and severe. Ketonuria is absent or minimal, in contrast to later-onset permanent diabetes mellitus. Insulin levels are inappropriately low for blood glucose concentrations. Management consists of correction of the dehydration and of the hyperglycemia with insulin. A few infants can be managed without continuation of insulin but the majority require regular insulin in dosage varying from 1 to 3 units/kg/day for periods as short as 14 days or as long as 18 months. These infants are extremely insulin sensitive. After initial correction of dehydration and establishment of enteral feeds they can usually be managed on a once or twice daily insulin regimen. In the majority, the dose of insulin can be tapered slowly before completely stopping.

In most instances, the condition is sporadic in occurrence although familial cases are reported with a few infants born to diabetic mothers. The etiology of transient diabetes mellitus is thought to be a temporary delay in maturation of β cell function and control. A few infants have been reported where there was an initial period of hypoglycemia, but within 3–14 days this gave way to hyperglycemia and transient diabetes mellitus. Permanent diabetes mellitus or later recurrence has been reported in a few individuals.

Leprechaunism. A constellation of mutations in the insulin receptor gene give rise to this syndrome of intrauterine growth retardation with minor dysmorphic features and characterized by insulin resistance, elevated plasma insulin levels and glucose intolerance. Infants usually die in the first year of life.

DISORDERS OF CALCIUM AND MAGNESIUM METABOLISM

Normal fetal and neonatal calcium homeostasis

In utero, there is an active movement of calcium from mother to fetus such that by term the concentrations of total and ionized calcium in fetal blood are approximately 10% higher than maternal values. This relatively hypercalcemic state suppresses fetal parathormone secretion and stimulates calcitonin release, conditions which favor fetal mineral deposition. After birth, the infant parathyroid remains suppressed and this transient hypoparathyroid state results in a fall in plasma calcium. In the normal term infant, the plasma calcium decreases during the first 24–72 h after birth, reaching values as low as 1.75–2.0 mmol/l. This state of relative hypocalcemia stimulates parathormone release and suppresses calcitonin secretion. Calcium levels gradually increase to within the normal range for infants by 4–5 postnatal days. This transition in calcium metabolism is usually without clinical features but symptomatic hypocalcemia develops if these mechanisms are delayed or exaggerated.

Hypocalcemia

Mild functional asymptomatic hypocalcemia occurs normally within the first few days of life but levels which constitute biochemical hypocalcemia can be defined as a corrected plasma calcium < 1.75 mmol/l or an ionized calcium < 0.625 mmol/l. Such infants are at risk of symptomatic hypocalcemia.

Calcium is present in plasma in three fractions: (a) protein bound (30–50%); (b) diffusible nonionized calcium chiefly in complexes with citrate or phosphate (5–15%); and (c) in an ionized state. The ionized state is the metabolically active form but dynamic equilibrium and interchange occurs between calcium in the various plasma fractions. Approximately 80% of protein-bound calcium is attached to albumin and the remaining 20% to globulin. Changes in pH influence calcium binding to albumin and acidosis results in an increased ionized calcium and alkalosis a decrease in ionized calcium.

Clinical assessment of ionized calcium can be made by electrocardiographic observations of the corrected QT interval (Q_0Tc interval) measuring the time from the origin of the Q wave to the origin of the T wave; it is prolonged > 0.19 s in full-term

Table 5.124 Causes of neonatal hypocalcemia

Neonatal hypocalcemia
    Early
    Late (neonatal tetany)

Primary hypoparathyroidism
    Sporadic
    X-linked, autosomal dominant or recessive
    DiGeorge syndrome

Maternal hyperparathyroidism
    Vitamin D deficiency
    Vitamin D dependency
    Rickets/osteopenia of prematurity
    Primary hypomagnesemia

infants and > 0.20 s in preterm infants who have a low ionized calcium value.

There are a number of clinical conditions where hypocalcemia is the presenting feature (Table 5.124) but the commonest of these is early neonatal hypocalcemia.

Early neonatal hypocalcemia

The onset of early neonatal hypocalcemia is typically in the first few days of life and most often between 24 and 48 h. At greatest risk are low birthweight infants, both premature and growth retarded, birth asphyxiated infants and the infant of the diabetic mother.

Pathogenesis. The etiology of early neonatal hypocalcemia is usually multifactorial. Most symptomatic infants will have had suboptimal postnatal calcium intake. The postnatal rise in parathormone may be delayed in preterm infants, and indeed most infants with early neonatal hypocalcemia have low or undetectable levels of immunoreactive parathormone. Calcitonin levels are normally elevated in the early newborn period but exaggerated concentrations have been documented in premature as well as in asphyxiated hypocalcemic infants. Hyperphosphatemia as a result of hypoxemic tissue damage or excessive catabolism releasing phosphate may lead to hypocalcemia. An intracellular movement of calcium can occur after hypoxic cell injury with depression of plasma calcium levels. Acute respiratory alkalosis can occur in ventilated infants resulting in reduced ionized calcium. Sodium bicarbonate administration or the use of citrated blood in exchange transfusions may create a metabolic alkalosis. Elevated plasma fatty acids generated from intravenous lipid infusions have been reported to lower ionized calcium levels.

Insulin-dependent diabetic mothers tend to have lower plasma magnesium levels throughout pregnancy, and infants have lower cord and 24-h postpartum plasma levels of calcium and parathormone. Chronic maternal hypomagnesemia may cause relative hypoparathyroidism in both mother and fetus. The majority of infants of diabetic mothers are asymptomatic but may show biochemical evidence of hypocalcemia and/or hypomagnesemia. In symptomatic infants with both biochemical abnormalities, the hypocalcemia and hypomagnesemia can be corrected with magnesium treatment.

Clinical features and course. The symptoms and signs of early neonatal hypocalcemia occur when the calcium falls to < 1.75 mmol/l and can be difficult to differentiate from those of associated pathologies, e.g. hypoxic-ischemic encephalopathy or intraventricular hemorrhage, or those of other metabolic abnormalities such as hyponatremia or hypoglycemia.

Management. Early enteral calcium supplementation has been shown to prevent early neonatal hypocalcemia in preterm infants. Gastrointestinal irritation and increased stool frequency are the only significant side effects. The vitamin D metabolites, 25-hydroxycholecalciferol and 1,25-dihydroxycholecalciferol, are also effective in raising plasma calcium levels but are rarely used.

Infants whose only pathology is early neonatal hypocalcemia and who have neurological symptoms should be treated as described for late neonatal hypocalcemia. Measurement of the Q_0Tc interval can be a useful screening procedure to determine whether low ionized calcium is present in a particular infant. Calcium gluconate 10% (1 ml/kg) can be given intravenously but cautiously over 10 min with ECG monitoring. Decreases in heart rate require slowing of the intravenous infusion or discontinuation. Maintenance calcium gluconate can be given continuously intravenously or orally (75 mg/kg/day). Peripheral i.v. infusions if they extravasate may result in skin slough, tissue necrosis and calcification. The preferred method of maintenance, where there is no central line, is by the enteral route and calcium gluconate 10% 1–2 ml/kg 4- or 6-hourly is usually tolerated.

Late neonatal hypocalcemia (neonatal tetany)

Late neonatal tetany can be regarded as a form of transitory hypoparathyroidism but usually symptomatic hypocalcemia and tetany are only problematic in infants subsequently exposed to high phosphorus intake.

Pathogenesis. Primary maternal hyperparathyroidism complicating pregnancy is rare but a temporary maternal hyperparathyroid state, secondary to vitamin D deficiency, may be more common. That this type of neonatal hypocalcemia is related to maternal vitamin D deficiency is supported by nutritional studies and a seasonal incidence in spring and early summer in the Northern hemisphere related to low sunshine exposure in the later months of pregnancy, with low levels of 25-hydroxycholecalciferol in both mothers and infants. Enamel hypoplasia is frequently found in affected infants and is indicative of disordered enamel formation during the last trimester of pregnancy. The mothers of infants with late hypocalcemia tend to be older, of higher parity and of lower social class than mothers of non-hypocalcemic infants.

Occurrence of neonatal tetany in a susceptible population is largely determined by the nature of the milk feed in the newborn period. Cow's milk contains three to four times as much phosphorus as human milk. Partially modified cow's milk formulae (particularly tinned evaporated milks), which still had a high phosphorus content, were used routinely until the mid-1970s when the incidence of neonatal tetany was as high as 1% of formula-fed infants. With the introduction of feeds with a calcium and phosphorus content approximating to that of human breast milk, neonatal tetany is now rare.

Clinical features. Late neonatal tetany usually occurs from the second half of the first week up to several weeks, classically in full-term infants born after a normal labor and delivery who are artificially fed. Although affected infants may have appeared a little jittery or tremulous with increasing tactile irritability of muscles, usually they have been otherwise well, feeding normally, responding normally and with a normal cry, before the sudden onset of convulsions.

Fits are usually transitory lasting for a few seconds and usually focal in nature and between convulsions the infant is alert. Jitteriness is evident on stimulation, the tendon reflexes are increased and increased muscle tone with extension, in the legs particularly, is usual. Trousseau's sign is seldom positive and Chvostek's sign, which can be elicited freely in the newborn infant, is of little value. Recovery may occur spontaneously, but in others fits may continue for several weeks unless treated.

Diagnosis. The diagnosis is based on a low serum calcium, < 1.75 mmol/l, and a high serum phosphorus, > 2.6 mmol/l. Occasionally the serum calcium is not markedly lowered and the raised phosphorus level is probably a more important diagnostic criterion. There is usually an associated hypomagnesemia but this is moderate in degree, in the range 0.5–0.6 mmol/l.

The differential diagnosis of neonatal tetany from other types of convulsions usually rests on the absence of an abnormal birth history, the normal behavior of the infant between the attacks, apart from muscular irritability, the absence of other signs which would indicate intracranial birth injury and the presence of normal or increased deep tendon reflexes.

Treatment. Treatment consists of calcium intravenously or orally usually in the form of calcium gluconate 10% solution 5 ml/kg/day. Vitamin D has also been used in a dosage of 5000 IU/day orally. Although hypocalcemia is the most obvious biochemical abnormality, the most effective treatment is intramuscular magnesium sulfate (0.2 ml/kg 50% solution per dose), particularly when convulsions are occurring; this can be followed with a further one or two doses at 12-hourly intervals. Intramuscular magnesium controls hypocalcemic tetanic fits more effectively than calcium, and calcium more effectively than phenobarbitone.

Prognosis. The prognosis of neonatal tetany per se is good, most cases making full recovery without sequelae. Where the hypocalcemia is secondary to an underlying disorder, the prognosis will be of that disorder.

Hypoparathyroidism

Primary hypoparathyroidism is a rare cause of hypocalcemia in the newborn. The diagnosis is confirmed by absent or low parathormone levels in the presence of hyperphosphatemia, hypomagnesemia and low alkaline phosphatase. Sporadic cases occur but most have a genetic basis, usually X-linked recessive, but autosomal recessive and dominant forms have been described.

DiGeorge syndrome is usually sporadic in occurrence and results from an embryological defect of the 4th branchial arch and derivatives of the 3rd and 4th pharyngeal pouches. The pattern of defects includes hypoplasia or absence of the parathyroids, hypoplasia or absence of the thymus and cardiovascular anomalies including aortic and truncal abnormalities with minor facial anomalies. The severity of the congenital heart disease usually determines the early prognosis and the degree of hypoparathyroidism may be variable and transient forms have been described. The etiology is heterogeneous. Several different chromosomal abnormalities have been described but deletions at 22q11.2 are most frequent. Teratogenic causes including retinoic acid and fetal alcohol syndrome are also described. Treatment of hypoparathyroidism consists of supplementation with vitamin D_2 or its analogues 1α-hydroxycholecalciferol or 1,25-dihydroxycholecalciferol.

Maternal hyperparathyroidism

Primary maternal hyperparathyroidism is a rare complication of pregnancy with parathyroid adenomas usually responsible but carcinoma has been described. The maternal diagnosis depends on the demonstration of persistently high plasma calcium, elevated plasma parathormone and low urinary calcium and phosphorus. Complications in pregnancy include hyperemesis gravidarum, weakness, renal calculi, spontaneous abortion and late fetal death. The most common neonatal complication is hypocalcemic tetany, observed in around 50% of infants born to mothers with untreated disease. The unexpected occurrence of neonatal tetany may provide the initial clue to the diagnosis of unsuspected maternal hyperparathyroidism. The etiology of neonatal hypocalcemia is thought to reflect prolonged parathyroid suppression from the chronic hypercalcemic state of mother and fetus. However, some infants have normal or elevated parathormone levels and the etiology may be more complex.

The clinical features, diagnostic criteria and treatment are those of neonatal tetany. Hypomagnesemia is a frequent occurrence. Most cases of neonatal hypocalcemia secondary to primary maternal hyperparathyroidism are transient but long-term congenital hypoparathyroidism has been described.

Maternal medullary carcinoma of the thyroid

Maternal medullary carcinoma of the thyroid is associated with high calcitonin levels. In the one reported case of this disease, several children born prior to maternal diagnosis exhibited radiological features of osteopetrosis.

Hypercalcemia

Plasma calcium levels > 2.75 mmol/l (corrected) are generally regarded as constituting hypercalcemia. Clinical manifestations include weakness, irritability, hypotonia, poor feeding, weight loss, polyuria, polydypsia, constipation and vomiting. The major causes are idiopathic infantile hypercalcemia (p. 1056), hyperparathyroidism (p. 1056), benign familial hypercalcemia (p. 1058) and vitamin D intoxication (p. 1058), and hypercalcemia associated with inadequate phosphorus intake in extremely immature infants (Lyon et al 1984).

Hypomagnesemia

Plasma magnesium levels in the newborn infant are relatively constant through the first week of life (range 0.59–1.15 mmol/l). Hypomagnesemia, < 0.6 mmol/l, does not usually occur during the first few days of life, nor in association with asphyxia, but most commonly occurs towards the end of the first week and later.

Isolated hypomagnesemia can occur as a primary cause of convulsions but is usually associated with concomitant lowering of the plasma calcium as in late neonatal hypocalcemia. Milk formulae with high phosphorus loads predispose to hypocalcemia and also to hypomagnesemia. Neonatal hypomagnesemia is also associated with maternal malabsorption, to parathormone deficiency in the infant, to a primary defect of magnesium absorption in the infant or to magnesium binding by citrate in exchange transfusions.

Treatment of hypomagnesemia is by intramuscular injection of magnesium sulfate 50% 0.2 ml/kg dose. This can be repeated for one or two further doses at 12-hourly intervals. If both hypomagnesemia and hypocalcemia are present, treatment with calcium alone may be ineffective. Improvement may only be achieved after magnesium is prescribed and this often results in the spontaneous rise in serum calcium level. The role of magnesium in relieving the symptoms of hypocalcemia may be due to its capacity to release ionized calcium for effective parathyroid function.

METABOLIC BONE DISEASE IN PRETERM INFANTS

Defective bone mineralization has been recognized in preterm infants for many years but the terminology used to describe this is confusing. The terms rickets of prematurity or osteopenia of prematurity have been used synonymously. Osteopenia of prematurity refers to hypomineralization of the skeleton of the preterm infant compared to that of the normal skeleton resulting from in utero accretion of minerals (Greer 1994). Rickets of prematurity implies the presence of radiologically detectable abnormalities, appearances which are historically related to vitamin D deficiency in children, but similar appearances can occur in preterm infants with severe metabolic bone disease. The term osteoporosis has been used to describe radiological rarefaction of bone and where this occurs without obvious rachitic changes represents a less advanced stage of metabolic bone disease, but substantial demineralization, quantified sensitively by means of photon absorptiometry or dual energy radiographic densitometry, can occur before radiological changes are obvious.

Pathogenesis

Bone formation is a complex process integrated by hormonal and growth factors and dependent on an adequate supply of calcium, phosphorus, magnesium, trace metals such as copper, and vitamin D. Matrix formation is as critical as that of subsequent mineralization, and deficiencies at any stage of bone formation may give rise to a common final presentation of disordered bone growth. The etiology of metabolic bone disease in preterm infants is probably multifactorial but a major component is likely to be as a consequence of a deficiency of calcium and phosphorus rather than vitamin D.

The vitamin D status of the infant at birth is largely dependent on the adequacy or otherwise of maternal vitamin D metabolism. In humans, 25-hydroxycholecalciferol crosses the placenta with a close correlation between maternal and cord blood levels both in term and preterm infants. Term infants approximate maternal values but preterm infant levels of 25-hydroxycholecalciferol may be significantly lower. Serum 1,25-dihydroxycholecalciferol levels show no correlation between maternal and cord blood samples, consistent with the concept that the fetoplacental unit is its own source of 1,25-dihydroxycholecalciferol in utero.

The newborn preterm infant may not have full expression of hepatic 25-hydroxylation of vitamin D but the majority of studies would support the concept that this ability appears to be achieved very early in postnatal life and adequate serum levels, by adult standards, can be achieved using vitamin D supplements as low as 400–500 IU/day for the first 1–3 months of life. Preterm infants are also capable of 1α-hydroxylation of vitamin D, based on serum estimation of 1,25-dihydroxycholecalciferol, which rises sharply during the first week of life when infants are supplemented with very high vitamin D intakes. On more physiological dosage regimens of vitamin D, 500 IU/day, lower increments of 1,25-dihydroxycholecalciferol are seen over the first week of life but gradually reach maximal values around 3–4 weeks postnatal age. The absorption of vitamin D is dose related and facilitated by bile salts; a low bile salt pool in preterm infants and a diet high in polyunsaturated fatty acids might predispose to a degree of malabsorption of vitamin D. The evidence of significantly increasing hydroxylated derivatives of vitamin D in vitamin D-supplemented preterm infants suggests that this ability is not significantly impaired.

Calcium, unlike phosphorus, is not well absorbed from formula milks. The higher bioavailability in human milk can result in 70% absorption provided that phosphorus and vitamin D contents are adequate. In term milks, the absorption of calcium is in the range of 30–60%, and 80–95% of this absorbed calcium can be retained. Calcium absorption increases with both gestational age and postnatal age. Postnatal age effects may be a reflection of gastrointestinal adaptation to calcium adequacy or deficiency. Absolute calcium retention increases with the amount of calcium ingested and with higher calcium intakes can be greater in preterm infants than occurs in utero. The concentration of calcium in the formula is therefore important, as is the quantity of milk consumed.

Preterm infants absorb phosphorus very efficiently (86–97% of intake) independent of the type of milk or the calcium or phosphorus concentration of that milk. Retention of absorbed phosphorus appears to be directly related to the rates of calcium and nitrogen retention. Calcium and phosphorus absorption are relatively independent. The renal absorption of phosphorus can be almost complete in preterm infants but fractional phosphorus excretion can be increased if phosphorus is supplied in excess, either in absolute terms or in conditions of relative excess, if calcium is deficient.

In utero calcium accretion rises exponentially in the last trimester from 114–125 mg/kg/day (2.89–3.12 mmol/kg/day) at 26 weeks to 119–151 mg/kg/day (2.97–3.77 mmol/kg/day) at 36 weeks' gestation. Phosphorus accretion over this gestational age range is 60–85 mg/kg/day (1.94–2.74 mmol/kg/day).

The calcium and phosphorus contents of human milk or term formulae cannot meet the requirements of the preterm infants if accretion of these elements is to continue at intrauterine rates. For example, an extreme preterm infant fed a commercial term formula at 150 ml/kg/day would have a calcium intake of 65 mg/kg/day (1.6 mmol/kg/day) and a phosphorus intake of 40 mg/kg/day (1.6 mmol/kg/day). If the infant typically absorbed 50% of the calcium intake and 90% of the phosphorus intake, then this would give an absorbed calcium of only 32 mg/kg/day (0.8 mmol/kg/day) and a phosphorus of 36 mg/kg/day (1.2 mmol/kg/day) available for retention. Comparison of these figures with the in utero accretion rates shows how wide the deficits can be between prenatal and postnatal life.

Histological studies have shown that metabolic bone disease in neonates differs from that of classical vitamin D deficiency rickets with markedly reduced matrix formation and decreased osteoblastic activity perhaps suggesting contributions from other deficiencies. However, more recent histomorphometric studies suggest increased bone resorption rather than impaired formation underlies the development of metabolic bone disease in preterm infants (Beyers et al 1994a). Copper deficiency in preterm infants could be easily confused where the radiological findings are of osteoporosis, flaring of anterior ribs, cupping and flaring of metaphyseal regions of long bones and subperiosteal new bone formation. It is equally possible that deficiencies in other nutrients may contribute to metabolic bone disease in preterm infants and, for example, when preterm infants are supplemented with calcium, magnesium absorption and retention decreases, with phosphorus having an additive effect. In these infants, magnesium supplementation can increase absorption and retention and dietary magnesium intakes may have to be higher (10–20 mg/kg/day) than those previously recommended (5–6 mg/kg/day) (Giles et al 1990).

The etiology of metabolic bone disease in preterm infants is probably multifactorial with the main deficiencies being those of calcium and phosphorus, rather than vitamin D.

Clinical features

The largest number of reports of metabolic bone disease are in extreme preterm infants. Skeletal mineralization may be compromised by several factors including prolonged intravenous nutrition with its inherent limitation of mineral intake as well as concerns about aluminum contamination, fluid restriction resulting in decreased intakes of calcium and phosphorus, prolonged immobility, chronic acidosis, treatment with dexamethasone or frusemide and the use of nonsupplemented human breast milk. Many of these factors are common to infants receiving prolonged intensive care and defective mineralization is not specific or more severe in groups with bronchopulmonary dysplasia as was thought in the past (Ryan et al 1987).

In the majority of infants with metabolic bone disease there are no overt findings on clinical examination and the diagnosis is dependent on the results of investigation. Occasionally, clinical features are present in preterm infants with well-established and severe rachitic disease (Fig. 5.76). Metabolic bone disease in preterm infants can be associated with impairment of linear growth, spontaneous fractures and chronic respiratory distress (Bishop 1989, Lucas et al 1989).

Investigation and monitoring

Bone mineral content, usually of the forearm, can be measured directly with photon absorptiometry and when specifically calibrated for small infants, can be precise and accurate (Greer & McCormick 1988). Bone mineralization is assessed relative to bodyweight or ulnar length and compared to a gestational age curve which represents in utero mineralization. Until recently, photon absorptiometry, although primarily a research tool, has been the only viable technique for the accurate assessment of the state of bone mineralization (Horsman et al 1989).

Photon absorptiometry is both sensitive and precise but it is expensive and the equipment bulk makes it impractical for routine use. The recent development of dual energy radiographic densitometry should overcome these difficulties (Lyon et al 1989). Radiographic densitometry has the advantage that bone mineral content can be assessed along the length of a bone or comparison easily made between bones. This may be important as bone mineralization is not uniform and wider assessment of the state of mineralization could be a major advantage (Tsukahara et al 1993).

The radiological changes of rickets in preterm infants, cupping and fraying of the metaphyses together with the loss of the provisional zone of calcification, have been well described (Fig. 5.76). Periosteal reactions and fractures of bone may also occur. Substantial demineralization has to occur before radiological changes become apparent and a dependence solely on radiological methods will seriously underestimate the extent of the spectrum of metabolic bone disease in a population. Measurement of cortical thickness as a means of studying bone formation similarly lacks precision in the study of bone mineralization.

In formula-fed infants, plasma calcium and phosphorus values are not good indicators of early metabolic bone disease with plasma calcium only falling significantly in the most severely affected infants with overt radiological rickets and phosphorus values often remaining unchanged. In infants fed human milk, phosphorus depletion is commonly recognized and characterized by hypophosphatemia, hypercalcemia, hypercalciuria, hypophosphaturia and elevated levels of plasma alkaline phosphatase. Prolonged absence of phosphorus from the urine with persisting calcinuria implies continued tissue phosphorus depletion and has been used sequentially in individual infants to assess the need for mineral supplementation.

Measurement of vitamin D metabolites has limited value in the diagnosis or management of rickets of prematurity.

The use and interpretation of plasma alkaline phosphatase activity as a marker of bone metabolism can be difficult in preterm infants. Reference values have been established for total plasma alkaline phosphatase activity in cord blood from preterm and term infants and it appears that the bone alkaline phosphatase is the predominant isoenzyme (Crofton & Hume 1987). The liver isoenzyme is undetectable in preterm and term infant plasma. Plasma fetal intestinal alkaline phosphatase is low at birth both in term and preterm infants but increases dramatically in preterm infants in the postnatal period, peaking at around 2 weeks of age when it may contribute up to 30% of the total activity in plasma. Thereafter peak plasma fetal intestinal alkaline phosphatase activity declines to negligible levels by 6–7 weeks postnatal age. The postnatal rise is related to gestation age and is marked in infants less than 34 weeks' gestation but rises only slightly in term infants. In preterm infants, total plasma alkaline phosphatase activity in the third trimester decreases with gestational age in infants 5–10 days postnatal age and total alkaline phosphatase has been correlated with the radiological features of rickets and used to monitor the effects of metabolic studies. There is no doubt that total plasma alkaline phosphatase activity can be a useful research tool with significant differences in mean values between groups. The wide variability between individual infants makes its usefulness limited on single samples (Lyon et al 1987) but sequential measurements from an infant increase its diagnostic value.

Total plasma alkaline phosphatase activity has limitations in the assessment of metabolic bone disease in individual preterm infants particularly in the first 2–3 weeks of life. In spite of these constraints, radiological appearances of rickets crudely correlate with total plasma alkaline phosphatase measurements although not with osteopenia (Lyon et al 1987) or with bone mineral content as measured by photon absorptiometry. Equally high total plasma alkaline phosphatase activity, representing metabolic bone disease in preterm infants, has been related to slower growth rates in the neonatal period and to a significant reduction in attained length at 9 months and 18 months post-term (Lucas et al 1989).

Management

The key to management of this disorder must be prevention, with a sufficient nutritive intake from early postnatal life to allow

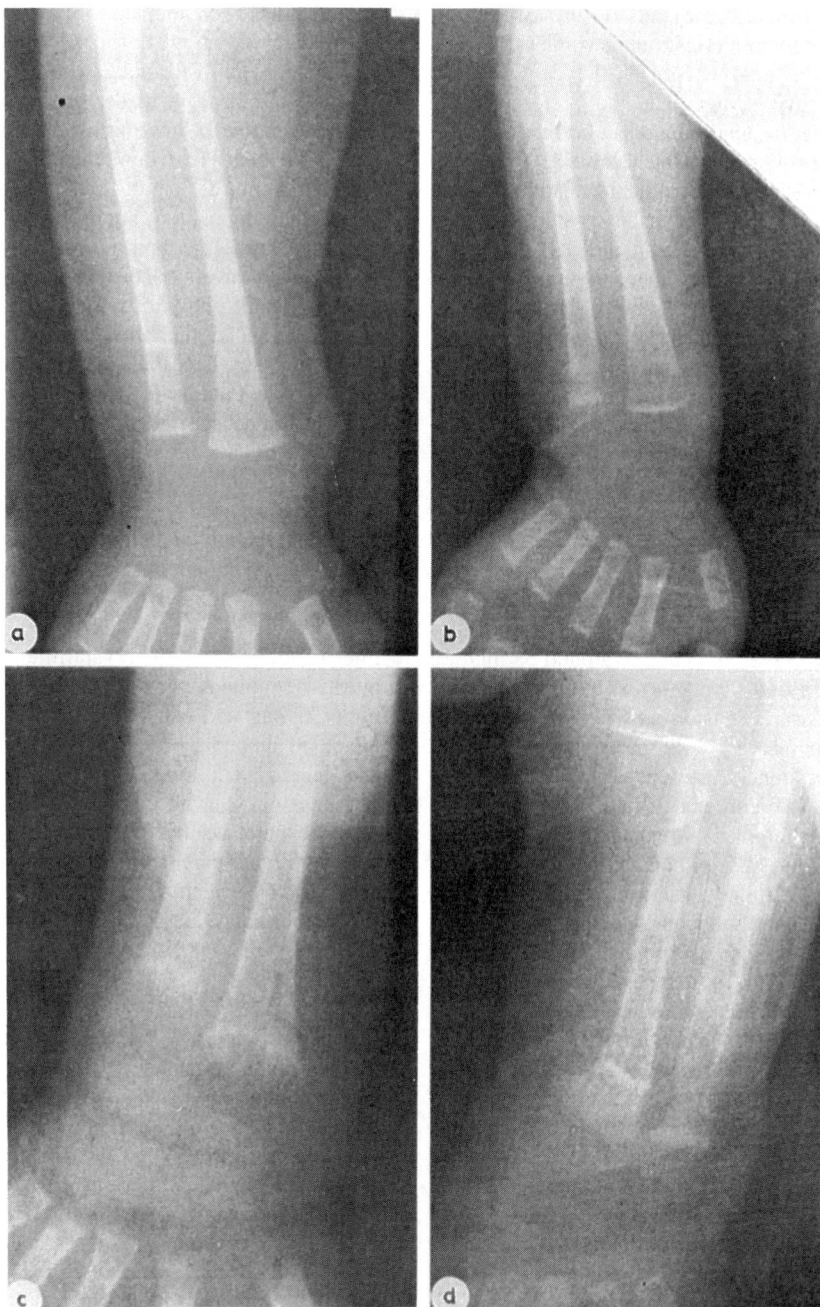

Fig. 5.76   X-ray grading of changes of rickets of prematurity at the wrist (Koo et al 1982): (**a**) grade 0 = normal; (**b**) grade 1 = osteopenia only; (**c**) grade 2 = cupping and fraying of ulnar metaphysis; (**d**) grade 3 = spontaneous fracture in association with grade 2 changes. (X-rays by kind permission of Professor N. McIntosh.)

mineralization to proceed in a manner which avoids clinical and overt radiological rachitic changes. Whether we should go further than this goal and attempt to achieve 'normal' mineralization in all preterm infants using in utero mineral accretion rates as our standard is an unresolved question (ESPGAN 1987).

Although vitamin D deficiency is not a major factor in the etiology of metabolic bone disease of preterm infants, it plays a critical role in facilitating normal mineralization and should be supplemented to around 500–1000 IU/day. In established metabolic bone disease, modest increases in vitamin D intake, 1000–2000 IU/day, are still used for short periods in conjunction with mineral supplementation. Regular monitoring is essential to avoid hypercalcemia, a particular problem with the hydroxylated derivatives of vitamin D – 1α-hydroxycholecalciferol and 1,25–dihydroxycholecalciferol – which are now rarely used.

Metabolic balance studies have shown that with calcium and phosphorus supplementation of term formulae, which have a mineral composition similar to that of human milk, postnatal retention of calcium and phosphorus can approximate intrauterine accretion (Giles et al 1987). Comparison of intrauterine accretion and postnatal retention of minerals depends on the assumption that the chemical growth of the preterm infant is similar to that of the fetus in utero. This is not necessarily the case. Photon absorptiometric studies have shown that the preterm infant approaching term may have a bone mineral deficit as much as 30% when compared with full-term infants. However, long-term studies have shown that these preterm infants have a rapid phase of mineral accretion between 40 and 60 weeks' postconceptional age which reduces perinatal mineralization deficits that might otherwise persist into childhood but there is no long-term evidence for mineral deficits in this population (Horsman et al 1989). Ziegler (1985) discusses this dilemma and emphasizes that the avoidance of overt bone disease should be the criterion for calcium and phosphorus need, rather than the necessity to achieve fetal accretion rates or in utero rates of mineralization. On this basis the requirement of the preterm infant for calcium and phosphorus is probably greater than the intake from human milk but less than that needed to achieve intrauterine accretion rates. The problem is how much calcium and phosphorus is required to avoid overt bone disease and how this need should be assessed.

The calcium and phosphorus concentrations in milk from mothers of preterm and term infants are similar and a premature infant fed 150 ml/kg/day receives an intake of around 55 mg/day (1.3 mmol/day) of calcium and 22 mg/day of phosphorus (0.5 mmol/day). Sequential measurements of bone mineral content in preterm infants fed human breast milk have shown that the postnatal increase in bone mineral content is significantly less than that expected in utero (Abrams et al 1988). Supplementation of maternal milk has been attempted with calcium or phosphorus or both (Gross 1987), addition of skimmed components of donor human milk, mixing maternal milk with formula containing high concentration of calcium and phosphorus and the use of proprietary powdered fortifiers. Indiscriminate fortification of human milk is to be avoided and reserved for extreme preterm infants where this type of nutrition is the major dietary source. Supplementation with calcium or phosphorus salts or sugars may result in increased osmolality, dilution of other constituents if mineral solutions are used, precipitation of salts and potentially undesirable intakes of other nutrients. Phosphorus supplements of up to 9 mg/dl (13 mg/100 cal) have been used to maintain the plasma phosphorus greater that 1.5 mmol/dl and avoiding excess urinary calcium losses. Calcium supplements should not be given without a proportionate amount of phosphorus in order to maintain the calcium : phosphorus ratio in the range of 1.4–2.0. Simultaneous additions of calcium and phosphorus salts to milks may result in precipitation. This can be avoided by adding the phosphorus first (usually disodium phosphate) and then calcium (usually calcium gluconate/glubionate). Diverse salts of calcium and phosphorus have been used to supplement preterm feeds and the absorption and retention properties vary. Mineral solubility may limit absorption and retention and absolute mineral content of the feeds cannot be the sole criterion on which selection is made and more attention should be focused on bioavailability.

The American Academy of Pediatrics (1985), on the basis of estimated fetal requirements, has advised enteral intakes of calcium 185–210 mg/kg/day (4.6–5.2 mmol/kg/day) and phosphorus 123–140 mg/kg/day (4–4.6 mmol/kg/day) for infants between 26 and 31 weeks' gestation. To achieve these intakes, assuming a fluid intake of 150 mg/kg/day, milk formulae would have a calcium content of 126–140 mg/dl (3.1–3.5 mmol/dl) and phosphorus 82–93 mg/dl (2.7–3.1 mmol/dl). A more cautious

approach has been adopted by ESPGAN Committee on Nutrition (1987), representing European opinion, where recommended calcium content of formulae would be between 56 and 112 mg/dl (1.4–3.8 mmol/dl) with a phosphorus content 40–72 mg/dl (1.3–2.3 mmol/dl). Low birthweight formulae currently available in the UK have calcium contents in the range 70–110 mg/dl (1.7–2.7 mmol/dl) and phosphorus 35–60 mg/dl (1.2–2.0 mmol/dl), compositions not optimal to meet mineral requirements if intrauterine accretion rates are to be attained but levels which should avoid overt bone disease. The number of studies using calcium- and phosphorus-supplemented milks, to the levels recommended by the American Academy of Pediatrics, are still small and they have only given limited information as to their efficacy, desirability or potential drawbacks. Excess dietary calcium can cause supermineralization in preterm infants, impede fat absorption as well as that of other minerals and lead to the risk of nephrocalcinosis.

Parenterally fed preterm infants are at particular risk of inadequate supply of calcium and phosphorus (Koo 1992). The solubility and stability of mineral substrate in parenteral solutions depends on a number of factors and precipitation of salts can occur readily, resulting in blocked lines and the potential for microembolization of crystalline particles. Most parenteral nutrition regimens can routinely achieve intakes of calcium of 1.5 mmol/kg/day and phosphorus 1.0 mmol/kg/day. By prescribing increased amounts of calcium and phosphorus only when fluid and amino acid intakes are appropriate, avoiding prolonged standing times, using the more soluble calcium gluconate rather than the chloride and only adding calcium and phosphorus to already diluted parenteral solutions precipitation can be avoided and intakes of calcium around 2.0 mmol/kg/day and phosphorus 1.7 mmol/kg/day can be achieved.

NEONATAL PRESENTATION OF INBORN ERRORS OF METABOLISM

Major advances have been made in the recognition and understanding of many inborn errors of metabolism. Prenatal diagnosis is available for a number of conditions allowing parents to avoid recurrence of serious disease or early management and treatment to avoid deleterious effects on the developing fetus or neonate. Increasingly successful treatment regimens are being devised but the outcome may depend on the earliest possible recognition and institution of therapy. Only a minority of inborn errors of metabolism are routinely screened for in the newborn and early recognition is often dependent on maintaining a high index of clinical suspicion and a low threshold for sometimes basic and sometimes complex biochemical investigations. This is particularly true where inborn errors can present as acute and serious illness in the newborn period (Saudubray & Charpentier 1995).

The aim of this review is to consider what inborn errors of metabolism can present in the newborn period and their clinical features. Although investigation and management will be discussed, details of individual inborn errors of metabolism will be found in Chapter 20 and will be cross-referenced.

Acute metabolic disorders

A number of metabolic disorders can present with acute overwhelming symptoms in the newborn period particularly the urea cycle defects, organic acidemias and certain

Table 5.125 Inborn errors of metabolism which may present as acute illness in the newborn period – see also Table 5.123 for metabolic diseases where hypoglycemia is a prominent feature

Disorders of amino acid metabolism
Maple syrup urine disease
Phenylketonuria
Tyrosinemia type I
Nonketotic hyperglycinemia
Hyper-β-alaninemia
Sulfite oxidase deficiency
5,10-methylene tetrahydrofolate reductase deficiency
Methylmalonic acidemia
Propionic acidemia
Isovaleric acidemia
β-methylcrotonylglycinuria
Multiple carboxylase deficiency
Hydroxymethylglutaryl-CoA lyase deficiency
β-ketothiolase deficiency
2-methylacetoacetyl-CoA thiolase deficiency

Urea cycle defects
N-acetylglutamate synthase deficiency
Carbamyl phosphate synthetase deficiency
Ornithine transcarbamylase deficiency
Citrullinemia
Argininosuccinic aciduria
Arginase deficiency

aminoacidopathies (Table 5.125). The majority of these disorders have no detrimental effects on fetal development because placental perfusion can correct the disordered metabolic accumulation. As a consequence, the majority of infants are full term, of normal growth, without dysmorphic features and asymptomatic at birth. An exception to this generalization is where the primary defect is in cerebral metabolism as occurs in nonketotic hyperglycinemia (p. 1112). These infants may be born with established brain damage and have clinical features of hypertonia, lethargy, poor feeding and seizures, both grand mal and myoclonic.

Many of the disorders are inherited as autosomal recessives and there may be a family history of previous perinatal loss or sudden and unexpected death in infancy. Autopsy findings may have been nonspecific and unrevealing unless specific biochemical investigations were done. A few inborn errors of metabolism have other patterns of inheritance, for example X-linked recessive in ornithine transcarbamylase deficiency (p. 1110).

Clinical features

The initial symptoms are usually nonspecific with lethargy, poor feeding, poor weight gain and vomiting. Diarrhea is less common but occurs in galactosemia (p. 1132) and hereditary tyrosinemia (p. 1106).

In the case of the infant who is well at birth, the onset of symptoms may be within a few hours of the first milk feed or may be delayed several weeks. The relationship to milk feeds and protein load may be further emphasized when the initial symptoms resolve with a period of intravenous fluids to recur again when milk feeds resume.

Progressive accumulation of intermediate metabolites may have neurotoxic effects and encephalopathic symptoms may accompany the presentation with apnea, periodic respirations, hypotonia, hypertonia, decerebrate rigidity, seizures and coma.

The clinical features may mimic the presentation of an acute neonatal infection. Indeed sepsis is a common accompaniment of acute exacerbations of metabolic disease as occurs in maple syrup urine disease (p. 1116) or the mitochondrial disorders of fatty acid oxidation (p. 1129). Certain metabolic disorders may predispose to the risk of infection, for example infants with type I glycogen storage disease (p. 1135).

Clinical examination may be unrevealing. Tachypnea may indicate an underlying metabolic acidosis. Hepatomegaly, if present, classically occurs in the glycogen storage disorders, galactosemia and fructose-1,6-diphosphatase deficiency (p. 1135), but has been described in some infants with urea cycle defects, disorders of mitochondrial fatty acid oxidation and some aminoacidopathies. Cataracts can occur in newborn infants with galactosemia. Dislocated lens, characteristic of homocystinuria (p. 1108) and sulfite oxidase deficiency (p. 1109), have been described in the first month of life. Abnormal hair fragility can be present in some infants with argininosuccinic aciduria (p. 1111).

The majority of infants with acute metabolic disease do not have congenital anomalies but dysmorphic features are characteristic of some metabolic disorders such as multiple acyl-CoA dehydrogenase deficiency (p. 1129). Ambiguous genitalia occur in association with congenital adrenal hyperplasia (p. 1061).

Abnormal urinary odors may accompany metabolic disorders: phenylketonuria, mousy or musty; maple syrup urine disease, maple syrup or burnt sugar; isovaleric acidemia and glutaric acidemia type II, sweaty feet and β-methylcrotonylglycinuria of cat urine.

Initial laboratory investigations

Infants suspected of acute metabolic disease require basic investigations not only for clinical management and resuscitation but to begin to determine the nature of the inborn error. Initial investigations should include blood gases, plasma electrolytes, plasma calcium and magnesium, blood glucose, blood ammonia and a full blood count. Valuable information can be gained by urine screening tests for pH, glucose (Clinistix), reducing compounds (Clinitest), ketones and keto acids with 2,4-dinitrophenylhydrazine and for the variety of compounds that react with ferric chloride. Urinary creatinine may be useful for standardization of subsequent investigations. These basic investigations should be available in all laboratories and be completed rapidly.

The differential diagnosis and the diseases which may be detected by Clinitest, ferric chloride and 2,4–dinitrophenylhydrazine testing of urine.

Metabolic acidosis. This is frequently present in acutely ill infants with galactosemia, gluconeogenic disorders, glycogen storage disease and particularly the organic acidemias (Tables 5.125 and 5.126). Infants with organic acidemias may have a significant anion gap.

Hyperammonemia. A high blood ammonia is present in the primary enzyme defects of the urea cycle (Table 5.125) and is exacerbated by high protein loads whether this is from milk or endogenous catabolism. Secondary hyperammonemia is often seen in the defects of mitochondrial fatty acid oxidation and the organic acidemias. Delayed ontogeny of the urea cycle in preterm infants, particularly those with high protein loads, may result in severe hyperammonemia. Blood urea may be inappropriately low in the presence of defects of the urea cycle.

Hypoglycemia. This is the predominant feature of the primary defects of carbohydrate metabolism and of mitochondrial fatty acid oxidation but can be present in disorders of amino acid metabolism or organic acidemias. Hypoglycemia is frequently present as part of the acute metabolic derangements in maple syrup urine disease, methylmalonic acidemia, glutaric acidemia type II and hydroxymethylglutaryl-CoA lyase deficiency (Tables 5.125 and 5.126). The list is not exhaustive but illustrates the overlap in presentations and the importance of blood glucose estimations in the investigation, monitoring and treatment of suspected metabolic disease.

Liver transaminases and direct hyperbilirubinemia. Elevated plasma alanine or aspartate aminotransferases are secondary to hepatotoxicity and may be found in galactosemia, type III glycogen storage disease, disorders of mitochondrial fatty acid oxidation and in the urea cycle defects (Tables 5.125 and 5.126). Indirect hyperbilirubinemia is a common accompaniment to a wide range of newborn illnesses. A direct hyperbilirubinemia occurs in those diseases which damage the liver, in particular galactosemia, fructose intolerance and tyrosinemia, but is also seen in the later stages of the presentation of urea cycle defects and hyperglycinemia.

Thrombocytopenia and neutropenia. These can be features of methylmalonic acidemia, propionic acidemia, isovaleric acidemia and lysinuric protein intolerance. In addition neutropenia has been described in carbamyl phosphate synthetase deficiency and nonketotic hyperglycinemia. Defective platelet function and bleeding may be a feature of type I glycogen storage disease (Tables 5.125 and 5.126). The presence of neutropenia and/or thrombocytopenia can be indices of sepsis in the newborn infant without an underlying inborn error of metabolism. The presence of either in the sick newborn infant should alert the clinician to the possibility of an underlying metabolic defect.

Anemia. Anemia can be found in association with methylmalonic aciduria and some of the aminoacidopathies.

Table 5.126 Metabolic storage disorders which may be suspected in neonates

Glycogen storage diseases
Type I, glucose-6-phosphatase system deficiencies
Type II, Pompe's disease, α-1,4-glucosidase deficiency
Type III, debrancher deficiency
Type IV, brancher deficiency

Lipid storage diseases
G_{M1} gangliosidosis type I
Gaucher's disease
Niemann–Pick disease
Wolman's disease
Farber's disease

Mucolipidoses
Type I, sialidosis
Type II, I-cell disease

Mucopolysaccharidoses
Type VII, β-glucuronidase deficiency

Glycoprotein storage disease
Fucosidosis

Detailed laboratory investigation

If hyperammonemia, unexplained metabolic acidosis or hypoglycemia is present then it must be assumed that the symptoms are secondary to an inborn error of metabolism and the infant thoroughly investigated (Burton 1987). This may require urine and plasma samples to be sent to a specialist laboratory. In general the full range of tests described below may have to be performed, but a priority order of investigations can be made on the basis of clinical features and the results of initial laboratory investigations, e.g. in the case of a vomiting infant with hypoglycemia and a urine positive for reducing substances, urine sugar chromatography will be the first priority to exclude galactosemia. Collaboration and discussion with personnel in a specialist center or laboratory is essential and a program of investigation can be agreed to the benefit of the patient. Not all sick newborn infants with metabolic disease need have hypoglycemia, metabolic acidosis or hyperammonemia. For example infants with nonketotic hyperglycinemia (p. 1112) may have severe encephalopathic features but unrevealing initial investigations. Detailed metabolic investigation can be worth pursuing even when initial laboratory results are unsupportive.

Semiquantitative analysis of urinary amino acids can be made relatively rapidly by thin layer or paper chromatography. A complete quantitative amino acid analysis of plasma, cerebrospinal fluid or urine is made by automated ion exchange chromatography and may take 12–24 h. Thin layer chromatography of sugars is semiquantitative but rapid and usually diagnostic. Urinary organic acids may initially be analyzed by gas–liquid chromatography but preferably by gas chromatography–mass spectrometry. Lactate and pyruvate are generally measured in plasma but urinary lactate measurements have been advocated for the differentiation of a primary from a secondary lactic acidosis (p. 1125). Carnitine and acylcarnitine are measured in plasma and urine samples.

These investigations may give a definitive diagnosis or one where there is a high index of suspicion of a known inborn error to allow specific treatment to begin. Complete characterization of an inborn error of metabolism may require enzyme studies on fibroblasts, leukocytes or tissue biopsies including DNA analysis.

Acute management of severe metabolic disease

The establishment of cardiorespiratory homeostasis and the correction of biochemical abnormalities are the priorities. The extent of resuscitative measures will depend on the clinical states of the infant and often must be instituted before a definitive diagnosis has been established.

Fluids are given intravenously as 10% dextrose solutions, the volume/kg/h will depend on the state of hydration and the presence of renal dysfunction. Hypoglycemia and hypocalcemia should be corrected. Hyperglycemia can potentiate the generation of lactate and should be avoided. This is particularly important for patients with pyruvate dehydrogenase complex defects (p. 1125) where a high carbohydrate load can dramatically accentuate the acidosis.

If the infant has a metabolic acidosis with no respiratory acidosis or a compensatory respiratory alkalosis, the metabolic acidosis should be corrected with sodium bicarbonate initially with boluses to raise the pH to around 7.25 and then maintained if necessary by a slow intravenous infusion. If the infant has a combined respiratory and metabolic acidosis with hypoventilation secondary to cerebral depression, the respiratory component is firstly corrected by ventilatory support and then the metabolic acidosis corrected. During this resuscitative phase, a mild respiratory alkalosis (PCO_2 4.0–4.5 kPa) can be induced by hyperventilation which may assist in correcting a very low pH as well as having beneficial effects on the control of cerebral edema. Oxygen should be given as required to maintain normal arterial saturation. Muscle paralysis with ventilatory support may have a specific role in severe lactic acidosis reducing the peripheral production. Blood gases and electrolytes should be monitored frequently.

Good tissue perfusion and oxygenation is essential to avoid secondary lactic acidosis. In correction of hypotension it may be more appropriate to use an inotropic agent such as dopamine rather than a high protein load of plasma or blood. As perfusion improves, the metabolic acidosis may worsen as peripheral lactate is brought into the circulation. Convulsive episodes may accentuate anaerobic metabolism and should be treated initially with intravenous phenobarbitone.

In the sick infant where severe metabolic acidosis persists or in spite of resuscitative efforts the clinical condition remains critical, exchange transfusion or peritoneal dialysis may result in an improvement. In hyperammonemic syndromes with blood ammonias > 600 µmol/l and with associated cerebral dysfunction, hemodialysis may be the preferred initial treatment.

Vitamins are essential cofactors for some enzymes and in certain conditions where cofactor function is abnormal reduced enzyme activity will result. Enzyme activity in some instances can be increased by prescribing vitamins in doses approximately 10–100 times the daily requirement. In the situation of the critically ill infant without as yet a specific diagnosis, the use of multivitamins is justified and should include thiamin (50–500 mg), riboflavin (20–50 mg), biotin (10–100 mg), nicotinamide (400–600 mg), pyridoxine (10–100 mg), vitamin B_{12} (1–2 mg), folic acid (15–30 mg), ascorbic acid (300–3000 mg), pantothenic acid (30–50 mg) and carnitine 100–150 mg/day. Multivitamin preparations for intravenous use are available

Protein catabolism can exacerbate most of these disorders and once the infant's condition is stable and the acute metabolic derangements have been corrected, calories can be increased by gradual increments of intravenous 20% dextrose. Hyperglycemia is to be avoided as it may exacerbate metabolic acidosis and insulin 0.05–0.1 IU/kg can be used to maintain blood glucose < 10 mmol/l. Insulin may also increase anabolism and can be used regularly 4- to 6-hourly. Once the infant is stabilized on this regimen and to maintain anabolism, protein and lipids are introduced either by the enteral or parenteral route. Protein can be commenced at 0.25–0.5 g protein/day and if tolerated increased by the same amount daily to reach 1.5 g/kg/day with an aimed caloric intake of 120 kcal/kg/day.

Specific treatments

Where investigations have led to a definitive diagnosis or where there is a high index of suspicion of an inborn error, specific treatment can be instituted. In urea cycle defects a combination of dietary therapy and the use of drugs to provide alternative pathways for nitrogen excretion can be successful. Arginine functions as an essential amino acid and supplementation will allow excretion of additional nitrogen. Amino acid nitrogen can be excreted as hippuric acid if sodium benzoate is given or as phenylbutylglutamine after administration of phenylbutyrate. Dietary modifications have been particularly successful in phenylketonuria (p. 1105) and galactosemia (p. 1132). Supplementations of vitamin B_{12} in methylmalonic aciduria (p. 1117), carnitine in organic acidemias (p. 1119), biotin in carboxylase deficiencies (p. 1126) and pyridoxine in homocystinuria (p. 1109) have been successful in some individuals. Alteration of the ratio of fat : carbohydrate : protein in the diet or the frequency of feeding have been used in the management of type I glycogen storage disease (p. 1136), fructose-1,6-diphosphatase deficiency (p. 1135) and the mitochondrial disorders of fatty acid oxidation (Roe & Coates 1995) (p. 1129).

Investigations where death is inevitable

The situation may arise where death is inevitable but where the exact diagnosis of an inborn error of metabolism has not been conclusively established. In these circumstances it is important that the fullest information be obtained to advise parents of the risks of recurrence in subsequent pregnancies. An autopsy is vital and should preferably be performed soon after death. The majority of parents, with skilled counseling, will give postmortem permission before the infant dies. At autopsy liver, kidney, skeletal muscle, cardiac muscle and areas of brain thought to be involved should be fixed for light and electron microscopy. Duplicate frozen tissue samples suitable for cryostat sections should be obtained. Skin or pericardial fibroblast cultures should be established. A substantial amount of each tissue should be snap frozen as 0.5 cm³ cubes in liquid nitrogen and stored at –70°C for subsequent enzyme analysis. Certain disorders particularly those of membrane-associated enzymes where there is a transport function or where the membrane is important for regulatory function or where the enzyme itself is sensitive to freeze–thaw may best be analyzed on fresh tissue. Specialist advice should be sought. Some parents will agree only to a limited postmortem, for example wedge biopsy or needle biopsy of liver with skin samples from the incision site. In these circumstances all available urine and plasma should be frozen and stored at –70°C.

Suspected metabolic storage disorders

Metabolic storage disorders which may present in the newborn period are shown in Table 5.126 but often symptoms and a diagnosis may be delayed into infancy or childhood depending on the severity of the enzyme deficiency or the rate of expression of pathognomonic features. Infants with glycogen storage disease may have hepatomegaly with or without obvious hypoglycemic symptoms. Pompe's disease, type II glycogen storage disease (p. 1138), is not associated with hypoglycemia but infants may have macroglossia, hypotonia, hepatomegaly and cardiomegaly with cardiac failure.

The clinical features of the mucopolysaccharidoses (p. 1158) are rarely fully expressed in the newborn period and a Hurler-like phenotype with coarse facies, macroglossia, limited growth and skeletal abnormalities is more likely to be a lipid or mucolipid storage disorder particularly GM1 gangliosidosis type I (p. 1162) or I-cell disease (p. 1170).

The acute infantile variant of Niemann–Pick disease (p. 1166), Gaucher's disease (p. 1165) and Wolman's disease (p. 1154) may present in the newborn period with hepatosplenomegaly, feeding difficulties, vomiting, choking, cyanotic episodes, failure to thrive and disorders of tone. Gastrointestinal symptoms are particularly marked in Wolman's disease with diarrhea and abdominal distention in addition to vomiting.

Metabolic disorders associated with dysmorphic features

Inborn errors of metabolism may be associated with dysmorphic features suggesting that metabolic derangements in utero have disrupted normal fetal ontogeny, for example congenital adrenal hyperplasia (p. 1061) in females is associated with ambiguous genitalia.

Peroxisomal disorders

Disorders of peroxisomal biogenesis as well as deficiencies in peroxisomal enzymes may present in the newborn period (Lazarow & Moser 1995).

Zellweger syndrome (cerebrohepatorenal syndrome) (p. 1172). This autosomal recessive condition has a number of characteristic clinical features. Craniofacial abnormalities may include a high forehead, flat occiput, wide sutures and fontanel, absent orbital ridges, micrognathia, redundant neck skin folds, external ear abnormalities and a high arched palate. The neurological features include hypotonia, poor feeding, nystagmus, hypo- or areflexia, psychomotor retardation and seizures. The brain is abnormal with disordered neuronal migration. Hepatomegaly is characteristic with prolonged jaundice, elevated transaminases and a progression to cirrhosis. The kidneys may show multiple cysts. Ocular abnormalities include cataracts, retinal pigmentation, optic disc pallor and Brushfield spots. Radiologically stippled calcification of the patella or acetabulum may be present. The clinical expression includes milder forms of the disorder (for review see Lazarow & Moser 1995).

Neonatal adrenoleukodystrophy (p. 1172). The clinical syndrome and symptoms may be indistinguishable from Zellweger syndrome (Lazarow & Moser 1995). The presence of skeletal stippling or renal cysts at autopsy have not been encountered in neonatal adrenoleukodystrophy (Monnens & Heymans 1987).

Infantile Refsum's disease (p. 1173). This condition was originally described as an association between elevated plasma phytanic acid in infants with craniofacial dysmorphism, ocular abnormalities, hepatomegaly and psychomotor retardation with peroxisomes absent or deficient.

Rhizomelic chondrodysplasia punctata (p. 1173). This condition is inherited as an autosomal recessive and is characterized by short stature, symmetrical rhizomelia with marked shortening of the humerus and femur and punctate calcification around the epiphysis with coarse irregularity of the metaphyses. Severe psychomotor retardation, hepatomegaly and craniofacial dysmorphism with cataracts and corneal changes complete the clinical picture (Heymans et al 1986, Lazarow & Moser 1995).

Hyperpipecolic acidemia (p. 1173). This syndrome is characterized by elevated pipecolic acid in plasma, minor dysmorphic features, optic disc pallor, retinal pigmentation,

psychomotor retardation and hepatomegaly with abnormal liver function progressing to cirrhosis. The postmortem findings show adrenal abnormalities, renal cysts, normal neuronal migration in the brain and normal peroxisomes in liver but a disturbance in multiple peroxisomal function (Budden et al 1986).

Zellweger-like phenotype with structurally intact peroxisomes (p. 1173). The biochemical defect in this group is confined to disorders of very long chain fatty acid oxidation or bile salt metabolism but with intact peroxisomes and include peroxisomal 3-oxoacyl-CoA thiolase deficiency (p. 1174) peroxisomal acyl-CoA oxidase deficiency (p. 1174) and peroxisomal bifunctional enzyme deficiency (p. 1174).

Mitochondrial electron transport chain defects

Multiple acyl-CoA dehydrogenase deficiencies (MAD) (p. 1130) *or glutaric acidemia type II*. MAD deficiency is classified into two variant forms, a severe (MAD-S) neonatal form or glutaric aciduria type II and a mild (MAD-M) variant with later onset.

In the severe neonatal form (MAD-S) two subgroups have been identified, those with congenital abnormalities and those without congenital abnormalities. In MAD-S deficiency with congenital abnormalities, characteristically the infants are born prematurely and may be growth retarded but develop a metabolic acidosis in the first 24 h of life with a characteristic odor of 'sweaty feet'. All patients have died in the first week of life. Neonatal MAD-S deficiency is associated with congenital abnormalities including facial dysmorphism, polycystic kidneys or some form of cystic dysplasia, cerebral abnormalities including disorders of migration, pulmonary hypoplasia, hypospadias and minor abnormalities of nail or palmar creases. At autopsy fatty infiltration of the liver, heart and kidneys is present. In MAD-S deficiency without congenital abnormalities the clinical course is similar with acidosis, hypoglycemia and odor with death occurring rapidly. Both types are a result of deficiencies of electron transport chain flavoprotein or its oxidoreductase. In MAD-M deficiency the clinical presentation is heterogeneous with first symptoms in the neonatal period, childhood or adulthood and characterized by vomiting, acidosis and hypoglycemia.

Riboflavin responsive defects of β-oxidation or riboflavin responsive multiple acyl-CoA dehydrogenase deficiencies (RR-MAD) (p. 1130). Some patients presenting with a Reye-like syndrome or hypoglycemia in the first years of life with defects in β-oxidation have been shown to be responsive to riboflavin. The biochemical etiology remains to be confirmed but a therapeutic trial with riboflavin should be attempted in all patients presenting with an organic aciduria suggesting a MAD deficiency. The perinatal implications are demonstrated by the case of Harpey et al (1983) when a 36-year-old woman had 11 children. Except for the first, all developed after birth a 'sweaty feet' odor and hypotonia and neurological distress, and seven died in the newborn period. In the ninth pregnancy, the maternal urinary organic acid profile showed a massive dicarboxylic and glutaric aciduria. The amniotic fluid profile was normal. Treatment with riboflavin normalized the organic acid excretion. Postnatally the infant was supplemented with riboflavin and a similar regimen was followed in the tenth and eleventh pregnancies. The last infant, treated with riboflavin since birth, has consistently elevated ethylmalonic and 2-methylbutyrylglycine excretion.

Miscellaneous conditions with newborn presentations

Crigler–Najjar syndrome (p. 1144); cystic fibrosis (p. 449), α1-antitrypsin deficiency (p. 1175); Menkes' kinky hair syndrome (p. 1146), hypophosphatasia (p. 1176); hereditary orotic aciduria (p. 1141); glucose-6-phosphate dehydrogenase deficiency (p. 1136); pyruvate kinase deficiency (p. 1131); pyridoxine-dependent convulsions (p. 1148); congenital erythropoietic porphyria (p. 1142); aminolevulinate dehydratase porphyria (p. 1142).

REFERENCES

Abramovich S J, Gregory S, Slemick M, Stewart A 1979 Hearing loss in very low birthweight infants treated with neonatal intensive care. Archives of Disease in Childhood 54: 421–425

Abrams S A, Schanler R J, Garza C 1988 Bone mineralisation in former very low birth weight infants fed either human milk or commercial formula. Journal of Pediatrics 112: 956–960

Abu-Osba Y K, Gafal O, Manasra K, Rejjal A 1992 Treatment of severe persistent pulmonary hypertension of the newborn with magnesium sulphate. Archives of Disease in Childhood 67: 31–35

ACTOBAT Study Group 1995 Australian collaborative trial of antenatal thyrotropin-releasing hormone (ACTOBAT) for prevention of neonatal respiratory disease. Lancet 345: 877–882

Adamkin D H 1986 Nutrition in very very low birth weight infants. Clinics in Perinatology 13: 419–443

Affleck G, Tenner H, Rowe J 1991 Infants in crisis: how parents cope with newborn intensive care and its aftermath. Springer-Verlag, New York

Agustsson P, Patel N B 1987 The predictive value of fetal breathing movements in the diagnosis of preterm labour. British Journal of Obstetrics and Gynaecology 94: 860–863

Alcorn D, Adamson T M, Lambert T F, Maloney J E, Ritchie B C, Robinson P M 1977 Morphological effects of tracheal ligation and drainage in the fetal lamb lung. Journal of Anatomy 123: 649–660

Alexander S, Keirse M J N C 1989 Formal risk scoring during pregnancy. In: Chalmers I, Enkin M, Kierse M J N C (eds) Effective care in pregnancy and childbirth. Oxford University Press, pp 345–364

Alfirevic Z, Neilson J P 1995 Doppler ultrasonography in high risk pregnancies; systematic review with meta-analysis. American Journal of Obstetrics and Gynecology 172: 1379–1387

Allan L D 1995 Echo cardiographic detection of congenital heart disease in the fetus: present and future. British Heart Journal 74: 103–106

Allen M C, Donohue P K, Dusman A E 1993 The limit of viability – neonatal outcome of infants born at 22–25 weeks gestation. New England Journal of Medicine 329: 1597–1601

Alon T, Hemo I, Itin A, Pe'er J, Stone J, Keshet E 1995 Vascular endothelial growth factor acts as a survival factor for newly formed retinal vessels and has implications for retinopathy of prematurity. Nature Medicine 1: 1024–1028

Als H, Lawhon G, Duffy F H, McAnulty G B, Gibes-Grossman R, Blickman J G 1994 Individualized development care for the very low-birth-weight preterm infant. Journal of the American Medical Association 272: 853–858

Altman R P, Randolph J G, Lilley J R 1974 Sacrococcygeal teratomata. American Academy of Pediatrics Surgical Section Survey 1973. Journal of Pediatric Surgery 9: 389–398

American Academy of Pediatrics 1985 Pediatric nutrition handbook. American Academy of Pediatrics, Chicago, Illinois, pp 66–87

American Academy of Pediatrics 1986a Committee on fetus and newborn. Use and abuse of the Apgar score. Pediatrics 78: 1148–1149

American Academy of Pediatrics 1986b Report of the Committee on Infectious Diseases. American Academy of Pediatrics, Chicago, Illinois, pp 181–189

American Academy of Pediatrics (Committee on Fetus and Newborn) 1995 The initiation or withdrawal of treatment for high-risk newborns. Pediatrics 96: 362–363

Amiel-Tison C 1995 Clinical assessment of the infant nervous system. In: Levene M I, Lilford R J (eds) Fetal and neonatal neurology and neurosurgery, 2nd edn. Churchill Livingstone, Edinburgh, pp 83–104

Amiel-Tison C, Grenier A 1986 Neurological assessment within the first year of life. Oxford University Press, New York

Amiel-Tison C, Stewart A L 1989 Follow up studies during the first five years of life: a pervasive assessment of neurological function. Archives of Disease in Childhood 64: 496–502

Anand K J S, Hickey P R 1987 Pain and its effects in the human neonate and fetus. New England Journal of Medicine 317: 1321–1329

Anderson G C 1991 Current knowledge about skin-to-skin (kangaroo) care for preterm infants. Journal of Perinatology 11: 216–231

Anderson P A M, Rickwood A M K 1991 Features of primary vesico ureteric reflux detected by prenatal sonography. British Journal of Urology 67: 267–271

Andersson S, Tikkanen I, Pesonen E, Meretoja O, Hynynen M, Fyhrquist S 1987 Atrial natriuretic peptide in patent ductus arteriosus. Pediatric Research 21: 396–398

Angell M 1983 Handicapped children: Baby Doe and Uncle Sam. New England Journal of Medicine 309: 659–661

Anand K J S, Hickey P R 1987 Pain and its effects in the human neonate and fetus. New England Journal of Medicine 317: 1321–1329

Annas G J 1984 The Baby Doe regulations: governmental intervention in neonatal rescue medicine. American Journal of Public Health 74: 618–620

Annibale D J, Hulsey T C, Engstrom P C, Wallin L A, Ohning B L 1994 Randomised, controlled trial of nasopharyngeal continuous positive airway pressure in the extubation of very low birthweight infants. Journal of Pediatrics 124: 455–460

Appleton R E, Lee R E, Hey E N 1990 Neurodevelopmental outcome of transient neonatal intracerebral echodensities. Archives of Disease in Childhood 65: 27–29

Archer N 1993 Patent ductus arteriosus in the newborn. Archives of Disease in Childhood 68: 58–61

Archer L N J, Levene M I, Evans D H 1986 Cerebral artery Doppler ultrasonography for prediction of outcome after perinatal asphyxia. Lancet ii: 1116–1118

Ashfaq M, Houston A B, Gnanapragasam J P, Lilley S, Murtagh E P 1991 Balloon atrial septostomy under echocardiographic control: six years' experience and evaluation of the practicability of cannulation via the umbilical vein. British Heart Journal 65: 148–151

Ashton N 1980 Oxygen and retinal blood vessels. Transactions of the Ophthalmological Societies of the UK 100: 359–362

Avery M E, Gatewood O, Brumley G 1966 Transient tachypnea of newborn. Possible delayed resorption of fluid at birth. American Journal of Diseases of Children 111: 380–385

Avery M E, Tooley W H, Keller J B et al 1987 Is chronic lung disease preventable? A survey of eight centers. Pediatrics 79: 26–30

Aylward G P, Pfeiffer S I, Wright A, Verhulst S J 1989 Outcome studies of low birthweight infants published over the last decade: a meta-analysis. Journal of Pediatrics 115: 515–520

Aynsley-Green A, Soltesz G 1985 Hypoglycaemia in infancy and childhood. In: Aynsley-Green A, Chambers T L (eds) Current reviews in paediatrics. Churchill Livingstone, Edinburgh

Bader J L, Miller R W 1979 US cancer incidence and mortality in the 1st year of life. American Journal of Diseases of Children 133: 157–159

Baley J E 1988 Neonatal sepsis: the potential for immunotherapy. Clinics in Perinatology 15: 755–771

Ballard P L 1984 Combined hormonal treatment and lung maturation. Seminars in Perinatology 8: 283–292

Ballard P L, Gonzales L K 1984 Mechanism of glucocorticoid and thyroid hormone action in fetal lung. In: Raivio K O, Hallman N, Kouvalainen K, Valimaki I (eds) Respiratory distress syndrome. Academic Press, London, pp 67–86

Barker D J 1988 Childhood causes of adult disease. Archives of Disease in Childhood 63: 867–869

Barlow A, McCance R A 1948 The nitrogen partition in newborn infants' urine. Archives of Disease in Childhood 23: 225–230

Barrington K J, Finer N N, Peters K L, Barton J 1986 Physiologic effects of doxopram in idiopathic apnea of prematurity. Journal of Pediatrics 108: 125–129

Barson A J 1978 Congenital neoplasia; the society's experience. Abstract. Archives of Disease in Childhood 53: 436

Bartholomew K M, Brownlee K G, Snowden S, Dear P 1994 To PEEP or not to PEEP? Archives of Disease in Childhood 70: F209–F212

Bartlett R H, Roloff D W, Cornell R G et al 1985 Extracorporeal circulation in neonatal respiratory failure: a prospective randomized study. Pediatrics 76: 479–487

Bax M, Nelson K B 1993 Birth asphyxia: a statement. Developmental Medicine and Child Neurology 35: 1023–1024

Becker P T, Grunwald P C, Moorman J, Stuhr S 1991 Outcomes of developmentally supportive nursing care for very low birth weight infants. Nursing Research 40: 150–155

Bell E F, Warburton D, Stonestreet B S, Oh W 1980 Effects of fluid administration on the development of symptomatic patent ductus arteriosus and congestive heart failure in premature infants. New England Journal of Medicine 302: 598–604

Berger J T, Gilhooly J 1993 Fibrin glue treatment of persistent pneumothorax in a premature infant. Journal of Pediatrics 122: 958–960

Berger M 1990 Complement deficiency and neutriohilic dysfunction as risk factors for bacterial infection in newborns and the role of granulocyte transfusion therapy. Review of Infectious Diseases 12: 401–412

Bergman I, Painter M J, Hirsch R P, Crumine P K, David R 1983 Outcome in neonates with convulsions treated in ICU. Annals of Neurology 14: 642–657

Bernbaum J C, Pereira G R, Watkins J B, Peckham G J 1983 Non-nutritive sucking during gavage feeding enhances growth and maturation in premature infants. Pediatrics 71: 41–45

Bernstein G, Heldt G P, Mannino F M 1994a Increased and more consistent tidal volumes during synchronised intermittent mandatory ventilation in newborn infants. American Journal of Respiratory and Critical Care Medicine 150: 1444–1448

Bernstein G, Mannino F L, Heldt G P et al 1994b Prospective randomised multicenter trial comparing synchronised and conventional ventilation (SIMV and IMV) in neonates. Pediatric Research 35: 216 (abstract)

Berseth C L, Nordyke C 1993 Enteral nutrients promote postnatal maturation of intestinal motor activity in preterm infants. American Journal of Physiology 264: G1046–1051

Bess F H, Paradise J L 1994 Universal screening for infant hearing impairment: not simple, nor risk-free, and not presently justified. Pediatrics 93: 330–334

Beyers N, Esser M, Alheit B, Roodt M, Wiggs B, Hough S F 1994a Static bone histomorphometry in preterm and term babies. Bone 15: 1–4

Beyers N, Alheit B, Taljaard J F, Hall J M, Hough S F 1994b High turnover osteopenia in preterm babies. Bone 15: 5–13

Bhutani V K, Abassi S, Sivieri E M 1988 Continuous skeletal muscle paralysis: effect on neonatal pulmonary mechanics. Pediatrics 81: 419–422

Birmingham Reflux Study Group 1983 Prospective trial of operative versus non-operative treatment of severe vesico-ureteric reflux. Two years observation in 96 children. British Medical Journal 287: 171–174

Bishop N 1989 Bone disease in preterm infants. Archives of Disease in Childhood 64: 1403–1409

Bishop N J, King F J, Lucas A 1993 Increased bone mineral content of preterm infants fed with a nutrient enriched formula after discharge from hospital. Archives of Disease in Childhood 68: 573–578

Bisset W M, Watt J B, Rivers J P A, Milla P J 1988 Ontogeny of fasting small intestinal motor activity in the human infant. Gut 29: 483–488

Bisset W M, Watt J B, Rivers J P A, Milla P J 1989 Postprandial motor response of the small intestine to enteral feeding in pre-term infants. Archives of Disease in Childhood 64: 1356–1361

Black V D, Lubchenco L O 1982 Neonatal polycythaemia and hyperviscosity. Pediatric Clinics of North America 29: 1137–1147

Bogdan R, Brown M A, Foster S B 1982 Be honest but not cruel: staff/parent communication on a neonatal unit. Human Organisation 41: 6–16

Bohin S, Draper E S, Field D J 1995 The impact of extremely immature infants on neonatal services. Archives of Disease in Childhood 74: F110–113

Bolande R P 1971 Benignity of neonatal tumors and concept of cancer repression in early life. American Journal of Diseases of Children 122: 12–14

Bolande R P 1974 Congenital and infantile neoplasia of the kidney. Lancet ii: 1497–1499

Boyer K M, Gotoff S P 1986 Prevention of early-onset neonatal group B streptococcal disease with selective intrapartum chemophrophylaxis. New England Journal of Medicine 314: 1665–1669

Boylan P 1987 Intrapartum fetal monitoring. In: Whittle M J (ed) Clinical obstetrics and gynaecology. Baillière Tindall, London, pp 73–95

Boyle M H, Torrance G W, Sinclair J C, Horwood S P 1983 Economic evaluation of neonatal intensive care for very-low-birthweight infants. New England Journal of Medicine 308: 1330–1337

Boynton B R, Hammond M D, Fredburg J J, Buckley B G, Villanueva D, Frantz I D III 1989 Gas exchange in healthy rabbits during high-frequency oscillatory ventilation. Journal of Applied Physiology 66: 1343–1351

Braddick O, Wattam-Bell J, Atkinson J 1986 Orientation-specific cortical responses develop in early infancy. Nature 320: 617–619

Brazelton T B 1973 Neonatal behavioural assessment scale. Clinics in Developmental Medicine, No 50. SIMP/Heinemann, London

British Paediatric Association 1992 Guidelines for the ethical conduct of medical research involving children. BPA, London

British Paediatric Association/Royal College of Obstetricians and Gynaecologists 1983 Standing joint committee of the British Paediatric Association and the Royal College of Obstetricians and Gynaecologists. Midwife and nurse staffing and training for special care and intensive care of the newborn. BPA/RCOG, London

British Paediatric Association Surveillance Unit 1994 9th annual report. BPA, London

British Paediatric Association Surveillance Unit 1995 10th annual report. BPA, London

Brothwood M, Wolke D, Gamsu H, Benson J, Cooper D 1986 Prognosis of the very low birthweight baby in relation to gender. Archives of Disease in Childhood 61: 559–564

Broadbent V A 1986 Malignant disease in the neonate. In: Roberton N R C (ed) Textbook of neonatology. Churchill Livingstone, Edinburgh

Broughton Pipkin F, Stephenson T J 1989 Plasma renin and renin substrate concentrations in the very premature human baby. Early Human Development 19: 71

Brouwers H A A, Ertbruggen I, Alsbach G P J, Van Leeuewen E F, Overbeeke M A M, Schausberg W, Van der Heiden C, Stoop J W, Englefriet C P 1988 What is the best predictor of the severity of ABO-haemolytic disease of the newborn. Lancet ii: 641–643

Brown M S 1988 Physiological anaemia of infancy. In: Stockman J A, Pochedly C (eds) Developmental and neonatal haematology. Raven Press, New York

Bryan A C, Froese A B 1991 Reflections on the HIFI trial. Pediatrics 87: 565–567

Bucher H C, Schmidt J G 1993 Does routine ultrasound scanning improve outcome in pregnancy? Meta-analysis of various outcome measures. British Medical Journal 307: 13–17

Budden S S, Kennaway N G, Buist N R M, Poulos A, Weleber R G 1986 Dysmorphic syndrome with phytamic acid oxidase deficiency, abnormal very long chain fatty acids, and pipecolic acidaemia: studies in four children. Journal of Pediatrics 108: 33–39

Buka S L, Lipsitt L P, Tsuang M T 1992 Emotional and behavioral development of low-birthweight infants. In: Friedman S L, Sigman M D (eds) The psychological development of low birthweight children. Ablex Publishing, Norwood NJ, pp 187–214

Burton B K 1987 Inborn errors of metabolism: the clinical diagnosis in early infancy. Pediatrics 79: 359–369

Bush A, Busst C M, Knight W B, Shinebourne E A 1988 Comparison of the haemodynamic effects of epoprostenol (prostacyclin) and tolazoline. British Heart Journal 60: 141–148

Bushnell I W R, Slater P C 1986 Concept formation in the preterm infant. Presentation at the Annual Conference of the British Psychological Society Developmental Section, Exeter, 17–20 September

Bussel J B, Berkowitz R L, McFarland J G, Lynch L, Chitkara U 1988 Antenatal treatment of neonatal alloimmune thrombocytopenia New England Journal of Medicine 319(21): 1347–1348

Cairo M 1989 Neonatal neutrophil host defence. American Journal of Diseases of Children 143: 10–46

Cairo M S, Plunkett J M, Mauss D et al 1990 Seven day administration of recombinant human granulocyte colony-stimulating factor in newborn rats. Blood 76: 1788–1794

Calame A, Fawer C-L, Claeys V, Arrozola L, Ducret S, Jaunin L 1986 Neurodevelopmental outcome and school performance of very low birthweight infants. European Journal of Pediatrics 145: 461–466

Calvert S A, Hoskins E M, Fong K W, Forsyth S C 1987 Etiological factors associated with the development of periventricular leucomalacia. Acta Paediatrica Scandinavica 76: 254–259

Campbell A G M 1995a Quality of life as a decision making criterion. In: Goldworth A, Silverman W, Stevenson D K, Young E W D, Rivers R (eds) Ethics and perinatology. Oxford University Press, Oxford, pp 82–103

Campbell A G M 1995b Government regulations in the United Kingdom. In: Goldworth A, Silverman W, Stevenson D K, Young E W D, Rivers R (eds) Ethics and perinatology. Oxford University Press, Oxford, pp 307–325

Campbell A N, Chan H S L, O'Brien A et al 1987 Malignant tumours in the neonate. Archives of Disease in Childhood 62: 19–23

Caplan A L, Blank R H, Merrick J C 1992 Compelled compassion: government intervention in the treatment of critically ill newborns. Humana Press, Totowa NJ

Carachi R, Lindop G B M, Leckie B J 1987 Inactive renin: a tumour marker in nephroblastoma. Journal of Pediatric Surgery 22: 278–280

Cardozo L, Fysh J, Pearce J M 1986 Prolonged pregnancy: the management debate. British Medical Journal 292: 1059–1063

Carlo W A, Chatburn R L (eds) 1988 Neonatal respiratory care, 2nd edn. Yearbook Publishers, Chicago

Carlo W A, Chatburn R L, Martin R J 1987 Randomized trial of high frequency jet ventilation in respiratory distress syndrome. Journal of Pediatrics 110: 275–282

Carlo W A, Siner B, Chatburn R L, Robertson S, Martin R J 1990 Early randomised intervention with high-frequency jet ventilation in respiratory distress syndrome. Journal of Pediatrics 117: 765–770

Carter B S, Haverkamp A D, Merenstein G B 1993 The definition of acute perinatal asphyxia. Clinics in Perinatology 20: 287–304

Carter J M, Gerstmann D R, Clark R H, Snyder G, Cornish J D, Null D M Jr, DeLemos R A 1990 High-frequency oscillatory ventilation and extracorporeal membrane oxygenation for the treatment of acute neonatal respiratory failure. Pediatrics 85: 159–164

Cartlidge P H T, Rutter N 1986 Serum albumin concentration and oedema in the newborn. Archives of Disease in Childhood 61: 657–660

Cartlidge P H T, Rutter N 1988 Percutaneous oxygen delivery to the preterm infant. Lancet i: 315–317

Castillo R A, Devoe C D, Hadi H A et al 1986 Non immune hydrops fetalis: clinical experience and factors associated with a poor outcome. American Journal of Obstetrics and Gynecology 155: 812–818

Catlin E A, Carpenter M W, Brann B S et al 1986 The Apgar score revisited: influence of gestational age. Journal of Pediatrics 109: 865–868

Chalmers I, Enkin M, Kierse M J N C 1989 Effective care in pregnancy and childbirth: a synopsis for guiding practice and research. In: Chalmers I, Enkin M, Kierse M J N C (eds) Effective care in pregnancy and childbirth. Oxford University Press, Oxford, pp 1465–1477

Chalmers J A, Chalmers I 1989 The obstetric vacuum extractor is the instrument of first choice for operative vaginal delivery. British Journal of Obstetrics and Gynaecology 96: 505–506

Chalmers R A, English N, Hughes E A, Noble-Jamieson C, Wigglesworth J S 1987 Biochemical studies on cultured skin fibroblasts from a baby with long-chain acyl-CoA dehydrogenase deficiency presenting as sudden neonatal death. Journal of Inherited Metabolic Disease 10: 260–262

Chan J C M 1983 Renal tubular acidosis. Journal of Pediatrics 102: 327–340

Chan V, Greenough A 1993 Randomised trial of methods of extubation in acute and chronic respiratory distress. Archives of Disease in Childhood 68: 570–572

Chan V, Greenough A 1994a Comparison of weaning by patient triggered ventilation or synchronous intermittent mandatory ventilation. Acta Paediatrica 83: 335–337

Chan V, Greenough A 1994b The effect of frequency on carbon dioxide levels during high frequency oscillation. Journal of Perinatal Medicine 22: 103–106

Chan V, Greenough A, Milner A D 1993 The effect of frequency and mean airway pressure on volume delivery during high frequency oscillation. Pediatric Pulmonology 15: 183–186

Chen Y-T, Burchell A 1995 Glycogen storage diseases. In: Scriver C R, Beaudet A L, Sly W S, Valle D (eds) The metabolic bases of inherited disease. 7th edn. McGraw Hill, New York, ch 24, pp 935–965

Chirico G, Rondini G, Plebani A et al 1987 Intravenous gammaglobulin therapy for prophylaxis of infection in high risk neonates. Journal of Pediatrics 110: 437–442

Christensen R D, Rothstein G, Astall H B et al 1982 Granulocyte transfusion in neonates with bacterial infection, neutropenia and depletion of mature marrow neutrophils. Pediatrics 70: 1–6

Chu A D, D'Angio G J, Favara B et al 1987 The working group of the histiocyte society. Histiocytis syndromes in children. Lancet i: 208–209

Cleary J P, Bernstein G, Mannino F L, Heldt G P 1995 Improved oxygenation during synchronised intermittent mandatory ventilation in neonates with respiratory distress syndrome: A randomised, crossover study. Journal of Pediatrics 126: 407–411

Cochrane Database of Systematic Reviews 1997 Update Software, Oxford

Colditz P, Murphy D, Rolfe P, Wilkinson A R 1989 Effect of infusion rate of indomethacin on cerebrovascular responses in pre term neonates. Archives

of Disease in Childhood 64: 1–12

Cole B R, Conley S B, Stapleton F B 1987 Polycystic kidney disease in the first year of life. Journal of Pediatrics 111: 693–699

Collaborative Dexamethasone Trial Group 1991 Dexamethasone therapy in neonatal chronic lung disease: an international placebo-controlled trial. Pediatrics 88: 421–427

Collaborative European Multicenter Study Group 1988 Surfactant replacement therapy for severe neonatal respiratory distress syndrome: an international randomized clinical trial. Pediatrics 82: 683–691

Colodny A H 1987 Antenatal diagnosis and management of urinary abnormalities. Pediatric Clinics of North America 34: 1365–1381

Colton T, Kayne H L, Zhang Y, Heeren T A 1995 meta-analysis of home uterine activity monitoring. American Journal of Obstetrics and Gynecology 173: 1499–1505

Committee for the Classification of Retinopathy of Prematurity (CCRoP) 1984 The international classification of retinopathy of prematurity. British Journal of Ophthalmology 68: 690–697

Committee for the Classification of Retinopathy of Prematurity (CCRoP) 1987 An international classification of retinopathy of prematurity. II The classification of retinal detachment. Archives of Ophthalmology 105: 906–912

Connell J, Oozeer R, de Vries L, Dubowitz L M S, Dubowitz V 1989a Continuous EEG monitoring of neonatal seizures: diagnostic and prognostic considerations. Archives of Disease in Childhood 64: 452–458

Connell J, Oozeer R, de Vries L, Dubowitz L M S, Dubowitz V 1989b Clinical and EEG response to anticonvulsants in neonatal seizures. Archives of Disease in Childhood 64: 459–464

Cooke R W I 1987a Early and late ultrasonographic appearance and outcome in very low birthweight infants. Archives of Disease in Childhood 62: 931–937

Cooke R W I 1987b Determinants of major handicap in post haemorrhagic hydrocephalus. Archives of Disease in Childhood 62: 504–507

Cooke R W I 1988 Outcomes and costs of care for the very immature infant. British Medical Bulletin 44: 1131–1151

Cooke R W I 1991 Trends in preterm survival and incidence of cerebral haemorrhage 1980–1989. Archives of Disease in Childhood 66: 403–407

Cooke R W I 1993 Annual audit of three year outcomes in very low birthweight infants. Archives of Disease in Childhood 69: 295–298

Cooke R W I 1994 Factors affecting survival and outcome at 3 years in extremely preterm infants. Archives of Disease in Childhood 71: F28–F31

Cooke R W 1996 Improved outcome for infants at the limits of viability. European Journal of Pediatrics 155: 665–667

Corcoran J D, Patterson C C, Thomas P S, Halliday H L 1993 Reduction in the risk of bronchopulmonary dysplasia from 1980–1990: results of a multivariate logistic regression analysis. European Journal of Pediatrics 152: 671–681

Costarino A, Baumgart S 1986 Modern fluid and electrolyte management of the critically ill premature infant. Pediatric Clinics of North America 33: 153–178

Costello A M de L, Hamilton P A, Baudin J et al 1988 Prediction of neurodevelopmental impairment at 4 years from brain ultrasound appearance of very preterm infant. Developmental Medicine and Child Neurology 30: 711–722

Cotton R, Seid A B 1980 Management of the extubation problem in the premature child. Anterior cricoid split as an alternative to tracheotomy. Annals of Otorhinolaryngology 89: 508–511

Cotton R B, Haywood J L, Fitzgerald G A 1991 Symptomatic patent ductus arteriosus following prophylactic indomethacin. Biology of the Neonate 60: 273–282

Coulter D L 1987 Neurologic uncertainty in newborn intensive care. New England Journal of Medicine 316: 840–844

Creasy R K, Gummer B A, Liggins G C 1980 A system for predicting spontaneous preterm birth. Obstetrics and Gynecology 55: 692–695

Crofton P M, Hume R 1987 Alkaline phosphatase isoenzyme in the plasma of preterm and term infants: serial measurements and clinical correlations. Clinical Chemistry 33: 1783–1787

Crowley P 1995 Antenatal corticosteroid therapy; a meta-analysis of the randomized trials, 1972–1994. American Journal of Obstetrics and Gynecology 173: 322–335

Crowley P, Chalmers I, Keirse M J N C 1990 The effects of corticosteroid administration before preterm delivery: an overview of the evidence from controlled trials. British Journal of Obstetrics and Gynaecology 97: 11–25

Cryotherapy for Retinopathy of Prematurity Cooperative Group (CRPCG) 1988 Multicenter trial of cryotherapy for retinopathy of prematurity: preliminary results. Archives of Ophthalmology 106: 471–479

Cullberg J 1972 Mental reactions of women to perinatal death. In: Morris N (ed) Psychosomatic medicine in obstetrics and gynaecology. 3rd International Congress, London, 1971

Cummins S K, Nelson K B, Grether J K, Velie E M 1993 Cerebral palsy in four northern California counties, births 1983 through 1985. Journal of Pediatrics 123: 230–237

Cunningham S, Fleck B W, Elton R A, McIntosh N 1995 Transcutaneous oxygen levels in retinopathy of prematurity. Lancet 346: 1464–1465

Curtis P D, Matthews T G, Clarke T A et al 1988 Neonatal seizures: the Dublin Collaborative Study. Archives of Disease in Childhood 63: 1065–1068

Davies P A, Gothefors L A 1984 Bacterial infection in the fetus and newborn infant. W B Saunders, Philadelphia

Davies P A, Robinson R J, Scopes J W, Tizard J P M, Wigglesworth J S 1972 Medical care of newborn babies. Clinics in Developmental Medicine Nos 44/45. Spastics International Medical Publications, William Heinemann Medical Books, London

Davignon A, Rautaharju P, Barselle E, Soumis F, Megelas M 1979/80 Normal ECG standards for infants and children. Pediatric Cardiology 1: 123–124

Davis C F, Carachi R, Young D G 1988 Neonatal tumours: Glasgow 1955–1986. Archives of Disease in Childhood 63: 1075–1078

Davis J M, Richter S E, Kendig J W, Notter R H 1992 High frequency jet ventilation and surfactant treatment of newborns with severe respiratory failure. Pediatric Pulmonology 13: 108–112

Dawes G S 1968 Foetal and neonatal physiology. Year Book Medical Publishers, Chicago, pp 141-159

de Louvois J, Harvey D 1988 Antibiotic therapy of the newborn. Clinics in Perinatology 15: 365–388

De Martino M, Tovo P A, Galli L et al 1991 HIV-1 infection in perinatally exposed siblings and twins. Archives of Disease in Childhood 66: 1235–1237

De Vries L M S, Dubowitz L M S, Dubowitz V et al 1985 Predictive value of cranial ultrasound in the newborn baby: a reappraisal. Lancet i: 137–140

De Vries L S, Connell J, Dubowitz L M S, Oozeer R C, Dubowitz V, Pennock J M 1987 Neurological, electrophysiological and MRI abnormalities in infants with extensive cystic leukomalacia. Neuropediatrics 18: 61–66

De Vries L S, Dubowitz L M S, Dubowitz V, Pennock J M 1990 A colour atlas of brain disorders in the newborn. Wolfe Medical Publications, Ipswich

De Vries L M S, Eken P, Groenendaal F, Van Haastert I C, Meiners L C 1993 Correlation between the degree of periventricular leukomalacia diagnosed using cranial ultrasound and MRI later in infancy in children with cerebral palsy. Neuropediatrics 24: 263–268

Dear P R F 1987 Monitoring oxygen in the newborn: saturation or partial pressure? Archives of Disease in Childhood 62: 879–881

Dear P R F, Conway S P 1984 Treatment of severe bilateral interstitial emphysema in a baby by artificial pneumothorax and pneumotomy. Lancet i: 273–277

Deaver J E, Leppert P C, Zaroulis K 1986 Neonatal allo-immune thrombocytopenic purpura. American Journal of Perinatology 3: 127–131

Dechant K L, Faulds D 1991 Colfosceril palmitate: a review of the therapeutic efficacy and clinical tolerability of a synthetic preparation (Exosurf® Neonatal™) in neonatal respiratory distress syndrome. Drugs 42: 877–894

Delgado-Escueta A V, Janz D 1992 Consensus guidelines: preconception counselling, management, and care of the pregnant woman with epilepsy. Neurology 42 (suppl 5): 149–160

Den Ouden A L, Kok J H, Verkerk P H, Brand R, Verloove-Vanhorick S P 1996 The relation between neonatal thyroxine levels and neurodevelopmental outcome at age 5 and 9 years in a national cohort of very preterm and/or very low birthweight infants. Pediatric Research 39: 142–145

Derycke M, Dreyfus M, Ropert J C, Tchernia G 1985 Intravenous immunoglobulin for neonatal iso-immune thrombocytopenia. Archives of Disease in Childhood 60: 667–669

Desci T, Koletzko B 1994 Polyunsaturated fatty acids in infant nutrition. Acta Paediatrica 395 (suppl): 31–37

Di Pietro M A, Brody B A, Teele R L 1986 Peritrigonal echogenic 'blush' on cranial sonography: pathologic correlates. American Journal of Radiology 146: 1067–1072

Diprose G K, Evans D H, Archer L N J, Levene M I 1986 Dinamap fails to detect hypotension in very low birthweight infants. Archives of Disease in Childhood 61: 771–773

Douglas G C, King B F 1992 Maternal–fetal transmission of HIV: a review of possible routes and cellular mechanisms of infection. Clinics in Infectious Diseases 15: 178

Drew J H 1982 Immediate intubation at birth of the very low birth-weight infant. Effect on survival. American Journal of Diseases of Children 136: 207–210

Dreyfuss D, Saumon G 1992 Barotrauma is volutrauma, but which is the volume responsible? Intensive Care Medicine 18: 139–141

Drummond M F, Stoddart G L, Torrance G W 1986 Methods for the economic evaluation of health care. Oxford University Press, Oxford

Drury P L, Doddridge M 1992 Pre-pregnancy clinics for diabetic women. Lancet 340: 919

Dubowitz L, Dubowitz L M S 1981 The neurological assessment of the preterm and full term newborn infant. Clinics in Developmental Medicine, No 79. SIMP/Heinemann, London

Dubowitz L M S, Mushin J, de Vries L, Arden G B 1986 Visual function in the newborn infant: is it cortically mediated? Lancet i: 1139–1140

Duff R S, Campbell A G M 1976 On deciding the care of severely handicapped or dying persons: with particular reference to infants. Pediatrics 57: 487–493

Dunn L, Hulman S, Weiner J, Kliegman R 1988 Beneficial effects of early hypocaloric enteral feeding on neonatal gastrointestinal function: preliminary report of a randomized trial. Journal of Pediatrics 112: 622–629

Dworetz A R, Moya F R, Sabo B, Gladstone I, Cross I 1989 Survival of infants with persistent pulmonary hypertension without extracorporeal membrane oxygenation. Pediatrics 84: 1–6

ECPPA Collaborative Group 1996 ECPPA randomised trial of low dose aspirin for the prevention of maternal and fetal complications in high risk pregnant women. British Journal of Obstetrics and Gynaecology 103: 39–47

Editorial 1994 Zidovudine for mother, fetus and child: hope or poison? Lancet 344: 207–209

Edwards A D, Wyatt J S, Richardson C, Potter A, Cope M, Delpy D T, Reynolds E O R 1990 Effects of indomethacin on cerebral haemodynamics in very pre term infants. Lancet 335: 1491–1495

EEC Working Group 1994 EEC trial of ethamsylate in prophylaxis against periventricular haemorrhage. Archives of Disease in Childhood 70: F201–F205

Eg-Andersen G 1989 Prediction of outcome in 164 infants born after 24 to 28 weeks gestation. Acta Paediatrica Scandinavica 360: 56–61

Eidelman A I, Hobbs J F 1978 Bicarbonate therapy revisited. American Journal of Diseases of Children 132: 847–848

Ekelund H, Finnstrom O, Gunnarskog J, Kallen B, Larsson Y 1993 Administration of vitamin K to newborn infants and childhood cancer. British Medical Journal 307: 89–91

Eken P, van Niuwenhuizen O, van der Graaf Y, Schalij-Delfos N E, de Vries L S 1994 Relation between neonatal cerebral ultrasound abnormalities and cerebral visual impairment. Developmental Medicine and Child Neurology 36: 3–15

Eken P, Toet M C, Groenendaal F, de Vries L S 1995 Predictive value of early neuroimaging, pulsed Doppler and neurophysiology in full term infants with hypoxic–ischaemic encephalopathy. Archives of Disease in Childhood 73: F75–F80

Elliott M, Bayly R, Cole T, Temple I K, Maher E R 1994 Clinical features and natural history of Beckwith–Wiedemann syndrome: presentation of 74 new cases. Clinical Genetics 46: 168–174

Emmanouilides G C, Riemenschneider T A, Allen H D, Gutgesell H P (eds) 1995 Moss and Adams: Heart disease in infants, children and adolescents: including the fetus and young adult, 5th edn. Williams & Wilkins, Baltimore, vol 1

Enkin M W, Keirse M J N C, Renfrew M J, Nielson J P (eds) 1995 The Cochrane pregnancy and childbirth database – Issue2. BMJ Publishing Group, London

Ens-Dokkum M H, Johnson A, Schrender M, Veen S, Wilkinson A R, Brand R, Ruys J H, Verloove-Vanhorick S P 1994 Comparison of mortality and rates of cerebral palsy in two populations of VLBW infants. Archives of Disease in Childhood 66: 204–211

Epstein L G, Berman C Z, Sharer L R, Khademi M, Desposito F 1987 Unilateral calcification and contrast enhancement of the basal ganglia in a child with AIDS encephalopathy. American Journal of Neuroradiology 8: 163–165

Ersley A J, Caro J G 1984 Secondary polycythaemia: a boon or a burden? Blood Cells 10: 177–180

Escobar G J, Littenberg B, Pettiti D B 1991 Outcome among surviving very low birthweight infants: a meta-analysis. Archives of Disease in Childhood 66: 204–211

ESPGAN Committee on Nutrition 1987 Nutrition and feeding of preterm infants. Acta Paediatrica Scandinavica 336 (suppl): 1–14

Estes J M, Harrison M R 1993 Fetal obstructive urology. Seminars in Pediatric Surgery 2: 129–135

European Collaborative Study 1992 Risk factors for mother-to-child transmission of HIV-1. Lancet 339: 1007–1012

Evans N 1993 Diagnosis of patent ductus arteriosus in the preterm newborn. Archives of Disease in Childhood 68: 58–61

Evans N J, Archer L N J 1990 Postnatal circulatory adaptation in healthy term and preterm neonates. Archives of Disease in Childhood 65: 24–26

Evans N J, Rutter N 1986 Reduction of skin damage from transcutaneous oxygen electrodes using spray on dressing. Archives of Disease in Childhood 61: 881–884

Evans P M, Alberman E 1985 Recording defects of children with cerebral palsy. Developmental Medicine and Child Neurology 27: 401–406

Evans D H, Levene M I, Archer L N J 1987 The effect of indomethacin on cerebral blood flow velocity in premature infants. Developmental Medicine and Child Neurology 29: 776–782

Ewer A K, McHugo J M, Chapman S, Newell S J 1993 Fetal echogenic gut: a marker of intrauterine gut ischaemia. Archives of Disease in Childhood 69: 510–513

Ewer A K, Durbin G M, Morgan M E, Booth I W 1994 Gastric emptying in preterm infants. Archives of Disease in Childhood 71: F24–F27

Ewighman B G, Crane J P, Frigoletto F D, Lefevre M L, Bain R P, McNeillis D 1993 Effect of prenatal ultrasound screening in perinatal outcome. New England Journal of Medicine 329: 821–827

Eyre J A, Nanei S, Wilkinson A R 1988 Quantification of changes in normal neonatal EEGs with gestation from continuous 5 day recordings. Development Medicine and Child Neurology 30: 599–607

Faber H K 1922 Food requirements in newborn infants – a study of spontaneous intake. American Journal of Diseases of Children 24: 56–60

Faerber E N (ed) 1995 CNS magnetic resonance imaging in infants and children. Clinics in developmental medicine No 134. MacKeith Press, Lavenham Press, Suffolk

Fajardo B, Browning M, Fisher D, Paton J 1990 Effect of nursery environment on state regulation in very-low-birth-weight premature infants. Infant Behavior and Development 13: 287–303

Fanaroff A A, Wright L L, Stevenson D K, Shankaran S, Donovan E F, Ehrenkranz R A, Younes N, Stoll B J, Tyson J E, Bauer C R, Oh W, Lemons J A, Papile L A, Verter J 1995 Very low birthweight outcomes of the National Institute of Child Health and Human Development Neonatal Research network, May 1991 through December 1992. American Journal of Obstetrics and Gynecology 173: 1423–1431

Farrell B for the Collaborative Low-dose Aspirin Study in Pregnancy 1994 CLASP: a randomised trial of low dose aspirin for the prevention and treatment of pre-eclampsia among 9364 pregnant women. Lancet 343: 619–629

Fawer C-L, Calame A 1991 Significance of ultrasound appearances in the neurological development and cognitive abilities of preterm infants at 5 years. European Journal of Pediatrics 150: 515–520

Faxelius G, Hagenevik K, Lagercrantz H, Lundell B, Irestedt L 1983 Catecholamine surge and lung function after delivery. Archives of Disease in Childhood 58: 262–266

Fazzi E, Lanzi G, Gerardo A, Ometto A, Orcesi S, Rondini G 1992 Neurodevelopmental outcome in very low birthweight infants with or without periventricular haemorrhage and/or leucomalacia. Acta Paediatrica 81: 808–811

Fenton T R, Bennett S, McIntosh N 1988 Air embolism in ventilated very low birthweight infants. Archives of Disease in Childhood 63: 541–543

Ferrara T B, Hoekstra R E, Couser R J, Gaziano E P, Calvin S E, Payne N R, Fangman J J 1994 Survival and follow up of infants born at 23 to 26 weeks of gestational age: effects of surfactant therapy. Journal of Pediatrics 124: 119–124

Ferrari F, Cioni G, Prechtl H F R 1990 Qualitative changes of general movements in preterm infants with brain lesions. Early Human Development 23: 193–231

Field D, Milner A D, Hopkin I E 1985 Inspiratory time and tidal volume during intermittent positive pressure ventilation. Archives of Disease in Childhood 60: 259–261

Fielder A R 1995 Disorders of vision. In: Levene M I, Lilford R J, Bennett M J, Punt J (eds) Fetal and neonatal neurology and neurosurgery. Churchill Livingstone, Edinburgh, p 565–589

Fielder A R, Mayer D L 1991 Delayed visual maturation. Seminars in Ophthalmology 16: 182–193

Fielder A R, Levene M I 1992 Screening for retinopathy of prematurity. Archives of Disease in Childhood 67: 860–867

Fielder A R, Foreman N, Moseley M J, Robinson J 1993 Prematurity and visual development. In: Simons K (ed) Early visual development, normal and abnormal. Oxford University Press, New York, pp 485–504

Finer N N, Etches P C, Kamstra B, Tierney A J, Peliowski A, Ryan C A 1994 Inhaled nitric oxide in infants referred for extracorporeal membrane oxygenation: dose response. Journal of Pediatrics 124: 302–308

Fishman R A 1991 The glucose transporter protein and glucopenic brain injury. New England Journal of Medicine 325: 731–732

Fitzgerald M, Millard C, McIntosh N 1988a Hyperalgesia in premature infants. Lancet i: 292

Fitzgerald M, Shaw A, McIntosh N 1988b Postnatal development of the cutaneous flexor reflex: comparative study of preterm infants and newborn rat pups. Developmental Medicine and Child Neurology 30: 520–526

Fleer A, Gerards L J, Aerts P et al 1985 Opsonic defence of *Staphylococcus epidermidis* in the premature neonate. Journal of Infectious Diseases 152: 930–935

Fleischman A R 1986 An infant bioethical review committee in an urban medical center. Hastings Center Report 16(3): 16–18

Flood R G, Pinelli R W 1949 Urinary glycocyamine, creatine and creatinine. 1. Their excretion by normal infants and children. American Journal of Diseases of Children 77: 740–745

Fraumeni J F Jr, Miller R W 1969 Cancer deaths in the newborn. American Journal of Diseases of Children 117: 186–189

Froese A B, Bryan A C 1987 High frequency ventilation. American Review of Respiratory Diseases 135: 1363–1374

Froese A B, McCulloch P R, Sugiura M, Vaclavik S, Possmayer F, Moller F 1993 Optimising alveolar expansion prolongs the effectiveness of exogenous surfactant therapy in the adult rabbit. American Review of Respiratory Disease 148: 569–577

Frostell C, Fratacci M-D, Wain J C, Jones R, Zapol W M 1991 Inhaled nitric oxide. A selective pulmonary vasodilator reversing hypoxic pulmonary vasoconstriction. Circulation 83: 2038–2047

Fuhrmann K, Reiher H, Semmler K, Glockner E 1989 The effect of intensified conventional insulin therapy before and during pregnancy on the malformation rate of offspring of diabetic mothers. Experimental and Clinical Endocrinology 83: 127–129

Fujimoto S, Togari H, Yamaguchi N, Mizutani F, Suzuki S, Sobajima H 1994 Hypocarbia and cystic periventricular leukomalacia in premature infants. Archives of Disease in Childhood 71: F107–F110

Fujimura M, Kitajima H, Nakayama M 1993 Increased leukocyte elastase of the tracheal aspirate at birth and neonatal pulmonary emphysema. Pediatrics 92: 564–569

Gal P, Oles K S, Gilman J T, Weaver R 1988 Valproic acid efficacy, toxicity, and pharmacokinetics in neonates with intractable seizures. Neurology 38: 467–471

Garcia L M 1972 Disorders of bilirubin metabolism. In: Assali N S (ed) Pathophysiology of gestation. Academic Press, New York, vol III, p 457

Gerdes J S 1991 Clinico-pathologic approach to the diagnosis of neonatal sepsis. Clinical Perinatology 18: 361–390

Gersony W M, Peakham G J, Ellison R C, Miettinen D S, Nadas A S 1983 Effects of indomethacin in premature infants with patent ductus arteriosus; results of a national collaborative study. Journal of Pediatrics 102: 895–906

Gerstmann D R, DeLemos R A, Clark R H 1991 High-frequency ventilation: issues of strategy. Clinics in Perinatology 18: 563–580

Giacoia G P, Neter E, Ogra P 1981 Respiratory infections in infants with idiopathic apnea. Pediatrics 63: 537–542

Gibb D, Arulkumaran S 1992 Fetal monitoring in practice. Butterworth-Heinemann, Oxford

Gibson K M, Breuer J, Nyhan W L 1988 3-hydroxy-3-methylglutaryl-coenzyme A lyase deficiency: review of 18 report patients. European Journal of Pediatrics 148: 180–186

Giles M M, Fenton M H, Shaw B, Elton R A, Clarke M, Lang M, Hume R 1987 Sequential calcium and phosphorus balance studies in preterm infants. Journal of Pediatrics 110: 591–598

Giles M M, Laing I A, Elton R A, Robins J B, Sanderson M, Hume R 1990 Magnesium metabolism in preterm infants: effect of calcium, magnesium, postnatal and gestational age. Journal of Pediatrics 117: 147–154

Gill A, Yu W Y H, Bajuk B, Asbury J 1986 Postnatal growth in infants born before 30 weeks' gestation. Archives of Disease in Childhood 61: 549–553

Gill A B, Weindling A M 1993 Randomised controlled trial of plasma protein fraction versus dopamine in hypotensive very low birth weight infants. Archives of Disease in Childhood 69: 284–287

Gilman J T, Gal P, Duchowny M S, Weaver R L, Ransom J L 1989 Rapid sequential phenobarbital treatment of neonatal seizures. Pediatrics 83: 674–678

Ginsburg C M, McCracken G H 1982 Urinary tract infections in young infants. Pediatrics 69: 409–411

Glass E, Avery G B, Subramaniou K N S, Keys M P et al 1985 Effect of bright light in the hospital nursery on the incidence of retinopathy of prematurity. New England Journal of Medicine 313: 401–404

Glass P, Miller M, Short B 1989 Morbidity for survivors of extracorporeal membrane oxygenation: neurodevelopmental outcome at 1 year of age. Pediatrics 83: 72–78

Goerke J, Clements J A 1986 Alveolar surface tension and lung surfactant. In: Macklen P T, Meads J (eds) Handbook of physiology. American Physiological Society, Washington, vol III, pp 247–261

Goldberg J H 1983 Neonatal convulsions – a ten year review. Archives of Disease in Childhood 58: 976–978

Goldberg R N 1981 Sustained arterial blood pressure elevation associated with small pneumothoraces: early detection via continuous monitoring. Pediatrics 68: 775–777

Goldberg P N, Moscoso P, Bauer C R 1986 Use of barbiturate therapy in severe perinatal asphyxia. Journal of Pediatrics 109: 851–856

Golding J, Paterson M, Kinlen L J 1990 Factors associated with childhood cancer in a national cohort study. British Journal of Cancer 62(2): 304–308

Golding J, Greenwood R, Birmingham K, Mott M 1992 Childhood cancer, intramuscular vitamin K, and pethidine given during labour. British Medical Journal 305: 341–346

Good W V, Jan J E, DeSa L, Barkovich A J, Groenveld M, Hoyt C S 1994 Cortical visual impairment in children. Survey of Ophthalmology 38: 351–364

Goodwin S R, Graves S A, Haberkern C M 1985 Aspiration in the intubated premature infant. Pediatrics 75: 85–88

Gorski P A, Huntington L, Lewkowicz D J 1990 Handling preterm infants in hospitals: stimulating controversy about timing of stimulation. Clinics in Perinatology 17: 103–112

Gould S J, Howard S, Hope P L, Reynolds E O R 1987 Periventricular intraparenchymal cerebral haemorrhage in preterm infants: role of venous infarction. Journal of Pathology 151: 197–202

Gourley C R, Arend R A 1986 Beta-glucuronidase and hyperbilirubinaemia in breast fed and formula fed babies. Lancet i: 644–646

Govindaswami B, Bejar R, Bernstein G, Heldt G P 1993 Reduction in cerebral blood flow velocity (CBFV) variability in infants <1500 gm during synchronised intermittent mandatory ventilation. Pediatric Research 33: 213A (Abstract 1258)

Graham M, Levene M I, Trounce J Q, Rutter N 1987 Prediction of cerebral palsy in very low birthweight infants. Lancet ii: 593–596

Grant A, Elbourne D, Valentin L, Alexander S 1989 Routine formal fetal movement counting and risk of antepartum late death in normally formed singletons. Lancet 11: 345–349

Grant A, O'Brien N, Joy M T, Hennessy E, MacDonald D 1989 Cerebral palsy among children born during the Dublin randomised trial of intrapartum monitoring. Lancet ii: 1233–1235

Graziani L J, Mitchell D G, Kornhauser M, Pidcock F S, Merton D A, Stanley C, McKee L 1992a Neurodevelopment of preterm infants: neonatal neurosonographic and serum bilirubin studies. Pediatrics 89: 229–234

Graziani L J, Spitzer A R, Mitchell D G, Merton D A, Stanley C, Robinson N, McKee L 1992b Mechanical ventilation in preterm infants: neurosonographic and developmental studies. Pediatrics 90: 515–522

Greaves M 1979 Molecular phenotypes: a new perspective on diagnosis and classification of leukaemias. In: Morris-Jones P (ed) Topics in paediatrics 1: haematology and oncology. Pitman Medical, Tunbridge Wells

Greenough A, Greenall F 1988 Patient triggered ventilation in premature neonates. Archives of Disease in Childhood 63: 77–78

Greenough A, Wood S, Morley C J, Davis J A 1984 Pancuronium prevents pneumothoraces in ventilated premature babies who actively expire against positive pressure ventilation. Lancet i: 1–3

Greenough A, Greenall F, Gamsu H R 1986 Selective paralysis of neonates – effects of fluid balance, catecholamine levels and heart rate variability. Abstracts of Paediatric Research Society (September)

Greenough A, Pool J, Greenall F, Morley C, Gamsu H 1987a Comparison of different rates of artificial ventilation in preterm neonates with respiratory distress syndrome. Acta Paediatrica Scandinavica 76: 706–712

Greenough A, Greenall F, Gamsu H 1987b Synchronous respiration: which ventilator rate is best? Acta Paediatrica Scandinavica 76: 713–718

Greenough W T, Black J E, Wallace C S 1987 Experience and brain development. Child Development 58: 539–559

Greenspan J S, Wolfson M R, Rubenstein S D, Shaffer T H 1990 Liquid ventilation of human preterm neonates. Journal of Pediatrics 117: 106–111

Greer F R 1994 Osteopenia of prematurity. Annual Review of Nutrition 14: 169–185

Greer F R, MacCormick A 1988 Improved bone mineralisation and growth in premature infants fed fortified own mother's milk. Journal of Pediatrics 112: 961–966

Gregory G A, Gooding C A, Phibbs R H, Tooley W H 1974 Meconium aspiration in infants – a prospective study. Journal of Pediatrics 85: 848–852

Grimes D A, Schulz K F 1992 Randomised controlled trials of home uterine activity monitoring; a review and critique. Obstetrics and Gynecology 79: 137–142

Gross S J 1987 Bone mineralisation in preterm infants fed human milk with and without mineral supplementation. Journal of Pediatrics 111: 450–458

Gruenwald P 1947 Surface tension as a factor in the resistance of neonatal lungs to inflation. American Journal of Obstetrics and Gynecology 53: 996–1007

Gryboski J D 1965 The swallowing mechanism of the neonate I: Oesophageal and gastric motility. Pediatrics 35: 445–452

Guignard J P, John E G 1986 Renal function in the tiny premature infant. Clinics in Perinatology 13: 377–401

Guin G H, Gilbert E G, Jones B 1969 Incidence of neuroblastoma in infants dying of other causes. American Journal of Clinical Pathology 51: 126–136

Guit G L, Van De Bor M, Den Ouden L, Wondergem J H M 1990 Prediction of neurodevelopmental outcome in the preterm infant: MR staged myelination compared with cranial ultrasound. Pediatric Radiology 175: 107–109

Gunn A J, Mydlar T, Bennet L, Faull R L M, Gorter S, Cooke C, Johnston B M, Gluckman P D 1989 The neuroprotective actions of a calcium channel antagonist, flunarizine, in the infant rat. Pediatric Research 25: 573–576

Hack M, Fanaroff A A 1988 Current controversies in perinatal care: how small is too small? Considerations in evaluating the outcome of the tiny infant. Clinics in Perinatology 15: 773–788

Hack M, Fanaroff A A 1989 Outcomes of extremely low birth weight infants between 1982 and 1989. New England Journal of Medicine 321: 1642–1647

Hack M, Horbar J D, Malloy M H, Tyson J E, Wright E, Wright L 1991 Very low birthweight outcomes of the National Institute of Child Health and Human Development network. Pediatrics 87: 587–597

Hack M, Wright L L, Shankaran S, Tyson J E, Horbar J D, Bauer C R, Younes N 1995 Very low birthweight outcomes of the National Institute of Child Health and Human Development Neonatal network, November 1989 to October 1990. American Journal of Obstetrics and Gynecology 172: 457–464

Hackett G A, Campbell S, Gamsu H, Cohen Overbeeke T, Pearce J M F 1987 Doppler studies in the growth retarded foetus and prediction of necrotising enterocolitis, haemorrhage and neonatal morbidity. British Medical Journal 294(1): 13–16

Haggard M P 1990 Hearing screening in children – state of the art(s). Archives of Disease in Childhood 65: 1193–1198

Halahakoon C H, Halliday H L 1995 Other acute lung disorders. In: Yu V Y H (ed) Pulmonary problems in the perinatal period and their sequelae. Baillière Tindall, London

Hall R T, Sgeoka A O, Hill H R 1983 Serum opsonic and peripheral neutrophil counts before and after exchange transfusion in infants with early onset group B streptococcal septicemia. Pediatric Infectious Disease Journal 2: 356–358

Halliday H L 1988 Neonatal patent ductus arteriosus. Pediatric Reviews and Communications 3: 1–17

Halliday H L 1989 Clinical experience with exogenous natural surfactant. Developmental Pharmacology and Therapeutics 13: 173–181

Halliday H L 1992 Other acute lung disorders. In: Sinclair J C, Bracken M B (eds) Effective care of the newborn infant. Oxford University Press, Oxford

Halliday H L 1993 Current views on the use of surfactant. Contemporary Reviews of Obstetrics and Gynaecology 5: 65–70

Halliday H L 1996 Natural vs synthetic surfactants in neonatal respiratory distress syndrome. Drugs 51: 226–237

Halliday H L, Hirata T 1979 Perinatal listeriosis – a review of twelve patients. American Journal of Obstetrics and Gynecology 133: 405–410

Halliday H L, Speer C P 1995 Strategies for surfactant therapy in established neonatal respiratory distress syndrome. In: Robertson B, Taeusch H W (eds) Surfactant therapy for lung disease. Marcel Dekker, New York

Hamada Y, Hayakawa T, Hattori H, Mikawa H 1994 Inhibitor of nitric oxide synthesis reduces hypoxic–ischemic brain damage in the neonatal rat. Pediatric Research 35: 10–14

Hamilton C M, Shaw J C L 1984 Changes in sodium and water balance, renal function and aldosterone excretion during the first seven days of life in very low birth weight infants. Pediatric Research 18: 91

Hamilton P A, Whitehead M D, Reynolds E O R 1985 Underestimation of arterial oxygen tension by transcutaneous electrode with increasing age in infants. Archives of Disease in Childhood 60: 1162–1165

Hammarlund K, Sedin G, Stromberg B 1983 Transepidermal water loss in newborn infants. VIII Relations to gestational age and post-natal age in appropriate and small for gestational age infants. Acta Paediatrica Scandinavica 72: 721–728

Hammerman C, Aramburo M J 1990 Prolonged indomethacin therapy for the prevention of recurrences of patent ductus arteriosus. Journal of Pediatrics 117: 771–776

Hamosh M, Scanlon J W, Ganot D, Likel M, Scanlon K B, Hamosh P 1981 Fat digestion in the newborn: characterization of lipase in gastric aspirates on premature and term infants. Journal of Clinical Investigation 67: 838–846

Hanley F L, Sade R M, Freedom R M, Blackstone E H, Kirklin J W 1993 Outcomes in critically ill neonates with pulmonary stenosis and intact ventricular septum: a multi institutional study. Journal of the American College of Cardiology 22: 183–192

Hann I M, Bodger M P, Hoffbrand A V 1983 Development of pluripotent haemopoietic progenitor cells (CFU-GEMM) in the human fetus. Blood 62: 118

Haque K N 1993 Indications for antimicrobial therapy in babies born after PROM: the Saudi experience. Postgraduate Doctor 16(9): 342–347

Haque K N 1995 Pitfalls of meta-analysis. Archives of Disease in Childhood 73: F196

Haque K N, Chagla A H 1989 Do gowns prevent infection in neonatal intensive care units. Journal of Hospital Infection 14: 159–162

Haque K N, Zaidi M H, Haque S K 1986 Evaluation of C-reactive protein by latex agglutination in neonatal sepsis. Pakistan Paediatrics Journal 4: 229–233

Haque K N, Chagla A H, Shaheed M M 1989 Half a decade of neonatal sepsis at King Khalid University Hospital, Riyadh, Saudi Arabia. Journal of Tropical Paediatrics 35: 31–34

Haque K N, Remo C, Bahakim H 1995 Comparison of two types of intravenous immunoglobulins in the treatment of neonatal sepsis. Clinical Experimental Immunology 101: 328–232

Harms K, Herting E, Kron M et al 1995 Randomized, controlled trial of amoxycillin prophylaxis for prevention of catheter-related infections in newborn infants with central venous silicone elastomer catheters. Journal of Pediatrics 127: 615–619

Harman C, Menticoglou S, Manning F, Albar H, Morrison I 1994 Prenatal fetal monitoring; abnormalities of fetal behaviour in high risk pregnancy. In: James D K, Steer P J, Wiener C P, Gonik B (eds) High risk pregnancies: management options. W B Saunders, London, pp 693–734

Harpey J P, Charpentier C, Goodman S I, Darbois Y, Lefebvre G, Sebbah J 1983 Multiple acyl-CoA dehydrogenase deficiency occurring in pregnancy and caused by a defect in riboflavin metabolism in the mother. Journal of Pediatrics 103: 394–398

Harrison H 1993 The principles for family-centred neonatal care. Pediatrics 92: 643–650

Harrison M R, Adzick N S, Flake A W et al 1993 Correction of congenital diaphragmatic hernia in utero: VI hard earned lessons. Journal of Paediatric Surgery 28: 1411–1418

Hart S M, McNair M, Gamsu H R, Price J F 1983 Pulmonary interstitial emphysema in very low birthweight infants. Archives of Disease in Childhood 58: 612–615

Hashimoto T, Tayama M, Miyazaki M, Fujii E, Harada M, Miyoshi H, Tanouchi M, Kuroda Y 1995 Developmental brain changes investigated with proton magnet resonance spectroscopy. Developmental Medicine and Child Neurology 37: 398–405

Hattori H, Wasterlain C G 1990 Posthypoxic glucose supplement reduces hypoxic–ischemic brain damage in the neonatal rat. Annals of Neurology 28: 122–128

Hauth J C, Goldenberg R L, Andrews W W, Dubard M B, Copper R L 1995 Reduced incidence of preterm delivery with metronidazole and erythromycin in women with bacterial vaginosis. New England Journal of Medicine 333: 1732–1736

Hawdon J M, Ward-Platt M P 1993a Metabolic adaptation in small for gestational age infants. Archives of Disease in Childhood 68: 262–268

Hawdon J M, Weddell A, Aynsley-Green A, Ward-Platt M P 1993b Hormonal and metabolic response to hypoglycaemia in small for gestational age infants. Archives of Disease in Childhood 68: 269–273

Hawdon J M, Aynsley-Green A, Bartlett K, Ward-Platt M P 1993c The role of pancreatic insulin secretion in neonatal glucoregulation. II. Infants with disordered blood glucose homeostasis. Archives of Disease in Childhood 68: 280–285

Hawgood S 1987 Surfactant deficiency in preterm infants. In: Yu V Y H,

Wood E C (eds) Prematurity. Churchill Livingstone, Edinburgh, pp 170–179

Hay P E, Lamond R F, Taylor-Robinson D, Morgan D J, Ison C, Pearson J 1994 Abnormal bacterial colonisation of the genital tract and subsequent preterm delivery and later miscarriage. British Medical Journal 308: 295–298

Heicher D A, Kasting D S, Harrod J R 1981 Prospective clinical comparison of two methods for mechanical ventilation of neonates: rapid rate and short inspiratory time versus slow rate and long inspiratory time. Journal of Pediatrics 98: 957–961

Heird W C, Driscoll J M, Schillinger J N, Grebin B, Winters R W 1972 Intravenous alimentation in paediatric patients. Journal of Pediatrics 80: 351–372

Helders P J M 1989 The effects of a sensory/range-finding program on the development of very low birthweight infants. Unpublished PhD Thesis, University of Utrecht, Utrecht, Netherlands

Hellstrom-Westas L, Westergren U, Rosen I, Svenningsen N W 1988 Lidocaine for treatment of severe seizures in newborn infants. Acta Paediatrica Scandinavica 77: 79–84

Hellstrom-Westas L, Rosen I, Svenningsen N W 1995 Predictive value of early continuous amplitude integrated EEG recordings on outcome after severe birth asphyxia in full term infants. Archives of Disease in Childhood 72: F34–F38

Hemming V G, Overall J C, Brett M R 1976 Nosocomial infections in a newborn intensive-care unit. New England Journal of Medicine 294: 1310–1316

Henderson-Smart D 1992 Pulmonary diseases of the newborn. Part I: Respiratory physiology. In: Roberton N R C (ed) Textbook of neonatology, 2nd edn. Churchill Livingstone, Edinburgh, pp 349–368

Henderson-Smart D J 1995 Recurrent apnoea. In: Yu V Y H (ed) Pulmonary problems in the prenatal period and their sequelae. Baillière Tindall, London

Hepper P G, Shahidullah B S 1994 Development of fetal hearing. Archives of Disease in Childhood 71: F81–F87

Herman S, Reynolds E O R 1973 Methods of improving oxygenation in infants mechanically ventilated for severe hyaline membrane disease. Archives of Disease in Childhood 48: 612–617

Hertz D E, Karn C A, Liu Y M et al 1993 Intravenous glucose suppresses glucose production but not proteolysis in extremely premature newborns. Journal of Clinical Investigation 92: 1752–1758

Hey E N 1975 Thermal neutrality. British Medical Bulletin 31: 69–74

Heymans H S A, Oorthnys J W E, Nelck G, Wanders R J A, Dingemans K P, Schutgens R B H 1986 Peroxisomal abnormalities in rhizomelic chondrodysplasia punctata. Journal of Inherited Metabolic Diseases 9: 329–331

HIFI Study Group 1989 High-frequency oscillatory ventilation compared with conventional mechanical ventilation in the treatment of respiratory failure in preterm infants. New England Journal of Medicine 320: 90–93

Hillier S L, Nugent R O, Eschenbach D A et al 1995 Association between bacterial vaginosis and preterm delivery of a low birth weight infant. New England Journal of Medicine 333: 1737–1742

Holtrop P C, Ertzbischoff L M, Roberts C L, Batton D G, Lorenz R P 1994 Survival and short term outcome in newborns of 23 to 25 weeks gestation. American Journal of Obstetrics and Gynecology 170: 1266–1270

Horsman A, Ryan S W, Congdon P J, Truscott J G, Simpson M 1989 Bone mineral content and body size 65 to 100 weeks postconception in preterm and full term infants. Archives of Disease in Childhood 64: 1579–1586

Howell J, Clozel M, Aranda J V 1981 Adverse effects of caffeine and theophylline in the newborn infant. Seminars in Perinatology 5: 359–369

Howie P W, Forsyth J S, Ogston S A, Clark A, Florey C D 1990 Protective effect of breast feeding against infection. British Medical Journal 300: 11–16

House of Commons Social Services Committee 1984 Perinatal and neonatal mortality report: follow up. HMSO, London

Hoyer J R, Anderson C E 1981 Congenital nephrotic syndrome. Clinics in Perinatology 8: 333–346

Hrabovsky E E, Mullett M D 1986 Gastroesophageal reflux and the premature infant. Journal of Pediatric Surgery 21: 583–587

Hudgins R J 1988 Natural history of fetal ventriculomegaly. Pediatrics 82: 692–697

Hudson I R, Gibson B E, Brownlie J, Holland B M, Turner T L, Webber R G 1990 Increased concentrations of D-dimers in newborn infants. Archives of Disease in Childhood 65: 383–384

Hughes C A, Dowling R H 1980 Speed of onset of adaptive mucosal hypoplasia and hypofunction in the intestine of parenterally fed rats. Clinical Science 59: 317–327

Hull J, Dodd K L 1992 Falling incidence of hypoxic–ischaemic encephalopathy in term infants. British Journal Obstetrics and Gynaecology 99: 386–391

Hume R, Burchell A 1993 Abnormal expression of glucose-6-phosphatase in preterm infants. Archives of Disease in Childhood 68: 202–204

Hume R, Lyall H, Burchell A 1992 Impairment of the activity of the microsomal glucose-6-phosphatase system in premature infants. Acta Paediatrica 81: 580–584

Hungerford J, Stewart A, Hope P 1986 Ocular sequelae of preterm birth and their relation to ultrasound evidence of cerebral damage. British Journal of Ophthalmology 70: 463–468

Hutto C, Parks W P, Lai S et al 1991 A hospital based prospective study of perinatal infection with human immune deficiency virus type 1. Journal of Pediatrics 118: 347–355

Ignarro L J 1989 Biological actions and properties of endothelium derived nitric oxide formed and released from artery and vein. Circulation Research 65: 1–21

Ikonen R S, Kuusinen E J, Janas M O, Koivikko M J, Sorto A E 1988 Possible etiological factors in extensive periventricular leukomalacia of preterm infants. Acta Paediatrica Scandinavica 77: 489–495

Ikonen R S, Janas M O, Koivikko M J, Laippala P, Kuusinen E J 1992 Hyperbilirubinemia, hypocarbia and periventricular leukomalacia in preterm infants: relationship to cerebral palsy. Acta Paediatrica 81: 802–807

Isaacs H 1985 Perinatal (congenital and neonatal) neoplasms: a report of 100 cases. Paediatric Pathology 3: 165–216

Isenberg S J (ed) 1994 The eye in infancy, 2nd edn. Year Book Medical Publishers, Chicago

Ito Y, Matsumoto T, Ohbu K et al 1988 Concentration of human atrial natriuretic peptide in cord blood and the plasma of the newborn. Acta Paediatrica Scandinavica 77: 76–78

Jacobson T, Grønvall J, Petersen S, Andersen G E 1993 'Minitouch' treatment of very low-birth-weight infants. Acta Paediatrica 82: 934–938

Jackson S K 1994 Endotoxin and septic shock – the antibiotic connection. Bayer, UK

Jakobsson I, Lindberg T, Lothe L, Axelsson I, Benediktsson B 1986 Human α lactalbumin as a marker of macromolecular absorption. Gut 27: 1029–1034

Jedeikin R, Primhak A, Shennan A T, Swyer P R, Rowe R D 1983 Serial electrocardiographic changes in healthy and stressed neonates. Archives of Disease in Childhood 58: 605–611

Jeffs R D 1987 Exstrophy, epispadias and cloacal and urogenital sinus abnormalities. Pediatric Clinics of North America 34: 1233–1257

Jobe A H 1993 Pulmonary surfactant therapy. New England Journal of Medicine 328: 861–868

Johanson R, Pusey J, Livera N, Jones P 1989 North Staffordshire/Wigan assisted delivery trial. British Journal of Obstetrics and Gynaecology 96: 537–544

Johnson A, Townshend P, Yudkin P, Bull D, Wilkinson A R 1993 Functional abilities at age 4 years of children born before 29 weeks gestation. British Medical Journal 306: 1715–1718

Johnson M A, Cox M, McKim E 1987 Outcome of infants of very low birthweight: a geographically based study. Canadian Journal of Medicine 136: 1157–1165

Jones R A K, Roberton N R C 1986 Small for dates babies: are they really a problem? Archives of Disease in Childhood 61: 877–880

Jones R W A, Rochefort M J, Baum J D 1976 Increased insensible water loss in newborn infants nursed under radiant warmers. British Medical Journal 2: 1347–1350

Kaiser A M, Whitelaw A G 1985 Cerebrospinal fluid pressure during post haemorrhagic ventricular dilatation in newborn infants. Archives of Disease in Childhood 60: 920–924

Kaiser A M, Whitelaw A G L 1988 Hypertensive response to increased intracranial pressure in infancy. Archives of Disease in Childhood 63: 1461–1465

Kaplan B S, Fay J, Shah V et al 1989 Autosomal recessive polycystic renal disease. Pediatric Nephrology 3: 43–49

Katz V L, Bose C L 1993 Improving survival of the very premature infant. Journal of Perinatology 13: 261–265

Keeley S R, Bohn D J 1988 The use of inotropic and afterload reducing agents in neonates. Clinics in Perinatology 15: 467–489

Keeling J W, Gough D J, Iliff P 1983 The pathology of non rhesus hydrops. Diagnostic Histopathology 6: 89–111

Keen D V, Pearse R G 1985 Birthweight between 14 and 42 weeks gestation. Diagnostic Histopathology 6: 89–111

Keirse M J N C, Grant A, King J F 1989 Preterm labour. In: Chalmers I, Enkin M, Keirse M J N C (eds) Effective care in pregnancy and childbirth. Oxford University Press

Kelly E J, Newell S J 1994 Gastric ontogeny: clinical implications. Archives of Disease in Childhood 71: F136–F141

Kelly E J, Newell S J, Brownlee K G, Primrose J N, Dear P R 1993 Gastric acid secretion in preterm infants. Early Human Development 35: 215–220

Kelly J R, Guntheroth W G 1988 Pansystolic murmur in the newborn: tricuspid regurgitation versus ventricular septal defect. Archives of Disease in Childhood 63: 1172–1174

Kennedy C R, Kimm L, Caferelli Dees D, Evans P I P, Hunter M, Lenton S, Thornton R D 1991 Otoacoustic emissions and auditory brainstem responses in the newborn. Archives of Disease in Childhood 66: 1124–1129

Kennell J H, Klaus M H 1971 Care of the mother of the high risk infant. Perinatal Biology 14: 926–954

Keszler M, Donn S M, Bucciarelli R L, Alverson D C, Hart M, Lunyong V, Modanlou H D et al 1991 Multicenter controlled trial comparing high-frequency jet ventilation and conventional mechanical ventilation in newborn infants with pulmonary interstitial emphysema. Journal of Pediatrics 119: 85–93

Kinmond S, Aitchison T C, Holland B M, Jones J G, Turner T L, Wardrop C A 1993 Umbilical cord clamping and preterm infants: a randomised trial. British Medical Journal 306: 172–175

Kinmond S, Hudson I R B, Aitchison T et al 1990 Placento-fetal transfusion in preterm infants. Early Human Development 22: 175

Kinsella J P, Neish S R, Shaffer E, Abman S H 1992 Low dose inhalational nitric oxide in persistent pulmonary hypertension of the newborn. Lancet 340: 819–820

Kinsella J P, Neish S R, Ivy D D, Shaffer E, Abman S H 1993 Clinical responses to prolonged treatment of persistent pulmonary hypertension of the newborn with low doses of nitric oxide. Journal of Pediatrics 123: 103–108

Kitchen W, Ford G W, Doyle L W, Rickards A L, Lissenden J V, Pepperell R J, Duke J E 1985 Cesarean section or vaginal delivery at 24 to 28 weeks gestation: comparison of survival and neonatal and two-year morbidity. Obstetrics and Gynecology 66: 149–157

Kitchens C S, Newcombe T F 1979 Factor XIII. Medicine 58: 413–429

Klaus M H, Kennell J H 1976 Maternal infant bonding. C V Mosby, St Louis

Klebanoff M A, Read J S, Mills J L, Shiono P H 1993 The risk of childhood cancer after neonatal exposure to vitamin K. New England Journal of Medicine 329(13): 905–908

Klein J O 1986 Recent advances in management of bacterial meningitis in neonates. Infection 12 (suppl): 546–554

Klein M, Stern L 1971 Low birthweight and the battered child syndrome. American Journal of Disease in Children 122: 15–18

Koelfen W, Freund M, Varnholt V 1995 Neonatal stroke involving the middle cerebral artery in term infants: clinical presentation, EEG and imaging studies. Developmental Medicine and Child Neurology 37: 203–212

Kogutt M S 1978 Systemic air embolism secondary to respiratory therapy in the neonate: six cases including one survivor. American Journal of Roentgenology 131: 425–429

Koh T H H G, Aynsley-Green A, Tarbit M, Eyre J A 1988 Neural dysfunction during hypoglycaemia. Archives of Disease in Childhood 63: 1353–1358

Kojima T, Hirata Y, Fukuda Y et al 1987 Plasma atrial natriuretic peptide and spontaneous diuresis in sick neonates. Archives of Disease in Childhood 62: 667–670

Kolacek S, Puntis J W L, Lloyd D R, Brown G A, Booth I W 1990 Ontogeny of pancreatic exocrine function. Archives of Disease in Childhood 65: 178–181

Koo N N I, Gupta J M, Nayanar V V, Wilkinson M, Posen R 1982 Skeletal changes in preterm infants. Archives of Disease in Childhood 57: 447–452

Koo W W 1992 Parenteral nutrition-related bone disease. Journal of Parenteral and Enteral Nutrition 16: 386–394

Koons A H, Mjoica N, Jadeja N et al 1993 Neurodevelopmental outcome of infants with apnea of infancy. American Journal of Perinatology 10: 208–211

Krantz M E, Wennergren M, Bengtson L G W, Hjalmarson O, Karlsson K, Sellgren U 1986 Epidemiological analysis of the increased risk of disturbed neonatal respiratory adaptation after Caesarean section. Acta Paediatrica 75: 832–839

Kraybill E N, Runyan D, Bose C L, Khan J 1989 Risk factors for chronic lung disease in infants with birth weights of 751 to 1000 grams. Journal of Pediatrics 115: 115–120

Kretzer F L, Hittner H M 1988 Retinopathy of prematurity: clinical implications of retinal development. Archives of Disease in Childhood 63: 1151–1167

Kroll H, Kiefel V, Giers G et al 1994 Maternal intravenous immunoglobulin treatment does not prevent intracranial haemorrhage in fetal alloimmune thrombocytopenia. Transfusion Medicine 4(4): 293–296

Lacy J B, Ohlsson A 1993 Behavioral outcomes of environmental or care-giving hospital-based interventions for preterm infants: a critical overview. Acta Paediatrica 82: 408–415

Lacy J B, Ohlsson A 1995 Administration of intravenous immunoglobulin for prophylaxis or treatment of infection in preterm infants: meta analysis. Archives of Disease in Childhood 72: F151–F155

Lagercrantz H, Nilsson F, Redham I, Hjemdal P 1986 Plasma catecholamines following nursing procedures in a neonatal ward. Early Human Development 14: 61–65

Lanska M J, Lanska D J, Baumann R J, Kryscio R J 1995 A population based study of neonatal seizures in Fayette County, Kentucky. Neurology 45: 724–732

Lawson E E, Brown E R, Torday J S, Madansky D L, Taeusch H W 1978 The effect of epinephrine on tracheal fluid flow and surfactant efflux in fetal sheep. American Review of Respiratory Disease 118: 1023–1026

Lawson K, Turkewitz G, Platt M, McCarton C 1985 Infant state in relation to its environmental context. Infant Behaviour and Development 8: 269–281

Lazarow P B, Moser H W 1995 Disorders of peroxisome biogenesis. In: Scriver C R, Beaudet A L, Sly W S, Valle D (eds) The metabolic bases of inherited disease, 7th edn. McGraw Hill, New York, ch 71, pp 2287–2324

Leach C L, Fuhrman B P, Morin F C III, Rath M G 1993 Perfluorocarbon-associated gas exchange (partial liquid ventilation) in respiratory distress syndrome: a prospective, randomised, controlled study. Critical Care Medicine 21: 1270–1278

Leach C L, Greenspan J S, Rubenstein S D et al 1995 Partial liquid ventilation with Liquivent: a pilot safety and efficacy study in premature newborns with severe respiratory distress syndrome (RDS). Pediatric Research 37: 220

Lebenthal E, Heitlinger L, Milla P J 1988 Prenatal and perinatal development of the gastrointestinal tract. In: Milla J P, Muller D P R (eds) Harries paediatric gastroenterology, 2nd edn. Churchill Livingstone, Edinburgh, ch 1, pp 3–29

Ledigo A, Clancy R R, Berman P H 1991 Neurologic outcome after electroencephalographically proven neonatal seizures. Pediatrics 88: 583–596

Leeson S C, Maresh M J A, Martindale E A et al 1996 Detection of fetal fibronectin as a predictor of pre-term delivery in high risk asymptomatic pregnancies. British Journal of Obstetrics and Gynaecology 103: 48–53

Leigh J R, Zee D S 1991 The neurology of eye movements, 2nd edn. F A Davis, Philadelphia

Leonard C H, Piecuch R E, Ballard R A, Coopler B A B 1994 Outcome of very low birthweight infants: multiple gestation versus singletons. Pediatrics 93: 611–615

Lester M D 1987 Developmental outcome prediction from acoustic cry analysis in term and preterm infants. Pediatrics 80: 529–534

Levene M I 1987 Neonatal neurology. Current reviews in paediatrics No 3. Churchill Livingstone, Edinburgh

Levene M I 1988 Management and outcome of birth asphyxia. In: Levene M I, Bennett M J, Punt J (eds) Fetal and neonatal neurology and neurosurgery. Churchill Livingstone, Edinburgh, pp 383–392

Levene M I 1990 Cerebral ultrasound and neurological impairment: telling the future. Archives of Disease in Childhood 65: 469–471

Levene M I 1992 Role of excitatory amino acid antagonists in the management of birth asphyxia. Biology of the Neonate 62: 248–251

Levene M I 1995 Birth asphyxia. In: David T J (ed) Recent advances in paediatrics, 13. Churchill Livingstone, Edinburgh, pp 13–27

Levene M I, De Crespigny L Ch 1983 Classification of intraventricular haemorrhage. Lancet i: 643

Levene M I, de Vries L S 1995 Neonatal intracranial haemorrhage. In: Levene M I, Lilford R J (eds) Fetal and neonatal neurology and neurosurgery. Churchill Livingstone, Edinburgh, pp 335–366

Levene M I, Evans D H 1983 Continuous measurement of subarachnoid pressure in the severely asphyxiated newborn.. Archives of Disease in Childhood 58: 1013–1015

Levene M I, Evans D H 1985 Medical management of raised intracranial pressure after severe birth asphyxia. Archives of Disease in Childhood 60: 12–16

Levene M I, Trounce J Q 1986 Neonatal convulsions: towards more precise diagnosis. Archives of Disease in Childhood 61: 78–87

Levene M I, Kornberg J, Williams T H 1985 The incidence and severity of post-asphyxial encephalopathy in full-term infants. Early Human Development 11: 21–26

Levene M I, Tudehope D, Thearle J 1987 Essentials of neonatal medicine. Blackwell Scientific, Oxford

Levene M I, Sands C, Grindulis H, Moore J R 1986 Comparison of two methods of predicting outcome in perinatal asphyxia. Lancet i: 67–69

Levene M I, Evans D H, Forde A, Archer L N 1987 Value of intracranial pressure monitoring of asphyxiated newborn infants. Developmental Medicine and Child Neurology 29: 311–319

Levene M I, Fenton A C, Evans D H, Archer L N J, Shortland D B, Gibson N A 1989 Severe birth asphyxia and abnormal cerebral blood-flow velocity. Developmental Medicine and Child Neurology 31: 427–434

Levene M I, Dowling S, Graham M, Fogelman K, Galton M, Phillips M 1992 Impaired motor function (clumsiness) in five year old children: correlation with neonatal ultrasound scan. Archives of Disease in Childhood 67: 687–690

Leversha A M, Wilson N J, Clarkson P M, Calder A L, Ramage M C, Neutze J M 1994 Efficiency and dosage of enalapril in congenital and acquired heart disease. Archives of Disease in Childhood 70: 35–39

Liggins G C, Kitterman J A 1981 Development of the fetal lung. In: The fetus and independent life. Ciba Foundation Symposium 86, Pitman, London, pp 308–335

Linder N, Aranda J V, Tsur M et al 1988 Need for endotracheal intubation and suction in meconium-stained neonates. Journal of Pediatrics 112: 612–615

Linshaw M A 1987 Potassium homeostasis and hypokalaemia. Pediatric Clinics of North America 34: 649–681

Lipper E G, Voorhies T M, Ross G, Vannucci R C, Auld P A 1986 Early predictors of one-year outcome for infants asphyxiated at birth. Developmental Medicine and Child Neurology 28: 303–309

Lipscomb A P, Blackwell R J, Reynolds E O R, Thornburn R J, Cusick G, Pape K E 1979 Ultrasound scanning of the brain through the anterior fontanelle. Lancet ii: 39

Lipscomb A P, Thorburn R J, Reynolds E O R et al 1981 Pneumothorax and cerebral haemorrhage in preterm infants. Lancet i: 414–416

Liu L M P, Cote C J, Goudsouzian N G et al 1983 Life-threatening apnea in infants recovering from anesthesia. Anesthesiology 59: 506–510

Lubchenko L O, Searls D T, Brazie J V 1972 Neonatal mortality rate: relationship to birth weight and gestational age. Journal of Pediatrics 81: 814–822

Lucas A, Cole T J 1990 Breast milk and neonatal necrotising enterocolitis. Lancet 336: 1519–1523

Lucas A, Gore S M, Cole T J, Bamford M F, Dossetor J F, Barr I, Dicarlo L, Cork S, Lucas P J 1984 Multicentre trial on feeding low birthweight infants: effects of diet on early growth. Archives of Disease in Childhood 59: 722–730

Lucas A, Bloom S R, Aynsley-Green A 1986 Gut hormones and 'minimal enteral feeding'. Acta Paediatrica Scandinavica 75: 719–723

Lucas A, Rennie J M, Baker B A, Morley R 1988a Low plasma triiodothyronine concentrations and outcome in preterm infants. Archives of Disease in Childhood 63: 1201–1206

Lucas A, Morley R, Cole T J 1988b Adverse neurodevelopmental outcome of moderate neonatal hypoglycaemia. British Medical Journal 297: 1304–1308

Lucas A, Brooke O G, Baker B A, Bishop N, Morley R 1989 High alkaline phosphatase activity and growth in preterm neonates. Archives of Disease in Childhood 64: 902–909

Lucas A, Brooke O G, Morley R, Cole T J, Bamford M F 1990a Early diet of preterm infants and development of allergic or atopic disease: randomised prospective study. British Medical Journal 300: 837–840

Lucas A, Morley R, Cole T J, Gore S M, Lucas P J, Crowle P, Pearse R, Boon A J, Powell R 1990b Early diet in preterm babies and developmental status at 18 months. Lancet 335: 1477–1481

Lucas A, Bishop N J, King F J, Cole T J 1992a Randomised trial of nutrition for preterm infants after discharge. Archives of Disease in Childhood 67: 324–327

Lucas A, Morley R, Cole T J, Lister G, Leeson Payne C 1992b Breast milk and subsequent intelligence quotient in children born preterm. Lancet 339: 261–264

Lucas A, Morley R, Cole T J, Gore S M 1994 A randomised multicentre study of human milk versus formula and later development in preterm infants. Archives of Disease in Childhood 70: F141–F146

Lucey J F 1993 Parent dissatisfaction with neonatal intensive care unit care and suggestions for improvement. Pediatrics 92: 724

Lupton B, Halliday H L, Thomas P S, McClure G, Reid G, Reid M McC 1987 Chronic lung disease in a neonatal intensive care unit: 8 years experience. Irish Medical Journal 80: 254–257

Lundström K E, Pryds O, Greisen G 1995 Oxygen at birth and prolonged cerebral vasoconstriction in preterm infants. Archives of Disease in Childhood 73: F81–F86

Luttkus A, Fengler T W, Friedmann W, Dudenhausen J W 1995 Continuous monitoring of fetal oxygen saturation by pulse oximetry. Obstetrics and Gynecology 85: 183–186

Lyall H, Burchell A, Howie P W, Ogston S, Hume R l994 Early detection of metabolic abnormalities in preterm infants impaired by disorders of blood glucose concentration. Clinical Chemistry 40: 526–530

Lyon A J, McIntosh N, Wheeler K, Brooke O G 1984 Hypercalcaemia in extremely low birthweight infants. Archives of Disease in Childhood 59: 1141–1144

Lyon A J, McIntosh N, Wheeler K, Williams J E 1987 Radiological rickets in extremely low birth weight infants. Pediatric Radiology 17: 56–58

Lyon A J, Hawkes D J, Doran M, McIntosh N, Chan F 1989 Bone mineralisation in preterm infants measured by dual energy radiographic densitometry. Archives of Disease in Childhood 64: 919–923

McClean P, Weaver L T 1993 Ontogeny of human pancreatic exocrine function. Archives of Disease in Childhood 68: 62–65

McCord F B, Curstedt T, Halliday H L, McClure G, Reid M McC, Robertson B 1988 Surfactant treatment and incidence of intraventricular haemorrhage in severe respiratory distress syndrome. Archives of Disease in Childhood 63: 10–16

McCormick B 1988 Screening for hearing impairment in young children. Chapman & Hall, London

McCracken G H Jr, Nelson J D (eds) 1983 Antimicrobial therapy for newborns. Grune & Stratton, New York

McCue C M, Martakas M E, Tingelstad J B, Ruddy S 1977 Congenital heart block in newborns of mothers with connective tissue disease. Circulation 56: 82–90

McDonagh A F, Palmer L A, Lightner D A 1982 Phototherapy for neonatal jaundice. Journal of the American Chemical Society 104: 6867

MacDonald D, Grant A, Sheridan-Pereira M 1985 Dublin randomized controlled trial of intrapartum fetal heart rate monitoring. American Journal of Obstetrics and Gynecology 152: 524–539

McDonald J W, Silverstein F S, Cardona D, Hudson C, Chen R, Johnston M V 1990a Systemic administration of MK-801 protects against N-methyl-D-aspartate and quisqualate-mediated neurotoxicity in perinatal rats. Neuroscience 36: 589–599

McDonald J W, Silverstein F S, Johnson M V et al 1990b Magnesium reduces N-methyl-D-aspartate (Non DA)-mediated brain injury in perinatal rats. Neuroscience Letters 109: 234–238

Macfarlane P I, Heaf D P 1989 Pulmonary function in children after neonatal meconium aspiration syndrome. Archives of Disease in Childhood 63: 368–372

Machin G A 1980 Persistent renal blastoma (nephroblastometosis) as a frequent precursor to Wilms tumour: a patho physiological and clinical review. American Journal of Pediatric Haematology and Oncology 2: 353–362

McIntosh N 1984 Rickets of prematurity. Bone 1: 26–27

McIntosh N 1988 Dry lung syndrome after oligohydramnios. Archives of Disease in Childhood 63: 190–193

McIntosh N, Mitchell V 1990 A clinical trial of 2 parenteral nutrition solutions in neonates. Archives of Disease in Childhood 65: 612–699

McIntosh N, Walters R O 1979 Effect of tolazoline in severe hyaline membrane disease. Archives of Disease in Childhood 54: 105–110

McIntosh N, Rodeck C H, Heath R 1984 Plasma amino acids of the mid trimester human fetus. Biology of the Neonate 45: 218–224

McIntosh N, Kempson C, Tyler R M 1988 Blood counts in extremely low birthweight infants. Archives of Disease in Childhood 63: 74–76

McIntosh N, Prakesh P, Smith A 1990 Air leaks and vasopressin release. Archives of Disease in Childhood 65: 1259–1262

McLain B I, Evans J, Dear P R F 1989 Comparison of capillary and arterial blood gas measurements in neonates. Archives of Disease in Childhood 63: 743–747

Maclennan A H, Green R I, O'Shea R et al 1990 Routine hospital admission in twin pregnancy between 26 and 30 weeks gestation. Lancet i: 267–269

McMahon P, Jewes L, de Louvois J 1990 Routine lumbar punctures in the newborn – are they justified? European Journal of Pediatrics 149: 797–799

Madansky D L, Lawson E E, Chernick V, Taeusch H W 1979 Pneumothorax and other forms of pulmonary air leaks in the newborn. American Review of Respiratory Disease 120: 729–737

Mahan J D, Mauer S M, Sibley R K, Vernier R L 1984 Congenital nephrotic syndrome: evolution of medical management and results of renal transplantation. Journal of Pediatrics 105: 549–557

Mahony L, Carnero V, Brett C, Heymann M A, Clyman R I 1982 Prophylactic indomethacin therapy for patent ductus arteriosus in very low birth weight infants. New England Journal of Medicine 306: 506–510

Maier R F, Obladen M, Scigalla P et al 1994 The effect of epoetin beta (recombinant human erythropoietin) on the need for transfusion in very low birth weight infants. New England Journal of Medicine 330(17): 1227–1228

Malcolm G, Ellwood D, Devonald K, Beilby R, Henderson-Smart D 1991 Absent or reversed end diastolic flow velocity in the umbilical artery and necrotising enterocolitis. Archives of Disease in Childhood 66: 805–807

Mann K G 1984 Membrane-bound enzyme complexes in blood coagulation. In: Spaet T H (ed) Progress in haemostasis and thrombosis. Grune & Stratton, New York, pp 1–23

Mann N P, Haddow R, Stokes L et al 1986 Effect of night and day on preterm infants in a newborn nursery: randomised trial. British Medical Journal 293: 1265–1267

Mannens M, Hoovers J M, Redeker E, Verjaal M, Feinberg A P, Little P, Boavida M, Coad N, Steenman M, Bliek J et al 1994 Parental imprinting of human chromosome region 11p15.3-pter involved in the Beckwith–Wiedemann syndrome and various human neoplasia. European Journal of Human Genetics 2: 3–23

Manning F A, Morrison E, Harman C R et al 1987 Fetal assessment based on fetal biophysical profile scoring: experience in 19,221 referred high risk pregnancies II an analysis of false negative fetal deaths. American Journal of Obstetrics and Gynecology 157: 880–884

Marret S, Gressens P, Gadisseux J-F, Evrard P 1995 Prevention by magnesium of excitotoxic neuronal death in the developing brain: an animal model for clinical intervention studies. Developmental Medicine and Child Neurology 37: 473–484

Martin E, Barkovich A J 1995 Magnetic resonance imaging in perinatal asphyxia. Archives of Disease in Childhood 72: F62–F67

Mason J, Drummond M, Torrance G 1993 Some guidelines on the use of cost effectiveness league tables. British Medical Journal 306: 570–572

Maternity Services Advisory Committee 1985 Maternity care in action – third report – care of the mother and baby (postnatal and neonatal care). HMSO, London

Mayne A J, Brown G A, Sule D, McNeish A S 1986 Postnatal maturation of disaccharidase activities in jejunal fluid of preterm neonates. Gut 27: 1357–1361

Mehta A, Wright B M, Callan K, Stacey T E 1986 Patient-triggered ventilation in the newborn. Lancet 1: 17–19

Ment L R, Oh W, Ehrenkranz R A, Philip A G S, Vohr B, Allan W, Duncan C C, Scott D T, Taylor K J W, Katz K H, Schneider K C, Makuch R W 1994 Low dose indomethacin therapy and prevention of intraventricular hemorrhage: a multicenter randomized trial. Pediatrics 93: 543–550

Meredith K S, DeLemos R A, Coalson J J et al 1989 Role of lung injury in the pathogenesis of hyaline membrane disease in premature baboons. Journal of Applied Physiology 66: 2150–2158

Merkatz I R, Peter J B, Barderr T P 1980 Ritodrine hydrochloride. A beta mimetic agent for use in preterm labour 1. Evidence of efficacy. Obstetrics and Gynecology 56: 7–12

Metcalf R, Dilena B, Gibson R, Marshall P, Simmer K 1994 How appropriate are commercially available human milk fortifiers? Journal of Paediatrics and Child Health 30, 350–355

Meyer E C, Coll C T G, Lester B M, Boukydis C F Z, McDonough S M, Oh W 1994 Family-based intervention improves maternal psychological well-being and feeding interaction of preterm infants. Pediatrics 93: 241–246

Miall-Allen V, de Vries L M S, Whitelaw A G L 1987 Mean arterial blood pressure and neonatal cerebral lesions. Archives of Disease in Childhood 62: 1068–1069

Mifsud A, Seal D, Wall R, Valman B 1988 Reduced neonatal mortality from infection after introduction of respiratory monitoring. British Medical Journal 296: 17–18

Millard D D, Shulman S T 1988 The changing spectrum of neonatal endocarditis. Clinics in Perinatology 15: 587–608

Miller M E 1969 Phagocytosis in the newborn infant: humoral and cellular factors. Journal of Pediatrics 74: 255–262

Miller O I, Celermajer D S, Deanfield J E, Macrae D J 1994 Guidelines for the safe administration of inhaled nitric oxide. Archives of Disease in Childhood 70: F47–F49

Milligan J E, Shennan A T, Hoskins E M 1984 Perinatal intensive care: where and how to draw the line. American Journal of Obstetrics and Gynecology 148: 499–503

Milner A D, Fox G 1995 Congenital abnormalities of the respiratory system. In: Yu V Y H (ed) Pulmonary problems in the perinatal period and their sequelae. Baillière Tindall, London

Milner A D, Boon A W, Saunders R A, Hopkin I E 1980 Upper airways obstruction and apnoea in preterm babies. Archives of Disease in Childhood 55: 22–25

Mitton S G, Burston D, Brueton M J 1988 Hyperphenylalaninaemia in parenterally fed newborn infants. Lancet ii 1497–1498

Modi N 1988 Development of renal function. British Medical Bulletin 44: 936–956

Mok J Y Q, McLaughlin F J, Pintar M, Hak H, Amaro-Galvez R, Levison H 1986 Transcutaneous monitoring of oxygenation: what is normal? Journal of Pediatrics 108: 365–371

Mok J Y Q, Hak H, McLaughlin F J, Pintar M, Canny G J, Levison H 1988 Effect of age and state of wakefulness on transcutaneous oxygen values in preterm infants: a longitudinal study. Journal of Pediatrics 113: 706–709

Moncada S, Gryglewski R, Bunting S, Vane J R 1976 An enzyme isolated from arteries transforms prostaglandin endoperoxides to an unstable substance that inhibits platelet aggregation. Nature 263: 663–665

Moniz C F, Nicolaides K H, Bamforth F J, Rodeck C H 1985 Normal reference ranges for biochemical substances relating to renal, hepatic and bone function in fetal and maternal plasma throughout pregnancy. Journal of Clinical Pathology 38: 468

Monnens L, Heymans H 1987 Peroxisomal disorders: clinical characterization. Journal of Inherited Metabolic Disease 10: 23–32

Morales W J, Schorr S, Albritton J 1994 Effect of metronidazole in patients with preterm birth in preceding pregnancy and bacterial vaginosis: a placebo controlled, double-blind study. American Journal of Obstetrics and Gynecology 171, 345–349

Morley R, Brooke O G, Cole T J, Powell R, Lucas A 1990 Birthweight ratio and outcome in preterm infants. Archives of Disease in Childhood 65: 30–34

MRC Vitamin Study Research Group 1991 Prevention of neural tube defects; results of the Medical Research Council Vitamin Study. Lancet 338: 131–137

MRC/RCOG Working Party on Cervical Cerclage 1993 Final report of the Medical Research Council/Royal College of Obstetricians and Gynaecologists Multicentre Randomized Trial of Cervical Cerclage. British Journal of Obstetrics and Gynaecology 100: 516–523

Mueller-Eckhardt C, Kiefel V, Grubert A et al 1989 348 cases of suspected neonatal alloimmune thrombocytopenia. Lancet i: 363–366

Mugford M 1995 The cost of neonatal care. Reviewing the evidence. Social and Preventive Medicine (Berne) 40: 361–368

Mujsce D J, Stern D R, Vannucci R C, Towfighi J, Hershey P A 1988 Mannitol therapy in perinatal hypoxic–ischemic brain injury. Annals of Neurology 24: 338

Muller D P R, Milla P J 1988 Selective inborn errors of absorption. In: Milla P J, Muller D P R (eds) Harries paediatric gastroenterology, 2nd edn. Churchill Livingstone, Edinburgh, ch 9, pp 211–238

Murdock N, Crighton A, Nelson L M, Forsyth J S 1995 Low birthweight infants and total parenteral nutrition immediately after birth. II. Randomised study of biochemical tolerance of intravenous glucose, amino acids, and lipid. Archives of Disease in Childhood 73: F8–F12

Murdoch D R, Darlow B A 1984 Handling during neonatal intensive care. Archives of Disease in Childhood 59: 957–961

Murphy D J, Hope P L, Johnson M A 1996 Archives of Disease in Childhood (in press)

Mustafa M M, Mertsola J, Ramilo O et al 1989 Increased endotoxin and interleukin 1b concentrations in CSF of infants with coliform meningitis and ventriculitis associated with intraventricular gentamicin therapy. Journal of Infectious Diseases 144: 302–311

Mutch L M M, Johnson M A, Morley R 1989 Follow up studies: design, organisation and analysis. Archives of Disease in Childhood 64: 1139–1402

Myers R E 1972 Two patterns of perinatal brain damage and their conditions of occurrence. American Journal of Obstetrics and Gynecology 112: 246–276

Naeye R L, Peters E C 1978 Amniotic fluid infections with intact membranes leading to perinatal death: a prospective study. Pediatrics 61: 171–177

Nelson K B, Ellenberg J H 1981 Apgar scores as predictors of chronic neurological disability. Pediatrics 68: 36–44

Nelson K B, Ellenberg J H 1984 Obstetric complications as risk factors for cerebral palsy or seizure disorders. Journal of the American Medical Association 251: 1843–1848

Newell S J 1995 Vitamin K and haemorrhagic disease of the newborn: now the dust has settled. Clinical Nutrition 4: 7–11

Newell S J 1996 Gastrointestinal function and its ontogeny: how should we feed the preterm infant. In: Ryan S (ed) Seminars in neonatology. W B Saunders, London

Newell S J, Sarkar P K, Durbin G M, Booth I W, McNeish A S 1986 Maturation of the lower oesophageal sphincter in the preterm baby. Gut 29: 167–172

Newell S J, Booth I W, Morgan M E, Durbin G M, McNeish A S 1989a Gastro-oesophageal reflux in preterm infants. Archives of Disease in Childhood 64: 780–786

Newell S J, Morgan M E, Durbin G M, Booth I W, McNeish A S 1989b Does mechanical ventilation precipitate gastro-oesophageal reflux during enteral feeding? Archives of Disease in Childhood 64: 1352–1355

Ng P C 1993 The effectiveness and side effects of dexamethasone in preterm infants with bronchopulmonary dysplasia. Archives of Disease in Childhood 68: 330–336

Ng P C, Dear P R F 1990 The predictive value of a normal ultrasound scan in the preterm baby – a meta-analysis. Acta Paediatrica Scandinavica 79: 286–291

Ng P C, Dear P R F, Thomas D F M 1988 Oral vancomycin in prevention of necrotising enterocolitis. Archives of Disease in Childhood 63: 1390–1393

Nicolaides K H, Berry S, Snijders R J M, Thorpe-Beeston J G, Gosden C 1990 Fetal lateral cerebral ventriculomegaly: associated malformations and chromosomal defects. Fetal Diagnostic Therapy 5: 5–14

Nishida H 1993 Outcome of infants born preterm, with special emphasis on extremely low birthweight infants. Baillière's Clinical Obstetrics and Gynaecology 7: 611–631

Northway W H, Rosan R C, Porter D Y 1967 Pulmonary disease following respirator therapy of hyaline membrane disease. Bronchopulmonary dysplasia. New England Journal of Medicine 276: 357–368

Nwaesi C G, Young D C, Byrne J M, Vincer M J, Sampson D, Evans J R, Allen A C, Stinson D A 1987 Preterm birth at 23 to 26 weeks' gestation: is active obstetric management justified? American Journal of Obstetrics and Gynecology 157: 890–897

Obladen M, Sachsenweger M, Stahnke M 1988 Blood sampling in very low birth weight infants receiving different levels of intensive care. European Journal of Pediatrics 147: 399–404

O'Driscoll K, Meagher D 1986 Active management of labour, 2nd edn. Henry Ling, Dorchester, pp 92–93

Ogata E S, Gregory G A, Kitterman J A, Phibbs R H, Tooley W H 1975 Pneumothorax in the respiratory distress syndrome: incidence and effect on vital signs, blood gases and pH. Pediatrics 58: 177–183

O'Hagan M, Reid E, Tarnow-Mordi W O 1991 Is neonatal inspired gas humidity accurately controlled by humidifier temperature? Critical Care Medicine 19: 1370–1373

Olsen P, Myrman A, Rantakallio P 1994 Educational capacity of low birthweight children up to the age of 24. Early Human Development. 36: 191–203

O'Rourke P P, Crone R K, Vacanti J P, Ware J H, Lillehei C W, Parad R B, Epstein M F 1989 Extracorporeal membrane oxygenation and conventional medical therapy in neonates with persistent pulmonary hypertension of the newborn: A prospective randomised study. Pediatrics 84: 957–963

Oski F A, Naiman J L 1982 Hematologic problems in the newborn, 3rd edn. W B Saunders, New York

Owen P, Donnet M L, Ogston S A, Christie S A, Howie P W, Patel N B 1995 Standards for ultrasound fetal growth velocity. British Journal of Obstetrics and Gynaecology 103: 60–69

Oxford Region Controlled Trial of Artificial Ventilation (OCTAVE) Study Group 1991 A multicentre randomised controlled trial of high against low frequency positive pressure ventilation. Archives of Disease in Childhood 66: 770–775

Palme-Kilander C 1992 Methods of resuscitation in low-Apgar-score newborn infants – a national survey. Acta Paediatrica Scandinavica 81: 739–744

Palmer C, Vannucci R C, Towfighi J 1990 Reduction of perinatal hypoxic–ischemic brain damage with allopurinol. Pediatric Research 27: 332–336

Palmer C, Towfighi J, Roberts R L, Heitjan D F 1993 Allopurinol administered after inducing hypoxia–ischemia reduces brain injury in 7-day-old rats. Pediatric Research 33: 405–411

Pandit P B, Dunn M S, Colucci E A 1995a Surfactant therapy in neonates with respiratory deterioration due to pulmonary hemorrhage. Pediatrics 95: 32–36

Pandit P B, Dunn M S, Kelly E N, Pearlman M 1995b Surfactant replacement in neonates with early chronic lung disease. Pediatrics 95: 851–854

Paneth N, Rudelli R, Kazam E, Monte W 1994 Brain damage in the preterm infant. Clinics in Developmental Medicine No 131. MacKeith Press, London, pp 119–137

Papiernik E, Bouyer J, Dreyfus J et al 1985 Prevention of preterm births; a perinatal study in Maguenall, France. Pediatrics 76: 154–158

Papile L, Burstein J, Burstein R, Koffler H 1978 Incidence and evolution of subependymal and intraventricular haemorrhage: a study of infants of birth weight less than 1500 g. Journal of Pediatrics 92: 529–534

Paryani S G, Arvin A M 1986 Intrauterine infection with varicella zoster virus after maternal varicella. New England Journal of Medicine 314: 1542–1546

Parker J C, Hernandez L A, Peevy K J 1993 Mechanisms of ventilator-induced lung injury. Critical Care Medicine 21: 131–143

Pascual J F, Lopez J D, Molina M 1987 Hemofiltration in children with renal failure. Pediatric Clinics of North America 34: 803–818

Patel J, Marks K A, Roberts I, Azzopardi D, Edwards A D 1995 Ibuprofen treatment of patent ductus arteriosus. Lancet 346: 255

Patz A 1980 Retrolental fibroplasia (retinopathy of prematurity). Transactions of Ophthalmology Society New Zealand 32: 49–54

Pearce J M, Campbell S 1987 A comparison of symphysis–fundal height and ultrasound as screening tests for light-for-gestational age infants. British Journal of Obstetrics and Gynaecology 94: 100–104

Peckham C S, Logan G S 1989 Cytomegalovirus infection in pregnancy. In: Cosmi E V, Renzo G C (eds) Proceedings of XI European Congress of Perinatal Medicine. Harwood Academic Publishers, London, pp 255–260

Peckham C S, Johnson C, Aden A, Pearl K, Chin K S 1987 The early acquisition of cytomegalovirus infection. Archives of Disease in Childhood 62: 708–785

Peliowski A, Finer N N 1992 Birth asphyxia in the term infant. In: Sinclair J C, Bracken M B (eds) Effective care of the newborn infant. Oxford University Press, Oxford, pp 249–279

Perlman J M, Tack E D 1988 Renal injury in the asphyxiated newborn infant: relationship to neurological outcome. Journal of Pediatrics 113: 875–879

Perlman J M, Tack E D, Martin T, Shackelford G, Amon E 1989 Acute systemic organ injury in term infants after asphyxia. American Journal of Diseases of Children 143: 617–620

Pharoah P O D, Cooke T, Cooke R W I, Rosenbloom L 1987 Trends in birth prevalence of cerebral palsy. Archives of Disease in Childhood 65: 379–384

Pharoah P O D, Cooke T, Cooke R W I, Rosenbloom L 1990 Birthweight specific trends in cerebral palsy. Archives of Disease in Childhood 65: 602–606

Pharoah P O D, Stevenson C J, Cooke R W I, Stevenson R C 1994 Prevalence of behaviour disorders in low birthweight infants. Archives of Disease in Childhood 70: 271–274

Philip A G S 1995 Neonatal mortality rate: is further improvement still possible? Journal of Pediatrics 126: 427–433

Phillips H M, Holland B M, Abdel-Moiz A et al 1986 Determination of red cell mass in the assessment and management of anaemia in babies needing blood transfusion. Lancet 1: 882–884

Pidcock F S, Graziani L J, Stanley C, Mitchell D G, Merton D 1990 Neurosonographic features of periventricular echodensities associated with cerebral palsy in preterm infants. Journal of Pediatrics 116: 417–422

Pike M G, Holmstrom G, de Vries L S, Pennock J M, Drew K J, Sonksen P M, Dubowitz L M S 1994 Patterns of visual impairment associated with lesions of the preterm infant brain. Developmental Medicine and Child Neurology 36: 849–862

Pinto-Martin J A, Riolo S, Cnaan A, Holzman C, Susser M, Paneth N 1995 Cranial ultrasound prediction of disabling and nondisabling cerebral palsy at age two in a low birthweight population. Pediatrics 95: 249–254

Plenat F, Vert P, Didier F, Andre M 1978 Pulmonary interstitial emphysema. Clinics in Perinatology 5: 351–375

Polin R A, St Gene J W III 1992 Neonatal sepsis. Advances in Paediatric Infectious Diseases 7: 25–34

Porter H J, Keeling J W 1987 Value of perinatal necropsy examination. Journal of Clinical Pathology 40: 180–184

Pourcyrous M, Leffler C W, Bada H S, Korones S B, Busija D W 1993 Brain superoxide anion generation in asphyxiated piglets and the effect of indomethacin at therapeutic dose. Pediatric Research 34: 366–369

Powell T G, Pharoah P O D, Cooke R W I 1988a Cerebral palsy in very low birthweight infants 1. Hemiplegia associated with intrapartum stress. Developmental Medicine and Child Neurology 30: 11–18

Powell T G, Pharoah P O D, Cooke R W I 1988b Cerebral palsy in very low birthweight infants II. Spastic diplegia associated with immaturity. Developmental Medicine and Child Neurology 30: 19–25

Prechtl H F R 1977 The neurological examination of the full term newborn infant, 2nd edn. Clinics in Developmental Medicine, No 63. SIMP/Heinemann, London

Prechtl H R F 1985 Ultrasound examination of human fetal behaviour. Early Human Development 12: 91–98

Prechtl H F R 1990 Qualitative changes of spontaneous movements in fetus and preterm infant as a marker of neurological dysfunction. Early Human Development 23: 151–158

Prechtl H F R, Bientema D 1964 The neurological examination of the full term newborn infant. Clinics in Developmental Medicine, No 12. SIMP/Heinemann, London

Prendiville A, Schulenberg W E 1988 Clinical factors associated with retinopathy of prematurity. Archives of Disease in Childhood 63: 522–527

Prendiville A, Thomson A, Silverman M 1986 Effect of tracheobronchial suction on respiratory resistance in intubated preterm babies. Archives of Disease in Childhood 61: 1178–1183

Procianoy R S, Giacomini C B, Oliveira M L 1988 Fetal and neonatal cortical adrenal function in birth asphyxia. Acta Paediatrica Scandinavica 77: 671–674

Puntis J W L, Edwards M A, Green A et al 1986 Hyperphenylalaninaemia in parenterally fed newborn babies. Lancet ii: 1105–1106

Quintero R A, Reich H, Puder K S et al 1994 Brief report: umbilical-cord ligation of an acardiac twin by fetoscopy at 19 weeks of gestation. New England Journal of Medicine 330: 469

Rai R, Clifford K, Regal L 1996 The modern preventative treatment of recurrent miscarriage. British Journal of Obstetrics and Gynaecology 103: 106–110

Raju T N K, Langenberg P 1993 Pulmonary hemorrhage and exogenous surfactant therapy: a metaanalysis. Journal of Pediatrics 123: 603–610

Ramji S, Ahuja S, Thirupuram S, Rootwelt T, Rooth G, Saugstad O D 1993 Resuscitation of asphyxic newborn infants with room air or 100% oxygen. Pediatric Research 34: 809–812

Ramsden C A, Reynolds E O R, Morley C J, Smith M, Milner A D 1987 Ventilator settings for newborn infants. Archives of Disease in Childhood 62: 529–538

Ransley P G, Risdon R A 1978 Reflux and renal scarring. British Journal of Radiology 14 (suppl): 1–35

Rascher W, Seyberth H W 1987 Atrial natriuretic peptide and patent ductus arteriosus in preterm infants. Archives of Disease in Childhood 62: 1165–1167

Ratner I, Perelmuter B, Toews W, Whitfield J 1985 Association of low systolic and diastolic blood pressure with significant patent ductus arteriosus in the very low birth weight infant. Critical Care Medicine 13: 497–500

Rees L, Shaw J C L, Brook C G D, Forsling M L 1984 Hyponatraemia in the first week of life in preterm infants. Part II. Sodium and water balance. Archives of Disease in Childhood 59: 423–429

Rennie J M 1995 Bacterial and fungal infections. In: Levene M I, Lilford R J (eds) Fetal and neonatal neurology and neurosurgery. Churchill Livingstone, Edinburgh, pp 473–499

Rennie J M 1996a Perinatal management at the margins of viability. Archives of Disease in Childhood 74: F214–F218

Rennie J M 1996b Neonatal cerebral ultrasound. Cambridge University Press, Cambridge

Rennie J M, Cooke R W I 1991 Prolonged low dose indomethacin for persistent ductus arteriosus of prematurity. Archives of Disease in Childhood 66: 55–58

Rennie J M, South M, Morley C J 1987 Cerebral blood flow velocity variability in infants receiving assisted ventilation. Archives of Disease in Childhood 62: 1247–1251

Rennie J M, Wheater M, Cole T J 1996 Antenatal steroid administration is associated with an improved chance of intact survival in preterm infants. European Journal of Pediatrics 155: 576–579

Rettwitz-Volk W, Scholosser R, Von Loewenich V 1993 One sided high frequency oscillatory ventilation in the treatment of neonatal unilateral pulmonary emphysema. Acta Paediatrica 82: 190–192

Reynolds E O R, Taghizadeh A 1974 Improved prognosis of infants mechanically ventilated for hyaline membrane disease. Archives of Disease in Childhood 49: 505–515

Rhoden N K 1986 Treating Baby Doe: the ethics of uncertainty. Hastings Center Report 16(4): 34–42

Rhodes P G, Graves G R, Patel D M, Campbell S B, Blumenthal B I 1983 Minimizing pneumothorax and bronchopulmonary dysplasia in ventilated infants with hyaline membrane disease. Journal of Pediatrics 103: 634–637

Riegel K, Ohrt B, Wolke D, Österlund K 1995 Die Entwicklung gefährdet geborener Kinder bis zum fünften Lebensjahr: die ARVO-YLLPÖ Neugeborenen – nachfolge Studie in Südbayern und Südfinnland. Enke Verlag, Stuttgart

Riesenfeld T, Hammerlund K, Sedin G 1987 Respiratory water loss in fullterm infants on their first day after birth. Acta Paediatrica Scandinavica 76: 647–653

Rietschel E T, Brade H 1992 Bacterial endotoxins. Scientific American 267(2): 54–61

Rigo J, Senterre J, Putet G, Salle B 1987 A new amino acid solution specially adapted to preterm infants. Clinical Nutrition 6: 105–109

Risdon R A 1987 The small scarred kidney of childhood: a congenital or an acquired lesion? Pediatric Nephrology 1: 632–637

Rivers R P A, Hathaway W E, Weston W L 1975 The endotoxin induced coagulant activity of human monocytes. British Journal of Haematology 30: 311–313

Roberton N R C (ed) 1986 Textbook of neonatology. Churchill Livingstone, Edinburgh

Roberts D S, Haycock G B, Dalton R N et al 1990 Prediction of acute renal failure after birth asphyxia. Archives of Disease in Childhood 65: 1021–1028

Roberts J A, Kaack M B, Morvant A B 1988 Vesico-ureteric reflux in the primate. IV. Infection as cause of prolonged high grade reflux. Pediatrics 82: 91–95

Roberts J D, Polaner D M, Lang P, Zapol W M 1992 Inhaled nitric oxide in persistent pulmonary hypertension of the newborn. Lancet 340: 818–819

Roberts R L, Szelc C M, Scates S M et al 1991 Neutropenia in an extremely premature infant treated with recombinant human granulocyte colony-stimulating factor. American Journal of Diseases in Childhood 145: 808–812

Robertson C M T, Etches P C, Kyle J M 1990 Eight year school performance and growth of preterm small for gestational age infants: a comparative study with subjects matched for birthweight or gestational age. Journal of Pediatrics 116: 19–26

Robertson C M T, Hrynchyshyn G J, Etches P C, Pain K S 1992 Population-based study of the incidence, complexity and severity of neuropathologic disability among survivors weighing 500g through 1250g at birth: a comparison of two birth cohorts. Pediatrics 90: 750–755

Robertson C M T, Sauve R S, Christianson H E 1994 Province based study of neurologic disability among survivors weighing 500g through 1240g at birth. Pediatrics 93: 636–640

Robertson C, Aldridge S, Jarman F, Saunders K, Poulakis Z, Oberklaid F 1995 Late diagnosis of congenital sensorineural hearing impairment: why are detection methods failing? Archives of Disease in Childhood 72: 11–15

Rochefort M J, Rolfe P, Wilkinson A R 1987 New fontanometer for continuous estimation of intracranial pressure in the newborn. Archives of Disease in Childhood 62: 152–155

Rodwell R L, Taylor K M, Tudehope D I 1995 Haematological scoring system in early diagnosis of sepsis in neutropenic newborns. Paediatric Infectious Diseases Journal 12: 372–376

Roe C R, Coates P M 1995 Mitochondrial fatty acid oxidation disorders. In: Scriver C R, Beaudet A L, Sly W S, Valle D (eds) The metabolic bases of inherited disease, 7th edn. McGraw Hill, New York, ch 45, pp 1501–1533

Rolleston G L, Shannon F T, Utley W L F 1970 Relationship of infantile vesico-ureteral reflux to renal damage. British Medical Journal 1: 460–465

Rosenberg A A 1992 Response of the cerebral circulation to hypocarbia in postasphyxial newborn lambs. Pediatric Research 32: 537–541

Roy R N, Pollnitz R P, Hamilton J R 1977 Impaired assimilation of nasojejunal feeds in healthy low birth weight newborn infants. Journal of Pediatrics 90: 431–434

Royal College of Ophthalmologists and British Association of Perinatal Medicine Joint Working Party 1995 Retinopathy of prematurity: guidelines for screening and treatment. BPA, London

Royal College of Physicians of London 1988 Medical care of the newborn in England and Wales. Royal College of Physicians, London

Ruth V J 1989 Prognostic value of creatine kinase BB-isoenzyme in high risk newborn infants. Archives of Disease in Childhood 64: 563–568

Ruth V, Autti-Ramo I, Granstrom M-L, Korkman M, Raivio K O 1988 Prediction of perinatal brain damage by cord plasma vasopressin, erythropoietin, and hypoxanthine values. Journal of Pediatrics 113: 880–885

Rutter N 1986 Temperature control and its disorders. In: Roberton N R C (ed) Textbook of neonatology, 1st edn. Churchill Livingstone, London, pp 148–161

Ruys J H, Verloove-Vanhorick S P, Den Ouden A L 1989 The viability of the preterm infant. European Journal of Obstetrics and Gynaecology and Reproductive Biology 33: 31–37

Ryan S, Congdon P J, Horsman A, James J R, Truscott J, Arthur R 1987 Bone mineral content in bronchopulmonary dysplasia. Archives of Disease in Childhood 62: 889–894

Saigal S, Rosenbaum P, Hattersley B, Milner R 1989 Decreased disability rate among 3 year old survivors weighing 501 to 1000 grams at birth and born to residents of a geographically defined region from 1981 to 1984 compared with 1977 to 1980. Journal of Pediatrics 111: 836–839

Saigal S, Szatman P, Rosenbaum P, Campbell D, King S 1990 Intellectual and functional status at school entry of children who weighed 1000g or less at birth: a regional perspective of births in the 1980's. Journal of Pediatrics 116: 409–416

Saigal S, Szatman P, Rosenbaum P, Campbell D, King S 1991 Cognitive abilities and school performance of ELBW children and matched term control children at eight years: a regional study. Journal of Pediatrics 118: 751–760

Saint-Anne Dargassies S 1977 Neurological development in full term and premature neonates. Elsevier/North Holland/Exerpta Medica, Amsterdam

St Gene J W III, Harris M C 1991 Coagulase-negative staphylococcal infection in the neonate. Clinical Perinatology 18: 281

Salmon A P, Keeton B R, Sethia B 1993 Developments in interventional catheterisation and progress in surgery for congenital heart disease: achieving a balance. British Heart Journal 69: 479–480

Samuels M P, Southall D P 1989 Negative extra-thoracic pressure in the treatment of respiratory failure in infants and young children. British Medical Journal 299: 1253–1257

Sanders R J, Cox C, Phelps D L, Sinkin R A 1994 Two doses of early intravenous dexamethasone for the prevention of bronchopulmonary dysplasia in babies with respiratory distress syndrome. Pediatric Research 36: 122–128

SANDS 1986 After stillbirth and neonatal death: what happens next. Stillbirth and Neonatal Death Society, London

Sarff L D, Platt L H, McCracken G H Jr 1976 Cerebrospinal fluid evaluation in neonates; comparison of high risk infants with and without meningitis. Journal of Pediatrics 99: 873–879

Sarman I, Tunell R 1989 Providing warmth for preterm babies by a heated, water filled mattress. Archives of Disease in Childhood 64: 29–33

Sarman I, Can G, Tunell R 1989 Rewarming preterm infants on a heated, water filled mattress. Archives of Disease in Childhood 64: 687–692

Sarnat H B, Sarnat M S 1976 Neonatal encephalopathy following fetal distress. Archives of Neurology 33: 696–705

Sasanow S R, Georgieff M K, Pereira G R 1986 Mid-arm circumference and mid-arm/head circumference ratio: standard curves for anthropometric assessment of neonatal nutritional status. Journal of Pediatrics 109: 311–315

Saudubray J-M, Charpentier 1995 Clinical phenotypes: diagnosis/algorithms. In: Scriver C R, Beaudet A L, Sly W S, Valle D (eds) The metabolic bases of inherited disease, 7th edn. McGraw Hill, New York, ch 5, pp 327–400

Sauer P J J, Dane H J, Visser H K 1984 New standards for neutral thermal environment of healthy very low birthweight infants in week one of life. Archives of Disease in Childhood 59: 18–22

Scanlon J E M, Chin K C, Morgan M E I et al 1992 Caffeine or theophylline for neonatal apnoea? Archives of Disease in Childhood 67: 425–428

Scanlon P E, Bamford J M 1990 Early identification of hearing loss: screening and surveillance methods. Archives of Disease in Childhood 65: 479–485

Scheifele D W 1990 Role of bacterial toxins in neonatal necrotising enterocolitis. Journal of Pediatrics 117: 544–551

Scher M S, Dobson V, Carpenter N A, Guthrie R D 1989 Visual and neurological outcome of infants with periventricular leukomalacia. Developmental Medicine and Child Neurology 31: 353–365

Scher M S, Aso K, Beggarly M E 1993 Electrographic seizures in preterm and full term neonates: clinical correlates, associated brain lesions and risk for neurologic sequelae. Pediatrics 91: 128–134

Schmidt R 1978 Bilirubin metabolism: the state of the art. Gastroenterology 74: 1307–1312

Schmitz J 1991 Digestive and absorptive function. In: Walker W A, Durie P R, Hamilton J R, Walker-Smith J A, Watkins J B (eds) Pediatric gastrointestinal disease. B C Decker, Philadelphia, pp 266–280

Schreiber M D, Heymann M A, Soifer S J 1986 Increased arterial pH, not decreased $pACO_2$, attenuates hypoxia-induced pulmonary vasoconstriction in newborn lambs. Pediatric Research 20: 113–117

Schulze A, Schaller P, Hehre D, Devia C, Nagoshi R, Suguihara C, Gerhardt T, Bancalari E 1995 Hemodynamic effects of proportional assist ventilation (PAV) in piglets before and after meconium instillation. Pediatric Research 38: 454

Schumacher R E 1993 Extracorporeal membrane oxygenation, will this therapy continue to be as efficacious in the future? Pediatric Clinics of North America 40: 1005–1022

Schwartz G J, Brion L P, Spitzer A 1987 The use of plasma creatinine concentration for estimating the glomerular filtration rate in infants, children and adolescents. Pediatric Clinics of North America 34: 571–590

Schwarz T F, Roggendrof M, Hottentrager B et al 1990 Immunoglobulins in the prophylaxis of parvovirus B19 infection. Journal of Infectious Diseases 162: 1214–1216

Schwersenki J, McIntyre L, Bauer C R 1991 Lumbar puncture frequency and CSF analysis in the neonate. American Journal of Diseases of Childhood 145: 54–60

Scottish Low Birthweight Study Group 1992a The Scottish Low Birthweight Study: I Survival, growth, neuromotor and sensory impairment. Archives of Disease in Childhood 67: 675–681

Scottish Low Birthweight Study Group 1992b The Scottish Low Birthweight Study: II. Language attainment, cognitive status and behavioural problems. Archives of Disease in Childhood 67: 682–686

Scottish Neonatal Consultants Collaborative Study Group and International Neonatal Network 1996 Trends and variations in use of antenatal corticosteroids to prevent neonatal respiratory distress syndrome: recommendations for national and international comparative audit. British Journal of Obstetrics and Gynaecology 103: 534–540

Seltzer E S, Ahmed F, Goldberg R N et al 1984 Exchange transfusion using washed red blood cells reconstituted with fresh frozen plasma for treatment of severe hyperkalaemia in the neonate. Journal of Pediatrics 104: 443–446

Shaffer T H, Tran N, Bhutani V K et al 1983 Cardiopulmonary function in very preterm lambs during liquid ventilation. Pediatric Research 17: 680–683

Shannon K M, Keith J F 3rd, Mentzer W C et al 1995 Recombinant human erythropoietin stimulates erythropoiesis and reduces erythrocyte transfusions in very low birth weight infants. Paediatrics 95(1): 9–10

Shannon K M, Naylor G S, Torkildson J C et al 1987 Circulating erythroid progenitors in the anemia of prematurity. New England Journal of Medicine 317: 728–729

Shaw J C L 1973 Parenteral nutrition in the management of sick low birth weight infants. Pediatric Clinics of North America 20: 333–358

Shaw J C L 1988 Growth and nutrition of the very preterm infant. In: Whitelaw A, Cooke R W I (eds) The very immature infant less than 28 weeks gestation. British Medical Bulletin 44(4): 984–1009, Churchill Livingstone, London

Shaw N J, Wilson N, Dickinson D F 1988 Captopril in heart failure secondary to left to right shunt. Archives of Disease in Childhood 63: 360–363

Shaw N J, Cooke R W I, Gill A B, Shaw N J, Saeed M 1993 Randomised trial of routine versus selective paralysis during ventilation for neonatal respiratory distress syndrome. Archives of Disease in Childhood 69: 479–482

Sheldon C A, Duckett J W 1987 Hypospadias. Pediatric Clinics of North America 34: 1259–1272

Sheldon R A, Partridge J C, Ferriero D M 1992 Postischemic hyperglycemia is not protective to the neonatal rat brain. Pediatric Research 32: 489–493

Shen E Y, Huang C C, Chyou S C, Hung H Y, Hsu C H, Huang F Y 1986 Sonographic findings of the bright thalamus. Archives of Disease in Childhood 61: 1096–1099

Shennan A T, Dunn M S, Ohlsson A, Lennox K, Hoskins E M 1988 Abnormal pulmonary outcomes in premature infants: prediction from oxygen requirements in the neonatal period. Pediatrics 82: 527–532

Short Report 1980 Perinatal and neonatal mortality. 2nd Report for the Social Services Committee. HMSO, London

Shortland D, Trounce J C Q, Levene M I 1987 Hyperkalaemia, cardiac arrhythmias and cerebral lesions in high risk neonates. Archives of Disease in Childhood 62: 1139–1143

Shortland D, Levene M I, Trounce J Q, Ng Y, Graham M 1988 The evolution and outcome of cavitating periventricular leukomalacia in infancy. A study of 46 cases. Journal of Perinatal Medicine 16: 241–247

Sidiropoulos D 1986 Immunoglobulin therapy in preterm neonates with perinatal infections: transplacental passage of IVIg. In: Morrell A, Nydeggar U E (eds) Clinical use of intravenous immunoglobulins. Academic Press, London, pp 163–166

Siegel J D 1985 Neonatal sepsis. Seminars in Perinatology 9(1): 20–28

Silverman W A 1980 Retrolental fibroplasia: a modern parable. Monographs in neonatology. Grune & Stratton, New York

Silverman W A 1985 Human experimentation: a guided step into the unknown. Oxford University Press, Oxford

Silverman W A 1992 Overtreatment of neonates? A personal retrospective. Pediatrics 90: 971–976

Simbruner G 1986 Inadvertent positive end-expiratory pressure in mechanically ventilated newborn infants: detection and effect on lung mechanics and gas exchange. Journal of Pediatrics 108: 589–595

Simpson J, Stephenson T J 1993 Regulation of extracellular fluid volume in neonates. Early Human Development 34: 179–190

Simsarian F P, McLendon P A 1942 Feeding behaviour of an infant during the first 12 weeks of life on a self demand schedule. Journal of Pediatrics 20: 93–98

Sinclair J C, Bracken M B (eds) 1992 Effective care of the newborn infant. Oxford University Press, Oxford

Skinner J R, Milligan D W A, Hunter S, Hey E N 1992 Central venous pressure in the ventilated neonate. Archives of Disease in Childhood 67: 374–377

Skoutelli H N, Dubowitz L M S, Levene M I, Miller G 1985 Predictors associated with survival and normal neurodevelopmental outcome in infants weighing less than 1001 grams at birth. Developmental Medicine and Child Neurology 27: 588–595

Slagle T A, Gross S J 1988 Effect of early low-volume enteral substrate on subsequent feeding tolerance in very low birth weight infants. Journal of Pediatrics 113, 526–531

Slater A 1989 Visual memory and perception in early infancy. In: Slater A, Bremner G (eds) Infant development. Lawrence Erlbaum, Hillsdale NJ, pp 43–71

Slater J E 1961 Retention of nitrogen and minerals by babies 1 week old. British Journal of Nutrition 15: 83–97

Sly P D, Drew J H 1981 Massive pulmonary haemorrhage: a cause of sudden unexpected deaths in severely growth retarded infants. Australian Paediatric Journal 17: 32–34

Smith C A, Nelson N M 1976 Physiology of the newborn, 4th edn. Charles C Thomas, Springfield, Ill

Smith N C 1987 Assessment of fetal acid–base status. In: Whittle M J (ed) Clinical obstetrics and gynaecology. Baillière Tindall, London, vol 1, no 1, pp 97–109

So B H, Tamura M, Mishina J, Watanabe T, Kamoshita S 1995 Application of nasal continuous positive airway pressure to early extubation of low birthweight infants. Archives of Disease in Childhood 72: F191–F193

Soll R F 1991 Overviews of the effects of exogenous surfactant. In: Chalmers I (ed) Oxford database of perinatal trials. Version 1.2. Disk Issue 5. Records 5253, 5252, 5207, 5206

Soll R F, McQueen M C 1992 Respiratory distress syndrome. In: Sinclair J C, Bracken M B (eds) Effective care of the newborn infant. Oxford University Press, Oxford

Soltesz G, Harris D, McKenzie I Z, Aynsley-Green A 1985 The metabolic and endocrine milieu of the human fetus and mother at 18–21 weeks of gestation: 1 plasma amino acid concentrations. Pediatric Research 19: 91–93

Soothill P W, Awayi R A, Campbell S, Nicolaides K M 1993 Prediction of morbidity in small and normally grown fetuses by fetal heart rate variability, biophysical profile score and umbilical artery Doppler studies. British Journal of Obstetrics and Gynaecology 100: 742–745

South M, Morley C 1986 Synchronous mechanical ventilation of the neonate. Archives of Disease in Childhood 61: 1190–1195

Southall D P, Bignall S, Stebbens V A, Alexander R, Rivers R P A, Lissauer T 1987 Pulse oximeter and transcutaneous arterial oxygen measurements in neonatal and paediatric intensive care. Archives of Disease in Childhood 62: 882–888

Stagno S, Brasfield D M, Brown M B, Cassell G H, Pifer L L, Whitley R J 1981 Infant pneumonitis associated with cytomegalovirus, chlamydia, pneumocystis and ureoplasma: a prospective study. Pediatrics 68: 322–329

Stahlman M T 1990 Ethical issues in the nursery: priorities versus limits. Pediatrics 116: 167–170

Standing Committee on Nutrition of the British Paediatric Association 1994 Is breast feeding beneficial in the UK? Archives of Disease in Childhood 71: 376–380

Stanley F J, Watson L 1992 Trends in perinatal mortality and cerebral palsy in Western Australia, 1967–1985. British Medical Journal 304: 1658–1663

Stapells D R, Kurtzberg D 1991 Evoked potential assessment of auditory system integrity in infants. Clinics in Perinatology 18: 497–518

Steel J M, Johnstone F D, Hepburn D A, Smith A F 1990 Can pre-pregnancy care of diabetic women reduce the risk of abnormal babies? British Medical Journal 301: 1070–1074

Steele B T, Vigneux A, Blatz S et al 1987 Acute peritoneal dialysis in infants weighing <1500 g. Journal of Pediatrics 110: 126–129

Steer P A, Lucas A, Sinclair J C 1992 Feeding the low birthweight infant. In: Sinclair J C, Bracken M B (eds) Effective care of the newborn infant. Oxford University Press, Oxford, pp 94–140

Steinberg S A, Shalev R S, Amr N 1986 Valproic acid in neonatal status convulsivus. Brain Development 8: 278–280

Stenson B J, Glover R M, Laing I A, Wilkie R A, Tarnow-Mordi W O 1995 Life threatening inadvertent positive end expiratory pressure. American Journal of Perinatology 12: 336–338

Stephenson T J, Broughton Pipkin F 1990 Atrial natriuretic factor: the heart as an endocrine organ. Archives of Disease in Childhood 65: 1293–1294

Stephenson T J, Broughton Pipkin F, Elias-Jones A C 1991 A study of factors influencing plasma renin and renin substrate concentrations in the premature human newborn. Archives of Disease in Childhood 66: 1150–1154

Stephenson T J, Broughton Pipkin F, Hetmanski D, Yoxall B 1994 Atrial natriuretic peptide in the preterm newborn. Biology of the Neonate 66(1): 22–32

Stevens C E 1991 Immunoprophylaxis of hepatitis B virus infection. Seminars in Paediatric Infectious Diseases 2: 135–145

Stevens J C, Webb H D, Hutchinson J, Connell J, Smith M F, Buffin J T 1989 Click evoked otoacoustic emissions compared with brain stem electrical response. Archives of Disease in Childhood 64: 1105–1111

Stevenson D K, Walther F, Long W A and the American Exosurf Neonatal Study Group 1992 1. Controlled trial of a single dose of synthetic surfactant at birth in premature infants weighing 500–699 grams. Journal of Pediatrics 120: S3–S12

Stewart A L, Reynolds E O R, Lipscomb A P 1981 Outcome for infants of very low birthweight: survey of world literature. Lancet i: 1038–1041

Stewart A L, Reynolds E O R, Hope P L, Hamilton P A, Baudin J, Costello A M L, Bradford B C, Wyatt J S 1987 Probability of neurodevelopmental disorders estimated from ultrasound appearance of the brains of very preterm infants. Developmental Medicine and Child Neurology 29: 3–11

Stinson R, Stinson P 1983 The long dying of baby Andrew. Little Brown, Boston

Stocker J T 1986 Sequestrations of the lung. Seminars in Diagnostic Pathology 3: 106–121

Stocker J T, Drake R M, Madewell J E 1978 Cystic and congenital lung disease in the newborn. Perspectives in Pediatric Pathology 4: 93–154

Stolar C J H, Snedecor S M, Bartlett R H 1991 Extracorporeal membrane oxygenation and neonatal respiratory failure: experience from the extracorporeal life support organisation. Journal of Pediatric Surgery 26: 563–571

Stonestreet B S, Rubin L, Pollak A, Cowett R M, Oh W 1980 Renal functions of low birth weight infants with hyperglycemia and glucosuria produced by glucose infusions. Pediatrics 66: 561–567

Strand C, Laptook A R, Dowling S, Campbell N, Lasky R E, Wallin L A, Maravilla A M, Rosenfeld C R 1990 Neonatal intracranial haemorrhage: I. Changing pattern in inborn low-birth-weight infants. Early Human Development 23: 117–128

Strome M, Donahoe P K 1982 Advances in management of laryngeal and subglottic stenosis. Journal of Pediatric Surgery 17: 591–596

Sugden R, Williams A 1978 The principles of practical cost–benefit analysis. Oxford University Press, Oxford

Swischuk L E 1976 Two lesser known but useful signs of neonatal pneumothorax. American Journal of Roentgenology 127: 623–627

Synnes A R, Ling E W Y, Whitfield M F, Mackinnon M, Lopes L, Wong G, Effer S B 1994 Perinatal outcomes of a large cohort of extremely low gestational age infants (twenty-three to twenty-eight completed weeks of gestation). Journal of Pediatrics 125: 952–960

Szymonowicz W, Yu V Y H, Bajuk B, Astbury J 1986 Neurodevelopmental outcome, periventricular haemorrhage and leukomalacia in infants 1250 g or less at birth. Early Human Development 14: 1–7

Szabo J S, Hillemeier A C, Oh W 1985 Effect of non-nutritive and nutritive suck on gastric emptying in premature infants. Journal of Pediatric Gastroenterology and Nutrition 4: 348–351

Taeusch H W, Boncuk-Dayanikli P 1995 Respiratory distress syndrome. In: Yu V Y H (ed) Pulmonary problems in the perinatal period and their sequelae. Baillière Tindall, London

Tarnow-Mordi W O 1991 Is routine endotracheal suction justified? Archives of Disease in Childhood 66: 374–375

Tarnow-Mordi W, Shaw J C L, Liu D, Gardner D A, Flynn F V 1981 Iatrogenic hyponatraemia of the newborn due to maternal fluid overload: a prospective study. British Medical Journal 283: 639–642

Tarnow-Mordi W O, Sutton P, Wilkinson A R 1986 Inadequate humidification of respiratory gases during mechanical ventilation of the newborn. Archives of Disease in Childhood 61: 698–700

Tarnow-Mordi W O, Griffiths P, Wilkinson A R 1989 Low inspired gas temperature and respiratory complications in very low birth weight infants. Journal of Pediatrics 114: 438–442

Tarnow-Mordi W O, Wilkie R A, Reid E 1994 Static respiratory compliance in the newborn 1: a clinical and prognostic index for mechanically ventilated infants. Archives of Disease in Childhood 70: F11–F15

Taylor D 1997 Paediatric ophthalmology, 2nd edn. Blackwell Scientific Publications, Oxford

Taylor M J, Murphy W J, Whyte H E 1992 Prognostic reliability of SEPs and VEPs in asphyxiated newborn infants. Developmental Medicine and Child Neurology 34: 507–515

Temple C M, Dennis J, Carney R, Sharich J 1995 Neonatal seizures: long term outcome and cognitive development among 'normal' survivors. Developmental Medicine and Child Neurology 37: 109–118

Ten Centre Study Group 1987 Ten centre trial of artificial surfactant (artificial lung expanding compound) in very premature babies. British Medical Journal 294: 991–996

Thomson A J, Searle M, Russell G 1977 Quality of survival after severe birth asphyxia. Archives of Disease in Childhood 52: 620–626

Thoresen M, Penrice J, Lorek A, Cady E B, Wylenzinska M, Kirkbride V, Cooper C E, Brown G C, Edwards A D, Wyatt J S, Reynolds E O R 1995 Mild hypothermia after severe transient hypoxia–ischemia ameliorates delayed cerebral energy failure in the newborn piglet. Pediatric Research 37: 667–670

Thornberg E, Thiringer K, Hagberg H, Kjellmer I 1995 Neuron specific enolase in asphyxiated newborns: association with encephalopathy and cerebral function monitor trace. Archives of Disease in Childhood 72: F39–F42

Thurlbeck W M 1979 Morphologic aspects of bronchopulmonary dysplasia. Journal of Pediatrics 95: 842–843

Toce S S, Keenan W J, Homan S M 1987 Enteral feeding in very low birth weight infants: a comparison of two nasogastric methods. American Journal of Diseases of Children 141: 439–444

Townsend C W 1894 The haemorrhagic disease of the newborn. Archives of Paediatrics ii: 559–565

Trounce J Q, Fagan D, Levene M I 1986 Intraventricular haemorrhage and periventricular leucomalacia: ultrasound and autopsy correlation. Archives of Disease in Childhood 61: 1203–1207

Trounce J Q, Shaw D E, Levene M I, Rutter N 1988 Clinical risk factors and periventricular leucomalacia. Archives of Disease in Childhood 63: 17–22

Tsang R C, Lucas A, Uauy R, Zlotkin S 1993 Nutritional needs of the preterm infant: scientific basis and practical guidelines. Williams & Wilkins, Baltimore

Tsukahara H, Sudo M, Umezaki M, Fujii Y, Kuriyama M, Yamamoto K, Ishii Y 1993 Measurement of lumbar spinal bone mineral density in preterm infants by dual-energy X-ray absorptiometry. Biology of the Neonate 64: 96–103

Tubman T R J, Halliday H L 1990 Surfactant treatment of respiratory distress syndrome following prolonged rupture of membranes. European Journal of Pediatrics 149: 727–729

Tuck S 1986 Fluid and electrolyte balance in the neonate. In: Roberton N R C (ed) Textbook of neonatology. Churchill Livingstone, London, pp 162–177

Tucker S M, Battacharya J 1992 Screening of hearing impairment in the newborn using the auditory response cradle. Archives of Disease in Childhood 67: 911–919

Tudehope D I, Smyth M J 1979 Is 'transient tachypnoea of the newborn' always a benign disease? Report of 6 babies requiring mechanical ventilation. Australian Paediatric Journal 15: 160–165

Tulloh R M R, Tansey S P, Parashar K, De Giovanni J V, Wright J G C, Silove E D 1994 Echocardiographic screening in neonates undergoing surgery for selected gastrointestinal malformations. Archives of Disease in Childhood 70: F206–F208

Tyrala E E, Chen X, Boden G 1994 Glucose metabolism in the infant weighing less than 1100 grams. Journal of Pediatrics 125: 283–287

UK Collaborative ECMO Trial Group 1996 UK collaborative randomised trial of neonatal extracorporeal membrane oxygenation. Lancet 348: 75–82

Van Bel F, Walther F J 1990 Myocardial dysfunction and cerebral blood flow velocity following birth asphyxia. Acta Paediatrica Scandinavica 79: 756–762

Van de Bor M, Guit G L, Schreuder A M, Wondergem J, Vielvoye G J 1989 Early detection of delayed myelination in preterm infants. Pediatrics 84: 407–411

Van de Bor M, den Ouden L, Guit G L 1992 Value of cranial ultrasound and magnetic resonance imaging in predicting neurodevelopmental outcome in preterm infants. Pediatrics 90: 196–199

Van de Perre P, Simonon A, Msellati P et al 1991 Postnatal transmission of HIV type 1 from mother to infant: a prospective cohort study in Kigali, Rwanda. New England Journal of Medicine 325: 593–601

Van Gelderen W F C 1992 Ultrasound diagnosis of an atypical pneumomediastinum. Pediatric Radiology 22: 469–470

Van Houten J, Long W, Mullet M et al 1992 Pulmonary hemorrhage in premature infants after treatment with synthetic surfactant: an autopsy evaluation. Journal of Pediatrics 120: S40–S44

Van Zeben A A, Verloove-Vanhorick S, Brand R et al 1989 Morbidity of very low birthweight infants at a corrected age of 2 years in a geographically defined population. Lancet i: 253–255

Van Zeben-Van der Aa D M, Verloove-Vanhorick S P, den Ouden L, Brand R, Ruys J H 1990 Neonatal seizures in very preterm and very low birthweight infants: mortality and handicaps at two years of age in a nationwide cohort. Neuropediatrics 21: 62–65

van-Goudoever J B, Sulkers E J, Chapman T E, Carnielli V P, Efstatopoulos T, Degenhart H J, Sauer P J 1993 Glucose kinetics and glucoregulatory hormone levels in ventilated preterm infants on the first day of life. Pediatric Research 33: 583–589

Vannucci R C, Mujsce D J 1992 Effect of glucose on perinatal hypoxic–ischemic brain damage. Biology of the Neonate 62: 215–224

Vannucci R C, Towfighi J, Heitjan D F, Brucklacher R M 1995 Carbon dioxide protects the perinatal brain from hypoxic–ischemic damage: an experimental study in the immature rat. Pediatrics 95: 868–874

Veen S, Ens-Dokkum M H, Schreuder A, Verloove-Vanhorick S P, Brand R, Ruys J H 1991 Impairments, disabilities and handicaps of very preterm and very low birthweight infants at 5 years of age. Lancet 338: 33–36

Ventriculomegaly Trial Group 1990 Randomised trial of early tapping in neonatal posthaemorrhagic ventricular dilatation. Archives of Disease in Childhood 65: 3–10

Ventriculomegaly Trial Group 1994 Randomised trial of early tapping in neonatal posthaemorrhagic ventricular dilatation: results at 30 months. Archives of Disease in Childhood 70: F129–F136

Verder H, Robertson B, Greisen G et al 1994 Surfactant therapy and nasal continuous positive airway pressure for newborns with respiratory distress syndrome. New England Journal of Medicine 331: 1051–1055

Verloove-Vanhorick S P, Verwey R A, Brand R et al 1986 Neonatal mortality risk in relation to gestational age and birth weight. Results of a national survey of preterm and very low birth weight infants in the Netherlands. Lancet 1986 i: 55–57

Verloove-Vanhorick S P, Verwey R A, Ebeling M C A, Brand R, Ruys J H 1988 Mortality in very preterm and very low birthweight infants according to place of birth and level of care. Pediatrics 82: 404–411

Victorian Infant Collaborative Study (VICS) Group 1991 Improvement of outcome for infants of birthweight under 1000g. Archives of Disease in Childhood 66: 765–769

Victorian Infant Collaborative Study (VICS) Group 1995 Neurosensory outcome at 5 years and extremely low birthweight. Archives of Disease in Childhood 73: F143–F146

Ville Y, Hyett J, Hecher K, Nicolaides K 1995 Preliminary experience with endoscopic laser surgery for severe twin–twin transfusion syndrome. New England Journal of Medicine 332: 224

Volpe J J 1989 Neonatal seizures: current concepts and revised classification. Pediatrics 84: 422–428

Volpe J J 1995 Neurology of the newborn, 3rd edn. W B Saunders, Philadelphia, pp 107, 730–768

Von Kreis R, Stannigel H, Gobe U 1985 Anticoagulant therapy by continuous heparin–antithrombin III infusions in newborn with disseminated intravascular coagulation. European Journal of Pediatrics 144: 191–194

Walshe M C, Klugman R M 1986 Necrotising enterocolitis: treatment based on staging criteria. Pediatric Clinics of North America 33: 179–199

Walters D V, Olver R E 1978 The role of catecholamines in lung liquid absorption at birth. Pediatric Research 12: 239–242

Wang E E L, Ohlsson A, Kellner J D 1995 Association of *Ureaplasma urealyticum* colonisation with chronic lung disease of prematurity: result of meta-analysis. Journal of Pediatrics 127: 640–644

Wariyar U, Richmond S 1989 Morbidity in preterm delivery: importance of 100% follow up. Lancet i: 387–388

Wariyar U, Richmond S, Hey E 1989a Pregnancy outcome at 24–31 weeks gestation: mortality. Archives of Disease in Childhood 64: 670–677

Wariyar U, Richmond S, Hey E 1989b Pregnancy outcome at 24–31 weeks gestation: neonatal survivors. Archives of Disease in Childhood 64: 678–686

Watanabe K, Miyazaki S, Hara K, Hakamada A 1980 Behavioural state cycles, background EEGs and prognosis of newborns with perinatal hypoxia. Electroencephalographic and Clinical Neurophysiology 49: 618–625

Watkin P M 1996 Neonatal otoacoustic emission screening and the identification of deafness. Archives of Disease in Childhood 74: F16–F25

Watkins A, Szymonowicz W, Jin X, Yu V Y H 1988 Significance of seizures in very low birthweight infants. Developmental Medicine and Child Neurology 30: 162–169

Wauer R R, Schmalisch G, Menzel K et al 1982 The antenatal use of Ambroxol to prevent hyaline membrane disease. A controlled double blind study. Biological Research in Pregnancy 3: 84–91

Way G L, Woolfe R R, Eshaghpour E, Bender R L, Jaffe R B, Ruttenberg H D 1979 The natural history of hypertrophic cardiomyopathy in infants of diabetic mothers. Journal of Pediatrics 95: 1020–1025

Weaver L T, Lucas A 1993 Development of bowel habit in preterm infants. Archives of Disease in Childhood 68: 317–320

Webber S, Wilkinson A R, Lindsell D et al 1990 Neonatal pneumonia. Archives of Disease in Childhood 65: 207–211

Weinberg R P 1986 Gastroenterology. I. Bilirubin physiology. In: Roberton N R C (ed) Textbook of neonatology. Churchill Livingstone, London, ch 18, pp 383–393

Weiner S P, Painter M J, Geva D, Guthrie R D, Scher M S 1991 Neonatal seizures: electroclinical dissociation. Pediatric Neurology 7: 363–368

Weiner Z, Farmakides G, Schulman H, Penny B 1994 Central and peripheral haemodynamic changes in fetuses with absent and diastolic velocity in umbilical artery; correlation with computerized fetal heart rate pattern. American Journal of Obstetrics and Gynecology 170: 509–515

Weisglas-Kuperus N, Heersema D J, Baerts W, Fetter W P F, Smorkovsky M, van Hof-van Duin J, Sauer P J J 1993 Visual functions in relation with neonatal cerebral ultrasound, neurology and cognitive development in very low birthweight children. Neuropediatrics 24: 149–154

Weisman L E, Stoll B, Kueser T et al 1992 Intravenous immunoglobulin therapy of neonatal sepsis. Journal of Pediatrics 121: 434–443

Weissman A, Jakobi P, Blazer S, Avrahami R, Zimmer E Z 1989 Survival and long term outcome of infants delivered at 24 to 28 weeks gestation by method of delivery and fetal presentation. Journal of Perinatology 9: 372–375

Welch J C, Bridson J M, Gibbs J L 1995 Endotracheal tolazoline for severe persistent pulmonary hypertension of the newborn. British Heart Journal 73: 99–100

Westgren M, Paul R 1985 Delivery of low birth weight infant by Caesarian section. Clinical Obstetrics and Gynaecology 28: 752–762

Wheater M, Rennie J M 1994 Poor prognosis after prolonged ventilation for bronchopulmonary dysplasia. Archives of Disease in Childhood 71: F210–F211

Whitelaw A, Rivers R P A, Creighton L, Gaffney P 1992 Low dose intraventricular fibrinolytic treatment to prevent posthaemorrhagic hydrocephalus. Archives of Disease in Childhood 67: 12–14

Whitley R J, Brasfield D, Reynolds D W, Stagno S, Tiller R E, Alford C A 1976 Protracted pneumonitis in young infants associated with perinatally acquired cytomegalovirus infection. Journal of Pediatrics 89: 16–22

Whyte H E, Fitzhardinge P M, Shennan A T, Lennox K, Smith L, Lacy J 1993 Extreme immaturity: outcome of 568 pregnancies of 23–26 weeks gestation. Obstetrics and Gynecology 82: 1–7

Widdowson E M 1980 Importance of nutrients in development with special reference to feeding the low birthweight infant. Proc. Ross Clinical Research Conference: Meeting the nutritional goals for low birthweight infants. Ross Laboratories, Tarpon Springs, pp 4–11

Wigglesworth J S, Desai R 1981 Use of DNA estimation for growth assessment in normal and hypoplastic fetal lungs. Archives of Disease in Childhood 56: 601–605

Wigglesworth J S, Desai R 1982 Is fetal respiratory function a major determinant of perinatal survival? Lancet i: 264–267

Wilcox D T, Glick P L, Karamanoukian H L, Leach C, Morin F C III, Fuhrman B P 1995 Perfluorocarbon-associated gas exchange improves pulmonary mechanics, oxygenation, ventilation, and allows nitric oxide delivery in the hypoplastic lung congenital diaphragmatic hernia lamb model. Critical Care Medicine 23: 1858–1863

Wilkins B 1986 The renal effects of aminophylline in very low birth weight neonates. Early Human Development 15(3): 184–185

Wilkins B H 1992a Renal function in sick very low birthweight infants: 1. Glomerular filtration rate. Archives of Disease in Childhood 67: 1140–1145

Wilkins B H 1992b Renal function in sick very low birthweight infants: 2. Urea and creatinine excretion. Archives of Disease in Childhood 67: 1146–1153

Wilkins B H 1992c Renal function in sick very low birthweight infants: 3. Sodium, potassium and water excretion. Archives of Disease in Childhood 67: 1154–1161

Wilkinson A R 1988 Cardiovascular adaptation in the very immature infant. In: Whitelaw A, Cooke R W I (eds) The very immature infant less than 28 weeks gestation. British Medical Bulletin 44(4): 935–956, Churchill Livingstone, London

Wilkinson J L, Cooke R W I 1986 Cardiovascular disorders. In: Roberton N R C (ed) Textbook of neonatology. Churchill Livingstone, Edinburgh, p 342

Wilmore D W, Dudrick S J 1968 Growth and development of an infant receiving all nutrients exclusively by vein. Journal of the American Medical Association 203: 860–868

Wilson C B, Lewis D B 1990 Basis and implications of selectively diminished cytokine production in neonatal susceptibility to infection. Review of Infectious Diseases 12: S410–S422

Windle W F 1966 An experimental approach to prevention or reduction of the brain damage of birth asphyxia. Developmental Medicine and Child Neurology 8: 129–140

Wiswell T E, Rawlings J S, Smith F R, Goo E D 1985 Effect of furosemide on the clinical course of transient tachypnea of the newborn. Pediatrics 75: 908–910

Wiswell T E, Tuggle J M, Turner B S 1990 Meconium aspiration syndrome: have we made a difference? Pediatrics 85: 715–721

Wiswell T E, Baumgart S, Gannon C M et al 1995 No lumbar puncture in the evaluation of early neonatal sepsis: Will meningitis be missed? Pediatrics 96(6): 803–806

Wojtulewicz J, Alam A, Brasher P, Whyte H, Long D, Newman C, Perlman M 1993 Changing survival and impairment rates at 18–24 months in outborn very low birthweight infants 1984–87 versus 1980–83. Acta Paediatrica Scandinavica 82: 666–671

Wolke D 1987 Environmental and developmental neonatology. Journal of Reproductive and Infant Psychology 5: 17–42

Wolke D 1991 Supporting the development of low birthweight infants. Journal of Child Psychology and Psychiatry 32: 723–741

Wolke D 1995 Verhaltensprobleme und soziale Beziehungen ehemals sehr kleiner Frühgeborener: Einfluesse des intensivmedizinischen Handlings. (Behaviour problems and social relationships of very preterm children: influence of neonatal intensive care handling.) Zeitschrift fuer Geburtshilfe und Neonatologie 199: 208

Wolke D 1997 The preterm responses to the environment – long term effects? In: Cockburn F (ed) Proceedings of the XVth European Congress of Perinatal Medicine 10–13 Sept 1996. Parthenon Publishing, Carnforth, ch 47

Wolke D, Meyer R, Ohrt B, Riegel H 1995 The incidence of sleeping problems in preterm and fullterm infants discharged from special neonatal care units: An epidemiological longitudinal study. Journal of Child Psychology and Psychiatry 36(2): 203–223

Wood B, Katz V, Bose C, Goolsby R, Kraybill E 1989 Survival and morbidity of extremely premature infants based on obstetric assessment of gestational age. Obstetrics and Gynecology 74: 889–892

Working Group on the Very Low Birthweight Infant 1990 European Community study of outcome of pregnancy between 22 and 28 weeks' gestation. Lancet 336: 782–784

Wright L, Horbar J, Gunkel H et al 1995 Evidence from multicenter networks on the current use and effectiveness of antenatal corticosteroids in low birthweight infants. American Journal of Obstetrics and Gynecology 173: 263–269

Wung J T, James S, Kilchevsky E, James E 1985 Management of infants with severe respiratory failure and persistence of the fetal circulation without hyperventilation. Pediatrics 76: 488–494

Wyatt J S 1994 Noninvasive assessment of cerebral oxidative metabolism in the human newborn. Journal of the Royal College of Physicians of London 28: 126–132

Wyatt J S, Edwards A D, Azzopardi D, Reynolds E O R 1989 Magnetic resonance and near infrared spectroscopy for investigation of perinatal hypoxic–ischaemic brain injury. Archives of Disease in Childhood 64: 953–963

Wyllie J, Wren C, Hunter S 1994 Screening for fetal cardiac malformations. British Heart Journal Supplement 71: 20–27

Wyszogrodski I, Kyei-Aboagye K, Taeusch H W, Avery M E 1975 Surfactant inactivation by hyperventilation: conservation by end-expiratory pressure. Journal of Applied Physiology 38: 461–466

Yeh T F, Torre J A, Rastogi A, Anyebuno M A, Pildes R S 1990 Early post-natal dexamethasone therapy in premature infants with severe respiratory distress syndrome: a double-blind controlled study. Journal of Pediatrics 117: 273–282

Young R S, Briggs R W, Yagel S K 1986 31-P NMR study of the effects of hypoxaemia on neonatal status epilepticus. Pediatric Research 120: 581–587

Yu V Y H, Ng P C 1995 Chronic lung disease. In: Yu V Y H (ed) Pulmonary problems in the perinatal period and their sequelae. Baillière Tindall, London

Yu V Y H, Loke H L, Bajuk B, Szymonowicz W, Orgill A A, Astbury J 1986 Prognosis for infants born at 23–28 weeks gestation. British Medical Journal 293: 1200–1203

Yu V Y H, Gomez J M, Shan J, McCloud P I 1992 Survival prospects of extremely preterm infants: a 10 year experience in a single perinatal centre. American Journal of Perinatology 9: 164–169

Zanjani E D, Poster J, Mann L I, Witsserman L R 1977 Regulation of erythropoiesis in the fetus. In: Fisher J W (ed) Kidney hormones Vol II. Erythropoietin. Academic Press, London, p 463

Zeigler J B, Cooper D A, Johnson R O, Gold J 1985 Postnatal transmission of AIDS-associated retrovirus from mother to infant. Lancet i: 896–897

Ziegler E E 1985 Nutrient requirements of the preterm infant: an overview. In: Tsang R C (ed) Vitamin and mineral requirements in preterm infants. Marcel Dekker, New York, pp 203–212

6 Infant feeding

A. F. Williams

Breast-feeding 326
    Prevalence of breast-feeding 326
    Is breast-feeding important? 326
    Establishing and maintaining breast-feeding 327
    Contraindications to breast-feeding 329
    Growth of breast-fed babies 330
    How long is breast milk sufficient on its own? 330
    Supplements for breast-fed babies 330
    Breast-fed babies who fail to thrive 331
Infant formula feeding 331
    Composition of human milk 332
    'Renal solute load' 333
    Milk consumption 333
    Soya formula and other milks 333

Weaning 333
    Weaning problems 334
    Vitamin supplements 334
    Dental health 334
    Drinks and water 334
    Pasteurized cow's milk 334
References 334

Feeding practices greatly affect growth rate and morbidity in infancy. More recently it has been suggested that nutritional state in infancy exerts a long-term effect on health and development through metabolic 'programming' (Lucas 1994). Optimizing nutrition is thus an important aspect of pediatric care; changing behavior requires not only an understanding of physiological and biochemical facets but an appreciation of the strong sociocultural influences underlying the enormous variation observed between and within countries.

BREAST-FEEDING

Prevalence of breast-feeding

In 1990 63% of mothers in Great Britain initiated breast-feeding, but 38% of these had stopped by 6 weeks and 61% by 4 months of age. Studies by the Office of Population Censuses and Surveys (e.g. White et al 1992) have consistently identified factors which affect the prevalence of breast-feeding (Table 6.1). Social class

Table 6.1 Factors affecting prevalence of breast-feeding in the UK

Factors which favor breast-feeding:
    Social class I
    Mother educated beyond 18 years of age
    Mother ≥ 25 years of age
    Live in London or southeast England
    First baby
    Breast-fed a previous baby

Factors which make breast-feeding less likely:
    Social class V
    Maternal smoking

Source: DHSS 1988.

Table 6.2 International comparison of breast-feeding rates (%)

	3 months	6 months
United Kingdom	26	22
Canada	53	30
United States	33	24
Australia	56	40
Sweden	47	23
Jamaica	95	82
Kenya	94	92

Source: UNICEF 1992.

and geographical gradients are particularly marked. For example, 86% of social class I mothers versus 41% in social class V chose to breast-feed their baby. Moreover, in London and southeast England 74% initiated breast-feeding, but only 50% in Scotland (White et al 1992). These figures contrast with much higher breast-feeding rates in other industrialized nations (Table 6.2), suggesting room for improvement.

Is breast-feeding important?

Breast milk is a living tissue. It consists of lymphocytes and macrophages suspended in a biochemically complex medium containing in addition to nutrients a host of compounds with trophic, immune, digestive and endocrine activity (Table 6.3). The function of many breast milk constituents is still not understood and it can reasonably be asked whether there is proof of biological benefit to the baby, or whether the presence of these substances is an accident of nature.

Table 6.3 'Non-nutrient' components of human milk

Passive immunity	
Cells	Lymphocytes
	Macrophages
Nonspecific immunity	Lactoferrin
	Lysozyme
	Lactoperoxidase
	Amino sugars
	Lipids
	Lipase
	Complement
Specific immunity	Immunoglobulin A
Growth factors	
Epidermal growth factor (urogastrone)	
Nerve growth factor-like substance	
Facilitators of nutrient assimilation	
Lactoferrin	
Bile salt-stimulated lipase	
Milk fat globule membrane	

Breast-feeding and infection. It has long been appreciated that breast-feeding is crucial to survival in less-developed countries. For example, a Brazilian study showed that infants fed formula were 14.2 times (95% CI 5.9–34.1) more likely to *die* of diarrheal disease in infancy than those breast-fed (Victora et al 1987). Debate has centered upon the potential contribution of breast-feeding to maternal and child health in the industrialized countries (British Paediatric Association, Standing Committee on Nutrition 1994). Randomized controlled trials – the 'gold standard' proof of cause and effect – are clearly unethical in this field and resort must be made to retrospective case control and prospective cohort observational methodology. Three problems beset the investigator: firstly, the variable duration of breast-feeding makes it difficult to define 'breast-fed'. Many infants are mixed fed; in 1990 over 40% of 'breast-fed' infants received some formula in the first week of life. Thus true exclusive breast-feeding is uncommon, at least in the UK. Secondly, many sociocultural factors correlated with method of feeding (e.g. smoking, alcohol, social class; Table 6.1) confound outcome. Thirdly, mothers who breast-feed might be less likely to report minor symptoms; a phenomenon known as 'detection bias'. A literature review (Bauchner et al 1986) concluded that most studies were methodologically flawed.

More recent studies have taken account of these criticisms. For example, a prospective cohort study in Dundee, Scotland concluded that bottle-fed infants were more likely to develop gastroenteritis, respiratory symptoms, and to be admitted to hospital than those breast-fed for 13 weeks or more, even after adjustment for confounding factors (Howie et al 1990). Infants who were partially breast-fed derived partial benefit. North American studies have confirmed the protective effect of breast-feeding, particularly against gastroenteritis and otitis media (Dewey et al 1995a, Duncan et al 1993). Using the Scottish data it has been calculated that each 5% increment in the prevalence of breast-feeding to 13 weeks of age would save the National Health Service in England and Wales £2.5 million annually solely by reducing the frequency of infantile gastroenteritis (DoH 1995).

Breast-feeding and allergy. Studies of breast-feeding and allergic disease have yielded conflicting evidence. Grulee & Sandford (1936) first proposed that artificial feeding increased risk for eczema. There have been many subsequent studies, though not all have substantiated this and one even suggested that eczema was commoner in breast-fed infants. This disparity may be attributable to several factors. Firstly, those with a history of allergy probably self-select for breast-feeding. Secondly, *exclusive* breast-feeding for as long as 6 months is uncommon in most industrialized countries and partial breast-feeding for short periods is not effective (Saarinen & Kajosaari 1995); even brief exposure to cow's milk formula may sensitize. A consensus is that any protective effect is probably strongest in those genetically at risk.

Breast-feeding and sudden infant death syndrome. Although many studies have shown sudden infant death syndrome (SIDS) to be more common among bottle-fed babies not all have addressed the confounding effects of smoking, low birth weight, and socioeconomic group. A large New Zealand study which controlled for these factors and sleeping position estimated the adjusted odds ratio for SIDS among babies bottle-fed at hospital discharge to be 2.45 (95% CI 1.32–4.55) (Ford et al 1993). A smaller British study observed an adjusted odds ratio of similar magnitude with evidence of graded risk among those partially breast-fed, though this was not statistically significant (Gilbert et al 1995).

Breast-feeding and long-term morbidity. The incidence of juvenile-onset, insulin-dependent diabetes mellitus (IDDM) is slightly decreased in children breast-fed as babies (Gerstein 1994) and diabetes can be induced by feeding cow's milk in strains of rat genetically at risk. Newly diagnosed diabetic children have antibodies to a 17 amino acid fragment of bovine serum albumin (BSA) which are not found in the serum of siblings or healthy children (Karjalainen et al 1992). Currently it is speculated that these antibodies form as a result of exposure to cow's milk in early life and precipitate the autoimmune process leading to diabetes. However, it is not yet clear when exposure to BSA is critical, or what dose and duration of exposure are important. Careful prospective studies in families at increased risk of IDDM will be needed to resolve this issue.

Breast-feeding and neurological development. Numerous studies have found a statistically significant association between breast-feeding and mental development in infancy and childhood (reviewed in British Paediatric Association, Standing Committee on Nutrition 1994) but potential confounding influences are numerous, e.g. alcohol intake, smoking, parental intelligence, 'parenting skills' (Florey et al 1995). The differences observed may be most marked in infants prematurely born (Lucas et al 1992) and in the majority of studies persist even after adjustment for identifiable confounding influences. Recently it has been suggested that they may be explained by differences in the fat composition of formula and breast milk (see p. 1942) (Crawford 1993) though this is currently unproven.

Breast-feeding and maternal health. Apart from contributing to child spacing through induction of lactational amenorrhea (see Endocrinology below) breast-feeding significantly reduces the mother's risk of premenopausal breast cancer. The effect is strongest in women who have breast-fed most babies for longest (UK National Case-Control Study Group 1993, Newcomb et al 1994).

Establishing and maintaining breast-feeding

Breast milk production. Prolactin and human placental lactogen induce hyperplasia and hypertrophy of the ducts and secretory structures of the breast during pregnancy. At birth the inhibitory influence of maternal progesterone is removed and milk production is stimulated by prolactin released in response to sucking. Sucking is therefore the primary stimulus to milk production and the means by which infant demand increases breast milk supply. Pregnancy is not an essential prerequisite to lactation which can be induced even after adoption by allowing the infant to suck ('*adoptive lactation*' or '*relactation*'; Auerbach & Avery 1980).

During the first 3–4 days of life the volume of milk gradually increases. This early milk (termed 'colostrum') is rich in protein, particularly secretory immunoglobulin A. As the volume of milk increases the protein and electrolyte content of the milk fall and the carbohydrate and fat content increase. By the fifth day the breasts usually produce more milk than the infant chooses to take at a feed and 5-day-old babies take significantly less milk from the second breast than the first if the breasts are presented in random order (left/right or right/left) at a feed. This confirms that the breasts are not actually 'empty' and the baby chooses to leave milk behind.

Many other experiments have confirmed that the *yield* (or volume of milk obtainable by expressing the breasts over a 24-hour period) usually exceeds the baby's *intake*. For example, Dewey et al (1991) estimated that an average 'residual volume' of 109 ml/day (range 0–457 ml/day) could be extracted from the breast in addition to the baby's normal intake. Regular pumping increases yield and an increment of 20% over intake can be achieved.

Such findings make it hard to understand why most British mothers who abandon breast-feeding in the early weeks of life believe they have 'insufficient milk'. They (and sometimes health professionals) probably fail to realize differences in the pattern of feeding between breast and bottle-fed babies. Breast-fed babies tend to feed frequently, particularly during the early weeks of life when milk production is rapidly increasing, effectively reaching a plateau between 1 and 3 months of age. This must not be interpreted as under-supply. The amount of time a baby spends sucking gives no useful information about the baby's intake as there is very pronounced variation between individual mother–baby pairs.

Breast-feeding management. Important features of breast-feeding management are shown in Table 6.4. These 'Ten Steps' were developed after extensive review of the scientific literature (Akre 1989) and are used by WHO/UNICEF's 'Baby Friendly Hospital Initiative' to assess breast-feeding practice in maternity hospitals internationally (WHO/UNICEF 1989).

Early feeding. Babies should be given an opportunity to breast-feed as soon as possible after birth when they are alert and will root vigorously. Supervision is important in order to ensure that the baby is both correctly *positioned* (i.e. head and shoulders facing the breast) and *attached*, showing slow, rhythmical jaw movements rather than rapid, shallow sucking with indrawing of the cheeks. It is important to understand the mechanics of breast-feeding (Fig. 6.1; Woolridge 1986a) if the importance of correct *attachment* (relationship between baby's mouth and mother's breast) is to be appreciated. As the baby attaches the nipple is drawn into the mouth, retained by suction, and elongated to about three times its former length. The lateral margins of the tongue curve upwards to enclose it and surrounding breast tissue in a cup formed by tongue and hard palate. Milk is then stripped by a peristaltic wave running anteroposteriorly along the tongue. In

Table 6.4 Steps which help to establish breast-feeding in hospital

Every facility providing maternity services and care for newborn infants should:

1. Have a written breast-feeding policy that is routinely communicated to all health care staff.
2. Train all health care staff in skills necessary to implement this policy.
3. Inform all pregnant women about the benefits and management of breast-feeding.
4. Help mothers initiate breast-feeding as soon as possible after delivery.
5. Show mothers how to breast-feed and how to maintain lactation even if they should be separated from their infants.
6. Give breast-fed newborn infants no food or drink *unless medically indicated*.
7. Practice rooming-in – allow mothers and infants to remain together – 24 hours a day.
8. Encourage breast-feeding on demand.
9. Give no artificial teats or dummies (pacifiers) to breast-feeding infants.
10. Foster the establishment of breast-feeding support groups and refer mothers to them on discharge from the hospital.

Adapted from WHO/UNICEF 1989.

this way milk is ejected from the lactiferous sinuses under the positive pressure created by nipple compression; negative pressure retains the nipple in the mouth and draws milk into the stripped lactiferous sinuses. This process is frictionless and the nipple should not be traumatized if the baby attaches correctly (Woolridge 1986a,b). The mechanics of breast- and bottle-feeding are different and babies may develop 'nipple confusion' if switched from one to the other (see below).

Incorrect attachment is a common cause of feeding problems. The baby may be fretful yet reluctant to take more than a few sucks; the nipple may be traumatized and bleed. Nipple pain should always prompt experienced assessment of feeding technique rather than resorting to ineffective remedies such as creams, sprays or nipple shields. The last may even exacerbate the problem by hindering milk flow. The midwifery skills necessary to resolve this problem are outside the scope of this chapter (see for example Woolridge 1986b, Royal College of Midwives 1988).

Supplementary feeds of formula or water are unnecessary for healthy, term breast-fed babies. There is no evidence that supplementary water or dextrose feeds accelerate resolution of neonatal jaundice in breast-fed babies and there is some data suggesting they *increase* the incidence of early jaundice.

Healthy breast-fed term babies do not require routine blood glucose monitoring. Blood glucose concentrations of such babies may fall below 2 mmol/l without clinical signs of neuroglycopenia, probably because ketone bodies are effectively mobilized and act as alternative cerebral fuels (Hawdon et al 1992). 'Symptomatic' hypoglycemia in a breast-feeding baby should never be attributed to starvation alone; there is likely to be an underlying illness such as infection. Simple supplementary feeding is not the solution.

Demand feeding. Babies should be allowed to feed until satiated whenever they are hungry. Limiting sucking time does not reduce the incidence of nipple trauma which is more likely to be attributable to poor attachment (see above). It is impossible to make rules about the frequency of feeds because babies vary greatly. They may feed only on a few occasions in the first 24 hours, becoming more active and hungry on the second and third days.

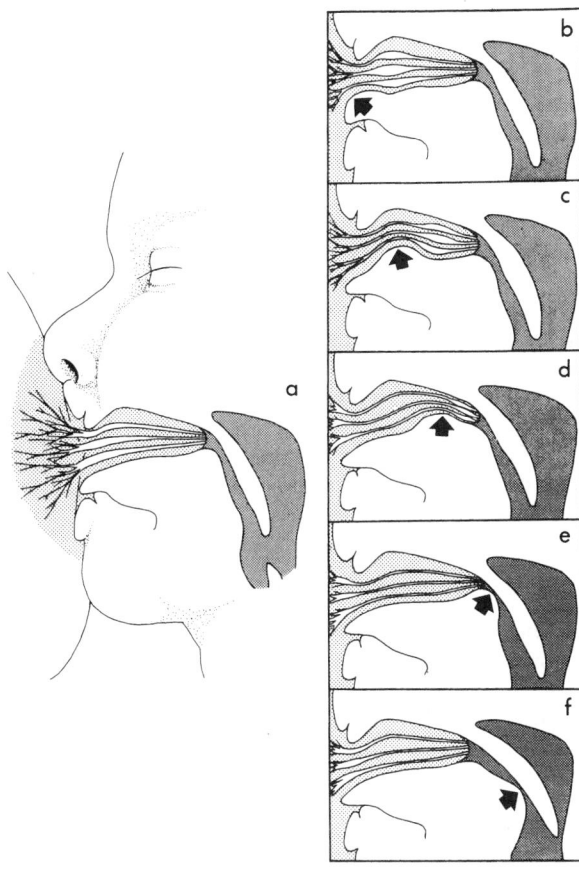

Fig. 6.1 Mechanism of sucking, from Woolridge (1986a) with permission. The figure shows a complete 'suck' cycle; the baby is shown in median section. The baby exhibits good feeding technique with the nipple drawn well into the mouth, extending back to the junction of the hard and soft palate (the lactiferous sinuses are depicted within the teat though these cannot be visualized on scans).

a. 'Teat' is formed from the nipple and much of the areola, with the lacteal sinuses, which lie behind the nipple, being drawn into the mouth with the breast tissue. The soft palate is relaxed and the nasopharynx is open for breathing. The shape of the tongue at the back represents its position at rest, cupped around the tip of the nipple.

b. The suck cycle is initiated by a welling up of the anterior tip of the tongue. At the same time the lower jaw, which had been momentarily relaxed (not shown), is raised to constrict the base of the nipple, thereby 'pinching off' milk within the ducts of the teat (these movements are inferred as they lie outside the sector viewed in ultrasound scans).

c. The wave of compression by the tongue moves along the underside of the nipple in a posterior direction, pushing against the hard palate. This roller-like action squeezes milk from the nipple. The posterior portion of the tongue may be depressed as milk collects in the oropharynx.

d, e. The wave of compression passes back past the tip of the nipple and pushes against the soft palate. As the tongue impinges on the soft palate the levator muscles of the palate contract raising it to seal off the nasal cavity. Milk is pushed into the oropharynx and is swallowed if sufficient has collected.

f. The cycle of compression continues and ends at the posterior base of the tongue. Depression of the back portion of the tongue creates negative pressure drawing the nipple and its milk contents once more into the mouth. This is accompanied by a lowering of the jaw which allows milk to flow back into the nipple.

In ultrasound scans it appears that compression by the tongue, and negative pressure within the mouth, maintain the tongue in close conformation to the nipple and palate. Events are portrayed here rather more loosely to aid clarity.

The duration of a breast-feed bears little relationship to the amount of milk consumed. Although a cross-sectional study suggested that, *on average*, 90% of the feed is consumed in the first 4 minutes, subsequent studies have shown that this conceals pronounced interindividual variation. It is impossible to formulate a rule applicable to all mothers and babies.

It is not necessary for babies to take both breasts at every feed. Babies adjust their milk intake to allow for variation in its fat (i.e. energy) content. When mothers were instructed to offer only one breast rather than both at each feed babies extracted more hindmilk, thereby consuming more fat and maintaining a constant total daily energy intake (Woolridge et al 1990). Moreover, if the mother curtails feeding at the first breast in order to offer both routinely there is a risk that the baby will consume excessive volumes of low-energy foremilk, leading to lactose overload with explosive, watery stools and 'colic'.

Maintaining lactation. Well babies need not be cared for in nurseries but disappointingly only two-thirds of babies born in British hospitals are with the mother continuously (i.e. 'rooming-in'; Table 6.4) in the postnatal period (White et al 1992). All breast-feeding mothers should be taught how to express milk by hand, though many prefer to use an electric pump. A mother should express milk about six times each day if separated from her baby, commencing as soon as possible after the birth. Expressed milk can be given by gavage, bottle or cup. The last is practicable for some babies of 30 weeks' gestation upwards (Lang et al 1994). Offering breast-fed babies supplementary feeds from a cup seems to cause less 'nipple confusion' than using a bottle though controlled studies have not been performed.

Contraindications to breast-feeding

There are few absolute contraindications to breast-feeding. Galactosemia is one, though with phenylketonuria it is usually possible to continue, supplementing with a low-phenylalanine formula according to blood phenylalanine concentrations. Maternal infections such as hepatitis B and tuberculosis do not contraindicate breast-feeding though in both cases the baby should be immunized (Akre 1989).

Human immunodeficiency virus (HIV) infection. HIV is present both in the cellular and aqueous fraction of breast milk of infected mothers. Transmission of HIV to the baby of a breast-feeding mother, herself known to have been postnatally infected by blood transfusion, is well described. In mothers infected antenatally the additional risk of vertical transmission attributable to breast-feeding has been estimated as 14% (95% CI 7–22%), whereas this rises to 29% (95% CI 16–42%) if the mother is infected postnatally (Dunn et al 1992). Currently, mothers in the UK known to be HIV antibody positive and those at risk of infection are counseled not to breast-feed. In countries with high infant mortality attributable to malnutrition or infectious disease the risk of bottle-feeding still outweighs the risk of vertical transmission of HIV and breast-feeding is recommended (WHO/UNICEF 1992).

Drugs in breast milk. There are very few instances in which maternal drug therapy need prevent breast-feeding; the decision should be based upon the toxicity of the drug, the quantity which the infant is likely to ingest, and the capacity of the infant to detoxify or excrete. Antimitotic agents are highly toxic and contraindicate breast-feeding even though the amount ingested may be small. The quantity of any drug passed into milk may either be measured or calculated from consideration of drug pK (milk pH = 7.2, i.e. < plasma pH) and lipid solubility. Passage of maternal drugs into breast milk has been comprehensively reviewed elsewhere (Atkinson et al 1988, Bennet 1988, American Academy of Pediatrics, Committee on Drugs 1994).

Growth of breast-fed babies

Growth charts in common use (such as the National Center for Health Statistics (NCHS) chart and Gairdner–Pearson chart) do not describe accurately the natural trajectory of the breast-fed infant who, in both industrialized and developing countries, grows rapidly in the first 2 months, slowing thereafter (Fig. 6.2; Dewey et al 1995b). This deceleration in weight velocity was once described as 'growth faltering' and speculatively attributed to a shortfall in energy intake from breast milk but it is now agreed that estimated energy requirements were then set too high. More recent recommendations probably still overestimate average requirements (Prentice et al 1988).

It is very important to note both that the apparent early weight spurt should not be interpreted as 'overfeeding' and that the deceleration after 2 months should not be construed per se as 'growth faltering' attributable to inadequate breast milk supply.

How long is breast milk sufficient on its own?

Several recent prospective studies have measured protein: energy intakes and growth during infancy. Bottle-fed infants consumed 66–70% more protein in the first 6 months than those exclusively breast-fed (Heinig et al 1993) and, unlike breast-fed infants, did not reduce their milk intake when weaning foods were introduced (Stuff & Nichols 1989). At 1 year old, bottle-fed infants were heavier and fatter than breast-fed though length and head circumference were similar (Heinig et al 1993; Dewey et al 1993).

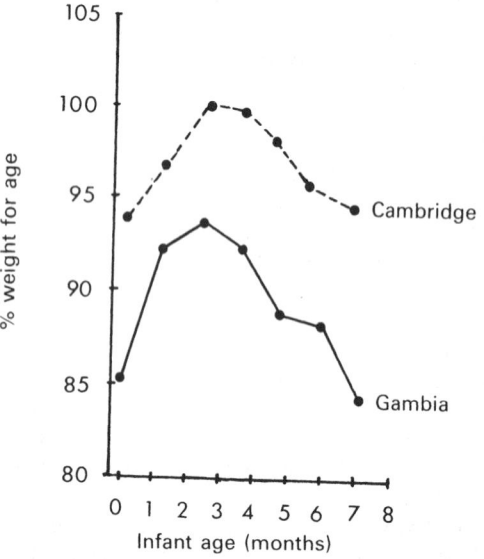

Fig. 6.2 The weight trajectory of breast-fed infants showing the normal acceleration relative to standard growth charts in the early months of life. (From Whitehead & Paul (1984), with permission.)

These growth differences may reflect the greater energy intake of bottle-fed babies and, perhaps, the insulinogenic stimulus of their greater protein intake. The long-term implications are not known.

Current recommendations of the World Health Organization are that babies be breast-fed exclusively for the first 4–6 months of life. When Honduran breast-fed babies were randomly allocated to receive solids at either 4 or 6 months both *total* daily energy intake and growth rate were comparable: breast milk intake simply fell in those weaned early as solid food intake rose (Cohen et al 1994, 1995). This suggests that breast-feeding alone is sufficient for at least the first 6 months of life but supply of other nutrients, particularly trace elements, requires further study. Moreover the adequacy of growth alone as a measure of nutritional adequacy is hotly debated for the reasons given above. Functional outcome measures (e.g. neurodevelopmental progress, immune function, long-term morbidity) need to be correlated with patterns of infant growth to address the unanswered question: 'Is bigger necessarily better?'.

Supplements for breast-fed babies

Vitamin K. Dietary deficiency of vitamin K may result in hemorrhagic disease of the newborn (HDN) (p. 230). Human milk contains less vitamin K than cow's milk or formula (Tables 6.5 and 6.6) and supplementation has been recommended for some years. An intramuscular injection of vitamin K (1 mg

Table 6.5   Composition of mature human milk

Total nitrogen	2.1 g/l
Protein	10.7 g/l
Casein	41% of total protein
α-lactalbumin	28% of total protein
Lactoferrin	14% of total protein
Serum albumin	2% of total protein
Lysozyme	1% of total protein
Secretory IgA	14% of total protein
Nonprotein nitrogen	0.4 g/l
Fat	42 g/l
Cholesterol	0.42 mmol/l
Carbohydrate	74 g/l
Total energy	700 kcal/l
Sodium (23)	6.5 mmol/l
Potassium (39)	15.4 mmol/l
Calcium (40)	8.8 mmol/l
Magnesium (24)	1.2 mmol/l
Phosphorus (31)	4.8 mmol/l
Chloride (35)	12.3 mmol/l
Iron (56)	13.6 μmol/l
Copper (64)	6 μmol/l
Zinc (65)	45 μmol/l
Vitamin A (retinol)	600 μg/l
Vitamin D	0.1 μg/l
Vitamin E	3500 μg/l
Vitamin K	15 μg/l
Thiamin (B_1)	160 μg/l
Riboflavin (B_2)	310 μg/l
Nicotinic acid	2300 μg/l
Pyridoxine (B_6)	59 μg/l
Vitamin B_{12}	0.1 μg/l
Folic acid	52 μg/l
Pantothenic acid	2600 μg/l
Biotin	7.6 μg/l
Vitamin C	38 mg/l

(DHSS 1977). Atomic weights of minerals in parentheses.

Table 6.6 Composition of cow's milk and infant formula

	Cow's milk	Formula
Major nutrients		
Protein	33	15–20* g/l
Casein:whey	79:21	80:20 or 40:60
Carbohydrate	48	48–100 g/l
Fat	38	23–50 g/l
Linoleic and linoleic acid		>1% of total energy
Minerals		
Sodium	50 (35–90)	15–35 mg/dl
Potassium	150 (110–170)	50–100 mg/dl
Chloride	95 (90–110)	40–80 mg/dl
Calcium	120 (110–130)	30–120 mg/dl
Phosphorus	95 (90–100)	15–60 mg/dl
Ca:P ratio	1.2:1	1.2–2.2:1
Magnesium	12 (9–14)	2.8–12 mg/dl
Iron	50 (30–60)	70–700 μg/dl
Zinc	350 (200–600)	200–600 μg/dl
Copper (see text)	20 (10–60)	10–60 μg/dl
Vitamins		
A (retinol)	31 (27–36)†	40–150 μg/dl
D	0.02	0.7–1.3 μg/dl
E (α-tocopherol)	0.09	>0.3 mg/dl
K	1–8.5	>1.5 μg/dl
C	2	>3 mg/dl
Thiamin (B_1)	40 (30–60)	>13 μg/dl
Riboflavin (B_2)	190 (150–230)	>30 μg/dl
Nicotinamide (B_3)	80(60–130)	>230 μg/dl
Pyridoxine (B_6)	40 (21–72)	>5 μg/dl
B_{12}	0.3	>0.01 μg/dl
Pantothenic acid	0.35 (0.2–0.5)	>200 μg/dl
Biotin	2 (1.0–1.3)	>0.5 μg/dl
Folic acid	5	>3 μg/dl

Data from DHSS (1980).
* May be <1.5 if casein:whey ratio 40:60.
† Summer–winter range for vitamins.

phytomenadione) offers the most effective prophylaxis (McNinch & Tripp 1991) but was associated in one study with an increased incidence of later childhood malignancy (Golding et al 1992). Although several other studies have not confirmed this association (Draper & McNinch 1994) there has been a move towards oral supplementation. Practice varies considerably but a common regimen involves giving 500 mcg orally at birth, repeated at 7–10 days and 4–6 weeks of age. An alternative may be to give further doses of 25 mcg daily or 1 mg weekly as in the Netherlands (Uitentuis 1990, Cornelissen et al 1993). There have been no controlled studies of alternative regimens but efficacy is currently being evaluated by case audit of HDN. A further problem has been lack of a vitamin K preparation licensed for oral administration.

Babies who have liver disease, malabsorption or receive prolonged broad spectrum antibiotics require continued supplementation in higher doses.

Vitamin D. Breast milk contains less calcium, phosphate and vitamin D than cow's milk or infant formula but rickets is rare among breast-fed babies in the UK. It is nevertheless occasionally seen in babies of dark-skinned ethnic minority groups, particularly if sunlight exposure is reduced or the mother has not received vitamin D supplements in pregnancy. The baby should be given a supplement of 400 iu/day (10 mg) under such circumstances.

Iron. Breast milk contains little iron but its bioavailability is high. The iron stores of 6-month-old breast-fed babies who had

been born at term were similar to those of babies fed iron-fortified infant formula. Thus breast-fed babies do not require iron supplements unless additional risk factors are present (e.g. low birthweight, delayed weaning). There are potential hazards in giving iron supplements to babies who do not need them: weight gain may be impaired (Idrajinata et al 1994) and zinc absorption reduced.

Water. Many studies have confirmed that it is unnecessary to offer water to breast-fed babies. The solute load of breast milk is low enough to permit free water availability even in tropical climates (reviewed by Martinez et al 1992).

Fluoride. See Dental health, page 334.

Breast-fed babies who fail to thrive

Physiological failure of milk supply is rare. Faulty breast-feeding technique more often underlies poor weight gain and expert midwifery counseling is essential. A history of early feeding difficulty or nipple pain may be obtained, the baby eventually becoming undemanding and sleepy. Breast engorgement or mastitis may have occurred, again indicating ineffective drainage. Physical illness in the baby needs to be excluded, particularly if change has been recent. Otherwise attention to technique and increasing the frequency of feeds, sometimes combined with expression may help to increase supply. There is no evidence that metoclopramide or other drugs more effectively increase supply than the physiological approach suggested.

Test-weighing using mechanical scales underestimates intake and is of no clinical value at all. Electronic scales improve weighing precision but may still undermine the mother's confidence and raise problems of interpretation. Firstly, test-weighing must proceed for *at least* 48 hours to take account of day-to-day and circadian variation. Secondly, the range of normal is very wide and the baby's milk consumption less than the mother's potential yield; the intake of one group of 3-month-old babies varied from 523–1124 g/day but, on average, a further 100 g could be obtained by expression (Dewey et al 1991). Finally, the baby's energy intake cannot be derived from weighed milk intake as the fat content of breast milk varies so much and tends to be inversely proportional to the volume of milk consumed (Woolridge et al 1990). For all these reasons test-weighing is of very limited value in the clinical context; it is much more important to diagnose and correct problems with breast-feeding technique.

INFANT FORMULA FEEDING

An '*infant formula*' is legally defined as a product which by itself meets the nutritional requirements of normal healthy infants in the first 4–6 months of life. The composition of infant formula is controlled by European Community and UK legislation (MAFF 1995). '*Follow-on formula*' is intended for use by normal healthy infants over 6 months of age (DoH 1994) as 'the principal liquid element in a progressively diversified diet'. It is not legally required to meet by itself the infant's entire nutritional needs.

Unmodified cow's milk is unsuitable for feeding infants. Amongst other things it generates a high *renal solute load* (p. 333), has an inappropriate calcium : phosphorus ratio, and is relatively low in iron and vitamin content. Some years ago a DHSS report set compositional guidelines for infant formula manufacturers. The philosophy underlying these was that the nutrient content of infant formula should match as closely as possible that of mature human milk, unless significant differences in nutrient bioavailability existed between breast milk and formula (as is the case, for example, with iron and protein; see below).

Although this principle has continued to influence formula manufacture a recent report (DoH 1996) has proposed that innovations should also produce demonstrable benefit in *outcome*, matching as closely as possible the nutritional optimum of the healthy breast-fed infant. This change has been stimulated by increasing appreciation of the molecular complexity of human milk and by the application of novel processes (such as recombinant DNA technology) to produce human milk constituents in vitro for addition to formula. It is essential to demonstrate that such developments will be both effective and safe.

Composition of human milk

The composition of expressed human milk has been extensively studied in view of its relevance to formula manufacture (Goedhart & Bindels 1994). Table 6.5 is based on a study of the composition of mature human milk expressed by British mothers. It is worth noting briefly the factors which affect milk composition and some important qualitative nutritional differences between human milk and formula (e.g. protein, fat, minerals and vitamins).

Factors affecting milk composition:

Gestation of baby. Most studies have found milk of mothers delivering prematurely to be higher in protein and sodium content but lower in lactose. Many differences can be explained by reduced milk output but serum leakage due to immaturity of mammary epithelial integrity might be relevant.

Maternal diet and nutritional state. The effect of maternal diet on the output and macronutrient content of breast milk has been overstated in the past. Lactational efficiency is unaffected by maternal body mass index (BMI) (Prentice & Prentice 1995) and nutritional supplementation of malnourished mothers is of little or no benefit.

Stage of lactation affects all milk constituents. Early milk is arbitrarily classified as *colostrum* (0–5 days) or *transitional* milk (5–10 days). Thereafter it is termed *mature*. Protein concentration changes greatly in the early stages, mainly because the immunoglobulin content of colostrum falls about 50-fold in the first week. The total output of immunoglobulin A nevertheless changes little because the volume of milk produced increases. Sodium concentration similarly falls in early lactation as the lactose concentration rises. Amongst the micronutrients, iron and copper concentrations fall slowly during lactation but zinc drops about 10-fold over a year. The changes in protein, lactose and sodium content reverse at weaning so that colostrum, weaning milk and 'preterm milk' are very similar in composition.

Changes within a feed. Fat concentration changes most, more than doubling during a feed. It has been observed that the fat content of cow's milk rises as it is squeezed from a sponge and it is proposed that within-feed changes in fat are attributable to this physical effect.

Time of day. Fat concentration shows most change and is inversely related to the time which has elapsed since the last feed; the longer the interval the lower the fat. Sociocultural variation in nursing patterns considerably affects circadian changes in fat concentration for this reason (Jackson et al 1988).

Protein and nonprotein nitrogen. Estimates of human milk protein concentration vary between 0.8 and 1.3 g/dl for methodological reasons. The *crude protein* content is total nitrogen (g) $\times$ 6.38 which is always higher than the true figure as 25% of total nitrogen is *'nonprotein nitrogen'*. Some of this, including urea (Jackson 1994), is incorporated into body protein together with the principal nutritional proteins, α-lactalbumin and casein. Many milk proteins (e.g. secretory immunoglobulin A, lactoferrin; Table 6.3) do not primarily function as nutrients and can be recovered from the stool though their digestibility increases with age. This difference in the digestibility of human and cow's milk proteins is one reason that the protein content of an infant formula does not straightforwardly equate with that of human milk.

A further reason is the difference in *protein quality*, i.e. the relative match between the amino acid content of a dietary protein and the requirement for growth and metabolism. Protein quality can be expressed numerically either by essential 'amino acid score' or 'net protein utilization', the proportion of ingested protein which is retained. Human milk is used as a reference protein in both cases, e.g.:

$$\text{Amino acid score} = \frac{\text{mg limiting essential amino acid in 1 g test protein}}{\text{mg limiting essential amino acid in 1 g human milk protein}} \times 100\%$$

By regulation an infant formula must be based on soya or cow's milk protein. The latter has broadly two classes: whey (or acid-soluble) proteins and caseins (acid-precipitable curd). As whey and casein differ in amino acid composition the quality of cow's milk protein can be manipulated by changing the whey : casein ratio from 20 : 80 to 60 : 40, closer to that of human milk. Such formulae are known as *whey dominant*. The claim that casein-dominant formula 'satisfies hungry babies' has no justification, though British babies commonly change to these within the first 6 weeks (White et al 1992). Crude soya protein has a low amino acid score because it contains relatively little methionine. Consequently it is supplemented with this amino acid for use in formula.

The plasma amino acid concentrations of babies fed cow's milk protein based formula containing 1.25 or 1.3 g/100 ml cow's milk protein as opposed to the usual 1.5–2.0 g/dl (Table 6.6) more closely approximate those of breast-fed babies. The whey : casein ratio also has less effect at these intakes (Janas et al 1987, Lonnerdal & Zetterstrom 1988). Thus the protein content of current formulae might be higher than necessary.

Fat. Breast milk contains long (LCT) and medium chain triglycerides (MCT). The fat composition of milk varies extensively with maternal diet. Until recently it was believed that provision of the essential polyunsaturated fatty acids (PUFA) (C_{18}-2ω6) and linolenic acid (C_{18}-3ω3) in formula generated sufficient docosohexaenoic acid (C_{22}-6ω3) for neural myelination but it is now believed that pathways involved in elongation and desaturation of C_{18} fatty acids are immature at birth, particularly before term.

The ω6 : ω3 fatty acid concentrations of breast milk vary little with maternal diet, perhaps to ensure a constant supply for the infant (Koletzko et al 1992). Differences in the PUFA intake of breast- and formula-fed babies affect the phospholipid composition of brain and other tissues (Farquharson et al 1992,

1995) and a study of 4-month-old babies observed an effect of PUFA supplementation on neurodevelopmental quotient (Agostini et al 1995) but whether differences persist is unknown. The ratio $\omega 3 : \omega 6$ PUFA must also maintain plasma arachidonic acid (C_{20}-4ω6) concentrations or growth may slow (Carlson et al 1992).

Iron. Cow's milk contains less iron than human milk and, furthermore, cow's milk iron is less bioavailable. Formulae are therefore enriched with iron salts, usually ferric ammonium citrate. Formulae sold in the US vary widely in iron content; so-called 'regular' formula contains < 1 mg/l iron whereas 'iron-fortified' formulae contain > 10 mg/l. A recent randomized trial showed that infants fed an iron-fortified formula showed iron status and psychomotor development at 9 and 12 months of age superior to those fed standard formula (Moffatt et al 1994). Infant formulae sold in the UK contain 5–7 mg/l iron and it is consequently not possible to extrapolate the results of the American study to British practice. If the mother is not breast-feeding, continued use of infant formula or follow-on formula to 12 months of age is nevertheless important in building iron stores and preventing iron deficiency in the toddler years.

Manufacture of infant formula in simple terms changes the composition of cow's milk (Table 6.6) as follows:

1. The protein and electrolyte content of cow's milk (see 'solute load' below) are reduced.
2. The whey: casein blend may be altered to improve protein quality and digestibility.
3. The calcium and phosphorus content is reduced and the Ca : P ratio altered.
4. The carbohydrate content is increased by addition of lactose or maltodextrins.
5. The fat blend is changed using vegetable oil to reduce saturated fat intake and increase intake of polyunsaturated fat, thus improving fat absorption.
6. Trace minerals are added, particularly iron and copper.
7. Vitamins are added.

'Renal solute load'

Both glomerular filtration rate and tubular concentrating power are reduced in the newborn (see Ch. 5). This limits the clearance and elimination of urea produced if protein intake exceeds growth demands. The *renal solute load* of a feed is the total quantity of unutilized dietary solute which must be eliminated in available water. It can be calculated by summing urea production* and sodium and potassium chloride intake surplus to growth and nonurinary losses. Human milk generates a solute load of 79 milliosmoles/l and unmodified cow's milk 221 milliosmoles/l. Thus, an infant with maximal tubular concentrating power of 600 milliosmoles/l of urine will require at least 370 (or $221/600 \times 1000$) ml of water for the safe elimination of the solute load generated by a liter of cow's milk. A high insensible water loss caused by diarrhea or fever may restrict water available for solute excretion and therefore give rise to hypernatremia. Energy density also has a bearing on solute load because it affects milk intake, and thus water available for urine formation.

---

*Each gram of dietary protein over growth and maintenance requirements generates a solute load of 4 milliosmoles.

Milk consumption

The normal intake of both breast- and bottle-fed babies is extremely variable. The oft-quoted requirement of 150 ml/kg per day is merely a guideline. Intakes of healthy 0- to 2-month-old infants fed ad libitum with a standard formula were 169 ± 25 (1 SD) ml/kg per day (boys) and 157 ± 22 ml/kg per day (girls). Similarly, although the average breast milk intake of 3-month-old infants is 700–800 ml/day, there is approximately 100% difference between the extremes of the normal range (Dewey et al 1991).

Consequently one cannot specify a 'normal' milk intake for any individual infant. Acceptable intake is guaranteed by satisfactory growth. If the baby is not growing, intake should be increased to the upper end of the normal range (mean + 2 SD).

Soya formula and other milks

Soya formula is probably overused. It is suitable for vegan infant feeding but has a dubious role in the prophylaxis or treatment of cow's milk protein allergy as cross-sensitivity to soya protein occurs in 15–43% of affected children. A formula based on cow's milk protein hydrolysate is preferable both in proven cow's milk protein intolerance (CMPI) and postgastroenteritis lactose intolerance because CMPI often coexists (Wharton et al 1988).

Goat's and sheep's milk present too high a solute load for infants. Goat's milk is also low in folic acid. A modified goat's milk (Nanny) is sold for feeding infants but technically cannot be described as an 'infant formula' (p. 331) because such products must contain protein only from a soya or cow's milk source (MAFF 1995). Its use has not been widely evaluated and a formula based on cow's milk protein hydrolysate or free amino acids is preferable for infants intolerant of standard formula.

WEANING

'Weaning' is the gradual introduction of foods other than breast milk or formula. It principally functions to increase the energy density of the diet when demands outstrip what milk alone can supply but weaning foods are also an important source of vitamins and trace minerals. The weaning process also contributes more generally to infant development by encouraging tongue and jaw movements in preparation for speech, introducing new tastes and textures, and increasing social interaction with carers. Many 'behavioral' eating problems have their origin in weaning mismanagement (see Douglas 1995 for review).

Weaning should commence no earlier than 4 months and no later than 6 months of age (DoH 1994). It is disappointing to note that over 90% of British infants are weaned early (DoH 1992), particularly as respiratory symptoms and eczema were more common in infants given solids before 12 weeks of age (Forsyth et al 1993). By 1 year old the infant should be taking three meals a day in addition to breast-feeds or approximately 500 ml of either infant formula or follow-on formula from a cup. Milk remains an important nutrient source; for example 500 ml of breast milk will supply almost a third of the 1-year-old's daily protein requirement.

The weaning diet is influenced by culture and the dietary habits of the family; in industrialized societies most infants receive commercially packaged weaning foods but those prepared at home (without added salt or sugar) may better achieve the social functions of weaning, viz. introducing the infant to tastes and meals shared by the family. Early weaning foods need to be smooth, e.g. baby rice mixed with milk, so that a minimum of chewing is required. Puréed fruit and vegetables may be given after a couple of weeks, progressing to meat and fish about a month later. Foods are best introduced one at a time so that likes and dislikes are noted; potentially allergenic items such as gluten and egg are probably best deferred until the second half of infancy.

Weaning problems

The largest share of weaning problems is borne by infants in less-developed countries placed at risk of gastrointestinal infection and energy dilution. Traditional gruels may be less nutritious than milk; programs encouraging use of locally produced bean/flour mixes have effectively reduced the incidence of childhood malnutrition.

Vegetarian and ethnic minority diets. Certain minority groups (e.g. vegans, Rastafarians) have limited choice of weaning foods. Protein quality, zinc, iron and vitamin B_{12} intake may be low. Phytates may reduce mineral availability (especially calcium and iron) and increase dietary bulk, compromising energy intake. Suggestions for a suitable vegetarian weaning diet are summarized in Table 6.7 (Poskitt 1988).

Iron deficiency has its roots in progressive depletion of iron stores during infancy though it may not present until the second year of life. The most effective prophylactic measures are prolonged breast milk or formula feeding (preferably into the second year of life), provision of heme iron (as meat or fish) and vitamin C with meals (as vitamin drops or fruit), and prescription of iron supplements for babies of low birth weight. Tea is an unsuitable drink for infants as tannins complex iron and reduce availability.

Vitamin supplements

Formula is fortified with vitamins, and supplementation is unnecessary until cow's milk is introduced. Breast-fed babies should receive vitamin supplements (e.g. Department of Health vitamin ACD drops;† Abidec; Dalivit) from 6 months of age or in some cases earlier (p. 154). Vitamin supplements should be continued until 2 years of age, and preferably until 5 (DHSS 1988, DoH 1994).

Dental health

Water fluoridation reduces the incidence of dental caries but fluoride supplementation (0.25 mg/day from 6 months of age) is required if the supply is unfluoridated and the risk of caries high. Excessive supplementation causes enamel mottling and must be avoided. Teeth should be brushed after eating or drinking, initially without toothpaste but later with only a small (less than pea-sized) amount. Fluoride supplements should be reduced to take account of intake from toothpaste. Minimizing intake of non-milk extrinsic sugars without sacrificing diet palatability, and using a cup rather than a bottle for liquids also help to prevent caries.

Drinks and water

Boiled tap water is sufficient if required for bottle-fed babies under 6 months of age. Flavored drinks are unnecessary. Natural mineral water, or water drawn through a domestic softener is of unsuitable electrolyte content and should not be given to babies.

Displacement of milk with flavored drinks during weaning is a common cause of failure to thrive. Moreover it may increase non-milk extrinsic sugar (e.g. sucrose) intake to the extent that it exceeds the recommended maximum of 10% of energy intake (DoH 1994).

Pasteurized cow's milk

Pasteurized whole cow's milk should not be given to infants under 1 year of age and semiskimmed milk should be avoided in children under 2 years. Other milk products, such as cheese and yogurt, may be used from 6 months onwards.

Table 6.7 Suggestions for vegetarian weaning diets

Nutrient	Problem	Solution
Energy	Energy density reduced by water absorption and fiber content. Most fruit low in energy	Use oils in cooking and spreading fats on food. Cereals, pulses, bananas and avocados are energy dense
Protein	Quality variable	Mix complementary food groups to achieve balanced intake, i.e. milk (dairy), legumes, grains, green vegetables
Vitamins	Low B_{12}, D and riboflavin	Use eggs, vitamin D-supplemented margarine or fish oils (if permissible). Consider oral B_{12} supplement
Minerals	Phytates reduce availability (especially of iron). Zinc and calcium intakes may be low	Green leaf vegetables rich in iron. Vitamin C increases uptake. Dairy products important as calcium/zinc source

†Department of Health vitamin drops contain (per ml): 5000 units vitamin A, 2000 units vitamin D, 150 mg vitamin C. Dose = 5 drops/day.

REFERENCES

Agostini C, Trojan S, Bellù R, Riva E, Giovanni M 1995 Neurodevelopmental quotient of healthy term infants at 4 months and feeding practice: the role of long-chain polyunsaturated fatty acids. Pediatric Research 38: 262–266

Akre J (ed) 1989 Infant feeding: the physiological basis. Bulletin of the World Health Organization 67 (suppl): 1–108

American Academy of Pediatrics, Committee on Drugs 1994 The transfer of drugs and other chemicals into human milk. Pediatrics 93: 137–150

Atkinson H C, Begg B J, Darlow B A 1988 Drugs in human milk. Clinical Pharmacokinetics 14: 217–240

Auerbach K G, Avery J L 1980 Relactation: a study of 366 cases. Pediatrics 65: 236–242

Bauchner H, Leventhal J M, Shapiro E D 1986 Studies of breast feeding and infections. Journal of the American Medical Association 256: 887–892

Bennet P N (ed) 1988 Drugs and human lactation. Elsevier, Amsterdam

British Paediatric Association, Standing Committee on Nutrition 1994 Is breast feeding beneficial in the UK? Archives of Disease in Childhood 71: 376–380

Carlson S E, Cooke R J, Werkman S H, Tolley E A 1992 First year growth of preterm infants fed standard compared to marine oil (*n*-3)-supplemented formula. Lipids 27: 901–907

Cohen R J, Brown K H, Canahuati J, Rivera L, Dewey K G 1994 Effects of age of introduction of complementary foods on infant breast milk intake, total energy intake, and growth: a randomised intervention study in Honduras. Lancet 344: 288–293

Cohen R J, Brown K H, Canahuati J, Rivera L, Dewey K G 1995 Determinants of growth from birth to 12-months among breast-fed Honduran infants in relation to age of introduction of complementary foods. Pediatrics 96: 504–510

Cornelissen E A M, Kollee L A A, de Abreu R A, Motohara K, Monnens L A H 1993 Prevention of vitamin K deficiency in infancy by weekly administration of vitamin K. Acta Paediatrica 82: 656–659

Crawford M A 1993 The role of essential fatty acids in neural development; implications for perinatal nutrition. American Journal of Clinical Nutrition 57 (suppl): 703S–710S

Department of Health 1994 Weaning and the weaning diet. Report on Health and Social Subjects 45. HMSO, London

Department of Health 1995 Breastfeeding: good practice guidance to the NHS. HMSO, London

Department of Health 1996 Nutritional assessment of infant formula. Report on Health and Social Subjects 47. HMSO, London

Department of Health and Social Security 1977 The composition of mature human milk. Report on Health and Social Subjects 12. HMSO, London

Department of Health and Social Security 1980 Artificial feeds for the young infant. Report on Health and Social Subjects 18. HMSO, London

Department of Health and Social Security 1988 Present day practice in infant feeding; third report. Report on Health and Social Subjects 32. HMSO, London

Dewey K G, Heinig M J, Nommsen L, Lonnerdal B 1991 Maternal versus infant factors related to breast milk intake and residual volume: the DARLING study. Pediatrics 87: 829–837

Dewey K G, Heinig M J, Nommsen L A, Peerson J M, Lonnerdal B 1993 Breast-fed infants are leaner than formula-fed infants at 1 year of age. American Journal of Clinical Nutrition 57: 140–145

Dewey K G, Heinig J, Nommsen-Rivers L A 1995a Differences in morbidity between breast-fed and formula-fed infants. Journal of Pediatrics 126: 696–702

Dewey K G, Peerson J M, Brown K H et al 1995b Growth of breast-fed infants deviates from current reference data: a pooled analysis of US, Canadian and European data sets. Pediatrics 96: 495–503

Douglas J E 1995 Behavioural eating disorders in young children. Clinical Paediatrics 5: 39–42

Draper G, McNinch A 1994 Vitamin K for neonates: the controversy. British Medical Journal 308: 867–868

Duncan B, Ey J, Holberg C J, Wright A L, Martinez F D, Taussig L M 1993 Exclusive breast-feeding for at least 4-months protects against otitis media. Pediatrics 91: 867–872

Dunn D T, Newell M L, Ades A E, Peckham C S 1992 Risk of human immunodeficiency virus type 1 transmission through breastfeeding. Lancet 340: 585–588

Farquharson J, Cockburn F, Patrick W A, Jamieson E C, Logan R W 1992 Infant cerebral cortex fatty acid composition and diet. Lancet 340: 810–813

Farquharson J, Jamieson E C, Abbasi K A, Patrick W J A, Logan R W, Cockburn F 1995 Effect of diet on the fatty acid composition of the major phospholipids of the cerebral cortex. Archives of Disease in Childhood 72: 198–203

Florey C du V, Leech A M, Blackhall A 1995 Infant feeding and mental and motor development at 18-months of age in first born singletons. International Journal of Epidemiology 24 (suppl 1): S21–S26

Ford R P K, Taylor B J, Mitchell E A et al 1993 Breastfeeding and the risk of sudden infant death syndrome. International Journal of Epidemiology 22: 885–890

Forsyth J S, Ogston S A, Clark A, du Florey V, Howie P 1993 Relation between early introduction of solid food to infants and their weight and illnesses during the first two years of life. British Medical Journal 306: 1572–1576

Gerstein H C 1994 Cow's milk exposure type I diabetes mellitus. A critical overview of the clinical literature. Diabetes Care 17: 13–19

Gilbert R E, Wigfield R E, Fleming P J, Berry P J, Rudd P T 1995 Bottle feeding and the sudden infant death syndrome. British Medical Journal 310: 88–90

Goedhart A C, Bindels J G 1994 The composition of human milk as a model for the design of infant formulas: recent findings and possible applications. Nutrition Research Reviews 7: 1–23

Golding J, Greenwood R, Birmingham K, Mott M 1992 Childhood cancer, intramuscular vitamin K, and pethidine during labour. British Medical Journal 305: 341–346

Grulee C G, Sandford H N 1936 The influence of breast and artificial feeding on infantile eczema. Journal of Pediatrics 9: 223–225

Hawdon J M, Ward Platt M P, Aynsley-Green A 1992 Patterns of metabolic adaptation for preterm and term infants in the first neonatal week. Archives of Disease in Childhood 67: 357–365

Heinig M J, Nommsen L A, Peerson J M, Lonnerdal B, Dewey K G 1993 Energy and protein intakes of breast-fed and formula-fed infants during the first year of life and their association with growth velocity: the DARLING study. American Journal of Clinical Nutrition 58: 152–161

Howie P W, Forsyth J S, Ogston S A, Clark A, Florey C du V 1990 Protective effect of breastfeeding against infection. British Medical Journal 300: 11–16

Idrajinata P, Watkins W E, Pollitt E 1994 Adverse effect of iron supplementation on weight-gain of iron-replete young children. Lancet 343: 1252–1254

Jackson A A 1994 Urea as a nutrient: bioavailability and role in nitrogen economy. Archives of Disease in Childhood 70: 3–4

Jackson D A, Imong S M, Silprasert A et al 1988 Circadian variation in fat concentration of breast milk in a rural northern Thai population. British Journal of Nutrition 59: 349–363

Janas L M, Picciano M F, Hatch T F 1987 Indices of protein metabolism in term infants fed either human milk or formulas with reduced protein concentration and various whey/casein ratios. Journal of Pediatrics 110: 838–848

Karjalainen J, Martin J M, Knip M et al 1992 A bovine albumin peptide as a possible trigger of insulin-dependent diabetes. New England Journal of Medicine 327: 302–307

Koletzko B, Thiel I, Springer S 1992 Lipids in human milk: a model for infant formulae? European Journal of Clinical Nutrition 46 (suppl 4): S45–S55

Lang S, Lawrence C J, Orme R L'E 1994 Cup feeding: an alternative method of infant feeding. Archives of Disease in Childhood 71: 365–369

Lonnerdal B, Zetterstrom R 1988 Protein content of infant formula – how much and from what age? Acta Paediatrica Scandinavica 77: 321–325

Lucas A 1994 Role of nutritional programming in determining adult morbidity. Archives of Disease in Childhood 71: 288–290

Lucas A, Morley R, Cole T J, Lister G, Leeson-Payne C 1992 Breast milk and subsequent intelligence quotient in children born preterm. Lancet 339: 261–264

McNinch A W, Tripp J H 1991 Haemorrhagic disease of the newborn in the British Isles: a two-year prospective study. British Medical Journal 303: 1105–1109

Martinez J C, Rea M, de Zoysa I 1992 Breastfeeding in the first six months British Medical Journal 304: 1068–1069

Ministry of Agriculture, Fisheries and Food 1995 Infant Formula and Follow-on Formula Regulations 1995. Statutory Instrument No. 77. HMSO, London

Moffatt M E K, Longstaffe S, Besant J, Dureski C 1994 Prevention of iron deficiency and psychomotor decline in high risk infants through use of an iron-fortified infant formula: a randomised controlled trial. Journal of Pediatrics 125: 527–534

Newcomb P A, Storer B E, Longnecker M P et al 1994 Lactation and a reduced risk of premenopausal breast cancer. New England Journal of Medicine 330: 81–87

Poskitt E M E 1988 Vegetarian weaning. Archives of Disease in Childhood 63: 1286–1292

Prentice A M, Prentice A 1995 Evolutionary and environmental influences on human lactation. Proceedings of the Nutrition Society 54: 391–400

Prentice A M, Lucas A, Vasquez-Velasquez L, Davies P S W, Whitehead R G 1988 Are current dietary guidelines a prescription for overfeeding in infancy? Lancet ii: 1066–1068

Royal College of Midwives 1988 Successful breastfeeding. Royal College of Midwives, London

Saarinen U M, Kajosaari M 1995 Breastfeeding as prophylaxis against atopic disease: prospective follow-up study until 17-years old. Lancet 346: 1065–1069

Stuff J E, Nichols B L 1989 Nutrient intake and growth performance of older infants fed human milk. Journal of Pediatrics 115: 959–968

Uitentuis J 1990 Toediening van vitamine K aan pasgeborenen en zuigelingen. Nederlands Tijdschrift voor Geneeskunde 14: 1642–1646

UK National Case-Control Study Group 1993 Breast feeding and risk of breast cancer in young women. British Medical Journal 307: 17–20

UNICEF 1992 The state of the world's children 1992. Oxford University Press, Oxford, pp 74–75

Victora C G, Smith P G, Vaughan J P et al 1987 Evidence for protection by breastfeeding against infant deaths from infectious diseases in Brazil. Lancet ii: 319–322

Wharton B A, Pugh R E, Taitz L S, Walker-Smith J A, Booth I W 1988 Dietary management of gastroenteritis in Britain. British Medical Journal 296: 450–452

White A, Freeth S, O'Brien M 1992 Infant feeding 1990. Office of Population Censuses and Surveys, HMSO, London

Whitehead R G, Paul A A 1984 Growth charts and the assessment of infant feeding practices in the western world and in developing countries. Early Human Development 9: 187–207

WHO/UNICEF 1989 Protecting, promoting and supporting breast-feeding: The special role of maternity services. World Health Organization, Geneva

WHO/UNICEF 1992 Statement on breastfeeding and HIV. Weekly Epidemiological Record 67: 177–184

Woolridge M W 1986a The 'anatomy' of infant feeding. Midwifery 2: 164–171

Woolridge M W 1986b The aetiology of sore nipples. Midwifery 2: 172–176

Woolridge M W, Ingram J C, Baum J D 1990 Do changes in pattern of breast usage alter the baby's nutrient intake? Lancet 336: 395–397

7 Preventive pediatrics

H. Campbell   W. A. M. Cutting

Principles of prevention   338
Preventive measures   338
Preconceptual prevention   338
Preventive measures during pregnancy   338
   Early pregnancy   338
   Late pregnancy   338
Prevention in the neonatal period   338
   Screening procedures   339
Prevention in infancy and childhood   339
Prevention in later childhood and adolescence   340
Prevention and protection through immunization   341
The importance and efficacy of immunization in prevention of disease   341
Vaccines – past, present and future   341
Adverse reactions and contraindications to immunization   342
   Side-effects of DPT vaccination   343

Contraindications to pertussis and other vaccines   343
Immunization schedules   343
   Basic principles   343
   Developing country schedules   344
Specific immunizations   345
   Measles and rubella in the UK   345
   Poliomyelitis vaccines   345
   Pertussis acellular vaccines   345
   Varicella vaccine   345
Immunization for international travel   345
Immunization coverage – improving uptake   345
   Causes of poor uptake   345
   Improving knowledge, information and training   346
   Operational measures   346
   Practical issues   346
References   347

Any child's health, development and welfare reflect the interaction of genetic endowment (see Ch. 3), family and social circumstances, and environment from conception, through pregnancy, childbirth and beyond. The provision of adequate, appropriate and hygienic food, water, housing, clothing and a healthy temperature are widely recognized as the basic rights of every child because they promote health and prevent disease (UNICEF 1989). Security, stability, a loving family and appropriate stimulation provide the necessary social environment for normal emotional and intellectual development (Inequalities in Health 1988). Social and economic policy can have an important impact on child health (Spencer 1991). In contrast, medical science and health services have made, and can make, only a limited contribution to prevention of ill health. The greater impact of political action, economic progress, improved education and social change is shown by falling morbidity and mortality long before antibiotics, vaccines and high-technology medicine became available (Fig. 7.1). The health of the child's mother is also an

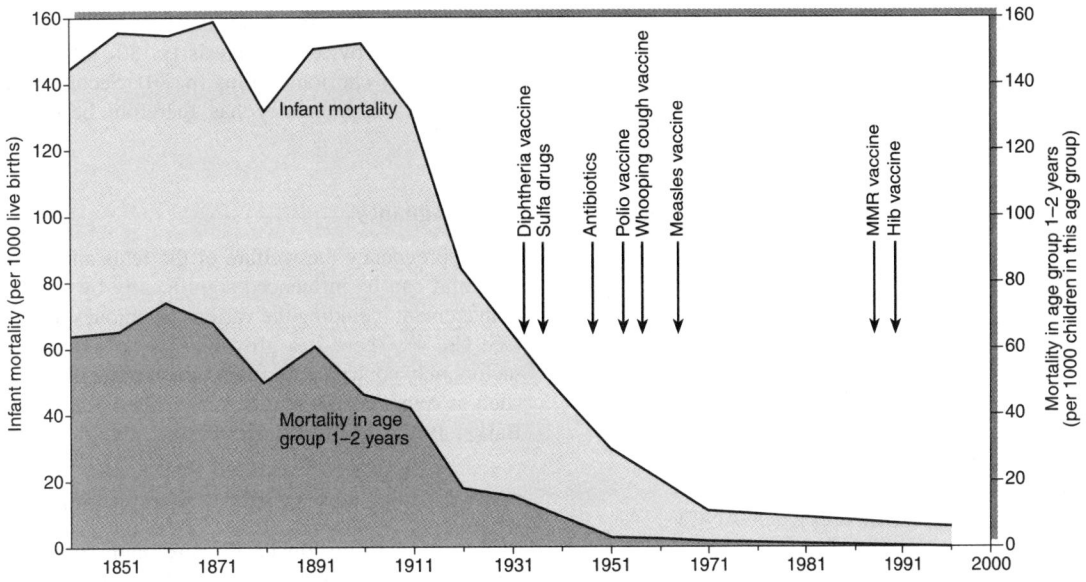

Fig. 7.1   Infant mortality in England and Wales and important developments in medicine.

important factor in determining the health of the child, whether this be, for example, in ensuring proper antenatal care of mothers with diabetes or treating and supporting mothers with psychiatric problems or alcohol addiction. It is in this context that this chapter presents the actions that can be taken principally by health services to promote child health and development and prevent childhood illness and handicap. Preventive medicine usually requires skilled teamwork to work with children and their families, often with colleagues outside the health services such as teachers and social workers. Preventive actions relevant to promoting child health in developing countries are presented in Chapter 35.

PRINCIPLES OF PREVENTION

Primary prevention implies specific measures which reduce the *incidence* of disease by controlling causes or risk factors (e.g. vaccination against poliomyelitis to prevent poliovirus infection and its attendant risks of paralysis, or the use of condoms to prevent HIV infection).

Secondary prevention aims to treat patients either in order to cure them or to reduce the more serious consequences of disease through early diagnosis and treatment. This reduces the *prevalence* of the disease (e.g. screening for hypothyroidism in neonates permits early replacement of deficient thyroxine and prevents the disabilities of cretinism). The term secondary prevention can also be applied to the termination of pregnancy to avoid the birth of a fetus with a recognized severe impairment.

Tertiary prevention aims to reduce the progress or complications of established disease. It consists of measures to reduce impairments and disabilities from the disease or injury and so minimize any handicap which may result. Thus after developmental screening (secondary prevention) has revealed motor, visual or hearing impairments before disabilities have become apparent, consequent early application of remedial measures (tertiary prevention) may limit the adverse effects of such impairments. For example, tertiary prevention through the rehabilitation of children with polio can enable them to take part in daily social life and bring about a great improvement in the well-being of these children.

PREVENTIVE MEASURES

PRECONCEPTUAL PREVENTION

Genetic factors in either parent, the present and past health of the mother, her age, her diet, her habits (e.g. smoking, alcohol), the frequency of her pregnancies, her previous immunizations (e.g. rubella and tetanus) and her social class are all factors which can potentially influence the health of her infant before it is conceived. Control or elimination of adverse factors will play an important part in prevention, e.g. the introduction of anti-D immunoglobulin for rhesus (Rh) negative mothers has significantly reduced the incidence of Rh incompatibility (see p. 232) and adequate consumption of folic acid before conception and during the first 2–3 months of pregnancy significantly reduces the risk of neural tube defects (MRC 1991, Czeizel & Dudas 1992).

PREVENTIVE MEASURES DURING PREGNANCY

Early pregnancy

In early pregnancy preventive measures include the avoidance of

teratogenic drugs and the prevention and cure of infections which might damage the fetus (p. 89). The following drugs and chemicals have been found to be associated with fetal defects: diphenylhydantoin (phenytoin), trimethadione, paramethadione, valproic acid, carbamazepine, thioureas, carbimazole, methimazole, isotretinoin vitamin A, etretinate, thalidomide, warfarin, methotrexate, corticosteroids, androgens, progestins, diethylstilbestrol, iodines, lithium, mercury and chlorobiphenyls. A number of other drugs and chemicals have featured in retrospective studies or case reports but associations with fetal defects have not been confirmed by subsequent investigations (see Stevenson 1993 for a further discussion). Exposure to abdominal X-rays should be avoided, but there is no evidence that ultrasound examinations are harmful to the fetus. The effects of a pregnant woman's smoking or alcohol (p. 91) consumption on her fetus are now well recognized and demand preventive action. Smoking can lead to intrauterine growth retardation, certain congenital anomalies and fetal loss. Excessive alcohol ingestion (above 1 oz absolute alcohol daily in early pregnancy) can lead to the fetal alcohol syndrome (Golding 1995). Routine screening for a number of conditions such as neural tube defects, rhesus hemolytic disease and maternal diabetes should be carried out (see Table 7.1). The 77% reduction in the birth prevalence of neural tube defects in the last 25 years is in part due to improved prenatal detection and selective termination of pregnancy. Recently, however, a link between low folate intake and neural tube defects has led to a national recommendation for all women to take oral folate supplements during pregnancy (Smithells et al 1980, Smithells 1996, Laurence et al 1981, MRC 1991). The risk of hyaline membrane disease can be reduced in preterm babies by the administration of steroids to the mother before or during preterm labor (Crowley 1993).

Individuals with a family history of a genetic disorder may undergo genetic testing. In the last 10 years there have been major advances in the understanding of the molecular basis of medical disorders and in the development of new techniques to identify genes associated with disease. Most of the genes for the more common inherited disorders have now been identified (see Ch. 3). This in turn often makes prenatal detection and genetic counseling possible (House of Commons 1995, Motulsky 1994). In conjunction with this there have been advances in prenatal diagnosis, e.g. by amniocentesis (p. 80), ultrasound techniques and biopsy of chorionic villus (p. 80). Secondary prevention by termination of pregnancy has therefore become more widely practiced.

Late pregnancy

In late pregnancy the welfare of the fetus and ultimate health of the child can be influenced significantly by competent obstetric management including the various techniques for fetal monitoring (see Ch. 4). There is a growing body of evidence that prenatal factors may contribute to important chronic diseases in adulthood such as hypertension and coronary heart disease (Barker 1995a, Barker 1995b, Law & Barker 1994).

PREVENTION IN THE NEONATAL PERIOD

Good intrapartum obstetric care and subsequent effective monitoring, investigation and treatment of the many disorders from which the newborn infant may suffer are important

Table 7.1 Current genetic screening programs in the UK (modified from Nuffield 1993)

Age group	Disease	Population screened	Type of screening test	Comments
Neonatal	Phenylketonuria	All newborn infants	Indirect	
	Hypothyroidism	All newborn infants	Indirect	
	Sickle-cell disease	All newborn in some areas; confined to certain ethnic groups in others	Indirect	Also detects carriers
	Cystic fibrosis	Some areas only (still at pilot stage)	Indirect	
	Duchenne muscular dystrophy	Pilot studies	Indirect	
	Other rare metabolic disorders	Family testing	Usually indirect	
Later childhood		NONE IN THE UK		
Premarital and prepregnancy	Cystic fibrosis	Pilot projects in general practice	Direct	Detects 85–90% of carriers
During pregnancy	Rhesus hemolytic disease	All mothers	Indirect	
	Diabetes mellitus	All mothers	Indirect	Fetuses have expert fetal anomaly scanning
	Congenital malformations	Most fetuses	Routine ultrasound	Confirm with fetal anomaly ultrasound
	Down syndrome	1. All mothers in some areas	Serum screening tests	Amniocentesis with chromosome tests on fetus required for confirmation
		2. All mothers over 35–37	Chromosome tests on fetus	
	Neural tube defects (spina bifida and anencephaly)	All mothers in many areas	Indirect	Confirm with fetal anomaly ultrasound
	Hemoglobin disorders	All mothers not of North European origin	Indirect	Detects carriers
	Cystic fibrosis	Pilot studies	Direct	Detects 85–90% of carriers

preventive measures. Such disorders include asphyxia, birth injury, low birthweight and hyperbilirubinemia (see Ch. 5). Vitamin K should be given to all babies at birth. The British Paediatric Association recommended oral vitamin K 500 μg at birth with a repeated dose at 4–6 weeks for breast-fed babies only (p. 230). However, there has been concern that although oral vitamin K is effective in preventing early hemorrhagic disease of the newborn, it is ineffective in preventing late disease in settings in which compliance in taking repeated oral doses is low (Zipursky 1996). Concerns about the possible increased incidence of childhood leukemia and cancer have been substantially allayed by the results of recent large case control studies which have shown no increased risk (Ansell et al 1996, Von Kries et al 1996, Zipursky 1996).

The promotion of breast-feeding is an important preventive measure. Breast-feeding reduces the risk of diarrheal disease, lower respiratory infections, otitis media, necrotizing enterocolitis and other serious neonatal infections (Campbell & Jones 1994). Recent evidence has linked lack of breast-feeding with poorer intellectual development, possibly due to the lack of certain long chain fatty acids, essential for normal brain development, in most breast milk substitutes (Lucas et al 1992, Florey et al 1995). Frequent breast feeds given over a prolonged period also significantly reduce fertility and the birth interval, with indirect benefits to both mother and infant (McNeilly 1979).

WHO and UNICEF are coordinating a global initiative (the Baby Friendly Hospital Initiative) to promote breast-feeding and to improve health service support for breast-feeding mothers. Many hospital routines and practices discourage women from breast-feeding or make it difficult for them to do so successfully (Anonymous 1994, Campbell et al 1995, Beeken & Waterston 1992). Good practice guidelines have been developed for maternity hospitals (see Table 6.4, p. 328). Improving hospital practices and staff skills in line with these guidelines has been shown to improve breast-feeding rates (Campbell & Jones 1994, Perez-Escamilla et al 1994).

Screening procedures

A number of preventive screening procedures are used in the neonatal period (see Table 7.1). These include: examination for congenital dislocation of the hips (p. 110); the careful routine examination of all newborn infants (Hall 1996); and a number of specific biochemical screening tests (e.g. for metabolic disorders such as phenylketonuria and galactosemia, and for congenital hypothyroidism (Table 7.1)). In some regions routine genetic screening for Duchenne muscular dystrophy (Wales) and cystic fibrosis (Victoria State, Australia; Wisconsin, USA) has been carried out for a number of years (Fenton-May et al 1994).

PREVENTION IN INFANCY AND CHILDHOOD

Breast-feeding should be maintained for at least 3 months. Its protective action against diarrheal and respiratory disease persists throughout the first year of life (Howie et al 1990). In infancy and childhood curative medicine can have an important preventive role. Early diagnosis and effective treatment of diseases such as meningitis, pneumonia, otitis media, osteomyelitis and patent ductus arteriosus can prevent chronic illness or permanent handicap in some children following these conditions.

Accidents cause nearly half of all deaths at ages 1–19 years in the UK (Jarvis et al 1996). The cause of the accidents, and therefore the preventive action, varies with the age of the child.

Important preventive measures include: using appropriate child car restraints; road safety education; child-proof containers for drugs; home safety devices such as stair gates and fire alarms; the design and installation of safe playground apparatus and surfaces; and the proper supervision of children near water (see Ch. 29).

Sudden infant death syndrome. Infants should be put to sleep on their backs and should not be overwrapped nor exposed to cigarette smoke in the home. These measures have been shown to substantially reduce the incidence of sudden infant death syndrome (DOH 1993). Recent studies, carried out in several countries after reductions in sudden infant death rates which followed health education campaigns promoting these messages, have highlighted the fact that further declines could be achieved by reducing maternal smoking (Dwyer & Ponsonby 1996, Blair et al 1996).

Immunization against polio, pertussis, tetanus, diphtheria, measles, mumps, *Haemophilus influenzae* type b, tuberculosis and, in some settings, hepatitis B continue to be important routine preventive measures for all children (see below).

Diet. A healthy diet should be promoted. Dietary guidelines have been published by many authorities (AAP 1976, DHSS 1984, BMA 1986, SHHD 1993). These combine concerns about achieving recommended daily intakes of selected essential nutrients with the need to reduce risks of chronic diseases of adulthood which are partly attributed to diet. In addition, in certain circumstances supplements may be necessary, e.g. iron for premature babies, iodine where specific deficiency is endemic, vitamins A, C and D for breast-fed babies after 6 months of age (Clark & Wharton 1995). The diet should contain adequate sources of available iron. Recent studies in the UK have shown a prevalence of iron deficiency anemia of up to 25% in young children, particularly in some ethnic minority communities. Effects on mental and motor development can be reversed if treatment is prompt (see Ch. 15). Much dental caries can be prevented by fluoride supplements where local water supplies are deficient (p. 334). There is evidence that diet and other factors in childhood can contribute directly to health problems in adult life (Falkner 1980).

Exposure to *harmful chemicals* in the diet, water or environment should be prevented or reduced, e.g. lead (p. 1708) and passive smoking (p. 493). In susceptible individuals the avoidance of food additives such as tartrazine derivatives (p. 1701) or allergens such as pollen or house dust mites may be attempted.

The prevention of *carcinogenesis* by chemicals or ionizing radiation has aroused scientific and political interest in recent years. The relative risks and potential for prevention require further study. Pediatricians should be aware of the relative amount of radiation involved in various diagnostic imaging techniques (p. 1895).

Preventive drug prophylaxis still has a place in the secondary prevention of meningococcal disease (Kristiansen 1996, Massell et al 1988), in the primary and secondary prevention of rheumatic fever (Massell et al 1988, Dajani et al 1988) (p. 632), protecting the heart from bacterial endocarditis (Table 13.8), preventing tuberculosis in susceptible contacts (p. 1340), malaria prophylaxis (p. 1448) and perhaps most commonly of all, in anticonvulsive therapy.

A structured program of child health promotion should be carried out to prevent disease and to detect problems affecting growth and development at an early stage. This should comprise both primary prevention through health promotion activities and secondary prevention through child health surveillance. Health promotion should incorporate a coordinated and determined effort to address issues such as accident prevention, good nutrition and dental care, and full immunization coverage. There should be sufficient flexibility in any program to allow health staff to give more attention and time to families with complex needs and to decide the specific input which is most appropriate to the needs of individual children. Child health surveillance should include only those activities which have been shown to be safe and effective, and which meet the well established criteria for screening tests (Wilson & Jungner 1968). Details of the latest (1995) recommendations of the UK Joint Working Party on Child Health Promotion should be consulted for further details (Hall 1996). It is important that there are good referral arrangements to specialist services when abnormalities are detected. At a district or regional level existing national child health surveillance policies should be adopted (Hall 1996) and local health promotion policies on the issues noted above should be developed. Personal child health records should be made available to all families and their use by both families and health staff encouraged.

All health professionals in contact with children should be alert to the possibility of *child abuse*, particularly in cases of repeated multiple or unusual trauma or burns, or in children with developmental delay (HMSO 1989). Prompt recognition can prevent future abuse and can identify the need for counseling or specific treatment (Green 1993, Glaser 1991).

The Education Act 1981 required that health authorities inform education departments of children who may have *special educational needs*. A full assessment of the child is then made and a statement of special educational needs produced. This system involves the parents of the child in the assessment and focuses on the needs of the child rather than on categorization of the child by diagnostic label. These children often require medical support also and this is usually best provided by a multidisciplinary team such as those found in child development centers or 'district handicap teams'. The aim of these procedures is tertiary prevention – to limit the handicap which can result from specific impairments by early recognition of the child's medical and educational needs and then appropriate intervention.

PREVENTION IN LATER CHILDHOOD AND ADOLESCENCE

The prevention of smoking, alcohol addiction, abuse of drugs and related substances, unplanned and unwanted teenage pregnancy, sexually transmitted diseases including HIV and AIDS, family breakdown, and child abuse and neglect is particularly challenging. Considerable medical, social, economic and, in the view of some, spiritual or moral resources are required to meet these challenges. In addition health professionals need to collaborate in school health promotion programs to promote healthy lifestyles in young people, including adequate regular exercise and a healthy diet.

The health risks of smoking are well recognized. In a national survey carried out in 1990 a quarter of 15-year-olds were found to be regular smokers. In recent years more boys than girls smoke in mid-teen years (Charlton 1995, Holland & Fitzsimons 1991). It has been estimated that there are over 500 000 smokers aged 11–15 years in Britain, with about 100 000 of them likely to die as a result of their tobacco consumption (Amos 1991). Health professionals should routinely ask about smoking in older children and their parents, and provide advice and help where necessary on stopping smoking. Parents who cannot stop smoking should be encouraged not to smoke in the house or in front of their children. Health services should actively support any effective and appropriate action against the promotion of cigarettes and tobacco (Power 1996).

A national study in 1989 showed that 26% of 16–17-year-olds in the UK drank more than 8 units of alcohol on at least one occasion during a 1-week period (Goddard 1991). Concern over alcohol use in adolescents is based not only on related health problems (for example, one-third of all accidental deaths in 16–19-year-olds are associated with alcohol) but also on drunkenness and its related social problems.

In addition:

1. The abuse of volatile substances and drugs such as marijuana, heroin and cocaine has increased among adolescents in recent years.
2. Approximately 1% of girls aged 14–15 years in Britain conceive each year and over half of these result in abortion.
3. Levels of physical activity decline in teenage years so that over one-third of young men aged 16–24 years and over half of young women do not take regular exercise.
4. National dietary surveys have shown that nutrient and energy intakes are generally adequate but that iron intake in teenage girls is low and the contribution of fat to energy intake is higher than currently recommended (Power 1996).

Responses to these problems require action in the early teenage years before the problem is fully manifest. A combination of interventions to reinforce negative views of the unhealthy behavior must be mixed with the promotion of a positive view of health and of healthy behaviors such as nonsmoking as the norm. Action needs to involve not only a wide range of health, education and social work professionals but also relevant voluntary agencies and young people themselves through peer projects and requires to be part of an overall strategy involving both national and local action. Health professionals who care for children should maintain a high level of awareness and know where and how to seek assistance when faced with these problems.

PREVENTION AND PROTECTION THROUGH IMMUNIZATION

THE IMPORTANCE AND EFFICACY OF IMMUNIZATION IN PREVENTION OF DISEASE

Immunization is the deliberate stimulation of an immune response in a person by giving a specific 'vaccine' to protect against an infectious disease (Ada 1990, Moxon 1990). The vaccine is usually a protein similar to part of a virulent infectious organism that can be recognized by the individual's immune system which then produces antibodies and cell-mediated immunity against the antigen in the vaccine.

Active immunity is the protection produced by the individual and the effects are usually long lasting. *Passive immunity* protects by injected antibodies either in the form of human immunoglobulin or produced by some other biological process. This produces immediate protection which only lasts for some weeks or months, until the donated antibodies are broken down or used up by the individual.

The immediate goal of immunization is to prevent disease in individuals, but the ultimate goal is to eliminate or even eradicate a communicable disease. *Herd immunity* exists if the number of

people in a community who have active immunity against an infection exceeds a critical level. Above this, susceptible individuals are unlikely to contact someone with the infection. In this way transmission falls or stops without universal immunity (Anderson & May 1990).

Immunization is a simple, economic and effective form of control for some infectious diseases. The efficacy of immunization depends on the vaccines available, the biological and social response of individuals, the epidemiology, modes of transmission and reservoirs of pathogens, and the health service infrastructure for delivering the immunization.

VACCINES – PAST, PRESENT AND FUTURE

A vaccine is a protein antigen, originally derived from or similar to a bacterium, virus or protozoon, used for active immunization. The term was previously used exclusively for smallpox vaccine derived from cowpox lymph (from Latin *vacca*, a cow). It is now used for all forms of vaccines.

Vaccines may be live, killed, toxoids or genetically engineered.

A *live attenuated vaccine* is one which produces active immunity by causing a mild 'infection'. A virulent organism is weakened, usually by multiple subcultures in unfavorable conditions, so that it produces an antigenic response without the serious consequences of a wild organism infection. Crossreacting organisms are another type of live vaccine which causes the body to produce a defense against the virulent strain. The BCG (bacillus Calmette–Guérin) vaccine is an example of this. The BCG is a strain of *Myobacterium bovis* which was isolated and attenuated by Calmette and Guérin in 1906 at the Pasteur Institute and is now used widely for vaccination against tuberculosis (Fine & Rodrigues 1990). There are new candidate organisms being tested to replace BCG against TB (WHO 1995).

Killed, or *inactivated vaccine* is prepared from virulent organisms or preformed antigen inactivated by heat, phenol, formaldehyde or some other means. Classical pertussis vaccine is an example of a whole cell killed and inactivated vaccine. Such vaccines usually require a series of spaced injections to produce an immune response.

Component vaccines use parts of pathogens as antigens and the newer pertussis vaccines are examples of this (Moxon & Rappuoli 1990, Edwards & Decker 1996). Meningococcal and pneumococcal vaccines are derived from the mucopolysaccharide coat of specific bacteria (Shann 1990). The response to polysaccharide vaccines is incomplete and unreliable and consequently these have sometimes been conjugated with other antigens in an attempt to improve the immunological response. An example is the linkage of *H. influenzae* polysaccharide with the pertussis antigen of DPT vaccine (Lepow et al 1984) and diphtheria toxoid (Lepow et al 1987) to produce a vaccine conjugate capable of stimulating T cells and thus eliciting immunological memory. An adjuvant is another product, for example an aluminum compound, combined with a vaccine to increase antigenicity and prolong the effect as in diphtheria and tetanus toxoids.

Toxoids also induce active immunity. A toxoid is an inactivated toxin preparation. The serious consequences of some diseases are due to toxins released by the organisms when they infect the patient. Diphtheria and tetanus toxins are examples of this. Toxoids from these produce antibodies which inactivate the toxins but do not kill the bacteria.

Vaccinology is the application of molecular biology to produce the vaccines of the future (Plotkin 1993). Conventional vaccine development depended upon the identification and isolation of an infectious agent, the production of that organism in a culture system, killing or attenuation of the organism and then the testing of the resulting antigen for potency and safety. Molecular biology has opened the way to the identification of key antigenic sites in organisms, an epitope or short sequence of amino acids which is responsible for the specific interaction between antibody and antigen (Brown 1990). It is possible to develop vaccines of small specific proteins, synthetic polypeptides or even 'naked' DNA, which can act as immunogens (Donnely et al 1994). There are also methods of synthesizing such specifically sequenced proteins and polypeptides by recombinant DNA techniques. These may be enhanced by using new adjuvants like viral liposomes, i.e. viral antigens attached to lipid spheres and immune stimulated complexes ('iscoms') which induce aggregates of viral protein.

Combination vaccines are being increasingly developed (Plotkin & Fletcher 1996). The internationally sponsored Children's Vaccine Initiative announced the goal of developing a vaccine that could immunize the newborn with one orally administered dose against the major vaccine-preventable diseases (Robbins 1993). More modest goals are the combination of six antigens in a single shot: diphtheria, tetanus, pertussis, *H. influenzae* b, hepatitis B and inactivated polio vaccine. Components must be very concentrated and compatible with each other and with preservatives and adjuvants (Insel 1995).

ADVERSE REACTIONS AND CONTRAINDICATIONS TO IMMUNIZATION

No child should be denied immunization without serious thought about the consequences, both for the individual child and the community. There are many false contraindications to immunization (see Table 7.2), as opposed to the true contraindications (Table 7.3) discussed below.

Table 7.2 FALSE contraindications to immunization

Illnesses or treatments
- Minor illnesses, e.g. mild upper respiratory infection
- Chronic diseases of heart, lung and kidneys
- Treatment with antibiotics or locally-acting corticosteroids, i.e. by topical application or inhalation
- Stable neurological condition such as Down syndrome, cerebral palsy, spina bifida
- Malnutrition or under a particular weight
- Dermatoses, eczema or localized skin infection
- Recent or imminent surgery

Personal or family medical history
- Personal or family history of allergy, asthma, eczema, hay fever, etc.
- Previous history of measles, pertussis, rubella, mumps, *Haemophilus influenzae*, polio or other specific infection
- Family history of adverse reaction to immunization
- Family history of convulsions
- Jaundice at birth or prematurity: do not postpone immunization
- Contact with an infectious disease
- Older than the usual age for immunization

Note: some of these conditions constitute priority or high risk groups for immunization, for example low birthweight infants, those with Down syndrome, asthma, congenital heart disease, chronic lung disease and infants with HIV-1 antibody positive mothers.

Adverse reactions may be due to faulty administration, for example abscesses due to unsterile needles or syringes, or to inherent properties of the vaccines.

Both minor and major side-effects of vaccination cause parental anxiety and undermine professional confidence in the benefits of

Table 7.3 TRUE contraindications to immunization

Summary of contraindications
1. Acute illness
2. Previous severe reaction to immunization
3. Immune deficiency or suppression, acquired or induced
4. Progressive or uncontrolled CNS disease
5. Specific situations with whole cell pertussis or some live vaccines

Definite contraindications – general
- Severe febrile illness. Immunization might superimpose adverse affects on the illness, or manifestations of the disease may wrongly be attributed to immunization. Postpone immunization

Definite contraindications – pertussis
- Definite history of severe adverse reactions from previous dose of the vaccine, usually DTP
- General reactions include fever above 39.5°C, anaphylaxis, bronchospasm, laryngeal edema, collapse, prolonged unresponsiveness or inconsolable screaming within 72 h
- Severe local reaction, implies extensive induration or inflammation around the injection site
- Definite convulsion within 72 h of administration of a previous dose of DPT
- Progressive neurological disease, e.g. uncontrolled epilepsy or tuberous sclerosis

Definite contraindications – live vaccines
- Patients with immune deficiency or those with impaired response due to leukemia, malignant disease and those with AIDS. Those who are HIV Ab positive with symptoms may be given killed vaccines
- Those being treated with large doses of corticosteroids or other immunosuppressive treatments, e.g. following organ transplantation
- Within 3 weeks of another live vaccine (but OPV, measles, rubella or BCG vaccine may be given simultaneously with another live viral vaccine)
- Within 3 weeks before or 3 months after a dose of normal immunoglobulin
- Allergy to hens' eggs if severe, e.g. anaphylaxis or generalized urticaria (these are relatively rare)
- BCG vaccine should not be given to those with:
  — generalized specific skin conditions; if eczema exists, vaccination should be in an area of healthy skin
  — positive skin sensitivity test to tuberculin protein; an interval of at least 3 weeks should be allowed between BCG and any live vaccine
- Patients with tuberculosis should not receive measles vaccine unless on full treatment for TB

Circumstances requiring individual consideration
- Children with a personal history of convulsions or 'febrile convulsions' (they can usually be immunized)
- Children with first degree relatives with epilepsy may have a fit after measles or MMR vaccine. However, the possibility of a fit is 10 times as great with an infection of measles. In these circumstances the matter should be discussed with parents, the vaccine should be given and they should be supplied with a pediatric dose of rectal diazepam and instructions about what to do if a convulsion occurs
- Documented evidence of cerebral damage in neonatal period including twitching and clonic episodes
- Stable abnormality of the CNS, including spina bifida and cerebral palsy
Note: previously these last two conditions were, but are no longer, accepted contraindications to DPT and measles immunization. Children in these categories do require special, individual consideration, a weighing of risk and benefit in each case
- In chronic heart, kidney and lung disease, including cystic fibrosis, failure to thrive and treated TB, MMR immunizations are recommended in the UK
- Diarrhea or vomiting is considered a reason to postpone OPV in the UK, but in many countries it is given, and an extra dose is recommended after recovery

immunization. The situation has been confused by anecdotal information, inadequate epidemiological studies and mass media speculation. Much debate has concerned the pertussis component of the DPT vaccine in the UK (Hinman & Orenstein 1990). Evidence indicates that the serious side-effects of both pertussis and measles vaccines are much less than the risks and morbidity of the clinical diseases in the first few years of life (Table 7.4; Galazka et al 1984). No case of SSPE has ever been attributed to measles vaccine. After 3 years of intensive case finding the British National Childhood Encephalopathy Study found so few cases that it 'could not say conclusively whether or not pertussis can cause permanent brain damage if such damage occurs at all' (Immunization Against Infectious Disease 1996). When the risk from a disease becomes very small, as with paralytic poliomyelitis in Europe, the small risk of vaccine associated paralytic poliomyelitis (VAPP) from live OPV becomes relatively more important and may warrant a reconsideration of vaccination policy (Beale 1990, Plotkin 1995).

Side-effects of DPT vaccination

Minor reactions

There are significantly different rates of these reactions between various vaccine lots and endotoxin content from reputable commercial manufacturers (Baraff et al 1989). Minor reactions are quite frequent in 20–50% of vaccines. Local reactions include inflammation, induration or a painless nodule at the site of injection. These are progressively more common after the first injection. Constitutional upsets include fever, screaming, crying more than usual or persistently (more than 5 hours in the first 12).

Serious reactions

In normal infants a neurological reaction such as a prolonged convulsion occurs after about 1 in 100 000 injections. Most result in no permanent damage. Encephalopathy and brain damage can occur in the first year of life in immunized and nonimmunized children. No completely reliable estimate can be made of the risk (Miller et al 1990).

Contraindications to pertussis and other vaccines

There is limited factual information about major side-effects and specific contraindications due to their relative rarity and underreporting. Moreover, confusion occurs because of background disease, emotion because of ignorance, guilt and fear of litigation. Doctors and health visitors are unsure about contraindications and in about 40% of the cases advised against pertussis and measles vaccinations, the reasons for withholding

were invalid (National Immunisation Study 1989). Table 7.4 gives the estimated rates of adverse reactions set out by the WHO EPI unit, compared with the risks from the relevant diseases.

There is general agreement about certain definite contraindications, but continuing uncertainty about other factors (Table 7.3). Even when a specific list of contraindications is given, there can be significant problems of interpretation of these. In the UK less than 5% of children have contraindications to DPT and less than 1% to measles vaccine with current guidelines (Nicoll & Jenkinson 1988).

IMMUNIZATION SCHEDULES

Immunization schedules are the basic framework for the delivery of immunizations to individuals and the community. No one schedule is applicable to all countries and communities of the world and several national programs are changing in response to local factors. The timing of the first immunizations is a compromise between the developing maturity of the infant's immune system and the risk of infection from virulent organisms (Anonymous 1990). Maternal transplacental IgG protects infants against many infections for the first few months of life. It is an incomplete protection, particularly against pertussis, but is satisfactory against measles and rubella. Consequently pertussis immunization should be provided early in situations where this disease is prevalent. The production of a satisfactory primary antigen response is vital. Unless this is achieved subsequent immunizations or infections will not produce an adequate recall response to effect protection. This is particularly relevant for inactivated vaccines.

Basic principles

The aim is to reach the majority of children before the age when exposure to natural infection occurs. Which vaccines are included and the ages at which they are delivered depends on the age-specific risks of disease, response to vaccines, risks of complications, potential interference from maternal antibody, cost of vaccine and health service infrastructure. No child should be denied immunization without serious thought about the consequences, both for the individual child and the community. The schedule should also be simple so that it can be remembered by staff and parents and should fit in with other aspects of health care such as developmental screening. The optimal age for starting immunization depends on both host immunological maturity and local disease epidemiology. In developing countries where tuberculosis and poliomyelitis may infect young children, immunization can be started soon after birth (WHO 1995, Hall et al 1990). In communities where pertussis is still a problem, this vaccine should be given early in the first year since cases before

Table 7.4 Estimated rates of adverse events following DPT and measles immunizations per 100 000 injections compared to complication rates of natural pertussis and measles per 100 000 cases (according to Galazka et al 1984 and World Health Organization Immunization Policy (WHO 1996))

Condition	Pertussis		Measles	
	Pertussis disease per 100 000 cases	DPT immunization per 100 000 injections	Measles disease per 100 000 diseases	Measles immunization per 100 000 injections
Encephalopathy or encephalitis	90–4000	0.2	50–400	0.1
Convulsions	600–8000	0.3–90	500–1000	0.02–190
Death	100–4000	0.2	10–10 000	0.02–0.3

Table 7.5 A comparison of three selected immunization schedules, recommended for use in the UK and USA and by the World Health Organization

Recommended age	United Kingdom* main schedule	United States†	WHO (1996) expanded program on immunization
Birth–neonatal period	BCG and Hep B-1 for special at-risk groups	Hep B-1	OPV-1 BCG Hep B-1a
2 months	DPT-1, OPV-1 Hib-1 Hep B-2	DTP-1, OPV-1 Hep B-2 Hib-1	OPV-2, DT-1 Hep B-1b
3 months	DPT-2, OPV-2 Hib-2		OPV-3, DPT-2 Hep B-2
4 months	DPT-3, OPV-3 Hib-3	DTP-2, OPV-2 Hib-2	OPV-4 DPT-3 Hep B-3
6 months	Hep B-3	DTP-3 OPV-3	(Measles MV‡)
7 months		Hep B-3	
8 months		Hib-3	
9 months			Measles (MV)
10 months			Yellow Fever (YF)
11 months			
12 months	MMR-1 at 12–15 months or at any age after 12 months	MMR-1	
15 months		Hib-4 Var	
18 months		DTP-4/DTaP	(DTP-4 in countries with good pertussis control)
2 years			
4–5 years	DT, OPV-4 MMR-2	DTP-5/DTaP, OPV-4 MMR-2 (or)	
10–14 years	BCG	MMR-2 Hep B (catch up) Var (catch up)	
14–16 years	Td OPV or IPV	Td	
Adult	RV OPV (IPV in special circumstances)		

* Immunization against Infectious Disease (1996)
Hib = *Haemophilus influenzae* b polysaccharide conjugate vaccine
RV = rubella vaccine
Td = tetanus, adult-type vaccine with low potency diphtheria vaccine
IPV = inactivated polio vaccine
Hep B = hepatitis B 1a = where perinatal risk is high 1b = standard regime
DTaP = diphtheria, tetanus and acellular pertussis (may replace DTP)
Var = live attenuated vaccine, varicella-zoster
† Advisory Committee on Immunization Practices of American Academy of Pediatrics 1996
‡ MV = measles vaccine, give early extra dose in situations of high risk
YF = yellow fever vaccine in all countries at risk

6 months of age have a higher morbidity and mortality. Where measles is a major threat in the first year of life, vaccine should be given early despite the fact that the response will be less than optimal. The most appropriate age for measles immunization depends on the age-specific attack rate in a particular community. In industrialized countries measles immunization may be deferred until 12–15 months of age since early risk of infection is not great and the vaccine works optimally only after 12 months. In countries where measles may occur much earlier the WHO recommends immunization at 9–12 months, preceded by an extra dose at 6 months of age in high risk situations.

The correct timing of immunizations of different vaccines is of great importance if an adequate primary immune response is to be obtained. Three current immunization schedules (for the UK, the USA and that recommended by the WHO) are set out in Table 7.5. The UK schedule completes primary immunization by 6 months of age, minimizing the number of drop-outs. The introduction of an Hib immunization program in the UK in 1992 has led to the rapid reduction of invasive cases of *H. influenzae* infection (Hargreaves et al 1996). In all countries, if an immunization schedule has been interrupted or has not been completed it is not necessary to start the schedule afresh. The course should be completed with the remaining doses administered at the recommended intervals.

Developing country schedules

In developing countries booster immunization schedules present financial and logistic problems so the main emphasis is on primary immunization as part of basic health care. The priority for the WHO is to deliver the primary immunization series to over 90% of infants and thus reduce the burden of these diseases. Low birthweight infants, whether due to premature birth or intrauterine growth retardation, or both, should generally be immunized with the same schedule as for normal weight, full-term infants (Anonymous 1990). In addition to the standard WHO schedule, other vaccines are available and recommended for use in specific geographic areas, for example Japanese encephalitis and pigbel vaccines. Others like Hib may not yet be affordable in some developing countries.

Mass immunization campaigns are an integral part of the global polio eradication strategy; they are now also recommended by WHO for use in measles elimination programs. They can have a dramatic impact as the first phase of an elimination strategy, especially where health infrastructure is limited. Such campaigns should not be isolated events, but part of the long-term strategy (WHO 1996).

In conclusion, a schedule should be epidemiologically relevant, immunologically effective, operationally feasible and socially acceptable.

SPECIFIC IMMUNIZATIONS

Measles and rubella in the UK

The earlier UK schedule for rubella immunization, targeting only schoolgirls, and the relatively poor uptake of measles vaccine in the 1980s left cohorts of older children susceptible to these diseases and outbreaks were predicted. In November 1994 there was a major campaign to immunize all children aged 5–16 years old with measles and rubella vaccine (MR). In England 92% of the target 7.1 million children received MR vaccine. Susceptible individuals were reduced to less than a third, and measles cases fell to a fifth of the number reported the previous year (Cutts 1996). Adverse reactions were reported as 1 in 2600, but serious neurological reactions were only 1 in 78 000 doses, and anaphylaxis or allergy within 24 h only in 1 in 65 000 doses. This may overestimate attributable risk. The serious reactions were significantly less than would have been expected with the diseases. There is need for better awareness of the benefits as well as the adverse reactions to sustain public confidence in immunizations.

Poliomyelitis (live oral, killed injectable or both) vaccines

WHO, in partnership with various groups, has set the objective of eradicating polio from the world by the year 2000. Eradication from the Americas was achieved in 1991, using oral polio vaccine (OPV). However, the Advisory Committee on Immunization Practices (ACIP) of the USA has recommended that the country adopt a sequential poliomyelitis immunization schedule – two doses of inactivated polio vaccine (IPV) followed by two doses of OPV (Frankel 1995, Plotkin 1995). This would prevent the 1 case per 2.5 million doses of OPV of vaccine associated paralytic polio (VAPP), but it will cost the USA $20 million annually. The WHO does not support this policy: it believes that global eradication is possible with OPV, and the US change in policy promotes a misconception that OPV is inadequate (Hull & Lee 1996). Recent epidemics indicate that the problem was a failure to vaccinate rather than OPV vaccine failure (Ward & Hull 1995). Moreover, IPV would be too expensive for many developing countries. Global eradication might cost $500 million by 2000, but thereafter there will be no risk of VAPP and an annual saving of $1500 million (Hull & Lee 1996).

Pertussis acellular vaccines

Whole cell vaccines, suspensions of killed *Bordetella pertussis* organisms, have been both effective in reducing the disease and unsatisfactory because of adverse reactions. The organisms contain a number of antigens; pertussis toxin, pertactin, filamentous hemagglutinin and several fimbrial antigens. These have been separated and used in combinations in acellular vaccines. Even whole cell vaccines have differences in composition due to different strains and manufacture. Many trials of acellular vaccines have been conducted (Edwards et al 1995, Edwards & Decker 1996). Although there are disputes about which combinations of antigens are best (Preston & Matthews 1996), the acellular vaccines had efficacies which approached and sometimes exceeded the comparison whole cell vaccines, and all had fewer and milder adverse reactions. It is likely that acellular vaccines will be widely used in the USA from 1997.

In the UK acceptance of whole cell vaccine is currently high and switching to acellular products will increase cost with little improvement in uptake. Other considerations may be more important; the purified acellular vaccines may be easier to mix with other antigens in the combined vaccines that seem likely in the future (Miller 1995). There is evidence of pertussis outbreaks in older children and adults in the USA, and acellular vaccines with lower reactogenicity will be more acceptable as boosters. Clinical trials in the UK are in progress to evaluate reactogenicity and immunogenicity of acellular pertussis and combined vaccines. It is probably only a matter of time before they are incorporated in the routine schedule.

Varicella vaccine

Varicella vaccine, from an attenuated varicella-zoster virus, has been licensed for use in healthy children in the USA. There are arguments about the costs and benefits, the immunization schedule and who it should be given to. Initially it is likely to be restricted to those at greatest risk, especially immunocompromised children (Gershon 1995, Ross & Lantos 1995).

IMMUNIZATION FOR INTERNATIONAL TRAVEL

Small children now travel with their parents to every corner of the globe. Such visits may expose children to infectious diseases no longer endemic in Europe and North America and to conditions which, although preventable, are not normally covered in a routine immunization program. As the disease incidence and health regulations are constantly changing, up to date advice should be sought from appropriate authorities. Basic preventive measures should always be observed: careful food hygiene, breast-feeding, protection from insects which transmit infections, etc.

Barnett & Chen (1995) reviewed recommendations for immunization of children involved in international travel. A list of immunizations to be considered for children traveling outside Europe and North America is shown in Table 7.6. Young children should have their full course of routine immunization appropriate to their home country. It may be advisable to give some immunizations at a rather earlier age than in the UK schedule. For example, BCG vaccine should be given in the first few months of life if the child is traveling to an area of high tuberculosis infectivity. If the risk from measles is high, this immunization may be given at 6–11 months of age and repeated between 12 and 15 months of age.

IMMUNIZATION COVERAGE – IMPROVING UPTAKE

Causes of poor uptake

In some communities immunization appears to have a low priority and false beliefs sometimes obstruct immunization. In parts of

Table 7.6 Vaccines and pretravel preparation for children

1. Make sure that routine immunizations are up to date
2. If going to a high risk area consider
    — BCG for neonates and children
    — Hepatitis B
    — Hepatitis A
    — Yellow fever
    — Typhoid
    — Cholera
    — Japanese encephalitis
    — Rabies
    — Meningococcal meningitis
    — Influenza

Southeast Asia measles used to be considered a disease which children had to have and overcome in order to grow up strong and healthy. In Europe there are many public fears about the dangers of adverse reactions from vaccines. Many of these are false and even what is true is sometimes exaggerated by the media. Professional fear of litigation in some countries encourages health workers to advise against vaccination in all cases where there is any doubt at all. Health workers in a number of countries, including the UK, are not entirely clear about the contraindications for immunization (Wood et al 1996). They then tend to extend contraindications to groups who really require immunization, such as children who fail to thrive or have recurrent infections (see Table 7.2). Conflicting advice undermines the confidence of both the public and the profession.

Improving knowledge, information and training

1. Use a simple schedule which is not changed more often than necessary.
2. Written guidelines should be available for staff and a simplified version for parents.
3. There should be a referral system for cases in which there is uncertainty about immunization.
4. Training specific to immunization counseling should be given to all those involved.
5. Clear instructions are required for dealing with anaphylaxis or other emergencies which are occasionally associated with immunization. (Nicoll et al 1989)

Operational measures

In any country an immunization policy with definite targets and clear allocation of responsibility is essential. The person in overall charge should be specified and also which members of the team are responsible for vaccines, supplies, recall of the children and the practicalities of immunization. Immunization should be clearly recognized as an activity of nurses and auxiliaries who are appropriately supported by a doctor trained and interested in the topic.

The immunization schedule should be coordinated with other activities of the health service. Times of developmental assessment and school entry examination are appropriate for reviewing the immunization status and 'sweeping up' any missed immunizations. Opportunistic immunization should also be available at outpatient and hospital services, accident and emergency departments and at school entry examinations.

Immunization clinics should be near to the community and held at hours which are convenient for the parents. In some services domiciliary and home visit immunizations may need to be available. A local back-up team is required for training, inquiries and emergencies. Those responsible for the service should respond quickly and with sensitivity to special needs and emergencies, such as alarm caused by severe side-effects. The public should be informed about the purpose and plan of immunization campaigns through local channels of communication. Conflict about immunizations in the media seriously damages confidence. Immunization records should be appropriate to the health service. Sometimes these are parent-retained, computerized or held by the doctors and clinics. Often a combination of record systems is required. It is essential that immunization uptake is recognized as a key indicator of health care. All those involved in the immunization service should receive regular feedback so they can understand how their particular part of the service is working in relation to the targets of child immunization.

Practical issues

Many practicalities are involved in running an effective immunization program. These include appropriate training, care of vaccines, maintenance of equipment and correct administration of the vaccines, when and how they should be given. Personnel need to know how to prepare for and conduct an immunization session. The health education opportunity of an immunization program needs to be utilized by appropriate preparation and materials. Finally, evaluating an immunization program both at a local and regional level is important. Many of these issues have been clearly and systematically set out in *Immunization in Practice – A Guide for Health Workers who Give Vaccines*, by the World Health Organization (WHO 1989), in which guidelines to improve vaccine coverage are set out (see Table 7.7).

Table 7.7 World Health Organization guidelines about immunization

Unnecessary restrictions on immunizations limit the coverage and effectiveness of a program. The WHO Global Program of Immunization urges health workers to consider the following points:

1. Health workers should use every opportunity to immunize eligible children
2. No vaccine is entirely without side-effects, but the risk of disease far outweighs the risks of vaccines, especially in developing countries
3. BCG and OPV can be safely and effectively given to newborns
4. DPT can be given from the second month of life
5. Measles vaccine, in countries where the disease affects many before 1 year, should be given at 9 months, possibly earlier for high risk
6. Do not give DPT to a child who had a severe reaction to a previous dose (see above). Complete the schedule with DT vaccine
7. Do not withhold OPV during diarrhea, but give an extra dose as soon as possible after recovery
8. Malnourished children particularly need protection
9. Low fever, mild respiratory infections, diarrhea and minor illnesses are *not* contraindications to immunization
10. Every hospitalized child should be individually considered for immunization. Some benefit from admission immunization, e.g. measles, if there are cases in the ward. Review the immunization status of all children at discharge, and give appropriate vaccines
11. The decision to withhold immunizations has potentially serious consequences. It should only be advised after careful consideration and usually a second opinion

REFERENCES

Ada A L 1990 Modern vaccines. The immunological principles of vaccination. Lancet 335: 523–526

Amos A 1991 Young people, tobacco and 1992. Health Education Journal 50: 26–30

American Academy of Pediatrics 1976 Committee on nutrition recommendations. Nutrition Reviews 34: 248

Anderson R M, May R M 1990 Modern vaccines. Immunization and herd immunity. Lancet 335: 641–645

Anonymous 1990 Editorial. Routine immunisation of preterm infants. Lancet 335: 23–24

Anonymous 1994 A warm chain for breastfeeding. Lancet 344: 1239–1241

Ansell P, Bull D, Roman E 1996 Childhood leukaemia and intramuscular vitamin K: findings from a case-control study. British Medical Journal 313: 204–205

Baraff L J, Manclark C R, Cherry J D, Christenson P, Marcy S M 1989 Analysis of adverse reactions to diphtheria and tetanus toxoids and pertussis vaccine potency and percentage of mouse weight gain. Pediatric Infectious Disease Journal 8: 502–507

Barker D J 1995a The fetal and infant origins of disease. European Journal of Clinical Investigation 25: 457–463

Barker D J 1995b Fetal origins of coronary heart disease. British Medical Journal 311: 171–174

Barnett E, Chen R 1995 Children and international travel: immunizations. Pediatric Infectious Disease Journal 14: 982–992

Beale A J 1990 Modern vaccines. Polio vaccines: time for a change in immunisation policy? Lancet 335: 839–842

Beeken S, Waterston T 1992 Health service support of breastfeeding – are we practising what we preach? British Medical Journal 305: 285–287

Blair P S, Fleming P J et al 1996 Smoking and the sudden infant death syndrome: results from 1993–5 case-control study for confidential inquiry into stillbirths and deaths in infancy. British Medical Journal 313: 195–198

British Medical Association 1986 Diet, nutrition and health. Report of the Board of Science and Education. Camelon Press Ltd, London

Brown F 1990 Modern vaccines. From Jenner to genes – the new vaccines. Lancet 335: 587–590

Campbell H, Jones I J 1994 Breastfeeding in Scotland. Scottish Needs Assessment Programme. Scottish Forum for Public Health Medicine, Glasgow

Campbell H, Gorman D, Wigglesworth A 1995 Audit of the support for breastfeeding mothers in Fife maternity hospitals using adapted Baby Friendly Hospital materials. Journal of Public Health Medicine 17: 450–454

Charlton A 1995 Smoking. In: Harvey D, Miles M, Smyth D (eds) Community child health and paediatrics. Butterworth-Heinemann, Oxford

Clark B, Wharton B 1995 Food and nutrition. In: Harvey D, Miles M, Smyth D (eds) Community child health and paediatrics. Butterworth-Heinemann, Oxford

Crowley P 1993 Antenatal steroids for the prevention of respiratory distress syndrome in preterm babies. In: Enkin M W, Keirse M J N C, Renfrew M J, Neilson J P (eds) The Cochrane pregnancy and childbirth database. Cochrane updates. Update Software, Oxford

Cutts F T 1996 Revaccination against measles and rubella. British Medical Journal 312: 589–590

Czeizel A E, Dudas L 1992 Prevention of the first occurrence of neural-tube defects by periconceptional vitamin supplementation. New England Journal of Medicine 327: 1832–1835

Dajani A S, Bisno A L, Chung K J et al 1988 Prevention of rheumatic fever. Circulation 78: 1082–1086

Department of Health and Social Security 1984 Diet and cardiovascular disease (COMA report). Reports on health and social subjects: number 28. HMSO, London

Department of Health 1993 The sleeping position of infants and cot death: report of the Chief Medical Officer's Expert Group. HMSO, London

Donnely J J, Ulmer J B, Liu M S 1994 Immunisation with DNA. Journal of Immunological Methods 176: 145–152

Dwyer T, Ponsonby A L 1996 Sudden infant death syndrome. British Medical Journal 313: 180–181

Edwards K M, Meade B D, Decker M D 1995 Comparison of 13 acellular pertussis vaccines: overview and serologic response. Pediatrics 96: 548–557

Edwards K M, Decker M D 1996 Acellular pertussis vaccines for infants. New England Journal of Medicine 334: 391–392

Falkner F 1980 The prevention in childhood of health problems in adult life. WHO, Geneva

Fenton-May J, Bradley D M, Sibert J R et al 1994 Screening for Duchenne muscular dystrophy. Archives of Disease in Childhood 70: 551–552

Fine P E M, Rodrigues L C 1990 Modern vaccines. Mycobacterial diseases. Lancet 335: 1016–1020

Florey C V, Leech A M, Blackhall A 1995 Infant feeding and mental and motor development at 18 months of age in first born singletons. International Journal of Epidemiology 24: S21–S26

Frankel D 1995 US group urges immunisation change. Lancet 346: 1151

Galazka A M, Lauer B A, Henderson R H, Keja J 1984 Indications and contraindications for vaccines used in the Expanded Programme on Immunization. Bulletin of the World Health Organisation 62: 357–366

Gershon A A 1995 Varicella vaccine: its past, present and future. Pediatric Infectious Disease Journal 12: 742–752

Glaser D 1991 Treatment issues in child sexual abuse. British Journal of Psychiatry 159: 769–782

Goddard E 1991 Drinking in England and Wales in the late 1980s. OPCS, HMSO, London

Golding J 1995 The environment and child health. In: Harvey D, Miles M, Smyth D (eds) Community child health and paediatrics. Butterworth-Heinemann, Oxford

Green A H 1993 Child sexual abuse: immediate and long term effects and intervention. Journal of Academy of Child and Adolescent Psychiatry 32: 890–902

Hall A J, Greenwood B M, Whittle H 1990 Modern vaccines. Practice in developing countries. Lancet 335: 774–777

Hall D M B 1996 Health for all children: a programme of child health surveillance. Oxford Medical Publications, Oxford

Hargreaves R M, Slack M P E, Howard A J, Anderson E, Ramsay M E 1996 Changing patterns of invasive Haemophilus influenza disease in England and Wales after introduction of the Hib vaccination programme. British Medical Journal 312: 160–161

Hinman A R, Orenstein W A 1990 Modern vaccines. Immunisation practice in developed countries. Lancet 335: 707–710

HMSO 1989 Effective intervention: child abuse. Guidelines on co-operation in Scotland. HMSO, Edinburgh

Holland W W, Fitzsimons B 1991 Smoking in children. Archives of Disease in Childhood 66: 1269–1274

House of Commons Science and Technology Committee 1995 Human genetics: the science and its consequences. HMSO, London

Howie P W, Forsyth S, Ogston S A, Clark A, Florey C V 1990 Protective effect of breastfeeding against infection. British Medical Journal 300: 11–16

Hull H F, Lee J W 1996 Sabin, Salk or sequential? Lancet 347: 630

Immunization against infectious disease 1996 HMSO, London

Inequalities in Health 1988 The Black report and the health divide. Penguin Books, London

Insel R A 1995 Potential alterations in immunogenicity by combining or simultaneously administering vaccine components. Annual New York Academy of Science 754: 35–47

Jarvis S, Towner E, Walsh S 1996 Accidents. In: Department of Health The health of our children. HMSO, London

Kohler G, Milstein C 1975 Continuous culture of fused cells secreting antibodies of predefined specificity. Nature, London 256: 495–503

Kristiansen B 1996 Secondary prevention of meningococcal disease. British Medical Journal 312: 591–592

Laurence K M, James N, Miller M H, Tennant G B, Campbell H 1981 Double blind randomised controlled trial of folate treatment before conception to prevent recurrence of neural tube defects. British Medical Journal 282: 1509–1511

Law C M, Barker D J 1994 Fetal influences on blood pressure. Journal of Hypertension 12: 1329–1332

Lepow M L, Peter G, Glode M P et al 1984 The response of infants to Haemophilus influenzae type b polysaccharide vaccine conjugate with diphtheria–tetanus–pertussis antigen. Journal of Infectious Diseases 149: 950–955

Lepow M L, Samuelson J S, Gordon L K 1987 Safety and immunogenicity of H. influenzae type b polysaccharide-diphtheria toxoid conjugate vaccine (PPP-D) in infants. Journal of Infectious Diseases 156: 591–596

Lucas A, Morley R, Cole T J, Lister G, Leeson-Payne C 1992 Breast milk and subsequent intelligence quotient in children born preterm. Lancet 339: 261–264

Massell B F, Chute C G, Walker A M, Kurland B G S 1988 Penicillin and the marked decrease in morbidity and mortality from rheumatic fever in the United States. New England Journal of Medicine 318: 280–286

McNeilly A S 1979 Effects of lactation on fertility. British Medical Bulletin 35: 151–154

Miller E 1995 Acellular pertussis vaccines. Archives of Disease in Childhood 73: 390–391

Motulsky A G 1994 Predictive genetic testing. Americal Journal of Human Genetics 55: 603–605

Moxon E R 1990 Modern vaccines. The scope of immunisation. Lancet 335: 448–451

Moxon E R, Rappuoli R 1990 Modern vaccines. *Haemophilus influenzae* infections and whooping cough. Lancet 335: 1324–1329

MRC Vitamin Study Research Group 1991 Prevention of neural tube defects: results on the MRC vitamin study. Lancet 338: 131–137

National Immunisation Study 1989 Factors influencing immunisation uptake in childhood. Action Research for the Crippled Child, Horsham

Nicoll A, Elliman D, Begg N T 1989 Immunisation – causes of failure and strategies and tactics for success. British Medical Journal 299: 808–812

Nicoll A, Jenkinson D 1988 Decision making for routine measles/MMR and whooping cough immunisation. British Medical Journal 297: 405–407

Nuffield Council on Bioethics 1993 Genetic screening: ethical issues. Nuffield Council on Bioethics, London

Perez-Escamilla R, Pollitt E, Lohnerdal B, Dewey K D 1994 Infant feeding policies in maternity wards and their effect on breastfeeding success: an analytical overview. American Journal of Public Health 84: 89–97

Plotkin S A 1993 Vaccination in the 21st century. Journal of Infectious Disease 168: 29–37

Plotkin S A, Fletcher M A 1996 Combination vaccines and immunization visits. Pediatric Infectious Disease Journal 15: 103–105

Plotkin S A 1995 Inactivated polio vaccine for the United States: a missed vaccination opportunity. Pediatric Infectious Disease Journal 14: 835–839

Power C 1996 Health related behaviour. In: Department of Health The Health of our Children. HMSO, London

Preston N W, Matthews R C 1996 Components of acellular pertussis vaccines. Lancet 347: 764

Robbins A 1993 The children's vaccine initiative. American Journal of Diseases in Children 147: 152–153

Ross L F, Lantos J D 1995 Immunisation against chickenpox. British Medical Journal 310: 2–3

Scottish Home and Health Department, Working party for the Chief Medical Officer of Scotland 1993 The Scottish diet. SOHHD, Edinburgh

Shann F 1990 Modern vaccines. Pneumococcus and influenzae. Lancet 335: 898–901

Smithells D 1996 Vitamins in early pregnancy. British Medical Journal 313: 128–129

Smithells R W, Shephard S, Schorah C J et al 1980 Possible prevention of neural tube defects by periconceptional vitamin supplementation. Lancet i: 339–340

Spencer N J 1991 Child poverty and deprivation in the UK. Archives of Disease in Childhood 66: 1255–1257

Stevenson R E 1993 The environmental basis of human anomalies. In: Stevenson R E, Hall J G, Goodman R M (eds) Human malformations and related anomalies, volume 1. Oxford Monographs on Medical Genetics, number 27. Oxford University Press, Oxford

UNICEF 1989 Facts for life. United Nations Children's (Emergency) Fund, New York

Von Kries R, Gobel U, Hachmeister A, Kaletsch U, Michaelis J 1996 Vitamin K and childhood cancer: a population based case-control study in Lower Saxony, Germany. British Medical Journal 313: 199–202

Ward N A, Hull H F 1995 Polio eradication. Lancet 345: 318

WHO 1989 Immunization in practice. A guide for health workers who give vaccines. Oxford University Press, Oxford

WHO 1995 (WHO/GPV/95.05) Report of the Scientific Advisory Group of Experts. WHO, Geneva

WHO 1996 (WHO/EPI/GEN/95.03 Rev.1) Global programme for vaccines and immunization. Immunization policy. WHO, Geneva

Wilson J M G, Jungner G 1968 Principals and practice of screening for disease. WHO, Geneva

Wood D, Halfron N et al 1996 Knowledge of the childhood immunization schedule and of contraindications to vaccinate. Pediatric Infectious Disease Journal 15: 40–45

Zipursky A 1996 Vitamin K at birth. British Medical Journal 313: 179–180

8 Physical growth and development

M. T. Dattani   M. A. Preece

Introduction   349
Normal growth   349
Prenatal growth   349
    Assessment   349
    Regulation   351
Postnatal growth   352
    The human growth curve   352
    Types of growth data   352
    Height and weight velocity charts   352
    Growth in the first 2 years of life   356
    Growth and development during adolescence 357
    Bone age   362
    Prediction of adult height   362
    Growth curves of different tissues and different parts of the body   363
    Other clinically useful measurements   363
    Catch-up growth and growth regulation   364
Endocrinology of growth – the hypothalamo-pituitary-somatotroph axis   364
GHRH/Somatostatin   364
The secretory pattern of hGH   364
The interaction of hGH with its receptor   365
The molecular heterogeneity of hGH   365
Insulin-like growth factors, their binding proteins and their receptors   365
Genetic control of growth and its disorders   366
Introduction   366
Genetic abnormalities in the action of GHRH   366
The hGH gene and the role of homeobox genes in the control of growth   366
The GH receptor gene   367

Environmental factors affecting growth   367
Nutrition   367
Ethnic differences in growth   367
Seasonal variation in growth   368
Disease   368
Psychological disturbance   368
Socioeconomic factors   368
Secular trend   368
Disorders of growth   368
Short stature   368
    Low birthweight   368
    Dysmorphic syndromes   369
    Turner syndrome   370
    Skeletal dysplasias   370
    Constitutional (familial) short stature   371
    Nutritional deficiency   371
    Psychosocial deprivation   372
    Chronic medical illness   372
    Constitutional delay of growth and puberty   372
    Growth hormone deficiency/insufficiency   372
    Laron-type dwarfism (GH receptor deficiency)   374
    Other endocrine conditions resulting in short stature   375
Tall stature   375
    Constitutional tall stature   375
    Tall stature with dysmorphic features   376
    Tall stature with disproportionate growth   376
    Pituitary gigantism   376
    Other endocrinopathies causing tall stature   376
Conclusion   377
References   377

INTRODUCTION

The process of growth is one that is shared by all organisms. In man, the process commences shortly after conception and continues until adulthood. Growth occurs as a result of hyperplasia, hypertrophy and differentiation. In childhood, these processes result in an increase in height and the maturation and differentiation of several structures, e.g. bone, permanent dentition, etc. These phenomena are unique to childhood. In later life, growth continues in certain tissues such as hair, skin and cells lining the gastrointestinal tract. However, there is no further increase in height.

Growth is largely determined genetically, with the modification of this genetic process by the environment. Any disease process interfering with normal growth and development in childhood may well have lifelong consequences. In this chapter, normal physical growth in childhood will be described in some detail. This will be followed by a description of the genetic control of

growth and finally, by the role of environmental factors on this process.

NORMAL GROWTH

PRENATAL GROWTH

Assessment

The prenatal period is the most crucial in determining a child's growth and future well-being, since growth is at its fastest during this time. Hence, the prenatal part of the growth process is the most vulnerable to adverse environmental circumstances and the time when such circumstances have the most profound effects. However, most of the events leading to growth during this time remain shrouded in mystery. The reason for this is the lack of access to the normal fetus between the time when social abortions are performed and term. Advances in ultrasound techniques and the study of prematurely born infants have significantly improved our knowledge.

An ultrasound scan is the most reliable method of monitoring the growth of a fetus. Repeated measurements are required to ensure that growth is satisfactory. Figure 8.1 shows the distance and velocity curves of body length, so far as it may be measured, in prenatal life and in the first year of life. In the distance chart, the crown–heel length in cm is plotted against the age in weeks; in the velocity chart, the velocity, calculated by dividing the increment in height by the time elapsed between two measurements, is plotted against the age. The peak velocity for body length is achieved at 18–22 weeks gestation. Fetal growth is exponential up to 12 weeks and linear thereafter. Crown–rump and crown–heel lengths increase proportionately in the early weeks although, as fetal age advances, the legs get relatively longer. Biparietal and occipitofrontal measurements of skull diameter correlate closely with measurements of length.

Fetal weight gain follows gain in length. However, the peak velocity for weight gain is achieved later, at 34 weeks gestation, compared with height, because of the varying contribution made to weight by different organs. Of these, the most significant is the brain, which grows extremely rapidly during mid-gestation and continues its growth postnatally. The great rate of growth of the fetus compared with that of the child is largely due to cellular proliferation. The proportion of cells undergoing mitosis in any tissue becomes progressively less as the fetus gets older and this is particularly marked in the central nervous system and the musculoskeletal system. Later weight gain is achieved principally by development and hypertrophy of cells.

From 34 weeks to birth, a dip in weight velocity occurs due to the influence of the maternal uterus, whose available space is by then becoming fully occupied. An additional contributory factor is the inability of the placenta to supply nutrients to maintain the rapid velocity, poor nutrition being an important cause of reduced birthweight worldwide. Twins slow down earlier, when their combined weight is approximately the 36-week weight of the singleton fetus. The velocity curve then shows an increase in the immediate postbirth period to make a peak which would quite naturally join with the prebirth peak to make a smooth velocity curve without the dip in the last few weeks before birth. The increase in velocity after birth represents catch-up growth following the uterine restriction on growth. Hence, there is a significant negative correlation between length and weight at birth and their respective increments during the first 6 months. In man, the correlation between length at birth and adult height is only approximately 0.3, but this value rises sharply during the first year. Between length at age 2 and adult height, the correlation is 0.8.

The actual weight at a given postmenstrual age depends somewhat on sex (boys being heavier than girls from about 34 weeks gestation), whether the child is first-born or later-born (first-borns are generally lighter), the height of the mother and her midpregnancy weight, nutrition before and during pregnancy, smoking and alcohol ingestion during pregnancy and, possibly, the genetic character of the population. Hormonal factors may play a very important role in fetal growth, as will be discussed in the next section. Standards of birthweight for different periods of gestation are available based on data from London and Cambridge.

Babies born with a weight of < 2.5 kg at term are described as low birthweight babies and they should be compared with the standards of birthweight for their gestation. The consequences of being small for gestational age are significant and may be lifelong. These will be discussed later.

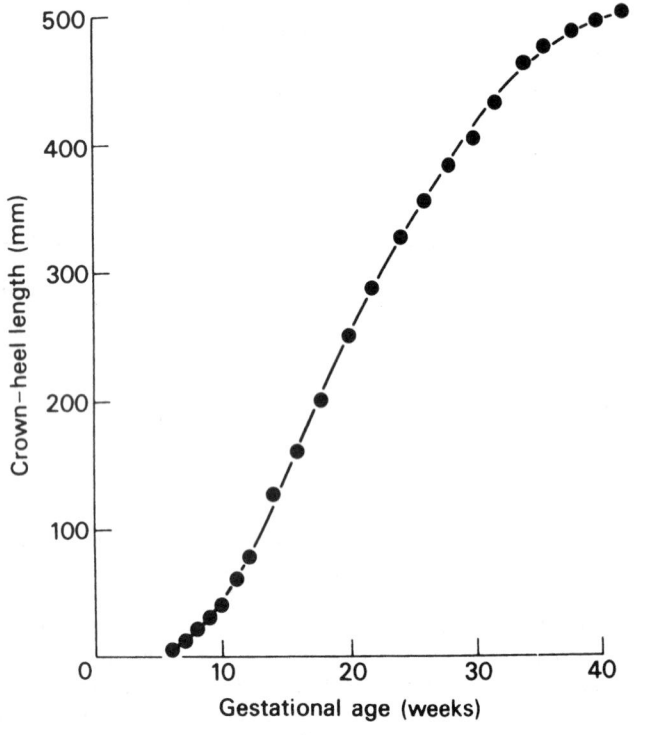

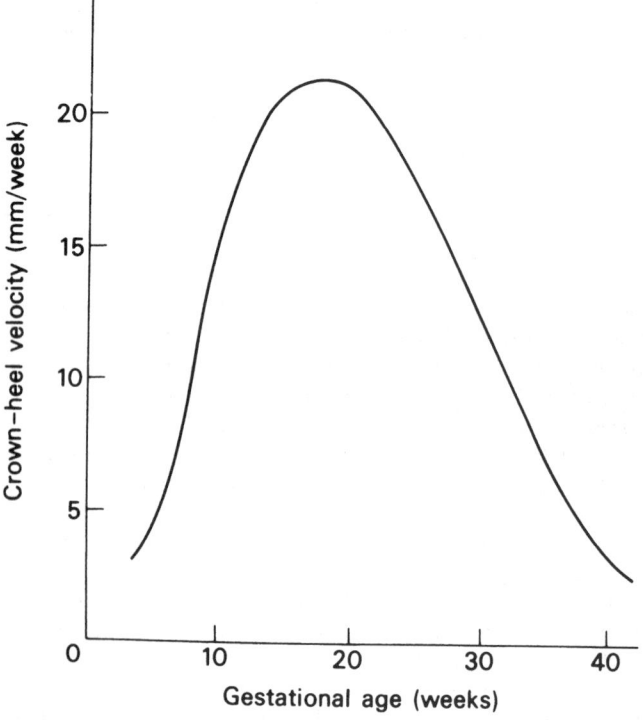

Fig. 8.1   Growth curve of human fetus. (a) Distance curve. (b) Velocity curve.

Regulation of prenatal growth

Embryonic and fetal growth is dependent on a complex interaction between various peptide growth factors. These factors are widely expressed at both the messenger (m) RNA and peptide levels in developing tissues. They bind to extracellular matrix, specific binding proteins and cell surface molecules other than high-affinity receptors and so they have limited access to target tissues for much of the time. They may rely on proteolytic processing from the target tissue to become bioavailable and they mostly interact with high-affinity cell membrane receptors which signal to the nucleus via tyrosine kinase phosphorylation events and the *ras* proto-oncogene signaling pathway (Hill & Hogg 1989).

The insulin-like growth factors (IGF-I and IGF-II; IGFs) share 50% homology with insulin. Both are present in human serum with molecular sizes of approximately 7.6 kDa. IGF-I, previously known as somatomedin-C, is a basic peptide of 70 amino acids whilst IGF-II is slightly acidic and contains 67 amino acids. The two peptides share 45 common amino acid positions, out of a total of 73 (Daughaday & Rotwein 1989, Humbel 1990). Liver is a major site of expression, although almost all tissues express these peptides in the human and animal fetus (Brown et al 1986, Hatikka & Hefti 1988), suggesting a predominantly autocrine or paracrine role. IGF-I is an important postnatal growth factor and its concentration increases at term and postnatally. Serum IGF-II levels remain detectable and are constant during the lifespan of human beings, although the postnatal role of this peptide is unclear.

IGFs bind with a low affinity to insulin receptors, accounting for their insulin-like activity. Two classes of IGF receptors have now been identified (Oh et al 1993). The type 1 receptor shares homology with the insulin receptor and high concentrations of insulin can bind to it, albeit with an affinity which is approximately 100-fold less than that of the IGFs. Both IGFs bind to the type 1 receptor with high affinity, with consequent activation of tyrosine kinase. The type 1 receptor is found in most developing tissues.

The type 2 receptor bears no resemblance to either the insulin or the type 1 IGF receptor. It binds IGF-II with high affinity, IGF-I with a greatly reduced affinity and does not bind insulin at all (Rosenfeld et al 1987). Several studies have shown that the mitogenic and metabolic actions of both IGF-I and IGF-II are mediated through the type 1 IGF receptor (Conover et al 1987, Adashi et al 1989). IGF-I is more potent than IGF-II as a mitogen since the receptor recognizes IGF-I with an order of magnitude greater binding affinity than it does IGF-II. In the fetus, however, IGF-II is the more important growth factor (Baker et al 1993). In addition to their mitogenic effects, IGFs support the differentiated function of many cell types and this includes the synthesis of extracellular matrix molecules such as fibronectin, collagens and glycosaminoglycans. The IGFs are mainly complexed in serum and in extracellular fluids to one of six distinct classes of specific binding protein, termed insulin-like growth factor binding protein 1 (IGFBP-1 – -6). They not only serve as carrier proteins to extend the biological half-life of the IGFs but also modulate their biological actions by either interacting or competing with the type I IGF receptors. The majority of IGF-I and -II in blood is carried on IGFBP-3. In the second half of the gestation period, IGFBP-3 is associated, together with an IGF molecule, with an acid-labile subunit in the circulation to generate a tertiary complex of 150 kDa. In this form, IGFs are restricted to the circulation.

The fibroblast growth factor (FGF) family contains at least nine members which are mitogenic for many cell types. They are potent mitogens for vascular endothelial cells and are angiogenic in vivo. Their actions are mediated by a family of at least four high-affinity receptors. Other growth factors present in embryonic and fetal tissues include epidermal growth factor (EGF), transforming growth factor (TGF)-α, TGF-β, platelet-derived growth factor (PDGF) and nerve growth factor (NGF). These growth factors stimulate DNA synthesis and mitogenesis. Each growth factor may act at different parts of the cell replication cycle and the different factors may synergize. Additionally, growth factors interact during cellular differentiation. Growth factors are widely expressed at mRNA and protein levels throughout the embryo and fetus. In the human fetus in late first and early second trimester, IGF-II and lower levels of IGF-I are widely expressed, but mostly localized to mesenchymal cells (Han et al 1987a). However, on immunohisto-chemistry, these peptides are present in epithelial tissues of the lung, gut, kidney, liver parenchyma, adrenal cortex and in differentiated muscle (Han et al 1987b). Thus the sites of synthesis and action differ. TGF-β1, -β2 and -β3 are expressed in the human fetus in a distinct spatial and temporal pattern during morphogenic events (Gatherer et al 1990).

The exact role of these growth factors in man remains undefined. Nevertheless, in the mouse embryo, mRNAs encoding TGF-α, TGF-β, activin and IGF-II are detectable shortly after fertilization. Using the technique of homologous recombination to disrupt either the IGF-I, the IGF-II or the type 1 IGF receptor gene loci in mice and subsequently interbreeding them, combination gene 'knockouts' have been obtained. Deletion of the IGF-1 gene yielded homozygotes with a birthweight about 60% that of normal and some died within 6 hours of birth (Liu et al 1993). IGF-II-deficient homozygotes had a similar growth deficiency at birth to animals lacking IGF-I (DeChiara et al 1990) and hence both IGFs are necessary for prenatal growth.

Deletion of the type 1 IGF receptor, which is primarily responsible for the signaling of both mitogenic and differentiation actions of both IGF-I and IGF-II, produced homozygote animals weighing only 45% of normal animals at birth. These mice died within minutes of birth as a result of widespread muscle hypoplasia, including that of the respiratory muscles (Liu et al 1993). Co-deletion of IGF-II and the type 1 receptor yielded animals with only 30% of normal birthweight at term and grossly retarded skeletal development. Hence, it would appear that a different receptor may be responsible for some of the actions of IGF-II.

In human infants suffering from intrauterine growth retardation, IGF-I concentrations are lower than in age-matched controls, whilst levels of IGF-II are similar (Lassarre et al 1991). On the other hand, in macrosomic infants of diabetic mothers, circulating levels of IGF-I are elevated (Delmis et al 1992). This would appear to indicate that the circulating concentrations of IGF-I may be closely related to growth rate in the last trimester. However, circulating concentrations of IGFBP-1 are significantly elevated in growth-retarded newborns and may therefore limit the availability of IGF-I to its high-affinity receptors (Wang et al 1991). Animal studies have demonstrated that tissue growth rate can be altered rapidly by a local or widespread change in IGFBP synthesis or by a limitation of the bioavailability of IGF-I and IGF-II (Iwamoto et al 1992, McLellan et al 1992).

Hence, although recent work has indicated the importance of growth factors in the regulation of fetal growth, we are only just beginning to understand the complicated process of fetal growth. The advent of sophisticated molecular biological techniques will shed further light on the subject over the next few years.

POSTNATAL GROWTH

The human growth curve

The human growth curve is clearly depicted in Figure 8.2, which describes the growth of the son of Comte Philibert de Montbeillard from 1759 to 1777, during which time he was measured at 6-monthly intervals. The top half of the figure shows the increase in height plotted every 6 months in the form of a distance chart. In the bottom half, the increment in height every 6 months has been converted into an annual figure by doubling and is plotted against the chronological age – a velocity chart. The velocity chart clearly describes the infancy–childhood–pubertal model of growth, which was first proposed by Karlberg et al in 1987. The three phases of growth are represented by the rapid and rapidly decelerating growth of the first 3 years (infancy phase), the steady and slowly decelerating growth of mid-childhood (childhood phase) and the pubertal growth spurt (pubertal phase). In a significant proportion of children, a growth spurt is clearly demonstrated between the ages of 6 and 8 years, as can be seen in

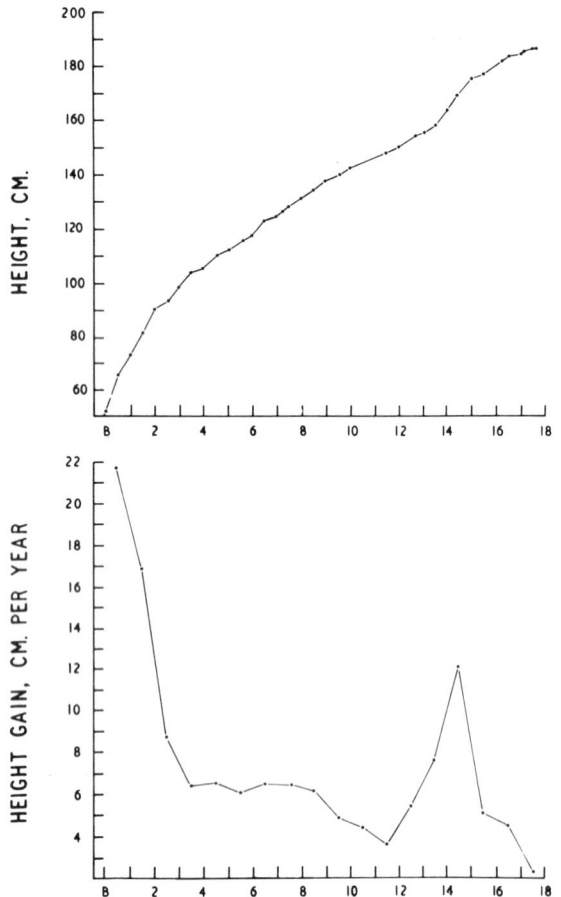

Fig. 8.2 Growth in height of Comte de Montbeillard's son from birth to 18 years (1759–1777) (**a**) Distance chart showing height (cm) attained at each age. (**b**) Velocity chart showing increment in height (cm/year). (From Tanner 1962 with permission.)

the velocity chart in Figure 8.2b. This feature of children's growth is more pronounced in boys, but also occurs in girls (Gasser et al 1985).

The height velocity or the rate of growth reflects the child's state at any particular time much more accurately than does the height attained, which is dependent upon the child's growth in the preceding years. The velocity actually decreases from the fifth month of fetal life. From birth till the age of 4 or 5 years, the height velocity declines rapidly. There then follows a period during which growth occurs at a steady rate between the ages of 5–6 years and adolescence. At adolescence, the growth spurt during puberty leads to a rapid acceleration and deceleration of growth.

Types of growth data

Curves representing growth can be fitted to data on single individuals. These will obviously differ from curves representing yearly averages derived from different children each measured once only. This distinction gives rise to the concept of longitudinal and cross-sectional data. Longitudinal standards are based upon a relatively small number of children measured on multiple occasions over many years; cross-sectional standards are based upon data from a large number of children each of whom is measured on a single occasion. A study may be longitudinal over any number of years; short-term longitudinal studies extend from age 4 to 6 for example, whereas longer term studies may extend from birth until the age of 20 years.

Both cross-sectional and longitudinal studies have their uses, but they do not give the same information and cannot be dealt with in the same way. Cross-sectional studies are cheaper and quicker but fail to reveal individual differences in the rate of growth or in the timing of particular phases of growth, e.g. the adolescent growth spurt. Longitudinal studies are laborious and time consuming; height measurements need to be very accurate, since in the calculation of a growth increment from one occasion to the next, two errors of measurement occur. Nevertheless, longitudinal studies are the basis of research and understanding of the growth process and essential for interrelating the dynamics of growth with endocrine or other controlling factors.

Cross-sectional data are particularly misleading in terms of the adolescent growth spurt. Figures 8.3a and 8.3b illustrate these effects. Figure 8.3a shows a series of individual velocity curves from 10 to 18 years, with each individual starting his growth spurt at a different age. The mean of these longitudinal curves, obtained by treating the values cross-sectionally and adding them up at different ages and then dividing them by 5, is shown by the heavy interrupted line. This line in no way characterizes the 'average' velocity curve, but is a total misrepresentation of a velocity curve. It smoothes out the adolescent spurt, spreading it along the time axis.

One way of circumventing this problem is by constructing curves whose 50th centile represents the actual growth of a typical individual, by taking the shape of the curve from individual longitudinal data and the absolute values for the beginning and end from large cross-sectional surveys. This approach has been used in the past to construct standards for height for clinical use.

Height and weight velocity charts

Recently, it has been suggested that the Tanner–Whitehouse growth charts which have been in use since 1966 do not represent

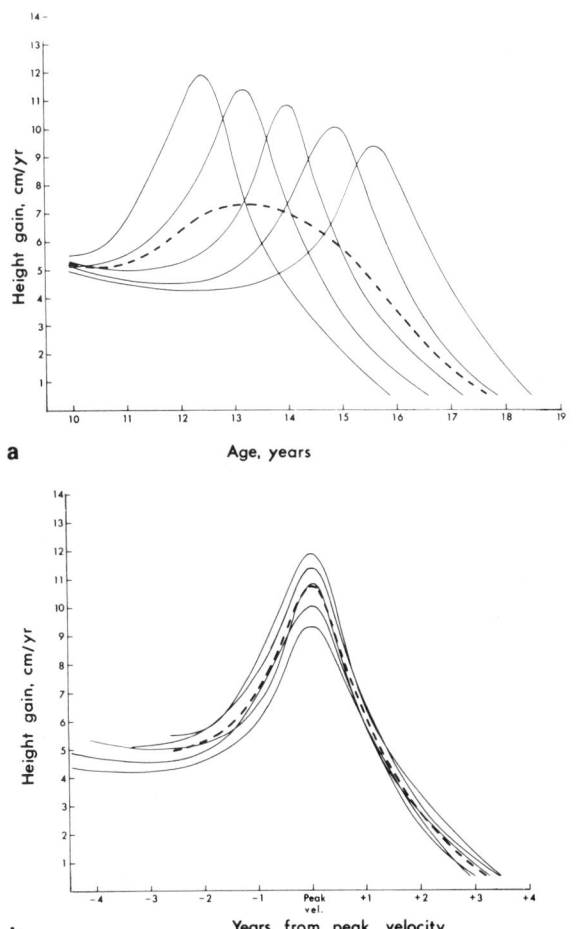

Fig. 8.3 The relation between individual and mean velocities during the adolescent growth spurt. (**a**) Individual height velocity curves of five boys from the original Harpenden Growth study (solid lines) with the mean curve (dashed) constructed by averaging their values at each age. (**b**) The same curves all plotted according to their peak height velocity. (From Tanner et al 1966 with permission.)

accurately the growth in stature and weight of present-day British children (Chinn et al 1989a). There are two potential reasons for this: the first is the secular trend towards earlier maturity and increased adult size (Chinn et al 1989b), the second that the data used to produce the charts were not nationally representative. In view of these concerns, new cross-sectional growth standards were constructed using data from several sources scattered throughout the UK between 1978 and 1990 (Freeman et al 1995). In clinical practice, using these cross-sectional standards rather than longitudinal charts makes little difference, provided that one remembers that normal individuals will probably cross centile lines at the time of puberty and that the growth pattern of each child should be individually assessed at this time. The advantage of using cross-sectional standards at this time lies in the fact that these standards can be regularly revised to reflect secular trends.

These newer cross-sectional data have shown that the 3rd, 50th and 97th centiles are greater than the Tanner–Whitehouse charts by up to 1.7 cm. Cole (1994) has suggested using an alternative set of nine centile curves for growth charts which are constructed by maintaining a constant 0.67 SD units between curves giving the 0.4th, 2nd, 9th, 25th, 50th, 75th, 91st, 98th and 99.6th centiles.

These charts provide a graded area for discussions about referral, as will be discussed in the section on growth disorders (p. 368).

Figure 8.4 shows the standard centile distance charts for boys and girls coupled with pubertal staging, which is a vital component in the assessment of growth. These charts show that girls are slightly shorter than boys at all ages till adolescence. On average, the pubertal growth spurt occurs 2 years earlier in girls than in boys and this means that girls are taller in early adolescence. This is reversed at the age of 14, when boys are well into their growth spurt and the growth spurt of girls may be complete.

The description of height at any age on a centile chart only compares the height of the individual with the heights of children in the reference population at the same age. It certainly gives no information as regards the diagnosis or management of growth disorders in individual children. Using the new centile charts, the percentage of children lying, say, below the 2nd centile is 2%. A proportion of these children will be normal, but the probability of any child being abnormal in this group is greater. A child whose height falls below the 0.4th centile (i.e. the shortest 4/1000 children in the population) is very unlikely to be normal. However, a child lying within the centile charts may also be growing abnormally because of a recently acquired growth disorder; a single point plotted on the distance chart will yield little useful information. Screening and investigating only children below the 0.4th centile for stature will lead to a failure to detect taller children with a growth disorder. Hence, sequential measurements of height are vital in the assessment of a short child. These are then plotted onto the distance chart.

The target height of a child is calculated by measuring the parents' heights and plotting them on the centile charts after the appropriate correction for the sex of the child and then calculating the mid-parental target height as follows:

MPH if male = [father's height + (mother's height + 14)]/2
MPH if female = [(father's height – 14) + mother's height]/2

The 2nd and 98th centiles for the family are defined by the MPH ± 10 cm. Following this, the expected distribution of heights of the children of parents of given heights is further narrowed down. Hence, all children assessed for growth problems should have their parents' heights transcribed onto the right-hand edge of the growth chart, after applying the appropriate correction of ± 14 cm for the parent of the opposite sex. It is important to note that the 14 cm figure is the mean difference between adult men and women in the UK and this figure should be adjusted appropriately in other populations according to local data. Generally, if a child's height falls outside the range defined by the parents' heights, an explanation should be sought.

Measurement of standing height up to the age of 2 years is virtually impossible. Hence, a supine measurement is performed One measurer holds the child's head in contact with a fixed board whilst a second measurer stretches the child out to their maximum length and then brings a moving board into contact with his or her heels. This supine length averages 1 cm more than the measurement of standing height performed on the same individual. Over the age of 2 years, measurements are based upon the use of the Harpenden stadiometer (Fig. 8.5). Using this instrument in trained hands, the accuracy of height is within ± 0.1–0.3 cm. It is important to ensure that the measurement is as accurate as possible, since any error will be reflected in the annualized height velocity. Standing height is measured as follows:

1. The child should stand straight and tall with heels firmly on the floor, shoulders relaxed and looking straight ahead.
2. The outer canthus of the eyes and the external auditory meati should be in the same horizontal plane.
3. The child should take a deep breath in and then out, whilst gentle upward pressure is exerted upon the mastoid process. The maximum height is then read off to the nearest millimeter.

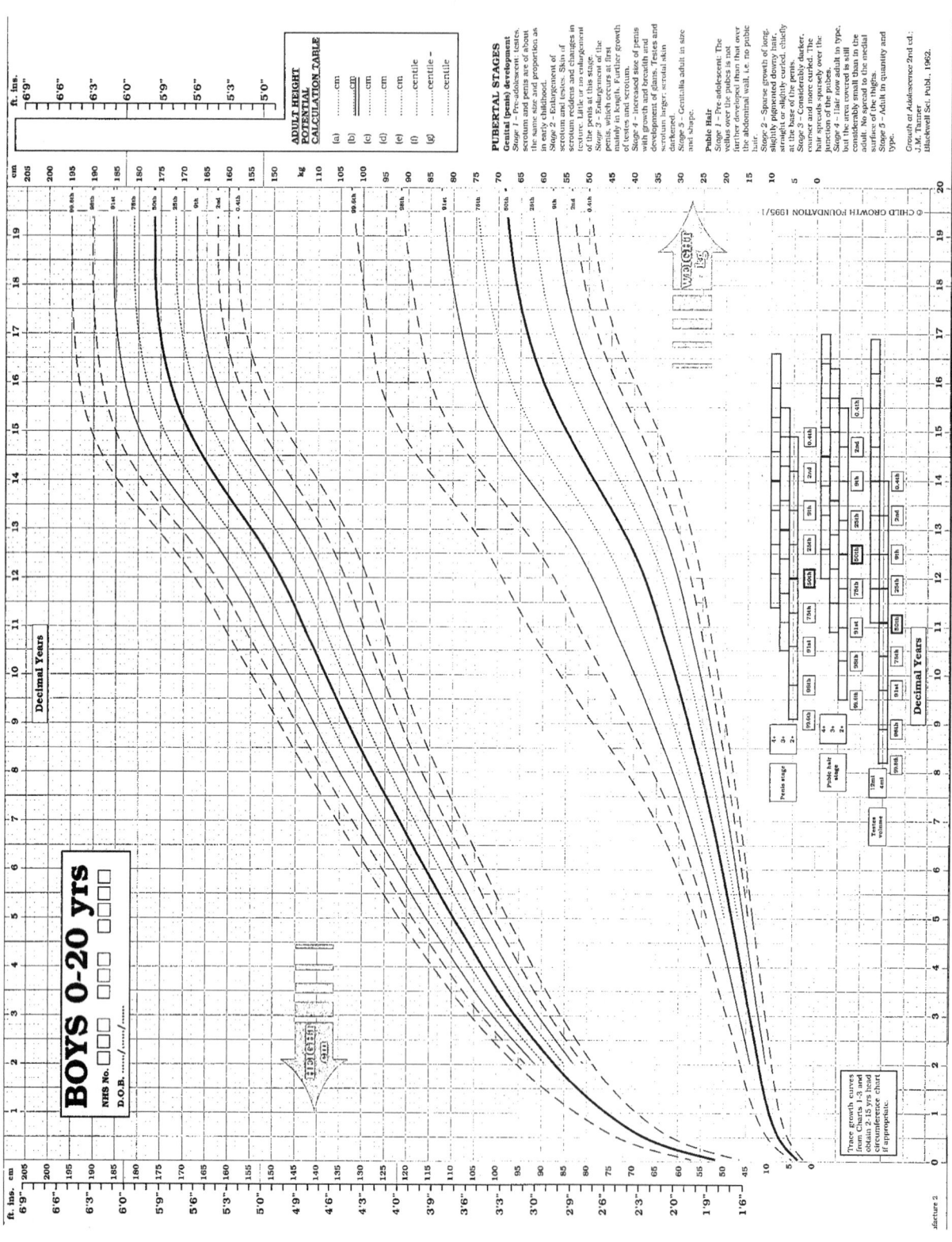

Fig. 8.4a Standard centile chart for height and weight in boys (© Child Growth Foundation 1995/1).

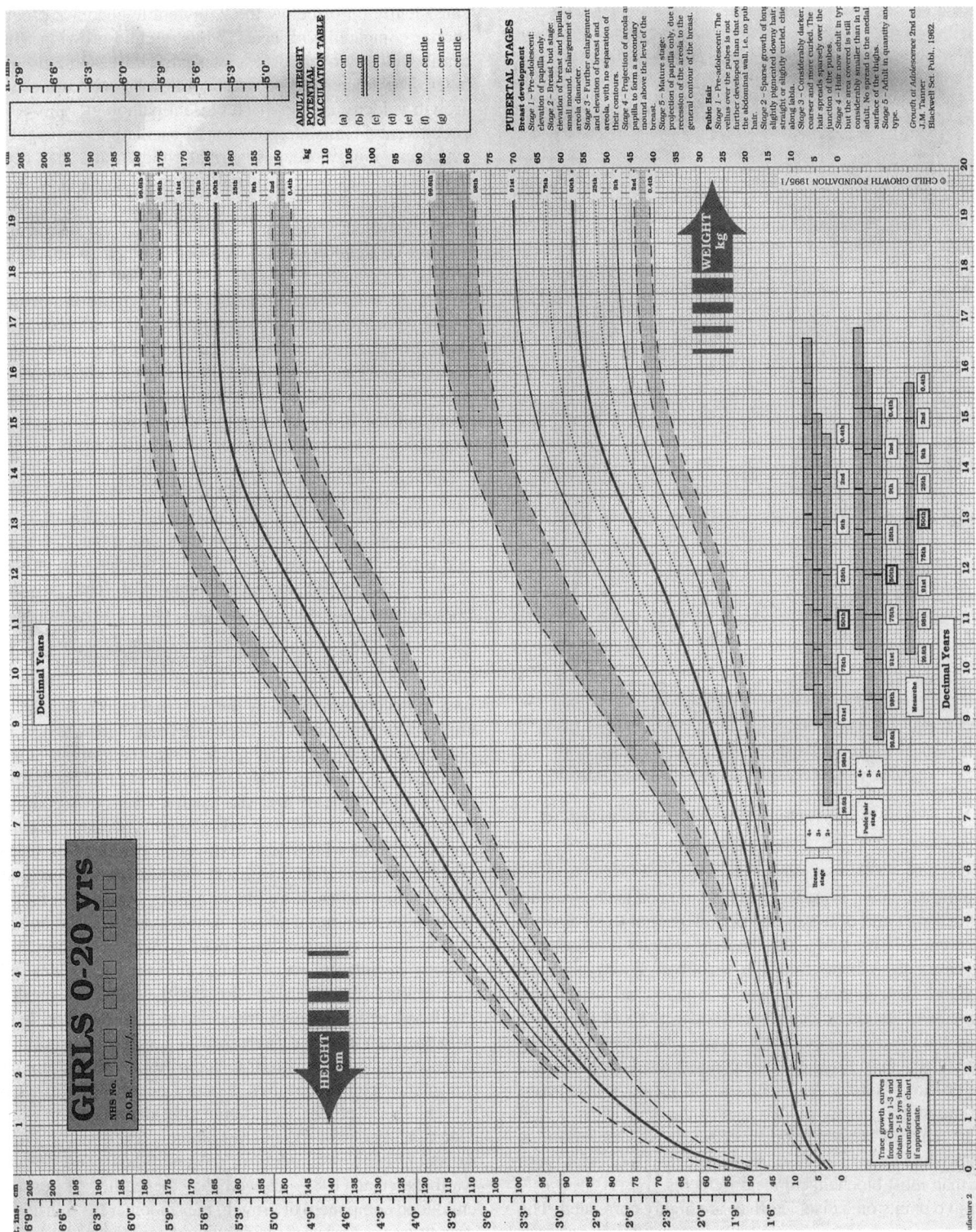

Fig. 8.4b   Standard centile chart for height and weight in girls (© Child Growth Foundation 1995/1).

Of paramount importance in the assessment of growth is the measurement of growth velocity. To estimate the rate at which a child is growing, it is essential to measure height on more than one occasion over a period of time, and divide the increment in cm by the time elapsed in years. It is important to ensure that the increment in height between two measurements is greater than the cumulative errors inherent in the two measurements. A reliable estimate of growth velocity is dependent upon the accuracy with

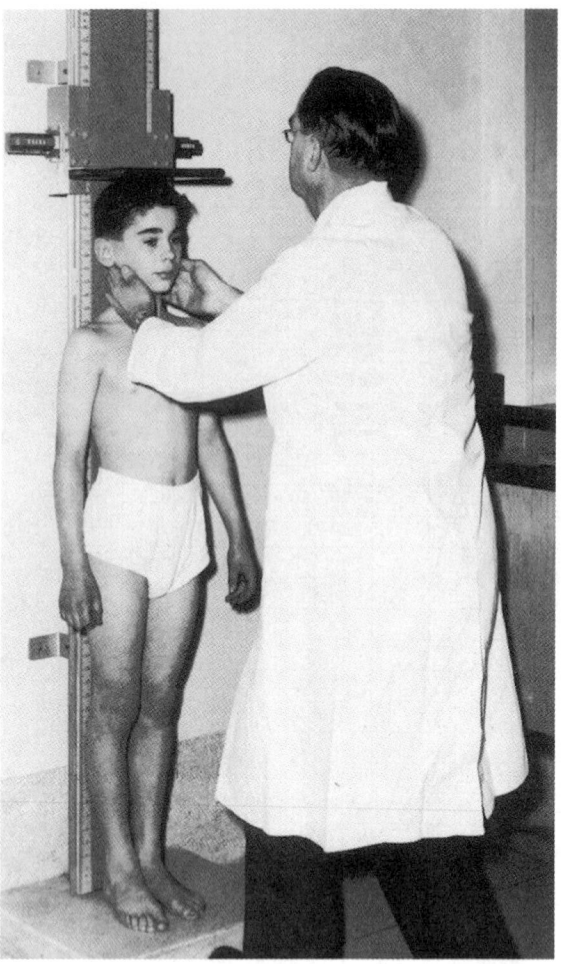

Fig. 8.5 Measurement of standing height using a Harpenden stadiometer.

consistently on or below the 25th centile becomes progressively shorter compared with peers, whilst a child growing with a 75th centile velocity over successive years will become progressively taller. The longer the period of follow-up, the more a reduced growth velocity is likely to represent pathology. This would also circumvent the misinterpretation of oscillations in height velocity which commonly occur in normal children and may actually be seasonal or may occur cyclically over intervals of about 2 years (Butler et al 1990).

Height velocity measured over an extended period is a good measure of a child's overall well-being. It detects abnormalities of growth regardless of stature achieved and this has a distinct advantage over distance charts. The exception is puberty, when height velocity means nothing without taking into account pubertal stage. For instance, in constitutional delay of growth and puberty, because puberty is delayed, the normal childhood velocity continues to decline, so that a child not entering a pubertal growth spurt until the 16th year may grow exceedingly slowly or may even stop growing and yet have a normal growth spurt in the end.

Growth in the first 2 years of life

Many disorders of growth present during infancy, when growth rate is particularly rapid. The rapid but decelerating growth of the first 2 years of life is a continuation of fetal growth and is predominantly nutrition dependent. Over- or undernutrition during this period may have lifelong effects on growth. Both weight and length should be considered in assessing the growth of a child in infancy. Centile charts exist for both parameters. Birthweight is predominantly controlled by the maternal uterine factors, so that a child who carries genes for large size cannot grow to his or her full potential until the postnatal period, when the restraint of the uterus is removed. At that time, there is a period of rapid catch-up growth. By 12–18 months of age, the catch-up period is complete and, subsequently, the child proceeds along his/her centile. During this period, a child with a low birthweight centile rises through the centiles, whereas a child with a higher birthweight centile may fall through the centiles. If a child with a low birthweight falls through the centiles, then further assessment is essential. Studies conducted in developing countries show poor growth alternating with rapid growth in infants postweaning and this correlates with the availability of food (Costello 1989). After the onset of the childhood period, growth proceeded at a normal rate. In children with growth hormone deficiency who have a growth hormone gene deletion, the growth pattern is compatible with a continuation of the infancy component (Wit & Van Unen 1992). This is because the childhood phase is predominantly dependent on the normal secretion of hGH by the anterior pituitary and in the absence of GH secretion, there is a failure of the childhood phase to take over. Karlberg et al (1987) showed that the earlier the onset of the childhood component of growth, the smoother the transition on the growth curve. Onset of the childhood component after the age of 12 months was extremely unlikely.

Preterm infants whose birthweight is appropriate for their gestational age grow normally given adequate postnatal treatment. Their weight and length should be plotted in relation to their postconception age. Small for dates babies do not, on average, reach the height and weight of normal children, even though they may have some initial catch-up growth. Their problems are often compounded by feeding difficulties in the first year of life which further compromise growth.

which the measurement is made; errors of 1 mm on measurements of height at either end of a 3-month period amount to an error of at least 1.6 cm/year if an annualized height velocity is calculated. This increases to 3.2 cm/year with errors of 2 mm on each measurement. Hence, great caution is required in interpreting measurements of height velocity over short periods of time. Use of purpose-built standard equipment by the same measurer at the same time of day minimizes errors. Each unit needs to perform a precision profile, whereby the coefficients of variation on a series of height measurements are plotted against the heights (Voss et al 1991). In careful hands, the coefficient of variation is considerably less than 1% and so this auxological tool is far more sensitive than most biochemical measurements.

Successive points on a distance chart are highly correlated. The child who is small on one occasion will almost certainly be small on subsequent occasions. The growth of a normal child is likely to follow a particular centile. Deviation from centile lines is only evident when growth is extremely slow or continues at a diminished rate over a long period of time. In this instance, plotting successive height velocities on a suitable velocity chart (see, for example, Tanner & Whitehouse 1976) gives valuable information. Successive velocities do not correlate and must oscillate about the 50th centile if the child is to keep up with his or her peers. The child whose velocity over successive years is

Growth and development during adolescence

Introduction

During the childhood phase, height growth occurs at a rate of 5–6 cm/year in a steady manner. Growth is dependent on GH during this phase. Prior to the adolescent growth spurt, the rate falls to 4–5 cm/year. Prepubertal growth occurs mainly in the limbs, as opposed to pubertal growth which occurs mainly in the trunk.

At puberty, a very considerable change in growth rate occurs. An increase in body size is accompanied by a change in shape and body composition and a rapid development of gonads. In boys, there is an increase in muscle bulk and strength. Additionally, various physical characteristics, known as secondary sexual characteristics, develop in both boys and girls.

The timing of puberty and hence the adolescent growth spurt, has undergone secular changes in the last 100–150 years and the age of menarche in the West has decreased by approximately 2–3 months per decade. The onset of menarche is very closely related to nutritional status. Moderate obesity is associated with earlier menarche, whereas delayed menarche is associated with strenuous physical activity, malnutrition and chronic disease.

Physical changes of puberty

The physical changes of puberty can be described objectively by using the standards formalized by Tanner to describe the maturation of secondary sexual characteristics.

BOYS The first sign of puberty in the boy is usually an acceleration of the growth of the testes and scrotum with reddening and wrinkling of the scrotal skin. There may be slight growth of pubic hair at this stage, although this is usually a later development. The spurts in height and penile growth usually occur a year after the first acceleration of testicular development. Testicular growth is mainly due to an increase in the size of the seminiferous tubules. Leydig cells are present at birth, regress rapidly shortly afterwards and then from 6 months until puberty, they are few, inconspicuous and inactive. They become more prominent at puberty and their full development is achieved in late puberty. The seminal vesicles, the prostate and the bulbourethral glands enlarge and develop at the same time as the growth of the penis. Spermatogenesis can be detected histologically at 11–15 years of age. Axillary hair appears approximately 2 years after the beginning of pubic hair growth. Facial hair develops at around the same time. Breaking of the voice is due to enlargement of the larynx as a result of the action of testosterone on the laryngeal cartilages and is a late and inconstant event. In 20–30% of boys, there is a distinct enlargement of the breast (often unilateral) in adolescence. This usually regresses after approximately a year.

GIRLS In girls, the appearance of the breast bud is the first sign of puberty, though the appearance of pubic hair sometimes precedes it. The uterus and vagina develop simultaneously with the breast. Menarche is a late event and occurs after the peak height velocity has been attained. The early cycles are often irregular and anovulatory.

Ratings of development for clinical use

BOYS In the male, ratings are expressed as stages of genital development, pubic hair development, axillary hair development and testicular volume. These standards are extremely important in

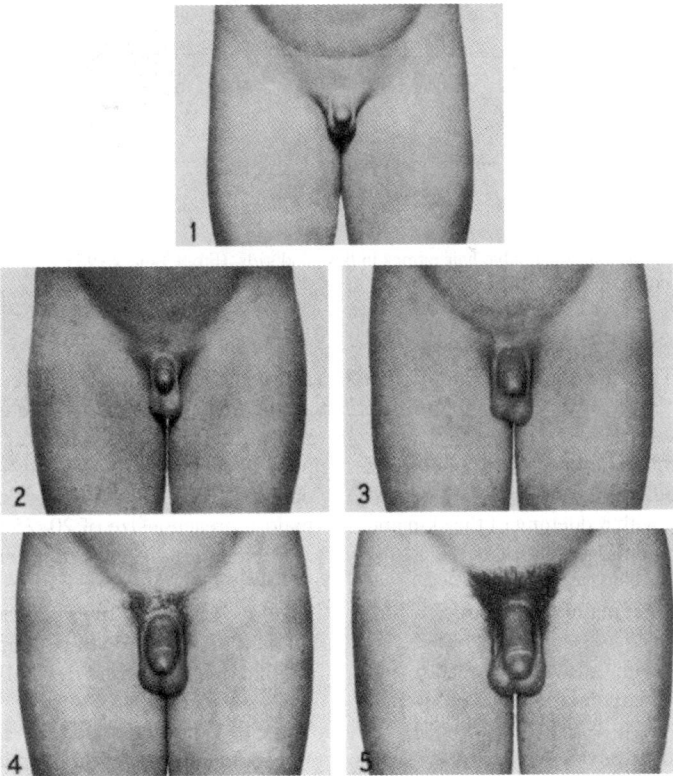

Fig. 8.6   Standards for genital maturity in boys. (From Tanner 1962 with permission.)

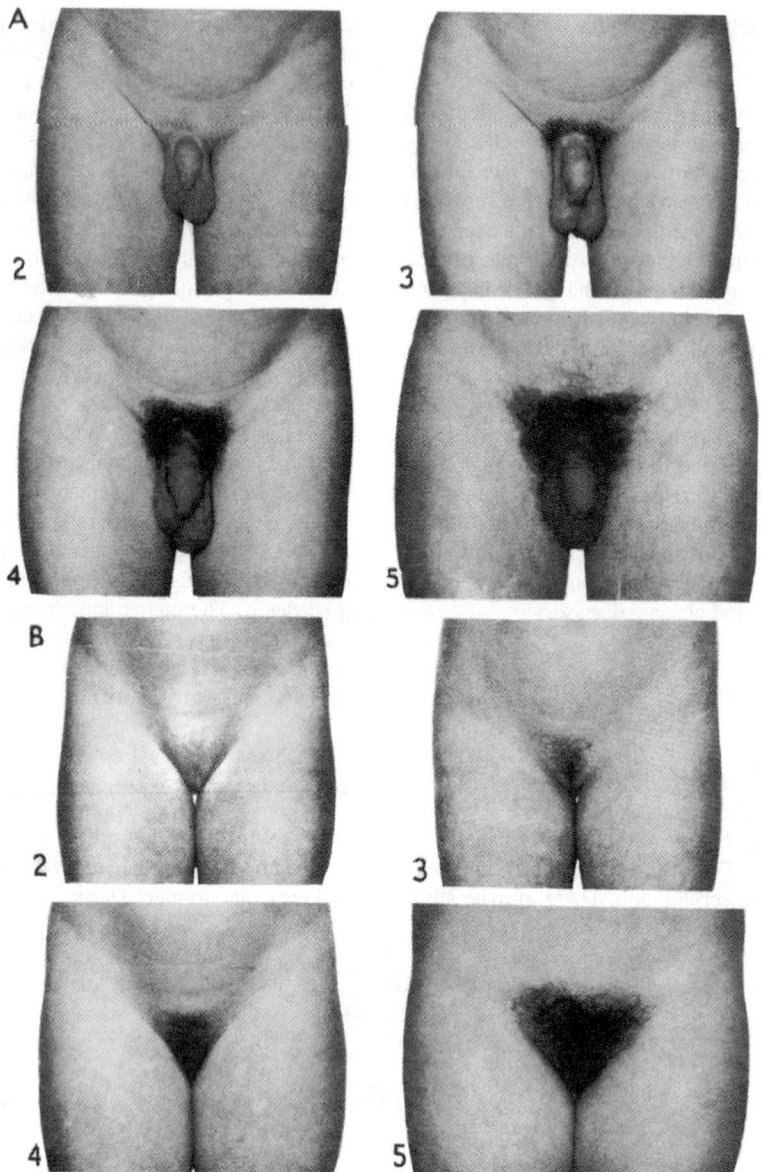

Fig. 8.7 Standards for pubic hair ratings in boys and girls. (From Tanner 1975 with permission.)

assessing growth in adolescents. They are shown in Figures 8.6 and 8.7 and are described below.

Genitalia

Stage 1: Preadolescent. Testes, scrotum and penis are about same size and shape as in early childhood.

Stage 2: Scrotum slightly enlarged, with reddening of the skin and changes in the texture. Little or no enlargement of penis at this stage.

Stage 3: Penis slightly enlarged, at first mainly in length. Scrotum further enlarged than in stage 2.

Stage 4: Penis further enlarged, with growth in breadth and development of glans. Further enlargement of scrotum and darkening of scrotal skin.

Stage 5: Genitalia adult in size and shape.

Testicular volumes are assessed by palpation in comparison with

a string of plastic models of testicular shape known as the Prader orchidometer. The models are marked according to their volumes in milliliters: sizes 1–3 are prepubertal, 4 signals the beginning of puberty and 10–12 are mid-pubertal and coincide with the pubertal growth spurt. A few individuals stop at 12 ml, but the majority reach a size of 20–25 ml in adulthood.

Pubic hair stages for boys and girls

Stage 1: Preadolescent. The vellus over the pubes is not further developed than that over the abdominal wall, i.e. no pubic hair.

Stage 2: Sparse growth of long, slightly pigmented downy hair, straight or slightly curled, chiefly at the base of the penis or along labia.

Stage 3: Considerably darker, coarser and more curled. The hair spreads sparsely over the junction of the pubes.

Stage 4: Hair now adult in type, but area covered is still considerably smaller than in adults. No spread to medial surface of thighs.

Stage 5: Adult in quantity and type with distribution of the horizontal (or classically 'feminine') pattern. Spread to medial surface of thighs, but not up the linea alba.

   GIRLS Breast development (see Fig. 8.8)
Stage 1: Preadolescent: elevation of papilla only.
Stage 2: Breast bud stage: elevation of breast and papilla as small mound. Areola diameter enlarged over stage 1.
Stage 3: Breast and areola both enlarged and elevated more than in stage 2, but with no separation of their contors.

Stage 4: The areola and papilla form a secondary mound projecting above the contor of the breast.
Stage 5: Mature stage: papilla only projects, with the areola recessed to the general contour of the breast.

Normal variations in pubertal development

There is considerable variability in children with respect to the rapidity with which they pass through various stages of puberty

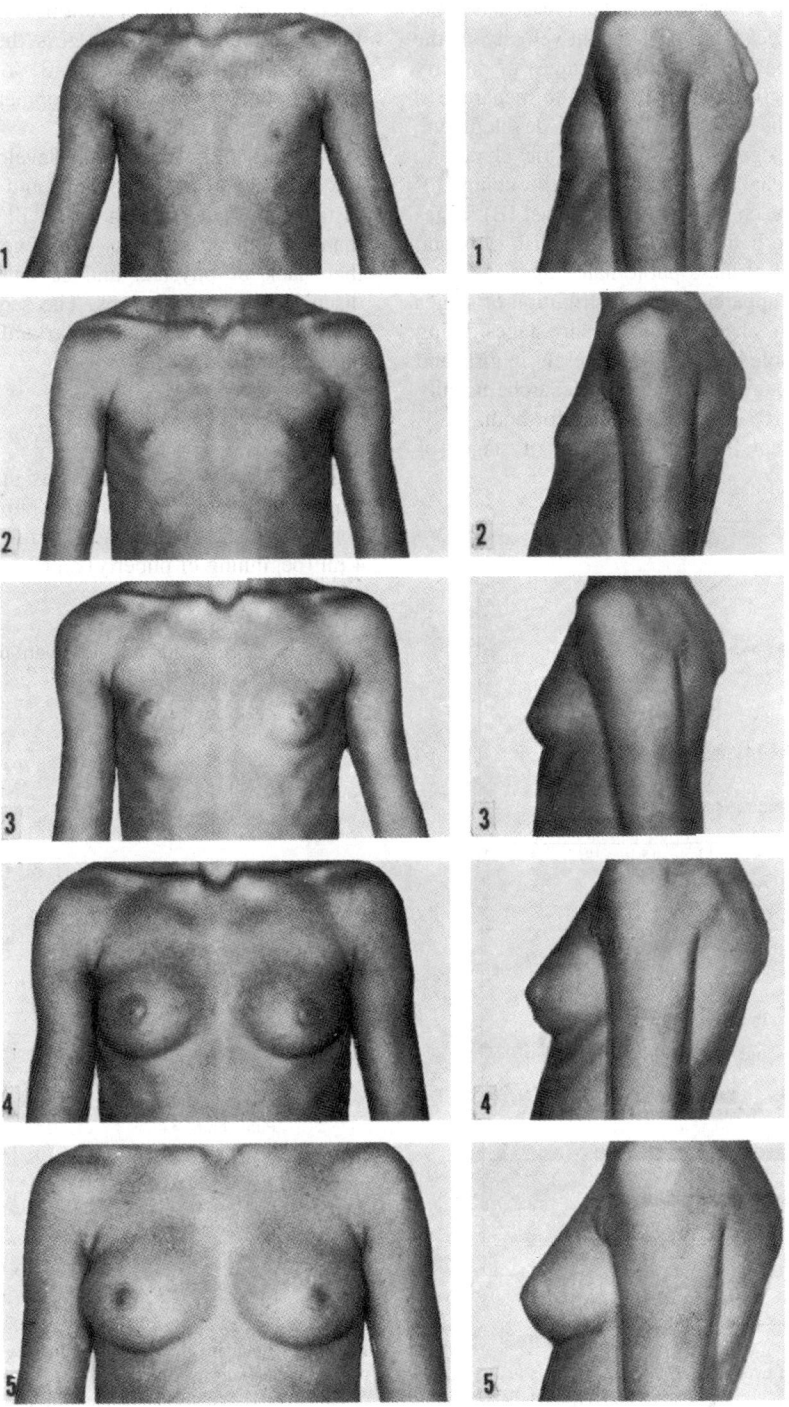

Fig. 8.8 Standards for breast development. (From Tanner 1962 with permission.)

and in the closeness with which the various events are linked together, as shown in Figure 8.9. The lines marked *breast* in the girls and *penis and testis* in the boys represent the period of accelerated growth of these organs and the lines and the rating numbers marked *pubic hair* represent its advent and development. The sequence and timings shown represent in each case average values for British boys and girls. To denote the variations from the means, figures for the range of ages at which the various events begin and end are inserted under the first and last point of the curves or bars.

At one extreme one may find a perfectly healthy girl who has not yet menstruated though she has reached adult breast and pubic hair ratings and is already 2 years postpeak height velocity. At the other extreme, a girl may have passed all the stages of puberty within the space of 2 years. To progress from B2 to menarche, a girl may take from 6 months to 5.5 years. Breast development, which is controlled by estrogen, and pubic hair development, which is controlled by adrenal androgens under the control of ACTH, are independent of each other. In girls, breast (B) stages 1–5 are represented at pubic hair stages 3–4 in British girls and stages B2–5 are represented at these pubic hair stages in Swiss girls. The same variation is apparent in the distribution of stages of pubic hair at B3, with all five pubic hair stages being represented. At stage B5, pubic hair is always present in girls and only 10% are at less than pubic hair stage 4. Menarche usually occurs at B4 and P4, but in 10% occurs at stage 5 for both.

Similar trends are apparent in the distribution of stages of genitalia and pubic hair in boys. Development of the genitalia may proceed from G2 to G5 over a time scale of 2–5 years. The acceleration of penile growth begins on average at the age of 12.5 years, but can occur at any age between 10.5 and 14.5 years. The completion of penile development usually occurs at the age of 14.5, but can occur at any age between 12.5 and 16.5. In a small proportion of boys, genitalia can develop to stage 4 before the growth of pubic hair.

The growth spurt occurs relatively later in boys than in girls. There is a difference of 2 years between boys and girls in terms of peak height velocity. The peak height velocity in boys usually occurs when a testicular volume of 10–12 ml has been attained, this corresponding to G4. In girls, the peak height velocity usually corresponds to breast stage 2–3. A few boys do not begin their growth spurts or penile development until the earliest maturers have entirely completed theirs.

The variability in pubertal development, particularly in boys, has profound psychological and social consequences. For instance, boys developing early will be stronger and more athletic than other boys, whereas late developers may be frustrated by their lack of physical and sexual development. This will be discussed in later sections. The sequence of normal puberty in children is, however, remarkably constant under normal circumstances.

Age standards for pubertal development

Figure 8.10 shows the standards in clinical use for the ages at which each genital, breast and pubic hair stage is observed in normal British children and also for the attainment of testes sizes 4 ml (beginning of puberty) and 12 ml (minimal adult size) from

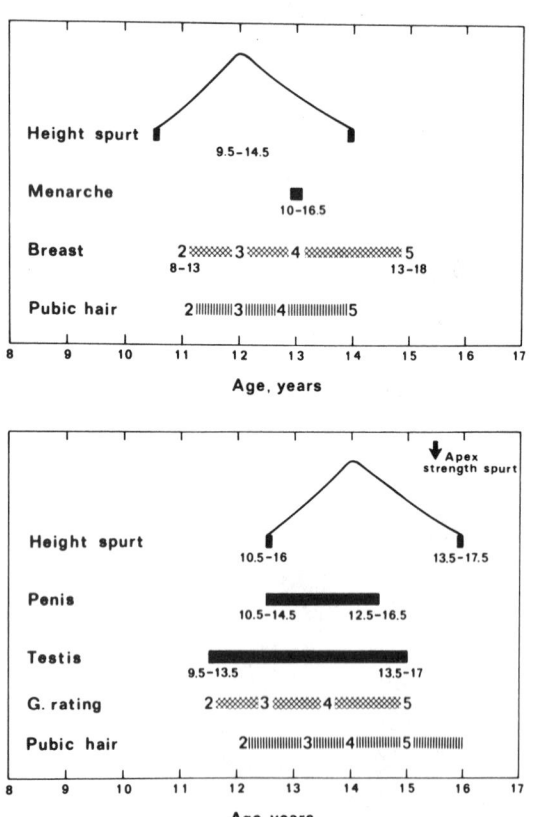

Fig. 8.9 Diagram of sequence of events in adolescence in boys and girls. The range of ages within which each event charted may begin and end is given by the figures placed directly below its start and finish. (From Marshall & Tanner 1970 with permission.)

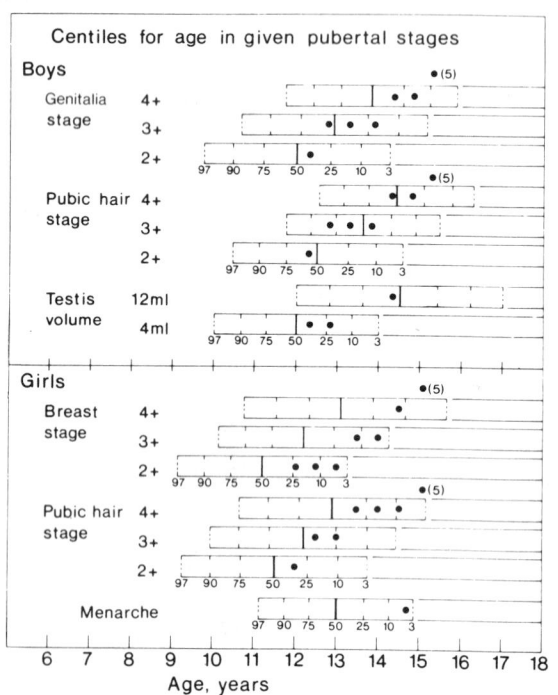

Fig. 8.10 Standards for age of occurrence of pubertal stages. Successive plots are made on successive visits and examination of the child at the times of the visits. The figures show the centiles for development of each stage and the vertical bars represent the 60th centile. (From Tanner 1975 with permission.)

a group of Swiss children. B2, for example, represents the instant in time when breast development is first noted. In practice, girls are usually seen when they are between B2 and B3 and this is referred to as either stage B2 or B2+. The standards refer to the age range at which each of the appearances is observed in healthy children, with appropriate designation of centiles.

The adolescent growth spurt

At puberty, there is a very considerable increase in growth rate along with the various physical and emotional changes. For a year or more, the height velocity practically doubles and so this is the most rapid rate of growth since the neonatal period. The growth spurt occurs in girls simultaneously with the onset of secondary sexual characteristics, compared with boys where the growth spurt is a late feature.

The peak height velocity (PHV) is approximately 10 cm/year in boys and 9 cm/year in girls (with a standard deviation of approximately 1 cm/year). This figure represents the instantaneous peak given by a smooth curve drawn through the observations. The velocity over the whole year encompassing the 6 months before and after the peak is somewhat less; during this year, a boy usually grows between 7 and 12 cm/year, whilst a girl grows between 6 and 11 cm/year. Children who have their peak early reach a somewhat higher peak than those who have their peaks late.

The average age at which the peak occurs varies between different population groups. For example, in British children, the mean age of PHV is 14 years in boys and 12 years in girls, with a standard deviation of 0.9 years in each case. This 2-year sex difference seems to be a constant feature in all groups. The earlier growth spurt in girls with a reduced period of prepubertal growth,

the shorter duration of the growth spurt and the reduced peak height velocity are the principal factors contributing to the average difference of 14 cm between men and women, as shown in Figure 8.11. Most of the adolescent spurt in height can be attributed to an increase in trunk length. The earliest dimensions to reach adult size are the head, hands and feet.

Following menarche, only about 6 cm growth remains. There is no such event in boys and bone age is the best indicator of the amount of growth still to come. The endocrine factors mediating the pubertal growth spurt are sex steroids and growth hormone. Increasing sex steroid production secondary to pulsatile gonadotropin secretion stimulates increased amplitude of growth hormone secretion at puberty, with subsequent increased production of IGF-I (Harris et al 1985). This then leads to the increase in height velocity which is characteristic of the pubertal growth spurt.

Changes in body composition at adolescence

Percentages of lean body mass and body fat are similar in prepubertal boys and girls, but this changes at puberty. The first change is an increase in lean body mass which starts at the age of 6 years in girls and 9.5 years in boys. By maturity, men have approximately 1.5 times the lean body mass of women, whilst women have twice the amount of fat. There is a marked increase in muscle bulk, this growth being greater in boys. Boys reach their peak at the time of the PHV, whereas girls reach their peak muscle development shortly after the peak height velocity. Hence, there is a narrow window of time, between 12.5 and 13.5 years on average, when girls have more well-developed muscles than boys. The increase in muscle size is naturally accompanied by an increase in muscle strength.

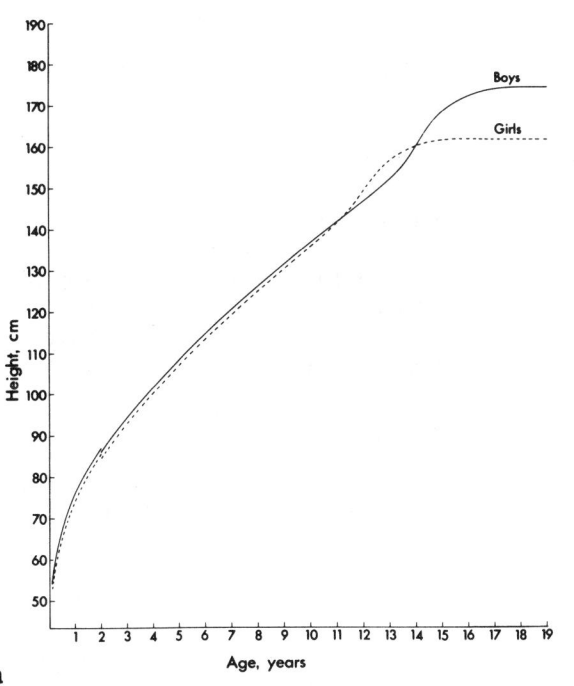

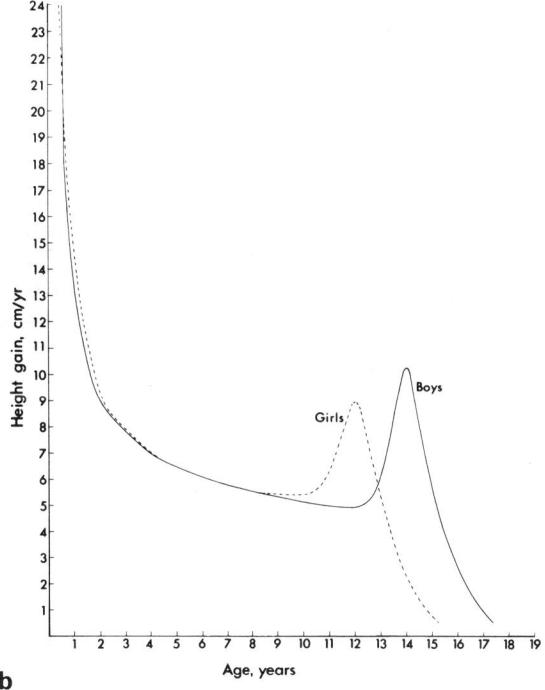

Fig. 8.11 Typical individual velocity curves for supine length or height in boys and girls. These curves represent the velocity of the typical boy and girl at any given instant. (From Tanner et al 1966 with permission.)

In contrast, adolescence is characterized by a loss of limb fat, especially in boys. The maximum rate of loss of limb fat is at the time of the peak height velocity in boys. In girls, there is a decrease in the velocity of fat accumulation; however, this does not translate itself into an absolute loss of fat.

Other changes include an increase in bone mineral density, total body water, intracellular water, the number of red blood cells and the concentration of hemoglobin. All of these changes are more marked in boys than girls.

Bone age

The maturation of the epiphyseal centers in the skeleton proceeds in an orderly fashion, each center going through relatively easily definable stages of radiographic change from the first appearance of the epiphyseal center to its fusion with the appropriate long bone. Skeletal maturity assesses how far the bones of an area have progressed towards maturity, not in size but in shape and in their relative positions to each other, as shown radiographically. The sequence of changes of shape through which each of the epiphyses passes is identical in all individuals. Hence, bone age can be estimated by the time of appearance of different epiphyseal centers or, when all are present, by the stage of maturity. Conventionally, X-rays of the hands and wrists are used for the estimation of skeletal maturity. The wrist is used because there is a large aggregation of long and round bones in a single area and it is easily X-rayed using minimal doses of radiation. Conventionally, the left side is used. The Greulich and Pyle system calculates the median of the skeletal maturities of each epiphyseal center in the hand and wrist. A set of radiological standards was compiled by taking hand radiographs in many children at different ages. For each epiphysis, a comparison is made with the standards and a bone age assigned. The bone ages for the epiphyses are then summated and a median overall bone age calculated. A disadvantage of this method lies in the comparison of an individual X-ray with a whole X-ray standard and identifying the best approximation, which can be misleading.

An alternative method is the Tanner and Whitehouse system (TW2). A series of standard stages is given for each individual bone and each epiphyseal center is assigned a score corresponding to the stage it has reached. The scores are mathematically weighted to produce the best overall estimate of total maturation. The scores are then added to give a bone maturity score. The score is then compared with the range of scores of a standard group at the same age and a percentile status is assigned. A skeletal age is also assigned, this being the age at which the given score lies on the 50th centile. The standards are those of Tanner et al (1983a) based on a large random sample of British children. These were 6–9 months less advanced than the North American well-off middle-class children used in the Greulich–Pyle standards.

In the TW2 version of the Tanner–Whitehouse system, bone age can be calculated using only 13 bones. These are the radius, ulna and the metacarpals and phalanges. This is called the RUS system for calculating skeletal age. In clinical practice it is preferable as the carpus reaches maturity by about 13 years and therefore provides no useful information in the middle and latter stages of puberty.

Skeletal age provides a true common scale of development, unlike 'height age', since all individuals reach the same skeletal age eventually. The information given by a bone age is, however, limited. It essentially assesses the amount of growth which has already taken place and the amount of growth which is left to come. It can also help in the prediction of final height, e.g. a boy aged 13 with a bone age of 11 years would have completed the majority of his growth and if he is short in relation to an average 11-year-old, his final height will be short. In certain pathological conditions, e.g. hypothyroidism, growth hormone insufficiency, the bone age may be delayed. In other conditions, e.g. precocious puberty and thyrotoxicosis, the bone age may be advanced.

The main usefulness of a bone age is in the monitoring of the treatment of a host of endocrine conditions, e.g. congenital adrenal hyperplasia, hypothyroidism, precocious puberty and growth hormone insufficiency. If the increment in height is exceeded by the increment in bone age, then the ultimate height prognosis is compromised. Inappropriate treatment of several conditions can result in such a scenario.

Prediction of adult height

It is important to note that the height centile of a child at any age does not translate directly into the final height centile. Differences in the duration of the growing period will alter the picture substantially; for instance, a delayed bone age will increase the final height centile (Fig. 8.12a), whereas an advanced bone age will lead to a final height centile which is lower than the original centile (Fig. 8.12b). An estimate of the final height can be achieved from the growth chart and will lie somewhere between the centile positions of height for chronological age and height for bone age.

The age at which growth ceases is closely related to the age at which adolescence occurs. In children with delayed puberty, growth in adolescence is somewhat less than would be expected and thus the final height will not lie on the centile for bone age. After the age of approximately 9 years, the amount of growth remaining, and hence final adult stature, can be better predicted by reference to skeletal age rather than chronological age. The use of height prediction is particularly important in the management of children with tall stature. It can influence decisions regarding therapy and, also, assess whether therapy is likely to be of any help in limiting final height. The prediction of adult height requires knowledge of chronological age, bone age and present height. Either the Greulich–Pyle skeletal age is used in conjunction with the Bayley–Pinneau tables (Bayley & Pinneau 1952) or the equation of Roche et al (1975) or the Tanner–Whitehouse skeletal maturity system, using RUS bone age and the equations given in Tanner et al (1983)

The accuracy of the latter is such that 95% (i.e. within 2 standard deviations) of predictions fall within ± 9 cm of true adult height in boys from 9 to 12, ± 7 cm at 13 and 14 and ± 6 cm at age 15. In girls, the prediction is more accurate if allowance is made for whether menarche has occurred. The TW method has a standard deviation of 3.0 cm for a premenarcheal 12-year-old girl and 1.8 cm for a postmenarcheal girl of the same age. All predictions are based on normal children and, strictly speaking, should only be used for normal children. However, height predictions are most often required for children with extremely advanced or delayed bone ages. In particular, height predictions are particularly important in treating tall girls with estrogens to induce early puberty and limit their adult height. It is necessary to bear in mind the limitations of these methods when applied to children with abnormal growth. In particular, these methods

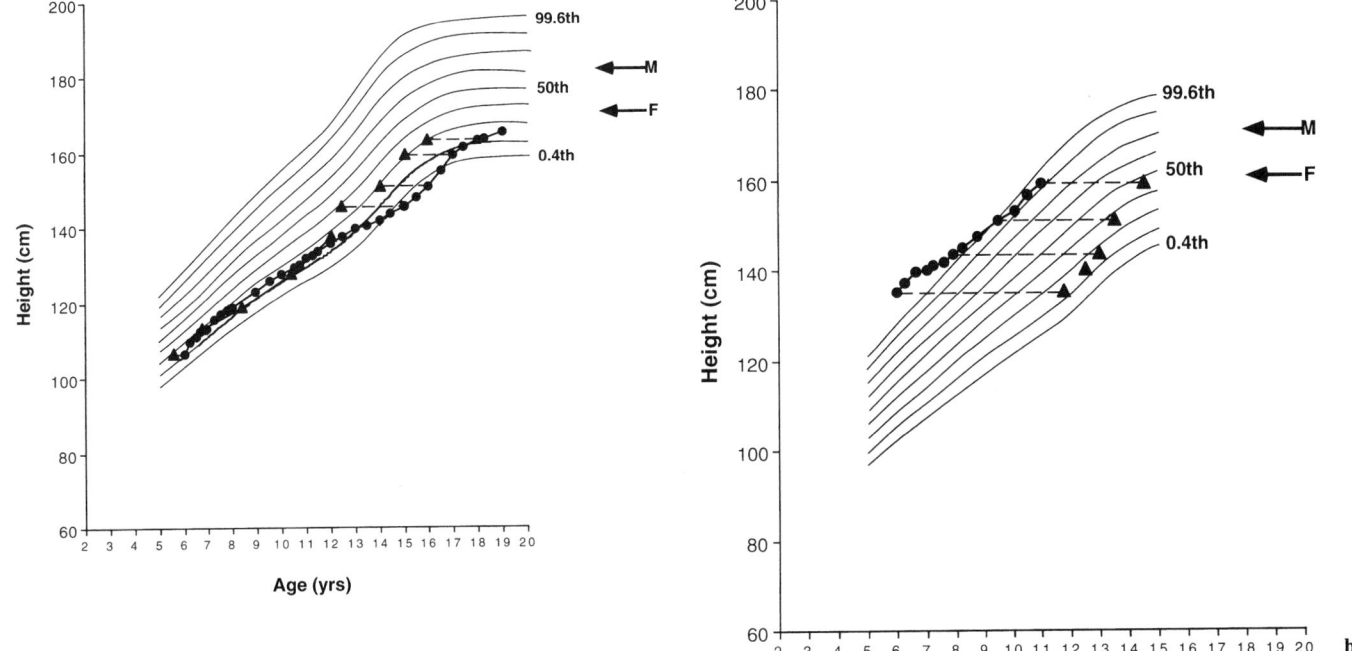

Fig. 8.12 Effect of (**a**) bone age delay and (**b**) bone age advance on final height.

should never be used in conditions where the bone morphology is grossly abnormal, such as in skeletal dysplasias.

The TW method included very tall and very short individuals in the data, making this method more suitable for children at the extremes of normality.

Growth curves of different tissues and different parts of the body

The majority of skeletal and muscular dimensions follow approximately the growth curve described for height and so also do the internal organs such as liver, spleen and kidneys. However, exceptions exist, most notably the brain and skull, the reproductive organs, the lymphoid tissue of the tonsils, adenoids and intestines, and subcutaneous fat. Figure 8.13 shows the differences between various tissues by plotting growth attained at each age as a percentage of the birth-to-maturity increment against the age in years. The reproductive organs grow slowly prepubertally, but in response to gonadotrophins, their growth is extremely rapid during puberty. The brain and skull grow extremely rapidly in the early part of life. At birth, the brain is 25% of its adult weight. By the ages of 5 and 10 years, it has attained 90 and 95% of its adult weight respectively. Lymphoid tissue reaches maximum growth before adolescence and then declines to its adult value.

Other clinically useful measurements

Head circumference

This is important in the assessment of neurological disorders, identifying potential hydrocephalus or microcephaly. The maximum circumference around the supraorbital ridges and the occipital protuberance is measured. Distance and velocity charts are available to monitor head growth.

Sitting height (crown–rump length) and subischial leg length

These measurements are particularly important in the assessment of bodily disproportion, e.g. in achondroplasia, hypochondro-

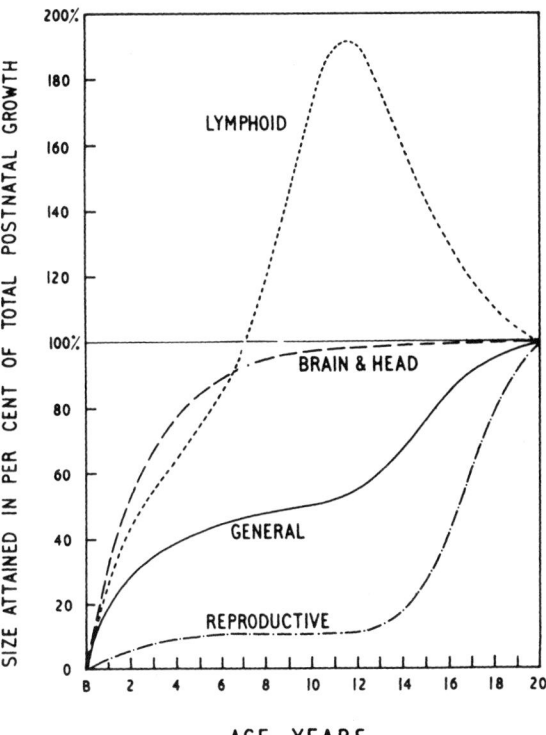

Fig. 8.13 Growth curves of different parts and tissues of the body. All the curves are of size attained and plotted as percent of total gain from birth to 20 years. (From Tanner 1962 with permission.)

plasia and Klinefelter's syndrome. Before the age of 2 years, the crown–rump length is measured. After the age of 2, sitting height is measured using a stadiometer. The subischial leg length is measured by subtracting the sitting height from the standing height. Standards exist for both of these measurements.

Weight

This is of limited use except in extreme thinness and obesity. It should be plotted separately on a weight centile chart.

Skinfold thicknesses

These are measured by using special calipers. Reliable sites include the triceps, the subscapular area and above the anterior superior iliac spine. Standards for the first two have been published and are in use. These measurements are important in the management of obesity. The body mass index, which is calculated by dividing the weight (in kg) by the height (in meters) squared, is useful in the assessment of obesity; new British reference data have recently been published (Cole et al 1995).

Catch-up growth and growth regulation

Growth in man is a very carefully regulated process. Children are meant to achieve a certain height, determined in large part by genetic factors. Each child therefore follows his or her own trajectory towards this target height. If the child's growth is interrupted by acute malnutrition or illness and this is then corrected, then the child catches up towards his or her original growth curve. Once this has been achieved, it then slows down again to adjust its path on to the old trajectory once again. The increased growth velocity following correction of the adverse circumstances is termed 'catch-up' growth, which is complete if the full genetic potential of an individual is achieved and incomplete if it is not. Complete catch-up growth may be achieved by either a rapid increase of velocity to supranormal levels or by a normal-for-age velocity but with growth prolonged beyond the usual time (catch-up with delay). This process is poorly understood. Additionally, there are sex differences in that girls slow their growth less in response to disease or malnutrition than do boys. Finally, the earlier and the more prolonged the stress, the more difficult it is for regulation to be fully effective in restoring the prestress situation.

ENDOCRINOLOGY OF GROWTH – THE HYPOTHALAMO-PITUITARY-SOMATOTROPH AXIS

GHRH/SOMATOSTATIN

In discussing the endocrinology of growth, the three phases of growth must each be addressed. Prenatal and early postnatal growth are mainly nutrition dependent, with growth factors playing an as yet undefined role. The childhood pattern of growth is largely dependent on the normal pulsatile secretion of human growth hormone by the anterior pituitary gland. This is in turn controlled by the secretion of two hypothalamic hormones, namely growth hormone-releasing hormone (GHRH) and somatostatin (SMS). GHRH controls the synthesis and release of GH whilst somatostatin is responsible for the pulsatile secretion of hGH.

Somatostatin was the first to be characterized and sequenced, following isolation of the peptide from ovine hypothalamic extracts. Although the existence of a stimulatory hypothalamic factor was proposed as early as 1960, it was only in 1982 that GHRH was isolated, characterized and sequenced from pancreatic islet cell tumors.

GHRH binds to a specific receptor on the cell membrane of pituitary somatotrophs (Gaylinn et al 1993) and acts as a mitogen via cyclic adenosine monophosphate (cAMP). This leads to proliferation of pituitary somatotrophs (Billestrup et al 1986), in addition to stimulating the expression of the growth hormone gene. The receptor is a 423 amino acid protein and is a member of the G-protein coupled family of receptors, with its seven transmembrane loops. Binding of GHRH to its receptor leads to an increase in intracellular cAMP, via a Gs regulatory protein. The cAMP then acts as a second messenger (Bilezikjian & Vale 1983, Labrie et al 1983, Struthers et al 1989). In certain situations, control of this system becomes pathologically abnormal. For instance, overactivation of the Gs regulatory protein action leads to uncontrolled hormone synthesis and release, e.g. pituitary somatotroph tumors (Landis et al 1989) and the McCune–Albright syndrome, where the unduly prolonged activation of Gs-α, which is due to a mutation in the gene for this G-protein subunit, leads to a variable phenotype consisting of precocious puberty, Cushing's syndrome, pituitary somatotroph tumors and thyrotoxicosis (Weinstein et al 1991).

Somatostatin exerts its actions via a specific membrane-bound receptor (Yamada et al 1992). It inhibits GH secretion by several mechanisms. These include a partial inhibitory effect on cAMP accumulation, an inhibitory effect via a calcium-dependent step in the GH release pathway (Ray et al 1986) and a cAMP-independent route via the phosphatidylinositol–protein kinase C system (Cronin et al 1984, Simard et al 1987). Somatostatin does not directly affect GH synthesis and any effect it may have on reducing GH gene transcription may be mediated via a suppression in GHRH release (Sugihara et al 1993). In male rodents and in man, it would appear that GH release takes place by a carefully regulated interaction between GHRH and somatostatin so that somatostatin sets the timing of the occurrence of the GH pulse and GHRH determines the magnitude of the pulse (Clark & Robinson 1988, Hindmarsh et al 1991). This pattern of GHRH and somatostatin secretion results in the typical pulsatile secretion of hGH observed in childhood. The integrity of this pulsatile pattern appears to be vital for linear growth.

THE SECRETORY PATTERN OF hGH

hGH is secreted by the anterior pituitary gland in a pulsatile fashion. This pattern of peaks alternating with troughs, where the GH levels are undetectable, appears to be vital for normal growth. Sleep-related peaks of GH appear in the first year of life in relation to the organization of sleep–wake cycles. An increase in the amplitudes of peaks is associated with the pubertal growth spurt, with a subsequent decline in pulse amplitude as time progresses (Mauras et al 1987).

During childhood, the stature of an individual is determined by the size which an infant has reached by the end of the first year of life, which is dependent on nutritional and genetic factors, and the rate of growth of the child subsequently. Data from cross-sectional studies suggest that the latter is related asymptotically to the

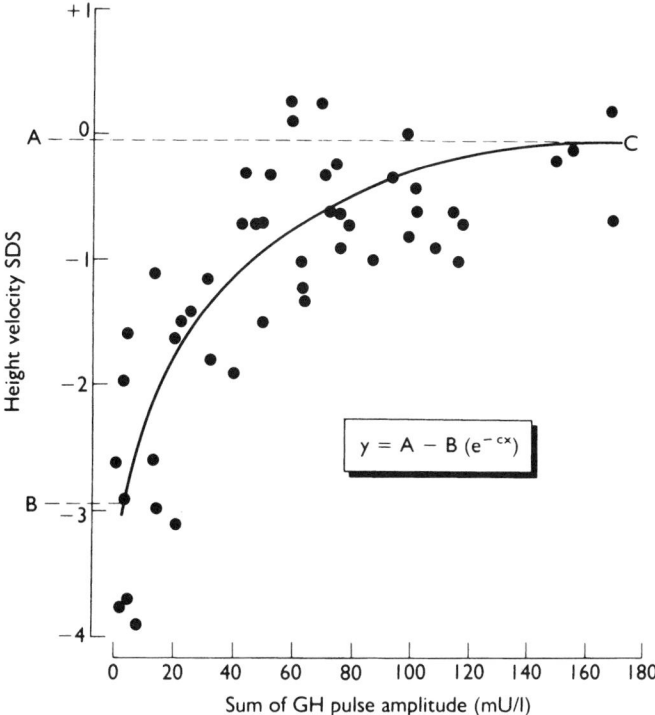

Fig. 8.14 Relationship between GH secretion and growth velocity expressed as a standard deviation score (SDS).

amount of hGH secreted (Fig. 8.14) (Hindmarsh et al 1987, Albertsson-Wikland & Rosberg 1988, Kerrigan et al 1990). Childhood growth is a GH pulse amplitude-modulated process. The frequency of GH secretion remains fairly constant after the age of 7 years until late adolescence. It is however increased during starvation, when the baseline of GH secretion is also elevated (Hartman et al 1992). At the age of approximately 7 years, a rise in GH pulse amplitude is also observed. These changes in GH secretion are in some way related to the process of adrenarche, whereby changes in the hypothalamo-pituitary-adrenal axis lead to the secretion of androgenic steroids, which may lead to the increase in GH peak amplitude.

THE INTERACTION OF hGH WITH ITS RECEPTOR

The hGH (somatogenic) receptor is a 620 amino-acid protein which is a member of the cytokine receptor superfamily, which also includes receptors for prolactin, erythropoietin and granulocyte-macrophage colony stimulating factor. These are single membrane-spanning receptors consisting of an extracellular ligand-binding domain, a short transmembrane domain and a cytoplasmic domain. Although hGH receptors are most abundant in the liver, they have also been identified in many other tissues, e.g. testis, heart, kidney, skeletal muscle, cartilage and adipose tissue (Kelly et al 1993). Human growth hormone can also interact with lactogenic receptors, which are also widely distributed, although the significance of the latter interaction is unknown.

The extracellular domain of the hGH receptor circulates in serum, where it is termed the high-affinity human growth hormone-binding protein (hGHBP). The hGHBP complexes

approximately 40–45% of circulating 22 kDa hGH under basal conditions (Baumann et al 1990). The biological role of the binding protein is at present the subject of much speculation. Degradation of bound GH is approximately 10-fold lower than free hGH and bound GH can therefore act as a circulating reservoir for the hormone. On the other hand, in vitro studies have clearly demonstrated the inhibition of the bioactivity of hGH by recombinant hGHBP (Dattani et al 1994). Reduced levels of the binding protein have been demonstrated in a variety of pathological conditions, e.g. hypothyroidism, Laron-type dwarfism, liver cirrhosis, insulin-dependent diabetes mellitus and uremia.

Various physicochemical studies (Cunningham et al 1991, Ultsch et al 1991, Wells et al 1993) have recently revealed that hGH binding to the extracellular domain of its receptor is followed by binding to a second receptor molecule which forms a dimer with the first receptor and only then does the process of signal transduction, and hence normal growth, occur. The postreceptor events following the formation of dimers are the subject of much research at present and involve several kinases.

THE MOLECULAR HETEROGENEITY OF hGH

Human growth hormone is a mixture of different isoforms (Baumann 1991). The most abundant (75% of circulating hGH) form is the 191 amino acid 22 kDa form of the hormone (22K hGH). Other forms include the 20 kDa alternative mRNA splice variant (the second most abundant form of hGH in the pituitary and circulation (Baumann et al 1987), accounting for approximately 10–15% of circulating hGH), deamidated and acyl forms and dimers and higher oligomers. All of these forms are believed to be secreted by the pituitary gland. Their biological roles are at present unknown. However, the 20 kDa form of hGH (20K hGH) has been shown to be biologically active in the rat, as shown by both in vivo and in vitro studies (Emoto et al 1987, Ohmae et al 1989, Dattani et al 1993). Although the in vivo studies suggest that 20K hGH has full growth-promoting and insulin-like growth factor-I-generating potency, in vitro studies suggest a relative potency of 20K hGH of only 10% that of 22K hGH. One possible reason for this discrepancy between in vivo and in vitro studies lies in the slower clearance of 20K hGH in vivo (Baumann et al 1985). Deamidated forms of hGH have a similar growth-promoting bioactivity to 22K hGH, as does the acylated form. However, dimers of hGH have approximately 10–20% of the growth-promoting activity of 22K hGH. Following acute stimulation of the pituitary gland, the distribution of the individual hGH variants in the circulation changes (Baumann & Stolar 1986). The implications of this phenomenon will be discussed in greater detail below (p. 366).

INSULIN-LIKE GROWTH FACTORS, THEIR BINDING PROTEINS AND THEIR RECEPTORS

The insulin-like growth factors (IGF-I and IGF-II) are related growth hormone-dependent peptide factors which are thought to mediate many of the anabolic and mitogenic actions of hGH. The level of IGF-I is reduced in growth hormone deficiency and in growth hormone receptor defects (Laron-type syndrome), leading to severe growth failure.

As discussed earlier, IGFs circulate in plasma complexed to a family of six binding proteins (IGFBPs). IGF levels can be measured in serum, but interference from the binding proteins can be a major problem (Daughaday et al 1986). Methods such as acid–ethanol extraction are now in use in order to separate the binding proteins from the growth factors.

In human fetal serum, IGF-I levels increase with gestational age and are approximately 30–50% of adult values in newborn serum. They increase during childhood and attain adult levels by the onset of sexual maturation. During puberty, they rise to levels which are 2–3-fold higher than those observed in adults (Cara et al 1987). It is generally believed that this rise in serum IGF-I levels in puberty is a direct effect of the action of sex steroids, since it has also been reported to occur in children with GH receptor defects, in whom GH cannot interact with the receptor to produce IGF-I (Vaccarello et al 1993). Subsequently, in adults, IGF-I levels decline in an age-related manner. On the other hand, IGF-II levels are approximately 50% of adult levels in human newborn infants and adult concentrations are attained by the age of 1 year, without an increase in the growth factor level at puberty. The GH dependence of serum IGF-I levels in man is well established and its use in the assessment of children with short stature will be discussed in further detail later (p. 374).

IGFBP3 is the major IGFBP in the circulation. It is clearly GH dependent (Martin & Baxter 1986). This molecule is thought to have a molecular weight of approximately 40–44 kDa, as demonstrated in Western ligand blots. However, in adult serum, it exists as part of a tertiary complex consisting of IGFBP3, IGF and an acid-labile subunit (Baxter 1988). IGFBP3 levels appear to correlate with spontaneous GH secretion (Hasegawa et al 1993) and are low in the serum of children with GH receptor deficiency (Savage et al 1993). The use of IGFBP3 levels in the diagnosis of GH deficiency will be discussed further in the section on growth disorders (p. 375).

GENETIC CONTROL OF GROWTH AND ITS DISORDERS

The rate of growth in any individual, and their final height, is dependent upon a complex combination of genetic and environmental factors. Environmentally produced changes in rate do not necessarily lead to alterations in final height because of the process of catch-up growth. The genetics of growth will be discussed below.

INTRODUCTION

The height of an individual is determined to a large extent by his or her genetic make-up, but the genetics of growth is poorly understood at present. Many genes are involved in the growth process, as evidenced by the way in which stature has all the characteristics of an attribute which follows the polygenic model, with a smooth Gaussian distribution of height at any age. In addition to this background, however, there are certain single gene factors which contribute to growth pathology.

The control of transcription of the growth hormone gene is currently the subject of much research. Hypothalamic factors such as growth hormone-releasing hormone (GHRH) and somatostatin are responsible for the control of the secretion of hGH. Abnormalities of these genes may be responsible for reduced secretion of hGH and hence growth hormone deficiency. Abnormalities of the hGH gene, its transcription factors and the gene for the receptor for hGH will be described below and these

defects lead to extreme short stature. Additionally, the age at which puberty commences and the age at which menarche is achieved in girls is largely determined genetically. Identical twin sisters growing up together under average West European economic conditions reach menarche an average of 2 months apart. Nonidentical twin sisters reach menarche on average 10 months apart. In boys with constitutional delay of growth and puberty, there is frequently a history of delayed puberty in the father.

GENETIC ABNORMALITIES IN THE ACTION OF GHRH

Activating mutations of the Gs-α subunit of the G-protein linked to the GHRH receptor have already been discussed. These can result in somatotroph proliferation and hypersecretion of hGH, either in isolation or as part of the McCune–Albright syndrome.

Animal models with naturally occurring mutations of the GHRH receptor have recently been described. In the *little* (lit/lit) mouse, a reduced number of somatotrophs contain only 10% of the normal GH content and reduced levels of mRNA. The somatotrophs are resistant to GHRH stimulation and homozygotes are growth hormone deficient and consequently growth retarded (Lin et al 1993). The mutation described in these animals leads to an impairment in signal transduction. An analogous nonsense mutation in the gene encoding the GHRH receptor in man, leading to a severely truncated GHRH receptor, has recently been described in two related children with severe growth hormone deficiency and an impaired response to exogenous GHRH (Wajnrajch et al 1996).

THE hGH GENE AND THE ROLE OF HOMEOBOX GENES IN THE CONTROL OF GROWTH

The human growth hormone (hGH)/placental lactogen (hPL) gene cluster is located on the long arm of chromosome 17. Among the five related genes are two which code for two hGH isoforms. Two of the genes code for hPL and the fifth may be either an hPL pseudogene or may encode an hPL-related protein of unknown function. The two hGH genes have been termed hGH 1 (hGH-N or hGH normal) and hGH 2 (hGH-V or hGH variant) genes. The two corresponding proteins (hGH-N and hGH-V) are highly homologous, differing by 13 out of 191 amino acids. The two genes give rise to several GH isohormones and variants. Whereas the hGH-N gene is expressed in the pituitary gland, the variant gene is expressed in the placenta. The role of the latter is at present unknown, although it has been postulated that this hormone may well have a role in fetal growth.

The hGH gene consists of five exons and five introns. Transcripts of the hGH-N gene are spliced into two different mRNAs. Two splicing sites, a 'regular' one at the boundary between intron B and exon 3 and an alternative one within exon 3, are used to produce mRNAs that code for 22 kDa hGH and 20 kDa hGH respectively (Cooke et al 1988). The 'regular' splicing site is preferentially used. The two corresponding proteins, named 22 kDa and 20 kDa GH, are produced in the pituitary gland. The former is a 191 amino acid single chain polypeptide containing two disulfide bridges, which gives the molecule its overall configuration of two loops. 20 kDa hGH differs from 22 kDa hGH by an internal deletion of a 15 amino acid sequence encompassing residues 32 to 46.

In man, the 22 kDa form of hGH is the most important form of hGH and accounts for most of the biological effects of hGH. Genetic causes of growth hormone deficiency (GHD) have been described. For example, mutations and deletions of the hGH-N gene (Goossens et al 1986) give rise to the classic early presentation of GHD with hypoglycemia and severe postnatal growth failure commencing at 6–9 months of age. The children have no detectable circulating growth hormone, and, although the initial response to hGH treatment is excellent, subsequent growth is blunted because of the development of high-affinity binding antibodies to the hGH molecule, as a result of the lack of immunological tolerance to the hormone (Schwartz et al 1987). This condition is called familial isolated GH deficiency type IA (IGHD-IA). Recently, a nonsense mutation in codon 20 of the hGH-N gene has been reported to cause IGHD-IA (Cogan et al 1993).

Other forms include an autosomal recessive form (type IB), an autosomal dominant form (type II) and an X-linked form (type III). These are forms of GH insufficiency, where insufficient amounts of hGH are produced in response to provocative stimuli and growth failure is not as extreme as in type IA. Antibody production in response to hGH therapy is not a problem in these cases. Splice-site mutations in intron III, which caused skipping of exon 3, have been described in children with IGHD-II (Binder & Ranke 1995).

Although the hGH gene is present in all cells in the human body, full expression of the gene only occurs in pituitary somatotrophs. This cell-specific expression is thought to be regulated in the pituitary gland by the homeobox gene PIT-1, which controls pituitary cell differentiation and function (Bodner et al 1988, Ingraham et al 1988) and is a member of the family of POU-domain DNA-binding transcription factors regulating mammalian development, so called because it consists of the anterior pituitary-specific transcription factor Pit-1, the B cell factor Oct-2, the ubiquitous octamer binding protein Oct-1 and the Caenorhabditis elegans unc-86 gene product. Homeobox genes govern embryonic development and gene expression and share a common DNA-binding domain. The product of the PIT-1 gene, the Pit-1 protein, is necessary for the embryonic development, proliferation and specialized function of GH-, prolactin- and thyrotrophin-producing cells. The DNA-binding domain of Pit-1 consists of the POU-specific and POU-homeodomain regions. When bound to DNA, Pit-1 activates GH, prolactin and TSH (thyroid-stimulating hormone) gene expression. Mutations in the PIT-1 gene have been described in two Dutch families in which each family contained two affected siblings with GH and partial thyrotrophin deficiency (Pfaffle et al 1992). Recent studies have reported the presence of mutations in exon 4 of the Pit-1 gene in other groups of patients (Cohen et al 1995). It is possible that mutations in genes encoding other proteins involved in the signaling cascade, such as cAMP response element binding protein and protein kinase A, may also lead to GH deficiency with somatotroph hypoplasia.

The hGH gene probably represents the final pathway for the expression of many of the factors which are important in GH control. IGF-I inhibits basal GH gene transcription (Yamashita & Melmed 1987), suggesting a negative feedback role of IGF-I in GH secretion. Thyroxine is also important in regulating GH gene expression. Hypothyroidism is associated with a decrease in GH mRNA levels in the pituitary, with a consequent reduction in pituitary GH content. This may account for the poor growth associated with hypothyroidism and the blunting of GH responses to various provocative stimuli (Katakami et al 1986). Stimulation of GH gene transcription is mediated by a thyroid hormone nuclear receptor which is a DNA-binding protein and which interacts with the GH gene (Ye & Samuels 1987). Glucocorticoids (Birnbaum & Baxter 1986) and estrogen have also been implicated in the regulation of GH gene transcription, although testosterone seems to have little or no effect.

THE GH RECEPTOR GENE

The gene for the human GH receptor is localized on chromosome 5p13.1–p12 and contains 10 exons. Exons 3–7 encode the extracellular ligand-binding domain of the receptor, containing 246 amino acids. Exon 8 encodes the 24 amino acid transmembrane domain of the receptor and exons 9 and 10 encode the 350 amino acid cytoplasmic domain and the 3′ untranslated region. Several different deletions and mutations in the GH receptor gene have been described (Rosenfeld et al 1994) and account for the clinical phenotype of Laron-type dwarfism (p. 374).

Recent reports have suggested that heterozygous mutations in the GH receptor gene may account for some cases of idiopathic short stature, in whom GH responses to provocation are normal but serum IGF-I and GH-binding protein concentrations are low (Goddard et al 1995).

ENVIRONMENTAL FACTORS AFFECTING GROWTH

NUTRITION

This is particularly important in determining early growth and influencing maturation. Early overfeeding leads to tall stature and growth advance, with consequent early pubertal maturation and the early achievement of final height. Obesity during the first 2 years of life leads to tall stature, whereas obesity or overfeeding later in childhood does not alter final stature.

Malnutrition, especially at a period of rapid growth, such as in utero or in the first year of life, also has lifelong consequences. It affects later height and weight and also neurodevelopmental outcome. Recently, it has been suggested (Barker 1992) that adults born with a low birthweight as a result of malnutrition in utero have an increased cardiovascular mortality and morbidity, in addition to an increased tendency to non-insulin-dependent diabetes mellitus. This is currently an active area of research and no doubt hormonal factors will be implicated in the scenario of low birthweight syndromes.

ETHNIC DIFFERENCES IN GROWTH

Ethnic differences are observed in the rate and pattern of growth and these can result in significant differences in final height. These may be determined genetically, but may also be due to nutritional differences. The African child matures earlier than the average Caucasian child, not only in terms of physical development but also in terms of motor development. In view of the variation between different population groups, growth standards should ideally be constructed for each population group. In practice, this is not easy to achieve. Hence, caution is required when comparing the height of an Asian child with standards derived from studies in Caucasian children. Nevertheless, it is of note that the shapes of growth curves are constant between different populations and that growth rate is remarkably constant between different populations. The topic has been extensively covered by Eveleth & Tanner (1990).

SEASONAL VARIATION IN GROWTH

Many children demonstrate a marked seasonal effect on growth velocity. They differ not only in the time of year at which they grow fastest, but also in the magnitude of the difference between one season and another.

DISEASE

Although minor and relatively short illnesses cause no measurable growth retardation, major chronic illnesses may lead to significant growth retardation, which may then be accompanied by a catch-up period when the disease is cured. Whether the genetic potential for height is then achieved depends upon the length of the illness and how long treatment was deferred.

PSYCHOLOGICAL DISTURBANCE

In 1957, Widdowson showed that the sadistic influence of a matron in a German orphanage was profoundly restrictive on children's growth, in spite of an adequate calorie intake. When the influence was removed, the children grew well, demonstrating the reversible nature of psychosocial deprivation, which will be described in greater detail below.

SOCIOECONOMIC FACTORS

Children in the upper socioeconomic groups are generally taller than those in the lower socioeconomic groups. In contrast, there is little difference in weight, although obesity is actually more common in older children from lower socioeconomic groups. The causes of the socioeconomic height difference are multiple. Differences in nutrition are important, as are home conditions. Those children from well-organized homes where the habits of regular meals, sleep and exercise have been followed are, on average, taller.

SECULAR TREND

During the last 100 years there has been a striking tendency for children to become progressively taller at all ages. The recent introduction of growth charts based upon data collected in 1990 shows an increase of up to 1.7 cm in the heights of British boys and girls since 1966 (Freeman et al 1995). The trend towards taller height in children also reflects a more rapid maturation. This is shown by the trend towards earlier menarche of 3–4 months per decade since 1850 in average Western European girls. The causes of this secular trend are probably multiple and include improved nutrition, although possible other factors remain unknown.

DISORDERS OF GROWTH

SHORT STATURE

This is the commonest reason for a child to be referred to an endocrinologist. Using the new growth charts, the referral criteria based upon either a single measurement or sequential measurements are as follows.

Single measurement All children with a height below the 0.4th centile should be referred. Referral should be considered for children with a height between the 0.4th and 2nd centiles and those children about whom parental or professional concern has been expressed or when there is a significant discrepancy between the mid-parental target centile and the child's present centile.

Sequential measurements All children should be referred if the growth curve crosses two centile lines, since this indicates a suboptimal height velocity with a high probability of underlying pathology. Additionally, referral should be considered if the growth curve crosses a single centile line between 2 and 5 years of age.

The flow diagram in Figure 8.15 gives an approach to the management of this condition.

The following sections will describe some of these conditions in more detail.

Low birthweight

This is defined as a low birthweight for a given gestation indicating a failure of growth in utero. It is important to realize that low birthweight is relative and is defined in relation to the birthweight of siblings within a family. One of the commonest conditions observed in clinical practice, children who are born with a low birthweight can be classified as follows:

1. Symmetrical – the length, weight and head circumference all lie within a similar centile range. Intrauterine growth failure probably commenced early in gestation and may have been due to chromosomal disorders, dysmorphic syndromes, teratogens, smoking, alcohol, drugs or intrauterine infections.
2. Asymmetrical – weight is on a lower centile than length or head circumference. This is usually due to poor weight gain in the last trimester of pregnancy. Placental insufficiency leading to poor nutrition and maternal hypertension are two of the commonest etiologic features.

Clinically, these children may present with hypoglycemia in the neonatal period. Later presentation is with short stature. They are usually thin. Feeding problems, often severe, in the first year of life are very common in this group of children.

The long-term outlook for height in these children has been the subject of several studies (Paz et al 1993, Tenovuo et al 1987, Sung et al 1993, Fitzhardinge & Inwood 1989). They fall into the following groups:

1. catch-up growth before 6 months of age in approximately 40%
2. catch-up growth before 3 years of age in a further 25%
3. catch-up after 3 years in 20%
4. no catch-up growth in approximately 15%.

The latter two groups never achieve their genetic potential. At present, little is known about the endocrinology of LBW babies and abnormalities in prenatal growth factors may be implicated.

No specific hormonal treatment is indicated. However, treatment may be required for complications such as hypoglycemia (frequent feeds). The prognosis for height is highly variable and a significant proportion (~40%) will have final heights which fall considerably short of their mid-parental target height. Growth hormone treatment has been used in this group of

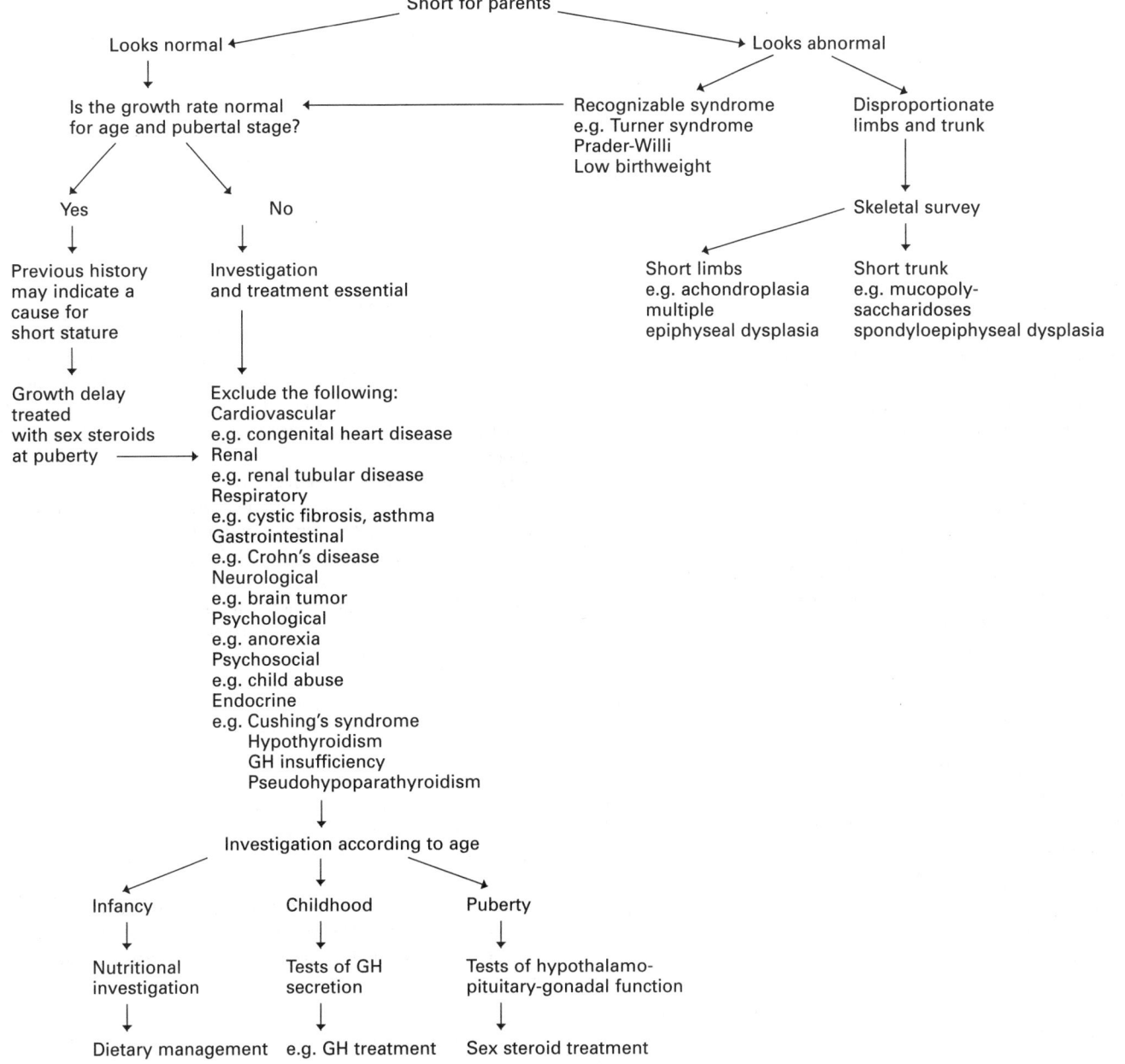

Fig. 8.15   Algorithm for the management of short stature.

children but has not improved height prediction in those children growing with a normal height velocity (Stanhope et al 1991). These children are prone to early pubertal development and growth hormone treatment could, in theory, accelerate pubertal progress and restrict the final height to a further extent (Darendelier et al 1990).

More recently, attention has focused on the long-term cardiovascular morbidity and mortality of children born with a low birthweight. An inverse relationship has been demonstrated between birthweight and adult outcomes including hypertension, coronary vascular disease and impaired glucose tolerance (Barker et al 1989, Barker 1992, Whincup et al 1995). Hence, in some way, birthweight may be implicated in the 'programming' of later blood pressure and cardiovascular morbidity and mortality.

Dysmorphic syndromes

Many dysmorphic syndromes are associated with short stature and a full treatise on the subject is beyond the scope of this chapter. The most frequently seen in the endocrine outpatient clinic are Silver–Russell syndrome (p. 1015), Noonan syndrome (p. 370) and Turner syndrome (p. 370). The latter will be dealt with separately.

The Silver–Russell syndrome is usually sporadic, but familial cases have been described. It is characterized by a striking degree of prenatal growth failure with poor catch-up growth and a mean height SDS of −3.6. Puberty may commence at a slightly earlier age and the peak pubertal growth spurt may be reduced (Davies et al 1988). In many ways, this syndrome behaves like a severe variant of low birthweight (or IUGR) children discussed above. Clinical features include thinness, clinodactyly, a triangular face with a prominent forehead, body asymmetry and cafe-au-lait spots. To date, no endocrine abnormalities have been consistently described, although occasional cases of GH insufficiency have been reported.

Noonan syndrome is characterized by a phenotype which is not unlike that of Turner syndrome. It is inherited as an autosomal dominant condition or may occur sporadically. Clinical features include short stature, delayed puberty, mild intellectual impairment, ptosis, low-set ears, neck webbing, pectus carinatum, cubitus valgus, right-sided heart lesions and cryptorchidism. The great majority of children lie below the third centile for height and reach a final height on or below the third centile (Ranke et al 1988). No consistent endocrine abnormalities have been described to account for the short stature, although IGF-I levels are reportedly low or low-normal, but with a normal mean GH and peak GH to stimulation (Ahmed et al 1991).

Turner syndrome (see p. 1032)

The incidence is reported to be 1 in 2500 live female births. The phenotype arises as a result of either the loss of one of the X chromosomes or an intrachromosomal rearrangement of an X chromosome. In 70–80% of cases, the retained X chromosome is maternal. Approximately 50% of cases have a 45XO karyotype with the remaining 50% demonstrating mosaicism with one 45XO cell line and another cell line often containing an abnormal X chromosome (or a Y chromosome).

Girls with this condition may present in the neonatal period with lymphedema (21–47%) of the hands and feet or with coarctation of the aorta or aortic stenosis (16–23%). There are four phases discernible in the growth pattern of children with this syndrome:

1. the birthweight may be low (~1 SDS below the mean)
2. Turner girls have feeding difficulties in the first year of life, with further loss of growth
3. they grow at a 25th centile height velocity during childhood, so that they fall further behind their peers. Hence, later presentation is usually with short stature for the family (88–100%)
4. these girls have a skeletal dysplasia with a coarse trabecular pattern in the long bones and tall vertebrae and, like all patients with skeletal dysplasia, growth during the pubertal years is extremely poor

Ovarian failure with streak gonads is observed in the vast majority of patients and this leads to amenorrhea (87–96%). Other clinical features include a broad, shield-shaped chest with widely spaced nipples (33–75%), anomalous auricles, epicanthic folds, micrognathia (60%), high arched palate (35–84%), short 4th and 5th metacarpals (35–77%), kyphoscoliosis (12–16%), low posterior hairline (40–80%), webbed neck (23–65%), cubitus valgus (27–82%), osteoporosis, narrow hyperconvex nails (43–83%), excessive pigmented nevi, renal anomalies (11–37%), recurrent middle ear infections (53%), sensorineural deafness, specific learning abnormalities, idiopathic hypertension, diabetes mellitus (34%), Crohn's disease and autoimmune hypothyroidism (21%). The mean final height of women with Turner syndrome is in the region of 143–146 cm in Western societies (Lyon et al

1985, Massa et al 1991, Ranke et al 1991) and is related to the parental heights. No difference in final height is observed between those with and without spontaneous onset of puberty (Massa et al 1990).

GH secretion is normal during childhood, but the usual increase in GH secretion and IGF-I production which ensues at puberty is blunted (Reiter et al 1991, Wit et al 1992). This may be due in part to the lack of pubertal development and in part to the relative obesity which occurs in the teenage years in many girls with Turner syndrome. However, these abnormalities do not explain the poor growth in mid-childhood.

The other main feature of the condition is ovarian dysgenesis; 10–20% of children with this syndrome will go into puberty spontaneously, with menarche occurring in 5–10%. Only 1% will be fertile (Massa et al 1991, Lippe 1991). Gonadotrophin levels will be elevated in the first 2 years of life, but will be normal between the ages of 3 and 10, with a further increase in the pubertal years if ovarian function is inadequate and puberty cannot be initiated.

Treatment of this condition entails the appropriate management of cardiac abnormalities, if present. Blood pressure should be regularly monitored. Growth promotion may be achieved with the use of low-dose anabolic steroids (oxandrolone), growth hormone and estrogen, although the timing of these interventions remains a source of much debate. Short and middle-term studies have demonstrated an increase in height velocity with the use of hGH (Rosenfeld et al 1988). However, higher doses of hGH than those used in GH insufficiency are required to achieve an increase in height velocity. Until final height data are available, the role and optimal timing of hGH treatment must remain uncertain. Pubertal induction with ethinyl-estradiol and the later addition of progestogens is required in the majority of cases at the appropriate age. Complications such as hypothyroidism are treated as they arise. If a Y chromosomal cell line has been demonstrated, the dysgenetic gonads should be removed because of the risk of gonadoblastoma at later ages.

The prognosis for final height is determined to a large extent by the parental heights. The use of in vitro fertilization and embryo implantation techniques has improved the prospects for childbearing.

Skeletal dysplasias

Several forms of skeletal dysplasia have been described, the commoner surviving forms being achondroplasia, hypochondroplasia, spondyloepiphyseal dysplasia and multiple epiphyseal dysplasia. The incidence of achondroplasia is 1 : 26 000 and it is inherited as an autosomal dominant condition with a fresh mutation rate of 90%. Hypochondroplasia is much commoner than was previously thought and can also be inherited as an autosomal dominant trait, as are spondyloepiphyseal dysplasia and multiple epiphyseal dysplasia.

Recently, mutations in the gene encoding fibroblast growth factor receptor 3 (FGFR3) on chromosome 4 have been identified in children with achondroplasia (Shiang et al 1994, Rousseau et al 1994). Hypochondroplasia is linked to the same region on chromosome 4 as achondroplasia and mutations of FGFR3 have also been described in this condition (Bellus et al 1995).

Clinically, skeletal dysplasias may present with extreme short stature or a height which is extremely short for the family. Achondroplastic children may present in the neonatal period with short limbs and characteristic craniofacial features. These include a large head with marked frontal bossing, a low nasal bridge and mild midfacial hypoplasia. Skeletal abnormalities include small cuboid vertebral bodies with short pedicles and progressive narrowing of lumbar interpedicular distance. Lumbar lordosis, mild thoracolumbar kyphosis, small iliac wings, short tubular bones and a short trident hand are other features of the condition. Mild hypotonia with some early motor delay is an occasional feature. Hydrocephalus secondary to a narrow foramen magnum is an associated feature. Spinal cord and/or root compression can occur as a consequence of kyphosis, spinal canal stenosis or disc lesions. It is also associated with upper airways obstruction and recurrent otitis media.

In hypochondroplasia, the presentation is usually with short stature in relation to the mid-parental target height centile. The growth rate is initially normal, with an extremely compromised pubertal growth spurt. Skeletal abnormalities are characteristic. Disproportion may only become apparent in puberty, although it may be seen earlier in more severe cases. Family history often reveals disproportionate short stature in one or both parents.

Spondyloepiphyseal dysplasia is characterized by prenatal onset growth deficiency, malar hypoplasia, cleft palate, short spine, lumbar lordosis, kyphoscoliosis, decreased arm span, weakness, talipes varus and congenital dislocation of the hip.

Multiple epiphyseal dysplasia presents with short stature. Skeletal survey reveals short metacarpals and phalanges and ovoid, flattened vertebral bodies. These children often have a waddling gait and growth is extremely poor. Early osteoarthritis may be a feature.

Diagnosis in all of these conditions is made by a skeletal survey which shows diagnostic radiological features. In achondroplasia, neuroradiological imaging may be indicated if hydrocephalus is suspected.

Treatment entails the correction of hydrocephalus and orthopedic abnormalities. The use of growth hormone to treat these conditions is the subject of clinical trials. Final height data are not as yet available, although the early response to hGH in achondroplastic children is often encouraging. In hypochondroplasia, hGH treatment may enhance the pubertal growth spurt, although the results are variable and uncertain. hGH treatment is of little use in pseudoachondroplasia, multiple epiphyseal dysplasia and spondyloepiphyseal dysplasia. Limb lengthening may be an option in achondroplasia and severe cases of hypochondroplasia. The gain in height needs to be balanced against the time and discomfort involved in these procedures. Without intervention, the height prognosis can be poor in achondroplasia and variable in hypochondroplasia.

Constitutional (familial) short stature

This is the commonest cause of short stature in most population groups. Usually one or both of the parents are short, although the history may not be so clear cut, with a grandparent or other more distant relative manifesting short stature. Underlying pathology which may be inherited needs to be excluded, e.g. growth hormone deficiency, skeletal dysplasia. It is possible that a number of these children and families will turn out to have abnormalities in one of the several genes controlling growth hormone secretion or later events in the GH/IGF-I axis, although none has been identified to date (Mullis et al 1991). It is clear, however, as discussed in the earlier sections, that our

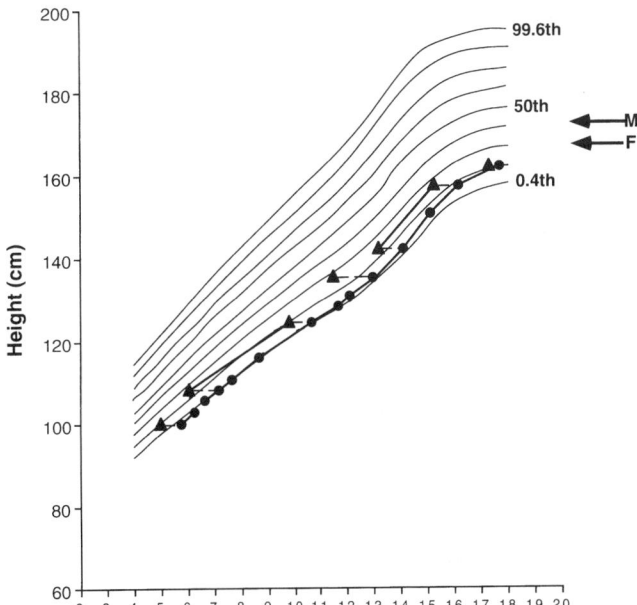

Fig. 8.16 Typical growth chart of a child with constitutional short stature. M=mother; F=father; triangle=bone age; circle=chronological age.

understanding of the genetic control of growth hormone secretion is in its infancy.

The bone age is not delayed in this condition and the height SDS usually lies within the mid-parental target range (Fig. 8.16). If the child is growing with a normal height velocity, there is little point in performing investigations. Similarly, no treatment is indicated in the constitutionally short child whose growth rate is normal (> –0.8 SDS). Growth hormone treatment has been attempted in groups of these children on a trial basis, but final height data are awaited and its use cannot be recommended in all children with constitutional short stature.

Nutritional deficiency (see also Ch. 21)

On a global basis, malnutrition is the commonest cause of poor growth and short stature. Kwashiorkor and marasmus are the commonest clinical syndromes and are due to protein–calorie and calorie insufficiency respectively. They are characterized by growth failure, lack of weight gain, edema, abnormal skin pigmentation, chronic diarrhea and recurrent infections.

In nutritional insufficiency, hormonal changes in the GH/IGF-I axis have also been described. These include an increase in mean GH secretion, with abnormal pulsatility such that the pulse amplitude is increased and trough levels are not observed. IGF-I and IGF-BP3 levels are low (Lifshitz & Moses 1985), implying a growth hormone-resistant state. These changes are reversed on refeeding.

In the developed world, frank malnutrition due to conditions of famine is rare, but may occur as part of more complex disease. For example, anorexia nervosa can present with growth failure and can be extremely difficult to diagnose. It is commoner in females, who present clinically with short stature, a paucity of subcutaneous tissue, increased body hair (lanugo) and delay in puberty. Self-induced vomiting may be a feature, along with other behavioral disturbances. Chronic medical conditions such as inflammatory bowel disease must be excluded.

Psychosocial deprivation

In children with this condition, an unsatisfactory child–parent relationship manifests itself as behavioral difficulties in the child, e.g. hyperphagia, polydipsia, enuresis, encopresis, theft of food, inappropriate formation of relationships with strangers, anxiety, etc., together with growth failure. Delayed bone age with a delay in pubertal development are other features of the condition. Decreased levels of hGH in spontaneous secretory profiles of GH secretion and following provocation and decreased levels of IGF-I in the serum may be documented. These endocrine abnormalities are reversible on removal of the child from the abnormal environment, e.g. by admission to hospital. The reversibility occurs over a period of 2–3 weeks. There is certainly no response to GH treatment (Blizzard & Bulatovic 1992, Stanhope et al 1988). Treatment may entail the removal of the child from the adverse environment, either temporarily or on a permanent basis.

Chronic medical illness

Children with chronic medical diseases such as celiac disease, inflammatory bowel disease, chronic renal failure, congenital heart disease and cystic fibrosis all tend to suffer from growth failure if the disease is undiagnosed or poorly controlled. A combination of decreased calorie intake and increased energy expenditure account for the growth failure. These children will usually be thin.

A careful history, physical examination and appropriate investigations are indicated. Bone age and puberty are usually delayed and GH levels may be high with low IGF-I levels. Once the diagnosis has been made, treatment should be directed at the primary condition.

Constitutional delay of growth and puberty (CDGP)

This is the commonest cause of short stature in the peripubertal years. The onset of puberty is delayed and there is often a strong family history of delay. The condition appears to occur much more commonly in males than females. Classically, an individual presents between the ages of 12 and 16 with short stature and a lack of pubertal development. The child continues to grow along the childhood curve and there is a failure of the pubertal growth spurt at the normal time, with consequent short stature in relation to the child's peers. The short stature may have been in evidence from mid-childhood, with a delay in the bone age. The height prognosis is appropriate for the parental heights. Since spinal growth occurs mainly during puberty, in CDGP boys have relatively long legs with a short trunk.

Diagnosis is made on clinical grounds, with short stature, a delayed bone age, lack of adequate pubertal development and a height velocity which is appropriately slow. Since boys experience their growth spurt when the testes are 10–12 ml in volume and since the prepubertal growth rate is inversely related to the age of the growth spurt (Riken & Wit 1992), the growth velocity in boys with CDGP can be extremely slow before puberty. Psychological problems are common in children with CDGP, particularly in boys (Crowne et al 1990). Deviant behavior and severe psychological problems may ensue, with consequent interference in education. Reassurance that the child's pattern of growth and development is normal and that expected height is within the normal range and appropriate for the parents' height may be sufficient in a proportion of children. However, in others reassurance may provide little consolation during the turmoil of adolescence and treatment may need to be considered in this situation.

Investigations are usually of little use. Serum gonadotrophins are low and do not respond to gonadotrophin-releasing hormone; the differential diagnosis is therefore one of hypogonadotrophic hypogonadism, where the pituitary gland is unable to secrete gonadotrophins. Growth hormone provocation tests will reveal low levels of hGH, since the pattern of GH secretion will parallel the low prepubertal growth velocity (Stanhope et al 1988). It is usually the accepted practice to prime a child with sex steroids at this age, in order to obtain a clear idea of the ability of the pituitary gland to secrete hGH. With priming, the pituitary responds normally to provocation.

Treatment is usually in the form of sex steroids or anabolic steroids. Anabolic steroids, e.g. oxandrolone, lead to an improvement in growth rate in children with CDGP without an advance in bone age if used for short-term periods (e.g. 3–6 months) in appropriate doses (Papadimitrou et al 1991, Tse et al 1990), whereas low dose sex steroids lead to both an improvement in growth and the development of secondary sexual characteristics. Neither has any effect on final height. It has nevertheless been reported that final height in children with untreated CDGP is on average 3–5 cm less than that predicted by the estimated mature height (Crowne et al 1990, 1991).

Growth hormone deficiency/insufficiency

The diagnosis of growth hormone deficiency or insufficiency constitutes one of the major dilemmas in pediatric endocrine practice. The diagnosis is usually based upon a combination of clinical features including auxology, biochemistry and genetics in a small proportion of cases (Hindmarsh & Brook 1995). The incidence of the condition is approximately 1 in 4000. The etiology is highly varied, as shown below. The term GH deficiency, implying complete absence of GH secretion, can only be applied to children with genetic abnormalities of the hypothalamo-pituitary-somatotroph axis. GH insufficiency then covers a multitude of other etiologies.

Etiology

The causes of GH deficiency/insufficiency are shown in Table 8.1.

Genetic forms of GH deficiency were described earlier. Idiopathic forms of GHD/GHI account for the majority of cases and usually present in early childhood. In these, the cause is often unclear, although a history of perinatal trauma is often present, with breech deliveries being more common in this group of children. Pituitary hypoplasia as seen on the MRI scan may be a factor in some of these cases (Marwaha et al 1992).

Growth hormone deficiency may be associated with midline defects, of which the commonest is septo-optic dysplasia, where there is absence or partial absence of the septum pellucidum, optic nerve hypoplasia and a variable degree of hypothalamo-pituitary dysfunction, often with an evolving endocrinopathy. These children often present in the first year of life with visual abnormalities including nystagmus, decreased visual acuity and optic nerve hypoplasia. Endocrine manifestations include early

Table 8.1 Causes of growth hormone deficiency/insufficiency (GHD/GHI)

Congenital

Genetic
Type IA
Type IB
Type II
Type III
Pit-1 gene deletion/mutation
GHRH receptor gene mutations

Associated with structural defects of the brain
Agenesis of the corpus callosum
Septo-optic dysplasia
Holoprosencephaly
Encephalocele
Hydrocephalus

Associated with midline facial defects
Single central incisor
Cleft lip/palate

Idiopathic

Acquired

Trauma
Perinatal tauma
Postnatal trauma

Infection
Meningitis/encephalitis

CNS tumors
Craniopharyngioma
Pituitary germinoma
Histiocytosis

Neurosecretory dysfunction

Postcranial irradiation

Pituitary infarction

Transient
Peripubertal
Psychosocial deprivation
Hypothyroidism

growth failure, diabetes insipidus, hypoglycemia and a micropenis with undescended testes in boys. Conjugated hyperbilirubinemia may be present, as may signs of hypothyroidism. The diagnosis is confirmed by appropriate biochemical testing and by neuroradiological imaging.

Other abnormalities such as agenesis of the corpus callosum, holoprosencephaly and hydrocephalus may be associated with multiple pituitary hormone deficiencies. Midline facial defects such as a nasal encephalocele, cleft lip and palate and a single central incisor may be associated with GH deficiency.

Craniopharyngioma is a congenital tumor which arises from remnants of Rathke's pouch, which is an invagination of the epithelium within the third pharyngeal pouch from which the anterior pituitary evolves. It may present in childhood or in adults and may arise within the pituitary fossa or in the suprasellar region. This tumor, which is classified as a benign tumor, can be extremely destructive because of its ability to invade surrounding structures. It is partly solid and partly cystic and the cystic component consists of cholesterol-rich fluid. It presents with visual disturbances, raised intracranial pressure and endocrine disturbances such as growth failure, diabetes insipidus, delayed puberty and secondary hypothyroidism. Examination reveals visual field deficits such as bitemporal hemianopia and optic

atrophy. Other neurological signs may be present. Investigations reveal a variable degree of hypothalamo-pituitary hormone deficiencies at presentation. Therapeutic maneuvers include surgery, radiotherapy and the instillation of radioactive substances into the cystic component. Morbidity and mortality are high in this condition. Complications include gross obesity and severe fluid balance problems with damage to the appetite and thirst centers in the hypothalamus. Intriguingly, several of these children continue to grow with a normal height velocity in spite of documented GH deficiency and low levels of IGF-I (Bistritzer et al 1988). Part of the explanation for this unusual phenomenon may lie in the hyperphagia demonstrated by these patients, with consequent hyperinsulinism (Sorva 1988), this being a potent mitogenic factor.

Langerhans cell histiocytosis (LCH) classically presents with diabetes insipidus, but anterior pituitary dysfunction may also be present. Other intracranial tumors such as pituitary germinomas and gliomata may also present with growth failure and growth hormone deficiency.

Owing to the improvement in the management of children with neoplasia, many children with brain tumors which have been treated with cranial irradiation now present with growth hormone insufficiency. The sensitivity of the hypothalamo-pituitary axis to damage by irradiation is dependent upon the dose of the radiation and the degree of fractionation. GH secretion is generally the most sensitive to damage, with 85% of children who have received 30 Gy of radiation manifesting GHD within 5 years of receiving irradiation (Shalet et al 1992). TSH, ACTH and gonadotrophin secretion, in order of increasing resistance to damage, can also be affected. Children who have received cranial irradiation may enter puberty earlier, with a blunted pubertal growth spurt (Moell 1988), leading to a further compromise in stature. Abnormalities in GH secretion have also been documented in children who have received 24 Gy as treatment for leukemia (Kirk et al 1987, Clayton et al 1988). In children who have received craniospinal irradiation for medulloblastoma and ependymoma, growth failure is further complicated by disproportion, since spinal growth will be suboptimal in comparison with growth of the limbs. Growth failure may also be a consequence of total body irradiation administered to children receiving bone marrow transplants (Ogilvy-Stuart et al 1992).

Clinical presentation

Most frequently, children with growth hormone deficiency present with short stature and a poor height velocity. The age of presentation ranges from 6 months to early adolescence. Children with GH deficiency due to a gene deletion may present early with hypoglycemia, a height velocity below the third centile for their age and a height standard deviation score of below −3 (p. 352). In an older child, the characteristic phenotypic features of GHD/GHI may be present. These include an immature face with a prominent forehead, midfacial hypoplasia, increased subcutaneous fat deposition, delayed dentition, a delayed bone age and a micropenis in boys.

Investigations

Investigation of the hypothalamopituitary axis should only be undertaken after exclusion of other systemic illnesses. A bone age is usually performed at the initial assessment. It is usually delayed, although its contribution to the diagnosis is minimal. A full blood count, ESR, urea and electrolytes, antigliadin antibodies and serum thyroxine should be performed in all children with growth failure, to exclude, for example chronic renal failure, Crohn's disease, celiac disease. A karyotype is indicated in all girls to exclude Turner syndrome. Should these all be normal, then further assessment should include an examination of the GH axis. Controversy rages over the most appropriate test of GH secretion (Rosenfeld et al 1995). Growth hormone secretion is pulsatile in nature and GH concentrations are low during the day. Physiological tests of GH secretion include the measurement of GH levels over a 24-hour period or specifically during periods of sleep. However, these tests are not cost effective in that the manpower required and the actual expense of performing the tests are considerable. Hence, provocation tests are used to test the ability of the pituitary gland to secrete GH. These include the insulin tolerance test, the glucagon test, clonidine and arginine tests (Hindmarsh & Swift 1995).

To date, the insulin tolerance test has been used as the 'gold standard' in terms of biochemical tests of GH secretion. However, the test is not without its dangers (Shah et al 1992) and should only be performed by trained personnel. Serum GH is measured using one of a number of immunoassays. When comparing GH values obtained in these different immunoassays, there were up to six-fold differences in serum GH concentrations between the different assays in the same samples (Celniker et al 1989). Hence, absolute values of serum GH concentrations vary depending upon the assay used. These differences arise because immunologically based assays utilize a variety of antibodies directed against different epitopes on the GH molecule, as well as using different GH standards. These differences appear to be more pronounced during provocative tests of GH secretion (Dattani et al 1995). Ideally, each laboratory performing GH assays should analyze its results carefully, with a view to adopting its own 'cut-off' value (Dattani et al 1992). In practice, however, the distribution of peak serum GH concentration responses to insulin is continuous in a large group of short children with varying growth rates. No clearly demarcated subpopulations exist, with considerable overlap between values observed in groups of short slowly growing children and short normally growing children.

Because of the differences between immunoassays for GH measurement during provocative tests and the dangers associated with these tests, it has been suggested that measurement of IGF-I and the IGF binding protein-3 (IGFBP-3) levels in serum may be an alternative method of assessing GH secretory status, since both are largely regulated by GH (Blum et al 1990, Cianfarani et al 1995). The former is, however, also nutrition and age dependent and must therefore be used cautiously. For children under the age of 6 years, the lower limit of the normal range for IGF-I is often close to the sensitivity of most assays and so discriminating a child with GHD on the basis of a low IGF-I is particularly difficult in this age group.

At present, there does not appear to be a single faultless test for the diagnosis of growth hormone deficiency and the diagnosis should therefore be based upon a combination of auxology, clinical assessment and biochemistry. Once a diagnosis of GHD has been made, imaging of the hypothalamo-pituitary region is indicated, preferably using MRI. This may shed light on the underlying etiology of GHD/GHI, e.g. an intracranial tumor or pituitary hypoplasia.

Treatment

Recombinant growth hormone treatment is indicated for the treatment of growth hormone deficiency or insufficiency. Virtually all children will grow faster if given GH (Moore et al 1993). However, this increase in growth rate has only been shown to translate into an increase in final height in GHD/GHI children. It is administered subcutaneously daily, the dose being dependent on body size.

The effect of GH treatment in GHI/GHD patients is dependent upon the pretreatment height velocity, the GH status of the subject and the dose used. The greatest increase in height velocity is in those children with the slowest pretreatment height velocity. Figure 8.17 shows the typical growth chart of a child with GHD who has commenced GH treatment.

GH treatment is usually continued until the child has achieved his or her pubertal growth spurt and the growth rate has slowed down to < 2 cm/year. However, recent work has focused on the use of GH treatment in adults with GHD, but this is beyond the scope of this chapter.

Laron-type dwarfism (GH receptor deficiency)

This rare autosomal recessive condition is caused by a defect in the growth hormone receptor leading to resistance to the actions of both endogenous and exogenous GH with a failure to generate IGF-I (Savage et al 1993) (p. 365). The condition is most frequently seen in oriental Jews and Ecuadorian subjects of Spanish descent.

Clinical features include a low birthweight and length, abnormal facies with a prominent forehead, midfacial hypoplasia and a depressed nasal bridge, hypoglycemia, micropenis, blue sclerae,

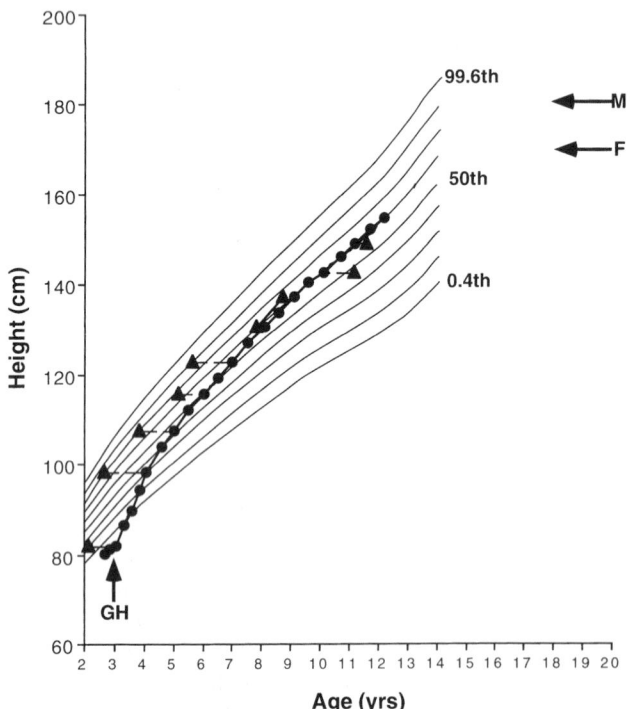

Fig. 8.17 Typical growth chart of a child with growth hormone deficiency treated with recombinant hGH. M=mother; F=father; triangle=bone age; circle=chronological age.

extreme short stature, a poor height velocity, excess subcutaneous fat, delayed skeletal maturation and delayed puberty.

Endocrine assessment reveals high levels of GH spontaneously and on provocation, with low levels of IGF-I, IGF-II and IGFBP-3. Although the pulsatile pattern of spontaneous GH secretion is maintained, GH levels fail to fall to normal undetectable levels in between pulses (Cotterill et al 1992). Growth hormone-binding protein may be present or absent, depending upon the site of the mutation (Savage et al 1993, Bauman et al 1987, Buchanan et al 1991). IGF-I levels fail to respond to the administration of exogenous GH.

Recently, recombinant IGF-I has been used to treat children with Laron-type dwarfism. Initial results are promising, with an increase in height velocity in one group of 26 patients from a mean pretreatment value of 3.9 ± 1.8 cm/year to 8.5 ± 2.1 cm/year after 12 months of therapy and a height velocity of 6.4 ± 2.2 cm/year in the second year in 18 out of the 26 children (Ranke et al 1995). Other effects include a reduction in skinfold thickness and a change in the facial appearance of these children. The treatment does, however, have some temporary side effects including hypoglycemia, hypokalemia and benign intracranial hypertension.

Other endocrine conditions resulting in short stature

Primary hypothyroidism (see also Ch. 19)

Hypothyroidism may present with short stature and a low height velocity. Primary hypothyroidism is mostly due to an autoimmune thyroiditis or congenital hypothyroidism. The latter is now usually detected by neonatal screening, before it can present with short stature. Other classic signs of hypothyroidism such as lethargy, hair loss, dry skin, constipation, coarse facies, delayed reflexes, cold intolerance, excessive weight gain and bradycardia are rarely present. Puberty may be delayed, although increased FSH secretion often leads to isolated early breast development in girls and testicular enlargement in boys. The diagnosis is revealed by a low free thyroxine level, with a high TSH level. Treatment should be commenced with half the replacement dose of thyroxine initially, increasing to full dosage over the following weeks.

The growth failure of hypothyroidism can be explained by the stimulatory effect of thyroxine on the transcription of the GH-N gene, thereby influencing the secretion of growth hormone. Low GH pulsatility has been documented at the time of biochemical hypothyroidism and this returns to normal on commencing thyroxine treatment (Buchanan et al 1988).

Cushing syndrome (see also Ch. 19)

This condition, which is due to glucocorticoid excess, frequently presents with short stature and a poor height velocity. The impairment of growth in Cushing syndrome is predominantly due to a direct effect at the growth plate. The commonest cause is iatrogenic, with pituitary and adrenal-dependent Cushing syndrome being much rarer. Ectopic Cushing syndrome is virtually unknown in childhood. Other clinical features such as excessive weight gain with truncal obesity, proximal myopathy, Cushingoid facies, hypertension, buffalo hump, purple striae, hirsutism, hypogonadism, glycosuria and susceptibilities to infection and bruising may be present. The diagnosis is based upon the lack of a diurnal variation in cortisol secretion and an elevated 24-hour urinary free cortisol level. Low and high dose dexamethasone suppression tests may help in elucidating the source of the excess glucocorticoid. Neuroradiological imaging may reveal a pituitary adenoma. Treatment will entail surgical removal of the tumor, although with pituitary adenomata, re-exploration is often necessary, since not all of the abnormal cells will have been removed at the first attempt.

TALL STATURE (see also Ch. 19)

This is a relatively uncommon problem in pediatric endocrine practice, compared with the issues of short stature. Children of tall parents tend to be tall themselves. Referral criteria for tall children based upon the new reference standards (see p. 1020) are as follows, depending upon either single or sequential measurements of height.

Single measurement All children with a height above the 99.6th centile should be referred to an endocrinologist. Additionally, referral should be considered for children with a height between the 98th and 99.6th centiles and those about whom parental or professional concern has been expressed or when there is a significant discrepancy between the mid-parental target centile and the child's present centile.

Sequential measurements All children should be referred if the growth curve crosses two centile lines, since this indicates an abnormally rapid rate of growth with a high probability of underlying pathology. Additionally, referral should be considered if the growth curve crosses a single centile line between 2 and 5 years of age.

Figure 8.18 shows an approach to the management of this problem.

The child's height should be compared with the mid-parental height. If the child is tall for the parents, then signs of any dysmorphic syndrome or endocrine disorder should be sought. In particular, the presence of sexual precocity should be sought. A bone age may be useful in giving a height prediction.

The most useful piece of information is the height velocity. Dickerman et al (1984) studied a group of 65 tall nonobese children and found that although the height velocity was maximal between birth and 6 months of age, it nevertheless remained above the 50th centile throughout childhood, giving rise to the concept that tall children are tall because they grow with an increased height velocity. Children with tall stature who have no signs of puberty ought to be investigated if their height velocity remains >98th centile for over a year. If the height velocity lies between the 75th and 98th centiles, then the child should be observed for a further 1-year period and investigated if the increased height velocity persists.

Children who become obese in the first year of life will generally be taller than those who achieve obesity after this time. In the latter group, the increase in height is usually accompanied by an advance in skeletal maturation and therefore little change in final height.

Constitutional tall stature

In this condition, the child presents with tall stature, but no dysmorphism or disproportion is noted. The child is otherwise well and there is a family history of tall stature. A bone age should be performed and a predicted height calculated. A height velocity should be obtained and if this is normal, then a decision should be taken in conjunction with the child and parents as to any possible

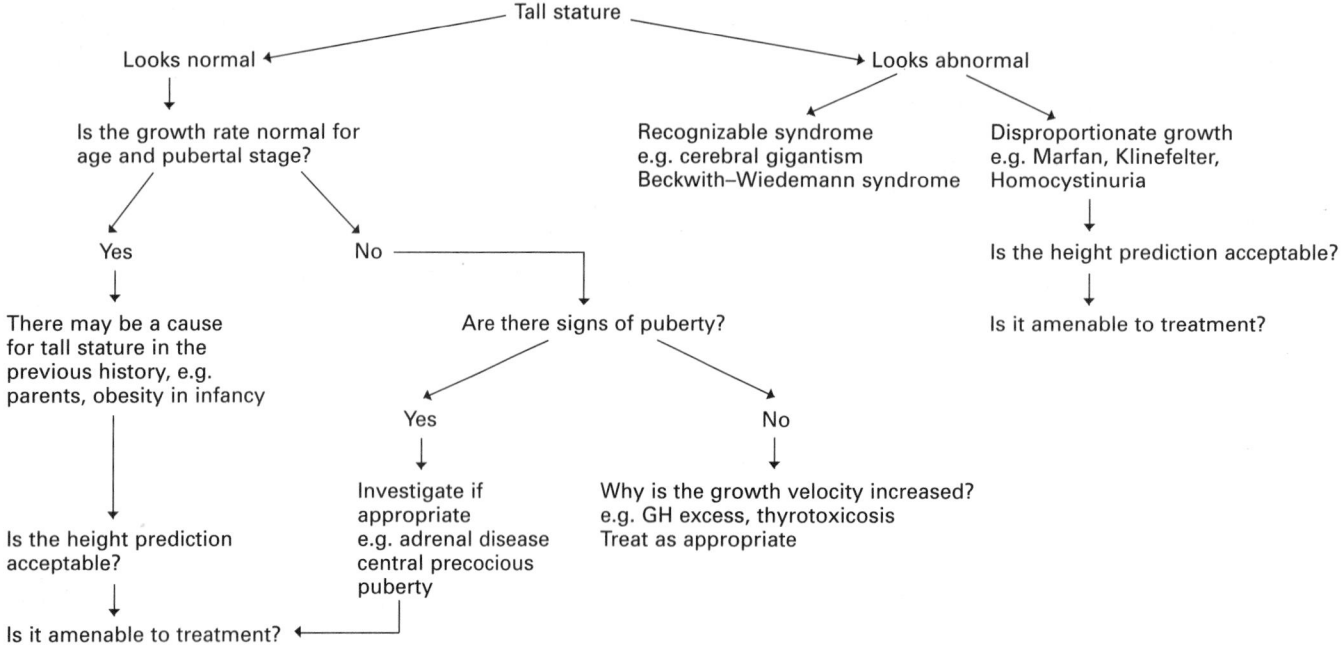

Fig. 8.18 Algorithm for the management of tall stature.

intervention to restrict the final height. Tall stature may have the same implications as short stature as regards acceptability by society. In particular, finding clothes and shoes may be a difficult and expensive business.

It is extremely difficult to manipulate the amount of growth which occurs in puberty, which is of the order of 25–30 cm. In the past, treatment has involved the use of appropriate sex steroids, usually in rather high doses to attempt to accelerate epiphyseal fusion. However, long-term results vary between reports and high dose estrogens are probably associated with unacceptable long-term risks. In young children destined for unacceptable final heights, the early induction of normal puberty with physiological doses of sex steroids may have a place.

Tall stature with dysmorphic features

Sotos syndrome and Beckwith–Wiedemann syndrome are characterized by a rapid intrauterine rate of growth which continues postnatally over the first few years of life, with dysmorphic features and tall stature. They are also associated with mental retardation. In the Beckwith–Wiedemann syndrome, exomphalos, polycythemia, an abnormal transverse crease in the pinna of the ear and hyperinsulinism leading to hypoglycemia are other features, together with a tendency to develop Wilms tumors of the kidney.

The genetic defect in Sotos syndrome is unknown, whilst in Beckwith's syndrome, abnormalities at chromosome 11p15 have been described. No endocrine abnormalities have been demonstrated to account for the tall stature observed in these two conditions.

Tall stature with disproportionate growth

Marfan syndrome is an autosomal dominant condition which is thought to be due to a mutation in the fibrillin gene on chromosome 15 (Tsipouras et al 1992). The syndrome is characterized by tall stature with excessively long limbs, upward dislocation of the lens of the eye, arachnodactyly, a high arched palate, hyperextensible joints and cardiovascular abnormalities, of which mitral valve prolapse is the commonest in childhood. Homocystinuria is an autosomal recessive condition due to a deficiency of cystathionine synthetase. It shares several phenotypic features with Marfan syndrome, but the lenticular dislocation is downward and mental retardation with a tendency to arterial and venous thrombosis is characteristic.

Klinefelter syndrome, with a karyotype of 47XXY, may also manifest itself with tall disproportionate stature. The clinical features include tall stature, long limbs, small testes, poor school performance, gynecomastia and infertility.

Pituitary gigantism

This is the pediatric equivalent of acromegaly and presents with tall stature and an excessive growth rate. Growth hormone levels are elevated and the baseline secretory rate may also be increased. There may be a paradoxical rise in GH levels following an oral glucose load. Additionally, GH may be released in response to exogenous thyrotropin-releasing hormone. However, the latter two phenomena may be observed in constitutionally tall adolescents and so are not particularly discriminatory. IGF-I is elevated in this condition. An MRI scan of the hypothalamus and pituitary may be required if a pituitary adenoma is suspected. If such a lesion is found, the definitive treatment involves transsphenoidal surgery.

Other endocrinopathies causing tall stature

If signs of precocious puberty are present, then this avenue should be pursued. Both gonadotrophin-dependent and gonadotrophin-independent precocious puberty can present with tall stature, a rapid growth rate and an advanced bone age, as can congenital adrenal hyperplasia and androgen-secreting tumors of the adrenals. Adrenarche, the process whereby the adrenal gland secretes excessive amounts of androgens, can also present with tall stature. The diagnosis can be established by assessing the gonadotrophin response to luteinizing hormone-releasing hormone and performing a 24-hour urinary steroid profile.

Thyrotoxicosis, a rare condition in childhood which is usually autoimmune in etiology, can also present with tall stature and an advanced bone age with a rapid height velocity. Elevated levels of free T3 and T4 levels, with a suppressed TSH level, are diagnostic.

CONCLUSION

This chapter has described some of the basic pathophysiological processes involved in the growth of man. With recent advances in molecular and cellular techniques, the way forward is exciting. In particular, we can look forward to important breakthroughs in the understanding of the genetic processes of growth. It is hoped that these will aid us in the management of children with disorders of growth.

Acknowledgment

We are grateful to the Child Growth Foundation for permission to reproduce the centile charts in Figure 8.4 a and b. Decimal and duodecimal versions of the charts may be purchased from Harlow Printing, Maxwell Street, South Shields NE33 4PU. The Child Growth Foundation, 2 Mayfield Avenue, Chiswick, London W4 1PW may be contacted for sources of growth measuring equipment, training and information.

REFERENCES

Adashi E Y, Resnick C E, Rosenfeld R G 1989 Insulin-like growth factor-I (IGF-I) hormonal action in cultured rat granulosa cells: mediation via type 1 but not type 2 IGF receptors. Endocrinology 126: 216–222

Ahmed M L, Foot A B M, Edge J A, Lamkin V A, Savage M O, Dunger D B 1991 Noonan's syndrome: abnormalities of the growth hormone/IGF-I axis and the response to treatment with human biosynthetic growth hormone. Acta Paediatrica Scandinavica 80 (suppl): 446–450

Albertsson-Wikland K, Rosberg S 1988 Analyses of 24-hour growth hormone profiles in children: relation to growth. Journal of Clinical Endocrinology and Metabolism 67: 493–500

Baker J, Liu J-P, Robertson E J, Efstratiadis A 1993 Role of insulin-like growth factors in embryonic and postnatal growth. Cell 75: 73–82

Barker D J P 1992 Fetal and infant origins of adult disease. BMJ Publishing Group, London

Barker D J P, Osmond C, Golding J, Kuh D, Wadsworth M E J 1989 Growth in utero, blood pressure in childhood and adult life, and mortality from cardiovascular disease. British Medical Journal 298: 564–567

Baumann G 1991 Growth hormone heterogeneity: genes, isohormones, variants, binding proteins. Endocrine Reviews 12: 424–448

Baumann G, Stolar M W 1986 Molecular forms of human growth hormone secreted in vivo: non-specificity of secretory stimuli. Journal of Clinical Endocrinology and Metabolism 62: 789–790

Baumann G, Stolar M W, Buchanan T A 1985 Slow metabolic clearance rate of the 20,000-dalton variant of human growth hormone: implications for biological activity. Endocrinology 117: 1309–1313

Baumann G, Winter R J, Shaw M 1987a Circulating molecular variants of growth hormone in childhood. Pediatric Research 21: 21–22

Baumann G, Shaw M A, Winter R J 1987b Absence of the growth hormone-binding protein in Laron-type dwarfism. Journal of Clinical Endocrinology and Metabolism 65: 814–816

Baumann G, Vance M L, Shaw M A, Thorner M O 1990 Plasma transport of human growth hormone in vivo. Journal of Clinical Endocrinology and Metabolism 71: 470–473

Baxter R C 1988 Characterization of the acid-labile sub-unit of the growth hormone-dependent insulin-like growth factor binding protein complex. Journal of Clinical Endocrinology and Metabolism 67: 265–272

Bayley N, Pinneau S R 1952 Tables for predicting adult height from skeletal age. Revised for use with the Greulich–Pyle hand standards. Journal of Paediatrics 40: 463–469

Bellus G A, McIntosh I, Smith E A, Aylsworth A S, Kaitila I, Horton W A, Greenhaw G A, Hecht J T, Francomann C A 1995 A recurrent mutation in the tyrosine kinase domain of fibroblast growth factor receptor-3 causes hypochondroplasia. Nature Genetics 10: 357–359

Bilezikjian L, Vale W 1983 Stimulation of adenosine 3′,5′-monophosphate production by growth hormone-releasing factor and its inhibition by somatostatin in anterior pituitary cells in vitro. Endocrinology 113: 1726–1731

Billestrup N, Swanson L W, Vale W 1986 Growth hormone-releasing factor stimulates proliferation of somatotrophs in vitro. Proceedings of the National Academy of Science USA 83: 6854–6857

Binder G, Ranke M B 1995 Screening for growth hormone (GH) gene splice-site mutations in sporadic cases with severe isolated GH deficiency using ectopic transcript analysis. Journal of Clinical Endocrinology and Metabolism 80: 1247–1252

Birnbaum M H, Baxter J D 1986 Glucocorticoids regulate the expression of a rat growth hormone gene lacking 5′ flanking sequences. Journal of Biological Chemistry 261: 291–297

Bistritzer T, Chalwe S A, Lovechik J C, Kowarski A A 1988 Growth without growth hormone, the 'invisible' GH syndrome. Lancet i: 321–323

Blizzard R M, Bulatovic A 1992 Psychosocial short stature: a syndrome with many variables. Bailliere Clinics in Endocrinology and Metabolism 6: 687–712

Blum W F, Ranke M B, Keitzmann K, Grauggel E, Zeisel H, Bierich J R 1990 A specific radioimmunoassay for the growth hormone (GH)-dependent somatomedin-binding protein: its use for diagnosis of GH deficiency. Journal of Clinical Endocrinology and Metabolism 70: 1292–1298

Bodner M, Castrillo J L, Theill L, Deerinck T, Ellisman M, Karin M 1988 The pituitary-specific transcription factor GHF-1 is a homeobox-containing protein. Cell 55: 505–518

Brown A L, Graham D E, Nissley S P, Hill D J, Strain A J, Rechler M M 1986 Developmental regulation of insulin-like growth factor II mRNA in different rat tissues. Journal of Biological Chemistry 261: 13144–13150

Buchanan C R, Stanhope R, Adlard P, Jones J, Grant D B, Preece M A 1988 Gonadotrophin, growth hormone and prolactin secretion in children with primary hypothyroidism. Clinical Endocrinology 29: 427–436

Buchanan C R, Maheshwari H G, Norman M B, Morrell D J, Preece M A 1991 Laron-type dwarfism with apparently normal high affinity serum growth hormone binding protein. Clinical Endocrinology 35: 179–185

Butler G E, McKie M, Ratcliffe S G 1990 The cyclical nature of prepubertal growth. Annals of Human Biology 17: 177–198

Cara J F, Rosenfeld R L, Furlanetto R W 1987 A longitudinal study of the relationship of plasma somatomedin-C concentration to the pubertal growth spurt. American Journal of Diseases in Childhood 141: 562–564

Celniker A C, Chen A B, Wert R M Jr, Sherman B M 1989 Variability in the quantitation of circulating growth hormone using commercial immunoassays. Journal of Clinical Endocrinology and Metabolism 68: 469–476

Chinn S, Price C E, Rona R J 1989a Need for new reference curves for height. Archives of Disease in Childhood 64: 1545–1553

Chinn S, Rona R J, Price C E 1989b The secular trend in primary school children in England and Scotland 1972–1979 and 1979–1986. Annals of Human Biology 16: 387–395

Cianfarani S, Boemi S, Spagnoli A, Cappa M, Argiro G, Vaccaro F, Manca Bitti M L, Boscherini B 1995 Is IGF binding protein-3 assessment helpful for the diagnosis of GH deficiency? Clinical Endocrinology 43: 43–47

Clark R G, Robinson I C A F 1988 Paradoxical growth-promoting effects induced by patterned infusions of somatostatin to female rats. Endocrinology 122: 2675–2682

Clayton P E, Shalet S M, Morris-Jones P H, Price D A 1988 Growth in children treated for acute lymphoblastic leukaemia. Lancet 1: 460–462

Cogan J D, Phillips III J A, Sakati N, Frisch H, Schuber E, Milner D 1993 Heterogenous growth hormone (GH) gene mutations in familial GH deficiency. Journal of Clinical Endocrinology and Metabolism 76: 1224–1228

Cohen L E, Wondisford F E, Salvatoni A, Maghnie M, Brucker-Davies F, Weintraub B, Radovic S 1995 A "hot spot" in the Pit-1 gene responsible for combined pituitary hormone deficiency: clinical and molecular correlates. Journal of Clinical Endocrinology and Metabolism 80: 679–684

Cole T J 1994 Do growth chart centiles need a facelift? British Medical Journal 308: 641–64

Cole T J, Freeman J V, Preece M A 1995 Body mass index reference curves for the UK, 1990. Archives of Disease in Childhood 73: 25–29

Conover C A, Misra P, Hintz R L, Rosenfeld R G 1987 Effect of an anti-insulin-like growth factor-I receptor antibody on insulin-like growth factor-II stimulation of DNA synthesis in human fibroblasts. Biochemical and Biophysical Research Communications 139: 501–508

Cooke N E, Ray J, Watson M A, Estes P A, Kuo B A, Liebhaber S A 1988 Human growth hormone gene and the highly homologous growth hormone variant gene display different splicing patterns. Journal of Clinical Investigation 82: 270–275

Costello A M 1989 Growth velocity and stunting in rural Nepal. Archives of Disease in Childhood 64: 1478–1482

Cotterill A M, Holly J M P, Taylor A M, Davies S C, Coulson V J, Preece M A, Wass J A, Savage M O 1992 The insulin-like growth factor (IGF)-binding proteins and IGF bioactivity in Laron-type dwarfism. Journal of Clinical Endocrinology and Metabolism 74: 56–63

Cronin M J, Hewitt E L, Evans W S, Thorner M O, Rogol A D 1984 Human pancreatic tumour growth hormone releasing factor and cyclic adenosine 3,5/-monophosphate evoke GH release from anterior pituitary cells: the effects of pertussis toxin, cholera toxin, forskolin and cycloheximide. Endocrinology 114: 904–913

Crowne E C, Shalet S M, Wallace W H, Eminson D M, Price D A 1990 Final height in boys with untreated constitutional delay in growth and puberty. Archives of Disease in Childhood 65: 1109–1112

Crowne E C, Shalet S M, Wallace W H, Eminson D M, Price D A 1991 Final height in girls with untreated constitutional delay in growth and puberty. European Journal of Paediatrics 150: 708–710

Cunningham B C, Ultsch M, de Vos A M, Mulkerrin M G, Clauser K R, Wells J A 1991 Dimerization of the extracellular domain of the human growth hormone receptor by a single hormone molecule. Science 254: 821–825

Darendelier F, Hindmarsh P C, Preece M A, Cox L, Brook C G D 1990 Growth hormone increases rate of pubertal maturation. Acta Endocrinologica 122: 414–416

Dattani M T, Pringle P J, Hindmarsh P C, Brook C G D 1992 What is a normal stimulated growth hormone concentration? Journal of Endocrinology 133: 447–450

Dattani M T, Hindmarsh P C, Weir T, Robinson I C A F, Brook C G D, Marshall N J 1993 Enhancement of growth hormone bioactivity by zinc in the eluted stain assay system (ESTA). Endocrinology 133: 2803–2808

Dattani M T, Hindmarsh P C, Brook C G D, Robinson I C A F, Marshall N J 1994 Inhibition of growth hormone bioactivity by recombinant human growth hormone-binding protein in the eluted stain assay (ESTA) system. Journal of Endocrinology 140: 445–453

Dattani M T, Hindmarsh P C, Pringle P J, Brook C G D, Marshall N J M 1995 The measurement of GH bioactivity using an eluted stain assay. Journal of Clinical Endocrinology and Metabolism 80: 2675–2683

Daughaday W H, Rotwein P 1989 Insulin-like growth factors I and II. Peptide, messenger ribonucleic acid and gene structures, serum and tissue concentrations. Endocrine Reviews 10: 68–91

Daughaday W H, Kapadia M, Mariz I 1986 Serum somatomedin binding proteins: physiologic significance and interference in radioligand assay. Journal of Laboratory and Clinical Medicine 109: 355–363

Davies P S W, Valley R, Preece M A 1988 Adolescent growth and pubertal progression in the Silver-Russell syndrome. Archives of Disease in Childhood 63: 130–135

DeChiara T M, Efstratiadis A, Robertson E J 1990 A growth deficiency phenotype in heterozygous mice carrying an insulin-like growth factor II gene disrupted by targeting. Nature 345: 78–80

Delmis J, Drazancic A, Ivanisevic M, Suchanek E 1992 Glucose, insulin, hGH and IGF-I levels in maternal serum, amniotic fluid and umbilical venous serum: a comparison between late normal pregnancy and pregnancies complicated with diabetes and fetal growth retardation. Journal of Perinatal Medicine 20: 47–56

Dickerman Z, Loewinger J, Laron Z 1984 The pattern of growth in children with constitutional tall stature from birth to age 9 years. A longitudinal study. Acta Paediatrica Scandinavica (suppl.) 73: 530–536

Emoto N, Tsushima T, Shizume K, Tanaka T, Saji M, Ohba Y, Wakai K, Arai M, Ohmura E 1987 Biological activities of human growth hormone and its

derivatives estimated by measuring DNA synthesis in Nb2 node rat lymphoma cells. Acta Endocrinologica (Copenh) 114: 283–291

Eveleth P B, Tanner J M 1990 World-wide variation in human growth, 2nd edition. Cambridge University Press, London

Fitzhardinge P M, Inwood S 1989 Long-term growth in small-for-dates children. Acta Paediatrica Scandinavica 349: 2–33

Freeman J V, Cole T J, Chinn S, Jones P R M, White E M, Preece M A 1995 Cross-sectional stature and weight reference curves for the UK, 1990. Archives of Disease in Childhood 73: 17–24

Gasser T, Kohler W, Muller H G, Largo R, Molinari L, Prader A 1985 Human height growth: correlation and multivariate structure of velocity and acceleration. Annals of Human Biology 12: 501–515

Gatherer D, TenDijke P, Baird D T, Akhurst R J 1990 Expression of TGF-β isoforms during first trimester human embryogenesis. Development 110: 445–460

Gaylinn B D, Harrison J K, Zysk J R, Lyons C E, Lynch K R, Thorner M O 1993 Molecular cloning and expression of a human anterior pituitary receptor for growth hormone-releasing hormone. Molecular Endocrinology 7: 77–84

Goddard A D, Covello R, Luoh S M, Clackson T, Attie K M, Gesundheit N, Rundle A C, Wells J A, Carlsson L M S 1995 Mutations of the growth hormone receptor in children with idiopathic short stature. New England Journal of Medicine 333: 1093–1098

Goossens M, Brauner R, Czernichow P, Duquesnoy P, Rappaport R 1986 Isolated growth hormone (GH) deficiency type IA associated with a double deletion in the human GH gene cluster. Journal of Clinical Endocrinology and Metabolism 62: 712–716

Han V K M, D'Ercole A J, Lund P K 1987a Cellular localization of somatomedin (insulin-like growth factor) messenger RNA in the human fetus. Science 236: 193–197

Han V K M, Hill D J, Strain A J, Towle A C, Lauder J M, Underwood L E, D'Ercole A J 1987b Identification of somatomedin/insulin-like growth factor immunoreactive cells in the human fetus. Pediatric Research 22: 245–249

Harris D A, van Vliet G, Egli C A, Grumbach M M, Kaplan S L, Styne D M, Vainsel M 1985 Somatomedin-C in normal puberty and in true precocious puberty before and after treatment with a potent luteinizing hormone-releasing hormone agonist. Journal of Clinical Endocrinology and Metabolism 61: 152–159

Hartman M L, Veldhuis J D, Johnson M L, Lee M M, Alberti K G, Samojlik E, Thorner M O 1992 Augmented growth hormone (GH) secretory burst frequency and amplitude mediate enhanced GH secretion during a two-day fast in normal men. Journal of Clinical Endocrinology and Metabolism 74: 757–765

Hasegawa Y, Hasegawa T, Aso T et al 1993 Comparison between insulin-like growth factor I (IGF-I) and IGF binding protein-3 (IGFBP3) measurement in the diagnosis of growth hormone deficiency. Endocrine Journal 40: 185–190

Hatikka J, Hefti F 1988 Comparison of nerve growth factor effects on development of septum, striatum and nucleus basalis cholinergic neurons in vitro. Journal of Neurosciences Research 21: 352–364

Hill D J, Hogg J 1989 Growth factors and the regulation of pre- and post-natal growth. In: Jones C T (ed) Clinical endocrinology and metabolism, perinatal endocrinology. Vol 3, No 3. Bailliere Tindall, London, p 579–625

Hindmarsh P C, Brook C G D 1995 Short stature and growth hormone deficiency. Clinical Endocrinology 43: 133–142

Hindmarsh P C, Swift P G F 1995 An assessment of growth hormone provocation tests. Archives of Disease in Childhood 72: 362–368

Hindmarsh P C, Smith P J, Brook C G D, Matthews D R 1987 The relationship between growth velocity and growth hormone secretion in short prepubertal children. Clinical Endocrinology 27: 581–591

Hindmarsh P C, Brain C E, Robinson I C A F, Matthews D R, Brook C G D 1991 The interaction of growth hormone-releasing hormone and somatostatin in the generation of GH pulse. Clinical Endocrinology 35: 353–360

Humbel R E 1990 Insulin-like growth factors I and II. European Journal of Biochemistry 190: 445–462

Ingraham H, Chew R, Mangalam H et al 1988 A tissue-specific transcription factor containing a homeobox domain specifies a pituitary phenotype. Cell 55: 519–529

Iwamoto H S, Murray M A, Chernausek S D 1992 Effects of acute hypoxia on insulin-like growth factors and their binding proteins in fetal sheep. American Journal of Physiology 263: E1151–1156

Karlberg J, Engstron I, Karlberg P, Fryer J G 1987 Analyses of linear growth using a mathematical model. Acta Paediatrica Scandinavica (suppl) 76: 478–488

Katakami H, Downs T R, Frohman L A 1986 Decreased hypothalamic growth hormone-releasing hormone content and pituitary responsiveness in hypothyroidism. Journal of Clinical Investigation 77: 1704–1711

Kelly P A, Ali S, Rozakis M, Goujon L, Nagano M, Pellegrini I, Gould D, Djiane J, Edery M, Finidori J, Postel-Vinay M C 1993 The growth hormone/prolactin receptor family. Recent Progress in Hormone Research 48: 123–164

Kerrigan J R, Martha P M, Blizzard R M, Christie C M, Rogol A D 1990 Variations of pulsatile growth hormone release in healthy short prepubertal boys. Pediatric Research 28: 11–14

Kirk J A, Raghupathy P, Stevens M M, Cowell C T, Menser M A, Bergin M, Tink A, Vines R H, Silink M 1987 Growth failure and growth hormone deficiency after treatment for acute lymphoblastic leukaemia. Lancet 1: 190–193

Labrie F, Gagne B, Lefevre G 1983 Growth hormone-releasing factor stimulates adenylate cyclase activity in the anterior pituitary gland. Life Sciences 33: 2229–2233

Landis C, Masters S, Spada A, Pace A, Bourne H, Vallar L 1989 GTPase inhibiting mutations activate the α chain of Gs and stimulate adenyl cyclase activity in human pituitary tumours. Nature 340: 692–696

Lassarre C, Hardouin S, Daffos F, Forestier F, Frankenne F, Binoux M 1991 Serum insulin-like growth factor binding proteins in the human fetus. Relationships with growth in normal subjects and in subjects with intrauterine growth retardation. Pediatric Research 29: 219–221

Lifshitz F, Moses N 1985 Nutritional growth retardation. In: Lifshitz F (ed) Paediatric endocrinology: a clinical guide. Marcel Dekker, New York, p 111–132

Lin S-C, Lin C R, Gukovsky I, Lusis A J, Sawchenko P E, Rosenfeld M G 1993 Molecular basis of the little mouse phenotype and implications for cell-type specific growth. Nature 364: 208–213

Lippe B 1991 Turner syndrome. Endocrinol Metab Clin N. America 20: 121–152

Liu J-P, Baker J, Perkins A S, Robertson E J, Efstratiadis A 1993 Mice carrying null mutations of the genes encoding insulin-like growth factor-I (Igf-I) and type 1 IGF receptor (Igf1r). Cell 75: 59–72

Lyon A J, Preece M A, Grant D B 1985 Growth curve for girls with Turner syndrome. Archives of Disease in Childhood 60: 932–935

McLellan K C, Hooper S B, Bocking A D, Delhanty P J, Phillips I D, Hill D J, Han V K 1992 Prolonged hypoxia induced by the reduction of maternal uterine blood flow alters insulin-like growth factor-binding protein-1 (IGFBP-1) and IGFBP-2 gene expression in the ovine fetus. Endocrinology 131: 1619–1628

Marshall W A, Tanner J M 1970 Variations in the pattern of pubertal changes in boys. Archives of Disease in Childhood 45:13-23

Martin J L, Baxter R C 1986 Insulin-like growth factor binding protein from human plasma: purification and characterization. Journal of Biological Chemistry 261: 8754–8760

Marwaha R, Menon P S N, Jena A, Pant C, Wethi A K, Sapra M L 1992 Hypothalamic-pituitary axis by magnetic resonance in isolated growth hormone deficiency patients born by normal delivery. Journal of Clinical Endocrinology and Metabolism 74: 654–659

Massa G, Vanderschueren-Lodeweyckx M, Malvaux P 1990 Linear growth in patients with Turner syndrome: influence of spontaneous puberty and parental height. European Journal of Paediatrics 149: 246–250

Massa G, Malvaux P, Vanderschueren-Lodeweyckx M 1991 Spontaneous growth in Turner syndrome: the Belgian experience. In: Ranke M B, Rosenfeld R G (eds) Turner syndrome and growth promoting therapies. Excerpta Medica, Amsterdam, pp 95–99

Mauras N, Blizzard R M, Link K, Johnson M L, Rogol A D, Veldhuis J D 1987 Augmentation of growth hormone secretion during puberty: evidence for a pulse amplitude modulated phenomenon. Journal of Clinical Endocrinology and Metabolism 54: 596–601

Moell C 1988 Disturbed pubertal growth in girls after acute leukaemia: a relative growth hormone insufficiency with late presentation. Acta Paediatrica Scandinavica (suppl) 343: 162–166

Moore K C, Donaldson D L, Ideus P L, Gifford R A, Moore W V 1993 Clinical diagnoses of children with extremely short stature and their response to growth hormone. Journal of Pediatrics 122: 687–692

Mullis P E, Patel M S, Brickell P M, Brook C G D 1991 Constitutional short stature: analysis of the insulin-like growth factor I gene and the human growth hormone gene cluster. Pediatric Research 29: 412–415

Ogilvy-Stuart A L, Clark D J, Wallace W H, Gibson B E, Stevens R F, Shalet S M, Donaldson M O 1992 Endocrine deficit after fractionated total body irradiation. Archives of Disease in Childhood 67: 1107–1110

Oh Y, Muller H, Neely E K, Rosenfeld R G 1993 New concepts in insulin-like growth factor receptor physiology. Growth Regulation 3: 113–123

Ohmae Y, Yano H, Umezawa S, Tanaka T, Hibi I, Miyamoto C, Furuichi Y 1989 Biological activities of synthesized 20K and 22K hGH in Nb2 bioassay and IM-9 radioreceptor assay. Endocrinologia Japonica 36(I): 9–13

Papadimitrou A, Wacharasindhu S, Pearl K, Preece M A, Stanhope R 1991 Treatment of constitutional growth delay in prepubertal boys with a prolonged course of low dose oxandrolone. Archives of Disease in Childhood 66: 841–843

Paz I, Seidman D S, Danon Y I, Laor A, Stevenson D K, Gale R 1993 Are children born small for gestational age at increased risk of short stature? American Journal of Diseases in Childhood 147: 337–339

Pfaffle R W, DiMattia G E, Parks J S et al 1992 Mutations of the POU-specific domain of Pit-1 and hypopituitarism without pituitary hypoplasia. Science 257: 1118–1121

Ranke M B, Heidemann P, Knupfer C, Enders H, Schmaltz A A, Bierich J R 1988 Noonan syndrome: growth and clinical manifestations in 144 cases. European Journal of Paediatrics 148: 220–227

Ranke M B, Chavez-Meyer H, Blank B, Frisch H, Hausler G 1991 Spontaneous growth and bone age development in Turner syndrome: results of a multicentre study, 1990. In: Ranke M B, Rosenfeld R G eds. Turner syndrome and growth promoting therapies. Excerpta Medica, Amsterdam, p 101–106

Ranke M B, Savage M O, Chatelain P G, Preece M A, Rosenfeld R G, Blum W F, Wilton P 1995 Insulin-like growth factor-I improves height in growth hormone insensitivity: two years results. Hormone Research 44: 253–264

Ray K P, Hart G R, Wallis M 1986 Effects of dopamine and somatostatin on phorbolester-stimulated prolactin and growth hormone secretion. Molecular and Cellular Endocrinology 48: 205–212

Reiter J C, Craen M, van Vliet G 1991 Decreased growth hormone response to growth hormone releasing hormone in Turner's syndrome: relation to body weight and adiposity. Acta Endocrinologica (Copenh) 125: 38–42

Riken B, Wit J M 1992 Prepubertal height velocity reference ranges over a wide age range. Archives of Disease in Children 67: 1277–1280

Roche A F, Wainer H, Thissen D 1975 Predicting adult stature for individuals. Monographs in Paediatrics 3: 1–114

Rosenfeld R G, Conover C A, Hodges D, Lee P D, Misra P, Hintz R L, Li C H 1987 Heterogeneity of insulin-like growth factor-I affinity for the insulin-like growth factor-II receptor: comparison of natural, synthetic and recombinant DNA-derived insulin-like growth factor-I. Biochemical and Biophysical Research Communications 143: 199–205

Rosenfeld R G, Hintz R L, Johanson A J et al 1988 Three-year results of a randomized prospective trial of methionyl human growth hormone and oxandrolone in Turner syndrome. Journal of Pediatrics 113: 393–400

Rosenfeld R G, Rosenbloom A L, Guevara-Aguirre J 1994 Growth hormone insensitivity due to primary GH receptor deficiency. Endocrine Reviews 15: 369–390

Rosenfeld R G, Albertsson-Wikland K, Cassorla F et al 1995 Diagnostic controversy: the diagnosis of childhood growth hormone deficiency revisited. Journal of Clinical Endocrinology and Metabolism 80: 1532–1540

Rousseau F, Bonaventure J, Legcai-Mallet L et al 1994 Mutations in the gene encoding fibroblast growth factor receptor 3 in achondroplasia. Nature 371: 252–254

Savage M O, Blum W F, Ranke M B et al 1993 Clinical features and endocrine status in patients with growth hormone insensitivity (Laron syndrome). Journal of Clinical Endocrinology and Metabolism 77: 1465–1471

Schwartz S, Berger P, Frisch H, Mancayo R, Phillips J A, Wick G 1987 Growth hormone blocking antibodies in a patient with deletion of the GH-N gene. Clinical Endocrinology 27: 213–224

Shah A, Stanhope R G, Matthews D 1992 Hazards of pharmacological tests of growth hormone secretion in childhood. British Medical Journal 304: 173–174

Shalet S M, Crowne E C, Didi M A, Ogilvie-Stuart A L, Wallace W H 1992 Irradiation-induced growth failure. Baillieres Clinical Endocrinology and Metabolism 6: 513–526

Shiang R, Thompson L M, Zhu Y-Z et al 1994 Mutations in the transmembrane domain of FGFR3 cause the most common genetic form of dwarfism, achondroplasia. Cell 78: 335–342

Simard J, Lefevre G, Labrie F 1987 Somatostatin prevents the desensitizing action of growth hormone-releasing factor on growth hormone release. Peptides 8: 199–205

Sorva R 1988 Children with craniopharyngioma. Early growth failure and rapid post-operative weight gain. Acta Paediatrica Scandinavica (suppl) 77: 587–592

Stanhope R G, Pringle P J, Brook C G D 1988a The mechanism of the adolescent growth spurt induced by low dose pulsatile GnRH treatment. Clinical Endocrinology 28: 83–91

Stanhope R, Adlard P, Hamill G, Jones J, Skuse D, Preece M A 1988b Physiological growth hormone (GH) secretion during recovery from psychosocial dwarfism: a case report. Clinical Endocrinology 28: 335–339

Stanhope R, Preece M A, Hamill G 1991 Does growth hormone improve final height attainment of children with intrauterine growth retardation? Archives of Disease in Childhood 66: 1180–1183

Struthers R, Perrin M, Vale W 1989 Nucleotide regulation of growth hormone-releasing factor binding to rat pituitary receptors. Endocrinology 124: 24–29

Sugihara H, Minami S, Okada K, Kamegai J, Hasegawa O, Wakabayashi I 1993 Somatostatin reduces transcription of the growth hormone gene in rats. Endocrinology 132: 1225–1229

Sung I, Vohr B, Oh W 1993 Growth and neurodevelopmental outcome of very low birth weight infants with intrauterine growth retardation: comparison with control subjects matched by birth weight and gestational age. Journal of Paediatrics 123: 618–624

Tanner J M 1962 Growth at adolescence, 2nd edn. Blackwell Scientific Publications, Oxford

Tanner J M 1975 Growth and endocrinology of the adolescent. In: Gardner L (ed) Endocrine and genetic diseases of childhood. W B Saunders, Philadelphia, pp 19-59

Tanner J M, Whitehouse R H 1976 Clinical longitudinal standards for height, weight, height velocity, weight velocity and the stages of puberty. Archives of Disease in Childhood 51: 170-179

Tanner J M, Whitehouse R H, Takaishi M 1966 Standards from birth to maturity for height, weight, height velocity and weight velocity: British children 1965. Archives of Disease in Childhood 41: 454, 613-635

Tanner J M, Whitehouse R H, Cameron N et al 1983a Assessment of skeletal maturity and prediction of adult height, 2nd edn. Academic Press, London

Tanner J M, Landt K W, Cameron N, Carter B S, Patel J 1983b Prediction of adult height from height and bone age in childhood. Archives of Disease in Childhood 58: 767–776

Tenovuo A, Kero P, Piekkala P, Korvenranta H, Sillanpaa M, Erkkola R 1987 Growth of 519 small for gestational age infants during the first two years of life. Acta Paediatrica Scandinavica (suppl) 76: 636–646

Tse W Y, Buyukgebiz A, Hindmarsh P C, Stanhope R, Preece M A, Brook C G D 1990 Long term outcome of oxandrolone treatment in boys with constitutional delay of growth and puberty. Journal of Paediatrics 117: 588–591

Tsipouras P, Del-Mastro R, Sarfarazi M et al 1992 Genetic linkage of the Marfan syndrome, ectopia lentis, and congenital contractural arachnodactyly to the fibrillin genes on chromosomes 15 and 5. The International Marfan Syndrome Collaborative Study. New England Journal of Medicine 326: 905–909

Ultsch M, de Vos A M, Kossiakoff A A 1991 Crystals of the complex between human growth hormone and the extracellular domain of its receptor. Journal of Molecular Biology 222: 865–868

Vaccarello M A, Diamond F B Jr, Guevara-Aguirre J et al 1993 Hormonal and metabolic effects and pharmacokinetics of recombinant human insulin-like growth factor I in growth hormone receptor deficiency (GHRD)/Laron syndrome. Journal of Clinical Endocrinology and Metabolism 77: 273–280

Voss L D, Wilkin T J, Bailey B J R, Betts P R 1991 The reliability of height and height velocity in the assessment of growth (the Wessex growth study). Archives of Disease in Childhood 66: 833–837

Wajnrajch M P, Gertner J M, Harbison M D, Chua S C Jr, Leibel R L 1996 Nonsense mutation in the human growth hormone-releasing hormone receptor causes growth failure analogous to the little (lit) mouse. Nature Genetics 12: 88–90

Wang H S, Lim J, English J, Irvine L, Chard T 1991 The concentration of insulin-like growth factor-I and insulin-like growth factor binding protein-1 in human umbilical cord serum at delivery: relationship to birth weight. Journal of Endocrinology 129: 459–464

Weinstein L S, Shenker A, Gejman P V, Merino M J, Friedman E, Speigel A M 1991 Activating mutations of the stimulatory G protein in the McCune-Albright syndrome. New England Journal of Medicine 325: 1688–1695

Wells J A, Cunningham B C, Fuh G, Lowman H B, Bass S H, Mulkerrin M G, Ultsch M, de Vos A M 1993 The molecular basis for growth hormone-receptor interactions. Recent Progress in Hormone Research 48: 253–275

Whincup P, Cook D, Papacosta O, Walker M 1995 Birth weight and blood pressure: cross-sectional and longitudinal relations in childhood. British Medical Journal 311: 773–776

Wit J M, van Unen H 1992 Growth of infants with neonatal growth hormone deficiency. Archives of Disease in Childhood 67: 920–925

Wit J M, Massarano A A, Kamp G A et al 1992 Growth hormone secretion in patients with Turner syndrome as determined by time-series analysis. Acta Endocrinologica (Copenh) 127: 7–12

Yamada Y, Post S, Wang K, Tager H, Bell G, Seino S 1992 Cloning and functional characterization of a family of human and mouse somatostatin receptors expressed in brain, gastrointestinal tract and kidney. Proceedings of the National Academy of Sciences USA 89: 251–255

Yamashita S, Melmed S 1987 Insulin-like growth factor-1 regulation of growth hormone gene transcription in primary rat pituitary cells. Journal of Clinical Investigation 79: 449–452

Ye Z S, Samuels H H 1987 Cell and sequence specific binding of nuclear proteins to 5'-flanking DNA of the rat growth hormone gene. Journal of Biological Chemistry 262: 6313–6317

9 Psychomotor and intellectual development

Ruth E. Day

Principles of development 381
Normal development 381
Motor skills 381
Cognitive or adaptive development 383
Language and communication 384
Personal–social 385
Factors which affect development 385
Psychosocial factors 385
Biological factors 386
Screening 386
Developmental assessment 386
The history 387
    The presenting concern 387
    Current functioning 387
    Developmental history 387
    General health 387
    Family history 387
    Social history 387
Developmental examination 387
    Up to 6 months 387
    6–11 months 392
    12–18 months 392

19 months to 5 years 392
Physical examination 393
    Hearing 394
    Vision 395
Evaluation and interpretation 396
Interpretation of developmental assessment 396
    Difficulties with developmental assessment 396
    Interpretation of abnormal development 396
Detection, assessment and management of the child with a handicap 399
    Child development centers 399
Psychometric tests in common use 400
    Complete profile 400
    Language 400
    Nonlanguage 400
    Tests for hearing impaired 400
    Tests for visually impaired 400
    Tests to analyze coordination difficulties 400
    Behavior scales 400
    Screening test 400
References 401

Developmental pediatrics is concerned with the maturational processes in structure and function of normal and abnormal children from fetal viability to full growth. There are three purposes:

1. to promote optimal physical and mental health for all children
2. to ensure early diagnosis and effective treatment of handicapping conditions of body, mind and personality
3. to discover the cause and means of preventing such handicapping conditions (Sheridan 1962).

This chapter will look at the process of development, how it can be observed and how abnormalities can be identified and interpreted.

PRINCIPLES OF DEVELOPMENT

Childhood marks the change from the entirely dependent fetus into the mature independent adult. During this period the child builds up a store of knowledge about the environment, he learns motor skills to survive and a language with which to communicate and think. This mental growth or development is dependent both on maturation of the nervous system and on experience.

The fetus at 5 months already has the full adult complement of 12 billion or more nerve cells. As the fetus and infant grow the developing interconnections between these cells result in patterns of behavior which are preconditioned and result in the general similarities and basic trends of child development. However, the acquisition of knowledge and the refinement of skills depends on the child's opportunity to observe, copy and experiment. Children actively construct their understanding of the world by interacting with it, thus developing schemes and strategies that can be applied to a wide variety of situations. Intelligence reflects the child's capacity to initiate and assimilate new experiences and to profit by past experience.

NORMAL DEVELOPMENT

In order to facilitate observation, it is traditional to describe child development as steps or stages in various fields of behavior (e.g. motor, adaptive, language and personal–social). This should not detract from the fact that a child's development at any specific age is an integrated whole and over time is a continuous process. Indeed a skill may fall into two or more areas of behavior, e.g. copying a horizontal line involves motor and adaptive behaviors and depending upon the accompanying emotional response may tell us something of the child's social development.

Table 9.1 gives a description of children's development at different ages. Sheridan (1975) has produced a useful booklet describing children's development to age 5 years. The following section looks at the sequence and process of development in different areas.

MOTOR SKILLS

The acquisition of motor skills depends on:

1. Loss of primitive reflexes. The fetus moves in utero and the newborn infant shows movements, some of which are reflexly determined. After birth, reflex movements which initially may be useful have to disappear before purposeful controlled movements can develop. The asymmetric tonic neck reflex, most evident at 2–3 months, may contribute to the development of visually directed grasping but its persistence, as in some children with cerebral palsy, interferes with bimanual manipulative skills.

2. The development of a body schema or image through interpretation of proprioceptive, vestibular, tactile and visual information.

3. The development of postural control which depends on reflex adjustment of tone in a large number of muscles in response to visual and proprioceptive feedback.

4. An increasing ability to interpret the visual information in the environment in order to judge, for example, distance, depth trajectory and weight correctly.

5. The development of movement patterns which are rapidly adjustable in response to environmental circumstances so that actions are smooth, refined and economical.

The child cannot develop sophisticated movements without first achieving postural control. All forms of movement are sequential postural adjustments, so that without resting tone or balance, movement is uncontrolled. Postural control develops in a cephalocaudal direction starting with head control, then progressing with sitting, standing, walking and running. At birth, the baby has little head control, but by 3 months he can hold his head up when held sitting. At 4 months he can control his head when pulled from supine to sitting. From the age of 6 months he can compensate well for trunk movement and with arm support he can sit with his back still somewhat curved and by 8 months sits independently. In the early months, he protects himself using limb reflexes (parachute responses) but later is able to adjust his trunk position to compensate for movement, thus enabling him to reach for an object without toppling (10 months). This improved postural control also allows the child to get from lying to sitting and to stand holding on (Fig. 9.1).

During the first half of the second year of life, most children learn to walk independently. Initially they walk with feet wide apart, hips and knees flexed, using arms for balance. The walking base decreases as balance improves and the arms are freed for pulling and carrying objects. By 2 years, children are extremely active; they run and climb and begin to kick a ball. By 3 years they can jump and stand on one leg momentarily and are able to catch a well-directed ball with arms out straight. At 4 years children can run, avoiding objects easily and can go up and down stairs. By 5 years they are able to skip, hop and dance, and can throw and catch a ball sufficiently well to join in group games. Catching with one hand, however, is not reliable until 9–10 years of age. Balance continues to improve as demonstrated by the length of time a child can stand on one leg and the number of times he can hop. By 10 years he can walk 'heel toe' backwards.

Once the child achieves reliable postural control he is able to develop increasingly accurate manipulative skills. Integration of visual input and motor output is essential for normal acquisition of these skills. At 3 months the child can look at and follow an object, but although he grasps and rattles an object placed in his hand he is not yet able to reach out and grasp it himself. Over the next 2–3 months the arm movements are better controlled and directed until he is able to pick up an object with a crude palmar grasp. Between 6 and 12 months reaching is smoother, distance is judged more accurately and the grasp becomes more refined so that at 1 year the child has a fine finger–thumb grasp and can also poke objects with his forefinger. Voluntary and accurate release is as essential as grasping for later manipulative skills. During the second half of the first year the child learns to transfer objects from one hand to the other and enjoys releasing objects voluntarily over his cot or chair side. In association with this, he learns that objects that go out of sight do not dematerialize, but are still there, and as a result he looks for fallen and later hidden objects. As release becomes more accurate he is able to place an object in the examiner's hand or in a cup. During the second year, refinement of release enables the child to build cubes to an increasing height and post objects accurately through holes (Fig. 9.2).

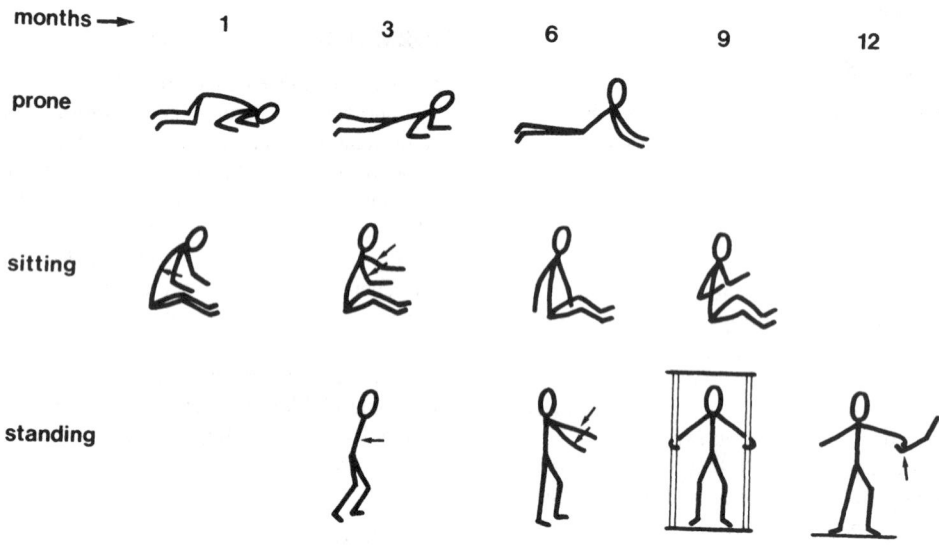

months → 1 3 6 9 12

prone

sitting

standing

Fig. 9.1 Gross motor development in the first year.

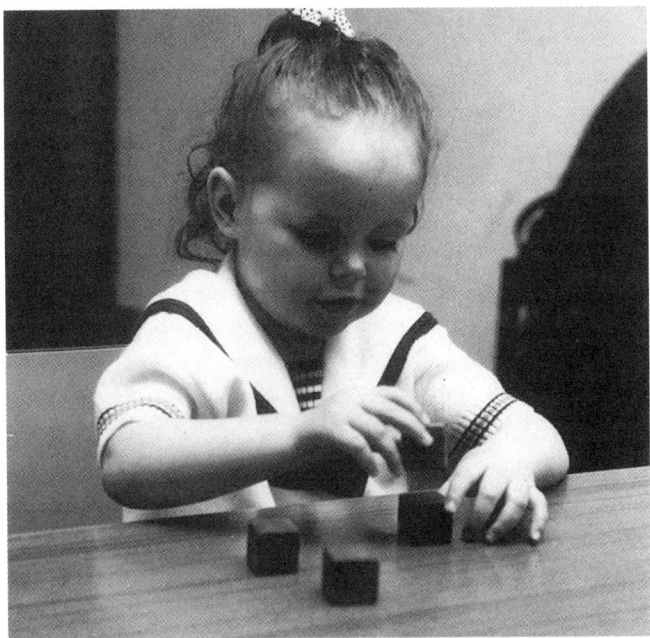

Fig. 9.2 Building cubes.

Increasing control of finger movements can now be used by the child to manipulate tools (e.g. spoon, crayon) (Fig. 9.3). Initially he holds both with a cylindrical palmar grip. During the third year of life he learns to use a more adult grip so that by 4 years he is holding his pencil in the adult way, the dynamic tripod. He is able to cut with scissors and thread beads. By 5 years the child shows great precision in hand movements and in the use of tools. He can cut a strip of paper neatly, and when building bricks holds the cubes with the ulnar fingers tucked in and his hand diagonal so that he has a better view of what he is doing. This increasing manipulative skill enables him to feed himself tidily with a spoon and fork, dress himself and brush his teeth.

Refinement of finger movements can be demonstrated by increasing speed at inserting pegs in a board and threading beads.

COGNITIVE OR ADAPTIVE DEVELOPMENT

Children learn about their world by listening, observing, copying and experimenting. The world of the infant is very small, his repertoire of skills limited and he learns about his world through observation, by reaching and grasping objects and by copying sounds and actions. In contrast, the toddler is mobile and his world large. His motor skills are greater and he begins to attempt constructional tasks thereby learning about size, shape, the properties of objects, space, etc. Make-believe play with dolls in which the child is reconstructing events he has observed is an important element of this period (Fig. 9.4). It indicates early symbolic representation and concept formation. The child begins to use language to direct or describe the action of his play, and as his command of language improves the need to act out the events decreases.

Perceiving shapes correctly and being able to reproduce them is essential for reading and writing (p,q,b,d). The ability to match shapes can be demonstrated by the use of form boards, which have different shapes (e.g. circles, squares and triangles) which have to be fitted into the appropriate space on the board. The ability to reproduce shapes is tested by asking the child to copy a three-brick bridge (3 years) and five-brick bridge (5 years).

The ability to copy shapes with a pencil starts with a vertical line (second year), horizontal line and circle (third year), a cross (fourth year), a square (fifth year), a triangle (sixth year) and a diamond (seventh year), progressing to letters and more complex shapes requiring juxtaposition of vertical, horizontal and oblique

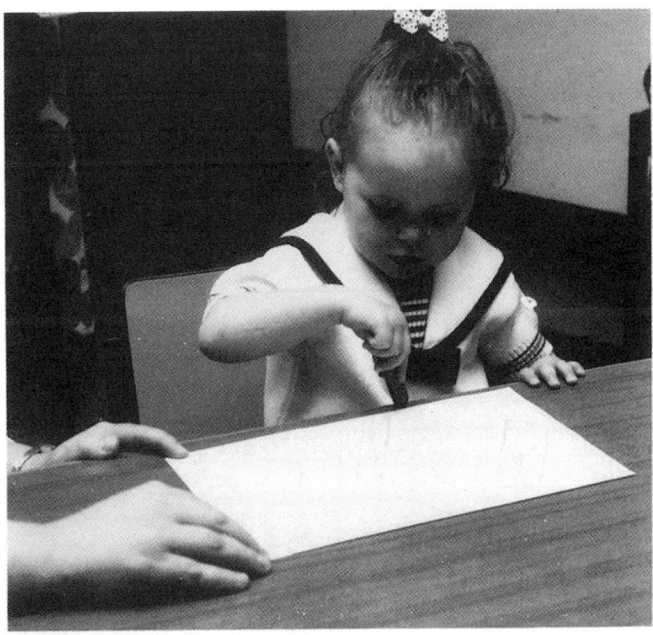

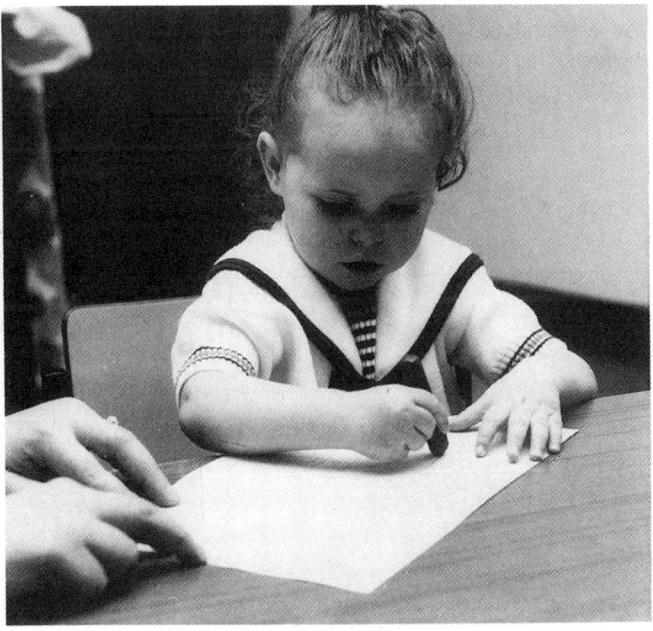

(b)

Fig. 9.3 Child aged 2 years holding crayon in (**a**) a cylindrical grasp, (**b**) a tripod grasp.

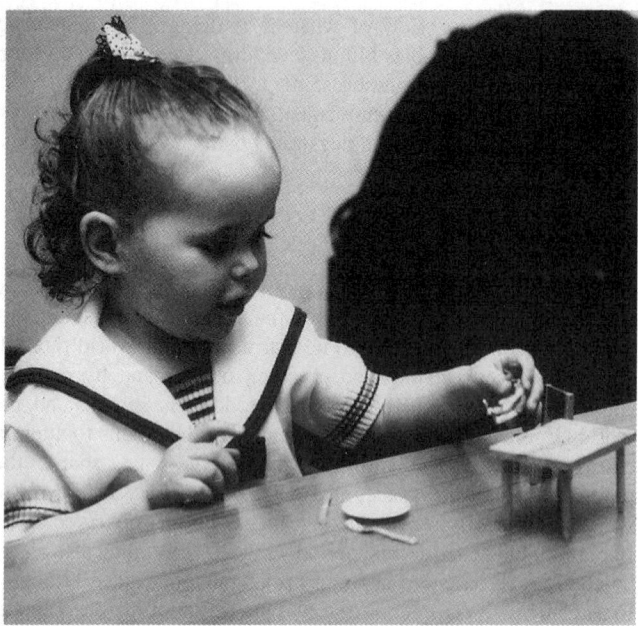

Fig. 9.4 Child placing doll on chair.

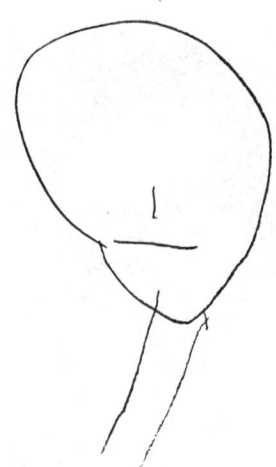

Fig. 9.5 'Draw a man' – age 3 years 4 months.

lines (Bender Gestalt test, p. 400). Goodenough (Harris 1963) has devised a scoring system giving age norms for the ability to draw a man. Such ability is related to control of pencil movement, ability to reproduce shapes and concept of body image. By 3 years the child has just learned to draw a circle and during the next year will add to this – vertical lines to represent legs, horizontal lines as arms and one or two features such as eyes and mouth (Fig. 9.5). It is not until 5 years that arms and legs are appropriately placed on a trunk (Fig. 9.6). At this age children can also draw a square and therefore a house with windows (some can do this at a younger age; Fig. 9.7).

LANGUAGE AND COMMUNICATION

An essential feature of human life is the use of a system of symbols for communication and thought. This attachment of

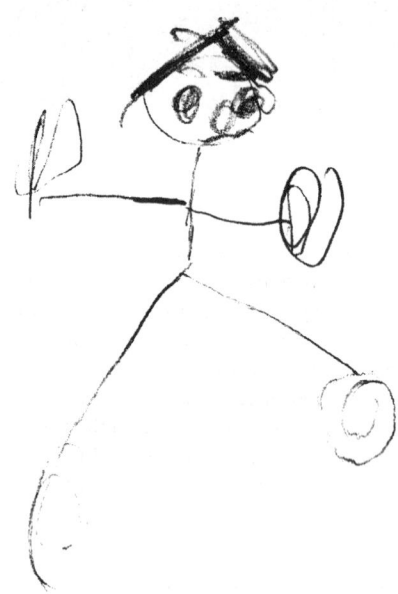

Fig. 9.6 'Draw a man' – age 5 years.

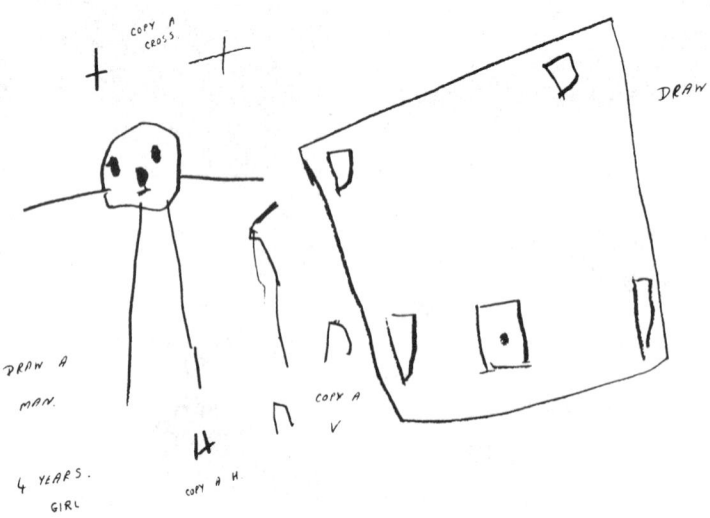

Fig. 9.7 'Draw a man and a house' – age 4 years.

names to objects and actions is an essential prerequisite not only for language but also for thinking. If we had no such system we would need to produce the object itself each time we wished to discuss it. This is just what an infant or child with a learning disability does.

It has been demonstrated that newborn infants show a preference for the human voice and face and are therefore programmed to develop an interest in human communication. The baby responds to facial expression and tone of voice (6 months) long before he understands the meaning of words. He uses sounds in a reciprocal or turn-taking manner before they are intelligible as words. Indeed his babbled sequence of sounds (10 months) have all the intonation and stress of speech but he has not yet got the correct code! The child's understanding that objects have labels is helped by the spontaneous behavior of adults who when they see children looking at or pointing to an object, will tend to name it, e.g. 'yes, that's the cat'. Children start to copy the words they hear and with practice improve the approximation to the correct sounds and this is reinforced by the object being produced. The development of grammar does not seem to depend on repeating adult structures; rather children seem to extract the rules of grammar and experiment for themselves sometimes to comical effect, e.g.

Lucy: Squeak, squeak – that's what mouses does.
Mother: That's what mice do.
Lucy: What do mices does?

(Crystal 1986)

Although prelanguage communication starts very early in life, it is only during the second and third year that the child uses speech to produce an effect and describe an event (i.e. for true communication). The answering of simple questions dealing with nonpresent situations presents difficulty as late as 3 years. Even the primary and junior school child still tends to be concrete in his way of thinking (i.e. real objects, here and now). Early in school life judgments are made intuitively on superficial appearances. With increasing experience and language at his disposal the child can imagine complex situations, think out the most appropriate solution and anticipate the outcome. Thus, the child has developed logical thinking from assimilating experience into schemes or general laws which he can apply to a range of situations.

PERSONAL–SOCIAL

This includes the child's social reactions to other persons and to groups and his mastery of skills such as feeding, elimination and dressing. It marks the change from a dim awareness of himself and his mother to an understanding of the complex rules of social behavior and interaction. Even neonates are socially competent in that they are able to elicit the attention of their parents. It has been shown that mothers respond to their babies behavior more often than the other way round. Babies respond to the human face and to objects quite differently. In response to a face their eyes widen, posture is relaxed and by 6 weeks a smile arises. The caretaker responds by smiling and gooing and sets in train a reciprocal social interaction quite clearly visible by 3 months. As the child's sounds increase in variety these are introduced into the 'conversation'. During the later half of the first year the baby loses his indiscriminate warm response to all people and begins to recognize familiar adults and to become wary of strangers. He develops a strong attachment to his caretakers and separation at

this time and during the second year of life is particularly distressing to a child. A securely attached child who is confident of his mother's warm presence is able during the second year to begin to explore and to achieve mastery of feeding and elimination. The child's increasing independence and awareness of self during the second and third year may also result in stubborn, negative behavior.

During the nursery years (3–5 years) the child's horizons widen as he is faced with a new social world of adults and other children. During this time the child becomes less egocentric and learns how to play with other children, taking into account their wishes and needs. He also obtains final mastery of self-help skills so that by 5 years he is ready for school. He is still essentially home based but during the primary school years the rules of the group become increasingly important so that by 10 years they are often quoted to parents in rather a rebellious way. At this age boys and girls tend to form separate groups or gangs and they are also very aware of rules although they cannot explain the principles behind them. The teenager is able to think in the abstract, work out the principles behind actions and is therefore able to become more independent. Freeing from parental authority is associated with a desire for acceptance and popularity in the peer group. However, developing sexual maturity is associated with concerns about sexual competence. They are also aware that they may be ridiculed and as a result may become more reticent.

FACTORS WHICH AFFECT DEVELOPMENT

It used to be thought that intelligence was determined entirely by the genes inherited from one's parents. It is now clear that there are both genetic and environmental contributions to intelligence and to personality. The contribution of each is complex as both the individual and the environment are continuously changing over time and the interaction between them which molds psychological growth is fluid and dynamic. The contribution of genetic inheritance is important and twin studies have suggested that up to 80% of the variance in intelligence in a population can be attributed to genetic transmission. Environmental factors may act in two ways: firstly by affecting the brain biologically – brain damage; secondly by altering the child's opportunity to learn by limiting or expanding his experience – psychosocial factors.

PSYCHOSOCIAL FACTORS

In general, people rather than physical elements are the most important factors in the environment of the young child. The parents are responsible for giving the child the opportunities to enable learning. Most crucially, if the infant does not develop a sense of trust in people from that first relationship with a parent then he is likely to have lifelong difficulties with relationships. There are various factors which affect the parents' capacity to cope well with the task of child rearing (Fig. 9.8).

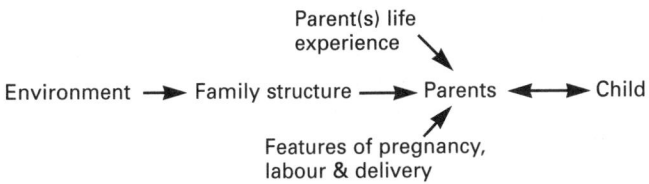

Fig. 9.8 Factors affecting parents' child-rearing capacity.

Children from depriving environments tend to show developmental delay, particularly of language. Children best learn the meaning of words when the word and the object are closely and frequently associated. The child deprived of simple play with adults does not have the opportunity to hear simple language related to his immediate environment. He may be surrounded by more complex visual and auditory stimuli from the television or older siblings but he will be unable to interpret and learn from these stimuli because of their complexity or because of direct interference from background noises. Children can only learn about actions and reactions if the responses are consistent. This applies particularly to behavior development. If the child does something naughty and on one occasion is smacked, on another laughed at and on yet another picked up by granny, he cannot learn acceptable behavior.

Children continue to practice skills if they are rewarded or the behavior is reinforced. A young baby hits an object during an involuntary action. If it makes a noise or looks attractive he is likely to try again and thus the process of exploring the environment starts. If when the baby waves his arms around and makes a noise there is no feedback or response from his environment or he gets shouted at, he is likely to stop exploring and keep quiet. It has been suggested that in this way severe deprivation in the first year of life can affect the child's ability to learn for the rest of his life. The more an infant has seen and heard the more he wants to see and hear later.

BIOLOGICAL FACTORS

A child's development may be affected by abnormalities of brain function, of special senses or of effector organs such as the muscles. Brain damage or dysfunction may affect all areas of function or only specific areas of function. Diffuse insults may produce specific dysfunction because of the vulnerability of a particular area of the brain at the time of insult (e.g. periventricular leukomalacia preterm, basal ganglia damage at term) and the skills being learned at any one time. The effects of an insult, e.g. cranial irradiation, may not be immediately apparent but only materialize when new learning is attempted. In many children with so-called developmental disorders (e.g. dyslexia, language disorder) there is no evidence of brain damage but often a strong family history. Presumably there is a genetic factor affecting the maturation of certain brain functions.

Defects of special senses most commonly affect vision and hearing and can result in a severe restriction of the information a child receives. Sensory defects interfere with the integration of information from various sources which is essential to normal development. Thus, the child with severe visual impairment may show delay in all areas of development. The normal stimulus which comes from seeing an object is absent and the child needs much more encouragement to explore his environment. Identifying and consequently labeling objects through touch, sound and smell is very much harder and therefore language acquisition is delayed. The congenitally profoundly deaf child will have severe language problems. Attaching labels in the form of signs and symbols to concrete objects is relatively easy but attaching labels to more abstract concepts (e.g. distance, size) and learning how to use the subtleties of language structure (e.g. tenses and word order) is much more difficult. There is evidence that milder degrees of sensory handicap can interfere with later development. The child who has been unable to learn about distance because of uncorrected myopia may remain clumsy and have difficulty throwing and catching even after the refractive error has been corrected. The child with intermittent hearing loss due to secretory otitis media may present later with reading and spelling difficulties as a result of interference with integrating sounds with symbols when younger.

Disorders of movement may be due to abnormality of the brain (cerebral palsy), spinal cord (paraplegia), nerves (spinal muscular atrophy) or muscles (dystrophy). These disorders have a direct effect on movement and also limit the child's experience. The child who cannot move independently does not experience space and distance and cannot reach things to manipulate them. It is important for parents and therapists to recognize this and to provide the child with compensatory experience.

When faced with a child showing delay or an abnormal pattern of development it is important to consider which of the above factors is contributing. There may well be more than one and biological and social factors may well interact. When there is a biological abnormality psychosocial factors become even more important determinants of the child's future, but it is precisely in this situation that parental resources are stretched. The child with a disability may have particular characteristics which are likely to make it harder for the parents to react to him, e.g. he may not smile or he may go rigid when picked up and thereby not elicit the normal mothering response. This can result in a vicious circle with the child becoming more disabled than originally expected. The severe visual impairment child may withdraw into self-stimulation, the rarely handled child with cerebral palsy becomes more rigid.

The more competent, less stressed parents may well have resources to consciously modify their reaction and provide for the child's special needs. The less competent or more stressed parents are less likely to be able to do this.

SCREENING

Screening involves the performance of tests on all children at certain ages to identify those who may have problems. Any child who fails a screening test needs a more detailed assessment to determine the nature of the problem, if any. Child health screening is now seen as part of a program of child health surveillance and health promotion. In Britain a working party chaired by Hall (1991) has set out what should be done at different ages. This is described in more detail in *The Child Surveillance Handbook* (Hall et al 1990). The Denver Developmental Screening Test provides a convenient summary of the age range at which abilities are usually acquired.

DEVELOPMENTAL ASSESSMENT

Knowledge of the normal patterns of child development enables us to assess the developmental level of a particular child. Gesell (1950) has stated that psychological/developmental examination should be regarded not as a series of achievement tests but as a means of eliciting significant behavior which calls for diversified analysis rather than a meager recording of success and failure. All developmental tests should be considered as a useful means of eliciting skills which can be recorded and compared with normal but failure must lead to a more detailed investigation of the nature of the child's difficulties.

The developmental examination should take place in a room with toys appropriate for the child and with one or both parents present. The number of toys displayed should be limited so that the child is not distracted. There should be a chair and table suitable for him to sit at. A history is then taken, all the time observing the child's behavior and interaction with parents. This period of talking to the parents enables the child to get used to his environment and to see that his parents accept this stranger, the doctor.

THE HISTORY

The general aspects of taking a history described in Chapter 2 apply to the child who presents with developmental problems. This section will comment on particular aspects of importance.

The presenting concern

It is useful to start by asking the parents what their areas of concern are as they may be different from those indicated in the referral letter and indeed some parents may say they feel nothing is wrong – it is extremely useful to be aware of this when discussing the results of the assessment. The presenting concern(s) can then be explored. General questions like 'how does he get around?' and 'what does he enjoy playing with?' can be useful to get an idea of his developmental level.

Current functioning

Current functioning in the different areas of development is elicited – play, language comprehension and expression, gross motor, social skills and behavior. It is important to inquire about all areas as some children's development is discrepant. Parents' interpretation of what their child does is often incorrect (e.g. he understands everything) but their observations are usually accurate (e.g. he will fetch his shoes only if they are visible).

Developmental history

Parents are unreliable in their recall of when milestones were passed, but it is important to determine the rate of development of skills in order to establish whether the child has always had a problem or whether there is any possibility of regression (deterioration or loss of skills). If the latter is suspected then the exploration of etiology follows a different path from that of a static nonprogressive disorder. If there is a suggestion of regression, it is useful to inquire at what age the child was at his best and to jog memories with questions such as 'what sort of things was he doing last Christmas that he cannot do now?'. Past history is directed at elucidating any cause for the problems, either real or wrongly attributed by the parents. Ruling out the latter (e.g. mother working or being depressed as a cause of autism) can reduce or remove parents' guilt and help them in accepting the child's difficulties. It is particularly important that problems are not wrongly attributed, e.g. to obstetric intervention or pertussis immunization which might result in missing a genetic problem. Such events as 'cord around the neck' rarely if ever cause problems and forceps delivery is done to protect the infant. What is important is the reason for intervention (e.g. fetal distress) which may have resulted in brain damage and the condition of the baby at birth (e.g. low Apgar, poor feeder, fits). These details must be elicited.

General health

The child's general health and any illnesses can be very relevant and must be inquired after and explored.

Family history

This is extremely important and inquiries must be made about parents, sibs, aunts, uncles and cousins. A diagnosis even if very definite must not be taken at face value and must be pursued if it might be relevant (e.g. a reported diagnosis of spina bifida in a male cousin turned out to be muscular dystrophy). In boys with learning disability a history of affected males on the mother's side must be very carefully pursued. The parents may need to be examined (e.g. child with hypotonia – mother myotonic dystrophy).

Social history

This is important not only because of its role in etiology, but also because social factors may well affect the family's capacity to cope with a child with a disability.

DEVELOPMENTAL EXAMINATION

From the history and unstructured observation it is possible to arrive at a rough estimate of the child's level of development. In order to confirm and refine this estimate more structured tests at around this developmental level can be applied. Material at this stage should be presented in a standard way but opportunities should be taken as they arise; for example, the Lowe and Costello symbolic play test (p. 400), which is essentially a nonverbal test of symbolic understanding consisting of miniature toys, is also an excellent medium for eliciting speech and testing comprehension of language. If the child is shy it is best to keep one's distance and administer the tests initially through the mother. Getting the mother to handle the young child to help demonstrate his sitting and walking has the added advantage that the doctor can sit back and observe.

The materials used at different ages will vary. The chart of development (Table 9.1) gives a wide range of tasks which may be looked at. The following is a guide to a few minimum observations and necessary materials. The ages given in parentheses are only rough guidelines as there are wide ranges over which children attain skills and there are also cultural differences to be considered.

Up to 6 months

Material – interesting rattle with stem handle that can be grasped by child (Fig. 9.9).
Position – seated on mother's knee.
Observe – alertness and interest in examiner's face, smiling (6 weeks), vocal responses. Alerting to own name (6 months) and responding to tone of voice (6 months).
– focusing on and following silent rattle horizontally (1 month) and vertically (3 months).
– looks at rattle placed in hand (3 months). Grasps rattle touching his hand (4 months) and when held away from him (5 months). Shakes it purposefully (6 months).

Table 9.1   Summary of normal development in the first 3 years (based largely on Gesell 1950)

Age*	Gross motor	Manipulation	General understanding	Expressive language and speech	Social behavior
4 weeks	Held in sitting position – may hold head up momentarily. Held in prone position with hand under abdomen (ventral suspension) – momentary tensing of neck muscles should be noted. Prone – momentarily holds chin off couch. Pulled to sit – almost complete head lag		Watches the mother when she talks to him. Opens and closes mouth as she speaks, bobs his head, quiets. (In next 2 weeks or so, before smiling begins, note the duration and intensity of this reaction in assessing a child.) Supine position – regards dangling toy when it is brought into his line of vision and will follow it, but less than 90°. Stops movements and whimpering when sound made nearby		
6 weeks	Ventral suspension – the head is held momentarily in line with the body. Prone – readily lifts chin off couch so that plane of face approaches angle of 45° to couch. Pulled to sit from supine – head lag not quite complete		Smiles momentarily when talked to by mother. Supine – looks at dangling toy when it is in midline; follows it to midline when it is moved from the side. Beginning to follow moving persons with eyes		Smiling henceforward becomes more and more frequent. The frequency of smiling and the ease with which it is elicited should be noted
8 weeks	Held in sitting position – head is held up but recurrently bobs forward. Ventral suspension – holds head up so that its plane is in line with that of the body		Supine – follows dangling toy from side to point past midline. (Always note the promptness with which child sees the ring.) Eyes show fixation, convergence, focusing		
12 weeks	Prone – lifts head and upper chest off couch, bearing weight on forearms. Held to sit holds head erect for several seconds. Pulled to sit from supine – only moderate head lag	Watches movement of own hands. Pulls at his clothes. No more grasp reflex. Holds rattle voluntarily when it is placed in his hand; retains it more than a moment. Desire to grasp objects seen – increased arm movements	Supine – follows dangling toy from one side to the other (180°) and also vertically, catches sight of it immediately. Not only smiles when spoken to but vocalizes with pleasure. (From now onwards it is essential to note the child's interest in what he sees. One must also note the obvious desire to grasp objects. This desire can be observed long before he can voluntarily go for them and get them. In another month his hands go forward for the object, but he misjudges the distance. By 5 months he can get the object)	Gurgles, squeals and coos with pleasure	
16 weeks	Held in sitting position– holds head well up constantly. He looks actively around, but head still wobbles if examiner causes sudden movement of trunk. Curvature of back now only in lumbar region as compared with rounded back of earlier weeks. Supine – head no longer rotated to one side as in earlier weeks	Hands come together and he plays with his hands. He pulls his dress over his face in play. Approaches object with hands, but overshoots the mark and fails to reach it. Plays with rattle prolongedly when it is placed in his hand, shakes and looks at it	General understanding becomes much more obvious. Excited when he sees toys. Shows considerable interest when he sees breast or bottle. Shows interest in strange room. Laughs aloud. Vocalizes pleasure when pulled to sitting position. Likes to be propped up in sitting position. Turns head towards a sound	Reciprocal vocalization in response to another person	

Table 9.1 *Cont'd*

Age*	Gross motor	Manipulation	General understanding	Expressive language and speech	Social behavior
20 weeks	Full head control. Held in sitting position – head stable when body is mildly rocked by examiner. Pulled to sit – no head lag	Now able to grasp objects deliberately – often two-handed scooping in approach. He splashes in the bath and crumples paper. (From this time onwards one must note the maturity of the grasp, the ease with which he holds objects and the size of the object which he is able to grasp. He cannot bring finger and thumb together to grasp a small object of the size of a thin piece of string till he is about 9 months old)	Smiles at image of self in mirror. When he drops his rattle he looks vaguely to see where it has gone. Visually insatiable		
24 weeks	Prone – weight borne on hands with extended arms, the chest and upper part of abdomen therefore being off the couch. Pulled to sit – head lifted off couch when about to be pulled up. Hands are held out to be lifted. Sits (supported) in high chair for a few minutes. Rolls from prone to supine. Held in standing position – bears large fraction of weight	Reaches and grasps object off table with whole hand, palmar grasp. He grasps his feet. Puts hands up to bottle. If he has one cube in hand he drops it when second one is offered	When he drops the rattle within his visual field he tries to recover it. May 'blow bubbles' or protrude tongue in imitation of adult. Laughs when head is hidden in towel in peep-bo game. Beginning to show likes and dislikes of foods	Produces a wide variety of recognizable speech sounds	May be shy with strangers
28 weeks	Prone – bears weight on one hand. Sits with hands forward for support. Rolls from supine to prone. Standing position – can maintain extension of hip and knees for short period when supported. He bounces with pleasure (previously sagged at hip and knees). Supine – spontaneously lifts head off couch	If he has one cube in hand he retains it when second cube is offered. Transfers objects from one hand to the other. Bangs objects on the table. Now goes for objects with one hand instead of two. Takes all objects to mouth. Feeds self with biscuit. Loves to play with paper	Pats image of self in mirror. Responds to name, recognizes tone of voice. Tries to establish contact with person by cough or other noise. May imitate movement, such as tongue protrusion	Says 'Da', 'Ba', 'Ka'	Drinks well from cup. Chews and so can take semisolids
32 weeks	Readily bears whole weight on legs when supported. Sits for a few moments when unsupported		Reaches persistently for toys out of reach. Responds to 'no'	Combines syllables, 'Da da', 'Ba ba'	
36 weeks	Stands holding on to furniture. Sits steadily for 10 minutes. Leans forward and recovers balance (cannot lean sideways). Prone – in trying to crawl may progress backwards. May progress by rolling	Can pick up small object such as currant between finger and thumb. When he has two cubes he brings them together as if making visual comparison between them	Puts arms in front of face to try to prevent mother washing his face. (From this age onwards note excitement when certain liked food stuffs are seen. Note particularly degree and maintenance of concentration in getting objects and playing with toys.) Plays peep-bo		Clearly distinguishes strangers from familiars

Table 9.1 *Cont'd*

Age*	Gross motor	Manipulation	General understanding	Expressive language and speech	Social behavior
40 weeks	Pulls self to standing position. Pulls self to sitting position. Goes forward from sitting to prone, and from prone to sitting. Sits steadily without risk of falling over (except for occasional accident). Creeps pulling self forward with hands, abdomen on couch	Goes for objects with index finger. Beginning to release objects, letting them go deliberately instead of accidentally as before. Clicks two bricks together in imitation	May pull clothes of another to attract attention. Plays 'patacake' (clapping hands). Copies ringing a bell. Holds arms out for sleeve or holds foot up for sock in dressing. (From this age the understanding of words should be observed. The child can understand the meaning of perhaps a dozen words by the age of a year, though he is only able to say two or three words at that age. At 9 months he alerts to such questions as 'Where is Daddy?')	Babbles sequence of different consonants and vowels, aa, ba, ga with speech-like stress and intonation	Slobbering and mouthing beginning to decrease
44 weeks	Prone – crawls (abdomen off couch). When standing holding on he lifts and replaces one foot. Sitting – can lean over sideways	Will place object into examiner's hand on request, but will not release it	Waves bye-bye. Covers own face with towel in peep-bo game. Drops objects deliberately in order that they will be picked up. (The maturity of the release behavior and the manipulative skill must be noted as he plays with his toys)	Says one word with meaning. Shakes head for no	
48 weeks	Walks sideways, holding on to furniture. Walks with two hands held. Sitting – can turn round to pick up objects	Rolls ball towards examiner. Gives and takes toy in play, releasing object into examiner's hand	Repeats performance laughed at. Now likes repetitive play, putting one cube after another into basket, etc. Anticipates with bodily movement when nursery rhyme being told. Shows interest when shown simple picture book. (This interest should be carefully noted from now onwards)		Apt to be shy, may cling to known adult
1 year	Walks with one hand held. Prone – walks on hands and feet like a bear. May shuffle on buttocks and hand. May stand for a moment	Can hold two cubes in one hand	May understand meaning of 'Where is your nose?' 'Where is your shoe?' May kiss on request. Gives toys to adult on request, e.g. 'Give it to me'. Looks for object hidden under cup	Says two or three words with meaning	Very little mouthing of objects
15 months	Can get into standing position without support. Creeps upstairs. Walks without help with broad base, high stepping gait and steps of unequal length and direction. (The maturity of the gait must be noted from now onwards)	Makes line or marks with pencil. Builds tower of two cubes (this requires some accuracy in release). Constantly throwing objects on to floor. Takes off shoes. Puts objects in and out of container	Looks at pictures with interest. Points to familiar objects on request. Obeys simple commands, e.g. 'Get your shoes'. Pushes car along. Feeds doll	Asks for objects by pointing and vocalizing. Jargon with words interspersed	Finger feeds, tries with spoon, uses cup, indicates that he has wet pants

Table 9.1 *Cont'd*

Age*	Gross motor	Manipulation	General understanding	Expressive language and speech	Social behavior
18 months	Walks well with feet only slightly apart. Pulls toys as he walks. Climbs stairs holding rail or a helping hand. Runs rather stiffly. Seldom falls. Seats self in chair, often by process of climbing up, standing, turning round and sitting down. Throws ball without falling	Builds tower of three cubes. Manages spoon without rotating it near mouth as previously. Turns pages of book two or three at a time. Scribbles spontaneously. Takes off gloves, socks and unzips fasteners. Replaces lid on box. Pulls cloth to get toy	Recognizes some miniature objects. Recognizes one or two clear pictures from a choice of three. Points to own or doll's nose, eye, hair on request. Copies mother in her domestic work, e.g. sweeping the floor, dusting	Uses 6–20 recognizable words. Names one or two simple objects	Alternates between clinging and resistance. Bowel control usually attained. Bladder more variable
21 months	Walks backwards in imitation. Picks up object from floor without falling. Walks upstairs, two feet per step	Builds tower of five or six cubes	Pulls people to show them objects	Names some pictures. Repeats things said. Ask for drink, toilet, food	Sleeping difficulties common. Sleep rituals beginning. Dry by day
2 years	Goes up stairs alone, and down holding on, two feet per step	Builds tower of six or seven cubes. Turns pages of book singly. Turns door knobs, unscrews lid. Puts on shoes, socks, pants	Imitates train with cubes, without adding chimney. Imitates vertical stroke with pencil.† Obeys simple orders, e.g. 'Give dolly a drink'. Imaginative play with dolls. (Much can be learnt by noting the maturity of the play and the imaginativeness shown)	May use words: me, you. Joins two words together, e.g. 'What's that', 'me go'	Dry at night if lifted out late in evening. Constantly demanding adults' attention. Parallel play – watches others play and plays near them, without playing with them
2 1/2 years	Jumps on both feet. Walks on tiptoe when asked. Kicks a large ball	Builds tower of eight cubes. Holds pencil in hand instead of in fist	Imitates train with cubes, adding chimney. Imitates vertical and horizontal stroke with pencil.† Relates two objects: 'Put the spoon in the cup'. Helps to put things away. Matches colors	Talks incessantly. 200 or more recognizable words. Speech may still show some immaturities. Gives full name	Often very active and rebellious. Washes and dries hands
3 years	Goes upstairs one foot per step, and downstairs two feet per step (goes downstairs with one foot per step at 4 years). Jumps off bottom step. Stands on one foot for a few seconds. Rides tricycle. Catches well-directed ball with arms out straight	Builds tower of nine cubes. Dresses and undresses self if helped with buttons, and advised occasionally about back and front and the right foot for the shoe. Unbuttons front buttons. Can be trusted to carry china and so to help to set the table. Cuts with scissors. Threads beads	Copies circle with pencil,† imitates cross (copies cross at 4, square at 5). Beginning to draw objects spontaneously (e.g. a man), or on request. Not always recognizable! Cubes – imitates building bridge of three cubes. Understands big and small, under and on. Recognizes objects by use – 'What do we sit on?' Knows some nursery rhymes. Vivid make believe. Dresses and undresses doll	Gives full name and sex. Carries on simple conversations. (Constantly asking questions 'what', 'where' 'who')	Attends to toilet without help. Eats with fork and spoon. More amenable, affectionate and confiding. Now joins children in play Understands sharing

* For mature babies; due allowance to be made for prematurity (i.e. if the baby is born at 36 weeks' gestation 'birth' is taken to date from 4 weeks of postnatal age).

† Copying a circle implies copying a representation of a circle on a card given by the examiner. When a child 'imitates' a circle he draws one after seeing the examiner do it.

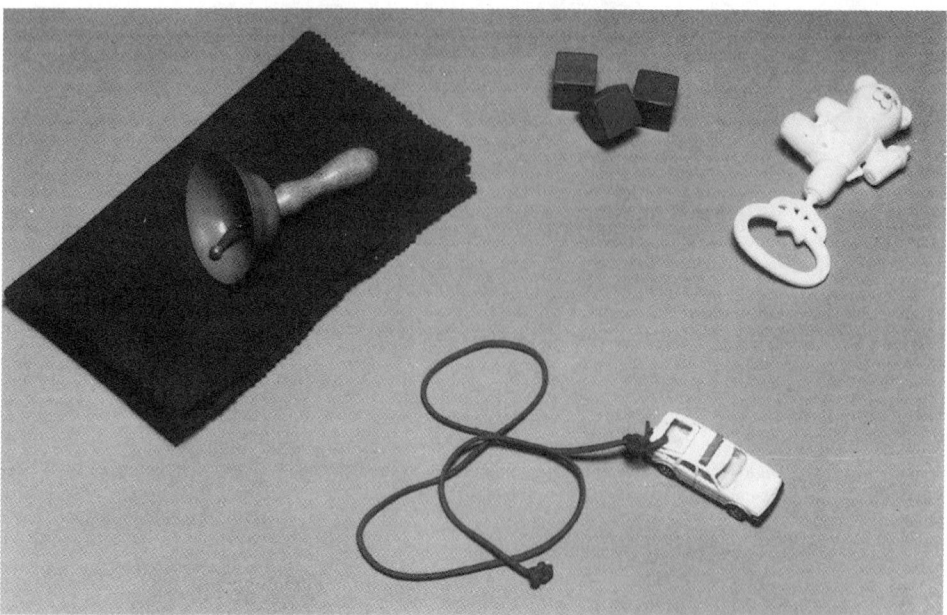

Fig. 9.9 Material for developmental observation – age 0–11 months.

– head control, limb position and trunk control in assisted sitting, prone and supine lying, prone suspension and assisted standing.

6–11 months

Material – 1-inch cubes, bell, cloth, car on a string, dolly mixture sweets (Fig. 9.9).

Position – seated on mother's knee or floor.

Observe – bricks on table – child reaches and grasps them with increasingly refined grasp (compare two hands). Will bang blocks together (10 months) or on the table (8 months). Will transfer objects from hand to hand (8 months) and will look after them when they fall (8 months). Refinement of finger–thumb grasp and first finger pointing can be observed using a small sweet. The child may volunteer to give up the object in your hand (10 months) but can't release it until around 11 months.

– socially around 9 months the child becomes more wary of strangers and a more cautious or gradual approach is required. The child may be encouraged to babble using an increasing variety of consonant sounds. By 11 months he enjoys playing peek-a-boo (cloth) and looks for an object placed under the cloth.

– placed on the floor to sit he becomes increasingly steady (8–9 months). He starts to move around actively by crawling (9–11 months) or bottom shuffling. He may be encouraged to pull to stand and then begins to cruise around the furniture (10–12 months). Some children will be walking independently by this age.

12–18 months

Material – doll and miniature spoon and cup, car, crayon and paper, cloth, 1-inch cubes and box with lid, simple picture book (Fig. 9.10).

Position – the child is still closely attached to mother and may sit on her knee but may be persuaded to sit on a small chair beside a table.

Observe – replaces cubes in box (13 months) and then places one on another (15 months), building increasingly high towers. By 18 months he will also be interested in putting the lid on the box. Given a crayon and paper he will scribble often needing a demonstration at 15 months but by 18 months doing so spontaneously. Pulls a cloth to retrieve an object placed on it (17 months).

– developing language and symbolic understanding is extremely important. At 12 months the child will relate the spoon to and possibly hug or kiss the doll on request. Increasingly he plays with miniature toys feeding the doll and running the car along with a suitable car noise. He starts this period by learning the names for some real objects and body parts and ends it by knowing the names of some miniature objects, some parts of the doll and even some clear pictures. He learns a variable number of words but at 18 months is beginning to use some of these to command the situation, e.g. 'up'. Use and understanding of language is often best demonstrated by the parents, the child being shy of the stranger.

– walking – most children learn to walk during this time and balance improves so that they are able to stoop, pick up an object and walk carrying it.

19 months to 5 years

Material – symbolic play material (Lowe and Costello symbolic play test, p. 405), pencil and paper, shapes' sorter or jigsaw, pegboard, 10 1-inch cubes of three different

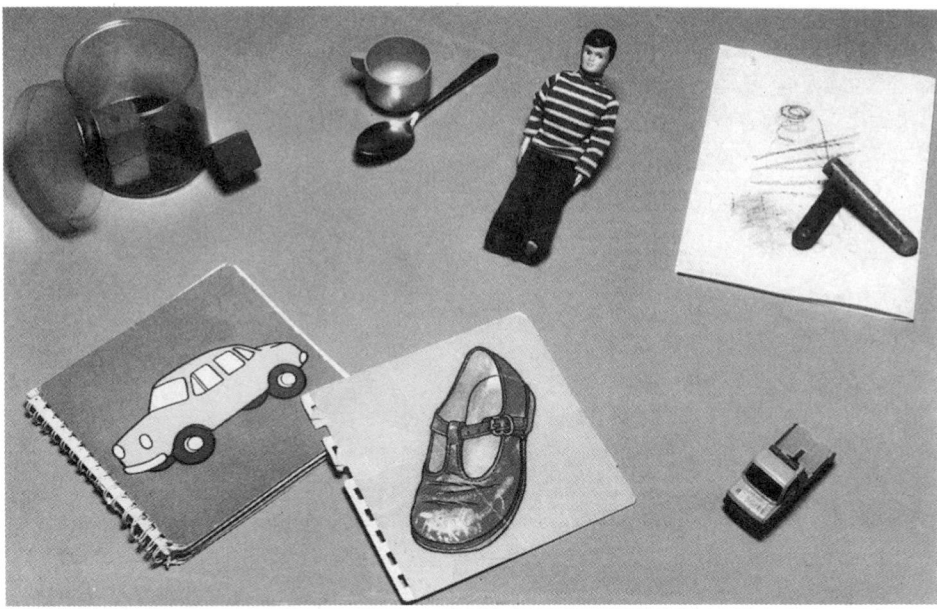

Fig. 9.10 Material for developmental observation – age 12–18 months.

colors with thread, clear pictures of objects and of scenes, tennis ball (Fig. 9.11).

Observe – symbolic play increases in complexity and is often accompanied by language. The 18-month-old can be asked to name objects, after 2 years he follows simple instructions (e.g. put the doll on the chair). By 3 years he recognizes objects by use (e.g. which one do we sleep on?) and identifies objects by size (e.g. give me the biggest doll). His expressive language consists of quite long sentences and is largely intelligible. Pictures may be used to try to elicit speech.

– pencil and paper are useful to observe the child's fine motor control and his ability to copy shapes (matching shapes can be observed using the shape sorter and jigsaw) and finally his ability to represent objects. At 2 years he can be encouraged to copy a vertical line, at 3 years a circle, at $3\frac{1}{2}$ years a cross, at 5 years a square. From 3 years he is able to produce increasingly sophisticated drawings (Figs 9.5, 9.6 and 9.7).

– the cubes can be used to observe motor and visuomotor skills (copying 3- and 5-brick bridges). If colored they can be used for color matching (3 years) and subsequently color naming. If they have holes in them threading can be demonstrated (3 years). At a later age they are useful for counting to 10 (age 5 years).

– motor skills become more sophisticated and the child can be asked to jump ($2\frac{1}{2}$ years), stand on one leg (3 years) and hop (4 years). He kicks and throws a ball with increasing refinement from 2 years. Catching is a difficult task and initially requires a well-judged throw from the examiner to succeed (3 years).

As well as recording whether the child does or does not perform a particular task, it is very important to record how he performs it. For example three infants can reach and grasp a toy car but one may reach for it as soon as he sees it, give it a casual glance and then throw it away. Another child may look at it carefully before picking it up and then do so with obvious interest, turning it around and turning the wheels with his forefinger; he may shake it to see if it makes a noise and then give it back. The third child may be visually very interested and make excited noises, but reach for and grasp the car in an awkward abnormal ways suggestive of motor problems: three very different qualitative performances which suggest different problems and require different investigation. The child's approach to the whole examination should be observed. How interested is he in the toys? Does he persist at one task or flit from one thing to another? What is the quality of the interaction between mother and child?

PHYSICAL EXAMINATION

A full examination should be done as described in Chapter 2. There are some aspects which are particularly important if the child has a developmental or neurological problem and these will be commented on. The physical examination is generally left to the end as the child may become upset and this would interfere with the developmental examination.

1. It is important to know whether the child has a motor disorder or whether any delay is just part of global learning difficulties This is best determined by observing the child's movement patterns and posture. This can be done during the developmental examination when the child is walking, speaking and handling material (e.g. tendency to keep the forearm pronated and rather deliberate finger movements in mild spasticity). Indeed after observing the child one should have a good idea of the nature and extent of any motor problem and examination of tone, reflexes and power is largely confirmatory.

2. It is useful to compare the two sides of the body and to determine the child's hand preference. The motor skill, tone, reflexes or the size of the limbs may be significantly asymmetrical suggesting hemisphere dysfunction and therefore focal pathology (mild hemiparesis and visuospatial difficulties).

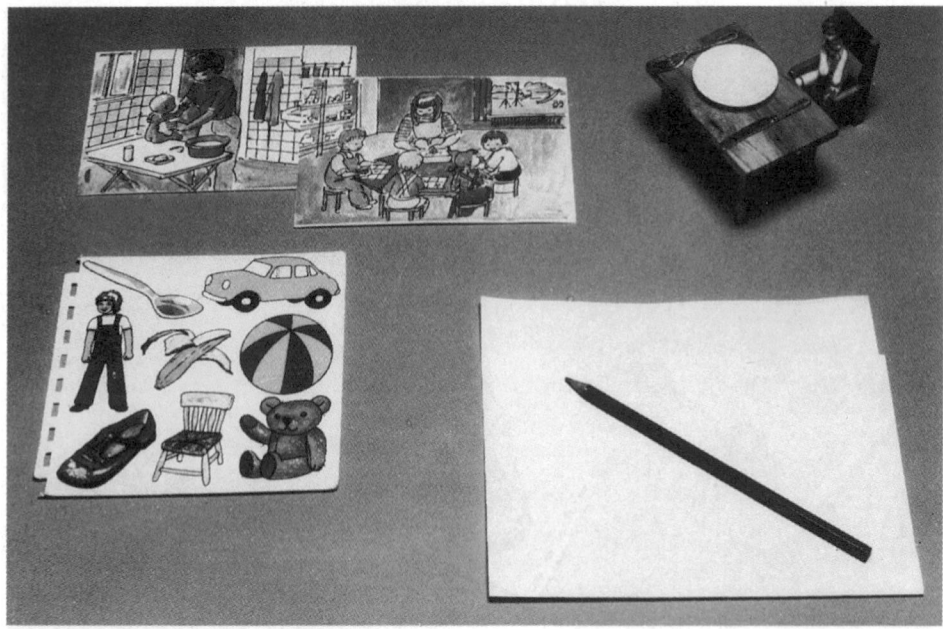

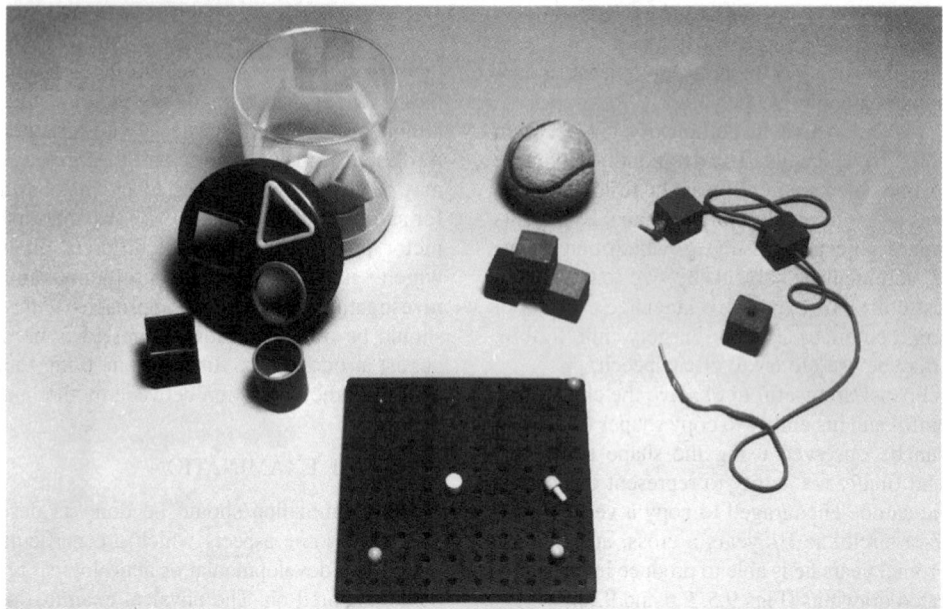

Fig. 9.11   Material for developmental observation – age 19 months to 5 years.

3. Head circumference must always be measured and plotted on a centile chart and compared with the child's height and, if there is any discrepancy, with the parents' head circumference.

4. Examination of the optic discs and fundi is difficult but can be very valuable in diagnosing particular disorders (septo-optic dysplasia) as well as raised intracranial pressure.

5. Dysmorphic features and congenital malformations must be looked for as they may suggest a particular syndrome or etiology (e.g. fetal alcohol syndrome).

6. The skin should be carefully examined for pigmented and depigmented spots.

7. Height, weight and growth rate should be determined (e.g. hypothyroidism).

8. The child's mental state should be observed, e.g. is he hyperactive, impulsive or does he concentrate well? Is he having absence or other seizures?

Hearing

Evaluation of a child's hearing is well covered in Chapter 14. It is extremely important to detect a hearing loss early so that the child with a hearing impairment can receive amplification and guidance to enable him to realize that sounds have meaning and that lip movements can help to decipher that meaning. Parents' or relatives' concern that their child is not hearing should always be taken seriously and assessment by an audiologist arranged. McCormick (1988) has devised a checklist of observations of response to sounds for parents to take home with their newborn child. This has been shown to be effective without creating a lot of anxieties or false positives. Hearing testing by health visitors at 8 months is more reliable if warble tone audiometers are used instead of the traditional high-frequency rattle, spoon and cup and tissue paper which produce sounds across a range of frequencies of undetermined loudness. Even if a child 'passes' his 8-month screening he may develop a hearing loss later due for example to secretory otitis media and therefore passing the screening test should not be seen as immutable. With increasing age and attention span hearing tests depending on more sophisticated responses can determine more accurately the child's level of hearing at different frequencies.

Vision

It is extremely important to evaluate the child's vision, as a significant visual impairment may affect all areas of development and alter the interpretation of data from other parts of the examination (e.g. naming pictures). Conversely a severe learning disability may affect the child's response to visually presented material giving the erroneous impression particularly in infancy that the child does not see.

Assessment of vision at any age should include asking the parents whether they feel the child sees all right and whether they have noticed any squint or turn in the eye. It should include examination of the eyes including the pupillary response to light and if indicated ophthalmoscopy. Eye movements should be observed in each eye separately and together. Squint should be tested for by looking to see whether the corneal reflection of a light is in the same position in the two eyes and by doing the cover test. In the cover test each eye is covered in turn whilst the child visually fixates on an object. Note is made of whether the uncovered eye moves to take up fixation. If the child objects to one eye being covered he is probably dependent for vision on that one eye. Visual acuity should be measured if possible in each eye separately.

Visual acuity is the ability to separate visual material, i.e. to discriminate detail. Accurate measurement depends on eliciting the minimum separation that can be detected by the person. The standard way of doing this is to use the Snellen letter chart at 6 m (20 feet). The letter size is expressed as the distance at which it would be seen by a normal person. The result is given as a pseudofraction – on top the distance tested at, and below the size of the letter seen, thus 6/6 is normal vision and 6/60 very poor vision. Similar charts with reduced type are used for near vision. These tests are dependent on the child naming the letters and this is generally only possible at 7 years and older.

Testing vision in the younger child is a matter of adapting the response (Sonksen 1993). Although he cannot name the letters, the younger child (from 3 years) can match the letters. Sheridan (1979) devised a test (STYCAR letter test) which involved the presentation of single letters of decreasing size at 3 m (10 feet). The child has a key card which has either five ($2\frac{1}{2}$–$3\frac{1}{2}$ years), seven ($3\frac{1}{2}$–$4\frac{1}{2}$ years) or nine (5–7 years) capital letters on it. In the 5–7 year age group the key card may be used with the Snellen letter chart at 6 m using only those letters which appear on the key card. This is valuable for some children with amblyopia for whom differentiation of one letter in a group may be more difficult than identifying single letters. To overcome this difficulty, Sonksen and Silver have devised a test of visual acuity using cards each with a single row of letters of one size (Sonksen 1993).

Below the age of $2\frac{1}{2}$ years it is difficult to get an accurate measure of visual acuity as the child is not interested in the fine discrimination required. However, it is possible to establish the size of the smallest object the child can see at a particular distance. This has been standardized by Sheridan using 10 white balls ($\frac{1}{8}$ to $2\frac{1}{2}$ inches in diameter) which are either rolled on a dark strip horizontal to the line of the infant's gaze at 3 m (10 feet) from the child, or mounted on sticks for presentation from behind a dark screen (STYCAR graded balls test). It is important to note that visualization of even the smallest ball does not denote perfect vision and rolling the ball considerably enhances its visibility. Near vision may be tested by placing small sweets of different sizes on the table and observing whether the child reaches for them (hundreds and thousands = 1.5 mm, saccharine tablets = 2 mm, cake decoration balls = 3 mm, Smarties = 15 mm diameter). Inability to locate the smallest of these suggests that the near vision is 6/36 or worse (Fig. 9.12).

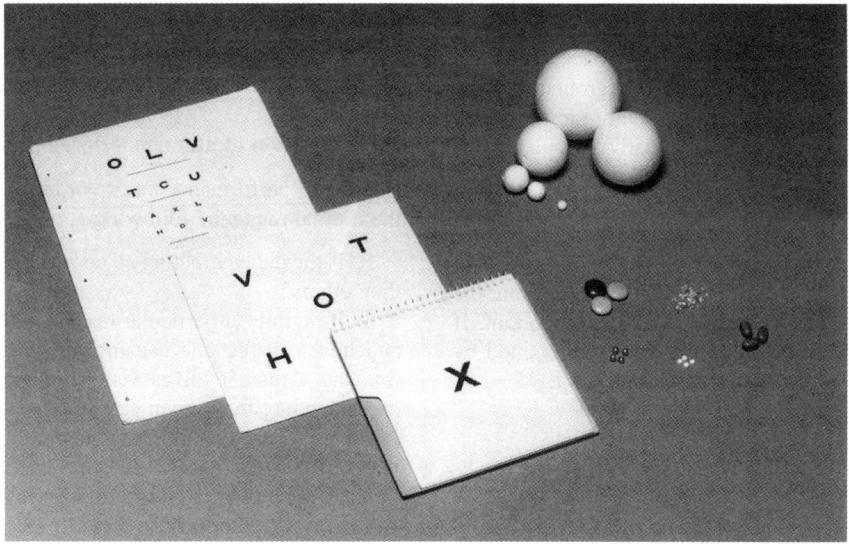

Fig. 9.12 Material for evaluating vision.

Sheridan (1979) also devised a test of vision which involves matching miniature toys. The child has a tray of seven small toys and the examiner standing at 3 m has a similar small set. The knife, fork and spoon are the objects that test fine visual discrimination. In normal children this can be used around 21 months and has only a short period of usefulness before the much more accurate letters can be used. However it may be useful until much older for some children with learning disabilities who are not able to do the letter tests.

The Kay Picture Test (1983) is similar to the STYCAR letter test but uses pictures and can be done by some children as young as 18 months. It is said to be accurate to within one line of Snellen's acuity and tests near and distance vision.

Evaluation of vision in the young infant may be observational – watching whether the child fixes and follows an object presented at about 12 inches ($\frac{1}{3}$ m) from the face (making sure that it does not produce sound) – or objective using forced choice preferential looking as on Keeler or Cardiff Acuity Cards (Teller et al 1986). Opticokinetic nystagmus may be demonstrated in the clinic setting using an opticokinetic drum with black and white stripes of varying diameter.

Assessment of vision in the child with a visual impairment

This presents considerable difficulties and standard tests of vision may be of no value. In particular the child with a visual handicap often shows the limited visual world similar to that of a younger child, i.e. he can see very much better near to and often no response can be obtained at more than 90 cm from the infant. The ability to see near objects may mislead people into overestimating vision. Most useful in the young child are functional tests which demonstrate what size of object at what distance and of what visual complexity the child can see. Thus fixed or rolling balls may be used at 3, 2 and 1 m and even on the table top, recording what size at what distance is seen. Life-sized and miniature objects, pictures and letters (Snellen or white on black 'Panda' letters) may be shown at 3, 2, 1, 0.5 and < 0.5 m, the child giving the name or an approximation or matching the object. It is important to start from a distance away and move in. The child should demonstrate that he knows the name for the object, picture or letter first using different material to prevent intelligent guesses. The test material should only be presented once. A child may recognize a clear picture of a dog on a white background but fail to pick out the same picture on a colored background or when part of a more complex picture. This is important to test as much educational material is presented in a visually complex way. Sonksen & Macrae (1987) devised a comprehensive assessment of the visually handicapped child which involves using selected Ladybird pictures.

If children have other disabilities as well as visual impairment it may be very difficult to determine what they see and the objective measures mentioned earlier become very important. If these fail then measuring the visual evoked response elicited by flash or pattern may be useful (Mackie & McCulloch 1995).

EVALUATION AND INTERPRETATION

Evaluation and interpretation of the historical, observational and test data is extremely important. It should lead to:

1. a profile of the child – both his assets and difficulties

2. a hypothesis about etiology which might need tests to confirm or refute
3. a description of the child's family, home and social setting.

INTERPRETATION OF DEVELOPMENTAL ASSESSMENT

Difficulties with developmental assessment

When interpreting a child's performance on informal or formal tests it is important to consider the following.

1. The child may not perform at his best and if this is suspected he will need to be seen again. Parents will often accept an opinion better if it is based on two periods of observation.

2. The range of normal for attaining some skills is so wide that children with handicaps may well fall within it and conversely many children whose milestones fall outwith the normal range (i.e. 97th centile) are normal. It may not be possible to diagnose mild learning difficulties or language disorder or clumsiness before 18 months to 2 years because the more complex skills involved are not exhibited earlier.

3. Some children may show abnormalities which disappear only for the child to have other associated difficulties later, e.g. language delay resolving but later reading and spelling problems; minor motor signs in the first year resolving but with clumsiness appearing later.

4. There are normal variants in development which result in delay in a later skill – classically bottom shufflers are late walkers.

5. The developmental assessment gives a picture of the child at one point in time. In order to refine prognosis and in particular to exclude regression it is important to determine the rate of development.

6. Some skills, e.g. symbolic play and language, reflect understanding of the environment and are therefore better indicators of intellectual ability than are for example purely motor skills.

7. If a significant difficulty with motor coordination or of the special senses is found then it is necessary to reassess findings in other areas in the light of this and some tests may no longer be of value in attributing intelligence (e.g. language subtests in a deaf child). Indeed it may be necessary to use specially devised tests in order to try to deduce intelligence (e.g. Reynell and Zinkin's test for blind children, p. 400).

Interpretation of abnormal development

If a child's performance on one or more skills is definitely outside the normal range the following approach is suggested:

1. Is the delay affecting all tasks equally or is he poorer at some than others?

2. If he fails at particular tasks what are the subskills required and how can the one causing the difficulty be elucidated, e.g. drawing a man involves vision, motor control and a cognitive understanding that a man can be represented in this way and the conventions used, and the praxic ability to produce the shapes. It may be apparent that the child has a tremor and that allowing for this he is doing an age-appropriate drawing (Fig. 9.13). Alternatively, although he has a mild tremor this cannot alone account for his immature drawing. It may be necessary to test his vision, and ask him to insert small pegs in a board, to match

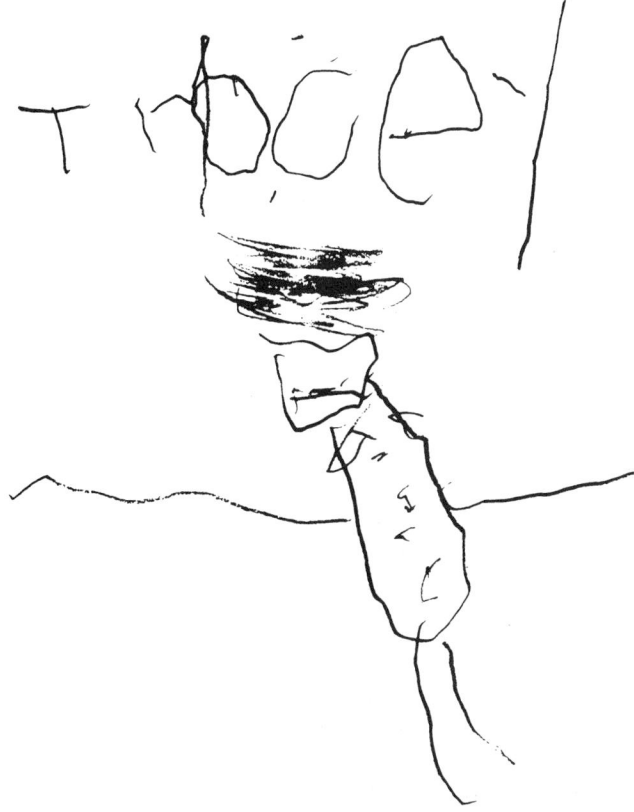

Fig. 9.13 Drawing by a child with tremor – age $4\frac{1}{2}$ years.

Table 9.2 Factors which may result in delayed walking

Site of disorder	Effect of disorder	Example
Environment	Lack of opportunity to practice	Child in pram or baby walker
Special senses	Interference with perception of environment	Visual handicap
Brain	Immaturity	Isolated delay
	Variant of normal	Bottom shuffler
	Lack initiative	Global learning disability
	Organization	Apraxia
	Control movement	Cerebellar ataxia, cerebral palsy
Motor output		
Spinal cord	Spasticity and weakness	Spinal dysraphism
Nerves	Weakness	Spinal muscular atrophy
Muscle	Weakness	Myopathies
Structural deformities	Mechanical	Talipes, amputation, hyperextensible joints, congenital dislocation of hip
General disorders	Pain, chronic hypoxia	Rickets, hypothyroidism, congenital heart disease, etc.

shapes and to do a simple jigsaw of a person before making a diagnosis.

3. Is there evidence of deviant development which would make a maturational delay or even simple learning disability unlikely, e.g. the delayed echoing of some children with a language disorder or autism?

4. What disorders present with this particular pattern of difficulties and how can this be pursued, e.g. hyperactivity, mild tremor, borderline IQ, ? fetal alcohol syndrome. Look for dysmorphology, short stature and history of alcohol consumption.

Example 1: The child of 20 months who is not yet walking

This places the child outside the 90th centile for British children

and while it may still be normal it is important to consider abnormality.

The different elements necessary for walking and the types of disorder that might be responsible are listed in Table 9.2. In order to determine what is the likely cause there are two questions that are discriminatory:

1. Is the motor pattern deviant, e.g. toe walking or pronated position of forearms suggesting spasticity or does it look normal for a younger child?
2. Is development in other areas normal or abnormal?

At this age language and symbolic play should be looked at. If the child has a significant motor disorder affecting hand function the methods used to determine intellectual ability will need to be modified, e.g. eye pointing to named objects. This analysis leads to four subgroupings (Fig. 9.14).

The nature of the disorder can be further elucidated by observing the nature of the child's movement pattern and by examining tone and reflexes, and looking for any persistent primitive reflexes, fasciculation, etc.

The underlying etiology of all the disorders can then be pursued through history, examination and tests, bearing in mind the most likely etiologies, for example:

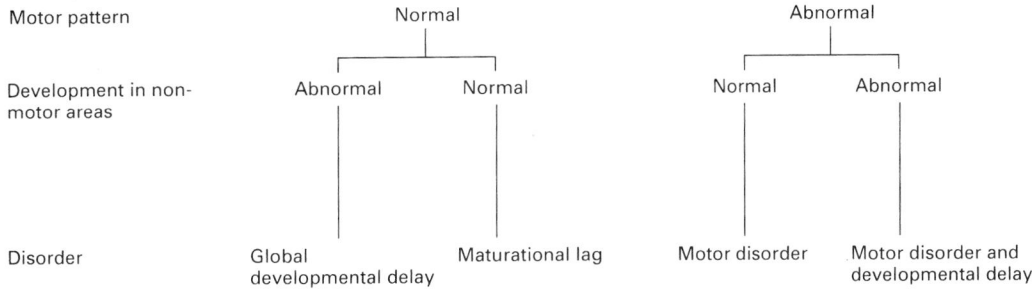

Fig. 9.14 Diagnostic approach to the child who does not walk.

- Global developmental delay + maternal male cousin with learning disability. Investigations would be fragile X chromosome ± creatinine kinase level.
- Spastic diplegia – preterm delivery, 2 days' ventilation, no family history, tended to sit with curved back, stood propped on toes with legs crossed. No need for further tests.

It is always extremely important to ascertain whether or not there is any question of regression as this would lead to another chain of inquiry and investigation.

Example 2: The child who is only saying a few single words by 30 months

At this age many children will be putting two or even three words together and most will have quite large vocabularies. The possible causes of language delay are: specific language delay or disorder, global learning disability, deafness, autism, environmental deprivation; a difficulty with speech (output unclear) may make evaluation difficult.

In order to discriminate between these it is necessary to determine what is the child's:

1. understanding of language
2. ability in nonlanguage areas – drawing, brick building, shapes, symbolic play
3. understanding and use of nonverbal communication, e.g. gesture, facial expression; is he a social child?
4. quality of speech – are the few words clear? Does he jargon using normal speech sounds and intonation?

5. pattern of development: is it following the normal lines or is it deviant in any way, e.g. use of the word rhinoceros before mum and dad?

Figure 9.15 shows how the most likely diagnosis can be reached using the above data.

It is necessary to determine from the history whether the child's environment is likely to be contributing. A family history of language delay might support a genetic predisposition which is common in developmental language disorder.

Hearing should be checked in all children – even if it is not the main cause, a mild loss may be making a child with a potentially mild developmental language disorder worse.

Example

John's profile on the Griffiths test (Fig. 9.16) showed that his ability in nonlanguage areas was normal, so he does not have a global learning disability. His symbolic play was also normal. He was a social child who understood and used pointing and some simple gestures. He was not therefore autistic. His understanding of language was a little delayed but not as much as his use of language. The words he had were clear and he used normal sounding jargon. There was nothing deviant about his language development, it was simply delayed. There was a history that his father had been slow to talk and later on had reading and spelling problems. The home environment was satisfactory. Hearing was tested and found to be normal.

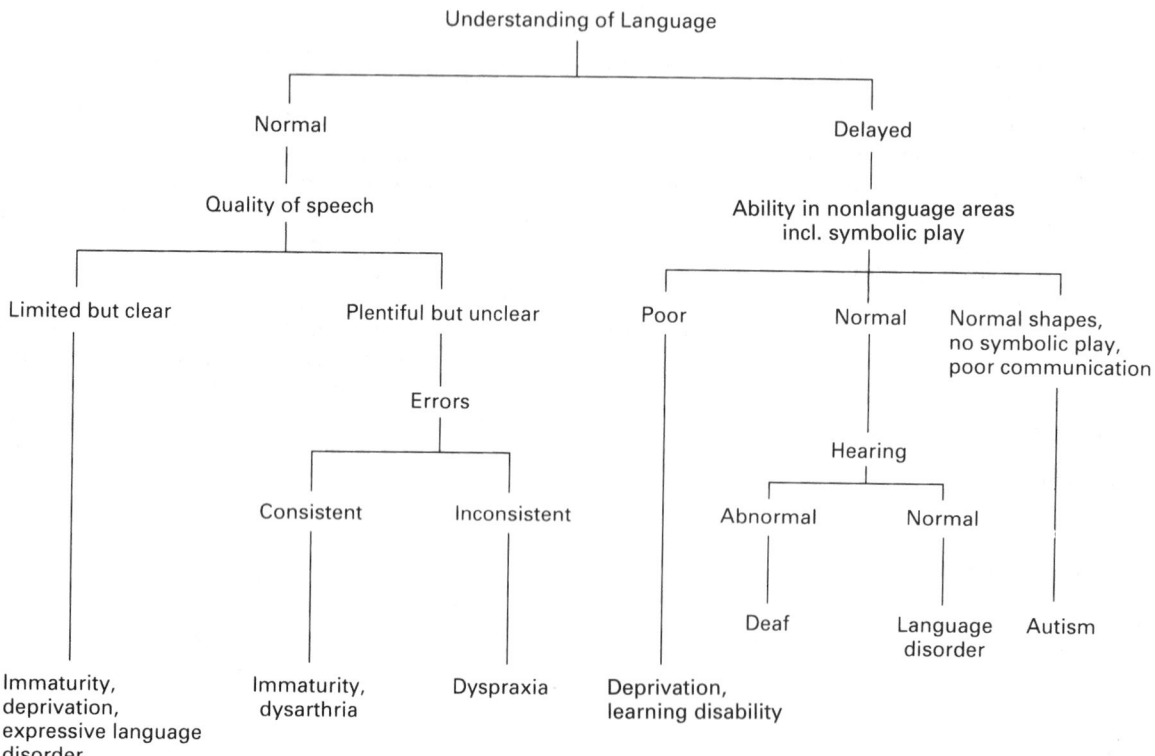

CHECK HEARING OF ALL CHILDREN

Fig. 9.15 Flow diagram to diagnose the cause of a child being slow with talking.

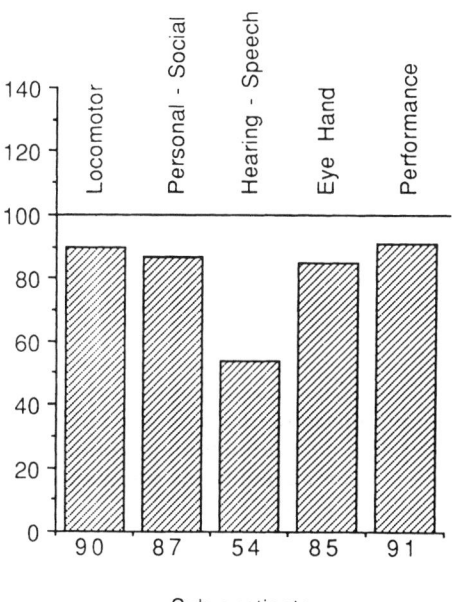

Fig. 9.16 Griffiths test profile, boy aged 30 months.

John therefore has a developmental language delay which is probably due to a genetic predisposition. As his language comprehension is reasonable and he is beginning to use words he is likely to make steady progress. It is possible he also will have reading and spelling problems at school. He should be reviewed by a speech and language therapist to make sure his progress is satisfactory and to offer parents advice on how to encourage language development.

DETECTION, ASSESSMENT AND MANAGEMENT OF THE CHILD WITH A HANDICAP

The child with a handicap often presents as a child with developmental delay. The full assessment given above should lead to a summary as follows.

1. A profile of the child:
   a. Neuromotor, e.g. spastic diplegia
   b. Sensory – hearing and vision
   c. Intellectual – allowing for a. and b.
   d. Functional – what can he do, any aids?
   e. Orthopedic
   f. Emotional/behavioral
   g. Epilepsy
   h. Medication.
2. An etiology and genetic implications.
3. The child's environment – parents, family, home, school, etc.

With this data it is possible to:

1. Discuss with the parents and if old enough the child:
   a. The nature of the child's difficulties and his abilities
   b. The cause and genetic implications
   c. The prognosis
   d. Management.
2. Plan management appropriate to the child's needs:
   a. Corrective treatment, e.g. thyroxine
   b. Ameliorative treatment, e.g. drugs, splints or surgery for spasticity
   c. Training
      (i) Reinforcing acquired skills
      (ii) Teaching developmentally appropriate skills
      (iii) Providing missed experience
      (iv) Making use of other skills to overcome difficulties
   d. Information about allowances, respite, etc.

Child development centers

Assessment and management of children involves a wide variety of professionals. Child development centers have been established in order that the professionals can work closely together and that children and parents need attend only one place. They generally serve a health district (child population 50 000 < 15 years). Staff should consist of the following.

Doctor

Often a consultant pediatrician in community child health (CPCCH).

Therapists

Following evaluation of the child, therapists advise the parents how best to promote their child's development. The physiotherapist deals largely with motor development, the occupational therapist with hand skills using appropriate toys and the speech therapist with language and speech. They often, however, work together and roles often overlap, e.g. feeding: physiotherapy to reduce tone and obtain good posture, occupational therapy advice on seating and cutlery, speech therapy advice on desensitizing the mouth and the type of food.

Psychologist

Many centers have both a clinical and an educational psychologist. The former is skilled in the assessment of the young child and in evaluating and treating behavior disorders. The latter is more skilled in the intellectual and educational assessment of the older child although there is great overlap in skills.

Nurses and nursery nurses

They look after the children's and parents' needs whilst at the center. They may well be in charge of the day-to-day running of the center and the nursery if present.

Health visitor and/or social worker

It is extremely important to have a member of the team who deals primarily with the parents and is able to listen to their concerns, preferably in their own home. S/he should also have practical knowledge of the services and allowances available.

Any child development center needs to be associated with an audiologist and ENT surgeon, orthoptist and ophthalmologist, orthopedic and orthotic service, medical genetics, child psychiatry, etc.

District handicap teams are being formed to supervise and indeed develop the service for children with disabilities both preschool and during the school years within the health districts. The members of the team may be the CPCCH and other staff from the district child development center but there are usually also representatives from social work and education.

PSYCHOMETRIC TESTS IN COMMON USE

The names of the tests are given with the mental age range over which they are used and the training required to be able to use them. Many are available from NFER – Nelson, Danville House, Windsor S14 1DF or The Psychological Corporation (PC), Kent, DA14 5HP.

1. Complete profile

a. The Bayley scales of infant development (2 months to $3\frac{1}{2}$ years). Professionals including pediatricians. Three areas tested: mental, motor and behavior (PC).

b. Griffiths scales (0–8 years). Clinicians trained to administer it. Five areas tested: locomotor, personal social, hearing and speech, eye–hand and performance.

c. British ability scales ($2\frac{1}{2}$–17 years). Psychologist.

d. WPPSI – Wechsler preschool and primary scale of intelligence (4–$6\frac{1}{2}$ years). WISC – Wechsler intelligence scales for children (6–16 years). Psychologists. Both have two scales, language and performance, with five subtests in each.

e. Stanford–Binet intelligence scale (Terman and Merril) (2 years to adult). Psychologist. (PC.)

f. Schedule of growing skills (0–5 years). Any professional Profile of development in nine areas (NFER).

2. Language

a. Reynell developmental language scale (1–7 years). Speech therapists, psychologists, some teachers. Assesses verbal comprehension and verbal expression separately so that comprehension scale can be used alone for children with severe articulatory difficulties (NFER).

b. Test of auditory comprehension of language (TACL) (3–10 years). Any professional. Assesses separate areas of verbal comprehension, i.e. word meanings in isolation and in relation to one another; grammatical structures; complex sentences. Child selects target picture from choice of three – no verbal responses required.

c. Picture vocabulary test (Peabody or British) ($2\frac{1}{2}$–8 years). Any professional. Tests single word vocabulary. The child selects picture most appropriate for the given word (NFER).

d. British language development scale (BLDS) (preschool). Any professional. Assesses language use in three areas – conversation (pragmatics), meanings expressed (semantics), form and structure (syntax) – (NFER).

e. CELF – clinical evaluation of language function (6–18 years). Any professional, usually speech therapist. Eleven subtests that probe different aspects of complex language functioning.

f. Speech/articulation tests. Edinburgh articulation test (EAT). Speech therapists.

3. Nonlanguage

a. Symbolic play test of Lowe and Costello (1–3 years). Any professional. Four groups of toys presented without verbal instructions. Results in an age equivalent score (NFER).

b. Goodenough–Harris drawing test (Harris 1963) (3–15 years). Any professional.. The child is asked to draw a man and a score is derived from the content and converted to a mental age (PC).

c. Ravens progressive matrices (5 years to adult). Any professional. A series of pictures or designs with one part missing (NFER).

d. Bender Gestalt test (4 years to adult). Test of perceptuomotor function. Nine designs for the child to copy (NFER).

e. Frostig – developmental test of visual perception (DTVP) (4–8 years). Five areas are tested: eye motor coordination, figure ground, constancy of shape, position in space and spatial relationships (NFER).

4. Tests for hearing impaired

a. Hiskey Nebraska test of learning aptitude (3–7 years). 11 subtests including bead stringing, block building, puzzle blocks, pictorial association, identification and analogies, completion of drawings and memory for colored objects and digits.

b. Ravens progressive matrices – see above.

c. The Reynell DLS and the BLDS are standardized for use with children who are deaf.

5. Tests for visually impaired

a. Reynell Zinkin scales (birth to 5 years). Any professional. Five subscales: social adaptation, sensorimotor understanding, exploration of environment, response to sound and verbal comprehension, expressive language. There is also a communication subscale for children with additional problems (NFER).

6. Tests to analyze coordination difficulties

a. Movement assessment battery (4–12 years). This looks at various aspects of motor skill including manual dexterity, static and dynamic balance and ball skills (PC).

b. Frostig – developmental test of visual perception (DTVP) (4–8 years). Five areas are tested: eye motor coordination, figure ground, constancy of shape, position in space and spatial relationships (NFER).

7. Behavior scales

There are several questionnaires available to be filled in by parents and/or teachers to try to measure various aspects of children's behavior. The most commonly used in the UK is perhaps that devised by Professor M. Rutter and available from the Institute of Psychiatry, University of London (Rutter et al 1970).

8. Screening test

Denver (revised) (birth–6 years). Any professional. Given age ranges at which children achieve certain skills. Test agency, Cournswood House, North Dean, High Wycombe, UK.

REFERENCES

Crystal D 1986 Listen to your child. Penguin Books, Middlesex

Gesell A 1950 The first five years of life. Methuen, London

Hall D M B 1991 Health for all children, 2nd edn. Oxford University Press, Oxford

Hall D M B, Hill P, Elliman D 1990 The child surveillance handbook. Radcliffe Medical Press, Oxford

Harris D B 1963 Children's drawings as measures of intellectual maturity. Harcourt, Brace & World, New York

Kay Picture Test 1983 P O Box 156, Coventry CV8 3LJ

McCormick B 1988 Screening for hearing impairment in young children. Croom Helm, London

Mackie R T, McCulloch D L 1995 Assessment of visual acuity in multiply handicapped children. British Journal of Ophthalmology 79: 290–296

Rutter M, Tizard J, Whitmore K 1970 Education, health and behaviour. Longman, London

Sheridan M D 1962 Infants at risk of handicapping conditions. Monthly bulletin. Ministry of Health, vol 21: 238

Sheridan M D 1975 The developmental progress of infants and young children, 3rd edn. HMSO, London

Sheridan M D 1979 The clinical assessment of visual competence in babies and young children. In: Smith V, Kean J (eds) Visual handicap in children. Heinemann, London

Sonksen P M, Macrae A J 1987 Vision for coloured pictures at different acuities. Developmental Medicine & Child Neurology 29: 337–347

Sonksen P M 1993 The assessment of vision in the preschool child. Archives of Disease in Childhood 68: 513–516

Teller D Y, McDonald M A, Preston K, Sebris L S, Dobson V 1986 Assessment of visual acuity in children: the acuity card procedure. Developmental Medicine and Child Neurology 28: 779–789

10 Fluid, electrolyte and acid–base disturbances

R. W. Logan

Body water   402
Total body water (TBW)   402
Distribution of body water   403
Water balance   403
The electrolyte composition of the body fluids   403
Extracellular fluids (ECF)   403
Intracellular fluids   404
Permeability of membranes and movement of water and solutes   405
Osmotic pressure, osmolarity and osmolality   405
Equivalent weight   405
Molarity   405
Molality   405
Osmolarity   405
Osmolality   405
Physiological water and electrolyte movement   406
Membrane potential   406
Donnan membrane equilibrium   407
Hydrostatic and colloid osmotic pressure   407
Individual cations   407
Sodium   407
Potassium   408
Magnesium   409
Dehydration and electrolyte disturbance   409
Homeostatic regulation of volume and osmolality of body compartments   409
Osmolal clearance   409
Free water clearance   409
Water depletion   410
Sodium depletion   410
Mixed water and sodium depletions   411
Potassium depletion and intoxication   411

The low sodium syndrome and water intoxication   412
Water intoxication   412
Edema   412
The syndrome of inappropriate antidiuretic secretion (SIADH)   412
Steady states   413
Treatment of fluid and electrolyte disturbance   413
Isotonic and hypotonic dehydration   413
Hypertonic dehydration (hypernatremia)   414
Hypokalemia   415
Potassium chloride-containing preparations   415
Hyperkalemia   415
Acid–base disturbances   415
Buffers   416
Maintenance of a normal pH   417
Plasma and whole blood buffers   417
The carbonic acid/bicarbonate system   417
The erythrocyte carbonic anhydrase system   417
Respiratory control of CO_2 tension   418
Renal hydrogen ion excretion and bicarbonate retention   418
The renal phosphate mechanism   418
Potassium deficiency and renal control of pH   418
Characterization of the blood acid–base status   419
Indices   419
Classification of disturbances   419
Mechanisms and sequences of events in acidosis and alkalosis   420
Treatment of acid–base disturbances   421
Alkalinizing agents   421
Acidifying agents   421
Clinical judgment and laboratory assessment   421
References and bibliography   422

The integrity of the whole organism depends upon the maintenance of a stable internal environment. This makes proper understanding of the principles underlying fluid and electrolyte treatment vitally important.

In most instances disturbance of fluid balance is not the primary cause of the patient's disorder but rather the result of the initial condition. It is worthwhile assessing the nature and magnitude of any such disturbance in a wide range of disorders since correction of these may well accelerate general recovery.

Although advances in laboratory techniques have enabled more precise determination of many of the biochemical indices of disturbed body function, the role of clinical assessment of the patient still cannot be overemphasized. Clinical and laboratory findings are complementary to each other and fluid therapy should not be prescribed on laboratory findings alone.

The normal content of water and electrolytes in the body will be considered before describing in detail the measurement of body fluids and electrolytes in disease.

BODY WATER

TOTAL BODY WATER (TBW)

The proportion of the body consisting of water varies with age, sex and the amount of adipose tissue present. Neonates have relatively the greatest body water content and obese adults the least. The percentage of water in the female tends to be lower than in the male but only after puberty and is due largely to the higher fat content of females. In both sexes the body water content falls with advancing age. Various substances may be used to determine total body water. The assumption is made that the material will diffuse rapidly throughout the water of the body without either being significantly metabolized or excreted during the period of equilibration. Among the many materials used are deuterium oxide (heavy water), tritium (^{3}H) oxide, antipyrine, and n-acetyl-4-amino antipyrine.

Deuterium dilution studies have shown that the water content of the newborn is 77%, falling to about 65% at the age of 6 months and 60% by 10–16 years. Using antipyrine, the corresponding result reported by Maclaurin (1966) for neonates was 72%.

DISTRIBUTION OF BODY WATER

It is convenient, although incorrect, to consider that body water is divisible into discrete compartments. This concept offers a reasonable basis for interpreting changes occurring in the fluid content. The intracellular fluid (ICF) is separated by cell walls from the extracellular fluid (ECF) which may be subdivided into intravascular and extravascular components. Specialized collections of transcellular fluids formed by secretory activity include such materials as biliary secretions, ocular and cerebrospinal fluids.

The principle utilized for measuring total body water applies also to ECF. Such compounds as thiocyanate, thiosulphate, sucrose and inulin have been employed for measuring total ECF. Plasma volume may be measured by human serum albumin labeled with ^{125}I. Red cell volume may be measured using radioactive chromium and, by use of a corrected whole body hematocrit (venous hematocrit × 0.91); the blood volume may then be calculated.

It is now the exception rather than the rule to employ these procedures in routine treatment of electrolyte and fluid imbalance.

Infants are vulnerable to loss of water because of the physiological inability of their renal tubules to concentrate urine. Their high metabolic rate and high ratio of body surface area to TBW also favor rapid fluid loss.

The distribution between the 'compartments' also differs between infants and adults (Table 10.1). During the first few days of life there is a transfer of water from ICF to ECF. This mechanism, which may protect the infant against the effects of dehydration, increases the already large ECF volume and could be a factor in the occurrence of edema sometimes observed at this time. In succeeding months the ratio of ICF : ECF volume increases from unity, nearing the adult value of 2 : 1 some time after the age of 1 year (see also Ch. 5, p. 139).

An infant exchanges about one-half of his extracellular fluid in the day whilst an adult exchanges only one-seventh.

WATER BALANCE

Maintenance of normal body water content depends on equilibrium between intake and output. Water loss occurs by various routes such as insensible perspiration, transpiration from lungs, and loss in urine, feces and sweat. Normally losses in feces and sweat are minimal. Insensible perspiration is essential to dissipate heat generated by metabolism and is augmented as required by sweating. Normal daily fluid intake must be related to calorie intake (Table 10.2), both on account of associated heat production and of the urinary solute load resulting from the diet. A normal infant requires 110 cal/kg body weight/day and approximately 150 ml fluid/100 cal expended (Table 10.3). Body temperature, environmental temperature and humidity greatly affect fluid balance. A rise in body temperature of 1°C is associated with an increment in metabolism of 13%, and hyperpnea may increase the loss of water vapor by the lungs fivefold.

THE ELECTROLYTE COMPOSITION OF THE BODY FLUIDS

EXTRACELLULAR FLUIDS (ECF)

The ECF is easily analyzed as plasma or serum. The electrolytes in these are representative of the ECF in most areas, possibly

Table 10.1 Partition of body fluids (average figures)

	Adult (70 kg; 1.85 m²)			Infant (3 kg; 0.2 m²)		
	% body weight	Liters	Liters/m²	% body weight	Liters	Liters/m²
Intracellular	40	28	15.2	38	1.14	5.70
Extracellular						
Interstitial*	16	11.2	6.0	33	0.99	4.95
Plasma	4	2.8	1.5	5	0.15	0.75
Total	60	42	22.7	76	2.28	11.4

* Includes transcellular fluids.

Table 10.2 Normal daily fluid and calorie requirements

Age	Water (ml/kg)	Calories/kg
First few days	50	0–100
Up to 1 year	160	110
1–2 years	120	110
3–4 years	100	100
10 years	50	70
Adults	30	45

(1 kcal = 4.18 kJ.)

Table 10.3 Water output per 100 calories expended in infants

		ml
Insensible loss	Skin	35
	Lungs	15
Sensible loss	Sweat	0–100
	Feces	5
	Urine	95
		150–250

Table 10.4 Composition of extracellular fluids

	(a) Intravascular fluid – plasma		(b) Interstitial fluid
	mEq/l plasma	mEq/l plasma water	mEq/l fluid*
Cations			
Sodium	140	150.0	142.5
Potassium	4	4.3	4
Calcium	5	5.4	?
Magnesium	2	2.1	?
	151	161.8	
Anions			
Chloride	103 (109†)	110.4	116
Bicarbonate	25 (18†)	26.8	28.2
Protein (electrical equivalents)	15	16.1	2
Phosphate	2 (3†)	2.1	?
Organic acid	6	6.4	?
	151	161.8	

* Assuming Donnan factor (see p. 407) to be 0.95 for monovalent cations and 1.05 for monovalent anions.
† Infants.

excepting tissues containing large amounts of collagen. All ECF is rich in sodium and chloride with relatively small amounts of potassium. The reverse applies to ICF where potassium, protein and phosphate predominate. The absolute electrolyte concentrations in ECF associated with bone, cartilage, tendon and skin vary considerably but in practice are of little clinical importance. The two divisions of ECF most frequently involved in the understanding of disease states are plasma and interstitial fluid.

The figures shown in Table 10.4 are averages for adults. Certain differences exist in infants, in whom the average plasma concentrations of chloride and phosphate are respectively 6 mmol/l (6 mEq/l) and 0.6 mmol/l (1 mEq/l) greater, whereas bicarbonate is correspondingly lower. Anion/cation balance must exist for electroneutrality to obtain. Age- and gender-related reference ranges should be available for each electrolyte being measured.

Normally, plasma water accounts for approximately 93% of the plasma volume. The remaining 7%, although predominantly proteins, includes lipids, electrolytes, glucose and urea. The water content of serum, in g/dl, is 98.4−(0.718 × protein concentration (g/dl)), e.g. for a protein concentration of 7.0 g/dl, water content = 93.4%.

The plasma volume occupied by electrolytes is always insignificant. In hyperlipemia, uremia or diabetes mellitus, the amount of lipids, urea or glucose may be large enough to produce a reduction in sodium concentration per unit volume. In hyperlipemia the concentration of water may be reduced to 75% and the concentration of sodium reduced to 111 mmol/l plasma, but when expressed per liter of water it is normal at 148 mmol/l.

INTRACELLULAR FLUIDS

Intracellular fluid is characterized by higher concentrations of potassium, phosphate and protein than ECF. The concentration of magnesium is greater in ICF, with 50% of the body's content being in the cells of soft tissue and most of the remainder in bone.

Analysis of ICF is extremely difficult. Any tissue sampled is a combination of both intracellular and extracellular phases.

Methods exist of estimating the amount of ECF present. These assume that almost all chloride is extracellular, then subtract the volume of ECF (calculated after measuring plasma chloride concentration) from the total water as estimated by weighing the tissue before and after desiccation. A particularly ingenious technique, was described by Graham et al in 1967. A correction is made for intracellular chloride by deriving this from the Nernst equation, assuming the membrane potential to be equal to − 85 mV. The ratio of extracellular chloride to intracellular chloride so calculated is approximately 24 : 1. Even if the membrane potential varies considerably from − 85 mV, there is still chloride present intracellularly. The problem also exists of referring intracellular electrolyte contents to some reference base unaffected by the degree of hydration. This can be accomplished in various ways, e.g. mmol/g fat-free tissue, mmol/g total nitrogen, mmol/g total phosphorus or mmol/g deoxyribonucleic acid phosphorus.

Typical ICF electrolyte concentrations are shown in Table 10.5.

The sum of anions and cations in ICF is greater than that in ECF. Normal osmotic equilibrium between the compartments requires equal numbers of osmotic particles in each. This is achieved by two factors. The first is the excess of divalent and polyvalent anions in ICF each contributing several electrical charges but only one osmotic particle. Secondly, some intracellular univalent ions (especially potassium) are not in free ionic form, but in combination with anions. This may also be inferred by measuring the membrane potential and extracellular concentration of potassium and calculating the concentration of 'active' potassium ion in the ICF.

Table 10.5 Intracellular fluid electrolytes (mEq/l ICF)

Cations		Anions	
Sodium	9	Chloride	4
Potassium	158	Bicarbonate	10
Calcium	3	Protein (electrical equivalents)	65
Magnesium	30	Phosphate	95
		Sulfate	22
		Organic acids	4
	200		200

PERMEABILITY OF MEMBRANES AND MOVEMENT OF WATER AND SOLUTES

The movement of substances between the different compartments in the body involves passage across membranes. Many factors govern such transport, including total osmotic pressure, hydrostatic pressure, colloidal (oncotic) pressure of proteins, Donnan equilibrium and the law of electroneutrality.

An 'ideal' membrane permits only water to pass through, and is impermeable to dissolved substances. Isolated cellular membranes are partially permeable. They are fully permeable to water and small crystalloid molecules but will not permit the passage of larger molecules such as proteins and mucopolysaccharides. They resemble molecular sieves with the added influence of solubility in the membrane lipids. The metabolic activity of the cell maintains differences between the intracellular and extracellular concentrations of various ions which will alter if the state of the cell is affected by cooling or poisoning.

Cell membranes are 50–100 Å thick, and carry negative internal and positive external charges. Substances cross the membrane in several ways. Water or solutes may simply flow through pores in the membrane. Solutes may also dissolve in the membrane and diffuse through it in solution or they may be actively transported from one side to the other. The membrane potential is governed by the ratio of internal to external concentration of certain ions. Potassium penetrates cells more rapidly than sodium, probably in part due to the smaller diameter of the potassium ion (3 Å), that of the sodium ion being 4.5 Å. At equilibrium the rate of movement of any material across a membrane is equal in both directions.

The rate of movement for water is governed by the chemical potential which depends on the number of collisions made by the water molecules per unit area of membrane. The chemical potential is increased by raising temperature or pressure and is reduced by adding solute to the water. With a difference in the chemical potential between the two sides of the membrane, movement of water or solute will tend to take place across the membrane to restore equilibrium. If the solute is not readily diffusible across the membrane, raising the pressure on the side to which the solute has been added prevents the expected movement of water. There is a corresponding pressure required to prevent movement of water for any given amount of solute. This pressure is called the osmotic pressure.

OSMOTIC PRESSURE, OSMOLARITY AND OSMOLALITY

Chemists define as colligative those properties determined mainly by the number and not by the nature of the particles present. Colligative properties include such characteristics as the lowering of vapor pressure, the elevation of boiling point, the reduction of freezing point and osmotic pressure, and the properties are interrelated.

Equivalent weight

The equivalent weight (gram equivalent) of an electrolyte

$$= \frac{\text{molecular weight in grams}}{\text{valency}}$$

e.g. sodium $= \frac{23}{1} = 23$, calcium $= \frac{40}{2} = 20$

In the SI system (Système International d'Unités) the preferred unit for chemical measurement is the mole (the amount of a substance with a mass equal to its molecular weight expressed in grams). According to this system concentrations are expressed in millimoles/liter (mmol/l) rather than as milliequivalents/liter. The relationship between the numerical values is:

$$\frac{\text{mEq/l}}{\text{valency}} = \text{mmol/l}$$

Molarity

Molarity is defined as the gram molecules (moles) of solute *per liter of solution*.

Molality

Molality is defined as the gram molecules (moles) of solute *per kilogram of solvent*.

At all body temperatures 1 kg of water may be equated with 1 liter with negligible error.

The terms molarity and molality should not be confused. For dilute aqueous solutions they are approximately equal, but in the body the distinction is marked.

Osmolarity

1 liter of solution containing 1 mole of undissociated solute represents an osmolarity of 1 osmol/l or 1000 mosmol/l. An aqueous solution of such concentration will exert an osmotic pressure of 22.4 atmospheres under ideal conditions and with an ideal membrane.

Osmolality

Osmolality is applicable when the concentration of solute is molal. This term, unlike osmolarity, takes account of the solute volume.

For undissociated nonelectrolyte solutions the molarity (molality) and osmolar (osmolal) concentrations are identical. For a substance dissociating fully into ions, however, each ion has the same osmotic effect as an undissociated molecule (i.e. dissociation increases the osmotic effect beyond that expected in terms of the molar content of the undissociated solute). A molar solution of sodium chloride (Na^+Cl^-) has, therefore, an ideal osmotic pressure of 2×22.4 atmospheres (2 osmoles). Calcium chloride ($Ca^{2+}2Cl^-$) yields three osmotically active ions if fully dissociated. In practice it is only with very dilute solutions that full dissociation occurs and the appropriate correction factor (osmotic coefficient) must be applied to calculate the osmolality when only the molality is known. Conversely association of macromolecules will result in a lowering of the theoretical osmotic pressure.

Solutions with the same osmotic pressure are termed isosmotic, and if separated by an 'ideal' membrane are termed isotonic when no net transfer of water occurs between them. Naturally most compartments in the body are in osmotic equilibrium although this does not apply to fluids such as urine and saliva. It is most convenient to determine osmolality by using an osmometer which

Table 10.6 Plasma – osmotic particles (mosmol/kg body water)

Sodium	150	Chloride	110.4			
Potassium	4.3			Sugar	4 (4 mmol/l)	TOTAL
Calcium	2.7	Bicarbonate	26.8			
Magnesium	1.0			Urea	5 (5 mmol/l)	
		Protein	2			
		Phosphate	1			
		Organic acids	3.8			
	158		144		9	311

actually measures the freezing point of plasma. Normal plasma osmolality is approximately 285 mosmol/kg body water. When the electrolyte concentrations per liter plasma water in Table 10.4 are considered, and allowance is made for valency but not for nondissociation, the number of osmotically active particles shown in Table 10.6 exists.

Assuming an osmotic coefficient of 0.925 the calculated osmolality equals 288 mosmol/kg, which is very close to the observed value.

Plasma and extracellular osmolality are closely related to the sodium concentration with a similar relationship between the osmolality of ICF and intracellular potassium concentration.

The polyvalent protein anions contribute about 16 electrical milliequivalents per liter of plasma water but they only represent approximately two osmotically active particles per liter.

PHYSIOLOGICAL WATER AND ELECTROLYTE MOVEMENT

When a solute is added to a solution on one side of a membrane there is a potential difference established between the phases and equilibrium can be established only by:

1. Free distribution of the solute on both sides of the membrane. This is possible only with a diffusible solute and permeable membranes.
2. Passage of water through the membranes, thereby eliminating the potential difference by equalizing the number of water molecules per unit area on each side of the membrane
3. By applying pressure to the solution to increase the potential again to that of pure water.

The addition of a diffusible solute to one compartment thus results in an increase of total osmolality in both compartments without net water transfer. A nondiffusible solute increases the effective as well as total osmolality and results in a transfer of water from one compartment to the other (Fig. 10.1).

Physiologically, urea may be regarded as being a freely diffusible (penetrating) solute, and increasing the concentration of urea in the body causes no transfer of water between the phases. An exception is when urea is rapidly removed from the plasma by hemodialysis, when, before outward diffusion of intracellular urea can occur, water moves into the ICF. In diabetes mellitus the elevated plasma glucose concentration causes intracellular water loss, because glucose is not a diffusible solute in the absence of insulin.

Although sodium, potassium and chloride are freely diffusible, the fact that most of the sodium and chloride are found in the ECF and that the potassium is mainly intracellular demonstrates that active mechanisms must exist for transporting at least some of the

ions across the cellular membranes. It is currently believed that sodium is actively expelled from cells by the expenditure of metabolic energy (the sodium pump), and that potassium diffuses passively into or out of the cells to maintain electroneutrality. The fixed intracellular anions (protein and phosphate) are unable to traverse the membrane and their concentrations will largely determine the concentration of potassium in the ICF. Inhibiting cellular metabolism by cooling or by enzyme inhibitors results in the disappearance of the sodium and potassium gradients normally present. The maintenance of a high intracellular potassium content by cells in a saline medium requires the presence of oxygen, glucose and L-glutamate. The absence of any one of these materials results in entry of sodium into the cell and diffusion of potassium into the ECF. Thereafter, application of Donnan equilibrium (see below) allows entry of water and further sodium ions, causing swelling, and finally rupture of the cell.

The diffusion of chloride ions into or out of the cell is intimately related to the membrane potential.

Membrane potential

The cell membrane may be regarded as being permeable to water, potassium and chloride, but impermeable to protein, phosphate and sodium. It is because of active expulsion of sodium that membrane impermeability to sodium may be assumed to obtain. A potential difference exists between the two sides of the membrane, referred to as the membrane potential. This has been measured in various cells and within experimental error the

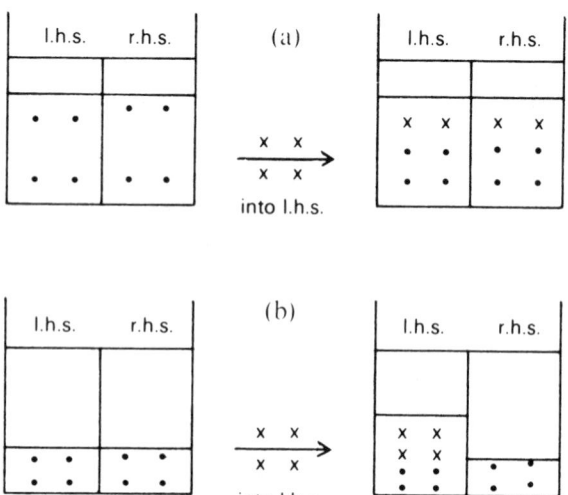

Fig. 10.1 Water distribution: (**a**) diffusible solutes; (**b**) nondiffusible solutes (l.h.s., left-hand side; r.h.s, right-hand side).

relationship for calculating its value depends upon the relative concentrations of diffusible ions in the ECF and in the ICF.

$$E_m \text{ (membrane potential)} = \frac{RT}{nF}\ n\ \frac{(Cl_i^-)}{(Cl_o^-)}$$

$$= 2.303\ \frac{RT}{nF}\ \log_{10} \frac{(Cl_i^-)}{(Cl_o^-)}$$

So, too:

$$E_m = 2.303\ \frac{RT}{nF}\ \log_{10}\ \frac{(K_o^+)}{(K_i^+)}$$

These expressions simplify to:

$$E_m = 58 \log_{10} \frac{(Cl_i^-)}{(Cl_o^-)}\ \text{millivolts}$$

$$\text{or}\ \ E_m = 58 \log_{10} \frac{(K_o^+)}{(K_i^+)}\ \text{millivolts}$$

A typical membrane potential is:

$$58 \times \log_{10} \frac{5}{150}$$

$$= 58 \log_{10} \frac{1}{30} = 58 \times -1.4771$$

$\ln$ = natural logarithm

R = thermodynamic gas constant

T = absolute temperature

F = Faraday

(Cl_o^-) = activity of chloride ion outside cell

(Cl_i^-) = activity of chloride ion inside cell

n = number of electrons involved

Activity, $(...)$, is approximately equal to concentration, $[...]$, in dilute solutions.

A potential difference exists across the membrane separating the intravascular phase of ECF (plasma) from the extravascular phase (interstitial fluid). This E_m is small since the gradients exhibited by sodium, potassium and chloride are not great. This is because sodium ions can penetrate capillary membranes freely, there being no active transport, and the electrolyte gradients result only from the presence of nondiffusible protein anions in plasma, and follow principles enunciated by Gibbs and confirmed experimentally by Donnan.

Donnan membrane equilibrium

When a diffusible solute, e.g. Na⁺Cl⁻ is added to water on one side (A) of a partially permeable membrane, rapid diffusion of the solute and water occur between the phases (A and B).

Donnan equilibrium

A	B	
Na_1^+	Na_2^+	$[Na_1^+] = [Cl_1^-] = [Na_2^+] = [Cl_2^-]$
Cl_1^-	Cl_2^-	

If, however, both diffusible and nondiffusible solutes are added to the water, e.g. Na⁺Cl⁻ and sodium proteinate (Na⁺Pr⁻), the following events occur.

Donnan equilibrium

A	B
Na_1^+	Na_2^+
Cl_1^-	Cl_2^-
Pr^-	

Thermodynamically:

$$[Na_1^+]\,[Cl_1^-] = [Na_2^+]\,[Cl_2^-]$$

Electroneutrality demands that:

$$[Na_1^+] = [Cl_1^-] + [Pr^-]$$
$$\text{i.e. } [Na_1^+] > [Cl_1^-] \text{ and } [Na_2^+] = [Cl_2^-]$$

The concentration of diffusible cation, $[Na^+]$, is thus greater at equilibrium on the side containing the protein. So, too, $[Cl_1^-] < [Cl_2^-]$.

These events cause:

1. development of a membrane potential
2. greater concentration of osmotically active particles in phase A, containing the nonpenetrating protein ion.

These conditions exist even in the absence of active transport such as between plasma and interstitial fluid but can be magnified or opposed by active transport, which can maintain an intracellular ion at a constant concentration as though it were a nonpenetrating ion. Unless opposed, there is a tendency for water to move into the compartment containing the constrained anion. The metabolic process preventing the entry of water to cells is directly related to the extrusion of sodium.

Hydrostatic and colloid osmotic pressure

Equilibrium in plasma is established between the formation and the reabsorption of interstitial fluid by the interplay of hydrostatic and colloid osmotic pressures.

The total osmotic pressure of plasma (285 mosmol/kg body water) is equivalent to about 6.5 atmospheres (5000 mmHg), but the proportion due to the colloid osmotic pressure of the proteins is small, being less than 30 mmHg. Since the interstitial fluid contains only small amounts of protein, the difference in colloid osmotic pressure (oncotic pressure) is equivalent to about 25 mmHg. Although it is small, this figure is of fundamental physiological importance in controlling the flow of water between plasma and tissue fluids (Fig. 10.2).

Since albumins have smaller molecular weights than globulins, approximately 80% of the plasma protein osmotic effect is due to albumin. Thus hypoalbuminemia predisposes to the formation of increased amounts of interstitial fluid, causing clinically detectable edema.

INDIVIDUAL CATIONS

SODIUM

The sodium content per kilogram body weight (Table 10.7) is 35 to 50% higher in the infant than in the adult due to the greater

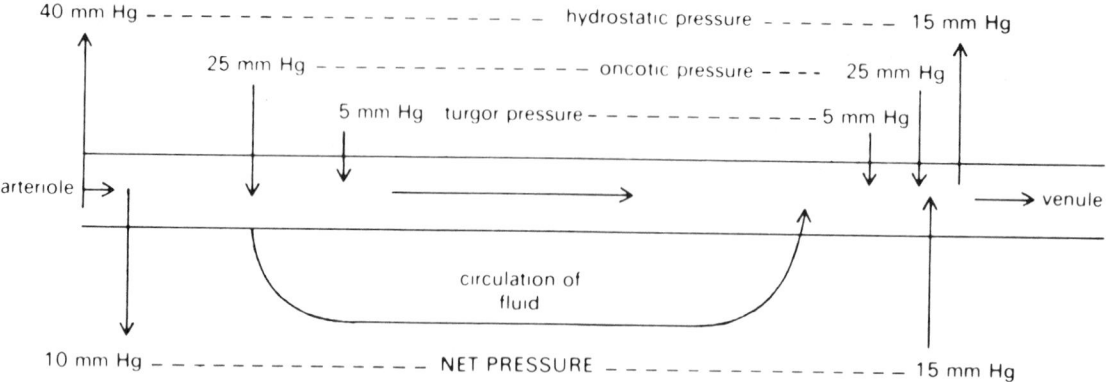

Fig. 10.2 The distribution of fluids between the intravascular and interstitial compartments.

Table 10.7 Amount and distribution of sodium (70 kg adult mean values)

	mmol/kg	(Total)	% total		Exchangeable
Extracellular fluid	25	(1770)	45	All	43 mmol/kg (3020) 77% of
Intracellular fluid	5	(350)	9	All	total. Wide normal range
Bone	26	(1800)	46	50%	
Total	56	(3920)	100		

(1 mmol Na = 23 mg.)

Table 10.8 Sodium balance (70 kg adult)

Dietary intake	Intermediary metabolism	Output
150 mmol	Secretion in intestinal juices = 900 mmol with almost total reabsorption Renal filtered load = 26 000 mmol but tubular reabsorption is almost complete	→ 10 mmol – feces (and sweat) → 140 mmol – urine ———— 150 mmol*

* In the growing child the output is slightly less than the intake.

amount of extracellular fluid. With the relative reduction of ECF with growth, adult values are reached at about 2 years of age. It is not possible to measure the total sodium content of the body directly, except by analysis of a cadaver. An estimate can be obtained by use of isotopes such as ^{24}Na (short half-life), or ^{22}Na (long half-life). The isotopic dilution method will measure only the readily exchangeable sodium. Since the exchangeable proportion is that readily available for metabolic purposes it may often be of as much interest to the clinician as the total body content.

A normal dietary intake ranges between 1 and 4 mmol (23–92 mg) per kg body weight per day, and equilibrium is maintained by renal regulation of sodium loss. A typical sodium balance is shown in Table 10.8.

Most of the sodium excretion from the body occurs via the kidney (Table 10.8) which can compensate within wide limits for variation in the dietary intake. Normal glomerular filtrate has an osmolality of 300 mosmol/kg but the osmolality of the urine excreted may range from 30 to 1200 mosmol/kg (specific gravity 1.001–1.035). The infant kidney is unable to form such concentrated or dilute urine, a more realistic range being 100–700 mosmol/kg (specific gravity 1.003–1.023). Sodium depletion (unlike water depletion) does not occur under conditions of

reduced intake but requires some abnormal loss – in sweat, alimentary secretions or urine.

POTASSIUM

Potassium is the predominant intracellular cation (Table 10.9), and its distribution among the organs of the body is related to their cell mass. In contrast to sodium, the potassium content per kilogram body weight increases from infancy to adult life. Average figures are 42.5 mmol/kg at birth, 46.4 mmol/kg at 1 year and 50 mmol/kg in the young adult. Total body potassium can be determined by measuring gamma ray emission from the naturally occurring isotope ^{40}K. The isotope ^{42}K affords a measure of

Table 10.9 Amount and distribution of potassium (70 kg adult mean values)

	mmol/kg	(Total)	% total
Extracellular	1	(70)	2
Intracellular	49	(3430)	98
Total	50	(3500)	100

(1 mmol potassium = 39 mg.)

Table 10.10 Potassium balance (70 kg adult)

Dietary intake	Intermediary metabolism	Output
70 mmol	Secretion in intestinal juices = 150 mmol with almost total reabsorption Renal filtered load = 940 mmol but tubular reabsorption is almost complete	→ 10 mmol – feces → 60 mmol – urine ——— 70 mmol

exchangeable potassium (K_e) which is only slightly less than total body potassium.

About 70% of the potassium is found in the muscles of the body.

The normal dietary potassium intake daily ranges between 1 and 3 mmol (39–117 mg) per kg body weight, the larger amounts being applicable to children. Equilibrium is attained mainly by the adjustment of renal loss (Table 10.10).

Renal conservation of potassium is efficient. The urine content normally falls to less than 20 mmol/day in the adult when there is restriction of dietary potassium intake and when the plasma concentration is less than 3.0 mmol/l. Potassium deficiency is usually caused by abnormal losses in alimentary secretions or in urine, rather than by a reduced intake.

MAGNESIUM

Second only to potassium, magnesium is the most important intracellular cation. The adult body contains about 14.5 mmol/kg or 1000 mmol (1 mmol = 2 mEq magnesium = 24 mg). The fetal content is higher per unit weight. Approximately half the magnesium is in bone and almost all of the remainder is in the cells of the soft tissues. Less than 1% is in the ECF.

The daily intake of the adult is about 12.5 mmol of which 4 mmol are absorbed and a similar amount excreted in the urine. The daily requirement of the child is 0.5–1.0 mmol/kg/day. The usual cause of deficiency is increased intestinal loss with or without a reduced dietary intake. Occasionally an increase in urinary excretion may result in deficiency.

Conversely, magnesium excess may be associated with a failure of renal excretion (anuria, chronic nephritis, Addison's disease), or with excessive dietary intake, or with release from damaged tissues. Calcium ions counteract the cardiotoxic actions both of hypermagnesemia and hyperkalemia.

The normal ranges for plasma magnesium, measured by atomic absorption spectroscopy, etc., are: infants, 0.6–0.9 mmol/l; older children and adults, 0.75–1.0 mmol/l.

DEHYDRATION AND ELECTROLYTE DISTURBANCE

Strictly speaking the term dehydration means loss or deprivation of water but it is employed loosely to include loss of water and various ions from the body, without specifying the source of either the water or accompanying ions. Clinically there are two distinct clinical syndromes, comprising water depletion and sodium depletion. The pure syndromes are uncommon and most cases present with features indicating deficiencies both of water and of sodium.

The major disturbances of water and electrolyte balance are:

1. water depletion (hypertonic dehydration)
2. sodium depletion (hypotonic dehydration)
3. mixed water and sodium depletion (may be isotonic, hypotonic or hypertonic)
4. potassium depletion and intoxication
5. the low sodium syndrome and water intoxication
6. acid–base disturbances.

There are other relatively rare or concomitant upsets not mentioned above, such as calcium or magnesium deficiency. A description of these deficiencies is included under the appropriate headings.

HOMEOSTATIC REGULATION OF VOLUME AND OSMOLALITY OF BODY COMPARTMENTS

The osmolality of ECF and hence of other body fluids is closely related to the concentration of sodium in plasma. Small alterations from the normal produce rapid changes in the secretion of the antidiuretic hormone, arginine vasopressin (AVP), by the posterior pituitary gland. This results in a prompt increase or decrease in the amount and osmolality of the urine produced, provided that the kidney is competent. The distal renal tubules and collecting ducts are responsible for this alteration in the osmolality of the urine, and ultimately cause the variation in 'free water clearance' (see below).

Osmolal clearance

The 'osmolal clearance' may be defined as the milliliters of plasma completely cleared per minute of osmotically active particles. In normal adults, this varies between 2 and 3 ml/min, and is largely independent of urine flow.

$$C_{osm} = \frac{U_{osm} \times V}{P_{osm}}$$

C_{osm} = osmolal clearance (ml/min)
U_{osm} = urine osmolality (mosmol/kg)
P_{osm} = plasma osmolality (mosmol/kg)
V = urine secretion (ml/min)

The following illustrations may serve to explain the concept: Under conditions of fluid restriction:

$$C_{osm} = \frac{1200 \times 0.5}{300} = 2.0 \text{ ml/min}$$

whilst following liberal water intake:

$$C_{osm} = \frac{30 \times 20}{300} = 2.0 \text{ ml/min}$$

Free water clearance

'Free water clearance' is defined as $V - C_{osm}$, and in the examples shown is – 1.5 ml/min where fluid is restricted, and + 18.0 ml/min

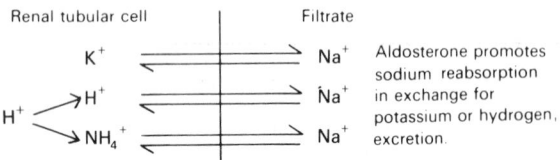

Fig. 10.3 The effect of aldosterone on renal tubular action.

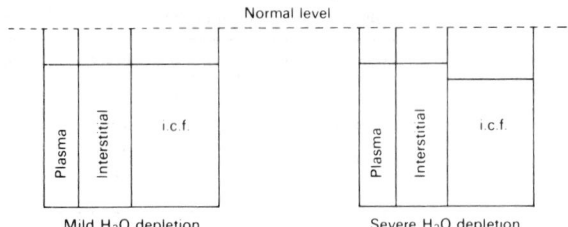

Fig. 10.4 Water depletion.

during liberal water intake. A negative value signifies water reabsorbed by the kidney and available for diluting body fluids. The kidney is much more efficient in shedding excess water from the body than it is in conserving water in times of shortage. Ultimately the sensation of thirst produced by the increase in plasma and ICF osmolality results in the individual increasing his water intake to compensate for any deficit (Kunau & Stein 1977).

Whilst the osmolality of the body is regulated by the plasma sodium concentration, the volume of the ECF is correspondingly regulated by the total amount of sodium present. A mechanism exists to prevent the ingestion of sodium being followed by a corresponding retention of water with a resultant increased volume of ECF of normal osmolality. The precise details whereby the excretion of sodium is regulated by the kidney are very complex, involving principally aldosterone and atrial natriuretic peptide (ANP). A decrease in plasma volume is known to cause an increase in the secretion of aldosterone. This hormone acts on the distal and collecting tubules of the kidney, enhancing the ionic reabsorption of sodium from the urinary filtrate (Fig. 10.3) (see also Ch. 17).

It is not possible to dissociate preservation of osmolality from preservation of ECF volume since the latter demands the regulation of the excretion of both sodium and water, and the former involves mainly the excretion of water. In normal circumstances the body endeavors initially to maintain its osmolality and is prepared to allow a reduction in ECF volume to accomplish this. With a progressive reduction in ECF, however, the volume receptors assume precedence over osmolality. The final result is a plasma compartment in which both the volume and osmolality are reduced.

WATER DEPLETION

Pure water depletion is comparatively rare and is seen more often in infants than in older children. This occurs in various clinical situations including esophageal lesions, infirmity, coma, high solute loads and impaired renal function. Since water is diffusible across the cell membranes, the initial extracellular loss is soon shared by the intracellular compartment (Fig. 10.4). The cardinal symptom is thirst and associated dryness of the mouth.

It should be noted that even if water intake is zero, water is produced by the oxidation of the hydrogen of those tissues undergoing catabolism.

$$
\begin{array}{ll}
100 \text{ g fat} & \left\{ \begin{array}{ll} \text{oxidation} & 72 \\ \text{release of tissue} \\ \text{water} & 35 \end{array} \right\} 107 \text{ ml water} \\
100 \text{ g protein} & \left\{ \begin{array}{ll} \text{oxidation} & 10 \\ \text{release of tissue} \\ \text{water} & 80 \end{array} \right\} 90 \text{ ml water} \\
100 \text{ g carbohydrate} & \text{oxidation} \qquad\qquad 60 \text{ ml water}
\end{array}
$$

Degrees of water loss and associated symptoms are listed in Table 10.11.

In water depletion, the packed cell volume (PCV) tends to remain normal, whilst the concentrations of hemoglobin and plasma proteins show only slight increases. Unfortunately the value of these observations is often obscured by the uncertainty of the pre-dehydration figures.

SODIUM DEPLETION

Pure sodium depletion (Fig. 10.5), like pure water depletion, is rare. It occurs where the body is losing fluid by various routes, e.g. sweat, intestine, kidney, and where fluid replacement is by ion-free water or dextrose. Initially the kidney loses water to maintain plasma osmolality. Thereafter the necessity of

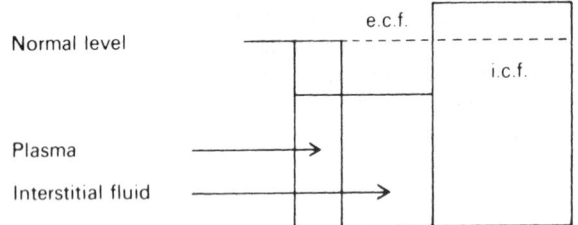

Fig. 10.5 Sodium depletion.

Table 10.11 Water depletion

| | % body weight | Liters | | Signs and symptoms |
		Adult (70 kg)	Infant (6 kg)	
Mild	3	2.0	0.18	Thirst; oliguria; dry mucous membranes
Moderate	6	4.0	0.36	Thirst; oliguria; restlessness, weakness and tachycardia
Very severe	7–14	5–10	0.42–0.84	Collapse, convulsions, blood pressure low; sunken eyeballs and fontanel; loss of skin turgor with 'doughy' feeling; plasma sodium, urea and osmolality all raised

Table 10.12 Sodium depletion

Sodium deficiency (mmol)		Signs and symptoms
Adult (70 kg)	Infant (6 kg)	
300	30	Just detectable. Cold, gray skin
300–600	30–60	Tachycardia, blood pressure low; dry mucous membranes, sunken eyeballs and fontanel, loss of skin turgor
600–1000	60–100	Severe shock, systolic blood pressure very low, uremia. Plasma sodium low. Plasma osmolality tends to be low

conserving plasma volume is of greater importance and hyponatremia occurs.

Degrees of sodium depletion and associated symptoms are indicated in Table 10.12.

Thirst tends to be absent since this symptom is primarily due to an increase in intracellular osmolality. Packed cell volume, hemoglobin and plasma proteins are often increased; but again may be masked by pre-illness deviations from normality.

MIXED WATER AND SODIUM DEPLETIONS

A loss of isotonic sodium-containing fluid results in the ECF bearing the reduction in volume, whereas a loss of (hypotonic) water is shared by both ECF and ICF. Since many of the clinical manifestations of dehydration are reflections of a reduction primarily in ECF volume, sodium deficiency and its attendant fluid loss produce more marked clinical signs than water deficiency of comparable magnitude.

One of the commonest forms of sodium and water depletion is that due to the loss of intestinal secretion (Table 10.13). This may be occasioned by intestinal obstruction, fistulae of the small intestine, enterocolitis, or an ileostomy. The composition of the fluid lost will vary, but with the exception of saliva all normal alimentary secretions are isotonic with plasma. Diarrheal fluid tends to be hypotonic and, as such, is liable to cause hypernatremia in infants where the fluid intake is relatively low, and the kidney is unable to produce a very concentrated urine. Conversely older children and adults suffering from diarrhea often present with hyponatremia since they ingest large quantities of hypotonic fluids and their kidneys can produce concentrated urine.

In an infant weighing 3 or 4 kg, the volume of alimentary secretions per 24 h is approximately 400 ml.

POTASSIUM DEPLETION AND INTOXICATION

After intestinal absorption, potassium is borne via the plasma and interstitial fluid compartments to its predominantly intracellular location. When cellular function is normal the content of potassium per gram of noncollagen nitrogen (K/N) can be shown to be fairly constant. For specimens of skeletal muscle the value is approximately 2.8 mmol potassium per gram of noncollagen nitrogen. Since about 70% of the body content of potassium resides in muscle tissue, it is obvious that any muscle wasting will result in loss both of potassium and water from the body. Naturally the exchangeable potassium (K_e) will diminish as muscle wasting progresses, but the K/N ratio often remains within normal limits. This state does not normally qualify for inclusion in the term 'potassium deficiency' (depletion) which is reserved rather for situations where the K/N ratio is reduced. It is doubtful whether a significantly increased K/N ratio ever exists for other than brief periods.

Extreme variations in the plasma concentration of potassium (1.0–12.0 mmol/l) have been observed in the living state, ranging both above and below the normal limits of 3.8–5.0 mmol/l in adults and 3.8–5.5 mmol/l in infants. Less than 1% of the potassium in the body is in the plasma and about 2% is in the ECF so that rapid changes in plasma concentration may occur following transfer between the extracellular and intracellular compartments. In many situations it is not valid to assume that hypokalemia indicates potassium deficiency, and hyperkalemia may be found with normal or reduced K/N ratios. In general, however, where the clinical condition justifies assuming potassium deficiency to be likely, hypokalemia can be used as an index for regulating potassium therapy.

Potassium deficiency occurs in a variety of situations but most often involves excessive loss via the intestinal and/or renal routes. Such conditions as vomiting, fistulae, diarrhea, Cushing's syndrome, primary hyperaldosteronism and the use of glucocorticoids or diuretics are particularly liable to induce potassium depletion with or without concomitant hypokalemia. An acidosis tends to cause renal excretion of hydrogen ions in exchange for sodium, whilst conserving potassium. Associated with this is the transfer of hydrogen into the intracellular space and the movement of potassium into the ECF. The final result is an increase in the plasma concentration of potassium. Conversely, an alkalosis will promote the production of hypokalemia without any immediate intracellular potassium deficiency occurring.

One situation where the result of these changes may manifest itself with potential danger to the patients is where intravenous therapy is employed to correct severe dehydration and possible associated acidosis. The initial plasma potassium concentration can be normal but falls rapidly as normal glomerular function is restored and potassium migrates intracellularly. In such circumstances, the use of potassium-free fluids should be avoided.

Table 10.13 Approximate volume and composition of alimentary secretions (adult, 70 kg)

Secretion	mmol/l					Liters/24 hours	pH
	H+	Na+	K+	Cl−	HCO3−		
Saliva	–	15	20	32	3	1.0–1.5	6.3–6.8
Gastric	80	50	20	150	–	2.0–3.0	1.0–1.5
Pancreatic	–	140	10	80	70	0.5–1.5	7.1–8.2
Biliary	–	140	10	120	30	0.5–1.0	7.0–7.6
Succus entericus	–	135	15	125	25	1.0–3.0	7.0–7.5

Most of the clinical upsets resulting from potassium depletion can be attributed to associated hypokalemia. One possible exception is the condition of adynamic ileus which seems to be due to intracellular potassium depletion. Balance studies have shown that in the adult, of a total body potassium of 3500 mmol, it is possible to have a deficiency as great as 1500 mmol (> 20 mmol/kg) following prolonged vomiting. Even with this magnitude of deficiency the membrane potential is affected less than where a change from 5 to 2 mmol/l occurs in the plasma concentration. The clinical symptoms of potassium depletion include muscular weakness, hypotonicity and paralysis, although tetany is occasionally observed. Polyuria due to renal tubular dysfunction is another well-recognized sign of potassium deficiency. Cardiac upsets occur including arrhythmias, tachycardia, hypotension and even ventricular fibrillation. Electrocardiographic changes observed comprise ST depression, prolonged Q–T interval and prominent U wave, T wave inversion and the appearance of bifid U waves.

Potassium intoxication is caused by the hyperkalemia almost invariably present rather than by an excess of total body potassium. This can be demonstrated by employing measures designed to cause the movement of potassium from the ECF to the ICF. Clinical improvement follows such therapy. The occurrence of hyperkalemia is always associated with a failure or overwhelming of the renal excretory mechanisms. The renal failure may be real as in glomerular or tubular disease or related to the lack of steroid hormones in Addison's disease. On the other hand it may be relative and due to excessive entry of potassium into the ECF. The latter situation is found in states of hemolysis, acidosis, infections, and injudicious potassium therapy. Cardiac arrest may occur if the plasma concentration exceeds 7.5 mmol/l, but this is very variable.

The electrocardiographic changes associated with hyperkalemia include peaked T waves, a prolonged P–R interval and ventricular slowing. These are valuable confirmatory signs of potassium intoxication but the clinical decision to employ treatment for hyperkalemia should be based largely on the result obtained for the plasma potassium determination. An exception to this statement is the description of electrocardiographic changes normally associated with hyperkalemia, but found in the presence of a normal plasma potassium concentration. These findings can be induced by administering potassium supplements too rapidly to patients with severe intracellular potassium depletion and hypokalemia. The hypokalemia is quickly corrected, but the intracellular potassium depletion persists. The membrane potential is altered to a value similar to that obtaining where a normal intracellular potassium concentration and hyperkalemia coexist.

THE LOW SODIUM SYNDROME AND WATER INTOXICATION

Whilst sodium depletion is often associated with hyponatremia, the occurrence of hyponatremia does not necessarily imply sodium depletion; it can be due to dilution. Unless this fact is appreciated, serious errors in therapy will result. The following are causes of hyponatremia:

1. true sodium depletion
2. water intoxication
3. diuretic-resistant edema, with or without uremia
4. inappropriate secretion of ADH
5. new 'steady states'
6. dilution of plasma sodium by excess glucose, fat or protein.

Categories 1 and 6 have already been mentioned.

Water intoxication

Water intoxication is the state which results when excretion of water is unable to keep pace with intake and production of water. It is especially liable to occur when prompt diuresis by the kidney fails to occur. It may be found in infants (relatively inadequate tubular function), following operations (increased ADH), in adrenocortical insufficiency (lack of cortisol), or when parenteral hypotonic fluid is given in excess of requirements. Clinical manifestations may appear when water amounting to between 5 and 10% of the body weight has been retained. The excess water is distributed between the ECF and ICF causing reductions in the concentration of plasma sodium and in plasma osmolality. Hypokalemia is also likely to be present unless renal failure is severe. The PCV is theoretically normal, whilst hemoglobin level and plasma protein concentration tend to be low. Anorexia, weakness, nausea, vomiting, headache, confusion and coma have all been reported in this syndrome. That these upsets are due to intracellular overhydration can be proved by infusing a small volume of hypertonic saline, following which water moves from the ICF to the ECF, and clinical improvement results. The finding of a normal plasma sodium concentration excludes the presence of water intoxication.

Edema

Diuretic-resistant edema may occur in renal or cardiac failure and implies that renal excretion is impaired in spite of the possible presence of an increased ECF volume. The total body sodium may be increased but water retention is even more marked, resulting in hyponatremia. The sequence of events leading to this syndrome is complicated and involves excessive secretion and/or diminished inactivation of aldosterone and ADH together with possible changes in capillary permeability. The outcome is an increase in the volume of interstitial fluid but a decrease in plasma volume. This results in pre-renal azotemia which is further aggravated by sodium restriction. The therapeutic use of hypertonic saline in this syndrome often causes improved renal function with a decrease in the uremia even if the edema may not be diminished.

The syndrome of inappropriate antidiuretic secretion (SIADH)

Inappropriate secretion of ADH produces a clinical picture similar to that observed in water intoxication. The fundamental fault is that the secretion of ADH persists even in the presence of a reduced osmolality. This may be associated with head injury where the ADH is of posterior pituitary origin, or it may be found with certain tumors where a vasopressin-like polypeptide is elaborated by the neoplastic tissue.

Treatment of this condition involves water restriction together with any specific therapy against the tumor if such is practicable.

Steady states

New 'steady states': there are some patients, especially in the older age group, whose plasma sodium concentrations are habitually about 132 mmol/l. They have no signs of sodium deficiency and are not suffering from water intoxication. Given hypertonic saline they neither achieve normal plasma sodium concentrations nor do they derive any benefit.

TREATMENT OF FLUID AND ELECTROLYTE DISTURBANCE

To sustain life, the basic principles involve the correction of deficit or excess of fluid and electrolytes, compensation for abnormal loss by whatever route and maintenance of a physiological balance. Where a patient has severe dehydration with attendant shock and peripheral vascular collapse the first move is to expand the plasma volume. To this end, immediate intravenous infusion of citrated plasma or suitable plasma substitute at 20 ml/kg may be life saving. Even in the above dramatic situation all fluids supplied to a patient will basically contain water, solutes and calories.

Water and solutes are usually required in more than normal amounts but when parenteral nutrition is limited to a few days an intake of 20–35% of the average calorie requirement will normally suffice.

The treatment of mild dehydration of the hypotonic, isotonic or hypertonic type does not necessarily require intravenous therapy. Mild gastroenteritis will yield to gastric lavage followed by oral half-strength physiological saline in liberal amounts, and the water-deprived hypernatremia to adequate oral intake of quarter-strength physiological saline. Moderate diarrhea may be treated away from hospital by reconstituted oral solutions such as those of WHO, Armour (Dioralyte) or Searle (Rehidrat). Their composition in mmol/l is shown:

	Sodium	Potassium	Chloride	Bicarbonate	Glucose (g/l)
WHO	90	20	80	30	20
Dioralyte	35	20	37	18	40
Rehidrat	50	20	50	20	16.4

Rehidrat also contains sucrose (32.3 g/l), citric acid (1.76 g/l) and fructose (1.76 g/l). The higher sodium concentration (WHO) is good for high sodium loss as in cholera, but less good for young infants for whom it may be diluted. Monosaccharides are beneficial but disaccharides less so and lactose may be harmful.

Provided that renal function is good it is relatively difficult to overload these infants and 150–200 ml/kg body weight/day are necessary save for the neonatal period when less is required. The widespread use of such 'stock' solutions has produced a dramatic fall in mortality in malnourished infants suffering from diarrhea. Recourse to the intravenous route demands knowledge of daily requirements of fluid and electrolytes. Normal daily requirements for water and electrolytes are listed in Table 10.14 but provided renal function is good, wide tolerance exists.

In a few patients parenteral magnesium (as magnesium chloride) at 0.5 mmol/kg/day in 5% dextrose is required, therapy being governed by measuring plasma magnesium concentration.

Over and above the need to maintain hydration is the need to correct existing deficits. In a considerably dehydrated child the water deficit will lie between 30 and 150 ml/kg body weight and

Table 10.14 Average daily requirements for maintenance of fluid and electrolytes per kg body weight at various ages

Age	Water (ml)	Potassium (mmol)	Sodium (mmol)
Day of birth	50	0	0
Infant	150	3	3
Older child	50	2	2

the deficit of sodium and/or potassium between 5 and 20 mmol/kg body weight.

Solutions for fluid and electrolyte replacement are given in Table 10.15.

ISOTONIC AND HYPOTONIC DEHYDRATION

These are by far the commonest patterns of dehydration resulting from sodium and water loss, with or without concomitant potassium loss. Fluids lower in sodium content are usually administered to infants as quarter- or half-strength physiological saline. Physiological (isotonic) saline tends to be used for older children. Energy is generally provided as 5% dextrose and a stock solution of half-strength physiological saline in 5% dextrose solution is a very useful fluid. The rate of infusion will be calculated to counteract continuing losses, to maintain fluid and electrolyte balance and to replace existing deficits. The aim should be to restore water and sodium deficiencies in 24–36 h and potassium deficit, if large, in 5 days.

It is important to stress to all attendants that because a target for administration over a 24-h period may be calculated this must not be divided by 24 and given at a standard rate for the first 24 h. Severe dehydration may require urgent partial correction, continuing diarrhea or vomiting increase the rate of flow required, or renal dysfunction mandate the reverse. The infusion should be started at a relatively fast rate for several hours at least, and progress reviewed on the clinical and biochemical findings.

Thus, in moderately severe dehydration a 1-year-old infant given 150 ml/kg body weight of half-strength 5% dextrose–saline in the first 24 h receives in this 150 ml water, 11.5 mmol sodium and 30 calories per kg body weight. For each of the first 6 h this infusion might run at 10 ml/kg body weight/h, being reduced to 5 ml/kg body weight as hydration improves. In addition, one might add potassium chloride to provide 3.0 mmol of potassium/kg/day. Severe diarrhea or vomiting would modify the rate of infusion in one direction and renal failure the reverse. Very young infants may require slower infusion and paradoxically more concentrated solutions (e.g. isotonic saline) initially to correct existing sodium depletion.

Clinical assessment of progress, tissue turgor, periorbital hydration, fontanel tension, urinary output and general appearances continues to yield remarkably helpful information.

In all but the most severe cases, continued small amounts of oral fluids to moisten the buccal mucosa are advised, and this route will gradually take over and replace the drip, which should be discontinued or reimplanted within 72 h.

The treatment of the basic cause of such dehydration will be undertaken synchronously with antimicrobials parenterally as indicated. When intravenous infusion is impracticable or impossible, smaller amounts of fluid may be given subcutaneously (with hyaluronidase) or intraperitoneally to supplement oral fluid therapy.

Table 10.15   Solutions for fluid and electrolyte replacement

	Approximate calories/liter	(MJ/l)
Dilute		
Dextrose 5%	200	(0.84)
Physiological ⎫ sodium chloride 0.9% (154 mmol/l)	–	
Isotonic ⎭		
Dextrose 5% in sodium chloride 0.45% (77 mmol/l)	200	(0.84)
Dextrose 5% in sodium chloride 0.225% (38 mmol/l)	200	(0.84)
Fructose 5%	200	(0.84)
Dextrose 4% in sodium chloride 0.18% (31 mmol/l)	160	(0.67)
Water	–	
Concentrated		
Potassium chloride (10%) 1.35 mmol/ml	–	
Sodium chloride (11.7%) 2 mmol/ml	–	
Ammonium chloride (5.35%) 1 mmol/ml	–	
Magnesium chloride (10.20%) 0.5 mmol/ml	–	
Calcium gluconate (10%) 0.22 mmol/ml	310	(1.3)
Sodium bicarbonate (8.4%) 1 mmol/ml	–	
Sodium lactate (11.2%) 1 mmol/ml	340	(1.4)
Fructose 10%	400	(1.7)
Fructose 20%	800	(3.3)
Dextrose 50%	2000	(8.4)

(1 kcal = 4.18 kJ)

HYPERTONIC DEHYDRATION (HYPERNATREMIA)

The association of hypertonic dehydration with hypernatremia, convulsions and brain damage has long been recognized. The dangers of overconcentrated feeds have been highlighted. Although infantile gastroenteritis with associated fever, hyperventilation and diarrhea may predispose to the development of hypertonic dehydration, the risk is enhanced by the use of overconcentrated feeds. All such infants displaying significant diarrhea should have solid food and milk removed from their diet for the first 24 h. Hypertonic dehydration is much less obvious than is hypotonic or isotonic dehydration and is now uncommon.

The condition usually affects infants aged less than 1 year and the serum sodium very often exceeds 150 mmol/l. Elevation of chloride, urea and potassium along with hypocalcemia and possibly hypomagnesemia are also usually present. Brain shrinkage and fall in CSF pressure while arterial pressure remains essentially intact are probably responsible for the dilation and rupture of cerebral vessels which is a pathological feature of hypernatremia. Approximately one-third of such cases are noted to convulse, generally within 24 h of admission to hospital and sometimes in relation to treatment. Most infants have diarrhea at some point of the illness and the plasma pH tends to be low, averaging 7.1–7.2. The cause of the convulsions is almost certainly related to renal dysfunction which leads to metabolic acidosis and to a continuing hyperosmolar state from a combination of the raised sodium and urea concentrations. Sudden alterations effected by treatment may trigger convulsions. This is probably due to cerebral edema which may also prove fatal. Rose (1984) stresses that as hyperosmolality develops, the brain responds in two ways. Initially water leaves the brain producing brain shrinkage and the symptoms described above. If this were the only response, rapid lowering of plasma osmolality would restore brain size to normal and there would be little danger to the patient. Unfortunately, the brain can also adapt to the hyperosmolal state by increasing intracellular osmolality by accumulating osmotically active Na^+, K^+ and Cl^- from the plasma and previously inactive cell stores. He stresses that in hypernatremia, brain size decreases initially and then returns to normal in 24 h. Once such adaptation has occurred, an acute reduction in plasma osmolality causes water to move into the brain and cerebral edema results. A low pH and a high blood urea level (or BUN) should alert the clinician to the likelihood of fits during the early treatment of hypertonic dehydration. Whilst the absolute level of serum sodium may not be related to the tendency to convulsions the same is not proven for subsequent brain damage.

Hypertonic dehydration is frequently present with and predisposes to renal venous thrombosis. Fluid orally or by intravenous infusion for hypertonic dehydration in infants should avoid the use of 50% dextrose solution alone since the cerebral disturbance during therapy seems likely to be due to intracellular overhydration from additional intracellular osmotic particles due to deranged metabolism.

A polyionic preparation may be employed as first suggested in 1968 by Bruck et al. Their suggestion was a fluid containing 57 mmol of sodium, 25 mmol of potassium, 3 mmol (6 mEq) of magnesium, 50 mmol of chloride, and 25 mmol of lactate together with 7 mmol of phosphate and 100 g glucose per liter. In practice, a solution of half- or quarter-strength saline in 5% dextrose is usually employed. If there is acidosis present, however, it may be desirable to give the sodium as $NaHCO_3$ and not as NaCl, and the number of mmol of sodium should be calculated. Thus 1 l of 5% dextrose plus 39 mmol of sodium bicarbonate is osmotically equivalent to quarter-strength saline in 5% dextrose.

The rate of infusion is variable but is usually 100–150 ml/kg body weight/day, provided that abnormal losses have ceased and renal handling of water is adequate. Ideally the water deficit should be restored slowly over a period of 3–5 days. It is thought that the added sodium prevents some of the water migrating osmotically into the cells. As normal cellular function returns, the smaller osmotic particles reunite and cellular volume tends to decrease to normal. The use of peritoneal dialysis for the grossly uremic, hypernatremic hyperosmolar cases offers what may prove to be the most successful therapy at present available.

Despite therapy, mortality and residual brain damage are common, each occurring to an extent of 8% of patients affected. Fortunately the use of lower solute and protein concentrations in infant formulae has led to a rapid and striking decrease in incidence, mortality and morbidity due to hypernatremic hyperosmolar dehydration (Arneil & Chin 1979).

Hypertonicity also occurs in diabetic ketosis but hypernatremia is not always a feature and rapid correction of dehydration is fairly safe. In adults with hypernatremia there is little danger of convulsions with rapid rehydration by 5% glucose solution.

HYPOKALEMIA

As already described, the causes of hypokalemia are many and varied, and the measures employed for its treatment depend to some extent on the primary upset. In any difficult or unusual situation therapy should be guided by frequent biochemical and electrocardiographic monitoring.

Potassium citrate mixture 30% (2.8 mmol/ml) is of particular importance in such conditions as the Fanconi syndrome where potassium deficiency is associated with renal bicarbonate loss and the presence of a systemic acidosis. Usual daily dosage is between 2 and 5 mmol/kg body weight. If necessary, supplementary sodium bicarbonate or Albright's solution (sodium citrate/citric acid) can be employed.

Potassium chloride-containing preparations

There are several forms in which this salt may be given and it is the compound of choice for all conditions where potassium loss is accompanied by concomitant chloride deficiency – typically encountered in vomiting due to pyloric obstruction.

1. Potassium chloride solution 10% (1.35 mmol/ml) may be administered in intravenous fluids to yield concentrations around 20 mmol/l. This is based on the assumption that fluid intakes will be between 100 and 200 ml/kg/day.
2. Potassium chloride syrup (Kay-Cee-L) 1.0 mmol/ml.
3. Effervescent potassium chloride tablets (Kloref) 6.7 mmol per tablet.
4. Potassium chloride tablets ('Slow K') 8.0 mmol per tablet.

HYPERKALEMIA

The causes of hyperkalemia have already been mentioned, and it remains only to state the emergency measures which can be adopted to counteract the elevated plasma concentration until such times as renal excretion can restore normokalemia. These are as follows:

Sodium bicarbonate (1 mmol/ml): 2–3 mmol/kg body weight may be given intravenously to promote entry of potassium into the ICF.

Dextrose solution (25%): 6 ml/kg of body weight of this solution, containing soluble insulin at 1 unit per 2 g dextrose should be administered intravenously. This has an action similar to sodium bicarbonate.

Calcium gluconate (10%): 1 ml/kg body weight given intravenously counteracts the cardiac effects of the hyperkalemia.

Sodium polystyrene sulphonate resin (Resonium A): this is usually administered orally or rectally four times per day to a total dose of 0.5–1 g/kg body weight. The resin is also available in the calcium form, where sodium absorption is not desirable.

Dialysis: where the other measures have been inadequate and glomerular failure persists, either peritoneal dialysis or hemodialysis may be employed. This is seldom required.

Corticosteroids: treatment of Addisonian crisis is by intravenous hydrocortisone, and fludrocortisone with adequate water, sodium, chloride and bicarbonate intake.

ACID–BASE DISTURBANCES

Most disturbances of fluid and electrolyte metabolism are associated with changes in the acid–base state of the blood. The appropriate treatment demands understanding of the physiological and pathological processes involved in their production.

Brønsted and Lowry defined 'acid' and 'base' in terms sufficiently embracing for clinical purposes in 1923, although extension has been necessary in chemistry. In the Brønsted–Lowry terminology an 'acid' is defined as any molecule or ion which tends to donate a proton (H^+) and a 'base' is defined as any molecule or ion which tends to accept a proton (H^+).

In general: $$HB \rightleftharpoons H^+ + B^-$$ (acid ⇌ proton + base)

B^- is referred to as the conjugate base of the acid HB (conjugate acid).

The more readily an acid donates a proton the stronger it is. The more readily a base accepts a proton the stronger is the base. This implies that the acidity of a solution is directly related to its hydrogen ion concentration. A number of acid–base pairs are illustrated in Table 10.16.

From Table 10.16 several interesting features emerge:

1. Biological acids may be neutral molecules, cations or anions.
2. Biological bases may be anions or neutral molecules.
3. Water is amphoteric (i.e. acts either as an acid or a base).

$$2H_2O \rightleftharpoons H_3O^+ \text{ (very strong acid)} + OH^- \text{ (very strong base)}$$

The equilibrium favors the production of water as shown.

Alternatively, where $K = \dfrac{[H^+][B^+]}{[HB]}$ (1)

[ ] = concentration
K = equilibrium constant

Table 10.16 Acid–base pairs (modified from Robinson 1972)

		Acid	⇌	Proton	+	Conjugate base		
	Very strong	HCl	⇌	H^+	+	Cl^-	Very weak	
	↑	OH_3^+	⇌	H^+	+	H_2O		
Increasing strength		H_2CO_3	⇌	H^+	+	HCO_3^-		Increasing strength
		$H_2PO_4^-$	⇌	H^+	+	HPO_4^{2-}		
		NH_4^+	⇌	H^+	+	NH_3	↓	
	Very weak	H_2O	⇌	H^+	+	OH^-	Very strong	

K is large for strong acids and small for weak acids.

This may be rewritten $[H^+] = \dfrac{K\,[HB]}{[B^-]}$ (2)

Sorensen introduced the term pH to simplify the appreciation of the concentration of hydrogen ions in solution.

pH = the negative logarithm (to base 10) of the molal hydrogen ion activity.

Hydrogen ion activity $(H^+) = [H^+] \times f$, where f = activity coefficient.

In dilute aqueous solution $f \rightarrow 1.0$ and $(H^+) \rightarrow [H^+]$. It is, therefore, justifiable to write as an approximation:

$$-\log [H^+] = -\log K + \log \frac{[B^-]}{[HB]}$$ (3)

$$pH = -\log K + \log \frac{[B^-]}{[HB]}$$ (4)

$$pH = pK + \log \frac{[\text{conjugate base}]}{[\text{conjugate acid}]}$$ (5)

(Henderson–Hasselbalch equation), where, by analogy with pH, $pK = -\log K$.

It is obvious that with increasing acidic strength the value of K increases but the value of pK decreases, and the value of $[H^+]$ increases but the value of pH decreases.

In the case of water and all aqueous systems:

$$K_w = \frac{(H^+) \cdot (OH^-)}{H_2O}$$ (6)

and since the dissociation of water is small, H_2O may be regarded as equal to unity.

$$\therefore (\,K_w = (H^+) \cdot (OH^-)$$ (7)

K_w at 25°C = 10^{-14}
K_w at 37°C = $10^{-13.6}$

and since in pure water which is neutral:

$$H^+ = OH^-$$
$$pH\ \text{at}\ 25°C = 7.00$$
$$\text{and pH at}\ 37°C = 6.8.$$

BUFFERS

A buffer is a substance which tends to prevent a change in pH occurring within a system when either an acid or a base is added.

Biological buffer systems are composed of a solution of weak acids together with their conjugate bases. The pH of the system is defined as shown by equation (5). The addition of an acid H^+ causes conjugate base → conjugate acid and vice versa. This alters the ratio $\dfrac{[\text{conjugate base}]}{[\text{conjugate acid}]}$ and hence the pH.

For any given addition of acid or base the change in ratio will be least when:

[conjugate base] = [conjugate acid],

i.e. when $\log \dfrac{[\text{conjugate base}]}{[\text{conjugate acid}]} = 0$

A buffer system is thus most efficient when operating at a value of pH = pK for that buffer (Fig. 10.6).

At any given pH, all the buffer systems present are in equilibrium. Biological buffer systems are illustrated in Table 10.17.

The relative importance of the systems depends both on their concentrations in the body compartments concerned and on the prevailing pH values.

The bicarbonate system is the most important in plasma, with proteins and phosphate making smaller contributions. Hemoglobin is the most important buffer in erythrocytes, whilst within other cells the major buffers comprise phosphates and proteins.

Most pH measurements have been made on whole blood or plasma. Plasma separated at 37°C from the erythrocytes yields the same pH value as that obtained using the whole blood sample at 37°C. The pH for arterial blood at 37°C is 7.40 (normal range = 7.36–7.42). This means that the concentration of hydrogen ions present is $10^{-7.4}$ moles (equivalents) per liter or 0.00004 mmol/l. This is a clumsy expression and it is more convenient to use the term nanomole.

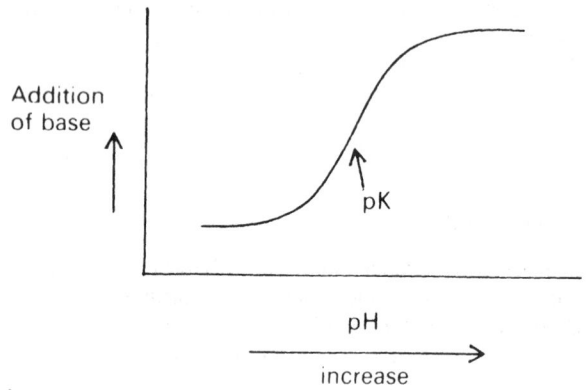

Fig. 10.6 Buffer systems.

Table 10.17 Biological buffer systems

Approximate % contribution to buffering of whole blood	Buffer acid (HB)	⇌ H⁺	+	Buffer base⁻ (B⁻)
64	H_2CO_3	⇌ H⁺	+	HCO_3^-
1	$H_2PO_4^-$	⇌ H⁺	+	HPO_4^{2-}
6	HPr	⇌ H⁺	+	Pr⁻ (Pr = protein)
29	HHB	⇌ H⁺	+	Hb⁻ (Hb = haemoglobin)
100				

1 nanomole = 10^{-9} mole

∴ pH 7.40 represents 40 nmol/l of hydrogen ions.
pH results expressed in this fashion are:

6.80 = 158 nmol/l
7.00 = 100 nmol/l
7.36 = 44 nmol/l } normal
7.42 = 38 nmol/l } range
7.80 = 16 nmol/l

} pH range which is compatible with life

Whereas the hydrogen ion concentration is fairly closely controlled under normal conditions, extreme concentrations can range from 40–400% of the normal mean. This indicates that the body is very tolerant of changes in hydrogen ion concentration. A change of 0.3 pH units is equivalent to a twofold change in the concentration of hydrogen ion.

MAINTENANCE OF A NORMAL pH

The long-term constancy of pH in any individual demands that the metabolic production of hydrogen ions be balanced by the respiratory and renal excretion of a similar amount of acid.

In an adult of 70 kg body weight some 660 liters of oxygen are utilized during the consumption of a normal diet containing 3150 calories. Since the respiratory quotient (volume CO_2 produced : volume of oxygen utilized) is about 0.8, the production of CO_2 is approximately 530 liters or 24 000 mmol/day. At the pH present in the body this would release 24 000 mmol of hydrogen ion if CO_2 were not excreted via the lungs. Clearly the control of respiration is of paramount importance in the regulation of pH.

Certain nonvolatile acids are produced during metabolism, derived principally from the sulfur contained in the methionine and cysteine of protein. On a normal protein intake the hydrogen ion from this source is excreted in the urine in combination with the conjugate bases, phosphate, creatinine and sulfate. This forms the titratable acid and ammonium in the urine, and accounts for about 80 mmol of hydrogen ion per day.

The body protects itself against pH change by:

1. dilution of any acid produced
2. buffering of any acid produced
3. regulation of respiratory rate to control plasma CO_2 tension
4. renal reabsorption of filtered bicarbonate, and excretion of excess hydrogen ion as titratable acid and ammonium salts.

PLASMA AND WHOLE BLOOD BUFFERS

The carbonic acid/bicarbonate system

Since all buffer systems are in equilibrium, it is convenient to discuss more fully the carbonic acid/bicarbonate system which is quantitatively the most important system in plasma and whole blood (see Table 10.17).

The Henderson–Hasselbalch equation applies:

$$pH = pK + \log \frac{[HCO_3^-]}{[H_2CO_3]} \qquad (8)$$

Since $CO_2 + H_2O \underset{\text{anhydrase}}{\overset{\text{carbonic}}{\rightleftharpoons}} H_2CO_3 \rightleftharpoons H^+ + HCO_3^- \qquad (9)$

the equation may be considered as:

$$pH = pK + \log \frac{\text{renal component}}{\text{respiratory component}} \qquad (10)$$

On the assumption that CO_2 dissolved in plasma is present entirely as H_2CO_3, a value $pK = pK' = 6.1$ may be taken. The equilibrium is such that only about 1/300 of the total CO_2 in physical form exists as H_2CO_3; but allowance is made for this in the value of 6.1.

Hence $\qquad pH = 6.1 + \log \frac{[HCO_3^-]}{[H_2CO_3]} \qquad (11)$

For plasma at 37°C the concentration of dissolved CO_2 + carbonic acid (= $[H_2CO_3]$ in equation (11)), expressed in mmol/l, is equal to $0.03 \times PCO_2$ (partial pressure of CO_2 in mmHg).

Thus when $\qquad PCO_2 = 40$ (5.3 kPa) $\qquad$ 1 kPa = 7.52 mm
$[H_2CO_3] = 0.03 \times 40$
$= 1.2$ mmol/l

So, if the pH = 7.40 (and $PCO_2 = 40$) then:

$$7.40 = 6.1 + \log \frac{[HCO_3^-]}{1.2} \qquad \text{from (11)}$$

∴ $\log \frac{[HCO_3^-]}{1.2} = 1.3 \qquad$ ∴ $\frac{[HCO_3^-]}{1.2} = 20,$

i.e. $[HCO_3^-] = 24$ mmol/l.
Total plasma CO_2 content

$$([H_2CO_3] + [HCO_3^-]) = 25.2 \text{ mmol/l}$$

The practical importance is that the total CO_2 content of the plasma can be measured manometrically or volumetrically and if the pH is also determined the PCO_2 may be calculated. The comparable expression in SI unitage, avoiding the use of logarithms is:

$$[H^+] \text{ (nmol/l)} = \frac{180 \times PCO_2 \text{ (kPa)}}{[HCO_3^-] \text{ (mmol/l)}} \qquad (12)$$

The erythrocyte carbonic anhydrase system

Plasma contains little carbonic anhydrase, but certain cells including erythrocytes are rich in this enzyme. This enables rapid occurrence of the reaction:

$$H_2O + CO_2 = H_2CO_3$$

in these tissues.

The importance of this in erythrocytes can be seen from the events occurring in tissues (Fig. 10.7).

The increase in CO_2 tension occurring in the transition from arterial blood (40 mmHg) to venous blood (46 mmHg) is partially offset by an increase in plasma bicarbonate. This tends to prevent the full pH change which would otherwise occur. If bicarbonate were the only buffer system present, increasing the PCO_2 experimentally from 40 to 80 mmHg would result in a fall in pH of 0.3 unit. With whole blood (in vitro) the actual pH change is approximately 0.2 unit.

The CO_2 in blood is present in physical solution (5%), as carbamino compounds (20%) and as bicarbonate (75%).

Oxyhemoglobin is more acidic than hemoglobin and for every mole of hemoglobin formed, 0.7 equivalent of hydrogen ions can be absorbed without change in pH. With a respiratory quotient of

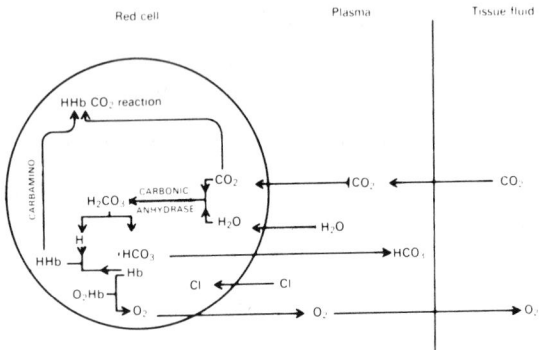

Fig. 10.7 Red blood cell carbonic anhydrase system and its importance to the tissues.

0.7, the hydrogen ions produced in the tissues could be absorbed by hemoglobin alone but the normal respiratory quotient exceeds 0.7 and use of the other buffer systems is mandatory to minimize pH change.

RESPIRATORY CONTROL OF CO_2 TENSION

Chemically, the carbonic acid bicarbonate buffer system is not ideal for maintaining pH = 7.40, since the $pK' = 6.1$ and the ratio of $\dfrac{\text{buffer base}}{\text{buffer acid}}$ at 20 : 1 is far from unity.

Fortunately the respiratory center is extremely sensitive to changes both in the CO_2 tension and the pH of plasma. This is the main reason why the system is effective physiologically in conserving blood pH within narrow limits.

RENAL HYDROGEN ION EXCRETION AND BICARBONATE RETENTION

In the renal absorption of filtered bicarbonate carbonic anhydrase

also plays a central role. Although CO_2 is fairly freely diffusible across the various membranes in the body, the bicarbonate ion may take several hours to attain access to all phases. The average adult filters about 5000 mmol bicarbonate per day at the glomeruli and if reabsorption of this is not complete, a fall in blood pH soon results. Renal tubular epithelium is rich in carbonic anhydrase. Currently it is believed that the renal cells of the proximal and distal tubules and collecting ducts are all capable of secreting hydrogen ion into the luminal fluid. The hydrogen ion is derived from tubular carbonic acid, and its secretion is related to the PCO_2 obtaining in the renal tubular cells.

Events are summarized in Figure 10.8.

Production of urine more acid or alkaline than the plasma is thus related both to the quantity of bicarbonate filtered at the glomeruli and to the amount of hydrogen ion secreted into the luminal fluid. Generally these mechanisms effectively minimize changes in the acidity of the plasma.

THE RENAL PHOSPHATE MECHANISM

In blood at pH = 7.40 the equation for the $HPO_4^{2-}/H_2PO_4^{-}$ buffer systems is such that:

$$7.40 = 6.8 + \log \frac{[HPO_4^{2-}]}{[H_2PO_4^{-}]}$$

i.e. $[HPO_4^{2-}] : [H_2PO_4^{-}] = 4 : 1$

whereas in a strongly acid urine:

$$4.6 = 6.8 + \log \frac{[HPO_4^{2-}]}{[H_2PO_4^{-}]}$$

i.e. $[HPO_4^{2-}] : [H_2PO_4^{-}] = 1 : 160$

POTASSIUM DEFICIENCY AND RENAL CONTROL OF pH

When potassium deficiency exists a paradoxically acid urine may be excreted in spite of a prevailing alkalosis in the blood. This

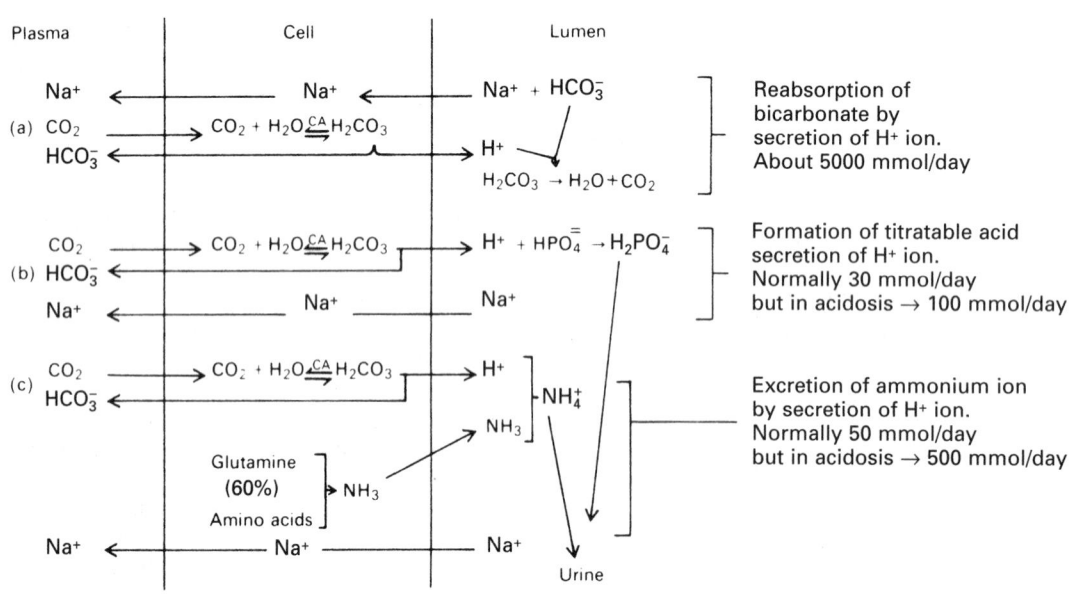

Fig. 10.8 Renal hydrogen ion secretion (CA = carbonic anhydrase).

occurs particularly when the need for renal sodium reabsorption is great.

1. Potassium depletion results in replacement intracellularly of the potassium by sodium and hydrogen ions. For every 3 mmol potassium lost from cells approximately 2 mmol sodium and 1 mmol hydrogen gain entry.
2. Intracellular acidity is increased but extracellular acidity is decreased.
3. Plasma sodium, and hence volume, tend to decrease resulting in enhanced aldosterone secretion.
4. Increased distal tubular reabsorption of sodium and bicarbonate occur in exchange for secretion of hydrogen ion and production of an acid urine ensues.

CHARACTERIZATION OF THE BLOOD ACID–BASE STATUS

The pH may be considered as being the resultant of two components, one metabolic and the other respiratory. It is important to know the respective contributions of each component in acid–base studies. The term 'buffer base' refers to the sum of the bases shown in Table 10.17. Nowadays it is usual to measure PCO_2 and PO_2 directly by means of suitable electrodes with other indices being derived by the analyzer by the use of suitable algorithms.

Indices

For the unambiguous assessment of disturbances of the acid–base metabolism, the following indices are used.

pH. Measured on arterial or arterialized capillary blood, this reflects the combined influence of metabolic and respiratory disturbances. Normal range = 7.36–7.42 (44–38 nmol H+/l) at 37°C.

Buffer base. Normal buffer base is defined as the sum of the buffer anions in the blood. At pH 7.40, PCO_2 40 mmHg and temperature 37°C it equals 41.8 + (0.4 × hemoglobin concentration in g/dl blood) = 48 nmol/l blood for hemoglobin concentration = 15.5 g/dl. Characteristic changes may occur in metabolic and respiratory disturbances.

Base excess. This is a measure of the metabolic component of blood pH. Normal range = ± 2.3 mmol/l blood. In a metabolic acidosis where nonvolatile acids such as lactic acid have accumulated to the extent of 18 mmol/l, the buffer base absorbs the hydrogen ions and falls from 48 to 30 mmol/l. The difference between the observed buffer base and the normal buffer base is called the base excess.

∴ Base excess = (30 – 48) mmol/l = – 18 mmol/l.

The negative base excess signifies an excess of nonvolatile acids. Conversely, in a metabolic alkalosis the buffer base may increase from 48 to 66 mmol/l, when the base excess = + 18 mmol/l.

In respiratory acidosis, for each moiety of H+ produced a corresponding increase in HCO_3^- occurs and total buffer base remains unaltered. A comparable situation occurs in metabolic alkalosis. Respiratory acidosis and alkalosis thus produce no change in the base excess unless renal compensation occurs.

PCO_2. This is a measure of the respiratory component of the composite acid–base status. Normal range = 35–45 mmHg (4.7–6.0 kPa).

Standard bicarbonate. This is an index of the metabolic component. It is the concentration of plasma bicarbonate in fully oxygenated blood at a PCO_2 of 40 mmHg and at 37°C. Normal range = 22–26 mmol/l plasma.

Actual bicarbonate (mmol/l plasma). This is the bicarbonate content of the plasma.

Total CO_2 content = actual bicarbonate + (PCO_2 mmHg × 0.03). This parameter is by definition a measure of both the metabolic and respiratory components of blood acid–base status. It is of interest to consider the possible effect of PCO_2 on the actual bicarbonate and total CO_2 content values, and to compare these with the unaltered standard bicarbonate (Table 10.18).

PO_2. Normal range = 80 – 100 mmHg (10.5–13.5 kPa).

Of the available indices, the most useful are pH, PCO_2, base excess and PO_2. Although it is customary to determine these indices on arterial blood, much useful information can be obtained using venous blood, provided that peripheral blood flow is reasonably good. Typical differences between arterial (capillary) and venous blood are shown in Table 10.19.

CLASSIFICATION OF DISTURBANCES

The indices already described allow any disturbance of the acid–base status to be defined both qualitatively and quantitatively (Table 10.20).

One primary cause may upset acid–base metabolism but compensation usually occurs fairly rapidly to alter the index not primarily involved. Consider a metabolic acidosis where the blood bicarbonate concentration is reduced. The pH is reduced, stimulation of the respiratory center results leading to a decrease in the PCO_2. Similarly, primary respiratory disturbances tend to be compensated by the various renal mechanisms already described. Compensation tends to offset any change in blood pH and, if fully effective, only the clinical history permits determination of the primary disturbance.

In certain circumstances more than one causal upset may be present, as in diabetes mellitus, where the initial metabolic acidosis (and respiratory compensation) are often complicated by a metabolic alkalosis occasioned by vomiting. Another multifactorial disturbance is the respiratory distress syndrome where the respiratory acidosis due to the hyaline membrane disease may be associated with a metabolic acidosis which is caused by intrapulmonary shunting of blood and resultant reduced

Table 10.18 pH versus PCO_2

PCO_2 (kPa)	2.66	5.32	10.64
H_2CO_3 (mmol/l plasma)	0.6	1.2	2.4
Actual bicarbonate (mmol/l plasma)	19	24	30.2
Total CO_2 content (mmol/l plasma)	19.6	25.2	32.6
Standard bicarbonate (mmol/l plasma)	24	24	24
pH	7.60	7.40	7.20

Table 10.19 Acid–base indices — arterial and venous bloods

	pH	PCO_2 (kPa)	Base excess (mmol/l)	PO_2 (kPa)	Oxygen saturation (%)
Arterial blood	7.40	5.32	0	12.63	96
Venous blood	7.37	6.11	+1.5*	5.32	66

* 0 if blood is arterialized in vitro, i.e. adjusted to PO_2 > 11.3 kPa.

Table 10.20   Classification of acid–base disturbances

Acidosis (excess acid or base deficit) pH = 6.80–7.36	Metabolic: base excess ≤ –2.3 mmol/l blood Respiratory: PCO_2 ≥ 45 mmHg (6.0 kPa)
Alkalosis (excess base or acid deficit) pH = 7.42–7.80	Metabolic: base excess ≥ 2.3 mmol/l blood Respiratory: PCO_2 ≤ 35 mmHg (4.7 kPa)

systemic arterial oxygen saturation. Another form of mixed primary disturbance is salicylate intoxication where the initial upset is respiratory alkalosis, and a metabolic acidosis is superimposed very soon due to the effect of salicylate on cellular metabolism. The actual acid–base status depends finally on the magnitude of each component.

Mechanisms and sequences of events in acidosis and alkalosis

The introduction or production of a nonvolatile acid (lactate, ketoacid anions, methylmalonate, etc.) causes a fall in the total buffer base. Successful respiratory compensation may occur and the pH will be normal at 7.40 but the total buffer base of the blood has been reduced, and the buffering capacity of the blood is now low (compensated metabolic acidosis). Restoration and repair of the buffer base take longer than simple compensation and are accomplished by introduction into the blood of additional bicarbonate either by the renal mechanisms previously described, or by conversion of the anion to bicarbonate when metabolism returns to normal. A rapid restoration of the buffer base content by the addition of sodium bicarbonate results in an increased plasma pH, increase in PCO_2, and a transient fall in the pH of cerebrospinal fluid. Relevant to these observations is the premise that although the control of the respiratory center is effected largely by blood PCO_2 and pH values, there may be some

contribution to this control by alteration in the pH of the cerebrospinal and intracellular fluids. This may explain why rapid correction of the metabolic acidosis in diabetes mellitus usually yields an elevated pH value due entirely to the presence of a continuing respiratory alkalosis.

By analogy, a metabolic alkalosis can be produced by the loss of hydrogen ion by vomiting, or by the introduction of bicarbonate-containing material into the body. In either event the blood pH tends to increase although the course of reactions is slightly different in each case.

$$\left. \begin{array}{l} H_2CO_3 \leftrightharpoons H^+ + HCO_3^- \\ HB \quad\quad \leftrightharpoons H^+ + B^- \end{array} \right\}$$

Loss of H^+ causes an increase in total buffer base and a reduction in H_2CO_3 (PCO_2).

$$HCO_3^- + HB \leftrightharpoons H_2CO_3 + B^-$$

Addition of bicarbonate causes an increase in total buffer base but an increase in H_2CO_3 (PCO_2).

Thereafter renal compensation causes a secondary increase or decrease in the bicarbonate and total buffer base of the blood.

In both the metabolic and respiratory upsets full renal compensation, if ever achieved, takes several days.

Listed in Table 10.21 are some of the clinical conditions associated with each disturbance.

Table 10.21   Acidosis and alkalosis – etiology

Metabolic acidosis			
Excess acid	Keto acids	{	diabetes mellitus starvation ketogenic diet
	Lactic acid	{	anoxia – cardiac arrest, RDS aerobic glycolysis – leukemia, inborn errors affecting the respiratory chain
	Sulfuric and phosphoric acids – glomerular insufficiency, with uremia unless on restriction protein intake		
	Hydrochloric acid – derived from NH_4Cl		
	Methylmalonic acid – metabolic error		
Base deficit	Loss of bicarbonate-containing fluid either via alimentary tract, by aspiration, fistulae and diarrhea or via the kidneys as in renal tubular acidosis		
Sodium chloride	Infusion of excessive amounts of saline. Although neutral, it should be remembered that the pH is acid compared to ECF		
Metabolic alkalosis	Loss of gastric hydrochloric acid (pyloric stenosis)		
	Excretion of acid urine associated with potassium depletion or following intensive diuretic therapy without overt potassium depletion		
	Ingestion of bicarbonate or other anions metabolized to bicarbonate, e.g. citrate, lactate		
Respiratory acidosis	Central or peripheral disturbances, e.g. head injury, barbiturates, morphine, poliomyelitis, asthma, cystic fibrosis, hyaline membrane disease		
Respiratory alkalosis	This is associated with hysteria, cerebral tumors, the early stages of salicylate poisoning, pulmonary edema and following certain thoracic operations		
Combined metabolic and respiratory acidosis	One of the combined types of, metabolic disturbance which can occur is associated with shock, pulmonary disease, hypothermia, cardiopulmonary bypass and cardiac arrest		

TREATMENT OF ACID–BASE DISTURBANCES

It must be decided from the history, diagnosis and the indices of blood acid–base status precisely what disturbance(s) exist(s). Therapy is then directed to cure the primary cause, e.g. pneumonia, vomiting, etc. Sometimes the clinical condition demands rapid restoration of blood acid–base status and for this purpose a variety of therapy is available.

Alkalinizing agents

Sodium bicarbonate is best administered intravenously as an 8.4% solution (1 mmol/ml), and may be added to water and saline. In emergencies it is given undiluted.

It has been shown that:

$$\text{Base excess (whole organism)} = 0.7 \times W \times \Delta \text{ total } CO_2 \text{ content} \qquad (13)$$

Δ = change in
W = body weight in kg

At constant PCO_2, Δ total CO_2
$$= \Delta \text{ standard bicarbonate} \qquad (14)$$

And Δ standard bicarbonate is approximately
$$= 0.8 \times BE \text{ (blood)} \qquad (15)$$

$\therefore$ As an approximation BE (whole organism)
$$= 0.5 \times W \times BE \text{ (blood)} \qquad (16)$$

Because of the slowness with which bicarbonate enters all compartments in the body it is inadvisable to administer rapidly the amount of bicarbonate calculated using formula (16). A similar relationship has been devised for correction of extracellular base deficits only:

$$\text{Base excess (extracellular phase)} = 0.3 \times W \times BE \text{ (blood)} \qquad (17)$$

Formula (17) provides a safe basis for the administration of bicarbonate in cases of metabolic acidosis although a paradoxical fall in the pH of CSF may occur and blood pH may enter the alkalemic range if organic acid radicals present are subsequently metabolized to bicarbonate. Certain physicians advocate treating diabetes mellitus, for instance, by supplying water, insulin, potassium and calories, and trusting that the restoration of normal metabolism will provide bicarbonate from the organic acid anions present. This is thought by some to be an injudicious form of therapy when the blood pH is less than 7.20, for the respiratory center becomes insensitive to the falling pH and there is antagonism to the action of insulin.

When hypernatremic dehydration coexists with metabolic acidosis the certainty of increasing the plasma sodium level must be weighed against the possible benefit of intravenous sodium bicarbonate as an alkalinizing agent.

Sodium lactate is normally administered as an M/6 solution prepared from a molar solution (1 mmol/ml) of 11.2%. This material must theoretically penetrate into cells before being converted to bicarbonate. Thus one of the known deficiencies of sodium bicarbonate is obviated. It is of no value when acidosis is due to increased concentrations of lactic acid, as in anoxia, when sodium bicarbonate should be employed.

The treatment of respiratory acidosis by alkali therapy poses some problems. In a partially compensated pure respiratory acidosis the base excess value is already positive and the only justification for bicarbonate is if the blood pH is still very low. This is unusual unless metabolic acidosis is also present.

Acidifying agents

Ammonium chloride is administered as a 5.35% solution (1 mmol/ml) and is generally added in the calculated dose to a solution of saline or glucose. The ammonia (NH_3) of the ammonium chloride (NH_4Cl) is metabolized in the body to urea and it is the hydrochloric acid remaining which corrects the alkalosis. Such therapy would be contraindicated in the presence of hepatic insufficiency. In pediatric practice it is seldom necessary to employ this agent since treatment with potassium chloride, although slower, is usually adequate.

When it is deemed advisable to correct the alkalosis more rapidly than can be accomplished using potassium chloride, the dosage of ammonium chloride can be determined from equation (17). Ammonium chloride corrects an alkalosis without renal involvement, the excess bicarbonate being converted to carbonic acid and the chloride remaining to maintain electroneutrality.

Potassium chloride is usually available as a 10% (1.35 mmol/ml) or 15% (2 mmol/ml) solution to be added to solutions of glucose or saline in the required amounts.

This treatment is especially useful when a metabolic alkalosis is accompanied by potassium depletion as occurs in vomiting with loss of gastric secretions. Severe potassium depletion can cause potassium deficiencies approaching 21 mmol/kg body weight. Theoretically the intracellular potassium so lost is replaced by sodium and hydrogen in the molar ratio 2 : 1. This means that restoration of the intracellular potassium will release 7 mmol/kg of hydrogen ion into the extracellular fluid. It is interesting to apply equation (17) in the case of a severe metabolic alkalosis with a base excess of + 25 mmol/l blood. The amount of hydrogen ion so calculated as necessary for therapy is 7.5 mmol/kg body weight.

In severe potassium depletion it is usually safe to administer potassium chloride in an amount not exceeding 3 mmol/kg body weight/day provided that urinary output is good. A larger dose may be required when excessive potassium loss continues, but therapy should be monitored by following the plasma potassium concentrations and by electrocardiography.

Clinical judgment and laboratory assessment

Careful assessment is an essential prerequisite to proper handling of electrolyte and water upsets. The first priorities are an adequate history of the disorder and skilled examination of the child. On this will depend the extent and celerity of investigation and the intensiveness of the treatment of that particular child. Investigation of the blood chemistry should be performed whenever intravenous therapy is considered necessary and should include the determination of urea, creatinine, electrolytes, pH, PO_2, PCO_2, base excess, osmolality, hemoglobin and PCV. The volume of the urine should be checked, and the electrolyte content, urea, pH and osmolality measured. Whilst it is helpful if accurate urine collections can be obtained to calculate electrolyte excretion, the simple expedient of relating sodium and potassium concentrations to urinary creatinine content can provide useful information when only casual urine specimens are available. In hypernatremia the state of the patient may mandate lumbar puncture, or potassium upset demand electrocardiography.

Further assessment both clinically and biochemically should be made when response to treatment can be assessed. One simple expedient is the practice of weighing the patient. An experienced clinician, given a good history of a child with reasonable renal function, can treat the majority of cases effectively with little or no laboratory help. In developing countries where gastroenteritis and other forms of diarrhea are rife this is the rule rather than the exception. On the other hand, by biochemical assessment invaluable information may be obtained on difficult problems and important and unexpected data provided in relation to the most apparently mundane case. Since delays often compound, one should never delay starting treatment in a seriously dehydrated or collapsed patient in order to obtain laboratory results. Commence with a plasma infusion or half-strength physiological saline in 5% dextrose pending the results of laboratory specimens.

REFERENCES AND BIBLIOGRAPHY

Arneil G C, Chin K C 1979 Lower-solute milks and reduction of hypernatraemia in young Glasgow infants. Lancet ii: 840

Astrup P, Jorgensen K, Siggaard-Andersen O, Engel K 1960 The acid base metabolism. A new approach. Lancet i: 1035–1039

Breyer M D, Ando Y 1994 Hormonal signalling and regulation of salt and water transport in the collecting duct. Annual Review of Physiology 56: 711–739

Bruck E, Guner A, Aceto T 1968 Therapy of infants with hypertonic dehydration due to diarrhea. American Journal of Diseases of Children 115: 281

Dluhy R G (ed) 1995 Clinical disorders of fluid and electrolyte metabolism. Endocrinology and Metabolism Clinics of North America 24(3): 459–662

Graham J A, Lamb J F, Linton A L 1967 Measurement of body water and intracellular electrolytes by means of muscle biopsy. Lancet ii: 1172–1176

Kunau R T, Stein J H 1977 Disorders of hypo- and hyperkalaemia. Clinical Nephrology 7: 173

Maclaurin J C 1966 Changes in body water distribution during the first two weeks of life. Archives of Disease in Childhood 41: 286–291

Robinson J R 1972 Fundamentals of acid–base regulation. Blackwell, Oxford

Rose B D 1984 Clinical physiology of acid–base and electrolyte disorders, 2nd edn. McGraw-Hill, New York

Sabolic I, Brown D 1995 Water channels in renal and nonrenal tissues. News in Physiological Sciences 10: 12–17

Shires G T 1988 Fluids, electrolytes and acid–base. Churchill Livingstone, Edinburgh

11 Disorders of the alimentary tract and liver

Chapter editor: W. M. Bisset

Introduction   423
Gastrointestinal function   423
The nature of gastrointestinal disease   424
The mouth   424
The esophagus   425
The stomach and duodenum   430
The small intestine   435
Malabsorption   439
Inborn errors of digestion and absorption   445
Investigation of the small intestine   447
Gastrointestinal tumors   448
The pancreas   449
Disorders of gastrointestinal motility   451
Acute infective diarrhea   451
W. M. Bisset
Protracted diarrhea in early infancy   454
The colon   455
Inflammatory bowel disease   456

Chronic gastrointestinal symptoms   460
H. R. Jenkins
Failure to thrive   465
Nutrition in patients with gastrointestinal disease   469
W. M. Bisset
Hepatic and biliary disease   470
Assessment of suspected liver disease   471
Hepatitis syndrome in infancy   473
Disorders requiring urgent surgical treatment   475
Viral hepatitis   476
Nonviral infections   478
Acute liver failure   478
Chronic liver disease   480
Cirrhosis   481
Liver tumors   484
Liver transplantation   484
A. P. Mowat   A. J. Baker
Self-help and research groups   485
References   485

INTRODUCTION

Optimum growth and development is dependent on the normal functioning of the gastrointestinal tract and of the liver. When this activity is deranged the child will develop symptoms of gastrointestinal disease and as a consequence will frequently fail to thrive.

The gastrointestinal tract extends from the mouth to the anus and is structurally and functionally divided into the mouth, oropharynx, esophagus, stomach, small intestine and colon (Table 11.1). Following the ingestion of food by the mouth the bolus is moved by the oropharynx into the esophagus which acts as a conduit for the transfer of food to the stomach where it is stored and mixed prior to its controlled passage into the small intestine. In the small intestine the food is digested and absorbed before moving on into the large intestine where salt and water are conserved prior to excretion. This simplified view of gastrointestinal function disguises the very complex nature of the many systems which interact to give normal intestinal function (Muller 1988).

GASTROINTESTINAL FUNCTION

DIGESTION

Ingested food consists almost exclusively of large macro-molecules which the intestinal tract is unable to absorb without prior digestion. Complex carbohydrates are broken down into their component monosaccharides, fats with the help of the emulsifying activity of bile salts are digested to free fatty acids and monoacylglycerol and proteins are dismantled into dipeptides and amino acids. The digestive enzymes act mainly within the lumen of the stomach and small intestine although the process is completed for carbohydrate and protein by small intestinal brush border disaccharidases and dipeptidases.

Table 11.1 The function of the gastrointestinal tract

Section of gut	Function
Mouth	Grinding of food by teeth Lubrication and partial digestion by salivary secretions
Oropharynx	Move food into esophagus Protect airway
Esophagus	Propulsive conduit for food Clearance of regurgitated food Prevention of reflux
Stomach	Store for food Gastric acid production Pepsin production
Small intestine	Digestion of food Absorption of food Immune tolerance
Terminal ileum	Absorption of vitamin B_{12} Absorption of bile salts
Pancreas	Digestive enzyme production Bicarbonate production
Colon	Reabsorption of luminal fluid Storage and excretion of feces

TRANSPORT

Discrete transport processes are present within the epithelial cells of the intestinal tract to promote the absorption of nutrients, salts and water by some cells and the excretion of salt and water by others. Many of these processes are dependent on the electrochemical gradient across the cell wall created by the Na^+/K^+ ATPase ion pump. This generates a low Na^+ concentration and a negative charge within epithelial cells and on transmembrane proteins, which facilitate the movement of specific ions and solutes across the lipophilic cell membrane.

MOTILITY

The movement of food along the gut is integrated with, and related to, the function of each section of the intestine. The rate of emptying of nutrients from the stomach is closely controlled to prevent overloading of the small intestine. Specific patterns of fasting motor activity have developed in the small intestine to clear the lumen of food debris after meals and highly developed control mechanisms are present to facilitate the controlled emptying of the distal colon and rectum at the time of defecation.

IMMUNITY

The gastrointestinal tract serves as the interface between ingested elements from the external environment and the internal milieu of the individual. By a combination of immunological and nonimmunological mechanisms the entry of noxious substances such as bacteria, viruses and undigested food protein is prevented. The development of tolerance to the foreign proteins of commonly ingested food is vital to the normal functioning of the gut.

ENDOCRINE

The gastrointestinal tract is a major endocrine organ and many regulatory peptides with endocrine, paracrine and neurocrine functions are released along the length of the intestine. The function of many of these peptides is poorly understood although it is clear that they have an important role in modulating intestinal secretion, growth and motor function.

A more detailed description of the anatomy and physiology of the intestinal tract is given in subsequent sections of this chapter.

THE NATURE OF GASTROINTESTINAL DISEASE

Normal intestinal function requires the combined action of each of the functional systems described above and if any one should break down intestinal function will be compromised. An understanding of the basic physiology of these systems is important when one is interpreting symptoms of gastrointestinal disease and planning the rational investigation of these problems.

Diarrheal disease will develop if, as a consequence of maldigestion or active secretion, there is an increased effluent of fluid passing into the colon from the small intestine or if the absorptive capacity of the colon is compromised by disease. Loss of normal intestinal motility will result in the development of symptoms of obstruction and where a defect of mucosal immunity is present recurrent enteric infection is likely to occur. Damage to

the digestive or absorptive capacity of the small intestine will result in failure of the patient to grow adequately.

The major gastrointestinal diseases of childhood are described in this chapter along with an outline of their management. The main symptoms of gut disease and their investigation are also discussed.

THE MOUTH

The mouth is responsible for the grinding of food into small fragments, through the voluntary action of the tongue and jaw, prior to its passage into the esophagus. In addition, the fragments are mixed with salivary secretions which help lubricate the food and initiate digestion, through the action of salivary amylase and lingual lipase. Any disease of the mouth which makes feeding painful or compromises the normal process of deglutition is likely to lead to difficulties with feeding.

While most oral lesions are the result of local disease, both gastrointestinal and systemic disease may result in abnormalities within the mouth (Rule 1991). It is therefore important to look closely at the mouth in all children undergoing physical examination.

THE LIPS

Unilateral or bilateral clefts of the upper lip are among the most common of congenital malformations and are frequently found in combination with a cleft of the palate (see Ch. 31). Dryness of the lips with cracking may be due to mouth breathing, and fissure formation at the angle of the mouth may result from chronic drooling in children with swallowing disorders. Nutritional deficiencies of iron, zinc and riboflavin may all produce an angular stomatitis.

Edema of the lips may occur as part of an immediate hypersensitivity reaction following the direct contact of the lips with a sensitized protein or as part of the systemic response in anaphylaxis. In Crohn's disease intermittent swelling of the lips may be associated with cobblestone ulceration of the buccal mucosa.

THE ORAL MUCOSA

Ulceration to the buccal mucosa occurs most commonly in healthy individuals as a result of recurrent aphthae. These may be precipitated by local trauma and heal spontaneously within 2 weeks. More persistent ulcers may occur in chronically debilitated patients, children with poor dental hygiene and as mentioned above in inflammatory bowel disease. Extensive ulceration of the oral mucosa in association with lesions on the perineum are seen in Stevens–Johnson syndrome and less commonly in Behçet's syndrome.

Abnormal pigmentation may be seen in Addison's disease and Albright's syndrome; in Peutz–Jeghers syndrome there is freckling of the lips and buccal mucosa and in lead, mercury and bismuth poisoning pigmented lines are sometimes seen near the dental margin of the gums. Koplik's spots are characteristically present in measles, palatal petechiae may be seen in rubella and oral vesicles in chickenpox can make feeding very uncomfortable.

The most common infections involving the mucosa are herpes stomatitis and thrush. Primary herpes infection occurs most commonly in children between the ages of 1 and 3 years and presents with pyrexia, lymphadenopathy and the eruption of vesicular lesions on the buccal mucosa, lips and on the skin below the mouth. The vesicles burst forming painful ulcers making the ingestion of solids and liquids very uncomfortable. Although the condition is self-limiting, with a course of 7–10 days, this may be shortened by treatment with oral acyclovir.

Oral candidiasis or thrush commonly occurs in young babies who become infected in the neonatal period but may also develop in patients on broad spectrum antibiotics, inhaled steroids or in patients who are immunosuppressed. Gut carriage may also lead to infection of the napkin area. Treatment is with a topical antifungal such as nystatin.

THE GUMS

Infection of the gums in children most commonly results from poor oral hygiene and leads to inflammation of the free margin of the gingiva. Hypertrophy of the gums is a common side effect of phenytoin treatment and may also be rarely seen in Langerhans cell histiocytosis (see Ch. 16). Bleeding of the gums may be secondary to local infection but will also occur in children with bleeding diatheses and in nutritionally compromised patients who are vitamin C deficient.

THE TONGUE

Macroglossia occurs in hypothyroidism, as part of generalized visceral enlargement in Beckwith's syndrome and in glycogen storage disease type II. A normal-sized tongue may appear to be enlarged if the oral cavity is small as in children with Down syndrome. The tongue can also be enlarged by a lymphangioma or a hemangioma and a mass in the region of the foramen cecum may be due to a lingual thyroid.

The surface of the tongue becomes coated in children with poor oral hygiene and in patients with dehydration. In scarlet fever the tongue is first white and coated and then becomes red, hence the name 'strawberry tongue'. In familial dysautonomia the tongue is smooth due to the absence of papillae and in congenital familial telangiectasia the vascular abnormality may be clearly seen. The focal loss of papillae leads to the so-called 'geographical tongue', a benign self-limiting condition.

THE TEETH

The primary dentition usually erupts at about 6 months but in hypothyroidism, hypopituitarism, rickets, congenital syphilis and cleidocranial dysostosis this can be delayed. Premature shedding of these teeth is likely to occur in hypophosphatasia and in mercury poisoning. The enamel of the teeth will become hypoplastic as a result of such insults as prematurity, kernicterus, vitamin D deficiency and from congenital infections such as rubella and syphilis. Similarly the shape of the teeth may be abnormal as a consequence of congenital infection (notched incisors in congenital syphilis) or in ectodermal dysplasias where the teeth may be peg shaped.

A black staining of the teeth can occur with oral iron, a brown discoloration occurs with congenital defects of enamel and dentine, in congenital porphyria the teeth are a purplish brown and in neonatal unconjugated hyperbilirubinemia a green staining may be left. The administration of tetracycline to a mother after the fourth month of pregnancy or to the infant in the first year of life will result in yellow discoloration of the primary dentition and administration up to the age of 7 years will effect the permanent dentition.

THE SALIVARY GLANDS

With the exception of mumps, inflammation or enlargement of the salivary gland is uncommon in childhood. Acute bacterial parotitis may occur in the neonate or debilitated child and is characterized by a unilateral swollen tender parotid gland. Infection with *Staphylococcus aureus* is generally responsible and treatment with flucloxacillin is required.

Recurrent parotitis either uni- or bilateral may occur where the symptoms are generally mild and not associated with systemic upset. Treatment with parotid massage and stimulants of salivary flow such as chewing gum along with oral penicillin are generally helpful. The condition is self-limiting and generally resolves by puberty. Less commonly, recurrent pain and infection may be precipitated by salivary stones.

THE ESOPHAGUS

STRUCTURE AND FUNCTION

The esophagus is a long narrow muscular tube which connects the oropharynx and stomach providing a conduit for the passage of food. The lumen of the esophagus is lined by a stratified squamous epithelium and is encircled by an inner circular and an outer longitudinal layer of muscle. The muscle of the upper third of the esophagus is striated and is dependent on extrinsic innervation from the vagus nerve while the muscle in the lower third is smooth muscle and is under the influence of both intrinsic and extrinsic controls. The muscle of the middle third forms a transitional zone. Two high pressure zones are found along the length of the esophagus, one at the proximal end forms the upper esophageal sphincter and the other at the distal end forms the lower esophageal sphincter.

Deglutition

After food has been chewed and mixed with saliva a bolus of food is isolated and pushed back, between the tongue and the hard palate, towards the pharynx at the same time as the soft palate is raised to close off the nasopharynx. As the food enters the oropharynx an involuntary reflex is initiated whose afferent limb is transmitted along the glossopharyngeal nerve and the superior laryngeal branch of the vagal nerve to the medulla. Efferent impulses from the facial, glossopharyngeal, vagus, accessory and hypoglossal nerves result in contraction of the pharyngeal muscles and relaxation of the upper esophageal sphincter with movement of the bolus of food onward into the upper esophagus. Entry of food into the larynx is prevented by cessation of respiration, elevation of the larynx and closure of the glottis.

Given the very complicated nature of this reflex and its reliance on many cranial nerve nuclei within the brainstem it is perhaps not surprising that central nervous system disorders which result in the development of bulbar or pseudobulbar palsies will disturb the swallowing reflex; similarly any anatomical disorder of the pharyngeal apparatus (i.e. Pierre–Robin or cleft palate) will disrupt normal feeding (Table 11.2). Disordered deglutition is also likely to result in the nasopharyngeal regurgitation of food and the

Table 11.2 A list of the causes of dysphagia

1. Anatomical abnormalities
    a. Cleft palate
    b. Micrognathia (Pierre Robin)
    c. Macroglossia
    d. Cysts, tumors and diverticulae of the pharynx
    e. Esophageal atresia
    f. Esophageal stricture
        (i) Anastomotic
        (ii) Corrosive
        (iii) Reflux esophagitis
    g. Esophageal compression
        (i) Aortic arch anomaly
        (ii) Mediastinal tumor
        (iii) Esophageal duplication

2. Neuromuscular
    a. Prematurity
    b. Cerebral palsy of any type
    c. Bulbar or pseudobulbar palsies
    d. Isolated cranial nerve paralysis or agenesis
    e. Familial dysautonomia (Riley–Day syndrome)
    f. Achalasia
    g. Esophageal dysmotility (i.e. spasm)
    h. Myasthenia gravis or dystrophica myotonica

3. Inflammatory/trauma
    a. Stomatitis
    b. Acute tonsillopharyngitis
    c. Esophagitis
        (i) Reflux
        (ii) Corrosive
        (iii) Infective (i.e. candida)
    d. Foreign body

4. Behavioral
    a. Rumination
    b. Globus hystericus

aspiration of ingested food into the lungs. This reflex develops in the neonate at approximately 34 weeks' gestation.

Oromotor coordination develops throughout the first year of life to accommodate the many food consistencies and textures experienced by the child after weaning. If inappropriate foods are given, which fail to match the child's oromotor development, feeding may become difficult and lead to the development of behavioral problems at meal times.

Esophageal peristalsis

During primary peristaltic activity pressure waves of 50–80 mmHg (7–11 kPa) propagate down the esophagus, pushing the bolus of food at a velocity of 2–5 cm/s. A marked reduction in magnitude and propagation velocity of this activity is seen in cerebral palsied children with severe gastroesophageal reflux. Secondary peristaltic activity which develops in response to distention of the esophagus and plays an important role in clearing regurgitated gastric contents back into the stomach is also compromised in children with neurological disease. Tertiary peristaltic activity occurs spontaneously and may be responsible for the pain induced by esophageal spasm.

Lower esophageal sphincter

The lower esophageal sphincter is a zone of raised pressure (20 mmHg (3 kPa)), just proximal to the gastroesophageal junction which has a central role in the control of the reflux of gastric

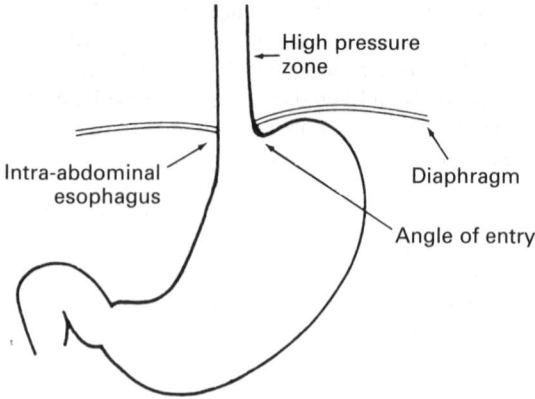

Fig. 11.1 The factors which contribute to the normal function of the lower esophageal sphincter. (From Brueton et al 1988, reproduced by kind permission of John Wiley and Son Ltd.)

contents into the esophagus. The lower esophageal sphincter shows maturational changes with pressures rising from as low as 5 mmHg (0.7 kPa) at 30 weeks' postconceptual age up to the adult level of 20 mmHg (3 kPa) by the first year of life (Newell 1988).

The effectiveness of the lower esophageal sphincter as an antireflux barrier depends also on a number of anatomical factors which assist the sphincteric smooth muscle. A length of intra-abdominal esophagus potentiates the high pressure zone of the sphincter, the acute angle between the esophagus and fundus of the stomach forms a flap valve which closes as the intragastric pressure rises and the crura of the diaphragm press on the lower esophagus. These mechanisms are illustrated in Figure 11.1. Loss of the normal anatomy of the gastroesophageal junction as occurs in patients with sliding hiatus hernias severely disrupts these mechanisms and increases the likelihood of gastroesophageal reflux.

DYSPHAGIA

Diagnosis

The diagnosis of dysphagia can be made by taking a detailed clinical history and by careful observation of the child feeding. Nasal regurgitation of liquids in the absence of vomiting is suggestive of nasopharyngeal reflux and coughing and choking during feeding is very suggestive of aspiration into the larynx. As a consequence the child may develop recurrent chest infections due to aspiration or, because of the difficulty in ingesting an adequate calorie intake, the child may fail to thrive.

Many of the anatomical abnormalities will be obvious on inspection (Table 11.2) and most neuromuscular disorders will be associated with other neurological sequelae such as cerebral palsy. Inspection of the mouth by a speech therapist will give insight into the level of oromotor coordination; video fluoroscopy (except esophageal atresia) will define the degree of pharyngeal coordination during swallowing and the motility of the esophagus and will determine whether aspiration or nasopharyngeal regurgitation has occurred. A chest X-ray will show signs of an aspiration pneumonia or mediastinal space occupation and laryngoscopy and esophagoscopy will allow direct visualization of any motor incoordination, foreign bodies or strictures that may be present.

Treatment

The management of dysphagia depends very much on the underlying cause. Great care and attention is needed with feeding technique but in some patients the airway has to be protected by instituting nasogastric or gastrostomy feeding. Neuromuscular disorders of swallowing are also frequently associated with severe gastroesophageal reflux and in conditions such as cerebral palsy and familial dysautonomia an antireflux procedure such as a Nissen fundoplication is frequently required in addition to a gastrostomy.

GASTROESOPHAGEAL REFLUX

Gastroesophageal reflux is the passive regurgitation of gastric contents into the esophagus and should not be confused with vomiting, which is an active process and requires the contraction of the diaphragm and abdominal muscles to initiate the event (Orenstein 1993). Gastroesophageal reflux will result if there is incompetence of the sphincteric mechanisms at the gastroeso-

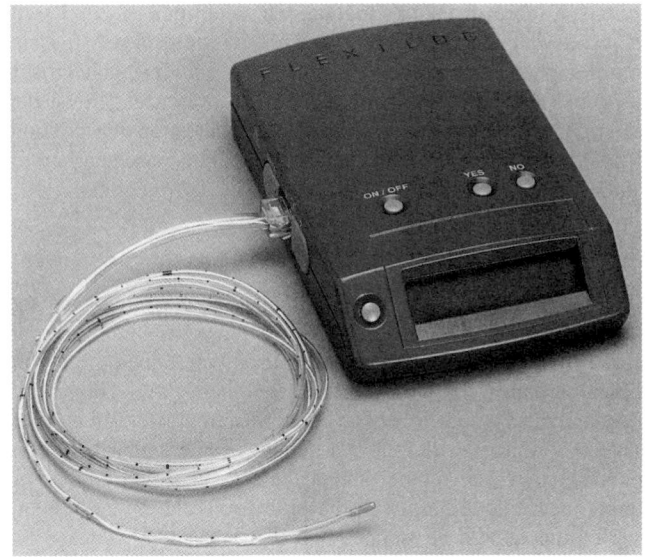

(a)

phageal junction or if raised intragastric or intra-abdominal pressures are able to overcome this mechanism. It is clear that the lower esophageal sphincter is poorly developed in the very young infant and that the formation of a sliding hiatus hernia severely limits the competence of the sphincter. Similarly in conditions where gastric emptying is delayed or in chronic respiratory diseases, such as cystic fibrosis, where coughing increases intra-abdominal pressure, gastroesophageal reflux is exacerbated.

With the recent development of prolonged ambulatory recordings of intraesophageal pH (Fig. 11.2) it has become clear that gastroesophageal reflux is a physiological phenomenon which occurs in all individuals for between 1 and 5% of any 24-h period with the majority occurring in the postprandial periods. Whether gastroesophageal reflux is deemed to be trivial or pathological is dependent on many factors of which the parents' perception of the problem, the absolute level of reflux and the development of any complicating sequelae are important (Glassman et al 1995).

It has been shown that in normal individuals reflux most commonly occurs as the child is swallowing and the lower esophageal sphincter is relaxing to allow the passage of food into the stomach (Mahoney et al 1988). During these brief 'unguarded moments' ingested food and acid pass into the lower esophagus where a secondary peristaltic wave promptly clears the food back into the stomach. If, however, esophageal peristalsis is deranged the contact time of gastric acid on the esophageal mucosa will be prolonged. In a patient with very severe reflux, spontaneous relaxations of the lower esophageal sphincter occur throughout the day leading to many more 'unguarded moments'. The most troublesome reflux occurs in patients with cerebral palsy or previous esophageal surgery where disordered innervation of the esophagus leads to increased spontaneous relaxation of the sphincter and poor peristaltic clearing mechanisms.

Clinical features

The passive regurgitation of milk occurs in the majority of newborn babies and is accepted by most mothers as being a normal feature of infancy. With time the problem steadily improves and with the introduction of solids and the development

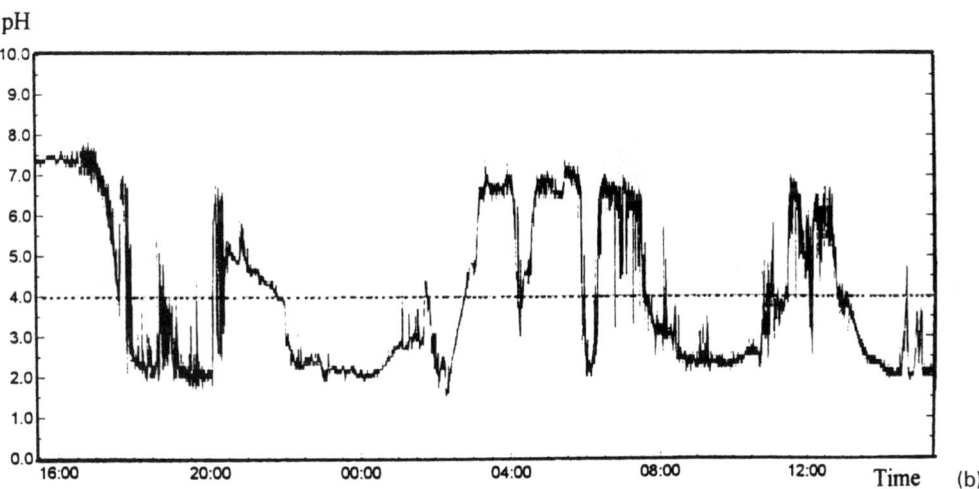

(b)

Fig. 11.2 (a) A solid state 24-h pH recorder with recording electrode. (b) A trace from a 24-h pH recording showing frequent reflux episodes with the pH dropping below 4.0. The time is shown along the base.

of a more upright posture the problem clears in almost all cases (Carre 1959, Johnston et al 1995). Problems, however, develop where the mother is inexperienced or stressed and has difficulty coping with the problem or where complications such as esophagitis, aspiration or failure to thrive occur.

In most children with reflux the volume of milk which is lost with each regurgitation is insignificant but in some children the intake is severely compromised and as a consequence weight gain is poor. With the prolonged contact of gastric acid on the esophageal mucosa an esophagitis may develop. This may present clinically as blood in the vomit or more insidiously with the development of anemia or stricture. Older children may complain of heartburn with reflux while smaller infants may develop feeding difficulties due to esophageal discomfort.

Aspiration in cerebral palsied children is very common, due to an inability to protect the upper airway from food during both swallowing and regurgitation. When considering the differential diagnosis for children with recurrent cough or respiratory tract infections, one must include gastroesophageal reflux. A bizarre presentation of gastroesophageal reflux has been described (Sandifer syndrome) where reflux episodes are associated with dystonic movements of the neck (Sutcliffe 1969). The clinical clue is that these episodes occur after meals and it has been postulated that stimulation of vagal afferents by the falling esophageal pH results in reflex stimulation of the spinal accessory nerve with the resulting contraction of the sternomastoid.

Although most children with reflux present in the first year of life there are some who present later with symptoms of heartburn or vomiting and a small group who though apparently symptom free through most of their lives present with a peptic stricture of the esophagus (Fig. 11.3). There is also the occasional child who will present outwith the first 2 years of life with the precipitous

development of severe gastroesophageal reflux in whom detailed investigation may reveal the presence of a posterior fossa tumor.

In children with reflux there may also be longer-term behavioral sequelae which can frequently lead to major management problems. Some children are reluctant to eat, particularly solids, and as a consequence feeding problems develop which may last long after the reflux has apparently cleared. Other children who find it easy to reflux are able to regurgitate at will and use this as a powerful attention-seeking tool. A small number of children develop the ability to ruminate, a condition which is generally associated with prolonged periods of reflux.

Diagnosis

In the majority of cases the diagnosis is made clinically from the history of effortless vomiting occurring after meals. Where this picture is unclear or where symptoms suggest a more severe problem, further investigation is required. Unfortunately no single investigation provides all the information which is required. A 24 h pH study will quantify the degree of reflux (Fig. 11.2) (ESPGAN 1993); a barium meal will tell you if there is a hiatus hernia or more distal obstruction (i.e. malrotation) but it will frequently fail to show reflux even when it is quite clearly present. A full blood count should also be done and if esophagitis is suspected an endoscopy is required. The presence of fat-laden macrophages in the sputum will help in the detection of aspiration. A fuller discussion of esophageal investigations is given later in this section.

Treatment (Table 11.3)

Although it is possible to differentiate between physiological and pathological reflux by using 24-h pH studies, it is likely that in most children treatment decisions will be determined largely on clinical grounds. In an otherwise well baby who is growing adequately and who is free of any complicating features it is likely that the condition will follow a benign course and will resolve spontaneously. The mother should be reassured and advised of simple measures to help with the problem. If the infant is being overfed this should be stopped and if over 3 months of age the introduction of solids should be encouraged. There is generally no need to alter the child's feed but where there is a strong family history of atopy or signs of eczema the introduction of a hypoallergenic feed may be indicated. As the consistency of the feed seems to influence the degree of reflux, thickening agents are found to be helpful in many babies. Alginate compounds are sometimes also found to relieve symptoms.

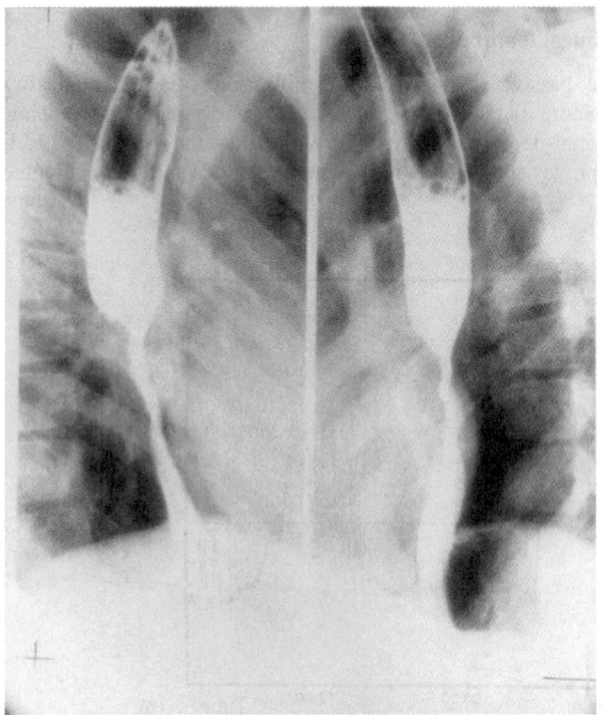

Fig. 11.3 A barium swallow showing a peptic stricture of the esophagus with the delayed passage of barium.

Table 11.3 Treatment for children with gastroesophageal reflux (see text for details)

Clinical condition	Treatment
Very mild reflux	Mother reassured Simple feeding advice
Moderate reflux	Thickened feeds Prokinetic drugs
Reflux with esophagitis	Add histamine 2 blockers Proton pump inhibitor
Failure of medical treatment	Fundoplication
Esophagitis with stricture	Fundoplication with dilation

Traditionally it was advised that children with reflux should be kept sitting upright in a chair but it is likely that this may increase intra-abdominal pressure and exacerbate the problem. More recently the prone position with the head raised (Vanderplas & Sacre-Smits 1985) has been suggested but in view of the fact that this position may increase the risk of sudden infant death syndrome it is clearly not to be recommended. The left lateral position has also been suggested but maintaining a small child for any length of time in any given position is likely to be very difficult.

Where these simple measures fail to reduce the reflux the use of prokinetic agents should be considered. Drugs such as domperidone or cisapride all appear to be of some clinical benefit in reducing reflux. They all increase the rate of gastric emptying and it has been postulated that they also increase the lower esophageal sphincter pressure. They do, however, have to be taken continuously to be effective.

In patients with esophagitis, measures in addition to those described above have to be taken. Histamine 2 (H_2) blocking drugs such as cimetidine or ranitidine, or proton pump inhibitors such as omeprazole, will raise the pH of the regurgitated food and seem to help in the healing of esophagitis. It is, however, unclear how long and in what dose this treatment should be continued as suitable controlled trials have yet to be carried out and a suitable formulation of proton pump inhibitor for children does not exist. Antacids have no place in the treatment of esophagitis as the amount required to adequately alkalinize the gastric juices would be likely to lead to salt overload.

Where medical management fails to control complications and gastroesophageal reflux persists, a surgical antireflux procedure is indicated (Kazerooni et al 1994). Where stricture formation has already occurred this should be combined with dilation of the stricture. It is important that these procedures are carried out by an experienced pediatric surgeon as the operation may be complicated by postvagotomy or gas bloat syndromes.

A suggested plan of treatment for patients with gastroesophageal reflux is shown in Table 11.3.

ACHALASIA

Achalasia of the cardia results from a failure of the lower end of the esophagus to relax with swallowing with the development of dysphagia, regurgitation, retrosternal discomfort and weight loss. This functional obstruction is caused by neurodegenerative changes in the enteric nerves of the esophagus.

The condition is very uncommon in childhood and may be confused with a peptic stricture in young children and anorexia nervosa in older children. An autosomal recessive form occurs which is associated with hypoadrenalism and absent tear production.

The diagnosis is confirmed by the barium swallow appearance of esophageal dilation with a funnel-shaped narrowing at the lower end and by esophageal manometry which demonstrates disturbed peristaltic activity in the body with increased basal tone and failure of relaxation of the lower esophageal sphincter.

The condition is generally progressive and is treated either by pneumatic dilation of the lower esophageal sphincter or by Heller's cardiomyotomy. Dilation procedures frequently have to be repeated more than once and effective treatment of the achalasia may lead to the development of gastroesophageal reflux. For this reason a myotomy and fundoplication procedure are frequently combined (Buick & Spitz 1985).

ESOPHAGEAL INVESTIGATIONS

A number of esophageal investigations are available but unfortunately no single test is likely to give all the information that is required to resolve a clinical problem. Each test gives information on a specific aspect of esophageal structure or function and it is necessary for tests to be combined for an overall picture to be obtained (Table 11.4).

Barium studies

Traditionally the barium swallow has been the investigation of choice in children with gastroesophageal reflux. While it is true that contrast studies give good information on the anatomy of the esophagus and the gastroesophageal junction it is a very insensitive test for reflux and the mucosal changes of esophagitis will only show if they are well advanced. Video studies are useful in detecting abnormalities of motor coordination and motility disturbances of the body of the esophagus. It is important that screening is continued until contrast has passed into the jejunum as abnormalities of gastric emptying or malrotation will otherwise be missed.

Gastroesophageal scintigraphy

Scintiscanning using technetium-99m-labeled milk has been shown to be more sensitive in detecting reflux than barium studies and with prolonged scans gastric emptying can be measured and bronchial aspiration of the milk can be detected. The method, however, requires the patient to remain still for up to 30 min on a gamma camera and gives very little anatomical information.

Esophageal manometry

This technique is presently available only in a few pediatric centers and its clinical uses are limited to the diagnosis of the less common conditions such as achalasia and esophageal spasm. The measurement of lower esophageal sphincter pressure is a very insensitive indicator of gastroesophageal reflux.

Esophageal pH monitoring

The prolonged ambulatory recording of esophageal pH using catheter-mounted electrodes has revolutionized the measurement of gastroesophageal reflux and is now accepted as the 'gold standard' for the detection of reflux in childhood (Fig. 11.2). Modern computerized systems allow the length of time and the number of episodes of reflux to be measured and their division

Table 11.4 Investigations of esophageal structure and function

Test	Uses
Barium studies*	Define anatomy of upper GI tract
Scintiscanning	For the detection of reflux and aspiration (not as sensitive as pH studies)
Manometry	Detect achalasia or esophageal spasm
pH monitoring*	Most sensitive test for gastroesophageal reflux
Esophagoscopy*	Detect esophagitis and mucosal biopsy

* Investigations of choice in gastroesophageal reflux.

between awake, asleep, postprandial and fasting periods can be derived. Recent research has suggested that shortening the test to a 6-h postprandial period does not result in a reduction in its sensitivity. This method does not, however, give any information on whether either a hiatus hernia or esophagitis is present.

Esophagoscopy

If significant reflux is found or esophagitis is suspected it is important that an esophagoscopy is carried out. This is the only method which allows accurate assessment of esophagitis both visually and histologically and mucosal inflammation can be detected at a very early stage long before any radiological changes are found. With modern pediatric endoscopes the procedure can be carried out as a day case under sedation or a short general anesthetic.

THE STOMACH AND DUODENUM
STRUCTURE AND FUNCTION

The stomach is a J-shaped organ which lies obliquely across the midline in the upper abdomen. It is covered by an inner oblique, middle circular and outer longitudinal layer of smooth muscle and is lined by a columnar epithelium which is indented with gastric pits. The muscular layer is thickened at the pylorus which acts as a valve to control the rate of emptying from the stomach. The columnar epithelium produces mucus which forms a protective layer over the mucosa. The pits in the antrum, body and distal fundus are short and contain the parietal cells which produce hydrochloric acid and intrinsic factor, the chief cells which synthesize and secrete pepsinogen, endocrine cells and mucus-producing cells which are located at the neck of the glands. The pyloric glands which also contain endocrine cells are more tortuous and secrete large amounts of mucus.

Gastric motility

Following the ingestion of food, the body and fundus distend greatly and act as a reservoir for the storage of food. In contrast the antrum is a more muscular organ which, working in concert with the pylorus, produces propagative, segmenting and retrograde activity to break the food down into small, easily digested pieces.

Liquids generally empty very rapidly from the stomach with the rate being determined by the pressure gradient across the pylorus. A typical half emptying time for a drink of orange squash is 15 min. Solids in contrast empty much more slowly with a half emptying time being more typically between 90 and 120 min. The rate of emptying is very closely controlled by mechanoreceptors in the antrum and chemorecepters in the duodenum which feed back to the gastric smooth muscle to limit the rate of emptying. As a consequence of this a homogenized meal will empty more rapidly than a solid meal and a low energy meal will empty faster than a more energy dense meal. The rate of emptying is also inhibited by the presence of undigested fat in the ileum and by distention of the rectum due to fecal loading. The nongastro-intestinal factors which influence gastric emptying are discussed further in the section on vomiting.

Digestion

Pepsinogen is released from zymogen granules in the chief cells of the gastric glands in response to the ingestion of food. Under the influence of hydrochloric acid and then by the autocatalytic action of free pepsin the active pepsin is formed. This enzyme has a pH optimum of 1.0–1.5 and initiates proteolysis in the stomach by hydrolyzing peptide bonds at the amino groups of aromatic or acidic amino acids.

It is also likely that triglyceride hydrolysis starts in the stomach with the activation of the acid-stable lingual lipase and possibly also by the action of gastric lipase. In the preterm infant, because of the very low activity of pancreatic lipase it is likely that this mechanism is of some importance.

Gastric acid production

Hydrochloric acid is actively secreted by the parietal cells of the gastric glands maintaining the pH of the stomach at approximately 1. The rate of acid production is modulated by circulating levels of the gut hormone gastrin which is produced by G cells within the antrum of the stomach The acid environment of the stomach has an important defensive role against ingested pathogens and as mentioned above provides the optimal environment for activity of the gastric digestive enzymes. The low pH facilitates the absorption of inorganic iron by preventing its precipitation and promoting its chelation by ascorbate and dietary carbohydrate. Excessive acid production, however, is likely to lead to an increasing incidence of duodenal ulceration.

The parietal cells are also responsible for the secretion of the glycoprotein intrinsic factor which stabilizes vitamin B_{12} during intestinal transit and binds to specific receptors in the terminal ileum prior to absorption. In autoimmune gastritis where the parietal cells are destroyed, hydrochloric acid and intrinsic factor production cease, resulting in achlorhydria and vitamin B_{12} deficiency.

The mucus protective layer

The acid environment of the stomach is a very hostile one and without a protective mucus layer the epithelium would soon become damaged (Table 11.5). With secretion of bicarbonate into this mucus layer from underlying cells a protective nonacidic milieu coats the lining of the stomach and duodenum (Crampton & Rees 1986). This barrier is enhanced by the rapid rate of mucosal repair and by the good gastric mucosal blood supply.

This layer can be deranged with ulceration of the underlying mucosa, by an increase in gastric acid output, by pepsin, by reflux

Table 11.5 The factors contributing to gastric mucosal damage

Damaging	Protective
Acid	Mucus
Pepsin	Alkali
Bile	Epithelial turnover
Mucosal ischemia	Tight intercellular junctions
Antiprostaglandin drugs	High mucosal blood flow
Helicobacter pylori	

of bile into the stomach and by the antiprostaglandin action of nonsteroidal anti-inflammatory drugs. It is likely also that bacterial agents such as *Helicobacter pylori* will disrupt this protective layer.

HELICOBACTER PYLORI

Since the identification of *Helicobacter pylori* in the mucosa of the gastric antrum (Warren & Marshall 1984) there has been an explosion of interest in the role of this small spiral organism and its causal relationship to gastritis, gastric ulcer, duodenal ulcer, lymphoproliferative disorders and gastric cancer. Our present understanding remains incomplete and many questions remain unanswered, concerning the best methods of detection, the selection of patients for treatment and the optimum treatment regimes (Rowland & Drumm 1995).

Pathogenesis

This organism is recognized as the most important cause of nonautoimmune gastritis in both children and adults. It may colonize either the antrum of the stomach, leading to increased acid production, or the body of the stomach where inflammation may lead to the development of an atrophic gastritis. Normal duodenal mucosa is not colonized unless gastric metaplasia has developed. *Helicobacter pylori* lies deep within the mucus layer which covers the gastric mucosa and through the action of the enzyme urease, which produces ammonia and the release of cytotoxins, the underlying mucosa becomes damaged and inflamed. During endoscopy a nodular inflammation of the antrum may be seen and hypertrophy of the gastric mucosal folds has been reported.

Epidemiology

It is thought that *Helicobacter pylori* is acquired in early childhood and once infected children are likely to remain colonized, despite the mounting of a host response, for the rest of their life unless they are inadvertently treated with antibiotics. Spread occurs though close physical contact either by oral–oral or fecal–oral routes with the prevalence increasing where there is social deprivation or institutionalization. In developed countries about 10% of children will have become infected by the age of 15 years, rising to 60–70% by the age of 60 years, while in developing countries levels as high as 80% may have been reached by adolescence.

Diagnosis

Serology

This test is based on the detection of specific IgG to *Helicobacter pylori* in serum samples. A number of commercial kits are available but each has to be independently validated against the population under study and false negatives may occur in the very young or the immunosuppressed who have failed to mount an adequate response to infection. The test generally has a sensitivity and specificity of about 90%. Tests using salivary antibodies have a poorer sensitivity and specificity.

Histology

The organism can be detected histologically by Giemsa staining of gastric mucosal biopsies. This test has a similar sensitivity and specificity to serology but requires endoscopy.

Culture

Culture of biopsy specimens in selective media for 10 days may fail to grow the organism in 20% of cases. A positive culture is very specific and, although not done as a routine, culture is essential if the sensitivity or the serotype of the organism is required.

Rapid urease (CLO) test

A single gastric biopsy is placed in the well of a CLO test slide. If *Helicobacter pylori* is present, its urease activity will cleave urea to produce ammonia which will turn the pH indicator red if left at room temperature for 24 h. See Figure 11.4.

C13 urea breath test

This noninvasive test involves the patient taking a small oral dose of C13-enriched urea following a test meal which delays gastric emptying. If *Helicobacter pylori* is present within the stomach the urea is cleaved, releasing C13-enriched CO_2 which is then exhaled in the breath. By collecting two breath samples, one before and the other 30 minutes after the oral urea, a rise in C13 levels in the breath signifies infection. This test has a sensitivity of 95% and a specificity of almost 100%. The sensitivity is reduced if antibiotics are not discontinued for 1 month prior to the test.

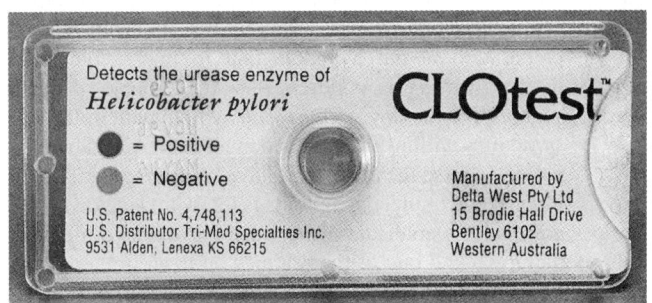

Fig. 11.4 (a) The CLO test used to detect *H. pylori* in mucosal biopsies. (b) The action of urease.

Symptoms

It is likely that the majority of children infected with this organism have no symptoms but, conversely, in children with evidence of chronic peptic ulceration, *Helicobacter pylori* is likely to have an important role in its pathogenesis. Why the majority of children have no symptoms and only a small minority develop peptic disease remains unclear. It is not possible to differentiate infected from noninfected patients on the basis of history alone and in infected patients only those with proven ulceration responded well to eradication therapy (Gormally et al 1995). This would suggest that *Helicobacter pylori* gastritis does not in isolation cause symptoms.

It is unlikely that this infection is a significant factor in children with recurrent abdominal pain.

Treatment

Clearly not all children infected with *Helicobacter pylori* require treatment. The majority will be asymptomatic and as outlined above, even when a gastritis is present, treatment may not be helpful in relieving symptoms. As *Helicobacter pylori* has been shown to be present and to be important in the pathogenesis in the vast majority of patients with duodenal ulcers, it is now advocated that eradication therapy is indicated at the time of primary treatment.

Many differing treatment regimes have been advocated for the eradication of *Helicobacter pylori* and only a minority of these have been tested in children. What is clear is that single therapy is ineffective and most regimes use two or three drugs. The combination of metronidazole, amoxicillin and bismuth subcitrate was advocated initially for a period of 2 weeks but compliance due to unpalatability was a problem. More recently the use of a proton pump inhibitor in addition to antibiotics has been advocated and eradication rates as high as 90% have been documented when combined with clarithromycin and either amoxicillin or metronidazole, for a period of 1 week.

Eradication can be confirmed by C13 breath testing but this has to be delayed for at least 4 weeks after antibiotic and proton pump inhibitor treatment has stopped. Antibody levels can take up to 6 months to fall after eradication and are therefore of little use in monitoring the response to treatment.

PEPTIC ULCERATION

Acute ulcers

Peptic ulceration can occur acutely in response to stress or the administration of ulcerogenic drugs. Stress ulcers can occur in either the stomach or duodenum and are most common in the neonatal period in response to birth asphyxia or respiratory distress but they can also occur in later childhood following severe burns, meningitis or other major stresses. In patients receiving nonsteroidal anti-inflammatory drugs for conditions such as juvenile arthritis or corticosteroids for severe asthma or inflammatory bowel disease, acute ulcers can also occur. It is unlikely that *Helicobacter pylori* plays a significant role in acute ulceration.

A stress ulcer is likely to present with intestinal bleeding or acute pain and should be treated with an H_2 blocker or proton pump inhibitor but where perforation occurs, surgery is required. In situations where stress ulceration is likely, prophylaxis with H_2-blocking drugs is indicated.

Chronic ulcers

Chronic peptic ulceration occurs most commonly in children over the age of 5 years but unlike acute ulcers which affect the stomach and duodenum equally, chronic ulcers occur 10 times more frequently in the duodenum (Nord 1988). As in adulthood there is very frequently a family history of peptic ulcer disease with a slight (3 : 2) male to female preponderance.

In many older children the classical ulcer symptoms of localized epigastric discomfort, nocturnal wakening and relief of symptoms with food or antacids are present. However, in younger children more nonspecific symptoms such as vague abdominal pain, vomiting and nausea may make the diagnosis less clear. Some children may present with an occult anemia or more acutely with a hematemesis or melena. Because of the vague nature of many of these symptoms it is very important to differentiate between peptic ulcer disease and the far more common 'nonorganic' recurrent abdominal pain of childhood. The presence of epigastric pain, nocturnal wakening, a progressive worsening of symptoms, an iron deficiency blood picture or a family history should alert one to the possibility of duodenal ulceration.

While the diagnosis can be made on a barium meal, carried out by an experienced radiologist, the relatively poor sensitivity of this test (50%) means that where a peptic ulcer is suspected upper gastrointestinal endoscopy should be the investigation of first choice (Wyllie & Kay 1994). In addition to visualizing the ulcer, endoscopy allows one to look for *Helicobacter pylori* infection in mucosal biopsies. Although the measurement of gastric acid output is a very insensitive way of diagnosing peptic ulcer disease, in the rare situation where multiple ulcers refractory to treatment are present it is important to measure fasting serum gastrin and basal and stimulated gastric acid output levels to exclude the possibility of a gastrin-secreting pancreatic tumor (Zollinger–Ellison syndrome).

Treatment

Most of the advice for treatment of peptic ulceration has been extrapolated from the adult experience as clinical trials in children have been limited by the small number of patients and by ethical constraints. It is likely, however, that one is dealing with the same disease in both groups of patients as the clinical experience of therapeutic regimes is similar in each.

The treatment of peptic ulcer disease is primarily aimed at reducing gastric acid production and removing any factors, such as *Helicobacter pylori*, which might lead to early recurrence. The former can be accomplished by the use of H_2-blocking drugs such as ranitidine or cimetidine or with proton pump inhibitors such as omeprazole. The proton pump inhibitors have the advantage that a single daily dose is required but unfortunately a pediatric preparation is not available and in many countries it is not licensed for use in children. A 6-week course of treatment with suppressive therapy will provide symptomatic relief of dyspeptic symptoms within 1–2 weeks in most patients and by the end of the 6-week course the ulcers will have healed in over 80% of patients. Recurrence of ulcer symptoms is likely to develop unless attempts are made to eradicate *Helicobacter pylori* and a course of triple therapy using one of the regimes outlined in the section on anti-Helicobacter therapy, is indicated at the time of initial treatment. If symptoms recur after treatment it is likely that the *Helicobacter pylori* has not been completely eradicated.

UPPER GASTROINTESTINAL BLEEDING

Bleeding from the upper gastrointestinal tract may present either as a hematemesis or melena depending on the site and severity of the bleeding. In the majority of cases the bleeding has little hemodynamic effect but major bleeds warrant urgent treatment. It is important, however, when taking a history to be sure that the child has in fact passed blood. The swallowing of bloodstained liquor, sucking on a cracked nipple, a recent nose bleed and the recent ingestion of beetroot can all mimic an intestinal hemorrhage.

Diagnosis

The most likely cause for a bleed can be determined from the age of the child and by searching for clues from the history and examination (Treem 1994). A history of previous gastrointestinal symptoms, recent drug ingestion, umbilical catheterization as a neonate, stigmata of chronic liver disease or a bleeding diathesis, or evidence of subcutaneous or cutaneous hemangioma should be sought (Table 11.6).

A full blood count will give an indication of the duration and severity of the bleed but may be misleading in the acute situation. A clotting screen will define the nature of any bleeding disorder that may be present. Direct visualization of the upper gastrointestinal tract by endoscopy should be carried out within 24 h of the bleed or whenever the patient is hemodynamically stable. This investigation will allow the detection of esophagitis, esophageal varices, gastric and duodenal ulcers and vascular malformations of the intestine proximal to the third part of the duodenum. If bleeding persists and these initial investigations are negative, a small bowel meal should be carried out to exclude intestinal polyps and where vascular malformation is suspected a selective angiogram should be carried out. If bleeding persists and no cause can be found a laparotomy may be indicated.

At times it can be very difficult to distinguish between upper and lower tract bleeding and it is suggested that this section is read in conjunction with the section on rectal bleeding (see p. 459).

Table 11.6 Causes of upper gastrointestinal bleeding

1. Hemorrhagic disease of the newborn
2. Stress peptic ulcer
3. Blood dyscrasia
4. Esophagitis
   a. peptic
   b. caustic
5. Esophageal varices
6. Mallory–Weiss tear
7. Chronic ulcers
   a. gastric
   b. duodenal
8. Gastric erosions
   a. salicylates
   b. nonsteroidal anti-inflammatory drugs
   c. corticosteroids
9. Infantile hypertrophic pyloric stenosis
10. Foreign body
11. Vascular malformations
12. Intestinal polyps

Treatment

The initial treatment of the shocked patient is resuscitation, ensuring the patient has a secure airway and is breathing adequately with maintenance of the circulation by the rapid infusion of 10–30 ml/kg of whole blood or other volume expander. Any bleeding diathesis should be corrected and attempts should be made to define the underlying cause. If varices are found the patient should be treated by a team experienced with this type of problem. A description of the management of a variceal bleed is given in the section on liver disease. Most patients stop bleeding with simple medical management, and treatment should be aimed at the underlying cause of the bleeding.

VOMITING

Vomiting is a very common symptom of disease in childhood and should not be confused with the regurgitation of food which occurs in conditions such as gastroesophageal reflux. The vomiting reflex is the body's response to noxious stimuli, which may reside within the gastrointestinal tract or result from some systemic disturbance and act directly or indirectly on the 'vomiting center' in the area postrema of the brainstem. The act of vomiting can be divided into three phases (Andrews & Hawthorn 1988). In the pre-ejection phase the patient feels nauseous, looks pale, salivates and through the action of visceral efferent nerves develops a tachycardia with relaxation of the proximal stomach. This is followed by a period of retching and then, with synchronous contractions of the intra-abdominal muscles and diaphragm with an open glottis, upper esophageal sphincter and mouth, the contents of the stomach are ejected.

In the neonate, vomiting may be the first symptom of an intestinal obstruction (see Chs 5 and 31), although any infection, metabolic disturbance or cerebral insult may present in an identical manner. The presence of bile in the vomit would suggest an obstruction distal to the duodenum. As the child becomes older the range of conditions causing obstructive and metabolic problems will change and in addition dietary indiscretions or intolerances may develop. The possibility of idiopathic hypertrophic pyloric stenosis should be considered in any baby of 1–4 months of age who develops projectile vomiting. In the older child drugs taken either accidentally or therapeutically may result in vomiting. A history of recurrent episodes of severe vomiting punctuated by asymptomatic periods should alert one to the possibility of cyclical vomiting. The symptoms of vomiting and diarrhea are frequently combined during enteric infections and it is likely that on a worldwide scale this is the most common cause of vomiting.

Diagnosis

A good history and examination will often give strong pointers to the most likely cause for the vomiting. A pyloric tumor or the mass of an intussusception may be palpable on abdominal examination. In some patients, particularly the very young, clues may be few and far between. and it must also be remembered that the differential diagnosis varies greatly depending on the age of the patient and on whether any associated features such as diarrhea are present (Table 11.7).

An erect and supine abdominal X-ray will show multiple air–fluid levels in intestinal obstruction but it must also be remembered that a functional obstruction due either to some

Table 11.7 Causes of vomiting in infancy

Cause	First week of life	After first week
Alimentary tract	Duodenal atresia Jejunal atresia Malrotation/volvulus Duplication of bowel Diaphragmatic hernia Meconium ileus Hirschsprung's disease Anal atresia Functional obstruction	Malrotation/volvulus Hirschsprung's disease Intussusception Strangulated hernia Pyloric stenosis Functional obstruction Peptic ulceration Appendicitis Bezoar Crohn's disease
Metabolic	Galactosemia Organic acidemia Hyperammonemia Hypercalcemia Hypoadrenalism	Organic acidemia Hyperammonemia Hypoadrenalism Diabetic ketoacidosis Drug intoxication Reye's syndrome Uremia
Dietetic	Cow's milk intolerance	Cow's milk intolerance Celiac disease Overeating
Infection	Any infection	Gastroenteritis Tonsillitis Otitis media Urinary infection Meningitis Septicemia
Cerebral	Birth trauma Hydrocephalus	Head injury Cerebral tumor Encephalitis Increased intracranial pressure
Others		Motion sickness Cyclical vomiting

intrinsic abnormality of the gut or to the toxic effect of sepsis or metabolic derangement may also give a similar picture. Barium contrast studies will define the nature of surgical causes of vomiting which are not clear from plain films. Where appropriate, detailed infection and metabolic screens should be carried out and signs of raised intracranial pressure should be sought. The serum electrolytes will give information on the extent of the vomiting and may even, as in the case of the hypochloremic hypokalemic alkalosis of pyloric stenosis, give clues to the underlying cause.

If a nonorganic cause for the vomiting is suspected or if a behavioral element is thought to be present, referral to a psychiatrist or psychologist for a diagnostic assessment should be considered.

Treatment

The treatment should be aimed at the resuscitation of the patient in the first instance and then more specifically at the underlying cause of the vomiting. Electrolyte losses should be corrected and oral fluids should be stopped. If vomiting persists a nasogastric tube should be passed and where an obstructive lesion seems likely a pediatric surgeon should be consulted. As an adjunct to the treatment of the underlying problem antiemetic drugs may be useful in modifying the emetic response. Given the wide variety of stimuli which can produce vomiting and the varying mode of actions of these drugs it is perhaps not surprising that these agents are not universally effective.

INFANTILE HYPERTROPHIC PYLORIC STENOSIS

Pyloric stenosis develops in approximately 3 per 1000 live births with a male to female preponderance of 4 : 1. The cause of the condition is unclear although a reduced number of cases occur in babies with blood group A and there is also a strong familial pattern of inheritance. A thickening of the pyloric muscle results in gastric outlet obstruction with resulting vomiting.

Symptoms of projectile vomiting occurring 10–20 min after a feed develop between the second and fourth week of life, although they can occasionally occur either sooner or at up to 4 months of age. With progressive vomiting the infants loose weight and may eventually become dehydrated and alkalotic. On clinical examination gastric peristaltic activity may be seen, and palpation of the right upper quadrant of the abdomen during a test feed will reveal the pyloric tumor in most cases. If the mass cannot be felt diagnosis can be aided by a barium meal which will show a narrow elongated pyloric canal or by ultrasound which should also define the mass.

The initial management of the patient after the diagnosis has been confirmed is intravenous rehydration and correction of any acid–base disturbance. The patient should then undergo a Ramstedt's pyloromyotomy where the pyloric muscle is split down to the mucosa. Oral feeds can be restarted 24 h after surgery (see Ch. 31).

Other surgical causes of vomiting are discussed more fully in Chapter 31.

PSYCHOGENIC VOMITING

Recurrent episodes of vomiting, sometimes referred to as cyclical vomiting, occur in children who are generally of school age. The attacks, which can occur as frequently as once a week in some children and as infrequently as every 6 months in others, are generally preceded by a prodromal phase when the child is pale and withdrawn with the attack lasting anything from 12 to 72 h. The vomiting may also be associated with a slight rise in temperature and in some children associated features of the periodic syndrome such as abdominal pain or headache are present (Lask 1988).

The vomiting may be exacerbated by the child's desire to drink large amounts of fluid; persistent vomiting can lead to Mallory–Weiss tears, dehydration, electrolyte imbalance and eventually coma. It is frequently difficult to define the factors which precipitate each attack but a careful psychological assessment frequently reveals stress factors, the most common being marital conflicts and school-based problems. Parents are sometimes reluctant to accept the diagnosis of a psychological problem and they have to be convinced that an organic cause for the problem has been adequately excluded. The children require a full blood count, the measurement of serum electrolytes and a urine culture; a barium meal examination will exclude a hiatus hernia or a malrotation. If gastroesophageal reflux is clinically suspected a 24-h pH study should be considered. In a small number of children an intercurrent viral infection may appear to initiate the episode.

If left untreated the majority of children will grow out of the problem but this may take many years. In others, headache may become a prominent feature and a picture of migraine may develop later (Abu Arafeh & Russell 1995). If stress factors have been revealed from the history, family therapy may be of benefit in preventing further attacks. During acute attacks the child may require hospital admission for intravenous fluids and a careful physical examination should be carried out to exclude any organic cause for the vomiting. Antiemetic drugs may be of limited use during acute attacks but the administration of psychotropic drugs long term is not helpful.

FOREIGN BODIES

Children between the ages of 1 and 4 are particularly liable to swallow foreign bodies. The majority of these cause very few problems and simply pass straight through the intestine but long pointed objects such as fish bones or needles can become lodged in the pharynx, esophagus or occasionally in the duodenal loop. If the foreign body becomes lodged in a high position, coughing and choking may occur but frequently there may be no initial symptoms. Perforation of the mucosa will result in the development of a mediastinitis or peritonitis and where a battery becomes lodged a caustic stricture or mucosal erosion may develop.

Bezoar

The repeated ingestion of hair or paper or fibers from clothing or blankets can result in the formation of a large nonopaque foreign body in the stomach. These masses can grow to quite a large size but frequently there are very few symptoms other than vague abdominal pain or halitosis. The bezoar may be felt by abdominal palpation or outlined on a contrast study where the barium adheres to the fibrous mass.

Treatment

Small foreign bodies without sharp edges should be left to pass through the intestine. If they do not appear within 72 h a plain X-ray should be taken to check on their position. Sharp foreign bodies should be removed endoscopically under direct vision. If endoscopic removal from the stomach is not possible a laparotomy will be required.

GASTRIC INVESTIGATIONS

Barium studies

In patients with chronic nausea and vomiting a barium meal will define the anatomy of the stomach and detect the presence of a hiatus hernia, reflux, if it occurs during the examination, malrotation or any space occupation due to a bezoar. Although duodenal ulcers may be detected, endoscopy is the investigation of choice where a mucosal lesion is suspected.

Gastroscopy

Fiberoptic endoscopy is the preferred investigation for detecting duodenal or gastric ulcers or the antral gastritis associated with *Helicobacter pylori* infection. The method can be used in infants of all ages allowing histological and microbiological confirmation of the suspected diagnoses (Ament et al 1988).

Gastric emptying

This is a useful functional measure of gastric contractile activity but unfortunately the traditional scintigraphic methods widely used in adults require the use of a gamma camera and exposure to radioisotopes. Newer noninvasive methods which rely on impedance or stable isotope methods are, however, now becoming available.

THE SMALL INTESTINE

STRUCTURE OF THE SMALL INTESTINE

In man the small intestine occupies the major length of the gastrointestinal tract and is the major organ of digestion and absorption. In the adult the small intestine varies in length from 3 to 5 m depending on the state of contraction, while in the term infant the length is probably nearer 1.5 m. The small intestine is divided into the duodenum which extends from the pylorus to the duodenal–jejunal flexure at the ligament of Treitz; and the remaining small intestine is arbitrarily divided into the jejunum and ileum which represent the proximal two-fifths and distal three-fifths respectively.

In cross-section the structure of the small intestine is grossly similar throughout. The inner circular lumen is lined by a highly convoluted mucosa which exposes a large surface area for the absorption of nutrients. Underneath the surface epithelium lies the submucosa which in turn is encircled by the muscularis which comprises an inner circular and an outer longitudinal layer. The outermost layer is the serosa which is in continuity with the peritoneum. The mesentery of the small intestine is inserted diagonally across the posterior abdominal wall from the ligament of Treitz to the cecum. When this mesentery is shortened by malrotation of the small intestine it becomes unstable and is liable to twist.

Mucosa

The mucosa consists of the surface epithelium and the lamina propria. The mucosal surface is covered by villi which project into the lumen and greatly increase the surface area and by the crypts of Lieberkühn which lie between the villi and form a depression in the mucosa (Fig. 11.5). In the jejunum the villous : crypt ratio is 3 : 1 but this decreases more distally to 1–2 : 1 in the ileum. Underneath the surface epithelium lies the lamina propria which contains a connective tissue core for the villi along with the vascular, lymphatic and neural networks which serve the nutrient and transport needs of the surface epithelium.

The surface epithelium

The crypts and villi should be thought of as the functional unit of the surface epithelium. The crypts contain paneth, goblet, endocrine and undifferentiated cell types. Goblet cells which lie on the lateral walls of the crypts produce large amounts of protective mucus, and the endocrine cells, which are neuroectodermal in origin, synthesize and secrete gastrointestinal hormones. Rapidly dividing undifferentiated cells migrate up the length of the crypts and on to the villi where they transform into mature villus cells (Fig. 11.5). The rate of division of these cells and their speed of migration is under the control of the trophic effect of enteral nutrients and a number of gut hormones. When

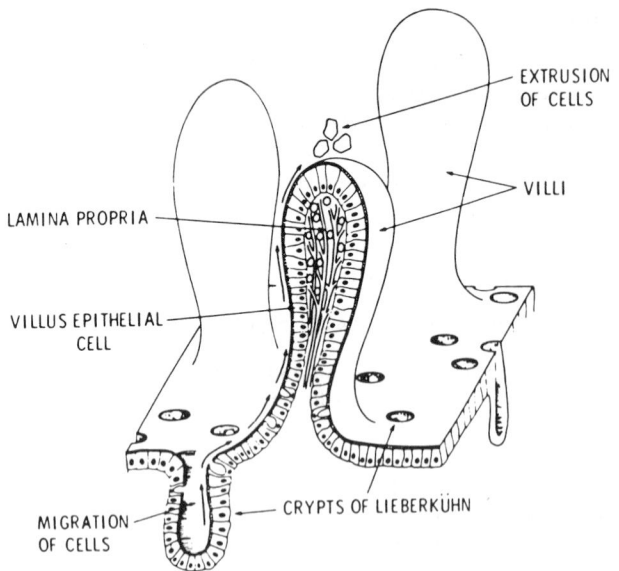

Fig. 11.5 A diagrammatic view of the surface of the small intestine showing the migration of newly dividing cells from the crypts to the tip of the villi. (Reproduced from *Harries' Paediatric Gastroenterology* by kind permission of author and publisher.)

enteral nutrients are removed as a result of starvation or the prolonged use of parenteral nutrition, mucosal hypoplasia results, while in the adaptation to small intestinal resection the rate of cell turnover increases resulting in mucosal hypertrophy and increased villous length.

As the epithelial cells reach the villous tip they degenerate and fall off into the lumen. This rapid turnover of the villous epithelium takes between 4 and 6 days and explains both why the intestinal mucosa is on the one hand very susceptible to the toxic effects of ionizing radiation and chemotherapeutic drugs and why on the other its rate of repair and recovery from serious insult can be very rapid. The enterocytes have a well-developed brush border which further increases the surface area of the mucosa to luminal nutrients and supports the enzymes responsible for the final digestion of nutrients prior to absorption (Fig. 11.6).

The cells in the crypts play an important role in the secretion of water and electrolytes into the lumen in contrast to the villous cells which largely absorb water, electrolytes and nutrients. In health the small intestine is a net absorber of water but in situations where the villous structure is damaged (i.e. celiac disease) or where mucosal inflammation stimulates the activity of the secretory crypt cells (i.e. Crohn's disease) this situation is reversed leading to active mucosal secretion. A similar situation occurs in rotavirus gastroenteritis where the rapid turnover of regenerative cells results in villi populated with immature cells which have yet to develop significant absorptive capacity.

The muscularis

The motor activity of the small intestine is provided by the inner circular and outer longitudinal muscle layers which are present along the whole length of the small intestine. Nerve fibers freely travel between these layers with extension distally on to the mucosa and proximally through afferent and efferent fibers which project both to and from the brainstem and cerebral cortex.

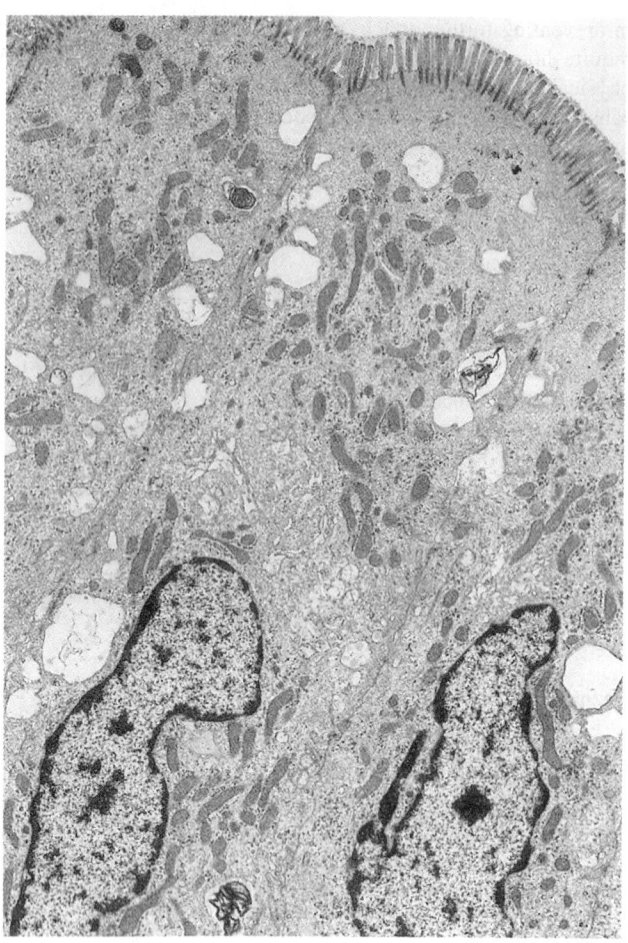

Fig. 11.6 An electron micrograph (magnified × 7800) showing a normal enterocyte with the microvillous membrane shown at the top of the cell and the nuclei towards the bottom. (Reproduced by kind permission of G. Anderson.)

DIGESTION

Digestion of carbohydrates

Starch, the main form of ingested carbohydrate, is a mixture of long chains of glucose units linked at the α-1,4 position (amylose) and shorter chains of α-1,4-linked glucose units connected by α-1,6 links to give a branched structure (amylopectin). As the intestine is only able to absorb monosaccharide units these large molecules require digestion by hydrolytic enzymes (Heitlinger & Lebenthal 1988).

This digestion takes place in two steps; the first, occurring within the lumen of the gut, breaks the starch into oligosaccharides and the second, which occurs on the brush border of the small intestine, further digests these carbohydrates to their component monosaccharides. The luminal digestion is carried out by amylase from the salivary glands and the pancreas, which hydrolyses α-1,4 bonds, breaking the amylose into maltose (two glucose units) and maltotriose, and amylopectin into limit dextrins with on average eight glucose units and one or more α-1,6 branching points. In the adult approximately 15% of duodenal amylase activity is salivary in origin but in the newborn infant, where pancreatic exocrine function is very poorly developed, this may increase to 50%.

Table 11.8 Carbohydrate digestion by the brush border

Enzyme	Substrate	Product
Lactase	Lactose	Glucose Galactose
Sucrase	Sucrose	Glucose Fructose
Maltase	Maltose	Glucose
Isomaltase	Isomaltose Limit dextrins	Glucose Glucose
Glucoamylase	Maltose Glucose oligomers	Glucose Glucose

Dietary disaccharides and the products of amylase digestion are further hydrolyzed by the enzymes of the enterocyte brush border membrane. These include the α-glucosidases sucrase, isomaltase, maltase and trehalase, the latter having no functional significance in the human. The β-galactosidase lactase is also present. The substrate and product of each of these enzymes is outlined in Table 11.8. These enzymes are all high molecular weight glycoproteins which are synthesized in the endoplasmic reticulum, processed in the Golgi apparatus and inserted into the plasma membrane. The sucrase and isomaltase activities originate from a large molecule which is synthesized in continuity and subsequently split, after insertion in the brush border, into two separate functional units. Damage to the villi results in loss of disaccharidase activity with lactase being the most susceptible enzyme.

Undigested carbohydrate is fermented by colonic bacteria and salvaged as short chain fatty acids. If, however, the carbohydrate load is large, the osmotic pull will draw fluid into the lumen causing diarrhea.

Digestion of proteins

Ingested proteins are all very large molecules which require to be broken down to their constituent amino acids or di- and tripeptides before absorption can occur (Schmitz 1991). The process of protein digestion involves the initial extraction of protein from food by mastication and the mechanical activity of the stomach and denaturation of the protein which is promoted by the low pH of the stomach. The subsequent hydrolysis of the denatured protein is brought about by four major groups of enzymes: the pepsins secreted by the chief cells of the gastric glands and trypsins, elastase and chymotrypsins which are all secreted by the acinar cells of the pancreas. All four enzymes are secreted as proenzymes with hydrogen ions promoting the activation of pepsin and the enzyme enterokinase and trypsin activating the other three (Fig. 11.7). The presence of enterokinase, which is found on the brush border membrane of the proximal small intestine, is vital for the activation of these pancreatic proteinases. Luminal digestion is completed by the action of amino- and carboxypeptidases which cleave the terminal amino acids of the peptides. This results in a mixture of small peptides and free amino acids being presented to the brush border membrane. The larger peptides are further hydrolyzed by brush border-bound peptidases leaving free amino acids, dipeptides and tripeptides for absorption.

Digestion of lipids

Dietary lipids are mainly in the form of triglycerides but

$$\text{pepsinogen} \xrightarrow{\quad H^+ \quad} \text{pepsin + peptide}$$

$$\text{trypsinogen} \xrightarrow[\text{trypsin}]{\text{enterokinase}} \text{trypsin + peptide}$$

$$\text{chymotrypsinogen} \xrightarrow[\text{trypsin}]{\quad} \text{chymotrypsin + peptide}$$

$$\text{proelastase} \xrightarrow[\text{trypsin}]{\quad} \text{elastase + peptide}$$

Fig. 11.7 The activation of proteolytic enzymes.

phospholipids and cholesterol esters are also present in smaller amounts. Lipid digestion occurs mainly in the small intestine under the influence of bile salts, which form an emulsion of the ingested fat, and of pancreatic lipase, which hydrolyses the ester links at the 1 and 3 position of the triacylglycerol to yield monoacylglycerol and free fatty acid (Lowe 1994).

The presence of an adequate concentration of bile salts in the lumen of the small intestine (> 2 mmol/l) is of vital importance, as a failure to form a fat emulsion with small micelles (approx. 1 μm in diameter) severely reduces the surface area of contact between the lipase and the fat with resulting maldigestion. Inadequate bile salt concentrations can occur where there is an obstruction to biliary flow, deconjugation by luminal bacteria or where the total bile salt pool is depleted by bile salt malabsorption due to ileal resection.

Pancreatic lipase is quantitatively the most important enzyme in the digestion of triacylglycerols but lingual and gastric lipase is also present. Gastric lipase may be important in the hydrolysis of lipids with short and medium chain fatty acids, and in the preterm and newborn infant where pancreatic exocrine function is very poorly developed it is likely that lingual and gastric lipase are the major enzymes of lipid digestion, helped in breast-fed babies by breast milk lipase. Ingested phospholipids are hydrolyzed by pancreatic phospholipase and cholesterol esters are hydrolyzed by pancreatic cholesterol esterases.

The resulting monoacylglycerols, free fatty acids and cholesterol are absorbed by the epithelial cells of the small intestine. The fat-soluble vitamins A, D, E and K are absorbed from micelles and where the production of micelles is compromised by low bile salt concentrations, fat-soluble vitamin malabsorption is likely to occur. Following the digestion and absorption of the lipid from the micelles the bile salts are reabsorbed by the terminal ileum and recycled through an enterohepatic circulation.

INTESTINAL ABSORPTION

The absorptive surface area of the small intestinal mucosa is greatly enhanced by the mucosal folds and by the presence of villi. The differentiated villous cells are responsible for the absorption of electrolytes and the products of the luminal and brush border digestion of food. Water is transported passively and moves down its osmotic gradient through a paracellular path. The epithelial cells are polarized with a brush border membrane facing the lumen of the intestine, a tight junction joining the lateral borders of adjacent enterocytes and a basolateral membrane which is in close contact with the vasculature of the villi (Fig. 11.8).

The membranes of cells are very rich in lipid and thus while

MUCOSA   SEROSA

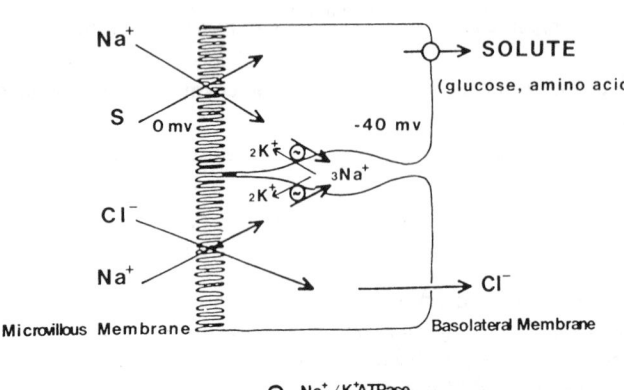

⊖ Na⁺/K⁺ATPase

Fig. 11.8 A diagrammatic view of Na⁺, Cl⁻ and solute absorption across the enterocytes of the small intestinal villi. Water moves passively between the cells down an osmotic gradient.

free fatty acids and monoacylglycerols can readily pass into epithelial cells, water-soluble compounds such as monosaccharides, amino acids, dipeptides and electrolytes all require specific transport processes to facilitate absorption.

Electrolyte absorption

The direction of movement of an electrolyte across a cell membrane is determined by the electrical and chemical gradient which exists across that membrane (Ghishan 1988). In the villous cells of the small intestine there is a strong electrochemical gradient for Na⁺ across the brush border membrane with the inside of the cell – 40 mV relative to the luminal surface and the intracellular Na⁺ concentration being much lower than that found externally (Fig. 11.8). This gradient is maintained by the activity of the basolateral membrane Na⁺/K⁺ ATPase which pumps Na⁺ out of the cell at the expense of the hydrolysis of ATP.

Sodium absorption may be either electroneutral when the absorption of Na⁺ and Cl⁻ is coupled, or electrogenic when it is linked to the absorption of a solute such as glucose or an amino acid. Once absorbed the Na⁺ is actively pumped out of the cell by Na⁺/K⁺ ATPase and the Cl⁻ is able to leave down its electrochemical gradient. K⁺ is transported across the small intestine by a passive process while HCO_3 is absorbed across the jejunum by a Na⁺-dependent process.

Solute absorption

The absorption of glucose and galactose across the brush border membrane occurs by a carrier-mediated process which is driven by the Na⁺ gradient across the cell, while fructose is absorbed by a Na⁺-independent mechanism. Similarly, group-specific active Na⁺-coupled cotransport is responsible for the absorption of free amino acids and unhydrolyzed short peptides.

The presence of a luminal solute enhances the absorption of Na⁺ and water by the small intestine. This explains the success of glucose electrolyte solution in the oral rehydration of children with diarrheal disease.

SMALL INTESTINAL MOTILITY

In the fasting state small intestinal motor activity is characterized by a highly organized band of propagative activity, which moves down the intestine from the stomach to the ileum, called the migrating motor complex (Milla 1988, Bisset et al 1988). This activity develops between 2 and 4 h after a meal and recurs, every 25 min in the term infant and every 90 min in the older child, until disrupted by the next meal. The exact role of the migrating motor complex is uncertain but it has been postulated that it helps clear the small intestine of undigested food debris between meals and this may in part explain the very high incidence of bacterial overgrowth in patients where this activity is absent.

Following the ingestion of food the rate of transit through the small intestine is slowed to allow the complete digestion and absorption of the luminal contents. The rate of slowing is dependent on the energy density of the meal with lipids exerting a greater inhibitory effect than carbohydrates or protein. If undigested lipid reaches the ileum a powerful entero-entero reflex called the 'ileal brake' reflexly decreases the rate of gastric emptying and the degree of propagated intestinal motor activity, a situation which might pertain in patients with cystic fibrosis. Mouth to cecal transit time as measured by the breath hydrogen method is increased from 60–90 min in the fasting state to 3–4 h postprandially.

IMMUNE DEFENSES

The gastrointestinal tract, as with other mucosal surfaces, acts as an important interface between the external environment and the internal milieu of the individual. On the one hand it has to allow the uninterrupted passage of nutrients while on the other it acts as a major barrier to the entry of toxic macromolecules derived from the microbiological flora of the gut or from ingested food (Castro & Arntzen 1993) (Table 11.9).

Nonimmunological mechanisms

Gastric acid has an important role in initiating the digestion of ingested protein and in activating the intraluminal proteases. The colonization of the small intestine by bacteria may be enhanced by reduced gastric acidity, and the failure to fully digest large macromolecules may facilitate the absorption of large unaltered proteins. Normal peristaltic small intestinal motor activity is required to clear the small intestine of food debris between meals

Table 11.9 Gastrointestinal defense mechanisms

1. Nonimmunological mechanisms
   a. Intraluminal
      (i)   Gastric acid
      (ii) Pancreatic proteases
      (iii) Intestinal motility
   b. Mucosal
      (i)   Mucin
      (ii) Microvillous membrane
      (iii) Lysozyme

2. Immunological mechanisms
   a. Mucosal immune system
      (i) Secretory antibody production
      (ii) Cellular immunity
   b. Systemic antibody production

and to prevent colonization by bacteria. The mucosal surface which comprises the microvillous membrane and overlying mucus acts as a physical barrier to the attachment and uptake of luminal antigen and bacteria.

Immunological mechanisms

The specific immunological response to absorbed antigen is expressed by the production of secretory antibodies, systemic antibodies and by activation of the cellular immune system.

The secretory response is initiated by the absorption of antigen across specialized epithelial cells (M cells) which overly lymphoid aggregates in the small intestine. This antigen is then passed to the underlying lymphoid tissue where, with the help of T lymphocytes, B lymphocytes are activated to become IgA-producing cells. These cells initially proliferate and then migrate through the thoracic duct into the systemic circulation. The plasma cells then move back into the lamina propria where dimeric IgA, and to a lesser extent IgG, is produced prior to processing by the epithelial cells and secretion into the lumen in their secretory form. Secretory IgA is also produced by the salivary and mammary glands. A systemic immune response will occur in response to some antigens with the production of IgG, IgE and IgD.

T cells are also activated by the absorption of foreign antigen and these follow a path similar to that described above, back into the lamina propria. Along with these activated lymphocytes, mast cells and macrophages are also available to initiate a cell-mediated response within the intestinal mucosa.

A failure of activation or conversely an overactivation of these immune defenses will result in the development of gastrointestinal disease.

MALABSORPTION

Malabsorption may result either from a failure of the intraluminal digestion of food or from a defect of mucosal function which prevents the absorption of nutrients. The range of conditions which can cause malabsorption is extensive and is listed in Table 11.10. The presenting signs and symptoms are also very variable and may include diarrhea, vomiting, abdominal distention and weight loss. Some children, however, do not have symptoms directly referable to the gastrointestinal tract and may present with evidence of nutritional or other deficiency states.

CELIAC DISEASE

Although first described in children over 100 years ago it was only in 1950 that Dicke noticed the association between celiac disease and the dietary protein gluten, and it was still later in 1957 that the enteropathy associated with this condition was first described following peroral jejunal biopsy (Sakula & Shiner 1957). The enteropathy associated with celiac disease involves predominantly the proximal small intestine and following the removal of gluten from the diet it resolves completely.

Etiology

Celiac disease is caused by the exposure of the small intestinal mucosa to the gluten component of the endosperm in wheat and rye, and possibly also in barley and oats. The β-gliadin component

Table 11.10 Causes of malabsorption

Disorders of intraluminal digestion
1. Congenital
   a. Pancreatic
      (i) Cystic fibrosis
      (ii) Shwachman's disease
   b. Hepatic
      (i) Neonatal hepatitis
      (ii) Hepatocellular failure
      (iii) Cholestasis
   c. Intestinal
      (i) Enterokinase deficiency

2. Acquired
   a. Pancreatic
      (i) Chronic pancreatitis
   b. Hepatic
      (i) Neonatal hepatitis
      (ii) Hepatocellular failure
      (iii) Cholestasis
   c. Intestinal
      (i) Bacterial overgrowth

Disorders of intestinal mucosal function
1. Congenital
   a. Carbohydrate absorption
      (i) Glucose/galactose malabsorption
      (ii) Sucrose isomaltase deficiency
      (iii) Alactasia
   b. Amino acid absorption
      (i) Cystinuria
      (ii) Hartnup disease
   c. Fat absorption
      (i) Abetalipoproteinemia
      (ii) Lymphangiectasia
   d. Electrolyte absorption
      (i) Chloride-losing diarrhea
      (ii) Primary hypomagnesemia
      (iii) Acrodermatitis enteropathica
   e. Enteropathies
      (i) Microvillous atrophy
      (ii) Idiopathic

2. Acquired
   a. Enteropathies
      (i) Celiac disease
      (ii) Food allergic
      (iii) Autoimmune
      (iv) Postgastroenteritis
   b. Infections
      (i) Tuberculosis
      (ii) Giardiases
      (iii) Hookworm
   c. Infiltrations
      (i) Crohn's disease
      (ii) Reticuloses
   d. Anatomical
      (i) Intestinal fistulae
      (ii) Short gut syndrome
   e. Drugs
      (i) Chemotherapeutic agents

of the gluten is the most toxic to the intestinal epithelium and once intolerance develops it is present lifelong. The exact mechanism by which gluten induces the enteropathic process is not clear, although immunological mechanisms are responsible (Tighe & Ciclitera 1993).

Alteration in both humoral and cellular immune mechanisms has been reported in celiac disease. Raised levels of IgA as a result of mucosal stimulation may occur and IgA-associated antigliadin, reticulin and endomysium antibodies are very frequently present.

It has also been found that following gluten challenge complement is activated and immune complexes are deposited within the lamina propria.

In patients with untreated disease or following a gluten challenge there is an increased infiltrate of intraepithelial lymphocytes of the suppressor cell type and an inflammatory infiltrate of the lamina propria, which is characterized by increased numbers of helper lymphocytes and macrophages. Activation of these cell-mediated mechanisms by exposure to gluten with an associated lymphokine-mediated inflammatory and cellular response may be the basis for the pathological features seen in this condition.

Although exposure to gluten is a prerequisite for the development of celiac disease there are also a number of genetic factors which determine the predisposition to this condition. The condition is well reported in European and American races although in black Africans and the Far East it is less clearly documented. There is also great local variation in the incidence of celiac disease with rates of between 1 in 2000 and 1 in 6000 reported in the British Isles compared to 1 in 300 in the West of Ireland. More recently the incidence of celiac disease has appeared to fall and this may in part be due to a reduction in the amount of gliadin in the diet of young children. The 30-fold increased incidence of celiac disease in Sweden compared to Denmark may relate to the fact that the Swedish weaning diet contains 40 times more gliadin than the Danish (Weile et al 1995). The increased incidence in first degree relatives of celiac patients, the high incidence in Down syndrome (Jansson & Johansson 1995) and in insulin-dependent diabetes mellitus and the association between the major histocompatibility antigens HLA-DR3 and DR4 and celiac disease emphasize the role of genetic factors in the etiology of the disease.

Pathology

As a consequence of the immunological assault on the intestinal villi with resulting loss of epithelial cells there is a compensatory increase in the rate of crypt cell replication. This explains the crypt hyperplastic subtotal villous atrophy which is characteristically seen in the proximal small intestine of untreated celiac disease. The proximal distribution of the enteropathy results from the digestion and destruction of the gluten as it passes down the lumen of the gut.

Under the dissecting microscope the loss of villi can be clearly seen with replacement by a flat featureless mucosa. With higher power magnification the increased mitotic activity of the hyperplastic crypts can be seen. There may be complete or near complete loss of villous architecture with an increase in intraepithelial lymphocytes and disruption of the columnar surface epithelial cells. In Figure 11.9 the normal small intestinal mucosa is contrasted with the flat mucosa seen in celiac disease.

Clinical features

The time of presentation is variable and probably depends to a large extent on the amount of gliadin in the diet. The classical presentation occurs between 9 and 18 months of age with the development of loose stools, anorexia and poor weight gain. This is now occurring less frequently, it being more usual for children to present between 3 and 5 years of age with more insidious symptoms such as iron-deficiency anemia or short stature. In Sweden where there are large amounts of gliadin in the weaning diet the classical presentation remains common while in Denmark a later presentation is more common (Weile et al 1995). With the increasing availability of antibody screening tests, asymptomatic sibling are also now more frequently diagnosed.

Diagnosis and investigations

In any child suspected of having celiac disease it is essential that a small bowel biopsy is carried out prior to starting on a gluten-free diet. In children who have been started on a gluten-free diet before biopsy it is impossible to make the diagnosis of celiac disease and a further gluten challenge is required. Serological screening tests have recently been developed with antireticulin, gliadin and endomysium antibodies being raised in the majority of subjects with celiac disease who are on a gluten-containing diet. The reliability of these tests varies between laboratories but generally when used in combination, a sensitivity and specificity as high as 90% can be reached. As with the small bowel biopsy, negative results will be obtained in patients on a gluten-free diet. Other screening tests such as the measurement of serum iron, fecal

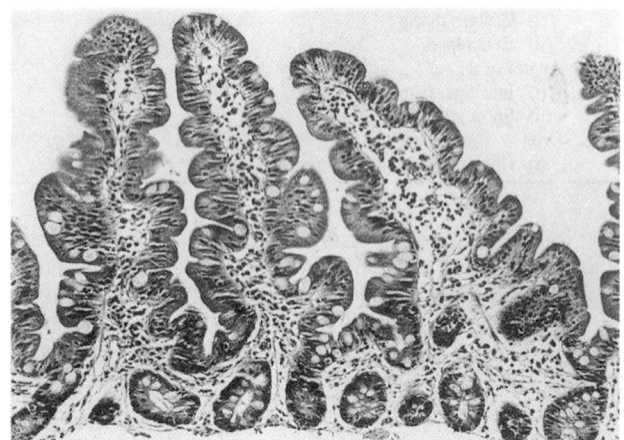
(a)

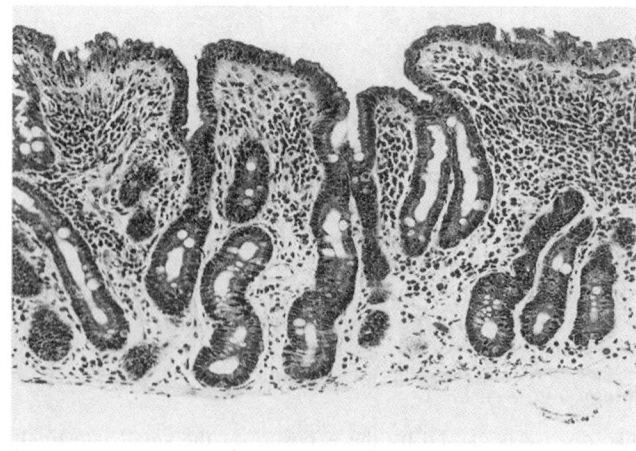
(b)

Fig. 11.9 A light micrograph (magnification × 240, stain hematoxylin and eosin) of a jejunal biopsy in (**a**) a normal child and (**b**) a child with untreated celiac disease. (Reproduced by kind permission of G. Anderson.)

fat, xylose absorption or mucosal permeability have all been suggested, but these tests are generally nonspecific and are no substitute for a small intestinal biopsy.

In a child with a classical presentation the finding of a subtotal villous atrophy makes the diagnosis of celiac disease highly likely but it must be remembered that such a presentation is now relatively uncommon and that a partial villous atrophy can also occur in cow's or soya milk protein intolerance, the postenteritis syndrome and less commonly in autoimmune and congenital enteropathies. For this reason and because the dietary treatment for celiac disease is lifelong it is important to be 100% certain of the diagnosis. A protocol for the diagnosis of celiac disease was outlined in 1979 by the European Society of Paediatric Gastroenterology and Nutrition (ESPGAN) (McNeish et al 1979) and has more recently been revised (Walker-Smith et al 1990) to take account of the increasing availability of serological testing.

The diagnosis of celiac disease is made in four stages.

Stage 1. An abnormal jejunal biopsy is found in a child on a gluten-containing diet. The biopsy will most commonly show a crypt hyperplastic subtotal villus atrophy and in the majority of subjects antibody testing will be positive.

Stage 2. Clinical response to a gluten-free diet.

Stage 3 (at least 1 year after start of diet). Where there has been typical presentation and histology with positive antibodies and a good response to dietary exclusion further jejunal biopsy may not be necessary if the antibodies now revert to normal on diet. When the presentation or biopsies have not been typical or the antibodies were negative at presentation a further biopsy is required to show that the jejunal mucosa has returned to normal. If the biopsy remains abnormal it indicates that either the initial diagnosis of celiac disease is incorrect or that the patient is not sticking to the diet.

Stage 4 (3 months after challenge or sooner if symptoms develop). The patient is challenged with gluten. The size of the gluten challenge will determine the severity of the enteropathy and it is essential that a dietitian checks that the patient has adequate gluten in the diet. Antibodies should now become positive and those who required a biopsy in stage 3 require a third biopsy which should now show a severely damaged jejunal mucosa. If the patient remains asymptomatic, with a normal biopsy or negative antibodies, the normal diet should continue and the investigation be repeated 2 years later. An abnormal biopsy confirms the diagnosis while a normal mucosa would make the diagnosis most unlikely.

Although in celiac disease the intolerance to gluten is lifelong there are some children who symptomatically improve following the removal of gluten from the diet but who fail to show the classical pathological features on jejunal biopsy. In some of these children there is evidence of other food intolerances or a family history of atopy, making it likely that the intolerance is due to a primary allergic etiology. Without serial jejunal biopsies it may be difficult to differentiate between celiac disease and transient gluten intolerance.

Management

Following a positive jejunal biopsy a gluten-free diet is started and a clinical response should occur within the first week or two of treatment. If there is no improvement on a strict diet the diagnosis of celiac disease should be seriously questioned.

Patients who are markedly hypoproteinemic with peripheral edema will require intravenous albumin infusion and if deficiency states are detected they should be corrected with appropriate vitamin and mineral supplements. It is important that the child is regularly reviewed so that the diet can be supervised, growth can be monitored and the appropriate follow-up investigations can be carried out.

It is our present understanding that the diet should be continued throughout life although it is not yet clear whether a strict adherence to a gluten-free diet reduces the reported increased long-term incidence of intestinal neoplasm in these patients.

TRANSIENT FOOD INTOLERANCE

Transient food intolerance is thought to result from an allergic reaction following the sensitization of the intestinal mucosa to dietary antigen (Patrick & Gall 1988, Vanderplas 1993). This characteristically develops in the first year of life and the most common culprit is cow's milk protein, although soya protein and a wide range of other dietary proteins may be responsible. This sensitization may occur under two differing circumstances. Firstly it develops in atopic individuals where frequently there is a family history of similar problems or clear evidence of other atopic symptoms such as eczema or urticaria. In many of these children, although their intolerance generally resolves between the age of 18 months and 5 years, symptoms of asthma and hay fever frequently follow. Low levels of circulating IgA are found in some of these patients, resulting in an increased antigen load to the mucosa with resulting sensitization. In the second group of patients sensitization follows an enteric infection and may add to the mucosal damage caused by the enteric pathogen.

The mechanism of mucosal damage is unclear and may vary from one individual to the next. In some patients an immediate hypersensitivity reaction appears to occur with vomiting, abdominal pain, urticaria and diarrhea developing shortly after exposure to the offending antigen. In other patients the symptoms are more insidious with evidence of poor weight gain and occasionally no overt gastrointestinal symptoms. In these children the presence of a partial villous atrophy with immune complex deposition in the lamina propria and intraepithelial lymphocytes would suggest a combined type III and type IV delayed hypersensitivity reaction. Equally unclear are the mechanisms by which most infants develop immune tolerance to the large number of foreign proteins they come in contact with in ingested food.

Cow's milk protein intolerance

This condition develops most commonly within the first 6 months of life and occurs predominantly in formula-fed babies or babies receiving cow's milk in weaning foods. Breast-fed babies are also at risk as cow's milk protein is secreted at lactation if the mother's diet contains cow's milk. The most common symptoms at presentation are of vomiting, diarrhea and poor weight gain with eczema frequently present in babies and asthma or hay fever in older children (Bock & Sampson 1994, James & Burks 1994).

Diagnosis

The diagnosis is made from the history and from the characteristic improvement in symptoms with exclusion of cow's milk protein from the diet. Jejunal biopsy is likely to reveal a patchy partial villous atrophy, although in some patients the enteropathy may be more severe and be difficult to distinguish pathologically from celiac disease. A full blood count may reveal evidence of a peripheral eosinophilia, serum immunoglobulins may show a raised IgE and a low IgA and skin test or RAST testing may reveal positive reactions to food and environmental allergens. These latter tests are all nonspecific with a high false negative rate and in many patients who are quite clearly food allergic they may still be negative. Jejunal biopsy is probably not required in most patients as the condition usually responds well to an exclusion diet and is self-limiting, but if there is severe failure to thrive or a failure to respond to a cow's milk-free diet a jejunal biopsy is essential to exclude any other more serious pathology.

Management

It is usual to exclude cow's milk protein from the diet and as many atopic children also react to egg protein a combined milk and egg exclusion is frequently required (Shaw & Lawson 1994). It is essential that the diet is supervised by a dietitian to ensure that adequate calories and calcium remain in the diet. A complete milk substitute based on soya protein or a whey or casein hydrolysate should be prescribed, and where the infant has been weaned the mother should be instructed on a diet containing milk- and egg-free solids. Many mothers put their babies on soya milk bought from a supermarket or health food shop, which may be nutritionally incomplete and should be substituted by a complete infant formula. While most children will do well on such a regime, up to a third of children who are cow's milk protein sensitive will subsequently become intolerant to soya protein and further dietary exclusions will be required. A small number of patients will even fail to tolerate a hydrolyzed formula and an elemental or chicken-based feed may be substituted. Some older children refuse to take these milk substitutes because of the taste and under such circumstances an oral calcium substitute should be prescribed.

Most children will improve quickly after starting their diet but it may take many months for full catch-up growth to occur in children who have been failing to thrive. The natural history of this condition is one of spontaneous remission but in some children further intolerances may develop.

Multiple food intolerances

Although cow's milk protein, soya and egg are most commonly responsible for food intolerances in children, wheat, colorings, preservatives and sugar have all been implicated. In the very atopic child almost any dietary intolerance is possible. In addition to the gastrointestinal and atopic symptoms described above for cow's milk protein intolerance, behavior disturbance and hyperactivity may occur in some children.

It should be possible to discover which foods are responsible for the symptoms by taking a good dietary history, and an appropriate exclusion diet should be devised. In some children, however, it is difficult to isolate which foods are causing the problem and under these circumstances two options are available. One can either put the child on a few foods diet and if this settles the symptoms add one new food at a time, or alternatively the mucosal allergic reaction can be suppressed by drug therapy. Oral sodium cromoglycate or beclomethasone may be helpful in some patients while histamine 1 and 2 blocking drugs or even systemic steroids may be helpful in the most severe cases.

Eosinophilic gastroenteritis

It is likely that a fair degree of overlap exists between the allergic conditions described above and eosinophilic gastroenteritis (Steffen et al 1991). The condition is characterized by an eosinophilic infiltrate which can involve the stomach and/or small intestine and which appears to be triggered by the presence of dietary antigens. Three forms of the condition, each involving a different layer of the intestine, have been described.

The mucosal form is characterized by protein loss with hypoalbuminemia and edema. Damage to the antral and duodenal mucosa will result in blood loss and anemia while jejunal damage leads to an enteropathy with malabsorption. Where the muscle layer is involved symptoms of intestinal obstruction occur and in the serosal form of the condition an eosinophilic ascites may develop. Most patient are likely to have the markers of atopy which are outlined above.

Diagnosis will be suggested by the history of atopy with abdominal pain, diarrhea, vomiting, weight loss and edema. Some patients, however, may have no abdominal symptoms. Barium contrast studies may show evidence of inflammation in the mucosal form or luminal obstruction in cases involving the enteric smooth muscle. Upper gastrointestinal endoscopy is invaluable for detecting antral and duodenal lesions and for confirming the diagnosis by mucosal biopsy. Jejunal biopsy will define the involvement of the small intestine but if the disease is patchy inflamed areas may be missed. Protein loss from the intestine may be detected by measuring the excretion of chromium-51-labeled albumin in the stool over a 5-day period or by measuring the stool α_1-antitrypsin.

Treatment is with dietary exclusion, supplemented if required by oral sodium cromoglycate, oral beclomethasone, histamine 1 and 2 blocking drugs and frequently also oral corticosteroids. The level of therapy required will vary from patient to patient but those with mucosal disease are likely to be the most responsive to therapy. Where intestinal obstruction occurs surgery with local resection is likely to be required.

POSTENTERITIS ENTEROPATHY

While most enteric infections are self-limiting and are free of long-term sequelae, some organisms damage the mucosal surface of the gut resulting in a persistence of symptoms long after the original infective organism has been cleared. This postenteritis syndrome can be caused by viruses such as adenovirus or by bacterial pathogens such as the enteropathogenic *Escherichia coli* which totally denude the mucosa of villi. The consequences of acute enteric infections and their management are discussed more fully later in this chapter (see p. 451).

CONGENITAL ENTEROPATHIES

Intractable diarrhea presenting from the time of birth may result from an enteropathy of the small intestinal mucosa. In the absence of any obvious acquired cause it has been proposed that the disruption to villous structure and function is congenital in origin. Because these disorders are frequently familial and are often associated with first cousin marriages, it is assumed that an inborn error of some major structural or functional enterocyte protein is present. Most of these congenital enteropathies, with the exception of congenital microvillous atrophy, have yet to be characterized (Davidson et al 1978).

Microvillous atrophy is characterized by a hypoplastic villous atrophy associated with depletion and shortening of the microvilli over the villous epithelium (Walker-Smith 1994). This condition can be differentiated from other congenital enteropathies by the presence of smudging of stains which outline the microvillous membrane and by electron micrographs which show the presence of characteristic microvillous inclusions in the villous enterocytes. Patients who survive with this condition are likely to remain dependent on parenteral nutrition as no specific treatment is known.

For children with the other forms of congenital enteropathy the lack of understanding of the underlying cause makes treatment and prognostication difficult. Nutritional support with predigested hypoallergenic feeds and intravenous alimentation can greatly prolong life but will frequently not alter the underlying disorder.

AUTOIMMUNE ENTEROPATHY

In a small number of patients with intractable diarrhea and an enteropathy the presence of autoantibodies to the cytoplasm of villous tip enterocytes has been described. In some of these patients other organ-specific autoantibodies or autoimmune diseases have also been found, making it likely that the intestinal disease is caused by an autoimmune process (Mirakian et al 1986). Treatment of these children with hypoallergenic diets, steroids and immunosuppressive drugs has been successful in some cases.

PROTEIN-LOSING ENTEROPATHY

Small amounts of albumin pass into the gut each day and under the influence of pancreatic enzymes are digested and reabsorbed. In response to an increased loss into the gut the liver is able to compensate by increasing the rate of albumin synthesis by up to a factor of two. Above this level, however, the patient becomes increasingly hypoproteinemic. Those proteins with the longest half-lives (albumin and IgG) are the first to fall and in severe protein-losing enteropathies between 10 and 50% of the plasma albumin pool may be lost into the gut each day (Schmitz 1988).

Etiology

Protein-losing enteropathy may arise either as a consequence of the increased permeability of the intestine to plasma proteins or as a result of disordered intestinal or mesenteric lymph flow which leads to the loss of lymphocytes and fat, in addition to protein, into the intestine. Protein loss owing to increased permeability is most marked in hypertrophic gastritis, eosinophilic gastroenteritis and in some forms of intestinal polyposis but any condition which results in severe damage or inflammation to the lining of the gut is likely to result in increased luminal protein loss. Lymphangiectasia is the most common cause of disordered lymph flow. The conditions associated with protein-losing enteropathy are listed in Table 11.11.

Clinical features and diagnosis

The clinical features are of peripheral edema and ascites, when the serum albumin falls below 20 g/l, in addition to those of the underlying condition. The diagnosis of a protein-losing enteropathy is confirmed by the detection of increased amounts of

Table 11.11 Causes of protein-losing enteropathy

1. Increased mucosal permeability to protein
   a. Hypertrophic gastritis
   b. Eosinophilic gastroenteritis
   c. Polyposis
   d. Inflammatory disease
       (i) Crohn's disease
       (ii) Ulcerative colitis
       (iii) Enterocolitis
       (iv) Pseudomembranous colitis
       (v) Radiation enteritis
       (vi) Graft-versus-host disease
       (vii) Autoimmune enteropathy
   e. Celiac disease
   f. Nephrotic syndrome
   g. Esophagitis

2. Altered lymph flow
   a. Primary intestinal lymphangiectasia
   b. Secondary intestinal lymphangiectasia
       (i) Congestive cardiac failure
       (ii) Constrictive pericarditis
       (iii) Lymphoma
       (iv) Tuberculous adenitis
       (v) Volvulus

protein in the stool in the face of a low serum albumin. The increased losses can be shown by the presence of > 4% loss of ^{51}Cr-albumin in the stool over a 5-day period and by increased levels of fecal α_1-antitrypsin. The cause of the protein loss, which may be from the stomach, small intestine or large intestine, can best be defined by endoscopy and biopsy and where this is not possible by jejunal biopsy.

The treatment is that of the underlying condition but 20% albumin infusion may be required in the short term to correct the hypoalbuminemia and edema.

INTESTINAL LYMPHANGIECTASIA

The lymphatics of the small intestine play a vital role in the absorption of fat, being responsible for the transport of chylomicrons from the mucosal cells, via the thoracic duct to the venous system. This lymphatic fluid is also rich in protein and in lymphocytes. In intestinal lymphangiectasia these lymphatic channels become blocked and as a consequence protein and lymphocytes are lost into the gut while fat and fat-soluble vitamins are malabsorbed.

The condition may be either congenital when it is frequently associated with other abnormalities of lymphatic development, such as peripheral lymphedema, or it may arise secondary to acquired lymphatic obstruction from congestive cardiac failure, constrictive pericarditis, malrotation or infiltration of the lymphatics by neoplastic processes. Examination of the jejunal mucosa under a dissecting microscope reveals pale villi of normal length. On higher magnification the lymphatics of the lamina propria and submucosa are distended and filled with lipid staining material (Fig. 11.10).

Patients are likely to present with diarrhea, abdominal distention with hypoproteinemia leading to edema and ascites. The loss of lymphatic cells will result in lymphopenia and an increased susceptibility to infections. Fat-soluble vitamin deficiencies are likely to lead to rickets and clotting abnormalities. The diagnosis is confirmed by the characteristic jejunal biopsy

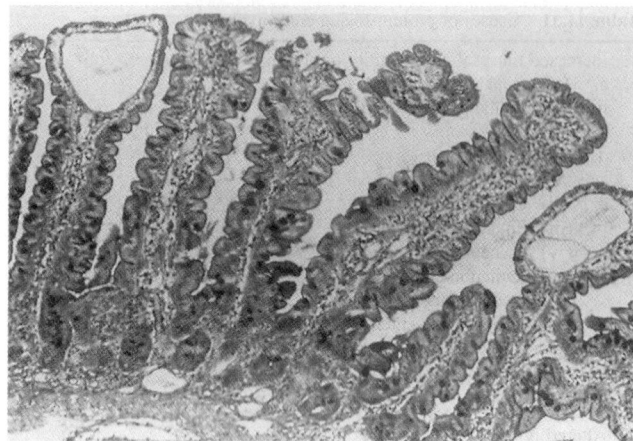

Fig. 11.10 A jejunal biopsy from a patient with lymphangiectasia showing lymphatic vacuolation of the villi (magnification × 240, stain hematoxylin and eosin). (Reproduced by kind permission of P. J. Milla.)

findings in a patient with lymphopenia and a protein-losing enteropathy.

If the primary cause of the lymphangiectasia cannot be remedied treatment involves the use of a high protein diet to compensate for the large stool losses and the substitution in the diet of long chain by medium chain fats which are absorbed directly into the portal venous circulation. In some patients regular albumin infusions may be required to control hypoproteinemia.

IMMUNE DEFICIENCY AND GUT DISEASE

The normal immune function of the small intestine plays a major part in preventing both the absorption of foreign proteins and the penetration of enteric pathogens across the lining of the gut. While the immunodeficiencies themselves very rarely cause any primary damage to the gut, the consequences of the sensitization of the gut to foreign proteins or of recurrent enteric infections can lead to structural damage to the small intestinal mucosa with the development of malabsorption and diarrhea (Gurbindo & Seidman 1991) and as a consequence, failure to thrive. The immunodeficiencies which can lead to compromised intestinal function are listed in Table 11.12.

While the majority of children with IgA deficiency may have no symptoms, the incidence of food allergy and of celiac disease is increased as is infection with *Giardia lamblia*. In agammaglobu-

Table 11.12 Immune deficiency leading to gastrointestinal disease

1. Antibody defect
   a. X-linked agammaglobulinemia
   b. IgA deficiency

2. Combined immunodeficiency
   a. Common variable immunodeficiency
   b. Severe combined immunodeficiency

3. Defect of phagocytosis
   a. X-linked chronic granulomatous disease

4. Immunodeficiency as part of a syndrome
   a. Wiskott–Aldrich syndrome
   b. DiGeorge syndrome

5. Acquired immunodeficiency syndrome

linemia and common variable immundeficiency (CVI), as well as giardiasis, bacterial overgrowth and nonspecific colitis can occur. Where T cell function is compromised in CVI, chronic fungal infection and a nonspecific enterocolitis may develop. Granulomatous disease can cause liver and perianal abscesses, and an enterocolitis which can mimic Crohn's disease; a granulomatous narrowing of the gastric antrum has also been reported.

In both Wiskott–Aldrich and DiGeorge syndrome there is T cell dysfunction, the former associated with severe eczema and thrombocytopenia and the latter associated with esophageal, parathyroid and cardiac defects. Acquired immunodeficiency syndrome frequently presents with opportunistic intestinal infection with *Cryptosporidium*, *Candida*, *Salmonella* or cytomegalovirus.

The diagnosis and treatment of these immune deficiencies is more fully described in Chapter 22. When gut disease occurs, therapy should be aimed at the primary disorder, at treating the enteric infection and at supporting nutrition with elemental feeds or even parenteral nutrition.

Immunodeficiencies may themselves occur as a consequence of primary gastrointestinal disease and this in turn can feed back to potentiate the initial disorder. This can occur in any severely malnourished child, in patients where gut protein loss results in hypoproteinemia and hypogammaglobulinemia and in acrodermatitis enteropathica where zinc deficiency suppresses immune function.

SHORT GUT SYNDROME

Resection of part of the small intestine is not uncommonly required in neonates who develop an acute surgical problem (Stringer & Puntis 1995) (Table 11.13). Similarly in the older child intestinal resection may be required following trauma or volvulus formation. The consequences of such a resection depend very much on the length of gut resected, the part of the small intestine resected, whether the ileocecal valve and colon are still present and on the nutritional state of the patient. Loss of more than 30 cm of intestine is likely to have nutritional consequences to the infant. The remaining bowel, however, has great powers of adaptation and it is possible for as little as 20 cm of small intestine with an intact ileocecal valve to adapt adequately to support life by enteral nutrition.

Clinical features

As a consequence of the loss of intestinal surface area the child develops diarrhea and the absorption of all nutrients, minerals and vitamins is reduced. This is likely to lead to weight loss and the development of specific nutritional deficiencies.

Table 11.13 Causes of the short bowel syndrome in the neonate

1. Small intestinal malrotation with volvulus

2. Jejunal and ileal atresias

3. Meconium ileus

4. Omphalocele or gastroschisis with volvulus

5. Internal hernias

6. Necrotizing enterocolitis

7. Congenital short small bowel

Loss of the terminal ileum will lead to malabsorption and depletion of the bile salt pool and failed vitamin B_{12} absorption will over a period of years lead to the development of a deficiency state. If duodenal bile salt concentration falls below 2 mmol/l micelle formation may be inhibited leading to malabsorption of long chain fats, and the passage of bile salts into the colon will result in intestinal secretion which will compound the diarrhea. The ileum is also rich in enteroglucagon, a potent trophic factor in intestinal adaptation, and where the ileum has been resected the adaptive response may be further delayed or blunted.

The ileocecal valve has a vital role in preventing the reflux of colonic flora into the small intestine and when the valve is resected bacterial overgrowth of the small intestine is an almost inevitable sequela. This leads to mucosal damage and the deconjugation of bile salts with resulting disruption of lipid solubilization and intestinal secretion. Without an ileocecal valve the length of gut that is needed to support life is probably more than doubled and this is further increased if the colon has also been extensively resected.

The small intestine also has an important role in the metabolism of gastrin and where a large length of jejunum is resected hypergastrinemia with increased gastric secretion can occur. This not only increases the fluid load on the intestine but also lowers the duodenal pH and as a result reduces bile salt solubility and the activity of the digestive enzymes.

Management

During the period of adaptation which follows an intestinal resection the turnover of regenerative cells in the crypts of the small intestine increases and as a consequence the length of villi increases. With time this leads to an increase in the absorptive capacity of the residual small intestine. This process, however, may take many months and the mainstay in management is the promotion of the adaptive response and the nutritional support of these patients during this period.

One of the most potent trophic factors in promoting adaptation is the presence of food within the gastrointestinal tract. Starvation is known to produce a partial villous atrophy which is reversed by refeeding. In the short gut syndrome it is therefore most important that enteral feeding is maintained at a level which is able to stimulate the adaptive response while at the same time not causing torrential diarrhea. Because of the reduced digestive and absorptive capacity of the small intestine it is usual to feed these infants with a predigested formula feed or a modular feed based on chicken meat (chix) to which carbohydrate and fat can be added individually as tolerated. Inevitably in infants with large resections this enteral input will need to be supplemented by parenteral nutrition.

There is also a need to control the many complications of the short gut syndrome in order to further increase the absorptive and digestive capacity of the gut. These treatments are listed in Table 11.14. In some infants where very little small intestine remains, or where the adaptive response has been blunted by loss of the ileum and ileocecal valve, the child may remain dependent on parenteral nutrition and under such circumstances efforts should be made to institute this therapy at home.

INBORN ERRORS OF DIGESTION AND ABSORPTION

Although most causes of gastrointestinal disease are acquired,

Table 11.14 Complications in short gut syndrome and their treatment

Complications	Treatment
Bacterial overgrowth	Antibiotics Resect stricture or stagnant loop
Gastric hypersecretion	Histamine 2 blockers
Rapid transit	Loperamide
Malabsorption of fats	Medium chain triglycerides in feeds
Bile salt diarrhea	Bile salt chelator: cholestyramine
Poor growth	Increase parenteral nutrition

there are a number of specific inborn errors of intestinal function which interfere with the normal digestion and absorption of nutrients. Although these disorders are generally uncommon it is important to be aware of their existence as failure to recognize their signs and symptoms may have severe consequences for the child. A knowledge of normal intestinal physiology is important if the clinical consequences of these defects are to be understood.

CARBOHYDRATE MALABSORPTION

Carbohydrates will be malabsorbed if there is a failure of luminal or brush border digestion or a defect in the transport proteins which facilitate the absorption of monosaccharides (Heitlinger & Lebenthal 1988). The most common inborn error involving carbohydrate digestion is cystic fibrosis in which luminal levels of pancreatic amylase are markedly reduced. Of the disaccharidases outlined in Table 11.8, specific defects of lactase, sucrase–isomaltase and trehalase have all been reported although the latter defect is of no clinical significance.

The presence of increased concentrations of disaccharides in the lumen of the small intestine leads to an osmotic diarrhea that results in abdominal distention with large water and electrolyte losses which can be life threatening in young infants.

Lactase deficiency

Primary lactase deficiency is very uncommon and presents with profuse watery diarrhea soon after the introduction of milk feeds. The diagnosis can be suspected from the clinical history and the response to a lactose-free diet, although it can only be confirmed by the measurement of brush border lactase activity. The condition is thought to be inherited in an autosomal recessive fashion.

In many African and Asian races, adult levels of lactase activity fall far below those found in European races. This has previously been labeled 'late onset lactase deficiency', but given that most of these individuals do not have any symptoms, it is probably incorrect to say that they are deficient. By far the most common cause of symptomatic lactase deficiency results from damage to the intestinal mucosa after some other primary infective or inflammatory process.

Sucrase-isomaltase deficiency

The incidence of this deficiency is probably very low although it is said to affect up to 10% of Greenland Eskimos. The condition probably occurs in a number of distinct genetic forms and this may in part explain the variability in its clinical presentation. Symptoms of diarrhea and failure to thrive usually develop following the introduction of sucrose or complex carbohydrate into the diet, but in some children the symptoms may be very mild and the condition goes undiagnosed. As sucrase also contributes to a large part of the brush border maltase activity the use of refined formula feeds which all contain glucose polymer invariably results in an increase in the diarrhea.

In response to an oral sucrose load, exhaled breath hydrogen rises and sucrose can be detected by sugar chromatography of the loose stools. Jejunal biopsy will show normal mucosal morphology but histochemical studies reveal low or absent enzyme activity. Dietary removal of sucrose and complex carbohydrate results in an immediate symptomatic recovery.

Glucose–galactose malabsorption

The condition results from a defect in the transport protein which is responsible for sodium–glucose and sodium–galactose linked cotransport. Diarrhea develops shortly after the first feed and persists until glucose and galactose are removed from the diet. In contrast fructose absorption is normal and sodium–amino acid cotransport is preserved. In some children the degree of glucose intolerance decreases with increasing age. The inheritance is autosomal recessive and is treated with the fructose-containing feed, Galactamin 19.

LIPID MALABSORPTION

Lipid malabsorption with steatorrhea will result from failed luminal solubilization and digestion of triglycerides, as occurs in pancreatic insufficiency, biliary disease and the short gut syndrome, and from failure of mucosal fat transport as occurs in abetalipoproteinemia and hypobetalipoproteinemia.

Abetalipoproteinemia

This autosomal recessive condition which was first described in 1950 is characterized by the presence from birth of steatorrhea, acanthocytosis on the peripheral blood film and failure to thrive; if diagnosis is delayed signs of ataxia and retinopathy may develop in the second decade.

Failure to synthesize apoprotein B means that chylomicrons cannot be manufactured and exported into the lymphatics. Lipid electrophoresis reveals absent serum low density lipoprotein (LDL), very low density lipoprotein (VLDL) and chylomicrons and as a consequence serum triglyceride and cholesterol levels are low. Jejunal biopsy reveals fat-laden enterocytes.

There is now strong evidence that the neurological signs result from chronic vitamin E deficiency and if treatment is started promptly with a low fat diet, large oral supplements of vitamin E (100 mg/kg/24 h) along with supplements of the other fat-soluble vitamins the development of ataxic symptoms and mental deterioration can be prevented.

PROTEIN MALABSORPTION

The digestion of proteins is dependent on the action of proteases which are secreted by the stomach, pancreas and the intestinal mucosa. Inborn errors of these enzymes are very uncommon although specific deficiencies of trypsinogen and enterokinase

have been reported. Both these conditions result in failure to thrive, hypoproteinemia, edema, anemia and neutropenia, and following the introduction of a protein hydrolysate feed with oral pancreatic supplements there is a marked improvement in symptoms.

Defects of brush border amino acid absorption tend to have few clinical consequences as the particular amino acid can still be absorbed as part of a dipeptide. This explains why cystinuria and iminoglycinuria do not result in the development of any nutritional deficiencies and why in Hartnup disease symptoms tend to develop only when the diet is otherwise compromised. Defects of basolateral transport appear, however, to have more severe clinical consequences.

Hartnup disease

A defect in the transport of free neutral amino acids across the brush border of the small intestine and the proximal renal tubules of the kidney lead to a pellagra-like skin rash in areas exposed to sunlight with associated diarrhea and a dementing psychiatric illness. These features are the result of low levels of tryptophan leading to the decreased production of nicotinamide. Treatment with nicotinamide supplementation controls the symptoms of pellagra which spontaneously become less severe with increasing age.

Lysinuric protein intolerance

In this disorder there is impaired absorption by the small intestine, liver and kidneys of the dibasic amino acids lysine, ornithine and arginine. Because peptide-bound lysine absorption is absent the patients present with severe failure to thrive, diarrhea, hepatosplenomegaly and mental retardation within the first 6 months of life. Hyperammonemia occurs following a protein load owing to the low level of urea cycle intermediates, and as a consequence treatment is with oral citrulline.

DISORDERS OF ELECTROLYTE AND MINERAL ABSORPTION

Congenital chloridorrhea

This condition is characterized by severe watery diarrhea with hypochloremia, hypokalemia and metabolic alkalosis (Kagalwalla 1994). This autosomal recessive condition is characterized by a defect in Cl^-/HCO_3^+ transport in the ileum and colon with the resulting loss of large amounts of Cl^- in the stool. Na^+ is also lost in the stool and as a consequence the patients develop secondary hyperaldosteronism with urinary sparing of Na^+ and loss of K^+. This secretion starts in utero and is associated with maternal polyhydramnios which frequently results in premature delivery. In the neonatal period the presence of diarrhea may be missed leading to confusion with Bartter's syndrome in which the Cl^- loss is primarily renal and not intestinal. If the salt losses are not corrected the infant will become increasingly dehydrated and may die. Alkalosis is not present at birth and only develops over the subsequent weeks. Those infants who survive without adequate electrolyte replacement are invariably growth retarded with hypotonia and developmentally delayed as a consequence of chronic salt depletion.

The diagnosis is made from the high Cl^- content of the stool with level > 90 mmol/l exceeding the sum of the Na^+ and K^+ concentrations. Blood gasses will show a metabolic alkalosis, serum Cl⁻ and K⁺ are low while the Na⁺ level is likely to be normal. Urinary electrolytes will show very low or absent Na⁺ and Cl⁻ excretion with markedly raised K⁺ losses in the face of hypokalemia.

Treatment is with oral electrolyte supplements in the form of both NaCl and KCl given in amounts large enough to suppress the hyperaldosteronism, maintain urinary Cl⁻ excretion and correct the electrolyte deficiency. This treatment does not influence the diarrhea but results in the normal growth and development of the child.

Acrodermatitis enteropathica (see also p. 1627)

This is an autosomal recessive condition characterized by a specific defect in the absorption of zinc by the histologically normal small intestinal mucosa. The resulting zinc deficiency leads to a florid rash over the perineum (Fig. 11.11), buttocks and oral region with associated diarrhea, infection, alopecia and behavioral disturbance. The clinical features are reversed promptly by treatment with oral zinc supplements which need to be taken lifelong.

Primary hypomagnesemia

This autosomal recessive condition results from the defective absorption of magnesium by the small intestine and leads in the first few weeks of life to tetany and generalized convulsions associated with hypomagnesemia and hypocalcemia. On a normal diet the patient is in negative magnesium balance but this can be reversed by giving oral magnesium supplements. These supplements increase serum levels of both magnesium and calcium but unfortunately frequently induce diarrhea.

INVESTIGATION OF THE SMALL INTESTINE

A wide range of tests are available to look at the structure and function of the small intestine. Each test has its own specific indications and limitations and with the correct choice of investigations the maximum relevant information can be obtained with the minimum of invasive investigations.

RADIOLOGY

Plain abdominal X-ray is of value in detecting intestinal obstruction and the presence of free gas will also be seen if perforation has occurred. The barium follow-through or small bowel enema is the investigation of choice to define the anatomy of the small intestine and to demonstrate the gross mucosal pattern. This examination will define the rotation of the small intestine and allow the detection of blind loops, strictures and duplication cysts. Contrast studies are also invaluable in detecting small bowel involvement in Crohn's disease, intestinal polyps and infiltrative lesions of the small bowel such as non-Hodgkin's lymphoma.

The ectopic gastric mucosa in Meckel's diverticulum can be outlined with a technetium-99 pertechnetate scan and mucosal inflammation can be detected with the autologous labeling of leukocytes with technetium-99 hexametazime (HMPAO).

Celiac axis angiography is only very rarely required to define the site of intestinal hemorrhage from a vascular malformation.

JEJUNAL BIOPSY

The development of peroral small intestinal biopsy using the Watson or Crosby capsule has led to major advances in the diagnosis and management of small intestinal disease in children (Fig. 11.12). With an experienced operator using a pediatric capsule good mucosal biopsies can routinely be obtained from any child over 4 kg in weight and occasionally smaller (Figs 11.9 and 11.10). Recently there has been an increasing use of upper gastrointestinal endoscopy for small bowel biopsy. This technique has the advantage that the area for biopsy can be directly visualized, other pathologies may be detected at endoscopy and with the development of small instruments, biopsies in preterm infants are now possible. A major limitation is that biopsies tend to be small and difficult to orientate but this problem can be overcome by taking multiple biopsies.

In addition, if the biopsy material is correctly stored it is possible to carry out the quantitative measurement of brush border disaccharides by histochemical methods, to characterize the infiltrate in the lamina propria with immunostaining, and with electron microscopy the characteristic lesion of microvillous atrophy can be seen.

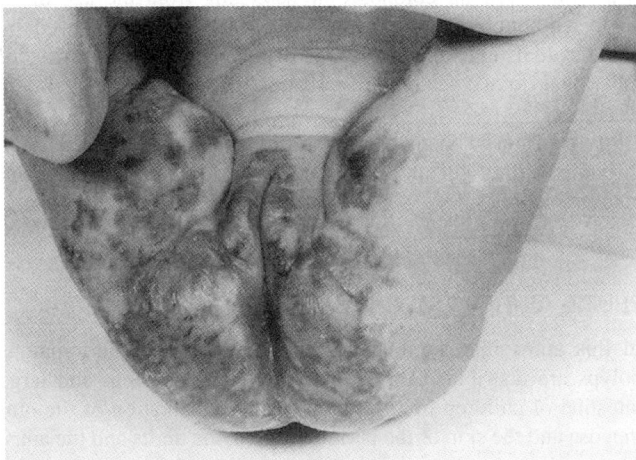

Fig. 11.11 The napkin area of a child with acrodermatitis enteropathica. (Reproduced by kind permission of P. J. Milla.)

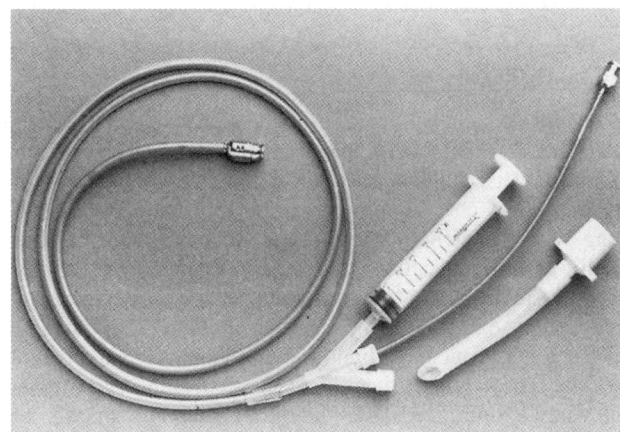

Fig. 11.12 The apparatus for a combined jejunal biopsy and pancreatic function test. The pancreatic secretions are aspirated through the overtube.

Serial mucosal biopsy is also valuable in monitoring the therapeutic response to a given line of therapy as has been described in the case of celiac disease.

NUTRIENT LOSS IN STOOL

Traditionally the loss of protein and fat in feces has been quantified by 5-day stool collections. Loss of protein labeled with chromium-51 albumin can be quantified by the measurement of radioactivity in the stool and the fat content can be directly measured. These techniques have now largely been replaced by simpler tests which rely on single stool samples. α_1-antitrypsin is a protein which is resistant to digestion by the gut and excretion in the feces is a reliable marker of stool protein loss. Fat loss can be quantified by the homogenization and separation of fat within fecal material by centrifugation of spot stool samples. The steatocrit refers to the fat content as a percentage of the total solid matter in the stool. Carbohydrate loss is detected by stool pH and clinitest measurement and quantified by chromatographic techniques.

BREATH HYDROGEN

When bacteria in the colon come in contact with undigested carbohydrate it is fermented with the production of hydrogen which is exhaled in the breath. By the use of a suitable carbohydrate load this phenomenon can be used to measure mouth to cecal transit time, the absorption of a range of mono- and disaccharides and to detect colonization of the small intestine by bacteria.

Lactulose is a naturally occurring carbohydrate which is not absorbed or digested by the human small intestine but is readily fermented by colonic bacteria to produce hydrogen. Therefore the time between an oral dose (250 mg/kg) and a rise in the basal level of breath hydrogen is an indication of mouth to cecal transit time. However, if an oral load of glucose (2 g/kg) is given to a healthy fasting subject the monosaccharide should be completely absorbed by the small intestine and no breath hydrogen peak will occur. In a patient with glucose–galactose malabsorption the glucose will pass straight into the colon causing a large peak in breath hydrogen along with abdominal pain and diarrhea. Finally, in a patient with bacterial overgrowth the glucose will be fermented almost immediately it leaves the stomach producing a very brisk and early rise in breath hydrogen.

STOOL CHROMATOGRAPHY

Whenever a patient has osmotic diarrhea it is likely that the stool will contain sugars. While these can be crudely detected using clinitest tablets, the quantification and characterization of these sugars by stool chromatography can be very useful, when taken along with the carbohydrate content of the child's feed or a specific oral load, in defining the cause of the underlying disorder. Two classic examples are the child with sucrase–isomaltase deficiency who, following the ingestion of complex carbohydrate, has loose stool containing limit dextrins, maltotriose and maltose and the baby with glucose–galactose malabsorption who, following a milk feed, has diarrhea containing glucose and galactose.

Specimens require immediate transport to the laboratory so that further digestion of sugars by colonic bacteria is prevented.

DUODENAL INTUBATION

When bacterial overgrowth is suspected, intubation with aspiration of duodenal juices is essential to confirm the diagnosis and define the sensitivities of the organisms present. Aspiration will similarly allow the concentration and pattern of luminal bile salts to be measured. The technique used to measure pancreatic function is described in the section on the pancreas.

GASTROINTESTINAL TUMORS

JUVENILE POLYPS

The most common polyp found in childhood is the juvenile polyp. These inflammatory lesions are found most frequently in the rectosigmoid but may develop more proximally and in 50% of cases more than one may be found. They present most frequently with painless rectal bleeding , in children between the ages of 2 and 5, although rarely they may present with recurrent abdominal pain and intussusception. These polyps do not undergo malignant change although if more than 10 lesions are seen, juvenile polyposis coli should be suspected. This condition can be differentiated from familial polyposis coli by the earlier age of onset and the presence of inflammatory, rather than adenomatous, polyps.

The diagnosis can be confirmed by flexible colonoscopy and at the same examination the polyps can be diathermied and removed for histological examination.

FAMILIAL ADENOMATOUS POLYPOSIS (FAP)

This autosomal dominant condition is characterized by multiple adenomatous polyps throughout the large intestine and is likely to present insidiously with diarrhea, blood and mucus in the stools (Foulkes 1995). The polyps which generally appear after puberty, slowly enlarge with time until they invariably undergo malignant change. The children of affected adults should be offered genetic screening and with the recognition of mutations in the FAP gene on chromosome 5q21 and the association with congenital hypertrophy of the retinal pigment epithelium, patients at high risk of developing the condition can be detected. Those at high risk require regular colonoscopic screening from the age of 10 years. Although the rate of polyp growth may be slowed by nonsteroidal anti-inflammatory drugs, for the majority of individuals total colectomy in early adulthood is still the treatment of choice.

In Gardner's syndrome adenomatous polyps are seen throughout the gut in association with bone osteomas and epidermoid cysts.

PEUTZ–JEGHERS SYNDROME

In this autosomal dominant condition multiple hamartomatous polyps are distributed throughout the jejunum, ileum and large intestine of children in association with pigmentation of the oral mucosa and the skin of the perioral region, the digits and the anus. The condition presents with anemia owing to blood loss or with obstruction secondary to intussusception. Malignant change is thought not to occur.

PSEUDOPOLYPS

In response to any inflammatory reaction the intestinal mucosa may become swollen and a polyp-like structure will be formed. As a result of enteric infections lymphoid hyperplasia with the formation of lymphoid follicles may occur and in conditions such as ulcerative colitis and Crohn's disease exuberant mucosal inflammation leads to pseudopolyp formation. The true nature of the lesions can be defined by mucosal biopsy.

HEMANGIOMAS

Intestinal hemangiomas which are frequently multiple are a well-recognized cause of rectal bleeding. Small colonic lesions can be sclerosed during endoscopic examination but laparotomy may be required for large angiomas and small intestinal lesions.

MALIGNANT TUMORS

Fortunately, malignant tumors of the intestine are very rare in childhood and in particular colonic and gastric neoplasms, which are so common in adult life, are hardly ever seen.

Small intestinal lymphoma of the non-Hodgkin's type is, however, occasionally seen. These tumors, which are of a B cell type, may be unifocal and present with obstruction or intussusception of the ileocecal region, or more commonly they are multifocal and present with ascites. Lymphoma occurs more commonly in immunodeficient children or following infection with the Epstein–Barr virus. If a laparotomy is required for intestinal obstruction the diagnosis can be made from the histology of the resected specimen but under other circumstances bone marrow aspiration and cytological examination of ascitic fluid is required.

THE PANCREAS

CYSTIC FIBROSIS

Cystic fibrosis is an autosomal recessive condition which affects approximately 1 in every 2000 live Caucasian births (Kopelman 1991). The underlying defect results from one of a number of possible mutations, in a chloride transporter protein which lines ductular epithelium. This results in inspissation of mucus in the ducts of the pancreas and in the bronchial and biliary trees with the resulting development of pancreatic insufficiency, chronic respiratory disease and biliary cirrhosis. In this section discussion will be confined to the effects of cystic fibrosis on the pancreas and intestine (Table 11.15) as the pulmonary (see Ch. 12) and hepatic (see p. 484) consequences are discussed elsewhere.

Pancreatic insufficiency

The inspissated concretions result in distention of the ducts and acini of the pancreas which with time progress to the formation of small cysts with destruction and fibrosis of the exocrine tissue. As a consequence of this the output of pancreatic enzymes and bicarbonate falls, leading to pancreatic insufficiency. In some patients endocrine pancreatic tissue is also damaged causing glucose intolerance in later life. Approximately 85% of patients with cystic fibrosis have pancreatic insufficiency with resulting malabsorption and steatorrhea, while in the remaining 15%, although not normal, the pancreas has adequate reserve capacity.

Table 11.15 Gastrointestinal manifestations of cystic fibrosis

1. Pancreas
   a. Pancreatic insufficiency
   b. Pancreatitis
   c. Diabetes mellitus

2. Hepatobiliary
   a. Biliary cirrhosis
   b. Lobular cirrhosis
   c. Cholelithiasis
   d. Biliary obstruction

3. Intestinal
   a. Meconium ileus
   b. Rectal prolapse
   c. Intussusception
   d. Esophageal reflux
   e. Distal intestinal obstruction syndrome

Signs of pancreatic insufficiency are usually present within the first 2 years of life with watery diarrhea progressing to foul, bulky pale stools. In the majority of children, growth is abnormal and fat-soluble vitamin deficiencies are likely to develop.

As a consequence of chronic steatorrhea bile salts are lost in the stool leading to depletion of the bile salt pool which may be further compounded if liver disease reduces the rate of synthesis. The resulting reduction in bile salt concentration will not only reduce the solubilization of lipids in the duodenum but may also reduce the solubilization of cholesterol and predispose to the formation of gallstones.

Meconium ileus

Cystic fibrosis may present in the first day or two of life with vomiting and abdominal distention due to meconium ileus. This obstruction to the small intestine with thick tenacious meconium may be complicated by volvulus, atresia or peritonitis. Plain abdominal X-ray will show dilated loops of intestine with meconium, outlined by trapped air, present in the obstructed segment of bowel and gastrografin enema will reveal a microcolon distal to the obstruction. The enema may be of benefit in the nonsurgical clearance of the meconium (see Ch. 31).

Difficulty in passing stool may also lead to rectal prolapse.

Distal intestinal obstruction syndrome

This condition, which is sometimes also referred to as meconium ileus equivalent, is a common problem known to occur in up to 15% of patients with cystic fibrosis. It is most common in adolescence and is characterized by recurrent episodes of subacute or occasionally acute obstruction with abdominal pain, vomiting and anorexia. Marked fecal loading may be detected by abdominal palpation or plain abdominal X-ray. If treatment with laxatives fails, the use of mucolytic drugs or balanced intestinal lavage should be considered.

Diagnosis of cystic fibrosis

The main diagnostic test for cystic fibrosis is the sweat test which measures the increased sodium content found in the sweat of children with cystic fibrosis. The vast majority of healthy children have a sweat sodium less than 45 mmol/l while in cystic fibrosis it is greater than 74 mmol/l in 99% of cases. A modification of this test measures the sweat osmolality which is greater than 125 mosmol/l in cystic fibrosis. The patient's DNA can be tested against a bank of known mutations of the cystic fibrosis gene but this in unlikely to be better than 90% accurate as many mutations have yet to be characterized. Where doubt still remains a formal pancreatic function test may be required to resolve the issue.

Treatment

As far as the intestinal complications of cystic fibrosis are concerned the main treatment for pancreatic insufficiency is with oral pancreatic supplements. Although only 10% of normal lipase activity is required to prevent steatorrhea, the majority of ingested supplements are inactivated by the low pH of the stomach and as a consequence symptoms may persist. This may be overcome by incorporating the pancreatic supplements within a pH-sensitive microsphere. The dose required by each patient is likely to vary greatly, although an inadequate dose will result in a failure to relieve symptoms while an excessive dose may lead to perianal excoriation or as recently reported, some children may develop thickening of the colonic mucosa, leading in some cases to obstruction.

The nutritional intake of patients with cystic fibrosis is frequently less than recommended for their age and given that their requirements may be up to 40% above average, it is perhaps not surprising that many children grow poorly. With improved dietary advice and the use of nutritional supplements children with cystic fibrosis are now growing better and as a consequence they are surviving longer. Where supplements cannot be given enterally, nasogastric or gastrostomy feeding may be helpful. Oral fat-soluble vitamin supplements, in particular vitamin E, are also required.

SHWACHMAN'S SYNDROME

After cystic fibrosis, Shwachman's syndrome is probably the next most common cause of pancreatic insufficiency in childhood (Berrocal et al 1995). This autosomal recessive condition is characterized by the presence of neutropenia with impairment of neutrophil function. The neutropenia may occur cyclically as may the thrombocytopenia which is seen in two-thirds of patients. Arrest in proliferation of the myeloid series may be seen on bone marrow aspiration and leukemic transformation has been reported in a number of patients. Bony abnormalities with metaphyseal chondrodysplasia are frequently seen with involvement of the femoral neck.

The diagnosis should be considered in any child with pancreatic insufficiency, a normal sweat test and neutropenia. Treatment is with pancreatic supplements while cimetidine or ascorbic acid may improve neutrophil function. The patients are particularly prone to recurrent infections and antibiotic prophylaxis may be of some benefit.

ACUTE AND CHRONIC PANCREATITIS

Pancreatitis is uncommon in childhood and frequently when it does occur no obvious precipitating cause can be found. Obstruction to the pancreatic duct, loss of vascular integrity and a direct insult to the parenchymal cells are all factors which can lead to the development of pancreatitis. Trauma, frequently as a consequence of child abuse, is one of the commonest causes of

Table 11.16 Causes of pancreatitis

1. Acute
   a. Trauma
   b. Infections
      (i) Mumps
      (ii) Coxsackie
      (iii) *Leptospira*
      (iv) *Ascaris*
   c. Gallstones
   d. Drugs
      (i) Valproic acid
      (ii) Cytosine arabinoside
      (iii) L-asparaginase
   e. Inflammatory bowel disease
   f. Metabolic
      (i) Reye's syndrome
      (ii) Refeeding malnutrition
      (iii) Parenteral nutrition
   g. Vasculitis
   h. Duodenal ulcer
   i. Idiopathic

2. Chronic
   a. Hereditary
   b. Metabolic
      (i) Hyperlipidemia
      (ii) Hyperparathyroidism
      (iii) Cystic fibrosis
   c. Duct malformations
   d. Idiopathic

acute pancreatitis (Mader & McHugh 1992) while hereditary causes are the most common reason for chronic pancreatitis (Perrault 1994). The causes of pancreatitis are listed in Table 11.16.

Presentation

Attacks of pancreatitis are characterized by severe epigastric or umbilical pain which tends to be constant rather than colicky and which can radiate to the back or shoulders. The pain is exacerbated by food and is not relieved by antacids. The patient will find abdominal movement uncomfortable and if the pancreatitis is severe, hemorrhagic bruising of the flanks with a paralytic ileus may develop. When the course is prolonged the condition may be complicated by circulatory collapse, hyperglycemia, hypocalcemia or by the formation of pleural effusions and pancreatic pseudocysts. The diagnosis is confirmed by markedly raised levels of serum amylase.

Treatment

The management of acute pancreatitis is conservative. All oral feeds should be stopped and intravenous fluids should be given to correct any fluid losses and to provide normal requirements. Acute pancreatitis can be very painful requiring adequate analgesia and where the patient is vomiting a nasogastric tube should be passed. An acute attack will normally last for between 3 and 5 days but if the attack is more prolonged total parenteral nutrition should be started and treatment with a somatostatin analogue should be considered. The patient should be monitored for the development of complications and serial abdominal ultrasounds will allow fluid collections to be detected at an early stage. Pseudocysts which fail to resolve spontaneously require to be drained.

In both acute and chronic pancreatitis if an underlying cause has been defined, this should be appropriately treated. Where a duct abnormality has been isolated reconstructive surgery may be of benefit and if a localized area of the pancreas is responsible for recurrent attacks, a partial pancreatectomy should be considered.

INVESTIGATION OF THE PANCREAS

The most commonly used indirect measure of pancreatic function in childhood is the sweat test which was discussed in the section on cystic fibrosis. The remaining investigations can be divided into blood tests which measure the level of pancreatic enzymes (i.e. amylase), tests which measure fecal fat or enzyme activity, more direct measures of pancreatic function and radiological imaging methods.

Pancreatic function tests

These tests can be divided into the traditional tests which require duodenal intubation and the newer tubeless function tests. The traditional tests remain the most accurate although they are also the most invasive. They involve the collection of duodenal juice (Fig. 11.12) during a basal fasting period followed by the stimulation of the pancreas with cholecystokinin (1–2 IU/kg) and then secretin (1–2 IU/kg) with the further collection of duodenal juice. In pancreatic insufficiency the stimulated levels of lipase and trypsin are reduced and the juice fails to alkalinize following stimulation with secretin. The tubeless tests rely on the pancreatic enzymes cleaving an ingested compound (bentiromide or fluoroscein dilaurate) and the amount subsequently collected in the urine is a measure of pancreatic function.

Radiology

Ultrasound is a very useful noninvasive imaging method in pancreatitis as it will show pancreatic edema during the acute attack, outline any fluid collections and allow gallbladder disease to be excluded. Where more detailed imaging is required of the structure of the pancreas, computerized tomographic techniques using X-ray and magnetic resonance may be used. In chronic pancreatitis where imaging of the pancreatic ducts is required to exclude a malformation or stricture, endoscopic retrograde cholangiopancreatography (ERCP) is invaluable. Any abnormality of the structure of the duodenum will be seen on a barium study.

DISORDERS OF GASTROINTESTINAL MOTILITY

Disorders of gastrointestinal motility are very common in childhood and are responsible for such diverse conditions as gastroesophageal reflux, the irritable bowel syndrome and chronic constipation (Milla 1988). Normal contractile activity relies on the coordinated action of the intestinal smooth muscle, its enteric and central neural connections and the humoral environment of the gut. Diseases exist in which damage to the enteric nervous system (Hirschsprung's disease) or smooth muscle (familial visceral myopathy) severely compromises the luminal transit of food and present with the symptoms of intestinal obstruction. The central nervous system has an important role in the modulation of intestinal motility with central insults commonly resulting in vomiting or even paralytic ileus. Lesser disturbances such as stress may lead to vomiting, abdominal pain and diarrhea.

ESOPHAGUS AND STOMACH

Motility disorders of the esophagus and stomach have already been discussed in their respective sections (pp. 425 and 426).

INTESTINAL PSEUDO-OBSTRUCTION

Intestinal pseudo-obstruction is a clinical syndrome characterized by the signs and symptoms of intestinal obstruction in a patient without any evidence of an obstructing lesion. Pseudo-obstruction occurs most commonly as a primary disorder in childhood; it may be familial, but may occasionally present in adolescence as a secondary manifestation of some other disease such as diabetes mellitus. The disorder tends to be generalized, involving either the smooth muscle or the enteric nerves of the entire length of the intestine.

A quarter of children present at birth and by 1 year two-thirds have developed symptoms of abdominal distention, vomiting, constipation and failure to thrive. Frequently it is only after an unnecessary laparotomy that the condition is diagnosed. Associated abnormalities of the urinary tract in some patients result in megacystis and megaureter and an association with malrotation of the small intestine has been reported. Diagnosis can be made from the history and from intestinal manometry which shows either a disruption or loss of cyclical fasting motor activity. A full thickness biopsy is required for a definitive diagnosis.

The condition is complicated by bacterial overgrowth of the small intestine and is punctuated by repeated episodes of obstruction. Nutrition is frequently compromised and in the most severe cases survival without total parenteral nutrition may not be possible.

LARGE INTESTINE

Colonic motility disorders will present in the neonatal period with the delayed passage of meconium and symptoms of intestinal obstruction if severe, or may be delayed for many months or years when they are more likely to present with chronic constipation. Hirschsprung's disease (see Ch. 31), hypo- and hyperganglionosis are now all well-recognized entities but unfortunately the nature of the structural or functional disorder in children with chronic constipation due to other causes is less well defined.

ACUTE INFECTIVE DIARRHEA

Acute infective diarrhea is one of the major causes of morbidity and mortality in childhood in the world today. It has been estimated that each year between 700 and 1000 million episodes of diarrhea occur in developing countries in children under 5 years of age and that this may result in up to 5 million deaths. This very high incidence results from the combined effect of contaminated water supplies, the preparation of bottle feeds under unhygienic conditions and from malnutrition which frequently occurs in these children at the time of weaning (Walker-Smith 1988).

In developed countries acute diarrheal illnesses occur most commonly in the first year of life and are second only to acute respiratory problems as a reason for hospital admission. Most acute diarrheal illnesses in well-nourished children are self-limiting and resolve within a few days. However, when frequent reinfection occurs, the child may develop a state of chronic diarrhea which will inevitably result in further malnutrition and an increased susceptibility to recurrent infection. It is this vicious cycle of events which along with the acute effects of dehydration leads to the significant mortality from this condition in developing countries.

ETIOLOGY AND PATHOGENESIS

The infective agent in acute diarrhea cannot always be isolated but with improvements in diagnostic techniques a pathogen can be isolated in up to 80% of cases. Viral agents are the most common cause of acute infective diarrhea in childhood, followed by bacteria and then protozoal infection. The causes of acute infective diarrhea are shown in Table 11.17 (Mehta & Lebenthal 1994).

In the young infant who is most at risk from the complications of acute diarrhea a number of protective mechanisms exist to limit the effect of infective pathogens. The acid content of the stomach and IgA secreted by the small intestine and in breast milk will limit the growth of bacteria in the upper small intestine and the resulting predominance of bifidobacteria in feces may inhibit colonization by enteric pathogens. These factors all lead to a reduced incidence of acute enteric infection in breast-fed infants.

Viral infection

The agent most commonly responsible for acute infantile gastroenteritis is the rotavirus. The rotavirus selectively attacks the mature enterocytes at the tips of the small intestinal villi which are killed and shed into the lumen. This leads to the increased production of immature crypt-like cells with shortening of the villi. These cells have greatly reduced absorptive and disaccharidase activity and this loss of normal small intestinal function leads to the production of diarrhea. Following the

Table 11.17   Causes of acute infective diarrhea

Bacteria
  Escherichia coli
  Vibrio cholerae
  Salmonella sp.
  Campylobacter sp.
  Staphylococcus aureus
  Yersinia enterocolitica
  Clostridium difficile
  Shigella sp.
  Aeromonas hydrophila
  Pseudomonas aeruginosa
  Bacillus cereus
  Enterobacter sp.
  Klebsiella sp.

Viruses
  Rotavirus
  Astrovirus
  Adenovirus
  Parvovirus-like (i.e. Norwalk agent)
  Coronavirus
  Small round viruses

Protozoa
  Giardia lamblia
  Entamoeba histolytica
  Cryptosporidium

clearance of the viral pathogen the functional mucosal abnormalities resolve.

Bacterial infection

Four major mechanisms are responsible for the effects of bacterial pathogens. Organisms such as *Vibrio cholerae* and some strains of *E. coli* synthesize proteins called *enterotoxins* which are able both to inhibit intestinal absorption and promote intestinal secretion. The preservation of electrogenic sodium-linked solute cotransport in these patients is exploited by the use of sodium- and glucose-containing oral rehydration solutions (ORS) which are able to promote net intestinal absorption in the face of active secretion.

Enteropathogenic organisms such as some strains of *E. coli* adhere to the brush border membrane of the small intestine (Fig. 11.13) causing severe mucosal damage which may take many weeks to recover and such children often require parenteral nutritional support during the intervening period. *Shigella* species and *E. coli* serotypes 0124 and 0164 possess enteroinvasive properties leading to the development of watery diarrhea and dysentery with bacterial invasion of the colonic mucosa, while some bacteria also produce *cytotoxins* which have a direct toxic effect on enterocytes.

CLINICAL FEATURES

Acute infective diarrhea characteristically results in a combination of nausea, vomiting, abdominal pain and diarrhea. In some children the symptoms may be relatively trivial while in others dehydration and metabolic disturbances may be life threatening. Symptoms appear generally to be most severe in younger and in malnourished infants who also run the risk of becoming septicemic from the enteric pathogen. Diarrhea and vomiting may also occur in a number of other medical conditions and it is important to consider systemic infection, metabolic disorders, surgical problems and other gastrointestinal disorders in the differential diagnosis of such patients.

The most serious consequence of acute diarrhea and vomiting is dehydration. In mild dehydration (2–5%) the child usually has a heightened thirst; when 5% dehydrated, oliguria develops with

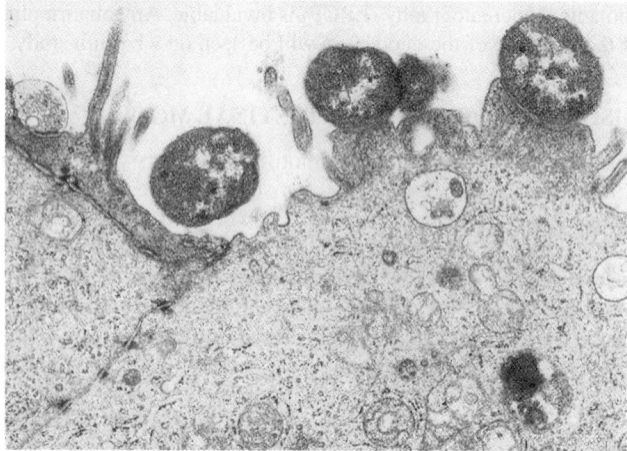

Fig. 11.13   An electron micrograph (magnification × 24 900) of an adherent enteropathic *E. coli* with destruction of the microvillous membrane. (Reproduced by kind permission of G. Anderson.)

reduced skin turgor, sunken eyes and sunken fontanel; and with increasing dehydration these symptoms become progressively more severe, with increasing apathy until the child is more than 10% dehydrated, when shock and anuria develop. Children on high solute diets, who develop diarrhea, may develop hypernatremic dehydration in which case the signs of dehydration are less obvious although lethargy and irritability may develop earlier.

Loss of bicarbonate and potassium in the stool, poor tissue perfusion, hypoglycemia, ketosis and renal failure may all lead to severe metabolic derangement. Symptoms of lethargy and irritability are particularly marked in hypernatremic dehydration and its rapid correction with i.v. fluids may lead to cerebral edema as a result of fluid shifts across the blood–brain barrier. This can result in convulsions or even death.

MANAGEMENT

The management of children with acute infective diarrhea hinges upon the treatment of their dehydration. The type of treatment required will depend very much on the severity of their dehydration and on the facilities which are available. Most mild cases can be treated at home by their family practitioner with oral rehydration therapy but where dehydration is more severe, social circumstances are poor or where other complicating medical factors are present, hospital admission is required. In developing countries where hospital facilities may be poor, the use of oral rehydration therapy has revolutionized the management of dehydrated infants (Lancet 1983). In addition to the management or the prevention of dehydration one has to consider how best to feed these infants during both the acute and recovery phase of their illness and whether drugs have any role in their therapy.

Dietary therapy

In patients with very mild or absent dehydration it is important that an adequate fluid intake is maintained to prevent the development of dehydration. In well-nourished children feeds may be reduced in strength for 24 h and fluids given as an oral rehydration solution. It has been suggested, however, that in children over the age of 9 months there is no need to reduce the strength of feed, as complications due to persistent diarrhea are relatively uncommon, and feeds should also be continued in breast-fed infants (Brown 1994). In poorly nourished children it is important to try to maintain food intake so that malnutrition is not further exacerbated, as fasting may prolong the diarrheal illness.

The use of oral rehydration solutions (ORS) has led to a large fall in mortality from acute infective diarrhea and has made it possible to treat moderate and severe dehydration without needing always to resort to intravenous therapy (Table 11.18). In 1980 the World Health Organization (WHO) published guidelines for the use of an ORS which contained a sodium concentration of 90 mmol/l and a glucose concentration of 110 mmol/l. There is some

concern that this sodium concentration is too high for children living in developed countries and a concentration of 60 mmol/l has been suggested as ideal for ORS solutions used in temperate climates. Where solutions need to be reconstituted with water prior to use, errors in dilution may lead to the production of hyperosmolar solutions which may further exacerbate the diarrhea.

When giving ORS solutions to prevent the development of dehydration, maintenance fluids should be given as a solution with a sodium concentration of 35–60 mmol/l or a 90 mmol/l sodium solution (WHO) in a ratio of 1 : 1 with water or breast milk. It has been suggested that in moderate and severe dehydration twice the estimated total fluid deficit is given orally over 6 h with two-thirds of this being given as 90 mmol/l ORS over the first 4 h and the remaining one-third as water over the next 2 h. If the infant is now rehydrated maintenance therapy should be started, as outlined above for the prevention of dehydration; if still dehydrated the regime should be repeated and if the dehydration is worse intravenous therapy should be started. This therapy is likely to be successful in up to 95% of cases. Where ORS solutions with a lower sodium concentration (i.e. 60 mmol/l) are used, all fluids should be given as ORS.

If the infant is shocked, is unable to tolerate the oral fluids or has evidence of an ileus, intravenous fluids should be initiated.

Intravenous therapy

If a child is severely shocked intravenous fluid in a volume of 15–20 ml/kg should be given rapidly over 10–15 min. In less severe cases it is more usual to give 40–80 ml/kg of fluid over 4 h as 0.45% sodium chloride/2.5% dextrose, although some of this fluid may be given as a plasma protein solution.

Once the child has been resuscitated, rehydration should be planned over the next 24 h for 5% dehydration and over 48 h for 10% dehydration. The volume required for rehydration = % dehydration/100 × weight (kg) × 1000 ml. The rehydration solution should be given as 0.45% sodium chloride/2.5% glucose and maintenance fluid should be given as 0.18% sodium chloride/4% dextrose. Potassium should only be added to the infusions once urine flow has started. Requirements for potassium will vary greatly (2–10 mmol/kg/24 h) depending on the extent of the losses.

In children with hypernatremic dehydration, rehydration should continue over 48 h to prevent sudden fluid shifts which might precipitate convulsions. The rehydration is similar to that described above for normonatremic infants except that after an initial period of half strength (0.45%) saline this can be reduced to one-fifth strength (0.18%). Where hyponatremia is present the total body sodium may paradoxically not be depleted and therefore 0.18% normal saline can be used for both rehydration and maintenance. However, when the sodium falls below 115 mmol/l extra sodium may be required. In severe cases intravenous bicarbonate should be given while in milder cases it is likely that the acidosis will correct spontaneously as the child is rehydrated. If urine flow is not re-established once circulatory volume has been restored, the possibility of acute renal failure should be considered.

Drug treatment

As a general rule drug treatment has very little part to play in the treatment of the majority of children with acute infective diarrhea. Opiate-derived antisecretory and antimotility drugs may under

Table 11.18 Major constituents of oral rehydration solutions (mmol/l)

	Sodium	Chloride	Potassium	Bicarbonate	Glucose
WHO–UNICEF	90	80	20	30	110
Dioralyte	60	60	20	10	90
Rehydrat	50	50	20	20	111

Table 11.19 Antibiotics used in the treatment of acute infective diarrhea

Infective condition	Antibiotic
Campylobacter enteritis	Erythromycin
Pseudomembranous colitis (*C. difficile*)	Vancomycin
Shigella dysentery	Co-trimoxazole
Typhoid	Co-trimoxazole or
Systemic salmonellosis	Chloramphenicol
Enteropathogenic *E. coli*	Gentamicin
Giardiasis	Metronidazole
Amebic dysentery	Metronidazole

some circumstances be harmful and should not be used. With certain pathogens treatment with antibiotics may be helpful although in the majority of cases treatment of the dehydration is all that is required. A list of antibiotics and their indications is shown in Table 11.19.

COMPLICATIONS

Acute infective diarrhea may be complicated by the extraintestinal spread of the infection with the development of intestinal perforation, abscess formation, septicemia and meningitis. If dehydration is pronounced acute renal failure may develop and if hypernatremia is corrected too rapidly cerebral edema with convulsions is likely to occur. This complication is less common when ORS is used as fluid shifts occur more slowly. In some children severe damage to the intestinal mucosa will lead to the development of diarrhea which persists long after the original pathogen has been cleared.

PROTRACTED DIARRHEA IN EARLY INFANCY

Protracted diarrhea may be defined as the passage of four or more watery stools per day persisting for at least 2 weeks. This definition encompasses a wide variety of disorders (Table 11.20) and a definitive diagnosis may only be made in approximately 70% of cases. In most instances, the protracted diarrhea appears to

Table 11.20 Causes of protracted diarrhea in early infancy

1. Food sensitivity/postenteritis syndrome
2. Cystic fibrosis
3. Celiac disease
4. Microvillous inclusion disease
5. Congenital chloride losing diarrhea
6. Congenital short bowel
7. Inborn error of carbohydrate absorption
   a. Sucrase–isomaltase deficiency
   b. Glucose–galactose malabsorption
8. Immunodeficiency
9. Hormone-secreting tumor (i.e. VIPoma)
10. Autoimmune enteropathy
11. Bacterial overgrowth
12. Nonaccidental injury (laxative administration)
13. Idiopathic

follow an episode of acute gastroenteritis in early infancy, although by the time of presentation to hospital it may be impossible to isolate an infective agent from the stool (Walker-Smith 1994). Furthermore, unless the situation is managed effectively at an early stage, a vicious cycle of malabsorption and malnutrition may result which will further compromise intestinal function and perpetuate the diarrhea.

One proposed sequence of events is that an acute infective insult may sensitize the intestine to foreign proteins (usually cow's milk protein), and subsequent ingestion of the offending food antigen causes further damage to the intestinal mucosa thus continuing the diarrhea. Although the resulting enteropathy may be caused primarily by the protein content of the milk feed, disaccharide intolerance (particularly lactose) may also develop and the institution of an appropriate exclusion diet will often result in resolution of the diarrhea. In this situation, an exclusion diet may be necessary only for 2 or 3 months after which a normal weaning diet can be reintroduced. In some cases, particularly in the developing world, bacterial overgrowth of the small intestine may be an added complication and bacterial toxins themselves may impair mucosal function.

Celiac disease, cystic fibrosis, selective inborn errors of absorption and immunodeficiency states may all present with intractable diarrhea of infancy. These conditions are discussed elsewhere in this chapter.

Although it is not possible to attach a diagnostic label to some 20–30% of cases of protracted diarrhea, over recent years several new causes of the condition have been described. Mirakian et al (1986) reported cases of protracted diarrhea in which autoantibodies to intestinal enterocytes were present as part of a polyendocrinopathy syndrome. In the remainder of cases of protracted diarrhea, a strong family tendency may be present and in these patients there is a high mortality (Candy et al 1981). Many of these children have true secretory diarrhea which may be evident from the large volume of stool passed and from analysis of the stool electrolytes. A proportion of these infants may suffer from congenital chloride losing diarrhea or intestinal microvillous inclusion disease (Phillips & Schmitz 1992). Where intestinal secretion is present in utero there may be a history of polyhydramnios or premature labor.

INVESTIGATIONS

Collection and examination of the stool is vital and a careful search for intestinal pathogens (bacteria, viruses, parasites) should be undertaken at an early stage. The stools should be analyzed for the presence of reducing substances (> 1%) and stool electrolytes and osmolality should be measured to determine whether the diarrhea is osmotic or secretory in nature (Table 11.21). Chromatography of a fresh stool specimen may help in the

Table 11.21 Stool analysis in osmotic and secretory diarrhea

	Osmotic	Secretory
Osmolality (mosmol/l)	400	290
Na^+ (mmol/l)	30	105
K^+ (mmol/l)	30	40
$(Na^+ + K^+) \times 2$	120	290
Solute gap (mmol/l)	280	0

diagnosis of inborn errors of carbohydrate absorption and in determining the osmotically active substances within the stool. Valuable information may also be obtained by fasting the child as this is likely to result in a marked diminution of osmotic diarrhea with little change in secretory diarrhea. It must be remembered, however, that in severe cases of osmotic diarrhea the child may be unable to absorb even endogenous secretions and thus the diarrhea will persist. It is essential to collect and measure the volume of all stools as this will influence the amount and the nature of fluid replacement therapy.

Jejunal biopsy is invaluable in detailing the morphology of the small intestinal epithelium and a sweat test can rule out cystic fibrosis. Blood tests are of limited value although peripheral blood eosinophilia may be present in children with food protein sensitivity and investigation of immune function may reveal specific abnormalities in the child with diarrhea due to immunodeficiency. Measurement of electrolytes and acid–base balance is important in the day-to-day management of fluid balance and may be abnormal in children with congenital chloride-losing diarrhea. If the cause of the diarrhea is not immediately evident serum should be sent for gut-autoantibody estimation to exclude gut autoimmune disease, and circulating gut hormones should be measured to exclude a hormone-secreting tumor. Serum and urine toxicology should be checked if laxative abuse by the mother is suspected.

Radiological studies are rarely informative but barium meal and follow-through will exclude malrotation and may occasionally demonstrate a blind loop. Endoscopic evaluation of the upper and lower gastrointestinal tract is often helpful and multiple biopsies may be taken for examination by light and electron microscopy in addition to obtaining fluid from the lumen of the gut, which should be screened for the presence of pathogens.

TREATMENT

The management of the infant with protracted diarrhea depends on the cause and the severity of the condition. In many cases dietary manipulation is the mainstay of management as appropriate exclusion diets often reduce the volume of diarrhea. A variety of hypoallergenic feeds may be appropriate either as a complete feed (e.g. Pregestimil, Mead Johnson, and Neocate, Scientific Hospital Supplies) or as a modular feed (e.g. comminuted chicken, Cow & Gate) when the protein, carbohydrate and fat contents of the diet can be varied independently. The assistance of an experienced pediatric dietitian is essential in the management of any infant with protracted diarrhea and details of appropriate diets may be found in a recent monograph (Shaw & Lawson 1994).

Those infants who are severely malnourished or who do not respond to enteral feeding and dietetic management may, in addition, need a period of intravenous feeding. In carefully selected cases of severe and intractable diarrhea, it may be possible to institute a regime of home parenteral nutrition so that the child may experience as normal an existence as possible (Puntis 1995, Bisset et al 1992).

In certain situations drug therapy may be beneficial. If there is evidence of bacterial overgrowth and bile salt degradation, cholestyramine and antibiotics may help the situation. Other agents such as corticosteroids or prostaglandin inhibitors may be used empirically with limited success, and antisecretory agents such as chlorpromazine and loperamide may be beneficial in some cases.

In general terms, for those children who present several weeks or months after birth the prognosis is good, while for those who present at birth with an intractable secretory diarrhea the prognosis is poor and the mortality high.

THE COLON

STRUCTURE

The colon is a long hollow tube which, with the exception of the sigmoid which has a short mesentery, lies retroperitoneally. Along its length from the ileocecal valve to the anus the mucosa is lined by a cuboidal epithelium which is indented with crypts. The mature colon has no villi and no brush border disaccharidase activity. Submucosal and myenteric nerve plexuses are present, similar to those in the small intestine, but the smooth muscle layers differ in that the longitudinal layer is incomplete forming three tenia coli.

FUNCTION

The large intestine fulfills both storage and salvage functions. The colon stores the intestinal contents prior to excretion, but it is also an organ of conservation which reduces liquid ileal effluent to solid feces excreted via the anus. It plays an important role in the salvage of electrolytes and water, and in addition, the salvage of nutrients in the form of short chain fatty acids.

Absorption

Although it is clear that the majority of water and electrolyte absorption occurs in the small intestine, it is often the adequacy of colonic function which determines whether the child experiences diarrhea, and whether or not there is net loss of water and electrolytes from the body. In small intestinal disease there is an increase in the volume of fluid arriving at the ileocecal valve but the colon has a reserve reabsorptive capacity which can adequately absorb the excess ileal effluent. When there is massive small intestinal secretion, the reserve reabsorptive capacity of the colon may be overwhelmed, resulting in diarrhea. In addition, in disorders which compromise colonic function such as inflammatory bowel disease, diarrhea may occur as a result of either reduced colonic absorptive capacity or frank colonic secretion (Jenkins & Milla 1993).

The importance of the colonic sodium absorptive mechanism is demonstrated clinically by the high rate of sodium supplementation necessary for normal growth in infants with ileostomies. The majority of sodium absorption occurs via an active, electrogenic mechanism, while chloride is absorbed down its electrochemical gradient. Potassium is secreted into the lumen largely in response to electrochemical gradients and, in older children, bicarbonate is secreted into the colonic lumen via an exchange mechanism with chloride (Jenkins & Milla 1988). Recently it has been shown that colonic sodium absorptive processes are already highly efficient in preterm infants and there is evidence that circulating aldosterone levels may be important in the regulation of these mechanisms (Jenkins et al 1990).

In addition to its role in the absorption of water and electrolytes, the colon may also salvage extra nutrient energy from the contents of the gastrointestinal tract via the absorption of short chain fatty acids such as acetate, butyrate and propionate. These are produced by colonic bacterial fermentation of unabsorbed dietary carbohydrate and studies have shown that they are rapidly absorbed from the large intestine, providing a significant additional source of energy, and also that they promote further colonic salt and water absorption (Jenkins et al 1993).

The salvage of electrolytes, water and nutrients requires sophisticated integration of the functions of bacterial digestion, epithelial transport and motor activity of the colonic muscle layers. Details of colonic motility patterns are scanty in childhood, although a major proportion of the total mouth to anus transit time occurs in the large intestine.

INFLAMMATORY BOWEL DISEASE

Although infective agents are the commonest cause of inflammatory bowel disease in a worldwide context, the term will be used in this section to describe chronic inflammation of the gastrointestinal tract in the absence of a detectable pathogenic agent. Included in this definition in descending order of importance are Crohn's disease, ulcerative colitis and allergic colitis. In addition, the term 'indeterminate colitis' has been employed to describe children with colitis which is impossible to precisely categorize at presentation: the final diagnosis may often only become evident in these patients with the lapse of time and further, or repeated, investigation.

EPIDEMIOLOGY

As in adults, the prevalence of Crohn's disease has increased dramatically over the last 30 years and in the UK stands at approximately 10–20 per 100 000 of the childhood population compared with a relatively constant prevalence of ulcerative colitis at 4–6 per 100 000 (Ferguson 1984, Cosgrove et al 1996).

There are two large peaks in incidence of inflammatory bowel disease, one in early and one in later adult life with a much smaller peak in infancy and early childhood. 25–40% of patients with Crohn's disease and only some 15% of patients with ulcerative colitis present before the age of 20 years (Booth & Grand 1988), and these diseases account for the peaks in adolescence and early adult life. Although Crohn's disease and ulcerative colitis present in early childhood, it now seems likely that many cases of colitis presenting in the first 2 years of life may be related to food allergy.

ETIOLOGY

The etiology and pathogenesis of Crohn's disease and ulcerative colitis are unknown despite many theories and much painstaking research work. There is an equal sex incidence and the disorders occur more frequently in north European, Anglo-Saxon races, European and North American Jews and urban dwellers (Booth & Grand 1988). Although there appears to be a genetic predisposition to develop the conditions, with studies reporting between 16 and 40% of patients' relatives also affected with inflammatory bowel disease, there is no evidence linking a particular HLA type to inflammatory bowel disease.

Multiple immunological abnormalities have been described in patients with inflammatory bowel disease but none has convincingly been shown to be a primary pathogenetic event. Infectious agents have been postulated as playing a major role but so far the evidence is inconclusive. Several bacteria and virus-like particles have been implicated and recently there has been interest that the measles virus may be a risk factor although this has not yet been proven (Thompson et al 1995). There is no good evidence to closely link environmental factors such as foodstuffs in the etiology of Crohn's disease or ulcerative colitis, although there is compelling evidence incriminating dietary allergens, particularly dairy produce and soya milk, in the pathogenesis of allergic colitis in younger children (Jenkins et al 1984). Studies have, however, shown that intestinal permeability may be increased in Crohn's disease and it is conceivable that this could result in an increase in absorption of antigens from the gut, which may be important in the pathogenesis of the disease. Finally, it has been suggested that psychosomatic factors may be important and a 'colitis personality' was previously defined. However, several studies have not supported this concept and it is hardly surprising that there may be a higher incidence of emotional problems and depression found in sufferers and their families as a consequence of their chronic, debilitating disease. Thus adequate psychological and emotional support from health care staff is of paramount importance in the management of children with inflammatory bowel disease. Adequate communication is vital, and several self-help groups publish helpful booklets and can provide additional support and information for the child and family. The contact addresses of the groups are shown at the end of the chapter.

CROHN'S DISEASE

Pathology

The disease may involve any part of the gastrointestinal tract from the lips to the perianal area, and normal bowel may be found in between affected areas. The inflammation is transmural, often extending from the mucosa to the serosal surface, resulting in sinus tracts or fistulae formation. In childhood disease, terminal ileitis is common with variable involvement of the colon in 50–70% (Griffiths 1992). Macroscopically, the bowel mucosa may look inflamed, and small shallow, aphthoid or linear ulcers may be present. Later on in the disease, deeper fissures may occur leading to the classic 'cobblestone' appearance of the mucosa, as well as stricturing of the bowel. Histologically, there is transmural inflammation and the diagnostic hallmark is the finding of noncaseating epithelioid granulomata with giant cells which may not be present in all affected tissues.

Clinical features

The insidious onset and subtle nature of the symptoms and signs of Crohn's disease often result in a considerable delay in diagnosis with left-sided colonic disease being usually diagnosed more rapidly than diffuse small intestinal disease. The manifestations of the disease depend upon the site of involvement (von Allmen et al 1995) but periumbilical, colicky abdominal pain, diarrhea with or without blood and growth failure are the commonest forms of presentation. Occasionally more subtle manifestations, such as oropharyngeal disease, perianal skin tags and fissuring or growth failure, may be the first signs of the disorder in the absence of overt gastrointestinal symptoms. The diarrhea in Crohn's disease is likely to be due to a combination of several factors which may include mucosal dysfunction, bile acid malabsorption, bacterial overgrowth and protein exudation from inflamed bowel.

On examination, it is important to ascertain whether extraintestinal manifestations of Crohn's disease are present. Thus there may be intermittent pyrexia, clinical anemia, arthralgia and arthritis, uveitis, finger clubbing, perianal disease (skin tags, bluish discoloration, fissures, fistulae), oral ulceration, skin manifestations (erythema nodosum and pyoderma gangrenosum), signs of liver dysfunction and evidence of growth failure and delayed sexual maturation. Examination of the abdomen may reveal generalized or localized tenderness and occasionally an ill-defined palpable mass. The importance of growth retardation and pubertal delay must be emphasized as it may occur in up to 30% of children with Crohn's disease and may be present well before the diagnosis is made (Kanof et al 1988). There is little evidence that this is due to a primary endocrine disturbance and the most likely reason for growth failure is nutritional deprivation or a direct effect of inflammatory molecules such as cytokines on the growing skeleton. Studies have indicated that children with Crohn's disease may ingest only 50–80% of recommended daily calories and there is increasing evidence that nutritional supplementation will promote growth in these patients (Belli et al 1988).

Diagnosis

Laboratory assessment involves the search for infective agents in the stools of patients with Crohn's disease presenting with diarrhea. Hematological investigation often reveals iron-deficiency anemia and acute phase reactants such as ESR and CRP may be elevated, although not universally. Thrombocytosis and hypoalbuminemia may also be present and these appear to be more reliable markers of disease activity. Plasma zinc levels are frequently low and liver function tests may be abnormal. It should, however, be remembered that alkaline phosphatase is a zinc-dependent enzyme which may be spuriously depressed in the presence of zinc deficiency.

Radiological assessment is important and plain abdominal X-rays may reveal evidence of intestinal obstruction or bowel dilation. A barium meal and follow-through is vital in order to assess the small bowel and, although a small bowel meal (via a transpyloric tube) is the most sensitive technique, this is not always acceptable as it may be particularly uncomfortable for the child. The presence of skip lesions, with narrowing of the lumen, thickening and fissuring ('rose-thorn ulcers') of the bowel wall and fistulae formation are all highly suggestive of Crohn's disease (Fig. 11.14). A technetium-labeled leukocyte scan is proving useful in the diagnosis and follow-up of disease and may become the first-line investigation (Jobling et al 1996).

The increasing usage of flexible endoscopes in pediatric practice has proved a safe method for assessing both the upper gastrointestinal tract and the colon (Rossi 1988). Using a pediatric colonoscope, it is possible to visualize the whole of the large intestine and the terminal ileum, and also to obtain multiple biopsies for histological assessment (Fig. 11.15).

In contrast to ulcerative colitis, the rectum in Crohn's colitis is normal in 50% of cases, but changes may be seen in the terminal ileum. If colonoscopy is not available, colonic Crohn's disease may be diagnosed by barium enema examination (preferably double contrast) looking for the suggestive features of discontinuous mucosal ulceration, loss of haustrations, and colonic narrowing with cobblestoning and fissures.

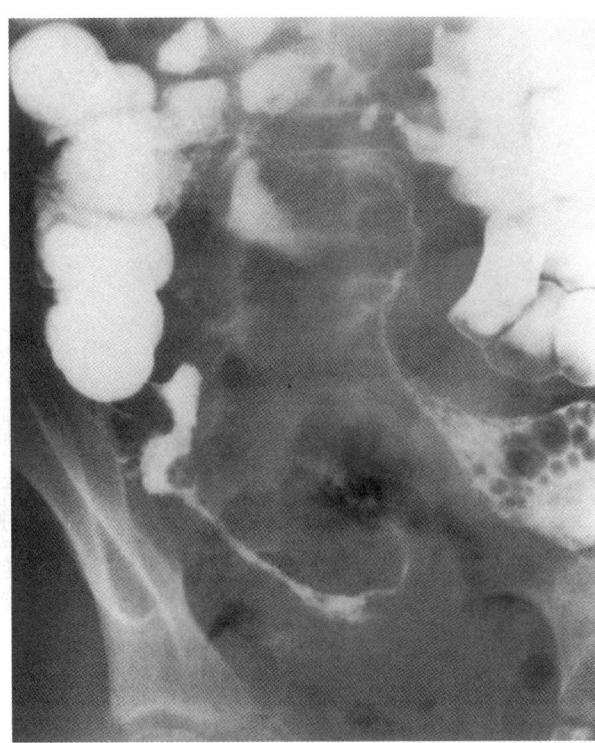

Fig. 11.14   Extensive narrowing of the ileum in a child with small intestinal Crohn's disease. (Reproduced by kind permission of P. J. Milla.)

Treatment

The goal of therapy is both to induce and maintain a remission of active disease and also to correct malnutrition and promote growth.

There is no convincing evidence that any drug alters the long-term natural history of Crohn's disease, but several agents have a place in the treatment of the disorder. Steroids may induce remission in over 70% of patients and prednisolone should be given in an initial dose of 2 mg/kg/day (max. 40 mg) with a gradual reduction after 2–4 weeks, preferably to an alternate-day regime in order to minimize the growth-suppressive side effects. There is no good evidence that low dose steroid therapy can maintain remission and, if possible, steroid therapy should be gradually reduced over a further 6–8 weeks and stopped if the disease is quiescent.

Sulfasalazine (50–80 mg/kg/day) is useful in the treatment of active Crohn's colitis in inducing remission, although there is little evidence that continuous therapy will maintain remission. The active moiety of sulfasalazine is 5-aminosalicylic acid and new preparations containing this drug may be effective alternatives in the future in those patients who experience side effects related to sulfasalazine (Leichtner 1995). Interestingly, immunosuppressive therapy (such as azathioprine or 6-mercaptopurine) may be useful in maintaining remission or reducing steroid requirements, although the use of these drugs is potentially hazardous and should be reserved for moderate to severe cases. Metronidazole may be effective in colonic and particularly perianal disease although peripheral neuropathy may develop with its long-term use. In children who are acutely toxic and systemically unwell on presentation, it is reasonable to start intravenous broad spectrum antibiotics, including metronidazole,

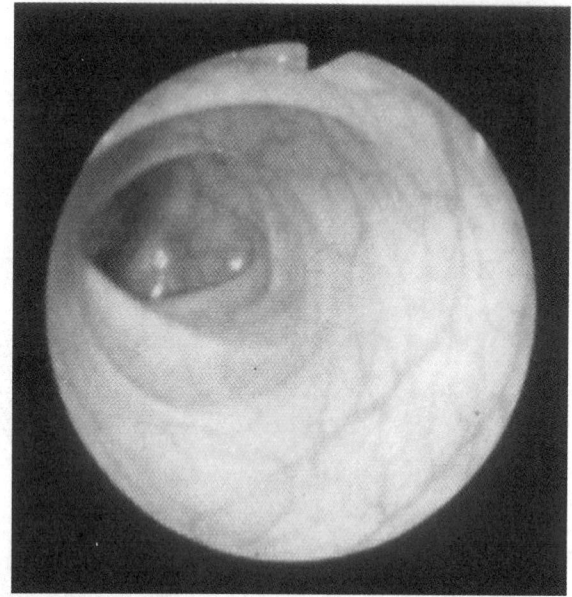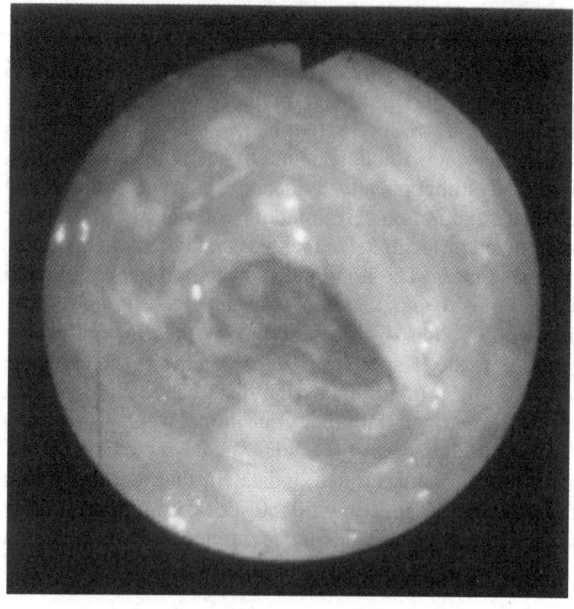

(a)   (b)

Fig. 11.15   The colonoscopic appearance in (**a**) a normal child with the mucosal blood vessels clearly seen and (**b**) in a child with Crohn's disease showing 'snail tract' ulceration and loss of the vascular pattern of the mucosa. (Reproduced by kind permission of P. J. Milla.)

in addition to intravenous steroids until the disease begins to remit.

Nutritional therapy has recently been recognized as a very important therapeutic modality in Crohn's disease, not only in the correction of specific nutrient deficiencies, but also in the reduction of disease activity and the reversal of growth failure. Patients may need specific therapy with iron, folate, vitamin B$_{12}$ and zinc in addition to ensuring an adequate energy intake via the oral or nasogastric route (with elemental feeds) or indeed via intravenous feeding. Furthermore, nutritional therapy has been shown to be effective in inducing remission of active disease (Griffiths et al 1995) and both enteral and parenteral routes may be used.

The indications for surgical intervention in Crohn's disease include intestinal obstruction, fistula formation, hemorrhage and perforation, and a failure of medical therapy, particularly where there is growth failure. The surgical results in Crohn's disease are most encouraging in children with localized ileal disease (Davies et al 1990), although children with both large and small bowel disease may require reoperation at a later date.

Prognosis

The prognosis for childhood Crohn's disease is reasonably optimistic and, although the morbidity is relatively high, the mortality is low (Ferguson & Sedgwick 1994). The outcome is dependent on the site of the disease with patients with colonic disease suffering more extraintestinal complications and more operations than those with small bowel disease.

The risk of colorectal carcinoma in childhood with Crohn's colitis is not well defined although there is a suggestion that the incidence is slightly increased when compared with a control population. Long-term follow-up studies are needed to clarify this point and the large intestine in patients with colitis should be inspected regularly by colonoscopy.

ULCERATIVE COLITIS

Pathology

Ulcerative colitis is an inflammatory disease of the large intestinal mucosa and the abnormal changes are seen most commonly in the rectum and distal colon, although the whole colon may be affected. Indeed, pancolitis is the most common form (62%) while disease of the left colon (22%) or rectum (15%) occurs less frequently. Unlike Crohn's disease, the inflammation is continuous and it is usually limited to the colonic mucosa. Macroscopically the mucosa is friable and granular, and ulceration may be present in association with a bloody or mucopurulent exudate. The ulceration, which is often patchy, may be interspersed with areas of regenerating epithelium, resulting in pseudopolyp formation. In addition, there may be an inflammatory reaction in the distal ileum, so-called 'backwash ileitis'. The characteristic histological features are an acute and chronic inflammatory cell infiltrate in the lamina propria, distortion of crypt architecture, the presence of crypt abscesses and goblet cell depletion.

Clinical features

The commonest presenting features are diarrhea, often associated with blood and mucus, and tenesmus with lower abdominal pain which is relieved by defecation. Attacks may be graded as mild, moderate or severe depending upon stool frequency, abdominal tenderness, fever and the degree of anemia and hypoalbuminemia. It is important to recognize that 5–10% of patients with ulcerative colitis may present with fulminating colitis associated with toxic megacolon, and a plain abdominal X-ray should be performed to look for the presence of a dilated colon (usually exceeding 6 cm in diameter).

On examination the only positive findings may be minimal lower abdominal tenderness, although in severe disease the child may be pyrexial, dehydrated, anemic and profoundly toxic. It is important to look carefully for evidence of extraintestinal manifestations which are similar to those of Crohn's disease, although growth retardation occurs less frequently in ulcerative colitis and affects less than 20% of patients at presentation.

Diagnosis

Infective agents such as *Shigella*, *Salmonella*, *Campylobacter*, *Yersinia* and *Entamoeba* may cause an acute or chronic colitis, and it is vital to look carefully for pathogens in the stool and perform appropriate serological tests. Further laboratory assessment may reveal anemia, raised levels of ESR and CRP, leukocytosis and hypoalbuminemia which may reflect the disease activity. Radiological investigations should include plain abdominal X-ray if the child is systemically unwell and endoscopic evaluation of the whole colon is very useful both in assessing the severity and the extent of the inflammation, and also to confirm the diagnosis histologically. However, the procedure should be deferred or at least limited in patients with acute severe colitis because of the risk of toxic megacolon and perforation.

A good colonoscopic examination makes barium enema examination unnecessary, although radiological changes may be seen on barium enema examination which range from superficial ulceration to loss of colonic haustrations, deeper ulceration with thickening of the bowel wall and eventually the finding of a shortened, featureless, tubular colon.

Treatment

Therapy is directed towards inducing and maintaining remission in mild or moderate disease and may be life saving in fulminating colitis. Patients with mild disease are best treated with sulfasalazine (50–80 mg/kg/day) and, in those children with disease confined to the distal colon, a topical steroid preparation may be useful. Moderately severe disease (bloody diarrhea five times/day, abdominal pain, fever) may require the addition of oral steroids (prednisolone 1–2 mg/kg/day, max. 40 mg) in order to induce remission, and this dose should be gradually reduced after 2 weeks if the child's condition is improving. Antispasmodic medication and agents which decrease gut motility should not be given as they may precipitate the development of toxic megacolon.

Severe, fulminating colitis is a medical emergency which is easily underestimated. The child should receive nothing by mouth and intravenous therapy is always indicated. The patient will usually need rehydration and blood transfusion, and regular albumin infusions are often required. All children should receive intravenous hydrocortisone (10 mg/kg/day) and broad spectrum antibiotics (penicillin, gentamicin, metronidazole) and, if malnourished, parenteral nutrition should be instituted at an early stage. Many children with severe colitis will respond to this aggressive medical therapy within 7–10 days, but if by this time there is no improvement, or the child develops a complication such as toxic megacolon, colonic hemorrhage or perforation, then surgery is necessary. In addition to emergency surgery for complications of acute disease, elective surgery may be required if there is a failure of medical therapy, severe growth retardation unresponsive to improved nutrition or severe colonic dysplasia with the risk of adenocarcinoma formation in long-standing colitis. The surgical procedures available for the child include a proctocolectomy with ileostomy or ileal reservoir, or a colectomy

with rectal mucosectomy and endorectal pull-through (Booth & Grand 1988).

As regards the maintenance of remission, there is good evidence that continued therapy with sulfasalazine (or its derivatives) is superior to placebo in preventing relapse although, in some patients, alternate-day steroids may also be required. Immunosuppressive drugs are proving to be useful in patients with intractable disease.

In contrast to Crohn's disease, there is little evidence that aggressive nutritional therapy alone, either enteral or parenteral, is effective in inducing remission in ulcerative colitis, although the correction of malnutrition and specific nutritional deficiencies is mandatory in all patients.

Prognosis

Approximately 90% of patients with ulcerative colitis presenting in childhood or adolescence will experience one or more relapses of their disease after initial treatment. The majority will be able to lead a relatively normal life despite chronic disease but some 20% will be chronically incapacitated. The prognosis is best for isolated, distal colitis, with only 10% progressing to pancolitis; overall, approximately 30% of patients will eventually require colectomy. There is an increased risk of developing large intestinal adenocarcinoma in patients with long-standing ulcerative colitis, although the risk is probably considerably less than previously thought (Fozard & Dixon 1989). The advent of flexible endoscopy has made possible careful, regular surveillance of the colonic mucosa and colonoscopy and biopsy should be performed at regular intervals in older patients with long-standing colitis.

RECTAL BLEEDING

The passage of small amounts of blood per rectum is not uncommon in childhood and is rarely of sinister significance, being often due to a simple anal fissure or self-limiting infective colitis. It is important to determine whether it is bright red blood that has been passed, around, after or mingled with the stool as in the case of bleeding from the colon, or whether the blood is altered, or indeed melena, which may signify a more proximal source of bleeding. It is also helpful to determine whether there is mucus or slime in the stool or if there is associated diarrhea or constipation, abdominal pain or perianal pain on defecation.

Clinical examination should attempt to assess the degree of blood loss and whether anemia is present. Adequate visualization of the perianal region is mandatory and the use of a pediatric proctoscope may yield important diagnostic clues. General examination includes a detailed examination of the skin for evidence of purpura and telangiectases, circumoral pigmentation, and evidence of arthritis and renal abnormalities should be sought. Although direct visualization of the stool may reveal fresh blood or melena, chemical testing may be required when occult bleeding from a more proximal source is present. A number of kits are available for the testing of occult fecal blood, although most are highly sensitive and are likely to give false positive results, particularly if the child is receiving vitamin C supplements or food high in peroxidase activity such as uncooked vegetables.

Etiology

Table 11.22 outlines some of the commoner causes of rectal bleeding in childhood. It is important at any age (particularly in the

Table 11.22 Causes of rectal bleeding in childhood

1. Anal fissure
2. Infective colitis
   a. *Shigella*
   b. *Salmonella*
   c. *Campylobacter*
3. Allergic colitis
4. Intestinal polyps
   a. Juvenile polyps
   b. Familial polyposis coli
   c. Peutz-Jeghers syndrome
   d. Gardner's syndrome
   e. Tuberous sclerosis
5. Generalized bleeding diathesis
6. Hemolytic uremic syndrome
7. Inflammatory bowel disease
8. Rectal prolapse
9. Intussusception
10. Meckel's diverticulum/gut duplication
11. Henoch–Schönlein purpura
12. Hemangioma/angiodysplasia/telangiectasia
13. Upper gastrointestinal bleeding

neonatal period) to exclude swallowed blood as a cause of rectal bleeding. The etiology of bleeding per rectum is influenced by the age of the patient and also by the mode of clinical presentation. Thus, a child with chronic constipation who passes bright red blood on the surface of the stool may have an associated anal fissure, while the infant with intussusception may present with colicky abdominal pain, shock and the passage of 'red currant jelly stools'. Acute vomiting and bloody diarrhea may herald the onset of intestinal infection and the presence of hematuria and proteinuria may suggest Henoch–Schönlein purpura or the hemolytic uremic syndrome. Chronic blood loss with the painless passage of bright red blood is suggestive of a colonic polyp or hamartoma and a detailed family history may be helpful.

Investigation and treatment

The pattern of investigation will depend upon the urgency of the clinical presentation. Thus an infant who is shocked and passing bright red blood per rectum will need resuscitation and an urgent plain abdominal X-ray and possibly a contrast enema to exclude intussusception. Usually the presentation is less acute and initial laboratory assessment should include a full blood count, ESR, serum iron and ferritin estimation, serum electrolytes and clotting studies. In cases of bloody diarrhea, stool culture is mandatory and plain abdominal X-ray may be helpful. The most useful investigation is colonoscopy, which after scrupulous bowel preparation will provide direct visualization of the colonic mucosa and allow multiple biopsies to be obtained for histology. Furthermore, the procedure may be therapeutic as smaller polyps may be removed at colonoscopy by diathermy (Douglas et al 1980).

Isotope scanning using technetium may identify ectopic gastric mucosa in either a Meckel's diverticulum or in a duplication of the intestine, and labeling of red blood cells with the isotope may also be useful in detecting the site of active, but occult, gastrointestinal blood loss. In the last resort, in selected cases of severe chronic unexplained iron-deficiency anemia associated with positive fecal occult blood, it may be necessary to perform angiography to localize the source of bleeding and rarely laparotomy and intraoperative endoscopy is indicated.

CHRONIC GASTROINTESTINAL SYMPTOMS

RECURRENT ABDOMINAL PAIN

Recurrent abdominal pain is a relatively common pediatric problem, occurring primarily in older children and adolescents. The term generally describes recurrent and moderately severe episodes of abdominal pain over a period of at least 3 months which may lead to absence from school and may affect the child's lifestyle. Typically the pain is nonspecific although most children describe colicky, periumbilical discomfort. Most importantly the child is healthy in between these episodes and physical examination is normal. Surveys of British and American populations have suggested that this disorder is very common, affecting some 10–20% of school children (Apley 1959, Oster 1972).

Etiology and pathogenesis

Although early studies showed that in only 7% of cases is an organic cause found to explain the pain (Apley 1959), it is increasingly recognized that many conditions may cause such pain, such as constipation, abdominal migraine (Symon & Russell 1995), gastritis and peptic ulcer associated with *Helicobacter pylori* (Wewer et al 1994) and the irritable bowel syndrome (Hyams et al 1995) (Table 11.23). As clinical examination is usually normal, it is vital to take a detailed and comprehensive history which may provide clues as to the etiology of the pain.

Although organic disease can cause recurrent abdominal pain, when investigations are normal, psychological disturbances including overreaction to life events and family dysfunction have often been considered important in the pathogenesis of the symptoms. However, studies have failed to show any psychological differences among children with recurrent abdominal pain compared with control subjects, although it is certainly true that a proportion of these children and their families may benefit from psychological or family therapy.

Table 11.23 Organic causes of recurrent abdominal pain in childhood

1. Gastrointestinal
   a. Constipation
   b. Peptic ulceration/gastritis
   c. Gastroesophageal reflux
   d. Anatomical abnormalities
      (i) Meckel's diverticulum
      (ii) Malrotation
   e. Inflammatory bowel disease
   f. Food intolerance
   g. Infection (e.g. *Yersinia ileitis*)
   h. Pancreatitis
   i. Hepatobiliary disease
2. Others
   a. Migraine
   b. Urinary tract disorder
      (i) Chronic infection
      (ii) Hydronephrosis
      (iii) Calculi

Management

Blanket investigation is no substitute for a careful history and examination although selective laboratory and radiological testing may be necessary, based on the pediatrician's clinical assessment. Routine urine testing and culture is mandatory and a full blood count and ESR may be helpful in excluding anemia and inflammatory conditions. If the child's symptoms are suggestive of pancreatitis, then a serum amylase may be useful when the child is experiencing pain, and liver function tests may be abnormal in children with pain due to hepatobiliary disease. Radiological investigations are usually unhelpful although a plain abdominal film will reveal calcification and gross constipation which may not be evident clinically. An abdominal ultrasound can be of use, particularly if urinary symptoms are suspected, but only rarely is it necessary to perform barium studies to exclude malrotation and inflammatory bowel disease. Screening for *Helicobacter pylori* infection by IgG serology may be appropriate and symptoms suggestive of peptic ulcer disease may merit upper gastrointestinal endoscopy.

Treatment will depend on the clinical assessment and on the results of investigations undertaken. It is important to exclude constipation as therapeutic intervention may cure the child's pain. In children where there is a typical history of abdominal migraine (Symon & Russell 1995), a trial of antimigraine prophylaxis such as pizotifen is sometimes justified, particularly if the child is missing a substantial amount of schooling. In the vast majority of cases, however, none of these measures is indicated and the most important therapeutic maneuver is to reassure the child and his parents that there is no serious organic disease present. It is often helpful to emphasize that the disorder is common in childhood and that the symptoms will almost certainly improve with age. It is important also to explain that although there is no obvious organic cause for the pain, it is not suggested that the pain is imaginary; rather it can be useful to admit that we as physicians do not understand why the pain is occurring, but do know that stress and emotional upheaval will tend to exacerbate the symptoms. In some children who present with intractable symptoms it is helpful to enlist the services of either a child psychologist or psychiatrist at an early stage so that a joint approach can be made in the exclusion of organic and nonorganic causes for the recurrent abdominal pain.

Prognosis

Prospective follow-up studies have been undertaken in children with recurrent abdominal pain and these suggest that a substantial proportion of children may continue to suffer in adult life from the symptoms of irritable bowel syndrome. Furthermore it has been suggested that in children who develop symptoms at an early age and in whom treatment is delayed, the prognosis may be worse. It is tempting to speculate that recurrent abdominal pain in childhood and the irritable bowel syndrome found in later life are manifestations of the same condition, although further large prospective studies are needed to clarify this point.

INFANTILE COLIC

Infantile colic is a condition which is difficult to classify and define. It is used to describe the baby who, in the first few weeks of life, has frequent spells of inconsolable crying, usually occurring in the evening, and often associated with excessive flatus. The infant appears to be suffering abdominal pain although the 'colic' is intermittent and usually self-limiting, often subsiding after 3 months of age. The disorder occurs equally in boys and girls and may occur in up to 20% of all babies in the first few months of life (Lothe & Lindberg 1989). The pathogenesis of the disorder is still unclear and several etiologic theories have been proposed including psychosocial factors, a failure of parent–infant interaction and milk allergy (Illingworth 1985).

Although the pathogenesis of the disorder is unclear, all the evidence points to an intestinal origin for the discomfort, and fundamental physiological and clinical research needs to be undertaken in order to understand the phenomenon more clearly.

As regards management, the most important therapeutic maneuver is to carefully examine the baby and reassure the parents that colic is common, self-limiting and without harmful long-term effects. Many remedies have been tried but the sheer number of treatment options testifies to the fact that none works particularly well. However, for the parents who are at the end of their tether, it may be worth a trial of simple measures such as gripe or peppermint water, and where a child is clearly atopic a cow's milk exclusion may be of benefit. Counseling and support of the parents, however, remains the mainstay of management (Taubman 1988).

Although the condition is usually self-limiting by 3 months of age, some children continue to experience colic throughout the first year of life and go on to develop recurrent abdominal pain and the irritable bowel syndrome in later life.

CHRONIC CONSTIPATION

Although often regarded as a less than glamorous and rather insignificant problem by many physicians, chronic constipation is of great importance to the child and his family. It should be stressed that early accurate assessment and prompt treatment of constipation is vital to the child's well-being and lifestyle, as delays in management will only exacerbate the problem and perpetuate the child's lack of self-esteem and feelings of hopelessness. Furthermore it has now been shown that constipation may cause reversible urinary tract abnormalities that may predispose the child to urinary tract infection and enuresis (Dohil et al 1994).

The term constipation is used to describe difficulty or delay in the passage of stools, which may progress to a chronic state where defecation is infrequent and the bowel motions passed are hard pellets or firm and very bulky; in addition there may be leakage of fecal liquid around the hard compacted stools in the dilated rectum causing soiling, which is distressing for the child and may result in inappropriate referral to a child psychiatrist. It is important to distinguish chronic constipation and associated overflow incontinence from true encopresis, which is the voluntary passage of normal stools in an inappropriate fashion or place. Normal bowel frequency varies widely although the average baby passes three to six stools per day in the neonatal period, one to two stools per day at 1 year of life and approximately one stool per day, or every other day, in the preschool years (Weaver & Steiner 1984).

Pathophysiology and clinical features

Although the vast majority of children presenting with constipation have no serious underlying organic pathology, it is generally true that the younger the child, the more likely it is that the problem is due to a congenital abnormality of the lower bowel. It is particularly important to diagnose Hirschsprung's disease (see Ch. 31) at an early stage, as the infant is at risk from developing an associated and severe life-threatening enterocolitis. Most children with chronic constipation, however, present in the preschool years with symptoms that may have been present for several months and sometimes several years. In these children it is unlikely that organic disease is present although the organic pathologies shown in Table 11.24 should be considered. A careful history and examination, particularly of the perianal region, is crucial in the evaluation of the problem, and the need for further investigation is dictated by the clinical assessment.

By the time most children present to the pediatrician, an enlarged megacolon full of hard feces is present. The child is usually otherwise well although abdominal pain and occasionally nausea and vomiting may be associated with chronic constipation. The original genesis of the constipation is often difficult to pinpoint and several factors may initially have been involved such as a loss of appetite during an acute illness, the prescription of constipating medications following a bout of diarrhea, pain from an anal fissure, a stressful life event, difficult toilet training made worse by inadequate facilities at school or aggressive management by parents determined to see their child toilet trained at a very early age. Interestingly, it has also become clear that chronic constipation may be a manifestation of food intolerance and this should be considered in a child or family with a strong history of atopy.

Almost certainly chronic constipation is the end result of a sequence of events which starts with an episode of acute constipation which is inadequately treated. Adequate bowel evacuation relies on the child experiencing the urge to defecate consequent on the distention of the rectum with feces. If this urge is suppressed, for whatever reason, a vicious cycle develops. Retained feces become hard and painful to expel and as they build up the rectum becomes distended, reducing rectal sensation and thus diminishing the urge to defecate. A consequence of this chain of events is persistent fecal loading, a capacious rectum and frequent overflow soiling caused by fluid stool passing around the hard feces and staining the child's pants. As a result of these

Table 11.24 Causes of constipation

1. Idiopathic
2. Dietary
3. Dehydration
4. Intestinal obstruction
5. Anal fissure/stenosis
6. Hirschsprung's disease
7. Hypo/hyperganglionosis
8. Cerebral palsy
9. Spinal cord lesion
10. Cystic fibrosis
11. Food allergy
12. Hypothyroidism
13. Hypercalcemia
14. Hypokalemia
15. Lead poisoning
16. Renal failure

symptoms the parents may adopt a punitive approach towards the child which may compound an already unfortunate situation.

The problem of chronic constipation in children with neurological disability such as cerebral palsy, or spinal cord abnormalities such as myelomeningocele, is especially intractable due to a combination of reduced sensation, weakness of the muscles of the pelvic floor and abdominal wall, and also particular abnormalities of gastrointestinal motility in these patients. These difficulties should be anticipated and appropriate measures taken at an early stage.

Management

Prompt management of children with acute constipation may prevent the development of chronic constipation and the vicious cycle outlined above. In the baby with delayed passage of meconium and continuing constipation, Hirschsprung's disease should be excluded by rectal suction biopsy at an early stage. Investigation of older children and exclusion of the rare organic causes of chronic constipation will depend on the clinical features following a careful history and examination. Laboratory assessment is usually not warranted, but a plain abdominal film may be very helpful in assessing the degree of constipation and the size of the rectum, and also to demonstrate the fact to the child and his parents (Blethyn et al 1995). General measures such as ensuring an adequate fluid and fiber intake are important and the advice of a pediatric dietitian is helpful in this regard. If anal stenosis is present, then repeated gentle anal dilation, or an anal stretch under anesthesia, may be of benefit. It is important to carefully examine the perianal region for the presence of an anal fissure as the application of local anesthetic preparations may encourage the child to open his bowels.

It is important to explain to the child and his parents the sequence of events leading to chronic constipation and to outline the aims of therapy which are designed, first, to clear the enlarged rectum and distal colon of feces, and second, to keep it empty. It should be stressed that the situation is not the child's or family's fault and that treatment may involve many months of therapy. It is vital to provide a reassuring approach that the situation will improve, although setbacks and further bouts of constipation may be encountered during this period. It is not adequate to prescribe a 2-week course of laxatives and tell the family that the situation will improve with time. In practical terms, the initial therapeutic goal is to empty the rectum and distal colon and this usually can be achieved only with daily, or twice-daily pediatric enema preparations. This may be undertaken on an outpatient basis if the general practitioner or health visitor is enthusiastic, but frequently it is necessary to admit the child to hospital for 1 or 2 days and check that the bowel is empty with an abdominal radiograph prior to starting laxative therapy. Once the large intestine is empty, oral laxatives should be prescribed in adequate doses to ensure that the child's bowels are open at least once a day. It is usual to combine a stool softener such as lactulose with a stimulant aperient such as senna. If the initial dose of laxatives is inadequate, it should be increased; if the laxatives result in diarrhea the dose should be reduced. With time, however, sensation will return to the rectum as its size decreases, and the amount of laxative medication can eventually be decreased and finally stopped.

In addition to medical therapy, it is usually beneficial to institute a behavioral program based on simple rewards such as a modified star chart, where the child is rewarded for a normal, daily bowel action. This is coupled with advice that the child should be able to visit the toilet in a relaxed atmosphere at regular times and it is helpful to see the child regularly in the outpatient clinic, initially at fortnightly intervals, to provide continuing support and encouragement.

Treatment of children with chronic neurological disease and spinal cord lesions poses particular difficulties and early institution of regular suppositories and oral laxative therapy may be helpful. Furthermore, the development of an enema continence catheter (Cardiomed catheter, Cambmac Instruments Ltd), whereby the colon is emptied on a regular basis, is providing a useful adjunct in patients with constipation and fecal incontinence who experience little or no rectal sensation (Shandling & Gilmour 1987).

Overall the long-term prognosis for functional chronic constipation is excellent and this should be emphasized to both the child, the parent and the physician.

Short segment Hirschsprung's disease

In a small proportion of children who present in childhood with a history of chronic constipation dating from birth, associated with the delayed passage of meconium, a diagnosis of short segment Hirschsprung's disease is made. In these children anorectal manometry is abnormal but rectal biopsy may be unremarkable. The term 'internal sphincter spasm' may be a more appropriate term for this condition with treatment involving a full anal sphincter stretch and internal sphincterotomy performed under general anesthesia.

In some children with chronic constipation rectal biopsy may show either an increase or decrease in the number of ganglion cells. Such hypo- or hyperganglionosis undoubtedly can result in altered colonic motility which leads to chronic constipation and the development of a megacolon.

TODDLER DIARRHEA

The syndrome of toddler diarrhea has been otherwise described as chronic nonspecific diarrhea, irritable colon of childhood or more graphically 'peas and carrots' syndrome. Although the condition is now recognized to be by far the commonest cause of diarrhea without failure to thrive in early childhood (Walker-Smith 1980), the mechanisms underlying the disorder are largely unknown and speculative, thus making it difficult to advise with confidence about management. It has been suggested that toddler diarrhea is self-limiting in 90% of cases, although others have reported a high incidence of constipation on follow-up and a significant history of functional bowel disorders in close family members (Davidson & Wasserman 1966). Indeed it seems likely that toddler diarrhea may be merely part of a spectrum of gastrointestinal motility disorders that includes colic in infancy, recurrent abdominal pain in older children and the irritable bowel syndrome in adults.

Clinical features

Children with toddler diarrhea present with loose stools usually between the ages of 6 months and 5 years. The condition is commoner in boys and a careful history will usually elicit the characteristic features of a variable pattern of stool consistency and frequency, often following an initial episode of acute gastroenteritis, with firmer stools passed in the morning and decreasing in consistency later in the day. Occasionally there may

be a history of alternating diarrhea and constipation and the presence of undigested foods (especially peas and carrots), with or without mucus, is typical of the disorder. The diarrhea is often exacerbated by a high roughage diet, fruit and sugary drinks. The absolute characteristic of the condition is the absence of failure to thrive, and it is of paramount importance to carefully document the child's height and weight on presentation and at subsequent follow-up. If the child is failing to thrive, the diagnosis must be suspect and further investigation is then warranted.

Etiology and pathogenesis

Although the precise pathophysiological mechanisms operating in toddler diarrhea are unknown, several possible etiologic factors have been suggested (Table 11.25). It is important to exclude excessive intake of fruit juices as a cause of diarrhea. Food allergy can cause similar symptoms in childhood and, although circumstantial evidence for this may be present in the form of a strong personal or family history of atopy, the most important diagnostic test is the response to an elimination diet and challenge. It has been suggested that a low dietary fat intake is a possible cause of toddler diarrhea as gastric emptying and gut transit time may be slowed by increasing dietary fat intake. It is thus conceivable that a diet low in fat causes rapid gastric emptying with increased propagative motor activity resulting in the formation of loose stools.

Abnormal intestinal secretion has been implicated in the causation of toddler diarrhea as has a primary motility disturbance. It has been suggested that some children with toddler diarrhea may demonstrate a significantly higher incidence of environmental indicators of personal or family stress compared with matched controls (Dutton et al 1985), which is in keeping with the anecdotal experience of many clinicians.

Diagnosis

Toddler diarrhea is primarily a diagnosis of exclusion although there are certain positive clinical features, already described, which may provide a pointer to the diagnosis. The prime feature is that the child is healthy and growing normally. In some children there may be a family history of functional bowel disorders, or indeed a personal or family history of food intolerance. It is important to exclude both urinary and enteric infection although food intolerance and the postenteritis syndrome are the main differential diagnoses. Any evidence of malabsorption, atypical clinical features or failure to thrive should prompt further investigation.

Treatment

In the majority of cases, simple reassurance is all that is required. It is important to explain to the parent that, apart from the loose

Table 11.25 Factors implicated in the pathogenesis of toddler diarrhea

1. Food intolerance
2. Low dietary fat intake
3. Increased intestinal secretion
4. Prostaglandins
5. Environmental stress
6. Primary motility disorder
7. Excessive intake of fruit juice

stools, the child is otherwise well and thriving, and the problem is likely to improve. It is also useful to explore the probable etiology of the disorder which may be explained in terms of deranged motility which will improve with time. It is very important to emphasize that growth and general health will be normal in the future, and there will be no delay in achieving continence. Most parents will accept with relief the fact that their child has no serious disease, but for parents who feel that the problem is too difficult to manage, further measures may be necessary.

It is important to advise the parents to avoid giving an excessive intake of fruit juices or squash. Dietary treatment may be beneficial and, in those children with a strong personal or family history of atopy or in whom chronic diarrhea was manifested following an episode of acute gastroenteritis, a trial of an exclusion diet (usually cow's milk and egg free) may be helpful. The services of an experienced pediatric dietitian are invaluable, and the diet must be adhered to for at least 1 month before any decisions are taken about its efficacy. If there is an improvement in symptoms, the diet is continued for at least 3 months before trying to gradually reintroduce the excluded foods. Some pediatricians have achieved success by increasing the child's fat intake so that 50% of the calories are derived from fat.

Although aspirin has previously been shown to be of benefit in some children with toddler diarrhea, it should not now be routinely used in view of the possible association with the development of Reye's syndrome. There is evidence that loperamide may provide symptomatic improvement and it can be used intermittently. All drugs, however, have significant side effects and they should be prescribed only in carefully selected cases. Recent reports of the benefits of stress reduction and environmental management in children with toddler diarrhea are intriguing and highlight that support and parental training in consistent, effective management of their child's behavior can alleviate some of the symptoms of toddler diarrhea.

Prognosis

Overall the parents can be reassured that the prognosis for the child with toddler diarrhea is very good. In the past, the condition has been described as benign and self-limiting and although it is known that diarrhea may persist after toilet training, it usually becomes less obvious to the parents who no longer have to change dirty nappies. It is possible that a proportion of children who manifest toddler diarrhea may represent one end of a spectrum of familial functional bowel disorders which will re-emerge as continuing gastrointestinal complaints as they become older.

INVESTIGATION OF THE COLON

Investigation of colonic anatomy and physiology has in the past been difficult, largely owing to the relative inaccessibility of the large intestine and the fact that investigation has involved the use of invasive techniques and exposure to radiation. Those investigative techniques in most common usage are described below.

Radiology

Plain abdominal film (supine and or erect) can be very useful in the investigation of acute and chronic gastrointestinal disease. Thus the presence of fluid levels may indicate intestinal obstruction, and free gas in the peritoneal cavity may represent intestinal perforation. Regular plain films are mandatory in cases of toxic megacolon associated with colonic inflammatory disease such as fulminant ulcerative colitis.

Barium enema examination is still the most widely used technique to study colonic anatomy, and it may yield useful diagnostic information as well as being potentially therapeutic in cases of intussusception. The indications for barium enema examination include neonatal intestinal obstruction, intussusception and, where colonoscopy is not available, it may be of help in patients with rectal bleeding or suspected inflammatory bowel disease. The use of double contrast barium enema technique is preferable for demonstrating colonic polyps or subtle mucosal disease, although it may be an uncomfortable examination for the child. The need for barium enema examination in Hirschsprung's disease has largely been superseded by the use of rectal suction biopsy.

Radioisotopic scanning after injection of technetium-labeled leukocytes may have a part to play in the diagnosis of the site and extent of inflammatory disease (Jobling et al 1996) and occasionally patients with unexplained lower gastrointestinal blood loss may require investigation by a ^{99}Tc-labeled red blood cell scan or selective angiography of the inferior mesenteric artery.

Rectal suction biopsy

Biopsy of the rectal mucosa and submucosa is the most useful technique for diagnosing Hirschsprung's disease but it also may be helpful in the diagnosis of neural lipidoses and amyloidosis. The technique is usually carried out under sedation, and multiple biopsies at varying intervals from the anal margin can be taken. The biopsies are studied for the presence or absence of ganglion cells and for the activity of cholinesterase (Qualman & Murray 1994).

Colonoscopy

The use of flexible endoscopy in pediatric practice has revolutionized the investigation of large intestinal disease in childhood (Rossi 1988). Using the technique it is possible to traverse and visualize the whole colon and also to obtain multiple biopsies for histological assessment.

Proctoscopy can be performed easily at the bedside in older children and the use of an auroscope may be useful in neonates. Rigid sigmoidoscopy is uncomfortable for the child and this technique has been superseded by the use of small diameter flexible pediatric colonoscopes. Colonoscopy may be performed under sedation using a premedication of chlorpromazine 1 h before, and a combination of pethidine and midazolam given intravenously immediately prior to the procedure. Alternatively a short general anesthetic may be more comfortable for the patient, easier for the operator and reduce recovery time. For an adequate inspection of the colon to be undertaken, it is vital that bowel preparation is effective and this may require the administration of 'clear fluids' for 24 h before the examination in addition to generous doses of laxatives and occasional recourse to rectal washouts. The procedure is generally well tolerated and the experience of centers using the technique in childhood has been that the complication rate is minimal (Rossi 1988).

Motility studies

Anorectal manometry is a useful technique for distinguishing the different causes of constipation and is particularly helpful in the diagnosis of short segment Hirschsprung's disease where the characteristic abnormality of failed internal sphincter relaxation is seen. Large bowel transit can be measured by the ingestion of multiple radio-opaque markers followed by a plain abdominal film at 48 and 72 h. More detailed investigation of colonic motility is at present only available in research centers.

FAILURE TO THRIVE

DEFINITION

A child is said to be failing to thrive when his or her rate of growth fails to meet the potential expected for a child of that age (Frank & Zeisel 1988). The expected growth rate for any one child, however, depends on many factors including the child's ethnic origins, the parental height and the birth weight. In the first few weeks of life the weight of a child will be more a reflection of intrauterine nutrition while subsequently environmental factors will have a more important influence on growth. Because the growth rate of a child is at its greatest during the first 2 years of life and during the early teens, it is at these times that children most commonly fail to thrive.

Standard growth charts are commonly used to define how the growth of a child compares to the norm. It must be remembered that these charts are constructed using a group of children, living in a given area at a given time and may not be appropriate for all populations. A single plot on a centile chart is of limited value and it should be possible with most children to obtain detailed information about weight gain over the first year of life from their child health clinic book. With this information plotted on a centile chart and a knowledge of parental height and racial background it should be possible to determine whether the child is failing to thrive or not (Fig. 11.16). When children have been failing to gain weight for only a few months, height and head circumference will continue to increase at a normal rate although when the nutritional insult is more prolonged linear growth and brain growth may both be compromised.

ETIOLOGY

Failure to thrive is not a diagnosis but simply a term which collectively describes the end result of a great number of different conditions (Maggioni & Lifshitz 1995). It will inevitably occur where there is an inadequate delivery of nutrients to the developing tissues and this may be due to any one of the problems listed in Table 11.26A. This medical classification includes conditions due to both gastrointestinal (1b, 1c, 2, 3) and nongastrointestinal disease (4, 5) which are clearly organic in origin. In contrast some children receive a reduced nutritional intake as a result of mismanagement or neglect by their parents and under such circumstances the cause is clearly nonorganic. There is also a third group of children in whom a combination of organic and nonorganic factors combine to produce failure to thrive (Table 11.26B).

DIAGNOSIS

History

Abnormalities in the obstetric history of the mother and the birth history of the child may point towards disease processes which have compromised nutrition before birth. Children who are born

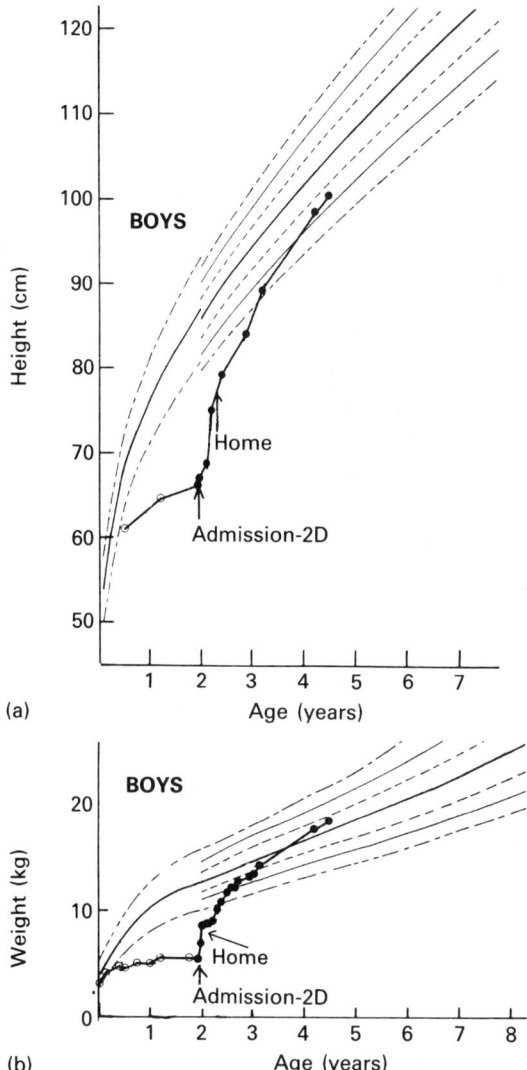

Fig. 11.16 The height (a) and weight (b) of a child with nonorganic failure to thrive showing the growth response to hospital admission and parental support at home. (Reproduced by kind permission of J. Grey.)

light for dates generally fall into one of two groups. There are those who are born small, presumably as a consequence of poor intrauterine nutrition during the third trimester of pregnancy, and who subsequently show good catch-up growth, while some children are born small and subsequently either fail to show any catch-up or fall further away from the centiles after birth. This first group are less of a worry but children in the second group are a much greater cause for concern. Some of these children, particularly those with small parents, will be constitutionally small, while the remainder includes children with chromosomal abnormalities, dysmorphic syndromes such as the Russell–Silver syndrome, and those exposed to serious intrauterine insults such as infection or prolonged nutritional insufficiency. Children within this latter group are frequently poor feeders and it is important to ascertain that a poor nutrient intake is not contributing to their poor growth. Children born prematurely or with birth asphyxia run an increased risk of long-term neurological sequelae and these may present indirectly with failure to thrive. Poor oromotor coordination and an increased risk

Table 11.26 Classification of failure to thrive

A. Medical
1. Reduced intake of nutrients
   a. Feeding mismanagement or neglect
   b. Anorexia
   c. Mechanical problem, i.e. bulbar palsy, cleft palate

2. Inability to digest or absorb nutrients
   a. Pancreatic insufficiency
   b. Small intestinal disease

3. Excessive loss of nutrients
   a. Vomiting
   b. Protein-losing enteropathy
   c. Chronic diarrhea

4. Increased nutrient requirements due to underlying disease
   a. Chronic cardiac or respiratory failure
   b. Chronic infection

5. Unable to fully utilize nutrients
   a. Metabolic disorder
   b. Dysmorphic syndrome

B. Psychological
1. Organic

2. Nonorganic

3. Mixed

of gastroesophageal reflux are likely to present with reluctance to feed, choking and regurgitation.

A full history detailing the child's health since birth may reveal symptoms suggestive of serious underlying disease. Gastrointestinal disease is likely to present with symptoms of vomiting, abdominal distention or diarrhea although it must be remembered that in some patients with gut disease, symptoms specifically pointing to the gastrointestinal tract may be absent. Chronic disease within any system is likely to lead to failure to thrive and the possibility of chronic infection, cardiac disease or an inborn error of metabolism must be considered. It is also of vital importance to take a good dietary history from the parent as an inadequate energy intake is probably the most common cause of failure to thrive in young infants. A newborn infant requires on average 490 kJ/kg/day (117 kcal) which should result in a weight gain of 200 g/week. This should be supplied by 160 ml/kg of breast or formula feed although if the feeds are diluted excessively or if the full volume is not given the child will fail to thrive. With formula feeds the calorie intake can be estimated but with breast-fed babies this can be very difficult to ascertain as the length of time the baby has been feeding or the number of feeds per day may mean very little if the mother's milk supply is poor. Most babies who are receiving an inadequate supply of milk from the breast will fail to settle after feeds and the problem will be remedied quickly by supplementing with a formula feed.

The timing of the introduction of solids can vary greatly from one child to the next but this usually occurs between 3 and 6 months of age. It should be checked that solids which are offered are of an appropriate consistency for the age of the child and that they are given in appropriate amounts. Many baby feeds are gluten free and this must be taken into account when a diagnosis of celiac disease is being considered. The relationship of the ingestion of certain foods to symptoms of vomiting or diarrhea should be checked if food intolerance is thought to be present and associated symptoms of eczema, asthma in older children and a positive family history would all support a diagnosis of food allergic disease. A detailed dietary history can be carried out by a dietitian as an outpatient but this may be open to error and a prospective 3-day assessment as an in-patient will give a much more accurate result.

The social and family history of the child should also be ascertained. Social deprivation is a major risk factor for nonorganic failure to thrive while in families with better circumstances, the mental state of the parents or their parenting abilities may be more relevant. Feeding mismanagement problems are much more common with first time parents, single parent families and in situations where the parents are unsupported by other family members. The progress of other children in the family has great relevance as a previous history of nonaccidental injury or unexplained failure to thrive would point very much toward a nonorganic problem, while a history of atopy, celiac disease or cystic fibrosis in other siblings might be more suggestive of an organic cause. It must, however, be remembered that organic disease is just as likely to occur in a deprived family and that neglect and child abuse occur across all social classes.

Examination

The physical examination of the child should reveal evidence of cardiac, respiratory or neurological disease if it is present. The child with gastrointestinal disease will frequently have no outward physical features although signs of recent weight loss or abdominal distention may be present. The general level of care and cleanliness of the infant should be noted and signs of physical abuse (i.e. burns or bruises) should be recorded.

Investigations

From the history and examination it should be possible to formulate a management plan for the child. All children who present with failure to thrive should have a urine culture with urinalysis, a full blood count and their electrolytes checked. More detailed organic investigation will depend on which underlying disorders are thought to be present.

Trial of feeding

There is inevitably a limit to the information which can be obtained from the history and examination and in children who are failing to thrive an inpatient admission allows the nutritional intake offered by the parent to the child to be prospectively assessed. Given that an inadequate intake is probably the most common cause of failure to thrive it may not be possible to accurately ascertain this from the history. A reduced intake may result either from parental neglect on the one hand or from difficulties that the infant has in feeding due to organic disease. The parent should be observed feeding the child by an experienced nurse as any difficulties that the infant has with feeding or the parent has with handling of the child will be noted. An admission will also allow the response of the infant to a good nutritional intake to be assessed as the child who is failing to thrive as a consequence of a poor intake should show prompt catch-up growth while a child with gastrointestinal disease will show no response. A brief summary of the diagnostic plan for children who fail to thrive is shown in Figure 11.17. In the remainder of this section gastrointestinal and nonorganic causes

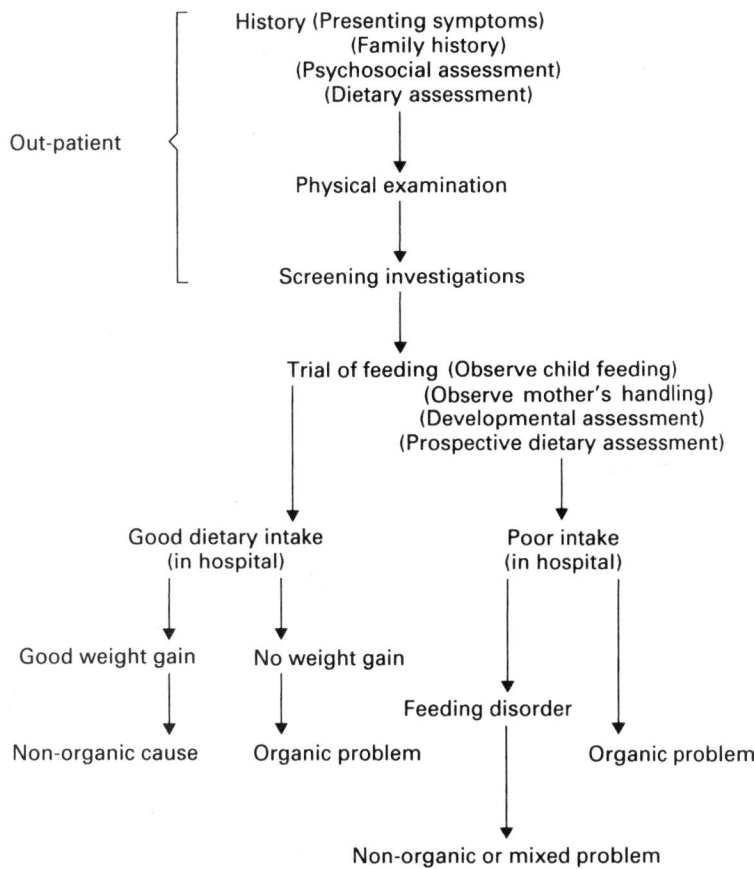

Out-patient
{
History (Presenting symptoms)
(Family history)
(Psychosocial assessment)
(Dietary assessment)

↓

Physical examination

↓

Screening investigations
}

↓

Trial of feeding (Observe child feeding)
(Observe mother's handling)
(Developmental assessment)
(Prospective dietary assessment)

Good dietary intake
(in hospital)   Poor intake
                                           (in hospital)

Good weight gain   No weight gain

                          Feeding disorder

Non-organic cause   Organic problem   Organic problem

Non-organic or mixed problem

Fig. 11.17 Diagnostic plan in failure to thrive.

of failure to thrive and feeding problems in children with gastrointestinal disease will be discussed. For further details on the diagnosis and management of children with organic nongastrointestinal problems please refer to the appropriate system chapter.

GASTROINTESTINAL CAUSES OF FAILURE TO THRIVE

Gastrointestinal disease can result in failure to thrive if the child's nutritional intake is compromised, if nutrients fail to be absorbed or digested, or if there are excessive losses of nutrients from the gut (Table 11.27).

Children with a cleft palate, neuromuscular incoordination of the pharynx or disordered esophageal function will have difficulty swallowing and may aspirate feeds. Anorexia is a common sequela to inflammatory bowel disease, enteric infection and disorders of the stomach and duodenum. This may be further compounded by therapeutic diets which are frequently unpalatable. Patients who are severely malnourished as a consequence of chronic anorexia and who have normal digestive and absorptive function are likely to show a marked rise in weight in response to enteral tube feeding.

Pancreatic exocrine insufficiency, which is most commonly due to cystic fibrosis, and disorders of the digestive and absorptive apparatus of the small intestine will result in poor weight gain in the face of an adequate nutritional intake. Recurrent vomiting resulting from severe gastroesophageal reflux may limit the amount of nutrients entering the small intestine and nutrient losses in the stool may occur in patients with chronic diarrhea.

Investigations

When it is felt that a child's failure to thrive is due to gastrointestinal disease it is important that the nature of the disease and any nutritional consequences are clearly defined.

Fall-off in weight and height in children with gastrointestinal disease is one of the best indications of significant malnourishment. Malabsorption of iron, calcium, zinc and vitamins will lead to anemia, poor bone mineralization, blood clotting abnormalities and an increased susceptibility to infection. A falling albumin level indicates either decreased protein synthesis as a result of lack of substrate or excessive losses into the gut. The measurement of the indices mentioned above will give an idea of the severity of the nutritional problem.

When the child is vomiting, barium studies will allow the anatomy of the upper gastrointestinal tract to be defined, a 24-h pH study will allow the degree of gastroesophageal reflux to be quantified and endoscopic examination will allow mucosal abnormalities to be defined. When pyloric stenosis is suspected a test feed should be done and where bilious vomiting is present erect and supine X-rays will ascertain whether the child has an intestinal obstruction.

Diarrhea may be either osmotic or secretory. In the former, which results from the osmotic effect of undigested food, the electrolyte content of the stools is likely to be low while sugars and fat, which can be quantified by stool chromatography or fecal fat measurement, will almost certainly be present in the stool. The pattern of sugars in the stool may also reflect the underlying

Table 11.27 Gastrointestinal causes of failure to thrive: expanded from sections 1b, 1c, 2 and 3 of Table 11.26

1. Anorexia
   a. Inflammatory bowel disease
      (i) Crohn's disease
      (ii) Ulcerative colitis
   b. Food allergic disease
   c. Gastroduodenal disease
      (i) Duodenal ulcer
      (ii) Idiopathic gastroparesis
      (iii) Gastritis
   d. Chronic enteric infection
      (i) Stagnant loop syndrome
      (ii) Small bowel colonization in malnutrition
   e. Iatrogenic
      (i) Therapeutic diets
      (ii) Drugs

2. Mechanical disorder of ingestion (see Table 11.2)
   a. Absent sucking
      (i) Neurodevelopmental delay
   b. Oral malformation
      (i) Cleft palate
      (ii) Pierre Robin syndrome
   c. Defective swallowing
      (i) Neuromuscular incoordination
          Cerebral palsy
          Brainstem tumor
   d. Dysphagia
      (i) Neuromuscular incoordination (as 2c(i))
      (ii) Esophagitis and stricture

3. Inability to digest or absorb nutrients (see Table 11.10)
   a. Pancreatic insufficiency
      (i) Cystic fibrosis
   b. Small intestinal disease
      (i) Celiac disease
      (ii) Food-sensitive enteropathy
      (iii) Inborn error of digestion or absorption
      (iv) Short gut syndrome

4. Excessive losses of nutrients
   a. Recurrent vomiting
      (i) Gastroesophageal reflux
      (ii) Pyloric stenosis
   b. Protein-losing enteropathy (see Table 11.11)

abnormality and can be of great value in diagnosing inborn errors of digestion and absorption. A fast will stop an osmotic diarrhea while a secretory process will result in the continued loss of electrolyte-rich fluid in the stool (Table 11.21). In any infant with diarrhea who is failing to thrive a sweat test and a jejunal biopsy will allow cystic fibrosis, celiac disease, cow's milk protein intolerance and a range of other disorders which result in an enteropathic process to be diagnosed. Signs of atopy, infection or immune deficiency should be sought if these seem clinically likely. In many conditions the clinical response to treatment is a useful confirmation of the suspected diagnosis. If colonic disease is suspected by the presence of blood or mucus, colonoscopy with biopsy will allow the nature of any inflammatory disorder to be defined.

Abdominal pain and colic are most frequently due to the irritable bowel syndrome which is not associated with failure to thrive. However, when poor growth does occur one must consider the possibility of duodenal ulcer disease, food allergy, pancreatitis, malrotation, inflammatory bowel disease and in particular Crohn's disease. Endoscopic examination of the stomach and colon along with a barium follow-through study

should help localize the problem while a raised amylase will support the diagnosis of pancreatitis and a raised ESR and platelet count will support an inflammatory cause.

Failure to thrive may be the only symptom of gastrointestinal disease in some patients and this frequently results in a long delay between the initiation of the disease process and the eventual diagnosis. When small intestinal disease is present the extensive reserve capacity of the colon allows excessive fluid entering the colon to be reabsorbed with the resulting passage of formed stools. This may occur in celiac disease, cow's milk protein intolerance and in older children this commonly occurs in Crohn's disease. Without an awareness of these conditions an early diagnosis is unlikely to be made.

Further information on the diagnosis and treatment of the conditions mentioned above can be found elsewhere in this chapter.

NONORGANIC FAILURE TO THRIVE

Etiology

During the assessment of a child who is failing to thrive it is very common to find no evidence of gastrointestinal or other organic disease. The mechanisms underlying such nonorganic failure to thrive are the subject of some controversy (Table 11.28) but it does appear most likely that this results from the child receiving an inadequate supply of nutrients. The prompt response of these children to an adequate nutrient intake would support this hypothesis (Frank & Zeisel 1988).

The inadequate supply of food to the child may result from poverty within the family, and indeed nonorganic failure to thrive most commonly occurs in lower social class families. This is frequently compounded by homelessness, inadequate food preparation facilities and insanitary conditions which will lead to an increased risk of recurrent infection.

Family dysfunction may also be a major contributing factor in the development of failure to thrive in children across all social classes. Stresses within the family resulting from marital discord, postnatal depression, chronic physical illness, alcohol or drug abuse, intellectual impairment or family bereavement may limit the ability of the parents to cope with their child. Such families may be able to handle a well-behaved, undemanding child but

Table 11.28 Factors responsible for nonorganic failure to thrive

1. Poverty
   a. Poor housing
   b. Unemployment
   c. Poor cooking facilities

2. Family dysfunction
   a. Marital discord
   b. Mental illness
   c. Alcohol or drug abuse
   d. Low intelligence of parent
   e. Single parent

3. Feeding disorder
   a. Inappropriate food
   b. Distractions during feeding
   c. Mealtimes chaotic
   d. Poor feeding technique

4. Maltreatment of child
   a. Physical abuse
   b. Withholding of food

when an increased load is put on their limited resources, by an ill or demanding infant, the family is unable to cope and as a result the child fails to thrive. In many cases the parents themselves may have come from a deprived family background and this may limit their ability to respond to the needs of their child.

The interaction between the child and his parent at the time of feeding is of great importance in determining whether he receives an adequate intake. When this interaction is poor, disorders of feeding behavior are likely to develop which will overwhelm the family compromised by poor social or family circumstances. It is frequently found that these children are receiving inappropriate food for their age or that their method of feeding is without structure or consistency or, conversely, follows an overly rigid pattern. The child who is malnourished and failing to grow may be developmentally delayed, lethargic and unresponsive to his parents at meal times, and this negative feedback will help to reinforce the vicious circle of factors which leads to nonorganic failure to thrive.

Most children with failure to thrive are not exposed to willful neglect or abuse but in a significant minority food is withheld and physical abuse and maltreatment may also occur. In this most worrying group of children chronic neglect and abuse results in significant long-term physical and psychosocial sequelae while in a small number there is a fatal outcome.

Assessment

Having undergone the general assessment for any child with failure to thrive, it is then important that the etiologic factors described above are explored to ascertain which may be relevant to the child in question. A detailed social history supported by discussions with the child's general practitioner, health visitor and the local social services department and any other relevant professionals will give information on the home and family circumstances and on any past history of nonaccidental injury. During the period of the 'trial of feeding' it will be possible to obtain information on interactions between the child and parent, on the quality and consistency of the food which is offered and on the manner in which it is given. Videotaping meal times can be useful in gathering this information and is also of value as part of a therapeutic program where the parents will be able to see for themselves how they are behaving during their child's feeding. Children who fail to thrive frequently show signs of developmental delay and the later this is recognized the more severe the delay is likely to be. It is therefore important that all children suspected of suffering from nonorganic failure to thrive should undergo formal developmental assessment as this allows both the extent of the delay to be measured and acts as a baseline against which future progress can be measured.

Management

The many factors which combine to cause nonorganic failure to thrive need to be defined in each patient so that an appropriate management program can be designed. It is likely, however, that this will be a time-consuming process which may require input from a variety of professionals including medical, nursing, dietetic, speech therapy, psychological and social work staff.

If the child feeds poorly or parents' feeding skills are lacking, in the first instance the parent(s) should be offered advice, adopting new techniques or modifying old ones. If this general support is insufficient, the next step would be to set up a feeding program which details what is to happen at meal and play times and who (parent/staff) is to carry out each aspect of this plan. Where family and social problems are present, a therapeutic program needs to be drawn up to address these specific problems, so that the family's functioning may be improved in order that their ability to undertake the care of the child is not compromised. It may be helpful to hold a meeting of those professionals (hospital and community) involved with the family to discuss and plan in detail any feeding therapeutic program.

Under most circumstances a period of sustained input will result in improved weight gain and development of the child who is living at home. However, not all families are able and/or willing to recognize the problem and utilize the help offered to them effectively. When a child thrives normally in hospital (Fig. 11.16), but repeatedly fails to do so at home, this raises major child care issues and referral to a statutory agency is indicated. Similarly, where physical abuse or neglect is suspected or diagnosed, the area child protection committee's procedure needs to be followed.

FEEDING PROBLEMS AND GASTROINTESTINAL DISEASE

The development of normal patterns of feeding behavior is dependent on interactions between the mother and child at the time of feeding (Graham 1986, Lask 1988). These patterns may fail to develop because of major psychosocial disturbances within the family (Table 11.28) or be due to disease within the gastrointestinal tract (Table 11.27). Frequently, however, organic and nonorganic factors combine to produce a feeding problem with a mixed etiology. It is likely that an infant with minor feeding problems and capable parents will ultimately do well and the problems will be adequately managed. However, an identical child living in a stressed noncoping family is likely to progress poorly and may ultimately fail to thrive because the parent is unable to maintain an adequate oral intake.

Feeding problems may take many forms. The child may fail to suck, reject the bottle or breast, or feeding may induce crying, vomiting or abdominal pain. In Table 11.2 the organic causes which are likely to limit the child's ability to feed normally are listed. The problem arises, however, when the clinical expression of these gastrointestinal problems is subtle, and frequently the feeding disorder may be the only sign that all is not well.

It is important that where organic causes are adversely influencing the feeding behavior of a child, they should be defined and treated at an early stage. Failure to do this may lead to persistent feeding problems and in some children these will be severe enough to compromise growth. Problems such as gastroesophageal reflux or food allergy resolve spontaneously in most children in the first 2 or 3 years of life but in many of these infants behavioral feeding problems may persist long after the primary triggering pathology has resolved. The longer the problem has been present the more difficult it is likely to be to treat.

NUTRITION IN PATIENTS WITH GASTROINTESTINAL DISEASE

Gastrointestinal disorders in childhood frequently have major nutritional consequences and dietary manipulation plays an important role in the treatment of such patients. An understanding of the nutritional requirements in childhood is of help both in planning the treatment of patients who are malnourished as a result of gastrointestinal disease and also in communicating with the pediatric dietitian who is responsible for the supervision of the child's dietary management (Shaw & Lawson 1994). Full details of nutritional requirements and the consequences of malnutrition are given in Chapter 21.

In children who are failing to grow adequately it is important to define whether their nutritional intake is adequate. Where deficiencies exist they should be corrected by giving adequate amounts of food but energy intake can also be boosted by the use of feeds fortified with added glucose polymer or fat. Diets low in vitamins and minerals should also be appropriately supplemented.

Therapeutic diets for the treatment of gastrointestinal disease should be closely supervised by a dietitian (Shaw & Lawson 1994). In celiac disease a gluten exclusion is all that is required but in food allergic patients multiple exclusion may be needed to prevent the development of atopic symptoms. It is usual to start with a cow's milk and egg exclusion but wheat, colorings, preservatives and soya are all frequently responsible for dietary intolerance in childhood. A milk substitute should be given which is complete with added vitamins and minerals and it is usual to prescribe a soya substitute initially but where this is not tolerated a predigested formula should be used. Many infants find these substitute feeds unpalatable and require to take oral calcium supplements instead.

Elemental diets which may be used in Crohn's disease are frequently administered by nasogastric tube because of their unpalatable taste. Similarly children who require energy supplements because of problems with swallowing will benefit from nasogastric feeds. Whenever possible the enteral route should be used to supplement nutrition and when an oral intake is not possible delivery directly into the stomach or duodenum by nasogastric tube or gastrostomy should be considered. Accurate enteral infusion pumps allow the steady delivery of feeds during the day or night and in many children this treatment can be continued safely at home.

In many of these children the gastrointestinal tract may be too severely damaged to tolerate a full enteral intake and under these circumstances parenteral nutrition will be required. It should be possible to maintain good nutrition in all children and this will invariably require the surgical placement of a tunneled silastic central venous catheter which will guarantee good venous access and allow the use of hyperosmolar solutions. When parenteral nutrition is prolonged it is important to closely monitor for vitamin or trace mineral deficiencies as requirements will frequently be increased in patients with gastrointestinal disease. An enteral intake, with its trophic effect on the gut, should be continued during periods of parenteral nutrition and increased as tolerance improves.

In a few children intestinal function may be so severely compromised that recovery may take many months or be unlikely ever to occur. Under such circumstances home parenteral nutrition should be considered. It is now technically possible to maintain normal growth and development over prolonged periods in children receiving this therapy at home.

The use of a nutrition care team, comprising a doctor, nurse, pharmacist, dietitian and biochemist, is of great help in supervising and monitoring the treatment of children with complicated nutritional problems managed both in hospital and at home.

HEPATIC AND BILIARY DISEASE

MICROANATOMICAL STRUCTURE AND FUNCTION OF THE LIVER

One major function of the liver is to maintain the concentration of macromolecules and solutes in the hepatic vein blood and bile within a very narrow range. A knowledge of the microanatomical relationships necessary for this and its other main roles is essential in appreciating some of the pathophysiological events that follow liver damage.

The structural organization of the liver and its vascular elements is designed to allow it to occupy a central place in metabolism while interposed as a guardian between the digestive tract (and spleen) and the rest of the body. Substrates are rapidly taken into the liver cells, metabolized, stored and their products transferred as required into the blood and bile. Blood-, bile- and lymph-containing channels transport nutrients, metabolites, antigens, antibodies, hormones and drugs to and from the hepatocyte, and also to the other specialized liver cells, the Kupffer cell, the sinusoidal endothelial cell, fat storage cell and to the cells of the biliary tree. The vascular arrangements ensure that each of the first three types of cells is in intimate contact with blood flowing through the liver.

The basic functional unit of the liver is the acinus, the mass of parenchyma receiving a blood supply from a single portal tract. Blood from terminal branches of the hepatic artery and portal vein in the portal tract enters and traverses the sinusoids, specialized capillaries lined by Kupffer and endothelial cells which contain fenestra which allow ready access of plasma and its contents to the surface of the hepatocyte. Some hepatic arterial blood reaches the sinusoids via a peribiliary capillary plexus which carries substances reabsorbed from the bile ducts thus completing a hepatobiliary recirculation (Fig. 11.18). The sinusoids drain to the central vein of the hepatic lobule, and ultimately into the inferior vena cava. Both endothelial and Kupffer cells are metabolically important having specific receptors for substrates in the circulation. The hepatocytes near the portal tracts receive more oxygen, nutrients and hormones, have a higher metabolic rate, synthesize more proteins and regenerate more rapidly than those nearer the central vein. Those near the central vein are particularly susceptible to cholestasis in the presence of hypoxia and to toxic necrosis. The hepatocytes are delicately suspended in plates one

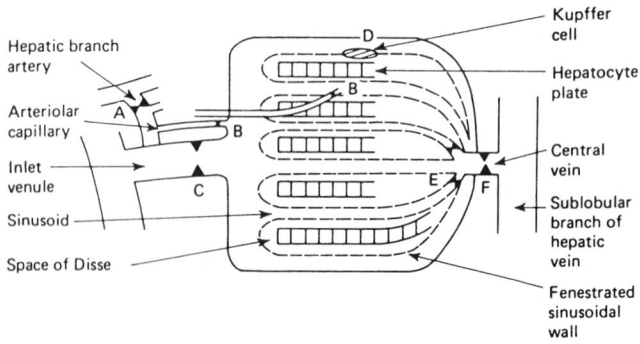

Fig. 11.18 A diagrammatic representation of the liver sinusoids and their blood supply. A–F represent sites of possible sphincters involved in controlling blood flow through the hepatic sinusoids. (Reproduced from *Liver Disorders in Childhood*, Butterworths, by kind permission of author and publisher.)

cell thick in a fine reticulin network penetrated by fenestra giving a sponge-like effect. Until 6 years of age many of the hepatocyte plates are two cells thick limiting passage of substrates.

This structure can regain its pristine condition when devastated by acute toxins such as paracetamol or type A viral hepatitis, but persisting injury with infiltration by migratory cells of the reticuloendothelial system sets in train a complex series of interactions which increase extracellular matrix components. These change the fenestrated sinusoids to capillaries with a plasma membrane, interact with receptors on the hepatocyte surface to modify their function, cause fibrotic distortion of the hepatic architecture with subsequent shunting of blood flow away from the hepatocyte, abnormal growth of the hepatocytes, cirrhosis and ultimately hepatocellular carcinoma. The prevention of such chronic injury, whether caused by genetic disorder, infections, environmental toxins or biliary abnormalities, is a major challenge in hepatology.

DEVELOPMENTAL CONSIDERATIONS

The liver has considerable reserve capacity for all its functions throughout childhood but a temporary hepatic insufficiency is a feature of the newborn, contributing to physiological jaundice. Some less obvious developmental changes in major hepatic functions are of equal or greater clinical and pathological significance. Although bile secretion commences between 12 and 16 weeks' gestation, full maturation of the transport mechanisms and enzymatic activities involved in bile formation does not occur until well after birth, contributing to impaired lipid absorption in newborn infants, particularly the premature. The few studies of development of hepatic function in man show different rates for different functions. Proteins involved in coagulation, however, are frequently at low concentration around the time of delivery but increase to normal levels within days. At birth the primary bile salt concentrations in serum are low but rise in a fashion similar to unconjugated bilirubin in the first week of life. Values remain elevated for 3–6 years and even at the age of 9 years chenodeoxycholic acid concentration may be elevated compared with adult values. Gluconeogenesis is impaired in the immediate postnatal period. Glycogen, normally deposited in the liver late in gestation, is rapidly mobilized immediately following birth. Hypoglycemia is a risk, particularly if there are inborn errors of either carbohydrate or amino acid metabolism. Protein synthesis is very active in fetal life and the newborn period. Nevertheless, premature infants given a high protein intake may be unable to metabolize amino acids efficiently and have dangerously elevated serum concentrations as a result. α-fetoprotein is the major serum protein in fetal life, having a concentration of 3 g/l at 13 weeks' gestation, falling linearly to around 70 mg/l in cord blood and to concentrations of 25 µg/l at 6 weeks of age. Albumin synthesis starts at 3–4 months' gestation and serum concentration is at adult values at term. Ceruloplasmin concentration is low at birth. It reaches its highest concentration at the age of 3 months and thereafter falls slowly to adult levels by the age of 2 years.

This lack of uniformity and the time course of changes in the concentration of these different proteins are mirrored by lack of uniformity in the rate of development of drug metabolism. In the first 2–4 weeks of life it is influenced by differences in the binding of drugs to serum proteins and renal function as well as developmental changes in hepatic metabolism that render drugs more soluble. Many of these metabolic reactions may not reach adult levels of activity until 3 months of age. Thereafter they may be more efficient. In early childhood it has been estimated that the hepatic metabolism of drugs such as theophylline is twofold higher than in adults.

ASSESSMENT OF AN INFANT OR CHILD WITH SUSPECTED LIVER DISEASE

Careful clinical assessment and standard liver function tests will usually detect the presence of liver disease but imaging, specific investigations and liver biopsy may be necessary to determine its nature and severity.

CLINICAL ASSESSMENT

Features pointing to the presence of liver disease are jaundice with bile pigments in the urine, pruritus, abdominal pain, abdominal distention, alimentary bleeding, or a generalized bleeding diathesis. Note that in infancy bile pigments produce a yellow urine which would be considered normal in color in an older child or adult. Initial signs maybe apparently unrelated to the liver, for example neurological dysfunction in Reye's syndrome, glycogen storage disease or Wilson's disease; skin lesions, e.g. papular acrodermatitis with hepatitis B infection; limb swelling or rickets in tyrosinemia.

PHYSICAL EXAMINATION

There may be no abnormal signs, for example in cirrhosis associated with asymptomatic hepatitis B infection detected by screening.

The liver in health extends from the level of the 5th intercostal space to 4 cm below the costal margin in infancy and 2 cm below the costal margin in older children. A small right lobe with an enlarged left lobe or a hard nodular surface suggests cirrhosis. A hard liver implies increased fibrosis or cirrhosis. Asymmetrical or focal enlargement may be due to tumors, cysts, abscesses, cavernous hemangiomata or focal nodular hyperplasia. Diffuse enlargement without alteration of its contour occurs in acute hepatocellular disease, storage disorders, infiltrative or congestive disorders and bile duct obstruction. A systolic bruit may be heard overlying tumors or hemangiomata. A cystic mass below the liver edge may indicate a choledochal cyst or a palpable gallbladder due to bile duct obstruction. Large kidneys suggest polycystic disease and possible congenital hepatic fibrosis. Splenomegaly may reflect portal hypertension, infective or infiltrative disorders. Hepatosplenomegaly may be due to metabolic (storage) disorders. Serial measurement of maximum abdominal girth and organ size is invaluable in following the progress of liver disorders.

Full examination of the skin, facial appearance, eyes (including slit lamp examination), neurological, cardiovascular, locomotor and central nervous systems with assessment of growth and developmental status may give a clue as to specific causes of liver disorder (Table 11.29).

Urine analysis and examination of stool color is essential.

LABORATORY INVESTIGATIONS

Tests listed in Table 11.30 may confirm the presence of a liver disorder and be of value in monitoring its progress. With the exception of direct serum bilirubin, serum bile salt concentration

Table 11.29 Abnormalities on physical examination in children with liver disease

Abnormal physical signs	Disorder
Skin lesions, purpura, choroidoretinitis, myocarditis etc.	Generalized viral infections
Cataracts	Galactosemia, hypoparathyroidism
Multiple congenital anomalies	Trisomy 21, 18 or 13
Cystic mass below the liver	Choledochal cyst
Ascites and bile-stained herniae	Spontaneous perforation of the bile ducts
Systolic murmur, abnormal facies, embryotoxin	Biliary hypoplasia
Cutaneous hemangiomata	Hepatic or biliary hemangioma
Situs inversus	Extrahepatic biliary atresia
Optic nerve hypoplasia or micropenis	Septo-optic dysplasia

Table 11.30 Relative specificity and sensitivity of commonly available 'liver function tests'

Investigation	Specificity	Sensitivity	Pertinent disorders
Elevated serum concentration Direct bilirubin	++++	+	All forms of acute and chronic liver disorders
Bile salts	++++	++++	All forms of acute and chronic liver disorders
Alanine aminotransferase	++	+++	All forms of acute and chronic liver disorders
Aspartate aminotransferase	+	+++	All forms of acute and chronic liver disorders
γ-glutamyltranspeptidase	++	++	All forms of acute and chronic liver disorders
Alkaline phosphate	+	++	All forms of acute and chronic liver disorders
Immunoglobulin	+	+++	Autoimmune chronic hepatitis, primary sclerosing cholangitis, Wilson's disease
Tissue autoantibodies	+	+++	All forms of acute and chronic liver disorders
Ammonia	++	+	Liver failure, urea cycle defects
α-fetoprotein	+++	+++	Malignant liver tumors, tyrosinemia
	+	++	Hepatitis in early infancy, bile duct hypoplasia
Low serum albumin	+	++	Liver disease of > 30 days duration
Prolonged prothrombin time	++	++	Cholestasis with fat malabsorption, Reye's syndrome, liver failure

and ammonia concentration, none are specific for liver disorders. They are of no value in differential diagnosis.

LIVER IMAGING

Ultrasound

Ultrasonic echography is extremely efficient allowing visualization of structures as small as 2 mm. Cysts appear as circular echo-free structures; abscesses and necrotic primary or secondary tumors appear as irregular cavitating lesions. Solid tumors appear as focal changes in the echo pattern. Hemangioendotheliomas produce irregular echo-free cavities. Dilation of the biliary tree occurs in choledochal cysts and tumors. Calculi, sludge and polyps in the gallbladder can be visualized. Calculi are frequently missed in the distal common bile duct. It is unhelpful in diagnosing biliary atresia other than it may show the gallbladder to be absent. Ultrasound findings in diffuse liver disease are nonspecific. Echogenicity is increased with fatty liver, in storage disorders and leukemic infiltration. Patency, diameter and, with Doppler, flow velocity can be demonstrated in the portal vein, hepatic vein and hepatic artery. It is useful in indicating spleen size but is of less value in demonstrating modest hepatomegaly.

Computed tomography

Computed tomography like ultrasound demonstrates anatomical features. Interpretation is easier. The disadvantages are the considerable radiation and sedation or anesthesia necessary for a small child. With intravenous contrast there is enhancement of vascular lesions.

Digital subtraction angiography

This technique allows visualization of the hepatic artery, portal venous system and intrahepatic vessels with visualization of vascular lesions. It is of value in planning surgical resection.

Radioisotope imaging of the biliary tree

Technetium-labeled iminodiacetic acid (IDA) derivatives are useful in demonstrating biliary excretion and abnormalities of the biliary system. Derivatives such as methylbromo-IDA or diisopropyl-IDA which have a relatively poor renal uptake and good hepatic uptake must be used. 5 days of preparation with oral phenobarbitone 5 mg/kg/day are required in neonatal cholestasis.

Cholangiography

Percutaneous transhepatic and endoscopic retrograde cholangiography are technically difficult and essential in the diagnosis of sclerosing cholangitis and in selected patients with biliary obstruction.

PERCUTANEOUS LIVER BIOPSY

Skilled histological interpretation, histochemical and biochemical analysis and bacterial, fungal or viral culture of liver biopsy tissue yields results which may be of crucial diagnostic importance (Ishak & Sharp 1987a). The most common indications in childhood are in identifying the causes of hepatitis syndrome in infancy, obscure hepatosplenomegaly, metabolic disorders and pyrexia of unknown origin which cannot be diagnosed by specific tests performed on the peripheral blood. It gives invaluable information on the severity of liver damage and structural change and also in assessing the requirements for therapy in chronic hepatitis. An ultrasound scan to exclude a focal liver lesion or bile duct obstruction is advisable before a biopsy. Contraindications are: INR (international normalized ratio for prothrombin time) greater than 1.3, platelet count of less than 70×10^9/l, hydatid cyst or abscess in the right lobe of liver biliary tract, angiomatous malformation of liver and α-fetoprotein-positive liver tumor (Ishak & Sharp 1987b).

HEPATITIS SYNDROME IN INFANCY

Hepatitis in infancy is characterized by clinical and laboratory features of hepatic inflammation and dysfunction, particularly conjugated hyperbilirubinemia. It must be suspected in any jaundiced infant particularly if the urine is yellow rather than colorless, or if jaundice persists beyond 14 days of age. If the stools contain no yellow or green pigment, cholestasis is complete and biliary atresia must be suspected.

Less commonly, infants will present with bleeding diathesis, hypoglycemia, fluid retention or malabsorption. The most important investigation is INR following administration of parenteral vitamin K which if it remains elevated indicates fulminant hepatic failure.

Standard biochemical tests for liver function confirm conjugated hyperbilirubinemia with elevation of serum aspartate aminotransferase, alkaline phosphatase and γ-glutamyltranspeptidase to values of between 1.5 and 6 times normal. Serum albumin is usually in the normal range but may be low if liver disease is severe or there is marked fluid retention. Serum lipids and cholesterol are usually normal in the first 4 months of life but increase thereafter, particularly in infants with bile duct hypoplasia.

PATHOLOGY

The prime pathological impact of disease may be on one of four sites:

1. hepatic parenchyma causing a hepatitis
2. portal tracts leading in some instances to paucity of interlobular bile ducts
3. intrahepatic bile ducts leading to sclerosing cholangitis or duct ectasia
4. extrahepatic bile ducts, most commonly as biliary atresia.

The prognosis in category 1 is dependent on the severity of liver damage and that of the associated disorder. Chronic liver disease rarely occurs in those associated with infection or whose disease remains cryptogenic after full investigation unless there is a positive family history or consanguinity. Of patients with α-1-antitrypsin deficiency, approximately 50% will develop cirrhosis with 25% dying or receiving liver transplantation in the first decade of life. Categories 2 and 3 may be followed by progressive intrahepatic cholestasis with cirrhosis. Two further groups with a poor prognosis are those with a normal serum γ-glutamyltranspeptidase activity in the presence of jaundice and abnormal biochemical tests of liver function and those who develop a sclerosing cholangitis.

Chronic liver disease of varying severity is almost inevitable in categories 2, 3 and 4 (Pittschieler 1994).

DIFFERENTIAL DIAGNOSIS

Priority in management is to identify infants with treatable bacterial, metabolic, endocrine or hematological disorders (Table 11.31) associated with hepatocellular disease or with surgically correctable disorders of the bile duct. Evidence of consanguinity

Table 11.31 Disorders associated with conjugated hyperbilirubinemia in infancy

1. Intrahepatic disorders
   a. Inherited disorders
   b. Endocrine abnormalities
   c. Vascular abnormalities
   d. Severe hemolytic disease
   e. Chronic hypoxia and circulatory abnormalities
   f. Chromosomal anomalies
   g. Intravenous nutrition
   h. Drugs
   i. Paucity of the interlobular bile ducts
   j. Sclerosing cholangitis
   k. Maternal systemic lupus erythematosus
   l. Idiopathic

2. Extrahepatic disorders
   a. Extrahepatic biliary atresia
   b. Choledochal cyst
   c. Spontaneous perforation of the bile duct
   d. Inspissation in the biliary system
      (i) hemolytic disorders
      (ii) cystic fibrosis
      (iii) total parenteral nutrition
      (iv) congenital infections
   e. Gallstones
   f. Malignant nodes
   g. Peritoneal bands
   h. Tumor of the duodenum or pancreas
   i. Hemangioendotheliomata
   j. Inflammatory infiltrate
   k. Duplication of the intestine

or liver disease in siblings suggests the possibility of familial, genetic, metabolic or hemolytic disease. Review of the perinatal case records and past medical history may reveal features suggesting uterine infection, exposure to toxins and drugs or intravenous nutrition. Most commonly the primary pathology is intrahepatic. Careful physical examination may reveal features of disorders listed in Table 11.32 but this is unusual and comprehensive systematic investigation is essential.

It is important to consider and exclude immediately coagulopathy due to vitamin K malabsorption, hypoglycemia,

Table 11.32 Inherited disorders associated with hepatitis syndrome in infancy

1. Galactosemia

2. Fructosemia

3. Tyrosinemia

4. α-1-antitrypsin deficiency

5. Cystic fibrosis

6. Niemann–Pick Type C

7. Gaucher's disease

8. Wolman's disease

9. Zellweger syndrome

10. Infantile polycystic disease

11. Erythrophagocytic reticulosis (Hirst et al 1994)

12. Neonatal hemochromatosis

13. Defects in synthesis of primary bile acids

septicemia, urinary tract infection, syphilis and herpes simplex infections, listeriosis and toxoplasmosis since effective treatment for these is available. Galactosemia (galactose-1-phosphate uridyl transferase activity), fructosemia (dietary exposure) and tyrosinemia (urinary succinylacetone excretion) should also be excluded immediately since dietary treatment is available. Urine analysis for hyperaminoaciduria and for nonglucose reducing substances is an important screening test. Consideration must then be given to excluding genetic disorders associated with this syndrome (Table 11.32). Recent additions to the differential diagnosis are inborn errors of bile acid synthesis (Suchy 1993). In the UK, α_1-antitrypsin deficiency, cystic fibrosis and Niemann–Pick Type C need to be excluded in all instances.

Specimens of stools must be saved in a container that excludes light and examined for pigment. An ultrasound examination is performed to identify dilation of the biliary tree indicating a choledochal cyst. Endocrine disorders associated with this syndrome (Table 11.33) must also be excluded on the basis of the clinical findings and appropriate laboratory investigations. A skillfully interpreted percutaneous liver biopsy is usually required for diagnosis. It is essential that some of the material obtained is frozen at $-70°C$ for subsequent biochemical analysis for inherited disorders (Table 11.32) if indicated by the liver histology or other investigations. The investigations for other conditions including congenital infections (Table 11.34) should not be allowed to delay consideration of biliary atresia or other surgically correctable disorders.

If percutaneous liver biopsy shows increased edema, fibrosis and bile duct reduplication in all portal tracts, biliary atresia is highly likely but this appearance can be found also in some

Table 11.33 Endocrine disorders associated with hepatitis syndrome in infancy

1. Hypopituitarism

2. Diabetes insipidus

3. Hypoadrenalism

4. Hypothyroidism

5. Hypoparathyroidism

Table 11.34 Infections causing hepatitis in infancy

1. Viral infections
   a. Cytomegalovirus
   b. Epstein–Barr virus
   c. Rubella virus
   d. Varicella zoster virus
   e. Hepatitis A
   f. Hepatitis B virus (+ delta virus)
   g. Non-A, non-B hepatitis
   h. Herpes simplex virus
   i. Coxsackie A9, B
   j. Echo virus 9, 11, 14, 19
   k. Adenovirus
   l. Reovirus Type III

2. Nonviral infections
   a. Bacterial infection
   b. Psittacosis
   c. *Listeria*
   d. *Treponema pallidum*
   e. *Toxoplasma gondii*
   f. Tuberculosis

genetic and endocrine disorders, in some infants who will ultimately develop bile duct hypoplasia and in disorders of the intrahepatic bile ducts. Radionuclide demonstration of bile duct patency using a ^{99}technetium-tagged iminodiacetic acid derivative (IDA) such as methylbromo-IDA may allow discrimination of biliary atresia from intrahepatic cholestasis. Repeated imaging up to 24 h after intravenous injection may be required to demonstrate isotope in the gut. Radionuclide studies are only of value in excluding atresia. Diagnosis is confirmed at laparotomy which should only be undertaken by an experienced surgeon who can assess changes in the porta hepatis and proceed to portoenterostomy (McClement et al 1985). Even with cholangiography hypoplastic extrahepatic ducts due to severe intrahepatic cholestasis may be considered atretic leading to an unnecessary destructive operation.

PAUCITY OF INTERLOBULAR BILE DUCTS (INTRAHEPATIC BILIARY HYPOPLASIA)

The diagnosis is based on a decrease in the number of interlobular bile ducts seen in portal tracts (ratio < 0.06). It is found in many conditions causing hepatitis in infancy and also occurs with cardiovascular, skeletal and ocular anomalies comprising Alagille's syndrome (syndromic paucity of the intrahepatic bile ducts; arteriohepatic dysplasia). The latter is probably inherited in an autosomal dominant fashion with variable expression. Mild cases may have intermittent pruritus only. The majority have jaundice from the neonatal period which in severe cases may persist but in others clears in late childhood or early adult life. The long-standing cholestasis causes jaundice, pruritus, hypercholesterolemia and xanthelasma. The long-term prognosis is uncertain but 15% may go on to develop cirrhosis and 5–10% die from liver disease. In one series 25% died from cardiac involvement, classically a peripheral pulmonary stenosis, or infection (Alagille et al 1987). Diagnosis is supported by the finding of the typical facies, deep-set eyes, mild hypertelorism, overhanging forehead, a straight nose which in profile is in the same plane as the forehead and a small pointed chin, posterior embryotoxon and vertebral arch defects on spinal radiographs. High serum cholesterol supports the diagnosis. The treatment is that of chronic cholestasis with particular emphasis on adequacy of vitamin E replacement and the control of pruritus (Deprettere et al 1987).

LIVER DISEASE ASSOCIATED WITH TOTAL PARENTERAL NUTRITION

Prolonged intravenous nutrition particularly in early infancy causes cholestasis and hepatocellular damage which may progress to cirrhosis and liver cancer if intravenous feeding cannot be stopped. The etiology remains unknown. Prevalence increases with the degree of prematurity, degree of growth retardation before birth, the duration of intravenous feeding and the absence of any enteral food intake. Sepsis, hypoxia, shock, blood transfusion, intra-abdominal surgery and potentially hepatotoxic drugs may aggravate the liver damage. Acute acalculous cholecystitis, biliary sludge, and cholelithiasis are complications.

Clinical features and laboratory findings

The first clinical indication of hepatic involvement is usually the appearance of conjugated hyperbilirubinemia. Hepatomegaly may be noted. Biochemical tests of liver function are elevated. It is important to consider other causes of cholestasis in this age group before concluding that the disorder is due to intravenous nutrition. If intravenous nutrition can be withdrawn the jaundice settles, although liver function tests may remain abnormal for 5 months and liver biopsy changes persist for up to 1 year.

DISORDERS REQUIRING URGENT SURGICAL TREATMENT

EXTRAHEPATIC BILIARY ATRESIA

In this disorder of unknown cause there is obstruction, destruction or absence of the extrahepatic bile ducts anywhere between the ampulla of Vater and the porta hepatis. A destructive sclerosing inflammatory process rapidly extends to the major intrahepatic bile ducts. If surgery is to be successful it must be performed before this occurs, usually by 60 days of age. In the liver substance the portal tracts become distended with edema, a mild inflammatory cell infiltrate and increased fibrous tissue deposition; proliferation of distorted bile ductules occurs around the periphery. By 6–10 weeks of age the portal pressure is increased. Cirrhosis rapidly develops. The mean age at death in untreated cases is 11 months with less than 5% surviving beyond 2 years.

Clinical features

The first sign of biliary atresia is prolongation of jaundice beyond the usual duration of physiological jaundice. It must be considered in any infant remaining jaundiced beyond 14 days of age. The incidence in the prematurely born or light-for-gestational age infant is the same as full term. The urine is always yellow. The stools contain no yellow or green pigment, but in up to 30% of infants with atresia stools are pigmented in the first weeks after birth before bile flow is completely obstructed. There may be hepatomegaly or splenomegaly. Investigations to confirm the diagnosis must be completed before signs of chronic liver disease develop. All too frequently the infant's apparent well-being causes pediatricians and other health workers to dismiss consideration of this disorder in the neonatal period (Mieli-Vergani et al 1989).

All of the following requirements need to be met to improve management of biliary atresia:

1. To identify asymptomatic jaundice; well-baby reviews should be at 4 rather than 6 weeks.
2. All infants jaundiced after 14 days of age should have urinalysis and total and direct serum bilirubin determination.
3. If conjugated bilirubin is present every infant should be referred to a pediatrician for urgent investigation.
4. If the stools have no yellow or green pigment every infant should be referred to a specialist center to exclude or treat biliary atresia.

Laboratory investigation

There is no single test which establishes a prelaparotomy diagnosis of biliary atresia. Percutaneous liver biopsy showing the features described above in all portal tracts is suggestive of atresia if α_1-antitrypsin deficiency, cystic fibrosis and arteriohepatic dysplasia (Alagille's syndrome) have been excluded. Radiopharmaceutical tests (^{99m}Tc methylbromo-IDA excretion) show complete cholestasis.

Laparotomy should be carried out by a surgeon with experience in assessing the bile ducts of infants at laparotomy and who can proceed to a portoenterostomy (Kasai operation). In this procedure an anastomosis is fashioned between the area of the porta hepatis from which the inflamed bile duct remnants have been resected and a Roux-en-Y loop allowing bile to drain directly from the main hepatic bile ducts directly into the bowel. Good bile flow can be achieved in 80% operated on by 60 days of age but in only 20–30% following later surgery. With a normal serum bilirubin a 90% 10-year survival has been reported with a good quality of life into the fourth decade (Kasai et al 1988, Ohkohchi et al 1989). If the bilirubin is not reduced the rate of progression of cirrhosis is not slowed. If bile drainage is partially effective death may occasionally be delayed to 10 years.

Complications

Cholangitis with a wide range of microorganisms occurs in over 50% of cases in the first 2 years after surgery. It is characterized by fever, recurrence or aggravation of jaundice and frequently features of septicemia. Blood culture, ascitic aspirate or liver biopsy to identify the organism responsible should precede intravenous antibiotic therapy which is continued for 14 days. Prophylactic antibiotics are of no proven value. Recurrent cholangitis may have a sustained adverse effect on liver function, indicating the need for early and aggressive treatment.

Portal hypertension is present in almost all cases at the time of initial surgery. Approximately 50% of those aged 5 years have esophageal varices but only 10–15% have alimentary bleeding. For these, injection sclerotherapy is the treatment of choice. All patients have a degree of malabsorption in the first year. They frequently require dietary supplements with medium chain triglycerides and glucose polymers. Supplements of fat-soluble vitamins K and A are essential and vitamins E and D in those whose jaundice persists beyond 5 months of age. In approximately 10% of cases in whom the serum bilirubin returns to normal, intrahepatic cholangiopathy progresses and complications of biliary cirrhosis ultimately develop. For these patients and those for whom surgery has not been effective liver transplantation is the only management.

CHOLEDOCHAL CYST

In this disorder there is enlargement or dilation of part or all the extrahepatic biliary system. There is reduced bile flow and intrahepatic changes similar to those of biliary atresia, progressing to cirrhosis. Cholangitis, rupture, pancreatitis, gallstones and carcinoma of the cyst wall are other important complications. In infancy it presents with features of a hepatitis of infancy or atresia. In older children there may be recurrent upper abdominal pain, recurrent jaundice and/or a palpable cystic mass but the classical triad is present in only a minority. Diagnosis is by ultrasonography and cholangiography (percutaneous transhepatic or endoscopic retrograde). The treatment is surgical removal with biliary drainage via a Roux-en-Y loop (Stringer et al 1995b).

SPONTANEOUS PERFORATION OF THE BILE DUCT

Perforation occurs at the junction of the cystic duct and common hepatic duct in infants who appear to have an obstruction low in the biliary system. Mild jaundice, acholic stools, failure to thrive and biliary ascites with bile-stained hernia are the clinical features.

The infants die of malnutrition or infection if the biliary system is not drained into a Roux-en-Y loop, usually via the gallbladder.

VIRAL HEPATITIS (see also Ch. 23)

Acute inflammation of the liver with varying degrees of hepatocellular necrosis may be caused by a wide range of viral infections. The term viral hepatitis is usually applied to infections caused by viruses with a high degree of hepatic trophism. Five distinct types can be identified at present although other agents of uncertain significance have recently been described.

ACUTE VIRAL HEPATITIS TYPE A (HAV)

This disorder is caused by ingestion of enterovirus type 72 (picorna). The virus becomes established in the liver, spills into the biliary system and is excreted in the stools. Stool concentration is highest 7 days before the onset of biochemical hepatitis. Thereafter it falls rapidly but virus may still be detected in small concentrations months later in patients who have an atypical relapsing course (Chiraco et al 1986). The diagnosis is confirmed by finding specific IgM antibodies to HAV which appear as early as 7 days after exposure, reaching peak concentrations at 20–40 days and usually clearing by 60 days. It is predominantly a disease of early childhood in areas with sewage-contaminated drinking water. In northern Europe only 10–15% become infected in childhood (Lemon 1985).

Clinical features

The incubation period varies from 15 to 40 days. There is a preicteric stage in which there may be anorexia, nausea, vomiting, fever, headache, lassitude, dull intermittent upper abdominal pain and loose stools, but the infection may be asymptomatic, particularly in children. The liver may be enlarged and tender, and the spleen may be palpable. After 5–10 days these features regress but jaundice and pruritus may develop with dark urine and pale stools. Jaundice usually lasts for 2 weeks, but it may persist for months or a relapsing course may occur (Sjogren et al 1987). Chronic liver disease has not yet been attributed to HAV infections. Rare complications include fulminant hepatic failure, bone marrow aplasia, pancreatitis, myocarditis and polyneuropathy.

Prevention

The provision of drinking water uncontaminated by fecal pathogens and the safe disposal of sewage is essential in the prevention of this disorder. Person to person spread may be minimized by scrupulous hand washing after defecation and before handling food. Two doses of hepatitis A vaccine 14 days apart provide over 95% protection and are extremely safe. There is no treatment for infection.

VIRAL HEPATITIS TYPE B (HBV)

The hepatitis B virus is a DNA-containing virus of the hepadna group. HBV DNA can integrate into the hepatocyte genome (Tiollais et al 1985). Unlike hepatitis A virus the immunological response is defective in up to 10% of those infected (up to 90% in the newborn) and a long-lasting, infective carrier state occurs. It may be associated with normal liver structure and function or a range of pathological abnormalities including cirrhosis and hepatocellular carcinoma. Patients infected by HBV may become superinfected by the delta virus (HDV).

Serological response in HBV infection

The response is variable both in time and density. Viral components and antibodies to them may be present so transiently that they are never detected or may persist in high concentrations for up to 30 years. The antigens and antibodies used in clinical practice are given in Table 11.35. Note that there may be an interval following the disappearance of an antigen before its antibody becomes detectable. Children who are immunosuppressed may have hepatitis B infection within the liver but without serological evidence.

Clinical features

The wide spectrum of acute and chronic responses to HBV infection in childhood are given in Table 11.36. The factors

Table 11.35 Serological markers in viral hepatitis type B

Marker	Clinical significance
HBsAg	Acute or chronic hepatitis B infection
HBsAb	Immunity to hepatitis B, postinfective or with active or passive immunization
HBcAb IgM	High titer: acute hepatitis Low titer: chronic infection
HBcAb IgG	Past exposure to hepatitis B
HBeAg	Highly infectious state
HBeAb	Less infective state in the HBsAb-positive patient
HBV specific DNA polymerase	Persisting viral infection
HBV DNA by direct DNA hybridization	A more sensitive indicator of viral replication

Table 11.36 Clinical expression of hepatitis B virus in childhood

1. Asymptomatic development of HBsAb
2. Acute hepatitis, anicteric or icteric
3. Papular acrodermatitis
4. Fulminant hepatic failure
5. Acute hepatitis proceeding to chronic hepatitis or cirrhosis
6. Disorders associated with circulating immune complexes
   a. Glomerulonephritis
   b. Periarteritis
   c. Pericarditis
   d. Arthritis
7. Chronic hepatitis
8. Cirrhosis
9. Hepatocellular carcinoma
10. 'Healthy' carrier state
11. Carrier state with immune disorders
    a. Down syndrome
    b. Malignant disease
    c. Renal failure
    d. Immunosuppression with transplantation

determining the outcome of infection are not understood. In all ages the reported carrier rate and frequency of serious sequelae is higher in males than in females. Carrier rate appears to be greatest in those infected in early infancy or by 3 years of age. Those with an anicteric hepatitis with minimal elevation of the transaminases appear to be at greater risk of becoming carriers. The carrier rate of the population varies from 0.1% in northern Europe and North America to 10% in southern European and Mediterranean countries and to as high 20% in parts of Africa and south-east Asia.

The clinical features of acute hepatitis type B are similar to those of type A but the incubation period ranges from 30 to 180 days and often the onset is more insidious. In many instances infection is asymptomatic and the carrier state is only detected by serological testing.

Natural history of hepatitis B infection

Over 80% of those infected in the first 6 months of life become carriers (i.e. HBsAg positive for more than 6 months) as opposed to less than 20% of those infected between 2 and 3 years. It has been estimated that 20–25% of those infected in infancy are still positive in the fourth decade. HBe clearance rate varies between 2% per annum for those infected in earlier infancy to 20% of children infected later in life. The conversion to anti-HBs in carriers is much rarer at between 0 and 2% per annum.

Only 5% of infections in early infancy are symptomatic, as opposed to 40% in later life. Neither the clinical features nor biochemical tests of liver function predict the histological response. Data on the long-term prognosis are sparse. Cross-sectional studies of carrier children in Europe suggest an incidence of chronic aggressive hepatitis (CAH) of over 50%, with chronic persistent hepatitis at 33%, the remainder having chronic lobular hepatitis or minimal changes. Histological diagnosis of cirrhosis is made in approximately 5% but if laparoscopy is used as many as a third are cirrhotic. Hepatocellular carcinoma, associated with HBV infections, accounts for 13% of childhood cancer in Taiwan occurring in children from 8 months upwards (Hsu et al 1987). Children with chronic persistent hepatitis or chronic lobular hepatitis usually have a good prognosis over a period of 15 years. Those with active CAH are more prone to develop cirrhosis and its complications, particularly if superinfected by D virus (Bortolotti et al 1988).

Prevention of hepatitis B

All blood and blood-derived products should be screened for hepatitis B and if positive, rejected. Close contacts of infected subjects may acquire infection from blood and possibly saliva, urine and other secretions. Wearing plastic disposable gloves and hand washing after handling blood or excretions appear to minimize the risk of infection. Highly immunogenic plasma-derived and synthetic vaccines are now available and should be used to protect family members where an index case has been identified. Medical and paramedical personnel may be similarly protected. Hyperimmune (to HBV) γ-globulin (HBIG) should be administered immediately after accidental inoculation of possibly hepatitis B-positive blood.

The combined use of HBIG in a dose of 200 IU, with active immunization starting within 48 h of delivery with further doses at 1, 2 and 12 months, is very effective in producing high anti-HBs titers. Further doses are recommended later if the anti-HBs titer falls below 100 IU/l. This schedule should be applied to all infants of mothers who are found to be HBsAg positive by screening during pregnancy, including those who are HBe antibody positive. In areas of high prevalence it is more cost effective to protect all newborns. Because of the high cost of such a regimen, it is likely that the vaccine alone will be used in many areas. In Africa and other localities where infection is acquired after the neonatal period, immunization at 3 months with other vaccines would seem to be most cost effective. Instead of the UK recommended dose of 20 μg doses as low as 2 μg given intradermally or intramuscularly are almost as efficacious (Milne et al 1987). Universal vaccination has been recommended by the World Health Organization.

Therapy of chronic hepatitis B

In European children, treatment with interferon 3 MU/m^2 for 3 months increased anti-HBe seroconversion rates over 12 months from 13% in controls to 40%. Pretreatment with steroids was not beneficial. The long-term clinical and histological benefit is assumed but unproven (Gregorio et al 1996).

VIRAL HEPATITIS DELTA (HDV)

Hepatitis delta virus is a defective RNA virus which can only replicate in the presence of HBV. It appears to be transmitted by direct parenteral inoculation or close body contact. All age groups simultaneously infected with HBV or who are already HBV carriers are susceptible. Knowledge of its epidemiology is sparse but its distribution appears to be worldwide (Farci et al 1985). When acquired simultaneously with HBV it may cause acute hepatitis varying in severity from asymptomatic infection to fulminant hepatic failure. Usually an HBV carrier state does not follow. Infection of HBV carriers causes a serious exacerbation of the hepatitis with progression to fulminant liver failure, chronic active hepatitis or cirrhosis. The diagnosis is confirmed by finding the delta agent in serum or liver tissue or by detecting antibodies to the delta virus. There is no treatment. HBV vaccination should limit its spread.

VIRAL HEPATITIS TYPE C (HCV)

Recent progress with serology and RNA polymerase chain reaction (PCR) tests have made the diagnosis of infection reliable. It has been shown that this 9500-RNA-base *Flavivirus* was responsible for up to 90% of post-transfusion hepatitis in North America prior to the screening of blood products. Infection in childhood occurs almost entirely through having received unscreened blood products, or rarely by vertical transmission. No vaccine is currently available.

The natural history of HCV infection

The consequences of infection for adults are becoming clearer and it is assumed that they are similar for children. A mild hepatitis typically follows infection and an incubation period of about 60 days. Only 30% are icteric and fulminant liver failure occurs exceedingly rarely. Perhaps 30–40% of immunocompetent patients will clear the virus while developing anti-HCV antibodies. The remainder will have chronic infection with anti-HCV antibodies and RNA PCR positivity. Of these the majority will have mild liver disease such as chronic persistent hepatitis with normal or occasionally abnormal transaminases. Liver disease is slowly progressive with cirrhosis developing over 5–30 years in 50%. Hepatocellular carcinoma occurs in 1–10% subsequently. Nonimmunocompetent patients are more likely to develop chronic infection but antibodies to HCV may remain negative. Interferon and ribavirin treatments have been used with benefit in adults, and are being evaluated in children (Alter 1995).

Other flaviviruses

During 1995 hepatitis G and three so-called 'GB agents' were identified. All have limited homology with HCV and may have similar epidemiology, being responsible for HCV-negative post-transfusion hepatitis. Their role in pediatric liver disease awaits clarification.

VIRAL HEPATITIS E (HEV)

This enterically transmitted 30 nm RNA virus is responsible for epidemics of hepatitis in the Middle East and Asia. Icteric disease occurs in 1–3% of infections. The prognosis is usually good but mortality is recognized in pregnant women (Skidmore 1995). Chronicity has not been documented.

NONVIRAL INFECTIONS

HEPATIC ABSCESSES

Hepatic abscesses may be caused by almost any bacteria or fungi. They occur in association with any septicemic state, particularly with portal pyemia. Patients at risk include those with primary or secondary immune depression, such as chronic granulomatous disease. Secondary infection of another hepatic lesion such as bile duct obstruction, tumor or sickle cell infarct may occur.

Clinical features

The clinical features are those of sepsis. There are frequently no clinical or biochemical features of liver disease. Diagnosis rests on ultrasonic detection of the lesion. The management is appropriate antibiotics as determined by culture of material aspirated from the lesion and ultrasonically guided drainage. Open liver biopsy may be required to obtain evidence of fungal infection. Surgical drainage is required if there is associated peritonitis, bile duct obstruction or if chronic abscesses with firm walls are present.

HEPATIC AMEBIASIS

This disorder has a high prevalence in children in insanitary areas. Fever, rigors and tender hepatomegaly in an ill child should suggest the diagnosis. It is unusual to obtain a history of diarrhea. Diagnosis is based on finding living ameba in the stools or gut biopsy and positive serological tests.

Treatment

Metronidazole (50 mg/kg/24-h in three doses for 10 days) is the treatment of choice. Therapeutic needle aspiration or surgical drainage may be necessary when rupture of the abscess seems imminent or the liver lesion enlarges in spite of drug treatment.

HYDATID DISEASE

Hydatid disease is usually caused by the larval stage of the dog tapeworm *Echinococcus granulosus*. Rarely the fox tapeworm, *E. multilocularis*, may be responsible.

Clinical features

Infection is usually acquired asymptomatically in early childhood. Discomfort in the right hypochondrium or hepatomegaly are presenting features. Rarely rupture into the biliary system may cause cholangitis or into the peritoneum a catastrophic collapse. A secondary bacterial infection may produce a liver abscess. The diagnosis is based on the typical appearance on ultrasonography and positive serological tests. Treatment is surgical resection. Patients with *E. multilocularis* infection or those too ill for surgery may respond to prolonged courses of mebendazole or albendazole.

SCHISTOSOMIASIS (p. 1507)

Hepatic features are firm hepatomegaly, portal hypertension with splenomegaly, ascites and or hematemesis. Liver disease may occur as early as 2 years after initial infection. The recovery of ova in stools or rectal mucosa proves schistosomal infection. Positive serology does not distinguish past from present infection. The treatment is praziquantel. Alimentary bleeding due to portal hypertension should be treated by injection sclerotherapy, not by portosystemic shunting.

LIVER INFESTATIONS (see Ch. 23)

The liver and biliary system may be damaged by infestation with *Fasciola hepatica* (sheep), *Clonorchis sinensis* (freshwater fish), *Opisthorchis felineus* and *Opisthorchis viverrin* (cat) and by larvae of the roundworm *Ascaris*. All cause cholangitis which may become suppurative and be complicated by bile duct obstruction, calculus formation, bile duct carcinoma, biliary cirrhosis and portal hypertension.

ACUTE LIVER FAILURE

Acute liver necrosis with hepatic encephalopathy starting within 8 weeks of the first sign of liver disease is termed 'fulminant' and between 8 and 24 weeks is termed 'late onset' (Gimson et al 1986). It is a rare, complex, multisystem disorder with a mortality of 30–70%. In infants severe liver failure may occur without apparent encephalopathy. The causes are given in Table 11.37. What factors determine the severity of hepatic injury or prevent hepatic regeneration are unknown. Life-threatening complications include septicemia especially from fungi, and cerebral edema progressing to raised intracranial pressure and impaired cerebral blood flow. If the patient survives, the liver usually regains normal histology and function

CLINICAL FEATURES

Hepatic encephalopathy is graded according to degree of severity as follows:

Grade 1   lethargy, minor reductions in consciousness or motor function, vomiting
Grade 2   stupor, irrational hyperactivity, combative behavior
Grade 3   unresponsive to command but responds to pain
Grade 4   unresponsive to command, extensor posturing and rigidity, brainstem depression with respiratory and vasomotor failure.

Table 11.37   Causes of fulminant liver failure

1. Infective
   a. Viral hepatitis
      (i) A, B, B+ Delta, C, enteric NANB
      (ii) EB virus
      (iii) Cytomegalovirus
      (iv) Herpes virus
      (v) Adenovirus
      (vi) Echovirus
      (vii) Yellow fever
      (viii) Lassa
      (ix) Ebola
      (x) Marburg
   b. Leptospirosis
   c. Septicemia

2. Toxic
   a. *Amanita phalloides*
   b. Carbon tetrachloride
   c. Paracetamol
   d. Halothane
   e. Valproate
   f. Carbamazepine
   g. Phenytoin
   h. Isoniazid
   i. Amiodarone
   j. Cytotoxics
   k. Monoamine oxidase inhibitors

3. Metabolic
   a. Galactosemia
   b. Fructosemia
   c. Tyrosinemia
   d. Familial erythrophagocytic reticulosis
   e. α_1-antitrypsin deficiency
   f. Neonatal hemochromatosis
   g. Wilson's disease
   h. Niemann–Pick Type C
   i. Respiratory chain defects

4. Ischemia
   a. Budd–Chiari syndrome
   b. Acute circulatory failure
   c. Septicemia with shock
   d. Heat stroke
   e. Leukemia

Shrinking liver size with the area of hepatic dullness on percussion reducing even within hours may be noted. Spontaneous hemorrhage, ascites and deepening jaundice are common features. Laboratory confirmation includes hyperammonemia, hypoglycemia and INR (international normalized ratio) uninfluenced by parenteral vitamin K, which if prolonged to more than 4.0 results in a mortality of 92%. The prognosis is particularly bad in children under 2 years and non-A non-B (non-C), drug-induced or late onset hepatitis.

TREATMENT

Intensive care aimed at preventing and treating complications is essential until the liver function recovers or transplantation can be performed. *Sedatives must not be given.* Other causes of coma must be excluded. Hypoglycemia must be prevented by intravenous glucose. Protein feeds are stopped. Lactulose may precipitate diarrhea without altering the outcome. Ranitidine and vitamin K both given intravenously may prevent bleeding from gastric erosions. Arrangements should be made to transfer the child to an intensive care facility with the experience to anticipate and control the multisystem complications and to proceed to liver transplantation if appropriate (O'Grady et al 1989).

REYE'S SYNDROME

Reye's syndrome is a rare, acute, frequently fatal encephalopathy of unknown cause occurring in children of any age. It is characterized by a self-limiting abnormality of mitochondrial structure and function lasting for 2–6 days, best documented in liver, with an acute catabolic state. Typically the disorder occurs during what seems to be an unremarkable viral infection of the respiratory or gastrointestinal tract or exanthema. Environmental factors such as aspirin may play a role (Forsyth et al 1989). It is essential to distinguish Reye's syndrome from an increasing range of inborn errors of metabolism presenting in a similar fashion, particularly urea cycle disorders, disorders of ketogenesis, e.g. medium chain acyl CoA dehydrogenase deficiency, organic acidemias and respiratory chain disorders. For some of these there may be specific treatment to prevent relapse, as well as important family implications.

The clinical features are pernicious vomiting with encephalopathy of all ranges of severity that may proceed over 4–60 h to brain death. There may be tachypnea. Typically there are no clinical features indicating hepatic involvement. Diagnosis must be suspected in any encephalopathy if there is laboratory evidence of liver involvement such as raised serum transaminases, ammonia, hypoglycemia or prolonged INR. The diagnosis is confirmed by liver biopsy, demonstrating swollen pleomorphic mitochondria with reduced activity of mitochondrial enzymes whilst cytoplasmic enzymatic activity is preserved. These changes are seen only in the first 2–5 days after the onset of encephalopathy. There is microvesicular fatty infiltration of the liver but this is nonspecific.

Treatment

Mortality rates are as high as 40% with a considerable proportion of survivors having permanent brain damage. The basis of treatment is to control increased intracranial pressure until the mitochondria recover. Tissue oxygenation must be maintained by mechanical 'overventilation' which helps to reduce cerebral pressure. Hypovolemia must be corrected. The blood sugar should be kept at the top end of the normal range by dextrose infusions giving 60% of normal fluid maintenance requirement. The patient should be nursed in a fashion which minimizes increases in intracranial pressure while being transferred to an intensive care unit. It is essential to collect and store (at $-70°C$) serum and urine at presentation in order to exclude metabolic disorders mimicking Reye's syndrome. Expert intensive care similar to that of acute liver failure is essential. Mannitol may be required if clinical features indicate increased intracranial pressure. A good outcome is most likely with early diagnosis and transfer to units with the expertise to carry out such treatment. Liver transplantation is not indicated as recovery of liver function is usual while encephalopathy may be progressive.

CHRONIC LIVER DISEASE

Chronic liver disease implies a long-standing irreversible change in the structure of the liver which may cause the complications of cirrhosis including premature death. The aim must be to identify the condition as early as possible so that further liver damage may be minimized by appropriate treatment. Chronic liver disease, including cirrhosis, may develop asymptomatically, insidiously and with no abnormal physical signs. Conversely, the presentation frequently appears acute. Chronic liver disease must therefore be suspected, however short the history, in any child with features of cirrhosis or in a child with apparent acute hepatitis unless an acute self-limiting infection has been confirmed by the presence of IgM antibodies to infectious causes of hepatitis or there is a history of recent exposure to hepatotoxic drugs. Such acute causes of liver inflammation may be superadded to chronic liver disease. Liver biopsy to define the pathology and aid in etiologic diagnosis should be performed without delay unless there is a specific contraindication or there is evidence of hepatitis B infection when it should be delayed for 6 months to allow spontaneous remission.

FEATURES SUGGESTING CHRONICITY

Chronic hepatitis should be suspected in a patient with a relapse of an apparent acute hepatitis, if clinical or biochemical features of serological proven hepatitis persist beyond 8 weeks, or if hepatitis occurs in a child with a history of conjugated hyperbilirubinemia in infancy. Signs indicating chronic liver disease include a small liver, an enlarged left lobe of liver, a hard liver, firm splenomegaly, ascites, cutaneous portosystemic shunts, large or numerous spider nevi. There may be growth failure or muscle wasting. Features associated with specific forms of chronic liver disease may be found, e.g. vitiligo in autoimmune chronic active hepatitis, diarrhea with mucus and blood in sclerosing cholangitis associated with inflammatory bowel disease, neurological abnormalities in Wilson's disease.

Investigation findings suggesting chronicity include a serum albumin of less than 35 g/l, prothrombin time prolonged by more than 3 s and raised serum immunoglobulins. A technetium-99 colloid liver scan may show poor hepatic uptake with increased splenic uptake and uptake in the bone marrow. Ultrasound abnormalities suggesting chronicity are heterogeneity of the parenchyma and demonstration by ultrasonically guided Doppler of reduced blood flow velocity in the hepatic artery or portal vein.

AUTOIMMUNE CHRONIC ACTIVE HEPATITIS (ACAH)

This disorder is characterized by an aggressive hepatitis with or without cirrhosis, high concentrations of serum immunoglobulins with an IgG commonly greater than 16 g/l, low concentrations of C4, and the presence of one or more non-organ-specific antibodies. Five types of autoantibody are seen: antinuclear, anti-smooth muscle, anti-liver/kidney microsomal, anti-gastric parietal cell and anti-liver/pancreas. There is impairment of T lymphocyte suppressor function. The etiology is unknown.

Clinical features

The patient may present with features of an acute hepatitis or of chronic liver disease as detailed above, or with complications of cirrhosis, such as ascites or hematemesis. There may be features indicating multisystem involvement in autoimmune processes, e.g. vitiligo, renal tubular acidosis, fibrosing alveolitis or polyendocrinopathy. Some children may have no clinical features of chronic liver disease. The differential diagnosis will include Wilson's disease, choledochal cyst, primary sclerosing cholangitis, chronic hepatitis B or C infection, α_1-antitrypsin deficiency and exposure to hepatotoxic drugs (Maggiore et al 1986).

Drug treatment

Prednisolone in a dose of 2 mg/kg/day up to a maximum 60 mg/kg/day is given initially and continued for 4 weeks during which time clinical features usually improve and the serum transaminase values fall. Over the course of 2–3 months the dose is gradually reduced to that which will have no side effects whilst maintaining a transaminase value at a level which is not more than twice the upper limit of normal. If the reduction of the steroid dose is associated with a rise in transaminase values or with a recurrence of symptoms, azathioprine at a dose of 0.5 mg/kg/day initially is added as a steroid-sparing agent. The dose, if necessary, is increased gradually to as much as 2.0 mg/kg/day. Weekly full blood counts and platelet counts are essential in the early weeks of azathioprine therapy.

Although the majority of patients with this disorder have cirrhosis at the time of diagnosis, over 90% can be maintained well over a 5-year period by immunosuppressive therapy. If this fails liver transplantation must be considered.

SCLEROSING CHOLANGITIS

Sclerosing cholangitis (SC) is a chronic obliterative inflammation in the intrahepatic and/or extrahepatic bile ducts. The characteristic features are irregularities in the outline of the ducts with areas of stricturing and dilation (beading) on cholangiography. The appearance must be distinguished from the 'attenuated' intrahepatic ducts seen in cirrhosis. The various types are listed in Table 11.38 (Debray et al 1994).

Table 11.38 Classification of sclerosing cholangitis

---

1. Primary (with or without chronic inflammatory bowel disease)
   a. With high serum immunoglobulins and non-organ-specific autoantibodies, C4 concentration normal and circulating T lymphocytes displaying IL-2R < 5%
   b. With normal serum immunoglobulins and no autoantibodies Following cholestasis in infancy (Amadee-Manesme et al 1987) (Neonatal sclerosing cholangitis)

2. Secondary (or with associated diseases)
   a. Langerhans histiocytosis
   b. Immune deficiency states
   c. Neutropenic states
   d. Cystic fibrosis
   e. Biliary surgery or trauma
   f. Choledochal cyst
   g. Congenital hepatic fibrosis
   h. Caroli's syndrome
   i. Ischemia after liver transplantation

Clinical features

In the primary form the majority present with nonspecific symptoms such as abdominal pain or fever. Less than 20% have had jaundice. Hepatomegaly, hepatosplenomegaly or abnormal liver function tests provoke further investigation and ultimately diagnosis. The age of presentation has ranged from 2 to 16 years with an equal incidence in males and females.

Laboratory findings are similar to those of ACAH except that the complement factor 4 is usually normal. Liver biopsy shows features of acute and chronic cholangitis, and frequently chronic aggressive hepatitis with or without cirrhosis (El-Shabrawi et al 1987).

Treatment

Symptomatic treatment includes adequate replacement of fat-soluble vitamins and cholestyramine to relieve pruritus. Dietary, drug and/or surgical treatment of associated bowel disease is necessary but does not appear to influence the biliary pathology. Corticosteroids and azathioprine, as used in the treatment of autoimmune chronic active hepatitis, produces a fall in transaminase and immunoglobulin levels but have not yet been proven to influence long-term prognosis. Ursodeoxycholic acid may be beneficial.

WILSON'S DISEASE

This inborn error of metabolism characterized by defective biliary copper excretion may present as virtually any form of liver disease from the age of 4 years onwards. The onset is usually insidious and few index cases are diagnosed before cirrhosis is well established. Nonspecific findings raising diagnostic suspicion are hemolytic anemia or evidence of renal tubular damage. The clinical features and laboratory investigations are identical to those of the above conditions except for features of neurological involvement in 20%. In 80% the serum ceruloplasmin value is less than 20 mg/dl (1.25 μmol/l). The urinary copper excretion is variable but usually more than 100 μg (1.6 μmol/24 h) increasing to more than 1000 μg (16 μmol/24 h) with 1 g of penicillamine. The liver copper concentration is > 250 μg/g of dry weight. Kayser–Fleischer rings may be identified by slit lamp examination in children over the age of 7.

Treatment

50% of those diagnosed in childhood have liver disease so advanced that liver transplantation is the treatment of choice (Table 11.39) (Nazer et al 1986). If the score is > 7, death within 2 months is almost invariable. Those with score < 6 should respond satisfactorily to low copper diet and penicillamine therapy (5 mg/kg/24 h increased by 5 mg/kg/24 h at 2-weekly intervals until a dose of 20 mg/kg/24 h is attained). Zinc sulfate in doses of 50–150 mg three times a day after meals given at different times from the penicillamine should be considered for those awaiting a liver donor (Caillie-Bertrand et al 1985). Patients with scores of 6 or 7 require close monitoring. Recovery on treatment may take 12 months or longer.

It is essential to screen siblings of patients with Wilson's disease or of children dying of liver disease of unknown cause so that therapy can be started before liver disease is advanced.

Table 11.39 Prognostic score in Wilson's disease

Bilirubin (μmol/l)	Aspartate amino-transferase (U/l)	Prothrombin time prolongation (s)	Prognostic score
N < 20	N < 40	N < 4	
< 100	< 100	4	0
101–150	101–150	4–8	1
151–200	151–200	9–12	2
201–300	201–300	13–20	3
> 300	> 300	> 20	4

Score < 6 – recovery likely with treatment.
Score > 7 – list for emergency liver transplantation.
Score 6 or 7 – regular review with list for emergency liver transplantation if deterioration occurs.

Genetic markers (Thomas et al 1995) have recently become available, which are most accurate once the status of the index case is known.

CIRRHOSIS

Cirrhosis is defined pathologically as a replacement of the normal hepatic structure by nodules of liver cells growing in a disorganized fashion in a vastly changed extracellular matrix with prominent fibrous tissue. The fibrous tissue frequently contains abnormal anastomoses between efferent and afferent vascular systems causing portosystemic shunting. The main pathophysiological effects are impaired hepatic function and portal hypertension. Hepatocellular carcinoma may develop. Although the diagnosis of cirrhosis implies an irreversible and usually progressive pathological change it may be compatible with normal growth and activity for many years.

There are two broad pathological categories, biliary cirrhosis and so-called postnecrotic cirrhosis. Genetic factors contribute to both pathological varieties (Table 11.40).

CLINICAL AND LABORATORY FEATURES

Clinical and nonspecific laboratory features are those described above under the heading chronic hepatitis. Laboratory abnormalities specific to the many causes may be evident. There may be features of the complications. Four disorders may cause diagnostic difficulty: extrahepatic portal hypertension, congenital hepatic fibrosis, constrictive pericarditis and infiltrative disorders such as reticulosis.

MANAGEMENT

On the basis of the history, examination findings and standard investigations listed in Table 11.41 it should be possible to limit the likely causes of liver damage prior to performing a liver biopsy. This is important because the limited liver tissue must be subjected to appropriate histological, electron microscopic, histochemical or biochemical analysis to determine the cause. In considering the genetic disorders, principal consideration must be given to those in which treatment, if started early, is effective, e.g. Wilson's disease, galactosemia or fructosemia. It is also similarly important to identify surgically correctable abnormalities of the biliary tree. Having made the histological diagnosis of cirrhosis and confirmed the etiology, the aim of management is to minimize further liver damage by treating the cause of liver disease if this is

Table 11.40 Causes of cirrhosis in childhood

1. Biliary
   a. Extrahepatic biliary atresia
   b. Intrahepatic biliary hypoplasia
   c. Choledochal cyst
   d. Cystic fibrosis
   e. Progressive cholestasis
   f. Familial intrahepatic cholestasis
   g. Bile duct stenosis or obstruction
   h. Choledocholithiasis
   i. Sclerosing cholangitis
   j. Ascending pyogenic cholangitis
   k. Cholangitis due to
      (i) *Fasciola*
      (ii) *Clonorchis sinensis*
      (iii) *Ascaris*
   l. Pancreatic fibrosis
   m. Pancreatic tumors
   n. Histiocytosis X

2. Postnecrotic
   a. Hepatitis in infancy, especially if α_1-antitrypsin deficient
   b. Chronic active hepatitis
   c. Acute viral hepatitis (viral hepatitis, B, C, delta, non-A non-B)
   d. Hepatitis due to drugs, e.g. actinomycin D, methotrexate
   e. Toxins, e.g. aflatoxin, copper

3. Genetic disorders
   a. Wilson's disease
   b. Galactosemia
   c. Fructosemia
   d. Glycogen storage disease Type IV
   e. Glycogen storage disease Type III
   f. Shwachman's syndrome
   g. Hurler's syndrome
   h. Cystic fibrosis
   i. Zellweger syndrome
   j. α_1-antitrypsin deficiency
   k. Tyrosinemia
   l. Cystinosis
   m. Ornithine carbamyl transferase deficiency
   n. Gaucher's disease
   o. Wolman's disease
   p. Abetalipoproteinemia
   q. Defects in fatty acid oxidation
   r. Sickle cell disease
   s. Thalassemia
   t. Hepatic porphyria
   u. Hemochromatosis, idiopathic
   v. Hemochromatosis secondary to chronic hemolytic disease
   w. Defects in primary bile salt synthesis
   x. Niemann–Pick disease Type C

4. Venous congestion
   a. Constrictive pericarditis
   b. Ebstein's anomaly
   c. Congestive cardiac failure
   d. Budd–Chiari syndrome
   e. Venacaval webs
   f. Veno-occlusive disease
   g. Radiation

Table 11.41 Investigation of children with suspected cirrhosis

1. Biochemistry
   a. Electrolytes and blood gases
   b. Serum proteins including electrophoresis
   c. Bilirubin
   d. Aspartate aminotransaminase, γ-glutamyltranspeptidase
   e. Alkaline phosphatase
   f. Cholesterol
   g. α-fetoprotein
   h. Ceruloplasmin
   i. Blood and urine metabolic screen

2. Immunology
   a. Serum immunoglobulins and tissue autoantibodies

3. Hematology
   a. Prothrombin time
   b. Full blood count

4. Imaging
   a. Radioisotope imaging of liver
   b. Chest radiography
   c. Ultrasonic scan
   d. Endoscopy or barium meal re varices

5. Histology
   a. Liver biopsy

Table 11.42 Complications of cirrhosis

1. Portal hypertension
2. Bleeding diathesis
3. Hypoxemia
4. Increased susceptibility to infection
5. Hyperdynamic circulation (cardiac failure)
6. Ascites
7. Spontaneous bacterial peritonitis
8. Pulmonary hypertension
9. Hepatoma
10. Malnutrition
11. Gallstone formation
12. Renal failure
13. Hepatic encephalopathy
14. Endocrine changes
15. Impaired hepatic metabolism of drugs and hormones
16. Impaired neurodevelopment, particularly gross motor

possible and preventing or controlling complications (Table 11.42).

The diet must contain sufficient protein, essential fatty acids, minerals, trace elements and vitamins for growth and normal activities. The calorie requirements may be up to 40% above standard for weight. Anorexia is frequently a problem which may be aggravated by restricted fluid and/or salt intake. Fat malabsorption of varying severity is usual. Water- and fat soluble vitamin supplements are frequently required. The latter may have to be given parenterally. If hepatic encephalopathy develops dietary protein intake should be stopped and gradually reintroduced up to the maximum tolerated, while lactulose is given to reduce absorption of nitrogenous toxins from the gut. There is no advantage in using branched chain amino acids.

Portal hypertension causes splenomegaly, ascites and alimentary bleeding. Splenomegaly and hypersplenism rarely require intervention. Ascites is best dealt with by restricting salt intake. If there is hyponatremia water restriction is essential. In an anorexic child it is rarely possible to reduce the sodium intake to less than 0.5 mmol/kg day. Diuretics in the form of spironolactone often control mild ascites. If these measures are unsuccessful albumin infusions with simultaneous frusemide may sufficiently expand the intravascular volume to improve urinary output and control of ascites by dietary and diuretic measures. Paracentesis may be necessary if there is severe abdominal distention or respiratory embarrassment with replacement of the protein removed by intravenous albumin. It is essential to monitor the patient's weight, abdominal girth, urinary output of water and sodium and to measure the serum urea and creatinine when managing ascites (Bernard et al 1985).

TREATMENT OF ALIMENTARY BLEEDING

However small the bleed the child should be immediately admitted to the nearest hospital with transfusion facilities. Following slow initial bleeds, sudden hematemesis may occur causing shock requiring rapid blood replacement to prevent death. Bleeding decreases hepatic perfusion with the possibility of hepatic encephalopathy and further deterioration of liver function. On admission, a baseline assessment of the clinical, hematological and biochemical state should be made, blood cross-matched, and a secure intravenous line established. Intravenous octreotide and a Sengstaken–Blakemore tube of suitable size should be available. Sedatives should be avoided. Lactulose should be given by fine nasogastric tube and ranitidine to reduce the risk of bleeding from gastric erosions. Intravenous vitamin K should be given if the prothrombin time is prolonged. As soon as the patient's condition has been stabilized arrangements should be made to transfer the child to a unit equipped to manage the causes and complications of portal hypertension. Endoscopy is essential to confirm the presence of varices and the source of bleeding, which may be gastric erosions or peptic ulceration rather than varices. It should be combined with injection sclerotherapy. Three or four varices may be injected (Howard et al 1988). If injection sclerotherapy cannot be performed and bleeding continues, the portal venous pressure may be lowered by intravenous octreotide. Emergency portosystemic shunting is rarely required.

SPONTANEOUS BACTERIAL PERITONITIS

This potentially lethal complication occurring in children with ascites requires early diagnosis and an antibiotic regimen effective against *Streptococcus pneumoniae* and Gram-negative organisms. It may present with clear signs of peritonitis. Frequently there are no such signs but the infection is manifest by a deterioration in hepatic, renal and/or neurological function. A blood culture and diagnostic ascitic tap are essential to identify the pathogen and select appropriate antibiotic therapy.

CHRONIC HEPATIC ENCEPHALOPATHY

Chronic hepatic encephalopathy is a complex neuropsychiatric syndrome occurring in association with ill-understood neurochemical changes in cirrhosis. It is characterized by intellectual impairment, personality change and clouding of consciousness which may progress to coma. Sleep patterns may be disturbed. A variety of neurological signs may appear indicating organic cerebral disease. Typically these vary from hour to hour. Causes of hepatic encephalopathy and compounding factors are given in Table 11.43.

Treatment

The objective of treatment is to prevent accumulation of ammonia and other vasoactive or false neurotransmitter substances in the

Table 11.43 Causes of hepatic encephalopathy

1. End stage chronic parenchymal disease
2. Fulminant or subacute liver failure
3. Liver disease with severe portosystemic shunting
4. Precipitating factors
    hypoglycemia
    hypokalemia
    hypovolemia
    sepsis
    GI bleeding
    hypoxia
    high protein or MCT diet

gut, to remove or correct identifiable precipitating factors and to try to improve liver function. Protein intake should be reduced to 0.5–1 g/kg of body weight initially but then increased if tolerated. Medium chain triglycerides should be avoided since they may increase short chain fatty acid concentration and thereby aggravate hepatic encephalopathy. Broad spectrum antibiotics such as neomycin, and lactulose, a nonabsorbable synthetic disaccharide, are both effective in preventing or treating recurrent encephalopathy.

Pulmonary complications

Hypoxemia is a relatively common complication of cirrhosis. It may be due to intrapulmonary shunting due to microscopic arteriovenous fistulae, ventilation/perfusion mismatch or a reduction in diffusion capacity. It may be aggravated by portopulmonary venous anastomoses connecting paraesophageal portosystemic collaterals with the pulmonary venous system. The degree of intrapulmonary change does not correlate with the severity of the liver damage or portal hypertension. Pulmonary hypertension may develop. These features cause exertional dyspnea and aggravate hepatic encephalopathy. They may be partially relieved by breathing an increased oxygen concentration and are cured by liver transplantation (Fewtrell et al 1994).

HEPATORENAL FAILURE

Oliguric renal failure without structural abnormalities in the kidney (functional renal failure) is frequently a terminal event in advanced cirrhosis. There is a slow development of azotemia, oliguria, hyponatremia with a low urinary sodium concentration. Glomerular filtration may show transient improvement with inotropes. Liver transplantation is the definitive treatment.

PORTAL HYPERTENSION DUE TO PORTAL VEIN OBSTRUCTION

The portal vein may be obstructed from without by infective or thrombotic disorders or by a congenital abnormality. The presenting features are asymptomatic splenomegaly, alimentary bleeding with portal hypertension, which can occur at any age throughout childhood or adult life, less commonly with ascites and failure to thrive. The diagnosis is suspected by the finding of portal hypertension or esophageal varices in a patient with splenomegaly and no clinical or biochemical evidence of liver disease. The diagnosis is confirmed by ultrasonography or angiography. The treatment is that of bleeding esophageal or rectal varices. Splenomegaly or hypersplenism rarely require intervention. Hepatic encephalopathy may occur in adult life.

CONGENITAL HEPATIC FIBROSIS

The unique pathological feature of this condition is the presence of wide bands of fibrous tissue, linking portal tracts but clearly demarcated from the hepatic parenchyma (Desmet 1992). The bands contain irregularly shaped spaces lined by bile duct epithelial cells. Portal veins are sparse. There is little inflammatory cell infiltrate unless there is associated cholangitis. There is frequently significant associated renal disease, particularly infantile polycystic disease and a wide range of dysmorphic syndromes. The clinical features are those of portal hypertension, hepatomegaly and occasionally cholangitis. Liver function is well preserved and liver function tests are usually normal although the alkaline phosphatase may be elevated. Diagnosis requires an adequate liver biopsy and renal excretion scans are essential to define renal involvement. Alimentary bleeding from varices is treated by injection sclerotherapy, cholangitis with appropriate antibiotics. Rarely liver transplantation is indicated for biliary cirrhosis secondary to chronic cholangitis.

CYSTIC FIBROSIS

The majority of patients with cystic fibrosis have pathological abnormalities in the form of expansion of the portal tracts with increased fibrosis and frequently fatty infiltration in the liver. Clinical syndromes include: (1) prolonged conjugated hyperbilirubinemia in infancy presenting as a hepatitis syndrome sometimes difficult to distinguish from biliary atresia; (2) massive hepatic steatosis which reverses as nutrition improves; and (3) cirrhosis with portal hypertension and variceal hemorrhage, hypersplenism or splenic pain. Biliary abnormalities take the form of microgallbladder present in up to a third, with gallstones in as many as 12%.

The treatment is aimed at improving nutrition, particularly deficiency of fat-soluble vitamins, controlling sepsis and the management of portal hypertension. Hepatic encephalopathy is possibly less frequent after portosystemic shunts in this disorder than in other forms of cirrhosis but can still occur and injection sclerotherapy is the treatment of choice for bleeding varices. Surgery may be required for symptomatic gallstones (Psacharopoulos & Mowat 1983). Liver transplantation has also been performed with improvement in the pulmonary status.

INDIAN CHILDHOOD CIRRHOSIS

This term is restricted to a form of cirrhosis occurring largely in the Indian subcontinent and characterized by necrosis of hepatocytes which contain Mallory's hyaline and orcein-staining granular material representing copper-associated protein. There is marked pericellular collagen deposition and a distinct lack of regeneration nodules except in chronic cases. The disorder starts insidiously in over 75% of cases with irritability, anorexia and hepatomegaly. Slight jaundice heralds the onset of decompensated cirrhosis with all its complications. Over 80% die within 6 months. The disease, which has an incidence of up to 1 in 4000 live births in some areas, appears to be due to an accumulation of copper in the liver. If exposure to dietary copper, mainly in the form of copper-containing vessels for storing buffalo milk, can be prevented, the disease may be eliminated. Penicillamine in a dose of 20 mg/kg/day if given to patients before the onset of ascites or jaundice gives a 50% survival (Tanner et al 1987). Non-Indian cases have been described both with and without excessive environmental exposure to copper. This has led to the hypothesis of a metabolic disease underlying some cases.

LIVER TUMORS

Primary liver tumors occur with approximately one-tenth of the frequency of neuroblastoma. Malignant tumors include hepatoblastoma and hepatocellular carcinoma, both of which are usually accompanied by a high α-fetoprotein level, fibrolamellar hepatoma, rhabdomyosarcoma and cholangiocarcinoma. Benign tumors include adenoma, teratoma, mesenchymal hamartoma, focal nodular hyperplasia and infantile hemangioendothelioma. The latter may present with cardiac failure. The others present with abdominal distention, hepatomegaly, abdominal pain or rarely complications of the tumor. Diagnosis is supported by the demonstration of a space-occupying lesion within the liver by scanning.

Treatment by resection, with appropriate chemotherapeutic agents for malignant lesions (Saxena et al 1993), or by hepatic artery ligation in congestive cardiac failure complicating infantile hemangioendothelioma (Davenport et al 1995) is best carried out in a specialist center.

LIVER TRANSPLANTATION

With 2-year survival rates as high as 90% and 5-year survival rates ranging from 64 to 78% (Iwatsuki et al 1988, Kalayoglu et a 1993), liver transplantation is a therapeutic option to be considered in any child with acute or chronic liver disease in whom early death is inevitable or when the quality of life has deteriorated to unacceptable levels, or if irreversible damage to the central nervous system is likely to occur. Full consideration must be given to other forms of treatment and the presence of relative contraindications to grafting (Paradis et al 1988). The recipient is likely to have one or more life-threatening complications in the perioperative or postoperative period. Lifelong immunosuppressive therapy with close medical and surgical supervision is required. The majority of survivors have a good quality of life. The longest survivor to date remains well 20 years after transplant. Supply of suitable donors remains a major limiting factor in liver transplantation in childhood despite improvements from reducing organs (de Ville de Goyet et al 1993), splitting organs between two recipients and using part of the liver of a live related donor. The precise indications and the optimum management of some of the intraoperative and postoperative problems including the control of rejection, remain the subject of ongoing research. The results are better in children transplanted in a good nutritional state and if the procedure is elective.

COMPLICATIONS

Complications are those of major surgery involving multiple vascular and biliary anastomoses, of rejection and the effects of long-term antirejection drugs. The risks of primary nonfunction and vascular thrombosis have been much reduced. Rejection occurs in up to 70% but is resistant to treatment with steroids in about 15%. In the first months after the procedure infections already present in the patient prior to transplantation and those related to the surgery are the major problems. In patients with poor graft function, opportunistic infections remain a high risk while those on modest doses of antirejection drugs are at risk of community-acquired infections such as pneumococcal infection. Between 1 and 6 months, cytomegalovirus, hepatitis B and non-A, non-B hepatitis and opportunistic infection with organisms such as *Nocardia* and *Pneumocystis* may occur. EB virus infection may lead to lymphoproliferative disease in patients who have received exceptional total immunosuppression for rejection. The use of cyclosporine has reduced the risk of infective complications but has major side effects including acute and

Table 11.44 Indications for liver transplantation

1. End stage chronic parenchymal disease – with likelihood of death within 12 months or evidence of deterioration which will worsen prognosis at transplantation or not amenable to more conservative management

2. Unacceptably low quality of life – e.g. severe pruritus in Alagille's syndrome

3. Fulminant or subacute hepatic failure – age < 2 years, INR > 4.0

4. Metabolic disorders – particularly those complicated by life-threatening crises
   a. α_1-antitrypsin deficiency
   b. Crigler–Najjar syndrome
   c. Wilson's disease
   d. Primary oxaluria
   e. Tyrosinemia
   f. Familial hypercholesterolemia
   g. Galactosemia
   h. Protein C deficiency
   i. Glycogen storage disease Type 0, I and IV
   j. Factor 8 deficiency
   k. Acyl Co-A dehydrogenase deficiency
   l. Urea cycle defects
   m. Cystic fibrosis

5. Liver tumors (rarely)
   a. Malignant – chemosensitive with unresectable primary but without extrahepatic spread (e.g. hepatoblastoma)
   b. Benign – life threatening but not amenable to more conservative treatment (e.g. infantile hemangioendothelioma)

chronic renal failure, hypertension, convulsions, tremor, paresthesia and hirsutism. Rejection is a major risk, particularly in the first month but may occur at any time.

In addition to end stage chronic parenchymal liver disease and poor quality of life, transplantation must be considered in fulminant or subacute hepatic failure and in selected children with an increasing range of metabolic disorders (Table 11.44). Orthotopic auxiliary transplants may be most suitable for some of these latter indications. Selecting the appropriate time for surgery is difficult. It is essential that patients who may become candidates for transplantation should be referred at the earliest possible stage to hepatology units with the expertise to advise on the optimum time for this procedure.

SELF-HELP AND RESEARCH GROUPS

Crohn's in Childhood Research Appeal, 48 Ewell Down's Road, Ewell, Epsom, Surrey KT17 3BN, UK

National Association for Colitis and Crohn's Disease, 3 Thorpefield Close, Marshalwick, St Alban's, Hertfordshire, UK

Ileostomy Association, Amblehurst House, Chobham, Woking, Surrey GU24 8PZ, UK

Coeliac Society, PO Box 222, High Wycombe, Buckinghamshire HP11 28Y, UK

Patients on Intravenous and Nasogastric Nutrition Therapy, 76 Stirling Close, Rainham, Essex, UK

Cystic Fibrosis Research Trust, Alexandra House, 5 Blyth Road, Bromley, Kent BR1 3RS, UK

Children's Liver Disease Foundation, 138 Digbeth, Birmingham

REFERENCES

Abu-Arafeh I, Russell G 1995 Cyclical vomiting syndrome in children: a population based study. Journal of Pediatric Gastroenterology and Nutrition 21: 454–458

Alagille D, Estrada A, Hadchouel M et al 1987 Syndromic paucity of interlobular bile ducts (Alagille's Syndrome or arteriohepatic dysplasia): review of eighty cases. Journal of Pediatrics 110: 195–200

Alter H J 1995 To C or not C: these are the questions. Blood 85(7): 1681–1695

Amadee-Manesme O, Bernard O, Brunelle F et al 1987 Sclerosing cholangitis with neonatal onset. Journal of Pediatrics 111: 225–229

Ament M E, Berquist W E, Vargas J, Perisic V 1988 Fiberoptic upper intestinal endoscopy in infants and children. Pediatric Clinics of North America 35: 141–156

Andrews P L R, Hawthorn J 1988 The neurophysiology of vomiting. Bailliere's Clinical Gastroenterology 2: 141–168

Apley J 1959 The child with abdominal pains. Blackwell Scientific Publications, Oxford

Belli D C, Seidman E, Bouthillier L, Weber A M, Roy C C, Plentinox M, Beaulieu M, Moring C L 1988 Chronic intermittent elemental diet improves growth failure in children with Crohn's disease. Gastroenterology 94: 603–610

Bernard O, Alvarez F, Brunelle F, Hadchouel P, Alagille D 1985 Portal hypertension in children. Clinics in Gastroenterology 14: 33–55

Berrocal T, Simon M J, al-Assir I, Prieto C, Pastor I, de Pablo L, Lama R 1995 Shwachman-Diamond syndrome: clinical, radiological and sonographic finding. Pediatric Radiology 25: 356–359

Bisset W M, Rivers R P A, Milla P J 1988 Ontogeny of fasting small intestinal motor activity in the human infant. Gut 29: 483–488

Bisset W M, Stapleford P, Long S, Chamberlain A, Sokel B, Milla P J 1992 Home parenteral nutrition in chronic intestinal failure. Archives of Disease in Childhood 67: 109–114

Blethyn A J, Verrier Jones K, Newcombe R, Roberts G M, Jenkins H R 1995 Radiological assessment of constipation. Archives of Disease in Childhood 73: 532–533

Bock S A, Sampson H A 1994 Food allergy in infancy. Pediatric Clinics of North America 41: 1047–1067

Booth I W, Grand R J 1988 Chronic inflammatory bowel disease. In: Milla P J, Muller D P R (eds) Harries' paediatric gastroenterology. Churchill Livingstone, Edinburgh, pp 137–169

Bortolotti F, Calzia R, Vegnente A et al 1988 Chronic hepatitis in childhood: the spectrum of the disease. Gut 29: 659–664

Brown K H 1994 Dietary management of acute diarrheal disease: contemporary scientific issues. Journal of Nutrition 124(8 suppl): 1455S–1460S

Brueton K J, Clarke G S, Sandhu B K 1988 Gastro-oesophageal reflux in infancy. In: Milla P J (ed) Disorders of gastrointestinal mobility in childhood. John Wiley, Chichester

Buick R G, Spitz I 1985 Achalasia of the cardia in children. British Journal of Surgery 72: 341–343

Caillie-Bertrand M V, Degenhert H J, Visser H K et al 1985 Oral zinc sulphate for Wilson's disease. Archives of Disease in Childhood 60: 656–659

Candy D, Larcher V F, Cameron D J S et al 1981 Lethal familial protracted diarrhoea. Archives of Disease in Childhood 56: 15–23

Carre I J 1959 The natural history of the partial thoracic stomach (hiatus hernia) in children. Archives of Disease in Childhood 34: 344–353

Castro C A, Arntzen C J 1993 Immunophysiology of the gut: a research frontier for integrative studies of the common mucosal immune system. American Journal of Physiology 265: G599–610

Chiraco P, Bortolotti F, Realdi G et al 1986 Polyphasic course of hepatitis type A in children. Journal of Infectious Disease 153: 378–379

Cosgrove M, Al-Atia R, Jenkins H R 1996 The epidemiology of inflammatory bowel disease. Archives of Disease in Childhood 74: 460–461

Crampton J, Rees W D W 1986 Gastroduodenal bicarbonate secretion: its role in protecting the stomach and duodenum. In: Pounder R E (ed) Recent advances in gastroenterology 6. Churchill Livingstone, Edinburgh, pp 35–50

Davenport M, Hansen L, Heaton N D, Howard E R, 1995 Haemangioendothelioma of the liver in infants. Journal of Pediatric Surgery 30(1): 44–48

Davidson G P, Cutz E, Hamilton J R, Gall D G 1978 Familial enteropathy: a syndrome of protracted diarrhea from birth, failure to thrive and hypoplastic villus atrophy. Gasterenterology 75: 783–790

Davidson M, Wasserman R 1966 The irritable colon of childhood (chronic non-specific diarrhea syndrome). Journal of Pediatrics 69: 1027–1038

Davies G, Evans C M, Shand W S, Walker-Smith J A 1990 Surgery for Crohn's disease in childhood: influence of site of disease and operative procedure on outcome. British Journal of Surgery 77: 891–894

de Ville de Goyet J, Hausleithner V, Reding R, Lerut J, Janssen M, Otte J B 1993 Impact of innovative techniques on the waiting list and results in pediatric liver transplantation. Transplant 56: 1130–1136

Debray D, Pariente D, Urvoas E, Hadchouel M, Bernard O 1994 Sclerosing cholangitis in children, Journal of Pediatrics 124: 49–56

Deprettere A, Portmann B, Mowat A P 1987. Syndromic paucity of the intrahepatic bile ducts: diagnostic difficulty; severe morbidity throughout childhood. Journal of Pediatric Gastroenterology and Nutrition 6: 865–871

Desmet V J 1992 Congenital diseases of intrahepatic bile ducts: variations on the theme 'ductal plate malformation'. Hepatology 16: 1069–1083

Dohil R, Roberts E, Verrier Jones K, Jenkins H R 1994 Constipation as a cause of reversible urinary tract abnormalities. Archives of Disease in Childhood 70: 56–57

Douglas J R, Campbell C A, Salisbury D M, Walker-Smith J A, Williams C B 1980 Colonoscopic polypectomy in children. British Medical Journal 281: 1386–1387

Dutton P V, Furnell J R G, Spiers A L 1985 Environmental stress factors associated with toddler diarrhoea. Journal of Psychosomatic Research 29: 85–88

El-Shabrawi M, Wilkinson M L, Portmann B et al 1987 Primary sclerosing cholangitis in childhood. Gastroenterology 92: 1226–1235

ESPGAN 1993 A proposition for the diagnosis and treatment of gastro-oesophageal reflux disease in children. European Journal of Pediatrics 152: 704–711

Farci P, Barbara C, Navone C et al 1985 Infection with delta agent in children. Gut 26: 4–7

Ferguson A 1984 Crohn's disease in children and adolescents. Journal of the Royal Society of Medicine 77 (suppl 3): 30–34

Ferguson A, Sedgwick D M 1994 Juvenile onset inflammatory bowel disease: predictions of morbidity and health status in early adult life. Journal of Royal College of Physician, London 28: 220–227

Fewtrell M S, Noble-Jameson G, Revell S, Friend P, Johnston P, Rasmussen A, Jamieson N, Calne R Y, Barnes N 1994 Intrapulmonary shunting in the biliary atresia/polysplenia syndrome: reversal after liver transplantation. Archives of Disease in Childhood 70: 501–504

Forsyth B W, Horwitz R I, Acanpora D et al 1989 New epidemiologic evidence confirming that bias does not explain the aspirin/Reye's syndrome association. Journal of the American Medical Association 261: 2517–2524

Foulkes W D 1995 A tale of four syndromes: familial adenomatous polyposis, Gardner syndrome, attenuated APC and Turcot syndrome. Quarterly Journal of Medicine 88: 853–863

Fozard J B J, Dixon M F 1989 Colonoscopic surveillance in ulcerative colitis – dysplasia through the looking glass. Gut 30: 285–292

Frank D A, Zeisel S H 1988 Failure to thrive. Pediatric Clinics of North America 35: 1187–1206

Ghishan F K 1988 The transport of electrolytes in the gut and the use of oral rehydration solutions. Pediatric Clinics of North America 35: 35–51

Gimson A E S, O'Grady J, Ede R J, Portmann B, Williams R 1986 Late onset hepatic failure: clinical, serological and histological features. Hepatology 6: 288–294

Glassman M, George D, Grill B 1995 Gastroesophageal reflux in children. Clinical manifestations, diagnosis and therapy. Gastroenterology Clinics of North America 24: 71–98

Gormally S M, Prakash N, Durnin M T, Daly L E, Clyne M, Kierce B M, Drumm B 1995 Symptoms in children before and after treatment of *Helicobacter pylori* infection. Journal of Pediatrics 126: 753–756

Graham P 1986 Feeding and growth. In: Child psychiatry: a developmental approach. Oxford University Press, Oxford, pp 52–63

Gregorio G V, Jara P, Hierro L, Diaz C, de la Vega A, Vegnente A, Iorio R, Bortolotti F, Crivelaro C, Zancan L, Daniels H, Portmann B, Mieli-Vergani

G 1996 Lymphoblastoid interferon-a with or without steroid pre-treatment in children with hepatitis B: a multi-centre controlled trial. Hepatology 23: 700–707

Griffiths AM, 1992 Crohn's disease. Recent Advances in Pediatrics 10: 145–152

Griffiths A M, Ohlsson A, Sherman P M, Sutherland L R 1995 Meta-analysis of enteral nutrition as a primary treatment of active Crohn's disease. Gastroenterology 108: 1056–1067

Gurbindo C, Seidman E G 1991 Gastrointestinal manifestations of immunodeficiency states. In: Walker W A (ed) Pediatric gastrointestinal disease. B C Decker, Ontario, pp 503–525

Heitlinger L A, Lebenthal E 1988 Disorders of carbohydrate digestion and absorption. Pediatric Clinics of North America 35: 239–255

Hirst W J R, Layton D M, Singh S, Mieli Vergani G, Chessels J M, Strobel S, Pritchard J 1994 Haemophagocytic histiocytosis: experience at two UK centres. British Journal of Haematology 88: 731–739

Howard E R, Stringer M D, Mowat A P 1988 An assessment of injection sclerotherapy in the management of 152 children with oesophageal varices. British Journal of Surgery 75: 404–408

Hsu H C, Wu M Z, Chang M H et al 1987 Childhood hepatocellular carcinoma develops exclusively in hepatitis B suffers antigen carriers in three decades in Taiwan. Journal of Hepatology 5: 260–267

Hyams J S, Treem W R, Justwich C J, Davis P, Shoup M, Burke G 1995 Characterisation of symptoms in children with recurrent abdominal pain: resemblance to irritable bowel syndrome. Journal of Pediatric Gastroenterology and Nutrition 20: 209–214

Illingworth R S 1985 Infantile colic revisited. Archives of Disease in Childhood 60: 981–985

Ishak K G, Sharp H L 1987a Metabolic errors and liver disease. In: Macsween R N M, Anthony P P, Scheuer P J (eds) Pathology of the liver, 2nd edn. Churchill Livingstone, Edinburgh, pp 99–180

Ishak K G, Sharp H L 1987b Developmental abnormalities in liver disease in childhood. In: Macsween R N M, Anthony P P, Scheuer P J (eds) Pathology of the liver, 2nd edn. Churchill Livingstone, Edinburgh, pp 66–98

Iwatsuki S, Starzl T E, Todo S et al 1988 Experience in 1,000 liver transplants under cyclosporin-steroid therapy: a survival report. Transplantation Proceedings 20S: 498–504

James J M, Burks A W 1994 Food hypersensitivity in children. Current Opinion in Pediatrics 6: 661–667

Jansson U, Johansson C 1995 Down's syndrome and celiac disease. Journal of Pediatric Gastroenterology and Nutrition 21: 443–445

Jenkins H R, Fenton T R, McIntosh N, Dillon M J, Milla P J 1990 The development of colonic sodium transport in early childhood and its regulation by aldosterone. Gut 31: 194–197

Jenkins H R, Milla P J 1988 The development of colonic transport mechanisms in early life: evidence for reduced anion exchange. Early Human Development 16: 213–218

Jenkins H R, Milla P J 1993 The effect of colitis on large intestinal electrolyte transport in early childhood. Journal of Pediatric Gastroenterology and Nutrition 16: 402–405

Jenkins H R, Pincott J R, Soothill J F, Milla P J, Harries J T 1984 Food allergy: the major cause of infantile colitis. Archives of Disease in Childhood 59: 326–329

Jenkins H R, Schnackenberg U, Milla P J 1993 In-vitro studies of sodium transport in human infant colon: the influence of acetate short chain fatty acids in the human infant colon. Pediatric Research 34: 666–669

Jobling J C, Lindley K J, Yousef Y, Gordon I, Milla P J 1996 Investigating inflammatory bowel disease – white cell scanning, radiology and colonoscopy. Archives of Disease in Childhood 74: 22–26

Johnston B T, Carre I J, Thomas P S, Collins B J 1995 Twenty to 40 year follow-up of infantile hiatus hernia. Gut 36: 809–812

Kagalwalla A F 1994 Congenital chloride diarrhea. A study in Arab children. Journal of Clinical Gastroenterology 19: 36–40

Kalayoglu M, D'Alessandro A M, Knechtle S J, Eckhoff D E, Pirsch J D, Judd R, Sollinger H W, Hoffmann R M, Belzer F O 1993 Long-term results of liver transplantation for biliary altresia. Surgery 114: 711–718

Kanof M E, Lake A M, Bayless T M 1988 Decreased height velocity in children and adolescents before the diagnosis of Crohn's disease. Gastroenterology 95: 1523–1527

Kasai M, Ohi R, Chiba T, Hayashi Y 1988 A patient with biliary atresia who died 28 years after hepatic portojejunostomy. Journal of Pediatric Surgery 23: 430–431

Kazerooni N L, VanCamp J, Hirschl R B, Drongowski R A, Coran A G 1994 Fundoplication in 160 children under 2 years of age. Journal of Pediatric Surgery 29: 677–681

Kopelman H 1991 Cystic fibrosis. 6. Gastrointestinal and nutritional aspects. Thorax 46: 261–267

Lancet Editorial 1983 Management of acute diarrhoea. Lancet i: 623–625

Lask B 1988 Psychological aspects of gastrointestinal disease. In: Milla P J, Muller D P R (eds) Harries' paediatric gastroenterology. Churchill Livingstone, Edinburgh, pp 290–294

Leichtner A M 1995 Aminosalicylates for the treatment of inflammatory bowel disease. Journal of Pediatric Gastroenterology and Nutrition 21: 245–252

Lemon S M 1985 Type A viral hepatitis. New England Journal of Medicine 313: 1059–1067

Lothe L, Lindberg T 1989 Cow's milk whey protein elicits symptoms of infantile colic in colicky formula-fed infants: a double blind crossover trial. Pediatrics 83: 262–266

Lowe M E 1994 Pancreatic triglyceride lipase and colipase: insights into dietary fat digestion. Gastroenterology 107: 1524–1536

McClement J, Howard E R, Mowat A P 1985 Results of surgical treatment for extrahepatic biliary atresia in the United Kingdom, 1980–1982. British Medical Journal 290: 345–347

McNeish A S, Harms H K, Rey J, Shmerling D H, Visakorpi J K, Walker-Smith J A 1979 The diagnosis of coeliac disease – a commentary on the current practices of members of the European Society for Paediatric Gastroenterology and Nutrition. Archives of Disease in Childhood 54: 783–786

Mader T J, McHugh T P 1992 Acute pancreatitis in children. Pediatric Emergency Care 8: 157–161

Maggioni A, Lifshitz F 1995 Nutritional management of failure to thrive. Pediatric Clinics of North America 42: 791–810

Maggiore G, Bernard O, Homberg J C et al 1986 Liver disease associated with anti-liver-kidney microsome antibody in children. Journal of Pediatrics 108: 399–404

Mahoney M, Migliavacca M, Spitz L, Milla P J 1988 Motor disorders of the oesophagus in gastro-oesophageal reflux. Archives of Disease in Childhood 63: 1333–1338

Mehta D I, Lebenthal E 1994 New developments in acute diarrhea. Current Problems in Pediatrics 24: 95–107

Mieli-Vergani G, Howard E R, Portmann B, Mowat A P 1989 Late referral for biliary atresia: missed opportunities for effective surgery. Lancet i: 421–423

Milla P J 1988 Gastrointestinal motility disorders in children. Pediatric Clinics of North America 35: 311–330

Milne A, Dimitrakakis M, Campbell C et al 1987 Low-dose vaccination against hepatitis B in children: one year follow up. Journal of Medical Virology 22: 387–392

Mirakian R, Richardson A, Milla P J, Walker-Smith J A, Unsworth J, Savage M O, Bottazzo G F 1986 Protracted diarrhoea of infancy: evidence in support of an autoimmune variant. British Medical Journal 293: 1132–1136

Muller D P R 1988 Structure and function. In: Milla P J, Muller D P R (eds) Harries' paediatric gastroenterology. Churchill Livingstone, Edinburgh, pp 30–51

Nazer H, Ede R J, Mowat A P, Williams R 1986 Wilson's disease: clinical presentation and use of prognostic index. Gut 27: 1377–1381

Newell S J 1988 Development of the lower oesophageal sphincter in the preterm infant. In: Milla P J (ed) Disorders of gastrointestinal motility in childhood. John Wiley, Chichester, pp 39–52

Nord K S 1988 Peptic ulcer disease in the pediatric population. Pediatric Clinics of North America 35: 117–140

O'Grady J G, Alexander G J M, Hayllar K, Williams R 1989 Early indicators of prognosis in fulminant hepatic failure. Gastroenterology 97: 439–445

Ohkohchi N, Chiba T, Ohi R, Mori S 1989 Long-term follow-up of patients with cholangitis after successful Kasai operation in biliary atresia: selection of recipients for liver transplantation. Journal of Pediatric Gastroenterology and Nutrition 9: 416–420

Orenstein S R 1993 Esophageal disorders in infants and children. Current Opinion in Pediatrics 5: 580–589

Oster J 1972 Recurrent abdominal pain, headache and limb pains in children and adolescents. Pediatrics 50: 429–436

Paradis K J G, Freese H T, Sharp H L 1988 A pediatric perspective on liver transplantation. Pediatric Clinics of North America 35: 409–433

Patrick M K, Gall D G 1988 Protein intolerance and immunocyte and enterocyte interaction. Pediatric Clinics of North America 35: 17–34

Perrault J 1994 Hereditary pancreatitis. Gastroenterology Clinics of North America 23: 743–752

Phillips A D, Schmitz J 1992 Familial microvillous atrophy: a clinico-pathological survey of 23 cases. Journal of Pediatric Gastroenterology and Nutrition 14: 380–396

Pittschieler K (ed) 1994 Deficiency of alpha$_1$-antitrypsin and the liver. Acta Paediatrica Supplement 393: 1–36

Psacharopoulos H T, Mowat A P 1983 The liver and biliary system. In: Hudson M E, Norman A P, Batten J C (eds) Cystic fibrosis. Baillière Tindall, London, pp 164–189

Puntis J W L 1995 Home parenteral nutrition. Archives of Disease in Childhood 72: 186–190

Qualman S J, Murray R 1994 Aganglionosis and related disorders. Human Pathology 45: 1141–1149

Rossi T 1988 Endoscopic evaluation of the colon in infancy and childhood. Pediatric Clinics of North America 35: 331–356

Rowland M, Drumm B 1995 Helicobacter pylori infection and peptic ulcer disease in children. Current Opinion in Pediatrics 7: 553–559

Rule D C 1991 The mouth. In: Walker W A (ed) Pediatric gastrointestinal disease. B C Decker, Ontario, pp 353–358

Sakula J, Shiner M 1957 Coeliac disease with atrophy of the small intestine mucosa. Lancet ii: 876

Saxena R, Leake J L, Shafford E S, Davenport M, Pritchard J, Mieli-Vergani G, Howard E R, Spitz L, Malone M, Salisbury J R 1993 Chemotherapy effects on hepatoblastoma. American Journal of Surgical Pathology 17(12): 1266–1271

Schmitz J 1988 Protein-losing enteropathies. In: Milla P J, Muller D P R (eds) Harries' paediatric gastroenterology. Churchill Livingstone, Edinburgh, pp 260–271

Schmitz J 1991 Digestive and absorptive function. In: Walker W A (ed) Pediatric gastrointestinal disease. B C Decker, Ontario, pp 266–280

Shandling B, Gilmour R F 1987 The enema continence catheter in spina bifida: successful bowel management. Journal of Pediatric Surgery 22: 271–273

Shaw V, Lawson M 1994 (eds) Clinical paediatric dietetics. Blackwell, London

Sjogren M H, Tanno H, Fay O et al 1987 Hepatitis A virus in stool during clinical relapse. Annals of Internal Medicine 106: 221–226

Skidmore S J 1995 Hepatitis E. British Medical Journal 310: 414–415

Steffen R M, Wyllie R, Petras R E, Caulfield M E, Michener W M, Firor H V, Norris D G 1991 The spectrum of eosinophilic gastroenteritis. Report of six pediatric cases and review of the literature. Clinical Pediatrics 30: 404–411

Stringer M D, Puntis J W 1995 Short bowel syndrome. Archives of Disease in Childhood 73: 170–173

Stringer M D, Dhawan A, Davenport M et al 1995 Choledochal cysts: lessons from a 20 year experience. Archives of Disease in Childhood 73: 528–531

Suchy F J 1993 Bile acids for babies? Diagnosis and treatment of a new category of metabolic liver disease. Hepatology 18: 1274–1277

Sutcliffe J 1969 Torsion spasms and abnormal postures in children with hiatus hernia: Sandifer's syndrome. Progress in Pediatric Radiology 2: 190–197

Symon D N K, Russell G 1995 Double-blind placebo controlled trial of pizotifen syrup in the treatment of abdominal migraine. Archives of Disease in Childhood 72: 48–50

Tanner M S, Bhave S A, Pradhan A N, Pandit A N 1987 Clinical trials of D penicillamine in Indian childhood cirrhosis. Archives of Disease in Childhood 62: 1118–1124

Taubman B 1988 Parental counselling compared with elimination of cows milk or soy milk protein for the treatment of infantile colic syndrome: a randomised trial. Pediatrics 81: 756–761

Thomas G R, Forbes J R, Roberts E A, Walshe J M, Cox D W 1995 The Wilson disease gene: spectrum of mutations and their consequences. Nature Genetics 9: 210–216

Thompson N P, Montgomery S M, Pounder R E, Wakefield A J 1995 Is measles vaccination a risk factor for inflammatory bowel disease? Lancet 345: 1071–1074

Tighe M R, Ciclitira P J 1993 The implications of recent advances in coeliac disease. Acta Paediatrica 82: 805–810

Tiollais P, Pourcel C, Dejean A 1985 The hepatitis B virus. Nature 317: 489–495

Treem W R 1994 Gastrointestinal bleeding in children. Gastrointestinal Endoscopy Clinics of North America 4: 75–97

Vanderplas Y 1993 Pathogenesis of food allergy in infants. Current Opinions in Pediatrics 5: 567–572

Vanderplas Y, Sacre-Smits L 1985 Seventeen-hour continuous esophageal pH monitoring in the newborn: evaluation of the influence of position in asymptomatic and symptomatic babies. Journal of Pediatric Gastroenterology and Nutrition 4: 356–361

von Allmen D, Goretsky M J, Ziegler M M 1995 Inflammatory bowel disease in children. Current Opinion in Pediatrics 7: 514–552

Walker-Smith J A 1980 Toddler's diarrhoea. Archives of Disease in Childhood 55: 329–330

Walker-Smith J A 1988 Gastroenteritis. In: Walker-Smith J A Diseases of the small intestine in childhood. Butterworths, London, pp 185–284

Walker-Smith J A 1994 Intractable diarrhoea in infancy: a continuing challenge for the paediatric gastroenterologist. Acta Paediatrica Supplement 83(395): 6–9

Walker-Smith J A, Guandalini S, Schmitz J, Shmerling D H, Visakorpi J K 1990 Revised criteria for the diagnosis of coeliac disease. Archives of Disease in Childhood 65: 909–911

Warren J D, Marshall B J 1984 Unidentified curved bacilli in the stomach of patients with gastritis and peptic ulceration. Lancet i: 1273–1275

Weaver L T, Steiner H 1984 The bowel habit of young children. Archives of Disease in Childhood 59: 649–652

Weile B, Cavell B, Nivenius K, Krasilnikoff P A 1995 Striking differences in the incidence of childhood celiac disease between Denmark and Sweden. Journal of Pediatric Gastroenterology and Nutrition 21: 64–68

Wewer V, Christiansen K M, Andersen L P, Henriksen F W, Hart Hansen J P, Trede M, Krasilnikoff A 1994 Helicobacter pylori infection in children with recurrent abdominal pain. Acta Pediatrica 83: 1276–1281

WHO 1980 World Health Organization. A manual for the treatment of acute diarrhoea.WHO/CDD/SER/80.2, Geneva

Wyllie R, Kay M H 1994 Applications of gastrointestinal endoscopy in infants and children. Current Opinion in Pediatrics 6: 568–573

12 Respiratory disorders

Chapter editors: Sheila McKenzie   Mike Silverman

Introduction 489
Sheila McKenzie
Culture and environment 492
Sheila McKenzie
Development of the respiratory system 494
Mike Silverman
**Respiratory physiology, pathophysiology and the
    measurement of respiratory function 497**
Mike Silverman
Clinical features 506
History and symptoms 506
Mike Silverman
Physical examination and physical signs 510
Sheila McKenzie
Special investigations 513
Imaging 513
Isky Gordon
Bronchoscopy 519
John Warner and Gary Connett
Special aspects of treatment 520
Mike Silverman

Resuscitation 522
David Zideman
Apnea and breathing disorders during sleep 528
Peter Fleming and John Henderson
**Respiratory defenses and infection in the compromised host
    531**
Duncan Matthew and Vas Novelli
Asthma 536
Mike Silverman
Cystic fibrosis 550
John Warner and Gary Connett
Respiratory infections 559
Sheila McKenzie
Inhalation of foreign material 570
Mike Silverman
Congenital abnormalities 572
Sheila McKenzie and Mike Silverman
Chronic lung disease 576
Sheila McKenzie
References 579
Further reading 583

INTRODUCTION

MORBIDITY AND MORTALITY

Mortality statistics for children are published annually by the UK Office of Population Censuses and Surveys (OPCS) (Tables 12.1 and 12.2). These are not only interesting records of deaths by age and cause but they also provide some insight into how disorders are perceived. Tuberculosis is classed as a disease caused by highly infectious agents but nevertheless is one which has occupied the attention of respiratory physicians for over half of this century. Bronchiolitis is a highly infectious disease but is classed in the respiratory section. This is probably because the causative organisms for bronchiolitis are not often sought since there is no good treatment for them. Children with bronchiolitis in the UK are rarely admitted to infectious disease units, probably because the illness is limited to the respiratory system and until recently has not been subject to infectious disease precautions.

Interpreting OPCS data is quite difficult and the reasons for changes in the incidence of specific conditions can at best only be speculative. For example, between 1978 and 1980 a new category 'epiglottitis' was added to the OPCS list and in the same period there appears to have been a dramatic increase in deaths from all categories of upper airway infections. This suggests that there was greater awareness of these diseases and not that there was necessarily an increase in their prevalence. Similarly the category 'bronchiolitis' has been in use since 1967 but even as late as 1988 most of the deaths recorded under the category 'bronchitis/bronchiolitis' were classified as bronchitis. By 1993 deaths in the category were nearly all called 'bronchiolitis'.

Only since 1971 has the OPCS included a category for sudden infant death syndrome (SIDS). Previously, many babies dying suddenly had been placed in the respiratory category. There has been a dramatic decline in postneonatal mortality due to respiratory causes even since 1980 (Table 12.2) and comparing 1980 and 1986 when the total numbers of postneonatal deaths were similar, the decrease in those registered as respiratory deaths is similar to the increase in the SIDS category. The dramatic drop in the postneonatal mortality rate since 1990 has been due to the reduction in SIDS associated with the advice to place young infants supine to sleep. The interpretation of mortality data is far from straightforward.

The marked reduction in the prevalence of respiratory disease in the Western world in the last 50 years reflects an improved standard of living, immunization against tuberculosis, pertussis, diphtheria and measles and the introduction of antimicrobial drugs. The improved mortality in the last decade is largely due to technological advances in the care of children with respiratory failure.

What is meant by an *improved standard of living* with respect to children's chest disease? Less crowded housing, reflecting both smaller family size and larger, houses, drier and better ventilated accommodation and, in the United Kingdom, the introduction of health care and education in hygiene, available to all, have made large contributions to respiratory health. Children of larger birthweights assumed to be born to better nourished mothers have better lung function as adults (Barker et al 1991). This is assumed to be because they have larger airways, less sensitive to the effects of infection and atopy (Taussig 1992). Unfortunately the problem of maternal cigarette smoking which adversely affects fetal lung growth has still to be addressed.

Table 12.1 Numbers of children 1 month to 14 years dying from respiratory disease and complications of other diseases (England and Wales)

	1978	1980	1982	1984	1986	1988	1990	1992	1993
Respiratory disease									
All deaths	1148	1005	825	509	438	454	337	215	298
Lower respiratory tract infections									
Bronchiolitis	349	206	182	134	111	81	59	31	44
Pneumonia	594	528	401	204	176	182	139	83	128
Total	943	734	583	338	287	263	298	114	172
Upper airway obstruction									
Laryngitis, tracheitis and pharyngitis	11	46	31	28	18	16	13	7	4
Epiglottitis		39	19	18	13	10	11	4	2
URTI – unspecified	24	33	34	13	23	. 7	13	7	10
Total	35	118	84	59	54	33	37	18	16
Asthma	43	40	44	39	26	38	37	20	19
Other diseases									
Cystic fibrosis	96	83	58	53	48	42	27	27	28
Pulmonary complications of infectious diseases									
Pulmonary tuberculosis	5	4	2	4	3	0	2	0	4
Pertussis	12	6	14	1	3	0	7	1	0

Data from Mortality Statistics (cause) for children. OPCS, HMSO

Table 12.2 Principal causes of death 1 month – 1 year (England and Wales)

	1980	1982	1984	1986	1988	1990	1992
All deaths	2803	2773	2430	2760	2849	2343*	1588*
Infections	103	81	74	98	85	100	77
Respiratory diseases	677	543	347	306	322	207	121
Congenital disorders	507	542	494	465	407	367	375
Diseases arising in the perinatal period	110	111	143	202	223	228	218
SIDS	929	1066	1002	1284	1390	1047*	434*
Injury	145	110	96	94	109	90	83

* The fall in 1990–92 is largely accounted for by the reduction in SIDS.
Data from Mortality Statistics (cause) for children. OPCS, HMSO.

Immunization has virtually eliminated tuberculosis as a cause of serious chest disease in both adults and children in developed countries. However, between 1978 and 1988 the previous fall in the notifications in the UK was less evident and there is a worrying rise in some areas in the USA. Immunization against pertussis has been extremely effective: in 1983 there were 600 000 reported deaths worldwide, in 1990 250 000 (Kim-Farley 1992). Similar changes in reported cases of diphtheria are not evident: 47 000 cases of diphtheria were notified in 1983 but in the epidemic in the New Independent States of the former Soviet Union alone, there were more than this in 1994. Approximately 30% of these were children. In 1983 there were 67 million cases of measles with 2 million deaths, falling to 800 000 in 1990, reflecting the improved uptake of measles immunization. Notifications of diphtheria in the UK are in single figures and respiratory deaths from measles are rare in immunocompetent and well-nourished children.

The role of *antimicrobial drugs* in the reduction of death from acute respiratory illness (ARI) is difficult to define although it is certainly considerable. Results of the World Health Organization's current programe (1984) to tackle ARI in developing countries has already shown benefit (Sazawal & Black 1992) with a 20% reduction in infant mortality and 25% reduction in under-5s mortality. This reduction is attributed to case management independent of other interventions such as immunization and oral rehydration. Drug and oxygen treatments seem to have played considerable roles.

The fall in deaths from respiratory causes in the United Kingdom since 1978 is indeed remarkable (Table 12.1). The biggest fall is from infections, although the standard of living and the availability of effective antimicrobial drugs has not changed commensurately. There can be no doubt that the development of *technological expertise* in the monitoring and ventilatory support of children in respiratory failure has had a major impact.

RECENT ADVANCES AND FUTURE NEEDS (Table 12.3)

The global fall in death rates due to *respiratory infections*, including those due to measles, is arguably the single most important advance in the delivery of health care in the last decade. When families can hope for their children's survival then fertility rates will fall, favoring a reduction in the rate of rise of the world population (Douglas 1991). Sustaining and expanding the WHO program (WHO 1984), together with the development of vaccines against pneumococcus and *Haemophilus influenzae* suitable for use in developing countries, are the next steps and developing a vaccine against respiratory syncytial virus is being pursued (Toms 1995). Tuberculosis is still the world's single most common infectious disease and the most challenging. Without a reduction in population growth and improved economic status for many poor areas in the world it is difficult to see how the toll that tuberculosis takes can be effectively addressed (Benatar 1995). Subjects with human immune deficiency virus are particularly at

Table 12.3 Recent advances and future needs

Some recent advances
- Worldwide reduction in mortality from respiratory infection
- Development of vaccine against *H. influenzae* type b
- Improved uptake of measles immunization
- Consensus management programs for asthma
- Understanding of atopy at a cellular level
- Understanding the role of parental smoking
- Lung function measurements in small children to enable longitudinal studies of respiratory health
- Prenatal screening for cystic fibrosis
- Development of intensive care
- Improved delivery systems for drugs to the lungs
- Heart-lung transplantation
- Extracorporeal membrane oxygenation
- Gene therapy

Some worrying developments
- Large very poor populations
- Resistance of common infections to antibiotics, e.g. tuberculosis, pneumococcus
- Diphtheria epidemics
- HIV coexisting with tuberculosis
- Rising incidence of asthma
- Increasing global pollution

Some needs
- Control against the spread of tuberculosis
- Vaccine for developing world against Hib and *Pneumococcus*
- Development of RSV vaccine
- Education about the responsible use of antibiotics
- Techniques for the better identification of common pathogens
- A consensus definition of asthma
- Validation of symptom questionnaires
- Treatment for wheezing disorders of infancy and early childhood
- How to prevent uptake of cigarette smoking
- Improved maternal nutrition

risk of infection with and reactivation of tuberculosis (De Cock et al 1992), putting children in the population at risk.

Although there is adequate treatment for bacterial respiratory infections very few, even in the developed world, have positive bacteriological diagnoses. The polymerase chain reaction is able to identify rhinoviruses and tuberculosis but only in a few highly specialized laboratories. Because bacteriological identification is not possible in well over 90% of respiratory infections, the blind use of antibiotics continues with the development of resistant organisms in alarming numbers (Ventakesan & Innes 1995). This is an area for urgent attention.

Asthma is a disorder about which much has still to be learnt. Despite the International Guidelines (Sheffer 1992) available for its management there is no consensus about the definition of the disease. Many diagnoses are made simply on parental reporting of symptoms. Precisely what parents understand of the symptoms listed in questionnaires is not clear and some method of objectively validating parents' reports needs to be worked out.

In the past 20 years advances in treatment have revolutionized the care of the asthmatic but it is possible that a disorder that was previously underdiagnosed is now overdiagnosed. It has been widely debated whether or not the prevalence of asthma is increasing. Two surveys in South Wales, 15 years apart, have indicated a rise in both symptoms and bronchial responsiveness (Burr et al 1989) and, even taking into account that there is no consensus on its definition, the prevalence of asthma seems to be increasing. The increased hospital admission rates for children in the late 1980s reflected more referrals from the community because of the increased severity of attacks (Anderson et al 1994).

Hospital admission rates in the mid-1990s seem to have plateaued and in some areas are falling. It seems likely that wheezing in the preschool nonatopic child has a different disease profile from classic atopic asthma (Silverman 1993). Mortality from asthma in childhood has only recently started to fall (Table 12.1) and it remains to be seen if the figures of 1990–93 are sustained. School absence allegedly due to asthma is still high but objective validation of the reasons for school absence is not available.

Major contributions to our understanding of asthma are emerging from several sources. The cell biology of the airways of adult asthmatics is now much better understood. Information about the airways of children, especially preschool wheezy children, now needs to be gathered for comparison. Markers of airway inflammation which can be reliably identified in the peripheral blood will aid the understanding of wheezing disorders in children. Such an understanding could be the basis of the development of a vaccine against asthma and other atopic disorders (Holt 1994). A number of genes related to the atopic status have now been identified (Le Souef 1995). Epidemiological methods, in particular those used in the longitudinal studies of respiratory health in children, are already providing important clues about the development of wheezing disorders.

The management of *cystic fibrosis* centered on diet, physiotherapy and antimicrobial treatment has meant that survival has improved so that ever more children reach adult life (Table 12.1). The identification of a genetic marker for this disorder where the parental genotype is informative has allowed the option of chorionic villous biopsy with a view to termination if the fetus is affected. Home care has revolutionized the quality of life for the young child with cystic fibrosis. Studies of gene therapy (Alton & Geddes 1995) to target the chloride defect are under way.

Why the prone position is an adverse factor in *SIDS* is still unknown. It is possible that lung function is fatally compromised when some infants sleep in this position but there is little to support a primary role of the respiratory system.

The proportion of babies who have *chronic lung disease of prematurity* has risen as more preterm infants have survived neonatal lung disease. Even uncomplicated prematurity or low birthweight are risk factors for chronic symptoms late in childhood (Chan et al 1989) and in adult life (Barker et al 1991). Babies who have required prolonged ventilatory support and have had increased oxygen requirements for prolonged periods are at increased risk of acute respiratory failure should they contract a respiratory infection. They and their families require specialist support in the community and need more hospital care in the first year or two. Oxygen therapy at home (and sometimes artificial ventilation) is now widely available.

Improvements in *technology* and *drug treatment* have meant that a greater proportion of children with previously fatal disorders is now surviving. Those with malignancies, chronic heart or renal disease or who have primary immunodeficiency or are immunosuppressed because of chemotherapy are at risk of serious chest infection. The management of such children is time consuming and costly. Not only is there risk from the usual array of respiratory pathogens but also from organisms such as *Pneumocystis pneumoniae*, cytomegalovirus, measles, fungi and so on. Heart–lung transplantation has become available, for example for end-stage lung disease in cystic fibrosis. Extracorporeal membrane oxygenation (ECMO) has been successfully used to treat respiratory failure where conventional support has failed. Replacement of the specific products of single gene disorders by packaged substitutes is possible, for instance in α-1-antitrypsin deficiency. Designer drugs targeted by aerosol technology may alter the outcome for disorders of the airways extending from the bronchus in asthma to the alveolar membrane in hyaline membrane disease.

The *prognosis* of respiratory disease in childhood is under examination by longitudinal studies in centers such as London, Perth (Australia) and Tucson. Children will be followed into adult life to try to define the role of childhood disease in the development of respiratory disease in adulthood. The relationship between bronchiolitis and asthma, the damage caused by neonatal lung disease and the long-term damage caused by atmospheric pollution are examples of problems which prospective studies address. The development of lung function testing in children from the newborn period onwards has allowed follow-up of cohorts of patients into adult life. This is now augmented by application of techniques belonging to cellular chemistry and molecular biology. Whatever new treatments for respiratory disease have to offer, it is still crucial that the fetus is offered an optimum environment where there is adequate maternal nutrition and good fetoplacental function.

CULTURE AND ENVIRONMENT

Relationships between cultural and environmental factors and respiratory disease have been examined by epidemiological studies. Such studies try to define the strength of associations between certain variables, such as quality of dwelling, air pollution, ethnic origin, etc. and illness. These associations may point to adverse risk factors and when there is a very strong, dose-related association between two factors, for example cigarette smoking and wheezing, a causal link can be proposed.

SOCIAL DEPRIVATION

Social deprivation, judged by unemployment rather than social class, is associated with increased prevalence and severity of respiratory disease, particularly in young children. This appears to be independent of passive smoking which is a separate risk factor (Colley et al 1973, Strachan 1992, Spencer et al 1996). Poorly ventilated housing may lead to indoor pollution where there is cigarette smoking and nitrogen dioxide from household gas fumes. Both increase the risk for respiratory symptoms. Dampness encourages mold and leads to high house mite populations and these appear to be associated with both cough and wheeze (Platt et al 1989, Brunekreff et al 1989, Dales 1991). Overcrowding increases the risk of respiratory infection. *Intrauterine growth retardation and smoking during pregnancy are* commoner in socially deprived groups. Babies from such pregnancies have smaller airways and are more at risk from respiratory illness (Rona et al 1993, Tager et al 1993).

The effect of living in cold housing and in a cold climate is unknown. However, the interesting observation that it is easier to catch a cold in a hut in the Antarctic than under similar conditions in the Common Cold Unit at Salisbury has led to the speculation that reflex rhinorrea, noticeable when first entering a warm atmosphere after coming in from the cold, may encourage the spread of virus-laden laden droplets (Lloyd 1988).

CHILDHOOD ENVIRONMENT AND OUTCOME FOR RESPIRATORY ILLNESS

It has been suggested that chronic obstructive lung disease in adults owes more to childhood infection than to cigarette smoking (Barker & Osmond 1986). The high rate of chronic bronchitis in Britain and its distribution within the country would seem to be a legacy of poor social conditions in the past (Barker 1988) mediated through poor lung growth in early childhood (Shaheen & Barker 1994). The relative contribution to lung disease in adulthood of small airways at birth and chest infection in early childhood should be answered by several longitudinal studies in progress.

Atopic disease related to environment has a different etiology. Atopic sensitization does not seem to be a feature of an underprivileged childhood. Comparison of atopic sensitization and asthma in East and West German populations – attractive because the similar genetic inheritance of the populations does not confound the effects of environment – suggests that children growing up in the poorer East, where they are likely to have been exposed to more viral respiratory infections, are less atopic and have no more asthma than their peers in the West (Von Mutius et al 1994). A good theoretical model based on the early development of lymphocyte populations in response to viral infection or to other allergens, and the balance of these populations, could explain this observation (Martinez 1994, Openshaw & O'Donnell 1994).

AIR POLLUTION

The risk of respiratory syncytial virus infections is much higher for infants living in industrial populations. Either this is a reflection of the social deprivation already mentioned or it could reflect damage to the airway due to pollutants which in turn predispose to the development of more severe effects of infection.

There is no doubt that air pollution adversely affects the respiratory health of children. Oxides of nitrogen and ozone are present in car exhaust fumes whilst sulfur dioxide and particulates are emitted from industrial pollution and diesel fumes. Children living in areas with high air pollution have more respiratory symptoms and measures to control environmental pollution appear to be beneficial. The study examining the effect of pollution in six communities in the eastern United States showed a strong association between frequencies of chronic cough, bronchitis and chest illness in preadolescent children and concentrations of airborne particulates, sulfur dioxide and nitrogen dioxide. Children with a history of wheeze or asthma had a much higher prevalence of respiratory symptoms (Dockery et al 1989). However, no association was found between pollutant concentrations and measures of pulmonary airflow. At least during the preadolescent years, there would appear to be no *evidence for permanent damage.*

Particulate matter and sulfur dioxide are related more strongly to cough, whilst nitrogen oxide and ozone are related to a worsening of asthma. Although evidence for long-term irreversible changes from chronic, low level exposure is not available, what is known justifies measures to control air pollution.

Pollution does not appear to cause asthma. Exacerbations are related to the atmospheric concentrations of ozone and nitrous oxide (Burr 1995). Respiratory symptoms in general and both asthma and rhinitis seem to be worse in city dwellers and in children living near high traffic flows (Weilland et al 1994). Interestingly a study of reported asthma in Skye, during a time when there was very low pollution of any kind, showed a high prevalence of symptoms and exercise-induced asthma, suggesting that pollution with chemical agents is not the whole story (Austin et al 1994).

SMOKING

Parental cigarette smoking has adverse effects particularly on the fetus and young infant (Couriel 1994). Airway growth is adversely affected, sudden infant death is increased by an odds ratio of at least 2 and wheezing illnesses are more prevalent in households where adults smoke. Salivary cotinine levels, which are a reasonable marker for passive smoking, correlate inversely with small airway function. Allergens and smoke appear to be synergistic in causing wheezing in asthmatics and although smoking is associated with more wheezing in preschool children, it is not related to atopic disease in 7-year-olds (Burr 1995).

The pediatrician's role in combating cigarette smoking is primarily advisory and should start at the first contact with parents or prospective parents. Ideally this should be undertaken at school (Polney 1995).

Eighty percent of adolescents who start smoking early will continue as regular smokers. If a young person has not smoked by the age of 20 years it is most unlikely to be taken up. The prevalence of smoking amongst adolescent girls has not changed in recent years and remains at 25–30%. Health professionals in all countries must take a lead to stop the promotion of the sale of cigarettes. This is a complex issue because several countries depend on growing tobacco for much of their economic survival.

ETHNIC DIFFERENCES AND RESPIRATORY ILLNESS

Confounding factors make it difficult to determine whether belonging to a particular ethnic group affects respiratory health. Several studies have reported differences in the prevalence of respiratory symptoms between ethnic groups in British cities. None has suggested that any differences are due to an inherent genetic factor in the groups studied. Apparent differences in the prevalence of respiratory symptoms and asthma are almost all explained by environmental factors. The interesting example of the very high prevalence of asthma in the Tristan da Cunha islanders illustrates this very well (Martinez 1994). Atopy is definitely inherited and it would be easy to believe that this accounted for the observation. However, asthma is much less frequent in those who have moved away from the islands. This can be explained by the effect of increased respiratory infections in childhood 'protecting' against the expression of atopy, a very good example of the effect of environment on genetics. Much remains to be learnt about genetic influence on lung growth in different ethnic groups.

RESPIRATORY DISEASE IN DEVELOPING COUNTRIES

Data from the Pan American Health Organization study of infant and child mortality in Latin America and the Caribbean (Puffer & Serrano 1973) indicated that two-thirds of postneonatal mortality occurs between 1 and 6 months, about half these deaths being due to diarrheal disease. A similar pattern has been found in other developing countries. Only in the last decade has serious attention been paid to respiratory infections as a major cause of the other early postneonatal deaths.

In 1984, a memorandum from the World Health Organization outlined the problem of acute respiratory disease and deaths and described a program for controlling acute respiratory infections in children. Registered death rates in children from influenza and pneumonia are often 20–50 times greater in developing countries than in the West. Malnutrition increases the incidence of pneumonia by a factor of 10–20 and bacterial infection plays a far greater role than in developed countries. The cornerstone of the WHO program is to develop a system of case management that can be used by semiliterate parents and primary health care workers: to facilitate the diagnosis of respiratory infection, to decide when to prescribe antibiotics, to know when to refer to higher levels of care and to know how to provide supportive treatment. Integral to all these measures is health education to promote timely immunization against measles, pertussis, diphtheria and tuberculosis, to promote breast-feeding and proper nutrition and to reduce parental smoking and other domestic air pollution. In many developing countries, in addition to increasing tobacco smoking, many homes contain high levels of smoke from biofuels such as wood, crop residues and animal dung used for cooking or heating. In about half the world's households such fuels are used daily, usually without a flue or chimney (Smith 1987). Exposures to indoor particulate levels in developing countries may be 20 times higher than in developed countries (Pandey et al 1989). The WHO Interim Program Report (1992) outlines progress and goals in all these areas.

ALLERGENS

There is close association between airborne allergens and asthma (p. 541). Sensitization to allergens in early infancy undoubtedly contributes to the development of atopic asthma (Peat et al 1990) but this is certainly not the whole story.

The house dust mite, so common in Europe, is rare in the New Guinea Highlands but in areas where there has been Westernization sensitization has increased (Dowse et al 1985). Variations in aerial mold spores due to damp housing already mentioned may explain differences in chest symptoms. Ownership of house pets seems to be a risk factor for children with troublesome asthma (Strachan & Carey 1995). The contribution of food allergens is very small and certainly does not warrant the introduction of expensive and tedious diets unless there is clear evidence that such a diet would make a considerable difference to symptoms. The number of patients likely to benefit from diet manipulation is tiny.

PSYCHOLOGICAL FACTORS

The role of psychotherapeutic intervention to help children and their families to come to terms with chronic respiratory complaints can be invaluable and an understanding of the fears and fantasies about such complaints can often aid management, for example by improving drug compliance. Unwarranted anxieties about side-effects from drugs, on behavior as well as growth, often need to be addressed (Bender & Milgrom 1995). Psychological issues are basically similar to those in other families where a child has a chronic or potentially life-threatening disorder (Chs 15 and 16). Anxiety can certainly precipitate a wheezing attack in an asthmatic child and doubtless there are physiological reasons for this. Psychological factors, however, do not cause asthma.

ALTERNATIVE THERAPIES

Hypnotherapy, acupuncture, homeopathy and even osteopathy have been considered for the treatment of respiratory illness, asthma in particular. There is no evidence that any of these are of value in the management of respiratory complaints. Occasionally, parents will want to try alternative treatments, often because they are unable to accept that their child has a disorder such as asthma which is incurable. Hostile reactions by medical practitioners are not likely to dissuade such families and more constructive measures such as facilitating the expression of anxiety about the complaint, the possible side-effects of drugs, the fear of stigma about a disorder and so on are far more likely to allow therapy of proven use to continue.

DEVELOPMENT OF THE RESPIRATORY SYSTEM

The links between development and disease are well illustrated in the respiratory system. The continuum of fetal and postnatal development will be considered in relation to anatomical changes, functional (physiological) adaptation and where information

exists, biochemical maturation. Although anatomically there is no sudden change at the time of birth, enormous alterations in function occur.

FETAL AND PERINATAL DEVELOPMENT

STRUCTURE (Jeffrey & Hislop 1995)

The endodermal foregut bud with its surrounding mesoderm arises at the fourth week of gestation. By 5 weeks the segmental bronchi are formed, 11 for each lung (Fig. 12.1), and by about 16 weeks the full complement of airways down to the terminal bronchi (generation 20) is complete. Each terminal bronchiole will eventually supply one acinus: a cluster of respiratory bronchioles, alveolar ducts and alveoli along which gas exchange can take place. Blood vessels form in parallel. All of the epithelial structures, including mucosal and submucosal glands, ciliated epithelium and ultimately alveolar lining cells, are derived from the endodermal epithelium. Their differentiation begins at about 16 weeks, as airway multiplication finishes. By 24 weeks the full complement of submucosal glands is present. Airway epithelium is sparsely ciliated; ultimately ciliated epithelium is found down to the respiratory bronchioles. Several major congenital anomalies have their origins before 17 weeks' gestation (Table 12.4). Experimental evidence suggests that amniocentesis may briefly disturb development. If this occurs at a critical time for airway growth, catch-up may not be possible.

Acinar development begins in the second trimester, at a time of

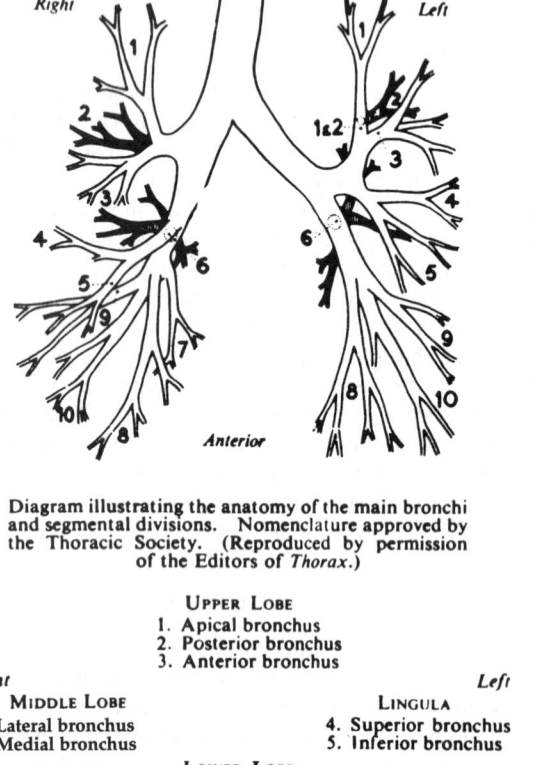

Diagram illustrating the anatomy of the main bronchi and segmental divisions. Nomenclature approved by the Thoracic Society. (Reproduced by permission of the Editors of *Thorax*.)

UPPER LOBE
1. Apical bronchus
2. Posterior bronchus
3. Anterior bronchus

Right / Left
MIDDLE LOBE / **LINGULA**
4. Lateral bronchus / 4. Superior bronchus
5. Medial bronchus / 5. Inferior bronchus

LOWER LOBE
6. Apical bronchus
7. Medial basal (cardiac) / 6. Apical bronchus
8. Anterior basal bronchus / 8. Anterior basal bronchus
9. Lateral basal bronchus / 9. Lateral basal bronchus
10. Posterior basal bronchus / 10. Posterior basal bronchus

Fig. 12.1 The segments of the lungs (from Sutton 1969).

Table 12.4 Anatomical development

Stage of gestation (weeks)	Embryonic (< 6)	Pseudoglandular (7–17)	Canalicular (13–25)	Saccular (24–40)	Alveolar (30 weeks to 2 years postnatal)
Developmental features	Segmental bronchi complete	Preacinar airways complete; cartilage developed; airway smooth muscle developing	Reduction in wall thickness of airways; submucosal glands complete	Double capillary bed; thinning of interstitium and blood–gas barrier; alveolar epithelium remains cuboidal; surfactant production	True alveoli (elastic fish net) with single capillary bed and thin membrane, and type I and II cells; intraepithelial lymphocytes appear; ciliated epithelium; diaphragm fiber types become more fatigue resistant
Disorders associated with abnormal or immature development	Agenesis/ aplasia Tracheal stenosis. 'Sequestration' complex. Congenital cysts	Possible hypoplasia from amniocentesis. Congenital diaphragmatic hernia: reduced acinar numbers. Abdominal wall defects	Hypoplasia, Potter's syndrome and prolonged membrane rupture	Hypoplasia due to reduced fetal breathing. Hyaline membrane disease. Pulmonary insufficiency of prematurity	Scoliosis: reduced alveolar numbers. Viral infection: Macleod's syndrome. Underdevelopment of alveoli in chronic bronchopulmonary dysplasia. Syndrome of ciliary dyskinesia. Respiratory failure of prematurity due to diaphragmatic weakness

great change in airway structure. By 24 weeks saccules have formed, shallow structures with a thinning, cuboidal, epithelial lining, capable of gas exchange. A number of disorders at this period may lead to pulmonary hypoplasia. Those which are associated with oligohydramnios cause anatomical, histological and biochemical immaturity. The DNA content (i.e. cellular complement) of the lungs of newborns who die with pulmonary hypoplasia due to renal agenesis is compatible with an onset before 16–20 weeks.

Alveolization begins at around 30 weeks. Arguments concerning the duration of alveolar development have depended on the distinction of saccules and alveoli and on techniques for counting alveolar number in post-mortem lungs. Current opinion suggests that about 50% of the final complement of alveoli is present at term, with 85% completion by around 2 years. The process of alveolization is accompanied by a reduction in interstitial tissue, remodeling of the pulmonary capillaries with a single network and enormous thinning of the blood–gas barrier. A network of elastin strands forms the 'skeleton' (likened to a fishnet) between which the new alveoli are formed. Normal breathing movements are important in promoting growth. The metabolic rate is a determining factor for lung size. Mild hypoxia (at altitude) enhances growth, whereas severe hypoxia may cause inhibition. Prematurity is associated with a reduced alveolar complement. Other factors known to affect lung growth in humans or animal models are maternal smoking, nutritional deficiency and infection. Postnatally, experimental hyperoxia inhibits alveolization.

The structure of airways deserves some comment. Cartilaginous structures appear in segmental bronchi at 10–12 weeks, but continue to develop in smaller bronchi until after birth. Generalized bronchomalacia or local disorders affecting trachea and bronchi are associated with several important disorders including tracheomalacia, stove pipe trachea and lobar emphysema. Airway smooth muscle, contrary to popular belief, is found at term down to the smallest terminal and respiratory bronchioles; failure of wheezy infants to respond to bronchodilators cannot therefore be ascribed to its absence.

At around term, the bronchus-associated lymphoid tissue becomes apparent, located at bronchial junctions, with intraepithelial lymphocytes. Whether the sparsity of this tissue in

preterm infants renders them more susceptible to inhaled substances is unknown. Ciliary dyskinesia presents in the newborn period, possibly as a result of failure to clear fetal lung fluid and bronchial mucus.

Vascular remodeling after birth may be disturbed as a result of widespread perinatal lung damage, such as chronic lung disease of prematurity, or in association with congenital heart disease (Ch. 13), leading to persistence of pulmonary hypertension. The double capillary alveolar network of fetal life often persists in Down syndrome.

The diaphragm becomes a complete membrane by 8 weeks of gestation and the abdominal wall is complete at 9 weeks, allowing the establishment of effective fetal breathing. At birth, however, the proportion of fatigue-resistant (type 1) striated muscle fibers in the diaphragm is 10%, much less than the 50% in adults. The proportion is even less in preterm infants and may explain the tendency of preterm infants to respiratory failure and apnea due partly to diaphragmatic fatigue.

A number of major developmental defects in the nasopharynx may lead to respiratory obstruction, infection or recurrent aspiration. These include choanal atresia or stenosis, palatal anomalies and, on a cellular level, ciliary dyskinesia. These, as well as mid-facial syndromes, Down syndrome and neuromuscular disorders, can lead to obstructive apnea or sleep-disordered breathing problems.

FUNCTIONAL DEVELOPMENT

Fetal breathing is essential to programmed lung development, as clinical and experimental evidence has shown. Neuromuscular disorders which affect fetal movements, such as severe myotonic dystrophy, lead to neonatal lung hypoplasia. Cigarette smoke is known to inhibit fetal breathing and experimentally causes alveolar hypoplasia. It is not known whether this is the mechanism by which smoking in pregnancy leads to childhood respiratory illness. In the presence of premature rupture of the amniotic membranes, reduced fetal breathing detected by ultrasound scanning is a poor predictor of severe lung hypoplasia and consequent respiratory failure.

Innervation of the airways is extensive by term. Details of the development of the vagal motor supply to glands and smooth muscle and of the sensory nerve plexus in larynx, trachea and bronchi are incomplete. Vagal myelination is incomplete in the preterm infant. Evidence of functional immaturity of vagally mediated, sensory, protective mechanisms has been obtained by observing changes in breathing pattern induced by tactile stimulation of the carina with a catheter in intubated babies. At less than 35 weeks apnea occurred, while more mature infants responded with increased respiratory effort or cough-like movements. Apnea of prematurity may in part be the result of immature tactile or chemoreceptor laryngeal reflex protective mechanisms.

Respiratory reflexes are important in the initiation and maintenance of breathing at birth (see Ch. 5). Vagal stretch receptors in the lungs and airways are responsible for Head's reflex, an inspiratory reflex which is normally confined to infancy, and for the Hering Breuer reflexes, which are maximal in infants and wane with age. Important changes in the rate and stability of breathing over the first 3 months of life could be important in relation to sudden, unexpected infant death (see Ch. 29 and p. 530).

Air breathing is a complex process. Fetal lung fluid secretion stops and is reabsorbed, surfactant is released and there is a great reduction in the pulmonary vascular resistance in order to match capillary perfusion with alveolar ventilation. Each of these processes can be defective, leading respectively to transient tachypnea of the newborn, hyaline membrane disease and persistent pulmonary hypertension. Surfactant composition alters during late fetal life and continues to do so thereafter. By 3 months of age the composition of surfactant phospholipids and the total quantity of surfactant present in the lungs reach adult proportions.

POSTNATAL DEVELOPMENT

ANATOMICAL GROWTH

After alveolar multiplication ceases at about age 3, the lungs grow simply as a result of increase in alveolar dimensions. The relative increase in size is great in relation to airway dimensions; this form of nonisotropic growth has been termed 'dysanaptic'. Central airways are relatively large in infancy and central airway conductance is relatively high. Peripheral conductance is low, providing one possible explanation for the severe nature of viral bronchiolitis in young infants. Following preterm birth and especially artificial ventilation, the structure of airways is affected, with increased smooth muscle and submucosal gland hypertrophy. The increase in peripheral conductance at about 5 years of age must be due to commensurate enlargement of peripheral airways along with the air spaces (isotropic growth). The sizes of the airways in children and adults are given in Table 12.5. There are sex differences in airway size relative to airspace size, girls having relatively wider airways in early childhood; the situation reverses during puberty.

The cartilaginous airways become stiffer with age (Penn et al 1989). For instance, the upper trachea deforms at low pressures in young infants, even during crying or mild struggling. Certainly some babies produce an inspiratory 'crow' when excited and breathing deeply.

Lung growth continues until the completion of skeletal growth in girls and for 2–3 years beyond in young men, probably because their greater muscularity and possibly their generally greater exercise performance provides the continued stimulus for lung expansion.

Table 12.5 Diameter of airways in various regions of the respiratory tract at different ages

Region of respiratory tract	Diameter of the airways (mm)		
	Infant	Child (6–8 years)	Adult
Trachea	5	10	16
Bronchioles	0.4	0.5	0.7
Terminal bronchioles	0.12	0.15	0.2
Alveoli	0.07	0.15	0.3

Growth can be affected by a number of childhood disorders. Infantile adenovirus pneumonia can cause severe peripheral lung damage with subsequent failure of alveolization. Radiation lung damage similarly disrupts growth. It is not known whether and up to what age true catch-up lung growth, rather than compensatory hypertrophy, can follow resection of the lungs.

The anatomy of the upper airway has received relatively little attention. The nasal sinuses pneumatize at a variable rate: the maxillary sinuses by about 2 years, frontal sinuses by 6 years and the ethmoid and sphenoid sinuses later. The nasal epithelium extends via the Eustachian tube to the middle ear. Nasal resistance accounts for 25–50% of the total airway resistance in infants; the nose acts as a filter and an air conditioner. Ciliary epithelium, a rich and dynamic submucosal vascular plexus and mucus-secreting glands probably subserve the same function in the nose and lower respiratory tract.

At a cellular level, there is experimental evidence for changes in the control of airway smooth muscle with age. At puberty in humans and some animals, airway responsiveness seems to decline. There is no explanation for this effect. There is no evidence for any alteration in the pattern of innervation of the airways with growth.

FUNCTIONAL DEVELOPMENT (Sly & Willett 1995)

Mechanical function

There is a wealth of information on lung mechanics in sedated infants and schoolchildren, but between ages 1 and 5 years it is difficult to make reliable measurements.

The pressure–volume characteristics (compliance) of the respiratory system change with age. The absolute elastic recoil pressure of the lungs increases with age, although there is probably very little change in recoil pressure when related to the growth in lung volume. More startling is the extremely compliant (floppy) chest wall of newborns compared with adults. Together these observations explain the low value for the relaxed lung volume (functional residual capacity, FRC) in the newborn, the small resting negative pleural pressure and the facility with which rib recession occurs with increased respiratory effort in infants.

The FRC adopted by newborns is greater than the truly relaxed value. This is because, at their normal breathing frequency, the expiratory time constant of the lungs (about 0.3 s) may be too long to permit full expiration. In both airway and alveolar disease, laryngeal braking (grunting) or pursed-lip breathing (in the elderly) are used to prolong the expiratory time constant and provide an energy-saving means of boosting FRC.

Although overall changes in airway resistance (R_{aw}) occur with growth, when normalized for lung volume specific resistance and conductance are remarkably constant with age. There are, however, relative changes in peripheral and central resistance (see above). During forced expiratory flow, young children and adults show flow limitation, frictional resistance in the airways being the limiting factor. In teenagers, flow is determined by chest wall compliance. Thus the forced expiratory flow volume technique in healthy children of that age is not a sensitive tool for detecting the early signs of airway disease.

Gas exchange

Remarkably, adequate gas exchange regularly occurs in the human infant after only 0.7 of gestation (28 weeks) has elapsed. The immediate process of adaptation takes about 5 h. Thereafter a large (A–a) DO_2 (see p. 504) persists for an indefinite period. This is mostly due to intrapulmonary anatomical shunt through nonalveolized vessels; about 25% is due to ventilation/perfusion imbalance and a negligible amount to diffusion limitation. Even in preterm infants, diffusion is not a limiting factor. Thus the mean PaO_2 for a term infant for the first week of life is 10 kPa, giving an approximate (A–a) DO_2 of 4 kPa compared with 1 kPa for an adult. Oxygen consumption per kg and hence alveolar ventilation in the newborn is double the adult value.

Developmental disorders of gas exchange are not common. Severe lung hypoplasia may impose limits in the newborn period which diminish with growth. Incomplete collateral ventilation (the canals of Lambert are not apparent in lungs from preschool children) may lead to atelectasis and hence impaired gas exchange in disease.

Airway caliber

The ontogeny of control of airway smooth muscle has been little studied in man. The walls of the intrathoracic airways contain a spiral layer of smooth muscle which is functionally a syncytium. On contraction, this smooth muscle produces narrowing and shortening of the airway. Under normal circumstances, the tone of the smooth muscle is under the direct influence of vagal activity which is balanced by the effect of circulating catecholamines on β2-adrenergic receptors. In addition, there is a nonadrenergic, noncholinergic (NANC) inhibitory system which is neurologically mediated and whose transmitters include polypeptides such as bombesin and substance P. The function of the airway smooth muscle in normal individuals is not clearly understood, but may be to stabilize the airways when transmural forces are great (coughing and exercise) and to help to optimize resistance and dead space.

Mature functional β-adrenoceptors are found in neonatal animals and humans, mainly in the respiratory epithelium. Functional airway smooth muscle reaches respiratory bronchioles by term. Whether the observed decline in bronchial responsiveness with age represents a real change in airway function or merely, an artefact (due to differences in aerosol deposition, geometric factors in the airways or techniques of measurement of lung function) is not clear and may never be settled. If true, it could explain the high frequency of wheeze in preschool children compared with older subjects.

Protective mechanisms against inhaled particles in the airways depend on filtration, impaction and mucosal clearance. Nasal filtration is extremely effective in infants, as judged by the tiny amount of jet-nebulized drug (less than 1%) deposited in the lower respiratory tract when presented by loosely fitting face mask.

Ciliary clearance in the lower airway has not been studied in normal children. Several disorders can break the integrity of the mucociliary 'escalator': chronic inflammatory conditions, dysplasia associated with tracheoesophageal fistula and severe asthma. All may lead to mucus retention with adverse consequences.

The integrity of the enormous area of the alveolar and airway epithelium is vital. It measures about 100 m^2 in adults, about 60 times greater than the body surface area. Its functional development is unknown. Particles of less than 300 Da, especially if lipid soluble, are readily absorbed. Breaks in the intercellular junctions may enhance absorption. Cigarette smoke is a potent cause of such breaches; exposure to environmental smoke in early childhood may lead to increased respiratory disease by this mechanism.

RESPIRATORY PHYSIOLOGY, PATHOPHYSIOLOGY AND THE MEASUREMENT OF RESPIRATORY FUNCTION

The principal function of the respiratory system is gas exchange: oxygenation of the blood and the removal of carbon dioxide. A knowledge of the means whereby this is achieved forms the basis for understanding many of the clinical features of respiratory disease and of lung function tests. The principles of disturbed pathophysiology are of course no different in children and adults. However, growth and development add further dimensions both to the interpretation of data and to the challenge of making the measurements in the first place. There are several good texts on applied respiratory physiology (see especially West 1992) and laboratory manuals (Stocks et al 1996, Quanjer et al 1989).

RESPIRATORY FUNCTION TESTS

GENERAL ASPECTS

Respiratory function may be measured as an aid to diagnosis or in the assessment of the severity of disease or its progress. In addition, some techniques are employed in research. In choosing any test, three criteria apply:

1. *sensitivity* – the ability of a test to identify particular pathophysiological processes in those with a particular disease;
2. *specificity* – the ability to identify the absence of disease in those who are free from it;
3. *repeatability* – expressed by the confidence interval or coefficient of variation, which describes just how well a significant change in lung function can be recognized within an individual.

A decision to carry out respiratory function tests will generally have followed clinical assessment and radiological, biochemical and immunological tests. Lung function testing can often usefully be combined with other investigations. The tests should be performed by an operator experienced in dealing with children, who can allay their anxiety and turn natural inquisitiveness and playfulness to advantage. A positive approach, with lots of encouragement and the insight to abandon a session before failure to cooperate turns into panic, are essential virtues.

For most simple procedures the equipment found in any adult lung function laboratory will be adequate. In infancy most measurements can only be made in specialized laboratories and will not be dealt with in this chapter. Preschool children form another difficult group, where specially adapted equipment may be needed and where the repeatability of measurements is poor. Spirometric measurements, for example, are rarely reliable below age 6; peak flow can occasionally be measured in 3–4-year-olds.

INTERPRETATION

In general, lung function is closely related to body length. There are small additional effects of age and sex, particularly around puberty, and of ethnic group. In the presence of scoliosis, arm span can be substituted directly for length. Body weight is a poor reference standard, since its variation in disease can be extreme. The significance of individual measurements in relation to the population is found by reference to a graph or table of predicted values. For sequential measurements in an individual, the confidence limits or coefficient of variation for repeated measurements must be sought. In asthma it is only appropriate to use the 'optimum' or maximum value for an individual rather than the population reference value as the target for home monitoring of peak flow.

RESPIRATORY FUNCTION

AIRWAYS

Physiology

The conducting airways extend from the tip of the nose to the terminal bronchioles. Although generally envisaged simply as a set of branching tubes, they are physiologically very active, varying their caliber and the nature of their secretions, for instance, in clinically important ways.

The airways condition the inspired air, bringing it up to 37°C at 100% relative humidity by the level of the segmental bronchi during quiet breathing. The volume of the conducting airways

constitutes a dead space (i.e. the volume of the lungs which although ventilated does not contribute to alveolar gas exchange, sometimes called wasted ventilation), measuring about 2.2 ml/kg throughout life. Disorders of airway structure such as bronchiectasis lead to an increase in anatomical dead space. In addition, the ventilation of underperfused regions of the lung, such as the apices in the erect posture, leads to another form of wasted ventilation referred to as physiological dead space.

Airway resistance (R_{aw}) is a function of gas flow and pressure drop: airway resistance = pressure drop/flow. The reciprocal of R_{aw}, airway conductance (G_{aw}), is often used, since its relationship with lung volume is linear, rather than curvilinear as with R_{aw}. In central airways, where flow is high, there is turbulence and resistance increases steeply with flow. In peripheral airways, because the total cross-sectional area of the enormous number of airways is large, linear flow is low and is normally laminar; resistance is low and less dependent on gas velocity. In the most distal respiratory bronchioles, alveolar ducts and alveolar spaces, gas molecules move by diffusive processes. During nasal breathing in infancy, about 50% of the total resistance is nasal, 25% is in the glottis and large central airways and the remainder in the peripheral airways. Thus infants are particularly prone to respiratory difficulty with upper airway obstruction. The resistance of the smallest peripheral airways falls with age. This may be one explanation for the fact that infants are also prone to small airway diseases (e.g. bronchiolitis) whereas in older children and adults the small airways represent a clinically 'silent zone'. Other predisposing factors to bronchiolitis include the smaller absolute dimensions of the airways (Table 12.5) and the lower elastic recoil (and hence supporting function) of the lungs of young infants in the tidal breathing range. Most importantly, obstruction in peripheral airways can, by upsetting the distribution of resistance along the airways, induce secondary expiratory narrowing in larger (proximal) airways, *dynamic airway narrowing*, which imposes a fixed limit on the maximum expiratory flow rate (Fig. 12.2).

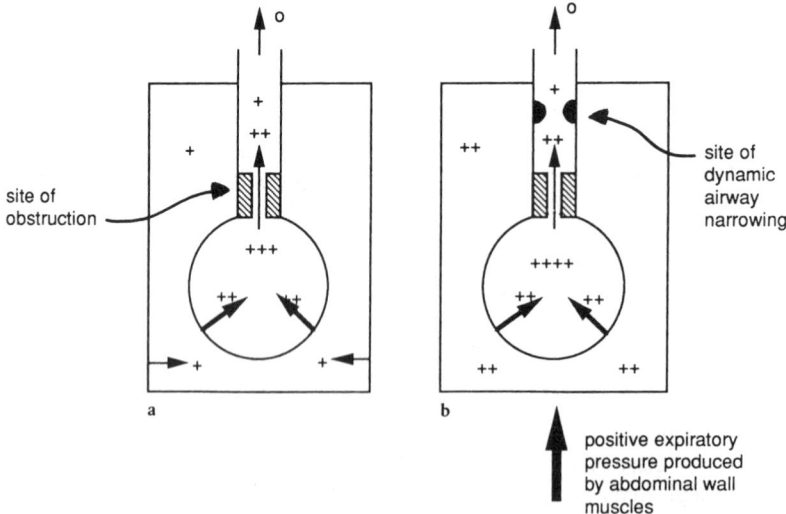

Fig. 12.2 Expiratory dynamic airways closure. (**a**) Passive expiration. Even in the presence of intrathoracic airway obstruction (the small hatched blocks) the elastic recoil of the lungs (++) and the chest wall (+) produces a positive alveolar pressure (+++) which drives air out of the airways. (**b**) Active expiration. During forced expiration, the pleural pressure may be raised to quite high values (++) and at increased flow rates the pressure gradient across the narrowed segment of the airways may be such that the pressure within the airways falls below the pressure within the surrounding pleural space. At or beyond this 'equal pressure point' the airways can deform (as shown by the indentation) producing a dynamic limitation to expiratory flow. Increased expiratory effort produces no increase in flow under these circumstances. This is referred to as 'flow limitation' or 'effort independence'.

Dynamic airway narrowing is important as a common cause of wheeze, as a cause of major airway obstruction in children with a wide variety of obstructive airway diseases and as the principle behind most of the tests of airway function which depend on maximal expiratory effort. Expiration is normally dependent on the elastic recoil of the lungs (Fig. 12.2a). In the presence of airway narrowing, expiration may be achieved by increasing lung volume ('hyperinflation') which has the double benefit of increasing the elastic recoil pressure and of distending the airways. Adults and older children can sometimes overcome quite severe obstruction (e.g. asthma, cystic fibrosis) this way. Infants, however, tend to respond to airway obstruction by exhaling actively, using abdominal muscles to raise the intrathoracic pressure. Under these circumstances, the pressure gradient across the obstructed segment of airway may be so steep that at some point downstream (i.e. towards the mouth), the pressure within the airway is less than the pleural pressure around it. Here, at the 'equal pressure point', depending on the floppiness of its wall, the airway may collapse causing flow limitation and an audible wheeze (Fig. 12.2b). This phenomenon can be seen through the bronchoscope!

Flow limitation implies that flow no longer increases with increased expiratory effort. This explains the fruitless effort expended by infants with acute airway obstruction, occasionally to the point of respiratory muscle fatigue and respiratory failure. Two other important factors apart from airway disease enhance flow limitation: reduced elastic recoil (e.g. early infancy, emphysema) and excessive floppiness of the large airways at the site of flow limitation (e.g. early infancy, bronchomalacia).

Inspiratory flow is normally limited only by effort. During inspiration, the intrathoracic airways are distended by tissue forces as the lungs expand and the intrathoracic airway resistance falls. Extrathoracic airway obstruction produces conditions of increased negative pressure in the upper airways, leading to indrawing and a pattern of flow limitation with inspiratory accentuation of stridor or snoring. Clinical patterns of inspiratory and expiratory flow limitation are shown in Figure 12.3.

Inflammation, excessive mucus secretion and active contraction of airway smooth muscle all lead to increased airflow obstruction. Although these processes may be part of normal defense mechanisms in the lungs, one of the characteristic features of asthma is an exaggerated airway responsiveness (i.e. reversible airway narrowing in response to either allergic or nonimmunological irritant factors). The degree of airway responsiveness can be measured by standardized challenge procedures based, for instance, on exercise or inhalation challenge with pharmacological agents such as histamine or methacholine (Fig. 12.4).

Measurement of airflow obstruction

Forced expiratory maneuvers, which require a maximum expiratory effort from total lung capacity, form the basis of the most useful tests of airways obstruction. The peak expiratory flow (PEF), the forced expiratory volume in the first second of expiration (FEV_1) and the indices derived from the maximum expiratory flow volume (MEFV) curve are the most commonly performed. In general, the best of three efforts (after two practice blows for novices) should be recorded, the single most important variable being the completeness of the maximum inspiratory effort at the start of each procedure. Most children from 5 years old can manage to perform a PEF maneuver, although the other

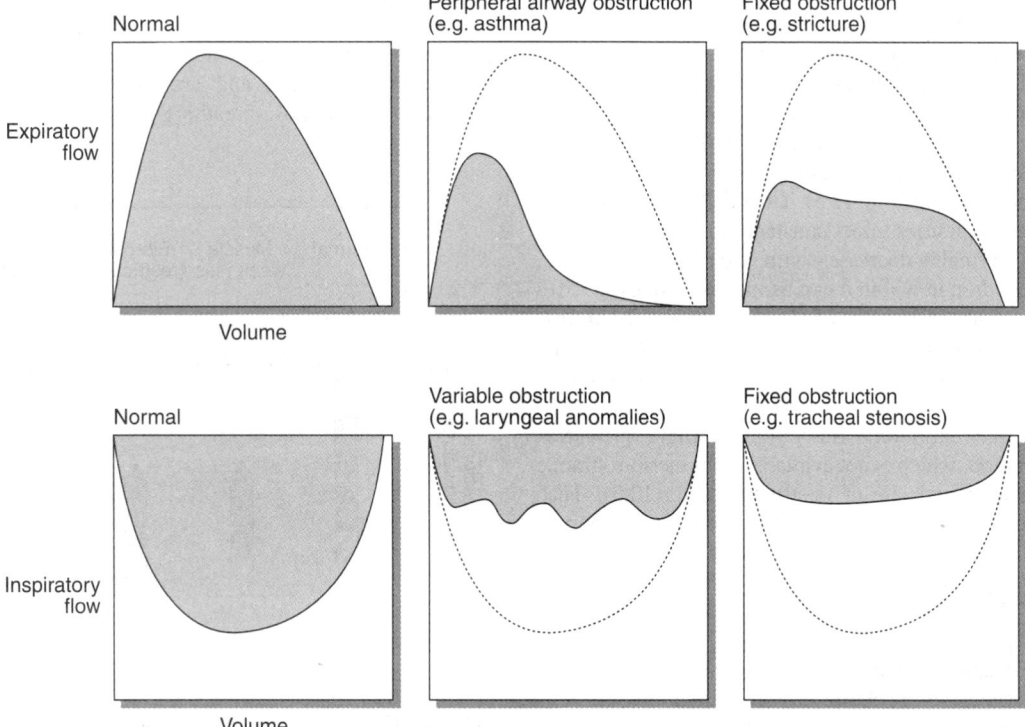

Fig. 12.3 Flow volume curves. Maximum forced expiratory and inspiratory flow volume curves, showing patterns characteristic of air flow obstruction at various sites.

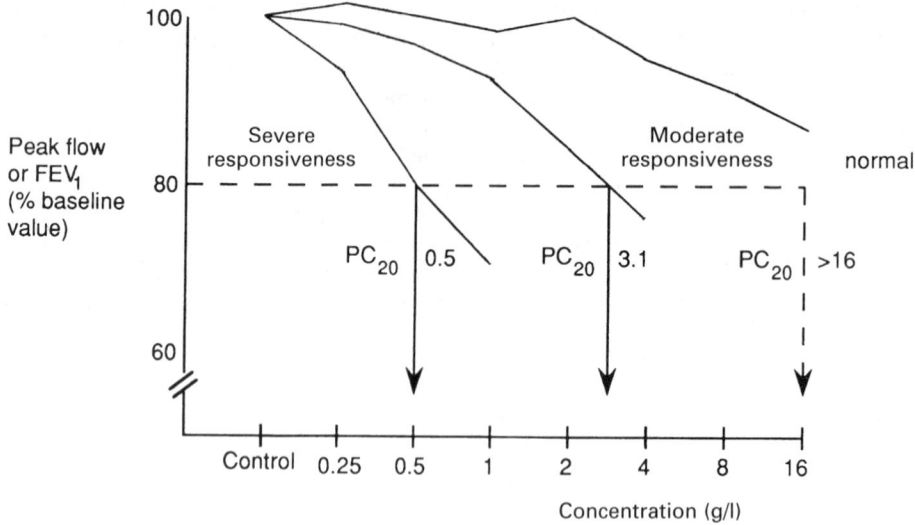

Fig. 12.4 Bronchial challenge test. Change in peak flow rate in response to increasing concentrations of histamine or methacholine administered by aerosol. Three subjects are shown. Their response is measured by the PC_{20} (g/l), the provoking concentration causing a 20% fall in peak flow rate (or FEV_1).

forced measurements (FEV_1, MEFV curve) cannot be relied upon in children under 7 or 8 years old. In children under 7, the whole vital capacity may be exhaled in under 1 s; in this group, the $FEV_{0.75}$ or $FEV_{0.5}$ are more sensitive indices of obstruction. Mini-peak flow meters are suitable for home monitoring, in spite of being a rather insensitive measure of airways obstruction. The PEF is rapid, repeatable, adaptable and portable and is the single most valuable measurement of lung function in childhood.

In pediatrics it is particularly important for quality control to be able to see the spirogram from which forced expiratory indices (the forced vital capacity, FVC and its derivatives) are derived. Its shape bears important information about both the technical quality of a test and the underlying pathophysiology. Airway obstruction is indicated by a reduction in the ratio FEV_1/FVC (or $FEV_{0.75}/FVC$) since airway obstruction will prolong the expiratory time constant of the lungs (see below) and therefore reduce that rate of emptying (Fig. 12.5). The FEV_1/FVC ratio is in effect the forced expiratory time constant of the lungs. The FEV_1/FVC ratio normally decreases with age, from over 90% in the youngest children in whom it can be measured to over 75% in young adults. The FEV_1 (or $FEV_{0.75}$), with contributions from the peak flow and the flow-limited sections of the expiratory maneuver, provides the best overall index of airway obstruction.

The shape of the expiratory flow volume curve provides additional information, which is not available from the spirogram, concerning the nature and site of obstruction (Fig. 12.3). The disadvantages of numerical analysis of the flow volume curve include very poor reproducibility, even in normal children. Compensatory changes in lung volume with airways disease or its treatment will minimize the apparent changes in forced flow rate. The maximal expiratory procedure itself may induce airway obstruction in asthmatics with very reactive airways. The effect is transient and is responsive to nebulized bronchodilators.

Flow volume curves have another important function, in the assessment of upper (extrathoracic) airflow obstruction. Use is made of the pattern of flow limitation produced on maximum inspiratory effort from residual volume as well as on the actual

maximal inspiratory flow rate at midvital capacity (MIF_{50}) in assessing extrathoracic airway obstruction (Fig. 12.3). Normally the ratio MIF_{50}/MEF_{50} is close to or greater than 1.

Methods for measuring airflow obstruction which do not depend on respiratory effort, and which have therefore been adapted for use in infants and young children, include the plethysmographic determination of airway resistance and the measurement of total respiratory system resistance (impedance) by a forced oscillation technique. Despite the many published reference values for normal children, these methods, requiring complex equipment and having poor repeatability, are of little proven clinical value. Like the PEF, they are influenced mainly by large airway function and are especially sensitive to glottic narrowing and (in nose-breathing infants) to nasal obstruction.

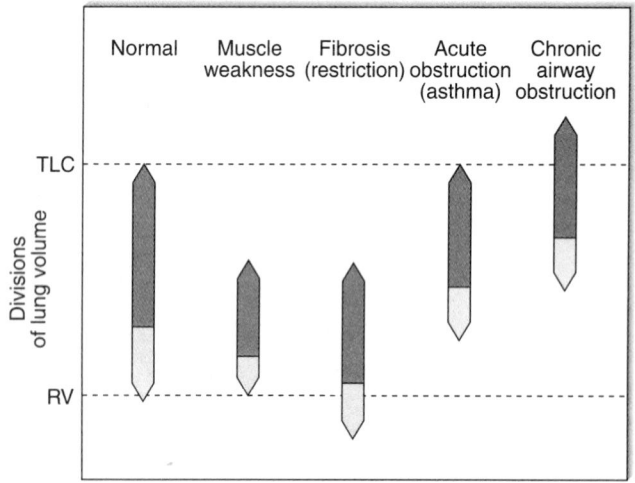

Fig. 12.5 Causes of reduced vital capacity. The length of the arrows indicates the vital capacity and the position indicates the changes in total lung capacity (TLC) and residual volume (RV) for each condition in relation to normal. The horizontal line across each arrow indicates the usual end-expiratory curve (functional residual capacity: FRC).

Measurement of bronchial responsiveness (bronchial provocation tests) (Wilson & Silverman 1995)

Bronchial provocation tests rarely help in the diagnosis of asthma because they are neither specific nor sensitive for asthma. They may be used in order to assess the importance of airway responsiveness in a patient with atypical symptoms (e.g. chronic cough) or in patients with other forms of airway obstruction (e.g. cystic fibrosis, bronchiectasis), although they are of extremely limited clinical value. Their main use is as a research tool for group population studies. Occasionally, the response to anti-asthma therapy may be measured using bronchial provocation tests. Children under the age of 6 can be tested only under the conditions of a research laboratory. Simple, repeatable measurement techniques (FEV_1, PEF) are normally used in bronchial provocation tests.

There are three broad categories of challenge test: pharmacological challenge by aerosol, bronchial provocation with aerosolized antigen and exercise (or isocapnic hyperventilation) challenge. In order to determine the degree of responsiveness, pharmacological or exercise challenge are usually used. Exercise is said to be specific for asthma, whereas a response to pharmacological challenge occurs in other lung disorders too. Antigen provocation is a risky procedure confined to research laboratories.

Pharmacological challenge with solutions of histamine and acid phosphate or methacholine is performed by administering increasing concentrations of aerosol by jet nebulizer at regular intervals, until at least a 20% fall in PEF or FEV_1 has been produced (or the maximum concentration has been reached). By interpolation on a graph the concentration which provokes a 20% fall in PEF or FEV_1 (PC_{20}) can be calculated (Fig. 12.4). The PC_{20} is an index of bronchial responsiveness. There is a continuum of values of PC_{20} from the lowest in severe, labile asthma to the highest in normal individuals. There is no clear separation. Many factors influence asthmatics, such as environmental antigen exposure (pollen, dust mite), time of day and recent medication. In children with other forms of chronic bronchial obstruction (e.g. cystic fibrosis), bronchial responsiveness appears to become greater as their airway obstruction worsens.

Exercise-induced asthma (EIA) can be reproducibly induced by having a child run for 5–6 min at a rate sufficient to produce a heart rate of >170 beats/min, ideally on a treadmill in an air-conditioned laboratory. The fall in PEF or FEV_1 can be expressed as a percentage of the baseline value, to provide an index of EIA (upper limit of normal about 15%). Again, a number of clinical variables (a recent cold) and laboratory conditions (air temperature and humidity) may affect the result; outdoor tests of a similar type are very poorly repeatable. Used as a diagnostic aid, EIA has poor sensitivity and specificity. Exercise tests can be used to study the protective effects of drugs given before challenge and to demonstrate their value to the child and family. They can also be used to show that some children get 'short of breath' when they exercise not because of EIA but simply because they are unfit!

THE AIRSPACES: LUNG VOLUME AND COMPLIANCE

Physiology

The elasticity of the lung and chest wall (i.e. compliance: change in volume for a given change in pressure) is such that at high volumes, the respiratory system tends to deflate and at low volumes to expand, reaching equilibrium at the functional residual capacity (FRC) when the forces balance. Alteration in the balance of forces between lungs and chest wall will alter the FRC. The outward recoil pressure of the chest wall is low in infancy so that FRC may be at a relatively lower level than in older age groups. Since airway dimensions are partly dependent on traction from tissues, this implies narrower airways; it is believed that some airways close completely toward the end of a normal expiration in infants. Perhaps this is another reason for the vulnerability of this group to acute airway obstruction and to segmental collapse during airway disease.

In pulmonary fibrosis where the lungs are less compliant (stiffer), the inward recoil forces of the lungs are greater and FRC is low. Conversely in emphysema and chronic asthma (where the lungs are 'stretched') the inward recoil forces are lower and hence FRC is increased. Removing the effect of the chest wall completely, as in pneumothorax, causes the lung to collapse.

Airway closure is a clinically important factor causing an increase in FRC. Airways tend to close during expiration, even at high lung volumes, leading to true 'gas trapping'.

The other 'static lung volumes', total lung capacity (TLC) and residual volume (RV), depend on several factors: lung compliance, chest wall compliance and the force of the respiratory muscles. These may all be important in relation to changes in the vital capacity (VC) in disease.

Measurement of lung volume and compliance

Lung volume is most commonly estimated by clinical examination aided by chest radiography. On formal laboratory testing, the distinction is often made between dynamic lung volumes produced by respiratory effort (e.g. vital capacity) and static lung volumes measuring absolute volume (e.g. FRC, RV and TLC). Static lung volumes and lung compliance are rarely measured and require a specialized lung function laboratory (Quanjer et al 1989).

The vital capacity is a most useful, repeatable measurement, although almost any disturbance of lung function will lead to a reduction in vital capacity (Fig. 12.5). Measured on an electronic spirometer (or as part of a flow volume maneuver), it is a simple means of monitoring progress in a number of rare or chronic disorders, especially neuromuscular disorders, interstitial lung disease and chest wall disorders such as scoliosis.

Lung volume may also be valuable in following the course of patients with these disorders. There are two methods: by the plethysmographic technique and by dilution of an inert nonabsorbable gas such as helium. The former technique measures all the gas in the thoracic cage, whether or not it is in communication with airways, using simple physical principles (Boyle's law) and extremely complex equipment. The latter technique, relying on equilibration between the gas in the lungs and in a bag containing a mixture of air and helium, tends to underestimate the volume of those parts of the lung which are very poorly ventilated (i.e. in the presence of obstructed airways). Both techniques require very cooperative subjects and are unreliable under the age of 8.

VENTILATION AND PERFUSION

Physiology

During tidal breathing, air is distributed within the lungs according to local variations in airway resistance and lung compliance. In the upright subject, because of the weight of the lungs (density about 0.2 g/ml), the pleural pressure is more negative near the apex so that the airspaces are relatively overdistended compared with those near the base. The ventilatory turnover is greater near the base, although because of the lower volume of the basal airspaces, the local airways are narrower and more readily close completely in disease. Disease may affect the regional distribution of ventilation by affecting the chest wall (e.g. spinal muscular atrophy, severe rickets in infancy), the diaphragm (e.g. congenital diaphragmatic hernia, eventration or paralysis), the airways (e.g. bronchiectasis, asthma) or the airspaces (e.g. lobar pneumonia, pulmonary edema).

The rate of filling or emptying of any part of the lungs (or the whole respiratory system) can be described by its time constant (time constant = compliance × resistance) and represents the time taken to achieve 63% of the steady state volume (which would be achieved given sufficient time) in a system which empties and fills exponentially. The respiratory time constant in a normal infant is about 0.3 s and in an adult about 0.5 s. The concept of the time constant is particularly important in relation to mechanical ventilation of the lungs.

The distribution of pulmonary blood flow is partly gravity dependent, tending to match the distribution of ventilation. During exercise and other states of high cardiac output, pulmonary perfusion becomes even. At a local level, pulmonary perfusion is actively controlled, so that a balance is maintained in the lungs between ventilation and perfusion, avoiding hypoxemia due to intrapulmonary shunting. An extreme example of this is illustrated by the almost total diversion of blood flow to the unaffected lobes of a child who has inhaled a foreign body, so that only mild hypoxemia ensues.

The matching of alveolar ventilation to pulmonary perfusion takes place at alveolar level. The airways also play a small part in this homeostatic mechanism. Alveolar hypoxia induces local pulmonary arteriolar constriction by a nitric oxide-dependent mechanism, cutting down the local blood supply. The effect is amplified by acidosis. The particular problems of the perinatal period are described in Chapter 5.

In older children, a sustained increase in pulmonary resistance, usually associated with severe chronic and generalized disease (e.g. chronic lung disease of prematurity, terminal cystic fibrosis), may lead to cor pulmonale.

Mismatching of ventilation (V) and perfusion (Q) occurs in acute lung disease before adaptation has occurred and in severe chronic disease, beyond the limits of adaptation. Its effects are wasted ventilation (excessive dead-space ventilation) on the one hand, and hypoxemia (due to right-to-left intrapulmonary shunting) on the other. Hypoxemia due to mild V/Q imbalance, as well as that due to alveolar hypoventilation, is largely corrected by increased inspired oxygen concentrations. Postural effects on the efficiency of regional ventilation may be important in babies. Unlike adults, where the chest wall is fairly rigid, in infancy chest distortion in the lateral posture reduces the ventilation of the dependent lung. In unilateral disease, it is important therefore to keep the good lung uppermost.

Tests of the distribution of ventilation and perfusion

Regional distribution of ventilation and perfusion can fairly simply be studied in standard nuclear medicine facilities, using X-ray emitting radionuclides and a gamma camera (see Ch. 36). Other tests remain research procedures.

GAS TRANSFER AND GAS TRANSPORT

Physiology

Within the alveoli, gas movement takes place by diffusion. Transfer of oxygen from alveolus (PaO_2 14 kPa) into the pulmonary capillary and of carbon dioxide in the reverse direction ($PaCO_2$ 5 kPa) take place by passive diffusion down concentration gradients.

The gradient of PO_2 can be thought of as running from alveolus to mitochondrion. Oxygen is transported as oxyhemoglobin. The quantity of oxygen carried depends on the PaO_2 (and its characteristic sigmoid relationship with oxygen saturation), the hemoglobin concentration and the cardiac output: oxygen delivered = oxygen content of blood × cardiac output. Thus oxygen delivery will be reduced by anemia, hypoxemia or diminished cardiac output. Metabolic acidosis (anaerobic metabolism leading to lactic acid production) is one consequence of impaired oxygen delivery.

The oxygen dissociation curve is also affected by a number of other factors: the dominant class of hemoglobin (e.g. HbF in the newborn), adaptive variations in intracellular 2.3 DPG concentration with chronic anemia and arterial pH and $PaCO_2$ (the Bohr effect).

The transport of CO_2 is much more robust, since the CO_2 content of blood is almost linearly related to PCO_2 over the clinical range. Respiratory acidosis results from hypercapnia.

Respiratory failure is a general term used to imply a breakdown of the supply of oxygen and removal of CO_2. A single definition which covers the whole pediatric range would be inappropriate, since for instance degrees of acute disturbance of blood gases which may have dire clinical consequences in a preterm neonate may have little effect on a chronically sick older child. In pediatrics, particularly in newborns when the labile fetal circulation shunts through fetal channels, a low PaO_2 may indicate a complex failure of ventilation and circulation which it would be inappropriate to label as 'respiratory'.

Terminology

Hypoxemia

Hypoxemia (PaO_2 at sea level in postneonates of less than 12 kPa) may have several causes (Fig. 12.6 and Table 12.6). At altitude the oxygen content of inspired air is reduced and the PaO_2 will fall. Acclimatization principally by hyperventilation and the development of polycythemia preserves the oxygen content of arterial blood at the expense of the reduction in PaO_2.

Alveolar hypoventilation may be due to mechanical factors (stiff or obstructed lungs), weakness of respiratory muscles or a defect of the control of breathing. Hypoxemia and hypercapnia result.

Shunt refers to systemic venous blood which effectively bypasses ventilated portions of lung. There are two main varieties of right-to-left shunt: intracardiac shunt and intrapulmonary shunt. In childhood, the main extrapulmonary cause of shunt is cyanotic congenital heart disease. Breathing 100% oxygen for at least 5 min (the nitrogen washout test) is useful for diagnosing this

Table 12.6 The oxygen waterfall in disease: hypoxia. Various causes of hypoxemia have their effect at different steps in the waterfall. Increase in inspired oxygen concentration (the hyperoxia test) will usually correct the first two causes of hypoxemia. The level of arterial PCO_2 depends on the degree of compensatory hyperventilation which is possible; in severe lung disease, hypercapnia may develop

Causes of hypoxia	Effect of increase in FiO_2	Value of $PaCO_2$
1. Decreased alveolar ventilation	Correction of hypoxemia	Increase
2. Impaired diffusion	Correction of hypoxemia	Decrease (unless severe imbalance)
3. Right–left shunt and ventilation/perfusion imbalance	No change if pure right–left shunt	Decrease (unless severe shunting)
4. Decreased oxygen delivery*	No change	Decrease (due to metabolic acidosis)
5. Demand for oxygen exceeding supply**	Depends on cause	Increased mixed venous PCO_2

FiO_2 = inspired oxygen concentration
$PaCO_2$ = arterial PCO_2
* PaO_2 may be normal under these circumstances; not true hypoxemia
** Refers to fall in mixed venous (pulmonary artery) PO_2; PaO_2 may be normal

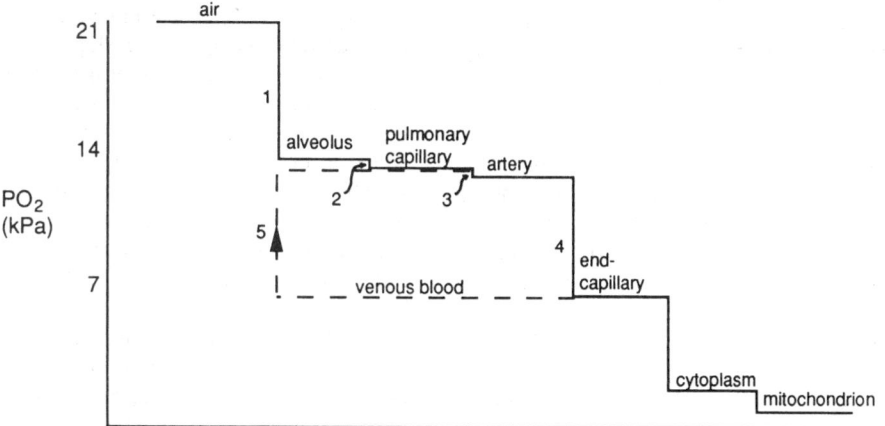

Fig. 12.6 The oxygen 'waterfall' in health and disease. Under normal circumstances oxygen is transported down a gradient between atmospheric air and the mitochondria where it is consumed.

'central' shunting. In order to understand this test, the shape of the hemoglobin–oxygen dissociation curve should be borne in mind. Even if the PO_2 of pulmonary venous blood is >400 mmHg the content of oxygen in that blood will be hardly greater than if the PO_2 is 100 mmHg. When mixed with shunted blood of low oxygen content the PaO_2 will fall dramatically. Even when the lungs are completely normal, the presence of a very small central shunt will prevent a significant rise in PaO_2 when breathing 100% oxygen. A rise in PaO_2 to 150 mmHg (20 kPa) makes cyanotic heart disease an unlikely cause of hypoxemia. On the other hand, if breathing 100% oxygen (for a minimum of 5 min) does successfully elevate the PaO_2 the hypoxemia in air is likely to have been due to intrapulmonary shunting (regions of low V/Q ratio) or hypoventilation. A specific exception to this rule is the situation of pulmonary hypertension in the newborn, when oxygen therapy, by reducing pulmonary vascular resistance, can abolish the extrapulmonary right-to-left shunt through fetal channels, causing the hypoxemia to resolve for 'vascular' rather than 'pulmonary' reasons.

Ventilation perfusion (V/Q) mismatching is by far the commonest cause of hypoxemia in pulmonary disease. Blood leaving alveolar units which are underventilated but well perfused will have a low O_2 content and a raised CO_2 content. For the reasons mentioned above the total PaO_2 will fall and hyperventilation results. CO_2 is washed out of the well-ventilated lung units. The CO_2 content of blood bears an almost linear relationship to $PaCO_2$. Thus the drop in CO_2 content of blood leaving well-ventilated units offsets the rise in that leaving poorly ventilated alveoli. However, no matter how good the ventilation of healthy alveolar units, the O_2 content of blood leaving them remains the same and does not offset the reduced content of those leaving poorly ventilated alveoli. Hypoxemia due to V/Q imbalance will therefore be unaltered by hyperventilation, an increased ventilatory drive will persist and the $PaCO_2$ may actually fall. (This is sometimes referred to as type I respiratory failure.)

This is the situation in the early stages of acute asthma and bronchiolitis. Increasing the inspired oxygen concentration will improve the oxygen content of poorly ventilated areas and the PaO_2 will rise as a result. Patients are able to compensate for the increase in dead space initially by increasing overall minute ventilation but eventually they may become exhausted or, because of worsening disease, the dead space may rise. In either case alveolar hypoventilation results and the $PaCO_2$ will eventually rise (type II respiratory failure).

Alveolar hypoventilation

Alveolar hypoventilation in the presence of normal lungs or severe ventilation perfusion mismatching, as described under hypoxemia, results in *hypercapnia*, a rise in $PaCO_2$. Hypercapnia should always be taken very seriously. In acute, respiratory disease the $PaCO_2$ may remain normal or low for some time but may eventually rise very quickly. Children in whom this happens are very often exhausted and may well require ventilatory support. With chronic hypercapnia, central insensitivity results as CSF pH is buffered by a rise in bicarbonate. Administration of an oxygen-enriched gas to a patient not receiving assisted ventilation may result in a further dangerous increase in $PaCO_2$ because of removal of hypoxia, the remaining drive to respiration. In practice this is extremely uncommon in children as chronic type II respiratory failure is rare. Oxygen should never be withheld from children with acute disease.

Alveolar–arterial PO_2 difference

(A–a) DO_2 is a measure of the degree of right-to-left shunt (of all types).

In respiratory failure of whatever cause the PaO_2 falls while the patient is breathing air. When accompanied by alveolar hypoventilation the $PaCO_2$ rises. An assessment of respiratory failure may be made by use of the alveolar air equation:

$$P_AO_2 = P_IO_2 - (P_ACO_2/R) + F$$

where P_AO_2 is the partial pressure of oxygen in the alveoli, P_IO_2 is the partial pressure of inspired oxygen (minus water vapor) (partial pressure: 6 kPa at body temperature), P_ACO_2 is the mean alveolar PCO_2, R is the respiratory quotient (approximately 0.8 in normal individuals) and F is a small correction factor which for clinical purposes can be omitted. P_ACO_2 in most clinical situations is equal to $PaCO_2$. Normally with a $PaCO_2$ of 5 kPa and a barometric pressure of 100 kPa breathing air (O_2 content = 0.21) and a water vapor pressure of 6 kPa, P_AO_2 = 0.21 (100 – 6) – (5/0.8) = 13.5 kPa.

In a normal child breathing air the difference between the P_AO_2 and the PaO_2 is 1–2 kPa. In pure alveolar hypoventilation this difference does not change or become smaller. In the presence of shunt or V/Q imbalance the difference rises. Hence the (A–a) DO_2 is an index of severity of mismatching of gas and blood.

Example 1. A baby with severe bronchiolitis may have a PaO_2 of 10 kPa in 70% oxygen. The $PaCO_2$ is, say, 8 kPa. The (A–a) DO_2 = 0.7 (100 – 6) – (8/0.8) – 10 = 46 kPa. He has both V/Q mismatching, resulting in a rise in (A–a) DO_2, and alveolar hypoventilation, resulting in a rise in $PaCO_2$.

Example 2. A child with infective polyneuritis breathing 30% oxygen has a $PaCO_2$ of 7 kPa and a PaO_2 of 18 kPa. The (A–a) DO_2 = 0.3 (100 – 6) – (7/0.8) – 18 = 1.5 kpa. This child has pure alveolar hypoventilation as the (A–a) DO_2 is normal and the $PaCO_2$ is raised.

In rare disorders which affect the alveolar membrane, where clinical disability is mainly reduced exercise tolerance and airway function is normal, oxygen transport across the membrane may be adequate at rest but not during exercise. The (A–a) DO_2 may become abnormally wide only during exercise.

Acid–base abnormalities

These relate to disturbed hydrogen ion homeostasis in body fluids. The maintenance of a normal blood pH is a function of lung and kidney which together control the buffering capacity of the blood. The most important physiological buffer is bicarbonate, because of its relationship with CO_2 which is excreted through the lungs. The Henderson–Hasselbalch equation describes the relationship:

$$H^+ + HCO_3^- \leftrightarrows H_2CO_3 \leftrightarrows CO_2 + H_2O$$

From this

$$H^+ \propto CO_2/HCO_3^-$$

and

$$pH = -\log H^+ \propto \log (HCO_3^-/CO_2)$$

Provided the ratio of HCO_3/CO_2 remains constant, the pH will remain constant.

When the acid–base balance is disturbed and the normal values of pH and PCO_2 are altered it is helpful to know something of the status of the buffering system in the blood in order to try to unravel the sequence of events. The *base excess* is a useful parameter which reflects the metabolic component of the abnormality under steady state conditions (*not* during rapid changes in acid–base status). When the blood gases are analyzed the pH of the sample is determined. The CO_2 electrode is calibrated with gases of high and low CO_2 concentrations and the $PaCO_2$ of the sample determined. Blood pH and log $PaCO_2$ have a linear relationship whose slope varies according to whether there is an excess or deficit of base. The line which describes the relationship when there is neither excess nor deficit is known as the 'normal buffer baseline'. The amount of base which has to be added to or removed from this 'ideal' sample to reach the line which describes the actual sample is referred to as the base excess or deficit (see also Ch. 10.).

In *respiratory acidosis* the $PaCO_2$ rises and the pH falls. In order to maintain the ratio HCO_3/CO_2 the kidney conserves bicarbonate.

Metabolic acidosis in pulmonary or cardiac disease reflects tissue hypoxia due to poor oxygen delivery, resulting in an increase in metabolic acid. There are, of course, several other important causes of metabolic acidosis (e.g. renal failure, severe infection, acute diabetic ketoacidosis). Bicarbonate falls as it buffers the rise in hydrogen ions. There is simultaneous increased drive to breathe, with increased CO_2 removal and a return towards normal HCO_3/CO_2 ratio.

Respiratory alkalosis occurs when the $PaCO_2$ falls due to voluntary or artifactual hyperventilation or hyperventilation due to CNS pathology (e.g. meningoencephalitis). The hydrogen ion concentration falls and to conserve the HCO_3/CO_2 ratio and hence the pH, the kidney sheds bicarbonate.

Metabolic alkalosis occurs in children when acid is lost through vomiting, as in pyloric stenosis. Hydrogen ions are lost and the bicarbonate rises. Hypoventilation produces a compensatory rise in CO_2.

Mixed respiratory and metabolic acidosis is a common situation in pediatric practice. Tissue hypoxia results in metabolic acidosis and inadequate ventilation results in respiratory acidosis. The $PaCO_2$ is elevated and the bicarbonate and pH are low. There will be a base deficit.

The administration of bicarbonate in this situation is tempting, particularly when the pH is below 7.2. In order for bicarbonate to correct the metabolic component, CO_2 must be formed and excreted from the lungs. In the presence of respiratory failure with an already elevated $PaCO_2$ this may not be possible. Administration of bicarbonate may elevate the $PaCO_2$ even further. The blood–brain barrier is much more permeable to CO_2 than it is to bicarbonate. Thus the effect on the CSF will be to paradoxically reduce pH and this can precipitate collapse in a child who is not receiving ventilatory support. Even in pure metabolic acidosis (e.g. diabetic ketoacidosis), rapid administration of bicarbonate can have this effect.

The treatment for mixed acidosis is the correction of the respiratory component first of all by increasing ventilation. The metabolic component may respond to better oxygenation, improved circulation or correction of anemia. When the $PaCO_2$ has returned to normal, bicarbonate may be given if the metabolic component persists.

Measurement of gas transfer

Gas transfer at alveolar level can be studied by measuring the diffusing capacity for carbon monoxide (D_{co}). By measuring the FRC by helium dilution simultaneously, the diffusing capacity can be normalized for variation in lung volume (K_{co}). The test has its main use in detecting the response to treatment of interstitial lung diseases (e.g. those associated with connective tissue disorders) in older children.

Measurement of arterial blood gases and acid–base balance

Oximetry has largely replaced arterial blood gas measurement for most children. Blood gas measurements are indicated for worsening acute lung disease where exhaustion (muscle fatigue) suggests the need for mechanical ventilation and in chronic lung disease as a guide to progress. Sampling of arterialized capillary blood (i.e. after warming or application of histamine cream) may be adequate for pH monitoring, but in general arterial sampling is preferable for postneonatal patients.

Blood should be collected from a radial artery cannula or, if impossible to site, by arterial puncture from the radial artery. This vessel is preferred for three reasons. First, the chance of sampling venous blood in error is small as no major veins lie nearby. Second, there is a good collateral circulation to the hand should circulation be compromised in any way as a result of the procedure. Third, the vessel is accessible. If pulsation is difficult to feel, as in shock, it may be approached blindly. The femoral artery, on the other hand, has a direct medial relation to the femoral vein. Infection may be introduced into the femoral sheath or into the hip joint from the groin. Collaterals will not compensate for femoral artery thrombosis, a particular hazard if the vessel is damaged in the presence of hypovolemia. It is also worth remembering that the femoral vessels may be used for cannulation at cardiac catheterization and it is particularly annoying for the cardiologist if the site has been traumatized.

As the walls of arteries are particularly sensitive and because more than one attempt may be necessary to obtain blood, local anesthetic cream should be applied to the site 30 min before starting and local anesthetic should be injected around the site. As well as being a kindness, this should allow the blood to be collected under conditions which are as stable as possible although admittedly anxiety is not always avoided. Hyperventilation will reduce the $PaCO_2$ and consequently the pH will rise; crying in a child who has a right-to-left intracardiac shunt may increase the shunt and reduce the PaO_2.

Noninvasive methods of measuring oxygenation include the transcutaneous PO_2 electrode, which is at best a trend indicator in postneonatal patients, and the pulse oximeter for monitoring oxygen saturation (e.g. in acute severe asthma and during sleep studies). For PCO_2, transcutaneous measurements again provide trends while end-tidal sampling using an infrared CO_2 meter gives a useful assessment of alveolar breath (and hence arterial) CO_2 only when lung disease is mild and during mechanical ventilation.

BREATHING

Physiology

The principal muscle of inspiration is the diaphragm, innervated by the phrenic nerve (C2–5). As with other skeletal muscles in general, within its usual working range the tension it can generate is proportional to its length. Because the diaphragm adopts a curved shape, when it contracts the pressure difference across it is proportional to the tension developed and inversely proportional to the radius of the curvature. Thus as a pressure generator, the diaphragm works best near its end expiratory position, where its radius of curvature is smallest. Hyperinflation by flattening the diaphragm, and hence increasing the radius of curvature, reduces the effective pressure generated for any particular muscle tension, reduces efficiency and may lead to muscle fatigue. The resulting alveolar hypoventilation, whose onset can be quite sudden, is the major contributory factor to respiratory failure in severe bronchiolitis.

The interaction of the diaphragm with the rest of the chest wall and abdomen is crucial. Because of its tangential insertion, normal diaphragmatic contraction causes the chest wall to expand laterally ('bucket handle' effect) and anteriorly ('pump handle' effect). Scoliosis, for example, disturbs normal integrated movements of diaphragm and chest wall and may lead to respiratory failure, presenting initially during sleep, when the diaphragm may be the sole muscle of breathing.

The phasic action of the intercostal muscles plays a part in stabilizing the chest wall, as illustrated by the indrawing (rib recession) which occurs during inspiration in patients with intercostal weakness (e.g. acute polyneuritis, spinal muscular atrophy) or in normal infants during rapid eye movement sleep (when the intercostal muscles remain passive). The diaphragm compensates for a floppy chest wall by increasing the amplitude of its contractions. This manifests itself as 'abdominal breathing' (i.e. large amplitude abdominal excursions) and may, if excessive, lead to muscle fatigue and respiratory failure. The stabilizing effect of the intercostal muscles is particularly important in infancy, when the chest is less rigid and when the expanding action of the diaphragm is less effective because it is flatter (because of its less acute insertion and because of the more horizontal arrangement of the ribs).

The distribution of inspired gas depends on regional lung mechanics. In health, posture may affect the distribution of ventilation.

Expiration is normally a passive function, dependent on the elastic recoil of the lungs and chest wall. The elastic work normally carried out by the diaphragm in expanding the lungs and chest is thus almost totally 'recovered' during deflation; the work expended in overcoming frictional forces (the resistance to air flow) is dissipated as heat. However, active expiratory effort, applied mainly by the muscles of the anterior abdominal wall, may be needed if ventilatory demands are great (e.g. during exercise), if there is increased resistance to expiratory airflow (e.g. laryngeal edema) or if the natural recoil of the lungs is reduced (as in emphysema). The diaphragm may be used as a brake during expiration, although when a more effective brake is required (e.g. in neonatal respiratory distress or infantile bronchiolitis), the variable resistance of the glottis may be used, resulting in the characteristic 'grunt'.

From the point of view of the respiratory physician, the brain is part of the respiratory system! Apart from recognized CNS disorders which can affect the respiratory centers (e.g. Leigh's disease) and primary hypoventilation ('Ondine's curse'), altered central respiratory drive is especially dependent on sleep state (see p. 530). REM sleep is normally associated with a small drop in PaO_2. However, when upper airway obstruction is present (e.g. due to weakness or to tonsillar or adenoidal hypertrophy) or in the presence of severe lung disease (e.g. cystic fibrosis, severe scoliosis) the degree of hypoventilation may be profound, leading to periods of extreme hypoxia. The consequences may be severe (pulmonary hypertension, hypoxic fits or brain damage) or limited to sleep disturbance as a consequence of repeated waking, leading to excessive somnolence (or paradoxically in children, hyperactivity) the following day.

Control of breathing may become clinically important in chronic respiratory failure with hypercapnia (e.g. terminal lung disease, chronic neuromuscular disorders) when renal compensation for respiratory acidosis leads to an increase in plasma and CSF bicarbonate concentration. This acts as a buffer, blunting the sensitivity of the respiratory center to further rises in PCO_2, again leading to severe hypoventilation during REM sleep, when the metabolic control of breathing is paramount.

Measurement of respiratory muscle strength

The function of the respiratory muscles is best assessed by clinical observations assisted (in the absence of gross lung disease) by comparison of supine and standing vital capacity. Diaphragmatic paralysis will be indicated by a fall in vital capacity of more than 10% accompanied by paradoxical respiratory movements in the supine posture. Direct measurements by mouthpiece and transducer of the maximum pressure which can be generated at the mouth during inspiratory effort from residual volume, and expiratory effort from total lung capacity, allow precise quantitations of respiratory muscle strength. Unfortunately, if weakness affects the facial muscles, children find it impossible to maintain an airtight seal around a mouthpiece.

The measurement of breathing pattern, breathing during sleep and control of breathing are dealt with on page 530.

CLINICAL FEATURES

HISTORY AND SYMPTOMS

HISTORY

Symptoms of respiratory illness generally draw medical attention directly to the respiratory tract or to the processes which regulate breathing. Thus cough, breathlessness or apnea are important clues to respiratory disease. There are, however, exceptions to this simple association. On the one hand, a few pulmonary disorders can become quite advanced before focal features develop. Pulmonary tuberculosis is such a disease. Occasionally, on the other hand, respiratory symptoms may draw attention to disorders which are largely nonrespiratory. Breathlessness due to heart disease and chest pain of neural origin are two examples. Finally, one must remember that nonrespiratory symptoms can be due to respiratory disease, fits secondary to hypoxemia and behavior disturbance secondary to obstructive sleep disruption, for instance.

Whatever their mechanism, a careful evaluation of clinical features is important in providing clues (or clinical hypotheses)

during the process of diagnosis and in providing the means to evaluate subsequent management. Techniques for recording symptoms may influence the outcome. For instance, direct questioning may be needed (Gold et al 1989).

The perception of illness by parents and child is articulated in their description of the symptoms. The subjective nature of symptoms and, in the case of infants and young children, their second-hand nature are both a problem and a challenge. For instance, when do parents consider their child's cough to be abnormal? The answer depends not only on the physical basis for the symptom and its quality, but also on the social context of the family. Chronic cough and nasal discharge, for instance, may be considered 'normal' in the winter months, in a large family living in overcrowded circumstances and is indeed evidence of normal host defense.

It is impossible to classify some clinical features separately as symptoms or signs; they are placed here for convenience.

COUGH

Under normal circumstances, coughing represents a protective response to the inhalation of a noxious substance or foreign body into the respiratory tract. Cough receptors are found from the external ear to the pleural surface! It is not normal for children to cough or clear the throat repeatedly. Preterm newly born infants rarely cough, relying on sneezing for this protective response. At that age, apnea may be induced by stimuli (such as milk in the larynx) which in older infants will lead to coughing. Infantile chronic cough suggests diagnoses such as cystic fibrosis, chlamydial pneumonia or recurrent aspiration. Ciliary dyskinesia and pertussis are rarer causes.

Mucus clearance in the major segmental bronchi, trachea and larynx is assisted by clearing the throat and coughing, which increase expiratory air flow rate.

Excessive coughing is the commonest presenting symptom of respiratory tract disease. Its chronicity, persistent or episodic nature, the quality of the sound and the presence or absence of mucus production are important diagnostic features (Table 12.7). Physical and radiological signs of a focal or generalized nature will help differential diagnosis. The relationship between chronic nasal symptoms (postnasal drip) and nocturnal cough is controversial. It is unclear whether postnasal drip triggers reflex coughing or whether chronic upper respiratory tract inflammation (allergic or infective) and chronic lower respiratory tract symptoms (cough) are merely manifestations of generalized respiratory disease.

There is no simple way to measure either the strength of the cough reflex or frequency of cough. Experimentally, the cough reflex has been studied by counting the frequency of coughing induced by the inhalation of increasing concentrations of aerosols of citric acid or capsicin (pepper extract). Diary cards filled in at home have been shown to be unreliable, by comparison with bedside tape recordings, as a means of assessing the severity of night-time cough in children (Archer & Simpson 1985).

The investigation of cough will vary with its clinical features (Table 12.7). Lung function tests may indicate the site of a focal lesion. Special radiological techniques such as fast CT imaging of the airways or fluoroscopy may help to identify the presence and site of a foreign body or the nature and site of focal inflammatory or anatomical disease. Sweat testing, monitoring of esophageal pH, tuberculin testing and studies related to specific infecting

Table 12.7 Major causes of cough

Onset	Periodicity	Sputum production	Cause and characteristic quality
Sudden (minutes)	Persistent or episodic	0	Inhaled foreign body; sudden choking
Subacute (hours)	Persistent	±	Acute infection (e.g tracheobronchitis): ± stridor Whooping cough: whoop; vomiting
Gradual	Persistent	0 +	Psychogenic: daytime; attention driven: 'honking' Bronchiectasis; cystic fibrosis; bronchomalacia
	Episodic	±	Asthma: exercise, night-time, with wheeze Recurrent aspiration: related to feeding or vomiting Focal lesions: tracheomalacia, repaired tracheoesophageal fistula, stricture, cyst: brassy cough ± stridor Nematode infections: ± wheeze, choking sensation
Lifelong	Persistent or episodic	±	Ciliary dyskinesia; host defense disorder; cystic fibrosis; anatomical anomaly

Most children with cough are basically healthy, do not have an identifiable cause and do not need investigation

organisms may be indicated if there is suggestive evidence to suspect an appropriate diagnosis. The treatment of cough should be directed at its cause.

Particular problems arise when the normal cough reflex is ineffective. Defective airway protection and poor mucus removal may lead respectively to recurrent aspiration or airway plugging and later to bronchiectasis or atelectasis. In neuromuscular disorders and conditions associated with pain (trauma, postoperative state), both ineffective cough and low expiratory flow rates contribute to poor mucus clearance. Children with tracheostomies seem to achieve adequate airway protection and mucus clearance.

Psychogenic cough or 'honking' is a troublesome tic. Characteristically the cough may well have been preceded by an upper respiratory tract infection. The child, however, continues to cough. This is almost always with the head thrown back and he will oblige with a demonstration if his 'cough' is casually mentioned. Diagnosis rests on absence of cough during sleep and a normal physical examination. The symptoms vary little in character from patient to patient. The family should be reassured that this will get better.

SPUTUM PRODUCTION

Mucus, secreted by mucosal goblet cells and submucosal glands, lines the respiratory tract. Swept towards the larynx by ciliary and convective forces, it provides an important defense against airborne particles. Awareness of mucus production is abnormal and indicates excess. Clearing the throat, productive cough or cough associated with vomiting of mucus are all abnormal.

Sputum, the visible sign of excess mucus production, is composed of airway mucus, inflammatory cells, bacteria and occasionally blood. Young children cannot voluntarily expectorate; they swallow sputum. Hence, sputum production is rarely a feature at that age.

Sputum production is important if it persists for more than a week after an acute chest infection, if it is purulent or if it is blood-stained. Excessive nasopharyngeal mucus secretion may lead to confusion since 'noisy breathing', cough and sometimes mucous vomiting may result.

Green (purulent) sputum generally indicates chronic suppuration, but up to 25% of chronic childhood asthmatics produce sputum which, if rich in eosinophils, may be yellow. Bronchial casts are now rare in asthma but may occur in bronchopulmonary aspergillosis.

Collection of sputum for microscopy and bacterial or fungal culture may be aided by postural drainage and percussion or by 'huffing' in practiced children. Nasophargyneal aspiration of such sputum by catheter, in very young children, is an alternative to expectoration. Some physiotherapists can pass a transtracheal catheter in the awake child. This is an unpleasant and potentially dangerous procedure which should be used only if essential, to avoid bronchoscopy. Special bacterial culture techniques may be needed to identify bacterial pathogenesis in mixed cultures (e.g. in cystic fibrosis).

Excessive sputum production is dealt with by tackling the cause. Where this is impossible, for instance in generalized bronchiectasis due to bronchomalacia or a defect of host defense, physiotherapy or possibly 'mucolytic' agents and nebulized antibiotic therapy may be helpful (see section on cystic fibrosis).

Hemoptysis is a rare childhood symptom which should always be taken seriously. However, the commonest cause is benign, due to superficial erosions in the upper airway (trachea, larynx or pharynx) associated with violent coughing in, for instance, acute tracheobronchitis or whooping cough. The distinction between hemoptysis, epistaxis and hematemesis is important. Recurrent hemoptysis (Table 12.8) warrants appropriate investigation. Major bleeding in the absence of a bleeding disorder is an indication for emergency bronchoscopy prior to surgery. If the cause is known to be unilateral, the child should be laid on the abnormal side.

NOISY BREATHING

The classification of noisy breathing is important to clinicians but quite foreign to most parents and children. It is important not only to elicit a description of the sounds but to ask parents to mimic them (or even to mimic them oneself). Whether the sounds

Table 12.8 Major causes of hemoptysis

Massive hemoptysis	Bronchiectasis (cystic fibrosis), endobronchial tuberculosis, vascular malformation
Recurrent hemoptysis	Pulmonary venous congestion, Goodpasture's syndrome, pulmonary hemosiderosis, arteriovenous malformation, coagulopathy

emanate from the upper or lower respiratory tract and whether, in the latter case, they occur predominantly during expiration or inspiration are the key features. Part of the problem in history taking is that there are few words to describe the respiratory noises.

Wheeze

The high-pitched, variable intensity, expiratory sound emanating from the lower respiratory tract which is called wheeze (or 'whistling in the chest') is difficult to describe but widely recognized. Many people (but not all) have heard the wheeze of an asthmatic or an elderly relative with chronic airway obstruction. Almost half UK preschool children are reported to have at least one episode of wheeze at some stage; reported recurrent wheeze affects about 15% at any time.

Wheeze is exceptionally unusual in the neonatal period. It then signifies a structural or functional congenital abnormality. In preschool children, wheeze is commonly accompanied by cough in episodes, triggered by viral infection. In older children, persistent or episodic wheeze is almost synonymous with asthma.

The symptom implies intrathoracic airway obstruction with one or more of the following elements:

1. intraluminal obstruction by, for instance, mucus or a foreign body;

2. fixed airway narrowing by, for instance, generalized inflammatory edema or a focal stricture;

3. variable (dynamic) narrowing of medium or large airways in, for instance, asthma (smooth muscle contraction) or bronchomalacia (loss of airway elastance);

4. small airway obstruction, in bronchiolitis, for example;

5. external compression in the presence, for instance, of a vascular ring or a 'bronchogenic' cyst. This is an extremely rare cause of wheezing.

The expiratory nature of the symptom is explained by the dynamic effects of forced expiration on airway caliber (Fig. 12.2). All these factors lead to turbulent expiratory flow and hence audible change.

Important features in the differential diagnosis (Table 12.9) include evidence about the focal or generalized origin of the sound, the nature of its onset and its chronicity or periodicity. Wheeze itself cannot be quantified. The degree of disturbance due to airway narrowing can be recorded subjectively on diary cards and measured by tests of airway obstruction or, if severe, by oximetry.

Stridor (Kilham et al 1987, Couriel 1988)

The inspiratory nature of stridor is easily confused with snoring noises emanating from the nose or pharynx during sleep. True stridor is caused by extrathoracic, inspiratory dynamic narrowing of the airway in the oropharynx, glottis or subglottic region or mid-trachea. Stridor and wheeze (with or without dysphagia) may coexist in the presence of mid-tracheal obstruction due, for instance, to vascular compression. Expiratory stridor, a harsh sound distinguishable from wheeze, may accompany inspiratory stridor if obstruction is severe.

Stridor is uncommon in the newborn period and when present indicates a congenital anomaly of the airway or its neuromuscular control (Table 12.10). They are not easy to differentiate without investigation.

The causes of stridor can be classified according to the duration of symptoms and age of the child (Table 12.11). In most cases a diagnosis can be reached without any investigation.

Acute or subacute stridor needs no special investigation, unless foreign body inhalation or recurrent aspiration is suspected. Then, direct laryngoscopy and bronchoscopy for foreign body or radiological investigations for recurrent aspiration are indicated. Persistent mild congenital stridor in an otherwise normal infant is generally caused by laryngomalacia and requires no investigation. It is worse during sleep, excitement and URTI. Parents need to be aware that severe recession may become critical during an URTI. Recurrent (spasmodic) croup in an older child is a benign condition and should not be further investigated.

All other children with chronic or recurrent stridor should be investigated; radiography and direct fiberoptic laryngoscopy (with bronchoscopy if necessary) are the two basic investigations. Plain radiographs of the neck and chest (including lateral views), to demonstrate the airways and soft tissues, may show strictures, cysts or compression of the airway. A barium swallow should be performed, attention being paid to the swallowing mechanism as well as to the contours of the esophagus in a lateral view and to the gastroesophageal junction. If a 'surgical' condition is suspected, the investigations should be discussed in advance with an ENT surgeon competent to deal with children. Emergency intubation may be required in acute epiglottitis or pseudomembranous croup (see p. 1308).

Upper respiratory noises

Snoring, snorting and rattly breathing are common during upper respiratory tract infections. Hypertrophied adenoids and large prolapsing tonsils are the commonest causes of this sort of

---

Table 12.9   Causes of childhood wheeze

Acute wheeze
Inhaled foreign body
Acute bronchiolitis

Persistent or episodic wheeze
Asthma
Inhaled foreign body
Recurrent aspiration
Chronic infection: cystic fibrosis, bronchiectasis, ciliary dyskinesia, immune
  deficiency
Postviral syndrome: obliterative bronchiolitis
Congenital airway anomaly: bronchomalacia, cyst
Perinatal infection

Table 12.10   Congenital causes of stridor

Micrognathia (Robin anomalad)

Laryngomalacia (infantile larynx)

Laryngeal web

Laryngeal cleft

Subglottic and tracheal stenosis

Hemangioma; cystic hygroma

Cyst of airway, tongue or esophagus

Vocal cord palsy

Vascular ring (tracheal compression)

Table 12.11   Causes of stridor. The most frequent are marked with an asterisk; other causes are all rare

	Onset and duration of symptoms		
	Acute (h)	Subacute (days)	Chronic (weeks)
Infancy (<2 years)	Epiglottitis* Infantile tetanus Aspiration (recurrent) Foreign body	Laryngotracheobronchitis*	Congenital anomalies* (see Table 12.10.) Postintubation stricture cyst* or granuloma Vocal cord palsy Angioma:cystic hygroma
Preschool (2–5 years)	Epiglottitis* Spasmodic croup (recurrent)* Foreign body Familial angioneurotic edema	Laryngotracheobronchitis* Diphtheria Pharyngitis* Quinsy and retropharyngeal abscess	Congenital anomalies* Tonsillar hypertrophy* Papilloma (tumor) Esophageal foreign body Tuberculosis Granuloma
Schoolchildren	Sensitivity reaction (angioneurotic edema)	Acute laryngitis* Acute pharyngitis*	Papilloma (tumor)

breathing. A history of snoring should alert the physician to the possibility of severe obstructive episodes during sleep (see p. 531). 'Rattly' noises indicate pooling of secretions in the hypopharynx and upper airways and are conducted to the chest, where they may be palpable and thus noticed by the parents. If these noises have been present since birth suspicion of a congenital narrowing of the nasal passages or nasopharynx should be aroused. Babies who are naturally nasal breathers may be severely compromised if an upper respiratory infection is superimposed.

APNEA; HYPOVENTILATION (see also p. 530)

Recurrent apnea is primarily a problem of neonates and infants. It may play a part in some cases of SIDS. In later infancy and childhood apnea and hypoventilation mainly occur secondary to chronic respiratory disease (obstructive apnea). Primary hypoventilation syndrome ('central' apnea) is very rare and confined to disorders of the CNS either recognized (e.g. Leigh's encephalopathy) or of unknown cause, 'Ondine's curse'; (see p. 530). All these disorders cause trouble mainly during sleep, perhaps because of reduced activity in the reticular formation. In most cases of sleep apnea, both 'central' and 'obstructive' elements are present but their relative contribution varies.

Although nocturnal hypoventilation may not be a primary complaint several clinical features may raise one's suspicions: a history of very irregular breathing in sleep, often punctuated by long pauses and loud snores or gasps; extreme restlessness at night; early morning headache, confusion or drowsiness; daytime somnolence. Cor pulmonale may eventually develop if chronic respiratory failure develops in persistent cases.

CHEST PAIN

This is not a particularly common symptom in childhood and is usually benign and self-limiting. It may be felt only on coughing or on deep inspiration. Most frequently it is due to trauma which has fractured a rib or bruised the chest wall. Bone disease with nerve root compression or infiltrative bone disease such as leukemia may rarely present in this way but there are usually other symptoms and signs pointing to the diagnosis. Bornholm disease

is a form of epidemic myalgia caused by coxsackie B virus and presents as chest pain with intercostal tenderness. The pain can be localized by the patient and is sufficient to prevent deep inspiration and effective coughing.

Herpes zoster is a rare disease of childhood but is responsible for the same severe burning root pain as it is in adults.

The most usual underlying respiratory disease in children is pneumonia with pleural involvement and the pain is associated with symptoms of cough or shortness of breath. Pneumococcal pneumonia used to be a common cause of this kind of pleural disease. Pneumothorax is rare outside the neonatal period but should not be forgotten as a cause of sudden chest pain and shortness of breath.

Frequently, no organic lesion can be identified.

BREATHLESSNESS

Awareness of the demand to breathe constitutes the symptom of breathlessness (dyspnea). As a primary symptom it is rare in childhood. We may infer the sensation in patients who are too young to speak by observing excessive respiratory effort, a raised breathing frequency or obvious distress. The sensation may be due to increased metabolic rate (e.g. fever, physical exercise), abnormal sensations arising in the lungs (e.g. acute pulmonary edema) or from stressed muscles (e.g. due to fatigue) or due to an abnormal awareness of breathing (e.g. anxiety or 'hysteria').

The severity of breathlessness in adults with chronic lung disease is assessed by their exercise tolerance. This may be appropriate in those few children with severe chronic disease for whom shortness of breath is a major handicap. It would be an inappropriate measure of disease severity in asthma or in acute lung disease.

Breathlessness of psychological origin may have its origins in a genuine but benign respiratory illness. Having excluded physical disease, simple measures (such as graded exercise on a treadmill) may reassure and cure the child. For more protracted cases or those with episodic overbreathing, psychiatric help is needed. Before referral for psychiatric help, it may be worth demonstrating the normal results of investigations to convince the parents and child who may have a very understandable reason for anxiety, such as the acquaintance of someone who has suffered from or died of chest disease.

PHYSICAL EXAMINATION AND PHYSICAL SIGNS

Skilled physical examination together with a careful history should identify most children with significant pulmonary disease. In acute lower respiratory tract disease when the history and physical examination suggest the same diagnosis a chest radiograph is rarely necessary. Where the two are inconsistent then a radiograph may be useful (Alario et al 1987). Similarly, good clinical evaluation of a child with acute asthma or croup should allow the physician to form a management plan which may or may not include further investigations.

Early signs of serious disease

In an effort to diagnose treatable illness early and so prevent sudden infant deaths it has been suggested (Valman 1985) that infants under 6 months of age should be referred to hospital if they demonstrate certain symptoms and signs, such as sudden onset of rapid and noisy breathing, poor feeding, drowsiness and irritability. A group of general practitioners concluded from a study of signs and symptoms in unwell babies under 6 months old who presented to them that the signs of rapid and noisy breathing did not distinguish those babies who needed hospital admission from those who did not and that signs and symptoms alone could not replace multifactorial clinical judgment (Wright et al 1987) In developing countries where field workers may not have had much medical training and where, because of the greater chance of bacterial infection, antibiotic treatment of chest infections can be justified, the identification of signs such as rapid breathing and chest retractions is very important in deciding who needs expensive treatment and who does not (Cherian et al 1988). Also important is the decision to refer a child to hospital, which may be many miles away. A rapid respiratory rate during sleep and chest retractions are probably the most useful signs in acute respiratory disease (Campbell et al 1989).

Adults and children

The difference between children's and adults' chests accounts for some of the differences in physical signs. The chest wall of the infant and young child is much more compliant than that of the adult. This explains the signs of intercostal and subcostal recession seen during severe respiratory illness. The chest wall is also thinner and the distance between the stethoscope and the large bronchi smaller. Thus there is less attenuation of the breath sounds which are normally heard throughout the entire respiratory cycle; in adults no noise is normally heard after the first part of expiration. A small child finds it difficult to 'take a large breath' and so crackles and wheezes which may be expected only during such a maneuver will not be heard. For the inexperienced examiner, crying and conducted noises from the upper airways can also make the interpretation of auscultatory findings difficult.

General observation

Much can be learnt by observation, during history taking for example. In the acutely ill child an alteration in the level of consciousness, restlessness, mouth breathing, flaring of the alae nasi, the presence and quality of cough, stridor, audible wheeze, an abnormal respiratory rate and pattern and the use of accessory muscles of respiration are abnormal signs which can be observed even before the child is undressed. Auscultation of the back of an infant or small child is best done by having a parent cuddle him/her over a shoulder.

Height and weight should be related to accepted standards for age and to the mid-parental height and ethnic origin. The velocity of growth is much more important than absolute measurements. Poor growth may reflect a primary problem, such as undernutrition, against which a respiratory illness is set or be a part of a multisystem disease, such as cystic fibrosis or immunodeficiency, or be related to chronic respiratory disease such as chronic lung disease of prematurity. Recent attention has been directed to the potential for inhaled steroids to cause poor growth.

Although *fever* is suggestive of infective illness it is not specific for it. The height of the fever is more helpful than previously thought in determining whether or not a respiratory infection is serious (Campbell et al 1989, Turner et al 1987). *Sweating* is associated with febrile illnesses but may also be associated with adrenergic stimulation, e.g. in shock or in cardiac failure or resulting from treatment with adrenergic agonists. In infants sweating is particularly noticeable over the head.

Skin rashes may accompany both viral and mycoplasmal respiratory illnesses. The rash of measles is rarely present in children with giant cell pneumonia. Erythema nodosum is an occasional accompaniment of primary tuberculosis in well-nourished children at the time the tuberculin test becomes positive but it is rarely seen in children who are undernourished. As well as accompanying some infectious diseases, scratch marks accompany atopic skin disease such as eczema. Even without eczema some asthmatic children develop localized itching in areas, such as the chest wall or scalp, at the onset of exacerbations of an acute attack (prodromal itch).

There are ever more children who have been the recipients of neonatal intensive care and thoracic surgery and who bear the scars associated with the insertion of pneumothorax drains, venous and arterial access and other cutaneous trauma. If the details of the past events have not been revealed in the history these signs should alert the examiner to the possibility of previous lung damage.

Disturbances of behavior and conscious level are important physical signs in acute respiratory disease. Signs of irritability or drowsiness should never be ascribed to tiredness or being frightened until the examiner is satisfied that the child is not hypoxemic or in respiratory failure. Meningitis can of course coexist with respiratory infection and be the cause of a change in either behavior or conscious level.

Drowsiness and tachypnea are also signs of severe metabolic acidosis which may accompany disorders such as diabetes and the organic acidemias.

Examination of the eyes can be helpful. Discolored puffy eyelids, desquamation of the periorbital skin because of rubbing and the thickened 'cobblestone' appearance of vernal conjunctivitis are all features of perennial or severe seasonal allergic disease affecting the eyes. These signs may coexist with asthma. Conjunctivitis often accompanies viral infections such as measles. Subconjunctival hemorrhages are associated with prolonged coughing spasms. The presence of phlyctenulae (pale conjunctival nodules) is a rare sign which may mark the onset of primary tuberculosis but can also be recurrent. Papilledema is an accompaniment of long-standing hypercapnia.

With severe respiratory distress or upper airways obstruction an infant may adopt a posture of *hyperextension* of the trunk and neck (Chidiac & Alexander 1990). This may sometimes be confused with meningism. Attempts to flex the trunk, to carry out a lumbar puncture for example, may precipitate collapse. In this position the accessory muscles of respiration are at their most efficient and the airways are held open. A child with epiglottitis prefers to sit up and forwards; indeed, lying down may result in complete occlusion of the airway.

Cardiovascular signs

Tachycardia accompanies fever, hypoxia and increased work of breathing and should not be attributed too readily to the effects of drugs such as bronchodilators or to excitement. A wide pulse pressure is an association of hypercapnia and patent ductus arteriosus. *Bradycardia* may be due to intense vagal stimulation and may accompany a long bout of coughing.

Pulsus paradoxicus is the difference between the systolic blood pressure measured in inspiration and expiration. Normally there is a fall in inspiration and a rise in expiration but the difference is no more than 5 mmHg. During inspiration intrathoracic pressure falls and there is an increased venous return to the right side of the heart, a shift of the ventricular septum to the left and a demand on the left ventricle to sustain the previous arterial pressure which it cannot meet; thus during inspiration the systolic pressure falls. In disorders where there is airway obstruction there is a larger than normal decrease in intrathoracic pressure in inspiration and so pulsus paradoxicus increases. Measurements of 20 mmHg or greater suggest hypercapnia in acute asthma.

In practice the measurement of pulsus paradoxicus in the presence of tachycardia is not easy. The best approach is to measure the interval between the pressure at which the Korotkoff sounds are first regularly heard at a slower rate than the heart rate and the pressure when the sounds are heard continuously at the same rate as the heart rate. In practice pulsus paradoxicus is rarely measured (Pearson et al 1993). If paradox is felt at the radial artery then it can be assumed that there is severe airway disease.

Finger clubbing is an unusual sign in children other than those with cystic fibrosis, bronchiectasis, fibrosing alveolitis or cyanotic congenital heart disease. It has not been recorded in children with chronic lung disease due to bronchopulmonary dysplasia. In the presence of empyema or infective endocarditis finger and toe clubbing can develop rapidly. Clubbing can also be familial.

Cyanosis

This is an unreliable sign at any time but particularly in artificial light. The color of the tongue should be assessed, rather than the lips or nail beds. Cyanosis implies >5 g/100 ml of desaturated hemoglobin but its absence does not imply that there is no hypoxemia. This is particularly true if there is anemia. A common and serious misconception is to assume that hypoxemia is not severe if there is no cyanosis on examination; treatment with additional oxygen should not await its development. If there is no method available for measuring arterial oxygen tension or saturation it is safer to assume that a child with tachypnea and other signs of acute respiratory disease is hypoxemic and thus deserving of oxygen therapy. This is especially true in an infant who is liable to become exhausted more quickly than an older child.

Upper respiratory tract

Examination of the *middle ear* reveals that redness of the drum is a frequent accompaniment of upper respiratory infections. The appearance of the eardrum does not distinguish between viral and bacterial otitis media although the presence of hemorrhagic bullae is suggestive of mycoplasmal infection. The appearance of the drum can be misleading in chronic middle ear disease. This is best assessed by an ENT expert, especially if there is hearing loss.

Examination of the *nose* in children with noisy, difficult breathing includes an assessment of the patency of the nostrils. If there is any doubt catheters should be passed to rule out choanal atresia. The anterior nares can be visualized by pressing the tip of the nose and inspecting the mucous membranes with a good light. The traditional nasal speculum requires some expertise and is unlikely to be tolerated. A boggy, swollen pale mucosa with a clear discharge is suggestive of allergic rhinitis, a purulent discharge accompanies viral coryza and a bloodstained smelly discharge may suggest a foreign body or a granulomatous or neoplastic condition. However, bloody discharges are more usually caused by nose blowing or picking. A deviated nasal septum compromises the patency of one side when there is additional mucosal swelling.

The *throat and mouth* should always be inspected except when a diagnosis of epiglottitis is suspected. Physical examination unfortunately cannot distinguish viral from bacterial pharyngitis as both can result in a red throat with a mucopurulent exudate on the tonsils. The presence of a membrane is suggestive of infections mononucleosis. A gray-green membrane is typical of diphtheria. Palatal hemorrhages are not specific to any particular infection.

During acute illness, especially asthma, the *neck* should be examined for surgical emphysema, suggesting an air leak not otherwise evident clinically. Enlarged nodes nearly always reflect local inflammation, past or present, but very rarely may be the clue to intrathoracic malignant disease or lymphoma. Tuberculous neck glands are nowadays extremely rare in childhood. Deviation of the trachea from the mid-line in a baby is not easy to determine but the position of the trachea should be easier to evaluate in older children.

Lower respiratory tract

The *counting of respirations*, and its meaning is still debated (Morley 1990, Berman et al 1991). Counting is best done before a child is disturbed by a general physical examination. In infants who are awake accurate counts are especially difficult because of movement, crying and so on. A rapid respiratory rate during sleep (>40/min) is of more significance in this age group. When tachypnea is present without other signs of respiratory disease such as chest recession or abnormal auscultatory findings, causes other than primary respiratory disease should be considered. These include metabolic acidosis and cardiac disease in the newborn. Brain disorders such as encephalitis sometimes cause tachypnea due to involvement of the respiratory center, resulting in respiratory alkalosis. The significance of respiratory rates in children with ARI is discussed on page 000.

Dyspnea or *difficulty with breathing* is generally considered to be a subjective sensation. However, in an infant the term is sometimes used to describe subcostal or intercostal recession. The infant's chest wall is more compliant than that of the older child. When the lungs are, 'stiff', as in hyaline membrane disease, the sternum is drawn in and there is intercostal and subcostal recession. In bronchiolitis, on the other hand, where airway narrowing is accompanied by hyperinflation, the chest wall appears prominent with intercostal and subcostal recession. The movements of the chest and abdomen appear out of phase, i.e. when the abdomen rises the chest falls and vice versa. 'Head-nodding' in an infant in time with respiration reflects use of the accessory muscles of respiration. In older children use of the accessory muscles, principally the scalenes and the sternomastoids, is seen in severe respiratory disease. Examination of chest movement with the child sitting or standing straight may reveal asymmetrical movement present, for example, in unilateral diaphragmatic paralysis or focal lung or chest wall disease.

A child's parents are often more worried about his *chest shape* than the child himself. Both pectus excavatum, where there is depression of the sternum, and pigeon-chestedness, where the sternum appears prominent, are relatively common and both may be familial. Poland's anomaly is a combination of absent pectoralis major with ipsilateral thumb anomaly and breast defect. This produces no other abnormal respiratory symptoms or signs.

The chest may also appear slightly asymmetrical. There is seldom underlying chest disease. In pectus excavatum, the heart may be displaced to the left if the deformity is severe. Bronchomalacia is one important associated abnormality which must be considered. Pigeon-chestedness is associated with chronic lung disease such as uncontrolled asthma or cystic fibrosis, heart disease or generalized disorders of the skeleton or spine, such as the mucopolysaccharidoses or idiopathic scoliosis. Congenital neuromuscular disorders, such as severe spinal muscular atrophy, produce abnormal chest shape and function. Noticeable asymmetry of the chest wall is most often associated with past trauma, scoliosis or an underlying small lung or abnormal diaphragm. Harrison's sulci, exaggerated grooves running parallel to the subcostal margins, are due to prolonged diaphragmatic traction, characteristically associated with chronic airway disease or rickets.

Pulmonary hyperinflation reflects gas trapping. The chest appears barrel shaped and the ribs become horizontal. In the presence of severe airways disease the volume in the lungs at the end of inspiration may reach twice normal and the residual volume at the end of expiration is also grossly elevated. However, the degree of hyperinflation as clinically assessed does not correlate well with the severity of disease.

A careful assessment of any skeletal abnormality, whether congenital or acquired, should be part of the clinical examination. This will need to be supplemented by radiographic measurements.

Neither *chest expansion nor percussion note* is particularly helpful in pediatric chest medicine. Chest expansion is reduced when there is pain, as in Bornholm's disease, generalized neuromuscular disease or decreased lung compliance, or in conditions when there is severe gas trapping, as in asthma, when the chest is already hyperinflated. Expansion of the chest may be asymmetrical in the presence of unilateral disease of the lung, diaphragm or chest wall. In the presence of neuromuscular disease, chest movements should be examined with the child in both the upright and supine positions. Diaphragmatic weakness leads to paradoxical abdominal movements in the supine position; these may be completely masked sitting or standing. A history of orthopnea and the finding of a reduced vital capacity in the supine position should lead on to fluoroscopy as the definitive investigation.

The percussion note is dull over solid lung, as in lobar pneumonia, or over a pleural effusion.

Breath sounds (Forgacs 1978) heard through the stethoscope in the normal patient are believed to be generated by turbulent flow in the large airways. The intensity of the sounds varies directly with the flow rate. Normally the second half of expiration is not heard through the chest wall because the flow rate is slow and the noise is filtered out. However, the smaller the child the less distance between the large airways and the chest wall and the longer sound will be heard through expiration. Similarly over upper lobes sound is filtered least and caution should be taken not to interpret the harsher expiratory sounds as bronchial breathing.

Over consolidated lung tissue, the breath sounds are less attenuated and are heard throughout inspiration and expiration. This has been described as 'bronchial breathing'. On the other hand breath sounds are heard very faintly when there is hyperinflation. This is believed to be due to reflection of sound at the pleural surface. Similarly when there is air or fluid in the pleural cavity sound is reflected at the separated pleural surfaces and the breath sounds are absent.

The nomenclature of *added sounds* has been subject to change. There has been much debate about the nature of *crackles* (previously referred to as crepitations). It is most likely that crackling is produced by explosive equalization of gas pressure between two compartments of the lung when a closed section of the airway separating them suddenly opens. Both the frequency of crackles and their timing in the respiratory cycle are important features.

In resolving lobar pneumonia crackling is heard in inspiration. There is a mixed population of alveoli and bronchioles, some of which are becoming re-aerated while others remain filled with exudate. The aerated alveoli receive disproportionately large volumes of gas through airways which snap open in the face of large pressure gradients during inspiration. Similarly in pulmonary edema, peribronchial edema is responsible for narrowing of the airways and their late opening. The fine high-frequency crackling heard in pulmonary edema is more likely due to this and not to the bubbling of intraalveolar fluid.

In primary airway disease such as asthma and bronchiolitis where airways are swollen and narrowed, generalized medium or coarse crackling is heard throughout both phases of respiration. Chronic suppurative disease of large airways, such as bronchiectasis or cystic fibrosis, leads to very coarse sounds which merge into wheezes. They may be focal and exaggerated by coughing.

The fine inspiratory crackling associated with lobar pneumonia or pulmonary edema originates in small airways and is of similar high pitch. The crackling associated with primary airway disease may originate anywhere along the airways which open and close at different times. The crackling is thus heard throughout inspiration and expiration.

Wheeze is a musical sound produced by turbulent airflow which causes oscillation of the bronchial wall. The pitch of the wheeze depends on the frequency of the oscillation which in turn depends on the flow velocity creating it.

The total cross-sectional area of the small airways of the lung is much greater than the total cross-sectional area of the large airways. The linear velocity of gas flowing in small airways is usually too slow to cause turbulent oscillation of narrowed airways. Wheeze originates in large airways which have been narrowed by compression or by intrabronchial or intraluminal obstructions, which cause an increase in flow velocity of gas through them with resultant oscillation.

In localized disease, such as that caused by a bronchogenic cyst, bronchomalacia or an inhaled foreign body, airway narrowing results in a wheeze whose pitch, although different in inspiration and expiration, is fixed and constant. The nearer the larynx the more resonance there will be in the supralaryngeal area and the inspiratory wheeze may take on the quality of stridor. Because noise is conducted well in a small chest it is often very difficult to be certain about the site of the lesion on auscultation alone.

When small airways are narrowed by mucosal edema, secretions or bronchospasm, the intrathoracic pressure rises in expiration in order to expel gas through them. The pressure outside the large airways exceeds that inside and the large airways are narrowed as a result. This is known as dynamic compression of the large airways and is the cause of wheezing in generalized small airways disease (Fig. 12.2).

Thus, on auscultation, wheeze of 'fixed' pitch occurring in inspiration and expiration suggests a localized abnormality. Wheezes of 'varying' pitch occurring predominantly throughout expiration reflect the narrowing of airways of different calibers, the result of dynamic compression associated with small airways disease. In practice children with localized disease, e.g. caused by an impacted foreign body, will have retained secretions peripherally and hence a 'mixed' pattern of wheezing may be heard.

A *pleural rub* is very difficult to distinguish from crackling. The sound is heard during inspiration and is mirrored in expiration. It is often accompanied by limited chest expansion due to pain.

Stridor may be classified as symptom or sign. It is sometimes confused with wheeze and, in practice, the two may occur together. The features and causes of stridor are dealt with above (p. 508 and Table 12.10).

SPECIAL INVESTIGATIONS

IMAGING (see also Ch. 36)

The chest radiograph continues to be an essential part of the full evaluation of the respiratory system despite the recent advances in imaging. Imaging has various roles: the first is to establish or substantiate the diagnosis and decide whether further more invasive examinations are required, the second is to determine the extent of the disease, its natural history and the effect of therapy. These imaging investigations should be considered in conjunction with the overall clinical picture, respiratory function tests and blood tests if they are to be interpreted correctly.

Apart from ultrasound examination (US) and magnetic resonance imaging (MRI), all imaging techniques involve radiation. Certain images involve an exceedingly low radiation dose, e.g. krypton 81m ventilation lung scan (81m Kr V); others are more invasive with a high radiation dose, e.g. cardiac catheterization or bronchography. It is therefore important to consider the invasiveness, the radiation dose and the potential discomfort to the patient when planning a detailed pulmonary investigation.

The importance of the esophagus cannot be overemphasized when chest disease is being investigated. Examination of the fully distended esophagus may reveal mediastinal pathology and/or diseases of the upper gut (e.g. hiatus hernia and/or recurrent inhalation) which may present with chest signs or symptoms.

Radiography of upper airways

The lateral neck/postnasal space (PNS) and sinuses are frequently included on the same radiograph. Frontal and lateral views are required. The frontal projection visualizes the facial sinuses but in children under 1–2 years of age the relatively small size of the facial bones makes it exceedingly difficult to interpret. The antra are usually aerated sufficiently by the age of 18–24 months to be seen on the radiograph. In older children the ethmoid and frontal sinuses, the nasal septum and turbinate bones should be seen (Kovatch et al 1984). The lateral view assists in visualizing the frontal sinus or in assessing its lack of development but there is a wide range of ages in the normal development of these sinuses. Aeration of the ethmoid/sphenoid air cells is also further aided by this view. The palatine tonsils as well as the adenoidal area must be studied. The relationship of the trachea to the cervical spine as well as the general tracheal caliber is well visualized. The lateral view has certain technical limitations and it is important to be sure that the projection is adequate, i.e. the floors of the anterior, middle and posterior fossae of the skull are overlapping, and that the cervical spine is truly lateral. The normal space between the trachea and the cervical spine is one vertebral body; an apparent increase in this space may be pathological but may also be due to the radiograph being taken in expiration – in this situation the trachea shows an acute angle.

Chest radiography

For a frontal posteroanterior (PA) chest radiograph (antero-posterior (AP) in younger children), the patient must be straight, best evaluated on the film by the relationship of the medial ends of the clavicles to the pedicle of the vertebral body. Even slight rotation can cause unusual appearances in a normal chest radiograph. The medial ends of the clavicles should lie at the level of the fourth vertebral body. Radiographs in inspiration are generally preferred, the degree of inspiration judged by counting either the anterior rib ends in the right mid-clavicular line down to the level of the diaphragm 'there should be 5–6 ribs present' or counting the posterior aspect of the ribs where one should see down to the 10th rib on inspiration. An expiration film is often regarded as being of little value but it demonstrates good compliance of the lungs suggesting that no overinflation or air trapping is present and this film may permit exclusion of lobar consolidation. The expiration film should not be disregarded but rather carefully reviewed to consider whether it needs to be repeated. Pathological conditions which result in a loss of compliance, e.g. opportunistic infection in the immune-suppressed child, cause repeated 'expiration films' to be obtained.

In the infant or sick child, supine AP chest radiographs are commonly carried out. The classic signs of well-known pathological conditions alter, e.g. pleural effusion may only be seen as an 'apical cap'; pneumothorax may not appear peripherally and a pneumomediastinum may appear only as a vague transradiancy in the mediastinum. A lateral chest radiograph with a horizontal beam is useful when doubt persists following the AP view.

The normal visualization of the cardiac outline as well as the diaphragm is due to an aerated lung being adjacent to a 'solid nonaerated organ'. Loss of the normal outlines means that the adjacent lung tissue is no longer aerated; this can occur with consolidation (i.e. fluid in the alveolar spaces due to infection, inflammation or pulmonary edema). If the airway remains patent throughout then consolidation without major collapse may occur. If there is collapse in a lobe of lung, i.e. loss of volume, then bronchial pathology, e.g. foreign body, mucus or extrinsic compression, must be borne in mind. When consolidation occurs first it is not possible for this solid pulmonary parenchyma to lose volume to any major extent. The diagnosis of a collapsed lobe is made by either identifying a displaced fissure, failing to identify the normal hilum or observing a displaced hilum with fewer vessels in the remaining lung parenchyma.

The lateral chest radiograph requires a greater exposure than the frontal film and because the two lungs are superimposed it makes interpretation difficult. This film should not be part of a 'routine' chest radiograph in pediatrics but rather reserved for certain clinical situations.

The presence or absence of overinflation may be best assessed on this view. Metastases in children with known solid tumors are less likely to be overlooked when the frontal and lateral films are taken together routinely. In a child with recurrent chest pathology undergoing investigation a lateral film at the time of the first chest radiograph is strongly recommended. In the long-term follow-up of chronic chest disease, e.g. cystic fibrosis, many would recommend that a lateral view is carried out whenever the PA film is obtained.

The normal lateral chest radiograph should show progressive transradiancy over the dorsal spine, i.e. the lower vertebral bodies are blacker than the upper ones. The lateral film may detect smaller volumes of pleural fluid than are seen on the frontal view by revealing obliteration of the posterior costophrenic angle. The trachea is well seen; displacement and narrowing are readily detected on this projection. Compression is rarely detected on the frontal view.

A filter view (Figs 12.8b and 12.9b) is a frontal (AP) coned view of the mediastinum using a high voltage (130–140 kV) technique and a copper/tin/aluminum filter very close to the radiograph tube (Deanfield & Chrispin 1981). Magnification is routinely employed. This gives good visualization of the trachea, carina and main bronchi on a single film. When the intrathoracic pathology results in shift of the mediastinum then the child must be positioned obliquely to allow the mediastinum to be visualized better. Narrowing of the airway due to either intrinsic pathology such as bronchomalacia or extrinsic pathology such as glands or vessels may be detected. Thoracic sites can also be assessed, important in the neonate with congenital heart disease.

For horizontal beam radiographs, the patient is placed supine or prone and the horizontal X-ray beam allows the effect of gravity to be maximized in order to demonstrate air–fluid interfaces or positional shifts of fluid. Either a frontal or a lateral film can be obtained. This technique is useful to demonstrate a small pleural effusion, the presence of pneumomediastinum or pneumothorax and, with intrapulmonary pathology, to demonstrate air–fluid interfaces.

The optimum degree of obliqueness on oblique chest radiographs is best judged by fluoroscopy and therefore should preferably be obtained under such circumstances. This film is most useful in the infant/child with the small lung and also in solitary masses in the chest.

Complex radiography

Tomography allows radiographic sections of the lung fields and mediastinum to be obtained. Tomography requires a cooperative child and is unsuitable for those under 2 years of age. Where computed tomography (CT) scanning and an appropriate high kV filter radiograph are available, traditional tomography has no role.

Bronchography

This examination is infrequently performed since surgical treatment for bronchiectasis is uncommon now and regional lung function can be assessed accurately by radioisotopes. With the use of CT in bronchiectasis, bronchography is very rarely undertaken. The major indication is suspected localized bronchomalacia. Bronchography is invasive and should only be undertaken by a trained experienced pediatric radiologist.

Cardiac catheterization/pulmonary angiography

This is the most invasive radiological investigation in the cardiorespiratory system and is therefore reserved for those patients in whom the diagnosis is unconfirmed by any other technique. Digital subtraction angiography allows a small volume of contrast to be used and provides high quality imaging with a lower radiation burden to the child (Fig. 12.7d and e). With the use of radioisotope ventilation/perfusion scans, ultrasound, CT and MRI the need for pulmonary angiography continues to decrease. However, certain conditions still require angiography, e.g. arteriovenous malformation.

Fluoroscopy

Fluoroscopy of thorax includes the lungs, diaphragm, pleura, mediastinum and the trachea. Whenever there is a complicated unexplained chest problem, valuable information can be obtained when an experienced radiologist fluoroscopes the thorax. Before beginning any fluoroscopic examination, the clinical questions to be answered should be well formulated and the previous and current chest radiographs reviewed.

Fluoroscopy should occur prior to any barium examination. The information available includes details of the movement of both hemidiaphragms with spontaneous and forced ventilation and the position of the mediastinum and the effect of respiration on both the mediastinum and trachea. If consolidation is present, its exact position, mobility and the presence of calcification can be ascertained. Fluid may be localized on fluoroscopy. If a diagnostic tap is thought necessary with small amounts of fluid, then both ultrasound and fluoroscopy may aid in a successful tap.

It is possible to look at all these features every time one fluoroscopes the chest, but since fluoroscopy does have a radiation burden, it is preferable to attempt to answer specific clinical problems in each case rather than to try to look at all aspects in every child.

Esophageal examination (Fig. 12.8c and d)

In the vast majority of cases this is simply a barium swallow. However, when an H-type tracheoesophageal fistula (TEF) is suspected, a normal swallow does not exclude the diagnosis.

A fully distended esophagus is essential for an adequate barium swallow examination. This examination is aimed at showing extrinsic lesions pressing on or displacing the esophagus. The aberrant left pulmonary artery may only be visible on the true

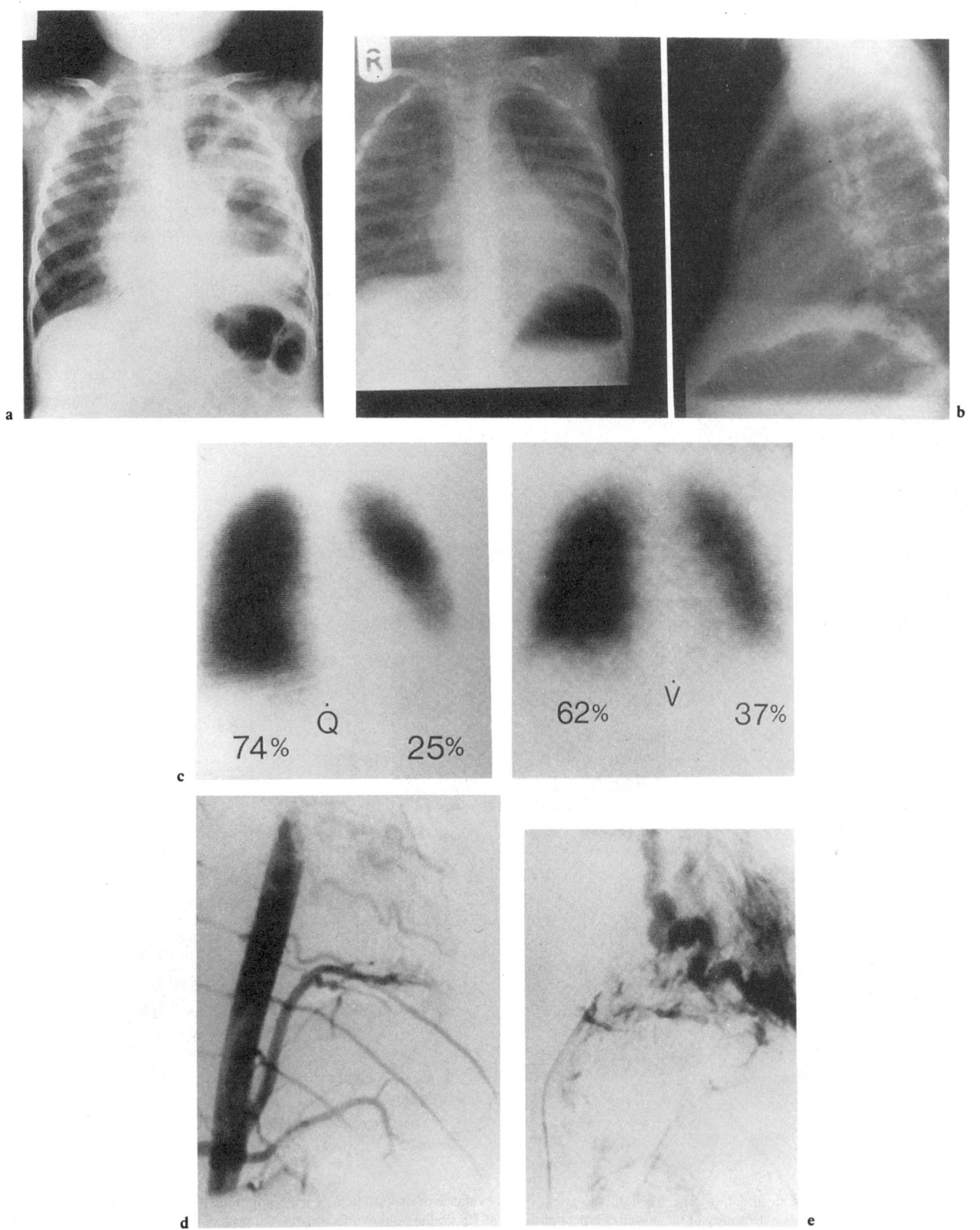

Fig. 12.7 A 3-year-old girl with unresolved pneumonia in the left lower lobe. (**a**) PA chest radiograph at 3 months of age. (**b**) Following recovery from the acute episode the routine follow-up chest radiograph 6 months later showed persistent shadowing in the left lower lobe. (**c**) A ^{99m}Tc macroaggregate perfusion scan (Q) and a krypton 81m ventilation scan (V) were obtained 1 year following the acute episode. The left lung shows decreased perfusion compared to the right with the left lung only contributing 25% of overall perfusion. On ventilation the left lung contributes 37% and there is a segment in the left lower zone which is relatively well ventilated but not perfused. The diagnosis of a sequestrated segment was suggested. (**d**) A digital subtraction angiogram was carried out. The arterial phase shows a vessel arising from the abdominal aorta going cranially into the thorax to supply the abnormal area on chest radiograph. (**e**) The venous phase shows the drainage from the sequestrated segment all going cranially. At surgery a sequestrated segment in the left lower lobe was resected.

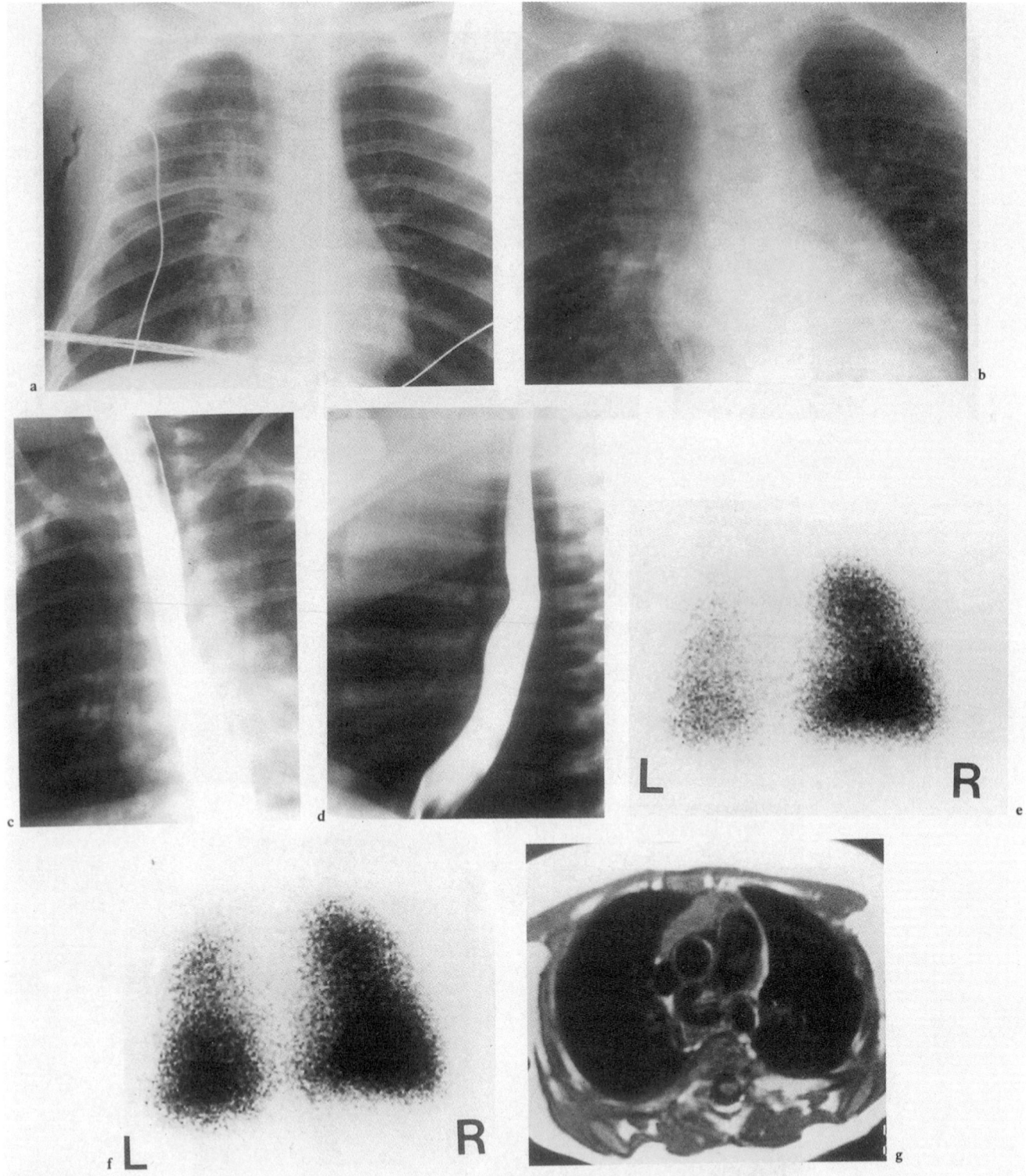

Fig. 12.8 A 6-month-old boy with stridor. (**a**) The PA chest radiograph shows evidence of overinflation of both lung fields. The left upper zone shows fewer vessels than on the right. There is a deformity of the posterior aspect of the right 7th rib but no previous surgery had been undertaken. (**b**) High kV filter image. The trachea, carina and major bronchi appear essentially normal. (**c**) Barium swallow. The frontal projection reveals a normal esophagus. (**d**) The lateral projection of the barium swallow shows clear indentation on the anterior wall of the esophagus at the level of the carina. This is a typical appearance of an aberrant left pulmonary artery which is only seen in the true lateral projection on barium. (**e**) Krypton 81m ventilation lung scan shows normal ventilation of the right lung with decreased ventilation of the left upper lobe. (**f**) ^{99m}Tc macroaggregate perfusion scan reveals a normal right lung with decreased perfusion of most of the left lung. The left lung contributed 32% to overall perfusion and 39% to overall ventilation. (**g**) MRI scan of the mediastinum shows the aberrant left pulmonary artery arising from the right pulmonary artery and curling around behind the trachea but in front of the esophagus. This child underwent resection and anastomosis of the left pulmonary artery to the main pulmonary artery. The postoperative V/Q lung scan revealed a normally perfused and ventilated left lung (not illustrated).

lateral projection. Intrinsic diseases, e.g. hiatus hernia, gastroesophageal reflux or incoordinate swallowing with aspiration, may be diagnosed.

The esophagogram is confined to those patients with a normal barium swallow, in whom an H-type TEF is still suspected. It requires an injection of water-soluble, nonionic contrast down an esophageal tube with the child in the prone position. A video recording of the fully distended esophagus in the lateral projection is essential since films are too slow to detect the small TEF.

Ultrasound (US)

The pathology must lie adjacent to the pleura or heart since aerated lung prevents the US waves from reaching the pathological area. In the opaque hemithorax on chest radiograph, i.e. lung white-out, US may distinguish between the presence of fluid, a mass or lung collapse. When a peripheral lung mass is present then ultrasound can determine if this is cystic, e.g. hydatid, or solid, e.g. tumor.

Occasionally in a child with pneumonia it is difficult both clinically and radiologically to assess how much fluid is present in addition to the consolidation; US is useful if the consolidation is basal, especially on the right. Effusion and empyema may require tapping or draining; US has been useful in defining the appropriate site. The diaphragm is well visualized by US especially on the right and therefore may be useful when defects are suspected. Antenatal diagnosis of thoracic pathology is no longer a rarity; diaphragmatic hernia, adenomatoid malformations as well as fluid collections in the lungs may alert the pediatrician to the birth of an infant who may require the facilities of a neonatal intensive care team (Cave & Adam 1984).

Children with stridor in whom the diagnosis of extrinsic compression is being considered should undergo US examination. US is sensitive in the detection of the aortic arch and may thus pick up the right-sided aortic arch and ligamentum teres or the double aortic arch. The detection of an aberrant left pulmonary artery arising from the right pulmonary artery and swinging back to the left between the esophagus and trachea may be missed on US.

In cases of suspected sequestrated segment US has been able to show the feeding vessel arising from the abdominal aorta.

Radioisotope investigation (Figs 12.7c and d, 12.8e and f, 12.9c, d, h and i)

Isotope scans provide a functional image which may be quantified; this contrasts with the anatomical information available from radiology and makes the two examinations complementary.

Krypton-81m (^{81m}Kr) Ventilation/technetium (^{99m}Tc) macroaggregate (MAA) perfusion lung scan (^{81m}Kr V/^{99m}Tc MAA Q)

Sequential images of both ventilation and perfusion can be obtained in children of any age. V/Q scans have been carried out in the newborn. Multiple views are obtained so that a three-dimensional image of the lungs is built up. ^{81m}Kr is an inert radioisotope gas with a half-life of 13 s. The inspired air/^{81m}Kr mixture never reaches equilibrium in the alveoli airspaces. The image is therefore of alveolar ventilation and not lung volume.

This holds true for all children over 1–2 years but in the neonate/infant the high respiratory rate may invalidate this situation so that the ^{81m}KrV scan may reflect a complex lung volume/specific ventilation situation. Xenon-133 (^{133}Xe) is used in many institutions where Kr is unavailable. The advantages of this gas are its free availability and relatively long half-life of 5.3 days; the disadvantages are the relatively high radiation dose. It is absorbed when given via i.v. infusion resulting in a high background activity and, most importantly, it requires very good patient cooperation so that it is used with difficulty in the child under 6 years old. Only a single posterior view can be obtained and therefore it is difficult to compare the ^{99m}Tc MAA Q scan images with the ^{133}Xe image. In the older cooperative child the ability to carry out a wash-in, equilibrium image and wash-out allows assessment of gas trapping.

The use of labeled particles to monitor mucociliary clearance requires a cooperative child breathing ^{99m}Tc-labeled microspheres. Relatively large particles are required and imaging must take place over some hours. In this circumstance a ^{99m}Tc MAA perfusion scan should be done 48 h preceding the mucociliary study.

^{99m}Tc MAA are injected i.v. and are stopped by the first capillary bed, normally the lungs. This gives images of pulmonary perfusion. In pulmonary hypertension caution should be exercised but a perfusion scan may be undertaken if clinically indicated. In the presence of right-to-left shunts perfusion lung scans have been used without ill effect; the ^{99m}Tc MAA are then seen in the systemic circulation (kidneys and brain).

The V/Q images reflect regional lung function. There is no other noninvasive method available to assess regional V/Q. Indications for V/Q scanning include establishing the diagnosis in children with suspected pulmonary artery pathology, e.g. absent pulmonary artery or segmental pulmonary artery stenosis. In the small lung/small hemithorax or a hyperlucent lung the final diagnosis may be made when the chest radiograph is taken in conjunction with the V/Q scan and fluoroscopy. Conditions such as congenital absence of the pulmonary artery, hypoplastic lung, sequestrated lung segment and Macleod's syndrome can be distinguished. The diagnoses of bronchiectasis or inhaled foreign body may be excluded by a normal lung scan. The extent of the disease may be established in certain chronic disorders, e.g. cystic fibrosis or bronchiectasis; the CT scan could provide similar information. The effect of treatment, both medical as in chronic lung disease and surgical for pulmonary arterial pathology, can be monitored. This is the only noninvasive means of following results of pulmonary arterial surgery.

The ^{81m}Kr V lung scan gives a very small radiation dose so that in a V/Q scan the majority of the dose is from the ^{99m}Tc MAA. The dose varies with age and is equivalent to 1.5 min screening by fluoroscopy.

Radioisotope milk scan

This is used for evaluation of gastroesophageal reflux and pulmonary aspiration. ^{99m}Tc sulfur colloid is added to a normal feed (5 µCi/100 ml). Following the feed a small volume of nonradioisotope fluid is given to clear any activity from the esophagus. Infants are cuddled for 5 min; all children are placed supine over the gamma camera. Continuous imaging for 1 h then takes place with delayed images of the lungs 3–5 h after completion of the feed. The Tc sulfur colloid has a particle size of about 50 µm

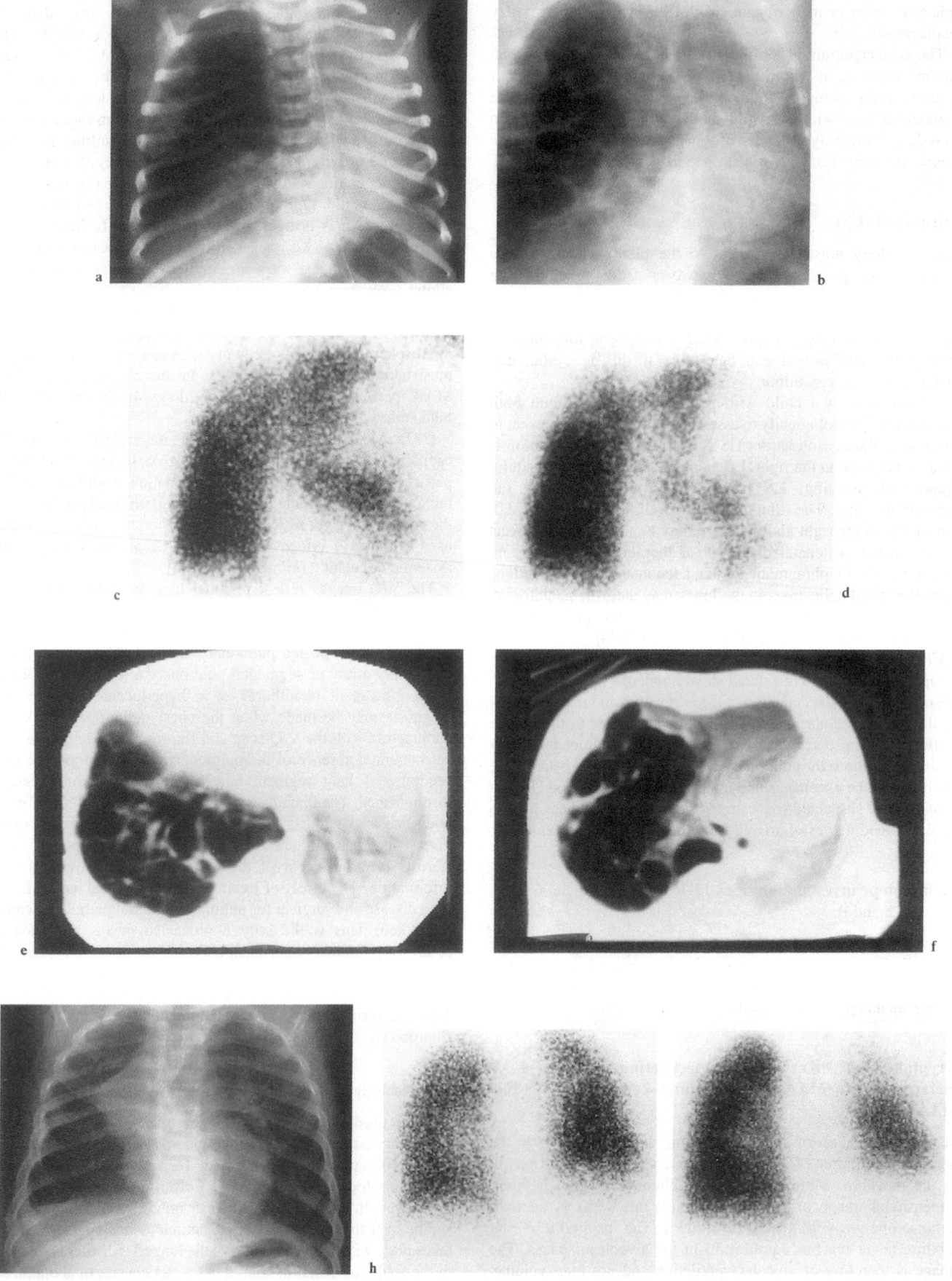

and is not absorbed by the gut mucosa. When aspiration occurs the activity may be seen in the lung. Ciliary movement and bronchial clearance seem to be relatively ineffective in removing the aspirated isotope. It is imperative to have the gamma camera linked to a computer system in order to analyze the results since one must be able to look at the esophageal area and lung fields independently of the high activity in the stomach.

This test is more sensitive than a barium swallow in detecting gastroesophageal reflux since the esophagus is studied for up to 60 min continuously. Quantification of the reflux permits assessment of therapy. Early reports suggested that this technique might be useful in detecting lung aspiration but this has not been substantiated.

Computed tomography (Fig. 12.9e and f)

Indications for CT include looking for lung metastases in children with known solid tumors. This should be done at presentation and also when there is suspicion of a lesion on the chest radiograph. Every child with a primary thoracic cage mass, e.g. Ewing's tumor, or tumor involving the pleura, e.g. small round cell tumor of uncertain origin, requires a CT scan. Certain solid tumors, e.g. osteogenic sarcoma and yolk sac tumors, require a CT scan at presentation and also for follow-up. Lung parenchymal pathology is well shown. CT is useful in certain cases of bronchiectasis. In other diffuse lung disease, e.g. cystic fibrosis, the role of CT is not well established. In cases of suspected sequestrated segment CT has been able to show the feeding vessel arising from the abdominal aorta but not always the venous drainage. Mediastinal pathology is well visualized and tissue characterization allows differentiation of solid from cystic lesions.

The high radiation burden of CT means that this examination should be carried out only when there is no other technique to obtain the information.

Magnetic resonance imaging (Fig. 12.8g)

MRI creates images by rapidly changing the strong magnetic field applied to the body; no radiation is involved. The images are very sensitive to motion artefact and so normal cardiac pulsation as well as respiratory movement create artefacts. With cardiac gating the cardiac motion can be removed but this is not yet true for respiration. This equipment is expensive and therefore not widely available. Its role in chest pathology is still being established. The technique is proving of great value in looking at the anatomy of the pulmonary veins and for certain pathology related to the pulmonary artery, e.g. aberrant left pulmonary artery. It may further reduce the indications for arteriography of the lungs.

BRONCHOSCOPY

The passage of instruments through the larynx to visualize, sample and manipulate the airways is a procedure with applications in many areas of pediatric practice. New diagnostic and therapeutic procedures continue to be described and the full potential of bronchoscopy has yet to be realized.

The first instrument to be developed was the rigid bronchoscope. Its use invariably requires children to be ventilated under general anesthesia. Its wide caliber enables good control of airway patency for prolonged periods and it remains the bronchoscope of choice for foreign body removal, tissue resection and the biopsy of tumor masses where there is a risk of copious hemorrhage. The placing of telescopic sites into the bronchoscope enables excellent visualization of the airway but access to the upper lobes and the distal bronchi is limited. The rigid scope enables good visualization of the posterior wall of the larynx and its use should be considered when looking for a laryngeal cleft or H-type tracheoesophageal fistula in this area. Subglottic edema as a result of the procedure can lead to worsening stridor.

The second type of instrument to become available was the flexible bronchoscope. Light is transmitted to visualize the airway through a solid bundle of glass fibers. The standard pediatric bronchoscope has a 3.4–3.7 mm external diameter with a 1.2 mm suction channel.

The channel can be used to perform saline bronchoalveolar lavage (BAL), bronchial brushings and bronchial biopsy in children as young as 1 month. The airways of neonates can be visualized with the 2.2 mm scope but this does not have a suction channel. The small adult 4.9 mm scope can be used in children aged over 7 years. Its larger working channel enables better suctioning of mucopurulent plugs and the passage of larger biopsy forceps to obtain tissue samples by fluoroscopically controlled transbronchial biopsy.

In most cases, flexible bronchoscopy can be safely performed using sedation and topical anesthesia (Raine & Warner 1991). Adequate sedation can be achieved in most cases by using up to 0.3 mg/kg of midazolam plus 1–2 mg/kg of pethidine. Two percent solutions of lignocaine are used for topical anesthesia above the cords and 1% solutions are used to anesthetize the trachea and main bronchi up to a maximum dose of 7 mg/kg. The topical vasoconstrictor oxymetazoline can be used to enlarge the nasal airway and ease the passage of the bronchoscope. Maintaining verbal contact with the child enables them to cooperate during the procedure whilst the operator gives appropriate instruction and reassurance. Allowing the child to breathe spontaneously enables a better assessment of dynamic function in situations where airway narrowing is suspected. Procedures should take place in a setting where there are facilities for oxygen and suction,

Fig. 12.9 This neonate had progressive respiratory distress at 4 h of age. The pregnancy and labour were uneventful. (a) PA chest radiograph shows the mediastinum deviated to the left with compression of the left lung. The right hemithorax is transradiant. (b) High kV filter radiograph shows numerous opacities through the transradiant right lung. The deviated mediastinum is again clearly demonstrated. These features suggested the diagnosis of cystic adenomatoid malformation of either the entire right lung or a lobe. (c) Krypton-81m ventilation lung scan. The left lung is normally ventilated whilst on the right there is a defect in the upper outer portion and also in the inferomedial aspect of this lung but the compressed right upper lobe is well ventilated as is the compressed middle lobe. (d) ^{99m}Tc macroaggregate perfusion scan. The left lung is normal. The right lung shows a similar appearance to that seen on the ventilation scan with quite good perfusion of the right upper and middle lobes only. (e) CT scan shows the cystic spaces within the overinflated right lobe to better advantage. (f) A higher CT scan cut shows the relatively normal right upper lobe which is displaced across the midline by the pathological right lower lobe. This child underwent right lower lobe lobectomy. (g) The postoperative chest radiograph at the age of 9 months shows the mediastinum is now central with obliteration of the right costophrenic angle and distortion of the mediastinum presumably by postoperative fibrosis. (h) The krypton-81m ventilation lung scan. The right lung shows good ventilation of the middle and lower zones but when taken in conjunction with the chest radiograph that part of the lung overinflated and lying immediately above the right hemidiaphragm is not participating in ventilation. (i) ^{99m}Tc macroaggregate perfusion scan shows the right lung not as well perfused as it is ventilated with the area of compensatory emphysema in the right lower zone being most affected.

equipment for monitoring of heart rate and oxygen saturation and facilities for full resuscitation. Personnel should include the bronchoscopist, an assistant and at least one other person to observe and monitor the patient's condition. A video camera and recorder are ideal for documenting clinical findings.

Bronchoscopy is contraindicated in circumstances where the relative benefits of the procedure are outweighed by its risks. Complications are more likely in children with unstable asthma, large hemoptysis, uncorrectable bleeding diatheses, severe airways obstruction, pulmonary hypertension, severe hypoxia and lung abscess where there is a danger of spreading pus throughout the lung following rupture of the cavity. When performed by properly trained personnel under carefully controlled conditions, bronchoscopy is a low-risk procedure. Complications include episodes of hypoxemia and bradycardia but these are usually transient and self-limiting. More serious problems include laryngospasm and pneumothorax but these are rare. Small hemoptyses commonly follow biopsy procedures and a transient pyrexia can be anticipated after bronchoalveolar lavage.

INDICATIONS FOR BRONCHOSCOPY (Wood & Postma 1988).

General

All infants with atypical, severe, progressive or biphasic chronic stridor should be investigated by flexible fiberoptic bronchoscopy under sedation to exclude lesions other than laryngomalacia. A complete bronchoscopy is mandatory. Up to 15% of children with upper airway problems as a cause of symptoms will also have significant lesions below the glottis. Bronchoscopy should also be considered when evaluating infants with recurrent obstructive apnea.

Persistent or recurrent wheezing and/or pneumonia might benefit from bronchoscopy to exclude anatomical abnormalities and the possibility of a foreign body. Lavage specimens should be obtained and sent for microbiology, virology and cytological studies. Acute atelectasis and obstructive hyperinflation that do not improve after antibiotics and physiotherapy might be resolved by the use of a flexible bronchoscope to aspirate mucous plugs or thick secretions. The local instillation of mucolytic agents such as DNase during such procedures might be of added benefit. Unfortunately the benefits from therapeutic bronchoscopies in children with cystic fibrosis and diffuse mucoid impaction are rarely sustained.

Bronchial biopsy is a useful clinical procedure that might provide diagnostic information when there is a suspicion of granulomatous disease (i.e. tuberculosis, sarcoidosis) and where there is unexplained inflammation of bronchial mucosa. However, there is conflicting evidence as to whether samples obtained by bronchoscopy are superior to gastric lavage in making a microbiological diagnosis of tuberculosis.

Transbronchial biopsy has been used to diagnose infiltrative lung disorders as an alternative technique to open or percutaneous lung biopsy but tissue samples might not always be sufficient to make a definitive diagnosis. Ciliary dyskinesia can usually be diagnosed using material obtained through nasal brushings without the need for brush biopsy of the lower respiratory tract.

Other indications for bronchoscopy include the evaluation of children with unexplained hemoptysis and the assessment of airway patency in children with tracheostomy tubes. More specialized uses include selective bronchography, laser ablation of endobronchial lesions, placement of bronchial stents, balloon dilatation of tracheobronchial stenoses and large volume lavage to treat alveolar proteinosis.

Immunocompromised patients (De Blic et al 1987)

Children with HIV infection and primary immunodeficiency and those receiving immunosuppressive agents are at risk of significant morbidity and mortality from pulmonary complications. When less invasive techniques are unsuccessful in diagnosing pulmonary lesions, BAL might usefully identify the causal agents. Specimens must be processed immediately after collection. The chances of making a positive diagnosis are increased when BAL is performed early in the course of pulmonary complications and before exposure to broad-spectrum antibiotics. The use of semiquantitative culture of BAL fluid can usefully distinguish true pathogens from contaminating organisms. Bronchial brush biopsy, especially when done with a protected brush, is a useful complementary method for obtaining specimens from the lower respiratory tract whilst minimizing upper airway contamination.

Transbronchial biopsy is a useful technique for diagnosing early signs of rejection in children who have undergone lung transplantation and for obtaining alveolar tissue when viral pneumonitis is suspected.

Intensive care (De Blic et al 1991)

Flexible bronchoscopy is useful to assess the airways of children who have failed a trial of extubation. Bronchoscopes have been used to facilitate difficult intubations and to check the positioning of endotracheal tubes without the need for X-ray confirmation. It is increasingly being used in the neonatal intensive care unit to investigate the complications of mechanical ventilation.

Research (Special Article 1991)

Aliquots of BAL fluid obtained by bronchoscopy for clinical indications should be retained for research purposes whenever possible. Consistent lavage and biopsy procedures should be carried out so that normal ranges for cell cytology, immunochemistry and histological appearances can be established for children of all ages.

Bronchoscopy is now established as a useful procedure in the management of cystic fibrosis. Lavage specimens provide information about the onset of inflammatory disease and the identification of lower respiratory pathogens in nonproductive patients (Khan et al 1995). Bronchoscopy might soon have a place in directing the need for therapy in children with asthma and many other chronic lung diseases. The development of new technology will continue to increase the uses of bronchoscopic techniques to the benefit of pediatric patients.

SPECIAL ASPECTS OF TREATMENT

MISCELLANEOUS

BEDSIDE SURGICAL PROCEDURES

Pleural tap and intercostal drainage

A pleural effusion (pus, exudate or transudate) should be tapped for diagnostic purposes. Effusions secondary to hypoalbuminemia can cause dyspnea and can be tapped for therapeutic purposes. This should be done after careful physical examination, chest radiograph (with lateral and penetrated views) and only if no major disorder of coagulation is suspected. If cloudy fluid or frank pus, is withdrawn, a tube can be inserted for closed tube drainage during the same procedure and streptokinase instilled. If an empyema is a serious possibility, the correct preparations (including ultrasound) should be undertaken and made ready before the tap (p. 568). Young children should be sedated orally, where safe to do so, with chloral (50–100 mg/kg) or trimeprazine (4 mg/kg). The surface markings should be used to locate a safe site over the effusion, with the infant lying or the older child sitting, arms raised and resting over a bed table.

A topical transdermal local anesthetic patch should be applied to the chosen site 30 min before starting. Local anesthetic (lignocaine 0.5% without adrenaline) is infiltrated down to the pleura. An intravenous cannula (size 16–20) is inserted over the inferior rib at the chosen intercostal site and the trochar removed and replaced with a 60 ml syringe and a three-way tap as the pleura is perforated. Fluid can then be safely aspirated and, using the three-way tap, ejected into sterile containers for analysis (bacteriology, cytology, protein estimation, etc.). If the effusion is chronic, no more than 1000 ml should be removed from a teenager (or the equivalent from young children); acute pulmonary edema or pulmonary hemorrhage may be precipitated.

Spontaneous pneumothorax can be drained if necessary using a similar procedure and repeated as needed. The operator should be sure that the lesion is indeed an air leak and not cystic disease before starting the procedure.

Insertion of an intercostal drain, ideally by a thoracic surgeon, may be required for empyema and for negative pressure, underwater seal drainage of a persistent, large or tension pneumothorax. If a loculated empyema is suspected on an ultrasound or CT scan, thoracotomy which allows adhesions to be broken followed by insertion of a wide-bore drain is usual (see section on empyema, p. 568).

A plain chest X-ray should be taken after needling the chest and inspected for pneumothorax as well as for diagnostic clues revealed by removal of the effusion.

Pleural biopsy

This procedure is occasionally used in pediatrics, in the diagnosis of chronic pleural effusion. Tuberculosis, neoplasia or a disorder of connective tissue may be diagnosed on histology. A pediatric Abrams pleural biopsy punch is available for young children. After sedation and local anesthesia, the procedure can be carried out at the same time as a diagnostic pleural tap. Brisk hemorrhage can ensue if an intercostal artery is torn. The procedure is best performed by an experienced operator.

PHYSIOTHERAPY

The main functions of physiotherapy are to facilitate removal of airway secretions and to promote re-expansion of collapsed lung. The physiotherapist is essentially a teacher, since only a small proportion of chest physiotherapy takes place in hospital. Recently, many physiotherapists have taken the role of advisors in asthma therapy, teaching children to use inhalation devices and peak flow meters.

Postural drainage followed by percussion is indicated on a regular basis (increasing in frequency to 4–6 times daily during exacerbations) in bronchiectasis, disorders of host defense, cystic fibrosis and temporarily following pneumonia (after the acute stage), whooping cough, aspiration or other conditions leading to focal collapse or consolidation. Postural drainage with 'huffing' is an effective alternative which requires no assistant. As an alternative to manual percussion, many teenagers with cystic fibrosis use electrical vibrators to administer their own 'percussion' (see section on cystic fibrosis, p. 550). This sort of physiotherapy has no part to play in asthma. During quiescent phases, children with cystic fibrosis benefit from regular energetic games as an adjunct to percussion drainage.

Breathing exercises have sometimes been advocated for asthmatics, as an aid to relaxation during acute attacks. They should never be used to replace or postpone drug therapy and have a role only in the management of older, cooperative children, subject to severe acute attacks, as a temporary means of allaying anxiety. There may also be a place for them in dealing with children with laryngeal dysfunction syndrome. Postoperative breathing exercises may be valuable in preventing basal collapse or consolidation after major abdominal surgery.

Formal chest physiotherapy has no role in acute pneumonia, asthma, bronchiolitis or croup. In fact, there may be adverse effects, leading in extreme cases to respiratory failure. During recovery from pneumonia, normal childhood activities are adequate.

Children with severe neuromuscular diseases, such as spinal muscular atrophy or terminal muscular dystrophy, commonly develop persistent chest infection, often accompanied by bronchial plugging and atelectasis. In addition to formal percussion drainage, positive pressure breathing, with or without nebulized bronchodilator therapy, may help. Bronchoscopy, followed by intensive physiotherapy and antibiotic therapy, is sometimes needed to re-expand a collapsed segment.

OXYGEN THERAPY

The amelioration of hypoxemia is a vital but often neglected part of respiratory therapy. Modern monitoring techniques permit accurate control of the inspired oxygen concentration. The trend towards deterioration or recovery can thus be easily determined and appropriate action taken. Oxygen therapy should be monitored by noninvasive methods. Pulse oximetry is most accurate at around 80–95% saturation and is the safest method. Transcutaneous oxygen monitors are trend indicators, since their accuracy is variable and diminishes with age beyond infancy. Direct arterial blood gas measurements (via an indwelling cannula) are essential if there is any suspicion of respiratory failure. Transcutaneous CO_2 measurements may thereafter provide an indication of trend. The need for resiting to prevent focal burns to the skin is a minor problem.

Oxygen may be administered by headbox or tent (up to 30%) in infants or by face mask in older children. A funnel over the child's face, supplied from a pipe coming over mother's shoulder, may be the best technique for a frightened toddler on mother's lap. A single nasal catheter such as an infant feeding tube passed along the floor of the nose to the nasopharynx or short nasal cannulae or 'spectacles' allow continuous low flow oxygen therapy for home or hospital use in acute disease (supplanting headboxes and tents) and in chronically oxygen-dependent children (e.g. chronic postneonatal lung disease, late-stage respiratory failure in cystic fibrosis). Fast flows may reduce the oxygen concentration by a

Venturi effect. If oxygen therapy is likely to continue for more than a few weeks, an oxygen concentrator should be installed in the home. Except where very low flow oxygen therapy is used, inspired gases should be humidified to prevent distressing nasal crusting. Only in chronic respiratory failure with hypercapnia may uncontrolled oxygen therapy, by removing hypoxic respiratory drive, exacerbate respiratory failure. This situation is very unusual in pediatric practice, except in end-stage disease or in chronic neuromuscular or skeletal disease (e.g. scoliosis).

RESUSCITATION (Respiratory support: see Ch. 32)

In infants and children the need for resuscitation is usually as a result of an airway or breathing problem. This is in contrast to the adult situation where collapse is most commonly as a result of an acute cardiac event. Trauma is the most common cause of death in the first four decades of life; sudden infant death syndrome is the most common cause in the first year. Circulatory hypovolemia from the sudden loss of blood or body fluids (gastroenteritis), congenital heart disease and septicemia are other notable causes of cardiac arrest in the young. Hypoxia is the precipitating factor and rapidly leads on to cardiac arrest in infants and children if not treated appropriately. The results of pediatric life support are poor and this is usually attributed to the different etiology with a prolonged hypoxic period prior to the final cardiac event. Resuscitation rates for infants and children are quoted at about 9% survival, but many of these have severe neurological impairment.

Collecting scientific data on pediatric life support events is difficult as the occurrences are infrequent. Many of the studies on which the resuscitation protocols have been based are small or, in an effort to collect substantial numbers, are spread over a number of years. The publication of the Utstein templates (Zaritsky et al 1995) for data storage and audit has resulted in the collection of standardized data using international definitions. This has allowed many small studies to be integrated so as to produce a sizable statistical cohort. The International Liaison Committee on Resuscitation (ILCOR) has reviewed the published scientific data and has published a series of advisory statements, including one on pediatric life support (Nadkarni et al 1997).

Definitions

Infant. An infant is a child under the age of 1 year.
Child. A child is aged between 1 and 8 years of age.

Children over the age of 8 years will still be treated as for a younger child but may require different techniques to attain adequate chest compressions.

BASIC LIFE SUPPORT (Fig. 12.10)

Immediate resuscitation performed without equipment is known as basic life support. It consists of the simple ABC maneuvers of opening and maintaining the airway, assessing breathing, providing expired air respiration, assessing the circulation and performing external chest compressions. Resuscitation must begin immediately and must not await a diagnosis or the arrival of resuscitation equipment. It is essential to commence basic life support and to maintain it until advanced cardiac life support, with its equipment and drugs, arrives.

Airway

Basic cardiac life support starts with opening the airway by tilting the head and supporting the lower jaw. Care must be taken not to overextend the neck of the child as this may cause kinking and obstruction of the trachea. In children where trauma has been the cause of the event, it is important not to tilt the head because of a potential cervical spine injury. In these cases the jaw thrust maneuver is recommended. Maintaining the airway requires careful attention to detail. Care must be taken not to push on the soft tissues in the floor of the mouth and only to 'lift' directly on the mandible.

Infectious diseases affecting the upper airway may cause serious or fatal consequences if not recognized or dealt with properly. An inspiratory stridor is usually the first sign and the child may prefer to sit up and lean forward to aid his airway maintenance and breathing. A humidified atmosphere is also helpful but further active intervention may worsen the situation. The child must be carefully moved, with adequate care and supervision, to a properly equipped hospital where expert staff are available.

Breathing

The three ways of checking for breathing are:

1. *looking* for chest movements
2. *listening* for breathing over the mouth
3. *feeling* for air movement over the mouth.

If no breathing is detected, expired air respiration must be commenced without delay. Mouth to mouth (for children) or mouth to mouth and nose (for infants) are the most effective methods. Expired air is blown into the child's lungs until the chest starts to expand and the child appears to have taken a deep breath. Up to five individual breaths are given. High airway pressures and hyperventilation must be avoided as gas will pass into the stomach and cause vomiting. Should the child only require expired air ventilation, this should be carried out at 15–30 breaths/min according to the size of the child.

If the chest of the child fails to rise then it must be assumed that the attempt at ventilation of the lungs has failed. Reposition the airway, ensuring that the neck is not overextended. Check the mouth for any visible foreign body. Removal of foreign bodies from the airway must also be performed with due care. Initially, simple and careful finger sweeps may remove the object. Blind probing of the airway or an indifferent technique may result in trauma, hemorrhage, edema formation, or further impaction of the foreign material. If these simple maneuvers are not sufficient to clear the airway, the child should be tilted head down and five back slaps applied to the centre of the back. These back slaps work in two ways, firstly by vibration, to loosen the object, and secondly by providing 'mini-coughs' or forced expirations, briefly squeezing the chest between the sternum and the vertebral column with each slap. If this fails the child should be turned back and five chest thrusts applied to the lower half of the sternum. The airway should then be inspected and, if the child is still not breathing, then rescue breathing should be attempted. Should ventilation fail again, then the sequence of back slaps, chest thrusts, airway inspection and ventilation should be repeated, but in children five abdominal thrusts should be substituted for five chest thrusts in alternate cycles. Abdominal thrusts are not recommended for infants as they may damage abdominal organs.

Pediatric Basic Life Support

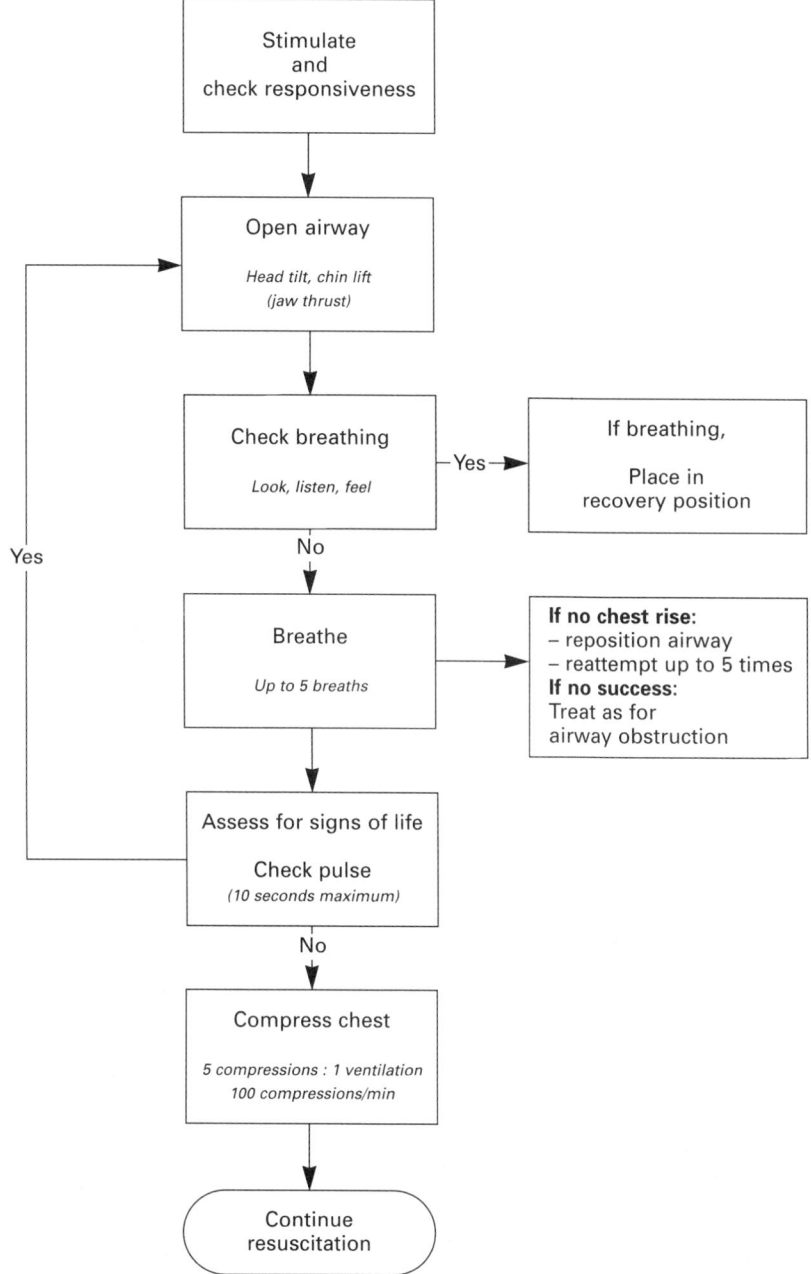

Fig. 12.10   Pediatric basic life support.

Circulation

Following the rescue breathing assess the child (swallowing, movement, breathing) and, if not present, check for a pulse. Check the pulse by feeling the brachial pulse in infants or the carotid pulse in children. Take no more than 10 secs for the pulse check. Bradycardia may be just as detrimental as asystole. A heart rate < 60 beats/min may indicate early hypoxia and must be treated immediately by effective ventilation and external chest compressions. If no pulse is felt or if there is a bradycardia, then external chest compressions must be performed. Compressions

are performed on the lower half of the sternum. For infants this position is identified as one finger breadth below the imaginary line joining the nipples. Compressions are carried out using the tips of two fingers, pressing vertically one-third of the resting diameter of the chest, at a rate of 100 compressions per min. Interpose one ventilation between every five chest compressions (compressions : ventilation ratio 5 : 1). For children place the heel of one hand over the lower half of the sternum, taking care not to compress on or below the xiphisternum, and compress to a depth of one-third of the resting diameter of the chest. The compression : ventilation ratio is still 5 : 1 and the compression rate is 100 compressions per min. The accuracy of the rate and depth of compression is not vitally important; again the rescuer should be confident enough to be able to adapt his technique to achieve the best result. In the older child, where the one-handed chest compression technique does not produce an adequate compression depth, use the 'adult' two-handed technique; place one hand on the lower half of the sternum placing the second hand on top of the first. Interlace the fingers so as not to press on the lateral chest wall. Compress the chest 4–5 cm at 100 compressions per min in a ventilation to compression ratio of 2 : 15.

Basic cardiac life support should be continued until the equipment for advanced cardiac life support has arrived. It should not cease at this point but should remain an ongoing procedure carried out until either recovery or the decision to terminate resuscitation is made.

ADVANCED LIFE SUPPORT (Fig. 12.11)

The use of equipment in pediatric resuscitation is fraught with difficulties. The variation in size of patients, from the infant to the average adolescent, requires the availability and the correct selection of suitable apparatus from a wide range of equipment together with an accurate knowledge of the appropriate doses of resuscitation drugs. Much of this knowledge together with the skills necessary to use the equipment can only be gained by repeated training and supervised practice.

Airway

The Guedel oropharyngeal airway is probably the simplest and best known airway device. The correct size must be selected (range from 000 to 4). If too small it will not overcome obstruction caused by the tongue, and if too large, it may damage the posterior pharyngeal wall. Some authorities are now recommending the laryngeal mask airway for resuscitation in adults, but the use of this device has yet to be evaluated in the pediatric context.

Tracheal intubation is the only way of providing a guaranteed airway. Intubation requires skills acquired only through training and repeated practice. To perform tracheal intubation, a complete range of size of tracheal tubes must be available. The selection of the correct size of tube is made by referring to a chart (Table 12.12) or can be approximated by using a simple formula: internal diameter of the tube (mm) is equal to (age divided by 4) + 4. Once selected the tracheal tube must be cut to the appropriate length to prevent inadvertent intubation of one or other main bronchus. Following intubation the chest must be auscultated to ensure equal ventilation of both lungs and the tube must be firmly fixed in position to prevent accidental movement or inadvertent extubation.

The appropriate size of tracheal tube connector must be at hand. The 15/22 mm British Standard connector will fit directly on to most self-inflating resuscitation bags. If other connectors are used then a suitable adaptor must be available to allow connection to the ventilation system. Intubation in children is usually carried out with a straight blade laryngoscope but in an emergency a curved adult blade could be used with extreme care. There are a wide variety of sizes and designs of straight blades but the overall need is for the operator to directly elevate the relatively long, floppy epiglottis with the flat tip of the blade, so as to be able to directly

Table 12.12 Tracheal tube size and length

Age	Tracheal tube internal diameter (mm)	Length (cm) Oral	Length (cm) Nasal	Suction catheter (FG)
Premature	2.5–3.0	11	13.5	6
Newborn	3.5	12	14	8
1 year	4.0	13	15	8
2 years	4.5	14	16	8
4 years	5.0	15	17	10
6 years	5.5	17	19	10
8 years	6.0	19	21	10
10 years	6.5	20	22	10
12 years	7.0	21	22	10
14 years	7.5	22	23	10
16 years	8.0	23	24	12

view the laryngeal opening. Finally a range of appropriately sized suction catheters must also be provided to keep the airway clear.

Breathing

The addition of oxygen to the inspired air will speed recovery and may, in some cases, prevent further deterioration. If the child is not breathing then a self-inflating bag–valve–mask system should be used. Clear plastic face masks are best as they allow direct observation of the child's color and airway without removal of the mask. The circular design of face mask is simple to use and one size will fit a wide range of sizes of children. Selection of the correct size of resuscitation bag depends on the age and weight of the child (Table 12.13). The two smaller bags are fitted with pressure limiting valves preset to allow up to 40 cmH$_2$O inspiratory pressure to prevent excessive pressurization in the child's lungs. This valve can be manually overridden to achieve higher pressures in noncompliant lungs or where there is a high airway resistance. Most self-inflating bag–valve–mask systems are fitted with a 22 mm connector which will directly accept the 15 mm male connector of a tracheal tube. Supplemental oxygen can be added to the resuscitation bag via an inspiratory reservoir system. The Jackson–Rees modification of the Ayre's T-piece is an anesthetic ventilation circuit which requires experience to achieve inspiration by occluding the tail of the bag at the same time as squeezing the ventilation bag. Accidental prolonged occlusion of the bag tail can lead to overinflation of the lungs and may cause a pneumothorax. This T-piece circuit should not be part of the routine resuscitation equipment.

Automatic resuscitators/ventilators are not recommended for use in acute resuscitation in children. Many adult automatic resuscitation models have been adapted to run at higher ventilatory frequencies and small tidal volumes, but unfortunately,

Table 12.13 Resuscitation bags

Age and weight	Bag volume (ml)	Tidal volume (ml)
<2 years (<7 kg)	240	205
2–10 years (7–30 kg)	500	350
>10 years (>30 kg)	1600	1000

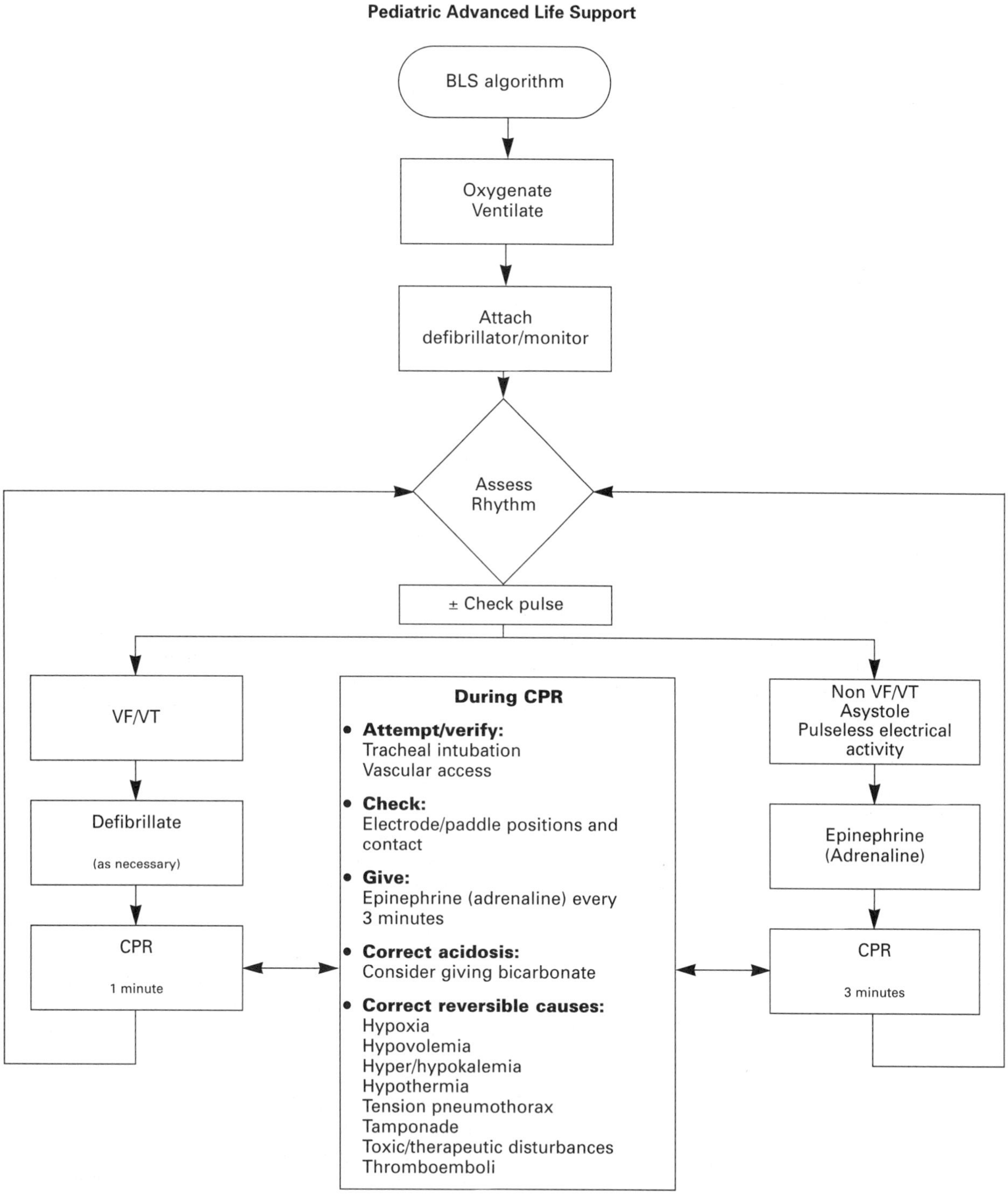

Pediatric Advanced Life Support

Fig. 12.11   Pediatric advanced life support.

Circulation

Cardiac rate and rhythm are best assessed using an electrocardiographic monitor (ECG) or via the paddles of a defibrillator. The procedures to be carried out next will depend on the electrocardiographic diagnosis. Hypoxia is usually associated these two features are often locked to a preset ratio which does not allow the flexibility required for children in emergencies.

with a bradycardia or asystole and ventricular fibrillation is rarely seen.

The procedures divide into those for asystole and pulseless electrical activity (non-VF/VT) and those for ventricular fibrillation and pulseless ventricular tachycardia (VF/VT).

Non-VF/VT

Treatment is based on the frequent administration of epinephrine (adrenaline) during maintained cycles of resuscitation. Epinephrine (adrenaline) is the only drug with proved benefit in a cardiac arrest. Spontaneous function of the myocardial pump can resume only if myocardial cells are perfused at an adequate rate with oxygenated blood. In animal experiments this perfusion pressure is at least 1.3–2.6 kPa. Epinephrine increases peripheral vascular resistance and thus aortic 'diastolic' pressure, which is the driving force for coronary perfusion in cardiac arrest. Animal studies show that it is the stimulation of the α-adrenergic receptor that is important in determining outcome in cardiac arrest.

An initial intravenous dose of 10 µg/kg epinephrine (0.1 ml/kg of 1 in 10 000 solution) should be followed by 3 minutes of cardiopulmonary resuscitation. If the rhythm persists then a further intravenous dose of 100 µg/kg epinephrine (1 ml/kg of 1 in 10 000 solution or 0.1 ml/kg of 1 in 1000 solution) should be given and repeated every 3 minutes during cardiopulmonary resuscitation. In addition any reversible cause of the arrhythmia should be looked for and treated. Such causes are hypoxia, hypovolemia, hyper- or hypokalemia, hypothermia, tension pneumothorax, tamponade, toxic disturbances, therapeutic disturbances or thromboemboli.

VF/VT

This is rarely seen in children but if diagnosed a defibrillation shock of 2 J/kg bodyweight should be attempted immediately. This should be rapidly followed by a further shock at 2 J/kg and a third shock at 4 J/kg. The precise calculation of the defibrillation energy is of less importance than a near estimate especially when using defibrillators with preset stepped energy levels. Pediatric paddles are available and the size selected should be that which produces best contact with the child's chest.

If ventricular fibrillation persists resuscitation should be carried out for 1 minute before a further three defibrillation attempts are made at 4 J/kg. The cycle is then repeated until defibrillation is successful. Epinephrine (adrenaline) should be given every 3 minutes during resuscitation to support the circulation.

Fluids and drugs

The administration of drugs and fluids is an essential part of pediatric resuscitation and venous access must be established. Direct venous access is the primary route but intraosseous access is a simple technique that will provide rapid and effective access to the circulation.

For direct venous access the selection of the type and size of cannula remains a matter of personal preference and experience. Establishing central venous access is not recommended during resuscitation as it is a time-consuming procedure which, in children, requires considerable skill. Peripheral venous access is the best route. It is the establishing of venous access which is important and not the route or size of the cannula. A 20 or 22 SWG cannula is perfectly satisfactory for pediatric resuscitation.

Intraosseous venous access is an alternative route of drug administration. An intraosseous cannula is inserted into the bone marrow of the tibia, 1 cm below the tibial plateau. All resuscitation drugs, except for bretylium tosylate, can be administered by this route and have rapid access to the circulation. The doses of drugs given via the intraosseous route are the same as for direct venous administration. Fluids can also be

Table 12.14 Resuscitation drugs

Drug	Dose	Route
Epinephrine (adrenaline)	10 µg/kg (0.1 ml/kg of 1 in 10 000)	Intravenous or endotracheal
Atropine	0.02 mg/kg (maximum 0.6 mg)	Intravenous or endotracheal
Sodium bicarbonate	1 mmol/kg (1 ml/kg of 8.4%)	Intravenous
Lignocaine	1 mg/kg (0.1 ml/kg of 1%)	Intravenous or endotracheal
Dextrose	1 g/kg	Intravenous
Frusemide	1 mg/kg	Intravenous

Infusions (usually in 5% dextrose solution): epinephrine 0.02–0.05 µg/kg/min, isoprenaline 0.05–0.1 µg/kg/min, dopamine 1–10 µg/kg/min (calculate by adding 3 × bodyweight in mg of dopamine to 50 ml of 5% dextrose – infusion in ml/h equivalent to µg/kg/min).

administered by this route but they must be given under pressure to achieve access to the circulation via the marrow cavity.

Drugs can also be given via the tracheal tube although there is some doubt about the effectiveness of drugs given by this route. Epinephrine (adrenaline), atropine and naloxone can be given down the tracheal tube for absorption into the pulmonary circulation. The dose of epinephrine for the tracheal route is 10 times the direct venous dose. A short period of hyperventilation should be used to distribute the drug throughout the lung fields. Direct intracardiac injections are not recommended except in extremis. They have a low success rate and their complication rate is high.

Resuscitation drugs are given according to bodyweight. All children should be weighed immediately on admission to hospital and the doses (and required volumes) of relevant resuscitation drugs precalculated for those children considered to be 'at risk'. In an emergency, the bodyweight may not be known and the following quick guide can be used: infants double their birthweight in 5 months; infants treble their birthweight in 1 year; between 1 and 9 years weight (kg) = (age + 4) × 2; between 7 and 12 years weight (kg) = age × 3.

Table 12.14 gives details of some of the drugs used (see also Ch. 38).

The use of a simple standardized pediatric resuscitation chart minimizes errors in drug administration. Figure 12.12 relates age, height and weight to tracheal tube sizes and the relevant dose of drugs required. By using a simple tape measure the accurate management of a child's resuscitation can be carried out with confidence. Alternatively the Broselow tape measure, a tape measure with precalculated doses of resuscitation drugs and fluids can be used.

Post-resuscitation

If resuscitation is successful the child will need to be carefully looked after in a pediatric high dependency or intensive care area. Medical and nursing care can only be carried out at this level in these specialized areas and this may require transporting the child to another hospital. A fully trained and properly equipped

Pediatric resuscitation chart

Endotracheal tube

Oral length (cm)	Internal diameter (mm)
18–21	7.5–8.0 cuffed
18	7.0 uncuffed
17	6.5
16	6.0
15	5.5
14	5.0
13	4.5
12	4.0
	3.5
10	3.0–3.5

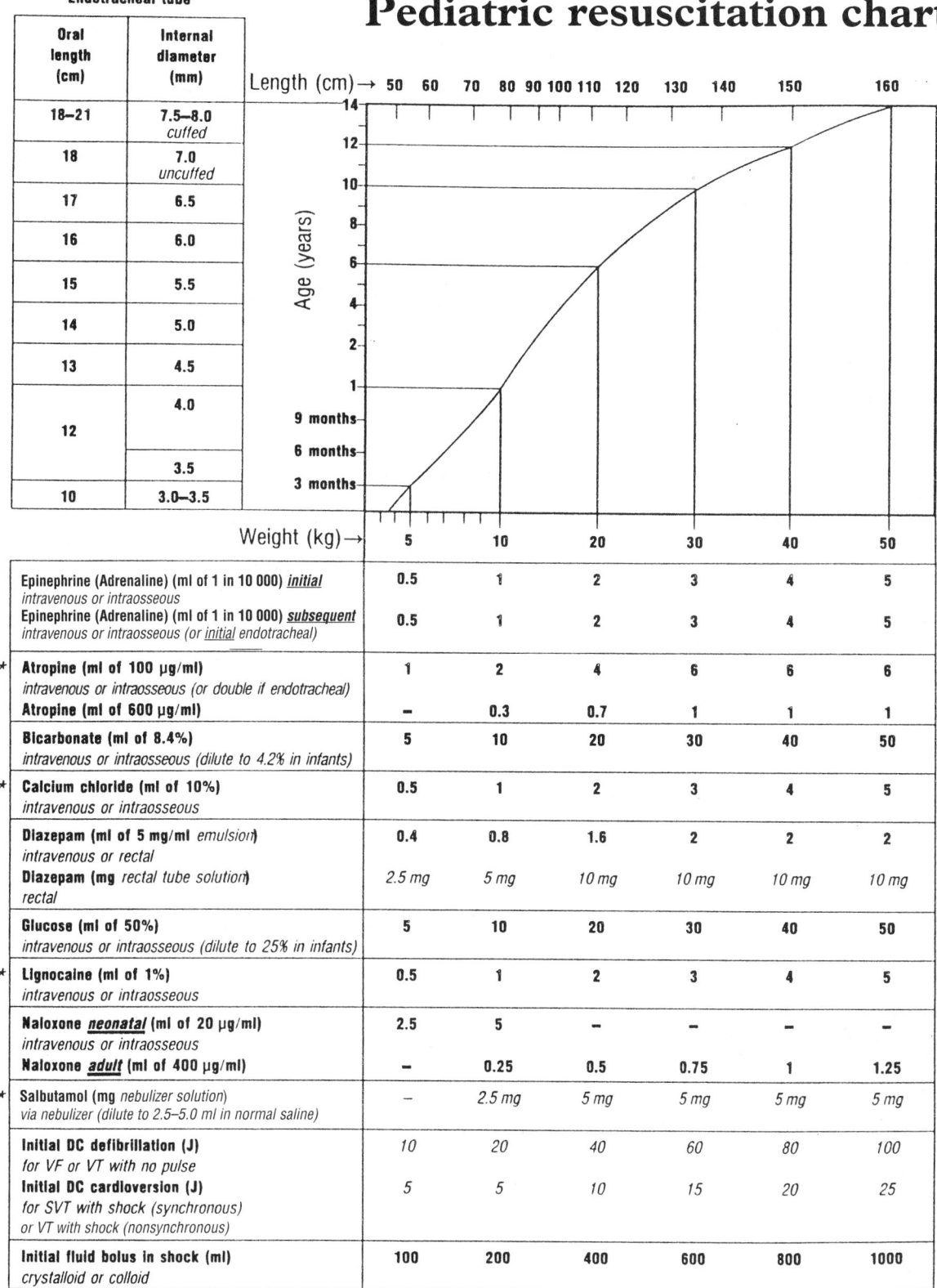

Length (cm) → 50 60 70 80 90 100 110 120 130 140 150 160

Age (years) — 14, 12, 10, 8, 6, 4, 2, 1, 9 months, 6 months, 3 months

Weight (kg) →	5	10	20	30	40	50
Epinephrine (Adrenaline) (ml of 1 in 10 000) *initial* intravenous or intraosseous	0.5	1	2	3	4	5
Epinephrine (Adrenaline) (ml of 1 in 10 000) *subsequent* intravenous or intraosseous (or *initial* endotracheal)	0.5	1	2	3	4	5
* **Atropine (ml of 100 μg/ml)** intravenous or intraosseous (or double if endotracheal)	1	2	4	6	6	6
Atropine (ml of 600 μg/ml)	–	0.3	0.7	1	1	1
Bicarbonate (ml of 8.4%) intravenous or intraosseous (dilute to 4.2% in infants)	5	10	20	30	40	50
* **Calcium chloride (ml of 10%)** intravenous or intraosseous	0.5	1	2	3	4	5
Diazepam (ml of 5 mg/ml emulsion) intravenous or rectal	0.4	0.8	1.6	2	2	2
Diazepam (mg rectal tube solution) rectal	2.5 mg	5 mg	10 mg	10 mg	10 mg	10 mg
Glucose (ml of 50%) intravenous or intraosseous (dilute to 25% in infants)	5	10	20	30	40	50
* **Lignocaine (ml of 1%)** intravenous or intraosseous	0.5	1	2	3	4	5
Naloxone *neonatal* **(ml of 20 μg/ml)** intravenous or intraosseous	2.5	5	–	–	–	–
Naloxone *adult* **(ml of 400 μg/ml)**	–	0.25	0.5	0.75	1	1.25
* **Salbutamol (mg** nebulizer solution) via nebulizer (dilute to 2.5–5.0 ml in normal saline)	–	2.5 mg	5 mg	5 mg	5 mg	5 mg
Initial DC defibrillation (J) for VF or VT with no pulse	10	20	40	60	80	100
Initial DC cardioversion (J) for SVT with shock (synchronous) or VT with shock (nonsynchronous)	5	5	10	15	20	25
Initial fluid bolus in shock (ml) crystalloid or colloid	100	200	400	600	800	1000

* **CAUTION!** *Nonstandard drug concentrations may be available:*
*Use **Atropine** 100 μg/ml or prepare by diluting 1 mg to 10 ml or 600 μg to 6 ml in normal saline.*
*Note that 1 ml of **calcium chloride** 10% is equivalent to 3 ml of **calcium gluconate** 10%.*
*Use **Lignocaine** (without adrenaline) 1% or give twice the volume of 0.5%. Give half the volume of 2% or dilute appropriately.*
***Salbutamol** may also be given by slow intravenous injection (5 μg/kg), but beware of the different concentrations available (e.g. 50 and 500 μg/ml).*

Fig. 12.12   Pediatric resuscitation chart.

transport team must be used to achieve this safely and without any undue risk to the child. A post-resuscitation chest X-ray, serum electrolytes and arterial blood gases may give some indication as to the cause of the arrest. More importantly, they may highlight various factors which need urgent corrective treatment to prevent the event recurring.

APNEA AND BREATHING DISORDERS DURING SLEEP

APPARENT LIFE-THREATENING EVENTS (ALTE)

The occurrence in a young infant of one or more episodes characterized by some combination of cyanosis, marked pallor, apnea, bradycardia and hypertonia or hypotonia is very frightening to parents who are commonly convinced that without some intervention their infant would have died. Since there is no evidence that such an episode would, without intervention, have progressed to sudden death and the great majority of such infants do not die from SIDS, the term 'near miss SIDS' is misleading. Similarly the term 'apnea of infancy' is inaccurate as many such infants do not experience apnea. Episodes of this type may have a wide range of possible causes, so the broad descriptive term 'apparent life-threatening event' is preferable. After investigation some such episodes may be shown to be secondary to a specific disorder (e.g. convulsions, cardiac arrhythmia, apnea, gastroesophageal reflux), but for many the precise cause is not found.

INCIDENCE

Because there is no universally accepted definition and because of the impossibility of being sure from parents' descriptions whether an episode is genuinely life threatening, estimates of the incidence of ALTE vary widely. A large US study of 757 SIDS cases and 1514 control infants found that 7% of parents of SIDS victims and 3% of parents of control infants had seen an ALTE or reported an episode of apnea or apparent lifelessness, whilst in a more recent study in the UK, 13% of 195 SIDS victims and 3.2% of 780 age-matched controls were reported as having had such an episode, though very few of these were of sufficient severity to result in medical attention being sought. Whether this incidence is real or represents selective recall by parents whose baby had died is unclear (Consensus Development Conference 1987). In the UK, ALTE severe enough to result in presentation or referral to a pediatrician have a frequency of around 1–2/1000 births. Very few of these infants will have required cardiopulmonary resuscitation for the initial episode. The fall in incidence of SIDS which has followed the UK 'Back to Sleep' campaign has been accompanied by a fall in incidence of severe ALTE, suggesting that, for at least some such episodes the pathophysiology is related to that of SIDS, though Kahn et al (1995) have described many differences in the epidemiology of the two conditions. The prone sleeping position is much less of a risk factor for ALTE than for SIDS.

PATHOGENESIS

Several conditions have been reported as occurring in association with ALTE (see Table 12.15). Certain infections, notably respiratory syncytial virus and pertussis, can lead to severe and prolonged episodes of apnea in young infants. Enterovirus infections (e.g. ECHO, coxsackie) can lead to marked hypotonia and severe apneic episodes may occur.

Gastroesophageal reflux is common in young infants and its relationship with ALTE or SIDS is not clear. Reflux of gastric contents or pharyngeal incoordination can provoke severe apneic spells via the laryngeal chemoreceptor reflex. Stimulation of laryngeal chemoreceptor in young animals causes apnea, bradycardia and central pooling of blood. The major determinants of whether infants with reflux have ALTE may be the coordination of swallowing and the infant's arousal threshold, together with the potency of the laryngeal chemoreceptor apnea reflex rather than the severity of the reflux (Jeffrey et al 1995).

Seizures may be accompanied by apnea, but the finding of an abnormal EEG or the subsequent occurrence of seizures after an ALTE does not prove that the initial episode was ictal in nature. It is possible that an initial severe hypoxic episode could cause hypoxic CNS damage leading to seizures. Some infants with normal EEGs between events have ALTE caused by seizures (Hewertson et al 1994).

Southall has described a clinical condition in which infants may exhibit repeated episodes of sudden onset of severe cyanosis with arterial hypoxemia. The infants are usually awake before the episode, but lose consciousness and may develop seizures. Apnea, with or without obstruction, may or may not be present. The pathogenesis is unclear. Episodes may recur over a period of many months (Southall et al 1990).

Some infants may present with ALTE as a consequence of being too warm. An excess of bedding or clothing (particularly if the head is covered) in a warm environment may lead to marked hypoventilation or apnea even in the absence of pyrexia. In an environmental temperature of 16–20°C, the appropriate total thermal resistance of bedding plus clothing for normal infants is in the range of 5–8 tog or less in the presence of an acute infection. Higher values of thermal insulation of bedding or clothing have been associated with ALTE and an increased risk of sudden infant death (Fleming et al 1993, 1996 Wigfield et al 1993). Kahn (1995) has noted the frequency of excessive sweating reported amongst infants who subsequently die suddenly and unexpectedly.

Table 12.15 'Causes' of ALTE in infants

Infection (e.g. RSV, pertussis, enteroviruses)

Seizures

Upper airway obstruction

Gastroesophageal reflux and laryngeal chemoreceptor reflex apnea

Cardiac disorders (e.g. arrhythmias, congenital heart disease)

Breath holding

Anemia

Central hypoventilation syndromes

Central nervous system tumors

Cyanotic spells with intrapulmonary shunting

Idiopathic ('apnea of infancy')

CLINICAL PRESENTATION AND INITIAL INVESTIGATION

A very careful history is essential. The parent or other caretaker should be asked to describe the incident or incidents in great detail, with particular reference to the infant's sleep or waking state just before the episode, the time relationship to feeding and the infant's position (see Table 12.16). A detailed perinatal history and a family history, particularly of sudden unexpected death, cardiac or respiratory disorders or convulsions, are also important.

If the infant presents for medical care shortly after the episode, blood gas analysis may give an indication of the severity of the episode. A capillary blood sugar should also be estimated immediately and the results verified by measuring true blood glucose concentration. If the infant is not seen immediately the severity of the episode (and its possible nature) may be inferred from the time after the episode before the infant was normally responsive.

Almost all infants should be admitted to hospital after an ALTE and observed closely with continuous monitoring of respiration and ECG for a period of 48–72 hours. Investigations on admission should be determined by the history, but will usually include full blood count, urea and electrolytes, chest radiograph, ECG, an EEG and cerebral ultrasound scan.

In the USA 'pneumograms' (recordings of respiration and ECG for 12–24 hours) have been widely used, but there is no good evidence that they are of value in predicting the risk of subsequent ALTE or death (Oren et al 1989). If the history or clinical course in hospital suggest that obstructive apnea, central hypoventilation, apneic seizures or cyanotic spells are possible diagnoses, then referral to a center with facilities for polygraphic physiological recordings including video monitoring during sleep ('polysomnography') should be considered. Alternatively, a recording of respiratory movements, expired and/or transcutaneous CO_2 and pulse oximetry is within the capabilities of many pediatric units (Lancet 1989a, Douglas et al 1992).

If the history and initial clinical assessment in hospital suggest an association between ALTE and gastroesophageal reflux, investigation by esophageal pH monitoring (possibly combined with respiratory and oxygenation recording) should be undertaken. Many such infants will improve on treatment of the reflux.

In up to 50% of infants with ALTE no explanation is found and no further episodes occur in hospital or after discharge home (Consensus Development Conference 1987, Kahn et al 1992).

Kahn et al (1995), reported 5435 infants with ALTE from a 10-year collaborative study in Belgium which included detailed clinical investigations and all-night polysomnographic recordings. For 68% of these infants a specific medical cause was identified (e.g. gastroesophageal reflux, seizure, airway abnormality, metabolic disorder, cardiac arrhythmia, imposed airway obstruction). In many cases the history was important in identifying the cause. In 32% no cause could be found. In this 'idiopathic' group the most frequent symptoms were apnea, hypotonia, hypothermia and intense pallor and these infants were on average 2–4 weeks older than the group with identified medical causes. In only 11% of the infants with 'idiopathic' ALTE was a major abnormality identified on the polygraphic recording (e.g. repeated upper airway obstruction during sleep, with drops in heart rate and saturation). In a detailed follow-up of 200 of these infants nursed on home cardiorespiratory monitors (Kahn et al 1992) the same authors reported that 10% had a further episode for which resuscitation was instituted by the parents, though all rapidly returned to normal appearance after resuscitation. It is not possible to say whether these were genuinely life-threatening events.

PROGNOSIS

A few infants are left with severe neurodevelopmental sequelae, but the great majority of infants are developmentally normal. The risk of further ALTE depends on the cause of the initial episode and on whether effective treatment is available (e.g. for gastroesophageal reflux, seizures, etc.).

Oren et al (1986) found that of 76 infants who presented with an initial ALTE severe enough to require mouth to mouth resuscitation and which was thought to be due to apnea of infancy, 25 (33%) had a subsequent episode which required vigorous stimulation or resuscitation and 10 (13%) died. Of those infants who developed seizures after the initial episode, four out of seven died. Almost all second episodes occurred within 2 weeks of the first. Infants with no further episodes within 2 weeks of the initial presentation may therefore be considered at low risk of future episodes.

All 200 infants with 'idiopathic' ALTE in Kahn's study (1992) survived to 1 year of age, as did all infants with an identified medical cause who were treated and all infants with apparently minor events who were not treated. The majority of these children were normal developmentally 7–10 years later.

Most studies have included many infants with less severe episodes. The mortality rate has been reported as being 0–4%, with higher rates from tertiary referral centers.

Table 12.16 Important aspects of the history of ALTE

What time of day did the episode occur?

How was it noticed and by whom?

Was the baby previously awake or asleep?

What happened during the episode?

What position was the baby in?

Any antecedent symptoms (e.g. URTI, cough, stridor, noisy breathing, choking)?

Any provoking factors?

How long did the episode last?

What color was the baby?

Any abnormal movement?

Were there any continued respiratory efforts?

Was the infant apparently alert or responsive during the episode?

How long was it until the baby become alert or responsive?

Was any intervention or resuscitation deemed necessary?

How long after the episode was it before the baby was back to normal?

Was the baby hot, cold or sweaty?

Was there any relationship to feeds?

Were there any previous episodes?

Was there anything different about the baby after the initial episode (e.g. dozy, less responsive than usual)?

SUBSEQUENT MANAGEMENT

Apnea monitors

The use of apnea monitors after discharge from hospital is controversial. There is no convincing evidence that the use of monitors influences the subsequent mortality, nor that combined ECG and respiration monitors, or those incorporating measures of oxygenation, together with recording devices are better than simple respiration or movement-sensing monitors. Most commercially available monitors will not reliably identify episodes of obstructive apnea and all are subject to problems with false alarms, which may add to parental anxiety (Keens & Ward 1993).

The reassurance provided by the audible and visible breath signals from a monitor helps some parents to cope in the aftermath of the terrifying experience of ALTE. This must be weighed against the disadvantages of false alarms and intrusion into normal care of the infant. The decision to use a home apnea monitor will be determined by many factors, including the assessed risk of recurrent ALTE, the availability of suitable monitors and the parents' wishes (Foundation for the Study of Infant Deaths and British Paediatric Respiratory Group 1990).

RELATIONSHIP BETWEEN ALTE AND SIDS

Based on data from several studies it seems likely that less than 10% of SIDS victims had been noted to have prolonged apneic episodes before death and less than 4% of infants presenting with ALTE will subsequently die of SIDS. The term ALTE describes the very general clinical syndrome and refers to a heterogeneous group of infants, including some of very high risk and some with very little or no increased risk of sudden infant death.

RESPIRATORY PROBLEMS IN SLEEP IN CHILDHOOD

THE CONTROL OF BREATHING AND SLEEP STATE

Respiratory pattern and the control of respiration are state dependent. In the awake state respiration is largely under conscious control, modulated by behavioral (e.g. speech) and postural requirements. The respiratory response to hypoxia and hypercarbia can to a certain extent be overridden by conscious effort in the awake adult. During rapid eye movement sleep (REM) respiration is quite irregular and, although influenced by chemoreceptor input, is not dependent upon it. The thermoregulatory system does have a marked effect on respiratory pattern in REM, however. Mild cooling causes a rise in metabolic rate and in minute ventilation, which is greater in REM than in quiet sleep (QS) in both infants and adults (Azaz et al 1992). The inhibition of tone in postural muscles (including the intercostals and genioglossus) in REM leads to a loss of coupling between the movements of the ribcage and abdomen and to increased upper airway resistance respectively. In QS the respiratory pattern is largely determined by autonomic (e.g. chemoreceptor) activity. Intercostal muscle tone is maintained in QS, thus the movements of the ribcage and abdomen are coupled and in phase (Hershenson 1992).

The respiratory pattern in both sleep states represents a complex series of interactions between multiple afferent inputs including those of the chemoreceptors, vagus, thermoregulatory and blood pressure control systems. Marked oscillations of respiration at 2–3 months are a normal feature of the respiratory control system at this age in both sleep states (Fleming et al 1988).

Thus damage or failure of the chemoreceptor control system of respiration (e.g. congenital central hypoventilation) leads to hypoventilation which is most marked in but not limited to QS. Obstructive sleep apnea, in which the loss of tone in genioglossus is an important factor, is most marked in REM. In conditions (e.g. phrenic palsy, diaphragmatic myopathy) in which damage is limited to or mainly present in the diaphragm, ventilation may be well maintained when awake and sometimes in quiet sleep, but in REM sleep there may be severe hypoventilation, because of the loss of intercostal and accessory muscle activity. Investigation of children with damage or disorders of any component of the respiratory musculature should therefore include measurements of respiration during sleep, particularly at the time of intercurrent illnesses, as abnormal respiratory muscles may not be able to sustain increased work loads.

DEVELOPMENTAL CHANGES IN SLEEP DURING CHILDHOOD

The newborn infant spends 16–20 hours/day asleep, of which 50–60% is REM and 40–50% quiet sleep (NREM). By 6 months total sleep time has fallen to 11–14 h, of which 30% is REM and 70% NREM sleep. Thus in the first 6 months there is an absolute increase in the amount of time spent in NREM sleep. From 6 months to adult life there is a progressive fall in the total sleep time to approximately 8 h with a further small reduction in REM sleep to 20% by age 18 (Scher et al 1992).

CONGENITAL CENTRAL HYPOVENTILATION SYNDROME (CCHS) ('ONDINE'S CURSE')

In this rare condition there is partial or complete failure of the chemoreceptor control system of respiration. The condition may be congenital or more rarely acquired, e.g. after viral encephalitis. There is variable hypoventilation most marked in QS. In the awake state the intact 'behavioral' control system usually maintains relatively normal levels of minute ventilation, but absent chemoreceptor reflexes make such children vulnerable to hypoxia during apneic spells which may occur when they are concentrating on something else. In REM sleep ventilation is very variable but it is commonly better maintained than in QS. The underlying pathological lesion is usually not identified, but the condition may be part of a generalized impairment of the autonomic nervous system. Associated conditions in some children with CCHS include Hirschsprung's disease, ophthalmological abnormalities and, occasionally, ganglioneuroblastoma. Seizures are common, some children have instability of body temperature and many have a reversal of the normal circadian rhythm of urine production, with a major diuresis occurring at night. Severe fluid retention (from increased ADH secretion) may complicate relatively minor infections. Severe pulmonary ventilation/perfusion mismatch is commonly present with severe hypoxemia complicating relatively mild hypoventilation during sleep.

Affected children may present with cyanosis, apnea or cor pulmonale, but hypoxic convulsions during sleep are not uncommon.

Investigations should include chest radiograph, ECG, EEG, echocardiogram, CT scan of the head and chest and polygraphic recordings of respiration and sleep state with continuous monitoring of blood gases. A rectal biopsy and barium enema should be performed if there is abdominal distention, vomiting or constipation.

Management

Theophylline, naloxone, imipramine and chlorpromazine are all ineffective. Doxapram and almitrine have both been shown to improve ventilation in sleep in this condition but major toxicity limits their use. Medroxyprogesterone has been used successfully but may cause pituitary/adrenal suppression.

Most children with CCHS will require long-term ventilatory support during sleep, usually by positive pressure ventilation via a face mask or tracheostomy or by a negative pressure ventilator. Up to half of affected children will also require ventilatory support when awake, particularly at times of intercurrent illnesses. Persisting ventilation/perfusion mismatch may necessitate oxygen treatment, which is sometimes necessary when awake and when asleep. Such treatment can commonly be managed at home for children more than 9–12 months of age.

Electrical pacemakers on the phrenic nerves have been used but are technically more difficult in young children and carry a significant risk of permanent damage to the phrenic nerves, leading to awake as well as sleeping hypoventilation.

Prognosis

Many children with CCHS can lead relatively normal lives and attend normal schools, though most show persisting hypotonia and delayed developmental progress. There is usually no improvement in sleeping ventilation with age. Many develop convulsions, though whether these are secondary to unrecognized hypoxic episodes is not clear. Respiratory infections may lead to the rapid onset of severe hypoxemia, fluid retention and cor pulmonale. Many affected children show poor growth and delayed puberty is common. Some affected children have survived to adult life, though many have died during childhood. Long-term life expectancy is unclear at present and is likely to be influenced by the development of pulmonary hypertension (Weese-Mayer et al 1992, Silvestri et al 1992).

OBSTRUCTIVE SLEEP APNEA

In the presence of any structural narrowing of the nasal airway or pharynx (e.g. enlarged tonsils or adenoids), the normal inspiratory narrowing of the oropharynx may be exacerbated, leading to partial or complete obstruction, which may be further exacerbated by the presence of an upper respiratory tract infection or by neck flexion. Such episodes are most marked during REM sleep. Without treatment episodes of obstructive sleep apnea may lead to cor pulmonale, systemic hypertension, growth failure or poor school performance. Symptoms commonly described by parents with children with obstructive sleep apnea include snoring, episodes of stopping breathing, difficulty in breathing when asleep, mouth breathing, restless sleep with frequent waking, abnormal sleep positions (e.g. on elbows and knees), sweating when asleep and daytime somnolence. Less common symptoms include nocturnal enuresis in older children, morning headaches, hyperactivity, nightmares, clumsiness and developmental delay. The symptoms are almost always worse at the time of upper respiratory infection.

Most children with obstructive sleep apnea are 2–8 years of age at the time of diagnosis but many have a history of symptoms suggesting onset of obstruction before 12 months of age and some may have presented in early infancy with apparent life-threatening events. Children with Down syndrome are especially prone to upper airway obstruction during sleep and this may contribute to the unexplained pulmonary hypertension seen in some. Other susceptible children are those with weakness or loss of tone due to neuromuscular disease (e.g. congenital myopathy) and anatomical, particularly craniofacial anomalies (such as Robin anomalad). Children with the Robin anomalad (Pierre Robin syndrome) of mandibular hypoplasia, relative macroglossia and posterior midline cleft palate may present with airway obstruction within hours of birth, but may be apparently well for a few weeks after birth and present with severe airway obstruction during sleep and apparent life-threatening events or severe feeding difficulties, most commonly at the age of 4–6 weeks.

Children with achondroplasia may present a diagnostic challenge as sleep-related breathing disturbances can occur as a result of total or partial airways obstruction or as a result of cervicomedullary compression leading to central hypoventilation or apneustic breathing.

The diagnosis of obstructive sleep apnea is strongly suggested by a history of frequent snoring and difficulty in breathing during sleep or obstructive apnea observed by the parents. A recording of respiratory movement, expired carbon dioxide and pulse oximetry during sleep is within the capabilities of many pediatric units and may confirm or refute the diagnosis. Nasal, laryngotracheal or other abnormalities must be sought by careful examination (e.g. by direct pharyngoscopy using a fiberoptic nasopharyngoscope) before assuming that obstructive sleep apnea is due to enlarged tonsils and adenoids. Detailed polygraphic recording of respiration and sleep state may be necessary to establish the diagnosis.

The removal of hypertrophied tonsils and adenoids in children with obstructive sleep apnea will commonly lead to marked improvement. However, associated problems such as an abnormally long soft palate or retroposition of the mandible may contribute to persistence of symptoms after adenotonsillectomy. In the absence of enlarged tonsils and adenoids, the use of a nasopharyngeal airway may alleviate symptoms, particularly for infants with the Robin anomalad. For others nasal continuous positive airways pressure (CPAP) may be effective and is the treatment of choice for children with persisting significant obstructive sleep apnea. For many children this can safely be used at home but should be re-evaluated on a regular basis as CPAP requirements are likely to change with growth. The presence of persisting severe obstructive sleep apnea not responsive to nasal CPAP may, rarely, necessitate tracheostomy (Lancet 1989a, Douglas et al 1992, Gaultier 1995, Guilleminault et al 1995).

RESPIRATORY DEFENSES AND INFECTION IN THE COMPROMISED HOST

More than any other organ, the lungs are exposed to both the external and internal environment, processing thousands of liters of air each day and receiving the total cardiac output. Complex defense systems exist for their protection and that these may fail is inevitable. Recurrent, persistent or unusual respiratory infection should suggest such a failure (Yoder 1994).

LUNG DEFENSE MECHANISMS

Protection against inhalation of particulate matter is provided first by the nose where turbulent flow encourages the deposition of particles by impaction. Particles penetrating into the bronchial tree are usually in the size range of 0.2–5.0 µg and are deposited by sedimentation as air flow decelerates.

Particulate or chemical stimulation may trigger the protective reflexes of sneeze, cough and bronchoconstriction. The bronchial tree, down to the terminal bronchioles at its 16th division, is lined by ciliated epithelium, each cell providing around 200 cilia which beat at about 20 cycles/s. The ciliated epithelium is covered by a layer of mucus produced by submucosal glands, epithelial goblet cells and serous cells. Mucus is divided into sol and gel layers. The cilia beat in metachronal motion in the sol layer, only their tips projecting into the viscous gel. The mucus is expelled towards the larynx, acting as a protective barrier. It contains specific and nonspecific protective agents including immunoglobulins, lysozymes and antiproteases such as α1-antitrypsin. Some small particles may penetrate beyond the ciliated epithelium to the gaseous exchange unit, the acinus, where they are cleared through phagocytosis by alveolar macrophages. These also ingest and clear bacteria, viruses, fungi, erythrocytes, cell debris and antigen–antibody complexes. As well as functioning as the major phagocytic cell of the normal lung, alveolar macrophages also act as antigen-presenting cells (APC) to lymphocytes, inducing their proliferation in response to invading organisms.

Lymphoid tissue is found throughout the length of the respiratory tract from the nose to the respiratory bronchiole, providing lymphocytes and plasma cells for the production of antibodies, particularly IgA and, to a greater extent peripherally, IgG. Although lymphocytes constitute a minor component of the total cellular population of lung cells obtained at bronchoalveolar lavage, they play a crucial role in defense mechanisms. CD4+ and CD8+ T-cells are present in the same proportions as in the blood, with a smaller proportion of B-cells, plasma cells and NK cells. Following activation of the CD4+ helper cells via APCs, IL-2 is secreted with subsequent clonal proliferation of T-cells; B-cells are also stimulated to produce immunoglobulin locally. There is an amplification of the immune response when activated CD4+ lymphocytyes produce γ-interferon which leads to activation of alveolar macrophages.

IMPAIRED FUNCTION

As more becomes known about abnormalities of host defense, it becomes easier to identify causes of predisposition to infection. Hence, children with unusually frequent or severe respiratory infection or those infected with unusual organisms should be suspected of and investigated for impairment of host defense. For example, except in cystic fibrosis, bronchiectasis is now a relatively rare problem in British children and a diligent search may reveal a significant predisposition in over half of cases. Similarly, a diagnosis of *Pneumocystis carinii* pneumonia in a young infant should lead to screening for a major T-cell deficiency syndrome (e.g. severe combined immune deficiency (SCID), AIDS, DiGeorge syndrome or hyper-IgM syndrome).

IMPAIRED MUCOCILIARY CLEARANCE

Abnormal ciliary function or ciliary dyskinesia, defined as a reduction in ciliary beat frequency, results in impaired mucociliary clearance. (Buchdahl et al 1988). This in turn results in retention of mucus with chronic or recurrent respiratory infection which may progress to suppurative lung disease and bronchiectasis. The normal cilium has circumferentially placed microtubules arranged in nine pairs, linked to each other by nexin strands and by radial spokes to two central microtubules. From each pair project an inner and outer dynein arm responsible for the flexing of the cilium. Ciliary activity is thought to determine the normal rotation of the archenteron to the left in the embryo. Absence of ciliary activity allows rotation to occur randomly to left or right, allowing situs inversus to occur in half the cases.

Abnormalities of the cilium include absence of dynein arms, radial spoke defects and microtubule translocations. Cilial aplasia may occur and ciliary function may be severely impaired despite no obvious abnormality in ultrastructure. Such abnormalities are usually primary and may be inherited recessively but secondary abnormalities do occur, particularly after respiratory tract infections. These may persist for many weeks. In addition, bacterial infection may produce factors which slow ciliary beating, without effect on ultrastructure. In primary dyskinesia symptoms of upper or lower respiratory tract problems are usually present from the first week of life. Most but not all patients will have chronic upper respiratory problems thereafter but the absence of chronic sinusitis does not exclude this condition. Diagnosis requires the examination of a nasal brush biopsy for normal beat frequency (greater than 10 Hz) and ultrastructure examination if the beat frequency is less than 10 Hz. The saccharin test of nasal mucociliary function is rarely possible under the age of 10 years. No specific treatment exists for ciliary dyskinesia but a program of physiotherapy, sputum culture surveillance and antibiotic treatment is indicated.

IMMUNODEFICIENCY (see also Ch. 22)

Disorders of the immune system adversely affecting the respiratory system may be primary or secondary. As a result of the respiratory tract's preeminent contact with antigen, deficiency states are often first mainifest as respiratory problems (Shyur & Hill 1991, Stieh n 1995).

Primary immunodeficiencies

These range from those which are severe with early onset of life-threatening respiratory infection to those which are milder, resulting in frequent respiratory tract infection with more insidious respiratory tract damage. The latter include IgG subclass deficiency and IgA deficiency. IgG is the major class of immunoglobulin in serum and all fluids, except mucosal secretions where IgA predominates. IgG consists of four distinct subclasses (IgG-1–4). The different classes have different functions (Ch. 22). Classes 1, 2 and 3 provide the response to viruses, vaccines and the protein antigens of bacteria, while class 2 responds to carbohydrate antigen and is important against polysaccharide-encapsulated organisms. Under the age of 2 years the IgG-2 response to polysaccharide is poor, predisposing this age group to infections caused by *Haemophilus influenzae, Pneumococcus* and *Neisseria meningitidis*. Recurrent and severe respiratory infections of the upper and lower respiratory tract are the most common manifestations of subclass deficiency, particularly where IgG-2 is lacking. While there may be an associated IgA deficiency, this is far from invariable.

It should also be noted that subclass deficiency, particularly IgG-2, IgG-3 and IgG-4, may occur with normal levels of total IgG. Some children may even have a specific inability to produce antibody to a particular organism despite having normal immunoglobulin and subclass levels. Subclass deficiency is thought to be common in some young asthmatics and may play a part in the pathogenesis of asthma. IgA deficiency has been similarly implicated in the pathogenesis of atopy as transient IgA deficiency is particularly common in atopic infants. Persistent IgA deficiency occurs in 1 in 500 of the general population, though most individuals are asymptomatic. IgA deficiency may also be caused by drugs such as phenytoin. IgA is the chief immunoglobulin of mucosal secretions and low levels of secretory IgA are almost always predicted by a low serum IgA. Deficiency may result in frequent upper and lower respiratory tract infection, particularly in those individuals unable to compensate for their IgA deficiency by producing an increase in secretory IgM and in those with associated IgG subclass deficiencies. Bronchiectasis and chronic otitis media may result. As with IgG subclass deficiency, symptomatic patients should be monitored for respiratory tract infection with early recourse to the use of antibiotics and, in some cases, use of prophylactic treatment such as co-trimoxazole over the winter. Because of recent guidelines issued by the Department of Health regarding the use of co-trimoxazole and the occurrence of Stevens–Johnson syndrome, some pediatricians may wish to use cefaclor or cefuroxime. When infection continues to be a major problem intravenous immunoglobulin treatment is indicated. Paradoxically, preparations low in IgA may be preferred as they are better tolerated.

More severe deficiencies of gammaglobulins such as Bruton's sex-linked agammaglobulinemia usually present with chronic or recurrent respiratory tract infection when levels of maternal antibody fall after the first few months. Persistent nasal sepsis is common, as is bilateral pneumonia often due to *Pneumococcus* or *H. influenzae*. Bronchiectasis often develops. Tonsils and lymph glands are small or absent. Immunoglobulin assay shows very low IgG and near absent IgA, IgM and IgE. Treatment is as for chronic suppurative lung disease (p. 576) plus regular gammaglobulin replacement treatment. Children with immunoglobulin deficiency and elevated IgM (hyper-IgM syndrome) behave similarly to children with X-linked agammaglobulinemia, but in addition are vulnerable to *Pneumocystis carinii* pneumonia (PCP).

Children with severe immunodeficiency involving cell-mediated immunity, such as SCID, tend to present within the first 6 months of life with lower respiratory tract infection, failure to thrive and diarrhea. They are particularly prone to viral, *Pneumocystis carinii* and fungal infections. Regular immunoglobulin infusions as well as prophylaxis with co-trimoxazole are indicated while awaiting definitive treatment via bone marrow transplantation.

Chronic granulomatous disease

This rare condition involves the failure of phagocytes to kill ingested microorganisms by oxidative mechanisms (Thrasher & Segal 1995). Affected children exhibit persistent or recurrent infection from an early age involving particularly skin, lungs, liver, gut, lymph nodes and bone. Organisms frequently involved are the catalase-positive bacteria such as *Staphylococcus aureus* and enteric Gram-negative rods such as *Klebsiella pneumoniae*, as well as various species of *Aspergillus, Candida* and *Nocardia*. The great majority of patients have chronic lung infections. Abscess formation with pleural and even rib involvement often occurs and hilar lymphadenopathy is invariable. There are characteristic histopathologic changes found in CGD, and consist of extensive granuloma formation in many tissues. Diagnosis is via the nitroblue tetrazolium (NBT) test which identifies those patients whose neutrophils fail produce a respiratory burst in the presence of NBT. Management consists of antimicrobial therapy for any acute infection, followed by long-term prophylaxis with co-trimoxazole, as well as itraconazole to prevent *Aspergillus* infection. Some patients may benefit by long-term administration of γ-interferon.

Secondary immunodeficiency

Worldwide the most common cause of death in early childhood is now acute respiratory infection (ARI). Many of these deaths occur because of immunodeficiency induced by malnutrition. All aspects of immune defense may be compromised by malnutrition leading to a failure to deal effectively with normal infections such as measles and a predisposition to opportunistic infections such as PCP. Infections themselves may cause immunosuppression, the anergic period which follows measles being an example of this. A second infection occurring within the anergic period may prove devastating.

HIV infection, occurring in children most commonly through vertical transmission from mother, also causes immunosuppression and result in a predominant T-cell immunodeficiency. Up to 60–70% of HIV-infected children develop lung disease, presenting as either chronic, recurrent or opportunistic respiratory tract infection. PCP is the most common AIDS-defining illness in HIV-infected children, reported in 30–40% of patients (Gibb et al 1994). However, the most frequently encountered illnesses are acute respiratory infections caused by common viruses and bacteria (*S. pneumoniae* and *H. influenzae*). Lymphocytic interstitial pneumonitis (LIP) is also commonly seen in children with HIV infection. This is a chronic condition characterized by the presence of bilateral, diffuse reticulonodular interstitial infiltrates on the chest X-ray. Most patients are asymptomatic, although some may develop progressive respiratory insufficiency. Corticosteroid therapy may be beneficial in this group of patients. Although lung biopsy provides a definitive diagnosis, this is rarely performed these days. The diagnosis is made on the clinical picture and also by excluding other major causes of an interstitial pneumonitis such as CMV, TB and *Pneumocystis carinii*. This may require bronchoalveolar lavage.

The most common cause of secondary immunodeficiency is immunosuppression by cytotoxic or immunosuppressant therapy. More aggressive cytotoxic regimens for oncological conditions are resulting in greater tumor cure rates but also in greater complication rates. The organisms involved depend on the type of immunosuppression induced. Neutropenia tends to favor bacterial and fungal infection whereas lymphopenia favors *Pneumocystis carinii* and viral infections (Pizzo et al 1991b, Pizzo 1993). Following bone marrow transplantation (BMT) for treatment of lymphoproliferative malignancies and some immunodeficiency disorders, an initial period of neutropenia induced by the conditioning regimen favors the development of bacterial or fungal pneumonias. Once there is engraftment, GVH becomes a major risk factor requiring continuing treatment with steriods and cyclosporin A; idiopathic interstitial pneumonitis and CMV pneumonitis may occur during this period (30–90 days post-BMT). Late pneumonias (> 4–6 months post-BMT) are usually accociated with persistent B-cell defects and are caused by encapsulated organisms; prophylactic antibiotics (penicillin V) are usually given during this period. Patients may also be rendered secondarily immunodeficient by antimicrobials and by loss of immunoglobulin and cells in the nephrotic syndrome, protein-losing enteropathy, intestinal lymphangiectasia and chylothorax

PNEUMONIA IN THE SEVERELY IMMUNOCOMPROMISED

These patients are predisposed to a wide range of infections, from common Gram-negative bacteria to rare fungi (Baughmann and Dohn 1995, Rivkin & Aronoff 1987). It must be remembered that although sometimes the organism may be rare, at other times the host response may be markedly altered, resulting in an unusual clinical presentation for a common organism (e.g. measles giant cell pneumonia). There are no pathognomonic symptoms or signs indicating infection with a particular organism but an accurate microbiological diagnosis at an early stage is of vital importance.

First it is necessary to recognize that a lower respiratory tract infection has occurred. The severely neutropenic patient may present with fever and dyspnea but few auscultatory signs and even fewer abnormalities on the chest radiograph. The patient with viral or opportunistic infection may often develop an interstitial pneumonitis, with a characteristic presentation. There is gradual onset of dry cough, tachypnea, dyspnea on exertion and then dyspnea at rest. On examination the patient may be breathless and cyanosed but may have good air entry bilaterally and no added sounds on auscultation. Blood gas analysis shows a type I respiratory failure with low oxygen and carbon dioxide tensions and the chest radiograph shows low volume lungs with a diffuse haze throughout both lung fields. This may mistakenly be reported as an expiratory film.

Secondly, it is important to remember that not all cases presenting in this manner are caused by infection and that the differential diagnosis may include pulmonary edema, pulmonary hemorrhage, drug- or radiation-induced pneumonitis and tumor infiltration. A low threshold of suspicion, a rapid start of empirical treatment and a thorough search for the causative organism(s) are of vital importance (Pizzo et al 1991a). The choice of empirical treatment will depend upon the clinical circumstances, but usually includes a broad-spectrum antibiotic to cover Gram-negative and Gram-positive organisms, erythromycin to deal with *Mycoplasma pneumoniae* and rare organisms such as *Legionella* and high-dose co-trimoxazole for *Pneumocystis carinii* pneumonia. Amphotericin B may be included in the severely neutropenic patient.

The search for causative organisms is hampered by the lack of sputum production. In the older child, the use of irritant inhalations of hypertonic saline (3%) or a mucolytic such as *N*-acetylcysteine may increase the yield of sputum and the chance of organism identification. The sputum should be examined by Gram stain and also stained for mycobacteria, fungi and *Pneumocystis carinii*. Monoclonal antibody stains for *Pneumocystis carinii* have greatly facilitated its identification. Sputum should be cultured for bacteria, viruses and fungi. Blood cultures should be taken for

bacteria and fungi and serology checked for evidence of any viral, *Mycoplasma*, *Chlamydia* or *Legionella* infection. Because of the limited antibody responses, serology is rarely helpful. Sensitive and specific tests to detect fungal antigens are still being developed. In the younger child, a nasopharyngeal aspirate should be obtained and urgent immunofluorescence requested for the presence of any respiratory viruses, CMV or *Pneumocystis carinii*.

Failure to respond to empiric therapy and failure to identify the causative organism(s) necessitates more invasive procedures. Bronchoscopy with bronchoalveolar lavage would be the preferred procedure and may lead to a diagnosis. In some centres, good results have been obtained using nonbronchoscopic bronchoalveolar lavage, requiring only intubation and the passage of a catheter through the ET tube for lavage and suction (Alpert et al 1992). Lung biopsy tends to be reserved for those patients who remain unresponsive to therapy and undiagnosed and in whom it is anticipated a histological diagnosis may prove helpful, e.g., pulmonary aspergillosis or lung GVH. In patients with diffuse interstitial pneumonitis, the most common cause is *Pneumocystis carinii* pneumonia, while cytomegalovirus and respiratory viruses such as influenza, parainfluenza, adenovirus and RSV are relatively common. Mixed infection with two or more organisms is not uncommon while in about 10% of patients, no specific cause is identified.

Pneumocystis carinii pneumonia

Although *P. carinii* is generally thought of as a protozoan, it has many features in common with a fungus and recently genetic analysis has confirmed this. By the age of 4 years, the majority of normal children have been infected and show evidence of seroconversion. In immuncompromised children, especially those with T-cell defects, it may produce a severe interstitial pneumonia. The clinical features, described in detail above, are of insidious onset of dyspnea and cyanosis with a nonproductive cough. Chest shows diffuse bilateral infiltrates, initially perihilar but spreading out to give a 'ground glass' appearance (Fig. 12.13).

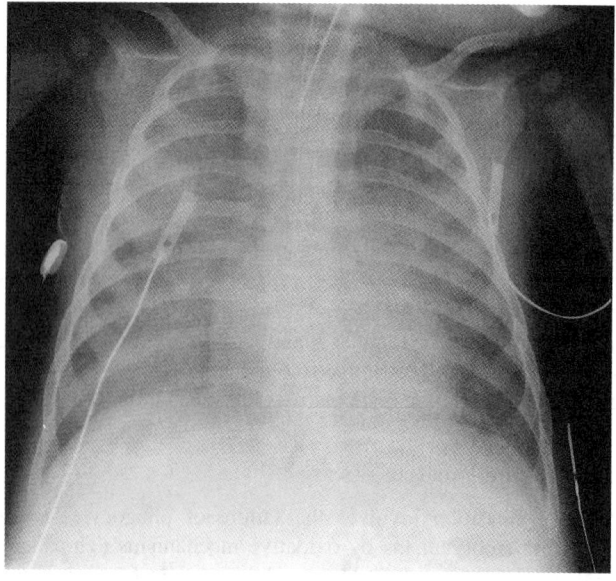

Fig. 12.13 Bilateral interstitial pneumonitis due to *Pneumocystis carinii* in an infant with vertically acquired HIV infection.

Characteristic cysts may be revealed by special staining (e.g. silver methenamine) of sputum, nasopharyngeal aspirate, bronchoalveolar lavage fluid or lung biopsy. Monoclonal antibody techniques improve identification rates, while polymerase chain reaction (PCR) for *Pneumocystis* is currently being evaluated.

Treatment should be with high-dose co-trimoxazole (trimethoprim component 20 mg/kg/day in four divided doses) for a period of 14–21 days. If there is no response within 5–7 days, therapy should be switched to intravenous pentamidine (4 mg/kg) and consideration should be given to performing a lung biopsy. Steroids have been shown to decrease mortality in patients with HIV and PCP and hence methylprednisolone should be added in full doses (1 mg/kg, 12-hourly) for 10 days, then weaned. Anecdotal reports have suggested surfactant therapy may also have a place in those patients not responding to the previous measures (Slater et al 1995). Prophylaxis is with co-trimoxazole, either daily or three times weekly; alternative drugs are dapsone or inhaled pentamidine though these are less effective.

Viral pneumonia

Cytomegalovirus

When it involves the lungs, CMV infection in the immunocompromised child carries a grave prognosis. Fortunately a greater awareness of its importance in transplant patients has led to preventive measures. Although reactivation of past infection can be a problem, primary infection is the more serious condition and carries the worse prognosis. Hence the CMV-negative patient must receive CMV-negative blood and blood products and ideally must have a CMV-negative transplant donor. Pulmonary involvement follows the pattern of interstitial pneumonitis. The clinical and radiological features are similar to those of *Pneumocystis carinii* pneumonia. A clue to CMV infection may be the presence of multisystem involvement, such as hepatitis, colitis or retinitis. Suggestive laboratory evidence may be via positive urine cultures, positive CMV immunofluorescence testing of nasopharyngeal aspirates, bronchoalveolar lavage fluid or buffy coat. A definite diagnosis of CMV pneumonitis is made via lung biopsy which shows the characteristic histological changes (e.g. cytopathic changes with presence of intranuclear and intracytoplasmic inclusions) and positive viral immunofluorescence. Quantative PCR for CMV plasma viral load is a technique increasingly being used to monitor BMT patients and to guide the physician in the treatment and prophylaxis of CMV infection. Therapy for established CMV pneumonitis has been disappointing and mortality may be as high as 80%. Some success has been reported with the use of hyperimmune CMV immunoglobulin and ganciclovir (10 mg/kg/day in two doses). Prophylaxis for high-risk patients (e.g. BMT patients) consists of either high-dose acyclovir (500 mg/m² dose t.d.s.) or low-dose ganciclovir (5 mg/kg once a day).

Varicella zoster

Primary infection with chickenpox in the immunocompromised, particularly lymphopenic, patient produces a life-threatening, disseminated disease in up to 30% of untreated patients. The varicelliform rash, which may be hemorrhagic, precedes the onset of respiratory symptoms of dry cough, dyspnea and chest pain. The chest radiograph often shows bilateral nodular infiltrates that may coalesce. Diagnosis is by examination of vesicular fluid by electron microscopy for the presence of a herpesvirus. Prevention of varicella is possible if VZIG is given to nonimmune immunocompromised patients within 72 hours of a varicella exposure. Varicella in the immunocompromised child should be treated promptly with intravenous acyclovir (500 mg/m² dose, 8-hourly) so as to prevent varicella pneumonitis. Respiratory support as well as antiviral therapy may be necessary for treatment of varicella pneumonia.

Herpes simplex

Mucocutaneous herpes simplex infection is common in severe immunodeficiency and may occur in as many as 50% of patients undergoing bone marrow transplantation. Infection is thought to be due to reactivation of latent virus. Upper airway ulceration and necrosis may progress through tracheobronchitis to pneumonia which may be focal or generalized. Chest radiographs show non specific bronchopneumonic signs. Diagnosis may be suggested by identification of viral inclusion bodies in epithelial cells but is established by viral isolation. Prophylactic therapy with acyclovir in at-risk groups has been shown to be effective; acyclovir is also effective treatment for established infection.

Measles giant cell pneumonia

Measles infection in the immunocompromised host may lead to this devastating condition. Prior exposure to measles or measles vaccine is usually protective for those undergoing severe immunosuppression. However, primary infection may follow an atypical course with an incubation period which may be prolonged, lack of the classic prodrome, a fleeting rash, no Koplik's spots, conjunctivitis or coryza. Instead patients may show high swinging fever, cough and dyspnea. Widespread inspiratory crepitations are heard. The chest radiograph shows widespread coarse nodular infiltrates and frequently evidence of air leak. Lung biopsy should be avoided as it is particularly poorly tolerated and the diagnosis can be more safely and effectively established by the identification of the virus on immunofluorescence of nasopharyngeal aspirate. No therapy has been shown to be effective though many, including antiviral agents, immunoglobulin, steroids and interferon, have been tried. The condition is often fatal. Fortunately, due to the generally good uptake of measles immunization, giant cell pneumonia is rare.

Fungal infection

As oncological regimens become more aggressive fungal pneumonias are more often encountered, most commonly caused by *Candida* or *Aspergillus*. The most sugnificant risk factor for these infections is prolonged neutropenia.

Candida albicans

Candida may be spread to the lungs by aspiration from the oropharynx or by hematogenous spread in candidemia. Aspiration often leads to a laryngotracheobronchitis with pneumonic changes in the lower lobes while hematogenous spread causes a widespread granulomatous pneumonia with generalized patchy soft shadows on the chest radiograph. Demonstration of *Candida* in the sputum or in nasopharyngeal secretions is not necessarily diagnostic as contamination may occur from the oropharynx. Growth of *Candida* from blood cultures and a positive serology for *Candida* antigen are strong pointers but in their absence a lung biopsy is sometimes required. Treatment requires the removal of any source of infection (e.g. Hickman line), followed by a prolonged course (6 weeks) of either amphotericin B, liposomal formulations of amphotericin or fluconazole. This latter drug is often used as prophylaxis for *Candida* infections in BMT patients.

Aspergillus

Insidious *Aspergillus* infection may occur in patients with chronic neutrophil defects such as chronic granulomatous disease but severe *Aspergillus* pneumonia, usually due to *A. fumigatus*, most often occurs in the immunosuppressed, profoundly neutropenic patient. It tends to be most common clinical presentation of invasive aspergillosis in immunocompromised patients (up to 60%). Such patients develop unremitting fever, cough and tachypnea. Rapid deterioration clinically and radiologically is often seen with radiographic changes of widespread opacifications which rapidly coalesce. In older patients CT scan of the chest may be helpful in the diagnosis; cavities may be demonstrable and a 'halo' sign is thought to be diagnostic. Bronchoalveolar lavage may also be helpful, but definitive diagnosis is by lung biopsy which shows fungal hyphae in tissues. There may be evidence of invasive *Aspergillus* in other organs such as brain, kidney, skin and bone.

Standard therapy consists of amphotericin B for 6 weeks. Early treatment is vital as mortality in advanced disease is high, often greater than 50–70%. New treatment strategies involve the use of liposomal amphotericin B and itraconazole, whilst adjunctive therapy may include the use of growth factors (e.g. G-CSF), γ-interferon or surgery. The following prophylactic regimen for patients undergoing BMT and significant immunosuppression is recommended: itraconazole (5 mg/kg day) or aerosolized amphotericin B. Construction in hospital facilities is associated with an increased incidence of aspergillosis in the hospitalized severely immunocompromised population; hence, the nursing of these patients in specially filtered, negatively pressure hospital rooms is essential.

ASTHMA

DEFINITION AND EPIDEMIOLOGY

Asthma is a condition characterized by variation in intrathoracic airway obstruction, occurring spontaneously or as a result of treatment. This definition is difficult to apply to young children in particular, because it is almost impossible to make accurate measurements of intrathoracic airway function. By default an operational definition of asthma in early childhood is: persistent or episodic wheeze, usually accompanied by cough where other conditions have been excluded. Although disorders such as 'wheezy bronchitis', 'the wheezy baby syndrome' and even 'chronic bronchitis' are generally classified under the general heading of asthma, it is clear that these conditions do not share a single mechanism. There is much evidence to suggest that 'wheezy bronchitis', a term denoting recurrent viral wheeze in the

first few years of life, is a disorder quite distinct from atopic asthma (Silverman 1993). Asthma is in fact an umbrella term, rather like the term 'hypertension'. Both asthma and hypertension represent clinically important syndromes, each of which may be brought about by several different mechanisms. Acute viral bronchiolitis is a separate disorder and is often a herald of recurrent wheeze.

About 10–15% of UK schoolchildren suffer from asthma at any time, although cumulative figures of up to 20–25% are reached if a single episode of reported wheeze is included within the definition. The prevalence and severity are steadily increasing in most of the industrialized nations of the world, presumably as a result of environmental change. Only in some rural areas of the developing world does childhood asthma appear still to be rare. Ethnic differences are largely explained by differences in environment and upbringing rather than genetics, although hereditary (familial) factors in asthma are well recognized.

A number of environmental factors are closely associated with recurrent chest symptoms in infancy. These include maternal smoking (particularly during pregnancy), the presence of older siblings in the family and gas cooking. Strong familial (hereditary) factors include parental history of asthma and other atopic disorders. Infant feeding practices have little effect on the development of asthma.

Asthma has been a major cause of childhood morbidity over the years. Its underdiagnosis and undertreatment have been responsible for much absence from school. In the UK about 3–4% of recognized asthmatic children are admitted to hospital each year, the peak months for admission being May–July and September–November. Overall, asthma is least troublesome in August and in winter. The changing density of aeroallergens (pollen, house dust mite, mold spores) and viral respiratory infections probably accounts for some seasonal variation. Clinical observations suggest that in contrast to older children, infants tend to be more frequently admitted with wheeze in the winter months, when respiratory viral infections are prevalent in the community; 50% of admissions to hospital for asthma at all ages in the UK occur in the under-5s. The mortality rate for childhood asthma has declined in the UK and currently stands at about 1 per 100 000 children per year (or 1 per 1000 asthmatic children per 10 years). In the first year of life, the death rate in the UK is declining, in spite of the apparent ineffectiveness of much asthma medication in young infants.

PATHOGENESIS

Both environmental and hereditary factors are important in the pathogenesis of asthma. The precise nature of the abnormalities which lead to airway narrowing is unclear. For instance, although it is known that atopy (Ch. 28) is a major hereditary predisposing factor, it is clearly insufficient, since some 30–40% of the UK population could be considered atopic in terms of their response to skin prick tests, though only one-third of these could be considered as having asthma at any stage in their lives. Bronchial inflammation is a major factor. Again, it is unclear why atopic asthmatics should respond to antigenic stimuli by developing florid inflammatory changes in airways. Finally, the nature of bronchial hyperresponsiveness, a concept which explains the exquisite short-term sensitivity of the airways of asthmatic subjects to common environmental triggers, is also unexplained. A tendency to develop hyperresponsive airways is probably inherited separately from atopy; both are necessary components of severe atopic asthma. In preschool wheezing children, atopy is no more common than in a random population sample and an inflammatory process can only be speculated.

HISTOPATHOLOGY

Most of the information on airway pathology in asthma has been obtained from examination of post-mortem material from patients who have died of asthma. Although the pathological features are striking, it is probable that most are potentially reversible. The increase in smooth muscle bulk and in the dimensions of the submucosal glands seen in chronic cases are, presumably, persistent features.

In fatal cases there may be plugging of the airways with mucus and widespread desquamation of the airway epithelium. There is subepithelial fibrosis and frequently inflammatory cell infiltration (particularly with eosinophils and lymphocytes) both in the airway lumen and in the epithelium and subepithelial layer. There may be hypertrophy of bronchial smooth muscle and edema of the bronchial wall. Hyperinflation due to air trapped behind obstructed airways is always found. In some cases of 'sudden' death from asthma in children who have previously received steroid therapy, adrenocortical atrophy has been demonstrated.

INFLAMMATION

Bronchoalveolar lavage (BAL) in mild stable adult asthmatics reveals the presence of increased populations of eosinophils and mast cells in the airways. These cells are active, as shown by high levels of their respective preformed products, major basic protein and histamine, in lavage fluid. The number of cells present seems to relate closely to the level of bronchial responsiveness. A wide range of cytokines and inflammatory mediators (including adhesion molecules, interleukins, PAF and prostaglandins) are present in increased amounts, leading to acute pathological changes and chronic airway remodeling.

Bronchial biopsies in volunteer asthmatic adults reveal, even in the mildest cases, thickening of the basement membrane, smooth muscle hypertrophy and increased numbers of inflammatory cells, including eosinophils, lymphocytes, neutrophils and mast cells, in the epithelium and submucosa. In more severe asthma, epithelial

stripping, collagenous thickening of the basement membrane and heavy infiltration with neutrophils and eosinophils is found.

The 'late reaction' to bronchial challenge in the inflammatory sequence is commonly associated with an enhancement of bronchial hyperresponsiveness which may persist for several days or even weeks (O'Byrne et al 1987). There is evidence that by blocking the late reaction with sodium cromoglycate or inhaled corticosteroids, given at the time of challenge, the subsequent enhanced bronchial responsiveness may be inhibited. This could provide an explanation for the effectiveness of these two drugs as prophylactic agents.

BRONCHIAL RESPONSIVENESS

The majority of research into bronchial responsiveness has concentrated on acute reversible changes in airways obstruction in response to pharmacological constrictors such as histamine or methacholine, which are likely to be due mainly to smooth muscle contraction. Although the airways of normal subjects can be made to respond, they are very poorly responsive compared with those of asthmatics. The role of the extensive submucosal plexus of veins in the airways has recently come to attention. By vasodilatation, this system has the capacity to cause sudden changes in airway caliber of the type previously ascribed to airway smooth muscle.

An understanding of the mechanisms of bronchial hyperresponsiveness is essential to the management of asthma. The steps leading from the exposure to a stimulus to airway narrowing have all been studied separately and abnormalities at one or more points along this pathway may be responsible for hyperresponsiveness (Fig. 12.14). There is evidence that the control of airway function in asthmatics may be both qualitatively and quantitatively different to that in normal subjects. There is also evidence that different mechanisms may coexist in individual patients and may interact to produce bronchoconstriction (Fig. 12.15).

Lesser degrees of bronchial responsiveness than are normally found in asthma occur in several other chronic respiratory disorders of childhood, such as cystic fibrosis, bronchiectasis and bronchopulmonary dysplasia. Whereas in asthmatic patients responsiveness is fairly independent of baseline lung function, in most of these other conditions it is proportional to the degree of baseline airways obstruction. Antiasthma treatment may be

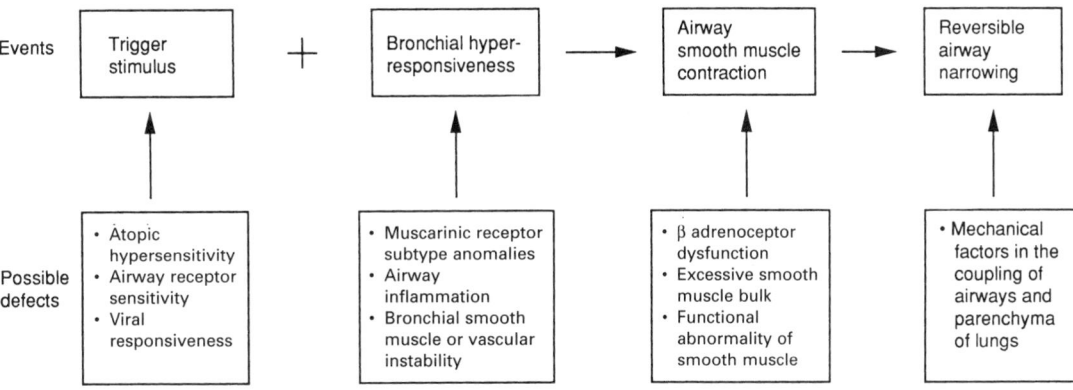

Fig. 12.14 Some of the abnormal mechanisms that have been proposed at each step in the pathway leading from exposure to a trigger stimulus to airway narrowing. It should be emphasized, however, that no single defect can explain the pathogenesis of asthma.

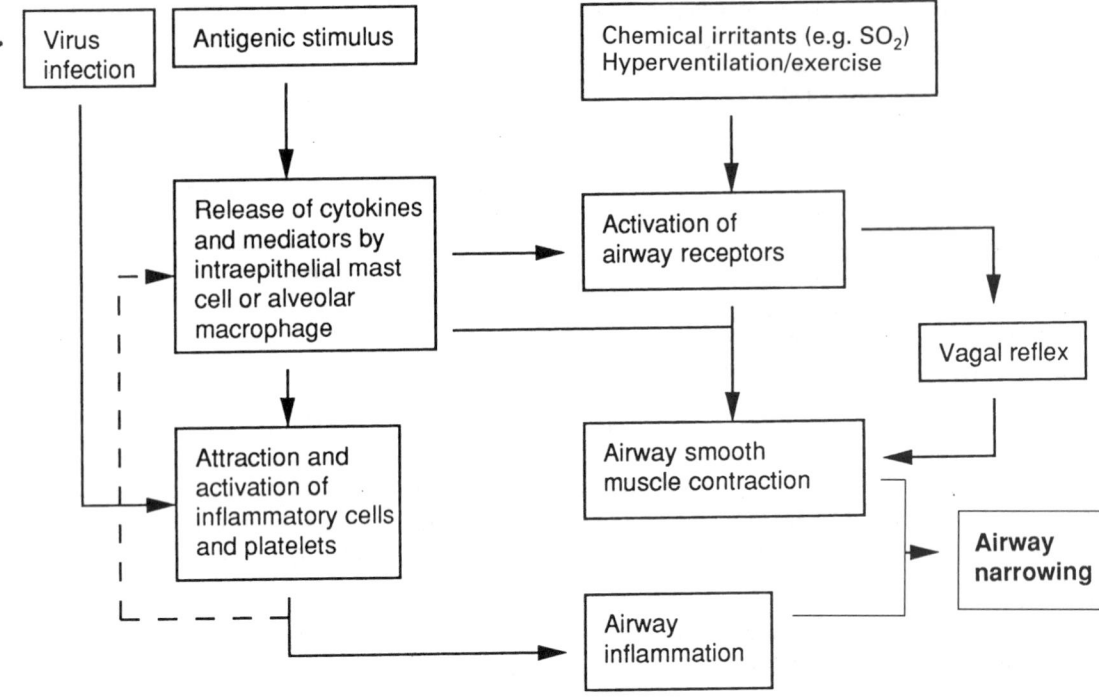

Fig. 12.15 The various neural, humoral and cellular mechanisms that interact to produce airway narrowing.

attempted in symptomatic patients with these conditions in whom hyperresponsiveness is demonstrated or suspected.

In spite of the fact that bronchial responsiveness as measured in the laboratory (p. 501) cannot explain the whole of clinical asthma, the concept is extremely important in understanding childhood asthma and its management. The measurement allows the physician to understand the problems of individual patients and to plan their management and also provides an insight into the natural history and mechanisms of airway obstruction in general and of asthma in particular. Most of the procedures for measuring bronchial responsiveness only provide information on the immediate response (i.e. within a few minutes of challenge). It is clear that the major inducers of childhood asthma (especially antigen exposure) may cause persistent bronchial hyperresponsiveness or airways obstruction over much longer periods.

The distribution of bronchial responsiveness in the population is unimodal, those with clinical asthma falling at one extreme of the range. In understanding the importance of trigger factors as precipitants of airway obstruction in asthmatics, the simple equation:

Trigger factor + bronchial responsiveness → airway narrowing provides a good basis for explanation to parents and children and for identifying and modifying important factors. Each of the processes in this equation (the avoidance of trigger factors, the use of drugs to modify bronchial responsiveness and the use of drugs to reverse airway obstruction) plays a part in management.

AIRWAY SMOOTH MUSCLE

Airway smooth muscle tone is controlled by neurohumoral mechanisms.

1. Vagal efferents (muscarinic, cholinergic mechanisms) are of major importance (Barnes 1989). The system of control is complex, as there appear to be at least five muscarinic receptor subtypes. It is speculated that a defect in one of these, the M_3 receptor which mediates an inhibitory feedback system onto vagal efferents, may be at least partly responsible for increased smooth muscle sensitivity in asthma.

2. Adrenergic mechanisms have direct and indirect influence. It is surprising, however, that the greatest density of β-2 receptors is found not on airway smooth muscle but on the epithelium. Nevertheless, there are β-2 receptors on airway smooth muscle as well as on vagal, cholinergic airway ganglia, the latter leading to reduced vagal motor activity. There is no direct sympathetic innervation of airway smooth muscle in humans so that β-adrenergic effects on this tissue are mediated by circulating catecholamines, not neurally.

3. The nonadrenergic, noncholinergic (NANC) inhibitory system, possibly relying on peptide neurohumoral transmitters such as bombesin and substance P, plays an active role in maintaining relaxation of airway smooth muscle. It is not yet clear whether any defect in the system is present in asthma.

LUNG FUNCTION

MECHANICAL CHANGES

The main physiological disturbance in asthma is episodic, intrathoracic airways obstruction. Its effects can be measured either by direct tests of airway resistance or by indirect tests of airway obstruction based on forced expiration, such as peak expiratory flow and spirometry. The latter are highly reproducible and their simplicity allows measurements to be made frequently – a great advantage in a condition as unstable as childhood asthma (see p. 499).

In addition to the well-recognized causes of airway obstruction in asthma (smooth muscle contraction, inflammatory edema,

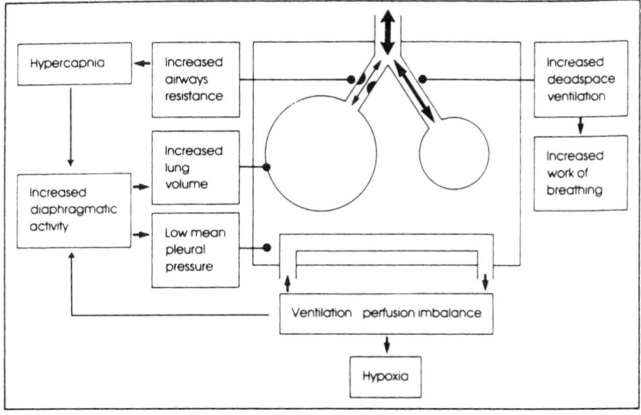

Fig. 12.16 The principal physiological features of asthma. All of these features are a consequence of uneven airways obstruction.

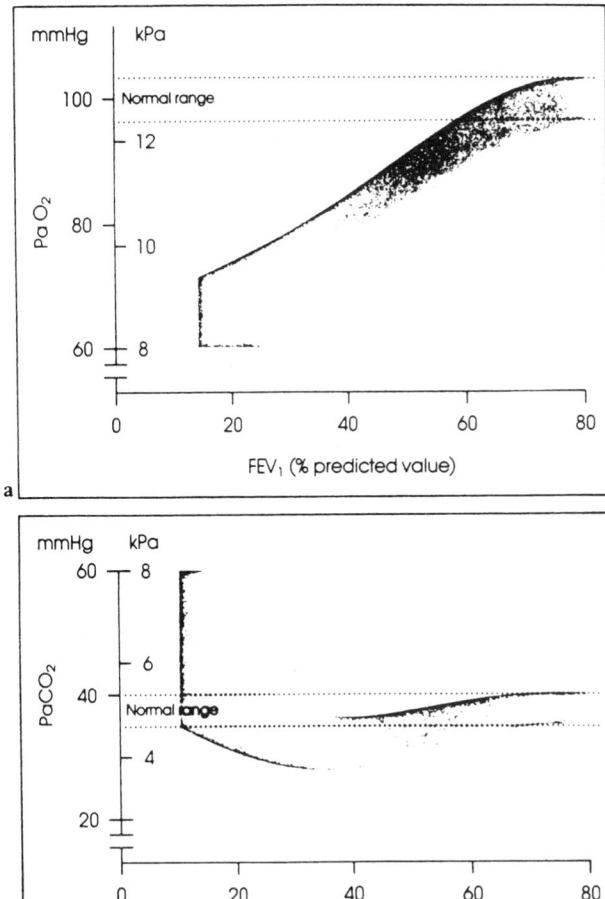

Fig. 12.17 The relation between lung function (FEV_1) and arterial oxygen (**a**) and carbon dioxide (**b**) tension (PaO_2 and $PaCO_2$ respectively). There is a progressive decline in PaO_2 as FEV_1 falls, but the situation is more complex for $PaCO_2$. Minor degrees of airway obstruction lead to relative hyperventilation with a small decline in $PaCO_2$, while severe airway obstruction causes CO_2 retention.

mucus secretion and venous congestion), variable airflow obstruction of a dynamic nature, particularly during forced expiration, should be remembered (p. 499). Variable glottic narrowing is also associated with and sometimes mistaken for asthma. In its extreme form it may constitute laryngeal dysfunction syndrome, a behavioral form of glottic obstruction which complicates management, especially in teenage girls.

One of the most obvious physiological consequences of airway obstruction is hyperinflation (Fig. 12.16). This may be brought about partly by passive 'air trapping' due to the closure of narrowed airways at fairly high lung volumes during expiration. However, the main cause of hyperinflation is active inspiratory muscle activity (increased diaphragmatic tone) which, by maintaining the lungs at a greater volume, provides greater traction on airways and thus increases airway patency, reducing the airways resistance.

CHRONIC AIRWAY OBSTRUCTION

Several groups have shown that abnormalities of lung function persist in the interval between acute attacks and even several years after clinical asthma has resolved. Evidence of minor degrees of hyperinflation, manifest as an increase in the residual volume of the lungs, and evidence of small airway dysfunction have been shown to be common in ex-asthmatics. The very sensitive indices of small airway function based on measurements of gas-mixing efficiency may be persistently abnormal. However, since bronchial hyperresponsiveness is known to persist even after clinical asthma has resolved, it is possible that these minor abnormalities of lung function represent subclinical episodes of reversible airways obstruction rather than fixed airway disease.

GAS EXCHANGE

Another consequence of airway obstruction is ventilation/perfusion imbalance. This leads to hypoxemia, the severity of which increases with the severity of airway obstruction (Fig. 12.17). Oximetry is a simple and satisfactory method of monitoring hypoxemia and the response to oxygen therapy. In the presence of mild airway obstruction, alveolar ventilation (and along with it dead-space ventilation) increases, leading to a slight reduction in arterial PCO_2 (Fig. 12.17). However, as airway

obstruction worsens, the ability of the respiratory muscles to cope with the increasing work of breathing begins to fail and, consequently, the arterial PCO_2 begins to rise. It is for this reason that the most valuable blood gas measurement in the assessment of severe asthma is the arterial PCO_2. As a general rule, an arterial PCO_2 of more than 6 kPa (45 mmHg) in a child with severe asthma indicates impending or actual respiratory failure, needing careful observation in a high-dependency area.

NATURAL HISTORY

INFANTS AND PRESCHOOL CHILDREN

The major inducer of reversible airway disease in infancy is viral respiratory tract infection, typified by recurrent episodic wheeze. This self-limiting condition has been labeled the wheezy baby syndrome or wheezy bronchitis. Clinical observations lend support to a distinction between episodic preschool wheeze and atopic childhood asthma. A difference in pathophysiology may explain the common failure of wheezy infants to respond to bronchodilator therapy which is so effective in older asthmatic children. If the pathological changes in fatal bronchiolitis (bronchiolar inflammation with epithelial desquamation and obstruction) are present in a milder form in the recurrent episodes of wheezing associated with viral infection in this group of children, then it is not surprising that drugs which act mainly on airway smooth muscle are ineffective in what is an acute inflammatory illness.

The atopic state is often present before the onset of asthma and may manifest itself as increased levels of IgE in cord blood in potentially atopic infants, as well as in symptoms such as infantile eczema or rhinitis which predate overt asthma by months or years. The level of exposure to inhalant allergens, especially house dust mite, in the first year of life may be critical in determining the likelihood of atopic asthma later in childhood in a susceptible infant. There is circumstantial evidence that food allergens from sources such as cow's milk may also predispose to atopic disease, especially eczema, in the infants of atopic parents, but asthma due to ingested allergens is very unusual. Atopy alone is not necessarily associated with increased bronchial responsiveness. In older children, atopic disease, manifested by a personal or first-degree family history of eczema, hay fever and asthma, is so closely associated with childhood asthma that it becomes increasingly difficult to dissociate increased bronchial responsiveness and atopic hypersensitivity.

A number of clinical and epidemiological observations suggest that episodic wheeze in preschool children and atopic asthma in schoolchildren can be considered as two distinct disorders. The natural history of these disorders over the first 6 years of life has been elegantly described by Martinez et al (1995).

1. Wheeze associated with viral infections accounts for most of the recurrent troublesome problems in the first year of life. At one extreme is acute viral bronchiolitis, due to infection with the respiratory syncytial virus (RSV) (p. 564). Common cold viruses (rhinovirus and coronavirus) are the other major precipitants of recurrent wheeze in this age group. Infants with this pattern of illness do not come preferentially from an atopic background and generally 'outgrow' their wheezing by their early school years, but may retain a tendency to be 'chesty with colds' into adult life.

2. Atopic asthma, a rare cause of infantile wheezing, increases in prevalence later in life, merging into the typical pattern of persistent childhood asthma. In this group there is usually a personal and family history of atopy, although viral infections again seem to be the trigger for severe attacks in the earlier years. Atopic features such as eczema may be related to ingested antigens in the first year of life, but aeroallergens predominate in later years. The risk factors for these two varieties of wheezing disease differ (Table 12.17).

SCHOOL CHILDREN

Most asthmatic children begin to develop symptoms of reversible airway disease by the age of 5 years, although not all of these are recognized as being asthmatic.

About 50% of children with asthma have relatively mild symptoms which regress spontaneously before puberty. About half receive continuous preventer therapy at some time during childhood and of these about half improve before and half during puberty. The most severe group of asthmatics, those requiring prophylactic therapy by means of high-dose inhaled or

Table 12.17 Risk factors for the two main wheezing syndromes of childhood

	Episodic viral wheeze	Atopic childhood asthma
Lung development		
Maternal smoking in pregnancy	+	+
Premorbid airway function	+	0
Premorbid bronchial responsiveness	+ (girls)	++
Atopy		
Personal features	0	++
Family history atopy	0	+
Family history asthma	+	++
Bronchial hyperresponsiveness	0	+++
Environmental factors		
Tobacco smoke	++	(+)
Communal childcare	++	0
Several older siblings	++	–

Key: + positive risk; 0 no known risk; – negative risk; (+) increases symptoms, not prevalence.

intermittent oral corticosteroid therapy, have the worse prognosis. Although almost all these patients show signs of improvement during puberty, few enter adult life symptom free.

It has been suggested (and proven in adults but not yet in children) that the long-term prognosis of asthma may be improved by the earlier introduction of inhaled corticosteroids (Agertoft & Pedersen 1994); the risk/benefit ratio has not been determined.

PUBERTY AND TEENAGE

A number of long-term prospective studies of childhood asthma have shown that symptoms usually decline at or before the onset of puberty. In association with symptomatic improvement, there is a decline in bronchial responsiveness. Puberty is delayed in atopic compared with nonatopic children, whether or not they have asthma. In one study, asthmatic boys entered puberty (stage II) 2 years later than expected. This may give the impression of growth failure (Fig. 12.18). Nevertheless, it is thought that except in the

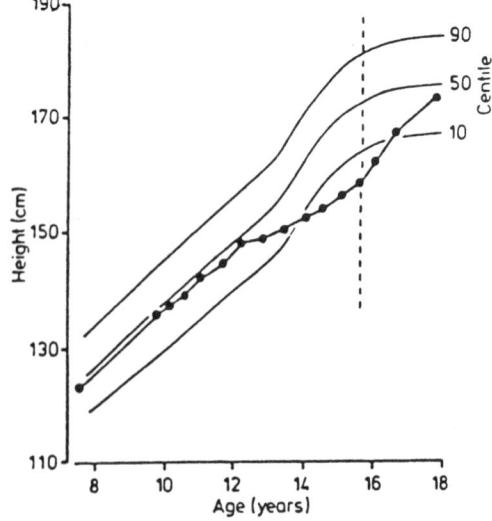

Fig. 12.18 Growth in a boy with non-steroid-dependent asthma, showing the deceleration of growth velocity which often precedes delayed puberty. The broken line represents onset of puberty. Final adult height was normal.

Table 12.18 Features of childhood asthma which predict continuation into adulthood

First-degree family history of atopy

Severe asthma during first 12 years of life

Eczema in first 2 years of life

Physical signs of chronic hyperinflation at puberty

Multiple positive skin-prick tests at puberty or IgE level > 90th centile for age

Failure to improve during puberty

Smoking

Table 12.19 Methods that can be used to identify allergic trigger factors

History supplemented by diary card

Other atopic features (e.g. seasonal rhinitis, food-induced symptoms, eczema)

Skin-prick tests (noting 'late' reactions)

Specific IgE measurement

Trial of allergen elimination
  Elimination diet
  House-dust mite or pet avoidance

Challenge tests
  Direct antigen inhalation challenge
  Indirect challenge

most severe, steroid-resistant cases, normal adult height can be expected. There is no explanation for either the delay in puberty or the amelioration of asthma during puberty.

It is now clear that the majority of childhood asthmatics who still have symptoms in their early teens will continue to have asthma of a similar pattern as young adults (Martin et al 1986). Episodic preschool wheezing does not cause permanent damage to growing lungs or lead to bronchial hyperreactivity (Godden et al 1994). The likelihood of childhood asthma continuing into adult life can be assessed from certain prognostic features (Table 12.18).

INDUCERS AND TRIGGERS

Some triggers can be avoided while others require active forms of management. It is therefore important to attempt to identify the main triggers responsible for attacks of asthma in individual patients. In general careful history taking is most rewarding, although some investigations are of value.

ALLERGY

The atopic state is an almost universal feature of asthma in children of school age (Zimmerman et al 1988). There are variations in the prevalence of important inhaled antigens in different parts of the world.

The first step in identifying an important allergen is a comprehensive case history (Table 12.19). The pattern of asthmatic symptoms may give a clue to the presence of an allergic trigger. Seasonal variations in pollen and mold spore exposure cause characteristic seasonal asthma in Europe and North America, although in some countries, such as Australia, pollen asthma is said to be rare. It is now recognized that there is a house dust mite 'season' at the end of summer in Western Europe. The presence of severe nocturnal asthma may provide a clue to house dust mite sensitivity. By using a daily record card, the association between symptoms of asthma and visits to particular places may become apparent.

Two groups of investigations are used in the identification of allergic triggers. Skin-prick testing is easy to perform, cheap and gives a quick answer. Although more than 30–40% of older children and adults are atopic (i.e. produce an immediate reaction to one or more common antigens on skin-prick testing), almost all schoolchildren with troublesome asthma are atopic and, in the UK, react to one or more of house dust mite extract, mixed grass pollen extract or cat dander. The relevance of these reactions is

difficult to ascertain, but it has been suggested that wheals of greater than 5 mm in diameter indicate that the allergen is probably of clinical significance. Skin-prick testing for food antigens provides a much poorer indication of clinical importance. Whenever skin-prick tests are carried out, the results should be used as a guide to likely clinical sensitivity and should be confirmed by careful history taking, challenge tests or avoidance. As well as the immediate (15–20 min) wheal-and-flare reaction to skin-prick testing, patients with a high degree of allergic sensitivity may develop a 'late' reaction after 3–6 h. This consists of a diffuse swelling in the area of the prick test and is much less easily defined than the early wheal, but is probably of equal clinical significance. It has been suggested that late reactions to skin testing can be used to identify particularly high degrees of sensitivity to important allergens.

By means of the RAST (radioallergosorbent test) procedure, the quantity of specific IgE antibodies against a range of common antigens can be determined. Values correlate well with the size of skin-prick test wheals. For inhaled allergens, there appear to be no advantages to these expensive and time-consuming laboratory tests. For young infants, however, and for individuals who may be sensitive to food proteins, RAST measurements can occasionally be helpful in the identification of important triggers. The other commonly performed measurement, the serum total IgE, is of no value in the identification of specific allergic triggers.

INFECTION

Rhinoviruses, coronaviruses and parainfluenza virus have frequently been implicated in acute severe asthma, but a range of other agents may also be responsible. In infancy, RSV epidemics lead to acute bronchiolitis, a predictor of recurrent wheezing in a small proportion of preschool children. The critical factor in the development of wheezing in response to a virus infection is individual predisposition. Those children who have a previous history of wheeze respond to virus infections with a further attack of wheeze. Bacterial infections play little or no part in asthma, but 'atypical' organisms such as *Mycoplasma pneumoniae* are occasionally found in older children.

EXERCISE

Exercise-induced asthma (EIA) is not a specific variety of asthma. Exercise is merely a trigger which will, in all moderate or severe asthmatic children, provoke brief and spontaneously reversible airway obstruction. Exercise-induced asthma is almost universal, but its severity varies, both between and within individual patients. While the importance of EIA in the individual patient can often be determined by careful history taking, a simple exercise test carried out on a treadmill or bicycle ergometer or even out in the open air is a useful confirmatory procedure (p. 501). The presence of EIA in a treated patient is a sign of poor control.

The mechanism of exercise-induced asthma is still unclear although many workers have shown that hyperventilation during exercise is of critical importance. It is probable that water loss by evaporation from the airways acts as the trigger, by producing either airway cooling or changes in local osmolality.

The ameliorating effects of warmed humidified air may partially explain the fact that swimming has less of an asthma-provoking effect than field sports, since the air immediately above the swimming pool is usually warmer and more humid than outdoor air. A period of relative refractoriness to further EIA occurs after a period of strenuous exercise and may persist for 2 h or so. Repeated exercise challenge produces progressively less EIA and it has been shown that, by performing a series of half-minute sprint warm-up exercises, asthmatic children can induce sufficient refractoriness to enable them to take part in strenuous sport without provoking an attack.

FOOD INTOLERANCE

The importance of food intolerance in childhood asthma has been a subject of debate for many years. There are several reasons for this. The first is the difficulty in obtaining (or believing) the histories provided by patients. There is no doubt, however, that when patients' histories are taken carefully there is ample evidence to suggest that many foods and drinks may be associated with cough and wheeze in asthmatic children. The interval between food ingestion and the onset of symptoms is so variable and the association between delayed symptoms and food ingestion is so difficult to fit into any current theories of asthma that patients' histories are often disbelieved.

Another important factor that has led to the doubt over the importance of food sensitivity is the rather poor outcome of objective challenge tests. In the past, these tests have relied on the detection of changes in lung function following ingestion of the suspected food, in a double-blind challenge. Even when there is no change in baseline airways obstruction, bronchial responsiveness may be enhanced by ingested allergens (e.g. eggs, peanuts), chemical agents (e.g. tartrazine, fried corn oil) or physical agents (i.e. ice, dilute hydrochloric acid) in sensitive individuals. This has been termed an indirect challenge procedure (Silverman & Wilson 1985).

In some children with intractable asthma, in whom it may not be possible to identify offending food antigens either by immunological tests or by bronchial challenge procedures, an elimination diet may be the only means of identifying major food intolerance. In order to avoid malnutrition, an expert dietitian must be involved in the supervision of such a diet.

PSYCHOLOGICAL FACTORS

Children with chronic perennial asthma are no more emotionally disturbed than any other group of chronically sick children. However, emotional disturbance may, like exercise, provoke an attack. Both laughter and crying are important triggers of airway obstruction, although they do not normally lead to any more than a brief and reversible attack of asthma. There are undoubtedly some children who can induce this form of attack.

GASTROESOPHAGEAL REFLUX

Claims that gastroesophageal reflux is an important trigger factor in asthma are controversial. There is, however, direct evidence implicating esophageal acid reflux. By infusing hydrochloric acid into the distal esophagus of asthmatic children with esophagitis, acute airway obstruction has been induced in up to half of the children tested. In experimental animals, airway changes induced by esophageal acid infusion have been prevented by cutting the vagus nerves, suggesting that a vagal mechanism is responsible.

The diagnosis of gastroesophageal reflux is remarkably difficult. Both upper gastrointestinal barium studies and radionuclide milk scans (looking for pulmonary aspiration) are unrewarding. Overnight monitoring of esphageal pH using a miniature probe has shown that minor degrees of gastroesophageal reflux are equally common in severely asthmatic children and controls. The mere presence of gastroesophageal reflux does not therefore imply any clinical relevance. The use of specific H_2-receptor antagonist drugs or proton pump inhibitors to control gastric acid secretion at night and prokinetic agents (cisapride) to enhance gastric emptying may improve symptoms.

MISCELLANEOUS TRIGGER FACTORS

It has been recognized since the 17th century that *air pollution* is important to respiratory health. The relationship with asthma is different in different environments. In general, pollution does not cause asthma but causes asthmatics to become symptomatic. In highly polluted environments, such as Los Angeles during the smog season, the prevalence of wheeze increases. However, atopy and asthma are *less* common in polluted Eastern Europe compared with Western Europe (von Mutius et al 1994). In some environments with no pollution at all (Skye) there is above average asthma. Air pollution is probably of greater significance in preschool episodic wheeze than in atopic asthma.

Several *drugs* can trigger airway obstruction in asthmatics. Some, such as nonselective beta-blockers, are rarely used in pediatrics while others such as aspirin, which are important triggers of asthma in nonatopic adults, are rarely implicated in childhood.

Coloring agents, such as tartrazine, which in the past have been added to medicines, are now generally being withdrawn, although some foods still contain potentially important triggers.

CLINICAL FEATURES AND DIAGNOSIS

The diagnosis of asthma is based mainly on the characteristic history of recurrent wheeze and cough. Occasionally, tests of lung function or bronchial responsiveness may be helpful but, where the history is not clearcut, these tests are also likely to give borderline results. Assessing the response to a trial of antiasthma therapy may be the final means of diagnosis in cases where doubt persists. There are particular difficulties in infants, who may be unresponsive to therapy, and preschool children whose major symptom may be cough. Recurrent cough in the absence of wheeze is probably not part of the asthma spectrum, but a therapeutic trial may be used to discriminate.

HISTORY AND PHYSICAL SIGNS

Patterns of asthma

Patterns of asthma in infants differ from the usual pattern of episodic wheeze found in older children and adults. Asthma tends to be less stable in young children, making diagnosis slightly easier but management more difficult. Episodic wheeze associated with virus infections, often with long, symptom-free intervals, is a common pattern (Fig. 12.19a). Episodic night cough, even in the absence of wheezing, may indicate preschool asthma and warrants a therapeutic trial; be sceptical! Interval symptoms between episodes may be absent or mild (Fig. 12.19b).

Schoolchildren with asthma are more likely to have chronic symptoms (such as EIA, sleep disturbance, seasonal exacerbations) as well as viral episodes (Fig. 12.19c). The pattern, severity and frequency of symptoms is important in management. Some children have unremitting symptoms, despite therapy (Fig. 12.19d).

Features in the patient's history which should arouse suspicion that the diagnosis may not be asthma include: intractable wheeze, wheezing associated with choking episodes or with feeding, the absence of a personal or first-degree family history of atopy in a

child of school age and a history of onset of symptoms in the perinatal period.

Physical examination

Physical examination is of some value in the diagnosis of asthma, but is most important in ruling out other causes of wheeze and other chronic respiratory symptoms in childhood. Asthma is a generalized disorder of intrathoracic airways and the physical signs should therefore be generalized. Hyperinflation and chest deformity (pigeon chest or Harrison's sulci) are useful in the assessment of severity and chronicity respectively, but they are not diagnostic. The presence of focal physical signs (crackles or wheezes) of a persistent or recurrent nature should arouse one's suspicion that structural lung disease such as bronchiectasis, obstruction due to a foreign body or airway compression are the cause of a child's symptoms. Clubbing does not occur in asthma and its presence suggests some form of chronic suppuration such as cystic fibrosis. Asthmatic children are often a little underweight, but marked growth failure should again suggest chronic hypoxia or chronic suppuration.

DIAGNOSTIC AIDS

Record card

The daily record card provides a systematic way of recording symptoms from day to day. Although there has been no objective validation, it is still used to assess the severity and pattern of symptoms and the response to therapy.

Peak flow measurements

Objective evidence of the severity and nature of airways obstruction in wheezy children of school age can be obtained by means of twice-daily peak flow measurements that can easily be made at home using a Wright peak flow minimeter. Values can be recorded on the diary card and, if necessary, displayed in graphical form to provide information about the variability of airway obstruction. Estimates of peak flow variability have been used in epidemiological studies of asthma but are of little value in the diagnosis of individual children. In contrast, peak flow measurements made at home can be of great value in providing objective evidence of the severity of asthma. A single isolated value of peak flow (or of any other measure of lung function) is of little use in the assessment of severity since variability, even within a 24-h period, is so great. However, single measurements of peak flow rate do have a part to play in assessing the perception of asthma.

Bronchodilator responsiveness

When airway obstruction is present, bronchodilator responsiveness can be a useful, simple test for asthma. An increase in peak flow or FEV_1 of more than 20% after an adequate dose of nebulized bronchodilator is diagnostic of asthma, but a negative result does not rule out the condition.

Bronchial responsiveness (see p. 537)

It has been suggested that, since bronchial hyperresponsiveness is a central feature of asthma, tests of bronchial responsiveness

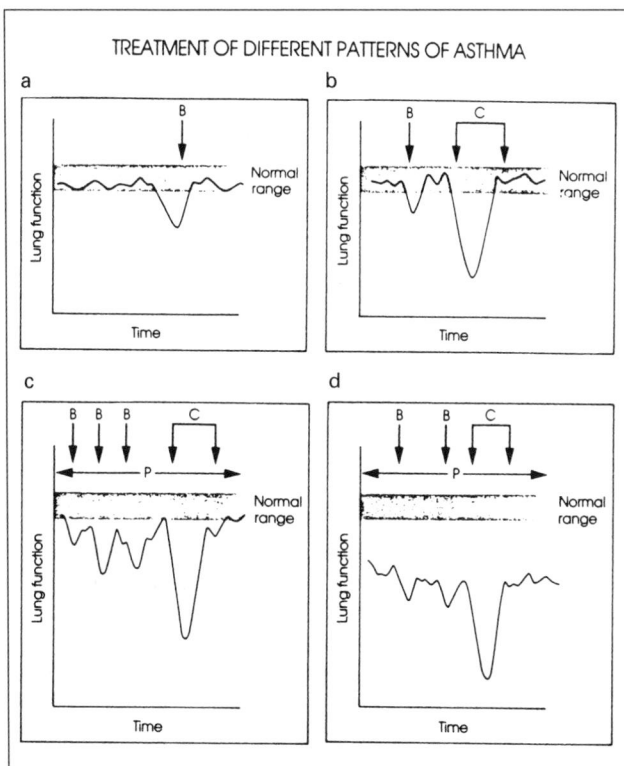

Fig. 12.19 The pattern of a patient's asthma largely dictates the drug treatment they should receive. This figure shows the basis for the use of bronchodilators (B), corticosteroids (C), and long-term prophylactic agents (P) in each of the four patterns of asthma: (**a**) mild episodic symptoms; (**b**) episodic with intercurrent symptoms; (**c**) chronic intercurrent and episodic symptoms fully reversible at times; (**d**) chronic intercurrent and episodic symptoms which never resolve completely.

could be valuable in the diagnosis of the condition. However, there are three reasons why this does not apply in childhood. First, tests of bronchial responsiveness are not at present feasible in children under the age of 6 years. Second, the degree of bronchial responsiveness in asthmatic children and normal children forms a continuum with a large 'gray area'. There is no single dividing line, so that where the diagnosis is in doubt on the basis of the history, tests of bronchial responsiveness are also likely to yield borderline results. Finally, it is quite clear that bronchial responsiveness is not constant in any individual asthmatic, but varies from time to time.

Chest radiograph

A chest radiograph should be taken of any child presenting with severe chronic respiratory symptoms. There are no characteristic radiological features of asthma but, like the clinical signs, the radiological changes in asthma are normally generalized: hyperinflation or bronchial wall thickening. Where there are focal radiological changes of a persistent or recurrent nature (localized bronchial wall thickening, hilar lymphadenopathy, unilateral hyperlucency or segmental atelectasis), the diagnosis of asthma should be in doubt. Acute severe asthma may be accompanied by pneumothorax or pneumomediastinum. Segmental or lobar atelectasis due to mucus plugging is another radiological feature. This occasionally occurs in the absence of wheezing in young children.

Other investigations

Other tests that are occasionally carried out in the investigation of asthma include hematological investigations, the measurement of serum immunoglobulins, including IgE and skin-prick tests for immediate hypersensitivity. In an atopic child with troublesome asthma and negative skin-prick tests for common allergens, (house dust mite, grass pollen, cat and dog) tests for specific IgE (RAST test or equivalent) may help. Antihistamines and oral steroids can suppress skin prick tests.

MANAGEMENT

The principal aim of management is to allow children to lead a normal life with the minimum possible interference from their illness.

ASSESSMENT OF SEVERITY

Asthma is much less stable in childhood than in adult life and therefore there is continuous need to assess the severity of the illness.

Home monitoring

The daily record card is a valuable means of assessment in children with asthma and a useful guide to further management. Some of the symptoms recorded are of greater significance than others. The amount of night disturbance is a very important indicator of the underlying severity of the condition. Even in the absence of overt daytime symptoms, cough and wheeze during the night indicate poorly controlled asthma. During the daytime, the presence of exercise-induced asthma, the number of days off school and the occurrence of obtrusive cough suggest poor control.

A record of the use of additional bronchodilators gives some idea of the overall severity of asthma, at least from the patient's point of view. Monitoring repeat prescriptions for bronchodilator therapy (e.g. inhalers) provides an additional safeguard and permits compliance with treatment to be assessed.

Recordings of home peak flow data are easily evaluated by inspection and an optimum for the individual derived. Because of the very wide range in population values, mean values from these charts are of little practical help. Peak flow rates of less than about 50–60% of the optimum value can be considered to represent severe airway obstruction and knowledge of 'own best' allows intervention long before this value is reached. Values between 50% and 80% represent moderate airway obstruction requiring less urgent action. By inspecting the records of peak flow on the record card, therefore, the physician can obtain a good idea of how variable and how severe a patient's asthma has been during the previous few weeks. It is certainly not necessary for children to record their peak flow daily when their asthma is under control and, in fact, this could lead them to acquire an unhealthy attitude towards their illness. The peak flow can be deceptively high first thing in the morning if the child has woken up during the night and taken an additional dose of bronchodilator.

In older children with unstable asthma, the provision of a peak flow meter for home use allows them to regulate their treatment according to the severity of airways obstruction during an acute attack. Patients can be instructed to seek urgent medical help, rather than to persist with possibly inadequate home therapy, when the peak flow falls to less than about 50% of the optimum and does not respond promptly to bronchodilator. At 25–30%, the child should be in a hospital.

Monitoring in the clinic or health center

The limitations of the patient's history in the assessment of severity can sometimes be largely overcome by using a record card system. Data storage spirometers for home use are a promising new development. Physical examination is of little value in assessing the severity of childhood asthma. Only where there are gross signs of airways obstruction, with chest deformity or hyperinflation and dyspnea, out of proportion to the child's or the parents' evaluation of his condition, does physical examination give particularly useful information.

Lung function tests are also of very limited value in the clinic, but the occasional measurement of lung function does have one extremely important function. This concerns the perception of the severity of asthma by the child and his parents on the one hand and the doctor on the other. The child who claims to be well and yet who has a severe degree of airways obstruction may be dangerously tolerant of his condition. Conversely, when the parents of a child express alarm about his condition and yet objective measurements of his lung function are normal, the physician might suspect a degree of exaggeration and overprotection bearing in mind the difficulty in determining the 'predicted' value. This sort of information is extremely important to the physician in the task of educating children and their parents about the condition. Such education is essential if the family are to be able to cope with the sort of responsibility for self-management which the condition necessitates.

TREATMENT

General measures

One of the most important aspects of the general management of childhood asthma is the education of both child and parents to understand the nature of the illness and thereby to be able to undertake guided self-management at home.

Avoidance of major trigger factors should be attempted provided that it does not interfere unduly with the child's lifestyle. House dust mite avoidance measures (removal of soft furnishings and carpets from the bedroom, vacuuming of the mattress and household carpets with a powerful cleaner fitted with fine filter, replacement of old blankets, quilts and pillows with synthetic materials, removal of teddy bears and other stuffed toys) have a limited role in diminishing nocturnal symptoms. Moisture-permeable fabric, mattress covers and pillow cases which exclude mite products from the patient and skin scales from the mites effectively reduce exposure. Acaricides are only temporarily effective, may be toxic and have not proved to be useful.

The removal of household pets is an even more contentious issue but should be advised if there is a clear clinical response to cats or dogs or a large immediate skin-prick test response. Even when there is clinical evidence of sensitivity, the decline in antigen load and clinical response is slow. A weekly bath for the cat and dog is a less traumatic means of reducing the household burden of antigen, but evidence as to its efficacy is lacking.

Parental smoking contributes significantly to ill health in asthmatic children. Maternal smoking during (the subsequent) pregnancy should be discouraged. Measures to remove house mites should probably be undertaken at the time the pregnancy is planned, to delay sensitization in highly atopic asthmatic families.

Of even less proven value is so-called hyposensitization by immunotherapy. This may have a part to play in very severe seasonal asthma, although the dangers of anaphylaxis during immunotherapy are greater in this highly sensitive group of individuals, and possibly in severe intractable asthma due to house dust mite sensitivity. For the run-of-the-mill asthmatic child, hyposensitization has no part to play.

Where a history of food intolerance is obtained, it is wise to avoid the food in question. The use of elimination diets or antigen avoidance (e.g. cow's milk avoidance) as a routine measure in nonatopic infants or older children with well-controlled asthma cannot be justified.

Psychological factors have been blamed for much of childhood asthma. As with any chronic illness, the interplay of anxiety on the one hand and the wish to avoid seeming troublesome on the other may lead to complications. With adequate pharmacological control, asthmatic children can have their behavior problems dealt with in the same way as other children. This can be tricky if there is nonadherence with treatment.

Sport and exercise should be positively encouraged, provided that adequate treatment is provided to prevent exercise-induced asthma. While there is no evidence that training reduces the severity of asthma, it can certainly make asthmatic children more fit and therefore more able to compete on equal terms with their fellows.

Physiotherapy and breathing exercises have in the past been advocated for asthmatic children. However, these procedures have virtually no part to play in patient management, since symptoms should be sufficiently controlled with adequate drug therapy. Rarely, a child who has overwhelmingly severe attacks exacerbated by panic or who has laryngeal dysfunction syndrome may benefit from controlled breathing exercises.

Drug therapy

Patterns of asthma

The choice of drug depends largely on the pattern of disease; the choice of device depends on age and dexterity. The pattern may be classified into one of four groups on the basis of the history or the symptom score or peak flow rate recorded on a daily record card (Fig. 12.19). It should be noted, however, that asthma in childhood is a changing condition and that children move from one pattern to another or even cease to have symptoms altogether.

Pattern a is the commonest and mildest form of asthma, requiring only intermittent bronchodilator therapy. *Pattern b* is commonly seen in preschool children who may be symptom free for much of the time but occasionally develop acute severe wheezing episodes with viral respiratory tract infection. In addition to intermittent bronchodilator therapy, short course oral steroid therapy should be available at home for administration by parents, provided that an adequate degree of understanding between the parents and the medical practitioner has been achieved. There is no evidence for any benefit from preventer therapy with inhaled steroids in this group, even if episodes are frequent (Wilson et al 1995).

Patterns c and *d* need continuous therapy. In *c*, there may be day-to-day symptoms (without persistent reduction in lung function), on which acute attacks are superimposed. Pattern *d* is characterized by long periods of persistent airway obstruction but, paradoxically, since these children often adapt quite well to their disability, their symptoms may be less pronounced than those in group *c*. Patients with either of these patterns need continuous long-term prophylactic therapy with sodium cromoglycate (if relatively mild or seasonal) or inhaled corticosteroids. Very occasional patients in group *d* may also need alternate-day steroid treatment if the above treatments are inadequate. In addition to these preventer treatments, intermittent bronchodilators may be required together with short course oral steroid therapy for acute exacerbations.

Route of administration (O'Callaghan & Barry 1997)

Drugs should be administered topically, by inhalation as dry powders or aerosols, whenever possible. Their action is rapid and systemic effects are few. The devices available for topical therapy include metered dose inhalers (MDI) used alone or together with a valved spacer (with soft face mask or mouthpiece), dry powder inhalers and wet aerosols generated by a jet nebulizer (with compressed air source) or an ultrasonic nebulizer and administered by loose face mask or mouthpiece. Under ideal conditions, none of these devices delivers more than 10–12% of the nominal dose to the lower respiratory tract. In the first 2 years of life, when administered by face mask, 1% or less is deposited in the lungs.

Oral β-agonists take about 1 h to exert their maximum effect and sometimes cause distressing systemic ill effects. Some drugs (theophylline, prednisolone) cannot be given topically.

Individual antiasthma preparations

Selective β2-adrenergic agonists (bronchodilators). Short-acting β2-agonists are the mainstay of symptomatic treatment in young children for intermittent or regular use and as additional rescue therapy during acute attacks. There are few side-effects with inhaled preparations and these should be used preferentially in children of all ages, since oral therapy is less effective, requires a higher dose and more frequently gives rise to side-effects such as troublesome tremor. It is possible to provide inhaled bronchodilator therapy for children of any age. The rise in asthma mortality in New Zealand in the 1980s was thought to be the result of chronic overreliance on β_2-agonists with consequent subsensitization (tachyphylaxis). There is evidence that chronic use does reduce the protective effects of β-agonists against bronchial challenge in adults (but not children), although the bronchodilator effect is preserved. The balance of opinion is that the contribution of β-agonist use to asthma mortality is negligible, but that exessive reliance is not advisable and indicates the need for more effective preventer therapy.

There is no generally applicable dose of bronchodilators. Their efficacy and duration of action depend on the severity of asthma. Moreover, the duration of protection against, for instance, exercise-induced asthma is a good deal shorter than the duration of the bronchodilator effect. Thus, both the dosage and the dose interval should be tailored to suit the needs of each individual patient. Generally, a 3–4 h drug interval proves satisfactory. However, where excessive reliance is being placed on bronchodilator therapy, it is more appropriate to move on to continuous preventer therapy.

Long-acting inhaled β2-agonists such as salmeterol and formoterol are effective for 12 hours or more. They are useful if nocturnal symptoms are troublesome and as regular twice-daily therapy for children who might otherwise need to go onto high doses of inhaled corticosteroids for poorly controlled asthma.

Sodium cromoglycate. Sodium cromoglycate was originally considered to be a mast cell stabilizer, inhibiting mediator release, but is now also thought to influence bronchial hyperresponsiveness, possibly through neural effects. In addition, the drug has been shown to reduce infiltration by inflammatory cells and mediator release. Sodium cromoglycate is only effective when given by inhalation and is available as a metered dose aerosol inhaler or dry powder inhaler. This drug has no significant side-effects. Its main use is as a regular prophylactic agent. For many years it has been the first-line prophylactic preparation in the UK, largely because of its very wide margin of safety. About 50% of children with mild pattern c asthma can expect good control from regular four-times-daily sodium cromoglycate. There is no evidence of efficacy in infancy.

The recommended dose (one 20 mg powder capsule or two 5 mg aerosol puffs four times daily) is adequate for most children. As with bronchodilator therapy, the interval between doses may also need to be adjusted because the duration of effect varies between individuals.

Corticosteroids. Corticosteroids inhibit the enzyme phospholipase A2, which is important in the production of membrane-derived mediators of bronchoconstriction (e.g. leukotrienes, thromboxanes) from mast cells and other inflammatory cells. In addition, they enhance β-adrenergic receptor responsiveness, perhaps by increasing the number of active receptors on smooth muscle cell membranes. By modifying the transcription of corticosteroid responsive genes, they reduce cytokine production and thereby inflammation. Corticosteroids can be given orally or by inhalation, but the indications for their use and their potential complications are different when given by these routes.

By the inhaled route, topically active, poorly absorbed corticosteroids are available in metered dose inhalers, dry powder inhalers or nebulizer suspensions for infant use. The delivery of suspensions by wet nebulization is uncertain. These preparations are indicated in patients with pattern c asthma, after first-line prophylactic therapy has failed. There are few significant adverse effects of inhaled preparations. In very high dose (over 20 μg/kg/day) there is some evidence of adrenal suppression, although this remains controversial. The short adrenal stimulation test (Synacthen test) is normal even on high dose therapy, although 9 am fasting serum cortisol levels and 24-h urinary cortisol breakdown products may be low. Oral candidiasis is unusual in childhood and may be prevented by the use of a spacer device. Dysphonia, thought to be due to a local steroid myopathy of the muscles of phonation, is also unusual in childhood. Inhaled corticosteroids in modest doses do not have any significant long-term adverse effects on growth. Knemometry (measurement of lower leg length) has been used to study short-term systemic effects of inhaled corticosteroids. There are undoubtedly short-term measurable effects, but these do not translate into long-term effects on statural height.

Oral prednisolone, given on an alternate-day basis (as a single dose in the morning), is occasionally required for chronic, poorly controlled asthma, for children who have other major, uncontrolled atopic disabilities, such as very severe eczema, and for some preschool children who cannot manage any form of topical, inhaled therapy. Doses of up to 20 mg on alternate days may be required for severe teenage asthmatics. When given on an alternate-day basis, hypothalamic-pituitary-adrenal suppression, peptic ulceration and hypertension are extremely unusual complications. Steroid cataracts have been described in this group of patients and evidence of their development should be carefully sought at regular intervals. Alternate-day therapy causes alternate day growth suppression, with adequate catch-up so that overall growth is unaffected at doses below 0.5 mg/kg/day. The main problem appears to be excessive weight gain due to appetite stimulation. Since adrenal suppression may be a feature of oral steroid therapy, children should carry a steroid card or a MedicAlert badge or bracelet.

Corticosteroids are generally introduced either when prophylaxis with sodium cromoglycate has failed or as the first preventer step for troublesome asthma. When used in acute severe asthma, their effects are measurable after about 4–6 h. However, when used in prophylaxis, an effect on exercise-induced asthma and on the acute response to inhaled antigen appears to take 1–2 weeks to develop. It is important to explain this fact to patients who otherwise tend to use metered dose corticosteroid inhalers in the same way as their metered dose bronchodilator inhalers.

Theophylline. Theophylline is traditionally thought to act by inhibition of phosphodiesterase, the active cellular enzyme that inhibits adenylate cyclase. This in vitro property may not explain its in vivo actions, since the concentration required for the effective inhibition of phosphodiesterase is far higher than that achieved during therapy. It is possible that theophylline has its effect on the nonadrenergic, noncholinergic inhibitory control of airways smooth muscle via adenosine receptors. It also has other actions on the central nervous system and on striated muscle. Recently, anti-inflammatory effects have been demonstrated at 50% of the previously recommended dose. There are several types of phosphodiesterase; selective inhibitors are likely in the near future.

In the home management of asthma theophylline has a minor

role, although until recently it had been the drug of first choice for prophylaxis in the USA. Slow release oral theophylline preparations given two or three times daily are able to produce controlled serum theophylline levels within the conventional range of 10–20 mg/l. In patients aged between 12 months and puberty, the maximum dose of theophylline should be about 25 mg/kg/day (in divided doses), falling to half this value in adults. Low-dose therapy has yet to be evaluated in children but the target range would be 6–10 mg/l. Theophylline has a very narrow therapeutic margin and it is impossible to increase the dose without risking toxic effects, which are common enough even within the therapeutic range. It has a very poor protective effect against exercise-induced asthma.

It is recommended that serum theophylline levels (or if facilities exist, salivary theophylline levels) are measured from time to time so that dosage adjustments can be made. Theophylline clearance is lower during acute respiratory infections and may be affected by concurrent antibiotic use.

Anticholinergic (antimuscarinic) drugs. Anticholinergic drugs which are poorly absorbed from the respiratory tract (oxitropium bromide, ipratropium bromide) act as competitive blockers of the muscarinic receptors on the vagus and airway smooth muscle. They are available effectively only by inhalation, since systemic atropine-like drugs have major side-effects. Side-effects are minimal by inhalation, but so too are the clear clinical benefits. Poorly controlled asthmatics, or those in whom bronchodilator therapy has only a short duration of action, may benefit by the addition of regular inhaled anticholinergic agents. There is undoubted synergism with inhaled, high-dose β-agonists in acute severe asthma. The advent of selective m_3 antagonists will render nonselective agents obsolete.

Other drugs. Several other drugs have been used in the management of childhood asthma. Antihistamines have no useful function in simple asthma, although they are sometimes beneficial in children with multiple atopy. Used in the daytime, 'cough medicines' cause more harm than good because of their sedative effects.

There is controversy concerning the role of gastroesophageal reflux in asthma and the place of antireflux therapy. Nocturnal asthma may be exacerbated by reflux and reflux itself may be made worse by hyperinflation and the relaxation of the distal esophagus brought about by bronchodilator and theophylline therapy. Recurrent gastroesophageal reflux may lead to esophagitis and is an indication for using more effective inhaled antiasthma therapy together with a selective proton pump inhibitor or H_2-antagonist, antacids and cisapride, if appropriate. For very severe or steroid-resistant cases, unusual forms of therapy are occasionally needed (Hill & Tattersfield 1995).

Home nebulizers

There are two indications for the use of nebulizers at home. First, preschool children who require continuous inhaled steroids as routine management, but who cannot manage the other inhaler devices may benefit enormously from a home nebulizer unit. Second, children who suffer from frequent severe attacks that are unresponsive to their normal inhalers may benefit from nebulized β2 bronchodilator treatment at home. This latter group is more controversial. Home nebulizers should be used only under regular medical supervision and written advice should be provided, but they may occasionally be life saving. Nebulizer provision should be regulated via a locality-wide service.

Insuring adherence to therapy

Careful explanation and education are essential, but there is no substitute for written, self-management guidelines with repetition at every contact with a health professional. An instruction/record card, such as that published by the UK National Asthma Campaign, serves as an aide-memoire for the patient and a means of communication between medical practitioners. Self-management plans should be based on local asthma guidelines, such as those published in the UK (Fig. 12.20).

ACUTE SEVERE ASTHMA

EMERGENCY MANAGEMENT

Assessment

The assessment of a patient with acute severe asthma is based on information provided by the history, physical examination and physiological measurements. A knowledge of the outcome of previous acute episodes is useful in planning management.

The history will provide little information about the severity of the asthma. However, it is vital to inquire into the patient's recent medication, particularly theophylline, since the addition of intravenous aminophylline in hospital could provoke fits in a child who already has a high serum theophylline level.

Physical examination is also of limited value. Studies have shown a poor correlation between most physical signs and the severity of airway obstruction. The most important physical signs are: extreme dyspnea, manifested by difficulty in speaking; the use of accessory muscles of respiration (the sternomastoid muscles); and, of course, cyanosis, which is a very late feature in childhood asthma and implies a critical degree of airway obstruction. The loudness of wheeze on auscultation does not provide a good indication of severity, but it is important to recognize a patient who has a 'silent' chest as this indicates critically severe asthma. Oximetry provides guidelines for action: $SaO_2 < 92\%$ after initial rescue therapy is an indication for admission to hospital.

One of the most important objective measurements for children over the age of 5 or 6 years is the measurement of the peak flow. A peak flow of less than 25–30% of the child's optimum (or failing this, the predicted value) indicates severe asthma requiring admission to hospital.

In extreme cases, only the most cursory assessment may be carried out in the A&E department while a nurse prepares a nebulizer. Even under these circumstances, it should be possible to bear in mind alternative diagnoses, particularly if the patient is not familiar to the medical and nursing staff. The few conditions that can mimic acute severe asthma include inhaled foreign body, severe laryngotracheobronchitis and the difficult condition of laryngeal dysfunction syndrome. Primary pneumonia in an asthmatic can be very confusing. Such children tend to be more profoundly hypoxemic than one would expect and show little response to asthma treatment. The use of inhaled adrenaline in the A&E department may mask the diagnosis.

Treatment (Warner et al 1989, Hargreave et al 1990)

Resuscitation with nebulized β2-agonist is almost always effective, even if the child appears to have received adequate doses of bronchodilator previously. However, the duration of bronchodilator effect may be as short as 20–30 min in a

- Avoidance of provoking factors where possible
- Working towards a self-management plan
- Selection of best inhaler device

Note
Patients should start treatment at the step most appropriate to the initial severity. A rescue course of prednisolone may be needed at any step (maximum daily dose 40 mg).

Prescribe a peak flow meter and monitor response to treatment where appropriate.

Stepping down

Regularly review the need for treatment. In older children use a peak flow record to assess the speed of withdrawal. Stop regular anti-inflammatory treatment after 6–12 months of few or no symptoms. If symptoms are seasonal consider stopping anti-inflammatory drugs at the end of the season.

Step 5

a: High dose inhaled steroids and bronchodilators

Inhaled steroids (800 µg daily) and other treatment as in step 4. Slow-release xanthines or nebulized β-agonists

b: Addition of regular steroid tablets
As in step 5a with the addition of alternate-day low-dose (5–10 mg) prednisolone. Consider regular ipratropium or subcutaneous infusion of a β-agonist.

Step 4

High dose inhaled steroids

Inhaled short-acting β agonists as required *plus:* beclomethasone or budesonide increased to 400–800 µg daily via a large volume spacer or dry powder divice. Consider short prednisolone course. Consider adding regular twice-daily long-acting β-agonist.

Step 3

Inhaled steroids

Inhaled short-acting β agonists as required *plus:* beclomethasone or budesonide 50–200 µg twice daily. Consider a 5-day course of soluble prednisolone 1–2 mg/kg/day or a temporary increase in inhaled steroids (double dose) for stabilization.

Step 2

Regular inhaled anti-inflammatory agents

Intermittent inhaled short-acting β agonists as required *plus:* cromoglycate as powder (20 mg thrice daily) or via metered dose inhaler and large volume spacer (10 mg thrice daily).

Step 1

Occasional use of relief bronchodilators

Short-acting β agonists "as required" for symptom relief but not more than once daily. Before altering a treatment step insure that the patient is having the treatment, the inhaler is appropriate and inhaler technique is good. Address any concerns or fears.

Fig. 12.20 Stepwise management plan for chronic asthma in children (from BTS 1997).

child with severe obstruction. This means that nebulized therapy should be repeated if necessary every 20–30 min until the child has been admitted to the emergency department of the nearest hospital.

Intravenous β-agonists may be needed. Subcutaneous terbutaline is preferable to adrenaline for emergency use, in the absence of a nebulizer. Ideally, all general practitioners should carry a small compressor pump and nebulizer unit so that bronchodilators can easily be provided as emergency treatment. An identical dose by MDI and spacer is as effective in children whose attack is not severe and who are old enough to cooperate.

Where possible, compressed oxygen rather than compressed air should be used in the nebulizer, since hypoxia is universal in acute severe asthma and may be transiently exacerbated by nebulized bronchodilator therapy.

FURTHER MANAGEMENT IN HOSPITAL

There should be no urgency to send an asthmatic child home after nebulizer treatment in the emergency department has been successful; the effect is frequently shortlived. Steroids are effective only after 4–6 h and the first dose should be given immediately following the nebulizer to any child with asthma severe enough to warrant attention at hospital. Where in doubt, admission should be arranged; if not, then at the least several hours' observation, a short course of steroids and a follow-up appointment should be arranged.

Assessment

A chest radiograph is not always necessary. It should be carried out for a first presentation if asthma is severe enough to need intensive care, if physical signs suggest an air leak or if the diagnosis of asthma is in doubt.

The least frequently performed but often the most critically important investigation is arterial blood gas estimation. Arterial blood gases should be measured when oximetry reveals severe hypoxemia in air ($SaO_2 < 85\%$) or when there is a progressive rise in oxygen requirements. Whenever the arterial PCO_2 is greater than the upper limit of normal (5.4 kPa, 40 mmHg) careful observation, with repeat blood gas measurements if necessary, should be carried out. A rising PCO_2 suggests the need for transfer to an intensive care unit. An arterial PCO_2 of greater than 10 kPa (75 mmHg) may be an indication for mechanical ventilation (Dworkin & Kattan 1989). Transcutaneous measurements are not reliable.

Treatment

Nebulized bronchodilator therapy (or an equivalent dose by MDI and spacer) is almost invariably used, given as frequently as necessary. Continuous nebulization has been advocated for the extreme case. Oxygen therapy should be given during and after nebulization. Very rarely, parenteral β2-agonist is indicated.

The use of intravenous aminophylline is reserved for patients who do not respond to β agonist treatment. The bolus dose should be omitted or reduced if the child has recently received a theophylline preparation before reaching the emergency department. It should never be necessary to use intravenous aminophylline outside hospital; frequently repeated nebulized β2 bronchodilator is preferable. However, in Third World countries it may be the only rescue drug available.

There is no doubt, despite previous controversy, that corticosteroid therapy is very effective. Whether intravenous hydrocortisone sodium succinate is necessary or whether oral prednisolone is likely to be sufficient depends on severity, history of vomiting and the need for intravenous fluid therapy. The usual dose of prednisolone is 1 mg/kg twice daily, up to a maximum of 40 mg daily for 3–4 days. It is rare to treat acute severe asthma for longer than this in childhood. Hyperreactivity and hyperphagia are often reported by parents, but are transient.

Other drugs are occasionally used. Nebulized ipratropium bromide is sometimes more effective than β2-agonists in infancy. In acute asthma in older children, it provides relief additional to maximal β-agonist therapy.

Nonpharmacological aspects of treatment are important. Parents should be able to remain with children in hospital. Young children may be best managed in their parents' arms, even in the intensive care unit. Vomiting or even acute gastric dilatation can be a problem, but most children are able to take oral fluids. Intravenous therapy should be used sparingly, especially in infants, in whom hyponatremia due to inappropriate ADH secretion exacerbated by overzealous fluid administration is a well-recognized complication of acute asthma.

Monitoring the response to treatment

Older children should record their peak flow before and after each dose of bronchodilator so that the rate and degree of improvement can be used to determine changes in treatment. When a steady improvement has been maintained without significant morning dips in peak flow rate, intravenous therapy can be terminated. The child's usual medication should be given together with regular 3- or 4-hourly nebulized bronchodilators and a short course of oral prednisolone. Oximetry should be used to monitor oxygen therapy. $SaO_2 > 90\%$ does not warrant continued oxygen therapy.

Where there is concern arterial blood gas measurements should be carried out.

Follow-up

Whenever a child has been admitted to hospital for management of acute severe asthma, an appropriate follow-up appointment should be arranged for 2–4 weeks later. Once the effect of the steroid therapy has worn off, there seems to be a particularly vulnerable period. Further follow-up arrangements should be decided jointly by general practitioner and pediatrician. One of the goals of management of all asthmatics, their families and primary care team is to prevent attacks. The reasons for every admission should be scrutinized with the family and lessons learnt. Triggers such as URTI or stepping out in the cold need to be preempted. 'The management of asthma is to keep ahead of the wheezing.' Patient education is integral to every admission or casualty visit and what has been discussed should appear in notes and summary in exactly the same way as the traditional documenting of history, examinations, investigations and management.

PARTICULAR PROBLEMS

EXERCISE-INDUCED ASTHMA

Appropriate preventive measures should be made available to all asthmatic children both during and outside school hours. Brief 30-s sprints at 2- or 3-min intervals repeated five or six times may induce temporary refractoriness to exercise-induced asthma. A more certain way of preventing exercise-induced asthma is to provide an inhaled β2-agonist bronchodilator for use immediately before exercise. This should provide effective protection for up to 2 h, although individual children with extreme responsiveness may only be protected for shorter periods. Remember, some children do not like exercise and may be happier in a chess club!

SEASONAL ASTHMA

Many asthmatic children are sensitive to pollens or molds which fluctuate seasonally. Such children can be identified by skin-prick testing or on the basis of a history of associated seasonal rhinitis. Preventer therapy should be provided to cover the season. Powerful antihistamines such as terfenadine given at bedtime are often useful during this period, although antihistamines are virtually ineffective for perennial childhood asthma. By providing adequate hay fever treatment (nasal sodium cromoglycate or steroid therapy, together with antihistamine/vasoconstrictor eye drops), the patient's well-being is improved and seasonal asthma seems to be more easily controlled.

The use of preseasonal hyposensitization therapy for seasonal asthma can be dangerous and is not recommended in Europe.

NOCTURNAL ASTHMA

Nocturnal symptoms are worrying in childhood asthma and their presence indicates that the disease is poorly controlled. A number of factors conspire to produce problems during the night (Barnes & Levy 1984). In adolescence, nocturnal asthma may be manifest as the 'morning dip', reflecting airway obstruction occurring in the early hours of the morning.

It is generally fruitless to try to identify the causes of nocturnal asthma but severe house dust mite sensitivity should be sought, since barrier methods may be effective in reducing exposure. Particular attention should be paid to therapy during the daytime, but if this fails to control symptoms then long-acting inhaled bronchodilator therapy or theophylline therapy at bedtime is often helpful. Nocturnal wheezing may respond to high-dose inhaled steroid therapy. Children who are prone to nocturnal symptoms should have ready access to inhaled bronchodilator therapy during the night.

EPISODIC WHEEZE IN VERY YOUNG CHILDREN

While the differential diagnosis of recurrent wheezing in infancy is wide, most wheezy babies will have episodic viral wheeze. Atopy is rarely a contributing factor. Parental smoking is a major cause. Unfortunately, particularly when wheezing is associated with recurrent viral infections, both rescue and preventer therapy are virtually ineffective during early infancy. In fact, a paradoxical increase in airway obstruction has recently been seen in wheezy infants after nebulized bronchodilator treatment. The failure of bronchodilator therapy in infants is due neither to the inability of infant airways to mount an acute response, nor to ineffective β-adrenoceptors. It seems likely that inflammatory processes are responsible for airway narrowing in infancy and that this is the reason for the poor response to bronchodilators. Failure to deliver an adequate dose of aerosol to the lungs of infants could also be a major factor.

Clinical observations suggest that those infants who have eczema and recurrent asthma as part of an atopic background are more likely to be responsive to regular antiasthma therapy and also more likely to proceed to chronic asthma. The only inhaled bronchodilator agent of proven value in wheezy infants is ipratropium bromide. Some but not all infants definitely benefit from this drug. If regular bronchodilator therapy is inadequate, regular nebulized corticosteroids may be tried, although of marginal value in infancy. Occasionally, additional alternate-day prednisolone treatment is required for severe symptoms. There is some evidence that bronchodilators become more effective during concurrent steroid therapy.

General measures, such as the avoidance of parental smoking at home, may be marginally beneficial in infancy. The importance of gastroesophageal reflux in infancy is always difficult to estimate. Food intolerance is a rare contributor to severe infantile asthma, usually in association with eczema. A trial of egg and dairy produce avoidance may then occasionally be justified.

RECURRENT SEGMENTAL COLLAPSE

Recurrent collapse of a segment, lobe or even a whole lung due to impaction of mucus is not infrequent in preschool asthmatic children and occasionally develops in the absence of overt airway obstruction. The symptoms are dyspnea and chest pain. Nebulized bronchodilators with physiotherapy are almost always effective in promoting reexpansion of the collapsed lobe. Bronchoscopy is rarely necessary but may be carried out to seek a treatable cause for recurrent segmental collapse (such as an inhaled foreign body or extrabronchial compression).

ALLERGIC BRONCHOPULMONARY ASPERGILLOSIS

This condition is rare in childhood, except in association with cystic fibrosis. It should be suspected if there is particularly intractable asthma associated with a high degree of eosinophilia or an immediate skin-prick test reaction to an extract of *Aspergillus fumigatus*. Radiological changes include flitting pulmonary shadows and in the later stages, signs of bronchiectasis. The diagnosis is confirmed by finding multiple precipitins against antigens of *Aspergillus fumigatus* in a serum sample. When troublesome, allergic bronchopulmonary aspergillosis can only be treated symptomatically by high-dose steroid therapy.

ADOLESCENT ASTHMA

Mild to moderate asthma usually resolves at or before the onset of puberty, only to recur in about 50% in early adult life. Of those few children whose symptoms persist during puberty, 80% can be expected to remain symptomatic as adults.

The common problems of adolescence complicate management. Denial of disease, irregular or inappropriate use of medication and rejection of advice from adults are frequent features. Taken to extremes, these trends sometimes have a fatal outcome. Smoking may exacerbate airway disease. Later, when advice is sought on the choice of career, referral to a specialist in occupational medicine may help.

The satisfactory management of the adolescent with asthma probably depends most of all on the strength of the direct relationship between physician and patient, as parental responsibilities for care give way to personal control. If home conditions are unsatisfactory, residential specialist schooling should be considered. Adolescent asthma is probably best managed in a separate adolescent clinic.

CONCLUSION

An awareness by doctors and by the public of the frequency of asthma in the community is an important prerequisite for adequate diagnosis. The recognition of asthma in individual children should not be considered as 'creating ill health' since there is good evidence that by treating previously undiagnosed cases, their quality of life can be markedly improved. Nevertheless the urge to label (almost) all that wheezes as asthma should not be allowed to induce diagnostic complacency. Not only must the impact of disease on physical and psychological development be considered, but the wider aspects of the interactions between the child, family and school have to be taken into account. It is clear that all of these factors can influence the pattern of symptoms, their recognition and the likelihood of compliance with effective treatment.

The long-term outcome of childhood asthma has not been fully determined. There is still no evidence that the more energetic treatment of childhood asthma can influence the long-term outcome. Research directed at the origins of asthma in early childhood may yield information which could lead towards the distant goal of the prevention of asthma.

CYSTIC FIBROSIS

INTRODUCTION

Cystic fibrosis (CF) is an autosomal recessive multisystem disorder. It is the most common cause of severe chronic lung disease in childhood and accounts for most cases of exocrine pancreatic insufficiency. The disease occurs in approximately 1 per 2500 children born in the United Kingdom. Those affected are homozygous for mutations within a gene on the long arm of chromosome 7. The gene codes for a protein called the cystic fibrosis transmembrane conductance regulator (CFTR), a molecule that facilitates the transport of chloride ions across apical cell membranes. Mutations in the CFTR gene cause reduced epithelial chloride ion permeability and lead to alterations in the concentration of electrolytes and the water content of fluids on cell surfaces. It is still not clear how abnormalities of CFTR cause many of the cellular defects and pathological processes that occur in CF patients. Heterozygotes are unaffected and can only be identified by genetic testing.

German folklore that 'a child who tastes salty on being kissed will surely die' was probably the first recognition of the disorder. A comprehensive medical description did not occur until 1938 when Dorothy Anderson linked pancreatic and lung manifestations, establishing CF as a separate diagnosis from celiac disease. During the 1948 New York heat wave, several CF patients suffered heat exhaustion because of excessive salt loss. This lead to the discovery of raised sodium and chloride concentrations in the sweat of CF patients and the subsequent development of the sweat test as a basis for diagnosis. "Mucoviscidosis" was coined by Faber in 1950 with reference to the thickened intestinal secretions of affected children but the term has fallen from use.

CF has a wide range of manifestations but the natural history is typically one of worsening malnutrition and progressive bronchiectatic lung damage leading to terminal respiratory failure in childhood. This gloomy outcome has been transformed in recent years and many affected individuals can expect to maintain good health well into adult life. This has been achieved through positive, aggressive management by multidisciplinary CF teams. Frequent follow-up and immediate treatment for any deterioration in clinical status have been essential in achieving this.

MECHANISMS OF DISEASE

GENETICS

One in 25 Caucasians in the UK is a carrier of abnormal CFTR genes. The gene frequency and types of gene mutation vary widely between different populations and racial groups. Disease frequency is 1 in 17 000 among American blacks and less than 1 in 90 000 among orientals. The high gene frequency among Caucasians suggests a selective advantage for heterozygotes or a very strong founder effect. Evolutionary benefits of maintaining abnormal CFTR genes in our gene pool have not been identified. It has been suggested that protection from salt-losing diarrheal illnesses such as cholera and resistance to *Mycobacterium tuberculosis* infection might occur among heterozygotes but these possibilities are unproven.

There is a slight selective advantage among the CF population favoring the male sex. A preponderance of male infants (105:100) suggests increased female mortality in utero. Age-specific mortality rates are higher for CF females and they have a shorter lifespan.

Since the isolation of the CFTR gene (Rommens et al 1989), more than 450 disease-associated mutations have been identified. The predicted protein structure of CFTR includes two membrane-spanning domains, each containing six hydrophobic regions, two nucleotide-binding folds and a regulatory domain. Abnormal genes can disrupt CFTR function in several ways. CFTR might get to the epithelium but not transport chloride efficiently, it might be unresponsive to regulatory signals, defectively processed so that it does not get to the epithelium or just not manufactured. The most common mutation is an "in frame" deletion of the amino acid phenylalanine at position 508 ($\triangle$F508), accounting for 70% of CF genes in North America and northern Europe (Cystic Fibrosis Genetic Analysis Consortium 1990). The mutation causes misfolding of the gene so that it does not pass through the normal biosynthetic processes to arrive at the cell membrane. Most other CF gene mutations involve a single nucleotide and result in either missense mutations, where a single amino acid is substituted, nonsense mutations, where an amino acid is substituted for a stop codon, or splice site mutations, where nucleotides crucial for the proper splicing of RNA are affected. Most other mutations cause frame shifts of the nucleotide sequence. Insertion or deletion of a small number of nucleotides causes a translational frame shift and the reading of premature stop codons. Several CFTR polymorphisms have been identified that do not cause disease. Studies relating genotype to phenotype suggest that $\triangle$F508 homozygosity invariably causes pancreatic insufficiency whereas mutations permitting partial CFTR function, such as R117H, R334W and R347H, are associated with prolonged pancreatic sufficiency. There is little correlation between genotype and lung disease suggesting that other factors are important in determining the development of pulmonary complications.

PATHOPHYSIOLOGY

While it is well recognized that CF cells have defective CFTR chloride channels (Rich et al 1990), the disease causes many other abnormalities of cellular function. Another channel known as the outwardly rectifying chloride channel (ORCC) also has impaired function and amiloride-sensitive sodium channels are hyperabsorbing. It is now clear that CFTR interacts with and regulates the operation of several other channels in controlling fluid balance on surface epithelia. The possibility of treatments to stimulate alternative chloride pathways and downregulate sodium absorption are under investigation.

The key abnormality in CF sweat glands is an increased concentration of sodium and chloride in surface sweat. CF patients do not produce increased volumes of sweat. Secretions are produced normally in the base of the sweat gland with electrolyte concentrations approximately isotonic with plasma. Failure of CFTR to facilitate chloride ion reabsorption and secondary retention of sodium in the proximal half of the gland causes salty sweat to emerge onto the skin surface.

In the pancreas the function of CFTR is to recycle chloride ions back onto the luminal surface following their exchange with bicarbonate. Bicarbonate is actively pumped out of pancreatic cells and draws water into the ductules to dilute pancreatic enzymes and flush them into the intestine. Without functional CFTR, chloride recycling does not occur, leading to secondary impairment of bicarbonate excretion. Concentrated enzymes accumulate in the ductal lumen where they damage the pancreatic acini, leading to gradual loss of exocrine function. CFTR is also expressed in intestinal mucosa where it causes isotonic fluid secretion to liquefy gut contents and facilitate digestion and absorption. Abnormal CFTR function in the small intestine contributes to the development of meconium ileus at birth in 10–15% of CF infants. Intestinal obstruction is caused by thickened viscid meconium blocking the ileal lumen. CFTR-dependent fluid secretion is critical for the patency of the epididymis and vas deferens. In males with CF there is progressive obstruction and secondary degeneration throughout childhood leading to infertility. Sexual potency is unaffected. Adults with congenital bilateral absence of the vas deferens (CBAVD) have a high incidence of CFTR mutations, suggesting that in many cases this condition is a mild variant of CF. Females have reduced fertility because of changes in cervical mucus and the nonspecific effects of chronic illness.

CFTR is very highly expressed in fetal lung tissues and there is a progressive decrease in expression postnatally with low levels only detectable in submucosal glands, type 2 pneumonocytes and clara cells. Despite this ontogeny of the molecule, there appear to be no abnormalities of lung development and the major impact of infection is initially in bronchioles rather than larger airways. While abnormalities in airway surface fluid composition and volume might lead to mucous plugging and secondary infection, the exact relationship between abnormalities in chloride transport and lung disease is not understood. It is possible that CFTR has unrecognized functions that are central to the integrity of important host defense mechanisms within the airways. The unprecedented upregulation of lung host defense by chronic airway bacterial infection is difficult to explain on the basis of the primary genetic defect and suggests the existence of secondary defects in the mechanisms responsible for downregulating airway inflammation. One alternative theory for the pathogenesis of lung damage proposes that CFTR is active intracellularly, controlling the pH within the Golgi apparatus. It has been suggested that mutant CFTR causes an increase in pH that decreases the activity of Golgi sialyltransferases. The increased numbers of sialylated receptors on the cell surface leads to increased adherence of *Pseudomonas* and upregulation of local immune responses.

Interestingly, CFTR is very highly expressed in the renal tubules but there is no evidence for a defect of tubular function in CF patients.

DIAGNOSIS

PRENATAL DIAGNOSIS

Prenatal diagnosis is most commonly performed in obligate carriers who have a child with CF and face a 1 in 4 risk of having another affected child in subsequent pregnancies. In up to 80% of CF families both gene mutations are identifiable and diagnosis can be carried out by direct gene analysis. In cases where the gene mutations are unknown and DNA is available from previous offspring, polymorphic markers and linkage analysis tests can be carried out to track the inheritance of each CF chromosome. Amniotic fluid analysis to detect the reduced level of microvillar enzymes characteristic of CF fetuses is rarely necessary.

Fetal material is most commonly obtained at 10–12 weeks by chorionic biopsy and is associated with an increased miscarriage rate of 1–4%. Miscarriage after diagnostic testing by amniocentesis is 0.5–1% but this procedure cannot be performed until the second trimester.

DNA amplification techniques have made possible preimplantation diagnosis of in vitro fertilized embryos using just one cell for testing. Carrier testing is increasingly being offered to extended family members of index cases and population screening has been performed in pilot studies. While the latter might benefit couples by increasing their reproductive choices, cost-effective screening will only occur if society deems acceptable the widespread abortion of affected fetuses. Benefits gained by prenatal diagnosis in enabling early treatment of nonaborted infants are more cost-effectively attained through neonatal screening.

NEONATAL SCREENING (Phelan 1995)

Screening tests include the detection of incompletely digested albumin in meconium and two stage assays to detect sustained elevations of immunoreactive trypsin (IRT) in serum or blood spots. More recently a one-stage IRT test, followed when positive by DNA analysis for the most common CF mutations, has been introduced. This latter screening process has a lower number of false positives prior to diagnostic confirmation by sweat testing. Early diagnosis eliminates the anger and frustration suffered by parents when their children suffer recurrent illness prior to the recognition that CF is the cause of symptoms. Expenditure on hospital admissions in the first 2 years of life is significantly reduced because of a decreased need to treat early complications of the disease. Evidence for improved survival among screened populations is difficult to demonstrate because of the overall improvement in prognosis in recent years, but there is good

evidence that airway inflammation occurs very early on in CF lungs and it remains common in many communities for children to have established bronchiectasis when diagnosed because of respiratory illness.

CLINICAL DIAGNOSIS

Diagnosis is based on clinical history and examination evidence of recurrent sinopulmonary infection with or without pancreatic insufficiency and raised levels of sodium and chloride in the sweat. The majority of patients fail to thrive with steatorrhea and recurrent respiratory infections in infancy. A few patients present in later childhood and early adult life with similar problems but there are many other presenting manifestations which should be regarded as indications for sweat testing (Table 12.20)

Sweat test

Although it is now possible to test for many of the gene mutations causing CF, the sweat test is still the most reliable tool for confirming a suspected diagnosis. Sweat test should be performed by persons skilled in the procedure. The most reliably established technique is the quantitative pilocarpine iontophoresis method. A weak electrical current aids the penetration of pilocarpine into the skin to induce maximal sweating. At least 100 mg of sweat is collected on a preweighed filter paper and the concentrations of sodium and chloride are measured by routine clinical methods. Two tests should be performed simultaneously with one on each arm.

The MACRODUCT system is an alternative sweat test device in which sweat is collected into capillary tubing and its osmolality measured. Simplified tests using chloride-sensitive electrodes and semiquantitative assays have also been devised but are not as reliable as iontophoresis.

Studies show that 98–99% of homozygous CF children have sweat chloride and sodium levels above 70 mmol/l. In CF the chloride levels are usually higher than the sodium levels. The reverse occurs in normals. Values between 50–70 mmol/l require further consideration. False-positive results may occur because of sweat evaporation and difficulties in obtaining adequate sweat

Table 12.20 Presentation of cystic fibrosis – indications for a sweat test

Pulmonary
Chronic or recurrent cough, pneumonia or bronchiolitis
Purulent sputum production
Difficult 'asthma'
Unexplained hemoptysis
Nasal polyps, chronic sinusitis

Gastrointestinal
Meconium ileus, meconium plug syndrome
Failure to thrive
Steatorrhea, malabsorption
Rectal prolapse
Atypical gastroesophageal reflux
Biliary cirrhosis, portal hypertension
Hypoproteinemia, edema
Neonatal hepatitis syndrome

Other
Pseudo-Bartter's syndrome
Heat exhaustion
Male infertility
Salty taste when kissed
Sibling with cystic fibrosis

volumes from dry or eczematous skin. Other conditions in which raised sweat electrolytes have been described are adrenal insufficiency, hypothyroidism, familial hypoparathyroidism, ectodermal dysplasia, type 1 glycogen storage disease, mucopolysaccharidoses, fucosidosis, nephrogenic diabetes insipidus, nephrotic syndrome, HIV infection, anorexia nervosa and severe malnutrition. Sweat electrolyte levels may be elevated in normal neonates during the first week of life. In practice it is technically difficult to obtain adequate quantities of sweat until 2–3 weeks of age. Profound hypoalbuminemic edema can cause misleadingly low results.

Sweat electrolyte levels normally increase during childhood and false positives become more likely after the age of 12 years. Electrolyte levels can be suppressed in this age group by administering 9-alpha-fludro-cortisone 3 mg/m^{-2} daily for 2 days. Individuals with CF are more resistant to the effects of the mineralocorticoid.

Whilst it is extremely rare for children to have typical features of CF and persistently normal sweat tests, there are a number of individuals with rare genotypes who have mild or variable disease expression and normal or only mildly elevated sweat electrolytes.

An alternative diagnostic test has been developed from the observation that CF patients have a markedly more negative potential difference across respiratory epithelia compared with controls. Measurements of nasal epithelial potential difference have proved useful in investigating older children and adults with borderline sweat tests and where there is uncertainty about the correct diagnosis.

Assessment of exocrine pancreatic function

Clinically significant pancreatic insufficiency occurs in 75–95% of children. Differences in incidence mostly reflect differences in the genetic make-up of the CF populations studied. In most cases, pancreatic insufficiency is manifest clinically. Tests of pancreatic function are useful when there is uncertainty about the presence of malabsorption and where there is a need to assess the adequacy of pancreatic enzyme replacement therapy. Simple tests on stools include microscopy for fat globules and measurement of fecal chymotrypsin. The latter test is only useful in patients not receiving pancreatic enzymes. A mean value should be calculated from testing at least three specimens. The steatocrit test measures the depth of the fatty layer in a sample of homogenized feces drawn up into a capillary tube. The test is widely used but is less accurate than the 'gold standard' 3–5-day fecal collection for measurement of fat balance. Stool weight has been shown to be a good indicator of fecal energy losses.

The modified N-benzoyl-1-tyrosyl p-aminobenzoic acid test (NBT-PABA), in which urine samples are analyzed for the excretion of PABA as an indication of chymotrypsin activity, is used in some centers. More invasive duodenal intubation and analysis of enzyme secretion following cholecystokinin/secretin stimulation are rarely necessary.

CLINICAL FEATURES

CF has a wide spectrum of manifestations. The course of the disease is unpredictable but with early diagnosis and good treatment most children should achieve normal growth with few signs of chest infection and malabsorption.

GASTROINTESTINAL

Meconium ileus causes intestinal obstruction in up to 15% of newborn children with CF (Fig. 12.21). Failure to pass meconium, abdominal distention and bile-stained vomiting are the hallmarks of the condition. Abdominal radiographs reveal distended loops of small bowel and ground glass opacification in the lower abdomen. Antenatal meconium peritonitis, volvulus and ileal atresia are rare complications. A Gastrografin enema typically demonstrates the presence of a microcolon and may also soften the meconium mass to relieve obstruction. The majority of cases require surgical intervention to flush out the impacted meconium and resect nonviable bowel. The condition tends to occur in familial clusters and has been described in children who have subsequently not required replacement pancreatic enzymes. Congenital ileal stenosis is a rare clue to the diagnosis of CF.

Clinically obvious pancreatic insufficiency occurs in up to 85% of cases during infancy. Affected infants often have a voracious appetite but are slow to gain weight. Malabsorption is exacerbated by abnormal duodenal acidity, intestinal mucosa dysfunction and impaired bile salt excretion. The result is steatorrhea manifested by the frequent passage of large, greasy and smelly stools which are difficult to flush down the toilet. Gaseous distention of the abdomen is a common feature and there may be recurrent vomiting. Very occasionally a voracious appetite compensates sufficiently for malabsorption to enable reasonable weight gain in early childhood with weight loss only occurring when respiratory infection leads to anorexia.

Recurrent rectal prolapse occurs in up to 10% of cases and may be the sole presenting feature. Salt deficiency is common at diagnosis and can result in severe hypochloremic metabolic alkalosis. Undiagnosed CF infants with loose stools and poor weight gain are sometimes treated by substitution of cow's milk with soy-based formula. Such children are at risk of developing hypoproteinemic edema, anemia and essential fatty acid deficiencies.

Inadequate absorption of fat-soluble vitamins have occasionally caused symptoms including bleeding disorders due to vitamin K deficiency, benign intracranial hypertension due to vitamin A

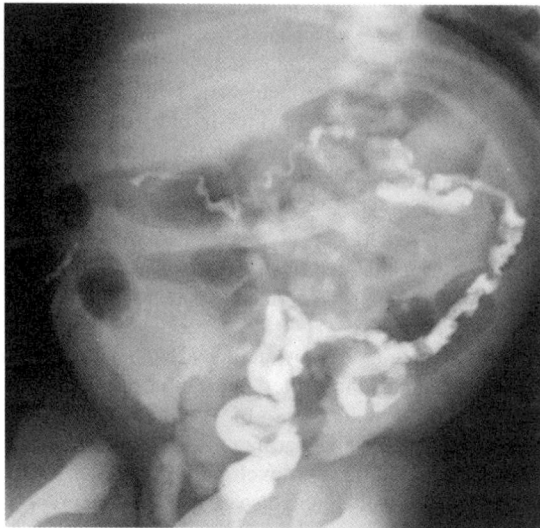

Fig. 12.21 Barium enema showing typical microcolon consequent to meconium ileus intestinal obstruction.

deficiency and hemolytic anemia or neurological symptoms due to vitamin E deficiency. CF must be distinguished from celiac disease. Although the latter is now uncommon it is important to note that it coexists with CF more frequently than would be expected by chance.

Distal intestinal obstruction syndrome (DIOS) occurs in older children and adults. The terminal ileum becomes occluded with sticky, mucofeculent material causing colicky abdominal pains, vomiting and abdominal distention. Typically, a fecal mass can be palpated in the right iliac fossa. Mild symptoms can be relieved with oral laxatives and adequate hydration but on occasions treatment with Gastrografin, N-acetylcysteine or balanced electrolyte intestinal lavage is necessary. Other causes of abdominal symptoms including constipation, appendicitis, pancreatitis, Crohn's disease, neoplasms and gynecological conditions should be considered. Occasionally a DIOS mass may form the apex of an intussusception. The etiology of DIOS is unknown. Inadequate dosing with pancreatic enzyme supplements is thought to be a contributory factor but DIOS does not occur in other conditions in which there is pancreatic malabsorption.

An apparently new CF-specific bowel abnormality was first described in 1994. A cluster of cases, all of them children, presented with subacute bowel obstruction and failed to respond to medical therapy. At surgery they were found to have marked thickening and stenosis but not inflammation in the ascending colon. The histology revealed extensive submucosal fibrosis. A large number of other cases have now been identified and there is a strong association between the phenomenon and the use of high-strength pancreatic enzyme minitab preparations. There are, however, a number of inconsistencies in the association and the mechanism is unknown.

The dietary management of cystic fibrosis frequently results in low fiber intake and as a result constipation with chronic fecal loading is a common problem.

RESPIRATORY (Zach 1990)

The age of onset and progression of respiratory symptoms varies considerably among CF patients. A persistent cough, often rattly and exacerbated by viral infections, is usually the first symptom. Occasionally the cough is paroxysmal and associated with vomiting, leading to the misdiagnosis of pertussis. Some infants present with a prolonged bronchiolitic type illness and many have recurrent wheezing illnesses suggestive of asthma. Sputum expectoration is usually only obvious in older children although some infants and young children vomit sputum that has been swallowed. Initially, sputum is relatively clear or creamy but with increasing infection becomes yellow and, with *Pseudomonas* colonization, green. Occasional blood streaking occurs during acute infections but massive fresh hemoptysis due to rupture of bronchial arteries is rare and confined to patients with more severe disease.

Hyperinflation, recognized by an increase in anterior–posterior chest wall diameter, is the earliest indication of airway mucous plugging. Progressive deformity of the compliant chest wall leads to sternal bowing (pectus carinatum), Harrison's sulci and kyphosis. Finger clubbing develops in parallel with the progression of suppurative lung disease and may be preceded by peeling of the skin overlying the nail beds.

Chest auscultation may be normal even in the presence of extensive respiratory disease but may reveal an increased expiratory phase, inspiratory and expiratory crackles of varying coarseness and polyphonic wheezing. Central cyanosis is a very late sign of respiratory disease.

RADIOLOGY

Initial findings on chest radiography are hyperinflation and peribronchial infiltrates. For unknown reasons changes are frequently predominant in the upper lobes and particularly on the right. With disease progression extensive peribronchial thickening is represented by tramline shadows and thick-walled circles in cross-section. Larger infiltrates become more prominent and extensive. Areas of atelectasis or consolidation may occur and peripheral rounded opacities 0.5 cm in diameter appear. These represent abscesses or infected bronchiolectatic areas and when drained appear as permanent ring shadows (Fig. 12.22).

High-resolution CT scanning is a sensitive means of detecting early bronchiectatic changes prior to those seen on the chest radiograph. Isotope ventilation scans are useful in assessing regional lung defects at a functional level, particularly in children who are unable to perform simple lung function tests.

LUNG FUNCTION

Most infants with CF identified by neonatal screening programs have normal measurements of lung dynamics at diagnosis. Infant lung volumes can be measured plethysmographically and expiratory flow rates assessed using the 'squeeze' or rapid thoracoabdominal compression technique.

From the age of 4–5 years children should be taught to perform maximal forced expiratory maneuvers so that spirometric measurements can be made from reliably reproduced flow-volume loops. Measurements of maximal mid-expiratory flow are most sensitive in detecting the early development of small airways obstruction but measurements have a wide coefficient of variation. Forced expiratory volume in the first second (FEV_1) is most commonly used in determining the need for changes in treatment and for predicting long-term prognosis in children with more advanced disease.

Plethysmography is useful in older children to assess hyperinflation and can be combined with gas dilutional measurements of lung volume to calculate the gas trapping index. Daytime oxygen saturation measurements are usually sustained until moderately severe lung disease occurs. Nocturnal hypoxemia occurs at an earlier stage and is more severe during respiratory exacerbations. Exercise tolerance can be usefully assessed by graded exercise testing under controlled conditions.

Bronchial hyperresponsiveness is common but variable within and between patients and not necessarily related to allergy or bronchodilator responsiveness. Bronchodilator responsiveness should be assessed regularly to determine the usefulness of bronchodilator therapy and because in some children these drugs can exacerbate airway obstruction.

BACTERIOLOGY

Patients with CF are susceptible to infection in the respiratory tract while having normal systemic immunity. Severe sepsis outside the respiratory tract is rare. It is not clear how the underlying defect initiates lung infection but the presence of organisms in the airways stimulates an excessive but relatively

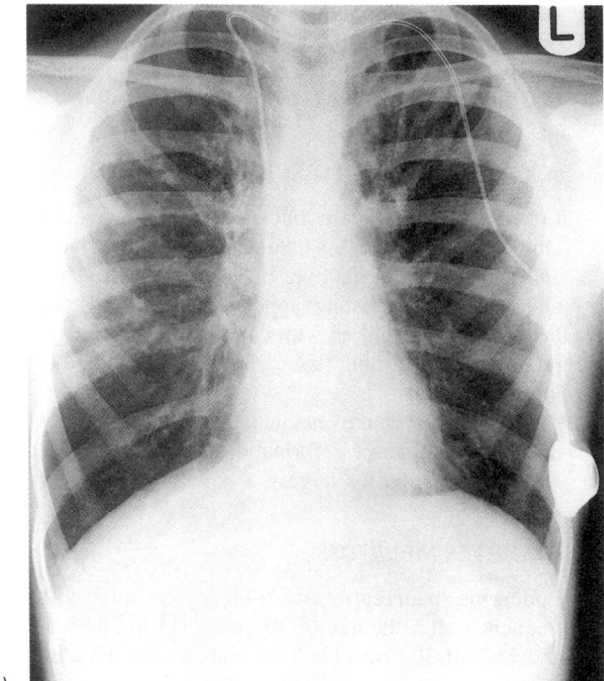

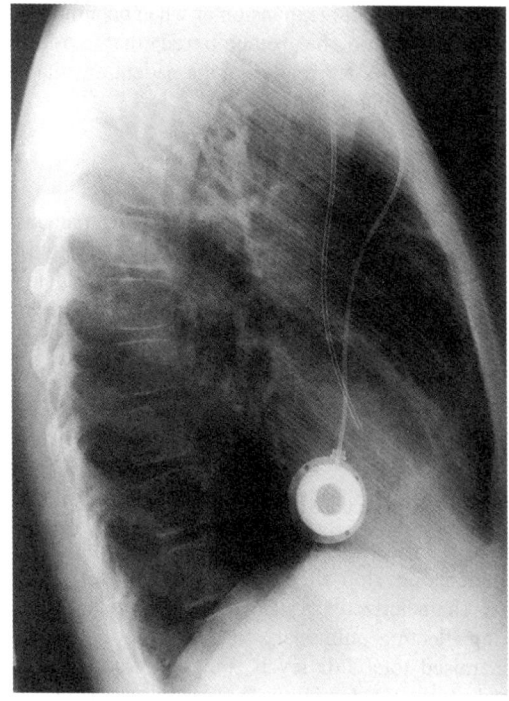

(a)

(b)

Fig. 12.22 (**a&b**) PA and lateral films showing bronchial wall thickening, cyst formation and peripheral small round opacities. The latter represent abscesses or bronchiectatic areas impacted with purulent secretions. A totally implanted venous access device is in situ.

ineffective neutrophil-dominated immune response that directly contributes to the progression of lung damage.

Staphylococcus aureus usually infects the airway during infancy followed closely by more fastidious noncapsular *Haemophilus influenzae*. These organisms continue to be important pathogens throughout life and recur intermittently, but as lung disease progresses the airways become continuously colonized with *Pseudomonas aeruginosa*. Viruses, *Mycoplasma* and *Chlamydia* can cause respiratory deterioration and also enhance the pathogenicity of *P. aeruginosa*.

Most patients who are colonized with *P. aeruginosa* tend to harbor just one genetic organism in their airways for most of their lives. However, *P. aeruginosa* undergoes remarkable phenotypic changes in the CF lung. These include the development of antibiotic resistance, release of toxins and the production of an exopolysaccharide called alginate. Occasional multiresistant pseudomonads have behaved epidemically and spread throughout CF clinics. Transition to the alginate-producing mucoid variants of *P. aeruginosa* leads to the formation of microcolonies in which the organisms are protected from phagocytosis and complement. Antibiotic access is inhibited and the bactericidal effects of neutrophils are blunted. Over the last 20 years *Burkolderia cepacia* has emerged as an endemic pathogen in some CF centers. Acquisition of this organism can result in asymptomatic carriage but in some cases it has resulted in progressive or rapidly fatal deterioration in patients who were previously mildly affected. Nontuberculous mycobacteria are isolated with increased frequency in older patients and there is accumulating evidence that these organisms behave as pathogens in some cases. Their treatment requires the prolonged use of multidrug regimens.

Bacterial cultures of swabs from the upper respiratory tract frequently fail to represent the organisms infecting the lungs

although the isolation of *P. aeruginosa* usually indicates its presence further down the airway. Pharyngeal aspirates using a soft catheter during induced coughing after physiotherapy may yield a useful specimen. In children who are productive there is reasonable correlation between organisms cultured in sputum and lung specimens.

NASAL POLYPS AND SINUSITIS

Sinus infection occurs in most children with CF. Sinus X-rays invariably show opacifications but acute purulent sinusitis causing symptoms is uncommon. Expanding sinus mucoceles causing bone deformity are a rare complication. Between 10% and 30% of patients develop nasal polyps. These can grow rapidly and often recur after surgical treatment.

ASTHMA AND ALLERGY

At least 20% of CF children have coexistent atopic asthma. However, positive allergy skin tests and bronchial hyperreactivity occur commonly in CF without this necessarily being related to asthma. A therapeutic trial of antiasthma therapy should be considered in cases where there is diagnostic uncertainty.

SPONTANEOUS PNEUMOTHORAX

This is a relatively rare complication in childhood but occurs in up to 20% of adults. It is more common in males than females. Small asymptomatic pneumothoraces can be treated conservatively. Larger pneumothoraces and those causing pleuritic pain or breathlessness require an intercostal chest drain. Surgical treatment should be considered in cases when conservative measures fail to bring about reexpansion or when pneumothoraces are recurrent. It should be remembered that widespread pleurodesis carries the risk of rendering the patient unsuitable for future heart–lung transplantation.

HEMOPTYSIS

Mild hemoptysis is common but up to 7% of older patients can have massive, even life-threatening hemoptysis. If significant bleeding occurs after appropriate antibiotic treatment and correction of any underlying coagulopathy, fiberoptic bronchoscopy should be performed to identify the bleeding site and angiographic bronchial artery occlusion attempted using gelatine foam. If this fails, thoracotomy and bronchial artery ligation or lobectomy should be considered.

ALLERGIC BRONCHOPULMONARY ASPERGILLOSIS

Simple allergy to *Aspergillus fumigatus* is common in CF but up to 10% of patients develop allergic bronchopulmonary aspergillosis. This is characterized by increased respiratory symptoms with wheezing, fleeting pulmonary shadows, blood and sputum eosinophilia, raised total IgE levels, raised IgE and IgG to *A. fumigatus* and positive *A. fumigatus* sputum cultures (Fig. 12.23). The condition causes worsening lung damage and treatment with prolonged high-dose steroids is essential. Relapses are common. Nebulized amphotericin and oral intraconazole might be of benefit in some cases. Mycetomas and invasive aspergillosis can occur in CF but are rare.

RESPIRATORY FAILURE AND COR PULMONALE

Patients with advanced lung disease causing severe hypoxemia are at risk of developing pulmonary hypertension and right ventricular hypertrophy. Doppler echocardiography usefully detects the early development of cor pulmonale. Overt signs of pulmonary heart disease do not occur until end-stage disease.

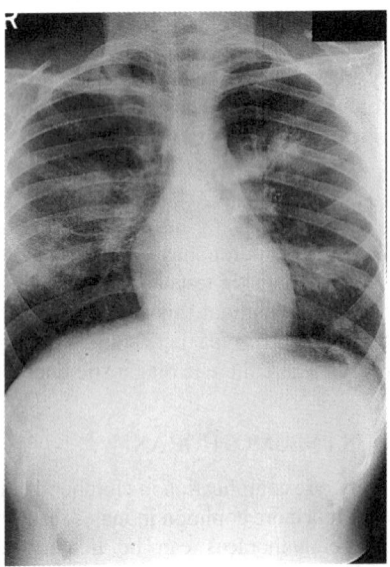

Fig. 12.23 Typical widespread nodular opacities caused by allergic bronchopulmonary aspergillosis.

Affected patients might benefit from long-term oxygen and diuretic therapy. Respiratory support using techniques such as overnight nasal ventilation might be of symptomatic benefit and buy time for patients selected for transplantation.

ATELECTASIS AND ABSCESS FORMATION

Lobar collapse is rare but occurs more frequently in early childhood. In most cases treatment with aggressive physiotherapy and antibiotics is effective. Bronchoscopy may be of benefit in children with persisting atelectasis after a week of intensive therapy. Those children with chronic symptomatic atelectasis and relatively normal lung tissue elsewhere should be considered for lobectomy.

Microabscesses are inevitable in the advanced stages of the disease. Large abscess formation is relatively rare but may be another indication for surgery.

DIABETES MELLITUS

Endocrine pancreatic insufficiency occurs with increasing frequency after the age of 10 years. Up to 24% of 20-year-olds and 76% of 30-year-olds have diabetes mellitus. Blood glucose, urinalysis and glycosylated hemoglobin measurements do not reliably identify diabetes compared with annual glucose tolerance tests. Ketoacidosis is rare. Most CF diabetics benefit from insulin therapy but should not change to a diabetic diet.

LIVER DISEASE (Nagel et al 1989)

A few patients with CF have prolonged neonatal jaundice. Neonatal hepatitis is a very rare presenting illness. Hepatomegaly secondary to fatty infiltration is well recognized in malnourished patients but can occur in those who are thriving. Liver disease in older children is usually occult and its prevalence increases with age. A high rate of familial concordance suggest that genes outside the CF loci play an important part in pathogenesis. Partial biliary obstruction leads to focal biliary fibrosis and cirrhosis. Common bile duct obstruction may contribute to the development of liver complications in a small proportion of patients. Incidental hepatomegaly, particularly affecting the left lobe, is the most common presentation. Liver function tests are poorly predictive. Acute variceal hemorrhage is the most serious complication of liver disease but rarely occurs in the absence of palpable splenomegaly. Hypersplenism can occur but rarely causes problems. Jaundice, ascites and encephalopathy occur very rarely in a small number of children with advanced disease. Treatment with ursodeoxycholic acid has been shown to improve liver function tests and increase bile flow in patients with CF liver disease but long-term benefits have not yet been demonstrated.

MISCELLANEOUS

Transient nonspecific arthritis occurs in some CF patients and most commonly affects the knee and ankle joints. The condition is possibly related to high levels of circulating immune complexes. It should be distinguished from hypertrophic pulmonary osteoarthropathy and other causes of arthritis. Oral fluoroquinolones cause joint pains in some patients. Vasculitic purpuric rashes, predominantly occurring below the knee joints, occur in a small number of patients with advanced lung disease.

Chronic lung inflammation has caused renal amyloid presenting as proteinuria, nephrosis and renal failure. There is an increased incidence of gastrointestinal malignancies among CF patients.

TREATMENT

DIET (Ramsey et al 1992)

Many infants thrive on breast milk provided enzyme supplements are given before each feed. Babies fed on modified cow's milk can be given supplements with glucose polymers if weight gain is poor. Infants should be weaned normally at around 3 months. Older children should eat a high-energy, high-protein diet without fat restriction. Patients should be encouraged to make high-fat food choices and establish good eating patterns.

Children have increased energy requirements partly due to increased metabolic activity related to the basic CF defect and many will have some energy losses from continuing intestinal malabsorption. Children with impaired pulmonary function have higher energy expenditure and calorie supplements should be provided to prevent weight loss during exacerbations of respiratory symptoms. Some children will not achieve optimal growth eating normal foods and will require regular oral dietary supplements. Those who fail to thrive despite these measures should be considered for artificial feeding. Parenteral nutrition can be of short-term benefit but is expensive and not practical on a long-term basis. Fine-bore nasogastric tube feeds are tolerated by some children but others find gastrostomy or jejunostomy feeding more acceptable. Tubes are inserted gastroscopically and their use achieves dramatic improvements in weight gain and growth in some cases. Enteral feeds are usually given over 8–10 hours at night and additional bolus feeds can be given during the day if necessary.

All children with malabsorption should receive routine supplements of vitamins A, D and E. Vitamin K supplementation is sometimes needed in children with liver disease and prolongation of their prothrombin time. Infants might benefit from additional salt supplements as might older children during the summer months.

PANCREATIC ENZYMES

Enteric-coated microsphere enzymes are the preparations of choice to treat pancreatic insufficiency. Enzymes are released when the spheres encounter a relatively high pH in the duodenum. They should be given before all meals and snacks. Microspheres can be emptied out of their capsules and mixed with puree immediately before feeds in children who are unable to swallow whole capsules. Initial doses of 3–4000 units of lipase/kg/day are adjusted to achieve normal stool frequency and absence of gut symptoms. Enzyme activity might be enhanced in some patients by the concomitant use of antacids, H_2-antagonists or proton pump inhibitors to increase gastrointestinal pH to a more suitable level for enzyme release and action.

PHYSIOTHERAPY

All patients with CF should receive daily chest physiotherapy. Treatment should be initiated and maintained as soon as possible after diagnosis even in the absence of overt respiratory symptoms. Infants and small children should be treated by postural drainage and chest clapping to produce coughing. Treatment sessions should be carried out before feeds for sufficient periods to clear secretions.

Older children are taught controlled breathing, thoracic expansion exercises and the forced expiratory technique. These components are brought together in the active cycle of breathing, an effective physiotherapy technique that can be carried out independently in postural drainage positions. Individuals should be taught to adapt their treatment sessions according to changes in their respiratory status. Adjuncts to physiotherapy include manual percussors and the positive expiratory pressure mask. Autogenic drainage, a regimen of breathing control and breaths at various lung volumes, is a physiotherapy technique used in some European centers. Physical exercise is encouraged but should not be considered a substitute for physiotherapy sessions.

ANTIBIOTICS

The main pathogens responsible for lung damage are S. aureus, H. influenzae and P. aeruginosa. Children who are not known to be colonized with P. aeruginosa and who have not had this organism recently isolated from their airways should receive oral antibiotics to treat the first two organisms mentioned above at the onset of any increase in respiratory symptoms. Drugs such as co-amoxiclav, co-trimoxazole, oral cephalosporins, macrolides and flucloxacillin plus amoxicillin would be good first-line choices although local resistance patterns might dictate otherwise. In vitro antibiotic sensitivity testing should be performed on respiratory specimens obtained at the onset of symptoms and routine specimens should be obtained at regular follow-up visits. Repeat isolates of S. aureus can often be eradicated by treatment with a combination of antistaphylococcal antibiotics including flucloxacillin, fusidic acid and clindamycin. Large doses should be prescribed for a minimum of 2–3 weeks on each occasion. Repeat specimens should be obtained in children showing a poor response to therapy and treatment adjusted according to culture results.

Later in the course of the disease chronic P. aeruginosa colonization occurs. Colonization might be delayed by repeated treatment with nebulized colomycin combined with oral ciprofloxacin when this organism is initially isolated from the respiratory tract. Acute respiratory symptoms in Pseudomonas-colonized patients causing a deterioration in lung function or chest X-ray appearances should be treated with intravenous antibiotics. Patients should receive a minimum of 10 days treatment or until a plateau of improvement has occurred. It is usual to give a combination of an aminoglycoside and either a carboxypenicillin, ureidopenicillin, a third-generation cephalosporin such as ceftazidime or a monobactam such as aztreonam or imipenem (Table 12.21). Aminoglycoside levels should be measured and the dosage adjusted to achieve safe therapeutic levels. Some units recommend intravenous antibiotics on a regular basis every 3 months irrespective of symptoms. Totally implanted subcutaneous venous access devices are increasingly used to facilitate treatment in children requiring frequent courses of intravenous drugs. Specialist nurses in many centers now provide the necessary support to families so that courses of intravenous antibiotics can be given at home Ciprofloxacin is an effective oral antipseudomonal agent but its frequent use leads to the development of drug resistance.

There is no consensus about the value of continuous oral antistaphylococcal prophylaxis although studies do suggest

Table 12.21 Antipseudomonal drugs for intravenous administration in cystic fibrosis

Drugs	Dose	Notes
Azlocillin	300 mg/kg/day Divide dose 8-hourly	More active than carbenicillin and piperacillin against *Pseudomonas*
Gentamicin	10 mg/kg/day Divide dose 8-hourly	Adjust dose according to levels: trough 1–2 mg/l; peak (1 h) 7–10 mg/l
Tobramycin	10 mg/kg/day Divide dose 8-hourly	More active than gentamicin against most strains of *Pseudomonas*. Adjust dose as above
Ceftazidime	150 mg/kg/day Divide dose 8–12-hourly	Potent antipseudomonal with Gram-negative bacilli activity
Aztreonam	200 mg/kg/day Divide dose 6-hourly	Inactive against anaerobes and Gram-positive cocci
Imipenem	90–100 mg/kg/day Divide dose 8-hourly Use max dose of 4 g/day in multiples of 500 mg	Broad spectrum activity. Requires infusion over 1–2 h
Colomycin	75 000 units/kg/day Divide dose 8-hourly	Use with caution. Serious side-effects can occur

benefits from using continuous prophylaxis in infancy. There is more agreement about the benefits of continuous aerosolized antipseudomonal antibiotics such as colomycin and aminoglycosides given twice daily after physiotherapy sessions.

BRONCHODILATORS (Tasker & Warner 1991)

Many patients with CF have bronchodilator responsiveness and it is therefore appropriate to give these drugs, particularly prior to chest physiotherapy and heavy exertion. Continued responsiveness should be assessed because some children develop paradoxical deterioration in lung function after bronchodilator therapy.

IMMUNE MODULATION

There is good evidence that host responses to lung infection are important in causing lung damage. This has led to the use of oral corticosteroids to suppress immune responsiveness. Whilst there is evidence of clinical benefit in controlled trials there are concerns about long-term side-effects after continued use in young patients (Auerbach et al 1985). Oral steroids are indicated to treat proven ABPA and progressive deterioration in pulmonary function, unresponsive to other measures. Preliminary studies also suggest clinical benefits from treatment with inhaled steroids. Long-term corticosteroid treatment in high dosages compromises the success of heart–lung transplantation because of an increased risk of breakdown at the site of tracheal anastomosis.

The unprecedented local host inflammatory response to chronic bacterial colonization in the airways has led to considerations of other forms of immunosuppression. Trials have suggested benefit with ibuprofen, a broad-spectrum nonsteroidal anti-inflammatory agent. There are anecdotal reports of benefits from the use of methotrexate and cyclosporin. There is a particularly notable improvement in lung function in CF patients who have received isolated liver transplants which might also be due to immunosuppression. Other agents being considered are intravenous immunoglobulin, vaccines to protect against *Pseudomonas* infection, antiproteases and humanized monoclonal antibodies against cytokines.

NOVEL THERAPIES

Infected sputum is viscous partly because it contains large amounts of DNA released from lyzed neutrophils. Recombinant human DNase I (rhDNase) is now available as a nebulized preparation to decrease the viscosity of sputum and improve airway clearance. Sustained improvements in lung function and well-being occur in up to one-third of patients receiving continuous treatment but values rapidly return to pretreatment levels when the drug is discontinued. It remains to be seen whether rhDNase has an impact on long-term prognosis.

Amiloride inhibits the reabsorption of sodium from epithelial lining fluid. It therefore increases sodium chloride and perhaps water content to reduce airway secretion viscosity. Studies have shown a diminution in the attrition of lung function when given by nebulizer four times daily. It does have a weak antibacterial effect which could also account for its clinical benefits. Trials are being conducted combining amiloride with the nucleotide UTP which increases calcium efflux from respiratory epithelial cells and might also stimulate alternative chloride channels.

HEART–LUNG TRANSPLANTATION (Madden et al 1992, Whitehead & De Leval 1994)

The development of heart–lung transplantation for those in irreversible respiratory failure has given new hope to a large number of patients and their families. It has been established that heart–lung transplantation can be successful in children. Currently only 15–20% of referrals to a heart–lung transplantation program benefit from this procedure. Up to three-quarters of those receiving a transplant can be expected to be alive after 1 year. Awaiting transplantation creates enormous emotional stresses for patients and their carers. Inclusion on a heart–lung transplant program should not detract from the delivery of appropriate care in the terminal stages of CF. Efforts must continue to ensure that patients are comfortable and are allowed to die with peace and dignity.

PSYCHOSOCIAL

A long-term chronic illness within a family takes an enormous emotional toll. In the toddler years, there are particular problems over eating and physiotherapy. Whilst there may be a period of relative stability in mid-childhood, these problems commonly recur in adolescence. At this age, there is often a rejection of many of the treatments, leading to anguish on the part of the parents and more rapid deterioration in the children. Needle phobia can be common if venesection is not handled sensibly. The needs of normal siblings in the family must also be considered. Jealousy is common because of the apparently excessive attention given to the affected child. Schooling problems may occur in relation to medication and particularly pre-meal pancreatic enzyme replacement. Bowel problems with offensive flatus will have an adverse effect on peer relationships and delayed adolescence with poor growth in the more severely affected will have an adverse effect on peer influence and self-confidence. Anticipation of problems and the availability of experienced psychological help is vital.

COMPREHENSIVE CARE

There is increasing evidence that CF patients cared for in specialist centers have a better life expectancy than those managed in the midst of other pediatric or respiratory clinics. Frequent supervision by a multidisciplinary team of experienced CF professionals including nurse specialists, physiotherapists, dietitians, social workers, psychiatrists and physicians is critical to achieving this outcome. The expertise of respiratory function laboratories, hematology, biochemistry and microbiology are all essential to good management. In such circumstances it can be expected that over 75% of patients will survive to 18 years of age and 50% to their late 20s.

RESPIRATORY INFECTIONS (see also Ch. 23)

Although, in developed countries, childhood mortality from respiratory infection has decreased spectacularly over the last 40 years, children with respiratory infections still account for a large number of hospital admissions, a half of all illness in the preschool child and a third of general practitioner attendances. In the UK, the fall in the death rate due to respiratory infection has been exaggerated in the OPCS data due to diagnostic transfer to SIDS after 1971. However, the death of a previously healthy child from respiratory infection is rare in the UK nowadays.

INFECTING ORGANISMS, HOST AND ENVIRONMENT

The variation in annual death rates due to respiratory infections (p. 000) is almost certainly a reflection of epidemics of RSV. The *virulence of the infecting organism* may be of more importance than previously recognized. The virulence of pneumococci, *Haemophilus influenzae*, influenza viruses and probably RSV and rhinoviruses varies according to type; types vary between and within countries (see below).

Independent of other factors, *living conditions* are important.

There is a close relationship between overcrowding and mortality due to respiratory infection. Children attending nurseries, starting school, in institutions, in overcrowded housing and in hospitals are at increased risk of becoming infected with respiratory pathogens, particularly viruses. *Atmospheric pollution* compounds the effects of respiratory infection (Lancet 1992).

The pattern and prevalence of infection also depends on *sex* and *age*. Boys are more likely to develop lower respiratory tract infections (LRTI) than girls. The perinatal period is a time of particular vulnerability. The pathogens acquired from the mother during this period, e.g. group B *Streptococcus* (GBS), *Chlamydia* and Gram-negative bacteria other than *Haemophilus influenzae*, rarely cause primary respiratory infection at any other time. The prevalence of GBS and *Chlamydia* in the female genital tract varies between populations and cultures. *Chlamydia* is much more prevalent in American women than in British women. Congenital viral infections such as cytomegalovirus may also cause neonatal pneumonia. Preterm infants, particularly those surviving respiratory distress syndrome (RDS), are at increased risk of being more severely affected by respiratory tract infections, particularly RSV. Bronchiolitis peaks at 3 months, the nadir of the protective effect of transplacental immunity, a phenomenon related to an age-related defect in the infant's immune response (Toms & Scott 1987). The disease pattern is influenced by the small caliber of the airways, babies with small airways being more severely affected than others. Both staphylococcal and pneumococcal pneumonia are most frequent in the first year of life but *Mycoplasma pneumoniae* and influenza infections mainly affect school children and adolescents.

Nutrition and feeding patterns play a role. Children with malnutrition have poor resistance to infection and those in developing countries are at particular risk of pneumonias following common acute infections of early childhood such as measles and pertussis. Obese babies appear to have a more severe illness when they contract respiratory infections but the reason for this is not known. Proof of a protective effect of breast-feeding for respiratory infections is difficult to establish because of confounding factors in any study. Bottle-fed infants in developing countries are four times more likely to die from pneumonia (Lancet 1994).

Children with *chronic lung disease*, e.g. cystic fibrosis (CF) and chronic lung disease of prematurity (CLDP), and those with *immunodeficiency* are at a greater risk of contracting severe LRTI. Those with chronic renal disease and heart disease are also at risk. Poor general nutrition and impaired host defense are probably the reasons. Children with primary immune deficiency can present with recurrent respiratory infection. Those with malignant disease, undergoing chemotherapy or with other diseases associated with immunodeficiency (p. 1264) have greatly improved survival times and organisms otherwise harmless are more likely to feature as respiratory pathogens in such children.

UPPER RESPIRATORY TRACT INFECTIONS

CORYZA

Rhino- myxo-, adeno-, rota-, corona, some types of ECHO and coxsackie viruses and *M. pneumoniae* are all associated with coryzal symptoms. The mode of spread of the common cold has been the subject of debate for many years. The evidence suggests that airborne spread is more important than spread by fingers or fomites (Lancet 1988a). Susceptibility seems to vary between subjects.

Symptoms and signs

As well as nasal discharge and conjunctivitis and sometimes fever, headache may be troublesome in the older child and diarrhea in the infant, especially with rotavirus and enteroviral infections.

Complications

Otitis media (p. 1680) is a complication in the preschool child and although the etiology is primarily viral, cultures of middle ear aspirates in children with otitis media suggest a high incidence of bacterial infection, presumably secondary. Poor feeding in infants should not too readily be ascribed to nasal obstruction; other more serious causes, such as septicemia, pneumonia and meningitis, must be considered. Those most at risk of developing serious lower respiratory illness are infants less than 3 months old and those with underlying chest disease. Upper respiratory tract infection (URTI) in these children may rapidly evolve into a LRTI.

Differential diagnosis

The child with a 'permanent cold' can be a worry. Allergic rhinitis is sometimes difficult to distinguish from viral rhinitis. Children may suffer from 3–6 upper respiratory tract infections each year, giving an impression of permanence. In allergic rhinitis the discharge is clear and watery and the nasal mucous membrane is pale. In the common cold the discharge becomes viscid and mucopurulent and the nasal mucous membrane is inflamed. Some other diagnoses should be kept in mind, such as measles, although now rare in the UK, and other infectious diseases where coryzal symptoms precede other signs. The discharge associated with an impacted foreign body is unilateral, purulent and sometimes foul smelling and bloodstained. A deviated nasal septum or complete or partial choanal atresia may result in noisy breathing, again giving the impression of a 'permanent cold'. Finally, some defects of host defense such as ciliary dyskinesia and IgG subclass deficiency may lead to repeated and troublesome URTI.

Management

Antipyretics and analgesics for fever and headache are usually sufficient. Vasoconstrictor nasal decongestants may give temporary relief but can be complicated by rebound mucosal swelling when treatment stops. Ephedrine nose drops are believed to be helpful in babies who have difficulty feeding but because tolerance to ephedrine develops rapidly, treatment should not continue for more than 36–48 hours. Antibiotics have no place in the treatment of the uncomplicated common cold. A purulent nasal discharge does not imply bacterial infection and does not warrant treatment with drugs.

PHARYNGITIS

Sore throat is a frequent accompaniment of viral URTI but the rarer causes should not be overlooked. Adenovirus is the commonest (Putto 1987) but *Streptococcus pyogenes* is the most worrying pathogen (p. 1330). *Corynebacterium diphtheriae* on the other hand is an extremely rare pathogen in developed countries but a most important cause of sore throat in Asia, Africa and countries of the former Soviet Union. Influenza and parainfluenza viruses are associated with pharyngitis and it is present in the pre-eruptive phase of measles. Coxsackie A and Epstein–Barr (EB) viruses are associated with herpangina and glandular fever respectively, both of which may present with severe acute pharyngitis.

Symptoms and signs

As well as the constitutional symptoms associated with URTI, dysphagia and the painful cough of an associated tracheitis may be distressing. A purulent exudate over the tonsils does not signify a bacterial etiology but a membrane is suggestive of EB virus or diphtheria. Leukemia can present with a persistent membranous pharyngitis. Punctate hemorrhages on the palate and cervical lymphadenopathy are nonspecific signs which often accompany pharyngitis. Vesicles on the fauces are suggestive of herpangina.

Diagnosis

Unfortunately *S. pyogenes* infection cannot be distinguished from viral pharyngitis by inspection. Children under 2 years of age are less likely to suffer from streptococcal infection. Identification of a virus is only of epidemiological importance but it seems important to identify and treat streptococcal pharyngitis. Recent endeavors to produce reliable, rapid test kits using immunological methods for the identification of *S. pyogenes* have not been successful. Because of the possibility of leukemia or infectious mononucleosis a differential white cell count is indicated if membranous pharyngitis persists.

Management

The effect of early treatment of sore throat caused by *S. pyogenes* is controversial (Markovitch 1990). Current conservative opinion is that early treatment reduces infectivity, the duration of symptoms and the incidence of suppurative complications. Whether the risk of nonsuppurative sequelae such as rheumatic fever and acute poststreptococcal nephritis is reduced is unclear. Penicillin is the traditional drug of choice with erythromycin as an alternative. The introduction of new cephalosporins which need only be given once a day should improve compliance. Treatment with amoxicillin 50 mg/kg once a day appears to be as effective as penicillin V four times a day for 10 days. All ampicillin derivatives can cause a rash in patients with infectious mononucleosis.

Infectivity

The infectivity of throat carriers of *S. pyogenes* is controversial. Many consider that asymptomatic carriers are neither a danger to themselves nor to the community. Nasal carriers pose a greater risk. The identification and treatment of patients with active pharyngitis seems to be the most efficacious way of preventing the dissemination and complications of streptococcal disease.

ACUTE OTITIS MEDIA (see also Ch. 27)

Middle ear infection is still an important cause of temporary and permanent hearing loss. Middle ear fluid aspirates have suggested that bacterial infection is frequent. The bacteria are considered to be secondary invaders following a viral upper respiratory infection. *H. influenzae* (usually noncapsulated but occasionally capsulated), *S. pneumoniae*, *S. aureus*, *M. pneumoniae* and occasionally gram-negative bacteria, particularly in neonatal infection, are the usual invaders. *H. influenzae*, previously believed to be important only in children under 3 years, has recently been demonstrated to be an important pathogen in older children with otitis media.

Symptoms and signs

Nonspecific symptoms such as fever, poor feeding, irritability, diarrhea and vomiting are associated in the infant with otitis media. Older children will complain of pain in the ear. The ears should always be examined in any child who presents with these symptoms. However, interpretation of the signs found on examination of the eardrum, not always an easy procedure, is not as straightforward as often suggested (Evans 1982). A red, dull, bulging drum suggests acute, suppurative otitis media. Hemorrhagic bullae on the surface of the drum are suggestive of *M. pneumoniae* infection. The drum may go on to rupture or may already have done so with relief of pain. Paradise (1987) has drawn up a scheme combining signs and symptoms to help with the classification of otitis media.

Complications

Meningitis and mastoiditis are unusual but important complications. Chronic disease has been considered to reflect inadequate treatment of acute disease but since recent studies have failed to demonstrate definite benefit from antibiotics the relationship remains unclear. Temporary hearing loss at all sound frequencies is common and routine hearing tests should not be carried out within 6 weeks of an upper respiratory infection, because of the possibility of otitis media.

Differential diagnosis

'Red ears' are an association of measles and pertussis but, more simply, they may just reflect prolonged crying or fever. In infants, who cannot indicate the source of pain, other causes of poor feeding, fever and irritability should be ruled out before otitis media is considered the primary diagnosis.

Management

Analgesia and antipyretic treatment should be used for symptomatic relief. Since there is no agreement about the role of antibiotics it is difficult to make recommendations. A number of studies show that their routine use does not make any difference to the development of bacterial otitis. If it is decided to use an antibiotic amoxicillin or a macrolide probably merit equal consideration. Decongestants such as ephedrine nose drops are of doubtful value in the prevention or treatment of acute otitis media. The proper treatment of effusions which do not resolve and which may compromise hearing is still unclear (Couriel 1995).

RESPIRATORY INVOLVEMENT IN INFECTIOUS DISEASES

DIPHTHERIA (see also p. 1305)

Because of recent epidemics and the migration of people from endemic areas the possibility of diphtheria should always be considered in the differential diagnosis of sore throat, especially in patients travelling from Bangladesh or Eastern Europe. Proof of immunity is not necessary for admission to the United Kingdom and since the incubation period is 1–6 days it is possible that travelers could arrive in the early stages of their disease. Diphtheria is rarely reported, the annual notification rates in the last decade in the UK being in single figures. Cutaneous lesions may be unnoticed but are highly infectious sources of the organism *C. diphtheriae*.

Symptoms and signs

These are caused by a membrane over the throat which extends forwards and backwards. The membrane becomes greenish-black and firmly adherent and when it involves the larynx causes stridor. In the days before immunization, laryngeal diphtheria used to be the commonest reason for tracheostomy in Britain. When the membrane involves only the nasal septum the disease is relatively mild. The patient presents with sore throat, stridor, fever and is generally unwell. The clinical features may be indistinguishable from epiglottitis so the throat should not be examined unless the precautions for epiglottitis are undertaken (see p. 1308).

Differential diagnosis

Glandular fever and leukemia may present with a faucal membrane and epiglottitis is also associated with stridor and sore throat. There is no membrane with streptococcal pharyngitis. Extra respiratory complications are dealt with in Chapter 23, page 1306).

Management

The child should be isolated and nursed in the same way as any child with stridor. Tracheostomy may be needed early. Antitoxin 5 000–30 000 units intravenously is recommended and systemic penicillin 250 mg 4-hourly. Erythromycin can be used to treat carriers.

PERTUSSIS AND PERTUSSIS-LIKE ILLNESSES

As well as *Bordetella pertussis*, adenovirus, *M. pneumoniae* and *Chlamydia trachomatis* have been associated with 'a whooping-cough-like' illness.

Symptoms and signs

A 'catarrhal' stage of fever and dry cough for 7–10 days precedes the onset of coughing spasms and apnea. When there is a coughing spasm of classic rising pitch terminated by a whoop, apnea and vomiting, the diagnosis is not difficult but if this is not present or witnessed the possibility of the diagnosis may be overlooked. Between coughing spasms the child without complications looks very well. When the child presents with the signs of hypoxia and tachypnea, suggestive of complicating lower respiratory infection, pertussis is rarely considered in the differential diagnosis (Sotomayor et al 1985). Respiratory viruses, such as RSV, may be isolated from patients with pertussis.

Complications

The secondary pulmonary problems are probably due to a combination of aspiration of vomit and preexisting airway disease. Respiratory failure due to bronchopneumonia is unusual except in babies with chronic lung disease of prematurity and undernourished children. Bronchiectasis, believed to result from inadequate treatment of lobar collapse, is now exceedingly rare in developed countries. Pneumothorax and subcutaneous emphysema may result from severe prolonged coughing even in the absence of obvious lung disease. Long-term follow-up – more than 20 years – has shown no measurable effect of pertussis on the respiratory system.

Differential diagnosis:

Whooping cough should always be considered in any child with nonspecific respiratory symptoms and incomplete immunization. In the early stages, during the 'spasmodic' phase, B. pertussis may be isolated from the nasopharynx using pernasal swabs and there may be a high lymphocyte count. This is one of the few occasions when a differential white cell count may be of diagnostic value.

Management

Ventilatory support (Ch. 32) may be needed for respiratory failure or prolonged apnea (Gillis et al 1988) and should not be left as a last resort. There has been some interest in the use of β-agonists for the reduction of the frequency and severity of coughing spasms but the precise place of these has not been fully evaluated. Salbutamol 0.1 mg/kg orally four times daily can be tried. Sedation has no place.

Infectivity

Pertussis is highly infectious and barrier nursing to prevent spread to attendants must be carried out for hospitalized patients. Older children and adults with waning immunity appear to be important disseminators of the disease. The illness in them is much milder and, although a 'whoop' is rarely heard, a severe and troublesome cough may persist for several weeks.

INFECTIONS CAUSING UPPER AIRWAY OBSTRUCTION

Acute inflammatory obstruction of the upper airways in children varies in severity from an almost trivial illness to a lethal disease. Fortunately, since immunization against H. influenzae type b has been available, mortality and morbidity from these disorders has decreased considerably. Unfortunately immunization is still not available in most developing countries and infections caused by H. influenzae are still common. Severe viral croup and bacterial tracheitis can still cause life-threatening upper airway obstruction (UAO). Bacterial tracheitis can be accompanied by septicemia and its complications.

Although there is much controversy about many of the aspects of management of these disorders (Couriel 1988), there is no doubt that a successful outcome depends on the recognition of when and how to intervene to establish an artificial airway.

EPIGLOTTITIS (see also p. 1308)

This is an inflammatory disease of the supraglottic tissues – the epiglottis, arytenoids and aryepiglottic folds. These are involved in varying degrees and the epiglottis may not be the most severely affected area. Characteristically, however, it is swollen, edematous and cherry red.

Etiology

Several bacteria have been associated with epiglottitis but H. influenzae type b is by far the most frequently linked to the condition. It is more often isolated from blood cultures than from swabs from the supraglottic area.

Signs and symptoms

Epiglottitis is usually of sudden onset and rapid progression and occurs in children between 2 and 7 years old. Sore throat, fever (a temperature above 38°C) and difficulty in swallowing precede stridulous and difficult breathing. The breathing is muffled and quiet, quite unlike that of croup, and is usually accompanied by the signs of airway obstruction – supraclavicular and subcostal indrawing. The child prefers to sit up and over a period of a few hours becomes very ill, hoarse or unable to speak and drools because swallowing is painful and difficult. The respiratory rate and heart rate increase in response to hypoxia and toxemia. Exhaustion leads to stupor and sudden respiratory arrest is a constant hazard. The reason for this is speculative and probably multifactorial. The swollen supraglottic area with pooling of secretions in the pharynx severely compromises the airway. Depression of the tongue during examination of the throat or other disturbing procedures such as venepuncture may induce intense vagal discharge, laryngeal spasm or airway occlusion.

Management

All children with a suspected diagnosis of epiglottitis should be transferred to a hospital with pediatric intensive care facilities. Transfer between home and hospital should be done with the child sitting on a parent's lap; lying a child down may provoke complete airway obstruction and ambulance staff should be advised of the importance of minimum disturbance. It has occasionally been advocated that medication should be given before transfer but the risk of the trauma of an injection probably outweighs any benefit conferred. The child should not be separated from the parents before the start of the intubation procedure and attending staff must be aware that any further distress is liable to result in complete airway obstruction. No investigations should be attempted before diagnostic laryngoscopy under anesthesia and intubation if the diagnosis is confirmed. Lateral neck radiographs are not necessary. Transfer between hospitals, should this be necessary, should be undertaken following intubation.

Following endotracheal intubation, blood for culture should be drawn and intravenous antibiotics for the treatment of H. influenzae given. Because of the increasing resistance to ampicillin, the antibiotic of choice is one of the cephalosporins. The role of corticosteroids in treating epiglottitis is unknown.

Progress and complications

Septicemia is an integral part of this disease and pneumonia and meningitis can coexist. Provided there are no problems associated with the endotracheal tube the disease is surprisingly short-lived and extubation can proceed after 24–36 hours.

VIRAL CROUP

Croup is a syndrome of stridor, a barking cough and respiratory distress due to upper airway obstruction. Laryngitis, tracheitis and bronchitis form a spectrum of anatomical diagnosis used in the past but all can be considered as 'croup'. Recurrent or spasmodic croup are terms more frequently used in North America and these describe recurrent stridor without fever possibly due to upper airway hyperreactivity in atopic children.

Etiology

Parainfluenza virus is the most frequent pathogen but rhinovirus and RSV can also cause croup.

Symptoms and signs

Coryzal symptoms are followed over 24–48 hours by a harsh, barking cough. Stridor is most evident when the child is disturbed and parents often report that it seems much worse at night. Restlessness, cyanosis, subcostal and intercostal indrawing suggest a severely compromised airway and impending obstruction. Although this happens infrequently it is important that these signs of severity are recognized early.

Differential diagnosis

Bacterial tracheitis and viral croup can each present with a similar harsh cough but bacterial tracheitis, like epiglottitis, is a much more severe illness. The onset of epiglottitis is more sudden than either. Table 12.22 sets out the comparisons. Retropharyngeal abscess, in the tissues of the posterior pharyngeal wall, although extremely rare, must not be forgotten. It occurs in young children, usually babies, with drooling and fever. Because of the obstruction the child holds his head back. Huge prolapsing tonsils are another cause of upper airway obstruction but this is likely to have been a recurrent or chronic problem. Bacterial croup, epiglottitis and retropharyngeal abscess are all diagnosed at laryngoscopy.

Stridor caused by an inhaled foreign body or acute laryngeal edema caused by burning, chemical inhalation or an allergic reaction can usually, but not always, be diagnosed from the history.

Management

Laboratory and radiological investigations are unhelpful. The decision to admit a child to hospital is difficult because it is impossible to know how the disease will progress. Continuous stridor, marked chest recession, restlessness, sustained tachycardia and irritability all suggest significant UAO and admission should proceed, without delay, to a high-dependency area at a site with intensive care facilities. The intensity of the stridor taken on its own is a poor indicator of the severity of the obstruction. Transcutaneous oxygen saturation measurements of <92% in air suggest additional oxygen is needed. Restlessness is a sign of hypoxemia and should not be confused with anxiety. Children who need oxygen may very soon need additional help and facilities for endotracheal intubation should be at hand.

A number of treatments have been recommended in the past – syrup of ipecac, cold mist, warm steam from a kettle or bath, sedatives – but none of these have any proven benefit. Burns from steam have been reported.

Nebulized adrenaline should only be used to buy time until the patient is admitted to an intensive care unit and preparation for intubation under way. Occasionally intubation can be avoided following the administration of adrenaline. The recommended dose is: adrenaline 1:1000, 2–3 ml nebulized over 10 min and administered by face mask. The effect may last for 10 minutes to 2 hours. Repeated doses have a diminishing effect.

Both dexamethasone and nebulized steroids are effective in reducing symptoms and it may be that corticosteroids will reduce the need for hospital admission or, if given early, the need for intubation (Doull 1995).

Table 12.22 Clinical presentations of upper airway obstruction due to infections

| | Croup | | Bacterial tracheitis | Epiglottitis |
	Viral	Spasmodic		
Age	<3 years	>1 year	>1 year	2–7 years
Cause	Para'flu viruses	?allergy	S. aureus S. pneumoniae H. influenzae	H. influenzae
Prodrome	Coryza	None	Coryza Sore throat	Sore throat Dysphagia
Fever	<38°C	None	>38°C	>38°C
Stridor	Barking cough Loud stridor	Variable stridor	Barking cough Variable stridor	Muffled stridor Stertorous breathing
Severity	<3% of hospitalized cases need intubation	Mild	>80% cases need intubation	All need intubation

BACTERIAL TRACHEITIS

This is a severe condition where an inflammatory, membranous exudate lines the trachea and subglottic area. Children of any age present with stridor and fever. The diagnosis is usually made at laryngoscopy. *S. aureus*, streptococci and *H. influenzae* are the commonest pathogens, often not in pure culture. The disease is thought to occur secondary to a viral infection. Severe systemic illness associated with septicemia can complicate the illness. A broad-spectrum antibiotic should be given systemically after collecting secretions or pus for culture.

LOWER RESPIRATORY TRACT INFECTIONS

BRONCHIOLITIS

This is the commonest LRTI of infancy and is associated with significant short-term morbidity, i.e. hospital admission, symptoms which can last for several weeks, feeding difficulty and pneumonia. The mortality is low in previously healthy babies but for those with previous cardiorespiratory disease mortality rates have been reported as high as 30% (McDonald et al 1982). The peak age at presentation is about 3 months. In the United Kingdom about 2% of the infected infant population requires hospital admission.

Etiology

RSV is isolated in up to 75% of cases. Adenovirus, rhinovirus and the myxoviruses can cause bronchiolitis too and some types of adenovirus – 7 and 21, for example – can cause a particularly severe illness, especially if associated with measles. The compounding effects of living in crowded conditions, cigarette smoking in the household and respiratory disease in the neonatal period and the prenatal effects on the airways of maternal smoking and poor fetal nutrition all operate to increase the severity of the illness. RSV can be contracted more than once. Subsequent illnesses are less severe. Those infants destined for atopy are more likely to suffer severe illness and require hospital admission (Martinez et al 1995, Sigurs et al 1995).

Pathophysiology

The mucous membrane of both large and small airways is inflamed and swollen. Fatal cases show widespread necrosis of the epithelium of the small airways with plugging of the lumen by inflammatory exudate. The result of this is a large increase in airways resistance and a corresponding increase in the work of breathing. The lungs become overinflated and as a result the diaphragms are depressed and flattened. In this position they function least efficiently. Fatigue of the respiratory muscles may be heralded by irregular breathing and this can proceed very rapidly.

Symptoms and signs

The illness begins with coryzal symptoms and low-grade fever. Cough, wheeze and tachypnea develop and the most severely ill babies become cyanosed with suprasternal and substernal recession. Inspiratory and expiratory crackles and wheezes are heard on auscultation. As the chest becomes hyperinflated the diaphragm pushes down the liver so that it becomes easily palpable and appears enlarged. The sign is sometimes mistakenly attributed to cardiac failure. This is extremely rare in previously well babies.

Physical signs bear little relationship to the degree of hypoxemia (Wang et al 1992). Cyanosis is unreliable. Nasal flaring correlates with hypoxemia but in a recent study of infants with bronchiolitis the respiratory rate did not correlate with severity as assessed by poor oxygen saturation values (Mulholland et al 1990). In a very ill baby who becomes exhausted the wheezing may lessen and the respiratory rate become irregular and slow just before collapse.

Differential diagnosis

This includes pneumonia, cardiac failure (CF), aspiration associated with reflux or tracheoesophageal fistula. *C. trachomatis* can cause LRTI in babies of less than 12 weeks but this is more associated with cough than wheezing. The possibility of CF must be considered in a child with a wheezing illness who is not thriving. RSV bronchiolitis can disclose CF and when it does the illness is usually severe and prolonged (Accurso 1991).

Rapid virus identification from nasopharyngeal swabs or nasal washings can be made using immunofluorescent methods which allow the result to be available on the day of admission. However, these methods are not totally sensitive and are especially dependent on good collection and transport techniques. The decision to isolate should not depend on positive identification. Culture of nasopharyngeal swabs and demonstration of a rising titer of serum antibodies is of interest for epidemiological and research work.

Radiology

Chest radiographs show hyperinflation and signs of segmental collapse in 25% of babies. Unless the baby has underlying disease or is likely to need ventilatory support a chest radiograph is not helpful (Dawson et al 1990).

Management

If an infant is too ill to feed then hospital admission and oxygen are necessary. Where there are facilities for measurement of oxygen saturation and blood gas analysis oxygen therapy will be guided by these measurements. Oxygen saturation of <92% suggests that additional oxygen is needed. Breast-feeding should continue for as long as possible. In developing countries this may be the most important source of calories when the infant improves and so should be preserved at all cost. Intravenous fluids can supplement this. Nasogastric feeding is often recommended as infants may be too short of breath to suck. However, the obstruction of a nostril by a tube will increase the work of breathing in babies who breathe through the nose (Sporik 1994). For a few the increase in total airways resistance will be followed by deterioration and apnea. Fluids should probably be given intravenously to infants too ill to suck.

Warmed, humidified oxygen can be given by nasal prongs but this will not be effective if the baby breathes by mouth or if the nose is blocked. Masks and headboxes are used less frequently nowadays but still have a place. Oxygen saturation measurements are now central in modern management. Mist was given in the past but there is good evidence that particulate water may actually induce bronchoconstriction (O'Callaghan et al 1991). There is no evidence that physiotherapy is helpful and indeed it may actually result in further hypoxemia and, in an exhausted baby, even apnea (Webb et al 1985).

Increasing heart and respiratory rates and the need for a higher inspired oxygen concentration suggests worsening disease with increasing ventilation/perfusion imbalance. As hypercapnia is a serious sign suggestive of exhaustion and indicating alveolar underventilation, the baby should be transferred to an intensive or high-dependency area. The decision to offer ventilatory support is largely clinical, based on an appreciation of increasing work of breathing and slowing and irregularity of breathing rather than any particular value of arterial PCO_2. Younger babies will need support before older, stronger infants. Of those children who require hospital admission for bronchiolitis, 1–2% need ventilatory support (p. 1817). Many of these are under 3 months or have preexisting heart or lung disease.

There has been much debate about the value of bronchodilators and corticosteroids in viral bronchiolitis (Rakshi & Couriel 1994). There is no clinically important benefit from either. Those babies who are likely to gain even a transient benefit are older and those who have atopic features such as eczema. These are the groups where a diagnosis of asthma is possible.

Ribavirin is an expensive antiviral agent which, until studies show benefit, should be reserved for babies with previous cardiorespiratory disease such as CF, CLDP or cardiac disease (Milner 1988). It is disputed whether even these groups benefit.

Secondary bacterial infection is unlikely in the majority of babies who do not need ventilatory support (Hall et al 1988) and so it is reasonable not to prescribe antibiotics as a routine measure. However, it is wise to consider that any sick infant could have a concurrent bacterial infection such as a urinary tract infection and to investigate appropriately. Pneumococcal and staphylococcal pneumonia can certainly coexist with bronchiolitis. This in practice is very rare and such children will have clinical features and radiographs which are atypical for simple bronchiolitis.

Infectivity and prevention

The respiratory viruses are highly infectious and spread principally by droplets and aerosols although transmission by fingers and fomites is also possible. Agah et al (1987) have shown that when nursing staff used masks and goggles in addition to ordinary barrier nursing techniques infection with RSV was dramatically reduced, suggesting that airborne transmission to nasal epithelium and conjunctivae is important. This is not as widely appreciated as it should be. In an epidemic it may not be possible to isolate all children with respiratory infections. Babies in hospital belonging to the high-risk group – those with chronic respiratory or cardiac disorders – should be isolated for their own protection and should be reviewed in their homes instead of as outpatients. Their families should understand how to protect them from respiratory infections.

Prognosis

Wheezing and hypoxemia may last for as long as 3 or 4 weeks. Most babies who have suffered bronchiolitis have recurrent wheezing episodes and long-term follow-up studies suggest that abnormal airways resistance is not uncommon. In the 3 years following admission, up to 80% have recurrent coughing and wheezing and even 10 years later there is double the risk of increased airways lability and asthmatic symptoms (Pullen & Hey 1982). It appears that those infants destined for atopy are likely to be worst affected by an RSV infection (Martinez et al 1995). The relationship between RSV and IgE in the pathogenesis of bronchiolitis is, however, unclear.

Obliterative bronchiolitis, a progressive chronic respiratory disorder, is a rare sequel of bronchiolitis due to adenoviral infection.

BRONCHITIS

In the past, bronchitis was a term reserved for children who cough with viral respiratory infections and who may also wheeze. Respiratory viruses – rhinovirus, RSV, adenovirus and parainfluenza virus in particular – cause a less severe illness in older children than they do in infants. This may be due to more competent host defense mechanisms in the older child and perhaps larger airways. The most important diagnosis to consider in a child of over 1 year who coughs and wheezes is asthma. Indeed, over the last few years children with recurrent wheeze are almost always diagnosed as asthmatic.

'Wheezy bronchitis' is certainly an illness in preschool children which is independent of later atopic asthma (Wilson 1989). Antibiotics are of no value in treatment and there is no proven value of 'cough mixtures' and 'expectorants'. Demulcent cough preparations contain substances such as syrup or glycerol and some patients believe these relieve a dry irritating cough (British National Formulary 1994). Simple linctus is harmless and inexpensive. There is no advantage in prescribing either alone or in combination drugs such as antihistamines and sedatives. β-agonists have a role in wheezy children but the value of steroids in the preschool nonatopic recurrently wheezy child is unclear.

COMMUNITY-ACQUIRED PNEUMONIA

The signs and symptoms of LRTI together with the radiological features of consolidation make up the clinical diagnosis of pneumonia. However, the radiological features of segmental consolidation are not always easy to distinguish from those of segmental collapse, apparent in about 25% of children with viral LRTI (Dawson et al 1990). Since in infants there is an overlap between the clinical picture of bronchiolitis and viral pneumonia, the term LRTI is possibly more appropriate. In older children the picture is usually much clearer but the terminology can still be confusing. Preschool children who wheeze with viral illness are sometimes considered asthmatic. Some have segmental or lobar collapse. Children with LRTI caused by *S. pneumoniae*, *H. influenzae* or *M. pneumoniae* more often have clinical and radiographic features which are unmistakably those of consolidation.

The term 'community-acquired pneumonia' suggests an infection acquired outside hospital and, it is assumed, in an immunocompetent patient. Perhaps this term could be replaced by 'LRTI (caused by …) in a previously healthy child'. This would cater for LRTIs diagnosed without chest radiography, would prompt consideration of the pathogen and a rational choice of treatment. It would also bring the terminology into line with the World Health Organization (WHO) terminology. Additional classification could identify patients who also wheezed.

Incidence and mortality

The WHO has estimated that in 1990 4.3 million children under 5 years died from acute respiratory infection, the single largest cause of death in childhood (Campbell 1993). It is also estimated that 60% of these infections are due to *S. pneumoniae* and *H. influenzae* (Lob-Levyt 1993). It should be very unusual for a previously healthy child to die from a LRTI in a developed country.

Common causes

Serotypes of *S. pneumoniae* may be of different invasiveness in different localities (Riley et al 1991) and infants in some cultures acquire *S. pneumoniae* very much earlier than in the West. This is thought to reflect early close exposure to many adult carriers. Similarly, in addition to *H. influenzae* type b other serotypes and nonserotypable strains of *H. influenzae* are responsible for LRTI in different localities. Whether these are primary or secondary invaders has yet to be determined (Moxon & Wilson 1991). Although uncommon in Britain even before immunization, LRTI caused by *H. influenzae* accounts for about 35% of LRTI in several countries (Peltola 1993).

The role of viruses in LRTI is more difficult to prove. RSV is comparatively easy to identify but rhinoviruses and coronaviruses are difficult outside specialist laboratories (Pattemore et al 1992). The severity of viral infection varies with subtype (MacConnochie et al 1990). Influenza A is associated with primary LRTI but like, measles predisposes to secondary infection (Markowitz & Nieburg 1991, Scheublauer et al 1992, Shann 1990). The presence of more than one organism probably occurs quite frequently in the community (Turner et al 1987, Lehmann 1992). The recent debate about the cause of LRTI in adults highlights the need for further clarification of the role of viruses as primary agents (MacFarlane et al 1993, Doull & Johnston 1993).

M. pneumoniae is more evident in developed countries (Broughton 1986) where it occurs in 4-yearly epidemics although it also occurs elsewhere (Shann et al 1986). In the first 3 months of life *C. trachomatis* is cited as the most common cause of pneumonia in the USA (Lancet 1988b) although it is reported less frequently elsewhere. Legionnaire's disease is unusual in children and a history of proximity to water coolers is associated. *S. aureus* is less common as a primary pathogen for LRTI even in developing countries. However, it can follow influenza or disclose an underlying disorder. Pulmonary tuberculosis remains common worldwide and tuberculous pneumonia is a severe complication.

In general it seems that the more adverse the environmental conditions and the greater the defect in host defense, caused by concurrent viral infection destroying local defense or by a general underlying defect, the more likely respiratory infections are to progress from the upper to the lower tract. An extreme example of the latter is the clinical picture of RSV infection in infants with acquired immune deficiency syndrome (AIDS) who have all the signs of classic pneumonia (Chandwani et al 1990). The invasiveness of the organism, whether bacterium or virus, varies with subtype and is an independent factor.

Clinical features

The signs of significant LRTI provided by the WHO were developed for fieldworkers so that they could judge when to admit children to hospital and when to prescribe antibiotics. These issues are important in all countries.

In infants chest indrawing and/or a respiratory rate >50/min gave a positive predictive value of 45% of radiological evidence of consolidation and a negative predictive value of 83% (Harari et al 1991). Respiratory rate is difficult to count in healthy children (Morley 1990) but in children with LRTI it is easier because they are sicker and quieter. Over the age of 36 months tachypnea and chest recession are not sensitive signs: children can have LRTI with lower respiratory rates (Cherian et al 1988).

A respiratory rate of over 50/min together with chest retractions are those signs which best distinguish LRTI from URTI and which can be used by fieldworkers who may not be medically trained. The presence of rapid breathing alone is likely to result in overuse of antibiotics. Campbell and colleagues (1989) in a field study in the Gambia indicated that, in addition to a rapid respiratory rate and indrawing, a fever of over 38.5°C, refusal to feed or persistent vomiting best distinguished mild from severe LRTI as defined by lobar consolidation on the chest radiograph and thus justified referral for hospital management as well as antibiotics. Many rural areas in developing countries have poor access to hospitals and the distinction between mild and severe pneumonia is important. The use of fever as a predictor will be confounded by the local incidence of other febrile diseases, particularly malaria, and so each community must set its own guidelines for the management of acute respiratory infections according to local circumstances. High fever in both infants and children has been considered to be another important sign in the community (Turner et al 1987).

Wheezing is not a useful sign for determining severity in infants and young children (Harari et al 1991). Wheezing occurs in 30% of *Mycoplasma* pneumonias (Broughton 1986). Because of this the clinical diagnosis of *Mycoplasma* LRTI in the absence of a chest radiograph is not always easy. Symptoms of a lower lobe pneumonia in older children may include abdominal pain, reflecting referred pain from the diaphragmatic pleura, and chest pain. The signs of bronchial breathing and pleural effusion are not present at the onset of symptoms. Occasionally abdominal distention reflects a paralytic ileus. Upper lobe consolidation may be associated with referred neck pain and apparent neck stiffness. Chest pain is common and is due to accompanying pleuritis.

Thus, serious consideration should be given to bacterial infection when the presentation is with recession and tachypnea, fever >38.5°C and cough, although in a young infant cough may not be very evident (Table 12.23). In developing countries these features should prompt health workers to prescribe antibiotic treatment. In developed countries, especially in the absence of wheeze, they should prompt chest radiography and measurements of oxygen saturation. Children who are feeding poorly, vomiting or needing additional oxygen require hospital admission. Wheeze is not considered a feature of primary bacterial pneumonia and if present, either a viral or mycoplasmal infection should be considered or an underlying condition which affects the airways, such as CF (Tables 12.23 and 12.24). Children with tuberculous pneumonia are severely ill. The radiographic appearances may provide clues that their illness is not a straightforward bacterial pneumonia (Ch. 23).

C. trachomatis pneumonia (see below) should be considered in infants <3 months.

Microbiological diagnosis

The identification of the organism(s) causing pneumonia is one of the most unrewarding tasks for the microbiologist. Without lung

Table 12.23 Bacterial lower respiratory tract infections (LRTI)

- Fever >38.5°C
- Respiratory rate >50/min
- Chest recession
- Wheeze not an early sign of primary bacterial LRTI
- Influenza, measles and other viruses can coexist
- Clinical and radiological signs indicate consolidation rather than collapse
- Co-trimoxazole first line of treatment in many countries
- Consider local resistance patterns before prescribing an antibiotic
- Consider underlying disorder if repeated bacterial LRTI

Table 12.24 Viral lower respiratory tract infections (LRTI)

- Cough
- Wheeze
- Fever <38.5°C
- Marked subcostal and intercostal recession
- Hyperinflation
- Respiratory rate normal or raised
- Chest radiograph shows hyperinflation and in 25% patchy segmental collapse
- Lobar collapse when severe
- Consider coexisting bacterial infection or underlying disorder if classic consolidation
- Consider aspiration of feed if recurrent collapse without infection

aspiration, the identification rate is about 50% (Turner et al 1987, Ramsey et al 1986) although in general pediatric practice in the UK this figure is certainly smaller. In Nigeria, 80% of lung aspirates yielded organisms (Silverman et al 1977).

Nasopharyngeal aspirates for viral diagnosis should be collected as soon as possible as viral shedding is maximal at the time of the onset of symptoms. Identification will be less successful the later material is collected. The presence of bacteria in the upper airway bears no relation to that in the lung.

Blood cultures are positive in about 10% of *S. pneumoniae* infections in the absence of previous antibiotic therapy. Recovery rates in invasive *H. influenzae* infection are probably higher. The more ill the child the more likely is a bacterial pathogen to be recovered from the blood.

Lung aspiration is the best way of identifying organisms causing pneumonia. This procedure is associated with low morbidity – hemoptysis and small pneumothoraces in 3–10% – and no deaths (Berger & Arango 1985). In countries where LRTI is common and where treatment with antibiotics is expensive accurate diagnosis is important (Ikeogu 1988).

Antigen detection is less rewarding in children than in adults. Pneumococcal antigen can be detected in sputum, blood, pleural fluid and urine. Antigen in sputum is believed to reflect antigen in the lung and not the upper respiratory tract (Venkatesan & MacFarlane 1992) but sputum is difficult to obtain from children. Urine has the greatest false-positive rate because of pneumococcal infections in other areas such as the middle ear and because of crossreactivity with other antigens (Ramsey et al 1986). Compared to blood cultures antigen screening is better for the identification of *Pneumococcus*.

Serum antibody detection is used to identify recent mycoplasmal, chlamydial and viral infections and should be collected at least a week following the onset of symptoms. Viruses such as rhinovirus and coronavirus, which may have an important role in respiratory infection, are not detected in this way. The polymerase chain reaction will have a role to play in the identification of both viruses and bacteria in the future (Johnston et al 1993).

Radiology

In children in whom a diagnosis of bacterial pneumonia is considered a chest radiograph is needed to identify air leaks, effusions, abscesses and the like. Most children with bacterial pneumonia will have segmental or lobar consolidation. The radiographic evidence of consolidation can lag behind signs. In staphylococcal pneumonia the chest radiograph shows widespread signs of pneumonia, occasionally with evidence of abscess formation, empyema, pneumothorax or pyopneumothoraces. Thinwalled cysts (pneumatoceles) are a characteristic feature, but also occur in other bacterial pneumonias and in aspiration pneumonias. They resolve spontaneously.

In *M. pneumoniae* infection, the radiographic features in 87% are usually in only one lung field; 34% have hilar adenopathy and there are pleural effusions in 20%. Radiographic features of *C. trachomatis* are bilateral areas of segmental collapse with mild hyperinflation. In uncomplicated pneumonia follow-up radiology is not needed (Gibson et al 1993). Complete resolution of radiographic changes may take several weeks.

Prevention

The WHO ARI program is directed to this and immunization programs are central to it (Table 12.25 and 12.26). The pathogenesis of infection due to *S. pneumoniae* and *H. influenzae* needs better understanding (Johnston 1991) and vaccines developed suitable for children in developing countries. The WHO is undertaking a program to establish the impact of reducing indoor smoke. Decrease in the incidence of HIV infection worldwide is thought to have little impact on LRTI and vitamin A supplementation has no beneficial effect on non-measles associated pneumonia. Antibiotic treatment of upper respiratory infections has no role in the prevention of LRTI (Lob-Levyt 1993).

Treatment

The severity of pneumonia cannot be well judged using clinical features. Generally if an infant is too ill to feed then hospital admission and oxygen are necessary. In developed countries a diagnosis of pneumonia in an infant is inconsistent with home care.

Table 12.25 ARI worldwide (Lob-Levyt 1993)

- > 4 million deaths/annum
- 60% *S. pneumoniae* and *H. influenzae*
- Measles and pertussis often associated
- Vitamin A affords no protection in non-measles related pneumonia
- Antibiotics for URTI do not prevent
- Reduction of HIV transmission has low impact on LRTI

Table 12.26   ARI in children – what's helpful?

Medical interventions
Immunization against measles and pertussis
Case management by fieldworkers
Appropriate prescribing of antibiotics

Poverty interventions and education
Better nutrition and birthweight
Promotion of breast-feeding
Maternal education about health and child spacing
Reducing overcrowding

Requirements
Better vaccines for *S. pneumoniae, H. influenzae*
RSV vaccine
Understanding of relationship of viral and bacterial infection
Reduction in pollution
   biofuel smoke indoors
   cigarette smoking
   atmospheric pollution

Where there are facilities for measurement of oxygen saturation and blood gas analysis treatment will be guided by these values. A saturation of <92% suggests additional oxygen is needed.

Supportive measures include adequate hydration and nutrition. In many areas hydration and nutrition during an acute respiratory infection and following recovery may be severely compromised because of parental ignorance and taboos about continuing to feed a sick child. Humidity may be increased by hanging wet clothing in the room. Where it is available, low-flow oxygen can be given by nasopharyngeal tube as this is considerably more economical than by mask and, provided the tube is inserted properly, should be perfectly safe (Shann et al 1988). The output from oxygen concentrators can be divided between several children, a cost-effective means of providing oxygen therapy.

Breast-feeding should continue for as long as possible as this may be the most important source of calories when the infant improves and should be preserved at all cost. Intravenous fluids can supplement this.

The WHO has promoted co-trimoxazole for the treatment of pneumonia in the community. This is cheap – a 5-day course from UNICEF costs <20 US cents (Lob-Levyt 1993) – and is as effective as procaine penicillin and ampicillin (Campbell et al 1988). Where a range of antibiotics is readily available, the very slight risk of side-effects from the sulfoxazole component of co-trimoxazole means this drug need not be considered. The treatment of pneumonia with trimethoprim alone has not been evaluated. The choice of antibiotic must depend on local patterns of antimicrobial resistance. Where resistance of *S. pneumoniae* to cheap and useful drugs is becoming a problem, antibiotics must be used more selectively (Venkatesan & Innes 1995). Penicillin penetrates lung tissue well and most isolates in the UK in the mid-1990s are of intermediate resistance with an MIC of 0.1–1 µg/ml, below the concentration in the lung or pleural fluid if penicillin is given intravenously (Pallares et al 1987). Resistance of *S. pneumoniae* to the macrolides is much more common. Macrolides are said to shorten the illness in patients with *M. pneumoniae*. There are worrying reports of developing resistance to cephalosporins (Klugman and Saunders 1993).

Physiotherapy has no place in uncomplicated pneumonia (Britton et al 1985). Simply encouraging the child to cough in the presence of pain may be all that is required to assist in the mobilization of secretions during resolution.

Further investigation

The isolation of *S. aureus* should suggest an underlying problem such as CF or primary immune deficiency but concurrent infection with influenza in a previously healthy child is probably more likely. Staphylococcal pneumonia is a disease which rarely affects children in developed countries.

Children with surface immune deficiency, such as CF, ciliary dyskinesia and CLDP, are at greatest risk from repeated severe LRTI due to viruses while those with sickle cell disease, nephrotic syndrome or functional asplenia are at increased risk of *S. pneumoniae* and mycoplasmal disease. Those with primary immune deficiency are at risk of bacterial infection and those with cellular deficiency at risk of severe illness with a range of micro-organisms. Chronic aspiration leads to a chemical pneumonia which should be considered in the differential diagnosis of recurrent collapse/consolidation with wheezing.

As in adults, chest infection may complicate underlying focal chest disease. Foreign bodies, congenital abnormalities and rare malignancies are the most likely causes in children and must be considered in all who present with unusual chest radiographs, particularly those with focal features slow to resolve.

Complications and outcome

Fifty percent of cases of *H. influenzae* pneumonia have associated otitis media, meningitis or epiglottitis and blood cultures are positive in the majority. The respiratory illness follows a similar course to other pneumonias. Staphylococcal pneumonia has a good outcome in spite of pyopneumothorax and other complications provided there is no malnutrition or underlying disease. Children with pneumococcal pneumonia also do well with the same provisos but this is more dependent on the subgroup of the organism. Adenoviral pneumonia is severe and can have long-term sequelae.

EMPYEMA

Any of the bacterial pneumonias can be complicated by an effusion or empyema (Hubbard & McKenzie 1996). Other associated conditions are physical handicap such as cerebral palsy which predisposes to aspiration, inhaled foreign body and hypogammaglobulinemia. In infants and in children following trauma or surgery chylothorax and hemothorax may need to be distinguished and this can often only be done at thoracentesis.

Children with untreated empyema look ill. Although cough and fever are the common presenting features abdominal pain may be quite misleading and represents referred pain from the diaphragm. Chest dullness and reduced breath sounds are the usual signs.

In about half of cases the pleural fluid is either sterile or grows more than one microorganism, including anaerobes. This is probably because treatment with antimicrobials has begun before aspiration. All but the smallest of pleural effusions seen on the plain chest radiograph should be aspirated in order to stage the effusion and to culture it. If the aspirate is purulent then an ultrasound scan should help in identifying loculation. Where there are no loculations, closed chest drainage or repeated daily aspirations with irrigation (Storm et al 1992) is the first treatment. Streptokinase should probably be instilled when pus is first identified (Rosen et al 1993). If in spite of this fever persists, CT scanning to identify loculation and followed by debridement will be needed. Thoracoscopy available in some centers (Stovroff et al 1995) avoids open surgical drainage. A telescope in the pleural space allows direct vision of breakdown of adhesions and aspiration using forceps and catheters introduced through an adjoining lumen. Decortication is needed when organization of the empyema has resulted in a thick pleural peel.

LUNG ABSCESS

Lung abscess has a similar etiology to empyema although aspiration probably plays a larger role and thus anaerobes feature more frequently. This is particularly the case in chronically ill and neurologically handicapped children who inhale food because of swallowing difficulties, regurgitation and difficulty with coughing. Undiagnosed foreign body inhalation in otherwise healthy children may also be complicated by abscess formation. Most abscesses resolve with antimicrobial treatment.

CHLAMYDIA PNEUMONIA

Chlamydia trachomatis can be recovered from 25% of infants of mothers who have been identified positive for chlamydial antigen (Preece et al 1989). This genital infection is more frequent in women of low socioeconomic status. It can be acquired across intact amniotic membranes and so babies delivered by cesarean section can be infected as well as those delivered vaginally.

About 15% of the infants have LRTI, from 4–6 weeks of age, with clinical symptoms and signs indistinguishable from those of pneumonia. A dry, 'staccato' cough in the neonatal period is a distinguishing feature. Crackles are described more frequently than wheeze. There is a history of sticky eye in 50%. Chlamydia is isolated by cell culture from respiratory secretions. The disease is generally mild and responds poorly to erythromycin. It is not a fatal illness in otherwise healthy infants. Respiratory symptoms can persist for at least 7 years afterwards but it is difficult to know whether this is because chlamydial infection identifies a host susceptibility or because it leads to permanent damage (Weiss et al 1986).

It is not known how often Chlamydia pneumoniae, identified in 1986, is responsible for respiratory infections in children. It has been suggested that it causes an illness similar to that caused by Mycoplasma pneumoniae but patients were more likely to be hoarse and afebrile (Marrie 1993). The spread of this strain is probably human to human rather than avian to human.

PSITTACOSIS (see also p. 1373)

This is a rare and potentially fatal zoonosis caused by Chlamydia psittaci. Most wild urban birds are infected but the infectivity of birds to man is variable: pigeons are poorly infective but parakeets and budgerigars are highly infective. Unlike the United States, psittacosis is not a notifiable disease in the United Kingdom. Much of the difficulty in making the diagnosis rests on the controversy about the specificity of chlamydia serological testing; many believe that the majority of chlamydial seropositivity is due to the strain of Chlamydia psittaci known as TWAR (TW for Taiwan where it was first identified and AR for acute respiratory). However, the increase in notification of the disease in North America has been associated with an increase in the importation of psittacine birds and the diagnosis rests on a history of contact with infected birds in the presence of respiratory infection and

with rising titers to chlamydial antigen. Extrapulmonary manifestations include myocarditis, nephritis, thrombophlebitis and meningoencephalitis. The symptoms and signs of pulmonary involvement are those of a mild to moderately severe pneumonia and the diagnosis may be suggested by the history of contact with sick birds.

MYCOPLASMA PNEUMONIA (see also p. 1374)

This is a common cause of pneumonia in schoolchildren and young adults (see above). In early school years it is responsible for about 12% of pneumonia, rising to 20% in older schoolchildren and over 30% in young adults. Recurrent infections with M. pneumoniae are not unusual and many are undoubtedly asymptomatic. The symptoms associated with pneumonia are often much worse than the physical signs would suggest. About half wheeze, but other often severe, systemic complaints such as weakness, headache, sore throat and chest or abdominal pain predominate. It is very much a 'flu-like' illness with cough and mucoid or yellow sputum. Signs in the chest are often insignificant but careful auscultation may reveal fine crepitations, either localized or multifocal. Extrapulmonary manifestations are discussed in Chapter 23.

A diagnosis of M. pneumoniae is suggested by a positive titer for cold agglutinins and a rise in titer of specific antibodies. The rise has frequently taken place before the child presents and a falling titer in convalescence is confirmatory. Culture of the organism takes about 3 weeks and is therefore not of clinical use. Chest radiograph changes are nonspecific and variable, from multifocal to lobar shadowing. Erythromycin is said to shorten the illness.

LEGIONNAIRE'S DISEASE

Legionnaire's disease is an unusual disorder in childhood. It occurs either sporadically or in epidemics in communities. Legionnella pneumophila is harbored in water supplies and water-cooled air-conditioning systems. Infected infants and children suffer from widespread pneumonia. The diagnosis is worth considering in any severe chest infection. Serological studies demonstrate raised titers to L. pneumophila and the organism can be identified at lung biopsy. Treatment is with erythromycin.

Q FEVER (p. 1374)

This is caused by Coxiella burnetii acquired from ticks which infest livestock. It is a frequent cause of pneumonia in the Basque country. It is usually a mild LRTI and responds to treatment with doxycycline or erythromycin.

RARE BACTERIAL PNEUMONIAS

Pneumonia caused by Streptococcus pyogenes is rarely seen nowadays. It has been described following viral respiratory infections and measles. The clinical course is similar to staphylococcal pneumonia. Group B hemolytic Streptococcus, however, is the most common cause of pneumonia in the newborn (see Ch. 5). The Gram-negative pneumonias are also very uncommon and are almost entirely confined to the newborn and to children with underlying disease.

FUNGAL INFECTIONS (see also p. 1470)

Despite the prevalence of fungi in the environment fungal disease is rare. Fungi cause both pathogenic and opportunistic infections and in the United Kingdom the latter, affecting children with altered host defense mechanisms, are by far the most prevalent.

Histoplasmosis, blastomycosis and coccidioidomycosis

These fungal infections are exceptionally rare in children outside the United States and South America. All cause illnesses which range from asymptomatic infection to disseminated disease and all have clinical features which are very similar to tuberculosis. In the lung, granulomas associated with hilar lymphadenopathy can progress to pneumonia, cavitating pulmonary lesions and pleural disease. The clinical features are those of nonspecific respiratory infection and diagnosis rests on appropriate skin testing and sputum culture. Amphotericin B is used to treat severe blastomycosis and coccidioidomycosis but the treatment of histoplasmosis is extremely difficult. These disorders should be considered in any child with a respiratory illness and features of tuberculosis who has recently arrived from the Americas.

Aspergillosis

Aspergillus causes two forms of respiratory disease in childhood: allergic disease and invasive pneumonitis. Much attention has been given to the role of *Aspergillus* hypersensitivity in both asthma (p. 536) and cystic fibrosis (p. 550). It is interesting to speculate about the evolution of mechanisms which protect *Aspergillus*, one of many fungi whose natural habitat is the soil, against the lung's defences. Killing of *Aspergillus* by macrophages is strongly inhibited by complement and this is likely to be present in large amounts in the inflamed airways of patients with asthma and cystic fibrosis. Invasive pneumonitis which occurs in the immunocompromised child is discussed on page 1361.

Actinomycosis

Many of the species of *Actinomyces* live in the mouth, in dental plaque and calculus. As mouth hygiene has become better actinomycosis, in which organisms reach the chest by inhalation, has become rare. Disease in children is confined to those at risk of inhaling food and of developing lung abscesses.

MYCOBACTERIA (see Ch. 23)

Tuberculosis is discussed on page 1334. The atypical *mycobacteria* infect human populations but the majority do not develop clinical disease. Lymphadenitis is usually the sole manifestation and pulmonary infection and dissemination are very rare. Skin tests to specific antigens are positive but the tuberculin test may also be positive. Final identification of the particular agent rests with its culture from biopsy material. Treatment if needed for symptomatic pulmonary disease is similar to that for tuberculosis.

PARASITES

Pulmonary eosinophilia or Loeffler's syndrome is believed to be caused by either parasites or drugs. *Ascaris*, *Toxocara*, the hookworms and *Strongyloides* are among those nematodes

responsible and aspirin, penicillin and the sulfonamides are among the drugs. Transitory symptoms and chest radiographic signs are believed to be due to the migratory phase of the life cycle of these parasites. More prolonged pulmonary disease causes cough, wheezing, shortness of breath, hemoptysis, fever and weight loss. Diagnosis is suggested by migratory pulmonary infiltrations and a high eosinophil count in the peripheral blood. Identification of the offending parasite can be made by stool examination and by serological methods. *Aspergillus* infection should be considered where appropriate. The disorder resolves when the cause is eliminated.

INHALATION OF FOREIGN MATERIAL

RECURRENT INHALATION

Recurrent inhalation of food or gastroesophageal contents may simply cause wheezing or may give rise to recurrent pneumonia or chronic inflammatory changes, with eventual airway narrowing, interstitial fibrosis and bronchiectasis. Handicapped children are particularly susceptible. The predominant site of pulmonary pathology depends largely on the patient's habitual posture: upper lobes for infants nursed supine; basal disease for older children propped in a semirecumbent position.

There are three main groups of causes of recurrent inhalation (Table 12.27). The anatomical abnormalities generally lead to pooling of food or saliva in the pharynx; abnormalities of coordination lead to aspiration during swallowing. In both groups, symptoms occur during feeds. Obstructive lesions of the esophagus characteristically cause dysphagia for solids. Similarly, fistulous connections between airway and esophagus tend to produce symptoms during feeds. Gastroesophageal reflux, on the other hand, leads to regurgitation or vomiting between feeds, particularly during sleep. Some patients with severe reflux have no symptoms referable to the gastrointestinal tract. Conversely, patients with gastroesophageal reflux identified in a gastroenterology clinic (i.e. with primarily gastrointestinal

Table 12.27   Causes of recurrent inhalation

Swallowing disorders
Anatomical abnormalities
  Cleft palate
  Macroglossia
  Laryngeal cleft
Neuromuscular disorders
  Cerebral palsy
  CNS degenerative disorders (e.g. leukodystrophies)
  Congenital muscle disorders (e.g. congenital myotonic dystrophy)
  Dysautonomia
  Prematurity

Esophageal lesions
Obstruction
  Stricture or compression
  Functional obstruction (e.g. following repair of esophageal atresia)
  Systemic sclerosis
  Megaesophagus
Tracheoesophageal fistula
Gastroesophageal reflux
Incompetent cardia
Hiatus hernia
Hyperinflation (severe asthma, cystic fibrosis)

complaints) do not as a group have more respiratory problems than control populations.

Respiratory symptoms include cough, wheeze and apnea directly related to episodes of inhalation and acute febrile illnesses with breathlessness and cyanosis if aspiration pneumonia develops. The features of bronchiectasis and of pulmonary fibrosis are found.

The diagnosis is achieved largely by awareness, careful history taking and physical examination. Observation of the child feeding is vital. Simple radiography will help in determining the extent rather than the cause of the disorder; barium swallow should be performed specifically to seek swallowing problems, hiatus hernia and tracheoesophageal fistula. Video recording of the swallow is essential. If a fistula is suspected, specific lateral views are taken while injecting contrast through a slowly withdrawn, lateral hole gastric tube. The main technique for the diagnosis of gastro-esophageal reflux is 12–24 h midesophageal pH monitoring. Radiolabeled milk scans, esophagoscopy and biopsy (for esophagitis) and the demonstration of fatladen macrophages in tracheal aspirate are sometimes useful. For some of these tests, there is no clear cut-off between normality and abnormality.

One of the most difficult areas of pediatric respiratory medicine is the relationship between gastroesophageal reflux and recurrent wheezing in infants and young children. Both are independently relatively common; when they occur in the same child, identifying a causal relationship is usually impossible. Therapeutic trials may effect improvement without necessarily giving the answer. Infants with chronic bronchopulmonary dysplasia and cystic fibrosis constitute another group in whom both reflux and recurrent respiratory symptoms commonly coexist.

The management clearly depends on cause. Gastric reflux, if minor, may be managed by thickening of feeds (using carob-based or agar-based substances) and posture. The supine posture is ineffective in preventing reflux. Only the prone posture (at 20–30°) will allow fundal air to be released without accompanying gastric fluid.

The prokinetic agent cisapride has been used with success to reduce gastroesophageal reflux in young children with lung disease. Occasionally, histamine 2-blocking drugs (e.g. ranitidine) or proton pump inhibitors may be temporarily needed if there is esophagitis. Fundoplication of the stomach should be reserved for intractable cases.

FOREIGN BODY INHALATION

This is common as an isolated episode, occurring predominantly in boys below the age of 4. Peanuts (ground nuts) and other nuts are the most common objects in the UK and among the worst irritant agents leading to florid local inflammation and necrosis of the bronchial epithelium. Grass seeds and seed husks are commoner in other parts of the world and may be especially troublesome, because their barbed nature prevents expectoration or removal by bronchoscope. Rarely, laryngeal obstruction may lead to rapid asphyxia. The most common site of impaction is a segmental bronchus, particularly the right intermediate bronchus.

The usual complaint is of sudden onset of choking, coughing or wheezing. After an initial fright, a symptom-free interval may ensue, but the persistence of physical signs (wheeze, diminished local breath sounds) and radiological changes (hyperinflation of the affected segment or, more rarely, collapse) will provide clues to the presence of a foreign body. A careful history will identify a choking episode in 80% of cases. If doubt persists, radiological screening (to look for mediastinal 'swing' away from the affected segment on expiration) or a ventilation lung scan (to seek segmental hypoventilation) can be helpful. Whenever strong suspicion of foreign body inhalation exists, bronchoscopy should be performed. Almost all foreign bodies are removable by this means, but occasionally thoracotomy and bronchotomy are required.

In about one-third of cases, there is delay of over a week in the diagnosis of inhaled foreign body, either because the episode was not witnessed or its significance not realized. Children may present later with persistent wheeze (mistaken for asthma), delayed resolution of pneumonia, chronic cough (occasionally with hemoptysis) or, very rarely, respiratory failure. In all cases, suspicion together with focal, persistent radiological signs should lead to bronchoscopy. Segmental resection of irretrievably damaged lung may be required. The long-term prognosis for inhaled peanuts is not necessarily benign.

DROWNING (Spyker 1985)

There is a bimodal age distribution of drowning in childhood. Teenage boys represent by far the greatest number. Preschool nonswimmers are also at risk. Ill-supervised infants, often left in the charge of older siblings, are at risk of drowning in the bath. In terms of management and prognosis, the difference between freshwater and seawater drowning is not important. The critical factors are duration of asphyxia and depth of coma which determine severity; hypothermia and 'dry drowning' (without aspiration) are protective.

Prolonged asphyxia and deep coma do not preclude full recovery if accompanied by hypothermia (core temperature less than 32°C). Normothermic individuals who arrive in the emergency department deeply unconscious with fixed pupils and no spontaneous respiration have a fatal outcome.

It is doubtful whether intracranial pressure monitoring is worthwhile, since the outcome for children with raised intracranial pressure requiring active management is uniformly bad.

The major pulmonary effects of drowning result from pulmonary edema and atelectasis. Patchy infiltrates with a perihilar distribution are seen on chest radiograph. Pulmonary edema is worse after seawater drowning. Hypervolemia always occurs, but electrolyte abnormalities are rarely severe. Hypoxemia, with circulatory, renal and neurological adverse consequences, is the major disturbance.

Full cardiopulmonary resuscitation should be followed by subsequent management in a high dependency or intensive care unit.

SMOKE INHALATION AND BURN INJURIES TO THE LUNGS

Direct and indirect injuries to the lungs occur in burn victims. Inhalation of smoke, steam or hot air can cause direct injury. Indirect effects of distant surface burns may lead to 'shock lung', while thermal damage to the chest wall can impair breathing. In addition, carbon monoxide poisoning may contribute to the ill effects of hypoxemia. This section concerns direct injuries.

Injuries to the upper airway predominate if hot air is inhaled. Steam and smoke inhalation may have additional effects in the lungs. Minor irritation may lead to cough and wheeze. Mucociliary clearance is impaired. More severe inflammation results in inflammatory bronchitis, bronchiolitis with epithelial shedding or pulmonary edema. Some of these effects may not be clinically apparent for several hours. Acute respiratory failure and bacterial pneumonia may develop. Late complications include obliterative bronchiolitis.

The presence of facial burns or of early respiratory symptoms should alert one to the likelihood of severe complications. Stridor or severe upper airway obstruction may be an indication for endotracheal intubation or tracheostomy with full respiratory support for progressive hypoxemia. Antibiotic and bronchodilator therapy are indicated, but corticosteroids are not useful in pulmonary injury. They may be required for purely upper airway edema or for the cerebral complications of severe hypoxemia. Hyperbaric oxygen therapy may be required if carbon monoxide poisoning is severe (i.e. hemoglobin CO saturation over 30–40%); for milder or suspected CO poisoning, humidified 100% oxygen should be administered as soon as possible. This increases the rate of dissociation of carboxyhemoglobin.

CONGENITAL ABNORMALITIES

Many abnormalities of the respiratory system coexist with abnormalities of other systems, especially the gastrointestinal, the cardiovascular and the musculoskeletal systems.

NASOPHARYNGEAL ABNORMALITIES

These are usually obvious in the neonatal period. Bilateral *choanal atresia* or *stenosis* compromises the baby who is an obligate nose breather, leading to apnea and cyanosis, or in milder cases there may be chest recession and aspiration during feeding. Diagnosis is suggested when nasal catheters cannot be passed. Management is surgical. Babies with marked breathing difficulty should have a large oral airway positioned or should be intubated until surgery is performed. Babies with unilateral stenosis present later with noisy and difficult breathing or with nasal discharge which is persistent and may be offensive. Glossoptosis associated with the *Pierre Robin syndrome* causes obstructed breathing. The baby should be nursed prone but if this is unsuccessful a carefully positioned nasopharyngeal tube or tracheostomy may be necessary until the mandible grows sufficiently to accommodate the tongue, usually before the age of 1 year. Congenital *tumors* and *cysts*, such as teratoma, hemangioma, ectopic thyroid and cystic hygroma, are unusual causes of pharyngeal obstruction, all of which require surgical treatment. Crowding of the pharynx occurs in Down syndrome and in disorders associated with a large or abnormally positioned tongue. Sleep-disordered breathing may result from airway obstruction as muscle tone falls during sleep.

CONGENITAL STRIDOR

LARYNGOMALACIA

This is the commonest cause of noninfective stridor and accounts for over 75% of stridor in infancy. The tissues of the larynx are flaccid so that the arytenoids, epiglottis and aryepiglottic folds fall inwards on inspiration. Stridor is usually evident in the first day or two of life but may not present until over 1 month. There is no cyanosis and abnormalities of cry and respiratory distress and

feeding difficulties are most unusual. The inspiratory stridor is worse during periods of agitation and upper respiratory tract infection. Some severely affected children may need hospital admission in case they tire and need oxygen during upper respiratory tract infections.

Although the clinical presentation is characteristic, endoscopy should always be carried out as other laryngeal abnormalities which are not benign may be missed. Sudden death in infants believed to have 'benign laryngeal stridor' has been reported. The stridor usually disappears by the age of 2 years but sometimes goes on until the child starts school.

LARYNGEAL STENOSIS

This is the second commonest cause of congenital stridor and may be caused by supraglottic, glottic or subglottic webs or subglottic stenosis.

Most *laryngeal webs* are glottic and present with stridor and a poor cry at or shortly after birth. The severity of the symptoms depends on the size of the web, which may indeed cause complete airway obstruction, a condition incompatible with life unless diagnosed and treated within minutes of delivery. Many of these babies have other severe abnormalities. Treatment is surgical.

Subglottic stenosis is usually the result of soft tissue thickening of the subglottic area, usually acquired following prolonged intubation during the neonatal period. Occasionally laser resection of the granulation tissue or tracheostomy is required but most improve as the larynx grows. Localized tracheo- or bronchomalacia resulting from damage in the neonatal period due to ventilatory assistance may also cause stridor with or without wheeze in the first few years of life. These babies are more likely to require hospital admission if they acquire a respiratory infection as they will almost certainly have associated lower respiratory tract damage. All babies who have needed intensive care during the neonatal period should have a clear route to effective medical help outlined before discharge from hospital.

SUBGLOTTIC HEMANGIOMATA

Subglottic hemangiomata become obvious before 6 months and 50% of babies have hemangiomata elsewhere, usually on the skin. Radiographs of the area show a subglottic soft tissue swelling which is confirmed at endoscopy. Regression during the first 2 years is the rule and thus a conservative approach is preferred. However, tracheostomy may be necessary in the neonatal period as the airway may be compromised and the hemangioma may enlarge before it regresses.

VOCAL CORD PARALYSIS

This can be unilateral or bilateral. Unilateral is more frequent. Paralysis may be associated with other abnormalities especially in the cardiovascular and respiratory systems. In most cases the paralysis is temporary with recovery within 4 weeks (Cotton & Richardson 1981). Birth trauma with stretching of the neck and the recurrent laryngeal nerve may be a factor. Bilateral paralysis is usually associated with central nervous system disorders, such as hydrocephalus, which may themselves have a poor prognosis. Diagnosis is made at laryngoscopy when cord paralysis is observed.

LARYNGEAL CLEFTS

Laryngeal clefts are associated with tracheoesophageal fistulae in about 20% and hydramnios in 30%. The infant presents with a toneless cry and has choking and cyanosis on feeding which sometimes results in aspiration pneumonia. Later in childhood a chronic cough may be the only clue. Diagnosis is at laryngoscopy and should be undertaken by an experienced laryngoscopist as less experienced operators may miss a mild cleft. Surgical repair can be extremely difficult.

LARYNGEAL CYSTS

Laryngeal cyst are very rare and cause stridor and a poor cry in the neonatal period. Endoscopy is hazardous as complete airway obstruction may be precipitated and removal of the cyst may be difficult without tracheostomy.

VASCULAR ABNORMALITIES

Vascular abnormalities include abnormalities of the vessels of the aortic arch which cause tracheal compression, usually presenting during the first year of life. Stridor, wheezing and a barking cough are the commonest presenting symptoms. Since the larynx is not involved, the tone of the cry is normal. Excessive secretions, difficulty with feeding and apneic episodes are sometimes associated. The commonest forms of 'vascular ring' are as follows: double aortic arch 50%, right aortic arch with left ligamentum arteriosum 20%, abnormal right subclavian artery 15%, abnormal innominate artery 10%. Most forms are seen as a posterior esophageal indentation on a barium swallow. An aberrant innominate artery is not associated with an abnormal barium swallow, however, but may be seen compressing the trachea anteriorly on a lateral chest radiograph. More precise anatomical diagnosis can only be determined at angiography.

If the airway is significantly compromised then surgery must be undertaken. This is usually necessary in double aortic arch, but the symptoms in childhood with aberrant innominate artery often improve with growth and surgery is not always needed. Because of distortion of the trachea by chronic compression respiratory symptoms may persist following surgery.

A rare cause of congenital stridor is a 'pulmonary sling'. This occurs when the left pulmonary artery arises from the right and passes between the trachea and esophagus, compressing the right main bronchus. This anomaly is frequently associated with other congenital abnormalities. It is the only vascular anomaly which produces anterior indentation of the esophagus on barium swallow. Tracheobronchial compression can also occur in children with a large left to right intracardiac shunt. The distended hypertensive pulmonary arteries and occasionally the left atrium cause airway compression resulting in localized or generalized pulmonary hyperinflation and wheezing. Symptoms improve when the size of the shunt is reduced. In absent pulmonary valve syndrome, distended pulmonary arteries may cause airway compression with eventual bronchomalacia.

TRACHEOESOPHAGEAL FISTULA (see also p. 1770)

The preoperative pulmonary problems associated with tracheoesophageal fistula (TEF) are related either to aspiration of secretions or food through the larynx if, as is usual, the upper end of the esophagus is blind or to reflux of stomach and duodenal secretions through the distal end of the esophagus into the tracheobronchial tree. Pulmonary disease in the immediate postoperative period may be compounded by leakage from the anastomotic site.

In the rare H-type fistula (4%) aspiration of food may cause recurrent chest infection. The underlying abnormality may even not be diagnosed until adult life. The diagnosis of the H-type TEF is not easy and rests on the demonstration of contrast medium flowing through the fistula (p. 1773). Seventy percent of lesions lie high in the esophagus and since the fistula passes obliquely upwards from the esophagus the procedure should be carried out with the child lying prone.

Prognosis is related to the maturity of the baby, the presence of pulmonary disease before surgery, the incidence of postoperative pulmonary disease and the association of other abnormalities. TEF has a reported association of congenital abnormalities of 50–70% and 2% of these are associated abnormalities of the respiratory tract.

Long-term follow-up of survivors of surgery suggests that small airway abnormalities are common. These may be related to disorders of esophageal motility and repeated small aspirations or they may be related to the severity of the initial respiratory disease. In addition, at the site of the fistula tracheal cartilage is inadequately formed or missing and there is an absence of normally ciliated respiratory epithelium. Tracheomalacia accounts for the brassy cough, worse during upper respiratory tract infections. Apneic episodes following feeding are a problem in a small number of babies and the incidence of sudden unexpected death is increased. Whether this is due to aspiration or associated with the tracheomalacia is debated.

BRONCHIAL AND LUNG ABNORMALITIES

There is a wide variety of abnormal bronchial branching patterns, many associated with other abnormalities, mainly of the heart and gut which may themselves determine the prognosis. Some do not present or cause symptoms until adult life whilst others severely compromise respiratory function in the neonate (Vogt-Moykopf et al 1992).

PULMONARY SEQUESTRATION AND RELATED CONGENITAL BRONCHOPULMONARY-VASCULAR MALFORMATIONS

The classification of these disorders proposed by Clements & Warner (1987) is based on a rational sequence of events in lung development; insults of different severity and timing could account for all lung anomalies that include 'malinosculation' of one or more components of the bronchopulmonary-vascular complex. Malinosculation is defined as an abnormal connection of one or more of the four major components of lung tissue – namely, tracheobronchial airway, lung parenchyma, arterial supply and venous drainage – which in various combinations make up a group of varied bronchopulmonary – vascular malformations.

Tracheal stenosis and bronchial stenosis

These have possibly resulted from a comparatively minor, localized insult during development which allows a local abnormality followed by normal development of the rest of the lung. They cause inspiratory stridor or wheeze with chest indrawing. Diagnosis is at bronchoscopy with or without bronchography. Distal bronchial stenosis may result in lobar collapse during a chest infection. If this does not resolve investigation should proceed so that the development of bronchiectasis distal to the obstruction is identified if present (p. 576). Local surgery may correct the local stenosis but lobectomy may be indicated if bronchiectasis has already developed and cannot be managed medically. Both these lesions in isolation are extremely rare.

Tracheal and bronchogenic cysts

These are fluid-filled cysts originating from the primitive foregut. They may be paratracheal, carinal, hilar or paraesophageal. The symptoms of inspiratory or expiratory wheeze result from compression of the airway. Pulmonary collapse and recurrent chest infection distal to the site of narrowing suggests there may be a focal bronchial abnormality. Chest radiography may suggest unilateral hyperlucency and a penetrated view may be helpful in defining the site of compression. Surgical removal is generally successful.

Cystic adenomatoid malformation

This results from an increase in terminal respiratory structures. Hydrops fetalis and maternal hydramnios are common. It is nearly always unilateral and symptoms are present at birth although occasionally much later, beyond infancy. In this case it should be distinguished from other causes of lung cysts (Table 12.28). Recently surgical removal shortly after birth has met with some success. The opposite lung can expand with compensatory emphysema.

Congenital lobar emphysema (CGLE)

This is caused either by localized bronchomalacia (see below) or a generalized abnormality in the acinar tissue of the whole segment. In about 50% of cases, symptoms are present in the neonatal period with respiratory distress and the radiographic features of CGLE. Most of the remainder are evident before the age of 6 months. The left upper and right middle lobes are most frequently affected but the disorder can be multilobar. The affected lobe usually has a normal pulmonary artery blood supply. Associated congenital heart disease occurs in 15–35% of cases.

Beyond infancy, CGLE may produce chest deformity or persistent wheeze or may be discovered incidentally. The history and investigations should be directed to excluding other causes of bronchial compression, such as bronchogenic cyst, or other causes

Table 12.28 Differential diagnosis of cystic-like lesions on the plain chest radiograph

Bronchopulmonary dysplasia
Infected sequestrated lobe
Cystic adenomatoid malformation
Solitary or multiple developmental cysts
'Congenital lobar emphysema'
Pneumatoceles following pneumonias – usually staphylococcal
Lung abscess
Encysted empyema
'Diaphragmatic hernia'

Other cysts are described many of which may be variations of cystic adenomatoid malformations

of the radiographic appearances of a hyperlucent lung (p. 514). It may not always be possible to distinguish lobar emphysema from a lung cyst. The need for treatment depends on the degree of respiratory distress. Conservative management is often successful, with spontaneous resolution. Provided there are no associated compromising abnormalities the outlook following surgery is good.

Lobar sequestration

This is a segment of lung parenchyma which has no connection with the bronchial system. It may be supplied by an aberrant artery arising from the aorta or one of its side branches. It is usually drained by the pulmonary veins. Intralobar sequestrations share the common pleura with the normal lung tissue; extralobar sequestrations are separated from the remaining lung tissue by a separate lining of pleura. Of these, most are on the left and are not usually cystic, 60% have related abnormalities, such as congenital diaphragmatic hernia, and about 75% are situated between the diaphragm and lower lobe.

Lung cysts with aberrant systemic arterial supply and congenital cystic bronchiectasis are probably developmentally related.

About 15% of sequestrations are discovered by chance on chest radiography and 10–15% occur in children with other congenital malformations (tracheoesophageal fistula, diaphragmatic hernia, congenital heart disease, skeletal abnormalities). Symptoms of cough, recurrent or unresolved pneumonia and sputum production occur in about 30% before the age of 10 years. Pneumothorax and hemoptysis are rare complications.

On plain chest radiography about 50% of intralobar sequestrations have cystic changes with fluid levels in a quarter of these. Bronchography shows lack of connection to the bronchial system and displacement of the bronchi of neighboring lobes. Aortography will define the arterial supply and venous drainage. This is important if surgery is contemplated as occasionally the supply may be by more than one vessel.

The scimitar syndrome

This describes the association of a hypoplastic right lung with systemic arterial supply and anomalous venous drainage, together with abnormal lobation and bronchial branching in the lower half of the right lung. A characteristic feature is the 'mismatch' between the aberrant systemic arterial supply and the anomalous venous drainage of the whole or major portion of the right lung. There are a number of variants of the combination of anatomical abnormalities.

OTHER BRONCHIAL ABNORMALITIES

Bronchomalacia and *tracheomalacia* describe localized or generalized changes in the quality or quantity of cartilage. The clinical presentation depends on the severity. Bronchomalacia can severely compromise infants with chronic lung disease of prematurity. Congenital lobar emphysema is usually associated with localized severe bronchomalacia. Pectus excavatum associated with wheeze in an older child should arouse suspicion. Diagnosis is at cine-bronchography when the bronchus is seen patent in inspiration and collapses on expiration. Children with

Table 12.29 Causes of bronchiectasis

Congenital	Acquired
Ciliary dyskinesia	Following foreign body aspiration
Williams–Campbell syndrome	Asthma (very rarely)
Cystic fibrosis	Persistent lobar collapse
Congenital cystic bronchiectasis	Postprimary tuberculosis (upper lobes)
	Allergic aspergillosis

Table 12.30 Associations of hypoplastic lungs

	Prognosis
Congenital diaphragmatic hernia	Depends on size of hernia
Congenital eventration of the diaphragm	Good
Fetal chylothorax	Good if successfully treated
Fetal hydrothorax	Poor
Renal agenesis/dysplasia with oligohydramnios	Lethal
Prolonged leakage of amniotic fluid	Depends on length and size of leak
Thoracic dystrophy	Poor
Obstruction of tracheobronchial tree	Good if localized
Abnormal pulmonary vasculature	Good
Primary	Usually lethal if bilateral

generalized deficiency of bronchial cartilage (Williams–Campbell syndrome) have highly compliant bronchi which collapse on coughing. Inspissated secretions become infected and eventually the normal structure of the airway mucosa becomes damaged. The patients have cough and wheeze from infancy with chest deformity, poor growth and finger clubbing developing in most because of chronic chest infection and bronchiectasis.

Children with tracheomalacia can be considered for tracheal stenting (Zinman 1995) but for those with bronchomalacia continuous positive airway pressure with a tracheostomy is necessary to hold the airways open until the lung grows and the airways become structurally and functionally more rigid during adolescence.

Bronchiectasis results from congenital bronchial abnormalities or follows acquired pulmonary disease (Table 12.29, p. 576).

Distended pulmonary vessels and mediastinal masses such as teratoma, cystic hygroma, hemangioma, lymphoma, neurogenic tumor, enteric or duplication cysts can all cause tracheobronchial narrowing by compression. Pulmonary capillary hemangiomatosis is a rare disorder characterized by the proliferation of small vessels with the connective tissue of the lung. The involvement of airways probably leads to hemoptysis. The prognosis is generally very poor.

OTHER LUNG ABNORMALITIES

Absence and *hypoplasia* are frequently associated with other congenital anomalies. These include vertebral defects, congenital heart disease, tracheoesophageal fistula, genitourinary and gastrointestinal anomalies and limb malformations. Absence of the right lung has a 50% associated mortality; left lung aplasia is more benign and is discovered incidentally. There may be no symptoms for years or tachypnea and recurrent chest infection due to spillage of infected secretions from the blind bronchial stump may be the reason for presentation. Postural drainage may control pooling of secretions in the stump.

There are many causes and associations of pulmonary hypoplasia (Table 12.30). Many present in the neonatal period. The small lung associated with Macleod's syndrome is discussed on page 576.

ABNORMALITIES OF THE DIAPHRAGM (see also p. 1769)

DIAPHRAGMATIC HERNIA

Diaphragmatic hernia occurs in about 1:3600 live births. Classification is according to position – 70–90% occur through the left diaphragm, most commonly posterolaterally between the lumbar and costal muscle fibers (the foramen of Bochdalek).

Usually the diagnosis is made at birth or on the first day of life when the infant presents with respiratory distress and physical examination suggests displacement of the heart, reduced air entry and bowel sounds in the chest. Bowel is seen in the chest on a chest radiograph.

Treatment is surgical but despite advances in the ventilatory management of neonatal respiratory failure, the survival rate after early surgery remains only 50%. Recently it has been suggested that surgery may be delayed (Bohn et al 1987), since it would appear that it is the degree of pulmonary hypoplasia that determines outcome and this would not be affected by surgical repair.

An initial nonsurgical approach may allow lung growth and improvement in function and thus provide a more favorable setting to proceed with surgery. In any event, if the baby does survive the neonatal period then the lungs will grow and, although small abnormalities can be measured, the long-term outlook for function is very good.

When the hernia is small presentation may be delayed. Such herniae are often anterior and appear cystic on the chest radiograph. The neck of the hernia may be wide and the contents slip in and out of the thorax. Previous chest radiographs may be normal. The possibility of this diagnosis should be considered in any child presenting with an air fluid level on a chest radiograph, cystic lesion or where the diaphragm is ill defined. A coexisting pneumonia may further confuse the issue. A barium swallow will confirm the diagnosis.

Operation should proceed immediately diagnosis is made as there is a very real risk of strangulation.

Long-term consequences of successful neonatal surgical repair show that although lung volumes may be normal, morphologically the lungs probably remain hypoplastic (with reduced alveolization). Pulmonary perfusion to the ipsilateral lung remains reduced even in adolescence.

EVENTRATION OF THE DIAPHRAGM

Eventration of the diaphragm is believed to result from failure of all or a portion of the normal muscularization of the developing diaphragm which remains thin and translucent. There is a frequent association with other abnormalities such as pulmonary hypoplasia, thoracic cage abnormalities and congenital heart disease.

Large eventrations may be associated with a varying degree of respiratory distress and it is important when considering surgical treatment to determine how much of the distress is caused by the eventration and how much by complicating pulmonary disease. The distinction between right-sided eventration and congenital diaphragmatic hernia can be difficult. An intraperitoneal injection of suitable contrast material may help.

Segmental eventrations seldom cause significant symptoms unless bilateral or complicating other problems, such as prematurity. The radiographic appearances may be confused with segmental pneumonia, mediastinal tumors, pulmonary sequestration and lung abscess. Fluoroscopy will help to distinguish phrenic nerve palsy where there is paradoxical movement of the diaphragm. In eventration there is little or no movement.

Plication of the diaphragm should be considered if the child is symptomatic.

DIAPHRAGMATIC PALSY

Diaphragmatic palsy is rarely congenital and usually either results from birth trauma or is secondary to intrathoracic surgery when the phrenic nerve is damaged. Diagnosis is at fluoroscopy when there is paradoxical movement of the diaphragm, i.e. up instead of down on inspiration and the mediastinum swings to the contralateral side. Recovery within 1–6 months is usual.

CHRONIC LUNG DISEASE

Asthma, cystic fibrosis and chronic lung disease of prematurity account for the majority of chronic lung disease in childhood. The disorders described in this section are all, by comparison, uncommon.

OBLITERATIVE BRONCHIOLITIS

This is a rare disorder which has been described in association with infections caused by adenovirus types 3,7 and 21, measles, pertussis, influenza A, mycoplasma and chronic aspiration due to a tracheoesophageal fistula or gastroesophageal reflux, for example. Often no cause can be identified. It is now a major complication of heart–lung transplantation with a cumulative risk at 3 years of nearly 50% (Madden et al 1992).

The clinical course is one of cough, wheeze and tachypnea in an infant or young child which may progress at a variable rate to respiratory failure and failure to thrive. Chest radiography initially shows generalized hyperinflation similar to that in acute bronchiolitis with neither focal changes nor changes suggestive of fibrosing alveolitis. High-resolution computed tomography (HRCT) scans more clearly demonstrate abnormalities but these bear no relationship to pulmonary function (Padley et al 1993). Lobar collapse may complicate up to one-third of children with adenoviral infection and focal hyperlucency involving a lobe or a whole lung represents the radiological appearance of Macleod's syndrome, in which the affected lung appears small and hyperlucent. This represents the long-term damage to lung development, both parenchymal and vascular, although it is difficult to understand why one lung should be so severely damaged following a generalized viral illness. This radiographic appearance should not be confused with other causes of hyperlucency such as hypoplastic pulmonary artery, congenital lobar emphysema or obstructive emphysema following foreign body aspiration. Radioisotope lung function studies examining both ventilation and perfusion of the lungs help to clarify equivocal radiographic features. In Macleod's syndrome the affected lung is both poorly perfused and ventilated and the images demonstrate that the lung is small.

Lung function studies indicate severe airway obstruction, increased lung volume but normal or near normal compliance, suggesting predominantly airway diseases. Underlying diseases such as cystic fibrosis, immunodeficiency, ciliary dyskinesia and chronic aspiration need to be ruled out. The main differential diagnosis is fibrosing alveolitis. In this the radiological appearances and lung function studies are suggestive of alveolar disease rather than airway disease and the lung volume is small.

Management is supportive. Steroids have no proven value. Individuals may find bronchodilators helpful.

The prognosis is most serious after adenoviral disease. Up to 50% go on to chronic respiratory failure and heart–lung transplantation is the ultimate option. The prognosis for the remainder seems to be more favorable but improvement may take many months.

BRONCHIECTASIS

Postinfective bronchiectasis, particularly that associated with tuberculosis, is nowadays rare in children. More often bronchiectasis is associated with congenital abnormalities of the lung (such as bronchomalacia or sequestration), aspiration of a foreign body which has gone unrecognized or chronic chest infection related to cystic fibrosis, ciliary dyskinesia or primary immune deficiency (Nikolaizik & Warner 1994). The rare Williams–Campbell syndrome (Jones et al 1993) is characterized by congenital defects in bronchial cartilage.

The symptoms are chronic cough, wheeze, poor weight gain, purulent sputum production, bad breath and recurrent chest infection. Finger clubbing indicates chronic suppuration. Radioisotope studies will determine the functional extent of the diseases. Bronchiectasis is unlikely in the presence of a normal chest radiograph. HRCT provides good anatomical information and has replaced bronchography in the initial assessment. Bronchoscopy should be undertaken if focal disease is found since occasionally an unsuspected foreign body can be removed. Conventional pulmonary function studies are unhelpful diagnostically but provide a baseline for follow-up. They demonstrate both a restrictive and obstructive defect.

Medical treatment is aimed at reducing further damage to the lung and allowing normal growth. Home physiotherapy and bronchodilator therapy may be beneficial. Sputum should be cultured regularly and antibiotics prescribed when necessary, i.e. when there is an increase in sputum volume or sputum is purulent. Children without underlying disorders and bronchiectasis which is neither generalized nor advanced will often respond to intermittent courses of oral antibiotics. Those with more severe disease may benefit from regular courses of intravenous antibiotics. *Aspergillus* is sometimes discovered in sputum cultures. Localized bronchiectatic segments can be resected with benefit (Cohen et al 1994).

SPONTANEOUS AIR LEAKS

Air leaks such as pneumothoraces, subcutaneous emphysema and pericardial and mediastinal air are very unusual outside the neonatal period. They may accompany trauma to the thorax, surgery or other medical procedures such as lung biopsy. Children who have chest infections, including tuberculosis, or who have underlying chest disease such as cystic fibrosis or asthma or have long bouts of coughing are at risk. Those receiving ventilatory support are especially at risk. A spontaneous pneumothorax in a previously healthy child is extremely rare and there is a recurrence risk of about 20%. Apical bullae or an isolated lung cyst are sometimes identified on a chest radiograph or CT scan. Presenting features include sudden chest pain and breathlessness. There are reduced breath sounds over the affected side. In the management of a first episode the options are observation alone, simple aspiration or tube drainage with pleurodesis (Lancet 1989b). Much will depend on the size of the pneumothorax and on risk factors such as distance from hospital or future air travel, as well as any underlying disease. The presence of established lung disease with lung overinflation would suggest a more active approach, since the consequences of a recurrent pneumothorax may be more serious in such patients. Conversely, a pneumothorax in association with cystic fibrosis, or in any child with advanced lung disease, should be treated less aggressively, since a pleurodesis increases the difficulty and risks of any future lung transplantation. In spontaneously breathing children with acute asthma, an air leak may be identified on a chest radiograph quite unexpectedly; the majority resolve without intervention. The positioning and management of drains in these circumstances is described on page 1844.

ALPHA-1-ANTITRYPSIN DEFICIENCY

This is an autosomal recessive disorder which usually presents in adult life with emphysema. In childhood, however, it presents as a neonatal hepatitis. Pulmonary disease is usually not evident until late in adolescence. Pulmonary function testing may show a loss of elastic recoil and small airways disease long before this. Children who are known to have this disorder should be advised never to smoke. Prognosis for pulmonary function is poor in smokers. Prenatal diagnosis is now possible (Abbot et al 1988). Gene therapy directly to the respiratory tract has shown transient benefit.

CILIARY ABNORMALITIES

Ciliary dyskinesia may be primary or secondary. In the primary syndromes abnormalities are functional with or without associated structural abnormalities. Respiratory infection is responsible for temporary dyskinesia.

The diagnosis should be considered in any child with chronic chest infection and in any neonate with unexplained respiratory disease. In the majority symptoms, such as nasal discharge and breathlessness due to delayed clearance of lung fluid, start in the neonatal period. Kartagener's syndrome – situs inversus, bronchiectasis and sinusitis – is associated with primary ciliary dyskinesia. Inheritance is believed to be autosomal recessive, affecting 1 in 15 000 people.

Investigations of ciliary function are undertaken by obtaining epithelium from the inferior turbinate of the nose using a cytology brush. When ciliary beat frequency is abnormal in the absence of purulent material further brushings are collected for ultrastructural examination (Buchdahl et al 1988).

Treatment is supportive and, as with all children with suppurative chest disease, is aimed at keeping sputum production at a minimum. Daily physiotherapy may delay the progression of chronic lung disease. Early aggressive treatment of sputum infection is important. In Kartagener's syndrome there is associated male infertility but the extent of this problem is not yet clear in patients with ciliary dyskinesia without situs inversus. As with cystic fibrosis there may be a spectrum of severity resulting in a variable outcome.

FIBROSING ALVEOLITIS

The predominant abnormal histological feature of fibrosing alveolitis is in the alveolar walls which are thickened and infiltrated with large mononuclear cells. There is a tendency to fibrosis within the alveolar spaces.

There are many causes and open lung biopsy may be required to establish a diagnosis (Sharief et al 1994).

INFECTIONS

Death from respiratory failure in young adults has been associated with the development of severe pulmonary fibrosis following an acute infection often accompanied by pleural effusion. In immunocompromised patients, viral agents such as cytomegalovirus, adenovirus and the herpes viruses, fungi, L. pneumophila and P. carinii have been documented by histological examination of lung biopsy tissue as causes of fibrosing alveolitis. They account for about 20% of such lung disease in these patients. Not only has P. carinii pneumonia been prevented and successfully treated by trimethoprim-sulfamethoxazole but this drug appears, at least in acute lymphoblastic leukemia, to have been reduced the incidence of nonspecific fibrosing alveolitis.

DRUGS AND POISONS

Where a causative agent cannot be identified in fibrosing alveolitis in the immunocompromised patient, presumptive etiologies have included unidentified viral infection in the face of chemotherapy and radiotherapy-induced immunosuppression, hypersensitivity pneumonitis and drug-induced idiosyncratic reactions. Bleomycin, cyclophosphamide, methotrexate and busulfan have all been incriminated. Paraquat poisoning has a mortality rate of 30–50%. The severity depends on the amount taken but even very small amounts can be fatal. Death is usually due to respiratory failure secondary to pulmonary fibrosis, whose onset is within the first 48 hours following ingestion. The role of steroids and immunosuppressive drugs is unclear.

DUSTS

Fibrosing alveolitis due to hypersensitivity to pigeon or budgerigar excreta or moldy hay has been reported rarely in children. In the case of bird-fancier's lung, a definite diagnosis rests on the production of symptoms 5–6 hours following inhalation testing with antigen. Positive serological testing for farmer's lung together with the knowledge of the clinical course and abnormal chest radiography confirm the diagnosis. Treatment in the acute stage is with steroids but once chronic lung disease has developed treatment has little or no effect.

IN ASSOCIATION WITH GENERALIZED DISEASES

Fibrosing alveolitis is a well-described feature of the *collagen diseases* in adults. It is, however, rare in children, although some with rheumatoid arthritis have evidence of small airway disease on pulmonary function testing. The association of pulmonary involvement with the 'rheumatic diseases' of childhood has been described in many instances in isolated case reports.

Sarcoid is more clearly associated with lung disease in children. As in adults, abnormal findings may be discovered at routine chest radiography in asymptomatic patients. Bilateral hilar adenopathy is usual and parenchymal disease is present in about 50%. Diagnosis is on lymph node biopsy and suggested by a high serum level of angiotensin-converting enzyme. Steroids are effective initially but their effect on the long-term prognosis in patients with sarcoid is unknown.

All forms of *histiocytosis* can affect the lungs. The lungs are affected in about 50% of children who have multisystem disease. Disease limited to the lung is very rare. Characteristically, the alveolar walls are infiltrated with granulomatous material and diffuse nodular mottling and hilar adenopathy are seen on the chest radiograph. If the disease progresses small cysts or bullae appear and eventually there is fibrosis and honeycombing. The other features of the histiocytosis syndromes (p. 925) should indicate the diagnosis but where disease is limited to the lung then lung biopsy will be necessary. This shows characteristic histiocyte cells on microscopic examination. No clear recommendations can be made for the treatment of isolated pulmonary histiocytosis although a therapeutic trial of steroids with or without chemotherapy seems reasonable. The long-term outcome is uncertain.

IDIOPATHIC FIBROSING ALVEOLITIS

Within this group where no etiological agent can be demonstrated there are wide variations in the degree of fibrosis and prominence and types of cells in the alveolar wall thickening and content of alveolar spaces. In the USA this group is divided into 'desquamative interstitial pneumonitis' and 'usual interstitial pneumonitis' because in the former the alveoli are filled with cells which were previously believed to be pneumocytes. These are now known to be macrophages and hence the adjective 'desquamative' is misleading. The diagnosis is made at lung biopsy and because the etiology is unknown and an immunological mechanism has been suggested, immuno-fluorescent staining and electron-microscopic examination as well as routine staining should be carried out on lung biopsy material. Tissue should be cultured for viruses, *Chlamydia* and fungi and stained for *L. pneumophila* and *P. carinii*. The presence of immune complexes should be sought.

About 50% of children with fibrosing alveolitis are aged less than 1 year. The chest radiograph shows a ground glass appearance in the early stages progressing to more distinct mottling and hilar streaking in the recovery stages. Occasionally the radiological features may progress to honeycomb lung. The clinical severity, histological features and response to therapy correlate poorly with the radiological features. The response to steroids in children (2 mg/kg/day for 4–8 weeks) is usually good initially. Chloroquine has also had apparent benefit (Avital et al 1994). The earlier the onset, the worse the prognosis. Before the availability of lung transplant, the mortality rate was 50% at 5 years.

ALVEOLAR PROTEINOSIS

This is a disorder of unknown etiology presenting usually in young adults but occasionally in children. There appears to be a separate, more severe, infantile form. In children it may be related to a form of immune deficiency such as thymic atrophy which has been discovered at autopsy, lymphopenia and immunoglobulin deficiency. The alveoli are stuffed with proteinaceous material which may be derived from pneumocytes and which is rich in surfactant lipids.

Clinically the course may be similar to that of fibrosing alveolitis with dyspnea, cough, fever and poor weight gain. The age of onset is usually less than 1 year and the disorder is almost always fatal.

The radiological appearance is similar to pulmonary edema which persists in spite of treatment with diuretics. Material obtained at bronchoalveolar lavage stains characteristically with PAS. Most cases, however, have been diagnosed at autopsy or lung biopsy.

Treatment with corticosteroids does not influence the outcome. In adults treatment under general anesthesia with bronchoalveolar lavage with heparin or acetyl cystinine has been successful. Although there is no published information about these methods in children it would seem appropriate to try such treatments with careful documentation of lung function before and after.

PULMONARY HEMOSIDEROSIS

This rare disorder where there is recurrent alveolar hemorrhage and anemia is of unknown etiology in most cases. Milk protein intolerance has been reported with response to an elimination diet. There is deposition of hemosiderin in the lung tissue. Tachypnea, cough, wheeze, hemoptysis and failure to thrive are the usual presenting features. Jaundice may occur secondarily to the breakdown of hemoglobin and occult blood found in the stools. Hepatosplenomegaly may be present in about 20% of children and finger clubbing can develop.

The diagnosis rests on the recovery of hemosiderin-laden macrophages from bronchial aspirates. Lung biopsy should not be undertaken because of the risk of bleeding. Chest radiography shows blotchy shadows in the perihilar areas which extend rapidly during a bleed.

There is a mean survival of 3 years. Death may occur early due to massive pulmonary hemorrhage but many patients survive into adult life. Fibrosing alveolitis and myocarditis can complicate the course in about 10%.

Steroids, azathioprine and splenectomy have been used. Their effect is uncertain.

MICROLITHIASIS

This disorder is usually asymptomatic and its etiology unknown. Calcium carbonate stones are formed within the alveoli and their presence only suspected incidentally at chest radiography. Pulmonary fibrosis may develop many years later when the patient becomes symptomatic.

ADULT RESPIRATORY DISRESS SYNDROME

Despite the title, this syndrome occurs in children in a similar form to adults and has been noted in neonates (Sarnaik & Lieh-Lai

1994). The syndrome results from injury to and increased permeability of the alveolar-capillary membrane that results in pulmonary edema. At post-mortem the pathology resembles that of neonatal hyaline membrane disease.

A wide range of insults is associated with the syndrome: pulmonary infection, toxic inhalation, aspiration, emboli, radiation, trauma, drug overdose, metabolic disorders, increased intracranial pressure and postcardiopulmonary bypass. The production of free radicals may be a common pathogenic pathway. Following the acute insult is a latent period of up to 48 hours followed in turn by acute respiratory failure.

Accumulation of edema in the alveoli and the interstitial space results in reduced lung compliance; ventilation/perfusion mismatching, especially of units with poor or no ventilation, results in hypoxemia due to intrapulmonary shunting. Thus the management of the respiratory failure is conceptually very similar to the management of severe hyaline membrane disease. The primary goal is to maintain adequate tissue oxygenation. Other organs may, of course, be damaged by the original insult or underlying disease or severe hypoxemia. Massive doses of surfactant and more recently nitric oxide have been used in management.

REFERENCES

Abbot C M, McMahon C J, Whitehouse D B, Povey S 1988 Prenatal diagnosis of alpha antitrypsin deficiency using polymerase chain reactions. Lancet 1: 763

Accurso F J 1991 Early respiratory course in infants with cystic fibrosis. Pediatric Pulmonology (supplement) 7: 42–45

Agah R, Cherry J D, Garakian A J, Chapin M 1987 Respiratory syncytial virus (RSV) infection rate in personnel caring for children with RSV infection. American Journal of Diseases of Childhood 141: 695–697

Agertoft L, Pedersen S 1994 Effects of long-term treatment with inhaled corticosteroid on growth and pulmonary function in asthmatic children. Respiratory Medicine 88: 373–381

Alario A J, McCarthy P L, Markowitz R, Kornguth P, Rosenfield N, Leventhal J M 1987 Usefulness of chest radiographs in children with acute lower respiratory tract disease. Journal of Pediatrics 111: 187–193

Alpert B E, O'Sullivan B P, Panitch H B 1992 Non-bronchoscopic approach to bronchoalveolar lavage in children with artificial airways. Pediatric Pulmonology 13: 38–41

Alton E, Geddes D M 1995 Gene therapy for respiratory diseases: potential applications and difficulties. Thorax 50: 484–486

Anderson H R, Butland B K, Strachan D P 1994 Trends in prevalence and severity of childhood asthma. British Medical Journal 308: 1600–1604

Archer L N J, Simpson H 1985 Night cough counts and diary card scores in asthma. Archives of Disease in Childhood 60: 473–474

Auerbach H S, Williams M, Kilpatrick J A, Colton H P 1985 Alternate day prednisone reduces morbidity and improves pulmonary function in cystic fibrosis. Lancet 2: 686–688

Austin J B, Russell G, Adam M G, Mackintosh D, Kelsey S, Peck D F 1994 Prevalence of asthma and wheeze in the Highlands of Scotland. Archives of Disease in Childhood 71: 211–216

Avital A, Godfrey S, Maayan C, Diamand Y, Springer C 1994 Chloroquine treatment of interstitial lung disease. Pediatric Pulmonology 18: 356–360

Azaz Y, Fleming PJ, Levine M, McCabe R, Stewart A, Johnson P 1992 The relationship between environmental temperature, metabolic rate, sleep state and evaporative water loss in infants from birth to three months. Pediatric Research 32: 417–423

Barker D J P 1988 Childhood causes of adult diseases. Archives of Disease in Childhood 63: 867–869

Barker D J P, Osmond C 1986 Childhood respiratory infection and adult chronic bronchitis in England and Wales. British Medical Journal 293: 1271–1275

Barker D J P, Godfrey K M, Fall C, Osmond C, Winter P D, Shaheen S O 1991 Relation of birth weight and childhood respiratory infection to adult lung function and death from chronic obstructive airways disease. British Medical Journal 303: 671–675

Barnes P J 1989 Muscarinic receptor subtypes: implications for lung disease. Thorax 44: 161–167

Barnes P J, Levy J 1984 Nocturnal asthma. Royal Society of Medicine International Congress and Symposium Series 73. RSM, London

Baughmann R P, Dohn M N 1995 Respiratory tract infections in the immunocompromised (non-HIV) patient. Current Opinion in Infectious Diseases 8: 110–115

Benatar S R 1995 Prospects for global health: lessons from tuberculosis. Thorax 50: 487–489

Bender B, Milgrom H 1995 Neuropsychiatric effects of medications for allergic diseases. Journal of Allergy and Clinical Immunology 95: 523–528

Berger R, Arango L 1985 The value and safety of percutaneous lung aspiration for children with serious lung infections. Pediatric Pulmonology 1: 309–313

Berman S, Simoes E A F, Laneta C 1991 Respiratory rate and pneumonia in infancy. Archives of Disease in Childhood 66: 81

Bohn D, Tamura M, Perrin D, Barker G, Rabinovitch M 1987 Ventilatory predictors of pulmonary hypoplasia in congenital diaphragmatic hernia, confirmed by morphologic assessment. Journal of Pediatrics 111: 423–431

British National Formulary 1994 Expectorant, demulcent, and compound cough preparations. British Medical Association and Royal Pharmaceutical Society of Great Britain, London

Britton S, Bejstedt M, Vedin L 1985 Chest physiotherapy in primary pneumonia. British Medical Journal 290: 1703–1704

Broughton R A 1986 Infections due to *Mycoplasma pneumoniae* in childhood. Pediatric Infectious Disease 5: 71–85

Brunekreff B, Dockery D W, Speizer F E 1989 Home dampness and respiratory morbidity in children. American Review of Respiratory Disease 140: 1363–1367

BTS 1997 British guidelines on asthma management. 1995 Review and position statement. Thorax 52 (suppl 1): 21

Buchdahl R M, Reiser J, Ingram N, Rutman A, Cole P J, Warner J O 1988 Ciliary abnormalities in respiratory disease. Archives of Disease in Childhood 63: 238–243

Burr M 1995 Pollution: does it cause asthma? Archives of Disease in Childhood 72: 377–378

Burr M, Butland B K, King S, Vaughan-Williams E 1989 Changes in asthma prevalence: two surveys 15 years apart. Archives of Disease in Childhood 64: 1445–1456

Campbell H 1993 Acute respiratory infections are main killer of under 5s. British Medical Journal 304: 335

Campbell H, Byass P, Forgie I M, O'Neill K P, Lloyd-Evans N, Greenwood B M 1988 Co-trimoxazole versus procains penicillin in the treatment of community-acquired pneumonia in young Gambian children. Lancet 1: 1182–1184

Campbell H, Byass P, Lamont A C et al 1989 Assessment of clinical criteria for identification of severe acute lower respiratory tract infection in children. Lancet 1: 297–299

Cave A P D, Adam A E 1984 Cystic adenomatoid malformation of the lung (Stocker type III) found on antenatal ultrasound examination. British Journal of Radiology 57: 176–178

Chan K N, Noble-Jamieson C M, Elliman A, Bryan E M, Silverman M 1989 Lung function in children of low birth weight. Archives of Disease in Childhood 64: 1284–1293

Chandwani S, Borkovsky W, Krasinski K, Lawrence R, Welliver R 1990 RSV and HIV infection. Journal of Pediatrics 117: 251–254

Cherian T, John T J, Simoes E, Steinhoff M C, John M 1988 Evaluation of simple clinical signs for the diagnosis of acute lower respiratory tract infections. Lancet 2: 125–128

Chidiac P, Alexander I S 1990 Head retraction and respiratory disorders in infancy. Archives of Disease in Childhood 65: 567–568

Clements B S, Warner J O 1987 Pulmonary sequestration and related congenital bronchopulmonary vascular malformations: a nomenclature and classification based on anatomical and embryological considerations. Thorax 42: 401–408

Cohen A J, Raifman C, Brendan J et al 1994 Localised pulmonary resection for bronchiectasis in hypogammaglobulinemic patients. Thorax 49: 509–510

Colley J R T, Douglas J W B, Reid D D 1973 Respiratory disease in young adults: influence of early childhood lower respiratory tract illness, social class, air pollution, and smoking. British Medical Journal 3: 195–198

Consensus Development Conference 1987 Infantile apnea and home monitoring. NIH Publication 87: 2905. US Department of Health and Human Services, National Institutes of Health, Bethesda, MD 20892

Cotton R T, Richardson M A 1981 Congenital laryngeal abnormalities. Otolaryngology Clinics of North America 14: 203–218

Couriel J M 1988 Management of croup. Archives of Disease in Childhood 63: 1305–1308

Couriel J M 1994 Passive smoking and the health of children. Thorax 49: 731–734

Couriel J M 1995 Glue ear: prescribe, operate or wait? Lancet 345: 3–4

Cystic Fibrosis Genetic Analysis Consortium 1990 Worldwide survey of ΔF508 mutation. American Journal of Human Genetics 47: 354–359

Dales R E 1991 Respiratory health effects of home dampness and molds among Canadian children. American Journal of Epidemiology 134: 196–203

Dawson K P, Long A, Kennedy J, Mogridge N 1990 The chest radiograph in acute bronchiolitis. Journal of Pediatrics and Child Health 26: 209–211

Deanfield J E, Crispin A R 1981 The investigation of chest disease in children by high kilovoltage filtered beam radiography. British Journal of Radiology 54: 856–860

De Blic J, Delacourt C, Scheinmann P 1991 Ultrathin flexible bronchoscopy in neonatal intensive care units. Archives of Disease in Childhood 66: 1383–1385

De Blic J, McKelvie P, Le Bourgeois M, Blanche S, Benoist M R, Scheinmann P 1987 Value of broncho-alveolar lavage in the management of severe acute pneumonia and interstitial pneumonitis in the immune compromised child. Thorax 42: 759–765

De Cock K M, Soro B, Coulibaly I M, Lucas S B 1992 Tuberculosis and HIV infection in sub-Saharan Africa. Journal of the American Medical Association 268: 1581–1587

Dockery D W, Speizer F E, Stram D O, Ware J H, Spengler J D, Ferris B G 1989 Effects of inhalable particles on respiratory health of children. American Review of Respiratory Disease 139: 587–594

Douglas N J, Thomas S, Jan M A 1992 Clinical value of polysomnography. Lancet 339: 347–350

Douglas R M 1991 Acute respiratory infections in children in the developing world. Seminars in Respiratory Infections 6: 217–224

Doull I 1995 Corticosteroids for the management of croup. British Medical Journal 311: 1244

Doull I, Johnston S 1993 Bacterial identification of adult lower respiratory tract infection. Lancet 341: 1160–1161

Dowse G, Turner K J, Stewart G A, Alpers M P, Woolcock A J 1985 The association beween Dermatophagoides mites and the increasing prevalence of asthma in the Papua New Guinea highlands. Journal of Allergy and Clinical Immunology 75: 75–83

Dworkin G, Kattan M 1989 Mechanical ventilation for status asthmaticus in children. Journal of Pediatrics 114: 545–549

Evans P 1982 Acute otitis media – then and now. Archives of Disease in Childhood 57: 326–327

Fleming P J, Levine M R, Long A M, Cleave J P 1988 Postneonatal development of respiratory oscillations. Annals of the New York Academy of Sciences 533: 305–313

Fleming P J, Levine M R, Azaz Y, Wigfield R 1993 The development of thermoregulation and interactions with the control of respiration in infants: possible relationship to Sudden Infant Death. Acta Paediatrica Scandinavica (supplement) 389: 57–59

Fleming P J, Blair P, Bacon C et al 1996 The environment of infants during sleep and the risk of the sudden infant death syndrome: results of the 1993–5 case-control study for the confidential enquiry into stillbirths and deaths in infancy. British Medical Journal 313: 191–195

Forgacs P 1978 Lung sounds. Baillière Tindall, London

Foundation for the Study of Infant Deaths and British Paediatric Respiratory Group 1990 Monitoring and sudden infant death syndrome: an update. Archives of Disease in Childhood 65: 238–240

Gaultier C 1995 Sleep related breathing disorders. 6 Obstructive sleep apnea syndrome in infants and children: established facts and unsettled issues. Thorax 50: 1204–1210

Gibb D M, Davidson C, Holland F, Novelli V, Walters S, Mok J 1994 Pneumocystis carinii pneumonia in children with vertically-acquired HIV infection in the British Isles. Archives of Disease in Childhood 70: 241–244

Gibson N A, Hollman A S, Paton J Y 1993 Value of radiological follow-up of childhood pneumonia. British Medical Journal 307: 1117

Gillis J, Gratton–Smith T, Kilham H 1988 Artificial ventilation in severe pertussis Archives of Disease in Childhood 63: 364–367

Godden D J, Ross S, Abdalla M et al 1994 Outcome of wheeze in childhood. American Journal of Respiratory and Critical Care Medicine 149: 106–112

Gold D R, Weiss S T, Tager I B, Segal M R, Speizer F E 1989 Comparison of questionnaire and diary methods in acute childhood respiratory illness surveillance. American Review of Respiratory Disease 139: 847–849

Guilleminault C, Pelayo R, Leger D, Bocian R C 1995 Home nasal continuous positive airway pressure in infants with sleep-disorder breathing. Journal of Pediatrics 127: 905–912

Hall C B, Powell K R, Schnabel K C, Gala C L, Pincus P H 1988 Risk of secondary bacterial infection in infants hospitalised with respiratory syncytial virus. Journal of Pediatrics 113: 266–271

Harari M, Shann F, Spooner V, Meisner S, Carney M, de Campo J 1991 Clinical signs of pneumonia in children. Lancet 338: 928–930

Hargreave F E, Dolovich J, Newhouse M T 1990 The assessment and treatment of asthma: a conference report. Journal of Allergy and Clinical Immunology 85: 1098–1112

Hershenson M B 1992 The respiratory muscles and chest wall. In: Beckerman R C, Brouillette R T, Hunt C E (eds) Respiratory control disorders in infants and children. Williams and Wilkins, Baltimore, pp 28–45

Hewertson J, Poets C F, Samuels M P et al 1994 Epileptic seizure-induced hypoxaemia in infants with apparent life threatening events. Pediatrics 94: 148–156

Hill J M, Tattersfield A E 1995 Corticosteroid sparing agents in asthma. Thorax 50: 577–582

Holt P G 1994 A potential vaccine strategy for asthma and allied atopic diseases during early childhood. Lancet 344: 456–458

Hubbard M, McKenzie S A 1996 Empyema in children. Current Paediatrics 6: 30–33

Ikeogu M O 1988 Acute pneumonia in Zimbabwe: bacterial isolates by lung aspiration. Archives of Disease in Childhood 63: 1266–1267

International Liaison Committee on Resuscitation 1997 Paediatric working group advisory statement. Resuscitation 34: (in press)

Jeffrey H E, Pag M, Post E J, Wood A K W 1995 Physiological studies of gastro-oesophageal reflux and airway protective responses in the young animal and human infant. Clinical and Experimental Pharmacology and Physiology 22: 544–549

Jeffrey P K, Hislop A A 1995 Embryology and growth. In: Brewis R A C, Corrin B, Geddes D M, Gibson G J (eds) Respiratory medicine. W B Saunders, London

Johnston R B 1991 Pathogenesis of pneumococcal infections. Review of Infectious Disease 13 (supplement 6): S509–517

Johnston S L, Bardin P G, Pattemore P K 1993 Viruses as precipitants of asthma symptoms. III Rhinoviruses: molecular biology and prospects for future intervention. Clinical and Experimental Allergy 230:237–246

Jones V F, Eid N S, Franco S M, Badgett J T, Budino J J 1993 Familial congenital bronchiectasis: Williams–Campbell syndrome. Pediatric Pulmonology 16: 263–267

Kahn A, Groswasser J, Kelmanson I 1995 Risk factors for SIDS: risk factors for ALTE? From epidemiology to physiology. In: Rognum T O (ed) Sudden infant death syndrome. New trends in the nineties. Scandinavian University Press, Oslo, pp 132–137

Kahn A, Rbuffat E, Franco P et al 1992 Apparent life-threatening events and apnea of infancy. In: Beckerman R C, Brouillette R T, Hunt C E (eds) Respiratory control disorders in infants and children. Williams and Wilkins, Baltimore, pp 178–189

Keens T G, Ward S L 1993 Apnea spells, sudden deaths and the role of the apnea monitor. Pediatric Clinics of North America 40: 897–911

Khan T Z, Wagener J S, Bost T, Martinez J, Accurso F J, Riches D W H 1995 Early pulmonary inflammation in infants with cystic fibrosis. American Journal of Respiratory and Critical Care Medicine 151: 1075–1082

Kilham H, Gillis J, Benjamin B 1987 Severe upper airway obstruction. Pediatric Clinics of North America 34: 1–14

Kim-Farley R G 1992 Expanded programme on immunisation for the 1990s. Vaccine 10: 940–948

Klugman K P, Saunders J 1993 Pneumococci resistant to extended-spectrum cephalosporins in South Africa. Lancet 341: 1164

Kovatch A L, Wald E R, Ledesma-Medina J et al 1984 Maxillary sinus radiographs in children with non-respiratory complaints. Pediatrics 73: 306–309

Lancet 1988a Editorial: splints and common colds. Lancet 1: 277–278

Lancet 1988b Editorial: pneumonia in childhood. Lancet 1: 741–743

Lancet 1989a Editorial: airway obstruction during sleep in children. Lancet (supplement) ii: 1018–1019

Lancet 1989b Spontaneous pneumothorax. Lancet 2: 843–844

Lancet 1992 Editorial: indoor air pollution and respiratory infections in children. Lancet 339: 396

Lancet 1994 Editorial: a warm chain for breastfeeding. Lancet 344: 1239–1240

Le Souef P 1995 Developmental processes in asthma: genetics. In: Silverman M (ed) Childhood asthma and other wheezing disorders. Chapman and Hall, London

Lehmann D 1992 Epidemiology of acute respiratory tract infections, especially those due to Haemophilus influenzae in Papua New Guinea children. Journal of Infectious Diseases 165 (supplement 1): S20–25

Lloyd E L 1988 Transmission of the common cold. Lancet 1: 597

Lob-Levyt J 1993 Prevention of pneumonia in children. Lancet 341: 821–822

MacConnochie K M, Hall C B, Walsh E E et al 1990 Variation of severity of RSV infection with subtype. Journal of Pediatrics 117: 52–62

MacFarlane J T, Colville A, Guion A, Macfarlane R M, Rose D H 1993 Prospective study of the aetiology and outcome of lower respiratory tract infections in the community. Lancet 341: 511–514

Madden B P, Hodson M E, Tsang V et al 1992 Intermediate term results of heart–lung transplantation for cystic fibrosis. Lancet 339: 1583–1587

Markovitch H 1990 Sore throats. Archives of Disease in Childhood 65: 249–250

Markowitz L E, Nieburg P 1991 The burden of acute respiratory infection due to measles in developing countries and the potential impact of measles vaccine. Review of Infectious Disease 13: S555–561

Marrie T J 1993 Chlamydia pneumoniae. Thorax 48: 1

Martin A J, McLennan L A, Landau L I, Phelan P D 1986 The natural history of childhood asthma to adult life. British Medical Journal 280: 1397

Martinez F D 1994 Role of viral infections in the inception of asthma during childhood: could they be protective? Thorax 49: 1189–1191

Martinez F D, Wright A L, Taussig L M et al 1995 Asthma and wheezing in the first six years of life. New England Journal of Medicine 332: 133–138

McDonald N E, Hal C B, Suffin S C, Alexson C, Harris P J, Manning J A 1982 Respiratory syncytial virus infection in infants with congenital heart disease. New England Journal of Medicine 307: 397–400

Milner A D 1988 Ribavirin and acute bronchiolitis in infancy. British Medical Journal 297: 998–999

Morley C J 1990 Respiratory rate and severity of illness in babies under six months old. Archives of Disease in Childhood 65: 234–237

Moxon E R, Wilson R 1991 The role of Haemophilus influenzae in the pathogenesis of pneumonia. Review of Infectious Diseases 13: S518–527

Mulholland E K, Olinsky A, Shann F 1990 Clinical findings and severity of acute bronchiolitis. Lancet 335: 1259–1261

Nadkarni V, Hazinski M F, Zideman D, Kattwinkel J, Quan L, Bingham R, Zaritsky A, Bland J, Kramer E, Tiballs J 1997 Paediatric Life Support: an advisory statement by the paediatric life support working group of the international liasion committee on resuscitation. Resuscitation 34: 115–127

Nagel R W, Westerby D, Javaid A et al 1989 Liver disease and bile duct abnormalities in adults with cystic fibrosis. Lancet 2: 1422–1425

Nikolaizik W H, Warner J O 1994 Aetiology of chronic suppurative lung disease. Archives of Disease in Childhood 70: 141–142

O'Byrne P M, Dolovich J, Hargreave F E 1987 Late asthmatic responses. American Review of Respiratory Disease 136: 740–751

O'Callaghan C L P, Barry P W 1997 Inhalational devices for young children. Pediatric and Perinatal Drug Therapy 1: 59–62

O'Callaghan C, Milner A D, Webb M S C, Searbrick A 1991 Nebulised water as a bronchoconstricting challenge in infancy. Archives of Disease in Childhood 66: 948–951

Openshaw P J, O'Donnell D R 1994 Asthma and the common cold: can viruses imitate worms? Thorax 49: 101–103

Oren J, Kelly D H, Shannon D C 1986 Identification of a high-risk group for sudden infant death syndrome among infants who were resuscitated for sleep apnea. Pediatrics 77: 495–499

Oren J, Kelly D H, Shannon D C 1989 Pneumogram recordings in infants resuscitated for apnea of infancy. Pediatrics 83: 364–368

Owen C A 1992 Recent advances in somatic gene therapy for hereditary respiratory diseases. Thorax 47: 315–316

Padley S P, Adler B D, Hansell D M, Muller N L 1993 Bronchiolitis obliterans: high resolution CT findings and correlation with pulmonary function tests. Clinical Radiology 47: 236–240

Paediatric Life Support Working Party of the European Resuscitation Council 1994 Guidelines for paediatric life support. British Medical Journal 308: 1349–1355

Pallares R, Gudiol F, Linares J, Ariza J, Rufi G, Murgui L 1987 Risk factors and response to antibiotic therapy in adults with bacteremic pneumonia caused by penicillin-resistant pneumococci. New England Journal of Medicine 3170: 18–22

Pandey M R, Boleij J S M, Smith K R, Wafula E M 1989 Indoor air pollution in developing countries and acute respiratory infection in children. Lancet 1: 427–429

Paradise J L 1987 On classifying otitis media as suppurative or nonsuppurative, with a suggested clinical schema. Journal of Pediatrics 111: 948–951

Pattemore P K, Johnston S L, Bardin P G 1992 Viruses as precipitants of asthma symptoms. I Epidemiology. Clinical and Experimental Allergy 22: 325–336

Pearson M G, Spence D P S, Ryland I, Harrison B D W 1993 Value of pulsus paradoxicus in assessing acute severe asthma. British Medical Journal 307: 659

Peat J K, Salome C M, Woolcock A J 1990 Longitudinal changes in atopy during a 4-year period: relation to bronchial responsiveness and respiratory symptoms in a population of Australian schoolchildren. Journal of Allergy and Clinical Immunology 85: 548–557

Peltola H 1993 Haemophilus influenzae in the post-vaccination era. Lancet 341: 864–865

Penn R B, Woolfson M R, Shaffer T H 1989 Developmental differences in tracheal cartilage dynamics. Pediatric Research 26: 429–433

Phelan P D 1995 Neonatal screening for cystic fibrosis. Thorax. 50: 705–706

Pizzo P A 1993 Management of fever in patients with cancer and treatment induced neutropenia. New England Journal of Medicine 328: 1323–1332

Pizzo P A, Rubin M, Freifeld A, Walsh T J 1991a I Empiric therapy for fever and neutropenia, and preventive strategies. Journal of Pediatrics 119: 679–694

Pizzo P A, Rubin M, Freifeld A, Walsh T J 1991b The child with cancer and infection. II Non-bacterial infections. Journal of Pediatrics 19: 845–857

Platt S D, Martin C J, Hunt S M, Lewis C W 1989 Damp housing, mould and symptomatic health state. British Medical Journal 298: 1673–1678

Polney L 1995 Health needs of school age children. British Paediatric Association, London

Preece P E, Anderson J M, Thompson R G 1989 Chlamydia trachomatis infection in infants: a prospective study. Archives of Disease in Childhood 64: 525–529

Puffer R R, Serrano C V 1973 Patterns of mortality in childhood. Pan-American Health Organistion Scientific Publications 262, Washington

Pullen C R, Hey E N 1982 Wheezing, asthma and pulmonary dysfunction 10 years after infection with respiratory syncytial virus in infancy. British Medical Journal 284: 1665–1669

Putto A 1987 Febrile exudative tonsillitis: streptococcal or viral? Pediatrics 80: 6–12

Quanjer P H, Helms P, Bjure J, Gaultier C 1989 Standardisation of lung function tests in paediatrics. European Respiratory Journal 2: 117s–265s

Raine J, Warner J O 1991 Fibreoptic bronchoscopy without general anaesthetic. Archives of Disease in Childhood 66: 481–484

Rakshi K, Couriel J M 1994 Management of acute bronchiolitis. Archives of Disease in Childhood 71: 463–469

Ramsey B W, Marcuse E K, Foy H M 1986 Use of bacterial antigen detection in the diagnosis of paediatric lower respiratory tract infection. Pediatrics 78: 1–9

Ramsey B W, Farrell P, Pencharz P B 1992 Nutritional assessment and management in cystic fibrosis: a consensus report. American Journal of Clinical Nutrition 55: 108–116

Rich D P, Anderson M P, Gregory R J 1990 Expression of cystic fibrosis transmembrane conductant regulator corrects defective chloride channel regulation in cystic fibrosis airway epithelial cells. Nature 346: 347–358

Riley I D, Lehmann D, Alpers M P 1991 Pneumococcal vaccine trials in Papua New Guinea: relationships between epidemiology of pneumococcal infection and efficacy of vaccine. Review of Infectious Disease 13 (supplement 6): S535–541

Rivkin M J, Aronoff S C 1987 Pulmonary infections in the immuno-compromised child. Advances in Pediatric Infectious Diseases 2: 161–180

Rommens J M, Ionuzzi M C, Kerem B-S et al 1989 Identification of the cystic fibrosis gene: chromosome walking and jumping (pp 1059–1065). Cloning and characterisation of complementary DNA (pp 1066–1072). Science 245

Rona R J, Gulliford M C, Chinn S 1993 Effects of prematurity and intrauterine growth retardation on respiratory health and lung function in childhood. British Medical Journal 306: 817–820

Rosen H, Nadkarni V, Theroux M, Padman R, Klein J 1993 Intrapleural streptokinase as adjunctive treatment for persistant empyema in pediatric patients. Chest 103: 1190–1193

Sarnaik A P, Lieh-Lai M 1994 Adult respiratory distress syndrome in children. Pediatric Clinics of North America 41: 337–364

Sazawal S, Black R E 1992 Meta-analysis of intervention trials on case-management of pneumonia in community settings. Lancet 340: 528

Scheiblauer H, Reinacher M, Tashiro M, Rott R 1992 Interactions between bacteria and influenza A virus in the development of influenza pneumonia. Journal of Infectious Disease 166: 783–791

Scher M S, Guthrie R D, Krieger D et al 1992 Maturational aspects of sleep from birth through early childhood. In: Beckerman R C, Brouillette R T, Hunt C E (eds) Respiratory control disorders in infants and children. Williams and Wilkins, Baltimore, pp 89–111

Shaheen S O, Barker D J P 1994 Early lung growth and chronic airflow obstruction. Thorax 49: 533–536

Shann F 1990 Pneumococcus and influenza. Lancet 335: 898–901

Shann F, Walters S, Pifer L L 1986 Pneumonia associated with infection with pneumoncystis, RSV, chlamydia, mycoplasma, and CMV in children in Papua New Guinea. British Medical Journal 292: 314–316

Shann F, Gatchalian S, Hutchinson R 1988 Naso-pharyngeal oxygen in children. Lancet 2: 1238–1240

Sharief N, Crawford O F, Dinwiddie R 1994 Fibrosing alveolitis and desquamative interstitial pneumonia. Pediatrics 17: 359–365

Sheffer A L 1992 International consensus report on the diagnosis and management of asthma. Clinical and Experimental Allergy 22 (supplement): 1

Shyur S D, Hill H R 1991 Immunodeficiencies in the 1990s. Pediatric Infectious Diseases Journal 10: 595–611

Sigurs N, Bjarnason R, Sigurbergsson F, Kjellman B, Bjorksten B 1995 Asthma and immunoglobulin E antibodies after RSV bronchiolitis: a prospective cohort study with matched controls. Pediatrics 95: 500–505

Silverman M 1993 Out of the mouths of babes and sucklings: lessons from early childhood asthma. Thorax 48: 1200–1204

Silverman M 1995 Childhood asthma and other wheezing disorders. Chapman & Hall, London

Silverman M, Wilson N M 1985 Bronchial responsiveness in children: a clinical review. In: Milner A D, Martin R (eds) Neonatal and respiratory medicine. Butterworth, London

Silverman M, Stratton D, Diallo A, Egler J 1977 Diagnosis of acute bacterial pneumonia in Nigerian children: value of needle aspiration of lung and counter current electrophoresis. Archives of Disease in Childhood 52: 925–931

Silvestri J M, Weese-Mayer D E, Nelson M N 1992 Neuropsychologic abnormalities in children with congenital central hypoventilation syndrome. Journal of Pediatrics 120: 388–393

Slater A J, Nichani S H, Macrae D, Wilkinson K A, Novelli V, Tasker R C 1995 Surfactant adjunctive therapy for Pneumocystis carinii pneumonitis in an infant with acute lymphoblastic leukaemia. Intensive Care Medicine 21: 261–263

Smith K R 1987 Biofuels, air pollution and health: a global review. Plenum, New York

Sotomayor J, Weiner L B, McMillan J A 1985 Inaccurate diagnosis in infants with pertussis: an eight-year experience. American Journal of Diseases of Children 139: 724–727

Southall D P, Samuels M P, Talbert D G 1990 Recurrent cyanotic episodes with severe arterial hypoxaemia and intrapulmonary shunting: a mechanism for sudden death. Archives of Disease in Childhood 65: 953–961

Special article 1991 Investigative use of bronchoscopy, lavage and bronchial biopsies in asthma and other airway diseases. Clinical and Experimental Allergy 21: 533–539

Spencer N, Logan S, Scholey S, Gentle S 1996 Deprivation and bronchiolitis. Archives of Disease in Childhood 74: 50–52

Sporik R 1994 Why block a small hole? Archives of Disease in Childhood 71: 393–394

Spyker D A 1985 Submersion injury. Epidemiology, prevention and management. Pediatric Clinics of North America 32: 113–125

Stiehm E R 1995 Immunologic disorders in infants and children, 4th edn. W B Saunders, Philadelphia

Storm H K R, Krasnik M, Bang K, Frimodt-Moller N 1992 Treatment of pleural empyema secondary to pneumonia: thoracentesis versus closed-tube drainage. Thorax 47: 821–824

Stovroff M, Teague G, Heiss K F, Ricketts R R 1995 Thoracoscopy in the management of pediatric empyema. Journal of Pediatric Surgery 30: 1211–1215

Strachan D P 1992 Causes and control of chronic respiratory disease – looking beyond the smokescreen. Journal of Epidemiology and Community Health 46: 177–179

Strachan D P, Carey I M 1995 Home environment and severe asthma in adolescence: a population based case-control study. British Medical Journal 311: 1053–1056

Sutton D (ed) 1969 Textbook of radiology. Churchill Livingstone, Edinburgh

Tager I B, Hanrahan J P, Tosteston T D et al 1993 Lung function, pre- and post-natal smoke exposure and wheezing in the first year life. American Review of Respiratory Disease 147: 811–817

Tasker R C, Warner J O 1991 Respiratory and allergic disorders. In: Barltrop D, Brueton M J (eds) Paediatric therapeutics. Butterworth Heinemann, London, pp 114–143

Thrasher A J, Segal A W 1995 Host defence disorders. Part III Inherited disorders of white cell function. Paediatric Respiratory Medicine 2: 30–34

Toms G L 1995 RSV – how soon will we have a vaccine? Archives of Disease in Childhood 72: 1–2

Toms G L, Scott R 1987 Respiratory syncytial virus and the infant immune response: annotation. Archives of Disease in Childhood 62: 544–545

Turner R B, Lande A E, Chase P, Hilton N, Weinberg D 1987 Pneumonia in outpatients. Cause and clinical manifestations. Journal of Pediatrics 111: 194–200

Valman B 1985 Preventing infant deaths. British Medical Journal 290: 339–340

Venkatesan P, Innes J A 1995 Antibiotic resistance in common acute respiratory pathogens. Thorax 50: 481–483

Venkatesan P, MacFarlane J T 1992 Role of pneumococcal antigen in the diagnosis of pneumococcal pneumonia. Thorax 47: 329–331

Vogt-Moykopf I, Rau B, Branscheid D 1992 Surgery for congenital malformations of the lung. Annales de Chirurgie 46: 141–156

Von Mutius E, Martinez F, Fritsch G T, Nicolai T, Roell G, Thiemann H-H 1994 Prevalence of asthma and atopy in two areas of West and East Germany. American Journal of Respiratory and Critical Care Medicine 149: 358–364

Wang E E R, Milner R A, Navas L, Maj H 1992 Observer agreement for respiratory signs and oximetry in infants hospitalised with lower respiratory infections. American Review of Respiratory Disease 145: 106–109

Warner J O, Gotz M, Landau L I, Levison H, Milner A D, Pedersen S, Silverman M 1989 Management of asthma: a consensus statement. Archives of Disease in Childhood 64: 1065–1079

Webb M S C, Martin J A, Cartlidge P H, Ng Y K, Wright N A 1985 Chest physiotherapy in acute bronchiolitis Archives of Disease in Childhood 60: 1078–1079

Weese-Mayer D E, Silvestri J M, Menzies L J et al 1992 Congenital central hypoventilation syndrome: diagnosis, management and long term outcome in thirty-two children. Journal of Pediatrics 120: 381–387

Weiland S K, Mundt K A, Ruckmann A, Keil U 1994 Self-reported wheezing and allergic rhinitis in children and traffic density on street of residence. Annals of Epidemiology 4: 243–247

Weiss S G, Newcomb R W, Beem M D 1986 Chlamydia and residual lung disease. Journal of Pediatrics 108: 659–664

West J B 1992 Pulmonary pathophysiology, 4th edn. Williams and Wilkins, Baltimore

Whitehead B F, de Leval M R 1994 Paediatric lung transplantation: the agony and the ecstasy. Thorax. 49: 437–439

Wigfield R E, Fleming P J, Azaz Y et al 1993 How much wrapping do babies need at night? Archives of Disease in Childhood 69: 181–186

Wilson N 1989 Wheezy bronchitis revisited. Archives of Disease in Childhood 64: 1194–1199

Wilson N, Silverman M 1995 Bronchial responsiveness and its measurement. In: Silverman M (ed) Childhood asthma and other wheezing disorders. Chapman & Hall, London

Wilson N, Sloper K, Silverman M 1995 Effect of continuous treatment with topical corticosteroid on episodic viral wheeze in preschool children. Archives of Disease in Childhood 72: 317–320

Wood R E, Postma D 1988 Endoscopy of the airway in infants and children. Journal of Pediatrics 112: 1–6

World Health Organization 1984 A programme for controlling acute respiratory infections in children: memorandom from a WHO meeting. Bulletin of the World Health Organization 621: 47–58

World Health Organization 1992 Programme for control of acute respiratory infections: interim programme report. WHO, Geneva

Wright A, Luffingham G H, North D 1987 Prospective study of symptoms and signs in acutely ill infants in general practice. British Medical Journal 294: 1661–1662

Yoder M C 1994 Development of respiratory defenses. In: Respiratory diseases in children: diagnosis and management. Williams and Wilkins, Baltimore, pp 35–46

Zach M S 1990 Lung disease in cystic fibrosis: an updated concept. Pediatric Pulmonology 8: 188–202

Zimmerman B, Chambers C, Forsyth S 1988 Allergy in asthma II the highly atopic infant and chronic asthma. Journal of Allergy and Clinical Immunology 81: 71–77

Zinman R 1995 Tracheal stenting improves airway mechanics in infants with tracheobronchomalacia. Pediatric Pulmonology 19: 275–281

FURTHER READING

Barbato A, Landau L I, Scheinmann P, Warner J O, Zach M 1995 The bronchoscope – flexible and rigid – in children. Arcari Editore, Treviso, Italy

Chernick V 1990 Kernig's disorders of the respiratory tract in children. W B Saunders, Philadelphia

Hilman B C 1994 Pediatric respiratory disease. W B Saunders, Philadelphia

Hodson M E, Geddes D M (eds) 1995 Cystic fibrosis. Chapman & Hall, London

McKenzie S A 1995 Clinical features and their assessment. In: Silverman M (ed) Childhood asthma and other wheezing disorders. Chapman & Hall, London

Perez C R, Wood R E 1994 Update on pediatric flexible bronchoscopy. Pediatric Clinics of North America 41: 384–400

Shaheen S O, Barker D J P, Sheill A W, Crocker F J, Wield G A, Holgate S J 1994 The relationship between pneumonia in early childhood and impaired lung function in late adult life. American Journal of Respiratory and Critical Care Medicine 149: 616–619

Silverman M (ed) 1995 Childhood asthma and other wheezing disorders. Chapman & Hall, London

Stocks J, Sly P D, Tepper R S, Morgan W J 1996 Infant respiratory function testing. Wiley Liss, New York

Taussig L M 1992 The conundrum of wheezing and airway hyperreactivity in infancy. Pediatric Pulmonology 13: 1–3

Warner J O (ed) 1992 Cystic fibrosis. British Medical Bulletin 48: 717–978

Zaritsky A, Nadkarni V, Hazinski M F, Foltin G, Quan L, Wright L, Fiser D, Zideman D, O'Malley P, Chameides L, Cummins R O, and the Paediatric Utstein Consensus Panel 1995 Recommended guidelines for uniform reporting of paediatric advanced life support: the Paediatric Utstein Style. Resuscitation 30: 95–115

13 Cardiovascular disease

Chapter editor: A. B. Houston

Principles of assessment of heart disease   584
History   584
Clinical examination   585
Chest X-ray   587
Electrocardiography   588
Ultrasound investigation   589
Cardiac catheterization   593
The asymptomatic child with a murmur   594
The innocent murmur   594
A. B. Houston
Congenital heart disease   595
Incidence   595
Etiology   596
Recurrence risk   597
Nomenclature of congenital heart disease   597
Medical care of congenital heart disease   598
The newborn infant with congenital heart disease   598
Heart failure   599
A. B. Houston
Acyanotic heart disease with arteriovenous shunt   599
Acyanotic heart disease without arteriovenous shunt   606
R. Lo
Cyanotic congenital heart disease   613
M. J. Godman

Disturbances of rate, rhythm and conduction   623
Investigation of arrhythmias   623
Disturbances of sinus node function   624
Supraventricular arrhythmias   624
Ventricular arrhythmias   625
Conduction disturbances   626
Management of arrhythmias and conduction disturbances   626
M. J. Godman
Acquired cardiovascular disorders   628
Rheumatic heart disease   628
Acute carditis   628
Chronic rheumatic heart disease   629
Infective myocarditis   630
Infective endocarditis   630
Endomyocardial fibrosis   631
Mucocutaneous lymph node syndrome   633
Heart muscle disease or cardiomyopathy   633
Dilated cardiomyopathy   633
Hypertrophic cardiomyopathy   634
Specific heart muscle disease   634
Pericarditis   634
Connective tissue disease   635
Cardiac tumors   636
Hypertension   636
A. B. Houston
References 638

PRINCIPLES OF ASSESSMENT OF HEART DISEASE

Patients with acquired heart disease are likely to present with symptoms, though not necessarily of cardiac involvement, as in acute rheumatic fever or Kawasaki disease. Congenital heart disease is more often recognized by the presence of clinical signs, the main ones being cyanosis, a murmur, cardiac failure or dysrhythmia. Assessment of the presence and severity of heart disease must include an appropriate history and examination to provide a provisional diagnosis before undertaking further investigations. Ultrasound examination has greatly simplified the precise diagnosis of cardiac defects but this is not often available to the pediatrician and much useful information is obtained from clinical examination with electrocardiography and chest radiology. Cardiac catheterization is not often required for diagnostic purposes but is essential in many patients when surgical intervention is thought to be necessary, and is increasingly undertaken as part of a transcatheter interventional procedure.

HISTORY

A detailed history is of limited importance in bringing the presence of congenital heart disease to attention, most cases being recognized from the presence of either cyanosis in the neonatal period, cardiac failure in infancy, or an asymptomatic murmur at any age. However, when a diagnosis of heart disease has been made some parents will subsequently comment on symptoms which they did not previously recognize or to which the medical attendants did not pay appropriate attention. On the other hand they may describe and worry about minor symptoms which would be dismissed in a normal child. In infancy cardiac failure can present with symptoms of breathlessness, feeding difficulty, and poor weight gain. Cyanosis may not be recognized by family members (or inexperienced medical observers) until it is moderately severe, but they are likely to be aware of episodes of increased cyanosis, as in hypercyanotic spells in tetralogy of Fallot. In the older child with cyanotic congenital heart disease the presence of symptoms is often important in deciding on the need for surgical intervention. Inquiry as to fainting episodes or palpitations should be made in certain situations. The family history and that of illness or exposure to teratogenic factors during pregnancy are appropriate in considering questions on etiology and possible recurrence. When rheumatic heart disease is a possibility inquiry should be made as to previous symptoms suggesting an episode of acute rheumatic fever, and present well-being and exercise capabilities.

CLINICAL EXAMINATION

Clinical examination remains the mainstay of the recognition, evaluation, and management of the child with heart disease. It must not simply be restricted to auscultation but should be performed in a systematic manner to include general examination for signs of cardiac or associated disease, palpation of the pulses, then precordial examination by inspection, palpation and auscultation. The means by which and the order in which these are performed may have to be adjusted depending on patient cooperation but it is essential that all are undertaken to ensure that no feature of diagnostic value is omitted. Inexperienced examiners may concentrate on a murmur; although this often provides the basic diagnosis, determination of the hemodynamic significance and subsequent management are largely decided by other clinical features on inspection and palpation.

Physical findings will depend not only on the basic lesion, its severity and hemodynamic effects but also on the possible presence of an associated abnormality. Thus, although there is a tendency to describe 'typical' findings there can be considerable variation. No single clinical feature or investigation should be taken in isolation and, in particular, it is essential that an ultrasound investigation is not performed or interpreted without clear knowledge of the clinical findings and their significance and the particular information which is being sought. Clinical findings are discussed with each specific lesion and excellent descriptions of physical signs and their cause have been detailed by Zuberbuhler (1981) and Perloff (1987).

General examination

This requires examination for specific syndromes, defects associated with heart disease, and other noncardiac abnormalities which might alter management. Thereafter, general features of congenital heart disease must be sought, in particular impressions of general health, growth and nutrition, cyanosis and clubbing, tachypnea and dyspnea and other evidence of cardiac failure.

Height, weight and nutrition

Although some infants and children with severe congenital heart disease show poor growth it must be remembered that often this is unrelated to the cardiac anomaly and is not in itself an indication for intervention.

Cyanosis

Cyanosis can be recognized when there is at least 5 g/100 ml of reduced hemoglobin in the skin capillaries and must be sought in the lips not the peripheries. Cyanosis can be less readily detected in newborn infants than in older children with the same lesion. Infants with conditions which later cause marked cyanosis may be acyanotic in the first few days of life when oxygenation is maintained by mixing at the level of an arterial duct or foramen ovale. The oxygen saturation level at which cyanosis can be detected clinically is related to the hemoglobin concentration; the higher the hemoglobin level, the higher the oxygen saturation at which cyanosis appears. Since the newborn infant has a relatively high hematocrit, cyanosis should be more readily apparent. However, the presence of fetal hemoglobin moves the oxygen dissociation curve to the left, providing a higher oxygen saturation

for any given PaO_2, with the result that a newborn infant with minimal cyanosis can have a PaO_2 of only 35–40 mmHg (5–6 kPa). Thus, where there is clinical suspicion of cyanosis an expectant policy is not appropriate and the PaO_2 should be measured. The normal newborn infant should have a PaO_2 of 60–70 mmHg (9–10 kPa) by 24 h.

It is not unusual for parents of normal young children to report intermittent episodes of 'going blue'. In these episodes the blueness is short lived (usually 5–10 minutes though occasionally longer), and often in the area around the mouth rather than the lips. Such episodes are probably the result of alteration in vascular tone but the exact mechanism is uncertain. Provided there are no abnormal cardiovascular findings further investigations are not necessary and the parents can be reassured.

Clubbing

Clubbing of the fingers or toes occurs in association with significant desaturation and cyanosis but does not become apparent until the latter part of the first year of life.

Jugular venous pulse

Examination of the jugular venous pulse is of little practical value in children since it is difficult to see and the relatively fast heart rate makes the distinction between the different wave forms difficult.

Cardiac failure

Cardiac failure in infancy presents with tachypnea, tachycardia, and hepatomegaly. These can also be signs of lung disease and one of the difficulties in the early recognition of heart disease lies in making a distinction between cardiac and pulmonary disease. In the full-term infant the resting heart rate is usually between 130 and 140/min although there is considerable variation. A sustained tachycardia of more than 160/min at rest would raise the possibility of underlying cardiac failure. Gallop rhythm is commonly heard on auscultation. Tachypnea, with a respiratory rate of more than 50/min in the full-term infant, is a nonspecific sign which may be the first indication of heart failure and may first become apparent on feeding. In the infant marked edema is unusual although some periorbital puffiness or pitting of the dorsal surface of the hands or feet may develop. Hepatomegaly is, however, a prominent finding, the liver size providing an indication of the severity of cardiac failure. In older subjects with right heart failure edema becomes more readily apparent.

Pulses

If the radial pulse is difficult to palpate in infants, the brachial or axillary arteries should be used. The right radial or brachial pulse is examined for rate, rhythm and volume and compared with that on the left, since aortic arch abnormalities may produce a discrepancy between the arm pulses. It is mandatory to palpate the arm and femoral pulses simultaneously. In a newborn with coarctation the femoral pulses may feel normal initially, but subsequently disappear as the arterial duct closes. Coarctation of the aorta in younger subjects is recognized from absence or decreased volume of the femoral pulses while in older ones with well-developed collateral arteries delay in pulse transmission tends to be more apparent. Bounding pulses are found with a large arterial duct, truncus arteriosus or aortic regurgitation. Low volume pulses occur with reduced left ventricular output in cardiac defects such as severe aortic stenosis or congestive cardiomyopathy.

Precordial examination

Inspection

With the exception of tachypnea and indrawing, this is of limited value in the infant, chest deformity occurring only with longstanding disease, following surgical intervention, or as the result of another associated abnormality. A median sternotomy (midline) scar usually indicates cardiac bypass surgery, and a lateral thoracotomy scar great artery surgery.

Palpation

Palpation is performed to determine three main features: the site and nature of the apex beat, the presence of a right ventricular heave, and the presence and site of a thrill. The position of the *apex beat* should be sought but it cannot always be felt or localized; in this circumstance it is likely that it is normal. It should be at or above the fifth interspace within the midclavicular or nipple line. With left ventricular hypertrophy it is displaced laterally and sustained ('heaving'); with right ventricular hypertrophy it is poorly sustained ('tapping'). The presence of a *right ventricular heave* is a most useful sign, often indicating pulmonary artery hypertension. It may be the only clinical sign of significant congenital heart disease in the infant and in this group it is often most easily felt in the subxiphoid position. In older subjects it is felt along the lower left sternal edge and is more prominent with right ventricular volume overload than with pressure overload, and thus more consistent with an ASD than with pulmonary stenosis.

A *thrill* should be maximal where the murmur is loudest and in most cases merely indicates a loud murmur. An exception is the thrill in the suprasternal notch which is most commonly associated with aortic stenosis, and may indicate the correct diagnosis when the murmur and other signs have been misinterpreted. A suprasternal thrill may also be felt with other lesions but in these circumstances the clinical diagnosis is usually readily apparent.

Auscultation

Heart sounds

These are usually best heard with the diaphragm of the stethoscope. The most important heart sound in the assessment of congenital heart disease is the *second* in the pulmonary area. In normal children both the aortic and pulmonary components are heard, the separation increasing with inspiration and virtually disappearing with expiration. A loud second sound in acyanotic congenital heart disease is associated with pulmonary artery hypertension, but in cyanotic congenital heart disease (and the rare acyanotic corrected transposition of the great arteries) this may be due to the closure of an anteriorly positioned aortic valve and can occur with normal or low pulmonary artery pressure. On the other hand, with severe aortic or pulmonary stenosis the respective component of the second heart sound is of diminished

volume and the sound may be single. A single second heart sound also occurs with cyanotic defects where there is only one semilunar valve, e.g. pulmonary atresia. With an ASD the second heart sound is classically widely and fixedly split, but this is not always the case.

The *first* heart sound is of less practical diagnostic value. It is loud if ventricular contractility is high (as with anxiety or exercise) or if mitral closure is relatively late when the first heart sound coincides with rapid rise in ventricular pressure (mitral stenosis, short PR interval). It will be soft if ventricular contractility is depressed (myocarditis, congestive cardiomyopathy) or if the mitral valve closes early, before ventricular contraction (long PR interval, severe aortic regurgitation).

A *third* heart sound, best heard at the apex, occurs shortly after aortic closure as the result of rapid ventricular filling and is heard in many normal children in whom it is of no clinical significance. It is common with mitral regurgitation, a slow heart rate, or anemia. When cardiac failure occurs a third heart sound may combine with the other sounds to produce a gallop rhythm.

A *fourth* heart sound, which occurs shortly before the first, is always pathological. It is not a common finding in children.

An ejection *click*, which occurs soon after the first heart sound, is audible with a mobile valve leaflet in aortic or pulmonary stenosis and with a bicuspid aortic valve. A similar though slightly later midsystolic click occurs with mitral valve prolapse.

Murmurs

Characteristics of specific murmurs are considered under individual lesions. A murmur should be described in terms of loudness, quality and pitch, timing, site and radiation. Of these, the most useful in making a basic diagnosis are the site and radiation followed by the timing, which should be accurately defined and not just stated as systolic or diastolic.

The *loudness* of a murmur should always be described, although it is not necessary for general purposes to use the conventional scale of 1–6 employed by most cardiologists. The loudness depends on the orifice size, pressure drop, volume of flow, distance from the chest wall and patient position. There is no clear relationship of the loudness or softness to the severity of a lesion.

The *quality* of a murmur can be difficult to describe and experience is needed to be confident about this. A high pitched murmur ('blowing') is heard with aortic or mitral regurgitation or a tiny VSD, a lower pitched one ('harsh' or 'rough') with outflow stenosis or a small VSD, and a very low pitched one ('rumble') with mitral stenosis.

In congenital heart disease most murmurs are systolic in *timing* and it is rare to have a diastolic murmur without an associated systolic one. However, with chronic rheumatic heart disease a diastolic murmur of aortic regurgitation or mitral stenosis is relatively common. An early to midsystolic murmur is usually due to aortic or pulmonary stenosis or is innocent, a pansystolic one to a restrictive VSD or mitral or tricuspid regurgitation, and a late systolic one to mitral valve prolapse. A diastolic murmur is almost always pathological. An early diastolic murmur occurs with aortic or pulmonary regurgitation, and a mid- to late diastolic one with stenosis of, or increased flow through, the mitral or tricuspid valve. The former are best heard with the diaphragm and the latter with the bell of the stethoscope. A continuous murmur, defined as one which continues through the second heart sound and into diastole, is heard when an artery communicates with a low pressure vessel or chamber, such as with an arterial duct, Blalock–Taussig shunt, an arteriovenous or coronary artery fistula. The length and timing of a murmur are related to the pressure differences across the defect producing the murmur and its size and nature. Thus, though a VSD is classically pansystolic, it can be much shorter when the defect is tiny or when there is marked right ventricular hypertension.

The *site of maximal intensity* of a murmur is perhaps the most useful observation in making a basic diagnosis, though it tells little of the hemodynamic significance of the lesion. To this end it is important to move the stethoscope to examine the whole precordium. A murmur results from turbulent blood flow and is loudest at the site of disturbed flow. Thus (with the exception of an atrial septal defect), it will be maximal over the position on the chest overlying the lesion. The classical sites of maximal intensity of the common systolic murmurs are summarized in Figure 13.1. A loud murmur may be conducted all over the precordium while others exhibit radiation to a specific site. The murmur of aortic stenosis is heard into the neck, that of pulmonary branch stenosis into the axillae and back, and of mitral regurgitation into the axilla.

Summary of clinical assessment

Although there are typical findings for each defect it is essential to realize that these will not always be as apparent as suggested in textbooks. Signs will depend on factors such as the severity of a lesion and the pulmonary pressure. For instance, in ductus arteriosus there is typically a collapsing pulse and continuous murmur; but pulses will be of normal volume if the duct is small or pulmonary pressure high and the murmur may be only systolic or absent with pulmonary hypertension. The specific features of individual lesions are discussed in detail under the lesion. Table 13.1 summarizes the typical classical findings in the common forms of acyanotic congenital heart disease.

CHEST X-RAY

The chest X-ray may provide information of diagnostic value where there is a significant cardiac defect but is of little practical

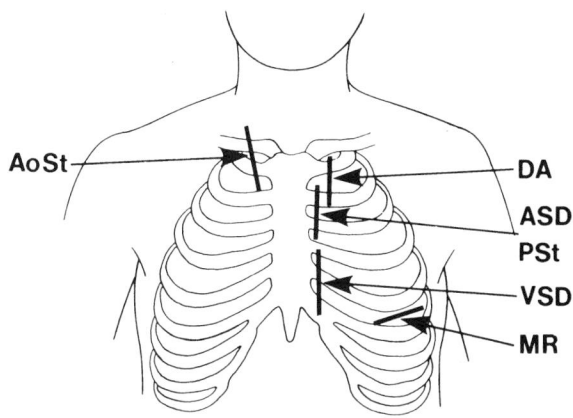

Fig. 13.1 Diagrammatic representation of the precordium showing the usual sites at which the murmur of the most common acyanotic lesions are heard. VSD, ventricular septal defect; ASD, atrial septal defect; DA, ductus arteriosus; AoSt, aortic stenosis; PSt, pulmonary stenosis; MR, mitral regurgitation.

value in trivial defects and none in distinguishing one of these from an innocent murmur. It is essential in postoperative management.

A chest X-ray should be examined for the cardiac size and configuration and pulmonary vascularity. In certain situations the thoracic situs and other abnormalities should be sought. Cardiomegaly is almost always found with a significant cardiac defect unless this is due to pressure overload (e.g. pulmonary stenosis). It is caused by enlargement or dilation of one or both ventricles from either volume overload associated with a shunt or valve regurgitation, or left ventricular dysfunction as in cardiac failure or cardiomyopathy. Cardiomegaly can also occur with pericardial effusion or occasionally atrial dilation, usually the right.

A semiquantitative assessment of the cardiac size can be calculated from the cardiothoracic ratio, the ratio of the cardiac diameter (measured as the sum of the distance from the midline to the most right and left margins of the cardiac shadow) to the maximal internal thoracic one (Fig. 13.2). However, this is not an absolute value and will be increased if the film is not taken in full

Table 13.1 Classical clinical findings in the most common forms of acyanotic congenital heart disease

Lesion	Pulses	Ventricular activity	Heart sounds	Murmur Systole	Murmur Diastole
VSD	Normal	Left (large shunt) Right (if PAH)	Accentuated II if PAH	Pansystolic Lower LSE	Apical mid-diastolic (if large shunt)
ASD	Normal	Right (large shunt)	II wide and fixed	Ejection Upper LSE	Mid-diastolic LLSE (if large shunt)
PDA	Collapsing or normal	Left (large shunt) Right (if PAH)	Accentuated II if PAH	Continuous, maximal in late systole Left clavicle to upper LSE	
Pulmonary stenosis	Normal	Right	Click if pliable valve	Ejection Upper LSE clavicle	
Aortic stenosis	Normal or reduced if severe	Left	Click if pliable valve	Ejection Upper RSE neck	
Coarctation of the aorta	Decreased or delayed femorals	Left Right in newborn	Click if bicuspid aortic valve	Mid-systolic Apex and back	

PAH = pulmonary artery hypertension; II = second heart sound; LSE = left sternal edge; RSE = right sternal edge.

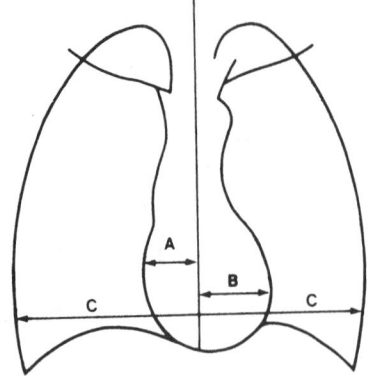

Fig. 13.2 Diagrammatic representation of the measurement of the cardiothoracic ratio:

$$CTR = \frac{A + B}{C} \times 100 \text{ where}$$

A + B = maximum transverse diameter of the heart
C = maximum transverse diameter of the chest.

inspiration or if it is an anteroposterior one, as in infants. In normal children the ratio is less than 0.5 but can be up to 0.55 in the first 2 years of life. The apex tends to be displaced downwards with left ventricular enlargement and directly to the left with right ventricular hypertrophy.

In infants the configuration of the superior aspect of the cardiac shadow will vary with thymic size and shape. A characteristic appearance may be found with certain cyanotic congenital defects but these are variable and are only suggestive of the diagnosis.

Increased pulmonary blood flow from a left to right shunt is manifest as large vessels passing outwards from the hilum. With pulmonary edema the hilar vessels are less easily identified but the bronchi become more easily seen and, if severe, linear septal shadows appear in the lower lateral aspects of the lung fields. Narrow pulmonary vessels with increased lucency of the peripheral fields occur with significant obstruction to pulmonary blood flow.

A penetrated film demonstrating the bronchi can help to establish the thoracic situs: the left main bronchus arises from the trachea at a less acute angle and its first branch arises more distally. Congenital skeletal abnormalities occurring with certain syndromes (e.g. VATERL) will be apparent. Rib notching may be seen with coarctation of the aorta, but not in the early years of life.

Chest radiology is important in distinguishing cardiac from respiratory disease, and essential in the peri- and postoperative management. However, it exposes the child to radiation and should be used judiciously. Frequently repeated chest radiographs are of little value in assessing progress of a lesion and worthless with minor defects.

ELECTROCARDIOGRAPHY

Electrocardiography remains an essential investigation in the evaluation of any child with a suspected cardiac lesion. It is the initial investigation in the analysis of rhythm and conduction disturbances (p. 626), and may provide information about the severity of an abnormality from the pattern of atrial or ventricular hypertrophy. Specific diagnostic patterns are associated with certain lesions, such as tricuspid atresia and atrioventricular septal defect, and on occasions the electrocardiogram may assist in the

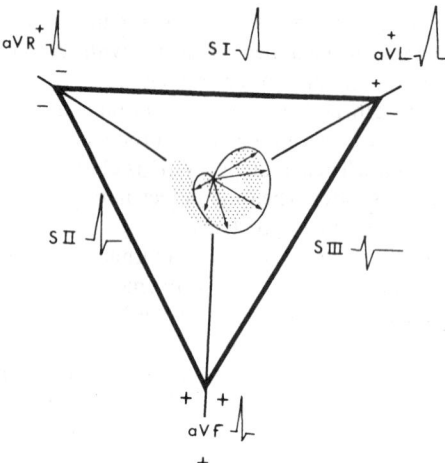

Fig. 13.3 The frontal vector loop related to the Einthoven triangle and the limb leads (standard and augmented) of the electrocardiogram.

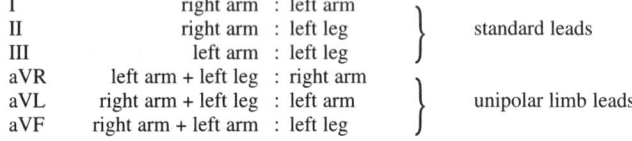

I	right arm : left arm	standard leads
II	right arm : left leg	
III	left arm : left leg	
aVR	left arm + left leg : right arm	unipolar limb leads
aVL	right arm + left leg : left arm	
aVF	right arm + left arm : left leg	

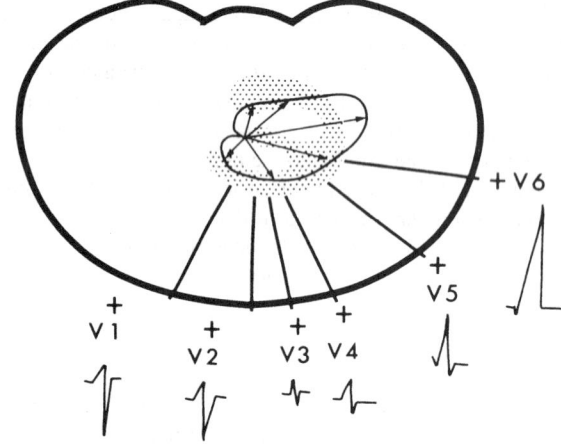

Fig. 13.4 The horizontal vector loop related to the unipolar precordial leads of the electrocardiogram.

detection of electrolyte abnormalities and some forms of drug intoxication.

The physiological principles of electrocardiography are beyond the scope of this section, but those points important to the pediatrician will be emphasized. More detailed information is available from some of the specialized texts (Park & Guntheroth 1981). An electrocardiogram (ECG) scans the electrical activity of the heart and plots it as voltage against time. Conventionally this is recorded from 12 arbitrary viewpoints, six in the frontal plane (the standard or unipolar leads) and six in the transverse or horizontal plane (the chest leads) (Figs 13.3 and 13.4).

The normal electrocardiogram

The approach to the analysis of an electrocardiogram should be systematic and start with consideration of the P wave, and progress to the PR interval, QRS complex, ST segment and T wave. The electrocardiogram of the infant or growing child undergoes dynamic processes, reflecting changes due to the anatomical growth of the heart and alterations in cardiac hemodynamics. In the first 6 months of life right ventricular dominance is normally present and regression may take 2–3 years although normally the left ventricle is dominant by the age of 6 months. With increasing age the R wave in V1 and the S wave in V6 become less, and the S wave in V1 and the R wave in V6 more prominent.

The *P wave* is a result of electrical activity which originates from the sinus node then spreads across the atria. Since the impulse spreads from right to left, the P wave is upright in leads I, II and aVF, inverted in aVR and can be upright, biphasic or inverted in leads III, aVL and V1. P waves should not be greater than 0.3 mV (3 mm at normal standardization of 10 mm to 1.0 mV) in the bipolar leads or 0.25 mV in the unipolar leads. The normal *PR interval* increases from 0.10 s in infancy to 0.16 s in adolescence.

The *QRS interval* represents depolarization of the ventricular muscle. The duration of the QRS complex is 0.06–0.08 s, and should not exceed 0.10 s. The Q wave is due to depolarization of the interventricular septum from the left side of the heart to the right. By definition, the Q wave is the negative deflection preceding the R wave and is usually not greater than 0.3 mV and if more than 0.4 mV is abnormal. Q waves may be found normally in all except the right precordial leads. In l-transposition of the great arteries, the septum is depolarized in a direction opposite to normal and in such cases Q waves may occur in V4R and V1 and be absent in V6. Large Q waves may occur in V5 and V6 in left ventricular or biventricular hypertrophy. The R wave is any positive deflection in the ECG. If there are two R waves, the second is denoted R′. An R wave of small voltage is denoted r. The size of the R and S waves in the different leads is determined by the thickness of the ventricular walls, and thus reflects right and left ventricular hypertrophy, the criteria for which are set out below.

The *T wave* results from repolarization of the ventricles. T waves are normally upright in the right precordial leads (V4R and V1) in normal newborns for 72 h, and if persistently upright beyond 7 days are abnormal. Inverted T waves in the right precordial leads are normal in infants and children, and can persist to 14–16 years of age. Slight upward displacement of the *ST segment* in the right precordial leads is common in normal children.

The *QT interval* is measured from the beginning of the Q wave to the end of the T wave and its duration varies with heart rate. Tables are available for normal QT intervals. It can be corrected for heart rate (QTc) using the RR interval from the formula, $QTc = QT/\sqrt{RR}$: this value should be less than 0.42 s. It may be lengthened in hypocalcemia and myocardial disease.

The electrical or *QRS axis* of the heart is the direction of the maximum electrical force during depolarization. An approximate method of deriving the mean frontal QRS axis is to find in which of the leads I, II, III, aVR, aVL and aVF, the deflections above and below the line are most nearly equal. The mean frontal QRS axis is at right angles to this lead. The normal QRS axis at birth averages 135° and changes gradually to a mean of about 60° at 1 year. Right axis deviation is usually due to right ventricular hypertrophy, but left axis deviation is usually the result of a conduction abnormality of the left ventricle and is found in atrioventricular septal defects and tricuspid atresia.

Criteria for chamber hypertrophy

Right ventricular hypertrophy (RVH) occurs principally in conditions associated with raised right ventricular pressure such as pulmonary stenosis, pulmonary hypertension, Fallot's tetralogy and transposition of the great arteries. The electrocardiographic features reflect the forces arising from the activation of increased right ventricular muscle mass, with increase in the voltage of the R waves over the right (V1 and V2), and the S waves over the left (V5 and V6) precordial leads. Voltage changes are helpful, but the evaluation should not be based solely on these.

The following features suggest right ventricular hypertrophy:

1. T waves positive in V4R and V1 after 72 h if R/S more than 1.0
2. R in V1 more than 2.0 mV at all ages, or greater than normal for age
3. S in V6 greater than normal for age: 0–7 days, 1.4 mV; 1 week to 6 months, 1.0 mV; 6–12 months, 0.7 mV; above 1 year, 0.5 mV
4. R/S ratio in V1: 0–3 months, 6.5; 3–6 months, 4.0; 6 months to 3 years, 2.4; 3–5 years, 1.6; 6–15 years, 0.8.

Left ventricular hypertrophy (LVH) occurs with volume or pressure overload of the left ventricle such as aortic valve disease, ventricular septal defect, persistent ductus arteriosus, coarctation of the aorta, mitral regurgitation and cardiomyopathy. Increased left ventricular forces are reflected by deepening of the S waves in V1 and increase in the R waves in V5 and V6.

The following features suggest left ventricular hypertrophy:

1. tall R waves in V5 and V6 or deep S waves in V1 for age (consult tables); in older children R in V5 or V6 > 2.6 mV
2. sum of S in V1 and R in V5 or V6 > 4.0 mV over 1 year or > 3.0 mV if under 1 year
3. Q wave 0.4 mV or more in V5 or V6
4. T wave inversion in V5 or V6.

Combined ventricular hypertrophy can be difficult to recognize and is most commonly a feature of large ventricular septal defects. The following features suggest biventricular hypertrophy:

1. criteria for RVH and LVH satisfied
2. RVH plus inverted T in V6
3. LVH plus wide or bifid R wave in V4R or V1 over 0.8 mV.

Right atrial hypertrophy is suggested by:

1. P waves 0.3 mV or more in bipolar leads
2. P waves 0.2 mV or more in unipolar leads

and *left atrial* hypertrophy by:

1. bifid P in any lead with P of more than 0.09 s duration
2. late inversion of P wave in V1 > 0.15 mV.

Criteria for hypertrophy in the premature infant are less certain than for the term infant or older child, but generally there is less right ventricular dominance than in the full-term infant (Thomaidis et al 1988).

ULTRASOUND INVESTIGATION

The combination of imaging ultrasound with spectral and color Doppler provides a very accurate assessment of cardiac anatomy, hemodynamics and function.

Echocardiographic imaging

The principles of imaging ultrasound are described elsewhere (Ch. 36; Allen et al 1978). Returning echoes are displayed as vertical displacement from a horizontal axis in the amplitude 'A' scan and a spot on its axis in the brightness 'B' scan. Where the echo producing structure is moving along the line of the ultrasound beam, motion of the returning echoes can be appreciated, but it is difficult to quantify or record. A motion (M-mode) recording is obtained by sweeping the 'B' scan at a constant rate across the oscilloscope; this allows the velocity of movement and the distance between the echo producing structures to be measured accurately (Fig. 13.5). By convention, in the M mode echocardiogram time is represented along the horizontal axis from left to right and distance from the transducer on the vertical one, the transducer being at the top (Fig. 13.6). A cross-sectional image is produced by mechanically or electronically rapidly sweeping the ultrasound beam across the field being imaged and writing each returning 'B' scan line of information in the appropriate position on an oscilloscope.

Figure 13.6a is an M-mode recording from an infant with a normal heart, taken through the body of the left ventricle. The ventricular septum and posterior left ventricular wall can be seen to move towards each other in systole as the left ventricle contracts. The left ventricle is larger than the right. The anterior mitral leaflet exhibits a characteristic M-shaped appearance, moving anteriorly in early diastole as it opens with ventricular relaxation and again in late diastole as a result of atrial contraction. The posterior mitral leaflet motion is a mirror image of the anterior leaflet, but with a lesser amplitude. The M mode is

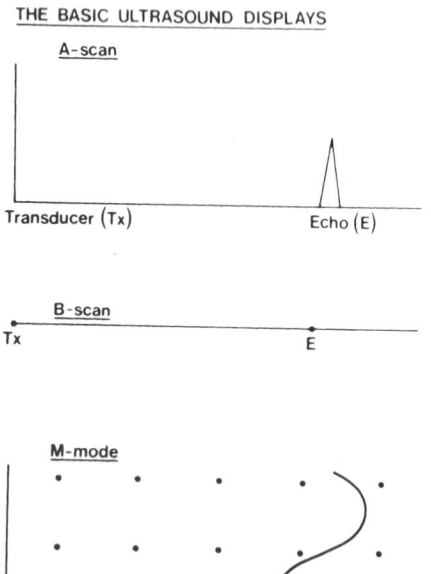

Fig. 13.5 Diagrammatic representation of the basic methods of displaying the ultrasound echoes. The returning echo is displayed as a vertical displacement from the horizontal axis in the A scan, as a spot on this axis on the B scan, and as a moving line on the M mode scan.

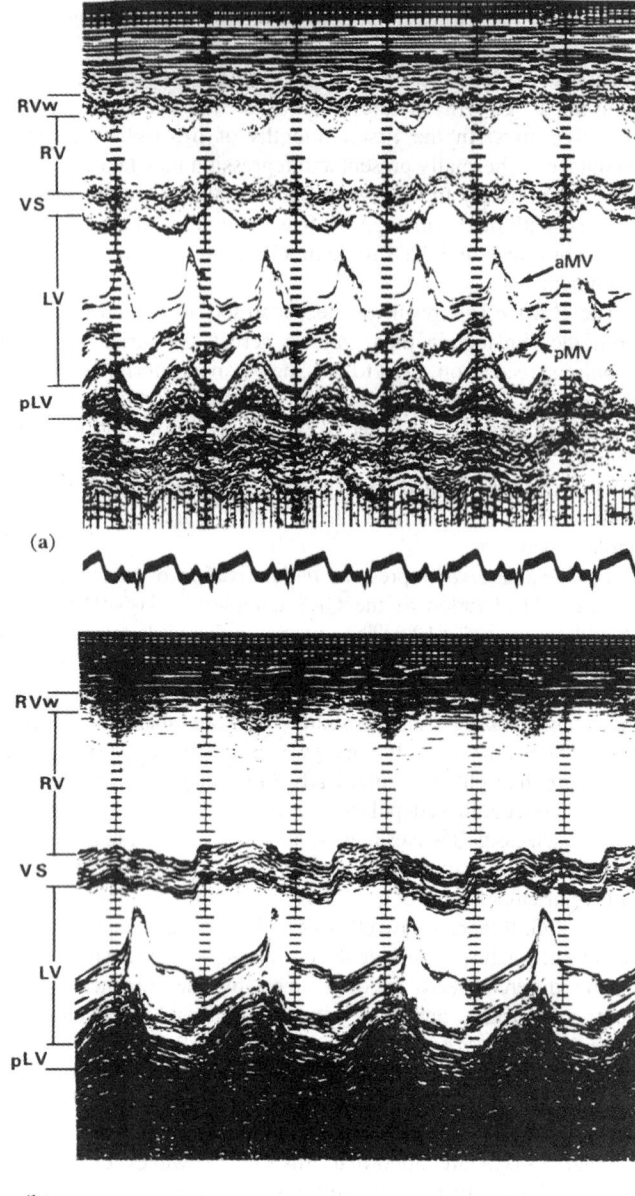

Fig. 13.6 (a) M mode recording through both ventricles and the mitral valve of an infant. The vertical markers are for both time and distance. RVw, anterior right ventricular wall; RV, right ventricular cavity; VS, ventricular septum; LV, left ventricular cavity; pLV, posterior wall of left ventricle; aMV, anterior mitral leaflet; pMV, posterior mitral leaflet. (b) M mode recording from a child with a secumdum ASD showing an enlarged right ventricle and paradoxical motion of the ventricular septum.

generally used for accurate measurement of chamber and vessel size and left ventricular function. By convention, measurement of left and right ventricular dimensions and the ventricular septal and wall thickness are made at the level of the tips of the mitral cusps and measurements of aortic root and left atrial size at the level of the aortic valve cusps. Normal values for these parameters for infants and children have been published (Allen et al 1978). Differences in size can be appreciated in Figure 13.6b, which shows a large right ventricle typical of an atrial septal defect. In addition, the septum moves anteriorly in systole; this is known as paradoxical septal motion and is characteristic of conditions with right ventricular volume overload.

Cross-sectional echocardiography provides detailed images of intracardiac structures and abnormalities. Scanning planes are based on standard views of the heart and not on transducer position on the chest (Tajik et al 1978). A long axis view through the left ventricle and aorta of a normal child is shown in Figure 13.7. Great artery size and relations are determined in a short axis view at the base of the heart. The aortic arch and head and neck vessels can be imaged from a high parasternal or suprasternal position. For many diagnostic purposes it is important to obtain a four chamber view which passes through the crux of the heart showing the junction of the ventricular and atrial septa and the mitral and tricuspid valves (Fig. 13.8). Abnormalities demonstrated in this view are exemplified by the atrial septal defect (Fig. 13.9) and single ventricle (Fig. 13.10). This view is of particular value in fetal echocardiography since it is relatively

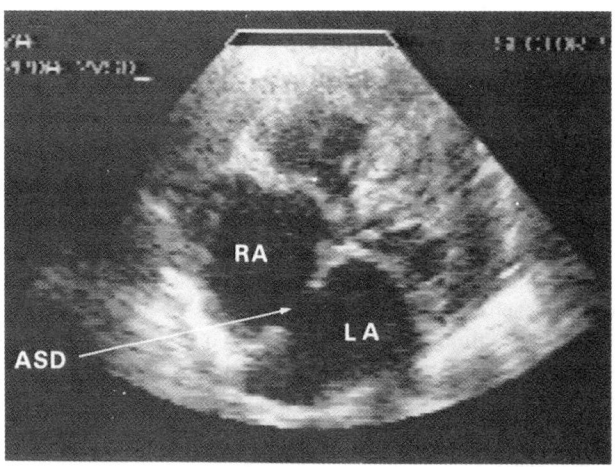

Fig. 13.9 View with the scanner adjusted to image the atrial septum and secundum atrial septal defect (ASD). Other abbreviations as before.

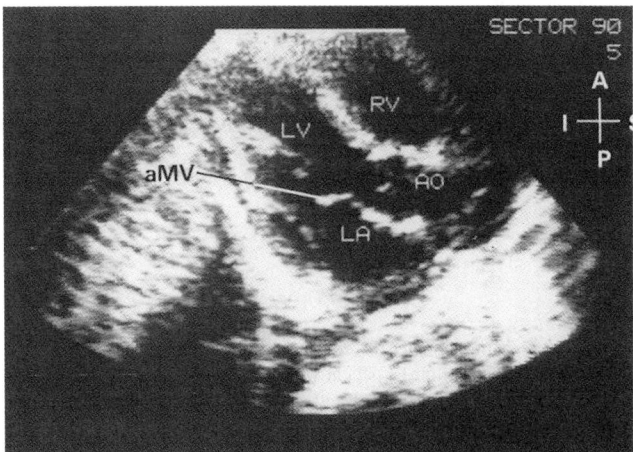

Fig. 13.7 Parasternal long axis view through the left ventricle and aortic root. AO, aortic root; LA, left atrium; A, anterior; P, posterior; S, superior; I, inferior. Other abbreviations as before.

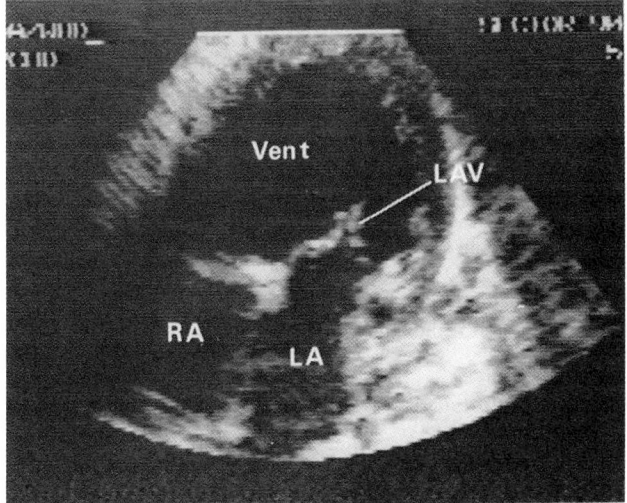

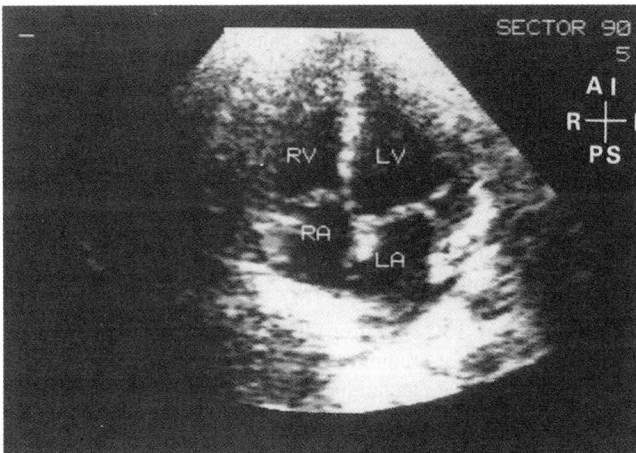

Fig. 13.8 Four chamber view. The ventricular and atrial septa are continuous with each other and the anterior leaflets of the mitral and tricuspid valves are inserted into the ventricular septum at different levels. RA, right atrium; AI, anteroinferior; PS, posterosuperior; R, right; L, left. Other abbreviations as before.

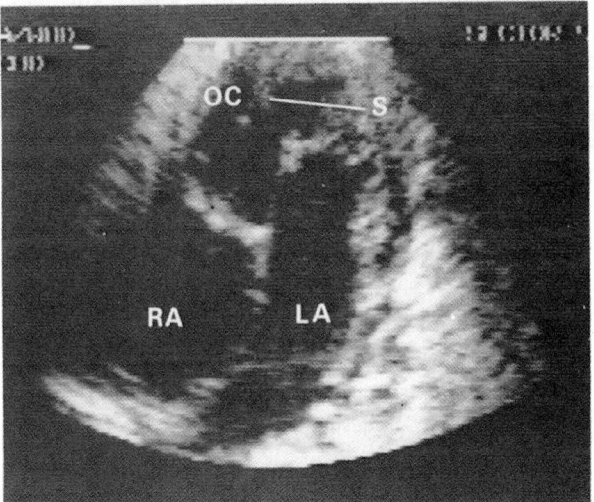

Fig. 13.10 Views from an infant with tricuspid atresia. The left atrioventricular valve (LAV) is closed (top) in systole but (bottom) opens and moves anteriorly in diastole but there is no evidence of a mobile right AV valve. Vent, ventricle; LAV, left atrioventricular valve; OC, outlet chamber; S, septum. Other abbreviations as before.

easy to obtain and allows a large number of complex and potentially serious defects to be diagnosed (Allan et al 1984).

Doppler ultrasound

The principles of cardiac Doppler ultrasound and its practical application have been well described (Hatle & Angelsen 1985, Houston & Simpson 1988). When a sound wave is reflected from a static target the returning and transmitted frequencies are the same. If there is relative motion of the transmitter and receiver towards each other the returning sound is of higher frequency, while if away from each other it will be of lower frequency. The relationship between this change in frequency and the velocity of relative motion is given by the Doppler equation:

$$f_t - f_r = \frac{2f_t V \cos\theta}{c}$$

where f_t = transmitted frequency, f_r = received frequency, V is the velocity of blood flow, θ is the angle of incidence of the sound wave to blood flow direction and c is the velocity of sound in blood (Fig. 13.11).

The frequency change is measured by the ultrasound equipment and the transmitter frequency and velocity of sound in tissue is known. Thus $V\cos\theta$ can be calculated electronically by the machine. Accurate angle measurement is impossible and the aim of the investigation is to obtain the highest frequency shift and presume θ is 0° and thus $\cos\theta$ = 1. If the angle of incidence of ultrasound can be kept within 15° of flow direction $\cos\theta$ is greater than 0.97 and can be considered to be 1, providing a measurement of V, the velocity of blood flow. Thus, although Doppler ultrasound can measure blood flow velocity there is a potential for underestimation if the angle is large.

Doppler spectral display

Spectral Doppler displays flow velocity with time along the X axis and flow velocity on the Y axis, flow towards the transducer being positive and away from it negative. Figure 13.12 (top) is the signal of normal pulmonary flow, obtained from a parasternal position over the right ventricular outflow tract. In systole, flow is away from the transducer (negative), starting just after pulmonary valve opening and reaching maximum velocity (0.8 ms⁻¹) in approximately midsystole and returning to the baseline with pulmonary closure. Characteristic patterns occur with flow through different valves.

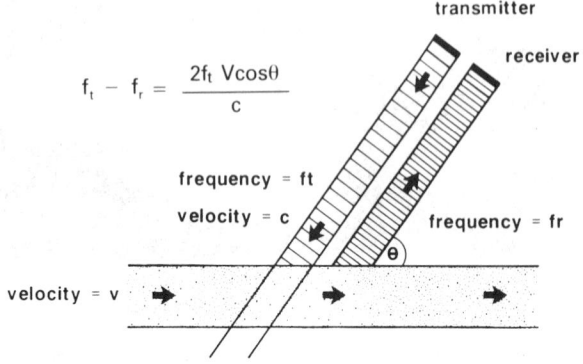

Fig. 13.11 The Doppler equation. See text for explanation.

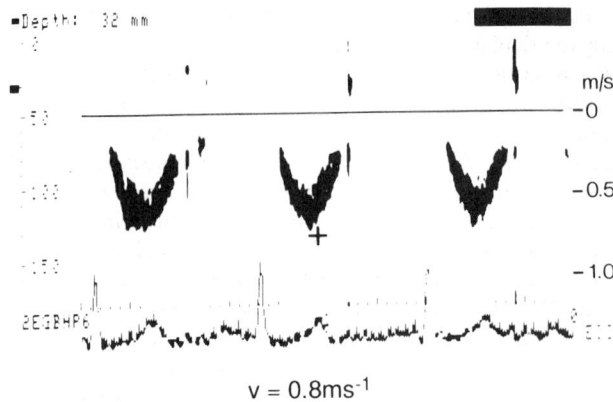

$$v = 0.8 \text{ms}^{-1}$$

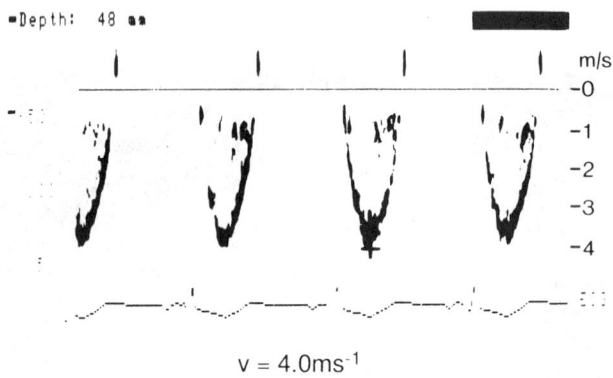

$$v = 4.0 \text{ms}^{-1}$$

Fig. 13.12 Spectral Doppler recordings of pulmonary flow from (top) a normal subject and (bottom) a patient with pulmonary valve stenosis. Time is represented along the X axis as with the ECG and velocity along the Y axis. Flow is away from the transducer and is thus represented below the base line by the U-shaped signal. The maximum velocity in the normal patient (top) is 0.8 m s⁻¹ but in the patient with pulmonary stenosis (bottom) is 4.0 ms⁻¹, equivalent to a pressure gradient of 64 mmHg.

The main clinical use of spectral Doppler ultrasound is in the assessment of the pressure drop across an obstruction or between different chambers or vessels; this allows valve gradients and pulmonary artery pressure to be calculated. It has also some application in the measurement of volumetric flow.

Pressure gradient. The pressure drop across a restrictive orifice is related to the maximum velocity across it by the modified Bernoulli equation:

$$P = 4V^2$$

where P = pressure gradient in mmHg
where V = maximum velocity in ms⁻¹.

Thus in Figure 13.12 (bottom) the maximum velocity of 4.0 m s⁻¹ is equivalent to a gradient of $4^2 \times 4$ = 64 mmHg. This can be an extremely accurate technique but may be subject to underestimation and it is not completely comparable to a gradient measured at catheterization. It should only be interpreted with full knowledge of the possible discrepancies and their significance.

Pulmonary artery systolic pressure can be estimated by application of the Bernoulli formula. Up to 80% of children with normal hearts have tricuspid regurgitation on Doppler. If the maximum velocity is measured with Doppler and translated to mmHg, this gives the pressure difference between the right ventricle and right atrium. Since the right atrial pressure is low, less than 10 mmHg, the right ventricular pressure is given by adding 10 mmHg to this value. In a ventricular septal defect the pressure drop between the ventricles can be measured. The left ventricular pressure is equivalent to the arm blood pressure. Thus the right ventricular pressure is given by the arm blood pressure minus the pressure drop across the septum. In the absence of pulmonary stenosis, which can be confirmed with Doppler, the right ventricular systolic and pulmonary artery pressures are approximately the same.

• **Volumetric flow**. The mean flow velocity can be measured from the spectral flow signal, most modern ultrasound machines having the facility to do this electronically. Theoretically, volumetric flow is then given by great artery area (measured with ultrasound) multiplied by the mean flow velocity. The major difficulty in this is accurate measurement of the area and since this is obtained by taking the great artery radius and squaring it, any error in determination of the radius is multiplied. The technique is of limited value in estimation of Qp/Qs. Doppler studies in neonates suggest a cardiac output (1 SD) of approximately 240 (±45) ml/kg/min and the technique has potential uses in intensive care (Hudson et al 1990).

Color Doppler flow mapping

Although the combination of imaging and spectral Doppler can allow the operator to determine the position from which the flow signal is obtained this is not always possible. In color Doppler flow mapping the flow velocity is measured from a number of different positions, color coded and then superimposed upon the cross-sectional image. This allows spectral Doppler to be more accurately positioned and permits areas of disturbed flow to be clearly shown and simplifies the demonstration of abnormalities that are difficult to show with imaging.

The application of imaging and Doppler to specific cardiac defects is considered with each individual lesion.

CARDIAC CATHETERIZATION

Diagnostic cardiac catheterization and angiocardiography are undertaken to obtain detailed information on the anatomical abnormality and its hemodynamic effects, such as pressure gradients, pulmonary artery pressure, shunt size and pulmonary vascular resistance. The requirement for this procedure has been reappraised in recent years with the use of ultrasound imaging to provide a basic anatomical diagnosis and the addition of Doppler ultrasound to give hemodynamic information. The indications for catheterization in different centers will depend on the availability of equipment and individual expertise with the noninvasive techniques and, most importantly, acceptance of them by the surgeons. Catheterization is increasingly undertaken not for diagnostic purposes but for treatment. Balloon dilation of the pulmonary valve (Tynan et al 1985) is an accepted technique though dilation for aortic stenosis (Bu'Lock et al 1993) and coarctation of the aorta (Rao 1995) are not universally accepted. Closure of an arterial duct (Lock et al 1987) is now an accepted routine procedure and closure of atrial (Hausdorf et al 1996) or ventricular septal defects is possible and may become the treatment of choice in certain subjects.

The procedure is performed with sedation and local anesthesia,

or general anesthesia if preferred and if facilities are available. The approach is generally percutaneous through the femoral vessels, the brachial or axillary ones occasionally being used. Arterial catheterization can frequently be avoided since the venous catheter may be passed into the left side of the heart through an atrial or ventricular septal defect, or patent foramen ovale. An atrial septostomy can be performed through the umbilical vein in the first few days of life but thereafter it becomes difficult to pass the catheter through the ductus venosus (Ashfaq et al 1991).

Catheterization should only be performed with a clear knowledge of the ultrasound and, if relevant, previous catheterization studies. The catheter course is of limited diagnostic value but, with angiography, may be important in establishing abnormal venous connections. The oxygen saturation is usually measured in the large veins, atria, ventricles and great arteries. A significant left to right shunt is suggested by a rise in oxygen saturation of 5% or more in the right atrium (atrial septal defect), right ventricle (ventricular septal defect) or pulmonary artery (ductus arteriosus). The arterial oxygen saturation gives an estimate of the severity of and the need for surgical intervention in cyanotic congenital heart disease. Systemic and pulmonary outputs can be calculated from the Fick principle and the pulmonary systemic flow ratio (Qp/Qs) is calculated from the oxygen saturation values in the aorta (Ao), pulmonary artery (PA), left atrium (LA) and the mixed venous saturation (MV) from the formula:

$$\frac{QP}{Qs} = \frac{Ao - MV}{LA - PA}$$

It must be remembered that while these figures give results sufficiently accurate for clinical management, they are not absolute values and will vary with time and hemodynamic status.

Pressures are measured in the atria, ventricles and great arteries. Mean pressure in the atria and great arteries is required for estimation of pulmonary or systemic vascular resistance and peak ones in the ventricles and arteries for measuring transvalve gradient. In children, the simple valve gradient rather than valve area is generally used in deciding on the need for surgical intervention. Pressure gradients show considerable variation with time or sedation and it now has to be considered whether a decision on the need for intervention should be based on a Doppler measurement with the patient awake rather than a lower one obtained at catheterization with the child sedated or anesthetized (Lim et al 1989).

The pulmonary vascular resistance rather than the pulmonary artery pressure is the main determinant of the prognosis and, indeed, the operability of a child with a left to right shunt. Where it is elevated it is appropriate to assess whether it is fixed or can be reduced by the administration of a pulmonary vasodilator such as 100% oxygen, tolazoline, or the newer therapies of prostacyclin or nitric oxide (Adatia & Wessel 1994).

Selective angiography is performed by the injection of radiological contrast into the chamber or vessel immediately proximal to the abnormality, e.g. left ventricle for ventricular septal defect, right ventricle for pulmonary stenosis, ascending aorta for coarctation. Angiography is now less important for the elucidation of intracardiac defects, but it remains necessary for abnormalities of the great arteries or veins, in particular the anatomy of the pulmonary artery and its branches in situations where they are reduced in size.

Although cardiac catheterization is a relatively safe procedure, death can occur, most commonly in those with severe pulmonary hypertension. Complications of catheterization include femoral artery occlusion, dysrhythmias, intramyocardial injection with pericardial effusion, cerebral embolus or thrombosis.

Interventional catheterization is now an important part of the management of heart disease in pediatrics (Bull 1986, Rao 1995). Balloon valvuloplasty is now the accepted treatment for pulmonary valve stenosis (Tynan et al 1985). It is relatively straightforward and safe and, with the exception of the dysplastic valve, effective in virtually all cases. Many centers also perform aortic valvoplasty but there is not universal agreement that this is appropriate; it may be that open surgical valvotomy will be a more precise procedure with less resulting aortic regurgitation (Bu'Lock et al 1993). Similarly, the risk of aneurysm formation following dilation of coarctation of the aorta (Wren et al 1987) has to be balanced against the relatively safe and effective surgical repair. Controlled comparative studies have not been reported but evidence suggests that balloon dilation may be equally effective (Rao 1995). Closure of an arterial duct with an 'umbrella' (Lock et al 1987) or 'coil' (Lloyd et al 1993) device is now accepted though long-term results are awaited. Catheter closure of atrial (Hausdorf et al 1996) or ventricular septal defects can be effective but detailed evaluation of the clinical place awaits further study. Interventional cardiology can be of value in patients with distal pulmonary narrowing. Where surgical intervention is difficult, stent placement may allow the narrowed area to be opened up. This is usually undertaken percutaneously but in some smaller subjects can be done as an intraoperative procedure (Mendelsohn et al 1993).

THE ASYMPTOMATIC CHILD WITH A MURMUR

The incidental finding of a murmur in an asymptomatic child is relatively common. The physician must then decide whether the child has:

1. a heart defect of hemodynamic significance, possibly needing surgical intervention and thus requiring referral to a pediatric cardiologist at that time or subsequently
2. a heart defect of little hemodynamic significance requiring only antibiotic prophylaxis against endocarditis and possible follow-up at infrequent intervals
3. an innocent murmur not requiring antibiotic prophylaxis or follow-up.

With a hemodynamically significant defect it is likely that either the murmur will be loud (semilunar valve stenosis), or there will be other abnormal physical signs as outlined for the individual defects. There is more difficulty in differentiating the soft murmur of a minor cardiac defect from an innocent one. In most cases where there is this uncertainty there will be no other physical findings and chest X-ray, electrocardiogram and echocardiogram will be normal, the only useful investigation being Doppler ultrasound.

A 'functional' rather than an 'innocent' murmur is usually heard at the aortic area as the result of a high output state, such as fever or anemia, in which there is no abnormality of cardiac structure.

THE INNOCENT MURMUR

An innocent murmur is a frequent finding in normal children and has been reported in over 90% of healthy children in one study

(Lessop & Brigden 1957). The diagnosis is made on the basis of its characteristic features after a significant defect has been excluded by the absence of other physical signs. Particular attention should be paid to ensuring that the femoral pulses are normal, that there is no parasternal or apical impulse, and that the second heart sound is not accentuated and is variably split. Innocent murmurs, with the exception of the venous hum, are early to midsystolic in timing, are soft (grade 2 or less), and are often altered by change in the patient's position. In addition, the murmur has specific characteristics which allow positive, rather than negative, identification that it is innocent (Zuberbuhler 1981, Coleman & Doig 1970).

Still's murmur

This murmur was first described in 1909 but its cause is as yet uncertain. It is the most common of innocent murmurs, is midsystolic, and of maximum intensity in the mid to lower left sternal edge with radiation towards the apex and occasionally to the base. Like all murmurs it is difficult to describe in words and an indication of this is given by the fact that it has been variously described as vibratory, buzzing, groaning, or twanging string. Although experience suggests its nature, it is not always possible to distinguish it from a small ventricular septal defect.

Carotid bruit

A carotid bruit is almost equally common. It is thought to arise in the carotid or subclavian arteries, is midsystolic in timing, and is best heard in the neck just above the clavicle, often radiating down to the aortic area. It should not be confused with aortic stenosis in which the murmur is louder below the clavicle than above.

Pulmonary flow murmur

An early to midsystolic murmur can often be heard at the upper left sternal edge, originating from flow through the pulmonary valve, and may raise the possibility of mild valve stenosis. In addition, in the first few months of life in premature infants a soft ejection murmur can be heard at the base with radiation into the axillae and even the back. This originates in the proximal pulmonary artery branches, disappears before 1 year of age, and does not represent true branch stenosis.

Venous hum

A venous hum is a continuous murmur heard at the base of the heart which is usually maximal just under the clavicle and radiates both above and below it. It is more often heard in the right than left side and most easily when the patient is upright, usually a toddler examined on the mother's knee. It can be identified (and distinguished from an arterial duct) by the demonstration that it disappears or is of altered intensity when the child lies flat or the neck is turned or gently compressed.

Apical murmur

An apical high pitched 'musical' midsystolic murmur may occur with little radiation to either the axilla or sternal edge.

Investigations

In the child with no other physical sign than a probable innocent murmur the chest X-ray is of little use and may simply subject the child to unnecessary exposure to radiation. An electrocardiogram is a worthwhile investigation and is of particular help with a basal murmur, where an RSR′ pattern will suggest an atrial septal defect which can, on occasions, be difficult to recognize clinically. Imaging echocardiography is also likely to be normal since it cannot detect a small ventricular septal defect or mild valve abnormalities. If there is doubt, Doppler ultrasound is a most useful investigation; it can be used to detect abnormal flow patterns associated with left to right shunts and valve regurgitation or stenosis. However, this technique is so sensitive that it can reveal abnormalities not detected clinically and full assessment of the patient requires consideration of clinical, electrocardiography and ultrasound findings. A normal Doppler study excludes virtually all minor cardiac defects. The parents can then be given a clear diagnosis and reassurance.

The use of sophisticated ultrasound techniques including Doppler has failed to determine the origin of the innocent murmur. Although there is a weak relationship to the presence of left ventricular muscle bands, heart rate and great artery flow velocity (Gardiner & Joffe 1991) further study is still required.

Management

For practical purposes a pediatrician has to decide whether the child requires referral to a pediatric cardiologist and, if not, whether there is need for antibiotic prophylaxis against infective endocarditis. When a child is seen in infancy it is worthwhile reassessing the situation at about 1 year of age. Thereafter, if the child is well, acyanotic with no other physical signs, growing satisfactorily, and the electrocardiogram shows no abnormality, it is unlikely that referral is necessary at that stage. If there is uncertainty such that subsequent follow-up necessitates attendance every 3–6 months it must be recognized that the physician has little confidence in his assessment and referral to a cardiologist might be appropriate. A cardiologist has the advantage not only of experience and knowledge, but also access to noninvasive assessment which can usually elucidate the exact anatomical and hemodynamic effects of a lesion of uncertain clinical significance. Echocardiographic study without assessment by a cardiologist is not appropriate or cost effective (Danford et al 1993). When the murmur is innocent, firm reassurance of the parents is necessary. It may be more reassuring to use the term 'normal' rather than 'innocent' murmur (Perloff 1987). The parents should be told that these murmurs may come and go and be heard at one examination and not at the next and vice versa, but it is of no relevance whether it is or is not heard at any individual examination.

When surgical intervention will be required and facilities are available this is undertaken in the early years in most lesions. The main exception is aortic stenosis which is almost the only situation in which long-term follow-up is usually necessary to decide the appropriate time for surgery. On the other hand there may be congenital heart disease which is not likely to require surgery, e.g. small ventricular septal defect. Antibiotic prophylaxis against infective endocarditis should be recommended, and depending on local circumstances, hospital follow-up may be indicated at annual or biannual intervals, simply to avoid further

worry when the murmur is subsequently heard at routine general practitioner or community clinical examinations.

CONGENITAL HEART DISEASE

INCIDENCE

The incidence of congenital heart disease is reported to be between 6 and 8 per 1000 live births with a higher rate in spontaneous abortions and stillbirths (approximately 1/10) (Hoffman & Christianson 1978). Differences in reported frequencies in different studies are likely to be due to the means of ascertaining and reporting the nature of defects, particularly the less severe ones. With the use of Doppler ultrasound, which allows exact noninvasive diagnosis of minor lesions not requiring surgery, it is likely that higher rates will be reported in the future. There is no certain evidence of racial differences in the incidence rate of congenital cardiac defects, although some differences in the type of lesion do occur (Fixler et al 1993). The relative frequency of the most common lesions varies with different reports, but some idea of this is given in Table 13.2 modified from the experience in Liverpool, England (Dickinson et al 1981).

The outlook for the infant and child with congenital heart disease depends on the nature and severity of the lesion, the presence of associated abnormalities, and the availability of surgical expertise. Some deaths are not the direct result of the cardiac lesion but are attributable to extracardiac malformations which occur with increased incidence in those with congenital heart disease. The mortality rate for untreated congenital heart disease is high, and prior to the introduction of modern surgery, a study of babies born live with heart disease reported that up to one-third would die from cardiac causes within the first month of life and 60% before the end of the first year (Macmahon et al 1953). Even now, 15–20% of those recognized to have heart disease in infancy die within the first year of life. However, figures for the total group have little practical meaning. Early deaths are related to the complexity of the defects, being uncommon in acyanotic lesions with the exception of coarctation of the aorta and atrioventricular septal defect, and more common in cyanotic lesions, though the outlook for many of these is now

Table 13.2 Most common congenital cardiac defects as a percentage of the total (from Dickinson et al 1981)

	%
Acyanotic lesions	
Ventricular septal defect	32
Arterial duct	12
Pulmonary stenosis	8
Coarctation of the aorta	6
Atrial septal defect	6
Aortic stenosis	5
Atrioventricular septal defect	2
Total	71
Cyanotic lesions	
Tetralogy of Fallot	6
Transposition of the great arteries	5
Single ventricle (including tricuspid atresia)	4
Hypoplastic left heart syndrome	3
Total anomalous pulmonary venous drainage	1
Truncus arteriosus	1
Total	21

good. Without surgical treatment most patients with cyanotic congenital heart disease will die in infancy or early childhood. Those who survive longer frequently have good mixing of systemic and pulmonary venous returns and moderate pulmonary stenosis which, while protecting the lungs from increased flow and the development of pulmonary vascular disease, is not so severe that the patient becomes very hypoxic.

The majority of those who have undergone successful surgical palliation or repair will remain well throughout childhood, but the prognosis for later life will not become clear until long-term studies become available.

ETIOLOGY

Environmental, genetic or multifactorial causes can be implicated as the cause of congenital heart disease, but with the exception of chromosomal abnormalities a specific etiologic factor is rarely identified.

Chromosomal abnormalities

There is a high incidence of cardiac defects in patients with trisomy 21, 13 or 18. Indeed it has been reported (Kenna et al 1975) that trisomy 21 accounts for 5% of all those with congenital heart disease. There appears to be no difference whether the chromosome abnormality is due to trisomy, translocation or mosaicism. Up to 40% of those with Down syndrome can have a cardiac defect, with atrioventricular septal defect and ventricular septal defect accounting for approximately 80% of lesions. It may thus be appropriate to undertake echocardiographic examination in all newborn infants with Down syndrome, even with apparently no clinical or electrocardiographic abnormalities; the presence or absence of congenital heart disease can then be considered in giving the parents a detailed account of likely management problems. Some physicians and surgeons have reservations about operating on cardiac defects in children with Down syndrome. Local facilities and circumstances must of course be considered, but if treatment is available it seems illogical to manage children with Down syndrome differently as they can look forward to many years of life. If they are physically incapacitated their quality of life will be diminished and the burden on those looking after them increased.

Cardiac defects are common in trisomy 18 (Edwards' syndrome) and 13 (Patau's syndrome). In both conditions the majority die early and since the few longer term survivors are severely retarded, surgical treatment will be indicated only in exceptional circumstances. Turner's syndrome, 45XO, has a clear association with left heart lesions with coarctation of the aorta being recognized in approximately 10% of cases.

Cardiac defects have been recognized with other rarer autosomal abnormalities causing low birthweight, mental retardation, small stature and dysmorphic features. It is thus appropriate to perform chromosomal analysis on infants with congenital heart disease with other malformations or marked dysmorphic features, or older children with significant developmental delay.

Single gene defects

Single gene defects are not a common association with heart disease but are increasingly being identified, and reviews of the subject have been published (Johnson et al 1995). Pompe's disease (p. 1138), which causes cardiomyopathy, has an autosomal recessive inheritance. Marfan's syndrome (p. 1587) has an autosomal dominant inheritance but frequently occurs with reduced expression in the parents or as a new mutation. Noonan's syndrome, which is most frequently associated with pulmonary valve or artery stenosis, has an autosomal dominant inheritance but since it is associated with decreased fertility most cases are due to new mutations. The abnormality resulting from deletion within chromosome 22 has been named the CATCH 22 syndrome: cardiac defects, abnormal facies, thymic aplasia, cleft palate, hypocalcemia. The cardiac defects take the form of conotruncal abnormalities and it is now recognized that DiGeorge syndrome is an extreme example and almost always results from a 22q11 deletion (Wilson D et al 1993).

Teratogens

In early pregnancy, maternal infection, illness or ingestion of certain drugs can result in cardiovascular abnormality. The clearest association is with the congenital rubella syndrome in which over one-third of patients have a cardiovascular malformation, most frequently peripheral pulmonary stenosis or an arterial duct. There is also an increased incidence (up to 4%) of a variety of lesions in the offspring of diabetic mothers, with the risk being minimized by good control of the diabetes in early pregnancy. Similarly, uncontrolled maternal phenylketonuria is associated with heart defects in 25–50% and a low phenylalanine diet should be introduced as early as possible, ideally before conception.

Maternal ingestion of some therapeutic drugs has been implicated in the cause of congenital heart disease. This has most frequently been reported with lithium (Ebstein's anomaly), phenytoin (semilunar valve stenosis, coarctation, arterial duct) and isotretinoin (Lammer et al 1985). Cardiac defects are recognized as a feature of the fetal alcohol syndrome (Beattie et al 1983) and in certain areas alcohol may be the commonest teratogenic factor.

Syndromes

Cardiac defects occur in a large number of syndromes, but, with the exceptions already discussed, they make a minor contribution to the incidence and prevalence of congenital heart disease. Other relatively common associations are de Lange (VSD, p. 830), Williams (supravalvar aortic stenosis, p. 833), Friedreich's ataxia (hypertrophic cardiomyopathy, p. 764), Jervell and Lange-Nielsen (prolonged QT, p. 626), Holt–Oram (atrial septal defect, p. 1546) and VATERL (VSD, p. 75).

Polygenic inheritance

It is often considered that congenital heart disease is due to polygenic or multifactorial inheritance in which as yet unknown inherited and environmental factors combine to cause the malformation. The polygenic model for inheritance of congenital heart disease has been supported by the correspondence between the theoretical predicted and reported recurrence risk for first degree relatives. However, the relatively high incidence in the offspring of those with significant congenital heart disease who now survive into adult life may indicate a greater importance for a single gene defect.

RECURRENCE RISK

Recurrence risk for a cardiac defect depends on the nature of the lesion and relationship of the affected person. The risk for another pregnancy rises to about 2% if one previous child is affected; this tends to be highest (3%) for VSD, arterial duct, and atrioventricular septal defect (Nora & Nora 1988). There is a tendency for a related anomaly to recur but this is not necessarily the case. If two previous children are affected the risk rises to 6–8% and recent studies of the offspring of parents with congenital heart disease have indicated a similar risk if the father has congenital heart disease. However, if the mother is affected there is an even higher risk (5–15%) depending on the lesion.

In counseling parents, consideration has to be given to known recurrence risks and exposure to possible teratogens, though this is rarely found. It is important to reassure them that there is no clearly known cause and that they have no reason to blame themselves. Fetal echocardiography provides an accurate means of diagnosing fetal cardiac abnormalities from about 18 weeks' gestation (Allan et al 1984). In the majority there will be no defect and the mother can be reassured. However, the implications for finding a defect, with the possibility of offering termination for severe defects, are major and should be discussed with the parents before the examination is carried out.

NOMENCLATURE OF CONGENITAL HEART DISEASE

The majority of congenital cardiovascular lesions can be regarded as simple and described as such, e.g. atrial septal defect or aortic valve stenosis. However, there can be difficulty in understanding the anatomical nature of complex cardiac abnormalities and this has been compounded by the extensive use of different terminology by different authors. Although a detailed understanding of congenital heart disease requires a thorough knowledge of cardiac morphology, a simple and useful approach is to regard the heart as having three basic components or segments – the atrial chambers, the ventricular mass, and the arterial trunks. If the nature, connections and relationships of these can be determined then the cornerstone of any malformed heart is in position (Anderson & Ho 1986, Anderson et al 1987). This approach is now generally accepted by most pediatric cardiologists and surgeons and is known as *sequential segmental analysis*. The basis of this analysis is the determination of how each of the three basic components or segments of the heart are connected. It is the type and mode of connection which determines the physiological derangement and the surgical approach if operation is required. It is usual firstly to determine the arrangement and connections of the atrial chambers and then to analyze the atrioventricular and ventriculoarterial junction. Any associated cardiac malformations are then catalogued, including any anomalous position of the heart itself.

Atrial arrangement

The atrial arrangement or situs has first to be determined. This does not always follow the situs of the abdominal viscera but usually that of the thoracic viscera and thus the bronchial morphology. The atrial position can therefore be inferred from analysis of the bronchial anatomy on X-ray, in particular with a penetrated film. The right main bronchus is more vertical and shorter than the left, branching above the lower lobe pulmonary artery while the left branches below it. The right atrium lies on the same side as the right bronchus. The usual atrial arrangement is described as *solitus* and its mirror image as *inversus*. When the atrial situs is uncertain it is frequently called *ambiguous* but in most cases careful analysis shows bilateral manifestations of right or left atrial morphology, which can then be described as right or left atrial *isomerism*. In the former, asplenia is the usual association and in the latter, polysplenia. Atrial arrangement or situs is summarized as follows:

solitus:	right atrium on right, left atrium on left
inversus:	left atrium on right, right atrium on left
isomerism – right:	bilateral right atria
isomerism – left:	bilateral left atria
ambiguous:	used if arrangement cannot be identified.

Atrioventricular connection

The atrioventricular connection then describes the way the atria communicate with the ventricles at the atrioventricular junction. If the connections follow the normal pattern they are said to be *concordant*, e.g. right atrium to right ventricle and left atrium to left ventricle, but *discordant* atria connect with the contralateral ventricle. When both atrioventricular valves enter one ventricular chamber, the connection is described as *double inlet* and if one or other atria is not directly connected to a ventricle, then that atrioventricular connection is said to be *absent*. Occasionally it may not be possible to state exactly the atrioventricular connection which is then described as *ambiguous*. These are summarized as follows:

concordant:	right atrium to right ventricle, left atrium to left ventricle
discordant:	right atrium to left ventricle, left atrium to right ventricle
ambiguous:	with atrial isomerism and one atrium entering each ventricle
double inlet:	both atria connect to the same ventricle
absent right or left:	no true or potential connection from the right or left atrium to a ventricle.

Ventriculoarterial connection

This describes the means by which the great arteries take origin from the ventricular chambers. If an artery overrides the septum, and thus arises from both ventricles, it is assigned to that from which more than half takes origin. Connections can thus be:

concordant:	pulmonary trunk from right ventricle, aorta from left
discordant:	aorta from right ventricle, pulmonary trunk from left
double outlet:	both great arteries from one ventricle
single outlet:	single great artery.

Three further steps are then necessary to complete the analysis: a statement of the relationship of structures; tabulation of associated lesions; and description of the cardiac position within the chest.

Relationships

These are described in simple spatial terms, such as right/left, anterior/posterior, superior/inferior, side by side. These relationships neither imply nor give any information on morphology or connections.

Additional abnormalities

These will include factors such as venous drainage, septal defects, stenosis or atresia of valves, and great artery anomalies such as coarctation.

Cardiac position

Abnormalities of cardiac position are discussed on page 612. When the heart is on the left side this is not usually stated if there is situs solitus, but should be described as levocardia where there is an abnormal situs. Dextrocardia simply describes the situation in which more than half of the cardiac shadow on X-ray is in the right side of the chest; it has no implications and makes no assumptions as to the atrial situs or intracardiac anatomy. Mesocardia is used when the heart appears to be in the center of the thorax.

Comment

To a physician who largely deals with more minor abnormalities this nomenclature may seem complicated and it is not required in the majority of patients who have normal chamber connections, morphology and relations. However, it greatly simplifies assessment and description of complex defects and prevents any ambiguity in communication between different cardiologists and surgeons. It is clear that such a detailed description is not required for most defects and in some of the less complex ones it is still appropriate to use the terms which have been in use for some time (such as transposition of the great arteries, tricuspid atresia), providing everyone in the group dealing with the patient agrees upon and understands these descriptions. Thus atrial situs solitus, atrioventricular concordance and ventriculoarterial discordance are understood as transposition of the great arteries.

MEDICAL CARE OF CONGENITAL HEART DISEASE

The treatment of significant congenital heart disease largely depends upon surgical expertise, and the surgical approaches to the infant or child with a cardiac defect are well established (Cohen 1992). The cardiologist will now use interventional catheterization techniques to undertake corrective procedures for some less complex lesions but otherwise the role of the physician is to provide general medical care, use the appropriate investigations to make an accurate diagnosis, and refer the patient to the surgeon at the appropriate time. There are some aspects of medical care which are worthy of individual consideration; the newborn infant, prostaglandin therapy, cardiac failure, and the management of arrhythmias (p. 626).

THE NEWBORN INFANT WITH CONGENITAL HEART DISEASE (see also Ch. 5)

The patient with congenital heart disease who survives beyond infancy has a relatively good outlook, with surgery generally carrying a low risk. However, even with modern surgery, up to 15–20% of liveborn children in whom a defect is recognized in infancy can die in the first year of life, usually in the early weeks or months. Thus the management of the newborn infant with heart disease is a major challenge to the pediatric cardiologist and

cardiac surgeon. The infant with congenital heart disease can show rapid progression to the stage of severe cardiac failure or cyanosis with hypoxia and acidosis. It is therefore essential that signs of heart disease are recognized as early as possible and the infant immediately referred to a center with full facilities for cardiac investigation and treatment.

Heart disease in the newborn is usually recognized by the presence of cyanosis or heart failure. Early detection of cyanotic heart disease is frequently difficult and has been discussed under General Examination (p. 30). The hyperoxic test is useful where there is uncertainty as to the diagnosis of congenital heart disease. It cannot always make a certain differentiation between heart and lung disease but in response to hyperoxia (80–100% oxygen) a PO_2 of over 150 mmHg (21 kPa) from the upper body excludes a major right to left shunt and a failure to rise suggests a cardiac defect. The most important early signs of heart failure are tachycardia (>160/min), tachypnea (>50/min) and hepatomegaly (General Examination, p. 30). Palpation of the pulses must include comparison of not only the right arm and the leg pulse but also the pulses in both arms. With coarctation of the aorta or hypoplastic left heart syndrome the femoral pulses may feel normal initially when the ductus is open. Low volume pulses occur with obstruction to left ventricular output such as hypoplastic left heart syndrome or severe aortic stenosis. A parasternal or subxiphoid heave may indicate the presence of a significant defect in a patient where there is no abnormality on auscultation. A single second heart sound should be considered abnormal after the first day of life. Gallop rhythm indicates cardiac failure. Many infants with significant heart disease have no murmur and when a murmur is heard it is often not diagnostic but merely suggests the presence of an underlying defect.

The ECG is often difficult to interpret in the first few days of life when right ventricular dominance is the normal finding and an infant with severe congenital heart disease can have a normal ECG. A straight chest X-ray is useful. When primary lung disease mimics heart disease this will generally be recognized. The contour of the heart and the great arteries and the effect of the anatomical abnormality on the pulmonary vascularity will generally be apparent, but typical appearances are not always found. A large thymus may cause difficulty in interpretation of the cardiac silhouette and increased pulmonary blood flow is not always reflected in the X-ray appearances. Echocardiography usually provides an accurate and detailed diagnosis and catheterization is usually only required for interventional procedures such as atrial septostomy. This is easily performed through the umbilical vein within the first 2 days of life.

Transfer to the cardiac centers should be as rapid as possible in a suitable transport incubator. General care of temperature, acidosis and electrolyte imbalance is essential.

Prostaglandin therapy

The use of E-type prostaglandins to dilate the ductus arteriosus is an essential part in the management of the newborn infant with a ductus dependent circulation. This occurs either when there is marked obstruction to pulmonary blood flow (such as pulmonary atresia) or an aortic arch abnormality (such as critical aortic stenosis or coarctation). Prostaglandin E_2, which is readily available in most obstetric hospitals, is cheaper than prostaglandin E_1, and equally effective (Olley et al 1976). Prostaglandins should be administered as a peripheral venous infusion, a suitable initial rate being 0.02 µg/kg/min with the dose being increased up to 0.05–0.10 µg/kg/min depending on the clinical response. The most serious complication of prostaglandin therapy is respiratory depression, but this is usually dose dependent with normal respiration rapidly returning when the infusion is stopped. It should then be restarted at a reduced dosage. Other well recognized side-effects include fever, tachycardia and jitteriness.

HEART FAILURE

The term heart failure describes the signs and symptoms which result from the inability of the heart adequately to deal with the venous return and maintain the cardiac output. Reviews of the pathophysiology and management have been published (Wilson N 1994). Cardiac failure in older children is relatively uncommon, usually results from acquired heart disease, and exhibits the clinical features of left or right heart failure as in the adult. Heart failure is more common with congenital heart disease and almost always occurs in the first few months of life, the commonest signs being tachycardia, tachypnea and hepatomegaly.

In infants combined ventricular failure occurs, with the first manifestations usually resulting from pulmonary venous congestion which produces tachypnea or dyspnea, more marked on feeding. Crepitations are not often heard. At this age cardiac failure does not produce marked edema though some facial puffiness or pitting of the dorsal surfaces of the hands or feet may develop. Hepatomegaly is a prominent finding, liver size providing an indication of its severity. Sweating at rest or on exertion may develop and chronic cardiac failure may cause feeding difficulties and growth retardation. Gallop rhythm may be detected by auscultation.

Investigation of the child with cardiac failure should be directed at determining its cause. Electrocardiography is of limited value. Chest X-ray will almost always show cardiomegaly and lung fields increased flow or venous obstruction. Kerley B lines are rare in young subjects. A small heart with increased lung markings in an infant with cardiac failure suggests a diagnosis of obstructed total anomalous pulmonary venous drainage.

The treatment of heart failure is directed at improving myocardial contractility, increasing the elimination of sodium, and undertaking general supportive measures. Diuretics are the mainstay of treatment of cardiac failure. The most widely used is frusemide in a dose of 2–3 mg/kg/24 h. Potassium depletion is not a common effect of oral frusemide therapy in infants and children but levels should be checked periodically and potassium supplements given for long-term therapy. If further diuretic therapy is required one acting at a different site in the renal tubule should be added. Spironolactone with its antialdosterone effects is a logical choice and some would suggest it be instituted before or with frusemide (Wilson N 1994), the initial dose being 2–3 mg/kg/24 h and any potassium supplementation stopped. Questions have been raised as to the efficacy of digoxin which has long been used for its positive inotropic effect, but it is now known also to reduce vascular tone. It can be of benefit where there is poor ventricular function, but it is of doubtful value in situations with volume overload, such as ventricular septal defect (Salmon et al 1989). Digoxin should be given as an initial loading dose over 24 h (as four divided doses) followed by a daily maintenance dose of about one-quarter of the loading dose in two divided doses daily.

A suitable initial loading dosage regime is:

preterm infant	20–30 µg/kg i.m.

with an oral dose in older children as follows:

term infant	50–70 µg/kg
1 month–2 years	60–80 µg/kg
over 2 years	40–60 µg/kg

with the parenteral dose being 75% of the loading dose.

Signs of toxicity are difficult to detect in infants, but will be suggested by vomiting and nausea in older subjects. The significance of blood levels in infancy is uncertain.

Cardiac failure from any cause results in neuroendocrine effects, with sympathetic stimulation and activation of the renin–angiotensin–aldosterone system (RAAS). The former produces increase in vascular tone (afterload) and thus increased work for the systemic ventricle, while angiotensin II increases vascular tone (afterload) and aldosterone increases water and salt retention and thus increases venous filling (preload). Angiotensin converting enzyme (ACE) inhibitors (captopril or enalapril) are widely used in heart failure in adults and can also be beneficial in congenital heart defects. These prevent the conversion of angiotensin I to angiotensin II and thus decrease vascular resistance and sodium and water retention. The reduction in vascular tone facilitates left ventricular function in cardiomyopathy and in VSD theoretically reduces the left to right shunt by reducing the systemic and thus left ventricular pressure. ACE inhibitors can be particularly helpful in conditions with diminished left ventricular function such as dilated cardiomyopathy, and may be of some value with volume overload. It is recommended that the starting dose of captopril should be 0.1 mg/kg three times daily up to a maximum of 2 mg/kg three times daily. Observation is required for possible hypotension immediately after the initial dose.

In an intensive care setting drug therapy with a number of other agents may be beneficial. Dopamine is given intravenously in an initial dosage of 2–10 µg/kg/min. Nitroprusside acts as an intravenous vasodilator which, by reducing systemic vascular resistance, and thus left ventricle afterload, can be useful in some cases. Hydralazine can be given parenterally in a dose of 0.25–0.5 mg/kg statim then 0.1–0.2 mg/kg/dose 4–6 hourly. It can also be used as an oral vasodilator in less acute cases, using doses of 0.2 mg/kg increasing gradually up to a maximum of 2.0 mg/kg twice daily.

A common problem with cardiac failure over a long period is the management of the infant who feeds poorly and fails to gain weight. Nasogastric tube feeding is often required and high calorie supplements should be added to the feeds (Unger et al 1992). However, cardiac failure is usually the result of an anatomical abnormality and if the infant does not improve and infant surgery is available it is not usually appropriate to persist with medical treatment. Surgical repair or palliation should be undertaken early rather than delay and risk deterioration in the infant's condition.

ACYANOTIC HEART DISEASE WITH ARTERIOVENOUS SHUNT

Ventricular septal defect

Anatomy

Ventricular septal defect is the most common congenital heart lesion, occurring in isolation in about 25% and in association with

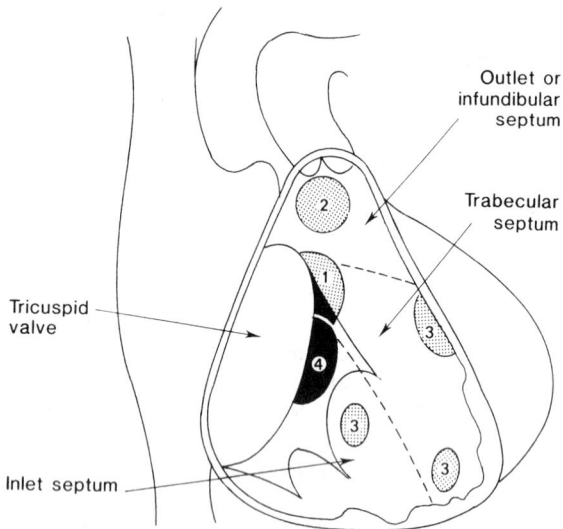

Fig. 13.13 Types of ventricular septal defect: (1) perimembranous; (2) outlet or subarterial; (3) muscular; (4) inlet.

other lesions in another 25% of patients with congenital cardiac malformations. Ventricular septal defects are usually classified according to their positions in the interventricular septum (Fig. 13.13). The commonest defect is in the membranous septum, usually extending into the muscular septum and thus termed a perimembranous ventricular septal defect. Inlet ventricular septal defects (the atrioventricular canal type) involve the inlet portion of the muscular septum and are usually an extension of a perimembranous defect. Muscular defects have entirely muscular rims and can be found in the inlet, trabecular or infundibular septum. Outlet (subarterial, subpulmonary or supracristal) defects involve the infundibular septum and are roofed by the contiguous aortic and pulmonary valves. Multiple defects may be present.

Physiology

The volume of the shunt across a ventricular septal defect depends on the size of the defect and the pulmonary vascular resistance. Since the latter is high at birth, the shunt is absent or minimal and the presence of the defect may not be recognized. With fall in the pulmonary vascular resistance flow across the ventricular septal defect occurs. The resultant increase in pulmonary blood flow in turn delays the normal postnatal fall of pulmonary vascular resistance so that the maximal shunting, and hence a hemodynamic disturbance, may not appear until several weeks after birth. Thus symptoms of a ventricular septal defect are not usually apparent until 3–6 weeks of age.

With large defects increased pulmonary blood flow and venous return to the left heart causes left atrial and left ventricular dilation and hypertrophy. Right ventricular hypertrophy will occur if the large pulmonary flow produces increased pulmonary artery pressure. With a large left to right shunt the pulmonary vascular resistance gradually increases and thet changes may become irreversible if the ventricular septal defect is not closed. On the other hand, defects may be so small that little shunting occurs. Spontaneous closure frequently occurs, mostly in the first 5 years of life. Even defects which cause congestive heart failure may close. Muscular defects are more likely and subarterial defects less likely to close spontaneously (Moe & Guntheroth 1987). A

pouch of the adherent tissue, often called aneurysm of the membranous septum or ventricular septal aneurysm, is frequently seen in perimembranous defects which close or reduce in size spontaneously.

Aortic regurgitation may develop in subarterial or perimembranous defects, usually due to prolapse of an aortic cusp into the defect which may become partially or even completely occluded. Aortic regurgitation often begins in adolescence and because of the risk of progression and increased incidence of infective endocarditis, surgical closure of the defect is indicated when significant regurgitation appears even in the presence of only a small left to right shunt (Leung et al 1987).

Acquired right ventricular outflow tract obstruction may develop in some patients with ventricular septal defects due to infundibular muscle hypertrophy, and serves as a natural protection from flooding of the lungs. Mild infundibular obstruction regresses with closure of the ventricular septal defect but it may progress and produce clinical features mimicking tetralogy of Fallot.

Clinical features

Symptoms and signs depend on the size of the left to right shunt across the ventricular septal defect. Large defects are usually manifest in early infancy, especially during the second or third month of life when the pulmonary vascular resistance drops and the pulmonary blood flow increases. Dyspnea at rest or during feeding and excessive sweating are the earliest symptoms, followed by failure to thrive or congestive heart failure. Recurrent respiratory tract infections are common and often precipitate acute deterioration in symptoms. As pulmonary hypertension develops and restricts pulmonary flow, improvement in the general condition of the child occurs, usually towards the end of the first year. If the ventricular septal defect is not closed progressive pulmonary vascular disease will develop and symptoms of reversed shunting or right heart failure will appear later in life. Small ventricular septal defects remain asymptomatic throughout life and are recognized incidentally by the presence of a murmur.

Clinical examination of the older infant or toddler with a large ventricular septal defect usually reveals a thin, dyspneic patient with a bulging precordium more prominent on the left side, and presence of the Harrison sulcus. Active cardiac pulsations may be seen over the left chest and epigastric region. The pulses are usually normal but may be weak in the presence of large left to right shunts or heart failure. Cardiomegaly is always present. The apex beat is well localized and thrusting, suggesting left ventricular hypertrophy. A left parasternal heave may also be palpable when pulmonary hypertension or infundibular stenosis is present. A systolic thrill may be felt over the lower left sternal border. The second heart sound is loud when pulmonary hypertension is present. There is typically a harsh, loud, pansystolic murmur widely conducted over the precordium, usually maximal over the lower left sternal border but higher with subarterial defects. A soft mid-diastolic murmur over the apex results from increased volume mitral flow representing relative mitral stenosis and is heard in patients with large left to right shunts. With small restrictive ventricular septal defects precordial findings are usually normal apart from a pansystolic murmur and possibly a systolic thrill. The murmur becomes ejection systolic and soft when the defect is very small.

In patients with severe pulmonary hypertension cardiomegaly is mild and a right ventricular impulse is dominant. The murmur becomes soft, midsystolic and is best heard over the second left intercostal space. The second heart sound is loud and there is sometimes an ejection click and a soft early diastolic murmur of pulmonary regurgitation. Cyanosis is a late feature of severe pulmonary vascular disease. On the other hand, presence of a right ventricular impulse and a soft second heart sound suggest coexisting or acquired right ventricular outflow tract obstruction.

Aortic regurgitation should be sought in the older child, especially one with a subarterial ventricular septal defect, and is detected by the appearance of a high pitch early diastolic murmur over the right upper or left middle sternal border.

Investigations

The chest X-ray is normal at birth but in large defects shows progressive cardiomegaly and pulmonary plethora as the left to right shunt increases. As pulmonary hypertension develops the pulmonary trunk becomes disproportionately dilated, and with severe pulmonary vascular disease the peripheral branches become less prominent ('peripheral pruning'). The heart size decreases as pulmonary blood flow reduces either due to increasing pulmonary vascular resistance or reduction in size of the defect. Late enlargement of the heart suggests aortic regurgitation or right heart failure.

The electrocardiogram is normal in small ventricular septal defects. Where there is a large shunt it characteristically shows left ventricular hypertrophy and, when pulmonary hypertension develops, right ventricular hypertrophy. Left axis deviation is seen in inlet or multiple defects. Progressive right ventricular hypertrophy and loss of left ventricular hypertrophy occurs with development of severe pulmonary vascular disease or right ventricular outflow tract obstruction.

Cross-sectional echocardiography permits visualization of the site of most ventricular septal defects (Sutherland et al 1982), septal aneurysm, right ventricular outflow tract obstruction, and prolapse of the aortic valve. Measurement of the left ventricular and atrial sizes reflects the magnitude of the left to right shunt. Small defects which are not visible can be demonstrated by Doppler studies. The pulmonary artery pressure can be estimated noninvasively by Doppler measurement of the pressure gradient between the left and right ventricles (Houston et al 1988).

At cardiac catheterization measurement is made of the increase in oxygen saturation in the right ventricle and the pulmonary artery pressure for calculation of pulmonary blood flow and vascular resistance. Angiocardiography in the left ventricle delineates the position, size and number of ventricular septal defects. Right ventricular or aortic angiography may be necessary when right ventricular outflow tract obstruction or aortic regurgitation has developed.

Treatment and prognosis

Small ventricular septal defects do not need any treatment and most are expected to close spontaneously. Antibiotic prophylaxis against infective endocarditis is required as long as the defect is present.

Symptomatic infants should receive medical treatment since spontaneous closure of large defects can take place. Evidence suggests that digoxin has no beneficial effect (Salmon et al 1989) and may reduce feeding intake. Diuretics and ACE inhibitors are the mainstay of medical management. Infants who still have intractable heart failure, failure to thrive, or recurrent respiratory tract complications should be operated upon before excessive wasting occurs. Where facilities for infant surgery are available,

primary repair of the defect is preferred to banding of the pulmonary artery followed by repair at a later age. Pulmonary artery banding may, however, be appropriate if such facilities are not available or there are multiple defects.

Patients who do not require operation in early infancy should be assessed at about 1 year for the development of pulmonary hypertension. In the second year of life surgery is certainly indicated if the pulmonary pressure is 75% or more of the systemic pressure and often at lower levels; any pulmonary vascular disease at this age is expected to regress after the defect is closed. To prevent further progress of pulmonary vascular disease closure is appropriate at 4–5 years of age for those with less marked pulmonary hypertension in whom the pulmonary arterial pressure is still elevated in the presence of left to right shunting. Some would undertake closure at 4–5 years in the absence of pulmonary hypertension if the shunt is more than 2 : 1, on the basis that it is unlikely that spontaneous closure of such defects will occur. Others might adopt an expectant policy. Defects with smaller shunt ratios are managed conservatively.

When a large defect has escaped earlier detection and severe pulmonary hypertension has developed, careful assessment of the pulmonary vascular resistance and its reversibility is essential before surgery can be considered (see Pulmonary Hypertension, p. 606). Patients who have developed significant infundibular stenosis or aortic regurgitation should be operated to prevent progression of these lesions.

Operative mortality for ventricular septal defects is low and most infants who have undergone surgery become asymptomatic and regain normal growth. Persistent pulmonary vascular disease is rare if pulmonary hypertension is detected early and repair of the ventricular septal defect performed before 12–18 months of age. Interventional closure is possible for some defects, particularly in the muscular septum, but experience of this is limited and long-term follow-up not yet available.

Atrial septal defect

Anatomy

Defects in the atrial septum are classified according to their sites in the septum (Fig. 13.14). An ostium secundum atrial septal defect is situated in the region of the fossa ovalis and is usually single but there may be multiple defects. An ostium primum defect is situated in the lower part of the atrial septum and is

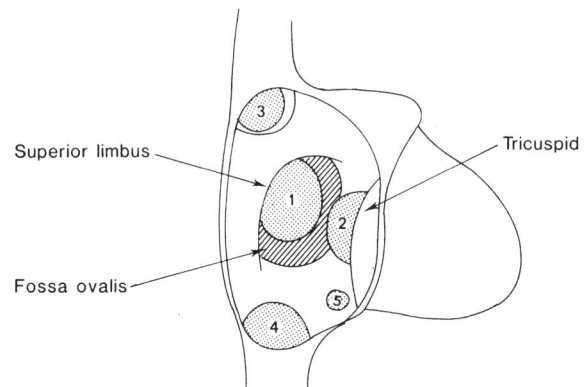

Fig. 13.14 Types of atrial septal defect: (1) ostium secundum; (2) ostium primum; (3) superior sinus venosus; (4) inferior sinus venosus; (5) coronary sinus.

classified as a partial atrioventricular septal defect. A sinus venosus defect is situated at the junction of the superior vena cava with the right atrium and is usually associated with anomalous connection of the right upper pulmonary vein. Mitral valve prolapse is reported in 8–37% of secundum atrial septal defects.

Physiology

The volume of the left to right shunt depends on the size of the defect and the compliance of the ventricles, and not on the pressure difference between the atria. In the neonatal period the pulmonary vascular resistance is high and the compliance of the two ventricles is similar and significant shunting takes several months or years to develop. Pulmonary hypertension usually does not appear during childhood, and severe pulmonary vascular disease is uncommon even in adults. Right atrial and ventricular dilation and hypertrophy develop as a result of volume overloading. Chronic distention of the right atrium predisposes to atrial arrhythmias in late adult life. Abnormal sinus node function and atrioventricular node conduction have been found in children.

Clinical features

Children with atrial septal defects are usually asymptomatic, although heart failure can occasionally develop in infants with sizable defects. Mild dyspnea or exercise intolerance and increased frequency of respiratory tract infections may be present.

The arterial and jugular venous pulses are normal. A slight prominence of the left precordium may be present in patients with a large left to right shunt. Mild cardiomegaly and a left parasternal impulse are present. The characteristic finding on auscultation is of wide splitting of the second heart sound that does not vary with respiration. Murmurs present in atrial septal defects are generated by high flow across the pulmonary and tricuspid valves and not through the interatrial communication itself. The typical murmur, an ejection systolic one over the upper left sternal border, is usually soft. A loud murmur suggests accompanying pulmonary stenosis. A mid-diastolic murmur over the lower left sternal border due to high tricuspid flow and relative tricuspid stenosis indicates a large shunt.

Investigations

The chest X-ray shows cardiomegaly with enlargement of the right atrium, and increased pulmonary vascularity.

The electrocardiogram shows sinus rhythm, atrial arrhythmias being rare in children. The QRS axis is normal or deviated to the right in ostium secundum or sinus venosus defects; left axis deviation is seen in ostium primum defects. An almost universal, and thus highly significant, feature is the RSR′ pattern in the right chest leads. Though often referred to as incomplete right bundle branch block, there is actually no conduction delay in the right bundle branch and the RSR′ pattern is more likely due to prolonged depolarization of a hypertrophied right ventricular outflow tract in response to chronic volume overload. The pattern is not specific for atrial septal defect since it is found in 5–10% of normal children and in patients with right ventricular hypertrophy from other causes.

The classical M-mode finding of an enlarged right ventricle and paradoxical septal motion (Fig. 13.6b) suggests right ventricular

volume overload but is not specific for an atrial septal defect. Cross-sectional echocardiography reveals both the size and site of the defect (Fig. 13.9) and where there is doubt color Doppler demonstration of flow through the defect should localize its site. Mitral prolapse and regurgitation can be demonstrated occasionally. In most children ultrasound provides a definitive diagnosis and catheterization is not required before surgery (Shub et al 1985). In older children and adults transesophageal echocardiography may be diagnostic when standard studies are inconclusive (Gnanapragasam et al 1991).

Cardiac catheterization shows increase in oxygen saturation from the venae cavae to the right atrium and equalization of pressures between the left and right atria. Angiography with contrast injection into the right upper pulmonary vein outlines the interatrial septum and the atrial septal defect. A left ventriculogram will demonstrate any mitral valve prolapse or regurgitation.

Treatment

Spontaneous closure of a secundum atrial septal defect is unusual though it has been reported to occur, mostly during the first few years of life (Ghisla et al 1985). Surgical closure of a large defect is recommended from the age of 2 and usually before school age. Operative risk is low and long-term results are excellent, although some patients may have persistent right ventricular enlargement or arrhythmias and conduction disturbances. A number of devices for transcatheter closure are being developed and this is likely to be practical for a number of defects (Hausdorf et al 1996).

Bacterial endocarditis complicating an atrial septal defect is very rare but some cardiologists believe that it is still worthwhile giving antibiotic prophylaxis until the defect is closed and also after surgery if prosthetic material is used.

Ductus arteriosus

Anatomy

The ductus arteriosus closes after birth by the contraction of its smooth muscle layer. Delayed closure occurs in the premature infant; the incidence varies from 20% to 60% and is higher in the more premature and smaller infants (Ellison et al 1983) but the ductus is likely to close by the time the infant reaches postconceptional maturity. The ductus arteriosus remains patent two to three times more frequently in females than males. There is some evidence that a ductus which remains patent is structurally different on histological examination from one that closes, but it is uncertain whether this is the cause or result of persistent ductal patency. A ductus arteriosus often coexists with other congenital heart defects and in cyanotic defects may serve as the only source of blood supply to the lungs at birth.

Physiology

Flow across a ductus arteriosus depends on its size and the difference in vascular resistance between the systemic and pulmonary circulation. If the ductus is large, pulmonary arterial pressure equalizes with aortic pressure and flow depends mainly on the resistance ratio. More often, the ductus is partially constricted and the pulmonary arterial pressure is less than systemic, producing continuous systolic and diastolic flow. The left atrium and left ventricle are enlarged because of increased pulmonary blood flow. In the longstanding large shunt, pulmonary hypertension develops and the flow becomes limited to systole or may even be reversed.

In the premature infant with a ductus arteriosus, increased pulmonary blood flow poses a special problem because the immature pulmonary vessels are less able to constrict against the volume overload, producing greater fluid leakage into the interstitial and alveolar spaces. Furthermore, cardiac reserve in the premature infant is reduced and ventricular failure can occur in the presence of modest shunts. Excessive run-off of blood from the aorta has also been implicated as a causative factor in cerebral hemorrhage and necrotizing enterocolitis (Bejar et al 1982).

Clinical features

Most children with a ductus arteriosus are asymptomatic and the condition is recognized by the detection of the characteristic murmur. Infants with large shunts may develop heart failure at 1–2 months when the pulmonary vascular resistance drops.

On examination, the peripheral pulses are characteristically easily palpable and brisk in the neonate and collapsing in the older child. Pulse pressure is widened with a low diastolic pressure. The heart is enlarged and displays a strong apical impulse. A left parasternal impulse of right ventricular hypertrophy is also palpable when pulmonary hypertension is present. The characteristic finding is a continuous or machinery murmur with its peak at the end of systole, best heard over the upper left sternal border or left infraclavicular region. With a small ductus, this may be the only positive physical finding on examination. In the neonate or premature infant, the murmur may initially be soft and is limited to systole. The heart sounds are usually inconspicuous and covered by the continuous murmur. With pulmonary hypertension, a loud second heart sound is heard, the diastolic component of the murmur disappears, and the systolic murmur becomes ejection in character.

Whenever the continuous murmur is heard over an area not typical for that of the persistent ductus arteriosus, other conditions causing a continuous murmur should be considered. These include the venous hum in the normal child, coronary or pulmonary arteriovenous fistula, aortopulmonary window, ventricular septal defect with aortic regurgitation, large collateral vessels associated with coarctation of aorta or pulmonary atresia, and ruptured sinus of Valsalva.

Investigations

On the chest X-ray the heart size and pulmonary plethora increase with the size of the ductus and left to right shunt. Both the aorta and pulmonary trunk are prominent. Sometimes a ductal bump can be seen as a separate convexity between the aortic knuckle and the pulmonary artery segment on the anteroposterior film. In the premature infant, often the left atrium and not the heart as a whole is enlarged and may lead to underestimation of the size of the shunt.

The electrocardiogram in the presence of a large shunt characteristically shows left ventricular hypertrophy. Right axis deviation and right ventricular hypertrophy occur with pulmonary hypertension. The electrocardiogram is less typical in the premature infant with coexisting pulmonary disease when right ventricular dominance is common.

The ductus arteriosus can be readily demonstrated with cross-sectional and Doppler echocardiography, so invasive investigations are seldom necessary for diagnosis. If performed, an oxygen rise will be found in the pulmonary artery and the catheter can be passed from the pulmonary artery across the ductus into the descending aorta. An aortogram shows the course and size of the ductus.

Treatment

Surgical or interventional closure of a ductus arteriosus has been considered to be indicated irrespective of its size unless there is established irreversible pulmonary vascular disease. Surgical ligation or division of the small ductus has been justified in view of the extremely low surgical mortality and morbidity, to prevent infective endocarditis which is estimated to have an incidence of 4–10 per 1000 patient years. Recanalization after ligation occurs in less than 1%. Closure should be undertaken as soon as possible for the symptomatic patient, and from the age of 6 months and certainly before school age for the asymptomatic child. Closure of the ductus with an occluding device using catheter techniques (Lock et al 1987) has become the accepted technique. The umbrella device is relatively expensive but the use of coil devices (Lloyd et al 1993) reduces the cost and these are appropriate where resources allow it. Recently, a clinical problem has arisen as to whether closure is appropriate for the tiny ductus which cannot be heard with the stethoscope but can be recognized by Doppler ultrasound (Houston et al 1991); there seems little clinical justification for closure and for the present it is correct to consider this a normal variant, and not recommend antibiotic prophylaxis.

For the symptomatic premature infant with delayed closure of the ductus, an initial trial of medical therapy is advocated with fluid restriction, diuretics, and if not improved, indomethacin (Evans 1995). Dosage regimes for indomethacin vary: 0.2 mg/kg/dose intravenously 12-hourly for 3 doses has been accepted but 0.1 mg/kg daily for 6 days may be more effective and have fewer side-effects (Rennie & Cooke 1991). Closure rate is lower in extreme prematurity. Surgical ligation is considered when there is no response. If the infant has few or no symptoms, spontaneous closure of the ductus can be expected and awaited.

Atrioventricular septal defect

Anatomy

Synonyms for this malformation include endocardial cushion defect, persistent atrioventricular canal and atrioventricular communis. The atrioventricular septum is the partition at the atrioventricular junction which separates the atria and ventricles from each other and the left ventricle from the right atrium. Failure of early embryological fusion of the endocardial cushions produces defects in atrial and ventricular septation and abnormalities in the formation of the atrioventricular valves with a single common annulus with the central atrioventricular valve leaflet shared between the left and right heart. Atrioventricular septal defects are usually classified into the partial or incomplete form with two separate atrioventricular orifices and no VSD, and the complete form with a large common atrioventricular orifice and a VSD (Fig. 13.15). In the partial form (ostium primum atrial septal defect) there is usually a defect on the left side of the

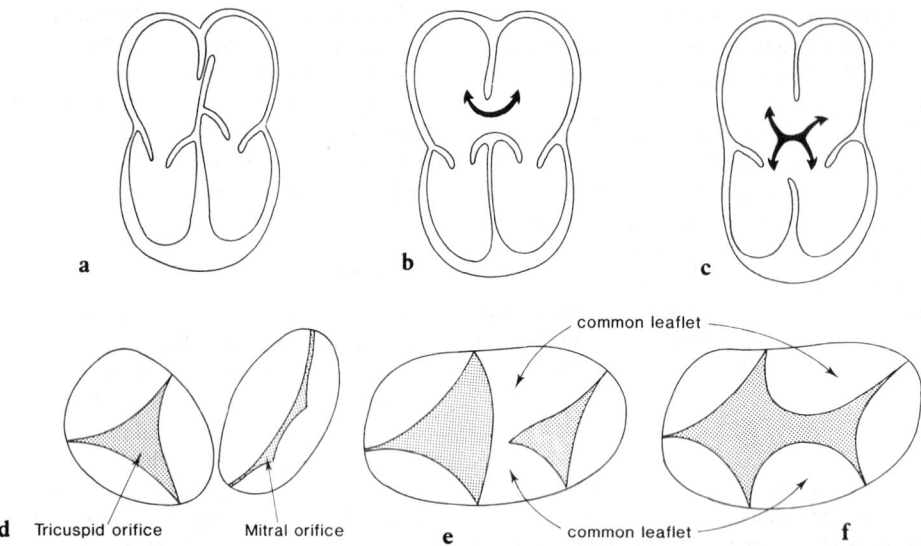

Fig. 13.15 Anatomy of the atrioventricular junction: (**a** and **d**) normal septation with no shunting and separate valve orifices; (**b** and **e**) partial atrioventricular septal defect with atrial shunting, two valve orifices and a 'cleft' anterior mitral leaflet; (**c** and **f**) complete atrioventricular septal defect with interatrial and interventricular shunting.

common central leaflet traditionally termed a 'cleft of the anterior mitral leaflet' (Penkoske et al 1985).

Atrioventricular septal defects frequently occur in patients with Down syndrome, asplenia or polysplenia. There is some evidence that the recurrence rate of atrioventricular septal defects in families is higher than for other congenital heart defects (Wilson L et al 1993).

Physiology

With a partial defect the effect is similar to that of a secundum atrial septal defect with additional left ventricular overload if there is mitral regurgitation through the cleft mitral leaflet. The regurgitant jet is often directed from the left ventricle towards the right atrium, augmenting the amount of left to right shunting. In a complete atrioventricular septal defect, shunting of blood occurs at both atrial and ventricular levels and there may be free atrioventricular regurgitation through the common orifice. Admixture of blood may render the patient cyanotic, especially when pulmonary hypertension is present. The physiology of a complete atrioventricular septal defect is similar to that of a large nonrestrictive ventricular septal defect with additional volume overloading to the right ventricle, which sometimes may be markedly dilated. Pulmonary vascular disease develops at a younger age than in simple ventricular septal defects, particularly in those with Down syndrome.

Clinical features

Clinical features depend on the relative size of the atrial and ventricular components of the defect. Thus a partial atrioventricular septal defect will have signs and symptoms of an atrial septal defect while a complete defect with a large ventricular component will be like a nonrestrictive ventricular septal defect. However, a clinical distinction between atrioventricular and simple atrial or ventricular septal defects may be inferred if there is evidence of mitral regurgitation. With a large ventricular component the murmur at the lower left sternal border may radiate towards the axilla and the mid-diastolic flow murmur may be heard better over the lower left sternal border rather than over the apex, representing excessive flow across the tricuspid valve.

Investigations

The chest X-ray in complete atrioventricular septal defects shows cardiomegaly from enlargement of both atria and ventricles, often producing a globular appearance of the heart. The pulmonary artery and its branches are also prominent and the lung fields are plethoric. In a partial atrioventricular septal defect with predominant atrial shunting it resembles the appearance in an ostium secundum atrial septal defect although left atrial enlargement is sometimes also present.

The electrocardiogram in both partial and complete atrioventricular septal defects characteristically shows left axis deviation. There may be prolonged PR interval or incomplete right bundle branch block. Biventricular hypertrophy or right ventricular hypertrophy alone is usual in the complete form.

Cross-sectional echocardiography gives reliable diagnostic assessment of the anatomical type of atrioventricular septal defect, the size of the atrial and ventricular septal defect components, and associated malformations (Silverman et al 1986). Echocardiography provides better definition of the anatomy than angiography.

Cardiac catheterization is required only to assess the pulmonary vascular resistance in older subjects. In the complete form, shunting may be detected at both atrial and ventricular levels and pulmonary hypertension is the rule due to excessive pulmonary blood flow and early onset of pulmonary vascular disease. Angiography can show the low position of the ostium primum atrial septal defect, any mitral regurgitation, and a classical 'goose neck' deformity in the left ventricular outflow tract.

Treatment

Complete atrioventricular septal defects nearly always require surgical correction before the age of 2 years, and often before 1 year, because of severe symptomatology or development of pulmonary hypertension. Surgery can be deferred until between 2 and 5 years for patients with the partial form of atrioventricular septal defects where there is no pulmonary hypertension. The common atrioventricular orifice has to be divided and the valve leaflets reconstructed to ensure competent mitral and tricuspid valves. Residual mitral regurgitation is an important sequel. For infants requiring surgery, primary repair is preferred but pulmonary artery banding may be beneficial for the very ill or small patient.

Other arteriovenous communications

Systemic arteriovenous fistulas

Fistulas between a systemic artery and vein are mostly congenital and can be present anywhere in the body. The common sites are between a cerebral artery and the vein of Galen, the subclavian artery and vein, the hepatic artery and portal vein, the internal mammary artery and the internal mammary vein or the ductus venosus. Cavernous hemangiomas can involve the skin, pelvis or the liver. Acquired arteriovenous fistulas are usually the result of trauma. Similarly, lesions in the lung may be congenital or result from chronic inflammatory diseases such as cystic fibrosis or bronchiectasis; these are likely to result in cyanosis.

The arteriovenous fistula allows run-off of blood from the aorta and increases systemic venous return, the magnitude depending on the size of the vascular communication. Small communications cause no symptoms or a localized swelling. Large communications produce increased arterial flow and circulating volume, resulting in so-called high output heart failure. A bruit or continuous murmur audible over the involved area, sometimes accompanied by a palpable thrill, is the characteristic finding. Other signs include bounding pulses, systemic venous congestion, cardiomegaly and hepatomegaly. Liver enlargement may be produced by hepatic artery fistulas or multiple hemangioendotheliomas. In any infant with heart failure and no obvious precordial or echocardiographic findings, a bruit suggestive of an arteriovenous fistula should be sought over the skull, chest wall and abdomen. Cranial bruits, however, are sometimes audible in the normal infant.

Cardiomegaly on the chest X-ray and biventricular hypertrophy on the electrocardiogram are associated with large fistulas. Echocardiography is useful in excluding cardiac pathology while ultrasound of the skull and abdomen may reveal dilated arteriovenous channels. Definitive diagnosis is obtained by catheterization showing increased oxygen saturation in the venous blood draining from the fistulous communication and angiogram on the arterial side showing the number and extent of fistulas.

Treatment traditionally required excision of the fistulous communication or ligation of the feeding artery. After surgery, recurrence is frequent and cure rate is low but the use of transcatheter embolization has recently improved the prognosis (Friedman et al 1993), although infants with symptomatic intracranial or hepatic fistulas still die and others may survive with brain damage.

Coronary artery fistula

A coronary artery fistula is usually congenital in etiology and occurs as an isolated malformation. The right coronary artery is more often involved and more than 90% of the fistulas drain into the right heart. The pulmonary to systemic flow ratio is seldom more than 2 : 1. Small fistulas are hemodynamically insignificant. Large fistulas may produce exercise intolerance, dyspnea or angina because of the 'stealing' of blood from the normal coronary circulation. Heart failure is rare. The characteristic finding is a continuous murmur best heard over the site of drainage into the heart. It is therefore maximal over the lower right or left sternal border when the fistula drains into the right atrium or right ventricle, and over the upper left sternal border when the fistula drains into the pulmonary artery or left atrium.

The chest X-ray and electrocardiogram are usually normal. With a large fistula the coronary artery involved is dilated and this is visible on echocardiography, and the drainage site may be detected by Doppler flow studies. Definite diagnosis is by demonstration of the fistula by aortography or selective coronary arteriography.

Treatment by surgical ligation or closure of the fistula is recommended for all patients to prevent the development of complications which include myocardial ischemia, heart failure, arrhythmias, progressive dilation or thrombosis and rupture of the fistula, and infective endocarditis.

Aortopulmonary septal defect

Aortopulmonary septal defect (aortopulmonary window or fenestration) is a direct communication between the ascending aorta and the pulmonary trunk, usually between the left side of the ascending aorta and the right side of the pulmonary artery.

Most defects are large and increased pulmonary blood flow and pulmonary hypertension are established early in life. Dyspnea, failure to thrive, and congestive heart failure are common in infancy. Examination shows collapsing pulses, cardiomegaly and biventricular cardiac impulses. On auscultation, the pulmonary second heart sound is accentuated and a systolic rather than continuous murmur is heard over the left sternal border. A mid-diastolic flow murmur over the apex may be present. The findings mimic a large ventricular septal defect or ductus arteriosus and pulmonary hypertension.

The chest X-ray shows cardiomegaly with prominent pulmonary trunk and pleonemic lungs. The electrocardiogram shows biventricular hypertrophy or left ventricular hypertrophy alone if pulmonary hypertension is mild. The defect may be visible on cross-sectional echocardiography and can be confirmed with contrast echocardiography or Doppler ultrasound. If considered necessary the precise site and size of the defect can be further defined with aortic root angiography and surgical closure of the defect should be performed early because of the high risk of pulmonary vascular disease developing.

Left ventricle to right atrium defect

A direct communication between the left ventricle and the right atrium may be due to a defect in the membranous atrioventricular septum above the tricuspid valve, or due to a perimembranous ventricular septal defect associated with an anomalous opening in the septal leaflet of the tricuspid valve such as perforation, fenestration, or cleft. Large volume shunting tends to occur because of the marked pressure difference between the left ventricle and the right atrium. Enlargement of the right heart is usual.

The clinical findings of a left ventricle to right atrium defect are essentially similar to those of a ventricular septal defect. The pansystolic murmur may be present at birth and not dependent on the postnatal fall in pulmonary vascular resistance. It may be heard over the sternum or the right sternal border. Evidence of right atrial enlargement may be present on the chest X-ray and electrocardiogram. Cardiac catheterization reveals increase in oxygen saturation in the right atrium and the left ventriculogram shows contrast passing from the left ventricle directly to the right atrium. Echocardiography with color Doppler is a more exact means of determining the exact nature of the defect and direction of the shunt.

Left ventricle to right atrium defects do not close spontaneously. Surgical closure is required if the shunt is large, the indications being as for ventricular septal defects.

Pulmonary hypertension

Pulmonary hypertension is considered to be present when the systolic pulmonary arterial pressure is above 30 mmHg or the mean pressure is above 20 mmHg. The main causes of pulmonary hypertension are listed in Table 13.3. The pathogenesis of pulmonary hypertension is still uncertain. Whatever the etiology, the pathology of pulmonary hypertension is similar and consists of a reduction in size and number of preacinar and intra-acinar arterioles resulting in a decrease in total pulmonary arterial luminal area (Table 13.4).

Those with primary pulmonary hypertension may present with

Table 13.3 Causes of pulmonary hypertension

1. Congenital heart diseases
   With increased pulmonary blood flow
   — left to right shunts, e.g. VSD, PDA
   — total anomalous pulmonary venous drainage, truncus arteriosus
   — transposition of great arteries
   With pulmonary venous obstruction
   — left ventricular inflow or outflow obstruction
   — obstructed total anomalous pulmonary venous drainage
   — pulmonary vein stenosis or veno-occlusive disease

2. Chronic lung diseases producing hypoxemia
   — airway obstructions, e.g. chronic asthma
   — parenchymal disorders, e.g. cystic fibrosis
   — restrictive disorders, e.g. kyphoscoliosis

3. Pulmonary vascular diseases
   — primary (idiopathic) pulmonary hypertension
   — persistent pulmonary hypertension of the newborn
   — collagen vascular diseases, e.g. systemic lupus erythematosus
   — thromboembolism, e.g. ventriculoatrial shunts for hydrocephalus

4. Others
   — high altitude
   — neuromuscular disorders producing hypoventilation
   — familial

effort intolerance or episodes of loss of consciousness. In patients with large left to right shunts, as the pulmonary vascular resistance rises the shunt decreases and features of pulmonary congestion and heart failure are reduced and the condition of the patient improves. This apparent 'recovery' lasts until exercise intolerance and right heart decompensation develop when the increasing pulmonary vascular resistance restricts pulmonary blood flow. The signs of the original shunt become less conspicuous or inapparent. When the pulmonary vascular resistance surpasses the systemic resistance, right to left shunting and cyanosis occur, a condition known as Eisenmenger's syndrome. The most suggestive physical finding is a loud pulmonary second heart sound. With severe pulmonary hypertension there is a strong right ventricular impulse, an early ejection click and nonspecific systolic murmur over the pulmonary area, and murmurs of pulmonary or tricuspid regurgitation.

The electrocardiogram in pulmonary hypertension typically shows right ventricular hypertrophy; right axis deviation and right atrial hypertrophy are also present in severe cases. The chest X-ray characteristically shows enlargement of the pulmonary trunk and its branches. In severe cases the proximal pulmonary arteries appear congested while the distal branches are diminished and the peripheral lungs clear, giving rise to the 'pruned' appearance of the pulmonary arterial tree. Doppler echocardiography can predict the magnitude of the pulmonary hypertension if tricuspid regurgitation can be recorded. Direct measurement of the pulmonary arterial pressure by cardiac catheterization carries a significant risk in this situation. Calculation of the pulmonary vascular resistance before and after inhalation of oxygen or administration of vasodilators such as tolazoline, prostaglandin or nitric oxide (Royston 1993) is required to determine reversibility of the pulmonary hypertension. When the ratio of pulmonary to systemic vascular resistance exceeds 0.7 it is generally believed that the pulmonary vascular disease is irreversible. In doubtful cases lung biopsy may be helpful.

There is no specific treatment for pulmonary hypertension itself. Early detection and correction of any causative disease are essential to prevent the development of irreversible pulmonary vascular changes. Heart and lung transplantation may be considered in some cases. Home oxygen therapy has been beneficial in some with primary pulmonary hypertension and this can produce symptomatic improvement in patients with Eisenmenger's syndrome.

ACYANOTIC DISEASE WITHOUT ARTERIOVENOUS SHUNT

Aortic stenosis

Anatomy

Left ventricular outflow tract obstruction can be at, below, or above the valve. Three-quarters of the cases are due to aortic valve

Table 13.4 Histological grading of pulmonary vascular disease

Potentially reversible	Grade I – medial muscle hypertrophy Grade II – intimal hyperplasia and thickening Grade III – occlusion of arteriolar lumen	Grade A – abnormal extension of muscle into peripheral arteries Grade B (early) – abnormal extension and mild medial hypertrophy Grade B (late) – abnormal extension and severe medial hypertrophy and decreased artery size
Usually irreversible	Grade IV – presence of plexiform and angiomatoid lesions Grade V – fibrosis of intima and media Grade VI – necrotizing arteritis	Grade C – above findings plus reduced artery number

stenosis resulting from fusion of the valve leaflets. The valve is most often bicuspid, but can be unicuspid, tricuspid or quadricuspid. Myxomatous degeneration and calcification develop in adult life, increasing the severity of obstruction. Poststenotic dilation of the ascending aorta is typically present in aortic valve stenosis. Subvalvar stenosis is due to a discrete membrane or fibromuscular ridge forming a crescent or complete ring below the aortic valve, which is often abnormal or becomes deformed by the high velocity jet of blood. Poststenotic dilation of the ascending aorta may or may not be present. Supravalvar aortic stenosis is caused by an hourglass narrowing or diffuse hypoplasia of the ascending aorta above the sinus of Valsalva. Poststenotic dilation is absent. Supravalvar stenosis may be sporadic or associated with congenital rubella or Williams syndrome (p. 833).

Clinical features

Children with aortic stenosis are usually asymptomatic and have normal growth. Those with severe obstruction may have symptoms of dyspnea, syncope or angina on exertion. Sudden death can occur but is rare and occurs during stressful exercise. The pulses are normal in mild or moderate stenosis but weak with reduced pulse pressure in severe stenosis. The heart is usually not enlarged and the apex beat is forceful or thrusting of the left ventricular type. A systolic thrill in the suprasternal notch is nearly always present, whatever the level of stenosis. On auscultation, an ejection systolic click, best heard over the apex or left sternal border, is characteristic of valvar stenosis with a pliable valve. With increasing severity of obstruction, the aortic closure sound becomes soft and delayed and the second heart sound appears single or, in an extreme situation, reveals paradoxical (expiratory) splitting. The murmur is ejection in nature and heard maximally at the aortic area with radiation into the neck.

In subvalvar or supravalvar stenosis there is no click, and the aortic closure sound is often loud in supravalvar stenosis. With subvalvar stenosis the murmur may be loudest over the mid-left sternal border, and a soft early diastolic murmur of aortic regurgitation may be present.

Infants with critical aortic valve stenosis usually become symptomatic within the first few months of life. Progressive dyspnea, congestive heart failure or frank pulmonary edema are common. The pulses are weak or impalpable and cardiomegaly is present. Gallop rhythm is usual and the ejection systolic murmur which may be heard over most of the precordium varies in intensity, depending on the contractility of the compromised left ventricle. An ejection click is rare as the valve is thick and immobile.

Investigations

The chest X-ray shows a normal heart size except in infants with congestive heart failure. The left heart border is often rounded near the apex suggesting left ventricular hypertrophy. Poststenotic dilation of the ascending aorta associated with valve stenosis is seen as a bulge on the upper right heart border.

The electrocardiogram shows a variable degree of left ventricular hypertrophy, but does not accurately reflect the severity of stenosis. However, the presence of ST depression and T wave inversion in the inferior and left chest leads signifies severe obstruction. Such changes sometimes become manifest only on exercise testing.

Cross-sectional echocardiography is useful in demonstrating the level of stenosis and nature of the aortic valve. Estimation of the pressure gradient across the stenotic site can be obtained by Doppler studies. Cardiac catheterization and direct pressure measurement is not essential. When performed, a left ventriculogram shows the anatomy of the obstruction and an aortogram shows any accompanying aortic regurgitation.

Treatment

Surgical valvotomy as an emergency procedure is required for infants with critical aortic stenosis and heart failure. Valvotomy is often palliative and reoperation for restenosis or aortic regurgitation, sometimes requiring aortic valve replacement, is frequently required. Surgery should generally be delayed as long as possible. Operation is indicated if the patient has symptoms of myocardial or cerebral ischemia, is asymptomatic but has electrocardiographic ST and T wave abnormalities at rest or on exercise test, or often if the systolic gradient on catheterization across the obstruction is greater than 50–60 mmHg. Balloon dilation of the aortic valve is an alternative to surgery; although some results are encouraging there is the possibility of significant regurgitation developing and its place is as yet uncertain. Aortic valve replacement is necessary in patients with a small aortic annulus, dysplastic valve or severe aortic regurgitation.

Patients who do not require intervention should be followed carefully since progressive increase in obstruction may occur. Restenosis and aortic regurgitation after surgery is frequent, demanding continued assessment.

Infective endocarditis complicates aortic stenosis at a rate of 2–3 per 1000 patient years. Antibiotic prophylaxis is mandatory before and also after operation. Sudden death is the most threatening complication and occurs in patients with clinical and electrocardiographic features of severe stenosis, although it has been reported in asymptomatic patients with normal resting electrocardiograms. The availability of cross-sectional and Doppler echocardiography should allow early detection of severe stenosis. Strenuous exercise should be restricted in patients with gradients above 50 mmHg; normal but not competitive sports can be allowed for patients with gradients between 25 and 50 mmHg, while exercise in those with lesser gradients need not be limited.

Bicuspid aortic valve

A bicuspid aortic valve occurs in about 1% of the general population and is considered the most common congenital cardiac malformation. It is also commonly associated with other congenital heart defects, particularly coarctation of aorta. It is seldom recognized in childhood unless accompanied by aortic stenosis or complications. Diagnosis is suggested by an ejection click over the apex conducted upwards to the right sternal border. There may be an ejection systolic murmur of mild aortic stenosis or a diastolic murmur of aortic regurgitation. Chest X-ray and electrocardiogram are normal. Echocardiography should show the valve morphology. No treatment is required, but antibiotic prophylaxis against infective endocarditis is recommended. Late complications include calcification and stenosis or regurgitation of the valve and valve replacement in later life may be required.

Congenital aortic regurgitation

Congenital aortic regurgitation is rare and is often due to intrinsic abnormalities of the aortic valve such as a bicuspid valve, fenestration of the valve, or an aorta to left ventricle tunnel. It may develop secondary to other congenital heart malformations such as an outlet ventricular septal defect or ruptured sinus of Valsalva aneurysm. Symptoms usually do not occur early in aortic regurgitation. The clinical features, investigation and management are similar to those in acquired aortic regurgitation (p. 629).

Sinus of Valsalva aneurysm

Congenital aneurysm of the aortic sinus (of Valsalva) most frequently involves the right coronary sinus. An aortic sinus aneurysm produces no symptoms unless rupture occurs, usually in adult life. An aortocardiac fistula results, usually draining into the right ventricle or right atrium and producing a significant left to right shunt. The characteristic finding is a continuous murmur over the mid-left sternal border. Other clinical features of aortic regurgitation and left to right shunt may also be present. The aneurysm and its site of rupture can be detected by ultrasound. An aortogram may be necessary to define the anatomy prior to surgery. Treatment consists of excision of the aneurysmal sac and closure of the aortic defect.

Pulmonary stenosis

Anatomy

Obstruction to the right ventricular outflow tract may be at the valve, below (infundibular) or above it. Pulmonary valve stenosis is produced by fusion of the commissures of the leaflets into a dome-shaped membrane with a small opening. Some cases are due to a dysplastic valve which is not fused but is grossly thickened by myxomatous tissue; obstruction results from immobility of the bulky leaflets, often associated with a small valve annulus. Infundibular stenosis may be due to a discrete fibromuscular ridge or more often hypertrophy of the infundibular muscle obstructing the right ventricular outlet; this usually develops in association with a ventricular septal defect which may even close spontaneously. Dynamic infundibular obstruction often occurs secondary to severe valve stenosis, the hypertrophied muscle constricting the right ventricular outlet during systole but relaxing during diastole. Supravalvar pulmonary stenosis is seen in patients with congenital rubella, Noonan's syndrome, Williams syndrome and tetralogy of Fallot. Poststenotic dilation of the pulmonary trunk is typically present in valve stenosis, sometimes in the dysplastic valve and not in infundibular stenosis.

Physiology

High right ventricular systolic pressure develops proximal to the obstruction and may exceed that of the left ventricle. In severe cases, reduced compliance of the right ventricle due to muscle hypertrophy causes elevation of the end-diastolic pressure and hence right atrial hypertension, and when there is an interatrial communication right to left shunting with consequent cyanosis.

Clinical features

Patients with mild to moderate pulmonary stenosis are usually asymptomatic and the lesion is recognized by the discovery of a heart murmur which may be detected soon after birth. Growth is normal and the body build is often stocky with a 'moon face', but these signs are neither invariable nor pathognomonic. Symptoms are rare, but infants with critical stenosis are cyanotic at birth and older infants and children may develop cyanosis, exercise intolerance and dyspnea. Heart failure is rare and is seen only in infants with severe stenosis.

The peripheral pulses and jugular venous pressure are usually normal. The heart is normal in size or slightly enlarged. The cardiac impulse is of right ventricular type. A systolic thrill may be palpable over the upper left sternal border and occasionally in the suprasternal notch. The second heart sound is widely split but varies with respiration with a soft pulmonary component. In valve stenosis an ejection click is usually heard preceding the murmur; it is produced by the restricted systolic opening of the valve and is absent in severe stenosis when the valve is quite immobile or fibrotic. The typical finding is a harsh ejection systolic murmur, best heard over the upper left sternal border at the second or third intercostal space and conducted towards the neck. The murmur is located in the third or fourth intercostal spaces in infundibular stenosis. In general, severe valve or infundibular stenosis is suggested by detection of an absent ejection click, a long systolic murmur with a late peak, loud intensity of the murmur, wide splitting of the second heart sound with a soft pulmonary component and presence of a fourth heart sound. In supravalvar stenosis or stenosis of the peripheral pulmonary arteries, the second heart sound is normal and the murmur is characteristically widely heard over the precordium radiating into the axilla and back. Rarely it may be continuous.

Investigations

The chest X-ray usually shows a normal heart size and pulmonary vascularity. Poststenotic dilation of the main pulmonary artery is characteristic of valve stenosis.

The electrocardiogram may be normal in mild to moderate stenosis, with evidence of right ventricular hypertrophy in moderate to severe stenosis. An RSR′ pattern is common in moderate stenosis while a tall R wave with increased R/S ratio or a pure R wave or qR pattern occurs as severity of obstruction increases. There is no distinction between valvar, infundibular or supravalvar stenosis, and only a rough correlation exists between electrocardiographic changes and the gradient across the obstruction.

Echocardiography will identify the site of obstruction and Doppler provides a reliable estimation of the pressure gradient across the right ventricular outflow tract and allows the selection of patients for balloon valvoplasty.

Cardiac catheterization measures the pressure changes from the pulmonary artery to the right ventricle and shows the level of the stenosis. However, the gradient will vary with time and sedation and it may be more important to take the Doppler gradient when the patient is alert and not sedated than at catheterization in deciding on the need for intervention (Lim et al 1989). A right ventriculogram will demonstrate not only the site of the stenosis but also the nature of the pulmonary valve, or the extent of infundibular or pulmonary artery stenosis.

Treatment and prognosis

Treatment to enlarge the stenotic site is indicated if the right ventricular systolic pressure is over 60 mmHg or the systolic gradient across the obstruction is in excess of 40 mmHg. Surgical operation consists of commissurotomy for valve stenosis, excision of hypertrophic fibromuscular tissue for infundibular stenosis, and reconstruction of the pulmonary artery for supravalvar stenosis. Balloon dilation valvoplasty (Tynan et al 1985) has become the preferred means of treatment for pulmonary valve stenosis. Early results are comparable to those of surgery, though long-term effects are pending. Balloon dilation is less successful in dysplastic pulmonary valves and pulmonary artery stenosis. Mild residual stenosis and regurgitation is the rule after either surgery or balloon dilation.

Patients with milder stenosis should be followed up throughout childhood since an increase in pressure gradient may develop as the child grows older.

Although infective endocarditis is rare in pulmonary stenosis (0.2 per 1000 patient years), antibiotic prophylaxis is best provided both before and after treatment, irrespective of the site and severity of the stenosis.

Idiopathic dilation of the pulmonary artery

This malformation is characterized by congenital dilation of the main pulmonary artery, and sometimes its branches, in the absence of associated heart disease. It is believed to be due to a developmental defect of the elastic tissue of the pulmonary artery. Patients are asymptomatic and initial suspicion is based on the radiological discovery of an enlarged pulmonary trunk or clinical detection of a heart murmur. There may be an ejection systolic click, a soft midsystolic murmur, and an early diastolic murmur of pulmonary regurgitation. The electrocardiogram is normal. The hallmark is a dilated main pulmonary artery on the chest X-ray indistinguishable from the poststenotic dilation seen in pulmonary stenosis. Ultrasound will demonstrate the dilated pulmonary artery and confirm there is no significant stenosis. A prominent pulmonary artery is also seen in patients with the straight-back syndrome, Marfan's syndrome, and partial absence of the pericardium. No specific treatment is necessary.

Congenital pulmonary regurgitation

Congenital pulmonary regurgitation is uncommon and is either associated with idiopathic dilation of the pulmonary artery or due to structural abnormality of the valve leaflets such as dysplastic or bicuspid valve, or 'absent valve'. The latter condition is seldom isolated and generally coexists with tetralogy of Fallot or ventricular septal defect. It is characterized in most cases by aneurysmal dilation of the pulmonary artery and its branches, causing bronchial compression and obstructive emphysema or atelectasis of the lungs, producing severe respiratory distress in the neonate or infant. Most patients with congenital pulmonary regurgitation are asymptomatic. Recognition of pulmonary regurgitation is based on the detection of the early diastolic murmur maximally heard over the upper left sternal border, usually with a midsystolic murmur, producing the characteristic to and fro murmur.

Surgical treatment is required for moderate or severe regurgitation, where there are respiratory symptoms and when absent pulmonary valve is associated with tetralogy of Fallot.

Left ventricular inflow obstructions

Anatomy

Obstruction between the pulmonary veins or left atrium and the left ventricle is rare and may be due to congenital mitral valve stenosis, a supravalvar stenotic ring, or cor triatriatum. The supravalvar stenotic ring consists of a circumferential ridge of endocardial tissue in the left atrium immediately above the mitral valve annulus in close proximity with the valve leaflets. It is commonly associated with a ventricular septal defect and ductus arteriosus. Cor triatriatum is produced by a fibrous diaphragm separating the left atrium into two chambers, usually with a small and obstructive communication between them.

Physiology

Significant left ventricular inflow obstruction from any cause produces elevation of the pressure proximal to the site of obstruction and hence pulmonary venous congestion or even edema. Pulmonary arterial and right ventricular hypertension are inevitable and right heart failure develops eventually. The hemodynamic consequences are often masked by coexisting malformations.

Clinical features

Patients with congenital mitral obstruction usually present with associated malformations such as coarctation of the aorta or ventricular septal defect and the mitral lesion is often not recognized. Isolated mitral valve stenosis, supravalvar ring or cor triatriatum produce similar manifestations when the obstruction is severe. Symptoms begin in early infancy with dyspnea, cough and failure to thrive. Right heart failure is common. Hemoptysis is rare compared to acquired mitral stenosis. Examination shows a strong right ventricular impulse and variable heart size. The first heart sound is normal or loud and an opening snap is only occasionally present. The second heart sound is always accentuated and often accompanied by other auscultatory findings of severe pulmonary hypertension. An apical diastolic rumble is more often audible in mitral valve stenosis or supravalvar ring than in cor triatriatum. Crepitations in the lungs and hepatomegaly are present when heart failure occurs.

Investigations

The chest X-ray shows cardiomegaly with enlargement of the left atrium producing a double density shadow at the right heart border. Pulmonary hypertension is reflected by a prominent pulmonary artery, and pulmonary venous congestion by a 'butterfly wing' distribution of vascular markings or ground glass appearance if pulmonary edema is present. The electrocardiogram almost always shows right ventricular hypertrophy. Right atrial hypertrophy is common in the presence of pulmonary hypertension. Left atrial hypertrophy is usually seen in mitral valve stenosis or supravalvar ring but not in cor triatriatum.

Cross-sectional echocardiography provides definitive diagnosis for the various stenotic lesions while Doppler flow studies help to assess the severity of obstruction and pulmonary artery pressure. Cardiac catheterization is not usually required. An end-diastolic pressure difference of 5 mmHg or more suggests significant obstruction. Angiography may show the site of obstruction but its diagnostic value is less than that of echocardiography.

Treatment

Surgical excision of the obstructive membrane is the definitive treatment for cor triatriatum and supravalvar ring. For congenital mitral stenosis, the deformity of the valve dictates the surgical approach; whenever possible, valvotomy with attempts to conserve the native valve is preferred to mitral valve replacement.

Mitral valve prolapse

Anatomy

Many synonyms have been used for this condition since its first description by Barlow in 1963, including billowing, floppy, or myxomatous mitral valve and the systolic click–late systolic murmur syndrome. It was originally a clinical diagnosis, but echocardiography has provided evidence of abnormal closure of the mitral valve and recognition of so-called silent prolapse. Its prevalence varies from 5% to 15% in the adult general population but only 1–2% in children. Silent prolapse is also rare in the young. Its incidence is higher in the female. Over one-third of cases in children are associated with other congenital heart defects. There is a high incidence in patients with pectus excavatum, hypokyphosis (straight-back) and Marfan's syndrome, suggesting the possibility of a connective tissue disorder.

Clinical features

Most patients are asymptomatic and the diagnosis is suggested by incidental auscultatory findings, usually in late adolescence or adult life. Nonspecific complaints such as chest pain, fatigue, dyspnea on exertion and nervousness may be present. Palpitations and syncope are rare in children.

The characteristic finding is auscultation of a midsystolic click, a late systolic murmur, or both, over the apex. These signs are more prominent, or only become manifest with the patient upright or lying in the left lateral position. A Valsalva maneuver, tachycardia or vasodilator administration shifts the click and murmur closer to the first heart sound, while squatting and bradycardia delay or abolish them. An apical pansystolic murmur typical of mitral regurgitation is uncommon in childhood.

Investigations

The chest X-ray is usually normal. Skeletal abnormalities mentioned earlier may be present. The electrocardiogram shows inversion of the T waves in the inferior leads in about half of children and adolescents with mitral valve prolapse. Arrhythmias such as premature atrial or ventricular contractions, supraventricular tachycardia and conduction abnormalities have been described at rest or during exercise, but the frequency is not significantly higher than in the normal population. Cross-sectional echocardiography demonstrates the systolic buckling or bowing of the mitral leaflets towards the left atrium. Multiple views should be taken to avoid false positive diagnosis. The presence of mitral regurgitation can be detected by Doppler study. Angiography is not necessary for the diagnosis of mitral valve prolapse; a left ventriculogram taken in the right anterior oblique view best demonstrates the prolapsing leaflets.

Management

No treatment is necessary for asymptomatic patients. Prognosis in children is usually good; progress to significant mitral regurgitation or sudden death is rare. The latter appears to result from ventricular tachycardia or fibrillation. Antiarrhythmia therapy is indicated in patients who are symptomatic with documented arrhythmias, or in the presence of frequent premature ventricular contractions, ventricular tachycardia or fibrillation. Bacterial endocarditis is estimated to occur in 0.1–0.3 per 1000 patient years and antibiotic prophylaxis is recommended. Patients who develop severe mitral regurgitation require antifailure treatment and surgical valvoplasty or mitral valve replacement.

Endocardial fibroelastosis

Endocardial fibroelastosis is a cardiomyopathy characterized by diffuse thickening of the endocardium by collagen and elastic tissue forming a pearly white layer. It is often confined to the left ventricle, but can involve other cardiac chambers and valves. It occurs as an isolated phenomenon or is associated with cardiac malformations, particularly left ventricular outflow obstructions and hypoplastic left heart syndrome. Its etiology is unknown. The overlying myocardium is hypertrophied but histologically normal apart from mild degenerative changes in the subendocardial region. The involved cardiac chambers are dilated and contract poorly.

Most patients with isolated endocardial fibroelastosis present with congestive heart failure during the first 3 months of life. Onset may be abrupt with rapid deterioration, often precipitated by a respiratory tract infection. Examination shows cardiomegaly with a bulging, active precordium. The second heart sound is usually loud and gallop rhythm is nearly always present. Characteristically there is no audible murmur but one of mitral regurgitation may be heard. The chest X-ray shows marked cardiomegaly and frequently pulmonary venous congestion or edema. The electrocardiogram characteristically shows tall voltages in the precordial leads, suggesting left ventricular or biventricular hypertrophy, and inverted or flattened T waves. Arrhythmias are common, especially in severe or chronic disease. Echocardiography reveals the dilated cardiac chambers and reduced contractile function. Cardiac catheterization and angiography are not essential and are often performed to obtain a diagnostic endomyocardial biopsy. Differential diagnosis for infants with congestive heart failure and no murmur include myocarditis, anomalous origin of the left coronary artery from the pulmonary artery, idiopathic calcification of the coronary arteries, metabolic cardiomyopathy such as Pompe's disease and carnitine deficiency, idiopathic dilated cardiomyopathy, and systemic arteriovenous fistula.

Treatment consists of control of heart failure and prolonged adequate digitalization. Prognosis in general is poor, most patients dying soon after presentation or after a period of fluctuating control. The earlier the symptoms appear and the greater the left ventricular impairment, the worse will be the prognosis. Some patients survive but have persistent symptoms, cardiomegaly and electrocardiographic abnormalities, while still others may have a complete clinical recovery but the long-term outcome remains guarded.

Right ventricular dysplasia

These are rare diseases of unknown etiology involving the myocardium of the right ventricle. The best known is Uhl's disease in which the myocardium of the right ventricle is extremely hypoplastic or absent with direct apposition of the epicardium and endocardium. Patients present at variable ages with heart failure, cardiomegaly on chest X-ray and absence of right ventricular forces on the electrocardiogram. Cyanosis is present if the foramen ovale is patent, allowing right to left shunting. Angiography shows a large noncontractile right ventricle. Most cases presenting in infancy or childhood die despite antifailure treatment. No operative treatment has been shown to be beneficial.

A rarer condition is hypoplasia of the apical trabecular region of the right ventricle. Patients may present with heart failure in infancy or remain asymptomatic. Investigations are often negative except for evidence of right atrial enlargement. Angiography shows absence of the apical trabecular component, giving a sausage-shaped instead of a triangular right ventricle.

Coarctation of the aorta

Anatomy

Coarctation of the aorta refers to narrowing of the aortic arch at its isthmus between the left subclavian artery and the origin of the ductus arteriosus, although constriction can occur at other sites such as the lower thoracic or abdominal aorta. Commonly it is produced by a shelf-like lesion but tubular hypoplasia of the aortic arch can occur. Discrete coarctations have been classified as preductal (infantile) or postductal (adult type) but terms such as 'juxtaductal' or 'paraductal' are perhaps better used to emphasize the close proximity of the coarctation to the opening of the ductus arteriosus. It is considered to be the result of an intrinsic maldevelopment of the primitive aortic arch itself together with extension of fetal ductal tissue into the aortic wall and its postnatal constriction producing or increasing the obstruction. Collateral arteries to the descending aorta usually develop but are inadequate in infancy.

Associated cardiovascular malformations are common. The aortic valve is often bicuspid. Males are affected twice as often as females. About 15% of patients with Turner's syndrome have coarctation of the aorta.

Physiology

Left ventricular overloading results from obstruction to aortic blood flow. With time, left ventricular function becomes depressed and left atrial and pulmonary venous and arterial pressures are raised. In the presence of a persistent ductus arteriosus or septal defects a large left to right shunt can develop, further increasing pulmonary hypertension. Systemic hypertension develops as a result of the mechanical obstruction and increased renin production and fluid retention due to reduced renal perfusion.

Clinical features

Most infants with symptomatic coarctation of the aorta present with heart failure in the first months of life, often during the first 2 weeks. Preceding symptoms of dyspnea or feeding problems are common but many newborns present acutely with severe respiratory distress and shock, presumably due to the postnatal closure of the ductus producing abrupt obstruction to aortic blood flow and left ventricular failure.

The diagnostic and pathognomonic sign of coarctation is weak or absent femoral pulses associated with strong upper limb pulses or a gradient between the blood pressure in the arms and legs. A discrepancy of 15–20 mmHg, lower in the legs, may be found in normal newborns. The difference in pulses might not be present in the first day or two after birth while the ductus is still open, but is always obvious when the infant becomes sick. The heart is enlarged and shows a right ventricular impulse; a strong apex beat suggestive of left ventricular hypertrophy is rare in infants. The second heart sound is loud because of pulmonary hypertension. An ejection systolic click over the left sternal border or apex may be present if there is a bicuspid aortic valve and is a useful diagnostic clue. Murmurs are nonspecific and may be absent.

Patients with less severe obstruction remain well during infancy and are recognized later in childhood or even adult life by the discrepancy in pulse and blood pressure between the upper and lower limbs, often following discovery of a heart murmur or hypertension. The heart size is usually normal but, unlike infancy, a strong left ventricular impulse may be present. The heart sounds are normal and an ejection click is frequently heard. An ejection systolic murmur is present in most patients with isolated coarctation and may be heard over the upper left sternal border though it is often best heard at the back between the scapulae. A mid-diastolic murmur may be heard at the back or the apex.

Investigations

The chest X-ray in the symptomatic infant shows cardiomegaly and pulmonary congestion. In the older child cardiomegaly is infrequent or mild. The diagnostic features of rib notching or a 'figure of 3' sign of the aortic knuckle may be present but usually do not develop until 5 years of age. The electrocardiogram in the young infant typically shows right ventricular hypertrophy and sometimes biventricular hypertrophy. Left ventricular hypertrophy is common in the older patients. Cross-sectional echocardiography can demonstrate the coarctation but is less satisfactory in older subjects. Pressure gradient across the obstruction can also be estimated by Doppler studies but correlation with measured gradients is poor. Cardiac catheterization and angiography are not necessary in most cases, particularly the sick neonate, and are performed only if the diagnosis is uncertain.

Treatment

Infants with coarctation and heart failure usually die unless the obstruction is relieved. Older patients with coarctation are at risk of infective endocarditis, severe hypertension, aortic dissection and cerebrovascular accidents. Surgery should be performed as soon as the diagnosis is made. The use of intravenous prostaglandin infusion to keep the ductus arteriosus open, in addition to inotropes, is helpful in the initial management of sick infants. Repair consists of excision of the coarctation segment and restoration of aortic patency by end-to-end anastomosis or left subclavian flap or patch aortoplasty. Major postoperative sequelae are recoarctation, which is mostly confined to patients operated upon in infancy, and persistent systemic hypertension, which is more common in patients operated at older ages. Balloon dilation angioplasty has been shown to be effective in relieving the obstruction, especially in the older patients and for recoarctation. Aneurysm formation has followed dilation of primary coarctation but recent evaluation of reported results suggests that in some patients balloon dilation may produce results equivalent to those of surgery (Rao 1995).

Vascular ring

Anatomy

A vascular ring is a malformation of the aortic arch or its brachiocephalic branches encircling and compressing the trachea and esophagus. Double aortic arch is the most common type; the ascending aorta divides into two vessels which reunite to form the descending aorta. A pulmonary artery sling is anomalous origin of the left pulmonary artery from the right pulmonary artery crossing the midline between the trachea and esophagus and producing severe tracheal compression. Intrinsic narrowing of the trachea often coexists.

Clinical features

Airway obstruction resulting from tracheal compression is the most important clinical problem and causes inspiratory stridor, which may be present soon after birth or delayed. Wheezing, cough and recurrent respiratory tract infections are common. Dysphagia due to esophageal compression is rare. The diagnosis is often delayed because of the failure to consider it in the child with respiratory difficulties.

Investigations

A barium swallow is the most useful investigation and demonstrates an indentation of the posterior aspect of the esophagus by a vascular ring. A double aortic arch is suggested by bilateral indentations, usually at different levels, in addition to the posterior indentation. A pulmonary artery sling characteristically produces an anterior indentation, sometimes accompanied by a posterior impression on the air column in the trachea at the same level. A more complete diagnosis of the vascular anatomy requires angiography but this is usually not required before surgery. Echocardiography may show a double arch or pulmonary sling but in most cases does not demonstrate the abnormality.

Treatment

Although spontaneous improvement of respiratory symptoms in patients with a vascular ring have been described, surgery is always indicated. Outcome is generally good although persistent respiratory symptoms may result from tracheal distortion.

Anomalous origin of the left coronary artery from the pulmonary artery

Anomalous origin of a coronary artery from the pulmonary artery is rare, the left coronary usually being involved. Perfusion of the left ventricle depends on the pressure in the pulmonary artery and the extent of collateral circulation from the right coronary artery. At birth, when the pulmonary pressure is still high, the left ventricular myocardium remains well perfused. Ischemia occurs with the postnatal fall in the pulmonary pressure, its severity depending on the amount of collateral circulation developing at the same time. Sometimes large fistulous communications are formed between the left and right coronary arteries producing an aortopulmonary shunt and diverting blood supply from the coronary artery branches. The manifestations can thus vary from minimal to severe congestive heart failure in early infancy.

The infant with inadequate left ventricular perfusion usually presents in the second month of life with 'anginal attacks', manifested as acute distress with crying, sweating, pallor or gray coloration, often during feeding or defecation. Subsequently, progressive heart failure appears. The heart is enlarged and gallop rhythm is common. Heart murmurs are nonspecific but there is often one of mitral regurgitation secondary to left ventricular dilation. X-ray shows marked cardiomegaly and pulmonary venous congestion. The electrocardiogram characteristically shows an anterior infarction pattern with T wave inversion and deep Q waves in the left chest leads, lead I and aVL. Echocardiography reveals a dilated and poorly contractile left ventricle with a dilated right coronary origin and the abnormal origin of the left coronary artery may be visualized. Angiography is necessary if ultrasound studies are inconclusive. An aortogram shows a large right coronary artery and its distal anastomosis with the left coronary artery which then drains into the pulmonary artery.

Patients who establish adequate collateral circulation early in life have few symptoms and may have evidence of mitral regurgitation or no cardiac findings. Ischemic symptoms on exertion may occur in adult life and sudden death has been described. Sometimes a continuous murmur representing the coronary aortopulmonary fistula may be heard.

Treatment consists of surgical anastomosis of the left anomalous coronary artery to the aorta.

Abnormal cardiac positions

Dextrocardia refers only to the situation in which more than half the heart is situated in the right side of the chest. It has no implication for the anatomy of the heart itself. Terms such as dextroversion, dextroposition and dextrorotation should be discarded because of controversial and confusing usage. Dextrocardia may thus be a primary abnormality of the heart or secondary to other thoracic pathology. Primary dextrocardia is often associated with abnormal positions of the abdominal organs. Complete situs inversus refers to the mirror image arrangement of the organs. It occurs with an incidence of 1 per 7000 to 1 per 10 000 and 90–95% of these individuals have a normal heart. When dextrocardia is associated with abnormal or ambiguous visceral arrangements the heart is usually abnormal, malformations including atrioventricular discordance, univentricular heart, anomalous pulmonary venous drainage and pulmonary atresia. About one-third of patients with asplenia or polysplenia have dextrocardia. The combination of situs inversus, bronchiectasis and paranasal sinusitis known as Kartagener's syndrome occurs in 10–15% of patients with mirror-image dextrocardia.

Mesocardia indicates the position of the heart in the center of the thorax, prominent neither to the right nor to the left. It is usually not recognized clinically and is apparent only from the chest X-ray. The term *levocardia* need be used only when the left-sided heart is associated with abnormal visceral situs.

The possibility of abnormal cardiac position should always be remembered. The cardiac apex and impulse should be palpated over the right chest if it is not apparent on the left side, and heart sounds should be auscultated on both sides. Abnormal location of the liver edge in the midline or the left side, or the stomach resonance on the right side of the abdomen suggests abnormal abdominal situs, often associated with cardiac malposition.

The straight X-ray confirms the position of the heart. The morphology of the bronchi will suggest the thoracic situs (p. 597), and the position of the stomach and liver the abdominal situs. Abnormal cardiac or visceral situs demands assessment for cardiac pathology. The electrocardiogram should be performed in the usual manner with the addition of right-sided chest leads (V3R to V7R). In dextrocardia, the QRS complexes are characteristically taller in the right chest leads and become progressively smaller from V3 to V7 in the left-sided chest leads. A negative P wave in lead I indicates reversed atrial arrangement (atrial situs inversus) but does not specify the position of the heart in the chest. Cross-sectional echocardiography using the segmental approach (p. 591) provides the best noninvasive means of identifying the arrangements and anatomy of the atria, ventricles and great vessels and any associated malformations.

Mesocardia and levocardia with abnormal visceral situs are commonly associated with asplenia or polysplenia. When asplenia or polysplenia is suspected, splenic ultrasound or scintiscan and examination of the peripheral blood for Howell–Jolly bodies are appropriate. Patients with asplenia should receive pneumococcal vaccine, and prophylactic antibiotic therapy with amoxicillin 25 mg/kg/24 h in divided doses is recommended.

CYANOTIC CONGENITAL HEART DISEASE

Cyanotic congenital heart disease accounts for less than 25% of congenital cardiac defects. However, many of these are life threatening in the first weeks of life and thus early recognition, diagnosis and treatment is essential.

The degree of cyanosis and mode of presentation can vary in conditions with the same basic diagnosis. Often the great arteries are in communication with the same ventricle or with both ventricles with an unrestricted ventricular septal defect between them. In such a situation the degree of cyanosis will depend on the severity of pulmonary obstruction. At its most severe (pulmonary atresia) the infant will depend on a ductus arteriosus for pulmonary blood flow and die when the duct closes. When there

is no pulmonary stenosis the pulmonary blood flow will increase as the pulmonary vascular resistance falls and if flow is very large cyanosis will be minimal and the patient will present with signs of cardiac failure.

Problems in nomenclature of complex congenital heart disease are discussed in the section on nomenclature (p. 597). Simple clinical features of the cyanotic patient are discussed in the sections Clinical Examination: Cyanosis (p. 585) and the Newborn Infant with Congenital Heart Disease (p. 198). Although there are typical findings in infants with cyanotic congenital heart disease there are considerable variations. These will be reflected in the clinical findings and they have different implications for patient management.

Ultrasound simplifies the diagnosis of cyanotic heart disease but for many pediatricians the assessment of the cyanotic infant has to be made without this. The integration of information available from the chest X-ray and electrocardiogram may allow the construction of a logic tree which allows the differential diagnosis of the cyanosed child to be narrowed and refined depending on whether the X-ray shows increased or decreased pulmonary blood flow, and whether the electrocardiogram shows right, left or biventricular hypertrophy (Table 13.5). A review and similar diagnostic algorithm has recently been published (Rigby 1994).

Complete transposition of the great arteries (TGA)

Transposition of the great arteries is the most common cyanotic congenital cardiac defect presenting in the newborn infant and accounts for about 5% of congenital heart disease. It is more common in males than females with a ratio of about 3 : 1.

Anatomy and pathophysiology

There has been disagreement amongst cardiac anatomists and pathologists as to how to describe the condition, the accepted definition now being an abnormality of ventriculoarterial connections in which the aorta is connected to the right ventricle and the pulmonary artery to the left. Employing the classification referred to earlier, complete transposition is therefore a

Table 13.5 Flow chart for the differential diagnosis of central cyanosis. Assessment of whether pulmonary blood flow is increased or diminished combined with the electrocardiographic findings helps to narrow the diagnostic possibilities

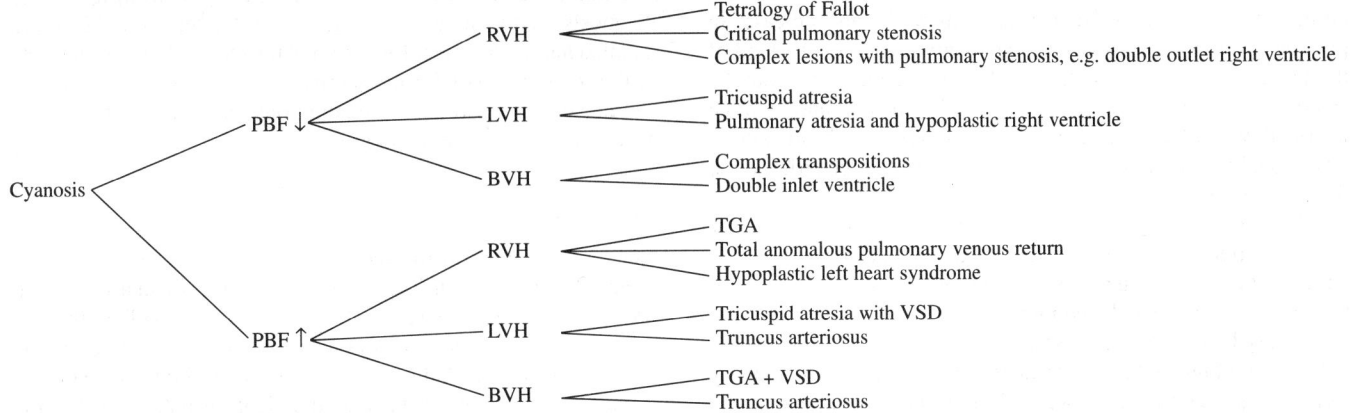

PBF = pulmonary blood flow; RVH = right ventricular hypertrophy; LVH = left ventricular hypertrophy; BVH = biventricular hypertrophy; TGA = transposition of great arteries.

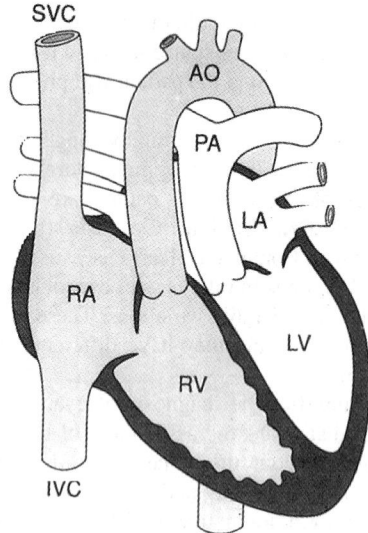

Fig. 13.16 Transposition of the great arteries (atrioventricular concordance, arterioventricular discordance). Shading indicates desaturated/unoxygenated blood. SVC, superior vena cava; IVC, inferior vena cava; AO aorta; LA, left atrium; PA, pulmonary artery; RA, right atrium; RV, right ventricle; LV, left ventricle.

combination of concordant atrioventricular and discordant ventriculoarterial connections (Fig. 13.16).

Since the pulmonary and systemic circulations are in parallel rather than in series as normally, it is essential for survival that there be an associated defect, such as a ductus arteriosus or ventricular or atrial septal defect, which permits mixing between the pulmonary and systemic circulations. The presence of one or other of these associated defects and the degree to which it permits mixing between the two circulations determines the clinical presentation and hemodynamic findings. In about 40% of cases a ventricular septal defect is present. Pulmonary stenosis (valvar or subvalvar) occurs in about a third of patients with a ventricular septal defect, and in a further 20% dynamic left ventricular outflow tract obstruction may occur without a ventricular septal defect.

Most commonly there is only a small communication at atrial level, a patent foramen ovale. These infants are usually severely cyanosed at or very shortly after birth. As a consequence of the low arterial PO_2 there is progressive unremitting metabolic acidosis with depression of myocardial function. As the pulmonary vascular resistance falls there is an increase in pulmonary blood flow and correspondingly a volume overload of the left atrium and left ventricle. The combination of metabolic acidosis with depression of myocardial function and volume overload of the left side of the heart may result in heart failure. Occasionally there may be a naturally occurring large atrial septal defect, and these infants fare better.

When there is a large ventricular septal defect there may be only minimal arterial desaturation and metabolic acidosis does not develop, the infant usually presenting with heart failure several weeks after birth when the pulmonary vascular resistance falls and pulmonary blood flow increases.

In those infants with a ventricular septal defect and pulmonary stenosis the ventricular septal defect is usually large and the severity of cyanosis is determined by the severity of the pulmonary stenosis. The presenting clinical features may simulate the tetralogy of Fallot or any other condition associated with a diminished pulmonary blood flow.

Clinical presentation and course

Most patients with transposition are cyanosed from shortly after birth, although in some the diagnosis may not be suspected until towards the end of the first week of life or beyond. Those with a small atrial septal defect/patent foramen ovale present earliest. Those with a large ventricular septal defect or ductus arteriosus may not be diagnosed until several weeks of age and frequently they are suspected of having another form of congenital heart disease dominated by left to right shunting.

The auscultatory findings are frequently unimpressive, particularly in those with an intact ventricular septum. The second heart sound may be single and accentuated, reflecting the anterior position of the aorta. In those patients with a ventricular septal defect there may be a systolic murmur which increases in intensity as the pulmonary vascular resistance falls. An ejection systolic murmur is usually present in those with left ventricular outflow tract obstruction.

The clinical course of patients born with transposition and not treated is invariably lethal, with 90% dying before the first birthday. Survival is longest in those who have a combination of a ventricular septal defect and pulmonary stenosis. Death is usually due to anoxia, acidosis, heart failure and complications associated with polycythemia including thromboembolic events.

Investigation

Arterial blood gas analysis with a hyperoxic test shows hypoxemia unresponsive to oxygen inhalation.

Right ventricular hypertrophy is almost always present on the electrocardiogram and in those infants with a large ductus arteriosus or ventricular septal defect or associated pulmonary stenosis there may be associated left ventricular hypertrophy, giving the appearances of biventricular hypertrophy. Radiologically there is an increase in the cardiothoracic ratio and pulmonary vascularity. With a significant degree of hypoxemia the thymus involutes to give a narrow cardiac pedicle.

Echocardiography rapidly provides a complete anatomical diagnosis by demonstrating the origin of the pulmonary artery from the left ventricle and the aorta from the right ventricle, and any associated anomalies (Houston et al 1978).

Cardiac catheterization and angiography add little to the diagnosis in the early newborn period but can provide more detailed hemodynamic information in the older infant, particularly in the more complex forms of transposition of the great arteries. Cardiac catheterization is also commonly combined with balloon atrial septostomy (see below).

Management

Once the diagnosis of transposition of the great arteries has been established by echocardiography the decision is usually taken to proceed to balloon atrial septostomy (Rashkind & Miller 1966). A balloon tipped catheter is passed into the left atrium through the foramen ovale, the balloon is inflated with fluid and then the catheter rapidly withdrawn into the right atrium, rupturing the floor of the fossa ovale and creating a defect in the atrial septum which allows interatrial mixing. This technique can now be performed very effectively under ultrasound control, though some cardiologists still prefer to combine it with cardiac catheterization and perform the procedure under fluoroscopic monitoring. If undertaken within the first 48 hours of life the umbilical vein can be used (Ashfaq et al 1991). This procedure usually results in a significant rise in arterial oxygen saturation which is usually sustained until definitive surgical treatment is undertaken.

If there is severe hypoxemia or metabolic acidosis a prostaglandin infusion can be used to reopen the ductus and improve the infant's situation while awaiting septostomy, or during transfer for this. Balloon atrial septostomy is successful in all but a few infants in the first few weeks of life. Beyond 1 month of age the atrial septum may be too thick and surgical intervention may be appropriate. Depending on surgical expertise this would usually take the form of arterial switch or inflow correction (see below). In centers where such facilities are not available for infants, surgical excision of the posterior part of the atrial septum without cardiopulmonary bypass may be performed (Blalock–Hanlon procedure).

A variety of definitive surgical procedures is now available for the different subsets of transposition of the great arteries. These may be divided into:

1. redirection of venous return at atrial level, the Mustard (Mustard 1964) or Senning operation
2. redirection of flood flow at ventricular level, the Rastelli operation (Rastelli et al 1969)
3. redirection of blood flow at great artery level – arterial switch operation (Quaegebeur et al 1986).

For those infants with transposition and an intact ventricular septum and no obstruction to pulmonary blood flow, the choice is between an intra-atrial repair or an arterial switch operation. In the Mustard procedure the pulmonary and systemic venous return are redirected at atrial level by using a baffle of pericardium (Fig. 13.17). The Senning procedure also redirects blood flow at atrial level but utilizes an atrial septal flap and the right atrial free wall to direct the pulmonary and systemic venous return. Both

procedures have their advocates and can be performed at any age but safely may be deferred to between 6 and 12 months of age if a good balloon septostomy has been performed. The mortality in the best hands is no more than 1–2%. Following the atrial redirection operation the aorta remains connected to the right ventricle which continues to function as a systemic ventricle. There is continuing uncertainty about the ability of the right ventricle to function in the long term as a systemic ventricle. Because of this fear most centers are now employing the arterial switch operation performed in the first week or two of life (Fig. 13.18). The early mortality for this operation is higher (0–20%) but the longer term outlook promises to be better since this is a more physiological operation. It has to be performed early in the newborn period when the left ventricular pressure is high. If the operation is deferred until the pulmonary vascular resistance has fallen, the pulmonary artery and left ventricular pressures will be low and the ventricle will be unable to function at systemic pressure if an arterial switch operation is performed.

For infants with an associated ventricular septal defect the operation of choice is usually the arterial switch procedure with closure of the VSD, since the left ventricular pressure is at systemic level and the left ventricle is well suited to an immediate adjustment to functioning at high pressure. When transposition is associated with a ventricular septal defect and severe pulmonary stenosis, left ventricular flow is directed to the aorta by placing an interventricular tunnel between the VSD and the aortic valve and a conduit between the right ventricle to the pulmonary artery (Rastelli procedure).

The outlook for infants born with transposition of the great arteries is now immeasurably better than 25 years ago. In those who have undergone an inflow correction there may be residual postoperative problems, such as arrhythmias, poor systemic ventricular function, early and late residual shunts, and obstruction to venous return. Arrhythmias and poor function can result in symptoms and sudden death in teenage or later life but the majority of infants born with transposition of the great arteries lead essentially normal, active lives during childhood. It is expected that those who have undergone an arterial switch

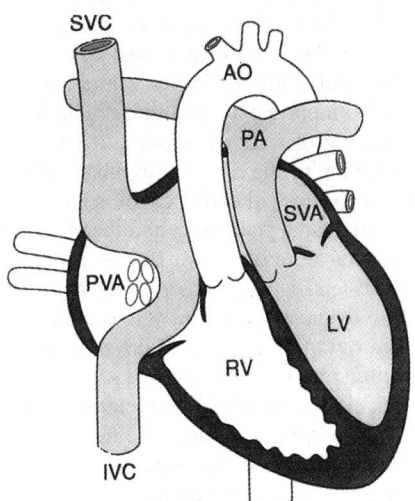

Fig. 13.17 Mustard procedure for transposition of the great arteries. Intra-atrial baffle of pericardium redirects pulmonary and system venous return so that SVC and IVC unoxygenated venous blood (shaded) is directed to LV and pulmonary venous blood to RV. SVA, new systemic venous atrium; PVA, new pulmonary venous atrium.

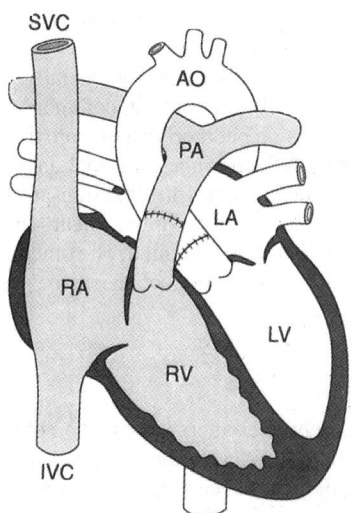

Fig. 13.18 Arterial switch operation for transposition of the great arteries. In addition to switching of the aorta and pulmonary arteries, the coronary arteries (not shown) are detached and anastomosed to the new aortic root.

procedure will have normal cardiac function in childhood and adult life.

Congenitally corrected transposition of the great arteries

This rare congenital cardiovascular lesion accounts for less than 1% of all defects. Patients with this lesion are not always cyanosed.

Anatomy and pathophysiology

This condition has a variety of eponyms including L-transposition (LTGA) and ventricular inversion. The condition is characterized by discordance of both the atrioventricular and the ventriculoarterial connection. The deoxygenated right atrial blood passes through the mitral valve into a morphological left ventricle from which the pulmonary artery arises, and the oxygenated pulmonary venous blood passes from the left atrium through the tricuspid valve into the morphological right ventricle and thence into the aorta. Thus although there is transposition, the anatomical fault is functionally corrected by the presence of atrioventricular discordance. The aorta is usually located anterior and to the left of the pulmonary artery (hence L- or levotransposition). Most patients have an associated cardiac lesion, although not necessarily one that results in cyanosis. Ventricular septal defect is the most frequent lesion and is commonly associated with pulmonary stenosis, which may result in cyanosis from shunting of deoxygenated blood into the aorta. A few patients have no functional abnormality but left sided atrioventricular valve (tricuspid) regurgitation may develop progressively over many years. Arrhythmias and heart block may occur at any time. The condition is commonly associated with dextrocardia.

Clinical presentation and course

The clinical presentation and course are usually dictated by the associated cardiac lesion. If a large ventricular septal defect is present heart failure develops early. Those patients with a ventricular septal defect and pulmonary stenosis may present with cyanosis and clinically resemble tetralogy of Fallot. In the absence of associated defects and arrhythmias, the patient may be completely asymptomatic and the condition not recognized clinically for many years.

There may be few signs to alert even the most careful clinician. A loud single second heart sound is common and may suggest pulmonary hypertension but it originates from the aortic valve, the increased intensity reflecting the abnormal anterior and leftward position of the aortic valve in corrected transposition. If the heart rate is slow, suggesting complete heart block, corrected transposition should be borne in mind. The other physical findings present are usually a reflection of the associated complicating lesions.

Investigations

Inversion of the ventricles alters the direction of ventricular septal depolarization and produces the characteristic electrocardiographic finding of the absence of Q waves in V_5 and V_6 and/or the presence of Q waves in V_4R or V_1. The electrocardiogram may also show varying degrees of heart block or arrhythmias and there is an association between corrected transposition of the great arteries and the Wolff–Parkinson–White syndrome. Radiologi-

cally the condition may be suspected by the presence of a straight upper left heart border produced by the left sided anterior aorta. Cardiac ultrasound examination will determine the abnormal atrioventricular and ventriculoarterial connections and define any associated cardiac abnormality.

Management

The management is usually that of the associated intracardiac lesion. Patients who are severely cyanosed may require a systemic to pulmonary arterial shunt. For those with heart failure secondary to a large ventricular septal defect, pulmonary artery banding may be indicated. Definitive closure of a ventricular septal defect in corrected transposition of the great arteries is associated with a high incidence of complete heart block, and the mortality for the condition is significantly greater than that for isolated ventricular septal defect. Cardiac pacemaker implantation may be required for complete heart block postoperatively or when it complicates the natural history of the condition.

Tetralogy of Fallot

Tetralogy of Fallot is the most common of the cyanotic congenital cardiac malformations, accounting for about 6% of all congenital defects.

Anatomy and pathophysiology

Tetralogy of Fallot has as its features a ventricular septal defect, pulmonary stenosis, overriding of the ventricular septum by the aorta, and right ventricular hypertrophy. The two most important abnormalities, however, are the pulmonary stenosis and ventricular septal defect. The ventricular septal defect is usually of the perimembranous type with extension into the outlet septum of the right ventricle, although other variations may be seen. It is usually large and nonrestrictive and allows equalization of pressure between the right and left ventricles. The pulmonary stenosis affects both the infundibulum and the pulmonary valve and artery. The infundibular stenosis is due partly to anterior deviation of the infundibular portion of the ventricular septum. The pulmonary valve is stenotic in almost all cases but only very rarely is it the only site of right ventricular outflow tract obstruction. It is important to recognize that the spectrum of severity in tetralogy of Fallot is determined principally by the degree of obstruction of the right ventricular outflow tract and it is this which determines the degree of right to left shunting through the ventricular septal defect and therefore the severity of any cyanosis detected clinically. If the infundibular and/or pulmonary valve stenosis is mild there is little, if any, right to left shunting and no cyanosis. Frequently it is only as the infant or child grows that right to left shunting develops as a consequence of increasing infundibular obstruction.

Right ventricular hypertrophy develops secondary to the increased right ventricular pressure. The degree of overriding of the interventricular septum of the aorta varies and this feature is of little importance in functional terms.

Clinical presentation and course

Infants with tetralogy of Fallot are usually not cyanosed at birth and only become so with the passage of time. They may be misdiagnosed clinically as either an isolated ventricular septal defect or pulmonary stenosis. In the majority, cyanosis develops by the end of the first year of life; occasionally its appearance is slower and associated symptoms therefore deferred. Some infants present with so-called 'hypercyanotic attacks' (hypoxic spells). These occur most frequently in the early morning after the baby wakens and may be initiated by irritability, crying, exertion and feeding. They commonly occur in infants who are normally pink. They can be life threatening, the infant can lose consciousness and they should never be ignored. They are probably due to spasm of the infundibular muscle as a consequence of which the pulmonary blood flow is greatly diminished. During attacks the heart murmur may lessen in intensity or disappear.

Children with the most severe forms of tetralogy of Fallot, in which there is a marked degree of right ventricular outflow tract obstruction (see pulmonary atresia with VSD), may present with cyanosis in the newborn period. The inadequacy of pulmonary blood flow under these circumstances is associated with severe hypoxemia.

The child with well-established cyanosis has finger clubbing. In contrast to pulmonary stenosis with an intact ventricular septum, a right ventricular heave is not commonly found. The second heart sound is usually single and the length and intensity of the systolic murmur reflects the degree of right ventricular outflow tract obstruction.

Where surgery is deferred beyond the first few years of life the child may adopt a squatting posture following exertion or when cyanosis deepens. This relieves distress by increasing systemic vascular resistance (and thus increasing pulmonary blood flow), and decreasing the return of reduced venous blood from the legs.

Investigations

The electrocardiogram usually shows right ventricular hypertrophy with right axis deviation, although the only clue to this in early infancy may be an upright T wave in V_1. The cardiothoracic ratio is usually normal. In about 25–30% of cases there is a right sided aortic arch. Depending on the severity of the right ventricular outflow tract obstruction, the pulmonary vascular markings will be decreased to a variable degree. Cardiac ultrasound examination demonstrates the position of the ventricular septal defect and the anatomy of the right ventricular outflow tract. The Doppler technique can be used to assess the pressure difference between the main right ventricular cavity and the pulmonary artery. Cardiac catheterization and angiography is usually still performed since additional information may be provided on the anatomy of the coronary arteries and of the pulmonary arteries.

Management

Without treatment 85% of infants born with tetralogy of Fallot die before they reach their teens. Medical management is important in avoiding complications and in having the child in an optimal state prior to surgery. Attention is required by the pediatrician to four aspects of management:

1. The hemoglobin and hematocrit should be monitored. Once the hematocrit is higher than 60% the viscosity rises sharply, with an increased risk of cerebral thrombosis and hemiplegia. Cerebrovascular accidents can also be the consequence of relative anemia and attention should therefore be paid to treatment with iron if hemoglobin is low.

2. Tetralogy of Fallot is the most common cyanotic abnormality likely to be associated with infective endocarditis, and patients who have had a systemic to pulmonary artery shunt (see below) are particularly at risk.

3. Deficiency in coagulation factors are more common in those with a high hematocrit.

4. Hypercyanotic attacks are usually self-limiting but may be fatal. During an attack the infant should be placed in the knee–elbow position and 100% oxygen given by mask. Metabolic acidosis may require to be corrected. Propranolol 0.1 mg/kg i.v. may reverse the increase in infundibular obstruction which has precipitated the attack. Thereafter it may be given prophylactically in a dosage of 0.5–1 mg/kg 3 or 4 times daily orally.

The definitive treatment of tetralogy of Fallot is surgical and the type of surgery and its timing is determined by the anatomy, the clinical symptoms and the experience and policy of the surgical team. When the pulmonary valve ring is of a good size and the main pulmonary artery well developed and the infundibular stenosis localized, surgical repair may be carried out in one stage. On the other hand, if the right ventricular outflow tract is profoundly hypoplastic with a small pulmonary valve ring and poorly developed pulmonary arteries with selective stenosis, one-stage repair may carry significantly higher risks and palliative surgery may be necessary. Palliative surgery takes the form of a shunt operation with an anastomosis between the systemic and pulmonary circulation. This is performed as the classical Blalock–Taussig operation (subclavian artery transected and anastomosed to pulmonary artery) or by the insertion of a Goretex graft between them (modified Blalock–Taussig procedure). Rarely the surgeon may choose to anastomose the ascending aorta to the right pulmonary artery (Waterston anastomosis). Following a palliative procedure, total repair is usually carried out electively between 2 and 4 years of age, depending on the child's symptoms and size. At operation the ventricular septal defect is closed with a patch and the right ventricular outflow tract enlarged with a vertical patch across the pulmonary valve ring although this can be confined to the infundibulum. Surgical results from tetralogy of Fallot are now good and most patients lead essentially normal lives with a good effort tolerance. There are usually residual systolic murmurs reflecting some mild remaining right ventricular outflow tract obstruction and frequently there is a diastolic murmur due to pulmonary regurgitation, especially in those in whom the patch has been extended across the pulmonary valve ring. Right bundle branch block is present in almost all patients. Patients continue to require follow-up because there may be a late incidence of ventricular arrhythmias and/or complete heart block.

Pulmonary atresia with ventricular septal defect

Pathology and hemodynamics

Pulmonary atresia with a ventricular septal defect represents the most severe end of the spectrum of tetralogy of Fallot. As a consequence of complete obstruction to flow from the right ventricle to the pulmonary artery, all the right ventricular blood enters the aorta. As well as complete interruption to the right ventricular outflow, the other feature which distinguishes pulmonary atresia with ventricular septal defect from tetralogy of Fallot is the severity of the deformity of the pulmonary artery and its branches which may be profoundly hypoplastic or atretic. The blood supply to the pulmonary artery is via a ductus arteriosus or aortopulmonary collateral arteries or both. Exact identification of these is important in management.

Clinical features and presentation

Infants born with this condition usually present shortly after birth with severe cyanosis, hypoxemia and metabolic acidosis. Those dependent entirely on a ductus for survival succumb when the ductus closes. If there is a well-developed aortopulmonary collateral circulation infants may present with heart failure rather than cyanosis. When an infant is dependent solely on a ductus arteriosus for pulmonary blood flow the auscultatory findings may be unimpressive, with only a single second heart sound and a continuous murmur which may be difficult to hear and must be sought posteriorly and laterally as well as anteriorly.

Investigations

On the chest X-ray the pulmonary artery segment is absent and there is usually marked pulmonary oligemia. The electrocardiogram shows right axis deviation with right ventricular hypertrophy.

On ultrasound examination the VSD and overriding aorta is seen as in tetralogy of Fallot but the outflow tract and main pulmonary valve are usually atretic. From a suprasternal view it may be possible to identify the presence or otherwise of a main pulmonary artery and whether or not there is confluence between the right and left pulmonary artery. The addition of color flow mapping may aid in identification of the anatomy of the pulmonary arteries and the blood supply to them. Angiocardiography is usually required to define the full extent and form of the pulmonary arteries and their blood supply, essential information for the planning of surgery.

Management

In the newborn period the management of these cases is difficult and is dictated by the pulmonary artery anatomy and the source of blood supply to the lung. Prostaglandin infusion may be invaluable in maintaining ductal patency and improving the infant's condition prior to surgery. When the pulmonary arteries are well formed and dependent on a ductus arteriosus, a shunt operation may be beneficial in maintaining blood supply to the lungs and encouraging further growth in the pulmonary arteries. At the other extreme of the spectrum, however, the pulmonary arteries may be very hypoplastic, and the major source of blood supply to the lungs derived from collateral circulation rather than the central pulmonary arteries. When the pulmonary arteries are confluent and of a good size and well distributed to all segments of the lung, a valve conduit can be connected from the right ventricle to the central pulmonary artery and the ventricular septal defect closed. The prognosis for many infants with this condition, however, must be regarded as poor, particularly when there are no central pulmonary arteries.

Pulmonary atresia with intact ventricular septum

It is important to distinguish between this condition and pulmonary atresia with VSD. In this condition the right

ventricular cavity is usually small and poorly developed. The right ventricular outflow tract is usually atretic but occasionally the atresia may involve only the valve. The cavity or sinus of the right ventricle is frequently obliterated by gross ventricular hypertrophy and the tricuspid valve is small and hypoplastic. In contrast to pulmonary atresia with VSD, the central pulmonary arteries are usually reasonably formed and are supplied by a ductus arteriosus rather than collateral arteries.

Clinical features and presentation

Cyanosis is present shortly after birth and increases in severity with closure of the ductus arteriosus upon which the infant survives. There may be no cardiac murmurs. Survival beyond a few weeks or months of life is unusual unless surgery is performed.

Investigations

A chest X-ray usually shows marked reduction in the pulmonary vascular markings. There may be cardiomegaly with a prominent right atrium. The electrocardiogram may display tall peaked P waves of right atrial hypertrophy. Because of the hypoplasia of the right ventricle the right precordial leads commonly show poorly developed right ventricular forces and this pattern may suggest the diagnosis of pulmonary atresia with intact septum in a cyanosed newborn infant. Cardiac catheterization is not usually required to make a diagnosis since cardiac ultrasound examination demonstrates the right ventricular morphology, and spectral and color Doppler flow mapping can determine ductal flow.

Management

Since survival in these infants is usually dependent on the ductus remaining patent, a prostaglandin infusion is started prior to surgery. If the atresia is confined to the pulmonary valve a transpulmonary valvotomy may be performed and in a small number of cases when the right ventricular cavity is a good size this may be all that is necessary. For most, however, a shunt operation is also required. Further surgery thereafter usually depends on the exact anatomy but in many it is possible to enlarge the right ventricular outflow tract and close the palliative shunt performed in the newborn period. For those infants in whom there is complete infundibular atresia and small right ventricular cavity, a Fontan procedure (see below) may be required. In certain cases the pulmonary valve may be opened by using radiofrequency energy to make a hole, allowing subsequent balloon dilation.

Ebstein's anomaly

This is a rare anomaly characterized by displacement of the posterior and septal leaflets of the tricuspid valve into the right ventricular cavity below the level of the normal tricuspid valve ring, the anterior leaflet arising normally. As a result, a portion of the right ventricle is 'atrialized'. The tricuspid valve may be both obstructive and regurgitant. There is usually an atrial septal defect or patent foramen ovale and because of the tricuspid valve regurgitation the right atrium is enlarged with right to left shunting at atrial level.

The spectrum of this disorder varies widely, with often only a minimal degree of displacement of the tricuspid valve leaflets (Fig. 13.19).

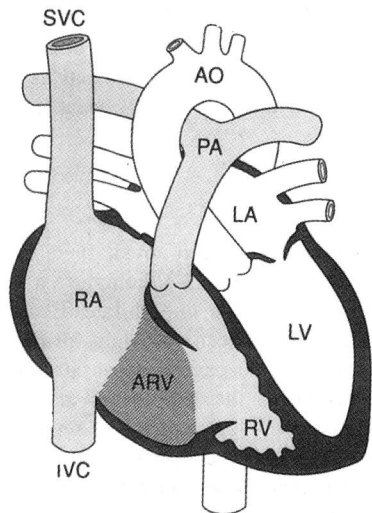

Fig. 13.19 Ebstein's anomaly. The hatched area represents the atrialized portion of the right ventricle (ARV) resulting from the displacement of the septal and posterior leaflets.

Clinical presentation and course

At birth a high pulmonary vascular resistance may impede forward flow from the right ventricle and the tendency to right to left shunting at atrial level is therefore greater. In many infants, however, there is a period of spontaneous improvement in the cyanosis, and those with a minor degree of Ebstein's malformation may be essentially asymptomatic in early childhood although later developing mild cyanosis and effort intolerance. On auscultation there may be a prominent triple or quadruple rhythm due to third and fourth heart sounds and this, combined with the presence of a systolic and scratchy diastolic murmur, produces a characteristic cadence to the auscultatory findings.

Investigation

Right atrial enlargement may be the only abnormal finding but in more severe degrees there is marked cardiac enlargement with pulmonary oligemia. The electrocardiogram may be diagnostic showing tall peaked P waves with a long PR interval and a pattern of incomplete or complete right bundle branch block. Type B Wolff–Parkinson–White syndrome is frequently seen (p. 625). Cardiac ultrasound examination defines the anatomy, demonstrating the tricuspid valve displacement into the right ventricular cavity. Doppler and color flow mapping studies may then be used to assess the degree of tricuspid regurgitation. Cardiac catheterization is not usually necessary in this condition.

Management

Abnormalities of rhythm, particularly atrial tachycardia, may require treatment. Plastic reconstruction of the tricuspid valve may be possible in some cases but in others the valve may have to be replaced and the atrial septum closed. Unfortunately, in the small infant who is severely symptomatic, treatment is still associated with a significant mortality.

Hypoplastic left heart syndrome

Hypoplastic left heart syndrome is a relatively common lesion presenting in the first week of life and accounts for up to 3% of all congenital cardiac defects. If not treated it usually results in death in the neonatal period. It was long considered to be inoperable but in the last decade treatment by palliative surgery or cardiac transplantation has become available and this is undertaken in some centers.

Anatomy and pathophysiology

The syndrome consists of a spectrum of differing degrees of hypoplasia of the left atrium, left ventricle and aorta, with stenosis or atresia of the aortic and mitral valves. In practical terms no blood is ejected from the left ventricle into the aorta; the pulmonary venous return passes through the atrial septum into the right atrium and then the right ventricle and pulmonary artery, with the systemic circulation being supplied through the ductus arteriosus. Since the pulmonary blood flow is high, cyanosis is not usually severe and the PaO_2 will show some rise on a hyperoxic test. The systemic circulation is initially maintained but decreases as the ductus closes, when the infant becomes very ill.

Clinical features

Infants are usually of normal birthweight and appear well initially. Within the first 2 or 3 days they become ill with tachypnea and cardiac failure and, as the duct closes, rapidly become shocked with poor peripheral pulses. The degree of cyanosis varies and is minimal in some. It is more severe if the atrial septum is restrictive and pulmonary vascular resistance high. Pulses are all poor if the duct is almost closed, but if it is still open (or the infant is on prostaglandins) the femorals may be of good volume with the arm ones less easily felt. There is usually a marked parasternal right ventricular heave, loud second heart sound, and a soft nonspecific murmur. Gallop rhythm is heard with severe cardiac failure.

Investigations

The chest X-ray shows cardiomegaly with plethoric lungs and the ECG shows right ventricular hypertrophy and low left ventricular voltages. Echocardiography provides a clear demonstration of the anatomical nature of the defect and will vary with the spectrum of mitral, left ventricular and aortic hypoplasia. The group which has pioneered the palliative surgical approach (Helton et al 1986) suggests a definition of features meeting the criteria for this diagnosis as an ascending aorta external diameter less than 7 mm and left ventricular end diastolic dimension less than 10 mm. Cardiac catheterization is not required for diagnosis but in some situations atrial septostomy may be required.

Management

The hypoplastic left heart syndrome has been considered inoperable and in many centers it is considered inappropriate or unethical to undertake surgery. However, palliative surgery is possible (Norwood et al 1983) and is successful in a number of centers, but in others the success rate is poor. Surgical intervention requires that the left and right pulmonary arteries are disconnected from the main pulmonary artery, which is then connected to the aorta by a tube graft; this means the right ventricle ejects to the aorta. A systemic–pulmonary shunt is then performed into the disconnected pulmonary arteries to supply the pulmonary blood flow. These patients can later undergo a Fontan-type procedure with the systemic venous blood being directed into the pulmonary arteries, leaving the right ventricle to supply the systemic circulation. Prior to undertaking surgery, the infant's condition can be improved or maintained by the use of a prostaglandin infusion. If no surgery is contemplated, it is inappropriate to undertake active measures and these infants usually die within a few days of presentation.

Double inlet (single) ventricle

This condition is more common than formerly appreciated and may account for up to 2–3% of all congenital heart disease. Understanding for the general pediatrician has been made difficult because of the variation in approaches to classification of the disorder. The term double inlet ventricle groups together a number of conditions which have in common the feature that there is a univentricular heart (nomenclature, p. 597). Within this overall large grouping, there are three subdivisions (Fig. 13.20):

1. double inlet atrioventricular connection, usually double inlet left ventricle
2. classical tricuspid atresia
3. absence of the left atrioventricular connection (mitral atresia).

Double inlet left ventricle

This is the most common variety of double inlet ventricle. There is a main ventricle with a morphology of a normal left ventricle and two inlet valves and the right ventricle is usually represented by a small rudimentary outflow chamber. The ventriculoarterial connection can vary but most commonly the aorta arises from the

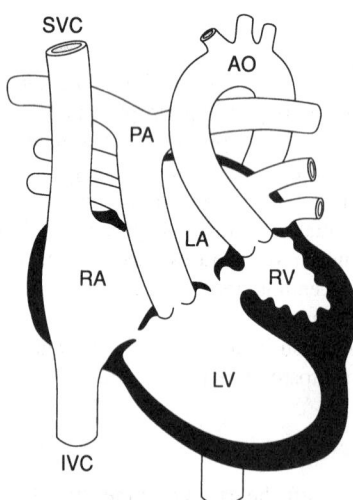

Fig. 13.20 Double inlet ventricle or single ventricle. In the most common variety as here both atrioventricular valves connect to a morphologically normal left ventricle (LV) and the right ventricle is represented by a small rudimentary outflow chamber from which the aorta arises. There is usually arterioventricular discordance.

rudimentary chamber and the pulmonary artery from the main ventricular chamber. The outlet chamber communicates with the main ventricular chamber via a ventricular septal defect. The severity of any associated pulmonary stenosis determines the presentation.

Tricuspid atresia

In the classical form of tricuspid atresia there is absence of the right atrioventricular connection, although occasionally the right atrioventricular valve may be imperforate. Because there is no direct communication between the right atrium and the right ventricle, right atrial blood passes via an atrial septal defect or patent foremen ovale to the left atrium and then to the left ventricle. There is usually a ventricular septal defect through which blood passes into the pulmonary outflow tract. Commonly there is a further degree of obstruction to the pulmonary blood flow in the form of pulmonary stenosis. Additionally there may be transposition, with the aorta arising from the right ventricular outlet chamber and the pulmonary artery from the left ventricle.

Mitral atresia

In this condition there is no communication between the left atrium and the left ventricle. Blood passes from the left atrium through the foramen ovale or atrial septal defect into the right atrium.

Clinical presentation and course

It is principally the presence of pulmonary outflow obstruction and its severity which determines the presentation and course of patients with double inlet ventricle. When there is no pulmonary outflow obstruction, the clinical picture is that of a high pulmonary blood flow simulating a large ventricular septal defect. When there is pulmonary outflow tract obstruction, cyanosis is the presenting feature and the clinical signs may simulate tetralogy of Fallot.

Investigation

The electrocardiogram may be particularly helpful in suggesting the diagnosis of tricuspid atresia as there is usually marked left axis deviation and absence of the normal degree of right ventricular dominance found in the newborn period. In double inlet left ventricle the axis can be normal.

The precise form of double inlet ventricle can usually be determined readily by cardiac ultrasound examination and the presence of associated abnormalities assessed by Doppler. It is important to decide whether there are one or two atrioventricular valves and the form of the ventriculoarterial connection and the degree of any outflow tract obstruction, as well as the ventricular morphology. If a good ultrasound study is obtained, cardiac catheterization may not be necessary if initial palliative surgery has to be considered. Detailed angiography and careful hemodynamic studies are usually required before definitive surgery.

Management

Most varieties of double inlet ventricle are not completely correctable although for selected patients radical surgery can improve the medium-term as well as the short-term prognosis. The long-term outlook for these patients, even after apparently successful radical surgery, is still uncertain, and the family must be made aware of this.

If the presentation is dominated by cyanosis, a palliative shunt is carried out. If, on the other hand, the pulmonary blood flow is high, then banding of the pulmonary artery to control excessive flow and alleviate heart failure, as well as preventing the development of pulmonary arterial vascular disease, should be performed. Definitive surgery can be undertaken under 2 years of age but is often left till 4 or 5 years of age. The most commonly considered operation has been the Fontan procedure (Fig. 13.21) (Fontan & Baudet 1971) in which the systemic venous return is directed directly into the pulmonary artery, bypassing the ventricular chamber which is left to eject the pulmonary venous

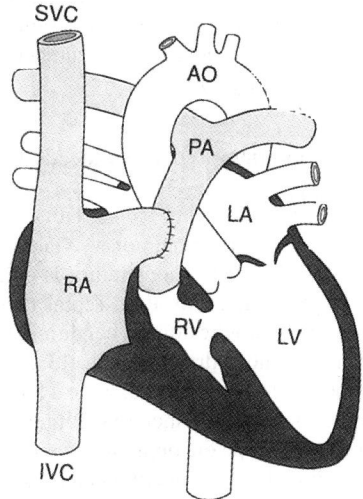

Fig. 13.21 Fontan operation. There are several variants of this procedure. Here the right atrium is anastomosed directly to the main pulmonary artery. The pulmonary valve/proximal main pulmonary artery are oversewn.

return to the aorta. More recently, surgical management has been to perform a total cavopulmonary connection (TCPC) (Stein et al 1991), anastomosing both the superior (SVC) and inferior (IVC) vena cava to the right pulmonary artery. This can be a single operation or a two-stage procedure with an initial bidirectional Glenn procedure (SVC to right pulmonary artery) (Pridjian et al 1993) and subsequent completion by anastomosing the IVC to the right pulmonary artery using an intra-atrial conduit.

Truncus arteriosus

Anatomy and pathophysiology

This condition results from failure of the primitive truncus arteriosus to divide into aortic and pulmonary arterial components. There is always a large nonrestrictive VSD sitting immediately below the single semilunar or truncal valve. The truncus arteriosus usually overrides both ventricles and the truncal valve may be stenotic or regurgitant. The condition can be subdivided into three types determined by pattern of origin of the pulmonary arteries from the common trunk; the right and left pulmonary arteries most commonly arise from the trunk from a common origin (type 1) but they may arise separately but close together from the back of the trunk (type 2) or separately from the lateral walls of the trunk (type 3) (Fig. 13.22).

In truncus arteriosus the magnitude of the pulmonary blood flow is determined by the size of the pulmonary arteries and by the pulmonary vascular resistance. Usually the arteries are large and as the vascular resistance falls in the first few weeks of life, increasing left ventricular volume overloading occurs with the development of the signs and symptoms of heart failure and it is these rather than the minimal cyanosis that may alert the clinician to the diagnosis.

Clinical presentation and course

At birth the newborn infant is usually well. Commonly symptoms appear at 2–3 weeks of age with increasing breathlessness and

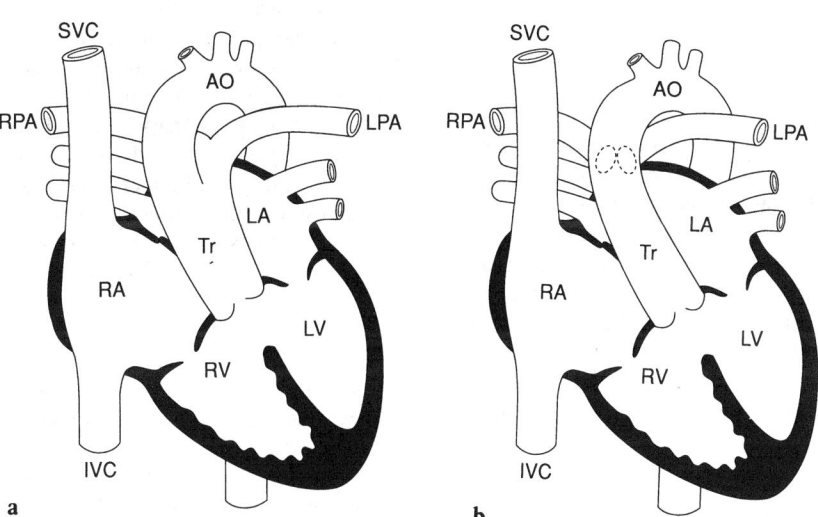

Fig. 13.22 Truncus arteriosus: (**a**) in type 1 the pulmonary arteries arise from the truncus (Tr) with a common origin; (**b**) in type 2 the pulmonary arteries arise separately from the back. In type 3 (not shown) the pulmonary arteries are more widely reported at origins and arise posteriorly/laterally from the trunk.

thereafter signs of heart failure. The degree of arterial desaturation present may not be sufficient to produce cyanosis. The peripheral pulses are usually bounding. The second heart sound is usually single but may appear split, probably because of asynchrony between closure of different parts of the common truncal valve. There is an ejection systolic murmur and when there is truncal valve regurgitation, an early diastolic murmur.

The outlook is poor and survival beyond 6 months of life is unusual. Pulmonary vascular disease can develop rapidly. Abnormalities of the truncal valve add to the early high mortality and the condition can also be associated with other complex abnormalities such as interruption of the aortic arch.

Investigations

The chest X-ray shows cardiac enlargement with increased pulmonary vascularity and a concave pulmonary artery segment. The aortic arch may be right sided. The electrocardiogram may be normal at birth but later shows right or combined ventricular hypertrophy. On ultrasound only one semilunar valve is identified with the common trunk usually overriding both ventricles. The origin of the pulmonary arteries from the trunk can usually be identified and Doppler studies allow assessment of the truncal valve itself. Cardiac catheterization may be required to assess the pulmonary blood flow and vascular resistance, particularly in the older infant.

Management

The initial management is that of heart failure. The surgeon normally prefers to defer operation till a few months of age since results in the newborn period, other than in few centers, remain poor. Definitive repair consists of detaching the pulmonary arteries from the common trunk and anastomosing them to the distal part of a homograft aortic conduit, the proximal end of which is sutured to the right ventricle. The ventricular septal defect is patched to direct the left ventricular blood into the aorta. As the child grows the conduit will require to be replaced.

Double outlet right ventricle

Anatomy and pathophysiology

In this condition the aorta and pulmonary artery both arise from the right ventricle. There are two common pathological or hemodynamic variations. In one variation there is a large ventricular septal defect with no pulmonary stenosis. This variety is commonly associated with a posterior pulmonary artery and an anterior aorta. The ventricular septal defect is related to the large pulmonary valve and has obvious similarities to transposition with a large ventricular septal defect (sometimes known as the Taussig–Bing malformation). In the other variation there is a large ventricular septal defect with pulmonary stenosis and the features mimic the tetralogy of Fallot.

Clinical presentation and course

There is no single clinical feature which suggests the diagnosis of a double outlet right ventricle. Depending upon the associated lesions the features mimic other lesions such as transposition, simple ventricular septal defect, or the tetralogy of Fallot.

The electrocardiogram and chest X-ray rarely display any diagnostic feature, although in the former a superior axis is not uncommon. Cardiac ultrasound examination allows a distinction to be made between the different varieties of double outlet right ventricle and other conditions which must be considered in the differential diagnosis.

Management

Those patients with high pulmonary blood flow and heart failure may require palliative surgery with banding of the pulmonary artery whereas those who present with severe cyanosis because of restrictive pulmonary blood flow may require a Blalock–Taussig shunt. In later life the form of definitive repair depends upon the site of the ventricular septal defect. Occasionally only an intracardiac patch may be required but in other patients switching of the great arteries and closure of a ventricular septal defect or major intracardiac and extracardiac reconstruction with the use of a conduit may be necessary. Under these circumstances, there may be late residua of major surgery.

Total anomalous pulmonary venous connection

Anatomy and pathophysiology

As the title suggests, none of the pulmonary veins connects to the left atrium and the pulmonary venous return is either directly or indirectly to the right atrium. An atrial septal defect is usually present. There are three varieties of the condition, defined by the site of the anomalous venous drainage (Fig. 13.23): in the supracardiac type the four pulmonary veins drain to a left sided superior vena cava (left vertical vein) and then to the innominate vein and right SVC; in the cardiac type the pulmonary veins empty into the right atrium either directly or indirectly via the coronary sinus; in the infracardiac type a common pulmonary channel receives the four pulmonary veins, passes below the diaphragm and drains into the hepatic vein, portal vein or inferior vena cava.

These three varieties may be subdivided into obstructive and nonobstructive, depending on whether or not pulmonary venous return is obstructed, and this to an extent determines the findings and clinical presentation. In the nonobstructive varieties the hemodynamics resemble those of a large atrial septal defect with diastolic volume overloading of the right ventricle. When there is obstruction to pulmonary venous return (most commonly the infradiaphragmatic type), there is pulmonary venous hypertension and secondary pulmonary arterial and right ventricular hypertension. Obstruction causes interstitial and alveolar edema and these infants tend to be more ill, tachypneic, and cyanosed than those without obstruction with a high pulmonary blood flow.

Clinical presentation and course

Infants with a nonobstructive variety of total anomalous pulmonary venous connection may be asymptomatic in the first few weeks of life. Thereafter, respiratory difficulties and failure to thrive may be the presenting features. On examination there is usually some degree of tachypnea and a right ventricular heave. There is a systolic ejection murmur at the upper left sternal edge because of increased flow through the pulmonary valve and there may be a diastolic flow murmur from the tricuspid valve. The second heart sound may show fixed splitting. Because of the large pulmonary blood flow there may be only minimal arterial desaturation.

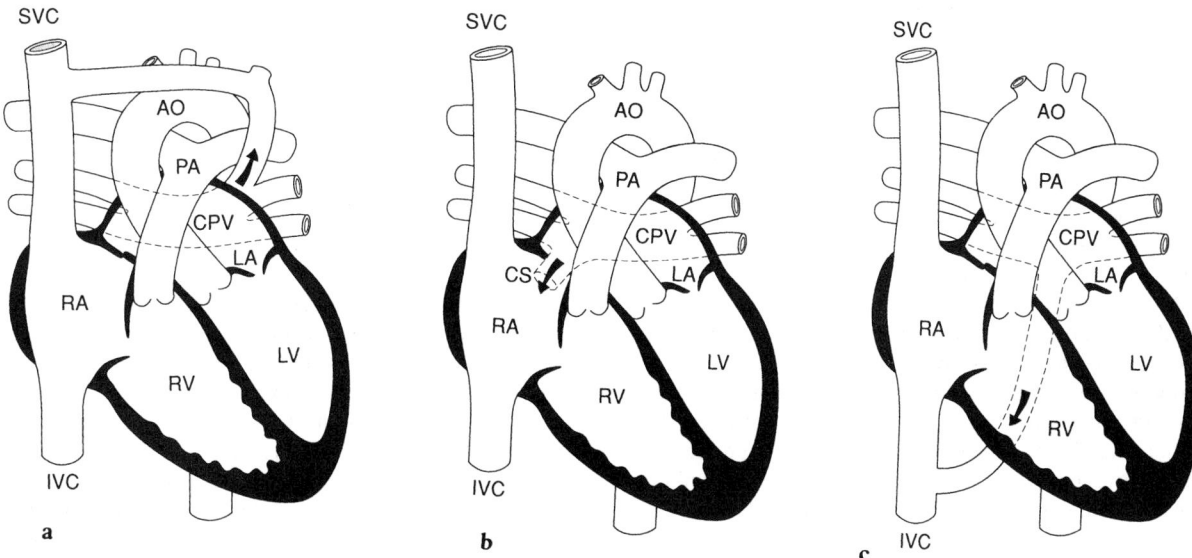

Fig. 13.23   Total anomalous pulmonary venous connection. The three common varieties are shown: (**a**) supracardiac with the four pulmonary veins draining into a common pulmonary venous channel (CPV) and then via a vertical vein to the innominate vein and the right heart; (**b**) cardiac with the pulmonary veins draining directly to the coronary sinus (CS) as shown or directly to the right atrium (not shown); (**c**) infracardiac draining into the inferior vena cava or portal vein.

Cyanosis may not be apparent if the arterial oxygen saturation is in the range of 80–90%. Those infants with obstructive anomalous pulmonary venous connection are usually cyanosed with severe respiratory distress because of pulmonary edema and poor mixing. The peripheral pulses may be poor because of a low cardiac output. Frequently there are no cardiac murmurs and the second heart sound is loud from pulmonary hypertension.

Investigations

In the nonobstructive variety the X-ray usually shows cardiomegaly and obvious increased pulmonary vascularity. The so-called snowman, or figure of eight, or cottage loaf appearance characterizes the supracardiac variety with pulmonary venous drainage to a left vertical vein but is not seen in the first months of life. In the obstructive variety the heart may be small and there may be intense interstitial and alveolar edema producing a ground glass appearance to the lung fields on the chest X-ray. Obstructed total anomalous pulmonary venous drainage is the only likely diagnosis in the newborn with cardiac failure but a small heart on X-ray. The electrocardiogram shows right axis deviation, right atrial and right ventricular hypertrophy. On cardiac ultrasound examination the left atrium and ventricle usually appear small and the right atrium, right ventricle and pulmonary artery enlarged. With careful attention to technique and examination from the subcostal and suprasternal view, it is usually possible to identify the type of anomalous pulmonary venous connection. If this cannot be achieved by echocardiography, angiography may be necessary. In the rare case there may be a mixed type of drainage with the pulmonary veins connected to several different sites.

Management

The outlook for infants born with the obstructive variety is poor and survival beyond a few weeks is unusual. Those with the nonobstructive forms survive longer but prognosis also remains poor without treatment. On cardiopulmonary bypass a wide anastomosis is usually made between the confluence of the pulmonary veins and the posterior wall of the left atrium. This technique is not applicable to the coronary sinus variety or that in which the veins connect directly to the right atrium. Results of surgery in the nonobstructive variety are excellent, but in the infradiaphragmatic form with obstruction there is a higher risk (Wilson W R et al 1992).

DISTURBANCES OF RATE, RHYTHM AND CONDUCTION

In childhood the electrocardiographic features of arrhythmias are similar to those seen in adults but there are important differences in etiology, symptomatology and frequency (Garson 1988). Many occur without any evidence of structural heart disease and indeed may be of no functional significance, while others may be associated with congenital lesions, most importantly Ebstein's anomaly and physiologically corrected transposition of the great arteries. Arrhythmias may follow cardiac surgery for a variety of lesions, either in the early postoperative period or many years after apparently successful surgical repair.

INVESTIGATION OF ARRHYTHMIAS

A standard 12-lead electrocardiogram may be of limited value in detecting an arrhythmia if it is transient and occurs infrequently, but may provide a clue to the underlying etiology such as a short PR interval in the pre-excitation syndrome or abnormal QT interval in any of the variants of the long QT interval syndrome.

Treadmill or bicycle exercise testing may be helpful in initiating certain types of arrhythmia, particularly ventricular arrhythmias and those following cardiac surgery.

Continuous ambulatory 24-h electrocardiographic monitoring is now a well-established technique and may be of particular value for the evaluation of transient events and those associated with symptoms such as syncope. With this method the electrocardiogram is usually recorded continuously for 24–48 h and is then scanned at high speed either visually (60 times normal speed) or by computer with a write-out of any irregularity. Two channel recordings are better than one and it is of value to have an event marker which can be used to correlate symptoms with electrocardiographic events. The use of this technique has clarified the variations in heart rate and rhythm that occur in normal healthy children. The heart rate may vary from 45 to 180/min and during sleep be as low as 30–70 beats/min.

Many rhythm disturbances occur very infrequently and the chance of detection from a single 24-h electrocardiographic recording may therefore be small. An alternative is to provide the family with an event recorder. These are activated by the child or parent when a symptom occurs. There are many different types but most record a short strip in solid state memory. The record can then be played back and analyzed by transmitting it by telephone or returning it to the cardiac center.

Complex cardiac arrhythmias may be further evaluated by intracardiac electrophysiological studies in which several electrode catheters are passed transvenously to the right side of the heart and intracardiac potentials are recorded from multiple sites, including the bundle of His. Simultaneous recordings of surface and intracardiac electrocardiograms help to determine more precisely the exact site of origin, delay, and direction of impulse conduction in complex arrhythmias. These techniques have their greatest value in defining the exact mechanism of tachycardia and may result in more appropriate therapy, particularly in children who have drug resistant tachyarrhythmias and who may be candidates for radiofrequency catheter ablation therapy of their arrhythmias (Kugler et al 1994).

DISTURBANCES OF SINUS NODE FUNCTION

Sinus tachycardia

Sinus tachycardia is sinus rhythm at a rate faster than normal. The usual rate per minute for a newborn is 110–150, for a toddler 85–125, for a 3–5-year-old 75–115; and after 6 years old the range is 60–100 beats. With fever the sinus rate in infancy may rise to 200–220/min. Sinus tachycardias may be differentiated from supraventricular tachycardia by variations in the rate from minute to minute and by transient slowing of the heart rate in response to carotid sinus pressure. In supraventricular tachycardia carotid sinus pressure produces no change or an abrupt reversion to normal rhythm.

Sinus bradycardia

A persisting slow heart rate is unusual in infants and rates consistently less than 80/min in this age may prompt consideration of some precipitating cause. With 24-h continuous tape monitoring, however, it is now recognized that in the majority of infants the heart rate, particularly during sleep, may fall transiently as low as 60 and in older children the minimal rate may vary between 30 and 70 beats/min.

Sinus arrhythmia

Variation in the rate of sinus node discharge is the commonest cause of an irregular heartbeat in childhood. The basic periodic slowing and acceleration of the heart rate which occurs is related to respiration, with the rate increasing on inspiration and slowing on expiration.

Sinoatrial block and sinus arrest

In sinoatrial block the sinus node fails to activate the atria. There is a dropped beat, which is shown on the electrocardiogram as complete absence of a complex. In sinus arrest the sinus node fails to initiate an impulse and usually, after a pause, an escape beat from the atrioventricular junction occurs. Sinoatrial block and sinus arrest are usually of little clinical importance though they can occur as features of digoxin intoxication. The term 'sick sinus syndrome' describes a disorder of the sinus node in which paroxysms of sinus bradycardia, sinoatrial block and sinus arrest may be associated with supraventricular tachycardia; syncope may result from too slow or too fast a heart rate. This may result from sinus node damage as a consequence of cardiac surgery or following myocarditis, but commonly no cause is found.

SUPRAVENTRICULAR ARRHYTHMIAS

Supraventricular rhythm disturbances can originate from the atrioventricular junction or the bundle of His.

Supraventricular ectopic beats (atrial and junctional)

Atrial and junctional ectopic beats are common and seldom give rise to symptoms. Older children may occasionally complain of being aware of an irregular heart beat. Ectopic beats are characterized by an abnormal P wave which may occur prematurely or, when the sinus node fails, as escape beats. The QRS morphology is usually normal but may be broad if intraventricular conduction is aberrant.

Supraventricular tachycardia (atrial and junctional tachycardia)

Supraventricular tachycardia is the most common abnormal tachycardia in infancy and childhood. It occurs more frequently in infants than in older children and the majority of patients do not have congenital heart disease. Two electrophysiological mechanisms underlie supraventricular tachycardia:

1. Enhanced automaticity in a localized focus in the atria or atrioventricular (AV) junction. Although this occurs in only about 15% of patients, this is approximately five times greater than that found in adults.

2. Re-entry circuit (reciprocating tachycardia). There may be an ectopic pacemaker in the atrial muscle or junctional tissue and the usual mechanism of onset is that an impulse originates in these areas and then re-enters the atrium via an accessory pathway and reactivates ectopic foci.

The clinical picture in supraventricular tachycardia differs in infancy from that found in the older child. In infancy most attacks occur before 6 months of age. They may be undetected or be associated with pallor and tachypnea. If an episode lasts for more than 24 h, heart failure usually ensues and treatment becomes urgent. These infants present with poor feeding and by the time they are seen by the pediatrician there is usually significant cardiorespiratory distress. Older children may complain of a rapid

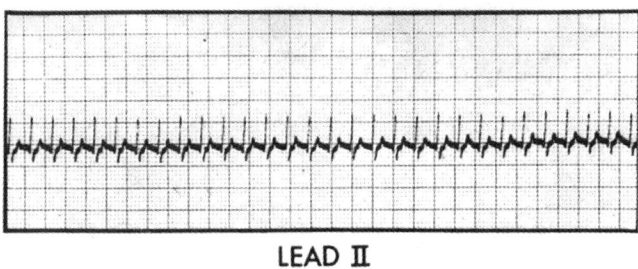

Fig. 13.24   Paroxysmal supraventricular tachycardia. No visible P waves. Normal QRS.

cardiac action, faintness or, uncommonly, chest pain. Clinical examination between paroxysms both in infancy and childhood is usually completely normal. During an attack the ECG shows a regular rate of 220–300/min with 1 : 1 atrioventricular conduction (Fig. 13.24). The QRS is usually narrow but there may be slurring and widening due to aberration from intraventricular conduction delay. The prognosis for attacks occurring in early infancy is usually excellent. In older children episodes may be repetitive over many years. Uncommonly, infants and children may present with a *chronic variety of atrial tachycardia* that persists unremittingly for weeks to years. This form may not be associated with any significant symptoms in many children and the basic rate is frequently slower. There may be, on occasion, marked cardiac dysfunction associated with the tachycardia.

Wolff–Parkinson–White syndrome

A significant number of infants and children with paroxysmal supraventricular tachycardia on return to normal rhythm show the electrocardiographic features of the Wolff–Parkinson–White (WPW) syndrome (Fig. 13.25). This eponym describes the association of the electrocardiographic features of a short PR interval, broad QRS complex and delta waves with a tendency to paroxysmal tachycardia. In this condition there is an accessory pathway bypassing the junctional tissue. This pathway may go from the left atrium to the left ventricle (type A WPW) simulating right bundle branch block, or from the right atrium to the right ventricle (type B WPW) simulating a left bundle branch block pattern. This accessory pathway allows a circuit to be formed which facilitates re-entry tachycardia. The degree of slurring of the QRS may vary from patient to patient and increases with age. During an episode of paroxysmal tachycardia the QRS duration is usually normal. The prognosis for most infants is good, although some continue to have attacks of tachycardia and persistence of the abnormal ECG pattern beyond infancy.

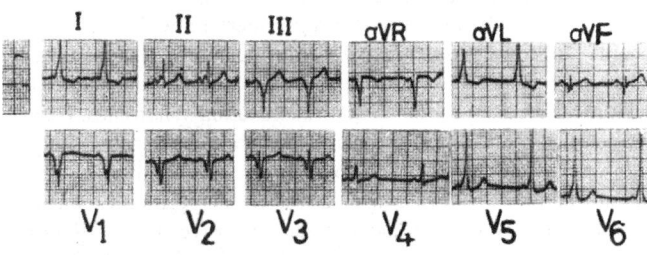

Fig. 13.25   Wolff–Parkinson–White syndrome. Note slurred QRS complexes with short PR.

Atrial flutter and atrial fibrillation

Atrial flutter and fibrillation are uncommon arrhythmias in childhood and are usually the consequence of severe longstanding heart disease in older children. They may complicate cardiac surgery, mitral valve disease, rheumatic or myocardial disease. In atrial flutter there is an atrial rate of 280/min or greater. The ventricles may respond only intermittently at ratios of 2 : 1 to 4 : 1 (Fig. 13.26). In atrial fibrillation the atrial activity is totally disordered and the ventricular response irregular.

VENTRICULAR ARRHYTHMIAS

Ventricular ectopic beats

Ventricular ectopic beats may arise as a result of myocardial disease, electrolyte disturbance or drug overdose, but it is important to recognize that they can also occur in healthy, asymptomatic children. Typically, the QRS complex in these beats is wide and bizarre with abnormal ST segments and T waves (Fig. 13.27).

Ventricular tachycardia

This is defined as four or more ventricular ectopic beats occurring in sequence. The heart rate is usually between 120 and 200/min (Fig. 13.28). The prognosis is usually poorer than that of supraventricular tachycardia and the patient may present with syncope, chest pain or dyspnea. Differentiation from supraventricular tachycardia with aberration is not always easy, and all broad QRS (>120 ms) tachycardias should be considered

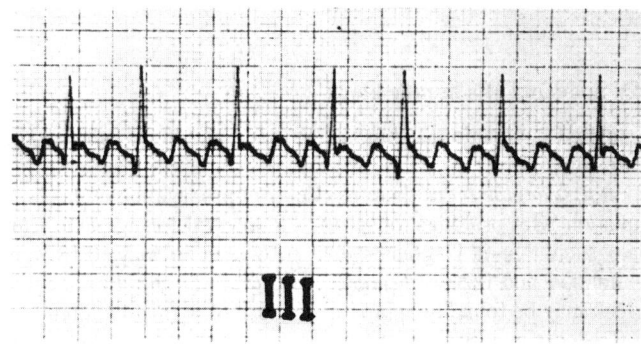

Fig. 13.26   Atrial flutter. Lead III shows rapid regular atrial flutter waves with variable ventricular response.

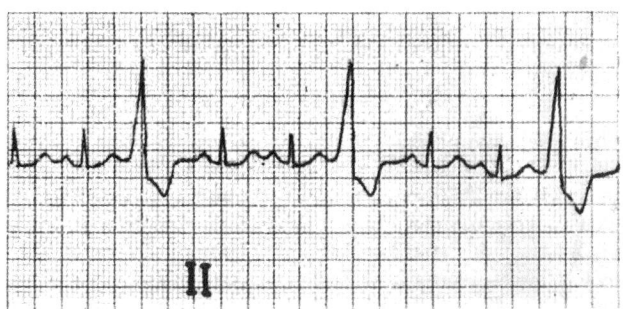

Fig. 13.27   Ventricular exrasystoles. Lead II. The third, sixth and ninth complexes show broad R waves with inverted T waves and a compensatory pause before the next QRS.

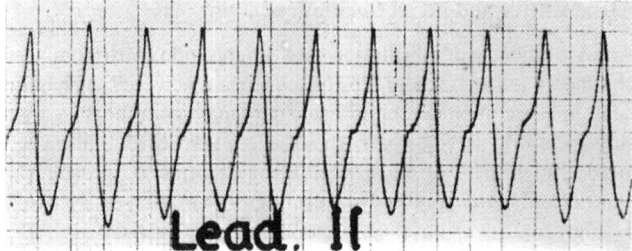

Fig. 13.28   Ventricular tachycardia.

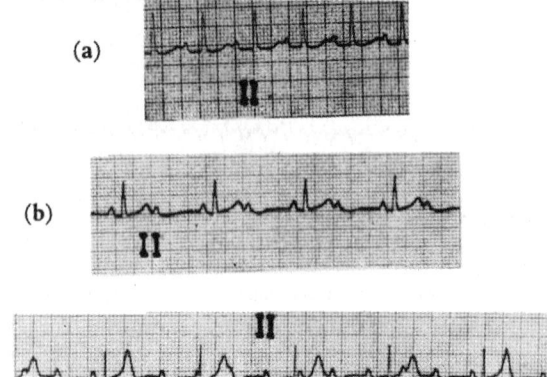

Fig. 13.29   Types of heart block: (**a**) first degree block, PR 0.24 s; (**b**) second degree block, 2 : 1 ventricular response; (**c**) third degree or complete heart block with complete dissociation between atrial and ventricular rates.

as ventricular tachycardia until proven otherwise. Ventricular tachycardia is a relatively rare arrhythmia in childhood and in approximately 50% of patients no underlying cause is identified. An uncommon etiology such as myocardial tumor, cardiomyopathy or drug toxicity should be considered. Rarely, recurrent attacks have a familial basis. The congenital long QT syndromes, some of which are associated with deafness, present with recurrent episodes of ventricular tachycardias/ventricular fibrillation and syncope (Jervell and Lange-Nielsen syndrome).

CONDUCTION DISTURBANCES

Bundle branch block

Complete block of conduction in either the right or left bundle is uncommon in childhood. Complete right bundle branch block is seen most often following open heart surgery in which a right ventriculotomy has been performed or a ventricular septal defect closed with damage to the right bundle branch. Left bundle branch block is rare in children and can be associated with myocardial disease.

AV node and His bundle block

Impaired conduction within the AV node and the bundle of His takes three forms.

In *first degree block* there is a delay in propagation at the A–V junction with prolongation of the PR interval for age and heart rate such that it is greater than 0.16 s in infancy, 0.18 s in childhood and 0.20 s in adolescence (Fig. 13.29). First degree block may be found in approximately 8% of normal children.

The commonest form of *second degree AV block* is known as the *Wenckebach phenomenon*. The PR interval becomes progressively more prolonged from beat to beat until one P wave is not succeeded by a QRS complex. The next atrial complex is followed at a normal or near normal interval by a QRS complex and the cycle of events recurs. Occasionally the QRS impulse may follow only every third or fourth atrial beat without any preceding prolongation of the PR interval.

In *third degree block* the atria and ventricles beat entirely independently of each other with the atrial rate higher than the ventricular rate (Fig. 13.29). Third degree or complete heart block may be congenital, or acquired following surgery or, more rarely, as a consequence of myocarditis. In congenital complete heart block the QRS complex is usually narrow in contrast to complete heart block following cardiac surgery. In congenital complete heart block without associated heart disease the prognosis is frequently good if there are no symptoms in early infancy. It may be associated with cardiac lesions such as corrected transposition of the great arteries,

atrioventricular or ventricular septal defects. There is an increasing recognition of the association between congenital complete heart block in infants of mothers who have a connective tissue disorder, particularly systemic lupus erythematosus. The fetal effect appears to relate to the passive transfer from the mother of anti-Ro or anti-DNA antibodies (Taylor et al 1986).

Many children with complete heart block are asymptomatic but syncopal episodes may develop (Stokes–Adams attacks). On clinical examination the pulse rate is usually slow and there may be intermittent 'a' waves in the jugular venous pulse and a systolic murmur over the precordium due to increased left ventricular stroke volume.

MANAGEMENT OF ARRHYTHMIAS AND CONDUCTION DISTURBANCES

Management of arrhythmias and conduction disturbances in infants and children depends on the establishment of a firm diagnosis, and then knowledge of the natural history of the disorder, the severity of symptoms and the efficacy of the proposed treatment. Many simple arrhythmias, such as supraventricular ectopic beats, require no treatment. Information and experience in dosage and metabolism in childhood of some of the newer antiarrhythmic drugs is limited. Table 13.6 details some of the drugs which are most widely used in the management of arrhythmias in childhood. Antiarrhythmic drugs have been classified on the basis of their cellular electrophysiological profiles in isolated tissue preparation (Vaughan Williams 1984), but before choosing a particular drug consideration must be given to its toxicity, the likely duration of use and careful consideration of the risk/benefit ratio in relation to treatment and symptoms.

Vaughan Williams Class I drugs interfere with the sodium channel to slow conduction and reduce membrane responsiveness. They are indicated for ventricular arrhythmias and the reciprocating tachycardias with pre-excitation syndromes. Class I drugs can be subdivided into groups Ia, b and c depending upon the degree of the effect upon the cell membranes. Beta adrenoceptor blocking drugs (Class II) act primarily through modification of the cardiac sympathetic drive. Class III drugs (amiodarone, sotalol) prolong repolarization by widening the action potential duration. The Class IV drugs and calcium

Table 13.6 Anti-arrhythmic drugs in childhood

Drug	Mode of action (Vaughan Williams 1984)	Dosage	Indications
Digoxin	–	See heart failure	Atrial flutter/fibrillation? Contraindication in WPW
Disopyramide	Ia	i.v. 1–2 mg/kg 10–20 mg/kg/day	Supraventricular tachycardia WPW syndrome
Verapamil	IV	Contraindicated < 1 year Over 1 year 0.1 mg/kg i.v. over 2 min (max. 5 mg)	Supraventricular tachycardia WPW syndrome
Propranolol	II	Under 1 year, orally 1 mg/kg every 6 h Over 1 year 5–10 mg t.i.d.	Long QT interval syndromes Supraventricular tachycardia
Lignocaine	Ib	1 mg/kg i.v. bolus Infusion 10–50 µg/kg/min	Ventricular tachycardia Ventricular fibrillation
Amiodarone	III	10–15 mg/kg loading dose orally 5 mg/kg orally maintenance	Atrial flutter/fibrillation Chronic ectopic atrial tachycardia Ventricular tachycardia
Flecainide	Ic	2 mg/kg i.v. infusion over 20 min 2–3 mg/kg/day orally in 2–3 divided doses	Supraventricular tachycardia WPW syndrome

antagonists (verapamil, diltiazem) affect conduction and calcium dependent tissues primarily via the atrioventricular node.

Paroxysmal supraventricular tachycardia may present as a true medical emergency in infancy when it has been prolonged and resulted in severe peripheral and central circulatory failure. Treatment should be instituted with urgency. Adenosine has proved to be an effective and safe form of treatment for some forms of tachycardia. It acts by preventing passage of the electrical impulse through the AV node. Thus it may stop the episode if there is a reciprocating tachycardia, and slows the ventricular rate and reveals the underlying atrial rhythm in atrial fibrillation or flutter. Its half life is only a matter of seconds and it can safely be administered in a larger dose after a few minutes if it is ineffective. Dosage should be given intravenously in an initial dosage of 0.05 mg/kg, increasing by 0.05 mg/kg every 2 minutes to a maximum of 0.25 mg/kg/dose. If adenosine is unavailable or unsuccessful, cardioversion rather than further drug therapy should be employed using a synchronized defibrillator with levels of 0.5–1.0 W/s/kg usually being adequate though higher levels may be required. For less acutely ill infants vagal maneuvers can be attempted but, with the exception of the diving reflex, rarely abort the attack. The diving reflex is most practically elicited by covering the infant's face with a small plastic bag filled with ice or immersing the infant's face in ice cold water. If this is ineffective intravenous digitalization is almost invariably effective. Thereafter the infant is usually maintained on digoxin until the end of the first year of life. If the electrocardiogram shows evidence of pre-excitation between attacks, many cardiologists would consider digoxin relatively contraindicated for it may shorten the antegrade refractory period, making the patient more susceptible to ventricular fibrillation. This is extremely rare, particularly in infancy as opposed to childhood, and digoxin is still therefore widely used as prophylaxis against SVT under 1 year of age. Disopyramide may also be effective in infants but verapamil should be avoided because it may have a more depressant effect on the neonatal infant myocardium than on the adult myocardium. In the older child presenting with a supraventricular tachycardia, vagal maneuvers, such as the Valsalva, are more likely to be effective in aborting short episodes but still do not have a high success rate. The chronic variety of supraventricular tachycardia can be very refractory to treatment and choice of drug may depend on expert evaluation of the mechanism of the tachycardia and other variables. In some cases consideration may be given to transcatheter radiofrequency ablation of an accessory connection (Kugler et al 1994).

Lignocaine is the drug of first choice in the management of ventricular tachycardia but can only be administered intravenously. For the long-term suppression of ventricular arrhythmias propranolol, flecainide, disopyramide and amiodarone may all have a role. Propranolol (or other beta-blocker) remains the appropriate drug for prophylaxis of dysrhythmia in the long QT interval syndrome. When there is no readily identifiable cause for the ventricular tachycardia, treatment should be supervised by a center or cardiologist experienced in the management of these problems.

As understanding of the anatomical substrate for many arrhythmias has improved, an increasing role for surgery or transcatheter ablation for some arrhythmias, particularly of the pre-excitation type, has been identified. Evaluation and treatment of this kind is available in only a few highly specialized centers. Other advances for intractable arrhythmias have included the development of specialized antitachycardia pacemakers and implantable cardiovertor/defibrillators but at present the role and scope of the application of these developments in childhood is limited (Campbell 1990).

For symptomatic bradycardia, atropine and isoprenaline may be effective in accelerating the heart rate. Atropine may overcome bradycardia due to excessive vagal activity and isoprenaline acts by increasing sinus node activity as well as junctional and ventricular pacemakers. With isoprenaline the rate of infusion must be carefully controlled. When a profound bradycardia associated with symptoms occurs as a result of complete heart block with a ventricular rate of less than 40/min, it may be necessary to stimulate the activity of the heart with an artificial pacemaker. Pacemaker insertion should be considered when there are symptoms such as syncope, heart failure, poor exercise tolerance, and in complete heart block following cardiac surgery. Intracardiac, endocardial or epicardial electrodes may be employed. A variety of cardiac pacemakers with a wide range of programmable facilities is now available and can be used even in newborn infants (Smith 1988). A modern pacemaker unit can be expected to have a life span of 8–10 years and although the complications of pacemakers in childhood are now much less than formerly, they can still occur. All patients with a pacemaker require regular follow-up at a clinic where the pacemaker parameters can be checked and altered if necessary.

ACQUIRED CARDIOVASCULAR DISORDERS

RHEUMATIC HEART DISEASE

In many developed countries acute rheumatic fever has become a rare and relatively mild disease, although outbreaks have been reported in the USA in the last decade (Ferrieri 1987). In the developing world it remains common and is the main cause of significant morbidity and mortality from heart disease in the pediatric age group. The pathogenesis and noncardiac manifestations of rheumatic fever are discussed in Chapter 24.

ACUTE CARDITIS

Carditis, the only manifestation of acute rheumatic fever which causes permanent sequelae, can occur in up to two-thirds of first attacks. The clinical diagnosis of carditis during an attack of rheumatic fever is suggested by the appearance of, or change in a significant murmur, pericarditis or cardiac failure. The development of a significant murmur is the prime indicator of carditis but it must be remembered that innocent murmurs are common in children, particularly associated with a febrile illness, and that an organic murmur may be due to pre-existing congenital heart disease. Thus the demonstration that a murmur has recently developed or, in a case with previous rheumatic heart disease, changed in character is more definite evidence of rheumatic carditis than its mere presence. The most common organic murmur in rheumatic carditis is the apical systolic one of mitral regurgitation, which may be due to myocarditis with dilation of the left ventricle and mitral valve ring, or endocarditis with swelling and cellular infiltration of the mitral valve cusps. A short apical mid-diastolic flow murmur may be associated with that of mitral regurgitation. Less commonly the high pitched decrescendo early diastolic murmur of aortic regurgitation is heard at the base and left sternal edge. The heart sounds are soft. Cardiac failure is not a common presenting feature but may result from valve regurgitation or ventricular dysfunction from myocarditis. Pericarditis, recognized by a characteristic superficial scratchy friction rub, never occurs in isolation and provides evidence of underlying myocardial disease. Sinus tachycardia is suggestive of carditis, particularly when it occurs during sleep in the afebrile patient. Occasionally a sinus bradycardia occurs.

Investigations

A variety of electrocardiographic (ECG) changes have been reported in acute rheumatic fever. Prolongation of the PR interval is frequently found but does not necessarily indicate carditis. Second degree or complete heart block can also occur. Measurement of the corrected QTc interval is of no practical value. Flattened or inverted T waves over the left precordium (leads V_4–V_6) are a characteristic finding of acute pericarditis.

With echocardiography a pericardial effusion can be demonstrated and cardiac chamber sizes measured. A dilated left ventricular cavity occurs with significant myocardial disease or valve regurgitation; contractility will be diminished with myocarditis but normal or increased with mitral or aortic regurgitation. Doppler ultrasound will demonstrate valve regurgitation but gives only a rough assessment of severity or change. It has been suggested that the demonstration of aortic or mitral regurgitation should be considered indicative of carditis (Folger et al 1992), but it must be recognized that minimal mitral regurgitation is a physiological condition and is shown with Doppler in up to 40% of normal subjects. The significance of mitral regurgitation must be interpreted with caution though aortic regurgitation is likely to indicate a nonphysiological situation. The antistreptolysin O titer is usually elevated above 200 units/ml and may be much higher for a long period. The ESR is increased unless heart failure occurs.

Prognosis

Figures obtained from patients suffering from the initial attack of rheumatic fever in the UK and USA in the 1950s indicated that 10 years after the initial attack the prevalence of heart disease increases from approximately 5% of those with no carditis at the start of treatment, to 25% of those with an apical systolic murmur, 40% of those with both an apical murmur and a basal diastolic murmur, and 70% of those with cardiac failure or pericarditis initially (UK and US Joint Report 1965). The marked decrease in the mortality and morbidity in the past 40 years in many countries may be the result of the use of penicillin in the treatment of group A streptococcal pharyngitis, emphasizing the importance of continued efforts to diagnose and treat it (Massell et al 1988). The disease has a much worse prognosis in less developed parts of the world where significant chronic rheumatic valve disease can develop in childhood.

Treatment

The treatment of acute rheumatic fever is described in Chapter 1599. Penicillin therapy, ideally parenteral benzathine penicillin G, must be given to eradicate streptococcal infection. Salicylate therapy (aspirin 75 mg/kg/24 h in four divided doses for the first 2 weeks with gradual reduction thereafter) is the usual routine and symptomatic treatment but has no effect on the rheumatic process. The value of glucocorticosteroid therapy in preventing the development of chronic rheumatic heart disease is not certain but this is generally recommended where there is evidence of carditis and certainly if heart failure occurs. To avoid a rebound of the disease when the steroid is stopped the dose should be gradually tailed off and salicylates given during this period and continued until all signs of the rheumatic process have disappeared.

Rheumatic fever is a recurring disease, the risk of recurrence being highest in young children and decreasing progressively with time after an attack. Each attack carries an increasing risk of a permanent valve defect developing and most chronic disability and deaths result from recurrent attacks. It is therefore essential that continuous antimicrobial prophylaxis against further streptococcal infection is started as soon as the initial therapeutic course of penicillin has been completed. Recommendations on both primary and secondary prevention have been published by the American Heart Association (Dajani et al 1988). The most effective form of prophylaxis is a monthly intramuscular injection of 1.2 megaunits benzathine penicillin. This is recommended for those who have had more than one attack of rheumatic fever, who have more than minimal heart disease, or who are likely to prove unreliable in taking oral antibiotics. For others oral medication can be given as either sulfadiazine 1.0 g once daily or phenoxymethylpenicillin (penicillin V) 250 mg twice daily, the dosage being halved for children less than 10 years old or less than 30 kg. Those sensitive to both penicillin and sulfadiazine should receive erythromycin 250 mg twice daily. Prophylactic therapy must be continued throughout childhood and adolescence. The decision whether to discontinue prophylaxis in adult life will depend on factors such as the severity of cardiac involvement, time since most recent attack, social circumstances and the increased risk of exposure to further streptococcal infections in some groups of people such as nursing staff, military personnel or school teachers.

CHRONIC RHEUMATIC HEART DISEASE

Well-established and life threatening chronic rheumatic heart disease occurs in childhood in the many countries where the incidence of rheumatic fever remains relatively high. The risk of this increases with increasing severity of initial cardiac involvement and decreasing age at the time of the initial attack. The mitral valve is affected in approximately 85% of cases, the aortic valve in 55%, and the tricuspid and pulmonary valves in less than 5%.

Mitral regurgitation is the most common lesion in children and adolescents with rheumatic heart disease. Where regurgitation is mild the child will be asymptomatic with an apical pansystolic murmur radiating to the axilla. In more severe cases the child may tire easily and experience effort dyspnea or palpitations. The apex beat will be of left ventricular type and displaced. The pulmonary second sound will be accentuated in the presence of pulmonary hypertension and a third heart sound may be prominent, its presence excluding the coexistence of tight mitral stenosis. The murmur is classically pansystolic and with severe regurgitation a mitral mid-diastolic flow murmur is heard because of the obligatory increase in diastolic flow through the mitral valve. With increasing severity of mitral regurgitation the X-ray and the echocardiogram will show enlargement of the left atrium and left ventricle, and the electrocardiogram demonstrates hypertrophy of these chambers. Doppler confirms the presence of regurgitation but can only give a semiquantitative assessment of its severity.

Rheumatic *mitral stenosis* can require surgical treatment in childhood in the parts of the world where rheumatic heart disease follows an accelerated course. There will be no symptoms initially, but effort intolerance and dyspnea may develop later and can progress to orthopnea, paroxysmal nocturnal dyspnea, cardiac failure or hemoptysis. The pulse is usually normal but may be of reduced volume. The apex beat will not be displaced unless there is also significant mitral regurgitation. The apical impulse is tapping and the first heart sound is loud. An opening snap early in diastole is followed by a low pitched rumbling mitral diastolic murmur, which is best heard using the bell of the stethoscope with the patient lying in the left lateral position, and can be accentuated by exercise. When there is no mitral regurgitation, increasing mitral obstruction causes progressive lengthening of the murmur resulting in the classical finding of presystolic accentuation. If atrial fibrillation occurs the presystolic component of this murmur (related to atrial systole) disappears. A right ventricular

parasternal impulse is palpable and the pulmonary second sound is accentuated when pulmonary hypertension occurs.

On chest X-ray the heart size is usually normal with left atrial enlargement apparent. Rise in the left atrial pressure causes increased perfusion of the upper lobes, dilation of the pulmonary veins and eventually edema of the interlobular septa which may be recognized as Kerley B lines. The ECG demonstrates the broad notched P waves of left atrial hypertrophy if there is moderate or severe mitral obstruction, and right ventricular hypertrophy when pulmonary hypertension develops. Atrial fibrillation is not commonly found in children. The M mode echocardiogram characteristically shows a large left atrium and a reduced closure rate of the anterior mitral valve leaflet, with the posterior leaflet usually moving anteriorly with it in diastole. The spectral Doppler signal shows a reduced rate of pressure fall across the valve throughout diastole, a quantitative assessment of which is given by the pressure half-time, the time taken for the pressure across the valve to reach half the initial maximum value. This provides some assessment of the severity of the obstruction and in normal adults is 60 ms and in those with mitral stenosis above 100 ms. This is less reliable in children.

Aortic regurgitation is the major form of rheumatic aortic valve disease in children and adolescents. There are no symptoms unless there is severe aortic regurgitation, when palpitations, excessive sweating and effort dyspnea may be experienced. The pulse pressure is wide, the pulse collapsing and the apical impulse of left ventricular type. The murmur of aortic regurgitation is high pitched blowing, occurs in early diastole, and is best heard at the upper and middle left sternal edge with the cooperative child leaning forward and holding his breath in expiration.

Although an aortic ejection systolic murmur is usually audible when there is marked regurgitation, this represents increased flow not aortic stenosis, which is usually congenital in etiology in this age group. An apical mid and late diastolic murmur (Austin Flint) can be heard with severe aortic regurgitation without mitral valve disease; it is due to forward flow through the closing mitral valve and clinically may be indistinguishable from organic mitral stenosis. In severe cases left ventricular failure may produce signs of pulmonary edema.

With moderate or severe regurgitation there will be left ventricular hypertrophy on ECG and enlargement on chest X-ray. The echocardiogram will demonstrate a dilated and hyper-contractile left ventricle and possibly flutter of the anterior leaflet of the mitral valve, and Doppler will show regurgitant flow and give a semiquantitative assessment of its severity.

Management

Patients with mild heart disease simply require follow-up. Antimicrobial prophylaxis against further attacks of rheumatic fever must be continued at least until early adulthood and prophylaxis against bacterial endocarditis is a lifelong requirement. If the defect is more than mild, competitive sport should be avoided. Indications for cardiac surgery include severe symptoms or heart failure. Where echocardiographic and Doppler facilities are available cardiac catheterization adds little to the noninvasive assessment of the severity of the valve lesion or pulmonary pressure.

Because of the possible need for valve replacement it is desirable to defer surgery if possible until the child is fully grown. A good result may sometimes be achieved with annuloplasty for mitral regurgitation or surgical or balloon valvotomy for mitral stenosis. Valve replacement is usually required for rheumatic aortic regurgitation.

INFECTIVE MYOCARDITIS

Viral myocarditis is most commonly due to the Coxsackie B virus, but it may result from infection with a variety of other agents including ECHO, mumps, influenza, adenovirus, rubella, cytomegalovirus, varicella and Epstein–Barr. This and other aspects of viral myocarditis have been fully reviewed (Woodruff 1980). Viral pericarditis is frequently associated with myocarditis. Myocarditis can be a rare complication of bacteremia or infections with *Toxoplasma* or *Candida* and toxic myocarditis is associated with diphtheritic infection.

Clinical features

Myocarditis frequently occurs during the course of an infection when other manifestations predominate and the diagnosis may not be apparent. Myocarditis may be suspected by the presence of a cardiac arrhythmia, tachypnea, persistent tachycardia or overt signs of heart failure. In myocarditis due to diphtheria exotoxin the conducting tissue is primarily affected, with the possible development of potentially fatal complete heart block.

The course and prognosis of viral myocarditis is variable. Death can occur either early or after a period of chronic illness. Survivors may recover completely, often after an illness of many weeks or months, or be left with a chronic disability (Weinhouse et al 1986) in the form of dilated cardiomyopathy (Levi et al 1988).

Investigations

The chest X-ray will generally show cardiac enlargement. ECG changes are relatively nonspecific. There may be an arrhythmia, often due to atrial or ventricular premature beats, or a variety of conduction disturbances. Decreased QRS voltage with T wave flattening and occasional inversion are commonly found. An echocardiogram will demonstrate a dilated and poorly contracting left ventricle. The ESR and cardiac muscle enzyme levels may be elevated. The diagnosis of viral myocarditis is uncertain in many cases. Virus isolation from myocardium or pericardial fluid is firm evidence for its etiologic association but failure to do so does not exclude it. Isolation from throat or feces does not definitely indicate they are of pathogenic significance. Serological demonstration of a significant viral infection by demonstrating a high titer, particularly if it is rising or falling, would be strong evidence for this. Such evidence of viral infection is most readily obtained in the early part of the disease but this is often before patients become symptomatic.

Management

The management of viral myocarditis has been reviewed (Rezkalla & Kloner 1989). Specific therapy is not available in most cases of infective myocarditis and treatment is largely supportive. In the initial stages bed rest and cardiac monitoring are advisable. Diuretics and digoxin are given for cardiac failure. Digitalization should be undertaken cautiously in view of a possible lower threshold to digoxin toxicity. Complete heart block

may necessitate electrical pacing. The value of specific drug treatment in viral myocarditis has been the subject of a number of studies. Experimental studies support the general recommendation that glucocorticosteroid (Tomioka et al 1986) or other immunosuppresive or nonsteroidal anti-inflammatory therapy should not be given in the first 10 days of an infection when it may have a deleterious effect, but steroids may be worthwhile if active disease continues in seriously ill patients who are deteriorating on supportive therapy.

INFECTIVE ENDOCARDITIS

The British Society for Antimicrobial Chemotherapy has published an extensive review of many aspects of infective endocarditis (Infective Endocarditis 1987). Infective endocarditis is usually superimposed on underlying congenital or rheumatic heart disease, particularly where there is a lesion associated with a high velocity jet of blood or an intracardiac prosthesis, but a child with a normal heart can also be affected. A predisposing factor, usually a dental or surgical procedure, can be identified in about two-thirds of children who have not undergone cardiac surgery (Karl et al 1987).

Bacteriology

Streptococcus viridans (alpha-hemolytic streptococcus) and *Staphylococcus aureus* are the main causes of infection in unoperated children. A wide variety of other organisms is found as the infecting agent on rare occasions. Gram-negative and fungal endocarditis occur in those with an intracardiac prosthesis or following cardiac surgery. In about 10% of cases of infective endocarditis no organisms can be isolated from blood culture. In neonates staphylococcal or candidal infections tend to occur and prognosis is poor (O'Callaghan & McDougall 1988).

Clinical features

The clinical features vary depending upon the infecting organism and the stage at which the child is seen. *Staph. aureus* endocarditis usually runs a subacute course in children. On occasions it may follow a fulminant course as a manifestation of a septicemia, particularly in the first 2 years of life and often in those with a previously normal heart. With *Strep. viridans* the onset is usually insidious. Unexplained fever in a child with organic heart disease may be the only finding. Anemia and leukocytosis are the rule with other early manifestations such as malaise, anorexia, weight loss and splenomegaly being relatively uncommon (Karl et al 1987). As vegetations increase in size, a murmur may appear or a change occur in the character of a pre-existing one. The ESR is almost always elevated. Hematuria is found in about one-third of patients. Petechiae may occur and are best seen on the oral mucosa, eyelids or optic fundi. Osler nodes, Janeway lesions and splinter hemorrhages are not usually found. Embolic phenomena have become relatively rare since antimicrobial therapy has been introduced. The skin lesions and hematuria are immune complex phenomena and not due to emboli.

Diagnosis

The early signs and symptoms of infective endocarditis are frequently mild, and early diagnosis depends on consideration of its possible presence in any child with heart disease with unexplained fever, even when there are no other features of endocarditis. In the majority of cases a specific diagnosis depends upon a positive blood culture. Three blood cultures should be performed within 24 h and a further three after 24 h if the initial ones are still negative (Washington 1987). Bacteremia is a steady feature in infective endocarditis making timing in relation to spikes of fever unimportant. Culture media should include those for aerobes, anaerobes and fungi and the media should be at a suitable temperature before use (25–35°C).

Six sterile cultures are strong evidence against infective endocarditis but do not preclude it, since about 10% of cases are negative on culture. Recent antimicrobial treatment is the most common explanation for this, but possible infection with nonbacterial agents such as fungi, coxiella, *Chlamydia* or rickettsia is worth considering. In these circumstances echocardiography may be of value in demonstrating the presence of vegetations but failure to do so does not rule out the diagnosis of infective endocarditis. Transesophageal echocardiography is a more sensitive technique (Erbel et al 1988) and if available may be appropriate in some older children.

Treatment

Where there is a strong suspicion of infective endocarditis and it appears to be following a fulminant course, antibiotic treatment should be started on the 'best guess' principle as soon as six blood cultures have been obtained. In less ill patients antimicrobials may be withheld until the results of blood cultures are available. Bactericidal drugs should be administered parenterally by bolus injection in a dose sufficient to provide a peak plasma concentration at least eight times the in vitro minimum bactericidal concentration. Therapy should be continued for at least 4 weeks and 6 or more weeks are recommended for certain bacteria such as *Staph. aureus* and enterococci.

The choice of antimicrobial, of dosage schedule, and of duration of therapy will depend on the organism and its sensitivity pattern. There is no general agreement on this specific antimicrobial therapy. Suggested doses of some commonly used antimicrobial drugs are given in Table 13.7 and in Chapter 38. The dosage should be adjusted according to the sensitivity of the organism and blood level of antimicrobial. For infections with a highly sensitive *Streptococcus viridans* benzylpenicillin (penicillin G) alone for 4 weeks is effective. If the organism is relatively insensitive then penicillin should be given for 6 weeks, the dose being increased depending upon blood levels and gentamicin therapy added. For staphylococci sensitive to cloxacillin or flucloxacillin either of these should be used in combination with fusidic acid. However, it has been found that some strains are now resistant not only to β-lactam antibiotics but also to aminoglycosides and many other antibiotics (Brumfitt & Hamilton-Miller 1989). Where the agent is unknown, a combination of benzylpenicillin, flucloxacillin and gentamicin can be used.

When endocarditis occurs following cardiac surgery in a patient with an intracardiac prosthesis, surgical removal of the foreign material is usually necessary. Active infective endocarditis is not necessarily a contraindication to cardiac surgery on the affected part; immediate valve replacement is indicated where a malformed valve causes moderate or severe heart failure or recurrent emboli occur. Fungal or coxiella infections respond poorly to medical therapy and surgery may be the only way to eradicate infection. Valve replacement within 1 week of diagnosis has been advocated for staphylococcal endocarditis regardless of the hemodynamic state.

Prophylaxis

Patients at risk of developing infective endocarditis must have antimicrobial prophylaxis for any procedure likely to cause bacteremia. This includes any dental treatment causing bleeding of the gums, abdominal surgery, surgery or instrumentation of the upper respiratory or genitourinary tract, and following burns and while receiving intravenous alimentation. It is not considered necessary for gastrointestinal endoscopy without biopsy except in those with intracardiac prostheses. There are some differences in the antimicrobial regimes recommended by the American Heart Association (Shulman et al 1984) and the British Society for Antimicrobial Chemotherapy (Report of a Working Party of the British Society for Antimicrobial Chemotherapy 1982, Report of the Endocarditis Working Party 1990; Simmons et al 1992). Table 13.8 details suitable antibiotic prophylaxis regimes taken largely from the latter recommendations. For dental treatment a single oral dose of amoxicillin or erythromycin is considered adequate for most patients. Particular care is required in the patient with an intracardiac prosthesis and parenteral antimicrobial prophylaxis is essential in this situation.

ENDOMYOCARDIAL FIBROSIS

Endomyocardial fibrosis is a progressive and usually fatal disease of unknown etiology occurring mainly in children and young adults living in specific regions of the tropics and subtropics, most frequently in Africa. The main pathological finding is an endocardial layer of dense fibrous tissue originating at the apex of one or both ventricles and spreading upwards to involve the papillary muscles, chordae tendinae and posterior cusp of the atrioventricular valves but not the semilunar valves. Intracardiac thrombi form, particularly in the right ventricle and its cavity may gradually be obliterated by organizing clot and fibrous tissue. Ventricular function becomes impaired and regurgitation of the mitral or tricuspid valve usually develops. Pericarditis occurs in about two-thirds of cases.

Clinical features

Children with endomyocardial fibrosis usually show general signs of chronic malnutrition with wasting and growth retardation. Signs relating to the cardiovascular system are of ventricular

Table 13.7 Suggested initial antimicrobial doses of commonly used antimicrobials for the treatment of infective endocarditis

	Total daily dose	Divided dosage: number of times daily
Benzylpenicillin	180 mg/kg to 6 g	6
Gentamicin	6 mg/kg up to 240 mg	3
Flucloxacillin	200–400 mg/kg up to 12 g	6
Fusidic acid	Equivalent to 20 mg/kg of sodium fusidate up to 1.5 g	3

Table 13.8 Antibiotic prophylaxis against infective endocarditis

A Dental extractions, scaling or peridontal surgery; surgery or instrumentation of the upper respiratory tract

1. *Under local anesthesia*
Patients not allergic to penicillin and not prescribed penicillin more than once in the last month:
— Amoxicillin as single oral dose taken under supervision 1 hour before procedure

Over 10 years	3 g
5–10 years	1.5 g
Less than 5 years	750 mg

Patients allergic to penicillin or prescribed penicillin more than once in the last month:
— Clindamycin as single oral dose taken under supervision 1 hour before procedure

Over 10 years	600 mg
5–10 years	300 mg
Less than 5 years	150 mg

2. *Under general anesthesia*
Patients not allergic to penicillin and not prescribed penicillin more than once in the last month:
— Amoxicillin orally 4 hours before and the same dose as soon as possible after the procedure

Over 10 years	3 g	followed by 3 g
5–10 years	1.5 g	followed by 1.5 g
Less than 5 years	750 mg	followed by 750 mg

OR

— Amoxicillin i.v. just before induction then oral dose 6 hours later (or i.m. in solution of 1 g in 2.5 ml 1% lignocaine hydrochloride)

Over 10 years	1 g i.m./i.v.	then 500 mg orally
5–10 years	500 mg i.m./i.v.	then 250 mg orally
Less than 5 years	250 mg i.m./i.v.	then 125 mg orally

Patients allergic to penicillin or prescribed penicillin more than once in the last month:
— Gentamicin 2 mg/kg to maximum of 120 mg ⎫
                                               PLUS ⎬   i.v. just before induction
— Teicoplanin 6 mg/kg to maximum of 400 mg ⎭

OR

— Clindamycin i.v. over 10 minutes as solution of 300 mg in 50 ml diluent

Over 10 years	300 mg i.v.	and	150 mg orally 6 h later
5–10 years	150 mg i.v.	and	75 mg orally 6 h later
Less than 5 years	75 mg i.v.	and	37 mg orally 6 h later

3. *Special risk patients (i.e. those who have had a previous attack of endocarditis or have prosthetic valves/intravascular prosthetic material)*
Patients not allergic to penicillin and not prescribed penicillin more than once in the last month:
(a) — Amoxicillin i.v. just before induction then oral dose 6 hours later (or i.m. in solution of 1 g in 2.5 ml 1% lignocaine hydrochloride)

Over 10 years	1 g i.m./i.v.	then 500 mg orally
5–10 years	500 mg i.m./i.v.	then 250 mg orally
Less than 5 years	250 mg i.m./i.v.	then 125 mg orally

PLUS

— Gentamicin 2 mg/kg bodyweight to maximum of 120 mg

Patients allergic to penicillin or prescribed penicillin more than once in the last month:
(b) — Gentamicin 2 mg/kg to maximum of 120 mg ⎫
                                               PLUS ⎬   i.v. just before induction
— Teicoplanin 6 mg/kg to maximum of 400 mg ⎭

OR

(c) — Vancomycin 20 mg/kg to maximum of 1 g by slow i.v. infusion over 60–100 mins

PLUS

— Gentamicin 2 mg/kg to maximum of 120 mg i.v. just before induction

B Genitourinary or gastrointestinal surgery or instrumentation

Cover is directed against fecal streptococci and should be 3(a) or 3(c) as above. For patients with infected urine prophylaxis should ensure coverage of the infecting organisms.

---

failure and atrioventricular valve regurgitation, and these vary according to whether one or other or both sides of the heart are affected. Thus with right sided involvement there may be raised central venous pressure, a large pulsatile liver, marked ascites, and a pansystolic murmur in the tricuspid area. In left sided involvement there are typical signs of mitral regurgitation, left ventricular failure and pulmonary hypertension.

When there is severe right sided endomyocardial fibrosis the chest X-ray shows an enlarged globular heart due to right atrial dilation. The ECG is nonspecific; there may be low voltage QRS complexes, bundle branch block, T wave inversion, or evidence of atrial hypertrophy. Echocardiography has been reported to show a variety of abnormalities including abnormally strong endocardial echoes, pericardial effusion and paradoxical septal motion. The coexistence of a pericardial effusion and tricuspid regurgitation is said to be pathognomonic of right ventricular endomyocardial fibrosis. The differential diagnosis includes any of the cardiomyopathies but when the clinical picture is considered in its geographic context the possibilities are limited largely to rheumatic or tuberculous disease, constrictive pericarditis and beriberi.

Management

The results of traditional supportive treatment with digoxin, diuretics and bed rest have been disappointing. More recent reports suggest that surgical treatment with endocardiectomy and atrioventricular valve repair or replacement is advisable for functionally disabled patients (Valiathan et al 1987, Martinez et al 1989) but the mortality rate is high and the procedure only palliative.

MUCOCUTANEOUS LYMPH NODE SYNDROME

The mucocutaneous lymph node syndrome (Kawasaki disease) is described in Chapter 23. In the early stages there may be myocarditis or pericarditis, but the only serious complication is coronary artery involvement with the development of aneurysms and areas of stenosis which may result in thrombosis with myocardial infarction or sudden death. Severe cardiac involvement usually becomes apparent early in the second week of the disease with a friction rub of pericarditis or gallop rhythm of cardiac failure or myocarditis. Myocardial ischemia may cause papillary muscle dysfunction and mitral regurgitation. Reported ECG findings include T wave changes and prolongation of the PR and QT intervals (Ichida et al 1988). Ultrasound may show a pericardial effusion, left ventricular dysfunction, and aneurysms of the proximal coronary arteries but cannot demonstrate stenotic lesions for which angiocardiography is required. In most cases complete recovery takes place with regression of the aneurysms (Chung et al 1988) and stenotic lesions. However, in about 1% of affected children sudden death from coronary thrombosis occurs, usually within the first 2 months of the illness.

Treatment

Glucocorticosteroids are contraindicated. High dose aspirin therapy (80–100 mg/kg/24 h) for the first 2 weeks may help reduce the incidence of coronary artery aneurysms (Koren et al 1985). Low dose aspirin therapy (3–5 mg/kg/day as a single dose), by reducing platelet aggregation, may decrease the incidence of coronary thrombosis and sudden death. Thus high dose aspirin therapy for 2 weeks should be followed by low dose therapy for at least 2 months, and where aneurysms are demonstrated, until they regress. There is evidence to suggest that high dose purified human gammaglobulin given in addition to high dose aspirin within 10 days of the onset of fever can reduce the incidence of coronary arterial lesions (Newburger et al 1986) and in particular giant aneurysms, the most serious of these abnormalities (Rowley et al 1988). It is suggested that the regime of a single dose of gammaglobulin 2 g/kg given intravenously over 10 hours is more effective than that of 400 mg/kg once daily for 4 days (Newburger et al 1991). It should be administered as soon as possible after the start of the illness, if possible within 10 days of its onset. Coronary artery bypass surgery is required in some children.

HEART MUSCLE DISEASE OR CARDIOMYOPATHY

Heart muscle disease or cardiomyopathy has been reported since the last century but has only been widely recognized in recent years. The term includes a number of different groupings of structural and physiological characteristics, and a functional classification was first suggested by Goodwin et al (1961). Subsequently the report of the WHO/ISFC Task Force (1980) defined cardiomyopathies as 'heart muscle disease of unknown cause' and classified them as dilated, hypertrophic, or restrictive although it was recognized that a few cases did not fit into this classification. The distinction has to be made between these cardiomyopathies and other heart muscle diseases of known cause or those associated with disorders of other systems and termed 'specific heart muscle disease'.

DILATED CARDIOMYOPATHY

Dilated cardiomyopathy is characterized by impaired systolic function of both ventricles, predominately the left in most cases. The left ventricle contracts poorly, becomes dilated and can cause dilation of the mitral valve ring producing mitral regurgitation. Congestive cardiac failure frequently develops.

The outcome is related to the severity of the dysfunction. Significant cardiomegaly, low cardiac output, and overt cardiac failure often suggest a poor prognosis. When a patient presents with findings of dilated cardiomyopathy a search should be made for a specific cause and this may alter the prognosis given to the parents.

Symptoms will vary with the severity of dysfunction and the level of activity of the child. In the acute state there will be marked dyspnea and cardiac failure while less severe states will produce easy fatigue and decreased exercise tolerance. Less commonly the patient may present with a cardiac arrhythmia or conduction defect.

Clinical examination may show signs of congestive cardiac failure with dyspnea, hepatomegaly, edema and poor volume pulses. The apical impulse may be displaced, gallop rhythm may occur and a murmur of mitral regurgitation develop.

Investigations

Chest radiology will show cardiomegaly with significant dysfunction and ECG variable changes of left ventricular hypertrophy and possibly ST changes. Echocardiography demonstrates a dilated, poorly contracting left ventricle with reduction of the indices of function such as the ejection fraction. Doppler ultrasound will demonstrate mitral regurgitation but gives only an approximate assessment of its severity. Since the clinical and echocardiographic features of dilated cardiomyopathy are nonspecific, it is appropriate to consider the possibility of any of the known conditions which produce similar findings and undertake investigation as appropriate.

Treatment

Since a true dilated cardiomyopathy is of unknown etiology treatment has to be symptomatic and nonspecific. It takes the form of accepted heart failure therapy, initially diuretics and digoxin. In severe cases captopril may be of value, and cardiac transplantation may have to be considered in the most severe. It has recently been suggested that high dose intravenous gammaglobulin may improve the prognosis of acute myocarditis (Drucker et al 1994).

HYPERTROPHIC CARDIOMYOPATHY

Hypertrophic cardiomyopathy is usually inherited by an autosomal dominant gene with incomplete penetrance. It is characterized by a nondilated hypertrophied left ventricle. This may involve the septum more than the free wall, which can result in a gradient low in the left ventricular outflow tract either at rest or on exercise. There is also left ventricular diastolic dysfunction with reduced distensibility and impaired relaxation. The condition is often not recognized until adult life but occurs at all ages, even infancy. A similar cardiomyopathy is found in patients with Friedreich's ataxia.

Symptoms are most often associated with a left ventricular outflow tract gradient. In older children dyspnea or excessive fatigue on exertion are most common but chest pain, dizziness, syncope and palpitations also occur. Infants may present with congestive cardiac failure, cardiomegaly or cyanosis. On clinical examination an ejection systolic murmur may be audible, maximal at the lower left sternal edge or apex and it may be possible to feel a 'jerky' arterial pulse or a double apical impulse.

There is no characteristic ECG abnormality. There may be left ventricular hypertrophy, ST and T wave abnormalities, deep Q waves, and prolongation of the QT interval. Echocardiography characteristically shows thickening of the septum and posterior left ventricular wall, often with asymmetric septal hypertrophy (ratio of thickness of ventricular septum to left ventricular wall 1.3 or greater) and systolic anterior motion of the mitral valve. Doppler ultrasound may demonstrate increased velocity low in the left ventricular outflow tract with a characteristic signal and an abnormal left ventricular filling pattern.

The course of the disease is variable. Sudden death can occur, probably from a ventricular arrhythmia and usually in symptomatic patients with left ventricular outflow obstruction. Although changes of ventricular hypertrophy may develop or progress in childhood and adolescence (Maron et al 1986), study of asymptomatic patients suggests that the prognosis may be relatively good for those are asymptomatic (Spirito et al 1989). Drug therapy with verapamil (Shaffer et al 1988), nefedipine or propranolol (or other beta-blocker) is indicated in symptomatic patients. These drugs have little influence on the incidence of sudden death but low dose amiodarone may be valuable in this context (McKenna et al 1988). Cardiac pacing can be of symptomatic benefit but its effect on long-term outcome is not yet known (Slade et al 1996).

Patients with severe left ventricular outflow gradients may also benefit from a septal myomyectomy. In general, children who are symptomatic or have signs of significant disease should have their activities restricted though it is worth noting that although severe exertion is considered a risk factor, in most cases sudden death is unrelated to exertion.

SPECIFIC HEART MUSCLE DISEASE

This is defined as heart muscle disease of known cause or associated with disorders of other systems. Myocardial disorders caused by systemic or pulmonary hypertension, valvular or congenital heart disease are excluded in the definition of this, but can produce similar findings and should be considered in reaching a diagnosis. Features similar to those of dilated or hypertrophic cardiomyopathy are produced by a number of different conditions and are considered in detail elsewhere.

Most commonly the presentation is that of a dilated cardiomyopathy; the cause most frequently encountered in pediatric cardiology is the result of anthracycline therapy. The more common of those possibilities which produce the effects similar to a dilated type of cardiomyopathy are outlined in Table 13.9.

Thickening of the ventricular walls which might mimic hypertrophic cardiomyopathy occurs in a number of specific heart muscle diseases. In most of these the thickening is concentric but this also occurs in hypertrophic cardiomyopathy and the ultrasound findings may be similar. Wall thickening can be found in the conditions detailed in Table 13.10.

The diagnosis of myocarditis should always be considered and if it is thought that there may be a specific heart muscle disorder related to a metabolic condition, the screening investigations given in Table 13.11 may be useful.

PERICARDITIS

A variety of inflammatory disease, both infective and noninfective, can involve the pericardium with the resultant production of an exudate which can be serous, fibrinous, hemorrhagic or purulent. Pericarditis often occurs as a manifestation of a more generalized illness. It may also be associated with myocarditis. Purulent pericarditis is rare in the developed countries but is not uncommon in the developing ones (Sinzobahamvya & Ikeogu 1987). Organisms most commonly isolated are *Staphylococcus aureus*, *Haemophilus influenzae b* and *Neisseria meningitidis*. Tuberculous pericarditis can result

Table 13.9 Conditions producing features of dilated cardiomyopathy

Other cardiac conditions (excluded in definition of specific heart muscle disease)
    Anomalous origin of left coronary artery
    Coarctation of the aorta
    Arrhythmias (SVT/VT)
    Systemic arteriovenous fistula
    Infections (myocarditis)

Drug therapy
    Anthracyclines

Infection
    Viral myocarditis
    Fungal/protozoal/metazoal myocarditis

Metabolic causes/storage
    Mucopolysaccharidoses
    Lipidoses (GM1 gangliosidosis)
    Sialic acid storage disorder
    Fucosidosis

Metabolic causes/energy production
    Carnitine deficiency
    Fatty acid oxidation defects (usually thick walls)
    'Mitochondrial' abnormalities (usually thick walls)
    Aminoacidemias (sick neonate/infant)

Neuromuscular disorders
    Muscular dystrophies (late, thin walls)
    Rare congenital myopathies ('floppy')
    (Friedreich's ataxia: mostly hypertrophic)

Chromosomal abnormalities (dysmorphic features)

Table 13.10 Specific heart diseases causing wall thickening

Other cardiac conditions
    Coarctation of the aorta
    Systemic hypertension
    Tumors

Metabolic causes/storage
    Glycogenoses (Pompe, GSDIII)
    Mucopolysaccharidoses (ASH in older children)

Metabolic causes/energy production
    Fatty acid oxidation defects
    'Mitochondrial' cardiomyopathies
    Organic acidurias

Endocrine
    Infant of diabetic mother
    Pancreatic tumors (severe neonatal hypoglycemia)
    Hypothyroidysm (ASH)

Neuromuscular disorders
    Friedreich's ataxia
    Rare congenital myopathies ('floppy')

Syndromes
    Noonan
    Leopard/neurofibromatosis/Williams
    Chromosomal abnormalities

ASH = asymmetric septal hypertrophy.

Table 13.11 Screening investigations for metabolic causes of heart muscle disease

Metabolic causes/energy production
    Carnitine
    Organic acids
    Amino acids
    Lactate
    Creatine phosphokinase

Metabolic causes/storage (for children < 1 year, or if there is strong suspicion)
    Blood vacuolated lymphocytes
    Urine glycosaminoglycans
    Urine oligosaccharides
    Creatine phosphokinase

from direct spread from nearby lymph nodes. Viral pericarditis is often associated with a myocarditis and is caused by a similar range of viruses. In the majority of cases where the clinical features suggest a viral pericarditis, no etiology can be ascertained; this has been termed acute benign pericarditis and may be related to a hypersensitivity reaction to a viral illness. Pericarditis occurs as part of the pancarditis of rheumatic fever and is also found in patients with chronic renal failure and collagen diseases, particularly systemic lupus erythematosus and rheumatoid arthritis. In children with leukemia or other malignancies pericardial effusion may occur early due to pericardial infiltration or later as a result of mediastinal irradiation.

Clinical features

The primary disease can overshadow the symptoms of pericarditis which may be overlooked, particularly in the infant. Signs of pericarditis can vary not only with the primary illness but also with the volume and rate of accumulation of pericardial fluid. Pain is not a common feature in children. Dyspnea and a nonproductive cough may develop as the effusion enlarges. Fever will be prominent with bacterial infection. Early signs include a friction rub which may be audible even in the presence of a fairly large effusion. If the effusion enlarges and produces cardiac tamponade neck vein distention, hepatomegaly, low pulse pressure, pulsus paradoxus and cardiac failure may become apparent. Significant pulsus paradoxus (which indicates tamponade) is generally considered to be present when there is a fall in systolic pressure on inspiration of more than 10 mmHg. Since signs and symptoms of purulent pericarditis may be minimal and nonspecific in the early stages or may be missed in the presence of a severe generalized illness, a high index of suspicion is necessary, particularly in the developing countries. The onset of cardiac failure in a child with bronchopneumonia, empyema or lung abscess may be the first sign of purulent pericarditis.

Diagnosis

Although the chest X-ray may demonstrate an enlarged globular cardiac shadow, and the ECG ST elevation with diminished QRS voltage, both these investigations may be normal. Echocardiography is the appropriate and most sensitive technique, readily showing the presence and size of a pericardial effusion.

Where infective pericarditis is suspected blood cultures should be performed and pericardiocentesis is mandatory. The fluid should be examined for cells and organisms and cultured for bacteria, viruses, mycobacteria and fungi. When appropriate, serological evidence of a viral infection should be sought.

Treatment

Purulent pericarditis is a medical and surgical emergency. Following pericardiocentesis and Gram stain of the fluid to establish the causal agent, high doses of appropriate antibiotics should be given intravenously. Pericardiocentesis to remove fluid is only a temporizing measure and prompt surgical drainage is essential. Treatment of viral and acute benign pericarditis is only symptomatic and the disease is self-limiting. The use of glucocorticosteroids has been advised where symptoms are severe or persistent and fail to respond to other therapy.

CONNECTIVE TISSUE DISEASE

Cardiac involvement can occur in all the connective tissue diseases but is most common in systemic lupus erythematosus (SLE). Pericarditis without tamponade is the usual presenting feature. The characteristic atypical verrucose endocarditis (Libman–Sacks) can cause valve regurgitation. Congenital complete heart block can occur in infants of mothers suffering from connective tissue disease who are seropositive for anti-Ro (Behan et al 1989).

In juvenile rheumatoid arthritis cardiac abnormalities as a rule occur in the acute systemic form of the disease with pericarditis, myocarditis and occasionally mitral regurgitation. Echocardiography may demonstrate a pericardial effusion in children with no clinical signs of heart disease. Cardiac failure is an uncommon complication but can be fatal.

Scleroderma can be associated with diffuse focal fibrosis within the myocardium producing ventricular dysfunction which may lead to left ventricular failure and death.

Polyarteritis nodosa is rare in infants and children, but in these age groups it follows a more fulminant course. Infantile polyarteritis is usually associated with coronary artery lesions which can result in myocardial ischemia, cardiac failure and death.

CARDIAC TUMORS

Primary cardiac tumors are rare in children. The majority are benign in the histological sense but, by compressing the conducting tissue or encroaching on the cardiac cavities, they may cause death from arrhythmia or from ventricular or valve dysfunction. A rhabdomyoma, fibroma or teratoma most frequently affects infants and young children, including the newborn, and a hemangioma or myxoma older children (Van der Hauwaert 1971). Rhabdomyomas are commonly multiple when associated with tuberous sclerosis.

Clinical features depend on the site and size of the tumor. Intramural tumors may be asymptomatic or cause an arrhythmia. Tumors within a cavity can cause ventricular outflow obstruction, or obstruction or regurgitation of the atrioventricular valves. A striking feature of a left atrial myxoma may be variation in the character of the mitral murmur with posture. Cardiac failure and embolic phenomena can also occur.

Echocardiography is the ideal technique for showing intracardiac tumors, particularly a left atrial myxoma where the echocardiographic appearance is diagnostic. Surgical therapy is indicated if there is an intractable arrhythmia or obstruction to the outflow or inflow tracts.

HYPERTENSION

Hypertension in children and adolescents has long been considered to be almost invariably secondary to other disease entities but it is now apparent that in the older child and adolescent it is at least as frequently of the primary or essential type. Furthermore, evidence suggests that primary hypertension has its origins in early life and those at risk may be identifiable in childhood or adolescence, allowing surveillance and management with the aim of preventing the later development of fixed hypertension. Measurement of blood pressure should be a routine part of the clinical examination of all children over 3 years old. There are difficulties in defining hypertension in children since blood pressure rises with age and exhibits considerable variability in an individual. The American Task Force on Blood Pressure control in Children (Report of the Second Task Force on Blood Pressure Control in Children 1987) has suggested that consistent diastolic values above the 95th centile should be considered to indicate hypertension. On this basis the prevalence of systemic hypertension in the pediatric age group is between 1% and 3%. Essential hypertension is most common in adolescents, particularly in those who have a hypertensive first degree relative or who are overweight. Renal disease accounts for about 95% of cases of secondary hypertension, the causes of which are outlined in Table 13.12.

Clinical features and evaluation

Hypertension is frequently discovered on routine examination of a patient who has no symptoms directly attributable to it. Symptoms, when they occur, result from complications. Thus

Table 13.12   Causes of secondary hypertension

Renal
Chronic glomerulonephritis
Reflux nephropathy
Obstructive uropathy
Polycystic disease
Dysplastic disease
Renal tumors
Collagen disease

Vascular
Coarctation of the aorta
Renal artery abnormalities
Renal venous thrombosis

Endocrine
Pheochromocytoma
Neuroblastoma
Cushing's syndrome
Primary aldosteronism
Congenital adrenal hyperplasia (17α-hydroxylase or 11-hydroxylase deficiency)

Miscellaneous
Intracranial tumors
Drugs (corticosteroids, oral contraceptives)
Lead poisoning
Familial dysautonomia
Porphyria
Turner's syndrome

raised intracranial pressure may cause headache or vomiting and eventually result in seizures or other neurological disturbances and left ventricular failure may cause dyspnea or cough. Physical examination may be normal initially but with established hypertension changes occur in the optic fundi and evidence of left ventricular hypertrophy may become apparent.

In a few patients with severe hypertension the diagnosis is beyond doubt but in many identification is dependent upon an arbitrary definition of the upper limits of normal blood pressure. Percentile charts of seated blood pressure for age from birth to 18 years have been published in the Report of the Second Task Force on Blood Pressure Control in Children (1987) and for height by a working party of the British Hypertension Society (de Swiet et al 1989) based on data published in the French literature. The American group suggested that levels greater than the 95th centile for age be considered abnormal and on this basis supine blood pressure values above the following should be regarded as indicating significant hypertension:

1 week–1 month:	104 systolic
1 month–1 year:	112/74
3–5 years:	116/76
6–9 years:	122/78
10–12 years:	126/82
13–15 years:	136/86
16–18 years:	142/92.

Blood pressure should be measured with the child lying or sitting comfortably with the sphygmomanometer at heart level. The cuff should be as large as possible and must cover at least two-thirds of the upper arm. Narrower cuffs give false high results. Blood pressure in children is labile and a single reading cannot be considered to indicate hypertension unless it is very high. The reading should be repeated and only if the level has been found to be elevated on at least three different occasions can the patient be considered to have hypertension. Larger children (heavier and taller) have higher blood pressures than smaller ones and if levels between the 90th and 95th percentiles are found height should be considered (de Swiet & Dillon 1989). An obese child with moderate hypertension should be encouraged to lose weight and the blood pressure subsequently repeated before undergoing investigation and possible treatment.

Investigation

Further management will depend on the patient's age, blood pressure level, and the history and physical findings. The history may suggest a renal cause (past or present kidney disease), pheochromocytoma (episodes of palpitations, excessive sweating, headache), aldosteronism (weakness, polyuria, muscle cramps) or drug ingestion (corticosteroid, oral contraceptive). Inquiry should be made for a family history of eclampsia, essential hypertension or premature coronary artery or cerebrovascular disease. Physical examination must include palpation of the femoral pulses and kidneys, and auscultation of the abdomen and flanks for a bruit suggesting renal artery stenosis. Fundoscopic and cardiac examination may demonstrate hypertensive changes. Every hypertensive patient should have a full blood count, urinalysis and urine culture, and serum electrolytes, urea, creatinine and uric acid concentrations performed. The presence of associated hyperlipidemia, a further risk factor in coronary artery disease, should be excluded. Other studies may be warranted on the basis of the history, or physical or laboratory findings.

Those with severe hypertension, symptoms, or advanced retinopathy require urgent investigation and treatment. In general, the younger the child and the higher the blood pressure, the more likely it is that the hypertension will be secondary and the more intense should be the search for an underlying cause. There are no clear guidelines on when to investigate and treat children with hypertension. It has been suggested that where the history is negative and the examination and preliminary laboratory tests are normal, further investigation is not indicated in children aged 3–12 years with a diastolic pressure less than 90 mmHg, or aged 13–18 years with a diastolic pressure of less than 100 mmHg. However, whereas the American Task Force has suggested investigation and treatment is appropriate for those with a diastolic above the 95th centile, others have made no firm recommendation.

Further evaluation should be carried out with the aim of excluding renal and endocrine disease, as detailed in Chapters 17 and 19 respectively. The search for a renal cause of hypertension requires estimation of serum creatinine concentration, and renal imaging with ultrasound, radioisotope scanning or micturating cystourethrography and measurement of peripheral plasma renin activity. Abdominal angiography is essential for identifying vascular lesions of the renal arteries and may demonstrate tumors such as pheochromocytoma. Where it is thought that there is a renal lesion contributing to hypertension which may benefit from surgery, samples for plasma renin activity should be taken from the inferior vena cava and both renal veins. Increased secretion by an affected kidney with suppression of secretion by the contralateral one suggests that corrective surgery will result in a reduction of blood pressure. Endocrine causes of hypertension are rare in children and their diagnosis requires specific biochemical tests. Screening tests should include measurement of hydroxymethoxymandelic acid (HMMA) (pheochromocytoma or neuroblastoma), metadrenaline (pheochromocytoma) and

homovanillic acid (HVA) (neuroblastoma) and urinary free cortisol and diurnal plasma cortisols (Cushing's syndrome). Hyperaldosteronism is suggested by hypokalemia but this is not a reliable screening test for aldosteronism in children, and plasma aldosterone and plasma renin activity should be measured.

Treatment and prognosis

The treatment of hypertension in children has recently been reviewed (Houtman 1994). The diagnosis of 'hypertension' has important psychological implications for the patient and family. Where the hypertension is borderline it is therefore advisable to avoid this label and instead use the term 'high normal blood pressure'. Borderline hypertension does not require drug therapy. All patients should be advised not to smoke and to avoid excessive salt intake and those who are obese encouraged to lose weight. Girls must be warned of the hypertensive effects of oral contraceptives. Thereafter the patient should be seen at least annually for blood pressure determination.

Those with undoubtedly high levels or symptoms or signs caused by the hypertension must be treated. For others it is difficult to know at what level of blood pressure to start specific drug therapy. Some would suggest a diastolic pressure of more than 90 mmHg for those under 13 years old and 100 mmHg for older subjects, while others suggest a diastolic pressure above the 95th centile. However, there can be difficulties in accurately measuring the diastolic pressure in children and in adults morbidity is more closely related to the systolic pressure so systolic pressure should also be considered in making therapeutic decisions (Weismann 1988). It seems appropriate where there is uncertainty to consult or refer the patient to a physician with specific training and experience in the investigation and management of hypertension.

The hypotensive drugs have a variety of side-effects and each should be introduced in a low dose which is then built up slowly to therapeutic levels (Table 13.13). Emergency treatment for severe hypertension should be intravenous labetalol or sodium

Table 13.13 Recommended dose of the more commonly used hypotensive agents

Oral therapy: minimum and maximum dose

Drug	Dose (mg/kg)	No. of times daily
Chlorothiazide	10–40	2
Frusemide	0.5–2.0	2
Propranolol	1–10	3
Atenolol	1–2	1
Labetalol	2–20	2
Hydralazine	1–8	2 or 3
Prazosin hydrochloride	0.1–0.4	3
Captopril	0.3–5	3
Minoxidil	0.1–2	2
Nifedipine	0.25–1	3–4
Phenoxybenzamine	1–4	2

Intravenous therapy

Diazoxide	2–5 mg/kg bolus over 15 min
Hydralazine	Initially 1–2 mg/kg bolus
	Maintenance 0.15–0.3 mg/kg
Labetalol	1–3 mg/kg/h
Nitroprusside	0.5–8 μg/kg/min

nitroprusside, although recent reports suggest sublingual nifedipine is effective. For less severe hypertension initial therapy is generally with a diuretic such as hydrochlorothiazide or frusemide. Potassium supplements or the addition of a potassium sparing diuretic may be necessary.

If diuretic therapy does not produce a satisfactory effect after 2 weeks on maximum dosage, a beta-blocker (e.g. propranolol or atenolol) should be added. In refractory cases the further addition of a vasodilator such as hydralazine will often provide satisfactory blood pressure control. If this is ineffective, treatment with angiotensin converting enzyme inhibitors (e.g. captopril) or calcium channel antagonists (e.g. nifedipine) should be used.

There is a general tendency for a child's blood pressure to remain at the same percentile level throughout childhood and adolescence. Since primary hypertension may have its onset in childhood it may be possible to identify a potentially hypertensive individual at an early age. However, on present evidence it is not always possible to predict which child will become a hypertensive adult. Indeed up to one-third of hypertensive children may become normotensive on follow-up for a few years. Furthermore, insufficient time has elapsed in prospective studies of hypertensive children to determine whether early recognition of mild or moderate hypertension will reduce the incidence of arteriosclerosis in later life.

REFERENCES

Adatia I, Wessel D L 1994 Therapeutic use of inhaled nitric oxide. Current Opinion in Pediatrics 6: 583–590

Allan L D, Crawford D C, Anderson R H et al 1984 Echocardiographic and anatomical correlations in fetal congenital heart disease. British Heart Journal 52: 542–548

Allen H D, Lange L W, Sahn D J et al 1978 Ultrasound cardiac diagnosis. Pediatric Clinics of North America 25: 677–706

Anderson R H, Ho S Y 1986 The diagnosis and naming of congenitally malformed hearts. In: Macartney F J (ed) Congenital heart disease. MTP Press, Lancaster

Anderson R H, Macartney F J, Shinebourne E A, Tynan M 1987 Terminology. In: Anderson R H, Macartney F J, Shinebourne E A, Tynan M (eds) Pediatric cardiology. Churchill Livingstone, Edinburgh, pp 65–82

Ashfaq M, Houston A B, Gnanapragasam J P, Lilley S, Murtagh E P 1991 Balloon atrial septostomy under echocardiographic control: six years' experience and evaluation of the practicability of the umbilical vein route. British Heart Journal 65: 148–151

Barlow J B, Pocock W A, Marchand P, Denny M 1963 The significance of late systolic murmurs. American Heart Journal 66: 443–452

Beattie J O, Day R E, Cockburn F et al 1983 Alcohol and the fetus in the west of Scotland. British Medical Journal 287: 17–20

Behan W M H, Behan P O, Reid J M et al 1989 Family studies of congenital heart disease associated with Ro antibody. British Heart Journal 62: 320–324

Bejar R, Merritt T A, Coen R W 1982 Pulsatility index, patent ductus arteriosus, and brain damage. Pediatrics 69: 818–822

Brumfitt W, Hamilton-Miller J 1989 Methicillin-resistant *Staphylococcus aureus*. New England Journal of Medicine 320: 1188–1196

Bull C 1986 Interventional catheterisation in infants and children. British Heart Journal 56: 197–200

Bu'Lock F A, Joffe H S, Jordan S C, Martin R P 1993 Balloon dilatation (valvoplasty) as first line treatment for severe stenosis of the aortic valve in early infancy: medium term results and determinants of survival. British Heart Journal 70: 546–553

Campbell R W F 1990 Investigation and management of cardiac arrhythmias. In: Lawson D H (ed) Current medicine, Vol 2. Churchill Livingstone, Edinburgh, pp 25–44

Chung K J, Fulton D R, Lapp R et al 1988 One-year follow-up of cardiac and coronary artery disease in infants and children with Kawasaki disease. American Heart Journal 115: 1263–1267

Cohen D M 1992 Surgical management of congenital heart disease in the 1990s. American Journal of Diseases of Childhood 146: 1447–1452

Coleman E N, Doig W B 1970 Diagnostic problems with innocent murmurs in children. Lancet 2: 228–232

Dajani A S, Bisno A L, Chung K J et al 1988 Prevention of rheumatic fever. Circulation 78: 1082–1086

Danford D A, Nasir A, Gumbiner C 1993 Cost assessment of the evaluation of heart murmurs in children. Pediatrics 91: 365–368

de Swiet M, Dillon M J 1989 Editorial. Hypertension in children. British Medical Journal 299: 469–470

de Swiet M, Dillon M J, Littler W et al 1989 Measurement of blood pressure in children. Recommendations of a working party of the British Hypertension Society. British Medical Journal 299: 497

Dickinson D F, Arnold R, Wilkinson J L 1981 Congenital heart disease among

160 480 liveborn children in Liverpool 1960 to 1969. British Heart Journal 46: 55–62

Drucker N A, Colan S D, Lewis A S et al 1994 Gamma globulin treatment of acute myocarditis in the pediatric population. Circulation 89: 252–257

Ellison R C, Peckham G J, Lang P et al 1983 Evaluation of the preterm infant for patent ductus arteriosus. Pediatrics 71: 364–372

Erbel R, Rohmann S, Drexler H et al 1988 Improved diagnostic value of echocardiography in patients with infective endocarditis by transoesophageal approach. A prospective study. European Heart Journal 9: 43–53

Evans N 1995 The neonate and the ductus arteriosus: importance, diagnosis and practical management. Current Paediatrics 5: 114–117

Ferrieri P 1987 Editorial. Acute rheumatic fever. The come-back of a disappearing disease. American Journal of Diseases of Children 141: 725–727

Fixler D E, Pastor P, Sigman E, Eifler C W 1993 Ethnicity and socioeconomic status: impact on the diagnosis of congenital heart disease. Journal of the American College of Cardiology 21: 1722–1726

Folger G M, Hajar R, Robida A, Hajar H A 1992 Occurrence of valvar heart disease in acute rheumatic fever without evident carditis: colour flow Doppler identification. British Heart Journal 76: 434–438

Fontan F, Baudet E 1971 Surgical repair of tricuspid atresia. Thorax 26: 240–248

Friedman D M, Verma R, Madrid M et al 1993 Recent improvement in outcome using transcatheter embolization techniques for neonatal aneurysmal malformations of the vein of Galen. Pediatrics 91: 583–586

Gardiner H M, Joffe H S 1991 The genesis of Still's murmurs. A controlled Doppler echocardiographic study. British Heart Journal 66: 217–220

Garson Jr A 1988 Advances in dysrhythmias: evaluation and treatment. In: Bricker J T, McNamara D G (eds) Pediatric cardiology. Its current practice. Edward Arnold, London, pp 69–98

Ghisla R P, Hannon D W, Meyer R A, Kaplan S 1985 Spontaneous closure of isolated secundum atrial septal defects in infants – an echocardiographic study. American Heart Journal 109: 1327–1333

Gnanapragasam J P, Houston A B, Northridge D B, Jamieson M P G, Pollock J C S 1991 Transoesophageal echocardiographic assessment of primum, secundum and sinus venosus atrial septal defects. International Journal of Cardiology 31: 167–174

Goodwin J F, Gordon H, Hollman A et al 1961 Clinical aspects of cardiomyopathy. British Medical Journal 1: 69–79

Hatle L, Angelsen B 1985 Doppler ultrasound in cardiology: basic principles and clinical applications, 2nd edn. Lea and Febiger, Philadelphia

Hausdorf G, Schneider M, Franzbach B et al 1996 Transcatheter closure of secundum atrial septal defects with the atrial septal defect occlusion system (ASDOS): initial experience in children. Heart 75: 83–88

Helton J G, Aglira B A, Chin A J et al 1986 Analysis of potential anatomic or physiologic determinants of outcome of palliative surgery for hypoplastic left heart syndrome. Circulation 74 (suppl 1): I70–I77

Hoffman J I, Christianson R 1978 Congenital heart disease in a cohort of 19 502 births with long term follow up. American Journal of Cardiology 42: 641–647

Houston A B, Simpson I A (eds) 1988 Cardiac Doppler ultrasound: a clinical perspective. Butterworth, London

Houston A B, Gregory N L, Coleman E N 1978 Echocardiographic identification of the aorta and main pulmonary artery in complete transposition. British Heart Journal 40: 377–382

Houston A B, Lim M K, Doig W B, Reid J M, Coleman E N 1988 Doppler assessment of pressure drop in patients with ventricular septal defects. British Heart Journal 60: 50–56

Houston A B, Gnanapragasam J P, Doig W B, Lim M, Coleman E N 1991 Doppler ultrasound and the silent ductus arteriosus. British Heart Journal 65: 97–99

Houtman P N 1994 The physiology and treatment of hypertension. Current Paediatrics 4: 77–82

Hudson I, Houston A B, Aitchison T et al 1990 Reproducibility of measurements of cardiac output in newborn infants by Doppler ultrasound. Archives of Disease in Childhood 65: 15–19

Ichida F, Fatica N S, O'Loughlin J E et al 1988 Correlation of electrocardiographic and echocardiographic changes in Kawasaki syndrome. American Heart Journal 116: 812–819

Infective Endocarditis 1987 Journal of Antimicrobial Therapy 20 (suppl A): 1–192

Johnson M C, Payne R M, Grant J W, Strauss A W 1995 The genetic basis of paediatric heart disease. Annals of Medicine 27: 289–300

Karl T, Wensley D, Stark J et al 1987 Infective endocarditis in children with congenital heart disease: comparison of selected features in patients with surgical correction or palliation and those without. British Heart Journal 58: 57–65

Kenna A P, Smithells R W, Fielding D W 1975 Congenital heart disease in Liverpool: 1960–69. Quarterly Journal of Medicine 44: 17–44

Koren G, Rose V, Lavi S et al 1985 Probable efficacy of high-dose salicylates in reducing coronary involvement in Kawasaki disease. Journal of the American Medical Association 254: 767–769

Kugler J D, Danford D A, Deal B J et al 1994 Radiofrequency catheter ablation for tachyarrhythmias in children and adolescents. New England Journal of Medicine 330: 1481–1487

Lammer E J, Chen D T, Hoar R M et al 1985 Retinoic acid embryopathy. New England Journal of Medicine 313: 837–841

Lessop M, Brigden W 1957 Systolic murmurs in healthy children and in children with rheumatic fever. Lancet 1957: 673–674

Leung M P, Beerman L B, Siewers R D, Bahnson H T, Zuberbuhler J R 1987 Longterm follow up after aortic valvuloplasty and defect closure in ventricular septal defects with aortic regurgitation. American Journal of Cardiology 60: 890–894

Levi G, Scalvini S, Volterrani M et al 1988 Coxsackie virus heart disease: 15 years after. European Heart Journal 9: 1303–1307

Lim M K, Houston A B, Doig W B et al 1989 Variability of the Doppler gradient in pulmonary valve stenosis before and after balloon dilation. British Heart Journal 62: 212–216

Lloyd T R, Fedderly R, Mendelsohn A M et al 1993 Transcatheter occlusion of patent ductus arteriosus with gianturco coils. Circulation 88: 1412–1420

Lock J E, Cockerman J T, Keane J F, Finley J P, Wakely P E, Fellows K E 1987 Transcatheter umbrella closure of congenital heart defects. Circulation 75: 593–599

McKenna W J, Franklin R C, Nihoyannopoulos P et al 1988 Arrhythmia and prognosis in infants, children and adolescents with hypertrophic cardiomyopathy. Journal of the American College of Cardiology 11: 147–153

Macmahon B, McKeown T, Record R G 1953 The incidence and life expectation of children with congenital heart disease. British Heart Journal 15: 121–129

Maron B J, Spirito P, Wesley Y et al 1986 Development and progression of left ventricular hypertrophy in children with hypertrophic cardiomyopathy. New England Journal of Medicine 315: 610–614

Martinez E E, Venturi M, Buffalo E et al 1989 Operative results in endomyocardial fibrosis. American Journal of Cardiology 63: 627–629

Massell B F, Chute C G, Walker A M et al 1988 Penicillin and the marked decrease in morbidity and mortality from rheumatic fever in the United States. New England Journal of Medicine 318: 280–286

Mendelsohn A M, Bove E L, Lupinetti F M et al 1993 Intraoperative and percutaneous stenting of congenital pulmonary artery and vein stent. Circulation 88: 210–217

Moe D G, Guntheroth W G 1987 Spontaneous closure of uncomplicated ventricular septal defects. American Journal of Cardiology 60: 674–678

Mustard W T 1964 Successful two stage correction of transposition of the great vessels. Surgery 55: 469–472

Newburger J W, Takahashi M, Burns J C et al 1986 The treatment of Kawasaki syndrome with intravenous gamma globulin. New England Journal of Medicine 315: 341–347

Newburger J W, Takahashi M, Beiser A S et al 1991 A single intravenous infusion of gamma globulin as compared with four infusions in the treatment of acute Kawasaki syndrome. New England Journal of Medicine 324: 1633–1639

Nora J J, Nora A H 1988 Update on counseling the family with a first-degree relative with a congenital heart defect. American Journal of Medical Genetics 29: 137–142

Norwood W I, Lang P, Hansen D 1983 Physiologic repair of aortic atresia: hypoplastic left heart syndrome. New England Journal of Medicine 308: 23–36

O'Callaghan C, McDougall P 1988 Infective endocarditis in neonates. Archives of Disease in Childhood 63: 53–57

Olley P M, Coceani F, Badach E 1976 E-type prostaglandins. A new emergency therapy for certain cyanotic congenital heart malformations. Circulation 53: 728–731

Park M K, Guntheroth W G 1981 How to read pediatric ECGs. Year Book Medical Publishers, London

Penkoske P A, Neches W H, Anderson R H, Zuberbuhler J R 1985 Further observation on the morphology of atrioventricular septal defects. Journal of Thoracic and Cardiovascular Surgery 90: 611–622

Perloff J 1987 The clinical recognition of congenital heart disease. W B Saunders

Pridjian A K, Mendelsohn A M, Lupinetti F M et al 1993 Usefulness of the bi-directional Glenn procedure as staged reconstruction for the functional single ventricle. American Journal of Cardiology 71: 959–962

Quaegebeur J M, Rohmer J, Ottenkamp J 1986 The arterial switch operation. An eight-year experience. Journal of Thoracic and Cardiovascular Surgery 92: 361–384

Rao P S 1995 Should balloon angioplasty be used instead of surgery for native aortic coarctation? British Heart Journal 74: 578–579

Rashkind W J, Miller W W 1966 Creation of an atrial septal defect without thoracotomy. A palliative approach to transposition of the great arteries. Journal of the American Medical Association 196: 991–992

Rastelli G C, McGoon D C, Wallace R B 1969 Anatomic correction of transposition of the great arteries with ventricular septal defect and subpulmonary stenosis. Journal of Thoracic and Cardiovascular Surgery 58: 545–552

Rennie J M, Cooke R W 1991 Prolonged low dose indomethacin for persistent ductus arteriosus of prematurity. Archives of Disease in Childhood 66: 55–58

Report of a Working Party of the British Society for Antimicrobial Chemotherapy 1982 The antibiotic prophylaxis of infective endocarditis. Lancet ii: 1323–1326

Report of the Endocarditis Working Party of the British Society for Antimicrobial Chemotherapy 1990 The antibiotic prophylaxis of infective endocarditis. Lancet 335: 88–89

Report of the Second Task Force on Blood Pressure Control in Children 1987. Pediatrics 79: 1–25

Rezkalla S H, Kloner R A 1989 Management strategies in viral myocarditis. American Heart Journal 117: 706–708

Rigby M L 1994 Diagnostic algorithm for cyanotic heart disease. Current Paediatrics 4: 68–72

Rowley A H, Duffy C E, Shulman S T 1988 Prevention of giant coronary artery aneurysms in Kawasaki disease by intravenous gamma globulin therapy. Journal of Pediatrics 113: 290–294

Royston D 1993 Inhalational agents for pulmonary hypertension. Lancet 342: 941–942

Salmon A P, Holder R, DeGiovanni J V et al 1989 Effects of digoxin in infants with ventricular septal defects and cardiac failure. British Heart Journal 61: 115

Shaffer E M, Rocchini A P, Spicer R L et al 1988 Effects of verapamil on left ventricular diastolic filling in children with hypertrophic cardiomyopathy. American Journal of Cardiology 61: 413–417

Shub C, Tajik A J, Seward J B, Hagler D J, Danielson G K 1985 Surgical repair of uncomplicated atrial septal defects without routine preoperative cardiac catheterization. Journal of American College of Cardiology 6: 49–54

Shulman S T, Amren D P, Bisno A L et al 1984 Prevention of bacterial endocarditis. A statement for health professionals by the Committee on Rheumatic Fever and Infective Endocarditis of the Council on Cardiovascular Disease in the Young. Circulation 70: 1123A–1127A

Silverman N H, Zuberbuhler J R, Anderson R H 1986 Atrioventricular septal defects: cross-sectional echocardiographic and morphological considerations. International Journal of Cardiology 13: 309–331

Simmons N A, Ball A P, Cawson R A et al 1992 Antibiotic prophylaxis and infective endocarditis. Lancet 339: 1292–1293

Sinzobahamvya N, Ikeogu M O 1987 Purulent pericarditis. Archives of Disease in Childhood 62: 696–699

Slade A K B, Sadoul N, Shapiro L et al 1996 DDD pacing in hypertrophic cardiomyopathy: a multicentre clinical experience. Heart 75: 44–49

Smith R T 1988 Advances in pacemaker therapy. In: Bricker J T, McNamara D G (eds) Current practice. Edward Arnold, London

Spirito P, Chiarella F, Carrantino L et al 1989 Clinical course and prognosis of hypertrophic cardiomyopathy in an outpatient population. New England Journal of Medicine 320: 749–755

Stein D G, Laks H, Drinkwater D C et al 1991 Results of total cavopulmonary connection in the treatment of patients with a functional single ventricle. Journal of Thoracic and Cardiovascular Surgery 102: 280–287

Sutherland G R, Godman M J, Smallhorn J F et al 1982 Ventricular septal defects: two dimensional echocardiographic and morphological correlation. British Heart Journal 47: 316–328

Tajik A J, Seward J B, Hagler D J et al 1978 Two-dimensional real-time ultrasonic imaging of the heart and great vessels. Technique, image orientation, structure identification and validation. Mayo Clinic Proceedings 53: 271–303

Taylor P V, Scott J S, Gerlis L M et al 1986 Maternal antibodies against fetal cardiac antigens in congenital complete heart block. New England Journal of Medicine 315: 667–672

Thomaidis C, Varlamis G, Karamperis S 1988 Comparative study of the electrocardiograms of healthy fullterm and premature newborns. Acta Paediatrica Scandinavica 77: 653–657

Tomioka N, Kishimoto C, Matsumori A et al 1986 Effects of prednisolone on acute viral myocarditis in mice. Journal of the American College of Cardiology 7: 868–872

Tynan M M, Baker E J, Rohmer J et al 1985 Percutaneous balloon pulmonary valvuloplasty. British Heart Journal 53: 520–524

UK and US Joint Report 1965 Natural history of rheumatic fever and rheumatic heart disease. Ten year report of a co-operative clinical trial of ACTH, cortisone and aspirin. British Medical Journal 2: 607–615

Unger R, DeKleermaeker M, Gidding S S, Christoffel K K 1992 Calories count: improved weight gain with dietary intervention in congenital heart disease. American Journal of Diseases of Childhood 146: 1078–1084

Valiathan M S, Balakrishnan K G, Sankarkumar R et al 1987 Surgical treatment of endomyocardial fibrosis. Annals of Thoracic Surgery 43: 68–73

Van der Hauwaert L G 1971 Cardiac tumours in infancy and childhood. British Heart Journal 33: 125–132

Vaughan Williams E M 1984 A classification of antiarrhythmic actions reassessed after a decade of drugs. Journal of Clinical Pharmacology 4: 129–147

Washington J A 1987 The microbial diagnosis of infective endocarditis. Journal of Antimicrobial Therapy 20 (suppl A): 29–39

Weinhouse E, Wanderman K L, Sofer S et al 1986 Viral myocarditis simulating dilated cardiomyopathy in early childhood: evaluation by serial echocardiography. British Heart Journal 56: 94–97

Weismann D N 1988 Systolic or diastolic blood pressure significance. Pediatrics 82: 112–114

WHO/ISFC Report 1980 Report of the WHO/ISFC task force on the definition and classification of cardiomyopathies. British Heart Journal 44: 672–673

Wilson D I, Burn J, Scambler P, Goodship J 1993 DiGeorge syndrome: part of CATCH 22. Journal of Medical Genetics 30: 852–856

Wilson L, Curtis A, Korenberg J R et al 1993 A large dominant pedigree of atrioventricular septal defect (AVSD): exclusion from the Down syndrome critical region on chromosome 22. American Journal of Human Genetics 53: 1262–1268

Wilson N 1994 Management of heart failure. Current Paediatrics 4: 62–67

Wilson W R Jr, Ilbawi M N, DeLeon S Y et al 1992 Technical modifications for improved results in total anomalous pulmonary venous drainage. Journal of Thoracic and Cardiovascular Surgery 103: 861–871

Woodruff J F 1980 Viral myocarditis. American Journal of Pathology 101: 427–429

Wren C, Peart I, Bain H et al 1987 Balloon dilation of unoperated aortic coarctation: immediate results and 1 year follow up. British Heart Journal 58: 369–373

Zuberbuhler J R 1981 Clinical diagnosis in pediatric cardiology. Churchill Livingstone, Edinburgh

14 Disorders of the central nervous system

Chapter editors: J. K. Brown R. A. Minns

Congenital disorders 641
Brain development 641
J. K. Brown
Congenital malformations of the central nervous
  system 645
J. K. Brown
Congenital abnormalities of the spinal cord 651
J. K. Brown
Hydrocephalus 657
R. A. Minns
Developmental disorders 666
J. K. Brown
Acute CNS disorders 671
Epilepsy 671
J. K. Brown and M. O'Regan
The epilepsy syndromes 679
Acute encephalopathies 693
R. A. Minns
Head injuries 699
J. K. Brown, R. A. Minns and A. J. W. Steers
Cerebrovascular disease and migraine 709
J. K. Brown

Chronic diseases of the nervous system 719
Diseases of the peripheral nervous system 719
J. K. Brown
Disorders of muscle 726
J. K. Brown
Disorders of movement 738
  Cerebral palsy 738
  Acute onset and progressive movement disorders 762
J. K. Brown, J. P. Lin and R. A. Minns
Degenerative brain disorders and the neurodermatoses 774
R. A. Minns
Disorders of higher cortical function 804
Speech and language disorders 804
A. O'Hare and J. K. Brown
Learning disorders 819
A. O'Hare and J. K. Brown
Mental handicap 826
R. A. Minns
References 842

CONGENITAL DISORDERS

BRAIN DEVELOPMENT

The concept of developmental neurology depends upon an understanding of brain development and the factors which affect it. Brain development can be divided into three stages:

1. formation of the neural crest and closure of the neural tube;
2. primitive vesicle formation;
3. differentiation of the primitive vesicles, especially the telencephalic vesicle, into the cerebral cortex (Alberts et al 1989).

CLOSURE OF NEURAL TUBE AND FORMATION OF NEURAL CREST

The neural tube becomes visible 22 days after conception and closure takes 4 days starting from the middle. The rostral and caudal ends of the neural tube will therefore be the last to close, i.e. the anterior and posterior neuropore. The cells at the margin of the neural plate and ectoderm form two longitudinal columns of cells, the neural crest cells.

Failure of fusion of the neural tube, i.e. rachischisis, occurs in the spina bifida complex along with more localized failures of closure such as meningoceles, meningomyeloceles or myelodysplasia. Failure of closure of the top end results in the Arnold–Chiari malformation or Dandy–Walker malformation. It is not known what controls neural tube closure though dopamine and noradrenaline are thought to be important: α-methyltransferase arrests catecholamine synthesis and causes the chick to develop spina bifida. In humans interference with closure in spina bifida is most often due to a combination of genetic factors with environmental factors such as folate deficiency. Other substances such as radiation, vitamin A, cytostatic drugs (especially antifolate drugs) and drugs such as sodium valproate may interfere with neural tube closure. In humans rubella, herpes simplex and toxoplasmosis infection in the mother will also occasionally interfere with neural tube closure and the effect of a heavy alcoholic binge at the time of closure is suspect (see p. 91). Agenesis of the sacrum with neural dysplasia may form part of the caudal regression syndrome seen in the infant of the diabetic mother. Meningomyelocele may be seen in chromosome abnormalities such as trisomies 8, 13 and 18.

There is a close relationship between neural crest cells and congenital malformation. Melanocytes are of neural crest origin and it is thought that cells in the pituitary producing melanocyte-stimulating hormone and catecholamine-producing chromaffin cells of the adrenal medulla are also formed from migrating neural crest cells. Other hormone-producing cells, such as those producing ACTH and the calcitonin-producing cells of the thyroid, most likely arise from the neural crest and the type 1 cells of the carotid body likewise originate from this tissue. These cells are referred to collectively as amine precursor uptake and decarboxylation cells (APUD cells). Diseases which involve abnormal neural crest cell migration, such as neurofibromatosis, show abnormal melanocyte migration and formation of depigmented areas and hamartomatous café-au-lait spots. Pheochromocytoma, thyroid tumors and the abnormal autonomic innervation seen in megacolon are all the result of abnormal neural crest migration.

DEVELOPMENT OF THE CEREBRAL VESICLES

The rostral end of the neural tube divides into three primitive vesicles: the prosencephalon, mesencephalon and rhombencephalon. In humans these are thought to be visible at around 28 days. The prosencephalon is subdivided into telencephalon and diencephalon. The telencephalon gives rise to the cerebral cortex and both the diencephalon and the telencephalon give rise to the thalamus. The diencephalon also gives rise to the third ventricle, hypothalamus, parts of the basal ganglia and the eye. The mesencephalon gives rise to the midbrain and the rhombencephalon to cerebellum, pons and medulla.

Development of the telencephalon

Cell division and migration

The vesicle is generally thin walled but with a thick layer of cells, the germinal plate, adjacent to the ependyma. There is a clear intermediate zone and an outer marginal zone. Cells divide in the subependymal germinal plate, then migrate outwards along guidewires provided by the processes of the Bergman glial fibers to form the 'cortical plate' of the marginal zone, i.e. the future cerebral cortex. The more recently the cell migrated, the more external its position in the cortical plate and hence the so-called 'inside out rule'. Cells do not undergo mitosis once they have left the germinal zone. Cell division in the subependymal zone remains active to about 28 weeks' gestation. Between 28 and 34 weeks the subependymal zone (germinal plate) undergoes rapid dissolution, but even at term a thin layer of subependymal cells can still be seen (Alberts et al 1989). The cells in the subependymal layer, although primitive, are already differentiated in that they are destined for certain areas of cortex. Several generations of young neuroblasts may migrate along the same glial fiber and so columns of cells form in the future cerebral cortex and this gives rise to grouping of cells in the cortex into cortical units or modules. Cells destined to be neurons tend to migrate before those which will give rise to glia.

It has been estimated that four generations of cells from the germinal layer would be necessary to give the total number of neurons and if a metabolic upset occurs it could theoretically drastically reduce the total number of neurons in the brain, resulting in microcephaly. Diseases such as neurofibromatosis, tuberous sclerosis and the cerebrohepatorenal syndrome of Zellweger and also cocaine addiction in the mother can be associated with abnormalities of migration so that the cortical architecture is disrupted and mental retardation and epilepsy result. The arrested cells show as heterotopia and these groups of cells are not under normal antimitotic control and may give rise to cerebral tumors.

Heterotopias in the temporal and occipital regions are quite common in the normal premature infant but usually disappear. Abnormal cells, however, may persist in some cases of temporal lobe epilepsy and are now thought to be a possible pathological basis for autism and dyslexia. Many of the diseases causing mental retardation, particularly those associated with chromosome abnormalities and the syndromes of mental handicap, are associated with cortical dysplasia, as are most of the infants suffering from intractable epilepsy, e.g. lissencephaly, laminar subcortical heterotopias, double cortex, hemimegalencepaly and opercular dysplasias. In these cases there may be abnormality in the actual number of cells or in the differentiation once they have arrived at the cortical plate. Fetal alcohol syndrome is associated with a failure of migration, the cells behaving as if drunk and either not arriving at the cortical plate or going too far and wandering out into the arachnoid.

Cell differentiation

There are six different types of neuron in the cerebral cortex and 60 different types of cell in the central nervous system. Blood vessels must penetrate the plate and the organization of the blood supply by mesenchyme invasion is not understood. In anencephaly one of the most obvious abnormalities on histological examination is a total disruption of vascular architecture with large areas of vascular malformation. A similar kind of vascular abnormality is seen in association with occipital encephaloceles.

Differentiation of neurons involves their correct orientation, i.e. with axons pointing downwards. In cortical dysplasias many neurons may be upside down. The axon develops from neurites which grow out from the cell body and move by ameboid movement. It is not known how the neurite is guided into its eventual effector site but there are chemicals which attract and some which repel the growing axon and many chemical substances such as lamellin and fibronectin are now known to be implicated.

The classic six cortical layers of the neocortex form in the order 5, 6, 3, 4, 2 and 1, granular cells of the fourth and second layer being particularly slow to mature. Evrard (1992) has shown that one can time an insult, e.g. if the fifth cortical layer is selectively involved in microcephaly.

Glial multiplication occurs between 28 weeks and term as the so-called second DNA spurt. Damage to the developing glia such as the oligodendroglia may result in a postnatal failure of myelination and this can now readily be seen on MRI imaging.

Up to the 28th week the cerebral cortex has been smooth and the insular open with the opercular lip and single central sulcus (Fig. 14.la). As cell numbers increase and the surface area of the cortical brain matter increases compared to the underlying future white matter, infolding is necessary to accommodate the greater surface area and this is seen in the formation of the gyral pattern (Fig. 14.1b and c).

Gross defects show as lissencephaly when no gyri form at all. An opening up of the sulci by stretching the cerebral cortex, as occurs in hydrocephalus, shows that there are other gyri normally not visible from the surface in the sulci and therefore normal gyral pattern disappears and is replaced by what is termed 'micropolygyria'. Ulegyria is due to atrophy or gliosis of normally formed gyri and is a cerebral deformation due to brain damage, not a malformation.

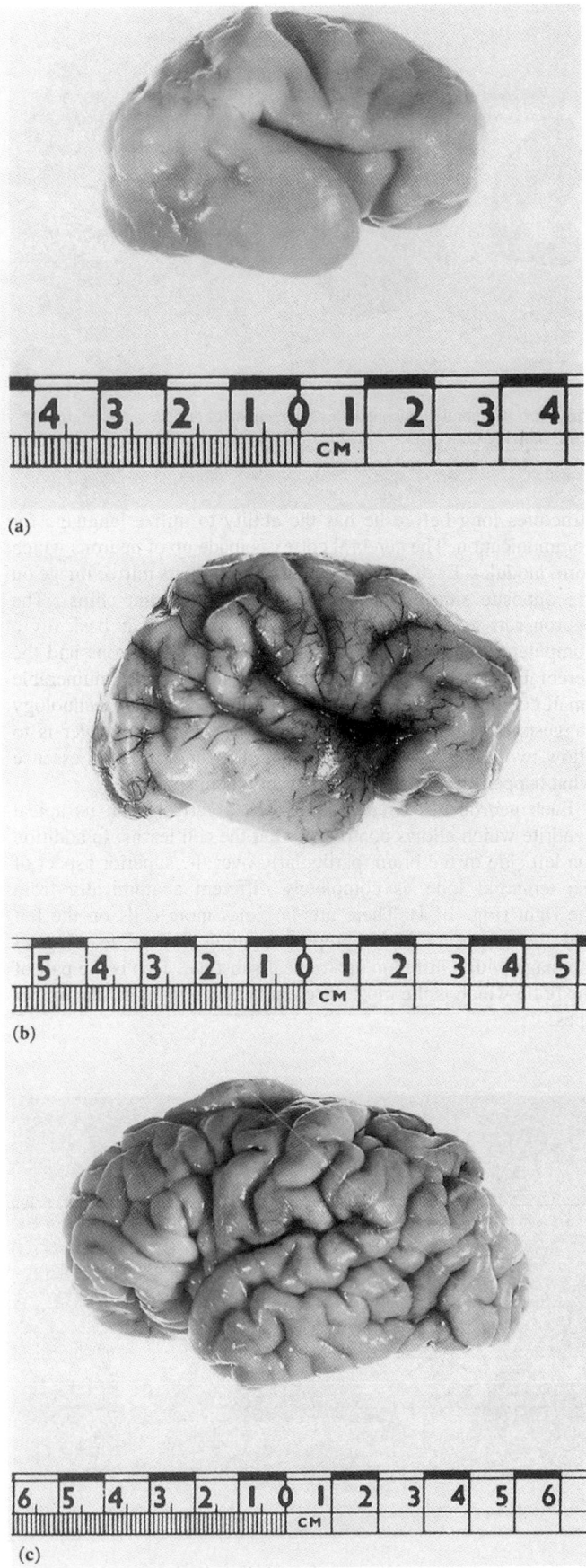

(a)

(b)

(c)

Fig. 14.1 Stages in the development of cortical gyral patterns.

Biochemical maturation

Once cell differentiation occurs certain specific substances may be produced, such as fetal glial-specific protein which appears as glial cells mature at 24 weeks. As neuronal membrane formation increases there is an increase in ganglioside formation. There is little ganglioside in the cerebral cortex during the phase of cell division but when processes start to form, with the need to form large amounts of membrane, there is a rapid increase in ganglioside concentration. The most rapid rise is from the time of birth until the first 2 postnatal months and it has leveled off by 4 months after birth. Synaptosomal membranes are particularly rich in ganglioside. The type of ganglioside changes; GT1 forms up to 40% of ganglioside in early fetal life and then GDla at the time of the ganglioside spurt. GM1 tends to be high but fairly constant during the whole period. GT1 falls away after 26 weeks leaving GM1 and GDla as the principal gangliosides at term. Ganglioside in the cortex differs from that in myelin by having 90% of its fatty acid content provided by stearic acid. After the first 4 weeks of postnatal life the astrocyte and the hepatocyte can synthesize certain essential fatty acids necessary for membrane formation from linoleic and linolenic acid in the diet. Before this time it is necessary to provide arachidonic and decosohexenoic acid in the diet. The fatty acid content of some of the structural brain lipids can therefore depend upon the type of milk that the infant is fed. This has led to speculation as to whether decosohexenoic acid which is present in breast milk but not in synthetic formulae should be added to infant formulae.

Enzymes differentiate in different patterns throughout the brain, e.g. succinic acid dehydrogenase appears in the visual cortex long before it does in the motor cortex. There appears to be a critical time for the development of many enzymes and thyroid hormone is also needed over a comparatively narrow band of time (critical period). There is a large influx of amino acids into the fetal brain during maturation to keep pace with the high rate of protein synthesis and this influx falls when the rapid phase of brain development is over. Amino acid imbalance can block protein synthesis within cells and inhibit mitosis. Phenylalanine in excess, for example, will block the entry of methionine, leucine and tryptophan into the brain. Amino acid imbalance produced either by inborn error of metabolism or by abnormal intravenous or enteral nutrition may produce impairment of brain development.

Cell process formation

Dendritic growth starts at 28 weeks' gestation and is maximal from 28 to 35 weeks. The formation of dendritic spines, i.e. connections between neurons, is vital to the development of modules which make up the learning units of the brain. Severe loss of spines is seen in chromosome disorders such as trisomy 18 and in the infant suffering from infantile spasms. More spines are formed than is necessary and at first they are thin but then thicken as synaptic contact is made. If no contact is made the thin ones are lost by 6 months after birth. Even in a short period of artificial ventilation of the premature infant, there may be abnormal dendritic spine formation.

Myelination

Myelin is produced in the central nervous system by the oligodendroglial cells and in the peripheral nervous system by the

Schwann cells. The cells form a membrane and wind round the axon in the well-known Swiss roll fashion. The first sheath is known as premyelin and it is only later that the lipids are laid down to produce the protein lipid sandwich of mature myelin. The purpose of myelin is to allow rapid conduction down the axon and to insulate it from ionic changes in the extracellular environment which would cause spontaneous depolarization. Conduction is faster the better myelinated the axon and this shows as the markedly increasing nerve conduction velocity in the premature infant between 28 and 46 weeks, when it increases at the rate of about 1 m/s per week.

The brain weighs around 350 g at birth and over the next 4 years will grow by a further 1000 g. This is largely due to myelination and the formation of dendrites, Nissl and association pathways. Myelination of brain occurs rapidly in the first 6 months after birth and then there is a slower phase over the next 4 years and a very slow phase up to 16 years of age (Fig. 14.2).

There are definite myelogenetic cycles. The leg area of the cortex myelinates before the arm area, yet upper limb function is accurate and well developed by the time the child takes his first clumsy steps (Fig. 14.3). Myelination of short association pathways such as the frontohypothalamic tract occurs gradually over the whole of childhood. It is possible that the timing of the onset of puberty and also the timing of abilities such as abstract thoughts (e.g. the ability to extract the meaning from physics experiments around the age of 12 years) are determined by the development of these association pathways.

PSYCHOGENESIS

The limbic system develops early and the small infant is capable of nonverbal communication involving limbic and temporal lobe

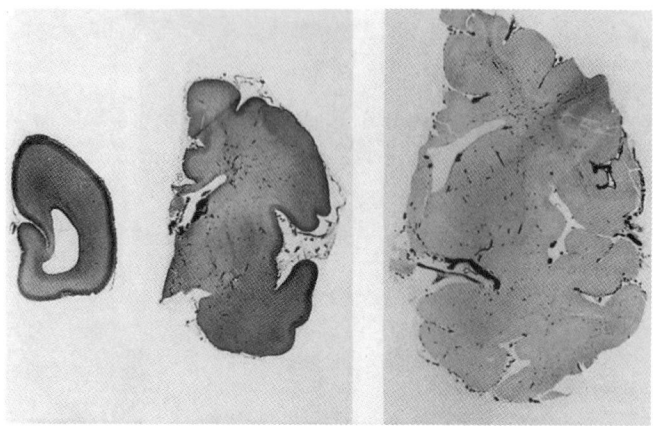

Fig. 14.3 Cerebral hemisphere development at 14 and 26 weeks and at term, showing (at term) myelination of the leg area.

structures long before he has the ability to utilize language for communication. The cerebral cortex is made up of neurons which form modules. Each module is connected with its mirror image on the opposite side and these form in effect 'brain chips'. The neuron acts as a memory and switch system and is basically a computer. Each module consists of some 2500 neurons and the cerebral cortex can be regarded as being made up of innumerable small computing or learning units. Modern computer technology suggests that the most effective way of improving power is to allow two computers to talk to each other and this is in essence what happens between the two cerebral hemispheres.

Each neuron has what is known as a cartridge on its apical dendrite which allows control of what the cell learns. In addition the left side of the brain, particularly over the superior aspect of the temporal lobe, is completely different anatomically from the right (Fig. 14.4). There are 17 times more cells on the left and there appears to be preprogramming for the learning of language with a different anatomical substrate. This is the part of the brain which is the most different between man and the higher apes.

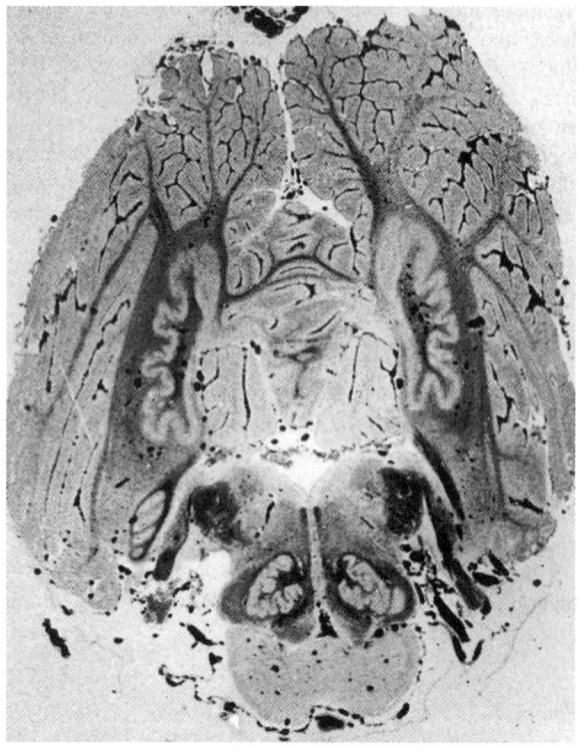

Fig. 14.2 Myelination of cerebellum and pons.

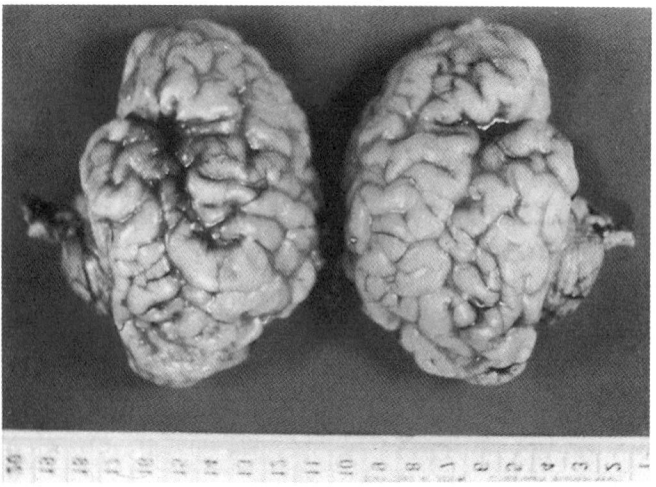

Fig. 14.4 Comparison of lateral surface of left and right cerebral hemispheres.

The development of modules, the connection of these modules one with another by association fibers and the preprogramming of these units for the learning of specific tasks is basic to the development of the brain as an organ of learning. If a module is damaged on one side of the brain it can be taken over by the opposite side. Normally one side is inhibited, i.e. there is reciprocal cerebral inhibition or 'dominance' so that there is no interference between one side of the brain and the other.

The left side of the brain develops more slowly than the right in boys. The parts of the brain on the left subserving language (the so-called tertiary zones) are amongst the last to mature under genetic control. This slower development in boys partly explains the higher incidence of developmental abnormality affecting speech, language, reading and writing which are five times more common in boys than girls.

CONGENITAL MALFORMATIONS OF THE CENTRAL NERVOUS SYSTEM

The term 'congenital malformation' signifies that there has been disruption in the normal process of organogenesis occurring before birth. A congenital malformation must be separated from a congenital deformation in which the organ has formed properly but then has been distorted or damaged as a result of a disease process, e.g. porencephaly, hydranencephaly. The earlier the insult, the more gross the malformation. Since organogenesis is dependent upon a timed sequence of events and the blueprint for this time schedule is held in the genes, it is not unexpected that abnormalities of genes, i.e. genetic disorders or chromosome disorders, are the most frequent cause of malformation.

A single malformation is not specific to a particular cause and so one may see neural tube defects which are of genetic origin, due to vitamin deficiency, associated with chromosome disorders or due to intrauterine exposure to infection, drugs or radiation.

Inheritance may be dominant as in some cases of neural tube defect, hydrocephalus complicating achondroplasia and myotonic dystrophy, they may be sex-linked dominant as in the case of Aicardi syndrome, sex-linked recessive as in some forms of hydrocephalus and aqueduct stenosis or autosomal recessive as, for example, in the Meckel–Gruber syndrome with occipital encephalocele.

Most of the chromosome disorders are associated with mental retardation and a degree of cortical dysplasia whilst others, notably chromosomes 8, 13, 17 and 18, are associated with gross malformations of the brain such as holoprosencephaly.

Malformations of the central nervous system used to be the commonest of all malformations with a perinatal mortality of about 2.5 per 1000 deliveries and an equal number of survivors. The use of α-fetoprotein screening in the blood, selected amniocentesis with assessment of α-fetoprotein and acetylcholinesterase, together with the more routine use of ultrasound in the more developed areas of the world, has allowed selective termination and so grossly diminished the number of babies being born with severe CNS malformations. The number of liveborn spina bifida infants is now only 10% of that seen 30 years ago. The histological malformations of the cortex presenting with intractable epilepsy and mental retardation are still a major problem in pediatric neurology and their diagnosis is becoming more common with better imaging with MRI.

TYPES OF CNS MALFORMATION

Malformation may take the form of absence of development of part of the brain, e.g. cerebellar agenesis, anencephaly, absence of the corpus callosum and absence of the cerebellar vermis. There may be failure of fusion (e.g. cranium bifidum and total rachischisis) or parts of the nervous system may fail to separate as seen in holoprosencephaly. The hemispheres may form but with gross disruption of the microscopic architecture; there may be abnormality of the gyral pattern as seen in lissencephaly and pachygyria. The commonest end result of failure of normal brain development is failure of brain growth. The brain should weigh 340 g at birth and 1340 g by 4 years. If the brain does not grow to its normal size, the result is microencephaly with a small cranial vault – microcephaly. Occasionally the brain grows too large, i.e. megalencephaly, when the head also is large to accommodate the enlarged brain, i.e. macrocephalus. The same type of abnormality of growth can also affect the cerebellum as in cerebellar hypoplasia.

DISORDERS OF THE CEREBELLUM

The cerebellum may be absent, i.e. cerebellar agenesis or severely underdeveloped, cerebellar hypoplasia. These abnormalities may be associated with other abnormalities of the brainstem or occur in isolation. They may be associated with congenital ataxia or in some cases with very little clinical abnormality. The Arnold–Chiari malformation usually occurs with the spina bifida complex but occasionally is seen in isolation when it may be the cause of congenital hydrocephalus or the hydrocephalus may only appear in later childhood (see p. 660) (Carmel 1986). Most abnormalities of the cerebellum are either genetic or metabolic and cerebellar hypoplasia can be autosomal recessive, autosomal dominant or sex-linked recessive in inheritance.

Aplasia of the cerebellar vermis

The Dandy–Walker syndrome

This is a syndrome consisting of agenesis of the midline vermis of the cerebellum together with failure of the roof of the fourth ventricle to perforate to form the foramina of Luschka and Magendi. The result is a cystic dilation of the fourth ventricle with a large posterior fossa, causing elevation of the torcula and the lateral sinuses. In most cases it is sporadic; occasional cases are reported with abnormalities of chromosome 9.

It presents with hydrocephalus in infancy and in the older child with signs of raised intracranial pressure and ataxia. There may be other associated malformations of the CNS such as agenesis of the corpus callosum, occipital encephalocele and brainstem dysplasia. Non-CNS malformations include median facial problems and cleft palate.

Diagnosis is easy with MRI scan, but differentiation is necessary from an arachnoid cyst of the posterior fossa, an isolated fourth ventricle in the premature infant following intraventricular hemorrhage or a megacistern. The hydrocephalus should be treated with a shunt rather than trying to remove the cyst. Provided the aqueduct is patent one should be able to prevent the cyst causing fatal medullary compression. There is an associated dysplasia of the cortex in many cases so that 50% may be mentally retarded (Raimondi 1986, Carmel et al 1977).

Isolated vermis aplasia

Congenital agenesis of cerebellar vermis

Dysequilibrium syndrome is transmitted by autosomal recessive inheritance. The patients tend to come from one geographical area of Sweden where consanguinity is common. The cerebellum is small, especially the vermis. There is also defective thymic dependent immunity, a low serum dopamine β-hydroxylase, cataract and mental retardation. This syndrome has to be differentiated from the Marinesco–Sjögren syndrome, also seen in Sweden, in which mental retardation, ataxia and cataracts are accompanied by a slowly progressive myopathy. The clinical presentation of the disequilibrium syndrome is of truncal ataxia with hypotonia and delay in postural development.

Orofacial digital syndrome

In this condition there are lingual hamartomas together with polydactyly and absence of the cerebellar vermis.

Vermis aplasia with facial nevus

This is a variation of the Sturge–Weber syndrome in which there is a hemangiomatous malformation over the face associated with absence of the cerebellar vermis.

Walker–Warburg syndrome

This syndrome consists of vermis aplasia with lissencephaly so that in addition to the disequilibrium and postural abnormalities from the vermis aplasia, fits and mental retardation are predominant due to the dysplasia of the cerebral cortex. There may also be an associated hydrocephalus which at first may mask the other findings. The syndrome is complete with a retinal dysplasia which may result in retinal detachment and also sometimes corneal opacities.

Joubert's syndrome

This autosomal recessive condition is associated with absence of the cerebellar vermis but without fourth ventricular dilation. There may be a wide gap between the cerebellar hemispheres on CT scan or there may be a narrow slit only demonstrable with MRI imaging.

The cerebellar defect is accompanied by abnormal respiration, especially episodic tachypnea and hyperventilation, which may be particularly marked during rapid eye movement sleep. Tachypnea of the order of 120/min may be seen soon after birth, causing diagnostic difficulty in the newborn period, and the infant may continue to have episodes of dog-like panting with a rate of up to 200/min. Periodic apnea instead of tachypnea occurs in some children. There is complete vermis aplasia, dysplasia of the cerebellar nuclei with heterotopia, abnormal inferior olives and an abnormal pyramidal decussation. Most of the infants show generalized psychomotor retardation with hypotonia, ataxia and abnormal eye movements. Some have other associated abnormalities such as hydrocephalus, agenesis of the corpus callosum or a meningocele. Differentiation from Leigh's encephalopathy is by CT scanning. It should be remembered that hyperventilation may cause a rise in lactate. Death is not uncommon before 3 years of age.

Partial agenesis of the corpus callosum and retinal colobomas resembles in part the Aicardi syndrome. The presence of renal cysts and retinopathy with an extinguished electroretinogram suggests overlap between other syndromes such as the Meckel–Gruber syndrome and Leber's congenital retinal amaurosis.

Meckel–Gruber syndrome

In this syndrome the child usually has a large occipital encephalocele associated with renal cysts and sometimes polydactyly. It is inherited as a Mendelian autosomal recessive condition. There may be abnormal vascular tissue in the sac of the encephalocele, making surgery difficult, and there may be associated agenesis of the cerebellar vermis or severe cerebellar aplasia. Removal of the encephalocele is undertaken in the neonatal period and any associated hydrocephalus shunted. Prognosis depends on the degree of associated dysplasia of the cerebellar cortex causing mental retardation (Fig. 14.5).

Chiari malformation

Although originally known as the Arnold–Chiari malformation and regarded as the typical hindbrain malformation associated with the spina bifida complex, most people now have reverted to original nomenclature described by Chiari who divided these anomalies into four types.

Type 1 Chiari malformation. The cerebellar tonsils are herniated through the foramen magnum without any displacement of the medulla itself. Hydrocephalus is usually associated but there may also be syringomyelia or syringobulbia. In later childhood abnormalities of eye movements and dysarthria together with bulbar weakness may complicate the signs of raised intracranial pressure from hydrocephalus. Straining, Valsalva

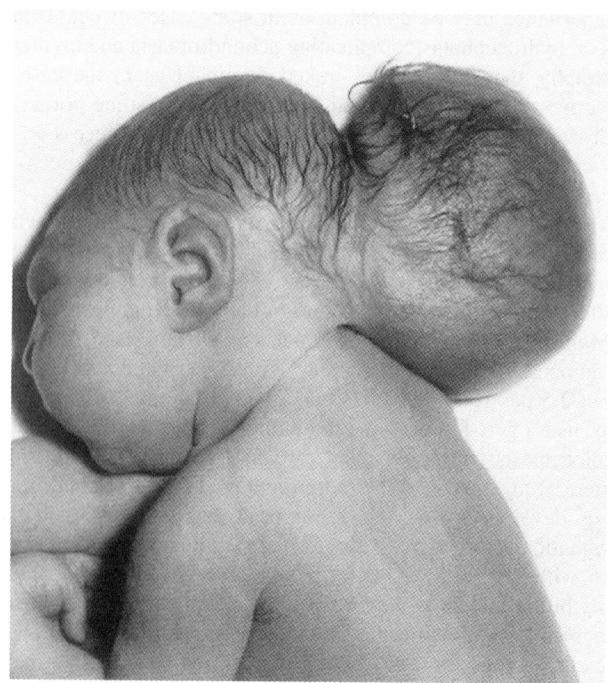

Fig. 14.5 Occipital encephalocele.

maneuver or raised central venous pressure may all bring on symptoms of dizziness, blurred vision, vomiting, vertigo or drop attacks. Treatment is by posterior fossa decompression.

Type 2 Chiari malformation. This is the common type of Chiari malformation which occurs in children with the spina bifida complex. It consists of the downward displacement of the cerebellar vermis as opposed to the cerebellar tonsils. The medulla is often displaced as well so that the lower cranial nerves course upwards through the foramen magnum. The posterior fossa is small due to displacement of a large portion of the cerebellum. Hydrocephalus is usually present. This type may be associated with tethering of the spinal cord and this has been suggested as initiating the problem by causing downward traction.

There may be respiratory abnormalities with laryngeal stridor or abnormal response of the brainstem respiratory centers to hypoxia and hypercarbia. Pain in the neck, a spastic gait, positional vertigo, weakness of the upper limbs with at times a bilateral Erb palsy type of pattern all appear due to foramen magnum impaction syndrome. Palatal weakness and nystagmus can also appear as crowding occurs in the posterior fossa and the foramen magnum. This type of abnormality is often called the Arnold–Chiari malformation. It may occur in patients without hydrocephalus and may also occur without myelomeningocele.

Type 3 Chiari malformation. This is when the cerebellum is herniated into an occipital encephalocele.

Type 4 Chiari malformation. This is in essence cerebellar hypoplasia and probably should not be considered a separate malformation from megacistern and vermis aplasia.

ABSENCE OF THE CORPUS CALLOSUM

Isolated absence of the corpus callosum

This may be a coincidental finding at post-mortem or MRI scan. It may be wrongly diagnosed by ultrasound or when there is poor myelination, as in some children with cerebral palsy. The corpus callosum may be partially or completely absent. The ventricles appear widely separated as though they have fallen sideways to produce a so-called bat wing or devil's horn appearance. The ventricles themselves may be enlarged due to reduction in the amount of white matter. It may be part of the spectrum of failure of separation of the two telencephalic vesicles with holoprosencephaly at the extreme end and failure of development of the corpus callosum at the other. Although the child may be of normal intelligence there is more often a degree of dysplasia of the frontal and parietal lobes resulting in the child being microcephalic and mentally retarded. Symptoms are usually due to the associated abnormalities of the cerebral cortex and they do not present as a simple disconnection syndrome as seen in the older child after corpus callosotomy. Isolated absence of the corpus callosum may be inherited as an autosomal recessive condition. It may also complicate abnormalities of chromosomes 13 and 18 or the basal cell nevus syndrome (Walsh 1986).

Aicardi syndrome

This is a sex-linked dominant condition occurring only in girls. Colobomas of the retina, partial or complete absence of the corpus callosum and a cortical dysplasia occur. The child presents retarded with onset of infantile spasms and the EEG may show a hemihypsarrhythmia due to failure of spread of the epileptic discharge from one hemisphere to the other (Chevrie & Aicardi 1986).

Median facial cleft syndrome

This is due to the frontonasal process being large and resulting in wide separation of the eyes (Fig. 14.6). It can be associated with:

1. marked hypertelorism with separation of the eyes;
2. anophthalmia or microphthalmia;
3. cleft palate or bilateral or central cleft lip;
4. hydrocephalus, deafness or abnormalities of the midline structures of the brain, e.g. cerebellar vermis, corpus callosum or medial septal structures (septooptic dysplasia);
5. peripheral abnormalities of the fingers such as polydactyly and clinodactyly.

Greig's syndrome of hypertelorism associated with abnormalities of the fingers, teeth and kidneys is probably not a separate entity.

Septooptic dysplasia

This is a sporadic disorder with midline abnormality in which there is hypoplasia of the optic nerves so that on fundoscopy it is often said the optic nerve head looks like a fried egg. There is also failure of development of the septum pellucidum and the septal nuclei. The child is blind and retarded but it is the associated abnormalities of the hypothalamus which often dominate the clinical picture. The child may have hypoglycemia in the neonatal period and poor temperature control. It may present later with hypothyroidism, growth hormone deficiency or with failure of gonadotropin secretion at puberty.

ABNORMALITIES OF THE CEREBRAL HEMISPHERES

Cranium bifidum

Like spina bifida there may be a superficial nevus such as a hairy tuft or capillary hemangioma, i.e. a cranium bifidum occulta or a

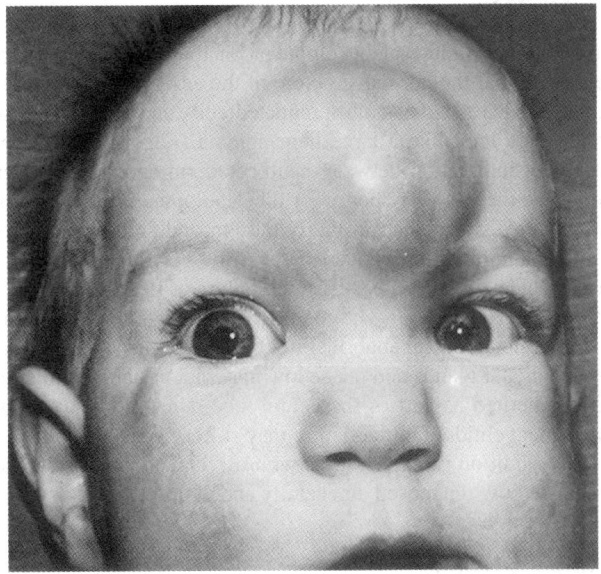

Fig. 14.6 Frontal encephalocele.

meningocele (with a skull defect through which protrudes a sac containing CSF), or brain tissue, i.e. an encephalocele (Fig. 14.5). Cases are usually sporadic and it is much less common than the spina bifida complex. Occasionally dominant inheritance is seen. It is more common in girls than boys. MRI scanning is essential to see if there are underlying brain or vascular abnormalities before dealing with the superficial cosmetic defect.

Craniomeningoceles

These are usually in the occipital area in the UK, USA and Europe whereas frontal or nasal meningoceles are more common in Burma, Thailand and Russia. The occipital meningoceles may occur anywhere from the parietooccipital region to the upper cervical region. Frontal meningoceles may be frontoethmoid and protrude above the nose (Fig. 14.6) or may be ethnoidosphenoidal and protrude into the nose when they may be associated with a cleft palate. There is a rare type of defect in which the sac protrudes into the orbit causing unilateral proptosis. Occipital meningoceles cause no problem in removal whereas diagnosis of the nasal variety can be difficult. They may pulsate and they swell with a Queckenstedt or Valsalva maneuver and when the child cries. Any attempt to aspirate results in a high risk of meningitis. Occasionally primitive brain tissue in the sac can cause a tumor so that one may see a so-called nasal glioma.

Encephaloceles

It may only be possible to differentiate a meningocele from an encephalocele after surgery when examination of the contents of the sac shows whether there was any primitive undifferentiated tissue or recognizable herniation of brain tissue. The primitive tissue is often very vascular and dysplastic but occasionally there may be herniation of occipital lobe into the sac. The brain underneath the encephalocele is usually abnormal so occipital cortical dysplasia, cerebellar agenesis or vermis aplasia are often associated. Hydrocephalus may complicate both meningoceles and encephaloceles.

Anencephaly

This signifies failure of development of the whole telencephalic vesicle so that the normal structure of the cerebral hemispheres is replaced by a mass of undifferentiated cells and aberrant vessels which may look like a large hemangioma (Fig. 14.7a). There is failure of integration between neuroectoderm and the mesoderm providing the vascular supply for the developing brain. Abnormal vasculature is also seen in the brainstem and spinal cord. There may be abnormalities of other parts of the nervous system which may include a total rachischisis with failure of fusion of the whole neural tube (Fig. 14.7b). The condition is more common in females and is associated with abnormalities of the kidneys and hypoplasia of the adrenal glands and hence low maternal urinary estriols. It is often inherited as part of the neural tube defect complex so that subsequent children in the family may suffer from spina bifida.

The condition is incompatible with survival and in the UK most cases are now diagnosed antenatally and aborted.

Hydranencephaly

This is really in most cases a deformation rather than a

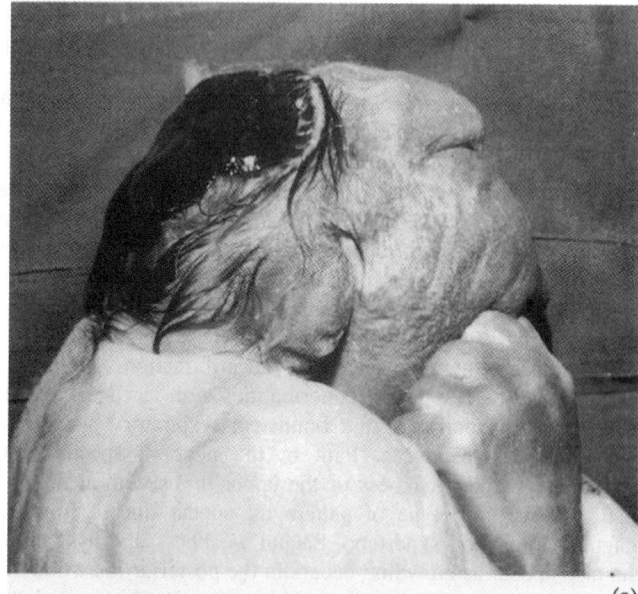

(a)

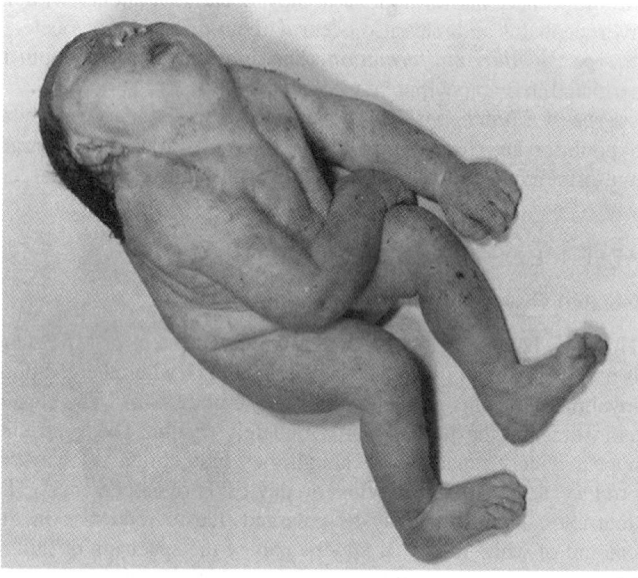

(b)

Fig. 14.7   (a) Anencephaly. (b) Iniencephaly.

malformation. It may be that the child has anencephaly but that the skull has developed over the surface. In these cases one finds a very rudimentary dysplastic brain surrounded by a large amount of fluid which is external to the dysplastic brain and not a gross hydrocephalus. In other cases it is really a very severe hydrocephalus with an extremely thin cortical mantle. The brain can be stretched providing its blood supply is not obstructed, causing secondary ischemia, and function may be remarkably good even with quite a thin layer of cortex. Once the cortex is less than 1.5 cm thick there is a tendency for intelligence to fall but this is not invariable. In other cases of hydranencephaly the brain is destroyed, e.g. due to infarction. It is thought that there may be bilateral carotid occlusion either from placental emboli or injury to the carotid arteries with resultant liquefaction of the infarcted brain. Intrauterine encephalitis may also be of a necrotizing type (e.g. toxoplasmosis). Abnormalities of other parts of the brain, e.g. absence of the cerebellar vermis, cerebellar agenesis and abnormality of the eyes, suggest that some cases are true congenital malformations.

Diagnosis is now by ultrasound and CT scan. This will give some idea whether there are associated malformations and whether the temporal lobe and anterior frontal area are preserved, i.e. whether it seems to be a severe form of hydrocephalus. The prognosis in severe hydrocephalus can be remarkable and brain appears to be reformed as the hydrocephalus is controlled. On the other hand severe destructive lesions of both hemispheres, e.g. with infarction and necrotizing encephalitis, result in a child with severe mental retardation, quadriplegia, blindness and a gross disability. The baby at birth may appear remarkably well and at times the severe degree of CNS lesion comes as a surprise since the macrocephaly is not great, there are no gross signs of raised intracranial pressure and the baby may appear to have reasonable flexor tone.

Signs of raised intracranial pressure such as increased pulsatility of the fontanel, scalp vein distention and sunsetting of the eyes are an indication that the child should have its intracranial pressure monitored. If there is any doubt a period on open ventricular drainage may help decide whether it is ethically justified to insert a shunt.

Holoprosencephaly

As the name suggests, the brain is a whole sphere, i.e. the telencephalic vesicle has not divided into the two cerebral hemispheres. There may be one large fused hemisphere with a single ventricle and one artery supplying it or the fusion may be restricted to the frontal region so that the brain has a horseshoe appearance with a single central ventricle with fusion of the thalami together with one anterior cerebral artery and two lateral middle cerebral arteries providing the blood supply (alobar holoprosencephaly) (Fig. 14.8).

Severe cases are also associated with cyclopia when there is one central eye or two eyes obviously fused together (Fig. 14.9). There may be a proboscis instead of a nose coming from between the eyes (ethmocephaly) or a nose with a single nostril (cebocephaly) and in others cleft palate or micrognathia. The brain may consist

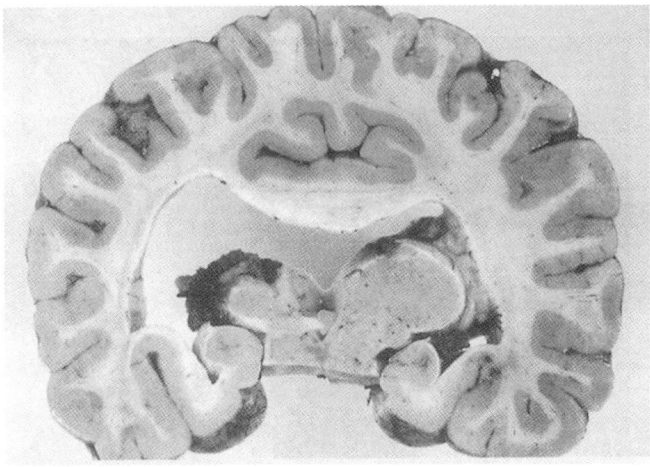

Fig. 14.8 Holoprosencephaly.

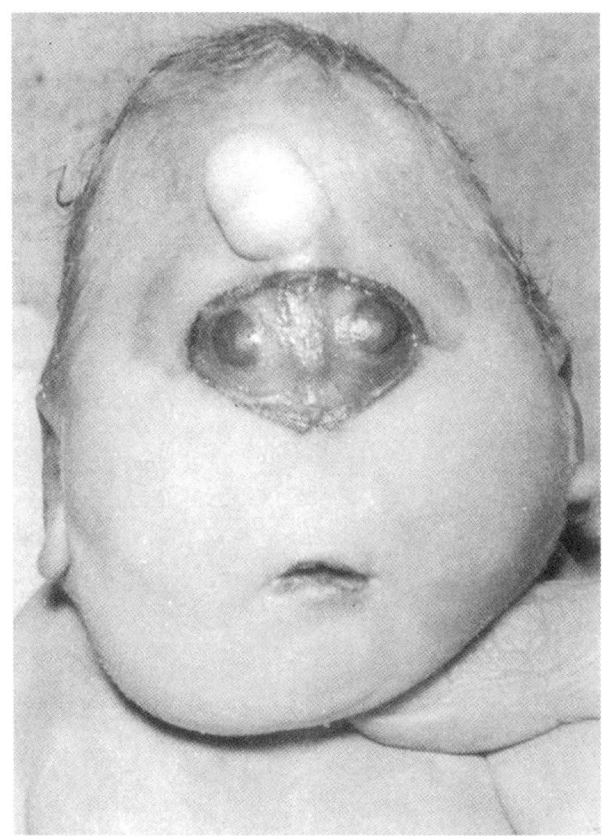

Fig. 14.9 Cyclops.

of one unfused hemisphere. In more moderate cases there may be hypotelorism together with colobomas of the iris and retina. In the mildest form one should probably regard absence of the corpus callosum and absence of the septum pellucidum as if it were a minimal fusion lesion (sometimes called lobar holoprosencephaly).

Apart from association with hypotelorism and facial abnormalities, there may be congenital heart disease (ASD, VSD or truncus), dysplastic testes and genitalia, cystic kidneys or malrotation of the gut. These associated abnormalities depend in part on whether the condition is an isolated CNS disorder or part of a general teratological problem due to abnormality of chromosome 13 or 18 which seem particularly liable to be associated with holoprosencephaly. Most cases are sporadic but occasionally intrauterine infections (toxoplasmosis, syphilis) and toxins can cause the disorder. Rare cases are familial autosomal dominant and recessive.

The child is nearly always severely mentally retarded with epilepsy and spastic quadriplegia, neuroendocrine problems and failure to thrive.

Cortical dysplasia

Microencephaly

Failure of brain growth results in a small, i.e. microencephalic brain. Any destruction of brain tissue resulting in cerebral atrophy and gliosis will result in a small scarred brain. Microencephaly therefore may be the result of a malformation – a histological

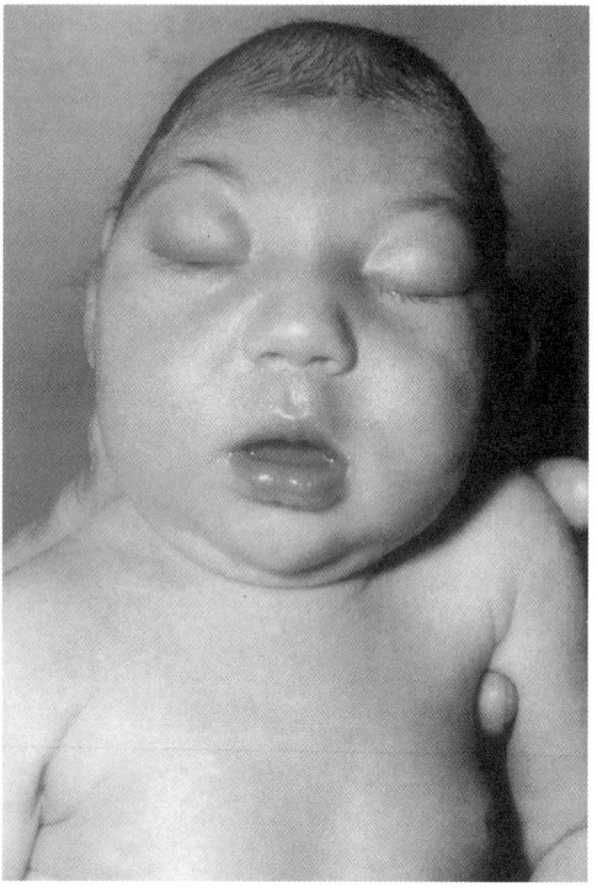

Fig. 14.10   Primary microcephaly.

cortical dysplasia – or due to a deformation, brain destruction and gliosis.

The skull normally grows to accommodate the brain unless there is a craniostenosis. Microcephaly (Fig. 14.10) with failure of the normal rate of growth of head circumference is therefore a sign that the brain itself is not growing and there is a microencephaly. The baby may have a normal head size at birth and as a result of damage from perinatal asphyxia, secondary microcephaly may occur.

The normal cerebral cortex consists of six horizontal layers with the cells stratified along these layers. In cortical dysplasia there is arrest in development and there may be only four layers of cortex with the cells remaining in columns. This failure of normal migration means that there may be heterotopic neurons in the white matter. Mental handicap and intractable epilepsy result and the heterotopic neurons may result in tumor formation. There are many conditions associated with cortical dysplasia (e.g. most of the chromosome disorders, Zellwegger syndrome, Aicardi syndrome, happy puppet syndrome, von Recklinghausen disease, tuberous sclerosis, Meckel–Gruber syndrome, Paine's syndrome, etc.), most having severe mental retardation and malignant intractable epilepsy such as infantile spasms or the Lennox–Gastaut syndrome.

Lissencephaly

The child may outwardly look normal apart from microcephaly. The brain may be smooth (agyria) with a few major sulci or show areas of abnormal fat flattened gyri, i.e. pachygyri. The cortex is thickened with incomplete stratification and neuronal migration. There are two pathological types of lissencephaly depending on the histological findings.

Type 1 has a small brain with a smooth surface, the vessels are very tortuous, the cortex is thick and white matter thin. There are only 4 layers on histological examination and neurons may be upside down and the cortex resembles an arrest at a fetal level. Most cases are sporadic and a few autosomal dominant. Lissencephaly may occur with chromosome 17p–, 17p monosomy or with ring 17 chromosomes. These children are dysmorphic with high narrow forehead, severe retardation, epilepsy and dystonia or diplegic cerebral palsy (Miller–Deiker syndrome). The EEG shows high amplitude fast activity of α or β frequency, while epileptic activity may resemble hypsarrhythmia. MRI is the method of diagnosis.

Type 2 Walker-Warberg syndrome lissencephaly may be associated with hydrocephalus, total disorganization of the cortical layering, retinal dysplasia and occasionally with an encephalocele. There are thick milky meninges. A variant seen in Finland is associated with muscle disease (the muscle–eye–brain disease). This may have features in common with the Japanese type of congenital muscular dystrophy (Fukuyama type) when congenital muscular dystrophy is associated with severe mental retardation and a leukodystrophy.

Hydrocephalus

This is discussed in detail later. Stretching of the cerebral cortical mantle results in an apparent increase in the number of gyri (micropolygyria) (Fig. 14.11). If the midline structures are also ruptured (Fig. 14.12) it may result in an erroneous diagnosis of congenital malformation, e.g. holoprosencephaly when the hydrocephalus may be a 'deformation' secondary to CSF obstruction following meningitis or an intracranial hemorrhage.

Porencephaly

This is a destructive and usually unilateral cystic area within the substance of the hemisphere which may or may not communicate with the ventricle. It is the result of liquefaction of an area of the brain as a result of hemorrhage, ischemia or infection.

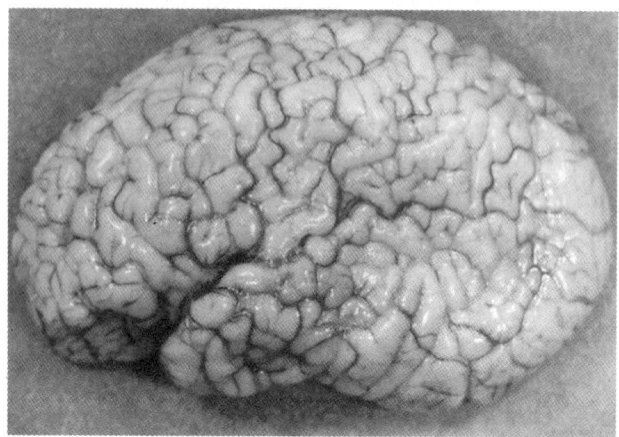

Fig. 14.11   Micropolygyria.

Hemorrhagic infarcts from middle cerebral thrombosis, emboli from the placenta, dissection from a subependymal bleed into an area of softened anoxic ischemic brain in the preterm infant or coalescence of a cyst resulting from infarction between the centrifugal and centripetal blood supply in periventricular leukomalacia (laminar necrosis) may all result in cysts within the substance of the brain itself.

Porencephalic cysts are often associated with hemiplegia and fits and the extent of associated brain damage and mental handicap are proportional to their extent. Tension in the cyst may worsen the fits and hemiplegia, which may thus improve with shunting.

Arachnoid cyst

This is a condition which has increased in importance though probably not in incidence with the advent of CT scanning (CT shows blood, bone and CSF better than MRI, which is best for brain). It consists of a localized collection of fluid within the subarachnoid space (Hanieh et al 1988). These cysts are more common in the anterior temporal region, suprasellar area in the region of the cisterna ambiens or in the posterior fossa though they are not confined to these sites. It is not known whether they are true malformations. Some are associated with head injury and subdural hematoma; others appear to be due to an adhesive arachnoiditis following meningitis or the presence of blood in the CSF. The temporal lobe cysts may be bilateral and appear to be associated with agenesis of the temporal lobe and used to be called the temporal lobe agenesis syndrome. This is now thought not to be the case but the mechanism by which they arise is not known for certain. They may achieve enormous size and be associated with signs of raised intracranial pressure and a large head whilst in other cases they do not appear to change in size over many years on sequential CT scan imaging. They are occasionally associated with metabolic diseases such as glutaric aciduria.

Temporal lobe arachnoid cysts may be associated with fits, headache and signs of raised intracranial pressure. There may be bulging of the temporal fossa or a large head. If the cysts are symptomatic or are very large then a cystoperitoneal shunt should be performed. If small, they should be watched by sequential CT scans. If there is any doubt whether a larger cyst is causing symptoms or progressing then a CSF access device may be inserted into the cyst and overnight pressure monitoring performed to see whether it is acting as a space-occupying lesion (Marinov et al 1989, Richard et al 1989).

Suprasellar cysts will usually require treatment as the symptomatology is much more obvious and includes loss of vision. This may not return with late treatment of the cyst. The child may present with unstable head control – the so-called bobble-headed doll. There is often associated hydrocephalus from obstruction of the third ventricle and endocrine disturbance from hypothalamic compression.

Interhemispheric cysts between the two cerebral hemispheres (most often between the parietal and occipital lobes) are usually due to a ventricular diverticulum as a result of successful shunting of a hydrocephalus. When the shunted ventricles contract the skull remains with a larger volume and the very thin area on the medial surface of the occipital region may herniate to give a diverticular cyst.

Cysts in the region of the cisterna ambiens are more often due to an adhesive arachnoiditis. Cysts in the posterior fossa need to be distinguished from the Dandy–Walker syndrome, isolation of the fourth ventricle and a mega cyst (giant cisterna magna).

CONGENITAL ABNORMALITIES OF THE SPINAL CORD

The term 'neural tube defect' or 'spina bifida complex' is used to cover a wide variety of disorders.

Mesodermal defects

There may be bony defects ranging from failure of fusion of the complete spine (total rachischisis) to simple deficiencies of the lower lumbar spinous processes as part of a spina bifida occulta. Hemivertebrae may give a scoliosis and the associated ribs may be absent or fused. Bony spurs occur in diastematomyelia. There may be absence of the sacrum or sacralization of the lower spine. Klippel Feil is fusion of cervical vertebrae with severe disruption of the cervical spine. This causes marked retroflexion of the head in iniencephalus.

Other mesodermal defects such as angiomas, lipomas, dermoids, renal abnormalities with pelvic kidney or horseshoe kidney may be added to the bony spectrum.

Ectodermal defects

A defect in the neuroectoderm is known as myelodysplasia. This may manifest as disruption of the histological architecture of the spinal cord (multiple anterior horns, several central canals, abnormal neurons), syringomyelia, failure of fusion of the cord so that there is a flat neural plaque rather than a fused tube (myelocele), double neural tube (diplomyelia), tethering of the cord or herniation through the bony defect as a meningocele or meningomyelocele.

Other ectodermal defects include dimples, sinuses, skin defects, hairy patches, tails and cutaneous capillary hemangiomas that can occur in any combination.

Incidence

The incidence of spina bifida was around 2.5 per 1000 births in the UK 30 years ago. This incidence has fallen by 90% so that in Edinburgh the number of liveborn infants with meningomyelocele is now only three per year. It appears to be much more common in communities of Celtic descent (Wales, Scotland and Ireland) and has always been very rare in the Far East where the incidence is in the order of 0.1 per 1000 live births.

Etiology

The neural tube is normally complete within 4 weeks of fertilization. Neural tube defects may be seen as a result of radiation, drugs (e.g. sodium valproate), as part of the congenital rubella syndrome and occasionally in alcoholic mothers and is an end result of many insults that occur during the period of neural tube closure. It can be produced experimentally by antifolate drugs, vitamin A, trypan blue but the possibility of folate deficiency in a genetically predisposed mother is now the most acceptable theory.

Folate and neural tube defects

The MRC periconceptional vitamin study in 1991, together with a Hungarian study (Czeizel & Dudas 1992), has shown that the occurrence and recurrence of neural tube defects can be prevented in 72% of cases by periconceptional folic acid. At the present time the recommendation to prevent recurrences is to take a 4 mg daily dose prior to conception and continue till the 12th week of pregnancy. To prevent the first occurrence extra folate is recommended for all women prior to conception and during the first trimester. This is achieved by:

1. extra dietary intake of folate-rich foods;
2. eating fortified foods;
3. taking an additional pharmacological supplement of 0.4 mg folate daily.

It is likely that a compulsory food fortification policy (grain products) will replace the voluntary scheme and ensure daily folate intake of 0.6 mg.

The findings of dominant inheritance in some families going back five or more generations suggest that there is a genetic background to many cases of neural tube defect. The fact that the condition clusters in time and space suggests that an environmental component aggravates a genetic predisposition. Hard water, soft water, fruit, tea, effluent from factories, blighted potatoes and subclinical vitamin deficiency in the mother have all been suggested as causes.

Although there can be no doubt that antenatal screening with α-fetoprotein and ultrasound has significantly reduced the incidence of neural tube defects, the number of infants aborted is not the same as the number that were liveborn in the past, suggesting a spontaneous reduction in association.

SPINA BIFIDA OCCULTA

Spina bifida occulta may attract attention in several ways.

1. Incidental radiological finding of a narrow split in the fifth lumbar or first sacral spinous process of no clinical significance. This is very common in young children and the incidence lessens with age.
2. A cutaneous lesion in the form of a small nevus, hemangioma, tuft of hairs, sacral pit or soft lipomatous swelling should be taken as a warning signal that there may be an underlying abnormality. This may consist of bony abnormality with bifid spinous processes but can also signify an underlying abnormality of the spinal cord with an associated myelodysplasia, lipoma, diastematomyelia or neuroenteric cyst. These cutaneous lesions should be taken as an indication for magnetic resonance imaging of the spine, whether or not there is any neurological deficit.

Myelodysplasia

This term is used to indicate that there is an abnormality in the histological development of the spinal cord. There may be several central canals, several anterior horns or disorganization of the 'muscle nuclei' so that specific muscles do not form properly. The characteristic clinical findings are often called the orthopedic syndrome of myelodysplasia. There is a cavovarus deformity of the foot; the foot is small so that shoe sizes are different. The leg on the affected side is shorter and appears to be the leg of a younger child. It is cold and often shows erythrocyanosis. It may be difficult to demonstrate definite weakness.

Tethering

Tethering of the cord may lead to damage from traction as the cord cannot ascend with growth of the spinal column. Tethering also means that repeated movements of the spine put the cord at risk. The child may present with weakness in one leg or with bladder problems and progressive neurological deterioration is a definite indication for surgery. Whether tethering without neurological deterioration in the legs should be operated upon remains an unanswered question. If operation is not undertaken then careful neurological follow-up is mandatory, especially at peak growth periods. With modern MRI scanning it is now possible to diagnose the condition with more accuracy and criteria for operation should become clearer. Serial somatosensory potentials also assist in diagnosis of progression.

Diastematomyelia

A further important cause of tethering is a bony or fibrocartilagenous spur which arises from a vertebral body and passes between the halves of a bifid cord – diastematomyelia. In some cases this fixes the cord and results in increasing traction with growth. In other cases the cord divides well above the spur and passes around the diastematomyelia in two separate dural canals, i.e. a diplomyelia.

Damage from tethering or compression may cause spastic paraplegia. More frequently, however, the child presents with more distal weakness of the foot with clawing of the toes and equinovarus posture and weakness of the peronei. Dribbling incontinence of urine may be an early feature and there may be sensory loss in the sacral territory, loss of ankle jerk and anal reflexes and trophic changes in the feet. Neurological deterioration in the presence of bony spur is an indication for removal (Chapman & Beyerl 1986). We would tend to favor removal of any bony spur demonstrated to put the cord at risk during growth and not wait for the development of neurological signs.

Intraspinal lipoma

The presence of a cutaneous lipoma or lipomeningocele may penetrate in dumb-bell fashion into the spinal canal. It may cause increase in pressure within the canal. Treatment of a lipoma can be difficult as the cord itself as well as nerve roots may be enmeshed in fatty tissue.

Infection

Infection may be the presenting feature of dermal sinuses. Blind pits over the coccygeal region are rarely associated with communication to the theca but focal infection with abscess formation may be a nuisance. Pits over the sacrum itself, especially at the site of the caudal neuropore, are much more of a concern as there may be a direct communication with the theca and therefore a risk of recurrent meningitis. These should be electively excised in the neonatal period.

SPINA BIFIDA CYSTICA

Meningocele

In this condition there is a defect in the spinous processes (spina bifida), together with herniation of the meninges through the defect to form a cystic mass on the back (Fig. 14.12). There may be cover by thick skin with little risk of rupture or infection or by a thin transparent membrane; there may be skin at the sides and a thin blue membrane over the top. There is no myelodysplasia or cord within the sac in the pure cases and the child is neurologically completely normal. Hydrocephalus is usually absent and simple repair of the defect can be carried out as a cold elective procedure. The result should be a normal child. Ultrasound of the head should be performed to be sure that there is not an associated hydrocephalus and ultrasound of the abdomen to be sure there is no associated renal abnormality.

Myelomeningocele

Spinal lesion

The spinal cord is an open flat plate on the surface of the bulging meninges. It is not known whether the developmental abnormality itself, intrauterine damage, secondary ischemia, trauma to neural tissue during delivery or postnatal infection is the principal cause of the neurological deficit. Exposure of neural tissue in normal fetal lambs to amniotic fluid results in neurological dysfunction of legs and bladder (Meuli et al 1995). Stimulation of the exposed neural plate shows that all the muscles of the legs have intact innervation to the exposed plaque. The lower motor neurons are intact but these are not connected to higher centers at the upper end of the plaque. These connections are lost as the plaque dries out or is infected.

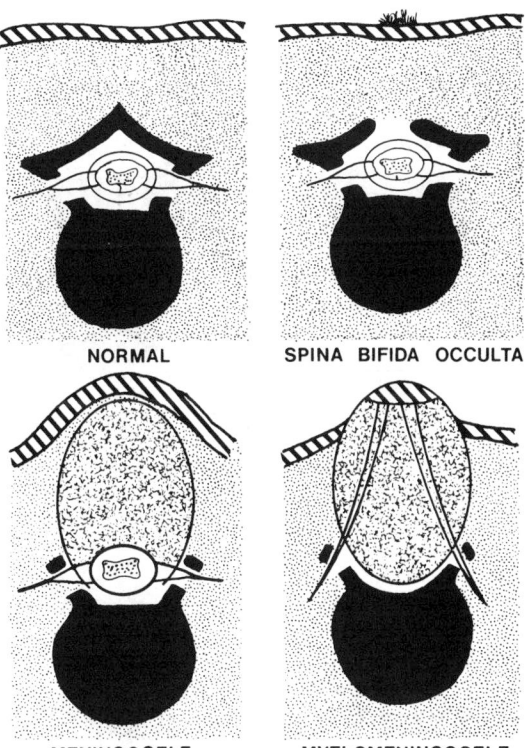

Fig. 14.12 Classification of spina bifida.

NORMAL   SPINA BIFIDA OCCULTA

MENINGOCELE   MYELOMENINGOCELE

There is no doubt that secondary postnatal injury may occur but the initial claim that immediate operation at birth reverses all the deficit is not true. The fetus at 12 weeks of gestation can be shown to have talipes and evidence of neuromuscular imbalance in utero.

A myelomeningocele is an open wound and therefore liable to infection (Fig. 14.13). Surface infection leads to meningitis or ventriculitis which is the usual cause of death in untreated patients. If the open lesion is not operatively closed and death from infection does not occur, there is gradual epithelialization of the lesion over a period of weeks or months. The end result is inferior to elective surgical closure as low-grade infection results in further loss of spinal cord function and more handicap and there is an ugly tender scar on the infant's back. Epithelialization may also result in tethering of nerve roots which can be very difficult to treat at a later date.

Patterns of spinal cord involvement

It is convenient to divide the type of cord lesion into types 1 and 2, type 2 being further subdivided into types 2a, 2b and 2c.

Type 1 cord lesion. In the type 1 lesion there is complete absence of function below a certain segmental level which results in a flaccid paralysis, loss of sensation and loss of all reflex movement and tendon reflexes below that level. Knowledge of the segmental innervation of the lower limb muscles allows the segmental level to be determined from examination of the lower limbs.

Type 2 cord lesion. In this type there is voluntary control of muscles which have normal innervation and are in direct communication with the long tracts of the brain above the level of the lesion. At the level of the lesion there may be a complete loss of all function, voluntary and reflex, and of sensation. This may extend over a very short area, i.e. one segment, or over several segments of the spinal cord. The cord then resumes reflex function, as an isolated cord segment. There will be no sensation and no voluntary movement of the muscles in this isolated cord segment. Muscles will, however, respond to dermatome stimulation tapping of the muscle, tapping of the tendon and pinprick.

Examination of the lower limbs is essential in determining the neurological level of paraplegia and also in prognosis of walking ability, type of deformity and degree of future handicap. The level of the lesion, level of vertebral abnormality and neurological level are not identical and one should not look at the back lesion and guess the neurology is the same.

Direct stimulation of the muscles which do not move is possible by dermatome-to-myotome stimulation, i.e. one strokes the corresponding dermatome and if there is reflex activity the muscle supplied by that segment will contract. In addition to testing the cremasteric reflex (L1), knee jerk (L3–4), ankle (S1–2), anal and bulbocavernosus reflexes (S4–5), one looks for exaggerated flexor withdrawal reflexes, contraction of the muscles of the perineum on stimulating the perianal region and contraction of the short toe flexors by flicking the toes. Reflexes not normally easily elicited, such as tendon jerks of the hamstring muscles, adductors and tibialis anterior, may be elicited and in very high lesions one may see adductor clonus and patella clonus.

If the isolated cord segment is long then complex reflexes such as flexor withdrawal responses may occur, making one think that the child is actually voluntarily moving the leg. This has led to confusion in the past as to the degree of paralysis and the tendency to give a misleadingly good prognosis in the neonatal period.

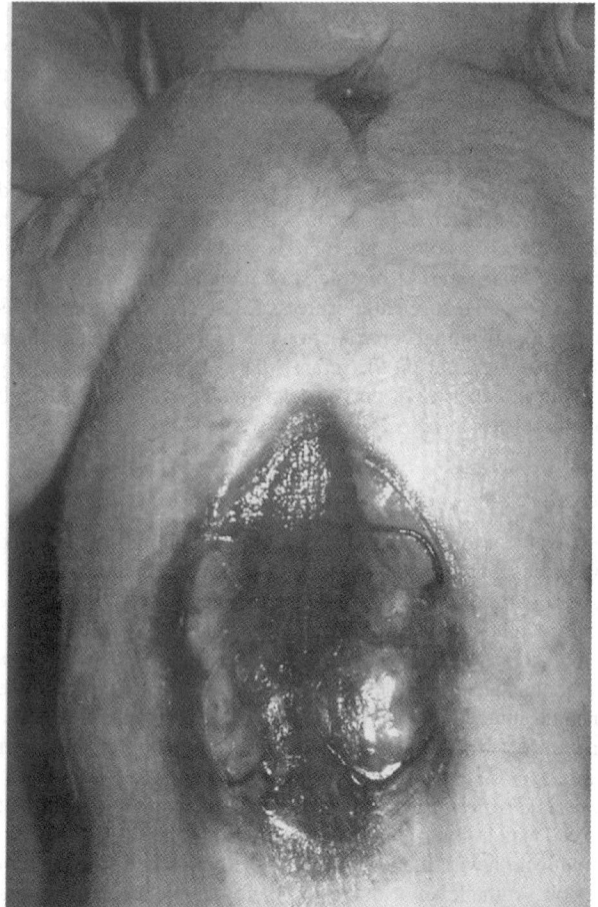

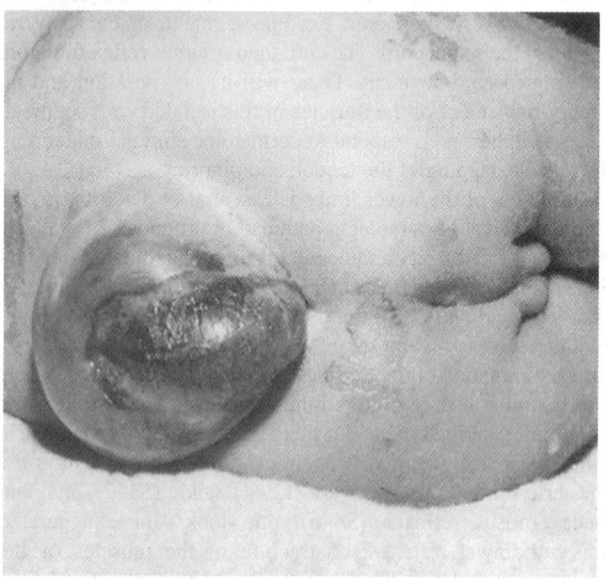

Fig. 14.13 (a) Meningomyelocele at birth. (b) Bulging meningomyelocele at a few hours of life.

If the area of isolated cord is limited to the sacral segments, then ankle clonus with a brisk ankle jerk and exaggerated anal reflex will be seen together with a spread of the response when stimulating the perianal region to cause toe flexion and flexion of the lateral hamstrings. Equally, tapping the toes in order to elicit the toe jerk

will produce flexion of the knee and a contraction of the anus. The segment of cord showing a lower motor neuron loss of activity is more often in the region of the abdominal muscles which may be completely paralyzed, causing a lumbar hernia and a pot belly.

Mechanism of deformity

The level of deformity often determines the neurological level, e.g. involvement below T8 is associated with paralysis of the abdominal walls and all the lower limb muscles. The lower limb deformities arise from two mechanisms. The first is due to muscle imbalance, e.g. dislocation of the hip when the flexors and adductors (L1–3) overcome the weak gluteal extensors and abductors (S1–2). Hip adduction is a potent cause of posterior hip dislocation. Involvement below L4 causes the lower limb muscles innervated from above this level (hip flexors, hip adductors, quadriceps and tibialis anterior) to be strong and under voluntary control whilst their antagonists are paralyzed. This causes the characteristic flexed hip, extended knee (genu recurvatum) and equinovarus foot (Fig. 14.14). If the tibialis anterior is active as a dorsiflexor (L4) whilst the calf muscles as plantar flexors (S1–2) are paralyzed, then dorsiflexion and inversion of the foot will occur.

The second cause of deformity results from immobility in utero. The fetus may present as a breech and the immobility results in secondary positional deformities adding to the neurogenic deformity (Fig. 14.15).

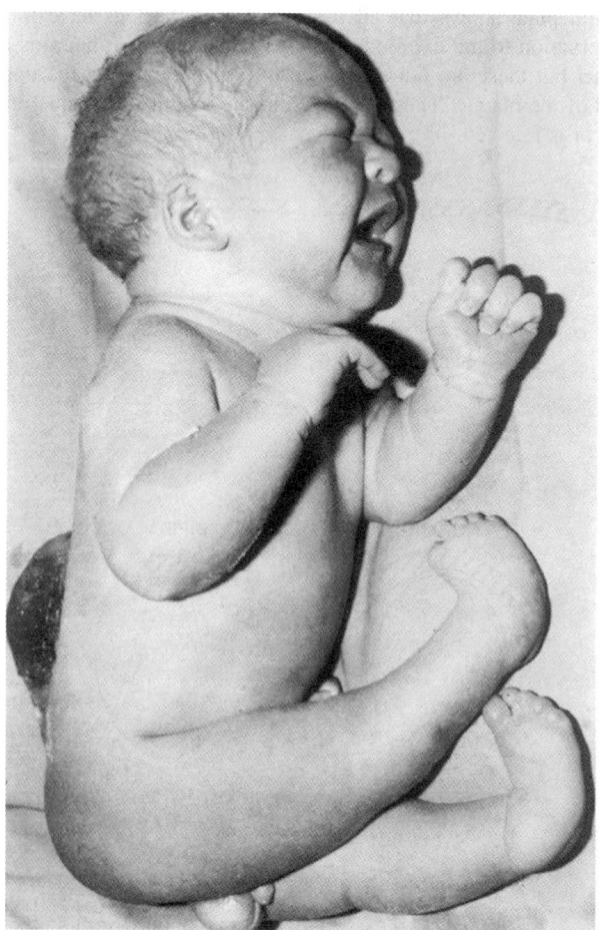

Fig. 14.14 Type 1 lesion: flaccid paralysis below fourth lumbar segment.

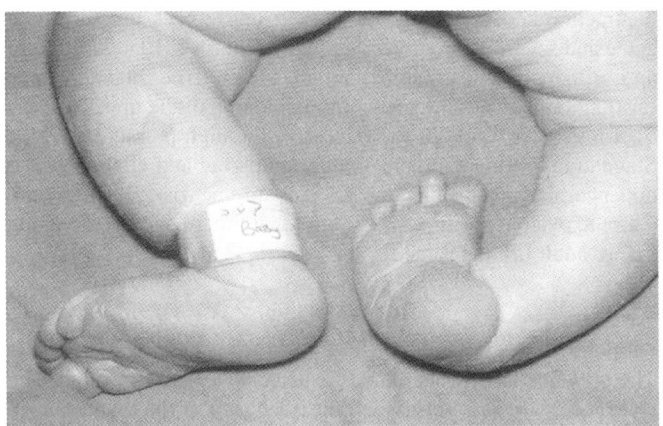

Fig. 14.15 Talipes due to muscle imbalance.

In 5% of cases the spinal cord is split with only one half of the cord exposed to the surface; the other half remains in the spinal canal and functions normally. In this case only one leg will have a neurological deficit.

NEONATAL MANAGEMENT OF THE CHILD WITH A NEURAL TUBE DEFECT

The general condition of the infant is assessed to insure there are no associated abnormalities such as chromosome disorder or other malformations of the heart and kidney. The face of a child with a meningomyelocele often has a suggestion of a Down syndrome appearance. The head circumference, sutures and fontanel are measured and cerebral and renal ultrasound are done routinely. X-ray of the spine will show hemivertebrae or gross disruption of the spinal architecture which would make even sitting eventually impossible.

The lesion is carefully examined for tears in the membranes or leakage of CSF suggesting that operation should be early because of the risk of meningitis. The hips are examined for dislocation.

Detailed neurological examination is carried out with the child warm and recovered from the immediate 'birth shock'. Sensory testing is carried out first with the child quiet; the skin is stimulated with the end of a straightened paper clip, starting in the saddle area and progressing through the sacral and lumbar territory. One observes facial grimace or a cry.

Following sensory testing and with the baby active and crying so that there is spontaneous movement of the upper limbs, one can determine the amount of spontaneous movement in the lower limbs as part of the baby's doggy paddling and cycling movements. It should be possible to give each muscle group an MRC grading of 1–5 and a voluntary motor level down to which the child can move in response to cerebral motor drive can be defined.

The factors identifiable at birth which are most predictive of severe disability are gross hydrocephalus, OFC more than 2 cm above the 90th centile or a cortical mantle less than 15 mm. Serious spinal deformity and absence of voluntary movement below L2 and other major defects are the factors which usually help in deciding whether early immediate operation should be performed or whether one should delay surgery to see how the child progresses over the first week or so.

If immediate closure is not undertaken and the spinal lesion granulates without meningitis developing, hydrocephalus may

progress. We regard it as unethical to let the child survive with impairment of intelligence which could be potentially reversible or preventable so would always shunt such a case. There is no good evidence that early repair of the back lesion will lessen the degree of paralysis in the lower limbs so that one is not jeopardizing the child's future by waiting to see what spontaneous progress occurs. Later plastic repair of the back that has granulated is still feasible.

While the infant is in hospital the parents should be encouraged to visit frequently and be given every opportunity to feed and handle their baby. During this period many questions can be answered, anxieties are allayed and genetic counseling undertaken. The support of a medical social worker is invaluable and the parents can be put in touch with one of the local parent support groups.

THE LATER MANAGEMENT OF THE CHILD WITH A NEURAL TUBE DEFECT

Motor problems

It should be possible to make a reasonably accurate prediction of the child's future mobility even in the neonatal period if an accurate clinical neurological assessment is made.

Prediction of walking ability in myelomeningocele

Voluntary motor level	Probable walking ability
T6–L2	Chair
	Crutches – swing through
	Parapodium
	Swivel walker
	RGO, HGO
L3	HKAFO
	RGO, HGO with sticks or tripods
L4	KAFO, HKAFO
	AFO
L5	AFO
	KAFO
Sacral	nil or AFO

RGO=Reciprocating gait orthosis, HGO = Hip guidance orthosis, HKAFO = Hip/knee/ankle/foot orthosis, KAFO = Knee/ankle/foot orthosis.

The child with a purely sacral lesion, as for example with sacral agenesis, or a very low meningomyelocele, will have problems with the feet due to paralysis of the intrinsic muscles of the feet, weak calf muscles and weak hip extensors. He will walk with a waddle and will need boots to support the ankles. He will also have a neurogenic bladder and will require a bladder regime.

Paralysis below L3–4 is compatible with walking unaided with sticks and below knee calipers. The spinal lesion may always be complicated by the effects of ataxia from the hydrocephalus or hemiplegia as a result of shunt malfunction, ventriculitis or puncture porencephaly. The child with a high lumbar lesion was in the past sentenced to immobility in a wheelchair but the use of reciprocating gait orthoses or hip guidance orthoses means that these children can now be mobile in the erect posture.

It may be necessary for an orthopedic surgeon to perform tenotomies in the neonatal period or later to correct muscle imbalance, e.g. the very tight tibialis anterior that may occur in an L4 lesion. Talipes will need correcting and hips will need to be released and put back into joint. Scoliosis may require surgery in adolescence.

Nonmotor neurological problems

Sensation

The sensory level in myelomeningocele, i.e. the lowest level of normal sensation, is usually within one or two segments of the motor level. As a result of cutaneous anesthesia there is a constant danger of painless ulceration. Pressure sores may develop over the sacral tuberosity, especially if incontinence has led to maceration of the skin. Sensory loss may become more of a problem in the future with the use of reciprocating gait orthoses when the risk of Charcot joints (i.e. neurogenic arthropathy) is added to the list of problems. The feet are often cold, blue and erythrocyanotic due to poor peripheral perfusion.

Burns may occur from hot-water bottles or sitting on radiators. Shoes which are too tight or failure to recognize the effects of intense cold in the winter can both result in gangrene of the toes. Fractures are painless and the use of reciprocating gait orthoses may lead to Charcot joints from a neuropathic arthropathy.

The neurogenic bladder

The bladder receives its nerve supply from three sources. First, the parasympathetic via the nervi erigentes from the sacral roots S2–S4 which controls detrusor contraction. Second, a sympathetic component supplies the trigone and internal sphincter and allows opening of the bladder neck during micturition. It is also important in sexual function when the internal sphincter is closed without any contraction of the detrusor. The third supply is via the pudendal nerve which carries the voluntary control of the striated external sphincter.

The bladder and bowel will be involved in most cases but the type of bladder involvement depends upon the type of lesion (Minns 1986).

If the lower limbs show signs of lower motor neuron denervation in the muscles innervated from S2–4 (type 1 lesion), e.g. calf, intrinsic muscles of the foot, anal sphincter and pelvic floor, then a weak or totally paralyzed bladder (acontractile) is to be expected. Lack of tone in the anal sphincter shows as a patulous anus, dribbling of urine and loss of the normal gluteal fold so that the anus appears wide open on top of a mountain rather than in a valley.

Depending on the degree of resistance of the bladder outlet, such infants may have constant dribbling of urine with an empty bladder or overflow incontinence from a distended bladder. Ureteric reflux may occur at low pressures from such inert bladders in which the valvular effect of the intramural ureter is lacking.

In infants with an isolated cord lesion (type 2 lesion) where examination of the limb shows purely reflex activity in S2–4 (i.e. spastic calves, toe flexors with exaggerated reflexes, a very brisk anal reflex), a reflex type of bladder (contractile) is to be expected. The ideal automatic bladder, i.e. one with periodic complete reflex emptying, is rare in myelomeningocele. At best an intermittent detrusor contraction results in voiding of up to 100 ml of urine; at worst persistent dribbling may result from constant poorly coordinated detrusor contractions. Despite an active detrusor which may generate pressures over 100 mmHg in a small infant, the bladder emptying may be poor because of a high urethral resistance. This outlet obstruction is probably due to failure of relaxation of the striated external sphincter which is normally under voluntary control via the pudendal nerve. This type of spastic bladder neck responds to stretching by further

contraction and very high pressures result in back pressure with acute and severe hydroureter and hydronephrosis. Bladder rupture and urinary ascites can occur in utero. True bladder neck obstruction is relatively uncommon. Dilation of the upper urinary tract may occur in both the flaccid or the high pressure bladder. Stagnation with incomplete bladder emptying and dilation of the upper urinary tract inevitably leads to the risk of infection. Chronic pyelonephritis may lead to renal failure and hypertension before adult life is reached.

Assessment of the upper renal tract

The presence of hydronephrosis is detected using ultrasound. The presence of ureteric reflux and the adequacy of the bladder neck and urethra can all be assessed using cystourethrography. Renal function is assessed using biochemical estimations such as urea electrolytes and creatinine together with a chromium or DMSA scan.

Assessment of the neurogenic bladder

Clinically the most important part of the assessment is to watch a child actually pass urine. If the urine can be passed in a stream one knows that there must be a coordinated detrusor contraction. If the stream is a good one, i.e. the child can 'pee in a parabola', there can be no serious bladder neck obstruction. In the older child the rate of passing urine can be measured as ml/unit time by getting the child to pass urine into a container with an electronic measuring device which draws out a graph of the rate of urination. This is a measure of detrusor contraction and bladder neck obstruction. The infant should be held up to see if there is any dribbling dependent on position and light suprapubic pressure applied to assess effective bladder neck contraction to allow continence and bladder filling.

Investigation of the bladder in the neonatal period is undertaken to answer the question whether the infant has a safe or dangerous bladder. If the upper renal tract is normal on ultrasound and the baby passes urine or it can be easily expressed, one can wait until 4 months of age for detailed urinary investigations. If, however, there appears to be bladder outlet obstruction, high pressure bladder and dilation of the upper renal tract then catheterization from birth may be necessary in order to preserve renal function.

Cystometrogram

This is performed either by a urethral catheter into the bladder when the effects of adding small aliquots of saline upon the pressure is monitored or, more physiological but more invasive, a suprapubic cystometrogram is performed using two catheters inserted into the bladder by suprapubic puncture. One of these is used to fill the bladder at the physiological rate of 2 ml/min and the second to measure pressure. The bladder volume, sensation and pressures at which urethral sphincters open can then be measured and it is possible to look at micturition and urethral resistance in a way that is not possible with a catheter per urethra.

Management of the neurogenic bladder

The infants are divided into those with a safe bladder and those with an unsafe bladder.

The safe bladder. By safe it is meant that there is a normal upper renal tract with normal renal function and no secondary pressure transmitted to the ureter or renal pelvis. There is a residual urine of less than 20 ml with normal pressures and no outlet obstruction. This may be due to the fact that the bladder is in fact completely normal and a toilet-training program is all that is required or it may be due to the fact that the child can safely empty the bladder by suprapubic manual pressure. This requires careful monitoring for urinary tract infection as well as regular monitoring of the upper renal tract to be sure that secondary damage is not occurring.

The unsafe bladder. In this situation there is already hydronephrosis and hydroureter, a high residual urine, a high intravesical pressure and/or the presence of outlet obstruction. There is a need for adequate bladder drainage to avoid progressive damage to the kidneys with resultant renal failure. The unsafe bladder may require catheterization in the immediate neonatal period. A silicone catheter may be changed every 4–6 weeks in the first few years of life after which intermittent self-catheterization can be taught once the child is old enough. Urinary diversions such as ureterostomy or a colonic loop are now only rarely indicated. Bladder neck obstruction can be treated by per urethral resection or pudendal neurectomy or bladder neck Y-V plasty may be required later to try and achieve relief of bladder neck obstruction without producing incontinence.

Toilet training is important in these children as one will occasionally achieve continence in the presence of a neurogenic bladder that was not thought to be under voluntary control. There is a need to regulate fluid intake, e.g. at night, and to go regularly to the toilet, utilizing the suprapubic crede maneuver, at first hourly. Constipation should be avoided, urinary tract infections carefully monitored and when there is voluntary control, double micturition should be practiced as a routine. Pelvic floor stimulators are unproven. They can be useful in selected cases in the short term but have many complications.

Most children are managed nowadays either by a simple toilet-training regime or with indwelling and then intermittent catheterization. One of the problems associated with intermittent catheterization is how to keep the child dry between catheterizations. Drugs may be used to increase or decrease bladder tone and capacity.

Cholinergic drugs such as carbachol, bethanechol chloride or ubretid will increase detrusor contraction whilst anticholinergic drugs such as propantheline, imipramine and oxybutynin will decrease detrusor contractions. α-adrenergic agonists such as ephedrine will increase the tone in the bladder neck whilst α-adrenergic blockers such as phenoxybenzamine will decrease the tone in the bladder neck. These have a useful but limited place in a small percentage of children.

Urinary tract infection is a constant hazard with the risk of pyelonephritis and this, together with the effects of back pressure on the kidney, may result in renal failure by teen age.

Sexual function

Motor problems are likely to lead to physical difficulty with sexual intercourse problems. Sexual function is also affected and in follow-up studies only small numbers of young adults with spina bifida have any sexual experience and very few females have children even though there is no reason why they should not become pregnant and have a normal delivery. In the male impotence will depend upon a sympathetic and parasympathetic involvement. Failure of closure of the bladder neck during ejaculation means that sperm enters the bladder and not the posterior urethra.

Bowel

Chronic constipation with gross dilation of the descending colon and overflow incontinence is common. Prolapse of the rectum may occur in infancy but rarely remains into school age. Chronic fecal retention may further impede bladder drainage. The anal sphincter, like the bladder neck, may either be patulous and incompetent or tight and spastic. Sensation may be absent so that severe constipation with retention of feces or fecal incontinence may occur. In spite of the neurogenic problems the bowel appears to be more amenable to training in the long run than the bladder. The child should take a high-fiber diet and it may be necessary to use stimulative laxatives such as senokot or fecal softeners such as dioctyl medo. One should find the time of day when the bowel would naturally empty. This need not necessarily be the morning and toilet training with abdominal pressure will be successful in at least half of the cases. Fecal impaction should be avoided as this presses on the bladder neck and may result in both urinary incontinence and secondary spurious diarrhea which can be cured by emptying the bowel. In occasional patients regular manual evacuation is necessary to maintain continence.

Teenage problems

As the pubertal growth spurt occurs several problems result. The sexual problems have already been discussed. The realization of the degree of handicap may cause profound reactive depression. The renal tract problems cause most anxiety, especially if renal damage has progressed to the point of considering the ethics of chronic dialysis or transplant. Scoliosis may be greatly aggravated by growth and pain at the site of the healed initial lesion may cause a lot of discomfort. Traction on the nerve roots due to tethering may cause downward pull at the foramen magnum. It is the medullary cervical junction which causes most problems and is the most difficult to deal with. Stretching of the medulla with obstruction at the aqueduct and the fourth ventricular foramina from the Arnold–Chiari may cause an isolated fourth ventricular hydrocephalus. This may require separate shunting. The pressure may be projected down the central canal of the spinal cord so that a hydromyelia results with gross distention of the cord, producing a string-of-sausages appearance. A localized dilation may occur as a syringomyelia. These brainstem and cervical spinal abnormalities present as drooling, swallowing difficulties, bilateral sixth and seventh paresis, Erb palsy posture, weakness of shoulder elevation or wasting, weakness and loss of use of the hands. Removal of tethering, shunting fourth ventricles, cerebellar tonsillectomy and removal of the arch of the atlas and part of the foramen magnum-impacted tissue may be attempted to try and prevent progressive loss of function.

HYDROCEPHALUS

DEFINITION

Hydrocephalus is a term of Greek origin which means the abnormal accumulation of fluid within the head. One could add to the definition 'with a secondary increase in the CSF spaces', so that in practical clinical terms, hydrocephalus is an increase in the ventricular or subarachnoid space seen on CT scan. It is important to recognize that hydrocephalus is a pathophysiological process and not a single disease and that the definition makes no reference to the level of intracranial pressure (ICP).

INCIDENCE

The incidence of hydrocephalus per 10 000 births around the world is particularly high in Alexandria (20.8), Belfast (12.5) and Dublin (35). A collaborative perinatal survey (Chung & Myrianthopolous 1975) found an incidence of 15 per 10 000 births, only half of whom were evident at birth. These figures are, however, now too high for the UK, as hydrocephalus associated with spina bifida, secondary to intraventricular hemorrhage in the premature infant and secondary to haemophilus meningitis and tuberculous meningitis have all declined. The ability to diagnose severe hydrocephalus antenatally by ultrasound means that some cases are prevented by termination.

PATHOPHYSIOLOGY

Factors that cause ventricular dilation

The normal intracranial pressure in the human represents a balance between the intracranial contents, i.e. blood, brain and CSF. For the CSF compartment, any increase in production or obstruction of flow or absorption will result in ventricular dilation.

Production of CSF

In normal subjects CSF is formed at a rate of 0.3–0.5 ml/min. In hydrocephalic patients on external drainage the CSF production rate is similar. CSF production occurs by two mechanisms.

1. That dependent on choroidal capillary blood flow which itself is a two-step process with, first, an ultrafiltrate of plasma produced hydrostatically through the lax choroidal capillary endothelium (blood–CSF barrier) and, second, an active process involving secretion of sodium into and out of the apical choroidal villi. The raised osmotic pressure causes water to follow passively.

2. The second mechanism is a direct neurogenic stimulation of choroidal villi (which have β2-adrenergic receptors, cholinergic receptors, GABA receptors), which is independent of choroidal blood flow. Stimulation of adrenergic fibers may reduce CSF flow by approximately one-third.

The production rate is similar in newborn and older children, despite the obvious difference in size of the choroid plexus. It is postulated that early maturation of enzyme systems may be responsible for the similar production rates.

A number of factors influence the CSF formation rate. Increased secretion may occur with a choroid plexus papilloma. Frusemide and acetazolamide reduce CSF production. Hypothermia will also reduce the rate of production and although the CSF formation rate is usually independent of the intracranial pressure, when high intraventricular pressures exist the production rate falls, due to decreased choroidal perfusion. Ventricular outflow rates appear to be pulsatile so that peaks and troughs of CSF evacuation occur from the ventricles when measured objectively in children undergoing closed ventricular drainage (Minns et al 1987).

Obstruction

A choroid plexus tumor may not only induce excessive CSF production but may also block the outlet of the ventricle. Intracranial hemorrhage or meningitis may cause leptomeningeal adhesions and obstruction to the CSF flow as well as impairing absorption by blocking arachnoid granulations. A common site for obstruction is the aqueduct of Sylvius. Congenital atresia may result in an inadequate lumen or a total blind-ending channel with forking of the upper and lower components of the aqueduct. Occasionally there is a filamentous or membranous obstruction which may be broken down either by an increase in the intraventricular pressure or by surgical bouginage from the fourth ventricle. This rarely results in an effective reduction of the hydrocephalus because inadequate development of the peripheral subarachnoid pathways, which has resulted from the noncommunicating hydrocephalus, means the dynamics are only changed from a noncommunicating to a communicating hydrocephalus. The aqueduct of Sylvius may also be occluded by organized blood clot after intracranial hemorrhage, inflammatory exudate following ventriculitis or from an aqueductitis resulting from mumps.

Obstruction to CSF flow at the outlet foramina of the fourth ventricle may be secondary to intracranial hemorrhage or infection or may be due to congenital failure of the foramina of Magendie and Luschka to open during development. Occlusion of the fourth ventricle foramina results in a fourth ventricular cystic dilation with atrophy of the cerebellum (the Dandy–Walker cyst). Tumors or clots, cysts or abscesses within or adjacent to the ventricular system may result in hydrocephalus. Thalamic tumors may obstruct the foramen of Monro and third ventricle and pontine or brainstem gliomas may distort the aqueduct of Sylvius, although frequently such pontine gliomas are invasive throughout the brainstem and do not usually cause a gross hydrocephalus. Cerebellar tumors will affect the CSF flow from the fourth ventricle. A choroid cyst of the third ventricle may give rise to intermittent high pressure and hydrocephalus by obstructing the foramen of Monro in a 'ballcock' fashion. During distention of the cyst or venous distention about it there is obstruction of CSF flow through the foramen of Monro. With a possible change of posture the obstruction may be rapidly released and the pressure decline. These children with cysts of the third ventricle frequently present with a 'bobble-headed doll' syndrome and progressive loss of intellect with a particular frontal horn dilation.

Decreased absorption

Decreased absorption may result from obstruction of the arachnoid villi or other peripheral subarachnoid pathways. Absorption (unlike formation) of CSF is a pressure-dependent phenomenon and increases linearly with CSF pressure. There are three types of absorptive defect. Normally CSF absorption begins at a mean pressure of 5 mmHg. In some patients the opening pressure for absorption is elevated, but the subsequent slope is normal. In others the slope alone is decreased and in the third group the resistance to absorption is increased as the pressure is raised.

Factors causing progression of hydrocephalus

Observations in experimental hydrocephalus suggest that after CSF obstruction the ICP rises acutely. This is followed by a stage of periventricular edema with expanded ventricles and subsequently by an increase in CSF absorption. Ventricular dilation and its eventual size depend on the external support of the brain. In infants up to 16 months of age the support of the brain is weak from the poorly myelinated soft parenchyma and there are unfused sutures. Clearly the level of pressure is important at first in the pathogenesis of ventricular dilation, together with the known increase in the outflow resistance (Jones 1987) and a higher 'pressure volume index' (PVI) than could be predicted from the volume of the cranial and spinal axis (Shapiro et al 1985).

In term and preterm infants we frequently see levels of intraventricular pressure of 5 mmHg (above normal for age) which are sufficient to interfere with the cerebral blood flow velocity and have the potential to cause ischemia.

A number of physiological buffers come into play in response to the hydrocephalus. There is collapse of cerebral veins, a shunting of CSF from the ventricular to the spinal CSF compartment, expansion of the skull and an increase in the CSF absorption from the raised pressure. There may also be increased CSF absorption about the spinal nerve roots and paranasal sinuses, etc. Once these compensatory mechanisms have been exhausted then further progression of the hydrocephalus will occur.

The sequence of events is that at first the pressure will increase. The dilation of the ventricles in response to this high pressure is termed 'active or progressive hydrocephalus'. Finally the pressure returns to the normal levels with severely dilated ventricles, a state of arrest (*compensated or arrested hydrocephalus*). Sometimes the active process may be followed by an intermittent pressure pattern with ventricular dilation until the arrested state is reached. This intermittent pattern may be reversible. However, significant elevation of the pressure with increasing ventricular dimensions to the point where brain perfusion is compromised necessitates CSF diversion procedures before shunt-dependent or compensated arrest occurs.

The effects of raised ventricular pressure

Raised intracranial pressure results in either ischemia or brain shift. The ischemia results from a reduced cerebral perfusion pressure (CPP) (mean arterial blood pressure minus intracranial pressure). At levels of CPP below 60 mmHg in the older child there is a progressive reduction in brain perfusion. At 40–50 mmHg profound ischemia results. In the newborn, cerebral perfusion pressures of 30 mmHg may be associated with a normal neurodevelopmental outcome (Raju et al 1982).

The subarachnoid space and the aqueduct are obliterated after shunting, presumably because they are used less, and the patient becomes totally shunt dependent.

Fourth ventricular entrapment, with ataxia, vomiting, cranial nerve disturbances and headache, is a result of outlet obstruction. Treatment is shunting of the ventricle itself. Fistulous communications and diverticulae of the ventricles are usually an accompaniment of severe ventricular dilation. This produces a complex CT scan appearance and intraventricular contrast studies are needed to distinguish these from primary subarachnoid cysts.

CLASSIFICATION AND ETIOLOGY

Terminology

Internal or noncommunicating hydrocephalus: excess of CSF within the ventricular system up to the level of the outlet foramina of the fourth ventricle. The common sites of obstruction are at the outlet foramina of the fourth ventricle, the aqueduct of Sylvius or at the foramen of Monro.

External or communicating hydrocephalus: an increase in the ventricular volume and the subarachnoid spaces of the cranium and spine. The sites of obstruction are at the arachnoid villi or in the basal cisterns.

Panventricular hydrocephalus: dilation of the lateral, third and fourth ventricles (in aqueduct stenosis the fourth ventricle is small or of normal size). An *isolated fourth ventricle* ('double compartment hydrocephalus' or 'trapped fourth ventricle') occurs when there is outlet obstruction from that ventricle and stricture of the aqueduct.

Unilateral hydrocephalus: abnormal dilation of the body, frontal and/or posterior horn of the lateral ventricle on one side. This may be due to compression of the ventricular system on the opposite side, obstruction to one foramen of Monro, slit ventricle syndrome or a hemiparenchymal atrophy.

Slit ventricles: a reduction in the size of the ventricular system seen on CT scan, usually in response to excessive CSF drainage. The slit ventricle *syndrome* is distinguished from radiological slit ventricles by the presence of symptoms and clinical signs attributable to this overdrainage. The etiology of hydrocephalus is given in Table 14.1.

DIAGNOSIS AND ASSESSMENT

Clinical features of progressive hydrocephalus

The symptoms and signs of progressive hydrocephalus in infants are shown in Table 14.2 (Kirkpatrick et al 1989). The symptoms of infantile progressive hydrocephalus are vague and consist of irritability and vomiting but about half are without symptoms. The most common clinical sign is an inappropriately increasing head circumference, followed by a tense nonpulsatile fontanel, then clinical and radiological separation of the sutures, scalp vein distention with taut skin over the scalp. It is important to realize that the classic adult presentation of raised intracranial pressure is rare in children (headache, vomiting, papilledema). Vomiting is a nonspecific symptom in childhood, as are behavioral changes (irritability).

The most common sign of hydrocephalus is really a sign of compensation for the raised ventricular pressure. 'Sunsetting' – the inability to look upwards – may initially be intermittent and later continuous (Fig. 14.16). It is due to pressure on the superior quadrigeminal plate against the free edge of the tentorium causing paralysis of the fourth nerve.

Neurogenic stridor is a result of deranged lower brainstem function caused by bilateral corticobulbar disruption and is a feature of pseudobulbar paresis. Abnormalities of sucking and feeding may also occur in hydrocephalic infants with seriously raised intracranial pressure.

Papilledema is rare but distended retinal veins are common.

The symptoms of *chronic hydrocephalus* are an insidious deterioration in school performance, intermittent headaches over many months, behavioral and personality changes, failure to thrive and dizziness. These are distinct from the signs and symptoms of *arrested hydrocephalus* of long standing which include features of ataxic and spastic cerebral palsy, precocious puberty, mental retardation and specific learning problems. The clinical features of hydrocephalus with raised intracranial pressure

Table 14.1 Etiology of hydrocephalus

Causes of prenatally determined hydrocephalus

Congenital (chromosomal) malformations
Maternal diabetes resulting in holoprosencephaly
Neural tube defects
Occipital meningocele and encephalocele
The Cleland–Chiari II malformation
Dandy–Walker syndrome
Hydranencephaly
Multicystic encephalomalacia
Schizencephaly
Achondroplasia
Arachnoid cysts
Quadrigeminal plate cysts, retrocerebellar cysts, cysts of the cerebellopontine angle and supracellar cysts
Congenital craniosynostosis (e.g. Apert's syndrome)
Agenesis of the corpus callosum and cysts of the cavum septum pellucidum and cavum vergae
Encephalocraniocutaneous lipomatosis
Isolated stenosis of the aqueduct of Sylvius
Sex-linked stenosis of the aqueduct of Sylvius
Hydrocephalus associated with giant hairy nevus (melanosis of the leptomeninges)
Aneurysm of the great vein of Galen
Hurler's disease
Basilar impression
Osteogenesis imperfecta (rarely)
Paget's disease
Colpocephaly
Lissencephaly
Say–Gerald syndrome

Causes of acquired hydrocephalus

Posthemorrhagic causes
   Neonatal intraventricular hemorrhage
   Subarachnoid hemorrhage
   Subdural hemorrhage
Postmeningitic
   Toxoplasmosis
   Mumps (aqueductitis, ependymitis)
   Pyogenic organisms (pneumococcus, haemophilus, etc.)
   Cytomegalovirus
   Other viral meningitides
   Rubella
   Tuberculous meningitis and tuberculoma
Space-occupying lesions
   Tumor
   Clot
   Cyst
   Abscess
Postasphyxial
   Injury

Other causes

Stenosis of the aqueduct of Sylvius
1. Due to raised intracranial pressure with secondary kinking of the aqueduct
2. Due to aqueductitis and ependymitis associated with mumps, toxoplasma, tuberculomas, pyogenic meningitis, rarely CMV, rubella and tumors
Dystrophia myotonia
Otitic hydrocephalus
Choroid plexus papilloma
Intrathecal contrast agents
Fungal infection (cryptococcus and blastomyces)
Cysticercosis
Sarcoidosis
Spinal tumor
Dural venous thrombosis
Isolated Chiari type I deformity

Table 14.2 Most common clinical features of progressive infantile hydrocephalus (50% of cases are asymptomatic)

Symptoms
Headache or irritability
Vomiting
Anorexia
Drowsiness or lethargy

Signs
Inappropriately increasing OFC (approx 75%)
Tense anterior fontanel
Splayed sutures
Scalp vein distention
Sunsetting (loss of upward gaze)
Neck retraction or rigidity
Pupillary changes
Neurogenic stridor
Decerebration

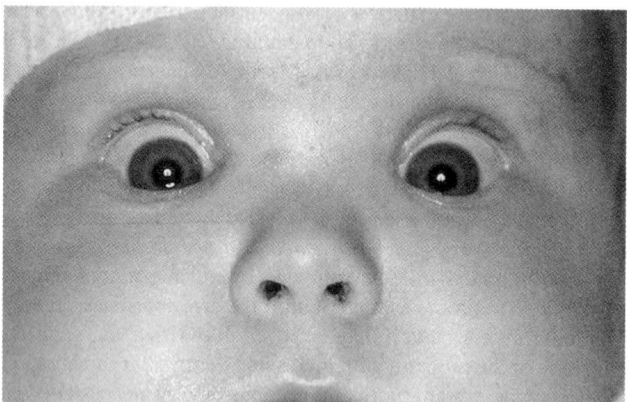

Fig. 14.16 'Sunsetting' due to loss of upward conjugate gaze.

may be extremely variable and any infant with a rapidly increasing head circumference should have a cranial imaging.

The older infant who presents with an enlarged head circumference but is otherwise asymptomatic is likely to have hydrocephalus if there is additional developmental retardation.

Clinical features of decompensated hydrocephalus

The possibility of a blockage of a shunted hydrocephalus is suggested by additional signs of raised pressure (Table 14.3). Our median survival time for a ventriculoperitoneal shunt is 4.31 years (Leggate et al 1988).

Unusual features of raised ventricular pressure include neurogenic pulmonary edema, profuse sweating, ptosis, neurogenic stridor, pseudobulbar paresis and skin rashes (Kirkpatrick et al 1989).

Imaging

X-ray examinations of the skull may show a 'copper-beaten' appearance, shallow orbits and splayed sutures. Computed axial tomography, ultrasound or magnetic resonance image scans will all define ventricular size. Although repeated ultrasound examinations may show progressive hydrocephalus, it is advisable to have a definitive CT or MRI investigation prior to any surgical intervention. The CT scan requires sedation or

Table 14.3 Clinical features of decompensated hydrocephalus (shunted patients)

Symptoms
Vomiting
Drowsiness or lethargy
Headache
Behavioral change
Anorexia
Valve malfunction
Sleep disturbance
Seizures

Signs
No clinical signs (approx 25%)
Decreased conscious level
Acute squint
Neck retraction
Distended retinal veins
Sluggish palpable valve mechanism

---

anesthetic for small children and provides information about the size and symmetry of the ventricles and whether there is any underlying pathology. A single CT scan, like a single ultrasound or MRI scan, may not reveal whether there is a progressive or an arrested hydrocephalus. When there is significantly elevated intraventricular pressure from progressive hydrocephalus, periventricular lucencies, rounding of ventricles, absence of a cortical subarachnoid space and a spherical appearance of the third ventricle (instead of the usual barrel appearance) are seen on CT scan. It is not sufficient to rely on the skull circumference measurements alone and repeated US scans are the most useful arbiter.

The most commonly used index of ventricular dilation is the V/P ratio, that is, the ventricular diameter at the mid-portion of the lateral ventricles divided by the biparietal diameter from inner table to inner table. Hydrocephalus is defined as a ratio higher than 0.26.

Antenatal ultrasound for assessment of fetal hydrocephalus is indexed slightly differently. The commonly used parameters are biparietal diameter and the ratio of the lateral ventricular width divided by the width of the head. The latter is approximately 0.61 at 14 weeks, 0.29 at 27 weeks and 0.29 at term. Absolute measurements of ventricular width are done using the atrium as reference point. Ultrasound estimates of ventriculomegaly in utero may be exaggerated by a factor of about 10% due to the distortion of sound signals passing through two fluids (amniotic and CSF). If hydrocephalus is suspected ultrasound is done weekly until elective cesarean section at 36 weeks (IVH is maximal before 34 weeks). Intracranial Doppler blood flow velocities should be measured in addition to the BPD.

Intracranial pressure

Ventricular CSF pressure monitoring is the only accurate way of assessing the activity of the hydrocephalus. This can be achieved by direct puncture of the ventricle via the anterior fontanel until it is closed at 18 months. Should repeated ventricular punctures be required then a frontal ventricular access device (Rickham or Ommaya reservoir) should be inserted into the frontal horn of the right lateral ventricle to allow sequential pressure measurements. Repeated brain puncture may cause a puncture porencephaly. A single measurement of intracranial pressure is of limited value.

The cerebral perfusion pressure (CPP) should be calculated by subtracting the intracranial pressure (mean ICP) from the mean systemic arterial pressure. For neonates the mean upper normal limit of intracranial pressure is 3.5 mmHg compared to 5.8 mmHg for infants up to 12 months, 6.4 mmHg from 1 to 3 years and 15 mmHg in adults (Minns et al 1989a).

For children who present with symptoms of shunt malfunction due to blockage or infection and who already have CSF shunting devices in situ, pressure measurements via a 'CSF access device' may be done continuously or overnight. This can indicate when raised pressure should be treated at the bedside and overnight measurements are a way of assessing whether the hydrocephalus is arrested or whether there is an intermittently active component. The rapid eye movement phase of sleep is associated with an increase of cerebral blood flow of about 40% in certain areas of the brain. This increase in intracranial volume has to be buffered if raised pressure is not to occur. In children with abnormal intracranial dynamics raised pressure is seen particularly during REM sleep and, to a lesser extent, during stage 2 non-REM sleep.

Cerebral blood flow

The cerebral perfusion pressure gives an indication of the potential for anoxic ischemic damage to the brain. There are a number of methods available for measuring the blood flow velocity or perfusion to the brain, including flow meters, electrical impedance, autoradiography, wash-out and wash-in techniques, microspheres, ultrasound, MRI, SPECT, PET and first pass (MTT). Our own studies of the first pass method measuring the net mean cerebral transit time use an isotope (sodium pertechnetate or technetium albumin) and were performed on 11 hydrocephalic children. The transit time values correlated with cerebral perfusion pressure values (Minns & Merrick 1989). Children with arrested hydrocephalus had transit times within the normal range, while those with progressive hydrocephalus had up to 15% of their sleep time with a cerebral perfusion pressure of less than 50 mmHg.

It is possible also to use a resistance index (systolic minus diastolic over systolic pressure $(S - D)/S$) or the area under the curve obtained by pulsed Doppler measurements of the major cerebral arteries as a measure of the cerebral blood flow velocity. The most useful vessel is the middle cerebral artery and an estimate of the velocity is best obtained through the squamous window of the temporal bone rather than via the open anterior fontanel. The resistance index correlates significantly with the intracranial pressure (Minns et al 1990) and the mean cerebral blood flow velocities fall with elevated ICP measurements. Doppler measurements can be performed intermittently or even continuously in hydrocephalic infants. Since the main effects of raised intracranial pressure are to produce ischemia and brain shifts, an increase in the ventricular pressure sufficient to impair blood flow is an indication for insertion of a CSF shunt. Despite the low values of ICP in normal newborn infants and the relatively low values in infantile and neonatal hydrocephalus, small rises may be sufficient to impair cerebral blood flow. It is our practice to measure both the pressure and the cerebral blood flow velocity sequentially on these infants and the volume of CSF which needs to be removed in order to produce and maintain a normal resistance index (normal equals 0.68); this will indicate whether the hydrocephalic process is arresting spontaneously or whether it is progressing (Minns et al 1990).

TREATMENTS

Shunts

The usual treatment of progressive hydrocephalus is to divert CSF from the ventricular system to another site. There are numerous valves and shunt systems available which take CSF out of the head to have it absorbed elsewhere (Spitz–Holter valve, Pudenz–Hakim, Raimondi, the Indian valve, the Denver, etc.). The author favors the unitized Pudenz with a proximal valve. There are now more sophisticated types (the Sophy programmable and multiprogrammable and the Cosman ICP telesensor) with various types of opening pressure device incorporated into the shunt system.

There are many variations on the basic shunt system which include a ventricular catheter with a flanged end to cause the choroid plexus to waft away from the drainage holes and so lessen proximal blockage. Some shunt systems have a twin valve, one arranged proximally and another distally, and some include a pump or flushing device. The valve usually has a distinct opening pressure, either 2–4, 4–6 or 6–8 cmH$_2$O, the CSF draining when this pressure is exceeded. In the newborn a device which opens at low pressure is advisable but as the child grows it may be necessary to replace this with one opening at a higher pressure to avoid the development of overdrainage and craniocerebral disproportion. A valve may be incorporated in the pump (Spitz–Holter system) or it may be a distal 'slit valve' at the peritoneal end. It may be a single continuous stiff tube with radiopaque gradations to avoid kinking, such as the Raimondi system. Many different valves and shunt system combinations therefore exist. Our reason for choosing the unitized system with a proximal valve is to avoid the overdrainage which frequently results by a siphon effect from a long distal catheter.

Various routes of drainage have been used. The earliest was the ventricular atrial route in which the distal tube was passed by the common facial vein into the right atrium. On occasions a ventriculoazygous route was employed. The potential complications from ventriculoatrial shunts were serious, with infection occurring in between 10% and 30% (Table 14.4). Acute infection with these shunts is automatically accompanied by septicemia and chronic infection may result in shunt nephritis or unexplained rashes of a vasculitic nature due to complement activation from chronic septic emboli. The other chronic effects are right heart failure from pulmonary hypertension (the end result of chronic embolic phenomena from the catheter tip lying in the right atrium) and bacterial endocarditis, thrombosis of the superior vena cava with superior vena caval syndrome arrhythmias and possible perforation of the myocardium. Most centers have now turned to the peritoneal route for drainage.

Ventriculoperitoneal shunts may also have complications and on at least one occasion shunt nephritis has been recorded (Table 14.4). More common is distal blockage due to pocketing of CSF from adhesions, preventing CSF spreading through the peritoneum. This may result eventually in pseudocyst formation. Other complications include penetration of the distal end into a viscus or through the gut wall and it has been known for ventriculoperitoneal shunts to appear per rectum. When infection of the shunt spreads distally, peritonitis may result.

Thecoperitoneal shunts or lumboperitoneal shunts have been largely replaced. They were useful in cases of communicating hydrocephalus following hemorrhage or infection but now are reserved for benign intracranial hypertension and occasionally posthemorrhagic hydrocephalus. Insertion of this shunt requires a

Table 14.4 Complications of CSF shunting

Blockage by choroid plexus, fibrin, neuroglia, blood clot and brain fragments causing raised intracranial pressure

Fractured tubing: fracture of the distal tubing may occur in the neck as a result of direct trauma or kinking of the tubing with repeated movements (fracture can also occur over the surface of the chest and exaggerated flexion/extension movements may result in a crack in the distal tube)

Infection (colonization and ventriculitis) with raised intracranial pressure

Shunt dependence

Slit ventricle syndrome

Other decompressive effects (e.g. subdural hematoma)

Migration of the tubing proximally or distally: cases have been reported of migration of the distal tubing through the gut wall or penetration of other organs. (Cases are known where the tubing has dramatically retracted from the abdominal cavity to the intracranial space. Migration of the distal tubing may cause a volvulus. Commonly if insufficient length is implanted initially, the tubing may retract subcutaneously over the chest with growth. Migration of the proximal tubing may result in the proximal catheter extending into a different ventricle or into subcortical structures)

Intestinal obstruction (volvulus)

Peritonitis and peritoneal fibrosis

Endocarditis (VA shunts)

Chronic pulmonary hypertension (VA shunts)

Superior vena caval syndrome (VA shunts)

Arrhythmias (VA shunts)

Shunt nephritis (VA shunts): a case has been reported of shunt nephritis following a VP shunt

Hyperlordosis (TP shunts)

Acute noncommunication (with TP shunts)

Product failure due to mechanical deficiency and a faulty valve

Surgical technique (malplacement or displacement)

Ventricular collapse from excessive drainage causing the tip of the catheter to impinge through the ependyma or brain substance

Pseudocyst formation with defective drainage

VA = ventriculoatrial; VP = ventriculoperitoneal; TP = thecoperitoneal.

laminectomy and hyperlordosis of the spine above the level of shunt insertion may develop. Recent studies also show there is a chronic distortion of the brainstem at the level of the foramen magnum. It is not nowadays considered a long-term option. It is advisable when these operations are used that additional supratentorial access is maintained by means of a reservoir into the frontal horn of the right lateral ventrical. On the positive side, shunting from the peripheries of the CSF fluid circulation encourages reopening of the subarachnoid pathways, which does not happen with VP anastomoses, and the risk of infection from thecoperitoneal shunts is about the same as for ventriculoperitoneal shunts but the technique avoids the need for cortical puncture. The opposite may occur with VP shunts, the aqueduct may close and the patient become totally shunt dependent. More recent lumboperitoneal shunt operations can be performed without a laminectomy.

Various other routes, such as ventriculopleural, ventriculothoracic duct, etc., have been used but are not a modern practical alternative.

Shunt and separate reservoir

Separate reservoirs have been used for acute surgical decompression since the early 1960s. They have been used to instill chemotherapeutic agents into the CNS in malignant disease and in the management of preterm intraventricular hemorrhage.

In Edinburgh the management of children with hydrocephalus has involved both the use of a shunt and a separate CSF access device (reservoir), which is inserted into the frontal horn of the right lateral ventricle at the same time as the primary shunt surgery. A study to assess the risks attendant on this policy showed no extra mortality or morbidity (Leggate et al 1988). There was less chance of the initial shunt blocking and a lesser incidence of visual and schooling handicap. The double cortical puncture did not result in an increased incidence of hemiplegia or epilepsy. The separate reservoir greatly eased the detection and management of raised intracranial pressure, shunt infection and ventriculitis. Children who only have shunts in situ may have optic discs that become scarred and unreliable as indicators of raised intracranial pressure and frequently the presentation may be subtle with, for example, a decline in school performance. Since there are no absolutely reliable signs or symptoms of raised pressure, the only means of detection is by direct measurement of the intraventricular pressure, which is easy when the reservoir is present.

Many children with shunted hydrocephalus will still present with the usual childhood illness and infections and symptoms of these are often impossible to differentiate from those due to shunt malfunction. With the facility for intracranial monitoring via a reservoir, the presence of raised pressure or infection can be detected in a matter of minutes rather than with prolonged inpatient observation and repeated CT scanning, etc. In our study, in 58% of admissions where a tap was thought necessary to exclude raised pressure or infection, normal values for both pressure and cell counts were obtained, thus avoiding the need for unnecessary emergency shunt surgery. If raised pressure is found it can be lowered by CSF removal via the reservoir. If repeated taps do not effectively normalize the pressure, closed external ventricular drainage can be easily instituted via the reservoir, allowing replacement of the shunt by elective rather than emergency surgery. This was the case in 60 admissions in the above series where the intracranial pressure was controlled by intermittent or continuous ventricular drainage.

The presence of a reservoir also has the advantage of an immediate diagnosis or exclusion of ventriculitis and therapy can be immediately instituted by direct instillation of the appropriate antibiotic into the ventricles, with monitoring of the CSF cell counts and antibiotic levels (Kontopolous et al 1986). In our series, in 28 admissions the reservoir was used to treat the infection while simultaneously controlling the raised intracranial pressure. With this method of management there is virtually no mortality from ventriculitis and one also expects a near zero infection rate from shunt and reservoir replacement.

Complications of CSF shunting (Table 14.4)

Shunt blockage

The Edinburgh series is shown in Table 14.5 (Leggate et al 1988). Survival analyses showed no significant relationship between the onset of mechanical blockage and the type of shunt, the age at reservoir insertion, the sex of the child, the etiology of

Table 14.5 Incidence of shunt problems before and after reservoir insertion

Period	Number episodes (episodes per child shunt year)			
	Serious shunt failure	Blockage	Infection	Ventriculitis
Prereservoir period 219 child shunt years	99 (0.45)	75 (0.29)	24 (0.11)	37 (0.17)
Postreservoir period 269 child shunt years	77 (0.29)*	55 (0.20)*	22 (0.08) ns	28 (0.10) ns

Figures in brackets = per child shunt year.
* = P 0.01 cf. pre- and postreservoir periods.

hydrocephalus or the time relationship of the shunt insertion to reservoir insertion. The reduction in complications with the introduction of the reservoir may be due to the ability to measure directly the intracranial pressure and so reduce the number of unnecessary shunt revisions (Table 14.5).

Ventriculitis

Ventriculitis is diagnosed on the basis of a positive ventricular CSF culture with or without pleocytosis.

Many factors influence the incidence of shunt infection, such as the length of operation, the skin preparation and the type of shunt, but infection remains a problem in a significant number of children with shunts. It can be difficult to diagnose and there is still controversy about the optimum management. Several different treatment regimes have been suggested, including vancomycin into the shunt and systemic therapy with oral trimethoprim and rifampicin. Others have advocated that infection can only be eradicated successfully by removal of the shunt.

It is our practice to subject the CSF to cytological techniques of cytocentrifugation and millipore filter collection. This improves the identification of cell types in the CSF. It is especially useful in cases of mild CSF pleocytosis. Routine biochemistry is also performed on the separated CSF specimen. Nineteen of 26 episodes of ventriculitis were due to *Staphylococcus albus* and two cases to *Escherichia coli* (Kontopolous et al 1986). Neurosurgical intervention increases the number of cells in the CSF transiently but infection may occur in the early postoperative period so the need for accurate cell type identification is clear. Macrophages can persist in the CSF for a long time (Kolmel 1977) and these need to be distinguished from the mild persisting pleocytosis of active infection when there are equal numbers of neutrophils, lymphocytes and macrophages. Macrophages indicate that there is an active repair process going on. Intrathecal penicillin and cephalosporins can also produce a CSF pleocytosis, i.e. a chemical ventriculitis.

It is imperative that treatment is begun immediately with intrathecal and intravenous gentamicin and cloxacillin at the same time that raised ventricular pressure is controlled. Occasionally there may be organisms present in the CSF which have not yet excited a cellular response and very few cells are found. In only three episodes of ventriculitis in our series were there less than 100 cells/ml. Shunt infections may also be associated with a negative organism culture. Because many of these children are highly shunt dependent, once the shunt is removed (which is necessary in ventriculitis because the organisms hide within mucoprotein colonies within the shunt tubing) it is imperative that their pressure is managed by tapping or draining CSF from the reservoir. It is also critical that shunt reinsertion is not done before the CSF is sterilized.

There is a significant discordance between lymphocytes and macrophages in the CSF. Neurosurgery may lead to a 20% increase in neutrophils on the first postoperative day with a progressive decline to a mean of 10 cells (range 7–12) on the fourth postoperative day. There is also a small decrease in the number of lymphocytes on the first postoperative day followed by an increase on the second day. Macrophages are reduced by 12% on the first postoperative day and then steadily increase from the second to the fourth day.

Slit ventricle syndrome

Effects of acute CSF decompression. This results in a low pressure headache, delayed valve pump refilling, a depressed fontanel and possibly an upward brainstem cone (apnea, bradycardia, syncope, hypotension, stridor and hemiparesis).

Effects of chronic CSF decompression. These include acquired craniosynostosis, skull deformity, a thickened skull vault, microcephaly, hyperpneumatization of the sinuses, pneumo-cranium (tension), subdural hematoma, hygroma, cephalocranial disproportion, slit ventricle syndrome (total or partial ventricular collapse), enlarged cortical vascular bed, partial stripped ependymal lining, gliotic scar tissue (subependymal and white matter), wide open Virchow–Robin spaces and decreased intracranial compliance.

In patients with normotensive hydrocephalus the normal ICP in the sitting position is negative and approximately 5 mmHg. Following a shunt insertion in the erect position, the pressures are approximately –18 mmHg. Therefore in most situations with the patient upright and mobile during the day, the pressures will be negative but when supine and during rapid eye movement sleep, there may be significant elevation of pressure. This has given rise to the concept of slit ventricles and the 'slit ventricle syndrome'. Our own studies suggest 10% have radiological slit ventricles, but only 1% were symptomatic.

The slit ventricle syndrome incorporates three components: intermittent or chronic headache secondary to episodic ventricular catheter obstruction; slit-like (Y shaped) ventricles on CT scan; and a slowed refill of the palpable valve mechanism.

The pathogenesis of the slit ventricle syndrome involves a siphon effect of continuing CSF flow down a shunt tubing (particularly with the ventriculoperitoneal route), excessive drainage from thecoperitoneal shunts in patients who are predominantly in the upright posture and the possibility that with ventriculoatrial shunts the diastolic phase of blood flow may encourage CSF withdrawal from the distal end of the shunt.

The management of slit ventricle syndrome has involved several procedures such as the use of high pressure valves, an antisiphon device, a valve upgrade together with an antisiphon device, a subtemporal decompression, a volume-regulated shunt system, an antisiphon ventricular catheter (that is incorporated into the shunt) and lastly the use of steroids and the head-down position.

Other treatments

Choroid plexectomy

This operation has been used to treat hydrocephalus, but in most cases hydrocephalus is due to an increased resistance to drainage

rather than an oversecretion of CSF and a reduction of over 50% of CSF production may not produce any substantial effect on the degree of hydrocephalus or pressure. Even patients showing relief of symptoms may relapse after a period of months. Animal experiments have shown that in those plexectomized the CSF production rate falls by about one-third.

Drug effects on CSF production

A number of drugs have been shown to have an effect on the rate of production of CSF but it is unlikely that even with a substantial reduction in CSF this could be a definitive management for progressive hydrocephalus. However, there may be additional measures to help control CSF pressure in different situations, e.g. with the patient on external ventricular drainage due to ventriculitis. Frusemide and acetazolamide reduce CSF production by virtue of their carbonic anhydrase inhibitory effect. Acetazolamide, while it reduces CSF production, has only a transitory effect and isosorbide (a sorbitol derivative), which acts as an osmotic diuretic, is unpalatable and may produce hypernatremia and metabolic acidosis. For any acute rise in intracranial pressure associated with hydrocephalus, mannitol may reduce the pressure sufficiently to prevent coning. Other drugs with receptor sites on the choroid plexus may also reduce CSF production without diminishing overall choroidal perfusion.

Other procedures

Third ventriculostomy (the opening of the ventricular CSF system into the subarachnoid space via the lamina terminalis) and ventriculocisternostomy (Torkildsen shunt) between the ventricle and the basal cisterns are reliant on a block being present in the CSF outflow from the ventricles with an intact subarachnoid space and surface CSF pathways.

Compressive head wrapping as a means of forcing alternative CSF pathways of absorption is not a method to be advocated because of the inevitable adverse effects on intracerebral blood flow.

When there is ventriculitis, meningitis, blood in CSF or other factors making the insertion of a CSF shunt impracticable, then a temporary measure may be necessary, such as ventricular tap through the anterior fontanel. As previously mentioned, a puncture may result in porencephaly and it is preferable to have neurosurgical assistance and have a temporary reservoir implanted.

SPECIFIC TREATMENT REGIMENS

Posthemorrhagic hydrocephalus

This is common in premature infants following periventricular hemorrhage (PVH) but may occur in other age groups as well. Posthemorrhagic ventricular dilation in prematures may be assessed by serial ultrasound to compare the ventricular index (above) to the centiles for age (Levene et al 1985). Approximately one-third of infants with a PVH will develop posthemorrhagic ventricular dilation and one-fifth of these will require a CSF shunt. Levene et al (1987) suggest that only 18% of cases of dilation are due to outlet obstruction at the fourth ventricle.

Distinguishing progressive hydrocephalus with high pressure, i.e. pressure-driven ventricular dilation, from brain atrophy in such circumstances requires ultrasound or imaging scans and pressure measurements. In atrophy the ventricles retain their usual configuration and do not have loss of the normal angles of the lateral ventricles.

There is no ideal or single method for managing posthemorrhagic hydrocephalus. Repeated lumbar punctures may prevent the need for shunting and will certainly ameliorate progressive ventricular dilation but the pressure should be measured at the same time with CSF removal to reduce the pressure level to normal.

Acetazolamide in a dose 25 mg/kg per 24 h, rising to a maximum of 100 mg/kg per 24 h orally may be of use for posthemorrhage hydrocephalus with raised pressure (Shinnar et al 1985). This drug may result in metabolic acidosis and blood gas monitoring is important.

Ventriculoperitoneal shunting is not done until the CSF hemorrhage has cleared sufficiently to avoid blocking the shunt.

The elective insertion of a ventriculostomy reservoir will allow measurement and treatment of raised pressure by sequential taps. The hydrocephalus may arrest or the patient may subsequently need a ventriculoperitoneal shunt.

Tuberculous meningitis

In this condition children frequently have an insidious prodrome and they may present in coma. Ventricular dilation is present in nearly 80% of these cases though it is uncommon in adult tuberculous meningitis. The immediate management is to have a CT scan done and to attend to the raised ventricular pressure. The child is unlikely to succumb from the tuberculous infection over the next 24 h but may suffer serious sequelae or die as a result of untreated or unrecognized pressure. Our routine is to have an emergency ventriculostomy reservoir inserted, which allows measurement of the ventricular pressure and decompression by CSF removal. A diagnostic lumbar puncture is then done. Pressure is measured at the time of lumbar puncture and comparison can be made with the ventricular measurement to see whether there is any spinal block (Froin's syndrome). CSF is then removed for cytocentrifuge cell count, protein, Ziehl–Neelsen, etc. in order to confirm the diagnosis of tuberculous meningitis.

The raised pressure, which may continue for many days, can be treated by intermittent taps of the reservoir or by closed external ventricular drainage against a pressure head of 10 mmHg. Routine antituberculous chemotherapy is commenced and both the infection and the pressure are monitored and treated carefully over the next 2 weeks. The use of intrathecal steroid preparations may be necessary if there is a spinal block or a basal adhesive arachnoiditis.

Early CSF shunting is an alternative way to control the pressure while treating the infection but the shunt will need to be replaced if it becomes colonized and shunt dependence continues. Alternatively a temporary shunt may be sufficient to control the pressure while attempting to sterilize the CSF. Although earlier practice was to routinely lumbar puncture suspected tuberculous meningitis patients (in most cases safely), there remains the possibility of coning at the time of diagnosis. These patients, and others who present in coma, must not have a lumbar puncture until a CT scan has been performed and the basal cisterns seen to be patent.

Benign intracranial hypertension

This is a clinical syndrome of symptomatic raised intracranial pressure, usually with papilledema, in a patient who is neurologically normal with normal CSF. There are numerous causes for this including endocrine causes, drugs, hematological causes, trauma, infections and other systemic conditions. Approximately half have no obvious cause. Headache is invariably present, nausea and vomiting and visual symptoms may occur. Papilledema is almost always present but may be unilateral. A sixth nerve palsy and enlarged blind spot are common but sudden visual loss is rare. The CT scan in these patients is normal or may show small ventricles and the EEG usually shows paroxysmal slowing. Those with a dural sinus thrombosis are easily recognized. CSF pressure is raised and this may be extreme despite the minor symptomatology. Pressures may be monitored variously, from the lumbar theca, from the ventricles or from the brain surface.

There are many theories about the pathophysiology of benign intracranial hypertension, perhaps the most popular being that of decreased CSF absorption. Benign intracranial hypertension is largely a self-limiting condition although a number of measures have been shown to be effective in reducing the intracranial pressure. Repeated lumbar punctures with CSF removal may initially be required daily and thereafter at reducing intervals. Steroids have not been properly evaluated for this condition but various single reports suggest that the pressure drops within 24 h. Acetazolamide is often given to patients who have an inadequate steroid response: large doses are required to be effective and sometimes the acetazolamide is combined with a loop diuretic. A lumboperitoneal or ventricular peritoneal shunt may be necessary for those who have failed medical treatment and symptomatic relief may occasionally be required by optic nerve decompression.

Fetal hydrocephalus

Fetal hydrocephalus has two broad etiologies. Firstly, those associated with other abnormalities (structural or chromosomal) which account for about 84% of cases (trisomy 18 and 21, Arnold–Chiari and spina bifida, Meckel–Gruber, Dandy–Walker, Bickers–Adams, porencephaly, holoprosencephaly). The second group have an isolated hydrocephalus, a congenital idiopathic and acquired communicating hydrocephalus or aqueduct stenosis, IVH or toxoplasmosis.

Detection of fetal hydrocephalus is now usually by ultrasound. The earliest one can detect hydrocephalus is 17–18 weeks and then only in severe cases. There is often associated polyhydramnios.

A ventricular amniotic shunt aimed at halting progression of the neurological deterioration and allowing normal development in the brain before birth has not been markedly successful. There have been many difficulties with shunt design and although clinical trials have been undertaken, patient selection is difficult and potentially this is likely to be of benefit to a minority only (Michejda 1985). Suitable cases have no associated defect with the hydrocephalus, are less than 32 weeks' gestation, with progressive ventricular dilation and a singleton pregnancy. The risks of precipitating labor or chorioamnionitis are significant.

Fetal hydrocephalus is associated with a 55–75% mortality which includes abortions carried out electively following diagnosis, intrapartum deaths and postnatal deaths. The prognosis is obviously better if there is no associated malformation. Of the survivors, 40% are severely abnormal and only 40% are normal (Serlo et al 1986, Chervenak et al 1984).

Prognosis

Natural history of untreated hydrocephalus

Several studies detail the course of untreated hydrocephalus. An average result from these studies indicates that approximately 50% survive and of the survivors, 25–30% have normal intelligence and 25–30% have severe motor and other handicaps.

Epilepsy

The frontal lobe is one of the most epileptogenic regions of the brain and there is therefore a theoretical risk of precipitating seizures from frontal reservoirs. Also with a reservoir there are two cortical insults. In our study seizure disorders occurred in nine children (16%) and this incidence is similar to that reported from a single cortical puncture (Machado et al 1985). The siting of a single VP shunt frontally (Dan & Wade 1986) was associated with a 54% incidence of seizures.

Hemiplegia

Hemiplegia is the commonest type of cerebral palsy complicating hydrocephalus associated with spina bifida. In a group of children with congenital hemiplegic cerebral palsy, biventricular hydrocephalus was present in seven cases (19%) (Claeys et al 1983). The hemiplegia in hydrocephalus may be due to the etiology (e.g. prematurity or meningitis) or may be a complication of the hydrocephalus as a result of parenchymal hemorrhage from brain puncture, traumatic puncture of the internal capsule, siting of the shunt to involve the motor strip, subdural hematomata as a result of overdrainage, cortical thrombophlebitis or basilar arachnoiditis or precipitation of status epilepticus with postconvulsive hemiplegia or puncture porencephaly. In our series hemiplegia was present in four cases of a total of 56 at follow-up. In no case was it associated with the insertion of a separate reservoir.

Vision

Blindness is not a problem of untreated hydrocephalus but sudden total blindness may result from raised pressure due to shunt malfunction. Gaston (1985), in studying a group of spina bifida children, found only 27% of 322 had normal visual function. Only one child in our series (n = 56 over 12 years) had severe visual handicap sufficient for blind registration and 88% had normal visual function. Visual impairment in children with hydrocephalus may result from optic atrophy secondary to chronic papilledema, distention of the third ventricle with chiasmal compression, posterior cerebral artery compression with ischemia to the optic radiation or calcarine cortex or gross thinning of the calcarine cortex because of selective posterior horn dilation. These are all due to raised pressure with hydrocephalus.

Intelligence

Fifty to sixty percent of shunted hydrocephalic children have normal IQs. In our study group 65% of children were in normal education, 29% in ESN placements and 6% in residential care for the severely handicapped. The pathophysiological mechanisms whereby learning is impaired include an associated cortical dysplasia, marked thinning of the cortical mantle (less than 15 mm), ventriculitis, chronically reduced cerebral perfusion pressure and coincidental parenchymatous brain damage (meningitis, asphyxia, etc.).

DEVELOPMENTAL DISORDERS

Introduction

Early insult to the brain results in an overt congenital malformation. The earlier the insult, the more generalized and profound the effect on the brain with the development of microcephaly and global motor and cognitive defects. Later abnormality disrupts cortical architecture with a microdysgenesis which may be generalized or focal. Such damage is likely to be more specific, affecting individual modalities of learning, e.g. dyslexia, dysgraphia, dyscalculia, etc.

The brain continues to grow postnatally under genetic control for about 17 years and throughout this time damage can interfere with brain growth and development. A slower rate of brain growth means that milestones and learning may be slowed. Both specific disorders with a basis of microdysgenesis and slowing of skills acquisition due to slow brain growth are encompassed by the term 'developmental disorder'.

The brain is the organ of learning. Damage or disease to the brain will therefore produce an abnormality in developmental learning even if it does not release hard neurological signs. It is expected that the child with an overt brain damage syndrome such as cerebral palsy will have slow development (e.g. the age of walking is independent of the neurological signs), but it can be more difficult to understand why a developmental disorder may occur without damage to the motor system producing overt signs. A developmental disorder cannot be separated from a neurological disorder. (It has therefore been suggested that pediatric neurology might be renamed 'developmental neurology'.)

Factors influencing the rate of brain development

1. Genetic or familial disorders
2. Chromosomal disorders (fragile X, XYY, XXY, etc.)
3. Damage during the phase of rapid brain growth (prematurity, asphyxia)
4. Sex – maleness
5. Less than 3rd centile – normal
6. Endocrine disorders (hypothyroidism, hypogonadism)
7. Environmental deprivation

NORMAL DISTRIBUTION OF ABILITIES

We accept when assessing height or weight that we should use percentile charts and consider that the child below the third or over the 97th centile is possibly abnormal. We should bear in mind that the 'rate of brain development' in any particular area also shows a normal distribution curve and there will be children who are fast or slow in that particular field. No one will suggest that a child who walked at 10 months is far more likely to become an Olympic athlete than one who walked at 14 months. It would be equally naive to think that the sexual prowess of a boy going through puberty at 9 years would be superior to a boy going through puberty at 15 years. Nevertheless we have ignored this fact in the development of speech, reading and numbers and assume that all children are the same at the same chronological age. Some children will be slow learners and some will be fast. Fast learners are not necessarily child prodigies or geniuses and their brain development may cease at an earlier age than the child with a slow rate of development. Children with rapid rates of brain development (gifted children) do not necessarily obtain first-class honors degrees.

ENVIRONMENTAL FACTORS

The brain will develop to a certain degree under genetic control after which environmental stimulation is necessary for the attainment of potential. We know that if one eye is occluded in a kitten and the other eye stimulated, the optic nerve on the stimulated side myelinates more quickly. In the child severe psychosocial deprivation results in a cessation of development and tender loving care can result in a massive developmental spurt. A child cannot have words in his vocabulary, develop manual skills (sewing, typing, tying laces, assembling a plug) or learn postural skills (swimming, riding a bike) that he has not experienced in everyday life.

INNATE DEVELOPMENTAL BEHAVIORS

The brain possesses a remarkable repertoire of preprogrammed strategies and behaviors. For example, the human fetus shows preprogrammed hatching behavior, moving into the vertex position and turning its head to the right in preparation for delivery in the left occipitoanterior position. We also show innate patterns of nesting, mourning, courting and maternal behavior so that our responses to particular situations are to some extent predictable and not necessarily the result of conscious thought.

Once a particular ability is developed to a stage where it is useful to the child there is a built-in preprogrammed behavior to make sure that this ability is used. Once visual fixation and following is established there is a period of forced visual fixation, usually around 3 weeks, when the child is compelled to look at objects and watch movement. With the development of hand function around 3 months there is a period of forced grasping and forced hand regard when the child must look at his hands and explore with them, pulling at his clothes and beginning to explore his environment. Around 6 months the feet become obvious and the child looks at them, bites them and sucks his toes. Children show active exploration as soon as they have started to walk. One is aware of babbling behavior and forced utterances in the small child who will not only imitate facial movement but also imitate sounds. The infant can be led to make sounds in response to an adult long before he has articulated speech.

COGNITIVE DEVELOPMENT

Specialist regional functions of the cerebral cortex have been demonstrated by anatomical ablation and stimulation studies. Cerebral metabolic and blood flow studies using positron emission tomography confirm these regions (see p. 1897).

The brain is not a sponge which, once developed, simply absorbs information in a random way. Information is stored in specific areas and needs to be classified into concepts in order that reasoning, thought and understanding can occur – the basis of cognitive development. This classification depends upon symbol systems, e.g. words, sounds, letters, numerical symbols, electronic symbols, chemical symbols or musical notation, all of which form

a brain 'computer language'. The ability of certain parts of the brain to use particular symbol systems in order to allow classification of memories into concepts requires a built-in 'strategy'. Each type of learning can be regarded as a modality (speech, reading, writing, numbers, spatial, praxic, music) and the strategy to allow learning in each of these modalities develops in a set chronological sequence. It is by examining the stage of development of this sequence that we are able to assess the child's stage of development or attainment. This forms the basis of the various tests of development (Griffiths, Vineland, Columbia mental maturity scale, Gesell, Bayley, Reynell, Portage, etc.) or intelligence (Stanford–Binet, Wechsler, etc.). Each modality can be lost in isolation, giving a specific learning disorder; alternatively there may be multiple learning disorders or a global cognitive learning disorder (mental handicap) (see p. 826). Each modality is specific and develops in a preset chronological order and is under genetic control. Thus genetic factors play an important part in many developmental disorders (familial late walkers, familial shufflers, familial slow speakers, familial enuresis, familial late puberty, familial dyslexia, familial dysgraphia and familial dysmusia).

DEVELOPMENTAL DISORDERS OF MOVEMENT

The child who is a slow walker frequently presents for pediatric opinion. If we consider the factors which cause slowing down of brain development outlined above then slowness in walking may be because the child is simply below the 3rd centile, that he is a perfectly normal child who will go through all the normal developmental milestones but at a slightly slower rate (Table 14.6). There may be a genetic component, a familial disorder associated with slow walking. The child may have slowed brain maturation from prematurity or asphyxia. Negro babies are ahead of white in motor development. Walking, though, is less dependent on environmental stimulation than cognitive development and so swaddled babies (e.g. Kurdish) still walk at the normal time. Slow walking may also be part of a definite disease process such as cerebral palsy, muscle disease or missed congenital dislocation of the hip.

The most characteristic developmental variant of movement is that of shuffling. The child is generally hypotonic and fits into the category of 'benign congenital hypotonia'. There are exaggerated joint angles and the child, when suspended, will not weight bear as his legs are held out in front of him perpendicular to his trunk and abducted (Foerster's sign). When one tries to put him on his feet he always lands on his bottom. The child may shuffle or hitch himself forward. This is a dominantly inherited characteristic and is the basis of some of the names in the north of England such as Shufflebottom, Hitchinbottom. These children may not walk until they are 20 months of age. It is thought that 7% of the population are bottom shufflers while 1% of children are rollers, mobile by rolling over rather than crawling. The crawling phase may be brief or absent and some may also exhibit generalized hypotonia. About 1% of the normal population also creep or crawl in the commando fashion by using their elbows with their feet out behind them and the abdomen still on the ground. They again tend not to walk until around 20 months. These shufflers, rollers, creepers and crawlers are normal children who have a genetic variation or deviant motor development but they are not going to have any significant motor handicap in later life. The child who shuffles on his bottom often shows a dislike of the prone position and there is a prone/supine

Table 14.6 Development of posture and mobility skills

Prone postures	
Headturning left/right (clears face)	Newborn
Head raised	6 weeks
Chest raised on forearms	4 months
Chest raised outstretched on hands (face vertical, hips extended, knees flexed)	6 months
Prone kneeling	8 months
Knee standing	9 months
Standing with support (e.g. furniture)	9 months
Pulls to standing	10 months
Standing with no support	1 year
Walks	10–14 months
Standing from bending to get object off the floor	16 months
Walking and jumping	
Round furniture	10 months
Two hands held	10 months
One hand held	11 months
Unsupported	12–14 months
Starts to run	18 months
Jump off step both feet together	3 years
Walk 6 steps on tip toes	3 years
Walks tandem along 4 foot line with little truncal sway	4 years
Hop 15 feet on right leg	5 years
Hop 15 feet on left leg	5 years
Tandem walk along a 4 foot line on the floor (mild truncal sway only)	4 years
Walk along a 3 inch beam 1 foot high – forwards	6 years
Walk along a 3 inch beam 1 foot high – backwards	8 years
Jump with both feet over a 10 inch height	5–6 years
Runs upstairs	5 years
Jump off 3 steps	3 years
Stairs	
Crawls upstairs	14 months
Up with rail or hand	20 months
Up two feet per step	2 years
Up one foot per step	3 years
Stairs down with rail	3 years
Down two feet per step	4 years
Down one foot per step	5 years
Later prowess	
Skips with rope (3 rounds)	7 years
Skips with rope (12 rounds)	8 years
Two wheeler bike (without stabilizers)	8 years

Note
Postural skills like manipulative skills depend upon exposure and practice so there are wide variations in normal. For example, a child may be able to ride a two wheeler bike without stabilizers before 5 years but it should not be regarded as abnormal unless he cannot learn after 8 years.

discrepancy in behavior. It is important to realize that other causes of hypotonia, such as the various types of congenital ataxia, may also shuffle without the benign course of the dominantly inherited genetic type. If a child has poor balance, in order to use his arms he either has to W sit or tripod sit, i.e. use his arms as props on each side (in which case he cannot use them for exploring). Because of the strain of internal rotation on the hips in W sitting, the child is often dissuaded from doing this and so cannot sit unsupported at all. Differentiation of simply deviant motor development from a neurological disease, e.g. an ataxia, may at

times be difficult. Children with metabolic diseases such as biotinidase deficiency, glutaric aciduria, early cases of ataxia telangiectasia, various forms of cerebellar hypoplasia and mild hydrocephalus can all present with late walking and shuffling.

Developmental coordination disorder

Once the child can walk he may still show slow or abnormal gross motor development, i.e. be a clumsy child. He may fall, not swing his arms, fail to develop heel strike in gait, cannot stand on one leg, cannot hop, cannot crouch without waving his arms around and falling over. For this reason one needs a test of posture and mobility. Motor development is not complete until 12 years of age when all associated movements between the arms and legs have disappeared (Fog test) (Table 14.6). One must look at the child in detail to be sure that he has not got mild cerebral palsy. All girls with slow motor development should have their hips X-rayed to exclude congenital dislocation of the hip and all boys with late walking should have their creatinine phosphokinase measured to exclude Duchenne muscular dystrophy. Any weakness, failure to move all limbs symmetrically, abnormal posture, retention of primitive reflexes, spinal curvature, Gowers' sign, Trendelenburg's sign or positive Thomas test are all indications that much more detailed study is required.

Walking occurs once the motor circuits in the brain have developed to a sufficient level. Practice is not necessary for walking to develop. Using the infant's primitive walking reflexes and practicing walking may improve muscle bulk but will not speed up the individual infant's ability to walk. When the child first starts to walk he has a broad base and flat feet, i.e. a physiological truncal ataxia. There are some children in whom this physiological ataxia is more obvious and lasts longer with corresponding delay in acquiring postural skills such as riding a bike and swimming. A number of children may toe walk and cause confusion with a mild diplegia. In some children this so-called 'ballerina syndrome' may persist until 4 years of age.

MANIPULATION

Normal

Table 14.7 shows the normal sequence or chronological strategy of the development of manipulation. At birth hand control is purely reflex so that any object placed in the palm of the hand and to which traction is applied results in a firm grasp reflex. If the dorsum of the hand is stimulated or if the arm is extended and the back of the hand placed against the buttock, the hand opens and remains open allowing the inspection of the palm. The hand also opens with the Moro reflex and one hand closes and the opposite opens often as part of an asymmetrical tonic neck reflex. The hand of the fetus can also be seen on ultrasound to open and close. From around 3 months the child develops hand regard and forced grasping and he begins to voluntarily release an object placed in his hand. By 4 months the grasp reflex is inhibited and there is voluntary opening and closing of the hands. At 5 months the infant can reach out for an object, hit his face and then by using his rooting reflex get an object into his mouth. At this stage he has no idea of distance; he simply hits the object and grasps it. Nor can he judge force, speed or direction of movement. By 6 months the hands are in the midline and he is able to pass objects from one hand to the other. Objects can be placed in the mouth without utilizing the rooting reflex

Table 14.7   The development of manipulation

Birth	Grasp and avoiding reflex
3 months	Forced grasping, hand regard, hold and release briefly
6 months	Picks up cube (voluntary grasp), transfers
7 months	Eats biscuit from hand
9 months	Uses sides of finger and thumb to uplift
10 months	Fingers objects with index finger, waves bye-bye, claps hands
12 months	Uses feeding cup, pincer grip, bangs bricks together
14 months	Pushes cars along, tries to help with dressing, puts lids on tins
18 months	Holds up one hand, scribbles, builds tower of three bricks, random stroke /
2 years	Tower of six bricks, turns single pages, copies \⁻
2.5 years	Closes fist, cuts with scissors
3 years	Threads beads, catches ball with two hands, builds ⊔⊓ , draws man ⅄ copies ○
4 years	Assembles biro, ties knot, copies + draws man (figure)
5 years	Ties laces, copies □ , draws man (figure)
6 years	Draws △ , builds blocks (blocks figure) , uses knife and fork
7 years	Draws ◇ , makes self a drink of squash, catches ball with one hand
8–14 years	Graphic skills increase: (series of shapes) and so do cursive writing skills; threads needle, plays piano, plays recorder, knits, sews, makes models and changes electric plug

which has now been inhibited and the distance an object should be placed in the mouth is more finely regulated. By 8 months of age the child can use one hand independent of the other and is able to hold and release an object in one hand independent of what he is doing with the other. Up to this stage the child has tended to grasp all his fingers in a rake and then gradually assume a radial grasp. At 10 months of age the index finger is released independently so that he explores with the index finger and is able to pick up objects between the finger and thumb (has no residual ataxia or incoordination). There are no involuntary movements and he has a well-established, neat, coordinated pincer grasp.

On top of this neurological maturation follows the development of hand skills. By 1 year the child can eat a biscuit, wave bye bye, clap hands and hold a cup with two handles and will pick up small bits of fluff or tiny objects accurately. He can put an object in a cup, take it out of the cup and will look under a cup when it is hidden. Neurological maturation of the hands is complete by 1 year and further development is of learned hand skills. Failure to develop these hand skills is developmental dyspraxia.

Dyspraxia

The ability to use one hand completely independently of the other and to use the fingers rapidly independently of each other without any associated movement is only acquired by 12 years. Recent studies of pyramidal tract conduction times utilizing magnetic induction techniques have confirmed this slow maturation. The ability to cut with scissors, use a knife and fork, tie shoe laces, catch a ball in one hand, etc. is developed in a specific sequence. A child can have a normal IQ and yet have the hand skills of a young child, i.e. manipulative retardation (developmental

dyspraxia). Children with hydrocephalus can have severe retardation in hand skills in the presence of a normal IQ and good cognitive development.

A dyspraxia relates to the inability to learn how to perform a motor skill which is commensurate with the child's age. Fine motor skills are learned according to a strategy in that the individual component movements are learned in isolation; they are then sequenced into a skill which is slow, clumsy and requires attention, i.e. it occupies a conspicuous part of consciousness. With practice there is a gradual increase in speed and the neatness of the skill until the skill becomes automatic or subconscious (overlearned). A skill, be it speaking, writing, typing, playing the piano, dancing, driving a car or using tools, is only fully learned when it no longer requires conscious effort. The learned skill produces an engram or motor memory (kinesthetic memory). This depends upon the motor association area, e.g. Broca's area for speech and the graphomotor area for writing. Eccles (1979) has been a proponent of the importance of the cerebellum in motor learning in the child as well as the cerebral cortex and children with congenital ataxia often have slow development of the hand skills and speech, which more resembles a dyspraxia than a coordination defect. Motor planning depends on past memories and experience but not on the ability to execute a movement, which requires an intact peripheral motor system. Learning of motor skills is also dependent upon a normal sensory system but the development and maturation of the cortical sensory system is very difficult to evaluate in the individual child. Finger agnosia occurs in 29% of normal 7–8-year-olds and inaccurate graphesthesia in 45%. Measurement of kinesthetic acuity and memory have proved difficult in young children and the results are controversial.

The child with a dyspraxia has difficulty in putting several movements together. This may take the form of sequencing the fingers, repeated tongue movements, postural sequences used in dancing or gymnastics or phonemes into a spoken or graphemes into a written word. It is possible to make the sound or copy the letter in isolation in all but the most severe cases. The child may not be able to carry out a constructional task after demonstration even though he has no weakness, spasticity, incoordination or involuntary movement (constructional dyspraxia). The child with isolated articulatory dyspraxia will always be able to bite, chew and swallow. The child with a manual dyspraxia will have good strong hands with no shaking and may be able to pour juice out of a jug without spilling any. The dyspraxia may be isolated for writing or involve all hand skills, e.g. cutting with scissors, coloring between lines, using feeding utensils, tying shoes and using tools. Speech may also be affected with slow development of phonology or developmental articulatory dyspraxia. A standardized test of hand function is necessary as although some IQ tests have components testing this ability, e.g. to fold a piece of paper or cut with scissors, they may miss children with very severe developmental dyspraxia. The child exhibiting a developmental dyspraxia should have the cause defined: is it genetic, is there an associated chromosome disorder, e.g. some of the sex chromosome disorders (XXY) or is it due to some form of brain damage? In children cerebellar damage may result not in intention tremor and dysmetria but in delayed motor learning. The speech disorders seen in cerebellar disease are also of a developmental type and not necessarily the dysrhythmic dysarthria seen in older patients. Children with hydrocephalus may have very significantly delayed motor skills and a developmental dyspraxia which is only revealed on specific testing. Environmental stimulation is important in developmental praxis; some children are encouraged to use tools or learn the piano at an early stage while others are not given this opportunity. When measuring such skills it is difficult to assess results in the context of previous experience and variations are extremely wide when it comes to children of secondary school age.

VISUOSPATIAL DEVELOPMENTAL DISORDERS

The nondominant hemisphere (usually the right) is responsible for the recognition of shape, faces, object concept and central color. The dominant hemisphere is responsible for the recognition of shapes that have a linguistic meaning, i.e. graphemes and written words. The built-in developmental strategy for visuospatial learning is the basis of many components of intelligence tests. Spatial learning may be assessed by looking at drawings. The child first of all can copy a line and does circular scribble. This is followed by the ability to copy a cross and a circle so that he can put lines at right angles.

A classic stage of development is the 4-year-old tadpole man which children draw irrespective of race or experience. The way the child subsequently draws a man is the basis of the Goodenough intelligence test. Children will often draw a human figure while saying to themselves 'eye', 'nose', 'hair' so that there is a linguistic component and it is not purely a test of spatial capabilities of the child. Children initially draw houses with the windows in a corner and then the windows gradually move to be independent. Later more subtle changes develop in the drawing, such as occlusion, where one object partially obstructs another, together with proportion, perspective and action. We tend to utilize children's ability to copy geometrical shapes in developmental testing (Fig. 14.17). The preprogrammed learning 'strategy' of the brain is such that children never learn to draw a diamond before they are able to draw a square.

Children can have severe disorders of space, shape and direction in isolation. They may not be able to draw and yet are able to write their names. They will not organize themselves on a page; they will not be able to hold to margins; they will slope across the page although their spelling and writing may be intact (see p. 821).

SPEECH DEVELOPMENT

This is considered in more detail on page 804. Children learn to speak following a defined developmental strategy so that they pronounce all the vowels and the simple consonants b, d, t, k. First baby talk develops – babba, mamma, ta ta, dadda, poo poo – independent of the basic languages. The child can only make fricative sounds and sounds which can be elongated, e.g. R, L, S, TH, SH, much later. Thus with slow speech development one gets led lolly for red lorry, poon for spoon and predictable phonemic errors.

The development of the past tense, plurals, the use of me for I and the length of utterance are all developed in sequence. The rule of thumb, i.e. age in years plus one, is a rough guide to the mean length of utterance of a child, so that a 3-year-old should have at least a 4-word average sentence, a 4-year-old at least a 5-word average sentence and so on.

Slow speech development, like other developmental disorders, may be genetic and familial, associated with chromosome

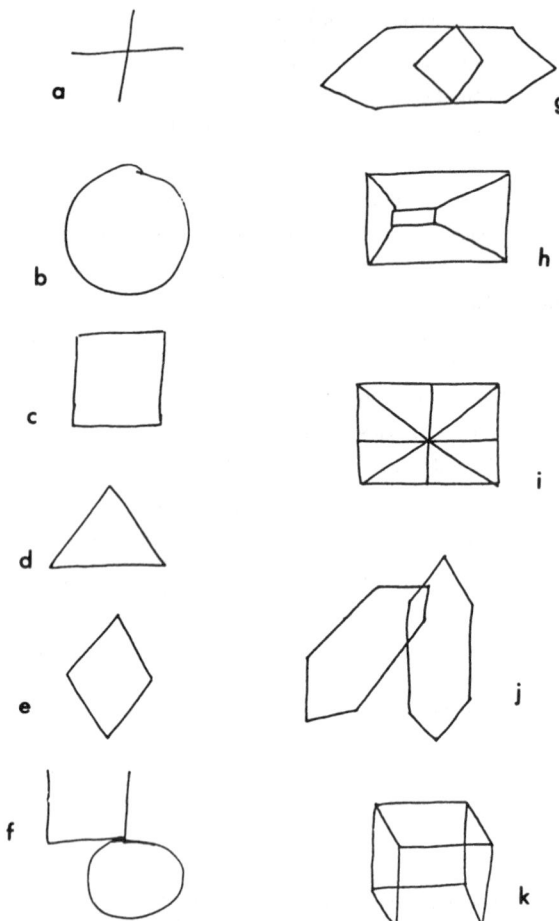

Fig. 14.17 Acquisition of drawing skills. (a) 4 years, (b) 3-3.5 years, (c) 5 years, (d) 6 years, (e) 7 years, (f) 8 years, (g) 9 years, (h) 10 years, (i) 11 years, (j) 12 years, (k) 13 years.

disorders, associated with minor brain damage and prematurity and asphyxia or due to environmental deprivation or the child may simply be below the third centile for the rate of development of speech at that particular age.

OTHER LEARNING DISORDERS

The way a child learns to read, write or spell again follows a particular sequence and these may be affected as discussed later in this chapter. It is usual to put the prefix 'dys', simply meaning 'difficulty with', before each ability and we then talk about *specific* learning disability such as articulatory dyspraxia, ocular dyspraxia, manual dyspraxia, writing dyspraxia, dyscalculia, dysmusia, dysphasia, dyslexia, dysgraphia, etc.

DEVELOPMENT AND PUBERTY

The onset of puberty has gradually come earlier during this century. This is thought to be due to better nutrition and general health. There is a normal variation in the onset of puberty with 3% of children developing puberty early and 3% who may be 15 years or older before its onset. The onset of puberty is determined by the hypothalamus in the brain. There is a biological clock of growth controlled by the diencephalon. Puberty tends to occur at a given stage of development which is best assessed clinically by the bone age rather than the chronological age. In hypothalamic disease puberty does not occur at all and infantilism results. The hypothalamus of the male is tonic and that of the female cyclical and it is thought that this is the result of early imprinting from the spurts of testosterone at 6 weeks postconception and 6 weeks postnatal life. Puberty can occur at any age and is not related to the ability of the pituitary to synthesize gonadotropins or the gonads to respond. Normally the hypothalamus is held in a state of inhibition probably by the habenular nuclei in the pineal region. In disease of the posterior end of the third ventricle, e.g. pinealoma, posterior ventricular cysts or third ventricular hydrocephalus, for instance, post-TB meningitis, impairment of this pathway causes precocious puberty. If, on the other hand, the lesion affects the hypothalamus or anterior part of the third ventricle then delayed puberty results.

It is thought that maturation of the frontohypothalamic pathways removes the habenular inhibition, thus allowing puberty to occur. Genetic disorders, often familial, and the effects of environment may influence the timing of puberty.

ACUTE CNS DISORDERS

EPILEPSY

INTRODUCTION

Epilepsy has been recognized since ancient times and although vast improvements have been made in management over this century compared to the previous 2000 years, there are still far too many children whose lives are crippled by poorly controlled seizures.

In childhood, seizures may occur on their own as primary epilepsy, but fits also occur and may be the presenting symptom in many neurological diseases, for example neuronal ceroid lipofuscinosis, birth asphyxia, cerebral palsy and tuberous sclerosis. Epilepsy of any type may be associated with other symptoms, particularly learning disorders and/or behavior problems.

Infants and children are more prone to have seizures than adults so whilst there are only 6/1000 adults who have epilepsy, 50/1000 children will have at least one fit at some time in childhood. This appears to reflect greater neuronal excitability at certain ages as the excitatory glutamate systems and inhibitory gamma amino benzoic acid (GABA) systems do not always balance each other. This also results in the tendency to exhibit symptomatic seizures related to high fever, virus infection, minor asphyxia, medication, bacterial toxins as from *Shigella* and *Campylobacter* infection and biochemical upsets such as hypo- or hypernatremia and hypocalcemia.

Childhood epilepsy differs from adult epilepsy since the brain is a developing organ. The clinical picture is not static and the pattern of fits may change with age, e.g. infantile spasms can evolve into Lennox–Gastaut syndrome. In addition many epileptic syndromes are restricted to childhood.

TERMINOLOGY

Most clinicians make little distinction between a fit, a seizure, a convulsion and epilepsy and use these terms interchangeably. To avoid confusion we would define them as follows.

1. A fit. This is the clinical manifestation of a cerebral dysrhythmia, which may be convulsive, as in generalized tonic or tonic–clonic convulsions, or nonconvulsive as in absence seizures or complex partial seizures.

2. A seizure. A seizure describes a paroxysmal alteration in behavior due to any transient brain pathology. It includes cerebral dysrhythmias, transient ischemic or anoxic attacks, the latter being referred to as 'faints', and a miscellaneous group of paroxysmal brain abnormalities usually grouped as 'funny turns'. The commonest examples of faints are reflex anoxic seizures (cyanotic breath-holding attacks) and reflex asystole seizures (pallid syncopal attack). The ischemic episodes of migraine would also be included in this group. They should not be treated as epilepsy despite their recurrent nature.

3. A convulsion. 'All that convulses is not epilepsy.' A convulsion is the term usually used when a child shows a sudden episode of decerebrate posturing which is followed by clonic jerking. The clonic phase is often intermittent decerebrate posturing rather than a rhythmic clonic jerking. Loss of control by the cerebral cortex over the brainstem reticular formation from any cause will cause release of extensor decerebrate rigidity.

A convulsion may be due to cerebral dysrhythmia, as a true grand mal convulsion (in reality an episode of electrical decerebration) or a transient ischemic attack (acute anoxic rigidity), raised intracranial pressure with tentorial herniation or a toxic state (e.g. from drugs such as metoclopramide or haloperidol).

4. Epilepsy. Epilepsy is recurrent fits due to repeated primary cerebral dysrhythmias.

THE DIFFERENTIAL DIAGNOSIS OF FITS, FAINTS, FUNNY TURNS

The child presents with a sudden transient change in behavior, which may affect awareness, motor, emotional or cognitive ability, i.e. he has a 'seizure'. All that twitches is not epilepsy, all that convulses is not epilepsy, all attacks of sudden paroxysmal decerebrate stiffness (tonic seizure), as in Table 14.8, are not epileptic. Such fits, faints and funny turns are very well described by Stephenson (1990).

Table 14.8 Causes of paroxysmal extensor hypertonus

Central causes
Pressure decerebration (tentorial herniation and cone)
Hypoxic ischemic decerebration.
Electrical decerebration – tonic–clonic seizure
Perinatal asphyxia – extensor phase
Drugs – phenytoin, maxolon, stemetil, fentanyl, etc.
Glutaric aciduria
Mitochondrial disease
Sandifer syndrome
Dystonic cerebral palsy
Metabolic decerebration – hypocalcemia, hyperbilirubinemia
Segawa syndrome
Krabbe's leukodystrophy
Carbon monoxide poisoning
Hydrogen sulfide poisoning (coal tips)
Wilson's disease

Peripheral causes
Hyperpyrexia rigidity syndrome – muscle diseases, scoline, etc.
Tetanus

TRANSIENT ISCHEMIC ATTACKS (TIAs)

There are many causes of recurrent episodes of impaired cerebral blood flow which occur in children (Table 14.9). These may be accompanied by focal symptoms of localized brain ischemia, e.g. aphasia, hemiparesis, hallucinations, blindness, or by one of two types of generalized nonepileptic seizure:

1. the child may suddenly become pale, very floppy, lifeless with loss of posture and loss of consciousness and the mother may think the child has died;
2. the child suddenly becomes stiff with tonic extension of neck and trunk (like a banana), the eyes roll upwards and the arms stiffen and extend in front of the child. There may be myoclonic jerks.

Anoxic seizures

When anoxia is severe, loss of consciousness may occur followed often by tonic extensor rigidity and there may be a few jerks of the limbs. The EEG features consist of slowing of the background rhythm as cortical anoxia develops followed by electrical silence with reappearance of slow waves at the time of return of oxygenation. Normal rhythms then rapidly recommence.

Syncope or fainting

This is common particularly in young teenagers, it may be familial and there may be a relation to migraine. The causal mechanism is a drop in systemic blood pressure which may be gradual or sudden. In many cases it appears to be a reflex vascular phenomenon or vasovagal attack. Attacks can be brought on by emotional upset, painful stimuli, such as a cut or injection,

Table 14.9 Causes of transient ischemic attacks in children

Migraine
Reflex anoxic seizure (blue breath-holding)
Reflex anoxic (ischemic) seizure (asystole)
Paroxysmal supraventricular tachycardia
Sick sinus syndrome
Long QT syndrome
Ball valve thrombus
Atrial myxoma
Prolapsed mitral valve cusps
Infundibular spasm – Fallot's tetralogy
Vasovagal attacks
Hyperviscosity syndromes
Mitochondrial metabolic diseases
Stokes–Adams attacks – rare congenital heart block
Nonaccidental smothering
Aortic stenosis
Pericardial effusion
Intra- and postcardiac surgery
Livedo reticularis and stroke-like syndrome
Proctalgia seizure syndrome
Mitochondrial encephalopathy with lactic acidosis and stroke (MELAS)
Fabry's disease
Alternating hemiplegia syndrome

sometimes even by the description of unpleasant things or the sight of blood. Sometimes faints occur on standing up from lying or when the child has had to stand still for a long period, particularly in warm or stuffy environments.

There is usually a subjective feeling of lightheadedness, nausea, sweating, difficulty focusing or sometimes a sense of clouding of vision. This is followed by loss of tone and falling. If witnessed at the onset, the patient is said to be 'as white as a sheet' and sweaty. The collapse may be followed by stiffening of the limbs and a few brief clonic jerks and incontinence but the attack is brief and recovery rapid. There is usually no postictal somnolence but the patient is often nauseated and weak after the episodes. The diagnosis can usually be made from the history and the parents and child can be reassured that no treatment is necessary. The child may also be advised to sit down with the head between the legs at the first sign of an attack, but this may not always be sufficient to abort it.

If attacks are frequent the parent can be shown how to take the pulse during an attack to try and determine the mechanism of syncope. If these are very frequent an ambulatory ECG and cardiology opinion should be sought as occasionally such attacks are symptomatic of a cardiac arrhythmia or congenital abnormality (such as the prolonged QT syndromes or sick sinus syndrome).

BREATH-HOLDING ATTACKS

Two types of breath-holding attacks can be distinguished: cyanotic and pallid.

Cyanotic breath-holding attacks. These are common in children under the age of 5 years. They are usually precipitated by minor trauma or an emotional upset such as being scolded and frequently occur as part of a tantrum. The child cries for a few seconds and then appears to stop breathing in expiration and become rapidly cyanosed. The child then loses consciousness and falls limply. Often this is the end of the attack or it may be followed by stiffening or a few clonic jerks. If the heart rate is observed during attacks it shows usually an initial tachycardia followed by bradycardia. Rapid recovery then occurs. Such attacks may occur infrequently or may be very frequent, occurring several times each day. The parents can be reassured that the attacks are harmless and that they will stop after a few months to 2 years. No specific treatment is necessary or effective.

Pallid breath-holding attacks (reflex anoxic seizures). These attacks are inappropriately named as they are not in fact breath-holding attacks but are a type of reflex asystole which has been called a reflex anoxic seizure (Stephenson 1978). These episodes start in a similar way and are often precipitated by minor trauma or a bump to the back of the head. The child becomes suddenly pale and limp, will fall if standing and loses consciousness. This is followed by stiffening and some clonic jerking of the limbs. The whole episode is brief, 30 s to 1 min and recovery is rapid. The appearance of the child during the episode is striking and parents often describe them as lifeless and sometimes think that they have died. These episodes are due to a reflex asystole due to increased vagal responsiveness. This can be induced during EEG by the unpleasant procedure of ocular compression which will be followed by a brief asystole and possibly by a clinical attack. This procedure is not usually necessary in order to make the diagnosis. Increased vagal tone seems to be familial. These attacks do not usually require treatment. However, if they are very frequent treatment with atropine has been shown to be effective.

FUNNY TURNS

'Funny turns' or paroxysmal behaviors which may initially resemble a fit are shown in Table 14.10. These may include frank malingering, pseudoseizures or falsified seizures by a parent as part of the syndrome of Munchausen by proxy. Children with true epilepsy may simulate seizures as a means of getting out of unpleasant situations.

Violent tics such as wild swinging of an arm in a hemiballismic manner may be due to a so-called 'tic convulsif'. In paroxysmal kinesiogenic dystonia there may be sudden involuntary movements when the child moves after a rest. The Segawa type of dystonia episodes of stiffening, may be treated with anticonvulsants for years before the true disease becomes apparent. Confusion from phenytoin, fentanyl or propofol-induced dystonia and severe jitteriness from water intoxication due to faulty fluid replacement may result in intensive care units increasing anticonvulsant medication.

Stereotypies in mentally retarded children may be self-mutilating or manneristic: in the latter there may be flicking and jerking of the arms with odd hand postures, rocking back and forward on the feet or sudden vocalizations.

Sleep abnormalities, such as the child awakening, screaming, not recognizing what is said to him, not recognizing parents, mouthing, hallucinating and reaching out into space, are similar to a temporal lobe seizure or benign rolandic seizure. They occur in 10% of children and can last from seconds to 10 minutes. Somnambulism occurs in 10% of 11–12-year-olds and there is a

Table 14.10   Miscellaneous CNS paroxysmal disorders

Psychological
Hysteria
Malingering
Munchausen by proxy
Voluntary pseudoseizures
Episodic dyscontrol – impulse disorder
Cataclysmic rage reactions (e.g. Prader–Willi)
Panic attacks
Hyperventilation syndrome
Schizoid psychosis with hallucinations

Physiological
Paroxysmal kinesiogenic dystonia
Paroxysmal choreoathetosis
Sandifer dystonia with esophageal reflux
Tics – *le tic convulsif*
Gilles de la Tourette syndrome
Mannerisms – paroxysmal stereotypies
Self-mutilating stereotypies
Toddler masturbation
Laughter – Angelman syndrome
Night terrors
Sleep apnea
Hypnogogic myoclonus
Toddler cataclysmic rages
Catatonia
Catalepsy
Spontaneous clonus – neonate and severe CP
Hyperplexia
Acute labyrinthitis with drop attacks
Cerebellar fits – tonic attacks with raised ICP
Benign paroxysmal vertigo
Acute toxic delirium – glue sniffing, etc.
Paroxysmal metabolic diseases (MCAD, MSUD)
Recurrent hypoglycemia
Dystonic attacks with poisoning
Nocturnal enuresis

vacant stare, with confusion and no memory after the event. Injury may occur. The peculiar behavior during the walk may therefore closely resemble a complex partial seizure.

Jitteriness from hunger, stretches, sleep startles and spontaneous clonus all cause confusion in the neonate and myoclonus can be very marked in the normal infant. Spontaneous hamstring and arm clonus in the child with cerebral palsy may look like a clonic fit: hamstring clonus may be at 3 beats per second, but this is relieved by passively flexing the child. Hypnogogic myoclonus, i.e. violent myoclonic jerks on going off to sleep, can be sudden and repetitive.

CEREBRAL DYSRHYTHMIA

The brain has a normal hierarchy of electrical rhythms. If a discharge occurs out of synchrony, is ectopic or spreads via an alternative pathway, an abnormal rhythm or dysrhythmia is said to occur. The EEG is essential in order to demonstrate disorders of electrocerebral activity. The dysrhythmia can be acute, chronic, recurrent or continuous. The source, the route of spread and whether the electrical discharge causes local irritation or local paralysis of function determine the very many clinical paroxysmal events which might constitute a fit.

A fit is accompanied by a spike on the EEG and this requires energy to generate. The 'fitting' part of the brain therefore has a high uptake of glucose and oxygen as shown by PET scanning or magnetic resonance spectroscopy. This increased cerebral metabolism is compensated for by an increase in cerebral blood flow of up to 400%. Systemic autonomic discharge and a hypercatecholaminemia cause dilated pupils, an increase in heart rate, blood pressure and cardiac output to maintain this increased demand. Blood glucose rises to give extra substrate and CSF and plasma lactate and hypoxanthine rise if this is not being met.

Muscles require energy to maintain a convulsion and also contribute to a rise in temperature, a high creatine phosphokinase and lactic acidosis.

The cerebellum as an obligatory inhibitor of the cerebral cortex may also be important in the brain's own anticonvulsant mechanism to stop fits once they have started.

What constitutes a fit?

There are four phases of a fit.

1. The early prodrome is usually indiscernible to a casual observer but often becomes the reliable herald of an impending fit for the patient or his parents. It is a behavioral or mood change; the child becomes irritable, expansive, overactive and apparently deliberately annoying. This may last for hours and no abnormality in electroencephalography (EEG) is detectable at this stage. This may, however, be important since any lesion, be it a genetic predisposition or brain tumor, is present 24 hours a day and this prodromal period represents the change in brain biochemistry which allows a fit to occur at a particular time on a particular day.

2. When the brain starts to generate a localized electrical disturbance, an aura occurs. It is usually brief and represents a circumscribed partial fit. Its presence indicates partial onset epilepsy. However, many patients cannot appreciate it due to its brevity and it is common that patients with complex partial seizures do not report auras. The absence of aura does not imply a generalized onset fit; on the other hand this localized disturbance

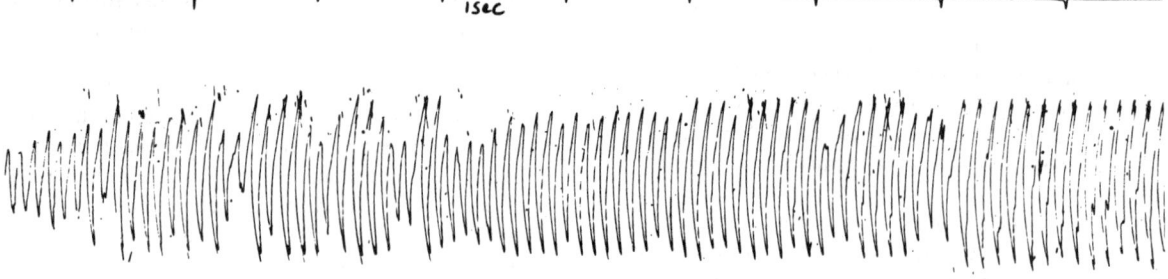

Fig. 14.18   Electroencephalogram showing 10 cycles/s ictal discharge.

may interfere with cognition which is not recognized by the child but affects learning as a transient cognitive impairment.

3. The phase of ictus then follows, which represents the fit itself. Its character depends on the spread of electrical disturbance. Most frequently it is an irritative event with positive symptoms like muscular twitching or hallucinations. But it can also be a paralytic event with negative symptoms such as loss of muscle tone or a release of inhibition over the primitive reflexes. For instance, infantile spasms are startle reflexes and adversive seizures are asymmetric tonic neck reflexes released from cortical inhibition. When the motor system is involved it becomes a simple partial seizure and when the reticular formation is involved bilaterally then consciousness is lost, i.e. a complex seizure. Fast spikes of 10 cycles per second or more 'tetanize' the brain, causing loss of cortical inhibition over the brainstem. When the midbrain centers are released a fit can manifest as doggy paddling, leg cycling or decerebrate rigidity (Fig. 14.18).

Generalized pulsed 3 per second discharge with a synchronous spike and wave in all areas is thought to arise from oscillation between the cerebral cortex and the thalamus as a result of genetic abnormality in the T type calcium ionophores in the thalamus. This blocks incoming perception with loss of awareness but the motor cortical areas are spared so that there is no loss of posture or jerking.

There is disagreement as to the importance of the cerebellum in the genesis of fits such as atonic fits where there is a sudden loss of muscle tone leading to violent falls. However, cerebellar dysfunction in the form of ataxia is a commonly seen feature of Lennox–Gastaut syndrome. Cerebellar pacing was proposed in the past as a means of controlling severe epilepsy. Experimental unilateral cerebellar ablation increases the epileptogenicity of the corresponding cerebral hemisphere. All these observations suggest the importance of cerebellum in the intrinsic antiepileptic mechanism of the central nervous system.

4. The postictal period is often marked by confusion and drowsiness. As a rule the patient should have no memory of the ictal event.

CLASSIFICATION OF EPILEPSY

Some form of classification is necessary so that therapy, prognosis and communication between professionals are possible. The most widely used and pragmatic classification of epileptic seizures is the 1981 classification of the International League Against Epilepsy (ILAE 1981) (Table 14.11). This is based on the clinically observed features of the attack and the accompanying EEG both ictally and interictally. It uses simultaneous video recordings of the seizures and the EEG to reach its conclusions.

Sadly this adds no light to the clinical situation in small children as up to 40% are difficult to classify. There are many different seizure types and a child may exhibit several at the same age (polymorphic epilepsy) or the type may change with age so that it appears as if the pediatrician could not make up his mind. We can therefore approach a classification system dependent upon type of fit, genetics, pathology or neurophysiology (Table 14.12).

This confusion has led to the development of a 'syndromic' approach to childhood epilepsy. Aspects such as seizure type, age, genetics, neurophysiology, imaging and response to medication that cluster together often enough in clinical practice suggest a specific entity or syndrome (Table 14.13).

Table 14.11   International League Against Epilepsy (1981) Classification

Partial seizures
Simple partial (focal) epilepsy
Complex partial epilepsy
   Loss of consciousness from start of fit
   Loss of consciousness after focal onset
Partial with secondary generalization
    Simple partial, then tonic–clonic
    Complex partial and then tonic–clonic

Generalized seizures
Simple absence
Complex absence
Myoclonic fits
Tonic–clonic fits
Clonic fits
Tonic fits
Atonic fits

Unclassified

Table 14.12   Classifications of epilepsy

Temporal – acute, recurrent, continuous

By syndrome

By age of onset (e.g. neonatal fits)

By type of fit (e.g. absence epilepsy)

By EEG (primary generalized, secondary generalized)

By presumed pathology (pyrexial convulsion, mesial temporal sclerosis and temporal lobe epilepsy)

By anatomy (temporal lobe, benign rolandic, benign occipital)

By etiology (idiopathic, cryptogenic, symptomatic, lesional, genetic)

By prognosis (benign epilepsies, malignant epilepsies, intractable epilepsies)

Table 14.13 Features assessed to place attacks within a particular epileptic syndrome

1. Clinical event (epileptic seizures)
2. Ictal and interictal EEG
3. Age of onset
4. Evolution and prognosis
5. Family history
6. Neurological findings, behavior or cognition
7. Determinable etiology on imaging or biochemistry
8. Precipitating factors
9. Specific response to medication
10. Anatomical locus

A CLINICAL CLASSIFICATION OF FITS (Table 14.14)

Partial seizures

Partial seizures are subdivided into simple, i.e. without alteration of consciousness; complex, with impairment of consciousness and partial seizures, which become generalized. Clearly, the most difficult aspect of this classification is the concept of altered consciousness which may be difficult to define in children. Simple partial seizures usually involve a motor event such as clonic jerking of one part of the body or may involve a sensory event such as paresthesia or an unusual taste or smell. Although psychic

Table 14.14 Clinical classification of fits

Tonic–clonic seizures (grand mal)

Tonic seizure

Clonic seizure

Simple absence seizure (including petit mal)

Complex absence

Myoclonic seizure

Infantile spasms

Astatic/atonic seizure (drop attacks)

Adversive seizure

Simple partial (focal) (includes jacksonian)

Complex partial (psychomotor)

Cognitive (transient cognitive impairments)

Reading epilepsy

Behavioral

Coprolalic

Orgasmic

Gelastic

Cursive

Happy clappers and pat-a-cake

Ictal amblyopia

Ictal eye deviation and pupil dilation

Autonomic tachycardia and hypertension

Respiratory arrhythmia, apnea, cyanotic attacks

symptoms have been described as the sole feature of a simple partial seizure in adults, such an occurrence in children is exceptional. Complex partial seizures may start with preservation of consciousness as a simple partial seizure and then progress or there may be alteration of consciousness from the onset. Both simple partial and complex partial seizures may spread to become generalized.

Generalized seizures

Generalized seizures must be defined by there being no evidence of a localized onset. It is possible that in some of these cases the seizure is arising from an undetectable locus, e.g. in medial temporal lobe, orbital surface of frontal lobe or cingulate gyrus.

Absence seizures

Absence seizures are those in which there is unresponsiveness and loss of consciousness from the onset without major motor accompaniments or loss of posture. They may be associated with phenomena such as blinking, slight decreases in tone or automatic behavior. Thus absences are subdivided into simple and complex depending on the duration and other associated motor phenomena. They are also classified as typical and atypical based on their speed of onset, length and on the presence or absence of 3 cycles/s spike and wave on the EEG. Such a distinction is not always possible and may be somewhat artificial (see below). Absence seizures occur in many different clinical settings (see Table 14.19).

Unclassifiable seizures are those in which either there is a lack of data or it is unclear whether the seizures are generalized or partial in onset (e.g. infantile spasms, gelastic seizures).

Acute dysrhythmias (Table 14.15)

These complicate acute diseases of the nervous system such as trauma (birth trauma, accidental and nonaccidental head injuries),

Table 14.15 Cause of acute cerebral dysrhythmias

1. Accidental trauma
2. Nonaccidental trauma
3. Birth trauma
4. Perinatal hypoxia/ischemia
5. Postcardiac bypass
6. Poisoning
7. Metabolic disease: hypocalcemia, hypomagnesemia, alkalosis, hyperventilation tetany (Rett's), hyponatremia, hypoglycemia, acute porphyria, biotinidase deficiency, holocarboxylase synthetase deficiency, carnisonase deficiency, hyperglycinemia, CSF hyperglycinorachia, MELAS (mitochondrial encephalopathy with lactic acidosis and stroke-like episodes), MERRF (myoclonic epilepsy with ragged red fibers), Leigh's encephalopathy (pyruvic dehydrogenase and decarboxylase), complex II (myoclonic epilepsy with progressive dementia and choreoathetosis), Menkes' disease, sulfite oxidase deficiency
8. Meningitis
9. Encephalitis
10. Febrile convulsions syndrome
11. Cerebral tumor
12. Drug induced
13. Stroke

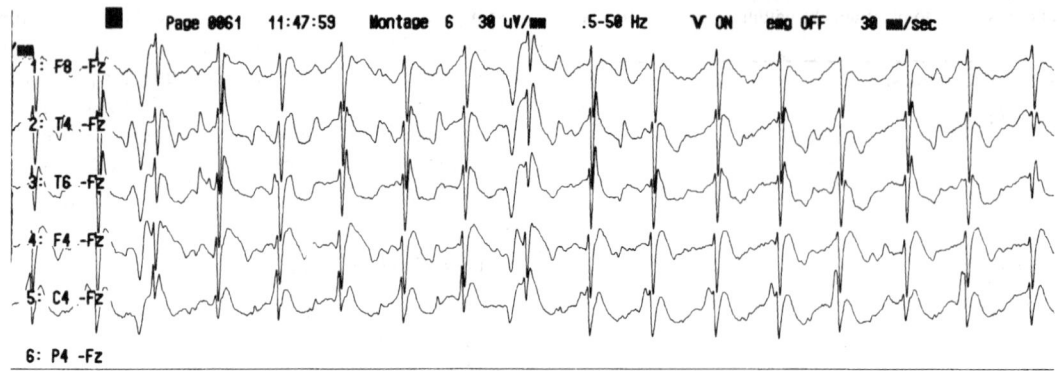

Fig. 14.19 Acute cerebral dysrhythmia induced by intrathecal injection of penicillin with 1 cycle/s spike and wave discharges.

acute asphyxial episodes (neonatal asphyxia, cardiac arrest and complications of cardiac surgery, drowning and smothering), meningitis, encephalitis, metabolic upset (e.g. hypocalcemia or hypoglycemia), inborn errors of metabolism (e.g. glycine encephalopathy, hyperammonemias, mitochondriopathies) and poisoning, including bacterial toxins such as from *Shigella* or *Campylobacter*.

The fits usually do not recur once the acute encephalopathy has settled. Fits are often a reason for anticonvulsant therapy during the acute illness but are not an indication for long-term therapy. The original pathology may itself cause a long-term chronic brain damage syndrome with epilepsy as an ongoing symptom. An acute dysrhythmia can be totally intractable, drug resistant or fatal as after the inadvertent injection of an overdose of intrathecal penicillin (Fig. 14.19).

Febrile convulsions in the young child can be regarded as such an acute dysrhythmia which occurs in response to an acute viral infection in a genetically predisposed child at a physiologically vulnerable age.

Chronic dysrhythmia

Chronic recurrent dysrhythmias

Recurrent clinical fits from recurrent cerebral dysrhythmia (not due to a recurrent pathology) is what we normally mean by the term 'epilepsy'. There may be a recurrent precipitant such as smells, sounds, flashing lights, television, video display unit, hyperventilation or strong emotion.

Continuous epilepsy (status epilepticus – Table 14.16)

A continuous cerebral dysrhythmia is status epilepticus. Any type of seizure disorder can become continuous and the concept of status epilepticus has in the past been too narrowly restricted to convulsive status. Nonconvulsive status lasting hours or days complicates many of the syndromes responsible for intractable epilepsy in childhood. Cognitive status epilepticus may occur in West's syndrome with severe autism and in Landau–Kleffner syndrome with aphasia. Difficulties in diagnosis arise when there is electrical status in sleep or when the clinical manifestations are subtle with slow reaction times, drooling, cessation of learning or speech abnormalities rather than motor fits.

DIAGNOSTIC TOOLS

EEG

No cardiologist would ever attempt to diagnose and treat a cardiac dysrhythmia without ECG assistance yet there are many pediatricians who happily treat presumed cerebral dysrhythmias without an EEG. It is our practice to carry out an EEG in all children known to have had an epileptic seizure and in those in whom the diagnosis is suspected.

Use of the EEG

1. It may give confirmation of the type of abnormality expected from the history, e.g. generalized 3 cycles/s spike and wave, rolandic spikes, hypsarrhythmia, photoconvulsive response, electrical status in sleep (ESIS).
2. It may suggest a focal abnormality where the history was that of a generalized seizure.
3. It may allow assessment of response to therapy, e.g. disappearance of hypsarrhythmia, abolition of 3 cycles/s spike and wave, the photoconvulsive response, benzodiazepine sensitivity testing, abolition of nonconvulsive status.

Table 14.16 Classification of status epilepticus

Convulsive status epilepticus
Generalized
   Primary generalized
   Secondary generalized
Partial
   Simple partial (jacksonian status or epilepsia partialis continua)
   Complex partial status
Myoclonic status

Nonconvulsive status epilepticus
Absence status
Lennox–Gastaut status
True petit mal status
Complex partial status (psychomotor fugue state)
Cognitive status
   Aphasia in Landau–Kleffner syndrome
   ? Some learning disorders
Behavioral status
   Some epileptic schizophrenic syndromes
   Autistic syndrome with West's syndrome
      Hyperkinetic cataclysmic rage reactions (Landau–Kleffner syndrome, left-sided epilepsy in boys)
      Gelastic laughing in hypothalamic hamartoma

4. It may show an abnormal background that suggests a diffuse disturbance of cerebral function underlying the seizures, e.g. tumor, or encephalitis, e.g. subacute sclerosing panencephalitis (SSPE).
5. A seizure may occur during the recording, which allows the site of origin to be made with more certainty than simply the presence of an interictal spike.
6. If epileptiform discharges are frequent it makes a diagnosis of clinical paroxysmal events much more likely to be that of epilepsy, but not certain.

Limitations of EEG

1. The recording lasts only 20–30 min and is a small sample of the patient's life.
2. In epileptic patients there is enormous variability from one recording to another.
3. The recording is usually interictal, i.e. fits are not usually recorded and thus the abnormalities seen are not necessarily those that occur with the seizure.
4. Epileptiform activity can occur in normal patients without seizures, but this is rare (perhaps 1% of the normal population).
5. An epileptic-looking EEG does not mean that the attacks the patient is having are epileptic seizures.
6. Normal EEGs can occur in epileptic patients, but this probably only occurs in up to 10% of cases.

Because of these difficulties various activation procedures are used to try and increase the yield of EEG abnormalities. These are:

1. *Hyperventilation.* If this is performed well for 2–3 min it leads to hypocapnia and cerebral vasoconstriction and this appears to increase cortical excitation. This may then precipitate paroxysmal activity, slow waves, spike and waves or a seizure. It is most useful in the diagnosis of absence epilepsy when it causes generalized 3 cycles/s spike and wave discharge. Hyperventilation in children normally causes a slowing of background and an increase in amplitude and this should not be regarded as abnormal.

2. *Intermittent photic stimulation.* In this procedure the child is asked to look at a bright light that is flashing at a varying rate from 1 to 50 cycles/s. The normal response is for there to be small amplitude rhythmical spikes detectable occipitally at the rate of the flash stimulus – flicker following. Some patients respond with a clear epileptiform discharge and may have a seizure (photoconvulsive response) (Fig. 14.20). The photoconvulsive response shows age-dependent expression, being most readily observed between the ages of 5 and 15, and is evidence of a lowered convulsive threshold that is genetically determined (see Photosensitive epilepsy below).

3. *Sleep.* Because of the tendency for both seizures and EEG abnormalities to be enhanced during sleep, recording a sleep EEG can increase the diagnostic yield of the procedure. Sleep can either be natural or drug induced. Advantage can be taken of young children's tendency for sleep during the day and the EEG arranged around that. Babies will often sleep after a feed. In older children a relaxing peaceful atmosphere in the EEG recording room can help them to fall asleep naturally. If these methods are not possible then induced sleep may be necessary with, for example, chlorpromazine, which has the added theoretical advantage of lowering the convulsive threshold. Benzodiazepines are

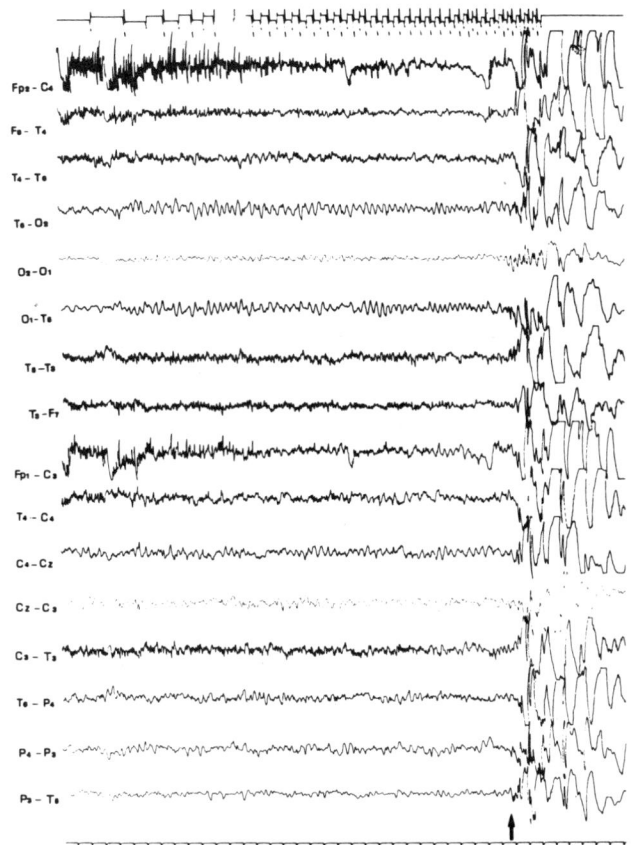

Fig. 14.20 Photoconvulsive response: paroxysmal activity induced by flashing light (arrow).

anticonvulsants and will abolish seizure activity. During sleep there are several types of paroxysmal activity which are physiological, e.g. sleep spindles, K complexes and vertex sharp waves. These must not be confused with epileptical activity (Fig. 14.21). A further type of activation that has been advocated is sleep deprivation.

If such routine EEG recordings fail to show any abnormalities and the diagnosis is in doubt then other more specialized or invasive procedures can be used. The most readily available technique is ambulatory monitoring where the EEG is recorded on to a small cassette recorder which the patient wears attached to a belt or clothing. Such recorders can record nine channels of EEG for 24 h to ordinary magnetic tape. The tape is then played back at high speed on to a VDU and the abnormalities can be further analyzed or recorded to paper if required.

For such a procedure to be useful it is essential that the parents or nurses keep an accurate diary of events and document any unusual behavior or seizures. If the paroxysmal events being investigated are occurring less than once every 24 h then it is wasteful of resources to carry out ambulatory monitoring as the chance of recording an event is low.

Video/EEG studies. The ideal is to record simultaneously both the clinical seizure and the EEG and to play them back synchronously. The indications for this type of intensive monitoring are similar to those for ambulatory monitoring and include particularly preoperative assessment of partial seizures where the site of origin of the seizures is uncertain.

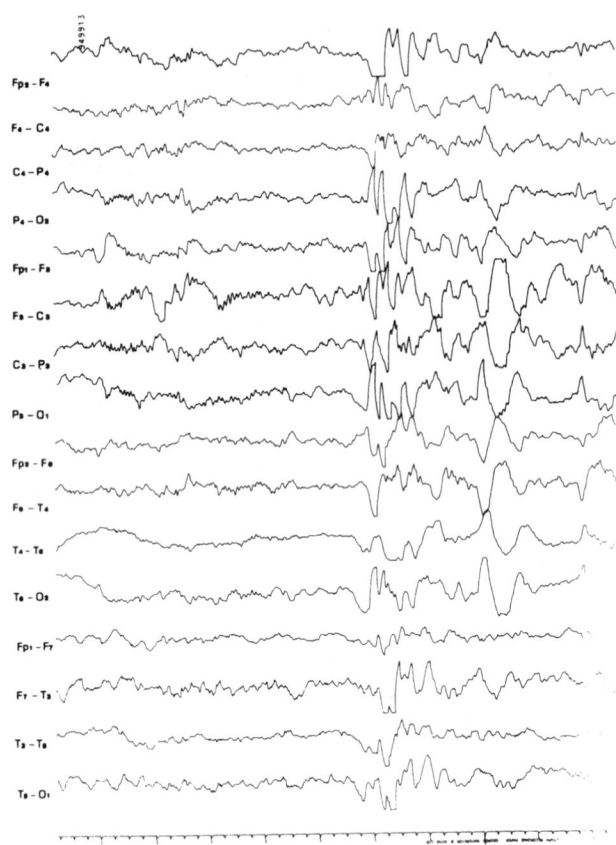

Fig. 14.21 Normal sleep EEG with sleep spindles and K complexes.

Special techniques. If localization is required more precisely than is available from scalp electrode recording, e.g. when contemplating surgery or investigation of bizarre behavior, special electrode techniques can be used. These include implanted surface electrodes, implanted depth electrodes and sphenoidal electrode recordings.

Neuroimaging

Skull X-ray

This has a very limited role in the neuroimaging of pediatric patients with epilepsy. In nonaccidental head injury presenting with fits the skull X-ray may reveal linear or expanding fractures. Skull X-ray can be used in the assessment of bone flaps and to visualize the position of grids, strips and depth electrodes after placement. A new use for skull X-ray has been created in screening patients suspected of having intracranial metallic materials prior to MRI.

Cranial ultrasound

Ultrasonography is a noninvasive, inexpensive, portable, real-time and multiplanar imaging modality well suited for the study of infants during the perinatal period and during the first year of life whilst the ultrasonic window (anterior fontanel) is patent. Imaging which does not depend upon ionizing radiation is desirable in children less than 4 years during the period of rapid brain growth. It has a place in preterm infants with apnea or seizures. It is useful in the diagnosis of neonatal hypoxic ischemic encephalopathy, suspected development malformation, hydrocephalus, infections and hemorrhage.

Computed tomography

The role of CT scan in the investigation of epilepsy is limited. CT scanning is superior to MRI in imaging blood (e.g. subdural, subarachnoid and intracerebral), CSF and bone. It is superior to conventional X-rays and MRI in detecting calcification. It is inferior to MRI in defining brain structure and pathology but is useful in the acute management of seizures, e.g. in confirming or excluding raised intracranial pressure prior to a lumbar puncture.

The strength of CT is its low cost, ready availability and its ease of use; it provides a relatively reliable imaging modality for physiologically unstable patients. The biggest disadvantage is the large amount of radiation to which the brain is exposed, especially when performing repeated scans as in the measurement of ventricular size with shunted hydrocephalus.

MRI

MRI is the imaging procedure of choice in the investigation of children with epilepsy (Jackson 1994). The advantages include the use of nonionizing radiation, high sensitivity and higher specificity than CT scan, multiplanar imaging capability, improved contrast of soft tissue and high anatomical resolution. This is particularly valuable in showing differences between white and gray matter and in highlighting differences between various types of tissue in the cerebral parenchyma. The technique enables sections to be made in any plane without moving the patient and bone artifact is ignored so that the posterior and temporal fossae show clearly. It is of great value in the diagnosis of malformations and tumors and for imaging structures such as the medial surface of the temporal lobe or the orbital surface of the frontal lobe which are often difficult to image on CT. It is important to recognize that MRI interpretation in the infant varies with the degree of myelination paralleling the normal development and maturational changes observed through the first 4 years of life. Patients with genetic epilepsies rarely have MRI scan abnormality.

Indications for MRI scan are as follows:

1. all children with epilepsy starting in the first year of life with the exception of febrile convulsions;
2. all children with focal neurological signs;
3. all children with partial seizures excluding those with benign partial epilepsy with central temporal spikes (see below);
4. all patients with intractable seizures or seizures that are becoming worse;
5. patients with bizarre but well-documented paroxysmal behavior (autism, aphasia, mood changes and aggressive outbursts) that may or may not be epileptic;
6. follow-up scans in patients with continuing poorly controlled epilepsy.

The scans of patients with epilepsy starting in the first year of life have been reported to be abnormal in 68% of cases. In patients with partial seizures between 40% and 70% of scans may be abnormal (Kendall 1988).

Positron emission tomography (PET)

PET scans allow determination of the intensity and site of metabolic processes within the brain. The patient is given an injection of a positron-emitting compound such as 18 fluorodeoxyglucose and after a period of time is scanned using a positron detector. A computed tomogram is then produced which allows quantification and localization of the metabolic processes in which the labeled compound is participating, e.g. glucose metabolism or oxygen consumption. Such a technique is at present a research tool and is unavailable in most centers. It is, however, being used in the preoperative assessment of patients going for epilepsy surgery. Such scans show hypometabolism at the site of the focus in the interictal state, with marked hypermetabolism during seizures. It is in the selection of infants with infantile spasms that a metabolic lesionectomy, i.e. of the hypometabolic area, usually parietooccipital, has been claimed to be most effective (Chugani et al 1990).

The use of PET scanning with labeled drugs such as benzodiazepines enables the localization of receptors within the brain.

Single photon emission computed tomography (SPECT)

SPECT images are created by recording emission of photons from radiotracers injected intravenously and trapped within brain tissue (English & Brown 1990). Sensitivity has improved markedly since the construction of gamma cameras with multiple detectors. The knowledge that metabolism and blood flow are coupled and that both blood flow and metabolism increase during ictal events and are decreased in the interictal state substantiates the application of cerebral blood flow imaging in epilepsy.

Interictal SPECT. Interictal measurement of cerebral blood flow by SPECT with (^{99}Tc)-HMPAO has been used in epilepsy for nearly a decade, almost exclusively as a method for localizing the epileptogenic zone in patients with refractory partial epilepsy considered for surgical treatment. When cerebral blood flow demonstrates regional reduction in a patient with partial epilepsy, it can help to confirm EEG localization of a lesion.

Ictal SPECT. The singular attraction of ictal SPECT remains the potential to image functional changes at the onset of an epileptic seizure by giving an injection of the radioligand at the time. This freezes the image; the scan itself can be performed later under more controlled conditions. This is being recognized as valuable because the clinical seizure does not always originate from the electrical focus seen on the EEG in the interictal period.

Receptor imaging with SPECT is in its infancy, but demonstration of reduction in benzodiazepine receptors in epileptic patients makes it of particular promise as a localizing method.

Newer techniques

These includes magnetic resonance spectroscopy (MRS), magnetic resonance relaxometry (MRR), functional magnetic resonance imaging and receptor PET studies.

Functional mapping

Established functional mapping techniques include the intracarotid amylobarbital procedure (WADA test) for identifying language dominance and adequacy of memory in both hemispheres. Mapping is also possible with direct intraoperative cortical stimulation.

THE EPILEPSY SYNDROMES

We can further classify epileptic syndromes into three main groups – genetic, lesional and malignant epilepsies. Although this does not produce a completely watertight classification, it helps in clinical management and seems to be helpful for treatment, e.g. genetic epilepsies by valproate, lesional epilepsies by voltage-gated sodium ionophore-mediated drugs and malignant epilepsies by GABA enhancement.

GENETIC EPILEPSIES (Table 14.17)

Introduction

These include various syndromes in which the primary cause is thought to be genetic. Genetic factors can, however, influence seizures in three different ways.

1. Genetic tendency to fits (threshold). The familial tendency is thought to be carried on chromosome 6 and to be age dependent in its manifestation. Unless EEG studies with hyperventilation and photic provocation are carried out between 3 and 15 years one may miss the dominant transmission as clinical fits may not occur. Precipitation of fits by computer games has reinforced this as an important area. Lennox 50 years ago showed that the number of close relatives with an epileptic EEG was six times higher with known epileptics than with normal controls.

2. Genetic epileptic syndromes. Diseases in which epilepsy is the only major manifestation include febrile convulsions, photoconvulsive epilepsy, the benign myoclonic epilepsy of infancy which occurs in identical fashion in identical twins and the severe form of myoclonic epilepsy of Dravet. Certain EEG patterns such as synchronization and generalization of 3 per second spike and wave activity, a photoconvulsive response, electrical status in sleep and a hyperventilation synchrony with spikes also all suggest a genetic tendency to fits.

3. Genetic diseases with epilepsy as a main symptom (Table 14.18). There are more than 200 Mendelian conditions with epilepsy as a main symptom.

Tuberous sclerosis is a good example of how a genetic disease may present as any one of the three clinical forms, i.e. genetic, lesional or malignant.

- There is incomplete penetrance so uncomplicated epilepsy may occur in members of the family without any other clinical manifestation of the disease.
- Single or multiple small gliomas, hamartomas and tubers act as focal 'lesions'.
- Malignant epilepsy such as West's syndrome or Lennox–Gastaut syndrome can occur in the infant of a tuberous sclerosis mother, especially after several generations. Dominant inheritance causes worse disease when acquired from the mother and may result in brain malformation with cortical dysplasia.

Some EEG studies in the siblings of children with generalized epilepsy or identical twin studies suggest that the generalized spike and wave EEG pattern is inherited as an autosomal dominant trait with age-dependent expression. Other workers have suggested that a polygenic inheritance is a better explanation of the data. The risk for siblings of patients with generalized epilepsy ranges from 4% to 8% which is substantially lower than

Table 14.17 The genetic epilepsies

Epilepsy	Age of onset	Seizure type	EEG/imaging	Genetics	Prognosis	Treatment	Neurology
1. Benign familial neonatal seizures	2–3 days of age. Rarely lasts more than 3 months	Short seizures, usually clonic +/– apnea. Occ tonic, focal or multifocal	No EEG criteria, imaging normal	AD, chromosome 20- nonsense mutation of acetylcholine receptor (Leppert et al 1989)	Good. Occasionally seizures later in childhood	Treatment not often required. Phenobarbitone, phenytoin or nitrazepam. Often resistant to medication	Normal development
2. Idiopathic partial epilepsy of infancy	Usually about 6 weeks age, several a day for few days	Simple partial seizures	Interictal EEG normal, ictal unilateral parietal or occipital spike discharges. Imaging normal	50% family history, ? related to dominant neonatal fits. Others on chromosome 19	Short duration. There may be several bouts. Excellent prognosis	No treatment is required as the condition is self-limiting	Neurology normal
3. Benign myoclonic epilepsy of infancy	Onset 6 months to 3 years – mean 10 months	Severe myoclonus in arms and upper torso	Photoconvulsive, 3/s spike and wave	AR seen in identical twins	Most normal or needing some learning support but may be overactive with major behavior problems	Very valproate sensitive	Normal development. Often mistaken for NAI
4. Childhood absence epilepsy (petit mal)	3–12 years, peak 6–7 years	Abrupt onset and finish; all actions stop and child freezes; conscious awareness lost, face looks blank of emotion, eyes are open and stare; no response to threat, no loss of posture, no incontinence, no forced grasping, no sniffing or lip smacking. Episodes rarely last > 15 s. Pyknolepsy = many absences close together (possibly 100+ in clusters especially when quiet and going off or awakening from sleep. More marked when bored, less when alert and attentive. Precipitated by hyperventilation and may be photoconvulsive	Normal background, bilateral synchronous symmetrical 3/s spike and wave. Imaging should be normal in true petit mal	AD, variable penetrance and age-dependent expression; 60–70% female	80% become seizure free. Occasionally tonic-clonic seizures develop 5–10 years after onset of absences. In 6% absence seizures persist there is an overlap with juvenile myoclonic epilepsy (p. 681)	Treatment of simple absence: (1) valproate; (2) ethosuximide; (3) combination or alternation of 1 and 2; (4) lamotrigine	Neurology normal, behavior usually normal with no severe learning difficulties (contrast with complex absences when behavior is usually abnormal and learning disorder common)
5. Photosensitive epilepsy	Median age onset 14 years, suggests puberty is a factor	Seizures may occur spontaneously or in response to flickering light or patterns. Seizures provoked are tonic-clonic or myoclonic absences. Partial seizures are rare	The basic EEG is normal, photoconvulsive response consists of spike and wave or polyspike and wave over all areas	Photosensitive epilepsy is genetically inherited and more common in females	The seizures are amenable to treatment but the photosensitivity persists	Valproate is the treatment of choice	Photosensitivity is found in five main groups: 1. Pure photosensitivity epilepsy 2. Epilepsy with photosensitivity 3. Eyelid myoclonia with absences 4. Self-induced epilepsy 5. Pattern-sensitive epilepsy
6. Epilepsy with myoclonic absences	7 years	Absences accompanied by severe bilateral rhythmical clonic jerks, often associated with tonic contractions	Ictal EEG; bilateral synchronous and symmetrical discharge of rhythmical spike-wave at 3 s, similar to childhood absences. Interictal EEG; normal background activity with superimposed generalized slow waves in one-third of cases	Male preponderance		High doses of both sodium valproate and ethosuximide. Lamotrigine is reported as effective in refractory cases	Neurology exam normal, mental retardation present in 45%. During the disease mental retardation occurs in a further 25%

Table 14.17 Cont'd

Epilepsy	Age of onset	Seizure type	EEG/imaging	Genetics	Prognosis	Treatment	Neurology
7. Juvenile absence epilepsy	Puberty	Overall frequency low. Usually absences but may have generalized tonic-clonic on waking	EEG – 3/s spike and wave		Good	Good response to valproate	Normal
8. Juvenile myoclonic epilepsy	Pre- to postpuberty	Predominantly on waking – bilateral jerking of upper arms and shoulders. Full consciousness. Frequently photosensitive and provoked by sleep withdrawal	Ictal; >3/s generalized often irregular spike-waves. Interictal; often polyspike waves	? Chromosome 6	Excellent response to treatment, but a high rate of relapse when medication withdrawn	Sodium valproate is the drug of choice (carbamazepine will exacerbate the seizures)	Normal
9. Benign Rolandic epilepsy (benign epilepsy with centrotemporal spikes)	Commonest form of epilepsy in children between 3 and 15, rare after 20 years	Fits likely to awaken from sleep with tingling in face mouth, lips, teeth and gums, and hand, speech arrest may be marked and drooling prominent. Consciousness usually preserved but can progress to generalized convulsion	High voltage, phase-reversing epileptic spike; often rather blunted, discharges focal and unilateral to central region (rolandic area) on one side. The side may change. Discharge accentuated by sleep (33% only in sleep). Imaging is normal	AD with variable penetrance very age dependent in its expression. Family history from 10 to 70%	Usually good, particularly for those with centrotemporal spikes where all cases resolve. But if the abnormal EEG discharge originates from areas other than this, the prognosis is slightly less favorable	Very sensitive to carbamazepine. Tendency to spontaneous remission. Treatment required if day seizures as well as nocturnal. Carbamazepine may precipitate continuous spike discharge in slow wave sleep (electrical status in sleep) in some patients. Nocturnal epileptic activity abolished by intravenous diazepam and so nitrazepam at night may suffice in some. Valproate may be useful	Absence of neurological and intellectual deficit. Recently families of benign rolandic seizures with articulatory dyspraxia have been described. Speech arrest may occur. Suggestion has been made that some cases of Landau–Kleffner syndrome who also developed electrical status in sleep may represent a not so benign variant (Scheffer et al 1995). Benign to malignant spectrum
10. Benign occipital with occipital spike-waves	Usually around 6 years of age	Transient scotomata, visual hallucinations which may be followed by partial or generalized motor seizure. Headaches closely resembling migraine may follow the seizure and cause problems in diagnosis	Interictal paroxysms of high amplitude spike-wave, recurring more or less rhythmically on the occipital and posterotemporal areas of one or both hemispheres and occurring only when eyes are closed		Usually remits in adolescence	This disorder is difficult to treat (drug resistant)	

Table 14.18 Known genetic markers and epileptic syndromes

1. Tuberous sclerosis (? 3 loci) – chromosome 9, 11, 12

2. Neurofibromatosis
   Peripheral – chromosome 17
   Central – chromosome 22

3. Juvenile myoclonic epilepsy – chromosome 6

4. Photic/absences – chromosome 6

5. Dominant neonatal fits – chromosome 20

6. Partial epilepsy with auditory symptoms – chromosome 10q

7. Frontal lobe epilepsy with nocturnal fits – chromosome 20q

8. Angelman syndrome – chromosome 15

9. Metabolic genetic epileptic syndromes

would be expected from a simple gene disorder. Partial epilepsies have often been regarded as nongenetic or lesional types of epilepsy. However, certain types do show clear genetic influence. These include benign partial epilepsies of childhood and posttraumatic epilepsy.

Siblings and offspring of affected probands have a three- to four-fold increase in febrile convulsion rate compared with the general population. Interpretation of family studies on febrile convulsions has resulted in conflicting conclusions: the inheritance has been said to be autosomal dominant, autosomal recessive or polygenic. The relationship of febrile convulsions to epilepsy is complex and there is some evidence that there may be two genetically distinct subtypes of febrile convulsions with different risks of subsequent epilepsy. In addition many children with febrile convulsions will subsequently show generalized spike and wave on EEG even though they do not have convulsions, as do a high proportion of siblings.

By discovering a linkage between juvenile myoclonic epilepsy and HLA markers, the gene responsible was successfully mapped to human chromosome 6p (Durner et al 1991). The locus was subsequently designated *EJM1*. Then by virtue of the close association of juvenile myoclonic epilepsy and other generalized epilepsy disorders (childhood pyknoleptic absence epilepsy (typical absence epilepsy), grand mal seizures on early morning awakening, photoconvulsive television or video game epilepsy), together with the high incidence of EEG abnormality in the close relatives, investigators concluded that the gene imparts a tendency for abnormal electrical activity to synchronize and generalize in histologically normal cerebral cortices.

The various epileptic syndromes are actually the different ways in which this tendency expresses itself (Delgado-Escueta et al 1990, Greenberg et al 1995). Juvenile myoclonic epilepsy can be considered the prototype which has a mixture of all three types of absence, myoclonic and generalized tonic–clonic fits, while the rest are milder variants or *forme fruste*. The expression of the gene is highly age dependent, just as childhood absence epilepsy tends to resolve after adolescence. Family screening cannot be reliably done by EEG alone as it may be absent in older individuals. Linkage or DNA analysis might be necessary.

A recent report of a linkage study showed no evidence for a locus on chromosome 6p in some British and Swedish families with juvenile myoclonic epilepsy and primary grand mal seizures (Whitehouse et al 1993). It is therefore reasonable to conclude that there is more than one gene carrying the tendency for

generalized fits. It is interesting to note that valproic acid is an effective antiepileptic drug for these syndromes. It is different from other drugs in that it is a fatty acid with eight carbon molecules. Eight-carbon fatty acids are anticonvulsants and 10-carbon fatty acids are anesthetic agents. Octanoic acid was thought to be the fatty acid with antiepileptic properties in the ketogenic diet. The fact that valproic acid appears specific for many genetic epilepsies suggests that it may correct an underlying metabolic abnormality. Hopefully gene cloning will provide insight into the mechanism of the fits as well as the antiepileptic action of valproic acid.

We would not include causes of hypoglycemia, hypocalcemia or hypomagnesemia in this group. These are acute dysrhythmias which complicate acute encephalopathy and it is the encephalopathy which may be recurrent and not simply the fits. Conditions such as mitochondrial encephalopathy with lactic acidosis and stroke-like episodes syndrome (MELAS syndrome) and myoclonic epilepsy with ragged red fibers (MERRF) are included. These disorders have either a known enzyme defect or morphological evidence of storage abnormality but the enzyme defect is still unknown. They are almost invariably associated with other neurological abnormality, particularly intellectual deterioration. Thus the presence of family history with a symptomatic combination of fits and mental retardation should trigger a search for inborn errors of metabolism as this has implications for treatment and genetic counseling.

Genetic epilepsy syndromes (Table 14.17)

There are many genetic epilepsy syndromes, some common, some rare (Table 14.17). The key features are outlined in the table but febrile convulsions are also detailed in the text below in view of their frequency.

Febrile convulsions

Febrile convulsions are the commonest type of genetic abnormality; 5% of all children will have a fit under 5 years, 3% of whom fulfill the criteria for febrile convulsions. The incidence is higher in Japan at 7–8%.

Definition and causation. A febrile convulsion is an acute cerebral dysrhythmia, usually in response to a *viral illness* in a *genetically predisposed child* at *a physiologically vulnerable age*. It is not strictly epilepsy as repeated seizures occur due to repeated and not persistent pathology. In some Third World countries a fit with fever can be the commonest cause of death.

Age of onset. Febrile convulsions are one of the most age-dependent types of epileptic syndrome. There are normal convulsant and anticonvulsant systems in the brain. It is thought the balance between these two systems varies at different ages, so that the convulsant threshold is not static throughout childhood. The age range shows a normal distribution curve from 6 months to 5 years with a mean of 20 months and 90% occurring before 3 years, with only 5% occurring less than 6 months of age or after 4 years. The incidence is slightly higher in boys than girls, but they tend to occur earlier in girls due to their more accelerated brain development.

Infection. By definition it is usual to exclude primary infections of the CNS, i.e. encephalitis and meningitis. However, in an epidemic of echo virus infection a seizure may be indicative of a mild encephalitis. A fit may be the only manifestation of acquired infection with Epstein–Barr virus or toxoplasma.

Gastroenteritis poses a particular problem. In a study by Avital (1982) of 117 children with *Shigella* gastroenteritis, 31% presented with convulsions and up to 25% of children with *Campylobacter* infections may present with convulsions. In these cases the fits are secondary to a toxic encephalopathy due to a circulating toxin from the gut organism. In a similar way Shiga or Vera toxins from *E. coli* 0157 may cause fits associated with the hemolytic-uremic syndrome. Fits in children with gastroenteritis may also be due to a secondary metabolic upset, e.g. hyponatremia, hypernatremia, hypocalcemia, hypomagnesemia. None of the above should be regarded as febrile convulsions. Pertussis immunization can cause a fit associated with fever, but there is dispute over whether this is a true febrile convulsion or a toxic encephalopathy from pertussinogen. It is thought that there are specific pertussinogen receptors on cells which activate cyclic AMP.

Evidence for virus infection can be found in over 90% of children with rigorous virus isolation techniques, rising antibody titers, changes in interferon or complement levels. In 85% of children the infection is in the upper respiratory tract.

Children with viral infections without fits often show EEG abnormalities, i.e. excess slow waves which are not seen with bacterial infection. Children who have had a febrile convulsion will have posterior slow waves for several weeks after the fit. Children with measles may show EEG abnormalities in over 90% of the cases. It is therefore postulated that viruses cause an encephalopathy due to their obligatory intracellular existence without causing encephalitis; bacterial infection is more likely to produce encephalopathy due to a toxin.

Pyrexia. The rate of rise and the maximum temperature have no influence on the occurrence of a seizure. A child may have a febrile convulsion at 38° and the following week may have a temperature greater than 39° and no convulsion will be precipitated. Higher fever from bacterial URTI may not cause a fit.

Genetics. Fifty percent will have a family history of fits and the commonest transmission is autosomal dominant with reduced penetrance. Eighty percent of monozygotic twins are concordant for febrile convulsions.

Type of seizure. Most febrile convulsions are short generalized tonic–clonic seizures but 4–18% will be unilateral. Only a few children will have more than one seizure during the same febrile episode; 4–30% of cases are long, lasting more than 30 min. Such long seizures are usually the child's first seizure and account for a quarter of all cases of status epilepticus in childhood. A postictal hemiparesis lasting for a few hours to a few days may occur in such a seizure. Febrile seizures can last for up to several hours and be followed by permanent hemiplegia: the hemiconvulsion, hemiplegia, epilepsy syndrome.

Investigations and management. The main differential diagnosis is meningitis, nonaccidental injury or metabolic disease. The history and examination may suggest an obvious source of the fever such as an otitis media or pharyngitis but this should not prevent a high index of suspicion for more serious infection, e.g. pneumococcal meningitis. Up to 25% of cases of pneumococcal meningitis may present with a fit, pyrexia and an otitis media. Under the age of 6 months a convulsion associated with fever should be considered as a sign of CNS infection. Between 6 and 18 months the signs of meningitis are nonspecific and our policy would be to do a lumbar puncture in all patients in this age range presenting with a first febrile convulsion. Over 18 months a selective policy is used: if the child appears well, fully conscious

with no signs of meningism and has an obvious source of infection lumbar puncture can be avoided. However, if such a decision is made and the child is not admitted to hospital the doctor must review the child over the next 24 h for change in condition.

If the child has not recovered consciousness on arrival in hospital the assessment is more difficult. If he has been given diazepam or phenobarbitone prior to admission then this may be the reason. Detailed examination needs to be performed looking for signs of raised intracranial pressure or focal neurological abnormality. If these are present then the management should be as for an acute encephalopathy with raised ICP and imaging must precede lumbar puncture.

EEG. An EEG carried out in the week after a febrile convulsion will be abnormal in a third of cases, showing posterior slow wave activity which may be bilateral or unilateral. Such abnormalities are not helpful for the prediction of subsequent epilepsy. The EEG at a later age, e.g. 5 years, often shows abnormality such as spike and wave activity which indicates a genetic predisposition but not that the child has epilepsy.

Prognosis. Excellent; less than 3% develop long-term epilepsy despite the strong genetic predisposition, but the prognosis is more guarded if the convulsion is prolonged or atypical. Up to 40% may have another convulsion and 15% a third episode. If the child suffers from multiple repeated febrile convulsions the possibility of an early malignant epilepsy such as myoclonic epilepsy of Dravet exists.

Subsequent epilepsy is more likely if:

● the child is less than 12 months old;
● a complex initial convulsion occurred with neurological signs;
● febrile convulsions are present in first-degree relatives;
● prolonged fits last more than 30 min;
● there are more than three episodes.

If two or more risk factors are present, the risk of subsequent epilepsy rises to 10%. The basis of the subsequent epilepsy is thought in many cases to be due to brain damage to the temporal lobes (mesial temporal sclerosis – see below) acquired during a prolonged or complicated seizure rather than due to the genetic low threshold.

Long-term management. Recurrences of febrile convulsions can be prevented by medication. The main reason for preventing recurrences would be to avoid a prolonged seizure. Most prolonged febrile seizures are first seizures and the risk for recurrence of a long seizure is low (1–4%).

Prolonged seizures can be prevented by the parents giving rectal diazepam when the seizure has lasted 5 min. In most cases prophylactic medication will not be required. Prophylactic oral medication may be used instead of rectal diazepam but prophylaxis does not give a guarantee that recurrence will not happen. Those children whose risk of recurrence is high should probably be started on continuous prophylaxis after the first febrile convulsion. These include children under 1 year old and those who have had a prolonged convulsion. These are not in themselves absolute indicators for continuous prophylaxis provided rectal diazepam is available to the parents. The final group that should have continuous prophylaxis is a small group who have very numerous recurrences of seizures with almost every febrile episode.

Continuous prophylaxis. Both phenobarbitone and sodium valproate have been shown to significantly reduce the rate of recurrences when taken continuously. Anticonvulsants which act on the voltage-gated sodium ionophore, such as phenytoin and carbamazepine, are not effective prophylaxis. Recurrence rates with effective drugs are around 8–12% compared with 30% for controls. Phenobarbitone has fallen into disfavor because of the high incidence (30–50%) of behavioral side effects in the form of hyperactive and aggressive behavior. Other problems are the possibility of seizures if the drug is discontinued suddenly by the parent, the possibility of acute poisoning in a child or siblings and concerns about the effect on learning in young children. For this reason sodium valproate has become the most widely used drug for continuous prophylaxis. It does not have any obvious effects on learning and is usually well tolerated although there have been reports of rare fatal hepatic toxicity (Dreifuss et al 1987). It is our policy to check plasma ammonia in children under 3 prior to the commencement of valproate, because of the risk that it may precipitate hepatotoxicity secondary to inborn errors of metabolism, such as ornithine carbamyl transferase deficiency. The risk of hepatotoxicity in the under-3 population is 1 in 500 whereas the incidence in adults is 1 in 30 000.

Intermittent prophylaxis. The rationale for this method is that regular diazepam suppositories or solution given at the start of the febrile illness will prevent convulsions occurring. This has been shown to reduce recurrence rates from 27% to 12% of cases. In some children the seizures occur before the parents realize that they are febrile. If fever occurs they should give paracetamol (orally or rectally) as an antipyretic, remove warm clothing and sponge the child down with a damp cloth. They should not use cold water or fans as these may make the child shiver and raise the core temperature. It must be emphasized that such measures will not guarantee the prevention of a seizure and some believe they are mainly of use to give the parent something to do. If a fit occurs, rectal diazepam is more likely to stop it and is easy for parents to use.

Genetic partial epilepsies

This group consists of benign Rolandic epilepsy, benign occipital epilepsy and benign temporal lobe epilepsy. The commonest of these benign epilepsies is the benign Rolandic with centrotemporal spikes. The list is expanding and, recently, further examples have been described, e.g. autosomal dominant frontal lobe epilepsy and episodic type 1 ataxia. The gene for benign neonatal myoclonus has been identified and is located on chromosome 20, the gene coding for the nicotinic acetyl choline receptor. In an Australian family with autosomal dominant frontal lobe epilepsy the gene has again been identified, located on chromosome 20. It is interesting in this group to try to explain how the genetic abnormality causes fluctuating focal epileptic discharge. The genetic background is further strengthened by the demonstration that family members without clinical seizures also show a high incidence of focal epileptic discharges.

We are now recognising that not all causes of benign Rolandic epilepsy are benign or self-limiting: there is a spectrum with more malignant forms, e.g. the Landau–Kleffner syndrome (? malignant Rolandic epilepsy). Scheffer et al (1995) have described a family with autosomal dominant Rolandic epilepsy and speech dyspraxia. There are also severe forms of occipital epilepsy, and mitochondrial disease can be associated with intractable occipital lobe epilepsies.

Table 14.19 Epileptic syndromes with absences

1.	Typical petit mal syndrome (childhood absence epilepsy)
2.	Complex absences of temporal lobe epilepsy
3.	Absences of juvenile myoclonic epilepsy (impulsive petit mal) (JME)
4.	Myoclonic petit mal (? different from JME)
5.	Absences of Lennox–Gastaut syndrome (petit mal)
6.	Absence of Dravet type polymorphic epilepsy
7.	Absences in SSPE
8.	Astatic petit mal of Doose
9.	Eyelid and perioral myoclonia with absences
10.	Absence with photoconvulsive epilepsy
11.	Absence with proven lesions

LESIONAL EPILEPTIC SYNDROMES OF CHILDHOOD (Table 14.20)

Epilepsy can be caused by virtually any lesion in the cerebral cortex. Lesions in the thalamus, basal ganglia, brainstem and cerebellum do not cause epilepsy as shown by the distribution of brain tumors which present with seizures. In the past it has been fashionable to talk about diencephalic epilepsy and although the thalamus is involved in the generation of the genetic 3 cycles/s spike and wave discharge, thalamic lesions do not cause epilepsy. Gillingham in Edinburgh made over 1000 stereotactic lesions in the thalamus and only one patient had a fit (personal communication). Traditionally 75% frontal, 50% temporal, 25% parietal and 5% of occipital lesions present as fits. The epileptic manifestation of lesional epilepsies depends on the locus of electrical disturbance. If it is circumscribed the seizure will be of a simple partial type without disturbance of consciousness. However, when the electrical activity spreads to other parts of the central nervous system, tonic–clonic, absence, complex partial or myoclonic seizures may occur. In other words, a generalized seizure does not preclude focal lesion.

Table 14.20 Lesional epilepsies in children

Mesial temporal sclerosis
Cerebral palsy
Cerebral infarcts
Focal dysplasias
Hamartomas
Sturge–Weber syndrome
Tubers – tuberous sclerosis
Subpial hamartomas
Gliomas in situ
Neurofibromatosis
Rasmussen's syndrome
Tumors
Arteriovenous malformations
Tuberculoma, cysticercosis
Congenital cytomegalovirus infection
Toxoplasmosis
Herpes simplex
After head injury (accidental and non-accidental injury)
Degenerative disease (lysosomal, peroxysomal, mitochondrial, etc.)

Table 14.21 MRI and lesional epilepsy in children

1. Tumors (gliomas not seen on CT)
2. AV malformations
3. Chronic focal encephalitis (herpes, Rasmussen's syndrome)
4. Hamartomas
   Hypothalamic hamartomas
   Temporal lobe hamartomas
   Subpial hamartomas
   Tubers
5. Focal dysplasias – opercular, occipital
6. Gross generalized gyral abnormality
   Lissencephaly
   Megalencephaly with heterotopias
   Microencephaly

If focal or multifocal abnormal activity is found on the EEG, it might be expected to be a *prima facie* case for lesional epilepsy. Unfortunately metabolic diseases such as hypocalcemia, hypomagnesemia and hypoglycemia or even a simple febrile convulsion may present with focal seizures. Lesional epilepsy has become easier to diagnose with brain imaging (MRI, SPECT or PET) (Table 14.21).

Epilepsy and cerebral palsy

The commonest lesional epilepsy in childhood is that associated with hemiplegic and quadriplegic cerebral palsy. Pure dyskinetic (e.g. postkernicteric) and ataxic cerebral palsy are only exceptionally associated with epilepsy. It is also uncommon in the pure diplegic cerebral palsy of prematurity. About one-third of hemiplegics and 90% of quadriplegics have fits.

Of 91 patients with cerebral palsy associated with seizures reviewed from Edinburgh, 87 patients suffered from continuing epilepsy which was characterized by an early age of onset and mixed seizure types (87% before the age of 5 years old, 61% mixed seizure types). A change in seizure type was noted in 43% of patients. EEG recordings showed focal and multifocal epileptiform activity in 44% of patients. Only 30% of patients were seizure free for at least 2 years. Polypharmacy was a common problem and associated with mixed seizure types. Factors associated with a poor outcome were the occurrence of status epilepticus and high seizure frequency. Some patients in this group might be potential candidates for epilepsy surgery. This study showed that one-third of our patients had daily or more frequent seizure attacks despite therapy and status epilepticus was common. Recurrent status epilepticus occurred in half the patients who had status epilepticus. Shinnar et al (1992) also concluded that the risk of recurrent status epilepticus in their symptomatic cerebral palsy group was almost 50%.

Cortical dysplasia

The neocortex develops by neuronal proliferation at 8–16 weeks gestation followed by migration at 12–24 weeks. Any interference in these processes will lead to disorganized brain growth with neurons in white matter, subpial neuronal collections, inverted neurons and vertical rather than horizontal laminar structure of the cortex. There may be macroscopic abnormality as in lissencephaly, microcephaly, pachygyria, polymicrogyria, heterotopias and hemimegalencephaly. Their recognition in clinical practice has

risen considerably with the advent of MRI scanning. Microscopic dysplasia (microdysgenesis) is also being found increasingly to be the cause of epilepsy, but requires histological examination and may escape detection even by the most sensitive neuroimaging technique.

In cortical dysplasia there may be a failure of migration with arrest of migrating cells in the future white matter, causing heterotopias. These may continue to grow as a future neoplasm. It is thought that the heterotopias, cortical dysplasias and high risk of cerebral neoplasms in tuberous sclerosis may be related to a defect in tuberin required for normal migration. The cells may breach the pia as subpial heterotopia, as seen floridly in fetal alcohol syndrome when the cells may continue to move into the subarachnoid space, causing CSF obstruction. Smaller degrees of pial breaching are seen in the dysplasias of epilepsy, dyslexia and autism.

Many neurocutaneous syndromes are associated with cortical dysplasia. Neurofibromatosis, tuberous sclerosis, Sturge–Weber syndrome and linear sebaceous nevus syndrome are the best known ones. Other examples include Zellweger syndrome, Miller–Dieker syndrome, Aicardi syndrome, Angelman syndrome and bilateral opercular dysplasia syndrome. Maternal abuse of alcohol and cocaine is also a known cause.

The failure of cortical differentiation may be gross with no gyral formation (lissencephaly), there may be retention of the cells in vertical columns, diminution in the normal six layers of cortex, neuron dispersal is abnormal and neurons may be upside down in the cortex. The overlying gyral pattern may show pachygyria (fat gyri) or ulegyria (small shriveled gyri). The overlying gyri can be normal and yet the brain show a microscopic focal dysplasia (microdysgenesis).

Cortical dysplasia causes partial fits with or without generalization and many malignant epileptic syndromes (discussed later). Apart from causing electrical instability, it will also disrupt the function of the affected parts of the brain. Mental retardation, speech difficulty and cerebral palsy are therefore common accompaniments. The epileptic fits are usually resistant to antiepileptic drugs.

Mesial temporal sclerosis

The medial temporal lobe is the junction of emotion, memory, consciousness and autonomic function. It connects the cerebral cortex, limbic system and the reticular formation of the brainstem. A lesion in this area can produce very complex symptomatology and affected children will also show behavioral and learning difficulties in addition to their epilepsy. The area may be the site of microdysgenesis or hamartoma. There may be collection of Langhans giant cells suggesting *forme fruste* of tuberous sclerosis. Small tumors may remain dormant for years or even decades. However, the commonest pathology is that of mesial temporal sclerosis.

Mesial temporal sclerosis has long been regarded as the most important cause of refractory complex partial epilepsy in adulthood. It is a disruption of the normal architecture of the hippocampal formation associated with neuronal loss and gliosis. Its strategic location in the hippocampus accounts for the limbic system involvement during seizures and their distinctive affective overtone, with hallmarks of sudden emotional change, distorted perception of self and environment and memory disturbance like amnesia and *déjà vu*. A vague abdominal sensation commonly heralds alteration in consciousness and automatism. Abdominal epilepsy, which represents the phase of aura in these seizures, seldom occurs without subsequent loss of consciousness. This is a useful distinguishing feature from recurrent functional abdominal pain. It is characterized by the presence of a firm, atrophic hippocampus and the presence on histology of neuronal loss and gliosis in some of the hippocampal subfields.

The medial temporal structures, like the basal ganglia and cerebellum, are very sensitive to hypoxia. They possess a high density of glutamate receptors and the possibility of excitotoxic damage is greatest in this part of the brain. Characteristic pathological findings are hypoxic ischemia lesions of varying ages and therefore some investigators have suggested that mesial temporal sclerosis is a progressive lesion. Antenatal and perinatal hypoxic and ischemia insults are also possible causes of mesial temporal sclerosis (Ounsted et al 1987) although a different part of the hippocampus is affected. Cerebral edema resulting in tentorial herniation can also cause ischemia of the mesial temporal structures (Brown & Hussain 1991).

Recent MRI studies have confirmed the early pathological findings (Harvey et al 1995). Up to 80% of adults with histologically proven mesial temporal sclerosis had a convulsion lasting for more than 30 minutes under the age of 3 and this is the major pathological entity one is attempting to define by MRI in epilepsy. The MRI features of hippocampal sclerosis include a small shrunken hyperdense medial temporal lobe with enlargement of the temporal horn.

Discharge from the deep structures in temporal lobe cannot always be readily picked up by conventional surface electrodes. Deep sphenoidal, foraminal, subdurally implanted electrodes and intraoperative electrocorticography are sometimes employed to localize the focus. The abnormality seen on surface EEG may not be the site of origin of the seizure and so an actual ictal EEG, provoked by stopping all anticonvulsant medication if necessary, may be justified.

There are two main messages for pediatricians: firstly, prolonged convulsion in small children should be avoided and secondly, mesial temporal sclerosis is the lesion *par excellence* which responds to surgery with an 85% cure rate.

Rasmussen's syndrome

This is a chronic progressive focal encephalitis characterized by intractable epilepsy, hemiparesis and usually a slow progressive dementia. The EEG shows diffuse and focal abnormalities and the MRI progressive hemispheric atrophy. There should be early consideration of hemispherectomy which may lead to complete remission and improvement of the child's long-term outlook. Immunoglobulins anecdotally have been shown to be helpful in management.

Other lesional epilepsies

Tumors are uncommon causes of epilepsy in children (compare adults). Astrocytomas and oligodendrocytomas, however, can cause epilepsy but hamartomata and vascular malformations are more common causes.

Medical treatment of lesional epilepsy syndromes

Lesional epilepsy responds favorably to antiepileptic drugs which act on voltage-gated sodium ionophores. These include carbama-

zepine, phenytoin and lamotrigine, which are the drugs of first choice. Sodium valproate and vigabatrin are also commonly used for partial seizures and gabapentin and oxycarbazine may be effective.

Surgical treatment of epilepsy

There are four main types of surgical procedure used in the treatment of epilepsy.

Lesionectomy

If a lesion is identified that corresponds to the site from which seizures are arising then removal of the lesion may cure or markedly improve the severity of the seizures. This is the case with arteriovenous malformations, tumors and abscesses. It is now thought that in conditions such as tuberous sclerosis one tuber may be causing most of the epilepsy and be worth removing.

Anterior temporal lobectomy

Complex partial seizures most commonly arise from the anterior temporal lobe. If this can be confirmed on EEG and the side of the habitual seizure determined, then removal of that anterior temporal lobe or amygdalohippocampectomy may cure or markedly improve the severity of the seizure. For this to be effective and safe, strict selection criteria are necessary. The seizures must be truly intractable and causing disruption to the patient's life. They must originate in a well-circumscribed region of the brain that can be removed without producing a major neurological handicap. Localization of the origin of the seizures can be determined from the history, clinical features of the attack and neuroradiological and EEG data. Surface EEGs may show a localized abnormality but this may be misleading. For this reason more intensive forms of EEG monitoring employing special electrodes such as sphenoidal, foramen ovale or chronically implanted depth electrodes may be necessary to demonstrate the focus. Ideally both ictal and interictal recordings should be done. The most difficult patients to evaluate are those in whom bilateral independent foci are demonstrated. PET or SPECT may be helpful in demonstrating interictal hypometabolism at the site of the focus. Prior to surgery detailed neuropsychological assessment is necessary to determine laterality of speech, handedness and memory function.

Hemispherectomy

Patients with dense hemiplegias and intractable epilepsy arising from the abnormal hemisphere may benefit markedly from removal of the abnormal hemisphere without significant deterioration in the degree of motor or intellectual function. Patients who may benefit from hemispherectomy are those with congenital or acquired hemiplegias and epilepsy, Sturge–Weber syndrome and chronic focal encephalitis of Rasmussen.

Division of the corpus callosum

Division of the corpus callosum has been shown to be effective in suppressing drop attacks and other secondarily generalized seizures. The mode of action is not clear but the limitation of spread of the seizure discharge from one hemisphere to the other is a likely mechanism. Although various neuropsychological abnormalities can be demonstrated after corpus callosum section, clinically significant problems are uncommon. The exact role of this procedure in the treatment of childhood epilepsy is not yet established. At present it is usually considered for intractable drop attacks, but it may also be of value in hemiplegic epilepsy where the hemiplegia is not dense and hemispherectomy is therefore not indicated.

Malignant epileptic syndromes (Table 14.22)

This distinctive group consists of Ohtahara syndrome, West's syndrome of infantile spasms, Lennox–Gastaut syndrome, Landau–Kleffner syndrome and polymorphic myoclonic epilepsy of Dravet (severe myoclonic epilepsy of infancy). All these syndromes are characteristically resistant to conventional antiepileptic treatment with high seizure frequency (Table 14.23). Cognitive impairment is common and there may be a progressive dementia suggesting an underlying degenerative disease. There is a high propensity to both convulsive and nonconvulsive status epilepticus. While the former will not be missed by parents and clinicians, the latter is often subtle and not recognized. Nonconvulsive status epilepticus may take the form of slight retardation of responsiveness or inappropriately altered affect. Motor seizure activity is limited to sporadic myoclonic jerks or eyelid flutter or is absent altogether. Ataxia and uncontrollable drooling are frequently observed signs. Autonomic changes like pupillary dilation and borborygmi occasionally happen. Nonconvulsive status can last for months without recognition and the external changes usually become less obvious with time. It is believed that the intellectual deterioration of these malignant epileptic syndromes is caused by prolonged spells of nonconvulsive status epilepticus. The brain is 'switched off' with the gross disturbance of electrical activity. Functional studies show hypometabolism of the cerebral cortex which therefore cannot acquire new experience.

About 30–40% of patients have an unknown etiology (the cryptogenic group), where histological section of resected brain often shows microdysgenesis.

Treatment of infantile spasms (West's syndrome)
(Table 14.22)

Only complete control is acceptable. Effective drugs act on the GABA A receptor which governs the opening of the chloride ionophore. Benzodiazepines, ACTH, B6 and vigabatrin all have an effect on the GABA A receptor and phenobarbitone binds to A and B receptors (all can be used for infantile spasms).

For most patients ACTH remains the treatment of choice. We would use ACTH in a dose of 40 units per day (0.5 mg synthetic corticotropin). We regard ACTH as mandatory to try and prevent subsequent dementia, particularly if the child has 'switched off' with reduced responsiveness, autistic features and a continuously hypsarrhythmic EEG suggestive of nonconvulsive status epilepticus.

Treatment

1. ACTH (40 units per day tailing off over 3–6 weeks).
2. Benzodiazepines (nitrazepam 0.25–1.0 mg/kg/day).
3. High-dose valproate (100–300 mg/kg/day).
4. Vigabatrin (40–80 mg/kg/day or 80–120 mg/kg).
5. Pyridoxine 100 mg i.v. stat then 100 mg per day oral.
6. High-dose pyridoxine 50 mg/kg/day (+ low dose ACTH 5–10 units per day).
7. Lesionectomy of hypometabolic area on PET scan.
8. Immunoglobulin infusions 0.4 kg per day for 5 days, repeated every 2 weeks for 3 months.

Tuberous sclerosis is an important symptomatic cause. Its identification is important as vigabatrin is now the drug of first choice though unfortunately dosage recommended varies from 20 to 120 mg/kg. It is also possible that it may help the spasms more than the hypsarrhythmia and thus not prevent the subsequent mental handicap. Valproic acid and nitrazepam are less effective alternatives. Surgical treatment is possible in some patients where hypometabolic lesions are identified on PET scan but show no abnormality on MRI.

PROGNOSIS OF EPILEPSY

Mortality

There is an excess mortality for epileptic children. This has been estimated as 5% during the first 10 years after onset of seizures with a further 3% risk over the next 10 years. There is an increased risk of accidents such as drowning, falling and road traffic accidents. Death is particularly likely in the first year when the fits are often symptomatic of an underlying disease and between 15 and 25 years when there is rebellion against medication and with loss of parental and pediatric supervision. The sudden unexpected death syndrome is now well recognized in epileptics and is postulated to be due to a cardiac dysrhythmia complicating the fit.

Morbidity

The prognosis of epilepsy is measured in terms of continuing seizures, social and emotional adjustment, educational attainment and employment prospects.

One of the most important prognostic indicators will be the type of epilepsy; a widely different prognosis may be expected, for example, between petit mal epilepsy and the Lennox–Gastaut syndrome.

Studies which have looked at large populations have not separated different epileptic syndromes and have included both adults and children. Some generalizations, however, are possible. Overall the likelihood of remission of seizures is between 50% and 70%. The best prognosis is in benign rolandic seizures and true petit mal (childhood absence epilepsy). With complex partial seizures about 33% will become seizure free and off medication, 33% seizure free on continuing medication and 33% still with problematic seizures despite medication at the age of 18. Malignant epilepsies such as Lennox–Gastaut and Dravet have the worst prognosis. It is not, however, the continuing seizures which are the main problem but the burnt-out dementia. Most relapses will occur during withdrawal of therapy or in the first 1–2 years after stopping treatment.

Individual factors that indicate a high chance of remission are absence of neurological abnormalities or brain lesion, normal intelligence, onset of seizure after the age of 3–4 years, low seizure frequency, brief duration of epilepsy prior to control, generalized tonic–clonic seizures, typical absence seizures or simple partial seizures, no episodes of status, normal EEG background and normalization of EEG after onset of therapy (Aicardi 1994).

Table 14.22 The malignant epilepsies

Epilepsy	Age of onset	Seizure type	EEG/imaging	Etiology	Prognosis	Treatment	Neurology
1. Ohtahara syndrome (early infantile epileptic encephalopathy)	0–3 months	Brief tonic seizures, simple partial or myoclonic jerks	Burst suppression pattern when infant is awake or asleep, with random multifocal spikes interspersed	Unknown, sometimes cortical dysplasia and microdysgenesis	Drug-resistant including ACTH. Severe developmental delay or death. If the child survives, West's and/or Lennox–Gastaut syndrome may develop	Try ACTH	Marked psychomotor retardation with intractable seizures
2. Infantile spasms (West's syndrome) A. 25% idiopathic cryptogenic B. 75% secondary, symptomatic	Before 1 year of age, peak onset between 3 and 7 months. Onset early in group B	Flexor spasms – arms extend and elevate, simultaneous flexion of neck and trunk (may be misdiagnosed as colic). Startle or hypnogogic myoclonus (sleep startles). Head nods. Occasional reversed spasms with extension trunk and legs (like Moro reflex). 'Switch off', become 'autistic' in nonconvulsive status with hypsarrhythmia	Interictal EEG; hypsarrhythmia in most cases, i.e. random or chaotic high voltage polymorphic delta slow waves with random spikes coming from all areas of brain (occasionally unilateral). Ictal EEG; flattening (electrodecremental response)	Cryptogenic 1 in 4000 births (normal exam and development, normal metabolic screen and cranial MRI). Group B: intrauterine rubella, CMV, toxoplasma cortical dysplasias (in tuberous sclerosis infantile spasms are the presenting feature in 68% of cases); Aicardi's syndrome, i.e. agenesis of the corpus callosum; choroid coloboma; hypomelanosis of Ito; perinatal ischemic encephalopathy; after cardiac surgery, focal tumors and porencephalic cysts; neonatal meningitis; metabolic disorders (untreated PKU); toxic – aminophylline poisoning	Prognosis depends on the etiology, with complete recovery confined to the cryptogenic group. It also depends on therapy. Spasms disappear by 5 years whether or not treatment has been given. Figures for mortality vary between 6 and 24%, with a mean figure of 16%	Only complete control is acceptable. Effective drugs act on the GABA A receptor which governs the opening of the chloride ionophore. Benzodiazepines, ACTH, B6 and vigabatrin all have an effect on the GABA A receptor and phenobarbitone binds to A and B receptors (all can be used for infantile spasms)	Depends on specific etiology. Associated behavior – irritable, autistic features, especially gaze avoidance
3. Lennox–Gastaut syndrome	1–8 years (mean 4 years)	Axial seizures with tonic elevation of the arms, neck retraction, head nods or arching. Tonic seizures often at night. Sudden axial or limb myoclonic. Atypical absences (eyes stare but also grimacing) and atonic seizure/drop attacks often described together as stare jerk and fall fits. Status epilepticus and nonconvulsive status are common	Interictal: slow ragged spike and wave (1.5–2.5 Hz) with abnormal slow wave background activity (epileptic encephalopathy). Occasionally hypsarrhythmia (even at school age). Ictal; in nonconvulsive status, random spike and wave with a background of high amplitude slow (delta) activity is continuous from all areas of brain	The three syndromes of Ohtahara, West and Lennox–Gastaut should be regarded as a continuum as they are age-dependent responses of the developing brain to cortical damage, most often microdysgenesis	Progressive mental retardation is common with dementia. After each episode of nonconvulsive status there is further deterioration in intellectual function. Behavioral problems are very common – aggression, sham rages and autistic behavior when in nonconvulsive status. The prognosis is very unfavorable with intractable drug-resistant epilepsy, poor educational progress, behavior and social independence	Resistant to conventional treatment (carbamazepine can cause deterioration in seizure control). Valproate, benzodiazepines and phenytoin are often used but vigabatrin, lamotrigine, steroids, immunoglobulin may result in improvement in the occasional case. If atonic seizures are the main problem, callosotomy can improve the quality of the patient's life and make management easier	Psychomotor retardation, neuropsychiatric symptoms and ataxia
4. Severe myoclonic epilepsy of Dravet	First year – mean 5 months (often misdiagnosed as pertussis immunization encephalopathy)	A severe polymorphic epilepsy. Suspect in any child with 3 or more febrile seizures. First general or unilateral febrile clonic seizures often with status: later generalized myoclonic seizures (second year); partial seizures may merge to complex partial seizures or complex absences with autonomic phenomena	Generalized spike and wave, polyspike and wave. Early photosensitivity and focal abnormalities	Positive family history of epilepsy in 33%, AD with incomplete penetrance	Psychomotor retardation develops with onset of myoclonic jerks. Language deficits common. Eventually severe regression with no independence and severe mental retardation. Sudden death in 16% (Dravet et al 1985). Seizures get less dramatic with age and more often at night. Ataxia may appear	Seizures very resistant to medication. Phenobarbitone, sodium valproate and benzodiazepines may decrease frequency and duration of afebrile seizures. Phenytoin may be useful. Immunotherapy is worth trying and steroids can give transitory improvement	Ataxia, pyramidal signs and interictal clonus

Table 14.22 *Cont'd*

Epilepsy	Age of onset	Seizure type	EEG/imaging	Etiology	Prognosis	Treatment	Neurology
5. Progressive myoclonic epilepsy syndrome	Depends on etiology	A myoclonic syndrome. Generalized tonic–clonic myoclonic and atonic seizures	Deterioration in background, alteration in sleep organization, paroxysmal abnormalities	Specific syndromes include Baltic myoclonus, Ramsay–Hunt syndrome, Lafora body disease, neuronal ceroid lipofuscinosis. Cherry red spot-myoclonus syndrome, mitochondrial encephalopathy, MELAS, MERRF	Progressive mental and neurological deterioration	No treatment for the underlying disorder	Cerebellar, corticospinal and extrapyramidal changes
6. Landau–Kleffner syndrome	Preschool years	Overt seizures only in 70%, status in 15%. Seizures may be nocturnal and polymorphic (generalized, tonic–clonic, atonic, absences, myoclonic jerks, facial myoclonia)	Normal basal rhythm, profuse nearly always bilateral spikes or spike-waves, variable in time and space but most often temporal/parietal and often continuous during slow or REM sleep	Males 2:1 but no family history. Etiology is unknown. Two theories: 1. the extreme end of the genetic epilepsies with centrotemporal spikes. 2. due to a localized vasculitis. Rarely, Rasmussen's chronic encephalitis can present similarly	Cessation of seizures and disappearance of EEG abnormalities is usual, speech improves but lasting communication and learning difficulty is common in 50% patients	The epilepsy may not be difficult to treat with conventional anticonvulsants, the main argument is whether the language problem is reversed by medication, especially steroids	Abrupt or gradual loss of language and inattentiveness to sound (there may be a receptive or expressive domination of the clinical picture). Speech development may not have been normal prior to the acute aphasia. Difficulty arises if the onset is between 18 months and 2 years before language is easily measured. The interruption in communication ability is temporally associated with seizure activity or EEG abnormality. Behavior may be autistic, hyperkinetic or odd personality
7. Epilepsy with electrical status in slow sleep	8 months to 12 years (mean 4.5 years)	Generalized tonic–clonic and simple partial	EEG – awake, diffuse spike and wave at 2–3/s. Asleep, continuous bilateral and diffuse slow waves appear (must involve 75% of sleep). EEG normalizes at puberty		Poor. Neuropsychiatric problems and moderate to severe learning difficulties	ACTH, benzodiazepines, clobazam	Associated learning difficulties and neuropsychic disturbance. DD benign epilepsy of childhood with centrotemporal spikes, Lennox–Gastaut, Landau–Kleffner

MELAS – Myoclonic epilepsy, lactic acidosis and stroke
MERRF – Myoclonic epilepsy and ragged redfibers
DD – differential diagnosis

Table 14.23 Intractable or severe drug-resistant epilepsy

1. Rasmussen's syndrome
2. Associated with quadriplegic cerebral palsy
3. Gelastic seizures with hypothalamic hamartoma
4. Complex partial with temporal lobe hamartoma
5. Angelman syndrome
6. Aicardi's syndrome
7. Ring 20 chromosome syndromes
8. Lissencephaly
9. Opercular dysplasias, etc.
10. Lafora body disease
11. Subacute sclerosing leukoencephalitis
12. Tuberous sclerosis
13. Landau–Kleffner syndrome
14. Following surgery to floor of third ventricle (craniopharyngiomas)
15. Late infantile Batten's disease

Prognosis for cognitive function in epilepsy

In general the same factors that indicate a good prognosis for seizure control will indicate a good prognosis for educational and social outcome. Patients with epilepsy will tend to score slightly lower on IQ tests when compared with normal siblings; 50–70% of patients will have normal IQ. IQ is also variable from day to day and reliance should not be placed upon a single test. Some patients show decreasing IQ as their epilepsy continues. This has particularly been noted in the Lennox–Gastaut syndrome but has been described in other children with epilepsy. Nonconvulsive status epilepticus in the dementia that occurs in the Lennox–Gastaut syndrome may be due to switching off the protein metabolism responsible for long-term memory in the neuron. Measurement of neuron-specific enolase, a specific marker for neurons, suggests that damage occurs in nonconvulsive epilepsy. Chronic toxic levels of anticonvulsants, particularly phenobarbitone and phenytoin, and also folate depletion may cause dementia.

Overall IQ scores can be misleading as a much larger proportion of children with epilepsy have specific learning difficulties. A study demonstrated significant difficulties in reading, spelling and arithmetic in up to 30% of epileptic children with normal or low normal IQ scores (Seidenberg 1989). Some have suggested that the problems relate to abnormal activity in the dominant hemisphere and correlate with left-sided spikes seen on the EEG. The brain has several built-in protection mechanisms and if one area is hyperexcitable and epileptic there is a mechanism for switching it to become hypometabolic. This could theoretically also switch off the normal function of that part of the brain and could mean that better control of the abnormal electrical activity by anticonvulsants would then improve learning. Others have suggested that the total number of spikes in a 24-hour period relates to the learning difficulty. It is difficult to know whether aggressive attempts to normalize the EEG will result in better learning or problems of toxic effects of anticonvulsants. The learning problem may be due to the same brain damage that causes the epilepsy, as in children with cerebral palsy and/or cortical dysplasia, and not a result of the seizures. Antiepileptic treatment with phenytoin, primidone or phenobarbitone may affect learning, benzodiazepines may disrupt memory and ethosuximide affects reaction times.

If the child is having multiple absences then consciousness has been peppered with unconsciousness. The child loses a few seconds of the teacher's sentence and so loses the meaning and appears inattentive in class. Boredom and lack of understanding will increase the number of absences, so creating a vicious circle.

The mesial temporal lobe structures in the hippocampus and amygdala are responsible for moving memories from short-term into long-term stores as well as affecting behavior. Epilepsy arising in this area could cause difficulty in learning new material (the left in storing verbal material and the right visual material). It is thought that left-sided epileptic foci are more likely to occur in boys and so are language-based learning difficulties such as reading and spelling.

Social and behavioral outcome

Around 20–30% of children with epilepsy will experience behavioral or psychiatric problems. Important factors are the degree of seizure control, type of epilepsy, the use of polytherapy and the family response. This illustrates that the behavioral outcome is the complex interaction between biological and psychosocial factors (Hermann et al 1989).

A poor outcome is often associated with a constellation of several problems, i.e. low intelligence, poor control of seizures and behavioral abnormalities. For optimal management of chronic epilepsy, therefore, three areas need to be evaluated each time the child is seen: fits, learning and behavior.

Autistic behavior. Loss of social awareness and ability to understand emotional cues in nonverbal communication occurs in West's, Lennox–Gastaut and Landau–Kleffner syndromes as well as in any cause of nonconvulsive status and in certain specific diseases such as tuberous sclerosis and Rett's syndrome.

Fight and flight responses and rage reactions. In the same way that there is a seizure threshold, there is equally a threshold for fight and flight or rage reactions and panic attacks. This threshold may be lowered so that minor frustrations cause either severe rages or panic. Boys with left-sided seizure discharges seem particularly prone to cataclysmic rages.

Attention deficit disorder. Overactivity, sleep disturbance, short concentration span and rage reactions may be seen in epileptic children and this is often combined with a deficit in cognitive learning.

Behavior disturbances in relation to the fit

Preictal behavior. The child may become irritable, expansive, annoying, and/or noisy so the parent realizes when the child gets out of bed in the morning that a fit will occur that day. The EEG at this time may be normal.

Ictal behavior. This commences with the aura and may consist of motor activities such as sniffing, lip smacking, running in circles, laughing or even imitating sexual intercourse. Speech may be lost or the child talks with words in a nonsense sequence. Loss of social awareness and autistic behavior may occur, as in West's syndrome or Landau–Kleffner syndrome.

Postictal behavior. This may consist of drowsiness with disorientation, staring into space or automatic behaviors for which the child subsequently has no recall.

Interictal behavior. This consists of overactive behavior, poor impulse control and learning difficulties.

Restriction in the epileptic child

The only sports which we restrict are rock climbing, lone canoeing, boxing and high diving. As most children do not wish to participate in these sports they are not upset by these recommendations.

Cycling on main roads should have the same restrictions as driving a car later, i.e. well-controlled epilepsy with no daytime seizures for 1 year. There may have to be a temporary restriction on cycling on main roads until seizure control is established. Bicycle helmets are for all children

All children should be encouraged to swim but the child with continuing seizures should never swim alone. The person who is supervising the child should never get out of his depth and should always be able to hold the child's head above water with his own feet on the ground. If a child has a fit while swimming they should be supported in the pool until the fit stops. A brightly colored cap helps keep tabs on the child in the pool when in a group.

Children who are photosensitive are advised to watch television in a well-lit room with a lamp on or beside the set, to sit 6 feet back from the television screen, to use a remote control to change channels and if it is necessary to approach the screen, to cover one eye. The child should not be allowed to play computer games when tired. High-resolution screens are safer than the lower 50 Hz type and hand-held games with liquid crystal displays do not appear to cause any problems.

There is an increased incidence of death among epileptic teenagers, partly from drowning in the bath. Showers are safer and allow the teenager privacy in the bathroom. The shower control should be of screw not lever type so it is not accidentally turned to very hot if the child falls against it.

Bright flashing strobe lights will induce a seizure in a susceptible child. However, sleep deprivation from an all-night rave, drugs and excess fluid intake are much more likely to precipitate a seizure than disco lights.

Alcohol can interfere with antiepileptic medication and will lower the seizure threshold.

Menstruation, the pill and pregnancy

Phenytoin and phenobarbitone will interfere with the metabolism of the contraceptive pill by hepatic enzyme induction and a higher estrogen content pill may be required.

During pregnancy phenytoin (an antifolate drug) can cause cleft lip and palate in the fetus. Sodium valproate causes a higher incidence of neural tube defects and increased incidence of complex cardiac lesions have also been reported. If at all possible any girl who is planning or even thinking about pregnancy should be weaned off valproate or changed to small frequent doses. Folate supplements must be taken.

Prepubertal girls may have exacerbation of seizures at puberty due to the unopposed action of estrogen which is a convulsant. This will improve when regular cycles are established as progesterone from the corpus luteum after ovulation is a natural anticonvulsant.

If pregnancy does not occur the possibility of polycystic ovaries, due to anticonvulsant medication, should be borne in mind and medical attention sought as to whether hormonal ovulatory help is needed.

Parents' problems

What do we tell the child?

Children need to know about their epilepsy. They have vivid imaginations and are capable of conjuring up all sorts of frightening fantasies. Children will also be aware that their parents are upset and anxious. They will have been seen by at least two doctors, had wires stuck on their head and are taking daily medicine. If an adequate and reassuring explanation is not given the child will become isolated with their fears and more likely to become rebellious over medication. Teenagers should know exactly what they are taking as they will have to learn to take responsibility for their own medication. If children are shown films of seizures or see other children having fits it may be reassuring although a number will then feign fits to get out of difficult situations. Teachers should be given a full explanation of the type of fit, what to do in an emergency, if swimming is allowed and how it might affect work or behavior in the classroom.

What to do in a fit

Tonic–clonic. Protect the child from any injury, remove any objects which may cause the child harm, extend the neck, support the jaw and cushion the head. The three-quarter prone position is ideal if it can be adopted. If the seizure is prolonged and lasts for minutes emergency medication may need to be given (rectal diazepam, etc.).

Complex partial seizure. If the child is wandering around in an acute state, guide him into a safe place.

Simple absence. Just wait until the seizure has passed.

Sleeping and monitoring at night

Many parents worry about their child having a seizure during the night. This is not unreasonable as some children are found in the morning to have convulsed for an hour or more at night. An intercom can help them feel more relaxed. There is no satisfactory monitor but if the child has prolonged seizures with a drop in oxygen saturation, a saturation monitor can be provided for home use. Parents should be taught basic first aid and in severe cases given a mucus extractor and Ambu bag.

Travel

There is no contraindication to traveling abroad or flying. Parents should be advised to carry an adequate supply of medication and particularly a supply of rectal diazepam if this has been prescribed (as hand luggage). The parents should know the generic names of the drugs as trade names differ around the world. Families traveling in European Community countries should insure they have their E111 form to receive free medical treatment if required.

CONTINUOUS CEREBRAL DYSRHYTHMIAS

Convulsive status epilepticus

Status epilepticus is defined as a continuous epileptic state. This can be further defined as a single continuous seizure or series of seizures between which the patient does not regain consciousness. The duration of a seizure defined as status epilepticus is generally taken to be from 30 min to 1 h.

Status epilepticus is more common in childhood than in adult life. At least 10% of children diagnosed as having epilepsy under the age of 15 years have an episode of status epilepticus. The majority of cases of status epilepticus occur in the first 2 years of life and 80% by 5 years. The episode of status epilepticus is often the first epileptic seizure.

The causes of status epilepticus can be divided into cryptogenic or symptomatic and the symptomatic cases further divide into acute and chronic. Overall 50% of cases will be cryptogenic, of which half will be cases of febrile convulsions. In other words 25% of cases of status epilepticus in childhood are due to febrile convulsions (Maytal et al 1989). Chronic CNS disorders such as cerebral palsy, ischemic anoxic brain damage, malformations, tumors and progressive diseases account in total for a further 25% of cases. The remaining cases are due to acute encephalopathies such as CNS infection, electrolyte disorders, metabolic and toxic causes, trauma and cerebrovascular accidents. Sudden withdrawal of antiepileptic drugs in epileptic patients is another important cause.

Effects of status epilepticus

During status there is often hypoventilation, hypoxia and hypertension (later hypotension). Tachycardia is present at first but bradycardia may ensue if the seizure is not controlled. Hyperthermia is common and hyperglycemia is usual unless seizures are due to hypoglycemia. Muscle ischemia and damage due to continuous muscle contractions will raise levels of lactate and CPK in the blood. Even if systemic factors are controlled there is much evidence that excessive neuronal activity itself will eventually lead to neuronal damage. There is a four-fold increase in cerebral blood flow and similar increase in cerebral metabolic rates. These may initially be compensated (stage 1 status) but eventually decompensation (stage 2 status) occurs leading to a series of metabolic derangements that may lead to further neuronal damage and death.

The mortality and morbidity from status epilepticus has decreased markedly over the last 20 years (11% of 239 children in 1970 compared to 3.6% of 193 in 1989; Maytal et al 1989). In this study all deaths occurred in patients with acute CNS insults or progressive CNS disease.

The morbidity has also changed – a 4% incidence of neurological sequelae and a 48% incidence of mental deterioration in 1970 compared to only 9% with new neurological or cognitive problems on follow-up in 1989. Approximately 10% of patients developed epilepsy following the status. The incidence of sequelae relates primarily to the cause of the status, the majority occurring in those with acute CNS diseases. The sequelae include hemiplegia, ataxic and extrapyramidal syndromes and mental retardation. Hemiplegia following a prolonged hemiconvulsion, which used to be a relatively common observation, has become rare (almost certainly due to better first aid management of seizures, particularly with widespread use of rectal diazepam and improved intensive care facilities for the patients after admission).

Management of status epilepticus

There are three stages to the management (Table 14.24). Rectal diazepam has revolutionized first aid treatment of status and has undoubtedly resulted in a reduced morbidity and mortality rate. It

Table 14.24 Management of status epilepticus

Emergency care (primary care)
1. Nurse in the 3/4 prone position
2. Clear airway, pull jaw forward, use a mucous extractor, do *not* put anything between the teeth
3. Facial oxygen 40%, even if the patient is not cyanosed the brain needs 400% more oxygen during status
4. Medication – rectal diazepam, sublingual lorazepam or nasal midazolam (rectal paraldehyde, intramuscular paraldehyde)

Secondary care hospital emergency room
1. Check airway
2. Record basic signs breathing, blood pressure, pulse
3. Obtain i.v. access
4. Check basic bloods: immediate BM stix then withdraw blood for electrolytes, Ca, anticonvulsant levels and save serum for later investigations
5. Intravenous diazepam (0.2–0.3 mg/kg over 1–2 min)

There are now three possibilities:
1. The convulsion resolves and does not recur (80%)
2. The fit may stop but then restart – repeat bolus dose of diazepam, and i.v. phenytoin
3. The fit may continue:
   a. Use i.v. phenytoin with ECG monitoring (10 mg/kg as slow i.v. (1 mg/kg/min) and repeat after 30–60 min: the peak brain penetration occurs within 5–6 min). If the child is on maintenance phenytoin use deep i.m. paraldehyde into the thigh, not the buttock (age in years = ml of paraldehyde). No more than 5 ml may be given in any one site i.m. This may need to be repeated every 2–4 h (in which case give PR diluted with equal volumes of arachis oil)
   b. If the fits stop but the child is unconscious it may be assumed that there is some degree of cerebral edema. Give 20% mannitol at a dose of 7 ml/kg over 20 min. Watch blood pressure very carefully
   c. If the child does not waken, further investigations must be performed, i.e. a CT scan

Third-line care
If the fitting continues, third-line management consists of:
1. Admit to ITU
2. Phenobarbitone
3. Paralyze and ventilate
4. Correct metabolic acidosis
5. Recheck electrolytes
6. Reconsider diagnosis, poisoning, encephalitis, meningitis, NAI
7. 2-hourly glucose monitoring
8. EEG monitoring
9. Beware of drug overdoses
10. Thiopentone infusion
11. Restrict fluid (treat inappropriate ADH secretion if present)
12. Monitor anticonvulsant levels
13. Monitor ICP if no improvement
14. Check for consumptive coagulopathy
15. If no response consider lignocaine
16. Remember anticonvulsants also have convulsant action, e.g. phenytoin
17. Propofol can cause involuntary movements that may be mistaken for convulsions but can also precipitate severe convulsions. Fentanyl may cause severe dystonia mistaken for tonic–clonic fits and cephalosporins may make fits worse

is absorbed rapidly and reaches peak levels within 4–10 min. A higher dose is needed rectally (0.5 mg/kg) than intravenously (0.1 mg/kg). If two doses of rectal diazepam have failed one further dose of intravenous diazepam is justified before a change to a different drug as respiratory depression can occur.

Never LP an unconscious child without a CT scan. It is essential to consider and rule out CNS infection, thus the decision about whether or not to do a lumbar puncture always arises. If the seizures stop and the child is showing signs of waking up and there are no other signs of raised intracranial pressure then a lumbar puncture should be done. If the seizure has been unilateral then a hemiplegia on that side is not a sign of structural cerebral damage and if there are no other indications of raised intracranial pressure it is not a contraindication to lumbar puncture. If the child does not wake up or does not stop fitting then he should be managed as for any other acute encephalopathy and a CT scan carried out before a lumbar puncture. This may mean treating with broad-spectrum antibiotics before the lumbar puncture (a retrospective diagnosis can be made using countercurrent immunoelectrophoresis when lumbar puncture is safe). Urine and blood should be sent for antigen testing against haemophilus, meningococcus and pneumococcus and a toxicology screen if the history is suggestive.

The management of status epilepticus involves prompt stopping of the seizure followed by the determination of the underlying cause, with treatment of this where possible.

In most cases of status our personal practice is to load the patient with phenytoin after the diazepam even if the seizures have stopped. This is to provide continued anticonvulsant cover over the next few hours. Status occurring in a patient already taking oral phenytoin is not a contraindication to intravenous phenytoin as long as ECG monitoring is in place. Paraldehyde is an extremely effective anticonvulsant and side effects or complications are very uncommon.

In some instances, particularly in an obese toddler where difficulties are encountered in finding veins and in whom rectal diazepam therapy has been tried, paraldehyde would be an appropriate first-line drug.

Although it is our practice to use diazepam as first-line anticonvulsant, there is evidence to suggest that lorazepam (Appleton et al 1995) may be the drug of choice in early status (bolus dose of 0.1 mg/kg). Its pharmacology and clinical effects have been extensively investigated in adults and neonates. It binds strongly to cerebral tissue and has a longer duration of action than diazepam. It is only moderately lipid soluble so there are fewer problems caused by redistribution than with other benzodiazepines but rapid tolerance develops. Initial injection is effective for 12 hours, but later administration seems less effective so maintenance antiepileptic drug therapy should always be given with lorazepam therapy. Lorazepam shares the same sedative side effects as the other benzodiazepines but sudden hypotension or respiratory collapse are less likely (Shorvon 1994).

There are very few seizures that paraldehyde will not stop. If after 20 minutes seizures are still present, phenobarbitone 10–20 mg/kg should be given by slow intravenous infusion. Although very effective, hypotension is a real risk and if intracranial pressure is raised this may have disastrous effects. Close attention should be paid to blood pressure and heart rate and respiratory rate and if hypotension occurs it should be treated aggressively with plasma or ionotropic drugs.

Seizures may cause rises in intracranial pressure that may persist after the seizure has stopped. Radiological evidence has shown cerebral edema in the acute phase of status epilepticus that disappears on recovery.

If the patient is anesthetized or paralyzed as part of third-line management (Table 14.24) EEG monitoring is essential to determine that seizure activity is abolished. In acute encephalopathies after control of clinical seizures, a stage of electroclinical dissociation may occur with continuous electrical seizures occurring without clinical accompaniment. This can be associated with continued raised intracranial pressure and if consciousness is not regained ICP monitoring may be required.

Treatment with lignocaine and/or chlormethiazole may be effective.

In our experience the use of diazepam, phenytoin, paraldehyde and mannitol allows the vast majority of cases of status to be treated outside the intensive care unit. Great care is needed as it is possible to lower cerebral perfusion pressure and depress respiration before controlling the electrical activity. We feel this should only be done under EEG control as we have seen extensive asphyxial damage in several children treated in this way. It is possible to use thiopentone infusions without ventilating the patients but this should be done only where facilities for easy intubation or ventilation are available.

If the patient is already on antiepileptic drugs then blood levels should be taken on arrival to hospital. Sudden withdrawal of antiepileptic treatment or loss from vomiting is a not uncommon cause of status in older children. If episodes are recurrent or the patient is not recovering then urinary organic acids, amino acids, blood lactate, ammonia and a blood gas test should be carried out to exclude a metabolic cause.

ACUTE ENCEPHALOPATHIES

DEFINITION AND CLASSIFICATION

Acute encephalopathy denotes a nonspecific brain insult in a patient manifested by a combination of coma, seizures, decerebration and, less commonly, ataxia, hemiplegia or cardiorespiratory arrest. Coma and seizures may be seen as neurological complications of many children's diseases, for example scalds and burns, cardiac bypass surgery, leukemia, hepatic failure in fibrocystic disease, diabetic ketoacidosis, celiac and nephrotic crises as well as gastroenteritis with 0157 E. coli, Shigella or Campylobacter infection.

Acute encephalopathies may be classified as:

1. hypoxic ischemic
2. infectious and parainfectious
3. hemorrhagic
4. traumatic (accidental and nonaccidental)
5. toxic
   a. exogenous
   b. endogenous
6. epileptic.

ETIOLOGY

Infection accounts for approximately one-third of cases presenting with acute encephalopathy and coma. The causes are seen in Table 14.25. Most organisms are capable of invading the nervous system (with the direct effects of cerebral edema, cerebritis, encephalitis, cerebral congestion, hydrocephalus, subdural effusion and empyemas, ventriculitis, thrombophlebitis and abscess), but encephalopathy may also result from the effects of extracranial infection by inappropriate ADH, inflammatory brain edema, thrombophlebitis, status epilepticus, severe endotoxemic shock and DIC. E. coli 0157, Shigella and Campylobacter may secrete a neurotoxin which causes fits and coma, a true toxic encephalopathy.

As an example, tuberculous meningitis may present as an acute hemiplegia resulting from vasculitis or as an acute encephalopathy with raised intracranial pressure from acute ventricular dilation or multiple tuberculomata.

Table 14.25 Causes of infectious encephalopathies

Bacterial or fungal meningitis/encephalitis

Cortical thrombophlebitis

Cerebral abscess (including immunocompromised patients)

Meningitis with septicaemia (*Meningococcus*/B hemolytic *Streptococcus*)

Viral encephalitis (e.g. herpes simplex encephalitis)

Parainfectious demyelinization

Subacute sclerosing panencephalitis (acute presentation)

Meningoencephalitis (protozoal, helminthic and rickettsial), e.g. *Toxoplasma*

Cerebral malaria

Acute disseminated encephalomyelitis

Viruses may result in an acute encephalopathy by virtue of their neurotropic nature or they may attack specific parts of the central nervous or peripheral system, e.g. polio and the anterior horn cells, chickenpox and the cerebellum or mumps and the aqueduct of Sylvius. Viruses may also produce an acute encephalitis or perivascular demyelination as a result of myelinoclastic antibodies produced by the leukocytes involved in perivascular cuffing.

A reversible encephalopathy from virus invasion of neurons may result in the 'pyrexial convulsion syndrome'. Virus infection may also lead to catabolic stress and precipitation of inborn errors of metabolism such as maple syrup urine disease, Leigh's syndrome (pyruvate decarboxylase deficiency), biotinidase deficiency, cytochrome oxidase deficiency or other complex mitochondrial cytopathies.

Hypoxic ischemia

This is a common and frequently irremediable cause of acute encephalopathy. The pathogenesis of hypoxic ischemic injury begins with hypoxia followed by a build-up of $PaCO_2$, lactic acid and a decreased pH. There follows a two-pronged insult.

1. To the brain cell membrane with inhibition of membrane ion pumps, resulting in accumulation of extracellular K^+ and intracellular Na^+ and Ca^{2+} and in depletion of ATP and phosphocreatine. The result is a cytotoxic edema which contributes to the raised intracranial pressure and infarction. The release of glutamate causes a rise in intracellular calcium and this activates proteases and can result in secondary or further cell death.

2. To the cardiac muscle (as well as lung, liver, kidneys and gut) with a resultant systemic pressure failure below the limits of cerebrovascular autoregulation. This results in failure of cerebral perfusion and infarction, i.e. ischemia is added to the hypoxia. The low systemic pressure additionally adds a degree of vasogenic brain edema.

The brain is able to withstand hypoxia without ischemia by anaerobic metabolism but is especially sensitive to ischemia when delivery of substrate fails and there is failure of removal of the lactic acid which causes a severe intracellular acidosis. In hypoxia alone there is reversion to anaerobic metabolism with glucose converted to lactate and pyruvate. If the circulation is intact these metabolites are removed and later converted back to glucose in the liver when oxygen becomes available. With ischemia (for example, from raised intracranial pressure and reduced cerebral

Table 14.26 Hypoxic ischemic causes of acute encephalopathy

Perinatal asphyxia

Pulmonary disease (upper airways obstruction, laryngeal TB, epiglottitis)

Alveolar hypoventilation

CO poisoning

Methemoglobinemia

Anemia

Status epilepticus

Near miss SIDS

Postcardiac arrest (any cause)

Cardiac bypass surgery

Near drowning

Cardiac dysrhythmia

Congestive cardiac failure

Hypotension

Disseminated intravascular coagulation

Hypoglycemia

Vitamin or cofactor deficiency (B_{12}, B_6, folate, etc.)

Anesthetic accidents

perfusion pressure), especially if there is plentiful glucose, glycolysis continues with an accumulation of lactate which is not cleared and causes intracellular acidosis. This prevents enzyme action and causes the lysosomes to rupture. Although status epilepticus is considered a separate cause of encephalopathies, the end result of uncontrolled and decompensated status epilepticus is cerebral edema and hypoxic ischemic injury with depleted ATP and PCr and increased lactate and diminished cerebral blood flow. The hypoxic ischemic causes of encephalopathy and coma are listed in Table 14.26.

Toxic and metabolic disorders

These may result in an exogenous or endogenous encephalopathy. The exogenous causes are seen in Table 14.27. Occasionally these may be nonaccidentally delivered as part of the Munchausen

Table 14.27 Causes of toxic encephalopathy (exogenous)

Antihistamines

Anticholinergics

Anticonvulsants

Antidepressants (tricyclics and phenothiazines)

Antimetabolites (vincristine, cyclophosphamide, methotrexate, asparaginase, vinblastine, cranial irradiation, cytosine arabinoside)

Hypnotics and analgesics (barbiturates, paracetamol, benzodiazepines and salicylates)

Antibiotics (penicillin, nalidixic acid)

Antiinflammatory agents (steroids, cimetadine)

Abused drugs (alcohol, solvents, amphetamines, etc.)

Environmental toxins (H_2S, CO, phosphates, DDT, iron, lead, hexachlorophane, aflatoxin, venoms, insecticides/pesticides, plants and minerals, heavy metals, hypothermia and heat stroke)

Table 14.28 Endogenous causes of acute encephalopathy

1. Fluid balance	Water intoxication
	Hypo- or hypernatremia
	Hypo- or hypermagnesemia
	Hypo- or hypercalcemia
	Hypo- or hyperphosphatemia
	Acidosis/alkalosis
	Trace metal deficiency
	Scalds
2. Endocrine	Diabetes mellitus/hypoglycemia
	Hypo- or hyperthyroidism
	Hypo- or hyperparathyroidism
	Hypopituitarism
	Hyperbilirubinemia
3. Organ failure	Liver
	Kidneys
	Pancreas
	Intestinal/volvulus
	Hypertensive encephalopathy
4. Inborn errors of metabolism	Aminoacidopathies – branched chain ketoacidosis
	Organic acidemia – propyl, malonyl, isovaleric and betaketothiolase
	Galactosemia
	Urea cycle defects
	Carnitine deficiency
	Porphyria
	Medium chain acyl dehydrogenase deficiency (MCAD)

syndrome by proxy (p. 1870). Endogenous sources of toxins include liver and renal failure, carbon dioxide narcosis and other causes given in Table 14.28.

Nontraumatic intracranial hemorrhage

This may be responsible for an acute encephalopathy, for example hemorrhage into a benign astrocytic cyst. Other causes are listed in Table 14.29.

Trauma

Trauma may be accidental or nonaccidental. Accidental head injury is discussed elsewhere (pp. 704–707). The young child who presents with an acute encephalopathy with retinal hemorrhages but little evidence of external trauma should be suspected of having had a 'whiplash shaking injury' (disciplinary injury). The shaking, with rotation of the head, results in subdural and

Table 14.29 Intracranial hemorrhage

Arteriovenous malformation

Ruptured aneurysm

Arteriovenous occlusion – thrombotic or traumatic
a. Infection (focal or widespread)
b. Cardiac
c. Hematological (sickle cell, polycythemia or idiopathic thrombocytopenic purpura)
d. Collagen (lupus erythematosus)
e. Metabolic (diabetes mellitus)
f. Moya moya

Intracranial venous thrombosis which may be sterile or secondary to thrombophlebitis

petechial brain hemorrhages, cerebral edema and retinal hemorrhages.

INVESTIGATION OF COMA

After the initial resuscitation of the cardiovascular and respiratory system and treatment of seizures, after a history has been obtained of the events leading to the coma and after an examination of the child, the clinician's approach to investigating the comatose child is two-fold. First, investigations are aimed at making a diagnosis (Table 14.30) and second, supportive investigations are necessary regardless of the etiology (Table 14.31). The coma state will require monitoring itself. Initially one of the coma scales is used, such as the original Glasgow coma scale (Table 14.35) or the modified Glasgow coma scale (Table 14.36). Alternatives are the Adelaide scale, the 0-IV scale (Table 14.32), the 'Jacobi scale', the children's coma scale and the children's orthopedic hospital and medical center scale. We favor the Adelaide scale and the 0–IV scale, but once the patient is paralyzed and ventilated, all scales are insufficient for following the progress of coma and the coma state then needs monitoring by means of:

1. ocular examination (pupils, eye movements, etc.);
2. bulbar reflexes;
3. temperature, pulse rate, respiratory rate and blood pressure.

MANAGEMENT OF ENCEPHALOPATHY

Whatever the cause of the encephalopathy, there are common factors responsible for the mortality and morbidity. These have led to a philosophy of management of 'treating the treatable':

1. treatment of infection;
2. control of seizures;
3. detection and treatment of raised intracranial pressure;
4. maintenance of cerebral blood flow;
5. maintenance of cerebral metabolism;
6. maintenance of homeostasis;
7. removal of circulating toxins.

Table 14.30 Strategy for coma management: diagnostic investigations

Obvious causes	Nonobvious causes
Hypoxic ischemic	CT – ultrasound
Diabetic ketoacidosis	LP (incl. immunofluorescence, etc.)
Poisoning	EEG
Infections	Toxicology (barbiturates, toluene, benzodiazepines, salicylates, iron, lead, anticonvulsants,
Drowning	antidepressants)
Burns/scalds	Metabolic (NH_3, LFTs, porphyrins, amino acids, dicarboxylic acids, urine sugars, lactate/pyruvate/
Cerebrovascular accident	acidosis, urea/creatinine, calcium, T_4/TSH)
	Tuberculin test
	Virology
	Technetium scan
	X-rays (skull, skeletal)
	Brain biopsy

Table 14.31 Strategy for coma management: supportive investigations (independent of cause of coma)

* Blood gases (4 hourly)
* Pulse oximeter (O₂ sat.)
  CVP −/+ Wedge
* Dextrostix/BMstix (4 hourly)
* Osmolality (8 hourly)
* Calcium and phosphate (bd)
  EEG (continuous)
  ICP/CPP (continuous) (mean pressure, pulse pressure, periodic waves)
* BP arterial (continuous)
  Coagulation (once then prn)
* Temperature
* Fluid balance (vs output, weight, labstix)
* Blood count and hemoglobin
* CXR (portable)
  Weight
  Anticonvulsant levels
* ECG (continuous)
* Urea and electrolytes (twice daily)
* Infection screen
  Visual-evoked potentials
  Brainstem-evoked potentials
  Liver function tests (once/day)
  Arteriovenous oxygen difference or jugular venous oxygen saturation
  Cerebral blood flow (initial + change) (autoregulation, CO₂ respiration and perfusion)
  Cerebral blood flow velocity (continuous, intermittent daily)
  Monitoring neurology and coma state
  1. Glasgow coma scale
  2. Ocular (pupils, external ocular movements, etc.)
  3. Bulbar reflexes
  4. Temperature, pulse rate, respiratory rate and blood pressure

* All coma regardless of cause.

Treatment of infection

The treatment of bacterial meningitis, cerebritis, encephalitis and thrombophlebitis is with appropriate high-dose intravenous antibiotic therapy or, in the case of herpes simplex encephalitis, acyclovir. It is common practice to give intravenous cefotaxime and acyclovir as initial treatment until detailed microbiological investigations are to hand.

Cytocentrifugation and millipore filter collection of cells has improved the identification of cell types in the CSF. The technique is useful in CNS leukemia, as well as in acute and chronic spinal meningitis (Kontopolous et al 1986). It is particularly useful in cases of mild CSF pleocytosis. There is a significant discordance between lymphocytes and macrophages in the CSF and the ability to recognize the recovery phase of pyogenic CSF infection by an increased macrophage count is useful while treating meningitis or ventriculitis.

Antibiotics vary in their ability to penetrate the CSF. Antituberculous drugs penetrate well but the aminoglycosides as a group show poor CSF penetration and need to be given intrathecally, e.g. for postoperative infections, shunt infections with *Staphylococcus albus* and the rare resistant pneumococcus. Antibiotic serum levels should also be routinely monitored. Low peak levels of antibiotic indicate that the frequency of administration needs to be increased while low trough levels indicate that the dose should be increased. It is important to insure the antibiotic is instilled at the appropriate locus to be effective, as antibiotics injected into the lumbar CSF may not reach the basal cisterns if there is loculation and very little will reflux back into the ventricles. In such situations a ventriculostomy reservoir may usefully be inserted for administration of the antibiotics.

In the case of tuberculous meningitis with coma the ideal management is first to obtain a CT scan and since tuberculous meningitis is frequently accompanied by an acute hydrocephalus in children, this is followed by the insertion of a ventriculostomy reservoir into the frontal horn of the right lateral ventricle. The intracranial pressure is then measured and relief of the

Table 14.32 Coma scales for use in children (see also Tables 14.35 and 14.36)

0-IV Scale		Adelaide Scale (Simpson & Reilly 1982) Children <5 years	
0	Arouses spontaneously and to stimuli	Eye opening	4 Spontaneous 3 To speech 2 To pain 1 Nil
I	Stuperose. Spontaneous arousal rare Roused readily but briefly by stimuli Cough/gag present		
II	Spontaneous arousal absent Semipurposive/avoidance motor response to stimuli Cough/gag depressed	Verbal response	5 Oriented 4 Words 3 Vocal sounds 2 Cries 1 Nil
III	Arousal in form of motor response only to intense, sustained, painful stimuli Cough/gag absent	Motor response	5 Obeys commands 4 Localizes pain 3 Flexion 2 Extension 1 Nil
IV	Not aroused even by intense/sustained painful stimuli Cough/gag absent		
		(Normal developmental milestones taken into account) 0–6 months >6–12 months >1–2 years >2–5 years >5 years	9 points 11 points 12 points 13 points 14 points

supratentorial pressure obtained by removal of CSF. With the intracranial pressure normal, a lumbar puncture is performed for lumbar CSF collection. The spinal meningitis is not necessarily accompanied by an increased cell count in the ventricular CSF. Persistent raised intracranial pressure needs to be treated by tapping the reservoir or by external drainage from the reservoir while at the same time sterilizing the CSF with the appropriate antituberculous medication.

Control of seizures

It is important to control seizures to prevent secondary hypoxic ischemic damage and routine EEG monitoring (preferably continuous display) should be carried out. A single fit during an acute encephalopathy requires only short-term prophylactic anticonvulsants. Phenytoin is the anticonvulsant of choice (see Ch. 38). For epileptic encephalopathy, intravenous diazepam and intravenous mannitol with or without paraldehyde may be required.

Paraldehyde can be given in modern plastic syringes. It is usually given intramuscularly in a dose of 0.05 ml/kg or 1 ml/year of age. The half-life is approximately 6 h (range 6–9 h). In an urgent situation it can be given well diluted intravenously, but this is not recommended. The dose should be reduced in the presence of hepatic or pulmonary disease. Much care is needed with intravenous injections because of serious hepatic necrosis or pulmonary hemorrhage which may result. The rectal route is a satisfactory alternative, if given in a 10% solution with normal saline or mixed with equal quantities of arachis oil. The dose of the 10% solution is 0.5 ml/kg. Estimation of blood levels of paraldehyde can be performed in some laboratories (therapeutic range is 300–400 mg/ml).

Intravenous phenytoin may be given as a slow or rapid regimen. For encephalopathies the rapid regime is required – 10 mg/kg intravenously at a rate of 10 mg/min, followed 1 h later by 5 mg/kg with a further 10 mg/kg in divided doses over the next 24 h. ECG monitoring is advised. The blood level must be measured daily and maintained in a therapeutic range. In the newborn there is a large dose range (between 2 and 25 mg/kg) and blood level should be regularly checked The dose required may change acutely in the second week of life. At high doses phenytoin may become epileptogenic and produce seizures which are resistant to benzodiazepines and paraldehyde. Prolonged thiopentone or chlormethiazole may result in enzyme induction and low phenytoin levels. The commonest reason for failure to control seizures in acute encephalopathy is failure to achieve adequate plasma concentrations of the drug.

Diazepam is useful to control seizures in the acute presentation of encephalopathies although some children may be diazepam resistant and have an exacerbation of seizure activity. With continuous EEG monitoring the benzodiazepine sensitivity can be readily assessed. There is a slight cerebral vasoconstrictor effect and therefore intracranial pressure is lowered. Following the first dose, if the fits have not ceased and provided the pupils have not dilated, the blood pressure is maintained and the child is not benzodiazepine resistant, it may be repeated. The intravenous preparation should not be diluted for injection or a white precipitate may form in the mixture, which is irritant. It should not be mixed with other drugs and should be injected at a rate of 1 mg/min. Fast injection may cause apnea or laryngeal spasm and hypotension. Other benzodiazepines, such as clonazepam, are more likely to produce hypotension and bronchorrhea. Peak brain

levels of diazepam occur 1 min after injection but the drug leaves the brain rapidly and fits may recur after 20 min. The dose is 0.25–0.4 mg/kg (age in years plus 1). An intravenous infusion is possible for those cases responsive to diazepam (0.1 mg/kg/hr).

Lignocaine, thiopentone and chlormethiazole are alternative anticonvulsants for use with encephalopathies. With thiopentone the aim is to stop seizures and not to produce anesthesia. Apnea, hypotension and laryngospasm may all occur from fast infusion of thiopentone.

Intracranial pressure

A common factor in children with encephalopathies and cerebral edema is the secondary brain shifts which cause ischemic brain damage. These are responsible for the mortality and the morbidity. They come about by a critical reduction in the vascular perfusion pressure to the brain produced usually by an increase in intracranial pressure.

Detection of raised intracranial pressure

The methods and sites for monitoring intracranial pressure are given in Table 14.33 (Leggate & Minns 1990). In children with encephalopathies, the preferred technique will depend on whether ventricular dilation is present or whether the ventricles are small and shifted as a result of the brain swelling.

For the infant with a patent anterior fontanel and with venticular dilation, the ventricles can be punctured percutaneously. If ICP monitoring is needed continuously and for long periods, then a ventriculostomy reservoir is neurosurgically inserted or a ventricular transducer placed in situ. For the infant with cerebral edema it is possible to continuously monitor the intracranial pressure by the use of a subdural or subarachnoid Teflon catheter placed percutaneously through the anterior fontanel. A ventricular transducer may be inserted which will record either the ventricular pressure (or if not in the ventricle, the brain parenchymal pressure). For the older child with acute ventricular dilation we either insert a ventriculostomy reservoir or, when the brain is edematous, monitor the intracranial pressure from the brain

Table 14.33 Sites for ICP monitoring

Ventricle	Catheter (percutaneous through the anterior fontanel)
	Catheter (via burr hole)
	Reservoir
	Transducer (camino)
	Telemetry (± inline with shunt)
Subarachnoid (and subdural)	Bolt (Beeds, Richmond, Newell, Philly, Bolt)
	Catheter (cordis via burr hole)
	Catheter (Teflon via anterior fontanel)
	Transducer (catheter tipped-gaeltec ICTb)
	Transducer (miniaturized, fitment to burr hole)
	Lumbar space (at LP or cannula)
Extradural	Catheter tip transducers
	Transducer (similar to subdural)
	Sensors (Ladd)
Brain parenchyma	Fiberoptic transducer (brain tissue pressure)
Fontanel	Fontanometers (aplanation especially pneumatic)
Tympanic membrane	Impedance test of tympanic membrane tension

surface by means of a 'Cordis fluid-filled catheter' coupled to a pressure transducer.

Because of the need to compare the intracranial pressure with arterial blood pressure the same units of measurement are usually used. These are mm of mercury (1 mmHg = 1.36 cmH$_2$O) or if SI units are used, ICP is expressed as kiloPascals (1 kPa = 7.5 mmHg). The normal ICP in adults is 0–15 mmHg (0–2 kPa). In children the upper limit of normal ICP is lower and for the newborn levels should not be in excess of 3.5 mmHg, for the older infant 5.5 mmHg and for the toddler 6.5 mmHg (Minns et al 1989a).

Brief rises in the intracranial pressure may occur during coughing, straining and crying, as well as other physiological activities that increase the central venous pressure. Sustained elevations or intermittent rises in pressure in the form of pressure waves may also occur (Fig. 14.22). Several wave forms have been described.

A waves or plateau waves. These show a rapid rise in ICP to 50 mmHg or more which last from 5 to 20 min.

B waves. These are sharply peaked waves lasting 30 s to 2 min. Both A and B waves are thought to result from cerebral vasodilation. In the A waves this occurs against a background of reduced craniospinal compliance in which small increments of volume result in large increases in pressure. B waves, on the other hand, may result from fluctuations in the cerebral vascular dimensions corresponding to alterations in arterial CO$_2$ tension.

C waves. Rapid sinusoidal fluctuations of about 6 per min corresponding to the Traube–Hering–Mayer fluctuations in the systemic arterial tree.

An increase in the intracranial pressure may come about as a result of increasing either the brain, blood or CSF contents of the skull. The actual increases in ICP that result from a given increment in volume will depend on the intracranial pressure–volume status. The pressure–volume response (PVR) is an increase in ICP in mmHg/ml of CSF volume added or withdrawn in 1 s. Normal values are 0–2 mmHg/ml; values of 3 mmHg or more at baseline ICP levels indicate reduced craniospinal compliance (or increased elastance). Marmarov et al (1975) defined a pressure–volume index (PVI) as a volume which if added to the CSF would produce a 10-fold increase in the intracranial pressure. The normal range of PVI in an adult is 25–30 ml. In a child it is from 12 to 25 ml.

The cingulate gyrus herniates under the lower margin of the falx as the midline is shifted. The medial part of the temporal lobe also herniates through the tentorial hiatus between the free edge of the tentorium and the midbrain. At the same time the brainstem is

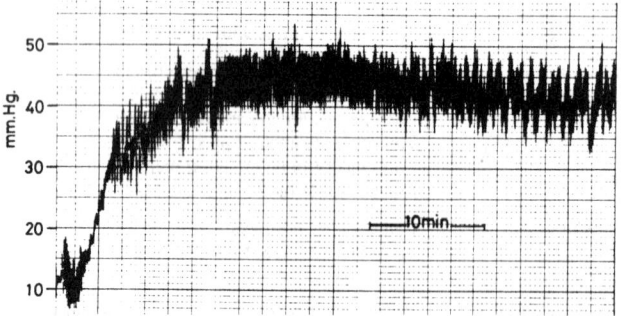

Fig. 14.22 Plateau or A-wave indicating reduced cerebral compliance in the presence of intact cerebrovascular autoregulation (mmHg = ventricular CSF pressure).

Table 14.34 Clinical features of brain herniations

Tentorial
  Sunsetting
  Dilated pupils
  VI nerve palsy
  Cortical blindness
  Hemiplegia
  Extensor motor pattern (decerebrate)
  Coma
  Respiratory irregularity
  Systemic hypertension
  Tonic seizures

Cingulate gyrus herniation
  Diplegia or hemiplegia
  Visual symptoms

Foramen magnum cone
  Cardiorespiratory arrest
  Bulbar palsy
  Neck stiffness
  Hypotonia
  Stridor
  Spinal flexion
  Hypotension
  Hyperthermia

shifted downward to the foramen magnum which tends to cut off the blood supply to the stem from the perforating branches of the basilar artery and results in ischemia. The signs of a cingulate gyrus herniation, tentorial herniation and foramen magnum cone are given in Table 14.34.

Cerebral perfusion pressure

With increasing ICP there is an increase in the cerebral venous pressure. This remains about 3 mmHg below the ICP so that cerebral circulation continues. The cerebral perfusion pressure is the difference between the mean systemic arterial pressure (MAP) and intracranial pressure (ICP), i.e. CPP = MAP – ICP.

The relationship between intracranial pressure and cerebral perfusion pressure is complex. Raised intracranial pressure may be caused by an increase in cerebral blood flow or it may be the limiting factor producing a reduction in cerebral blood flow. In encephalopathies the brain is frequently pale and devoid of blood flow as a result of the raised intracranial pressure producing ischemia. A cerebral perfusion pressure of 60–70 mmHg is normal and there is a progressive fall in perfusion to the brain with decreasing cerebral perfusion pressures down to 40 mmHg. Below this there is an absolute fall in the brain perfusion and levels of less than 18–20 ml/100 g of brain per min will result in ischemic infarction.

Cerebral blood flow

The earliest measurements of blood flow utilized the Fick principle with a method which involved inhalation of a metabolically inert gas that diffused freely in and out of brain tissue. The normal value in man is 50 ml/100 g per min. The normal cerebral arteriovenous oxygen content difference is 6 ml/100 ml of blood and therefore the normal cerebral oxygen uptake rate is 3 ml oxygen/100 g per min. Ordinarily there is coupling between cerebral blood flow and brain metabolism but in coma the cerebral metabolic rate consuming oxygen falls as well as the cerebral blood flow.

The determinant of cerebral blood flow is the arterial $PaCO_2$ level. Increases in the arterial $PaCO_2$ increase the cerebral blood flow and a fall in arterial $PaCO_2$ reduces the cerebral blood flow due to cerebral vasoconstriction. Changes in cerebral blood flow cause changes in the cerebral blood volume and this influences the ICP. Inducing hypocapnia by hyperventilation can reduce ICP (if the raised ICP had been due to cerebral vasodilation). If, however, the cerebral blood flow is already low from cerebral edema then hyperventilation will result in worsening ischemia. CO_2 responsiveness may be lost globally or regionally.

The cerebral blood flow remains constant over an arterial pressure level of 60–140 mmHg in normal adults. With low systemic arterial pressures, below the limits of cerebrovascular autoregulation there is a fall in cerebral blood flow and with blood pressure rises above 140 mmHg there is a breakthrough of autoregulation (break point) with progressive cerebral edema. Autoregulation, therefore, can be defined as a maintenance of the cerebral blood flow by alteration of the cerebral blood volume in response to large changes (increases or decreases) in the systemic perfusion pressure. Autoregulation can also be lost globally or regionally.

Treatment of raised intracranial pressure

Removal of CSF is possible if a ventricular cannula is in situ but this is not always possible with small shifted ventricles and cerebral edema. Despite this, for some conditions such as tuberculous meningitis this may be the optimal method of managing the raised intracranial pressure.

Steroids have a number of important actions on the brain – an immunosuppressant effect, an antiinflammatory effect and the reduction of CSF formation. At a cellular level the endothelial junctions of the blood–brain barrier are tightened, there is stabilization of lysosomal activity and restoration of the microcirculation. Other effects include inhibition of the release of free radicals, fatty acids, prostaglandins and the products of catecholamine metabolism. Steroids also cause glial uptake and transcapillary efflux of water with resolution of edema. Steroids cross the blood–brain barrier to reach neuronal receptor sites. There is an additional direct effect on cerebral metabolism with increased neuronal function and stimulation of glucose consumption.

Steroids are of little use in controlling the raised intracranial pressure in Reye's syndrome. They are most useful in reducing the perifocal edema surrounding mass lesions. They may be positively harmful in hypoxic ischemic brain damage and their use in herpes simplex encephalitis is debatable. Mannitol in combination with dexamethasone will prevent the unwanted escape of mannitol across the blood–brain barrier. Mannitol reduces brain water by controlled hyperosmolar dehydration, it reduces blood viscosity and increases cerebral vasoconstriction (the cerebral blood flow remains normal while the cerebral blood volume is decreased). Mannitol also scavenges free radicals. If mannitol and frusemide are used together, the circulating volume is decreased and, depending on the central venous pressure, volume expansion may be necessary. Mannitol is given in a dose of 7 ml/kg of a 20% solution or 0.21 g/kg per dose.

Hyperventilation should not be used prophylactically in encephalopathies to control raised intracranial pressure. Its use should be restricted to episodic increases in intracranial pressure because the cerebral vasoconstriction, changes in pH, bicarbonate

and CO_2 reactivity are not maintained if hyperventilation is continued for longer than 24 h. Prolonged hyperventilation can lead to ischemia. During episodes of raised intracranial pressure the $PaCO_2$ level should be reduced no lower than 3.5–4.0 kPa.

Barbiturates produce a concomitant reduction in the cerebral metabolic rate and cerebral blood flow. Their use is restricted to those patients unresponsive to mannitol, hyperventilation and steroids. It is important to carefully monitor the systemic blood pressure during their use for fear of reducing the cerebral perfusion pressure.

Other measures, such as decompression craniotomy or hypothermia, have some support in some units but, as with barbiturates, their use where first-line methods have failed is less likely to be successful.

HEAD INJURIES

Head injuries in children occur in three distinct categories which are age and mechanism specific:

1. birth injury – compression head injury;
2. nonaccidental head injury – shaking whiplash injury;
3. accidental head injury – acceleration and deceleration injuries.

BIRTH INJURY – COMPRESSION HEAD INJURY

The classic model for compression head injury in childhood is birth injury. The head is most compressed if there is malpresentation (occipitoposterior, deep transverse arrest or extended neck) or disproportion from too big a head (e.g. infant of diabetic mother, Sotos syndrome) or too small an outlet (pelvic contraction). The brain is mainly water and will not compress but is elastic, deformable and will easily mold. In breech presentation the head has to be squeezed and molded very rapidly with a much greater chance of rupturing vessels. In vertex presentation the head may mold in the anteroposterior diameter to give a 'Magoo head' when there is no forehead but a large amount of skull behind the ears. This stretches the falx and tentorium beyond their elastic limits so they tear. The vein of Galen and major sinuses in these dural reflections then tear causing severe tentorial hemorrhage, middle fossa subdural and posterior fossa bleeding. Transfontanel ultrasonography fails to reveal 50% of the hemorrhages but they show readily on CT scan (Faillot et al 1990). MRI is now the method of choice and will delineate injuries well. The head also is compressed laterally so that the parietal bones override and pull the sagittal sinus between them (sagittal sinus entrapment syndrome). This puts traction on the veins entering the sinus and tears them so that a hemisphere subdural and subarachnoid hemorrhage results. The head ossifies rapidly after 40 weeks gestation and will not mold and so obstructed labor with the infant failing to descend and skull fractures and cephalhematomas is then more common.

Compression head injury in the past was also associated with cephalhematomas, brachial plexus lesions, fractures, cervical spinal injuries and metaphyseal injuries. The intracranial bleeding associated with compression injury used to be a common cause of acute and chronic subdural hematomas. The latter presented with a big head, irritability, fever, vomiting at several months of age, i.e. the same time as nonaccidental injury.

NONACCIDENTAL HEAD INJURY

Incidence

Figures of 2000 children murdered and 1 700 000 punched or bitten each year in the USA were given by Solomons (1979). Kempe (1971) suggests an incidence of 6/1000 of the childhood population. Less than 10% of all physically abused children will have significant head injury with brain involvement. If head injuries under 2 years are considered then a high prevalence of abuse is found: of 100 children studied in a carefully controlled prospective study (Duhaime et al 1992), 24% were presumed inflicted and these carried a higher mortality and risk of permanent brain damage than true accidental injuries.

In approximately 75% there are bruises, burns in 20%, fractures in 40% and intracranial damage in 40%.

Neurological presentation of child abuse

The neurological presentation is not specific and may not immediately suggest abuse. The child may present as a recurrent encephalopathy when encephalitis or metabolic disease may be suspected rather than repeated poisoning or shaking. Fabrication of symptoms, especially fits (fictitious epilepsy), is a form of child abuse in Munchausen by proxy. A seizure is a common presentation of nonaccidental head injury; the child may present as an isolated fit from shaking or as status epilepticus. Odd turns, fits, apneic attacks, cyanotic attacks, rigidity or coma can be due to repeated attempts to suffocate the child. Video recordings have shown that a parent may carry a rolled-up item of clothing to put over the child's mouth and they will do this in hospital or intensive care unit (Southall et al 1987). Polygraphic studies using ambulatory monitoring show the child struggling on the EMG, apneic, bradycardiac and the EEG flattens from hypoxemia rather than showing epileptic spikes. The greatest difficulty is in separating the rare child who presents as a cot death from nonaccidental suffocation.

The child may present as a true head injury with bruising, swelling, lacerations, fractured skull and neurological signs and symptoms. Injuries remote from the head can present with fits and coma (e.g. scalds encephalopathy). In the shaking injury there may be no evidence of trauma to the head unless there has been an associated impact.

The commonest presentation is as a nonspecific unwell child, irritable or excessively quiet, refusing feeds, vomiting, with seizures, tonic extensor episodes, breathing difficulties, periodic breathing and cyanotic attacks (Duhaime et al 1987). The infant is often hypothermic, pale and shocked with low blood pressure and tachycardia, a presentation which does not immediately suggest severe intracranial bleeding and raised intracranial pressure.

Nonaccidental skull fractures

Most accidental fractures are simple linear fractures, usually parietal and over the vertex or coming from the coronal suture. If the fracture line branches, crosses suture lines, is bilateral, stellate, multiple with separate fractures, more than 5 mm wide at presentation or expands as a growing fracture, then nonaccidental fracture is more likely. A depressed fracture, especially of the occipital bone in a child under 3 years, also suggests abuse. Any of these features merits a full skeletal survey.

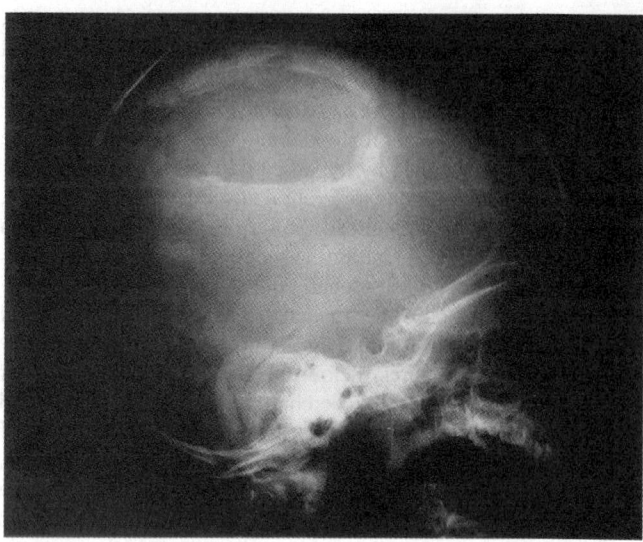

Fig. 14.23 Extensive growing skull fracture requiring rib graft.

The minimum radiological survey in this instance should include AP and lateral skull, chest, spine and pelvis on one large film plus an AP of arms and legs looking for associated fractures of ribs and long bones (Carty 1989).

Growing skull fractures or cephalohydroceles are very typical of nonaccidental skull fractures, often wide at presentation, in the first year of life. They occur in the rapid phase of skull growth, 50% occurring under 1 year and all under 3 years. The possible mechanisms may be:

1. a dural tear with trapping of dura between the fracture ends;
2. pulsation of the dura (i.e. a meningeal hernia or cephalohydrocele);
3. the formation of a pseudoarthrosis, i.e. a neosuture (Scarfo et al 1989).

The edges gradually become smooth and eroded as the center expands to several centimeters (Fig. 14.23) and the deficit may become so large that a bone graft may be necessary to fill in the hole. The ventricle on the affected side expands and shifts towards the deficit.

A skull fracture by itself is only medically important if:

- it is depressed into brain;
- it goes through the anterior fossa and cribriform plate, allowing CSF rhinorrhea and a risk of meningitis;
- it goes through the petrous temporal into the ear with a risk of meningitis;
- it enters the sinuses or is across the base with brainstem injury.

Skull fractures are legally important as they suggest impact and the use of possible premeditated force rather than simple disciplinary shaking. The excuses that the infant fell off a couch, etc. can then assume great importance.

Shaking whiplash injuries

An injury characteristic of child abuse is the whiplash shaking injury. The full picture, originally described by Caffey, consists of a subdural hematoma, massive cerebral edema, hemorrhagic retinopathy, fractured ribs and metaphyseal injury. One may see any combination, e.g. fractured ribs and retinopathy, retinopathy and fits, cerebral edema and retinopathy without subdural hematomas, retinopathy and subdural without fractured ribs. The classic picture occurs without any skull fracture, bruising of the scalp, edema or evidence of direct head trauma but impact of the head against a surface whilst shaking may give additional features of an impact injury.

The commonest age for shaking injury is 5 months. Of 30 children with nonaccidental head injury with brain involvement seen by the authors and in whom there is adequate follow-up, 17 were thought to be due to shaking, 12 due to impact with fractures and one to impact without fracture. In 16 of the 30 a subdural hematoma was diagnosed, in three subarachnoid hemorrhage alone and in four an intracerebral hemorrhage; 11 cases developed posthemorrhagic hydrocephalus. Jacobi (1986) described 62 battered children, 22 of whom were shaking injuries.

Mechanism of shaking

The child is usually shaken by the shoulders and upper arms, which may cause spiral humeral fractures or periosteal avulsion. Humeral fractures in very young children, excluding supracondylar fractures, were all found to be due to child abuse (Thomas et al 1991). Alternatively the smaller child is held by the rib cage which is often severely squeezed, leaving fingermark bruising and fractured ribs and causing a high central venous pressure which causes a retinopathy.

Rib fractures are thought to be due to chest compression; they may be unilateral or bilateral and may be more severe on the left side in a right-handed abuser. The fractures are more commonly posterior near the costovertebral junction, especially fourth to seventh rib. The rib is anchored posteriorly and may lever against the transverse process and so when pressed anteriorly, it is most likely to snap at its posterior convexity. Rib fractures are very rare in young infants due to falls, cough or birth injury; even very vigorous cardiac massage and resuscitation do not normally fracture any ribs (Feldman & Brewer 1984).

Other methods such as holding the abdomen and squeezing with the fingers during shaking can result in tearing of the mesentery with fatal hemorrhage into the peritoneal cavity. Holding the child by the ankles and swinging him round or holding him upside down and hammering the feet will also cause a high central venous pressure and retinopathy in addition to metaphyseal injuries.

Metaphyseal injuries, an integral part of the shaken baby syndrome, occur from twisting the limb as a disciplinary injury. The tendency to slap, shake the child or to grab a limb and twist it appear to be part of the same compulsive act by an exasperated adult (slap, shake and twist injuries).

Sufficient numbers of parents have admitted the manner of shaking to establish it as a cause (Kleinman et al 1989, Duhaime et al 1987, Aoki & Masuzawa 1986). Associated impact injury may be due to the head being banged against a hard surface repeatedly during the shaking; the child may be thrown or dropped on the floor after the shaking or his head hit against the wall. Concurrent injuries to the cervical spine with epidural spinal hemorrhage and bruising of the cervicomedullary junction are probably underestimated; they were found in five of six fatal cases of whiplash shaking injury by Hadley et al (1989).

The young infant has a relatively large heavy head in relation to the body (the brain represents 10% of the infant's and 2% of the

adult's weight). The neck muscles are weak with little head control so that even picking the infant up requires a hand behind the occiput to prevent the head flopping back. The force required is only sufficient to overcome the neck muscles and allow the head to whiplash with each shake. As with impact injuries, the acceleration or velocity is an important component as well as the duration. Many parents, if exasperated, will shake the infant slowly a couple of times but the serious abuser goes on in blind fury. It is thought that repeated minor shakings could be cumulative, in the same way as a boxer becomes demented with repeated knock-outs.

As the child gets older his bodyweight increases in relation to the head and the neck muscles are stronger. The head therefore moves with the body and it takes more force to accelerate him so that shaking whiplash injuries are rare after the second year of life and characteristic of the small child.

Pathophysiology of brain injury from shaking

Shaking causes the brain to swirl first in one direction and then the reverse. This sets up shearing forces within the skull and within the brain itself and is equivalent to repeated knock-outs by a boxer. The brain and skull have different inertial properties so the brain rotates at a different acceleration and timing, i.e. starts and stops rotating, from the skull. The shearing force causes tearing of bridging veins running from the surface of the brain to the sagittal sinus and this in turn causes a surface and interhemispheric subdural and subarachnoid bleeding without any fracture being present. Gray matter is firm and cellular whilst poorly myelinated, more gelatinous white matter is of different density and so they swirl at different velocities. This can be demonstrated on ultrasound imaging (Jaspan et al 1992).

CSF acts as a buffer and the brain floats in it, adding inertia to any movement but allowing the brain to carry on moving once the external force is removed.

The tentorium anchors the brainstem and the mid-brain acts as a pivot upon which the cerebral hemispheres can rotate. This can cause a primary brainstem injury with concussion. Sudden acceleration of the head must cause rotation in order to be concussional. In impact injuries associated with concussion, the sudden coma is due to rotation of the brain within the skull.

In child abuse tears in the white matter of the orbital, first and second frontal convolutions and temporal lobe are common. Axons can withstand enormous compressive forces but are easily sheared by traction. It is suggested that the poorly myelinated axons of the young child may stretch more than fully myelinated adult fibers. Shaking may cause slit-like cavities in white matter, called gliding contusions, and the ependyma may be torn so that necrotic brain extrudes into the ventricles (Rorke 1990). Blood vessels may stretch and if they do not themselves rupture, they can act like a cheese cutter and cause local cutting of white matter tracts. Shearing injuries occur in white matter of the hemispheres, particularly the corpus callosum, superior cerebellar peduncle and in the mid-brain. Lesions in the latter may be unilateral or bilateral but are usually asymmetrical and often multiple.

Cerebral edema

In impact and shaking injuries cerebral edema is often very severe. It is thought to take about 6 hours to appear after the injury. Cerebral edema has many different mechanisms of production, e.g. vasogenic, osmotic, hydrostatic, cytotoxic or necrotic (Brown 1991). The cause of the edema in the shaken infant is probably multifactorial with vascular damage (as in the eye) causing vasogenic edema, white matter damage, venous damage from shearing the venous drainage, damage to the blood–brain barrier, high central venous pressure from chest compression, brain necrosis from shock and impaired perfusion and secondary hydrocephalus causing hydrostatic edema from obstruction of the arachnoid granulations by blood.

Retinopathy of nonaccidental injury

Retinal hemorrhages are most characteristic of nonaccidental shaking injuries with chest compression. In Duhaime's series nine out of 10 children with retinal hemorrhage had been subjected to physical abuse; the one other case was a fatal high speed impact injury in a car (Duhaime et al 1992). Retinopathy can occur without subdural hemorrhage or cerebral edema but is seen in 50–70% of subdural hematomas. Retinal hemorrhages alone can be due to accidental injury, resuscitation or possibly prolonged fits. It is when combined with subdural hemorrhage, cerebral edema and fractured ribs that the syndrome becomes reliable as a pointer to nonaccidental injury.

Purtscher's retinopathy is a retinal angiopathy with paravenous hemorrhages secondary to sudden thoracic compression in adults (Kaur & Taylor 1992). In a typical angiopathic retinopathy the hemorrhages are not around the disc or flame shaped but tend to be paravenous petechiae, throughout the retina bilaterally and extend to the periphery, though one eye may be much more seriously affected than the other. In severe cases the retinal hemorrhage is extensive and confluent and not petechial.

The bleeding involves all retinal layers and is also preretinal, extending into the vitreous or backwards, i.e. subretinal, to cause retinal detachment. Exudates appear and the lens can dislocate. If one adds to this the optic atrophy from raised intracranial pressure and calcarine infarction of the visual area from tentorial herniation compressing the posterior cerebral arteries, it is not surprising that severe visual defect (about 60%) is common in survivors.

Subdural hematoma

Subdural hematomas are classified as acute (within 3 days of injury), subacute (3 days to 3 weeks) and chronic (Choux et al 1986). An acute subdural is usually associated with shock and a severe contusional brain injury progressing to severe necrotic cerebral edema. The brain is covered with a layer of 'redcurrant jelly' which may not itself be of great space-occupying volume yet it is fatal in 50% of cases due to the associated brain injury. In contrast a chronic subdural is insidious in onset with few signs of pressure despite a large space-occupying volume and an excellent prognosis (80% for complete recovery, 10% morbidity, 7% with seizures) and a low mortality, about 3%. The subacute subdural is intermediate to these two extremes.

A subdural hematoma is not a common accompaniment of head injury in children, apart from birth injury (now rare) or nonaccidental injuries, and in 6700 children with head trauma described by Choux et al (1986) it was present in only 4.3% of all cases.

If one considers all types of child abuse a subdural is only present in 8% of cases. Selection of cases will increase the percentage, as in Smith & Hanson's series (1974) where subdurals occurred in 60% of 134 cases of child abuse.

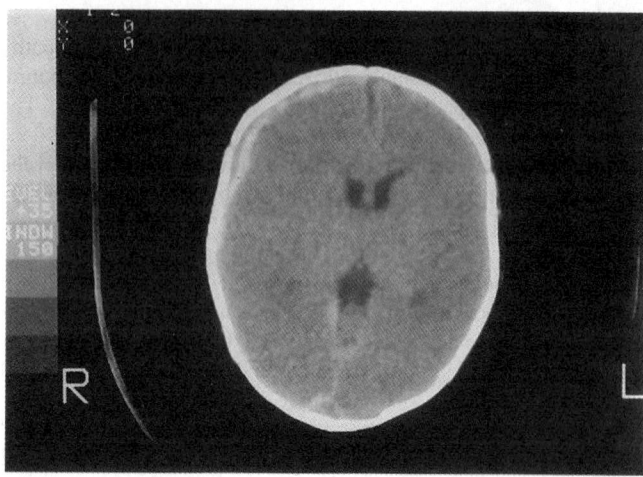

Fig. 14.24   Acute subdural hemorrhage over right hemisphere with hemispheric swelling and poor gray-white differentiation and some shift of midline.

Subdural hematomas in the first 2 years of life are more commonly acute and due to child abuse than birth injury or accidental injury. Only one case of subdural hematoma was found in a series of 536 children who had accidentally fallen a distance of 20–60 inches while 67% interhemispheric hematomas are thought to be the result of being shaken. Most fatal nonaccidental head injuries and many of those with persisting handicap have a subdural hematoma (Fig. 14.24).

Seventy-five percent of subdural hematomas are bilateral, 90% are supratentorial and 10% infratentorial. In nonaccidental injury they are most likely to be posterior, i.e. parietooccipital or interhemispheric in site, and 80% of interhemispheric subdural hematomas also have a retinopathy. An extradural hematoma is seen as an easily recognized biconvex disc on CT scan but the crescentic subdural is more easily missed.

Mechanism of subdural hematoma formation

An extradural hematoma is usually due to arterial bleeding and a subdural to venous bleeding. The extradural is commonest in true accidental injuries with skull fractures from falls with direct impact, which damages the meningeal artery. Although the child is shocked with acute brain compression, the outlook is excellent with no residual brain damage if treatment is rapid.

A subdural is virtually always a traumatic lesion produced by rotation between brain and dura. Rotation of the brain causing shearing of bridging veins is the mechanism in most shaking and impact injuries; depressed skull fractures penetrating vessels, a primary penetrating injury hitting a sinus or contusion causing oozing of surface veins appear less important. A depressed fracture is a rare cause of subdural hematoma (Choux et al 1986).

Arteriovenous malformations can bleed into the subdural space and hemorrhagic diatheses can cause spontaneous subdural bleeding, but this is rare without trauma. Scurvy, aspirin, hypoprothrombinemia from vitamin K deficiency (common in adult alcoholics or during warfarin therapy), congenital platelet abnormalities, genetic coagulation disorders and virus-induced thrombocytopenia are all possible causes.

Treatment of subdural hematomas

Small acute subdural hematomas without mass effect (the majority) will usually resolve spontaneously. In larger or persisting hematomas there is general agreement that the volume should be lessened by aspiration through the fontanel or by burr hole (Kotwica & Brzezinski 1991, Drapkin 1991). Flushing of the cavity between two burr holes is advocated by some. There should be no attempt to remove any membrane. A 3-day period of closed external drainage is recommended by some authorities. If there is secondary craniocerebral disproportion or a persisting external hydrocephalus a temporary subduroperitoneal drain may be required. The use of steroids in prevention of chronic inflammation is still contentious, with only 15 of 109 neurosurgeons questioned using them routinely (Byrne & Bartlett 1991).

Medicolegal aspects

Timing of injury

Often a lawyer will push the doctor for the timing of an incident, with a demand for accuracy that is not possible. Several factors can be helpful.

A CSF sample should be taken whenever possible (from ventricle or at surgery) and divided into several aliquots for cells, culture, biochemistry, cytospin examination and spectrophotometry. Following an intracranial hemorrhage the centrifuged specimen becomes hemoglobin tinged within 6 h and at this stage contains oxyhemoglobin on spectrophotometry, little methemoglobin or bilirubin. Arachnoid cells break down the liberated hemoglobin from lysed red cells to bilirubin which makes the fluid xanthochromic within 12–24 h. Xanthochromia persists for 3 weeks in the absence of further bleeding but for months in a chronic subdural hematoma. The oxyhemoglobin is replaced by methemoglobin and the color of the CSF (or subdural fluid) changes from red to brown. By 24 h the red cells are crenated and by 3 days there should be no intact red cells on microscopy of the noncentrifuged specimen.

Cerebral edema causes raised intracranial pressure, loss of cerebral perfusion and brain infarction. This takes about 6 h from injury to signs of tentorial herniation and 12 h to brain death but edema may come on quicker. Pressure will build up more rapidly with an intracranial hematoma. Secondary brainstem hemorrhage can change the clinical picture at any time (Brown 1991).

Massive cerebral edema causes loss of body homeostasis due to brainstem failure. This causes loss of body temperature control and infants are often hypothermic when they are first seen. Central body temperature is said to fall by 2.5°C per hour in a normal environment. After the first 5 h there is a plateau of slow cooling. Infants, however, have a large surface area to volume ratio and can cool very quickly, especially if wet, so care should be taken in using data derived from adult studies too strictly.

Callus in rib fractures, calcification in periosteal hemorrhage and rounded smooth edges of skull fractures suggest an injury at least 2 weeks old. Fractures of a different age from the recent head injury are the most important observation from a timing point of view. In long bone and rib fractures periosteal reaction occurs early at 4–10 days, soft callus appears at 14–21 days and hard callus at 3–6 weeks. Rib periosteal reaction cannot be seen till 10–14 days after injury on X-ray, but is seen more easily on radionuclide scan (Carty 1989). One cannot accurately date many skull or metaphyseal fractures.

On CT scan a subdural hematoma is at first hyperdense compared to brain and CSF but after 2–4 weeks it becomes isodense (Faerber 1995). The presence of hydrocephalus suggests an injury several days or weeks old.

At autopsy one can use brain repair processes as a guide to timing. There may be evidence of repeated injuries. The oligodendroglia swell within 1 h of brain tissue death; microglia begin to stream by 12 h; compound granular corpuscles appear by 24 h; hemosiderin appears in macrophages by 1 week; astrocytic glial processes are aligned around 2 weeks with a frank gliotic web by 1 month. Fibroblasts begin to grow into a subdural hematoma by the third day.

Management of the suspected case of child abuse

The organization of services for the abused child will vary from country to country and town to town.

There is general agreement that no matter how trivial the injury, the child should be admitted to hospital, if necessary on a temporary place of safety order.

Careful clinical examination must include charting all bruises, their configuration and color. The presence of clinical fractures, local bruising and tenderness is important but metaphyseal and skull fractures may be painless and so absence of clinical signs does not exclude the need for full radiological examination. Retinoscopy should be performed in all cases and if there is retinopathy, retinal photography is desirable.

The skeletal survey may need to be repeated after 10–14 days or supplemented with an isotope scan.

Photographs must be taken of all clinical injuries. All times and dates must be entered and every entry in the notes signed and X-rays numbered in sequence.

CT and US scans are now mandatory but MRI is likely to be used increasingly in place of CT to assess the extent of injury, edema and subsequent damage.

The parents should be interviewed, preferably separately, and asked how the injuries arose. If there are inconsistencies about the injury and the proposed mechanism or if the story changes or the parents give different versions or disagree, this must be carefully documented.

'At-risk' registers should be searched for any previous injury in child or siblings. If the injury amounts to unequivocal assault the police should be informed and police registers searched for any known violent offender in the household.

Most areas now have specialist social workers in child abuse who have a 24-hour service. These should be notified immediately.

The physician can only say that an injury has taken place, that it is suggestive of nonaccidental injury, possibly how, possibly when, but only rarely by whom. This may depend upon dental impressions, blood grouping, DNA fingerprinting of blood, saliva or semen and hence there is a need to involve the police and forensic service early.

The child will usually remain in hospital until after the case conference has decided whether it is safe for him to return home.

The management of the actual head injury is no different from that due to accidents. These infants should be nursed in a pediatric intensive care unit rather than a neurosurgical head injury unit but full imaging, EEG and intracranial pressure monitoring facilities with a combined pediatric and neurosurgical approach must be available (Leggate & Minns 1991). Less severe cases admitted under pediatricians must again have full imaging and proper neuro-observations with regular Glasgow coma scale observations. Cases managed by neurosurgeons must have proper documentation of the medicosocial and medicolegal aspects.

Nearly all deaths are due to uncontrollable raised intracranial pressure. Necrotic edema does not respond to hyperventilation or mannitol. Barbiturates lower the intracranial pressure often by lowering the perfusion pressure which maintains the ICP. If a craniotomy is performed, the subdural is often small but the necrotic brain edema may be so great that the dura and skull cannot be closed without performing a lobectomy.

Long-term effects of nonaccidental head injury

The child with bruises, fractures of long bones and ribs or even malicious body injuries but no head injury can be expected to make a full physical recovery if hemorrhage does not occur and can be placed in a loving home to try and forget his horrifying experience. There may not, however, be a full psychological recovery as abused children as a group are shy, have fewer friends and show disturbed behavior, poor self-esteem and lower ambitions over a long period of time.

Head injury of all types in children carries a significant morbidity and mortality, so a pediatric pathologist experienced in fatal child abuse cases is very important. In accidental head injury the duration of unconsciousness, decerebration, posttraumatic amnesia and rate of recovery in the first days all correlate with outcome. Results for accidental head injury are significantly better than those for nonaccidental head injuries.

Zimmerman et al (1979) found that all children who presented initially with interhemispheric subdural hematomas from child abuse (Fig. 14.25) subsequently developed cerebral atrophy and 50% developed brain infarcts. It has been suggested that up to 400 children per year in the United Kingdom could suffer from chronic brain damage as a result of nonaccidental head injury.

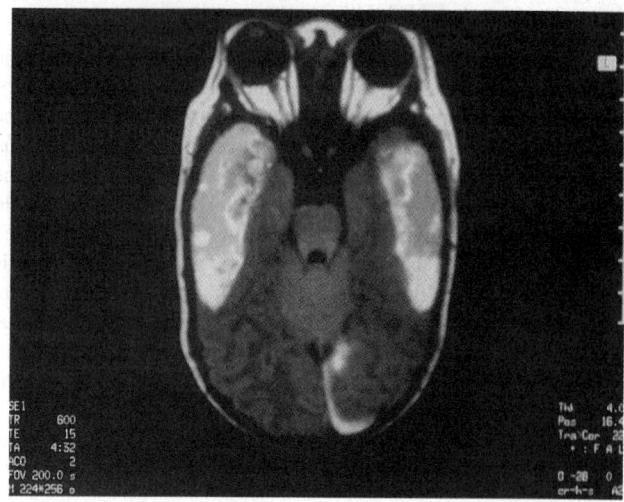

Fig. 14.25 MRI scan of 2-month-old child with bilateral temporal hemorrhage, evident tissue loss and posterior interhemispheric hemorrhage as a result of nonaccidental head injury.

ACCIDENTAL HEAD INJURIES

Accidental head injuries are common in children and the majority will have a straightforward course with a good outcome. A small number will sustain brain injury with the potential for more serious complications. All significant head injuries should have their levels of consciousness carefully evaluated by a coma scale (Tables 14.35, 14.36).

Epidemiology

Most reports on the epidemiology of head injuries in children obtain their data from recordings of hospital admissions, attendances at

---

Table 14.35 Glasgow Coma Scale

Eyes	Score	Best motor response	Score	Best verbal response	Score
Open		*To verbal command*			
Spontaneously	4	Obeys	6	Orientated and converses	5
To verbal command	3	*To painful stimulus*		Disorientated and converses	4
To pain	2	Localizes pain	5	Inappropriate words	3
No response	1	Flexion – withdrawal	4	Incomprehensible sounds	2
		Flexion abnormal	3	No response	1
		Extension	2		
		No response	1		

GCS total 3–15.

Table 14.36 Children's Coma Scale (modified Glasgow Coma Scale)

Eye opening	Score	Best motor response	Score	Best verbal response		Score
Spontaneous	4	Spontaneous (obeys verbal command)	6	Smiles, orientated to sound, follows objects, interacts		5
Reaction to speech	3	Localizes pain	5	*Crying*	*Interacts*	
Reaction to pain	2	Withdraws in response to pain	4	Consolable	Inappropriate	4
No response	1	Abnormal flexion in response to pain (decorticate posture)	3	Inconsistently consolable	Moaning	3
		Abnormal extension in response to pain (decerebrate posture)	2	Inconsolable	Irritable restless	2
		No response	1	No response	No response	1

CCS total 3–15.

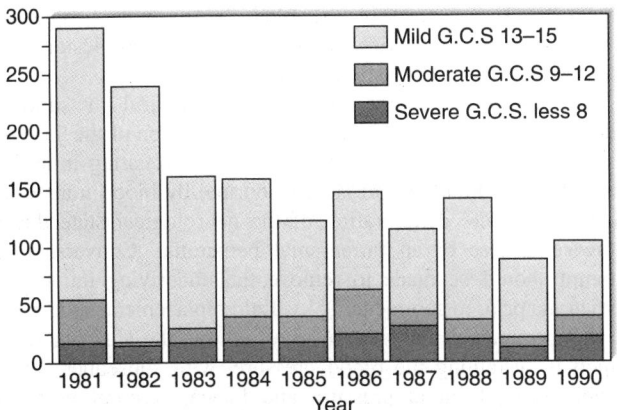

Fig. 14.26 Head injury in children under 16 years over a 10-year period. (GCS = Glasgow Coma Scale.)

accident and emergency departments or from returns on death certificates giving mortality rates. However, many factors will affect these figures such as the degree of access to local hospitals, the provision of local health care facilities, medical admission policy, socioeconomic status of the patients, the local environment (city or rural) and the amount of preventive legislation. It is probable that published figures for both incidence and mortality of head injury are an underestimate of the true figures.

Preventive measures are leading to a gratifying reduction in accidental head injury (Fig. 14.26). These include compulsory seat belts, back-facing baby restrainer seats, speed control by cameras and traffic calming by sleeping policemen, drink/driving laws, spot breathalyzer tests and cycle helmets and modification of children's playgrounds with a forgiving surface such as forest bark and rails on slides.

Causes

The causes of head injury in children will vary with the age of the child. Males at all ages show a higher prevalence of head injury compared to females. In our own practice, in children under 2 years of age, falls account for 85% of the cases of extradural hematoma. Road traffic accidents are a major cause of severe, fatal head injury in older children but direct trauma, either accidental or as a result of an assault, accounts for less than 4% of all head injury admissions (Fig. 14.27).

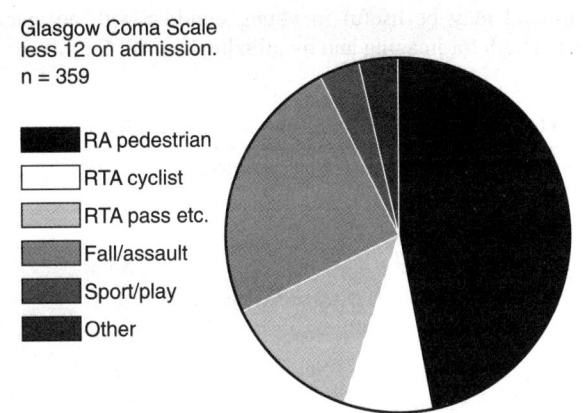

Glasgow Coma Scale less 12 on admission. n = 359

- ■ RA pedestrian
- □ RTA cyclist
- ▨ RTA pass etc.
- ▨ Fall/assault
- ▨ Sport/play
- ■ Other

Fig. 14.27 Causes of accidental head injury in children under 16 years.

Mechanism of injury

The primary injury can be due to four different mechanisms.

1. Penetrating or missile injuries

These are high-velocity, high-energy injuries acting over a small area with penetration of bone. The most obvious is a gunshot wound which in the UK is rarely nonaccidental in children. Knife and scissor blades or screwdrivers can penetrate the vault of the skull in malicious assault. Accidental penetrating injuries of the orbits with sticks, knitting needles, pencils and toy railway lines are seen. The stick may be broken off leaving a piece still in the frontal lobe as a source of infection. The pathophysiology of this type of injury is laceration and bleeding with secondary infection. Objects in the mouth may penetrate the tonsillar fossa and cause carotid artery injury. There may be a delay of a day or more before the onset of neurological signs as a dissecting aneurysm forms. Cavernous sinus thrombosis or caroticocavernous fistulae can result from intracranial injuries to the carotid.

2. Compression head injuries (see birth injury p. 122)

3. Impact injuries

These may be accidental or nonaccidental and one cannot say from a study of the injury whether the infant accidentally fell or was pushed out of a window or thrown down the stairs.

Acceleration injuries. This is when a moving force hits the child and so imparts acceleration to the child. This is seen when the child is hit with a moving vehicle, fist, foot, etc. If the child flies through the air some of the force is dissipated as the imparted motion.

Deceleration injuries. Conversely, in this situation the child is moving and comes to a sudden halt, as in a head-on car crash. They occur in children who fall or are pushed or thrown from windows, beds, etc. Impact injuries can only be dissipated by bounce or a very forgiving surface. If the impact force cannot be dissipated these deceleration impact injuries form the most devastating type of head injury.

4. Whiplash shaking injuries (see nonaccidental injury pp. 700, 1897)

The primary injury occurs as a direct result of the force that has been applied to the head. This may result in:

- damage to the cranial skeleton in the form of fractures and extradural hematomas;
- damage to the underlying dural sac with subsequent CSF leakage either via the nose (CSF rhinorrhea) or ear (CSF otorrhea);
- damage to the underlying brain tissue which may result in subdural hematomas, intracerebral hematomas, cerebral contusions or deep white matter shearing injuries (diffuse axonal injury).

There is very little that can be done to minimize this damage once the primary injury has occurred. The major aim of modern head injury management is the prevention of the secondary injury.

Management

1. Documenting the primary injury.
2. Preventing the secondary injury (Table 14.37)

Table 14.37 Causes of secondary brain injury

Hypoxia

Ischemia

Raised intracranial pressure (with reduced cerebral perfusion pressure)

Infection

Loss of metabolic homeostasis

Epilepsy

3. Setting up rehabilitation facilities and helping the patient and family adapt to any permanent disability that may result.

Children have a relatively small blood volume and a scalp laceration or intracranial hematoma may represent a large percentage of their blood volume. They may be at risk of circulatory collapse and shock if this is not recognized.

Criteria for admission

For most patients presenting without altered consciousness, without focal neurological deficit and with only evidence of minor scalp trauma, e.g. clean laceration or minor grazes and without the presence of a scalp hematoma, admission to hospital is not indicated. If there is any possibility of loss of consciousness at the time of head injury, altered sensorium at the time of examination, focal neurological deficit or the presence of extensive external signs of head injury, e.g. large scalp hematomas, extensive skin/scalp lacerations or skin loss, the child should be admitted to hospital.

In general, the management of head-injured patients will depend on their conscious state and will always commence with the ABC of resuscitation, viz. maintenance of the Airway, adequacy of Breathing, which may or may not require ventilatory support under full paralysis and sedation, and support for the Circulation (see Table 14.38). Scalp lacerations should be dealt with as a priority. Simple compression bandaging is usually sufficient to stem the blood loss but if necessary, a temporary continuous suture can be placed into large scalp lacerations in the accident and emergency department to stop bleeding.

Drowsiness, vomiting and irritability are all important clinical signs of an intracranial problem and whilst drowsiness is of more importance in the younger age group, irritability is of more

Table 14.38 Elements to consider in the management of head injury

Airway

Breathing

Circulation

Fractures
  Linear
  Depressed
  Compound
  Growing

Hematoma
  Intracerebral
    Extradural
    Subdural
    Intracerebral
  Extracranial
    Subperiosteal
    Subgaleal

prognostic significance in the older age group. It must be remembered that in children, large intracranial mass lesions may exist without any neurological deficit.

The possibility of an underlying extradural or subdural hematoma cannot be ruled out until CT evaluation of the head has been carried out. Care must be taken in resuscitating infants as restoration of the blood pressure to normal by blood transfusion may cause acute deterioration of the neurological state due to increase in size of an intracranial hematoma. Conversely, no attempt should be made to remove the underlying intracranial hematoma prior to commencing i.v. fluid replacements as removal of the intracranial mass lesion may remove the Cushing reflex which is sustaining the blood pressure, with subsequent catastrophic loss of blood pressure and hence, cerebral perfusion pressure.

Imaging

CT scanning

The advent of axial tomography (CT scanning) revolutionized the management of head injuries. CT has maintained its place since it is excellent for visualizing blood, bone and CSF. The main advantages are precise anatomical location of an intracranial hematoma and the accuracy in diagnosis and differentiation between intracerebral, subdural and extradural hematomas. In the absence of loss of consciousness or neurological deficit, a skull X-ray is still used as the initial screening test. Children who have been fully conscious and have no skull fracture do not merit further investigation by CT scanning unless there is a focal neurological deficit. If a fully conscious child has persisting drowsiness, vomiting and/or anemia or a neurological deficit, a CT scan should be carried out independent of the presence or absence of a skull fracture. If there is a diminished conscious level as measured on the Glasgow coma scale (Table 14.35) or, for children under 3 years of age, the children's coma scale (Table 14.36) there should also be an urgent CT scan. The indications for CT scanning are shown in Table 14.39. The problem of CT scanning children with head injuries too early has provoked much discussion, as an intracranial hematoma has appeared on a subsequent scan in some cases. The presence of a normal CT scan initially should not mean that further CT scanning is not indicated should the clinical condition of the patient alter.

Ultrasound

Ultrasound may be useful in young children with an anterior fontanel both for imaging and by utilizing Doppler for monitoring

Table 14.39 Algorithm for CT scanning head-injured children

Glasgow Coma Scale	Presence of fracture	Clinical features	CT scan indicated
15	No	None	No
15	Yes	None	No
15	Yes	Signs/symptoms	Yes
13/14	No	None	Nonurgent but yes
13/14	Yes	None	Yes
≤12	Yes/no	Signs/symptoms	Yes
		or none	Yes

possible raised intracranial pressure and its subsequent response to treatment. There are great advantages in a portable, bedside and easily repeatable investigation with no radiation risk. The main disadvantages are the need for a 'window' through the skull through which to operate. The modern 4–8 MHz probe makes it possible to clearly differentiate periventricular lesions and identify subdural collection.

Raised intracranial pressure may affect the resistance index of the intracranial vessels on Doppler examination. Normally there is an inverse relationship of cerebral blood flow and resistance index and a high index reflects a slow or reduced blood flow.

Magnetic resonance imaging

At this time it is mainly used as an investigative tool in order to correlate neuroradiological abnormalities with functional disability in those children with residual neurological or neuropsychological deficits (Levin et al 1989).

SKULL FRACTURES (Table 14.40)

Forty percent of infants hospitalized with cranial trauma will have a skull fracture, but sequelae in the form of intracranial hematoma will only develop in between 8% and 22% of such patients. Leggate et al (1989) showed that all infants under 6 months of age operated on for an extradural hematoma had either a skull fracture or suture separation seen on X-ray, and in a group of 40 infants an abnormal X-ray was present in 90% of those with an extradural hematoma. Most skull fractures are linear.

The skull in the neonate consists of poorly mineralized membrane bone which can easily be cut at autopsy with a pair of scissors. Linear fractures due to birth trauma occur but are rare in the compressive head injuries of birth unless postmature. Under these circumstances it offers little protection to the underlying brain which is easily compressed in a ping-pong ball or Pond fracture where severe local bruising and hemorrhage into the brain is then seen with minimal fracture. Splintering (i.e. a cranial greenstick fracture) may be seen under a cephalhematoma. In a Hemsath fracture, there is indentation of the occipital bone (which arises from eight ossification centers) by the maternal pubis. This particularly occurs in breech extraction and causes osteodiastasis. Little may be seen on X-ray, but splintering may be seen at autopsy with severe cerebellar hemorrhage.

Skull fractures do not heal by callus formation and so dating of an injury is difficult. If the edges are rounded and smooth, it is more than 2 weeks old. At autopsy the margins are heaped, smooth and discolored with hemosiderin. A skull fracture normally heals in 2–3 months and has disappeared on X-ray by 6 months. In small infants the fracture site may not heal but form a growing skull fracture as described below. There may be no bruising at all over the scalp even with a severe impact.

Table 14.40   Incidence and types of fractures

Linear	73–80%
Depressed	7–10%
Compound	1%
Growing	1%
Basal	<1%

In a study of 100 consecutive children less than 2 years of age the skull fractures were linear in 27, depressed in eight, multiple in three, stellate in one, bilateral in three and basilar in four (Duhaime et al 1992).

Compound fractures

Compound fractures secondary to penetration injuries may be obvious or subtle (e.g. orbital trauma from an object such as a pencil or sharp pointed stick penetrating the medial aspect of the orbit, passing into the ethmoid sinus and through the cribriform plate into the intracranial cavity in its subfrontal compartment). Another typical site for a penetrating injury is the temporal region. In all such cases, extensive preoperative investigation is required, including CT scanning and MRI angiography, prior to a thorough exploration of the penetrating tract with debridement of damaged brain and formal closure of dura. The use of antibiotics is controversial but our habit is to use intravenous cefotaxime.

Growing fractures

At follow-up X-ray, a simple linear fracture will sometimes appear to have enlarged. Typically, the child presents with a palpable and pulsating skull defect. A third of cases will present with epilepsy and some will develop late neurological deficits. Management consists of closure of the underlying dural defect with natural or artificial membrane and closure of the bony defect with either acrylic or the patient's own bone harvested by using either partial thickness skull grafts or split rib grafts.

Basal skull fractures

Basal skull fractures are uncommon in pediatric head trauma but when present, manifest in the same way as in adults, with CSF leaks, otorrhea, or rhinorrhea. In the case of fracture of the petrous temporal bone there may be an ipsilateral facial nerve palsy. Management is conservative, the main complication being meningitis. Once again, the routine use of antibiotics is controversial. Careful observation is required, however, to detect the onset of meningitis. CT scan confirms the safety of performing a lumbar puncture. In a large proportion of cases, there will be a traumatic subarachnoid hemorrhage and the development of the cardinal signs of meningitis (neck stiffness, pyrexia, headache, nausea, vomiting and photophobia) may all be a result of blood in the CSF rather than an infective meningitis.

RAISED INTRACRANIAL PRESSURE

In children under 12–18 months the open sutures enable the skull volume to increase and large intracranial masses may accumulate without rapid or large rises in ICP. After 2 years of age the cranial cavity behaves more like the adult with a fixed volume. The development of cerebral edema as a normal response of the central nervous system to injury causes an increase in the volume of the brain. With the volume of the skull cavity fixed there will inevitably be either diminution in the total volume of CSF spaces and/or diminution of the pool of venous blood within the skull. As intracranial pressure increases there will be an increased resistance to inflow of arterial blood and thus a fall in the cerebral perfusion pressure. (Cerebral perfusion pressure (CPP) = the mean systemic blood pressure (SBP) – the mean intracranial pressure (ICP).) This fall in CPP leads to a fall in the cerebral blood flow and if this is below 20 ml/100 g of tissue per min, brain ischemia will develop. The brain ischemia further increases the formation of cerebral edema and leads to a further rise in intracranial pressure. A fall in cerebral blood flow below 10 mg/100 g per min leads to electrical dysfunction of the neurons and loss of intracellular ion homeostasis.

Generalized rises of ICP will initially cause transtentorial and eventually transforaminal herniation. Unilateral increases in ICP secondary to hematoma will cause ipsilateral uncal herniation and nipping of the third nerve against the free border of the tentorium with ipsilateral pupillary dilation secondary to loss of parasympathetic constrictor tone to the ciliary muscles. Uncontrolled further herniation will cause in addition a contralateral third nerve palsy.

Potent causes of raised pressure such as hypoxia and ischemia should be corrected by adequate resuscitation and ventilation to try and keep an oxygen saturation in the region of 95% and $PaCO_2$ between 3.0 and 4.0 kPa.

Primary brain injury resulting in cerebral edema is treated by a combination of therapies. The head-injured child should be nursed in a 15–20° head-up position to optimize venous drainage. In the short term acute rises in intracranial pressure can be managed by hyperventilation to a $PaCO_2$ of 2.5 kPa or less. This will reduce the intracranial pressure for long enough for other maneuvers to be performed, e.g. evacuation of intracranial hematoma. Hyperventilation should not be continued for a long period as it may render the child's brain more ischemic by reducing cerebral blood flow. Where ICP is still high after primary maneuvers have been carried out, treatment with mannitol (initially in a dose of 1 g/kg bodyweight and subsequently with 0.5 g/kg to a total of 2 g/kg per 24-h period) will usually reduce ICP. This last figure may be exceeded provided plasma osmolalities do not exceed 320 mosmol/l when further addition of mannitol may possibly have a detrimental effect. Care must be exercised that the osmotic diuretic effect of mannitol removing crystalloid does not result in a sudden drop in blood pressure. Supportive colloid is used routinely in some centers.

The use of the diuretic frusemide combined with aliquots of plasma is a helpful adjunct in controlling intracranial pressure which is proving resistant to single therapy maneuvers. In all these regimens, the aim is to maintain the intracranial pressure below or equal to 20 mmHg although in very young children, this level must be reduced still further and in infants pressures of greater than 12–15 mmHg are pathological.

Correction and maintenance of electrolyte homeostasis is carried out continuously and the hematocrit is maintained between 30% and 35% (providing an optimal ratio of viscosity and oxygen carriage).

Temperature has a marked effect on intracranial pressure and in patients who are pyrexial, the temperature should be reduced by either fanning or antipyretics. If there is poor peripheral perfusion then the periphery can be dilated using pharmacological agents (e.g. chlorpromazine).

Intensive monitoring is needed in a severely head-injured child. A standard monitoring set-up for such a patient would be: arterial line, central venous pressure line, two large bore peripheral venous cannulae, urinary catheter, rectal and peripheral temperature probes, ECG and oximetry. Optimal additional monitoring depending on the facilities would include: intracranial pressure monitor (either subdural, intraventricular or intraparenchymal) and brain electrical monitoring by full electroencephalography (EEG). This is still woefully deficient in most centers.

In patients in whom the head injury is associated with chest or myocardial injury or in whom the exact fluid balance state is unclear, the central venous pressure line may be replaced by a Swann–Ganz catheter with facilities for measuring cardiac output and left ventricular function.

Finally, as an indirect measurement of the coupling of the cerebral metabolic requirements for oxygen ($CMRO_2$) and cerebral blood flow (CBF), there is a place for monitoring the arterial jugular venous oxygen difference (A-JDO_2). This is carried out by placing a catheter in the internal jugular vein in the neck running in a cranial direction until it lodges inside the jugular bulb. Sampling of venous oxygen content from this catheter will indicate the oxygen content of the cerebral venous blood uncontaminated by scalp or facial venous blood. In this way the difference between the arterial oxygen content and the jugular venous oxygen content can be measured (normal range 4–8 ml/100 ml). Levels below 4 ml indicate a hyperemic state of the cerebral circulation following the head injury and levels above 8 ml would suggest ischemia. In this way, valuable information can be obtained as to the state of the cerebral blood flow in the child and its response to different forms of treatment for raised ICP. It may also prevent continuation of detrimental treatment, e.g. the use of mannitol in a child with a hyperemic state.

Cerebral protection

This technique relies on a reduction in intracranial pressure by reduction of the cerebral metabolic rate for oxygen ($CMPO_2$). This is best evaluated by continuous electrical monitoring using the EEG (CFM or CFAM) which should be kept at burst suppression levels. Short-acting anesthetic agents such as γ-hydroxybutyrate can also be used. The place of nitric oxide and antiglutamate drugs is a subject of intense current interest but they are not yet of proven value.

INFECTION

Many of the clinical signs of meningitis will also result from the presence of blood within the CSF. A high index of suspicion must always be maintained for the development of meningitis in an unconscious child with an open head injury. A persistently raised core temperature with an infectious picture in the peripheral white count and a persistent tachycardia are important signs of a possible meningitis. The possibility can only be eliminated confidently by lumbar puncture but this should only be carried out after CT examination has confirmed the presence of open CSF cisterns and free communication between the supra- and infratentorial compartments. If there is any doubt about the safety of a lumbar puncture, it should NOT be carried out. CSF can then be obtained either from a ventricular tap or by swabbing the cerebral cortex after making a small burr hole (note that a clear ventricular tap does not exclude the diagnosis of meningitis in the subarachnoid spaces). Where a high index of suspicion for meningitis exists and CSF cannot be safely obtained from a lumbar puncture and facilities do not exist for ventricular sampling, then blind antibiotic cover may be instigated. Metronidazole, gentamicin and a third-generation cephalosporin are given intravenously in large doses.

EPILEPSY

The use of continuous electrical monitoring of brain activity either by CFM, CFAM or intermittent full EEG examinations will help detect seizure activity. In an unconscious or paralyzed ventilated child there may be clinical warning signs such as surges in the systemic blood pressure, intracranial pressure, accompanied by tachycardia with or without pupillary dilation. In the conscious child or nonparalyzed child, seizures will usually be clinically obvious. Treatment consists of loading with phenytoin (dose 20 mg/kg bodyweight) and maintaining blood levels in the therapeutic range by regular daily doses. Immediate control of the seizure may be effectively obtained with diazepam given intravenously or rectally. Seizures which prove resistant to this treatment may require control with barbiturate infusion. This is subsequently tailed off when adequate blood phenytoin levels have been obtained and seizure activity has ceased.

DIABETES INSIPIDUS

Diabetes insipidus may be seen with basal skull fractures. Most cases are transient and therapy consists of maintenance of normal plasma osmolality using the vasopressin analog DDAVP. In other cases diabetes insipidus develops as a result of profound and prolonged increase in intracranial pressure. This is a poor prognostic indicator and is often accompanied by incipient brain death. Management consists of maintenance of the systemic blood pressure by adequate fluid replacement and DDAVP to reduce the continuing urine output.

BRAIN DEATH

In cases of severe primary brain injury and in those cases in which ICP has not responded to treatment, then one may be faced with the situation of brain death in a ventilated child. Following the recommendation of the Royal Colleges of Surgeons and Physicians (1976, 1979), after exclusion of all narcotics, sedative or paralyzing drugs and in the absence of hypothermia or metabolic derangements, formal testing for brain death can be carried out by two senior doctors. There must be no movement, reflex or other, in the upper limbs. The child must be unconscious with no change in state and no sleep wake cycles. There must be an internal and external ophthalmoplegia with fixed cadaveric pupils. The heart rate is usually fixed about 135 and does not change on painful stimulus. There are no gag, cough or oculocephalic reflexes and absent caloric reflexes. The EEG will be flat and isoelectric at high gain. An apnea test is carried out (5–8 min of apnea without any attempt at ventilation at the end of which the $PaCO_2$ should be equal to or greater than 6.7 kPa or 56 mmHg). Adequate oxygenation is provided throughout the test by oxygen introduced at 6–10 l/min via a tracheal cannula. If the brain death criteria are satisfied then ventilation may be terminated or, where indicated by the relatives and where there is no objection from the legal authorities (coroner in England and Wales, Procurator Fiscal in Scotland), beating heart organ donation may take place.

OUTCOME

The prognosis for a head-injured child bears a direct relationship to the initial Glasgow coma score. Modern imaging techniques and easy access to neurosurgical units should diminish the mortality of treatable lesions such as acute extradural hematomas. The mortality of extradural hematoma in the pre-CT scan era was between 10% and 30% but is now reduced to zero.

Overall, most series of severely head-injured patients show a combined mortality and morbidity of approximately 30%. About 10% will die, 5% at the accident scene and 5% in the first few days, with a further 20% showing a motor disability on follow-up. Ten percent have persistent difficulties affecting cognition and behavior. The prognosis may be much more favorable than the initial impression and hemiplegias improve, aphasia in most cases will recover but there will be residual language problems showing as difficulties in spelling at school. Improvement is most rapid in the first 6 months and measurable improvement will continue to 18 months but one cannot say that residual handicap is permanent and will not improve further till 5 years have passed. Concentration may be poor and memory deficiency may be severe enough to class as a posttraumatic Korsakoff's syndrome. Personality changes and rage reactions may make the parents' lives unbearable and yet little may be found on a superficial neurological examination. The use of SPECT scanning has shown that many children with predominantly learning or behavior problems do have very definite residual pathology. This disability may be behavioral, requiring neuropsychological management, educational, requiring the need for special schooling or learning support in normal schools, or there may be difficulties with communication, gross or fine motor dysfunction or epilepsy.

Decerebrate or decorticate motor activity may persist due to extensive anoxic ischemic cortical damage which may also produce a severe posttraumatic dementia and total dependence for feeding (by tube or gastrostomy), tracheostomy for chest toilet and dedicated nursing care. This is often termed the persistent vegetative state.

CEREBROVASCULAR DISEASE AND MIGRAINE

Intracranial and intracerebral hemorrhage is a common problem at the extremes of life in the neonatal period and in old age. In the neonatal period subependymal and intraventricular hemorrhage of prematurity, subdural hematoma and tentorial tears of birth trauma, thalamic hemorrhage following asphyxia or hemorrhage into an infarct from a presumed placental embolus are all seen.

In the postneonatal period the commonest cause of intracranial hemorrhage is head trauma and this is considered on page 699. Cerebrovascular disease presenting as either stroke or an acute intracerebral hemorrhage is relatively rare and affects only about 2 per 100 000 of the childhood population. Intracranial hemorrhage is usually either subarachnoid or intracerebral with subdural bleeding being extremely rare other than from trauma. Infarction of the brain may result from many causes and may be due to vascular thrombosis, cerebral embolism, watershed zone lesion infarction, vascular compression or vascular injury.

The presentation is usually that of acute hemiplegia with a stroke or sudden-onset headache and vomiting with meningism or coma.

In 27 cases of intracerebral hemorrhage presenting after the neonatal period arteriovenous malformations were responsible for hemorrhage in 37% and aneurysm in 11%. Hemophilia and coagulopathies result in individual cases. Hypertension is a rare cause of primary intracerebral hemorrhage in children but hemorrhage into a tumor, particularly cerebellar astrocytomas, is responsible for 20% of cases. This may be the presenting feature so that hemorrhage into a benign astrocytic cyst may mask the underlying neoplasm.

INTRACRANIAL HEMORRHAGE

Subarachnoid hemorrhage

Subarachnoid hemorrhage is most commonly due to a bleed from an arteriovenous malformation or an aneurysm. It presents classically in the older child with sudden onset of headache, vomiting, loss of consciousness with bilateral sixth nerve palsy and possibly subhyloid hemorrhages in the fundus.

Although diagnosis rests on finding bloodstained CSF on lumbar puncture it should be stressed that lumbar puncture should never be performed on a child presenting with decreased conscious level without a prior CT scan. Since computed tomograms are the most useful way of diagnosing subarachnoid hemorrhage in most cases one can demonstrate the bleed on the scan without the need for a lumbar puncture. The CT is best for blood, bone and CSF and MRI for brain. Only very small leaks may not show enough change in the density pattern of the CSF to be picked up on a CT scan and lumbar puncture is then necessary.

The CSF is found to be bloodstained and after 6 h xanthochromia appears, the red cells are crenated and if there is any doubt as to whether one is dealing with a true subarachnoid hemorrhage or a traumatic puncture, then spectrophotometry of the fluid is indicated. This will show a bilirubin peak together with hemoglobin in a true subarachnoid hemorrhage whilst the oxyhemoglobin peak will predominate in a traumatic tap. There are still cases of subarachnoid hemorrhage in children missed with a label of traumatic lumbar puncture who then have a fatal second bleed before the diagnosis is established.

In addition to arteriovenous malformations and aneurysm one can have the presentation of subarachnoid hemorrhage or a primary intraventricular hemorrhage in conditions such as hemorrhagic disease of the newborn, thrombocytopenia and rarely hemophilia secondary to bleeding from a coagulation disorder. Subarachnoid bleeding can also be prominent in nonaccidental shaking injury.

Cerebral aneurysms

An aneurysm is a weakness in the wall of a blood vessel such that the intraluminal pressure causes the wall to stretch either along a segment as a fusiform aneurysm or as a local outpouching, a saccular (berry) aneurysm. These are situated on arteries and are most commonly the saccular type but fusiform aneurysms can occur when there is a uniform dilation of the blood vessel from softening of the wall, as with infection with a mycotic basis.

Aneurysms may occasionally be familial and some cases may have a congenital defect in collagen III. Mycotic aneurysms secondary to bacterial endocarditis should be borne in mind and a complete examination inclusive of the cardiovascular system is always mandatory. Aneurysms are associated with coarctation of the aorta, Marfan's syndrome, Ehlers–Danlos syndrome, polycystic disease of the kidneys and occasionally with abnormalities of the cerebral vessels themselves, such as a common trunk anterior cerebral artery with aneurysm of the pericallosal vessels. Vasculopathies occur in pseudoxanthoma elasticum. Although Kawasaki disease is associated with a vasculopathy and secondary aneurysm formation in the heart it is a rare cause of cerebral aneurysms.

Between 1% and 3% of all aneurysms occur in children. They tend to occur under 2 years or over 10 years of age. In 23 aneurysms described by Heiskenen (1989), 10 were at the carotid bifurcation and eight on the anterior communicating artery. Those on the middle cerebral artery are often on the distal part of the vessel and may achieve much larger proportions than in the adult.

Diagnosis is nearly always because of presentation with a subarachnoid hemorrhage or hemorrhagic stroke. Occasionally calcification in an aneurysm is seen on a plain skull film. Local pressure on the third nerve presenting as an isolated third nerve palsy or on the hypothalamus with diabetes insipidus can occur but is unusual. The bleeding may occasionally be intracerebral as well as subarachnoid.

Bleeding into the subarachnoid space results in intense vasospasm which can itself result in secondary cerebral infarction. Occasionally posterior fossa aneurysms of the basilar artery or posterior inferior cerebellar artery occur in children and are more common in children than adults. Multiple aneurysms are rare, but in very young children under 2 years of age the aneurysms may reach quite a large size.

Diagnosis rests upon arteriography and this is much more accessible now with MRI angiography although some people feel that CT angiography is better for demonstrating aneurysms such as posterior communicating ones presenting with an isolated third nerve palsy.

Arteriovenous malformation

These are of several types.

The capillary or telangiectasia type of capillary hemangioma. Characteristic of the Sturge–Weber syndrome. Although this lesion may be extensive it rarely bleeds. Rarely, as a result of status epilepticus, it may thrombose and so cause infarction of the hemisphere with onset of a hemiplegia. This type of lesion has no large feeding vessels and due to sluggish flow may not show at all on angiography, but is shown well on isotope scan or MRI imaging.

Sudden unexpected intracerebral hemorrhage, especially a cerebellar hemorrhage, is often blamed upon a small telangiectatic vascular malformation which is destroyed by the bleed and so is often impossible to verify.

Cavernous hemangiomas. These occur particularly in the neonatal period and may be part of a syndrome of multiple hemangiomas. They have small feeding vessels but large blood-filled sinusoids reaching 1 mm in diameter which form a honeycomb with little brain between vessels (Herter et al 1988). The vessels may calcify. They may leak before a large bleed as shown by hemosiderin in surrounding tissue. There may be a familial occurrence of hemangiomas or blood vessel abnormalities elsewhere such as the eye, skin or viscera. These lesions have no capsule but have well-defined limits. They are not invasive and do not metastasize. They behave as hamartomas and may grow with the child so that presentation may be of a space-occupying lesion with headache, focal signs and raised intracranial pressure with papilledema as well as with the classic features of hemorrhage, which may be intracerebral, subarachnoid or intraventricular. Fits are often a symptom before a bleed occurs. Seventy-five percent are supratentorial and 25% infratentorial and they are most common in the territory of the middle cerebral artery.

When removed at surgery, nearly all show evidence of repeated small bleeds with hemosiderin deposits and cyst formation so that recurrent small bleeds may herald a large bleed. CT scan shows a hypo- or hyperdense area. Angiography may not show the lesion because of stagnation with little flow and because the feeding vessels are small, unlike the commoner arteriovenous malformation (see below) (Suarez & Viano 1989).

Venous arteriovenous malformations. These usually constitute an abnormal plexus of veins at the base of the brain which may form one large sinus such as an aneurysm of the vein of Galen. The blood flow in this type of malformation may be torrential so that the child presents with a large head, hydrocephalus, a loud bruit and high output heart failure. Diagnosis is by MRI angiography and treatment is ideally by occlusion or embolization of feeding vessels although the torrential flow makes this difficult without causing venous infarction.

Arteriovenous fistulae. These are the more common type of arteriovenous malformation and consist of a direct arterial to venous connection with no capillary between, i.e. 'bag of worms'. They usually have large feeding vessels, are unilateral and occur more in males than females. More than 50% are in the parietal area with the frontal lobe and basal ganglia next in frequency. They may occur in the posterior fossa or brainstem. Presentation is by fits or a sudden subarachnoid and intracerebral bleed though a history of migraine may precede the bleed. A stroke is a more likely presentation than subarachnoid hemorrhage. An intracranial bruit is not a reliable sign as it may be absent in the presence of large arteriovenous malformations. A loud bruit may be heard in the head of normal children and any cause of a rise in intracranial pressure results in a systolic bruit over the fontanel and orbits.

Diagnosis is by MRI angiography but four-vessel direct angiography is needed and precedes surgical occlusion. This will demonstrate the extent of the abnormality and the feeding vessels. If the child presents with fits there is a 25% chance of a bleed during childhood and the mortality if a bleed occurs is between 10% and 20% so that treatment is always warranted. Even without seizures the presence of an arteriovenous malformation means that there is a 2–3% chance per year of a bleed. The mortality from surgery is thought to be less than 2% (Fong & Chan 1988).

Management of intracranial hemorrhage

1. Hypertension should be avoided and if present, treated.
2. Straining at stool and anything producing a Valsalva maneuver should be avoided.
3. There should be bed rest with no exercise.
4. Sedation with diazepam is useful and an antiemetic should be given if vomiting is occurring.
5. Analgesia is important for the headache.
6. Control of seizures with intravenous phenytoin may be indicated.
7. Monitoring of intracranial pressure is performed in almost all neurosurgical centers.
8. The use of antifibrinolytic agents is not recommended in children.
9. Surgery: in children who present with a subarachnoid or intracerebral bleed due to an aneurysm or arteriovenous malformation, surgery is the management of choice. If the child is in coma, if angiography shows the aneurysm is fusiform or if there is any question of a mycotic aneurysm then conservative medical management is indicated. In the case of berry aneurysms surgery should be carried out preferably within the first week using microsurgical techniques in order to get a clip round the neck of the sac. If it is impossible to clip the base of the aneurysm then it is sometimes wrapped or the feeding vessel itself is clipped. Large surface arteriovenous malformations can have their feeding vessel clipped and completely removed. Obliteration by intravascular techniques will probably gradually supersede open surgery.

10. Arteriovenous malformations or large fusiform aneurysms may nowadays be treated by inserting a balloon catheter into the feeding vessel and embolizing it or occluding it using a detachable balloon or a suitable glue.

The prognosis overall for cerebral hemorrhage in childhood is poor with a 54% mortality. Aneurysms presenting with subarachnoid hemorrhage without intracerebral extension carry a 30% mortality (Livingston & Brown 1986, Heiskenen 1989).

Stroke in childhood

An acute cerebrovascular accident may be caused by a sudden intracerebral hemorrhage as already discussed, but more frequently may be the result of a vascular occlusion (Wanifuchi et al 1988, Roach & Riela 1988). The many possible causes are listed in Table 14.41.

Vascular lesions

The vessels in the neck can be traumatized at birth, by blows on the shoulder, accidental hanging, following puncture at angiography or by falls on objects, e.g. a pencil in the mouth which penetrates the tonsillar fossa. In these cases there is often an interval between the injury and onset of hemiplegia, probably due to formation of a thrombus at the site of the trauma which eventually loosens and becomes a cerebral embolus. In some cases when the child falls on an object in the mouth, the tear of the vessel wall causes a dissecting aneurysm to form and secondary occlusion may then follow.

Roughened areas of endothelium may be seen on angiography of the internal carotid artery in the tonsillar fossa. It is postulated that arteritis secondary to adjacent tonsillitis roughens the endothelium, allowing platelet adhesion and subsequent embolization.

The carotid artery can occasionally be elongated into redundant loops and these may kink with neck movement.

Arteritis due to immune mechanisms is rare in childhood but large vessels are involved in Takayasu's disease, polyarteritis and in disseminated lupus erythematosus. The vessels are abnormal in Menkes' disease which, along with homocystinuria and Fabry's disease, represents metabolic diseases which can present with cerebrovascular accidents. Certain of the mitochondrial disorders may also present with seizures and stroke (e.g. MELAS syndrome). Moya moya is the name given to a peculiar leash of small vessels which is seen on angiography in children who have sustained a stroke. This is said to resemble a puff of smoke and is much more common in Japanese children. It may be seen in any child who has a stenosis or occlusion in the terminal carotid or proximal middle cerebral artery. An idiopathic fibromuscular hyperplasia may be seen in Japanese children which may affect the cerebral vessels in the same way as the more commonly

Table 14.41 Causes of hemiplegia or stroke

Genetic and malformational
1. Focal ulegyria and pachygyria
2. Porencephalic cysts
3. Sturge–Weber syndrome
4. Tuberous sclerosis with fits
5. Progeria
6. Cockayne's syndrome
7. De Lange syndrome
8. Seckel bird-headed dwarfs
9. Hemimegalencephaly

Metabolic and toxic
1. Ornithine transcarbamylase deficiency
2. MELAS syndrome
3. Menkes' syndrome
4. Complex 1 and 3 deficiency
5. Protein C deficiency
6. Protein S deficiency
7. Fabry's disease
8. Methylmalonicaciduria
9. Isovalericaciduria
10. Homocystinuria
11. Marfan's syndrome
12. Cyclosporin toxicity
13. *E. coli* 0157 toxemia
14. Endotoxemia with DIC
15. Hypernatremic dehydration
16. Salt poisoning
17. Diabetic hyperlipidemia
18. Familial hypercholesterolemias

Traumatic
1. Birth trauma with subdural hematoma
2. Accidental contusional injury
3. Accidental penetrating injury
4. Accidental compressive injury
5. Nonaccidental injury
6. Puncture porencephaly
7. Carotid trauma
8. Fall onto object in mouth
9. Intravascular catheters, angiography
10. Ventricular puncture/cannulation

Infections
1. Cerebral abscess
2. Subdural empyema
3. Basal meningitis with carotid thrombosis
4. Infectious vasculitis
5. Encephalitis – herpes simplex
6. Tuberculoma
7. Cysticercosis
8. Toxoplasmic encephalitis
9. DIC and septicemia
10. AIDS
11. Papova and measles in immunosuppression

Tumors
1. Gliomas
2. Leukemia
3. PNET
4. Lymphoma

Vasculitis
1. Radiotherapy
2. Disseminated lupus erythematosus
3. Polyarteritis
4. Chickenpox vasculitis with delayed stroke
5. *Haemophilus* cerebritis
6. DIC and septicemia
7. Kawasaki disease
8. Takayasu disease
9. Japanese moya moya
10. Menkes' syndrome
11. Mitochondriopathies (see above)
12. Anticardiolipid antibodies with cardiomyopathy and stroke

Cerebral embolism
1. Fat embolism
2. Vegetations (SBE)
3. Atheromatous plaques
4. Mural thrombus
5. Following cardiac surgery (clot, bubble, vegetation)
6. Congenital heart disease
7. Atrial thrombus – atrial fibrillation
8. Paradoxical emboli in CHD from pelvic veins or legs
9. Tumor emboli – atrial myxoma
10. Placental embolus
11. Embolus in neonate from venous umbilical catheters

Cerebral hemorrhage
1. Hemophilia
2. Christmas disease
3. Thrombocytopenia
4. Hemorrhagic disease – vitamin K
5. Trauma (see above)
6. Choroid plexus hemorrhage in full-term neonate
7. Neonatal thalamic hemorrhage
8. Intraventricular, germinal plate hemorrhage
9. Hemorrhage into preexisting infarct
10. Hemorrhage into neonatal PVL
11. Arteriovenous malformations
12. Hypertensive hemorrhage
13. Ruptured berry aneurysm

Cerebral thrombosis
1. Thrombocythemia
2. Thrombotic thrombocytopenia
3. Postsplenectomy thrombocythemia
4. Macro, cryoglobulinemia
5. Dehydration – any loss plasma water
6. Polycythemia
7. Overdose clotting factors
8. Atheroma
9. Endothelial diseases – see trauma, metabolic, etc.
10. Sickle cell disease
11. Thalassemia
12. Cyclosporin toxicity
13. Diabetic hyperlipidemia and hyperviscosity
14. Vasospasm – postsubarachnoid hemorrhage
15. Migraine
16. Alternating hemiplegia syndrome

Vascular compression
1. Thoracic outlet syndrome
2. Raised intracranial pressure and tentorial cone
3. Cervical spondylosis
4. Foramen magnum cone
5. Tuberculous nodes neck
6. Woody change in tuberculous meningitis
7. Prolonged vascular spasm of electrocution

described lesions in the renal arteries. It can present with transient ischemic attacks or as an established stroke.

Arteriosclerosis is rare in children except in familial hypercholesterolemia.

Vascular spasm is a more difficult diagnosis to prove with certainty although in cases of spasm following subarachnoid hemorrhage, one can now demonstrate this with pulsed Doppler. Whether this will be applicable in migraine remains conjectural.

Migraine is a classic model for recurrent spasm and hemiplegic migraine certainly occurs in children. The alternating hemiplegia syndrome is a separate entity which is familial. The occasional occurrence of a hemiplegia after severe exercise such as swimming or after minor trauma is often only explicable on the basis of vascular spasm.

Thrombosis

Thrombosis in an otherwise normal vessel may occur in hyperviscous and hypercoagulable states. Polycythemia in the neonatal period secondary to placental insufficiency may cause vascular occlusion and infarction.

Polycythemia vera is extremely rare in childhood and the commonest cause of polycythemia is cyanotic congenital heart disease or chronic chest disease (e.g. cystic fibrosis). Primary thrombosis may occur in the presence of a high hematocrit in cyanotic congenital heart disease but separation of primary thrombosis from embolism can be difficult. The possibility of a cerebral abscess in these cases must always be borne in mind. Postoperative complications of cardiac surgery are more likely in the presence of a severe preoperative hyperviscous state. Hyperviscosity is also seen in severe gastroenteritis with dehydration; cerebral vessel occlusion is far more likely to occur in the presence of complicating hyperosmolality when a persistent hemiplegia is not uncommon. Poorly controlled diabetes with persistent ketoacidosis is accompanied by hyperlipidemia, hyponatremia and hyperviscosity so that sludging or frank occlusion and cerebral infarction may occur. Disseminated intravascular coagulation with vascular occlusion is seen particularly in the hemolytic uremic syndrome, meningococcal septicemia and other Gram-negative septicemias: sudden hemiplegia may complicate the clinical state. In pneumococcal and tuberculous meningitis, the basal exudate may surround the middle cerebral artery causing a vasculitis with secondary thrombosis, so that an acute hemiplegia may appear at a time when the meningitis appears to be getting better. Hypercoagulable states may be seen postsplenectomy and in idiopathic thrombocytosis, macroglobulinemias, thalassemia and sickle cell disease, all of which may be complicated by cerebrovascular occlusions. In sickle cell disease a cerebrovascular accident may be the first presentation of the condition. Many children who were thought to have an idiopathic stroke presenting with a middle cerebral artery thrombosis for no obvious cause are now suspected of having an abnormality of the plasma proteins, C and S. These affect blood coagulation and may be responsible for many of the cases of idiopathic stroke in children. There is also a condition of lactic acidosis, basal ganglia calcification, stroke-like episodes and cortical blindness which may be due to cytochrome reductase deficiency. Other mitochondrial disorders including OTC deficiency may present as stroke and fits.

Embolization

Emboli may consist of blood clot, fat, air, atheromatous plaque, vegetations from the heart or foreign bodies. The heart and neck vessels are the usual source but paradoxical emboli from the placenta via the physiological intracardiac shunt can occur in utero. In congenital heart disease with a septal defect paradoxical emboli may occur associated with sepsis from the pelvic veins. Thromboembolic infarction occurs in approximately 17% of brains studied at autopsy in children with congenital heart disease and this is five times more common following surgery or cardiac catheterization. Embolization has also been reported in association with prolapse of the mitral valve cusps, cardiac arrhythmia, severe burns and Q fever endocarditis.

Any child presenting with a sudden stroke should have a cardiac ultrasound examination prior to cerebral angiography. This will also pick up rare conditions such as atrial myxoma.

Intracerebral hemorrhage

This has been fully discussed above and with the advent of the CT scan it has been shown that intracerebral hemorrhage is not as rare in children as was previously thought. Post-mortem findings suggested that hemorrhages into cerebral substance were rare in the neonatal period whilst subdural, subarachnoid and intraventricular hemorrhages were well documented. We now know that intracerebral hemorrhage sometimes and for no apparent reason does occur in the neonate. Hypertension in children from acute nephritis, coarctation of the aorta, pheochromocytoma, polycystic disease of the kidneys or renal vascular hypertension is not in our experience a significant cause of cerebrovascular disease in children. Massive intracranial hemorrhage may complicate chickenpox treated with steroids (fulminating hemorrhagic chickenpox), hypernatremic dehydration (complicated by hyperviscosity, hyperosmolality and venous thrombosis) and pertussis (also complicated by cerebral thrombosis).

Infection

Acute hemiplegia may be the presenting feature in *Haemophilus influenzae* meningitis when there is in addition to the meningitis a true bacterial encephalitis with perivascular infiltration within the brain substance. This can be shown as a vasculitis on microangiography. The result is acute brain swelling, fits and neurological signs such as a hemiplegia or choreoathetosis. Secondary thrombosis of the middle cerebral due to organization of the basal exudate in pneumococcal and tuberculous meningitis has been described. The virus encephalitides are discussed on page 1375–1376. The commonest seen in Britain is herpes simplex with a predilection for the temporal lobe but occasionally the mode of presentation may be the rapid onset of a hemiplegia. Abscess from middle ear infection or congenital heart disease can also present with hemiplegia. Subdural empyema can complicate an ethmoid sinusitis and be very subtle in presentation. The complicating cortical thrombophlebitis results in the onset of hemiplegia. Another subacute encephalitis which can present in a relapsing course with hemiplegia is acquired toxoplasmic encephalitis. This may disappear with steroids and may appear each time they are discontinued. Hemiplegia may also be a feature of parainfectious encephalomyelitis, infections with Coxsackie virus or Q fever which may cause an endocarditis with resultant stroke. Carotid arteritis from tonsillar bed infection has already been described. Virus infections may cause febrile convulsions. The convulsing brain requires many hundred percent more oxygen and a vast increase in blood supply. If this is not met, e.g. due to airway obstruction or due to competition for oxygen by the convulsing muscles or prolonged seizures themselves interfering with respiration, a consumptive asphyxia may result. The part of the brain giving rise to the convulsions will be the most damaged, as it has the greatest oxygen demand, so a permanent hemiplegia can result from inadequately treated convulsions.

Trauma

Birth trauma has been discussed as a cause of congenital hemiplegia but trauma occurring in postnatal life from nonaccidental injury may also cause hemiplegia. Shaking an infant with the head unsupported can cause tears of the bridging veins with a resultant acute subdural or subarachnoid hemorrhage and retinal hemorrhages. Hemiplegia with visual difficulty is the commonest long-term neurological sequel to nonaccidental injury.

Iatrogenic trauma from attempts to needle the lateral ventricle may cause bleeding into the internal capsule. A rise in intraventricular pressure in the presence of a ventriculoperitoneal shunt may result in a puncture porencephaly with a hemiplegia that may appear only at the time of raised pressure.

Accidental injury is the commonest cause of acquired hemiplegia in children and may be due to pressure from an external clot such as an extradural or subdural hematoma. An acute subdural hematoma is nearly always associated with a severe contusion of the underlying cortex and persistent focal neurological signs are more likely to follow than following an extradural hematoma. Cerebral contusion or contracoup injury can cause a cortical hemiplegia. A tentorial cone from any cause of raised intracranial pressure may compress one of the cerebral peduncles causing an ipsi- or contralateral brainstem hemiplegia. Occasionally rare conditions such as a pneumatocele from a fracture into the frontal sinus or obstruction of the foramen of Monro on one side may cause a hemiplegia with an easily remediable cause.

Hypoxic ischemic encephalopathy

With abnormal anatomy of the circle of Willis there may be differential flow in the six main vessels supplying the cerebral cortex. These are end arteries so that in hypotensive states the territory between the adjacent arterial territories (watershed zones) are more liable to infarction. Thus a generalized insult such as hypotension will not affect all regions of the cerebral cortex equally. Fits further compound the effect by increasing local demand and localized edema also interferes with the microcirculation. Once the damage has occurred loss of vessel reactivity to carbon dioxide as well as release of thromboplastin from damaged brain (causing thrombosis in the veins draining the area) create a complex set of intermediate pathological mechanisms whereby hypoxic ischemic damage can cause a focal cerebral infarction. Later in life anoxic ischemic brain damage is likely to occur from status epilepticus, head injury, cardiac arrest, poisoning, drowning, carbon monoxide poisoning, anesthetic accidents, acute hypotension from blood loss or endotoxic shock, cardiac bypass surgery or respiratory obstruction from foreign bodies or laryngeal obstruction. In most cases when hemiplegia occurs this is against a picture of more widespread damage with ataxia, dystonia, mental handicap and epilepsy with or without cortical blindness.

Neoplasia

A glioma may rarely present with acute hemiplegia when hemorrhage occurs into it. Although this can occur in a benign tumor (cystic astrocytoma), hemorrhagic necrosis is usually a sign of severe malignancy. Leukemia is the commonest malignancy of childhood and with modern treatment prolonged survival is possible so that neurological complications are common. Hemorrhage in leukemia may occur in the acute or terminal stages from thrombocytopenia. Multiple hemorrhagic infiltrations can cause a 'cherry cake' brain and following treatment, when a very high CSF white cell count exists, there may be a hyperviscosity syndrome which may cause multiple infarcts.

Meningeal leukemia was common prior to the use of radiotherapy which has almost abolished CSF leukemia. Now, however, radiation vasculitis and late stroke must be added to the list of complications along with possible risk of microgliomas of the brain. Immunosuppressive drugs may predispose to infections with cytomegalovirus, toxoplasma and measles virus. Malignant glands in the neck may rarely infiltrate the internal carotid artery to give a hemiplegia.

Management of the child with acute-onset hemiplegia

In this section we will confine ourselves to the management of the acute focal ischemic brain insult.

Fits. Fits must be treated energetically but ensuring that no drop in cerebral perfusion pressure is caused from drug-induced hypotension. It is essential that an EEG is performed in all cases. In ideal circumstances continuous EEG monitoring will provide early warning of cerebral dysrhythmia. Electrical status epilepticus with a resultant increase in oxygen requirement of the convulsing brain may occur with only minor clinical ictal activity. Diazepam should be given intravenously during the EEG if there is any abnormality to see whether it is due to infarction or an arrhythmia. Intravenous diazepam has a duration of action of less than half an hour so that phenytoin should also be commenced as background therapy. Paraldehyde given intramuscularly should be used if the fits are not benzodiazepine sensitive and in intractable seizure activity, may be given on a regular basis by the rectal route mixed with arachis oil.

Raised intracranial pressure. The three common types of cerebral edema, i.e. vasogenic, toxic and osmotic, may all be present together in the same patient. The area infarcted from ischemia is associated with opening of tight endothelial junctions which allows fluid and protein into the intercellular space.

Steroids are now back in favor in the management of meningitis. They are thought to stabilize lysosomal membranes to inhibit cell lysis, tighten endothelial junctions to prevent albumen escaping and to have a vasodilator effect, possibly improving microcirculation. Fluid should be restricted to 50–60% of calculated requirements to prevent water intoxication from inappropriate antidiuretic hormone secretion. If there is hyperosmolality and hyperviscosity which require fluids the circulation must be maintained by use of plasma expanders and extracellular dehydration treated with normal saline so that there is no change in osmolality. If the child has any impairment of consciousness or change in neurological state, intracranial pressure should be monitored. If it is found to be raised treatment with mannitol, hyperventilation, frusemide and colloid may be given appropriately.

Maintain the microcirculation. Blood pressure is maintained by the use of plasma expanders or dopamine depending on the cause of shock. Polycythemia is treated by venesection, plasma exchange or mannitol. In the experimental situation anemia is extremely beneficial as a low hematocrit improves the microcirculation far better than any other measure provided blood pressure and oxygenation are maintained. Mannitol may exert its beneficial effect not only as an osmotic diuretic reducing cerebral edema but also as a plasma expander improving the microcirculation. It is thought in addition to have an antioxidant effect. Some centers try and maintain hemodilution in cerebrovascular disorders over several days by the use of low molecular weight dextrans. Hyperviscosity from hyperlipidemia requires urgent treatment in diabetes. Acidosis should be corrected and there is a theoretical preference for tris-hydroxyamino-methane (THAM) as it will treat the intracellular acidosis in the damaged area and not cause hypernatremia, which may occur with the overzealous use of sodium bicarbonate.

The adhesion of platelets to damaged endothelium causing local thrombosis may further block the microcirculation. Liberation of thromboplastin from the damaged brain also tends to encourage secondary thrombosis in the veins draining the damaged area, further aggravating the situation. Aspirin can be given in very small doses to try and prevent platelet stickiness and in the cases of vascular damage (e.g. in neck trauma or recurrent vascular spasm) it can be continued on a long-term basis. Anticoagulants such as warfarin or heparin are only rarely indicated in children unless there is a known focal arterial lesion or possibly in protein C or S deficiency. They are contraindicated once cerebral infarction has actually occurred because of the risk of bleeding into the infarct.

Cerebral protection. Barbiturates reduce the cerebral metabolic demands and reduce cerebral edema. Theoretically they should reduce neuronal oxygen demands, stabilize membranes, reduce fits and prevent local edema. If intracranial pressure is being monitored one can give a test dose of thiopentone in order to see whether this will reduce the intracranial pressure but if there is any depression of blood pressure one is likely to lose more by reducing cerebral perfusion pressure than one gains by reducing metabolism. Large doses of barbiturates in many cases drop the intracranial pressure directly proportional to the drop in blood pressure. If the child is breathing spontaneously they may depress respiration and continuous PCO_2 monitoring is desirable. One cannot use the EEG to monitor barbiturate dose in small infants as burst suppression may not occur before dangerous doses have been given.

Maintain homeostasis. The sick child may show the syndrome of inappropriate antidiuretic hormone secretion inability to excrete a water load. Water intoxication with edema and hyponatremia may result if intravenous fluids are given at the normal rate. Hypoglycemia may occur at any stage and blood glucose estimation must be done 3-hourly in any child with an acute neurological problem. Alternatively, raised intracranial pressure causing secondary brainstem compression may result in hyperglycemia, i.e. cerebral diabetes. The blood glucose may also rise in the presence of seizures to levels seen in diabetes. Insulin must be avoided in children showing central hyperglycemia as severe hypoglycemia may result. Hypocalcemia is a common problem in infants with acute neurological disease and this may itself aggravate the situation by causing seizures. Respiration may be depressed or there may be central neurogenic hyperventilation. There may be vasoparalytic shock requiring dopamine or severe hypertension which may cause fits and retinal hemorrhage. Regular monitoring of blood gases is necessary due to the potent cerebral vasodilator effect of carbon dioxide which will cause severe intracranial hypertension. Monitoring should also include

electrolytes, osmolality, hematocrit, acid–base status and continuous blood pressure.

Surgery. Surgery is the treatment of choice in children with bleeding from aneurysms or arteriovenous malformations. Subdural hematoma, abscess or hemorrhage into tumors also merits early surgical intervention. The use of surgery in the established stroke and cerebral thrombosis is limited.

HEADACHE AND MIGRAINE IN CHILDREN

Headache is common in children with about 10% of children at the age of 10 years complaining of a periodic headache.

Classification of headache

Headache can be divided into four main varieties.
1. Vascular headache (used synonymously with migraine)

2. Organic neurological headache

This is usually worse after sleep or upon awakening in the morning. It is aggravated by lying down, tends to be a daily occurrence and not periodic, there is no family history and one would expect other neurological abnormalities. The commonest concern when a child is referred to hospital with a headache is to exclude a cerebral tumor. Certain tumors such as cystic astrocytoma or hemangioblastoma may be very chronic and may cause a headache over a period of a year or more. Raised intracranial pressure characteristically causes a headache which may be worse when the child wakens in the morning or may awaken him in the night as a result of the rise in pressure that occurs with rapid eye movement sleep. Apart from cerebral tumor, hydrocephalus, chronic subdural hematoma and benign intracranial hypertension may all result in a child presenting with a headache. One must be aware of benign intracranial hypertension in the obese child at puberty which can easily be falsely labeled as migrainous or psychogenic in origin. The other disorders which may cause a vascular-type headache on the basis of an organic pathology are arteriovenous malformations. These may cause a headache in their own right or as a result of small bleeds, raised intracranial pressure or as a result of pain from the blood vessels themselves.

MRI imaging is indicated in the following disorders:

1. neurological lateralizing signs;
2. persisting visual problems;
3. increase in occipitofrontal circumference;
4. deterioration in school performance;
5. change in behavior;
6. early morning headache;
7. association with seizure disturbance;
8. complicated migraine, e.g. temporal lobe ischemia;
9. amblyopic attacks;
10. cough headache;
11. transient global amnesia.

3. Psychogenic headache/tension headache

This is usually continuous (not episodic) and is reported as occurring every day and there is no family history. The headache is often described as a tightness or pressure around the head. There may be pain in the muscles at the back of the neck. There is no vomiting, fortification spectrum or visual disturbance. One should always look for the possibility of a learning disorder as a source of stress and it is becoming accepted that depression in childhood is more common than was previously thought. A tension headache or psychogenic headache should not simply be dismissed without considering it as a sign of either a learning disorder or a depressive illness in the child.

4. Manifestation of systemic illness (see Table 14.42)

Migraine

Migraine was described by Socrates 25 centuries ago and the name 'migraine' is derived from 'hemicrania'. It is thought that the Abbess Hildegard in 1180 illustrated her visions of the celestial city during migraine hallucinations. Alice in Wonderland is said to have been stimulated in the mind of Lewis Carroll during the micropsia or Lilliputian hallucinations of temporal lobe ischemia from migraine.

The incidence is approximately 50 per thousand school-age children. Up to 10% of 10-year-olds and 20% of women over 20 years may have some migrainous phenomena. Migraine increases in frequency with age and is rare under 2 years of age. In the prepubertal period boys outnumber girls by 2:1. At puberty migraine lessens in boys and increases in girls, resulting in the established female preponderance in adults.

Classification

The accepted classification of migraine is:

1. Classic migraine with defined aura and hemicranial type of headache.
2. Common migraine with less well-defined aura, more diffuse headache, associated with nausea, vomiting and general feeling of being unwell.
3. Cluster headaches, migrainous neuralgia (histamine cephalgia) when repeated bouts of unremitting pain in the orbit are accompanied by edema, lacrimation and conjunctival

Table 14.42 Differential diagnosis of chronic headache in children

Typical migraine
Atypical migraine
Tension headache
Cerebral tumor, e.g. pilocytic astrocytoma
Chronic subdural hematoma
Hydrocephalus
TB meningitis
Sarcoidosis
Pseudotumor cerebri
Hypertension (rare in children)
Refractive errors
Sinusitis
Lead poisoning
EB virus or *Mycoplasma* infection
Alcohol hangover headache
Histamine headache
Chronic carbon monoxide poisoning

injection. It is probable that cluster headache is not truly a migrainous phenomenon as a family history of migraine is exceptional and even in adults it affects males more than females. The episode also rarely lasts more than an hour.

4. Complicated migraine and migraine equivalents which include cyclical vomiting, paroxysmal vertigo, ophthalmoplegic migraine, hemiplegic migraine, abdominal migraine, convulsive migraine, basilar migraine and psychomotor migraine.

Pathophysiology

Migraine is thought to be due to increased reactivity of the blood vessels to multiple stimuli. There is a vasoconstrictor phase which precedes a vasodilator phase. The vasoconstrictor phase may occur in the intracranial vessels and the vasodilator phase in the extracranial vessels. Spasm in the intracranial vessels is thought to determine the particular clinical picture, dependent upon whether it is the retinal artery, internal carotid or basilar artery. Blood flow can be shown to be reduced to the corresponding area of the brain with ischemia causing a decrease in oxygenation and a rise in CSF lactate. The vasoconstriction can be demonstrated in the fundus when spasm can be visualized and vessels can also be shown to be in spasm on angiography. It may be severe enough to result in cerebral infarction. The brain responds in a peculiar way by a spreading wave of depression (wave of Leao) and it is thought that this may account for some of the neurological symptoms rather than ischemia alone. All the vasoactive neurotransmitter substances and peptides have been incriminated (histamine, bradykinin, prostaglandin, serotonin and noradrenaline) but the exact mechanism is not yet understood. The vasoconstrictor phase can be abolished by amyl nitrite and can be prolonged by ergotamine or adrenaline. This must be borne in mind when trying new medications such as sumatriptan which cause vaso-constriction and chest pain. It is thought that the vasodilator phase affecting the extracerebral vessels is mainly responsible for the headache. The superficial temporal vessels may be very tender and there may be edema around them in the scalp. Biopsy at this stage may show edema of the vessel wall and digital pressure over the artery will temporarily relieve the discomfort.

Etiology

Ninety percent of children with typical migraine will give a positive family history in one of the immediate family. This is an autosomal dominant tendency with more complete penetration in the female. Hemiplegic migraine may show a definite dominant inheritance; migrainous neuralgia does not have a genetic basis. Common and classic migraine both often show a dominantly inherited susceptibility to some environmental precipitant such as trigger foods (cheese, chocolate and bananas which contain vasoactive substances such as tyramine, phenylethylamine and serotonin), red wine (which releases serotonin from platelets) and other foods (e.g. gluten, milk and eggs). Monosodium glutamate is also vasoactive and may precipitate attacks following a Chinese meal. Cold food may occasionally cause 'ice lolly headache'.

Exercise may induce attacks in some children so that an excruciating headache may follow competitive sports such as a game of rugby. Mild trauma may also be the first trigger and this can cause anxiety about more severe intracranial damage from a relatively trivial injury.

There is no doubt that anxiety and stress, particularly secondary to schooling difficulties, may precipitate attacks of migraine. Differentiation from simple tension headache may be difficult.

Hormones have an additional effect to the genetic predisposition. Puberty changes the susceptibility in males and it is thought that androgen may suppress and estrogen aggravate the tendency to migraine. The contraceptive pill will produce severe migraine in certain individuals and menstrual migraine may be eased by giving progesterone.

Virus infection may also precipitate attacks of migraine when differentiation from sinus infection may not be easy. Eye strain is often suspected, but rarely proven, as a primary cause of headache but some individuals are very susceptible to certain visual patterns and a particular carpet or wallpaper may bring on an episode of migraine.

Clinical features

The headache is classically described as throbbing or pulsating. It is only typically hemicranial in distribution in 25% of children. It is classically periodic and it is usual to have at least five episodes before accepting the diagnosis of migraine, lasting from 10 min to most of 1 day (average 1–3 h). In status migrainosis the headache may last several days and may be associated with cyclical vomiting. In a typical attack an aura may precede the headache and this may be due to either retinal ischemia or ischemia of the visual or calcarine cortex from basilar migraine. The vision may merely be blurred or the child may temporarily become blind. Scotomas may appear in the visual field. They may be static or they may flash six or 12 times per second. Colored lights, flashes, zigzag lines or fern-like shadows may flash or move across the visual field (phosphenes, teichopsia, fortification spectra). If the temporal lobe is ischemic in cases of basilar migraine then micropsia, macropsia, derealization and hemianopia all occur associated with cinematographic vision in which the whole visual field flashes as in an old film. Objects may appear to be moving very slowly or very fast. There may be hallucinations, both visual and auditory. Holes may appear in the paper when the child is writing or the blackboard may appear to be moving. Visual features are associated with migraine in approximately 30% of children.

Another common feature is nausea which occasionally goes on to intractable vomiting, i.e. cyclical vomiting. The child may feel unsteady. Travel or motion sickness is said to occur in up to 40% of children with migraine. There may be abdominal pain (abdominal migraine) and it has been suggested that some of these cases are due to a milk intolerance with deficiency of intestinal lactase and the headache is part of the toxic syndrome.

If the basilar artery is predominantly involved, the very young child may have sudden attacks of vertigo during which he drops to the floor and may mimic epilepsy. The vision may be blurred or the child may be very ataxic in the episodes. Involvement of the temporal lobe in basilar migraine may result in a psychomotor syndrome very similar to that seen in psychomotor epilepsy. Rarely there may be complete loss of memory for a short period, i.e. transient global amnesia. The condition is further complicated by a relationship between migraine and epilepsy (the migraine epilepsy syndrome) when spikes on the EEG and true seizures may complicate the ischemia phase of migraine.

In hemiplegic migraine the internal carotid territory is mainly involved and a hemiplegia occurs lasting several hours. There may be associated parasthesia of one half of the body or transient aphasia. Occasionally an established stroke results from the reduction in cerebral blood flow below a critical level. Other rare phenomena are pseudoangina and ophthalmoplegic migraine.

Management of the child with migraine

Any child with confirmed migraine is managed with advantage in a migraine clinic (Table 14.43).

Investigation. In a typical case of a school-age child presenting with headache associated with visual phenomena and a positive family history who is neurologically completely normal on examination and in whom the headache is classically periodic and ceases after lying down, no further investigation is necessary. If

Table 14.43 Management in the migraine clinic

1. Reassure that the problem is not brain tumor or investigate to reassure

2. Investigate whether there is a learning disorder

3. Recommend anxiolytic relaxation and feedback for stress

4. Start a dietary diary – cheese (tyramine), chocolate (phenylethylamine), bananas (5-HT), red wine (release 5-HT from platelets), gluten flour, milk, etc.

5. If exercise induced, medicate prior to exercise. Use a mild analgesic, e.g. paracetamol 12 mg/kg/dose × 4 or 50 mg/kg/24 h (Calpol pink has 120 mg paracetamol per 5 ml; Calpol 6+ orange has 250 mg paracetamol per 5 ml; Paramax sachet is paracetamol 500 mg with metoclopramide 5 mg). Ibuprofen – 5 mg/kg/dose or 20 mg/kg/24 h. Codeine phosphate – 3 mg/kg/24 h to maximum 240 mg in adult. Rectal (if vomiting): paracetamol suppositories or aspirin suppositories – 300 mg. Migraleve: pink tablet – paracetamol 550 mg, codeine 8 mg, buclizine 6.25 mg; yellow tablet – paracetamol 500 mg, codeine 8 mg (10–14 years – one pink at start then one yellow 4-hourly, double dose after 14 years)

6. Analgesic/antiplatelet adhesive – aspirin 5–10 mg/kg over 12 years, 6-hourly

7. Antiemetic (cyclical vomiting): stemetil orally 250 µg/kg bodyweight two or three times per day (not under 2 years)

8. Pizotifen: 0.5–3.0 mg nocte (or divided up to 4.5 mg max)

9. Propranolol: 1.0–1.5 mg/kg per day

10. Cafergot suppositories: ergotamine 2.0 mg, caffeine 100 mg

11. Sumatriptan (never with ergotamine) 5-HT$_1$ agonist. Only over 12 years. Full dose is 100 mg at onset or autoinjector of 6.0 mg at onset.

12. Clonidine: 25 µg tablet. Start one b.d., after 2 weeks two b.d., after 4 weeks three b.d. No serious side-effects and should not be hypotensive at this dose

13. Elimination diet

14. Ergotamine – may make vomiting worse. Never give in hemiplegic migraine. Does not help aura, visual disturbance or vasoconstrictive phase. Medihaler 360 µg per metered dose. Suppository: Cafergot – ergotamine 2.0 mg and caffeine 100 mg; sublingual tablet: Lingraine – ergotamine 2.0 mg; tabs: Migril – ergotamine 2 mg, caffeine 100 mg and cyclizine 50 mg; Cafergot – ergotamine 1 mg, caffeine 100 mg

15. Antidepressants – amitriptyline 10.0 mg nocte

16. Calcium channel blockers: verapamil; nifedipine: 1.0 mg/kg/24 h; flunarizine: once daily dose of 5.0–7.5 mg

17. Cyproheptidine (antihistamine, anti-5-HT and calcium channel blocker): dose 0.2–0.4 mg/kg/day

18. Severe vomiting: buclizine; prochlorperazine; domperidone; metoclopramide; ondansitron

there are psychomotor features or changes in conscious level then an EEG will be indicated to exclude an associated seizure disorder.

Imaging. MRI or CT scanning is indicated with any neurological abnormality, absence of family history or early morning headaches. The pubertal child with the possibility of benign intracranial hypertension presenting with intractable headache may show papilledema or may have raised pressure without papilledema and lumbar puncture following CT scan would be indicated with monitoring of the intracranial pressure by a nondisplacement transducer method.

In all cases the child's school performance should be examined as long periods of unnecessary medication may be prescribed when remedial teaching would be more effective.

The parents should be encouraged to keep a diary of the attacks together with a dietary history of all the foods taken for the 24 h prior to attacks. If one can identify trigger foods then avoidance of these is preferable to longer term medication. In children with abdominal migraine a trial period without milk or gluten may be indicated. In severe intractable drug-resistant migraine with status migrainosis it may be necessary to give a low antigenic diet for a period before reverting to a chicken-based diet and gradually increasing the variety of foods offered.

Many attacks can be managed simply by the child lying down for 20 min in a darkened room. Photophobia and phonophobia are not uncommon during the attack and a short sleep may abort the episode.

Drug therapy (Table 14.44)

Since migraine is likely to persist for several years, drug therapy on a regular basis should be reserved for the minority of sufferers who have such severe or frequent attacks that they interfere with normal life, i.e. it is a handicapping condition.

If nausea and vomiting are pronounced or the child becomes anxious about the condition, a small dose of prochlorperazine often helps. Caffeine has stimulant and anticonvulsant effects, but also appears to have a specific effect in improving the absorption of ergotamine from the gut, so it is included in preparations such as Cafergot (1 mg ergotamine, 100 mg caffeine). Some people find that a cup of tea or coffee will help alleviate their attacks, so the vasoactive properties of caffeine may have some effect in their own right.

Analgesics. Aspirin has many theoretical advantages with its effects on platelet stickiness and prostaglandins. Concern over the association of salicylates with Reye's syndrome has lessened its general use but it should not be abandoned in migraine especially if there are focal neurological signs, e.g. hemiplegia. Paracetamol

or other mild analgesics such as ibuprofen have largely taken its place. The failure to respond to one analgesic does not mean that others should not be tried. In severe cases other nonsteroidal analgesics which inhibit prostaglandin synthesis such as indomethacin, naproxen, ketoprofen, flufenamic acid and mefenamic acid may help the individual child.

Antiemetics. These may be given if vomiting is a major problem. Stemetil is commonly used but there are preparations which include an analgesic and antiemetic such as Migraleve. Dystonic reactions can occur which respond to procyclidine. Antiemetics should be taken with the first warning of an impending attack as there is gastric dilation during the actual attack so medication will not be absorbed until the episode has ended spontaneously. Stemetil may be given regularly for several weeks if the child starts to group attacks and particularly if cyclical vomiting is a prominent feature.

Vasoactive drugs

Sumatriptan. This is a 5-HT$_1$ receptor agonist that has a selective vasoconstrictor effect on the cranial vasculature of the carotid bed. It can be used in children over 12 years. Absorption after subcutaneous, oral and intranasal administration is rapid. Bioavailability is nearly 100% after subcutaneous administration and 14% after the oral route. Peak plasma concentrations are achieved within 15 minutes of intranasal administration. Elimination is predominantly by metabolism to a nonactive indoleacetic acid analog in the liver. Plasma half-life is 2 hours. It is generally well tolerated but may produce a number of minor adverse events, namely heavy-headedness, tingling, heaviness, pressure, warmth in various parts of the body, chest discomfort and tightness across the chest, all of which are of mild to moderate severity, occurring after all routes of administration and usually short-lived (few minutes following parenteral administration and up to 1 h after the oral route). No behavioral effects are recorded and no effects on CNS function. No interactions are seen with other drugs but it should not be taken with ergotamine. Nausea and photophobia are significantly reduced.

Ergot. Ergot preparations, the mainstay of treatment in the adult, are used only sparingly in children since the vasoconstrictor phase is often more marked than in the adult and ergot preparations may prolong the vasoconstrictor phase or give a hemiplegia.

Propranolol. Propranolol is a β-antagonist affecting both β1 and β2 receptors in the smooth muscle of blood vessels. It may aggravate concurrent bronchial asthma. Children on high-dose propranolol may feel extremely weak. Propranolol prevents the breakdown of glucose and may also affect the ability to increase muscle blood supply so that poor exercise tolerance may be due to a combination of failure to increase cardiac output, failure to increase blood sugar and failure of muscle blood supply. It should only be used if the migraine is severe, with school absence or if there is complicated migraine with basilar or internal carotid artery symptomatology. Our own dosage schedule is to start with 10 mg twice a day up to a maximum of 20 mg three times per day in the 10- to 12-year-old age group but others start with a dosage of 10 mg t.d.s. and increase to as much as 80 mg t.d.s. in those adolescent patients who have attained adult proportions. The drug is initially used for 3 months but it is suggested that there should be a summer drug holiday. Improvement can be expected in 70% of patients. A few children feel light-headed or nauseous or have sleep disturbances but these effects are usually relatively mild.

Table 14.44 Drug therapy for migraine

Acute attack	Maintenance therapy	Status migrainosus
Analgesic	Pizotifen	Sumatriptan
Antiemetic	Propranolol	Antigen-free comminuted
Ergotamine	Clonidine	chicken diet
Sumatriptan	Calcium channel blocker	Parenteral antiemetics –
	Cyproheptidine	dramamine, cyclizine
		Parenteral fluids
		Ergotamine
		Ondansitron
		Dexamethasone

Pizotifen. This tricyclic drug blocks the effects of serotonin. Pizotifen can be given as a once-daily dose in the evening before the child goes to bed. It is usual to give a 3-month course to try and break the cycle. The commonest side-effect apart from mild sedation is increased appetite which can cause unwelcome obesity in adolescents.

Other drugs. Clonidine has not lived up to initial expectations. In cluster headaches with severe migrainous neuralgia indomethacin or carbamazepine may warrant a trial. In tension headache associated with depression imipramine or amitriptyline would be indicated. In children with migraine epilepsy syndrome carbamazepine may serve also as an antimigraine preparation and should be tried alone in the first instance. Cyproheptadine can also be used as prophylaxis especially in the presence of asthma when propranolol cannot be used.

Behavior modification

Various types of relaxation therapy and biofeedback have been tried, occasionally successfully, in migraine and psychogenic headache. The importance of recognizing the child with learning disorders and so relieving the stress and anxiety of chronic failure has already been emphasized. Biofeedback techniques depend upon measurement of skin resistance and trying to influence skin blood flow. Biofeedback techniques and elimination diets should be considered in children in whom simple medication and dietary advice have not worked rather than embarking on long-term dangerous polypharmacy.

CHRONIC DISEASES OF THE NERVOUS SYSTEM

DISEASES OF THE PERIPHERAL NERVOUS SYSTEM

The peripheral nervous system consists of the anterior horn cell, peripheral nerve, neuromuscular junction and muscle on the motor side together with the sensory receptors, sensory nerve fibers, dorsal root ganglion and posterior root on the sensory side.

DISEASE OF THE ANTERIOR HORN CELL

The anterior horn cell may be affected by the same types of pathology as any other cell, i.e. congenital problems, traumatic, infective, metabolic conditions and degenerative.

Congenital

Congenital abnormalities of the anterior horn cell consist of dysplasia or aplasia of the cells. This may take the form of aplasia of motor nuclei in the brainstem, e.g. the sixth and seventh motor nerve nuclei in Moebius' syndrome. The extended Moebius' syndrome is when other groups of anterior horn cells are also involved. Each muscle is represented within the spinal cord by a group of anterior horn cells, i.e. there is a spinal motor nucleus for each muscle. These may be abnormal so that individual muscles may be absent. A particular dysplasia involves the anterior horn cells particularly to the legs, resulting in paralysis, muscle imbalance across the joints and deformity with severe talipes, dislocated knees and dislocated hips at birth and severe intrauterine contractures, i.e. a form of neurogenic arthrogry-

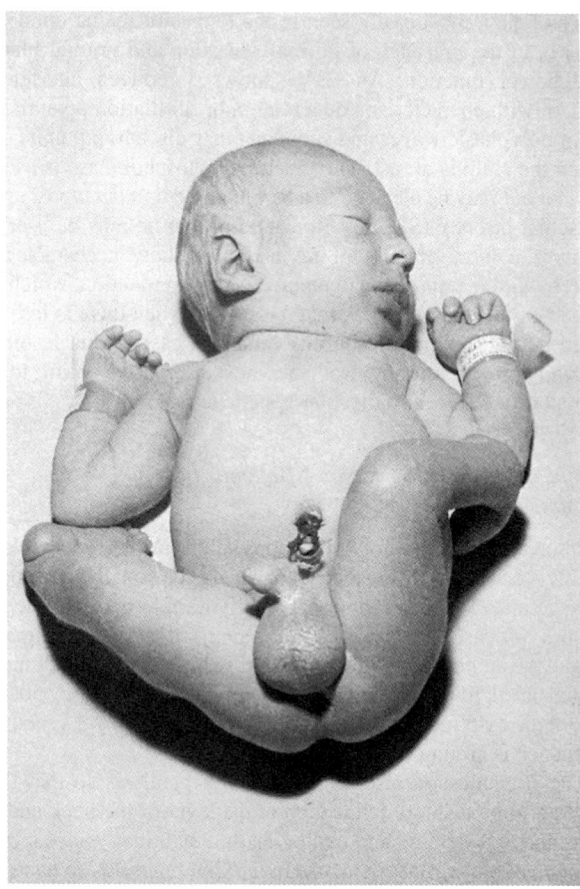

Fig. 14.28 Intrauterine positional deformity.

phosis (Fig. 14.28). Although muscle biopsy shows denervation this is not progressive and is not a form of intrauterine spinal muscular atrophy.

The anterior horn cells are selectively affected with infections such as polio virus and Coxsackie B virus. It is thought there may be a specific genetic factor which allows a cell to be resistant to polio virus. This is discussed in more detail on page 1378.

Metabolic disease affecting the anterior horn cell is typified by acute intermittent porphyria and lead poisoning (see p. 1708).

Degenerative disease of the anterior horn cells

Progressive degeneration with death and loss of anterior horn cells is characteristic of the group of disorders known as spinal muscular atrophies. Although regarded by some as a single disease with a broad clinical spectrum, there is mounting evidence that spinal muscular atrophy is a group of more or less discrete disease entities. There are three main types of spinal muscular atrophy dependent upon the age and acuteness of presentation and these are probably all carried at the same gene locus on chromosome 5q(13). There are two genes at this locus – neuronal apoptosis-inhibitor protein gene (NAIP) and survival motor neuron gene (SMN). Both are deleted in patients with SMA. NAIP is disrupted in 45% of patients with SMA 1 and 18% of SMA 2 and 3. Deletions of exons 7 and 8 of the SMN gene occur in 98% of SMA 1.

The clinical diagnosis of an anterior horn cell lesion depends upon the clinical presence of weakness, wasting and often fasciculation, most easily seen in the tongue or thenar eminence. This is in the presence of normal sensation and normal bladder and bowel function. An EMG shows a reduced interference pattern with characteristic denervation or fibrillation potentials or giant polyphasic waves and spontaneously discharging units even when the child is at rest. The creatinine phosphokinase is usually normal but may be elevated to a few hundred units in type 2 spinal muscular atrophy (SMA). Ultrasound of muscle may be useful if there is a large amount of fat and may show a characteristic pattern with increased echogenicity. Nerve conduction, which one would expect to be normal, may be slowed when there is loss of a large number of motor neurons in severe cases. Muscle biopsy showing group atrophy was the most useful test prior to the availability of recent molecular genetic tests.

Spinal muscular atrophy type 1 (infantile type, Werdnig–Hoffman disease)

This presents as a profoundly floppy infant in the first weeks of life. It is occasionally present at birth and occasionally may appear to have an acute onset in an apparently normal baby. In the vast majority of cases it is obvious by 3 months of age. Approximately 33% have an onset in utero and 50% by the end of the first month of postnatal life. This is a rapidly progressive disease, 50% of whom die by 6 months, 95% by 18 months and all by 3 years. The incidence is around one in 25 000 live births.

The floppiness is also associated with paralysis so that there appears to be a sharp delineation at the level of the neck and the arms and legs lie limp and unmoving. It may initially appear more obvious in the legs and is worse in proximal muscles so hand and finger movements may persist. The child has an alert expression with normal facial muscles and at first is able to swallow normally with normal bulbar muscles (Fig. 14.29). The presentation sometimes raises the question of birth injury to the cervical spine. Tendon reflexes are absent. There is normal sensation and the bladder shows normal detrusor contraction and urine is passed in a jet. Fasciculation is visible in the fingers and the tongue but this is not easy to separate from the normal tremor seen in infant tongues. Progress can be rapid, the child never sits, has no head control and there is total paralysis of all axial muscles, leaving the child totally paralyzed and unable to move either arms or legs.

There is progressive chest deformity which flattens in the anterioposterior diameter with paralysis of the intercostal muscle so that respiration depends upon the diaphragm with increasing paradoxical breathing, giving the so-called 'bell-shaped chest'. Pooling of secretions, inability to cough and aspiration from gastroesophageal reflux leads to death in respiratory failure.

The disease is inherited as an autosomal recessive but the basic metabolic defect in the anterior horn cell is not yet known and it may vary in severity within a sibship. The heterozygote is normal. The disease is now known to be carried on chromosome 5q. Modern DNA technology has identified the exons 5, 7 and 8 as being diagnostic of SMA 1 in over 90% of cases. The specific test for homozygosity of exon 5 and 7 has lessened the need for EMG and muscle biopsy in diagnosis.

Spinal muscular atrophy type 2

This is a more subacute or chronic type of disorder. It usually comes on after the age of 3 months but is obvious in most cases by the end of the first year of life. The child shows generalized

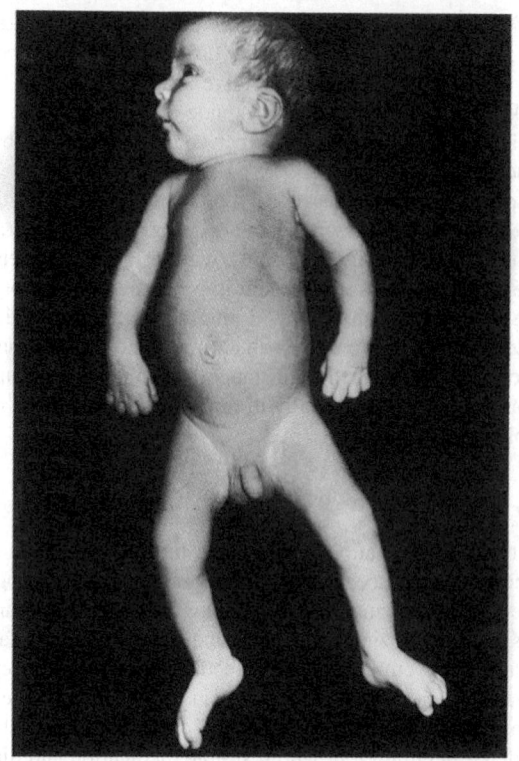

(a)

(b)

Fig. 14.29 Infantile spinal muscular atrophy illustrating gross hypotonia: (a) in supine, (b) in ventral suspension.

hypotonia with exaggerated joint angles, absent reflexes and weakness. The infant may appear to be making normal motor development, can often sit and may even get to the standing stage before regression begins. Twenty-five percent die before the age of 5 and 60% by their 10th birthday.

The condition is associated with severe wasting, together with loss of subcutaneous fat (Fig. 14.30). It is not known why fat is preserved in certain lower motor neuron lesions such as spina bifida, whilst it is lost in others such as polio and chronic spinal muscular atrophy. The hands, diaphragm, facial and eye muscles and myocardium are not affected. There is marked tremor of the fingers due to fasciculation in the muscles. Intelligence is usually

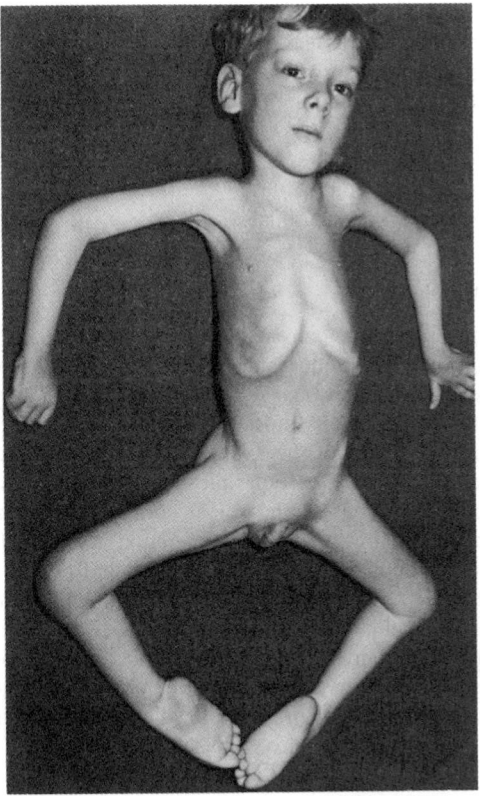

(a)

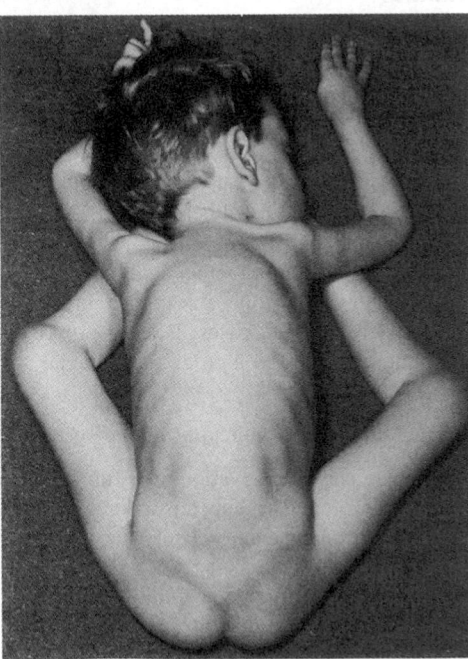

(b)

Fig. 14.30 Chronic infantile spinal muscular atrophy.

normal. The immobility together with growth and gravity leads to severe deformities with scoliosis, rib asymmetry, pelvic tilt, windsweeping of the legs, hip flexion contractures and contractions at the knees and talipes of the feet.

There is chest deformity with prominence of the sternum, an increase of anterior posterior diameter of the chest or else the chest is completely flattened, appearing in some children dramatically thin in the anterior posterior diameter. The diaphragm is preserved but the intercostals may be severely affected. There is a risk of esophageal reflux and repeated aspiration.

A small number may be able to walk with calipers or reciprocating gait orthoses but the majority lead a wheelchair existence. Scoliosis should be treated early before severe restriction of ventilation.

SMA type 2 in most cases shows classic EMG changes of denervation. Muscle biopsy is characteristic with group atrophy of fibers. Occasionally the creatinine phosphokinase may be raised and fibrosis in muscle may make differentiation from a muscular dystrophy difficult.

It is inherited as an autosomal recessive but consanguinity is strangely unusual.

Juvenile spinal muscular atrophy type 3 (Kugelberg–Welander)

This more benign variety is a less genetically pure disease than the other two types. Although most cases are autosomal recessive in inheritance, autosomal dominant and sex-linked recessive forms have also been recognized.

These children will walk normally and after the age of 2 years pelvic girdle weakness results in a waddling gait, difficulty climbing stairs or getting up after a fall, thus mimicking Duchenne muscular dystrophy. Shoulder girdle weakness occurs with winging of the scapulae but the chest deformity seen in the other types does not occur. There is gradual loss of the ability to walk, tendon reflexes are lost and there may be fasciculation of the tongue and hands. The disease appears to come in episodes rather than progressing steadily. If clinical arrest occurs for more than 2 years further deterioration is unlikely but scoliosis may become a major problem. A mean survival of 30 years after onset and a mean age of death of 51 years has been reported (Fig. 14.31). The basic biochemical defect is not yet known. Hexosaminidase A deficiency has been reported with a picture of spinal muscular atrophy but is not typical of Kugelberg–Welander disease.

Distal spinal muscular atrophy

Degeneration at the anterior horn cells affecting the peripheral muscles below the knee presents as peroneal muscular atrophy. Biopsy of the peroneal muscles shows classic neurogenic atrophy. There are a mixture of other diseases in which spinal muscular atrophy may be a feature which can be associated with retinitis pigmentosa, mental retardation, bulbar palsy, spastic diplegia, deafness or cerebellar ataxia.

There is also a type of amyotrophic lateral sclerosis which in children may be either genetic or a young onset of the adult type. In these cases proximal wasting is combined with an upper motor neuron paraplegia together with a progressive bulbar palsy. This is related to adult motor neuron disease. The genetic basis may be similar to some chronic polyneuritis with wasting and weakness which are now known to be due to an abnormality in superoxide dismutase (SOD).

DISORDERS OF THE PERIPHERAL NERVES

The commonest lesion of the peripheral nervous system in childhood is trauma. The brachial plexus and its branches may be

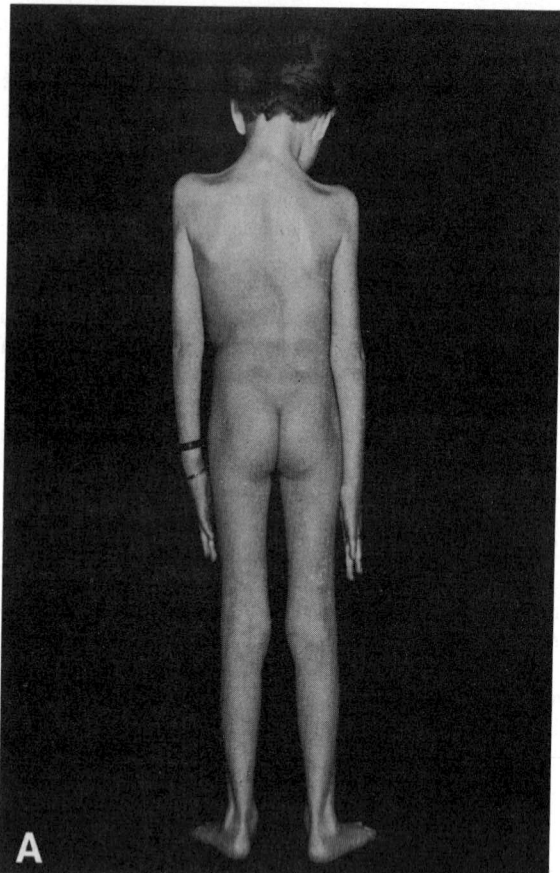

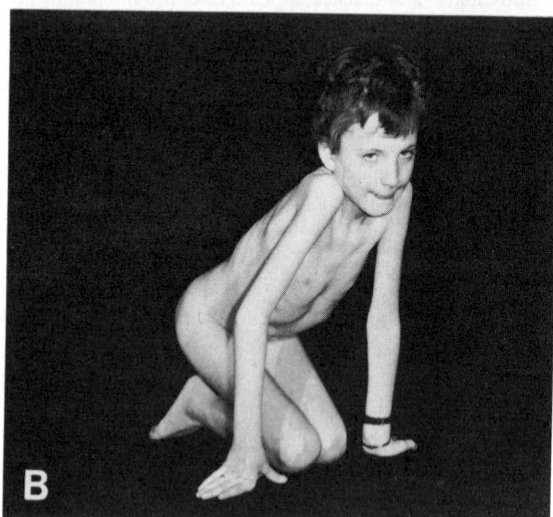

Fig. 14.31 Juvenile spinal muscular atrophy: (**a**) limb girdle wasting and scoliosis; (**b**) method of rising from floor.

1. hereditary degenerative neuropathies:
    a. hereditary motor and sensory neuropathies (HMSN)
    b. hereditary sensory neuropathies;
2. metabolic neuropathies;
3. toxic neuropathies;
4. deficiency neuropathies;
5. parainfectious neuropathies;
6. idiopathic chronic neuropathy.

Pathophysiology

The peripheral nerve consists of the axon together with the Schwann cell which produces the myelin. Diseases may therefore affect the axon, the Schwann cell or myelin. Axonal degeneration affects the longest axons most severely, i.e. those to the distal extremities. Nutrition of the axon, which may be up to 1 m in length, is dependent on cytoplasmic transport mechanisms from the anterior horn cells in the spinal cord. Recovery in axonal degenerations is slow, requiring regeneration of axon cylinders.

Demyelination may result from destruction of myelin which is already formed or disease of the Schwann cell which maintains a segment of myelin between two nodes of Ranvier. Break in continuity of the myelin sheath impedes saltatory conduction causing slowing of nerve conduction velocity as an early feature. It is, however, destruction of the axon which results in denervation of muscle with group atrophy of muscle fibers.

Clinical features

These consist of motor and sensory phenomena. Sudden wrist drop or foot drop is the commonest presentation of the acute neuropathies. Talipes with cavovarus deformity of the feet, wasting below the knee and the peroneal muscular atrophy syndrome is characteristic of the more chronic neuropathies. There is wasting and distal weakness with absent tendon reflexes.

If the sensory nerves are involved then there may be sensory loss of a glove and stocking distribution or paresthesia or anesthesia. Loss of sweating together with cold blue feet and a delayed capillary return from autonomic involvement may dominate the picture in some cases. Loss of proprioception can cause the presentation to be by a progressive ataxia.

Investigation of peripheral neuropathies

Muscle biopsy may show denervation. Creatinine phosphokinase is usually normal. Diagnosis depends upon the estimation of motor nerve conduction time and sensory nerve conduction time or somatosensory evoked potentials. Biopsy of a peripheral nerve is sometimes undertaken, usually the sural nerve, but it should be remembered that this is essentially a sensory, not a motor, nerve.

Hereditary motor and sensory neuropathies (HMSN)

As the name suggests, this group of disorders affects both the motor and sensory nerve fibers.

HMSN type 1

The clinical picture is not specific with distal weakness in the legs and a peroneal muscular atrophy type of picture. This Charcot–Marie–Tooth, distal wasting or peroneal muscular

damaged at birth, particularly with delivery of the anterior shoulder in large babies. Postnatal injury of the radial ulnar and median nerve may be associated with fractures or lacerations. Ischemic neuropathy of the sciatic nerve may follow injections into the umbilical artery or the nerve itself may be injected with irritants such as paraldehyde or penicillin. This section will be confined to the more generalized disorders of peripheral nerves, i.e. the polyneuropathies. They can be classified as follows:

atrophy is not specific but caused by several different diseases. Pes cavus, weakness in the forearm muscles and ataxia pose the main motor problems. Sensory loss occurs in 60% of patients and if present, helps to differentiate from an anterior horn disease. Walking is not usually lost and progress is very slow. The child walks with a 'steppage' foot drop gait. The peronei, then the calf and then lower thigh show symmetrical atrophy to give the champagne bottle leg. Ankle jerks are lost early.

Pathologically there is hypertrophy of the nerves which may sometimes be clinically palpable – 'hypertrophic peripheral neuropathy' (Fig. 14.32). This is due to segmental demyelination with remyelination giving layers of myelin reminiscent of an onion – 'onion bulb formation' (this is not a specific diagnostic finding for this disease). Large-caliber myelinated fibers are most affected. Motor and sensory nerve conduction will be markedly reduced early in the disease. There may be degeneration in the posterior horns of the spinal cord and anterior horn cells.

The autosomal dominant form is thought to be due to a gene locus on chromosome 1. Onset is usually before 10 years but it may be very early in the first years of life and there may be asymptomatic members of the family from variable penetrance, making the genetics not always obvious. It may be necessary to perform nerve conduction studies in both parents. There is also an autosomal recessive form with onset around 10 years of age with pes cavus, ataxia and distal wasting (associated with chromosome 17). If tremor is marked along with ataxia it is classified as the Roussy–Lévy syndrome.

HSMN type 2

Nerve biopsy shows axonal degeneration, not demyelination and no onion bulbs. It may be inherited as an autosomal recessive or autosomal dominant and so is probably a heterogeneous collection of diseases. Abnormal motor and sensory nerve conduction may be present in the family without clinical signs, those with clinical signs may not show particularly slowed conduction and the EMG shows a denervation pattern. The presentation is of weakness and wasting of the distal limbs in a school-age child, i.e. again as peroneal muscular atrophy. It has a later onset, in the second decade, and an slower course than type 1. Ataxia and spinal complications are less common.

HSMN type 3 (Dejerine–Sottas disease)

There is poor myelination of the peripheral nerves which may be thickened and palpable with onion bulbs on biopsy. Nerve conduction studies show markedly slowed motor and sensory nerve conduction velocities and in severe cases no conduction may be measurable. There is often a rise in CSF protein which may clinically help differentiate this form from HMSN type 1.

The inheritance is in most cases autosomal recessive. The onset is in infancy and the child may present with slow motor development with delay in walking and is never able to achieve any 'athletic mobility'. Pes cavus occurs, with distal wasting, scoliosis and absent reflexes which may cause confusion with Friedreich's ataxia. These children may need a wheelchair for community mobility when they become young adults.

Hereditary sensory neuropathies (HSN)

As the name suggests, the dominant symptom in these children is insensitivity to pain with the risk of ulceration of the feet. Burns and other injuries occur because the children do not take the normal precautions against injury. There may be complete loss of pain and temperature sensation. Shooting pains may occasionally occur. Muscle power is preserved although tendon reflexes may be diminished due to interference with the afferent arc. Denervation of the joints can result in a destructive arthropathy, i.e. Charcot joints.

HSN type 1

There is severe loss of pain sensation in this autosomal dominant condition, which is occasionally associated with sensory neural deafness. There is degeneration in the posterior roots and dorsal root ganglia. Progressive loss of sensation occurs in the second decade in the lower extremities with ulceration and cellulitis. Nerve conduction and EMG are normal.

HSN type 2

Nerve biopsy shows loss of myelin in this autosomal recessive condition. Clinically loss of tendon reflexes is the rule with touch and pressure sensation more affected than pain and temperature.

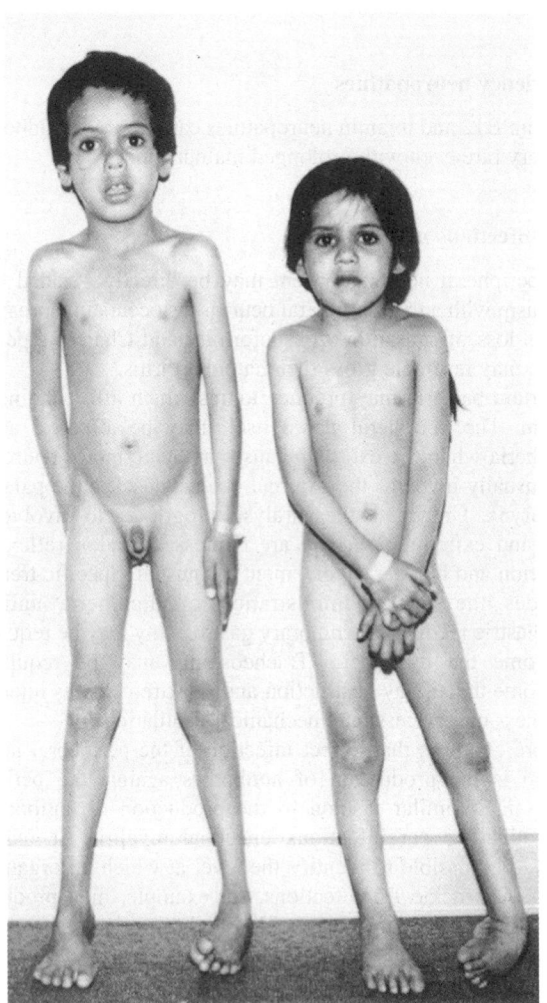

Fig. 14.32 Hypertrophic interstitial neuropathy in a brother and sister.

They present as burns or painless fractures in infancy. Deafness is again seen and in some instances bladder involvement causes worry about spinal cord tumors.

Some children with sensory neuropathy may also have abnormalities of sweating with attacks of hyperpyrexia which may be fatal. These children may be mentally retarded and with the absence of pain sensation, self-mutilation and repeated injuries from overactivity may be a major problem.

Sural nerve biopsy shows abnormality, confirming a peripheral nerve lesion.

HSN type 3 (familial dysautonomia; Riley–Day syndrome)

This is the commonest of the sensory neuropathies and is more common in Jews. In addition to the peripheral sensory neuropathy, which causes insensitivity to pain, there is an autonomic neuropathy.

It is present from birth in a floppy baby with feeding difficulty, vomiting, failure to thrive and a poor cry. Unstable blood pressure, unstable temperature, apnea, vomiting, blotchy skin, absence of tears, all point to the autonomic nervous system. There is poor esophageal motility and reflux.

There are no fungiform papillae on the tongue, no axon flare with the triple response, meiosis occurs following metacholine instillation in the eye and deep reflexes are absent. Prognosis is poor and death may occur during childhood.

HSN type 4

This is a congenital insensitivity to pain with absent sweating present from birth. Fever occurs with the absent sweating and many are mentally retarded.

Metabolic neuropathies

Diabetic neuropathy

Diabetes rarely causes a clinical neuropathy in childhood but subclinical features such as loss of ankle jerk, impairment of vibration sense and slowing of nerve conduction velocities can be encountered in up to 10% of diabetic children. Since diabetes may be diagnosed as a toddler there may be 15 years of good or bad control during childhood.

Uremic neuropathy

This is extremely rare in childhood.

Refsum's syndrome

This is due to the storage of a C16 fatty acid (phytanic acid) and involves all levels of the nervous system with ataxia, retinitis pigmentosa, night blindness and peripheral neuropathy (see p. 785). It presents around 5 years but may not be recognized till after puberty and is sometimes included as HMSN type 4.

α-lipoprotein deficiency (Tangier disease)

This metabolic disease is associated with tonsillar enlargement and peripheral neuropathy from accumulation of cholesterol esters (see p. 790).

Others

Peripheral neuropathy also complicates other metabolic diseases such as metachromatic leukodystrophy (see p. 776), abetalipoproteinemia (see p. 790), Krabbe's disease (see p. 777), argininosuccinic aminoaciduria (see p. 1111), tyrosinemia (see p. 1106), cerebrotendinous xanthomatosis, acute intermittent porphyria (see p. 790), Fabry's disease (see p. 776), Cockayne's syndrome and adrenoleukodystrophy (see p. 785–786).

Toxic neuropathies

The peripheral nerves may be affected in subacute poisoning due to heavy metals – lead, mercury, arsenic and thallium. Lead poisoning in childhood is more likely to result in encephalopathy whilst the peripheral nervous system may be affected in the older age group. Mercury intoxication which produced Pink disease in the past is now only of historical interest. Other exogenous toxins include drugs such as vincristine, cisplatin, nitrous oxide, ethambutol, thalidomide, metronidazole and isoniazid. Solvents such as N-hexane may affect the peripheral nervous system in children who sniff glue.

Deficiency neuropathies

Vitamin B12 and thiamin neuropathies can occur in childhood but are very rare even with prolonged malnutrition.

Parainfectious neuropathies

The peripheral nervous system may be directly invaded by the organism with a true peripheral neuritis, as occurs in leprosy. This causes loss of sensation with deformity and Charcot-type joints which may resemble gross rheumatoid arthritis.

Certain bacteria may produce toxins which affect the nervous system. The peripheral nerve itself may be affected, as with diphtheria when the exotoxin causes an acute motor neuropathy. This usually involves the external ocular muscles, the palate and the larynx. Untreated, the paralysis progresses to involve face, neck and extremities. There are depressed tendon reflexes but sensation and bladder involvement is unusual. Specific treatment includes the early administration of diphtheria antitoxin. Nasogastric feeding or temporary gastrostomy may be required to overcome the dysphagia. Tracheostomy may be required to overcome the airway obstruction and in extreme cases intercostal weakness may necessitate mechanical ventilation.

More common than direct infection of the peripheral nervous system is the production of antibodies against the peripheral nerves in a similar fashion to the production of antibodies in demyelinating parainfectious encephalomyelitis. It may not always be possible to identify the level at which an organism is acting. Coxsackie B5 infections, for example, may produce an acute myositis with extremely high levels of creatinine phosphokinase and sudden onset of severe muscle pain but Coxsackie virus can also cause peripheral nerve involvement which resembles the Guillain–Barré syndrome or an acute myelitis with a picture identical to poliomyelitis.

Acute parainfectious mononeuritis

Bell's Palsy

Many virus infections may be followed after 1–3 weeks by demyelination of the peripheral nerves. Bell's palsy in most cases is a parainfectious mononeuritis and may be seen in association with many viruses (especially mumps) or Lyme disease. Some cases of Bell's palsy are due to edema of the nerve as it comes through the sternomastoid canal and this adds an ischemic component to the demyelination. It can occasionally be seen as the presentation of multiple sclerosis. Facial palsy may also be the presenting feature of a pontine glioma or Fisher's syndrome.

Clinical features. The whole of one side of the face is involved, the eye does not close, the nasolabial crease is lost and the face on that side does not move with either voluntary, associated, reflex or emotional movements. Tears tend to overflow, food lodges between the gums and cheeks, speech is slurred and the cheek on the affected side balloons with respiration. There may be pain in the face at the time of onset, as with the other 'neuralgic amyotrophies'. Localized tenderness and some swelling over the region of the sternomastoid foramen is not uncommon. Two-thirds of cases will settle down spontaneously with no treatment, improvement being noted within 3 weeks. In other cases mild asymmetry persists, the face being symmetrical at rest but not on smiling. Rapid facial movements may be more poorly executed on the affected side. Denervation in a minority of cases causes the syndrome of crocodile tears, i.e. tears upon eating. A few cases remain with disfigurement, either hemifacial atrophy or marked asymmetry which requires a plastic surgical sling procedure to restore facial symmetry.

Treatment. Treatment in the acute phase is to relieve pain if present and prevent conjunctival infection, corneal abrasion or drying out of the eye. Closure with Sellotape and artificial tears or chloramphenicol eye drops are more likely to be required in chronic facial palsy from brainstem tumors or postoperatively when, in addition to regular artificial tears, tarsorrhaphy may be required. Before treatment of the acute Bell's palsy, hypertension, leukemia, brainstem tumor, middle ear disease, etc. must be excluded from the diagnosis. In children this means full blood count and a careful clinical examination with audiometry. These are mandatory if steroids are to be used. The rationales for prescribing steroids are:

1. the immunosuppressant effect;
2. the antiinflammatory effect – the hope of reducing edema and so subsequent ischemia and permanent damage to the nerve.

There is always anxiety over possible exacerbation of a geniculate herpes infection. Steroids must be given early and in big doses, e.g. 40 mg prednisolone or dexamethasone equivalent for 3 days, rapidly tailing off over the rest of the week. Only a small number of cases tend to be seen early (within 48 h) and since so few have marked long-term sequelae only a minority tend to receive any therapy. Since the outcome cannot be predicted in the first 3 days (electrophysiological tests are no help at this stage) evaluation of early therapy is difficult. Exploration and release of the facial nerve in the sternomastoid foramen as an emergency procedure is not recommended unless more evidence from controlled trials becomes available. Galvanic stimulation, much used in adults, will rarely be tolerated in children. Birth trauma as a cause of facial palsy is discussed on page 122.

Optic neuritis

Parainfectious optic neuritis results in pain in the eye, blurring of vision, loss of acuity and scotoma. The relationship between parainfectious optic mononeuritis and subsequent risk of multiple sclerosis is still not clear.

Isolated sixth nerve weakness

Some children appear to get a sudden abducens palsy in relationship to infection. This may lead to a sudden paralytic squint with loss of abduction of the affected eye. If this occurs in very young children loss of visual fixation on the macula and parallelism of the visual axis may leave the child with a concomitant squint once the paralytic component has resolved. Differential diagnosis is from raised intracranial pressure when a sixth nerve palsy is a frequent false localizing sign, brainstem glioma often presents with a sixth nerve weakness and benign intracranial hypertension may also present with a sixth nerve weakness.

Acute radial nerve palsy

This presents as a sudden onset of wrist drop and may be a type of parainfectious mononeuritis.

Lateral popliteal palsy

This presents as a sudden onset of a foot drop. Differentiation from a microvascular disease such as a collagenosis or a toxic peripheral neuropathy will be required.

Bell's nerve palsy

The long nerve of Bell has nothing to do with Bell's palsy affecting the face. This is a parainfectious mononeuritis affecting the long thoracic nerve which causes sudden unilateral scapular winging.

Neuralgic amyopathy

This is the name given when the C5 root is affected. This is a very common root to be involved. It is thought that C5 is a watershed zone in the vascular supply to the cord and roots. This condition may follow known infections such as glandular fever or the use of antitetanus serum. Pain is a feature of many of the infectious neuritides and the child here presents with pain in the shoulder and upper limb. He will not move the arm and it may take some time before it is realized that this is not antalgic paresis but due to severe weakness of the deltoid and biceps muscle on that side. This may be complete with severe wasting and denervation on the EMG. Recovery is slow and sometimes incomplete. The value of steroids has not been proven and it should be regarded as a localized form of Guillain–Barré syndrome.

Acute parainfectious polyneuritis (Guillain–Barré syndrome)

This condition may follow different infectious agents though it is unusual to isolate any organism from the CSF. Exceptions to this are in the case of Coxsackie B infections and Lyme disease which can produce an acute infective rather than an acute parainfectious type of myeloradiculitis. The same applies to the polio virus. There may be features of neuralgic amyotrophy and pain may be very severe with bilateral facial palsy. Wrist drop or foot drop show that it is a most severe variant with multiple nerves being involved, i.e. polyneuritis as opposed to mononeuritis.

Pathophysiology. An antigen–antibody reaction to a nonspecific virus infection has been postulated. It is also interesting that in Italy, where brain-extracted ganglioside is injected into children, it has been suggested that this causes an increase in incidence of Guillain–Barré syndrome (Figueras et al 1992). Demyelination occurs, affecting mainly the motor nerve roots and the peripheral nerves, and degenerative changes may be found in the anterior horn cells. Evidence for an immune basis has come particularly from the rapid reversibility of symptoms using plasmapheresis. Viruses involved are Epstein–Barr and cytomegalovirus in particular but also Coxsackie, ECHO virus, influenza, viral hepatitis and the mycoplasma agent. More recently chronic infection of the upper gut with *Campylobacter* is being recognized as a possible precipitating cause. An identical condition can also occur in Lyme disease and after certain types of swine influenza vaccine or insect bites. The long terminal latency suggests a conduction block and rapid reversibility in some cases together with normal nerve conduction in many suggests a reversible antibody reaction may be as important as demyelination. There may be macrophages and lymphocytes around the nodes of Ranvier and localized demyelination. It is thought that lymphocytes are sensitized to peripheral nerve protein, macrophages contribute to the inflammatory reaction and damage and then Schwann cells multiply to remyelinate.

Clinical features. School-age children are mainly affected but even young infants may develop the disease. A history is often obtained of a preceding mild febrile illness such as an upper respiratory tract infection. There is sudden onset of weakness but pain in the limbs may be very severe and totally mask the other symptoms. Meningeal irritation occurs in almost one-third of children. The onset of neck stiffness and pain without cells in the CSF may cause initial diagnostic confusion. Weakness is symmetrical and usually most marked in the lower limbs and in distal rather than proximal muscles. In some children the proximal muscles may predominate. Tendon reflexes are absent and the limbs are hypotonic. In severe cases bilateral facial palsy and bulbar muscle involvement occurs. There is a more isolated form of parainfectious polyneuritis when only the lower cranial nerves may be involved with palatal paresis and facial paresis. Respiratory paralysis has necessitated mechanical ventilation in 10–25% of cases. In mild cases muscle tenderness and parasthesia may occur with little paralysis. Sensory involvement is usually minimal or absent. Bladder and bowel control is usually preserved, thus differentiating the condition from spinal cord paralysis.

The weakness progresses for up to a week before recovery begins. 'Landry's paralysis' is a particularly severe variant with rapidly progressive ascending paralysis.

Differentiation is from an acute myeloradiculitis, from poliomyelitis or Coxsackie infection, spinal cord trauma from spinal cord concussion, especially in the presence of any congenital abnormality of the spinal column, and metabolic disease such as acute intermittent porphyria or lead poisoning. Familial motor neuron disease or amyotrophic lateral sclerosis may be due to an inborn error of metabolism involving superoxide dismutase (SOD) and may mimic an infectious polyneuritis.

Diagnosis. Diagnosis is helped by the finding of an increased CSF protein with a normal cell count. The protein can, however, be normal in the CSF during the first few days of symptoms. There is slowing of peripheral nerve conduction velocity which often involves the terminal parts of the nerve (prolonged terminal latency). F waves may be absent or very slow. Evidence of denervation only appears in chronic cases and is of poor prognostic significance.

Treatment. There is no evidence that steroids such as methylprednisolone shorten the duration or course of the disorder. Plasmapheresis given as early as possible and certainly within 2 weeks can be dramatic; reflexes may reappear during the plasmapheresis. Several plasmaphereses over 7 days are usually necessary. It should be considered in all severe cases, in acute ascending paralysis or when there is impaired ventilation. More recently, however, discussion has centered around the use of immunoglobulin in all cases. The Dutch study has shown that improvement is more rapid after plasmapheresis than with supportive therapy alone. They then compared the simpler treatment with intravenous human immunoglobulin (400 mg/kg/day for 5 days) with plasmapheresis and found it just as effective with a significant increase in power in cases of respiratory failure (van der Meche et al 1992). If one treatment fails there is no contraindication to then proceeding to the other; some authorities believe the relapse rate is higher after immunoglobulin than with plasmapheresis.

It has been suggested that mild immunosuppression may alleviate the chronic disorder. Some cases go on to a chronic form of Guillain–Barré syndrome which may have a more subacute onset or have a relapsing course.

The child should have regular assessment of capillary gases (PCO_2) and some measure of ventilation such as peak expiratory flow or forced vital capacity is desirable to give warning of hypoventilation and the need for ventilatory support.

Fisher's syndrome

This is a localized form of polyneuritis involving the extraocular muscles which presents as an ophthalmoplegia, bulbar palsy and ataxia. The pupils may be affected so that it is an internal and external ophthalmoplegia.

DISORDERS OF MUSCLE

As a tissue, muscle is relatively free from acquired diseases. It is, however, subject to numerous genetic, degenerative and metabolic disorders (Dubowitz 1995a). These can be divided into:

1. disorders of the neuromuscular junction;
2. muscular dystrophies;
3. myotonic syndromes;
4. myopathies;
5. inflammatory myopathies (myasthitis).

DISORDERS OF THE NEUROMUSCULAR JUNCTION

These are typified by myasthenia gravis, but certain toxins such as botulinus toxin may affect the neuromuscular junction causing a severe and prolonged paralysis. Such toxins may be a cause of the floppy baby syndrome, e.g. from botulinus colonization of the gut. In older children toxins from dog tick bites, certain snake bites and organophosphate poisoning in addition to botulism can all present as neuromuscular paralysis. More recently, acute toxic paralysis has been seen from eating shellfish which have fed on poisonous algae.

Neonatal myasthenia

This is due to antiacetylcholine receptor antibodies passing across the placenta. Neonatal myasthenia gravis is rare but about 15% of infants born to myasthenic mothers suffer from transient myasthenia with an average duration of 4–6 weeks. The severity of disease in the mother and whether it is active or quiescent does not relate to the presence or severity of the disease in her infant. Onset is within hours of birth and certainly in the first day the infant is weak and floppy with a feeble cry, shallow respiration, difficulty swallowing and liability to apneic attacks. The face is immobile with lower facial weakness and the eyes wide open and staring as ptosis is infrequent. The condition may be mistaken for birth asphyxia, Prader–Willi syndrome, the infant of a mother with dystrophia myotonica, Werdnig–Hoffman disease or a congenital muscular dystrophy.

The diagnosis can be confirmed by the response to edrophonium given subcutaneously or intramuscularly 1.0 mg or slowly intravenously after a test dose of 0.03 mg/kg followed by small fractional doses over 5 min to a total of 0.15 mg/kg (Dubowitz 1995b). Therapy is by neostigmine 0.25 mg intramuscularly followed by an oral maintenance therapy of 1–5 mg with each feed which causes regression of the symptoms. The disease itself gradually disappears over the first few weeks of life and gradual reduction in dosage is necessary to avoid toxicity. In severe cases an exchange transfusion may have a rapid and lasting effect. Ventilation may be needed for the first few days and tube feeding for a longer period. Recovery is complete by 3 weeks and they do not develop myasthenia in later life.

Congenital myasthenia

There is also an autosomal recessive form of myasthenia which may appear in the newborn period and is more resistant to therapy. It is thought that the disease is due to an abnormal acetylcholine receptor. There are no circulating antibodies and the mother does not have the disease. Severe weakness and hypotonia requiring artificial ventilation, feeding difficulty and repeated apneic attacks contrast often with no ophthalmoplegia or ptosis (there is, however, a rare variant in which the latter are prominent). The weakness tends not to improve dramatically with edrophonium and only mild improvement occurs with large doses of pyridostigmine. It may follow a fluctuating course with remissions and exacerbations. It is possible that there are several presynaptic disorders such as a defect in the synthesis and mobilization of acetylcholine, a defect in release of acetylcholine, absence of acetylcholinesterase and abnormal ion channels. The motor end plate in all cases shows fatiguability on repeated stimulation.

Myasthenia gravis

This is now known to be the result of an IgG antibody against acetylcholine receptor protein. This binds to the receptors on the postsynaptic membrane of the synapse and the number of receptors may be diminished. There is lymphoid hyperplasia in the thymus and lymphocytic aggregates in the muscles, suggestive of a cell-mediated immune response. There is an increase in the incidence of other autoimmune disease in patients with myasthenia gravis so that thyroid disease occurs in 5%, but thyroid antibodies may be present in 33%. There is often clinical and immunological evidence of other autoimmune diseases such as rheumatoid arthritis and systemic lupus erythematosus. HLA studies have shown an increase in HLA-B8 in female patients with myasthenia gravis and an increase in HLA-A3 in male patients. There may in association be antibodies to striated muscle itself. It would appear that some individuals have a genetic predisposition to autoimmune disease of which myasthenia gravis is one type. The ability to measure antiacetylcholine receptor antibody in the serum has greatly aided diagnosis. The use of plasmapheresis to remove antibody and reverse the disease has also confirmed the autoimmune basis. The peripheral nervous system is very susceptible to autoimmune disease as antiperipheral nerve antibodies cause Guillain–Barré syndrome, antiacetyl receptor antibodies cause myasthenia gravis and muscle antibodies polymyositis.

Clinical features

The condition is four times more common in girls than boys. The onset may be acute and appear as a complication of a current infection but the most common presentation in childhood is ophthalmic with ptosis and squint. Eye movements may be limited but the pupils usually react normally. Rarely there may be difficulty in accommodation with the child having difficulty in seeing the blackboard from intraocular myasthenia. Myasthenia confined to the ocular muscles has a 30% chance of spontaneous remission.

Difficulty in chewing and swallowing, dysarthria and nasal speech are common early features with palatal and facial involvement. Generalized weakness and hypotonia involving the limb girdles is less common and respiratory failure is less common in children than in the late teenage groups. The paresis need not be symmetrical and involvement of the palate or eyes in an asymmetrical way with ptosis and squint can arouse fears of a brainstem tumor. There is no muscle wasting, tenderness or fasciculation and tendon reflexes are often normal. Fatigue with effort or at the end of the day is characteristic but often not a prominent feature. Chewing does, however, show fatigue.

Diagnosis

Diagnosis is confirmed by the immediate response to intravenous injection of edrophonium (Fig. 14.33). Atropine given before the edrophonium will prevent the muscarine effects of the cholinergic drug. Electromyography may demonstrate fatigue in limb muscles on repetitive nerve stimulation which is not evident clinically, i.e. clinically it may appear confined to eye muscles but be demonstrable in the extensor muscles of the forearm. The fatiguability is reversed by edrophonium. Direct assay of acetylcholine receptor antibody should be done to check the diagnosis; this is positive in 80% of cases. Imaging of the mediastinum should be performed to detect any associated thymoma.

Treatment

Initial therapy consists of a cholinesterase inhibitor in a dosage adjusted to control weakness without causing warning signs of toxicity, i.e. colic, diarrhea, blurred vision or excessive salivation

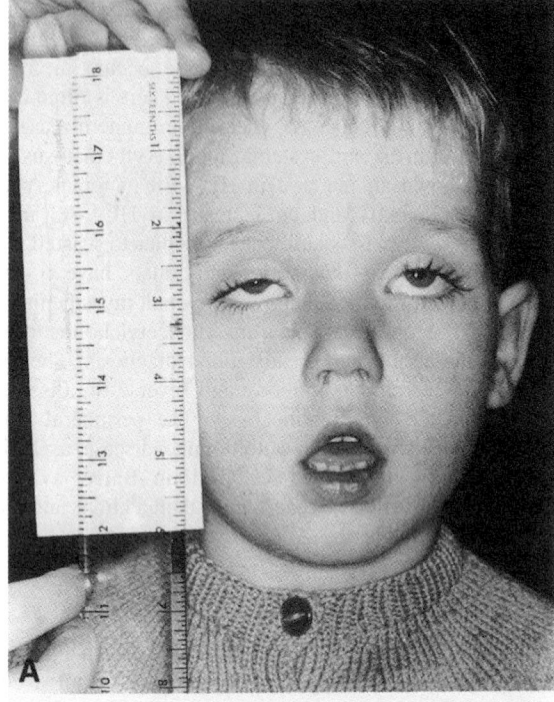

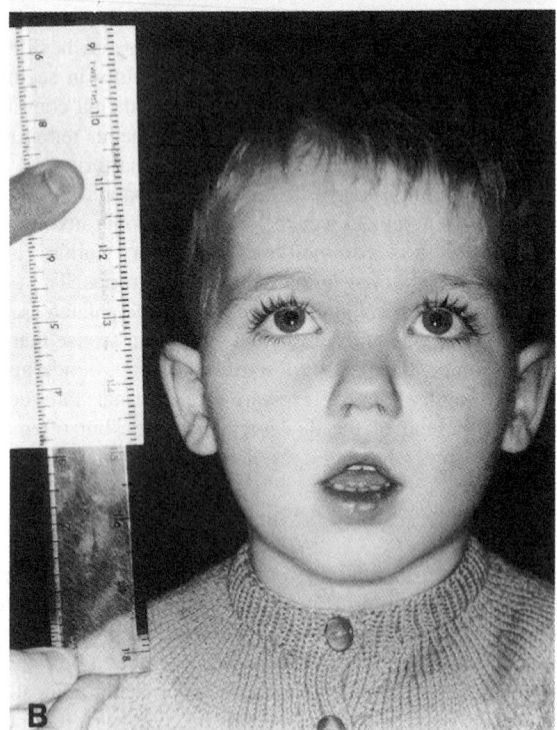

Fig. 14.33 Myasthenia gravis: (a) before and (b) after intravenous edrophonium.

and sweating. A period of pyridostigmine is given 4-hourly during waking hours with a starting dose of approximately 1 mg/kg – this is usually preferred to neostigmine which must be given at least 3-hourly (starting dose approximately 0.25 mg/kg). Hospital admission may be required during intercurrent illness and is mandatory for dental extraction.

Sudden increase in weakness may be due to myasthenic crisis or cholinergic overdose. These are differentiated by injection of edrophonium 0.5–1 mg. Myasthenic crisis indicated by transient improvement is treated with intramuscular neostigmine (0.04 mg/kg) and an increase in the oral medication. Cholinergic crisis which is aggravated by edrophonium may necessitate tracheotomy and assisted ventilation. Improved understanding of the pathogenesis of myasthenia gravis has encouraged early resort to thymectomy in children with bulbar but not ophthalmic presentations. This may result in a total cure with substantial reduction in anticholinesterase drug dosage in more than 70% of patients and complete removal of the need for continuous therapy in some.

Drugs which cause neuromuscular block, such as phenytoin and the aminoglycoside group of antibiotics, must be avoided in myasthenic patients. Although 25% of patients can be expected to improve or 'cure' after 2 years this should not hold back consideration for thymectomy. Antiacetylcholine antibodies are reduced following thymectomy. In patients with acute respiratory failure plasmapheresis will improve the child for surgery and shorten the period of ventilatory support. Steroids can be used in the short term during acute exacerbations which are not anticholinesterase responsive and in preparation for surgery. Chronic cases may need immunosuppressive treatment, e.g. with cyclosporin.

Eaton–Lambert syndrome

This is a type of myasthenia which is not always sensitive to neostigmine and arises as a complication of malignant diseases (particularly carcinoma of the bronchus) in adults. It is extremely rare in childhood but has been reported in association with leukemia, rheumatoid arthritis and disseminated lupus erythematosus.

MUSCULAR DYSTROPHY

The term 'muscular dystrophy' covers a group of primary muscle diseases which are genetically determined and usually progressive. Progression of the disease may be relentless and fatal as in the Duchenne form of sex-linked recessive muscular dystrophy or with a severe presentation and yet slow or negligible progression as in some cases of congenital muscular dystrophy. Onset may be in utero or at any time up to adult life.

The term 'dystrophy' suggests a degenerative disease of muscle. Muscle fibers form normally and then undergo a degenerative process, die and are removed by phagocytosis and are replaced by either fat or connective tissue.

Congenital muscular dystrophy

Congenital muscular dystrophy presents either as a very floppy baby or as an infant born with joint contractures and the myopathic form of arthrogryphosis. The latter may present as any form of talipes, posterior subluxation of the knee, bilateral dislocation of the hip or club hand (Fig. 14.34). These types of deformity occur in any type of weakness or paralysis and may occur in children with spina bifida, intrauterine anterior horn cell disease, myotonic dystrophy, congenital myopathy such as central core disease or congenital muscular dystrophy. There may be a history of arrest of fetal movements or of very poor fetal

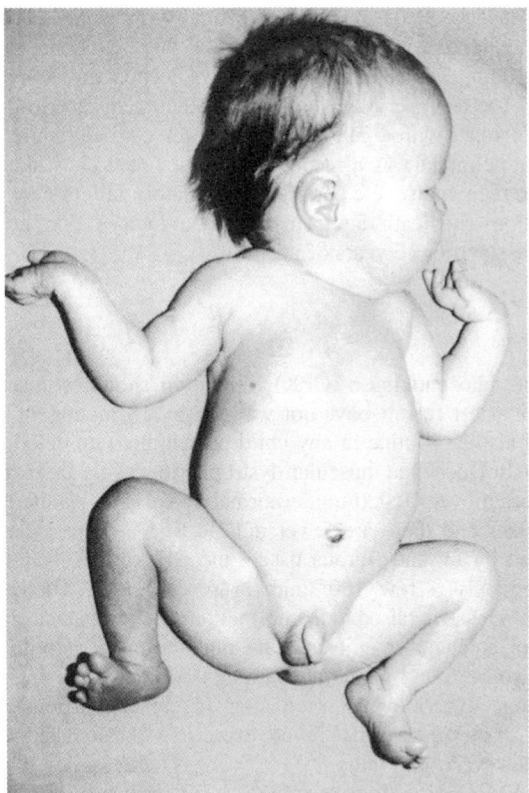

Fig. 14.34 Congenital myopathy (congenital muscular dystrophy).

movements. Weakness may result in difficulty in establishing independent respiration at birth. There is a severe form of congenital muscular dystrophy which may be fatal and this needs to be separated from myotubular myopathy and severe forms of myotonic dystrophy. There is a more benign form which may be associated with contractures and extreme floppiness and immobility at birth and yet does not appear to progress so that the child may eventually learn to walk at several years of age. Orthopedic complications such as severe scoliosis and secondary hip dislocation with muscle contractures may dominate the picture in later childhood. Respiratory symptoms with weakness of intercostal muscles and hypoventilation in sleep can occur by school age.

The creatine phosphokinase is unreliable in the newborn period and may be extremely high in normal infants: it is not particularly high in congenital muscular dystrophy and may be normal. EMG is also often not helpful and muscle biopsy is needed to prove the diagnosis. The biopsy may reveal very marked changes suggesting extremely severe progressive dystrophy and this may not predict the clinical course. The biopsy may show muscle loss with florid fibrosis – the sclerosing form of congenital muscular dystrophy. Alternatively there may be only islands of muscle fibers with fibrous tissue and fat appearing to replace most of the muscle or finally, the only finding may be marked variation in fiber size with central nuclei. The congenital muscular dystrophies are now classified as merosin deficient and merosin normal on biopsy and the merosin gene is thought to be carried on chromosome 6.

The variant form of congenital muscular dystrophy which occurs in Japan, known as the Fukuyama type, is differentiated from the more common types of muscular dystrophy seen in the United Kingdom in that the brain is also affected. There is leukodystrophy on CT scan as well as microgyria, pachygyria and a cortical dysplasia. Treatment is of the arthrogryphosis, scoliosis and ventilatory failure.

Duchenne muscular dystrophy

This is the commonest type of muscular dystrophy, occurring with an incidence of one in 3000 male births. It is inherited as a sex-linked recessive character with a high, 33%, new mutation rate. The lesion is now known to be on the short arm of the X chromosome in the region of Xp21. The gene is thought to be 2 500 000 base pairs in size. It is therefore the largest locus so far characterized and contains at least 65 exons. The size of the gene is thought to account for the frequency of new mutations. There are a lot of nontranslated base pairs (introns) (Buller & Goodfellow 1989).

Proteins are not unvarying structures and actin which forms the thin filament or Z line of the contractile unit in a sarcomere has six isoforms (α cardiac, α skeletal, α smooth, γ smooth, together with β and γ cytoplasmic actin). These are very similar to spectrin in the red cell membrane. Myosin is even more diverse and has a different fetal and neonatal form together with differences in different skeletal muscles. This might explain why some muscular dystrophies affect particular muscles, suggesting that if a genetic disease can isolate certain groups of muscles they must be metabolically different from other muscles. Acetylcholine receptors also have fetal and adult subunits (Emery 1988).

Duchenne muscular dystrophy is one of the triumphs of modern molecular biology. By isolating the gene as a result of studies in, for example, X autosome translocations at Xp21 and then carrying out detailed studies of the gene it was possible to find out which protein was produced by the gene locus. This turned out to be a previously unrecognized protein which is now known as dystrophin.

Dystrophin is encoded by a 14 kb gene. The formed protein is found in muscle cells at a concentration of only 0.01% of all cellular protein. It is even lower in quantity in Duchenne muscular dystrophy. The protein is the same in animals and man and has been well conserved in evolution. It is thought that dystrophin occurs in the membrane of T tubules of myofibers and forms a net between the T tubes and the plasma membrane. It is part of the cytoskeleton of muscle cells, is 3600 amino acids in length and is very rich in the amino acid cysteine. It is now thought that the cytoskeleton of neurons also contains dystrophin and that this may account for the mental handicap and CT scan changes seen in association in cases of muscular dystrophy (Buller & Goodfellow 1989).

Duchenne muscular dystrophy in females

Duchenne muscular dystrophy can occur in females with Turner's syndrome. It can also occur with a balanced translocation between the X chromosome at Xp21 and one of the autosomes. It may occur in a milder form due to lyonization, i.e. loss of the normal chromosome as a Barr body in the majority of maternal cells. It has been postulated that there may also be an autosomal recessive form of muscular dystrophy which has in the past been confused with the Duchenne form.

Clinical presentation

The disease usually presents between the ages of 1 and 4 years. The child may be slow to walk, falls frequently and in particular has difficulty getting up, climbing stairs or getting in and out of a car. When he falls he tends to get up in a characteristic way, climbing up his legs, i.e. Gower's sign (Fig. 14.35). Weakness begins in the pelvic girdle, so the child waddles as he walks. The disease gradually progresses so that the extensor muscles of the back are affected, the child assuming a position of lordosis in order to stabilize his spine by bony opposition. He cannot bend forward without falling. Muscle imbalance across the hip encourages hip flexion contractures and it is then necessary for the child to toe walk as a compensation for the hip flexion contractures and lordosis (Fig. 14.36). There may also be toe walking as a result of the hypertrophy of the calf muscles with a true tightening of the tendo Achillis. If the tendo Achillis is cut when the child is toe walking as a compensation for hip flexion contractures and weak extensor muscles of the back, he may lose the ability to walk altogether.

By the age of 8 years walking is in most cases extremely inefficient and tiring for social or community mobility and the need for a chair gradually increases till over 95% are in a wheelchair by the age of 12 years. The knee jerks disappear early in the course of the disease but the ankle jerks may be preserved. Very occasionally the plantar responses may appear to be extensor, causing confusion in early diagnosis.

Once the child is in a wheelchair loss of lumbar lordosis prevents stabilization of the spine and there is a tendency for him to tilt to one side. This encourages the rapid development of scoliosis. The pressure on the lateral side of the feet as a result of the weight of the leg often results in very severe varus deformity of the feet.

With the development of scoliosis (bunching of the ribs), there is a marked reduction in forced vital capacity. Distortion of the diaphragm may result in esophageal reflux with acute esophagitis and hematemesis, together with the risk of repeated aspiration pneumonitis which is made worse by the poor cough reflex.

The brain is affected with mental retardation occurring in 30% of cases. This is not progressive and may be present before the muscle disease is diagnosed. It does not correlate with the severity of the muscle disease.

Cardiac muscle is also affected so that ECG changes occur early. Because of the movement difficulty the child is unable to run or undertake severe exercise so that there is no stress on the myocardium. The electrocardium shows deep Q waves and tall R waves. The teenager may show a persistent tachycardia of 140 or more together with a gallop rhythm. Frank cardiac failure is rare but cor pulmonale as a result of the associated chest deformity may be seen and severe peripheral circulatory failure may follow aspiration. The death rate from cardiorespiratory failure increases relentlessly after 16 years of age.

Diagnosis

Creatine phosphokinase (CPK) estimation should be used as a screening test for all boys not walking by 18 months of age. It should also be routine in any child presenting with deterioration of gait. In Duchenne muscular dystrophy the levels are extremely high, often over 10 000 units (normal up to 150). As the disease progresses and there are fewer muscle fibers, the muscle being replaced by fat and fibrous tissue, the CPK gradually falls and may be only a few 100 units in severe cases. The creatine phosphokinase is raised in the normal fetus in utero and cannot be used for antenatal diagnosis. Care must be taken as high levels may also be found in the neonate and levels equally high as in Duchenne dystrophy are seen after severe convulsions and in acute Coxsackie myositis. Severe exercise will also raise the CPK value to several 100 units.

An EMG will show a reduced interference pattern with characteristic myopathic units in most cases, though it may be normal.

Muscle biopsy is needed to confirm the diagnosis. There is variation in fiber size and the normal polygonal shape of muscle fibers is lost as they become more rounded. There may be occasional central nuclei. Degeneration of muscle fibers with local macrophage reaction to remove the dead fiber is characteristic of a dystrophy. The dead fibers are then replaced by adipose tissue and fibrous connective tissue. Eventually only islands of very sick-looking muscle fibers may remain in a mass of connective tissue. Diagnosis is most difficult in the very young infant.

The proteins were first extracted and identified by Western blot technique. Immunohistochemical staining of biopsy material for dystrophin in the sarcolemmal membrane is nowadays the

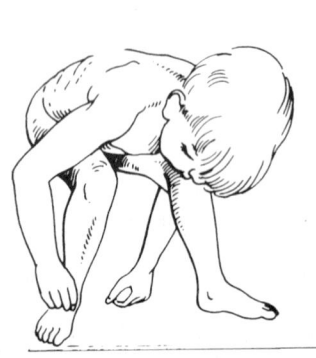 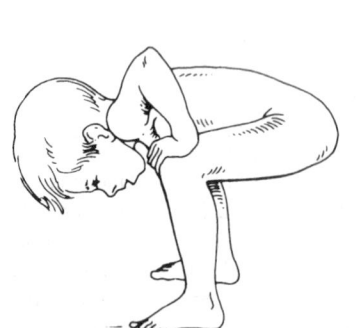 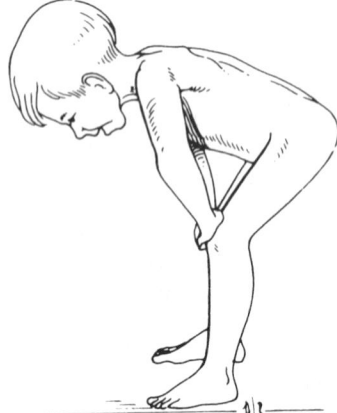

Fig. 14.35 Manner of rising from the floor in child with Duchenne-type muscular dystrophy. The boy climbs up his legs (Gower's sign).

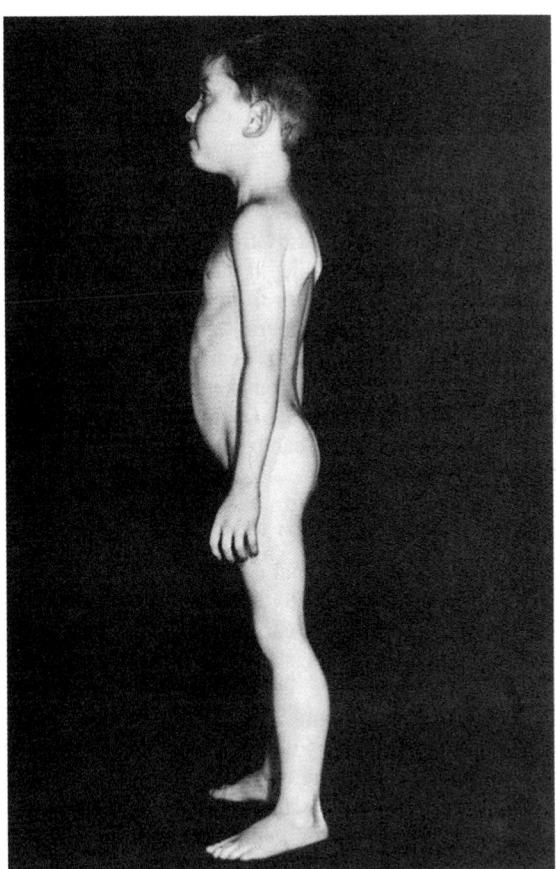

Fig. 14.36 Duchenne muscular dystrophy. Note limb girdle wasting and hypertrophy of calves.

benchmark for diagnosis. This shows absent dystrophin in Duchenne muscular dystrophy, an abnormal intensity of staining which is variable and patchy compared to the continuous staining in the normal or non-Duchenne/Becker dystrophies. Carriers show a normal pattern (Dubowitz 1995c).

DNA technology looking for specific deletion of exons within the DMD gene using cloned DNA has shown several exon deletion patterns.

Electrocardiography should be performed to assess the severity of myocardial involvement together with a cardiac ultrasound examination. Baseline respiratory function studies are also necessary and an assessment of the degree of spinal curvature.

Some form of structured assessment of posture and movement helps to follow the rate of deterioration and compare interventional treatments. This may be a simple timing of the Gower maneuver or a more standardized assessment.

1. Walk and climb stairs without assistance.
2. Walk and climb stairs using the handrail.
3. Walk and climb stairs with handrail with difficulty (i.e. less than eight steps in 25 s).
4. Walk and get out of chair but cannot climb stairs.
5. Walk but not get out of chair.
6. Walk with help or independently with braces.
7. Walk in long leg braces but not independently.
8. Stand in long leg braces but cannot walk.
9. Cannot walk or stand.

Management of Duchenne muscular dystrophy

Pharmacological. Many treatments, including calcium-blocking agents and attempted ATP replacement, have been tried to no avail. Whether it will be possible to replace dystrophin as a structural protein and stabilize the cell membranes is conjectural. Controversy still exists as to the effect of cyclical steroids since anabolic steroids build up muscle power but catabolic steroids are known to cause a myopathy in their own right. There is still a suggestion that cyclical (10 days each month) use of catabolic steroids such as prednisone (0.75 mg/kg/day) reduces the rate of deterioration in Duchenne muscular dystrophy (Dubowitz 1995d). Care also needs to be taken not to cause excess weight gain and osteoporosis. Cyclosporin is also undergoing study to try and slow the rate of deterioration.

Exercise. Physical exercise should be encouraged and inactivity avoided as weakness may appear to progress after periods of being confined to bed, for example due to intercurrent illness. Active exercise such as swimming is to be encouraged on a regular basis. Formal physiotherapy is aimed at preventing muscle contractures, in particular hip flexion contractures and contracture of the tendo Achillis.

Wheelchair versus orthosis. All children will eventually require a wheelchair. It is possible initially at around 6 years to maintain ambulation using orthopedic surgery to release contractures, e.g. of the tendo Achillis, hamstrings and iliopsoas (Rideau et al 1986), with the child then being managed in a full-length knee–ankle–foot orthosis or a reciprocating gait orthosis. The child needs his arms for support, trying to sit and getting on and off the toilet which can become a time-consuming exercise. Arguments vary between different major centers as to whether it is better to psychologically accept that the child is going to need a chair and to provide this as soon as his community mobility is reduced to a point that his social activities are being restricted or to try and maintain him on his feet at all costs. Our own policy is that mobility is the main objective and the child must be able to lead as normal a life as possible, able to move where he wants to, when he wants to (Heckmatt et al 1989).

Obesity. The muscle is replaced by fat, the paralyzed limbs are obese and immobility can lead to a marked truncal obesity. Whilst the child is still mobile with weak muscles it is undesirable to be carrying extra weight and dietary advice should be given early in management. It is more difficult to control obesity when the child is chair bound, especially if he obviously enjoys good food.

Scoliosis. This can be successfully treated by the use of the Luque procedure which is successful in 90% of cases of paralytic scoliosis providing the vital capacity is not less than 30% of that predicted for age. Scoliosis usually appears once the child has become wheelchair bound. The lordosis of the ambulant child appears to stabilize the spine and prevent scoliosis. Since death is often due to cardiorespiratory failure from cor pulmonale, chest infection, aspiration syndrome, failure to cough and decreased vital capacity, it is of prime importance to prevent the rib and chest deformity.

Studies are urgently needed to show whether elective fusion of the spine as soon as the child becomes wheelchair bound preserves respiratory function and prolongs life. There is no evidence that one can improve respiratory function by operating on the scoliosis once the vital capacity is reduced.

Psychological. The psychological problems of the child gradually going off his feet and not being able to keep up with his peers are considerable. The necessity for special education where he may meet other children with the condition has to be emphasized. The realization in adolescence that his friends are dying and that he is also progressively deteriorating means that psychological support is of considerable importance.

Education. One might ask why education is needed since none of the boys are going to benefit in terms of employment. Since life has eventually got to be mental rather than physical one should not reduce the educational demands or expectations. Achievement at school may be one of the few areas where the child can feel that he has really succeeded.

Respiratory. We have already discussed the effects of scoliosis with deformity on vital capacity. More recently it has been appreciated that sleep apnea is much commoner in Duchenne muscular dystrophy and Becker muscular dystrophy than was previously thought. Periods of hypoxia may occur in the night and again debate continues as to whether some form of assisted external ventilation, e.g. by a Curasse ventilator, is required (Heckmatt et al 1989).

Antenatal diagnosis

The ideal for the future must be to try and eliminate this dreadful disease by carrier detection and intrauterine diagnosis of affected children and carriers. Until recently one could only offer termination of all male pregnancies with the resultant termination of 50% of normal male children. This approach does not decrease the female carrier rate. Because of genetic heterogeneity, DNA should now be collected on all indexed cases. Two-thirds of cases exhibit deletion in one of the 65 exons. One needs the index case number to show which exon and then one can test the fetus accurately in nearly 100% of cases. Those who do not show a deletion need more time-consuming linkage studies, but we now possess many more accurate probes to make clinical diagnosis possible.

One can demonstrate dystrophin in muscle biopsy tissue by immunofluorescent techniques. This shows that there is dystrophin deficiency in dystrophic muscle. This can be valuable in very young children with a high CPK when the biopsy is not typical but diagnosis is essential so that genetic counseling, carrier detection and antenatal diagnosis can be carried out. Immunofluorescent dystrophin staining of the muscle is then valuable. In cases where a fetus has been aborted it is also a useful way of showing whether the fetus was affected or not, muscle biopsy being difficult to interpret. More detailed description of carrier detection and antenatal diagnosis is given on page 77.

Becker muscular dystrophy

This occurs in one in 60 000 births. It is a sex-linked recessive condition and is milder than Duchenne muscular dystrophy. It breeds true but is due to a mutation in the same gene as Duchenne, i.e. it is an Xp21 gene dystrophy. It is due to deletion at the same end of the gene as Duchenne but in exons 45–48. There is no mental retardation in most cases of Becker muscular dystrophy. The onset is later, progress is slower and cramps or muscle pain may be prominent. Walking is preserved but some may lose walking in their 20s while others may walk to 40+ years. There is no difference in the creatine phosphokinase which is very high, EMG is myopathic, biopsy findings are not a reliable means of differentiating Duchenne and Becker, dystrophin on staining is

present but diminished and there is patchy distribution. The usual division between the two diseases rests upon whether the child is still walking or in a wheelchair at the age of 12 years. Cardiac muscle may be affected on ECG and echocardiography.

Emery–Dreifuss muscular dystrophy

This is a contractural muscular dystrophy that particularly affects the elbows and tendo Achillis. It has a sex-linked recessive inheritance. Toe walking occurs from contractures at the tendo Achillis. Wasting of the humeral and peroneal muscles is complicated by involvement of the heart muscle which can result in heart block requiring a pacemaker and can cause sudden unexpected death (Emery 1989). Dystrophin is normal and the gene is at Xq 28 region. CPK can be normal.

Facioscapulohumeral muscular dystrophy

This is inherited as an autosomal dominant characteristic carried on chromosome 4q. It is a relatively benign dystrophy with very little progression over many years. It does, however, like most autosomal dominant disorders, show marked variation in severity within families. Intelligence is normal. There is no cardiac involvement. Electromyography and creatinine phosphokinase are often unhelpful and diagnosis depends upon the clinical picture, family history and muscle biopsy findings. The biopsy may not show gross dystrophic changes, there may be split fibers and often a lot of cellular reaction in the interstices. Differential diagnosis from a polymyositis can be difficult. Other complications include sensory neural deafness together with a retinopathy, i.e. Coat's retinopathy, or even a retinoblastoma.

Clinical wasting of the upper arm, facial droopiness and winging of the scapulae and particular difficulty in abducting the arms are the main features, together with weakness in closing of the eyes or pursing of the lips with a poverty of expression so that the child tends always to look sad (Fig. 14.37). Articulation is impaired and the voice may have a nasal quality from palatal weakness. Hypertrophy and contractures are rare.

Rigid spine syndrome

The fibrosis of muscle which occurs in a muscular dystrophy can result in the child presenting with a very rigid spine, a lordosis with fixed flexion contractures at the hip, a scoliosis, bilateral dislocation of the hip or onset of contractures at the elbow and foot as in the Emery–Dreifuss type of muscular dystrophy. Mild forms of pelvic or femoral girdle dystrophy may have an orthopedic presentation. The rigid spine syndrome appears to be a specific clinical entity with various muscle diseases presenting as a stiff as opposed to a floppy baby with muscle fibrosis and contracture and may be complicated by fatal cardiac muscle involvement or nocturnal respiratory failure.

There is also the so-called hereditary 'stiff baby syndrome' when the infant may necessitate cesarean section because of stiffness, preventing normal vaginal delivery. The stiffness may come on hours after birth and be associated with swallowing difficulty and aspiration with apneic and cyanotic episodes. Increased muscle spasms resembling tetanus may come and go over the first year of life and then the condition appears to settle down. The muscle spasms are diazepam sensitive.

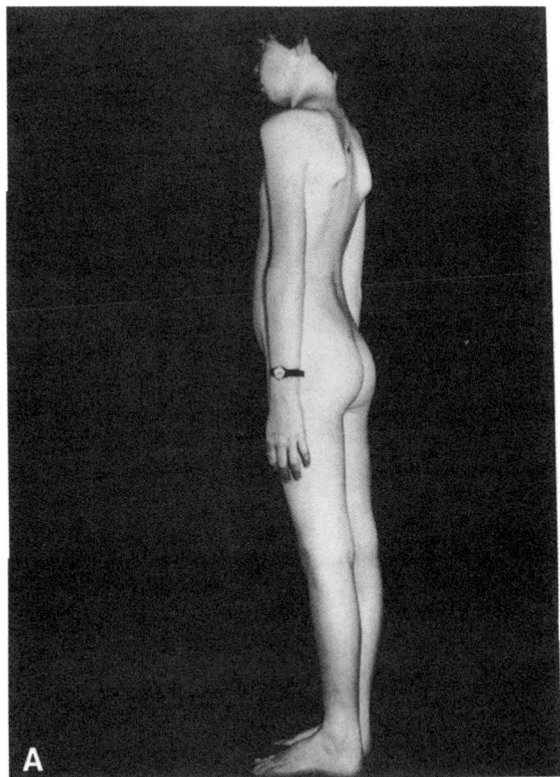

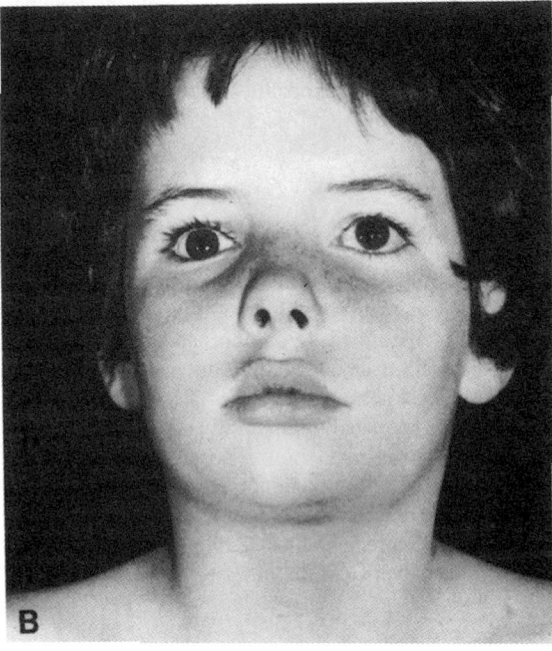

Fig. 14.37 Facioscapulohumeral muscular dystrophy: (a) wasting of shoulder girdle with scapular winging; (b) expressionless face with pouting lips.

Autosomal recessive limb girdle dystrophy

This usually presents as a progressive muscular dystrophy with wasting weakness and difficulty walking, together with a high creatine phosphokinase and a biopsy picture typical of dystrophy

in girls. It is likely that the boys will be misdiagnosed as a Becker type of Duchenne muscular dystrophy.

MYOTONIC SYNDROMES

Myotonia may complicate metabolic disease of muscles such as the muscle glycogenoses. It needs to be differentiated from cramps which may themselves be seen in mitochondrial myopathies and carnitine deficiency states.

Myotonia means failure of the muscle to be able to instantly relax after a contraction. The failure of relaxation occurs not only with voluntary contraction but also upon percussion of the muscle. A similar phenomenon is seen in the myotonic ankle jerks of myxedema. In the extreme form contractions occur and persist as the 'stiff man' or 'stiff baby' syndrome. This can be at its most alarming when it occurs as a response to muscle relaxant agents during anesthesia. An injection of scoline may result in total opisthotonus, with muscle contraction producing enormous heat with hyperpyrexia and extreme difficulty in ventilating or intubating the child. The possibility of this reaction must always be borne in mind when anesthetizing any child with a muscle disease. The only way to relax the muscle is by dantrolene sodium which acts on calcium within the muscle.

Paramyotonia

This is a syndrome in which there is inability to relax muscle after contraction in very cold weather. It is inherited as an autosomal dominant disorder and permanent contractures may develop.

Myotonia congenita (Thomsen's disease)

These children have myotonia without any dystrophy, i.e. without wasting or weakness. The persistent muscle contraction results in muscle hypertrophy so that the child presents as an infant Hercules. There is failure to relax the grasp or to be able to suddenly initiate change in movements. Intelligence is normal. The condition does not progress. There may be difficulty suddenly starting to run but once going there is good muscle power. The neonate may show feeding difficulties and an abnormal cry. Intention myotonia may appear to root the child to the spot and children have been stuck in the classroom during fire drill. The child may be unable to let go of a door handle or a railing on a bus. The EMG will demonstrate the classic myotonic discharge. Muscle biopsy is usually unhelpful.

Dystrophia myotonica

This is the commonest of the myotonic syndromes. Many mothers suffering from dystrophia myotonica have the diagnosis made as a result of having an affected infant. They may have regarded themselves as being a bit stiff or having a 'touch of rheumatism', demonstrating that many cases exist undiagnosed in the community.

The classic description of the male in his 40s with bald head, cataract, testicular atrophy, progressive weakness of sterno-mastoids and pectoral girdle muscles and myotonia belies the clinical picture seen by the pediatrician. The mother of the infant with dystrophia myotonica will usually be in her mid-20s, may have a droopy, myopathic facies, be unable to bury her eyelids and be mildly mentally retarded. Other cases may appear to have good facial expression and only apparent awkwardness when trying to relax with rapid flexion and extension of the fingers. EMG of the small muscles of the hand will, however, demonstrate the classic 'dive bomber' myotonic discharges.

The infant of the mother born with dystrophia myotonica shows a much more profound picture, suggesting that there is some transplacental humoral factor. It has been suggested that since all infantile cases have occurred when the mother has been affected and not the father, there may be a mitochondrial DNA component (donated by the ovum and not the sperm). The fact that the neonatal symptomatology is in part reversible would support some form of chemically mediated transplacental factor. The condition is inherited as an autosomal dominant with variable penetrance and with the locus on the long arm of chromosome 19. The condition is now known to belong to the trinucleotide or triple codon repeat type of disease, with a cytosine, thymine, guanine repeat on chromosome 19, the gene product being myotonin protein kinase. Anticipation due to expansion of the CTG repeat occurs in succeeding generations, especially following female meiosis.

There may be polyhydramnios due to the fetus being unable to swallow. The muscle in lower esophagus and rectum may be affected so swallowing difficulty with reflux or chronic constipation may be prominent. The infant may require resuscitation at birth and congenital abnormalities of the diaphragm may necessitate ventilation or the infant may appear to have respiratory distress syndrome. Respiratory insufficiency requiring ventilation may last 3 months and yet be reversible. Talipes of the feet or club hand may be severe. The very floppy child with bulbar palsy often requires tube feeding for the first weeks of life. Swallowing appears to improve over the first few weeks of life. There is a characteristic, droopy myopathic, rather shiny face, an open carp mouth with drooling and jaw laxity. The hypotonia persists but most of the children eventually walk unaided. Mental retardation of moderate severity, i.e. IQ about 60, is the rule but intelligence can be normal (Fig. 14.38). The ventricles are often dilated but a true hydrocephalus requiring shunting is relatively rare. Myotonia, mental retardation and constipation are often the main problems in late childhood.

Diagnosis depends upon family history. Examination of the mother should include electromyography of the small muscles of the hand. If clinical doubt exists examination of the lens for multicolored lens opacities may be helpful – these are thought to be specific. Muscle biopsy on the infant will show small type 1 fibers (type 1 hypotrophy) together with an increase in muscle acid phosphatase. The creatine phosphokinase may be normal or elevated. Electromyography is the most helpful investigation.

Tube feeding is often necessary in the neonatal period but after a period of feeding difficulty oral feeding is usually established and gastrostomy is not necessary. The child needs his joint deformities treated and all children with congenital myotonic dystrophy should receive intense physiotherapy. The majority of children eventually manage to walk. Myotonia is not usually a major problem in the child so that specific drug therapy is not usually indicated (procainamide or phenytoin). Mental retardation requires special educational help. DNA analysis and detailed

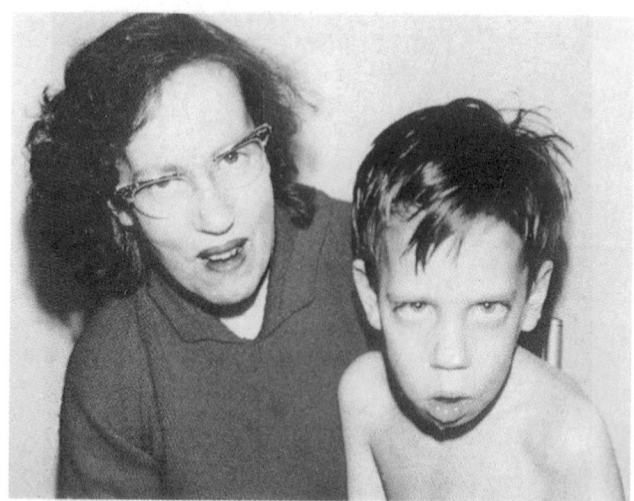

Fig. 14.38 Congenital dystrophia myotonica showing typical facies of patient with affected mother.

genetic counseling should be carried out together with contraceptive advice from the immediate neonatal period.

MYOPATHIES

This term encompasses developmental disorders of muscles such as central core disease and myotubular myopathy, together with metabolic diseases of muscle such as the muscle glycogenoses, carnitine deficiency, the mitochondrial myopathies, the periodic paralyses and endocrine myopathies (Table 14.45). They often present as a differential diagnosis of the floppy infant (Dubowitz 1980).

Central core disease

This is inherited as an autosomal dominant. It shows variable penetrance and may be so mild that it is missed. The infant presents with generalized hypotonia and joint contractures, talipes, hip dislocation and spinal deformity. The parent may show ptosis and mild weakness.

CPK and EMG are usually unhelpful and routine staining with hematoxylin and eosin may show a normal muscle biopsy. It is only when the activity of mitochondrial enzymes is estimated that central areas of the muscle fiber are shown to be devoid of enzyme activity, i.e. central core. The muscle biopsy appearance does not correlate with the severity of the disease.

Myotubular myopathy

This sex-linked recessive myopathy presents in the neonatal period with profound hypotonia, paresis and inability to swallow. Weakness of the intercostal muscles and diaphragm may make resuscitation difficult and there may be a misdiagnosis of perinatal asphyxia. Muscle biopsy shows that the muscle has not developed beyond a primitive myotube stage.

A less severe autosomal dominant form presents with limb girdle weakness and involvement of the extraocular muscles and is nonprogressive.

Table 14.45 Congenital myopathies

Disease	Inheritance	Pathology	Clinical features
Central core disease	AD	Muscle fibers have functionless central cores devoid of enzyme activity. Type I fibers predominant and mainly affected	Floppy baby with motor delay. Face involved. Relatively benign
Nemaline myopathy	AD	Rod bodies derived from Z-band protein (trichrome stain)	Floppy baby with motor delay. Very thin with 'marfanoid' features. Facial + respiratory weakness which may be fatal
Myotubular (centronuclear) myopathy	AD	Central nuclei surrounded by clear area without myofibrils (resembling fetal myotubes)	Floppy baby with motor delay. Facial weakness, ptosis + ext. ophthalmoplegia. Later scoliosis
Severe, X-linked myotubular myopathy	X-linked	Central nuclei surrounded by clear area without myofibrils (resembling fetal myotubes)	Severe weakness + hypotonia from birth; facial weakness, ptosis + ext. ophthalmoplegia. Respiratory involvement often fatal
Myotubular myopathy with type 1 fiber hypotrophy	?	Central nuclei in small type 1 fibers	Floppy baby with motor delay ± ptosis ext. ophthalmoplegia. May be severe, progressive
Multicore (minicore) disease	?AR	Multiple, minute foci lacking enzyme activity. Type 1 fiber predominance	Floppy baby with motor delay or later mild proximal weakness. Benign.
Congenital fiber type disproportion	?AD	Type 1 fibers small: type 2 normal or enlarged	Floppy baby. CDH or contractures at birth. Later scoliosis
Congenital type 1 fiber dominance	?	>60% of fibers of type 1	Floppy baby with motor delay. Benign
Congenital muscular dystrophy	AR	Striking dystrophic features with prominent fibrosis; apparently arrested at birth	Floppy baby with motor delay. May be contractures at birth, facial weakness, later scoliosis. CPK ↑ early, later normal
Oculocraniosomatic syndrome	?	'Ragged red' fibers on trichrome staining. Abnormal subsarcolemmal mitochondria	Mild proximal weakness + progressive ptosis and ext. ophthalmoplegia. Retinopathy, deafness, ataxia, heart block, growth + developmental retardation. CSF protein ↑
Hypermetabolic myopathy	?	Large, abnormal mitochondria (uncoupled oxidative phosphorylation)	Slight weakness, marked fatigue. Weight loss, sweating, hyperphagia, ↑ BMR (normal T_4)

AD = autosomal dominant; AR = autosomal recessive.

Metabolic myopathies

Glycogenoses

Glycogen storage disease and its classification are discussed elsewhere. In this section the types affecting skeletal muscles will be briefly considered. These disorders, inherited by autosomal recessive mechanisms, are rare but must be considered in the differential diagnosis of the floppy infant and the child with limb girdle weakness or muscle cramps.

Type 2 (Pompe's disease). In this disorder glycogen accumulates in vacuoles adjacent to the lysosomes as a result of deficiency of the lysosomal enzyme amylo-1,4-glucosidase (acid maltase). Many tissues are affected but the clinical syndrome is related mainly to the involvement of cardiac and skeletal muscle. Affected infants are weak and hypotonic from birth with failure to thrive. Death usually occurs in the first year from cardiac and/or respiratory failure. A milder form without cardiac involvement presents as a muscular dystrophy. Diagnosis depends on histochemical study of muscle biopsy or demonstration of the enzyme defect in leukocytes.

Type 3 (limit dextrinosis). Deficiency of the debranching enzyme amylo-1,6-glucosidase leads to deposition of an abnormal glycogen with short side chains. This substance, limit dextrin, accumulates in liver and muscle. Weakness and hypotonia are less severe than in type 2 but the clinical picture is dominated by hepatomegaly associated with attacks of hypoglycemia and metabolic acidosis. The enzyme defect can be recognized in liver, muscle and leukocytes.

Type 5 (McArdle's disease); myophosphorylase deficiency. This presents in adolescence or early life with muscle stiffness and cramp-like pains after exercise. It is rare in childhood but may cause fatiguability at this time. The more severe attacks are accompanied by myoglobinuria. The condition results from deficiency of muscle phosphorylase which controls glycogen breakdown during muscular activity and thus there is no increase in blood lactate following ischemic exercise. Electromyography is helpful in diagnosis, in contrast to the other types of muscular cramps. There is electrical silence with no motor unit activity during the attack. Muscle biopsy is necessary for confirmation of the diagnosis.

Type 7 (Tarur's disease). Deficiency of the enzyme phosphofructokinase is clinically indistinguishable from McArdle's disease.

Lipid myopathies

During fasting and in prolonged exercise long chain fatty acids such as palmitic acid are a major source of energy for muscle. Before they can cross the mitochondrial membrane for oxidation they must be linked to carnitine by the enzyme carnitine palmityl transferase (CPT). Inborn errors of metabolism affecting this pathway or deficiency of carnitine result in the accumulation of lipid in vacuoles within the cell. This produces the characteristic vacuolar myopathy on muscle biopsy. If it is not appreciated that the vacuoles are the hallmark of the disease they may be thought to be artifactual in preparation of the specimen.

Carnitine deficiency. This condition usually begins in childhood with a slowly progressive weakness of proximal limb, neck and facial muscles. In some cases weakness is preceded by bouts of vomiting and metabolic acidosis. It usually results from a hereditary (probably recessive) defect in hepatic synthesis of carnitine. Low levels of carnitine are found in serum, muscle and liver. On muscle biopsy type 1 fibers in particular are peppered with minute lipid droplets. The EMG and CPK are normal. Symptoms may be improved with steroids or oral carnitine 2–3 g/day.

Systemic carnitine deficiency. There may be systemic carnitine deficiency when the concentration is low or absent in liver and serum as well as in the muscle. The deficiency can be confined to muscle carnitine.

Carnitine palmityl transferase deficiency. In carnitine palmityl transferase deficiency there are muscle cramps and pain in the muscle with myoglobinuria after severe exercise. The attacks are made worse by fasting. The creatine phosphokinase is very markedly elevated during the episode and there is myoglobinuria which may be severe enough to cause renal failure. The serum cholesterol and triglycerides are increased and there is a conspicuous absence of ketonuria on fasting. The enzyme defect is detectable on muscle biopsy. Symptoms can be prevented by a high carbohydrate diet and avoidance of exercise whilst fasting.

Myoadenylate deaminase deficiency

This is possibly a not uncommon disease as a cause of cramps on exercise. It is benign and nonprogressive without any myopathic weakness. The muscle will not metabolize ammonia normally with an abnormal anaerobic exercise test.

Mitochondrial myopathies (Table 14.46)

The energy supply to all cells requires the production of ATP. This can proceed as far as the production of pyruvic acid by anaerobic metabolism. Anaerobic metabolism produces only a few molecules of ATP. Complete oxidation of glucose depends upon subsequent aerobic oxidation of pyruvate which in turn rests upon

Table 14.46 Neurological diseases based on mitochondrial disorders

1. Mitochondrial myopathy, encephalopathy with lactic acidosis and stroke (MELAS)
2. Myoclonic epilepsy with ragged red fibers (MERRF)
3. Neurogenic weakness, ataxia and retinitis pigmentosa (NARP)
4. Leigh's disease (p. 1125)
5. Alpers–Huttenlocher (p. 1125)
6. Kearns–Sayre disease
7. Chronic progressive external ophthalmoplegia
8. Sensorineural deafness
9. Benign infantile myopathy
10. Fatal neonatal myopathy
12. Leber's optic atrophy

the enzyme chains found in mitochondria as the Krebs cycle and the respiratory chain. The enzymes required for the respiratory chain depend upon DNA in the nucleus but also the specific DNA in the mitochondria which always comes from the oocyte in the mother. This means than Mendelian genetics may not seem to apply to the inheritance of these diseases. The clinical features of mitochondrial cytopathies are variable and often involve the CNS and muscle.

In diseases of the mitochondrion muscle, either cannot produce energy for contraction or utilizes large amounts of energy and generates an enormous amount of heat so that there is muscle weakness, easy fatigue with sometimes cramps or even myoglobinuria.

Kearns & Sayres (1958) described an ocular craniosomatic neuromuscular disease. In this condition there is paralysis of eye movements, i.e. a progressive ophthalmoplegia, together with retinitis pigmentosa, mental retardation, ataxia and deafness and this is associated with muscle weakness of the limbs and cardiac conduction defects. The onset is usually of a gradually progressive ophthalmoplegia starting with a ptosis in the early school years and the children are often of short stature. Muscle biopsy shows characteristic ragged red fibers when the muscle is stained with the special trichrome stain. The fibers show strong staining with special histochemical stains for succinate dehydrogenase and the mitochondria can be shown to be abnormal on electron microscopy. MRI may show spongy degeneration of the brain's white matter. Visual evoked potentials are abnormal. Resting lactic acid may be normal and cannot be used as a screening test. The cardiomyopathy may present as syncope and require pacing. The disorder is thought to be due to a deletion in mitochondrial DNA.

MELAS

This may present from preschool to adult life as a stroke. Cortical blindness may occur together with focal or simple partial seizures, dementia and deafness. Diabetes also complicates many mitochondrial diseases. MRI shows focal lucencies in basal ganglia as well as ischemic events. Resting lactic acid concentrations are raised. The same syndrome may arise from complex 1 deficiency.

MERRF

Myoclonic epilepsy accompanied by ataxia and a myopathy. Deafness is also frequently associated. CSF and blood lactate are raised but not necessarily markedly. Cerebral and cerebellar atrophy is seen on MRI. Complex 1 and iv defects may cause the syndrome. Muscle biopsy shows ragged red fibers.

Alper's disease

An autosomal recessive disease of infancy with progressive gray matter degeneration and dementia which may be due to disordered pyruvate metabolism or respiratory chain (see p. 1125).

Leigh's encephalopathy (see p. 1125)

Endocrine myopathies

Weakness, wasting and abnormal fiber type proportions on biopsy are seen in children on long-term steroids. Hypokalemia in

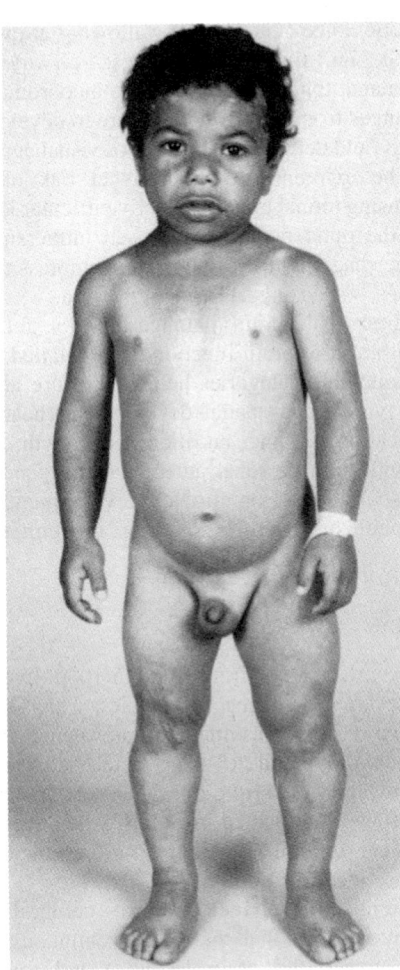

Fig. 14.39 Kocher–Debré–Séméliegne syndrome: a 9-year-old untreated congenital cretin with muscular hypertrophy and serum CPK of 1600 IU/1.

Cairn's syndrome can cause a vacuolar myopathy with weakness. In hypothyroidism fatigue with myotonic jerks is well recognized but there is a rare syndrome of cretinism with a myopathy associated with high plasma CPK concentrations (the Kocher–Debré–Séméliegne syndrome – Fig. 14.39). A myopathy with wasting and weakness may also be a feature of thyrotoxicosis.

INFLAMMATORY DISEASE OF MUSCLE, POLYMYOSITIS AND DERMATOMYOSITIS

Muscle can be involved in systemic diseases such as acquired toxoplasmosis, toxocariasis, sarcoidosis and *Trichinella* infection as well as in the various types of arthritis or polyarteritis. An inflammatory response in muscle can be seen in adults with cancer. The commonest type of inflammatory disease of muscle seen in childhood is polymyositis. It is thought to be a hypersensitivity reaction with a microvasculitis precipitated by a viral infection. There appears to be an immune-dependent inflammation which progresses in a similar way to that seen in rheumatoid arthritis and ulcerative colitis. Immmunological studies suggest Coxsackie virus may be important in some cases but there may be a familial predisposition to such conditions indicated by the HLA-B8 haplotype.

Onset

Onset can be at any age from infancy to adult life. Weakness is the predominant symptom with pain and wasting. Pain may be predominant in the shoulder girdle or pelvic girdle and the weakness may only become apparent once the pain has been controlled. Any group of muscles, proximal or distal, may be involved. The quadriceps are commonly involved early. Absence of pain with predominant weakness may make clinical differentiation from a primary muscular dystrophy difficult without muscle biopsy.

It may be difficult to separate polymyositis from the Guillain–Barré syndrome or cases of polio in which pain may be a prominent feature. The young child is likely to present as refusal to walk and one may not even be able to establish with certainty whether the pain is in muscle or joint.

Skin involvement, i.e. dermatomyositis, makes the diagnosis obvious in the more chronic case. There is a so-called violaceous or purple-colored rash over the eyelids and often over the cheeks and there may be localized areas of erythema over the knees and bony prominences. Calcification occurs in the subcutaneous tissues which often produces sheets of hard indurated skin which may ulcerate to discharge the calcified tissue. Vasculitis may be visible in the vessels in the fundi of the eye or the nail bed. Ulceration of the skin due to focal infarction may also occur.

The child feels unwell, listless, febrile and anorexic and there may be gastrointestinal involvement or swallowing problems.

Diagnosis

The creatine phosphokinase is usually but not invariably raised, as is the erythrocyte sedimentation rate. The EMG may be normal, but characteristically an established case shows the splintered polyphasic short duration potentials of a myopathy combined with a denervation pattern showing fibrillation and evidence of reinnervation with giant polyphasic potentials.

The diagnosis rests on muscle biopsy which shows perivascular inflammation with inflammatory tissue spreading between the fascicles of fibers. There may be perifascicular atrophy. Electron microscopy shows abnormality in the endothelial cells of the small blood vessels in keeping with a primary vasculitis.

Treatment

Treatment with steroids lessens the degree of long-term wasting and contracture. The usual regimen consists of prednisolone in moderate dose, i.e. 30 mg/day (1 mg/kg bodyweight per 24 h), the response being judged by the ESR and creatine phosphokinase levels. The dose can be weaned down after 2 weeks and then by further reducing the dose every 2 weeks providing improvement continues. Dubowitz (1995e) feels that the dose of steroids should be tailed down as soon as possible. One must be aware of the possibilities of producing a steroid myopathy in place of the weakness of polymyositis. Potassium depletion must be avoided. Others suggest that low doses of steroids should be continued for years after the initial high-dose treatment.

Failure to respond to steroids means that second-line drugs to produce immunosuppression such as cyclosporin, methotrexate or cyclophosphamide should be tried. Although 5% may die, a satisfactory response can be expected in 75% cases. A poor initial response to steroids may herald a chronic course. Immunoglobulin or plasmapheresis may be tried in resistant cases. Vigorous physiotherapy to maintain joint range and prevent muscle wasting is very important. Wasting, muscle contracture and muscle fibrosis do not respond to drug therapy. The severe form may lead to a chairbound child with marked wasting and fixed deformities.

DISORDERS OF MOVEMENT

CEREBRAL PALSY

Introduction

Modern accounts of cerebral palsy (CP) begin with the attribution of CP to difficult deliveries by William Little (1843), i.e. to perinatal causes. Fifty years later, Freud speculated that CP could represent the effects of 'deeper-lying influences' on the development of the fetus, i.e. antenatal causes. Because of the medicolegal implications controversy still rages as to how much prenatal and how much intrapartum factors contribute (Kuban & Leviton 1994).

Definition

CP is a dynamic (changing) disorder of posture and mobility being the 'motor manifestation of nonprogressive brain damage (static encephalopathy) sustained during the period of brain growth in fetal life, infancy or childhood'. This definition emphasizes several points.

Firstly, all children with cerebral palsy have suffered some form of brain damage and this has involved the motor pathways. The term 'cerebral' palsy differentiates such children from those with muscle palsies, orthopedic palsies and 'spinal' palsy as seen in the spina bifida complex, traumatic paraplegia or familial paraplegias, etc.

Secondly, it indicates that the pathology is nonprogressive, thus excluding conditions such as cerebral tumors, the degenerative brain diseases (e.g. the gangliosidoses) or the progressive multisystem diseases (e.g. Friedreich's ataxia). It does, however, include nonprogressive genetic disease or congenital malformation.

This does not mean that cerebral palsy is a static condition; the clinical pattern changes as brain maturation continues throughout childhood, resulting in a dynamic clinical pattern despite a static pathology.

The child with CP and damage to the motor mechanisms would be expected to have damage to other parts of the brain as well and this may be manifest as epilepsy, specific learning problems, organic behavior disturbances, speech problems or mental handicap. Equally a child with cerebral palsy may not have epilepsy or mental retardation.

Epilepsy accompanies one-third of all cases: 33% in the case of hemiplegic CP and even 90% in quadriplegic CP. The risk of subsequent *learning difficulties* is much higher if CP is complicated by epilepsy and conversely, the prognosis for educational development is far higher in the absence of fits. As a distinct group, cases with pure basal ganglia (extrapyramidal) syndromes, though severely motor impaired, rarely have fits and may have normal intelligence. Mixed forms of CP, on the other hand, do worse. *Speech* and *feeding* are particularly difficult in the quadriplegic and dyskinetic (extrapyramidal) groups. The dyskinetic CP children have difficulty initiating voluntary movements as well as suppressing unwanted movements. This

produces chaotic voice control and swallowing at every level of motor control, i.e. disorganized chest, airway, laryngeal, pharyngeal, palatal, tongue and lip muscle incoordination. *Visual impairment* ranges from squints with failure to develop conjugate vision, through field deficits and degrees of visual agnosia to total amblyopia. The ex-premature infant is at risk of *retrolental fibroplasia* causing retinal blindness, periventricular leukomalacia may destroy the optic radiation or raised intracranial pressure from posthemorrhagic hydrocephalus can compress the posterior cerebral arteries, so causing calcarine infarction.

Most children with brain damage do not fall into neat categories. All areas of brain function need detailed assessment. We find the following categories helpful: posture and mobility; manipulation; vision and spatial development; hearing, speech and communication; feeding, nutrition and growth; activities of daily living with both personal and social independence skills; behavioral, social and emotional development; epilepsy; education–global or specific learning difficulties; musical abilities.

Epidemiology

The prevalence data vary from 1.5–2.5/1000 live births for moderate or severe CP. Prospective studies, which include mild CP cases, have a higher estimate of prevalence than service registers, which only tend to see severely affected children. Figures have always varied from one country to another. Rates as low 0.74 per 1000 were quoted in Belfast when the rate in New York was 5.9 per 1000. These figures raise suspicion as to the accuracy of case identification.

Determinations of the incidence of cerebral palsy are complicated by the fact that there is a continuously changing relationship between the brain lesion(s) and the functional impairment. The diagnosis may not be clear until the end of the first or second year. In the Collaborative Perinatal Project, two-thirds of the children with 'spastic diplegia' and half of all children with signs of 'cerebral palsy' at their first birthday outgrew their symptoms by the age of 7 (Nelson & Ellenberg 1982). As a result of this it is often several years before data on the incidence of CP in a given birth cohort can be ascertained. Some people are more sensitive to the ataxic child and some exclude ataxics if there is an identifiable cause such as an occipital encephalocele or Joubert's syndrome.

Despite changes in obstetric care practices, including the identification of at-risk mothers and the establishment of neonatal units for the care of the newborn, the prevalence of CP has changed little over the past 30 years, suggesting nonobstetrical causes for CP. Jaundice, which used to be a cause of kernicterus and severe choreoathetoid cerebral palsy, is now seldom seen outwith countries who have a major G6PD problem. Birth injury with compression head injury has been virtually eliminated by obstetric practice which avoids postmaturity and prolonged labor so that the incidence of subdural hematoma has dramatically reduced. Intrapartum asphyxia, the major cause of severe morbidity, has not lessened with better fetal monitoring. On the other hand, the complications resulting from the survival of more very low birthweight infants are now replacing some of the older etiologies.

Although the premature infant is 50–70 times more at risk of developing CP than his term counterpart and there is no doubt that the absolute incidence of CP in the lowest birthweight groups has increased in parallel with the increased survival of such infants, the *relative incidence* remains unchanged since it is also the case that many more low birthweight infants survive without motor disability as well (Forfar et al 1994). That is to say if there are 100 very low birthweight infants and the morbidity stays at 10% but survival increases from 20% to 70% then there will be twice as many children with cerebral palsy. This also suggests that neonatal intensive care does not 'produce' brain-damaged infants.

Although the total prevalence has remained stubbornly in the region of 2.0/1000 live births for 30 years, there is no doubt that this hides major changes in etiology over the same period. There has recently been a clinical suggestion that with better monitoring and support of blood pressure, antenatal steroids and artificial surfactants, periventricular leukomalacia and intraventricular hemorrhage are lessening.

Etiology of cerebral palsy

It is usual to divide the cerebral palsies into congenital and acquired types. The acquired cerebral palsies account for about 10% of the total and are due to a whole miscellany of problems such as trauma (accidental and nonaccidental), infection, stroke, hypoxic ischemic events such as postcardiac bypass and resuscitated near miss cot deaths. Arguments as to whether a static encephalopathy after 2 years or 4 years constitutes cerebral palsy is a sterile argument and hence we have used 'the growing brain' as part of the definition. This emphasizes that the clinical picture will change during brain growth in childhood; brain growth is what divides pediatric from adult neurology.

The correlation between observable brain damage on neuroimaging (CT scanning) and functional impairment is not necessarily tight (Wiklund & Uvebrandt 1991, Lin et al 1993). Severe CP may be present with normal imaging and vice versa. MRI scanning is proving to be more discriminating in revealing neuronal migration defects and disordered white matter.

In congenital cerebral palsy damage may arise by any means (e.g. genetic defects, migrational defects, cerebral malformation, hypoxic ischemic encephalopathy, nutritional deficiency, trauma, infection, infarction, hemorrhage). In a series of 100 children referred consecutively to the Scottish Council for Spastics in the 1970s 18% were thought to be due to genetic factors, 10% due to postnatal acquired disease, 7% due to unknown causes and 65% due to perinatal abnormalities. In the 1980s and 1990s the figures are as in Tables 14.47 and 14.48.

There are a vast number of causes of cerebral palsy but four stand out as most important: prematurity, asphyxia in the full-term

Table 14.47 Etiologic grouping of cases of cerebral palsy

	1970 n = 92	1980 n = 100	1990 n = 100
Prenatal causes	18	38	31
Perinatal stroke	–	9	10
Intrapartum asphyxia	25	18	15
Low birthweight	29	24	37
Postnatal	9	9	7
Kernicterus	6	0	0
Birth injury	6	0	0
Unclassified	7	2	0

Table 14.48 Antenatal causes of cerebral palsy (n = 41) (1990 series)

Stroke from presumed placental embolus	10 cases
Intrauterine infection	1 case
Genetic diplegia	2 cases
Prenatal unknown cause (? placental)	7 cases
Intrauterine growth retardation (? cause)	2 cases
Congenital malformation	15 cases
Holoprosencephaly	3 cases
Hydrocephalus with hemiplegia	3 cases
Porencephalic cyst	5 cases
Primary genetic microcephaly	2 cases
Megalencephaly	1 case
Aicardi syndrome	1 case
Other causes perinatal stroke	4 cases

infant, perinatal strokes and genetic conditions. In the case of the premature infant we can now recognize three distinct pathologies related to different modes of brain damage:

1. subependymal bleeding with intraventricular hemorrhage and hydrocephalus;
2. cystic, infarctive, periventricular leukomalacia;
3. perinatal telencephalic leukoencephalopathy.

The well-recognized effects of trauma, meningitis, encephalitis, intrauterine infections, etc. occur as sporadic causes of brain damage and are less important numerically than the big four when directing research to try and reduce the maximum number of cases of cerebral palsy.

We will consider the potential causes for each of the major types of cerebral palsy in the relevant section.

Classification (Tables 14.49 and 14.50)

There are many ways of classifying the cerebral palsies according to:

1. *Pathology*: genetic syndrome, malformation, infective intrauterine encephalitis or vasculitis, hemorrhage, infarction, hypoxic ischemic damage, periventricular leukomalacia (PVL) or the noninfarctive telencephalic leukomalacia (see below).
2. *Site of brain injury*: cortical, subcortical–periventricular white matter, basal ganglia, cerebellar, brainstem, global.
3. *Topography of signs*: monoplegia, diplegia, triplegia, quadriplegia, hemiplegia, double hemiplegia (arms worse than legs).
4. *Neurology*: spastic, dystonic, dyskinetic (choreoathetoid), hypotonic and/or ataxic.
5. *Severity*: mild, moderate, severe.

Topographical cerebral palsy syndromes

Hemiplegia

Hemiplegia in children may be congenital or acquired. Thirty-five years ago hemiplegia was responsible for one-third of over 650 cases of cerebral palsy. More recent data for Edinburgh show that this has not changed, 36% of 114 cases of cerebral palsy born in 1972–1977 being hemiplegic and a similar percentage in the mid-1980s. A similar incidence in black children (35%) has been reported from Cape Town. Approximately 90% of cases of cerebral palsy of hemiplegic type are congenital.

Table 14.49 Previous classifications of cerebral palsy

1. *Little 1862*
   Hemiplegic rigidity
   Paraplegic rigidity
   Generalized rigidity
   Disordered movement without rigidity

2. *Freud 1897*
   Hemiplegia
   Diplegia (bilateral cerebral palsy)
     Generalized rigidity
     Paraplegic rigidity
     Bilateral hemiplegia
     Generalized chorea
     Double athetosis

3. *Little club 1959*
   Spastic cerebral palsy
     Hemiplegia
     Diplegia
     Double hemiplegia
   Dystonic cerebral palsy
   Choreoathetoid cerebral palsy
   Mixed forms of cerebral palsy
   Ataxic cerebral palsy
   Atonic diplegia

4. *Ingram 1964*

Neurology		Extent		Severity
Hemiplegia	{	Right Left	{	Mild Moderate Severe
Bilateral hemiplegia			{	Mild Moderate Severe

Diplegia
  Hypotonic
  Dystonic
  Spastic
	}	{ Paraplegic
		Triplegic
		Tetraplegic
			{	Mild
				Moderate
				Severe

Ataxia	{	Unilateral Bilateral	{	Mild Moderate Severe

Dyskinesia
  Dystonic
  Choreoid
  Athetoid
  Tension tremor
	}	{ Monoplegic
		Hemiplegic
		Triplegic
		Tetraplegic
		Mixed types
			{	Mild
				Moderate
				Severe

5. *Swedish – Hagberg 1984*
Spastic
  Hemiplegic*
  Tetraplegic
  Diplegic

Ataxic
  Simple
  Diplegic (overlap and counted together)

Dyskinetic
  Dystonic – mainly
  Choreoathatoid (overlap and counted together)

*Hemiplegias with abnormalities on the opposite side are not counted as asymmetrical double hemiplegias but simple hemiplegia.

General features of congenital hemiplegia. In most series males outnumber females by 3:2. Right hemiplegia is twice as common as left hemiplegia in congenital but not in acquired cases. Right preponderance applies to both males and females. The easiest way to gauge severity is to compare good and bad hand

Table 14.50   Research classification of cerebral palsy

Topographical	Neurological	Severity
Monoplegia	Spastic Rigid	Mild
	Hypotonic Dyskinetic	Moderate
	Ataxic	Severe

Hemiplegia
left/right
	Spastic
	Rigid
	  Flexor dystonia
	  Extensor dystonia
	Hypotonic
	Dyskinetic
	  Hemichorea
	  Hemiballismus
	  Hemiathetoid
	  Ataxic	

Diplegia (cerebral paraplegia)	Spastic
	  Proximal
	  Distal
	Dystonic/rigid
	Ataxic (hypotonic)	

Triplegia (diplegia with superimposed hemiplegia)
  Arm – spastic/rigid/hypotonic, dyskinetic/ataxic
  Leg – spastic/rigid/hypotonic		

Tetraplegia (quadriplegia)		

1. Symmetrical spastic double hemiplegia
2. Asymmetrical spastic double hemiplegia
3. Leg > arm type (diplegia + arms less involved, leg dominant)
4. Rigid tetraplegia – flexor (neonatal posture)
5. Rigid tetraplegia – extensor (classic dystonic posture)
6. Dyskinetic arms spastic legs (dyskinetic diplegia)
7. Choreoathetoid tetraplegia
8. Ataxic, hypotonic tetraplegia (pithed frog posture)
9. Asymmetrical – positional (windswept deformities)
10. Decerebrate tetraplegia (opisthotonus)
11. Spinal tetraplegia

Topographical	Neurological	Severity
Both arms	Ataxia Tremor Dystonia	
Truncal	Ataxia (hypotonia)	
Simple developmental delay		
Unclassifiable		

function in some form of standardized test (Brown et al 1987). In 50 children examined in this way 42% were classified as mild (hemiplegic hand 75% function compared with good hand), 12% as moderate (50–75% function), 20% severe (25–50% function) and 26% very severe (less than 25% ability in the affected compared to the unaffected hand).

Etiology of congenital hemiplegia. Hemiplegia is due to destruction of brain tissue, most commonly at the level of cerebral cortex. This results in the secondary atrophy seen on MRI with marked attenuation of the internal capsule and the pyramids in the medulla. Brain lesions in hemiplegic children vary in size and in site and the only consistent feature is that it is always in the opposite cerebral hemisphere to the clinical hemiplegia.

Although the lesion can occur antenatally, genetic factors are not important in hemiplegia (there is a very rare form of congenital absence of the pyramidal tract). Evidence from computed tomograms shows that in more than 70% of cases there is an obvious lesion which is either classic infarction or a porencephalic cyst, usually in the distribution of the middle cerebral artery. This has resulted in widespread acceptance of the fact that although the etiology may not be clear, congenital hemiplegia is in many cases the result of a perinatal stroke. Nevertheless, hemisyndromes may have no obvious neuroradiological manifestations.

Causes of congenital hemiplegic cerebral palsy. Of 121 cases of hemiplegia seen in the cerebral palsy clinic in Edinburgh, 100 were congenital and 21 postnatally acquired. Of the 100 cases of congenital hemiplegia males outnumbered females – there were 62 males and 38 females. A right hemiplegia was present in 70% and a left in 30% in keeping with the accepted predominance of right hemiplegia in congenital cases. Twenty-eight percent of congenital hemiplegias are born preterm and 19% postterm, 26% are delivered by cesarean section, 26% by breech extraction, 10% by forceps and 42% are induced. In 50 consecutive cases of congenital hemiplegia, birth trauma was presumed to be the cause in 6%, a preterm hemorrhage or periventricular leukomalacia in 20%, symptomatic asphyxia in 20%, a genetic cause in 8%, catheters and exchange transfusion in 4%. No cause was obvious in 42%: these are the cases one would now class as perinatal strokes from a presumed placental embolus so they merit a closer look. Preeclamptic toxemia or hypertension was present in 53%, induced labor in 49%, a placental abnormality, e.g. infarct, in 28%. Twenty-four percent were postmature, 14% small for gestation (mean birthweight 2980 g and mean gestation 39.2 weeks, range 36–43 weeks). If we cumulate PET, hypertension, recognized placental abnormality, growth retardation and postmaturity, then 86% were suggestive of a placental dysfunction and only three cases could be regarded as having a completely normal pregnancy and delivery.

Behavior in the neonatal period was in contrast usually normal; two were hypothermic, one sleepy and a poor feeder and one irritable. Fits were recorded in only one infant, there were no apneic attacks, need for tube feeding or other major neurological symptoms.

Asphyxia with a low Apgar score and the need for resuscitation was found in 50%, twitching in the newborn period in 32%, apnea, cyanosis, fits, hypothermia or some newborn problem in 82%. Fetal distress had been noted in 26% of the labors. Hemiplegia is associated with a high perinatal problem rate which can roughly be divided into three categories – prematurity, asphyxia and placental insufficiency. Birth trauma previously formed a fourth group of perinatal insult resulting in congenital hemiplegia, but with modern obstetrics, a compression head injury from malpresentation and disproportion followed by difficult, often instrumental delivery with resulting cerebral contusion, subdural hematoma or neck trauma to the major vessels is now a rarity.

Clinical picture in congenital hemiplegia

Neonatal. The only localizing feature which has any significance from the point of view of a cortical lesion in the neonate is a focal clonic seizure. Focal cortical seizures may also arise from benign biochemical disorders such as hypocalcemia and do not signify a definite structural abnormality of the brain.

An EEG may show localized high amplitude focal spike and slow waves if the infant is over 36 weeks' gestation. Focal seizures are rare in the preterm infant. Eighty percent of infants who will develop a hemiplegia will show some abnormality of neonatal behavior with fits, apnea, cyanotic attacks and hypothermia after birth, but in the early neonatal period such infants may show symmetrical movements, equal flexor tone, symmetrical grasp reflexes and symmetrical tendon reflexes even in the presence of a gross cortical lesion. This is because all infants have in effect a double hemiplegia with an apraxia, obvious grasp reflexes, brisk tendon reflexes, ankle clonus and extensor plantar responses, their movements consisting mainly of extrapyramidal-type progression movements or neonatal athetoid movements.

Hemisyndromes. A hemisyndrome is not the same as a hemiplegia and may in fact appear on the opposite side from a future hemiplegia.

Hemisyndromes may be of three types:

1. *Aparalytic hemisyndrome*: when there is weakness with poverty of movement or inability to reflexly support the weight on that side. This is often due to a cervical cord or brachial plexus lesions (e.g. trauma, myelodysplasia, neuroblastoma, neonatal polyneuritis).

2. A *reflex hemisyndrome* may affect either phasic reflexes, giving asymmetrical tendon reflexes and ankle clonus, or postural reflexes such as the Moro, ATNR, crossed extensor or trunk incurvation reflexes or may be associated with asymmetric movements and tone.

3. *Asymmetrical muscle tone*, usually consisting of extensor hypertonus on one side, with relative hypotonia on the other so that recoil, scarf signs, popliteal angles and range of dorsiflexion are asymmetrical.

All these asymmetries are more commonly seen in recovery from extensor hypertonus which may be either postasphyxial rigidity or decerebration due to cerebral edema or hydrocephalus and so are commonest following intrapartum asphyxia. A true hemisyndrome may occur in the neonate as a *Todd's paresis* following severe focal fits.

Children who have been immobile in utero may show asymmetrical postures which override the normal neonatal flexor tone.

The developing true hemiplegia. As the brain continues to develop in the postnatal period it soon becomes obvious that certain parts are damaged and the developing abilities which that particular part of the brain controls fail to emerge. The movement of the upper limbs becomes more asymmetrical with a lessening of movement on the affected side. At 3 months hand regard and forced grasping will be reduced on the affected side. Although the child will reflexly hold an object placed in his hands by the grasp reflex, he cannot release it on the affected side which is normally possible by 3–4 months once the obligatory grasp reflexes have diminished. At 5 months the normal child reaches, holds an object, hits his face with it, then slides it into his mouth with a marked physiological dysmetria. This will be absent on the affected side in the hemiplegic infant. There may be no spasticity. Since ankle clonus is normal in some infants up to 4 months of age its absence or presence is not significant and the hemiplegic infant will stand with feet flat even though later the leg may be severely spastic with an equinus deformity. By 6 months the arm will be obviously abnormal with failure of development of manipulative skills but it may be thought to be a monoplegia and even careful examination at this stage may reveal little neurological abnormality in the leg. In the arm, parachute responses do not develop, spasticity of the pronators increases with persistence of the grasp reflex and adduction of the thumb across the palm with the fingers closed over it. In the leg, spasticity and a tendency to equinus appear in the second half of the first year.

The established true hemiplegia. The muscles of the trunk have bilateral representation and are not affected in a hemiplegia so that scoliosis, or asymmetry of erector spinae muscles, is not an important feature. The face is also bilaterally represented and facial weakness is usually less obvious with a congenital than an acquired hemiplegia. There is no bulbar weakness so bite, chew and swallow are normal and there is normal bladder and bowel control.

1. The upper limb. Weakness of movement is not a total paralysis but a loss of volitional skilled movements which are more distal than proximal (the pyramidal tract in man is thought to innervate mainly the distal part of the limbs). Voluntary grasp is weak but the muscles will still function reflexly as shown by the spastic response to stretch and the grasp reflex. Proximal muscle movements are preserved so that fly swatting or windmill movements of the affected arm may be well performed. The child may swim with the hand fisted and with reasonable shoulder movements. Dyspraxia (inability to learn skilled movements) is common and is independent of the degree of spasticity so that some children with a lot of spasticity can learn trick movements and others with practically no spasticity have a useless arm. The hand is kept closed (Fig. 14.40) and there is sustained grasp. If the position of the arm is reversed and the limb is extended and internally rotated with the back of the hand on the buttock, the hand opens and the grasp is released. Reaching is clumsy and the adductor pollicis muscle is usually very spastic. In order to abduct the thumb the metacarpophalangeal joint is often dislocated so that the phalangeal part of the thumb abducts whilst its metacarpal stays adducted. The fingers themselves flex at the metacarpophalangeal joints and extend at the interphalangeal. There is no pincer grasp and the child extends the fingers and abducts the thumb as best he can and then uses his better proximal movements to project his hand till it hits the object (Fig. 14.41). Fine individual finger movements are lost and the child cannot oppose each finger and thumb in turn. The wrist is often flexed so that there is a poor functional position of the hand. The thumb may protrude between the second and third fingers. The upper limb is usually maintained in a flexed posture at elbow, wrist and fingers with increased resistance to extension due to spasticity but this is not the only reason as the leg is extended even though the spasticity affects mainly the flexor muscles. The flexed posture of the upper limb and extended lower limb is due to labyrinthine influences on an α pathway and is not determined by spasticity alone.

Some children with no spasticity always keep the arm flexed and do not swing it. The same applies to the rotation at the shoulder, the arm usually being internally rotated in congenital hemiplegia, but in some children with acquired hemiplegia there is marked external rotation of the flexed arm. The severity of spasticity does not equate with function and this must be borne in mind when attempting to reduce spasticity.

There are, therefore, several components to a hemiplegia which are to some extent independent and so different children may show a different constellation of signs in addition to different grades of severity. The arm may show hypertonia of spastic or rigid type. In a few children severe dyspraxia and brisk tendon reflexes may be associated with a hypotonic arm. This will allow

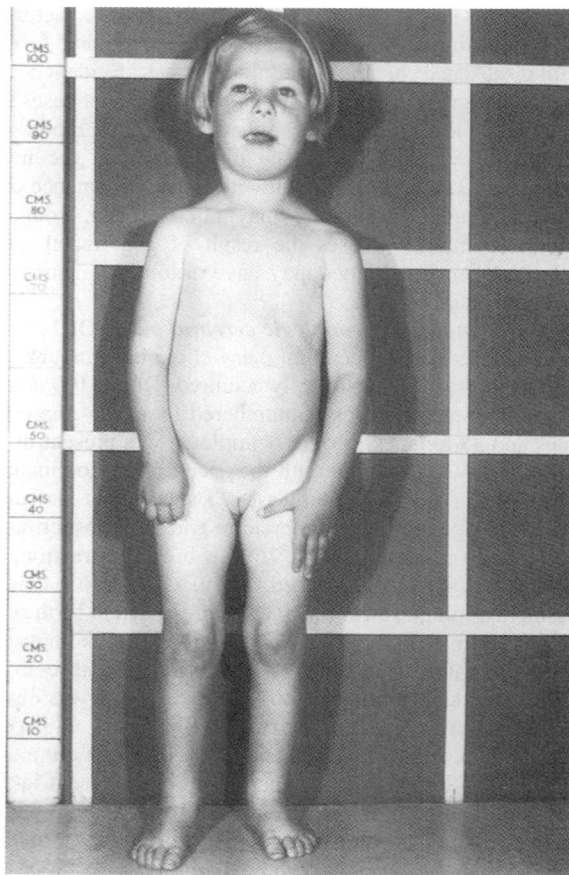

Fig. 14.40 Congenital hemiplegia showing dwarfing of affected limbs. Note 'fisting' and edema of hand.

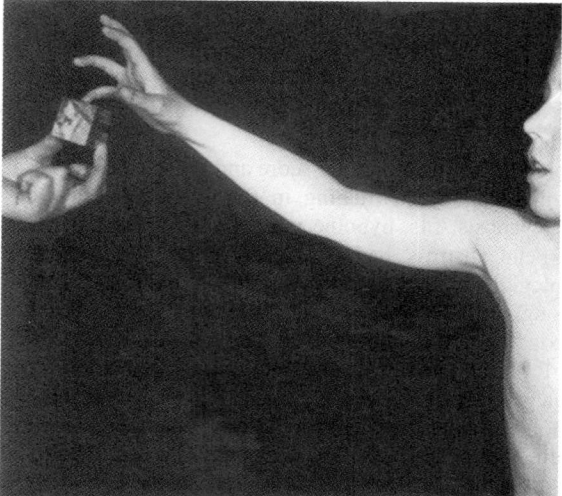

Fig. 14.41 Congenital hemiplegia: attempted voluntary grasping.

excess joint ranges to passive movement (e.g. hypersupination and hyperextension at the elbow). Rigidity (which is discussed later) may be of extensor or flexor type. In the former the arm is rigidly extended in the so-called dystonic or avoiding posture

(Fig. 14.42). It may present in this way in the first year of life and be diagnosed mistakenly as Erb palsy. Flexor rigidity is made worse with anxiety or attention being drawn to the limb, resulting in fluctuating muscle tone. Both these types of rigidity, most likely due to associated basal ganglia involvement, are seen in postasphyxial hemiplegias and may be accompanied by hemiathetosis (but rarely chorea) in the older child. Occasionally the hemiplegia consists of a unilateral dystonia with minimal pyramidal involvement affecting arm and leg and reminiscent of torsion dystonia. The asymmetrical tonic neck reflex may then influence muscle tone on the affected side. Spasticity with increased resistance to stretch and a tendency to muscle shortening and fixed contracture is seen in the biceps, forearm flexors of wrist and fingers, pronators and adductor pollicis. Brisk reflexes usually accompany the spasticity with a finger jerk and wide afferent field with overspill to other muscle groups. Overflow is also seen as associated movements so that when the good hand is used the hemiplegic hand closes and the grasp tightens. The Fog test shows increased flexion in the arm when the child walks with his feet inverted: equinus of the foot may result in associated movements of the upper limb so that operation on the foot may subsequently change the posture of the arm.

2. The lower limb. The leg is often stated to be less affected in a hemiplegia than the arm. In most cases this is untrue. The distal fine movements of the toes are just as weak as in the fingers. A hemiplegic cannot use his toes instead of his hands as is possible,

for example, in children suffering from thalidomide embryopathy. The leg functions as a support and proximal circumducting movements are needed for progression: it is extended, as is the arm, via labyrinthine pathways and this overcomes the flexed position which would be imposed by the pattern of spasticity and which would cause the child to collapse. Walking is always possible with an uncomplicated hemiplegia utilizing the retained proximal flexion and adduction movement at the hip in the swing phase of gait.

Spasticity is of two types, phasic and tonic. In the phasic type increased muscle contraction accompanies rapid stretch and is accompanied by brisk reflexes and no tendency to contracture; this type is often seen in quadriceps and calf and may be the first spasticity to appear in the young infant. It contrasts with tonic spasticity of the leg in which there is restricted lengthening, even with very slow stretching, no brisk tendon reflexes and ready occurrence of contractures. The phasic spasticity of the quadriceps may help to support the child, the stretch reflexes being activated as the child tends to collapse. Tonic spasticity causes reciprocal inhibition of the antagonist muscle and as a result the quadriceps and dorsiflexors of the ankle may appear correspondingly weak. The child walks with foot in equinus, flexed at the hip and knee with a circumducting gait (Fig. 14.43). Even after tendo Achillis

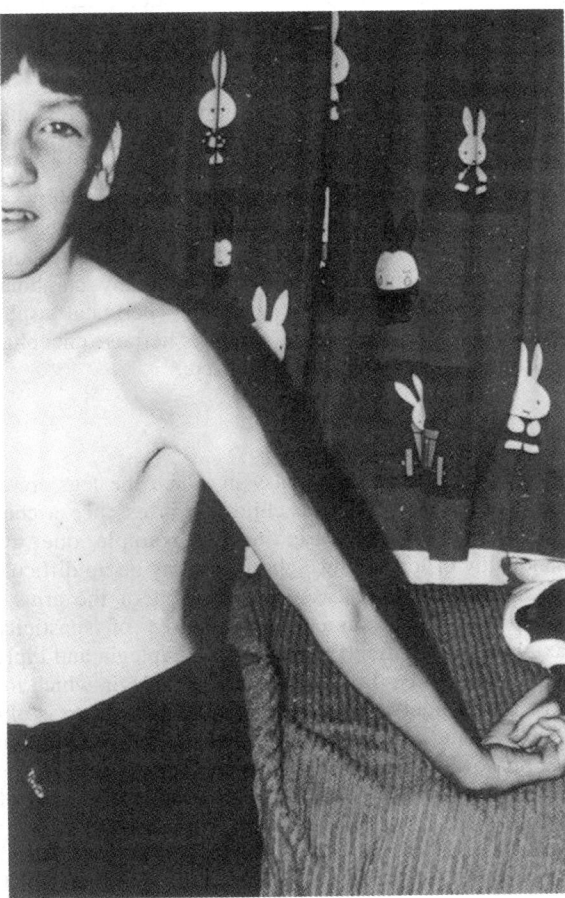

Fig. 14.42 Hemiplegia – arm held in avoiding posture.

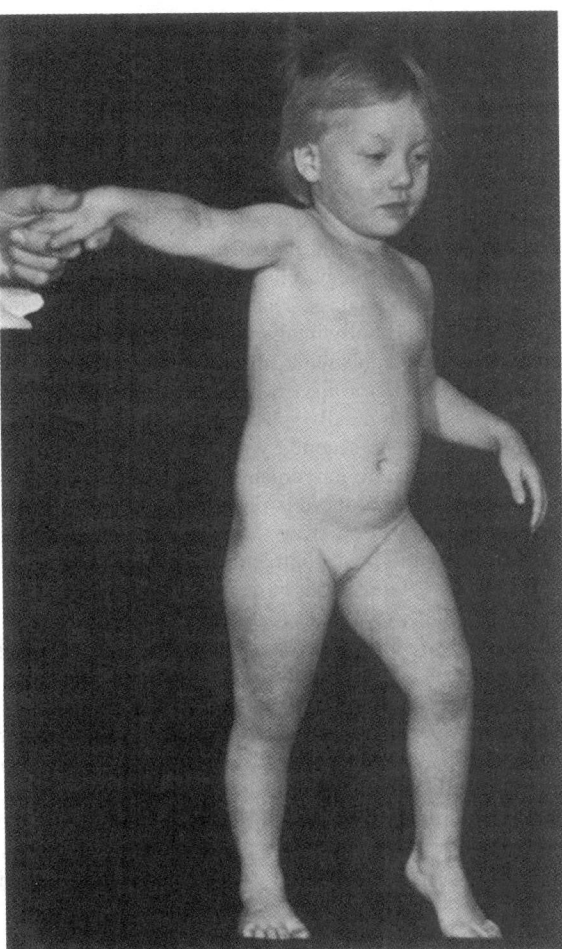

Fig. 14.43 Characteristic gait in hemiplegia. Equinus position of foot and hemiplegic posture of affected upper limbs.

lengthening he cannot walk heel-toe toe-heel and loses heel pivot and toe spring in the stance phase of gait. As in the upper limb, there is often a superimposed pattern of internal rotation but in acquired hemiplegias this may be replaced by predominant external rotation so that the knee rotates laterally and there is an equinovalgus instead of the more common equinovarus. Another variation seen at the knee in mild cases of equinus is a severe back knee or genu recurvatum posture on the hemiplegic side, in the stance phase of gait due to a toe–heel gait.

Other abnormalities. Growth disturbance is common (Fig. 14.40) and shows more obviously in the leg as shortening than in the arm when comparison of finger nails will more easily demonstrate smaller fingers on the affected side. In 48% of hemiplegias dwarfing is present in the lower limb and the short leg imposes secondary changes such as pelvic tilt or a compensatory forefoot equinus.

Vasomotor changes show as a cold blue leg and foot with poor capillary return and chilblains in winter. Using the back of the hand as a sensor, the foot is commonly found to be colder on the affected side. In an acute hemiplegia, on the other hand, the leg may be warmer, pinker and swollen.

The skin is thin, shiny, heals poorly and the nails may be thickened and shrunken. It is not known whether these are autonomic effects with sympathetic excess due to loss of pyramidal inhibition.

Sensory defects such as impaired pain, temperature, position and vibration sense are rare in congenital hemiplegia. Loss of two-point discrimination, texture sense, dysgraphesthesia (recognition of shapes traced on the hand), astereognosis and finger agnosia are more common. Sensory abnormalities may be found on the normal side. Such sensory defects occur in about 25% of cases but the incidence depends upon the age at which testing is performed. A normal child of 7 years cannot tell shapes, textures, etc. placed on his hand: such recognition is developmentally determined so that to examine a hemiplegic child at 8 years and say he has a sensory defect is meaningless. There may be delay in maturation on the affected side. If body image is tested throughout childhood the number of hemiplegias with difficulty gets progressively less.

Contractures and deformity in hemiplegia are usually due to muscle shortening in tonically spastic muscles or else rotation. In some children there is a secondary change in muscle proteins so stiffness and resistance to movement occur without any electrical activity on the EMG, i.e. there is plastic change in muscle, these muscles show a relaxation over time, e.g. 20 seconds, and are easily confused with fixed contractures or tonic spasticity (see later). Positional deformities are rare (see later) and hip dislocation secondary to spasticity is very uncommon. Scoliosis is unusual apart from some pelvic tilt associated with a very short leg or rotation at the shoulder. The commonest deformities requiring help are equinus at the ankle and wrist flexion.

Sixty percent of hemiplegics have normal *intelligence* and the 40% who are mentally retarded are so because of a more generalized insult such as perinatal asphyxia or prematurity. The side of the hemiplegia does not influence IQ. The frequency of epilepsy varies according to etiology and genetic predisposition from 16% to 43%. Hemianopia is rare in congenital hemiplegia (present in less than 25% of other cases). Since 70% of cases affect the presumed dominant hemisphere speech retardation would be expected to be common. It is thought that the opposite hemisphere can take over speech function in congenital hemiplegia and the incidence of speech retardation is the same as that of mental retardation. In hemiplegics with slow speech the usual 2:1 right:left ratio is present so that it does not appear that the side of damage is important in determining whether speech retardation is present or not. Classic dysphasia is not seen and it is always a delayed developmental pattern of speech which occurs. The displacement of other types of learning by speech is seen in the discrepancy found on formal psychometric testing whereby the child functions less well in concepts of space, shape and direction (i.e. so-called visuospatial defects) than verbally.

Schooling problems may occur despite an intelligence quotient in the normal range: 60% of children with cerebral palsy and IQs over 90 are not up to their grade. The mean IQ for hemiplegics as a whole is shifted to the left by just over one standard deviation (15 points). Reading retardation and especially number difficulty may be attributed to poor attention and poor psychosocial adjustment but in many cases they are due to a specific learning problem; 25% of children with severe prematurity or birth asphyxia will have some form of schooling difficulty even without a hemiplegia. Conversely many children with a severe hemiplegia and marked abnormality on CT scan may attend normal school and make excellent progress.

Behavior problems are not a complication of the hemiplegia but depend upon family and social stresses, specific learning problems, presence of epilepsy and male sex – not the side of the hemiplegia.

The minimal hemiparesis. The mildest degree of hemiplegia shows as difficulty with fine individual finger movements, such as fastening top or cuff buttons, a mild pronator catch, excessive associated movement especially on the Fog test, weak grasp on dynamometry, failure to swing the arm and excessive flexion when running or using the opposite limb. The nails on the affected side may be slightly narrower, the foot slightly colder. Hopping and standing on the leg on that side will be less effectively performed than on the opposite side. The foot may slap down, causing an audibly asymmetric gait. The tendo Achillis shows less lengthening from the point where the tendon just tightens to full dorsiflexion. Brisker reflexes, a spontaneous Babinski response or equivocal plantar reflex may be present in any combination. Minimal hemiparesis may be seen after perinatal asphyxia, apparent recovery from head injury, herpes encephalitis, hypernatremic dehydration, meningitis, etc.

Diplegia

Diplegia is a spastic cerebral palsy in which the legs are more affected than the arms and the child has in essence a cerebral paraplegia. In the pure case, as for example due to the encephalopathy of low birthweight, there may be no difficulty in diagnosis whilst in other cases involvement of the arms with athetoid posturing or some milder degree of spasticity or dyspraxia makes it difficult to delineate tetraplegia and diplegia. Diagnosis may also be difficult in cases of diplegia which follow upon low birthweight or intrapartum asphyxia as there is often a so-called 'dystonic phase' which precedes the spastic phase. In the dystonic phase all four limbs and the trunk may be involved, even though the spasticity will eventually, by the age of 5, only affect the legs.

A further source of diagnostic difficulty is to differentiate a true paraplegia from a diplegia. Children with brain damage from meningitis may also have spinal cord damage so that they may have a true paraplegia complicating their meningitis rather than diplegia. Cases of familial spastic paraplegia may be difficult to separate from some of the types of genetic diplegia. They may present early and may not appear to progress over several years. It is not uncommon to see children with diastematomyelia, various types of myelodysplasia or neurenteric cysts of the spinal canal misdiagnosed as cases of cerebral diplegia before the true paraplegic nature of the illness is recognized. Careful examination to find involvement of the upper limbs together with the history of a dystonic phase of development and the presence or absence of bladder and sphincter involvement are helpful in diagnosis.

Etiology of diplegia. The distribution of diplegia in children according to the maturity at birth is distributed in two separate peaks, one related to prematurity and one possibly due to asphyxia in full-term infants. We can divide the causes of a static diplegia, i.e. diplegic cerebral palsy, into five groups (Table 14.51).

The low birthweight infant is at risk of many patterns of brain damage from different causes; for example, he may be of low birthweight because of abnormalities before birth (genetic, chromosome, infection, alcohol). There is risk of brain damage from hyperbilirubinemia, intraventricular hemorrhage, birth trauma, metabolic disturbances, asphyxia, nutritional problems, etc. and although spastic diplegia is very characteristic of low birthweight, there are many other ways in which the low birthweight infant may sustain brain damage and many other

Table 14.51 Causes of diplegic cerebral palsies

1. Little's disease of prematurity – encephalopathy of low birthweight or perinatal telencephalic leukoencephalopathy

2. Postasphyxial complex diplegia with infarctive periventricular leukomalacia

3. Abnormalities of pregnancy
   Fetal alcohol syndrome
   Congenital rubella
   Neonatal hepatitis
   Maternal phenylketonuria
   Cytomegalovirus infection

4. Genetic diplegic syndromes
   Diplegia with osteogenesis imperfecta
   Diplegia and photoconvulsive epilepsy and mental handicap
   Diplegia and T lymphocyte dysfunction
   Autosomal recessive ataxic diplegia with mental handicap
   Dominant spastic diplegia with normal intelligence
   Diplegia with ichthyosis
   Diplegia and myotonic dystrophy
   Diplegia with cystinosis
   Diplegia with phenylketonuria (older patients)
   Paine's syndrome – microcephaly and diplegia – sex linked
   Diplegia with X-linked hydrocephalus*
   X-linked MASA syndrome of mental retardation, aphasia, diplegia with shuffling and adducted thumbs*
   X-linked familial spastic paraplegia (diplegia) type 1*
   Diplegia with Segawa DOPA-sensitive dystonia
   Autosomal recessive diplegia with microcephaly (Middle East syndrome)

5. Acquired causes of diplegia
   Parasagittal dysplasias
   Parasagittal lipomas, hemangiomas and nonprogressive tumors
   Dehydration and superior sagittal sinus thrombosis
   Ataxic diplegia with hydrocephalus (nongenetic)
   Parasagittal trauma, e.g. severe molding and tearing sagittal veins
   Diplegia with Lyme disease

* Note all three X-linked diplegias are linked to a single gene locus on X chromosome coding for matrix glycoproteins with fibronectin. Mixtures of these occur within a family.

types of cerebral palsy, e.g. hemiplegia due to perinatal strokes, ataxic diplegia secondary to hydrocephalus of intraventricular hemorrhage, tetraplegia due to severe brain destruction from ischemia and intraventricular hemorrhage. Spasticity in diplegia of low birthweight is characteristically preceded by an extrapyramidal type of dystonia identical to that seen in dyskinetic cerebral palsy due to kernicterus.

Encephalopathy of low birthweight (Little's disease) Little described this syndrome 150 years ago and also ascribed it to prematurity. Clinically, it produces symmetrical weakness and spasticity of the legs, i.e. diplegia, occurring in low birthweight infants. Twenty-five percent are twins and there is often a history of a poor reproducing mother shown as involuntary infertility, previous miscarriage and previous premature births. The infant may have grown poorly in utero (SGA) and then take more than 2 weeks postnatally to regain its birthweight, suggesting that there may be a nutritional component to causation. Dystonia involving the upper limbs and trunk is evident by 6 weeks and is replaced by spasticity, which first appears at about 1 year, over the first 4 years. Most walk between 4 and 6 years and they have a low normal IQ. They are often myopic with a convergent squint and a degree of dyspraxia of the upper limbs. Fits are rare and there is no sensory loss, bladder or bowel problem. The CT is normal in over 80% but the ultrasound in the neonatal period may show flares but not cystic infarction. The MRI shows dilated posterior horns and poor myelination of the cerebral hemispheres in the trigone area.

In contrast, children with severe periventricular hemorrhages tend to be mentally retarded, have hydrocephalus, fits and a hemiplegic or tetraplegic form of cerebral palsy, which contrasts very markedly with the bright, nonconvulsing children with normal CT scans with classic Little's disease. Thus diplegia of prematurity appears to be due to some form of encephalopathy of low birthweight which does not seem to be due to subependymal hemorrhage, hypoglycemia, hyperbilirubinemia, hypoxia, ischemia or birth trauma.

The low birthweight infant examined on its expected date of delivery, i.e. at the age of 2–3 months, does not behave like the normal full-term infant but is stiff, with extensor hypertonus, the so-called dystonic syndrome of low birthweight. It would appear that the later reading problems, behavior problems and nearly all the cases of diplegia occur in the group of children who have shown this dystonic pattern of maturation. Not all children with dystonia, however, go on to long-term overt handicap.

This dystonic pattern of maturation has fluctuated over the last 30 years and in the 1970s dropped from 46% to 10% and the incidence of diplegia was correspondingly reduced. In the 1980s there was, however, a return of diplegia for unknown reasons. The fact that the pattern is changing is against the hypothesis that these children are genetically abnormal and are born small and early because they are genetically predisposed to be abnormal and favors some abnormality in the preterm infant which is potentially preventable, e.g. nutrition.

Clinical features of diplegia. Diplegia as a result of intrapartum asphyxia or from the encephalopathy of low birthweight tends to be associated with a dystonic phase followed by the spastic stage of the diplegia (Fig. 14.44). Children with a so-called ataxic diplegia from hydrocephalus tend to be very floppy before pyramidal signs appear in the legs and the spasticity is not as marked as it is in the other types of diplegia, the ataxia of much more of a clinical problem. Most difficulty aris

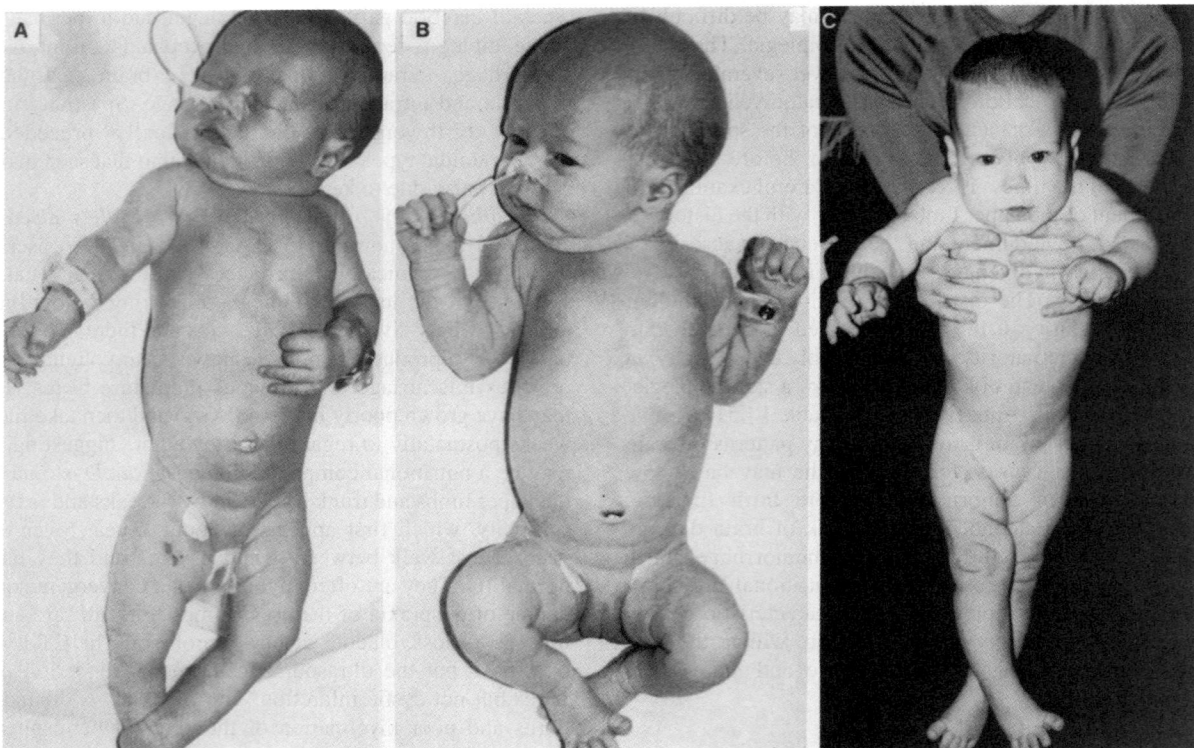

Fig. 14.44   Development of cerebral diplegia after asphyxia at birth. (**a**) Extensor hypertonus at 72 h. (**b**) Flexor tonus at 14 days (feeding difficulties). (**c**) Cerebral diplegia at 10 months.

genetic diplegias, as these children may not show any abnormalities of muscle tone until the end of the first year when spasticity appears without a preceding dystonic phase and it may be very difficult to be sure at first whether this is a progressive disease or not. The dystonia which occurs in the common types of diplegia in the first few weeks of life is an alerting sign that all is not well and that these infants may develop long-term problems. Infants of 4–6 months, however, can show marked extensor hypertonus and at this stage it may not be possible to say whether they will go on to frank cerebral palsy or show resolution and this forms one of the groups of children in whom miracle claims for the effects of physiotherapy have been made. That is not to say that with an immobile infant, because of the risk of positional deformities, physiotherapy should not be started (especially an intensive positioning program) as soon as there is suspicion about the infant's development. Caution should be exercised, however, before prognosticating on the basis of dystonia as many low birthweight infants will not proceed to a long-term motor handicap significantly affecting their posture and mobility.

Dystonic stage of diplegia. The infant shows extensor hypertonus which is maximum when lying supine or when suspended vertically under the armpits, i.e. there is a labyrinthine component. If placed prone the child may resume the fetal position of flexion, i.e. the legs flexed at the hip and knee and tucked under the abdomen. The position of the head in relationship to the body also affects the muscle tone so that extension of the neck causes both arms to be rigidly extended in front of the child, the hands fisted and the arms showing internal rotation. Flexion of the neck abolishes this posture. In severe cases tonic opening of the mouth occurs in association with

extension of the arms. Rotation of the head on the trunk will be associated with retention of the asymmetrical tonic neck reflex (Fig. 14.45), the trunk incurvation reflex (Galant reflex) and the so-called progression reflexes, walking, stepping, crawling and cycling. Contact with a surface is the third factor which will enhance muscle tone so that if the child lies supine in contact with a hard surface he will arch into opisthotonus (Fig. 14.46). Any pain, anxiety or sudden startling may greatly enhance the tone, as may attempts to feed the child with stimulation, especially with a metal spoon around the perioral region. All these factors may result in attacks of opisthotonic posturing or 'dystonic attacks'. Extension of the legs is associated with equinus posture and the big toe extends in the spontaneous Babinski response with fanning of the small toes. At this stage there is no ankle clonus and no fixed deformity. Lengthening reaction of the muscles, once the rigidity is overcome by positioning the child to inhibit this, will be found to be normal. When the feet are allowed to touch the floor with the child suspended the progression reflexes cause the child to run rapidly on tiptoe like a ballet dancer with one foot treading on the other. The corresponding postural development of sitting, rolling and standing will be delayed. Attempts to pull the child into a sitting position result in him coming up like a log into standing. This pattern of dystonia appears soon after the expected date of delivery and is usually very obvious by 4 months of age. Primitive reflexes such as the Moro, grasp (Fig. 14.47), asymmetrical tonic neck and walking, which have normally disappeared by 4 months, persist.

The dystonic phase of development may last until 7 or 8 months and then disappear or it may last the whole of the child's life. In most cases the dystonic rigidity gradually merges into the spastic

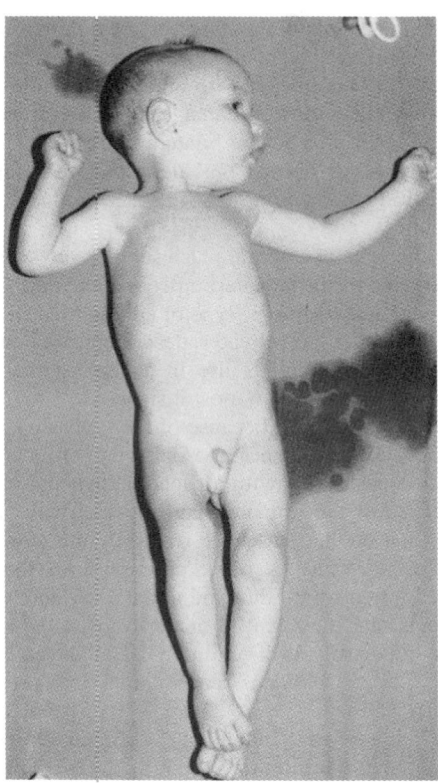

Fig. 14.45 Asymmetrical tonic neck reflex in dystonic phase of cerebral diplegia.

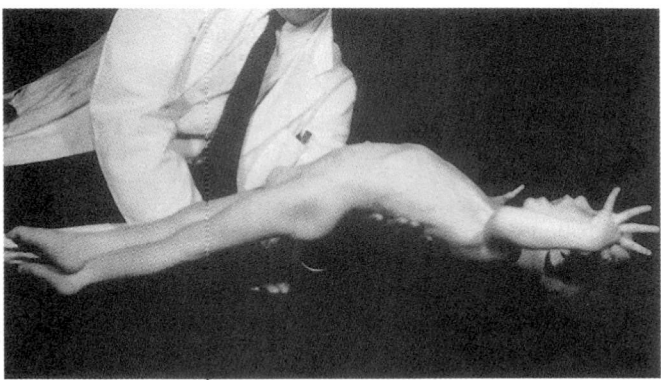

Fig. 14.46 Decerebrate rigidity.

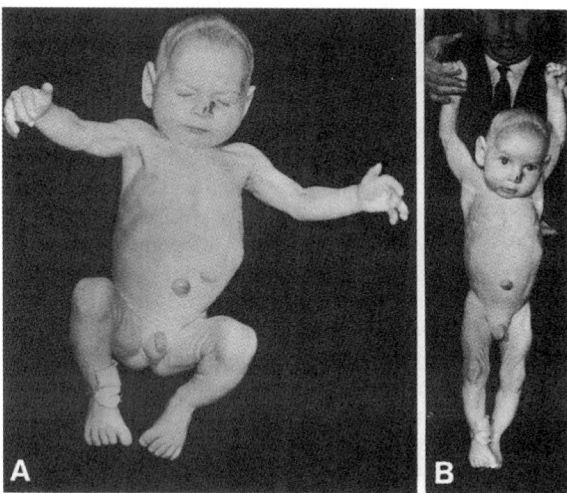

Fig. 14.47 Retained primitive motor reflexes in a diplegic child aged 11 months. (**a**) Moro reflex; (**b**) grasp reflex.

phase so that the child goes through a mixed so-called rigid/spastic phase before developing the characteristic spasticity confined to the legs. Since the dystonia affects the neck and trunk extensor muscles and the upper limbs and causes retention of primitive reflexes, with disappearance of the dystonia the child often appears to put on a developmental spurt and will develop head control, increase his hand manipulative skills, learn to sit up and to control the upper part of his body. At the same time, increasing adductor spasticity and flexor spasticity in the lower limbs is likely to result in a flexed rather than an extended posture with much more fixed deformity.

Spastic phase of diplegia. One of the mysteries of clinical neurology, in spite of a vast quantity of basic research in neurophysiology, is the nature of spasticity. It is based on exaggeration of peripheral stretch reflexes but not all spastic muscles have exaggerated tendon reflexes. There are various types and levels of spasticity which may be organized at spinal cord, brainstem or cortical level. From the point of view of cerebral palsy, it is a cortical pattern of spasticity which affects mainly the flexor muscles in 'tonic' spasticity; extensor muscles such as the triceps and quadriceps may be affected by 'phasic' spasticity. It is the phasically spastic muscle which shows very brisk reflexes and often shows the clasp knife reaction. Tonically spastic muscles show decreased lengthening reactions and rapidly develop contractures. The hip flexor muscles, hamstrings and calf muscles, together with the adductor muscles, form the main tonic groups in the lower limbs, thus causing the child to be flexed at hip, knee and in equinus at the ankle, with the legs usually internally rotated and the characteristic scissoring reaction (Fig. 14.45). When the upper limbs are affected in a double hemiplegia or spastic tetraplegia, they are flexed at the elbow and wrist and the fingers are flexed across the adducted thumb with marked spasticity of the pronators. Increasing spasticity of the muscles around the hip causes the legs to scissor increasingly from adduction with flexion and secondary dislocation of the hip may occur. At the ankle the equinus becomes fixed with only 10° or so of lengthening of the calf muscle compared to the normal 35°. In diplegia the knee and ankle jerks are brisk with bilateral ankle clonus and the plantar responses are extensor. A painful plantar stimulus is associated with a flexor withdrawal reflex as opposed to the spontaneous Babinski reflex in association with rigid extension seen in the extensor dystonic phase. The knee jerks show all the characteristics of a pathological reflex with a wide afferent field so that the jerk can be elicited from the tibia. A low amplitude stimulus is required, there is a very markedly exaggerated response and wide spread of the reflex with adductor responses spreading to the opposite limb. Tonically spastic muscle is associated with reciprocal inhibition of its antagonist so that the spastic hip flexor muscles are associated with apparent weakness of the extensor muscles of the hip, the spastic hamstrings with apparent quadriceps weakness and the spastic heel cord with apparent weakness of the dorsiflexors. This can cause the child to have a characteristic waddling gait or occasionally to show a collapsing gait due to the quadriceps being unable to hold the baby upright. As the dystonic phase disappears and the child develops sitting balance there is also the risk that with increasing spasticity the hips will dislocate or fixed contractures will develop at knee and ankle. He should be encouraged on to his feet using a rollator or tripod. Many of the less severely affected children eventually will walk independently in equinus with the legs internally rotated and with a waddling gait. Problems of surgery in children with spastic diplegia are discussed later.

Associated features. As a general rule the more severely the arms are affected, the lower will be the intelligence. Most children with predominant leg involvement have an intelligence quotient in the lower range of normal with a mean of 75. This often, however, hides severe learning problems in that the child may have delay in learning to read and difficulty with arithmetic. The hands may not appear to be involved with spasticity but severe dyspraxia with difficulty in learning skilled manipulative tasks is not unusual. Taking all cases of diplegia, epilepsy occurs in 25% (but in diplegia from encephalopathy of low birthweight, only 3%). Mental handicap and choreoathetosis, as well as epilepsy, are frequent complications of children with diplegia from perinatal asphyxia. Squints, both paralytic due to fourth nerve palsy and concomitant, are common. Short-sightedness and central visual cognitive difficulties may all add to the child's problems in school.

Quadriplegic cerebral palsy

The greater the skill required to execute a movement, the more lateralized it becomes within the brain. In children with a hemiplegia there is a loss of learned volitional hand skills with preservation of functions of the axial musculature, i.e. bite chew, swallow, control of micturition and defecation; 100% speak and 100% walk if the damage is strictly unilateral. Immediately a bilateral lesion of the cerebral cortex is made the result is devastating and the effects on function far worse than simply a double hemiplegia. Walking is lost, bowel and bladder control is lost, bulbar muscles are affected making speech and feeding very difficult and intelligence is markedly decreased and most will have fits (Minns et al 1989b).

Whereas one expects 100% of children with a hemiplegia to walk, less than 10% of children with quadriplegia will achieve any independent mobility and those that do are more likely to be diplegias with arm involvement than true double hemiplegias.

Etiology of quadriplegia. The commonest cause of severe bilateral brain damage is either gross malformation with cortical dysplasia or generalized severe bilateral damage following hypoxic ischemic conditions. This latter includes perinatal asphyxia, uncontrolled status epilepticus, drowning, poisoning, postcardiac bypass catastrophes and survival from a near miss cot death. Destructive lesions from the cerebral cortex may occur with hydranencephaly, severe hydrocephalus or necrotizing encephalitis, such as from toxoplasmosis, rubella, cytomegalovirus and herpes simplex.

Abnormalities in the structure of the cerebral cortex, i.e. the cortical dysplasias such as lissencephaly and holoprosencephaly, may also be associated with profound mental handicap, epilepsy and a quadriplegic type of cerebral palsy.

In children with severe head injury the damage is usually secondary with hypoxic ischemic damage secondary to uncontrolled raised intracranial pressure or failure to maintain the airway and adequate oxygenation. The persistent vegetative state is really a severe tetraplegia with amentia. In cases of nonaccidental shaking injury diffuse damage to the microvasculature of the brain can result in a severe bilateral brain damage syndrome. The end stage of a 'burned out' degenerative disease such as metachromatic leukodystrophy, SSPE, etc. produces an identical clinical picture.

Some of the genetic cerebral palsies which are seen from first-cousin marriages result in severe microcephaly, epilepsy, mental retardation and a quadriplegic type of cerebral palsy.

Clinical features. As already described, the child will be immobile and expectation is life in a chair with only passive mobility, i.e. being pushed in most instances.

Feeding will be difficult because of the bulbar palsy present in 95%. There is a high incidence of esophageal reflux and aspiration syndromes. A spastic jaw with a pseudobulbar palsy means bite, chew and swallow are impaired with poor airway protection so nasal regurgitation and tracheal overspill are common. Tube feeding or gastrostomy is often necessary. In the past these children were often small, thin and undernourished. Gastrostomy feeding shows that they can be made to grow but great care is needed to avoid obesity as the children need to be constantly lifted and carried. Cortical blindness and deafness are present in 40% (Minns et al 1989b).

Epilepsy may be intractable and difficult to control with episodes of status epilepticus and relative anticonvulsant resistance. Absence of bladder or bowel control with incontinence and chronic constipation are common. The prevalence of medical problems in a group of 21 children all with severe quadriplegic CP was as follows:

Contractures	47%
Scoliosis/windswept	66%
Nasogastric feeding	28%
Hiatus hernia	28%
Reflux esophagitis	33%
Epilepsy	76%
Recurrent aspirations	19%
Recurrent chest infections	14%
Constipation	76%
Growth failure	52%
Anemia	10%

The 'positional deformities' often result in the child windsweeping, with dislocation of the hip, a pelvic tilt, scoliosis, rib deformities and these horrific positional deformities may completely override the underlying neurological spasticity.

Positional deformity

In cerebral palsy the type of deformity may be produced by many different mechanisms:

1. as a result of tonic spasticity and true muscle shortening;
2. postures which may be imposed upon the child from the primitive reflexes;
3. dystonic postures, e.g. from extensor rigidity;
4. the effects of labyrinthine reflexes causing the upper limb to flex and the lower limb to extend;
5. abnormal limb growth;
6. biomechanical change in muscle, i.e. plasticity;

7. soft tissue contractions as in joint capsules, e.g. knee or secondary joint dislocations, e.g. hip, thumb and ankle.

Growth disturbances may exaggerate any deformity: the affected limb may not grow and may be shorter than the normal limb; spastic muscle may not develop at the same rate as the normal muscle; ill-considered orthopedic surgery may add to the deformity as in tendo Achillis lengthening causing an exaggeration of crouch gait (Brown & Minns 1989).

Children with severe motor disorders who are not able to change their own position during a period of growth develop a particular constellation of deformities due to immobility, growth and gravity. These include plagiocephaly with bat ear, facial asymmetry, orbital asymmetry and asymmetrical neck movements. The chest shows asymmetrical flattening of the ribs on one side, a rigid segment of spine, pelvic tilt and windsweeping of the lower limbs (Fig. 14.48). The leg on the abducted side shows that the positional deformity can override the neurologically imposed deformity as the leg remains in abduction even though the adductor muscles are still spastic. The leg on the abducted side, most commonly the left, is especially likely to undergo secondary hip dislocation which may be painful. The rigid spinal segment, pelvic obliquity and asymmetrical ribs often progress so that especially at puberty, a true rotational scoliosis is added. Often the legs cannot be separated properly for hygiene and toilet purposes. The asymmetrical chest and ribs appears to affect the gastroesophageal junction so that esophageal reflux or even massive hematemesis may be seen. The scoliosis and chest deformity mean that chest infections tend to occur. This positional deformity is similar to the so-called squint baby syndrome seen in some normal infants in the first 6 months of life. The importance of positional deformity is that attempts to correct it by derotation osteotomy for the windswept leg, major spinal surgery to correct the spinal scoliosis and hip surgery to correct the secondary dislocation of the hip are rarely successful. Thus prevention is the ideal and early diagnosis is essential, before the child has started to develop positional molding and windsweeping which can occur by 6 months of age if the infant has been totally immobile and has not developed the ability to roll or change his position. A positioning regime in order to keep pelvic and pectoral girdle

aligned and prevent asymmetry is essential. This may mean turning 2-hourly during the day and 4-hourly at night and positioning with pillows or special U-shaped foam wedges. The child needs to be in different positions, prone, standing or even suspended for a time. Thus the prevention of positional deformity involves a 24-h regime with, in addition, more active physiotherapy sessions carried out by the parents who need to be trained for this role (Minns et al 1989b).

Children with 'total body involvement' type of quadriplegia pose enormous problems in nursing by their parents. Improvement with therapy programs is often minimal and in our own experience very few ever achieve a developmental level above 4 months of age. Ethical issues arise, such as whether a gastrostomy should be performed in order to allow adequate nutrition. How often should one treat pneumonia in a child with gross scoliosis, chest deformity and esophageal reflux despite repair? It is also in these children that parents are likely to 'doctor shop' and be offered false hope of miracle cures by different systems of therapy. Death is likely to be by aspiration or during a bout of status epilepticus; about 3–5% of cases die per year so 50% die before school-leaving age. Death is more likely the more functionally disabled the child (Hutton et al 1994).

Ataxic cerebral palsies (chronic nonprogressive ataxias)
(Table 14.52)

Like the hemiplegias, nonprogressive ataxias can be divided into congenital or acquired types but this is not a particularly useful division in clinical practice. More useful is the division into acute ataxia, intermittent ataxia, progressive ataxia (see later) and nonprogressive ataxia (cerebral palsy).

Clinical aspects of ataxic disorders in children

The term 'ataxia' is usually accepted as indicating incoordination of postural control and gait and of the skilled movements which are involved in hand manipulation and speech. Movement requires that there is a plan or engram which must then be translated into a movement pattern. It is thought that the cerebellum is vital for this latter component and that there are certain prelearned movement patterns which can be used to allow speed in the learning of new tasks. The cerebellum is thought to be involved in motor learning as well as in the coordination of those movements. Coordination means judgment of the speed required, the amount of force and the distance to be moved, stabilization of the limb or trunk during the movement and gradual relaxation of antagonists during agonist movement.

Anatomy of the cerebellum

The cerebellum is immature at birth and it is thought to be particularly vulnerable to insult. There is some dispute as to when cell division actually stops in the human cerebellum and whether it continues into the first 18 months of postnatal life, but when fully mature it has a surface area of about 1000 cm^2 and like the cerebral cortex, is folded into folia, only one-sixth of the surface being actually visible. There are phylogenetically distinct elements to the cerebellum.

The *archicerebellum* (*vestibular cerebellum*) consists of the vermis, the oldest part of the cerebellum with strong vestibular connections.

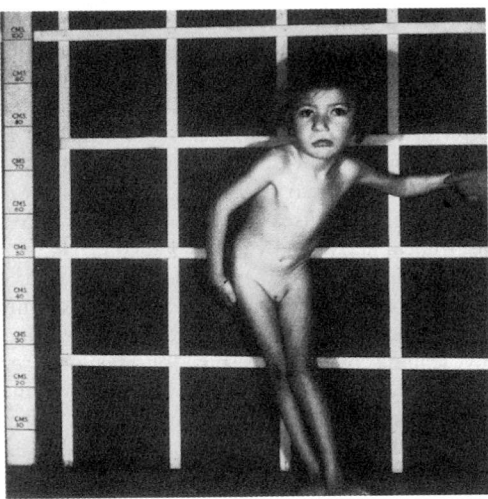

Fig. 14.48 'Windswept' deformity of lower limbs in cerebral palsy.

Table 14.52 Causes of nonprogressive cerebellar ataxia: the ataxic cerebral palsies

Congenital malformations
1. Chiari malformation:
   Type 1 (tonsils only herniated)
   Type 2 (with spina bifida)
   Type 3
   Type 4
2. Dandy–Walker malformation
3. Meckel–Gruber malformation
4. Occipital encephaloceles (sporadic)
5. Genetic vermis aplasia (AR)
6. Joubert's syndrome (AR)
7. Cerebellar hypoplasia (AR)
8. Sex-linked recessive hydrocephalus
9. AR – hydrocephalus
10. Cerebellar agenesis
11. Orofacial digital syndrome with vermis aplasia
12. Facial nevus with vermis aplasia
13. Vermis aplasia with lissencephaly
14. Cerebellar and renal cystic disease
15. Glutaric aciduria with arachnoid cysts
16. Cavernous hemangioma, cerebellar hypoplasia, and coarctation of aorta (3C syndrome)

Genetic ataxic cerebral palsies
1. Ataxia with retinal and choroid coloboma (AR)
2. Ataxia with cataracts and myotonia
3. Ataxia with macula degeneration
4. Ataxia, retinitis pigmentosa, deafness, mental retardation
5. Ataxia – ocular dyspraxia and mental retardation (AD) COMA
6. Ataxia, aniridia mental retardation – Gillespie syndrome (AR)
7. Ataxia, cataracts, mental retardation – Marinesco – Sjögren syndrome (AR)
8. Ataxia, cataracts, deafness, dementia, ulcerated skin, epilepsy, bone cysts – Flynn–Aird (AD)
9. Thyrocerebrorenal syndrome – ataxia, myoclonus, goiter, high uric acid, progressive nephropathy and deafness
10. Ataxia, nephritis, retinitis pigmentosa, skeletal abnormalities
11. Cockayne's syndrome
12. Biemond syndrome – ataxia, short 3 and 4 metacarpals, nystagmus and proprioceptive ataxia
13. Cerebrohepatorenal syndrome – Zellweger
14. Hypogonadism and ataxia (sex linked)

Genetic ataxic cerebral palsies (cont'd)
15. Prader–Willi syndrome (chromosome 15)
16. Angelman syndrome (chromosome 15)
17. Coffin–Siris syndrome
18. Trisomy 4pS
19. Trisomy 20pS
20. Von Hippel–Lindau syndrome
21. Xerodermic idiocy syndrome, microcephaly, mental retardation, ataxia, xeroderma, photosensitivity and hypogonadism (De Sanctis–Cacchione) (AR)

Trauma
1. Birth injury tentorial tears and cerebellar damage
2. Birth injury vertebral arteries (Yates)
3. Permanent postaccidental injury damage
4. Postoperative

Hydrocephalus
1. Postmeningitic
2. Posthemorrhagic
3. Posttraumatic (nonaccidental or accidental)
4. Posttumor
5. Isolated 4th ventricle

Endocrine
1. Cretinism

Vascular
1. Infarction cerebellum – embolic
2. Germinal layer hemorrhage
3. Following inferior cerebellar artery compression in raised intracranial pressure

Hypoxic ischemic
1. Birth asphyxia
2. Near miss cot death
3. Poisoning
4. Near drowning
5. Status epilepticus
6. Following cardiac bypass

Epilepsy
1. Lennox–Gastaut syndrome

The *paleocerebellum* (*spinal cerebellum*) consists of the anterior lobe of the cerebellum and part of the vermis and has strong spinal connections. The main input is proprioceptive from the spinocerebellar tracts, but also from the eyes and the labyrinths. It is concerned with muscle tone, posture and gait.

The *neocerebellum* forms 90% of the cerebellar surface in man. Evolutionally it has developed most recently and is concerned with coordination of skilled movements forming a feedback loop with the cerebral cortex.

The cerebellum is a vast computer of information and has 40 times more afferent than efferent fibers and has more sensory input than the cerebral cortex itself although it is a motor organ. It analyzes the current situation of the muscles of the body from the information it receives via the muscle spindles, joint receptors, pressure receptors, position of the head and its relationship to the body, motion of the body via the labyrinths, information from the eyes and body image and parietal cortex. This allows a total picture of the body's position in space, motion, head position and limb position, as well as the state of contraction of different muscles, to be available if needed to allow a cortical movement to occur. It also allows the movement to be adjusted in speed, force or direction and other parts of the body stabilized against imbalance produced by that movement.

Clinical aspects of cerebellar disease

Disorders of posture and gait may result from an abnormality of input to the cerebellum, disease of the cerebellum itself or interruption of the output. Ataxia will occur in peripheral nerve lesions such as those of the Roussy–Levy syndrome and in spinal cord disease such as Friedreich's ataxia affecting the spinocerebellar tracts and tabes dorsalis or subacute degeneration of the cord interfering with the proprioceptive information arriving at the cerebellum. Vestibular disorders result in gross disequilibrium and frontal lobe lesions may be accompanied by ataxia.

Clinically cerebellar disease can be divided into two main subgroups, truncal ataxia and volitional ataxia.

Truncal ataxia. This is a disorder of posture (standing, turning), tone, locomotion (walking, crawling, swimming) and equilibrium (standing up from lying, rolling, changing center of gravity by leaning over). This type of ataxia is seen in the disequilibrium syndrome, congenital absence of the vermis, vermis tumors (such as medulloblastomas) and some cases of hydrocephalus following perinatal asphyxia.

Clinical disorder of posture. There is poor head control, slow sitting, slow standing without support and inability to get the center of gravity right (head and bottom nonaligned). They cannot stand on one leg or hop and crouch with arms out, touching the floor and may wobble over. There is titubation and head tilt. There is a static tremor and dysynergia with outstretched arms. They cannot walk toe to heel. If the problem is unilateral, the shoulder on the affected side droops. They have difficulty standing still as the center of gravity changes – overswing. If concentration goes or they are distracted, they may suddenly sit.

Truncal ataxia occurs commonly not as an isolated type of ataxia but in association with limb ataxia as part of the generalized cerebellar disorder. The child is floppy, showing exaggerated joint angles so that the arms can be wrapped around the neck in the so-called scarf sign. The elbows can be made to touch behind the back and extension at the elbow is limited by bone and not by muscle tone so that there is hyperextension. The forearms hypersupinate so that the hands can be placed back to back with the thumbs touching each other. In the legs the hips will show passive abduction of 150° or more, straight leg raising is increased and the popliteal angles are increased up to 180°. The heels can be placed at the side of the head or the nose tickled with the big toe. There is slow weight bearing. The tendon reflexes are usually present and because of poor damping secondary to the poor postural muscle tone, are often pendulous. A degree of weakness may be present but this is not as marked as in a myopathy, spinal muscular atrophy or a peripheral neuromotor disease. Development of posture is always retarded so that at first there is poor head control, then gradually truncal control improves so that with support to the thorax and then the pelvis and then without support the child achieves sitting and standing. In severe cases this may mean that the child is 10 or 12 years old before he finally walks. Because of the poor balance the child characteristically takes a long while walking round furniture. Prior to that only one finger held may give sufficient support for the child to stand or take a few steps. Walking round furniture with the hand held and pushing a truck or pram for a long period of time is characteristic of the child with truncal ataxia. The feet tend to be flat with the heel in the valgus position; there is also an associated genu recurvatum. The child staggers when he walks and may suddenly sit on his bottom if his attention is distracted; turning corners is difficult and he tends to sway or wobble and may even get stuck in a corner and not be able to turn round and get out of it. The gait is broad based with the arms out sideways as balancing poles (Fig. 14.49); retropulsion may occur if pushed or walking backwards instead of forwards.

As improvement occurs the base narrows, the arms are no longer held sideways but the child cannot stand on one leg or crouch on his haunches without constantly overbalancing or having to just touch the floor to regain his balance. The speed of walking is slower than normal, the stride length tends to be reduced and double support time is increased. All the parameters of gait vary from step to step, i.e. how long the stride, how high the steppage and the speed of hip acceleration. There is more associated truncal and head sway whilst walking. If standing still there is constant adjustment of posture and sway. If the child has an associated cortical lesion, for example spastic diplegia, the combination of ataxia and diplegia results in paralysis of the tonic γ component which normally causes spasticity, so that he still walks with difficulty, shuffling without a toe-to-heel gait, but showing very brisk reflexes and ankle clonus but not the contractures normally seen in the spastic form of diplegia.

As already discussed, the child may be 10 before he achieves independent walking and in reality he has to 'learn' to walk as opposed to this being a natural innate ability.

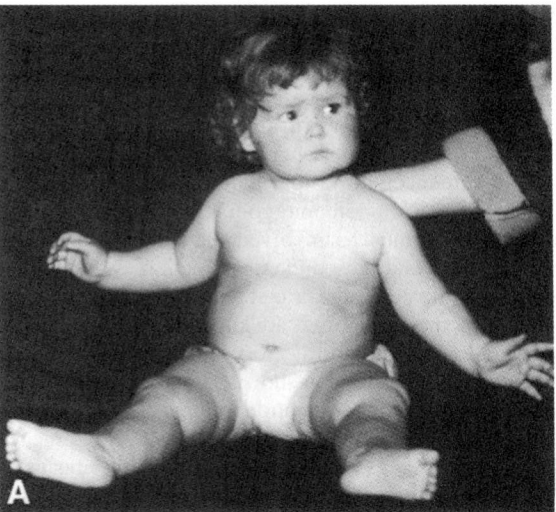

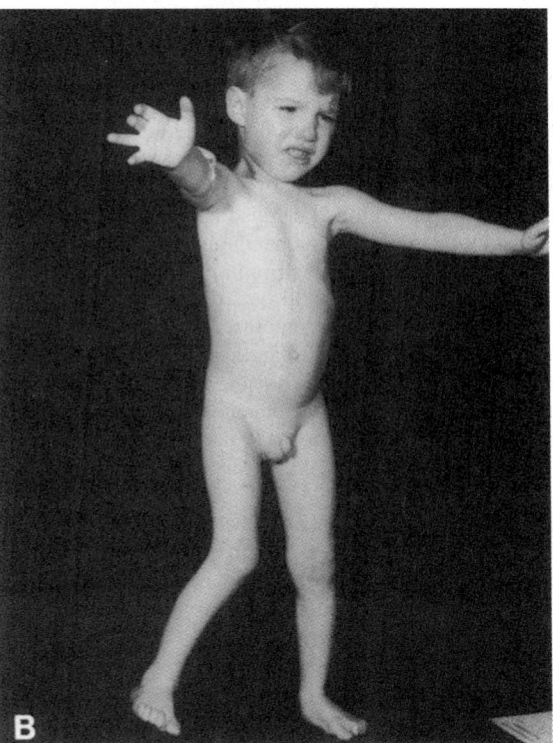

Fig. 14.49 Compensatory balancing movements of the upper limbs in ataxic children: (**A**) sitting; (**B**) walking. (Note broad-based gait.)

The child with an acquired truncal ataxia, for example due to a midline vermis tumor, may appear perfectly normal when lying in bed since the clinical disorder is one of posture and mobility and not one of limb incoordination. A droopy face with drooling is a frequent accompaniment but dysarthria or slow speech development need not necessarily occur with a pure truncal ataxia. Righting reactions may be specifically affected in some children, that is, the ability to roll, get up from lying to sitting and standing up. In these cases the child will walk if lifted on to his feet but cannot get himself up to a standing position if placed lying flat on his back. Another odd feature is that riding a tricycle, climbing wall bars and swimming require less balance than walking and may be achieved and enjoyed by the child prior to independent gait.

Volitional ataxia. The large input from the cerebral cortex via the corticopontine pathways to the cerebellum and then back to the cortex allows the motor engram in the cortex to be converted into a movement with a particular speed, force, distance, direction, relaxation of antagonist and regulation of the lengthening of the muscles involved and stabilization of the body. If the cerebellum is diseased the movement may still be executed but is clumsy with poor adjustment of force, so things are dropped or broken, and speed, so things are knocked over, and in direction, so objects are missed, the trajectory often requiring the constant correction and overcorrection shown as intention tremor.

This shows clinically as intention tremor, which in the adult and older child is tested by the finger/nose test and in the younger child by putting pegs into a board, threading beads onto a shoelace, assembling a Biro or drawing a spiral. Difficulty in judging distance is shown as dysmetria and past pointing. The child tends to grab at an object with the hand approaching at too great a speed, the thumb and fingers abducted until he hits the object and often knocks it over, i.e. misjudges the force and distance required. Speed is abnormal, being too fast and jerky, but there is also difficulty in controlling speed as shown in poor fast tapping of one hand on the other. Starting and stopping a movement rapidly is also difficult, as seen with rapidly alternating pronation and supination, i.e. dysdiadochokinesia. This is also seen as lack of damping in the pendular jerks. Constant correction and overcorrection are seen as rippling contractions of muscles to try and maintain the arms held outstretched in front of the body. This causes jerking of the unsupported limbs which may resemble choreiform movements. More marked jerking is seen as intention myoclonus or as opsoclonus of the eyes in certain cerebellar diseases, especially acquired degenerative diseases such as in Hunt's cerebellar degeneration, the dancing eye syndrome and in the parainfectious encephalopathy described as Baringer's syndrome.

Similar difficulties are seen in speech, as this is explosive and staccato with slurred consonants and a dysarthria.

The other accompaniment in acquired ataxia but absent in congenital ataxia is nystagmus. The limbs are hypotonic but not to the same degree as in the truncal ataxia.

There is an additional component in congenital ataxia in children which relates to the learning of motor skills. Since the cerebellum is part of the motor circuit necessary for the execution of skilled movements, it is not surprising that in the child still acquiring basic skills, diseases of the cerebellum can interfere in motor learning. This is seen especially in speech when the usual speech defect in a congenital ataxia is not a dysarthria but a developmental delay in articulation. The hands also, apart from showing clumsiness, show difficulties in learning as seen with attempts to fasten buttons and laces, assemble objects or learn to use tools. These difficulties are not simply due to clumsiness but to a dyspraxia.

Physiological developmental ataxia

Many of the signs which in the adult would be taken as indicating disease of the nervous system can be normal in children at certain stages of their development. As the cerebellum is a postnatal maturing organ it is not surprising that cerebellar ataxia can be a normal finding at a certain stage of development. A child of 5 months reaches out with a classically dysmetric grasp, bangs his hand against the object then closes the fingers, aims generally in the direction of his face then slides the object down his face using his rooting reflex to put it in his mouth. He misjudges the distance and gags and chokes as he pushes it too far into his throat. Tremor while performing tasks such as trying to put a peg into a hole is normal until 30 months or so. Equally, when starting to walk the child has a broad-based staggering gait with the arms widely abducted and his feet flat. The normal child cannot stand on one leg until the age of 3 years, hop until 5 years or crouch without wobbling until 6 years. Dysdiadochokinesia is normal until 7 years of age. Slowing up of this normal maturation process will result in developmental ataxia. This may be familial or brain growth may be slowed down as a result of prematurity, mild asphyxia or possibly hyperbilirubinemia. Although the child will be slow in the development of walking and postural skills, he will eventually achieve these without any lasting physical disability.

Perinatal causes of nonprogressive ataxia

Damage to the cerebellum resulting in lasting ataxia is especially likely with asphyxia and hydrocephalus. The vertebral arteries may be damaged during delivery of the head, hypoglycemia may affect the cerebellum and bilirubin will affect the maturation of the cerebellar cells. The use of albumin and exchange transfusion for hyperbilirubinemia left a persisting ataxia rather than the choreoathetosis of full kernicterus. Hemorrhage into the cerebellum can occur from tight bands around the occipital region in the neonatal period or from fracture when the occipital bone is bent inwards against the maternal pubis during breech delivery if the trunk is extended before the occiput has descended. Occasionally hemorrhage can also occur in the germinal layers of the cerebellum in a similar way to that seen in the subependymal matrix.

Thyroid hormone is required for cerebellar maturation. Ataxia and myxedema may be seen in older patients. Children with hypothyroidism during the rapid phase of cerebellar maturation in the first 3 months of life may remain with a permanent chronic ataxic syndrome. Intrauterine hypothyroidism may result in permanent damage to the cerebellum so that even diagnosis at birth by TSH screening may be too late to restore completely normal cerebellar growth and development. A further recent interesting association between thyroid and cerebellum is the suggestion that thyrotropin-releasing hormone reverses cerebellar symptomatology in some progressive ataxias.

While asphyxia will cause a severe persisting ataxia this is not common in a pure form and is usually mixed with spasticity and some involuntary movement. Pure ataxic cerebral palsy occurred in only seven of 174 cases of cerebral palsy due to perinatal asphyxia seen in Edinburgh.

Congenital malformation and cerebellar ataxia

Genetic factors appear to be more important in ataxic forms of cerebral palsy than in any other. Difficulties arise in the diagnosis of primary cerebellar hypoplasia.

Malformation of the cerebellum is a common accompaniment of occipital encephalocele or the Meckel–Gruber syndrome (occipital encephalocele with renal cystic dysplasia). Cerebellar hypoplasia is also described in association with noncerebral neurological diseases such as Werdnig–Hoffman disease. The Dandy–Walker malformation (consisting of cystic dilation of the fourth ventricle due to dysgenesis of the foramina in the roof) is associated clinically with an ataxic syndrome. The Arnold–Chiari malformation results in hydrocephalus and causes clinical ataxia–how much is due to the malformation and how much to hydrocephalus is difficult to determine.

Hydrocephalus may be due to other malformations such as platybasia or basilar impression of the skull and is an occasional complication of achondroplasia. There is also a sex-linked recessive form. Certain chromosome disorders such as those affecting chromosome 8 or trisomy 18 may be associated with cerebellar hypoplasia, malformation of the brain and hydrocephalus. The fetal alcohol syndrome may cause posterior fossa malformation and hydrocephalus. Other rarities are familial hydrocephalus with blue sclera, familial nephrotic syndrome and the so-called HARDE syndrome consisting of hydrocephalus, agyria, retinal dysplasia and encephalocele which is of autosomal recessive inheritance. Hydrocephalus can follow intracranial hemorrhage or neonatal meningitis. All causes of hydrocephalus can be associated with an ataxia. This is improved by CSF shunting and blockage of the shunt with resultant raised intracranial pressure can show itself as a sudden increase or reappearance of the ataxia.

There appears to be a peculiar association between the cerebellum and the kidney. Cerebellar cystic disease and renal cystic disease occur together as a syndrome, cystic renal disease and occipital encephalocele occur in the autosomally recessively inherited Meckel–Gruber syndrome, the cerebrohepatorenal syndrome of Zellweger and the association of cerebellar pathology with familial nephrosis has just been described. In the von Hippel–Lindau syndrome retinal angiomas are associated with cerebellar hemangioblastoma and with hypernephromas of the kidney. Both hypernephroma and cerebellar hemangioblastoma are complicated by polycythemia and a metastasis from a hypernephroma in the cerebellum may look like a hemangioblastoma. There is a rare thyrocerebrorenal syndrome consisting of myoclonus, deafness, goiter and progressive nephropathy with a high uric acid and an equally rare syndrome of familial ataxia nephritis with retinitis pigmentosa and skeletal abnormalities.

Complete cerebellar agenesis may occur with very little clinical upset. This is in keeping with the neurosurgical observation that a diseased and malfunctioning cerebellum causes more problems than a cerebellar hemispherectomy.

Genetic causes of nonprogressive cerebellar ataxia

Many of the congenital malformations just described are genetically determined. There is an even larger group of genetically determined cerebellar ataxias not based on obvious anatomical malformations. There is one group of ataxic 'cerebral palsy' which may be dominantly or autosomally recessively inherited. Many syndromes of mental retardation are also accompanied by slow cerebellar and slow cerebral development. Cerebellar ataxias may be associated with eye lesions – for example, cataracts in the Marinesco–Sjögren syndrome, the Flynn–Aird syndrome or the syndrome of cerebellar ataxia, myotonia and cataracts. Abnormal eye movements are seen with Joubert's syndrome, Biemond syndrome, dominantly inherited ataxia and oculodyspraxia with mild mental retardation. Other abnormalities of the eyes are seen in the syndrome of aniridia, ataxia and mental retardation; retinitis pigmentosa often has deafness, ataxia, coloboma of the retina and iris; macular degeneration may be accompanied by ataxia and optic atrophy with ataxia and mental retardation.

Postnatally acquired causes of nonprogressive cerebellar ataxia

The cerebellum is a metabolically active organ. Purkinje cells contain secretory granules which disappear following hypoxic insults, hypoglycemia or severe toxic states such as chronic phenytoin administration, thiamin deficiency, thyroid and autoimmune states. The cerebellum may also show fairly acute atrophy with onset ataxia which remains static for the rest of the child's life, when complicating certain malignancies such as Hodgkin's disease in children. Ataxia may be seen after any prolonged hypoxic episode, status epilepticus, poisoning, drowning and cardiac arrest. Head injury may result in secondary brainstem hemorrhages which may damage the cerebellar pathways and cerebellar hemorrhage into the peduncles and olives resulting in permanent ataxia. Surgery for posterior fossa lesions may leave the child with permanent nonprogressive ataxia after the cause has been successfully treated. Certain disorders may be difficult to classify: for example, is the broad-based, wobbly gait associated with hypotonia seen in celiac disease an ataxia? Certainly the association of the abnormality of gait with the intense irritability suggests that there may be a true toxic encephalopathy (as well as a toxic enteropathy) which may improve on a gluten-free diet.

Dyskinetic cerebral palsy

Dyskinetic cerebral palsy represents less than 10% of all cases of cerebral palsy in childhood in Britain but up to 33% of cases in countries where G6PD deficiency is a major problem. Dyskinetic CP is seen more frequently in a mixed form with varying degrees of spasticity following perinatal asphyxia; 80% of cases are due to perinatal brain damage following jaundice, asphyxia and prematurity. As a rule of thumb it could be said that jaundice produces a pure choreoathetoid form, asphyxia a choreoathetoid form associated with spasticity while prematurity produces rigidity without choreoathetosis.

Causes of dyskinesia include:

- bilirubin encephalopathy;
- hypoxic ischemic encephalopathy;
- neonatal hypoxic ischemic damage;
- carbon monoxide poisoning;
- postcardiac bypass surgery;
- mitochondrial diseases – Leigh's disease/glutaric aciduria;
- genetic syndromes;
- autosomal recessive striatonigral dysplasia;
- DOPA-sensitive dystonia (Sagowa);
- dystonia of prematurity.

Posticteric choreoathetosis

Hyperbilirubinemia in the newborn period has many causes (p. 216). The blood–brain barrier consists of the capillary endothelial junctions together with the astrocytes acting as an intermediary between the bloodstream and the neuron. Any disease which interferes with the endothelial junctions and astrocytes may allow molecules to pass into the brain extracellular space. This occurs with ischemia, acidosis and anoxia, all conditions known to be associated with kernicterus. In asphyxiated neonates yellow staining may be seen in infarcted areas not normally affected in classic kernicterus, e.g. in the region of the caudate and periventricular white matter.

In prematurity an immature glucuronyl transferase system, a low serum albumin, a low pH and a poor blood–brain barrier are claimed to result in kernicterus at low serum bilirubin concentrations, e.g. 200 µmol or less. Some infants who die and have never had any clinical symptoms of kernicterus are found to have yellow staining at autopsy. One does not, however, see clinical neonatal kernicterus or the classic long-term sequelae of kernicterus in the low birthweight infant. The susceptibility to hyperbilirubinemia, a mitochondrial toxin, may only develop when that part of the brain becomes aerobic and oxygen dependent. This only occurs in the cerebral cortex in the last few weeks of pregnancy starting with layer 5 and the basal ganglia after about 30 weeks.

Pathology. The subthalamic nucleus is particularly affected and this may account for the more vigorous choreiform or ballistic movements in kernicterus compared with asphyxia. Less intensely stained are the globus pallidus, dorsomedial thalamic nucleus, corpora quadrigeminae, dentate nucleus, inferior olive, vestibular nucleus, cochlear nucleus and cranial nerve nuclei in the floor of the fourth ventricle. The caudate, putamen and other thalamic nuclei are not usually affected. Any associated areas of infarction will be deeply stained. The pigment begins to fade after a week to 10 days. The staining of cells is eventually replaced by dense gliosis. Cell loss in the subthalamic nucleus is usually early whilst heavily stained areas such as dentate and olive show no eventual cell loss. Children who die subsequently with established dyskinetic cerebral palsy show a dense gliosis of the globus pallidus and subthalamic nucleus.

Clinical features.

Neonatal. As the jaundice deepens, the infant's feeding deteriorates, he becomes irritable and resents handling which may provoke extensor spasms. Ultimately the infant becomes fixed in total opisthotonos. Eye movements are often bizarre with gross sunsetting. Doggy paddling of the arms and cycling of the legs may be continuous, feeding may become impossible due to bulbar paresis and hyperpyrexia, hypoglycemia and respiratory failure culminate in death within a week.

Hypotonic phase. If the infant survives, opisthotonos and tonic fits stop after about a week and the infant begins to regress, behaving as a more immature infant with hypotonia. He is lethargic and there is little spontaneous movement. Visual fixation or following is slow to develop and the infant may be thought to be blind. The development of head control is poor, feeding remains difficult, the infant showing rapid and persistent infantile feeding reflexes and tending to push food out of the mouth so that weaning becomes impossible. The primitive reflexes persist beyond 6 months of age.

Dystonic phase. This tends to appear about 4 months of age or later and is associated with an increase in extensor tone so that the infant adopts primitive obligatory extensor postures. There is sudden extensor rigidity turning to opisthotonos with the legs rigidly extended in equinus when the child is held erect, put on to his back on a firm surface or has the head extended. The arms are extended at the elbow, adducted, pronated and flexed at the wrist. Loud noises, bathing or sitting in a chair may all cause the child to have arching attacks. There is no head control and the child cannot sit without support. Attempts at voluntary movement produce a dystonic response, but this gradually becomes less, mass movements tending to become more discrete and changing from proximal to distal as involuntary movements begin to appear. Changes in muscle tone also become more discrete, affecting one limb rather than the whole body. As the dystonia lessens the child moves into the phase of more discrete involuntary movements and head control and sitting balance begin to improve. Tendon reflexes are usually present, but sluggish. There is no ankle clonus. At the end of this stage the child learns to sit and he can get an object near his mouth without causing generalized dystonic arching.

Stage of involuntary movements. There is still a tendency to go into extension of the legs when suspended with marked extensor thrust when placed erect on the feet, with reciprocal progression movements. Unaided walking is rare before 2 years and the child may be over 7 before he achieves walking without support. Athetosis, with slow writhing, distal movements, fluctuating between hemiplegic and avoidance postures, gradually becomes more and more obvious as the child's sitting and standing balance improves and the mass extensor pattern of muscle tone diminishes.

The classic, fully developed picture is one of a child able to walk, reeling all over the place with gross choreoathetoid movements of the upper limbs, deaf with loss of upward conjugate deviation, marked enamel dysplasia of his teeth which tend to break off at the jaundice line leaving little black stubbles (permanent dentition is not necessarily affected). He remains severely dysarthric and has difficulty with hand manipulation. Intelligence may be well preserved and these are the children who respond dramatically to use of alternative communication systems such as the Bliss symbol system or computer-aided communication. Classic kernicterus or classic choreoathetoid cerebral palsy as a result of uncontrolled hyperbilirubinemia should never be seen with modern perinatal care. It has been suggested that more subtle learning disorders and behavior problems that arise in the premature infant could be due to bilirubin affecting the brain at lower concentrations. This has not been proved and there are many other possible pathological substrates.

Postasphyxial dyskinesia

Carbon monoxide poisoning is associated with cystic necrosis of the basal ganglia with a choreiform syndrome; dyskinesias may follow cardiac bypass surgery and severe dystonia may result from a cardiac arrest. The most frequent cause of dyskinesia is secondary to perinatal asphyxia.

Metabolically and structurally, the infant brain is designed to withstand a certain amount of asphyxia during a normal labor. Oxygen saturation may be very low during a normal labor yet the infant is born crying with a normal Apgar score. Compensation by anaerobic metabolism depends upon availability of glucose or ketones. The infant with intrauterine malnutrition may be deficient in both glycogen and fat so is particularly at risk.

There is more glycogen in the fetal than the adult brain and it can utilize ketones. There are fewer synapses and a smaller area of cell membrane to keep depolarized and it can therefore withstand very low PO_2 concentrations. The brain, however, cannot withstand impairment of its blood supply at any age and ischemia is far more devastating than hypoxia. Hypoxic ischemic episodes in utero are more likely to be prolonged and may last hours or days whereas postnatally they are accompanied by apnea and cyanosis which would demand immediate resuscitative intervention.

Pathology. Perinatal asphyxia may cause mental handicap, epilepsy, learning disorders, perceptual disorder, organic behavior problems, speech or communication difficulties and any type of cerebral palsy (i.e. a hemiplegia, diplegia, ataxia or dyskinesia). There may be any combination of these difficulties which can be mild, moderate or severe. The only way in which a single etiology, e.g. a prolapsed cord, could cause such a widely divergent clinical picture would be by setting up a cascade of different intermediary pathological mechanisms so that different patterns of brain damage could occur even although the etiology is the same. Thus cerebral edema, selective vulnerability, intraventricular hemorrhage, watershed zone infarction, kernicterus or failure of brain growth can all be the clinical manifestations of asphyxia. The basal ganglia are susceptible to asphyxia causing status marmoratus. The 'marbled' state of the basal ganglia is due to an excess of myelinated fibers in what is usually a mass of gray matter (i.e. the putamen, caudate and thalamus) associated with loss of cells and gliosis and it is thought that the excessive myelin is due to an abnormal response of the oligodendroglia which, at term, are just starting to lay down myelin in the area of the internal capsule. If the neurons and their axons are destroyed the oligodendroglia will myelinate any fiber that happens to be there so that the myelination of residual astrocytic processes is thought to be the reason why myelin is laid down in an area of brain that normally consists of cell bodies. The failure of perfusion between the external penetrating vessels and the deep vessels coming up from the perforating vessels and Heubner's artery means that ischemic infarction is particularly likely in the periventricular region (see below). The head of the caudate nucleus could be involved in this, as well as commonly being the site of a subependymal bleed in the small premature infant.

Clinical features.

Neonatal. The infant at birth is usually hypotonic with no response to pharyngeal stimulation, bradycardia and with poor or no respiratory effort. The time to establishment of respiration will vary, but the time to first gasp and to the onset of spontaneous respiration are important pointers to the degree of intrauterine asphyxia. The manifestations of hypoxic ischemic encephalopathy are discussed in Chapter 5.

Postneonatal stage. The mother will usually find that on getting her infant home from the maternity hospital he continues to be a slow feeder and may take up to an hour over feeds. He is irritable, unresponsive, awakens frequently in the night, is slow to fix and slow to smile. No abnormality on examination may be found until about 4 months of age when extensor hypertonus again becomes obvious with fixed 'obligate' asymmetrical tonic neck reflexes, snout reflexes, Galant and progression reflexes. Muscle tone gives apparently good head control in the prone position but is poor in the pull to sit. Moro and grasp reflexes persist. There is failure of appearance of rolling, sitting and parachute responses and at 6 months the infant is classically dystonic, dependent upon position in space, contact with a surface and relationship of head to body to determine posture. This may persist for months or years dependent upon the severity.

The stage of established cerebral palsy. There is continuing feeding difficulty and gradually the picture of a bulbar palsy appears with speech, chewing and biting all affected. The extensor tone pattern becomes broken up in the second year. The arms adopt athetoid postures and movements, the legs remain dystonic with brisk reflexes and ankle clonus and adductor spasticity heralds the appearance of the spastic phase of diplegia. The head may fail to grow after birth. Mental handicap may be mild with a 'locked in' child or it may be profound so that it is very difficult to assess in the first 2 years exactly what level of cognition a 'bright-eyed' child actually possesses. In a few cases a purer choreoathetosis develops without spasticity. These are the exception. In most cases the end result is a mixed spastic dyskinetic cerebral palsy associated with bulbar palsy, mental retardation and microcephaly.

Management of the child with cerebral palsy and chronic motor disability

Assessment and objective measurements of 'muscle tone'

Children with cerebral palsy were often labeled as 'spastics'. This term of abuse suggested increased resistance to stretch of a muscle.

Pitfalls in the treatment of CP arise from the fundamental assumption that the problems of CP are caused by *spasticity* alone, while failing to understand that CP is a comprehensive disorder of the development of movement, posture and 'muscle tone', including dystonia and reflex excitability (Lin & Brown 1992, Lin et al 1994a,b).

Muscle tone is the product of a number of different physical factors acting in concert but constantly changing. Clinically, the appreciation of muscle tone is obtained by assessing the resistance upon passively stretching a muscle which involves rotating a limb about a joint. The factors resisting stretch may be nonelectrical (biophysical) and electrical (neurological) phenomena (Lin et al 1994a) (Table 14.53).

The various ways the muscle is stretched allow measurement of each of these factors. The measurement of tone encompasses many techniques.

Clinical nonparametric rating. Is the tone normal, raised (hypertonic) or depressed (hypotonic)? Does it fluctuate (dystonia) or is it constant (as in physical contracture and lead pipe type parkinsonian rigidity) or is it only evident when the limb is rapidly stretched (spasticity)? The presence or absence of clonus (and its frequency) can be measured. It is important to

Table 14.53 Factors contributing to muscle tone

Nonelectrical (biomechanical) factors
  Elasticity – length dependent
  Viscosity – velocity dependent
  Inertia – acceleration dependent
  Plastic – time dependent
  Contracture – short muscle/short tendon

Electrical (intramuscular and neural) factors
  Myotonia – a slowness to relax due to intramuscular electrical discharges
  Spasticity – increased resistance upon speed of stretch (velocity-dependent stretch reflexes, i.e. tendon jerks)
  Dystonia – fluctuations with changes in labyrinthine input, body contacts and nonspecific afferent inputs
  Posture – voluntary and involuntary, e.g. hemiposture
  Movement – voluntary and involuntary

know whether the abnormal tone and posture persist in sleep, which would indicate the presence of brainstem involvement of a fixed contracture. Rapid eye movement sleep abolishes the influence of the basal ganglia and cortex on the spinal cord. Brainstem damage not only produces abnormal sleep patterns but also affects the diurnal variation in muscle tone: many parents will testify that their hypertonic children become floppy or like rag dolls in sleep, the hypertonic pattern returning each morning. This phenomenon is quite often exploited by the observant parent and physiotherapy team who will use the periods of normal tone in sleep to position the child in ways which offset the production of contractures.

Length–tension measurements. As the stretch torque is increased, so the muscle length increases. This increase can be gauged by measuring the joint angle and plotting this against stretch torque.

Work of stretch and plastic properties of muscle. There is invariable hysteresis in the joint angle–torque plot, the joint angle being greater for any given torque as the torque is incrementally decreased. The area of the hysteresis represents the work absorbed by the 'plastic properties' of muscle. It is thought that this represents the work required to break weak chemical bonds between the sliding filaments and possibly also the noncontractile elements in the muscle.

Stress relaxation, creep and molding (the plastic properties of muscle). Using a constant torque, the muscle appears to reach a given length and then to gradually creep to a longer length (Walsh et al 1994). The increase in joint angle can be very considerable. To prevent creep in the joint angle, i.e. to maintain the muscle at a constant length, it would be necessary to keep reducing the stretch torque over time: this is stretch relaxation. If the stretch torque is removed completely, the muscle only gradually returns to its original length, a process which may take many seconds (muscle molding).

Measurement of muscle stiffness (resonant frequency). A nonspecific measure of muscle stiffness can be obtained by measuring the resonant frequency (RF) of the muscle obtained by sinusoidally oscillating a limb about a joint at gradually increasing frequencies (chirps). Resonant frequency measures can be obtained in hypotonic or hypertonic states (Brown et al 1991), i.e. regardless of whether the muscles are myotonic, spastic, dystonic, involuntarily or voluntarily activated. However, the oscillation is usually perceived as quite pleasurable and may actually be therapeutic in its own right. Also the stiffness will be altered by the history of movement of the muscle owing to changes in the *thixotropic* or plastic properties of muscle (Lakie et al 1984).

Ramp stretching and sinusoidal stretching. Standard pulsed torques can be used to apply stretches at graded velocities which allow measurements of the *reflex velocity threshold* and *velocity gain* of the EMG response generated both monosynaptically and polysynaptically. This can be used as a measure of *reflex excitability.*

Contractile properties of muscle following an ankle jerk. The mechanical contraction and relaxation of the muscle in response to a tendon tap involves the muscle spindles, afferent nerves, α motor neurons in the spinal cord and the voluntary muscles. Isometric measurements of these allows the noninvasive physiological assessment of the interaction between muscle spindle, spinal cord and voluntary muscle in the short and long term. Slow relaxation times of the soleus muscle in children compared with adults have already been reported (Lin et al 1994c, 1996).

A note on the definition and measurement of spasticity in CP

The term 'spasticity' refers to a clinical neurological syndrome characterized by an injury to the central nervous system (CNS) which produces heightened velocity-dependent stretch reflexes, clonus, an extensor Babinski response as well as distal weakness and loss of fine motor dexterity (Lin et al 1994a,b). The mode of onset and the mechanism(s) of this spasticity remain elusive. A 'pyramidal lesion' may occur at any point along the course of a corticospinal fiber: the exact site of the lesion may produce a flaccid or spastic state and the natural history may be to stay flaccid or to become spastic over time. This may arise from damage to associated 'extrapyramidal structures' or to damage to corticospinal collateral projections to brainstem and spinal cord.

Cerebral palsy syndromes comprise a disorder of *movement*, of *posture* and of *muscle tone*. The disturbance of tone may be *dystonic, spastic* or relate to intrinsic *biomechanical* changes in the properties of the muscles, i.e. both the well-understood viscoelastic and the less well-known *plastic* properties of muscle.

The *ideal theory* of spasticity should be capable of describing the phenomenon in clear operational terms, explaining why it takes days or often weeks for spasticity to emerge after spinal or cerebral injury, and finally to offer clues for the rehabilitation of the patient which are likely to be beneficial.

The *ideal measurement(s)* should be simple and relate to the pathological process as well as predict the likely effects of intervention for planning a course of treatment.

The classic models for spasticity have involved the study of the roles of the muscle spindle (intrafusal fibers), type Ia and type II sensory nerve afferents, α-motor neuron, γ-motor neuron (fusimotor) and spinal interneurons. Such studies have established that there is no change in muscle spindle sensitivity to stretch and no evidence for fusimotor overactivity in the production of spasticity. Studies using muscle vibration have established the likelihood of a loss of presynaptic inhibition between the dorsal root afferents and the α-motor neuron, resulting in a lowering in the reflex velocity threshold and an increase in reflex gain to a given velocity of muscle stretch as measured by the electromyographic (EMG) response of the muscle.

Recent studies indicate that changes in the contractile properties of the muscle proper contribute to the clinical manifestation of reflex excitability in relation to short-term muscle stretches in healthy as well as spastic individuals. Muscle unloading results in fast twitchy muscle and increased reflex excitability and clonus (Lin et al 1997), whereas muscle loading produces the opposite effect, i.e. is 'antispastic' and reduces or abolishes clonus. These studies go some way to explaining the natural history of spasticity after acute neurological injury. According to this model, paresis results in muscle unloading and muscular transformation at the level of the sarcoplasmic reticulum and myosin ATPase isoforms to produce fast-twitch muscles, brisk reflexes and clonus over the first few weeks. This phenomenon of muscular change, over both short and long term, can be measured and altered in a variety of ways both to the benefit and detriment of the patient (Barry et al 1994).

Treatments in cerebral palsy

The overall objective of treatment in cerebral palsy is to *improve function* and *prevent deformity*. The improvement in function if they can walk must mean that as a result of treatment they can

Table 14.54 Summary of treatments in cerebral palsy

1. Physical therapies – Bobath, Voitja, Doman-Delicato, Peto, Temple Fay, PNF, high resistance exercise
2. Orthotics – solid and hinged
3. Plaster immobilization – serial casting
4. Drugs – diazepam, baclofen: oral and intrathecal, dantrolene, L-DOPA, nerve blocks
5. Botulinum toxin – intramuscular injections
6. Therapeutic and functional electrical stimulation
7. Orthopedic surgery – single and multiple soft tissue releases with or without bone surgery
8. Selective dorsal rhizotomy – multiple divisions of dorsal sensory afferent rootlets
9. Aids for posture and mobility
10. Positioning program
11. Neurosurgery

PNF = proprioceptive neuromuscular facilitation (Kabat method)

walk further, faster or more efficiently, i.e. using less energy. Prevention of deformity is important as otherwise there is deterioration in function. Not all deformity needs treatment and the 'straightening out' of children with cerebral palsy may seriously decrease function. The successful outcome of any intervention depends on a number of factors and the many therapies, most never scientifically verified, illustrate the fundamental gaps in our understanding of the pathophysiology of CP (Lin et al 1994a,b) (Table 14.54).

The use of physical therapies combined with orthotics with occasional plaster immobilization and orthopedic surgery remain the pillars of interventional management in CP, although much remains to be learned regarding the effects of such treatments (Lin et al 1994c, Barry et al 1994).

Physiotherapy

In the physiotherapy of cerebral palsy many systems have been adopted with religious fervor and yet objective assessments are lacking. Systems include those described by Peto and Bobath and various methods designated as Temple Fay, Brunnstrom, PNF, Rood and Vogt. These methods have the advantage that they offer the young inexperienced therapist specific techniques that can be applied when faced with a young child with cerebral palsy. Each technique can readily be shown to reduce muscle tone, e.g. positioning to reduce primitive reflexes, the local application of vibration or ice to spastic muscles, the avoidance of pressure over extensor surfaces. Certainly anyone dealing with children with cerebral palsy and seeing cases from countries where no treatment is available cannot doubt the value of physiotherapy in preventing the gross contractures which can result from the absence of therapy. Any system should be used in conjunction with a knowledge of appliances, the management of postoperative cases, serial plastering, splinting and the prevention of positional deformity. The physiotherapist is also the person who is seen to actually offer practical help and is therefore more acceptable to the parents than other professionals and may be in a particularly good position to provide support to the family as a whole.

Manipulative methods. Various methods of influencing muscle tone are utilized by the physiotherapist. It must always be remembered that 'cerebral' palsy means that the abnormality in

muscle power and tone are due to release of lower centers and that something, i.e. function, is also lost so changing muscle tone will not necessarily restore that function.

Muscle tone can be inhibited in a child with rigid extrapyramidal dystonia by counteracting the factors which enhance the tone, i.e. contact with surface, relationship of head to body and position in space. If the child is put in a position of flexion with no contact over extensor surfaces and the head is kept flexed in the neutral position muscle tone will be inhibited, making it easier to feed the child, to change nappies and to carry him. This position also allows him to make more use of such voluntary activities as he has by lessening the superimposed involuntary extensor rigidity. Relaxation in children with dyskinetic cerebral palsy can also have a similar effect, as may rhythmic activities such as performing movements to a metronome or a drum or getting the child to walk over footsteps or lines painted on the floor. Inhibition of excess muscle tone in individual limbs can also be achieved by techniques such as stroking or icing the limb or by utilizing reciprocal inhibition (e.g. by using some form of vibrator or vibrating pad) which can be used, for example, to produce contraction of the quadriceps muscle which will then reflexly inhibit the hamstrings and allow increasing extension of the knee. These techniques can be combined with exercises to increase the power of the quadriceps and methods to try and increase the lengthening of the contracted muscle. Intermittent stretching exercises have been the mainstay of the management of equinus deformities for many years. If a muscle is splinted in a shortened position it will adapt to that new length and if splinted in a hyperextended position the muscle will actually lengthen by increasing the sarcomere size and possibly by increasing the number of sarcomeres. Such adjustment of muscle to produce the best functional position is the basis of serial plastering of limbs, e.g. serial plasters can be applied below the knee to prevent increasing heelcord contractures.

Orthotics

Night splints can be expected to work in the same way, i.e. by stretching a muscle over a prolonged period. The muscle needs to be relaxed during the stretch so sleep, medication or botulinus toxin may allow a period of stretch without the muscle fighting back: it is thought that at least 8 hours of stretching over a 24-h period are necessary to encourage increase in muscle length. These measures can also be used to improve the position of the wrist by gradually increasing the range of dorsiflexion.

One management problem common to hemiplegic and diplegic ambulators is equinus at the ankle with toe walking (Table 14.55). This has been revolutionized by the use of plastic ankle foot orthoses.

The newer materials available have increased the range of orthoses available, e.g. the ankle–foot orthosis (AFO) worn within the shoe to control equinus deformity. A good orthotist is essential in the management of cerebral palsy as decisions as to the best material, e.g. polyethylene or polypropylene, the length of the foot plate, the calf height, degree of dorsiflexion, calf cut out or whether hinged are all decisions which, if wrong, may hinder walking rather than help it. Calipers are only rarely indicated in cerebral palsy and are of most use in lower motor neuron lesions, as with polio or spina bifida, or following surgical overlengthening in diplegia. Other forms of splinting include Plastezote jackets to try and prevent positional deformities and to

Table 14.55 Treatment of the equinus foot in cerebral palsy

Stretching exercises

Night splints

In-shoe orthosis – Ankle/foot orthosis (AFO), calflet

Serial casting

Caliper

Baclofen

Nocturnal electrical stimulator

Neurotrypsy

Alcohol into muscle or motor end plate

Botulinus into muscle

Operative lengthening of Tendo Achillis (TA)

Aponeurectomy

Muscle transfer

Table 14.56 Prognosis for walking related to type of cerebral palsy

Hemiplegia	100%
Diplegia (paraplegic)	90%
Ataxic diplegia	88%
Ataxia	88%
Dyskinesia	80%
Quadriplegia	18%

Table 14.57 Prognosis for walking in cerebral palsy related to other milestones

Sit unsupported before 2 years	97%	walk
Sit unsupported 2–4 years	50%	walk (less efficiently ± aids)
Sit unsupported after 4 years	3%	walk unaided
Asymmetric tonic neck reflex and dystonia at 4 years	0%	walk

try and hold the child in acceptable posture during the pubertal growth spurt, particularly to prevent collapsing scoliosis.

Inflatable splints are useful in athetoid children to obtain standing in total body involvement. Various methods of weighting and damping limbs are used in children with impaired extrapyramidal and cerebellar function. Most centers will use a combination of methods: for example, initially a small dose of nitrazepam to relieve the dystonic spasms and later a combination of baclofen with serial plastering and tendo Achillis lengthening together with an intense positioning program. Each child will require a different program personalized to his own needs and generalizations that say children with diplegia should be treated in a particular way are inappropriate as the deformities and their mechanisms will differ between children with the same type of cerebral palsy.

Exercise and mobility

Many children with cerebral palsy are physically unfit. In previous times strengthening of muscle was frowned upon in the false belief that a strong muscle was more spastic. In fact one can exercise a spastic muscle and greatly increase its power without increasing the spasticity. Many children will develop independent walking. This may be with an abnormal gait or with aids such as tripods or a rollator. Other children may only be able to achieve very limited independent mobility, for example getting on and off the toilet, in and out of the bath or around the house, whilst they remain too slow and ponderous for independent ambulation. In the past a wheelchair was often regarded as a sign of failure of therapy but one has only to see the total change in personality of a young child given an electric wheelchair and made independent for the first time to realize that mobility is needed at two different levels. Social mobility may necessitate some form of vehicle but for basic biological activities and movements within a house a chair may be useless, too cumbersome or limiting. A child with cerebral palsy may become mobile in the swimming bath and be able to ride a tricycle before he can walk. Just as the concept of 'total communication' has developed with the deaf child so 'total mobility' packages should be considered in the physically handicapped. He can enjoy horse riding, using the horse's legs instead of his own over rough ground, use a wheelchair in crowded streets where he would get knocked over and tripods or

rollator at school whilst rolling, knee walking or commando crawling may be effective at home. Mobility depends on the type of cerebral palsy and the age at which certain milestones are achieved (Tables 14.56 and 14.57). One would expect all children with a pure hemiplegia to walk unsupported. If there is an associated ataxia or mild abnormalities on the other side then only supported walking may develop. Children with diplegia, if below knee, will all walk with a waddling gait but the more proximal the diplegia, the later walking is achieved (i.e. 4–6 years) and the more support will be needed with rollator, arrow walker or tripods. Eighty percent can be expected to achieve useful mobility. The child with dyskinesia is most difficult. Certain rules apply to all children with CP. If the child sits independently by 2 years most can be expected to walk independently; if sitting is achieved by 3 years 50% will walk with or without support and by 4 years very few and if there is still a persistent asymmetrical tonic reflex, probably none. Children with ataxia may be late and yet achieve independent walking after years of supported walking. Quadriplegic children with a double hemiplegia will rarely walk but diplegias with arm involvement may.

Drugs

The marked extensor spasms which occur with the onset of the dystonic type of rigidity in the small baby may make handling very difficult. As soon as the infant is put into the bath, opens his bowels or experiences anxiety, rigid arching of the back occurs. This can often be lessened by small regular doses of benzodiazepine, such as nitrazepam. Over the years many drugs have been claimed to reduce the amount of spasticity in muscle.

Baclofen reduces the severity of spasticity and the increased muscle tone of dynamic deformities. It will not affect fixed deformities for which some form of plastering or orthopedic surgery is usually required. The main difficulty with drugs such as baclofen is knowing the age at which treatment should start, whether they are safe drugs during the period of rapid brain growth in the first 4 years of life, whether they influence synaptic development and whether they effect sufficient improvement in function to warrant medication in young children over many years. The decrease in muscle tone may result in the child developing different deformities such as increasing internal rotation or being unable to stand when previously he could.

Sodium dantrolene has received less widespread acceptance in children because of the risk of producing severe paralysis or acute hepatic dysfunction. It can also reduce muscle tone and may have beneficial effects in selected cases. Regular assessment and preferably the periodic introduction of a placebo is required to make sure that the drug is still having definite effects.

L-DOPA and tetrabenazine are discussed in the section on dyskinetic disorders and these may have beneficial effects in specific circumstances. It has been claimed that L-DOPA will occasionally produce dramatic results in children with athetoid cerebral palsy. The majority of cases, however, show little response and there may be an increase in involuntary movements as a side-effect. There is no clinical way of predicting whether an individual child belongs to the minority who show a response. Dramatic response should question the diagnosis as to whether a Segawa-type dystonia has been missed.

The use of alcohol injected into the motor end plate was one method of treatment. It has a transient action lasting for several weeks but can lead to quite a dramatic improvement, e.g. the relief of a spastic equinus so that the child is able to undergo a period of intensive physiotherapy whilst able to get his heel to the ground. More recently it has been suggested that alcohol injected into spastic muscles will have a similar effect without causing any muscle necrosis or fibrosis in the muscle and that the injection need not be into the motor end plate.

New treatments for hypertonus in cerebral palsy

Intrathecal baclofen. Baclofen, a GABA-B receptor agonist, was first used in the treatment of spasticity in 1970 at the Prince Henry Hospital in Australia in two quadriparetic and four quadriplegic adults over a 3-month period. The study concluded that baclofen reduced the dynamic sensitivity, reducing muscle spasms in 3/6 and clonus in 2/4 cases without causing weakness. Overall, baclofen proved superior to diazepam (a GABA-A receptor agonist) in 5/6 cases. A further open trial in patients with spinal and cerebral lesions, using larger doses for up to 6 years, demonstrated that baclofen was largely beneficial to those patients with spinal spasticity in whom 87% had improved and in 52% spasticity was 'no longer a problem' so that the limiting factors to mobility were the underlying weakness produced by the paraparesis or paraplegia.

Complications included: dreams, hallucinations or visual illusions 7%, drowsiness 7% and depression, paranoia, headache, blurred vision, nausea and tremor (2% each), i.e. cumulative side-effects were noted in 20% of cases receiving treatment. There were no biochemical or hematological side-effects, but one case attempted suicide by taking 1000 mg of baclofen which produced coma requiring ventilation for 6 hours associated with hypotonia, areflexia and flexor plantar responses. All the features of spasticity returned as the baclofen wore off.

Intrathecal infusions (IT) of baclofen emerged as a strategy of overcoming the central effects produced by large doses and chronic use. The first report showed improvements in six adults who had programmable pumps implanted (Penn & Kroin 1985). Technical difficulties included problems of pump implantation, programming, overdosage causing light-headedness, weakness, drowsiness and loss of consciousness requiring ventilation. Catheter blocks and leaks were also reported.

Trials of IT baclofen have been reported by Armstrong et al (1992) in two ventilator-dependent children with chronic posttraumatic mixed cranial and spinal spasticity, spasms and rigidity. Both children had been given trials of oral baclofen but developed symptoms of sedation. The first case showed evidence of gradual tolerance to IT baclofen which culminated in doubling the daily IT dose from 600 µg/day to 1200 µg/day over a 16-month period. The second case died following a bolus infusion of 800 µg of IT baclofen after a partially beneficial trial of IT baclofen which had necessitated many revisions of the infusion pump concentration and infusion rate over an 18-month period.

Both cases illustrate the complexity surrounding continuous IT baclofen infusions along with the associated morbidity and possible mortality arising from overdosage. These problems cast doubt on the advisability of IT baclofen therapy in cerebral palsy.

Selective dorsal rhizotomy. Unlike IT baclofen, there have been no reported deaths using rhizotomy which has been principally targeted at the child with cerebral diplegia who has already attained walking mobility, is free from cognitive impairments or seizures, has well-motivated parents, access to good physical therapy facilities and shows no evidence of extrapyramidal manifestations (Peacock & Staudt 1990, Park & Owen 1992).

One overt aim of rhizotomy is to treat spasticity 'once and for all' while at the same time preventing the need for multiple orthopedic procedures over many years. Neither aim has been fulfilled as increasing numbers of studies reveal the return of spasticity in as little as a year and the need for repeated orthopedic interventions (Bretas & Dias 1991, Sienko et al 1994).

The prospective follow-up in an observational study of 34 children with 'spastic CP' (24 diplegic, 10 quadriplegic), while showing a reduction in spasticity, also showed 'considerable variability' (McLaughlin et al 1994). Another randomized control study of 24 children, 12 of whom were randomized to SDR, showed no statistical differences in the gross motor function scores of children undergoing SDR: while improvements in stride length, stride time and velocity were noted, the significance of these findings was weak (Shiel et al 1994, Wright et al 1994).

The popularity of SDR is virtually confined to North America. The surgery, which may last up to 8–10 hours, is costly. The target group is that in whom one would expect the best prognosis for walking and the aim of preventing repeated orthopedic interventions or the use of orthotics and aggressive physiotherapy has not been fulfilled.

Botulinum toxin. The use of botulinum toxin, which began with the treatment of blepharospasm, laryngospasm and torticollis in patients suffering from dystonia, appears ideal for the management of dynamic deformities and postures.

Botulinum toxin inhibits the release of acetylcholine from the presynaptic nerve ending of the neuromuscular junction. This effect reaches a maximum over a few weeks but lasts several months. It has the potential benefit of being repeatable if and when signs recur.

An additional advantage is that since the muscle is the final common pathway of all motor activity, botulinum toxin abolishes voluntary and involuntary movements, dystonia, spasticity and reflex excitability. It is therefore suitable for the treatment of dynamic hypertonus of any origin. However, by definition, treated muscles will become weak, if not paralyzed.

Whether or not botulinum toxin prevents contractures remains to be fully established, though early studies of its use in the lower limb for dynamic equinus (Cosgrove et al 1994, Sutherland et al

1994) and for use in the upper limb (Corry et al 1994) appear promising. Long-term effects on the muscle are not yet determined as one is actually trying to produce secondary muscle atrophy and some patients have been shown to develop antibodies which may limit effectiveness.

This chronic 'poisoning' of the muscles is a relatively new form of treatment but botulinum does provide the ability to tailor treatments individually at relatively low cost in a way which proves impossible with conventional orthopedic surgery or rhizotomy.

The risk of systemic poisoning with respiratory failure is small but nonetheless exists, particularly in cases in whom respiratory function is already compromised by poor coordination and spinal deformities.

There seems little point in giving injections every 3 months in order to hold off orthopedic surgery, unless botulinus can be shown to prevent a fixed contracture, as both will weaken the muscle. The main use is in dystonic, i.e. dynamic, equinus when it allows the proper fitting of an AFO or allows stretch by orthoses and night splints on a relaxed rather than contracting muscle.

Surgery (Table 14.58)

Surgical operations have been devised which interrupt structures involved in movement, ranging from the central nervous system down to the muscle itself.

Neurosurgery has only a limited place in the child with cerebral palsy. Great hopes were raised with the use of stereotactic surgery, especially in dyskinetic disorders, but results were disappointing. The cerebral atrophy and diffuse nature of the disease make siting of the lesion difficult and even with modern neurophysiological methods of identifying the particular nucleus in the thalamus, stereotactic thalamotomy has not proven to be of any definite value. Operations on the cerebellum including stereotactic lesions of the dentate nucleus and more recently pacemakers have been used to stimulate the cerebellum. While muscle tone can be

Table 14.58 Principles of surgery in cerebral palsy

- Surgery will not make a child walk
- Surgery may prevent a child from ever walking
- Deformity need not stop a child walking
- Tenotomy may relieve spasticity but grossly weakens the muscle
- Surgery is better for fixed deformity
- Surgery has little part to play in dystonia, athetosis or ataxia
- The primary aim is to improve function, not increase range at a joint
- Combined iliacus and psoas surgery can stop a child walking
- There is a high chance of recurrence if operation undertaken under 4 years
- Always use intense postoperative physiotherapy
- If the operation is for pain, e.g. in hip, the outcome must be absence of pain, not radiological correction of a deformity
- Start at the top of the patient's body and work down, e.g. do not start with surgery for equinus deformity in diplegia as this will cause severe crouch gait, dropped pelvis and lordosis
- Surgery at one joint will have effects on distant joints which may not be predictable. It is better to do a little surgery often
- Soft tissue surgery alone will *not* correct a bony deformity or dislocation
- Obturator neurectomy in a walking child will cause the legs to fly apart and walking is made worse

influenced by stereotactic dentatomy the effects tend not to be long lasting and do not appear to improve function: postural muscle tone may be abolished so that the child may lose, for example, head control. Cerebellar stimulation has not lived up to the initial claims and expectations.

Selective dorsal rhizotomy has already been discussed separately. Peripheral nerve lesions (e.g. neurectomy which is used specifically in the obturator nerve to weaken the adductor muscles) or crushing the nerves (i.e. neurotripsy which can be used in the muscles to the calves to weaken the muscle for a short time) are usually used as adjuncts to some other form of more definitive orthopedic surgery.

Orthopedic surgery can realign the pull of muscles by osteotomy (derotation osteotomies of the femur). The stretch reflexes in muscles can be reduced by tenotomy, e.g. of the Achilles tendon. The most frequent use of orthopedic surgery is, however, for muscles with fixed contractures producing deformities. This is most likely to involve the hip flexors, hip adductors, hamstrings and the calf. Lengthening of the tendo Achillis was by far the commonest operation performed in children with cerebral palsy and whilst this will have a very beneficial effect when performed unilaterally on a fixed deformity in a hemiplegic child, it can have a disastrous effect if performed bilaterally on a dynamic deformity in a diplegic child when the result will be that the child gradually collapses at the knees and may become unable to walk. Toe walking has many causes including dynamic deformity of the calf, spastic deformity of the calf, pes cavus, forefoot equinus or compensatory hip flexion contracture.

Orthopedic surgery in cerebral palsy is used to improve ambulation, improve seating, help nursing and to treat pain or discomfort. Deformity which might lead to irreversible loss of function may be prevented (e.g. scoliosis on ventilation, hip dislocation with secondary acetabular dysplasia) and treated.

Dynamic deformities, i.e. rigid muscles that do not show fixed contractures, or deformities which disappear with anesthesia pose a much more difficult problem and in these cases muscle slide or transfer operations, e.g. transferring the tibialis posterior or half the gastrocnemius muscle to the front of the leg to act as a dorsiflexor, are useful. Orthopedic surgery is considered for all bony and joint problems such as knee capsular problems, dislocated patella, gross valgus at the ankle, hallux valgus, hip dislocation and scoliosis. It should always be considered for fixed deformities. Whilst tenotomy is usually performed for fixed contracture of the psoas, hamstrings, adductor muscles and calf, tendon lengthening or aponeurectomy can be used at the ankle. Excessive lengthening of the tendo Achillis in a nonfixed deformity can result in secondary flexion at the knee and hip and if this is treated by further surgery to the hamstring muscles, increasing hip flexion contracture, increasing lordosis and decreasing function may result.

Measurement of outcome in treatment of CP

1. Technical outcome – X-ray better, reduced tone on measurement, joint straighter with improved range of movement.
2. Functional outcome – improved mobility, communication and independence with the absence of pain. Parents put mobility as the first priority and children (later) communication.

3. Statistical outcome – treated compared to control group.
4. Patient satisfaction – everything possible being done

Associated disorders

Behavior disturbances

In the early months of life a child with brain damage often shows a reverse sleep pattern. This may persist into later childhood with the child at first wanting to sleep during the day and then appearing to require less total sleep, awakening in the night, being difficult to get off to sleep and showing resistance to hypnotic drugs. The infant is also likely to be irritable and slow at feeding. The older child will show a poor concentration span and a decreased threshold for fight and flight so that he may have violent attacks of cataclysmic rage over minor frustrations or panic attacks over mild anxieties.

Educational problems

Many area education authorities have appointed preschool educational visitors to increase the amount of environmental stimulation received by cerebrally palsied children with particular emphasis on the development of concepts of color, number, positions, size, weight, time, etc. A nursery placement is desirable by 3 years of age and it may be possible then to transfer some of the therapy to the nursery. The Warnock Committee recommended that as many handicapped children as possible should be educated in normal schools. Most children with hemiplegias fall into this category. Difficulties arise if a child has a mobility problem, epilepsy, specific learning difficulties or requires physiotherapy, speech therapy or alternative communication systems. These requirements may disrupt normal school life. The child may sit out of PE and games without any alternative provided and may not get the amount of remedial help that he needs. Unfortunately many schools still have difficulty coping with children with simple epilepsy and specific learning difficulties and find it impossible to cope with more severely handicapped children. Unless there is willingness to provide schools with the facilities which are already available in schools for physically handicapped children, improvement is unlikely. For this reason most children with moderate or severe cerebral palsy need to be educated in special schools. The majority of such children are also of subnormal intelligence – in most series only about a third are found to be of average or superior intelligence and between a quarter and a third have an IQ of less than 55. Children with bilateral hemiplegia or a diplegia with involvement of the upper limbs are less intelligent than those with hemiplegia, diplegia confined to the lower limbs or dyskinesia.

In addition to overall decrease in intellectual function, many of the children show specific learning difficulties, especially in arithmetic, and do not attain the level of competence predicted from their IQ.

Visual problems

Squint is very common in children with cerebral palsy and may be paralytic. In 25% of low birthweight infants squint associated with myopia occurs. Optic atrophy is a common finding but is not usually associated with severe loss of vision or visual acuity. A significant percentage of multiply handicapped children have a major degree of cortical blindness, however. Specific difficulties with concepts of space, shape and direction are characteristic of the brain-damaged child and give rise to the classic verbal performance discrepancy on IQ testing. The child will experience difficulty in copying shapes, as in the Bender Gestalt test.

Visuospatial problems by themselves are not a common cause of reading or writing difficulties but produce untidiness (see section on learning disorders, p. 819). Visuomotor disorders are also common. These may include the inability, in the absence of spasticity, to imitate gestures (which may be important if the child is trying to learn a manual sign system), difficulties with fine finger coordination such as fastening buttons or tying shoe laces. This is primarily an associated dyspraxia rather than a visual or proprioceptive problem.

Sensory disorders

A normal child cannot tell differences in weights placed in his hands and does not recognize shapes drawn on his hands or recognize which fingers are touched (finger agnosia). Sensory inattention is common until about 7 years of age. Brain-damaged children are much older before they acquire these abilities so that sensory defects may be diagnosed in a child and yet subsequently disappear. Rejection of a limb and failure to learn volitional tasks have often been attributed to failure of sensory feedback. There is no doubt that children with chronic motor disorders may experience a disordered body image and unlike normal children, will not get the normal feedback from utilizing the limb during the critical periods of parietal maturation in infancy by exploring objects, textures, etc. It is for this reason that many programs include this type of sensory stimulation, e.g. to a hemiplegic limb. The limbs may also show growth disturbance and be blue and cold so that in cold weather, a pair of shoes a size larger than the child needs (to accommodate an extra pair of socks) may be required to prevent chilblains or in extreme cases, loss of toes secondary to ischemia.

Epilepsy

The incidence of epilepsy in children with cerebral palsy ranges between 20% and 50% and it occurs in the majority of patients who suffer from bilateral hemiplegia and in about 50% of patients who suffer from a hemiplegia. It is rarest in children with pure diplegia, ataxia or dyskinesia.

Communication problems

These are outlined in detail in the section on dysarthria (p. 810). The child may suffer from pseudobulbar, hyperkinetic, hypokinetic or ataxic bulbar palsy or a combination of these. Dysarthria occurs in 100% of children with dyskinetic cerebral palsy. In children with ataxia or diplegia following prematurity, a speech disorder is more likely to be developmental than a true dysarthria. The speech therapist should be involved in positioning and feeding from an early age, trying to encourage proper lip closure and bite. Formal speech therapy will be required later and the child may need an alternative communication system such as one of the sign languages, e.g. the Makaton, Paget Gorman or Bliss symbol system, or the Possum type of communication aid. The speech therapist can also help the child with severe drooling in whom a combination of exercises, the use of drugs such as propantheline, biofeedback systems, orthodontic appliances such as palatal lifts or plastic surgical operations such as pharyngoplasty may be needed in individual cases.

Personal and social independence

Along with independent mobility and ability to communicate, independence forms the third element of the triad which we should try to achieve. It is usual to consider independence under the two headings of personal and social. By personal independence is meant the ability to dress, undress, look after personal hygiene, toileting and, in girls, to be able to cope with periods at adolescence. By social independence we mean the ability to use the telephone, go to shops, cook and use kitchen aids. All these skills require training and are helped by a good occupational therapist. Clothing may need to be modified for ease of putting on or taking off, e.g. shoes should be slip-on rather than lacing, buttons replaced by Velcro fasteners. Toilets may need to be adapted with rails, electric flushing devices or self-wiping aids. The house may need modifying with downstairs toilets and bathrooms, ramps or stair lifts, etc.

Assessment

Assessment of every child is necessary in order that a therapeutic program can be worked out for his needs. It is for this reason that assessment units have been established in most pediatric departments. Assessment should always follow diagnosis and should precede therapy and there should be a period of reassessment following therapy to try and evaluate the success or otherwise of the program prescribed and modify it accordingly.

ACUTE ONSET AND PROGRESSIVE MOVEMENT DISORDERS

Acute ataxias

The presentation of ataxia may be acute and dramatic; the child may suddenly be unable to walk. Alternatively reeling and staggering may be so severe that the child cannot sit up unsupported. If the limbs are affected then shaking, dysmetria and incoordination may range from mild clumsiness to complete inability to feed. Nystagmus is a usual accompaniment of the acute onset ataxias and speech is usually dysarthric. Tremors may be coarse and titubation of the head a prominent feature.

Etiology of acute ataxias (Table 14.59)

Infections. An abscess of the cerebellum may occur from middle ear disease or as a metastatic abscess in pyemia or cyanotic congenital heart disease. The eighth nerves, labyrinth and cerebellum may all be damaged in pyogenic meningitis and ataxia may result from postmeningitic hydrocephalus. The classic acute cerebellar ataxia of childhood, which presents with alarming suddenness in an otherwise well child usually under the age of 5 years, is most commonly due to a so-called virus cerebellitis. The child is usually free of headache and may be apyrexial with no meningism. Whether the disorder is due to virus within the Purkinje cells or to parainfectious demyelination is not certain. In some cases there is definite demyelination in the brainstem which may be seen on a CT scan as a low density area. The commonest

and most typical of the parainfectious group is caused by chickenpox (varicella zoster) virus. The ataxia may appear before, during or after the rash and in nearly all cases recovers after about 3 weeks. Occasionally it may persist for a few months and rarely results in permanent sequelae. Other viruses such as polio 1 virus, Coxsackie group B, Epstein–Barr virus, ECHO viruses and influenza viruses have all been incriminated in outbreaks of ataxia. In the case of chickenpox, ataxia is thought to complicate only about three of every 1000 cases. The latest in the list of possible causes of acute ataxia is legionnaire's disease.

Some viruses cause a so-called rhombencephalitis in which ataxia may be present, but lower cranial nerve palsies, especially those affecting eye movements with a degree of ophthalmoplegia and less frequently bulbar palsy, may complicate the picture (Fisher's syndrome). Mumps, measles or the Epstein–Barr virus are the most commonly implicated and the prognosis is not as favorable, with more permanent neurological defects sometimes persisting. Difficulty may occur in differentiating rhombencephalitis from a pontine glioma.

In a typical case of acute cerebellar ataxia of childhood the CSF is clear and may have only a few lymphocytes when associated with mumps, ECHO or polio viruses.

Acute ataxia may occur in certain bacterial diseases when it should be regarded as a toxic encephalopathy, for example in association with diphtheria, scarlet fever and other streptococcal disease and pertussis. A rare cause of cerebellar ataxia with prominent myoclonus, which may persist for 6 months or so, is thought to be a type of parainfectious encephalopathy.

Toxic and metabolic causes of acute ataxia. The classic acute toxic cerebellar ataxia follows alcohol ingestion, but many of the metabolic diseases which cause mental retardation also cause a chronic ataxia and a smaller group may produce an intermittent acute ataxic syndrome, usually precipitated by infection or a sudden increase in protein intake. This latter group of disorders includes Hartnup disease, argininosuccinic aminoaciduria and the intermittent form of maple syrup urine disease, all of which may present with acute ataxia and myoclonus before lapsing into coma in more severe cases. Argininosuccinic aminoaciduria may present as paroxysmal ataxia in an otherwise normal child with only mild cerebellar signs occurring between acute exacerbations. Disorders of the urea cycle associated with hyperammonemia, for example ornithine transcarbamylase deficiency, may also present with recurrent ataxia or fits. Hypoglycemia may present with ataxia or fits before coma supervenes. Of the organic acidurias, disorders of lactate and pyruvate appear specifically to cause an ataxia, for example in Leigh's encephalopathy, when abnormal eye movements, ataxia and extrapyramidal signs are the usual presentation of the acute form. The metabolic basis of Leigh's encephalopathy is not known for certain and it is really an autopsy diagnosis dependent upon finding the Wernicke-type vascular hypoplasia rather than specific metabolic findings at the time of the neurological presentations.

A child under treatment for threadworms may develop acute ataxia from piperazine. Anticonvulsant drugs, especially phenytoin and mysoline, can cause cerebellar ataxia, but CT scans have shown that cerebellar atrophy is much more common in patients on long-term phenytoin than the frequency of ataxia suggests. Exogenous toxins, e.g. lead or glue, must also be borne in mind. Diphtheria toxin may cause an irreversible ataxia. Almost any drug taken in overdose will cause ataxia as well as impaired consciousness.

Table 14.59 Causes of ataxia

---

1. Causes of an acute-onset ataxia

Exogenous toxic causes
1. Alcohol
2. Phenytoin
3. Piperazine
4. Primidone
5. Lead encephalopathy
6. Toluene encephalopathy
7. Diphtheria toxin
8. Tick paralysis
9. Chronic thallium poisoning
10. Histidine with zinc deficiency (treating scleroderma)
11. Organic mercury poisoning (wheat, Minamata Bay disease – fish)

Neoplasms
1. Cerebellar astrocytoma
2. Medulloblastoma
3. Other primitive neuroectodermal tumors
4. Ependymoma
5. Hemangioblastoma
6. Pontine glioma
7. Hand–Schüller–Christian histiocytosis
8. Lymphoma in immunosuppressed

Trauma
1. Secondary brainstem hemorrhage
2. Peduncular shearing injuries
3. Posttraumatic hydrocephalus

2. Causes of intermittent ataxia
1. Mitochondrial encephalopathies
2. Basilar migraine
3. Basilar insufficiency from other causes of basilar insufficiency
4. Cardiac arrhythmias
5. Dominant, familial diamox-sensitive
6. Vestibular neuronitis
7. Lennox–Gastaut syndrome
8. Glutaric aciduria
9. Argininosuccinic aminoaciduria
10. Hartnup disease
11. Hyperammonemia
12. Occipital epilepsies

Endogenous toxic causes
1. Maple syrup urine disease
2. Ornithine transcarbamylase deficiency
3. Argininosuccinic aminoaciduria
4. Biotinidase deficiency
5. Hartnup disease
6. Leigh's encephalopathy
7. Mitochondriopathies – cytochrome oxidase
8. Thiamin deficiency
9. Lesch–Nyhan syndrome
10. 3-methylgutaconic aciduria
11. Kearns–Sayre syndrome
12. MERRF
13. Triosephosphate deficiency

Vascular
1. Basilar migraine
2. Arteriovenous malformations
3. Micro-arteriovenous malformation with hemorrhage
4. Familial, dominant, intermittent diamox-responsive ataxia

Raised intracranial pressure
Acute hydrocephalus from any cause

Infections
1. Cerebellar abscess – congenital heart disease, middle ear
2. Paraviral cerebellaritis:
   poliovirus
   ECHO virus
   Coxsackie virus
   influenza virus
   varicella-zoster virus
   Epstein–Barr virus
3. Baringer syndrome
4. AIDS
5. Postmeningitis
6. Epidemic labyrinthitis
7. Acute ataxia with *Legionella* pneumonitis
8. Acute rhombencephalitis – mumps
9. Tuberculoma

Hypersensitive/immune
1. Multiple sclerosis
2. Hyperimmune thyroiditis
3. Paraneoplastic degeneration
4. Kinsbourne's syndrome
5. Post-Hodgkin's ataxia
6. Parainfectious demyelination

Other
Benign paroxysmal upward tonic gaze with ataxia

Tumors/raised intracranial pressure. The onset of ataxia in a child should always raise the strong suspicion of an intracranial tumor until proved otherwise. Brain tumors are the second most common of the malignancies seen in childhood and posterior fossa tumors are common. Medulloblastoma, cystic astrocytoma of the cerebellum, hemangioblastoma, fourth ventricular ependymomas and pontine gliomas all occur in childhood and ataxia is one of the most common clinical presentations. The histiocytic reticuloses may metastasize to the cerebellum, e.g. Hand–Schüller–Christian disease. Leukemia associated with raised intracranial pressure and cerebellar bleeding can be complicated by an ataxic illness. Long-term immunosuppression used to treat malignancies (such as leukemia and Hodgkin's disease) can result in carcinoma, microgliomas or odd lymphoid tumors. Sarcoidosis of the central nervous system is associated with meningeal infiltration, strangulation neuropathies of the cranial nerves (for example, bilateral seventh nerve palsy) and ataxia. Certain genetically determined conditions, for example Fanconi's anemia, Bloom's syndrome or ataxia telangiectasia, are associated with abnormal DNA repair mechanisms and with chromosome breaks, especially of chromosomes 7 and 14; these

conditions have a high incidence of malignancy so that cerebellar tumors such as medulloblastoma can complicate a condition such as ataxia telangiectasia when there is already an explanation for the child's ataxia. Raised intracranial pressure for whatever reason (including cerebellar tumors) will cause ataxia and this may be relieved by shunting. Neuroblastoma in young infants may also be associated with a paraneoplastic syndrome of ataxia, opsoclonus and choreiform movements, the so-called dancing eye syndrome. This syndrome is thought to be so characteristic that, even if catecholamine studies are normal, a body scan should be performed to examine the region of the suprarenal gland, as the syndrome may be seen in association with a maturing ganglioneuroma.

Miscellaneous causes of acute ataxia. Vascular causes of ataxia in children are uncommon, although arteriovenous malformations and cerebellar hemorrhage from microvascular malformations are seen. Hemorrhage into a benign astrocytoma may be responsible for an acute and possibly fatal cerebellar syndrome. Basilar embolism in congenital heart disease will result in cerebellar infarction that, if not immediately fatal, will cause acute ataxia. Basilar migraine, especially in the preschool years, can present as recurrent vertigo, drop attacks and ataxia. Head injury with secondary brainstem hemorrhage is a common cause of ataxia which may persist for 6 months or more but has a good tendency to recover in the young child. In the older child disseminated sclerosis must be borne in mind and is a difficult diagnosis to substantiate with the first episode.

Familial paroxysmal ataxias. A dominantly inherited familial disorder starting as early as 2 years and tending to be worst in the childhood years than after the age of 15 is described. There is a sudden onset of a reeling gait with intention tremor and dysarthria, occasionally accompanied by vomiting and nystagmus. The attack lasts from several days to a month and then clears completely. In adults the episodes are briefer and last only a couple of days. One family contained 206 members in five generations and 35 had ataxic episodes. Virus infections or mild trauma may precipitate attacks in predisposed individuals. No biochemical abnormality has been recognized in the dominant form of the disease.

A subgroup of this type of hereditary, autosomal dominant, paroxysmal ataxia last minutes to several hours and occur several times a week or a few times per year and may show marked diamox (acetazolamide 250 mg b.d. or t.d.s.) sensitivity which abolishes the ataxia. The presence of diplopia, vertigo, vomiting and ataxia means that it is easily confused with basilar migraine or paroxysmal vertigo.

Progressive ataxias

Progressive ataxia in children may present a difficult diagnostic problem. There are a vast number of rare diseases, many of which even in a specialist unit may be seen only once in a professional lifetime (Table 14.60). It is important to continue to study these

Table 14.60 Conditions with chronic progressive ataxia in childhood

1. Friedreich's ataxia
2. Marie's ataxia
3. Olivo Ponto cerebellar degeneration
4. Fazio–Londe syndrome
5. Hunt's cerebellar degeneration with myoclonus
6. Leigh's encephalopathy
7. Pyruvate dehydrogenase deficiency
8. Lipoamide deficiency
9. Abeta-lipoproteinemia
10. Metachromatic leukodystrophy
11. Late infantile Batten's disease
12. Adult type GM1 gangliosidosis
13. Type 3 GM2 gangliosidosis
14. Menkes' cerebral and cerebellar degeneration
15. Déjérine–Sottas proprioceptive ataxia
16. Roussy–Levy syndrome
17. Refsum's syndrome
18. Pelizaeus–Merzbacher syndrome
19. Central pontine myelinosis
20. Hippel–Lindau syndrome with hemangioblastoma
21. Ataxia telangiectasia
22. Progressive neuraxonal dystrophy with spheroids
23. Juvenile tabes dorsalis
24. Lennox–Gastaut syndrome

diseases as only in this way will prevention through antenatal diagnosis or treatment become possible. Some conditions may have an acute onset and leave the child with a nonprogressive ataxia (i.e. cerebral palsy) and others may progress so slowly, for example Pelizaeus–Merzbacher disease, that it is not recognized for many years as being progressive so that again the child is considered to have 'cerebral palsy'. Other progressive disorders may eventually appear to burn out, for example ataxia telangiectasia.

Heredodegenerative ataxias

These genetic disorders are associated with a progressive clinical ataxia. Problems in classification have arisen because it has now been discovered that some have a biochemical basis. In some diseases several parts of the nervous system undergo degeneration together, so that it may be difficult to classify conditions as peripheral neuropathy, ataxia, familial paraplegia, anterior horn cell degeneration, optic neuritis, progressive deafness or progressive dyskinesia. Each part of the central nervous system may undergo a pure degenerative disorder, as in Leber's optic atrophy, peroneal muscular atrophy, progressive dentate degenerations and familial spastic paraplegia, or else may be involved as part of a multisystem degenerative disease in which literally any combination may occur.

The clinical ataxia, which is the basis of classification of the progressive degenerative group of ataxias, may be due to lesions in the cerebellum with loss of Purkinje cells in the cerebellar nuclei such as the dentate degenerations, olivary atrophy, spinocerebellar tract degeneration, posterior column demyelination and peripheral nerve lesions with a sensory neuropathy. In other conditions when eighth nerve damage, deafness and disequilibrium result, unsteadiness may be due to loss of afferent vestibular input. It is thus necessary to investigate vestibular, cerebellar, proprioceptive and peripheral nerve function in all cases.

Friedreich's ataxia

Since Friedreich described an ataxic syndrome in 1863, there has been difficulty in defining its limits. Charcot–Marie–Tooth disease and Roussy–Levy syndrome are frequently confused with Friedreich's ataxia and this is made more difficult as there are many families with their own variants (for example the French-Canadian variant). This may not have made any great difference to routine clinical practice in the past, but among these disorders the genetics and prognosis are different and if we are to try and identify the biochemical basis of these different types, we need to be sure we are comparing like with like.

Genetics. Although a dominant form of Friedreich's ataxia has been described in the past, only autosomal recessive inheritance is now accepted. The dominantly inherited form is most likely the Roussy–Levy type of hereditary motor and sensory neuropathy (HMSN type 1, p. 722) identified with a gene on chromosome 9 in the pericentromeric region. Antenatal diagnosis using linkage analysis is possible.

Pathology. The main pathology is in the spinal cord with degeneration and demyelination in the posterior columns, corticospinal pathways and the spinocerebellar tracts.

Clinical features. Although ataxia in a child in puberty (mean 10–12 years) is the common presenting feature it may come on for the first time in the preschool years and very rarely after the teens.

Occasionally cardiomyopathy or scoliosis may present before the ataxia. Incoordination affects both limbs and gait: it is accompanied by nystagmus in only 20% of cases but speech is affected eventually in 100% (46% have a moderate or severe dysarthria early in the disease). The corticospinal pathways are involved in 90% of cases with extensor plantar responses and weakness but absent knee and ankle jerks. The absent jerks are now regarded as a hallmark of Friedreich's disease and any patient with brisk tendon reflexes would be regarded as having some form of variant. Posterior column involvement shows as loss of position and vibration sense but although this is an absolute finding in a patient with long-standing disease, these signs may be absent on initial presentation. The limbs also show distal wasting, affecting the calf muscles in the leg and small muscles of the hand. This is common in the late stage of the disease but if marked at presentation, peroneal muscular atrophy should be suspected. Pes cavus with clawing of the toes and forefoot equinus is usual (Fig. 14.50). Scoliosis is present in more than three-quarters of cases and can be extremely severe and the cause of death from secondary cardiorespiratory embarrassment.

The heart is not uncommonly involved and may be the presenting feature with angina, palpitations and dyspnea on exertion accompanied by an abnormal ECG which shows left ventricular preponderance and supraventricular extrasystoles. The myocardium shows interstitial fibrosis with little cellular reaction and secondary fiber-type hypertrophy resembling chronic ischemia or hypertrophic cardiomyopathy. Sudden chest pain, a rise in enzymes such as creatine phosphokinase and an infarct pattern on the ECG may occasionally be seen in young teenage children with Friedreich's disease. Murmurs are common and may arouse suspicion of left ventricular outlet obstruction or ruptured papillary muscles.

Although optic atrophy (finding pale discs) on ophthalmoscopy is present in 33% of cases, visual symptoms are not usually a major complaint. Deafness may be a rare complication due to peripheral sensory nerve involvement.

Prognosis. The patient is usually chairbound by the mid-20s but

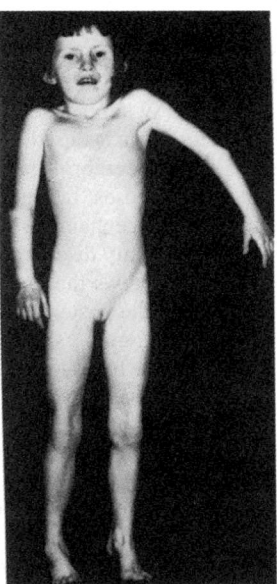

Fig. 14.50 Friedreich's ataxia showing ataxic stance and foot deformity.

survival to the late 60s is possible. Death is more likely from chest complications and severe scoliosis. Heart failure is unusual. The mean age of death is 37 years with a range of 21–69 years.

Biochemistry. The fact that Friedreich's disease is inherited as an autosomal recessive trait strongly suggests that it has a metabolic basis; 10% of cases develop diabetes mellitus. Disorders of carbohydrate metabolism, especially at the site of entry of the pyruvate into the Krebs cycle, have been suggested as the basic cause, especially as enzymes such as pyruvate dehydrogenase, pyruvate carboxylase, oxoglutarate dehydrogenase and thiamin inhibitors have all been associated with various types of progressive ataxia. In view of the similarity to abetalipoproteinemia, lipid metabolism has been extensively investigated but no conclusive abnormalities found. Vitamin E deficiency has been implicated in certain families and vitamin E levels should be checked. Because of the known rise in alanine concentration in certain metabolic disorders associated with intermittent ataxia, amino acid metabolism has been looked at in great detail. No unequivocal biochemical system has so far been incriminated and there is no biochemical marker that can be used as a diagnostic criterion or for antenatal diagnosis. Full biochemical investigation should, however, be performed in children presenting with Friedreich's ataxia as the difference between Friedreich's disease and abetalipoproteinemia or some of the disorders of lipoamide metabolism cannot be made on a clinical basis. Nerve conduction studies show that there is a normal rate of motor nerve conduction but a definite reduction in sensory conduction velocity. Brainstem auditory evoked potentials are abnormal in many more patients than show clinical deafness and these may be helpful additional investigations in arriving at a diagnosis.

Management. Various diets have been suggested in the light of presumed biochemical basis for the disease, but there is no convincing evidence of their efficacy. The management is that of a progressive motor handicap, the most difficult decision being usually when or if surgery for the scoliosis should be attempted. Care must be taken to avoid hypovolemia during surgery in the presence of cardiomyopathy. The question of the use of β blockers in cardiomyopathy is discussed on page 634. As with other ataxias, once gait has deteriorated to the point of wheelchair mobility the condition appears to become more static provided secondary skeletal deformity is controlled.

Metabolic disease and cerebellar degeneration

A progressive spinocerebellar degeneration has been described as the presenting feature of chronic GM2 gangliosidosis. All cases were Ashkenazi Jews and all had β-hexosaminidase A deficiency. Abetalipoproteinemia mimics Friedreich's disease. Lipoamide dehydrogenase has been described as a possible cause of a similar Friedreich-like disease. The enzyme is low in fibroblasts and in fresh platelet-enriched fractions of blood. Ataxia is a prominent symptom of pyruvate dehydrogenase and pyruvate carboxylase deficiencies. Dehydrogenase deficiency may be restricted to the brain when hypotonia, myoclonic epilepsy, marked ataxia, delay in walking, marked nystagmoid movements and Cheyne-Stokes types of respiration form the clinical constellation of signs and symptoms. In this pure cerebral form the CSF lactate and pyruvate are increased and only the gray and white matter of the brain show grossly abnormal metabolism, whereas in the usual type of metabolic acidosis plasma lactate and pyruvate are increased in association with abnormal pyruvate metabolism in the liver and fibroblasts. There is also a slowly progressive form of pyruvate dehydrogenase deficiency when an elevated plasma lactate and pyruvate together with a raised plasma alanine may present as spinocerebellar degeneration in the 5–15 age group.

Progressive ataxia in association with peripheral neuropathies

Roussy–Levy syndrome (HMSN type 1). See page 722.
Metachromatic leukodystrophy. See page 776.
Déjérine–Sottas syndrome (HMSN type 3). See page 723.
Peroneal muscular atrophy. See page 722.
Refsum's syndrome. See page 785.
Mitochondrial myopathy. See page 787.

Central progressive cerebellar ataxias

Most of the ataxic syndromes so far considered have been due to failure of proprioceptive information reaching the cerebellum as a result of peripheral nerve or spinocerebellar degeneration. In the degenerative diseases such as metachromatic leukodystrophy, GM1 gangliosidosis, GM2 gangliosidosis and Batten's disease, all levels of the nervous system are affected and sooner or later dementia with ataxia will dominate the picture. Neuroblastoma and Hodgkin's disease may be associated with persistent ataxia and show cerebellar atrophy on CT scanning. Macroglobulinemias can also be a cause of progressive ataxia.

There are a group of spinocerebellar degenerations, olivopontine degenerations and pontocerebellar atrophies which are more common in adults and are based on triple codon repeats. Spinocerebellar ataxia type 1 is a CAG repeat, normally 30–35 and in disease 40–80 repeats, on chromosome 6 with a gene product called ataxin 1. Dentatorubral-pallidoluysian atrophy is also a CAG repeat on chromosome 12.

Ataxia telangiectasia. Ataxia telangiectasia clinically shows a mixture of telangiectasia (particularly of the conjunctiva) and ataxia. The finding of a very low level of IgA in the blood, together with the recurrent chest infections common in the syndrome and a very high risk of neoplasia, have led some authors to include it as an immunological deficiency state rather than a neurodermatosis.

Pathology. In the central nervous system the main finding is the loss of Purkinje cells in the cerebellum. There may also be demyelination in the posterior columns of the spinal cord, but this does not seem to be associated with clinical loss of position and vibration sense and the ataxia seems definitely cerebellar and not proprioceptive in type. There may be enlarged venules in the cerebellar meninges.

Ataxia telangiectasia is inherited as an autosomal recessive character and there is now known to be a defect on chromosome 11q22–23. There are reported cases with aminoaciduria and abnormal carbohydrate metabolism. Immunological deficiencies in ataxia telangiectasia are varied. Immunoglobulins may be normal or there may be a reduction in IgA, IgG or IgE. The thymus is hypoplastic and thymic hypoplasia with abnormal T cells causes cellular immunity to be impaired. There may be an abnormal macroglobulin in the serum. The response of cultured lymphocytes to blast transformation by phytohemagglutinin is also impaired. There does not appear to be a clear relationship between clinical infections and immunological state. Thymec-

tomy in rats results in ataxia with low IgA levels. IgA may be low in Still's disease, disseminated lupus erythematosus and some cases of malabsorption, as well as in one in 700 normal people. In ataxia telangiectasia there is an increased risk of tumor formation, particularly reticuloses (lymphosarcoma, Hodgkin's disease, reticulum cell sarcoma) and medulloblastoma. There may be chronic ulcerated skin granulomas. On tissue culture there are odd breaks in chromosomes 7 and 14 and translocations at the points coding T cell and immunoglobulins in white cells which could predispose to neoplasia. There may be associated abnormalities of testes or ovaries.

Clinical findings. The ataxia is present from early childhood and is often mainly truncal at first so that the child is slow in walking independently, but may walk around furniture for a long time. He is hypotonic. The ataxia increases very slowly. Intention tremor appears but the child is usually 4–5 years of age before any progressive disease is suspected. Recurrent chest infections or infections of the upper respiratory tract are common but are not invariable. The ataxia is made worse by the appearance of involuntary movements around school age. The child may be thought to have a nonprogressive ataxic cerebral palsy. He may be referred because his writing and drawing are deteriorating. The involuntary movements progress to frank choreoathetosis. The intellect is initially normal, but appears to regress as the disease progresses. There is no loss of voluntary power although there is coordinating defect. The plantar responses are usually flexor. There is a severe dysarthria. The children themselves are usually pleasant, equable and good-natured. There are marked defects in eye movements with poor conjugate gaze, nystagmus and sometimes ophthalmoplegia. The commonest ocular finding is, however, an oculomotor apraxia which is always very suggestive of ataxia telangiectasia. Although conjunctival telangiectasia may appear at any time in childhood it usually shows itself at the age of 5 years or more. Once it has appeared it steadily increases in extent. It begins on the bulbar conjunctiva as prominent tortuous vessels and eventually spreads into a butterfly distribution on the cheeks, ears, elbows and popliteal fossa. It is thought to be predominantly a venous telangiectasis. Confusion can occur in the occasional case who also presents with *café-au-lait* spots.

Diagnosis and differential diagnosis. Diagnosis is easy with the fully established picture. The low IgA levels may be diagnostic after the neonatal period but are low in normal children in the first year of life. There is defective switching from IgM to IgA and IgG with infection. Serum α-fetoprotein is raised. Differential diagnosis is from hypotonic forms of cerebral palsy, spinocerebellar degeneration, other neurodermatoses, tumor and other brainstem degenerations such as Leigh's encephalopathy. The aminoaciduria may raise the possibility of Hartnup disease, but the skin features are different. MRI or CT scan shows that the cerebellum is small and there is increase in CSF in the posterior fossa. Tomograms of the chest show that the thymic shadow is diminished. Chromosomes may show multiple breaks with 7–14 translocations. The chromosomes show great sensitivity to X-rays or bleomycin.

Treatment is aimed at control of the recurrent infections. The ataxia and choreoathetosis progress so that the child is very often chairbound by adolescence. There is wide variation between families in the rate of progression of the ataxia, some being still mobile at 30. In some families all sibs develop malignancies, in others, all get infections. These children are very sensitive to radiotherapy and careful consideration should be given before this is embarked upon to treat secondary malignant disease. A careful diary should be kept of the amount of radiation from diagnostic imaging which should be kept to a minimum; MRI must now be used instead of CT. The sensitivity of the cells in tissue culture to irradiation is being investigated as a possible means of antenatal diagnosis and a confirmative test in difficult cases.

α-lipoprotein deficiency (p. 1150). This is a genetically determined disorder involving cholesterol storage. A neuropathy has been described with peripheral nerve involvement resulting in weakness, wasting and diminished reflexes; electromyographic abnormalities show denervation. Numbness is also present with sensory loss.

Abetalipoproteinemia (p. 790). The neurological picture in this disease may resemble Refsum's syndrome with cerebellar ataxia, posterior column loss, peripheral neuropathy and retinitis pigmentosa. The electromyogram may show slowed nerve conduction and denervation. It has been suggested that the steatorrhea results in poor vitamin E absorption and since vitamin E is carried by β-lipoprotein, it may be absent from the blood. The neurological signs could be associated with this. A clinical difficulty is that children with celiac disease often appear to have a truncal ataxia with hypotonia which may be part of the celiac toxic encephalopathy.

Extrapyramidal disorders: dyskinesias

In clinical practice there are a large number of diseases which affect specifically the basal ganglia, in which there is no spasticity or loss of underlying volitional movement, but in which involuntary movements and abnormal muscle tone are prominent (Table 14.61).

Anatomical considerations

The extrapyramidal system in classic neurology consists of part of the cerebral cortex anterior to the motor strip and several masses of gray matter deep in the white matter of the hemisphere and the upper brainstem. The nomenclature has been rather confusing as words such as basal ganglia, striatum, corpus striatum, lenticular nucleus are either synonyms or groupings of nuclei. The corpus striatum is a name given to the lentiform nucleus (i.e. the combined putamen and globus pallidus) and the caudate nucleus. It is more appropriate to think in terms of the caudate, putamen and globus pallidus in the cerebral hemisphere together with the substantia nigra in the upper brainstem and the subthalamic nucleus of Luys as constituting together the basal ganglia.

Table 14.61 Choreiform conditions

1. *Acute-onset choreiform disease*
    Sydenham's chorea
    Toxic dystonic/chorea
    Phenothiazines – chlorpromazine (Largactil), trifluoperazine (Stelazine), fluphenazine (Moditen), thioridazine (Melleril)
    Phenytoin
    Carbamazepine (tics and dystonia)
    Maxolon
    Prochlorperazine (Stemetil)
    Lithium
    Tricyclics – amitriptyline
    Manganese poisoning
    Thallium poisoning
    Hydrogen sulfide
    Fentanyl
    Propofol
    Serotonin reuptake inhibitors – paroxetine
    Bethanecol
    High estrogen contraceptive pill
    Lamotrigine
    Chorea gravidarum
    Chorea and the contraceptive pill
    Chorea and lupus erythematosus
    Chorea and Henoch–Schönlein purpura
    Hemolytic uremic syndrome
    Hypoparathyroidism
    Paroxysmal kinesiogenic dystonia
    DOPA-sensitive dystonia (Segawa)
    Carbon monoxide poisoning
    Following cardiac bypass surgery
    Postdialysis dyskinesia
    After burns – burns shakes
    Metabolic diseases – Leigh's disease
    Familial paroxysmal choreoathetosis
    Infections
    Encephalitis lethargica
    Toxoplasmic encephalitis
    Coxsackie, echo and varicella encephalitis
    Haemophilus influenzae B meningitis
    AIDS encephalopathy
    Neurosyphilis
    Epidemic rubeola

2. *Progressive diseases*
    Huntington's chorea
    Idiopathic torsion dystonia
    DOPA-sensitive dystonia of Segawa
    Metabolic
    Wilson's disease
    Glutaric aciduria
    Phenylketonuria
    Leigh's encephalopathy (see later)
    Mitochondrial diseases MELAS, MERRF
    Homocystinuria
    Triosephosphate isomerase deficiency
    Sulfite oxidase deficiency
    Methylmalonic acidemia
    Dihydropteridine reductase deficiency
    Hexosaminidase A and B deficiency (onset 10 years with dystonia)
    Lesch–Nyhan syndrome
    Lysosomal enzyme disorders – G_{M1}, G_{M2}, Krabbe and metachromatic leukodystrophy
    Fahr's syndrome (basal ganglia calcification)
    Hypoparathyroidism
    Infectious origin
    SSPE
    AIDS encephalopathy
    Infantile bilateral striatal necrosis
    Hallervorden–Spatz disease
    Ataxia telangiectasia
    Ataxia with ocular dyspraxia (Aicardi)
    Pelizaeus–Merzbacher disease
    Familial dystonic paraplegia
    Paroxymal dystonia with myoclonus
    Paroxymal sleep dystonia
    Neuraxonal dystrophy
    Parkinson's disease
    Hunt's juvenile parkinsonism (striatonigral degeneration)
    Hunt's pallidocerebellar degeneration
    Pilocytic astrocytoma

3. *Chronic nonprogressive disease (cerebral palsies)*
    Bilirubin encephalopathy
    Hypoxic ischemic encephalopathy
    Autosomal recessive striatonigral dysplasia
    Dystonia of prematurity

The basal ganglia can be regarded as a major motor computation center receiving information from the cortex about movements being planned together with information from the parietal cortex about body image and from vision. They receive input regarding the force, speed and direction of movement planned by the cerebellum together with information on the position of the head and eyes from the labyrinth and information about body contact and visual information on the position of the body in space. The basal ganglia and extrapyramidal motor cortex inhibit certain primitive brainstem reflexes such as the asymmetrical tonic neck reflex, primitive walking and swimming reflexes.

Biochemistry and the basal ganglia

The basal ganglia are particularly susceptible to hypoxia. This is seen in carbon monoxide poisoning, neonatal asphyxia or postbypass states. Heavy metals also appear to have a special affinity for this part of the brain (e.g. copper deposition with Wilson's disease, iron deposition in Hallervorden–Spatz disease or the dyskinesias of manganese, molybdenum or thallium poisoning). Metabolic diseases such as untreated phenylketonuria, Leigh's encephalopathy and glutaric aciduria may present with a predominant dyskinetic clinical picture. The main interest in biochemistry of the basal ganglia stems from the discovery of the dopaminergic pathways from the substantia nigra, the effects of L-DOPA in parkinsonism and the study of the extrapyramidal side effects of drugs like the phenothiazines.

Classic parkinsonism has three components – tremor, bradykinesia and rigidity – and although the symptoms and signs of basal ganglia disease will be discussed in more detail later, it is necessary to consider some aspects to understand the role of dopamine and L-DOPA in normal basal ganglia function and in disease. The three components appear independently determined because the tremor may be made worse by L-DOPA but helped by surgery; the bradykinesia is helped by L-DOPA but surgery has no effect; the rigidity is helped by L-DOPA and surgery and is especially helped by anticholinergics. Current evidence suggests that cholinergic, serotonergic and gabanergic pathways are normally balanced (inhibited) by dopamine and that while dopamine is important in inhibiting rigidity, it is involved in the causation of the hyperkinetic dyskinesias. In tardive dyskinesia and chorea there should be inherent dopamine excess or drugs that directly stimulate dopamine receptors could be responsible. Drugs which cause tardive dyskinesias such as the phenothiazines are known to have anticholinergic, antiserotonin and antihistamine effects and to leave dopamine unopposed. Drugs which reduce dopamine action such as tetrabenazine, haloperidol and reserpine will reduce the involuntary movements in chorea, but are more likely to induce a parkinsonian picture as a side-effect. Parkinsonism can be induced either by depleting the brain's production of dopamine, as occurs with reserpine and tetrabenazine when the dopamine receptors remain free, or alternatively it can be caused by blocking the dopamine receptors by such drugs as haloperidol when L-DOPA cannot reverse the parkinsonism so produced.

Some of the other effects of drugs are also important. Thus multiple tics may appear as a complication of chronic amphetamine use or chronic overdose by methylphenidate (Ritalin). Both of these drugs increase brain dopamine as well as having a noradrenergic effect. 5-hydroxytryptophan has been given to patients with Lesch–Nyhan syndrome when it appears to lessen self-mutilation. It has also been given to children with Down syndrome in the hope that it would improve their muscle tone and motor performance, but it was found to produce marked rigidity and myoclonic jerks. Cholinergic drugs such as physostigmine will make parkinsonism worse, but will lessen choreiform movements. In the basal ganglia we see an amalgam of anatomy, physiology, biochemistry and pharmacology which to some extent explains a clinical maze of signs and symptoms.

Clinical features of extrapyramidal disorders

The possible clinical features seen in extrapyramidal disease are tremors, tics, akathisia, myoclonus, hemiballismus, chorea, athetosis, torsion dystonia, parkinsonism, tardive orofacial dyskinesias or various types of rigidity. In clinical practice it is often difficult to define the difference between a tic, choreiform movement and a myoclonic movement. Hemiballismus is really a severe form of unilateral chorea. There is a release of primitive reflexes. It is easiest to classify all these syndromes into hyperkinetic or hypokinetic movement difficulties (i.e. dyskinesias). For the sake of this chapter we shall divide the disorders of the basal ganglia into three categories, hyperkinetic dyskinesias, hypokinetic dyskinesias and rigidities, even though there is a degree of overlap.

Hyperkinetic dyskinesias. These are typified by the choreas, hemiballismus, akathisia, tics and orofacial dyskinesias. This group is most often associated with a reduction in muscle tone and the movements disappear in sleep or if the child is totally relaxed and lying down. Symptomatically there is a close link between this group of disorders and cerebellar dysfunction, e.g. myoclonus can occur in both. In the hyperkinetic dyskinesias the child is restless, fidgety, cannot sit still, stamps his feet, grimaces, shakes his head, may get a constant urge to run, may grunt, make clucking noises and show respiratory irregularity. This group tends to be associated with high levels of dopamine or noradrenergic substances.

Differentiation from epilepsia partialis continua may at times be difficult except that the latter continues into sleep and the EEG clinches the diagnosis. True choreiform movements tend to be jerky, unpredictable and random and differ from tics in that they have no pattern of repetition, but the so-called convulsive tic with repeated wild flinging movements of the arms and lateral jerking of the head may resemble hemiballismus. The sudden wild flinging of the arm or the head in chorea is made semipurposive by pretending to scratch the head or straighten the hair.

The child may sit on his hand or hold his tongue between his teeth to try and lessen the movements. Walking and feeding may become impossible due to the repeated jerkings of the head and limbs together with involvement of the lips, tongue and palate.

Orofacial dyskinesia is typical of the tardive drug-induced dyskinesias but is also seen in severe chorea or in the Gilles de la Tourette syndrome of multiple tics. The face may be drawn up into a grimace or risus sardonicus, there may be twitching of the mouth and eyes, quivering of the chin, rolling of the tongue, repeated tongue protrusion, sudden mouth opening, titubation of the head, pursing of the lips or mouthing as if the child was speaking. Some of these facial contortions are so grotesque that the child's life is made a misery due to teasing at school. This is especially likely in the maladie de tics in which the clucking and respiratory noises are further exacerbated by coprolalia. The borderland between the tic, the fit and the myoclonic jerk is blurred in subacute sclerosing panencephalitis when the same sudden repeated movements of an arm may be so violent that the head is repeatedly struck and there may be gross local bruising. This may be preceded by symmetrical jerking of the arms (metronomic myoclonus).

True choreiform movements can be appreciated most easily by getting the child to stand still with his arms outstretched when the jerkings appear as a gross caricature of the milder constant readjusting movements seen in pure cerebellar disease as if there was a total absence of damping, with wild overswings of correction. The head and upper limbs are affected more than the trunk and lower limbs and total relaxation in the supine position lessens the movements as maintenance of posture and initiation of voluntary movement seems to be important in triggering them off. The face and bulbar muscles are involved when there are bilateral choreiform movements of the arms (a tic may be unilateral and have bulbar involvement). The restless leg syndrome of Ekbom could be regarded as a mild form of hyperkinetic dyskinesia limited to the legs.

Hypokinetic dyskinesia. In the most severe cases there is akinesia and the patient cannot initiate any movement even though not paralyzed. Less severe cases with bradykinesia are associated with difficulty in initiating a movement, e.g. difficulty in running is characteristic. Facial movements are affected so that the expression is often one of misery, sadness or is totally impassive. The patient may not be able to get his hand out quickly enough to shake hands when someone offers theirs. He has great difficulty in initiating walking and when he gets started he has small, slow, shuffling steps which gradually get faster (festination). There is no spring in the gait and the arms do not swing. In severe cases walking is lost altogether. Writing is slow, small and laborious with micrographia. Speech is slow and monotonous with constant loss of features (i.e. no expression) and is slurred. There is in a normal person a natural cadence for walking, writing and speaking and although this varies between different people, its loss is one of the early signs of basal ganglia disease. The choreas may be regarded as being associated with total loss of damping of movements whilst in a bradykinesis there is complete damping to the point of cessation (akinetic mutism). The most characteristic hypokinetic state is parkinsonism which is classically associated with dopamine depletion.

Rigidities – abnormalities of muscle tone. Changes in muscle tone can be considered under several headings, i.e. flexor dystonia, extensor dystonia, hemiplegic dystonia and athetosis. Abnormal patterns of muscle tone can be constant or fluctuating and the latter may be slow, as in torsion dystonia and tensions, or more rapid as in athetosis.

Flexor dystonia is a feature of carbon monoxide poisoning, head injury and encephalitis. The patient may lie curled up with marked flexor dystonia and complete akinesia. In less severe cases the patient is stooped, flexed at elbows, knees and hips with the head bent forward. Classically in flexor dystonia the arms are flexed and resist passive extension and the legs are flexed on the abdomen with the toes tending to claw. The asymmetrical tonic neck reflexes and progression reflexes are absent. The glabella reflex is positive. This flexed posture with akinesia is known as the pallidal syndrome. It is not influenced by anxiety and does not disappear in sleep. Chorea and athetosis are not seen. L-DOPA will release the patient from his flexor rigidity.

Extensor dystonia is seen much more commonly in children as the dystonic phase of cerebral palsy. It does not correspond to a

known neurotransmitter imbalance but may be seen as part of some of the very acute dystonic reactions described later as side-effects of certain neuroleptic drugs, in which case they are rapidly abolished by anticholinergics. Extensor dystonia corresponds to the physiological second stage of extension seen in normal child development between 6 weeks and 4 months after birth. In the abnormal or diseased state it is an obligatory exaggeration or caricature of this normal physiological developmental state. It is the hallmark of the postkernicteric cerebral palsies before any choreoathetosis makes its appearance or of dystonia associated with prematurity or due to basal ganglia damage following perinatal asphyxia.

Extrapyramidal rigidity is not associated with shortening or contracture of muscles: there is a normal lengthening reaction. The muscle spindles are not involved so that stretching need not be applied to affected muscles and dorsal root section does not abolish it (thus the opposite of spasticity). The rigidity disappears with anesthesia or diazepam leaving a full range of movement at the joint. In the leg there is a dynamic as opposed to a fixed spastic equinus. Lengthening of the heelcords in these cases is strongly contraindicated. In the acute dystonic reactions which come immediately after starting drugs such as haloperidol or maxolon there is retrocollis, torticollis, opisthotonus, dystonic extension of the arms, tonic mouth opening (Fig. 14.51) and oculogyric crises, which may be dramatically relieved in minutes by diazepam or anticholinergic drugs. Benzodiazepine drugs will also relieve the extensor hypertonus of dystonic cerebral palsy and nitrazepam prevents the gross extensor thrust which can make management of these children so difficult. It is not clear which receptors are being blocked or stimulated by these drugs. (Benzodiazepine receptors and GABA receptors are allied.)

In the classic dystonic child there is neck retraction so that when in the prone position, there appears to be excellent head control which contrasts with the marked head lag in the 'pull to sit' position. Extensor hyperactivity of the muscles of the trunk and of the hip and knees may induce opisthotonic posturing. The

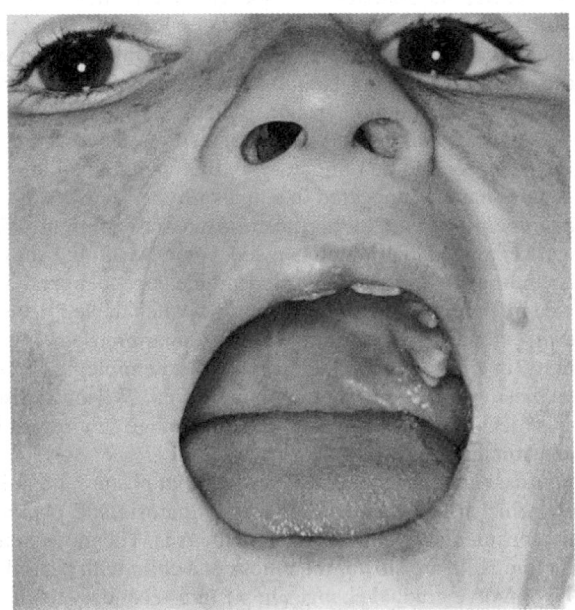

Fig. 14.51 Involuntary movements of the mouth in dyskinesia.

arms are internally rotated and rigidly extended with the wrists flexed, the fingers extended when beside the body but showing a tight grasp reflex when the arm is flexed to the side of the head. The extension of the legs is accompanied by equinus and a rigid calf and with a spontaneous Babinski response.

This extensor posture is not constant and disappears in sleep. The child can be positioned to lessen or heighten the exaggerated muscle tone. Anxiety, performing mental arithmetic or a sudden noise all heighten the extension. Pressure over the nose (trigeminal area, i.e. the snout reflex) or perineum will throw the child into total extensor rigidity associated with vigorous doggy-paddling movements of the upper limbs as long as the pressure is maintained.

Extensor hypertonus is accompanied by exaggeration and invariable elicitation of all the so-called extensor reflexes, e.g. asymmetrical tonic neck reflex, tonic neck reflex, etc. Contact reactions are seen in the child with dystonic extension, e.g. lying on the back increases the tone bilaterally whilst lying on the left side will heighten the tone in the left arm and leg. Stroking an extensor surface, e.g. the paraspinal region, heightens the tone in the erector spinae muscles on that side but also the leg on that side will abduct and extend, the arm will extend and abduct and the head will rotate to that side. This trunk incurvation or Galant reflex produces an asymmetrical tonic neck reflex posture in prone suspension. The Perez reflex, i.e. stroking along the spinous processes, causes the trunk to extend and the hips to flex. Suspension of the child in space enhances labyrinthine stimulation and the tone will increase with a tendency to go into rigid extension of the lower limbs with a degree of scissoring and spontaneous Babinski responses. Lying prone will inhibit the extensor tone and the child will often go into a flexed neonatal position. Flexion and extension of the head (symmetrical TNR) or rotation to one or other side (asymmetrical TNR) causes increases in the tone in the arm and leg on both sides or one side according to the head movement used. Unilateral torsion dystonia with torticollis and extension of the arm with internal rotation, of the leg with equinus and of the big toe is a classic pattern, usually in an older child, but bilateral extensor dystonia is more commonly a feature in the development of cerebral palsy. It is also a prominent feature of Leigh's encephalopathy, Hallervorden–Spatz disease and some cases of Huntington's chorea. It is thought that the subthalamic nuclei are responsible for the primitive progression (i.e. walking and stepping) reflexes. These are usually easy to elicit, tend to be obligatory and are maintained long after they should have disappeared in extensor hypertonus.

Hemiplegic dystonia. In this, posturing consists of tightly flexed arms and extended legs which is made worse by tilting backwards or suspending. This response is labyrinthine dependent and can be reversed by holding the child upside down when the leg flexes and the arm extends. This posture can be superimposed upon the spasticity in typical hemiplegia or double hemiplegia. It is the typical posture seen in Huntington's chorea, Wilson's disease, Hallervorden–Spatz disease and cortical damage syndromes from hypotension and asphyxia.

Athetosis. Athetosis literally means without posture, i.e. it is the posture which is constantly changing. Athetosis and chorea are usually considered together as choreoathetosis. The movements in the athetoid child are slower than those in a child with pure chorea and they involve gradual changes in posture secondary to changes in muscle tone. The upper limbs appear to be constantly moving between the primitive extensor posture and the hemiplegic flexor

posture. The fingers start in the hemiplegic position with the hand closed across the adducted thumb and flexed at wrist and elbows. The fingers then extend and the arm extends, abducts and internally rotates into the extended (also called avoiding) position. Since the leg is extended in both postures it remains in equinus and does not show the same movements as occur in the arms. In bilateral lesions the face is also involved: with a pattern of total extension, the mouth is held tonically open with the tongue protruding and there is usually retention of the baby feeding reflexes (rooting and sucking) and cardinal point reflexes. Later trismus may occur. Feeding, especially chewing, is difficult and speech is always affected. Walking may be possible with a reeling gait with contortions of the trunk and yet surprisingly few falls.

Athetosis of the hands, dilation of the alae nasae and fanning of the toes is often seen in normal infants at birth and may become very obvious after relatively mild asphyxia. Pathological athetosis rarely appears in the first year of life in brain damage syndromes. Dystonic extension appears at about 4 months of age and athetosis may not occur for a further 2 or 3 years. Grimacing, laughing, crying and inappropriate emotional responses can accompany the fluctuating muscle tone.

Classification of basal ganglia diseases

These can be considered in two ways. Firstly, anatomically, it is sometimes considered that lesions of the globus pallidus cause parkinsonism, lesions of the putamen cause athetosis and lesions of the caudate cause chorea but this is a gross oversimplification. Secondly, basal ganglia disorders can be classified on the basis of clinical presentation, i.e. whether there is an acute dyskinesia, progressive dyskinesia or chronic nonprogressive dyskinesia (Table 14.62).

Types of basal ganglia disease

Parkinsonism. The clinical picture of tremor, bradykinesia and flexor rigidity has already been outlined. Parkinsonism is a form of dyskinesia rarely seen in children (Table 14.63).

Treatment of parkinsonism consists of L-DOPA combined with inhibition of the peripheral tissue breakdown by a specific carboxylase which increases the concentration of L-DOPA in the brain. This is often combined with an anticholinergic such as benztropine. Surgery does not have a place in most of the cases of childhood parkinsonism.

Tremor. Physiological tremor is faster than the 5/s shake in parkinsonism. It is present to some degree in all individuals and can become more obvious in anxiety, thyrotoxicosis or the administration of β-mimetic drugs such as salbutamol. It may be a prominent side-effect of lithium or sodium valproate treatment. Hypoglycemia causes adrenaline release and is associated with a very coarse tremor. Certain families have a coarse dominantly inherited tremor present from early childhood, so-called benign or essential tremor. This does not progress to incapacitation but may get worse at puberty. In a few cases marked head tremor may be a nuisance, but on the whole it interferes surprisingly little with hand skills. Alcohol, which may cause tremor in delirium tremens, tends to abolish essential tremor and care must be taken to see that adolescents do not resort to this as a remedy. Essential tremor can often be abolished by a small regular dose of β-blockers such as propranolol. Drug addiction, especially on withdrawal, causes a

Table 14.62 Dyskinesias

Acute dyskinesias in children
1. Carbon monoxide poisoning
2. Cardiac bypass surgery
3. *Haemophilus influenzae* meningitis
4. Encephalitis lethargica, mumps encephalitis
5. Familial paroxysmal choreoathetosis
6. Postdialysis dyskinesia
7. Burns encephalopathy, scalds shakes
8. Hypernatremic dehydration
9. Heavy metal poisoning – manganese, thallium, etc.
10. Drug-induced dyskinesias
11. Extrapyramidal epilepsy
12. Tumors of the third ventricle
13. Convulsive tics
14. Gilles de la Tourette syndrome
15. Familial striatal necrosis
16. Leigh's encephalopathy and mitochondrial encephalopathies
17. Intermittent maple syrup urine disease
18. Subacute sclerosing panencephalitis
19. Sydenham's chorea
20. Chorea gravidarum

Chronic nonprogressive dyskinesias (cerebral palsies)
1. Asphyxia
2. Hyperbilirubinemia
3. Familial non progressive dyskinesia
4. Autosomal recesssive nonprogressive dyskinesia
5. Familial (dominant) nonprogressive dyskinesia
6. Familial striatonigral dysphasias

Chronic progressive dyskinesias of childhood
1. Huntington's chorea
2. Hallervorden–Spatz disease
3. Wilson's disease
4. Ataxia telangectasia
5. Fahr's syndrome
6. Pelizaeus–Merzbacher disease
7. Encephalitis lethargica
8. Jakob–Creutzfeld disease
9. Subacute sclerosing panencephalitis
10. Striatonigral degeneration (Hunt's, juvenile parkinsonism)
11. Hunt's pallido/cerebellar degeneration
12. Lesch–Nyhan syndrome
13. Late infantile or juvenile Leigh's disease
14. Glutaric aciduria
15. Dystonia musculorum deformans
16. Piloid astrocytoma basal ganglia
17. Sulfite oxidase deficiency
18. Familial striatal necrosis

Table 14.63 Causes of parkinsonism in children
1. Familial striatonigral degeneration of Hunt
2. Postencephalitic
3. Drug induced – haloperidol, reserpine, phenothiazine
4. Subacute sclerosing panencephalitis – measles
5. Batten disease
6. Phenylketonuria – lack of tyrosine
7. Head injury, e.g. boxers
8. Lewy body idiopathic
9. MPTP toxicity
10. Manganese toxicity

profound tremor and this is seen in the newborn infant with narcotic or phenobarbitone withdrawal symptoms. Flapping tremor may be seen in hepatic failure, the genetically determined hyperammonemias secondary to enzyme defects in the urea cycle or Wilson's disease and in CO_2 narcosis. A very peculiar coarse head tremor called the 'bobble-headed doll syndrome' is characteristic of third ventricular tumors.

Stereotypes. Many normal children develop repetitive habits such as rocking, head banging and, in the older age group, tics. Adults under stress will often show particular mannerisms such as coughing, constantly adjusting spectacles, brushing the hair with the hand, twiddling the thumbs or always making the same utterance under stress. Mentally retarded children show very marked stereotypes which are usually divided into two main groups – mannerisms and self-mutilating stereotypes. The mannerisms consist of head nodding, hand regard, flicking objects with the fingers, vocal stereotypes such as grunting or screaming, turning round and round, jumping up and down, running backwards and forwards on tip toe, touching objects or at times standing with arms outstretched in very athetoid postures so that one may be led to make a misdiagnosis of athetoid cerebral palsy. Self-mutilating stereotypes include forced head banging, lip biting, finger biting and these may occur in association with nonspecific mental handicap or very prominently in association with overt choreoathetosis in the Lesch–Nyhan syndrome. It is claimed that self-mutilating stereotypes do sometimes respond to therapy with 5-hydroxytryptophan.

Tics (see p. 1745). Tics may be idiopathic or due to discernible causes.

Simple developmental tic. This is the common tic which is seen in the normal child, 8–12 years of age, often associated with a family history suggesting dominant inheritance and clearing spontaneously. It nearly always involves the head and shoulders and tends to be simple, i.e. one group of movements always repeated.

Manneristic tics. These occur in the mentally retarded or autistic child.

Maladie de tics, Gilles de la Tourette syndrome. This is a much more severe disorder in which multiple tics affect different groups of muscles. The condition may come on at 2 or 3 years of age and last many years into adult life. These are gross facial distortions, sometimes violent ballistic movements and characteristically a vocal component which may start as grunting and clucking but progresses so that the child may bark like a dog, make apparent muttering movements with his lips and eventually with the tics make forced utterances which are usually coprolalic consisting of most of the Anglo-Saxon four-letter swear words. It is thought that Gilles de la Tourette is an organic syndrome in that it can be caused by drugs and tends to respond to dopamine receptor blockade with drugs such as haloperidol.

Multiple tics. These can be caused by L-DOPA, by chronic amphetamine poisoning which releases endogenous dopamine and noradrenaline in the brain and by overdosage with methylphenidate (Ritalin), carbamazepine or pemoline. The incrimination of dopamine as a cause for the multiple tic syndrome as well as the effect of blockage of dopamine receptors by haloperidol is one of the strongest pointers to an organic basis for the condition. It may be that the balance between dopamine and noradrenergic receptors is important as drugs such as amphetamine and Ritalin have a noradrenergic as well as a dopamine-releasing effect and clonidine, a noradrenergic receptor stimulant, has been found to have a beneficial effect in the treatment of some cases of multiple tics.

Multiple tics, which could be accompanied by coprolalia, were seen in the past in the acute stages of encephalitis lethargica and can be presenting features of subacute sclerosing panencephalitis.

Tics may occur in association with Sydenham's chorea and it can be difficult to know if the chorea has cleared and the tic is the result of a previously imposed movement, i.e. a true habit spasm or whether it is part and parcel of the chorea persisting in a mild form of chorea minor.

Drug reactions and extrapyramidal syndromes. Extrapyramidal syndromes are one of the commonest toxic manifestations of drugs. Tremor may occur with β-mimetic drugs, tics with amphetamine and Ritalin and choreoathetosis with phenytoin. There are four other types of drug reaction.

1. Drug-induced parkinsonism, which occurs as a consequence of depleting brain dopamine with reserpine or tetrabenazine or due to blocking dopamine receptors as with phenothiazines and butyrophenones. Rigidity and bradykinesia are more obvious than tremor along with the mask-like facies, inappropriate emotion and gait disturbance.

2. Acute dystonic reactions are not uncommon in children, especially from the use of drugs such as haloperidol and maxolon, overdose of fluorine-containing phenothiazines, stemetil and stelazine. Acute dystonic reactions can come on soon after starting treatment. The child may go into total opisthotonus with risus sardonicus, trismus, fits, torsion spasms, torticollis, catatonia, oculogyric crisis and severe dysarthria. Lack of awareness that these drugs have been given (e.g. as a suppository for sedation) may result in a diagnosis of tetanus, tetany or encephalitis being entertained. Although the child is often drowsy the fact that he can be aroused and the presence of decerebration with reacting pupils should alert to the possibility of a toxic encephalopathy. A rare association is a respiratory abnormality similar to the so-called Ondine's curse with the child losing automatic ventilation, though he will breathe if told to do so. This abnormality can be reversed by naloxone.

Response to treatment of acute dystonia is often dramatic. Anticholinergic drugs such as procyclidine or benadryl will reverse the dystonia within minutes, suggesting that cholinergic pathways are important in the maintenance of the acute dystonia.

3. Akathisia. The child becomes restless and intensely fidgety, cannot sit down or sit still, stamps, runs, taps with his fingers, shows facial mannerisms or tics. This tends to start weeks or months after starting therapy and can be combined with parkinsonism or tardive dyskinesia.

4. Tardive dyskinesia. As the name suggests, involuntary movements are tardy in appearance, coming on after months or years of treatment. They may appear for the first time after a drug is discontinued and may be suppressed by increasing the dose still higher; such suppression of tardive dyskinesia may cause increasing parkinsonism. Cessation of drug therapy can also be associated with vomiting, sweating and weight loss or alternatively with overactivity and euphoria to the point of psychosis. In mentally retarded children withdrawal of chronic neuroleptic medication can cause aggression and increase in stereotypes and self-mutilation. It has been suggested that there is good reason for giving repeated drug holidays of 12 weeks at a time in all patients with chronically administered neuroleptics.

The classic tardive dyskinesia affects the face with chewing movements, facial grimacing and tongue protrusion. There may occasionally be more frank choreiform movements or even a picture resembling Huntington's chorea. Phenothiazine drugs are the most commonly incriminated. Reserpine and tetrabenazine are not associated with tardive dyskinesia. High-dose haloperidol may cause the condition and it is no service to replace a tic with a tardive dyskinesia. Carbamazepine may also cause an orofacial dyskinesia. Similar types of dyskinesia appear with L-DOPA which will make tardive dyskinesia worse. The movements are reduced by tetrabenazine or reserpine. Anticholinergic drugs have no effect. It is thought that chronic blocking of dopamine receptors could result in a supersensitivity. It has been postulated that there may be two populations of dopamine receptors, one involving parkinsonism and one tardive dyskinesias. There is a rare form of orofacial dyskinesia mainly affecting adults which is not related to neuroleptic medication, known as Meige's syndrome, which is probably familial.

If a normal person is given barbiturates for a long period of time and suddenly stops, withdrawal fits will occur. Long-term blocking of endorphin receptors by narcotic addicts and the subsequent withdrawal has similar effects. Children, supposedly hyperkinetic, treated with large doses of sympathomimetic amines for a long period of time develop irritability and overactivity on withdrawal which is often thought to show that the drug was needed to suppress the symptoms when in fact the symptoms are due to the withdrawal. Infants exposed to phenobarbitone, narcotics or sympathomimetic amines in utero can develop neurotransmitter imbalance which may show as fits, bradycardia, intense restlessness, tremor, irritability and constant motion with exaggeration of the progression reflexes lasting several weeks after birth. The balance of neurotransmitters can thus be altered if drugs are given over a long period of time. Whether this is more likely to be permanent in the case of the developing brain when synapses are forming for the first time is not known. Some cases of tardive dyskinesia are permanent. It is possible that long-term caffeine and nicotine could act in a similar way. On the other hand there is little conclusive evidence to support the suggestion that a chronic intake of natural salicylates, cadmium and food dyes causes a form of restless akathisia.

Chorea. Chorea is seen in its purest form in diseases such as Sydenham's chorea and chorea gravidarum. It may appear in many other diseases such as Huntington's chorea, drug-induced choreoathetosis, ataxia telangiectasia, Wilson's disease, Hallervorden–Spatz disease, glutaric aciduria, Lesch–Nyhan syndrome and the late form of Leigh's encephalopathy. It occurs in association with athetosis in the dyskinetic cerebral palsies, postasphyxial states and hyperbilirubinemia. Chorea may be seen transiently for a few days or at most a few weeks following cardiac bypass surgery, meningitis (especially *Haemophilus influenzae* meningitis) or hypernatremic dehydration.

Sydenham's chorea. See page 1598.

Paroxysmal choreoathetosis. This is an odd condition with grimacing and choreiform movements with abnormal posturing which comes in episodes. It may be difficult without a continuous 24-h EEG recording to differentiate sporadic cases from the rare basal ganglia epilepsies. The condition does not progress over the years and is not associated with dementia. Onset may be as early as 6 months of age. Examination between episodes is normal and the EEG in the classic attack is also normal. It is dominantly inherited and no biochemical abnormality has been recognized. Sudden movement or a particular movement may precipitate bouts of choreoathetosis. The episode may be brief or may last several hours. Consciousness is usually maintained even in paroxysmal choreoathetosis lasting hours or days. Paroxysmal choreoathetosis can also occur from organic basal ganglia lesions as a form of basal ganglia epilepsy, e.g. in very low grade astrocytomas. In this epileptic type of paroxysmal choreoathetosis the EEG may show only slow waves rather than a spike focus. Dystonia or athetoid posturing precipitated by movement, i.e. paroxysmal kinesiogenic dystonia, may be very sensitive to carbamazepine.

Treatment is with anticonvulsants in the first place and this may have some success but in the prolonged episodes treatment with anticholinergics such as benztropine is likely to be effective.

Familial striatal necrosis. Leigh's encephalopathy has been described on page 788. There is a variant disease in older children with a progressive dyskinetic presentation, a CT scan showing longitudinal slits in the basal ganglia and cystic necrosis at autopsy. A further group of children have bilateral symmetrical necrosis of the neostriatum (putamen and caudate) presenting with dysarthria, abnormal gait, abnormal postures, myoclonic jerks and involuntary movements, coming on usually after trivial febrile illnesses. This progresses gradually over the years and is inherited as an autosomal recessive disorder.

Huntington's chorea. This dominantly inherited condition characteristically appears in adults around 30 years with dementia, rigidity and chorea as well as psychological and behavior changes. Ten percent of cases start in childhood and inheritance is usually from the father. It is another triple codon repeat disease; 35–90 repeats of trinucleotide CAG are diagnostic on chromosome 4p 16.3. Diagnosis of suspected childhood cases is now possible. Presentation can be with fits in 50% of cases, thus differing from the adult who presents with dementia or dystonia. MRI scans may show selective atrophy of the head of the caudate nucleus.

Glutaric acidemia (p. 1113). Episodes of crying, cyanosis, pallor, lethargy and hypotonia may commence in the first year of life. Episodes of tachypnea, acidosis and stiffness following minor infections which can be associated with fits may suggest a diagnosis of pyrexial convulsions or encephalitis in the first instance. The episodes tend to be repeated and dystonia and choreoathetosis gradually appear. The caudate and putamen show a loss of nerve cells and gliosis. Treatment has been tried with a low lysine and tryptophan diet without dramatic clinical improvement. Choreoathetosis can also be a symptom of other disorders such as d-glyceric acidemia and sulfite oxidase deficiency.

Hallervorden–Spatz syndrome. The basal ganglia are very rich in iron. The function of this is not known nor the reason why the basal ganglia are so selectively vulnerable to heavy metal toxicity. Hallervorden–Spatz syndrome transmitted by autosomal recessive inheritance is associated with an increase of the amount of stainable iron. The globus pallidus and substantia nigra are affected with accumulation of iron pigments, a decrease in myelin and axonal swellings (spheroids). The clinical picture is one not of parkinsonism but of spasticity with brisk reflexes, extensor plantar responses and increasing extrapyramidal rigidity with a hemiplegic dystonic type affecting all four limbs. The child may be thought to have cerebral palsy when the progression is very slow. Usually by the age of 10 years there is fixation of posture with varying degrees of choreoathetosis. Death usually occurs in the early 20s. There is no definite diagnostic test. Brain biopsy does not help unless one is fortunate enough to see spheroids and

iron metabolism as judged by the estimation of serum iron, transferrins or iron absorption is normal. No treatment is of any avail. The disease is rare and differentiation from metachromatic leukodystrophy, Alexander's disease or Pelizaeus–Merzbacher disease can be clinically difficult. All these in the first instance may be misdiagnosed as cases of cerebral palsy.

Wilson's disease. See page 1145.

Lesch–Nyhan syndrome (p. 790). This is an inborn error in uric acid metabolism inherited as a sex-linked recessive character and is due to a deficiency in the enzyme HGPRT. The basal ganglia are known to have high concentrations of this enzyme. Choreoathetosis, spasticity, mental retardation and particularly self-mutilation are characteristic of the condition with gouty tophi and renal calculi as possible additional features. Death may occur from a nephropathy secondary to the raised urinary uric acid. The plasma uric acid is raised. The enzyme can be assayed to establish the diagnosis.

Dystonia musculorum deformans. A severe dystonia may occur in many of the diseases already described. The term is usually restricted, however, to unilateral torticollis extension of the leg, torsion of the trunk, extension and internal rotation of the arm (Fig. 14.52). Although this can be seen in some cases of dyskinetic cerebral palsy and in some children with a more pure form of dyskinetic hemiplegia, there are two genetic forms,

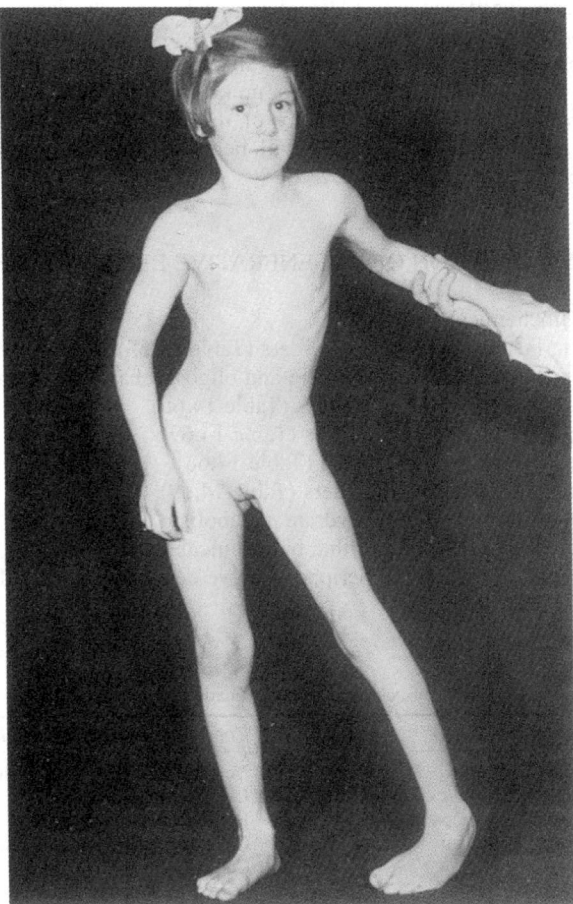

Fig. 14.52 Characteristic posture of the left lower limb in dystonia musculorum deformans. Mother and an uncle also suffered from the condition.

autosomal recessive and autosomal dominant, the former being more common in Ashkenazi Jews. No specific enzyme system has so far been identified in the causation.

A group of children with onset of a paroxysmal dystonia which is better in the mornings and worse as the day wears on has been described. Rest will not lessen the dystonia but REM sleep results in alleviation for a short time. This condition may be associated with severe extrapyramidal dystonia with brisk reflexes and extensor plantar responses and may progress to the point where the child cannot walk. The importance of this subgroup is that these children are extremely sensitive to L-DOPA and 25 or 50 mg of the drug together with a peripheral carboxylase inhibitor results in very dramatic improvement in the child's condition.

Basal ganglia calcification

With the advent of modern imaging a not uncommon finding is calcification of the basal ganglia. This has many causes (Table 14.64) and may be asymptomatic in terms of the movement disorders described.

DEGENERATIVE BRAIN DISORDERS AND THE NEURODERMATOSES

Progressive degenerative disorders can be broadly defined into those for which there is a biochemical basis, e.g. storage disorders, peroxisomal disorders, mitochondrial disorders, etc., and those in which there is as yet no known biochemical basis. It seems likely that in time many of the conditions in the latter group, e.g. Batten's disease, will be found to have a specific biochemical abnormality.

CLASSIFICATION OF DEGENERATIVE BRAIN DISEASE

1. Biochemical
   a. lysosomal storage disorders (Table 14.65)
   b. disorders of glycoprotein and oligosaccharide metabolism including mucolipidoses (Table 14.66)
   c. mucopolysaccharidoses (Table 14.67)
   d. peroxisomal disorders (Table 14.68)
   e. mitochondrial disorders (Table 14.69)
   f. disorders of carbohydrate metabolism (Table 14.70)
   g. other conditions with a biochemical defect (Table 14.71)
2. Spinocerebellar and peripheral nerve degenerations (Table 14.72)

3. Tumors (Table 14.73)
4. Infections (Table 14.74)
5. Epileptic (Table 14.75)
6. Psychological (Table 14.76)
7. Reversible (Table 14.77)
8. Apparent (Table 14.78)
9. Miscellaneous (Table 14.79)

While storage disorders may result in neurological deterioration and dementia as a direct result of the stored substance, in other conditions intermediates in the biochemical pathways may be responsible for the deterioration.

There are several different patterns of clinical presentation of degenerative brain disease. There may, for example, be a sudden loss of skills and intellect or a more gradual decline in psychomotor functioning. The onset may follow normal development or delayed development. In the early stages there may simply be a slowing down in the acquisition of skills.

During infancy the regression is seen as a loss of motor skills and a loss of interest which may be visual or in nonverbal communication.

In the toddler, changes are seen in speech and behavior as well as motor irregularities.

The school-age child demonstrates regression with a decline in school performance, concentration, penmanship, etc. New learning is difficult because of a poor memory and coordination is defective.

INVESTIGATION OF NEURODEGENERATIVE DISEASE

The clinical history including the age of onset of the condition, the tempo of the disease, together with specific clinical features referable to the nervous and other systems, may suggest a differential diagnosis of causes. The investigation of degenerative brain disease is summarized in Table 14.80. For further details of these conditions the reader is referred to standard works on the subject such as Scriver et al (1989).

THE NEURODERMATOSES

This is a group of disorders which have in common the association of a skin lesion with a neurological lesion and in many cases there is also a high risk of tumor formation. Certain other diseases such as Hartnup disease (p. 799) or Refsum's syndrome (p. 785), which also involve lesions of skin and a neurological tissue, have been considered elsewhere. The main features of the neurodermatoses are given in Table 14.81.

Table 14.64   Causes of basal ganglia calcification

Endocrine	Congenital and metabolic disease	Infection	Neoplasms
Hypoparathyroidism	Mitochondrial encephalopathies	Toxoplasmosis	Craniopharyngioma
Pseudo hypoparathyroidism	Leigh's encephalopathy	SSPE	Optic nerve glioma
Pseudopseudo hypoparathyroidism	Hallervorden–Spatz disease	Cytomegalovirus infection	Radiotherapy
Hyperparathyroidism	Chronic methemoglobinemia	Congenital rubella	Methotrexate therapy for leukemia
Hypothyroidism	Carbon monoxide poisoning	AIDS	
	Lead poisoning	Systemic lupus	
	Cockayne's syndrome		
	Down syndrome		
	Tuberous sclerosis		
	Neurofibromatosis		

Table 14.65 Lysosomal storage disorders – lipidoses and sphingolipidoses

Disorder	Genetics	Stored substance	Enzyme defect	Age of onset	Neurology	Visceral involvement	Other clinical features	Diagnostic sample	Prenatal diagnosis
Generalized gangliosidosis (GM1 gangliosidosis)	AR (chromosome 3)	GM1 ganglioside (brain, liver), oligosaccharides (urine)	β-Galactosidase	Infantile (0–6 months) (type I)	Mental and motor retardation, fits, hypotonia, blindness	Hepatosplenomegaly	Coarse facies, skeletal changes, cherry red spot (~50%), edema, startle response, vacuolated lymphocytes, foam cells	Leukocytes,* fibroblasts	Yes
				Juvenile (6–20 months) (type II)	Mental and motor retardation, fits, ataxia	None	Mild skeletal changes, startle response, vacuolated lymphocytes, foam cells	Leukocytes, fibroblasts	Yes
				Adult (teens) (type III)	Mental and motor retardation, progressive spasticity and ataxia, dysarthria	None	Mild skeletal changes	Leukocytes, fibroblasts	Yes
Sandhoff disease (GM2 gangliosidosis, O variant)	AR (chromosome 5)	GM2 ganglioside (brain), globoside (viscera), oligosaccharides (urine)	Total hexosaminidase	Infantile (3–6 months)	Mental and motor retardation, fits, early blindness, hypotonia	No hepatosplenomegaly but histological involvement of viscera	Doll-like face, cherry red spot, foamy histiocytes in kidney, lung, spleen, etc., startle response	Leukocytes, fibroblasts	Yes
				Juvenile and adult forms also reported	Juvenile/adult forms with progressive cerebellar ataxia and spinocerebellar degeneration, mild dementia				
Tay-Sachs (GM2 gangliosidosis, B variant)	AR common in, but not confined to Ashkenazi Jews where carrier frequency is 1/30 (chromosome 15)	GM2 ganglioside (brain)	Hexosaminidase A	Classically infantile (3–6 months)	Mental and motor retardation, fits, early blindness, hypotonia and hyperplexia	None	Doll-like face, cherry red spot at macula, startle response	Leukocytes, serum, fibroblasts	Yes
				Juvenile and adult variants reported	Spinocerebellar degeneration, spinal muscular atrophy	None		Juvenile and adult forms may have normal fundi	
GM2 gangliosidosis, B1 variant	AR Some patients may be genetic compound with Tay-Sachs	GM2 ganglioside (brain)	Hexosaminidase A mutation at natural substrate binding site and different from Tay-Sachs	Similar to Tay-Sachs (3–6 months) or more juvenile in presentation	Similar to Tay-Sachs	None	Patients with B1 variant probably rare – B/B1 genetic compound more common, especially where B variant (Tay-Sachs) gene frequency high	Leukocytes, serum fibroblasts	Yes

Table 14.65 *Cont'd*

Disorder	Genetics	Stored substance	Enzyme defect	Age of onset	Neurology	Visceral involvement	Other clinical features	Diagnostic sample	Prenatal diagnosis
GM2 gangliosidosis, AB variant	AR (chromosome 5)	GM2 ganglioside (brain)	Activator for GM2 ganglioside	Similar to Tay-Sachs (3–12 months)	Similar to Tay-Sachs	None	Few cases studied but infantile and juvenile types reported	Fibroblasts	Yes
Fabry (angiokeratoma corporis diffusum)	X-linked recessive (X chromosome)	Ceramide trihexosides and ceramide dihexoside (kidney, urine)	α-Galactosidase	Usually in childhood or early adulthood	Cerebrovascular disease	Cardiac and renal complications	Progressive accumulation of lipid in vascular epithelium leads to increasing morbidity; excruciating pain especially at extremities, angiokeratomas particularly distributed around umbilicus, knees, flanks and scrotum; corneal opacity seen on slit lamp; mild disease may be expressed in heterozygous females	Leukocytes, fibroblasts	Yes
Wolman	AR (chromosome 10)	Cholesterol esters, triglycerides (liver, spleen)	Acid lipase	Infancy	Nonspecific progressive mental deterioration	Hepatosplenomegaly	Diarrhea, vomiting and marked failure to thrive, anemia, vacuolated lymphocytes and foamy histiocytes in marrow; adrenal calcification a pathognomonic feature not present in the milder variant, cholesterol ester storage disease	Leukocytes, fibroblasts	Yes
Metachromatic leukodystrophy	AR (chromosome 10)	Sulfatides (brain, kidney and gall bladder)	Arylsulfatase A	Late infantile form ~2 years	Unsteady gait and slow learning – blindness, loss of speech, quadriparesis, bulbar palsy, peripheral neuropathy, ataxia, dementia	No hepatosplenomegaly but metachromatic storage material may be seen histologically in kidney, liver and gall bladder	Loss of white matter may be seen on CT scan of brain as diffuse symmetrical loss in density; demyelination of peripheral nerves with metachromatic granules present; high CSF protein and delayed nerve conduction velocity; increased sulfatide excretion in urine; metachromatic deposits may be found on staining	Leukocytes, fibroblasts. NB: a pseudoenzyme deficiency is not uncommon and in such instances sulfatide loading test should be carried out on fibroblasts	Yes

Table 14.65 Cont'd

Disorder	Genetics	Stored substance	Enzyme defect	Age of onset	Neurology	Visceral involvement	Other clinical features	Diagnostic sample	Prenatal diagnosis
Metachromatic leukodystrophy (Cont'd)							freshly collected urine cells with cresyl violet or certain other stains		
	AR	Sulfatides	Arylsulfatase A	Juvenile type ~4–6 years	Difficulties with mental ability, ataxia, spasticity; extrapyramidal dysfunction–pseudobulbar palsy, seizures	No hepatosplenomegaly but visceral storage may be seen histochemically	Usually presents with a fall off of attention and mental ability at school, associated with clumsiness; other features as for late infantile type	Leukocytes, fibroblasts (but note above)	Yes
	AR	Sulfatides	Arylsulfatase A	Adult type 16 years–adulthood	Behavioral changes – psychosis, dementia, ataxia, spasticity	No hepatosplenomegaly	CSF protein may or may not be raised and nerve conduction velocity normal or delayed	Leukocytes, fibroblasts (but note above)	Yes
Krabbe	AR infantile (chromosome 17)	Galactocerebroside (in globoid cells in the white matter) galactosyl-sphingosine (white matter)	Galactosylceramide β-Galactosidase	3–6 months but late onset (2–6 years) and adult forms are reported	Irritability, hypertonia with psychomotor neuropathy, fits and optic atrophy; deaf and blind; loss of deep tendon reflexes due to demyelinating neuropathy	No hepatosplenomegaly, pathology confined to nervous system	Not a true storage disease; galactocerebroside is an essential component of myelin but with the breakdown of myelin, glycolipids are lost from white matter; an accumulation of the toxic deacylated galactosylphingosine (psychosine) may be responsible for the pathogenesis and lead to the accumulation of characteristic multinucleate globoid cells in the white matter; CSF protein raised in infantile patients and possibly in later-onset form; delayed nerve conduction velocity and loss of white matter on CT scan	Leukocytes, fibroblasts	Yes

Table 14.65 *Cont'd*

Disorder	Genetics	Stored substance	Enzyme defect	Age of onset	Neurology	Visceral involvement	Other clinical features	Diagnostic sample	Prenatal diagnosis
Gaucher	AR type I adult nonneuropathic form common in Ashkenazi Jews	Glucocerebroside (spleen, liver)	β-Glucosidase	Childhood/adulthood	Normally no neurological involvement	Hepatosplenomegaly	Bone infiltration – pain/osteomyelitis/collapse of femoral head; hematological complications, characteristic foamy macrophages (Gaucher cells) in blood marrow	Leukocytes, fibroblasts	Yes
	AR type II infantile neuropathic form	Glucocerebroside (spleen and liver as well as brain, where glucosylsphingosine may be toxic metabolite)	β-Glucosidase	Infancy	Fits and psychomotor retardation, pyramidal tract dysfunction – hypertonic, brisk reflexes; bulbar signs – strabismus, apathy, dysphagia, etc; loss of saccadic eye movements	Progressive hepatosplenomegaly	Lung infiltration, hematological complications, Gaucher cells in marrow, pale optic discs; may present as hydrops fetalis	Leukocytes, fibroblasts	Yes
	AR type III juvenile form common in Sweden as Norrbottnian type (chromosome 1)	Glucocerebroside (spleen, liver and probably brain, glucosylsphingosine also in brain)	β-Glucosidase	Childhood	Subacute neuropathy, retarded psychomotor development which may be more progressive after splenectomy; ataxia and strabismus; defective horizontal saccadic eye movement	Hepatosplenomegaly	Bleeding tendency but complications often more marked after splenectomy, pale optic discs, skeletal involvement leading to fractures	Leukocytes, fibroblasts	Yes
Niemann-Pick	AR type A, common in Ashkenazi Jews (chromosome 17)	Sphingomyelin (spleen, liver, brain)	Sphingomyelinase	Infancy	Neurological deterioration – hypotonia, blindness; areflexia, slow motor nerve conduction velocity suggests demyelinating neuropathy	Massive hepatosplenomegaly	Rapidly progressive with marked failure to thrive leading to emaciation with thin extremities; skin often discolored waxy yellow/brown; cherry red spot in eye, with corneal opacification; characteristic foamy histiocytes (may be sea –blue) especially in bone marrow	Leukocytes, fibroblasts	Yes

Table 14.65 *Cont'd*

Disorder	Genetics	Stored substance	Enzyme defect	Age of onset	Neurology	Visceral involvement	Other clinical features	Diagnostic sample	Prenatal diagnosis
	AR type B, non-neuropathic form	Sphingomyelin (spleen, liver)	Sphingomyelinase	Childhood	No neurological involvement	Marked hepatosplenomegaly	Hematological complications, lung infiltration and histiocytes in bone marrow	Leukocytes, fibroblasts	Yes
	AR type C, juvenile subacute neuropathic form	Sphingomyelin, cholesterol, glucocerebroside (spleen, liver)	Defect in cholesterol esterification	Variable from infancy to adulthood	Neurological deterioration with variable time course; hypotonia, mental and motor regression, pyramidal tract involvement; in others unsteady gait and cerebellar ataxia, lack of coordination, dysarthria, cataplexy, fits, dystonia, supranuclear ophthalmoplegia with loss of saccadic eye movements in the vertical plane (cataplexy in humorous situations)	Moderate splenomegaly is common but marked (hepato-) splenomegaly also found	Prolonged neonatal cholestatic icterus and ascites in some patients; (sea-blue) histiocytes in bone marrow; this condition has also been called by other names such as 'juvenile dystonic lipidosis', 'neurovisceral storage disease with (vertical) supranuclear ophthalmoplegia'	Fibroblasts	Yes
	AR type D, Nova-Scotia variant	Cholesterol and sphingomyelin (in spleen)	Possible defect in cholesterol esterification	Similar to type C (above)	Similar to type C (above)	Similar to type C (above)	Similar to type C (above)	Fibroblasts	No
Farber	AR rare condition	Ceramide (nodules, kidney)	Ceramidase	Infants generally	Progressive psychomotor impairment	No marked hepatosplenomegaly but visceral storage on histology	Striking clinical features include: numerous subcutaneous nodules, arthritis with painful and deformed joints, hoarseness due to laryngeal involvement which may lead to breathing and swallowing difficulties	Leukocytes, fibroblasts	Yes

AR = autosomal recessive

Table 14.66 Disorders of glycoprotein and oligosaccharide metabolism including mucolipidoses

Disorder	Genetics	Stored substance	Enzyme defect	Age of onset	Neurology	Visceral involvement	Other clinical features	Diagnostic sample	Prenatal diagnosis
Aspartyl-glucosaminuria	AR rare but more common in Finland	Aspartyl-glucosamine (esp. urine)	Aspartyl-glucosaminidase	About 6 months onwards	Mental retardation from almost 5 years of age, behavioral problems	Generally no hepatosplenomegaly	Coarse featured with loose skin, mild dysostosis multiplex, short stature, lens opacity, acne, vacuolated lymphocytes	Leukocytes, fibroblasts	Yes
Fucosidosis	AR rare but common in Italy (chromosome 1)	Fucose-rich oligosaccharides glycoproteins and glycolipids. Note H-antigen (with terminal fucose residue) (urine, liver, brain)	α-Fucosidase	Two phenotypes: type I 3–18 months, type II 1–2 years	Psychomotor retardation, more marked deterioration in type I	Hepatosplenomegaly may be present	Mildly coarse featured, short stature, dysostosis multiplex but less marked in type II; increased sweat NaCl in type I and angiokeratoma in the longer surviving type II; vacuolated lymphocytes in both types	Leukocytes, fibroblasts. Note low serum α-fucosidase activity polymorphism in unaffected healthy individuals	Yes
Mannosidosis	AR rare (chromosome 19)	Mannose-rich oligosaccharides (urine, tissues)	α-Mannosidase	Two phenotypes: type I 3–12 months, type II 1–4 years	Psychomotor retardation, deafness	Hepatosplenomegaly	Coarse featured, dysostosis multiplex and characteristic corneal and lens opacities, especially in type I; vacuolated lymphocytes in types I and II	Leukocytes, fibroblasts	Yes
β-Mannosidosis	Probably AR	Mannose-rich disaccharide (urine)	β-Mannosidase	Variable	Mental retardation, deafness	No hepatomegaly	Only three families reported so far, all with different phenotypes	Leukocytes, fibroblasts	Probably yes
α-N-acetyl-galactosaminidase deficiency	AR	N-acetyl-galactosamine containing oligosaccharides (urine)	α-N-acetyl galactosaminidase	~9 months	Severe psychomotor retardation, cortical blindness, myoclonic seizures, neuroaxonal dystrophy	No hepatomegaly	Recently described disease, only in one family so far	Leukocytes, fibroblasts	Probably yes

Table 14.66 Cont'd

Disorder	Genetics	Stored substance	Enzyme defect	Age of onset	Neurology	Visceral involvement	Other clinical features	Diagnostic sample	Prenatal diagnosis
Sialic acid storage disease	AR	Free sialic acid (urine, tissues)	Lysosomal sialic acid transport protein	1–2 months	Mental retardation, slow regression	Hepatosplenomegaly	Coarse facies and short stature, dysostosis multiplex but clear corneas; hypopigmentation (fine wispy hair); vacuolated lymphocytes and punctate calcification; beware, some features like Zellweger syndrome; may present as hydrops fetalis; a milder variant known as Salla disease is common in Finland	Urine fibroblasts	Yes
Mucolipidosis I (sialidosis)	AR (may be more common in Italians) (? chromosome 10)	Sialyloligosaccharides (urine, tissues)	α-Neuraminidase	Type 1 8–20 years, type 2 variable, infancy–late childhood	Type 1 myoclonic seizures, cherry red spot in eye, psychomotor retardation in some. Type 2 cherry red spot, seizures	Type 1 no hepatosplenomegaly Type 2 hepatosplenomegaly	Considerable variation in phenotype; type 1 patients not dysmorphic, but type 2 patients, dysmorphic and coarse featured, short stature with dysostosis multiplex; vacuolated lymphocytes in both types	Fibroblasts	Yes
Galactosialidosis	AR (chromosome 20)	Sialyloligosaccharides (urine and tissues)	α-Neuraminidase and β-galactosidase	Variable	Similar to mucolipidosis I (type 2)	No hepatosplenomegaly	Similar to mucolipidosis I (type 2) but with angiokeratoma in some patients; primary defect in combined enzyme protective protein. May lead to hydrops fetalis	Fibroblasts	Yes

Table 14.66   *Cont'd*

Disorder	Genetics	Stored substance	Enzyme defect	Age of onset	Neurology	Visceral involvement	Other clinical features	Diagnostic sample	Prenatal diagnosis
Mucolipidosis II (I-cell disease)	AR (chromosome 4)	Various mucopoly-saccharides and oligosaccharides (urine, certain cells)	N-acetyl-glucosamine-1-phosphotransferase	Neonates and infants	Psychomotor retardation	Usually hepatosplenomegaly and cardiomegaly	Coarse facies, marked skeletal deformities including gibbus and kyphoscoliosis, short stature; joint contractures, 'puffy' eyes and gingival hyperplasia; little or no corneal clouding; characteristic intracellular inclusions (hence I-cell) in certain cell types, especially cultured fibroblasts; primary defect in Golgi enzyme responsible for phosphorylation of lysosomal glycoproteins including most lysosomal hydrolases; defect results in failure of receptor mediated uptake into lysosomes	Serum fibroblasts	Yes
Mucolipidosis III (pseudo-Hurler polydystrophy)	AR (chromosome 4)	Various mucopoly-saccharides and oligosaccharides (urine, certain cells)	N-acetyl-glucosamine-1-phospho-transferase (same as mucolipidosis II, above)	About 4–5 years	Slow psychomotor retardation	Possibly mild hepatosplenomegaly	Mild phenotype of MLII; usually presenting features include stiff joints	Serum fibroblasts	Yes
Mucolipidosis IV	AR	Phospholipids and gangliosides (tissues)	Ganglioside sialidase but not confirmed	In the first year	Marked psychomotor retardation, visual impairment	No hepatosplenomegaly	Corneal opacities with retinal degeneration; short stature; foamy histiocytes in bone marrow	Fibroblasts	Yes

AR = autosomal recessive.

Table 14.67 Mucopolysaccharidoses – MPS disorders

Disorder	Genetics	Stored substance	Enzyme defect	Age of onset	Neurology	Visceral involvement	Other clinical features	Diagnostic sample	Prenatal diagnosis
MPS I Hurler–Scheie	AR all forms (chromosome 22)	Dermatan sulfate and heparan sulfate (urine, tissues)	α-Iduronidase	2/3 phenotypes (i) Hurler – onset in first year and death usually by 10 years	Marked psychomotor retardation, hydrocephalus	Hepatosplenomegaly and cardiomegaly	Coarse features, stunted growth, dysostosis multiplex, lumbar lordosis, stiff joints and claw hand; characteristic radiological changes (skull, vertebrae, ribs and clavicle); umbilical hernia and progressive corneal clouding	Leukocytes, fibroblasts	Yes
				(ii) Scheie – onset during childhood or adulthood (formerly designated MPS V)	No neurological deficit	No visceromegaly normally seen	Milder clinical phenotype than in Hurler; mildly coarse facies and skeletal deformities but normal stature; corneal opacities; note: an intermediate phenotype, Hurler–Scheie may result from a genetic compound	Leukocytes, fibroblasts	Yes
				(iii) Hurler–Scheie intermediate type					
MPS II Hunter	X-linked recessive (X chromosome)	Heparan sulfate and dermatan sulfate (urine, tissues)	Iduronate 2-sulfatase	Usually between 2–5 years, but milder types survive to late adulthood	Slowly deteriorating mental retardation	Hepatosplenomegaly Cardiac defects due to infiltration into valves and arterial walls	Normally no corneal clouding but papilledema may lead to blindness; also differs from Hurler in absence of gibbus; pale nodular skin lesions, especially over scapulae; recurrent respiratory infections, cardiac abnormalities (murmurs) stunted growth, dysostosis multiplex, claw hands, coarse featured, hernias, progressive deafness; note: milder variant surviving into late adulthood – carpal tunnel syndrome	Serum, leukocytes, fibroblasts	Yes

Table 14.67 *Cont'd*

Disorder	Genetics	Stored substance	Enzyme defect	Age of onset	Neurology	Visceral involvement	Other clinical features	Diagnostic sample	Prenatal diagnosis
MPS III Sanfilippo	AR all forms (chromosome 12)	Heparan sulfate (urine, tissues)	Four types: MPS III A heparan N-sulfatase MPS IIIB N-acetyl-α-glucosaminidase MPS IIIC acetyl-CoA: α-glucosaminide N-acetyltransferase MPS IIID N-acetyl-α-glucosaminide-6-sulfatase	All types similar usually between 2–6 years	Severe and progressive mental deterioration, usually impairment of complete extension of the fingers	Mild or no hepatosplenomegaly	All four types are clinically indistinguishable; in the UK, the most common appears to be MPS IIIA, and MPS IIID the least frequent; relatively mild skeletal and somatic involvement and generally no corneal clouding; often main feature is behavioral disturbance with hyperactivity and sleep problems; many become institutionalized	Serum, and/or leukocytes (depending on type), fibroblasts	Yes
MPS IV Morquio	AR both forms (chromosome 3)	Keratan sulfatase, chondroitin sulfate (urine, tissues)	Two types: MPS IVA galactosamine-6-sulfatase MPS IVB β-galactosidase	Usually first years of life	No primary neurological involvement in either type but quadriplegia and myelopathy may result from compression of the cervical cord	Mild, no hepatosplenomegaly	Characteristic skeletal deformities, corneal clouding, dwarfism, thin dental enamel	Leukocytes, fibroblasts	Yes
MPS VI Maroteaux-Lamy	AR (rare) (chromosome 5)	Dermatan sulfate (urine, tissues)	Arylsulfatase B	Usually first years of life	No primary neurological involvement but secondary problems as in MPS IV	Hepatosplenomegaly	Marked skeletal abnormalities with corneal clouding, characteristic leukocyte inclusions	Leukocytes, fibroblasts	Yes
MPS VII Sly	AR (rare) (chromosome 7)	Dermatan sulfate, heparan sulfate (urine, tissues)	β-Glucuronidase	Variable (only few patients)	Variable but may have mental retardation	Hepatosplenomegaly	Few patients described; spectrum of severe (hydrops fetalis) to adult forms	Leukocytes, fibroblasts	Yes
Multiple sulfatase deficiency	AR	Mucopoly-saccharides (especially heparan sulfate), sulfatides and steroid sulfates (urine)	Various sulfatases	1–2 years usually	Marked psychomotor deterioration, deafness and abnormal gait	Hepatosplenomegaly	Combines features of mucopolysaccharidosis with those of metachromatic leukodystrophy; mildly dysmorphic, high CSF protein and ichthyosis present; no corneal clouding; enzyme deficiency may be variable in expression and both leukocytes and fibroblasts should be studied for several sulfatase activities	Leukocytes, fibroblasts	Yes

AR = autosomal recessive

Table 14.68 Peroxisomal disorders

Disorder	Genetics	Stored material	Enzyme deficiency or defect	Age of onset	Neurology	Visceral involvement	Other clinical features	Diagnostic sample	Prenatal diagnosis
Zellweger (cerebro-hepatorenal syndrome)	AR (chromosome 7)	Very long chain fatty acids, bile acid intermediates (plasma), also phytanic acid, pipecolic acid, (plasma) dicarboxylic acids (urine) but more variable	Not known, but several peroxisomal enzymes, one of which may be used for diagnosis (dihydroxyacetone phosphate acyl-transferase)	At birth/neonate, most succumb by 6 months	Severe hypotonia, seizures, psychomotor retardation, areflexia, deaf and blind, flat ERG	Hepatomegaly, renal cysts, adrenal atrophy, no peroxisomes seen on liver microscopy	Multiple abnormalities: characteristic facies, high forehead, flattened nasal bridge, epicanthus, low set ears and high arched palate; large fontanel; cataract/retinal pigmentation and/or pale optic disc; failure to thrive, jaundice, raised LFT and diminished response to ACTH; punctate calcification especially in neonate, simian crease, cryptorchidism; these patients appear to lack peroxisomes in all cells	Plasma, platelets, fibroblasts	Yes
Neonatal adreno-leukodystrophy	AR	Similar to Zellweger (above) but mainly saturated very long chain fatty acids	Similar to Zellweger (above)	At birth/neonates, most succumb by 6 years	Similar to Zellweger but less marked; severe neuro-degeneration	Similar to Zellweger (above)	Similar to Zellweger but less marked craniofacial abnormality, but generally blind and deaf. More marked adrenal atrophy but less marked renal cysts. Punctate calcification not usually found. Numerous foamy macrophages esp. in adrenal, with characteristic lamellar inclusions. Patients appear to lack peroxisomes	Plasma, platelets, fibroblasts	Yes
Infantile Refsum	AR	Similar to Zellweger (above) but phytanic acid more evident with dietary intake	Similar to Zellweger (above)	Usually in the first months but generally not in neonatal period; may survive into teens	Neurological symptoms become more evident after 6 months when regression develops, with psychomotor delay and hypotonia; autistic behavior with impaired vision and hearing	Only mild hepatomegaly	Only mildly dysmorphic like Zellweger	Plasma, platelets, fibroblasts	Yes
Zellweger-like syndrome	Probably AR	Similar to Zellweger	Peroxisomes present but many enzyme activities deficient	Neonate	As for Zellweger	As for Zellweger	Apart from the presence of peroxisomes, this condition appears to be similar to Zellweger	Plasma, fibroblasts	Probably yes

Table 14.68 Cont'd

Disorder	Genetics	Stored material	Enzyme deficiency or defect	Age of onset	Neurology	Visceral involvement	Other clinical features	Diagnostic sample	Prenatal diagnosis
Peroxisomal β-oxidation defects									
(a) Pseudo-Zellweger	AR (chromosome 3)	Very long chain fatty acids and bile acid intermediates	3-Oxoacyl-CoA-thiolase	Neonate	Severe hypotonia similar to Zellweger	Mild hepatomegaly, renal cysts present	Presents like Zellweger but peroxisomes present and dihydroxyacetone phosphate acyltransferase activity normal; no punctate calcification and no simian crease	Plasma, fibroblasts	Yes
(b) Pseudo-neonatal adrenoleukodystrophy	AR	Very long chain fatty acids	Acyl-CoA-oxidase	Neonate	Similar to neonatal adrenoleukodystrophy	No, or mild hepatomegaly	Similar to neonatal adrenoleukodystrophy but peroxisomes present as above; not markedly dysmorphic	Plasma, fibroblasts	Yes
(c) Bifunctional enzyme deficiency	AR	Very long chain fatty acids	Bifunctional enzyme	Neonate	Similar to neonatal adrenoleukodystrophy	See (b)	Similar to (b)	Plasma, fibroblasts	Yes
Rhizomelic chondrodysplasia punctata (type of Conradi syndrome)	AR	Phytanic acid (plasma) and plasmalogens (tissues)	At least two peroxisomal enzyme deficiencies (dihydroxyacetone phosphate acyl-transferase and phytanic acid oxidase)	At birth but usually succumb in first year	Marked psychomotor retardation and failure to thrive	No hepato-splenomegaly reported	Severe and symmetric dysmorphology; microcephaly; prominent forehead and flattened nasal bridge; proximal limb shortening and joint contractures; punctate calcification especially of epiphyses; cataracts and ichthyosis; several peroxisomal defects but peroxisomes present. Normal levels of very long chain fatty acids and bile acid intermediates	Plasma, platelets, fibroblasts	Yes
Adrenoleuko-dystrophy (Addison disease with cerebral sclerosis, Schilder disease)	X-linked recessive	Very long chain fatty acid (>C22 length) (plasma, fibroblasts esp. adrenal, CNS), fatty acid ratio of C26:C22 increased	Peroxisomal very long chain fatty acyl-CoA synthetase	Usually 4–8 years but milder adrenomyelo-neuropathy at 20–30 years	Progressive psychomotor deterioration, ataxia, dementia, loss of vision and hearing	No hepato-splenomegaly	CT-symmetrical white hypodensities especially in occipital poles; CSF protein increased; oligoclonal bands commonly present; affected males have neurological symptoms with loss of adrenal function; bronzing of skin, characteristic curvilinear storage bodies especially in adrenal cortex, peripheral nerve and CNS; the milder adrenomyeloneuropathy may present with leg stiffness and peripheral neuropathy	Plasma, fibroblasts	Yes

Table 14.68 Cont'd

Disorder	Genetics	Stored material	Enzyme deficiency or defect	Age of onset	Neurology	Visceral involvement	Other clinical features	Diagnostic sample	Prenatal diagnosis
Refsum (heredopathia atactica polyneuritiformis)	AR	Phytanic acid (plasma)	Phytanic acid oxidase	1–20 years	Polyneuropathy, ataxia, loss of vision (retinitis pigmentosa), loss of hearing and smell	No hepato-splenomegaly	Skeletal changes, e.g. shortened metatarses, cardiac arrhythmias and ichthyosis (which may respond to dietary restriction of phytanate); anosmia is one of the first and most consistently presenting features	Plasma, fibroblasts	Yes — but treatable condition

AR = autosomal recessive

Table 14.69 Mitochondrial disorders and Leigh's encephalopathies

Disorder	Genetics	Stored substance	Enzyme or protein defect	Age of onset	Neurology	Visceral involvement	Other clinical features	Diagnostic sample	Prenatal diagnosis
Kearns-Sayre	AR or mitochondrial	Lactate (in some patients)	Possible respiratory chain defects: cytochrome c oxidase (complex IV) but may be deficient in other conditions (Leigh's, etc.)	Before 15 years	Cerebellar involvement, ophthalmoplegia and retinal degeneration, ataxia	Cardiomyopathy with arrhythmias	High CSF protein; myopathy of skeletal, including occulomotor, and cardiac muscle; ragged red muscle fibers; weakness of facial muscles, short stature, possibly a heterogeneous group of disorders, including some with mitochondrial respiration chain defects	Muscle	No
Mitochondrial encephalo-myopathy, lactic acidosis and stroke-like episodes (MELAS)	Possibly mitochondrial (maternal)	Lactate in some patients	Possible respiratory chain defects, e.g. NADH-CoQ reductase	Childhood	Cortical blindness, hemiparesis and deafness, seizures	None reported	Stunted growth, episodic vomiting, ragged red muscle fibers and spongy degeneration of brain at PM; probably a heterogeneous group of disorders including patients with respiratory chain defects	Muscle	No
Myoclonic epilepsy with ragged red fibers (MERRF)	Possibly mitochondrial (maternal)	Lactate in some patients	Possible respiratory chain defects – none known	Before 20 years	Myoclonus, ataxia, weakness and seizures	None reported	Some patients may present as Friedreich's ataxia but this is probably a heterogeneous group of disorders; ragged red muscle fibers found but no specific enzyme deficiencies yet identified	Muscle	No

Table 14.69 *Cont'd*

Disorder	Genetics	Stored substance	Enzyme or protein defect	Age of onset	Neurology	Visceral involvement	Other clinical features	Diagnostic sample	Prenatal diagnosis
Leigh's subacute necrotizing encephalopathy	AR ?mitochondrial	Lactate	In some patients specific deficiency (a) pyruvate carboxylase or (b) pyruvate dehydrogenase or (c) cytochrome c oxidase or (d) biotinidase	Early childhood	Marked neurodegeneration, deaf, blind and progressive spasticity, eye movement control, control of respiration, ataxia, possible peripheral neuropathy	None	Appears to be a heterogeneous group of conditions often associated with specific enzyme deficiencies; deficiencies are not specific to Leigh's and many patients have no known enzyme defect; deficiencies may be tissue/cell specific; CT: low densities in putamen, cerebellum and brain stem	Fibroblasts, muscle	Yes, only expressed in fibroblasts
Fumarase deficiency	Probably AR	Fumarate (urine)	Fumarase	Infancy	Developmental delay, hypotonia and cerebral atrophy	None	Progressive neurological disorder which may present as 'mitochondrial myopathy', with lethargy and failure to thrive	Muscle, liver	No

AR = autosomal recessive

Table 14.70 Disorders of carbohydrate metabolism

Disorder	Genetics	Stored substance	Enzyme defect	Age of onset	Neurology	Visceral involvement	Other clinical features	Diagnostic sample	Prenatal diagnosis
Glycogenosis type I (Von Gierke)	AR	Glycogen (liver)	Glucose-6-phosphatase	Usually in infancy	Secondary to hypoglycemia as convulsions, coma	Massive hepatomegaly and enlarged kidneys	Primarily liver and kidney involvement with short stature; usually marked hypoglycemia, with raised lactate, blood lipids and uric acid; three variants: type Ia — glucose-6-phosphatase deficiency; type Ib — microsomal glucose-6-phosphate transporter, more severe disorder with neutropenia; type Ic — microsomal phosphate translocase	Fresh liver	No
Glycogenosis type II (Pompe)	AR infantile (chromosome 17)	Glycogen (liver, muscle), oligosaccharides (urine)	Acid maltase (α-glucosidase)	Two types: generalized infantile form and adult myopathic form (infant–adult onset)	Marked hypotonia in infantile form. Progressive muscle weakness in adults	Marked cardiomegaly with hepatomegaly	Severe and generalized condition with cardiorespiratory involvement and failure to thrive; patients are grayish, pale and listless, and tongue may be enlarged; vacuolated lymphocytes present; most patients succumb in first year. Variable presentation in children and adults; skeletal and respiratory muscle involvement especially in trunk and proximal limits	Fibroblasts, lymphocytes	Yes

Table 14.70 Cont'd

Disorder	Genetics	Stored substance	Enzyme defect	Age of onset	Neurology	Visceral involvement	Other clinical features	Diagnostic sample	Prenatal diagnosis
Glycogenosis type III (Cori)	AR	Glycogen (limit dextrin) (liver, muscle), oligosaccharides (urine)	Amylo-1, 6-glucosidase (debrancher)	Usually in infancy	Muscle wasting and myopathy in some patients	Massive hepatomegaly and moderate splenomegaly	Infants may appear to be obese with rosy cheeks; muscle involvement may extend to heart and lead to hypertrophy and sudden death; hypoglycemic generally only after fasting; different variants without muscle involvement known	Blood (erythrocytes and leukocytes), liver	Yes in some cases
Glycogenosis type IV (Anderson)	AR	Glycogen (amylopectin)	α-1, 4-glucan-α-1, 4-glucan-6-glucosyltransferase	Infancy	Poor development, hypotonia, muscular atrophy	Hepatosplenomegaly	Marked failure to thrive with ascites and progressive cirrhosis; abnormal storage bodies in CNS and peripheral nerves	Leukocytes, fibroblasts	Yes
Glycogenosis type V (McArdle)	AR (chromosome 11)	Glycogen (muscle)	Muscle phosphorylase	Childhood and young adults	Muscle weakness, cramps on exercise	No visceromegaly	No increase in venous lactate after ischemic exercise; myoglobulinuria; a severe infantile type has been reported; muscle phosphofructokinase deficiency (Tarui disease) is clinically similar	Muscle	No
Glycogenosis type VI	AR (chromosome 14) or X-linked recessive	Glycogen (liver)	Liver phosphorylase (AR) or more usually phosphorylase b kinase, deficiency (X-linked form)	Infants	No neurological symptoms, usually	Hepatomegaly	This type should not present as a neurological problem	Liver or erythrocytes	No

AR = autosomal recessive

Table 14.71 Other conditions with biochemical defects

Disorder	Genetics	Stored substance	Enzyme or protein defect	Age of onset	Neurology	Visceral involvement	Other clinical features	Diagnostic sample	Prenatal diagnosis
Cerebrotendinous xanthomatosis	AR	Cholestanol and cholesterol	Steroid 26-hydroxylase	Childhood onwards	Cerebellar ataxia; dementia	None	Tendon xanthomas; cataracts	Serum fibroblasts	Possible
Cerebrotendinous xanthomatosis	AR	Cholestanol and cholesterol	Steroid 26-hydroxylase	Childhood onwards	Cerebellar ataxia; dementia	None	Tendon xanthomas; cataracts	Serum fibroblasts	Possible

Table 14.71 Other conditions with biochemical defects

Disorder	Genetics	Stored substance	Enzyme or protein defect	Age of onset	Neurology	Visceral involvement	Other clinical features	Diagnostic sample	Prenatal diagnosis
Abeta-lipo-proteinemia	AR (chromosome 2)	Low blood cholesterol	Apoprotein B	Childhood onwards; common in Jews	Progressive spinocerebellar ataxia; peripheral neuropathy; pigmentary retinopathy	Not usually involved	Acanthocytosis of erythrocytes; hematological complications; fat malabsorption with gastrointestinal manifestations of celiac disease	Plasma	No
Tangier disease	AR	Cholesterol esters in tissues, low blood cholesterol	HDL	Childhood onwards	Relapsing polyneuropathy; sensory loss; muscle weakness and wasting	Hepatosplenomegaly	Enlarged orange tonsils; extensive foamy histiocytic infiltration	Plasma	No
Acute intermittent porphyria	AD	Porphobilinogen (urine and plasma)	Porphobilinogen deaminase	Latent condition, with attacks after puberty	Acute neuropathic episodes; muscle weakness; mental disturbance	None	Acute abdominal pain; vomiting; tachycardia, attacks precipitated by drugs	Urine, erythrocytes	Possible
Lesch-Nyhan	X-linked recessive (X chromosome)	Uric acid	Hypoxanthine-guanine phosphoribosyl transferase	3–6 months	Choreoathetosis; spasticity; mental retardation; self-mutilation	None	Renal stones and obstructive neuropathy; gouty arthritis	Erythrocytes, fibroblasts	Yes
Succinyl-purinemic autism	Possibly AR	Succinylpurines	Adenylosuccinase	Infancy	Autism, hypokinesia; may self-mutilate	None	Few cases studied	Urine, liver	No
Nonketotic hyperglycinemia	AR	Glycine	Glycine cleavage enzyme	Neonate	Muscular hypotonia; marked seizures; apneic attacks; lethargy and coma	None	Generally fatal condition but some milder phenotypes have been reported	Liver, placenta	Yes
Homocystinuria	AR (chromosome 21)	Homocystine	Cystathionine β-synthase or defects in B_{12} metabolism	Early childhood	Mental retardation and convulsions; cerebrovascular accidents	None	Lens dislocation is common; osteoporosis and marfanoid features with elongated long bones; thromboembolism a major cause of morbidity	Fibroblasts	Yes
Phenylketonuria	AR (chromosome 4)	Phenylalanine	Phenylalanine hydroxylase or defects in biopterin metabolism	If missed in neonatal screen onset ~6–12 months	Seizures and increased muscle tone; agitated behavior	None	Fair hair, blue eyes and eczema	Plasma	Yes, by DNA
Biotinidase deficiency	AR	3-Hydroxyiso-valeric acid and several other organic acids	Biotinidase	3–6 months	Seizures; hypotonia, ataxia; developmental delay	None	Skin rash, alopecia	Plasma	No

Table 14.71 *Cont'd*

Disorder	Genetics	Stored substance	Enzyme or protein defect	Age of onset	Neurology	Visceral involvement	Other clinical features	Diagnostic sample	Prenatal diagnosis
Menkes' disease (kinky or steely hair disease)	X-linked recessive (X chromosome)	Copper (intracellular)	Copper transport protein	2–4 months	Neurological degeneration, fits, hypothermia	No hepatosplenomegaly	Abnormal hair (pili torti) hence kinky/steely hair syndrome; unusual face, bony changes and fractures, tortuosity of blood vessels and aneurysms	Fibroblasts (low blood copper and ceruloplasmin levels)	Yes
Wilson disease (hepatolenticular degeneration)	AR	Copper (in liver)	Not known	8 year–adulthood	Neurological involvement often later in onset, as dysarthria, uncoordinated movement; pseudobulbar palsy	Liver disease, often acute; renal stones	Characteristic Kayser-Fleischer rings in cornea of eye, esp. in neurologically affected patients; bone and joint disorders; low serum copper and ceruloplasmin common but not diagnostic	Liver increased copper on biopsy	No
Combined sulfite oxidase and xanthine oxidase deficiency	AR	Sulfite, taurine thiosulfate and S-sulfocystine (urine); low uric acid in blood and urine, with high xanthine and sulfite in urine	Molybdenum cofactor	Neonate	Severe psychomotor retardation and regression, tonic seizures; lens dislocation and dysmorphism	None	A rapidly degenerating leukodystrophy, most patients die by 18 months; biochemical defect recently described	Fibroblasts	Yes
Canavan (spongy degeneration of CNS)	AR (more common in Jews)	N-acetyl-aspartate	Aspartyl-acylase	Early infancy	Megalencephaly, visual loss, marked degeneration of white matter; severe mental deficit, blind, atonic neck muscles and hyper-extension of legs	None	A rapidly degenerating leukodystrophy, most patients die by 18 months; biochemical defect recently described	Fibroblasts	Possible
Sjögren-Larsson syndrome	AR (more common in Sweden)	Long chain alcohols, e.g. hexadecanol	Fatty alcohol: NAD oxido-reductase	Skin lesions at birth, neurological deficit around 3 years	Mental retardation, spasticity	None	Ichthyosis of skin and glistening spots in ocular fundus	Fibroblasts	Possible

AR = autosomal recessive

Table 14.72 Spinocerebellar and peripheral nerve degenerations

Disorders	Genetics	Age at onset	Neurology	Other clinical features	Diagnosis
Dentatorubral atrophy (Ramsey Hunt syndrome)	Familial	Late childhood to adolescence	Myoclonic epilepsy; cerebellar ataxia		Involvement of dentate nucleus, dentatorubral tract and spinocerebellar tract and superior cerebellar peduncle
Friedreich's ataxia	AR (chromosome 9)	Mean 10.5 years (range 2–16 years)	Presenting: ataxia (limbs and trunk), scoliosis, tremor, cardiomyopathy (T inversion and LVH). Later: dysarthria, pyramidal signs with extensor plantars and diminished reflexes, proprioceptive loss, pes cavus, distal amyotrophy (distal fasting and weakness), optic atrophy and nystagmus, deafness CCF or arrhythmias, gradually progressive	Diabetes mellitus; sudden cardiac death in the 30s	
Familial spastic paraplegia	AR 11.5 years AD 18.5 years		Slow learning to walk; mild spastic paraplegia; stiff gait; scissoring of legs; slowly progressive (variable)		Spinal cord degeneration of lateral pyramidal tract, corticospinal, lateral cerebellar and posterior columns
Progressive cerebellar ataxia	AR	Mean 9.4 years	Dysarthria, pyramidal signs, absent ankle jerks (others normal); sensory loss	Better prognosis than Friedreich's ataxia	Sensory action potentials reduced in size; cerebellar atrophy on CT scan
Familial spastic-ataxic syndrome	AR		Progressive insidious involvement with signs relative to cerebellum, corticospinal tract and occular signs	Death over 5–20 years	
Olivopontocerebellar atrophy (OPCA) (Types I–V)	AD … OPCA (Types I, III, IV, V) AR … OPCA (Type II)		With retinal degeneration progressive cerebellar ataxia; parkinsonian rigidity; resting tremor; impairment of speech		Atrophy of cerebellar ponds and inferior olives
Ataxia telangiectasia (Louis-Barr syndrome)	AR (chromosome 11)		Progressive neurological deterioration with ocular and cutaneous telangiectasia. Early: cerebellar ataxia (often less than developmental progress). Later: Decreased IgA, dysarthria, choreoathetosis; titubation. Sometimes progressive dementia. Telangiectasia of conjunctiva, pinnae, face, V of the neck, and flexures begins after 3 years; occulomotor dyspraxia	Growth retardation; wheelchair by 10–12 years; survivors show distal weakness, wasting, posterior column signs after 10 years; death before adulthood. Immunological: tonsils hypoplastic, abnormal IgM, thymic hypoplasia. Neoplasia: lymphomas, sarcomas, lymphosarcomas, leukemia, Hodgkin's cerebellar neoplasms, ovarian and gastric tumors. Blood: lymphocytopenia. Endocrine: abnormal carbohydrate metabolism	Increased AFP; increased in vitro radiosensitivity of chromosomes; chromosome breaks especially 7–14; DNA repaired defect in fibroblasts

Table 14.72 *Cont'd*

Disorders	Genetics	Age at onset	Neurology	Other clinical features	Diagnosis
Huntington's chorea in childhood	AD	Usually 30–50 years, 5–12% present in childhood		Dementia (withdrawn and disturbed); seizures (early); akinetic – rigid; cerebellar ataxia; horizontal saccadic eye movements	L-DOPA provocation in presymptomatic cases; abnormal monoamines (decreased GABA and GAD); ventricular enlargement with atrophy of caudate nucleus and putamen; necropsy shows shrunken caudate and putamen due to a loss of small nerve cells and astrocytic proliferation
Idiopathic torsion dystonia (dystonia musculorum deformans)	AR 4–16 years (rapid) AD Variable onset (slow)		Progressive abnormal dystonic postures; difficulty in the use of legs and arms; abnormal gait; torticollis or tortipelvis; speech abnormality; intellect mostly preserved	Progressive for 5–10 years; mostly static beyond 35 years; one-third need wheelchair	Elevated blood dopamine-β-hydroxylase in some cases
Hereditary progressive dystonia with diurnal variation	AD (low penetrance)	16 months–9 years	Progressive dystonia (spreads in an 'N' fashion); worse by day	Especially in Japan	Trial of L-DOPA
Juvenile parkinsonism	Rare in childhood		Akinetic – rigid; tremor		
Infantile neuroaxonal dystrophy	AR	6 months–2 years	Loss of motor and mental milestones with regression; early visual involvement (ocular wobble); symmetrical pyramidal tract signs; marked hypotonia; anterior horn cell involvement (peripheral motor and sensory defect); dementia and decerebration	Death less than 10 years	Axonal spheroid bodies in peripheral nerve, skin, conjunctiva, and brain; iron pigment in basal ganglia; axonal neuropathy (EMG denervation); normal NCV; EEG high voltage beta waves; VERs reduced or absent; CSF protein normal
Multiple sclerosis in childhood		12–13 years	Remitting course (1–2 episodes in childhood); optic/retrobulbar neuritis bilaterally (a quarter of childhood cases subsequently develop MS); gait disorder (with spasticity or ataxia)		Increased CSF protein (first or mid-zone colloidal gold); CSF moderate pleocytosis; MRI/CT demyelination; active-E-rosette test is positive on lymphocytes
Neuromyelitis optica (Devic's disease)			Optic neuritis; spinal cord symptoms (transverse myelitis)		
Giant axonal neuropathy	AR	Early school years	Chronic peripheral mixed neuropathy; regression of gait, movement and IQ; fits; nystagmus	Precocious puberty; pale, slightly reddish tightly curly hair	Axonal swellings (spheroids) in spinal cord, brainstem, cortex, peripheral nerves; demyelination in peripheral nerves and increased cytoplasmic filaments in nerve cells; diagnosis on skin biopsy of filaments in the cytoplasm of fibroblasts; EEG (spike and wave/disorganized); decreased motor and sensory nerve conduction velocity

Table 14.72   *Cont'd*

Disorders	Genetics	Age at onset	Neurology	Other clinical features	Diagnosis
Hallervorden–Spatz disease	AR	About 10 years	Progressive impairment of gait by pes equinovarus; spasticity with atrophy of distal muscles; athetosis and extrapyramidal rigidity; seizures (some); dementia; retinitis pigmentosa or optic atrophy (occasional); impaired speech	Death in early 20s	?Primary axonal dystrophy of substantia nigra and locus caerulus; destruction seen as low density areas in putamen and globus pallidus — low density on CT; in neurones and glia there is increased stainable iron in basal ganglia with demyelination and spheroids

AR = autosomal recessive; AD = autosomal dominant

Table 14.73   Tumors

Disorders	Genetics	Age of onset	Neurology	Other clinical features	Diagnosis
Amyloidosis		Late childhood	Peripheral neuropathy, cerebrovascular disease and dementia	Cardiomyopathy, hepatomegaly, splenomegaly, nephrosis, macroglossia	Congo red tests; gum or liver biopsy
Hand–Schuller–Christian disease	Nongenetic	Childhood	Cerebellar ataxia (rare presentation); proptosis; diabetes insipidus (the latter two due to infiltration of the base of the skull)	Lymphadenopathy, hepatosplenomegaly, lung infiltration; skull lesions; xanthoma and skin lesions	Foam cells on biopsy
Craniopharyngioma			Hallucinations; regression; growth failure; endocrine abnormalities		
Frontal lobe glioma			Headache; declining school performance		

Table 14.74   Infections

Disorders	Genetics	Age of onset	Neurology	Other clinical features	Diagnosis
Subacute sclerosing panencephalitis		5–15 years Male:female ratio 2.5:1	Stage 1 (months): insidious deterioration of behavior and intellectual performance; involuntary movements (falling or staggering backwards). Stage 2: mental deterioration; symmetrical metronomic myoclonus with frozen movements every 4–20s; spasticity; cortical blindness or hemianopia, focal chorioretinitis at maculae; nystagmus, optic atrophy; raised intracranial pressure (occasionally papilledema); rare cases arrest in this stage. Stage 3: extrapyramidal/pyramidal dysfunction (including ballismic movements); severe dementia; seizures. Stage 4: 1 year or more from onset; decerebrate rigidity; coma		Early measles (6–8 years before); EEG burst suppression; ERG normal; VER diminished; intranuclear and intracytoplasmic inclusions show bright fluorescence when stained with measles labeled antibody; incidence after measles vaccine, 10 times lower; high measles antibody (CF and HI); high levels of antibody in CSF to measles; protein in the CSF normal or slight increase; IgG increased (first zone colloidal gold); CSF cells normal or increased mononuclears; CT-slit ventricles; brain inflammation and degeneration

Table 14.74 *Cont'd*

Disorders	Genetics	Age of onset	Neurology	Other clinical features	Diagnosis
Progressive rubella panencephalitis	Following congenital rubella, rarely after ordinary rubella	Abour 10 years +	Progressive dementia; pyramidal and extrapyramidal and cerebellar signs; myoclonic seizures	Slower than SSPE; incubation 10–15 years	Increased rubella antibodies in serum and CSF; some increase in CSF protein and an oligoclonal pattern of globulins; no periodic complexes on EEG
Progressive multifocal leukoencephalopathy	Rare, male:female 15:1		Papova virus (polyomavirus JC strain); underlying malignancy	Fatal in 12 months	Multifocal demyelination in the cortex; virus (nuclear) in oligodendroglia; circular low attenuation on CT scan
Juvenile paretic neurosyphilis		Mean 13 years	Mental retardation then deterioration (with confusion, flattened affect, and restless purposive behavior); chorioretinitis and optic atrophy; cerebellar defects; spasticity; seizures; spinal cord involvement (taboparesis); facial nerve and other cranial nerve palsies	Death in 2–5 years	Tabes is rare in congenital syphilis; CSF has few lymphocytes; some increase in CSF protein; paretic Lange curve; serological test for syphilis is positive on CSF
Lyme disease			*Borrelia burgdorferi*; later dementia following treatment		Raised borrelia specific IgG antibody in serum and CSF
HIV dementia		Infantile (severe): 90% have evidence of encephalopathy and 50% die before 3 years. The older child (>2 years) less susceptible to encephalopathy	Delay or regression; seizures (rare); spasticity; acquired microcephaly	Occurs regardless of the root of the infection	HIV virology; CT shows nonspecific atrophy or calcification basal ganglia; CSF normal

Table 14.75 Epilepsy

Disorders	Genetics	Age of onset	Neurology	Other clinical features	Diagnosis
Lafora body (progressive myoclonic epilepsy)	?Familial	7–10 years	Grand mal and myoclonic fits (myoclonic status); mild intellectual deterioration worsening to dementia; spasticity; ataxia	Death in 10–15 years	Lafora bodies (concentric amyloid bodies found in the cytoplasm of ganglion cells especially in the dentate, substantia nigra, reticular formation, and hippocampus). They are also detectable in the cortex and muscle. There are PAS-positive polyglucosan bodies which are not invariably present. They may also be detected in sweat glands. EEG abnormal (bilateral spike and wave); large SSEP response; no abnormal ERG
Unverricht's disease (Baltic myoclonic epilepsy)			Progressive intellectual deterioration and myoclonic seizures; grand mal seizures as well as myoclonic (photoconvulsive inducement early then easily induced). Later: cerebellar ataxia and terminal spastic quadriparesis with myoclonic status; dementia if treated with phenytoin, no dementia if treated with valproate		No Lafora bodies; EEG bilateral sharp and synchronous spikes; phenytoin or carbamazepine may exacerbate myoclonic epilepsies
Lennox-Gastaut syndrome (myoclonic astatic epilepsy)		2–7 years	Myoclonic and atonic fits (stare, jerk and fall); fluctuating course with clouding of consciousness and polymyoclonia; mental retardation (present in one-half of cases initially, and 80% eventually)		EEG slow spike wave of 1–2.5 Hz; heterogeneous group often follows West's syndrome and acquired brain insults postnatally; 40–50% no obvious brain damage

Table 14.76   Psychological conditions

Disorders	Age of onset	Neurology	Diagnosis
Rett's syndrome	Girls 6 months –2¹/₂ years	Normal development until regression begins; isolation (autistic-like); profound mental handicap; characteristic handwringing (stereotypes – tense clasping or squeezing of fingers) with loss of purposeful hand function and frequently accompanied by bursts of hyperventilation; ataxic, jerky gait; develop a secondary microcephaly; neuromotor signs develop slowly over years with seizures	Later EEG shows slow, disorganized spike and sharp waves in sleep
Disintegrative psychosis	Males 4–7 years	Normal development until onset of progressive dementia (loss of social and scholastic skills); no psychotic features	May be idiopathic or symptomatic of metabolic, or organic brain condition with CT abnormalities, etc.

Table 14.77   Reversible regression

Disorders	Neurology
Blocked CSF shunts	Chronic symptomatology raised intracranial pressure (intellectual deterioration, personality change, fatigue, precocious puberty, etc.)
Anticonvulsants and psychotropic drugs	Particularly multiple anticonvulsants for long periods in large doses

Table 14.78   Apparent regression

Disorders	Neurology	Diagnosis
Foramen magnum tumor	Extension and irritability similar to neurodegeneration	
Sandifer's syndrome		Infant with a static disorder appears to regress with dystonic extension of the neck due to reflux through a hiatal hernia

Table 14.79   Miscellaneous regression

Disorders	Genetics	Age of onset	Neurology	Other clinical features	Diagnosis
Batten's disease (neuronal ceroid lipofuscinosis)	AR (chromosome 16)	Late infantile form (Bielschowsky and Jansky) 22 months	Slowing of development (may be masked by seizures); seizures (especially myoclonic); cerebellar ataxia; increasing spasticity; pigmentary maculae and retina; optic atrophy	Death 6–7 years	Increased urinary dolichols; cerebral atrophy; flat ERG; grossly enlarged VER; suction rectal biopsy without general anesthetic (curvilinear inclusions which are PAS positive, sudanophilic material showing autofluorescence on UV light); similar curvilinear inclusions seen in myenteric plexuses, vascular and smooth muscle cells, glands from skin biopsy and brain biopsy – they may also be seen in lymphocytes (buffy coat) with EM
	AR	Juvenile form (Speilmeyer-Vogt), age of onset 5–7 years	Progressive visual failure (pigmentary retinopathy and later optic atrophy); seizures (later); dementia; extrapyramidal and cerebellar signs (later)	Death 13–20 years +	'Finger print bodies' on EM of biopsy from rectum, appendix, smooth muscle; vacuolation in lymphocytes in 15%; ERG reduced or absent
	AR	Infantile form, age of onset 8–18 months	Progressive mental deterioration with microcephaly; ataxia; visual failure (optic) atrophy and brown discoloration of maculae; myoclonic jerks; pyramidal signs and	Rapid course, especially Finland. Death 8–9 years	Granular osmiophilic deposits in biopsies from skin, appendix, rectum, smooth muscle and lymphocytes. Rectal biopsy using UV autofluorescence and fat stains and EM for 'snow storm' inclusions. ERG reduced

Table 14.79 *Cont'd*

Disorders	Genetics	Age of onset	Neurology	Other clinical features	Diagnosis
			contractures (later); 'hand knitting' behavior; autistic appearance		then absent; VER (occipital) reduced; EEG slowing with irregular bursts of sharp, slow and spike wave abnormality becoming flat later; cerebral atrophy
Alper's disease (Huttenlocher's disease)	AR	1–3 years	Probable group of disorders with degeneration of gray matter; convulsions (myoclonic); dementia; spasticity; opisthotonos	Sclerosis and coagulation defects; death in 10 months	Increased CSF protein; associated with complex IV cytochrome oxidase deficiency in muscle and brain; abnormal cortical cytoarchitecture; EEG high voltage, later runs of spike and wave
Alexander's leukodystrophy and spongiform degeneration	Sporadic	Infancy-childhood	Insidious, slowly progressive dementia; seizures; spasticity; megalencephaly	Persistent hiccup; emaciation (late)	CT scan shows ventricular enlargement and low attenuation in white matter particularly anteriorly; brain biopsy shows diagnostic Rosenthal fibers (fibrillary tangles) with demyelination and rarefaction of white matter; at PM soft cavities in the white matter, degeneration of spinocerebellar tract, atrophy of the dentate nucleus, pallor of the superior cerebellar peduncle
Alzheimer's disease		Rarely less than 10 or 20 years, females predominate	Onset dysmnesia; seizures		Cholinergic deficit; neurofibrillary tangles on brain biopsy; absolute decrease in brain CAT; loss of ganglion cells in the frontal and temporal region and generalized atrophy
Fahr's syndrome	Probable autosomal recessive	Early in life	Calcification in basal ganglia in the absence of overt parathyroid disease; fits; dementia; chorioathetosis and rigidity; cerebral edema; subacute combined degeneration; psychosis	Microscopic involvement of kidney; stridor; tetany; cataracts; monilial infection; abnormal teeth and nails; abdominal cramps	Normal calcium and phosphate; basal ganglia calcification especially lenticular and dentate; the calcification is perivascular and related to local high concentration of alkaline phosphatase; if hypoparathyroid, calcium reduced and phosphate increased; in pseudoparathyroidism there is failure of urinary cyclic AMP to PTH
Central pontine myelinosis			Palatal palsy; dysarthria; ophthalmoplegia; ataxia; decerebrate postures; return of primitive reflexes; tetraplegia; respiratory difficulty		Central degeneration of myelin with cavitation in the central ponds; triangular in shape and stains with Sudan stains; may result from malnutrition, dehydration, vitamin deficiency, leukemia, renal failure, and following surgical removal of carniopharyngiomas
Aicardi–Goutiéres syndrome			Spasticity; dystonia; nystagmus; secondary microcephaly; global regression		CSF lymphocytosis without infection; later, symmetrical basal ganglia calcification
Pelizaeus–Merzbacher disease	Infancy – sex-linked recessive (more common); autosomal dominant – later onset		Slowly progressive in a previously normal infant; nystagmus and roving eye movements; dystonia; rotatory head movements and ataxia with arrhythmic trembling and poor head control; tetraplegic spasticity (later)		Demyelination in CNS may be seen on MRI (abnormality on T2 weighted images of white matter) and on biopsy or at PM there may be sudanophilic features with islands of myelination around small blood vessels; a reduction in cerebrosides in gray matter and abnormal long chain unsaturated fatty acids

Table 14.80   The investigation of neurodegenerative disease

Urine	*Plasma*
Phenistix	T3, T4, TSH
Dolichols	Ammonia
Renal epithelial metachromatic	Organic acids
granules	Amino acids
Amino acids	Copper
Ehrlichs	Ceruloplasmin
Aldehyde test for urobilinogen	Lactate and pyruvate
and porphyrobilinogen	Uric acid
Uric acid	Cholesterol
Succinylpurines	Alpha-lipoprotein
	Very long chain fatty acids
Leukocyte and fibroblast culture	Immunoglobulins
Lysosomal enzymes	VDRL and TPHA
HGPRT-ase (on fibroblasts)	HIV
Fibroblast sensitivity to UV light	Measles IgM
Electron transport chain enzymes	Rubella IgM
G1 UPD	Borrelia titers
FIP aldolase	Anticonvulsant levels
	Alphafetoprotein
	Chromosomes
CSF	
Protein	*Neurophysiology*
Immunoglobulins (oligoclonal bands)	EEG
Cells (cytospin)	VEP
Uric acid	ERG
Glycine	Motor NCV
Succinylpurines	SSEP
Measles IgG	EMG
Rubella IgG	ECG
Imaging	
CT scan	*Biopsies*
MRI	Blood film microscopy
X-ray skull	EM of buffy coat
Angiogram	Active-E-rosette test
	Skin biopsy
	Peripheral nerve biopsy
	Muscle biopsy
	Rectal biopsy
	Bone marrow biopsy
	Brain biopsy (conjunctiva, tonsil)

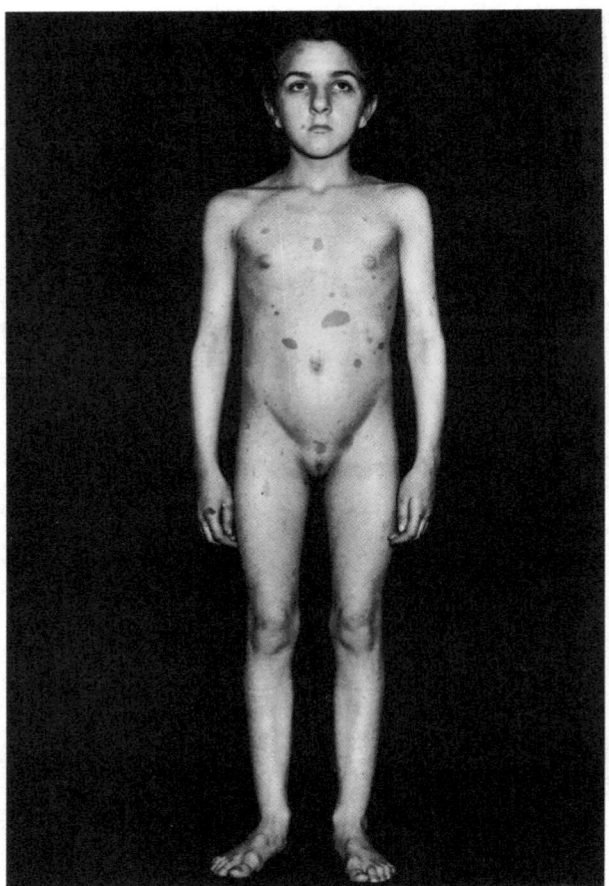

Fig. 14.53   *Café-au-lait* spots in neurofibromatosis.

Neurofibromatosis (von Recklinghausen disease)

This is the most commonly seen member of the group of neurodermatoses. It may be manifest clinically by abnormality of virtually any part of the body, due to cellular migration or tumors (multiple) arising from the sheaths of spinal, cranial or sympathetic nerves, cutaneous pigmentation, abnormalities of bone and frequently defective development of the nervous system. Thus the clinical picture tends to be a complex one. The incidence is one per 2500 births. It is inherited as an autosomal dominant disorder. Diagnosis rests upon a positive family history and the skin manifestations, usually consisting of one or more *café-au-lait* patches (Fig. 14.53).

Ten percent of normal adults have 1–5 *café-au-lait* spots of more than 1.5 cm. In people with proven neurofibromatosis, 75% have more than six spots of this size. Only 0.75% of normal children less than 5 years of age have more than two. Five spots or more make the diagnosis mandatory. Axillary freckling associated with *café-au-lait* patches is also strong presumptive evidence of the disease.

Neurofibromatosis consists of two distinct genetic diseases. The first is peripheral neurofibromatosis, a single gene disorder which is dominantly inherited and appears in children from 1 to 10 years of age. The gene locus is 17q 11.2. The gene product has

been named neurofibromin. The milder affected have multiple *café-au-lait* spots and subcutaneous neurofibromas and the more severely affected developmental and neoplastic abnormalities in tissues derived from the neural crest or neuroectoderm with consequent bone, blood vessel and endocrine disorders.

The second distinct genetic type is central neurofibromatosis which is likewise dominant and begins after the age of 20. The gene locus for NF2 is 22q12 and the gene product is a protein called merlin. These individuals have bilateral acoustic neuromas and few *café-au-lait* spots or subcutaneous neurofibromas. Malignant transformation is not seen in this type and apart from the hearing loss, imbalance and tinnitus they may also develop raised intracranial pressure and adjacent cranial nerve dysfunction. This type is exacerbated by pregnancy.

There are qualitative differences in 'nerve growth factor' (NGF). In the peripheral variety the functional activity of NGF is increased whereas the antigenic activity of NGF is increased in the central type.

Pathology

The cells of the cerebral cortex form from the primitive neuroblasts in the subependymal regions and migrate outwards in fetal life and early infancy. The melanocytes of the skin are formed from neural crest cells. One of the lesions in

Table 14.81   The neurodermatoses

Disorder	Cutaneous	Neurological	Tumor	Other lesions	Biochemical	Genetics
Neurofibromatosis (chromosome 17)	*Café-au-lait* fibromas; plexiform neurofibroma	Epilepsy; mental retardation; dementia; paraplegia; deaf; blind; tumor	Glioma; ependymoma; meningioma; acoustic neuropathy; optic glioma; neuroblastoma; pheochromocytoma; thyroid carcinoma	Proptosis; glaucoma; scoliosis; bone cysts; elephantiasis; megacolon; renal artery stenosis; phakoma	Raised urinary VMA with neural crest tumors	AD
Tuberous sclerosis (chromosomes 9, 11)	Adenoma sebaceum; vitiligo; Shagreen patches; *café-au-lait* spots; ichthyosis; telangiectasia	Epilepsy (TLE); mental retardation; dementia; infantile spasms	Glioma; glioblastoma; rhabdomyoma; hypernephroma; renal sarcoma	Phakoma; honeycomb lung; hemangioma liver, spleen; intracranial Ca	None	AD
Sturge-Weber syndrome	Cutaneous angioma trigeminal area; telangiectasia of sclera	Epilepsy; mental retardation; behavior disturbance; hemiplegia	Angioma of cerebral cortex; hemangioma of choroid	Glaucoma; retinal detachment; limb gigantism intracranial Ca	None	? Nongenetic
Von Hippel-Lindau syndrome (chromosome 3)	Retinal angioma	Ataxia	Hemangioblastoma cerebellum; hypernephroid tumor kidney	Cysts—cerebellum, liver, pancreas, kidney; retinal detachment	None	AD
Ichthyosis with diplegia (Sjögren–Larsson) (Rud's variant)	Ichthyosis	Diplegia; mental retardation	—	Epilepsy; dwarfism; infantilism	Low gonadotrophin in urine	AD
Incontinentia pigmenti	Bullae at birth; dystrophic hair, nails, teeth; slate-gray skin pigmentation; warty skin	Convulsions; feeding difficulty; apathy; epilepsy; mental retardation; cerebral palsy	Tumors post. chamber eye	Eosinophilia vesicle fluid; up to 50% eosinophils in peripheral blood	None	?Sex-linked dominant males die in utero
Encephalocraniocutaneous lipomatosis	Lipoma skin and skull	Convulsions; mental retardation	Lipoma eye, viscera and intracranial	Calcification on plain X-ray	None	?
Ataxia telangiectasia (chromosome 11)	Telangiectasia sclera, cheeks, ear lobes, elbow; popliteal fossa	Ataxia; choreoathetosis; abnormal eye movements; dysarthria; falling IQ	Lymphosarcoma; Hodgkin's; reticulum cell sarcoma; medulloblastoma	Chest infection; occasionally granulocytopenia; small stature	Low IgA; aminoaciduria; abnormal CHO metabolism	AR
Hartnup disease	Photosensitive pellagra-like dermatitis	Ataxia; psychosis	None	Short stature	Aminoaciduria; H type indoles urine	AR
Refsum's syndrome	Ichthyosis	Ataxia; peripheral neuropathy	None	Retinitis pigmentosa; deaf; visual impairment; abnormal EEG; skeletal abnormality	Copper, serum phytanic acid and CSF protein raised	AR
Linear sebaceous nevus	Midfacial nevus sebaceous; hyperpigmentation; hyperkeratosis	Epilepsy	Basal cell epithelioma; nephroblastoma; renal hamartomas	Cortical atrophy; cloudy cornea; colobomas; lipodermoid of conjunctiva; VSD, coarctation	None	?
Hypomelanosis of Ito	Hypomelanosis	Epilepsy	—	Face/limb asymmetry; toe/finger malformation	—	—

AR = autosomal recessive;   AD = autosomal dominant

neurofibromatosis appears to be an abnormality of cell migration. Heterotopic groups of cells are found in the brain. These cells do not function normally but also do not seem to be under the normal restraining tissue influences and may become neoplastic or may be hamartomatous. Anatomical lesions such as anterior meningoceles, especially in the thoracic region, or syringomyelia may also be found in neurofibromatosis.

Clinical features

There are two peaks of clinical problems for those with peripheral neurofibromatosis. The first is in infancy or early childhood when the disease is first noted and the second is in middle age when there is malignant transformation of tumors.

The *café-au-lait* patch is a flat, lightly pigmented, nonhairy spot. These are multiple over the trunk and inner aspects of limbs (Fig. 14.53). They increase in number and size as the child gets older but behave usually more like hamartomas and do not become malignant. They are best seen in natural light or with a Wood's lamp, since some are large and only lightly pigmented. Giant pigment granules or macromelanosomes in DOPA-dependent melanocytes are specific for the *café-au-lait* spots of peripheral neurofibromatosis but are not always seen in children or in the central type of disease. The skin overall may be rather darker than the rest of the family. Fibromas are small, pink, pedunculated skin tumors which usually only appear at puberty. They may range in size from small mm size papules to large pedunculated lesions. They generally do not interfere with function but the occasional patient may complain of pain due to compression. They are especially likely to develop just outside the intervertebral canals and are thus not palpable, but they may be associated with others in the spinal canal and give rise to polyneuritic symptoms. They may undergo sarcomatous degeneration.

The plexiform neurofibroma is characteristic and consists of an overgrowth of the peripheral nerve elements; the local overgrowth of nerve tissues may produce elephantiasis. This may affect a whole limb; it may affect the tongue and cause macroglossia; it may affect the appendix or the colon when a type of megacolon results from replacement of the myenteric plexus by plexiform proliferation. The mandibular region and cheek are common sites for plexiform neurofibromas to form and the whole ramus of the mandible may be eroded. The breast may be replaced by large redundant folds of thickened, rough plexiform neurofibromatous tissue. There is a high risk of carcinoma breast which can be bilateral in the mothers of children with neurofibromatosis.

The peripheral nerves may show swelling and be palpable over bony prominences or subcutaneously. Schwannomas occur on the eighth nerve and gliomas may form on the optic nerves. On spinal nerves or in the cauda equina, tumors may present, sometimes as 'dumb-bell' tumors with one half inside the spinal canal and one half in the chest or abdomen, communicating through the intravertebral foramina.

Other tumors in the chest and mediastinum have been described, as has megacolon, giant appendix, papillary adenomatosis of the intestinal mucosa and tumors of splanchnic and pelvic nerve plexuses.

Scoliosis is the commonest bony lesion; this may be due to erosion by a neurofibroma on a nerve root, a plexiform neurofibroma of the bone, a hemivertebra or fibrosa cystica of the body. In most cases no cause can be found for the scoliosis other than a leg length discrepancy. Fibrous replacement of the bones to form cysts may occur and result in pathological fractures which heal poorly and may cause pseudoarthroses. Bone erosion may occur into the orbit from adjacent tumors.

Proptosis is quite a common presenting sign. It may be due to an associated glaucoma with buphthalmos, an optic nerve glioma, retroorbital plexiform neurofibroma, erosion of the orbital wall by adjacent tumor or metastatic neuroblastoma. There may also be tumors of the iris, choroid, retina, ciliary body or retina. Occasionally the posterior wall of the orbit may be absent or cystic replacement of a temporal lobe may push the orbit forward.

Vascular diseases may occur. Pulmonary valve stenosis or other congenital heart disease and systemic vascular occlusive disease including renal artery stenosis are also encountered. Occasionally the occlusive vascular disease affects the cerebral vasculature.

Neurological signs and symptoms

Neurological symptoms and signs are many and vary greatly in their clinical manifestations in different patients. Although they can have normal intelligence, mental defect or epilepsy may result from disruption of the architecture of the cortex. Dementia, megalencephaly or epilepsy may result from a diffuse proliferation of glial tissue. Epilepsy is not as common as often thought with less than 10% of cases having a major seizure problem. Any constellation of neurological signs or symptoms may present as a result of tumors on the cranial or spinal nerves or tumors of brain and spinal cord. There are a wide variety of tumors – ependymomas, meningiomas, gliomas, acoustic neuromas or gliomatosis. A neurological syndrome similar to progressive muscular atrophy may occur. Myelodysplasia with several spinal canals and disruption of the normal two anterior and two posterior horn pattern of the spinal cord is also described.

Central neurofibromatosis with bilateral acoustic neuromas may be suggested by a positive family history, some skin lesions or nodules in the periphery of the iris – 'Lisch spots'. Magnetic resonance imaging will define the tumor but it will be necessary in addition to perform definitive tests of hearing and vestibular function. Drowning is a potential hazard for these patients due to a loss of direction under water. Unilateral acoustic neuromas need to be differentiated from ependymomas, hemangiosarcomas, gliomas or arachnoid cysts.

Other developmental abnormalities include meningoceles, spina bifida occulta, abnormalities of the fingers and scapulae, asymmetries, particularly of the face and skull, and absent long bones.

Neural crest tumors. Melanocytes, the sympathetic system and the adrenal medulla arise from migration of neural crest cells. Neuroblastoma and pheochromocytoma can both occur in neurofibromatosis. Thyroid disorders such as myxedema and thyroid carcinoma also seem to be more common. It is interesting to note that all the cells involving the metabolism of DOPA are involved, i.e. melanin, thyroxine and adrenaline. The catecholamines are raised in the urine in neuroblastoma, pheochromocytoma and retinoblastoma and may cause hypertension. Hypertension in children with neurofibromatosis has also been described due to stenosis of the renal arteries.

Imaging

The advent of MRI has greatly eased the diagnosis of brain involvement in neurofibromatosis and the definition of tumors and optic nerve gliomas has been greatly helped. Specific changes known as unidentified bright objects have been discovered in the brains of many children who were clinically asymptomatic. These may represent hamartomas but although they may appear to be getting bigger during childhood, they may regress at puberty. Multiple bilateral lesions may be seen in the basal ganglia and extensive brainstem lesions may be seen with remarkably little clinical symptomatology. Diffuse changes in white matter, calcification, arachnoid cysts and hydrocephalus may also be seen. An acquired form of megalencephaly from diffuse gliosis makes differentiation from a very low grade glioma difficult.

Prognosis and treatment

The disease runs a long course dependent on the extent and site of the tumors. Treatment is restricted to removal of the presenting tumor, the shunting of hydrocephalus if present and the control of seizures. Radiotherapy is of little use. Genetic counseling is very important since the condition is almost always of autosomal dominant inheritance.

Tuberous sclerosis (epiloia, Bourneville's disease)

Tuberous sclerosis used to be regarded as a variant of neurofibromatosis and von Recklinghausen himself described tuberous sclerosis lesions in the brain of a newborn child. It is now proven to be a separate member of the group of neurodermatoses. It is inherited as an autosomal dominant character but not as regularly as neurofibromatosis. The incidence is also much less; one in 50 000 of the population. Seventy-five percent of cases have a positive family history but this is rarely detectable when the child is born. *Formes frustes* and incomplete penetrance mean that MRI on the parents may be needed to be sure of a new mutation.

Pathology

The characteristic cell is the large tuberous sclerosis giant cell which is a primitive one not very different in appearance from a neuroblast. It can develop glial or neuronal characteristics. These cells may be the only manifestation of the disease or may give rise to hamartomas, frank gliomatous tumors or to a diffuse gliosis. The usual finding is of multiple nodules which project into the ventricles and this is said to resemble candle gutterings. This may be present at birth even in the premature infant. Calcification may occur and show on plain X-ray films (Fig. 14.54) or better by computed axial tomography or ultrasound. Malignant change may occur as a progressive enlargement to form a glioma or malignant spongioblastoma, glioblastoma or ependymoma. The diffuse type can give rise to dementia with megalencephaly. The tubers are the tumors described but as the name suggests there is sclerosis, i.e. an overgrowth of astrocytic fibrils, as well.

Clinical features

The characteristic features of tuberous sclerosis are mental retardation from birth and epilepsy starting usually before 2 years of age. It may present as infantile spasms with autistic behavior. Autism is more likely if imaging shows anterior and posterior hemisphere hamartomas but is also the result of poorly controlled

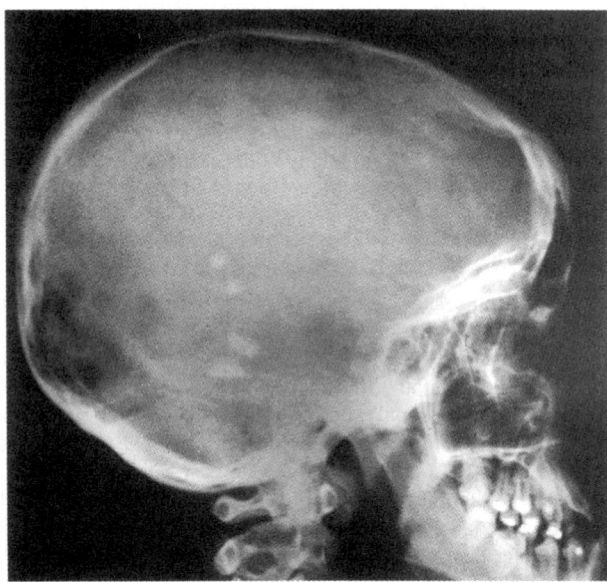

Fig. 14.54 Tuberous sclerosis. Skull showing thickened internal table in frontal region with nodular intracranial opacities representing adenoma formation.

epilepsy with nonconvulsive status. The sleep disturbances, also common, appear to relate to the control of the epilepsy.

It may present in the newborn or preterm infant with multiple rhabdomyomas of the heart producing cyanotic attacks, malrotation of the intestine and diaphragmatic hernia. Other associated defects include spina bifida, hare lip, agenesis of the corpus callosum, omphalocele and splenic sinus histiocytosis. True polycystic kidneys may occur and it is thought that this may be due to involvement of an adjacent gene. The fits may be of grand mal type or focal jacksonian fits. The temporal lesions may cause psychomotor disturbance, sometimes associated with a marked psychotic component. Adenoma sebaceum (p. 1625) is commonly present but in infancy depigmented macules on the skin may be of more diagnostic value. Dementia can occur in the course of status epilepticus or as a result of progression of the disease. Dementia in an epileptic patient with poor control of the seizures may also suggest the diagnosis. Signs of raised intracranial pressure may indicate a tumor or blockage of part of the cerebrospinal fluid pathway by a tuber. *Formes frustes* of the condition are probably more common than realized and relatives of known cases show the greatest variation in clinical severity. Intellect may be normal with intracranial calcification or seizures. Tubers of the retina may be seen as phakomata. Heart tumors can present as cyanotic attacks.

The classic clinical triad consists of adenoma sebaceum, epilepsy and mental retardation. This is the triad seen in the older institutionalized case but not necessarily in the young child presenting with fits, as the rash does not develop fully until the sebaceous glands hypertrophy at puberty. It may only consist of telangiectatic dilation of vessels over the nose or the full warty, elevated reddish yellow lesion over the cheeks and bridge of the nose, consisting of small 2 mm tumors of sebaceous glands with hyperkeratosis. Other skin lesions found are the Moroccan leather shagreen patches over the sacrum and back, ichthyosis, *café-au-lait* spots, subungual fibromas, telangiectasia and vitiligo.

Renal tumors consist of sarcomas or hypernephromas. Rhabdomyomata of the heart, either single or multiple, usually in the left ventricle, are also common. Cystic lesions in the lung may give rise to a honeycomb lung and cause cough and dyspnea. Hemangiomas of liver or spleen are also sometimes associated. This, together with the facial telangiectasia, links the disease with Sturge–Weber and other nevoid neurodermatoses.

Diagnosis

Diagnosis is easy if all the features of the syndrome are present. Siblings may present with epilepsy or a child with an affected parent or there may be a family history of specific mental retardation. Intracranial calcification, candle guttering on air encephalography or renal abnormalities on intravenous pyelography may suggest the diagnosis in the absence of adenoma sebaceum. *Café-au-lait* patches may suggest neurofibromatosis. Angiomata or telangiectasia of the face may suggest one of the other neurodermatoses. Retinal phakomata also are a valuable sign if present. The young presenting case may be diagnosed by examination for depigmented macules with a Wood's light.

Imaging

The calcified periventricular hamartomatous tumors, heterotopia, white matter lesions, foramen of Monro astrocytic giant cell tumors and hydrocephalus are nowadays all better delineated by MRI. It is now thought that the epilepsy arises from the cortical hamartomas and not the more obvious subependymal ones. These may be clustered, e.g. in a frontal lobe, and this is important as surgical removal may then alleviate the fits.

Cytogenetics

This is complicated and not due to a single gene on one chromosome. Chromosome 16p 13.3 with a gene product called tuberin appears a major site but 11q22–23 and possible linkage to chromosome 9 are implicated.

Treatment

This consists of control of the seizures and the management of any hydrocephalus. The relation between seizures and intelligence is strong and so every effort should be made to control fits in the very young child. Forty percent of children presenting with infantile spasms are thought to be due to tuberous sclerosis and it is suggested that in these cases vigabatrin is particularly helpful. A giant astrocytic tumor in the region of the foramen of Monro is particular to tuberous sclerosis and presents with unilateral hydrocephalus. Repeat MRI scans will be needed with any change in symptomatology.

Encephalotrigeminal angiomatosis (Sturge–Weber syndrome)

Encephalotrigeminal angiomatosis consists of an angiomatous malformation of the skin usually in the distribution of one of the branches of the trigeminal nerve (Fig. 14.55) and a similar vascular anomaly of the occipital area of the ipsilateral cerebral hemisphere. The resultant cerebral ischemia gives rise to mental retardation, epilepsy and hemiplegia. It is only when the upper

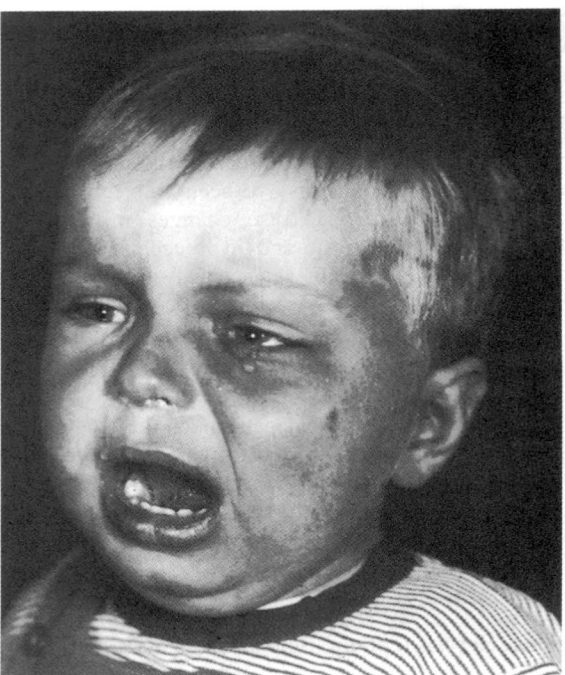

Fig. 14.55   Sturge–Weber syndrome.

part of the face and forehead are affected that changes in the meninges are also found. Rarely the cerebral nevus has been found in the frontal lobe. The cerebral lesion is very similar in appearance to the facial nevus and consists of a 'feltwork' of small abnormal vessels in the pia-arachnoid. Deep to these and within the cerebral cortex are linear zones of calcification which tend to follow the contours of the gyri and therefore show characteristic patterns (e.g. double 'tramlines') on X-ray (Fig. 14.56). There may be associated anomalies of the eyes such as congenital glaucoma, buphthalmos, marked telangiectasia of the conjunctiva and varicosities of the retinal vessels. There may be hemangioma

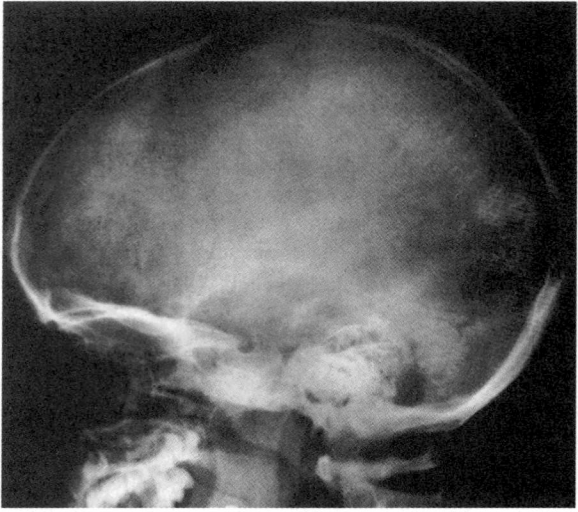

Fig. 14.56   Sturge–Weber syndrome. Skull with parallel lines of calcium deposited in perivascular tissues in posterior parietal and occipital region.

of the choroid as an isolated lesion. The fundus may be a dark red color and the retina may detach. The cutaneous angioma may follow the distribution of a peripheral nerve in the trunk or a limb. The blood supply of the retina and face comes from the inner layer of the primordial vascular system and the skin and meninges are supplied by a common vascular supply with the retina and face. The facial angioma is present at birth and does not spread. Abnormal vessels are also found in the spinal cord and in lung and pancreas. The cortex shows displacement of cells and again there may be heterotopic islands of cells that have not migrated in the white matter. It is not known whether deterioration is due to progression of a primary cortical dysplasia or a vascular lesion or to intractable fits causing anoxic brain damage but Garcia et al (1981) have described recurrent thrombotic episodes producing a gradual loss of function, which has obvious implications for possible use of antiplatelet agents. Histologically lesions can be seen in the trigeminal nucleus. There is a shrinkage of the hemisphere and neuronal cell loss under the angioma. The atrophy only occurs after birth. Hemiplegia only occurs after a series of fits and is not due to the angiomatous lesion itself.

Clinical features

In its complete form the syndrome is shown by a child with facial nevus and epilepsy. The epileptic attacks may be generalized or focal, confined to or originating in the side of the body opposite to the nevus. The attacks may be intractable, leading to progression in the mental retardation which is present in approximately 60% of cases. Because of the site of the cerebral lesion there is hemianopia and there may be hemiparesis, both being contralateral to the vascular anomalies. Severe behavior and schooling problems may occur in the absence of a frank hemiplegia. Buphthalmos and glaucoma may occur. There is characteristic calcification (Fig. 14.56). A cranial bruit is uncommon. Rarely heart failure may occur due to shunting through intracranial angiomas. Subarachnoid and subdural hemorrhage may occur but are uncommon.

Treatment

If epileptic attacks are not satisfactorily controlled by antiepileptic drugs occipital lobectomy is recommended with a view to making attacks more amenable to drug therapy and arresting or slowing progressive intellectual deterioration. However, frequently when the brain is exposed, the nevus proves to be extensive, involving parietal and temporal lobes as well. Under such circumstances selective resection under electrocorticographic control or, rarely, hemispherectomy should be employed. Angiography will not outline the capillary nevus which shows better on a radioactive brain scan. The facial nevi can be considerably improved by laser treatment.

Von Hippel–Lindau syndrome

The von Hippel–Lindau syndrome consists of retinal angioma with a cerebellar, brainstem or spinal cord hemangioblastoma. The retinal hemangioma is a focal red nodule with large tortuous feeding vessels. It is bilateral in 50% of cases. There may be massive secondary retinal exudates. The spinal cord is frequently involved with the hemangioblastomas at the pontomedullary level. Visceral cysts in liver, pancreas and kidney may occur.

Hypernephroid tumors of kidney may occur and the hemangioblastoma of the cerebellum may at times look like a metastasis from a hypernephroma when there is no renal lesion. Both these tumors are known to be associated with polycythemia. There may also be angiomas in the bones, epididymal tumors of the testis and pheochromocytomas.

It is thought that it clusters in some families and may relate to multiple lesions on a complex gene on chromosome 3p.

Symptoms are either visual from the angioma or retinal detachment or cerebellar with progressive ataxia. The signs of raised intracranial pressure may be paroxysmal and a fluctuating syndrome of basilar insufficiency with episodes of vertigo, nausea, vomiting and sometimes ataxia may occur.

Spinal cord angiomas can also be associated with cutaneous ones over the corresponding dermatome. These can thrombose and give rise to an acute paraplegia. Multiple hemangiomas of skin or face can be associated with intracranial aneurysms or arteriovenous malformations.

Gadolinium-enhanced MRI will delineate the cerebellar lesion and repeat scans may be indicated in children at risk. Regular retinal examination should be performed after 2 years.

Ichthyosis with Diplegia (Sjögren–Larsson syndrome)

The Sjögren–Larsson syndrome presents with progressive mental retardation, congenital ichthyosis and a spastic diplegia. In a variant of the syndrome (Rud's syndrome) there is associated dwarfism, infantilism, low gonadotropin in the urine and no spermatogenesis. The condition of the Sjögren–Larsson syndrome is of autosomal recessive inheritance. It is commoner in the Scandinavian countries.

Incontinentia pigmenti (Bloch–Sulzberger)

Incontinentia pigmenti is a syndrome that presents in infancy as a bullous eruption (p. 1626). It occurs especially in females as it is thought that the majority of affected male infants die in utero. The condition is usually diagnosed initially as pemphigus neonatorum due to staphylococcal infection. The high eosinophil count in the blood and vesicle fluid which is sterile help to distinguish these conditions. It is a familial condition, up to eight cases being reported in a single family. Apathy, feeding and swallowing difficulties, failure to thrive and convulsions are associated. There may be dystrophic changes in the hair, nails and teeth. Epilepsy, mental retardation and cerebral palsy are present in up to one-third of cases, but are not progressive after infancy. The name derives from the slate gray pigment spots which appear as the bullous lesions settle. The bullae last about 4 months when the skin may appear warty before the pigment appears. Steroids seem to have a beneficial effect on the rash. The brain shows micropolygyria with small cavities in the white matter and patchy foci of neuronal loss, especially in the cerebellum. In many cases there may be retinal lesions which can be mistaken for retinoblastoma due to a mass in the posterior chamber.

Encephalocraniocutaneous lipomatosis

Encephalocraniocutaneous lipomatosis may present as convulsions in the neonatal period with developmental retardation and later severe mental retardation. There are lipomata of the skin and skull and the eye and viscera may be involved. The skull lipomata can be mistaken for a cephalhematoma. There may be multiple intracranial lipomas which tend to be on the same side as the skull lipomata. There may be calcification seen on plain X-rays of the skull due to calcium in the affected cerebral cortex.

Ataxia telangiectasia (Louis–Bar syndrome) (see page 1253)

Other neurodermatoses

Feuerstein–Mims syndrome

This consists of a sebaceous nevus of the face and upper trunk associated with fits and mental retardation. It may be associated with vitamin D-resistant rickets.

Other disorders

Other disorders with a dermatological and neurological component such as Wolman's disease (p. 1154), Fabry's disease (p. 1164), Hartnup disease (p. 799), Refsum's disease (p. 785) and Fanconi's anemia (p. 854) are considered elsewhere. Another such condition is the giant pigmented hairy nevus (bathing trunks nevus) associated with melanocytosis of the meninges. Linear sebaceous nevus can be associated with fits, mental retardation or cerebral palsy.

Hypomelanosis of Ito

This condition is characterized by hypomelanosis, epilepsy, face and limb asymmetry and malformations of the fingers and toes. The hypomelanosis is the reverse of pigmentary changes seen in incontinentia pigmenti (above). This condition is more easily recognized in dark-skinned people but for lighter skin colors a Wood's light may be a useful aid.

DISORDERS OF HIGHER CORTICAL FUNCTION

SPEECH AND LANGUAGE DISORDERS

Speech and language, although closely related, are not synonymous. Language, which is the basis of cognitive development, is a systematic symbol system used to develop concepts and so allow understanding. It is usually expressed through speech, but it can just as readily be conveyed through other means such as sign language and musical notation. It is possible for a child to have normal 'inner language' in the absence of speech, e.g. akinetic mutism. It is also possible for a child to develop speech without a commensurate level of inner language, e.g. 'cocktail party chatter' of hydrocephalics and Williams' syndrome. These children recall by rote whole pieces of conversation, which they do not understand, but which are produced in social situations and give rise to a false impression of language competency (pragmatics as opposed to cognition).

Speech is a phonological system. Phonology refers to the rules which govern the way sounds are combined in speech. Syntax, which is closely related developmentally, refers to the grammatical structure of speech and semantics refers to the underlying meaning.

The development of speech is the most sophisticated motor skill demanded of the preschool child. Its normal progress depends on the integrity of the bulbar musculature, brainstem motor pathways, basal ganglia, cerebellum and cortical motor pathways. The development of speech may be impaired independently of cognitive development. However, if there is a primary language disorder (dysphasis) or a global delay in cognition (mental handicap), the child will be slow to speak – secondary speech disorders.

DEVELOPMENT OF SPEECH

The first year

By the time children produce their first word with meaning (50th centile 12 months, 90th centile 18 months) they have already developed complex preverbal communication and have all the sounds required for speech. During their first 6 months, infants learn to distinguish between speech and nonspeech sounds and can differentiate intonation (auditory discrimination). They can produce consonant/vowel single syllable babble. During the second 6 months, they start to distinguish their name and those of other family members and babbling becomes increasingly complex. By the end of the first year they use many consistent sound sequences to represent meaning, 'protowords', and these, combined with increasing use of nonverbal features such as eye gaze and gesture, increase their ability to communicate.

The second and third years

Between 12 and 18 months children's understanding relies heavily on context and nonverbal cues, but they can identify familiar items and follow simple commands. By the end of the second year they can understand simple 'what, where, when' type questions. By the end of the third year they understand concepts such as preposition, quantity, color and size. During the second year, vocabulary is small and 'overextensions' occur, e.g. all animals are called cat. The third year their vocabulary rapidly increases to an average of 1000 words.

The third to fifth years

Between 3 and 5 years comprehension becomes increasingly complex, e.g. adjectives and descriptive words are recognized (large/small, beside/inside) and the function of objects is understood. At school entry, normal children can understand three-part instructions, are less dependent on context and are developing abstract understanding, e.g. time.

Phonology

Phonological development proceeds in a predictable manner and thus, the pediatrician can recognize normal patterns of omissions, e.g. 'poon/spoon', substitutions, e.g. 'lolly/lorry', insertions, e.g. 'plegs/pegs', and reversals, e.g. 'aminals/animals'. Between 12 and 18 months, children can only sequence a limited range of consonants, i.e. p/b/t/d/m/n, whereas by 2–3 years they can sequence a wider range, i.e. k/g/s/f/h/w/i/j. Between 3 and 4 years, phonology matures but some normal children continue to show difficulties with consonant clusters, e.g. ch/sh. By the age of 5, the phonological development is largely complete and although there may still be problems with r/l/th, the speech is entirely intelligible.

Syntax

Children have to learn the syntactical rules that govern their language but the speed at which they do this is closely related to phonological development, suggesting that syntax depends more on motor circuitry than cognitive. During the second year children progress from 'holophrastic' speech, where one word represents a whole sentence, e.g. 'up', through the 'open/pivot' system, e.g. 'Mummy juice', to producing three- or four-word sentences (50th centile 23 months, 90th centile 30 months (girls), 32 months (boys)). During this time, children generalize simple syntactical rules, e.g. plurals 'mouses/foots', past tense 'goed/comed'. In the third year, possessives are used and correct pronoun use develops. Three- to four-year-old children continue to show many syntactical errors as they start to link clauses together and produce longer sentences. However, by the age of 5 they will be largely fluent and correct.

ETIOLOGY OF SPEECH DISORDERS

During the first 4 years of life, the brain increases in size from 350 to 1000 g, reflecting the increasing sophistication and 'wiring' of the 'human computer'. The motor learning of speech is slower than that of sensory skills or comprehension. The speed of learning is influenced by both the environment and the maturation of the brain. The majority of children with significant delay in speech and language development have delayed neurological maturation of the brain as the single most important factor and this rate of maturation is largely determined by inherited factors and heavily influenced by male sex (Bishop & Edmundson 1987).

Brain damage may also slow up the maturation of areas of the brain governing speech, e.g. in 25–30% following symptomatic birth asphyxia and in 40% of children with hemiplegia.

EPIDEMIOLOGY

The reported incidence of slow speech development in the childhood population depends on the criteria used. If all children are included, then 1.8% of boys and 0.9% of girls will remain unintelligible at the age of 7 years with a preponderance from lower income groups and large families. However, 50% of children who are language delayed by 30 months will be generally retarded in nonverbal abilities on follow-up. The incidence of severe specific speech and language disorder, defined as only a few single words at 3 years, limited connected speech at 5 years, but average intelligence, is one per 1000. Against all these figures it must be remembered that speech development follows a normal distribution curve with 10% of children falling below the 10th centile and these children are not necessarily 'abnormal' in relation to their peers.

DEVELOPMENTAL DISORDERS

Developmental disorders of speech and language do not as readily separate into primary and secondary disorders of speech relating speech to language, as do the acquired disorders or those in which there is an identifiable neurological cause. To reflect this, Table 14.82 distinguishes between the different developmental disorders on the basis of whether abnormalities of speech or language predominate.

Table 14.82   Classification of speech and language disorders

1. Developmental disorders
   a. Speech
      (i) Dysrhythmia
      (ii) Phonological delay (dyslalia)   ± syntactical delay
                                           ± receptive/expressive language delay
      (iii) Articulatory (verbal) dyspraxia

   b. Language
      (i) Receptive and expressive language delay, e.g. lexical-syntactical deficits
      (ii) Verbal auditory agnosia/central deafness
      (iii) Semantic–pragmatic disorder

2. Neurological and/or acquired disorders
   a. Speech
      (i) Dysphonia: anatomical
                         neurological, e.g.   recurrent laryngeal nerve
      (ii) Dysrhythmia: e.g. cerebellar disease   palsy, brainstem lesions
      (iii) Dysarthria: anatomical, e.g.
                         cleft palate
                         neurological,
                         bulbar palsy: flaccid
                                                   pseudobulbar/spastic
                                                   extrapyramidal
                                                   hyperkinetic and
                                                   hypokinetic ataxic
      (iv) Acquired articulatory dyspraxia

   b. Language
      (i) Dysphasia: expressive receptive
                         transcortical
                         conduction
      (ii) Acquired auditory agnosia/central deafness, e.g. Landau-Kleffner

3. Secondary speech and language disorders
      (i) Peripheral deafness
      (ii) Mental handicap
      (iii) Autism
      (iv) Psychosocial deprivation
      (v) Miscellaneous

Speech

Dysrhythmias

During normal speech the voice is switched on and off, lips, tongue and palate take up constantly changing positions and the air stream is either directed into the nasal cavities for resonance or the nasal cavities are shut off. This requires a very rapid sequence of motor instructions. Someone speaking very quickly can achieve 300 words/min so that an enormous number and variation of impulses must be transmitted from the brainstem to the various articulatory muscles. The speed of speaking varies with the individual and either from excitement or in order to stress certain words or emphasize a piece of information, the speech may increase. The change in speed, pitch, stress of syllables and of words, together with the phrasing, all help to give meaning and to communicate nonverbal emotional cues. While slow speech may be used deliberately to create a feeling of importance or gravity, a rate of speech of less than 60 words/min sounds very slow and becomes difficult to hold in short-term memory in order to extract meaning. Speeds over 300 words/min (as may happen in the case of racing commentators) cause difficulty in sustaining attention and the speech may become incomprehensible. Children with dysarthria and dysphasia (see below) will tend to have telegrammatic speech. Very rapid speech, i.e. tachylalia, may occur in some children when the child 'falls over himself in speech', so-called cluttering.

The commonest abnormality of rate, rhythm and flow of speech is seen in the condition of stammering (stuttering). Many children in the 2–4-year age group go through a period of physiological dysfluency when their ideas come at a greater rate than their motor skills can express. It shows itself as repetition of sounds, syllables or words; in about 1% of cases this becomes more severe with prolongation of a sound or actually blocking of speech, so that there is both a tonic and a clonic component to the stammer. It is not known why certain children with physiological dysfluency develop a permanent dysrhythmia of speech. The 1% of children who develop a persistent stammer, which continues into the school years, constitute the majority of the adult stammerers. The dysfluency starts in most cases before puberty, 90% before 8 years. Occasionally the child may speak normally and then have an 'onset' stammer. It is not known why this should occur at a particular time or what precipitates it. A minority of cases seem to be related to emotional stress or neurological insult. The child most commonly has difficulty in starting a new word or phrase and he will either block, so that no sound comes out, prolong the first syllable or repeat the first syllable or whole word (stammer). Repetitions tend to develop before the blocks and prolongations. Most patients come to recognize particular words in a sentence that will cause them difficulty. Long words giving meaning at the beginning of a sentence are most likely to cause problems, but there is no particular group of words in the English language which is common to all stammerers as likely to cause particular difficulty. Speaking in public, using telephones or anxiety-provoking situations can make the stammer worse and it is least likely to occur with people who know the child and know that he has a stammer. In severe cases the child's life becomes ruled by his stammer and the anxiety produced by his communication difficulty or imitation and ridicule by his classmates may cause secondary behavior disturbances and produce an anxiety state which in the past was often blamed as the cause of the stammer. In severe cases there is an obvious struggle to get words out with an overflow of associated movements which can cause grimacing, head nodding, abnormal breathing control and even movements of the hands and feet.

Treatment of stammering. When faced with a young dysfluent child the decision to treat or not treat can be a delicate one. The transition from transient persisting dysfluency is often largely aided and abetted by the child's increasing awareness of the phenomenon as a 'fault' so that counseling of parents and discussion of their attitudes may be more important than therapy to the child in the first instance. If the parents of a preschool child, who appears to be going through a period of normal physiological dysfluency, are particularly anxious it may be helpful for them to be referred to the speech therapist for discussion before their anxiety transmits itself to the child.

For the older primary school or teenage stammerer, therapy will become more formal. Many speech therapists now run intensive group courses for stammerers. These may take the form of 1 or 2 weeks of all-day sessions, usually during the school holidays, with periodic follow-up thereafter. Intensive group treatment has advantages not only in helping to establish new techniques but also in going some way to providing a more natural setting for the practice of new communication modes. It is well recognized that stammering rarely occurs during singing, reading in unison or talking to pets and babies, largely because of the reduced level of 'communication' involved.

Techniques taught may include the imposing of a controlled pacing of syllables, using deliberate slowing and regulating each syllable to the time of a metronome, i.e. so-called syllabic timed speech. More direct work on the reduction of articulatory tension and relaxation techniques may be used. An electronic aid which masks the speaker's own voice can in some cases bring dramatic relief to a chronic older stammerer, suggesting that the motor disorder is in some way related to an abnormality in the auditor's feedback. Some patients find that if they tap a foot or tap a finger with their hand in their pocket they can maintain the flow of speech. On the whole such mechanical aids are crutches rather than cures. All these methods need to be combined with a behavior modification approach to decrease the child's anxiety and to teach him to stand up in class and to speak and to read in front of children, to speak in a group, buy things in a shop or use the telephone.

Phonological delay/disorder (developmental speech retardation, dyslalia)

These children are characterized by a constant lag in the onset of various stages of speech development. The majority have a good prognosis for speech and there are many different reasons why their speech development is slow: male gender, genetic influence (there is frequently a positive family history in first-degree male relatives), sensory deprivation from chronic secretory otitis media, impoverished linguistic environment, slow acquisition of cerebral dominance and minimal brain damage from asphyxia and prematurity (Fig. 14.57) (Largo et al 1986).

Many children will have some associated delay in expressive and receptive language but the most striking clinical feature is their unintelligibility, even though they may be fluent, know what they want to say and try to say it. A subgroup of these children will have marked syntactical difficulties with dysfluency. Their speech lacks 'function' word, e.g. articles, prepositions and pronouns and word endings denoting past tense, number and possession and their speech sounds telegrammatic.

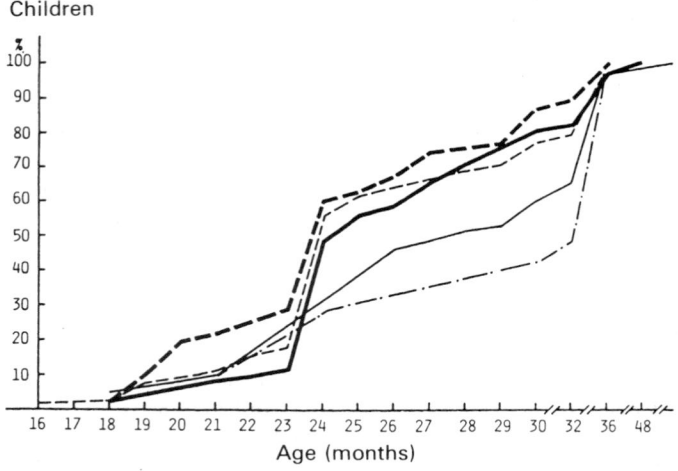

Children

Fig. 14.57 Onset of four-word sentences. Term boys —, term girls – – ; preterm boys — and girls – – without CP; boys and girls with CP —.—. (From Largo et al 1986.)

Articulatory dyspraxia

Development of the primary motor area of the cortex and corresponding association areas is essential for the learning of the sequenced motor skills of speech, i.e. placing the lips, tongue and palate in the correct sequence. When phonology is severely disturbed, the clinical picture of dyslalia merges into that of an articulatory dyspraxia. There is decreased blood flow in the lower part of the premotor cortex (Broca's area) in such children. Children with articulatory dyspraxia are distinguished by their poor prognosis for the development of speech.

In a minority of cases there may be some nasal escape in speech but the palate will move well with 'ah' and the gag reflex is normal. However, the soft palate does not close off the nasopharynx during connected speech and this may cause misdiagnosis of mild pseudobulbar palsy. The pattern of speech is often deviant with bizarre omissions and substitutions which are inconsistent and may involve vowels as well as consonants. By school age the child may be able to make most of the 46 speech sounds in isolation but cannot sequence them into words. Once the child is of an age when developmentally he should be able to make all the speech sounds, the specific difficulty of sound sequencing or 'word synthesis' becomes increasingly apparent. In trying to repeat a sentence after the examiner he may be able to produce the correct pattern of words and syllables thus showing that he has an inner representation of the correct syntactical pattern. There will be some words that he learns and articulates well, i.e. he may overlearn a few words or phrases. When anxious his speech will disintegrate further and when speaking quickly it will become even less understandable. A specific speech sound may be used in one word and not in another. In very severe cases he may not even be able to imitate certain individual sounds. He may learn to say a simple word such as cat and yet when trying to say catapult cannot even pronounce the cat distinctly. In severe cases the child may circumvent his severe articulation problem by contracting his sentences so that speech becomes telegrammatic, often consisting of one- or two-word utterances. Some children may have oromotor dyspraxia, e.g. they cannot imitate rapid repetitive lateral movements of the tongue. In addition they may have an upper limb dyspraxia which presents problems when learning a manual signing system to augment communication. However, there is not always a strict relationship between the two and such methods are always worth considering (McEwan & Lloyd 1990).

Language

Receptive and expressive language delay (congenital dysphasia)

Language is fundamental to thought and intelligence and utilizes most parts of the cerebral cortex. A child may be able to name an object by retrieving the word from their lexical store (motor memory or 'engram' for the word), but only if the child can access all the memory banks that relate to that word will they hold in consciousness the total concept in order to reason. A primary disorder of language therefore has a major effect on learning. Some children will have associated abnormalities of speech but others will have normal phonological development and yet be echolalic without comprehension. They may be able to recognize and name objects but be unable to carry out more complex language tasks such as classifying or categorizing. They cannot cope with abstract notions such as time, e.g. today, yesterday, now, later. Children with lexical-syntactical deficits show greater effects on expressive language and characteristically have severe word retrieval (anomic) difficulties. They rarely initiate conversation or relate a competent story because of their problems with connected language. This type of difficulty may be pronounced in children with Klinefelter's syndrome.

Auditory/verbal agnosia and word deafness

Sound is bilaterally represented in the brain as neural connections from both ears project via crossed and uncrossed pathways to the primary auditory cortices in the temporal lobes. The dominant auditory cortex has a predilection for speech as opposed to nonverbal sounds but if this is damaged in a young child the opposite side is capable of taking over. Therefore, in congenital word deafness there must be bilateral interference with temporal lobe function.

In clinical practice it may be impossible to distinguish between central word deafness and auditory agnosia (where the association area is affected). Such children show gross auditory inattention to speech and clearly great care must be taken to exclude a peripheral hearing loss. Ability to comprehend language through a visual mode is preserved. The children are typically mute or severely dysfluent. If they do speak, their articulation is grossly defective.

It may be difficult to differentiate these conditions from mental handicap and autism, unless the child can be shown to have normal development in nonverbal skills, e.g. formboards, drawings and jigsaws.

Semantic-pragmatic disorder

These children may be 'chatty' and articulate but closer inspection of their language reveals echolalia, perseverations, circumlo-cutions and semantic paraphrasias and errors. Their comprehension is delayed compared to their expression and they fail to understand much of their own speech. Their pragmatic use of language is impaired; they do not take turns in conversation or maintain a topic, they do not understand the nature of sarcasm or the adjustments required in language depending on the other person, e.g. to a sibling compared to an adult in authority such as the teacher. The clinician may be struck by their bizarre behavior and overlook their language disorder despite the sensation of tangential conversation and the impression that most of the work is being done by the listener when trying to establish a theme to the communication. If nonverbal communication is grossly disturbed the disorder merges into autism or Asperger's syndrome (severe abnormalities of social behavior and clumsiness) (Bishop & Edmundson 1987).

Diagnosis

Children with mild delay in phonological development form the majority of those who are slow to speak. Provided they are of normal intelligence, their progress is good, although some will show difficulties later on in reading and spelling. The thrust of their management is towards encouraging communication both at home and in the nursery.

Diagnosis of moderate to severe communication disorders is facilitated by a multidisciplinary approach with the speech therapist and psychologist. Referral to a speech therapist should be made early so that the child's performance in areas such as language comprehension and expression, syntax and articulation can be assessed with progression to further assessment, e.g. auditory memory, receptive vocabulary and naming as indicated. Diagnosis can be very difficult in the noncommunicating young child. Priority should be given to excluding a peripheral deafness which, with neurophysiological methods, is possible even in the uncooperative child. The presence of autistic features is particularly disruptive to the parent–child interaction and it can be very difficult to establish whether the child's nonverbal skills are normal. In these circumstances the pediatrician may be unable to give a clear prognosis to the parents and reassure them, although he must offer practical management.

Many children with a developmental disorder of communication will have no other abnormalities on examination, but the range of possible etiologies is so wide that a detailed history and examination is essential in anything other than a mild phonological delay. As genetic influences are so important, inquiry should be made not only towards detecting family members with speech problems, but also towards detecting those with literacy difficulties which are closely related.

General examination should include body habitus, height and weight, presence of cutaneous stigmata and dysmorphism. Neurological examination includes not only examination of bulbar musculature, but also a general assessment of motor function looking for long tract or other specific neurological signs, including signs of cerebral dominance, associated movement, immature Fog test, finger agnosia, dysgraphesthesia, sensory inattention, disorders of weight and texture discrimination, mirror movement or choreoid movements.

Investigations

Hearing must be examined (see p. 1683) and should include impedance tympanometry to evaluate conductive middle ear disease. Analysis of karyotype, particularly for sex chromosome disorders, may be indicated. Delayed speech development occurs in nearly half of boys with XXY and XYY sex chromosome disorders and XXX girls (Ratcliffe 1994). The decision as to whether to investigate further, e.g. CT of the brain or electroencephalography, depends on the likelihood of associated brain damage, e.g. hydrocephalus or porencephaly following intraventricular hemorrhage of prematurity and other factors such as periodicity of symptomatology. In cases of developmental language disorder the brain CT scan is usually normal, but the SPECT scan may reveal areas of hypoperfusion in the inferior frontal convolution of the left hemisphere in impairment of language expression and in the left temporoparietal region when there are additional receptive difficulties (Denays et al 1989).

Management

For normal intellectual growth the child must develop inner language. Therefore, even if in the early stages after presentation the diagnosis and prognosis remain unclear, some form of language program for the communication-disordered child must be implemented, e.g. 'Portage' Parent Guidance Program.

Children with phonological disorders will require formal articulation therapy often into the early school years. By the age of 7 years, most children with developmental defects of articulation will be largely intelligible but they often have difficulty with phonics in reading and spelling and this propensity should be communicated to the school to avoid the effects commonly seen from the chronic failure in this area.

Children with a severe and persisting language disorder may need special schooling. There are a few schools for speech and language-disordered children and an increasing number of language units are being established. These are usually attached to normal primary schools and admission guidelines are established (Invalid Children's Aid Nationwide 1988).

Certain children with severe language disorders may be taught a system of nonverbal communication, not so much to compensate for unintelligible speech as to provide an alternative framework for building up meaningful language. The system of choice will depend on several factors which can be assessed jointly by the speech therapist and educationalist.

NEUROLOGICAL/ACQUIRED DISORDERS

Dysphonia

The normal voice

The larynx has two functions: firstly a sphincter action to protect the respiratory tract from aspiration of food and secondly, phonation. Phonation can occur without a larynx, however (as is seen in esophageal speech). The lungs act as a pair of bellows producing an air stream under pressure which determines the volume of the voice. Sound is produced by a vibrating air stream as a result of the vibrations set up in the vocal cords. The cords themselves do not produce speech, merely a noise which, without resonation of the nasal cavities, pharynx and chest, sounds quite thin and reedy. Vocal cord vibration is constantly switched on and off. Vocal cords are necessary for sounds such as b, d, g, z, j, l, m, n and all the vowels but not for p, t, k, s, th, ch and h. The voice shows obvious pitch differences between male and female, particularly after puberty and normal speech shows wide swings of pitch. The volume of a voice also varies in normal speech. Apart from producing sound which is then modulated by the articulators into spoken speech, the voice also, as a result of the changes in pitch and volume, gives clues to the emotional accompaniment (prosody) of speech. Phonation also varies with nationality or dialect.

The breath stream pressure makes the cords vibrate only when they are proximate and when they are contracted; it is not a free vibration of loose cords in the air stream. The tension in the cord will vary the pitch and changing breath stream pressure will alter the volume. The cricothyroid muscle is the main muscle which causes lengthening of the vocal cord and the thyroarytenoid (which includes the vocalis muscle) shortens the cords. Other movements of importance in the larynx are:

1. dilation of the glottis, i.e. to allow an increase in air flow during breathing (posterior cricoarytenoid muscle);
2. closure of the glottis and approximation of the cords (lateral cricoarytenoid and aryepiglottic muscles) to produce a sphincter action to prevent aspiration.

All the intrinsic muscles of the larynx are supplied from the medulla, having their origin from the nucleus ambiguus. The cricothyroid muscle takes its innervation from the superior laryngeal nerve which is a branch of the vagus nerve in the neck and sometimes has some fibers from the spinal accessory nerve, whilst all the other muscles of the larynx are supplied by the recurrent laryngeal nerve which branches from the vagus, on the right side of the body looping around the right subclavian artery whilst on the left it loops at the level of the left ligamentum arteriosum. Both nerves in the neck lie in the groove between the trachea and the esophagus.

Anatomical dysphonia

Dysphonia can result from an anatomical abnormality of the larynx (Table 14.83) or from a neurological lesion affecting its innervation or the muscles themselves. The cords may be involved in tumors, such as malignant tumors of the larynx, or benign polyps and cysts. They may be thickened and have nodules as a result of excessive use of the voice, so-called singer's nodules, which in children are more likely to be due to constant screaming and shouting. Acute laryngitis results in hoarseness, loss of high tones, a drop in pitch, loss of pitch swings, eventual aphonia and in severe cases stridor. Chronic involvement of the cords occurs in tuberculosis; they may be thickened in myxedema when the voice is deep and sounds as though the patient is talking through a mouthful of food. Tumors such as hemangiomas of the subglottic region may splint the vocal cords, preventing free movement and causing dysphonia. Trauma to the larynx can occur from accidental hanging, prolonged intratracheal intubation or drinking caustics. The larynx may be congenitally abnormal as with a glottic web or in some of the craniofacial syndromes such as the Goldenhar syndrome and occasionally in the Treacher Collins syndrome. There is a rare familial type of dysphonia inherited as an autosomal recessive condition in which there may be no phonation and the child communicates by whispering. Dysphonia with a harsh gruff, low-frequency voice is a common manifestation in children with Down syndrome.

Neurological dysphonia

The laryngeal muscles will weaken with prolonged use of the voice in myasthenia gravis. The recurrent laryngeal nerve may be injured in the neck during surgery (especially thyroid surgery or removal of a cystic hygroma) or in chest surgery, being especially vulnerable on the left side where it runs round the aortic arch. It can be trapped in suppurating hilar lymph nodes. The vagus nerve is more likely to be involved in compression by tumors of the nasopharynx spreading into the base of the skull through the jugular foramen – this could result in complete paralysis of the pharynx with associated dysarthria and dysphagia. The nucleus ambiguus, from which all the fibers controlling articulation and laryngeal function arise, lies at the level of the olive on each side of the midline in the brainstem, being about 1.5 cm long. Both nuclei can be affected in brainstem infarction and secondary brainstem hemorrhage, as in children with head injuries or pontine gliomas. In cases of recurrent laryngeal nerve palsy the abductor muscles of the larynx are affected first (Semon's law), so that the vocal cord on the affected side moves towards the midline. As the recurrent laryngeal nerve palsy becomes complete, the cord comes to lie in the so-called cadaveric abducted position. If the lesion is unilateral, the opposite cord gradually manages to oppose the paralyzed cord so that the hoarseness will diminish, but if the paresis is bilateral, persistent aphonia will result.

Aphonia may rarely arise as a hysterical symptom especially in teenagers.

Investigation

The breadth of investigation for dysphonia is wide and is clearly directed in large part by the associated features, e.g. MRI scan to demonstrate brainstem tumors, tensilon (edrophonium chloride) test in myasthenia gravis. Most children will require laryngoscopy with or without bronchoscopy to visualize the involved structures. Rarely electromyography of the larynx may be helpful.

Treatment of dysphonia

The treatment of organic conditions causing dysphonia is discussed in Chapter 27. Removal of nodules, tumors and polyps requires skilled surgery. Relaxation techniques, breath control and phonatory exercises may be required in cases of vocal abuse or when cords have been chronically inflamed. In some cases of unilateral vocal cord paralysis, controlled exercises can encourage the opposite cord to cross the midline and effect a compensatory closure.

It is rare for a child to undergo total laryngectomy for malignancy, but teenage cases are known and where possible the child will be taught to produce esophageal speech by injecting a small amount of air into the upper esophagus which is then allowed to vibrate outwards. This produces a fundamental sound equivalent to vocal cord phonation which can then be modified intraorally as before to produce speech. Children with permanent tracheotomies pose a particular problem in that they are not able to phonate and a total communication approach may be necessary. Total loss of voice has psychological effects and psychological readjustment may be an important part of any therapy program. Functional loss of voice, during which the vocal cords are usually abducted, requires careful discussion with the patient in an attempt to ascertain the cause rather than blindly treating the symptoms. Injury to the cords from intubation can be treated with laser therapy.

Dysrhythmia

Dysrhythmia of speech accompanies basal ganglia disease ('festinant' speech, as in gait) and acquired disease of the cerebellum. Ataxia interferes with the smooth stopping/starting of speech and the judgment of force and staccato or explosive speech results.

Table 14.83 Anatomical dysphonia

1. Tumors, e.g. hemangioma, papillomata

2. Nodules, polyps, cysts

3. Cord thickening, e.g. myxedema, tuberculosis

4. Congenital abnormalities,
   e.g. atresia, web
   e.g. associated syndromes, Goldenhar's, Treacher Collins

5. Laryngitis
   acute
   chronic

6. Iatrogenic
   tracheostomy, laryngectomy

7. Familial dysphonia

8. Functional paralysis (hysterical)

Dysarthria

Dysarthria is a term used to convey difficulty with articulation and although it refers mainly to the movement of lips, tongue and palate, in many cases there will also be dysphonia and dysrhythmia. The muscles of articulation modify the air stream in order to produce vowels and consonants. If there is a disorder of the muscles of articulation the consonants will be imprecisely articulated, the speech may be slow, slurred and difficult to understand, the voice is often harsh and monotonous with no intonation, phrases are short, speech comes in bursts and shows excessive hyper- or hyponasality. Speaking is also obviously associated with an increased effort and consciousness of the act of articulation, which is normally subconscious. Respiratory control is also poor so that a breath is taken in the middle of a word or phrase.

Classification of dysarthria

Dysarthria can be classified into two main subdivisions:

1. anatomical dysarthria;
2. neurological dysarthria.

The neurological causes are conveniently subdivided according to the neurological type of lesion into:

1. spastic dysarthria (pseudobulbar palsy);
2. flaccid dysarthria (true bulbar palsy and myopathies);
3. extrapyramidal or dyskinetic dysarthria:
   a. hypokinetic
   b. hyperkinetic;
4. ataxic dysarthria.

Anatomical causes of dysarthria

The commonest cause of dysarthria due to an anatomical lesion is the cleft palate syndrome. If the palate is not intact, the soft palate does not close off the nasal cavity completely and intrabuccal pressure cannot then be increased to produce certain sounds such as p, b, t, or those requiring a sustained air flow such as s. Instead, the air escapes through the nose and may be heard during speech as nasal escape. Slow and difficult feeding, especially with regurgitation through the nose, should suggest the possibility of a cleft or submucous cleft palate. The palate itself may be congenitally short as part of the malformation or an inadequate repair or postoperative infection may have caused fibrosis and subsequent contraction. Acquired palatal disorders, such as injury from falling on a sharp object whilst holding it in the mouth, can result in contraction from scarring. Penetrating injury or chronic diseases such as syphilis may result in secondary fistulae of the hard or soft palate. If the palate does not close completely, the eustachian tubes may not be protected so that reflux or obstruction will predispose to chronic secretory otitis and conductive deafness which further aggravates the speech disorder.

The palate may be congenitally short with or without a submucous cleft, often associated with a bifid uvula. The classic signs of a submucous cleft palate are a bifid uvula, translucent central zone and notched hard palate with anterior insertion of the palatal muscles but not all may be present. Alternatively, the maxilla may be very long in children with rather scaphocephalic heads, so that the soft palate only approximates to the posterior pharyngeal wall provided there is a pad of adenoids. Removal of the adenoids may then result in nasal escape and hypernasal speech. This latter condition is often referred to as the palatal disproportion syndrome. The opposite to hypernasal speech is hyponasal speech or hyporhinophonia, which occurs when there is obstruction to the nasopharyngeal air passage. Adenoids are the most obvious cause when mouth breathing, snoring, poor resonance to the voice and eustachian obstruction causing deafness are the usual presenting features.

Palatal disproportion may operate in the opposite direction to that described above. For example, in the Treacher Collins syndrome there is maxillary hypoplasia and there may be a very narrow nasopharynx. Tumors of the nasopharynx such as rhabdomyosarcoma, angiofibroma or even carcinomas do occur in children and may be missed or thought to be due to adenoids until lower cranial nerve palsies or proptosis point to the true nature of the disease.

Abnormalities of the tongue are usually overemphasized as a cause of speech disorders. Children with congenital abnormalities of the tongue may have hemiglossectomies and still have completely normal speech. It has been suggested that even aglots can have fairly intelligible speech. In spite of this, tongue tie is still given as a cause of developmentally slow speech. True tongue tie, which causes the tongue to furl when the child attempts to protrude it so that it cannot be protruded between the lips, does occur and may be helped by division of the frenum, but it is very rare as a cause of speech disorder.

Investigation. There are a large number of associated syndromes with clefts of the lip and palate and these may dictate the need for additional investigations, e.g. Stickler's syndrome with associated eye defects of myopia and retinal detachment and the velocardiofacial syndrome. For examination of the palatal function a lateral X-ray of the neck combined with palatogram or videofluoroscopy during vocalization will demonstrate the soft palate, tongue, larynx, adenoidal pad and nasopharynx and movement and closure of the soft palate. Pernasal endoscopy combined with vocalizations allows definition of the movement of the palate.

Management. Children with anatomical dysarthria should be jointly managed with the plastic surgeon, ENT surgeon, orthodontist, audiometrician and speech therapist.

Improvements in plastic surgery over recent years have resulted in very acceptable cosmetic results in the treatment of the harelip but children with severe anatomical dysarthria from the cleft palate are still seen. Research is now directed towards trying to achieve better speech from the palatal repair. The use of palatal obturators to try and improve alveolar alignment and to prevent turning out of the edges of the cleft while awaiting repair may help. Early closure of the palate at 4 months of age rather than waiting until 18 months of age may also help. Modern techniques of nasal endoscopy and videofluoroscopy help to give a more dynamic approach to studies of palatal function in order to try and assess whether a pharyngoplasty would further improve speech (Sommerlad 1994).

Neurological causes of dysarthria

Flaccid bulbar palsy (dysarthria). Included within this subgroup are all diseases which affect the lower motor neuron, viz. anterior horn cell, i.e. bulbar nucleus, peripheral nerve, neuromuscular junction and the muscle itself. There may be involvement of all the muscles of mastication, articulation and swallowing or of individual cranial nerves, causing a more localized lesion. The muscles of mastication, which are not major muscles of articulation, include temporalis, masseter and the two pterygoid muscles and these have their own masticatory nucleus in the brainstem, the innervation being carried by the motor branch of the trigeminal nerve. The muscles of the soft palate, pharynx and larynx are innervated via the vagus nerve from the nucleus ambiguus and also the motor part of the glossopharyngeal nerve, which also rises from the nucleus ambiguus in the brainstem. The motor supply to the tongue is by the hypoglossal nerve, which has its nucleus on each side of the midline in the floor of the fourth ventricle and is a pure motor nerve supplying only the muscles of the tongue. The muscles of the lips, especially the orbicularis oris, are supplied by the facial nerve and this is responsible for lip closure and pursing. Sensory feedback is mainly via the trigeminal, glossopharyngeal and the chorda tympani branch of the facial nerve.

The clinical presentation of a flaccid bulbar palsy is that the child has a lax open mouth with jaw muscle atonia together with weakness and wasting. There is drooling, feeding is difficult, the jaw and gag reflexes are absent and there is no cough reflex. The absence of protective reflexes means that food may be aspirated into the lungs or come down the nose and there is often a severe dysarthria or anarthria. The tongue will be wasted, will not protrude and will show fasciculation. Stridor may occur if the vocal cords are affected; the voice itself will be weak and breathy. The palate will not move with the gag reflex or upon saying 'ah'. If isolated cranial nerves are involved the tongue may only be wasted on the affected side and deviate on protrusion or alternatively, one-half of the palate may rise with the gag reflex and the uvula move to that side. Many of the disorders which affect the lower motor neuron are progressive so that there may be clinical deterioration from mild dysarthria and drooling with tongue deviation to a total anarthria, the need to tube feed and distressing accumulation of secretions leading to aspiration, pneumonia and death.

The bulbar muscles may be affected in the congenital form of dystrophia myotonica (Fig. 14.58) when severe feeding problems present at birth, gradually improve, but are followed by slow speech development which is aggravated by the associated mental retardation. The Prader–Willi syndrome may present as congenital bulbar palsy with drooping, drooling facies and slow speech development associated with mental slowness. Bulbar muscle function will improve as the infant gets older in both of these conditions, so that normal feeding is eventually possible. Myasthenia gravis in childhood may have an oculopharyngeal presentation and this can be acute, precipitated by a virus infection; the abnormal eye movements may be asymmetrical, as may palatal movements and the condition may mimic a brainstem tumor if the possibility of myasthenia gravis is not entertained and an edrophonium (tensilon test) performed. The facioscapulo-humeral form of muscular dystrophy affects the face which is droopy and expressionless and the child cannot purse the lips or whistle. There is also a rare form of oculopharyngeal muscular dystrophy which is not usually seen in childhood. The so-called whistling face syndrome may also be associated with facial muscle involvement and a nonprogressive or only slowly progressive myopathy.

The neuromuscular junction or peripheral nerve can be attacked by certain toxins in botulism and diphtheria with resultant palatal and pharyngeal paralysis. The malignant form of hyperphenylala-

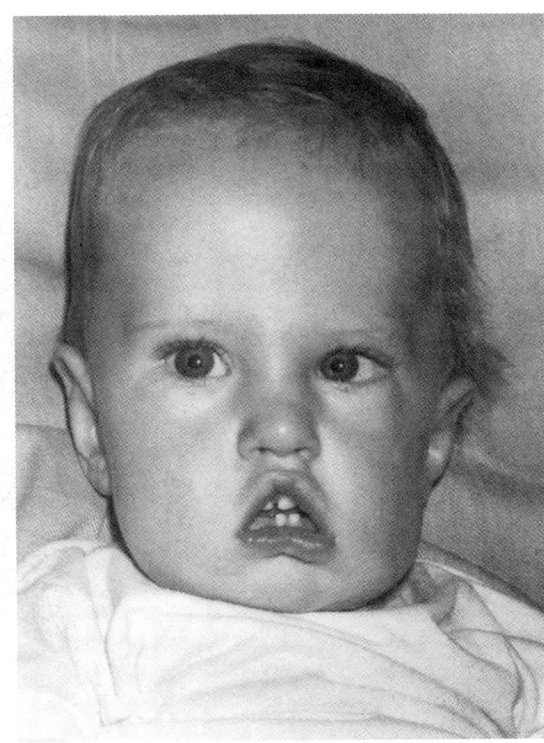

Fig. 14.58 Flaccid bulbar palsy: dystrophia myotonica.

ninemia also presents with bulbar weakness and progresses to a flaccid totally areflexic infant with complete bulbar paresis. The peripheral nerves, i.e. the cranial nerves supplying the bulbar musculature, may be involved by compression as they come through the various foramina of the skull. Tumors of the nasopharynx such as rhabdomyosarcoma may present with dysarthria as the tumor infiltrates through the jugular foramen into the skull. The facial nerves may be affected bilaterally with compression from dural tumor deposits in leukemia or sarcoidosis. Alternatively, the bony canals themselves may be narrowed in certain bone diseases such as osteopetrosis or juvenile Paget's disease. The nerves to the bulbar musculature can be selectively damaged or as part of a more generalized parainfectious polyneuritis (Guillain–Barré syndrome).

The anterior horn cells in the medulla, which form the cranial nerve nuclei, can be involved in disease processes such as bulbar poliomyelitis, acute intermittent porphyria, rhombencephalitis or in pontine gliomas. Congenital dysplasia of the brainstem (Moebius' syndrome) results in agenesis of the sixth and seventh motor nerve nuclei (Fig. 14.59). Other bulbar nuclei can also be affected with complete bulbar palsy which may necessitate long-term tube feeding or gastrostomy and is associated with a persisting anarthria. The anterior horn cells in the spinal cord supplying the limbs may also be involved as an 'extended Moebius syndrome' with complicating arthrogryposis. The Moebius syndrome is nonprogressive but there is a comparable group of disorders seen in childhood with progressive degeneration, e.g. Fazio–Londe syndrome and von Laere syndrome. Vascular lesions of the brainstem are more likely to be secondary to raised intracranial pressure (for example after head injuries with secondary brainstem hemorrhage) than due to

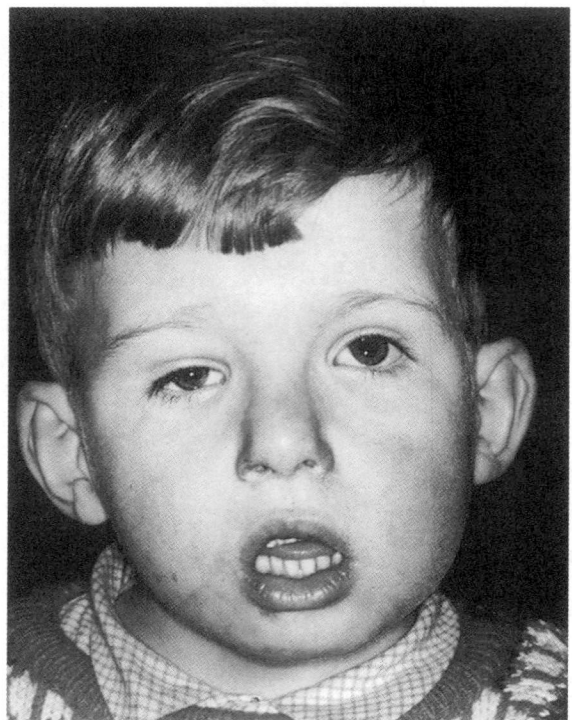

Fig. 14.59 Moebius syndrome in a child, affecting speech – flaccid dysarthria.

primary vascular disease of the brainstem which in children is more often embolic (for example from congenital heart disease) or, rarely, hemorrhagic into the cerebellum from a microvascular malformation. The disastrous prognosis of these conditions means that onset of dysarthria in a child must always be taken as an indication for a full and detailed neurological examination and investigation.

Spastic dysarthria (pseudobulbar palsy). This is an upper motor neuron type of bulbar palsy with release of the brainstem reflexes from cortical and mid-brain control. The jaw is stiff, the mouth difficult to open fully, the jaw jerk is brisk and often accompanied by jaw clonus. The tongue is small and bunched and rapid movements such as protruding and moving from side to side are difficult although some movement of the tongue is usually possible. Chewing is difficult due to the spastic masseter muscles, there is no wasting, for example of the temporalis muscle, the gag reflex is brisk, the cough reflex is present, inhalation is not common as the airway retains its reflex protection. Feeding difficulty is common; the child cannot easily bite or chew. Drooling is often a frequent and distressing problem.

Speech, if there is any, is slow and labored with poor variation in pitch; it is hypernasal, the voice is harsh and the rhythm may be explosive. Consonants are imprecise and slurred; emphasis is absent or is applied in the wrong place. The child finds it difficult to control his breathing for speech, thus interfering with normal phrasing.

The bulbar muscles involved in speech have bilateral cortical representation so that although a unilateral cortical lesion can cause speech dyspraxia, a bilateral lesion is necessary to cause a pseudobulbar palsy. Dysarthria is not therefore seen with a hemiplegia but is the rule with a tetraplegia. The commonest causes of pseudobulbar palsy seen in childhood are therefore associated with cerebral palsy and especially following perinatal asphyxia. Any severe anoxic ischemic episode, as may result from uncontrolled status epilepticus, drowning, poisoning, cardiac arrest, etc., may cause a pseudobulbar palsy. The brainstem of the neonate is selectively vulnerable to asphyxia so that occasionally two associated pathological lesions, one in the cortex and one in the stem, cause hemiplegia and bulbar palsy. Encephalitis (Fig. 14.60) and brainstem tumors may cause a mixed upper and lower motor neuron picture, as may amyotrophic lateral sclerosis.

Disseminated sclerosis, which is a common cause of pseudobulbar palsy and dysarthria in adolescents and young adults, is not common in prepubertal children. Brainstem ischemia with infarction can result from embolization. Degenerative brain diseases not uncommonly present with dysarthria and spastic bulbar palsy, especially conditions such as subacute sclerosing encephalitis, metachromatic leukodystrophy, Alexander's disease, Batten's disease or the adolescent form of GM_2 gangliosidosis. An onset bulbar palsy has a much more sinister prognosis than a congenital bulbar palsy, which is usually associated with a nonprogressive cerebral palsy. Another common cause of pseudobulbar palsy in children is head injury with mid-brain or upper brainstem damage associated with deceleration or acceleration and secondary brainstem ischemia due to tentorial herniation causing impairment of the vascular supply to the central parts of the brainstem and consequent secondary hemorrhage. Dysarthria can be extremely severe after a head injury in children but often makes a surprisingly good recovery.

There is a very unusual form of pseudobulbar palsy which may present in early infancy with feeding difficulties and then appears to recover. There is then delay in speech development with dysarthria accompanied by drooling, poor control of fast tongue

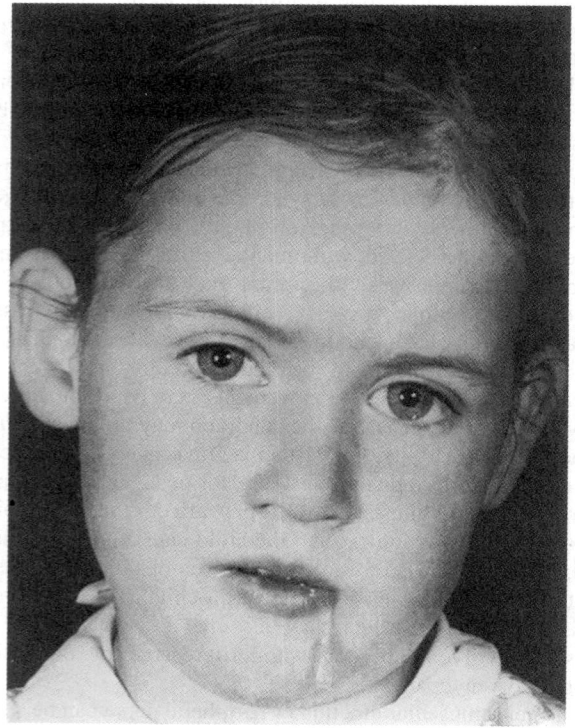

Fig. 14.60 Postencephalitic mixed flaccid and spastic dysarthria.

movements, poor palatal movements and a very brisk jaw jerk, but little feeding difficulty by the time the child is 3 or 4 years of age, although still marked difficulty with speech. This occurs in isolation without any obvious cause and must be differentiated from bulbar weakness secondary to perinatal asphyxia; it is often known as the Worster Drought syndrome and is thought to be a developmental, probably genetically determined condition.

A congenital bulbar palsy with feeding difficulties in the newborn period which appears to improve but is associated subsequently with severe persisting dysarthria accompanied by varying degrees of mental handicap and abnormalities of the fingers and toes is also seen in the dominantly inherited condition of Pfeiffer's syndrome.

Extrapyramidal or dyskinetic dysarthria. Dyskinetic bulbar palsies have been divided into two forms, hyperkinetic and hypokinetic. The hypokinetic form is seen most commonly in the adult with parkinsonism and only seldom in children. The face is expressionless, the voice slow, monotonous, of little volume and sometimes accompanied by festination of speech. Hyperkinetic bulbar palsy is much more common in children. There are many unwanted movements which interfere with normal articulation. These movements are both reflex and involuntary in type and are seen in association with choreoathetosis affecting limb and trunk muscles. The hallmark of the hyperkinetic as opposed to pseudobulbar palsy is the retention in the former in an obligatory manner of all the infant feeding reflexes, so that rooting, reflex bite, cardinal points, lip reflexes, sucking and tonic mouth opening are all easily elicited. Tonic opening of the mouth which the child cannot overcome occurs if the head is extended, traction applied to the hands or the perioral region stimulated with a metal spoon or else it forms part of a mass extensor response to a sudden shock or anxiety. The tongue is often protruded in a tonic manner or may show rolling rhythmic movements. The gag reflexes and cough reflexes are retained so that aspiration of food is uncommon and the airway remains protected. The jaw jerk is present but not exaggerated unless there is a mixed lesion, as in the spastic dyskinetic picture, which may complicate perinatal asphyxia. Chewing and biting are difficult, feeding is messy and particular care must be taken not to trigger the various reflexes.

As the child gets older, lips, tongue and palate will become progressively more involved in involuntary movements so that grimacing, chewing movements, tongue rolling, clucking and pharyngeal movements become very obvious. These are seen in their most manifest form in the isolated, so-called orofacial dyskinesias and tardive dyskinesias which may follow prolonged use of phenothiazine drugs, especially haloperidol.

The causes of dyskinesia are discussed in the section on cerebral palsy (see p. 753). Kernicterus, which used to be the commonest cause of a pure extrapyramidal syndrome in childhood, is now rare and more mixed spastic dyskinetic patterns following perinatal asphyxia are more common. Anoxia, as from carbon monoxide poisoning, uncontrolled status epilepticus or cardiac bypass surgery, may result in dyskinetic bulbar paresis with an associated marked dysarthria. There is a group of metabolic degenerative diseases which can also selectively affect the basal ganglia, as is seen for example in Fahr's syndrome, Leigh's encephalopathy, glutaric aciduria, Hallervorden–Spatz disease, etc.

In children with hyperkinetic bulbar palsy speech is difficult to understand and is associated with a lot of facial grimacing and torsion movements of the head and limbs. It is often very explosive, slurred and coming in rushes, sometimes on an ingressive air stream. The pitch is monotonous, the voice is harsh and vowels may be distorted as well as consonants. Intelligence may be well preserved or above average so that this condition includes one of the most important groups of noncommunicating children or so-called 'locked-in' children, in whom mental retardation may be wrongly diagnosed in early childhood due to the communication difficulties. These severely anarthric children are the ones who par excellence are helped by alternative communication systems. In children with postkernicteric hyperkinetic bulbar palsy, although the intelligence is preserved, the condition is aggravated by an associated sensorineural deafness.

Ataxic dysarthria. Children with acquired destructive lesions of the cerebellum such as occur with cerebellar tumors, for example astrocytomas or hemangioblastoma of the cerebellum, may develop dysarthria. On the other hand, children with congenital ataxia secondary to cerebellar hypoplasia or agenesis rarely have dysrhythmic or staccato speech; they are often hypotonic and may have the open mouth and drool so that they may be diagnosed as having flaccid bulbar palsy. The cerebellum regulates the length of the muscle, the starting and stopping of a movement, the force to be used in order to execute skilled movement and is involved in childhood motor learning. Children with ataxia from infancy due to hydrocephalus, perinatal asphyxia or the various genetic syndromes have a developmental pattern of delayed articulation, i.e. a delay in motor learning. Disorders such as Friedreich's ataxia, with gross incoordination of limbs and trunk, are associated with a gross dysarthria but not usually until the later teens, whilst other causes of degenerative ataxia such as ataxia telangiectasia may have an early dysarthric component. As a general rule, cerebellar pathology present under 3 years of age tends to be associated with a slowing up of the development of articulation whilst lesions developing after this age result in a true dysarthria.

Investigation. The child who presents with an onset dysarthria is of particular concern and the clinician must consider the range of investigations for metabolic disease, neurodegenerative disease, imaging of the brainstem and possible sites of emboli. The imaging described in dysphonia may be applicable to the dysarthric child and MRI may be particularly useful to image brainstem and posterior fossa (Faerber 1995).

Management. The management of the dysarthric child poses many problems. Progress depends not only on the etiology and the severity of the dysarthria, but also on the child's intelligence, motivation and associated neuromuscular disorders, e.g. cerebral palsy.

Feeding difficulties are often prominent and date from the neonatal period. Since control of lips, tongue and soft palate is a prerequisite for speech, the speech therapist is often asked to advise on the various aspects of oral control for feeding. Therapy will aim to help the child to acquire good lip closure, to inhibit reflex tongue thrusting and to encourage biting and chewing movements. Exercises for drooling control may also be included in the program. The position of the child during feeding, in order to prevent mass extensor patterns from causing tonic mouth opening and tongue thrust, together with the avoidance of utensils such as metal spoons which may trigger off primitive reflexes all need to be explained to the parents.

For the older child exercises of breathing control, phonation, articulation and nasality may improve speech.

For the child with no useful speech but good understanding of language it is important for the speech therapist to decide at what point an alternative medium for communication should be introduced in order to prevent frustration and stagnation of expressive language skills. The choice of system should be based on a number of considerations such as level of intelligence, age, whether hand function is normal and the opinion of the classroom teacher.

In children with normal hand function sign language, such as that used by the deaf, may be preferred or one of the other sign systems, e.g. Makaton. It is essential that the school staff and the family are all willing to learn the child's sign system. For the physically handicapped child many of these sign language systems require the ability to imitate gestures which are beyond his capability. In such a situation a pictographic system, e.g. the Bliss symbolics system where small pictograms based directly on meaning rather than on sounds, is used. By various combinations of symbols, existing vocabulary can be augmented to provide a fairly sophisticated communication system. Bliss symbols can be learned considerably more easily than the written word. The Bliss system also has the advantage that the board used by the child has the word printed underneath it so that parents and teachers have no difficulty in interpreting the symbols if they themselves do not know them. The child may point to the Bliss symbols by various additional devices from head pointers to more sophisticated microchip-based indicators.

Flexible communication may be increased on combining the pictograms with a computer 'concept' keyboard with speech 'Introtalker' (Fig. 14.61). Computer technology has also increased communication horizons for older physically disabled children who can read and spell. Word processors, accessed through interfaces, can be tailored for their individual needs.

Acquired articulatory dyspraxia

In its fully developed form this is very similar to the congenital form. There is difficulty with speech sounds, especially consonant blends with inconsistent substitutions or omissions. Word synthesis is slow, problems occurring more with the beginning of words than the end. Long words cause particular difficulty; individual syllables may be pronounced in isolation but cannot be sequenced together. The child's comprehension is normal, he does not have any word-finding difficulty, unless there is an additional expressive dysphasia, he knows what he wants to say and knows that his pronunciation is abnormal. Acquired articulatory dyspraxia is usually caused by small lesions in the region of the inferior frontal gyrus of the dominant hemisphere due to vascular lesions, small tumors, bullet wounds, etc. Augmentative communication may be required.

DISORDERS OF LANGUAGE

Dysphasia

Speech is localized to the left hemisphere in 95% of dextrals and 60% of sinistrals. The sensory association area for speech (Wernicke's) area lies in the posterior temporal lobe next to the primary auditory area (Heschl's gyrus). Wernicke's area is connected by long intra- and intercortical fibers. The most prominent of these are those forming the arcuate fasciculus which connects to Broca's motor speech area in the left third frontal convolution.

Acquired aphasias in childhood differ in a number of respects from those which characterize adult pathology. Although aphasia is commoner after left-sided lesions, it also occurs relatively frequently after right-sided lesions in young children. Typically the aphasia is motoric/expressive and mutism dominates the clinical picture irrespective of the site of the lesion. Recovery is typically rapid as the nondominant hemisphere has the potential for speech, although this is increasingly less so the older the child at the time of the CNS insult. Left hemisphere lesions sustained by infants under 1 year of age have a more pervasive effect on intellectual development.

Expressive dysphasia

This most frequently follows trauma from road traffic accidents or, more rarely, cerebrovascular disease (Fig. 14.62). There are some similarities to Broca's aphasia in adults. Initial mutism is followed by word-finding difficulties, syntactical disorganization and pronunciation difficulties which affect spontaneous speech, sentence repetition and reading aloud. Paraphrasias may occur with substitutions of well-articulated phonemes or words (verbal paraphrasias). If substitutions become numerous following the mutism, jargon aphasia may result with words becoming unrecognizable neologisms.

There is usually a good degree of recovery although complex language tasks remain affected with lexical poverty and persisting dysgraphia with adverse effects on educational progress. In adult expressive aphasics, an adverse prognosis is related to damage to the most rostral portion of the medial subcallosal fasciculus in the lateral angle of the frontal horn (deep to Broca's area and affecting projections from the cingulate gyrus and the premotor strip to the caudate nucleus) and this may have some relevance in children (Naeser et al 1989).

Receptive dysphasia

Dominant temporal lobe damage produces a receptive dysphasia. The etiologies include post-head injury with extradural

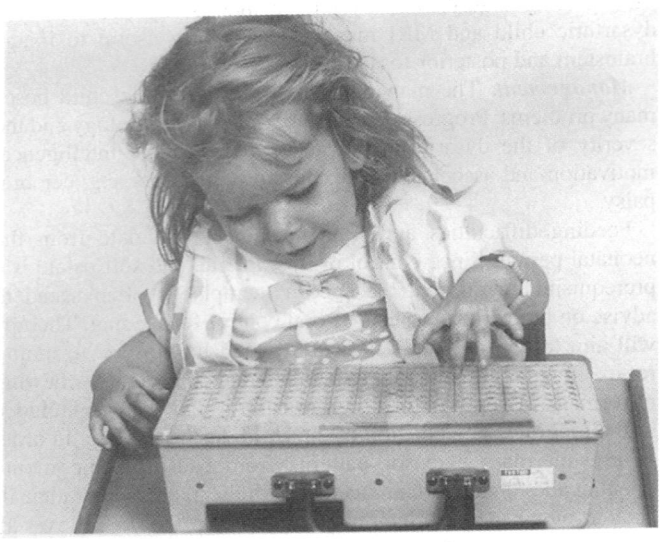

Fig. 14.61 Augmentative communication with Reybus Introtalker (pictograms) being used by an anarthric child with severe mixed cerebral palsy.

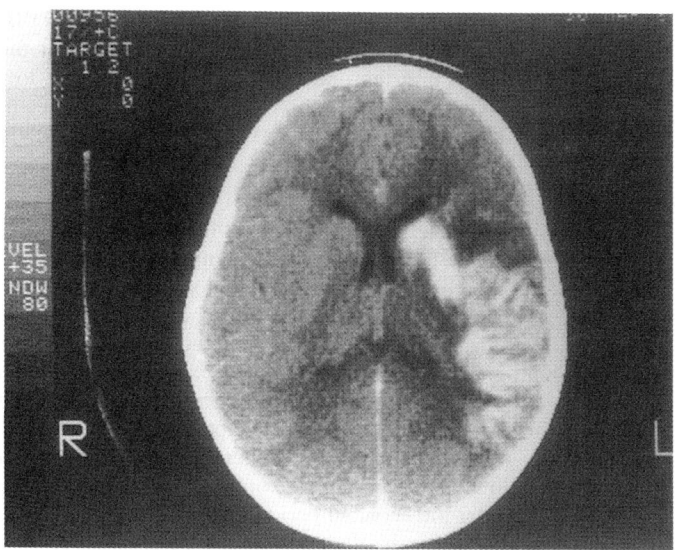

Fig. 14.62 Expressive dysphasia: CT scan appearances of cerebral infarct in 8-year-old child.

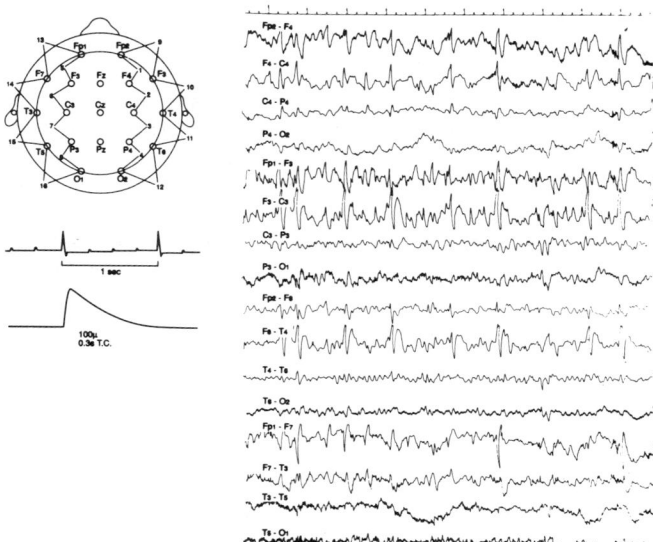

Fig. 14.63 Bilateral temporal lobe epileptic discharges in Landau-Kleffner disorder.

hematoma, direct contusional injury, contrecoup injury or swirling of the brain against the edge of the sphenoidal wing, epileptic dysphasis, temporal lobe abscess from middle ear infection, emboli, cortical thrombophlebitis, herpes simplex encephalitis, meningitis or temporal lobe tumor. In the adult (Wernicke's aphasia), a fluent aphasia results with jargon speech and neologisms but the clinical picture in childhood is dominated by mutism. As the mutism resolves, the comprehension difficulties persist and include the child's understanding of his own speech. Reading skills are usually lost.

Transcortical aphasias

If the arcuate fibers are interrupted, sensory and motor aspects of speech would be expected to be independent and this gives rise in the older child to what has been described as a transcortical aphasia and is usually divided into a transcortical motor and a transcortical sensory aphasia. The important feature about this group of speech and language disorders is that there is retention of the ability to repeat a sentence. Transcortical sensory aphasia is like classic sensory aphasia – there is inability to understand what is said and spontaneous speech is well pronounced.

Conduction aphasia

This is an unusual type of dysphasia in children, characterized by fluent paraphrasic speech, good verbal comprehension and striking difficulty in sentence repetition. Short-term auditory verbal memory is impaired. It is associated with a lesion in the auditory association area, supramarginal gyrus and arcuate fasciculus.

Acquired central deafness and auditory agnosia

A pure word deafness may follow damage to the superior temporal lobe in older children and etiologies include focal tumors, trauma and embolic vascular events. However, more commonly the adjacent association area is involved and a receptive dysphasia results.

Auditory agnosia and a receptive dysphasia may follow the onset convulsive disorder of Landau–Kleffner. In this disorder language regresses in association with EEG spike activity in one or both temporal lobes (Fig. 14.63). Overt clinical seizures occur but are not invariable. Prognosis relates to the age of onset with a worse outcome for children with onset before the age of 5 years. It is thought that the clinical symptomatology results from disruption of auditory input into Wernicke's area.

Investigation

Investigations may include imaging of the brain with MRI following, for example, trauma, CNS infection or vascular disease. EEG may be indicated to evaluate the temporal lobe, e.g. Landau–Kleffner, herpes simplex encephalitis. Neurophysiological measurement of peripheral and central auditory pathways may be necessary.

Management

Children with aphasis frequently have associated neurological disorders, e.g. right hemiparesis or brainstem injury and these will have an impact on their ability to communicate. A child with a brainstem injury, with an ophthalmoplegia and quadriplegia, will be an akinetic mute with no way of expressing his needs. Mute dysphasic children may or may not have comprehension problems. A detailed assessment in conjunction with the speech therapist will indicate how the child's communication can be augmented. Even the simple expedient of a yes/no facility, e.g. a flashing light, can go a long way towards alleviating the child's distress. As previously mentioned, dysphasic children can experience persisting difficulties which hamper their educational progress and long-term follow-up from the speech therapist may be indicated. In Landau–Kleffner syndrome the recovery of language may be promoted by corticosteroids and they merit consideration even though the effects may be disappointing.

SECONDARY SPEECH AND LANGUAGE DISORDERS

Peripheral hearing loss

A full assessment of hearing is mandatory in children with disturbed speech and language development. This must include the minimum decibel thresholds across all the major frequencies (250–8000 Hz). A hearing loss in the low to middle frequencies (125–2500 Hz) interferes with the perception of vowels and prosody in speech and the higher frequencies (2000–8000 Hz) affect the consonants. The latter situation can be particularly deceptive because the child may respond to sound but he will perceive speech as indistinct and will not be able to understand it.

Conductive deafness

The commonest cause of deafness is the conductive type secondary to secretory otitis media ('glue ear'). Up to a third of preschool children experience at least one episode in a bimodal distribution at 2 and 5 years (Zielhuis et al 1989). Over half of these episodes will resolve spontaneously within 3 months but the chronic condition produces a persisting hearing loss of the order of 20–40 dB across all frequencies and can affect speech development (Rach et al 1988).

Sensorineural deafness (Table 14.84)

Without appropriate intervention, the child with a congenital sensorineural deafness will not develop inner language and will

Table 14.84   Etiology of peripheral sensorineural deafness

Congenital
1. Genetic
   a. Isolated: autosomal recessive
               autosomal dominant
               sex-linked

   b. Associated syndromes:
      (i) ophthalmological; 25 types, e.g. Usher's
      (ii) ectodermal/pigmentary, e.g. Waardenburg's
      (iii) skeletal/craniofacial, e.g. Treacher Collins
      (iv) chromosomal, e.g. Turner
      (v) metabolic/endocrine/renal, e.g. Pendred (hypothyroidism), Alport's (renal), Jervell-Neilsen (prolonged QT interval)
      (vi) neurological, e.g. Cockayne

2. Acquired
   a. Teratogenic: thalidomide
                  quinine

   b. Intrauterine infection:
               cytomegalovirus
               rubella
               toxoplasmosis
               syphilis

Acquired
a. Perinatal asphyxia
b. Neonatal hyperbilirubinemia
c. Toxic: aminoglycoside antibiotics, streptomycin
d. Infection: bacterial meningitis, mumps, measles
e. Petrous temporal bone fracture
f. Neurodegenerative disease; Fazio-Londe
g. Neurocutaneous disease; neurofibromatosis

function as dysphasic. Severe (65–80 dB) and profound (85 dB) sensorineural hearing loss affects one in 1000 children but the incidence can be as high as one in 40 in ventilated very low birthweight survivors.

Etiology of congenital loss

The ear develops between the sixth and 14th gestational weeks when it is vulnerable to teratogens, e.g. quinine and thalidomide and congenital infection, e.g. rubella, cytomegalovirus and later, toxoplasmosis (toxoplasmosis exerts most effect in the last trimester). Rubella embryopathy has been reduced by effective vaccination programs (Banatvala 1987) whereas cytomegalovirus remains a common cause of intrauterine infection. Following primary maternal infection, 30% of symptomatic and 10% of asymptomatic neonates will develop a hearing loss. In common with losses following rubella and toxoplasmosis infections, the loss may occur after the neonatal period and be progressive.

Sensorineural deafness is often genetically determined usually through autosomal recessive transmission, although sex-linked and dominant inheritance occurs. There are also a large number of syndromes associated with deafness, many of which have ophthalmological abnormalities; 2.3% of congenitally deaf children have the autosomal dominant condition of Waardenburg. In addition to their deafness, they may show a range of dysmorphic features which include broad nasal root, lateral displacement of the medial canthus, hyperplasia of the medial portions of the eyebrows, white or gray lock of hair (usually forelock) and heterochromia of the irides. Three to six percent of congenitally deaf children have the autosomal recessive condition of Usher's syndrome in which the child develops a progressive retinitis pigmentosa with devastating implications for the child who already has a serious sensory deficit. Posterior subcapsular cataracts and vestibular deficiency may accompany the disorder.

Acquired sensorineural deafness (Table 14.84)

Perinatal asphyxia can selectively damage the cochlear nuclei and inferior colliculi. Kernicterus may similarly affect the cochlear nuclei and lower auditory pathways. However, peak levels of free bilirubin or measurement of serum bilirubin-binding capacity does not predict hearing loss, presumably because the integrity of the blood–brain barrier is an important additional factor. Aminoglycoside antibiotics, used in recommended doses and monitored by serum levels, do not contribute to neonatal deafness.

Damage to the eighth nerve occurs in the course of bacterial meningitis in 33% of infections with *Pneumococcus*, 9% with *Haemophilus influenzae* and 5% with *Meningococcus*.

Diagnosis

In the UK, infants are routinely screened at 7–8 months of age by distraction audiometry. In many areas babies at risk are identified at an even earlier stage by checklists of hearing, e.g. 'Can your baby hear you?'. Screening distraction audiometry is carried out by presenting a sound stimulus on the horizontal plane, at an angle of 30–40° from the back of the infant's ear and at arm's length from the mother. A sound stimulus of 35 dB(A) is presented in low frequencies (humming human voice), high frequencies 2–4 kHz (repetitive consonant 's') and higher frequencies 8–10 kHz

(Manchester rattle), whilst an assistant 'distracter' holds the baby's attention with a visual stimulus.

Diagnostic audiometry is mandatory in the presence of delayed speech development even if a child passed his screening test in infancy. Although distraction audiometry is very effective if carried out with scrupulous attention to detail, there are potential pitfalls from visual, tactile or olfactory clues and other children may develop a later hearing loss. Techniques for establishing hearing include cooperative testing, performance testing (the child is conditioned to respond to very quiet levels of low and high frequencies in a simple play situation) and pure tone audiometry. A toy discrimination test is helpful. A child with normal hearing can discriminate the verbal toy stimuli at 40 dB(A) at 3 feet. Impedance audiometry, e.g. tympanometry which measures the compliance of the tympanic membrane in relationship to alterations of air pressure, produced by a sealed external auditory canal, can determine the contribution of a conductive loss.

Particularly in circumstances where the child is unable to cooperate with testing, electrophysiological measurements of brainstem evoked responses (ABSER), electrocochleography and cortical auditory evoked potentials will demonstrate the integrity of the auditory pathways. Around 40% of cases of significant sensorineural deafness requiring hearing aids occur in high-risk infants, i.e. those with admission to a neonatal unit for more than 48 hours, a positive family history of sensorineural hearing loss, head and neck anomalies and strongly suspected intrauterine infection. Neonatal screening programs targeting these high-risk infants could be expected to diagnose these children to allow 'aiding' before the age of 6 months. Screening by BSER audiometry or otoacoustic emission is possible; although the latter is of little use in determining the severity of hearing loss, it has great potential as a screening test (Richardson 1995).

Investigations and management

Conductive. The management of chronic bilateral serous otitis media usually involves surgery and without this, fluid will persist in over 70%. Grommet insertion benefits the child in the short term and more persisting benefit follows adenoidectomy (Maw 1995). Optimum management remains controversial.

Sensorineural. Evidence of TORCH intrauterine viral infection can be difficult to demonstrate, particularly as all these infections can suppress the immune response. CMV virus isolation in the first week of life is the only definite indication of intrauterine CMV infection. Rubella IgM (enzyme immunoassay) persists in the infant for 6–12 months and in the mother for 1 month (rarely 1–2 years) and toxoplasmosis ELISA infant titers persist for 6–12 months. In some children a retrospective diagnosis of intrauterine rubella infection can be inferred from in vitro lymphocyte responsiveness. Ophthalmological stigmata of these diseases may occur. Such an examination has revealed a previously unsuspected cause of deafness in 8%. Disturbances in peripheral visual fields and electroretinograms (ERG) suggest Usher's syndrome whereas the ERG associated with the retinitis in rubella embryopathy is normal.

In view of the associated syndromes the deaf child should also have a urinalysis, measurement of thyroid status and QT interval. Radiological investigation of the inner ear can be satisfactorily achieved by a plain film in young infants and severe dysplasias of the semicircular canals are nearly always associated with poor cochlear function.

Children with bilateral sensorineural deafness require an amplified auditory input (Figs 14.64 and 14.65). Experience has shown that children with severe to profound losses derive most benefit from a radio transmission aid where the amplified output of the remote microphone is transmitted to the child by frequency modulated radio transmission. With appropriate support from members of the hearing impaired, many children can be integrated into ordinary school using oral/aural communication. Some children, particularly those in whom maximum amplification does

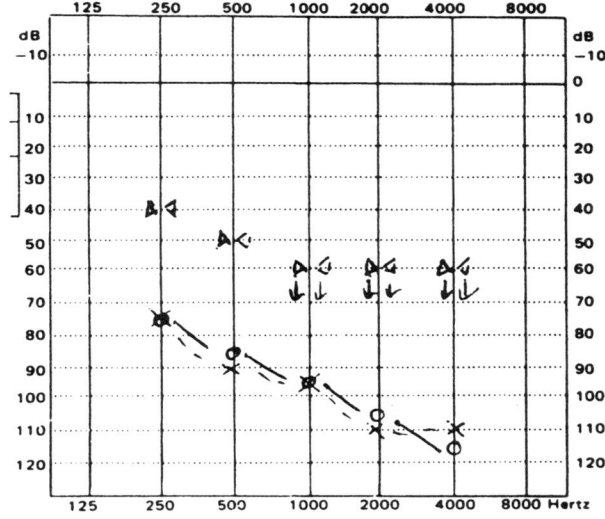

Fig. 14.64 Pure tone audiogram: severe sensorineural hearing loss.

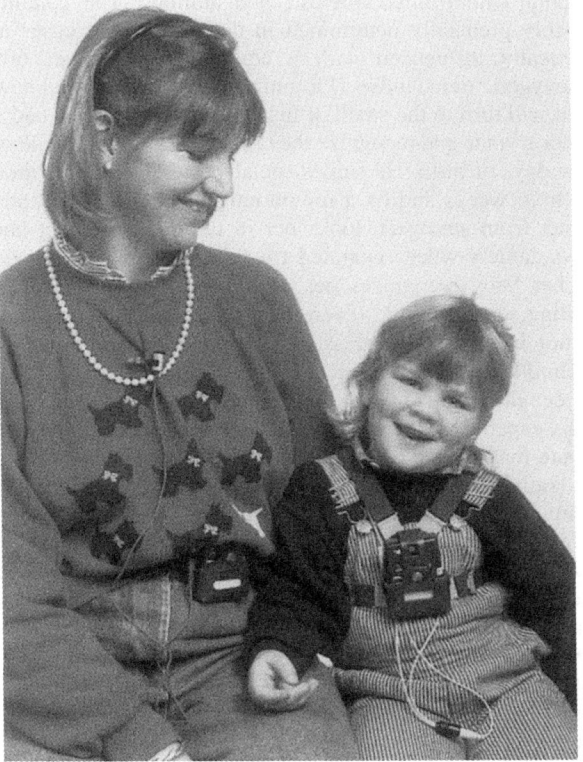

Fig. 14.65 Deaf child wearing radio transmission aid.

not bring their hearing levels into an adequate range to perceive speech, may benefit from a manual signing language. Better sound amplification for these children may be achieved by a cochlear implant. This is an electronic device which is inserted into the inner ear of a totally deaf person to introduce or restore perception of sound. The sooner sound can be introduced into a child's developing auditory system the better will be the linguistic result, but at present 2 years of age appears to be the ideal because of accuracy in diagnosis of the degree of hearing loss (Ramsden & Graham 1995).

Mental handicap

Slow speech and language development is a common presentation of a mentally handicapped child, i.e. global delay in cognitive development, and it is therefore not surprising that long-term follow-up of children who present in this way reveals a high proportion with low nonverbal IQs. Children with specific delay in speech and language can be distinguished by demonstrating normal development in nonverbal cognitive areas.

Many mentally handicapped children have not only the expected delay in their speech and language milestones, but additional deviant development, e.g. in phonology. This may be characteristic of the particular syndrome, e.g. articulatory dyspraxia in fragile X syndrome or 'cocktail party chatter' in Williams' syndrome.

Autism

Children with autism have a triad of impairments affecting social development, communication and cognition. They have restricted imagination and display repetitive and stereotyped patterns of behavior with limited interests and abilities. The condition is probably prenatally determined in the majority of cases and is genetically influenced with a concordance of over 60% in monozygotic twin studies (Plomin et al 1994). A normal newborn infant will turn to the smell of his own mother's breast pad or his mother's voice and recognize the taste of his mother's milk within a few days of birth. He smiles socially and looks at his mother's face by 6 weeks and by a few months will recognize mother as distinct from strangers, looks her in the eye, smiles at her and shows anxiety when separated from her. No mother is in doubt that her baby recognizes her as a person, shows love to her, cuddling in, babbling (even deaf children) and so showing emotion in his facial expression and body language. Even though the child has no verbal lexicon, he is communicating his feelings and recognizing his mother as a person as distinct from an object and is capable of interpreting his mother's facial expression (a neonate may mimic facial expressions) and realizes that it is her face rather than some other part of her anatomy which communicates most and that is the area he will watch.

This is a nonverbal and to some extent preprogrammed system by which communication occurs. The system may depend on an intact temporal lobe and limbic system. The limbic system is a primary area and amongst the first to develop. Later, this nonverbal communication system shows as intonation of voice, sparkle in the eyes, hand gestures associated with speech, sprightliness of gait and the nonverbal pattern of acceptance or rejection in sexual approach. This system is abnormal in autism and the child will be apparently aloof, will not look his mother in the face or show any emotion, although he may show interest in inanimate objects. Thus he may not recognize people as being any more worthy of emotion than inanimate objects, although children with autism and normal intellect may show affection to their parents, but no interest in peers. By the age of 18 months autistic children fail to develop pretend play and joint-attention behavior such as protodeclarative pointing, showing objects to others and gaze monitoring (Baron-Cohen et al 1992). Autism is the most severe of the neuropsychiatric disorders of childhood and 70% of affected children have an accompanying mental handicap. Prognosis is difficult to determine in the individual child but is favorably influenced by normal intellect and the development of speech by the age of 5 years. Some authorities explain the behavioral and cognitive abnormalities of autism as a 'theory of mind' deficit whereby the autistic child lacks an appreciation of other people's capacity for independent thought and thus is unable to appreciate their perspective. These theories can influence treatment programs which are predominantly behaviorally based and of mixed success.

Investigation

A number of genetically determined neurodevelopmental disorders may give rise to a behavioral phenotype of autism, e.g. tuberous sclerosis, fragile X syndrome, congenital rubella and some metabolic and structural brain abnormalities. The skin should be examined under Wood's light. There should be a karyotype including DNA fragile X analysis. Brain imaging should be considered in all cases. Hypoplasia of a portion of the cerebellum and cerebral hemisphere asymmetries have been described in populations of autistic children but are difficult to interpret in individuals. EEG studies are indicated if there is accompanying epilepsy.

Psychosocial effects on language development

If a child is not spoken to he will not acquire language, as he will not understand or use words he has never heard. The parent is, in essence, programming a computer and no matter how good the child's potential, if the quality of the language that he hears, the sophistication of the grammar and the variety of vocabulary is restricted, this must show in the child's language skills. In addition frank abuse or neglect has an adverse effect on children's speech and language development (Law & Conway 1992). There is a very marked difference between the language skills of children in social classes I and II and those in IV and V. Children from working class families, however, tend not to speak much in front of strangers and not to ask many questions. This applies in school and may give a false impression, so that care must be exercised in making assessments of children's language in places other than the home.

There is now mounting evidence that slowness in language development secondary to poverty of environmental stimulation can be quite dramatically improved despite several years of suboptimal stimulation, providing that the child is subsequently placed in a verbally rich environment.

Miscellaneous

For the sake of completeness a miscellaneous group of disorders should be considered. In true schizophrenic psychosis there may be delusions, hallucinations, thought insertions and flights of ideas, all of which show in an abnormal or inappropriate content of speech. Children with psychomotor epilepsy may hear voices or talk in English words which are not joined together in any meaningful sentence. The delirious child or the child poisoned by drugs, plants or glue sniffing may appear to be dysphasic in the acute stage and may lose the reality of thought so that he has difficulty in distinguishing what is imagination or fantasy from what he is really seeing or hearing. Korsakoff's psychosis can occur in children after head injury or severe anoxic ischemic episodes, e.g. cardiorespiratory arrest. The child will perform normally in intelligence testing, will remember all events up to the time of the acute brain damaging event, will speak normally but cannot store new memories and may confabulate. Some children, rather than confabulation, may appear cheeky and learn to answer back and this may mask the severity of the memory defect so that it is only when the child returns to school that it is realized that he is learning nothing new and stays at his premorbid level of attainment.

LEARNING DISORDERS

We conclude that learning has taken place when we can elicit certain behaviors in children. We can think of learning at three levels. At its most primitive level, learning is reflex and depends solely on the neurological maturation of the brain. Such 'preprogrammed' reflex behavior is seen in the positive and negative feeding reflexes of the newborn infant which constitute his feeding behavior. However, once the brain has reached a certain point of development, children must interact with their environment through looking, listening, manipulating and moving for continued development of a skill.

The second level of learning is 'conditioned' reflex learning where a given behavior is always triggered by the same environmental stimulus without accompanying understanding. The child shows a learned response and such conditioned responses can be developed in the mentally handicapped child to achieve activities of daily living such as toileting. These learned behaviors also show in stereotypic phenomena, e.g. echolalia and 'barking' at print (i.e. reading without comprehension).

It is the third level of cognitive learning, where there is understanding, which concerns us most in the school-age child. The brain is obviously the organ of learning and its rate of maturation influences the expression of cognitive learned behaviors. The terminal zones, such as the frontal lobes which are essential for forward planning and motivation and the angular gyrus which is important for reading, are the last areas to mature in childhood. Therefore problems in these areas are only going to be manifest when they would have been otherwise expected by virtue of the child's chronological age and environmental experience. We cannot necessarily diagnose the etiology of the learning disorder by simply describing how the behavior is disturbed. We also need to remember that motor learning, although developing in parallel with cognitive learning, can be affected independently of it. Difficulties in these areas can adversely affect a child's educational progress, e.g. dyspraxia affecting penmanship.

INFLUENCES ON LEARNING

Progress in learning is influenced by many factors which can be broadly separated into the learning environment, i.e. parents and home, teachers and school, and the child's innate learning potential.

Environment

Children from lower social class homes, particularly in the presence of crowding and poor amenities, have low scores on academic achievements in reading and mathematics. The parents' interest in their child's progress and preschool exposure to books, colors and numbers will influence their child's educational progress. Children in care have lower academic achievements and this is more marked the earlier they were received into care.

The teacher's expertise, interest and rapport with the child, along with factors such as the organization of the classroom, nature of the curriculum and attendance at school, all have to be taken into account.

Motivation

Feelings of satisfaction and sense of achievement are considered to be mediated by endogenous brain endorphin release and they promote learning. Failure, criticism and denigration, particularly when the child has a learning difficulty and has had to put a lot of effort into a piece of work which nevertheless falls short of the standard normally expected for the child's age, will create anxiety and undermine motivation.

Attention

Attention is the focusing of conscious awareness upon a particular sensory input or motor act whilst rejecting ('gating out') unwanted stimuli and it is considered to arise from the intralaminar thalamic nuclei. Anxiety from stress at home will disrupt attention. Attention will be lost if the material is boring or beyond the child's understanding. This is seen at its most extreme in the aimless wandering and handling of toys displayed by the mentally handicapped child.

A child with a specific learning disorder may not be able to participate fully in the lesson and he may be anxious and aware of failure. He may wander about in the classroom and become disruptive. A short attention span, distractibility, poor concentration on teaching materials, school phobia and 'acting-out' behavior may all mask the true diagnosis.

Attention deficits are therefore generally secondary to the learning disorder rather than the cause of it. Although true hyperkinetic syndromes do occur in brain-damaged children, e.g. boys with left-sided temporal lobe epileptic foci with overactivity, distractibility, aggression and rage reactions, sleep disturbances and learning difficulties, they are rare and the majority of children with specific learning difficulties have congenital developmental types. In some parts of the world, notably the USA, this was not accepted and many such children were diagnosed as having minimal brain damage and attention deficit disorders. It was considered that the condition was exacerbated by diet and children were treated with sympathomimetic amines and modified diets. Such manipulations where substances such as food dyes and additives were excluded and multivitamins administered gave questionable benefit.

Sympathomimetic amines should be reserved for those children, very few in number, who have genuine hyperactivity complicating brain damage, e.g. postneonatal asphyxia, whereas the other children will be better served by addressing their learning difficulties directly.

Memory

Memory involves the short-term store, transfer from this into the long-term store, the capacity of the long-term store and retrieval. Bilateral damage to the anterior temporal lobes and hippocampi, which can follow the uncal herniation seen with raised intracranial pressure or bilateral epilepsy, can severely interfere with the laying down of new memories and the child has to rely on those already present before the insult.

Consciousness and arousal

This is a function of the reticular system and if this is disturbed, secondary to subclinical status epilepticus or frequent 3/s spike and wave discharges, the child may present with learning difficulties.

Sensory perception

Naturally, a child has to have adequate hearing and vision to participate fully in the classroom. However, in clinical practice deficits in these areas, e.g. refractive visual deficits, rarely occur as previously unrecognized disorders in children with learning difficulties.

Intelligence

Intelligence is an empirically based measure of a child's performance on a multiplicity of tasks which relates to the expected range for that child's age. As such, it gives insight into a child's learning ability but it is not synonymous. However, children with global cognitive delay, i.e. mental handicap, will score below normal on an IQ test. When a child presents with a learning difficulty, a measure of the child's intelligence will help to determine whether the child's difficulties are unexpected, i.e. a child of well below average intelligence may be behind the rest of the class in their academic achievements but be succeeding well within his potential.

Brain damage and acquired disorders

Children with epilepsy may show specific difficulties in written language skills and mathematics, which cannot be explained by their level of intelligence and school experience. Specific learning difficulties may also be expressed following brain damage, such as in the delay in reading that follows the slow speech development in survivors of prematurity or perinatal asphyxia or the dysgraphia which persists after childhood acquired dysphasia.

Congenital/developmental learning disorders

These constitute the greater number of children with specific learning disorders. There is selective delay in the maturation of the brain subserving a particular function and in some children this delay persists into adult life and takes more the form of a permanent disorder. Children may have single or multiple specific learning disorders (Table 14.85). The theories proposed as to why

Table 14.85 Specific learning disorders

1. Central deafness
2. Receptive aphasia
3. Expressive aphasia
4. Articulatory dyspraxia
5. Dyslexia
6. Dysgraphia
7. Dyscalculia
8. Dysmusia
9. Dysprosodia
10. Manual dyspraxia
11. Postural dyspraxia
12. Visual agnosia

these children are affected in this way will be expanded within the framework of dyslexia.

SPECIFIC LEARNING DISORDERS

Specific reading retardation and dyslexia

In 1968 the World Federation of Neurology defined dyslexia as 'A disorder in children who despite conventional classroom experience fail to attain the language skills of reading, writing and spelling commensurate with their intellectual abilities'. By convention we accept a delay of 2 years in the acquisition of these skills as significant. There are many different terms used in the literature to describe dyslexic subgroups, e.g. surface/deep, dysphonetic/dysdietic, but we have chosen to describe the children by clinical syndromes. Population studies suggest that 3–7% of children demonstrate selective difficulty in learning to read.

Developmental dyslexia secondary to slow speech development

Children show a developmental progression through understanding of speech, expression of speech, reading, writing and spelling. Not surprisingly, therefore, as many as 50% of children with developmental dyslexia have previous slow speech development. A third of children with developmental language delay will be slow to read. Males exceed females by 4:1 and a positive family history is common. The literary problems arise from the child's inability to analyze syllables into smaller phonological units. Children who have severe expressive phonological impairments at the time they start school are at particular risk for reading and spelling problems (Bird et al 1995).

Specific developmental dyslexia with delayed cerebral dominance

Features attributed to delayed cerebral dominance occur in 33% of dyslexic children with or without a prior history of slow speech. Such features are termed 'interference phenomena'. These interference phenomena would be normal if the child were younger but it is their persistence in the older child which is abnormal, e.g. b/d confusion (strephosymbolia) which is present in the writing of 1% of 7–year-olds (Temple 1986). Interference phenomena include reversals seen in block design and matrices, confusion between right and left and difficulty with crossed commands. Some children have neurological immaturity of the motor system with associated movements on synkinetic Fog gaits and choreiform movements of the outstretched limbs and present as clumsy children.

Reading is a skill which is lateralized to the dominant left hemisphere along with speech and writing whilst musical ability, concepts of space, shape and direction are lateralized to the nondominant right hemisphere. As discussed in dysphasia, young children have the ability to develop language-based skills in the nondominant hemisphere if the dominant hemisphere is damaged. However, in the normal course of events, the left hemisphere becomes dominant for language and it is thought that the 'mirror' areas in the right hemisphere are inhibited. If this developmental dominance is delayed, interference phenomena are seen (Geschwind & Galaburda 1985). The left hemisphere is preferentially developed for language, demonstrated with positron emission tomography, and the rate of maturation of the left hemisphere is slower than the right, reflected in the maturation of the EEG α rhythm.

The contribution of the delayed hemisphere dominance per se to the child's literary difficulties is unclear and it may be simply a marker for the phonological linguistic problems which underpin the dyslexia. Most dyslexic children learn to read and during development show reading errors which are indistinguishable from normal younger readers but many of them will continue into adult life with spelling and syntax difficulty in written language.

Specific developmental dyslexia (congenital word blindness) (Table 14.86)

Children characterized by a very severe reading disorder amounting to word blindness were described by the ophthalmologist Hinschelwood as early as 1902. Many of the reading problems which they show have features in common with those seen in general reading retardation and the specific developmental dyslexias but they are distinguished by their severity. The dyslexia persists into adult life, despite skilled remedial teaching. Spectral analysis of brain activity reveals differences in activity of the angular gyrus and Wernicke's and Broca's areas in the left hemisphere in these children. The cytoarchitecture of the angular gyrus can be abnormal. There is a strong genetic predisposition of autosomal dominant type with variable penetrance and a major gender influence (the disorder is

Table 14.86 Common reading errors

Letter difficulties

1. Spatial (static) reversal of letters, e.g. b/d, p/q, u/n
2. Confusion of hard and soft consonants, e.g. dekide/decide
3. Difficulty with consonant cluster graphemes, e.g. ough, sh
4. Substitutions, as in phonological development, e.g. l/r or for similar anatomical articulation, e.g. m/n

Word difficulties

1. Slavishly phonetic
2. Guesses according to shape of the word
3. Semantic substitutions
4. Letter position (kinetic) reversals, e.g. dna/and, was/saw
5. Word blindness

much commoner in boys). In some families, the disorder has been mapped through generations in association with chromosome 15 (Pennington et al 1987).

Acquired dyslexia

Cerebral lesions of the cortex or neuronal dysconnections may produce alexia. Often the alexia is overshadowed by the accompanying dysphasia, as in the sensory impairment of reading that follows damage to the superior temporal gyrus. Dyslexia may occur with dysphasia and dysgraphia, when damage extends from the angular gyrus down to the underlying white matter. A child may be unable to learn to read following damage to the dominant temporal lobe.

Pure alexia without dysgraphia follows a lesion of the paraventricular white matter of the left occipital lobe. This may follow interference with blood supply in the territory of the posterior cerebral artery and there may be an accompanying right hemianopia.

A rare form of reflex 'reading' epilepsy occurs in which epileptic discharges, either generalized or focal to the dominant hemisphere, are triggered by the complex cerebral activity that accompanies the language function of reading. There is often a family history with onset of the disorder in the teens.

Writing disorders (dysgraphia)

Dysgraphia is retarded development or an acquired loss in the skill of writing. This difficulty may be subdivided into three groups:

1. abnormalities in motor learning and execution, i.e. penmanship;
2. difficulties with the syntactical aspects of written language, i.e. spelling, sentence construction (grammar) and punctuation;
3. abnormal content of what is written, i.e. semantic aspects of dysgraphia.

The latter is often not specific as the dysgraphia is then secondary to a disorder of inner language. This may itself be specific, i.e. a dysphasia, or be part of a more global cognitive learning disorder, i.e. mental handicap. Thus the time-honored division of writing skills into penmanship, spelling and composition still holds good.

Ontogenically, writing is the last language skill to develop in the child (comprehension, speech, reading and writing) and is, therefore, the abnormality which is likely to persist the longest in disorders of language development or be lost most easily in acquired brain disease. The child who has brain damage acquired after the development of speech, reading and writing may show a persisting disorder of writing even after there has been an otherwise good recovery. A dysgraphia is also the disability most likely to persist into secondary school in the child with developmental slow speech followed by dyslexia and dysgraphia.

Definition of groups

Figure 14.66 shows a flow diagram of the three main categories of dysgraphia. Motor disorders affecting writing (penmanship) are further divided into several subgroups (O'Hare & Brown 1989a,b).

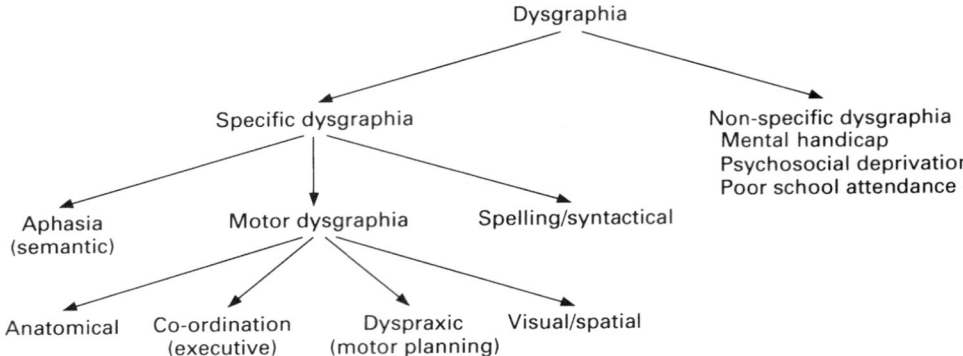

Fig. 14.66 Classification of dysgraphia.

Anatomical motor dysgraphia. Children who have an anatomical defect of the upper limb, such as phocomelia, will often devise alternative ways of bypassing the difficulty, e.g. by using the feet. A pincer grip with very accurate praxic skills, e.g. writing or threading a needle, is perfectly possible using the feet provided that there is no brain damage. This was seen at its most impressive in children with phocomelia from thalidomide embryopathy when the toes were far more efficient than the most sophisticated arm prosthesis. Trick movements can be used so children with lower motor neuron lesions, such as brachial plexus palsies or neurogenic arthrogryposis, can develop impressive skills provided that the motor engram (praxis) in the brain, i.e. the ability to plan and remember the movement, is intact. Any trick movement which allows the child to hold a pen will often demonstrate surprisingly little impairment of spelling or syntax although writing may be large and untidy depending upon the mechanical disadvantage in getting positioned over the paper.

Visual perceptual/visuospatial motor dysgraphia. Perception is the conscious awareness of input to the brain from the five senses (smell, touch, taste, vision and hearing) and also the appreciation of limb position through proprioception, movement through kinesthetic sense and the awareness of pain and temperature. Several of these perceptual inputs are vital to writing competence, such as hearing for the development of inner language and comprehension, as well as establishing a word store or lexicon. Vision is necessary to see the letters and words in order to read and copy as well as orientation upon the page. The motor skill at first depends upon visual monitoring but once the task is learned, the movement is stored as a movement memory, i.e. kinesthetic memory. This is then very dependent on proprioceptive feedback, not from position and vibration sense as usually measured, but from muscle spindles and tendon organs which do not normally reach conscious awareness.

There are several types of visual agnosia, e.g. the inability to recognize shapes, objects, faces, places, geometrical shapes, musical notation and letters. These can be lost in isolation or in different combinations. The ability to recognize faces, shapes, objects, places and direction is generally accepted as being dependent upon normal functioning of the occipital and parietal lobe on the nondominant side. The recognition of graphemes as shapes with a linguistic (word) and sound (phonemic) association indicates a linguistic spatial function of the left or dominant hemisphere.

Visual copying of letters is a primary skill in learning to write, but as the motor engram becomes established it becomes less important, i.e. one can write and spell with the eyes closed, albeit with poor spatial arrangement on the page. Alternatively one can execute the motor skill with a toe in the sand, a pen in the mouth or the opposite limb (in mirror fashion). As the motor skill is learned it becomes subconscious (see below) and becomes more strongly associated with visual and auditory imagery and the developing knowledge of language.

A child with a severe visuospatial difficulty may be unable to organize himself on the page yet writes and spells acceptably. The converse is also true; children with severe reading and writing problems may have normal or superior spatial skills.

Examination of the writing of a child with visuospatial problems reveals that the margins vary, the writing tends to slope down diagonally from left to right, one line runs into another, letters are omitted, the end of the line is misjudged so that one runs out of the page in the middle of a word and there is poor spacing between words. The difficulties occur with equal expression in copying, writing to dictation and original composition, although greatest difficulty may be observed in the copying exercise. The term 'visuomotor difficulty' is vague and may refer to a child with blindness, cerebral palsy, spatial difficulty or dyspraxia and is often all-embracing for hand skills in dressing, drawing, writing, construction, block designs and the ability to perform well with jigsaws.

Motor dysgraphia: executive/coordination. The movement is planned by the cerebral cortex dependent upon motor memories (engram) from past experience and practice. The execution of this planned movement in a smooth coordinated way is dependent upon the precentral motor cortex, pyramidal tract, extrapyramidal and cerebellar systems. In pyramidal lesions, the child can plan but not execute the movement. The degree of distal weakness correlates well with the loss of function. The speed of movements is decreased and this loss of speed also correlates well with the loss of skill (Brown et al 1987). The child has an immature grasp and may, in severe cases, have retention of the primitive grasp reflex.

The extrapyramidal system regulates the natural speed of a movement and so the cadence of speech, gait and writing. In cases of hypokinetic dyskinesia (e.g. parkinsonian complex), writing is small (micrographia) and slow (bradygraphia), whilst the converse is the case in hyperkinetic dyskinesias. Involuntary movements may cause sudden unexpected jerks, sudden angulation of letters, blotching or drawing of the pen across existing script. This is seen best in choreoathetosis. A typewriter will immediately overcome this problem (Fig. 14.67).

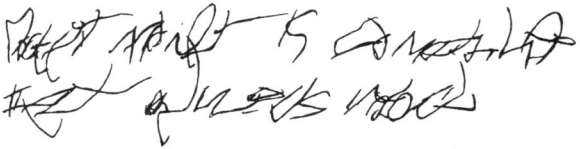

"POCKET MONEY IS SOMETHING THAT ALWAYS INTERESTS..."

Fig. 14.67 Incoordination dysgraphia: hyperkinetic dyskinesia, writing and typing.

Coordination is a measure of the accuracy of judging the distance, force, speed and direction of muscle movement required to execute the planned movement. Abnormalities produce clumsiness, with dropping and breaking of objects and loss of fine neat adjustment producing clumsy untidy writing.

Dyspraxic dysgraphia. This may occur in any child with brain damage and can complicate any type of cerebral palsy so that, for example, a child with a spastic diplegia but little or no increase in muscle tone may have quite gross dyspraxic difficulties with his hands. As with so many developmental disorders, there is a condition of pure dyspraxic dysgraphia which appears to be genetic in origin and not based on any neurological damage. There may be interference phenomena from the opposite side if dominance is not established so 'p' will be written 'q', b/d, was/saw, god/dog. This may occur in a pure form without any difficulty in actually writing the letters down but if the child has additional spatial problems, there will be irregularities and the script may slant across the page.

Dyspraxic dysgraphia is a disorder of motor learning involving the graphomotor center which has the same relationships to hand movements as Broca's area has to movements of lips, tongue and palate. The child is slow when writing, he cannot remember which way to move his hands to make the letters, he will make a stroke, see how it looks, half make the letter then correct it when it looks wrong, so that he is constantly correcting by visual means on a trial and error basis, crossing out and making the writing appear very untidy. There is also difficulty with spacing, one word often running into another (Fig. 14.68).

Some children have additional difficulties in that they do not only have a dyspraxia for writing but may have difficulties with other hand skills, such as fastening buttons or laces, dressing, using a knife and fork, wiring an electric plug, i.e. manipulative or constructional dyspraxia which shows as particular difficulty in sequencing (Dewey 1991). Manipulative dyspraxia and writing dyspraxia are not interdependent but may be seen together in the clumsy child with schooling difficulties.

Dysgraphia: spelling/syntactical

Spelling can be defined as the production of a correct sequence of graphemes to correspond to a word of spoken speech as dictated by the rules of the particular language. Speech is the same, substituting phoneme for grapheme. It should not, therefore, surprise us that syntactical and spelling dysgraphia should so often follow a developmental speech retardation syndrome (Fig. 14.69). Mastery of spelling requires a high degree of linguistic competence and is the last language skill to develop. There are cases of isolated familial spelling dysgraphia without any preceding abnormality in speech development, again suggesting

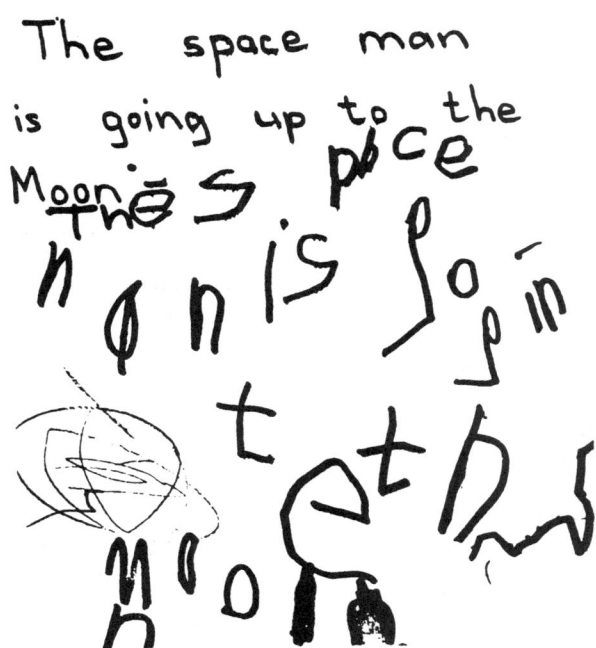

Fig. 14.68 Dyspraxic dysgraphia.

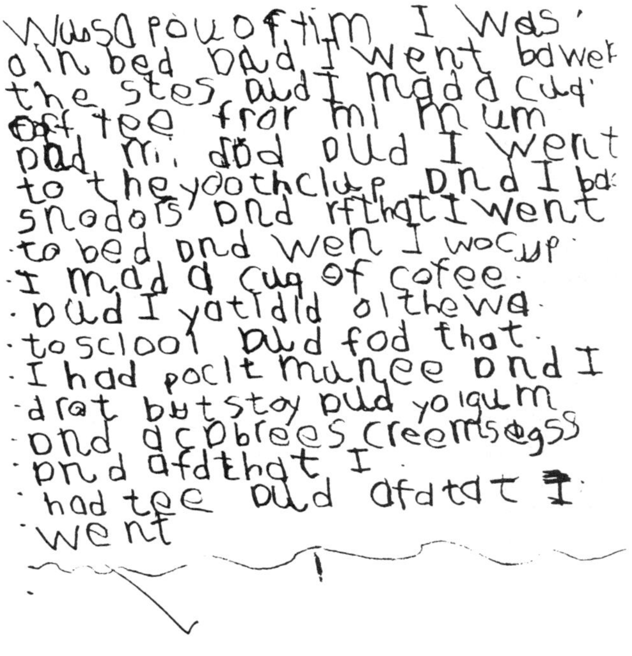

Fig. 14.69 Spelling dysgraphia.

that there must be genes acting during childhood governing the maturation of individual systems within the brain.

With a spelling dysgraphia, writing speed is slow and there is difficulty retrieving words from spelling vocabulary. Words are written in a slavishly phonetic way (sodeam/sodium, matilic/metallic, dimonds/diamonds, pepol/people) or according to dialect (reet doun for right down) and very occasionally as the child speaks them with immature speech (led lolly/red lorry, doddy/doggy). Complex graphemes such as ph, ch, sh, th, ough, cause particular difficulties. Spelling age is retarded on standardized tests and mirror writing, with god/dog, was/saw, b/d, adds confusion to what at first may appear an unintelligible muddle. The child has no idea of punctuation, phrase or sentence and spacing may be absent between words. They cannot read what they have written, even though they can read the same passage from a book. They can copy well and neatly but writing to dictation and spontaneous composition is very poor, with short, poorly constructed, simple sentences. The child will deliberately search out words he can spell in order to try to get his ideas down on paper. This is slow and very frustrating.

The learning of syntax in speech follows the development of the phonetic system and that in the writing system follows graphemic skills, so sentence construction is more related to motor than cognitive learning. The child may have an IQ over 130, i.e. excellent cognitive development, and yet have very severe syntactical dysgraphic difficulty. Acquired brain damage, which causes a Broca's aphasia, will in most cases also cause a dysgraphia since the motor association area of Broca, controlling motor learning in lips, tongue and palate, is adjacent to the graphomotor area on the left which controls motor learning of the right hand required for writing. In children, head injury, encephalitis, tumor, epilepsy or stroke can all cause an acquired dysgraphia. The spelling dysgraphia may remain when the motor aphasia of speech has cleared.

Nonspecific and semantic dysgraphias

Children who show a semantic or linguistic dysgraphia do not usually have a specific disorder as their problem is part of a more global cognitive learning disorder, i.e. mental handicap.

There are, however, children with a specific receptive aphasia who have severe language difficulty with little understanding of speech and with severe reading and writing problems. Semantic dysgraphia is, therefore, not an isolated or single specific disorder, but part of a wider language disorder which dominates the picture more than the writing defect.

Dyscalculia

Many children have difficulties with mathematics that reflect their low intelligence and are therefore not specific. However, over a third of epileptic children show academic underachievement in this area which cannot be explained on the basis of their IQ. Children with Gilles de la Tourette syndrome frequently have specific difficulty with mathematics. Dyscalculia may also arise from the right hemisphere cognitive difficulties which occur in Asperger's syndrome.

Most children who have the specific learning difficulty of dyscalculia have other associated specific learning difficulties, e.g. dyspraxia and dysgraphia. In the developmental form of dyscalculia, the child presents with a 'virtually insurmountable problem in learning the primary elements of calculation'.

There is a very wide range of normal in the speed of acquisition of mathematical skills. The ability to recognize, understand and produce numbers appears to be independent of the calculation system and these functions can break down in isolation in pathological states in adults. From these considerations, we have proposed guidelines to the development of arithmetical skills in children (Fig. 14.70).

Developmental dyscalculia may occur in association with nondominant hemisphere dysfunction (Weintraub's syndrome), i.e. low performance IQ constructional dyspraxia, poor visual motor skills, dysprosodia and disturbances of emotions and interpersonal skills, slow motor skills in left hand and hypoplasia of left-sided limbs (Weintraub & Mesulam 1983). Other forms of developmental dyscalculia are accompanied by dysgraphia, finger agnosia and left–right disorientation and more closely resemble the acquired left hemisphere Gerstman complex from damage to the superior angular gyrus and posterior supramarginal gyrus.

Acquired cerebral disorders in older children may present with features more familiar in adult pathological states, e.g. dominant frontal lobe lesions that impair writing numbers and planning calculations, dominant temporal lobe lesions where reading of numbers is preserved but there is impaired comprehension of mental and written arithmetic and dominant parietal lobe lesions that produce strephosymbolia and writing of higher order numbers in mirror order.

Investigations

Many children with developmental specific learning disorders are managed effectively within school and do not present to pediatricians. However, there are a number of circumstances where a pediatric opinion is sought: where the presentation masks the primary learning disorder, e.g. migraine, behavior disturbances, anxiety or depression, where the child was known to have premorbid risk factors, e.g. slow speech development or where there is thought to have been CNS insult or congenital anomaly and where the disorder is severe and intractable and not responding to remedial teaching.

The breadth of specific learning disorders is large and only a detailed history and examination will point to appropriate investigations which might include chromosomes, EEG and CT scan. Most children will not need further investigation but their clinical neurodevelopmental examination must be comprehensive and include vision, visuospatial and visuomotor skills, hearing, auditory memory, auditory discrimination, lexicon development, language comprehension, posture and mobility and hand skills (O'Hare & Brown 1989b).

Management

The needs of these children are best met when the pediatrician contributes as part of a multidisciplinary team which might include the psychologist, teacher and therapists. The doctor is well placed to explain the nature of the disorder to the child and family and this will often be therapeutic in its own right. Much of the remedial treatment is the province of the education system but there are several principles which the doctor must bear in mind.

Reduce anxiety

The child often has low self-esteem and low morale and may be teased at school if he is not good at physical activities due to his clumsiness, as well as being poor at academic subjects. He may show acting-out behavior, buy favors, become the class buffoon, develop school phobia or other anxiety states. The anxiety may manifest as migraine, punishment behavior at home with the parents (he goes berserk when released from school), enuresis or

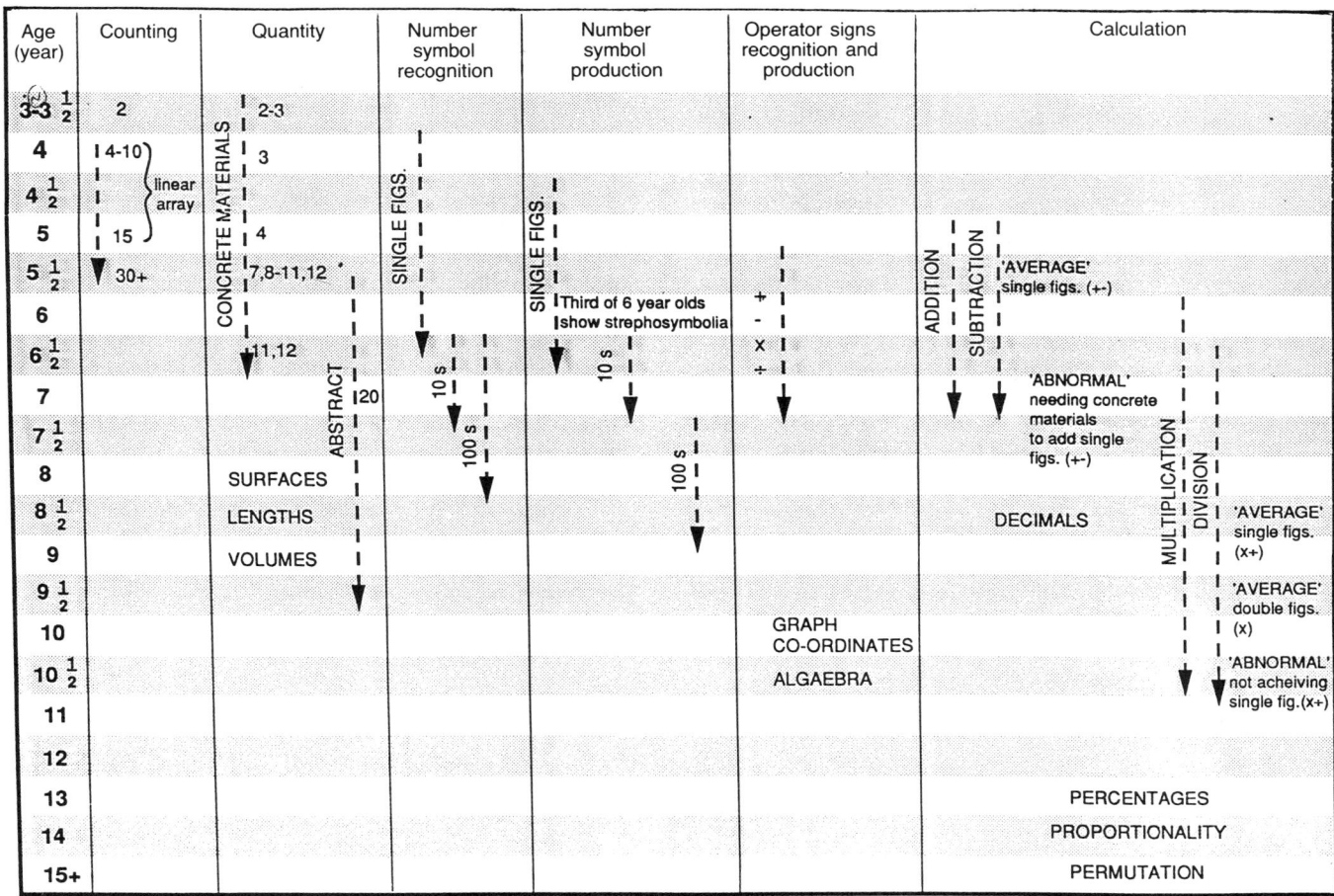

Fig. 14.70 Guidelines to the development of arithmetical skills.

deliberate provocative behavior. Anxiety may be obvious with fear, pallor, tachycardia and panic in relation to certain lessons. During testing the child will cooperate whilst succeeding but will fidget and become restless and say he wants to go home as soon as an area of difficulty is tested in which he knows he is going to fail.

It is easy then to blame the learning difficulty upon poor concentration and restless overactivity, i.e. blaming the effect as the cause. The anxiety engendered will block further learning and the teacher must allay this and not simply present the child with a program to practice all the things he knows he cannot do (Morris 1989).

Circumvent the handicap

The child who cannot read is missing out on information and the way around this is to read to him and buy taped stories and not practice reading material which is emotionally much too young for him. The child with a dysgraphia needs to be given some way of putting his ideas down in some form of retrievable store. The use of a keyboard with a typewriter or word processor may not only alleviate the demands on the child's 'secretarial skills' but actually promote development in penmanship and composition. Oral answers should be accepted where possible. In severe cases, with a combined executive motor and syntactical dysgraphia, so

that the child's spelling precludes use of a word processor, the decision may have to be made to allow a totally oral method with the use of a hand-sized tape recorder with notes being kept on tape and not in a book.

Handicap may be bypassed where appropriate with facilities for scribing, typing, oral answering and tape recording, with an emphasis on communication. An assessment of the optimum methods of help in the light of the child's difficulties should be undertaken well in advance of formal examination demands.

Practice areas without disability

The child's morale, as well as his continuing education, depends upon stimulation of learning in areas where the child has no disability. He should not be punished in subjects such as history, geography, physics or chemistry for his poor graphic skills. 'Untidy, careless, could do better' when referring to his writing makes things worse and criticism should be leveled at the subject being taught when the teacher knows that the child can do better. The child should be encouraged to take up swimming, golf, horse riding, skiing or some physical activity where he can succeed and if possible outstrip some of his classmates to restore self-esteem. Computer work appears to be particularly appealing to children and apart from circumventing the handicap, may allow them to develop skills above the level of their classmates.

Prepare a remedial program

The prognosis for acquiring useful writing skills may be very poor, especially in children with dyspraxias. Children who are simply below the third centile for the development of the particular skill will show steady improvement with remedial help. Those following head injury, encephalitis or focal infarcts, if persisting for more than 18 months after the acute insult, are usually permanent. The familial dyspraxias and those associated with chromosome disorders are also usually persistent. The child with slow speech will usually be speaking well by 7 years but be dyslexic; this will improve by 11 or 12 years but the dysgraphia will often persist into secondary school and professional exam time.

It is because the disorder is long standing with often very slow improvement or slow response to remedial education that we place the remedial program as number four and not the first stage of management. It is not that it is not important, nor that any child will learn to write and spell without continued practice, but that we cannot have an emotionally disturbed child who then fails in a subject in which he does not have a disability, because his whole world has revolved around his disability.

A program aimed at the child's motor proficiency should be developed independently of a spelling program. It is not, however, clear to what extent children transfer remedial pencil skills into their everyday writing. Nevertheless, some children with executive writing difficulties may benefit from attention to pencil skills with, for example modification of pencil design to improve grip and the use of nonslip material on the desk or taping the paper to the desk.

Children with spelling problems may restrict their spontaneous output and decreasing the emphasis on spelling may allow them to express themselves and communicate their ideas. The spelling difficulties themselves can then be addressed. Affirming motor patterns with oral spelling may help. The types of spelling errors can be delineated and a program of remediation planned to practice the types of spelling giving problems.

MENTAL HANDICAP

DEFINITION

Mental handicap is a term used to describe a condition of lifelong intellectual impairment and accompanying disabilities in social functioning. It is not simply a clinical diagnosis; it is a social process of changing expectations, labeling and families coming to some, perhaps idiosyncratic, understanding of what handicap means.

People with an IQ of under 50 are now referred to as 'people with severe mental handicap' or as having 'severe learning difficulties'. Those with intelligence test scoring in the 50–70 range are termed mildly mentally handicapped or as having moderate learning difficulties. Children who function at a level below 50 are almost invariably still educated within special schools or in classes for children with severe learning difficulties.

The current diagnostic criteria of mental handicap are in the third edition of the Diagnostic and Statistical Manual (DSM III) of the American Psychiatric Association (1987):

1. Significant subaverage intellectual functioning – an IQ of 70 or below – on an individually administered IQ test (in the case of infants, a clinical judgment of significant subaverage intellectual functioning).

2. Concurrent deficits or impairments in adaptive behavior, taking the person's age into consideration.

3. Onset of intellectual impairment before the age of 18 years (when the impairment occurs after the age of 18 years this is classified in DSM III as dementia and includes brain damage after head injury, chronic psychosis and presenile dementias).

Here we shall define mental handicap as a learning disorder in which the abilities of the brain necessary for memory recall, thought and reasoning are impaired. Thus, mental handicap is global delay in the development of cognitive learning. In order to differentiate it from the specific learning disorders – dysphasia, dysgraphia, dysmnesia, dyscalculia, dyslexia and dyspraxia – a distinction is drawn between learning with understanding and rote or memory learning without understanding, e.g. parrot fashion learning of simple nursery rhymes or tunes. Considering learning with understanding, it is also necessary to differentiate other noncognitive learning, such as learning to sit, crawl and walk which really depend upon the stage of brain maturation. In practical terms, this means that a mentally handicapped child may be able to sit, crawl and walk at the correct times, which 15–20% of severely mentally handicapped achieve. Often, mental handicap and delay in achieving any motor activities (motor milestones) are closely associated in the early stages of development. It is this frequent association which justifies seeking to detect mental handicap at an early stage. By emphasizing mental handicap as a learning disorder it is hoped to stress that all mentally handicapped children pose an educational problem, many a social problem and only a few a medical problem. Thus, with a mentally handicapped child teaching approaches are of primary importance.

PREVALENCE

The prevalence of the generally accepted three grades of mental handicap (mild, severe and profound) are 30 per 1000, three per 1000 and 0.5 per 1000. In developed countries 0.3 per 1000 will still be in (and seem to require) hospital-type environments (Minns et al 1989b). The profoundly retarded stretch the concept of what is meant by educability as they include a small number who are so brain damaged that they are literally ament, i.e. without mental ability and with a learning ability of nil. Clarke & Clarke (1984) have pointed out the need for care in making predictions about the development of disadvantaged young infants. However, even the most profoundly handicapped and disadvantaged child is likely, given the correct environment and stimulation, to show apparent increment in development. Without this promise it would make motivating staff to work with such problem children even more difficult.

INTELLIGENCE

At the end of the last century Binet in Paris was asked to devise some method of testing children to sort out those who would benefit from schooling. He devised a series of graded test items to assess range of abilities in language, drawing, spatial concepts, number, hand skills, etc. and this formed the basis of the Stanford–Binet intelligence scale. These tests were carried out on large numbers of children to establish what the normal child should be able to do at different ages. So standardized, the test could then establish the mental age of a patient and when compared with the chronological age and expressed as a percentage, this gave an intelligence quotient, i.e.:

$$IQ = \frac{\text{mental age} \times 100}{\text{chronological age}}$$

Several points of importance emerge from this. Firstly, it is the intelligence quotient which is constant and not intelligence: intelligence increases with age and is a function of a child's brain development and life experience. Secondly, intelligence is not a static innate function of the individual but is very dependent upon the environment in which he has been reared as well as upon the integrity of the sensory and coordinating mechanisms through which stimuli from the environment can reach him. That the intelligence quotient will vary with environmental stimulation can be seen in the child suffering from psychosocial deprivation or institutional neurosis. With love and stimulation his intelligence will rise. Language ability plays a very important part in all IQ tests of general ability and so a mildly deaf child, for example with glue ear, or a child from a linguistically poor environment or different racial group is unlikely to perform as well as one with normal hearing or one from a linguistically fluent home. Motivation to learn will often be poor in the anxious child from the broken home so although the learning potential of his brain may be normal and the opportunity to learn present, he may not in fact learn. Intelligence quotients may also vary quite erratically in the epileptic child and from test to test he may range from above average to mentally subnormal. Despite these limitations the IQ test remains a good overall screening test to determine whether a child can learn in a normal school setting with 30 other children in the class and using normal teaching methods. If he scores poorly he will probably need extra help in school.

The value of intelligence tests is that they allow a comparison of a child with his peer group and enable those in need of special help to be selected out before they are demoralized by failure. Most IQ tests, however, do not try and pick out areas of great strength or weakness but test overall ability. Some children are better than others at solving arithmetical problems, some have larger vocabularies and use more sophisticated grammatical constructions, some are good at solving specialized problems demanding complex thought processes.

Distinctions have to be drawn between intelligence, social competence and personality. The majority of educationally subnormal children look perfectly normal, are toilet trained, able to bath and feed themselves and can eventually marry and rear a family – thus they are socially competent. They respond to other people in a warm way and are not violent, aggressive or destructive – thus they have a normal personality. On the other hand, severely brain damaged, mentally handicapped children can have gross problems of social competence and maladjustment.

In summary, intelligence is the increasing ability of the child to understand and reason, think rationally and learn skills and knowledge which allow him to adapt and deal with changing situations.

Intelligence tests for children

1. WISC iii (Wechsler Intelligence Scale for Children) – applicable 6–17 years, not suitable for severely retarded children.
2. WAIS (Wechsler Adult Intelligence Scale) – revised for age 16+.
3. Stanford–Binet – international scale, 4th edition, 2 years to adult, useful for handicapped children.
4. Kaufman Assessment Battery for Children – 2–12 years. Not used for severely retarded.
5. McCarthy Scales of Children's Abilities – 2–8 years. May underestimate IQ in severely learning retarded.
6. Wechsler Preschool and Primary Scale of Intelligence – revised, 3–7 years, not appropriate for severely affected.
7. Bayley Scale of Infant Development – mental and motor scores 2–30 months, but poor predictor of IQ.
8. Merrill Palmer Scales of Mental Development – 2–5 years, appropriate for severely cognitively impaired and language-retarded children. Standardization is dated.
9. Peabody Picture Vocabulary Test revised – 2 years to adult, not a test of general intelligence.
10. Raven's Progressive Matrices – 5 years to adult, test of nonverbal problem solving but useful when combined with 9.

SUBCULTURAL MENTAL RETARDATION

Comparing the social class distribution of children with brain damage with that of children suffering from subcultural mental retardation, there is among the former no social class bias. The subcultural group, on the other hand, is almost confined to social class V. There is an increased incidence of subcultural retardation in the poorer areas of large towns with overcrowding and poverty and within known problem families (parents in debt, rent arrears, prison and careless with property). Most children attending special classes will have a sibling or parent who also needed special education. The educationally subnormal child will usually have crawled and walked at the correct age, will not be subject to fits and will not have an abnormal appearance. The parents will not have sought help prior to schooling and will not regard the child as abnormal for the family. IQ will only rarely be less than 50.

Subcultural retardation is not itself a homogeneous group and there are various mechanisms whereby social factors may affect learning ability.

Genetic factors

Intelligence, like height and weight, is inherited on a polygenic basis. Some perfectly normal people can happen to have lower intelligence than normal, just as there are a small number of geniuses at the other end of the scale. The lower intelligence group of people is often referred to as the 'submerged tenth', i.e. those below the 10th centile. Because of poor job prospects they are likely to show social mobility in the sense that they are likely to drift into social class V. It is not known whether they have fewer neurons or a less complex pattern of dendritic connections. They have no disease and usually only present a problem when they go to school, hence the apparently much lower incidence of mental handicap in the adult than in the child population.

Psychosocial deprivation

The brain of the human infant at birth is poorly developed as far as cortical function is concerned. The neurons have few dendritic connections, there is practically no myelination of the axons, no association pathways have been formed and no Nissl substance has been laid down. The whole cerebral cortex is therefore 'unwired'. This accords with the observation that the mesencephalic anencephalic infant can perform all the reflex functions of the normal full-term infant.

The brain continues to develop after birth at a very rapid rate, especially during the first 3 years of life, continuing until around the age of 18 years. The increase in abilities as a result of progressive brain development is the basis of developmental pediatrics. Thus disease processes have a different effect at different stages of development. At certain early stages an insult, be it metabolic, endocrine, drug or infection, may have a permanent damaging effect which would not have occurred at a later stage.

There is mounting evidence that not only is the correct metabolic (chemical) environment necessary for normal brain development but also the brain must receive stimulation of the developing pathways. One optic nerve is more rapidly myelinated if it is stimulated while the other eye is kept covered. Much more important than myelination is the possibility that the actual dendritic connections which are established in the cortex of the visual area are determined once and for all at the time of rapid postnatal development and are dependent upon visual stimulation at the time. If this is true, severe deprivation of environmental stimulation and experience during the first 3 years of life may set up an organic pattern in the brain which cannot later be reversed by increased stimulation (teaching). This would support the contention that emotional deprivation at this time results in permanent stunting of the affect with subsequent difficulties in maintaining interpersonal relationships in later life. Emotional, physical and linguistic stimulation tend to go together, particularly in the home. Lack of them is likely to result in an intellectually retarded individual with antisocial behavior.

Gross psychosocial deprivation may arise when the parents are inadequate, not only because they are intellectually retarded but because they are very poor parents, uncaring, unloving and having little or no bond with their children. A child in such a family is not picked up and cuddled, is fed with his bottle propped up in his pram, left with neighbors and siblings and may eventually be abandoned. The clinical picture is of a dwarfed deprivation (dwarfism, a pot-bellied, floppy, disinterested child retarded in all aspects of development including gross motor development). He may be apparently deaf or a visual defect may be suspected because he will not look at people's faces. He may lie in his cot indifferent to procedures such as venepuncture. There is a secondary hypopituitarism which affects especially ACTH and growth hormone production. If admitted to hospital and given tender loving care and no other therapy, with the same calories offered as previously, he will exhibit a striking development spurt. Deprivation has held back normal brain growth and love and stimulation alone have caused 'catch-up' brain growth. It has even been shown that pseudotumor cerebri may occur as a result of this process with splaying of the sutures and papilledema. Severe developmental retardation, diencephalic failure to thrive and hypopituitarism are extremes and more minor variants may often pass undiagnosed. Attempts to keep this type of family together without offering the infant an alternative mother figure are likely to be in the infant's worst interests.

Restrictive childrearing practices

Perhaps the purest form of subcultural mental retardation relates to defective childrearing practices. The parents involved are likely to be very caring and devoted but to have a different cultural pattern from the middle-class 'establishment' who tend to act as normal controls for the standardization of IQ tests in a community. The group includes many colored families and different ethnic groups. The parents, although caring for their children, may not read bedtime stories to them, there are few books in the house, the culture may frown upon toys and the language used in the home may not be English or may belong to what is often called a 'restricted code' type of English. As Trevarthen (1987) shows, the early language of children is sensitive to the human environment. Social class differences in children's speech demonstrate this. As infants in different social worlds begin to grasp acts of meaning in the second 6 months of life they may receive different responses from their mothers. Just as two different geographical areas have different dialects, so different social classes use different language codes and the 'subcultural' mentally handicapped child commonly uses a 'restricted language code' of the working class. The socially deprived, mildly mentally handicapped child may not form long phrases or complete sentences; he may not know some essential words; he may speak with more emphasis on rapport than on logic and keep to familiar topics. Language is for him more for the purpose of communicating emotion and achieving solidarity than for information. He may break his speech with lots of repetitions, with hesitation phrases such as 'D'you know?'. Trevarthen & Marwick (1986) compared working-class and middle-class mothers in Edinburgh when their infants were 16–41 weeks and starting to share tasks. It was noted that working-class mothers were much more ready to praise or criticize their infant and that middle-class mothers made many more statements of fact than working-class mothers and they used more questions. Thus, working-class mothers were more interpersonal and middle-class mothers more ideational, encouraging experiences of the environment. This compares with the articulate open code to which the middle-class child is exposed. No matter what his 'native wit intelligence' is in the sense of learning potential, a child brought up in a poor environment starts school with an inferior vocabulary and ability to express himself. Such children are normal in appearance, in reaching motor milestones and in behavior, but they perform poorly on IQ testing and may be competing with children whose vocabulary may be thousands of words superior at 5 years of age. These children may well be motivated to learn but if placed in a school in a poor area with low standards and low expectation and if mixed with a delinquent group, they suffer further education deprivation. It is this group of children that the preschool nursery education program and comprehensive schooling are hoping to benefit. The parents of these children will have good standards for acceptable behavior and will want their children to do well, in contrast to the disinterest and lack of parental discipline seen in parents responsible for psychosocial deprivation.

Further, mothers with families too large for them to cope with and with financial worries may require all their resources to feed the children and are unlikely to be able to buy books or have much time to sit and talk.

Organic factors

It may seem inappropriate to discuss organic factors in an account of an essentially socially determined handicap. However, mothers in social classes IV and V are less likely to attend for antenatal care, more likely to have premature babies and more likely to abuse their children. Thus handicap primarily due to an adverse psychosocial situation may be compounded by organic factors. Other risks derive from a larger family size and concomitant risk of complications in the grandmultiparous mother or the risk of brain damage due to hypernatremic dehydration when a mother of low intelligence does not make up feeds correctly. Drug addiction, alcoholism and heavy smoking during pregnancy may cause additional brain damage. In situations such as this expert family planning must be available and it may be necessary actually to search out the mothers to make sure that they do get antenatal care.

Nutritional deprivation

Mental handicap due to nutritional deprivation is rare in the UK but is a problem in developing countries. The developing brain requires all its nutrients at given critical times for different aspects of brain development. The last trimester of pregnancy and the first 6 months of life are of prime importance from the point of view of total nutrition. If a mother suffers from malnutrition her infant will be smaller than it would have been if she had had a normal adequate diet. Intrauterine starvation followed by immediate postnatal malnutrition may cause a permanent impairment of brain development so that the child is mentally retarded and microcephalic. Poor intrauterine growth of the small-for-dates infant due to placental insufficiency or the effects of heavy smoking on placental function are not yet well enough documented by follow-up studies to know if they are significant causes of handicap in this country.

Summary

Mentally handicapped children with so-called subcultural retardation do not fall into absolutely differentiated subgroups, but there are different patterns of social pathology, several of which may operate in any one child. Prevention is the ideal and much to be preferred to special educational provision at a later age. This group of children is numerically far larger than the group associated with gross pathology.

MENTAL RETARDATION RELATED TO ORGANIC DISEASE (Table 14.87)

Children suffering from organic mental handicap show no social class preference and span the whole range of IQ from ament to

Table 14.87 Disorders associated with mental retardation (after Aicardi 1992)

	Severe%	Mild to moderate %
Cerebral palsy	21	9
Epilepsy	37	12
Deafness	8	7
Blindness	15	1
Hydrocephalus	5	2
One or more of above	40	24
Autism	8	4
Other psychological abnormalities	56	53

normal range. The paradox of mental handicap and normal IQ arises in children who, as a result of adverse perinatal factors such as asphyxia, birth trauma or prematurity, have suffered brain damage which may have reduced their potential IQ by anything up to 50 and yet not brought them below the lower limit of the normal range. Such retarded children within a family of higher intelligence may suffer relative mental handicap and exhibit in addition other abnormalities attributable to brain damage such as squints, clumsiness, overactivity, poor impulse control, sleep disturbance, fits, slow speech development and specific learning disorders. All of this the parents may find socially extremely embarrassing so that a psychosocial factor may be added to an organic one. Even conditions such as Down syndrome may have a range of intelligence from the normal down to the severely subnormal.

Many inborn errors of metabolism and endocrine abnormalities are genetically determined, for example phenylketonuria, homocystinuria, argininosuccinic aciduria, histidinemia and some types of cretinism. A number of syndromes of mental deficiency associated with physical stigmata, e.g. the Prader–Willi syndrome (chromosome 15) and Down syndrome (mongolism, trisomy 21), are due to a chromosomal abnormality. Other causes of mental retardation occur in the stage of organogenesis of the fetus and are related primarily to maternal disorder. The unborn child may be affected by rubella encephalopathy or radiation damage to the brain at this stage. In pregnancy toxoplasmosis, cytomegalic inclusion disease and syphilis may cause brain damage from infection or during labor and delivery there may be hypoxia or traumatic damage. Severe postnatal metabolic disorders such as hypoglycemia and hyperbilirubinemia can also cause brain damage.

In later childhood brain damage resulting from meningitis, encephalopathy associated with severe metabolic disorders, hypernatremia, virus infection or hypoglycemia may cause acquired mental defect which may often but not inevitably be associated with cerebral palsy and epilepsy.

Mental retardation may be progressive or nonprogressive. Progressive mental retardation tends to be associated with continuing activity of the causative factor, e.g. a biochemical factor as in the sphyngolipidoses. Nonprogressive mental retardation usually results from a once-for-all blighting of brain development, as in a congenital defect or birth injury.

MEDICAL ASCERTAINMENT OF MENTAL RETARDATION

Patterns of presentation

The ascertainment of mental retardation depends on the stage of development at which the child presents. A number of disorders may be diagnosed at birth because of physical stigmata of specific type. These include Down syndrome, trisomy 13/15 and 17/18, the de Lange syndrome (Amsterdam dwarfism), bird-head dwarfism, the Smith–Lemli–Opitz syndrome, the Sotos syndrome, Lowe's syndrome and congenital rubella. In other disorders the characteristic physical stigmata only become apparent later, e.g. cretinism and Turner's syndrome (ovarian dysgenesis) where the classic facies, neck webbing, increased carrying angle in the upper limbs and dwarfism may not be obvious at the time of birth and only become apparent towards the end of the first year of life. Table 14.88 shows the more common dysmorphic syndromes associated with mental handicap. Hydrocephalus, whether or not associated with spina bifida, may

Table 14.88   Features of major retardation syndromes

Syndrome	Etiology/genetics	Major features	Other features/course	Mental retardation
Aicardi	Mostly females (chromosome 21)	Severe mental retardation, infantile spasms, choroidoretinopathy, agenesis corpus callosum, hypotonic, fused vertebrae, hemivertebrae	Microcephaly	Severe psychomotor retardation
Angelman syndrome (happy puppet)	Chromosome abnormality (15p-inherited from mother)	Inappropriate bouts of emotion/laughing, stiff puppet-like gait, vertical ataxia (of limbs equivalent to puppet), prognathism and tongue protrusion, hooked nose (viz Punch), horizontal occipital depression, hypotonia, absence of choroid pigment and blue eyes, small OFC and brachycephaly	Abnormal EEG – characteristic spike and wave 2 Hz and 5–6 Hz activity uninfluenced by eye opening	MR
Apert's syndrome (acroscaphocephaly)	AD (older paternal age in sporadic cases)	Irregular craniostenosis (short AP diameter – brachycephaly) also high forehead and flat occiput. Facies: flat, shallow orbit, downward slant of the eyes, small nose. Limbs: syndactyly (II-IV fingers), broad thumbs		Severe MR although may be normal
Beckwith syndrome	Mostly sporadic, occasional AR (chromosome 11)	Macrosomia, macroglossia (with feeding problems), prominent eyes, linear fissures in lobules of external ear, renal dysplasia (enlarged or abnormal kidneys), pancreatic hyperplasia, fetal adrenocortical cytomegaly, interstitial cell hyperplasia of gonads, pituitary hyperplasia (accelerated growth), diaphragmatic eventration, cryptorchidism	Neonatal polycythemia, neonatal hypoglycemia (due to hyperinsulinemia) – prediabetic older patients – omphalocele or umbilical abnormality – occasional hepatomegaly – thymic or thyroid enlargement – skeletal asymmetry – Wilms' tumors – micro- or hydrocephaly – uterine abnormalities	MR (mild-moderate)
Bonnevie-Ullrich's	Mostly sporadic, either sex, normal karyotype	Phenotypically Turner's syndrome	Right-sided cardiac defects	IQ < 50 in some (usually diminished)
Cat eye syndrome	Abnormal small acrocentric extra chromosome	Coloboma of iris, preauricular fistula/pit, anal atresia	Eyes: hypertelorism, downward slant	MR (mild-moderate)
Conradi's disease	AR	Short stature, vertebral abnormalities ± scoliosis. 'Koala' facies. Limbs: hypoplastic (short) long bones with transient punctate mineralization in the developing cartilage, joint contractures, syndactyly or polydactyly	Large fontanel (anterior) craniostenosis	MR (50%)
Cri-du-chat syndrome	Partial deletion of short arm of chromosome 5	Slow growth (from birth on), cat-like cry, hypotonia, microcephaly	Facies: round epicanthus, low set ears. CHD. Simian crease	MR
De Lange syndrome (Amsterdam dwarfism)	Chromosome abnormality in some patients, sporadic in others	Brachycephalic small head, hirsutism (dark hair and low hairline), synophysis (eyebrows bushy meet in mid-line), antimongoloid slant of eyes, broad nasal bridge, anteverted nares, wide philtrum, low set ears, tone abnormalities, nystagmus, microcephalic brain with abnormal gyral pattern, seizures in 10%, basophils may be absent in the pituitary	Prominent veins of face, short stature (deficient GH). Limbs: proximally inserted thumb or syndactyly or phocomelia or other limb abnormalities. Pyloric stenosis, renal and urological anomalies, malrotation of gut, duplication and duodenal atresia, CHD, abnormal ACTH, thyroid, sugar, serum cholesterol high, curious cry	MR – severe
Down's syndrome (trisomy 21)	Full trisomy 94%; 21 trisomy/normal 46 mosaicism 2.4%; translocation D/G, G/G 3.3% (most common malformation in man)	Relatively small stature, hypotonia (mouth open and tongue protruding, diastasis of recti, hyperreflexibility of joints), awkward gait (femoral acetabular dysplasia and incoordination) brachycephaly with flat occiput, hypoplasia of frontal sinus (and flat facial profile), small nose and low nasal bridge, upward slant of palpable fissures, inner	CHD (40%) (AV canal, VSD, PDA, ASD, abnormal subclavian), infertility (100%), leukemia 1%, C1–2 instability, ear and finger anomalies, excess skin back of neck	MR

Table 14.88 *Cont'd*

Syndrome	Etiology/genetics	Major features	Other features/course	Mental retardation
		epicantic folds, speckling of iris (Brushfield's spots), lens opacity (59%) and refractive error. Simian crease		
Ellis-van Creveld	AR	Short extremities, polydactyly, atrial septal defect, alveolar ridge dysplasia, partial anodontia, hypoplastic nails, small thorax, mental retardation, cryptorchidism, hypospadias, foot deformities, cone-shaped metaphysis	Short stature, hand function difficulties, 50% die in infancy	
Fanconi syndrome	AR	Pancytopenia and multiple anomalies, microcephaly, (brown) skin pigmentation. Deafness, ptosis, strabismus, nystagmus, dwarfism	Skeletal abnormalities – hypoplasia of thumb – retarded bone age Splenic hypoplasia, small genitalia and UDT's, leukemia	MR in 20% +
Incontinentia pigmenti	XLD	Irregular pigmented skin lesions on trunk or extremities begin as inflammatory, vesicular or veruccous and go on to pigmented lesions. Microcephaly, fits and spasticity	Eye and osseus abnormalities, patchy alopecia, hypodontia	MR
Joubert	AR	Episodic hyperpnea (resembles panting of dog), abnormal eye movements, ataxia, wide mouth, tongue protrusion, epicanthic folds, strabismus	Agenesis cerebellar vermis, dysplasia and heterocerebellar nuclei, enlarged fourth ventricle on CT scan	50% die before 3 years
Lawrence–Moon–Biedl syndrome	AR	Obesity (especially after puberty), retinitis pigmentosa (± nystagmus, squint or anophthalmia), hypogonadism, dwarfism, occasional deafness and spinocerebellar ataxia, polydactyly (postaxial) and syndactyly	CHD – especially males, VSD, ASD, PDA, PS. Renal anomalies	MR (mild-moderate)
Lightwood's (infantile hypercalcemia)	Sporadic	Elfin facies, short stature, hypotonia in infancy. Hypertension, valvular heart disease, renal deposition calcium osteosclerosis base skull, CDH	After infancy calcium normalizes, progressive renal impairment	IQ 40–75
Lowe (oculocerebrorenal)	XLR	Hypotonia, hyperactivity, cataract ± glaucoma, undescended testes, renal tubular dysfunction. Fits, craniostenosis, pectus excavatum	Diffuse EEG abnormality, hyperchloremic acidosis, organic aciduria, general aminoaciduria, osteoporosis, growth retardation	MR (moderate-severe)
Marinesco-Sjögren syndrome	AR	Small for dates infant. Cerebellar ataxia with nystagmus, hypotonia and dysarthria. Cataracts leading to blindness	Short stature, kyphoscoliosis	MR (moderate-severe)
Opitz syndrome	AD	Ocular hypertelorism, hypospadias	Congenital heart disease, lipomata, osteochondritis	MR (mild-moderate)
Pierre Robin	Sporadic (X-linked and AD also)	Micrognathism, cleft palate, glossoptosis. Cardiac, ocular, skeletal	Urgent respiratory support as neonate	
Prader-Willi syndrome	Sporadic or chromosome abnormality (15p-inherited from father)	Hypotonia (walk around 30 months) and poor coordination. Obesity – insatiable appetite and hyperphagia. Hypogonadism, cryptorchidism and hypoplastic scrotum. Narrow bifrontal forehead diameter. Scratching and picking of skin. Strabismus and refractive errors	Small hands/feet, increased incidence of diabetes mellitus. Cardiac problems, scoliosis, some with growth hormone deficiencies (short)	MR IQ about 70. Poor at maths
Renpenning (fragile X chromosome)	XLR	Tall stature, prominent ears low set, facial hair, seizures, fair hair, macroorchidism, prominent jaw, slight spasticity, eye defects	Prenatal diagnosis on cultured fibroblasts, physically strong	Most IQ < 40

Table 14.88   *Cont'd*

Syndrome	Etiology/genetics	Major features	Other features/course	Mental retardation
Riley-Day syndrome (familial dysautonomia)	AR	Indifference to pain (Charcot joints), feeding difficulties in newborn – difficulty swallowing, cyclical vomiting, diarrhea and failure to thrive. Cyanotic attacks, aspiration and breath holding, chronic pneumonia, slow developmental progress and poor coordination, absent corneal reflex, no tears, corneal ulcers, marked blotching with emotion. Hypotonia and hyporeflexia, hypothermia and poikilothermia, positional hypotension and unstable blood pressure, hypo- and hyperglycemia. Fungiform papillae absent – defective taste	No flare with histamine, urinary frequency, loss of cells/degeneration in reticular formation, loss of ganglion cells in sympathetic ganglia and celiac plexis, increased homovanilic acid	MR in some
Rubella syndrome	Rubella virus infection of fetus in first trimester of pregnancy	Deafness, eye (cataract, corneal opacity, 'pepper and salt' chorioretinitis). PDA (PS and septal defects), microcephaly, growth deficiency (including IUGR)	Early infancy: thrombocytopenia, anemia, hepatosplenomegaly, obstructive jaundice, pneumonia, osteolytic lesions, genitourinary abnormalities, encephalopathy	MR
Rubinstein-Taybi syndrome	Sporadic	Broad thumbs and toes (great), IUGR and postnatal growth limitation. Eyes: antimongoloid slant, ptosis, cataract, colobomata. Facies: hypoplastic maxilla and mandible, beaked nose, hypertelorism, epicanthus, posterior rotation of ears	Epilepsy, enlarged skull foramina, high arched palate (frequent URTI), abnormal dermatoglyphics, associated spina bifida, UDTs, CHD and horseshoe kidney	MR (IQ < 50)
Seckel's syndrome	AR	Growth deficiency, microcephaly (from synostosis), prominent nose, ear, finger and joint abnormalities	Hyperkinesis, UDTs, dislocations scoliosis	MR
Silver syndrome	Unknown	Short stature, skeletal asymmetry, incurved fifth finger	Down-turned angle of mouth, triangular facies, altered sexual maturation (30%) and hypospadias, syndactyly (30%) joint dislocations	MR
Sjögren-Larsson	AR	Congenital ichthyosiform erythroderma, spastic diplegia, short stature, flexion contractures, macular degeneration, seizures, basilar impression	Demyelination in spinal cord and pyramidal tracts, cortical cell loss, < tenth centile for height	IQ 30–50
Smith-Lemli-Opitz syndrome	?AR	Congenital dwarfism, pyloric stenosis with FTT, ptosis with broad nasal bridge, upturned nose and micrognathia, microcephaly	Hypospadias, cryptorchidism and epispadias, syndactyly 2nd–3rd toes, simian creases, low set ears	MR (moderate-severe)
Sotos syndrome		Cerebral gigantism, large birth weight (average 4 kg) and excess growth in early years. Tremor, dysarthria/clumsy, inappropriate socially, friendly hyperkinetic behavior. Persistent tachycardia, some ventricular dilatation	Seizures. Drooling saliva, flushing, prognathism and supraorbital overgrowth, large eyes and nose, advanced bone age, insensitive to pain	MR (mean IQ 60)
13 Trisomy (D group 13–15) Patau	Older maternal age	Holoprosencephaly (mid-face and brain), seizures, microcephaly, deafness, eyes – microphthalmia; mouth – cleft; ears – low set; skin – capillary hemangiomas; hands and feet – abnormal joints, nails	CHD (80%), VSD, PDA, ASD, dextrocardia, genitalia abnormal and UDTs, single umbilical artery, 18% survive to 1 year	MR – severe
18 Trisomy syndrome (Edwards)	2nd most common malformation. Male:female 3:1 (older maternal age)	Feeble newborn and failure to thrive, altered gestational timing, polyhydramnios, growth deficiency, hypoplasia (of muscle, fat, subcutaneous tissue). Facies: narrow bifrontal diameter, low set malformed ears, micrognathia. Clenched hands with hypoplastic nail	Survival 10% at 1 year, hernias, UDTs, CHD (VSD, PDA), short sternum	MR – severe

Table 14.88 *Cont'd*

Syndrome	Etiology/genetics	Major features	Other features/course	Mental retardation
Turner's syndrome	XO (female) (Bonnevie–Ullrich's syndrome in male or female with phenotypic Turner's but normal karyotype)	Short stature, broad chest with widely spaced hypoplastic nipples, lymphedema (of fingers and toes in infancy)	Gonadal dysgenesis and sexual infantilism, webbing of neck and redundant skin of neck, cubitus valgus, coarctation of aorta, excessive pigmented nevi, hearing and renal anomalies	MR in approx. 10%, mean IQ = 95
Williams		Prominent lips and mouth, anteverted nares, dysphonia	Supravalvular aortic stenosis, mild neurological features	

UDTs = undescended testicles

be present at birth or its appearance may be delayed for a period of weeks or even months and since it is frequently associated with mental retardation and cerebral palsy, its early recognition is important.

In some syndromes the diagnosis is made as a result of the routine biochemical screening of newborn infants whether they appear to be normal or not. Children suffering from phenylketonuria, homocystinuria, galactosemia and maple syrup urine disease may be diagnosed in this way by Guthrie testing.

In a high proportion of children suffering mental defect there is no positive family history to raise the suspicion that the child may be mentally retarded and there are no characteristic physical, biochemical or chromosomal stigmata. In these circumstances the doctor suspects mental retardation on the basis of the history he obtains, the observations he makes of the child's behavior and the physical examination. The types of history which give rise to a suspicion that mental retardation may be present have already been described. There may be a history of mental retardation in other relatives or of the mother having had an excess of stillbirths and infant deaths amongst her offspring. Pregnancy, labor and delivery may have been abnormal or have been followed by an abnormal neonatal course. The child may have been delivered prematurely or have been asphyxiated at birth. He may have behaved as if 'birth injured', showing a picture of undue apathy, hypotonia and difficulty in feeding or of extensor hypertonus with jitteriness. There may have been convulsions, especially in the first 48 hours with temperature instability and apneic attacks. If any of these manifestations have been observed it is likely that the baby will be included in a long-term follow-up program by the maternity hospital.

In many cases the doctor has to rely upon his history taking and examination first to suspect and then to confirm the presence of mental defect. Fifteen percent or more of children later found to be mentally retarded have a history of normal motor development although almost invariably the milestones of speech, adaptive and social behavior have been reached late. A suspicion of mental defect will be further reinforced by finding abnormalities which are commonly associated with mental defect. These include convulsions, an infant who is 'too good', sleeps a lot and does not waken for feeds, reversal of the sleep pattern, difficulties in feeding, asymmetries of movement observed by the parents or suspicions that the child may have defects of vision or hearing.

After the first year the child may present with delay in achieving the normal milestones of development. Speech development is a good guide to intellectual maturation and in any child with slow language development who is not deaf there is a possibility of mental retardation. Psychological assessment must form part of the investigation of all language-disturbed children.

In the latter, high tone deafness, central deafness and autism have also to be considered and the differentiation between these and mental defects may be difficult. A proportion of children, especially those in the subcultural group, may first be diagnosed because of failure to learn at school and a small percentage present at a later stage before the courts with delinquency.

Examination

In the course of his examination the doctor first confirms the parents' account of the child's motor, linguistic, adaptive and social development and then proceeds to a careful examination of the baby, including assessment of his hearing and vision and detailed neurological study. He may find that there is clinical evidence of neurological conditions often associated with mental defect such as cerebral palsy, an early hydrocephalus, squints, bulbar palsy, etc. Certain findings may help to pinpoint the diagnosis, such as abnormal eye signs, hepatosplenomegaly or associated congenital heart disease. It should be remembered that the classic syndromes of cerebral palsy only emerge gradually and that for many months children who will later manifest the typical clinical picture of cerebral palsy show only slowness in reaching their milestones of motor development and often also their milestone of adaptive and social development. In dyskinetic cerebral palsy, for example (see p. 753), there is frequently a latent period during which the child superficially appears to be normal for 2–3 months. Following this, the doctor will find not the involuntary movements and tension so characteristic later of the child suffering from dyskinesia, but merely delayed motor development and possibly persistence of primitive reflexes (e.g. Moro and grasp) which should have disappeared.

In the majority of infants with retarded development, however, no other specific abnormalities are found and the presumptive diagnosis must be one of mental retardation unless evidence of severe systemic disease or gross environmental neglect in early infancy can be shown to have been present.

Height and weight

Growth generally is under hormonal control but innervation is also essential for normal growth (e.g. dwarfing of a hemiplegic limb). The profound effects on growth which neurological disturbance can have are seen also in gigantism, acromegaly, cerebral gigantism, the diencephalic syndrome, anorexia nervosa and pituitary dwarfism. Growth of mental defectives is thought to be at a slower rate than normal and to continue for a longer period. The symphysis to heel height is lower the lower the IQ. In most cases mentally defective children have a later onset of puberty. A large number of the syndromes of mental retardation are associated with dwarfism and this may present at birth when the infant appears small for dates. Mongolism, Turner's syndrome, the Prader–Willi syndrome, the Rubinstein–Taybi syndrome, Amsterdam dwarfs, cretins, bird-headed dwarfs and Cockayne's syndrome are all of short stature as part of the syndrome. The child with subcultural handicap may also be small due to 'deprivation dwarfism'.

Head size

This is measured as occipitofrontal circumference but this does not always reflect cranial volume. Tables of normals with the two standard deviation upper and lower limits are essential for the population being studied. The head grows to accommodate the brain except in craniostenosis; if the skull is small then microcephaly is found. A large head is not synonymous with hydrocephalus and may be due to megalencephaly, subdural hematoma or other space-occupying lesions. Megalencephaly may be due to storage disorders such as GM1 gangliosidosis, Sandhoff's disease, Tay–Sachs disease, Canavan's disease and astrocytic abnormalities, e.g. Alexander's disease or von Recklinghausen's disease. Equally hydrocephalus need not be associated with an increased head size. Enlarged ventricles may be evident on CT or ultrasound scanning in a head of normal size and even microcephaly can coexist with hydrocephalus, carrying a bad prognosis. Most cases of megalencephaly of the familial type associated with the neurodermatoses are mentally retarded. In most cases microcephaly is a significant finding in suspected mental retardation but 10% of people with significant microcephaly have a normal IQ. The most important finding is a head circumference which on serial measurement falls away from its percentile. In malnutrition in the first 6 months of life brain growth may be affected and a degree of microcephaly result. After this period there is brain sparing and so comparisons of height, weight and occipitofrontal circumference may be useful in detecting the relative roles of malnutrition, dwarfism or cerebral causes for growth failure.

Minor dysmorphic stigmata

If any group of mentally subnormal children is examined a high proportion are found to have minor abnormalities which do not add up to any definite syndrome. They do suggest that the cause of the subnormality is either genetic or due to abnormalities in early pregnancy rather than abnormalities at the time of birth or in the neonatal period. These stigmata include such findings as hypertelorism (telecanthus), epicanthic folds, abnormal palmar creases, double hair whorls, low-set ears, abnormal pinna of the ear or syndactyly. These must be differentiated from acquired lesions such as a flat occiput or plagiocephaly due to immobility after birth (see p. 21).

It is particularly in the face that these stigmata may be evident so that many disorders in which mental defect is a major component have characteristic facies. Other stigmata may be evident in eyes, heart and liver (Table 14.89).

BEHAVIOR IN MENTAL HANDICAP

The learning difficulties of a mentally handicapped child can usually be accepted by the parents. It is behavior abnormalities

which cause more distress. Children with organic brain dysfunction have a high incidence of psychological disturbance. About 50% of mentally handicapped children have a psychological disturbance (Table 14.90). The factors which underlie these disorders are the mental retardation itself, brain damage where it has occurred and maladjusted behavior due to environmental factors in someone who is psychologically vulnerable. The mentally handicapped child has a poor attention span and his imagination is limited or slow in developing. He has difficulty, especially if severely mentally handicapped, in understanding his environment because of his communication difficulties. Parents frequently bring to parent–baby interactions a negative set of expectations as to the communicative competence of developmentally disabled or 'at-risk' infants, a proposition most clearly supported in respect of premature infants (Stern & Hildebrandt 1986). Developmentally disabled infants create problems for adults attempting to communicate with them by their passivity and their unpredictability, as well as their sometimes unattractive appearance; these behaviors make it difficult for parents and other adults to 'read' their infants' communications. Parents particularly then strive, sometimes too hard, to obtain optimum levels of behavior from their infants, resulting in intrusiveness and withdrawal by the child. The child himself feels that his intentions are not noticed and, because of lack of effectiveness, becomes increasingly helpless. Lastly, it is proposed that 'learned' helplessness further exacerbates infants' inappropriate or bizarre attempts at sociocommunicative behaviors and leads the parents to feel helpless too.

It is now considered that many of the socially unacceptable behaviors typical of the severely mentally handicapped and autistic children have communicative intentions underlying them and that many of the tantrums and mannerisms exhibited by the mentally handicapped are primitive, clumsy, failed attempts to communicate. The result is a vicious circle of 'learned' helplessness and increased useless mannerisms – rocking, rolling things between their fingers, running on tiptoes, touching objects, choreoathetoid movements of the hands, persistent hand regard, flicking shoelaces. These behaviors are more common in 'institutionalized' environments. Removing such behaviors requires skilled psychological help and markedly different approaches from those applied in institutions in the past.

The most distressing behaviors are severe aggression and self-mutilation. Some, such as the self-mutilation of Lesch–Nyhan syndrome, are probably organically based but the condition is so widespread that it is most profitably viewed as a failed sociocommunicative action. The child may bite his lips and his hands and cause profuse bleeding and head banging may even cause subdural hematomas and further brain damage. These painful, compulsive acts are not generally attention seeking and the child is relieved and prevented from injuring himself by restraint. Time out and seclusion generally worsen the condition.

PERVASIVE DEVELOPMENTAL DISORDERS

The imprecision of the terms 'autism' and 'childhood psychosis' has led the compilers of the DSM III to introduce the diagnostic category 'pervasive developmental disorders' to describe children in whom multiple distortions of development have occurred. In the DSM III distinction is made between pervasive developmental disorders (PDD) and specific developmental disorders (e.g. the

Table 14.89 Minor dysmorphic stigmata associated with mental defect

Characteristic facies
1. Mongolism
2. 17/18 trisomy
3. Amsterdam dwarfs
4. Hunter–Hurler syndrome
5. Cretinism
6. Hypercalcemia
7. Hydrocephalus
8. Craniostenosis, craniofacial dysostosis
9. Apert's syndrome
10. Bird-headed dwarfs (Seckel)
11. Sturge–Weber syndrome
12. Tuberous sclerosis
13. Homocystinuria
14. Phenylketonuria
15. Smith–Lemli–Opitz syndrome
16. Sotos syndrome
17. Happy puppet syndrome
18. Cockayne's syndrome

Eye defects
Cataracts
1. Rubella
2. Lowe's syndrome
3. Galactosemia
4. Hypoparathyroidism
5. Dystrophia myotonica
6. Marinesco–Sjögren syndrome
7. Infants of PKU mothers
8. Mongolism
9. 13/15 trisomy
10. Cretinism
11. Diabetes
12. Werner's syndrome
13. Incontinentia pigmenti
14. Cerebrotendinous xanthomatosis

Retinopathy
1. Rubella
2. Toxoplasmosis
3. Retinitis pigmentosa
    a. Refsum's syndrome
    b. Juvenile amaurotic idiocy (Batten's disease)
    c. Laurence–Biedl–Moon syndrome
    d. A-β-lipoproteinemia
    e. Spastic paraplegia
    f. Familial
    g. San Filippo mucopolysaccharidosis

h. A mixed group of basal ganglia degeneration, ophthalmoplegia, ataxia and muscular atrophy in individual families
    i. Hyperpipecolic acidemia
4. Phakomata of neurodermatoses
5. Associated with colobomata, e.g. Aicardi syndrome

Other eye defects
1. Dislocation of lens in Marfan's syndrome and homocystinuria
2. Telangiectasia of the conjunctiva in Sturge–Weber and ataxia telangiectasia
3. Buphthalmos or glaucoma in neurofibromatosis and Sturge–Weber syndrome
4. Corneal changes in Fabry's disease and gargoylism
5. Anophthalmia or microphthalmia in 13/15 trisomy, microphthalmia in congenital rubella syndrome
6. Brushfield spots in mongolism

Congenital heart disease
1. Mongolism
2. 13/15 trisomy
3. 17/18 trisomy
4. Congenital rubella
5. Hypercalcemia
6. Amsterdam dwarfs
7. Turner's syndrome
8. Myocardium involved in mucopolysaccharidoses
9. Myocardium infiltrated in glycogenoses
10. Tumors in tuberous sclerosis
11. Fetal alcohol syndrome

Hepatosplenomegaly
1. Glycogenoses (types 1 and 3)
2. Mucopolysaccharidoses
3. Galactosemia
4. Congenital rubella
5. Cytomegalovirus infection
6. Toxoplasmosis
7. GM1 gangliosidosis
8. Niemann–Pick disease
9. Argininosuccinic aminoaciduria
10. Gaucher's disease
11. Lactosyl ceramidosis

Associated neurological damage
1. Cerebral palsy
2. Epilepsy

Others
1. Dermatoglyphics
2. Hair whorls

Table 14.90 Psychiatric disorders in Camberwell children with severe mental retardation ($n = 140$) (Corbett 1979)

Adjustment reaction	6%
Conduct disorder	4%
Neurotic disorder	4%
Isolated habit disorders	2%
Severe stereotypes and pica occurring in isolation	10%
Hyperkinetic behavior disorder	4%
Childhood psychosis	17%
No additional psychiatric disorder	53%

Reprinted from James F E , Snaith R P (eds) 1979 Psychiatric illness and mental handicap. The Royal College of Psychiatrists.

developmental language disorders). Subdivisions of pervasive developmental disorder include infantile autism (IA) where gross abnormalities of speech, language and relationships occur in the first 30 months of life (Table 14.91), atypical pervasive developmental disorder (Table 14.92) which does not meet all the criteria of autism but occurs in the first 30 months and childhood onset of pervasive developmental disorders (COPDD) which may meet the criteria but occurs later.

Recently the American Psychiatric Association published a revised third edition of the DSM which notes that the age of onset differentiating infantile autism from other PDDs is not valid and we now have 'autistic disorder' embracing IA and COPPD and a category of 'atypical cases – pervasive developmental disorder not otherwise specific' (PDDNOS). The known etiologies of PDDs include prematurity, multiple congenital anomalies, phenylketonuria, congenital rubella, fragile X syndrome, meningitis, infantile spasms, tuberous sclerosis, neurofibromatosis, Albright's hereditary osteodystrophy, agenesis of the corpus callosum, Pfeiffer's syndrome and various degenerative illnesses. Wing & Gould's (1979) classification of childhood psychosis is based on a degree of social impairment found on clinical examination independent of the history of the child. They identify three groups:

Table 14.91 DSM III diagnostic criteria for infantile autism

A. Onset before 30 months of age

B. Pervasive lack of responsiveness to other people (autism)

C. Gross deficits in language development

D. If speech is present, peculiar speech patterns such as immediate and delayed echolalia, metaphorical language, pronominal reversal

E. Bizarre responses to various aspects of the environment, e.g. resistance to change, peculiar interest in or attachments to animate or inanimate objects

F. Absence of delusions, hallucinations, loosening of associations, and incoherence as in schizophrenia

Reproduced with the permission of the Journal of Mental Deficiency Research.

Table 14.92 DSM III diagnostic criteria for childhood onset and atypical pervasive developmental disorder

A. Gross and sustained impairment in social relationships, e.g. lack of appropriate affective responsivity, inappropriate clinging, associality, lack of empathy

B. At least three of the following:
1. Sudden excessive anxiety manifested by such symptoms as free-floating anxiety, catastrophic reactions to everyday occurrences, inability to be consoled when upset, unexplained panic attacks
2. Constricted or inappropriate affect, including lack of appropriate fear reactions, unexplained rage reactions and extreme mood lability
3. Resistance to change in the environment (e.g. upset if dinner time is changed), or insistence on doing things in the same manner every time (e.g. putting on clothes always in the same order)
4. Oddities of motor movements, such as peculiar posturing, peculiar hand or finger movements, or walking on tiptoe
5. Abnormalities of speech, such as question-like melody, monotonous voice
6. Hyper- or hyposensitivity to sensory stimuli, e.g. hyperacusis
7. Self-mutilation, e.g. biting or hitting self, head banging

C. Onset of the full syndrome after 30 months of age and before 12 years of age

D. Absence of delusions, hallucinations, incoherence or marked loosening of associations

Atypical pervasive developmental disorder in these studies defined patients who had symptoms before 30 months of age but did not meet criteria for autism. Since symptom onset before 30 months of age excludes a diagnosis of childhood onset the atypical category was utilized.
Reproduced with the permission of the Journal of Mental Deficiency Research.

1. infantile psychosis – the commonest group;
2. disintegrative psychosis – a rare group where abnormalities usually begin after the age of 3;
3. childhood schizophrenia where the child – usually of school age – starts to develop signs of adult schizophrenia, e.g. delusions and hallucinations.

Positive prognostic features in children with pervasive developmental disorders include the presence of useful speech before the age of 5 years and Gilles de la Tourette syndrome.

LANGUAGE AND THE MENTALLY HANDICAPPED CHILD

Not all mentally handicapped children have a behavior disorder but no mentally handicapped child can have normal language function. Language is the most fundamental aspect of cognitive learning. Language is used by most people as the system of symbols by which information is coded, stored and categorized within the brain. It is not therefore the same as speech. The child may have very impaired language function and yet speak at a simple level, as seen with echolalia, or at a more sophisticated level, as seen in the reciting of nursery rhymes or the parroting of the whole of previously heard conversations as in the 'cocktail party' syndrome. The mentally handicapped child may have a good memory for an object or picture and its name and so may appear to score quite well on passive vocabulary tests as in the Peabody picture vocabulary or the picture vocabulary of the Stanford–Binet test. On the other hand vocabulary as tested by asking the child to define a word, such as 'What is an orange?', will be poor. When tested on language comprehension, as with the Reynell tests, he will also score poorly. Because he cannot classify information he is unable to develop concepts such as time, space, texture, size, weight, etc. He may be able to identify several animals by name but will not be able to grasp that they were all animals (or kitchen utensils or clothes, etc.). Since he cannot categorize and bring back related previous experiences from memory stores which are relevant to thought at that moment, he cannot reason. The language disorder therefore shows as a disorder of concept formation, reasoning and imagination and therefore also of the ability of the child to understand the world around him and to play in it. Speech may be affected by delay in development, as in the developmental speech disorder syndrome (p. 805). Dysarthria will result if there is any neurological impairment of bulbar function.

Syntax is usually primitive with telegrammatic speech for a prolonged period and of simple grammatical structure. The mean length of sentence will be shorter than in children of similar age. The very severely mentally handicapped child with no understanding of any words, i.e. with a complete word deafness or auditory agnosia, may nevertheless show a sensitivity to intonation of the voice and this together with other forms of nonverbal communication such as facial expression is very important. Elaborate attempts to 'teach' language and condition learning may inadvertently abolish the very cues necessary for the child's limited understanding, hence the importance of the mother as a teacher rather than the structured group.

Language

Most medical practitioners are criticized for their faltering attempts to communicate with mentally handicapped people of all grades of intelligence and are also bewildered when they fail to achieve rapport with the parents of mentally handicapped children. Communicating with the mentally handicapped is detailed elsewhere (McLean et al 1987, Fraser et al 1990) but good practice for talking to the mildly/moderately handicapped includes the following maxims:

1. Cue them by name; insure that the handicapped person is looking (if they are not looking, they are not likely to be listening).
2. Use simple grammatical constructions and short precise input.
3. Use consistent words or labels, e.g. one word for toilet.
4. Use other channels of communication; as well as speech, gestures should be employed clearly, even flamboyantly.
5. Give the handicapped person time to answer.
6. Make the interaction interesting and enjoyable for the handicapped child.
7. The onus is on you to insure you are understood.

In the case of the more severely handicapped, often without speech, firstly the clinician should either understand basic Makaton (a signing system derived from British sign language) or be accompanied by a colleague, e.g. speech therapist, who can signal to the handicapped person in Makaton or other effective signing system. The clinician should assume that the profoundly handicapped person is trying to mean something by his strange noises, gestures, etc., i.e. the clinician should assume *intentionality*. The handicapped person's behavior should be the starting point of the communication and the clinician should scrutinize the patient's vocalizations and movements to see if they mean something (pain, distress, etc.). Communication with the profoundly handicapped is more thoroughly documented in McLean et al (1987). With the more profoundly handicapped the clinician's interaction cannot be quite so goal orientated (to get answers to questions) and must be much more interaction orientated (simply creating a setting in which some intentions of the handicapped person may be discerned). It is noteworthy here that the most recent fashionable philosophies of normalization, e.g. Wolfensberger's (1983) that the mentally handicapped person ought to be treated as if he were a normal person of equivalent chronological age, are not feasible and the original normalization philosophy of Nirje (1969), that the mentally handicapped person should be treated as normally as possible within the limitations of his handicaps, is much more sensible, i.e. one should communicate with the person at his obvious mental age rather than follow some sociophilosophical concept of dignity by addressing him at his chronological age equivalent.

SCREENING FOR MENTAL RETARDATION

The very large number of comparatively rare causes of mental retardation means that to exclude every one requires a vast array of biochemical, radiological and microbiological tests. Any condition with therapeutic possibilities must be included in the schedule of investigation, but it is impossible to test for every known inborn error of metabolism. Examples are given in Table 14.93.

Urine tests

Many ward urine tests have also been traditionally performed on children with mental retardation.

Reducing substances in the urine

By Clinitest – if positive, a full sugar chromatogram is needed.

Cyanide nitroprusside test

This is used primarily for the detection of homocystinuria. It is a test for sulfhydryl groups and so may be positive in cystinuria, Fanconi's syndrome and Wilson's disease.

Ehrlich's aldehyde test

1 ml of Ehrlich's reagent is added to 5.0 ml of fresh urine and examined after 10 min. A pink color is found with porphyrobilinogen or urobilinogen and the urobilinogen can be extracted by shaking with chloroform. Indoles, as in Hartnup disease, may also give a positive reaction.

Table 14.93 Tests used in children with mental retardation

Neurophysiology
Electroencephalogram
Electroretinogram and visual evoked potentials
Brainstem auditory evoked potentials
Nerve conduction studies

Imaging
Ultrasound
MRI
CT
Bone age

Cytogenetic
Chromosome analysis
Specific DNA test for fragile X

Serology
Toxoplasmosis
Cytomegalovirus
Herpes
Chickenpox
AIDS
Syphilis
Rubella

Metabolic study
Plasma and urinary amino acids
Urinary organic acids
Ammonia
Lactate
Lead
Uric acid
Copper
Very long chain fatty acids
Calcium, phosphate, alkaline phosphatase
Creatine phosphokinase

Endocrine
Thyroid hormone and TSH

In selected difficult cases
Peroxysomal enzymes
Lysosomal enzymes
Mucopolysaccharides
Specific mitochondrial
DNA tests

Tests for mucopolysaccharides

There are two side-room tests available – the CTAB test (cetyltrimethyl ammonium bromide) and the toluidine blue test. For the CTAB test six drops of CTAB reagent are added to 1.0 ml of urine: a cloudy flocculent precipitate is a positive reaction and is seen in all the mucopolysaccharidoses except the Morquio type. In the toluidine blue test 5, 10 and 25 ml of urine are spotted on to a Whatman number 1 filter paper. The paper is then dipped into 0.04% aqueous toluidine blue solution for 1 min and then rinsed in 95% ethanol: a purple spot against a pale blue background is positive; a spot of known concentration of chondroitin sulfate should be added for comparison. Infants in the first week of life may give a false positive.

MANAGEMENT OF THE MENTALLY HANDICAPPED CHILD

In the past 30 years there has been a change in society's view of the mentally handicapped. In most countries there is general acceptance that the care of the mentally handicapped should no longer be regarded as the sole responsibility of one discipline and that the institutionalization of mentally handicapped children on the grounds of mental handicap alone is unacceptable. The use of ordinary environments, living at home and ordinary services wherever possible is encompassed in the normalization philosophy which entails minimizing the effect of handicap and maximizing the similarities to other people. It means more than that – central to the idea of normalization is that the mentally handicapped person is regarded as a respected and valued member of the community in which he lives.

The problems with this very reasonable idea include:

1. overzealous ignoring of special needs;
2. a fashion, especially prevalent in the 1970s, of vilifying all professionals who work in institutions, whatever their concern for personalized care;
3. unfeeling pressure on parents, whatever their resources, to undertake forms of home training whose value has often been unsubstantiated or to participate intensely in the construction of community support services.

The balance has now, fortunately, been regained and almost all professionals regard their relationship with parents as that of partnership.

There are four basic principles which apply to the management of all types of handicap, including mental handicap and these are in strict order:

1. relieve the anxiety and stress of the handicap, i.e. the demoralizing effect of failure;
2. seek a way to circumvent the handicap;
3. encourage development in areas least affected by the handicap;
4. try to produce a therapeutic program which *may* help to reduce the handicap.

No one would expect that attending a 'blind school' could enable a blind child to develop normal vision and yet we expect the physiotherapist to make the spastic child walk and the teacher to enable a mentally handicapped child to speak, read and write. The purpose of a multidisciplinary assessment team is to find the areas in which the child experiences least difficulty so that he can achieve success, rather than pinpoint and emphasize his weaknesses till he has completely lost motivation to learn by other means. The spastic child, for example, needs to try to achieve mobility by whatever means are open to him, not to spend hours every day with a physiotherapist on exercises which will never overcome the direct effects of his atrophied internal capsule. The mentally retarded child has a cognitive learning defect and if we try to develop language by sitting him in a group and showing him objects and repeating the name he will have a concentration span of only seconds and may merely revert to stereotypes. His area of least handicap is in gross motor activities and if he is placed in a swimming pool, in a gymnasium or on horseback then when he is relaxed and succeeding we will get far more spontaneous speech than in the formal setting. It is therefore a paradox that the physiotherapist probably has more part to play with the mentally handicapped than the spastic child. There is no reason why many mentally handicapped children should not be first rate swimmers, athletes, gymnasts or riders.

Circumvention of the handicap means that if the child cannot read then read to him, if he cannot tie shoe laces give him slip-on shoes, if he cannot walk then let him get in a wheelchair and learn to do wheelchair dancing, wheelchair basketball, racing, etc. rather than struggle between parallel bars with long leg calipers. In the past we put our treatment in the reverse order and we practiced the handicap so that if the child could not speak he had articulation exercises by a speech therapist, if he could not walk he had daily physiotherapy, if he could not read he had remedial reading and if he had visuospatial difficulties, he had a Frostig program. The evidence that any one of these therapies is successful is difficult to find. A remedial program should certainly be planned for the child but not so that it interferes with learning and motivation in other areas or produces secondary behavior disturbances. Failure is bad for child, parent and therapist and a happy child living as normal a life as possible within the range of his abilities and overcoming his handicap should be our aim.

In addition to gross motor skills, the mentally handicapped child can learn by conditioning (rote learning) and so toilet training, bathing, feeding and table manners can all be taught, i.e. personal and social independence skills. The best therapist is the child's mother. The mentally handicapped child learns more by sitting on his mother's knee with her speaking to him in normal everyday English rather than in a structured language group with a teacher using simple English with repetition and reinforcement.

The mother should not get conflicting advice from general practitioner, hospital specialist, health visitor, psychologist, social worker, physiotherapist, speech therapist, occupational therapist, nursery nurse and teacher.

Services for mentally handicapped children

The pediatrician should insure that certain broad objectives are being met in the area that his practice serves.

1. That there is a form of register or identification of children with mental handicap.
2. That there are basic support services.
3. That there is an infrastructure for coordinating service delivery.
4. That there is a staff development strategy to prepare staff to work in the services.

Early counseling should be available from community mental handicap nurses working with the area mental handicap team – the pediatrician, psychologist, psychiatrist and social worker. The success of this depends on the accumulation of knowledge on practical baby care, child development and practical ways in which a mother can cope with a mentally handicapped child's behavior and feeding, toilet training, etc. A specialist social worker post with a brief to provide counseling advice and information to families of children with a handicap is invaluable. Alternative family placements ought to be available where families are no longer able to offer children a home. Respite care should be immediately available to families to provide children with a flexible service using a range of facilities from ordinary homes to hospital facilities which would extend children's horizons and keep them in touch wherever possible with nonhandicapped peers. Support is necessary for families and other informal carers in their own homes with specialized babysitters, specialized home help schemes, home–school liaison, preparation for adult services for children with behavioral problems and preparation for adulthood schemes (which, for example, would consist of an ordinary three-bedroomed staffed house to increase independence).

The family

Parents are often realistic about developmental retardation but very resistant to the idea of mental retardation and may refuse to accept the diagnosis when it is made. The period of denial can last for many months or years before it is replaced by the reactions described below.

There are three times when parents may be told that their child is not normal. First, during the first few days after birth when the child is born with obvious congenital abnormalities. This, if we could choose, would be the worst possible time to impart bad news. Parents, however, want to know as soon as the facts are known. Second, a diagnosis of increasing suspicion, where the handicap is gradually evolving during early childhood, the child is not reaching his milestones and gradually it becomes apparent that he is mentally retarded. Sometimes, to spare the parents anxiety, the diagnosis is withheld until certain. Parents insist again they would prefer to be involved from the moment the pediatrician suggests all is not normal. The third typical time is after an illness such as encephalitis or an accident in childhood. The child is likely to have been admitted to an intensive treatment unit seriously ill and parents are faced no longer with the prospect of their child's death but an unpredictable developmental future.

A bereavement response is necessary in coming to terms with the loss of significant objects or persons. In mental handicap the bereavement response is modified. After the stage of *shock* and emotional paralysis, *panic and rejection* may occur which, after the initial period of weeping and sadness, sleeplessness and agitation, are directed inwardly as *guilt* or outwardly as *anger*. Anger is particularly likely to be directed against professionals – 'Why didn't my doctor suggest genetic counseling?', 'Why was I allowed to deliver the child at home?' – and by never having registered the pediatrician's explanations. A revision of memory occurs, attributing insensitivity to the pediatrician. The value of the baby may be questioned by friends and grandparents. The child may be rejected, even abandoned. *Bargaining* commonly occurs – 'I'll look after him if the authorities, nurses, etc. teach him to be clean and dry, to walk, to speak, to earn his living' and this gives way to acceptance and reality. *Acceptance* will never be reached if there is a continued shopping around attracted by the claims of fringe medicine and 'new' therapies which are springing up in ever-increasing numbers. A state of debilitating and enduring depression may pervade the entire family – the major life events for the family and the handicapped person are indicated in Table 14.94.

Pediatricians must pay heed to the concerns expressed by parents. Parents quickly sense something is wrong, even before a diagnosis is made, and may pick up negative attitudes from other parents towards their child. Parents are extremely sensitive to other people's reactions to their new baby at this stage and they particularly note any suggestion that the baby is not worth bothering about or is of little value. It is essential that professionals show the parents that they value the baby while honestly and realistically evaluating the handicapping condition. If the professional cannot feel any value in the infant it would be essential to delegate the disclosure in early interviews to someone who does.

Parents ought to be told together. They need time and privacy to talk to each other and to the staff. Many parents value the opportunity to talk again to the doctor who made the initial disclosure as they have often not been able to take in what was said. Some 60% of parents would value the opportunity early on to talk to another experienced parent. It should be clear from the initial disclosure that counseling will continue. Many parents later state that they often do not know where to get help or how to get the immediate advice and support required. When a referral is received by a particular agency, then from lack of knowledge of other services or through lack of coordination, the result may be a 'feast or famine' phenomenon, sometimes with large numbers of professional staff involved, increasing parents' anxieties, eroding their confidence and inundating the family with conflicting advice. Conversely, no service at all may be forthcoming. 'Famine' families are less common nowadays but can still occur in immigrant populations. The importance of some central referral point is crucial for management.

Long-stay provision for the profoundly mentally handicapped

Attention has been drawn to the basic needs of profoundly mentally retarded children with multiple handicaps by Hagberg et al (1988) and Minns et al (1989b). The indications are that there is a need for 10–12 beds per 300 000 of the population for this group of children. This number represents one-third of the total number of children in the population with profound mental handicap.

In an Edinburgh study of 21 profoundly and multiply handicapped children in full-time residential care, five were males and 16 female. Their ages ranged from 23 months to 17.75 years and the mean duration of residence was 5.9 years ± 2.6 years. The criteria for admission had been medical and social in all cases. Half of the families involved had been divorced and one had been divorced twice. Nineteen of the 21 children had continuing contact with their family.

The etiology in this group was acquired brain damage in 12 cases, brain malformation in seven cases and a degenerative brain disease and a mental handicap syndrome.

A detailed neurodevelopmental examination revealed that at a mean chronological age of 10.8 years the developmental postural level was 3.8 months, manipulative function 4.2 months, visual function 4.0 months and verbal communication 4.3 months. In addition, 42% were cortically or peripherally blind, 38% cortically deaf and 95% had a bulbar palsy. Their medical problems are seen in Table 14.95. Their medical problems were minor in comparison with their nursing difficulties as none of them could talk, walk, change their own position, self-feed, dress

Table 14.94 Life events for the handicapped person and their family

Diagnosis: labeling which will often remain with the handicapped person for life

Separation experiences: frequent admission for short-term care when intellectual function does not enable understanding of the temporary loss

Breaking of friendship ties: frequent and particularly in adolescence when loneliness is particularly distressing

Sexuality: emerging sexuality may be awkward for the mentally handicapped person and their family

Family death: the mentally handicapped person is commonly excluded from bereavement rituals

Moving to residential care: this must be a positive experience and not a guilt-ridden one

Table 14.95   Medical problems (after Minns et al 1989b)

1. Contractures	47%
2. Scoliosis/windswept	66%
3. N/G feeding	28%
4. Hiatal hernia	28%
5. Reflux esophagitis	33%
6. Epilepsy	76%
7. Recurrent aspirations	19%
8. Chest infections (recurrent)	14%
9. Constipation	76%
10. Growth failure (less than third centile)	52%
11. Anemia	10%

or bath. All were doubly incontinent and tetraplegic and many had intractable epilepsy. The professional contact with these children is continuous for nursing staff, daily or weekly for the physiotherapist and the various medical specialties (pediatric, mental handicap, orthopedic surgeons, etc.) and speech and occupational therapists when required. Teachers see these children daily and medical social workers have close contact with the group and their families.

Genetic counseling

Most of the genetically determined conditions associated with mental subnormality show autosomal recessive inheritance. Screening procedures in many cases are not so much to make a diagnosis for the purpose of treatment but to enable the risk to further children to be assessed and explained. If one member of the family is already suffering from a particular disease several courses of action are open to the parents. If the disorder is treatable, as with phenylketonuria or galactosemia, they may be willing to take the risk and very careful screening at birth will insure early diagnosis. Sterilization and adoption is another possible option. The risk with dominant inheritance must be stated clearly and truth should not be confused with any misguided attempt not to be too pessimistic. Two developments which have made genetic counseling more pertinent for some families have been first, improved advice on and availability of contraception and second, the possibility of antenatal diagnosis by amniocentesis and termination of an affected pregnancy.

The physician's greatest dilemma is when he is confronted with parents demanding to know the risk of other children being mentally handicapped after having one affected child who does not manifest any known syndrome. In this case the clinician cannot always even be sure that the condition is genetically determined and not due to some unidentified abnormality in early pregnancy. He may, on general grounds, guess at autosomal recessive inheritance and give a pessimistic view of a one in four chance. The fact that it is a guess must be stressed and a frank confession that the risk may be one in many hundreds and that true guidance is impossible is all that is usually possible.

Nursery

Nursery placement is essential for the retarded child so that he can experience social contact with other children of his own age and allow his mother to do her housework, shopping and see her friends. Residential care is often necessary for short periods. This shows the mother that the child is not totally dependent upon her. From the child's point of view it should also have a positive value with activities of daily living such as toilet training, washing, feeding and dressing (vital at this stage) being taught with skilled nursery care. The nursery period may be extended to 6 or 7 years of age and should start at about 2 years. The child at this stage may also be taught concepts that normal children learn readily such as time/space, self/reality, size/weight, number and color. Language stimulation is also a major role of the nursery through structured play under the guidance of a speech therapist.

Education

The ascertainment of handicap is a responsibility placed upon the local authority. Arrangements should be made for appropriate education before the child's fifth birthday. Parents can ask the local authority to examine their child for handicap after the age of 2. The Mental Health (Scotland) Act 1960 demands that the education authority report on any child coming to their notice between 2 and 5 years who is considered to be mentally retarded. The 'slow learner' poses more educational than medical problems. If there are no associated defects then walking and speech should not be a problem. The child may be slow in acquiring speech, but with a prolonged nursery placing and speech therapy this should mature in time. Readiness for reading, writing and arithmetic will be delayed and the child may not be ready for formal education in the subjects till after 7 years of age. Excess pressure should not force a child to learn before he is developmentally ready. With an enormous amount of effort and conditioning it is often possible to teach a child to read without understanding, but noncognitive learning of this type is of no value to the child. The teachers of slow learners at a normal or a special school need to be highly trained in learning theory, child development and teaching methods.

The child who is uneducable and severely retarded may not require medical or nursing help but will require special methods to impart knowledge and understanding to him. The application of learning theory to include learning on physical, social and emotional planes is of great importance. The child must be encouraged to communicate with play therapy and training the child to accomplish as much as possible to make himself sufficient in daily living is important. Independence in personal hygiene, toilet training, table manners and the ability to dress and undress will enable the child later to be managed under shelter. This has given rise to a broader view of education. Training centers are now under local education authority control and using a developmental approach, it should be possible to assess each child's needs independently with the formulation of an individual training program.

Employment

The aim of the pediatrician must be to produce an individual who is socially independent, who can keep employment and has sufficient academic achievement to be able to budget his finances. The educationally subnormal child should be able to manage this unless he is emotionally so immature and sociopathic that he cannot integrate into society. The trainable child is likely at best to achieve sheltered hostel care with some form of industrial therapy.

Medical care

The physician's role in the care of the mentally handicapped child in the community is early diagnosis, parent guidance and supervision of the child for the first few years of life. He will work in conjunction with the speech therapist, occupational therapist and physiotherapist to help with feeding problems, speech problems or associated physical handicap.

Certain specific disorders such as phenylketonuria and hypothyroidism need constant medical care though if this is successful the child should not be mentally subnormal. The services of a psychiatrist are essential in disturbed subnormal children, as well as those with autistic features.

Trivial conditions should never be disregarded as they may loom very large to the mother. Dental caries may make feeding difficult. Constipation can be troublesome because of the necessity for a semifluid diet with little roughage. Mothers should be reassured that an infrequent bowel motion does not matter. Vomiting is not uncommon and may be associated with hiatus hernia.

Management of behavior disorders in mentally handicapped children

If the child is in a normal happy, secure and stable home he is less likely to have behavior abnormalities and crises than if he is in a poor quality home or institution. Many mentally retarded children have never learned how to behave and have never had any guidelines drawn so they can find themselves in mental deficiency hospitals because of poor social circumstances and inadequate parents. A poor quality environment may lead to long periods of sensory deprivation with resultant deterioration and the development of delinquent behavior.

Modern methods of behavior modification using methods of reinforcing desirable behavior (positive reinforcement) may for the first time offer guidelines to some of these children as to what is socially acceptable behavior. Positive reinforcement can be used to suppress violence, swearing, bad manners or antisocial acts and the results are good. To get the child to learn activities of daily living the best punishment or reward is the natural one of praise or disapproval of the mother. Although restraint is a thing of the past, some form of light elbow splint with pastazoate and Velcro which can be quickly applied may be necessary in self-mutilation syndromes. It may produce relaxation and not anxiety in the child.

Drugs play only a small role in the management of the mentally handicapped child. Anticonvulsants are necessary to control seizures but the effect of phenobarbitone in aggravating hyperkinesis should be remembered.

Hyperkinetic behavior should be regarded as indicating possible epilepsy or emotional vulnerability. The child usually does best with a stereotyped and ritualistic structured timetable. Rage reactions can have bad effects on staff and other children but parents and house staff should be warned that coercion measures will not help the child. If the child has an attack of catastrophic rage, the drug of choice is 1–5 mg of intravenous haloperidol. If haloperidol is continued it carries a high risk of extrapyramidal side-effects and should be combined with benzhexol (Artane) (2–4 mg/day in divided doses). In milder cases when overactivity, rather than rage reactions, is the main problem, amphetamine or methylphenidate may be tried (5–30 mg in early morning). In psychotic behavior or with hyperkinesis not associated with epilepsy, phenothiazines may be used.

The low serum concentrations of 5-HT in Down syndrome have been increased with antidepressant therapy. This lessens the hypotonia but does not influence the mental subnormality and may cause infantile spasms.

Future problems

Although better understanding of etiology, earlier recognition and improved treatment of diseases causing mental retardation is likely to continue, the most difficult problems raised are of a social and moral character. If the mentally subnormal person is freed from custodial care in hospital he or she may be more likely to marry and the question of long-term contraception or sterilization must be raised if the subnormality is from a heritable disease.

PREVENTION OF MENTAL HANDICAP

With advances in pediatrics and obstetrics over the past few years the possibility of preventing some mental handicap has become a practical reality. Genetic counseling has become more relevant in that reliable methods of contraception are available. Antenatal diagnosis of chromosome abnormalities is possible when there is known to be a recurrent risk as with certain translocations. In order to prevent Down syndrome, amniocentesis can be offered to all mothers over 35–40 years of age. There are a large number of metabolic diseases such as lipidoses, aminoacidopathies, mucopolysaccharidoses, etc. which, if there is an index case in the family, carry a definite risk within the particular marriage. Amniocentesis may enable diagnosis in the first trimester. Termination in pregnancy may be sought in cases of sex-linked recessive diseases (muscular dystrophy, Fabry's disease, Menkes' syndrome, Lowe's syndrome, Lesch–Nyhan, Pelizaeus–Merzbacher, etc.) when the fetus has been shown by amniocentesis to be male. In a similar way α-fetoprotein examination of liquor from amniocentesis (following screening of maternal blood) enables certain major CNS malformations (e.g. open spina bifida) to be diagnosed in families at risk.

The avoidance of drugs during pregnancy, not smoking, only social drinking, avoidance of X-radiation and adequate nutrition will all contribute in part to lessening the risk of handicap. In Scotland the perinatal mortality may range from nine to 40 per 1000 in areas of good and bad social conditions. The premature infant, who is at greater risk of mental handicap, is more likely to come from a lower social class. Serious morbidity of infants weighing less than 2000 g at birth has fallen dramatically with the advent of neonatal intensive care units. Modern obstetric care has reduced by half the incidence of asphyxia and birth trauma has dramatically lessened.

The use of exchange transfusion and more recently the rhesus immunization program and phototherapy have virtually abolished kernicterus. Routine rubella immunization has prevented further serious pandemics. The possibility of a vaccine for cytomegalovirus is being explored. Routine screening by the Guthrie test has been extremely successful in the early detection of phenylketonuria with treatment before brain damage has occurred. The other metabolic diseases tested for by the Guthrie test are less impressive in numbers but are important. Screening for hypothyroidism is important to prevent mental handicap, as long-term follow-up studies suggest that cretins do not fare well. Certain diseases in the mother, such as phenylketonuria, can result in all her children being mentally handicapped and this is preventable by diet during pregnancy.

Following birth the most important preventive measure is to reduce the number of accidents to children (e.g. road traffic accidents and the battered baby). Meningitis must be diagnosed early and arguments over antibiotic regimes are less important than continually stressing that children do still have acute illnesses and failure to see the child until the next morning may mean permanent mental handicap. The same applies to status epilepticus in which there appears to be a disturbing increase in the number of children permanently brain damaged from poorly controlled status. Primary care physicians must treat status epilepticus as an emergency (even in the middle of a busy surgery). The possibility of children's hospitals developing either open casualty departments or 'fit flying squads' will need to be considered.

Recent changes in infant feeding regimes and the recent increase in breast feeding will both reduce hyperosmolar dehydration. Lead poisoning, although not a major problem in the UK, represents a completely preventable cause of mental handicap.

It is unfortunate that children in whom mental handicap has been prevented do not stand out in the community and so the really beneficial effects of modern obstetrics and pediatrics are difficult to count compared with the failures. What has been achieved with the organic type of mental handicap is in no way matched in the larger group of subculturally handicapped children.

THE ATTAINMENT OF ADULTHOOD

The laudable objective of care in the community of all mentally handicapped children and adults who do not require continuous nursing care raises as many questions as it answers. The costs of care in the community have not yet been addressed though health economists have stated that the NHS can never afford 'Rolls Royce' care in the community (Maynard 1986). However, with the exception of those who have severe behavior disturbance and a tiny minority of the profoundly handicapped, it is a practical and not overwhelmingly expensive solution, given adequate support from the health services. The parents of mentally handicapped children are very aware of the uncertainties about where their children will live when they are too old to look after them and whether the service promised by social services will be sustainable. The traditional mental deficiency hospitals are planned, with few exceptions, to close within the next 5–10 years.

Who will take over the medical care from the pediatrician when the child becomes an adult? It is quite common in many European states for the pediatrician just to continue indefinitely as the mentally handicapped person's general physician. For the profoundly and multiply handicapped adult this approach has some attractions – no other type of specialist is better equipped to oversee the handicapped person's medical needs. As the profoundly handicapped person gets older and presents the social and behavioral problems not only of adolescence but also of mid-life, the pediatrician's interest, competence and suitability must come into question.

In the UK the specialist medical care of the profoundly mentally handicapped adult is largely nonexistent. There is no formal training or career structure for 'adult developmental disability' and unless there is an enthusiastic general practitioner, neurologist or community medical officer with a special interest, the consultant psychiatrist in mental handicap has to fill the gap. The evolution of the psychiatry of mental handicap as a subspecialty of psychiatry has been at the price of the demise of the specialist in mental deficiency. The medical care of the mentally handicapped adult in the community (no longer in the care of their parents) presents considerable problems for the health service. It is hoped that the UK will follow examples such as New South Wales where health promotion and maintenance clinics for the adult developmentally disabled have been set up (Beange & Bauman 1990).

REFERENCES

Alberts B, Bray D, Lewis J, Raff M, Roberts K, Watson J D 1989 The cell. Garland, New York

Aicardi J 1992 Mental retardation. In: Diseases of the nervous system in childhood. Clinics in developmental medicine no 115/118, 25. MacKeith Press, London, pp 1286–1294

Aicardi J 1994 Epilepsy in children, 2nd edn. Raven Press, New York, pp 381–394

American Psychiatric Association 1987 Diagnostic and statistical manual of mental disorders. Revision. American Psychiatric Association,Washington DC

Aoki N, Masuzawa H 1986 Subdural haematomas in abused children: report of six cases from Japan. Neurosurgery 18: 475–477

Appleton R, Sweeney A, Choonara I, Robson J, Molyneux J 1995 Lorazepam versus diazepam in the acute treatment of epileptic seizures and status epilepticus. Developmental Mental Medicine and Child Neurology 37: 682–688

Armstrong R W, Steinbok P, Farrell K, Cochrane D, Norman M G, Kube S 1992 Continuous intrathecal baclofen treatment of severe spasms in two children with spinal cord injury. Developmental Medicine and Child Neurology 34: 731–738

Avital A, Maayan C, Goitein K J 1982 Incidence of convulsions and encephalopathy in childhood Shigella infections: survey of 117 hospitalized patients. Clinical Pediatrics 21: 645–648

Banatvala J E 1987 Measles must go and with it rubella. British Medical Journal 295: 2–3

Baron-Cohen S, Allen J, Gillberg C 1992 Can autism be detected at 18 months? British Journal of Psychiatry 161: 839–843

Barry J A, Cotter M A, Cameron N E, Patullo M C 1994 The effect of immobilisation on the recovery of rabbit soleus muscle from tenotomy: modulation by chronic electrical stimulation. Experimental Physiology 79: 515–525

Beange H, Bauman A 1990 Health care for the developmentally disabled. Is it necessary? In: Fraser W (ed) Key issues in mental retardation research. Routledge, London

Bird J, Bishop D V M, Freeman N H 1995 Phonological awareness and literacy development in children with expressive phonological impairments. Journal of Speech and Hearing Research 38: 446–462

Bishop D V M, Edmundson A 1987 Specific language impairment as a maturational lag: evidence from longitudinal data on language and motor development. Developmental Medicine and Child Neurology 29: 442–459

Blair E 1993 A research definition of birth asphyxia. Developmental Medicine and Child Neurology 35: 449

Bretas C T, Dias L S 1991 Selective dorsal rhizotomy. Developmental Medicine and Child Neurology 33, suppl. 64: 46

Brown J K 1991 Mechanism of production of raised intracranial pressure. In: Minns R A (ed) Problems of intracranial pressure in childhood. Clinics in developmental medicine nos 113/114. MacKeith Press, London, pp 13–37

Brown J K 1991 Pathological effects of raised intracranial pressure. In: Minns R A (ed) Clinics in developmental medicine nos 113/114. MacKeith Press, London, pp 38–76

Brown J K, Hussain I H M I 1991 Status epilepticus. 1 Pathogenesis. Developmental Medicine and Child Neurology 30: 121–125

Brown J K, Minns R A 1989 Mechanisms of deformity in children with cerebral palsy. In: Minns R A (ed) Seminars in orthopaedics. W B Saunders, Philadelphia, pp 236–255

Brown J K, Van Rensburg F, Walsh G, Lakie M, Wright S W 1987 A neurologic study of hand function of hemiplegic children. Developmental Medicine and Child Neurology 29: 287–304

Brown J K, Rodda J, Walsh E G, Wright G W 1991 Neurophysiology of lower limb function in hemiplegic children. Developmental Medicine and Child Neurology 33:1037–1047

Byrne P, Bartlett J 1991 Chronic subdural haematoma. British Journal of Neurosurgery 5: 459–460

Buller A J, Goodfellow J 1989 In: Newson-Davies J M (eds) Molecular genetics of muscle disease. Duchenne and other dystrophies. British Medical Bulletin, Vol 45, No 3, Churchill Livingstone, Edinburgh

Carmel P W 1986 The Chiari malformations and syringomyelia. In: Hoffman H J, Epstein F (eds) Disorders of the developing nervous system: diagnosis and treatment. Blackwell Scientific Publications, Oxford, pp 133–151

Carmel P W, Antunez J L, Hilal S K 1977 Dandy-Walker syndrome: clinico-pathological features and re-evaluation of modes of treatment. Surgical Neurology 8: 132–138

Carty H 1989 Skeletal manifestations of child abuse. Bone 6: 3–7

Chapman P H, Beyerl B 1986 The tethered spinal cord, with particular reference to spinal lipoma and diastematomyelia. In: Hoffman H J, Epstein F (eds) Disorders of the developing nervous system: diagnosis and treatment. Blackwell Scientific Publications, Oxford, pp 109–131

Chervenak H A, Duncan C, Ment L T et al 1984 Outcome of fetal ventriculomegaly. Lancet ii: 179–181

Chevrie J J, Aicardi J 1986 The Aicardi syndrome. In: Pedley T A, Meldrum B S (eds) Recent advances in epilepsy. Churchill Livingstone, Edinburgh, pp 189–210

Choux M, Grisoli F, Peragut J C 1975 Extradural haematomas in children: 104 cases. Child's Brain 1: 34–37

Choux M, Lena G, Genitori L 1986 Intracranial haematomas. In: Raimondi A J, Choux M, di Rocco C (eds) Head injuries in the newborn and infant. Springer-Verlag, Heidelberg, pp 203–216

Chung C S, Myrianthopolous N C 1975 Factors affecting risks of congenital malformations. Report from the Collaborative Perinatal Project. Birth Defects 11: 1–22

Chugani H T, Shields W D, Shewmon D A, Olson D M, Phelps M E, Peacock W J 1990 Infantile spasms. I. PET identifies focal cortical dysgenesis in cryptogenic cases for surgical treatment. Annals of Neurology 27: 406–413

Claeys V, Beonna T, Chrzanowski R 1983 Congenital hemiparesis: the spectrum of lesions. A clinical and computerized tomographic study of 37 cases. Helvetia Paediatrica Acta 38: 439–455

Clarke A D B, Clarke A N 1984 Constancy and change in the growth of human characteristics. Journal of Child Psychology and Psychiatry 25: 191–210

Corbett J A 1979 Psychiatric morbidity and mental retardation. In: James F E, Snaith R P (eds) Psychiatric illness and mental handicap. Gaskell Press, London, pp 28–45

Corry I S, Cosgrove A P, Walsh E G, McLean D, Graham H K 1994 Botulinum A toxin in the hemiplegic upper limb: a double blind trial. Developmental Medicine and Child Neurology 36, Suppl. 70: 11

Cosgrove A P, Corry I S, Graham K 1994 Botulinum toxin in the management of the lower limb in cerebral palsy. Developmental Medicine and Child Neurology 36: 386–396

Czeizel A E, Dudas I 1992 Prevention of the first occurrence of neural tube defects by periconceptional vitamin supplementation. New England Journal of Medicine 327: 1832–1835

Dan N G, Wade M J 1986 The incidence of epilepsy after ventricular shunt procedure. Journal of Neurosurgery 65: 19–21

Delgado-Escueta A V, Greenberg D, Weissbecker K et al 1990 Gene mapping in the idiopathic generalized epilepsies: juvenile myoclonic epilepsy, childhood absence epilepsy with grand mal seizures and early childhood myoclonic epilepsy. Epilepsia 31, Suppl. 13: S19–S29

Denays R, Tondeur M, Foulon M, Verstracten F, Ham H, Piepsz A, Noel P 1989 Regional brain blood flow in congenital dysphasia: studies with technetium-99m HM-PAO SPECT. Journal of Nuclear Medicine 30(ii): 1825–1829

Dewey D 1991 Praxis and sequency skills in children with sensorimotor dysfunction. Developmental Neuropsychology 7(2): 197–206

Drapkin A J 1991 Chronic subdural haematoma: pathophysiological basis for treatment. British Journal of Neurosurgery 5: 467–473

Dravet C, Roger J, Bureau M 1985 Severe myoclonic epilepsy of infants. In: Roger J, Dravet C, Bureau M, Dreifus F E, Wolf P (eds) Epileptic syndromes in infancy, childhood and adolescence. John Libbey Eurotext, London, pp 58–67

Dreifuss F E, Santilli R N, Langer D H, Sweeney K P, Moline K A, Menander

K B 1987 Valproic acid hepatic fatalities: a retrospective review. Neurology 37: 370–385

Dubowitz V 1980 The floppy infant, 2nd edn. Clinics in developmental medicine no 76. Spastics International Medical Publications and Heinemann, London

Dubowitz V 1995a Diagnosis and classification of neuromuscular disorders. In: Dubowitz V (ed) Muscle disorders in childhood. W B Saunders, London, pp 1–33

Dubowitz V 1995b Myasthenia. In: Dubowitz V (ed) Muscle disorders in childhood, 2nd edn. W B Saunders, London, p 411

Dubowitz V 1995c The muscular dystrophies. In: Dubowitz V (ed) Muscle disorders in childhood, 2nd edn. W B Saunders, London, p 55

Dubowitz V 1995d The muscular dystrophies. In: Dubowitz V (ed) Muscle disorders in childhood, 2nd edn. W B Saunders, London, p 61

Dubowitz V 1995e Inflammatory myopathies. In: Dubowitz V (ed) Muscle disorders in childhood, 2nd edn. W B Saunders, London, p 444

Duhaime A C, Gennarelli T A, Thibault L E, Bruce D A, Margulies S S, Wiser R 1987 The shaken baby syndrome. Journal of Neurosurgery 66: 409–415

Duhaime A C, Alario A J, Lewander W J et al 1992 Head injury in very young children: mechanisms, injury types and ophthalmological findings in 100 hospitalized patients younger than 2 years of age. Pediatrics 90: 179–185

Durner M, Sander T, Greenberg D A, Johnson K, Beck-Mannagetta G, Janz D 1991 Localization of idiopathic generalized epilepsy on chromosome 6p in families of juvenile myoclonic epilepsy patients. Neurology 41: 1651–1655

Eccles J C 1979 The human mystery. Springer, Berlin

Emery A E H 1988 Duchenne muscular dystrophy. Oxford University Press, Oxford

English R J, Brown S E 1990 Single photon emission: a primer. Society of Nuclear Medicine, New York

Evrard P, Miladi N, Bonnier C, Gressens P 1992 Normal and abnormal brain development. In: Rapin I, Regalowitz S J (eds) Handbook of neuropsychology. Elsevier, Amsterdam, pp 11–44

Faerber E N 1995 Intracranial tumours. In: Faerber E N (ed) CNS magnetic resonance imaging in infants and children. Clinics in developmental medicine no 134. MacKeith Press, London, pp 165–172

Faillot T, Zerah M, Comoy J 1990 Obstetrical head injuries. Review of 30 cases. Child's Nervous System 6: 143–147

Feldman K W, Brewer D K 1984 Child abuse, cardiopulmonary resuscitation and rib fractures. Pediatrics 73: 339–342

Figueras A, Morales-Olivas F J, Capella D, Palop V, Laport J-R 1992 Bovine gangliosides and acute motor polyneuropathy. British Medical Journal 305: 1330–1331

Fong D, Chan S 1988 Arteriovenous malformation in children. Child's Nervous System 4: 1999–2003

Forfar J O F, Hume R, McPhail F M, Maxwell S M, Wilkinson E M, Lin J P, Brown J K 1994 Low birthweight: a 10 year outcome study of reproductive casuality. Developmental Medicine and Child Neurology 36: 1037–1048

Fraser W, Green A, MacGillivray R 1990 Caring for people with mental handicaps, 8th edn. Butterworth, London

Garcia J C, Roach E S, McLean W T 1981 Recurrent thrombotic deterioration in the Sturge-Weber syndrome. Child's Brain 8: 427–433

Gaston H 1985 Does the spina bifida clinic need an ophthalmologist? Zeitschrift fur Kinderchirurgie 40, suppl 11: 45–50

Geschwind N, Galaburda A M 1985 Cerebral lateralisation biological mechanical associations and pathology: a hypothesis and a program for research. Archives of Neurology 42: 428–459

Greenberg D A, Burner M, Resor S, Rosenbaum D, Shinnar S 1995 The genetics of idiopathic generalized epilepsies of adolescent onset: differences between juvenile myoclonic epilepsy and epilepsy with random grand mal and with awakening grand mal. Neurology 45: 942–946

Hadley M N, Sonntag V K H, Rekate H L, Murphy A 1989 The infant whiplash-shake injury syndrome: a clinical and pathological study. Neurosurgery 24: 536–540

Hagberg B, Edebol-Tysk K, Edstrom B 1988 The basic care needs of profoundly mentally retarded children with multiple handicaps. Developmental Medicine and Child Neurology 30: 287–293

Hanieh A, Simpson D A, North J B 1988 Arachnoid cysts: a critical review of 41 cases. Child's Nervous System 4(2): 92–96

Harvey A S, Grattan-Smith J D, Desmond P M, Chow C W, Berkovic S F 1995 Febrile seizures and hippocampal sclerosis: frequent and related findings in intractable temporal lobe epilepsy of childhood. Paediatric Neurology 12(3): 201–206

Heckmatt J, Rodillo E, Dubowitz V 1989 Management of children with muscular dystrophy. British Medical Bulletin 45(3): 788–801

Heiskenen O 1989 Ruptured intracranial arterial aneurysms of children and adolescents. Surgical and total management results. Child's Nervous System 5: 66–70

Hermann B P, Whitman S, Dell J 1989 Correlates of behaviour problems and social competence in children with epilepsy aged 6–11. In: Hermann B P, Seidenburg M (eds) Childhood epilepsies: neuropsychological, psychosocial and intervention aspects. John Wiley, Chichester, pp 143–158

Herter T, Brandt M, Szuwart U 1988 Cavernous haemangiomas in children. Child's Nervous System 4: 123–127

Hutton J L, Cooke T, Pharoah P O D 1994 Life expectancy in children with cerebral palsy. British Medical Journal 309: 431–435

ILAE Commission on Classification and Terminology 1981 Proposal for revised clinical and electroencephalographic classification of epileptic seizures. Epilepsia 22: 489–501

Invalid Children's Aid Nationwide 1988 Units for primary school children with speech and language disorders. Suggested guidelines

Jackson G D 1994 New techniques of MRI in epilepsy. Epilepsia 35, Suppl. 6: S2–S13

Jacobi G 1986 Damage patterns in severe child abuse with and without fatal sequelae. Monatsschrift fur Kinderheikunde 134: 307–315 (German)

Jaspan T, Narborough G, Punt J A G, Lowe J 1992 Cerebral contusional tears as a marker of child abuse – detection by cranial sonography. Pediatric Radiology 22: 237–245

Jones H C 1987 The pathophysiology of congenital hydrocephalus. Journal of Pediatric Neurosciences 3(1): 9–20

Kaur B, Taylor D 1992 Fundus haemorrhages in infancy. Survey of Ophthalmology 37: 1–17

Kearns T P, Sayres G P 1958 Retinitis pigmentosa, external ophthalmoplegia and complete heart block. Archives of Ophthalmology (Chicago) 60: 280

Kempe C H 1971 Paediatric implications of the battered baby syndrome. Archives of Disease in Childhood 46: 28–37

Kendall B 1988 Neuroradiology. In: Laidlaw J, Richens, A, Oxley J (eds) A textbook of epilepsy. Churchill Livingstone, Edinburgh, pp 307–349

Key E A H, Retzius G 1875 Studien in der Anatomi des Nervensystems und des Bindegewebes. Samson and Wallin, Stockholm

Kirkpatrick M, Engelman H A, Minns R A 1989 Symptoms and signs of progressive hydrocephalus. Archives of Disease in Childhood 64: 124–128

Kleinman P K, Blackbourne B D, Marks S C, Karellas A, Belanger PL 1989 Radiological contributions to the investigation and prosecution of cases of fatal infant abuse. New England Journal of Medicine 320: 507–511

Kolmel H W 1977 Atlas of cerebrospinal fluid cells. Springer, Berlin

Kontopolous E, Minns R A, O'Hare A E, Eden O B 1986 Sedimentation cytomorphology of the CSF in ventriculitis. Developmental Medicine and Child Neurology 28: 213–219

Kotwica Z, Brzezinzki 1991 Chronic subdural haematoma treated by burrholes and closed system drainage: personal experience in 131 patients. British Journal of Neurosurgery 5: 461–465

Kuban K C K, Leviton A L 1994 Cerebral palsy. New England Journal of Medicine 330: 188–195

Lakie M, Walsh E G, Wright G W 1984 Resonance at the wrist demonstrated by the use of a torque motor: an instrumental analysis of muscle tone in man. Journal of Physiology (Lond.) 353: 265–285

Largo R H, Molinari L, Comenale Pinto L, Weber M, Duc G 1986 Language development of term and preterm children during the first five years of life. Developmental Medicine and Child Neurology 28(33): 33–35

Law J, Conway J 1992 Effect of abuse and neglect on the development of children's speech and language. Developmental Medicine and Child Neurology 34: 943–948

Leggate J R S, Minns R A 1991 Intracranial pressure monitoring – current methods. In: Minns R A (ed) Problems of intracranial pressure in childhood. Clinics in developmental medicine nos 113/114. MacKeith Press, London, pp 123–140

Leggate J R S, Baxter P, Minns R A et al 1988 Role of separate subcutaneous cerebrospinal fluid reservoir in the management of hydrocephalus. British Journal of Neurosurgery 2: 327–337

Leggate J R S, Lopez-Ramos N, Genitori, Leena G, Choux M 1989 Extradural haematoma in infants. British Journal of Neurosurgery 3: 533–540

Leppert M, Anderson V E, Quattlebaum T et al 1989 Benign familial neonatal convulsions lined to genetic markers on chromosome 20. Nature 337: 647–648

Levene M I, Williams J L, Fawer C-L 1985 Ultrasound of the infant brain. Spastics International Medical Publications and Heinemann Press, London

Levene M I, Evans D H, Forde A, Archer L N J 1987 The value of direct intracranial pressure monitoring in asphyxiated newborns. Developmental Medicine and Child Neurology 29: 311–319

Levin H S, Eugenio G A, Eisenberg H M et al 1989 Magnetic resonance imaging after closed head injury in children. Neurosurgery 24(2): 223–227

Lin J-P, Brown J K 1992 Peripheral and central mechanisms of hindfoot equinus in childhood hemiplegia. Developmental Medicine and Child Neurology 34: 949–965

Lin J-P, Goh W, Brown J K, Steers A J 1993 Heterogeneity of neurological syndromes in survivors of grade 3 and 4 periventricular haemorrhage. Child's Nervous System 9: 205–214

Lin J-P, Brown J K, Brotherstone R 1994a Assessment of spasticity in hemiplegic cerebral palsy. I: Proximal lower limb reflex excitability and function. Developmental Medicine and Child Neurology 36: 116–129

Lin J-P, Brown J K, Brotherstone R 1994b Assessment of spasticity in hemiplegic cerebral palsy. II: Distal lower limb reflex excitability and function. Developmental Medicine and Child Neurology 36: 290–303

Lin J-P, Brown J K, Walsh E G 1994c Physiological maturation of muscles in childhood. Lancet 343: 1386–1389

Lin J-P, Brown J K, Walsh E G 1996a Soleus muscle length, stretch reflex excitability and the contractile properties of muscle in children and adults: a study of the functional joint angle. Developmental Medicine and Child Neurology (forthcoming)

Lin J-P, Brown J K, Walsh E G 1996b The maturation of motor dexterity: or why Johnny can't go any faster. Developmental Medicine and Child Neurology 38: 244–254

Lin J-P, Brown J K, Walsh E G 1997 Ankle clonus and muscular transformation after heel-cord lengthening: clues to the pathophysiology and peripheral management of clonus. Developmental Medicine and Child Neurology (forthcoming)

Livingstone J H, Brown J K 1986 Intracerebral haemorrhage after the neonatal period. Archives of Disease in Childhood 61: 538–544

Machado H R, Machado J C, Contrera J D et al 1985 Ultrasonographic evaluation of infantile hydrocephalus before and after shunting. A study in 20 children. Child's Nervous System 1: 341–345

Marinov M, Undjian S, Wetzkap 1989 An evaluation of the surgical treatment of intracranial arachnoid cysts in children. Child's Nervous System 5(3): 177–183

Marmarov A, Shulman K, La Morgese J 1975 Compartmental analysis of compliance and outflow resistance of the cerebrospinal fluid system. Journal of Neurosurgery 43: 523–534

Maw A R 1995 Glue ear in childhood. Clinics in developmental medicine no 135. MacKeith Press, London, p 11

Maynard A 1986 The economics of health care. Royal Society of Medicine, London

Maytal J, Shinnar S, Moshe S L, Alvarez L A 1989 Low morbidity and mortality of status epilepticus in children. Pediatrics 83: 323–331

McEwan I R, Lloyd L L 1990 Some considerations about the motor requirements of manual signs. Augmentative and Alternative Communication 6(3): 207–215

McLaughlin J F, Bjornson K F, Astley S J, Hays R M, Hoffinger S A, Armantrout E A, Roberts T S 1994 The role of selective dorsal rhizotomy in cerebral palsy: critical evaluation of a prospective clinical series. Developmental Medicine and Child Neurology 36: 75–769

McLean J, Schneider J, McKlean L 1987 Form and function of communicative behaviour among persons with severe developmental disabilities. Australia & New Zealand Journal of Developmental Disabilities 13: 83–98

Meuli M, Meuli-Sommen C, Hutchins G M, Yingling, C D, McBiles Hoffman K, Harrison M R, Adzick N S 1995 In utero surgery rescues neurological function at birth in sheep with spina bifida. Nature Medicine 1: 342–347

Michejda M 1985 The fetal neural tube: is intervention progress? Zeitschrift fur Kinderchirurgie 40, Suppl. I: 53–57

Minns R A 1986 The management of children with spina bifida. In: Gordon N, McKinlay I (ed) Neurologically handicapped children. Blackwell, Oxford

Minns R A, Merrick M V 1989 Cerebral perfusion pressure and net cerebral mean transit time in childhood hydrocephalus. Journal of Pediatric Neurosciences 5(2): 69–77

Minns R A, Brown J K, Engelman H M 1987 CSF production rate: 'real time' estimation. Zeitschrift fur Kinderchirugie 42, suppl. I: 36–40

Minns R A, Engelman H M, Stirling H 1989a Cerebrospinal fluid pressure in pyogenic meningitis. Archives of Disease in Childhood 64: 814–820

Minns R A, Wong B, Brown J K, Fraser W I 1989b Neuro-developmental study of profoundly mentally handicapped children in hospital care. Journal of Mental Deficiency Research 33: 439–454

Minns R A, Goh D, Pye S, Steers J 1990 A volume-blood flow relationship derived from CSF compartment challenge as an index of progression of infantile hydrocephalus. Proceedings of International Symposium on Hydrocephalus, Japan, November

Morris H 1989 'Don't look at the penguins.' Article on offering help with literacy skills. Special Children 29: 7–10

Naeser M A, Palumbo C L, Helm-Estabrooks N, Stiassny-Eder D, Albert M L 1989 Severe nonfluency in aphasia: role of the medial subcallosal fasciculus and other white matter pathways in recovery of spontaneous speech. Brain 112: 1–38

Nelson K B, Ellenberg J H 1982 Children who outgrew cerebral palsy. Pediatrics 69: 529–536

Nirje B 1969 The normalisation process and its human management implications. In: Kugel R, Wolfensberger W (eds) Changing patterns in residential services for the mentally retarded. President's Committee on Mental Retardation, Washington DC

O'Hare A E, Brown J K 1989a Childhood dysgraphia Part 1: an illustrated classification. Child Care, Health and Development 15: 79–104

O'Hare A E, Brown J K 1989b Childhood dysgraphia Part 2: a study of hand function. Child Care, Health and Development 15: 151–166

Ounsted C, Lindsay J, Norman R 1966 Biological factors in temporal lobe epilepsy. Clinics in developmental medicine no 22. Spastics International Medical Publications and Heinemann Press, London

Park T S, Owen J H 1992 Surgical management of spastic diplegia in cerebral palsy. New England Journal of Medicine 326: 745–749

Peacock W J, Staudt L A 1990 Spasticity in cerebral palsy and the selective dorsal rhizotomy procedure. Journal of Child Neurology 5: 179–185

Penn R D, Kroin J S 1985 Continuous intrathecal baclofen for severe spasticity. Lancet ii: 125–127

Pennington B F, Smith S D, Kimberling W J, Green P A, Haith M M 1987 Left handedness and immune disorders in familial dyslexics. Archives of Neurology 44: 634–639

Plomin R, Owen M J, McGruffin P 1994 The genetic basis of complex human behaviours. Science 264: 1733–1739

Rach G H, Zielhuis G A, Van Der Brock P 1988 The influence of chronic persistent otitis media with effusion on language development of 2–4 year olds. International Journal of Pediatric Otorhinolaryngology 15: 253–261

Raimondi A J 1986 Cystic transformation of the IV ventricle (the Dandy-Walker cyst). In: Hoffman H J, Epstein F (eds) Disorders of the developing nervous system: diagnosis and treatment. Blackwell Scientific Publications, Oxford, pp 235–246

Ramsden R, Graham J 1995 Cochlear implantation. British Medical Journal 311: 1588

Raju T N K, Doshi U V, Vidyasager D 1982 Cerebral perfusion pressure studies in healthy pre-term and term newborn infants. Journal of Pediatrics 100: 139–142

Ratcliffe S G 1994 The psychological and psychiatric consequences of sex chromosome abnormalities in children based on population studies. In: Poustka R (ed) Basic approaches to genetic and molecular biological developmental psychiatry. Quintessenz, Berlin, pp 99–122

Richard K E, Dahl K, Sanker P 1989 Long-term follow-up of children and juveniles with arachnoid cysts. Child's Nervous System 5(3): 184–187

Richardson J 1995 Otoacoustic emissions. Archives of Disease in Childhood 73(4): 284–286

Rideau Y, Duport G, Delaubier A 1986 Premieres remissions reproductibles dans l'evolution de la dystrophie musculaire de Duchenne. Bulletin de l'Academie Nationale de Medicine 170: 605–610

Roach E S, Riela A R 1988 Paediatric cerebrovascular disorders. Futura, New York

Rorke L B 1990 Neuropathology of homicidal head injury in infants. Child's Nervous System 6: 295 (abstract)

Royal Colleges of Surgeons and Physicians 1976 Conference of Medical Royal Colleges and their Faculties in the UK. Diagnosis of brain death. British Medical Journal i: 1187–1188

Royal Colleges of Surgeons and Physicians 1979 Conference of Medical Royal Colleges and their Faculties in the UK. Diagnosis of death. British Medical Journal i: 322

Scarfo G B, Mariottini A, Tomaccini D, Palma L 1989 Growing skull fractures: progressive evolution of brain damage and effectiveness of surgical treatment. Child's Nervous System 5: 163–167

Scheffer I E, Jones L, Pozzebon M, Howell R A, Saling M M, Berkovic S F 1995 Autosomal dominant rolandic epilepsy and speech dyspraxia: a new syndrome with anticipation. Annals of Neurology 38: 633–642

Scriver R C, Beaudet L A, Sly W S, Valle D (eds) 1989 The metabolic basis of inherited disease, 6th edn. McGraw-Hill, New York

Seidenberg M 1989 Academic achievement and school performance of children with epilepsy. In: Hermann B P, Seidenberg M (eds) Childhood epilepsies. Neuropsychological, psychosocial and intervention aspects. John Wiley, Chichester, pp 105–118

Serlo W, Kirkinen P, Jouppila P et al 1986 Prognostic signs in fetal hydrocephalus. Child's Nervous System 2: 93–97

Shapiro K, Fried A, Marmarou A 1985 Biomechanical and hydrodynamic characterisation of the hydrocephalic infant. Journal of Neurology 63: 69–75

Shiel E, Wright F V, Naumann S, Drake J, Wedge J 1994 Randomized control trial of selective dorsal rhizotomy: biomechanical evaluation. Developmental Medicine and Child Neurology 36, suppl. 70: 19–20

Shinnar S, Gammon K, Bergman E W, Epstein M, Freeman J M 1985 Management of hydrocephalus in infancy: use of acetazolamide and furosemide to avoid cerebrospinal fluid shunts. Journal of Pediatrics 107: 31–37

Shinnar S, Maytal J, Krasnoff L, Moshe S L 1992 Recurrent status epilepticus in children. Annals of Neurology 31: 589–604

Shorvon S 1994 Status epilepticus, its clinical features and treatment in children and adults. Cambridge University Press, Cambridge, pp 238–243

Sienko S, Aiona M D, Buckon C E 1994 Does gait continue to improve two years following selective dorsal rhizotomy? Developmental Medicine and Child Neurology 36, Suppl. 70: 20

Simpson D, Reilly P 1982 Paediatric coma scale. Lancet 2: 450

Smith S M, Hanson R 1974 134 battered children: a medical and psychological study. British Medical Journal 3: 666–670

Solomons G 1979 Child abuse and developmental disabilities. Developmental Medicine and Child Neurology 21: 101–108

Sommerlad B C 1994 Management of cleft lip and palate. Current Paediatrics 4: 189–195

Southall D P, Stebbens V A, Rees S V, Lang M H, Warner J D, Shinebourne E A 1987 Apnoeic episodes induced by smothering: two cases identified by covert video surveillance. British Medical Journal 294: 1637–1641

Stephenson J B P 1978 Reflex anoxic seizures (while breath-holding). Non-epileptic vagal attacks. Archives of Disease in Childhood 53: 193–200

Stephenson J B P 1990 Fits and faints. Clinics in developmental medicine no 109. MacKeith Press, London

Stern M, Hildebrandt K 1986 Prematurity sterotyping effects on mother-infant interaction. Child Development 57: 308–315

Suarez J C, Viano J C 1989 Intracranial arteriovenous malformations in infancy and adolescence. Child's Nervous System 5: 15–18

Sutherland D H et al 1994 Effects of botulinum toxin on gait of patients with cerebral palsy: preliminary results. Developmental Medicine and Child Neurology 36, suppl. 70: 11–12

Temple M 1986 Developmental dysgraphias. Quarterly Journal of Experimental Psychology 38A: 77–110

Thomas S A, Rosenfield N S, Leventhal J M, Markowitz R I 1991 Long bone fractures in young children distinguishing accidental injuries from child abuse. Pediatrics 88: 471–476

Trevarthen C 1987 Sharing makes sense: intersubjectivity and the making of an infant's meaning. In: Steele R, Tredgold T (eds) Language topics: essays in honour of Michael Halliday. John Benjamins, Amsterdam

Trevarthen C, Marwick H 1986 Signs of motivation for speech in infants and the nature of a mother's support for development of language. In: Lyneblum, Zetterstom R (eds) Precursors of early speech. Wenner-Gren Center international symposium series, vol 44. Macmillan, Basingstoke, pp 279–308

Van Der Meche F G A, Schmitz P I M, and the Dutch Guillain-Barré Study Group 1992 A randomised trial comparing intravenous immune globulin and plasma exchange in Guillain-Barre syndrome. New England Journal of Medicine 326(17): 1123–11229

Walsh E G, Lin J-P, Brown J K, Dutia M B 1994 Muscular creep in juvenile hemiplegia. Proceedings of the Physiological Society (Lond.), Bristol meeting

Walsh J W 1986 Agenesis of the corpus callosum. In: Hoffman H J, Epstein F (eds) Disorders of the developing nervous system: diagnosis and treatment. Blackwell Scientific Publications, Oxford, pp 225–233

Wanifuchi H, Kagawa M, Takeshita M, Isawa M, Kitamura K 1988 Ischaemic stroke in infancy, childhood and adolescence. Child's Nervous System 4: 361–364

Weintraub S, Mesulam M 1983 Developmental learning disabilities of the right hemisphere. Archives of Neurology 40: 463–468

Whitehouse W P, Rees M, Curtis D et al 1993 Linkage analysis of idiopathic generalized epilepsy and marked loci on chromosome 6p in families of patients with juvenile myoclonic epilepsy: no evidence for an epilepsy locus in the HLA region. American Journal of Human Genetics 53: 652–662

Wiklund L M, Uvebrandt P 1991 Hemiplegic cerebral palsy: correlation between CT morphology and clinical findings. Developmental Medicine and Child Neurology 33: 512–523

Wing L, Gould J 1979 Severe impairments of social interaction and associated abnormalities. Journal of Autism and Developmental Disorders 9: 11–29

Wolfensberger W 1983 Social role valorisation: a proposed new term for the principle of normalisation. Mental Retardation 21: 234–239

Wright F V, Shiel E, Naumann S, Drake J, Wedge J 1994 Gross motor function following selective dorsal rhizotomy – results of a randomized control trial. Developmental Medicine and Child Neurology 36, suppl. 70: 18

Zielhuis G A, Rach G H, Van Der Brock P 1989 Screening for otitis media with effusion in pre-school children. Lancet i: 311–313

Zimmerman R A, Bruce D, Schut L, Uzzell B, Goldberg H I 1979 Computerised tomography of craniocerebral injury in the abused child. Radiology 130: 687–690

15 Disorders of the blood and reticuloendothelial system

Derek J. King (following Ian M. Hann)

Normal blood production 847
The ontogeny of blood formation 847
The origin of circulating blood cells 848
Other significant changes in fetal/neonatal blood 849
Regulation of hemopoiesis 849
Hematological assessment in childhood 849
Anemia 850
Deficiency anemias 850
Iron deficiency 850
Folate deficiency 851
Vitamin B$_{12}$ deficiency 853
Other causes of megaloblastic anemia 853
Aplastic anemias 854
Etiology and classification 854
Constitutional aplastic anemias 854
    Fanconi's anemia 854
    Familial marrow dysfunction 854
    Dyskeratosis congenita 854
    Shwachman–Diamond syndrome 855
    Amegakaryocytic thrombocytopenia 855
    Reticular dysgenesis 855
Acquired aplastic anemia 855
Pure red cell aplasia 856
Leukoerythroblastosis 856
Hemolytic anemias 856
Hereditary hemolytic anemias 857
Acquired hemolytic anemias 863
Methemoglobinemia 864
Secondary anemias 865
Chronic infection and inflammation 865
Chronic renal failure 865

Malignant disease 865
Endocrine disorders 865
Liver disease 865
Drugs 865
Defects of heme synthesis 865
    Congenital erythropoietic porphyria 865
    Lead poisoning 865
    Sideroblastic anemias 866
Neutropenia 866
Other white cell disorders 868
Eosinophilia 868
Leukemia 868
Classification of leukemia 868
Clinical manifestations 869
Diagnosis and laboratory findings 871
Treatment 872
Disorders of hemostasis 875
Nonthrombocytopenic purpuras 875
Thrombocytopenic purpuras 876
    Thrombocytopenia secondary to infection 878
    Drug-induced thrombocytopenia 878
    Congenital and neonatal thrombocytopenia 878
Disorders of platelet function 879
    Hereditary 879
    Acquired 879
Coagulation disorders 879
Hereditary coagulation defects 879
Acquired coagulation defects 881
Thrombosis in children 882
References and Bibliography 882

NORMAL BLOOD PRODUCTION

THE ONTOGENY OF BLOOD FORMATION

Within a few days of implantation of the egg, angioblastic tissue separates from the wall of the blastocyst and spreads into the developing body stalk and yolk sac wall. Solid masses of cells ('blood islands') form within the yolk sac and by the 14th day of gestation they have hollowed out, with peripheral cells forming the vascular endothelium and central cells making up the first blood cells. Clefts then develop between the blood cells to form the vascular lumen. By the 25th day these differentiation processes within the mesenchyme make up the vascular system of the embryo.

Studies in mice have shown that the development of hemopoietic organs, i.e. liver spleen and bone marrow (Fig. 15.1), is probably dependent on colonization by cells derived from the yolk sac. Supportive evidence for the existence of this process in humans comes from the demonstration of high levels of circulating hemopoietic progenitors in fetoscope-obtained blood samples and from mid-trimester abortuses (Hann et al 1983).

Subsequent stages in hemopoietic development are illustrated in Figure 15.1. Following the yolk sac stage, the liver takes over between the 6th and 10th weeks. Its importance diminishes after the mid-trimester and ceases at term except when extramedullary hemopoiesis persists because of excessive demands, e.g. hemolytic disease of the newborn. Large numbers of pluripotent and committed hemopoietic progenitor cells can be demonstrated in cultures from fetal liver throughout the mid-trimester.

The initiation of bone marrow activity varies from the 7th or 8th (clavicle) to the 18th or 19th (sternum) week of gestation. The blood cell-forming marrow consists of a vascularized stromal matrix derived from perichondral cells and hemopoietic parenchyma. It becomes populated with progenitor cells at some stage between the 11th and 15th week of gestation. The relative contribution of various bones is shown in Figure 15.1. One practical point is that it is usually possible to obtain good marrow samples from the pelvis of a neonate and it is not usually necessary to attack other sites.

The spleen is a densely packed mass of mesenchymal cells at 8 weeks of gestation but by the 12–14th week they form a syncytial

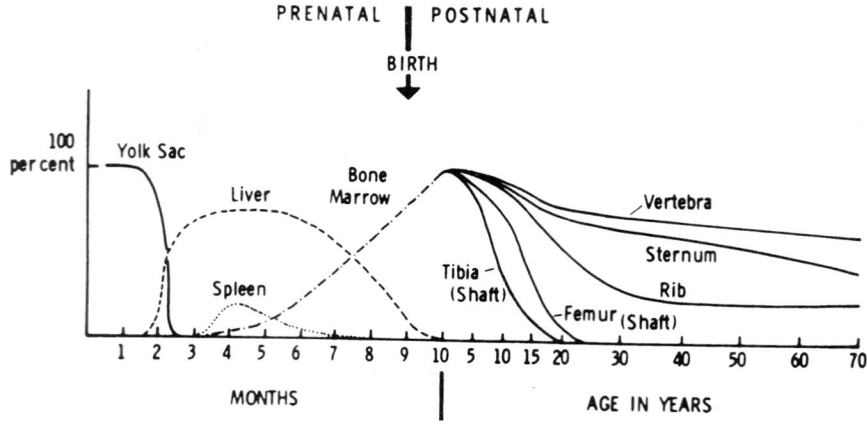

Fig. 15.1   The sites of hemopoietic tissue in the fetus and adult life. The other flat bones, e.g. skull and pelvis, are also hemopoietic similar to the vertebrae and sternum. The ordinate refers in the fetus to the contribution to total hemopoiesis. It refers in postnatal life to the proportion of the bone marrow at the various sites which are hemopoietic (the remainder being fat). (From Hoffbrand & Lewis 1981 with permission.)

network with erythroblastic islands, megakaryoctyes and scattered lymphocytes. Splenic hemopoiesis has been shown to begin between 12 and 16 weeks and continues throughout the second trimester.

THE ORIGIN OF CIRCULATING BLOOD CELLS

It is likely that all hemopoietic cells are derived from pluripotent stem cells (Fig. 15.2). Using in vitro culture techniques it is possible

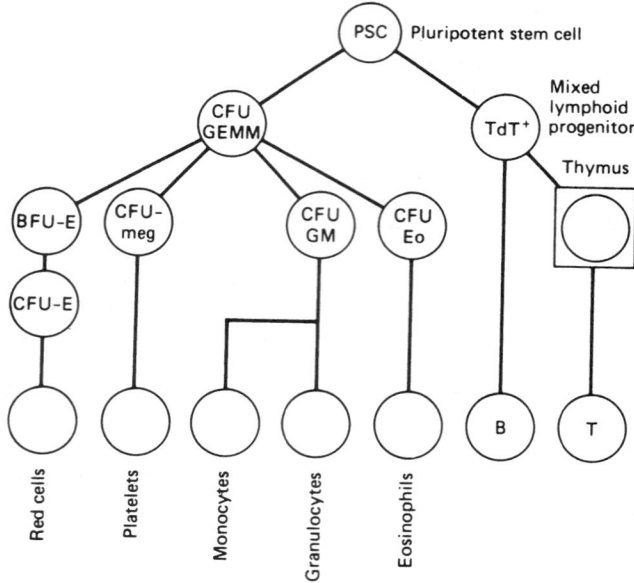

Fig. 15.2   A scheme of hemopoiesis. The pluripotent stem cell (PSC) gives rise to a series of committed progenitors defined by culture characteristics in semisolid medium. CFU-GEMM = colony-forming unit, granulocyte, erythroid, megakaryocyte, monocyte; BFU-E = burst-forming unit, erythroid; GM = granulocyte/monocyte; meg = megakaryocyte; Eo = eosinophil; TdT = terminal deoxynucleotidyl transferase. (From Hoffbrand & Lewis 1981 with permission.)

to study human hemopoiesis and investigate its controlling factors both cellular and humoral. Identification of growth factors has clinical implications for therapy as discussed later.

Primitive megaloblastic red cells constitute nearly all the nucleated blood cells from the 4th to the 8th week of gestation. The proportion of these cells falls off rapidly from then onwards and they are not found in the blood after 12 weeks. The concentration of nonnucleated red cells in fetal blood increases from 1×10^{12}/l at 12 weeks to 3.5×10^{12}/l at 40 weeks (see Table 15.1). These changes are paralleled by the hemoglobin content which is at a mean of 6 g/dl at 10 weeks and 18 g/dl at term. The packed cell volume (PCV) rises from 20% to 50% over this period. The mean red cell volume in the fetus is large and is 108 fl in full-term neonates, falling to 78 fl at 1 year of age (Table 15.1).

Granulocytes circulate in very small numbers in early fetuses. Band forms and neutrophils only really begin to appear at 9–10 weeks and form 4% of nucleated cells by 12 weeks. At term they rise to a mean of 6×10^9/l. Eosinophils and basophils begin to appear at 14–16 weeks and monocytes are present at from 4 to 6 weeks. Large lymphocytes make up 3–5% of nucleated blood cells from the 11th week but small lymphocytes are present in much larger numbers from 9 weeks of gestation. The lymphocyte count at 20 weeks is at a mean of 1.5×10^9/l rising to 2.5×10^9/l at term. Megakaryocytes are present in the yolk sac at 5 weeks and platelets are present in the blood from about this time.

After the first 2 days of postnatal life the neutrophil leukocytosis and erythroblastosis seen at birth disappears. Until the age of 4 years there is a preponderance of lymphocytes (Fig. 15.3). The eosinophil concentration may be relatively high during the first year of life and tends to be generally higher in young children than in teenagers or adults although the differences are small. Monocyte levels are high during the first year of life and then return to levels equivalent to those in adults (Fig. 15.3). The platelet count of normal term infants is similar to that of adults. Earlier claims of 'physiological thrombocytopenia' in premature infants probably arose because the studies included babies with other problems such as infection. A platelet count below 150×10^9/l is abnormal and warrants further investigation.

Table 15.1 Normal hematological values in infancy and childhood

Age	Red cell count (× 10^{12}/l)	Hb (g/dl)	PCV	MCV (fl)	MCH (pg)	MCHC (g/dl)	Average reticulocytes (%)	Total WBC range (× 10^9/l)	Absolute neutrophil count (× 10^9/l)	Absolute lymphocyte count (× 10^9/l)	Absolute monocyte count (× 10^9/l)	Absolute eosinophil count (× 10^9/l)
Newborn, full term	5.1 ± 1.0	18.4 ± 2.2	0.60 ± 0.07	108 ± 9	35 ± 4	36 ± 2	3.2	9 –30	4.5–13.2	2.7–11.0	0.4–3.1	0.2–0.9
7 days	5.1 ± 1.0	17.9 ± 2.5	0.56 ± 0.09	99 ± 11	32.5 ± 4	35 ± 2	0.5	5 –21	1.5–10.0	2.0–17	0.3–2.7	<0.7
3 months	4.5 ± 0.7	11.3 ± 0.5	0.33 ± 0.03	88 ± 8	29 ± 5	33 ± 3	0.7	6 –15	1.5–7.0	4.0–12	0.2–1.5	<0.7
1 year	4.5 ± 0.7	11.8 ± 0.5	0.39 ± 0.02	78 ± 8	27 ± 4	32 ± 3	0.9	6 –15	1.5–7.0	5.0–10	0.2–1.5	<0.7
3–6 years	4.5 ± 0.7	12.7 ± 1.0	0.37 ± 0.03	87 ± 8	27 ± 3	33 ± 2	1.0	5 –12	2.0–6.0	5.5–8.0	0.2–1.5	<0.7
10–12 years	4.6 ± 0.6	13.2 ± 1.0	0.39 ± 0.03	86 ± 8	27 ± 3	33 ± 2	1.0	5 –12	2.0–6.0	1.5–4.0	0.2–1.5	<0.7
Male adult	5.2 ± 0.8	16.0 ± 2.0	0.47 ± 0.05	85 ± 8	29.5 ± 2.5	33 ± 2	1.0	4.3–10	2.0–7.5	1.5–4.0	0.2–0.95	<0.7
Female adult	4.8 ± 0.6	14.0 ± 2.0	0.42 ± 0.05	85 ± 8	29.5 ± 2.5	33 ± 2	1.0	4.3–10	2.0–7.5	1.5–4.0	0.2–0.95	<0.7

This table is compiled from several studies. Race may affect normal values; thus Negroes frequently have Hbs 0.5 g/dl lower than whites even after correction of iron deficiency.
Prematurity affects values, e.g. MCV of 118 fl at 34 weeks; total WBC up to 30% lower than value at term.
Abbreviations: PCV = packed cell volume, MCH = mean corpuscular hemoglobin, MCHC = mean corpuscular hemoglobin concentration, WBC = white blood cell count, MCV = mean corpuscular volume.

OTHER SIGNIFICANT CHANGES IN FETAL/NEONATAL BLOOD

The susceptibility of neonatal red cells to oxidant injury leads to glutathione instability, methemoglobinemia and Heinz body formation. The reason for this is uncertain, although it is probably the result of a number of factors: inappropriately low levels of glutathione peroxidase for the metabolic age of the red cells, reduced levels of methemoglobin reductase and catalase and reduced levels of membrane –SH groups associated with low levels of membrane antioxidants such as vitamin E.

Interest in fetal hemoglobin synthesis has been aroused because of the availability of blood samples obtained at fetoscopy and by other methods, which can be used in antenatal diagnosis. Moreover, the possibility of 'switching on' hemoglobin F (HbF) synthesis as a means of treating severe inherited disorders of hemoglobin synthesis, e.g. β-thalassemia major, continues to excite research throughout the world. However, what causes initiation of adult hemoglobin production is still unknown. A variety of globins, each molecule comprising four polypeptide chains, are synthesized throughout fetal and postnatal life. HbF ($\alpha_2\gamma_2$) accounts for about 30% of hemoglobin in the earliest fetal studies and the rest is made up of Hb Gower ($\alpha_2\epsilon_2 + \zeta_2\epsilon_2$) and Hb Portland ($\zeta_2\gamma_2$). For the remainder of intra-uterine life HbF is the major type. After 36 weeks, there is a gradual increase in the proportion of adult hemoglobin ($\alpha_2\beta_2$). At term about 50–65% is fetal and the rest is of the adult type with a small amount of HbA$_2$ ($\alpha_2\delta_2$). At 3 months after birth only 5% is fetal and little can be detected after 1 year from birth. As a consequence there is a shift to the right of the oxygen dissociation curve with increased oxygen availability to the tissues. After the first week of life there is a virtual cessation of erythropoiesis resulting in a gradual fall of hemoglobin over the next 3 months (Table 15.1). Erythropoietin is detectable in the baby's plasma at birth and then disappears until stimulated to re-emerge by the increased off-loading of oxygen to the tissues at 2–3 months. Because of the changes described, it has been clearly shown that clinical abnormalities such as tachycardia, tachypnea and poor feeding are more useful indicators of 'available oxygen' than hemoglobin values alone in neonates and hence better indicators for transfusion needs.

REGULATION OF HEMOPOIESIS

Research over recent years has demonstrated the complexity of factors controlling hemopoiesis. While lymphocytes have an important role in regulating blood cell formation, it involves the interaction of a great variety of humoral factors (cytokines) including stem cell factor, interleukins and colony stimulating factors. These act at different stages of hemopoiesis, influencing cell division and differentiation. Erythropoietin was one of the first cytokines identified and plays a major role in controlling red cell production. The genes for cytokines such as erythropoietin and granulocyte-colony stimulating factor (G-CSF) have been sequenced and factors produced by recombinant DNA technology are available now for clinical use. Erythropoietin has become established in the management of the anemia of renal failure and may have a role in treating the anemia of prematurity. G-CSF has a role in the management of certain types of congenital neutropenia and in reducing the duration of neutropenia after chemotherapy and bone marrow transplantation. Current research is exploring the use of combinations of cytokines in bone marrow failure syndromes and improving bone marrow function after chemotherapy. It is likely that there will be considerable expansion in the clinical application of cytokines.

HEMATOLOGICAL ASSESSMENT IN CHILDHOOD

The advances in automated laboratory instruments make it possible to carry out most tests on small volumes of blood such as from expertly collected capillary samples. This is particularly important in neonatology and the development of diluted assays has revolutionized the investigation of coagulation disorders (Andrew et al 1988). A full range of coagulation tests, factor assays and a blood count can be carried out on properly collected heel prick or finger prick samples. Although there are slight differences between blood counts taken by venepuncture and capillary methods, these are of no clinical significance. With the development of micromethods for ESR estimation and RIA methods for B$_{12}$, folate and ferritin estimations, the volume of blood required for hematological testing has been dramatically reduced, to the benefit of the patient.

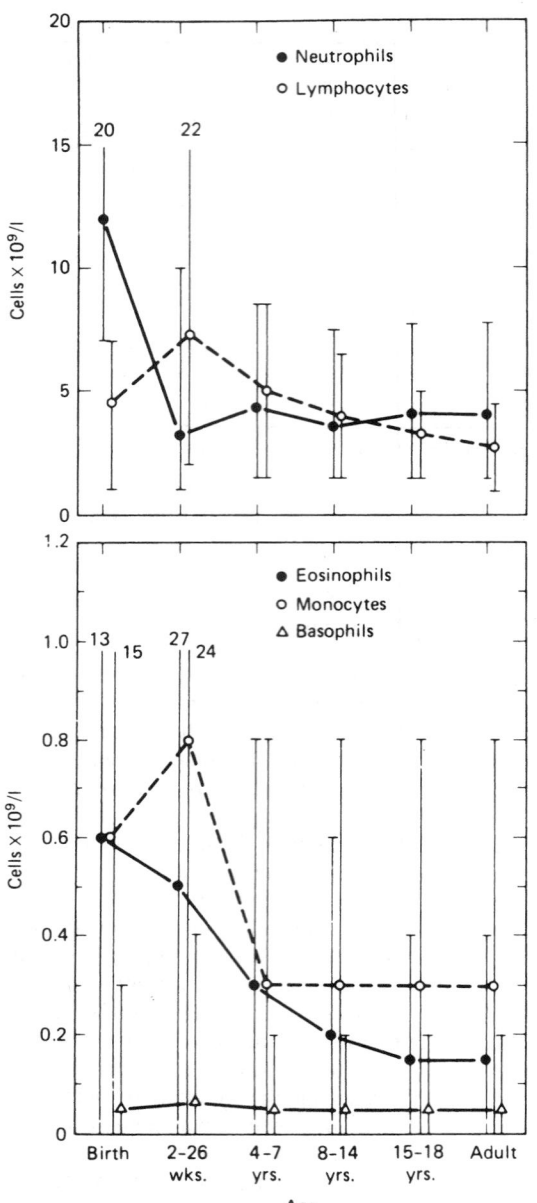

Fig. 15.3 Values for blood concentration of neutrophils and lymphocytes (above) and of monocytes, eosinophils and basophils (below) during infancy and childhood. (Collected from data of Kato and of Weshburn for infants, and of Osgood and coworkers for older children. See Wintrobe et al 1981, p. 51. Fig. 3.10 for original references. With permission of Lea and Febiger.)

Bone marrow aspirations (sometimes with percutaneous trephine biopsy) are sometimes required in the elucidation of hematological disorders in children. Techniques for these procedures are simple and can be carried out under ketamine anesthesia, formal general anesthesia or sometimes under local anesthesia or hypnosis. It is very rarely necessary to use other than the very safe approach to the anterior or posterior superior iliac spines even in neonates and the techniques are reviewed in a text of practical procedures (Hinchcliffe & Lilleyman 1987). Specific investigation schemes will be discussed under the appropriate headings (see below).

ANEMIA

APPROACH TO ANEMIA

It is suggested that the following approach should be used in the assessment of a child who may be anemic and this should guide subsequent appropriate investigations. After the history and examination are performed and the result of the blood count is known three questions are asked.

1. Is the child anemic? This requires the result of the hemoglobin level and knowledge of the normal ranges for the age of the child.
2. What is the morphological description of the red cells? The laboratory will report on the blood film and this will suggest potential diagnoses and initial investigations (Table 15.2).
3. What is the pathophysiological mechanism of the anemia? This requires synthesis of the clinical and laboratory findings, and consideration of the mechanisms shown in Figure 15.4.

DEFICIENCY ANEMIAS

These disorders commonly present to general pediatricians and are a major health problem worldwide. They frequently reflect disorders in systems other than the blood or deficiencies in nutrition. It should be emphasized that deficiency of a factor important in red cells production can have greater effects in children as growth and development can be adversely affected, e.g. the importance of vitamin B_{12} in the development of the central nervous system.

IRON DEFICIENCY

Etiology

This is the commonest cause of anemia in childhood. It should be appreciated that iron deficiency is not a diagnosis but a description of a type of anemia. The underlying cause has to be identified and corrected. Most cases occur during the second half of the first year of life when neonatal iron stores are fading and increasing red cell mass is not compensated by adequate dietary intake. Very often the diet taken during this period of life does not contain the required 7–8 mg elemental iron/day. Human and cow's milk contain negligible amounts of iron, and fruit, eggs, milk and vegetables are the usual source. Thus, iron-fortified cereals or milk are required after the first 6 months. There are also higher risk groups such as premature babies, those from multiple births and children who have been anemic in the neonatal period, e.g. due to hemolytic disease of the newborn. Supplementation is required for these patients along with those who have malabsorption, e.g. celiac syndrome, or occult gastrointestinal loss, e.g. parasitic gut infestation. In older children, the question of occult intestinal blood loss should be more formally investigated. Some details of supplemental therapy and other useful facts and figures are given in Table 15.3.

Clinical features

Presenting signs and symptoms are varied and often nonspecific. Irritability, anorexia, listlessness, gastrointestinal upsets, pica and susceptibility to infection can all be presenting features. The pallor may be incidental to another illness. There is now some evidence

Table 15.2 Morphological diagnosis of anemia

Red cell appearances	Hypochromic microcytic		Normochromic normocytic		Macrocytic	
Discriminatory test	Serum ferritin		Reticulocyte count		B_{12}/Folate assay	Bone marrow examination
Result	Reduced	Normal or increased	Reduced	Normal or increased	Megaloblastic	Nonmegaloblastic
Possible diagnoses	Iron deficiency	Thalassemia Hemoglobinopathy Sideroblastic anemia	Bone marrow hypoplasia Red cell aplasia	Hemolysis Blood loss Secondary anemia	Deficiency of B_{12}/folate Abnormality of B_{12}/folate metabolism	Liver disease Thyroid disease Congenital dyserythropoietic anemia

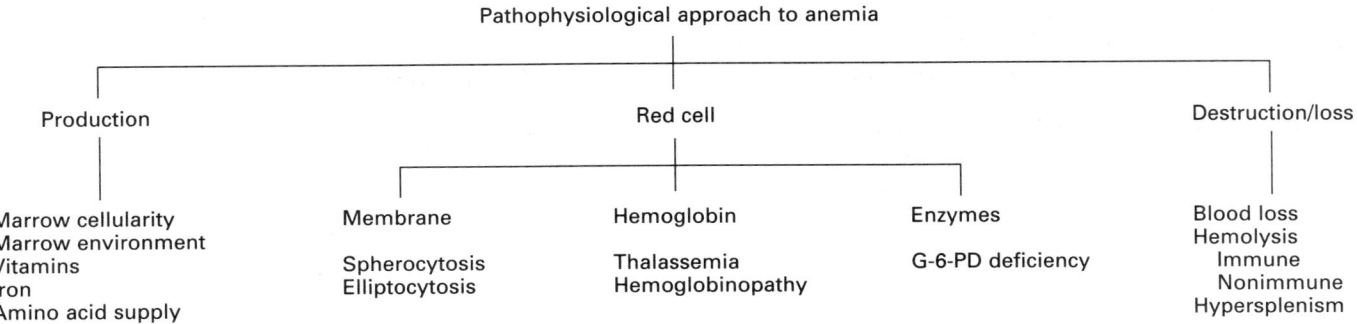

Fig. 15.4 Pathophysiological approach to anemia. Consider the possible mechanisms of anemia as a guide to appropriate investigations and management.

that intellectual function may be significantly impaired. In children, mucosal pallor is the most reliable sign and atrophic glossitis, dysphagia and koilonychia are much less frequently seen than in adults. Slight splenomegaly may occasionally be found and rarely heart failure can occur at low levels of hemoglobin, especially if there has been an episode of acute blood loss. A soft apical systolic 'hemic' flow murmur may also be present. In children it is remarkable how well tolerated are quite severe degrees of anemia.

Diagnosis

Most children are overinvestigated. With modern, accurate automated blood counters many cases are picked up at an early stage and the red cell indices are often diagnostic. A low

Table 15.3 Useful facts and figures

Blood volume
Mean blood volume 75 ml/kg
Mean plasma volume 48 ml/kg

Transfusion
4 ml/kg packed cells or 6 ml/kg whole (anticoagulated) blood raises the Hb by 1 g/dl
Exchange transfusion 175 ml/kg
Storage of blood 4 ± 2°C

Coagulation therapy dosage
Fresh frozen plasma (FFP) 15–20 ml/kg raises factors by about 20%
Cryoprecipitate (Cryo) 30 ml/kg raises factor VIII by approximately 30%
Factor VIII: 15 units/kg raises level by approximately 30%
Factor IX: 15 units/kg raises level by 15%

Heparin therapy
Loading dose 100 units/kg i.v. followed by 25 units/kg/h i.v. Adjust dose to keep PTT twice normal

Iron therapy
5 mg elemental iron/kg oral daily until Hb normal and for further 3 months

hemoglobin (outside the ranges of Table 15.1) associated with a normal or low red cell count, low MCH and low MCV should be enough to establish the diagnosis. However, nonwhite children and especially those with a high normal or raised red cell count must be investigated to see whether they have a thalassemia trait. There is always the risk of missing a mixed folate/iron deficiency which will tend to normalize the MCV and MCH, but careful inspection of a blood film should rule out most of these cases. Final confirmation of the diagnosis can be made by demonstration of a low serum ferritin level, the serum ferritin being an accurate reflection of body iron stores unless there are hepatic disorders or chronic inflammatory disorders.

When iron deficiency is due to blood loss it is frequently associated with a 'reactive' picture, i.e. a high platelet count and reticulocytosis. Occult blood stool testing should be performed and other investigations as indicated, for example the search for a Meckel's diverticulum.

It is important to have an assessment of the child's diet as high consumption of cow's milk with little solid food is probably the commonest cause of iron deficiency in infants and toddlers.

Treatment

By the time iron deficiency anemia is diagnosed there is marked depletion of tissue iron stores. The management of iron deficiency involves correcting the underlying cause and giving sufficient iron replacement therapy to return the hemoglobin and the red cell indices to normal, then replenish the depleted iron stores. Thus, oral iron should be continued for 3 months after correction of the hemoglobin and the underlying disorder. Ferrous iron is more efficient than ferric, with 4 mg/kg/day of dietary iron an appropriate intake to prevent deficiency for infants with a birthweight below 1000 g and 3 mg/kg/day for those between 1000 and 1500 g. The requirement for full-term infants is 1 mg/kg/day (maximum total daily dose 15 mg) starting no later than 4 months of age until 3 years of age. Between 4 and 10 years, the requirement is 10 mg/day and above 11 years and through adolescence, 18 mg/day. Therapeutic doses of oral iron are usually given as 3 mg/kg/day in three divided doses and the importance of ensuring a response to treatment should be emphasized.

Ferrous sulfate is the cheapest and simplest preparation and it can be given with milk or cereal feeds with consequent less intestinal intolerance. It is rarely necessary to resort to other formulations. One very important point is that iron tablets look remarkably like popular sweets and thus they must always be dispensed in containers with secure tops and with warnings about overdosage. Sodium iron edetate ('Sytron') is a liquid preparation of iron which may be more easily given to young children After a lag period of 7–10 days it should be possible to demonstrate a reticulocytosis and hemoglobin rise. If not, the patient should be reassessed for compliance/malabsorption/blood loss. It is rarely necessary to transfuse a child with simple iron deficiency and this is usually contraindicated because of the inherent risks of transfusion.

FOLATE DEFICIENCY

Etiology

All causes of megaloblastic anemia in children are rare but when it does occur it is most commonly due to folate deficiency. Unlike iron, folate stores are relatively labile and in constant need of replenishment. It is required for nucleic acid synthesis and 1-carbon unit transfer in all cells of the body, particularly growing tissues (Fig. 15.5). Breast milk from a folate-replete mother contains about 25 µg/l of folate and provides enough folate for the normally developing child. However, if preterm babies are not supplemented with oral folate about a third will develop low serum folate levels by 6 weeks of age and 10% develop megaloblastic anemia by 8 weeks of age when the hepatic stores have been depleted. It must be remembered that heating of milk results in a 40% loss of folate and reheating of pasteurized milk causes an 80% loss. In short, all babies are in a precarious state of folate balance during the first weeks of life. Rapid growth, fever, infection, diarrhea or hemolysis all increase folate requirements and may further deplete the stores to the level of clinical deficiency.

Folate is absorbed in the upper jejunum by an active transport mechanism which is impaired in malabsorption states, particularly celiac syndrome. In these disorders the deficiency does not usually produce a frank megaloblastic anemia. Other malabsorptive disorders such as tropical sprue, Crohn's disease, multiple diverticulae of the small intestine and blind loop syndrome will frequently produce folate deficiency.

Increased requirements for folate and subsequent deficiency occur in chronic hemolytic anemias, where low levels can result in pancytopenic 'aplastic crisis'. Various drugs are associated with deficiency of folate, e.g. phenytoin, barbiturates, methotrexate, pentamidine and trimethoprim. Congenital deficiency of the following enzymes can produce deficiency: dihydrofolate reductase, glutamate formiminotransferase, N^5-methyltetrahydrofolate cyclohydrase and homocysteine methyltransferase (see Fig. 15.5).

Clinical features

In infancy this deficiency leads to anorexia, failure to thrive, weakness with liability to infections and gastrointestinal

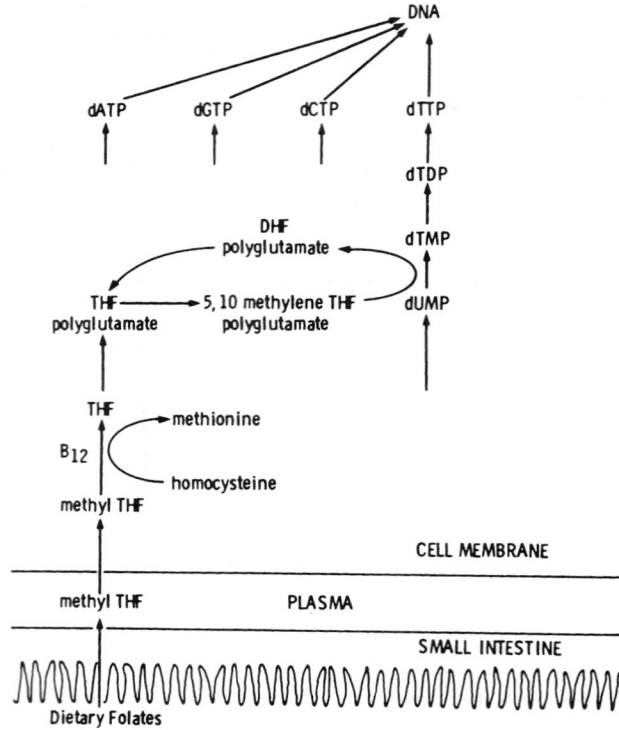

Fig. 15.5 Role of vitamin B_{12} and folate in DNA synthesis. Dietary folates are converted to methyltetrahydrofolate (methyl THF) by the small intestine. Inside marrow and other cells, methyl THF transfers a methyl group to homocysteine to form methionine. Vitamin B_{12} (B_{12}) is needed for this reaction. The THF formed is conjugated to the polyglutamate form possibly after formulation. 5,10-methylene THF polyglutamate is coenzyme for thymidylate synthetase, responsible for the methylation of the pyrimidine deoxyuridine monophosphate (dTMP). The folate coenzyme is oxidized to dihydrofolate (DHF) polyglutamate which is recycled to the fully reduced (THF) form by the enzyme dihydrofolate reductase (DHFR). dTMP is phosphorylated to thymidine triphosphate (dTTP). This is polymerized with the other three deoxyribonucleoside triphosphates, dA (deoxyadenosine) TP, dG (deoxyguanosine) TP, and dC (deoxycytidine) TP to form DNA. (From Hoffbrand 1983 with permission.)

disturbance. In older children, symptoms directly attributable to the anemia may predominate. However, now that most patients with excess requirements usually receive supplements, the most common presentation is a low red cell folate level demonstrated during routine investigation of failure to thrive.

Diagnosis

A presentation with pancytopenia and megaloblastic anemia is rare. In children there is an additional hazard in that iron and folate deficiency (due to malabsorption or poor diet) frequently coexist. This tends to balance out the red cell indices which may thus not demonstrate the typical macrocytosis. A further clue may be given by the presence of hypersegmented neutrophils which can easily be seen in the ordinary blood film. The red cell folate by radioimmunoassay gives an accurate measure of folate stores unaffected by concomitant antibiotic therapy. The normal range is between 160 and 640 µg/ml and the only potential confusing factor is the presence of a high reticulocytosis (e.g. in hemolytic anemia) when a falsely high level occurs. In vitamin B_{12} deficiency there will be a low red cell folate in 60% of cases. Bone marrow examination is rarely required except for the congenital disorders of folate synthesis.

Treatment

Successful treatment, as for all deficiency anemias, depends upon correction of the underlying disorder plus supplementation. A dose of oral folic acid 5 mg daily is usually more than enough and should be continued for several months. Where demand for the folate remains high (e.g. in chronic hemolytic anemias) lifelong supplementation will be necessary. There is often a dramatic clinical response within a few days and a reticulocytosis can be demonstrated by the end of a week.

VITAMIN B_{12} DEFICIENCY

Etiology

The causes of vitamin B_{12} absorption defects are summarized in Table 15.4. Intrinsic factor deficiency is a rare disorder in childhood with less than 50 cases reported. The majority develop a megaloblastic anemia in the first 3 years of life and show an isolated deficiency of intrinsic factor with a strong family history, normal gastric acidity and histology and no antibodies to intrinsic factor or gastric parietal cells (congenital pernicious anemia (PA)). Even fewer cases occur later in childhood or adolescence and these cases of juvenile PA show achlorhydria, gastric atrophy and absent intrinsic factor. As with the disorder in adults, they often show antibodies to parietal cells and intrinsic factor and they also have a high incidence of endocrinopathies. An isolated and specific defect of vitamin B_{12} absorption also occurs and these infants have normal gastric acid and intrinsic factor secretion. The association of this defect with proteinuria was described as a syndrome by Imerslund and Gräsbeck. Other cases of vitamin B_{12} malabsorption may be due to more generalized defects or surgical blind loops etc.

A variety of other very rare defects can lead to vitamin B_{12} deficiency. The fish tapeworm *Diphyllobothrium latum* competes with the host for the vitamin. In the rare event of maternal deficiency either due to PA or veganism, the infant may develop a deficiency if breast-feeding is prolonged. A very rare and treatable cause of mental retardation is caused by congenital deficiency of the carrier protein transcobalamin II (TCII). Finally, methylmalonic aciduria with homocystinuria is associated with vitamin B_{12} deficiency.

Clinical features

There is usually an insidious onset of pallor, lethargy and anorexia. In some cases neurological defects may predominate and occasionally there is a lemon-yellow discoloration of the skin due to excessive breakdown of dysplastic red cells.

Diagnosis

The red cell and white cell changes are indistinguishable from those associated with folate deficiency. The serum vitamin B_{12} level, usually measured by radioimmunoassay, will be low (less than 100 µg/ml) except in the deficiency of TCII. This latter finding occurs because the assay measures mainly vitamin B_{12} bound to TCI. The serum folate level will be high or normal and the red cell folate misleadingly low. The Schilling test is valuable in distinguishing the various absorptive defects (Table 15.4).

Treatment

The usual dose of vitamin B_{12} (as hydroxocobalamin) for children is 100 µg, given intramuscularly, three times a week until the hemoglobin is normal, followed by 100 µg monthly thereafter. It is to be noted that the neurological defects may take longer to recover. In TCII deficiency very large doses are required.

OTHER CAUSES OF MEGALOBLASTIC ANEMIA

The following are all very rare and details can be obtained from standard texts (Chanarin 1990): orotic aciduria, Lesch–Nyhan

Table 15.4 Cause of defects of vitamin B_{12} absorption

| Type of anemia | Age of onset (years) | Familial incidence | Stomach | | | Schilling test | | Serum antibodies | | Associated features |
			Histology	IF	HCl	+ IF	− IF	IF	Parietal cell	
Congenital PA	< 3	Autosomal	Normal	Absent	Normal	↓	Normal	Absent	Absent	None
Juvenile PA	> 10	Absent	Atrophy	Absent	Absent	↓	Normal	Present	Present	Occasional SLE, IgA deficiency, moniliasis, endocrinopathy in siblings
Juvenile PA with endocrinopathies	> 10	Absent	Atrophy	Absent	Absent	↓	Normal	Present	Present	Hypothyroid, hypoparathyroid, Addison's, moniliasis
Specific B_{12} malabsorption	Infancy	Present	Normal	Present	Normal	↓	↓	Absent	Absent	Benign proteinuria and aminoaciduria
Generalized malabsorption	Any age	Absent	Normal	Present	Normal	↓	↓	Absent	Absent	Malabsorption syndromes
Acquired intestinal lesions	Any age	Absent	Normal	Present	Normal	↓	↓	Absent	Absent	Findings of associated disease/surgery

PA = pernicious anaemia, HCl = hydrochloric acid, IF = intrinsic factor.
Adapted from Nathan & Oski (1992) with permission.

syndrome, thiamine responsive, congenital dyserythropoietic anemia Type I.

APLASTIC ANEMIAS

ETIOLOGY AND CLASSIFICATION

Bone marrow failure is usually characterized by reduced production of red cells, platelets and white blood cells with consequent pancytopenia. In certain conditions one or two of these elements are decreased. Neutropenia will be discussed later, but red cell aplasias are dealt with in this section. Decreased numbers of mature blood cells may be due to reduced number or function of their progenitors, e.g. in aplastic anemia or Blackfan–Diamond anemia. In other conditions there is ineffective hemopoiesis with increased numbers of precursors seen in the marrow. Examples of this are the neutropenias and myelodysplastic disorders. A useful classification is shown in Table 15.5.

CONSTITUTIONAL APLASTIC ANEMIAS

Patients with these disorders have a genetic propensity for bone marrow failure presenting at birth or developing later. In the Boston Children's Hospital series of 134 patients with aplastic anemia over 20 years, 30% fell into this category, and half of these had Fanconi's anemia (Alter et al 1978).

Fanconi's anemia

Almost 600 cases have now been described. The disorder can present from birth to 35 years of age although mostly within the first 13 years of life. It is slightly commoner in boys than girls and it may present with aplastic anemia, leukemia, deficiency of white cells or platelets alone, or tumors. Half have typical physical findings especially hyperpigmentation, café-au-lait spots, microsomy, microcephaly, thumb anomalies, hypergenitalia, renal anomalies, ear anomalies, other skeletal anomalies, microphthalmia and mental retardation. This is inherited in an autosomal recessive fashion with a heterozygote frequency of about 1 in 300 people.

It is to be noted that patients often present with thrombocytopenia or leukopenia before pancytopenia, which is usually mild or

Table 15.5 Classification of aplastic anemia

Constitutional aplastic anemia
Fanconi's anemia
Familial marrow dysfunction
Dyskeratosis congenita
Shwachman-Diamond syndrome
Amegakaryocytic thrombocytopenia
Reticular dysgenesis

Acquired aplastic anemia
Drugs, toxins, infections
Idiopathic
Paroxysmal nocturnal hemoglobinuria

Pure red cell aplasias (PRCA)
Congenital (Blackfan-Diamond)
Acquired
Transient erythroblastopenia of childhood (TEC)
Congenital dyserythropoietic anemias (CDA)
Parvovirus induced

moderate at first and becomes severe later. Thus, one must always think of the diagnosis when for instance a young child with dysmorphic features and thrombocytopenia presents. The red cells are usually macrocytic (MCV > 100 fl) and are associated with fetal characteristics, i.e. a raised HbF and increased manifestation of i red cell antigen. The bone marrow may have areas of hypercellularity initially but these disappear as aplasia progresses. The diagnostic test is the identification of breaks, gaps, rearrangements, exchanges and endoreduplications (Fig. 15.6) in stimulated blood lymphocytes, similar to those seen in Bloom's syndrome which is also associated with a high leukemia risk. This is thus one of the DNA repair disorders and all of the features of the disease are presumably related to this defect although the mechanism is not entirely clear.

Treatment of Fanconi's anemia was unsuccessful in the past and a review of 300 cases in 1980 showed a median survival of 5 years, with all patients dead by 25 years from diagnosis. The androgen oxymethalone does produce virilizing and stunting effects but probably prolongs survival. However, the only curative treatment at present is allogeneic bone marrow transplantation which is associated with significant problems of graft-versus-host disease. Patients with DNA repair defects do not tolerate irradiation therapy well and thus highly modified preparative regimens are required. When a histocompatible sibling is not available, transplant from a matched unrelated donor is usually justified although experimental at the present time. As with all cases of pancytopenia, supportive care with red cell and platelet transfusion and antibiotics is essential until more specific therapy can be instituted.

More than 15% of Fanconi's anemia patients develop a malignancy sooner or later. Half will be leukemias of the myeloid variety and the other half are liver and other tumors. Androgens may well exacerbate a genetic risk for liver tumors. Whether or not the risk of malignancy persists after 'curative' bone marrow transplantation remains to be seen.

Familial marrow dysfunction

This is a large group of very rare disorders defined by their associated disorders. The inheritance pattern is of various types and both adults and children are affected. The anomalies seen in association with pancytopenia include: hand anomalies, radial hypoplasia, deafness, vascular occlusions, immune deficiency, ataxia and X-linked lymphoproliferative syndrome. The patients have variable degrees of pancytopenia and red cell macrocytosis with hypocellular bone marrows. Androgens can provide temporary relief from the problems and bone marrow transplantation should be considered.

Dyskeratosis congenita

Ectodermal dysplasia and X-linked recessive inheritance characterize this disorder. Skin manifestations begin during the first decade and progress. Features include reticulated hyperpigmentation of the face, neck and shoulders; dystrophic nails; mucous membrane leukoplakia; epiphora; hyperhidrotic palms and soles; poikiloderma; thin sparse hair; early loss of teeth; esophageal strictures and dysphagia; subnormal intelligence and hypogenitalia. 56% of cases develop hematological manifestations, usually after the dermatological problems at a mean age of 17 years. There may be single cell deficiencies or

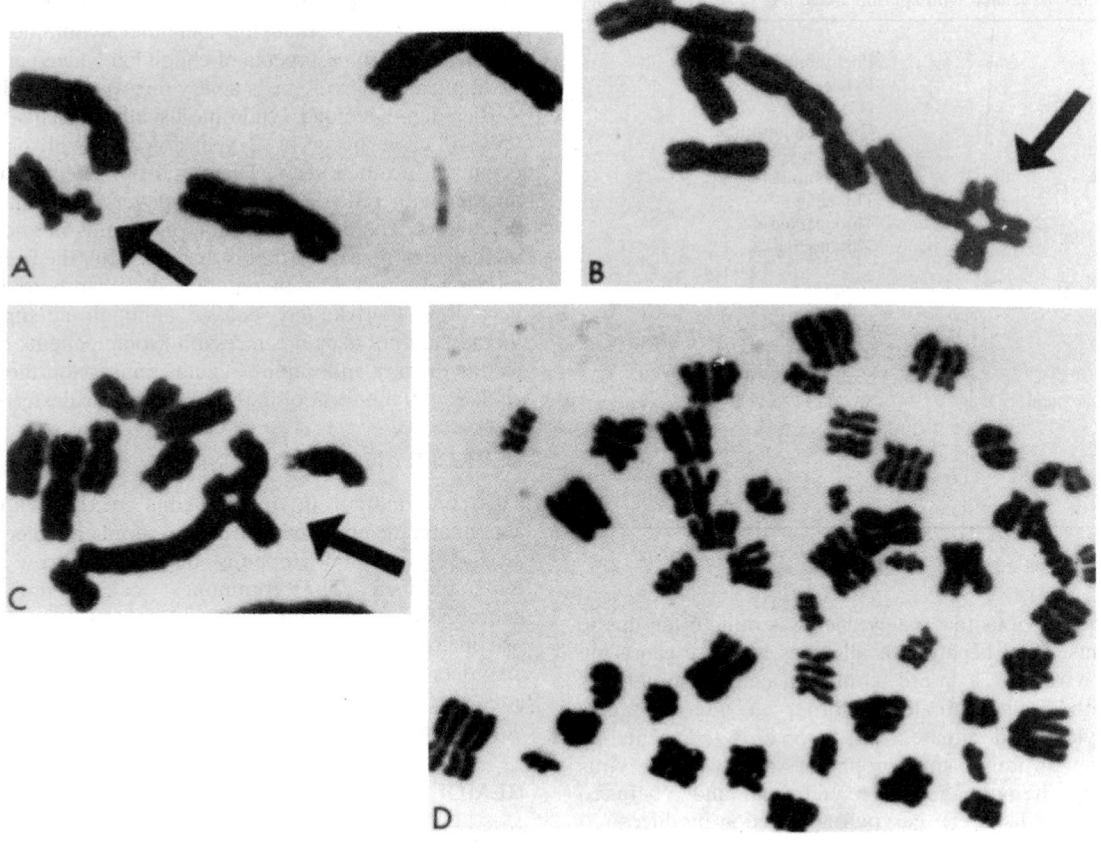

Fig. 15.6   Cytogenetic findings in Fanconi's anemia: (A) chromatid breakage; (B, C) chromatid exchanges, (D) endo-reduplicated metaphase. (From Bloom 1972 with permission.)

pancytopenia and the bone marrow may show hypercellularity at the onset with progressive loss of cellularity. Macrocytosis and elevated HbF levels are found. In reported series the overall death rate is about 33% at 20 years with 45% death rate in those with pancytopenia. 13% of cases develop a malignancy which can be buccal cancer (associated with leukoplakia), stomach cancer and pancreatic tumors. A variety of other rare malignancies have also been reported. Treatment is the same as for other constitutional aplastic anemias and bone marrow transplantation has been carried out successfully although the dermatological and malignant sequelae will probably not be affected.

Shwachman–Diamond syndrome

The features are of pancreatic insufficiency with neutropenia usually detected in infancy. Anemia or thrombocytopenia or both develop in many patients and pancytopenia in a quarter. More males than females are affected and it is probably autosomal recessive. Occasional cases have sideroblastic anemia with vacuolization of marrow precursors. It is to be noted that patients with cartilage–hair hypoplasia also have metaphyseal dysostosis and neutropenia but normal pancreatic function. Laboratory findings are similar to other constitutional aplasias along with the pancreatic function abnormalities. Supportive care and pancreatic enzyme replacement are the mainstay of therapy. As with other constitutional aplasias this is a premalignant condition with a

number of leukemias (both lymphoblastic and myeloid) occurring. The median survival is greater than 20 years but patients do die of infection, bleeding and leukemia.

Amegakaryocytic thrombocytopenia

Patients with this very rare disorder develop thrombocytopenia and pancytopenia later in life. Most cases are in males and some are of subnormal intelligence with neurological abnormalities. The marrow shows absence of megakaryocytes and later on generalized hypoplasia. Median survival is only 3 years and there is again a predisposition to leukemia.

Reticular dysgenesis

This is a rare absence of granulocytes and lymphocytes with absent cellular and humoral immunity. Survival is short without an allogeneic bone marrow transplant.

ACQUIRED APLASTIC ANEMIA

Most cases of aplastic anemia in children are of unknown cause. Table 15.6 lists those agents which may be associated with aplastic anemia. In many cases it is not possible to be certain about their etiologic role. Withdrawal of these agents may lead to improvement in the pancytopenia.

Table 15.6 Agents associated with aplastic anaemia

Drugs	
Acetazolamide	Phenylbutazone
Amodiaquine	Pyrimethamine
Arsenicals	Quinacrine
Barbiturates	Quinidine, quinine
Chloramphenicol	Streptomycin
Chlordiazepoxide	Sulfonamides
Cimetidine	Thiazides
Colchicine	Thiocyanate
Hydantoins	Thiouracils
Meprobamate	
Phenothiazines	
Insecticides	*Solvents*
Chlordane	Benzene
DDT	Carbon tetrachloride
Gamma benzene hexachloride	Stoddarts solvent
Parathione	Glues
	Toluene
Radiation	
Trinitrotoluene	

Adapted from Alter et al (1978).

It is becoming obvious that pancytopenia is quite often due to infectious agents. Viral hepatitis of all types is a rare cause but Epstein–Barr virus is a more common cause, sometimes associated with a disseminated disorder in which macrophages/histiocytes predominate. This probably represents an immune defect with failure to appropriately deal with the virus (viral-associated hemophagocytic syndrome and X-linked lymphoproliferative disorder). Parvovirus infection produces red cell aplasia usually in patients with hemolytic anemia but other cell lines can be affected.

Paroxysmal nocturnal hemoglobinuria is a disorder of red cells, white cells and platelets in which these cells fix excessive amounts of complement with consequent cell lysis. Pancytopenia occurs in some cases and bone marrow transplantation has provided apparent cures.

Decisions about management of patients with aplastic anemia are made difficult by problems of analysis of the various reported trials and studies of therapy (Young & Barrett 1995). The major difficulty is in the definition of 'aplastic anemia' and relating this to the risks of morbidity and mortality from infection and bleeding balanced against the risks of the potential treatments. If severe aplastic anemia (defined as pancytopenia with neutrophils $< 0.5 \times 10^9/l$, platelets $< 10 \times 10^9/l$ and reticulocytes $< 1\%$, and documented bone marrow hypocellularity) is considered in children there is good evidence that the treatment of choice is allogeneic bone marrow transplantation from a matched sibling donor. This gives actuarial survivals of 60–80% at 5 years, possibly higher in children. If a sibling donor is not available the most appropriate treatment is intensive immunosuppression using antilymphocyte globulin combined with cyclosporine. This type of treatment results in responses in over two-thirds of patients but there is a higher relapse rate compared with bone marrow transplantation (Bacigalupo et al 1995, Rosenfeld et al 1995).

The use of unrelated donor bone marrow transplants is not yet of proven value.

PURE RED CELL APLASIA

In the absence of infection (often due to parvovirus) and folate deficiency the commonest causes of red cell aplasia are the congenital variety, Blackfan–Diamond syndrome, and cases of transient erythroblastopenia of childhood where parvovirus cannot be implicated. Thymoma is a very rare association in children.

Blackfan–Diamond syndrome usually presents in infancy and 95% of cases occur by 2 years of age, with occasional cases occurring up to 6 years. Diagnosis is made by the presence of anemia with reticulocytopenia and very few marrow erythroid precursors. The early institution of steroids is said to reduce the incidence of resistance to this therapy. After the first few weeks of moderately high dose therapy, the dose can be reduced, often to very low alternate-day dosage although attempts to remove therapy are not usually successful. Some patients do not respond to this therapy and require regular transfusion therapy with iron chelation in the form of daily subcutaneous desferrioxamine.

LEUKOERYTHROBLASTOSIS

This is a condition in which anemia coexists with erythroblasts and immature granulocytes in the peripheral blood. There may also be thrombocytopenia due to marrow invasion or hypersplenism. The commonest causes are tumors, e.g. neuroblastoma, infections, e.g. tuberculosis, storage disorders and osteopetrosis. This picture can also exist in the myeloproliferative disorders and leukemias (see below). Treatment consists of control of the underlying disorder and in osteopetrosis this implies bone marrow transplantation.

HEMOLYTIC ANEMIAS

GENERAL FEATURES

The hemolytic anemias are those which result from an excessive rate of red cell destruction. The marrow is capable of compensating for this loss by increasing its erythrocyte production 6- or 8-fold before anemia develops. The level of hemoglobin is a balance of the increased red cell destruction and the ability of the bone marrow to compensate. Red cell survival is reduced from a mean of 120 days to only a few days in severe cases. A simplified classification of causes is shown in Table 15.7. In most cases the excessive red cell destruction leads to a raised blood unconjugated bilirubin and urine urobilinogen. Where intravascular hemolysis occurs the carrier protein for hemoglobin is saturated resulting in a reduction in free plasma haptoglobin, hemoglobinuria and the detection of free hemoglobin in the plasma. A proportion of the hemoglobin released is oxidized to the trivalent iron form, released from the cell and binds to plasma albumin, forming methemalbumin which is readily detectable. Hemosiderinuria also occurs and is particularly useful in the diagnosis of paroxysmal nocturnal hemoglobinuria. The bone marrow shows an excess of normal marrow which is only grossly dysplastic in the congenital dyserythropoietic anemias.

The patient with hemolysis may show pale mucous membranes, jaundice which is usually mild and can fluctuate, and splenomegaly. In some situations the fluctuating course can be very pronounced, suggesting some exacerbating factor such as intercurrent infection in hereditary spherocytosis or drugs in G6PD deficiency. Pigment gallstones may complicate the disorder and hemolytic anemia should always be considered when they present in childhood. Aplastic crises may occur, usually precipitated by parvovirus infection or folate deficiency, both of which are characterized by 'switching off' of erythropoiesis,

Table 15.7   Causes of hemolytic anemia

	Defect	Disease
Hereditary	Membrane	Hereditary spherocytosis
		Hereditary elliptocytosis
	Metabolism	Embden-Meyerhof pathway, e.g. G6PD and pyruvate kinase
	Hemoglobin	1. Abnormal – HbS, HbC, unstable hemoglobin
		2. Defective synthesis – thalassemias
Acquired	Immune	Autoimmune hemolytic anemia, Evans' syndrome.
		Isoimmune – hemolytic disease of the newborn and transfusion reactions
		Drugs, e.g. methyldopa
	Red cell destruction	Microangiopathic – HUS and TTP
		Heart valves, patches' etc.
	Hypersplenism	
	Secondary	Renal disease, liver disease
	Miscellaneous	Drugs, toxins, infections, chemicals, burns

HUS = hemolytic uremic syndrome,
TTP = thrombotic thrombocytopenic purpura.
Modified from Hoffbrand & Pettit (1993) with permission.

producing reticulocytopenia and anemia. In folate deficiency there will be a megaloblastic picture and for this reason all children with hemolysis are treated with folate throughout the period of disease activity.

HEREDITARY HEMOLYTIC ANEMIAS

Membrane defects

Hereditary spherocytosis (HS)

This is the commonest hereditary hemolytic anemia in north Europeans. The primary defect is complex and involves the spectrin structural protein in the red cell membrane. It is a dominantly inherited disorder with variable expression and investigation of other family members may identify asymptomatic persons who may have a mild phenotype. In the blood the typical finding is of multiple small dense cells termed microspherocytes. The marrow produces normally shaped biconcave cells and progressive loss of membrane results in the spherical shape and their increased osmotic fragility (Figs 15.7 and 15.8).

The anemia is very variable in severity and can present at any time between infancy and old age. The jaundice fluctuates and splenomegaly and gallstones frequently occur. The diagnostic tests are appearances of the blood film and osmotic fragility curve. It is necessary to perform the osmotic fragility (OF) test with 24-h incubation in order to detect the abnormality in some cases, especially in the very young.

Splenectomy is not indicated in all cases of hereditary spherocytosis and should be avoided in all but the most severe cases during the first 10 years of life when the risk of postsplenectomy sepsis is highest. The recommendations for management of patients undergoing splenectomy are continually being revised as the risks of infection with encapsulated bacteria appear to be lifelong. Currently patients should be immunized with pneumococcal, haemophilus and meningococcal vaccines before splenectomy to allow maximal response. It is suggested that oral penicillin or amoxicillin should be given on a long-term basis although realistically there are likely to be problems with compliance. Patients should be issued with a medical card indicating they have had a splenectomy and warned about the importance of early reporting of symptoms of infection.

Attitudes towards splenectomy have changed and most patients are followed to see whether any evidence of failure to thrive, gallstones or other clinical abnormalities ensue. It is by no means certain that a blanket approach to this problem is the best one and many fully informed parents will not accept the small risk of

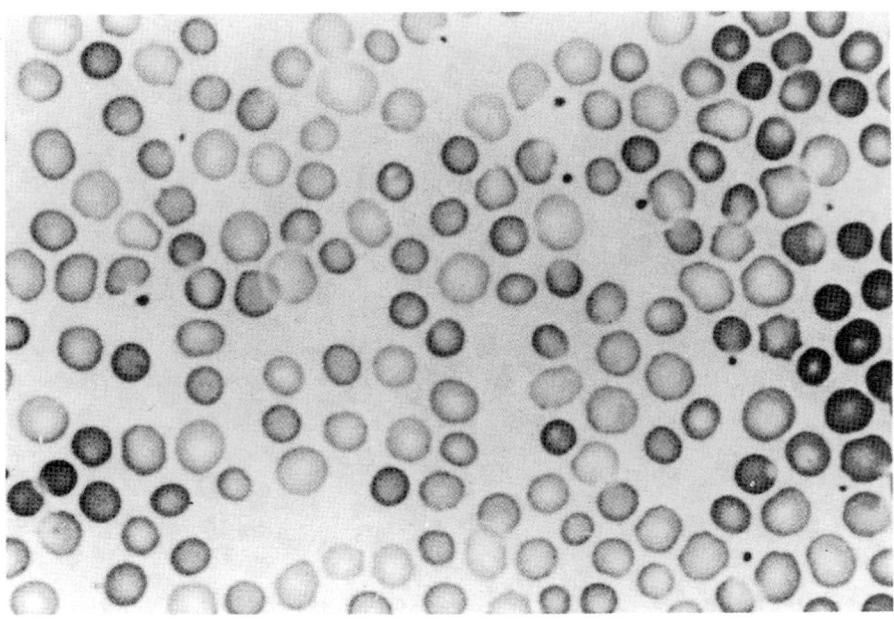

Fig. 15.7   The peripheral blood film in hereditary spherocytosis. The spherocytes are densely staining and of small diameter. (From Hoffbrand & Pettit 1993 with permission.)

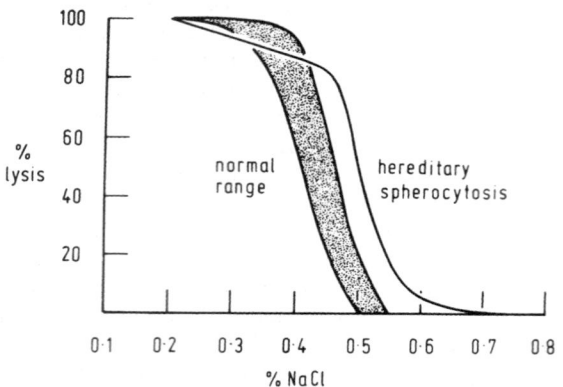

Fig. 15.8   The osmotic fragility curve in hereditary spherocytosis. The curve is shifted to the right of the (shaded) normal range, but a tail of more resistant cells (reticulocytes) is also present. (From Hoffbrand & Pettit 1984 with permission.)

surgery when they are aware of asymptomatic cases diagnosed very late in life. Careful follow-up and balancing of risks is required. Clinical acumen is still important in this and other hematological disorders. When the operation is performed the biliary tree should be assessed for the presence of gallstones and appropriate action taken. All cases probably respond to splenectomy and failure to do so indicates a wrong diagnosis and the need for detailed red cell membrane studies.

Hereditary elliptocytosis (HE)

This common disorder is usually inherited as an autosomal dominant trait but rare homozygous variants have been described in which chronic severe hemolysis occurs. The usual blood picture is shown in Figure 15.9 and consists of many cells which are neither elliptical nor oval although they are closer to the latter

shape than the former. Most cases are asymptomatic or have very mild chronic hemolysis requiring no further therapy. In the rare severe homozygous cases splenectomy usually provides symptomatic improvement.

Hereditary stomatocytosis

A very rare and moderately severe hemolytic anemia has been described in which the red cells show central pallor similar to a mouth or stoma. However, it must be remembered that this can be a variant of normal especially in Mediterranean peoples and can be drug induced.

Red cell enzyme defects

Figure 15.10 shows the pathways of glucose metabolism and energy production in the red cell. Pure fetal blood from the mid-trimester obtained at fetoscopy is now available, has allowed the establishment of normal values (Lestas et al 1982) and should allow the prenatal detection of severe enzyme deficiencies, e.g. triose phosphate isomerase. Deficiencies of almost all of the enzymes involved in the Embden–Meyerhof pathway and hexose monophosphate shunt can be associated with significant hemolysis. This is also true of the enzymes of ATP metabolism, pyrimidine 5'-nucleotidase and adenosine deaminase and also of superoxide dysmutase deficiency. This section will deal with the most common of these disorders.

Glucose-6-phosphate dehydrogenase (G6PD) deficiency

The effect of this enzyme is to maintain glutathione in its reduced state and consequently it is one of the vital mechanisms for protecting red cell membranes from oxidant stress. Thus, enzyme deficiency is associated with hemolysis when such a stress is produced usually by certain drugs or chemicals (Table 15.8). The gene for G6PD is on the X chromosome and many different

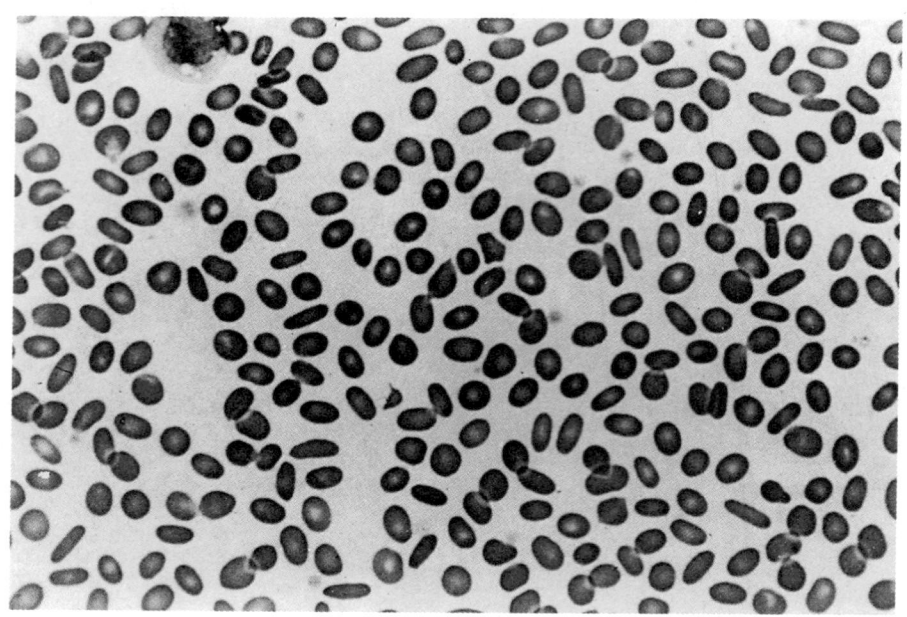

Fig. 15.9   Typical blood film appearances of hereditary elliptocytosis.

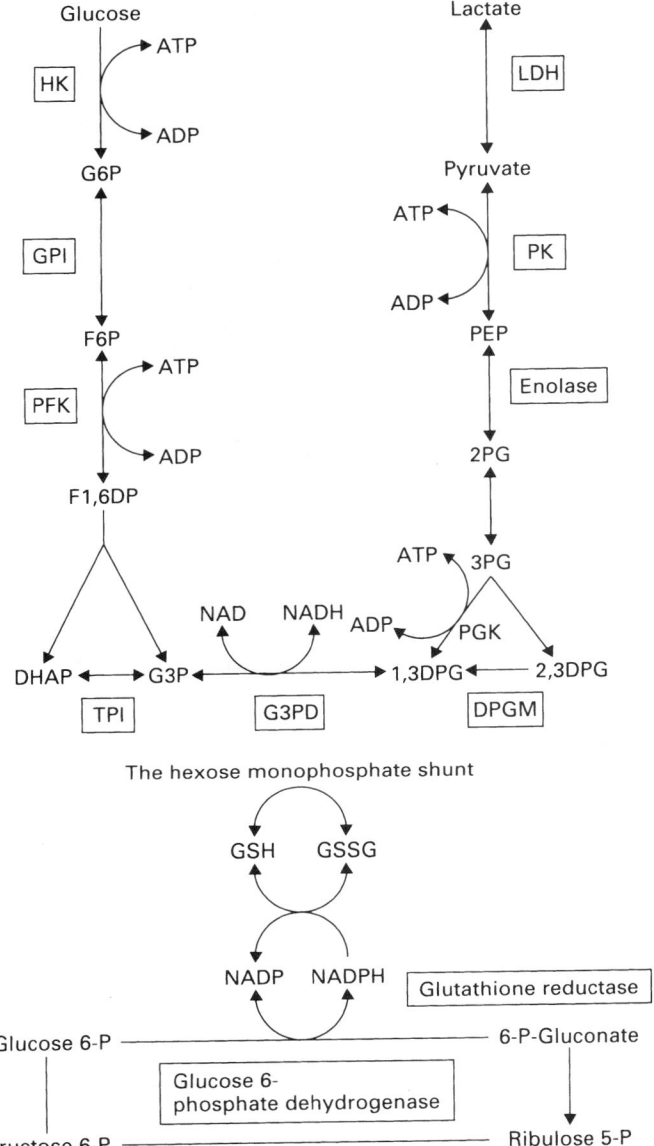

Fig. 15.10 The Embden–Meyerhof pathway and hexose monophosphate shunt. Enzymes: HK = hexokinase, GPI = glucose phosphate isomerase, PFK = phosphofructokinase, TPI = triose phosphate isomerase, G3PD = glucose 3-phosphate dehydrogenase, PGK = phosphoglycerate kinase, DPGM = 2,3-diphosphoglycerate mutase, PK = pyruvate kinase, LDH = lactate dehydrogenase. Intermediates: G6P = glucose 6-P, F6P = fructose 6-P, F1,6DP = fructose 1,6 di-P, 3PG = 3-P glycerate, 1,3DPG = 1,3-diphosphoglycerate, G3P = glyceraldehyde 3-P, PEP = phosphoenolpyruvate, DHAP = dihydroxyacetone P.

mutants of G6PD occur in different racial groups, all carried on the X chromosome. They differ according to enzyme activity, electrophoretic mobility, etc. The racial incidence varies greatly from extreme rarity in northern Europeans through 1–35% in different Mediterranean races, up to 10% in African Negroes. Deficiency leads to a number of syndromes; neonatal jaundice is more common in oriental male babies and this is particularly so if infections or acidosis occur or if oxidant drugs are given to the mother in late pregnancy or to the neonate. Infections can precipitate hemolysis at all ages and diabetic ketoacidosis has also

Table 15.8 Drugs and chemicals associated with hemolysis in G6PD deficient subjects

Group	Drugs
Antimalarials	Primaquine, pamaquine, quinacrine, quinine
Sulfonamides	Sulfapyridine, sulfisoxazole, salicylazosulfapyridine
Nitrofurans	Nitrofurantoin, furaltadone
Analgesics and related compounds	Acetylsalicylic acid, para-aminosalicylic acid
Miscellaneous	Synthetic water-soluble vitamin K analogues, chloramphenicol, phenylhydrazine, naphthalene, aniline dyes, nalidixic acid

been reported to do so. Favism produces severe hemolysis, is related to eating cooked broad beans and is commonest in Mediterraneans and in the Middle East although it does occur in Orientals and Europeans. Cases of chronic hemolysis in northern European races have also been described.

When hemolytic crises do occur they vary in severity and degree of fulminant onset. Favism is associated with the most explosive course and all the classical signs of intravascular hemolysis. A typical sign is the dramatic darkening of the urine with hemoglobin and urobilinogen to produce so-called 'Coca-Cola' urine. This may lead to renal dysfunction which can be severe. Diagnosis of the disorder depends on an assay for the enzyme but it must be remembered that reticulocytes nearly always have higher levels of all red cell enzymes and thus caution must be observed in interpretation during hemolytic crises. It is as well to think before ordering this investigation as it is almost useless following recent blood transfusion and the likelihood of finding abnormal levels in northern European girls is vanishingly small. Despite these obvious points many unnecessary requests are made.

Exchange transfusion therapy may be required during the neonatal period. At other times all that is necessary is to be aware of the problem in appropriate ethnic groups and thereafter to avoid the precipitating factors. Patients should be schooled in the hazards and usually far too little time is spent on this most important aspect of their care. If a crisis does occur then supportive care is all that is possible.

Pyruvate kinase (PK) deficiency

Autosomal recessive inheritance characterizes this deficiency which produces widely variable and persistent hemolysis. Neonatal jaundice does occur and at other times infection can precipitate more severe hemolysis. Parvovirus infection can, as in other red cell enzyme deficiencies, produce dramatic aplastic crises. Splenomegaly is usually present. Drugs do not precipitate crises.

The blood film in PK deficiency does not have any specific diagnostic features although irregularly contracted cells are seen especially after splenectomy. Diagnosis depends on measurement of the enzyme level which must be carefully corrected for the usually very high reticulocytosis. Unfortunately some poorly functioning variants of PK can produce normal assay results; this can be sorted out by measurement of the intermediate products of the Embden–Meyerhof pathway in order to demonstrate a block at the appropriate point.

Because of its position in the energy pathway, PK deficiency causes a rise in 2,3-DPG levels and thus a shift to the right in the oxygen dissociation curve and a consequent improvement in oxygen availability. For this reason, patients with PK deficiency can tolerate very low hemoglobin levels and conversely hexokinase-deficient patients may require blood transfusion at relatively high hemoglobin levels. Thus, it is very important not to transfuse PK-deficient patients unless they are clinically unwell, failing to thrive or are otherwise genuinely symptomatic. Many patients are transfused unnecessarily on the basis of a perfectly acceptable hemoglobin level of about 5–6 g/dl. However, occasional patients do require regular transfusions with iron chelation. In these children, splenectomy usually produces a beneficial reduction or abolition of the need for blood transfusion and it is part of the mythology of medicine that it is not effective.

Hemoglobinopathies and thalassemia

Etiology

Hemoglobin is composed of two alpha globin chains and two nonalpha globin chains; Table 15.9 shows the globin chain constitution of normal and abnormal hemoglobins. Hemoglobinopathy results from the production of an abnormal globin chain with the pathological forms of adult hemoglobin resulting from the substitution of a single amino acid, e.g. valine for glutamine in position 6 of the β chain for HbS. The substitution may occur in the β chain as in HbI, and other β chain variants are HbC and E.

Thalassemia results from impaired synthesis of either normal α chains or normal β chains, referred to as α- and β-thalassemia, respectively.

The type of globin chain affected by either type of disorder is important because HbF contains α and γ chains and is thus only affected by α chain or γ chain disorders. Disorders affecting α and, in particular, β chains thus tend to manifest later in life but may be seen at birth or in utero, e.g. the homozygous form of α-thalassemia causes fatal hydrops fetalis due to cardiac failure. The β chain disorders do not present until HbF production reduces in the early postnatal period. Similarly, γ chain variants are only manifest when HbF is in action.

Inheritance

The polypeptide chain structure is determined by a pair of autosomal allelomorphic genes. The β, γ, δ and ϵ chains are carried on chromosome 11 and the α chain types are on chromosome 16. Each type of hemoglobinopathy may exist in the heterozygous or homozygous state, e.g. sickle trait and sickle cell disease. The former usually has an intermediate severity of phenotypic expression. Since different hemoglobinopathy genes for the same chain are allelomorphic, mixed hemoglobinopathies such as HbS and C can occur. When both abnormalities affect the same chain, such as β-HbSC, the severity is greater than when they affect different chains. Thalassemia genes are also allelomorphic with the hemoglobinopathy genes; hence mixed hemoglobin substitution variants/thalassemias do occur, e.g. HbE/thal, HbS/thal (Table 15.10). The combination may produce a much more severe anemia than for instance HbE homozygous state. An additional complication occurs in the α-thalassemias where two sets of allelomorphic genes come into play. The most severe form (Bart's hydrops) consists of a lack of four genes, HbH disease is a deficiency of three and the two types of trait are due to lack of two or one genes.

Geographical distribution and incidence (Fig. 15.11)

The main reservoir of HbS is tropical Africa and Madagascar where the incidence may be as high as 40%. It is also relatively common in Turkey, Greece and other Mediterranean countries including North Africa. The distribution in the Old World is similar to that of malignant tertian malaria. Heterozygotes for HbS have some protection against the worst ravages of falciparum malaria and this more than compensates in genetic terms for the mortality of the HbSS state. Thus persistence of the gene probably occurred and produced what is grandly called a 'balanced polymorphism'. The main occurrence of HbC is in West Africa, of HbD in western India and HbE in Burma and Thailand. β-thalassemia occurs characteristically among races bordering on the Mediterranean (*thalas* = inland sea). The incidence reaches 20% in Turkey and Greece, 10% in Sicily and the Po delta and 4% in southern Italy. There is also a high incidence in Burma and Thailand and a lower incidence in China, India and central Africa. α-thalassemia has the reverse distribution compared with the β form since its main occurrence is in the Far East and in Negroes, with a low incidence in Mediterraneans.

Pathogenesis of the clinical features

In many cases this is imperfectly understood. In the thalassemias there is impaired globin chain production of one type with a consequent excess of the other. In β-thalassemia major the excess of α chains is deposited in the red cell and may cause damage to the membrane and lysis. The primary defect is the gene mutation in both α- and β-thalassemia. Consequent upon these primary and secondary events there is a feedback inhibition of hemoglobin synthesis and an accumulation of intracellular iron. Thus

Table 15.9   Constitution of normal and abnormal hemoglobins

Hemoglobin containing normal α, β, γ or δ chains	
Normal adult hemoglobins	
Hb A	$\alpha_2 + \beta_2$
Hb A2	$\alpha_2 + \delta_2$
Normal fetal hemoglobins	
Hb F	$\alpha_2 + \gamma_2$
Hb Barts	γ_4
Hb H	β_4
Normal embryonic hemoglobins	
Hb Gower 1	ϵ_4
Hb Gower 2	$\zeta_2 + \epsilon_2$
Hb Portland	$\zeta_2 + \gamma_2$

Abnormal hemoglobins due to β chain substitutions
C, D, E, G, J, N, O, P, S M Saskatoon, M Milwaukee

Abnormal hemoglobins due to α chain substitutions
D_a ST Louis, I, K, Q, Hopkins No. 2, Norfolk, M Boston

Abnormal hemoglobins due to γ chain substitutions
Hb F Alexandra, F Aegina, F Rome, F Texas

Abnormal hemoglobins due to δ chain substitutions
Hb Lepore, Flatbush, Sphakia

The subscript numeral indicates the number of such chains present.
The suffix A indicates that the chain is that of the normal adult variety.

Table 15.10   Hemoglobin types in different hemoglobinopathies and thalassemia

Disease	Genetic status	Hemoglobin types present	Other tests
Sickle cell disease	S/S	S + F	Sickling
Sickle cell trait	S/A	S + A	Sickling
Hb C disease	C/C	C	
Hb C trait	C/A	C + A	
Hb D disease	D/D	D	
Hb E disease	E/E	E + F	
Sickle cell – Hb C disease	S/C	S + C + F	Sickling
β-thalassemia major	Thβ/Thβ	$F + A_2 \pm A$	Kleihauer
β-thalassemia minor	Thβ/A	$A_2 + A \pm F$	
α-thalassemia	Th/A	H + A (+ Hb Barts at birth)	Inclusion bodies
Sickle cell – thalassemia	S/Thβ	$S + F \pm A$	Sickling
Hb C – β-thalassemia	C/Thβ	$C + A \pm F$	
Hb E – β-thalassemia	E/Thβ	E + F + A	Sickling

hemoglobin is not made and the cells become hypochromic and 'ghost-like' with a shortened survival.

Additional factors accentuate the anemia in other hemoglobinopathies. The high intracellular concentration of HbS in sickle cell disease causes intermolecular aggregation in the reduced state and consequent severe distortion of the red cell envelope to form the sickled cell. This leads to intravascular red cell aggregation and vascular obstruction in tissues such as spleen or bones during sickling. The degree of anemia is less marked in the other hemoglobinopathies, occurring in decreasing order of severity as follows: HbS, C, E, D. The effect of a double 'dose' of abnormal hemoglobin such as SC, or combination with the thalassemia gene such as S/thal or E/thal, increases the degree of hematological abnormality.

Hemoglobins with an amino acid substitution adjacent to the heme plate, e.g. Hb Zurich and Hb Köln, result in increased sensitivity of the heme grouping to oxidative damage from drugs, producing a Heinz body hemolytic anemia. Other, relatively unstable hemoglobins are designated HbM since they show an increased liability to methemoglobin formation. Certain hemoglobins of which Hb Chesapeake is an example, result in familial polycythemia and should be looked for as the potential

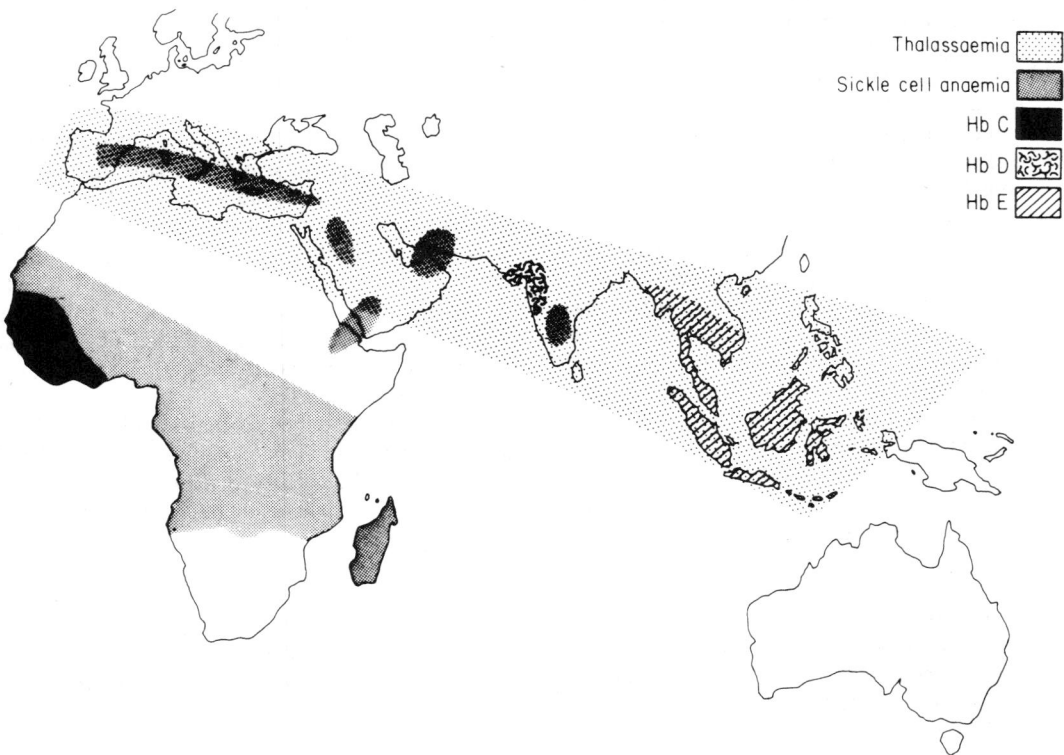

Fig. 15.11   The geographical distribution of the thalassemias and more common inherited structural hemoglobin abnormalities. (From Hoffbrand & Pettit 1993 with permission.)

cause of this disorder. An amino acid substitution near the heme grouping causes an abnormally high oxygen affinity with chronic tissue anoxia similar to that producing high altitude polycythemia. Finally, several variants such as HbG San Jose produce no clinical or hematological abnormality.

Clinical manifestation

Sickle cell disease presents after the age of 6 months. There is a high mortality in the first 5 years of life, as high as 25% in some series. The cause is often infection due to *Pneumococcus*, *Haemophilus* or *Salmonella* with bacteremia, osteomyelitis or meningitis. The mortality has been reduced by the use of oral penicillin prophylaxis along with pneumococcal and *H. influenzae* vaccines. Most importantly, the family must be educated from the outset to detect signs and symptoms of infection including abdominal examination for splenomegaly, which is present in the dangerous sequestration crisis. This latter is characterized by signs of infection, rapid splenic enlargement and a dramatic fall in hemoglobin. Aplastic crises with reticulocytopenia occur usually as a consequence of parvovirus infection. Aplastic crises due to folate deficiency are rare now that routine supplementation is used. Painful crises can affect joints, back, long bones or abdomen and are frequently associated with fever. Infection, dehydration and acidosis are all potential precipitating factors. In younger children, pain and swelling of the short bones of the hands and feet due to infarction cause the characteristic hand–foot syndrome (Fig. 15.12). Children with sickle cell disease are susceptible to osteomyelitis which may be due to the usual bone-infecting organisms or to *Salmonella* or *H. influenzae*. Infarction may be very difficult to differentiate from infection and pyrexia does not help. A high white cell count may be indicative but one usually has to rely on clinical acumen and be particularly aware that abdominal pain mimics appendicitis and that unnecessary laparotomies have been carried out in the past.

Hemoglobin SC disease is different from HbSS in that it is associated with less infection and painful crises and has better survival. However, it is associated with avascular necrosis of the femoral head and retinal vascular problems (especially during pregnancy). Individuals with HbSA or sickle trait usually have no specific problems so long as they are maintained with good oxygenation, e.g. during anesthesia. For this reason, sickle cell screening must be carried out routinely in any child from the appropriate ethnic background. They may also have mild renal tubular derangement and hyposthenuria. The latter defect is a consistent problem in HbSS patients and persistent enuresis is a real difficulty.

β-thalassemia major patients usually present during the first year of life with pallor and failure to thrive. There is evidence that the later they present the better and this has important connotations for management because the late-presenting cases may be milder (thalassemia intermedia) and may not require frequent transfusion. Splenomegaly is always present due to extramedullary hemopoiesis. In the past, untreated thalassemia was associated with severe bone problems (see Fig. 15.13). These changes are due to chronic tissue hypoxia leading to stimulation of the bone marrow to expand in the skull and other bones. Nowadays, these problems may be delayed by hypertransfusion programs with iron chelation but we are still likely eventually to see the problems of 'bronzed diabetes', multiple endocrinopathies, liver cirrhosis and cardiac failure. Long follow-up is necessary to determine the incidence of these features with modern treatment.

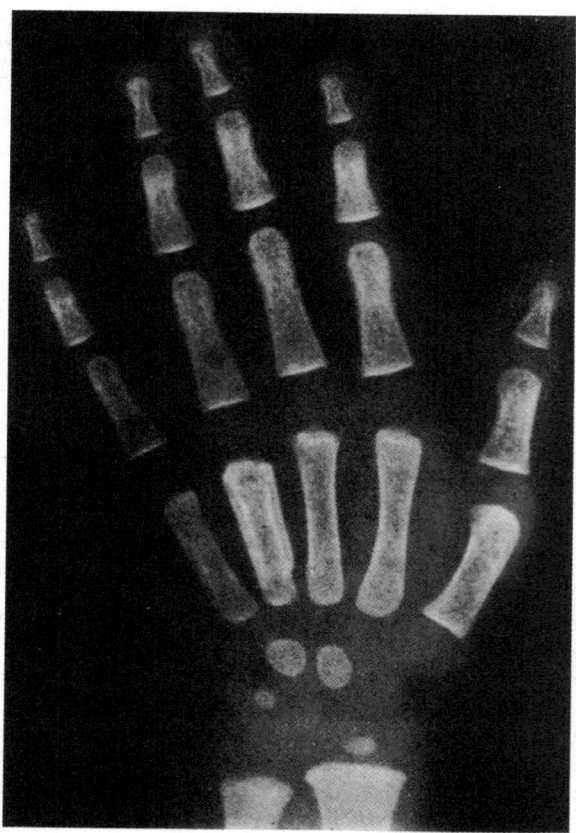

Fig. 15.12 Hemoglobinopathy. Hand showing dactylitis of fourth metacarpal with extensive subperiosteal new bone formation widening shaft – infarction with or without infection. Nigerian baby with homozygous sickle cell disease showing 'hand–foot' syndrome with symmetrical changes in fourth metacarpals and first metatarsals.

Meanwhile, all children with hemoglobinopathy require regular careful follow-up with eye checks (for vascular problems in HbSC and desferrioxamine-induced problems), audiometry (for desferrioxamine-induced hearing defects), and to detect endocrine deficits, cardiac dysfunction, gallstones, liver dysfunction and abnormalities of growth. An integral part of the management of all of these cases is patient and parent education with regard to the genetic aspects of the disease in particular. Antenatal diagnosis is available in most instances and national referral centers have been set up in most countries.

As already described, α-thalassemia is a 'four-gene' disorder and lack of all four is incompatible with life – Bart's hydrops. The three-gene defect, HbH disease, is of varying severity and children may be transfusion dependent.

Hemoglobins of the M group (methemoglobins) produce problems following drug exposure, especially to agents such as sulfonamides, aniline dyes and nitrates. In some cases there is cyanosis from birth which can prove disfiguring. The high affinity hemoglobins produce problems with polycythemia and most cases require regular venesection to reduce the risk of thrombosis.

Diagnosis

Most children with significant hemoglobinopathy are anemic with a blood reticulocytosis. The diagnosis is usually made by

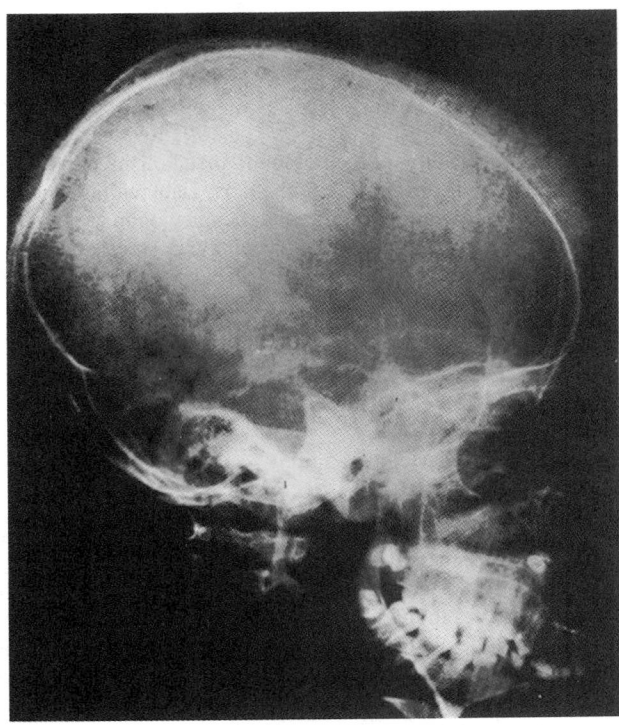

Fig. 15.13 β-Thalassemia major. Skull showing widening of diploic space and atrophy of outer table with radial striation giving 'hair-on-end' appearance associated with chronic marrow hyperplasia.

combination of the hemoglobin and red cell indices along with hemoglobin electrophoresis. A Heinz body and unstable hemoglobin preparation may assist. It is important to recognize that the diagnosis of thalassemia major is usually only clinched by demonstrating the carrier state in both parents and correcting possible concomitant severe folate deficiency. The diagnosis of thalassemia intermedia states depends upon *clinical* severity and not the measurement of globin chain levels of production. Antenatal diagnosis depends upon the application of gene probes, which may be oligonucleotide in nature, to chorionic villus samples and occasionally upon the measurement of globin chain synthesis rates in fetal blood samples.

Treatment

Management of sickle cell disease depends at first upon the early institution of penicillin prophylaxis and parental education about sequestration and other crises, the role of infection in precipitating crises and the importance of adequate hydration in limiting the effects of a crisis. Most painful crises are managed with copious intravenous fluids and, for example, subcutaneous diamorphine. Too often inadequate analgesia has been used. Patients who do not respond to simple analgesia and increased oral fluids at home require hospital admission and intensive treatment. It is not necessary to treat every patient in crisis with antibiotics even though they are usually pyrexial. However, vigilance for infections such as mycoplasma pneumonia or salmonella osteomyelitis is vital. Severe problems such as intracerebral sickling and the chest syndrome require exchange transfusion urgently to reduce the HbS level to values equivalent to that in

sickle trait (20–30% approximately). Care must be taken in preparing a patient with sickle cell disease for surgery and exchange transfusion may be indicated. Recently the use of hydroxyurea has been evaluated in patients with sickle cell disease and has been shown to reduce the incidence of painful crises by increasing the production of HbF (Charache et al 1995). Further work is required with longer follow-up to assess the effects of this cytotoxic agent on the rest of bone marrow function.

Patients with β-thalassemia major require to be on regular transfusion regimens which keep their hemoglobin level over 11 g/dl. The aim of this regime is to maintain tissue oxygenation and reduce stimulation of bone marrow activity, thus limiting the skeletal abnormalities. This results in a considerable iron load; thus at the same time iron chelation with daily subcutaneous desferrioxamine and oral vitamin C should be instituted, noting that compliance with this protocol is a major problem (Brittenham et al 1994). If desferrioxamine is used early in a transfusion regime and proportional to the transfusion iron load it has been shown to reduce the risk of impaired glucose tolerance, overt diabetes mellitus, cardiac disease and death (Olivieri et al 1994). The search for an effective oral iron chelating agent is on-going and trials of deferiprone have shown activity but with neutropenia as a significant side-effect (Olivieri et al 1995). Splenectomy is indicated at a stage dictated by age and transfusion requirement with the operation being indicated when transfusion of packed red cells exceeds 180–200 ml/kg/year. After splenectomy certain patients with thalassemia intermedia require very infrequent transfusions; the need for these can be judged by growth patterns and general health and not just by the hemoglobin level. Patients with thalassemia are susceptible to certain infections such as *Yersinia enterocolitica* and the usual precautions against postsplenectomy sepsis must of course be observed.

Bone marrow transplantation is potentially curative in thalassemia major. In the series reported from Italy (Lucarelli et al 1995) risk factors for the outcome for bone marrow transplantation were hepatomegaly, liver fibrosis and quality of iron chelation treatment. In 'Class I' patients who lacked any risk factors the overall survival was 96% at 10–11 years with an event-free survival of 92%, whereas 'Class III' patients with all three risk factors had an overall survival of 76% with an event-free survival of 53% at 10–11 years because of increased transplant-related morbidity and mortality. These results suggest that if bone marrow transplantation is to be undertaken it should be in young children before there has been significant transfusion iron overload.

ACQUIRED HEMOLYTIC ANEMIAS

Unlike the inherited hemolytic anemias caused by abnormalities intrinsic to the red cells, the great majority of acquired abnormalities are caused by factors affecting the environment extrinsic to the red cells. Other than hemolytic disease of the newborn this type of anemia is rare in children.

Autoimmune hemolytic anemias (AIHA)

In this disorder, autoantibodies to red cell antigens attach to the erythrocytes and cause red cell destruction, either through fixation of complement or ingestion by the macrophages of the reticuloendothelial system. In most cases the primary process is unknown but a positive direct Coombs' test which detects the cell-bound antibody is present in generalized autoimmune disorders

FORFAR AND ARNEIL'S TEXTBOOK OF PEDIATRICS

such as systemic lupus erythematosus (SLE). AIHA also occurs with certain drug-induced hemolysis such as that due to methyldopa. It is very rarely associated with lymphoproliferative disorders in childhood. It is quite useful to divide AIHA into 'cold' and 'warm' types depending on the temperature at which the antibody is best detected in vitro. On the whole, IgM antibodies react best in the cold and IgG in the warm. The cold type of AIHA is chiefly found after viral or mycoplasma infection and the warm type is associated with SLE and methyldopa. In the latter type, steroids may be beneficial and sometimes splenectomy is necessary because it removes the prime site of red cell destruction. Occasionally neither maneuver is successful and immunosuppressive therapy is necessary. In the cold variety the disorder is usually short lived except in paroxysmal cold hemoglobinuria when avoidance of low temperature stress and treatment of the primary disorder are important.

Isoimmune hemolysis is discussed in detail elsewhere (see hemolytic disease of the newborn, Ch. 5) but the pathogenetic process is similar. A form of autoimmune hemolysis associated with autoimmune thrombocytopenia, often occurring in young infants, has been named Evans' syndrome (Evans et al 1951).

Microangiopathic hemolytic anemia (MAHA)

The characteristic features are a rapidly developing hemolytic anemia with distorted fragmented red cells and thrombocytopenia. The underlying process is red cell shredding through fibrin strands deposited in small blood vessels and consumption of platelets within the resultant microthrombi. There is also oxidant damage to the red cells. A similar blood picture can occur with disseminated intravascular coagulation, septicemia and mechanical heart valves. The classical example in childhood is hemolytic uremic syndrome (HUS) described elsewhere (Ch. 17).

Hemolytic anemias secondary to other causes

Hypersplenism

Any of the causes of marked splenic enlargement, such as portal hypertension, leishmaniasis and storage disorders, is liable to produce a shortening of red cell survival due to excessive sequestration in the expanded reticuloendothelial system. The anemia is mild and usually associated with mild leukopenia and thrombocytopenia.

Infections

Malaria is an infection in which microorganisms are present within red cells at the time of hemolysis. Mild hemolysis may occur with many other infectious processes. Septicemia, particularly due to clostridial organisms, may produce an acute hemolytic process usually as part of a consumptive coagulopathy. Bartonella infection is another documented cause of hemolysis (Ch. 23).

Miscellaneous causes of hemolysis

Hemolysis may be caused by extensive burns, chemical poisoning (e.g. lead chlorate or arsine) and snake and spider bites. Hyperphosphatemia during intravenous feeding leads to hemolysis due to impaired glycolysis. An intermittent hemolytic anemia develops in a proportion of patients with Wilson's disease.

Abetalipoproteinemia leads to hemolysis due to membrane lipid peroxidation upon oxidant stress.

METHEMOGLOBINEMIA

This is an abnormality of hemoglobin metabolism consequent upon oxidation of its ferrous iron to the ferric state within intact red cells. It may arise because of enzyme deficiency or an abnormality of the hemoglobin molecule. The enzyme methemoglobin reductase (diaphorase) is important in the production of NADH which maintains hemoglobin in its reduced state. This is a side-shoot process of the main Embden–Meyerhof pathway:

$$\text{Glyceraldehyde-3P} \xrightarrow[\substack{\text{MetHb} \quad \text{Hb} \\ \text{NADH} \quad \text{NAD} \\ \hline \\ \text{Methemoglobin} \\ \text{reductase}}]{} \text{1,3-diphosphoglycerate}$$

A second group of patients have an abnormal hemoglobin molecule which renders it more liable to oxidative injury even in the presence of normal methemoglobin reductase levels. The abnormality resides in the part of the globin molecule close to the heme plate and the abnormal states are designated heme plate M hemoglobinopathies (HbM). They are inherited as dominant traits.

Sulfhemoglobinemia needs to be considered as a very rare cause of undiagnosed cyanosis. The porphyrin moiety of hemoglobin contains a sulfur atom with reduced oxygen affinity. One congenital case has been described and clinical associations have been made with ingestion of phenacetin and sulfur-containing compounds.

Clinical manifestations

Dusky or slate-gray cyanosis involving skin and mucous membranes develops in the absence of respiratory or cardiac causes. Those HbM which affect the γ chains present at birth whereas those affecting the β chain do not present problems until after 2–4 months of age. In the acquired toxic forms, such as that due to the drug dapsone, the onset will clearly be related to exposure. In these cases the prime diagnostic clue is that the cyanosis occurs in a patient who is otherwise well.

Laboratory diagnosis

A strong indication of the diagnosis occurs upon taking blood when it can be noted that the blood is a brown color and does not redden on exposure. The only other situation where this happens is when large amounts of cold antibody produce red cell aggregation. Spectroscopic examination shows a peak absorption at 634 nm which disappears with cyanide. Quantitative methods will allow an accurate measure of methemoglobin as a percentage of the normal hemoglobin. In premature babies the upper limit of normal is 4.4%, in full-term babies 2.8% and in later life 1.9%. The value is 10–70% in cyanotic infants with methemoglobinemia. Assays of methemoglobin reductase and detection of HbMs are required to confirm the specific diagnosis.

Management

The enzyme deficient, toxin- and drug-induced varieties may respond to intravenous methylene blue (1–2 mg/kg as a 1%

solution in saline). The HbM varieties do not. The methylene blue is reduced to leukomethylene blue which produces nonenzymatic reduction of hemoglobin. Oral ascorbate 300–400 mg/day may be useful in chronic therapy where rapid reversal of causative factors is not possible.

SECONDARY ANEMIAS

Many of the anemias seen in clinical practice occur in patients with common systemic disorders which are the primary problem. Many of the factors causing the blood problems are common to several diseases, e.g. the anemias of chronic disorders, iron deficiency and folate deficiency, but some are particularly associated with one or other body system.

CHRONIC INFECTION AND INFLAMMATION

Any chronic infection which lasts for more than a few weeks is liable to produce anemia of moderate severity which will not respond to hematinic therapy but gets better when the underlying infection, e.g. tuberculosis, is cured. Chronic inflammatory disorders such as rheumatoid arthritis, other connective tissue disorders and rheumatic fever produce similar problems. However, the connective tissue diseases often produce a mild generalized cytopenia. In all of these disorders the main finding is usually the anemia of the chronic disorder. The anemia is normocytic and normochromic with usually a low serum iron and transferrin and normal ferritin. The problem is one of iron utilization and not deficiency and it is illogical and unnecessary to give these patients iron supplements. However, some of the patients may become genuinely iron deficient because of poor diet or blood loss from the gut (possibly due to nonsteroidal anti-inflammatory drugs). Rheumatoid arthritis is particularly complex because the patients may also develop marrow hypoplasia due to drugs, e.g. gold therapy. They also develop folate deficiency and hypersplenism (Felty's syndrome). Patients with connective tissue disorders should be investigated for the presence of autoimmune hemolysis if they become anemic.

CHRONIC RENAL FAILURE

The main contributory factors include reduced erythropoietin, anemia of chronic disorders, folate and iron deficiency and hemolysis with 'burr' cells. Additional factors in some patients are blood loss and microangiopathic hemolysis. Recombinant erythropoietin has a role in maintaining the hemoglobin at a level adequate for relieving symptoms and improving the quality of life of these patients.

MALIGNANT DISEASE

Anemia at presentation of malignant disease is quite common and the usual cause is the anemia of chronic disorders. Tumors which involve the marrow, such as neuroblastoma and lymphoma, along with the leukemias will consistently produce anemia. However, leukemic blasts will be present in the blood and leukoerythroblastic change occurs in the solid tumor cases.

ENDOCRINE DISORDERS

A high proportion of patients with hypothyroidism develop an anemia which is often macrocytic. However, the picture may be colored by the presence of iron deficiency and in adults by an association with pernicious anemia. Addison's disease and hypopituitarism also frequently present with a mild anemia. The anemia in these endocrinopathies will not usually respond until appropriate endocrine replacement is instituted.

LIVER DISEASE

Contributing factors include blood loss, hypersplenism (which usually produces a mild to moderate pancytopenia), folate deficiency and the rare association with autoimmune hemolytic anemia. Patients with liver disease are also more likely to bleed because of thrombocytopenia due to hypersplenism and the deficiency of clotting factors synthesized by the liver, i.e. II, V, VII, IX and X.

DRUGS

Blood abnormalities are amongst the most frequent systemic side effect of drugs and these are discussed in the appropriate sections, e.g. marrow hypoplasia, methemoglobinemia, Heinz body anemia, neutropenia, sideroblastic anemia and thrombocytopenia.

DEFECTS OF HEME SYNTHESIS

Whereas the hemoglobinopathies refer to abnormalities affecting the globin portion of the hemoglobin molecule, anemias can also result from defects affecting the heme portion. These can be further subdivided into defects of synthesis of the porphyrin group of heme and defective iron incorporation into the porphyrin moiety to form heme (see Fig. 15.14). Congenital erythropoietic porphyria belongs to the first category, lead poisoning and the sideroblastic anemias to the second.

Congenital erythropoietic porphyria

The clinical manifestations are fully described elsewhere (Ch. 20). The biochemical disorder is a defect of protoporphyrin synthesis in the erythroblasts which leads to an excess of abnormal copro- and uroporphyrin-1 accumulation. There is a hemolytic anemia which does not usually become manifest until after the neonatal period and may lead to a requirement for splenectomy at a later stage.

Lead poisoning

Excessive lead ingestion from whatever cause leads to a disturbance of porphyrin synthesis with coproporphyrinuria and hypochromic anemia with an increase in stainable iron-producing siderocytes and sideroblasts. There is some evidence of abnormal globin chain production and there may also be a hemolytic element to the general picture. In addition, there is interference with the breakdown of RNA by inhibition of the enzyme pyrimidine 5′-nucleotidase, causing accumulation of denatured RNA in red cells. This gives the classical appearance of punctate basophilia on the ordinary blood film. Ringed sideroblasts are red cell precursors with iron accumulation in a ring around the nucleus within the mitochondria. They may be present in lead poisoning.

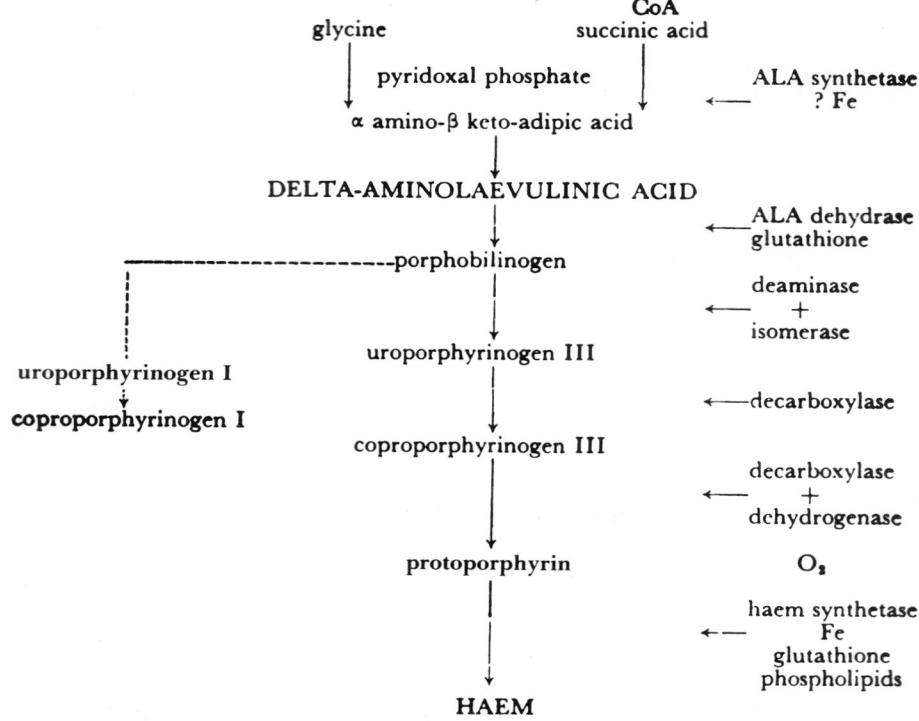

Fig. 15.14   The synthesis of heme. (From Hoffbrand & Lewis 1981 with permission.)

Sideroblastic anemias

This group of anemias is characterized by erythroid hyperplasia and the presence of ringed sideroblasts in the bone marrow. There are two main types depending upon whether they are inherited or acquired. In the hereditary form the anemia is hypochromic and microcytic and is due to deficiency of the enzyme δ-amino-levulinic acid synthetase (ALA synthetase). This form occurs in males and is transmitted by females in an X-linked fashion, but it also rarely occurs in females who are double hemizygotes.

The primary acquired form, which occurs in either sex mainly in middle and old age, is due to a somatic mutation of the red cell progenitor cells causing defects in both heme synthesis and defects in DNA synthesis with megaloblastic and other dyserythropoietic features and frequently a raised MCV. This type sometimes transforms into acute myeloblastic leukemia after many years of follow-up and is now classified with the myelodysplastic syndromes (MDS) (see below). Very rare cases do occur in children.

In the hereditary and primary acquired sideroblastic anemias more than half of the marrow red cell precursors are ringed sideroblasts. It is important to note that lesser numbers occur in other marrow disorders such as the myeloproliferative disorders and myelodysplastic syndromes. They can also be induced by certain drugs such as cycloserine and also alcohol. Vitamin B_6 (pyridoxine) deficiency is a rare cause but isoniazid is a pyridoxine antagonist which can produce a sideroblastic anemia. In some patients there is a response to pyridoxine therapy which is always worth a try. Pyridoxal phosphate has also worked in a few patients who fail to respond to pyridoxine.

In patients with the hereditary type of sideroblastic anemia, the degree of anemia is not severe and regular phlebotomy is necessary to counteract the problems of tissue iron overload which occur in these patients. Iron chelation may also be necessary in some cases especially where blood transfusion proves necessary.

NEUTROPENIA

The neutrophil count in the blood varies greatly with factors such as time of day and exercise, and between racial groups, with the normal neutrophil count in Negro races being lower than in Caucasians. Interpretation of the neutrophil count should take account of the clinical findings in the patient, in particular the incidence and severity of infections. In general neutropenia is likely to be significant if the neutrophil count is persistently less than $1 \times 10^9/l$, and severe infections occur if the count is less than $0.2 \times 10^9/l$. It is also important to decide if the neutropenia is 'isolated' or part of a pancytopenia likely to reflect a more generalized bone marrow disorder. This section is concerned mainly with isolated neutropenia. (see Table 15.11).

The commonest cause of neutropenia is infection, which can lead to problems in defining which came first. However, the neutropenia associated with viral infection, for example, is transient and an appropriate history and patience on the part of the clinician should clarify the clinical significance of the neutrophil count.

DRUG-INDUCED NEUTROPENIA

Many drugs can cause neutropenia and it is thus mandatory to take a very careful drug history in any newly presenting case. If the patient has recently received medication then the records of the relevant drugs control authority should be examined to see whether there is a previously known association and in all cases the authority must be informed of possible causative drugs. The drugs listed in Table 15.11 are examples of those which produce neutropenia only in a proportion of cases. Excluded from the list are drugs known to cause neutropenia as part of a general bone marrow suppression, e.g. cytotoxic agents used in the treatment of malignant disease.

In the majority of instances the cause of the neutropenia in idiosyncratic cases is marrow depression. However, a few drugs such as amidopyrine produce neutropenia by a mechanism related to a hypersensitivity type of reaction, following the development of antibodies to protein–drug complexes which, in the presence of the circulating drug on subsequent exposure, causes leukoagglutination. In this situation there is a dramatic onset of neutropenia. The bone marrow will show lack of myeloid precursors in the former situation and may actually show increased cellularity when immune destruction is the underlying process.

Clinically, drug-induced neutropenia is usually asymptomatic although if it is severe enough there may be infections of the mouth and throat with ulceration which is often painful and intractable. In addition, infection of all types may occur at other sites with a predilection for bacterial and possibly fungal infections.

Treatment is to remove the causative substance and provide supportive care, usually with broad spectrum intravenous antibiotics until recovery ensues. In cases of prolonged neutropenia associated with significant infection the use of G-CSF (granulocyte-colony stimulating factor) might be considered.

CHRONIC BENIGN NEUTROPENIA

An increase in the marginating blood pool of neutrophils with a consequent reduction in the circulating fraction occurs in many normal Africans and other races and also, rarely, as a familial abnormality in other parts of the world. Although a majority spontaneously remit with time a proportion have a persistently low count, but there is rarely any evidence of increased susceptibility to infection.

Table 15.11   Causes of neutropenia

Congenital	Kostmann's syndrome	
	'Benign' neutropenia	
	Cyclical neutropenia	
	Reticular dysgenesis	
	Schwachman's syndrome	
Acquired	Drug-induced*	Anti-inflammatory drugs
		Anti-bacterial drugs
		Anticonvulsants
		Anti-thyroids
		Phenothiazines
		Others
	Infection	Viral (hepatitis, influenza, HIV, EBV, CMV)
		Severe bacterial infection
	Immune	Autoimmune neutropenia

Adapted from Hoffbrand & Pettit (1993) with permission.
* For details of specific drugs consult reference, data sheet on drug or Committee on Safety of Medicines literature.

CYCLICAL NEUTROPENIA

This is a rare disorder which may present in infancy or later in childhood. The clinical course is punctuated by repeated infections, sometimes trivial but sometimes more serious, such as peritonitis, pneumonia or osteomyelitis. Also, there may be cyclical malaise, aphthous ulcers and arthralgia coincident with the periods of neutropenia which recur at 14–21 day intervals. The cycles can continue unabated for many years and at times of maximal depression the peripheral blood may show total agranulocytosis along with a monocytosis. Treatment in the past has been symptomatic but G-CSF is now indicated for those patients with recurrent severe infections.

INFANTILE GENETIC AGRANULOCYTOSIS (KOSTMANN SYNDROME)

This disorder is characterized by severe pyogenic infections, neutropenia and early death. The inheritance is autosomal recessive and neutrophil counts less than $0.5 \times 10^9/l$ are usually present. Bone marrow examination reveals overall normal cellularity with absent mature granulocytes and often a preponderance of promyelocytes and myelocytes. Bone marrow cultures may show in vitro colony growth but failure to develop mature forms. Without treatment the prognosis is poor with more than 70% mortality from infection and only 50% survival to 1 year of age. There is also a predisposition to develop myeloid leukemia in those who survive long enough. It is very important to differentiate these cases from reticular dysgenesis where there is also a failure of the stem cells to produce lymphoid cells, and from those cases associated with other disorders of T and B lymphocytes. Thus, full immunological testing is required in each new case of severe neutropenia. Shwachman's syndrome can be differentiated because these patients have pancreatic dysfunction and the rare disorder of myelokathexis is obvious from the blood film which shows neutrophils with cytoplasmic vacuoles and abnormal nuclei with very thin filaments connecting the nuclear lobes.

The advent of recombinant growth factors makes these the treatment of choice in Kostmann syndrome. The value of G-CSF is shown by the chart of one of the author's patients with congenital neutropenia who, in the first 3 years of her life, spent a significant number of days as an inpatient for the management of infection including lung abscesses (Figure 15.15). After starting G-CSF she has had virtually no admissions to hospital and minimal antibiotic requirement. Although G-CSF is expensive the overall economic balance seems in its favor, especially when patient well-being and improved growth and development are accounted for. The reservation about G-CSF is related to the potential development of leukemia and all patients on this therapy are monitored regularly with bone marrow examination including cytogenetic analysis.

OTHER CAUSES OF NEUTROPENIA

Low neutrophil counts are frequently seen in autoimmune disorders, often along with low platelets and hemoglobin. Occasionally this may be the only manifestation of an autoimmune disorder. Lower neutrophil counts may be seen in children of Negro racial background and in premature babies.

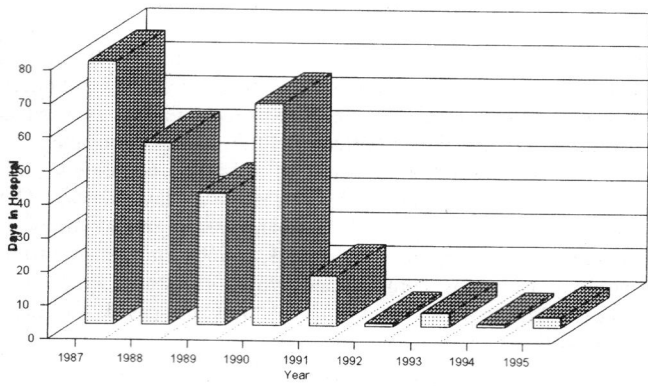

Fig. 15.15 Use of G-CSF in the treatment of congenital neutropenia. Demonstration of effect in reducing inpatient stays for management of severe infections. G-CSF was started in April 1991.

OTHER WHITE CELL DISORDERS

EOSINOPHILIA

An arbitrary level of $0.5 \times 10^9/l$ is taken as the level above which eosinophilia is said to exist. The commonest cause is the presence of allergic disease, especially atopy. Parasitic diseases such as hookworm, ascariasis, tapeworm and schistosomiasis should be sought when eosinophilia persists. A good history of overseas travel is essential. Eosinophilia is seen in patients recovering from antimalignancy chemotherapy and in recovery from acute infections. A number of skin diseases other than atopic eczema have been associated with eosinophilia, and the best examples are psoriasis, pemphigus and dermatitis herpetiformis. Drug sensitivity rarely produces an eosinophilia but it is seen in association with various lymphomas including Hodgkin's disease. The rarer causes include polyarteritis nodosa, Schulman's fasciitis, pulmonary hypereosinophilic syndrome and leukemias with eosinophilia – especially myelomonocytic varieties.

LEUKEMIA

ETIOLOGY

The etiology of childhood leukemia is a highly emotive subject because of its possible association with radiation and apparent clustering of cases in relation to certain nuclear establishments in the UK and elsewhere in the world (Beral et al 1993). While there is a documented association of the increased incidence of leukemia in the survivors of the atomic bomb explosions in Japan at the end of the second World War, in patients with ankylosing spondylitis treated with spinal radiotherapy and in the babies of mothers who had abdominal X-rays during pregnancy, the risk of environmental radiation is not known. Viruses can cause leukemias in animals such as cats (feline leukemia virus), and the human T cell leukemia virus (HTLV) has been implicated in a particular adult type of leukemia/lymphoma found particularly in Japan and the Caribbean. The epidemiological investigation of Burkitt's lymphoma suggests a role for Epstein–Barr virus infection. In keeping with other cancers it is unlikely that there is one 'cause' for leukemia but an interaction of at least two factors – the 'Two-hit' hypothesis of Knudson.

The majority of childhood leukemia is lymphoblastic in type, with 80–85% being of B lymphocyte precursor origin. This has

lead to theories of an infective cause of leukemia, possibly an aberrant response to a common infecting agent, supported by the 'new town' clustering of cases (Greaves 1988, Kinlen 1988). In the UK a national case-control study investigating the etiology of childhood leukemias and other cancers is completing recruitment after 5 years and is looking particularly at environmental factors. By the time the next edition of this book is published the results may be available but it is perhaps overoptimistic to think there will a definite answer to the 'cause' of leukemia.

The incidence of leukemia is increased in Down syndrome and this is usually of the acute lymphoblastic variety. There are also reports of increased incidences of acute leukemia in association with D trisomy and Turner's syndrome. What is certain is that the DNA repair syndromes, Fanconi's anemia, ataxia telangiectasia and Bloom's syndrome have a high risk of leukemia. Other bone marrow failure syndromes are also associated with a high risk.

Exposure to certain chemicals has been linked to leukemias especially in adults, e.g. benzene compounds. For this reason there is current interest in the potential role of various environmental pollutants.

INCIDENCE

The incidence of acute leukemia in childhood seems to vary throughout the world; for every million children in the UK, about 35 new cases of acute leukemia will present per annum. This equates to a 65 in 100 000 risk for a boy throughout childhood up to 14 years of age and a 46 in 100 000 risk for girls. Despite all the changes in the environment and large fluctuations with time, there is no evidence of a general upward trend in incidence over recent years.

CLASSIFICATION OF LEUKEMIA (Table 15.12)

Leukemias are classified according to clinical presentation and morphological type. The clinical classification of acute or chronic refers to the speed of progression of the illness without treatment, with acute leukemia demonstrating the clinical features of rapidly advancing bone marrow failure. In contrast chronic leukemias are more slowly progressive but only chronic granulocytic leukemia is seen in children. The myelodysplasias are a group of conditions of increasing importance in children as they are the precursor states of some cases of leukemia and may be seen after treatment of various cancers by chemotherapy, particularly alkylating agents, with or without radiotherapy.

The morphological classifications of acute lymphoblastic leukemia (ALL) and acute myeloblastic leukemia (AML) have been described by the French–American–British (FAB) group, and pediatric myelodysplasias by Passmore et al (1995) (Table 15.12).

The immunological subtype of the acute lymphoblastic leukemias represents clonal expansion of a cell 'arrested' at a normal stage of development. The use of various antibodies to identify cell-surface and cytoplasmic antigens allows separation of B cell precursor (null, pre-B and common), T cell and true B cell leukemias. It is important to identify the true B cell leukemias as patients with this type require chemotherapy appropriate for B cell non-Hodgkin's lymphoma, not standard ALL therapy.

Acute myeloblastic leukemias are more complex and less easily divided because monoclonal antibodies are less frequently of help in this context. Most cases can be subdivided simply by studying

Table 15.12   The leukemias and myelodysplastic syndromes

Main group	Subtypes
Acute lymphoblastic leukemia	Common Pre-B Null } immunophenotype T B L1 L2 } morphological L3
Acute myeloblastic leukemia	M0 undifferentiated M1 without maturation M2 with granulocytic maturation M3 promyelocytic M4 myelomonocytic M5 monocytic/monoblastic M6 erythroleukemia M7 megakaryoblastic
Myelodysplasia	RA refractory anemia RARS refractory anemia with ringed sideroblasts RAEB refractory anemia with excess blasts (5–20%) RAEBT refractory anemia with excess blasts in transformation (blasts 20–30%) JCML juvenile chronic myeloid leukemia Imo7 infantile monosomy 7 CMML chronic myelomonocytic leukemia EOS eosinophilia

From Bennett et al (1982) and Passmore et al (1995).

the ordinary stained bone marrow aspirate film. Specific cytochemical staining with Sudan black, nonspecific esterase and acid phosphatase can give additional information. The FAB classification is based on identifying the predominant cell type and the degree of differentiation of the cells. Certain types have characteristic associations such as M3 (promyelocytic) with disseminated intravascular coagulation, M5 (monoblastic) with gum hyperplasia and skin rash, and M7 (megakaryoblastic) with Down syndrome.

The myelodysplastic syndromes (MDS) are rare in childhood and have gone under a wide variety of synonyms in the past – preleukemia, subleukemia, smoldering leukemia, sideroblastic anemias, etc. The original FAB classification was not designed with children in mind and thus two particular disease entities, juvenile chronic myeloid leukemia and monosomy 7 syndrome, are not really accommodated. Refractory anemia (RA), in which there are myelodysplastic features and a few ringed sideroblasts, and refractory anemia with ringed sideroblasts (RAS) are very rare in childhood, but carry a much better prognosis than other MDS in adults. The other types are basically variants of AML in children and current evidence is that they should be treated as such. The only difference between refractory anemia with excess blasts (RAEB), RAEB in transformation (RAEBT) and AML is the percentage of blasts (5–20%, 20–30%, more than 30%) along with more marked myelodysplastic features in the former two types. The proposed classification of Passmore et al expanded the FAB suggestions and developed a scoring system of 'FPC' based on level of HbF, platelet count and complexity of karyotype. A favorable score gives a 5-year survival of approximately 60% with all of those with an unfavorable score being dead within 4 years of diagnosis.

The increasing use of cytogenetic analysis of the leukemic blast cells and more sophisticated molecular genetic techniques can help:

- *in diagnosis*, e.g. the t(15;17) translocation in M3 AML and the t(9;22) translocation (Philadelphia chromosome) in CGL
- *in prognosis*, e.g. hyperdiploidy in ALL for good prognosis and the t(9;22) translocation (Philadelphia chromosome) in ALL for poor prognosis
- *in detection of residual disease*, e.g. bcr-abl oncogene in CGL or ALL.

One of the areas of greatest interest in the management of leukemia is the concept of minimal residual disease. Conventional methods of detecting residual leukemia cells in bone marrow include microscopy, immunophenotyping and detection of chromosomal translocations, these all being relatively crude. Improvements in molecular technology can allow detection of one leukemia cell in 100 000 or 1 000 000 (Campana & Pui 1995). Currently these techniques are being used in prospective studies to assess the significance of minimal residual disease as a risk factor for relapse, then subsequently study whether changes in therapy can influence outcome.

CLINICAL MANIFESTATIONS

Acute myeloblastic leukemia has a steady low incidence throughout childhood although the monoblastic/monocytic types tend to occur relatively more often in infancy. Acute lymphoblastic leukemia is most common between the ages of 2 and 5 years with a preponderance of males at about 1.5 : 1. Rare cases of congenital leukemia do occur and these are usually malignancies of early B cells. Juvenile chronic myeloid leukemia and monosomy 7 tend to occur in infants.

The clinical features of leukemia are due to:

1. bone marrow failure – anemia, neutropenia and thrombocytopenia

2. tissue and organ infiltration
3. metabolic effects.

Hemorrhage

This is a frequent presenting feature and can be catastrophic. This is still the commonest cause of the rare deaths which occur during the first few hours in hospital and there is a strong association with very high blast cell counts in the blood. In these cases, leukostasis (i.e. sludging of the microcirculation due to the very high blast cell count) and bleeding are closely associated. Most bleeding episodes are milder and thrombocytopenia is by far the commonest cause. Typically there is epistaxis, gum bleeding and bleeding from the gut. One particularly important feature is severe retinal hemorrhage which may be associated with leukemia infiltrates. Significant impairment of vision is usually avoided by constant vigilance and intensive platelet support therapy. All new patients should be investigated with a coagulation screen because hepatic dysfunction and disseminated intravascular coagulation (DIC) do occur, the latter frequently in association with M3 acute promyelocytic leukemia or bacteremia.

Anemia

This occurs in most cases and is often the reason for referral. Some of the commoner symptoms and signs such as pallor, lethargy, anorexia and breathlessness are caused by the low hemoglobin. Cardiac failure is uncommon even at very low levels of hemoglobin but tachycardia and cardiac flow murmurs are very common.

Infection

Susceptibility to infection may occur for an extended period before presentation and some patients have a serious infection at diagnosis. Pyrexia at presentation can be due to the disease process itself, but all episodes in newly presenting patients must be treated seriously and broad spectrum intravenous antibiotics instituted. In neutropenic leukemia patients at any stage of their illness the accepted policy is always to institute this type of therapy empirically before the results of blood cultures allow more specific treatment, otherwise early deaths will occur. The best regimen is a synergistic combination of an aminoglycoside and ureidopenicillin or ceftazidime. Thereafter an intensive search for the cause of the infection is mandatory, bearing in mind that chest X-ray changes and cutaneous manifestations may not occur because of the grossly impaired inflammatory response.

Bone and joint involvement

Orthopedic surgeons and rheumatologists frequently see children with bone pain and/or arthralgia and when these symptoms occur a blood count should always be checked along with a careful physical examination for hepatosplenomegaly and lymphadenopathy. Two-thirds of children with acute lymphoblastic leukemia (ALL) present with bone pain and at least half of these have radiological bone changes (Fig. 15.16), the most frequent of which are radiolucent bands across the ends of long bones. In acute megakaryoblastic (M7) and other types of leukemia osteosclerosis can occasionally occur. The bone pain responds rapidly to antileukemic therapy. 'Starting' of the cranial sutures and other radiological evidence of raised intracranial pressure can sometimes be seen in the presence of meningeal leukemia (Fig. 15.17).

Hepatosplenomegaly, lymphadenopathy and other organ enlargement

Splenomegaly exists in about 80% of new cases of leukemia and is particularly marked in certain variants such as chronic granulocytic leukemia (CGL) and juvenile chronic myeloid leukemia (JCML). The enlargement is smooth, firm and nontender unless it is chronically enlarged as in CGL when infarction can cause pain and tenderness. Hepatosplenomegaly is

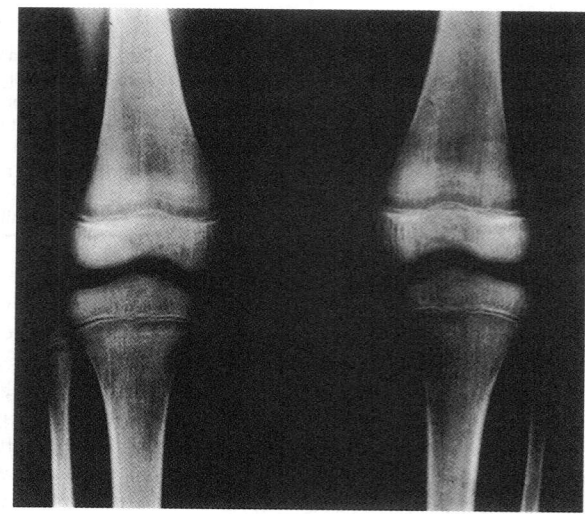

Fig. 15.16 Lymphoblastic leukemia. Knees showing generalized osteoporosis with transverse radiolucent bands across long bone metaphyses adjacent to metaphyseal bone ends, found in malignant infiltration of bone marrow.

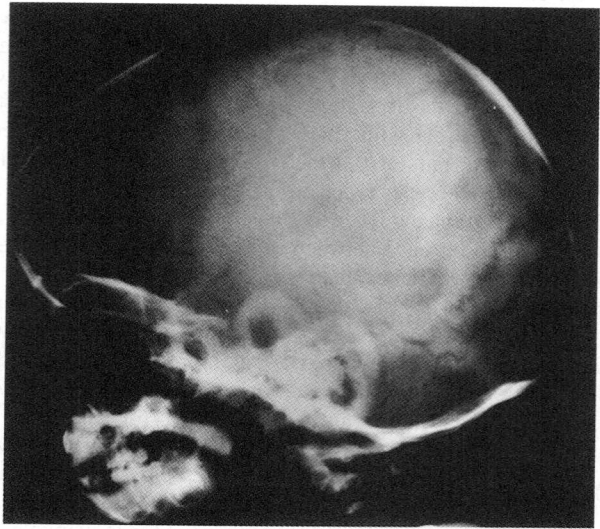

Fig. 15.17 Leukemia. Started cranial sutures associated with raised intracranial pressure at onset of leukemic meningitis.

common although less frequent and occasionally the kidneys can be felt, although abdominal ultrasound will show nonpalpable renal enlargement quite often in ALL. Ovarian and testicular enlargement are rarely felt at diagnosis but regular careful examination of the testes throughout follow-up is essential as relapse in this site is quite common.

Enlarged lymph nodes are the cause of many referrals to hematologists. The cervical glands are the most commonly involved in leukemia. They are typically discrete, painless and rubbery and may sometimes be very large without associated hepatosplenomegaly. Hilar lymphadenopathy is sometimes seen and large anterior mediastinal masses of either thymic or lymphatic origin occur in several types of ALL but typically the T cell variety (Fig. 15.18).

Gum hypertrophy does occur with all types of leukemia but is particularly common with M4 and M5 type. Skin infiltration with

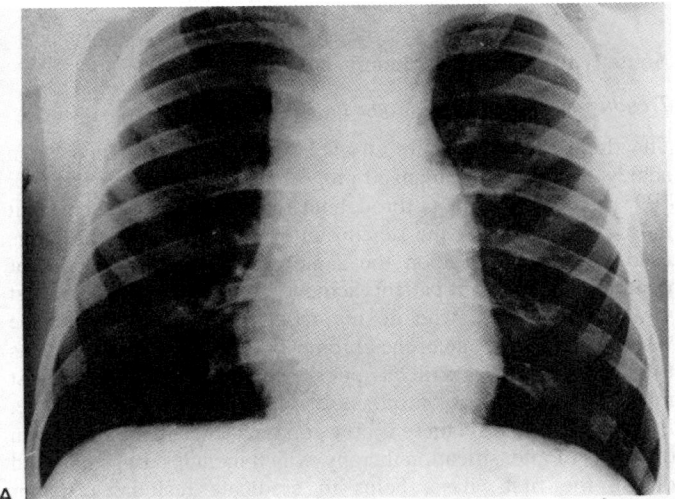

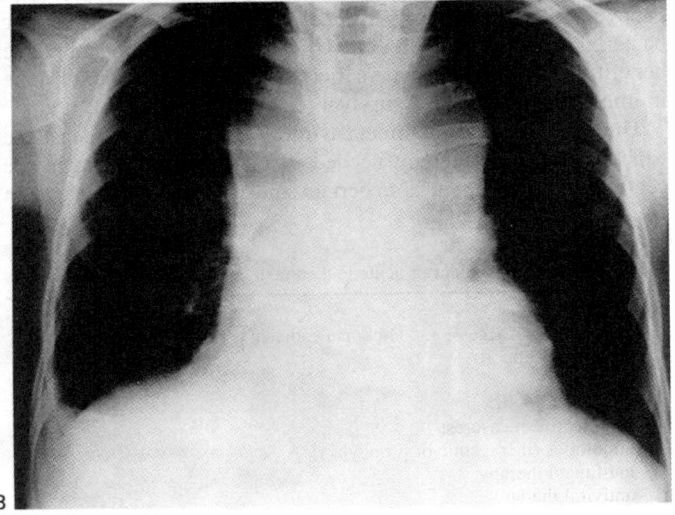

Fig. 15.18 Chest in T cell leukemia, early and advanced. (A) Widened superior mediastinal shadow consistent with thymic enlargement, normal hilar shadows and no lung lesion. (B) Wide superior mediastinal shadow with convex borders and lobulated hilar shadows consistent with thymic enlargement and bronchopulmonary lymphadenopathy. Secondary collapse at right cardiophrenic angle and trace of fluid obstructing right costophrenic angle.

leukemia is rare but does occur in the neonatal variety when it produces bluish blebs and it is also seen sometimes in M4 and M5. Juvenile chronic myeloid leukemia is associated with 'pustular' facial rashes.

Masses of abdominal leukemia/lymphoma tissue not related to the liver and spleen typically occur in the B-ALL cases and breakdown of these masses of tissue, as in other instances where there is a high leukemia mass, can lead to the tumor lysis syndrome. This is characterized by hyperkalemia, hyperphosphatemia, hyperuricemia and renal failure. Treatment is designed to prevent this problem with a forced diuresis and allopurinol and if this fails there is a need to institute renal dialysis at an early stage. All leukemic children are in fact susceptible to hyperuricemia and oral allopurinol is given prophylactically during the first 1–2 weeks of treatment.

An unusual complication of acute leukemia is leukostasis which occurs when the white cell count in the peripheral blood is extremely high and causes obstruction of flow in the microvasculature. This tends to occur more with AML than ALL, and the author has seen one child die within hours of admission with a white cell count of $940 \times 10^9/l$ and postmortem examination demonstrated extensive microvasculature obstruction.

Meningeal leukemia

Most cases occur when planned therapy has been stopped, usually after about 2 years of treatment. However, a proportion first present with blast cells in the cerebrospinal fluid and this is associated with a particularly poor prognosis despite more intensive treatment than usual in the form of craniospinal irradiation and extra intrathecal methotrexate. The usual presenting symptoms of CNS relapse are referable to raised intracranial pressure with vomiting in most and also severe headaches along with papilledema and sometimes signs of the so-called 'hypothalamic syndrome', with voracious appetite and excessive weight gain. Cranial nerve palsies especially of VI are common. However, none of these signs is usually present at diagnosis although occasionally a patient can have gross neurological disturbance and decreased level of consciousness.

DIAGNOSIS AND LABORATORY FINDINGS

The most constant finding at presentation of leukemia is changes in the peripheral blood. However, 1 in 100 children with leukemia presents with a perfectly normal blood count. 99% of children presenting with acute leukemia will have circulating blasts and/or thrombocytopenia. Two-thirds are neutropenic and nearly 90% are anemic. Thus one can nearly always infer the diagnosis on a blood count and physical examination alone although a specific diagnosis depends upon examination of the bone marrow by simple microscopy along with cytochemistry and immunophenotyping of the marrow cells. ALL blasts tend to be positive with the periodic acid Schiff (PAS) stain and negative with Sudan black. T cells are positive with blocks of acid phosphatase and AML cells are positive with Sudan black. Nonspecific esterase is positive in the M5 varieties. Criteria for classification of the varieties of acute leukemia have already been described.

Cerebrospinal fluid is best examined in cytospin preparations and the usual criterion is that more than five blasts per high-power field constitute leukemic meningeal infiltration. However, it is possible to be more precise than this, particularly in ALL wherein one can use the antibody to the enzyme terminal deoxynucleotidyl transferase to differentiate blasts from reactive or normal lymphocytes.

There is really no relationship between chronic granulocytic leukemia (CGL) in childhood, which does not differ from the adult variety, and so-called juvenile chronic myeloid leukemia (JCML). The frequent efforts to compare and contrast the two are really pointless. In fact there is a move to change the name of the latter to 'myelomonocytic syndrome' but this is likely to confuse it with chronic myelomonocytic leukemia in adults. As with adult patients the bone marrow cells in childhood CGL show a translocation of part of the long arm of chromosome 22 to another, usually number 9 chromosome, to produce the Philadelphia chromosome. The blood and bone marrow show a massive expansion of the total body granulocyte mass. The blood shows a high total white cell count, usually over $100 \times 10^9/l$, and the predominant cell types are myelocytes, metamyelocytes and neutrophils with smaller numbers of eosinophils, promyelocytes and basophils. Typically, the basophils are degranulated. There may be a very low percentage of blood and marrow blasts and if these are more prominent than usual it suggests that a blastic transformation or myelodysplastic syndrome may be present.

JCML is associated with a reversion to a fetal type of hemopoiesis with a high HbF and i red cell antigen. There is also a higher percentage of blasts in the blood with an excess of dysplastic monocytes and eosinophils. A related syndrome exists in association with a monosomy 7 chromosomal constitution.

Chromosomal changes are in fact found in most cases of leukemia when carefully investigated with modern banding techniques and a full discussion can be found in standard texts. Examples are the 8;21 translocation seen in many cases of M2 AML and the 8;14 translocation seen in B-ALL. There is evidence that hyperdiploidy in ALL is associated with a better prognosis and that a loss of chromosome 7 in AML cases is associated with a poorer prognosis. Total numbers of chromosomes per malignant cell seem less important than the presence of genetic rearrangements.

Making a precise diagnosis in leukemia not only helps to subdivide the cases but can also be very useful prognostically and in deciding what type of therapy should be given. Thus, in ALL the poor prognostic factors are: white cell count greater than $50 \times 10^9/l$, age less than 1 year, B cell type, 4;11 chromosomal translocation and 4;19 translocation and CNS disease at diagnosis. Good risk features are age 2–5 years, white cell count less than $20 \times 10^9/l$ and common ALL immunophenotype. The prognostic factors in AML are much less well defined except that patients with CNS disease and high white cell counts at diagnosis do worse.

TREATMENT

In the management of acute leukemia the basic assumption is that there is a population of normal hemopoietic stem cells in the bone marrow which can restore normal marrow function if the leukemia cells are eliminated. The mainstay of treatment is the use of a combination of chemotherapeutic drugs, with or without radiotherapy, to reduce the number of leukemic cells in the body, allow recovery of marrow function and arguably permit immunological mechanisms of the body to eliminate residual leukemia cells. The problems of detection of minimal residual

disease and how such knowledge might be put to clinical use have been discussed above. At present the length and intensity of chemotherapy can only be planned in the light of randomized clinical trials and the knowledge gained over the years about prognostic factors.

Advances in antileukemic therapy have to a large extent been paralleled and facilitated by improvements in supportive care applied in major treatment centers. In the UK most children are treated within United Kingdom Children's Cancer Study Group (UKCCSG) centers and results from these centers have proved superior to ad hoc therapy elsewhere. The intensive chemotherapy needed to eliminate leukemic cells initially aggravates the bone marrow failure and it is essential that adequate supportive care is available particularly with transfusion of platelets and red cells, and the prompt identification and aggressive treatment of infections. 20 years ago very few children recovered from leukemia, now more than half survive. Table 15.13 summarizes the principles of management of acute leukemia.

Acute lymphoblastic leukemia

Treatment of patients at diagnosis

The dramatic increase in survival rates from ALL have been achieved by carefully planned progressive randomized trials (Pui 1995). Not all regimens throughout the world are the same but most are based upon the schema in Figure 15.19 and the drugs used are variations upon the same theme. With this type of treatment over 97% of patients achieve a remission within the first 4 weeks and those who do not require reinvestigation to see whether they have one of the chromosomal translocations such as t(4;11) associated with a poor prognosis. As with most malignancies, speed of response is related to eventual outcome. Following this period there is now good evidence that the addition of blocks of intensification therapy, which includes drugs not used during the first phase, helps to eradicate residual resistant leukemia clones. Both phases are associated with profound pancytopenia and a high risk of serious infections, usually bacterial or fungal in nature. The UKALL X trial demonstrated the benefit of two blocks of intensification therapy over one or none in improving relapse-free survival (Chessells et al 1995).

The third phase of treatment is more controversial in that the exact modality of therapy needed to eradicate leukemia in the central nervous system is uncertain and is being investigated in

Table 15.13 Management of acute leukemia

General
  Reliable venous access, e.g. Hickman catheter
  Transfusion support:
  – red cells
  – platelets
  Anti-infective measures:
  – antibiotics (therapeutic or prophylactic)
  – antifungal therapy
  – antiviral therapy
  – immunoglobulin
  – ? G-CSF
  Good communication with patient and family

Specific
  Chemotherapy
  Radiotherapy
  Bone marrow transplantation

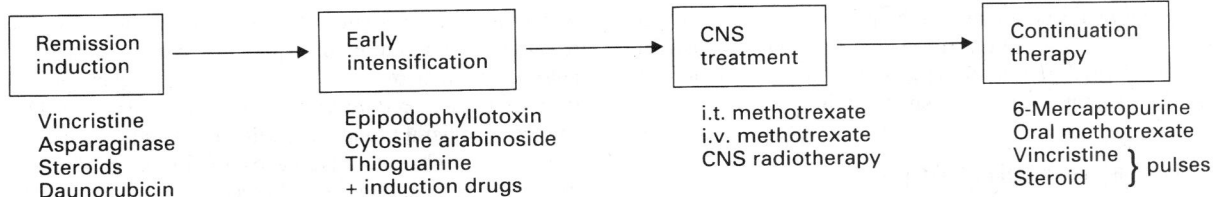

Fig. 15.19 Scheme for treatment of acute lymphoblastic leukemia. Drugs listed are only examples of those which can be used.

many current randomized studies. What is known for certain is that treatment directed to the CNS is required and that conventional therapy with cranial irradiation 18 Gy and six doses of intrathecal methotrexate is associated with an incidence of late sequelae to the nervous system. These usually take the form of specific and often subtle learning difficulties which are more marked in children aged less than 3 years at the time of irradiation. The current UKALL XI trial is investigating whether patients at low risk of CNS disease (i.e. those with initial white cell blood counts less than $50 \times 10^9/l$) can be treated with intrathecal methotrexate rather than cranial irradiation. Conversely, those patients at higher risk are being investigated to see whether high dose intravenous methotrexate with its known CNS penetrative effect can be substituted for cranial irradiation while still reducing the risk of relapse. An important part of the trial is a psychometric study to assess the intellectual impact of the types of treatment in relation to late sequelae.

Much time has been spent looking at the next phase of treatment, which is the continuation phase. However, there is no evidence that anything is better than daily oral 6-mercaptopurine, weekly oral methotrexate and monthly vincristine with 5 days of steroids. This is well tolerated providing neutrophil and platelet counts are monitored at weekly to fortnightly intervals. A very important development has been the involvement with shared care hospitals wherein local pediatricians manage the majority of therapy closer to the patient's home. The best length of continuation therapy is not certain at the present time and 2 years is the current recommendation in the UK with no advantages having yet been shown for shorter or longer periods of treatment. An important aspect of this phase of treatment is that the doses of mercaptopurine should be pushed to maximum tolerance as it has been demonstrated that those children having periods of neutropenia during continuation treatment have a better prognosis.

Patients with the previously described high risk factors can be considered for allogeneic transplantation during first remission of the disease but this is controversial because these patients are faring considerably better with modern chemotherapy schedules.

Management of relapse in ALL

Nowadays most relapses occur following cessation of all therapy. Most of these occur in the first year after stopping treatment but there is a diminishing risk throughout the 8 years from initial diagnosis. Any type of relapse which occurs whilst treatment is still being given carries a very poor prognosis and allogeneic transplantation from a histocompatible donor should be considered in these patients. The role of high dose therapy with autologous marrow rescue is not defined in this situation and is under investigation at present.

The commonest type of relapse is that occurring in the bone marrow following cessation of therapy. In a number of cases, further investigation reveals disease in other sites, either the CNS or testicles or both. Ovarian relapse is very uncommon and carries a poor prognosis. Bone marrow relapse occurring at any stage is almost invariably fatal although the second remission can be as long as or occasionally longer than the first. More usually, further relapse and death occur within a matter of months. The usual plan is to use the standard four-drug induction therapy and then to introduce intensified treatment with different drugs in high dosage in an attempt to eradicate the residual resistant disease. If a donor is available for an allogeneic bone marrow transplant it is likely that this approach will result in a higher leukemia-free survival, for example 40% compared with 17% for continuing chemotherapy (Barrett et al 1994) but there are no randomized trials available to confirm this and the results for both bone marrow transplantation and chemotherapy can vary between centers. When a donor is not available there is some evidence that high dose therapy with autologous transplant rescue may produce cures but this remains to be confirmed. The developments in unrelated donor bone marrow transplantation have increased the use of this method of treatment in children with relapsed leukemia. Although individual centers claim leukemia-free survivals similar to sibling transplants (Casper et al 1995) the value of this remains to be proved. Currently the Medical Research Council is organizing a randomized trial to assess the use of unrelated donor transplant in children with relapsed ALL who do not have a sibling donor.

Central nervous system relapse is associated with the chance of long survival although no more than 10% are cured. There is also a high risk of late CNS and hormonal sequelae because of the treatment required as well as damage from the disease itself. Because of these features the role of allogeneic transplant and high dose therapy with autologous marrow rescue is being assessed. The more conventional approach is to give a further 2 years of reinduction and continuation therapy to counteract the high risk of systemic relapse and also to reirradiate the whole neuraxis. The duration of continuation therapy for marrow and CNS relapse is very uncertain at the present time and there is a feeling that this phase of treatment in many cases is merely 'damping down' the disease.

The one situation in which nontransplant retreatment has been associated with appreciable numbers of cures is isolated testicular relapse following cessation of therapy. Although this is seen much less frequently now that more effective primary systemic therapy is given, about 1 in 10 boys develops this complication in the first year after stopping treatment. Almost three-quarters of these patients will achieve long survival following 2 more years of systemic induction, continuation therapy and intrathecal therapy, along with 24 Gy testicular irradiation.

Relapse at other sites is rare although one does occasionally see disease recurring in skin and bone. Relapse in the eye usually presents as an obvious hypopion and the prognosis is poor with disease usually present elsewhere, especially in the CNS.

Acute myeloblastic leukemia (AML)

In AML, prognostic factors are not well enough refined to allow specification of therapy for each of the M1 to M7 subtypes. Children with high white cell counts and CNS disease at diagnosis do badly but there is no evidence that any type of therapy is better than another at treating these or any other varieties of AML. The possible exception to this is the use of all-trans retinoic acid in the treatment of the M3 subtype – acute promyelocytic leukemia. The last 10 years have seen a dramatic and significant improvement in survival from AML and this is due to several factors. Supportive care has improved dramatically and consequently much more intensive regimens of therapy can now be used. This has resulted in complete remission rates in the region of 80–90% in children. In addition, allogeneic bone marrow transplantation has definitely improved the outlook for children with AML in first remission. The best current estimate is that 60–70% of children survive following marrow transplantation in first remission and 30–40% following conventional chemotherapy. It is noteworthy that 10 years ago only 10% of children survived.

In the previous edition a number of questions were posed that were to be addressed in the then current Medical Research Council Trial AML10. The value of autologous bone marrow transplantation in first or second remission, or the use of epipodophyllotoxin in induction have not yet been clarified. However, combined with experience from other countries, certain prognostic groups can be identified. In particular the M3 type, characterized by the t(15;17) translocation, has a good prognosis with chemotherapy alone and such patients should not be exposed to the toxicity of bone marrow transplantation. The M3 type can respond to all-trans retinoic acid as an adjunct to conventional chemotherapy.

The value of interleukins and other biological response modifiers needs to be evaluated. Continuation therapy is of no proven value in AML management. The role of CNS-directed therapy is also uncertain and most patients are given six doses of intrathecal therapy with methotrexate, cytosine arabinoside and hydrocortisone. Some children present with CNS disease at diagnosis and they are treated with either craniospinal irradiation or bone marrow transplantation. The best approach is still being evaluated.

Bone marrow transplantation (BMT)

The principle of bone marrow transplantation is the provision of a source of hemopoietic stem cells to repopulate the bone marrow after high doses of chemotherapy, with or without radiotherapy, have destroyed the patient's own bone marrow cells (Armitage 1994). The term bone marrow transplantation is becoming outdated as alternative sources of hemopoietic stem cells are found, e.g. peripheral blood stem cells and cord blood stem cells.

Donors

At the present time the best evaluated approach is the allogeneic type using a histocompatible sibling and the rare syngeneic type when an identical twin is fortuitously available. A great deal of research is continuing into the use of high dose therapy with autologous marrow rescue although the question of residual disease in the stored marrow has not been answered. The potential role of peripheral blood stem cells harvested on a cell separator is great with apparent advantages of lower contamination with malignant cells and more rapid recovery of marrow function. The mechanical problems related to the volume of blood needed to prime the cell separator may limit its application in small children. Matched unrelated donors (MUD) would considerably widen the availability of BMT and very large panels of potential donors are being set up with the hope that genetic probing may facilitate the present extremely cumbersome matching process. If the control of transplant-related problems such as graft-versus-host disease can be improved the use of MUD transplants will be extended. The use of partially matched family donors has only been addressed in the context of immune deficiency disorders where it is showing some success.

Preparation of recipient

A commonly used regimen is cyclophosphamide given over 2 days followed by total body irradiation (TBI). There are many other approaches and non-TBI regimens such as the combination of busulphan and cyclophosphamide are being investigated and may be particularly applicable to young children where TBI is not feasible. The idea of this treatment is to make marrow 'space', eradicate the underlying disease and to 'condition' the patient's immune system to accept the donor marrow.

Harvest procedure

Under general anesthetic a minimum of 2×10^8 nucleated cells/kg recipient body weight is removed by multiple bone marrow needle aspirations. Only the pelvic sites are usually required. The volume is replaced by blood which can be stored from venesection of the donor 1 week previously. The marrow is then transfused into the recipient or stored in liquid nitrogen when used for HDTAMR. If there is ABO incompatibility between donor and recipient the red cells can be removed using a cell washer.

Graft-versus-host disease

This is a disorder in which the T cells from the donor marrow attack the patient causing hepatitis, maculopapular and desquamating skin disease and severe gastrointestinal problems. It may be controlled using high dose steroids but may prove fatal. In children the frequency of severe cases is very low if one uses a regimen of cyclosporine and methotrexate conditioning. Another approach is to use T cell depletion of the marrow which may be indicated particularly in MUD transplants although this procedure produces a higher risk of graft rejection. Rejection is otherwise uncommon in BMT for leukemia.

Infections and other problems

BMT recipients are especially susceptible to *Aspergillus* infection and thus should be nursed in a filtered air environment. Laminar air flow is probably not necessary. One of the other major problems is with cytomegalovirus (CMV) infection which can be reduced to a much smaller problem in children by the use of CMV-screened antibody-negative blood products. The use of prophylactic CMV immunoglobulin is still under evaluation and the antiviral agent ganciclovir is available as treatment for active CMV infection. Acyclovir can reduce the high risk of herpes simplex reactivation and it is now used routinely for this purpose. If carried on for long enough it may even reduce the risk of varicella zoster reactivation.

As in other situations whereby the patient is severely immunocompromised, all pyrexial episodes should be treated empirically with a combination such as an aminoglycoside and ureidopenicillin. However, as most of these patients have indwelling i.v. catheters, there is often a need to add in vancomycin to deal with the consequent resistant Gram-positive infections. There is also a high risk of disseminated fungal infection and a febrile patient not responding to antibiotic therapy by 48 hours must be treated with intravenous amphotericin B. It is extremely difficult to find the causative organism in fungal infections. The use of prophylactic antifungals such as oral amphotericin reduces the risk of oropharyngeal candida and oral fluconazole and itraconazole are now being evaluated as alternatives. Gut sterilization is of unproved value in children and is very poorly tolerated. Co-trimoxazole is used routinely as it will prevent *Pneumocystis carinii* infection.

Late sequelae of leukemia therapy

Irradiation of children's brains is associated with learning difficulties in a proportion of cases and in some instances, especially in the youngest patients, this can be severe. Precocious puberty is seen in some children who have been treated for ALL. The evidence at present is that late teratogenicity is not a major problem and many survivors of leukemia treatment are now having normal babies. Total body irradiation is associated with cataract formation, hypothyroidism and deficiencies of growth and sex hormones. There is some evidence that the new fractionated regimens will reduce the problem. Total body irradiation invariably produces sterility. For all of these reasons, drug-only regimens are being evaluated but in most situations these are experimental. It is incumbent upon us to follow up all survivors of malignant disease so that we can learn lessons to help us modify therapy for current and future generations of patients.

DISORDERS OF HEMOSTASIS

The normal hemostatic mechanism comprises the reaction of the vessel wall, the formation of the platelet plug and activation of coagulation with the formation of fibrin to stabilize the platelet plug. Subsequently fibrinolysis limits the extent of fibrin formation and maintains the patency of the vessels. Clinical problems with bruising or bleeding can be caused by abnormalities of any part of the hemostatic mechanism.

NONTHROMBOCYTOPENIC PURPURAS

These vascular disorders primarily affect the blood vessels or their adjacent connective tissue and cause relatively localized hemostatic defects with petechiae, purpura and ecchymoses.

Occasionally bleeding from mucous membranes occurs. The coagulation screening results are typically normal.

Hereditary hemorrhagic telangiectasia (Osler–Weber–Rendu disease)

This is an uncommon disorder transmitted as an autosomal dominant trait in which dilated microvascular swellings appear during childhood and become more numerous in adult life. The telangiectasia characteristically appear on the skin of the face, lips, palmar surface of the fingers and hands, under the fingernails, on the ears and on the mucous membranes of the nasal septum, tip and dorsum of the tongue. The gut, lungs, kidneys and brain may be involved. The cutaneous lesions are small, slightly elevated, red to purple and blanch on pressure. Because these blood vessels do not have muscle or connective tissue in their walls, hemostatic control is poor and mucosal bleeding, especially epistaxis, is common. Recurrent gastrointestinal tract hemorrhage may lead to iron deficiency anemia.

Ehlers–Danlos syndrome and related disorders

Patients with this disorder have abnormal elastic tissue possibly due to a defective fibronectin. Similar problems occur in pseudoxanthoma elasticum and Marfan's syndrome. Both Ehlers–Danlos and Marfan's have been associated with platelet dysfunction with reduced aggregation to ADP, collagen and noradrenaline. Patients with Ehlers–Danlos syndrome develop elastic scars, particularly at the knees and elbows, and hyperextensibility of joints (Fig. 15.20). There is a lifelong tendency to excessive bruising and hematoma formation together with increased bleeding and poor wound healing after surgery. There is no specific treatment.

Henoch–Schönlein purpura (HSP) (anaphylactoid purpura)

The underlying problem in patients with HSP is an immune complex type III hypersensitivity reaction often following an acute infection. This produces a vasculitis with exudation and a perivascular infiltration which includes eosinophils. The coagulation times and platelet count are normal. The rash is typical (Fig. 15.21) and is raised and maculopapular due to the vasculitic changes. In the early stages it can resemble urticaria but it becomes erythematous with a central area of hemorrhage and finally it fades to brown due to denaturation of the extravasated hemoglobin. Initially it is itchy or painful and appears in crops predominantly on the buttocks and extensor surfaces of the arms and lower legs. Accompanying the rash are joint and gastrointestinal symptoms and localized edema in the majority of patients. Overt renal damage with hematuria occurs in one-third of patients (Chs 17 and 24).

Scurvy (vitamin C deficiency)

Deficiency of vitamin C still does occur in malnourished children. It presents with pain and tenderness of the limbs due to subperiosteal hemorrhages. Epistaxis, hematuria, gastrointestinal bleeding, petechiae and ecchymoses may appear. There are often characteristic perifollicular hemorrhages and bleeding from the friable gums with loosening of the teeth. The primary defect is thought to reside in the intercellular substance.

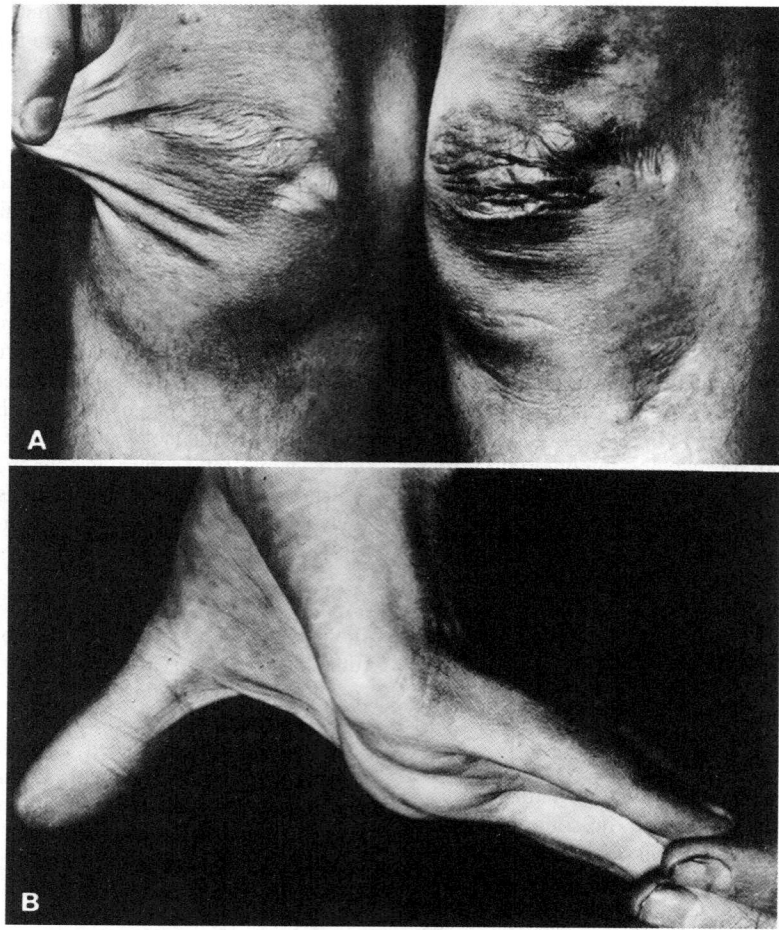

Fig. 15.20 Ehlers–Danlos syndrome: (A) scar tissue on knees; (B) hyperextensibility of joints.

Purpura associated with infections

Mild transient nonthrombocytopenic purpura occurs in the course of many infections and examples include measles, scarlet fever, typhoid, rickettsial infections and meningococcal septicemia. A severe form of rapidly spreading skin hemorrhage can occur, particularly in meningococcemia, and must be distinguished from that due to protein C deficiency (see below). Gangrene of the extremities and facial prominences may occur. This is primarily a vasculitic condition but a consumptive coagulopathy with secondary thrombocytopenia may also develop. This is one of the rare instances when continuous heparin infusions (adjusted to keep the partial thromboplastin time approximately twice normal) may be of value in preservation of tissue.

Steroid purpura

Long-term steroid therapy is associated with purpura caused by defective vascular supportive tissue.

THROMBOCYTOPENIC PURPURAS

There are many causes of low platelet count, which have been classified (Table 15.14). Both in terms of classification and differential diagnosis it is useful to make a primary subdivision into those with normal or increased numbers of megakaryocytes in the marrow and those with reduced or absent numbers. This differentiates between increased peripheral destruction and reduced production as the cause of the thrombocytopenia. Generally, there is no significant hemostatic defect until the platelet count falls below $100 \times 10^9/l$ and widespread spontaneous purpura rarely develops above $25 \times 10^9/l$. The hemostatic defect is mainly due to failure of formation of an adequate platelet 'plug' at the site of damaged capillaries, small arterioles and venules. Coagulation screening tests such as the prothrombin time, thrombin time and partial thromboplastin time will be normal. The standardized template bleeding time will be prolonged usually to over 10 min if the platelet count is low, but it is rarely necessary to perform this in the presence of severe thrombocytopenia.

Differential diagnosis

The first step is to take a careful clinical history and examination. There may be a family history of bleeding in cases of congenital thrombocytopenia. These cases are often very mild and often picked up at a later age because of the family history, length of history and sometimes because of characteristic blood film

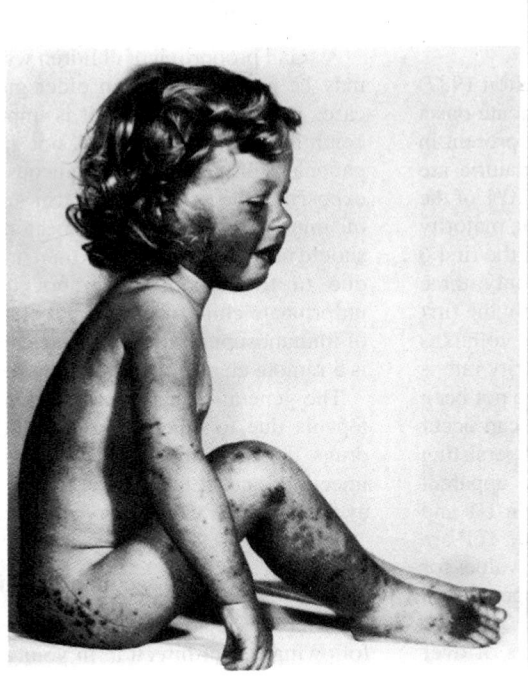
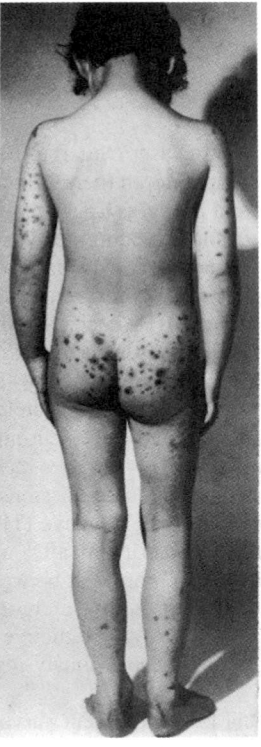

Fig. 15.21   Rash of anaphylactoid purpura. Two patients showing characteristic distribution of the rash on buttocks, shins and extensor surfaces of arms.

Table 15.14   Causes of thrombocytopenia in childhood

A. Failure of platelet production		
1. Congenital	TAR syndrome	
	Megakaryocytic hypoplasia	
	Bernard-Soulier syndrome	
	May-Hegglin anomaly	
	Wiskott-Aldrich syndrome	
	Metabolic disorders, e.g. isovaleric acidemia	
	Trisomy 13 or 18	
2. Acquired	Aplastic anemia	
	Marrow infiltration – tumor/infection	
	Drug or radiation induced	
	B_{12}/folate deficiency	
B. Sequestration	Hyperthermia	
	Hypothermia	
C. Dilutional	Massive transfusion	
D. Increased destruction		
1. Immunological	ITP	
	Drug induced	
	Infection	
	Post-transfusion purpura	
	Autoimmune disorders	
	Neonatal immune	
2. Non-immunological	Hemolytic uremic syndrome	
	TTP and DIC	
	Kasabach-Merritt syndrome	
	Heart valves/patches	

ITP = idiopathic thrombocytopenic purpura,
TAR = thrombocytopenia with absent radii, TTP = thrombotic
thrombocytopenic purpura, DIC = disseminated intravascular coagulation.

findings especially in *Bernard–Soulier syndrome* and the *May–Hegglin anomaly*. If the blood film is normal apart from an almost complete lack of platelets and there is no family history, no previous history of bruising, and examination reveals no abnormality other than bruising, the most likely diagnosis is idiopathic thrombocytopenic purpura. It may not be necessary to perform a bone marrow in every case if there are no unusual features. However, in all other cases it is necessary to subdivide the causes as already stated.

Coagulation screening tests are not usually indicated unless there is a possibility of consumptive coagulopathy or there is hypersplenism, when there may be hepatic dysfunction. Finally, a history of drug ingestion is very important in determining potential causative factors.

Idiopathic thrombocytopenic purpura (ITP)

This is the commonest example of an immune type of thrombocytopenia. They are almost always characterized by increased amounts of IgG on the platelet although there is not always a correlation between the amount of antibody and severity of the disease. The reticuloendothelial (RE) cells within the spleen are the most important sites of clearance of IgG-coated platelets. A history of recent infection especially of the upper respiratory tract is common and it is postulated that IgG binds to viral antigen absorbed on to platelets. The annual incidence of symptomatic childhood ITP is estimated to be four per 100 000 children. Thus there should be just a little over 40 cases in a country the size of Scotland each year. However, this is probably an underestimate on account of the number of mild cases and the lack of centralization of management. The age distribution is very similar to ALL with the peak between 2 and 5 years of age and an equal sex incidence.

Clinical manifestation

Recent reviews of a large number of cases (Stuart & Kelton 1987) have clarified the picture. In most children there is an acute onset with easy bruising, petechiae and purpura. Epistaxis is present in about a quarter and gastrointestinal bleeding and hematuria are less common. Minimal splenomegaly occurs in only 5–10% of the symptomatic cases and this may be an overestimate. The majority of cases of intracranial hemorrhage (ICH) occur within the first 6 months and a review of 1800 ITP cases showed only three occurring after this age with the majority occurring within the first month. The median time to recovery of normal platelet counts is 1 month and 75% recover within 6 months. The chronicity rate is difficult to determine because most series of cases have not been followed for long enough and spontaneous remissions can occur for many years after diagnosis. Less than 5% have ITP persisting for several years. Occasionally ITP can recur after an apparent complete recovery and this has been reported in between 1% and 4% of cases. Response rates for splenectomy in chronic ITP are between 75% and 88%, and there is no predictive value for response as to whether or not they had previously responded to steroids.

Overall mortality from ITP is low and recent surveys of over 1000 patients show an approximately 0.5% fatality rate in symptomatic patients. The mortality of established ICH cases is approximately one-third.

Hematological findings

In most cases the only abnormal finding is a very low platelet count although anemia may ensue in children (less than 10%) where significant bleeding occurs. If a marrow is performed it shows normal or increased numbers of megakaryocytes but no specific diagnostic features. It is not usually necessary to perform any other tests except autoantibody screening in atypical cases to exclude SLE. A direct Coombs' test is worth carrying out because it is straightforward and a negative result rules out autoimmune hemolysis as part of Evans' syndrome (see above).

Management

ITP is a relatively benign disease with the majority of children making a complete recovery, therefore it is important not to overtreat. There is no evidence that bed rest in the early stages of the illness is of benefit. The majority of patients do not require any specific therapy and it should be emphasized that one treats the child and not the platelet count. If the child has generalized petechiae and purpura, especially if there is mucosal bleeding, fundal hemorrhage or gut bleeding, it is reasonable to treat with a 2-week course of prednisolone 2 mg/kg/day tailing it off rapidly over the third week. This will allow assessment of the response to steroids but limit the side effects. There is no indication for long-term steroid therapy. Although intravenous immunoglobulin has been demonstrated to improve the platelet count rapidly in ITP it is not recommended as first-line therapy because it means using a blood product with potential risk of transmission of infections and it is expensive.

After a course of prednisolone is completed it is common for the platelet count to fall then progressively recover, so that restarting steroids is not indicated, neither is resorting to intravenous immunoglobulin. A moderate amount of skin bleeding does not require therapy.

A small proportion of children will develop chronic ITP and this may be more common in older girls. The management of such cases can be difficult but it is important to consider the clinical condition of the child and not just the platelet count. Some patients will have late spontaneous recoveries and should not be exposed to the risks of long-term steroid therapy, repeated courses of immunoglobulin or splenectomy. The last two treatments should only be considered if there is clinically significant bleeding due to the chronic thrombocytopenia. For the even rarer unfortunate child who does not respond to this approach, the use of immunosuppressive agents or danazol may be justified as there is a remote chance that they may be successful.

The general management of children with ITP, or thrombocytopenia due to other causes, includes avoiding aspirin or other drugs that can impair platelet function, avoiding intramuscular injections and, if the platelet counts are very low, children should avoid situations which carry significant risks of severe trauma.

Thrombocytopenia secondary to infection

Mild thrombocytopenia of the order of $50–100 \times 10^9/l$ is common following recent infection in young children. Sometimes there is accompanying splenomegaly and both resolve within a week or two. The infection is often a simple upper respiratory tract infection but is sometimes due to specific causes such as glandular fever, cytomegalovirus or toxoplasmosis. Many of the more serious infections produce consumptive coagulopathy.

Drug-induced thrombocytopenia

Drugs such as alkylating agents and antimetabolites used in leukemia treatment regularly produce a dose-dependent general marrow suppression. The other main type of drug-induced thrombocytopenia is that produced by immunological mechanisms, usually of the drug–hapten variety. This has been shown to occur with sedormid, quinidine, quinine, sulfamethazine, antazoline and other drugs. This emphasizes the importance of the drug history in patient assessment.

Congenital and neonatal thrombocytopenia

Neonatal thrombocytopenia can be caused by any severe infection and is frequently seen with toxoplasmosis, CMV and herpes simplex. Maternal problems such as SLE, ITP and ingestion of thiazide diuretics can also lead to low platelet counts in the baby. Isoimmune thrombocytopenia occurs by an identical mechanism to isoimmune hemolysis. The most common antigen involved is PlA1. Emergency treatment of this disorder is with PlA1-negative platelets either from a donor or from the mother. Intravenous immunoglobulin is effective in raising the platelet count in affected babies and its use antenatally in the mother is being evaluated.

Bernard–Soulier syndrome is an autosomal recessive disorder with giant platelets on the blood film and usually a moderate bleeding tendency. The defect is caused by an inherited deficiency of platelet membrane glycoprotein Ib leading to absent aggregation with ristocetin which does not correct with normal plasma. *Wiskott–Aldrich syndrome* is X-linked recessive and is characterized by severe eczema, thrombocytopenia and immunological deficiency. The *May–Hegglin anomaly* has been described under white cell disorders. *Thrombocytopenia with absent radii* (TAR) presents in the neonatal period and is probably inherited in an autosomal recessive fashion. There is a 35% mortality from bleeding during the first year of life.

DISORDERS OF PLATELET FUNCTION

These can be hereditary or acquired and present typically with a normal platelet count, skin and mucosal bleeding and a prolonged template bleeding time.

Hereditary

These are all rare. *Glanzman's disease* or thrombasthenia shows autosomal recessive inheritance and the absence of platelet membrane IIb/IIIa complex with resultant lack of aggregation with all stimulants except ristocetin. The bleeding is generally mucosal and can be severe. The only specific therapy is platelet transfusion which should be used sparingly because of the potential development of antibodies to IIb/IIIa.

In a number of platelet storage pool diseases there is defective release of platelet nucleotides owing to an intrinsic deficiency in the number of dense granules or alpha granules. The association with tyrosinase-positive albinism is called *Hermansky–Pudlack syndrome* and the bleeding problems are usually mild.

Acquired

Aspirin causes inhibition of prostaglandin synthetase and impaired thromboxane A2 synthesis. There is a failure of the release reaction and aggregation with adrenalin and ADP. A single small dose can have an effect for more than a week and this can be useful in the management of thrombocytosis. However, it is a nuisance when trying to investigate bleeding disorders and a very careful drug history must be taken before performing platelet aggregation.

Uremia and liver disease are associated with platelet dysfunction as are the myeloproliferative disorders. Other drugs such as nonsteroidal anti-inflammatory drugs, sulfinpyrazone, dipyridamole and ticlopidine have been linked with platelet dysfunction.

COAGULATION DISORDERS

The steps in normal coagulation are illustrated in Figure 15.22. The disorders can be conveniently divided into hereditary and acquired types.

HEREDITARY COAGULATION DEFECTS

The three most common serious defects are due to deficiency of factors VIIIc and IX and von Willebrand's disease. The other disorders are either very rare or they do not produce significant

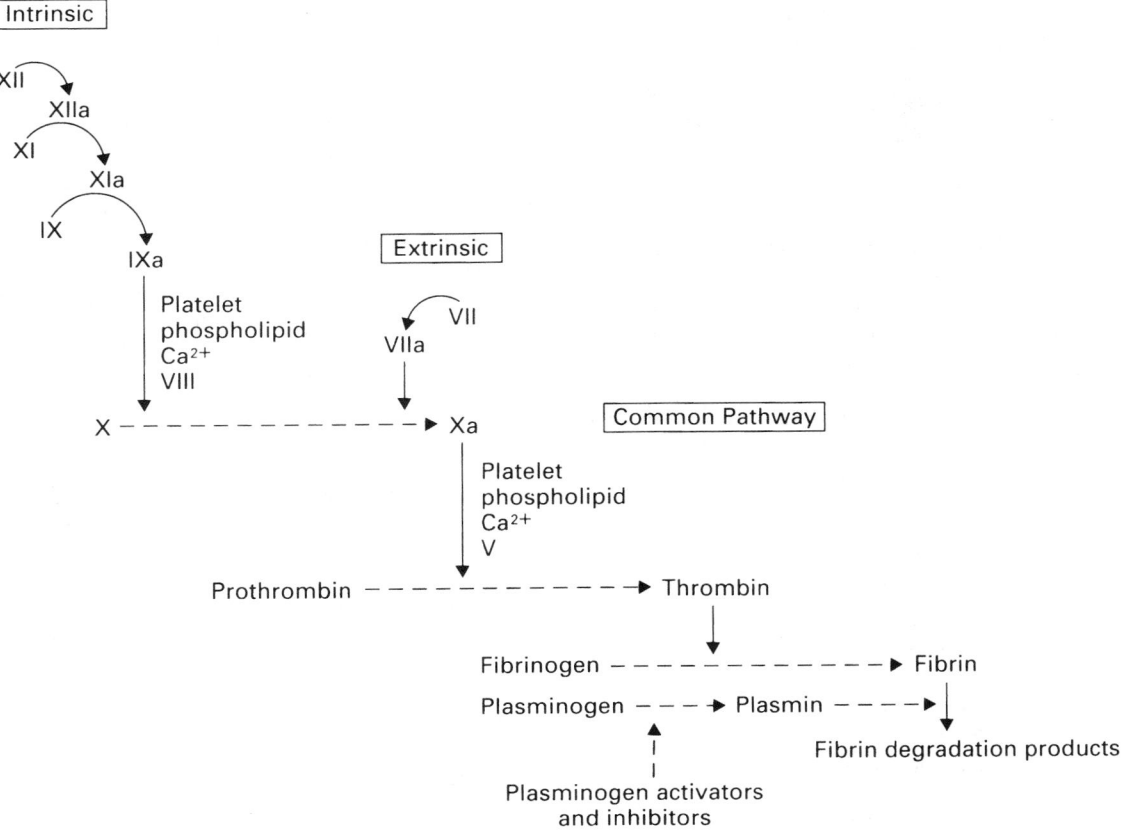

Fig. 15.22 Normal blood coagulation. Prothrombin time (PT) measures extrinsic and common. Partial prothrombin time (PTT) measures intrinsic and common. a = active form.

Table 15.15 Hemorrhagic disorders

Deficient factor	Site of production	Synonym	Inheritance	Approximate incidence
VIIIc	Liver	Hemophilia A	X recessive	1:30 000
IX	Liver	Christmas	X recessive	1:150 000
VIII VWF	Endothelial cell and platelets	von Willebrand's	Autosomal dominant	1:30 000
XI	Liver	PTA	Autosomal recessive	1:150 000
X	Liver	Stuart Prower	Autosomal recessive	1:500 000
VII	Liver	Proconvertin	Autosomal recessive	1:1 000 000
I	Liver	Fibrinogen	Autosomal recessive	Very rare
II	Liver	Prothrombin	Autosomal recessive	Very rare
XII	Liver	Hageman	Autosomal recessive	Very rare
XIII	Liver or platelets	Fibrin stabilizer	Autosomal recessive	Very rare

C = coagulant activity, PTA = plasma thromboplastin antecedent, VWF = von Willebrand's factor.

bleeding problems. Inheritance patterns and incidence are detailed in Table 15.15.

Hemophilia A (classical hemophilia)

This is one of the commonest hereditary bleeding disorders and a family history can be obtained in two-thirds of cases. The other third probably result from new mutations. Absence or low levels of factor VIII coagulation activity (VIIIc) is the basis of the disorder. Immunological studies reveal a normal amount of factor VIII related antigen (VIII RAG) which is separately synthesized in endothelial cells. The factor VIII component concerned with the platelet adhesion mediating function, factor VIII von Willebrand's factor (VIII VWF) is also unaffected.

Clinical features

The age and type of presentation correlates well with the level of factor VIIIc in a particular patient and will depend on the nature of any hemostatic challenge (Table 15.16). Severely affected individuals (with a level less than 2%) can present in early infancy with easy bruising (often confused with nonaccidental injury) or with spontaneous hemarthroses when they become more mobile. More severe manifestations, particularly intracranial hemorrhage, can occur following traumatic delivery and severe internal injuries at any age may well produce problems. However, they do not usually bleed excessively from cuts or from mucosal surfaces unless raw areas (e.g. tooth sockets) exist. Recurrent painful hemarthroses and muscle hematomas dominate the clinical course. In the past this led to progressive deformity with crippling

Table 15.16 Hemophilia A and B–level of clotting factor related to clinical features

Level of clotting factor (% of normal)	Clinical features
< 2%	Severe disease Spontaneous bleeding into joints and muscles
2–5%	Moderate disease Bleeding after trauma Occasional spontaneous bleeding
5–20%	Mild disease Bleeding after trauma

and painful ankylosed joints. Nowadays, this can largely be prevented by appropriate therapy. Operative and post-traumatic hemorrhage can be life threatening both in severely and 'mildly' affected patients with VIIIc levels of 5–30%. Hematuria is quite common; gastrointestinal hemorrhage less so.

Some hemophiliacs develop liver disease due to episodes of hepatitis mainly due to hepatitis C virus now that all patients are vaccinated against hepatitis B.

Diagnosis

The clinical history is crucial in the diagnosis of bleeding disorders and a family 'tree' should be constructed in any case where there is a history of bleeding in other family members. Particular aspects to look out for are bleeding or lack of it after dental extraction, circumcision, tonsillectomy and childbirth, all of which are severe hemostatic stresses. In hemophilia A, there will be a prolonged partial thromboplastin time (PTT) with a normal thrombin time (TT), prothrombin time (PT) and fibrinogen. The bleeding time is normal or near normal and the factor VIIIc assay is low with normal factor VIII RAG and VWF. Carrier females can now be detected by measuring the factor VIIIc : RAG ratio along with the family history and gene probe analysis. Antenatal diagnosis is thus feasible using gene probes on chorionic villus samples or by factor VIIIc analysis on fetoscopic blood samples where this is not feasible.

Management

Mild or moderate hemophiliacs may respond to treatment with desmopressin (DDAVP) sufficiently to cover minor procedures such as tooth extraction. Major procedures can also be managed in this way although failure of response after several days (tachyphylaxis) is a genuine problem.

Severe hemophilia is best treated with a factor VIII concentrate which has been sufficiently heat treated to reduce the risk of hepatitis and HIV transfer to minimal levels. 15 units of factor VIII per kg body weight raises the circulating factor VIII level by 30%, which is hemostatic for most clinical circumstances. This level will arrest spontaneous bleeding such as hemarthrosis, but a sustained level of over 50% is required to deal with severe bleeding episodes such as intracranial hemorrhage or to cover surgery such as appendectomy. This usually requires twice daily or even thrice daily treatment. Until recently the available factor

VIII concentrates were derived from human plasma and were treated to minimize the risk of transmission of viral infection. The characterization of the gene for factor VIII has allowed the manufacture of a recombinant factor VIII concentrate which should virtually eliminate the infection risk. Initial clinical use of this product has demonstrated its efficacy in treatment of episodes of bleeding. Currently this product is expensive and criteria for appropriate use are being worked out, most likely newly diagnosed hemophiliacs, most children and those with milder disease who are treated infrequently. Ultimately it is likely that recombinant products will become the treatment of choice.

There is insufficient space to deal with the many problems facing doctors caring for children with hemophilia. Some of the more important will be mentioned here. Bleeding around the throat or at the base of the tongue must be dealt with as an extreme emergency because of the risk of respiratory tract compression which is extremely difficult to manage. Similarly, compartmental compression of arteries in the forearm and leg can lead to severe problems of ischemia in the hand and foot if not dealt with promptly. Iliopsoas bleeding leads to hip flexion and femoral nerve dysfunction, usually because of intra-abdominal bleeding which must be treated with high doses of factor VIII and bed rest. Hemarthroses require prompt treatment at the first sign of swelling or onset of pain. Prophylactic therapy, giving factor VIII concentrate three times per week, has been shown to reduce long-term joint damage in severe hemophilia and should be considered in all severely affected boys from the age of 12–18 months (Nilsson et al 1994). This usually means insertion of a reliable means of venous access such as a 'Portacath' so that the parents can give the treatment at home. Hematuria needs to be treated promptly but tranexamic acid (a fibrinolytic inhibitor) must not be used as it can cause clotting in the ureters. This drug is, however, very useful in managing mucosal bleeds including tooth sockets. Hemophiliacs should never be given aspirin nor intramuscular injections but vaccines may be given subcutaneously or intradermally. Excellent dental care is essential to avoid the need for extractions.

The psychosocial problems of hemophiliacs are immense and should be at the forefront of management plans if the children are to integrate fully into 'normal' society.

HIV and hemophilia

All blood products carry a potential risk of HIV and other blood-borne virus infections. Thus they must never be used unless absolutely necessary. The proportion of hemophiliacs infected with HIV is falling as the newer factor VIII concentrates are safer and recombinant products will improve this further. The future for the patients who are HIV-positive is uncertain but it is beyond the scope of this chapter to deal with the extremely difficult problems they face. Azidothymidine (AZT) therapy in the early stages holds out some hope of delaying further progress of the disease and newer approaches are being developed.

Hemophilia B (Christmas disease)

This is caused by deficiency of factor IX and many of the manifestations of the disease are indistinguishable from those of hemophilia A. Some patients produce an abnormal molecule which is immunologically detectable (IXCAg). Diagnosis rests upon the features described for hemophilia A, along with a long PTT, normal PT, TT, fibrinogen and bleeding time and low factor IX level. It is very important to make sure that the patient does not have a hepatic disorder as a low factor IX may present in this way. If there is any doubt, assays of other vitamin K-dependent factors II, VII and X, if they are normal, will confirm the specific deficiency. Christmas disease does tend to have a milder clinical phenotype than hemophilia A but general management policies are the same. Treatment is with heat-treated factor IX concentrate, which has a longer half-life than factor VIII, and daily therapy for bleeds usually suffices.

Von Willebrand's disease (VWD)

The actual incidence of this disorder is uncertain because better diagnostic tests have only been available for a few years and many children are very mildly affected. Because of its autosomal inheritance, homozygous cases do occur; these are severely affected but usually still with mucocutaneous bleeding as the predominant problem. The defect is a failure of synthesis of factor VIIIc, VIII RAG and VIII VWF all of which can now be measured. The bleeding time is usually grossly prolonged as is the PTT, with normal PT, TT and fibrinogen. Ristocetin-induced platelet aggregation is impaired because factor VIII VWF potentiates platelet adherence to the subendothelial connective tissue. Clinically, the bleeding is mucocutaneous and following trauma.

Epistaxes can be a persistent problem in VWD patients and nasal cautery, tranexamic acid and DDAVP are all useful in therapy. DDAVP is effective in raising the level of VIII VWF in most types of VWD. Cryoprecipitate is rich in VIII VWF but is not heat treated; however, certain factor VIII concentrates contain therapeutically useful amounts of VIII VWF. A heat-treated concentrate containing VIII VWF is likely to be developed to avoid the potential infective risks of cryoprecipitate.

Other hereditary bleeding disorders

Congenital deficiencies of fibrinogen and factors V, VII, XI, XII and XIII are all rare and autosomally inherited. In general, the severity of the hemorrhagic state is mild and produces a familial bruising tendency, or bleeding following surgery. However, severe factor X deficiency with undetectable levels is a very severe disorder for which treatment is now available with lyophilized concentrate. Congenital afibrinogenemia is also severe and presents within the first 2 years of life. Factor XI deficiency is mild and more common amongst Jewish people. Factor XII deficiency is a very mild clinical disorder. Factor XIII is the fibrin-stabilizing factor and in deficiency typically produces delayed hemorrhage 24–36 h after injury, with delayed wound healing and sometimes scarring. Bleeding from the umbilical stump and delayed separation of the cord also occur and give a clue to the diagnosis. Specific assays define the diagnosis of all of these disorders.

ACQUIRED COAGULATION DEFECTS

Deficiency of vitamin K-dependent coagulation factors

The prothrombin complex, factors VII, IX, X and prothrombin itself (factor II) are all synthesized in the liver. The vitamin is fat soluble and obtained from green vegetables and bacterial synthesis in the gut. Deficiency may present in the newborn, when it is called hemorrhagic disease of the newborn (see Ch. 5, p. 230), or in later life. The prothrombin time, which can be performed on capillary blood samples, or the capillary thrombotest measures the vitamin K-dependent factors and specific assays will confirm the diagnosis where necessary. The PTT will also be prolonged.

Vitamin K-dependent factors are low at birth and fall further in breast-fed infants in the first few days of life. Liver cell maturity and lack of gut bacterial synthesis can contribute to deficiency which used to present on the second to fourth days of life. However, it can present later if routine supplementation has not been given or when these etiologic factors persist. Premature and ill babies are prone to deficiency and should always be supplemented. Oral supplements can be used where absorption is likely to be normal and before giving up routine supplementation it should always be remembered that the bleeding can be very severe. When this occurs, fresh frozen plasma can be used to supplement levels of deficient factors.

Vitamin K deficiency in older children can result from obstructive jaundice, pancreatic and small bowel disease. Prophylaxis can be achieved with 5 mg vitamin K oral daily.

Liver disease

Multiple hemostatic defects occur with liver disease and can worsen the bleeding from esophageal varices. Biliary obstruction results in impaired absorption of vitamin K. Severe hepatocellular disease also causes loss of production of factor V and fibrinogen. Hypersplenism causes thrombocytopenia and abnormalities of platelet and fibrinogen function occur in liver disease.

Consumptive coagulopathy – disseminated intravascular coagulation (DIC)

Platelets, fibrinogen, factor V and factor VIII are consumed in a variety of clinical situations, examples of which are promyelocytic leukemia, meningococcemia, falciparum malaria, snake bites and hemolytic transfusion reactions. The process is often accompanied by an acute hemolysis characterized by fragmentation of red cells which are damaged by the fibrin strands laid down in the microvasculature by the intravascular coagulation process. A similar pathogenesis occurs when this picture occurs in patients with heart valves and patches. Because of consumption of these coagulation factors the PT, PTT and TT will be prolonged with a low fibrinogen and raised fibrin degradation products (FDP). All of these abnormalities may also exist in liver disease (FDPs are cleared by the liver) and it may be necessary to measure factor V and VIII levels to differentiate between the two. The pathogenesis is complex and probably includes (a) entry of procoagulant material into the circulation, (b) widespread endothelial damage and collagen exposure and (c) widespread intravascular platelet aggregation.

Treatment of DIC is primarily to treat the precipitating disorder and replace the deficient factors with fresh frozen plasma, cryoprecipitate and platelets. The role of heparin therapy is controversial and there is little evidence that it works except possibly in promyelocytic leukemia and peripheral gangrene occurring in meningococcemia. The usual method of monitoring heparin therapy is to keep the PTT approximately twice normal with protamine sulfate used to reverse the effect when necessary.

THROMBOSIS IN CHILDREN

The control of the coagulation mechanism is complex with numerous inhibitors of activated procoagulant factors. It is increasingly recognized that deficiency of one of these naturally occurring anticoagulants can increase the risk of thrombosis. The recently described activated protein C resistance is thought to be the commonest of these thrombophilic states and deficiencies of antithrombin III, protein C and protein S are recognized. There may also be abnormalities of fibrinolysis with failure of plasmin generation.

Antithrombin III is the main physiological inhibitor of coagulation and in addition it is essential as a cofactor for heparin therapy. Thus, deficiency produces heparin resistance. It was named thus because it neutralizes thrombin but it also acts at other stages of the coagulation pathway and is the main physiological inhibitor of activated factor X. It is responsible for about 50–80% of the inhibitory capacity of plasma and the rest is provided by a_2-macroglobulin and α_1-antitrypsin. It is made in the liver and decreased levels occur in liver disease and pregnancy. Congenital deficiency leads to thrombosis usually occurring first in the teens and associated with a strong familial tendency. Oral anticoagulant therapy and specific replacement concentrates can control the disorder.

Protein C is vitamin K dependent and is another important regulating protein. It inactivates factors Va and VIIIa with protein S as a cofactor and in the presence of the thrombin/thrombomodulin complex on the endothelial cell surface. Deficiency of protein C is inherited as an autosomal dominant trait. Heterozygotes have a level of about 50% and are at risk of thromboembolic disease. The homozygous state has been associated with recurrent purpura fulminans and most children have died of thrombosis in infancy. Therapy with protein C concentrates and anticoagulants holds out hope for these patients as well as the heterozygotes. Protein S deficiency produces levels of 35–50% in heterozygotes with a consequent risk of venous thrombosis.

REFERENCES AND BIBLIOGRAPHY

Alter B P, Potter N U et al 1978 Classification and aetiology of the aplastic anaemias. Clinical Haematology 7: 431–466
Andrew M, Paes B, Milner R et al 1988 Development of the human coagulation system in the healthy premature infant. Blood 72: 1651–1657
Armitage J O 1994 Bone marrow transplantation. New England Journal of Medicine 330: 827–838
Bacigalupo A, Broccia G, Corda G et al 1995 Antilymphocyte globulin, cyclosporin, and granulocyte colony-stimulating factor in patients with acquired severe aplastic anemia (SAA): a pilot study of the EBMT SAA Working Party. Blood 85: 1348–1353
Barrett A J, Horowitz M M, Pollock B H et al 1994 Bone marrow transplants from HLA-identical siblings as compared with chemotherapy for children with acute lymphoblastic leukemia in a second remission. New England Journal of Medicine 331: 1253–1258
Bennett J M, Catovsky D, Daniel M T et al 1982 Proposals for the classification of the myelodysplastic syndromes. British Journal of Haematology 51: 189–199
Beral V, Roman E, Bobrow M (eds) 1993 Childhood cancer and nuclear installations. British Medical Journal Publishing Group, London

Bloom G E 1972 Disorders of bone marrow production. Pediatric Clinics of North America 19: 983–1008

Brittenham G M, Griffith P M, Nienhuis A W et al 1994 Efficacy of deferoxamine in preventing complications of iron overload in patients with thalassemia major. New England Journal of Medicine 331: 567–573

Campana D, Pui C-H 1995 Detection of minimal residual disease in acute leukaemia: methodologic advances and clinical significance. Blood 85: 1416–1434

Casper J, Camitta B, Truitt R et al 1995 Unrelated bone marrow transplants for children with leukemia or myelodysplasia. Blood 85: 2354–2363

Chanarin I 1990 The megaloblastic anaemias, 3rd edn. Blackwell, Oxford

Charache A, Terrin M L, Moore R D et al 1995 Effect of hydroxyurea on the frequency of painful crises in sickle cell anemia. New England Journal of Medicine 332: 1317–1322

Chessells J M, Bailey C, Richards S M 1995 Intensification of treatment and survival in all children with lymphoblastic leukaemia: results of UK Medical Research Council trial UKALL X. Lancet 345: 143–148

Cline M J 1994 The molecular basis of leukemia. New England Journal of Medicine 330: 328–336

Evans R S, Takahashi K et al 1951 Primary thrombocytopenic purpura and acquired haemolytic anaemia: evidence for a common etiology. Archives of Internal Medicine 87: 48–65

Greaves M F 1988 Speculations on the cause of childhood acute lymphoblastic leukemia. Leukemia 2: 120–125

Hann I M, Bodger M P, Hoffbrand A V 1983 Development of pluripotent haemopoietic progenitor cells in the human fetus. Blood 62: 118–123

Hinchcliffe R F, Lilleyman J S 1987 Practical paediatric haematology. Wiley, Chichester

Hoelzer D 1994 Acute lymphoblastic leukaemia. Clinical Haematology 7: 2

Hoffbrand A V 1983 Pernicious anaemia. Scottish Medical Journal 28: 218–227

Hoffbrand A V, Lewis S M (eds) 1981 Postgraduate haematology, 2nd edn. Heinemann Medical Books, London

Hoffbrand A V, Pettit J E 1993 Essential haematology, 3rd edn. Blackwell, Oxford

Hoyer L W 1994 Hemophilia A. New England Journal of Medicine 330: 38–47

Kaspir D O, Luban N L 1987 Pediatric transfusion medicine. CRC Press, Florida

Kinlen L 1988 Evidence for an infective cause of childhood leukaemia: comparison of a Scottish new town and with nuclear reprocessing sites in Britain. Lancet ii: 1323–1327

Lestas A N, Rodeck C H, White J M 1982 Normal activities of glycolytic enzymes in the fetal erythrocytes. British Journal of Haematology 50: 439–444

Lilleyman J S, Hann I M 1992 Paediatric haematology. Churchill Livingstone, London

Lucarelli G, Giardini C, Baronciani D 1995 Bone marrow transplantation in thalassaemia. Seminars in Hematology 32: 297–303

Lusher J M 1994 Transfusion therapy in congenital coagulopathies. Hematology/Oncology Clinics of North America 8: 1167–1180

Madhok R, Forbes C D, Evatt B L 1987 Blood, blood products and AIDS. Chapman & Hall, London

Nathan D G, Oski F A 1992 Haematology of infancy and childhood, 4th edn. W B Saunders, London

Nilsson I M, Berntorp E, Ljung R, Lofqvist T, Pettersson H 1994 Prophylactic treatment of severe hemophilia A and B can prevent joint disability. Seminars in Hematology 31(2)(suppl 2): 5–9

Olivieri N F, Nathan D G, MacMillan J H et al 1994 Survival in medically treated patients with homozygous beta-thalassemia. New England Journal of Medicine 331: 574–578

Olivieri N F, Brittenham G M, Matsui D et al 1995 Iron-chelation therapy with oral deferiprone in patients with thalassemia major. New England Journal of Medicine 332: 918–922

Passmore S J, Hann I M, Stiller C A et al 1995 Pediatric myelodysplasia: a study of 68 children and a new prognostic scoring system. Blood 85: 1742–1750

Pui C-H 1995 Childhood leukemias. New England Journal of Medicine 332: 1618–1630

Rosenfeld S J, Kimball J, Vining D, Young N S 1995 Intensive immunosuppression with antithymocyte globulin and cyclosporine as treatment for severe acquired aplastic anemia. Blood 85: 3058–3065

Stuart M J, Kelton J G 1987 The platelet: quantitative and qualitative abnormalities. In: Nathan D, Oski F (eds) Haematology of infancy and childhood. W B Saunders, London, pp 1343–1428

Wintrobe M M et al 1981 Clinical haematology, 8th edn. Lea and Febiger, London

Young N S, Barrett A J 1995 The treatment of severe acquired aplastic anemia. Blood 85: 3367–3377

16 Oncology and terminal care

O. B. Eden

Incidence and prevalence 885
Factors influencing survival 885
Etiology 885
Congenital disorders 887
Chromosomal deletions/rearrangements 887
Environmental factors 889
    Ionizing radiation 889
    Electricity and electromagnetic fields 890
    Drugs 890
    Chemicals 890
    Viruses 891
Epidemiological conclusions 891
General principles of diagnosis 891
Pathology 891
Radiology 891
Biochemical markers 891
Molecular and cytogenetics 891
Bone marrow examination 892
Principles of therapy 892
Tumor cell resistance 892
    Primary resistance 892
    Secondary resistance 892
Surgery and irradiation 893
Monitoring tumor response 893
Specific effects of treatment 893
    Ionizing irradiation 893
    Chemotherapy 893
    Hematological toxicity 894
    Neutropenia and infection 894
    Immunosuppression 895
    Bleeding 895
    Local tissue toxicity 895
    Nausea and vomiting 895
    Mucositis 896
    Bowel dysfunction 896
    Renal toxicity 896
    Cardiotoxicity 896
    Neurotoxicity 896
    Ototoxicity 897
    Hepatotoxicity 897
    Biochemical disturbance 897
    Acute psychological effects 897
Long-term sequelae 897
    Late recurrence 897
    Second tumors 898
    Growth impairment 898
    Educational and psychological 899
    Cardiorespiratory 899
    Life prospects 899
    Conclusions on sequelae 899

Central nervous system tumors 899
Symptoms and signs 900
    Infratentorial lesions 900
    Supratentorial lesions 900
Diagnosis 901
General principles of treatment 901
    Surgery 901
    Radiotherapy 901
    Chemotherapy 901
Medulloblastoma (PNET of cerebellum) 901
Ependymoma 902
Cerebellar astrocytomas 902
Supratentorial astrocytomas 903
Brainstem gliomas 903
Optic gliomas (optic nerve, chiasma and tracts) 904
Pineal tumors 904
Craniopharyngioma 905
Choroid plexus neoplasms 905
Supratentorial PNETs 906
Spinal cord tumors 906
Non-Hodgkin's lymphoma (NHL) 906
Origins of lymphoma 906
Classification 907
Presentation 907
    Lymphoblastic lymphomas 907
    Small noncleaved tumors 907
    Localized disease 907
    Pharyngeal involvement 908
    Isolated testicular disease 908
    CNS involvement 908
Diagnosis 908
Staging 908
Prognostic factors 908
Management 908
Hodgkin's disease 909
Cell biology and classification 909
Clinical presentation 909
Diagnosis 909
Staging and therapy 910
Neuroblastoma 910
Presentation 911
Investigations 911
Staging 912
Management 912
Screening 913
Nephroblastoma (Wilms' tumor) 913
Mesoblastic nephroma 915
Soft tissue sarcomas (STS) 915
Rhabdomyosarcoma 915

Osteosarcoma   917

Ewing's sarcoma   918

Germ cell tumors   920

Teratomas   920

Germinoma (seminoma in testis, dysgerminoma in
    ovary)   920

Embryonal carcinoma   920

Endodermal sinus tumor (yolk sac)   921

Choriocarcinoma   921

Gonadoblastoma   921

Polyembryoma   921

Sacrococcygeal tumors   921

Mediastinal teratomas   922

Abdominal germ cell tumors   922

Intracranial teratomas   922

Gonadal tumors   922

Management   922

    Benign germ cell tumors   922

    Immature germ cell tumors   923

    Malignant germ cell tumor   923

Retinoblastoma   923

Liver tumors   924

Hepatoblastoma   924

Hepatocellular carcinoma   924

Diagnosis   924

Staging and histology   924

Management   925

    Hepatoblastoma   925

    Hepatocellular carcinoma   925

Histiocytoses   925

    Class I histiocytosis   925

    Class II histiocytosis   926

    Class III histiocytoses   927

Terminal care   927

Telling the truth   927

Symptom control   928

    Pain   928

    Itching   928

    Bowel dysfunction   928

    Urinary retention   928

    Transfusion   928

Explanations   928

Conclusion   929

References   929

INCIDENCE AND PREVALENCE

Childhood cancer is relatively rare in the United Kingdom with an overall estimated incidence during the first 15 years of life of 1.36 per 1000 live births. Relative and absolute incidence figures for individual tumor types are shown (Tables 16.1 and 16.2) (Parker et al 1988, Obioha et al 1989). Variations in incidence around the world relate to methods of diagnosis as well as genetic variations (e.g. retinoblastoma and nephroblastoma) and environmental factors which explain the very high incidence of B cell lymphomas in equatorial Africa. There are other as yet unexplained phenomena such as the very low incidence of Ewing's sarcoma amongst American blacks (Olisa et al 1975). The different incidence of some tumors (e.g. non-Hodgkin's lymphoma (NHL) as seen in Table 16.2) between the sexes has not as yet been fully explained. Tumors now constitute the commonest cause of childhood deaths after accidents and congenital abnormalities in the UK, but that may alter with progressively improving disease-free survival for many childhood cancers (Table 16.3). Hawkins (1989) demonstrated a marked improvement in disease-free survival which has occurred since 1970 for acute lymphoblastic leukemia (ALL), Hodgkin's disease, nephroblastoma, medulloblastoma, ependymoma and malignant ovarian germ cell tumors. For other tumors, e.g. acute nonlymphoblastic leukemia (ANLL), the trend for improvement has only occurred in the last 5 years. Although there is not a significant overall increase in incidence of childhood cancer in the UK, certain tumors, e.g. Hodgkin's disease, medulloblastoma, neuroblastoma, and germ cell tumors, show national or regional increases over the last decade (Blair & Birch 1994). At the same time, the prevalence of survivors in society is increasing rapidly with recent estimates that by the year 2000 one in every 900 individuals aged between 16 and 44 years will have survived a childhood tumor and consequently the quality as well as the quantity of survival now requires detailed consideration (Young et al 1986).

FACTORS INFLUENCING SURVIVAL

Prognostic factors for each tumor type will be discussed elsewhere, but some general factors are relevant. The improvement from 10% to 60% overall disease-free survival for ALL over the last 20 years has been achieved by the use of multiagent chemotherapy. The associated morbidity requires intensive nursing support, an adequate blood transfusion service and laboratory back-up. Given the rarity of these diseases, centralization of care has enabled the rational use of such facilities. Improvement in disease-free survival has occurred because patients have been entered into strict therapeutic protocols (Eden et al 1991) and are mainly treated in specialized pediatric oncology centers. Centralization of care has also been demonstrated to improve survival for ANLL, non-Hodgkin's lymphoma, nephroblastoma, osteosarcoma, Ewing's sarcoma and rhabdomyosarcoma (Table 16.3) (Stiller 1988). There is still a tendency for low stage Hodgkin's disease and nephroblastoma to be treated in district hospitals while more advanced disease is referred to specialized centers. This may obscure the significance of the overall improving trends. Treatment in nonexperienced centers may be excessive (Pritchard et al 1989). Failure to recognize the true extent of disease and to modify treatment appropriately can lead to undertreatment and death, or conversely overtreatment and excess toxicity.

ETIOLOGY

Compared with adult cancers relatively little is still known about the etiology of pediatric cancers but the widespread search for causative factors is motivated by the concept that prevention

Table 16.1   Crude relative incidence figures for childhood cancers (%) and related conditions

	England and Wales*	Eastern Nigeria†	USA* White	USA* Black
Leukemias	33.6	12.9	31.0	23.1
Lymphomas				
NHL Burkitt's	0.3	26.5	1.5	0.4
NHL all other	5.8	6.2	5.7	4.4
Hodgkin's disease	4.3	6.6	5.6	4.9
Brain and spinal tumors	23.5	9.7	19.0	21.0
Neuroblastoma (+ other sympathetic nervous system tumors)	6.8	3.0	8.2	8.6
Nephroblastoma (+ other renal)	5.2	14.0	6.1	10.8
Bone tumors				
All tumors	5.1	?	4.9	4.7
(Ewing's sarcoma)	(1.9)	?	(2.1)	(0.3)
Germ cell tumors	2.4	?	3.3	4.0
Retinoblastoma	2.7	6.2	2.5	4.1
Liver tumors	0.9	2.3	1.1	1.2
Histiocytoses	0.5	?	0.2	0.2
Other	1.3	7.8	4.2	4.4

* Data derived from Parker et al (1988).
† Data from Obioha et al (1989).
NHL = non-Hodgkin's lymphoma.

Table 16.2   Crude rates per million children aged 0–15 of childhood malignancies (and related conditions) by sex

	England and Wales M	England and Wales F	USA White M	USA White F	USA Black M	USA Black F
Leukemias	38.7	30.5	44.2	35.9	22.9	25.6
Lymphomas	16.0	7.4	21.7	12.7	15.0	6.2
Non-Hodgkin's Burkitt's	(0.3)	(0.2)	(3.6)	(0.4)	(0.7)	(–)
NHL (all other)	(8.5)	(3.7)	(9.6)	(4.1)	(5.5)	(3.1)
Hodgkin's	(6.3)	(2.7)	(7.5)	(5.9)	(8.2)	(2.1)
Brain and spinal tumors	26.1	22.1	26.1	23.1	21.1	22.5
Soft tissue sarcomas	7.0	5.3	9.0	8.2	9.6	7.6
Sympathetic nervous system (including neuroblastoma)	6.6	5.3	10.7	10.4	8.5	9.3
Renal (including nephroblastoma)	6.0	6.4	6.9	8.6	10.2	12.5
Bone tumors						
All types	5.6	4.7	6.2	6.4	4.8	5.2
(Ewing's)	(2.1	1.7	2.9	2.5	0.3	0.3)
Germ cell tumors	2.2	2.7	3.8	4.4	2.7	5.5
Retinoblastoma	2.7	2.8	3.0	3.5	4.1	4.5
Liver tumors	0.8	0.9	1.8	1.0	1.0	1.4
Total	114.1	91.9	137.8	121.5	104.4	105.2

Data derived from Parker et al (1988).
NHL = non-Hodgkin's lymphoma.

Table 16.3 Actuarial 3-year percentage survival rates for children at each type of treatment center with results of log rank tests for heterogeneity of survival curves among types of treatment center allowing for age and year of diagnosis

Diagnostic group	Treatment center and years of diagnosis						X^2 (2 df)	P value
	Pediatric oncology center		Other teaching		Other nonteaching			
	1977–1980	1981–1984	1977–1980	1981–1984	1977–1980	1981–1984		
Acute nonlymphoblastic leukemia	28	32	23	(21)	9	(6)	8.29	< 0.05
Hodgkin's disease	90	98	91	85	88	100	0.69	NS
Non-Hodgkin's lymphoma	56	70	32	(56)	43	(58)	10.8	< 0.01
Neuroblastoma	32	49	52	(54)	(25)	*	4.09	NS
Nephroblastoma	83	80	81	(77)	81	*	0.31	NS
Osteosarcoma	39	54	32	24	38	37	4.39	NS
Ewing's sarcoma	46	50	24	(33)	(43)	(45)	8.04	< 0.05
Rhabdomyosarcoma	63	63	25	(36)	46	*	21.0	< 0.0001

Figures in parentheses are % for fewer than 20 patients.
* Fewer than 10 patients in group.
Data from Stiller (1988).

would be preferable to intensive therapy. For many childhood cancers at least a component of genetic predisposition is considered likely.

CONGENITAL DISORDERS

Tables 16.4–16.6 show some of the well-recognized congenital disorders with an increased risk of malignancy. Mulvihill (1977) and McKusick (1988) have defined over 300 chromo-somal or genetic conditions in which there is a neoplastic tendency. A wide range of somatic and germ cell chromosomal disorders predispose to childhood malignancy. Down syndrome is the best

recognized and, even in phenotypically unrecognized mosaicism, leukemoid reactions can be seen in the neonatal period. Follow-up is required since approximately 15% of those with such reactions subsequently develop leukemia. ALL is still the most common form of leukemia occurring in the trisomy 21 patient although there is a higher incidence of ANLL than in other children.

CHROMOSOMAL DELETIONS/REARRANGEMENTS

DNA rearrangements are increasingly recognized in a wide variety of tumor types. Retinoblastoma is the most carefully documented genetically determined tumor. A two mutation

Table 16.4 Some constitutional chromosomal abnormalities associated with malignancy

Chromosome involved	Defect	Childhood tumor	Estimated risk
21	Trisomy (Down)	Acute leukemia Testicular Retinoblastoma*	1 in 74 (15 × normal) ?
13	Trisomy	Teratoma, leukemia Neurogenic	?
	Deletion q14	Sporadic retinoblastoma (± birth defects), osteosarcoma, pinealoblastoma	?
11	Deletion q13	Sporadic aniridia with/without Wilms' tumor	?
8	Trisomy	Preleukemia	?
X	Monosomy	Postestrogen endometrial carcinoma in Turner's syndrome ? Neurogenic ? Leukemia	?
X	Extra	Breast carcinoma Acute leukemia + NHL } in Extragonadal germ cell } Klinefelter's syndrome	?
Y	Present (in XY gonadal dysgenesis)	Gonadoblastoma Dysgerminoma	?
Sex chromosome aneuploidy	Present (XXYY, XXXY, XXX)	Retinoblastoma*	?
2Y	Mosaicism + XYY	Osteosarcoma Medulloblastoma CML Acute leukemia	?

* Often in Trisomy 21 associated with sex chromosome aneuploidy.

Table 16.5 Some genetic instability and DNA repair disorders predisposing to malignancy

Clinical disorder	Inheritance	Site of gene/defect	Tumor	Risk
Fanconi's anemia	AR	Gene at 20q (chromosomal breaks)	AML Squamous cell carcinoma Hepatic adenomas and carcinomas (? following androgen use)	1 in 12
Bloom's syndrome	AR	15q 26.1 chromosomal breaks + sister chromatid exchanges	Leukemia Gastrointestinal NHL	1 in 8
Ataxia telangiectasia (variants now being identified)	AR	Gene at 11q22 + (chromosomal breaks)	Lymphomata Leukemia Stomach carcinoma Brain Hodgkin's ? Other carcinomas (marked radiation sensitivity, ? also carriers)	1 in 8
Xeroderma pigmentosa	AR	(? Encode for helicases) (Failure to repair) (UV damage)	Basal and squamous cell Melanoma Tongue carcinoma	

Modified from original table by Strong (1984).
AR = autosomal recessive.

Table 16.6 Some examples of single gene defects predisposing to childhood tumors

Hereditary disorder	Inheritance	Site of genetic defect	Tumor types
Neurofibromatosis Type 1	AD	17q11.2	Sarcoma, neuroma, schwannoma, meningioma, optic glioma, pheochromocytoma, ALL + AML, neuroblastoma, nephroblastoma, melanoma, hepatic
Neurofibromatosis Type II	AD	22q	Bilateral acoustic neuromas, meningioma, spinal neurofibroma

Retinoblastoma	AD	13q14	In germ line:
			  retinoblastoma, pinealoblastomas, sarcomas (bone + soft tissue) carcinomas
			In somatic retinal cells:
			  retinoblastoma

Li–Fraumeni cancer family syndrome	AD	17p (P53 gene)	Sarcomas, breast carcinoma in young, brain, leukemia, lung carcinoma, adrenal cortical carcinoma
Wilms' tumor	AD	11p13 (loss of heterozygosity)	Wilms'
	AR	11p15.5	Wilms' with Beckwith–Wiedemann (ACC, hepatoblastoma, brain, sarcoma)
Familial polyposis coli and Gardner's syndrome	AD	5q21	Carcinoma of colon, hepatoblastoma, gastrointestinal polyps, osteosarcomas, fibromas, carcinoma of ampulla of Vater, pancreas, thyroid and adrenal
Gorlin's syndrome (nevoid basal cell carcinoma)	AD	9q22	Basal cell carcinoma, medulloblastoma, ovarian fibroma

AD = autosomal dominant; AR = autosomal recessive.

hypothesis has been proposed which would explain retinoblastoma oncogenesis. In the dominantly inherited form the first mutation occurs in germinal cells prezygotically and is present in all cells of the body. A second mutation in the somatic retinal cell is necessary to create the tumor. In the nonhereditary form two or more events are required within the somatic retinal cell itself. The first event may be a new mutation in the germinal cell so that all the infant's cells are affected or it may be a somatic mutation within the retinal cell. In the first two instances the affected child will then pass on the mutation to any future offspring he/she may have, but where both events have occurred in somatic cells there will be no hereditary component. The retinoblastoma gene has been isolated to chromosome l3 (13q14). Development of a tumor has been shown to be due to loss or inactivation of wild type retinoblastoma alleles at this locus. Loss of both alleles is required for tumor formation. Mutant genes such

as Rb1 which interrupt the function of the partner normal allele are known as tumor suppressor genes. The changes at this locus can result from nondisjunction, a mitotic recombination event or gene conversion as well as a point mutation. The same sequence of DNA is deleted in some patients with osteosarcoma. In the genetically predetermined form there are DNA changes in all tissues, not just the retina. All bilateral and 20% of unilateral retinoblastoma are of this inherited type. These patients are not only susceptible to retinal tumors, but also radiation-induced sarcomas and tumors remote from the primary site (sarcoma, melanomas, brain tumors and leukemia). There is also a strong association with the development of pineal tumors ('third eye'). Interestingly, new mutations are shown most often to be of paternal origin. Another tumor suppressor gene increasingly recognized as being involved in pediatric and familial cancers (germ line mutation) is the P53 gene at 17q12–13.

Increasingly, other deletions or rearrangements are being identified as modern cytogenetic and molecular techniques are perfected (e.g. 11q13 deletion in sporadic aniridia with and without nephroblastoma, and 1p32–p36 deletion in familial neuroblastoma). As DNA sequencing has become increasingly precise it is evident that certain rearrangements are consistently associated with specific leukemic processes (Emery 1984). A 9 : 22 translocation is consistently found in the 'adult type' of chronic myeloid leukemia when it occurs in childhood and in a small percentage of ALL and indicates very poor prognosis. The cleavage points are very constant. We do not know whether this represents an inherited defect of the host's pluripotential stem cell or whether it occurs in response to specific, but unknown, oncogenic agents. More recently, involvement of the ALL1 or MLL gene at 11q23 in both infant and secondary leukemia has fueled considerable new research into basic mechanisms of leukemogenesis.

In the 1970s it was discovered that RNA tumor viruses could take up cellular genes and activate them. This caused infected cells to undergo malignant transformation. These cellular genes were know as proto-oncogenes and, in their activated form within the viral genome, as oncogenes. It is now known that some oncogenes encode for growth regulatory functions (Bishop 1987). It has been shown that oncogenes can be transferred into normal cells in culture and produce malignant changes (Land et al 1983). The products from some proto-oncogenes have biochemical activities, e.g. abl located on chromosome 9 for tyrosine kinase while n-ras combines guanine nucleotides and has some involvement in GTP-ase activity. The fact that chromosomal rearrangements have been shown to occur in the region of proto-oncogenes and that some of these appear to produce growth factors has led to considerable speculation that they are involved in cancer formation (Yunis 1986). The full details of this activation and its importance remain to be clarified. A list of oncogenes and associated tumors includes c-myc and Burkitt's lymphoma, abl and chronic myelogenous leukemia, N-myc and neuroblastoma, rel and rhabdomyosarcoma and ets-1 with Ewing's sarcoma and neuroepithelioma. All of these known oncogenes are thought to act in a dominant fashion. Activation of proto-oncogenes may result from gross structural rearrangement (abl in CML), point mutation (N-ras in thoracic neuroblastoma), amplification (N-myc in neuroblastoma), or regulatory changes (myc in Burkitt's lymphoma). As yet the full mechanisms by which altered gene products affect normal cellular processes has not been clarified for most pediatric tumors. Specific genetic rearrangements associated with individual tumors will be mentioned under tumor headings.

Some of the genetic instability syndromes are listed in Table 16.5 (Strong 1984). These disorders have a high risk for the development of malignancy, particularly of lymphoid tumors. New syndromes involving both genetic instability and immune dysfunction are now being described. There is renewed interest in ataxia telangiectasia and its variants now that the gene has been identified, since although the syndrome is rare 1–2% of the population may be carriers. It has been postulated that the severe radiosensitivity seen in the homozygous state may be present to a lesser extent in heterozygotes and that they may be at increased risk of developing cancer. This line of research highlights the close interplay of genetic predisposition and environmental factors (e.g. in ataxia telangiectasia, ionizing irradiation). Table 16.6 shows the commonest of the hereditary disorders predisposing to tumor formation in childhood. For all of them there may be a long latent period between manifestations of the syndrome, e.g. neurofibromatosis, and the development of tumors. Other factors, e.g. colonic flora or chemicals, may be necessary to precipitate the malignant change seen in familial polyposis.

Where immune competence is impaired there is a high risk of leukemia and lymphoma development (Table 16.7). Greaves (1988) has postulated that an abnormal or exaggerated response to infection at a time of maximal normal B cell proliferation might explain the peak incidence of ALL at 3–6 years in the developed world. This may not be a reflection of an inherent immune defect but rather a failure to be exposed to infection at a younger age. Acquired immunodeficiency secondary to chemotherapy (e.g. cancer or chronic renal disease) and infection with HIV does predispose to tumor formation (Purtilo & Sakamoto 1984).

As interest in epidemiology has grown, more associations have been identified. Li & Fraumeni (1982) described a family syndrome of soft tissue sarcomas, breast cancer and other neoplasms occurring in children and young adults and Birch et al (1984) showed a 13-fold increase in the risk of breast cancer in mothers of children with soft tissue sarcoma. The majority but not all of these familial carriers are associated with P53 germ line mutations. Some familial and community clustering is related to shared environmental factors.

ENVIRONMENTAL FACTORS

Relatively few childhood cancers to date have a definite link to an environmental influence.

Ionizing radiation

Prenatal exposure

Stewart et al (1956) reported an approximately 1.5-fold increase in childhood cancer for fetuses exposed to X-rays performed on the maternal abdomen and pelvis during the first trimester of

Table 16.7 Some of the immunodeficiency disorders predisposing to childhood tumors

Immunodeficient condition	Inheritance	Tumors
Purtilo syndrome (hyperlymphoproliferative)	XR	Burkitt + other lymphomas
Bruton/agammaglobulinemia	XR	Lymphoma Leukemia Brain
Severe combined immuno-deficiency (SCID)	XR	Lymphoma Leukemia
Wiskott–Aldrich	XR	Lymphoma Leukemia
Chediak–Higashi	AR	Pseudolymphoma
True IgA deficiency	? AD	Lymphoma Leukemia Gastrointestinal Brain

XR = X-linked recessive; AR = autosomal recessive; AD = autosomal dominant.
(See Table 16.5 for ataxia telangiectasia.)

pregnancy. This apparent dose-related phenomenon has not been confirmed in all studies. No such effect was noted for the offspring of mothers exposed to the atomic bomb at Hiroshima and Nagasaki, but there was an effect on fetal head size among the Hiroshima bomb survivors (Jablon & Kato 1970, Miller & Mulvihill 1976).

Postnatal exposure

Children who were within 1 km of the epicenter of the Hiroshima bomb experienced an excess of acute and chronic myelogenous leukemia and ALL 3–10 years after the exposure. Young people surviving the atomic bomb are still developing thyroid and other adult cancers after 50 years.

Therapeutic (low dose) external irradiation delivered to the scalp for tinea capitis or to the thymus have both been associated with significant increases in leukemia, brain tumors and thyroid carcinoma (Modan et al 1977, Upton et al 1986). Dosages to the infant thyroid as low as 0.2 cGy have been reported in association with the development of carcinoma 12–17 years later. Speculation about the effects of radionucleotide ingestion from fallout has mostly centered on military personnel observing nuclear tests, although there is an alleged excess of childhood leukemia in Utah following exposure to fallout from atmospheric nuclear detonations (Lyon et al 1979).

Recently an increased risk of childhood malignancy (specifically leukemia) has been reported around nuclear reprocessing plants in the UK, both at Sellafield and Dounreay (Black 1987, COMARE 1986, 1988, 1996, Heasman et al 1987). Studies of known, environmental nuclide levels, routes of access and associated exposure to chemicals have failed to explain this risk, although Kinlen et al (1990) have postulated extreme population mixing, and Greaves (1988) abnormal infection response as possible etiologic factors in these remote and unusual communities. Irradiation (and chemotherapy) for a primary malignancy carries with it a definitive risk for development of a second tumor (see Late effects sections). It is important to remember that some children (e.g. with retinoblastoma gene, ataxia telangiectasia, nevoid basal cell carcinoma syndrome) are particularly sensitive to ionizing irradiation.

Ultraviolet radiation

Sunlight is the most common known cause of cancer in adults, with an increasing UK incidence as a result of more sunshine holidays and sunbed usage. The risk begins in childhood with unprotected and excessive sun exposure. The actual incidence of skin tumors during childhood is low.

Electricity and electromagnetic fields

Both proximity to high voltage electricity cabling and the effect of electromagnetic fields have recently joined the list of factors under investigation as contributing to childhood cancers.

Drugs

Prenatal

Maternal ingestion of diethylstilbestrol is associated with clear cell carcinoma of the vagina and cervix in the female offspring, maternal phenytoin with neural crest tumors, alcohol with adrenal,

neural crest and liver tumors and teratomas and barbiturates possibly with brain tumors. There may be a long latent period, e.g. the vaginal tumors did not occur until age 14–23 years when exposure was before 20 weeks of gestation. Other sedatives taken in pregnancy are also under scrutiny (Melnick et al 1987). The effect of phenytoin may be related to its immunosuppressive effect.

Postnatal exposure

Intensive immunosuppression as in renal transplantation is associated with a 20- to 40-fold increased risk of lymphoma development, especially intracerebral tumors with a short latent period. Modern intensive leukemia therapy carries an increased risk of inducing secondary leukemia (ANLL) and other neoplasms (e.g. brain). Chronic malnutrition, by inducing immune paralysis, coupled with chronic infective antigenic stimulation may be important in the induction of B cell neoplasias in tropical Africa.

There is an increased risk of developing ANLL for those treated with alkylating agents for other tumors (at the rate of 5–10% over the 10 years following exposure in adults). The most commonly used, cyclophosphamide, especially when hemorrhagic cystitis has been induced, has also been incriminated as causing bladder cancer (Tucker et al 1987). The exact risk for children treated for either cancer or glomerulonephritis has not been quantified, but the avoidance of combined irradiation and alkylating agent chemotherapy, especially when the bladder is involved, appears wise. Long-term use of androgens and other anabolic steroids has been associated with the development of hepatomas in patients with Fanconi's anemia. Most tumors are benign, but hepatocellular carcinoma has been described. Such tumors have been reported in other conditions and in athletes taking long courses of anabolic steroids without any known underlying genetic instability.

Phenytoin in children can induce a benign lymphadenopathy, a self-limiting pseudolymphomatous condition; and rarely a true lymphoma. Barbiturates used in early infancy have also been incriminated in brain tumor formation.

Chemicals

Table 16.8 shows some of the parental occupations or exposures which have been incriminated in childhood tumor formation. The exposure may be maternal or paternal, e.g. solvent exposure in the aircraft industry may act on the male germ cell line which is then

Table 16.8 Possible parental occupation associations with childhood cancers

Occupation	Substance	Tumor type
Petroleum Lead } industry	Hydrocarbons	Nephroblastoma ? Other tumors
Aircraft Painting } industry	Organic solvents	Brain tumors
Paper/pulp mill working	? Organic solvents	Brain, urinary tract tumors
Farming	Insecticides Phenoxy herbicide ? N-nitroso compounds	Brain tumors (? only adults)

Modified from Strong (1984).

transmitted to the fetus. Although close exposure to asbestos mines in childhood was associated with the development, in later life, of mesotheliomas in South Africa, the rare mesotheliomas of childhood do not appear to be related to asbestos exposure.

Viruses

None of the common viral agents leading to intrauterine infection have yet been shown to be oncogenic. Postnatal exposure to Epstein–Barr virus (EBV) is associated with B cell lymphoid malignancies (Burkitt's lymphoma and leukemia) in malarial areas of Africa where they comprise up to 50% of all childhood tumors (Magrath 1993). African Burkitt's lymphoma occurs almost exclusively in areas of endemic malaria where early exposure (almost the whole population has been exposed by the age of 3 years) and high titers to EB virus are expected. Most of the tumors in endemic areas show evidence for the inclusion of viral DNA and the most consistently detectable antigen is the EB surface capsid antigen. Infection early in life is thought to increase the size of certain pre-B and B cell populations and maintains them in a proliferative state making them more likely to genetic change. Alternatively EBV may produce an immortal cell clone with genetic translocation already present. Repeated infection, in particular with malaria (itself a T cell suppresser and B cell mitogen), and malnutrition lead to a major degree of T cell immunosuppression, and B cell hyperplasia, with tumor formation likely. We do not know whether the initial infection or subsequent events lead to the very characteristic translocation of DNA from chromosome 8 into the immunoglobulin coding sites on chromosomes 14, 2 or 22. The role of other cofactors, such as plant extracts, in promoting proliferation has not yet been fully evaluated. Outside equatorial Africa where exposure to EBV is usually much later, B cell tumors, especially extensive abdominal lymphomas, have been shown to contain viral antigen but in a *lower* percentage of cases. There are other differences between the endemic and sporadic cases, but the same genetic translocation may be found in both forms. EBV has also been associated with nasopharyngeal carcinoma in nonmalarial areas and rare familial cases of both Burkitt's lymphoma and nasopharyngeal carcinoma have been observed in tropical Africa. Recently the same virus has been implicated in other immunoregulatory and lymphoprolife-rative disorders (Magrath 1993) and in Hodgkin's disease (see below).

Retroviruses alter the growth and differentiation of cells from various hemopoietic lineages. Abelson murine leukemia virus can induce nonthymic lymphomas in mice while feline leukemia is associated with another retrovirus. There is a clear relationship between infection with the retrovirus HTLVI and adult T cell leukemia and lymphoma (Yoshida et al 1982) and although there has been recent speculation about in utero transmission no childhood case has yet been reported. HIV infection, presumably as a result of its profound effect on helper T cells, predisposes to the development of a particularly virulent lymphoma in young adults. An increasing incidence of Kaposi's sarcoma has been reported in African children.

EPIDEMIOLOGICAL CONCLUSIONS

Clearly a number of children with chromosomal defects, genetic rearrangements or immune deficiency are genetically susceptible to the development of tumors. Such children may be especially susceptible to environmental factors (e.g. ataxia telangiectasia and irradiation, Fanconi's anemia and anabolic steroids). These and other environmental factors may affect all of us if we are exposed in a high enough concentration or over a long enough period. All of these are now the subject of intense international research.

GENERAL PRINCIPLES OF DIAGNOSIS

A complete history and thorough clinical examination will suggest a diagnosis in most childhood malignancies. Investigations are designed to confirm the histology, determine the extent of disease, identify markers by which therapeutic response can be monitored and identify biochemical status as a baseline prior to therapy. Some tumors are very specifically associated with biochemical disturbance (e.g. tumor lysis syndrome in extensive lymphomas) prior to commencement of treatment.

PATHOLOGY

Prior to any biopsy the pathologist should be consulted in order to optimize use of the specimen. Nowadays routine histology is complemented by immunocytochemistry, cytogenetics, DNA studies for specific rearrangement or oncogene expression and electron microscopy. The pathologist is a key member of the team identifying unfavorable histological features and without whom true incidence and survival figures would not be possible. In these rare tumors central review has enabled audit and consistency of diagnosis. Biopsies are frequently now possible under ultrasound or CT scan guidance but whatever technique is used an adequate sample must be obtained.

RADIOLOGY

Specific radiological investigations will be discussed under each tumor heading but some general principles are important. Plain X-rays may be very suggestive of a specific diagnosis, e.g. suprarenal calcification and neuroblastoma, or onion skin periosteal reaction and Ewing's sarcoma, but are never diagnostic. As far as possible investigations should be rapid, noninvasive and avoid the need for general anesthetic (not always possible in the very young). The new CT scanners and MRI technology enable very precise tumor delineation. MRI is especially helpful for brain, spinal and liver tumors.

BIOCHEMICAL MARKERS

A few tumors secrete specific markers which can assist in diagnosis and in monitoring the response to treatment. Re-emergence of identifiable markers frequently precedes clinical relapse. Examples are catecholamine excretion in neuroblastoma (total catecholamines, VMA and HVA), serum α-fetoprotein (AFP) in hepatoblastoma and teratomas and human chorionic gonadotropin in some germ cell tumors. Nonspecific markers, such as the ESR and serum copper levels in lymphomas are modified by too many factors to be useful.

MOLECULAR AND CYTOGENETICS

Banding techniques, and *in situ* hybridization studies have revolutionized routine karyotyping and tumor cytogenetics respectively. Increasingly, application of probes for specific breakpoints or cloned genes, coupled with polymerase chain reaction amplification of nucleic acid sequences are enabling oncologists to better define tumors. It is essential to combine tumor studies (appropriate specimens required) with karyotype to exclude constitutional defects.

BONE MARROW EXAMINATION

Most childhood tumors are highly malignant and likely to be disseminated at presentation, with many (e.g. neuroblastoma, lymphoma, rhabdomyosarcoma, Ewing's sarcoma, retinoblastoma) potentially metastasizing to the bone marrow. To exclude infiltration two aspirates and two trephines from different sites are considered a minimum requirement. The posterior iliac crest is normally more cellular in children. The use of immunophenotyping with a battery of specific monoclonal antibodies has enhanced tumor recognition (especially in lymphomas and neuroblastoma).

PRINCIPLES OF THERAPY

Malignant childhood tumors must always be presumed to be disseminated, and require chemotherapy. Most chemotherapeutic agents are poorly active against resting (G_0) cells but have potentially lethal effects upon normal proliferating cells, especially the gastrointestinal mucosa and hemopoietic cells (especially marrow progenitor cells which can be destroyed by injudicious drug therapy). For most tumors there is some difference in cell cycle duration and this is usually longer than for normal cells even within the same organ. Tumors continue to grow because they appear to overcome normal apoptotic (programmed cell death) mechanisms. Some tumor cells will undergo a degree of differentiation, some will go into resting phase while the majority in pediatric tumors will be recruited into the active growth fraction. For any specific tumor a complex interaction of specific gene expression (e.g. BCL2, BAX), growth factor activation by oncogene amplification and cytokine stimulation will determine the proliferative rate. Therapy must destroy dividing, resting and maturing cells, and should assist the normal processes of limiting nutrition, vascular supply and oxygenation to the tumor bulk. Normal immune surveillance appears to be overwhelmed by tumor presence. Sometimes within tumors or surrounding nodes, lymphoid hyperplasia, although apparently increasing tumor bulk, is antitumor in effect and caution must be used so as not to completely destroy normal immune responses. Some drugs, for example vincristine, cytosine or hydroxyurea, are phase specific (for the DNA-specific phase) in the cell cycle and should be given at intervals greater than the median duration of the cell cycle in order to kill all the cells passing through the S phase. Other drugs, for example the alkylating agents or external beam irradiation, are cytotoxic at all phases of the cell cycle (cycle specific). Such drugs are best given as a single maximally tolerated dose with a gap between doses to allow for host cell recovery.

One of the major obstacles to the effective kill of all tumor tissue is the presence of hypoxic and nutritionally depleted cells which remain nonproliferative at the time of therapy but retain proliferative capacity and only start to divide when more favorable circumstances prevail. Although the true resting G_0 cell may be as sensitive to radiation as proliferating cells, it is relatively untouched by most antimitotic drugs. Another major

reason for failure of therapy in childhood tumors is the use of local therapy without taking into account the fundamentally disseminated nature of all childhood tumors. Tumor cells may metastasize to pharmacological sanctuaries where drugs penetrate poorly, e.g. the brain in leukemia.

Greater understanding of the cellular mechanisms particularly of apoptosis and cellular triggers for proliferation will in the future enable a much more subtle approach to antitumor therapy.

TUMOR CELL RESISTANCE

There are a number of mechanisms that operate to prevent tumors being effectively killed by drugs (Erttmann 1989).

Primary resistance

This may be either extrinsic or intrinsic. Extrinsic means that the drug does not reach the tumor cells in adequate concentration. This can arise from poor bioavailability of a drug, or its metabolism or excretion, or from inbuilt barriers to drug penetration such as the blood–brain barrier. There may be limited drug diffusion into a very large tumor or it may be that the concentration needed to kill the tumor produces excessive host toxicity and therefore cannot be used. In ALL therapy where at least 2 years of continuing oral therapy is utilized, recent studies have shown that poor patient compliance as well as variable drug metabolism do contribute to worsened prognosis (Davies et al 1993). As tumors develop, mutation, deletion, gene amplification, translocation or chromosomal rearrangement can lead to the spontaneous generation of drug-resistant cells which clearly have a survival advantage (e.g. wild type P53 gene appears to inhibit multiple drug-resistant gene expression (see below) but mutant P53 enhances it). Inherent primary resistance of this type is not prominent in pediatric tumors.

Secondary resistance

This is more common in pediatric tumors. Relapse follows a good initial response to treatment and is often after cessation of chemotherapy. The failure of adequate dose therapy to kill leukemic cells, for example within the brain, can lead to secondary resistance. As the cells within pharmacological sanctuaries begin to replicate any mutation which produces resistance, particularly to low levels of cytotoxic agents, will have selective advantage. Resistance may be against a single cytotoxic mechanism or against a battery of cytotoxic agents with different mechanisms. To prevent such resistance developing, pediatric oncologists have developed the strategy of exposing tumor cells to a battery of agents in as short a time as possible with complementary or synergistic combinations delivered in quick succession. A number of mechanisms for the development of tumor cell resistance are now known:

1. *Tumor cell overproduction of the drug target.* For example the enzyme dihydrofolate reductase is the target for methotrexate within the cell. Overamplification of the gene for this enzyme has been demonstrated. In addition an enzyme with low affinity for methotrexate has also been demonstrated. In both circumstances the efficacy of methotrexate will be affected.

2. *Transport resistance.* There may be diminished intracellular transport or enhanced outward transport of a drug from the cell.

Methotrexate inhibits folate-specific transmembrane transport, polyglutamation (essential for effective action) and activation of thymidine salvage pathways (used to counteract methotrexate effect). Enhanced outward transport has been demonstrated with many drugs ranging from the vinca-alkaloids to the anthracyclines. Juliano & Ling (1976) and Roninson et al (1984) demonstrated the activation of a multiple drug resistance gene. Initially identified in Chinese hamster cells, this gene encodes for a membrane transport glycoprotein (p-glycoprotein) which enhances the elimination of drugs from cells. Kartner et al (1985) demonstrated activation of this gene in multiple cell lines. This appears to be the principal mechanism of pleiotropic resistance development whereby there is decreased intracellular drug accumulation and an increase in the activity of an energy-dependent efflux pump protein (p-glycoprotein). Other mechanisms and other resistance genes have been identified. Mdr-1 gene (which encodes for p-glycoprotein) expression has been identified in normal liver, kidney, colon, adrenal and blood vessel endothelial cells as well as in the cells of ALL, neuroblastoma, rhabdomyosarcoma, and some bone sarcomas. Although rarely significant at initial presentation, it increases in response to therapy and whenever present confers a worsened prognosis on the patient.

3. *Enhanced biochemical detoxification.* Anthracyclines, alkylators and radiation all produce active antigenic metabolites which the metathione redox system renders harmless. Overproduction of glutathione within cells inactivates these agents.

4. *Activation of DNA repair system.* This occurs with alkylating agents, anthracyclines and radiation. Tumor cells developing resistance to these agents have been shown to have enhanced DNA repair.

To overcome resistance the Goldie–Goldman model can be utilized with rapid alternating drug therapy. High dose chemotherapy potentially toxic to normal cells can be used with peripheral stem cell (± growth factor stimulation) or marrow transplantation (autologous or allogeneic) to rescue the normal hempoietic cells (Hartmann et al 1988). In vitro partial reversal of mdr-1 expression has been possible with calcium channel blockers such as verapamil. This is cardiotoxic and more success has been obtained using cyclosporine. New in vitro and in vivo studies with nonimmunosuppressive cyclosporine analogues are looking promising.

SURGERY AND IRRADIATION

As a general principle surgery can remove large masses of tumor (which may be insensitive to drugs and irradiation) with minimal toxicity. Irradiation can effectively deal with microextensions of malignant cells which have spread to adjacent tissues or nodes. Both surgery and irradiation are effective in sites such as the lung, brain or bone, especially with isolated deposits where drugs may be ineffective. Since most childhood tumors are disseminated at diagnosis the principal place for surgery is in obtaining material for diagnosis though there are notable exceptions which will be mentioned later. The main limitation of irradiation is the ill-effect on normal tissues. The therapeutic ratio depends on the sensitivity of the tumor and the tolerance of neighboring tissues and organs. Megavoltage therapy has a sharper beam edge, better depth of penetration and can give a more even dose distribution avoiding damage to skin and overlying tissues when administered to deep

organs. When therapy is planned, careful clinical and radiological assessment of the tumor is undertaken so that radiation fields can be drawn up with plans to shield vital organs such as the kidney or liver if they are not actively involved in disease. New radiation technology is facilitating much more focused therapy with sharp cutoff to minimize damage to surrounding normal tissues. When irradiation is included with chemotherapy in treatment protocols there is a potential for additive toxicity as well as efficacy. The most worrying combination is that of alkylating agents and irradiation, where there is increased risk of the development of secondary neoplasms.

Enhancement of normal cell-mediated immunity using immunotherapy, for example BCG immunization, has proved disappointing for pediatric cancers. Other agents although toxic such as α-interferon, and the cytokines (e.g. IL2) may have some place in treatment of resistant disease.

MONITORING TUMOR RESPONSE

Standardization of tumor response criteria is essential to facilitate comparison of treatment protocols. What constitutes each category of response is not always easy in any specific tumor.

1. *Complete regression* (CR): complete macroscopic regression of all apparent tumor.

2. *Partial regression* (PR): more than 50% reduction, but less than 100% of any single measurable lesion without any new lesions appearing or growth of other identifiable lesions.

This category is sometimes split into good partial response and poor partial response.

3. *Stable disease*: no change in any tumor as defined by less than 50% reduction of any single measurable lesion without any new lesions appearing. In pediatric tumors stable disease represents an unacceptable response.

4. *Progressive disease*: enlargement of at least one measurable lesion and/or the development of new lesions while on therapy.

SPECIFIC EFFECTS OF TREATMENT

Ionizing irradiation

Ionizing irradiation may kill or severely damage a cell. Sublethal cell damage, particularly to normal tissue surrounding a tumor, can cause tissue aging, malformation, growth impairment or induce carcinogenesis. Irradiation is generally given in daily fractions to facilitate normal cell recovery but hopefully not that of tumor cells. As cells in the periphery of the tumor mass are killed, more centrally placed and hypoxic cells will undergo a reoxygenation process and will become susceptible to therapy, particularly if there is an interval between radiation exposures.

Multiple fractions of radiation produce the same effect as a single large dose, but are better tolerated and more efficacious for most tumors. Tolerance curves can be produced for normal and malignant tissues. It is sometimes possible to calculate split course therapy during the intervals of which normal tissues can repair and some tumor cells will be recruited into the proliferative phase where they will be more susceptible to therapy.

Chemotherapy

Table 16.9 shows some adverse drug effects. Most produce alopecia, some gastrointestinal upset and myelosuppression.

Table 16.9 Specific drug toxicity effects of some commonly used chemotherapeutic agents

Drug	Myelosuppression	Immunosuppression	Tissue irritant	Nausea + vomiting	Cystitis	Nephrotoxicity	Cardiotoxicity	Neuropathic	Ototoxicity	Pulmonary	Hepatotoxicity
Anthracyclines (adriamycin + daunomycin)	++	+	+++	++	–	–	+++	–	–	–	Radiation recall effect
Actinomycin	++	+	+++	++	–	–	–	–	–	–	Radiation recall effect
Bleomycin	–	+/–	+	+/–	–	–	–	–	–	++	–
Alkylating agents											
Cyclophosphamide	++	++	+	++	++	+	+ (high dose)	+ (IADH)	–	+	–
Ifosfamide	++	++	+		+++	++	? ++	++ (>in adults)	–	+	–
(Nitrosoureas' e.g. CCNU)	+++ (cumulative)	(++)		(++)	–	++ (cumulative)	–	+ (rare)	–	++	
Nonclassical alkylating											
Cisplatinum	+	+	+/–	+++	–	+++	–	++	+++ (cumulative)	–	–
Dacarbazine (DTIC)	+	+/–	+ (+ pain)	++	–	–	–	–	–	–	++ (+ veno-occulusive)
Antimetabolites											
Methotrexate (oral, i.v., i.m., i.t.)	++	++	–	Mucositis ++ (high dose)	–	++ (high dose)	–	++ (high dose systemic + chronic i.m.)	–	+ (acute + chronic)	++
6-mercaptopurine (oral + i.v.)	+	+	–	Rarely	–	–	–	–	–	–	+
Cytosine (i.v./i.m.)	++	++	–	++ (diarrhea)	–	–	–	Cerebellar in (high dose)			
Vinca alkaloids											
Vincristine	+/–	++	+++	–	–	–	–	+++ (+ IADH)	–	–	–
Vinblastine	++	++	+++	+/–	–	–	–	+/–	–	–	–
Epipodophyllotoxins, etoposide	++	+	+	+/– + Mucositis	–	–	± (hypotension)	+ (mild peripheral)	–	–	+ (enzymes)
Steroids	–	+++	High dose pain	–	–	–	–	–	–	–	–
Asparaginase	++	++	–	–	–	–	–	Encephalopathy	–	–	++

In addition epipodophyllotoxins, asparaginases, bleomycin, and rarely cytosine + cisplatinum are associated with acute life-threatening hypersensitivity reactions.
+ → +++ denotes varying degree of toxicity.
– denotes no recorded toxicity of type.

Patients worry about the nausea and vomiting, physicians about infection risks and hemorrhage.

Hematological toxicity

The degree and duration of neutropenia increases the risk of sepsis with leukemia patients at greater risk than those with solid tumors. The risks are greater before remission has been achieved. Regular monitoring of counts and careful education of parents as to the risks are essential (Prentice 1984).

Neutropenia and infection

Neutropenia secondary to marrow infiltration or treatment leads to a significant risk of bacterial and fungal sepsis when the total neutrophil count is less than $1.0 \times 10^9/l$ and grave risk to life when less than $0.2 \times 10^9/l$. The patient's own skin, mucosal surface and gastrointestinal flora may penetrate local defense mechanisms and produce septicemia. In most series the commonest isolated organisms are Gram-positive skin flora, including *Staphylococcus albus*, *Staph. aureus* and *Staph. epidermidis*, but the gravest threat to life comes from the Gram-negative bowel organisms including *Escherichia coli*, *Proteus*, *Klebsiella* and *Pseudomonas*.

Meticulous hand washing techniques by all staff prior to patient contact can reduce nosocomial infection including colonization with some pathogens. Good oral hygiene reduces secondary infection in drug-induced mucositis, although there is still controversy as to whether oral antiseptic gargling is not as effective as antifungal agents, e.g. nystatin or fluconazole. The avoidance of vigorous tooth brushing reduces gum trauma.

The increased use of central venous lines has been associated with a rise in Gram-positive sepsis, some of which can be avoided by expert placement (tip in right atrium or low SVC) when the patient is not neutropenic, and by meticulous care thereafter. All rectal procedures should be prohibited during neutropenia unless absolutely unavoidable. The only prophylactic antibiotic of proven value in pediatric practice is oral co-trimoxazole to prevent *Pneumocystis carinii* pneumonitis (Darbyshire et al 1985).

The rapid introduction of intravenous antibiotics for any child with less than $1 \times 10^9/l$ neutrophils and a sustained fever (> 2 h)

of 38.5°C has reduced mortality. Clinical signs of infection without fever necessitate a similar response. The antibiotic regimen chosen must take into account hospital and unit infection and sensitivity profiles (require careful monitoring) but must cover both Gram-negative and Gram-positive organisms (e.g. an aminoglycoside and third generation cephalosporin or uridopenicillin). In a recent survey of our unit 50% of leukemia patient admissions and 34% for patients with solid tumors were for infection. With more use of broad spectrum antibiotics fungal infection rates have increased. Whether effective oral prophylaxis to reduce GI tract colonization reduces systemic infection is unproven. Failure of resolution of pyrexia after 48–72 h of effective i.v. antibiotics or if there is clinical deterioration are indications for systemic antifungal therapy with amphotericin (or its liposomal equivalent).

Prior to antibiotic therapy bacterial cultures should be taken from blood, throat, nose, any superficial skin lesion and urine. Stool cultures are useful in the presence of gut dysfunction. Fungal and viral cultures plus serology should be performed if there is poor response. Chest X-ray is indicated in the presence of respiratory symptoms or lack of resolution of fever. An aggressive search for the culpable organism is necessary.

Altered vital signs, and signs of shock necessitate the addition of plasma expanders and i.v. dopamine to maintain renal perfusion. Junior medical staff and nurses require expert training to respond to such life-threatening crises.

Immunosuppression

Both chemotherapy (especially leukemia treatment) and radiotherapy can induce lymphopenia and impaired T and B cell function. Viral infections may not be adequately cleared and common viruses may be excreted for months. Chickenpox and measles pose major risks. De novo or reactivated varicella infection formerly carried a 10% mortality but aciclovir therapy given prophylactically on contact history (200–400 mg q.d. for 21 days) or therapeutically 5–10 mg/kg i.v. 8-hourly for at least 5 days followed by at least 2 weeks of oral therapy to prevent recrudescence has dramatically reduced the risk. Immunosuppressed patients contracting measles and developing either immune encephalitis (weeks or months postinfection) or giant cell pneumonitis have a near 100% mortality (Gray et al 1987). Human immunoglobulin in a dose of 1 g/m^2 given i.m. within 72 h of contact may reduce the risk of the patient contracting the infection, although this has never been proved by a controlled trial. Higher titer immunoglobulin and interferon have been used for neurological and pneumonic signs but clear evidence of benefit is not available (Simpson & Eden 1984). Prevention of measles in the patient with malignancy is best achieved by high community uptake of measles vaccination and avoidance of close contact with cases at school or in the community. Although immunization programs have reduced measles prevalence, only uptake rates in excess of 90% will make epidemics a feature of the past. Herpes simplex (HS) and cytomegalovirus (CMV) infections can be very troublesome after bone marrow implantation. Prophylactic aciclovir may reduce the risk for both organisms. CMV infection can significantly impair marrow engraftment after transplantation.

Pneumocystis carinii pneumonitis may occur during periods of profound lymphopenia. It presents with intractable fever and tachypnea often with no clinically detectable chest signs despite florid radiographic changes. It can be prevented by the use of oral long-term co-trimoxazole. Treatment of the pneumonitis requires a higher dose (trimethoprim 20 mg/kg/day and sulfamethoxazole 100 mg/kg/day given in two divided doses daily). About 80% of patients respond, with some doing so only on the addition of steroids (Darbyshire et al 1985). A small percentage of patients respond only to i.m. pentamidine which is nephrotoxic and can produce marked hypoglycemia. Aerosol pentamidine can be used in those hypersensitive to sulfonamides but has had disappointing results in leukemic patients. Cytomegalovirus may coexist with pneumocystis and can produce a similar pneumonitis. Ideally lung biopsy should be performed to confirm the diagnosis, certainly if there is poor response to therapy. Disease infiltration, fungi and drug reactions can all mimic *Pneumocystis carinii* pneumonitis.

Live vaccines, including measles and polio, must be avoided during therapy but killed vaccines such as those for diphtheria, pertussis and tetanus are permitted although they may be less effective than in the normal child because of the immunosuppression.

Bleeding

The development of efficient blood transfusion services has facilitated the advances made in the therapy of childhood cancer over the last 20 years. Red cells and platelets for transfusion have reduced morbidity and mortality from bleeding. Children have more efficient platelets and good blood vessel wall support when compared with adults and only tend to bleed overtly at very low platelet counts ($< 10 \times 10^9$/l) except in the presence of severe infection. There is little evidence in favor of prophylactic 'platelets' given at specific levels. Indications for platelet transfusion should be mucosal bleeding and/or florid skin petechiae with counts less than 20×10^9/l or at higher counts if fever is present. If invasive high risk procedures, such as lumbar punctures, are to be carried out, it is advisable to keep counts above 50×10^9/l for 24 h. Extradural hematomata have been reported when counts are not maintained. Frequent platelet transfusion leads to antibody development with poor increases in platelet number. (Children receive blood products from three to six donors for each platelet transfusion.) The CMV immune status should be assessed for all patients at diagnosis and only CMV-negative donors used for those with no immunity.

Local tissue toxicity

Many antimitotics are tissue toxic if they extravasate (e.g. vincristine and anthracyclines). Use of central lines has decreased the risks although these are associated with an increase in infections. For both central and peripheral lines, only experienced fully trained staff should give cytotoxics and correct line placement should always be checked prior to injection (good blood flow back, easy flushing with saline and no pain).

Nausea and vomiting

Many drugs, e.g. the alkylators and platinum analogues, can produce profound nausea and vomiting. Control has been greatly enhanced by use of the 5-HT$_3$ receptor antagonists which apart from occasional headaches avoid the central effects (e.g. extrapyramidal) of agents such as the phenothiazines (Pinkerton et al 1990). 70–80% of vomiting can be controlled by regular dosing starting before or just after chemotherapy. The addition of i.v. dexamethasone yields nearly 100% control in children, although hypertension and glycosuria must be checked for. Metoclopramide is an alternative but because of its short half-life really requires frequent (every 3–4 h) administration which can induce 'dystonia'. High dose regimes used in adults are not well tolerated in children. Initial bad experiences with chemotherapy may induce anticipatory vomiting especially in older children, for which oral anxiolytics (e.g. benzodiazepines) 12 h prior to therapy and even added to the ongoing regimen, relaxation and/or abreaction therapy or even hypnosis may be necessary (Zeltzer et al 1984). Late or persistent vomiting can be a problem with the platinum compounds but also should alert the physician to possibilities of infection, hepatotoxicity or ongoing anxiety and psychological problems (Wang 1985). Repeated emesis can clearly cause significant fluid and electrolyte imbalance which requires correction.

Mucositis

Methotrexate, the anthracyclines and actinomycin all induce mucositis which is frequently complicated by secondary infection especially candida. Oral herpetic infection and neutropenia can mimic drug-induced ulceration. Good oral hygiene (mouthwash ± prophylactic nystatin) can reduce the risks.

Bowel dysfunction

High dose chemotherapy (e.g. melphelan, or busulphan and cyclophosphamide pretransplantation) can produce profound watery diarrhea as can continuous infusion or twice-daily cytosine arabinoside. Mucositis and such diarrhea can produce significant (> 10% of body weight) weight loss for which parenteral nutrition is required. In the absence of diarrhea such weight loss is due to tumor cachexia and loss of appetite is an indication for enteric feeding.

The vinca alkaloids produce severe constipation and ileus. This autonomic neuropathy may be complicated by enterocolitis, bowel wall edema and even intussusception. Regular use of bowel softeners (e.g. lactulose) may decrease the risk but when established it may require bowel stimulants, suppositories or enemas which carry infection risks in the neutropenic. Prevention by attention to fluid intake, maximizing activity, avoidance of excess narcotics and stool softeners is preferable.

Renal toxicity

Cisplatin causes progressive tubular and glomerular deterioration with increasing cumulative dosage and occasionally acute tubular necrosis. Vigorous hydration (saline and mannitol) can protect to some degree. Concomitant diuretics and aminoglycoside antibiotics should be avoided. Hydration should be continued for 24 h after cisplatinum. Glomerular function should be monitored regularly and no further cisplatinum should normally be given if the GFR falls below 60 ml/min/1.73m². Profound leakage of magnesium and calcium can produce weakness and tetany and require careful replacement. Systemic methotrexate and melphelan if given when renal function is impaired can cause further nephrotoxicity, delaying their own clearance and producing severe myelosuppression.

Cyclophosphamide and ifosfamide cause hemorrhagic cystitis if their metabolites are not voided from the bladder. Regular voiding and hydration for 24 h after administration are essential. The metabolites can be inactivated by concomitant equivalent doses of 2-mercaptoethane sulfonate sodium (Mesna).

The alkylators and vincristine can have an antidiuretic hormone effect with resultant fluid overload and dilutional hyponatremia. Seizures can result especially in the very young. Urinary flow must be maintained, if necessary with diuretics. Ifosfamide also can produce long-lasting renal tubular defects with hypophosphatemia, clinical rickets and reduction in glomerular filtration rate with cumulative dosage.

Cardiotoxicity

The anthracyclines produce cardiotoxicity. Acute toxicity with arrhythmias, conduction defects and fall in left ventricular output is relatively rare, transient and does not absolutely prevent future use of the drugs. Late cardiomyopathy is related to cumulative dosage with the incidence of congestive cardiac failure increasing steeply beyond 450 mg/m² with doxorubicin. Doppler M mode echocardiography and endomyocardial biopsies have, however, demonstrated functional abnormalities and loss of myofibrils at much lower cumulative dosages (Hausdorf et al 1988). Dose rate and infusion time both affect toxicity (Bielack et al 1989). Studies have reported echocardiographic changes in children who have received only 200–250 mg/m² of doxorubicin (Lipshultz et al 1991) and late-onset congestive cardiac failure is being reported (Steinherz et al 1991). Careful monitoring of ventricular end diastolic function and cessation of drug when abnormal, concomitant use of cardioprotectants such as ICRF 187 (chelates iron, which is a cofactor in the anthracycline free radical reaction inducing the damage) (Speyer et al 1988) and altering peak concentrations have all been tried in adults and more recently in children. Weekly scheduling of lower drug dose fractions or continuous infusions may offer a solution, although in adults infusion times beyond 96 h were necessary to provide significant benefit (Hortobagyi et al 1989). New analogues (e.g. idarubicin or epirubicin) may be less cardiotoxic especially those where the anthraquinine moiety can be omitted or modified. We do not yet know what the true long-term risk will be.

Neurotoxicity

Vincristine can produce peripheral neuropathy (ranging from loss of ankle jerks during therapy, through foot drop (5%), wrist drop (2%) to slapping gait and paresthesia of extremities), and rarely convulsions and encephalopathy (Weiss et all 1975). The central effects may be complicated by an antidiuretic hormone effect with dilutional hyponatremia and seizures. Encephalopathy has most often been recorded with leukemic induction therapy of weekly vincristine. However, such patients receive concomitant l-asparaginase (can produce cerebral hemorrhage, thrombosis, high ammonia levels and asparagine depletion) and intrathecal methotrexate both of which can induce seizures and encephalopathic features.

CNS-directed therapy in leukemia can cause a leukoencephalopathy, most commonly if intrathecal or systemic methotrexate is administered after cranial irradiation. The least toxic modality is continuing intrathecal methotrexate alone (see below); ifosfamide produces an encephalopathy more commonly in adults than children (Pratt et al 1986).

Ototoxicity

Platinum analogues especially cisplatinum cause progressive high tone deafness with increasing cumulative dosage. Tinnitus and, especially if combined with cranial irradiation, rapid deterioration of hearing can occur (Brock et al 1987).

Hepatotoxicity

Oral methotrexate can induce a cirrhotic state and mercaptopurine cholestatic jaundice. High dose i.v. methotrexate can induce florid hepatic disturbance with mucositis and severe myelosuppression (more likely if combined with other drugs cleared by the liver). Actinomycin and anthracyclines should be avoided if possible for the first 4–6 weeks following abdominal (liver encroachment) irradiation. These and busulphan/cyclophosphamide conditioning for transplantation have been associated with a veno-occlusive condition.

Biochemical disturbance

Either spontaneously or following treatment, tumor cell breakdown can result in a lysis syndrome, most commonly in T and B cell lymphoblastic disorders. Hyperkalemia (from cell death), hyperphosphatemia (high content in lymphoblasts) and consequent hypocalcemia, hyperuricemia (and oxypurines from nucleic acid breakdown), renal tubular urate deposition, and azotemia can occur. The risks can be reduced by phased drug introduction, avoidance of citrated blood (exacerbates hypocalcemia), control of any infection, high fluid intake (2.5–3 $l/m^2/day$), allopurinol (10 mg/kg/day in divided doses, i.v. if necessary) and careful urinary alkalinization with i.v. bicarbonate. The aim is to keep the urine at pH 6.5–7.0 to keep urate and xanthine in solution. At higher pH values phosphate may precipitate in the renal tubules. Blood phosphate levels can be reduced by oral aluminum hydroxide. Intravenous calcium should be avoided (it will be tissue deposited) and careful i.v. injection of magnesium preferred to relieve tetany.

Acute psychological effects

Painful procedures and toxic therapy can become intolerable for the child unless reduced to a minimum by a closely coordinated team of doctors and nurses. The family need to make the child realize the absolute need for such treatment, and must tolerate but not overindulge the natural reaction to the treatment and show that they care for their child as a special individual. Displays of personal warmth by the pediatrician can be amazingly effective in defusing emotional crises. The pediatric oncologist must support and help not only the child but the whole family. The parents must know and understand the diagnosis, the nature of cancer and the effect of treatment if the child is to come through emotionally intact. It is essential from the start to explain repeatedly in everyday language what is happening, the likely diagnosis and what it means to the child. The initial shock or numbness at the news precludes 'real' hearing and, subsequently, phases of anger at the apparent injustice are often misdirected at the staff (Eden et al 1994). This must be tolerated and emphasis placed on the team

approach necessary to help their child through. Excess optimism or pessimism must be avoided but if treatment is offered and accepted, some feeling of hope must be conveyed. Involvement in the simpler aspects of nursing their child often provides a sense of purpose for parents. As they come to terms with the shock of the diagnosis, parents frequently ask more searching questions which must be answered truthfully. If more than one member of staff explains matters, it is essential to stress that words used may be different but the meaning is the same. The caring team must be both seen to be and in fact coordinated, and unit meetings are essential for this purpose. There are a few genuine circumstances where the extent of disease or nature of tumor diagnosis precludes cure. For such a child where there is no realistic treatment option and if parents agree, support for the whole family is even more important. Parents must realize that they are always told the truth, 'good' means good and the converse is true about any bad news. Parents may wish their child to be protected from the facts of the disease and diagnosis, but for the majority of children this is a mistake. Children are usually much more resilient than adults and provided appropriate words are used, and they have confidence in the person conveying the problem, they can cope admirably with even the worst of news. Time is necessary to build up confidence for the child and parents, and if such time is not spent at the beginning, management will become fraught with problems. Secrets about the disease within the family, especially keeping facts from siblings, is also unwise. When trust has developed, even if treatment fails and the patient becomes terminal, the team can usually support the patient and family through the final illness more adequately.

For teenagers striving to find themselves and naturally rebellious against parental and other authority, the news of cancer and its necessary treatment can be particularly hard as it inevitably requires compliance with and dependence upon those from whom they are striving to emotionally separate. They require great understanding and sometimes even a little support in their rebellion.

The involvement of a dedicated child psychiatrist in the team who can help staff to understand family interactions and can guide both staff and family through specific crises has proved very useful in many oncology centers. It may be that help is required by specific families where stress has become too great or where previous psychopathology is present. Cancer does not select specific families but affects the spectrum of the population independent of intelligence, insight and behavior.

LONG-TERM SEQUELAE

Table 16.10 lists the potential long-term sequelae seen in childhood cancer survivors.

Late recurrence

Patients and parents worry most about disease recurrence Hawkins (1989) studied over 11 000 3-year cancer survivors over 10 years (Table 16.11). He found no excess late deaths and consequently cure was possible in non-Hodgkin's lymphoma and nongenetic retinoblastoma. The late excess deaths in ALL were largely confined to boys with recurrent leukemia. Young age was a definite advantage in nephroblastoma and neuroblastoma, and late relapses in both tumors were rare (< 1 in 200). Over 75% of late deaths were due to primary disease. Second tumors caused the

Table 16.10 Potential long-term sequelae of childhood cancer

Late recurrence

Secondary neoplasia

Growth impairment

Endocrine dysfunction

Infertility

Educational and psychological dysfunction

Other organ toxicity, e.g. cardiopulmonary

Problems with jobs, insurance, adoption

Table 16.11 Long-term survivors in childhood cancer

Tumor type	% of survivors at 3 years still alive at + 10 years	Excess deaths (per *n* survivors at + 10 years)
Acute lymphoblastic leukemia	60%	1 in 100
Hodgkin's disease	74%	< 1 in 100
Non-Hodgkin's lymphoma	85%	None
Neuroblastoma	89%	< 1 in 200
Nephroblastoma	94%	< 1 in 200
Retinoblastoma Genetic Nongenetic	93% 100%	1 in 200 None

Data derived from Hawkins (1980).

excess deaths in genetic retinoblastoma and Hodgkin's disease. A more recent follow-up study shows continuing improvement in survival.

Second tumors

The Late Effects Study Group studied 9000 tumor patients (1936–1979) and reported a second neoplasm incidence of 8% at 20 years (15 times higher than the general population) (Table 16.12). Retinoblastoma (genetic) and Hodgkin's disease were the most frequent primary tumor, identifying genetic susceptibility and likelihood of treatment with irradiation and alkylators respectively (Meadows et al 1985, Meadows 1988). Certain other genetic disorders predispose to multiple malignancies, e.g. neurofibromatosis, nevoid basal cell carcinoma syndrome and Li–Fraumeni syndrome (germ line P53 mutation). In the series two-thirds of all second solid tumors occurred in radiation fields, with 30% being soft tissue or bony sarcomas. Secondary leukemia was most consistently associated with previous receipt of alkylators. Recently, secondary AML with a short latency period has been increasingly described with use of the epipodophyllotoxins (e.g. VP16, VM26), which involve the MLL gene at chromosome 11q23. This risk appears to be dose and schedule dependent (Pui et al 1989).

Growth impairment

The tumor itself, poor nutrition and infection as well as treatment all impair growth and cause weight loss but there is usually catch-

Table 16.12 Second neoplasms developing in 353 children treated for malignancy

Type of tumor	First tumor (*n*)	Second tumor (*n*)	
		Radiotherapy associated	No radiotherapy
Retinoblastoma	57	0	0
Hodgkin's disease	51	0	0
Soft tissue sarcomas	41	46	16
Nephroblastoma	40	0	0
Brain	38	20	20
Neuroblastoma	29	0	0
Bone sarcomas	23	63	18
Leukemias	23	30	10
Non-Hodgkin's lymphoma	19	9	12
Thyroid carcinoma	0	28	3
Skin carcinoma	0	20	3
Melanoma	0	2	10
Breast carcinoma	0	8	3
Others	32	17	22
Total number	353	243	117

Data derived from Meadows (1988).

up once remission is achieved. Cranial irradiation (leukemia or CNS tumors) will impair growth hormone production or release and, in higher total dosages (also fraction dependent), gonadotropin and adrenocorticotropin production (Shalet et al 1988). Disproportionate growth (spinal versus limbs) occurs. Spinal irradiation will significantly impair final height achievement (5–6 cm at 10 years). For leukemic patients 18–25 Gy cranial irradiation may induce premature and foreshortened puberty in girls, further reducing final height. Replacement of irradiation by intensive chemotherapy may reduce this growth impairment but not completely prevent it. Total body irradiation is associated with poor response to growth hormone therapy because of concomitant spinal shortening, thyroid deficiency, epiphyseal plate damage, chronic GVH and malnutrition. Abdominal irradiation will impair lumbar spinal growth. Replacement with recombinant GH is now possible and safe provided the patient is in full remission and at least 1 year has elapsed since treatment. At this time the evidence does not support a significant effect on tumor reactivation or induction of secondary malignancy (Redman et al 1988). Puberty can be delayed by use of gonadotropin releasing hormone analogues. Regular assessment of linear growth, pubertal status and weight are required both on and for a long term off therapy.

Other endocrine dysfunction

Thyroid radiation damage results in a rise in TSH and then hypothyroidism. This follows TBI, craniospinal irradiation, and local neck irradiation (e.g. Hodgkin's disease). Low doses (100 Gy) may be enough to induce damage and even after cranial irradiation (up to 7.5% scatter may impinge on gland) thyroid adenomas and carcinomas have been induced. Tumors are thought to result from prolonged overdrive by TSH. Persistent TSH elevation on follow-up requires replacement even in the absence of clinical or biochemical hypothyroidism. Chemotherapy may enhance irradiation damage.

Gonadal dysfunction and infertility

From spinal irradiation there will be a scatter to ovaries (90–1000 cGy dependent on field and dosage) and testes (40–1020 cGy) potentially affecting fertility. Direct testicular therapy in leukemia (20–24 Gy) ablates the germinal epithelium (leading to infertility) and the younger the patient the more likely it will damage Leydig cell function (raised basal levels of FSH and LH, low testosterone and impaired response to HCG). If present, androgen replacement will be required from age 12–13. TBI will impair spermatogenesis, and have a variable effect on endocrine function depending on total dose, fraction and any gonadal boost given. Ovarian function is dependent on dose delivered, with variable endocrine and oogenic consequences. TBI invariably causes secondary amenorrhea in postpubertal females from which there may be some recovery.

Drugs have a variable impact on gonadal function. The nitrosoureas (BCNU and CCNU) and procarbazine produce primary gonadal failure with elevated basal FSH and sometimes LH levels. Girls achieve puberty at a normal age with regular menses but whether these are ovulatory cycles or whether reproductive life may be shortened is unclear. Testicular size is reduced postpubertally with oligospermia and, in some, total infertility. There is no evidence of recovery for the boys. Chemotherapy compounds irradiation effects. Testicular germinal epithelial damage is particularly common with cyclophosphamide and cytosine, although some recovery of spermatogenesis may occur with time. Leydig cell function is minimally affected by these agents. In standard Hodgkin's disease therapy including alkylating agents, the germinal epithelium of boys may be severely and apparently irreversibly affected while Leydig cell function may be near normal. In adolescents and young adults sperm banking is now recommended before treatment (Shafford et al 1993). In young girls ovarian damage is not clinically obvious but for postpubertal women, ovarian failure may occur in up to 60% of patients. This demonstrates the complexity of endocrine disorders, and an endocrinologist should be involved in the long-term follow-up and management of childhood cancer survivors.

Educational and psychological

Time lost from schooling especially at critical stages of learning (e.g. peak age for ALL is 3–6 years) may impair educational achievement. CNS-directed therapy in leukemia and even more so for CNS tumors produces neuropsychological sequelae with the youngest (especially under 3) most affected (Kun et al 1986). These effects are irradiation associated, but alternative strategies of high dose methotrexate or intrathecal therapy alone in ALL treatment may not be totally innocent. A UK Medical Research Council psychometric study in parallel with a trial of different treatment modalities will report in 1997–8. With irradiation the impairment is principally of cognitive function, short-term memory and problem solving.

The incidence of long-term psychological problems appears remarkably low, although the impact of 'waiting for a relapse' cannot be overestimated (Meadows et al 1989).

Cardiorespiratory

Acute cardiac effects after anthracycline drugs have been mentioned but late sudden death from endocardial muscle damage has been reported (Van Hoff et al 1979). Pulmonary function tests in leukemia survivors 5 years or more after treatment showed that 65% had one or more of the following defects; low vital capacity, total lung capacity, residual volume or transfer factor (Shaw et al 1989). Few were symptomatic. The most likely explanation is impairment of lung growth which may have significance in later life, especially for smokers. Among solid tumor survivors, chest wall growth impairment restriction defects and/or fibrosis are more frequently identified, especially where the lungs have been irradiated (Shaw et al 1991, Attard-Montalto et al 1992).

Life prospects

Given these sequelae, it would not be surprising if childhood cancer survivors had problems functioning within society. In fact the vast majority complete normal education, and, if anything, have slightly higher employment prospects than peers (Malpas 1988). There is some evidence of social and occupational underachievement related to outdated knowledge and attitudes by some employers and some insurance and pension schemes who treat or weight these survivors unfairly. They should be given the same chance as nonsufferers and not suffer double jeopardy as a result of the childhood cancer over which they had no control.

Conclusions on sequelae

Without intensive treatment most children with cancer died 30 years ago. Now over 50% survive long term and most have good quality of life. Some sequelae such as gonadal failure and infertility may be an acceptable, if regrettable, price for life but second tumors and late cardiac deaths are not. It is essential that all childhood cancer patients are followed for life so that lessons can be learnt and therapy modified where appropriate without any loss of efficacy.

CENTRAL NERVOUS SYSTEM TUMORS

Central nervous system tumors constitute the commonest solid tumors of childhood. The commonest, embryonal medulloblastomas are quite distinct from the common adult glioma (Cohen & Duffner 1984). Recognized etiologic factors are shown in Table 16.13, and Table 16.14 shows the incidence of different childhood brain tumors. Agreement about classification is lacking. Most modern schemes divide them into four broad categories (Rorke et al 1985): (1) glial, (2) neuronal, (3) primitive neuroectodermal tumor (PNET) and (4) pineal cell tumors. Attempts to grade tumors by the degree of anaplasia have only been partially successful. With modern immunohistochemistry and molecular biological methods it is possible to more accurately identify the cells within CNS tumors (Coakham & Brownell 1986). Markers include antibodies detecting glial fibrillary acidic protein, S100 protein, neuron specific enolase and neurofilament protein. These are coupled with nonneuronal markers such as cytokeratin, vimentin, desmin and AFP to enable the pathologist to more accurately determine the cellular nature of the tumors. More than 60% of childhood brain tumors are infratentorial and nearly half are undifferentiated embryonal tumors (Table 16.15).

Only modification of the WHO classification takes all these pediatric features into account (Rorke et al 1985).

The primitive neuroectodermal tumor (PNET) which occurs almost exclusively in childhood, in or around the cerebellum, is usually identified as a medulloblastoma. Similar tumors may occur in the cerebrum, the pineal region, the brainstem or in the cord where they may be labeled ependymoma, pinealoma, retinoblastoma or even infratentorial-cerebral neuroblastoma. Controversy exists as to whether all these tumors should be called PNET and how the differentiation between them should be made.

SYMPTOMS AND SIGNS

The presenting symptoms and signs of brain tumors in childhood depend more on the site than on type of tumor. Neurological features are due to infiltration, compression of neuronal structures or by raised intracranial pressure secondary to obstruction of CSF pathways. Raised intracranial pressure presents early in the majority of the infratentorial tumors with the classic triad of morning headache, vomiting and visual disturbance. There may be more vague symptoms of tiredness, falling school performance, personality change and nonlocalized headache for a variable period before the classic triad presents.

Headaches in young children should always be taken seriously and investigated. In infants presenting symptoms may be irritability, loss of appetite and developmental delay or even the loss of acquired skills. Even with large tumors full neurological examination may yield few signs. Infants under 2 years may develop an increase in OFC with springing of the sutures as intracranial pressure increases and in babies the setting sun sign may be seen. Fundi are frequently pale with just the early signs of papilledema. Fundal examination particularly in the infant can be very difficult and sedation and pupillary dilation may be appropriate. Developmental assessment should be part of the full examination. Specific signs depend on the site of the tumor.

Infratentorial lesions

Raised intracranial pressure and disturbance of balance (truncal and extremity) and specific cranial nerve dysfunction are the cardinal signs of the well-established tumor. Midline medulloblastomas may present only with raised intracranial pressure and truncal unsteadiness and without localizing features while the cerebellar hemisphere lesions (e.g. astrocytomas) may present with lateralizing features before intracranial pressure is evident. It is, however, usually not possible to distinguish between astrocytoma and medulloblastoma clinically. Sixth nerve palsy may be a false localizing sign arising from intracranial pressure. When present bilaterally and especially when in combination with 5th, 7th or 9th nerve palsies, brainstem involvement is likely. Head tilt is frequently seen together with cochlear nerve palsy and vertical or horizontal diplopia when cerebellar tonsillar herniation occurs.

Supratentorial lesions

Both the site and the size of the tumor determine the presenting signs. With these lesions nonspecific headaches, seizures of all types and long tract signs may predominate. Raised intracranial pressure may be the first sign of tumors in relatively silent areas of the cortex (frontal, parietal or occipital) and the tumor may be very large. Raised pressure may be an early feature in small 3rd ventricular lesions. Visual field defects may help to localize tumors. In primitive neuroectodermal tumors such as medulloblastoma, dissemination throughout the CNS via the cerebrospinal fluid may lead to symptoms and signs far removed from the

Table 16.13 Etiologic factors for CNS tumors

Heritable syndromes
  Neurofibromatosis (visual pathway tumors + gliomas)
  Tuberous sclerosis (glial ependymomas)
  Von Hippel–Lindau (cerebellar + retinal + pheochromocytomas)

Familial clustering without identifiable genetic factor (various tumors including pinealomas)

Familial with autosomal dominant inheritance: astrocytoma

Retinoblastoma and pinealoblastoma (13q–)

Rhabdoid renal tumors and PNETs of brain

Monosomy 22: meningiomas + acoustic neuromas

Ionizing irradiation: after low dose scalp and possibly dental treatment

Immunodeficiency (intracerebral lymphomas) especially:
  a. postrenal transplantation
  b. Wiskott–Aldrich
  c. ataxia telangiectasia

Parental exposure to organic compounds such as nitrosamines and polycyclic hydrocarbons

Table 16.14 Relative incidence of CNS neoplasms in childhood (1971–1980)

	Boys	Girls
Astrocytoma (all types)	34.5%	40%
Medulloblastoma	22.9%	15.7%
Ependymoma	12.3%	12.1%
Other gliomas	15.0%	18.6%
Other and unspecified	15.3%	13.6%
Total numbers	1489	1196

Data from Parker et al (1988).

Table 16.15 World Health Organization classification of pediatric brain tumors

A. Glial tumors
  1. Astrocytic *astrocytoma*
  2. Oligodendroglial tumors
  3. Ependymomal tumors (including *ependymoma*)
  4. Choroid plexus tumors
  5. Mixed gliomas
  6. Glioblastoma multiforme

B. Neuronal tumors
  1. Gangliocytoma ⎫ including primary
  2. Ganglioglioma ⎬ intracranial neuroblastoma
  3. Anaplastic ganglioglioma ⎭

C. Primitive neuroectodermal tumors (PNET)
  1. PNET not otherwise specified = *medulloblastoma*
  2. PNET with differentiation
  3. Medulloepithelioma

D. Pineal cell tumors
  1. Pineocytoma
  2. Pineoblastoma (PNET)

primary lesion with consequent diagnostic confusion. Careful documentation of all signs and symptoms in the order that they appear is important and their disappearance with treatment should be monitored for response rates.

DIAGNOSIS

CT and MR scanning have revolutionized the diagnosis of pediatric brain tumors. CT is useful for rapid identification of hydrocephalus and mass effect but MRI is preferred for precise tumor definition in multiple planes prior to surgery (especially for brainstem gliomas and spinal tumors (Packer et al 1986). Positron emission tomography (PET) may prove useful in detecting variations in metabolism between residual tumor and normal brain. For the PNETs, exclusion of spinal deposits by myelography or MR scanning postoperatively is essential.

GENERAL PRINCIPLES OF TREATMENT

Surgery

Preoperative steroids to reduce edema, external decompression of hydrocephalus and new scanning techniques have facilitated more complete surgical removal of visible tumor without increased morbidity. Extent of excision is a determinant of outcome especially in the PNETs. Midline posterior fossa tumors more frequently require long-term ventriculoperitoneal shunting.

There is no evidence that this increases the likelihood of extracerebral metastases. Surgeons reduce peripheral damage by use of operative microscopes, ultrasonic aspirators and lasers. Operative mortality for most tumors has been reduced to under 1% although morbidity may be as high as 20%. For some (e.g. cerebellar astrocytomas) excessive attempts to excise all of the tumor initially may be contraindicated (see below).

Radiotherapy

Fields and volumes treated should be limited to minimize normal tissue damage. Astrocytomas of Grade III and IV do require whole brain irradiation and medulloblastomas, ependymomas, PNETs and some germ cell tumors, craniospinal irradiation. Although local areas can tolerate total dosages as high as 50–55 Gy, whole brain dosages over 35 Gy are associated with significant sequelae. Fraction size, number of fractions and duration of treatment all influence toxicity. Hypoxic cell sensitizers have not yet found a place in pediatric practice.

Acute radiation side effects include headache (hot head), vomiting, skin erythema, alopecia and otitis externa. Lymphopenia is universal and may persist for 6 months. Profound myelosuppression may follow spinal irradiation and make subsequent chemotherapy difficult to deliver. 5–10 weeks after cranial irradiation 'somnolence syndrome' can occur (profound sleepiness, mild pyrexia, and some have GI upset) owing to a temporary disturbance of myelination. A similar effect on the spine produces Lhermitte's sign (shooting arm pains). Long-term effects are described above.

Chemotherapy (Blasberg & Groothuis 1986)

The blood–brain barrier limits access to the brain of most drugs. At the margins of tumors, the tight capillary endothelial junctions persist, while neoplastic neovascularity makes the core of tumors more accessible. Lipid solubility, molecular size, protein binding and plasma concentration all determine the ability of a drug to penetrate the CNS. Lipophilic drugs (e.g. nitrosoureas) will penetrate tumor margins and water-soluble agents (e.g. cisplatinum) the core.

MEDULLOBLASTOMA (PNET OF CEREBELLUM) (20% of CNS tumors)

This is a midline vermis PNET arising adjacent to the roof of the fourth ventricle. The peak age incidence is 5 years (some series show a second peak at 10–12 years). There is a male preponderance.

Presentation

Obstruction of the fourth ventricle leads to raised intracranial pressure, progressive ataxia of the lower limbs, diplopia, and V, VII and other cranial nerve deficits. Long tract signs appear rather later. Nuchal rigidity and/or head tilt suggests cerebellar tonsillar herniation and necessity for rapid relief. The differential diagnosis includes cerebellar astrocytoma, ependymoma, brainstem glioma, and infectious encephalitis (although the last is usually of more acute onset). CT scan shows a solid homogeneous, iso- or hyperdense lesion which is enhanced by contrast but these features are not unique to medulloblastoma. An MR scan may more easily differentiate a medulloblastoma from the other tumors by clearly showing the site of origin (Packer et al 1986). Lumbar CSF examination should *not* be performed before surgery.

Prognostic features

In 1969 Chang devised a staging system based on tumor size, local extension and presence of metastases (Harisiadis & Chang 1977). Degree of resection other than size of tumor per se may influence prognosis. Any subarachnoid spread and of course extraneural disease significantly worsens prognosis but isolated positive CSF cytology does not. Young age (under 5 but especially under 2) is adverse with likelihood of large tumor bulk and treatment modification to prevent neuronal damage. A diploid DNA content within tumor cells worsens prognosis (35% at 4 years compared with 85% in hyperdiploidy in one series). c-myc oncogene amplification and differentiation within the tumor may prove to be adverse features.

Pathology

This is a highly cellular soft and friable tumor full of small round undifferentiated cells with hyperchromatic nuclei and abundant mitoses. There can be variable glial or neuroblast differentiation which may be of prognostic significance.

Management

Complete macroscopic resection is achievable in about 50% of cases. 1-year disease-free survival figures appear to be 30–50% better for those with complete resection, but at 5 years the improvement is down to about 10%. Provided there is no evidence of morbidity during the procedure, complete removal should be attempted. These tumors are the most radiosensitive of the primary CNS childhood tumors and radiotherapy is required to the whole neuraxis with at least 50 Gy to the posterior fossa. Attempts to reduce whole craniospinal dosages by use of chemotherapy have resulted in worsened prognosis.

Historically the best unselected series survival figures for surgery plus radiotherapy are 35–40% disease free at 10 years. These patients have high morbidity from whole CNS irradiation (intellectual impairment and growth). Medulloblastoma has been shown to be chemosensitive in relapse schedules and in vitro. Single-center nonrandomized studies have reported 96% 2-year total survival with CCNU, vincristine and cisplatinum (26 patients) or 81% disease-free survival at 6 years with vincristine and cyclophosphamide (21 patients). (Packer et al 1988, McIntosh et al 1985). However, in large international randomized trials pre- and postradiation chemotherapy has not significantly improved long-term survival. Trials using the most effective agents from single arm studies, including vincristine, cisplatinum or carboplatin, cyclophosphamide and CCNU are in progress. Whether all or only high risk patients will benefit remains to be answered. The aim is to improve the current 50% 5-year disease-free survival and reduce the need for such toxic whole CNS irradiation dosages.

EPENDYMOMA (5–10% of CNS tumors)

These arise from the lining of the ventricular system and central canal of the spinal cord (75% in the posterior fossa, 25% in the cord). The peak age of onset is in the first 2 years of life. Like the medulloblastomas they may be a heterogeneous group; most are well demarcated but with areas of hemorrhage and cyst formation internally. There is considerable variation in anaplasia, pleomorphism and differentiation. The *subependymoma* is often silent and found coincidentally at autopsy. The ependymomas spread locally and disseminate. Spinal subarachnoid space involvement is much more likely with infratentorial tumors (20–30%) than with the supratentorial tumors (3–8%). High grade ependymomas may disseminate within the CNS through the CSF but systemic spread is rare.

Presentation

Raised intracranial pressure is common in all posterior fossa tumors. There may be some cerebellar dysfunction. Local cranial nerve deficits are more commonly seen than in medulloblastoma because of local infiltration and invasion of the floor of the 4th ventricle and brainstem. Supratentorial ependymomas more commonly present with seizures and long tract signs. The duration of the history depends on the site and the grade of the tumor ranging in high grade tumors to just 3 or 4 weeks and in lower grade ones, up to 1 year. The differential diagnosis will include astrocytomas, medulloblastomas, brainstem gliomas and, where they arise in the lateral or 3rd ventricles, choroid plexus tumors or astrocytomas.

Diagnosis

CT scans will show a hyperdense and contrast-enhancing tumor with hydrocephalus. Internally there will frequently be hemorrhage and cysts, MR scanning will delineate infiltration. CSF examination is needed postoperatively along with myelography or MR scanning.

Prognostic features

Spinal cord and especially myxopapillary cauda equina tumors fare better but otherwise site is not of prognostic significance. It is unclear for ependymomas whether histology (anaplasia) or degree of resection are of significance. Young age (< 5 years) and brainstem invasion do adversely affect outcome.

Management

Attempts at primary total resection are indicated and usually possible for supratentorial tumors, less so in the posterior fossa where brainstem infiltration increases perioperative morbidity (5%–10%). With surgery alone 5-year survival is 15–20%. For supratentorial tumors extended local field irradiation to a total dose of 50–55 Gy (tumor + 1- to 2-cm margin) and for posterior fossa lesions a field to extend down to C3–4 are indicated. Most relapses are local but 10–15% have subarachnoid spread. This may be greater in posterior fossa and anaplastic tumors; for them, craniospinal irradiation has been recommended. For low grade tumors, surgery and extended field radiotherapy yield 50% 5-year survival. Intramedullary spinal cord tumors may be cured by complete microsurgical resection. Chemotherapy has not yet been shown to significantly improve survival, although ependymoma has been shown to be chemosensitive especially in infants. The platinum compounds appear the most active (Gaynon et al 1990).

CEREBELLAR ASTROCYTOMAS (10–20% of CNS tumors)

These occur throughout childhood without an obvious age peak but there is a slight male preponderance. Four-fifths are pilocytic with areas of loose cellularity or cyst formation intermixed with more compact cellular areas. The remainder are termed diffuse astrocytomas. These more solid tumors appear to have a poorer prognosis. Most cerebellar astrocytomas are well localized although occasional reports of noncontiguous spread have occurred even in the pilocytic tumors. It is possible that some of these deposits represent multifocal disease. Very rarely high grade astrocytomas do arise in the cerebellum.

Presentation

Because of their usual slow growth, these tumors are often associated with less acute clinical onset and symptoms present for longer than in medulloblastoma. Presentation is usually with the symptoms and signs of raised intracranial pressure, although involvement (pressure or invasion) of the cerebellar peduncles and brainstem may give cranial nerve and long trait signs.

Diagnosis

Distinction from medulloblastoma is often difficult although on CT astrocytomas are usually less dense and often have a cystic component (the wall and nodule of which contrast enhance). MR scans usually show sharper demarcation of tumor margins.

Management

Lateral tumors should be removed as completely as possible. While this may be more difficult for midline or peduncular tumors, between 80% and 90% of all low grade cerebellar astrocytomas can be fully resected with less than 1% mortality. Some patients require preoperative and some long-term CSF shunting. After complete resection about 90% of patients in most series remain alive and well, requiring no further treatment ever. More controversial is what should be done for patients with incompletely resected tumor and what their survival is like. Radiotherapy does not significantly influence survival following surgical resection particularly if there are no adverse prognostic features. The current recommendation is to consider whether no surgery or radiotherapy would be the most appropriate management if the tumor regrows. With improved surgical techniques, smaller residual loads remain and survival figures for those with incomplete resection and no radiotherapy are now reported at 60–70% compared with the more variable results ranging from 40 to 80% when radiotherapy is used. Local control has been obtained in large cystic lesions by the use of intracavity ^{32}P. There would appear to be little or no place for chemotherapy in treatment of low grade tumors (Gjerris & Klinken 1978) unless brainstem extension prohibits surgery or radiotherapy.

SUPRATENTORIAL ASTROCYTOMAS (up to 35% of CNS tumors)

There is a peak age incidence of these tumors at 3 years and a second peak in adolescence with twice as many males affected as females. Cystic tumors often occur in the diencephalon and ventricles and have a good prognosis. Fibrillary tumors with more dense cellularity and less cystic change occur particularly in the cerebral hemispheres. They are mostly low grade, grow slowly and have a fair prognosis. Anaplastic tumors including glioblastoma multiforme and anaplastic astrocytoma are rapidly growing aggressive tumors also most frequently found in the hemispheres. Glioblastomas in particular will spread widely within the CNS and even systemically (Gjerris 1978).

Presentation

For all sites the predominant presenting features (75%) are those of raised intracranial pressure. Seizures are seen in 25% of supratentorial tumors especially low grade ones (may precede all other symptoms/signs). 25–50% may have visual disturbances, weakness, hemiplegia or cranial nerve deficit. Diencephalic tumors may present with the classic syndrome of emesis, emaciation and even euphoria or with CSF obstruction. Dysmetria and chorea is seen in basal ganglia and optic atrophy with neuroendocrine disturbance in hypothalamic tumors Neurofibromatosis is associated with 10–20% of diencephalic lesions.

Diagnosis

Low grade astrocytomas on CT scanning are usually of low density with minimal enhancement in contrast to high grade tumors which have more variable density, marked enhancement and greater mass effect. MR scanning always defines more tumor than CT and is better able to distinguish edema from infiltrating neoplasia.

Prognostic features

Low grade (I and II) especially pilocytic varieties fare better than high grade (III and IV) and fibrillary tumors which are more common. Children fare better than adults, except infants where higher grade tumors and greater surgical risks coexist. Degree of resection influences outcome. Site is not a significant independent prognostic variable.

Management

Complete resection should be attempted (40–80% possible in supratentorial, less than 40% in diencephalon). In low grade tumors complete resection may lead to 80% survival at 7 years (Loftus et al 1985); with incomplete removal survival is only 14–48% at 10 years even with radiotherapy. Whether there is long-term benefit for radiotherapy is unclear; in partially resected low grade tumors it may be reasonable to delay radiotherapy in children under 5 years until there is tumor regrowth. High grade tumors do require postoperative radiation although 5-year survival in Grade IV tumors is poor. (5–25% at 5 years). Extended field irradiation with a tumor bed dosage of 50–55 Gy are used in Grade III and IV lesions (90% of recurrences are local). Because of the poor survival rates chemotherapy especially with vincristine and cyclophosphamide or CCNU and prednisolone have been tried. 40–50% response rates are reported but long-term survival may only be marginally improved on surgery plus radiation. High dose chemotherapy (thiotepa, VP16 ± BCNU) with autologous marrow rescue is giving early promising response rates but follow-up is awaited (Finlay et al 1990).

BRAINSTEM GLIOMAS (10–20% of CNS tumors)

These have a peak incidence between 5 and 8 years but no sex difference. 75% occur in the pons and the rest in the medulla and midbrain. About 50% are of low grade malignancy, graded I or II mostly with a fibrillary histology, and a few are pilocytic. 35–40% are high grade anaplastic astrocytomas or glioblastoma multiforme. 10% are ependymomas and primitive neuroectodermal tumors.

Presentation

Raised intracranial pressure and hydrocephalus develop slowly with nonspecific, nonlocalizing features of headache, nausea and vomiting but only with late papilledema. Emesis may be related to infiltration of local nuclei. Cranial nerve palsies (III, V, VI, VII, IX and X) are common and cerebellar and long tract signs may all be found. Pontine tumors may cause behavioral and emotional changes.

Diagnosis

On CT most are hypo- or isodense, and poorly enhancing while MR TI weighted images show hypodensity and T2 images a hyperdense mass. MR much more accurately defines tumor extent especially exophytic components.

Prognostic features

Low grade tumors have improved survival (50–60% at 2 years for Grade I + II; 0–15% for Grade III and IV). The presence of calcification, Rosenthal fibers and no mitoses are favorable features. Midbrain and medullary sites have improved outcome compared with pontine tumors (more likely low grade). Pontine tumors present rapidly, with cranial nerve defects. Patients with diffuse infiltrating tumors fare very badly (< 10% 2-year survival) while those with dorsal exophytic tumors have gradual onset and do well (up to 90% survival at 4–5 years).

Management

Attempts at resection are hazardous. For dorsal exophytic, cervicomedullary junction, and nonenhancing cystic or small tumors subtotal resection should be attempted. In the rest even stereotactic biopsy should be performed with great care (Hood et al 1986). With radiation (45–50 Gy to tumor field) in the majority of pontomedullary tumors, the best survival is 30% at 3–5 years. Hyperfractionated therapy (total dose up to 72 Gy) has proved disappointing. To date no optimal or appropriate chemotherapy has been found.

OPTIC GLIOMAS (OPTIC NERVE, CHIASMA AND TRACTS) (5% of CNS tumors)

Three-quarters occur before 10 years but chiasmal tumors tend to occur in older children. There is no sex difference. Neurofibromatosis is seen in up to 75% of patients with optic nerve tumors but is less frequent in those with more central lesions. The tumors tend mostly to be astrocytomas of low grade malignancy with a tendency for local infiltration along the optic tracts but also into the frontal lobes, hypothalamus, thalamus and other midline structures especially from the chiasma. Growth tends to be erratic but slow.

Presentation and diagnosis

Clinical features depend on the site and the age of the patient. The young usually present with squint, nystagmus, mild proptosis or developmental delay rather than loss of vision. The discs may be pale and atrophied but signs of raised intracranial pressure may occur in large chiasmal or hypothalamic tumors. Visual loss can be very profound, intraorbital lesions leading to central vision loss, chiasmal lesions to temporal hemianopia. In addition there is often a very fine and rapid unilateral or bilateral nystagmus. Lesions that spread to the hypothalamus may be associated with endocrine disorders or growth failure and even the diencephalic syndrome. Differential diagnosis will include rhabdomyosarcoma and neuroblastoma in the orbit; angiomas, lymphangiomas and meningiomas of the optic sheath; and in infants spasmus mutans (for chiasmal lesions). Gliomas, craniopharyngiomas and other suprasellar tumors may be confused with lesions in the optic tract. CT scanning will show an isodense mass with contrast enhancement especially in chiasmal tumors. Hydrocephalus may be present with the intracerebral lesions. MR scans often show much greater spread due to local infiltration. Careful ophthalmological evaluation of fields and acuity is required in conjunction with CT scans for follow-up. Visual evoked responses may be required to assess vision in the young.

Prognostic features

Intracranial site carries a worse prognosis. Chiasmal tumors have a 10-year survival of around 50% compared with 90–100% for intraorbital tumors. Those with chiasmal tumors and preceding neurofibromatosis may have a better prognosis.

Management

The natural history of the optic gliomas is variable. Even without treatment some patients may remain stable for long periods of time while others may progress quite rapidly. Only surgical biopsy will confirm the diagnosis although CT or MR scanning is probably adequate for most. There may be a place for attempted surgical resection in those with isolated intraorbital lesions but deeper intracranial tumors need a biopsy to exclude other tumors which might be more radiosensitive. Complete resection is usually impossible. For optic nerve lesions there seems to be little difference in outcome between those who are observed compared with those given initial radiotherapy. The aim of radiotherapy even for optic nerve lesions is to reduce tumor mass to improve vision although it may improve survival for large chiasmal lesions. Radiotherapy, particularly with chiasmal lesions, may cause intellectual, neuropsychological or endocrine sequelae. Actinomycin and vincristine have been shown to arrest at least temporarily the progression of optic gliomata in up to 80% of cases. More recently, regimens using nitrosoureas and/or platinum analogues have shown favorable responses. Such an approach may have a place in the very young in whom radiotherapy would cause major toxicity.

PINEAL TUMORS (0.5–2% OF CNS tumors)

These fall into two categories:

1. 20–40% are pineal parenchymal tumors (pinealoblastomas or pinealocytomas) and occur in the first 10 years and more frequently in girls.
2. The remainder are germ cell tumors, seen much more commonly in boys and girls in the second decade of life.

Pinealoblastomas have all the appearances of medulloblastoma and are best categorized as PNETs, often showing some differentiation resembling retinoblastoma. Pinealocytomas are generally more differentiated. The germ cell tumors are a heterogeneous group. The commonest is the germinoma, then teratoma and the rarer embryonal carcinoma, choroid carcinoma and endodermal sinus tumor (see below). Pineal tumors spread locally and pinealoblastomas and germinomas may disseminate, but teratomas tend to remain localized. Systemic non-CNS metastases occur with pinealoblastoma, germinoma and the rarer embryonal carcinoma and choroid carcinoma.

Presentation

Raised intracranial pressure from 3rd ventricular outflow obstruction is the most common presenting feature. Other signs will depend on the site and the degree of extension of the tumor. Encroachment on the midbrain will produce vertical gaze paralysis, on the thalamus will produce hemiparesis, incoordination, visual impairment and movement impairment, and suprasellar extension particularly in germ cell tumors will produce neuroendocrine disorders. CT scanning will identify the lesion but not differentiate the type since both germ cell and parenchymal tumors tend to have irregular mixed density mass lesions but with a fairly uniform contrast enhancement. Both of them may have calcification. The more mature teratomas often have a mosaic pattern with variable density and contrast enhancement with irregular calcification. CSF examination is needed following decompression particularly in pinealoblastoma and germinoma. Elevation of AFP in the CSF and possibly in the serum in germ cell tumors is a useful marker.

Prognosis

This is determined by histology with germinomas having the best prognosis at 60–85% 5-year disease-free survival, and teratomas 50%. Pineal parenchymal tumors fare badly with at least 50% dead within a year of diagnosis. The remaining rare germ cell tumors have an even worse prognosis. About 10% of pineal parenchymal tumors and germinomas show leptomeningeal spread. Extracranial metastases are rare but include bone, lung and nodes.

Management

Biopsy is recommended to clarify the diagnosis. It is associated with a high morbidity (though low mortality), with frequent impairment of the vision. In well-circumscribed teratomas excision may be possible but for the rest, where local infiltration is quite common, biopsy with some debulking and relief of hydrocephalus is all that can be achieved with surgery. The primary treatment for the majority is radiotherapy with whole brain irradiation in the region of 35–45 Gy and a boost of 10–15 Gy to the tumor area for germ cell tumors and pinealoblastomas. There is controversy as to who actually needs spinal irradiation. It should probably be judged by the presence or absence of cells in the CSF and abnormal myelographic features but some recommend routine whole neuroaxis radiation in pinealoblastoma. There is no blood–brain barrier in the pineal region and drugs such as vinblastine, bleomycin, cisplatinum and VP16 have all been shown to have some efficacy in pineal tumors. The intensive chemotherapy used for non-CNS germ cell tumors including vinblastine, bleomycin and cisplatinum or carboplatin yield similar improved results for these with CNS tumors. There is some evidence that high dose methotrexate may be effective for choriocarcinoma.

CRANIOPHARYNGIOMA (about 6% OF CNS tumors)

Two-thirds of these tumors occur before the age of 20 with a median age of 8 years. There is no sex difference. Most of the tumors are suprasellar but some occur in the sella itself. They may be solid, mixed or cystic with or without calcification. Although they are frequently well differentiated and benign histologically they cause erosion of surrounding tissues.

Presentation

Obstruction of the 3rd ventricle and the foramen of Monro leads to hydrocephalus and raised intracranial pressure. The optic discs are often pale showing signs of atrophy from slow tumor growth. Papilledema is occasionally present. Other signs result from the tumor impinging on the optic chiasma producing visual disturbances (homonymous hemianopia or bitemporal hemianopia) or from pressure on the pituitary and the hypothalamus leading to hormone deficiency (growth hormone, adrenocorticotropic hormone, TSH, TRH or ADH). Hormonal changes occur in 80–90% of patients. The patient may present with diabetes insipidus and short stature.

Diagnosis

Plain skull X-rays will identify the large distorted sella with or without calcification. CT scanning will show a cystic low density lesion with contrast enhancement and often considerable calcification. The MR scan may define the solid and cystic components of this tumor better and identify the surrounding anatomy.

Prognosis

Total resection and cystic tumors are favorable; large poorly resectable tumors and age under 5 years are adverse features.

Management (Amendola et al 1985)

For this low grade tumor with visual and neuropsychological disturbances the efficacy of treatment is often difficult to evaluate. With preoperative steroids to reduce pressure and vasopressin to control diabetes insipidus, morbidity and mortality have decreased. 75–80% of tumors can be completely removed with recurrence rates of 20–25% (most in the first 2 years). Morbidity is high with secondary bleeding and local tissue damage. Periodic CT or MR scanning plus endocrine follow-up are essential. If scans show no disease and no calcification postsurgery there is a 70% 10-year event-free survival. If there is residual tumor or calcification, radiotherapy (50–55 Gy local field) is required. Many now recommend subtotal resection and radiotherapy rather than radical surgery. Intracystic radiocolloid injection has been used successfully in recurrent cystic lesions. No role has yet been established for chemotherapy.

CHOROID PLEXUS NEOPLASMS (3% of CNS tumors)

Most occur in the lateral ventricles and are intraventricular papillomas which secrete CSF, but they can seed. About 15% are slow-growing carcinomas which can reach huge dimensions and can truly metastasize.

Presentation

This is usually with raised intracranial pressure and hydrocephalus (they can produce CSF up to four times the normal rate) owing to ventricular obstruction with or without hemorrhage. Arachnoiditis may also occur. Other more specific neurological effects will depend on the site of the tumor. The differential diagnosis will include ependymomas and midline astrocytomas. A plain skull X-ray will show sutural diastases in 70% (20% of these patients are in their first year of life). CT scan will show hydrocephalus and an isodense to hyperdense intraventricular tumor with contrast enhancement, MRI will show where the fronds of the tumor extend into the ventricles.

Management

Surgery is the treatment of choice but there is a high mortality and morbidity. For papillomas, curative complete resection appears to be possible in between 75% and 100%. Shunting may be necessary to relieve persistent hydrocephalus. For the papillomas there is no need for further therapy. For carcinomas there is a worse prognosis with only an occasional long-term survivor. Radiotherapy has not been of benefit; chemotherapy may have a role but the optimal specific drug regimen has not yet been defined.

SUPRATENTORIAL PNETS (2–3% of CNS tumors)

This heterogeneous group of tumors may represent medulloblastomas or similar tumors in a supratentorial position. 90% occur within the cerebral hemispheres and less than 10% in the midline. Although they may appear well circumscribed there is frequently microscopic infiltration which may be quite extensive and there is a high risk of leptomeningeal spread.

Presentation

This is usually with raised intracranial pressure, seizures and motor signs. The time from symptom onset to diagnosis may be quite long (up to 10 months). CT scanning will show hydrocephalus plus the mass with or without calcification and cysts and with variable enhancement. Myelography and CSF examination will be required once the pressure has been relieved.

Management

This is by surgical reduction of bulk followed by craniospinal radiotherapy to the tumor bed in doses of 50–60 Gy. There is some evidence that dosages less than 45 Gy worsen prognosis but the whole craniospinal axis will require radiation. The prognosis is generally poor for the majority with 5-year survival in the region of 25%. Radiotherapy does appear to prolong survival. Chemotherapy is undergoing evaluation but as yet no clear-cut evidence in favor of specific agents or combinations has emerged. Cisplatinum or carboplatinum look most promising.

SPINAL CORD TUMORS

These comprise about 5% of primary CNS tumors and can occur throughout childhood. Two-thirds are astrocytomas and most of the rest are ependymomas. The majority are well differentiated and of low grade malignancy often with cystic change and slow growth with local infiltration. Leptomeningeal spread has a low incidence but multifocal disease may be seen in patients with neurofibromatosis.

Presentation

This is often insidious in onset with weakness, pain, sensory change, change in gait and eventually sphincter dysfunction. About 10% of patients have raised intracranial pressure secondary to either high cervical spinal canal obstruction or to spinal block and rise in protein. Plain X-rays are abnormal in about 50% of patients. MR scanning is the ideal modality to define spinal tumors.

Management

Biopsy is essential for diagnosis and wherever possible resection should be attempted using ultrasonography and laser scalpels. Careful follow-up of spinal growth and development is necessary in children. Where resection is complete, no radiotherapy is needed but if it is incomplete, dosages in the region of 45–50 Gy to the affected area are necessary.

Prognosis

For low grade astrocytomas survival appears to be about 55% at 10 years for those incompletely resected and treated with radiotherapy, but near 100% if resection is complete. For ependymomas of low grade malignancy 10-year figures vary between 50% and 70% but for high grade tumors progression and death is quite rapid. Consequently chemotherapy is now being explored.

NON-HODGKIN'S LYMPHOMA (NHL)

There is considerable worldwide variation in incidence (Table 16.1). NHL is twice as common in boys as girls and histologically predominantly diffuse, not nodal and overwhelmingly disseminated. The pattern of dissemination which determines the mode of presentation follows the layout of the lymphoid immune system.

ORIGINS OF LYMPHOMA

The immune system in childhood consists of many different end stage functional cells and an array of precursor and stem cells (Magrath 1987). Malignancy can occur at any stage. Using monoclonal antibodies we can define the differentiation processes of normal and malignant cells. Children constantly exposed to antigens are required to respond to this antigenic attack without having a significant immune memory. A high proportion of lymphoid cells are in an active state undergoing molecular rearrangements in order to produce immunoglobulin and other factors needed for a normal immune response. For B cells to respond properly to antigen, the genes which regulate the different components of immunoglobulin have to be rearranged. In T cells, T cell antigen receptor genes similarly need to be organized.

Immunoglobulin heavy chain genes are on chromosome 14 (q24), lambda light chains on chromosome 22 (q11) and kappa on chromosome 2 (p11). For the cells to function appropriately, there is an ordered sequence required for the rearrangement. For malignant change to occur, genetic rearrangements occur secondary to deletion, mutation or translocation at the chromosome level (i.e. interruption of the normal orderly process). What initiates the disorganization is not clear but evidence incriminates viruses in some. For example, products from HTLV1 retrovirus rearrange genes within the host cell thereby stimulating production of interleukin 2 and its receptor which can activate T cell proliferation. Clonal or polyclonal proliferation provides the opportunity for the second strike necessary to produce a malignant clone. Epstein–Barr virus involvement in the etiology of Burkitt's lymphoma has been described earlier. The characteristic 8 : 14 chromosome translocation seen in this tumor follows a specific pattern. The breakpoint on the chromosome 8 corresponds to the proto-oncogene c-myc and that on chromosome 14 to the immunoglobulin heavy chain gene. In many instances the c-myc gene is translocated from chromosome 8 to chromosome 14. In a few, a part of the light chain gene, either the kappa light chain locus on chromosome 2 or the lambda on chromosome 22, is translocated to chromosome 8 distal to the c-myc gene. In all cases the c-myc gene lies adjacent to immunoglobulin constant region sequences. The c-myc oncogene appears to be necessary for proliferation and by its translocation is activated resulting in cell proliferation. What initiates the abnormal translocation is not clear, but the band Q24 on chromosome 8 is a fragile site. Some have speculated that Burkitt patients may have an inherited defect in DNA repair. Translocations have not been so consistently found in other lymphomas. The T cell receptor genes are on chromosome 14 (q11) (α locus) and chromosome 7 (q35–6 β locus). A complete molecule requires two chains – an α from chromosome 14 and β from chromosome 7. In normal health the rearrangement process needed to produce the product of the receptor gene is very similar to that for the immunoglobulin genes. It is thought that translocations occur when there is inappropriate recombination between chromosomes. The enzyme terminal deoxynucleotidyl transferase (TDT) appears to be involved in T cell gene rearrangements. This enzyme is persistent in lymphoblastic lymphomas and in ALL but not other types of lymphoma. B cell malignancies appear to have completed their rearrangements so the enzyme is absent. TDT is therefore a useful marker to distinguish T from B cell diseases. In childhood the thymus is large and active and T cell leukemia and NHL occur in precursor T cells commonly with a thymic origin. B cell tumors are of precursors of the B cell lineage and disease tends to arise in primary lymphoid sites. These origins are in contrast to adult NHL which is more commonly nodal and of more mature cells. Although most lymphomas in childhood are of early and immature cells, paradoxically Burkitt's lymphoma is a malignancy of Epstein–Barr virus memory B cells.

All childhood lymphomas are rapidly growing tumors with a large growth fraction (nearly 100% in some), but often with a high natural cell death rate. As a result tumor lysis syndrome is not uncommon even before therapy is started. Tumor doubling time may only be 2–3 days. The rapid growth has the advantage that chemotherapy is likely to be quite successful. There are specific features in the epidemiology of NHL which put those with immune deficiency at special risk. Lymphomas also occur commonly as second malignancies particularly if alkylating agents have been used.

CLASSIFICATION (Rappaport & Braylen 1975, Lukes & Collins 1975, Nathwani et at 1976)

A confusing array of classifications exists for NHL. In childhood these bear little relationship to our understanding of the cell of origin or pattern of behavior (Kingston 1987).

For childhood NHL it is best to define the tumors according to the National Cancer Institute Working Formulation:

1. *Lymphoblastic lymphomas*, convoluted and nonconvoluted, mostly of T cell origin (though some are pre-B) which are diffuse and of high grade malignancy. The histology is indistinguishable from ALL although T cell ALL usually arises from early thymocytes whereas lymphomas are more frequently of intermediate or late T cell type. There is considerable overlap. T cell lymphomas have a high propensity for marrow infiltration and CNS involvement.

2. *Noncleaved types* (50%). These include Burkitt's and non-Burkitt's type. They are again diffuse and high grade B cell tumors.

3. *Large cell lymphomas* (15–20%). Half of these are of intermediate grade malignancy, the rest are diffuse and high grade. Most are of B cell origin but a few are T cell. Some lymphomas have surface expression of the Ki-1 antigen. They are classified as immunoblastic but they are lumped with the large cell lymphomas. Characteristically these involve lymph nodes and present with skin lesions and lymphadenopathy. A few large cell lymphomas are truly histiocytic and not lymphoid malignancies.

Monoclonal antibody screening of lymphoid malignancies continues to help reclassification. Some of the lymphoblastic lymphomas have been found to have natural killer cell characteristics and the distinction between lymphoblastic lymphoma and leukemia is quite arbitrary. Even if lymphomas infiltrate the bone marrow, they are still classified as lymphomas by international agreement provided there is less than 25% marrow infiltration. Above that, blood changes appear and they are termed leukemia. This fairly arbitrary cutoff point is currently under review and for B cell lesions 70% may be a more accurate cutoff. Current management is based more on the cell of origin than specific histological considerations. No consistent correlation between histology and survival has been recorded for childhood NHL.

PRESENTATION

Although the scope for presentation is endless depending on the site of the primary lymphoid mass and features of dissemination such as fatigue, pain and anemia, there are some very characteristic presentations (Magrath 1990).

Lymphoblastic lymphomas

Up to two-thirds present with a mediastinal mass (with or without pleural effusion, superior venacaval obstruction, dysphagia and dyspnea). Lymphadenopathy associated with the mediastinal mass is usually confined to the neck and axillae. Spread to abdominal nodes is rarer but hepatosplenomegaly is common as is the propensity for bone marrow (in more than 50%) and CNS involvement. Occasionally, lymphoblastic lymphomas present peripherally with primary skin or bone disease. They are frequently found to have a more mature T cell phenotype.

Small noncleaved tumors

In Europe small noncleaved tumors present as abdominal masses with pain and swelling. There are two commonly recognized types (Magrath 1990):

1. Localized tumors of bowel wall (usually terminal ileum) thought to arise in Peyer's patches leading to a mass with intussusception or bleeding. Patients often have a right iliac fossa mass and are thought to have an appendix abscess.

2. Diffuse abdominal disease: spread throughout the abdominal cavity often involving the kidney, the liver and the spleen. Bone marrow (20%) and CNS disease is common. Non-African Burkitt's presents with jaw involvement in less than 20% of cases. In Equatorial Africa the same tumor presents most frequently with multiple quadrant jaw involvement but also orbital tumors (often maxillary bone). Abdominal involvement is present in 50% but is of the diffuse rather than the localized type.

Localized disease

Lymphoid swellings can occur anywhere but are most common in the neck and can be of any cell type. There appears to be a fairly low risk of any CNS spread in these localized tumors.

Pharyngeal involvement

Most often of B cell disease.

Isolated testicular disease

Isolated testicular disease which rapidly disseminates, is rare and usually of lymphoblastic type. These unusual site lymphomas frequently have large cell histology.

CNS involvement

CNS involvement, particularly in lymphoblastic and Burkitt's lymphoma, leads to headache, vomiting, papilledema, cranial nerve dysfunction and seizures. It is much more common at the time of diagnosis if the bone marrow is also infiltrated and requires specific therapy. The risk of such spread appears to be much lower in localized disease and large cell histology.

DIAGNOSIS

The aim of investigation is to confirm the diagnosis rapidly and determine extent of disease. A chest X-ray is required to exclude mediastinal mass and/or pleural effusions.

Investigations

For localized disease total excision biopsy is indicated; in disseminated tumors the most accessible tumor should be biopsied (extensive surgery is contraindicated). Cytogenetic, molecular and immune markers should be performed on all biopsies. At least two marrow aspirates and trephines from different sites are required to assess marrow involvement. Lumbar puncture should be performed. If cranial nerve deficit or papilledema is present a CT or MR scan should first be performed to exclude nodal deposits. Diffuse meningeal infiltration is not a contraindication to careful LP.

Ultrasonographic or CT scanning of abdominal masses and organs is needed. Bone scans or focal X-rays are indicated for localized bone pain or swellings.

Blood tests must include a full blood picture, liver and renal function tests, LDH levels (prognostic in B cell disease) and electrolyte profile (for tumor lysis).

STAGING

Table 16.16 shows the most commonly used staging system for childhood NHL (Murphy 1980). It is important to note that all primary mediastinal tumors and diffuse abdominal tumors are at least Stage III. Spread in NHL, unlike Hodgkin's (see below), is not orderly and contiguous from node to node. There is no place for routine staging laparotomy in NHL nor for lymphangiography.

PROGNOSTIC FACTORS

Tumor load is the most significant prognostic indicator. Historically the worst prognosis was seen in advanced stage B cell disease especially with CNS disease at diagnosis (see below).

Table 16.16 St Jude modified staging system for non-Hodgkin's lymphoma

Stage		Approximate by stage seen in UK
I	Single tumor (extranodal) or single anatomic area (nodal) (not mediastinum or abdomen)	5%
II	Single tumor (extranodal) with regional node involvement. Primary gastrointestinal tumor with or without involvement of associated mesenteric nodes only. On the same side of diaphragm: (a) two or more nodal areas (b) two single (extranodal) tumors with or without regional node involvement	20%
III	On both sides of the diaphragm: (a) two single tumors (extranodal) (b) two or more nodal areas. All primary intrathoracic tumors (mediastinal, pleural, thymic); all extensive primary intra-abdominal disease; all primary paraspinal or epidural tumors regardless of other sites	50%
IV	Any of the above with initial CNS or bone marrow involvement (<25%)	25%

MANAGEMENT

Chemotherapy is the preferred modality for childhood NHL since all are capable of or have already disseminated.

Chemotherapy protocols

Localized lymphomas

Biopsy excision should be followed by short duration chemotherapy. The simple COMP (cyclophosphamide vincristine, methotrexate, prednisolone) regimen was shown early to be as effective as more intensive protocols. 91% of 63 children treated on UK8501 protocol (pulsed CHOP-cyclophosphamide, adriamycin, vincristine, prednisolone based chemotherapy) are alive at 5 years. Given this result the next UK protocol attempted to reduce duration and long-term toxicity (infertility, second tumors and cardiomyopathy) by eliminating cyclophosphamide, restricting total adriamycin received to 200 mg/m^2 and cutting duration to 23 weeks. CNS directed therapy was only included (I/T methotrexate) for head and neck primaries. Six out of 51 patients followed for at least 1 year have relapsed or progressed (M. Gerrard, personal communication, 1997). Only longer-term follow-up will show if certain subgroups do require more intensive therapy. Certainly lymphoblastic and large cell anaplastic histology types seem to require different strategies (T cell leukemia type and intensive B cell therapy respectively).

Lymphoblastic lymphomas

Intensive multiagent chemotherapy yields 60–80% survival for disseminated lymphoblastic NHL (Stage III + IV) (Müller-Weihrich et al 1985). Leukemia type therapy with induction, intensification modules, CNS directed therapy (CNS irradiation or high dose systemic methotrexate) and 2 years of continuing therapy are now preferred (Eden et al 1992). Surgical resection in mediastinal primaries is contraindicated at diagnosis; occasionally a small incision is required for biopsy (if this is the only evidence of disease). Airway compromise must be guarded against, while initial investigations (bone marrow, LP and biopsy) are being performed.

Residual masses on X-ray after 60 days of treatment may be worth biopsying. True nonremission at this stage carried a 7% reduction in survival for 95 patients treated on UKCCSG 9004 (Eden et al, unpublished work, 1996). Tumor lysis is common even before therapy (Tsokos et al 1981) and effusions may require drainage if they are compromising function. CNS disease at diagnosis requires weekly I/T methotrexate to clear the CSF and then cranial irradiation. Cranial nerve lesions require urgent radiotherapy to maximize recovery. Low stage lymphoblastic tumors at any site appear to require the same intensive chemotherapy as more advanced disease.

B cell lymphomas

Apart from the low stages, B cell lymphomas required intensive pulsed chemotherapy. The French LMB group have demonstrated dramatic results for advanced B cell tumors (Patte et al 1991). The LMB '89 protocol used an initial COP (cyclophosphamide, vincristine, prednisolone) (to reduce too rapid cytoreduction and lysis), 2 × COPADM (COP plus adriamycin and methotrexate), 2 × CYM (cytosine arabinoside and methotrexate) and a third COPADM with over 90% event-free survival for Stage III B NHL (predominantly abdominal primaries). More intensive and varied therapy using extra high dose cytosine and cranial irradiation but still cyclophosphamide and methotrexate-based has yielded almost as favorable results for B ALL and Stage IV disease (Patte et al 1992). High fluid input, allopurinol (i.v. if necessary), forced alkaline diuresis and even dialysis are required on occasions. Now that results are so improved re-evaluation of what is essential in the therapy is occurring. Most patients with large cell anaplastic lymphomas are treated on B cell lymphoma protocols.

HODGKIN'S DISEASE (Kingston 1987, Selby & McElwain 1987)

Hodgkin's disease has a peak incidence in young adults and a second in old age (> 50 years). The early peak is prepubertal, with a male preponderance. Epidemiological features include greater risk in: higher socioeconomic groups, siblings of patients, association with some immunological disorders (e.g. SLE, rheumatoid arthritis, and ataxia telangiectasia.) and a pattern suggesting infective etiology. In up to 60% of patients EBV DNA has been detected in Reed–Sternberg cells especially in mixed cellularity disease (Grufferman & Delzell 1984, Weiss et al 1989).

CELL BIOLOGY AND CLASSIFICATION

The malignant cell in Hodgkin's disease is the Reed–Sternberg (RS) cell. Its exact origin is unclear but it may be derived from an interdigitating reticulum cell involved in antigen presentation to T cells (Fisher 1982). In cell cultures the Reed–Sternberg cell produces a wide range of mediators and if this is similarly true in Hodgkin's disease it might explain the variable cellular patterns seen. R–S cells are not pathognomonic of Hodgkin's disease but seen in some NHLs, in Epstein–Barr virus infection and some carcinomas. Hodgkin's disease, however, cannot be diagnosed in the absence of such cells. They are large (15–45 mm) with

abundant cytoplasm and multiple or multilobed nuclei, frequently with a prominent and characteristic halo around the nucleoli.

The Rye classification is universally used. Types 1 and 2 are commoner in young children. Prognosis appears to be related to the proportion of lymphocytes present in 1–3.

1. Lymphocyte predominance: Reed–Sternberg cells may be quite scarce, fibrosis is rarely seen and the prognosis is good.
2. Mixed cellularity: Reed–Sternberg cells are usually profuse (5–15 per high power field), often with fine fibrosis and focal necrosis.
3. Lymphocyte depletion: large mononuclear abnormal cells are often seen as well as Reed–Sternberg cells with few lymphocytes. Fibrosis and necrosis is common and often quite diffuse – rare in childhood.
4. Nodular sclerosis: lacunar cells are a characteristic finding with a thickened capsule and bands which divide the tissue into nodules. This histology is especially common in lower cervical, supraclavicular and mediastinal Hodgkin's disease of childhood.

Hodgkin's disease generally follows an orderly pattern of spread from node to contiguous node. In the spleen, the infiltration starts as small nodules. Splenic enlargement does not necessarily mean that it is actually involved. Liver infiltration is also usually focal. Progression of the disease tends to go from lymphocyte predominance to mixed cellularity and then lymphocyte depletion if inadequate treatment is given.

CLINICAL PRESENTATION

In childhood most present with painless swelling of the cervical or supraclavicular glands which feel firm or rubbery on palpation – they may be quite tender.

Two-thirds of children with Hodgkin's disease have mediastinal involvement. It may be found coincidentally on X-ray but may compromise the airway and present with dyspnea and wheeze. Involvement of pleura or pericardium may worsen the chest symptoms.

Axillary or inguinal node involvement is less common, the latter occurring in less than 5% of childhood cases. The finding of a large spleen or liver with symptoms of a full abdomen is an indication of advanced disease. 30% of patients have nonspecific features of tiredness and anorexia. Fever, weight loss (more than 10%) and night sweating indicate a worse prognosis and are designated B disease (e.g. Stage II B). In the absence of these symptoms the patient is designated A. Generalized pruritus and unexplained pain on taking alcohol do not affect prognosis. Anemia may be present, either from hemolysis (Coombs' negative) or from iron utilization problems. Thrombocytopenia secondary to a platelet-associated antibody is seen in a small number of cases. Lymphopenia is a sign of advanced disease. The blood picture may change considerably if there is significant splenomegaly and hypersplenism. Patients may have problems with infection both before and during treatment or for many years afterwards due to T cell dysfunction.

DIAGNOSIS

Differential diagnosis includes infective causes of lymphadenopathy (infectious mononucleosis, toxoplasmosis and atypical TB) and non-Hodgkin's lymphoma (particularly in lymphocyte predominant disease). NHL usually has a more rapid onset and tumor growth. In childhood the differential diagnosis is most often between reactive hyperplasia after viral infection. Metastatic disease from nasopharyngeal primaries or from rhabdomyosarcoma have to be considered. Diagnosis is confirmed by a series of investigations.

1. *Clinical assessment* for any node or organ enlargement and documentation of any symptoms.

2. *Chest X-ray* (PA and lateral). If the ratio of any mediastinal mass to maximum intrathoracic diameter exceeds 30%, radiotherapy will be required post-chemotherapy.

3. *Node biopsy* to confirm diagnosis, subtype and molecular/infective studies.

4. *CT or MR scan* of chest and primary site to define precise dimensions and assist response assessment. CT scan of abdomen for organ and nodal assessment. Small retroperitoneal nodes (1–2 cm) may be difficult to visualize due to absence of fat in children. The para-aortic area at the level of the pancreas poses particular assessment problems. Ultrasonography may assist.

Lymphangiography is now rarely performed but in experienced hands still probably provides the clearest visualization of pelvic and para-aortic nodes. Improved MRI techniques will replace it. Gallium scanning is not specific but can be used to monitor response in known disease areas.

5. At least two *marrow aspirates* and two *trephines* are required to exclude infiltration.

6. *Blood tests* required include full blood count, ESR (to monitor response), liver and renal function, alkaline phosphatase, EBV serology, immune status for measles and chickenpox, T and B cell numbers and immunoglobulin levels. Nonspecific markers are used by some to assess progress (serum copper, ferritin, fibrinogen, alkaline phosphatase, interleukin-2 receptor).

7. *Laparotomy* is now rarely required to stage disease in childhood. Splenectomy carried with it a lifelong risk of overwhelming sepsis. Since all but very localized disease receive intensive chemotherapy, scanning alone is adequate for staging.

STAGING AND THERAPY

Table 16.17 shows the Ann Arbor staging system most frequently used throughout the world. With the increasing use of chemotherapy for all but Stage I disease the meticulous staging of the past has been less strictly followed and it is more difficult now to compare results between series when different methods are used to stage patients. Since results are so good this is only really important as attempts to modify therapy are made to avoid late sequelae.

Management

Hodgkin's disease is very radiosensitive but its previous use was associated with unacceptable local tissue growth problems. Combined modality therapy was adopted to minimize the toxicity of both radiation and intensive chemotherapy but maximize cure. There are international variations in approach to therapy. In the UK confirmed Stage I disease (usually high neck) has long been treated with involved field irradiation (35 Gy). Overall survival is 95% at 10 years, with the overwhelming majority of relapsing patients being salvaged with chemotherapy. Most patients can thus be saved from needing chemotherapy.

MOPP combination chemotherapy (mustine, vincristine,

Table 16.17　Ann Arbor staging system for Hodgkin's disease

Stage I	Involvement of a single lymph node region (I) or of a single extralymphatic organ or site (I_E)
Stage II	Involvement of two or more lymph node regions on the same side of the diaphragm (II) or localized involvement of an extralymphatic organ or site and one or more lymph node regions on the same side of the diaphragm (II_E)
Stage III	Involvement of lymph node regions on both sides of the diaphragm (III) which may be accompanied by involvement of the spleen (III_S) or localized involvement of an extralymphatic organ or site (III_E) or both (III_{SE})
Stage IV	Diffuse or disseminated involvement of one or more extralymphatic organs or tissues with or without associated lymph node involvement

(+B – presence of fever, night sweats or weight loss >10% in previous 6 months; +A – none of above.)

procarbazine and prednisolone) was first shown to be effective in 1970. Since then various alternatives have been introduced to decrease acute and long-term toxicity (vomiting, infertility, second neoplasms). In the UK, CLVPP (chlorambucil, vinblastine, procarbazine and prednisolone) was introduced as outpatient therapy and well tolerated. 93% survival for Stage II, 88% for Stage III and 66% for Stage IV disease are reported at 10 years in the UK series but this included relapse rates of 16% with Stage II, 24% in III and 38% with Stage IV which therefore required further treatment. The salvage rate (with alternative drugs ± irradiation) was clearly adequate for Stage II and III disease (M. Radford et al, personal communication, 1996), but the results for Stage IV disease are disappointing. For all but the latter the results are as good as other reported series using MOPP (mustine, vincristine, procarbazine and prednisolone), MVPP (mustine, vinblastine, procarbazine and prednisolone) and the ABVD (adriamycin, bleomycin, vincristine and DTIC) regime devised to avoid alkylators. Some have recommended fewer courses of chemotherapy with involved field radiation in Stage II and III disease. Large mediastinal primaries all require 35 Gy irradiation following chemotherapy and there are anxieties about cardiomyopathies and lung damage with such therapy in those who have received anthracyclines. Hybrid regimens (initially MOPP alternating with ABVD but subsequently a variety of combinations) are based on the Goldie–Coldman (Goldie et al 1982) theory that delivering the maximum number of active drugs as early as possible after diagnosis with the maximum dose intensity will reduce the emergence of resistant clones. Such combinations theoretically also enable total dose reduction of any specific toxic agent (e.g. alkylators or anthracylines). Early response to treatment does appear to predict for outcome especially in advanced disease.

For all but Stage IV disease the efficacy of therapy has to be balanced against long-term toxicity (especially infertility and second tumors).

NEUROBLASTOMA

Although most frequently presenting as a large abdominal mass, this tumor has metastasized in 70% of patients at diagnosis. Common primary sites are the adrenal gland (40%), other abdominal sites (25%), the chest (15%), pelvis (5%) and neck (5%). The thorax is more frequently involved in those under 1 year. Neuroblastoma arises from primordial neural crest cells which form part of the sympathetic and rarely the parasympathetic nervous system. 1 in 250 neonates dying of other causes is found to have small foci of adrenal neuroblasts but disease occurs only in 1 in 10 000 live births. These foci may represent tumors in situ or may be a reflection of a normal stage of adrenal development which regresses in health but persists in malignancy. Spontaneous regression of malignant neuroblastoma to benign ganglioneuroma has been recorded particularly in infants with quite widespread disease (see below).

Age under 1 improves prognosis. Neuroblastoma occurs slightly more frequently in boys and occasional familial clusterings have been reported. Genetic rearrangement involving the short arm of chromosome 1 has been described and it is possible that 20–25% of cases may be heritable. Geographical variations may reflect genuine genetic or environmental factors or may be a reflection of low detection rates. Neuroblastoma occurs with increased frequency in Beckwith–Wiedemann syndrome, neurofibromatosis, nesidioblastosis and in fetal phenytoin syndrome.

PRESENTATION

The features of neuroblastoma are protean because of early dissemination and origin anywhere along the sympathetic chain. Although there will always be a primary (often asymptomatic) this may not always be identified. Localized disease is most likely to be in the neck, or less commonly in the pelvis or chest. Neck lesions will present as a mass, while pelvic lesions often present as obstruction to the bowel or bladder outflow. Silent masses can occasionally be found on routine examination for other reasons. Most abdominal tumors have metastasized, most commonly to the bone marrow or liver or skin by the time of diagnosis. The commonest presentation is with a large firm abdominal mass often crossing the midline but with the features of marrow infiltration including anemia, bruising, fever, lethargy and irritability. Anemia is present in approximately 90% of cases even in the absence of marrow infiltration. Bony disease gives characteristic deep-seated intractable pain in one or more limbs and often causes a limp.

Proptosis and/or periorbital bruising is a characteristic feature due to disease either within the orbit or in the sphenoidal bone. Local infiltration through an intervertebral foramen can produce spinal extradural tumors, (sometimes of great length), with cord compression at any level. They are more common in congenital disease. The spinal canal may be widened as it has grown to accommodate a mass present from early in embryonic or fetal life (such patients have a good prognosis provided they do not have neurological signs). Approximately 1–2% of tumors produce vasoactive intestinal peptide which gives an intractable diarrhoea. Most (90%) tumors secrete catecholamines and although blood levels may be very high they do not normally cause hypertension. Hypertension does occur but is usually renovascular. Urinary levels of catecholamines are used to monitor disease. A syndrome of opsoclonus/myoclonus in which the patient has acute cerebellar and truncal ataxia with rapid eye movements may be seen. CNS disease is rare although increasingly described as length of survival improves.

Cervical disease often produces a unilateral Horner's syndrome. Large abdominal tumors involving the liver may present with elevation of the diaphragm and respiratory symptoms secondary to both pleural effusions and a splinted diaphragm but actual pulmonary disease is rare. Nontender bluish, mobile subcutaneous nodules are most often seen in infants with neuroblastoma. In older patients even quite extensive abdominal masses may be missed and the patient presents with weight loss, change in behavior and vague generalized pain.

INVESTIGATIONS

The diagnosis must be confirmed and extent of disease evaluated.

Biopsy

All should have histological confirmation from the most easily accessible tumor deposit. In addition to routine histology, immunocytochemistry and molecular/genetic studies are required. Deletions of the short arm of chromosome 1 are found in 70–80% of near diploid cells (rarely 1p – is found in constitutional karyotype) and can assist in differentiation from other small round cell tumors. DNA content overall is of prognostic significance (pseudodiploidy associated with advanced disease and poorer survival). N-myc amplification is associated with advanced disease. Consequently, tumor cytogenetics, ploidy and N-myc amplification studies are all required. Histologically, neuroblastoma consists of small blue round cells with fibrillary bundles, hemorrhage, necrosis, calcification and attempts at rosette formation. Maturation to ganglion cells with fibrils may be diffuse (ganglioneuroma) or patchy (ganglioneuroblastoma). Table 16.18 shows ways in which small round cell tumors of childhood may be distinguished.

Bone marrow

Multiple site aspirates and trephines are necessary to exclude involvement since it is the commonest metastatic site. When present, infiltration may be very heavy and mimic *all* or show patchy clumps or rosettes. Monoclonal antibodies (e.g. UK13A) may identify equivocal infiltration.

Diagnostic imaging

CT, MR and ultrasound scans can all be used to define primary tumor extent. It is essential to have three-dimensional assessment of tumor size to document response accurately. MR is optimal to determine any spinal extension. CXR is probably adequate to exclude thoracic extension or involvement from primary abdominal tumors. Bony involvement should be assessed by technetium bone scan (the isotope may also be taken up by the primary). Iodine-131 (or -123) metaiodobenzylguanine scans (taken up by secretory vesicles) is frequently a good marker of disease. Plain bone X-rays may show mixed lytic and sclerotic areas especially in skull and long bones (especially around knees). There is often marked periosteal elevation (osteomyelitis mistakenly diagnosed in a limping child).

Urinary catecholamines

85–90% of patients have detectable excess in their urine and the total levels of catecholamines and vanillyl mandelic acid (VMA) and homovanillic acid (HVA) can be used to monitor tumor response. Elevated levels of cystathione are reported to predict a

Table 16.18 Useful markers in the differentiation of small round cell tumors of childhood

Tumor	Tdt	Cytoplasmic immunoglobulin	Markers (now identified immunologically)				Intermediate filament proteins			
			Actin	Myosin	Neuron-specific enolase	S100 protein	Desmin	Vimentin	Neurofilament	Cytokeratins
Rhabdomyosarcoma	–	–	+	+ (if differentiated type)	+/– (rare)	+/–	+	+	–	+/–
Neuroblastoma	–	–	–	–	+	+	–	–	+	–
Askin tumor	–	–	–	–	+	–/+	–	+/–	?	+/–
Peripheral PNET	–	–	–/+	–	+	+	–/+	+/–	+/–	+/–
Ewing's sarcoma 'typical'	–	–	–	–	–(+) (occasional)	–	–	+	–	+/–
NH lymphoma	+T –B	In B cell	–	–	–	–	–	+	–	–
ALL	+ (95%)	In pre-B (10–15%)	–	–	–	–	–	–	–	–

This battery of markers should be combined with specific antibodies to detect surface antigens, e.g. UJ13A for neuroectodermally derived cells or UJ181A from fetal brain cell origin. Tdt = terminal deoxynucleotidyl transferase.

poor outcome. Catecholamines should ideally be measured on 24-h specimens but can be done on spot specimens provided they are related to creatinine levels. Plasma dopamine levels can also be monitored.

Blood tests

Full blood count, liver and renal function, serum ferritin (nonspecific elevation associated with advanced disease) neurone-specific enolase (elevated in 95% of advanced but not localized disease) should all be performed. Serum levels of GD2 ganglioside can be a useful marker. Constitutional karyotyping should be arranged.

STAGING

Brodeur et al (1988) published an international neuroblastoma staging system (Table 16.19). Standardization will enable comparison of treatment results which has been difficult in the past. All previous criteria were based on clinical, radiological and

Table 16.19 New international staging system for neuroblastoma

Stage 1	Localized tumor confined to the area of origin, complete gross excision, with or without microscopic residual disease, identifiable ipsilateral and contralateral lymph nodes negative microscopically
Stage 2A	Unilateral tumor with incomplete gross excision, identifiable ipsilateral and contralateral lymph nodes negative microscopically
Stage 2B	Unilateral tumor with complete or incomplete gross excision, with positive ipsilateral regional lymph nodes, identifiable contralateral lymph nodes negative microscopically
Stage 3	Tumor infiltrating across the midline with or without regional lymph node involvement; or unilateral tumor with contralateral regional lymph node involvement; or midline tumor with bilateral regional lymph node involvement
Stage 4	Dissemination of tumor to distant lymph node, bone, bone marrow, liver and/or other organs (except as defined in IVS)
Stage 4S	Localized primary tumor as defined for stages 1 and 2 but with dissemination limited to liver, skin and/or bone marrow

bone marrow examination but now staging includes the division of Stage 2 into those with and without lymph node involvement (alters prognosis and may indicate the need for a change in therapy). The overall distribution by stage is approximately 10–15% Stage 1, 8–10% Stage 2, 15–20% Stage 3 and 60% Stage 4. In those under 1 year almost 30% have Stage 1 disease. Nearly 40% of infants (< 1 year) affected have localized disease compared with 20% of older children. Stage 4S (Stage 1 or 2 with dissemination limited to liver, skin and/or bone marrow) is almost exclusively seen in infants. Table 16.20 shows recognized prognostic features.

MANAGEMENT (Look et al 1991, Nitschke et al 1991)

Low risk group (Stage 1 and 2A all ages, Stages 2B and 3 in those under 1 year, and 4S disease; see Table 16.20)

Surgery only is recommended for Stage 1 and 2A disease (90% and 85% survival respectively). Chemotherapy is reserved for any recurrence. For infants with 2B and 3, surgery followed by short course chemotherapy yields 85–90% survival. Optimal chemotherapy is not yet clear. In Europe, the European Neuroblastoma Study Group (ENSG) alternating OJEC and OPEC pulses (vincristine (O), carboplatinum (J), etoposide (E), cyclophosphamide (C), and cisplatinum (P)) are used (Shafford et al 1984) but in the USA, cyclophosphamide and adriamycin are given to a maximum of 4–6 pulses. The aim is to cure without acute or long-term significant toxicity. An occasional infant with Stage 3 circumscribed disease has been cured by complete excision. For 4S disease there is no standard approach. Sometimes a rapidly enlarging liver may require low dose irradiation (100–300 Gy may be adequate) and progressive disease may require limited chemotherapy as for 2B and 3 Stages. Stephenson

Table 16.20 Prognostic features in neuroblastoma

Good	Adverse
Age under 1 year	Age > 1 year
Stages 1, 2 and 4S	Stages 3 and 4
Primary neck and thorax	Abdominal primary
Low serum ferritin	High ferritin

et al 1986 defined a higher risk 4S group of patients who were under 6 weeks of age and without skin involvement who had a survival of 38% compared with 86% for the complete series. These patients may need more aggressive therapy.

Intermediate risk group (all with Stage 2B and 3 over 1 year and infants with Stage 4)

6 months of chemotherapy with OPEC/OJEC, cyclophosphamide and doxorubicin, or cisplatinum/etoposide, followed by radiotherapy to any residual disease post-chemotherapy is considered optimal (50–60% survival). Controversy still exists as to the benefit of post-chemotherapy surgery and results of current trials are awaited. Intensive multiagent chemotherapy can produce remission rates of 75%. Again the optimal regimen is not clear. Some guide to intensity and duration may be drawn from speed of response to initial therapy. The newly identified adverse prognostic features of N-myc amplification, low DNA index and Ip deletion predict for poor response and the need to intensify treatment. Their absence may be an indicator for downgrading therapy. Stage III patients with adverse features have under 30% 5-year survival.

High risk group (all over 1 year with Stage 4 disease)

This forms the majority of patients with survival of only 10–15%. Using platinum-based regimens the European Neuroblastoma Study Group has been performing a dose intensification study (OPEC/OJEC versus rapid COJEC) with the same total dosages in both arms but rapid delivery according to the Goldie–Coldman theory in one arm (dose intensity 1.83 in rapid arm) (A. D. Pearson, personal communication, 1996).

No results are yet available but overall survival is superior to previous studies at this stage. For patients achieving near complete or good partial remission surgical debulking of residual tumor is recommended, followed by high dose chemotherapy (usually melphelan 180–200 mg/m^2) and autologous marrow rescue. In the European Neuroblastoma Study Group trial, 65 patients were randomized to receive such treatment or not (Pinkerton et al 1987). For those receiving melphelan, median event-free survival was 25 months compared with 7 for those not receiving autologous bone marrow transplant ($P = 0.03$). There are 23 surviving patients at least 7 years from treatment, with survival to death longer in those receiving ABMT (40 months) compared with those not (14 months). Whether this improved response rate will translate into long-term cure remains unsure.

Since neuroblastoma is radiosensitive, a place for total body irradiation or targeted radiotherapy (radiolabelled metaiodo-benzylguanidine (MIBG)) in the above plan has been suggested. The optimal timing of such therapy remains unclear.

SCREENING

Since the prognosis for localized disease is good and that for advanced disease is so very poor and there is a readily obtainable marker for disease (urinary catecholamines) attempts have been made to carry out urinary screening of infants. An extensive screening of 6-month-old infants pioneered in Japan initially showed promise but this study may be picking up neural crest rests at 6 months which would disappear later as well as genuine neuroblastoma. Initial enthusiasm has consequently faltered.

NEPHROBLASTOMA (WILMS' TUMOR)

The incidence is about 1 in 10 000 live births with no sex predominance and a peak at 3 years (90% occur under 7). There is an association between aniridia, urogenital abnormalities and Wilms' tumor which has been demonstrated to be linked to a deletion on chromosome 11 (11p13) involving a tumor suppresser gene. The initial loss of heterozygosity (LOH) which leads to tumor formation is most often of the maternal allele. Subsequently Wilms' has been associated with three other syndromes; Drash syndrome with pseudohermaphroditism and a congenital nephropathy; hemihypertrophy (localized or generalized) not necessarily on side of tumor and Beckwith–Wiedemann syndrome (organomegaly, large tongue, omphalocele). Some Wilms' tumors without aniridia have been shown to have LOH at 11p13, and they are frequently associated with intralobar nephroblastomatosis (disordered embryogenesis). A second gene at 11p15.5 is involved in the Beckwith–Wiedemann syndrome and other tumor suppresser genes have now been incriminated in nephroblastoma. About 1% of patients have a family history of such tumors, and it is possible that all bilateral (5%) and up to 20% of unilateral forms might be genetic in origin. Nephroblastomatosis is seen in various forms and may show different patterns with different forms of the tumor.

PRESENTATION (Byrd 1988)

Presentation is usually with an enlarged abdomen and a mass although the child may be very well. The mass may be found coincidentally on routine examination. Fever is present in about 25% and may be due to unrelated causes, hematuria is seen in 25%, abdominal pain in 40% and hypertension in 5–10%. Usually the dilated mass is smooth, nontender and may be surprisingly large for the well-being of the child. A child can rarely present with 'peritonitis' following rupture of the tumor.

INVESTIGATIONS

1. Plain abdominal films will show the soft tissue mass, peripheral calcification (less dense than neuroblastoma) and displaced bowel. Noninvasive ultrasonography will define the mass and enable assessment of the contralateral kidney and vena caval patency. Ultrasound has replaced intravenous pyelography in most centers. The increasing availability of CT and MR scanning enables even more precise definition of tumor spread and anatomy.

Posteroanterior (PA) and lateral chest X-rays must be carefully scrutinized for pulmonary metastases (commonest secondary site). Equivocal shadows require CT scanning. Small metastases seen on CT but not on chest X-ray do not affect staging or outcome on current treatment programs.

Bone scans are indicated if there is focal or diffuse bone pain or if histology confirms a clear cell sarcoma (bone metastasizing tumor). Rhabdoid tumors require CNS visualization for metastases or concomitant primary CNS tumors.

2. Peripheral blood and tumor cytogenetics and molecular studies should be performed for the Wilms' tumor associated genes.

3. Very careful clinical review is required to exclude the congenital syndromes associated with tumor formation.

HISTOLOGY

Tumors are separated into favorable and unfavorable categories (Beckwith 1988). There is little correlation between the very diverse histology and outcome except for the presence of large hyperchromatic nuclei with multipolar mitotic figures (anaplasia) which occur in about 5% of patients. This change is rare before 2 years of age and reaches a peak between ages 5 and 7. The presence of anaplasia in just one small focus within a tumor conveys an adverse prognosis so multiple sectioning of all of the renal tumor is required. Formerly two other types of histology, namely clear cell sarcoma and rhabdoid histology, were linked with anaplasia in the unfavorable group, but they are now recognized as quite separate entities. Clear cell sarcoma comprises 5–7% of childhood renal tumors and is associated with a very high risk of bony metastases (e.g. 76% of 38 cases, Marsden et al 1978). These tumors are quite cystic and there are very characteristic cellular appearances with a fairly evenly spread fibrovascular network. With aggressive treatment these bone metastasizing tumors have a better prognosis and it is therefore particularly important to recognize this even in a localized Stage I tumor.

Rhabdoid tumors comprise just 2% of childhood renal tumors, and are very malignant with a poor prognosis. They occur more in the first year of life and in younger males than either Wilms' or clear cell sarcoma type. They metastasize to the brain and there is also an increased risk of developing a primary PNET (usually in the posterior fossa). These patients may have hypercalcemia. Anaplasia, clear cell sarcoma and rhabdoid histology account for more than 50% of deaths from renal tumors (Beckwith 1988).

PROGNOSIS

Stage and tumor histology (see above) influence outcome. Table 16.21 shows the usual staging system (Breslaw et al 1986). 60% are Stage I and II, 20% Stage III, 10–20% Stage IV. Comparison with historic reports are becoming difficult. The UKCCSG first Wilms' tumor study (1980–86) yielded 10-year event-free survival (EFS) results by Stage of: I 95% (88), II 87% (81), III 81% (80), IV 62% (50), V 73% (73) (Pritchard et al 1995).

These proportions are changing with increasing preoperative chemotherapy.

MANAGEMENT

The aim of therapy is to cure without excessive toxicity in Stage I to III, and improve long-term disease control in Stage IV disease. Controversy still exists as to whether initial surgery or preoperative chemotherapy (formerly radiotherapy) is optimal. The International Society of Pediatric Oncology Studies have shown that presurgical therapy reduces the risk of tumor rupture, downstages tumors and consequently reduces the numbers requiring flank or whole abdominal irradiation. With such overall good survival for low stage disease, such considerations are of great importance. In the UK and USA except in Stage IV disease, the classic approach has been for initial surgical excision. With CT and MR scanning it is much easier to detect truly localized Stage I tumors which can be fully resected and where very limited postoperative chemotherapy (10 weeks of vincristine) can cure over 90% of patients. There may indeed be patients (under 1 year Stage I) who do not require postoperative chemotherapy but as yet these have not been defined. For all other stages, following careful radiographic staging and exclusion of IVC or even cardiac thrombus, biopsy can be followed by chemotherapy (vincristine and actinomycin for Stage II, vincrinstine (V) and alternating adriamycin (Ad) and actinomycin (A) for Stage III, and VAAd all together for Stage IV). Interval surgery is then performed, followed by further chemotherapy according to stage with radiotherapy for any tumor extension within the abdomen. For bilateral (Stage V) disease, the usual approach has been nephrectomy for the largest tumor and partial nephrectomy for the smaller but bilateral partial nephrectomies are now being considered. (Zucker et al 1986, Pritchard et al 1995). Lung irradiation for pulmonary metastases may improve long-term survival.

SPECIFIC LATE EFFECTS

Chronic nephritis and renal failure is clearly seen in the Drash syndrome but also following abdominal irradiation involving the contralateral kidney. Kidney shielding and reduced total dosage has lowered the risk. Scoliosis, and asymmetrical soft tissue wasting were once very common. Fields including the full vertebral width have reduced bony anomalies and lower dosages reduced muscle atrophy. Hepatitis and especially late enteritis (vascular) have been reduced by lowering dosage to 20 Gy from 30 Gy. An acute veno-occlusive syndrome is occasionally seen when right-sided flank irradiation (liver involved) is combined with actinomycin or adriamycin (both should be avoided for 6 weeks post-radiation). Lung irradiation for residual pulmonary metastases (or even whole abdominal) can cause an acute pneumonitis, fibrosis and impairment of lung function (Shaw et al 1991). Meadows et al (1985) described 24 second tumors amongst Wilms' tumor patients, with 22/24 having received radiotherapy and 10/24 both chemotherapy and radiotherapy. As for Hodgkin's disease, increasingly attempts are made to avoid radiation and chemotherapy wherever possible, hence the increasing trend towards presurgical chemotherapy to reduce tumor rupture and the enforced need for radiotherapy.

Table 16.21 Staging system for nephroblastoma

Stage I	Tumor limited to one kidney and totally excised. The renal capsule intact with no rupture pre- or during surgery. No residual tumor is apparent beyond the margins of excision. Tumor may have been biopsied
Stage II	Tumor extension beyond the kidney but totally excised. The extension is regional referring to renal vessels outside kidney infiltrated or containing thrombus. There may be penetration through the capsule to the outer surface and into the perirenal soft tissue. Biopsy may have been performed with local flank spillage. No residual tumor beyond margins of excision
Stage III	Residual nonhematogenous tumor confined to abdomen. Any one or more of the following may be present: 1. Extension beyond surgical margins micro- or macroscopically 2. Diffuse peritoneal contamination by spread or spillage 3. Involved nodes (renal hilar nodes previously) 4. Tumor not fully resectable because of local infiltration into vital organs, e.g. liver
Stage IV	Blood-borne metastases, e.g. lung, liver, bone and/or brain
Stage V	Bilateral kidney tumors initially or subsequently

MESOBLASTIC NEPHROMA

This tumor forms only a small percentage of childhood renal tumors but it is the commonest in the neonatal period with a mean age at diagnosis of 3–4 months. It is a quite distinct entity from Wilms' tumor. The kidney may be large with no pseudocapsule. Hemorrhage, cysts and necrosis are rare but the tumor may appear to infiltrate into the normal kidney and the perinephric connective tissue. The mass is most commonly felt coincidentally at the time of an examination for other reasons. Occasionally there is hematuria, hypertension secondary to a rise in renin and even congestive cardiac failure. Babies with this tumor can have increased risk of preterm delivery (polyhydramnios). Prenatal diagnosis has occurred using ultrasound. The differential diagnosis is hydronephrosis and multicystic kidney. Ultrasound can distinguish between these but cannot distinguish a nephroma from a nephroblastoma. The treatment of choice is nephrectomy; recurrence is rare and usually only in children presenting beyond 3 months of life. Adjuvant treatment is only required for recurrence or significant rupture or if the patient is older than 3 months with marked mitoses on histology. There are rare reports of mesoblastic nephroma metastasizing but doubt is cast as to whether the diagnosis was correct in those circumstances.

SOFT TISSUE SARCOMAS (STS) (D'Angio & Evans 1985)

Sarcomas can arise from primitive mesenchymal cells anywhere in the body and can develop in bone, cartilage, muscle and fibrous tissue. They are the sixth most common form of childhood cancer.

RHABDOMYOSARCOMA

These are the commonest soft tissue sarcomas and arise from tissue which imitates striated muscle. They make up over 75% of the soft tissue sarcomas. Males slightly predominate. There is no recorded worldwide variation in incidence. Bladder and vaginal rhabdomyosarcomas predominantly occur in infancy and the young and are principally embryonal or botryoid in type. Older children most commonly have truncal and extremity lesions which more frequently have undifferentiated and alveolar histology. Intra-abdominal tumors can occur at any age.

Specific etiologic factors

Rhabdomyosarcoma has been reported in association with congenital lung cysts, nevoid basal cell carcinoma syndrome (Gorlin's), fetal alcohol syndrome, neurofibromatosis and Rubenstein–Taybi syndrome. Li & Fraumeni (1969) first described the association of breast cancer and STS. Birch et al (1984) reported that the risk of mothers having breast cancer when their child had STS was as high as 13.5-fold. The risk is due to germline mutations of the p53 tumor suppresser gene on chromosome 17. Tumor cytogenetics have yielded an amazing array of chromosomal rearrangements, including a putative rhabdomyosarcoma gene locus on the short arm of chromosome 11(p) but also consistent t(2;13) translocations have been described in alveolar histology tumors. Amplification of both N-myc and c-myc oncogenes has been reported in some tumors. A genetic basis of rhabdomyosarcoma seems increasingly likely with possible environmental factors including maternal alcohol consumption, ionizing irradiation, paternal smoking and exposure to solvents.

Clinical presentation

Rhabdomyosarcomas can arise at any site in the body as mass lesions. They are usually nontender and the presentation depends on the site of the tumor.

Head and neck (40% of all rhabdomyosarcomas)

About 10% of tumors arise in the orbit producing proptosis and ophthalmoplegia. These usually present early, before the tumor has metastasized. There is little lymphatic spread from the orbit and the prognosis is good. Parameningeal tumors (about 20%) arise from the nasopharynx, paranasal sinuses, middle ear, mastoid and pterygopalatine fossa, producing nasal airway and ear symptoms often with signs of secondary purulent or even bloody discharge. There is a high risk of cranial nerve or meningeal involvement by contiguous spread. If this has occurred, headache, vomiting and raised intracranial pressure may be the presenting features. These tumors frequently have hematological spread. Before the high risk of central nervous involvement was realized these patients had an extremely poor prognosis and treatment must include CNS treatment. Other head and neck sites including scalp, face, oral mucosa, oropharynx, larynx and neck do not carry the same risk of CNS spread and present as mass lesions; they tend to be of low stage and nonmetastatic.

Genitourinary tract (20%)

These usually arise in the bladder and prostate (12%) presenting as a polypoid mass inside the bladder leading to hematuria, urinary obstruction or even extrusion of the tumor into the urethra in females. They tend to be localized. Prostatic tumors lead to bladder outlet obstruction. Constipation may arise from obstruction of the rectum. Bladder tumors tend to occur in younger patients. Prostatic tumors have a higher risk of dissemination (especially lungs). Vaginal and uterine rhabdomyosarcomas make up 2% of the total. Most are botryoid (grape-like) and present with a mucusy and sometimes bloody discharge as would a foreign body. Paratesticular tumors make up about 6% of the total and usually present as painless swellings in the scrotum or inguinal canal – often with nodal involvement. The genitourinary tract tumors tend to have embryonal histology.

Extremity lesions

These comprise 20% of the total and present as mass lesions with or without pain. The majority have alveolar histology and some nodal involvement. Spread can be extensive locally and they metastasize via lymphatics and blood.

Truncal (10%)

On the trunk the mass may reach massive proportions before diagnosis. Local recurrence and distant spread is more likely than lymphatic or nodal involvement.

Other sites (10%)

Intrathoracic and retroperitoneal tumors may reach large dimensions before diagnosis. Intrathoracic primaries may present with airway obstruction or other respiratory symptoms and abdominal tumors with gastrointestinal obstruction. Perineal lesions are rare but can present like an abscess or a polyp. They often have alveolar histology and nodal spread. Biliary tract and liver tumors are rare but can mimic hepatoblastoma and hepatocellular carcinoma though more frequently presenting with jaundice. Differential diagnosis for rhabdomyosarcoma includes almost any other tumor and may be infrequently mistaken for traumatic bruising and soft tissue damage. It is not uncommon for a history of trauma to bring a mass to the attention of the patient, family and doctors.

Diagnosis

Careful assessment of primary tumor extent and regional node involvement (clinical and radiological with CT and MR scanning) is required as a baseline. A truly localized lesion should have a full excision biopsy attempted but most will have diagnostic biopsy, with material sent for routine histology, EM studies, extensive immunocytochemical staining (see Table 16.18), cytogenetics and DNA studies. In parameningeal sites, investigations should include full CNS visualization by CT or MR plus CSF examination if there is no intracerebral mass lesion. All patients require PA and lateral chest radiographs, and CT chest scans if the X-rays are equivocal, and bone scans. Bilateral marrow trephines and aspirates are required to exclude involvement.

Three distinct forms (although hybrids are seen) of rhabdomyosarcoma are recognized (Marsden 1985).

1. *Embryonal* – tumor simulates skeletal muscle – most head and neck, and genitourinary tumors. Tendency to arise where there is no covering mucosa. These are the most favorable tumors.

2. *Botryoid* – more loosely arranged than embryonal – arise in structures with mucosa close to a body cavity (e.g. bladder or vagina).

3. *Alveolar* – classically resemble pattern of lung parenchyma but a few lacunae only may be seen (solid alveolar variant) – occur on extremities and trunk most commonly; least favorable outcome.

About 10–20% of STS are labeled undifferentiated.

Investigations should also include full blood count, assessment of liver and kidney function and levels of blood calcium, phosphate and uric acid.

Although rhabdomyosarcoma is the commonest sarcoma, there are other tumors including extraosseous Ewing's sarcoma, fibrosarcoma and primitive neuroectodermal tumors of peripheral type which may need to be differentiated. Identification on light and electron microscopy of cross-striations will facilitate a specific diagnosis. Immunocytochemistry as outlined in Table 16.18 has enabled easier differentiation of rhabdomyosarcoma from other tumors (Kemshead 1989). Desmin is the most useful marker but caution is required for its interpretation. Multiple monoclonal antibodies may help to confirm the diagnosis. It is the pattern of positivity rather than any single marker which determines the diagnosis.

Staging

The system used by the Intergroup collaborators (IRS) is the most

Table 16.22 Intergroup rhabdomyosarcoma study clinical grouping system

Clinical group	Definition
I	A. Localized, completely resected, confined to site of origin
	B. Localized, completely resected, infiltrated beyond site of origin
II	A. Localized, grossly resected, microscopic residual
	B. Regional disease, involved lymph nodes, completely resected
	C. Regional disease, involved lymph nodes, grossly resected with microscopic residual
III	A. Local or regional grossly visible disease after biopsy only
	B. Grossly visible disease after > 50% resection of primary tumor
IV	Distant metastases present at diagnosis

widely accepted (Table 16.22) but attempts are now being made to adapt the TNM system (Lawrence et al 1987) and relate it to site, and extent of disease. A new grouping system is under trial in most recent trials.

Prognostic variables

The single most important prognostic feature is the group or extent of disease. For those with localized tumors, complete excision (Group 1/A) yields better survival than those with microscopic residual tumor or regional extension (Group II/B). Even poorer survival is seen for those with macroscopic Group III/C residual tumor and the worst for those with metastatic disease (IV/D). The site of the primary influences the lag time between first symptoms and diagnosis, the likelihood of metastatic spread and the possibility of surgical excision, and is also related to histological type (see above). Rate of response to treatment and achievement of complete response closely predict for outcome.

Management

The International Society of Pediatric Oncology MMT 95 Study has the following management strategy by risk grouping (SIOP MMT Committee, personal communication, 1995):

1. All patients with localized, completely resected tumors (no microscopic residual) at any site except orbit (TNM classification = T1 N0 M0 (pT1)) with embryonal or botryoid histology receive, post-excision, a 9-week course of vincristine (eight doses) and actinomycin (four doses). Complete excision must be verified and no paratesticular tumor excised through a scrotal incision can be included because of uncertainty about inguinal extension. These have an excellent prognosis.

2. The standard risk group includes localized tumors not completely removed (or biopsy only) or regionally extended tumors which have been microscopically resected (but which carry increased risk of dissemination) and similar tumors which have been incompletely removed. This incorporates groups (T1 N0 M0), Stage IpT3ab; (T1 N0 M0), Stage IpT2; and (T2 N0 M0), Stage IIpT3ab; but only applies to the special sites of vagina, uterus and paratestis with embryonal histology. These tumors have a good prognosis. Their chemotherapy consists of vincristine, ifosfamide

(6 gm/m²/course) and actinomycin (IVA) for three (every 3 weeks) courses, with re-evaluation. If the tumor has shrunk more than 50%, three more courses are given; if it has not, chemotherapy is changed to carboplatin, epirubicin and vincristine (CEV) alternating with ifosfamide, vincristine, etoposide. Re-evaluation again occurs after three more courses of alternating chemotherapy and local treatment have been given. This strategy incorporates the policy of modification of therapy in slow responders.

3. All other patients with local or low stage regional disease but without distant metastases including all Stage I–III tumors with alveolar histology and any with pleural effusions, and parameningeal disease are randomized between an IVA regimen and a 6-drug protocol (IVA + CEV). Re-evaluation after three pulses again occurs and subsequent therapy is modified according to speed of response. Local therapy is included. Total duration of therapy is 27 weeks. Certain tumor groups are allocated IVA (Stage I and II orbital), whilst young children with parameningeal disease and with Stage III nodal disease receive the more intensive 6-drug regime.

4. All patients with distant metastases receive a very intensive 6-drug, pulsed regime, proceeding to high dose chemotherapy with marrow rescue for good responders. All of these strategies have resulted from a series of trials, most notably that of the SIOP MMT 89 study (Stevens et al 1994), emphasizing the need for good local as well as distant control, recognizing the influence of site and histology and altering therapy when there is slow tumor response to chemotherapy.

OSTEOSARCOMA

The childhood incidence is approximately 5–6 cases per million and accounts for about 60% of malignant bone tumors in childhood. It arises from primitive bone-forming mesenchymal stroma. Ewing's sarcoma is slightly more common in the first decade of life. For osteosarcoma there is a male preponderance and a peak age incidence in the second decade around puberty (maximum growth spurt). It usually occurs at the metaphyses of the most rapidly growing bones (distal femur, proximal tibia, proximal humerus). Trauma frequently draws attention to the tumor but is probably not causative. Ionizing irradiation is implicated in about 3% of all osteosarcomas secondary to therapeutic irradiation (latency 10–15 years). Osteochondromas and chronic osteomyelitis can predispose to osteosarcoma and there is a strong association with retinoblastoma. (50% of second tumors are osteosarcomas within or without the radiation fields.) With the same chromosome 13 defect in both tumors it is thought that cells at the proliferating region of long bones may be particularly susceptible to mitotic errors and lead to homozygosity of the retinoblastoma alleles within the cells at this site. A number of other familial clusterings have also been described, including in families with demonstrated p53 germline mutations.

PRESENTATION

Most osteosarcomas present with an associated soft tissue swelling. Symptom duration is usually about 2–3 months. A more delayed presentation is commoner in *periosteal sarcoma* when symptoms may even be present for many months or even years. The most common sites are the distal femur (33–35%), proximal tibia (15%), proximal humerus (9–10%), mid-femur (5%) and proximal femur (4–5%). Axial flat bones can be affected

especially in the pelvis (15–20%) but tumors in these sites are seen less often in children. Up to 20% have metastases at diagnosis (especially the lungs). Spread is usually hematogenous and rarely lymphatic. Occasionally multifocal disease is seen in childhood (poor prognosis). Symptoms of weight loss, malaise and fever denote the presence of metastases.

DIAGNOSIS

Plain X-rays of the primary tumor site usually show destruction of the normal trabecular pattern with irregular margins and no endosteal bone reaction. There is usually surrounding soft tissue swelling. Periosteal elevation and new bone formation is common producing the classic X-ray appearances of Codman's triangle. The appearances are characteristic in about two-thirds of cases particularly in association with a metaphyseal site. Lesions are sclerotic in 45% of cases, lytic in 30% and mixed in 25%. In contrast, Ewing's sarcomas are usually diaphyseal, lytic and more often involve flat bones

CT or MR scans are essential to define the extent accurately, especially in the medullary cavity; MR is superior to CT. CT scanning of the chest should also be performed as PA and lateral chest X-rays alone are not adequate for the exclusion of metastases (10–20% will be missed on plain X-ray). False positive nodules may be seen on CT scanning but the exact percentage is not clear. The presence of metastases will alter management. 90% of all metastases are pulmonary.

Technetium bone scanning can show the extent and vascularity of the tumor, the latter extending beyond the tumor. This will identify safe margins for surgical excision. It will also enable identification of any multifocal lesions or metastases within bone (10% of metastases).

Arteriography may help define operability, especially when limb salvage is to be considered.

Blood tests should include estimations of alkaline phosphatase (elevated in about 40% of cases). This does not correlate with the extent of the disease but can be a useful marker if elevated at diagnosis. The serum lactate dehydrogenase may be elevated in about 30% of patients even without metastases and may be a useful marker for response to treatment.

Biopsy: once the extent of the disease has been assessed a biopsy should be performed. Most often an open biopsy is recommended with the site of incision carefully chosen to facilitate limb salvage. A frozen section is necessary to ensure adequacy of the tissue material obtained. The surgeon should manipulate the limb as little as possible and try to limit bleeding to decrease the risk of seeding of tumor. In addition to routine histopathology, ploidy (DNA content) studies are helpful.

PATHOLOGY

The characteristic features of osteosarcoma are a malignant sarcomatous stroma with variable tumor osteoid and bone formation. The two tumors with which osteosarcoma is most confused, namely chondrosarcoma and fibrosarcoma, lack the production of osteoid. Chondrosarcoma tends to affect the trunk and proximal limbs and has a longer history with metastases occurring late and less often. Both chondro- and fibrosarcoma tend to occur in older patients.

A number of pathological types of osteosarcoma exist. The most common in childhood is the *conventional osteosarcoma* of which 50% are osteoblastic with active osteoid. 25% are chondroblastic with some differentiation to cartilage but osteoid is always present. It may be difficult to distinguish from true chondrosarcoma. 25% are fibroblastic and can be confused with fibrosarcoma but again osteoid is present. These are all high grade tumors. Less common in children are *telangiectatic tumors* where there is lysis and some calcification (the lesions frequently look like aneurysmal bone cysts or giant cell tumors). A further diagnostic dilemma is that of *malignant fibrohistiocytoma*. This is often difficult to distinguish from conventional osteosarcoma but has a poorer prognosis.

Other forms, for example *parosteal*, occur in the distal femur in older patients and have a longer history. Parosteal osteosarcomas tend to encircle the bone with a risk of local recurrence but metastases are late. *Periosteal* osteosarcomas do not extend into the medulla, occur most commonly in the 10–15 age group and in the upper tibia and are of high grade. Local recurrence is common but metastases late and rare. There is also a low grade *intraosseous osteosarcoma* with slow growth, local infiltration and a low metastatic rate.

STAGING

The usual scheme for bone tumor staging by grade of malignancy, site within bone and metastases is as follows: I, low grade; II, high grade; III, metastatic with (a) intramedullary or (b) extramedullary primary (Enneking et al 1980). Almost all pediatric cases are high grade and extramedullary or metastatic. 90% of metastases are in the lung, with 10–30% also in bone. Less common sites include the pleura, pericardium, kidneys, adrenal and brain. Lymph node involvement is rare. Patients usually die from the pulmonary complications of the metastases.

PROGNOSIS

The most important nontherapy-related prognostic factor is extent of disease. Those with metastases at diagnosis have little chance of cure. Favorable histological features include parosteal and intraosseous well-differentiated tumors; the telangiectatic type is unfavorable. The degree of lymphocyte infiltration of tumor may be related to better outcome. Tumor DNA content appears to relate to outcome (near-diploid more favorable than hyperdiploidy). Since subsequent surgical excision is so important, certain sites, e.g. skull or vertebrae, have proved difficult to treat although new surgical techniques may improve their outcome. In general the more distal the site the more favorable the outcome. Tumor size, e.g. involvement of more than one-third of affected bone, or greater than 15 cm in diameter or extent of local infiltration (Spanier et al 1990), may influence outcome. Multifocal tumors and/or skip lesions worsen survival. The longer the duration of symptoms the more favorable the outcome. Age under 10 is an adverse feature. Girls fare better than boys. Elevated serum and tumor alkaline phosphatase levels predict for metastatic disease. High LDH levels predict poor outcome.

MANAGEMENT

To achieve long-term survival adequate surgical removal is essential. Historically, this was achieved by amputation but most (80%) still developed metastases (50% within the first 6 months) with a 5-year event-free survival of only 20% (10-year 15–20%).

Since 80% died with metastases it was assumed that the majority had micrometastases at diagnosis. Strategies were developed using primary chemotherapy post-biopsy to reduce tumor bulk and facilitate surgery as well as eliminate micrometastases.

The most effective agents are cisplatinum, adriamycin (doxorubicin) and methotrexate, with the first two having been shown to be as effective as regimens including high dose methotrexate in a randomized trial. Ifosfamide has more recently been shown to be a promising agent. Intensive chemotherapy has been used to reduce bulk and enable time to fashion personalized prostheses (Lewis 1986) as part of limit salvage procedures (to avoid amputation). Degree of response to presurgical therapy (histologically) appears to relate to outcome. Some have changed chemotherapy postsurgery based on degree of tumor necrosis (Rosen et al 1982, Jaffe et al 1978). Studies using growth factors (e.g. G-CSF) to increase dose intensity of optimal drug combinations such as doxorubicin and cisplatinum are now in process.

Traditionally, amputation was associated with about 20% cure but at some sites (e.g. shoulders) it was not possible. Stump recurrences occurred. In young children such surgery is devastating and increasingly wide soft tissue and bone excision with graft replacement either from cadaveric or more recently endoprosthetic replacement have proved successful (Lewis 1986). An expandable prosthesis to facilitate growth can now be inserted. There is no evidence of a significant local relapse. Grafts of bone and endoprostheses may have a limited life span and repeated surgery may be necessary for growth. There is no doubt that endoprostheses have a great advantage for the upper limb but for the lower limb they are more controversial. Unless intensive physiotherapy is incorporated in the postoperative plan they may not be functional. Alternative surgery for the lower femur using rotation-plasty has been functionally successful (Kotz & Salzer 1982). For nonmetastatic osteosarcoma 5-year event-free survival is now 60–65%. Whether all of these patients will be cured remains unclear. Although mobility has been improved by limb salvage procedures it is not yet certain whether they are better tolerated psychologically in all patients.

The treatment of metastatic disease is more controversial. The appearance of chest secondaries formerly predicted death within 1 year. Surgical removal by thoracotomies was rarely successful in the long term. CT scanning has enabled earlier recognition of small lesions leading to earlier intervention. Even though the CT scan is more accurate the surgeon usually finds more lesions than those identified on scans. A wide margin of removal is necessary in any patient appearing with lung metastases so a careful search for nonpulmonary deposits must be made prior to any decision about thoracotomy. If the lesions are sizable then initial chemotherapy and/or radiotherapy can be used to shrink them prior to planned thoracotomy.

With these new aggressive approaches to pulmonary metastases 30–40% of patients may be alive 5 years from the time of relapse; their long-term survival remains unclear but may be as high as 25%. Regular chest X-rays are needed for up to 5 years from diagnosis as metastases may appear late with more recent intensive chemotherapy regimes.

EWING'S SARCOMA (D'Angio & Evans 1985)

This is the second most common malignant bone tumor of childhood. The malignant cell may be of primitive, neural origin. The peak age is 10–15 years and there is a slight male predominance. Racial variations are shown in Table 16.1 with a low risk amongst American blacks and Chinese. A few associated congenital features have been reported but there is no obvious pattern of inheritance. A reciprocal translocation t/11; 22 (q24,q12) has been identified in this, Askin tumors and peripheral primitive neuroectodermal tumors suggesting a common neural crest cell of origin. The hybrid transcript resulting from the translocation can be employed as a diagnostic marker. Further understanding of tumor genesis will result from exploration of the DNA configuration.

Although trauma (as for osteosarcoma) frequently brings the patient to medical attention, it is thought to be coincidental not causative.

PRESENTATION

The commonest presentation is with a painful swelling of an affected bone and adjacent soft tissue. If metastases are present, tiredness, anorexia, weight loss and fever can be expected. Both X-ray appearances and the presence of fever may lead to the mistaken diagnosis of osteomyelitis and delay appropriate therapy. The most common sites are the pelvis, proximal humerus and femur but any bone can be involved. The axial skeleton is more frequently involved than with osteosarcoma where extremity lesions are commoner. In long bones metaphyseal and diaphyseal sites are the rule. Rib primaries may present with pleural effusion and respiratory difficulties. Sacral tumors may present with sacral nerve compression and either limb or bladder signs and symptoms.

DIFFERENTIAL DIAGNOSIS

This includes osteomyelitis, arthritis, traumatic injury to bone, osteosarcoma, neuroblastoma, primitive neuroectodermal tumors especially a skin tumor of the chest wall, bony lymphomas and even leukemia and chondrosarcoma. Sometimes the precise definition of a small round cell tumor can be very difficult and often the diagnosis of Ewing's sarcoma is by exclusion of other tumor types. Few other tumors have a diffuse mass of undifferentiated round cells infiltrating into bone marrow and out into soft tissue. Ewing's sarcoma does not have a collagenous stroma like most of the other tumors and stains for reticulin will usually be negative. In rhabdomyosarcoma secondary bone involvement and erosion can occur but both light and electron microscopy studies may identify cross-striations. More undifferentiated sarcomas may be quite difficult to distinguish from Ewing's sarcoma but cytochemical differences such as PAS staining, immunocytochemistry and the use of monoclonal antibodies will prove useful.

There are no unique antigen determinants for Ewing's sarcoma, the diagnosis of which is therefore often a matter of exclusion, matched with the clinical picture, although PCR-based diagnostic tests should be available soon.

DIAGNOSIS

X-ray of the local mass determines the extent of disease but MR scanning or CT are preferable for full determination of the extent of intramedullary and soft tissue involvement. Good PA and lateral chest X-rays are mandatory and, if there is doubt, CT scan of the chest is performed to exclude metastases at diagnosis. A technetium bone scan will help to determine the extent of vascularity with clear margins before a diagnostic biopsy. Great care must be exercised to obtain an adequate specimen yet avoid creating a pathological fracture and, if radical surgery is anticipated, the incision must be in the position where it can be excised at the time of definitive surgery. A frozen section should be carried out at the time of biopsy to ensure adequacy of material. It is usually possible to make the diagnosis on soft tissue rather than disrupting the bone excessively. Light microscopy, electron microscopy and immunocytochemistry will be required together with cytogenetic studies on the tumor and peripheral blood. Bone marrow aspiration from two sites and trephines from two sites should be performed at the same time as the tissue biopsy. Blood tests should include a full blood count, biochemistry for hepatic and renal function, calcium, electrolyte and LDH levels. High levels of c-myc RNA, with or without amplification but no N-myc amplification can help to distinguish from neuroblastoma (in which the reverse is true).

STAGING AND PROGNOSTIC FEATURES (Gehan et al 1981)

No staging system has proved universally acceptable. As for osteosarcoma the Enneking system is used by some.

The presence of overt metastases at diagnosis (15% of patients) confers a poor prognosis. The most common site is lung, then bone and bone marrow. Lymphatic spread is much less common. There is a low incidence of cerebral disease both at diagnosis and subsequently (about 10%) but spinal and paraspinal spread is quite common and may cause cord compression. Bone and bone marrow metastases worsen the prognosis while patients with lung metastases at diagnosis, especially if treated aggressively, can be salvaged by intensive chemotherapy.

The site of the primary appears to affect prognosis. Distal extremity disease is most favorable while pelvic and sacral tumor sites have a poorer prognosis. The humerus, femur and rib sites have an intermediate outlook.

The extent of extraosseous soft tissue extension may significantly affect prognosis. If only bone is involved there is over 80% survival but involvement of soft tissue reduces this to 20% 5-year survival. A volume estimated at less than 100 ml is reported by Gobel et al (1987) as having 3-year disease-free survival of 75–80% compared with only 17% for those larger than 100 ml.

A filigree pattern within the tumor is also associated with a worse prognosis.

An elevated LDH at diagnosis appears to correlate with a poor outlook.

The initial response to chemotherapy may correlate with prognosis as it does for osteosarcoma. Girls have improved survival compared with boys (Craft 1990) and younger patients seem to fare better (under 10 years).

MANAGEMENT

Surgery

Poor long-term survival was obtained with surgery alone. Improvement has resulted from the use of intensive chemotherapy coupled with local control obtained either with radical tumor removal or high dose radiotherapy. For all but the most localized tumors, biopsy is recommended followed by chemotherapy which may render the tumor resectable. There is some evidence that long-term sequelae, in particular second tumors, are less common if chemotherapy and surgery are used rather than chemotherapy and radiotherapy. However, certain sites (the sacrum and spine) are not amenable to radical surgery and for them radiotherapy is essential. Amputation of certain bones such as ribs or the small bones of the feet is possible and associated with minimal loss of function. Proximal fibula lesions can be removed with the distal bone left to stabilize the ankle joint. By and large, attempts are made to treat all other long bone lesions with limb-sparing procedures. These might include removal of bone segments and, as for osteosarcoma, replacement with increasingly ingenious prostheses. Sometimes amputation becomes necessary either when pathological fractures develop at a previous tumor site sterilized by radiotherapy or when soft tissue sequelae follow extensive field radiotherapy.

Radiotherapy

Ewing's sarcoma is radiosensitive. Primary treatment must be with chemotherapy to control dissemination but local control can then be achieved with local radiotherapy. Delivery of chemotherapy may be compromised as a result of myelosuppression secondary to extensive pelvic and spinal marrow radiation. Therefore intensive early chemotherapy is essential to try to sterilize the tumor. The radiation fields should include the entire affected bone plus soft tissue extension with a 3- to 5-cm margin if possible although in the pelvis this may have to be reduced to 2 cm. The Ewing's sarcoma Intergroup showed some benefit for the extra use of radiotherapy to areas of gross metastatic disease, particularly in the lung. Total body irradiation and high dose chemotherapy with autologous marrow transplantation is now being tried in patients who have metastases at diagnosis.

Chemotherapy

Before the introduction of chemotherapy most series using surgery with or without radiotherapy reported 5-year survival figures of less than 10%. A number of drugs have been shown to be effective including cyclophosphamide, adriamycin, ifosfamide, VP16, actinomycin, vincristine, 5FU and melphalan, as single agents. It is only with the use of combination therapy that survival has improved. Nesbit et al (1981) reported the results of the first Intergroup Ewing's sarcoma study in which VAC (vincristine, adriomycin and cyclophosphamide) with adriamycin gave 2-year disease-free survival figures of 74% compared with only 35% for VAC only in nonmetastatic disease. Intensive chemotherapy seemed to have greatest benefit for those with pelvic disease where the prognosis previously was so bad. In Rosen's (1981) series, 53 out of 67 patients with localized disease were alive after a median follow-up period of 41 months including 95% survival for patients with distal lesions. The most effective agents were cyclophosphamide and adriamycin. Radiotherapy without surgery was associated with a higher incidence of local recurrence.

Most centers are now using intensive initial chemotherapy incorporating vincristine, high dose cyclophosphamide or ifosfamide with adriamycin and actinomycin, then local treatment, either surgery wherever possible or radiotherapy followed by ongoing chemotherapy with alkylating agents and adriamycin until the limits are reached for that drug and then reverting to actinomycin. For high risk patients etoposide is added to treatment regimens. In most multicenter studies 3-year disease-free survival is in the region of 60–70% for distal extremity lesions and 30–35% for pelvic and proximal extremity disease. The initial response is better with the new intensive regimes but whether improved long-term survival will result remains unclear. Overall results from the first United Kingdom Ewing's protocol (Craft 1990) shows 8-year survival rates of 11% and 40% for those with and without metastases, respectively. These results are comparable with other unselected series.

GERM CELL TUMORS

They are derived from primordial germ cells and can arise both within the gonads and at other sites as during embryonal development cells may miss their targets during migration and be deposited adjacent to the midline in the sacrococcygeal, retroperitoneal, mediastinal, neck or pineal regions. These nests of misplaced cells can form benign or malignant tumors. The malignant ones account for 3% of all childhood cancers. A number of structural chromosomal changes have been detected in germ cell tumors, most consistently an isochrome 12p and a deletion on 12q (del(12)q14). A small number of families with multiple affected individuals have been reported. Klinefelter's syndrome is strongly associated with mediastinal tumors (20% of males so affected) and at other sites. 46XY gonadal dysgenesis is frequently complicated by germ cell tumors. Ataxia telangiectasia and Li–Fraumeni syndrome families have also been reported in association with such tumors.

TERATOMAS

These are tumors with tissue arising from all three germinal layers, with a lack of organization and variable maturation. They may be solid or cystic and are most often found in the sacrococcygeal region. There are three subtypes: *mature*, with well-differentiated tissues, e.g. brain and skin; *immature*, with embryonic components; and malignant with disorganized embryonic tissue and malignant germ cell elements (e.g. germinoma, choriocarcinoma, endodermal sinus tumor or embryonal carcinoma). In the newborn a sacrococcygeal teratoma may consist of either mature, immature or a mixture of both types of cells. Neonatal tumors outside the sacrococcygeal region, e.g. in the nasopharynx, the jaw or the mediastinum, do not normally contain malignant components.

GERMINOMA (SEMINOMA IN TESTIS, DYSGERMINOMA IN OVARY) (Dehner 1983)

The commonest sites for these tumors in childhood are the ovary, anterior mediastinum and pineal region. 10% of all ovarian tumors and 15% of all germ cell tumors are germinomas and they are the commonest in undescended testicles. There is a characteristic histological appearance of large round cells, vesicular nuclei and clear eosinophilic cytoplasm. Serum levels of AFP and HCG levels are not elevated in pure germinoma.

EMBRYONAL CARCINOMA

This is a poorly differentiated tumor usually with an epithelial appearance (although it may look more like an anaplastic carcinoma with necrosis). Apparent pathological maturation to teratoma has been noted after chemotherapy. These tumors stain markedly for AFP and HCG. In pediatric practice it is rare to find the tumor in a pure form but more commonly in association with teratomatous and endodermal sinus tumor deposits. In young males, the commonest site is the testis.

ENDODERMAL SINUS TUMOR (YOLK SAC)

This tumor occurring alone or in combination with teratoma is the most common malignant germ cell tumor in childhood. The sacrococcygeal region is the usual site in infancy but later the ovary and testes are more frequently affected, although it can occur elsewhere. The tumors are often soft and friable with a papillary, reticular or a solid pattern.

CHORIOCARCINOMA

This highly malignant tumor is rare in childhood and arises from nongestational extraplacental tissue. The commonest sites are the mediastinum, ovary and pineal region. Beta-HCG but not AFP is markedly elevated in serum. Histology shows large round cells with vesicular nuclei (cytotrophoblasts) and large, usually vacuolated, cells which form syncytia (syncytiotrophoblasts). Hemorrhage and necrosis are common.

GONADOBLASTOMA

This tumor is most frequently found in dysgenetic gonads. 30% of patients with gonadal dysgenesis develop a gonadoblastoma which is bilateral in 40% of cases. Local invasion is seen within the gonads but if elements of germinoma are present it is more likely to spread. AFP and HCG are not produced by this tumor.

POLYEMBRYOMA

This is a rare tumor of the ovary or anterior mediastinum. Both AFP and HCG are elevated. The tumor contains elements resembling small embryos.

Ovarian granulosa and theca cell and testicular Sertoli and Leydig cell tumors arise from the true sex cords and stroma of the developing gonad and are not classified as germ cell tumors.

Biochemical markers

Three markers may help with diagnosis and monitoring of therapy.

Alphafetoprotein

Alphafetoprotein (AFP) production from the yolk sac is maximal at about 12–15 weeks of gestation. Normal adult blood levels are not reached until 6–12 months postpartum. Tumors arising from the pluripotential germ cells of the yolk sac secrete high concentrations with the exception of pure dysgerminoma, pure choriocarcinoma, mature teratomas and gonadoblastoma. Monitoring of serum levels can be useful, especially for evidence of resistant or recurrent disease. Staining of tumors for AFP is a useful diagnostic tool.

Beta-human chorionic gonadotropin

This glycoprotein is produced by specialized placental cells so that tumors with trophoblastic elements (choriocarcinoma and hydatidiform moles) have high levels. The half-life is extremely short (45 min) so rapid normalization occurs with tumor kill.

Lactate dehydrogenase isoenzyme 1

Elevation of this isoenzyme is seen in tumors derived from the yolk sac. It can be used to monitor response to therapy.

SACROCOCCYGEAL TERATOMAS

The incidence is 1 in 35 000 live births with 65% being benign, 30% malignant and 5–10% having an immature appearance. Approximately 40% of all germ cell tumors occur in this area. There is a marked female sex preponderance (70%). The mode of presentation will depend on the precise site of the tumor.

1. The buttocks with a minimal presacral component. This is the commonest site in the newborn (186 out of 398 in a series by Altman et al 1974). They are unlikely to be malignant but may become so if not fully excised.
2. External but with a significant intrapelvic component (138 out of 398 in Altman's series).
3. External with most of the mass intrapelvic extending into the abdomen (35 out of 398 in Altman's series). This is the group most likely to be malignant de novo.
4. Entirely presacral with no external component or significant pelvic extension (39 out of 398). These are likely to be missed clinically and more frequently give rise to constipation, less commonly to urinary frequency or lower limb weakness from sacral nerve compression. Any young child with a history of persistent constipation should have a rectal examination as well as careful pelvic ultrasonography or radiology.

In types (1), (2) and (3) the diagnosis is usually made on clinical grounds from the presentation of an external mass, although in (2) the external component can be quite small and may be missed.

Diagnosis

The early detection and surgical removal of even benign tumors is necessary because of the risk of malignant change. If the diagnosis is made before 2 months of age the chance of malignancy is low (10% in boys and 7% in girls). After 2 months, the risk of malignancy is over 60% in boys and 45–50% in girls. Essential investigations include AP and lateral X-rays of the pelvis along with pelvic ultrasound in teratomas (calcification is frequently seen). The estimation of AFP and HCG levels is mandatory and urinary catecholamines can be measured to exclude a pelvic neuroblastoma. A chest X-ray must be performed to exclude pulmonary metastases prior to surgery. CT or MR scanning will help to determine the exact extent of the tumor and also identify any spinal extension.

Staging

Staging in this site is postsurgical. Stage I: a completely excised mass which was localized; Stage II: an excised tumor which extended to adjacent structures or ruptured at surgery; Stage III: a mass which was resected but with residual microscopic (A) or macroscopic (B) tumor; Stage IV: a tumor with metastases.

MEDIASTINAL TERATOMAS

These almost always arise in the anterior superior mediastinum along the urogenital ridge which extends from C6 to L4. They are sometimes found coincidentally on chest X-ray or they may present with airway obstruction, cough, wheeze and dyspnea. Many histological types have been reported, ranging from pure teratoma to embryonal carcinoma and endodermal sinus tumor. Appearances on chest X-ray are of a well-rounded mass often with calcification. Sometimes teeth may be identified in a mature teratoma. CT or MR scanning is essential to determine the extent of the tumor. The differential diagnosis will include thymoma, cyst, lymphoma and neurogenic tumor. A full blood count including platelet count and bone marrow aspiration will exclude advanced stage lymphoma. AFP, HCG levels and urinary catecholamines should be measured. Ultrasonography of the abdomen is necessary to exclude an intra-abdominal mass. It is important to exclude other diagnoses because, for a mediastinal teratoma, complete surgical excision is necessary for cure whereas in other tumors (especially lymphomas) chemotherapy is the treatment of choice.

ABDOMINAL GERM CELL TUMORS

Most arise in the retroperitoneal area but they can occur within the gastrointestinal tract, omentum or liver. In the stomach they may present as obstruction or hemorrhage and in the liver as a mass or jaundice. The retroperitoneal area is the third commonest site after the sacrococcygeal and mediastinal regions in those under 2 years. Pressure from the mass causes pain, constipation or urinary difficulties. Ultrasonography and plain X-rays will often identify calcification or the presence of bone or teeth within the lesion. Investigations to distinguish other tumors should include abdominal ultrasound, CT scan and measurement of urinary catecholamines and serum AFP levels.

INTRACRANIAL TERATOMAS

These account for about 6% of germ cell tumors. Most arise in the pineal region but they can also arise in the suprasellar and infrasellar regions, more frequently leading to CSF pathway obstruction at 3rd ventricular level. A wide variety of histological types including germinomas, embryonal carcinoma and pure teratoma are reported and it is important to distinguish between them since the treatment will be different. For teratoma, surgical excision is the treatment of choice; for embryonal carcinoma, which is more likely to be highly malignant, a biopsy is followed by intensive chemotherapy and radiotherapy.

Other sites for extragonadal germ cell tumors are the oral cavity, the pharynx, the orbit and the neck, collectively making up about 6% of germ cell tumors. These are mostly found at birth and are of benign histology though they can cause death from airway obstruction. Vaginal tumors, mostly of the endodermal sinus tumor type, usually present with bloody discharge. The differential diagnosis will be with rhabdomyosarcoma of botyroides type or a clear cell carcinoma.

GONADAL TUMORS

Ovarian tumor

These account for about 30% of all germ cell tumors. 65% are benign teratomas, 5% are immature teratomas and about 30% are malignant. In children epithelial carcinoma of the ovary is rare. Most malignant germ cell tumors within the ovary occur around the time of puberty. Presentation is usually with pain which may be acute, secondary to tumor torsion or necrosis or it may be chronic associated with some gastrointestinal upset such as nausea and vomiting. There may be fever. These tumors are not infrequently misdiagnosed as appendicitis and at laparotomy a mass is found within the ovary.

The mass may reach a surprising size with omental seeding before clinical symptoms related to the bowel or urinary tract bring the patient to attention. If beta-HCG secretion is marked, pregnancy may be misdiagnosed. The tumors can spread locally to the adnexae, throughout the abdomen (with ascites), to nodes or via the blood. Investigations of a suspected ovarian mass should include plain X-rays of the pelvis and abdomen plus ultrasonography. Malignant tumors less commonly show calcification. MR and CT scanning will give better identification of the exact extent and site of the tumor. CT scanning should be combined with chest cuts to exclude any metastases. AFP levels will be elevated if the tumor is an endodermal sinus tumor or a teratoma and beta-HCG if it is an embryonal carcinoma or choriocarcinoma. Other potential sites for metastases include bones and brain.

Stage I tumors are localized to the ovary with no cells in the peritoneal fluid; Stage II extend beyond the ovarian capsule but only locally without invasion of retroperitoneal nodes (peritoneal fluid negative); Stage III has either positive retroperitoneal nodes, cells in the ascitic fluid or abdominal extension; and Stage IV has extra-abdominal extension.

Testicular tumor

These comprise about 7% of all germ cell tumors and about 70% of all testicular tumors in childhood. 80% are malignant and nearly 20% are pure teratomas. The most common malignant tumor is endodermal sinus tumor. The presentation is with a slowly growing painless testicular mass, with or without accompanying hydrocele (25%) and/or inguinal hernia (20%). These tumors may be misdiagnosed as either epididymitis or hydrocele. If the testis is undescended the risk of malignancy is 20–40 times greater. There may be an inherent problem within the testes since the risk of malignant change is also higher in the contralateral descended testis in a patient with unilateral cryptorchidism. Investigations include ultrasonography of the abdomen and pelvis with CT scanning of abdomen, pelvis and chest; and measurement of AFP and HCG levels. Einhorn's simple staging system for carcinoma of the testis is sufficient. Stage I is tumor localized to testis only; Stage II testis plus retroperitoneal nodes; and Stage III indicates supradiaphragmatic involvement.

MANAGEMENT

Benign germ cell tumors

The optimal treatment for mature teratomas is surgical excision and complete removal is necessary for cure. Recurrence can occur many years later as a mature teratoma or as an endodermal sinus tumor (malignant). The benign tumors need no radiotherapy or chemotherapy but the AFP should be followed long term to identify any recurrence. External sacrococcygeal tumors require a transacral approach but if the pelvis is involved an abdominal combined approach is needed. Removal of the coccyx is essential if recurrence is to be avoided. Spillage from cysts must be avoided and the surgeon should ensure that there is no intraspinal extension of the tumor.

Immature germ cell tumors

Controversy exists about the ideal treatment of immature teratomas. For localized but immature forms, most authorities still recommend surgery and follow-up, as the diagnosis is often only made after tumor removal. If a higher grade of immaturity is reported or if the tumor is more extensive, primary chemotherapy is recommended (see below).

Malignant germ cell tumor

Einhorn et al (1981) showed that cisplatinum, bleomycin and vinblastine (BVP) were superior to all previous chemotherapy for malignant ovarian and testicular germ cell tumors. More recently the UKCCSG has demonstrated that pulsed carboplatin etoposide and bleomycin (JEB) is as effective and less toxic for all malignant extracranial nongonadal tumors. 5-year event-free survival was 64% (95% confidence intervals 48–79%) and overall survival 89%. Renal toxicity and deafness in cisplatinum-based regimens was high (15–20% and 25–30% respectively) but no significant abnormalities have been reported with the JEB protocol (J. R. Mann on behalf of UKCCSG, personal communication, 1996). The role of surgery has changed given the improvement in chemotherapy results. For all it is essential to have adequate material to make a reliable assessment of all cellular components of the tumor. For ovarian tumors wherever possible total excision without spillage should be attempted but extensive pelvic exenteration is contraindicated. If necessary, further residual disease surgery after intensive chemotherapy is to be preferred. In localized testicular tumors, excisional biopsy is recommended through an inguinal approach, and for malignant tumors in that site, radical orchidectomy with high ligation of the cord. For all but the most localized testicular tumors and benign teratomas, intensive chemotherapy should be given. Duration of therapy can be determined by normalization of AFP where that is elevated initially. For relapsing patients high dose chemotherapy with autologous bone marrow rescue and radiotherapy are being tried.

RETINOBLASTOMA (Donaldson et al 1993)

This malignant embryonal tumor occurs predominantly in the first 2 years of life. There is a family history in about 10% of cases, the remaining 90% apparently being sporadic. 20–30% of all tumors are bilateral and clearly 'genetic' (even if there is no family history) and about 10–12% of unilateral ones are also inherited. This means that overall about 40% are 'genetic' either from an affected, surviving parent, from a nonaffected carrier parent (sometime they have regressed retinomas) or as the result of a new germinal mutation in a parent. 60% are 'nonhereditary' or 'non genetic' and result from spontaneous somatic cell mutations (within retinal cells only). They are always unilateral and have no family history. Knudson (1971) proposed that in the 'genetic' form the first mutation occurred prezygotically, while a second event triggers the tumor in the retina or in fact elsewhere. In nongenetic types the two events occur within the retinal cells. Carriers of the retinoblastoma gene (13q14) can develop single or

multiple retinal tumors and/or neoplasms at other sites. The cloned gene encodes for a 928 amino acid protein, which is a nuclear phosphoprotein with DNA-binding activity, thought to play a critical role in cell growth regulation. Loss of both alleles at this locus is required for tumor formation. The wild type allele is probably a tumor suppresser gene. In view of all this knowledge, very accurate genetic counseling is possible from the mode of presentation, family history and search for evidence of the gene in parents. Any child of a surviving parent has a 50% chance of developing a tumor. If normal parents have one affected child, the next one has a 1% risk if the first child had unilateral disease and 6% if it was bilateral. As with all tumor suppressor genes sequencing has demonstrated heterozygous point mutations along the 27 exons of the Rb gene. Prenatal and postnatal prediction using such sequencing, although cumbersome at present, clearly enables even more accuracy.

PRESENTATION

Nowadays most children are identified with the tumor still intraocular. The commonest presenting feature is leukocoria or the 'cat's eye reflex'. The tumor shows as a creamy to pinkish mass through the iris. Strabismus is common if the tumor arises in the macula. Occasionally, patients may show inflammatory changes or even a fixed pupil. A common reason for delay in diagnosis is a mistaken diagnosis of uveitis or endophthalmitis. The tumor is not painful unless there is secondary glaucoma or inflammation. If the involvement is unilateral the child will probably not complain of visual loss. Metastatic symptoms occur if the disease has spread outwith the orbit but this is rare at diagnosis. Most often parents note the eye abnormality and seek help. A full ophthalmological examination under general anesthetic is required (with pupillary dilation). Ultrasonography, CT and MR scanning have enabled better visualization of the tumor. Skull X-rays may show calcification. Bone marrow aspiration and lumbar puncture should also be performed under general anesthetic (necessary for a good ophthalmological examination) to exclude dissemination. Hemorrhage and calcification are quite common and pieces of tumor may break off and seed either into the vitreous or elsewhere on to the retina. External layer disruption can lead to choroid involvement and a greater risk of blood-borne metastases. The iris may be pushed forward by a mass effect or the trabecular network infiltrated leading to glaucoma. Spread can occur along the optic nerve to invade the brain and CSF. Blood-borne spread commonly goes to bone, brain and other organs. Lymphatic spread to the preauricular and submandibular nodes is rare. A staging system based on size of tumor, site of tumor on retina, extension to involve choroid, optic nerve or vitreous and presence/absence of metastases is now employed.

MANAGEMENT

All patients require treatment in highly specialized multidisciplinary centers (e.g. Glasgow and St Bartholomew's Hospital in UK).

The general principles which guide therapy are:

1. For nongenetic tumors near 100% cure is possible by enucleation.

2. Further treatment (radiotherapy or more recently chemotherapy) of nongenetic tumors is only indicated if there is

evidence of extraorbital spread or if on histology, choroidal or nerve head infiltration is present.

3. For those with small unilateral lesions (4 disc diameters) cryotherapy and photocoagulation offer an alternative, but very careful expert follow-up is required.

4. For 'genetic' disease, enucleation in unilateral disease, and the worse eye in bilateral disease, is usually performed.

5. With the high risk of tumors developing in the other eye, if not already present, radiotherapy and/or chemotherapy is used as well to try to conserve some vision in those with genetic disease.

6. Vincristine, cyclophosphamide, adriamycin, ifosfamide, cisplatinum, carboplatin and etoposide have all been shown to produce shrinkage. Limited dosage JOE (carboplatin, vincristine and etoposide) has been used successfully with the least toxicity and lowest rate of secondary tumors to date. Careful attention to scheduling and total dosage must be paid.

7. Even with bilateral disease, event-free survival at 5 years can be 90% unless there is orbital or CNS invasion, but with germline Rb carriage it would appear that secondary neoplasm is almost inevitable over the ensuing 30–40 years. All planned combined modalities should attempt to minimize this (e.g. avoidance of irradiation and alkylators).

LIVER TUMORS

Liver tumors make up about 1% of childhood tumors; 60% are malignant, with hepatoblastoma being slightly more common than hepatocellular carcinoma (HCC). 40% are benign hamartomas or hemangiomas. Both malignant types occur more often in males. Hepatoblastoma has a peak at 18 months, and rarely occurs beyond 10 years while HCC has a median age of onset of 12 years. Predisposing conditions for hepatoblastoma are Beckwith–Wiedemann syndrome and hemihypertrophy (2% of cases) and Wilms' and concurrent hepatoblastoma have been reported. Loss of heterozygosity at both 11p13 and 11p15.5 (see Wilms' tumor) has now been reported within some such hepatoblastomas. Other clonal anomalies, rare sibling pairs and an association with familial adenomatous polyposis (gene on 5q) strongly imply that a variety of gene disturbances can lead to tumor formation. Possible environmental associations have included maternal ingestion of oral contraceptives, and fetal alcohol syndrome. Hepatocellular carcinoma is associated with hepatitis B infection and patients have a greatly increased hep.B surface antigen carrier rate than controls. Recently hepatitis C has also been incriminated. Other causes of cirrhosis including hereditary tyrosinemia, α-1 antitrypsin deficiency, extrahepatic biliary atresia and progressive familial cholestatic cirrhosis predispose to HCC. Prolonged use of anabolic steroids can induce adenomas and multifocal hepatocellular carcinomas. In young patients these are most often seen in Fanconi's anemia. HCC has also occurred in association with familial adenomatous polyposis, ataxia telangiectasia and neurofibromatosis.

PRESENTATION

Hepatoblastoma

This tumor usually presents as an abdominal mass in a child under 2 years with some having weight loss, anorexia, vomiting and pain but symptoms are less prominent than in hepatocellular carcinoma. Occasionally a tumor has ruptured and the patient

presents with an 'acute' abdomen. Not infrequently the tumor is found on examination for general malaise. Abdominal distention with a big liver is the most common finding. Jaundice is rare but the patient may be anemic. There may be splenomegaly and finger clubbing. Rarer associated features include sexual precocity if beta-HCG secretion is high. Up to one-third have severe osteopenia with bone pain and even vertebral fractures.

Hepatocellular carcinoma

Right upper quadrant distention is the most common presentation, often with features of underlying cirrhosis (or tyrosinemia). It is common to find splenomegaly with finger clubbing and spider nevi. Pain is more common than in hepatoblastoma as are nausea, vomiting, fever, weight loss and anorexia. These tumors may also rupture. Jaundice is reported in up to 25% of cases. There may also be associated thrombocytosis and polycythemia due to raised erythropoietin and probably thrombopoietin levels.

DIAGNOSIS

PA and lateral chest X-rays should exclude metastases, significant elevation of the diaphragm and reactive effusions; abdominal X-rays and ultrasound are needed to define the mass, up to 10% of which may show calcification. Benign tumors tend to be poorly echogenic and much more commonly cystic. Ultrasonography is also useful to inspect the inferior vena cava, hepatic and portal veins. CT scanning shows lower attenuation in the tumor than in normal liver and can define the anatomic extent of the tumor. Both hepatoblastoma and hepatocellular carcinoma are deeply infiltrative and may be multicentric. MR scanning is superior to CT for definition of tumor margins. Hepatoblastoma occurs most commonly in the right lobe of the liver. Angiography is necessary to define the vascular supply. Blood tests should include a full blood count and platelet count. Mild normochromic normocytic anemia is quite common but, particularly in hepatocellular carcinoma, increased erythropoietin production may lead to polycythemia. The platelets may be elevated in excess of 1000×10^9/l in childhood liver tumors. The most useful marker is AFP, produced exclusively in the liver in postnatal life. The normal adult range (3–15 ng/ml) is reached by approximately 1 year; the half-life is between 5 and 7 days and is raised in about two-thirds of patients with hepatoblastoma. It is less commonly elevated in those with embryonal type of histology than in the fetal type and is useful for monitoring the course of the disease. Failure to fall along the usual gradient or a late rise suggests persistent or recurrent disease. This may occur prior to any clinical evidence of relapse. AFP levels are raised in about 50% of patients with hepatocellular carcinoma. In those with precocious puberty beta-HCG levels can be monitored for tumor response. Liver function should be evaluated and monitoring of calcium, phosphate and alkaline phosphatase levels are necessary particularly if there is any significant osteopenia. Hepatitis B serology is often positive in hepatocellular carcinoma but rarely in hepatoblastoma.

STAGING AND HISTOLOGY

Staging is based on assessment before and after surgery. Cure only appears to be possible if complete resection occurs at some stage. The consensus approach now is that, apart from highly isolated lateral disease, most hepatoblastomas and probably all hepatocellular carcinomas should be treated with primary chemotherapy. Surgical staging is therefore no longer possible. New schemes have been developed for staging based on site and extent within the liver. The extent is measured by CT scanning. With the increasing use of primary chemotherapy a biopsy is necessary and is safest done as wedge biopsies through a small abdominal incision. More recently 'true cut' biopsies have been shown to be safe in experienced hands.

There are two morphological forms of hepatoblastoma: a pure epithelial (70%) of either fetal or embryonal cells, or a mixture of both, and a mixed tumor with mesenchymal tissue as well as epithelial elements (Weinberg & Finegold 1986). Even osteoid production may be present in these. It is doubtful if the histological type truly predicts outcome, although which epithelial type (i.e. fetal or embryonal) predominates may determine resectability. Hepatoblastoma most often metastasizes to lungs and nodes at the porta hepatis and rarely to bone. Hepatocellular carcinoma similarly metastasizes to the lungs, nodes and later to bone.

MANAGEMENT

Hepatoblastoma

Hepatoblastoma requires total surgical excision for cure. Historically 50–60% of tumors could be primarily resected of which about 60% lived long term giving at best a 30–40% cure for all tumors. Up to 85% of the liver can be removed and residual liver regenerates. Adjuvant postoperative chemotherapy increases survival to 80% in patients where the tumor is fully resected and the most effective drugs are cisplatinum and adriamycin (Douglas et al 1985). Preoperative chemotherapy has increased the numbers of patients who can have complete tumor resection and some patients with lung metastases at diagnosis who are treated in this way can also probably be salvaged. In the first SIOP liver tumor trial 95% of patients showed some response to cisplatinum and adriamycin, enabling 100/134 to have complete resection. 83 of the 100 are alive free of disease (at 4–67 months). Only 10/34 not resected are alive disease free (E. Shafford, personal communication, 1996). Longer follow-up to assess curability is needed. A small number of patients have early death (4%) or progress on treatment (4%). About 10% of truly lateralized disease can have primary resection with good cure rates. The site within the liver and the presence of metastases predict for outcome.

Hepatocellular carcinoma

Historically less than 30% were amenable to primary surgical resection, and one-third of these had long-term survival. Cisplatinum, doxorubicin and etoposide have all been shown to produce shrinkage. In the SIOPEL-1 study, preoperative therapy (cisplatinum, doxorubicin) was given to 36 of whom 12 had complete resection, and 2 incomplete. 22 were still unresectable. Fibrolamellar hepatocellular carcinoma is more often circumscribed, and consequently more amenable to surgery. Radiotherapy may benefit residual disease after chemotherapy and surgery. In multifocal nonresectable HCC in childhood, liver transplantation may also have a place.

HISTIOCYTOSES

This heterogeneous group of diseases causes confusion exemplified by the wide range of conflicting classifications. Delineation is essential as the management required for each type is different. All share an increase in mononuclear phagocytic cells (histiocytes derived from bone marrow). These cells accumulate in a variety of tissues. There are other conditions in which such cells also infiltrate including graft-versus-host reaction, X-linked lymphoproliferative syndrome and some lipidoses.

It is useful to consider the development of the histiocyte to understand this group of conditions. The pluripotential marrow stem cell develops into a committed granulocyte and macrophage stem cell and these differentiate into colony-forming stem cells producing myelocytes and monocytes. When monocytes are produced they are released into the blood and undergo terminal differentiation into macrophages or histiocytes in many tissues, e.g. Kupffer cells in the liver and Langerhans cells in the skin. Monocytes and these terminally differentiated cells can be divided into:

1. *Antigen-processing or phagocytic cells.* These include tissue histiocytes or macrophages, monocytes in the blood, lymph node follicle macrophages, sinusoidal histiocytes and epithelioid histiocytes.

2. *Antigen-presenting or dendritic cells.* These include dendritic reticulum cells in the node follicles, interdigitating reticulum cells in the node cortex and Langerhans cells. These cells present antigen to the circulating T and B cells. All of the antigen-presenting cells and in particular Langerhans cells have a strong affinity for class 2 antigens which the T4 or helper T cells recognize. In addition, Langerhans cells contain structured organelles called Birbeck granules (rod-like structures with central striations and a terminal vesical expansion which looks like a tennis racket under E. M.).

CLASSIFICATION (Writing Group of the Histiocyte Society 1987)

In the group of conditions known as 'Langerhans cell histiocytosis' the normal Langerhans cell is immunologically stimulated to proliferate. This accumulation leads to a failure of normal immune mechanisms, including autocytotoxicity (the body kills its own fibroblasts and red cells in culture) and an altered thymus appearance. In viral or other infection associated with hemophagocytic syndromes, the proliferation of histiocytes results from reaction to a foreign antigen or from excessive lymphokine production by lymphocytes (probably T4). If the patient has an underlying or acquired T cell dysfunction (e.g. from the effects of infection), the lymphokine (phagocytosis inducing factor) leads to continued proliferation and 'self'-phagocytosis.

In familial erythrophagocytic lymphohistiocytosis (FEL), plasmaphoresis can remove a factor which causes proliferation so that the cell-mediated immune system can revert to normality at least temporarily.

There is a further group of conditions in which there is a true neoplastic clonal proliferation of histiocytes. In some of these there may also be erythrophagocytosis. Table 16.23 shows the classification of histiocytoses.

Class I histiocytosis

The generic name Langerhans cell histiocytosis (LCH) is used to encompass the entities formerly called eosinophilic granuloma (single or multiple), Hand–Schuller–Christian triad and

Table 16.23   Classification of histiocytoses

Class I	Class II	Class III
Langerhans cell histiocytosis (histiocytosis X)	1. Infection associated	True malignant proliferation
1. All have Birbeck granules	2. Familial erythrophagocytic lymphohistiocytosis	1. Malignant histiocytosis
2. Cell surface antigens S100 and CDI positive	Normal macrophages proliferate but show erythrophagocytosis throughout the reticuloendothelial system	2. Acute monocytic leukemia
3. Variable eosinophils + giant cells		3. True histiocytic lymphoma
4. Proliferation of the normal Langerhans cell		

Letterer–Siwe disease. These are proliferations probably secondary to defects of immunoregulation. The Langerhans cell seen in them is identified by S100 protein positivity, T6 antigen surface expression and Birbeck granules (the key feature for diagnosis). The cells often have extra antigenic expression, especially to CD11 and 14 monoclonal antibodies on their surface. In addition to the histiocytes in the granulomas, there will be variable numbers of eosinophils (especially in bone), lymphocytes and multinucleated giant cells. This group of conditions presents in a wide variety of ways from nonspecific aches and pains to specific lytic bone lesions, found coincidentally on X-ray, to widespread lymphadenopathy, hepatosplenomegaly and skin rash. Chronic otitis media, diabetes insipidus and weight loss are common in some forms.

The old term 'histiocytosis X' has been modified into a form of staging system: Stage I, single lytic bone lesion; Stage II, multiple lytic bone lesions (both formerly termed eosinophilic granulomata); Stage IIIA, bone plus soft tissue lesions, often associated with diabetes insipidus (pituitary involvement) or exophthalmos (previously termed Hand–Schuller–Christian triad); Stage IIIB, soft tissue only, disseminated form (previously termed Letterer–Siwe disease). The categories are not exclusive and overlap and progression is seen. Stage IIIB is most often seen in young infants and although overall Langerhans cell histiocytosis has a low mortality, those aged under 6 months with IIIB disease have a mortality of 50–60%. They often have wasting, adenopathy, hepatosplenomegaly, anemia and pancytopenia with red to purple skin rashes, a high incidence of seborrheic dermatitis and multiple organ involvement. Children under 2 years are at higher risk of dissemination and more advanced disease.

In most cases of Langerhans cell histiocytosis the disease appears to be self-limiting so that minimal intervention is optimal except where the disease is clearly progressing (Broadbent 1986). For Stage I and II bone disease excisional biopsy or curettage for diagnosis with the intralesional injection of steroids is the favored treatment. Local low dosage irradiation has been used for deposits which cannot easily be treated by curettage. Chemotherapy has no real place for these lesions. For Stage III disease the crucial determinant is whether there is organ dysfunction in addition to infiltration (particularly for those under 2 years at diagnosis). Evaluation should include full blood count, renal and liver function, pulmonary function tests, investigation for diabetes insipidus, bone marrow aspirates and hearing tests. Less than 15% of patients have dysfunction (Broadbent 1986). Aggressive chemotherapy may in the past have contributed to morbidity and mortality particularly in those under 1 year of age. In an International Histiocyte Society Study, patients with Stage III disease received an initial short course of steroids and were then randomized between weekly vinblastine or 3-weekly etoposide for 6 months. Response by 6 weeks predicted outcome, and to date no significant difference has been reported between the two drugs for survival or reactivation of disease (V. Broadbent, personal communication, 1996). For those responding to steroids and vinblastine with minimal late toxicity the outlook appears as good as with more intensive therapy. The problem is how to manage progressive disease, especially in the very young. A new trial has commenced for such patients using etoposide, cyclophosphamide and busulphan conditioning and allogeneic marrow transplantation (where sibling match) or antithymocytic globulin, prednisolone and cyclosporine where there is no donor. Those with such progressive disease have a 50–60% morbidity.

Class II histiocytosis

Class II histiocytosis includes a whole range of nonmalignant conditions in which normal macrophages and/or monocytes proliferate. These cells do not show atypical features or malignant change and lymphocytes may also be increased in numbers. In lymph nodes, total infiltration may be present and proliferation of the histiocytes may occur throughout the reticuloendothelial system. The familial type must be distinguished from infection-associated histiocytosis as the prognosis is very different. No Birbeck granules are seen in the cells of this form of histiocytosis. Other rare conditions are also fitted into this class of histiocytoses (sinus histiocytosis with massive lymphadenopathy and Kikuchi's necrotizing lymphadenitis).

Infection-associated hemophagocytic syndrome IAHS (Risdall et al 1979)

This is reported in association with immunodeficient conditions (congenital or acquired), in T cell malignancies and in angioimmunoblastic lymphoproliferation. Patients usually have fever, malaise, liver and coagulation dysfunction and anemia. Both the production and consumption of coagulation factors are affected. The cells involved are normal macrophages. Bone marrow aspiration is useful for diagnosis with the macrophage showing all the surface antigen activity of normal macrophages and not that of Langerhans cells. There are no cellular malignant characteristics. Epstein–Barr virus infection has been incriminated as causative in some. Since this is most frequently associated with secondary immunosuppression, recommended treatment is to tentatively withdraw the immunosuppressives agents. Acyclovir has been used in some patients with EBV infection and IAHS. Etoposide which appears to interfere with monocyte–macrophage function may reduce toxicity while the infection resolves but in such benign conditions caution must be stressed about using this known leukemogen unless the disease is out of control.

Familial erythrophagocytic lymphohistiocytosis

This is a rare, rapidly fatal condition with an apparent autosomal recessive mode of inheritance. Clinically the patients present in the first 4 years of life with fever, weight loss, failure to thrive, hepatosplenomegaly, a characteristic rash (yellow-brown color), CNS dysfunction (with coma and sometimes seizures), hyperlipidemia, low fibrinogen levels in blood and cellular immune dysfunction.

Erythrophagocytosis may be very marked leading to pancytopenia and even jaundice. Node, liver, bone marrow or lung biopsies will all assist in the diagnosis but the clinical features and the family history are usually adequate except for the first family member involved. Although the course is rapidly downhill this is not a true malignancy. Plasma exchange has been associated with some improvement in immune defects but relapse appears almost invariable. Recently, very aggressive application of treatment similar to LCH, particularly use of steroids, etoposide, cyclosporine and intrathecal methotrexate (high rate of CNS involvement), is under trial by the Histiocyte Society. A few have tried allogeneic marrow transplantation but the outcome is unclear at this time.

Sinus histiocytosis and massive lymphadenopathy

This is usually seen in patients of African origin and presents with cervical lymphadenopathy which may be quite massive, mediastinal enlargement and fever. There is a polyclonal increase in immunoglobulins and a neutrophil leukocytosis. The disease spontaneously regresses in most. Occasionally, progression has been arrested by the use of chemotherapy and/or radiotherapy.

Class III histiocytoses

These are true malignant processes, and include:

1. Acute monocytic leukemia, a malignant proliferation of the bone marrow monoblasts in both bone marrow and blood with a high incidence of skin and gingival involvement and usually hepatosplenomegaly.
2. Malignant histiocytosis with proliferation of macrophages intermediate between monoblasts and the fixed tissue histiocyte. There is a clear overlap between these two conditions. The most common sites to be involved in malignant histiocytosis are nodes, spleen and liver, bone marrow and then skin and bone. Erythrophagocytosis may be seen but is not as prominent as in the class II histiocytosis.
3. True histiocytic lymphoma is rare but can occur as a primary disease affecting any reticuloendothelial site as well as the skin and bone. These lymphomas are very often classified as large cell immunoblastic lymphomas. In these malignant conditions the most useful cytochemical marker is nonspecific esterase: Birbeck granules are not seen.

True malignant histiocytosis is rare, in older children presenting with fever, wasting, lymphadenopathy, hepatosplenomegaly, raised skin lesions and sometimes subcutaneous inflammatory infiltrates. It may be quite difficult to distinguish from familial erythrophagocytic histiocytosis or infection-associated histiocytosis. A node biopsy with full immunophenotyping is necessary for diagnosis. The use of intensive chemotherapy regimens, including drugs such as cyclophosphamide, adriamycin, vincristine and prednisone (CHOP) has increased the median survival from less than 6 months in historical series to more than 40 months. This regimen may also be useful for true histiocytic lymphoma.

TERMINAL CARE (Goldman et al 1990)

There are nearly 11 000 childhood deaths in the UK every year of which 4000 are in the neonatal period, 50% are acute and unexpected (e.g. accidents) and about 1600 are from degenerative disorders and cancer.

Sudden or unexpected death is the most difficult for families and health workers to cope with and it is often the case that those dealing with the family acutely will have had little or no previous contact with them and have no knowledge of personalities or relationships. Frequently, follow-up care and bereavement facilities are lacking or inadequate. The onus will fall on general practitioners and community services for whom training has been lacking or inadequate. In 1988 the National Association of Health Authorities recommended that in every health district in the UK, there should be an official to take overall responsibility for the training and organization of terminal care and bereavement services. In addition, it was recommended that a 24-h home nursing service and respite facilities should be available. Some but not all areas have activated such services for children. Pediatric oncologists feel that it is imperative to build and foster a caring, supportive and empathetic relationship with the child and family from the time of diagnosis so that if curative therapy fails, emotional support will be available. A separate terminal care team is not necessary if the previous therapists have the time to manage the final stages of illness, preferably at home. Less often it may be necessary to use respite in hospital for cancer victims but the ideal of excellent palliation of symptoms at home should be sought. Hospitalization away from family and familiar surroundings is particularly contraindicated in young children. Dying at home is an increasingly preferred option for most children and their families, but with respite available in a pediatric hospice or hospital.

Children are much more resilient and aware than we credit. Quite frequently children realize that they are dying and indicate what they want done for their family and friends.

TELLING THE TRUTH

Each patient and family must be individually assessed; rules to tell or not must be flexible and pragmatic. Children under 5 or 6 years of age may well be aware of death but see it as a separation from loved ones and loved objects that is not necessarily unpleasant or permanent. Going to be a star in the sky, to heaven to join Jesus, or to paradise has often been taught as a not unpleasant experience and if it means escaping needles, pain, bleeding, chemotherapy, etc. it may be preferable for them at that time. Time does not hold the same significance as for adults but children must be reassured that they will never be left alone wherever they are. The older child may be much more aware of self and loss with feelings of rejection or may view death as a punishment for things said or deeds done. In the 6- to 12-year-old age group, decisions about telling the truth can be very difficult for everyone although direct questions must be answered appropriately. 'I am going to die, aren't I?' needs a 'yes' and a lot of support while, 'I am not going to die, am I?' suggests a need to support with denial. Most often that question means, 'I am not going to die right now' and can lead on to further discussion. Caring staff must above all be good listeners. Dying teenagers present the most difficulties. The full realization of the permanence of death frequently leads to regression, anger and tantrums and the whole family needs to be supported through such a crisis and beyond.

SYMPTOM CONTROL

Pain

While the emotional support of the patient and family is important, equal attention must be given to the control of unpleasant symptoms, especially pain. Initially, aches or general discomfort may be controlled by regular 4-hourly paracetamol. Bone pain is sometimes well relieved by the addition of mefenamic acid in a dosage of 250 mg t.i.d. or q.i.d. However, there should be no hesitation at any stage in proceeding to diamorphine or morphine to ensure pain relief (Burne & Hunt 1987). Slow-release morphine sulfate (starting with 1 mg/kg/dose) can be given orally twice a day and usually provides good pain relief. Dosage may need to be adjusted quite frequently to fit the patient's needs. At the outset it may be necessary to use regular 3- to 4-hourly oral diamorphine or morphine elixir (5 mg/5 ml) until pain relief is obtained, to be continued with slower-release morphine. A shorter acting opioid can usually be omitted once the morphine sulfate slow-release tablet achieves control but there should be no hesitation in reintroducing regular diamorphine if there is any question of failure to obliterate pain. Morphine slow-release medication appears to be less emetic than diamorphine given every 3–4 h. Sometimes patients cannot tolerate oral medication or cannot swallow tablets and then either continuous i.v. diamorphine through a central line or subcutaneous diamorphine by pump can be utilized with dose adjustment as necessary. Patients often initially need 0.5–1 mg/h to control pain under these circumstances. The use of subcutaneous infusions has revolutionized therapy and, of course, can easily be managed effectively at home. There is a degree of tachyphylaxis with systemic opioids so that to achieve equiefficacy, dosages may need to be adjusted every few days or at least weekly depending on symptom control. An alternative mode of administration currently under trial is the use of transdermal patches containing fentanyl, a synthetic opioid previously used in anesthesia and intensive care. The patches give steady drug delivery over 72 h and different sizes are available to deliver different dose rates. Their place may be in those unable to swallow and where more invasive routes are not desired or acceptable.

Good treatment is the obliteration of pain. The initial somnolence on opioids disappears after about 24–36 h after which the patient is much more alert and able to lead quite an active life. Such therapy does not shorten life, indeed evidence suggests that symptom-free, such patients may live longer. Addiction is neither a problem for children with painful symptoms nor should it even be a consideration although parents frequently require assurance on this point. This author's record for time on diamorphine sulfate is 18 months for a boy with an extensive and inoperable liver cancer who led a very active outdoor life once his previously intractable pain was controlled.

Vomiting may be worsened by analgesia. Oral chlorpromazine added to diamorphine elixir or given separately usually controls the drug side effects but is sometimes excessively sedative. Alternatives include low dose metoclopramide, or the newer 5HT$_3$ antagonists.

Itching

In some tumors intractable itching occurs during the terminal phase and an antihistamine such as chlorpheniramine or promethazine is indicated. This is opiate-induced usually and slow-release preparations seem less culpable.

Bowel dysfunction

Evacuation of the bowels becomes a problem due to poor fluid and dietary intake, debility, and opiate analgesics. Considerable discomfort may be experienced. It is better to avoid the need for suppositories and painful enemas by the early and regular use of stool softeners such as lactulose or a gentle laxative such as sodium picosulfate.

Urinary retention

Considerable pain and anguish can be caused by a full bladder and an inability to void. Debility, sedation, neurological damage and pelvic tumors predispose to this problem. Although invasive intervention is, in general, to be avoided during childhood terminal illness, sometimes urinary catheterization is preferable to the struggle of attempted but unsuccessful voiding.

Transfusion

To transfuse or not is often a vexed question. Symptoms rather than blood counts or actual pallor will determine the need. Many children would prefer not to come into hospital for a transfusion and with a well-organized home care team it should be possible to transfuse them if necessary at home. Apart from when overt bleeding occurs, the routine use of platelets should be avoided.

EXPLANATIONS

Many patients and all families will ask frequently, 'How will it happen'. They want to know the timing, about symptoms and signs, particularly any pain, bleeding, infection, fits, etc. It is essential to be honest and not omnipotent in predictions, but to promise maximum symptom relief and allow the child who is fully aware, as much as possible, to have a say in what is done to him or her. It is important for the dying child's sake that both the parents and oncology team anticipate problems and plan how to cope with them (e.g. nose bleeds, bowel problems). This avoids acute dramas or mercy dashes to hospital. Most eventualities can be predicted and facilities made available in the home to deal with them.

Many parents will feel guilty if they actually look forward to the end. They must be reassured that it is normal and natural to feel that with death their child will no longer be suffering. They may feel very angry if the patient rejects them but often this is a defense mechanism by the child to protect those closest from the worst features of death. Alternatively, grief by the parents and relatives may lead to them almost appearing to reject the child. It is particularly difficult for nurses and junior doctors to understand why parents spend more time with other children than with their own dying child. This escape or denial must be understood and the parents helped to cope with their grief. Even when long expected, reactions at the actual time of death cannot always be predicted. Bereavement takes a long time, although most people pass through phases of numbness, anger and rejection to acceptance and devastation and then to a stage of putting all in perspective. Some never accept death fully and may need very long-term support. During bereavement counseling (which should be available for all families) certain parental activities appear to predict poor adjustment. A premature change in lifestyle (rapid change of job, house, emigration, etc.), retention of all the child's possessions for more than 1 year (like building a shrine), a too early next pregnancy (replacing the child) and early plus prolonged involvement in disease-related charities are all features which either suggest a rapid denial of the realities and rejection or

excessive holding on to the lost one. Siblings may present with problems from neglect, rejection, their own fears and guilt at things they have said or thought. Frequently, mothers support the whole family with no time to come to term with events themselves. They may present years later with symptoms of severe anxiety or breakdown. Visual or auditory hallucinations by parents are not rare and require reassurance and explanation. They do not indicate psychosis.

CONCLUSION

The terminal illness of a child must be managed with as much meticulous care and dedication as the active treatment of the disease. Each child must be allowed to die peacefully, with dignity and without painful or unpleasant symptoms.

REFERENCES

Altman R P, Randolph J G, Lilly J R 1974 Sacrococcygeal teratomas. Journal of Pediatric Surgery 9: 389–398

Amendola B E, Gebarski S S, Bermudez A G 1985 Analysis of treatment results in craniopharyngioma. Journal of Clinical Oncology 3: 252–258

Attard-Montalto S P, Kingston J E, Eden O B, Plowman P N 1992 Late follow up of lung function after whole lung irradiation for Wilms' tumour. British Journal of Radiology 66: 1114–1118

Barnes N D 1988 Effects of external irradiation on the thyroid gland in childhood. Hormone Research 30: 84–89

Beckwith J B 1988 Pathological aspects of renal tumours in childhood. In: Broecker B H, Klein F A (eds) Pediatric tumors of the genitourinary tract. Alan Liss, New York, pp 25–48

Bielack S S, Erttman R, Winkler K, Landbeck G 1989 Doxorubicin: effect of different schedules on toxicity and antitumor efficiency. European Journal of Cancer and Clinical Oncology 25: 873–882

Birch J M, Hartley A L, Marsden H B, Harris M, Swindell R 1984 Excess risk of breast cancer in the mothers of children with soft tissue sarcomas. British Journal of Cancer 49: 325–331

Bishop J M 1987 The molecular genetics of cancer. Science 235: 305–311

Black D 1987 New evidence on childhood leukaemia and nuclear establishments. British Medical Journal 294: 591–592

Blair V, Birch J 1994 Patterns and temporal trends in the incidence of malignant disease in children. European Journal of Cancer 30A: 1490–1511

Blasberg R, Groothuis D 1986 Chemotherapy of brain tumours. Physiological and pharmacokinetic considerations. Seminars in Oncology 13: 70–82

Bodey G P, Buckley M, Sathe Y S, Friereich E J 1966 Quantitative relationships between circulating leukocytes and infection in patients with acute leukaemia. Annals of Internal Medicine 64: 328–340

Bonadonna G, Zucali R, Monfardini S, De Lena M, Uslenghi C 1975 Combination chemotherapy of Hodgkin's disease with adriamycin, bleomycin, vinblastine and imidazole carboxamide versus MOPP. Cancer 36: 252–259

Breslow N E, Beckwith J B 1982 Epidemiological features of Wilms' tumor. Results of the National Wilms' Tumor Study. Journal of the National Cancer Institute 68: 429

Breslow N E, Churchill G, Nesmith B et al 1986 Clinicopathologic features and prognosis for Wilms' tumor patients with metastases at diagnosis. Cancer 58: 2501–2511

Broadbent V 1986 Favourable prognostic features in histiocytosis X: bone involvement and absence of skin disease. Archives of Disease in Childhood 61: 1219–1221

Brock P R, Pritchard J, Bellman S C, Pinkerton C R 1987 Ototoxicity of high-dose cisplatinum in children. Medical and Pediatric Oncology 16: 368–369

Brodeur G M, Seeger R C, Barrett A et al 1988 International criteria for diagnosis, staging and response to treatment in patients with neuroblastoma. Journal of Clinical Oncology 6: 1874–1881

Bryant B M, Ford H T, Jarman M, Smith I E 1980 Prevention of isophosphamide induced urothelial toxicity with 2-mercaptoethane sulphonate sodium (Mesnum) in patients with advanced carcinoma. Lancet ii: 657

Burkitt D 1958 A sarcoma involving the jaws in African children. British

Journal of Surgery 46: 218–223

Burne R, Hunt A 1987 Use of opiates in terminally ill children. Palliative Medicine 1: 27–30

Byrd R L 1988 Wilms' tumour – medical aspects. In: Broecker B H, Klein F A (eds) Pediatric tumors of the genitourinary tract. Alan Liss, New York, pp 61–73

Coakham H B, Brownell B 1986 Monoclonal antibodies in the diagnosis of cerebral tumours and cerebrospinal fluid neoplasia. In: Cavanaugh J B (ed) Recent advances in neuropathology. Churchill Livingstone, Edinburgh, Vol 3, pp 25–53

Coburn M 1982 The alkylating agents. In: Chabner B (ed) Pharmacologic principles of cancer treatment. Saunders, Philadelphia, pp 276–308

Cohen M E, Duffner P K 1984 Brain tumours in children. International Reviews of Child Neurology. Raven Press, New York

Committee on Medical Aspects of Radiation in the Environment (COMARE) 1986/1988 Bobrow M (Chairman) HMSO Report 1 (West Cumbria, 1986), HMSO Report 2 (Dounreay, 1988)

Committee on Medical Aspects of Radiation in the Environment (COMARE) 4th Report 1996 The incidence of cancer and leukaemia in young people in the vicinity of the Sellafield site, West Cumbria. HMSO, London

Craft A 1990 Results of 1st United Kingdom Children's Cancer Study Group. Ewing's Sarcoma Study 1978–86. UKCCSG Scientific Report 1990

Craft A W, Reid M M, Gardner P S et al 1979 Virus infections in children with acute lymphoblastic leukaemia. Archives of Disease in Childhood 54: 755–759

Crist W, Raney R B, Ragal A et al 1987 Intensive chemotherapy including cisplatinum with or without etoposide for children with soft-tissue sarcoma. Medical and Pediatric Oncology 15: 51–57

Dahlen D, Unni K 1977 Osteosarcoma of bone and its important recognisable varieties. American Journal of Surgical Pathology 1: 61–72

D'Angio G J, Evans A E (eds) 1985 Bone tumours and soft tissue sarcomas. Edward Arnold, London

D'Angio G J, Evans A, Breslow N et al 1981 The treatment of Wilms' tumor. Results of the Second National Wilms' Tumor Study. Cancer 47: 2302

Darbyshire P, Eden O B, Jameson B, Kay H E M, Lilleyman J, Rankin A 1985 Pneumonitis in lymphoblastic leukaemia in childhood. European Journal of Paediatric Haematology and Oncology 2: 141–147

Davies H A, Lennard L, Lilleyman J S 1993 Variable mercaptopurine metabolism in children with leukaemia: a problem of non-compliance? British Medical Journal 306: 1239–1240

De Vita V T, Hellman S, Rosenberg S A 1989 Cancer: principles and practice of oncology, 3rd edn. Lippincott, Philadelphia

Dehner L P 1983 Gonadal and extragonadal germ cell neoplasia of childhood. Human Pathology 14: 493–511

Dohrmann G J, Farwell J R, Falnnery J T 1976 Ependymomas and ependymoblastomas in children. Journal of Neurosurgery 45: 273–283

Donaldson S S, Egbert P R, Lee W H 1993 Retinoblastoma. In: Pizzo P A, Poplack D G (eds) Principles and practice of pediatric oncology, 2nd edn. Lippincott, Philadelphia, pp 683–696

Dosoetz D E, Blitzer P H, Wang C L 1980 Management of glioma of the optic nerve and/or chiasma. Cancer 45: 1467–1471

Douglas E C, Green A A, Wrenn E et al 1985 Effective cisplatin based chemotherapy in the treatment of hepatoblastoma. Medical and Pediatric Oncology 13: 187–190

Eden O B, Shaw M P, Lilleyman J S, Richards S 1990 Non-randomised study comparing toxicity of *Escherichia coli* and *Erwinia* asparaginase in children with leukaemia. Medical and Paediatric Oncology 18: 497–502

Eden O B, Lilleyman J S, Richards S, Shaw M P, Peto J 1991 Results of the Medical Research Council Childhood Leukaemia Trial UKALL VIII. British Journal of Haematology 78(2): 187–196

Eden O B, Hann I, Imeson J, Cotterill S, Gerrard M, Pinkerton C R 1992 Treatment of advanced stage T-cell lymphoblastic lymphoma: results of the United Kingdom Children's Cancer Study Group protocol 8503. British Journal of Haematology 83: 310–316

Eden O B, Black I, Mackinlay G A, Emery A E H 1994 Communication with parents of children with cancer. Palliative Medicine 8: 105–114

Einhorn L H, Williams S D, Troner M et al 1981 The role of maintenance therapy in disseminated testicular cancer. New England Journal of Medicine 305: 727–731

Emery A E H 1984 Molecular pathology of cancer. An introduction to recombinant DNA. Wiley, Chichester

Enneking W F, Spanier S S, Goodman M A 1980 Current concept reviews: the surgical staging of musculo-skeletal sarcoma. American Journal of Bone and Joint Surgery 62: 1027–1030

Erttmann R 1989 Tumour cell resistance against cytostatic drugs. In: Borsi J D (ed) The role of clinical pharmacology in pediatric oncology. Proceedings of Workshop at International Society of Paediatric Oncology, Prague, pp 84–96

Evans A E, Lund V J, Newton W A et al 1982 Combination chemotherapy in the treatment of children with malignant hepatoma. Cancer 50: 821–826

Farquhar J W, Claireaux A E 1952 Familial hemophagocytic reticuloses. Archives of Disease in Childhood 27: 519–525

Feldman S, Hughes W T, Daniel C B 1975 Varicella in children with cancer. Pediatrics 56: 388–397

Finlay J L, August C, Packer R et al 1990 High-dose multi-agent chemotherapy followed by bone marrow 'rescue' for malignant astrocytomas of childhood and adolescence. Journal of Neuro-oncology 9: 239

Fisher R I 1982 Implications of persistent T cell abnormalities for the aetiology of Hodgkin's disease. Cancer Treatment Reports 66: 681–687

Gatti R A, Good R A 1971 Occurrence of malignancy in immunodeficient disease. Cancer 28: 89–98

Gaynon P S. Ettinger L J, Baum E S 1990 Carboplatin in childhood brain tumours: a Children's Cancer Study Group Phase II trial. Cancer 66: 2465

Gehan E A, Nesbit M E, Busgent E O et al 1981 Prognostic factors in children with Ewing's sarcoma. National Cancer Institute Monographs 56: 273–278

Gilles F 1983 Cerebellar tumors in children. Clinical Neurosurgery 30: 181–188

Gjerris F 1978 Clinical aspects and long-term prognosis in supratentorial tumors of infancy and childhood. Acta Neurologica Scandinavica 57: 445–470

Gjerris F, Klinken L 1978 Long term prognosis in children with benign cerebellar astrocytoma. Journal of Neurosurgery 49: 179–184

Gobel V, Jurgens H, Etspuler G et al 1987 Prognostic significance of tumour volume in localised Ewing's sarcoma of bone in children and adolescents. Journal of Cancer Research and Clinical Oncology 113: 187–191

Goldie J H, Goldman A J, Gudanskas G A 1982 Rationale for the use of alternating non-cross-resistant chemotherapy. Cancer Treatment Reports 66: 439–449

Goldman A, Beardsmore S, Hunt J 1990 Palliative care for children with cancer – home, hospital or hospice. Archives of Disease in Childhood 65: 641–644

Gralla R J, Itri L M, Pisko S E et al 1981 Antiemetic efficacy of high dose metoclopramide. New England Journal of Medicine 305: 905–909

Gray M, Hann I M, Glass S, Eden O B, Morris-Jones P, Stevens R F 1987 Mortality and morbidity caused by measles in children with malignant disease. British Medical Journal 295: 19–22

Greaves M F 1988 Speculations on the cause of childhood acute lymphoblastic leukaemia. Leukaemia 1: 120–125

Grufferman S L, Delzell E 1984 Epidemiology of Hodgkin's disease. Epidemiology Reviews 6: 76–106

Harisiadis L, Chang C H 1977 Medulloblastoma in children: a correlation between staging and results of treatment 1977. International Journal of Radiation Oncology, Biology and Physics 2: 833

Hartmann O, Pinkerton C R, Philip T, Zucker J H, Breatnach F 1988 Very high dose cisplatin and etoposide in children with untreated advanced neuroblastoma. Journal of Clinical Oncology 6: 44–50

Hausdorf G, Morf G, Beron G, Erttmann R, Winkler K, Landbeck G, Keck E W 1988 Long term doxorubicin cardiotoxicity in childhood: non-invasive evaluation of the contractile state and diastolic filling. British Heart Journal 60: 309–315

Hawkins M M 1989 Long term survival and cure after childhood cancer. Archives of Disease in Childhood 64: 798–807

Heasman M A, Urquhart J D, Black R J, Kemp I W 1987 Leukaemia in young persons in Scotland. A study of its geographical distribution and relationship to nuclear installations. Health Bulletin 45/3: 147–151

Holmes G E, Holmes F F 1975 After 10 years what are the handicaps and lifestyles of children treated for cancer? Clinical Pediatrics 14: 819–823

Hood T W, Gebarski S S, McKeever P E et al 1986 Stereotaxic biopsy of intrinsic lesions of the brain stem. Journal of Neurosurgery 65: 172–176

Hortabagyi G N, Frye D, Buzdar A U et al 1989 Decreased cardiac toxicity of doxorubicin administered by continuous intravenous infusion in combination chemotherapy for metastatic breast cancer. Cancer 63: 37–45

Houghton J A, Cook R L, Lutz P J, Houghton P J 1985 Melphalan: A potential new agent in the treatment of childhood rhabdomyosarcoma. Cancer Treatment Reports 69: 91–96

Hughes W T, Price R A, Kim H et al 1973 Pneumocystis carinii pneumonitis in children with malignancies. Journal of Pediatrics 82: 404–415

Israel M A 1993 Cancer cell biology. In: Pizzo P A, Poplack D G (eds) Principles and practice of pediatric oncology, 2nd edn. Lippincott, Philadelphia, pp 57–80

Jablon S, Kato H 1970 Childhood cancer in relation to prenatal exposure to atomic bomb radiation. Lancet ii: 1000–1003

Jaffe N, Frei E, Watts H, Traggis D 1978 High dose methotrexate in osteogenic sarcoma. A 5-year experience. Cancer Treatment Reports 62: 259–264

Jaffe N, Smith E, Abelson H, Frei E 1983 Osteogenic sarcoma: alterations in the pattern of pulmonary metastases with adjuvant chemotherapy. Journal of Clinical Oncology 1: 251–254

Juliano R L, Ling V 1976 A surface glycoprotein modulating drug permeability in Chinese hamster ovary cell mutants. Biochimica et Biophysica Acta 455: 152–162

Kalifa C, Lemerle J, Cailland M M, Valayer J 1984 Resectability of childhood hepatoblastoma is improved by primary chemotherapy. Proceedings of the American Society of Clinical Oncology 3: 308

Kartner N, Evernden Porelle D, Bradley G, Ling V 1985 Detection of P-glycoprotein in multi-drug resistant cell lines by monoclonal antibodies. Nature 316: 820–823

Kellerman J, Varni J W 1982 Psychosocial aspects of paediatric hematology. In: Willoughby M, Siegel S (eds) Hematology and oncology. Butterworths, London, pp 14–26

Kemshead J T 1985 Monoclonal antibodies. Their use in the diagnosis and therapy of paediatric and adult tumours derived from the neuroectoderm. In: Baldwin R W (ed) Monoclonal antibodies for cancer detection and therapy. Academic Press, London, p 281

Kemshead J T 1989 Pediatric tumors: immunological and molecular markers. CRC Press, Florida

Kingston J E 1987 Special aspects of treatment of paediatric lymphomas. In: McElwain T, Lister T A (eds) Clinical haematology – the lymphomas. Baillière Tindall, London, Vol 1, pp 223–233

Kinlen L J, Clarke K, Hudson C 1990 Evidence from population mixing in British new towns 1946–85 of an infective basis for childhood leukaemia. Lancet 336: 577–582

Kinumaki H, Takeuche H, Nakamura K 1985 Serum lactate dehydrogenase isoenzyme-1 in children with yolk sac tumor. Cancer 56: 178–181

Kissane J M, Askin F B, Faulkes M et al 1983 Ewing's sarcoma of bone: clinicopathologic aspects of 303 cases from the Intergroup Ewing's Sarcoma Study. Human Pathology 14: 773–779

Knudson A G 1971 Mutation and cancer: statistical study of retinoblastoma. Proceedings of the National Academy of Sciences USA 68: 820–823

Knudson A G, Strong L C 1972a Mutation and cancer. A model for Wilms' tumour of the kidney. Journal of the National Cancer Institute 48: 313

Knudson A G, Strong L C 1972b Mutation and cancer. Neuroblastoma and pheochromocytoma. American Journal of Human Genetics 24: 514–532

Kotz R, Salzer M 1982 Rotation-plasty for childhood osteosarcoma of the distal part of the femur. American Journal of Bone and Joint Surgery 64: 959–969

Kun L E, Mulhearn R K, Crisco J J 1986 Quality of life of children treated for brain tumours: intellectual, emotional and academic function. Journal of Neurosurgery 58: 1–6

Kwa S L, Fine L J 1980 The association between parental occupation and childhood malignancy. Journal of Occupational Medicine 22: 792–794

Lahey M E 1981 Prognostic factors in histiocytosis X. American Journal of Pediatric Hematology and Oncology 3: 57–65

Land H, Pasada L F, Weinburg R A 1983 Tumorigenic conversion of primary embryo fibroblasts requires at least two compensating oncogenes. Nature 304: 596–601

Lashford L S 1989 The development of targeted radiotherapy for the treatment of small round cell tumours of childhood. In: Kemshead J T (ed) Pediatric tumours: immunological and molecular markers. CRC Press, Florida, pp 95–104

Lawrence W, Gehan E A, Hays D M, Beltangady M, Maurer H M 1987 Prognostic significance of staging factors of the UICC staging system in childhood rhabdomyosarcoma. A report from the Intergroup Rhabdomyosarcoma Study (IRS II). Journal of Clinical Oncology 5: 46–54

Lewis M M 1986 The use of an expandable and adjustable prosthesis in the treatment of childhood malignant bone tumors of the extremity. Cancer 57: 499–502

Li F P, Fraumeni J F 1969 Soft tissue sarcoma, breast cancer and other neoplasms. A familial syndrome. Annals of Internal Medicine 71: 747–752

Li F P, Fraumeni J F 1982 Prospective study of a family cancer syndrome. Journal of the American Medical Association 247: 2692–2694

Liebner E, Pretto J, Hochauser M et al 1964 Tumors of the posterior fossa in childhood and adolescence: their diagnostic and radiotherapeutic patterns. Radiology 82: 193–201

Lipshultz S E, Colan S D, Gelber R D et al 1991 Late cardiac effects of doxorubicin therapy for ALL in childhood. New England Journal of Medicine 324: 808–815

Loftus C M, Copeland B R, Carmel P W 1985 Cystic supratentorial gliomas: natural history, and evaluation of modes of surgical therapy. Neurosurgery 17: 19

Look A T, Hays F A, Shuster J J et al 1991 Clinical relevance of tumour cell ploidy and N-myc gene amplification in childhood neuroblastoma: a Pediatric Oncology Group Study. Journal of Clinical Oncology 9: 581

Lukes R J, Collins R D 1975 New approaches to the classification of the lymphomata. British Journal of Cancer 31: 1–28

Lyon J L, Klauber M R, Gardner J W, Udall K S 1979 Childhood leukaemias associated with fallout from nuclear testing. New England Journal of Medicine 300: 397–402

McIntosh S, Chen M, Sartain P A 1985 Adjuvant chemotherapy for medulloblastoma. Cancer 6: 1316

McKenna R, Schwinn C, Soong K, Higginbotham N 1966 Sarcomata of the osteogenic series. An analysis of 552 cases. Journal of Bone and Joint Surgery (American) 48: 1–26

MacKinney A A, Booker H E 1972 Diphenylhydantoin effects on human lymphocytes in vitro and in vivo. An hypothesis to explain some drug reactions. Archives of Internal Medicine 129: 988–992

McKusick V A 1988 Mendelian inheritance in man, 8th edn. Johns Hopkins University Press, Baltimore

Magrath I T 1987 Malignant non-Hodgkin's lymphomas in children. Hematology and Oncology Clinics of North America 1: 577–602

Magrath I T (ed) 1990 The non-Hodgkin's lymphomas. Edward Arnold, London

Magrath I T 1993 Malignant non-Hodgkin's lymphoma. In: Pizzo P A, Poplack D G (eds) Principles and practice of pediatric oncology, 2nd edn. Lippincott, Philadelphia, pp 537–575

Malpas J S 1988 Cancer: The consequences of cure. Clinical Radiology 39: 166–172

Marsden H B 1985 The pathology of soft tissue sarcomas. In: D'Angio G J, Evans A E (eds) Bone tumours and soft tissue sarcomas. Edward Arnold, London, pp 14–46

Marsden H B, Steward J K 1976 Tumours in children. Springer–Verlag, Berlin

Marsden H B, Lawler W, Kumar B U 1978 Bone metastazing renal tumor of childhood. Morphological and clinical features and differences from Wilms' tumor. Cancer 42: 1922–1928

Meadows A T 1988 Risk factors for second malignant neoplasms: report from the Late Effects Study Group. Bulletin of Cancer 75: 125–130

Meadows A T, Kramer S, Hopson R, Lustabader E, Jarrett P, Evans A E 1983 Survival in childhood acute lymphocytic leukaemia: effect of protocol and place of treatment. Cancer Investigation 1: 49–55

Meadows A T, Baum E, Fossati-Bellani F et al 1985 Second malignant neoplasms in children: an update from the Late Effects Study Group. Journal of Clinical Oncology 3: 532–538

Meadows A T, Mckee L, Kazak A E 1989 Psychosocial status of young adult survivors of childhood cancer: a survey. Medical and Pediatric Oncology 17: 466–470

Melnick S, Cole P, Anderson D, Herbst A 1987 Rates and risks of diethylstilbestrol related clear cell adenocarcinoma of the vagina and cervix. An update. New England Journal of Medicine 316: 514–516

Miller R W 1974 Susceptibility of the fetus and child to chemical pollutants. Science 184: 812–814

Miller R W, Mulvihill J J 1976 Small head size after atomic irradiation. Teratology 14: 355–357

Miller R W, Fraumeni J F, Manning M 1964 Association of Wilms' tumour with aniridia, hemihypertrophy, and other congenital malformations. New England Journal of Medicine 270: 922–927

Miser J S, Pizzo P A 1985 Soft tissue sarcomas in childhood. Pediatric Clinics of North America 32: 779–800

Modan B, Ron E, Verner A 1977 Thyroid cancer following scalp irradiation. Radiology 123: 741–744

Müller-Weihrich S, Henze G, Odenwald E et al 1985 B.F.M. trials for childhood non-Hodgkin's lymphomas. In: Cavalli F, Bonadonna G, Rosenswieg M (eds) Malignant lymphomas and Hodgkin's disease. Experimental and therapeutic advances. Martinuus Nijhoff, Boston, p 633

Mulvihill J J 1977 Genetic repertory of human neoplasia. In: Mulvihill J, Miller R W, Fraumeni J F (eds) Genetics of human cancer. Raven Press, New York, pp 137–143

Mulvihill J J, Ridolfi R L, Schultz F R, Borzy M S, Haughton P B T 1975 Hepatic adenoma in Fanconi anaemia treated with oxymetholone. Journal of Pediatrics 87: 122–124

Murphy S B 1980 Classification. Staging and end results of treatment of childhood non Hodgkin's lymphoma: dissimilarities from lymphomas in adults. Seminars in Oncology 7: 332–339

Nathwani B N, Kim H, Rappaport H 1976 Malignant lymphoma, lymphoblastic. Cancer 38: 964–983

Nesbit M E, Perez C A, Tefft M et al 1981 Multimodal therapy for the management of primary non-metastatic Ewing's sarcoma of bone. An Intergroup Study. National Cancer Institute Monographs 56: 255–262

Ninane J, Chessells J M 1981 Serious infections during continuing treatment of acute lymphoblastic leukaemia. Archives of Disease in Childhood 56: 841–844

Ninane J, Pritchard J, Morris-Jones P H et al 1982 Stage II neuroblastoma. Adverse prognostic significance of lymph node involvement. Archives of Disease in Childhood 57: 438–442

Nitschke R, Smith E I, Altshuler G et al 1991 Treatment of grossly unsectable localised neuroblastoma. A Pediatric Oncology Group study. Journal of Clinical Oncology 9: 1181

Oakhill A (ed) 1988 The supportive care of the child with cancer. Wright, London

Obioha F I, Kaine W N, Ikerionwu S E, Obi G O, Ulasi T O 1989 The pattern of childhood malignancy in Eastern Nigeria. Annals of Tropical Paediatrics 9: 261–265

Olisa E G, Chandra R, Jackson M A et al 1975 Relative incidence of childhood cancer. Journal of the National Cancer Institute 55: 281–284

Ozols R, Cunnion R E, Klecker R W, Hamilton T C, Ostchega Y, Porillo J E, Young R 1987 Verapamil and adriamycin in the treatment of drug resistant ovarian cancer patients. Journal of Clinical Oncology 5: 641

Pack G R, Islami A H 1965 Surgical treatment of hepatic tumours. In: Popper H, Schaffner F (eds) Progress in liver diseases. Grune and Stratton, New York, Vol 2, pp 499–511

Packer R J, Siegel S R, Sutton L N et al 1985 Lepto-meningeal dissemination of primary central nervous system tumours of childhood. Annals of Neurology 18: 217–227

Packer R J, Zimmerman R A, Bilanuik L T 1986 Magnetic resonance imaging in the evaluation of treatment related central nervous system damage. Cancer 58: 635–640

Packer R J, Siegel K R, Sutton L N 1988 Efficacy of adjuvant chemotherapy for patients with poor-risk medulloblastoma. Annals of Neurology 24: 503

Parker D M, Stiller C A, Draper G J, Bieber A, Terracini B, Young J L (eds) 1988 International childhood cancer incidence. IARC Scientific Publications No. 87. International Agency for Research in Cancer, Lyon

Patte C, Philip T, Rodany C et al 1991 High survival rate in advanced stage B-cell lymphomas and leukaemias without CNS involvement with short intensive polychemotherapy. Results from the French Pediatric Oncology Society of a randomised trial of 216 children. Journal of Clinical Oncology 9: 123–132

Patte C, Levergen G, Robert A et al 1992 Results of the LMB-89 protocol on B-cell leukaemia: a study of the SFOP. Medical and Pediatric Oncology 20: 405 (Abstract)

Pearson D 1982 Radiotherapy in paediatric oncology. In: Willoughby M, Siegel S (eds) Hematology and oncology. Butterworths, London, pp 30–46

Perlin E, Engler J E, Edson M et al 1976 The value of renal measurements of both human chorionic gonadotrophin and alpha-fetoprotein for monitoring germ cell tumors. Cancer 37: 215–219

Peters J M, Preston-Martin S, Yu M C 1981 Brain tumours in children and occupational exposure of parents. Science 213: 235–237

Phillips S L 1993 Occupation and employment issues in pediatric oncology. In: Pizzo P A, Poplack D G (eds) Principles and practice of pediatric oncology, 2nd edn. Lippincott, Philadelphia, pp 1209–1211

Pinkerton C R, Pritchard J, de Kraker J et al 1987 ENSGI: randomised study of high dose melphelan in neuroblastoma. In: Dickie K, Spitzer G, Jugannoth S (eds) Autologous bone marrow transplantation. University of Texas Press, Houston, p 401

Pinkerton C R, Williams D, Wooton C et al 1990 5HT3 antagonist ondansetron — an effective outpatient antiemetic in cancer treatment. Archives of Disease in Childhood 65: 822–825

Pochedly C (ed) 1982 Neuroblastoma: clinical and biological manifestations. Elsevier Biomedical, New York

Pratt C B, Green A A, Horowitz M E et al 1986 Central nervous system toxicity following the treatment of pediatric patients with ifosfamide/mesna. Journal of Clinical Oncology 4: 1253–1261

Prentice H G (ed) 1984 Infections in haematology. Clinics in Haematology, Vol 13(3)

Price R A, Jamieson P A 1975 The central nervous system in childhood leukaemia. II: subacute leukoencephalopathy. Cancer 35: 306

Pritchard D J 1980 Indications for surgical treatment of localised Ewing's sarcoma of bone. Clinical Orthopaedics 153: 39–43

Pritchard J, da Cunha A, Cornbleet M et al 1982 Alpha-fetoprotein (AFP) monitoring of response to adriamycin in hepatoblastoma. Journal of Pediatric Surgery 17: 429

Pritchard J, Stiller C A, Lennox E L 1989 Overtreatment of children with Wilms' tumour outside paediatric oncology centres. British Medical Journal 299: 835–836

Pritchard J, Imeson J, Barnes J et al 1995 Results of UKCCSG First Wilms' Tumour Study. Journal of Clinical Oncology 13: 124–133

Pui C, Behm S G, Raimondi S C et al 1989 Second acute myeloid leukaemia in children treated for acute lymphoid leukaemia. New England Journal of Medicine 321: 136–142

Purtilo D T, Sakamoto K 1984 Immunodeficiency as a factor in lymphomagenesis. Perspectives in Pediatric Pathology 8: 181–191

Raney R B, Donaldson M H, Sutow W W, Lindberg R D, Maurer H M, Tefft M 1981 Special considerations related to primary site in rhabdomyosarcoma. Experience of the Intergroup Rhabdomyosarcoma Study 1972–6. National Cancer Institute Monographs 56: 69–74

Rappaport H, Braylan R C 1975 Changing concepts in the classification of malignant neoplasms of the haematopoietic system. International Academy of Pathology Monographs 16: 1–19

Redman G P, Shu S, Navis D 1988 Leukaemia and growth hormone. Lancet 1: 1335

Risdall R J, McKenna R W, Nesbit M E et al 1979 Virus-associated hemophagocytic syndrome – a benign histiocytic proliferation distinct from malignant histiocytosis. Cancer 44: 993–1002

Robbins K C, Antionades H N, Devare S G et al 1983 Structural and immunological similarities between simian sarcoma virus gene product(s) and human platelet derived growth factor. Nature 305: 605–608

Roninson I B, Abelson H T, Housman D E, Howell N, Varshavsky A 1984 Amplification of specific DNA sequences correlates with multi-drug resistance in Chinese hamster cells. Nature 309: 626–628

Rorke L B, Giles F H, Davis R L 1985 Revision of the World Health Organization classification of brain tumours for childhood brain tumours. Cancer 56: 1869–1886

Rosen G, Caparros B, Nirenburg A et al 1981 Ewing's sarcoma: ten year experience with adjuvant chemotherapy. Cancer 47: 2204–2213

Rosen G, Caparros B, Huvos A G et al 1982 Pre-operative chemotherapy for osteogenic sarcoma. Selection of post-operative adjuvant chemotherapy based on the response of the primary tumor to pre-operative chemotherapy. Cancer 49: 1221–1230

Sawada T, Kidowaki T, Sakamoto I et al 1984 Neuroblastoma: mass screening for early detection and its prognosis. Cancer 53: 2731–2735

Selby P, McElwain T J 1987 Hodgkin's disease. Blackwell, Oxford

Selby P J, Jameson B, Watson J G, Morgenstern G, Powles R L, Kay H E M 1979 Parenteral acyclovir therapy for herpes virus infections in man. Lancet ii: 1267

Shafford E, Rogers D, Pritchard J 1984 Advanced neuroblastoma improved response rate using a multi-agent regimen (OPEC) including sequential cisplatin and VM26. Journal of Clinical Oncology 2: 742–747

Shafford E A, Kingston J E, Malpas J S, Plowman P N, Pritchard J, Savage M O, Eden O B 1993 Testicular function following the treatment of Hodgkin's disease in childhood. British Journal of Cancer 68: 1199–1204

Shalet S M 1989 Endocrine consequences of treatment of malignant disease. Archives of Disease in Childhood 64: 1635–1641

Shalet S M, Clayton P E, Price D A 1988 Growth and pituitary function in children treated for brain tumours or acute lymphoblastic leukaemia. Hormone Research 30: 53–61

Shaw N J, Tweeddale P M, Eden O B 1989 Pulmonary function in childhood leukaemia survivors. Medical and Pediatric Oncology 17: 149–154

Shaw N J, Eden O B, Jenney M E M, Stevens R F, Morris-Jones P H, Craft A W, Castillo L 1991 Pulmonary function in survivors of Wilms' tumour. Paediatric Haematology and Oncology 8(2): 131–137

Simpson R McD, Eden O B 1984 Possible interferon response in a child with measles encephalopathy during immunosuppression. Scandinavian Journal of Infectious Diseases 16: 315–319

Spannier S S, Shuster J J, Vender Griend R A 1990 The effect of local extent of the tumour on prognosis in osteosarcoma. Journal of Bone and Joint Surgery (American) 72: 643–653

Speyer J L, Green M D, Kramer E et al 1988 Protective effect of the bispiperazinedione ICRF-187 against doxorubicin induced cardiac toxicity in women with advanced breast cancer. New England Journal of Medicine 319: 745–752

Stehelin D, Varmus H E, Bishop J M, Vogt P K 1976 DNA related to the transferring gene(s) of avian sarcoma viruses is present in normal avian DNA. Nature 260: 170–173

Steinherz L J, Steinherz P G, Tan C T, Murphy M L 1991 Cardiac toxicity 4–20 years after completing anthracycline therapy. Journal of the American Medical Association 266: 1672–1677

Stephenson S, Cook B, Mease A, Ruymann F 1986 The prognostic significance of age and pattern of metastases in Stage IV-S neuroblastoma. Cancer 58: 372–375

Stevens M C G et al 1994 Non metastatic rhabdomyosarcoma: experience from the SIOP MMT89 study. Medical and Pediatric Oncology 23: 171

Stewart A, Webb J, Giles D, Hewitt D 1956 Malignant disease in childhood and diagnostic radiation in utero. Lancet ii: 447

Stiehm E R 1979 Standard and special human immune serum globulin as therapeutic agents. Pediatrics 63: 301–319

Stiller C A 1988 Centralisation of treatment and survival rates for cancer. Archives of Disease in Childhood 63: 23–30

Strong L C 1984 Genetics, etiology and epidemiology of childhood cancer. In: Sutow W W, Fernbach D J, Vietti T J (eds) Clinical pediatric oncology. 3rd edn. C V Mosby, St Louis, pp 14–41

Tsokos G E, Balow J E, Spiegel R J, Magrath I T 1981 Renal and metabolic complications of undifferentiated and lymphoblastic lymphoma. Medicine 60: 218

Tucker M A, Meadows A T, Borie J D et al 1987 Leukaemia after therapy with alkylating agents for childhood cancer. Journal of the National Cancer Institute 78: 459–464

Upton A C, Albert R E, Burns F J, Shore E 1986 Radiation carcinogenesis. Elsevier, New York

Van Hoff D D, Layard M W, Basa P et al 1979 Risk factors for adriamycin induced congestive heart failure. Annals of Internal Medicine 91: 710–717

Vanel D, Henry-Amar M, Lumbroso J 1984 Pulmonary evaluation of patients with osteosarcoma. Roles of standard radiography, tomography, CT, scintigraphy and tomoscintigraphy. American Journal of Radiology 143: 519–523

Wang S C 1985 Emetic and antiemetic drugs. In: Root W S, Hofmann F G (eds) Psychological pharmacology. Academic Press, New York, Vol 2, pp 255–328

Weinberg A G, Finegold M J 1986 Primary hepatic tumors in childhood. In: Finegold M J (ed) Pathology of neoplasia in children and adolescents. Saunders, Philadelphia, pp 333–372

Weiss H D, Walker M D, Wiernik P H 1975 Neurotoxicity of commonly used antineoplastic agents. New England Journal of Medicine 291: 75–127

Weiss L, Movahed L A, Warnke R A et al 1989 Detection of Epstein-Barr viral genomes in Reed–Sternberg cells of Hodgkin's disease. New England Journal of Medicine 320: 502–506

Winkler K, Beron G, Kotz R et al 1984 Neoadjuvant chemotherapy for osteogenic sarcoma. Results of a cooperative German/Austrian Study. Journal of Clinical Oncology 2: 617–624

Wollner N, Burchenal J H, Lieberman P H et al 1976 Non-Hodgkin's lymphoma in children. A comparative study of two modalities of therapy. Cancer 37: 123–134

Womer R B, Pritchard J, Barratt T M 1985 Renal toxicity of cisplatin in children. Journal of Pediatrics 106: 659–663

Writing Group of the Histiocyte Society 1987 Histiocytosis syndromes in children. Lancet i: 208–209

Yoshida M, Miyoshi I, Hinuma Y 1982 Isolation and characterisation of retrovirus from cell lines of human adult T-cell leukemia and its implication in the disease. Proceedings of the National Academy of Sciences USA 79: 2031–2035

Young J L, Ries L G, Silverberg E 1986 Cancer incidence, survival and mortality for children younger than age 15 years. Cancer 58: 598–602

Yunis J J 1986 Chromosome rearrangements, gene fragile sites in cancer. Clinical and biological implications. In: De Vita V T, Hellman S, Rosenberg S A (eds) Important advances in oncology. Lippincott, Philadelphia, pp 93–128

Zeltzer L, Le Baron S, Zeltzer P M 1984 The effectiveness of behavioural intervention for reduction of nausea and vomiting in children and adolescents receiving chemotherapy. Journal of Clinical Oncology 2: 683–690

Zucker J M, Cailaux J M, Vanel D et al 1980 Malignant histiocytosis in childhood: clinical study and therapeutic results in 22 cases. Cancer 45: 2821–2829

Zucker J M, Tournade M F, Vorite P A et al 1986 Report on SIOP 6 nephroblastoma trials. Proceedings of the International Society of Paediatric Oncology 18: 31–34

17 Disorders of the urinary system

Chapter editor: Alan R. Watson

Development of the renal tract   934
Antenatally detected urinary tract abnormalities 935
Antenatal detection   935
Investigation of infants postnatally   936
Renal cystic disease   940
Alan R. Watson
Renal physiology   941
Assessment of renal function   942
Renal tubular disorders   944
Fanconi's syndrome   944
Renal tubular acidosis   945
Hypokalemic alkalosis   946
C. Mark Taylor
Urinary tract infections   949
Vesicoureteric reflux   956
Wetting problems   957
Hematuria   958
Glomerulonephritis   960
Acute glomerulonephritis   961
Mesangial IGA nephropathy   962
Membranoproliferative glomerulonephritis   963

Membranous glomerulonephritis   964
Henoch–Schönlein (anaphylactoid) purpura nephritis   964
Systemic lupus erythematosus   964
Rapidly progressive (crescentic) glomerulonephritis   965
Goodpasture's and Goodpasture-like syndrome   965
Hereditary nephritis (Alport's syndrome)   965
Familial recurrent hematuria syndrome   966
Other systemic disorders associated with glomerular disease   966
Proteinuria   966
Nephrotic syndrome   968
Idiopathic nephrotic syndrome   968
Focal segmental glomerulosclerosis (FSGS)   971
Congenital nephrotic syndrome   971
Renal hypertension   972
Alan R. Watson
Acute renal failure   973
Hemolytic uremic syndrome   977
Chronic renal failure   978
Mary McGraw
References   982
Recommended reading   984

DEVELOPMENT OF THE RENAL TRACT

The human kidney derives from the metanephros, the third and final excretory organ to be formed from the embryonic mesoderm. During the fifth week of embryonic development the ureteric diverticulum develops as an outgrowth of the mesonephric duct from a point near to the cloaca. Growing headwards into the nephrogenic cord the ureteric bud becomes surrounded by the mesodermal tissue which will give rise to the metanephros (Fig. 17.1). Whether the bud induces nephron formation or whether the reverse is the case, primitive nephrons differentiate in close proximity to it (Evan & Larsson 1992).

The ureteric bud in turn divides and subdivides while growing towards the periphery of the metanephros. Thus the first nephrons to be formed are those most deeply situated in the kidney. As each branch of the duct is surrounded by nephrogenic tissue, the fetal kidney assumes a lobulated appearance which generally disappears before birth in mature infants but may persist longer as an innocent abnormality. New nephrons continue to form in the human infant only until the 36th week of gestation; thereafter, increase of nephron mass is by increase in tubular length and glomerular size. Histological examination of the kidney of a newborn infant commonly reveals a small proportion of sclerosed glomeruli, especially in the subcapsular zone of the cortex. This 'fetal sclerosis' occurs in the youngest glomeruli when their tubules fail to communicate with the ureteric bud as its growth ceases in the later stages of fetal life. In addition, other glomeruli show signs of immaturity varying from unvascularized clumps of epithelial cells to occasional cuboidal epithelium and limited lobulation of the tufts. Microdissection studies have shown that tubular immaturity is probably even more profound than that of the glomeruli, for the ratio of glomerular surface area to tubular volume is much greater than in later childhood.

The ureteric bud, by a process of subdivision followed by coalescence, gives rise to the renal pelvis, calyces and collecting ducts. During this process the oldest, deepest nephrons are lost, although occasionally glomeruli in 'aberrant' positions beneath the pelvic mucosa or within the arterial walls will survive.

The urinary bladder is formed from the ventral and cephalic portion of the cloaca after this has been separated from the rectum by the urorectal septum. Into this are incorporated the caudal ends of the mesonephric tubes and ureteric buds. Together these form the bladder and urethra.

The anatomical evidence of renal immaturity at birth is mirrored physiologically by the glomerular filtration rate and by renal bicarbonate and glucose reabsorption which, despite correction for body size, are markedly diminished compared with the adult. Glomerular filtration rate at birth is about one-third of the value expected for size, and takes from 9 to 18 months to attain adult values, the time taken depending on the method of correction for size employed. With such a low filtration rate it seems surprising that the infant can maintain a normal blood urea, until it is appreciated that less urea is produced by the rapidly growing baby. Relatively more dietary nitrogen is deposited as protein in the tissues, and anabolism and growth as well as renal clearance are responsible for maintenance of normal blood urea

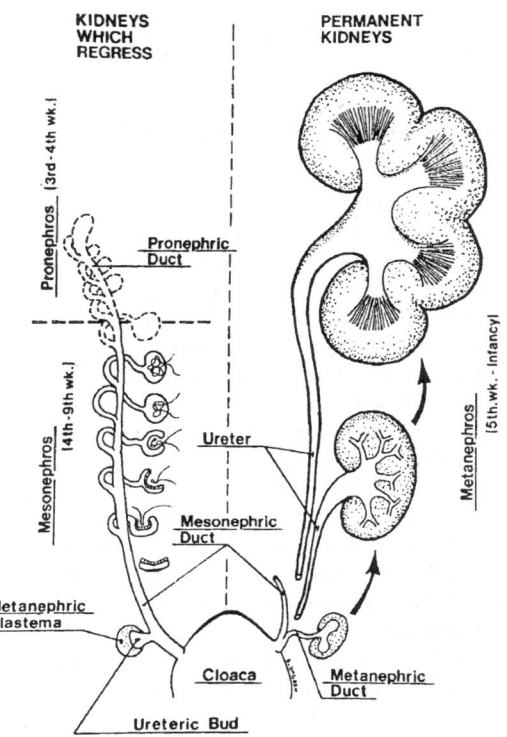

Fig. 17.1 Mammalian renal development. On the left the initial events of pronephric and mesonephric development are illustrated. These structures involute early in gestation. The definitive kidney results from a series of reciprocal interactions between the ureteric bud and the mesonephric blastema or mesenchyme. (From Evan & Larsson 1992, with permission.)

levels in the small infant. Excessive quantities of dietary protein, growth failure or tissue catabolism (for instance in acute infections) can all lead to urea synthesis in excess of the kidney's excretory capacity. Thus, a raised level of blood urea in the infant, while 'abnormal', does not necessarily indicate renal functional impairment. Diminished urea excretion is mainly responsible for the poor concentrating capacity of the newborn's kidney. When deprived of fluid, the infant's urine contains almost as high a concentration of nonurea solutes as the adult. The ability to produce a dilute urine is not impaired, although the rapidity with which a given water load is excreted is diminished.

Although an anatomical basis for these physiological changes is available, it seems probable that functional adaptation to extrauterine life involves a more complex interplay of structure and function than is yet understood.

It is known, for instance, that the lamb fetus (and probably the human fetus too) actively excretes large volumes of urine and much sodium before birth. The human baby, deprived by birth of a virtually limitless transplacental supply of water and sodium, must suddenly conserve both of these. That its kidney is able to achieve water and sodium balance within a few days of birth says much for the functional integrity of the renal tubules, 'immature' though they may be.

These sudden changes in renal function, as well as some part of the more gradual 'maturation' which occurs in the following weeks, reflect hemodynamic adjustments as well as histological changes. There is now ample evidence that maturation of glomerular function is mainly a consequence of increased blood flow to the kidney and a redistribution of flow within it, so that the cortical (glomeruli-rich) areas receive a larger proportion of the total (Corey & Spitzer 1992).

ANTENATALLY DETECTED URINARY TRACT ABNORMALITIES

DEVELOPMENTAL ABNORMALITIES

A large number of congenital abnormalities may be found in the urinary tract. They are of importance because they lead to either: urinary obstruction with increase of pressure in the pelvis and renal tubules, and so interfere with renal function; or retention of urine which predisposes to recurrent and prolonged infection. By a combination of these factors there is a risk that the renal parenchyma, perhaps already malformed, may be further damaged and so lead to chronic progressive renal failure.

Urinary tract abnormalities often come to light in the wake of the investigation of a patient with urinary tract infection or chronic renal failure. A few will be found because the kidneys may be visualized when children with congenital heart disease or other anomalies are investigated.

It should be emphasized that a unique opportunity to detect urinary tract and renal abnormalities occurs in the newborn baby. The neonatal abdomen is thin, soft and easy to palpate. With practice, even normal kidneys can often be felt, and careful routine abdominal examination will allow the detection of moderate numbers of asymptomatic but potentially important renal and bladder abnormalities.

ANTENATAL DETECTION

Many abnormalities of the urinary tract are now being recognized prenatally because of obstetric ultrasound scans. This is particularly the case in recent years with the resolution of ultrasound scans improving and many units offering the mother a detailed scan of the fetus between 16 and 20 weeks' gestation. In a study of 105 542 total births in two Nottingham hospitals between January 1984 and December 1993, 201 abnormalities of the urinary tract were detected (James & Watson unpublished observations). In the years 1984–88 the incidence was 1 in 964 compared to 1 in 364 total births in the years 1989–93. The large increase was due to the advent of detailed fetal scanning in 1989 which significantly increased the percentage of early detected abnormalities (<20 weeks) from 12% to 62% without an apparent increase in termination of pregnancy rate. Although urinary tract abnormalities may accompany other congenital abnormalities and be associated with chromosomal disorders, most of the abnormalities detected affected only one kidney (see Table 17.1).

Very rarely is intervention contemplated antenatally by the placement of a vesicoamniotic shunt in male fetuses with obstructive uropathy due to posturethral valves. Such problems require very detailed assessment in specialist centers (Quintero et al 1995).

Since the natural history of many of these antenatally detected urinary tract abnormalities still needs to be defined, it is important that parents are given appropriate information and counseling (Watson et al 1988). From Table 17.1 it will be noted that 14% of the 201 conditions detected were 'transient'. This means that although there was significant pelvic dilation noted antenatally in the fetus, the postnatal ultrasound failed to reveal an abnormality.

Table 17.1 Antenatally detected urinary tract abnormalities – spectrum of conditions in 201 fetuses, Nottingham 1984–1993

	%
Pelviureteric junction obstruction	26
Multicystic dysplastic kidney	18
Vesicoureteric junction obstruction	8
Vesicoureteric reflux	7
Duplex systems	6
Posterior urethral valves	5
Others, e.g. renal agenesis, single kidney	16
'Transient'	14

Our current practice is not to investigate these infants further unless there is a family history of vesicoureteric reflux or other urological problems. However, the parents should be warned that the child should be seen again if there is any suspicion of a urinary tract infection.

INVESTIGATION OF INFANTS POSTNATALLY

A scheme for investigation of infants with antenatally detected urinary tract abnormalities is shown in Fig. 17.2. After the initial ultrasound it may be appropriate to discuss management with a pediatric nephrologist or urologist if bilateral obstructive uropathy is recognized or if there is a single large hydronephrotic kidney which may require drainage.

Many parents are increasingly concerned about the exposure of their asymptomatic infant to imaging investigations. We have found that contact and reassurance from a member of the nursing staff who streamlines the postnatal investigations has been invaluable.

Pelviureteric junction (PUJ) and vesicoureteric junction obstruction (VUJ)

These two conditions cause hydronephrosis and have provided one of the biggest dilemmas in respect of postnatal management. PUJ and VUJ can occur at any time of life in association with intermittent abdominal pain, hematuria, urinary tract infection and asymptomatic flank mass. Such symptoms or signs are justification for a pyeloplasty or reimplant operation.

However, most infants with antenatally detected hydronephrosis have little in the way of signs or symptoms postnatally. If there is a large tense kidney with very diminished function then an initial nephrostomy is undertaken. Most infants are assessed by a combination of ultrasound, micturating cystourethrogram (to exclude associated reflux) and a radionuclide scan which is either MAG 3 (^{99m}Tc-labeled mercaptoacetyltriglycine) or DTPA (^{99m}Tc-labeled diethylenetriamine-pentaacetic acid). The general consensus is that a combination of significant calyceal as well as pelvic dilation accompanied by a reduction of function below 40% on the radionuclide scan are indicators for an operative approach (Figs 17.3a and 17.3b). However, the results of controlled trials are awaited and the issue remains controversial (Najmaldin et al 1991).

Multicystic dysplastic kidney

The most common cystic lesion recognized antenatally is a multicystic dysplastic kidney (MCDK) disease. In this disorder renal dysplasia is associated with a variable number of cysts and

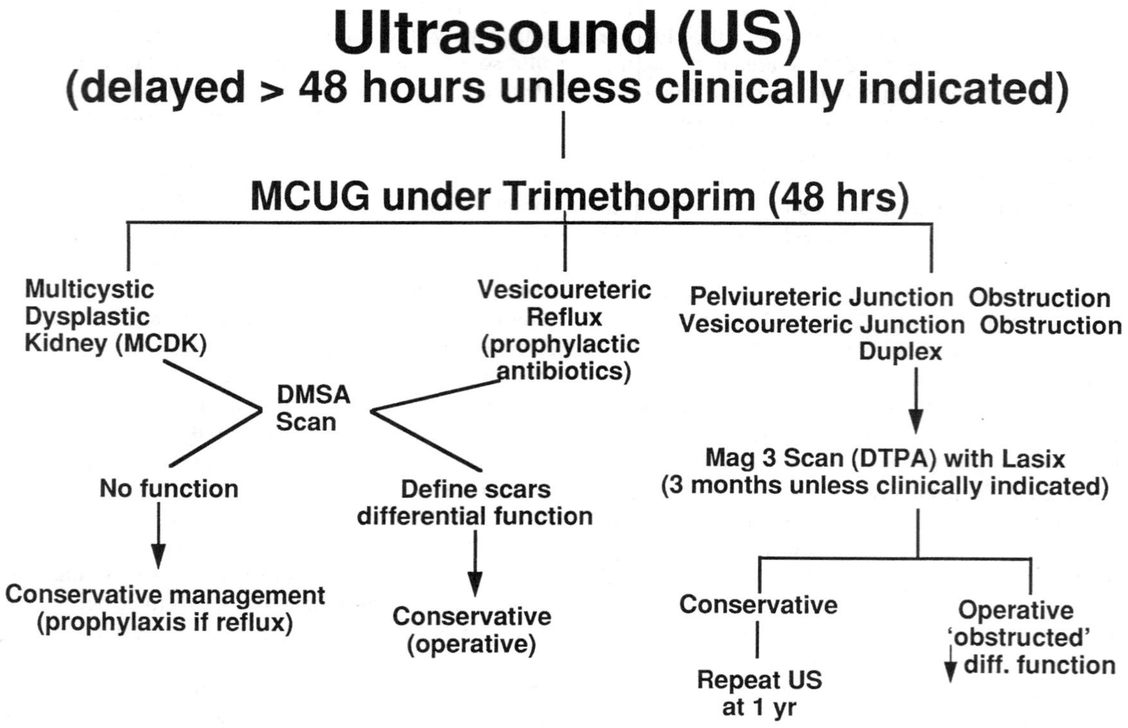

Ultrasound (US)
(delayed > 48 hours unless clinically indicated)

MCUG under Trimethoprim (48 hrs)

Multicystic Dysplastic Kidney (MCDK)

Vesicoureteric Reflux (prophylactic antibiotics)

Pelviureteric Junction Obstruction
Vesicoureteric Junction Obstruction
Duplex

DMSA Scan

No function

Define scars differential function

Conservative management (prophylaxis if reflux)

Conservative (operative)

Mag 3 Scan (DTPA) with Lasix (3 months unless clinically indicated)

Conservative

Operative 'obstructed' diff. function

Repeat US at 1 yr

Fig. 17.2 Scheme of postnatal investigations for antenatally detected urinary tract abnormality.

Vesicoureteric reflux

Even minimal hydronephrosis may be associated with gross degrees of reflux on the MCUG. Care should be taken in neonates where gross reflux is detected to ensure the urine is kept sterile with a 5-day course of full dose antibiotics as instances have occurred of urosepsis if prophylactic antibiotics have been inadequate.

It is now obvious that many children with gross reflux at a very early age already have very poorly functioning kidneys at the outset, even in the absence of infection (Figs 17.5a and 17.5b) (Anderson & Rickwood 1991). Many of these kidneys are already probably severely dysplastic. Although there is no controlled trial in this young age group, the management of infants with reflux is generally conservative (see later under Urinary Tract Infections).

Duplex systems

Varying degrees of duplication occur. Double and completely separate pelves may occur (on one or both sides), draining via separate ureters to separate ureteric orifices in the bladder. There may be two pelves and one ureter or the two ureters may unite in Y fashion during the descent to the bladder. Such duplication is sometimes associated with vesicoureteric reflux or other abnormalities and this gives rise to problems such as recurrent infection.

However, duplex kidneys is probably one of the commonest abnormalities detected on imaging of the urinary tract and in the absence of other urinary tract disease requires no treatment. Occasionally one of the ureters is associated with a ureterocele which can lead to obstruction and hydronephrosis (Figs 17.6a and 17.6b).

The ureter leading from the lower pelvis to the upper ureteric orifice is most often the abnormal one. Either ureteric orifice may open ectopically elsewhere in the bladder, urethra or vagina. It can give rise to the problem of continued wetting and is one of the conditions to consider when a child is referred with a wetting problem and has never apparently had a dry day.

Posterior urethral valves

Even with antenatal detection and, occasionally, intervention many fetuses do not survive to term or die in the neonatal period because of the associated oligohydramnios and the severe lung abnormalities. However, posterior urethral valves is a spectrum disorder with some neonates presenting with bladder outflow obstruction, infection and acute renal failure in the newborn period in association with urosepsis (Fig. 17.7). Other children present later with apparently minor symptoms. Most severe cases are managed in conjunction with a pediatric urologist and the prognosis will depend upon the degree of associated renal dysplasia and bladder abnormality.

Other developmental abnormalities

Bilateral renal agenesis is incompatible with prolonged extrauterine life due to the associated pulmonary hypoplasia and oligohydramnios sequence, such as Potter's facies with large low-set ears.

Unilateral renal agenesis occurs in about 0.1% of the infant population, is more common in males and has been described as associated with abnormalities of the external ear on the ipsilateral side. Failure of formation or atresia of the corresponding ureter is

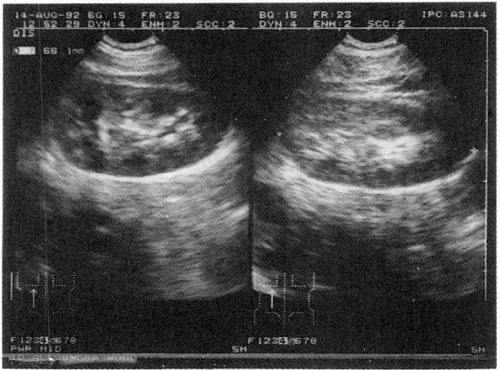
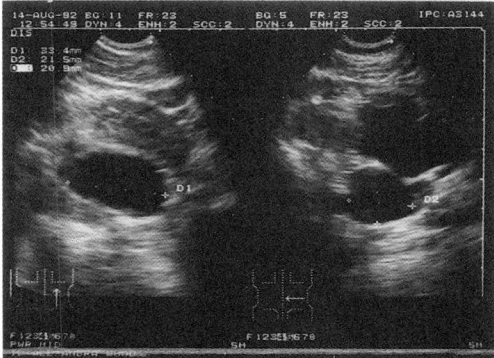
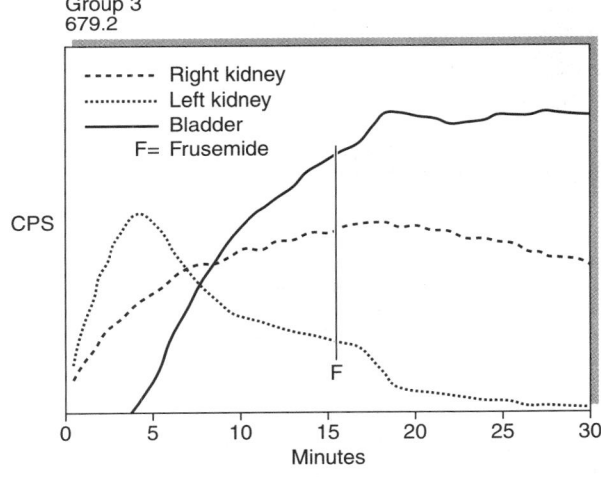

Fig. 17.3 (a) Ultrasound of 1-month-old infant with antenatally detected right hydronephrosis showing normal left kidney and dilation of pelvis and calyces on right side. (b) Excretion curves of MAG 3 scan in the same infant showing normal excretion left kidney and delayed excretion right side with poor response to frusemide. Differential function: right 36%, left 64%.

is believed to result from failed coordination development of the metanephros and the branching ureteric bud. Al-Khaldi et al (1994) reported 44 fetuses with MCDK disease. In 14 the disease was bilateral and there were associated lethal abnormalities or syndromes. All 30 surviving infants had unilateral disease, 6 (20%) having significant reflux into the normal contralateral kidney. Although there have been occasional reports of sepsis, hypertension and even malignancy in association with cystic dysplastic kidneys, current management is conservative as many MCDK kidneys involute with time (Figs 17.4a and 17.4b).

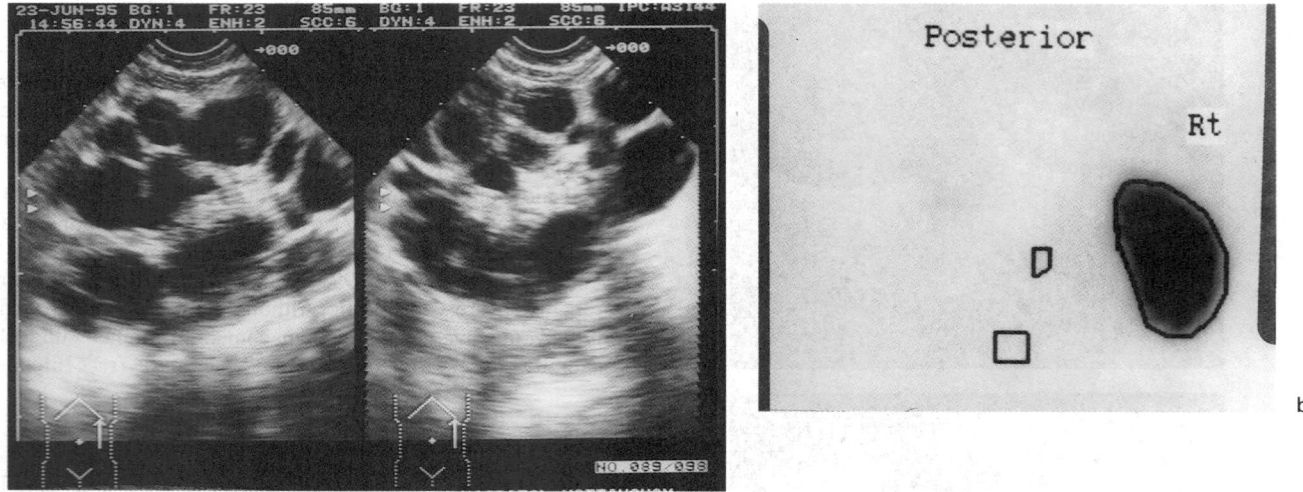

Fig. 17.4   (**a**) Postnatal ultrasound of infant with left MCDK showing numerous cysts in enlarged kidney. (**b**) Non function confirmed on DMSA scan.

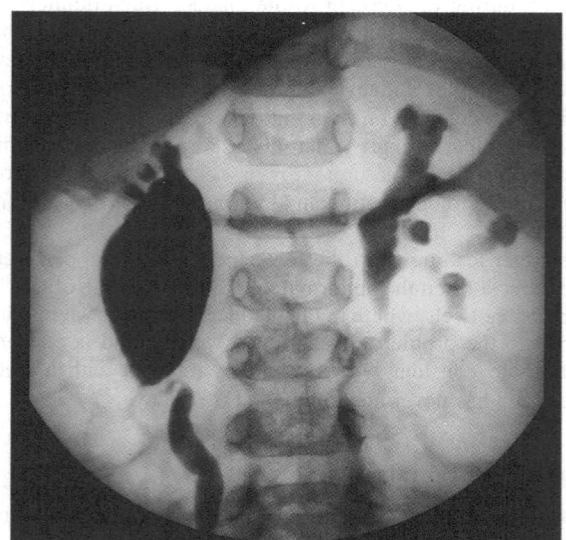

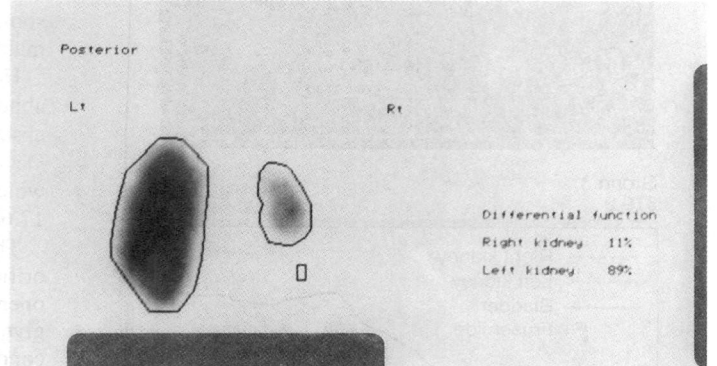

Fig. 17.5   (**a**) Postnatal MCUG on infant with antenatally detected hydronephrosis showing gross reflux bilaterally with pseudo PUJ appearance on right side. (**b**) DMSA scan in same infant showing very poor function on right side suggesting dysplastic kidney (no history of infection).

frequent and supports the view that unilateral renal agenesis is commonly the result of failure of formation of the ureteric bud or its inability to stimulate differentiation of the nephrogenic mesoderm. Ultrasound and DMSA scan, including views of the whole abdomen to exclude ectopic location, should be undertaken. The presence of a normal hypertrophied kidney on the contralateral side should lead to reassurance and there is no need for long term follow-up unless there are other associated abnormalities.

Renal dysplasia and hypoplasia

It is difficult to know whether these two conditions should be separated. True hypoplasia (i.e. a normally developed but unduly small kidney) is rare. It is best identified by its small size and diminution of the number of papillae and calyces present. Most cases are associated with some degree of dysplasia as well. Renal dysplasia may produce diminution or increase in total renal size, but its characteristic is the presence of pluripotent undifferentiated mesenchyme which may give rise to aberrant tissue such as cartilage and smooth muscle within the kidney. Cyst formation is common and has been attributed to premature cessation of branching by the ureteric bud which, being unable to induce nephron formation, degenerates and becomes cystic. Obstruction to the ureter in fetal life is also a factor in pathogenesis, and causes well marked dilation of Bowman's capsule in some cases. The dysplasia may be unilateral when the opposite kidney functions normally, or may be bilateral.

Renal hypoplasia and dysplasia contribute significantly to the causes of chronic renal failure in childhood, especially now that dialysis and transplantation is possible for even small infants. Many children may go undetected but progress into chronic renal failure at the end of the first decade when their body size begins to outgrow their kidney reserve.

Oligomeganephronia is one form of dysplastic kidney when there is a reduced number of very large nephrons which undergo progressive focal sclerosis (see later).

Renal fusion and ectopia

The metanephric blastema is originally sited in the pelvis and ascends to its subdiaphragmatic position during early fetal life. During the ascent some rotation occurs so that the renal pelvis, which originally lies anterior to the disc-shaped pelvic metanephros, comes to lie medial to the lumbar kidney. Moreover, the kidney assumes its reniform shape by virtue of its lumbar position and the rotation it undergoes. An ectopic nonascended kidney is therefore likely to be nonreniform in shape, being usually discoid, and to have a pelvis and ureter arising anteriorly. The ureter may have a normal vesical opening but may also open in an ectopic position in the bladder, bladder neck, urethra or vaginal vault. The blood supply is derived from nearby arteries such as the common iliac. A frequent site for the ectopic kidney is in the pelvis but it may be higher up the posterior abdominal wall or crossed to the opposite side. Such 'crossed' ectopia is more often than not fused with the normal kidney – 'crossed fused ectopia'. Fusion of normally placed kidneys may also occur – commonly at the lower poles – and gives rise to the 'horseshoe kidney' (Fig. 17.8). The fusion of such kidneys prevents normal medial rotation, and the ureters arise from an anterior or lateral, rather than medial, position relative to the renal parenchyma.

The site of an ectopic kidney may render it more vulnerable to trauma or liable to obstruct the delivery of an infant (although most pelvic kidneys do not). The usual route of the ureter may impede urinary drainage and lead to stasis and dilation with subsequent infection. Dysplastic tissue is not infrequently also found, increasing the risk of infection. An ectopic ureteric orifice in the bladder may lead to vesicoureteric reflux. If the ureter opens into the urethra or vagina there may be incessant urinary incontinence. Despite these problems many malpositioned or fused kidneys function well and are quite unproductive of symptoms.

Diagnosis is made by appropriate radiological investigations, particularly ultrasound and radionuclide imaging.

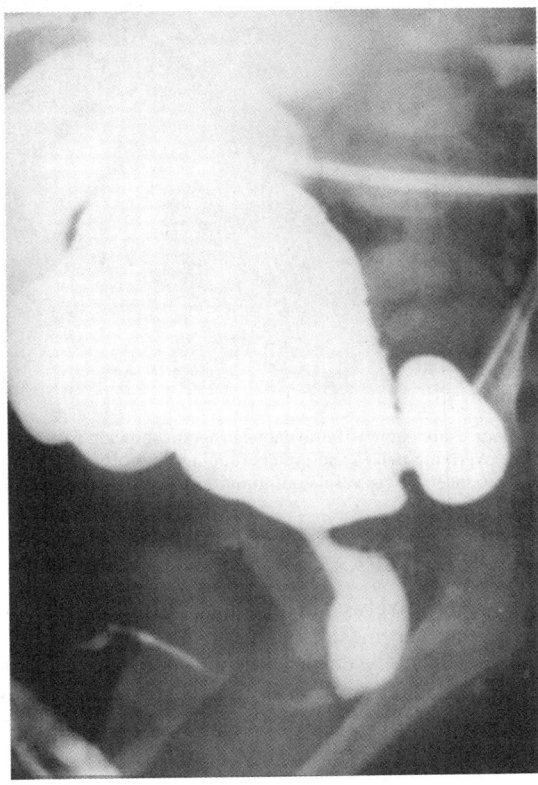

Fig. 17.7 MCUG in a male infant presenting with septicemia and acute renal failure. Gross dilation of posterior urethra, bladder diverticulum and reflux into dilated ureter.

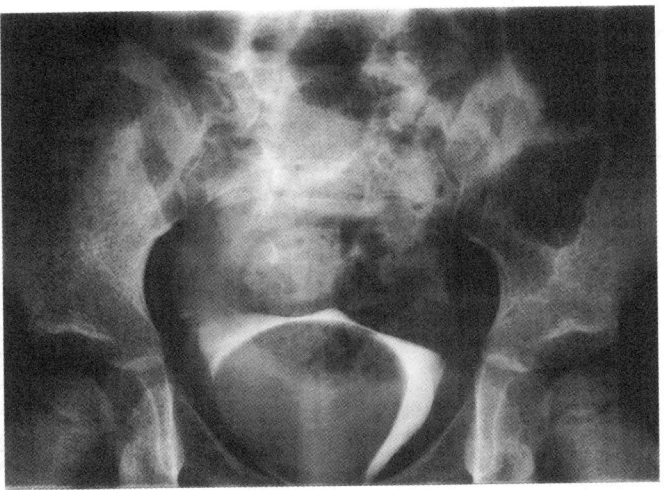

Fig. 17.6 (a) IVU in 3-year-old girl with urinary tract infection, duplex system of left side and gross hydronephrosis on right side. (b) Hydronephrosis associated with large ureterocele seen as filling defect in bladder.

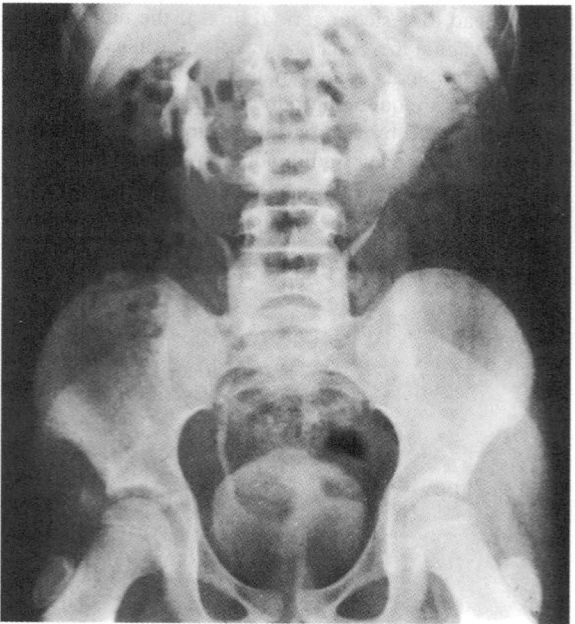

Fig. 17.8 Horseshoe kidney. Intravenous urogram showing rotated kidneys with calyces overlying pelves and ureters running inferiorly and then medially to produce 'flower vase' configuration.

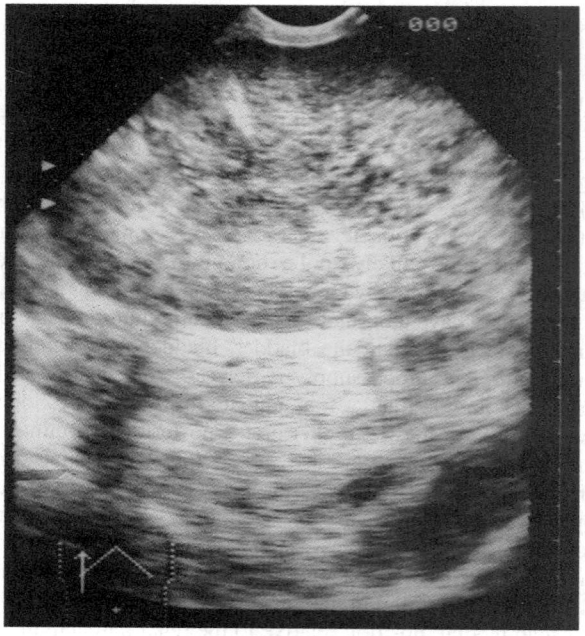

Fig. 17.9 Ultrasound showing diffuse increase in echogenicity. Bilateral enlargement in newborn with ARPKD.

RENAL CYSTIC DISEASE

Renal cysts are relatively common lesions. They may be single or multiple, cortical or medullary, sporadic or familial (Kissane 1990) (Table 17.2). Cystic disease may occur in hereditary or malformation syndromes such as tuberous sclerosis, Zellweger cerebrohepatorenal syndrome, Von Hippel–Lindau and trisomy 13 syndromes.

Polycystic disease

Autosomal recessive polycystic kidney disease (ARPKD)

The so-called 'infantile' form commonly presents at birth (or before it) with massively enlarged kidneys which on ultrasound are hyperechoic (Fig. 17.9), but with cysts too small (as a rule) to be separately identifiable. Intravenous urography shows a characteristic 'streaky' nephrographic pattern but after a delay of many hours. The cysts are fusiform and radially orientated so that the overall 'reniform' shape is preserved. The liver always exhibits fibrosis if biopsied, and sometimes cysts: these hepatic abnormalities may be detectable by ultrasound. Characteristically, life-threatening renal failure is present at birth, and it is the degree of lung hypoplasia that will determine immediate outcome. If the child has sufficient lung function then a decision about chronic dialysis can be undertaken after prolonged discussion with the family and renal team members. Unilateral or bilateral nephrectomy may be required.

Again this is a spectrum condition and sometimes it presents only in later childhood with hypertension, chronic renal failure or the consequences of portal hypertension caused by the hepatic fibrosis.

Autosomal dominant polycystic kidney disease (ADPKD)

The 'adult' type of polycystic kidney disease may appear in neonates and has even been identified on antenatal scans, although characteristically ADPKD gives rise to symptoms of renal failure in middle age and there is often a clear family history, usually of highly penetrant autosomal dominant inheritance. The kidneys become distorted by roughly circular and randomly distributed cysts which are easily recognized on ultrasound (Fig. 17.10). The cysts may be due to embryological failure of union of collecting duct and nephron, or to cystic dilation of the earliest generation of nephrons which ordinarily undergo degenerative changes and disappear.

It is uncommon for this type of cystic disease to be symptomatic during childhood, though the occasional baby with the condition perhaps has a worse prognosis and hypertension can occur in infancy. However, the cysts may be demonstrable by ultrasound or CT scanning and can be observed to become more numerous and larger through childhood. One cannot be confident

Table 17.2 A classification of renal cysts

I.	Polycystic kidney disease
	  a. Autosomal recessive (ARPKD)
	  b. Autosomal dominant (ADPKD)

II.	Glomerulocystic renal disease

III.	Medullary renal cysts
	  a. Medullary cystic disease (juvenile nephronophthisis)
	  b. Medullary sponge kidney

IV.	Renal cystic dysplasia
	  a. Multicystic kidney (total renal dysplasia)
	  b. Cystic dysplasia with urinary tract obstruction
	  c. Diffuse cystic dysplasia (with teratogenic syndrome and nonsyndromal)

V.	Localized segmental and unilateral renal cysts a. Simple renal cysts (solitary and multiple)
VI.	Acquired renal cystic disease

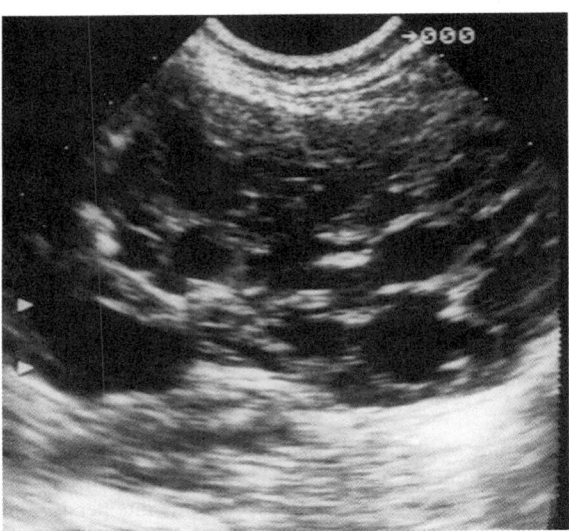

Fig. 17.10 Ultrasound showing features of ADPKD (multiple cysts in large kidney) in 18-month-old infant with hypertension.

that cysts will not develop in a patient genetically at risk until they are in the 25–30 year age group.

Hypertension and progressive renal failure will ensue but the age of onset is variable, commonly the third or fourth decade but sometimes in adolescence.

ADPKD is a good example of an hereditary disease caused by mutations at different genes with most families having abnormalities of the PKD1 gene on chromosome 16 and others PKD2 on chromosome 4 (Breuning & Peters 1996).

Familial juvenile nephronophthisis

This condition is inherited as an autosomal recessive gene. It is uncommon, but diagnostic difficulties make its incidence uncertain. Histological changes are nonspecific in the early stages, but later there is patchy glomerular sclerosis, tubular atrophy and interstitial fibrosis and chronic inflammatory infiltration of the cortex with cysts mainly at the corticomedullary junction.

The clinical presentation is insidious, usually in later childhood (around 8–10 years), with poor growth, anemia and polyuria and polydipsia. Other symptoms of chronic renal failure occur, and progression to end-stage renal failure is inevitable within a few months or years. No treatment is effective in preventing this, though conservative and, later, renal support treatment is perfectly feasible.

Diagnostically the histological, radiological and clinical features are nonspecific; the existence of a sibling with the disease is often the clinching feature, taken together with the absence of an alternative reason for the chronic renal failure. Additional diagnostic clues obtained from nonrenal features sometimes associated include tapetoretinal degeneration, cerebral and cerebellar abnormalities and, occasionally, hepatic fibrosis.

Medullary cystic disease

This is a very similar condition to familial juvenile nephronophthisis, with a very similar pathology, but presenting usually in adult life and inherited as an autosomal dominant gene.

Medullary sponge kidneys

Again this condition more commonly comes to light in adult life, when calcification in the renal pyramids may give rise to calculi, abdominal pain and hematuria. It is occasionally identified in childhood for the same reasons, but more often because of the urographic appearance of streaky opacification of the renal pyramids. It is also frequently asymptomatic.

RENAL PHYSIOLOGY

The main function of the kidney is the regulation of water and electrolyte homeostasis, and excretion of nitrogenous and other waste products. Hormonal function is also important and includes the regulation of erythropoiesis, vitamin D and parathyroid hormone, as well as arterial blood pressure through the renin and angiotensin system. Water homeostasis is achieved by the nephrons and for simplicity their function can be considered in four parts:

1. *Glomerular filtration.* This refers to the bulk flow of plasma water across the glomerular capillary wall into Bowman's capsule. The process is rapid so that an amount of water equivalent to the entire plasma volume is cleared every 25–30 min. Filtration is passive and is driven by the glomerular intracapillary pressure, the work for which is generated by the left ventricle. The glomerular filtration rate (GFR) is closely regulated by adjusting intracapillary pressure through afferent and efferent arteriolar tone. Autoregulation keeps the GFR constant over a wide range of blood pressure. Superimposed on this there is also a circadian rhythm with an amplitude of about 25% and physiological increases after a high protein meal and during pregnancy. In early infancy the GFR, whether standardized for body surface area or weight, is a fraction of that in older children and adults. Outside of the neonatal period it is convention to express GFR per body surface area as this relationship holds constant from about 3 years of age until late adulthood, the normal being between 85 and 140 ml/min/1.73 m².

2. *Isosmotic salt and water reabsorption.* At least 80% of the filtered salt and water is recovered in the proximal tubule in the cortex of the kidney. Although this requires energy expenditure through Na⁺-K⁺-ATPase, the process is facilitated by the fact that plasma in the peritubular capillaries has a high oncotic pressure. Glomerular filtration is a selective process and proteins such as albumin are retained in the circulation. The plasma leaving the glomerulus which goes on to supply the peritubular capillaries is hyperoncotic and contributes an additional driving force for water reabsorption.

The active export of sodium from the basolateral surface of the proximal tubular cells by Na⁺-K⁺-ATPase creates an ionic and sodium gradient across the epithelium. This gradient is responsible for the cotransport systems which recover glucose, phosphate and amino acids. Hydrogen ion secretion by the proximal epithelium is essential for the recovery of filtered bicarbonate. In the presence of apical carbonic anhydrase, H^+ and HCO_3 combine to form carbonic acid. This dissociates to carbon dioxide which can readily enter the cell and is converted back to bicarbonate. The essential luminal hydrogen ion secretion which permits this process also depends on the sodium gradient. Failure of the sodium gradient for any reason gives rise to the Fanconi syndrome of impaired proximal tubular reabsorption of bicarbonate, glucose, phosphate and amino acids (see Fanconi's syndrome).

3. *Urine dilution*. In the thick ascending limb of the loop of Henle sodium is actively pumped into the renal interstitium. However, owing to the water proofing effect of Tamm–Horsfall protein, uniquely secreted into the lumen of this part of the nephron, water cannot follow. Nascent urine flowing along this section of the nephron therefore becomes increasingly dilute, achieving an osmolality of <80 mosmol/kg. Meanwhile the renal interstitium becomes hyperosmolar, reaching 1400 mosmol/kg in the renal papillae, the deepest part of the medulla.

An important anatomical feature is that at the end of the diluting section, the nephron is reflected back to pass by the hilum of its own glomerulus. Here the specialized tubular cells of the macula densa relate intimately with the juxtaglomerular apparatus and both the afferent and efferent arterioles. At this site tubular performance is policed, and filtration regulated by a process referred to as tubuloglomerular feedback. If there is a major failure of tubular reabsorption upstream of the macula densa there will be increased sodium chloride delivery to this site which in turn signals for down regulation of filtration. The kidney fails safely. One can appreciate that the low GFR observed in infancy is an appropriate response to the smaller capacity for salt and water recovery by the relatively short proximal tubules. Newborns are much more dependent on the distal nephron for electrolyte reabsorption. This is one of the reasons why mineralocorticoid deficiency has such profound effects in the newborn compared to older subjects.

4. *Urine concentration*. Beyond the macula densa the distal nephron, derived originally from the ureteric bud, has two special properties. One is the presence of aldosterone sensitive Na^+-H^+-K^+-ATPase. This system allows fine tuning of sodium balance by reabsorbing sodium in exchange for hydrogen ion and potassium. Healthy children exposed to salt restriction can almost fully recover sodium in the nephron. However, newborns commonly have a fractional excretion of 1%, and in preterm infants as much as 5% of the filtered sodium load. Aldosterone is stimulated not only by the renin–angiotensin system but also directly by the plasma potassium concentration, a feature which assists in excretion of a potassium load. The second feature is the presence of aquaporins, membrane bound molecules which under the influence of vasopressin permit the passage of water. In this case water moves down an osmotic gradient from the dilute urine arriving in the distal nephron to the hyperosmolar medullary interstitium surrounding the collecting ducts. The maximum urine concentration capacity thus depends on the presence of vasopressin, the integrity of vasopressin-2 receptor and aquaporin assembly, as well as a high medullary interstitial solute (sodium and urea). In breast-fed infants whose dietary protein is efficiently used for anabolism there is proportionately less for urea generation. Thus the maximal medullary concentration and urine concentration capacity is reduced. In health, and with adequate protein intake, children over 6 months of age can generate urine concentration >870 mosmol/kg and figures approaching this can be achieved from the early weeks of life.

ASSESSMENT OF RENAL FUNCTION

MEASUREMENT OF GFR

There is no direct way to measure the bulk flow of plasma water into Bowman's capsule. However, by assuming that small molecules traverse the capillary wall as easily as water, and using a low molecular weight marker-substance which is neither absorbed or excreted by the tubule, nor bound to proteins or lipids, one can calculate GFR. A time honored marker is inulin, an inert sugar with a molecular weight of 5500 which can be measured with accuracy in plasma and urine. After an intravenous loading dose, an infusion is maintained to provide a constant plasma concentration of inulin (P). One then needs to know either the mass of inulin excreted over a fixed time (urine volume × urine concentration, UV), or assuming a steady state the dose of inulin infused, which should be the same. One can then deduce the theoretical volume of plasma that contains the mass of inulin excreted per minute using the formula:

$$\frac{UV}{P}$$

The volume of plasma cleared of its inulin can then be regarded as the net volume of water that has been filtered; the glomerular filtration rate. It is convention to express this rate per 1.73 m^2, the average body surface area of an adult man. This allows comparison of rate between individuals of different stature and holds true down to 3 years of age.

In clinical practice one seldom requires the precision of inulin clearance methods and such tests are best reserved for specialist departments. The same can be said for slope clearance methods, although they have the important advantage that timed urine collections are not required. In slope clearance methods a bolus of a marker (inulin, ^{51}Cr edetic acid, or ^{99m}Tc DTPA) is injected rapidly into a vein. Following this there is a complex distribution into the extracellular fluid space as well as clearance from the circulation by glomerular filtration. After approximately 1 h the plasma concentration falls exponentially. Two or more plasma samples are then taken over the next few hours and from the slope of the declining concentration one can estimate the theoretical volume of distribution at the moment of injection and the half-time when 50% of the marker has been cleared. From this information GFR can be estimated. Precision of this method is excellent except at very high filtration rates.

Endogenous creatinine is a useful, although imperfect, marker with which to measure clearance. Formal creatinine clearance studies relying on timed urine samples have poor precision, probably because children are unable to void to completion on demand. There is *no* place for such tests in routine pediatric practice. More accurate, reproducible and user friendly is the interpretation of plasma creatinine in relation to a child's height. In the steady state creatinine excretion (UV creatinine) is matched by creatinine synthesis in muscle and is thus related in turn to muscle mass and bodyweight. Bodyweight and height also feature in the calculation of surface area in the denominator of the GFR expression. Although the logic is tortuous this conveniently resolves to the formula:

GFR/body surface area = (body height/plasma creatinine) × constant

Much hinges on the accuracy of plasma creatinine measurement, especially at the low concentrations of normal range. New automated methods overcome errors from drugs or non-creatinine chromogens. Using these methods, and with the child's height in cm and plasma creatinine expressed in µmol/l the constant in the above equation is approximately 40. Put another way, in children outside infancy, if the body height/creatinine ratio is >2 cm/µmol/l, GFR is likely to be normal; if < 1.5 it is certainly reduced and there is uncertainty between these two ranges. The formula performs well when used sequentially to follow GFR in an individual.

Given that tubular performance upstream of the macula densa governs filtration rate by tubular glomerular feedback mechanisms, clinicians are able to use estimates of GFR as a guide to whole kidney performance. It is not surprising that some of the most abrupt and severe reductions of GFR are caused by interstitial or tubular injury rather than isolated glomerulonephritis. The corollary of this is that extensive glomerular destruction may occur with little if any change in plasma creatinine. In a disorder which gives a progressive loss of nephrons over time, surviving nephrons will exhibit hyperfiltration. Thus considerable nephron loss has to occur before there is any downward trend in GFR; renal impairment is a late indicator. It is helpful to correlate impaired GFR with kidney size as determined, for example, by ultrasound. If kidney size is normal, or perhaps increased, while GFR is impaired, it is likely that the nephron population is intact but parenchymal injury has induced a shutdown of filtration. The causes may be inflammatory, drug induced, metabolic as in hypoxia or recent ischemia, or secondary to malignant infiltration. By contrast, if both kidneys are small it is likely that the nephron population is reduced because of some previous destructive process. Small echobright kidneys with normal contours might suggest a previous glomerulonephritis. Small kidneys with an irregular outline are seen following the coarse scarring of pyelonephritis or secondary to renal dysplasia.

PROXIMAL TUBULAR FUNCTION

In normals, urinary *glucose* is not detected by conventional glucose oxidase strip reagent until the plasma glucose concentration exceeds 10 mmol/l, the renal threshold for glucose. Glycosuria occurring at a lower threshold may indicate an isolated transport defect, idiopathic renal glycosuria. If this occurs in conjunction with other markers of proximal tubular dysfunction it implies either renoparenchymal injury, chronic renal failure or the Fanconi syndrome.

90% of filtered *amino acids* are absorbed proximally by five separate cotransport systems:

1. basic amino acids and cystine
2. glutamic and aspartic acids
3. neutral amino acids
4. imino acids
5. glycine.

At very high plasma concentrations an amino acid may overspill into the urine. With normal plasma concentrations, newborns frequently have mild generalized aminoaciduria as a transient event. Otherwise, generalized aminoaciduria with normal plasma concentrations indicates tubulopathy in exactly the same way as glycosuria (above). Specific patterns of aminoaciduria imply isolated transport defects, e.g. cystinuria.

Phosphate is extensively recovered in the proximal tubule. However, the amount of phosphate filtered is close to the maximum rate of recovery, so that small changes in recovery rate govern plasma phosphate concentrations. Under normal conditions phosphate reabsorption will exceed 80% and the fractional excretion will therefore be less than 20% of filtered load. The fractional excretion can be calculated easily for any

compound freely filtered at the glomerulus by comparing its clearance with that of creatinine:

Fractional excretion of x (%) = (urine x/plasma x) ÷ (urine creatinine/plasma creatinine) × 100

50% of plasma *calcium* is bound to protein and therefore not available for filtration. In the proximal tubule calcium reabsorption is proportionate to salt and water reabsorption. Thereafter there is both passive and active reabsorption in the loop of Henle. 10% of the filtered calcium then reaches the distal nephron and of this two-thirds will be reabsorbed. Hypercalciuria can be readily diagnosed by urine calcium/creatinine ratio. The normal upper limit in children is given below:

Age range	Urine calcium/creatinine (molar)
0–6 months	<2.4
7–18 months	<1.7
1½>–6 years	<1.2
7 years–adult	0.7

DISTAL TUBULAR FUNCTION

Although the ability to excrete a water load can be tested, it has little clinical relevance. By contrast, *tests of urine concentration capacity* are important. A simple screening test is to measure the urine osmolality on the first urine sample voided in the morning after fluids are restricted at bedtime. A urine osmolality value of 600 mosmol/kg is generally taken as excluding significant impairment of urinary concentration. However, in a recent study in 318 apparently healthy children with a median age of 9.8 years the median osmolality was 845 mosmol/kg (range 275–1344). Only 82% of males and 75% of females had an osmolality of 600 mosmol or more (Skinner et al 1996).

If the diagnosis of diabetes insipidus is entertained a water deprivation test should only be undertaken in hospital with close observation of hydrational status. The end point is either a urine concentration capacity >800 mosmol/kg or a 3% bodyweight loss, by which time the plasma osmolality should be rising and in excess of 295 mosmol/kg. If the latter, the final urine osmolality would be accepted as the concentration capacity. In fully expressed diabetes insipidus a urine osmolality will remain lower than that of plasma. As well as the obvious risks, young children find water deprivation disagreeable. A screening test for the ability to concentrate urine is to administer DDAVP 20 µg nasally (10 µg for infants) in the normally hydrated state. At 1 h children are asked to void and that urine sample is discarded. Between 1 and 5 h after DDAVP normal children will produce a urine osmolality in excess of 800 mosmol/kg (infants <600 mosmol/kg). Patients with pituitary diabetes insipidus will respond to this test either normally or they will achieve osmolalities close to normal. Failure to respond implies either nephrogenic diabetes insipidus, in which case the urine osmolality will be below that of plasma, or chronic renoparenchymal disease, where the urine osmolality will be similar to plasma concentrations. Normality and fully expressed diabetes insipidus are easy to distinguish. Problems arise when the urine osmolality falls between 300 and 870 mosmol/kg. Often this is because the water deprivation study has not been conducted rigorously. Also habitual water drinkers, especially those with poor dietary protein intake, have a reduced medullary solute concentration and underachieve for this reason. Reductions in maximal urine concentration capacity may be seen in any renoparenchymal disorder, including recent upper urinary tract infection. As chronic renal failure progresses concentrating and diluting capacity is lost and urine osmolality approaches that of plasma.

TESTS OF RENAL TUBULAR ACIDOSIS

The kidney is responsible for the excretion of a small proportion of the total acid production of the body, this being those acids which cannot be metabolized to carbon dioxide and water and eliminated by respiration. Thus in severe renal failure patients develop a moderate acidosis with an *increased* anion gap. The acidosis of chronic renal failure is readily corrected by 1–2 mmol/kg/day of administered bicarbonate. Renal tubular acidosis describes the hyperchloremic acidemia with a *normal* anion gap, $(Na + K) - (Cl + HCO_3) = <20$ mmol/l, which occurs with normal glomerular function. There is either a failure to recover filtered bicarbonate, an inability to secrete hydrogen ion or both.

Complex tests of *urine acidification* are seldom required in clinical practice. In the renal tubule, hydrogen ion (H^+) is pumped against an actual or potential gradient. In the proximal tubule H^+ is buffered by bicarbonate and leads to net bicarbonate recovery via the formation of carbon dioxide. Less than 10% of the filtered bicarbonate is presented to the distal nephron. In the distal nephron, where luminal bicarbonate is at a low concentration, two other buffering systems are proportionately more important. One is the tubular secretion of ammonia (NH_3) generated by the deamination of glutamine. In the presence of H^+ an ammonium (NH_4^+ ion) forms which is unable to diffuse back across the tubular epithelium. The second is the conversion of filtered alkaline phosphate HPO_4^{2-} to acid phosphate $H_2PO_4^-$. These buffers allow the urine to 'carry' more hydrogen ion. In health the actual H^+ gradient becomes apparent in that the urine can be made acid with a pH as low as 4.5. A simple overnight fast would be a sufficient stimulus in most people to induce a urine pH <5.5 in the first voided urine in the morning. However, a recent study in healthy schoolchildren demonstrated that only eight children had a urine pH of 5.4 or less on the first morning sample (Skinner et al 1996).

To test the maximum H^+ gradient delivered by the distal nephron it may be necessary to induce a metabolic acidemia by administration of ammonium chloride enterically. In distal renal tubular acidosis (*type 1 RTA*) urine pH remains above 6.5 even if the plasma bicarbonate is reduced to <22 mmol/l. This test is seldom required as type 1 RTA patients typically present with sufficient systemic acidosis to observe the inappropriately alkaline urine. Moreover, correction of acidosis occurs at modest doses of sodium bicarbonate such as 3–5 mmol/kg bodyweight per day.

90% of bicarbonate is recovered in the proximal tubule, the remainder distally, so that normally the threshold at which bicarbonate starts to appear in the urine is a plasma concentration of 25–26 mmol/l. In infants this threshold is rather lower at approximately 22 mmol/l. An isolated failure to recover bicarbonate is known as proximal or *type 2* renal tubular acidosis. Proximal renal tubular acidosis may also occur as part of a generalized tubulopathy. If the plasma bicarbonate concentration falls below the threshold for bicarbonaturia it is possible for normal distal mechanisms of urinary acidification to produce an acid urine. A simple clue to proximal renal tubular acidosis is the very large requirement for replacement bicarbonate to improve the acidemia. Often this amounts to more than 10 mmol/kg/day

which is quite unlike that required to control the acidemia of chronic renal failure or distal (type I) renal tubular acidosis. In patients presenting with hyperchloremic acidosis in whom proximal renal tubular acidosis is suspected, sodium bicarbonate is infused intravenously to lift the plasma concentration of bicarbonate. The bicarbonate concentration in paired plasma and urine samples are plotted, thus determining the renal threshold.

RENAL TUBULAR DISORDERS

FANCONI'S SYNDROME

The Fanconi syndrome consists of a generalized failure of proximal tubular reabsorption. This leads to glycosuria, phosphaturia, calciuria, bicarbonaturia and generalized hyperaminoaciduria. Proximal sodium reabsorption also fails and the distal nephron, driven by aldosterone, attempts to recover sodium, but only at the expense of potassium and hydrogen ion secretion. Hypokalemia results and is often severe. The salt and water wasting gives rise to polyuria, polydipsia and failure to thrive. Usually children exhibit a metabolic acidosis secondary to the urinary loss of bicarbonate (type 2 renal tubular acidosis). However, distal hydrogen ion secretion in most forms of Fanconi's syndrome is normal, and during periods of hypovolemia and reduced glomerular filtration, the pH of urine may actually fall below 5.5. In states of extreme dehydration hypokalemic alkalosis may be seen. At other times hypokalemia with *acidosis* is a strong pointer to a proximal tubular lesion. The hypokalemia itself may aggravate the proximal tubular nephropathy as well as giving rise to muscle weakness, growth retardation and constipation. The glycosuria and aminoaciduria themselves have little in the way of clinical sequelae. The hypercalciuria is not associated with urinary stone formation, probably because of the very high urine flow rate. Plasma calcium concentrations tend to be normal. By contrast hypophosphatemia is the principal cause of the osteopenia and rickets of the Fanconi syndrome.

In clinical practice Fanconi's syndrome is rare. The causes are legion and include primary disorders, sometimes familial with a variety of inherited patterns. Some of these are likely to prove to be secondary to respiratory chain defects and one type has been described in which the brush border of the proximal tubular cell is absent. The condition can arise secondarily due to intoxication by heavy metals or drugs and in relation to other inborn errors of metabolism (see Table 17.3). However, by far the commonest single cause of the Fanconi syndrome is *nephropathic cystinosis* and this condition is therefore dealt with in more detail.

Table 17.3 Associations with Fanconi's syndrome

Inborn errors of metabolism
Nephropathic cystinosis
Lowe's syndrome (oculocerebrorenal dystrophy)
Glycogen storage
Galactosemia
Fructose intolerance
Tyrosinemia type 1
Wilson's disease (hepatolenticular dystrophy)

Tubulotoxic events
Drugs, e.g. tetracycline, ifosfamide
Heavy metals, e.g. lead, cadmium, uranium, mercury, thallium
Maleic acid (experimental)

Cystinosis

Cystinosis is a rare metabolic disorder inherited as an autosomal recessive trait, the gene defect being located on chromosome 17p. Cystine is stored intracellularly in lysosomes and there appears to be a defect in the ability to transport cystine back into the cytoplasm. Various patterns of cystinosis have been described. In the benign adult form cystine crystals are deposited only in the cornea, bone marrow and leukocytes; there appears to be no renal involvement. A juvenile form of the disorder includes a slowly progressive nephropathy which becomes manifest in the second decade of life. By contrast, infantile nephropathic cystinosis is the most severe form. These infants appear normal at birth and the disorder becomes apparent at around 6 months of age with failure to thrive, polyuria, polydipsia, episodes of dehydration and unexplained fever. Rickets occurs early.

Over the first few years the glomerular filtration rate remains normal, and it is during this early stage that abrupt episodes of dehydration and electrolyte disturbance precipitated by intercurrent infective illnesses can prove fatal. The GFR declines with time so that end-stage renal failure is reached in untreated patients within 10 years of diagnosis. There is profound growth retardation and photophobia is a universal complaint. In later childhood children have biochemical evidence of hypothyroidism.

The diagnosis is confirmed by the positive identification of cystine deposition. In the first months of life the kidneys look histologically normal but later the birefringent crystals of cystine can be seen in the interstitial tissue between tubules. Interstitial fibrosis then occurs so that the kidneys in time become small and contracted. Crystals can be seen in the cornea by slit lamp examination of the eye. The cystine concentration of leukocytes can be measured, and this test can be applied shortly after birth. Antenatal diagnosis is also possible, cystine measurements being made on fibroblasts obtained from amniotic fluid or chorionic villus sampling.

Cystinosis patients are difficult to manage and require careful electrolyte supplementation. Many need tube feeding to ensure an adequate salt, water and calorific intake. Attempts to reduce the glomerular filtration rate, and thus the electrolyte loss, using indomethacin are advocated. Cysteamine treatment can mobilize intralysosomal cystine and deplete cystine in cells. Cysteamine has a foul taste and compliance with this therapy is often poor. However, where cysteamine therapy or phosphocysteamine therapy has been given early with good compliance, children have retained kidney function longer than expected (Van't Hoff & Gretz 1995).

Once end-stage renal failure is reached, renal transplantation is an effective treatment. The transplant may become colonized by host cells which will store cystine but the tubular cells of the donor do not have the underlying biochemical defect and long term kidney function is satisfactory. Concern is raised, however, that long-term survivors risk previously unrecognized complications such as corneal degeneration, diabetes mellitus, hypercholesterolemia and cerebral atrophy.

RENAL TUBULAR ACIDOSIS

Renal tubular acidosis refers to conditions in which there are defects in the tubular reabsorption of bicarbonate, the excretion of hydrogen ion or both (Rodriguez-Soriano & Vallo 1990). They can be primary disorders, or secondary to a wide range of

Table 17.4 Classification of renal tubular acidosis

Type 1–Distal RTA
Primary
   —sporadic, familial (autosomal dominant)
   —transient infantile

Secondary
   —interstitial nephritis, hypergammaglobulinemia, transplant rejection
   —hypercalciuria, nephrocalcinosis
   —drugs, lithium, amphotericin

Type 2 – Proximal RTA
Primary
Secondary – Fanconi's syndrome

Type 3 – Mixed proximal and distal RTA

Type 4 – Hyperkalemic RTA
Hypoaldosteronism, Addison's disease, congenital adrenal hyperplasia
Pseudohypoaldosteronism
Distal tubular dysfunction, e.g. obstructive uropathy
Hyperreninemia, hypoaldosteronism in chronic renal failure
ACE inhibitors
Early childhood hyperkalemia RTA (transient)

pathogenic insults to the tubular cells. Four types are described (see also Table 17.4).

Permanent distal renal tubular acidosis

Permanent distal renal tubular acidosis (*type 1 RTA*) is more often a sporadic disease, although families with autosomal dominant inheritance are well described. The nature of the cellular defect is not known. Infants present with growth retardation, vomiting, polydipsia, constipation and dehydration, although these symptoms may be mild and the diagnosis is often not made until the child is more than 2 years of age. Osteomalacia and rickets do not occur, but nephrocalcinosis is an early complication secondary to the accompanying hypercalciuria and hypocitraturia. Treatment demands lifelong therapy with bicarbonate or citrate. High compliance with therapy is essential if progressive nephrocalcinosis is to be avoided. The long-term stability of renal function depends on control of nephrocalcinosis.

Proximal renal tubular acidosis

Proximal renal tubular acidosis (*type 2 RTA*) occurs because of failed bicarbonate reabsorption in the nephron. As a primary inherited disorder both autosomal recessive and autosomal dominant inheritance patterns have been described. A transient form of *type 2 RTA* occurs in infants. In any child suspected of having *type 2 RTA* it is important to look for other evidence of proximal tubular dysfunction as bicarbonate wasting occurs as part of the Fanconi syndrome. Patients with *type 2 RTA* present with growth retardation and vomiting. Because they have normal urine acidification mechanisms in the distal nephron, nephrocalcinosis does not occur. The low bicarbonate threshold means that the more one increases the plasma concentration therapeutically, the greater the urine loss. Thus massive bicarbonate replacement is needed to control the acidemia, often more than 10–15 mmol of bicarbonate/kg bodyweight/day.

The term *type 3 RTA* is used to describe a mixed picture of both proximal and tubular defects and can occur with almost any renoparenchymal injury.

Type 4 RTA is probably the most common subtype in children. In this there is hyperchloremic acidosis with hyperkalemia and an acid urine during acidosis. The pathogenesis is linked to $H^+/K^+/Na^+$ exchange in the collecting duct. It is therefore seen in states of mineralocorticoid deficiency such as congenital adrenal hyperplasia and Addison's disease. Similarly it is seen in pseudohypoaldosteronism in which there is end organ unresponsiveness to aldosterone, or occasionally in conditions where there is direct damage to the distal nephron such as in obstructive uropathy. In all these cases there is accompanying salt wasting which is most evident in the very young child who relies heavily on the distal nephron for physiological sodium reabsorption. *Type 4 RTA* can also occur with hyporeninism and hypoaldosteronism in chronic renal failure patients who are not volume depleted. An isolated early childhood form of *type 4 RTA* has been described. This occurs without salt wasting and the condition resolves by 5 years of age. Both sexes are affected and the disorder appears in siblings. High dose alkaline therapy may be required (up to 20 mmol/kg/day), but this dose independently corrects the hyperkalemia. Nephrocalcinosis does not occur and the underlying nature of the defect is not known.

HYPOKALEMIC ALKALOSIS

Severe potassium chloride wasting can occur from either the gastrointestinal tract or from the kidney. In the former, causes include pyloric stenosis, familial chloride diarrhea or laxative abuse. In these situations the kidney responds appropriately by conserving electrolytes unless potassium deficiency has become so profound that proximal tubular cells become vacuolated and lose their ability to reabsorb salt and water. In this situation there can be an additional proximal tubular defect causing inappropriate salt and water loss – hypokalemic nephropathy. Renal potassium wasting occurs in covert diuretic abuse, notably with frusemide, or as a group of primary disorders generally referred to as *Bartter's syndrome*. The hypokalemic alkalosis of all of the above disorders is accompanied by various degrees of extracellular fluid volume depletion. It is this feature that distinguishes them from the hypokalemia and alkalosis of actual or apparent mineralocorticoid excess in which there is enhanced sodium and water reabsorption in the distal nephron giving rise to sodium expansion and hypertension (see below).

Bartter's syndrome

Bartter's syndrome is a rare disorder, either familial or sporadic, which can affect both children and adults. The pathogenesis is best explained by a failure of chloride reabsorption in the thick ascending limb of the loop of Henle, thus resembling the pharmacological effect of frusemide. Mutations in the Na-K-2 Cl co-transporter or the potassium channel regulator have been described (Simon et al 1996 a,b). As a secondary event there is activation of the renin–angiotensin–aldosterone pathway in an attempt to recover sodium chloride in the distal nephron. This is achieved at the expense of increased potassium and hydrogen ion secretion which is part of the explanation for the hypokalemic alkalosis.

Children present with failure to thrive, hypotonia, lethargy, poor feeding, polydipsia and polyuria. There is a wide spectrum of disease expression with a severe form presenting in the neonatal period. Such infants are usually born prematurely after a pregnancy complicated by polyhydramnios. In early life they may become so volume depleted as to experience secondary oliguric renal failure, during which time the hypokalemic alkalosis is masked. Dehydration also gives rise to episodes of fever and developmental delay. In this group there is hypercalciuria and bone demineralization which may be secondary to the increased production of prostaglandins PGE_2 and PGI_2 which is found in this and other forms of Bartter's syndrome. Nephrocalcinosis is a serious and early complication. The neonatal form of Bartter's syndrome, first described by Fanconi in 1971, has at times been inappropriately titled calcium losing tubulopathy, or primary hyperprostaglandin E syndrome.

Management consists of potassium, sodium and chloride replacement. Prostaglandin inhibitors such as indomethacin 3 mg/kg daily in divided dose are indicated, and angiotensin-converting enzyme inhibitors such as captopril may give additional control.

Bartter's syndrome presenting in older children may run a relatively mild course without hypercalciuria or nephrocalcinosis. Simple potassium supplementation may be all that is required.

Gitelman's syndrome

Gitelman's syndrome is a distinct disorder in which there is renal loss of both potassium and magnesium so that hypokalemia and hypomagnesemia result. These patients present with muscle weakness, particularly after exercise. They may also come to medical attention incidentally when they are investigated for intercurrent illnesses such as diarrhea. Away from these events they maintain normal renal function and grow appropriately. They do not experience hypercalciuria. Potassium and/or magnesium supplements ameliorate symptoms.

Hypokalemic alkalosis

Hypokalemic alkalosis with *volume expansion* and *hypertension* can occur because of mineralocorticoid excess, as in Conn's syndrome. Other conditions in which plasma aldosterone concentrations are suppressed or normal may mimic this and are referred to as disorders of *apparent mineralocorticoid excess*. One of these is 11β-hydroxysteroid dehydrogenase deficiency, a rare inherited disorder in which the conversion of cortisol to cortisone is defective. Cortisol directly operates the mineralocorticoid receptor in the collecting duct, thus driving distal sodium reabsorption. Children present with severe labile hypertension. The hypertension itself is sufficient to cause failure to thrive. Hypercalciuria and nephrocalcinosis occur. The condition is inherited as an autosomal recessive. Another is *Liddle syndrome*. In this there is constitutive activation of the amiloride-sensitive sodium channel in the distal renal tubular epithelium, brought about by mutation in the beta or gamma subunit. The syndrome is familial and can present clinically either in childhood or adult life. Treatment of both these disorders consists of amiloride to reverse the salt and water retention. This controls blood pressure and normalizes plasma potassium.

Renal tubular hyperkalemia

This refers to the failure of the tubules to secrete potassium in conditions other than chronic renal failure. This can occur if there is a failure in the renin–angiotensin–aldosterone pathway.

Examples would include treatment with angiotensin-converting enzyme inhibitors such as captopril and the failure to synthesize mineralocorticoid in the salt-losing forms of congenital adrenal hypoplasia.

Primary pseudohypoaldosteronism is an autosomal dominant disorder with variable penetrance. The distal tubule is insensitive to the high circulating concentrations of aldosterone. Infants present in the neonatal period with failure to thrive, vomiting and dehydration. There is acidemia and hyperkalemia. They do not respond to synthetic mineralocorticoids but are treated with sodium supplements. Once past 2 years of age the salt wasting improves as the kidney becomes less dependent upon the distal nephron for sodium recovery.

Gordon's syndrome (*pseudohypoaldosteronism type II, or 'chloride shunt' syndrome*) is a rare disorder of hyperkalemia, hyperchloremic metabolic acidosis, volume expansion and hypertension. Plasma renin activity and aldosterone concentrations are suppressed. Patients may also have hypercalciuria and a tendency to stone formation. The mechanism of the disorder at a cellular level is unknown beyond the concept that there is unregulated chloride reabsorption. Treatment is with thiazide diuretic.

Early childhood hyperkalemia describes a transient disorder in infants presenting with hyperkalemia and type IV renal tubular acidosis. They present with failure to thrive and vomiting. Hypertension is not described in this condition and salt wasting is variable being absent in some cases. There appears to be an end organ unresponsiveness to aldosterone as plasma concentrations of aldosterone may be elevated. Treatment consists of bicarbonate and, if necessary, a controlled potassium intake or even potassium ion exchange resins. Growth appears to normalize by 6 months and therapy can be discontinued at about 5 years of age.

Cystinuria

Cystinuria is a complex genetic disorder involving at least three alleles governing dibasic amino acid (lysine, orthnithine, arginine) and cystine transport (Byrd et al 1991). It is more common in Japanese and Caucasians, with an incidence of 1 : 18 000 in Japan and 1 : 20 000 in the UK. Defects are seen in both renal tubular and intestinal epithelial transport. Nutritional disturbances probably do not arise because amino acids are absorbed from the gut as oligopeptides rather than free amino acids. Renal tubular cells demonstrate an inability to take up cystine from their brush border, but can do so from the basolateral surface. Because the excretion of cystine can exceed the amount filtered, there is evidence of net cystine secretion by the tubule.

The clinical manifestations are confined to individuals in whom the cystine concentration in urine exceeds its solubility product and leads to calculus formation. This occurs in homozygotes, and in those heterozygous for the type II allele. Family studies show that heterozygotes excrete different amounts of cystine depending on the allele type (see below). Almost all untreated homozygotes will experience calculi at some time in their lives, a quarter of them before 20 years of age. The lasting damage to the urinary tract is caused by obstruction and infection. Patients present with renal colic or episodes of hematuria. The stones are radiopaque because of their high sulfur content. Ultrasound is a good way of identifying calculi in both the renal collecting system and the bladder. Microscopy of the urine reveals flat hexagonal birefringent crystals under polarized light, and the nitroprusside test for urinary disulfides is positive. Confirmation is by quantification of urinary cystine secretion:

Cystine excretion as urinary cystine/creatinine ratio

Normal		<12 mmol/mmol (<24 mg/g)
Heterozygote	type I	<12 mmol/mmol
	type II	35–140 mmol/mmol
	type III	12–70 mmol/mmol
Homozygous cystinuria		>120 mmol/mmol (>240 mg/g)

The mainstay of treatment is to keep the urine volume sufficiently high that cystine is kept below its solubility maximum of 1.25 mmol/l (300 mg/l). This necessitates fluid loading, especially at night to overcome the normal nighttime antidiuresis. The solubility maximum of cystine increases to 2.0 mmol/l (500 mg/l) where the urine pH exceeds 7.5. A second line of treatment, additional to and not a substitute for the first, is to prescribe bicarbonate or citrate to ensure that the early morning urine pH is alkaline.

Family members should be screened so that presymptomatic affected members can be treated early. It is easier to prevent stone formation than to dissolve existing stones. In difficult cases with existing calculi a further increase in cystine solubility can be achieved by forming a thiol-cysteine disulfide with agents such as D-penicillamine.

Oxalosis

Oxalosis is the final stage of primary hyperoxaluria (PH) when reduction of glomerular filtration rate produces systemic oxalate accumulation. PH1 is an autosomal recessive disease characterized by the deficiency of alanine glyoxylate aminotransferase (AG) activity in the liver resulting in excessive production of oxalate leading to nephrocalcinosis, recurrent urolithiasis and progressive renal insufficiency (Broyer et al 1996). Primary hyperoxaluria type II corresponds to another enzymatic defect and the glyoxylate reductase is expressed in leukocytes. It seems to be a rare form of oxalosis as does as hyperoxaluria due to increased oxalate reabsorption from the gut.

When the GFR falls below 40 ml/min/1.73 m^2 calcium oxalate crystals become deposited in bone resulting in a severe and incapacitating bone disease with spontaneous fractures. The oxalate may also deposit in muscles, artery walls leading to ischemia, eyes, skin and nerves.

The management of oxalosis attempts to prevent the progressive nephrocalcinosis and renal failure by diluting the urine with daily water intake estimated between 3 and 4 l/m^2/day. In addition, crystallization of calcium oxalate can be reduced by inhibitors such as citrate, orthophosphate and magnesium. Some cases of PH1 are partially or completely responsive either to small or pharmacological doses of pyridoxine. Dietary advice should aim to avoid high oxalate foods and beverages such as black tea or cocoa as part of a high fluid intake.

Although some groups have reported successful kidney transplantation using detailed protocols aimed at reducing the risk of oxalate accumulation in the graft, these patients remain at risk because of the persistent genetic defect responsible for persisting oxalate production. Combined liver transplantation appears the most effective approach and the European Transplant Registry recently reported 64 liver kidney transplantations in this condition with a 5-year patient survival of 80% and progressive healing of oxalosis.

Oculocerebrorenal (Lowe's) syndrome

Oculocerebrorenal (Lowe's) syndrome describes a rare syndrome of mental retardation, excess organic aciduria, cataract and glaucoma. This is thought usually to be a sex-linked recessive disease of males transmitted by women carriers who are normal or at worst have early onset of cataract, but several female cases have been reported. The basic causal mechanism is not known, but abnormality of Krebs cycle, and particularly of ornithine arginine metabolism, has been postulated.

Clinical features

Boys present from 2 months of age with the facial features of large ears, prominent forehead, flattened nasal bridge and prominent scalp veins in a pale skin. Cataract is typical and in the early stages may only be detected by slit lamp examination. The severity of the cataract varies as does its distribution. Buphthalmos and congenital glaucoma may be present.

Intermittent pyrexia and failure to thrive are usual, and growth retardation, osteoporosis and rickets often occur. The mental deficiency is usually severe, with loss of muscle tone, hypermobility of joints and absent or greatly diminished tendon jerks. The eyes are often roll in pseudonystagmus and it is commonly noted that children press on their eyeballs with their fingers to produce visual 'hallucinations'. The EEG may show the fast 24 cycle per second general activity. The blood pressure is normal and ultrasound of the kidneys is often normal. Proteinuria occurs with complex tubular dysfunction which may not manifest itself until the second year of life. Tubular acidosis, usually of classical 'distal type' is present and there is hyperphosphaturia with hypophosphatemia, normocalcemia and elevated levels of alkaline phosphatase.

Treatment

Treatment is supportive with adequate replacement of bicarbonate, potassium, phosphate and vitamin D metabolites. As with all rare conditions, parents may obtain benefit from contact with other families.

Hereditary hypophosphatemic rickets (vitamin D-resistant rickets)

The disease is usually inherited as a sex-linked dominant gene so that affected fathers have no affected sons and all their daughters are abnormal. Half the sons and half the daughters of affected females are affected. Thus the disease is twice as common in females as in males. Males tend to be more seriously afflicted, perhaps because they are hemizygotes with respect to the gene, whereas the female carries a normal gene on the other X chromosome. The Lyon hypothesis suggests that only one of the female's two X chromosomes is active in a given cell, and that inactivation of one or the other is a random process; in consequence, the female heterozygote may have an active gene for the disease in only half her cells and may or may not show actual rickets, but only hypophosphatemia. The onset of the disease is usually from 6 months to 5 years. In the young infant the plasma level of phosphate may not be excessively low for some months after the onset of the phosphaturia, and even after X-ray changes are visible in long bones. In the established case, hyperphosphaturia and hypophosphatemia are always present; hypocalcemia is not seen. No other tubular defects can be found and usually not even the aminoaciduria associated with nutritional rickets.

Treatment of hypophosphatemic rickets aims to increase the extracellular phosphate concentration continuously, by which bone mineralization should be improved and bony deformities prevented. Oral neutral phosphates (Phosphate Sandoz) should be pushed to the limit of tolerability (high doses produce diarrhea) in a dose of 50–100 mg/kg/day in at least 4, preferably 5 doses. Alfacalcidol is also introduced in an initial dose of 20–40 ng/kg/day but a careful watch must be kept for hypercalcemia and hypercalciuria (Reusz et al 1990).

Renal diabetes insipidus

Renal diabetes insipidus is an inherited condition, due to a sex-linked recessive gene and therefore confined to males, in which there is deficiency of renal concentrating capacity and consequent polyuria and polydipsia. Some of the female heterozygotes may show lesser degrees of deficiency in urine concentration The pathogenesis is uncertain, but resistance of the collecting tubule to the effect of antidiuretic hormone is the most probable explanation. Qualitatively abnormal antidiuretic hormone blocking the tubular acceptor sites while remaining physiologically inert, or a torrential flow of fluid from defective proximal tubules which overwhelms the collecting tubules have both been suggested.

Clinical features

The condition usually presents in infancy but a later onset can occur. Polyuria and polydipsia are prominent features but difficult to recognize in infancy; a preference for water rather than milk feeds may be evident. Uncompensated polyuria leads to recurring episodes of dehydration with consequent fever, constipation and vomiting. There is failure to grow normally, retardation both of skeletal maturation and of intellectual development. The defect is permanent, but with increasing age water intake spontaneously increases to compensate for the persistent polyuria so that episodes of dehydration are avoided.

Diagnosis and differential diagnosis

Serum sodium and chloride concentrations are increased and, when dehydration is severe, renal plasma flow falls leading to raised blood urea and serum creatinine levels. The osmolality of the urine is commonly around 15 mosmol/kg. Fluid restriction must be carried out very carefully as a test of renal concentrating power, for quite severe dehydration may rapidly ensue. DDAVP has no effect on urine concentration and this forms the basis for the diagnosis.

Treatment

Replacement of urinary water losses by increasing the fluid intake is the basis of treatment; this may need to be intravenous in the initial stages. Extra aqueous fluids between feeds of milk may be taken quite avidly even when appetite is poor. Paradoxically, thiazide diuretics have been shown to decrease free water clearance and urine flow rate in this condition. This action depends on the induction of a state of salt depletion which causes an increase in proximal tubular reabsorption and therefore diminished excretion of sodium and water. The effect can be maintained by a low-salt diet when thiazide diuretics are stopped. Unfortunately, the urine volume may decrease only by about one-third, sometimes a useful result and sometimes too little to be of much importance. The addition of prostaglandin synthetase inhibitors such as indomethacin to this treatment causes a further and much more worthwhile fall in urine volume; it does not enhance urine concentration but, by enhancing tubular sodium reabsorption, restricts salt (and thus water) delivery to the collecting duct, reducing total water losses. Provided adequate supplies of water are maintained from early infancy, mental development is preserved but physical growth often remains a problem. The overall outlook is thus fairly good but only after early diagnosis and with great devotion to the feeding of extra water by the parents.

In later childhood it is often preferable to discontinue the thiazide/indomethacin therapy because it carries significant hazards, particularly from peptic ulceration and hemorrhage. At this stage the increased polydipsia/polyuria is merely an inconvenience which most children adapt to well; of course, the therapy can be reintroduced for longer or shorter periods as needed – for example during a holiday to a hot climate where excessive thirst could be a serious problem.

URINARY TRACT INFECTIONS

FREQUENCY AND DYSURIA SYNDROMES

Although frequency and dysuria are commonly associated with urinary tract infection, only 25% of children who have these symptoms have significant bacteriuria based on 10^5 organisms/ml ($> 10^8$/l) which is the diagnostic standard for voided specimens of urine. Viral infections may play a part and acute vulvitis or balanitis may be associated with poor hygiene, perineal candidiasis or contact sensitivity to nylon pants. Attention should be paid to the possibility of pin worm infestation or constipation.

There is a small group of children where pathological causes such as infection or stone have been excluded and frequency persists. It is possible that emotional factors are at work and generally the condition is self-limiting. Occasionally anticholinergic drugs such as oxybutynin may be required to improve bladder stability. Recurrent urinary tract symptoms associated with anogenital signs may be a pointer to sexual abuse.

URINARY TRACT INFECTION (UTI)

UTI in childhood is important because of its association with:

1. *morbidity* such as septicemia and failure to thrive, enuresis and poor school attendance
2. unsuspected *congenital abnormalities* of the urinary tract such as posterior urethral valves, pelviureteric junction obstruction, ureterocele and other obstructive uropathy
3. *vesicoureteric reflux* (VUR) with its potential for renal scarring, hypertension and chronic renal failure in later life.

It is concern about these late outcomes coupled with debate about the sensitivity of the different imaging techniques available that has led to some of the current controversy on the management of children with UTI (White 1987, Rickwood et al 1992).

There is a strong association between urinary tract infection and vesicoureteric reflux (VUR) with subsequent scarring of the kidneys, termed chronic pyelonephritis or *reflux nephropathy*. This condition has been quoted as causing up to 25% of end-stage renal failure in childhood and adults. These children are also at risk of developing hypertension with a quoted risk of at least 10%. Obviously these adverse outcomes are of concern and have long term implications for monitoring of blood pressure and future pregnancies (Jacobsson et al 1989). However the risk of such adverse outcomes may have been overstated as:

1. Many children had VUR as a cause of their end-stage renal failure in *association* with obstructive uropathy and other abnormalities of the urinary tract (Alexander et al 1990).
2. The postnatal investigation of neonates with antenatally recognized hydronephrosis has shown that gross vesicoureteric reflux can result in dramatic reduction in renal function on isotope renography in the *absence* of infection in such infants, suggesting underlying dysplasia (Elder 1992). These children with 'congenital' reflux nephropathy need to be distinguished from those whose kidneys were originally normal and where vesicoureteric reflux and infection resulted in acquired scars.
3. The incidence of hypertension in association with renal scars may be overstated as the reports are from specialist centers. Although hypertension may develop during long term follow-up and the rare child with renal scarring has malignant hypertension (Goonasekera et al 1996), Wolfish et al (1993) found *no* hypertension in a retrospective study of 146 children with renal scarring and primary vesicoureteric reflux.

So although it is accepted that UTI is associated with reflux nephropathy it must be remembered that in some children the damage has already occurred prenatally and reflux need not always be or have been present to achieve renal damage (Gordon 1995).

Young age at first infection appears to be an important risk factor with a higher prevalence of vesicoureteric reflux (VUR) and potential for damage in the growing kidney (Watson 1994). Older children being followed for VUR can have progression of, but rarely new scar formation. Such new scars appear mostly in children who have suffered further UTIs or in those with a history of delayed diagnosis and treatment (South Bedfordshire Practitioners' Group 1990, Smellie et al 1985).

It would appear that we should concentrate more of our efforts on the detection and treatment of UTI in *infants* and those with *recurrent infections*. The balance is between over-zealous investigation and reluctance to investigate with the proper selection of the imaging procedure(s) (see later).

Epidemiology

It is estimated that at least 1% of boys and 3% of girls experience their first UTI during the first decade. The true prevalence is uncertain as urine collection methods are still inadequate. It is only during the first 12 months of life that both symptomatic UTI and asymptomatic bacteriuria affect males more than females (Wettergren et al 1985). Nosocomial urinary tract infections associated mainly with urinary catheters are an important cause of hospital morbidity.

Circumcision and urinary tract infection

A number of studies have suggested an association between UTI and the uncircumcised state, but these studies have been criticized on methodological grounds. A more recent case control study in the setting of a large ambulatory pediatric service in 144 boys <5 years of age who had a microbiologically proven symptomatic UTI confirms circumcision as decreasing the risk of symptomatic UTIs (Craig et al 1996). This is not a strong indication for circumcision but it does emphasize that particular care should be taken with the foreskin in male infants who are known to have obstructive uropathy or an anatomical abnormality which might predispose to UTI.

Urinary tract infection and breast-feeding

There is a strong suggestion that breast-feeding may reduce the risk of UTI (Pisacane et al 1992). The mechanism by which breast milk may be protective is unclear but a preliminary report suggests that neutral oligosaccharides found in breast milk inhibit bacterial adhesion to uroepithelial cells.

CLINICAL PRESENTATION OF UTI

The younger the child the more nonspecific the symptoms:

1. Prolonged *neonatal* jaundice is a classical association of bacteriuria in the newborn where a high index of suspicion is being maintained in any baby 'going off' or who has abdominal distention, disturbance of temperature regulation, changing ventilation requirements or metabolic disturbance.

2. *Infants* may present with vomiting, diarrhea, poor feeding and failure to thrive or fever. UTI should be excluded in any infant with an unexplained temperature. Suprapubic aspiration of urine should always be attempted in children presenting as sick and septicemic as part of the 'septic workup'.

3. Young infants can present with *acute renal failure* and gross electrolyte abnormalities when infection occurs in an abnormal urinary tract.

4. *Cystitis-like* symptoms such as frequency and dysuria are common symptoms in the older child. There may be mild lower abdominal discomfort and hematuria. Such symptoms do not exclude involvement of the upper urinary tract.

5. *Acute pyelonephritis.* The classical symptoms of high fever, abdominal or loin pain and rigors in the child who is very unwell is an uncommon clinical presentation in children. The presence of such symptoms or septicemia in a young infant does influence subsequent management and intensity of the investigations. A raised ESR, white blood count and C-reactive protein levels along with reduced renal concentrating capacity have been used to distinguish upper from lower tract involvement, but there is no certain diagnostic test.

Examination

This should include palpation for renal masses and fecal loading as there is a strong association between UTI and constipation. A palpable bladder combined with a poor urinary stream suggests obstructive uropathy due to posturethral valves in a male infant or neurogenic bladder. Examination of the spine and lower limb reflexes should be included. Examination of the anal and genital areas might suggest signs of sexual abuse in a female infant. A rare abnormality such as ureterocele may even be noticed at the vaginal introitus. There are a number of syndromes associated with urinary tract abnormalities such as Prune belly and anorectal anomalies.

Diagnosis of urinary tract infection

The classical definition of significant bacteriuria (10^5 organisms per ml (10^8/l) of urine) is still applied in childhood with the proviso that any bacteriology reports should always be interpreted in the clinical context. It is important to remember that the original criteria were based upon midstream urine collections in adult females when two such samples increased the probability to 96%. It is possible that a lower colony count, especially with a pure growth on repeated samples, is clinically important, but bacteriology labs still apply the same diagnostic criteria. Any growth obtained on a suprapubic urine sample is regarded as significant.

Urine collection

Since there is a large focus on infants with UTI, greater attention needs to be given to *urine collection methods* in this group of infants both in primary care and hospital practice:

Different types of *urine collection bags* are now available but are prone to provide contaminated specimens if not applied properly and not removed as soon as the urine is passed. Recent work has suggested that urine could be collected from infants using a urine collection pad and removing the urine by syringe from the pad (Vernon 1995). This method needs to be assessed further before it can be recommended for general use.

Clean catch urine. In some young infants micturition occurs as a reflex action stimulated by bladder fullness. Micturition can be encouraged by tapping in the suprapubic region, stroking alongside the spine or even exposure to cold while undressing. Sterile trays should always be to hand and parents should be encouraged to participate in this method of urine collection.

Midstream urine collection. The older continent boy can easily introduce a sterile container into the urinary stream and there is no need for specific cleansing of the glans or withdrawal of the prepuce. Similarly the vulva does not require cleansing (antiseptics are to be avoided) in older girls, but cleaning with sterile water may be required in younger girls where a sterile container placed inside a potty is usually employed. Using the child's own potty is not satisfactory and is a common reason for erroneous results in general practice.

Suprapubic aspiration of urine (SPA) is a safe and reliable method of obtaining urine in infants and young children in whom the distended bladder is an abdominal organ. The procedure should be taught to the junior staff and an important practice point is to aspirate while advancing the needle other than on withdrawal to minimize the risk of contamination. If an ultrasound machine is available then bladder size can be checked before attempting the procedure.

Catheter specimen of urine. Catheterisation is only resorted to if there has been a failed SPA or in a sick older child where urine cultures need to be obtained before commencing antibiotics. Instrumentation of the lower urinary tract does carry the risk of introducing infection or traumatizing the urethra.

Microscopy

Although the finding of pyuria is good supportive evidence of UTI, up to 50% of patients with significant bacteriuria will not demonstrate a significant number of white cells (> 5 white cells per high powered field) in the centrifuged urine specimen. A recent study confirmed that pyuria may occur in 9% of febrile children *without* a urinary tract infection (Turner & Coulthard 1995). We no longer request routine microscopy of urine for white cells on children referred to outpatients, but it may still have a role in the child admitted to hospital acutely unwell where the presence of bacteria and white cells on a fresh urine microscoped on the ward is strong evidence to support UTI and commence appropriate antibiotic therapy.

Dipsticks

Urine dipsticks which incorporate strips for the detection of white blood cells (leukocyte esterase) or the production of nitrite by reduction of nitrate are increasingly favored for the diagnosis of UTI. White cells might be misleading and the nitrate might not be reduced to nitrite if there is frequent bladder emptying, dilute urine, inadequate dietary nitrate or infection with enzyme deficient bacteria. Nevertheless these dipsticks can be employed in certain clinical situations such as the outpatient setting where the presence of an obviously clear urine and negative dipstick in an asymptomatic child no longer results in the urine sample being cultured routinely.

This enables the laboratory to concentrate on the more important specimens from symptomatic patients and should have significant cost savings.

Dip slides

Dip slides for transmitting urine specimens or bottles containing boric acid have been promoted as a means of collecting specimens at home where there are transport difficulties to the laboratory. However, technical failures with dip slides may be disappointingly high and if the container with boric acid is not filled with urine to the appropriate level then growth may be inhibited (Jewkes et al 1990).

Handling of urine culture specimens

Since we are so reliant upon urine culture to confirm the UTI, it is important that all urine cultures should be submitted to the laboratory with the minimum delay. If there is any delay, storage at 4°C will permit accurate diagnosis for 24 h and possibly longer.

Guidelines published by the Royal College of Physicians for the management of acute urinary tract infection in childhood (Royal College of Physicians 1991) emphasized the importance of urine culture methods and this is still a key factor. A recent study in our unit of 251 referrals to the children's clinic from primary care showed that only 66% of urine cultures had been taken by appropriate methods, and only 39% of parents had been given appropriate instructions on how to collect the urine sample. If we are to stress the importance of investigating *every* child with a first UTI, then we must pay attention to obtaining the proof that such an infection has occurred.

MICROBIOLOGY

E. coli is responsible for at least 80% of UTIs in childhood. Other organisms that commonly cause infection include *Proteus*, *Enterococcus*, *Pseudomonas* and *Klebsiella* species. *Staphylococcus aureus* and *Staphylococcus epidermidis* are

urinary pathogens in small children. Any organism may cause sepsis in this young age group, with the kidney and urinary tract becoming involved by hematogenous spread from a generalized septicemia.

Pathophysiology

A symptomatic or covert bacteriuria occurs more frequently than symptomatic UTI at all ages. It must be remembered that many young infants are sitting in nappies filled with feces. Infection of the urinary tract must be related to both the characteristics of the invading bacteria and those of the host urinary tract. Virulence factors have been well studied in *E. coli* and most strains isolated from patients with suspected upper UTIs have pili or fimbriae which are polypeptides with tubular receptors specific for glycolipid components of human cell membranes. Such fimbriae allow attachment to the receptors which are expressed on uroepithelial cells. Over 90% of *E. coli* isolated from children with a first episode of pyelonephritis expressed P. fimbriae compared with 19.2% of isolates of children with cystitis. The role of other virulence factors are reviewed elsewhere (Stull & LiPuma 1991).

TREATMENT

Parenteral antibiotic therapy is required in any child with systemic symptoms. Initial therapy in neonates is usually intravenous ampicillin and gentamicin or a cephalosporin such as cefotaxime in the older child (Sherbotie & Cornfeld 1991). The duration of intravenous therapy is always controversial: a minimum of 5 days is generally recommended but it would depend upon the child's symptoms, such as fever, and whether obstructive uropathy is suspected. A total of 10–14 days' therapy should be completed with a switch to oral antibiotics as appropriate. A check should always be made that the urine culture is sterile.

Suitable oral antibacterial drugs used in the treatment of UTI are shown in Table 17.5. Information should be available from the local microbiology laboratory about changing pattern of *antibiotic resistance* locally. 50% of *E. coli* isolates locally are resistant to ampicillin and the level of trimethoprim resistance is approximately 20%. The recent prescription of broad spectrum antibiotics to a child may dramatically alter the bowel flora and select resistant organisms such as *Klebsiella*. Although not generally recommended for children, ciprofloxacin (8–15 mg/kg/day) has proven to be a useful oral antibiotic for the treatment of *Pseudomonas* infections and avoids the need for parenteral therapy. The dosage of all drugs should be carefully checked in children with known renal impairment.

The duration of treatment for a child with an uncomplicated urinary tract infection treated by the oral route should be for 5–7 days. The child under 1 year of age, those who require intravenous therapy or who have an abnormal initial ultrasound should be continued on prophylactic therapy until investigations are completed. In both groups urine culture should be taken to ensure resolution of the infection.

Single doses of 48 h of antibiotics are not advised in any child presenting with a first infection on an uninvestigated urinary tract.

Treatment and investigation of UTI go hand in hand. Children with obstructive uropathy such as posterior urethral valves should be managed in centers where there is both nephrology and urology expertise.

Table 17.5 Antibiotics used in the treatment and prophylaxis of urinary tract infections

	Treatment (dose in mg/kg/day)	Dose interval (h)	Prophylaxis (dose in mg/kg/day)
Co-amoxiclav	75 mg i.v.	8	NR
	20–40 oral amox content	8	NR
	25–45 oral amox content	12 (duo suspension)	NR
Amoxicillin	25 oral	8	NR
Trimethoprim	8 oral	12	2
Nalidixic acid	50 oral	6	12.5
Nitrofurantoin	3–5 oral	6	1
Cefotaxime	100 i.v.	12	NR
Cephradine	25–50 oral	8–12	NR
Cefuroxime	60 mg i.v.	8	NR
	6.25–25 oral	12	NR
Gentamicin	2 mg/kg/dose i.v.	Depends upon renal function and levels	NR

NR = Not recommended for prophylaxis

PREVENTION OF UTI

Recurrence of UTI is common in children, even in those who do not have a demonstrated structural abnormality of the urinary tract. This may be due to abnormal Gram-negative colonization of the introitus and periurethral areas in girls. It is important to provide the child and family with information about trying to reduce the number of urine infections and part of the outpatient consultation should be the provision of an information sheet such as the example below:

PREVENTION OF URINARY TRACT INFECTIONS

When your child has a urinary tract infection, the doctor will prescribe antibiotics. As well as the antibiotics, there are also some things you can do to help the infection to get better and also prevent another infection.

1. AVOID CONSTIPATION. You can do this by giving your child a high fiber diet to include wholemeal bread, whole-wheat cereals and fresh fruit and vegetables. Ensure that your child drinks a lot and has regular exercise. The doctor may also give your child a medicine to soften the stools.
If your child has any problems with WORMS let the doctor know.
2. In young girls the tube to the bladder is very close to the back passage. WIPING should be done in a front to back direction.
3. It is better to take a shower rather than a bath. Always avoid irritating soaps and bubble baths. CLEANLINESS is very important to help prevent infection.
4. EMPTYING THE BLADDER PROPERLY IS VERY IMPORTANT. Encourage your child to use the toilet regularly and empty the bladder every 2–3 hours. Sometimes we ask that your child will double empty the bladder. The child will pass water then wait a few minutes before trying to pass water again.
5. Always encourage your child to DRINK as much as possible during the day, and to EMPTY THE BLADDER PROPERLY LAST THING AT NIGHT.

6. CORRECT UNDERWEAR. Avoid tight underpants or pantihose. They prevent air from circulating freely and encourage the warm, moist environment which favors infection. Soft cotton briefs, changed daily, are a far better choice. Consider changing the washing powder you use for the panties if irritation persists.
7. When taking antibiotics the full course must be taken at the time required. Any PROBLEMS such as burning when passing water, going to the toilet often, or blood in the water SHOULD BE REPORTED to the doctor. We hope that these ideas will help you to help your child. Please do not hesitate to ask questions or contact us if you are worried.

INVESTIGATIONS OF CHILDREN WITH UTI

At present the consensus is that all children, boys and girls, should undergo appropriate investigations after the *first* proven urinary tract infection. However, opinions differ about appropriate investigations at different ages, especially when children are referred for investigation and urine cultures have been taken by dubious methods. This is particularly relevant to one of the high risk groups, namely infancy. The nature and extent of investigations depend to a large extent upon the age of the child, clues from the history and the examination, and the availability of local imaging facilities and expertise. One is more inclined to investigate fully a child who presents with a septicemic illness than a child referred to the outpatient department with dysuria and frequency with a culture taken inappropriately. The following imaging techniques are employed for the investigation of children with proven UTI:

Ultrasound (US) (all age groups)

Ultrasound will reveal anatomical information even in the kidney without function. It will give basic information on the structure of the urinary tract, and kidney sizes should be recorded with reference to centile charts based on the child's height. US will also reveal problems of obstruction and bladder abnormality as well as stones. It is relatively cheap and requires no radiation (Fig. 17.11).

However, US is operator-dependent and is difficult in unco-operative children. It may only show gross scarring. Significant vesicoureteric reflux may be present with a normal ultrasound.

Initially it was suggested that a *plain abdominal X-ray* was always required with the ultrasound. However, unless stones are suspected from the history, or there is the suggestion of a spinal abnormality on abdominal examination, a plain X-ray is now not *routinely* performed. We did originally use it to highlight to the child and the family the presence of fecal masses implying constipation, but there is a poor correlation between clinical and X-ray features of constipation and children are now not routinely reviewed in the clinic if they have had an uncomplicated UTI and the US is normal.

In skilled hands the ultrasound may suggest renal scarring but is generally regarded as less sensitive than the dimercaptosuccinic acid (DMSA) scan in this respect.

Intravenous urogram (IVU)

This has been superseded by the US but may be requested if there is an ill defined abnormality on the ultrasound examination, if DMSA is not readily available, or if detailed upper tract imaging is required prior to surgery (Fig. 17.6).

Although intravenous urography is widely available it does require an i.v. injection and the radiation dose can be high unless the number of films are limited. It also gives poor visualization of scars in infants.

Micturating cystourethrogram (MCUG)

A micturating cystourethrogram (MCUG) is still routine in children under 1 year of age with a proven UTI as this is the major risk period for scarring from vesicoureteric reflux. This examination is only required in those *over* 1 year of age who have recurrent infections or abnormalities on the ultrasound or (IVU) or a strong family history of vesicoureteric reflux (VUR) and/or renal scarring. An MCUG is requested more readily in boys, particularly if there are any reported difficulties with the urinary stream.

The MCUG is the most traumatic of the imaging investigations for UTI (Phillips et al 1996) and it is important that the technique is performed by experienced radiologists so that the procedure does not need to be repeated in referral centers for failure to visualize problems such as the posterior urethra in male infants. A study performed in our department has recently shown the benefit of proper preparation of the child and family for this procedure using stories and play preparation. At least 48 h antibiotic cover should be prescribed to cover the MCUG (usually trimethoprim twice a day) and if the child is discovered to have reflux then he should be immediately commenced on antibiotic prophylaxis if he is not already on it.

Direct isotope cystography

Direct isotope cystography (technetium pertechnetate) gives lower radiation dose than contract cystography but still requires catheterization and the bladder structure and urethra are not visualized.

Dimercaptosuccinic acid (DMSA) scan

Dimercaptosuccinic acid (DMSA) scan demonstrates acute renal involvement in UTIs and is the best technique for scars (Fig. 17.12). It provides a measure of the differential renal function and

the use of this imaging technique has provided one of the major dilemmas in current imaging as the closer to the infection the DMSA is performed, the more abnormalities are detected, some of which resolve (Verber & Meller 1989, Jakobsson et al 1992). If possible, the DMSA should be delayed for 6 weeks.

Isotope renography (MAG 3 or DTPA) (see Plate 17.13)

These isotopes are good for confirming obstruction and calculation of differential kidney function as the radionuclide is taken up by the kidney and excretion curves are generated (Fig. 17.3b). Initial curves are not comparable to DMSA for definition of renal cortical anatomy or scarring, although the resolution is better with the MAG 3 scan which is now favored. The technique does require intravenous injection.

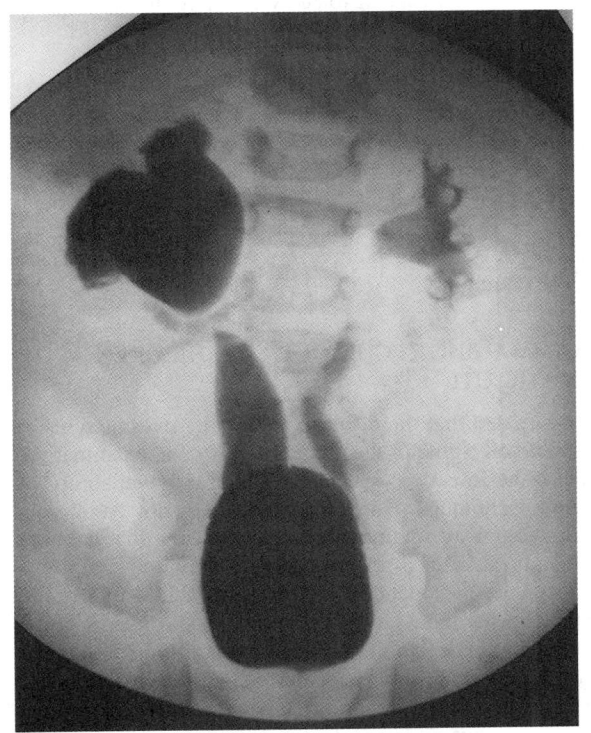

b

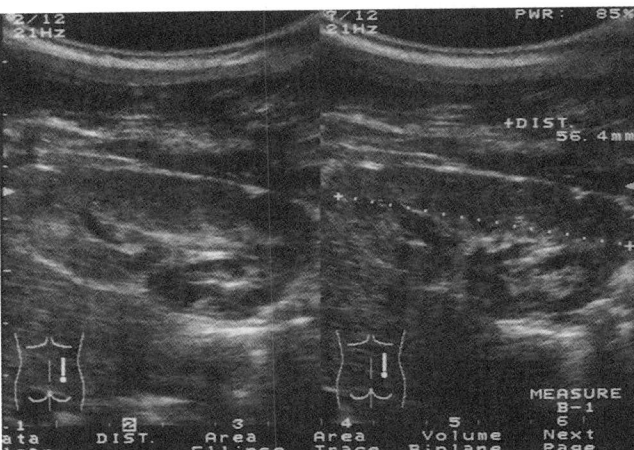

a

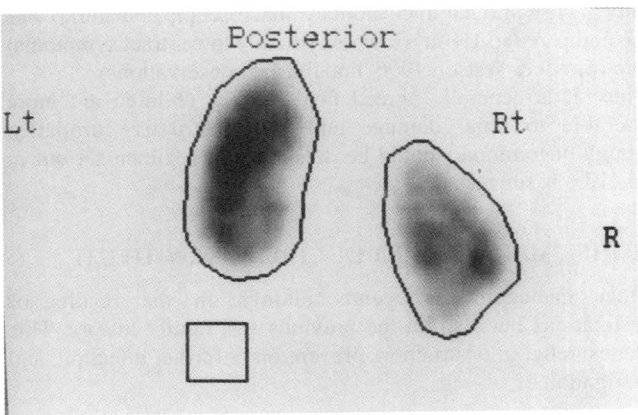

c

Fig. 17.11 Investigation in a 2-year-old boy with proven UTI: (**a**) ultrasound revealed normal left kidney (6.6 cm) with right kidney (shown) 6.2 cm and extensively scarred, especially at upper pole; (**b**) MCUG showed bilateral vesicoureteric reflux, gross right side; (**c**) DMSA shows scarring at both poles laterally of right kidney (40% of differential function).

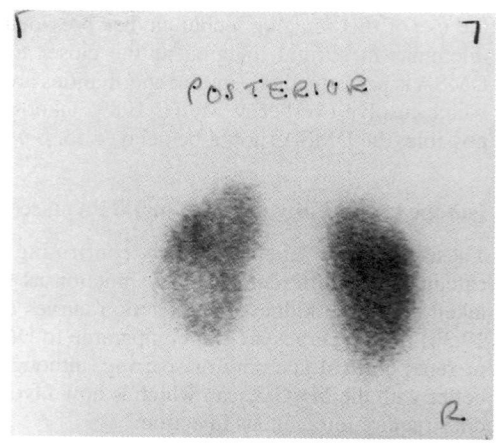
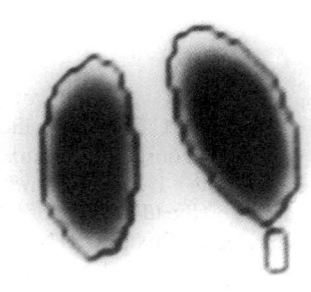

Fig. 17.12 (a) DMSA scan showing parenchymal defects in left kidney of 3-year-old with pyelonephritis. (b) DMSA scan in the same child 4 months later showing resolution of acute changes.

In the cooperative child over 4–5 years of age the scanning can continue as the child empties his or her bladder. This is the basis of *indirect micturating cystography* with obviously a lower radiation dose than the direct MCUG (Fig. 17.13). Although catheterization is avoided, the technique still requires i.v. injection of isotope. False negatives in comparison with a direct MCUG are believed to be common.

CHOICE OF IMAGING TECHNIQUES IN CHILDREN WITH SYMPTOMATIC UTI

It should be stressed that the decision to initiate investigations in any child should take note of the clinical history and examination, proof of the urine infection, age of the child and availability of local imaging techniques. Clinical history may not be closely related to radiological findings but nevertheless one is more inclined to investigate a child presenting with symptoms suggestive of acute pyelonephritis rather than a child referred to the outpatient department with frequency and dysuria. In a prospective study of 257 children referred to our *outpatient* clinic by primary care physicians the incidence of significant radiological findings in a high risk group (symptoms suggesting upper tract involvement, recurrent urinary infections, less than 2 years old, family history of renal tract anomaly, macroscopic hematuria) was 7.5% compared to 1% in a low risk (mainly lower tract symptoms) group (Savill & Watson 1996, unpublished observations).

Since it is generally agreed that younger children are more vulnerable to renal damage and that obstructive uropathy, although uncommon, should be detected, the regimen set out in Table 17.6 is suggested.

FURTHER MANAGEMENT OF CHILDREN WITH UTI

Further management depends mainly on the results of investigations but also on the previous and family history. This includes: relief of obstruction; prevention of further infection; and investigation of siblings.

Relief of obstruction

The uncommon child with an obstructive uropathy or stones will require surgical consultation. Children with suspected neurogenic bladder will require further imaging such as MRI scans of the spine and urodynamic evaluation of the bladder (O'Donnell 1991).

Prevention of further infection

Even in the child presenting with a first UTI it is important to stress preventive measures (see above). It is particularly important to stress a normal bladder emptying routine and to treat constipation. Dietary advice should be given on increasing fiber in the diet and the use of mild laxatives such as lactulose

Table 17.6 Investigation of children with proven UTI – choice of imaging techniques

0–1 year of age
- Ultrasound of the urinary system (kidneys, ureters and bladder)
- Direct micturating cystourethrogram (catheterization should be delayed until the urine is free from infection but delay for up to 6 weeks is not necessary)
- If there is significant hydronephrosis on the ultrasound in the absence of reflux on the MCUG then a pediatric nephrology or urology opinion should be sought to plan the need for further imaging such as isotope renography with MAG 3 or DTPA
- DMSA scan (or limited IVU if DMSA not available)

The timing of DMSAs is controversial at present as the closer to the infection it is performed then the more abnormalities are detected. However, some of these abnormalities will resolve, and, if possible, DMSA should be delayed for *6 weeks* after infection.

1–5 years
- Ultrasound of the urinary system
- MCUG *only* if ultrasound/DMSA shows abnormality, or if there are recurrent proven infections and/or strong family history. The detection of VUR will warrant prophylactic antibiotics
- DMSA scan if the child has had suspected pyelonephritis, abnormal US or if the MCUG shows evidence of reflux (to better define scarring)

Over 5 years
- Ultrasound of the urinary system
- DMSA scan if abnormal ultrasound or severe systemic symptoms
- Isotope renography with indirect micturating cystography to define reflux if scarring present on ultrasound/DMSA
- Direct MCUG only if surgery contemplated or recurrent symptoms despite negative indirect micturating cystography

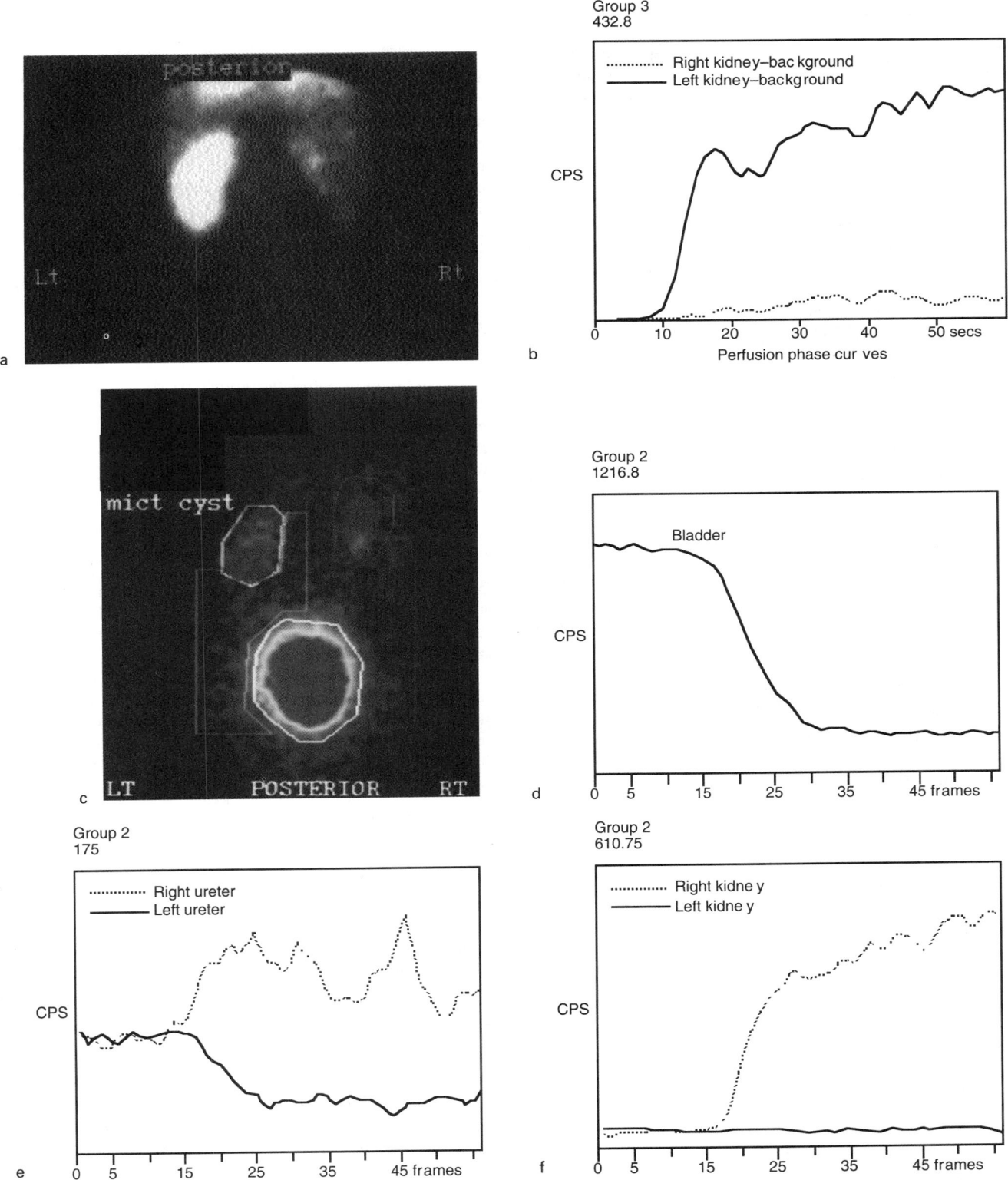

Fig. 17.13 (a) MAG 3 scan in 6-year-old boy with history of UTI and (b) small right kidney on scan (see Plate 17.13). (c–f) Indirect micturating cystogram showing gross reflux right side, as bladder empties, reflected in increased counts over right ureter and kidney.

(occasionally stronger ones such as Senokot may be required for short periods).

There is a group of children with dysfunctional voiding patterns (see under wetting) who are prone to recurrent infections. Such children may require assessment of bladder emptying by ultrasound and stressing double or triple voiding. In addition, some are best managed with prophylactic antibiotics from 6–12 months to break the vicious cycle of reinfection.

Investigation of siblings

Vesicoureteric reflux is known to occur in 20–30% of siblings (Aggarwal & Verrier-Jones 1989) and VUR behaves as an autosomal dominant condition with variable penetrance. In any family where VUR is detected the parents are advised to keep a close eye out for UTI in other children. When moderate to gross reflux is noted in one child an ultrasound is requested on siblings and if abnormal, an MCUG is requested. Although others have advocated an MCUG on all, it is felt that this more conservative approach is a useful compromise in view of the potentially traumatic nature of the MCUG and radiation dose.

VESICOURETERIC REFLUX (Fig. 17.14)

MANAGEMENT OF CHILDREN WITH VESICOURETERIC REFLUX

In recent years the pendulum has swung to conservative medical management with surgical reimplantation of the ureters being reserved for those children with obstructive uropathy or recurrent symptomatic urine infections despite prophylaxis. This approach has been confirmed by both the Birmingham and International study comparing conservative versus operative management, where the incidence of new scars, progression of existing scars, overall kidney function and frequency of breakthrough urinary tract infections was no different in the two groups (Birmingham 1987, International Reflux Study 1992).

MEDICAL REGIMEN

This includes repeated discussion with the child and family about

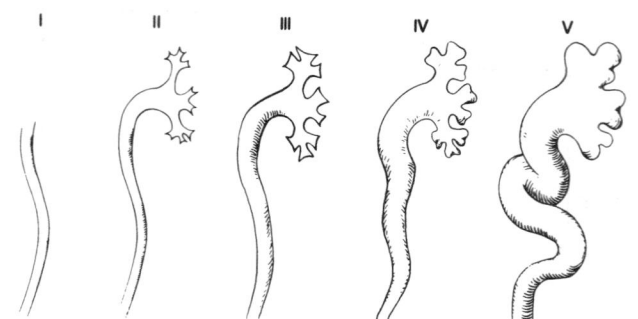

Fig. 17.14 International classifications of grades of reflux: **I** ureter only; **II** ureter, pelvis and calyces, no dilation; **III** mild or moderate dilation and/or tortuosity of the ureter and mild or moderate dilation of renal pelvis but no, or only slight, blunting of the fornices; **IV** moderate dilation and/or tortuosity of the ureter and moderate dilation of renal pelvis and calyces. Complete obliteration of sharp angle of fornices but maintenance of capillary impression in majority of calyces; **V** gross dilation and tortuosity of ureter, gross dilation of renal pelvis and calyces, capillary impressions are no longer visible in majority of cases.

general preventive measures, including regular, frequent repeat-voiding and avoidance of constipation. Low dose antibiotic prophylaxis should be taken in a single evening dose and urine cultures should be taken if the child has any symptoms. We no longer encourage the *routine* culture of urine samples from asymptomatic children but emphasize the need for cultures if *symptomatic*. Urine specimens obtained at the clinic that are negative on dipstick are also not routinely cultured. An explanatory booklet is given to the family and they are asked to record details of any positive urine culture results taken in the primary care setting. When the child is taking prophylactic antibiotics we stress to the family:

1. Try to avoid *missing* any doses.
2. Do *not* double up the dose if your child has a suspected urine infection. *Do* obtain a urine culture and take it to your doctor or clinic.
3. If your child is given another antibiotic for an infection such as a sore throat, then *continue* the prophylactic antibiotic.

The duration of antibiotic prophylaxis is debatable but in our unit it is given for a 2-year period. After such time it is appropriate to reassess kidney growth and evidence of scarring by ultrasound and DMSA scans. This will determine the planning of long term follow-up. Urinary prophylaxis is discontinued after the 2-year period if the child has been free of infections and if there is:

1. No evidence of scars on DMSA/ultrasound. Discharge to primary care and see again if recurrent infections.
2. Scarring in *one* kidney. Review annually and reinstigate prophylaxis if further documented infection. May repeat ultrasound and/or DMSA in further 2 years. If child remains normotensive after 10 years of age refer to general practitioner for blood pressure measurements yearly.
3. *Bilateral renal scarring.* These children are at greater risk of chronic renal insufficiency and/or hypertension and should be under long term follow-up by a pediatric nephrologist. Further assessment may include annual blood pressure checks and a MAG 3 scan with indirect cystography combined with ^{51}Cr EDTA GFR measurement at 5-year follow-up.

From the above regimen it should be noted that the direct MCUG is *not* repeated without good reason as we know from previous studies that a great deal of reflux resolves and the damage is done early. The exception is in the child with recurrent *symptomatic* infections where surgery may be contemplated. There may be an element of noncompliance resulting in recurrent infections or the antibiotic sensitivity of the local organisms may have changed.

SURGICAL REGIMEN

Difficult cases with complex anomalies of the urinary tract and those children with recurrent symptomatic infections are best referred to a unit where there is joint discussion between a pediatric urologist, nephrologist and radiologist. The standard reimplantation procedure is the Cohen or Leadbetter Politano technique which involves changing the intramural segment of ureter through the bladder wall. Operative success rates are 90–95% in centers with pediatric urological expertise.

There has been a great deal of interest recently in the 'sting' procedure with the submucosal injection of substances such as polytetrafluoroethylene paste or, more recently, microsilicone particles alongside the ureter. This can be done as a day case procedure. Although there may be good success rates in experienced hands there have been concerns raised about long term consequences of injection of foreign material and the need in some cases for repeated injection and cystograms to check the effectiveness of the procedure.

WETTING PROBLEMS

This is a common symptom which can cause much distress and anxiety to the child and parents. *Enuresis* can be defined as the involuntary voiding of urine in a child over 5 years of age without structural or neurological disease of the bladder or urinary tract, whereas *incontinence* is the leakage of urine in a child with structural or neurological disease of the bladder or urinary tract.

Enuresis is far more common than incontinence and the two should be distinguished from the history, physical examination and limited investigations, as shown in Table 17.7.

IDIOPATHIC (PRIMARY) NOCTURNAL ENURESIS

This can affect up to 10% of 7-year-old children and there is usually a family history in close relatives. Epidemiological studies show that if one parent has a history of nocturnal enuresis, his/her children are five to seven times more likely to have the disorder than those without an affected parent. Recent genetic studies in families with nocturnal enuresis have located two markers known as ENUR1 which flank the enuresis gene on chromosome 13 (Eiberg et al 1995).

As well as the inherited tendency, environmental factors such as stress, emotional disturbances and low social class are also contributing factors. The history should attempt to identify any environmental factors; potential physical disorders that may lead to wetting should be excluded on thorough physical examination and urinalysis.

Spontaneous resolution of nocturnal enuresis occurs at the rate of 15% per annum. If the child is distressed by the wetting or it is leading to distress within the family, then treatment should be

considered. An interested and sympathetic health care professional can certainly help to support the family and between 5 and 7 years the strategy of explanation, reassurance, star charts and praise or small rewards for dry nights is usually all that is necessary. For older children conditioning therapy with an enuresis alarm is the most effective treatment. However, this requires families to be closely supervised and supported. The role of medication remains controversial but may give some short term relief. Desmopressin, a synthetic analogue of antidiuretic hormone, can be given as a nasal spray. The tablet form is being evaluated. Imipramine is also effective but has a higher incidence of side-effects and is potentially lethal to children in accidental overdose.

DIURNAL ENURESIS DUE TO BLADDER INSTABILITY

This problem is usually classified as enuresis because there is no structural or neurological deficit. The wetting results from a functional disturbance of the detrusor muscle which intermittently contracts during the filling/storage phase of the bladder at a time when the muscle is normally relaxed. The child has difficulty suppressing these contractions (normally an involuntary reflex) which therefore results in leakage of urine and urgency/urge incontinence before the child contracts the pelvic floor to stop micturition. The condition has a strong association with urinary tract infection and constipation, and emotional stresses may precipitate the problem in some children.

Treatment is again aimed at providing information and support along with establishing a routine of complete and regular emptying of the bladder to restore the child's confidence. Star charts and rewards may be helpful. Constipation must be vigorously treated and urine infection eradicated. If infections are proven then the child will justify an ultrasound of the urinary tract with a check on bladder emptying. An anticholinergic drug such as oxybutynin is usually effective but more conservative measures should be tried first.

NEUROPATHIC BLADDER

Myelomeningocele is the main cause of neuropathic bladder in the pediatric population. Although children with myelomeningocele are usually born with normal kidneys, the function of the obstructed neuropathic bladder can result in chronic kidney damage if unrecognized (Borzykowski & Mundy 1988). Neuropathic bladder/sphincter dysfunction is complex and these children require careful assessment in specialist centers with expertise in urodynamics. The detrusor and/or striated pelvic floor muscles may lack spinal motor innovation (inactivity); with lesions above the level of the spinal motor neuron pelvic floor muscles are over active during filling and voiding. This dyssynergic pelvic floor activity constitutes a functional infravesical obstruction during voiding implying a high risk of kidney damage because of high emptying pressures.

Clean intermittent catheterization has been the major advance in the management of children with neuropathic bladders. It provides a means of both promoting continence as well as safeguarding kidney function. Oxybutynin to inhibit detrusor overactivity is often combined with intermittent catheterization. Patients and families derive great benefit from close support by a specialist nurse.

Table 17.7 Differential diagnosis of enuresis

Diagnosis	Clinical indicators
Urinary tract infection	Other urinary tract symptoms, secondary onset wetting
Detrusor instability	Daytime symptoms of urinary frequency, urgency and urge incontinence usually with a minor degree of wetness and worse in the afternoons
Neuropathic bladder	Constant severe daytime wetting, soiling, lumbosacral dimple or nevus, abnormal gait, abnormal perianal or lower limb neurology, palpable bladder
Ectopic ureter	Constant dribble of urine between voidings
Posterior urethral valves	Poor urinary stream, daytime wetting, palpable bladder
Chronic renal disease	Chronic ill health, hypertension, palpable kidneys or bladder, anemia, polydipsia
Diabetes mellitus	Recent illness with weight loss, thirst and polydipsia

HEMATURIA

Children may present with gross (or macroscopic) hematuria, in which case they are usually quickly brought to medical attention, or they may be found to have microscopic hematuria on routine urinalysis using one of the many types of urinary testing strips (dipsticks). The degree of hematuria is a poor guide to the severity of any underlying disease, but careful examination of the urine is an important noninvasive diagnostic tool.

Urinary dipsticks are very sensitive for blood and it is important that the manufacturer's instructions are followed closely and the test repeated on further samples. Microscopic hematuria may be transient and can occur in the context of exercise or stress. Urine could also be contaminated with blood from the external genital area, urethral meatus or menstrual blood.

Gross hematuria may be described as coke- or tea-colored due to the oxidized heme pigment, but it may also be bright red suggesting an extrarenal or lower urinary tract source. Inquiry should be made of other possible causes of red urine, such as foods (beetroot, berries and food dyes) and drugs (e.g. rifampicin). Hemoglobinuria and myoglobinuria should also be considered. Urate crystals may give the urine a pinkish tinge when present in high concentration, particularly in young infants.

URINE MICROSCOPY

Microscopy of fresh urine should be performed in all cases of hematuria to confirm the presence of red blood cells. Red cells hemolyze in standing urine, and fresh urine is also better for the identification of red cell or heme granular casts which are a strong pointer to a renal source for the hematuria (Fig. 17.15). Microscopy may also reveal pyuria and/or motile bacteria (suggesting infection) or crystals (using contrast microscopy). It may be possible to differentiate glomerular bleeding, when the red cells appear dysmorphic, from bleeding originating from the lower urinary tract, when the red cells tend to be of uniform shape and size (Shichiri et al 1986).

CAUSES OF HEMATURIA

The causes of hematuria are listed in Table 17.8. Many of the causes can be differentiated on the basis of the history, examination and urinalysis. If gross hematuria is reported, then the child or observer should be asked if it is more prominent in the initial or terminal parts of the urinary stream. Initial hematuria suggests an urethral cause, but this line of questioning is unlikely to be as relevant as it is in the adult patient, where bladder tumors and stones are much more prominent causes of hematuria.

Infection

Hematuria associated with dysuria, frequency, enuresis and suprapubic discomfort suggests a hemorrhagic cystitis, while systemic upset, fever, abdominal pain or loin tenderness suggest pyelonephritis. Urinary tract infection, either proven or suspected, remains a common cause of hematuria. Since other symptoms and signs may be minimal, it is essential that appropriate urine cultures are taken before treatment is initiated.

Viral infections can result in acute hemorrhagic cystitis, particularly adenovirus types 11 and 21. This is usually a self-limiting illness with resolution towards the end of the first week.

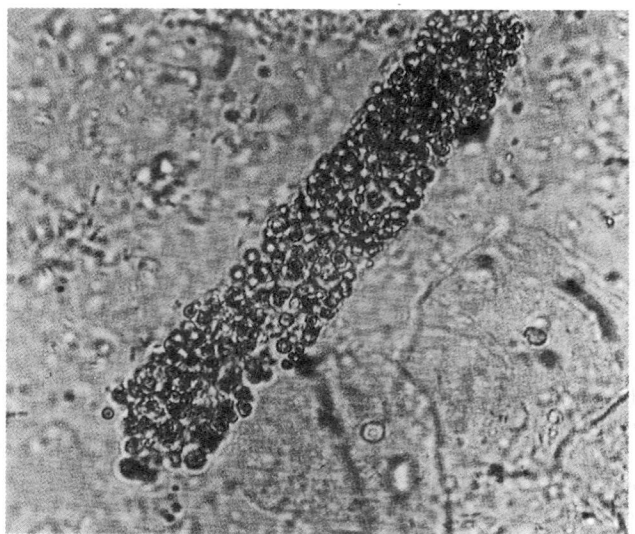

Fig. 17.15 Red cell granular cast. The outlines of many erythrocytes could still be made out clearly. (× 400)

Table 17.8 Causes of hematuria

1. Infection	a.	Bacterial
	b.	Viral
	c.	Schistosomiasis
	d.	Tuberculosis
2. Glomerular diseases		
3. Stones	a.	Urolithiasis
	b.	Idiopathic hypercalciuria
4. Trauma		
5. Anatomic abnormalities	a.	Congenital abnormalities, e.g. pelviureteric junction obstruction
	b.	Polycystic kidneys
	c.	Tumor
6. Vascular	a.	Arteritis
	b.	Infarction and thrombosis
	c.	Loin-pain hematuria syndrome
7. Hematological	a.	Coagulopathies
	b.	Sickle-cell disease
8. Drugs	e.g. Cyclophosphamide	
9. Exercise-induced		
10. Factitious		

Persistent dysuria, hematuria and sterile pyuria would suggest tuberculosis in the right clinical context, but this would be a very rare cause of hematuria in children in western countries. Infection with *Schistosoma haematobium* is an important cause of hematuria in endemic areas such as the Middle East and Africa. The ova can cause a granulomatous reaction in the bladder wall and lower ureter, and prompt treatment is essential (see Chapter 23).

Glomerulonephritis (see also p. 960)

The history of an upper respiratory tract or other infection, particularly if associated with gross hematuria, is suggestive of some form of acute postinfectious glomerulonephritis. Recurrent macroscopic hematuria in the older child raises the suspicion of Berger's disease (IgA nephropathy).

A positive family history of renal disease with or without deafness suggests the possibility of hereditary nephritis.

Stones

Stones or calculi in the urinary tract (urolithiasis) and/or deposition of calcium salts in the renal parenchyma (nephrocalcinosis) are uncommon in children in the UK, with an incidence of approximately 2 per million population compared to 2 per thousand for older men (Chambers & Moss 1994). However, urolithiasis is much commoner in other parts of the world, and this is probably attributable to high infection rates and dietary factors. Stones may be asymptomatic or result in hematuria, abdominal pain and urinary infection. Rarely, acute renal failure results from stones obstructing a single kidney or both kidneys. Any associated abdominal pain is usually unilateral and can be due to the stone itself or, rarely, the colic is due to clots of blood passing down the ureter.

Idiopathic hypercalciuria without hypercalcemia and overt stone formation has recently been recognized as an important cause of asymptomatic gross or microscopic hematuria in childhood (Stark et al 1988). It can be screened for by measuring the calcium/creatinine ratio (normal < 0.7 mmol/mmol) on the second morning urine sample, and confirmed by a 24-h urine collection (normal < 0.1 mmol Ca/kg per day) (Shaw et al 1990). As well as recommending the general advice of a high fluid intake and low calcium diet, treatment with thiazide diuretics may be considered.

Children with obvious stones will need investigation in conjunction with a pediatric surgeon. Stones causing obstruction or persistent infection will require removal by operation or dissolution by extracorporeal shock wave lithotripsy.

Trauma

Hematuria is associated with an obvious history of a damaging event. There is often bruising and other signs of external injury. With increasing recognition of the spectrum of sexual abuse, it is important that a careful history be taken if the injury involves the anogenital region.

Anatomic abnormalities

Although it is sometimes hard to equate abnormalities on X-ray with hematuria, there is no doubt that problems such as hydronephrosis, due for example to pelviureteric junction obstruction, can be a cause of hematuria. Although autosomal dominant polycystic kidney disease is increasingly recognized in childhood by the use of ultrasound scanning, it very rarely results in hematuria in the pediatric population.

The major kidney tumor of childhood is nephroblastoma (Wilms' tumor), and this usually presents as an abdominal mass with one-third of patients having associated hematuria, mainly microscopic. Bladder tumors are very rare in childhood (Rayner et al 1988) and so cystoscopy is rarely indicated, unlike the case in the adult population.

Vascular and hematological causes

Hematuria may occur in the context of any child with a problem such as hemophilia, leukemia or sickle-cell disease. The hematuria in the latter condition is presumably due to sickling of erythrocytes in the hypertonic, hypoxemic medulla, with resulting local papillary infarcts. It is unlikely to be the initial presentation.

Gross hematuria associated with a palpable mass in a newborn infant would suggest renal vein thrombosis. Hematuria may be part of the symptom complex in a multisystem disorder such as polyarteritis.

The loin pain–hematuria syndrome, which predominantly affects young women, is rare in childhood and requires renal angiography in suspected cases.

Drugs

There is an extensive list of drugs, poisons and ingested substances which can give rise to hematuria (Meadow 1994). Cyclophosphamide is a well-recognized cause of a sterile hemorrhagic cystitis, and a high fluid intake should be maintained during the use of this drug. Other drugs such as sulfonamides can cause crystalluria.

Exercise-induced

Hematuria may occur after severe exercise and has usually disappeared within 48 h. It would appear to have a glomerular origin and is an accentuation of the small amount of blood excreted by a number of people after heavy exercise.

Factitious hematuria

This may be part of the spectrum of Munchausen syndrome by proxy, where the child's carer (usually the mother) adds blood to the urine sample after it has been passed. There may be other pointers in the history or behavioral observations which suggest this diagnosis (Rinaldi et al 1993). A forensic laboratory may be able to determine whether the origin of the blood is from the parent or child.

INVESTIGATIONS IN A CHILD WITH HEMATURIA

The tests performed will depend upon the information provided from the history, examination and urinalysis. Again, it should be stressed that *microscopy* on a fresh urine sample can be invaluable, as identification of dysmorphic red cells and hemegranular or red cell casts (the urine should be centrifuged for 3 min at 3000 rev/min) strongly suggests a nephritic process and the child will be investigated accordingly. A *familial* condition may be detected by testing the urine of all immediate family members, particularly in cases of persistent microscopic hematuria.

Urine culture

A proven bacterial infection will lead to the appropriate investigations. Urine is rarely cultured for viruses, but should be considered in epidemics.

Hematology

Full blood count and film. Coagulation tests if appropriate.

Biochemistry

1. plasma urea, electrolytes, calcium, phosphate, alkaline phosphatase, albumin, total protein
2. urine calcium/creatinine ratio on second morning sample (if >0.7 mmol/mmol confirm with a 24-h collection).

Radiology

1. Plain abdominal X-ray and abdominal ultrasound. The ultrasound may fail to detect small areas of calcification visible on the plain abdominal X-ray.
2. An intravenous urogram may be ordered to confirm any suspicion raised on the initial screening ultrasound or to define the level of obstruction.
3. A micturating cystourethrogram or cystoscopy is *rarely* necessary in childhood, but may be indicated based on the history. If there is recurrent or persistent gross unexplained hematuria then cystoscopy during an episode may localize the bleeding to one kidney (in which an anatomic abnormality is probably present) or to both kidneys (making glomerulonephritis more likely).
4. Further radiological investigations may include CT scanning for renal masses, radionuclide scans or rarely renal arteriography.

Further tests for glomerulonephritis

Glomerulonephritis should be suspected if there are characteristic urinary changes or if the hematuria is persistent and no other cause can be found. The appropriate investigations will be discussed in detail later but should include:

1. throat swab for bacteria and viruses
2. antistreptolysin 0 titer and other streptococcal antigens
3. complement studies
4. autoantibody screen including antinuclear factor antibody
5. viral titers including screening for hepatitis B surface antigen.

Hearing test

In cases of suspected familial nephritis.

Renal biopsy

This is never routine and is only performed when there are indications of a more serious and potentially progressive disease, such as: progressive or persistent renal impairment; hypertension; persistent hypocomplementemia; heavy proteinuria; a familial disease that has not been characterized; a systemic disorder where therapy may be influenced by the histopathological findings, e.g. SLE. Renal biopsies are also carried out in children with persistent microscopic hematuria (usually of greater than 1 year's duration), often because of the family's request to know a specific diagnosis and prognosis (Fig. 17.16).

A renal biopsy should only be carried out by nephrologists experienced in the technique, who have access to expert pathology advice based on light and electron microscopy as well as immunofluorescence (or immunohistochemistry). In most instances, the biopsy is performed under ultrasound (or IVP) guidance in the sedated child. The biopsy can be carried out as a

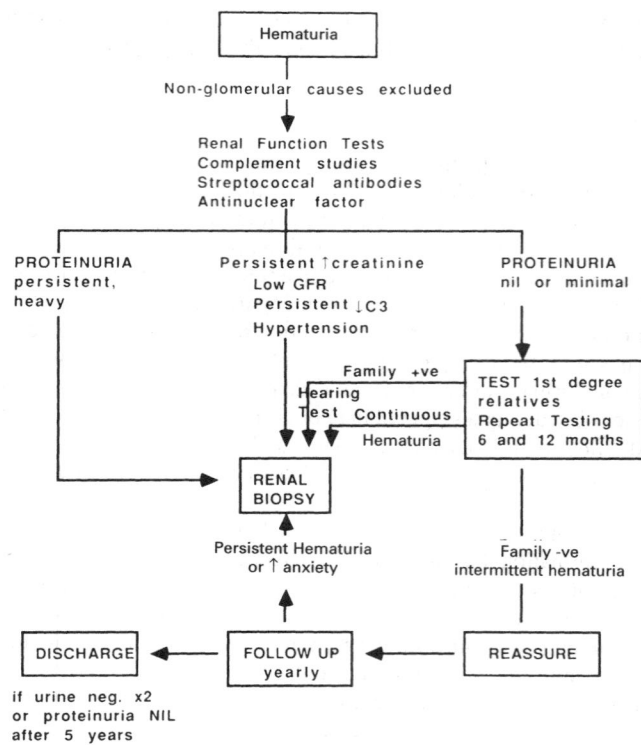

Fig. 17.16   A scheme for the management of children with hematuria.

day case procedure with appropriate preparation of the child and family (Tomsett & Watson 1996). An open renal biopsy under general anesthetic is only necessary in the very young child. In expert hands the morbidity associated with renal biopsy is low.

GLOMERULONEPHRITIS

Glomerulonephritis, or more simply nephritis, is both a generic term for several diseases, and a histopathological term signifying inflammation and proliferation of cells within the glomerulus. In many instances the inflammatory changes are initiated by immunological mechanisms, but in others the pathogenesis is unknown.

Injury may be limited to the kidney alone, or the immune or nonimmune mechanisms may be part of a systemic disorder (Table 17.9).

We still understand very little of the specific events involved with glomerulonephritis, and so when therapy has been employed it has tended to be 'blunderbuss' in nature, with broad spectrum immunosuppressive drugs such as corticosteroids, azathioprine and cyclophosphamide, or other therapies such as plasma exchange (Haycock 1988).

Pathology

Many of the categories of so-called primary glomerulonephritis (Table 17.9) are based on histopathological descriptions obtained from renal biopsy specimens. The terminology is derived from changes that are found on light, electron and immunofluorescent microscopy (Figs 17.17 and 17.18).

Clinical patterns of glomerulonephritis

Patients with glomerulonephritis may present with:

1. *Asymptomatic hematuria* and/or proteinuria.
2. *Acute nephritic syndrome* characterized by hematuria, oliguria, edema and hypertension. The hematuria is heavy with red cell casts on microscopy. Proteinuria is variable.
3. *Nephrotic syndrome* characterized by heavy proteinuria leading to hypoalbuminemia and edema with hyperlipidemia. The urinalysis shows heavy proteinuria (+++ or >5 g/l) with variable hematuria. Microscopy may show fatty casts and free fat droplets.

Table 17.9   Classification of glomerular disorders

PRIMARY GLOMERULONEPHRITIS
1. Immune complex glomerulonephritis
   a. Postinfectious acute glomerulonephritis
   b. Mesangial IgA nephropathy (Berger's disease)
   c. Membranoproliferative glomerulonephritis (types I to III)
   d. Membranous glomerulonephritis (idiopathic)

2. Anti-GBM-antibody-mediated glomerulonephritis

3. Uncertain etiology, e.g. minimal lesion glomerulonephritis, focal segmental glomerulosclerosis

GLOMERULONEPHRITIS ASSOCIATED WITH SYSTEMIC DISORDERS
1. Immunologically-mediated
   a. Henoch–Schönlein purpura
   b. Systemic lupus erythematosus and other collagen disorders, e.g. scleroderma
   c. Polyarteritis nodosa, Wegener's granulomatosis and other vasculitides
   d. Mixed cryoglobulinemia
   e. Systemic infections (subacute bacterial endocarditis, shunt nephritis, syphilis, malaria, hepatitis B)

2. Hereditary disorders
   a. Familial nephritis, e.g. Alport's syndrome
   b. Sickle-cell anemia

3. Other conditions
   a. Diabetes mellitus
   b. Amyloidosis

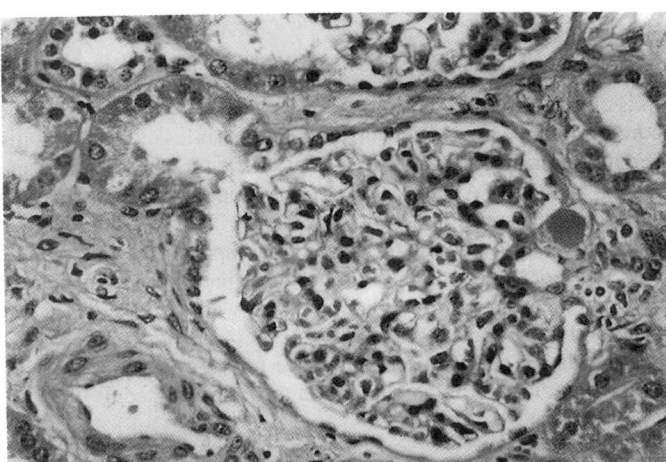

Fig. 17.17   Light microscopy of a normal glomerulus. Part of the proximal tubule at upper left hand corner and hilum on the right.

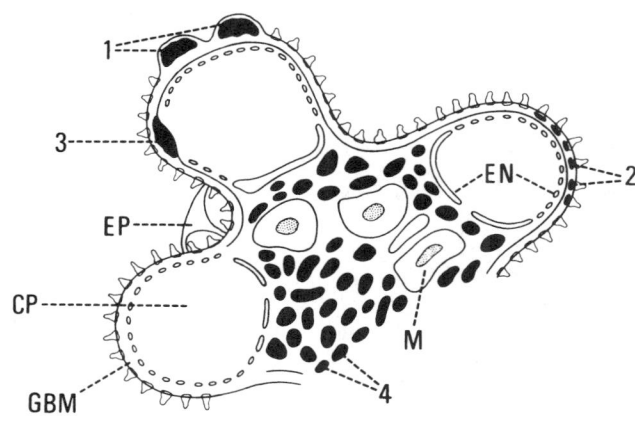

Fig. 17.18   Schematic depiction of the anatomy of the glomerulus and possible sites of immune complex deposition (EP = epithelial; EN = endothelial; M = mesangial cell; CP = capillary space; GBM = glomerular basement membrane). Deposits are in the following locations: 1 = subepithelial lumps; 2 = intramembranous; 3 = subendothelial; 4 = mesangial.

It is important to appreciate that there is a spectrum of clinical presentation and patients may have a mixed picture of nephritis/nephrosis. For example, the majority of children with Henoch–Schönlein purpura have a nephritis with asymptomatic hematuria and/or proteinuria, which usually resolves but may progress into a nephritic syndrome. If the proteinuria is so heavy that hypoalbuminemia results, then the patient may have the clinical picture of nephrotic syndrome.

ACUTE GLOMERULONEPHRITIS

Acute glomerulonephritis is associated with dark urine, diminished urine output, edema, hypertension and varying degrees of renal insufficiency.

It is the classical example of an acute nephritic syndrome. Some of the family contacts may exhibit a milder form with asymptomatic hematuria.

In children, the majority of cases will be postinfectious, with group A β-hemolytic streptococcus being the organism most commonly implicated. Acute poststreptococcal glomerulonephritis (APSGN) may follow nasopharyngeal or skin infection.

Although the disease is now uncommon in western countries, it is still very prevalent in many parts of the world where overcrowding, poor nutrition and widespread skin sepsis still prevail. As APSGN has diminished in developed countries, other postinfectious causes of acute nephritis are being recognized. These include infection with staphylococcal, pneumococcal, salmonella and mycoplasma species, as well as viral infections such as Coxsackie, ECHO, Epstein–Barr and influenza viruses.

Clinical features

Poststreptococcal glomerulonephritis is most common in the younger school-age child but can occur at any age. The acute nephritis typically develops 1–2 weeks after an upper respiratory tract infection with sore throat (Fig. 17.19). The latent period associated with pyoderma-related APSGN is more variable. The severity of renal involvement may vary from asymptomatic hematuria with normal renal function to acute renal failure.

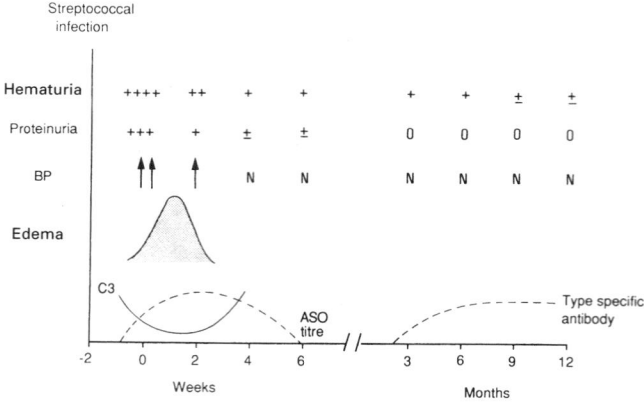

Fig. 17.19 Course of acute poststreptococcal glomerulonephritis.

Facial swelling may be the first symptom, and is often attributed to oversleeping or allergic problems. However, increasing edema or the occurrence of gross hematuria will bring the child to medical attention earlier.

There may be a variety of nonspecific symptoms, such as malaise, abdominal pain, anorexia, headaches and weakness. Oliguria may only be revealed on direct questioning.

Edema and hypertension may be noted on physical examination. The degree of hypertension is variable and not proportional to the degree of edema, which may be sufficient to cause pleural effusions and, rarely, congestive cardiac failure. The rare patient may also develop hypertensive encephalopathy, with headaches, alteration of mental state, convulsions and coma.

Diagnosis

Urinalysis will show heavy hematuria and variable proteinuria, with microscopy revealing numerous dysmorphic red cells and heme granular casts in the florid case. Casts may only be found on centrifuged urine in the mild case. Blood should be taken for full blood count and platelets (a mild normochromic normocytic anemia due to dilution is usually present) and renal function tests, which will include plasma electrolytes, bicarbonate, urea, creatinine, serum albumin and total protein levels.

The diagnosis is confirmed by finding evidence of recent streptococcal infection along with hypocomplementemia. Throat swabs from both the patient and family should be cultured, and the patient's blood is sent for antibody titers to streptococcal antigens. Since the antistreptolysin O (ASO) titer may not rise after streptococcal skin infection, a request should be made for anti-DNase B and antihyaluronidase titers which may show a significant rise in this context. Total hemolytic complement and the components C3 and C4 should also be measured, along with antinuclear antibodies (to exclude lupus nephritis). Other immunological tests may include viral, antineutrophil cyto-plasmic antibody (ANCA), antiglomerular basement (anti-GBM), immunoglobulin and cryoglobulin titers as appropriate.

The very edematous child may justify a chest X-ray (pleural effusions and cardiomegaly), and a renal ultrasound may be considered.

The combination of an acute nephritic syndrome, evidence of recent streptococcal infection and a low C3 level are sufficient evidence to support the diagnosis of APSGN. A renal biopsy is indicated *when* there is evidence of: worsening renal failure; development of nephrotic syndrome; a normal C3 level in the acute phase; or the persistence of marked hematuria and proteinuria with hypocomplementemia for several weeks.

The complications of APSGN are those of any child with acute renal failure (p. 973), and include hypertension, fluid overload, hyperkalemia, uremia, hypocalcemia, hyperphosphatemia, acidosis and seizures.

Treatment

A 10-day course of penicillin is prescribed to the patient and any culture-positive family members. There is no evidence that it affects the natural history of glomerulonephritis but it is known to limit the spread of the nephritogenic strains. Activity need not be restricted, and dietary and drug management will depend upon the degree of renal function and the need to control hypertension. Fortunately, in most children with APSGN, the illness is mild and manageable by conservative treatment without resort to acute dialysis.

Prognosis

Complete recovery occurs in over 95% of children with poststreptococcal glomerulonephritis (Clark et al 1988). In a small minority there may be a rapid progression of the renal disease with extensive crescent formation ('rapidly progressive glomerulonephritis') leading to glomerular hyalinization and chronic renal insufficiency. There is little evidence that progression to a chronic glomerulonephritis occurs following APSGN. However, some patients with a preexisting chronic glomerulonephritis may have an exacerbation precipitated by a streptococcal illness. Second attacks of APSGN are very rare, and there is no indication for penicillin prophylaxis or tonsillectomy. Children with APSGN can usually be quickly discharged from hospital if their renal function is satisfactory or improving and there is no hypertension. Repeat blood tests will be required to check that the complement levels have returned to normal and to confirm a significant rise in ASO titers. Microscopic hematuria may persist for 1–2 years, but if the urinalysis, blood pressure and creatinine are normal then the patient can be discharged from long-term follow-up.

MESANGIAL IGA NEPHROPATHY

This clinical/pathological entity is now recognized as probably the commonest cause of recurrent, symptomless, macroscopic hematuria and persistent microscopic hematuria in children and young adults (D'Amico 1985). There appears to be a marked geographical variation in its incidence, being commoner in Southern Europe, South East Asia and Japan. This may reflect both the more frequent use of biopsies in patients with persistent microscopic hematuria in some units, as well as possible dietary factors (Takebayashi & Yanase 1992).

There is a 2 : 1 male predominance for IgA nephropathy, with the peak incidence in late childhood through early adult life.

Clinical features

The major modes of presentation are macroscopic hematuria or the incidental finding of hematuria and proteinuria on routine urinalysis. The blood pressure, creatinine and complement levels are typically normal, and less than 50% of patients are reported to have raised serum IgA levels. The clinical diagnosis is further supported by episodes of *recurrent* macroscopic hematuria occurring 1–3 days after an upper respiratory tract infection. This is in contrast to APSGN, where the latent period is usually 7 days. Microscopic hematuria usually persists in IgA nephropathy between the episodes of macroscopic hematuria. Rarely, the presentation is with a nephrotic syndrome or a picture of acute glomerulonephritis with hypertension, acute renal insufficiency and crescents on renal biopsy indicative of a rapidly progressive glomerulonephritis.

Diagnosis

The condition is often recognized from the clinical pattern and after other causes of hematuria and postinfectious nephritis have been ruled out.

The renal biopsy usually reveals focal and segmental mesangial proliferation and increased mesangial matrix, with occasional patients showing diffuse disease with crescents and scarring. The electron microscopic findings of mesangial deposits is nonspecific, but the diagnosis is supported by immunofluorescent deposits of mesangial IgA and lesser amounts of IgG and IgM.

Mesangial deposits of IgA also occur in Henoch–Schönlein purpura but this is usually distinguishable on the clinical features. However, it has been well documented for IgA nephropathy and a Henoch–Schönlein syndrome to occur in the same patient separated in time by several years, suggesting the two conditions have a common immunopathological basis.

Normal levels of C3 complement and anti-DNA antibodies will distinguish IgA nephropathy from poststreptococcal glomerulonephritis and lupus nephritis respectively.

Treatment

No therapy has been shown to alter the course of IgA nephropathy.

Prognosis

IgA nephropathy is generally a benign disease in childhood, but some children may have a progressive course and in adult series up to 25% of patients have ultimately developed renal failure, and the process may also occur in transplanted kidneys. Neither the number of episodes of gross hematuria nor the persistence of microscopic hematuria between episodes correlates with the likelihood of progressive disease.

Activity need not be restricted. Patients will need to be monitored in the outpatient clinic for signs such as hypertension, diminished renal function and heavy proteinuria which might portend progressive disease.

Since the prognosis of IgA nephropathy is generally so good, and there is no specific treatment, routine renal biopsy may be deferred unless there is a suggestion of progressive disease. However, some would advocate a renal biopsy in any child with persistent hematuria after 12–24 months of observation, even if the renal function is normal. The biopsy will help to establish a diagnosis on which a firmer prognosis may be based. It should help to allay child and parental anxiety even though no specific treatment may be available. The information may be relevant for future employment counseling, particularly with respect to the Armed Forces.

MEMBRANOPROLIFERATIVE GLOMERULONEPHRITIS

This type of chronic glomerulonephritis was first recognized in 1965, and was originally described as chronic lobular glomerulonephritis, mesangiocapillary glomerulonephritis, or chronic hypocomplementemic glomerulonephritis. However, since not all patients have hypocomplementemia and since the glomerular pathology refers to thickened membranous-like glomerular capillary walls and mesangial proliferation, membranoproliferative glomerulonephritis (MPGN) is now the accepted term. Three histological types have been described.

Type 1 MPGN

This is the most common form, with the glomeruli revealing an accentuation of the lobular pattern due to a generalized increase in mesangial cells and matrix. The glomerular capillary walls appear thickened and in some areas duplicated or split due to interposition of mesangial cytoplasm and matrix between the endothelial cells and glomerular basement membrane. Crescents may be present, and MPGN is one form of a rapidly progressive glomerulonephritis. Deposition of C3 and a lesser amount of immunoglobulin is shown on immunofluorescence, and electron microscopy confirms the presence of deposits in the subendothelial and mesangial regions.

Type 2 MPGN

In this type, the capillary walls demonstrate irregular, ribbon-like thickening due to dense deposits. Electron microscopy reveals extensive homogeneous electron-dense material in the glomerular basement membrane in the region of, but distinct from, the lamina densa.

Type 3 MPGN

In type 3 disease there are contiguous subepithelial and subendothelial deposits associated with disruption of the basement membrane.

Clinical features

Membranoproliferative glomerulonephritis is most common in the second decade of life. The clinical onset is variable, with either gross hematuria, nephrotic syndrome or asymptomatic proteinuria and microscopic hematuria. In about one-third of patients, hypertension and an elevated serum creatinine are evident at presentation.

Both MPGN and acute poststreptococcal glomerulonephritis may present with a nephritic syndrome, low C3 and elevated ASOT levels (coincidental in MPGN). The distinction may have to be made on natural history grounds.

Most patients with APSGN recover within 4 weeks, with return of complement levels to normal. A persistently low C3 with a nephrotic state or heavy hematuria would be an indication for renal biopsy to exclude MPGN.

There is an association between partial lipodystrophy, low

concentrations of C3, the presence of a C3 nephritic factor and type 2 MPGN.

Treatment and prognosis

Evaluating therapeutic regimes in a chronic disease with such a variable course as MPGN has been difficult. Success may depend upon the degree of histopathological change and the stage at which treatment is initiated (McEnery & Coutinho 1994). Success in stabilizing the clinical course has been reported in patients receiving long-term alternate-day prednisolone therapy or inhibitors of platelet function. The actuarial kidney survival curves have shown 50% of patients to be in end-stage disease at approximately 10 years.

Membranoproliferative glomerulonephritis associated with systemic disease

The features of MPGN can be seen in the renal biopsies of patients with a number of systemic conditions, such as systemic lupus erythematosus, polyarteritis nodosa and Henoch–Schönlein purpura.

MPGN features may also accompany chronic infections such as subacute bacterial endocarditis, infected ventricular–atrial shunts, syphilis, hepatitis B, candidiasis and malaria. The infecting organisms usually have low virulence and the host is chronically seeded with foreign antigen. The combination with host antibodies results in complexes being deposited in the glomerular mesangium, producing mesangial proliferation and interposition. Immune deposits are subendothelial and in the mesangium. Hence, the disease is like type 1 MPGN with hypocomplementemia. If elimination of the infecting agent is achieved, then the lesion may heal but with scarring and there is the possibility of progression to end-stage renal failure.

Chronic infections may also produce the pathological changes of membranous glomerulopathy, focal glomerulosclerosis, and focal and segmental proliferative glomerulonephritis.

MEMBRANOUS GLOMERULONEPHRITIS

Membranous glomerulonephritis (MGN) is the commonest cause of nephrotic syndrome in adults, but is uncommon in childhood. It very rarely causes hematuria alone. Membranous glomerulonephritis is defined by the histological appearances on light microscopy of diffuse thickening of the glomerular basement membranes without significant proliferative changes. On silver staining, the continuous subepithelial deposits give a spike appearance to the glomerular basement membrane, and immunofluorescent microscopy demonstrates granular deposits of IgG and C3 which can be also identified by electron microscopy.

Clinical features

The disease can occur at any age but is most common in the second decade of life. The presentation may be covert with disease discovered at routine urinalysis, or it presents with nephrotic syndrome and, less often, macroscopic hematuria. The blood pressure and C3 levels are normal.

It is usual practice to biopsy children who present with nephrotic syndrome over 10 years of age because of the likelihood of finding a condition other than minimal lesion glomerulone-phritis, such as MGN. This type of glomerulonephritis may occasionally be seen in association with systemic lupus erythematosus, drug therapy such as gold or penicillamine, syphilis, hepatitis B virus infection and some cancers.

Treatment and prognosis

Spontaneous remission is quite common with this pathology, and the present consensus is that children who are not clinically nephrotic are at only slight risk of developing renal failure in the long term and do not require treatment. However, children with a prolonged nephrotic syndrome may have a poor prognosis and alternate-day steroid therapy has been suggested. The nephrotic state is best controlled with salt restriction and diuretic agents.

HENOCH–SCHÖNLEIN (ANAPHYLACTOID) PURPURA NEPHRITIS

Henoch–Schönlein purpura is one of the commonest systemic diseases with renal involvement encountered in children. It is a vasculitis of the smallest blood vessels (capillaries, arterioles and venules), with characteristic skin involvement, gastrointestinal symptoms and joint manifestations in a large percentage of patients.

Renal involvement is present in 70% of children and is usually manifest within the first months but can be delayed up to 3 months after the rash. It is mainly mild and asymptomatic, with microscopic hematuria and low grade proteinuria. Renal biopsy would only be undertaken if there were signs of persistent or progressive renal impairment or the development of heavy proteinuria or nephrotic syndrome. The histological appearances may vary from mild mesangial proliferation through to diffuse proliferation with a large percentage of crescents or membrano-proliferative changes. Immunofluorescence reveals mesangial IgA deposits, and presumably the process is of an immune-complex-mediated disease, but the precise etiology is unclear.

Rapidly progressive glomerulonephritis with crescents may justify immunosuppressive therapy but there are no conclusive studies. Children with persistent urinary abnormalities following Henoch–Schönlein purpura should continue to be followed in the outpatient clinic to detect the late development of hypertension and renal impairment (Berg & Widstan-Attorps 1993).

SYSTEMIC LUPUS ERYTHEMATOSUS

Systemic lupus erythematosus (SLE) is a multisystem immune-complex-mediated disorder which has a wide spectrum of clinical manifestations and renal involvement. This may vary from microscopic hematuria and mild proteinuria through to renal insufficiency and nephrotic syndrome. Since the overall prognosis of childhood and adult SLE is closely correlated with the nature of the pathological renal lesions, it has been recommended that a kidney biopsy be performed on all patients presenting with renal involvement to establish the severity of the histological changes. These may vary from normal to mesangial lupus, proliferative (focal and diffuse) and membranous appearances.

Treatment and prognosis

Clinical symptoms, such as malaise, skin rash and arthritis, are controlled with the lowest doses of corticosteroids possible.

Laboratory monitoring of parameters such as complement levels and anti-DNA antibody titers are also useful. More aggressive therapy is prescribed for major organ involvement with renal, cardiac or central nervous complications, and may include high dose methylprednisolone or cyclophosphamide pulses (Balow et al 1996). Plasma exchange therapy has also been advocated, while azathioprine has been used as a steroid-sparing agent in the long term to prevent steroid toxicity.

The prognosis for survival in patients with SLE has improved considerably over the past two decades. The 10-year survival figure is approximately 90%. The object is to achieve a balance between suppressing the disease process without invoking complications of the therapy itself. The majority of patients with lupus nephritis can be successfully treated and will maintain normal renal function. In a few patients, the active renal disease progresses and irreversible renal involvement with glomerular scarring and interstitial fibrosis may result. Renal transplantation can be quite successful in this group.

RAPIDLY PROGRESSIVE (CRESCENTIC) GLOMERULONEPHRITIS

Rapidly progressive glomerular nephritis (RPGN) is a description of the clinical course of several forms of nephritis where there is acute renal insufficiency associated with the presence of extensive crescents on the renal biopsy. Such crescents may be found in poststreptococcal, membranoproliferative, lupus and Henoch–Schönlein purpura nephritis, as well as the glomerulonephritis of Goodpasture's disease.

After the above forms of glomerular nephritis have been excluded, there remains a small group of patients with so called idiopathic rapidly progressive disease. Often there is no evidence for immunological mechanisms and the C3 level is normal. All forms of RPGN have crescents which are found on the inside of Bowman's capsule and are composed of fibrin, proliferating epithelial cells of the capsule, basement-membrane-like material and macrophages. The stimulus for crescent formation is believed to be the deposition of fibrin in Bowman's space as a result of necrosis or disruption of the glomerular capillary wall.

Severe crescentic nephritis is associated with acute renal failure in association with a nephritic or nephrotic syndrome. Although there have been well-documented spontaneous recoveries of renal function with poststreptococcal and Henoch–Schönlein purpura nephritis, many patients will progress to end-stage renal failure within weeks or months after onset. With such a rare condition it is hard to mount a controlled trial, but it is claimed that some patients have improved with aggressive therapy combining immunosuppressive agents with anticoagulation and plasma exchange.

GOODPASTURE'S AND GOODPASTURE-LIKE SYNDROME

This refers to a combination of pulmonary hemorrhage and glomerulonephritis associated with antibodies against lung and glomerular basement membrane. It is one form of a rapidly progressive glomerulonephritis, with immunofluorescence showing a continuous linear pattern of IgG along the glomerular basement membrane. Goodpasture's syndrome is extremely rare in childhood but a similar clinical picture of pulmonary hemorrhage and glomerulonephritis may occur in association with SLE, anaphylactoid purpura, polyarteritis nodosa and Wegener's granulomatosis.

Hemoptysis is the usual presenting complaint and pulmonary hemorrhage can result in death. Antiglomerular basement antibodies (Goodpasture's) or antineutrophil cytoplasmic antibodies (C-ANCA in Wegener's) support the diagnosis.

As well as ameliorating the renal injury, a combination of plasma exchange and immunosuppressive therapy early in the disease may even be life saving (Rondeau et al 1989).

HEREDITARY NEPHRITIS (ALPORT'S SYNDROME)

Hereditary nephritis is not a homogeneous entity, as the clinical expression of the disease and the mode of inheritance can vary widely between families. The classic description of Alport's syndrome was of a progressive hematuric nephritis associated with sensorineural deafness and ocular abnormalities such as anterior lenticonus and cataracts. The gene in Alport's has been located to X chromosome ($X_q21.2–_q22.2$) and it is hypothesized that the basic genetic defect lies in the gene for the α 5 chain of type IV collagen (Tryggvason et al 1993). The condition is generally more severe in male members of the family, with most (but not all) females remaining in good health throughout life. The prognosis is best based upon the progress of other affected family members, as there is a strong correlation between deafness, ocular abnormalities, proteinuria and chronic renal failure.

Renal biopsy in the early stages of Alport's syndrome shows only focal mesangial hypercellularity. There is progressive glomerular sclerosis, tubular atrophy, interstitial inflammation and foam cells (nonspecific lipid-laden tubular or interstitial cells). Immunofluorescence is unrewarding, but electron microscopy may reveal irregular thickening, thinning, splitting and layering of the basement membrane of the glomeruli, with a lattice work appearance described as 'basket weave'. (Fig. 17.20) These findings are very suggestive of Alport's syndrome of the classical type but may occur in patients without an abnormal family history, suggesting a new mutation.

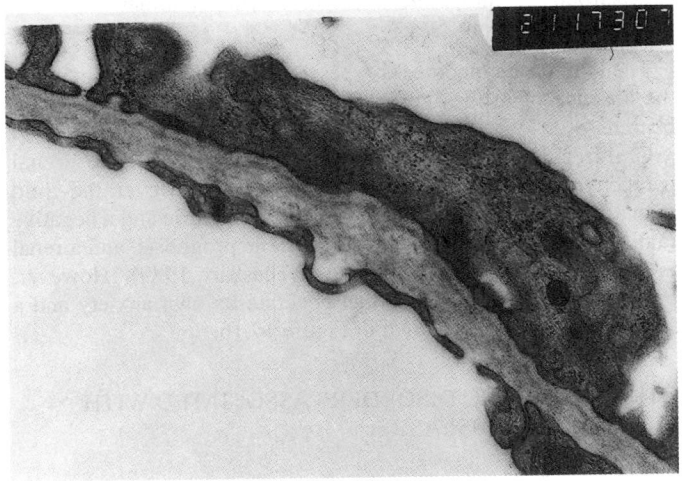

Fig. 17.20 Electron microscopy of basement membrane in child with Alport's syndrome. Lattice work appearance.

Clinical features

The disease is characteristically silent during childhood, but microscopic hematuria and proteinuria may be identified in affected family members after the first few years of life. There is progression in the second decade of life as sclerosis proceeds and the proteinuria becomes heavier with hypertension and renal failure. Nephrotic syndrome can occasionally occur at presentation or late in the disease process. There is no effective treatment, and dialysis and transplantation will be required as early as the second or third decade of life.

The deafness is initially high frequency but is progressive and may ultimately be quite profound, especially in males. It is wise to carefully assess the hearing of children with any type of inherited nephritis. This may be of more initial importance than the renal disease.

FAMILIAL RECURRENT HEMATURIA SYNDROME

In any child with persistent microscopic hematuria it is important to test the urine of all first degree family members even though there is no clear history of familial nephritis. A familial recurrent hematuria syndrome is generally inherited as an autosomal dominant trait, but recessive examples may occur. The microscopic hematuria may sometimes be accompanied by shortlived episodes of frank hematuria with mild proteinuria. However, there is usually no impairment of renal function.

The condition is generally regarded as benign (synonym: benign familial hematuria) and hence not all children have been subjected to renal biopsy. Part of the reluctance to do so is because of the absence of therapeutic measures and the lack of a history of progressive nephritis.

However, even if the biopsy is normal on light microscopy and immunofluorescence it may be possible to demonstrate changes in the glomerular basement membrane (GBM) on electron microscopy (Lang et al 1990). Basement membrane nephropathy has been grouped into:

1. Group 1. Lamellation type with features indistinguishable from Alport's syndrome.
2. Group 2. Extensive thinning commonly found in children with mild microscopic hematuria.
3. Group 3. Idiopathic hematuria with minimal basement membrane alteration.

The long-term outcome for types 2 and 3 is still uncertain but in the absence of a positive family history is usually regarded as benign.

Children with hematuria *and* proteinuria have renal parenchymal disease until proven otherwise. However, the child with asymptomatic, low degree, isolated hematuria and a negative family history is likely to have a favorable prognosis, and a renal biopsy is not initially warranted (Vehaskari 1989). However, prolonged clinic supervision can generate its own anxiety and a suggested approach is shown in Figure 17.16.

OTHER SYSTEMIC DISORDERS ASSOCIATED WITH GLOMERULAR DISEASE

Scleroderma

Scleroderma, or progressive systemic sclerosis is a rare multisystem disorder in children. Renal involvement is unusual at the outset but can occur with progression of the disease, and is characterized by proteinuria, hypertension and renal insufficiency. Scleroderma renal crisis occurs with the abrupt onset of malignant hypertension and oliguric renal failure. The angiotensin-converting enzyme inhibitor, captopril, has been used successfully in its treatment.

Vasculitis

Vasculitis is characterized by inflammation of medium or small blood vessels. Classification is difficult because of the heterogeneous nature of many of these conditions and the overlapping clinical features. Vasculitis of small vessels occurs with Henoch–Schönlein purpura and conditions such as serum sickness, whereas vasculitis with granuloma formation is found in Wegener's granulomatosis. Vasculitis of medium and large arteries with giant cells is characteristic of systemic or temporal arteritis and also Takayasu's arteritis.

Polyarteritis nodosa

This is a necrotizing vasculitis of small and medium-sized muscular arteries. There is multiple organ involvement with angiographic features of aneurysms in hepatic, renal and abdominal vessels. Elevated antineutrophil cytoplasmic antibodies (P-ANCA) are present in 80% of patients with 'pauci-immune' vasculitis. The prognosis will depend upon the organ systems involved, and can be improved with the use of corticosteroid and immunosuppressive therapy such as cyclophosphamide.

Diabetic nephropathy

Diabetic nephropathy accounts for 25% of adult patients developing end-stage renal failure. However, diabetes mellitus in childhood is rarely associated with significant clinical manifestations of renal disease. It is apparent that injury to the kidneys occurs shortly after the onset of the diabetic state, and a great deal of research has therefore centered on the detection of microalbuminuria as a marker of early diabetic nephropathy (Davies et al 1985). Tight glycemic control will prevent the mild physiological derangements of increased glomerular filtration rate and microalbuminuria, but established diabetic nephropathy with extensive basement membrane thickening cannot be reversed.

Amyloidosis

Juvenile rheumatoid arthritis (JRA) has become the most common cause of secondary amyloidosis in children following the eradication of tuberculosis and chronic osteomyelitis in western countries. However, it is very rare in childhood and only occurs after many years of severe disease. Renal vein thrombosis is a well documented complication of renal amyloidosis. Confirmation of the diagnosis requires biopsy material. Immunosuppressive agents such as busulphan may be of benefit.

PROTEINURIA

Although proteinuria is one of the cardinal features of renal disease, its isolated occurrence may be a transient finding in healthy children. Proteinuria combined with hematuria is much more significant.

Plasma proteins can cross the glomerular barrier depending upon their molecular size and charge. The glomerular capillary wall contains sialoproteins and proteoglycans, such as heparan sulfate, that are negatively charged. Proteinuria may result from increased glomerular permeability due to:

1. loss of the negative charges in the basement membrane
2. an increase in the effective pore size or number due to direct damage to the basement membrane, or possibly a change in the structure of the basement membrane resulting from loss of the anionic proteins
3. the hemodynamic effects of angiotensin II and other vasoactive amines which may explain the mild proteinuria seen with heart failure.

Albumin (MW = 69 000) is the predominant protein lost in the urine, but globulin excretion may also be increased.

Another type of proteinuria, *tubular* proteinuria, occurs when there is increased excretion of the normally filtered low-molecular weight proteins, such as immunoglobulin light chains and β2-microglobulin (MW <50 000). Tubular proteinuria occurs when proximal tubular reabsorption is impaired, as in the Fanconi syndrome, or when the production is increased to a level exceeding tubular reabsorption capacity, e.g. in multiple myeloma.

NORMAL VALUES

Most of the filtered protein is reabsorbed, and the normal daily protein excretion in a child is <4 mg/h/m^2, or <150 mg/24 h in an adult. Albumin accounts for about 25% of the normal protein excretion and after severe exercise proteinuria may increase several fold with the albumin excretion representing up to 80% of total urinary protein. 40% of normal urinary protein is of tissue origin, and the major protein in this group is uromucoid or Tamm–Horsfall protein which is produced in the distal tubule.

DETECTION

Testing for proteinuria has been simplified by the use of dipsticks which are impregnated with a dye, tetrabromophenol blue, which changes color according to the quantity of protein present. The strips detect predominantly albuminuria, but a negative dipstick does not exclude the presence in the urine of low concentrations of globulins, hemoglobin, Bence Jones protein or mucoproteins. These would be detected by 3% sulfosalicylic acid, which detects all proteins. However, dipsticks predominate in clinical practice. It is important to appreciate that false-negative results can also occur with very acid or dilute urine, whereas false-positive results may occur in the presence of highly concentrated or alkaline urine (pH >8) along with gross hematuria, pyuria and contamination with antiseptics, such as chlorhexidine.

Dipsticks are highly sensitive and cannot accurately measure protein excretion, which is best quantified using timed (preferably 24-h) urine collections. However, obtaining accurate 12- or 24-h urine collections in children can be difficult to accomplish. Single voided urine samples which relate the concentration of both the protein and creatinine in the same sample have a high correlation with 24-h urine excretion rates. The urine protein : creatinine ratio can be used to estimate the severity, and follow the progress, of proteinuric patients. The normal urine protein : creatinine ratio is <20 mg/mmol in the early morning urine sample (Elises et al 1988).

Protein selectivity index

This has usually been measured by comparing the clearances of small and large molecular weight proteins on the basis that diseases such as glomerulonephritis, which cause severe histological change to the glomeruli, are more likely to result in the urinary loss of large plasma proteins than are diseases such as minimal change nephrotic syndrome in which there is no obvious glomerular injury. However, there is considerable overlap in the results and the test is no longer performed routinely. It is preferable to rely on clinical features and/or the response to corticosteroids in children with nephrotic syndrome.

The causes of proteinuria are listed in Table 17.10.

INTERMITTENT PROTEINURIA

Transient proteinuria may be found in patients with high fevers in excess of 38.5°C. The mechanism is unknown and the proteinuria usually resolves as the fever abates.

Proteinuria, like hematuria, may also follow vigorous exercise and again usually resolves within 48 h of rest.

Postural or *orthostatic* proteinuria is important because it is a relatively frequent cause of referral to pediatric clinics. It is suggested by finding normal protein excretion in the supine position and increased protein excretion in the upright collection. It is best to confirm the diagnosis with accurately timed urine collections or protein : creatinine ratios on appropriate samples. Long-term follow-up has suggested that orthostatic proteinuria as an isolated finding is benign. These patients do not need prolonged follow-up in the clinic. However, it is important to note that patients with glomerular disease will often have an orthostatic component to their proteinuria, so that true orthostatic proteinuria

Table 17.10   Causes of proteinuria

INTERMITTENT PROTEINURIA
1. Postural (orthostatic)

2. Non-postural
   a. Exercise
   b. Fever
   c. Anatomic abnormalities, e.g. urinary tract
   d. Glomerular lesions, e.g. Berger's disease
   e. Random finding; no known cause

PERSISTENT PROTEINURIA
1. Glomerular
   a. Isolated asymptomatic proteinuria
   b. Damage to glomerular basement membrane, e.g. acute or chronic glomerulonephritis
   c. Loss or reduction of basement membrane anionic charge, e.g. minimal change and congenital nephrosis
   d. Increased permeability in residual nephrons, e.g. chronic renal failure

2. Tubular
   a. Hereditary, e.g. cystinosis, Wilson's disease, Lowe's syndrome proximal tubular acidosis, galactosemia
   b. Acquired, e.g. interstitial nephritis, acute tubular necrosis, post renal transplantation, pyelonephritis, vitamin D intoxication, penicillamine, heavy metal poisoning (gold, lead, mercury, etc.), analgesic abuse, drugs

should not be diagnosed unless the urine collected in the supine position has no protein detectable by routine methods.

PERSISTENT PROTEINURIA

In these patients, the amount of protein present in the individual samples may vary considerably, but is persistent unless it resolves as in acute glomerulonephritis. If the proteinuria is associated with additional evidence for renal disease, e.g. microscopic hematuria, then these patients are most likely to have significant pathology in the kidney or urinary tract.

GLOMERULAR PROTEINURIA

In the majority of cases, persistent proteinuria is of glomerular origin. The degree of proteinuria may range from >4 mg/h/m^2, to more than 400 mg/h/m^2 when it is usually associated with altered levels of protein in the plasma and nephrotic syndrome. Acute and chronic glomerulonephritis are believed to produce proteinuria as a result of damage to the glomerular basement membrane which increases the permeability to plasma proteins to a degree which overwhelms the tubular absorptive mechanisms. In conditions such as minimal change or congenital nephrotic syndrome it is usually a highly selective loss of albumin as a result of loss of the glomerular anionic charge for reasons still to be elucidated.

There has been a great deal of recent interest in patients who develop proteinuria with a reduced renal mass. Evidence has accumulated that the remaining nephrons in such patients are subject to hyperfiltration damage which produces progressive glomerulosclerosis (Fogo & Kon 1994).

TUBULAR PROTEINURIA

The amount of protein in the urine resulting from tubular damage is usually not as great as with glomerular disease but it has occasionally been sufficient to result in a nephrotic syndrome. Transient overflow proteinuria may occur after repeated blood or albumin infusions, and increased secretion of tubular proteins may occur with urinary tract infection or transiently in the neonatal period. Many hereditary causes of tubular proteinuria are part of a Fanconi-type syndrome.

PERSISTENT ASYMPTOMATIC PROTEINURIA

This is defined as proteinuria in apparently healthy children, occurring without hematuria but persisting on repeated testing over 3 months. Significant proteinuria (Uprot/Ucr >20 mg/mmol) is usually an indication for proceeding with further investigations. These would include urine culture, full blood count, blood chemistry including electrolytes, urea, creatinine, albumin and an accurate measurement of glomerular filtration rate. The serological tests are performed at the same time and will include antistreptolysin O. antinuclear antibodies, immunoglobulins and complement studies. A renal tract ultrasound and plain abdominal X-ray will usually exclude any significant urinary tract pathology. A renal biopsy will only be considered in those with confirmed proteinuria or when there are other abnormal tests, such as a decreased GFR, abnormal urinary sediment, hypocomplementemia or evidence of generalized vascular disease.

NEPHROTIC SYNDROME

The nephrotic syndrome is characterized by:

1. heavy proteinuria (>40 mg/h/m^2 or protein/creatinine ratio >200 mg/mmol)
2. hypoalbuminemia (<25 g/l)
3. edema.

The incidence of all forms of nephrotic syndrome in childhood is 2–4 per 100 000 population, but this figure will vary according to the ethnic mix of the population. For instance, the incidence amongst Asian children in two cities in the UK was reported as ranging from 9–16 per 100 000 respectively (Sharples et al 1985).

The predominant pathology is minimal change disease (MCD), with contributions from other pathologies such as FSGS and membranoproliferative glomerulonephritis. This applies only in Caucasian populations, as around the world the pathology varies. For instance, the predominant lesion in West Africa is quartan malaria nephropathy, with schistosomiasis being responsible for the majority of the cases in South America.

Nephrotic syndrome could be subdivided into congenital, idiopathic (primary) or secondary. Many of the secondary causes have already been mentioned, and include Henoch–Schönlein purpura nephritis; connective tissue disorders (e.g. SLE); toxic causes (e.g. drugs and heavy metal poisoning); sickle-cell disease; and amyloidosis.

IDIOPATHIC NEPHROTIC SYNDROME

Minimal change disease accounts for approximately 85% of cases presenting in childhood but only 10% of cases in adults. The other histological types of mesangial proliferative and focal segmental glomerulosclerosis may well represent the spectrum of a single disorder with varying histological features. There are familial cases of MCD, but these appear to be very rare in the UK, and there is no true inheritance pattern.

The cause of minimal change nephrotic syndrome remains unknown. It is more prevalent in families with an atopic history, and some studies have suggested an abnormality of T cell function. Although broad spectrum immunosuppressive drugs have been used to control the disease, there is lack of evidence for classical mechanisms of immunological injury.

In minimal change disease, the glomeruli appear normal or show a minimal increase in mesangial cells and matrix. The immunofluorescence studies are negative, and electron microscopy reveals gross epithelial cell process fusion which is a nonspecific finding in any patient with heavy proteinuria.

Clinical features

Minimal change nephrotic syndrome is more common in boys than girls (2 : 1) and usually occurs between the ages of 2–6 years. There may be an antecedent history of an upper respiratory tract infection and, certainly, these are well known to precipitate relapses in this condition. The presenting feature is usually edema which is first noticed around the eyes (Fig. 17.21). Since the condition is so uncommon in general practice, many children are treated for allergic conditions before the true nature of the condition is appreciated. The edema may become generalized, with swollen limbs, ascites and pleural effusions with diminishing

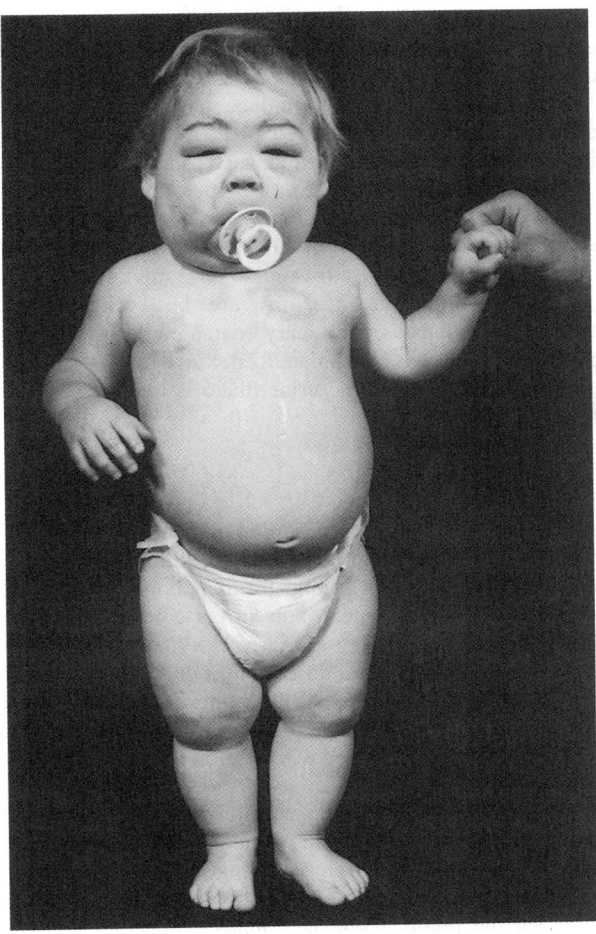

Fig. 17.21   17-month-old male infant with nephrotic syndrome and gross generalized edema (anasarca).

urine output. There may be lethargy, poor appetite, mild diarrhea and sometimes abdominal pain.

Investigations

The diagnosis is suggested by simple urinalysis which will show heavy proteinuria (+++ or >5 g/l). About 30% of patients will have transient microscopic hematuria, but gross hematuria is rare. Heavy proteinuria can be confirmed by timed urine collections or by early morning urine protein/creatinine ratio (>200 mg/mmol). Renal function is usually normal, but there will be a low serum albumin (<25 g/l) with raised serum cholesterol and triglyceride levels. Swabs should be taken from the throat and any skin lesions as well as a urine culture. Overt or covert infection can be the cause of steroid resistance. Serological tests such as complement studies, an ASO titer, hepatitis B surface antigen and antinuclear factor antibodies should be measured in selected cases especially when there is a mixed nephritic/nephrotic picture. The traditional urine protein selectivity index can be omitted because in terms of prognosis the response to corticosteroids is more important.

Children between the ages of 1 and 10 years are very likely to have *steroid-responsive minimal change disease* and so prednisolone therapy is usually initiated without a renal biopsy.

This latter procedure is recommended *before* treatment with corticosteroids when the nephrotic syndrome occurs:

1. onset at less that 6 months of age (congenital nephrotic syndrome types)
2. initial macroscopic hematuria (in the absence of infection) at any age
3. persistent microscopic hematuria if associated with hypertension and/or low plasma C3, especially if female and/or adolescent.

A biopsy may be *considered* in children with nephrotic syndrome and:

1. onset between 6 and 12 months of age
2. persistent hypertension, microscopic hematuria, or low plasma C3
3. renal failure – persistent and not attributable to hypovolemia.

Complications

Children with nephrotic syndrome still have a 1–2% mortality rate. The two major complications are infection and thrombosis.

Peritonitis is the most frequent type of infection and *Streptococcus pneumoniae* is the most common organism. Gram-negative bacteria are also encountered. The reasons for the susceptibility may be multifactorial and include decreased immunoglobulin levels, ascitic fluid acting as culture medium and immunosuppressive therapy. While on corticosteroids the clinical findings may be masked, and so any child with nephrotic syndrome and abdominal pain should be carefully evaluated in conjunction with a surgeon. Although there are instances where an unnecessary laparotomy has been carried out on a child with primary peritonitis before the edema and nephrotic state has been recognized, there are also instances of children with nephrotic syndrome and appendicitis. In the very edematous state penicillin prophylaxis may be considered but antibiotics to cover Gram-negative organisms should be used for any suspected peritonitis until the cultures and sensitivities are known. Some authors have advocated polyvalent pneumococcal vaccine when the child is in remission, but this does not appear to be fully effective as not all the serotypes are covered.

Chickenpox and measles are major threats to the immunocompromised child. The varicella-zoster and measles immunity status should be checked as part of the routine evaluation. Zoster immune globulin should be given if there is chickenpox exposure while taking high dose prednisolone or alkylating agents and acyclovir given promptly if the condition develops.

Nephrotic children also have a tendency to arterial and venous thrombosis. The nephrotic syndrome is a hypercoagulable state with high levels of fibrinogen, factor VIII: R: AG and $\alpha2$-macroglobulin with a decrease of both functional and immunological antithrombin III (Hoyer et al 1986). The greatest risk of thrombosis appears to be when the albumin level is very low. Children with nephrotic syndrome should be seen for prompt assessment if they have a potentially dehydrating state such as vomiting and diarrhea.

Treatment (Fig. 17.22)

Hospitalization should only be required for the initial attack, when the diagnosis can be established, treatment initiated and the

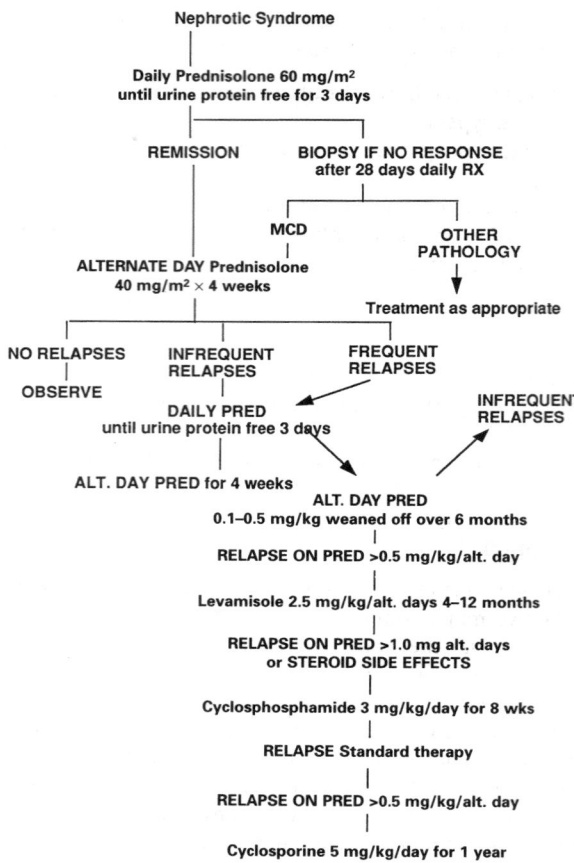

Fig. 17.22   Scheme for the management of children with nephrotic syndrome.

several days to act) can be used to control the edema until there is a diuretic response to the corticosteroids. Occasionally, metolazone (0.2–0.4 mg/kg per 24 h) in combination with frusemide may be needed to induce a diuresis, but careful biochemical monitoring is required.

If there are signs of hypovolemia, such as abdominal pain (due to a contracted plasma volume), hypertension, oliguria or evidence of renal insufficiency, then an intravenous salt-poor albumin infusion (1 g/kg) given over 1–2 h with careful monitoring and followed by frusemide (1–2 mg/kg) may reverse the situation. Albumin infusions are both expensive and potentially hazardous as pulmonary edema could be precipitated if the volume status has been misjudged. Since most of the infused albumin is rapidly lost in the urine, there is little place for their routine use.

Corticosteroid therapy

Minimal change nephrotic syndrome is characteristically steroid responsive, and after completion of the initial investigations, prednisolone (usually the soluble form) is commenced. Dosage regimes vary between centers, but current consensus suggests a regimen of prednisolone 60 mg/m² per 24 h (based on appropriate weight for height; maximum dose 80 mg) divided into two doses throughout the day (Consensus 1994). Intravenous methylprednisolone in equivalent dosages may be used in the vomiting child, but this therapy should be used with caution because of the greater risks of hypertension.

Daily prednisolone is maintained until the urine is protein free (negative or trace) for 3 days (based on dipstick testing of the first morning urine), when the dosage is changed to single dose therapy on alternate days of 40 mg/m² per 24 h. This is maintained for 28 days, when the prednisolone is stopped. There is usually little gastric upset from the use of soluble prednisolone, and the more expensive enteric coated forms or drugs to control gastric acidity are not routine.

85% of patients will lose their proteinuria within 4 weeks of the therapy. If there has been no response to daily steroids after 4 weeks then a change to alternate-day therapy and discussion with a pediatric nephrologist is warranted, as a renal biopsy is usually indicated to determine the underlying pathology. Before this, it is important to exclude occult infection such as urinary tract infection as a cause of the steroid resistance.

The parents should be told that daily steroids may well alter the child's behavior as well as increasing the appetite. General dietary advice about excess consumption of snacks, etc. should be given. A steroid warning card should be issued, and the parents should report if the child is exposed to infections such as measles or chickenpox while on daily steroids. Immunization using live vaccines should be avoided until the child has been off daily steroids for at least 3 months, but are permissible if the child is on alternate-day steroids (<0.5 mg/kg bodyweight/day). Killed vaccines are best given when the child is in remission, and inactivated rather than live polio utilized.

Steroid-responsive patients

The family are instructed in the use of dipsticks for recording the first morning urine protein results which should be carefully logged in a diary. This can serve as an individual record of the child's condition over a number of years.

response evaluated. It will also give an opportunity to educate the patient and the family in what may be a frustrating chronic illness. Good education and efficient communication should enable further problems to be assessed and treated on an outpatient basis.

Bed rest does not need to be enforced, and activity level can be determined by the child.

Dietary advice

The traditional high-protein, no-salt-intake diet should be abandoned in favor of trying to maintain the recommended daily allowances of calories and protein in a child whose appetite is likely to be markedly diminished until on steroids (Watson & Coleman 1993). When edema is present, a no-added-salt diet is advised with avoidance of foods known to be high in sodium, particularly snack or processed foods.

Diuretics

A moderate fluid restriction of 750–1000 ml is advocated in the edematous state. Diuretics should be used with caution in plasma-volume-depleted nephrotic patients, as they may be predisposed to fluid and electrolyte disturbances. Thiazide diuretics have little effect. Cautious use of loop diuretics such as frusemide (1–2 mg/kg per 24 h) in combination with an aldosterone antagonist such as spironolactone 0.5–5 mg/kg per 24 h (which may take

When there is a relapse of proteinuria (three consecutive days of heavy proteinuria (++ or greater)), treatment may be withheld for up to 5 days or possibly 10, unless the child becomes edematous. This is because some children will spontaneously remit during this period. If proteinuria persists, then remission is induced with daily steroids as before until the urine is protein free for 3 days, and then alternate-day corticosteroids are continued for 28 days. More than 75% of children with minimal change nephrotic syndrome will have at least one relapse.

Frequent relapses or steroid dependency

If the child has two or more relapses within 6 months of initial treatment or four or more relapses within any 12-month period (frequent relapser) then a slow weaning dose of alternate-day prednisolone may be considered after inducing remission with daily steroids as above. The prednisolone may be weaned off over 6 months, and by this means steroid toxicity may be minimized.

Steroid dependency may be defined as those who relapse on two consecutive occasions as prednisolone is being decreased, or within 2 weeks of it being discontinued. If a child requires more than 0.5 mg/kg of prednisolone on alternate days to remain protein free, and particularly if there are signs of steroid toxicity, then alternative therapy should be considered. Such steroid side-effects would include stunting of growth, cataracts, obesity and behavioral changes, but alternative therapy to corticosteroids and/or the advice of a pediatric nephrologist will, preferably, have been sought before many of these side-effects are manifest. Alternative therapy consists of levamisole, cyclophosphamide, chlorambucil and cyclosporine (Fig. 17.22).

Cyclophosphamide

When cyclophosphamide was originally used in MCNS it was prescribed for 6–12 months and achieved 90% long-term remission. However, this was before gonadal toxicity was appreciated, and many young men were subsequently rendered oligo- or azoospermic. Consequently, the course of cyclophosphamide had been restricted to 8 weeks and is given after remission has been induced with daily steroids which are then usually tapered off over 4–6 weeks. The restriction to shorter courses of 8 weeks means the remission rate has been reduced to approximately 50% at 2 years.

The potential toxic effects of bone marrow depression, hemorrhagic cystitis and mild alopecia can be minimized by close monitoring of weekly blood counts and clinic visits. Although there is no firm guarantee of future fertility, restriction of therapy to less than 16 weeks or 300 mg/kg bodyweight appears to be safe (Watson et al 1985, 1986). Nevertheless, this point needs to be discussed at length with the parents, as a prolonged remission cannot be guaranteed and there may still be long-term effects from the use of this drug. Chlorambucil does not appear to be superior to cyclophosphamide and its use has been more limited.

It was once customary to perform a renal biopsy on all nephrotic children *prior* to cyclophosphamide therapy. However, this is probably no longer justifiable if the patient is still *steroid responsive*. Even if focal segmental glomerulosclerosis changes are found on biopsy, the best prognostic indicator remains *steroid responsiveness*.

Psychosocial

We have found it helpful to provide the family of a child with nephrotic syndrome with an information booklet about the condition, as a great deal of anxiety can result with the clinical course of relapse and remission. In addition the parents have benefited from attending a local parents' group where they can discuss and share many of their anxieties (Moore et al 1994).

If a nephrotic child has been free of relapses for 5 years, then there is a strong chance of a long-term remission. However, some children may continue to relapse into adult life, and those who develop nephrosis earlier in life are likely to relapse more often (Lewis et al 1989). With a decreasing relapse rate the urine tests can be performed less frequently, but the family should be cautioned to test at times of stress such as incidental infection.

FOCAL SEGMENTAL GLOMERULOSCLEROSIS (FSGS)

This is characterized on light microscopy by sclerosis or hyalinosis of glomeruli in a focal and segmental distribution. The involved area obliterates Bowman's space and is adherent to the capsule without epithelial cell proliferation. Epithelial foot process fusion is similar to that seen in MCD and electron microscopy should confirm the sclerosing nature of the lesion. There may be nonspecific deposition of IgM and C3 in the affected segments. Tubular atrophy and interstitial fibrosis are proportional to the extent of glomerular damage.

The typical features of FSGS may be missed if the renal biopsy is too superficial, as the changes are more likely to be seen in the juxtamedullary region. Focal segmental glomerulosclerosis usually carries with it an entirely different prognosis from minimal lesion, especially if the patient is steroid resistant. Again, the important practice point is that if the patient responds to steroids then whether the histology shows MCD and FSGS is generally irrelevant as long as steroid resistance does not develop. Even when the patient is steroid resistant, some authors have advocated the use of immunosuppressive agents such as cyclophosphamide (Cortes & Tejani 1996). This agent may reduce the proteinuria sufficiently for the patient to remain edema free, with all its attendant benefits.

CONGENITAL NEPHROTIC SYNDROME

Nephrotic syndrome is very rare during the first year of life, and an onset before 3 months of age implies an inborn basis for this disorder. Congenital nephrotic syndrome was predominantly described in children of Finnish extraction (hence 'Finnish type') and is an autosomal recessive disorder. The major pathological feature is dilation of the proximal convoluted tubules (microcystic disease), but this is very variable. The glomeruli may initially appear quite normal by light microscopy, but later show mesangial hypercellularity with an increase in matrix. Most glomeruli are immature. Both sexes are equally affected, and prematurity with a placenta which weighs more than 25% of the infant's birthweight is typical. Proteinuria is usually present at birth, and a frank nephrotic syndrome is usually apparent within 3 months of life. The clinical course is one of persistent edema and recurrent infections.

This condition was previously almost invariably fatal before 2 years of age. However, more aggressive feeding regimes with unilateral or bilateral nephrectomy and the appropriate management for end-stage renal disease has resulted in increasing numbers of children being successfully transplanted with normal growth and development (Holmberg et al 1996). Genetic counseling is very important, as antenatal diagnosis is possible by measuring the α-fetoprotein level in the amniotic fluid as early as 15 weeks of gestation. The gene for the Finnish type has been mapped to the long arm of chromosome 19.

Other histological types have been described in association with nephrotic syndrome in the first year of life (Table 17.11). Diffuse mesangial sclerosis is a steroid-resistant lesion with progressive loss of renal function, and renal replacement therapy may be required in the second year of life. Patients with the histological appearances of focal segmental glomerulosclerosis and minimal change have also been described in very young patients. Biopsy is therefore essential, because minimal change may respond to a course of steroids.

In any female infant with early-onset nephrotic syndrome, chromosome analysis should be considered as there is an association between nephrotic syndrome, pseudohermaphroditism and Wilms' tumor (Drash syndrome). There appears to be a distinctive kidney lesion characterized by fibrillar sclerosing of the mesangium, thickening of the glomerular capillary walls and mesangial deposits of IgM.

Secondary causes of infantile nephrotic syndrome are shown in Table 17.11. Syphilis can cause a membranous type of glomerular nephropathy, while cytomegalovirus and toxoplasmosis may be coincidental rather than causative agents. Mercury intoxication can cause a nephrotic syndrome which usually responds to withdrawal of the toxic agent.

RENAL HYPERTENSION

The prevalence of hypertension in childhood is not clearly defined but is believed to be between 1 and 3%. About 10% of such children will have a secondary cause for their hypertension (Dillon 1987). Reference needs to be made to appropriate centile charts of blood pressure for the child's sex and height when deciding whether a child is hypertensive (de Man et al 1991). Sustained hypertension, especially if severe, is likely to be due to renal disease.

Causes

The causes of renal hypertension are listed in Table 17.12.

Renal parenchymal disease is the largest category. The hypertension may occur acutely as with acute renal failure from any cause (particularly hemolytic uremic syndrome), acute glomerulonephritis and Henoch–Schönlein nephritis. Hypertension in these situations is often accentuated by fluid overload,

Table 17.11 Causes of infantile nephrotic syndrome

Primary	a.	Congenital nephrotic syndrome – 'Finnish' microcystic disease
	b.	Diffuse mesangial sclerosis
	c.	Minimal change nephrotic syndrome
	d.	Focal segmental glomerulosclerosis
	e.	Drash syndrome
Secondary	a.	Syphilis
	b.	Toxoplasmosis
	c.	Cytomegalovirus
	d.	Mercury
	e.	Nail–patella syndrome

Table 17.12 Causes of renal hypertension

1. Chronic renal failure and post renal transplant

2. Renal parenchymal disease
   a. Scarring due to reflux nephropathy or obstructive uropathy
   b. Acute or chronic glomerulonephritis
   c. Hemolytic uremic syndrome
   d. Renal dysplasia
   e. Polycystic kidneys

3. Renovascular disease
   a. Renal artery stenosis
   b. Renal artery thrombosis
   c. Renal artery aneurysm
   d. Arteriovenous fistula
   e. Vasculitis, e.g. polyarteritis nodosa

4. Renal tumors
   a. Nephroblastoma
   b. Hamartoma
   c. Hemangiopericytoma

but in many other cases the renal parenchymal disease is associated with the excess production of renin. The most important cause in this category is scarring associated with reflux nephropathy (formally called chronic pyelonephritis) or obstructive uropathy. One of the reasons for following children for coarse renal scarring associated with reflux, either in the clinic or in general practice, is to detect the 8–10% who may well develop hypertension (Goonasekara et al 1996). The onset of hypertension in such children can be quite explosive, with the first manifestation being headaches, central nervous disturbance and convulsions.

Investigations

In moderate (blood pressures consistently above the 95th centile for age and sex) and severe hypertension, investigations will include urinalysis, urine culture, full blood count, electrolytes, creatinine, calcium, phosphate and a peripheral vein renin and aldosterone measurement. The chest X-ray, ECG (preferably echocardiogram) and 24-h urine for vanilylmandelic acid (VMA) and catecholamines (or urine VMA : creatinine ratio) should also be considered. However, investigations must include imaging of the renal tract, which initially will be with plain abdominal X-ray, ultrasound and chest X-ray. Further imaging may include radionuclide imaging such as ^{99m}Tc dimercaptosuccinic acid (DMSA) scanning and further investigation of a renal mass may include computer tomographic scanning. If renal vascular disease is considered then angiographic investigation in a specialist center will be required. (Fig. 17.23) If a small shrunken kidney is found on investigation, then its removal may be considered if it contributes less than 10% to the overall kidney function and it is proven, by measuring the renin levels from both renal veins, to be the source of excess renin production.

Treatment

The list of hypertensive agents is shown in Table 17.13. The pharmacokinetics and exact dosing schedules of many of these drugs have not been fully evaluated in children, as many drugs are not licensed for use in children. It is important to consider compliance, particularly in the long term with adolescent patients. The favored combination is a beta adrenergic blocker such as

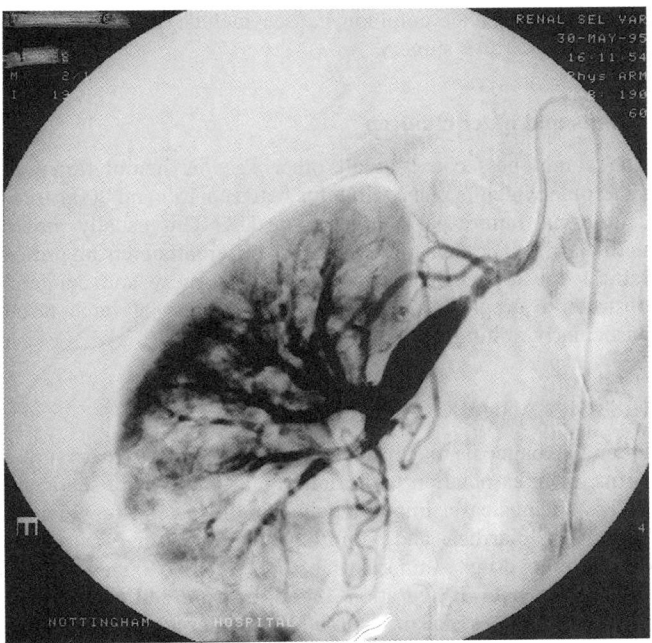

Fig. 17.23   Renal angiogram in 13-year-old female with sustained hypertension and abnormal spectral Doppler flow on ultrasound. 33% stenosis of the mid portion of the main renal artery.

Table 17.14   Maintenance oral therapy for treatment of hypertension

Vasodilators		
Nifedipine	0.25–2 mg/kg per 24 h	2 divided doses
Hydralazine	1–8 mg/kg per 24 h	2–3 divided doses
Prazosin	0.05–0.4 mg/kg per 24 h	2–3 divided doses
Minoxidil	200 µg–1.0 mg/kg	Single dose
Beta-blockers		
Propanolol	1–10 mg/kg per 24 h	2–3 divided doses
Atenolol	1–4 mg/kg per 24 h	Once/day if adequate renal function
Diuretics		
Frusemide	1–5 mg/kg per 24 h	1–2 divided doses
Spironolactone	1–3 mg/kg per 24 h	1–2 divided doses
ACE inhibitors		
Captopril	0.5–5 mg/kg per 24 h	2–3 divided doses
Enalapril	0.1 mg–1 mg/kg per 24 h	Single dose

propanolol in two to three divided doses or once daily atenolol (if renal function is adequate) with a vasodilator such as slow-release nifedipine (Table 17.14). The angiotensin converting enzyme inhibitor, captopril, has proved very useful in patients with renin-dependent hypertension and, again, the equivalent once daily enalapril should help with long-term compliance and ease of administration.

Nephrectomy or heminephrectomy may be considered in some instances. Success has been achieved by percutaneous balloon angioplasty or direct vascular surgery in patients with renal artery stenosis.

ACUTE RENAL FAILURE

Acute renal failure (ARF) is a sudden decrease in renal function resulting in an accumulation of nitrogenous wastes and associated with fluid and electrolyte imbalance. A urine output of 300 ml/m^2/24 h (or 0.5 ml/kg/h in infants) is required to excrete the daily solute output. Acute renal failure is therefore usually associated with oliguria, although it may be associated with

polyuria, particularly in the neonate. The incidence of acute renal failure in children varies according to the population studied. In the UK the incidence based on those children referred to regional nephrology units for further management suggested an incidence of 7.5 children per million population per year (BAPN 1995).

PATHOGENESIS

Prerenal

If renal perfusion pressure falls, renal blood flow and glomerular filtration rate (GFR) decline but there is excretion of good quality urine (see Table 17.15). Causes include:

1. excess losses
—gastroenteritis
—diabetes
—burns
—ileus
—hemorrhage
  These children appear dehydrated with signs including sunken fontanel, poor peripheral perfusion with wide peripheral core temperature gap, tachycardia, and hypotension.
2. impaired cardiac output
—congestive heart failure
—pericardial tamponade
—sepsis/shock
3. hypoalbuminemic states
—nephrotic syndrome
—liver failure
  These children are often edematous but have intravascular volume depletion with signs including poor peripheral perfusion

Table 17.13   Drug therapy of hypertensive crisis

Drug	Administration	Onset of effect	Side effects
Nifedipine	Sublingual hourly p.r.n. 0.2–0.5 mg/kg	Minutes	Headaches, tachycardia
Sodium nitroprusside	0.5–10 mcg/kg/min as infusion	Seconds/minutes	VERY rapid effect, titrate dose, cyanide accumulates after 48 hours of use
Labetalol	1–3 mg/kg/hr	10–30 min	Postural hypotension
Hydralazine	Slow i.v. 0.1–0.5 mg/kg	10–30 min	Tachycardia, flushing, headaches
Phentolamine	0.02–0.1 mg/kg	Minutes	Use in catecholamine excess states

Table 17.15   Biochemical urine indices in renal failure

	Prerenal	Renal
Urine osmolality	> 500	< 350
Urine Na	< 20 mmol/l	> 40 mmol/l
U/P creatinine	> 40	< 20
U/P urea	> 15	< 5

with wide peripheral core temperature gap and tachycardia. Blood pressure, particularly in nephrotic syndrome, is variable.

Renal

Intrarenal causes of renal failure may be vascular, glomerular or tubular. These children are more likely to present with oliguria and signs of fluid overload, although those with tubular damage may present with polyuric renal failure. Causes include:

1. vascular
—renal vein thrombosis
—arterial occlusion
—arteritis
—hemolytic uremic syndrome
2. glomerular
—acute glomerulonephritis
3. tubular
—nephrotoxins (especially drugs)
—acute interstitial nephritis
—myoglobinuria
—hemoglobinuria
—crystal nephropathy
—secondary to prerenal failure.

Postrenal

Many children with obstructive causes present acutely with infection associated with obstruction and have signs of septicemia. A poor urinary stream or a palpable bladder is highly suggestive of bladder outflow obstruction. Causes include:
—posterior urethral valves
—pelviureteric junction obstruction
—vesicoureteric junction obstruction
—neuropathic bladder
—nephrolithiasis.

AGE AT PRESENTATION

The cause of renal failure varies according to the age group of the child.

Neonates

The commonest cause in neonates is perinatal asphyxia. The frequency of acute renal failure in association with asphyxia is unclear as this depends on the definitions used and the population studied. Although up to 60% of severely asphyxiated infants in one study were shown to have renal failure none of these required dialysis (Karlowicz & Adelman 1995). Renal failure in association with asphyxia is usually polyuric renal failure which can be managed conservatively with appropriate fluid

management. Other common causes include posterior urethral valves and cardiac surgery.

Infants and older children

The commonest cause at all other ages is hemolytic uremic syndrome which is responsible for between 150 and 200 cases of acute renal failure per annum in the UK. This usually presents with diarrhea and thus may need to be differentiated from prerenal failure due to diarrhea losses. Cardiac surgery and congenital obstructive uropathy remain important causes of renal failure, particularly in infancy.

HISTORY AND EXAMINATION

Often the diagnosis may be clear, e.g. after cardiac bypass surgery, burns, or in association with multiorgan failure as in septicemia. In less obvious cases important clues in the history may include a history of diarrhea and vomiting, a poor urinary stream or exposure to drugs. Important features to note on examination include the state of hydration, blood pressure and other features including the presence of enlarged kidneys or a palpable bladder.

INVESTIGATIONS

Initial investigations should include full biochemical indices, including renal function and acid base status together with hematological indices, including a blood film, and in many cases a blood culture. Dipstick urinalysis for blood and protein, microscopy and culture of the urine should also be performed and in some cases urine electrolytes may be helpful in differentiating prerenal and renal failure (see Table 17.15). A renal tract ultrasound will give information on renal size and will exclude obstruction.

All other investigations ordered will depend on these initial screening results. If the ultrasound suggests bladder outflow obstruction a micturating cystogram will be necessary to demonstrate the presence of urethral valves. If the ultrasound suggests pelviureteric obstruction a percutaneous nephrostomy together with a nephrostogram (or antegrade pyelogram) will be both therapeutic and diagnostic.

If the clinical picture is that of acute glomerulonephritis then further serological investigations and a renal biopsy will help to elucidate the cause and also guide further management with respect to immunosuppressive therapy (see Glomerulonephritis).

MANAGEMENT

Fluids and circulation

Volume depletion with a low blood pressure, low central venous pressure and a wide peripheral core temperature gap requires resuscitation with either volume expanders, e.g. isotonic saline, or plasma 20 ml/kg. If the low blood pressure persists despite adequate volume an inotrope may be indicated. Dopamine 2 µg/kg/min improves renal perfusion but doses of 5–10 µg/kg/min may be required to elevate systemic blood pressure. If poor peripheral perfusion remains, i.e. a wide peripheral core temperature gap, despite an adequate circulating volume and perfusion pressure, a vasodilator, hydralazine 0.2 mg/kg, may reverse the peripheral vasoconstriction.

Volume overload with hypertension, raised central venous pressure and edema may be treated with a diuretic frusemide 1–5 mg/kg/intravenously. If there is no response dialysis is indicated.

Maintenance fluids should be calculated as insensible losses together with continuing losses. Daily fluid requirements are directly related to energy expended. In practice, insensible losses are calculated as approximately 400 ml/m² body surface area or 20 ml/kg bodyweight. Modifications are required in the presence of fever (an increase of 12% of calculated insensible losses per degree above 37.5°C), tachypnea (an increase of 20–25%), or in neonates nursed under radiant heaters (an increase of 25%).

Electrolyte disturbances

Hyperkalemia

- 10% calcium gluconate 0.5 ml/kg over 5–10 min antagonizes the effect of hyperkalemia on cells and is useful for prevention, or treatment of cardiac dysrhythmias.
- 8.4% sodium bicarbonate 1–2 mmol/kg may lower serum potassium in the presence of acidosis.
- Glucose 0.5 g/kg/h with insulin 0.1 u/kg/h intravenously acts rapidly (within 1 h) to lower potassium but has been superseded by:
- Salbutamol (β2 adrenoceptor stimulant) as the first choice treatment (McClure et al 1994). Salbutamol can be given intravenously (4 µg/kg in 10 ml of water over 10 min) or by nebulizer (2.5 mg <25 kg bodyweight or 5 mg >25 kg bodyweight).
- Calcium resonium 1 g/kg orally or rectally acts more slowly.

The above measures should only be regarded as temporary until dialysis can be established.

Hyponatremia

Hyponatremia may be associated with neurological disturbances and convulsions particularly with values less than 120 mmol/l. This is often due to fluid overload and therefore treatment should be aimed at fluid removal. However, excess losses, particularly gastrointestinal, are associated with true sodium deficits which should be replaced. Sodium deficit may be calculated as follows: mmol sodium deficit = (140 – actual serum sodium) × 0.6 × bodyweight in kg.

Half the deficit should be replaced in the first 24 h and the situation reviewed.

Hypocalcemia

Symptomatic patients may be given a bolus of 10% calcium gluconate 0.5 ml/kg intravenously over 5–10 min. Slower correction may be achieved by an infusion of 10% calcium gluconate 0.1 mmol/calcium/kg bodyweight/h. The dose should be adjusted by frequent blood monitoring at least 6-hourly. Reduction of high phosphate levels may also improve plasma calcium levels.

Hypomagnesemia

50% magnesium sulfate 0.1 ml/kg intramuscularly.

Acidosis

Sodium bicarbonate 2 mmol/kg intravenously as immediate treatment. The total deficit may be calculated as follows:
(24 – the actual bicarbonate) × 0.6 × bodyweight in kg

Half this amount may be given as an infusion over 4–6 h, and the acid base status rechecked. Sodium bicarbonate needs to be given with caution, particularly in neonates and infants, as it may cause sodium, and thus fluid overload as well as precipitating hypocalcemic symptoms.

Hyperuricemia

Uric acid levels are elevated in ARF and no specific treatment is usually given. *Tumor lysis* syndrome with grossly elevated uric acid levels can occur in the treatment of lymphomas and leukemia and a high fluid intake, allopurinol and an alkali therapy are usually employed (Jones et al 1995). However, the production of uric acid may be switched to that of xanthine and hypoxanthine which can also cause a crystalline nephropathy.

Convulsions

Convulsions may be due to electrolyte disturbances, uremia, hypertension, or the underlying disease such as hemolytic uremic syndrome. Many anticonvulsants tend to accumulate in renal failure. The safest emergency treatment is diazepam 0.25 mg/kg intravenously.

Hypertension

Hypertension may be due to fluid overload which should be treated appropriately. Severe hypertension should be treated with labetalol 1–3 mg/kg/h as an intravenous infusion which will lower blood pressure in a controlled manner. Nitroprusside 0.5–0.8 µg/kg/min intravenously is a suitable alternative although cyanide levels need to be monitored after 24 h. If intravenous access is difficult sublingual nifedipine 0.25 mg/kg is an effective alternative. For sustained moderate hypertension a suitable regimen is a beta-blocker (e.g. propranolol) with or without a vasodilator (e.g. hydralazine) and/or calcium channel blocker (e.g. nifedipine).

Nutrition

Adequate nutrition is essential to prevent catabolism and the child should receive at least the estimated average requirement (EAR) for energy for chronological age. Energy is best provided as a combination of carbohydrate and fat, often using glucose polymers exclusively or in combination with fat emulsions. Protein intake will depend upon whether the child is being managed conservatively or is on dialysis (Watson 1995a). Enteral feeding should be used whenever possible, although intravenous feeding may on occasions be necessary. Fluid restriction may limit the amount of nutrition that can be administered and this may be an indication to institute dialysis or increase ultrafiltration on dialysis. Specialized renal feeds often contain a high energy density and may need to be introduced gradually to prevent gastrointestinal intolerance. The protein, phosphate, sodium and potassium content of feeds need to be analyzed carefully as many are unsuitable for use in renal failure.

Anemia

This is inevitable in ARF but transfusion is only indicated if there are symptoms or the hemoglobin concentration is less than 6 g/dl or falling rapidly. Caution is required in transfusing a child who is not on dialysis as hyperkalemia and fluid overload may be precipitated.

Dialysis

The need for dialysis will in part be guided by the anticipated prognosis for recovery. If a quick return of renal function seems likely then the child may be managed conservatively. However, if a prolonged period of oliguria seems likely it is better to dialyze earlier and be able to ensure adequate nutrition as well as maintain metabolic balance. Guidelines on the indications for dialysis may be:

1. uncontrollable fluid overload/hypertension
2. uncontrollable acidosis
3. symptomatic electrolyte disturbances not controlled by above measures
4. symptomatic uremia
5. presence of a dialyzable toxin
6. established anuria, even if 1–5 not present, provided obstruction excluded.

Peritoneal dialysis

Peritoneal dialysis is the preferred option for most patients and particularly useful in the hemodynamically unstable patient who may tolerate hemodialysis, or even hemofiltration, poorly.

A soft Silastic or a more rigid polyethylene catheter is inserted percutaneously into the abdomen using a Seldinger technique. Commercially available dialysis solutions containing electrolytes, and glucose as an osmotic agent, are then introduced into the abdominal cavity. The volume and duration of the cycles of fluid are adjusted according to the ultrafiltration and clearance requirements of the patient.

Hemodialysis

Hemodialysis may be used in patients in whom there are technical difficulties encountered in running peritoneal dialysis, for example catheter blockage or leakage. It may also be used in those children in whom peritoneal dialysis is contraindicated, for example children with intra-abdominal sepsis, major intra-abdominal pathology or following recent abdominal surgery. Vascular access is usually obtained via a venous catheter inserted percutaneously into a large vessel (either subclavian or femoral vein), to permit the necessary rapid blood flow rates required. Commercially available filters and lines are available to enable hemodialysis to be undertaken even in neonates.

Hemofiltration

Hemofiltration is an alternative therapy in the critically ill, immobile child as it is usually well tolerated (Kierdorf & Sieberth 1995). It involves an extracorporeal procedure whereby plasma is ultrafiltered by hydrostatic pressure across a highly permeable hemofilter. In conventional continuous arteriovenous hemofiltration (CAVH) hydrostatic pressure is generated by the patient's

own arteriovenous gradient (Fig. 17.24). However, if there is difficulty in obtaining arterial access then continuous venovenous hemofiltration (CVVH) can be undertaken, often using the standard double lumen catheters used for hemodialysis. A blood pump is then required in the exit venous line. The most important use of hemofiltration is for safe removal of fluid often from unstable critically ill patients. Convective transport of solutes does however also occur and can be increased by running dialysis fluid countercurrent across the filter, a procedure known as continuous hemodialfiltration (Fig. 17.25) CAVH does not require the use of specialized equipment and can therefore be run by most trained intensive care staff. CVVH or hemodialfiltration (CVVHD), however, require the expertise of hemodialysis trained staff.

Drugs

The kidney is the major route of elimination of many drugs and their metabolites. Decreased renal function leads to both predictable and unpredictable changes in the pharmacokinetic profiles of various drugs. Many drugs will also be removed by dialysis although as peritoneal and hemodialysis remove different sized molecules, the elimination of drugs may be different with the two forms of dialysis. It is therefore essential to refer to either drug data sheets or a reference text (Wong et al 1994) to ensure the correct dosages of drugs are administered.

Family support

Acute renal failure is an uncommon problem in developed countries. When dialysis is anticipated or a biopsy is necessary the child is transferred to a designated pediatric nephrology center which can be some distance away from the patient's home, which adds to the stress. Appropriate information and psychosocial

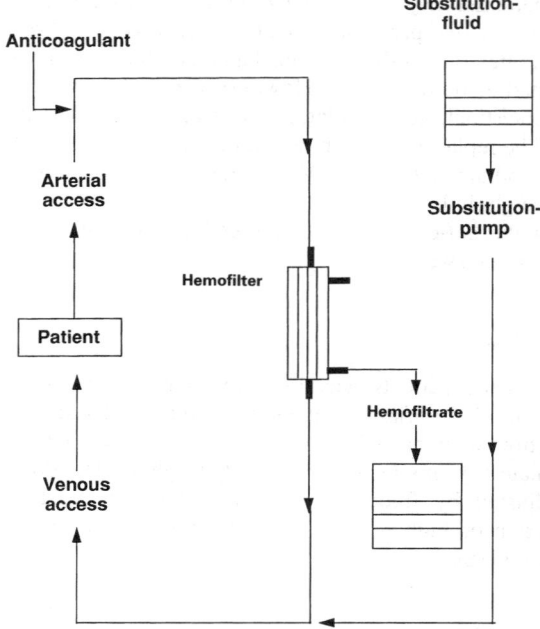

Fig. 17.24 Schematic diagram of continuous arteriovenous hemofiltration (CAVH).

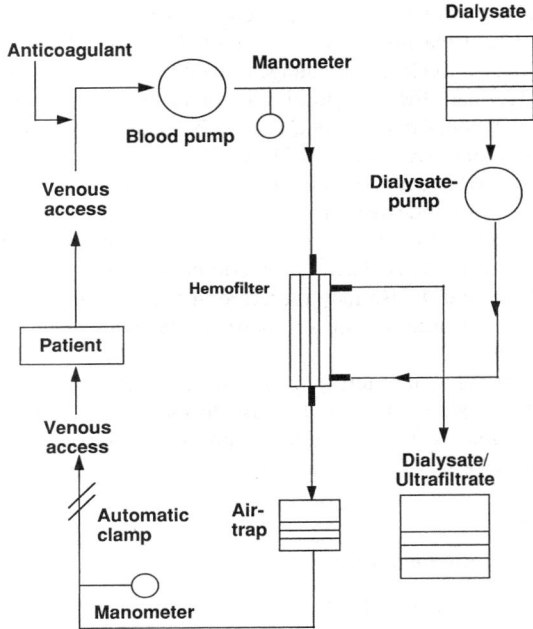

Fig. 17.25 Schematic diagram of continuous venovenous hemodiafiltration (CVVHD).

support from the center's multidisciplinary team are very necessary.

HEMOLYTIC UREMIC SYNDROME

The hemolytic uremic syndromes (HUS) comprise a heterogeneous group of disorders in which a triad of features, microangiopathic hemolytic anemia, thrombocytopenia and acute renal failure occur together. They are a major cause of acute renal failure in childhood responsible for around 150–200 cases per annum in the UK and can be classified into two categories, the epidemic and sporadic forms.

The epidemic form occurs most commonly in the summer months, affects younger children and is associated with a prodromal illness usually of bloody diarrhea. The majority of these cases are associated with infections, the commonest etiologic agent being the verocytotoxin producing *E. coli*. A variety of other bacteria, viruses and *Rickettsiae* have also been described in association with the syndrome. The prognosis for a full recovery in this group is excellent and 85% can be expected to make a full recovery.

The sporadic form is much rarer and accounts for only 5% of the total number of cases. There is no seasonal incidence nor a prodromal illness. This group includes those rare relapsing and familial cases. 70% of this group progress to renal failure.

Clinical features

The commonest presentation is with gastrointestinal symptoms, usually bloody diarrhea. This prodrome may last for up to 2 weeks before the onset of the triad of features comprising the syndrome. Increasing pallor and mild jaundice due to hemolysis are noted, together with decreasing urine output. Typical hematological features are then present, the blood film revealing a microangiopathic hemolytic anemia, with thrombocytopenia and the presence of fragmented red cells. Biochemical changes indicative of renal dysfunction together with macroscopic or microscopic hematuria and variable proteinuria are indicative of renal dysfunction. There is often no correlation between the severity of the hemolysis and the renal failure. Other nonrenal features include:

Gastrointestinal

Colitis is a feature of the disease and it may be difficult to distinguish between the prodrome and the onset of the disease itself. The presence of abdominal pain, and the passage of blood and mucus per rectum may lead to misdiagnosis as intussusception, ulcerative colitis or even Henoch–Schönlein syndrome. The acute colitic phase is usually self-limited although, when severe, complications such as rectal prolapse, bowel necrosis with perforation, or intussusception can occur.

Cardiorespiratory

Most of the cardiovascular manifestations are due to volume overload. However, there are reports of cardiac involvement with thrombotic microangiopathy resulting in myocarditis, cardiomyopathy and cardiac failure.

Neurological

Minor neurological disturbances of irritability, drowsiness, myoclonic jerks and tremor or ataxia are common. These may be due to metabolic derangements, or accelerated hypertension as well as a result of neurological involvement in the disease. More major neurological involvement such as coma, focal neurological deficit or decerebrate rigidity occurs less frequently although seizures may occur in up to 30% of patients (Gallo & Gianantonio 1995). Although children who have neurological involvement may have severe neurological impairment many will recover completely or with only minor deficits (Siegler et al 1991).

Pathogenesis

The endothelial cell is the main site of injury in hemolytic uremic syndrome and a variety of mechanisms have been postulated (Kaplan et al 1990).

Verocytotoxins

The association of a verocytotoxin producing *E. coli*, most commonly serotype 0157: H7, with the epidemic form of HUS was first described in 1983. Verocytotoxin has been shown to be cytopathic to cultured endothelial cells. Other observations have suggested that neutrophils may also have an important role in this pathogenesis. A high neutrophil count, $> 20 \times 10^9$, is associated with an adverse prognosis (Coad et al 1991) with 93% of patients having a neutrophil count $< 20 \times 10^9$ having a good outcome compared to 33% of those with a neutrophil count $> 20 \times 10^9$. Neutrophils from patients with HUS have been shown to have increased adhesion to endothelium and able to induce endothelial injury in vitro. It is postulated that these activated neutrophils degranulate onto endothelium causing damage by local release of proteases such as elastase, which has been found to be elevated in patients with HUS.

Verocytotoxin also causes the release of von Willebrand factor (factor VIII related antigen) which mediates platelet adhesion to the endothelium and promotes the formation of platelet thrombi. Raised factor VIII related antigens together with an abnormal multimer pattern have been shown in HUS. These abnormalities return to normal on recovery but have been shown to persist in patients with recurrent episodes or in patients with progressive disease.

Prostacyclin

Prostacyclin is produced by normal endothelial cells and is a powerful inhibitor of platelet aggregation. Its precise role in the pathogenesis of HUS remains controversial although prostacyclin activity has been shown to be low, either due to accelerated prostacyclin degradation or due to a reduction in production of prostacyclin in some patients with HUS.

Neuraminidase

Neuraminidase is an enzyme produced by a number of microorganisms, although in many it is cell bound and not released. It removes sialic acid from erythrocytes, platelets and glomeruli exposing the hidden Thomsen–Friedenreich antigen (T-cryptantigen). Anti-T, an IgM antibody present in most adult plasma can then react with this exposed antigen leading to all the clinical manifestations of HUS. This phenomenon has been described in association with sporadic HUS in association with, most commonly, *Streptococcus pneumoniae* but also other infections including influenza, parainfluenza, *Clostridium perfringens*, and *Bacteroides fragilis*.

Management

Many children with hemolytic uremic syndrome can be successfully managed with supportive therapy and careful attention to fluid balance without the need for dialysis. However, it is essential to arrive at the diagnosis as soon as possible as much morbidity can be induced by inappropriate fluid therapy in patients whose renal function is compromised. Therefore the diagnosis should be suspected in any child with acute bloody diarrhea, and biochemistry, hematology and fluid balance monitored appropriately. Children with deteriorating renal function, oliguria/anuria or poor prognostic features should be referred early to a pediatric nephrology center. Poor prognostic features would include older children without a diarrheal prodrome, evidence of nonrenal involvement including encephalopathy or cardiomyopathy, or those children with a high neutrophil count $> 20 \times 10^9/l$. A prospective study of children with HUS showed that 57% of children received dialysis (Milford et al 1990). Treatments other than careful supportive therapy together with dialysis should be reserved for those children with the more severe disease who would be predicted to have a poorer outcome.

A wide variety of treatments have been used in HUS but none have been shown by controlled studies to affect prognosis, with the exception of the use of plasma infusion in a multicenter study (Loirat et al 1988). Unfortunately this study is disadvantaged by the inclusion of children with epidemic HUS, who would be expected to have a good prognosis, together with those with sporadic HUS who would be expected to have a poorer prognosis. The benefits of plasma, therefore, need to be weighed against the disadvantages. Such disadvantages would include the risk of volume overload, the transmission of blood-borne viral diseases and the worsening hemolysis that may be seen in those patients with neuraminidase associated HUS. Plasma exchange has also been advocated and although it has been shown to be of benefit in thrombotic thrombocytopenic purpura in both the acute illness and in patients with recurrent episodes, there are insufficient data on children with HUS. There are theoretical reasons why it may be beneficial and its use may therefore justified in the child with a severe deteriorating course, particularly with neurological involvement.

The observed abnormalities of prostacyclin metabolism seen in some patients with HUS has led also to the use of prostacyclin infusions. Studies have produced conflicting results although again it may be justified in the patient with a severe deteriorating course.

Influencing long term outcome

The acute mortality of HUS is around 5% in most series. The long term consequences are, however, less well documented and although the majority of survivors recover completely, a small proportion do develop a secondary decline in renal function. Evidence of hypertension or impaired glomerular filtration rate may be seen in between 11–25%. A positive correlation between microalbuminuria and systolic blood pressure and a negative correlation between microalbuminuria and glomerular filtration rate (Fitzpatrick et al 1991) suggests that those children with albuminuria should receive longer and closer follow-up to identify occult nephropathy earlier. A normal urine-protein/creatinine ratio at 1 year appears to be a good discriminator between those with a good outcome compared to those with a poor outcome (Milford et al 1991). The full implications of the long-term sequelae of HUS may not yet have been realized, as a study on renal functional reserve demonstrated that all patients who had apparently made a complete recovery presented abnormalities in their renal functional reserve similar to that seen in children with a single kidney. However, the patients with HUS showed in addition an increase in microalbuminuria after a protein load, which may imply a poorer long-term prognosis (Perelstein et al 1990).

CHRONIC RENAL FAILURE (Tables 17.16 and 17.17)

Data on the prevalence of chronic renal failure is uncertain, at least in part as a result of the differing definitions of the level of renal dysfunction.

European data (BAPN 1995) suggests a prevalence of between 25 and 50 children per million child population with a glomerular filtration rate (GFR) less than 25–50 ml/min/1.73 m².

Table 17.16   Stages of chronic renal failure

	GFR (ml/min/1.73 m²)	
Mild	50–75	Asymptomatic
Moderate	25–50	Metabolic abnormalities
Severe	< 25	Progressive growth failure
End-stage renal failure	< 10	Require renal replacement therapy

Table 17.17 Primary renal disease of 2372 children <15 years requiring renal replacement therapy in Europe 1981–1985 (Brunner et al 1988)

	EDTA* (%)
Glomerulonephritis	25.8
Focal segmental glomerulosclerosis	6.8
Other glomerulonephritis	19.0
Pyelonephritis/interstitial nephritis	24.2
Obstructive uropathy	10.8
Vesicoureteric reflux	7.8
Other causes	5.6
Hereditary/familial nephropathy	15.6
Polycystic kidney disease	1.6
Medullary cystic disease, including nephronophthisis	6.3
Hereditary nephritis with nerve deafness	1.6
Other hereditary nephritis	0.6
Cystinosis	3.2
Primary oxalosis	0.9
Congenital nephrotic syndrome	–
Other causes	1.4
Congenital hypoplasia/dysplasia	13.5
Aplasia/hypoplasia/dysplasia	10.0
Prune belly syndrome	0.8
Other causes	1.8
Multisystem disease	10.2
Lupus erythematosus	0.8
Henoch–Schönlein purpura	2.4
Hemolytic uremic syndrome	4.8
Systemic immunological disease	–
Other multisystem disease	2.2
Renal vascular disease	1.6
Miscellaneous	3.5
Kidney tumor	0.7
Drash syndrome	–
Others	2.8
Chronic renal failure	5.7
Unknown cause	

*European Dialysis Transplant Association

End-stage renal failure is defined as the stage at which dialysis and renal transplantation are required. There is no absolute level of renal function at which this is required although in practice it is usually a GFR < 10 ml/min/1.73 m^2. The European Dialysis Transplant Association (EDTA) register of children under 15 years of age accepted for renal replacement therapy each year suggests an incidence increasing from 4.6 per million child population in 1971 to 7–8 per million child population per annum in 1991 (Broyer et al 1993). In the UK the acceptance rate in 1992 was 9.7 per million child population. The number of patients receiving treatment is increasing as the treatment criteria broaden and, in particular, younger children being now accepted for renal replacement therapy. The proportion of treated children below the age of 6 years has risen from 14% to 21% over the past decade, with a third of these being under the age of 2 years at the start of treatment (Rizzoni et al 1989).

The etiology of renal failure varies according to the child's country of origin, and age at presentation. In Europe the three commonest causes are chronic glomerulonephritis, pyelonephritis (reflux nephropathy) and malformations of the renal tract. Hereditary renal diseases and hemolytic uremic syndrome are also important causes of end-stage renal failure.

CLINICAL PRESENTATION

In many children chronic renal failure will be the end result of known progressive renal disease. More recently, antenatal diagnosis has led to detection of renal tract malformations before symptoms develop. Other children may present with signs and symptoms associated with renal failure. These may be nonspecific symptoms, including lethargy, poor appetite and nausea, together with urinary symptoms, including polyuria or enuresis.

Growth

Growth failure is a major problem for children with chronic renal failure. The severity of the growth failure is related to the age at presentation: 50% of children with renal failure since infancy have growth failure, with a height of > 2 SD below the mean height for age, in contrast to 10% of those with acquired disease. Important factors contributing to the growth failure include: acidosis, salt depletion, other biochemical abnormalities, renal osteodystrophy, and energy malnutrition. Estimation of renal function would be a routine investigation in a child presenting with unexplained growth failure.

Renal osteodystrophy

Phosphate retention, secondary hyperparathyroidism and skeletal resistance to parathyroid hormone, intestinal malabsorption of calcium leading to hypocalcemia and altered vitamin D metabolism all contribute to the disturbances in bone and mineral metabolism associated with renal osteodystrophy. The severity of the bone disease is related to age at onset and underlying renal disease together with the level of renal function and duration of renal failure. It is more common with the congenital and obstructive uropathies and rarely manifests clinically with a GFR of above 25 ml/min/1.73 m^2 although biochemical abnormalities are seen with a GFR between 50 and 80 ml/min/1.73 m^2. Symptoms may include poor growth, bone pain, skeletal deformities, and slipped epiphyses.

Anemia

Anemia secondary to a lack of erythropoietin is also a well recognized complication of renal failure and may be the presenting feature of the condition.

Hypertension

Renin dependent hypertension is the commonest cause of hypertension in childhood and may be associated with renal failure. The presentation of renal failure may therefore be with the symptoms of hypertension including headache, visual disturbances or hypertensive encephalopathy.

MANAGEMENT

Fluid and electrolyte therapy

Many children with congenital renal diseases, in particular dysplasia, obstructive uropathy and nephronophthisis, have poor renal concentrating capacity with polyuria and salt loss. Salt supplementation is often necessary and salt deficiency is an important cause of poor growth in these infants. Children with acquired diseases, in particular focal glomerulosclerosis and other forms of glomerulonephritis, may have salt and water retention and therefore require salt restriction. Acidosis is common and should be corrected with sodium bicarbonate.

Infection

Urine cultures should be checked, especially in those with abnormalities of the urinary tract, as repeated infection may hasten progression of CRF.

Renal osteodystrophy

The impairment of renal production of 1,25-dihydroxycholecalciferol is a major factor in the development of renal osteodystrophy. Pharmacological replacement with 1α-hydroxycholecalciferol should be commenced when there are biochemical features of altered mineral metabolism (hypocalcemia, hyperphosphatemia, rising alkaline phosphatase or hyperparathyroidism) or if the GFR falls below 25 ml/min/1.73 m^2. An initial dose would be 10 ng/kg/per 24 h increasing according to clinical and biochemical parameters up to dosages of 50 ng/kg/per 24 h. Hyperphosphatemia also plays an important role in the development and maintenance of secondary hyperparathyroidism. Initially, dietary phosphate restriction may be sufficient to control hyperphosphatemia although this can be difficult in young infants on a predominantly milk diet. Phosphate binders may become necessary in addition and calcium carbonate would be the drug of choice. Aluminum hydroxide, although an effective phosphate binder, is best avoided in children because of its potentially neurotoxic effects.

Erythropoietin

The production of human erythropoietin (rhEPO) by recombinant DNA techniques has made possible the treatment of the anemia of chronic renal failure and significantly improved the quality of life for many patients. The use of rhEPO, usually given subcutaneously, has been shown effective in raising the hematocrit of children with end-stage renal failure. It is also effective in predialysis patients. There is, however, concern that administration of rhEPO may increase the blood viscosity, causing glomerular hypertension and glomerular hyperfiltration with acceleration in functional renal decline. RhEPO may result in hypertension and it is not known if effects on renal function are independent or consequent upon changes in blood pressure. Despite these concerns, erythropoietin should be considered for all patients with severe anemia. Blood pressure and renal function should be monitored closely.

Growth hormone

Short stature is a serious problem for children with chronic renal failure. Endogenous growth hormone secretion is normal, as are serum levels of insulin like growth factors I and II. However, exogenous growth hormone has been shown to increase the height velocity in a number of conditions in which growth hormone secretion is not impaired and more recently its efficacy in children with chronic renal failure has been studied. It has been shown that growth hormone does increase the short term growth velocity of prepubertal children with chronic renal failure and is now licensed for use. The effect on final height is not known but its use in 20 prepubertal children for 5 years led to a significant improvement in standards of height without excessive advancement of bone age and minimal clinical adverse events (Fine et al 1996). Of most concern is that growth hormone may accelerate renal functional decline by increasing renal plasma flow and glomerular hyperfiltration. In view of the possible side-effects its use should be restricted to children who are below the third centile for height and in whom all other abnormalities such as electrolyte and acid base balance, renal osteodystrophy and nutritional deficiencies have been corrected.

Nutrition

General recommendations for children with chronic renal failure suggest that children should have at least the estimated average requirement (EAR) for chronological age for energy, although many will need additional energy to promote growth. Protein intake should be based on the reference nutrient intake (RNI) for height age. However, individual dietary and biochemical assessment will determine requirements as well as the stage of management (Coleman 1994). Large reliance is placed upon nutritional supplements to achieve nutritional goals in infants and children with chronic renal failure and the assistance of an experienced pediatric dietitian is essential. In many infants and young children the supplements are delivered either nasogastrically or preferably via the gastrostomy route if long term feeding is required.

Phosphate restriction naturally follows protein restriction but the majority of children require phosphate binders in the form of calcium carbonate to control serum phosphate and parathyroid hormone levels in advancing chronic renal failure. Each child will also need assessing individually with respect to fluid and electrolyte needs along with adequacy of micronutrient intake. These children require frequent and repeated assessments of their dietary prescriptions if growth is to be maintained or promoted.

Over the last decade considerable attention has focused on dietary modifications to retard the progression of chronic renal failure. Of particular interest has been the role of restriction of dietary phosphate and protein in retarding the progression of chronic renal failure. Both the efficacy and safety of severe protein restriction in growing children requires evaluation because of the concern regarding the effect of protein restriction on growth. The results from trials using protein restriction of 1 g/kg/day have shown conflicting results in the effect on GFR although no adverse effect on growth has been demonstrated (Wingen et al 1991). Compliance with dietary manipulations in childhood is often poor and in the European study on protein restriction only 76% of children adhered to their dietary prescription. Further studies are needed before such treatments are recommended for widespread clinical use in children.

Dialysis

Dialysis does achieve satisfactory control of fluid and biochemistry but is an incomplete form of renal replacement therapy and is therefore considered a stepping stone to renal transplantation in most children. There are three main forms of dialysis available:

Continuous ambulatory peritoneal dialysis (CAPD)

Access to the peritoneal cavity is by way of a surgically implanted permanent Silastic catheter. Dialysis fluid remains in the abdomen throughout the 24-h period, the fluid being exchanged three or four times with exchange of water and solutes between the blood and fluid occurring continuously.

Continuous cycling peritoneal dialysis (CCPD)

The principle is similar only an automated cycling machine delivers and exchanges fluid frequently, usually overnight. CCPD produces better clearances and ultrafiltration than CAPD and is particularly suited to the needs of infants in whom rapid glucose absorption from the peritoneum favors shorter cycles.

The disadvantages of both techniques are the risk of peritonitis and other abdominal complications such as hernias. Both procedures are, however, carried out at home by the families and offer the child the opportunity to attend school full time and participate in all the usual activities.

Haemodialysis

Haemodialysis requires adequate vascular access either via an arteriovenous fistula, or more commonly, via an indwelling vascular catheter, usually in the subclavian or jugular vein. Although the technical principles of hemodialysis are similar in adults and children, because of the challenges presented by the smaller intravascular volumes of children and the potential hemodynamic instability, together with the psychological issues it is recommended that children be treated in units with pediatric expertise. Difficulties with vascular access, including infection, are a disadvantage of the technique.

The choice between peritoneal dialysis and hemodialysis will depend on patient preference, geographical and practical considerations. Since its first introduction in 1978 the popularity of peritoneal dialysis has increased and in the UK over two-thirds of the patients on dialysis are on peritoneal dialysis, with CCPD being increasingly favored.

Transplantation

Renal transplantation is the best mode of renal replacement therapy for children and adolescents (Watson 1993). At all ages pediatric renal transplant recipients have better survival than do dialysis patients of the same age. Moreover, successful transplantation confers a degree of physiological and psychological rehabilitation not seen with any form of dialysis. Some patients may be fortunate enough to receive a transplant without dialysis with preemptive transplant rates of around 10% in Europe and over 20% in North America.

Graft survival

Graft survival rates in the UK suggest 1-year graft survival of 80% for cadaveric renal transplantation with over 90% survival for live donor grafts. Longer term follow-up results need to be interpreted with caution as treatment modalities and immunosuppressive regimens have changed considerably over the last decade. However, 10- and 13-year survival rates of 52% and 61% have been reported. The use of live donor grafts between countries is very variable. In the UK less than 10% of grafts are from live donor, in North America 50% and in Scandinavia as high as 70%.

Graft success rates are dependent on a wide variety of factors including tissue matching, donor age, storage time of the kidney, immunosuppression regimens, previous transplantation and original and associated diseases. Of recent concern, as more young children are accepted onto renal replacement programs, is the outcome in the younger renal transplant recipient. Both European and North American data tend to suggest that graft survival is lower in children under 2 years compared to older children (Avner et al 1995, Ehrich et al 1992). However, there is a tendency to use young donors in young recipients and when stratified for donor age, recipient age does not seem to influence outcome. Results of live donation are comparable with other age groups. It is anticipated that policies involving not using organs from young donors in young recipients will improve the outcome of this group.

Immunosuppression

All transplanted children will remain on immunosuppressive therapy with cyclosporine, usually with steroids and, in some, also azathioprine. It is important to consider the side-effects of these medications, including risk of infection, hypertension, hirsutism and other cosmetic side-effects which may influence compliance, particularly in adolescents.

Rehabilitation

Growth is improved after renal transplantation, with a significant increase in growth velocity in prepubertal children. However, perhaps one of the most important issues when considering the quality of life following renal transplantation is the neurodevelopmental and the psychological outcome.

Early reports of children with chronic renal failure, particularly those who had had renal failure since infancy, showed a worrying proportion of those children having significant developmental delay. The etiology was felt to be multifactorial, including: poor biochemical control; inadequate nutrition; the use of aluminum-containing phosphate binders; and psychosocial factors. However, more recent studies from the same institutions (Geary & Haka-Ikse 1989, Davis et al 1990) have been more encouraging and the authors concluded that the marked improvement in neurodevelopmental outcome compared to their own previous reports was due to a shift in emphasis in renal failure management with a more aggressive approach to nutrition and biochemical parameters. They therefore recommended that early aggressive treatment for infants with renal failure improves neurological outcome.

Studies on older children with renal failure have demonstrated effects on cognitive development but despite these deficits there is no difference in grades achieved at school. Studies on the psychosocial adjustment of adult survivors of pediatric dialysis and transplant programs have shown that although the educational and employment achievements of those with renal disease are less than those of controls, two-thirds of the patients leave school with qualifications and two-thirds are in employment. (Reynolds et al 1991).

In conclusion, therefore, dialysis and transplantation enable the majority of children with end-stage renal failure to enter adulthood in good physical health and well adjusted socially.

However, the burden for families caring for children with renal failure, as with many other chronic illnesses is considerable. It is essential that such families have the benefits of support from an experienced multidisciplinary team which includes nursing and medical staff, dietitians, social workers, teachers, play leaders, psychologists and psychiatrists, who are able to work not only in hospital but also support the families in their own communities (Watson 1995b).

REFERENCES

Aggarwal V H, Verrier-Jones K 1989 Vesicoureteric reflux – screening of the first degree relatives. Archives of Disease in Childhood 64: 1538–1541

Al-Khaldi N, Watson A R, Zuccollo J, Twining P, Rose D H 1994 Outcome of an antenatally detected cystic dysplastic kidney disease. Archives of Disease in Childhood 70: 520–522

Alexander S R, Arbus G S, Butt K M H et al 1990 The 1989 Report of the North American Pediatric Renal Transplant Cooperative Study. Pediatric Nephrology 4: 542–553

Anderson P A M, Rickwood A M K 1991 Features of primary vesicoureteric reflux detected by prenatal sonography. British Journal of Urology 67: 267–271

Avner E D, Chavers B, Sullivan E K, Tejani A 1995 Renal transplantation and chronic dialysis in children and adolescents: the 1993 annual report of the North American Pediatric Renal Transplant Cooperative Study. Pediatric Nephrology 9: 61–73

Balow J E, Boumpas D T, Fessler B J, Austin II H A 1996 Management of lupus nephritis. Kidney International 49(53): S88–S92

Berg U B, Widstam-Attorps U C 1993 Follow-up of renal function and urinary protein excretion in childhood IgA nephropathy. Pediatric Nephrology 7: 123–129

Birmingham Reflux Study Group 1987 Prospective trial of operative versus non-operative treatment of severe vesico-ureteric reflux in children: five years' observation. British Medical Journal 295: 237–241

Borzykowski M, Mundy A R 1988 The management of neuropathic bladder in childhood. Pediatric Nephrology 2: 56–66

Breuning M H, Peters D J M 1996 Genetic heterogenicity of autosomal dominant polycystic kidney disease. In: Watson M L, Torres V E (eds) Polycystic kidney disease. Oxford Medical, Oxford, pp 391–403

British Association for Paediatric Nephrology 1995 Report of a Working Party : the provision of services in the United Kingdom for children and adolescents with renal disease.

Broyer M, Chantler C, Donckerwolke, Ehrich J H H, Rizzoni G, Scharer K 1993 The paediatric registry of the European Dialysis and Transplant Association: 20 years' experience. Pediatric Nephrology 7: 758–768

Broyer M, Jouvet P, Niaudet P, Daudon M, Revillon Y 1996 Management of oxalosis. Kidney International 49(53): S93–S98

Brunner F P, Broyer M, Brynger H et al 1988 Demography of dialysis and transplantation in children in Europe. Nephrology Dialysis Transplantation 3: 235–243

Byrd D J, Lind M, Brodehl J 1991 Diagnostic and genetic studies in 43 patients with classic cystinuria. Clinical Chemistry 37: 68–73

Chambers T L, Moss G 1994 Hypercalciuria, stones and nephrocalcinosis. In: Postlethwaite R J (ed) Clinical paediatric nephrology. Butterworth Heineman, Oxford, pp 389–398

Clark G, White R H R, Glasgow E F et al 1988 Poststreptococcal glomerulonephritis in children: clinicopathological correlations and long-term prognosis. Pediatric Nephrology 2: 381–388

Coad N A G, Marshall T, Rowe B, Taylor C M 1991 Changes in the postenteropathic form of hemolytic uremic syndrome in children. Clinical Nephrology 35: 10–16

Coleman J E 1994 The kidney. In: Shaw V, Lawson M (eds) Clinical paediatric dietetics. Blackwell Scientific, London, pp 125–142

Consensus statement on management and audit potential for steroid responsive nephrotic syndrome 1994 Report of a workshop by the British Association for Paediatric Nephrology and Research Unit, Royal College of Physicians. Archives of Disease in Childhood 70: 151–157

Corey H E, Spitzer A 1992 Renal blood flow and glomerular filtration rate during development. In: Edelman C M (ed) Pediatric kidney disease. Little, Brown, Boston, pp 49–77

Cortes L, Tejani A 1996 Dilemma of focal segmental glomerular sclerosis. Kidney International 49(53): S57–S63

Craig J C, Knight J F, Sureshkumar P, Mantz E, Roy L P 1996 Effect of circumcision on incidence of urinary tract infection in preschool boys. Journal of Pediatrics 128: 23–27

D'Amico G 1985 Idiopathic IgA mesangial nephropathy. Nephron 41: 1–13

Davies A G, Price D A, Postlethwaite R J 1985 Renal function in diabetes mellitus. Archives of Disease in Childhood 60: 299–304

Davis I D, Chang P N, Nevins T E 1990. Successful renal transplantation accelerates development in young uraemic children. Pediatrics 86: 594–600

de Man S A, Andrea J L, Bachmann H et al 1991 Blood pressure in childhood: pooled findings in six European studies. Journal of Hypertension 9: 109–114

Dillon M J 1987 Investigation and management of hypertension in children. Pediatric Nephrology 1: 59–69

Ehrich J H H, Rizzoni G, Brunner F P et al 1992 Renal replacement therapy for end stage renal failure before two years of age. Nephrology Dialysis and Transplantation 7: 1171–1177

Eiberg H, Berendt I, Mohr J 1995 Assignment of dominant inherited nocturnal enuresis to chromosome 13g. Nature Genetics 10: 354–356

Elder J S 1992 Importance of antenatal diagnosis of vesicoureteral reflux. Journal of Urology l48: 1750–1754

Elises J S, Griffiths P D, Hocking M D, Taylor C M, White R H R 1988 Simplified quantification of urinary protein excretion in children. Clinical Nephrology 30: 225–229

Evan A P, Larsson L 1992 Morphologic development of the nephron. In: Edelman C M (ed) Pediatric kidney disease. Little, Brown, Boston, pp 19–48

Fine R N, Kohaut E, Brown D, Kuntze J, Attie K M 1996 Long-term treatment of growth retarded children with chronic renal insufficiency, with recombinant human growth hormone. Kidney International 49: 781–785

Fitzpatrick M M, Shah V, Trompeter R S, Dillon M J, Barratt T M 1991 Long term renal outcome of childhood haemolytic uraemic syndrome. British Medical Journal 303: 489–492

Fogo A, Kon V 1994 Pathophysiology of Progressive renal disease. In: Holliday M A, Barratt T M, Avner E D (eds) Pediatric nephrology, 3rd edn. Williams & Wilkins, Baltimore, pp 1228–1240

Gallo G E, Gianantonio C A 1995 Extrarenal involvement in diarrhoea associated haemolytic uraemic syndrome. Pediatric Nephrology 9: 117–119

Geary D F, Haka-Ikse K 1989 Neurodevelopmental progress of young children with chronic renal disease. Pediatrics 84: 68–72

Goonasekera C D A, Shah V, Wade A M, Barratt T M, Dillon M J 1996 15-year follow-up of renin and blood pressure in reflux nephropathy. Lancet 347: 640–643

Gordon I 1995 Vesico-ureteric reflux, urinary-tract infection, and renal damage in children. Lancet 346: 489–490

Haycock G B 1988 The treatment of glomerulonephritis in children. Pediatric Nephrology 2: 247–255

Holmberg C, Laine J, Ronnholm K, Ala-Houhala M, Jalanko H 1996 Congenital nephrotic syndrome. Kidney International 49(53): S51–S56

Hoyer P F, Gonda S, Barthels M, Krohin H P, Brohedy J 1986 Thromboembolic complications in children with nephrotic syndrome. Acta Pediatrica Scandinavica 75: 804–810

International Reflux Study in Children: European Group 1992 Five year study of medical and surgical treatment in children with severe reflux: radiological renal findings. Pediatric Nephrology 6: 223–230

Jacobsson S H, Eklof O, Eriksson C G, Lins L E, Tidgren B, Winberg J 1989 Development of hypertension and uraemia after pyelonephritis in childhood. 27 year follow up. British Medical Journal 299: 703–706

Jakobsson B, Nolstedt L, Svensson L, Soderlundh S, Berg U 1992 99mTechnetium-dimercaptosuccinic acid scan in the diagnosis of acute pyelonephritis in children: relation to clinical and radiological findings. Pediatric Nephrology 6: 328–334

Jewkes F E M, McMaster D J, Napier W A et al 1990 Home collection of urine specimens – boric acid bottles or dipslides? Archives of Disease in Childhood 65: 286–289

Jones D P, Mahmoud H, Chesney R W 1995 Tumour lysis syndrome: pathogenesis and management. Pediatric Nephrology 9: 206–212

Kaplan B S, Cleary T G, Obrig T G 1990 Recent advances in understanding the pathogenesis of the hemolytic uremic syndromes. Pediatric Nephrology 4: 276–283

Karlowicz M G, Adelman R D 1995 Nonoliguric and oliguric renal failure in asphyxiated term neonates. Pediatric Nephrology 9: 718–722

Kierdorf H, Sieberth H G 1995 Continuous treatment modalities in acute renal failure. Nephrology Dialysis Transplantation 10: 2001–2008

Kissane J M 1990 Renal cysts in pediatric patients. Pediatric Nephrology 4: 69–77

Lang S, Stevenson B, Risdon R A 1990 Thin basement membrane nephropathy as a cause of recurrent haematuria in childhood. Histopathology 16: 331–337

Lewis M A, Baildom E M, Davis N, Houston I B, Postlethwaite R J 1989 Nephrotic syndrome: from toddlers to twenties. Lancet I: 255–259

Loirat C, Sonsino E, Hinglais N, Jais J P, Landais P, Fermanian J 1988 Treatment of the childhood haemolytic uraemic syndrome with plasma. Pediatric Nephrology 2: 279–285

McClure R J, Prasad V K, Brocklebank J T 1994 Treatment of hyperkalaemia using intravenous and nebulised salbutamol. Archives of Disease in Childhood 70: 126–128

McEnery P T, Coutinho M J 1994 Membranoproliferative glomerulonephritis. In: Holliday M A, Barratt T M, Avner E D (eds) Pediatric Nephrology, 3rd edn. Williams & Wilkins, Baltimore, pp 739–753

Meadow R 1994 Haematuria. In: Postlethwaite R J (ed) Clinical paediatric nephrology. Butterworth Heineman, Oxford, p 6

Milford D V, Taylor C M, Guttridge B, Hall S M, Rowe B, Kleanthous H 1990 Haemolytic uraemic syndromes in the British Isles 1985–8: association with verocytotoxin producing E. Coli. Part 1: clinical and epidemiological features. Archives of Disease in Childhood 65: 716–721

Milford D V, White R H R, Taylor C M 1991 Prognostic significance of proteinuria one year after onset of hemolytic uraemic syndrome. Journal of Paediatrics 118: 191–194

Moore E A, Collier J, Evans J H C, Watson A R 1994 Information needs of parents of children with nephrotic syndrome. Child Health 2(4): 147–149

Najmaldin A S, Burge D M, Atwell J D 1991 Outcome of antenatally diagnosed pelviureteric junction hydronephrosis. British Journal of Urology 67: 96–99

O'Donnell P D 1991 Pitfalls of urodynamic testing. Urological Clinics of North America 18: 257–268

Perelstein E M, Grunfield B G, Simsolo R B, Gimenez, Gianantonio C A 1990 Renal functional reserve in haemolytic uraemic syndrome and single kidney. Archives of Disease in Childhood 65: 728–731

Philips D, Watson A R, Collier J 1996 Distress and radiological investigations of the urinary tract in children. European Journal of Pediatrics (in press)

Pisacane A, Graziano L, Mazzarella G, Scarpellino B, Zona G 1992 Breast-feeding and urinary tract infection. Journal of Pediatrics 120: 87–89

Quintero R A, Johnson M P, Romero R et al 1995 In-utero percutaneous cystoscopy in the management of fetal lower obstructive uropathy. Lancet 346: 537–540

Rayner R J, Watson A R, Bishop M C 1988 Haematuria in an adolescent due to bladder carcinoma. European Journal of Pediatrics 147: 328–329

Reusz G S, Hoyer P F, Lucas M, Ehrich J H H, Brodehl J 1990 X-linked hypophosphataemia: treatment height gain and nephrocalcinosis. Archives of Disease in Childhood 65: 1125–1128

Reynolds J M, Garralda M E, Postlethwaite R J, Goh D 1991 Changes in psychosocial adjustment after renal transplantation. Archives of Disease in Childhood 66: 508–513

Rickwood A M K, Carty H M, McKendrick T 1992 Current imaging of childhood urinary tract infections, prospective study. British Medical Journal 304: 663–665

Rinaldi S, Strologo L D, Montecchi F, Rizzoni G 1993 Relapsing gross haematuria in Munchausen syndrome. Pediatric Nephrology 7: 202–203

Rizzoni G, Ehrich J H H, Brunner F P et al 1989 Combined report on regular dialysis and transplantation in children in Europe 1988. Nephrology Dialysis and Transplantation Supplement 4: 31–40

Rodriguez-Soriano J, Vallo A 1990 Renal tubular acidosis. Pediatric Nephrology 4(3): 268–275

Rondeau E, Levy M, Dosquet P et al 1989 Plasma exchange and immunosuppression for rapidly progressive glomerulonephritis: prognosis and complications. Nephrology, Dialysis and Transplantation 4: 196–200

Royal College of Physicians 1991 Guidelines for the management of acute urinary tract infection in childhood. Report of a working group of the Research Unit, Royal College of Physicians. Journal of the Royal College of Physicians, London 25: 36–42

Sharples P M, Poulton J, White R H R 1985 Steroid responsive nephrotic syndrome is more common in Asians. Archives of Disease in Childhood 60: 1014–1017

Shaw N J, Wheeldon J, Brocklehurst J T 1990 Indices of intact serum parathyroid hormone and renal excretion of calcium, phosphate and magnesium. Archives of Disease in Childhood 65: 1208–1212

Sherbotie J R, Cornfeld D 1991 Management of urinary tract infections in children. Medical Clinics of North America 75: 327–338

Shichiri M, Oowada A, Nishio Y, Tomita K, Shilgai T 1986 Use of autoanalyser to examine urinary-red-cell morphology in the diagnosis of glomerular haematuria. Lancet I: 781–782

Siegler R L, Milligan M K, Burningham T H et al 1991 Longterm outcome and prognostic indicators in the haemolytic uraemic syndrome. Journal of Paediatrics 118: 195–200

Simon D B, Karet F E, Hamdan J M et al 1996a Bartter's syndrome, hypokalaemic alkalosis with hypercalciuria, is caused by mutations in the Na-K-2Cl cotransporter NKCC2. Nature Genetics 13 (June): 183–187

Simon D B, Karet F E, Rodriguez-Soriano J et al 1996b Genetic heterogeneity of Bartter's syndrome revealed by mutations in the K+ channel, ROMK. Nature Genetics 14(Oct): 152–155

Skinner R, Cole M, Pearson A D J, Coulthard M G, Craft A W 1996 Specificity of pH and osmolality of early morning urine sample in assessing distal renal tubular function in children: results in healthy children. British Medical Journal 312: 1337–1338

Smellie J M, Ransley P G, Normand I C S, Prescod N, Enwards D 1985 Development of new renal scars: a collaborative study. British Medical Journal 290: 1057–960

South Bedfordshire Practitioners' Group 1990 Development of renal scars in children: missed opportunities in management. British Medical Journal 301(6760): 1082–1084

Stark H, Tieder M, Eisenstein B, Davidovits M, Litwin A 1988 Hypercalciuria as a cause of persistent or recurrent haematuria. Archives of Disease in Childhood 63(3): 312–313

Stull T L, LiPuma J J 1991 Epidemiology and natural history of urinary tract infections in children. Medical Clinics of North America 75: 287–297

Takebayashi S, Yanase K 1992 Asymptomatic urinary abnormalities found via the Japanese school screening program: a clinical, morphological and prognostic analysis. Nephron 61: 82

Tomsett A, Watson A R 1996 Renal biopsy as a day case procedure. Paediatric Nursing 8(5): 14–15

Tryggvason K, Zhou J, Hostikka S C, Shows T B 1993 Molecular genetics of Alport syndrome. Kidney International 43: 38–44

Turner G M, Coulthard M G 1995 Fever can cause pyuria in children. British Medical Journal 311: 924

Van't Hoft W G, Gretz N 1995 The treatment of cystinosis with cysteamine and phosphocysteamine in the United Kingdom and Eire. Pediatric Nephrology 9: 685–689

Vehaskari V M 1989 Asymptomatic haematuria: a cause for concern? Pediatric Nephrology 3: 240–241

Verber I G, Meller S T 1989 Serial ^{99m}Tc dimercaptosuccinic acid (DMSA) scans after urinary infections presenting before the age of 5 years. Archives of Disease in Childhood 64: 1533–1537

Vernon S 1995 Urine collection from infants: a reliable method. Paediatric Nursing 7(6): 26–27

Watson A R 1994 Urinary tract infection in early childhood. Journal of Antimicrobial Chemotherapy 34(A): 53–60

Watson A R 1993 Renal transplantation in children. Current Paediatrics 3: 151–155

Watson A R 1995a Nutrition in renal disease. In: Davies D P (ed) Nutrition in child health. Royal College of Physicians, London, pp 133–142

Watson A R 1995b Strategies to support families of children with end-stage renal failure. Pediatric Nephrology 9: 628–631

Watson A R, Coleman J E 1993 Dietary management in nephrotic syndrome. Archives of Disease in Childhood 69: 179–180

Watson A R, Rance C P, Bain J 1985 Long term effects of cyclophosphamide on testicular function. British Medical Journal 291: 1457–1460

Watson A R, Taylor J, Rance C P, Bain J 1986 Gonadal function in women treated with cyclophosphamide for childhood nephrotic syndrome: a long-term follow-up study. Fertility Sterility 46(2): 331–333

Watson A R, Readett D, Nelson C S, Kapila L, Mayell M J 1988 Dilemmas associated with antenatally detected urinary tract abnormalities. Archives of Disease in Childhood 63: 719–722

Wettergren B, Jodal U, Jonasson G 1985 Epidemiology of bacteriuria during the first year of life. Acta Pediatrica Scandinavica 74: 925–933

White R H R 1987 Management of urinary tract infection. Archives of Disease in Childhood 62: 421–427

Wingen A M, Fabian-Bach C, Mehls O 1991 Low protein diets in children with chronic renal failure. Pediatric Nephrology 5: 496–500

Wolfish N M, Delbrouck N F, Shanon A, Matzinger M, Stenstrom R, McLaine P N 1993 Prevalence of hypertension in children with primary vesicoureteral reflux. Journal of Pediatrics 123: 559–563

Wong A F, Bolinger A M, Gambertoglio J G 1994 Pharmacokinetics and drug dosing in children with decreased renal function. In: Holliday M A, Barratt T M, Avner E D (eds) Pediatric Nephrology, 3rd edn. Williams & Wilkins, Baltimore, pp 1305–1314

RECOMMENDED READING

Edelman C M Jr (ed) 1992 Pediatric kidney disease, 2nd edn. Little, Brown, Boston

Holliday M A, Barratt T M, Avner E D (eds) 1994 Pediatric Nephrology, 3rd edn. Williams & Wilkins, Baltimore

Postlethwaite R J (ed) 1994 Clinical Paediatric Nephrology, 2nd edn. Butterworth Heineman, Oxford

18 Gynecological diseases

Anne Garden

Introduction 985
Problems in prenatal life 985
Problems at birth 986
　　Ambiguous genitalia 986
　　Other congenital abnormalities 987
Problems in early childhood 987
　　Vulvovaginitis 987
　　Other vulvar disorders 988
Problems of puberty 989
　　Precocious puberty 989
　　Amenorrhea 989
　　Primary amenorrhea with absence of secondary
　　sex development 990
　　Primary amenorrhea with normal sexual
　　development 990

Problems in adolescence 991
　　Dysfunctional uterine bleeding 991
　　Dysmenorrhea 992
　　Secondary amenorrhea 992
Gynecological tumors 993
　　Ovarian lesions 993
　　Cervical/vaginal lesions 993
Pregnancy in teenagers 994
Contraception for teenagers 994
　　Methods of contraception 994
References 995

INTRODUCTION

Gynecological disorders in childhood are not uncommon but are often poorly managed. Adult gynecologists may not appreciate the difference in the physiology and pelvic anatomy of prepubertal girls compared to adult women. Pediatricians may not feel comfortable dealing with hormonal, menstrual or sexual problems of their adolescent patients. Although not uncommon, gynecological problems in girls are rarely discussed, leading to feelings of isolation and bewilderment among mothers who often believe that their daughters are the only ones to have these problems. Care and explanation by pediatricians who have a sound knowledge of gynecology, or by gynecologists experienced in pediatrics, are necessary in the management of these families. Pediatric gynecology is a subspecialty where communication between the separate disciplines, perhaps in the form of joint clinics, is of great benefit.

Gynecological problems in childhood may be relatively short-lived in that they affect only one epoch of a girl's development, often related to the physiology of that stage of development. Alternatively, they may be more long-standing, resulting from either tumors or congenital abnormalities. Other problems related to the girl's social circumstances may include that of child sexual abuse, which will be covered in greater detail in Chapter 32. This and other gynecological problems may cause continuing problems in adult life, the consequences of which may be seen in adult gynecology and psychiatry clinics.

PROBLEMS IN PRENATAL LIFE

The increase in the use of ultrasound in the management of pregnancy, with the continuing improvements in image resolution,

has led to several gynecological problems being diagnosed in prenatal life and even the management of these problems prior to delivery. Fetal ovarian cysts are not an uncommon finding, mainly in the third trimester of pregnancy. A review of the pathology of these fetal ovarian cysts found them to be either follicular or theca-lutein cysts (Landrum et al 1986). High circulating levels of maternal human chorionic gonadotropin are the likely cause. Treatment of these cysts is expectant, with the size of the cyst being monitored by ultrasound. They rarely cause problems although in one case reported the size of the cyst was such that it was believed that there was a significant risk of thoracic compression with resultant pulmonary hypoplasia (Landrum et al 1986). This cyst was drained prenatally. There are risks, however, with such surgical antenatal management, and in the majority of cases drainage of the cyst can be delayed until delivery (Purkiss et al 1988).

In the neonatal period, management of such cysts is also expectant. Widdowson et al (1988) found that complications such as torsion or rupture occurred only in cysts of greater than 5 cm diameter. They recommended simple aspiration with ultrasound follow-up, with surgery being required only for those cysts that were recurrent or underwent torsion.

Prenatal diagnosis has also been used in conjunction with medical management of gynecological disorders diagnosed in utero. The first case of congenital adrenal hyperplasia treated in utero by the maternal administration of dexamethasone was described in 1984 (David & Forest 1984). Since then, DNA probes have been developed which facilitate first trimester diagnosis (Strachan et al 1987). This will allow more families the option of prenatal diagnosis and the possibility of therapy to suppress the masculinization of the genitalia, thus preventing the need for such extensive corrective surgery.

PROBLEMS AT BIRTH

Ambiguous genitalia

The most common gynecological problem which appears at birth is that of uncertain gender or ambiguous genitalia. It is essential that this problem is dealt with accurately and sensitively if the girl and her family are to be spared many years of emotional trauma.

The external genitalia develop from mesodermal thickenings on either side of the urogenital sinus, the genital folds. In the absence of testosterone, or in the absence of the ability of the genital tissues to respond to testosterone as in the androgen insensitivity syndromes, the genital folds fuse anteriorly to form the genital tubercle which then enlarges slightly to form the clitoris. Production of dihydrotestosterone from the Leydig cells of the testis results in greater enlargement of the genital tubercle and the formation of a penis. The genital swellings in the female develop into the labia while in the male they fuse in the midline to form the urethra and scrotum. Under the influence of androgens, overgrowth of the perineum to form a single perineal opening with the vagina and urethra opening on to it may also occur.

Congenital abnormalities

Congenital abnormalities resulting in ambiguous genitalia may result from masculinization of a female fetus or, less commonly, inadequate masculinization of a male fetus or true hermaphroditism.

The external features of the three conditions are very similar. The child presents with an enlarged clitoris/phallus with the urethral opening anywhere on the ventral surface from the tip to the base, abnormalities of the genital swellings to form labia/scrotal sacs, and, rarely, a small vaginal opening. Palpation of testes in the scrotal sacs or in the inguinal canal will eliminate masculinization of a female fetus, but otherwise no real distinguishing features are to be found on clinical examination. It is extremely important when managing a child with ambiguous genitalia that the parents appreciate that their child does have a definite sexual identity and is not going to remain somewhere between the two sexes.

Masculinization of the female fetus

Congenital adrenal hyperplasia. The commonest cause of ambiguous genitalia is congenital adrenal hyperplasia. It is important that this diagnosis is made as early as possible because of the risk to the child if the enzyme deficiency is complete. If undiagnosed, the salt loss and resultant dehydration may cause death in the neonatal period (see p. 1061).

Congenital adrenal hyperplasia results from a variety of possible enzyme disorders, the commonest of which is 21-hydroxylase deficiency. This causes a reduction in the conversion of 17α-hydroxyprogesterone to C-11-desoxycortisol, and of progesterone to desoxycorticosterone. The reduced cortisol production causes increased production of ACTH, which stimulates production of all the adrenal hormones including the androgens. Raised levels of androgens during development of the external genitalia result in masculinization of the female fetus, although the development of the uterus, tubes and vagina is unaffected as their development is not hormone dependent.

Diagnosis. The initial step in diagnosis is the confirmation of the 46XX karyotype by chromosomal examination and hormone assays. Accumulation of 17α-hydroxyprogesterone (normally less than 20 nmol/l) and raised testosterone (normally less than 1.8 nmol/l) are found. Raised levels of pregnanetriol also indicate accumulation of 17α-hydroxyprogesterone. A reduced serum sodium and raised serum potassium are found in the salt-losing syndrome.

Treatment. This is by suppression of ACTH production with the administration of adequate doses of mineralocorticoids and glucocorticoids. If the chromosomes confirm a 46XX karyotype, the parents should be assured that despite the appearance of her genitalia the girl is completely female and potentially fertile. Surgical correction of the genitalia is probably best carried out as a two-stage procedure. Reduction of the clitoris, with conservation of the glans, should be carried out early, in the neonatal period. Correction of the vagina can be postponed until later, usually in adolescence. More extensive surgery will be required if there is overgrowth of the perineum with associated narrowing of the lower third of the vagina. The degree of correction is best assessed when the maximum growth has occurred. Growth of the tissues around puberty produces more labial skin which can be mobilized to form reconstructive flaps. Estrogenization of the tissues after puberty also results in better wound healing.

Congenital adrenal hyperplasia is an autosomal recessive disorder and parents should be offered genetic counseling prior to a further pregnancy. The possibility of prenatal diagnosis and therapy has already been mentioned (see also p. 1062). The risk of a woman with congenital adrenal hyperplasia having a child with the condition varies with the incidence of the gene in the population, and is usually in the order of 1 : 100 to 1 : 200.

Other causes. Other causes of masculinization of a female fetus are less common. They include maternal ingestion of androgenic or potentially androgenic drugs in early pregnancy, maternal Cushing's syndrome or maternal arrhenoblastoma. The latter two causes are extremely rare. Potentially androgenic drugs include progestogens such as norethisterone, often used for dysfunctional uterine bleeding, or danazol given for maternal endometriosis. The degree of masculinization depends on the dosage and the gestation at administration. Diagnosis can be made from the history. Doctors prescribing such drugs should be aware of the potential effects. Management is by surgical correction, as for congenital adrenal hyperplasia, although the masculinization effects are not usually so marked.

Inadequate masculinization of the male fetus and true hermaphroditism

Less commonly, ambiguous genitalia may result from inadequate masculinization of a male fetus or true hermaphroditism. The differentiating feature between the two conditions is the presence of both ovarian and testicular tissue in the child with true hermaphroditism, but only testicular tissue in the undermasculinized male. The diagnosis, therefore, can only be made after examination under anesthetic, laparotomy and gonadal biopsy. Prior to this, congenital adrenal hyperplasia should be excluded and the karyotype known. Laparoscopy is not sufficient to examine and biopsy the gonads and the technique is a hazardous one unless the operator has experience of the procedure in neonates.

True hermaphroditism. Under anesthesia, the genitalia should be closely inspected to assess the size of the vagina, the position of the urethra and the size of the phallus. On the basis of this, a decision can be made as to the sex in which the child should be reared. Unless the phallus is of comparable size to a normal penis, it is probably preferable that the child is reared as a female, as the success of reconstructive vaginal surgery is much greater than that of reconstructive surgery to the penis. Laparotomy allows careful inspection of the gonads. Biopsies should be taken from representative areas of both gonads, as a combination of tissues may only be found in one gonad. Any area of the gonad which has a different appearance from the rest should also be biopsied. The gonadal tissue which is not associated with the sex decided on by the external examination should be removed before puberty. Hormone replacement therapy (p. 1064) will be necessary for those girls with inadequate functional ovarian tissue to initiate puberty.

Other congenital abnormalities

More extensive malformations may also present at delivery. Abnormalities in the separation of the cloaca into the anterior urogenital part and the posterior rectal part result in a range of anomalies, from the minor anterior displacement of the rectum to the more serious common cloaca with the urethra, vagina and rectum opening into a single cavity. The management of this condition is discussed in Chapter 31.

Hydrocolpos

A less serious but frequently missed or misdiagnosed abnormality is hydrocolpos. This presents in neonates as a bulging membrane which can be easily seen on parting the labia. The condition results from failure of breakdown of the membrane between the urogenital sinus, which forms the lower third of the vagina, and the Müllerian duct, which forms the upper two-thirds. Accumulation of fluid from vaginal secretions stimulated by maternal hormones occurs. The amount of fluid varies and if slight in amount may not be noticed. Under these circumstances, the fluid is gradually absorbed and the imperforate vagina will not be diagnosed until menarche, when the girl presents with cryptomenorrhea and hematocolpos.

If the diagnosis is made, treatment is by excision of the membrane and drainage of the fluid. In some cases, the hydrocolpos may be very large and may present as an abdominal mass. Examination of girls with an abdominal mass in the neonatal period must include inspection of the vagina. Although the study is an old one, unnecessary laparotomy in these girls has been associated with a perioperative mortality as high as 35% (Gravier 1969).

It is important to remember that congenital abnormalities of the genital tract are associated with renal tract abnormalities, and an intravenous urogram should be performed.

PROBLEMS IN EARLY CHILDHOOD

Most of the problems of the early childhood years relate to inadequate estrogen production. At birth, the child has raised levels of circulating estrogen as a result of transplacental passage from the mother. This produces quite marked estrogenic stimulation of the genital tract. The labioscrotal swellings are well developed, the hymen is prominent, the vaginal walls are thick and rugose and a clear white vaginal discharge may be present. In rare cases, the maternal estrogenic stimulation is sufficient to cause endometrial proliferation with resultant withdrawal bleeding following delivery. The bleeding is slight and usually of short duration but will cause parental alarm if the cause is not understood. Breast enlargement may also result from intrauterine hormone stimulation and, similarly, a small amount of clear fluid discharge from the nipple may occur. The effect of maternal hormones usually resolves quickly and certainly by 6 weeks of neonatal life.

Following this, estrogen levels fall. Initially, FSH and LH levels are high, similar to those found in the postmenopausal period, but by the age of 3 months fall by a mechanism which is poorly understood but which is frequently referred to as 'resetting of the gonadostat'. Pulsatile secretion of gonadotropin-releasing hormone (GnRH) appears before the onset of puberty causing release of FSH and LH with corresponding increase in estrogen production. The factors involved in the onset and control of puberty are considered more fully in Chapter 19.

Prior to the onset of puberty, however, the girl is hypoestrogenic. The uterus is small, the vulva is flat with thin attenuated labia minora. The vaginal epithelium is thin and red. There is a little vaginal secretion, which is relatively alkaline.

Vulvovaginitis

These anatomical changes of attenuation of the external genitalia, and the physiological changes of decreasing amount and acidity of the vaginal secretions result in the girl being susceptible to vulvovaginitis. The symptoms of vulvovaginitis vary from minor discomfort to intense perineal pruritus which may prevent the girl from sleeping. On examination, the vulva and introitus are red and inflamed. This is accompanied by vaginal discharge which varies in amount and which may be serous but is more usually purulent and green/brown in color. Vulvovaginitis is usually due to recurrent bacterial infection; a study from Liverpool showed the most common organisms to be *Haemophilus influenzae* and fecal organisms. Gonococcus, gardnerella and candida were rare causes of infection (Pearce & Hart 1992).

Differential diagnosis. Other conditions which may cause vulvar and vaginal irritation are pinworm infestation, which can be diagnosed by the Sellotape test, dermatological conditions such as lichen sclerosis et atrophicus (LS&A) and allergies – particularly to detergents and fabric softeners. Vaginal discharge due to a foreign body is extremely heavy, foul smelling and is usually bloodstained. Botryoid sarcoma may also present with bloodstained vaginal discharge.

Investigation. Investigation is usually limited to clinical examination to confirm the presence of discharge and to exclude dermatological conditions. A gentle separation of the vulva will allow inspection of the introitus and hymenal orifice. Bacteriological swabs from the introitus are unhelpful as they are usually contaminated by fecal flora; swabs from higher in the vagina should not be obtained from a prepubertal girl without a general anesthetic. In most cases, identification of specific bacteria is of academic interest and is usually only required if there is a suspicion of sexual abuse or of a sexually transmitted infection.

In girls with bloodstained discharge, examination under anesthesia is mandatory.

Treatment. In the first instance, this consists of advice on perineal hygiene, daily baths or showers and wearing of loose-fitting cotton pants. Explanation to the mother as to the cause of the condition, and reassurance that it will improve as the girl approaches puberty, is necessary. Salt baths, with the girl being encouraged to sit for about 10 minutes in a basin of warm water to which two tablespoons of salt have been added, are often helpful, especially when the girl is particularly uncomfortable. The use of bland emollient creams such as Sudacrem or E45 may be of benefit as a barrier. Antibacterial cream such as Sultrin may also be helpful. Estrogen cream applied to the vulva will improve the condition by increasing the resistance of the vagina to infection, but its use must be strictly controlled. Estrogens are easily absorbed through the skin and systemic affects of local therapy are not rare. If estrogen therapy is to be used, the girl's mother must be warned of the risks of indiscriminate use. Instructions should be given to apply the cream sparingly.

Prepubertal girls with proven Candida infections should be screened for diabetes.

Other vulvar disorders

Labial adhesions

In very young girls, usually < 3 years of age, fusion of the labia is not uncommon (Fig. 18.1). It is important to differentiate this from congenital absence of the vagina. In the latter, the vulva can be easily seen, with the urethral meatus and clitoris. The hymen is seen as irregular rugae where the introitus should be. In a child with labial adhesions, the vulva is flat and no structures are seen beyond it. The adhesions usually begin at the posterior vulva and move forward until only the urinary meatus can be seen. They result from chronic irritation causing excoriation of the labia which then adhere together.

Treatment. This is simple and involves the application of a small amount of estrogen cream twice daily for 2 weeks. The adhesions will usually then separate spontaneously. If necessary, subsequent courses can be given after a break of 2 weeks. When separated, advice about vulvar hygiene and salt baths will reduce

the risk of further episodes of vulvovaginitis and adhesions. Surgery to separate the adhesions is not required.

Vulvar warts

The presence of vulvar or perianal warts (Fig. 18.2) in a young girl must be managed very sensitively. Although they may be indicative of child sexual abuse, they are more likely to have been transferred quite innocently from a relative. The presence of warts on the hands of the mother, father, siblings, grandparents, baby-sitter – anyone who may have washed the child or changed her nappies – must be ascertained before sexual abuse is considered. If there is any suspicion of sexual abuse, it is worth carrying out DNA typing of the human papilloma virus (HPV) isolated from the wart before taking the matter further.

Treatment. Warts are best treated with podophyllin, taking care not to damage the normal surrounding skin. In girls under 5 years of age, podophyllin 10% should be used for a maximum of three applications; in those 5–10 years of age podophyllin 20% for three treatments; and in older girls podophyllin 20% weekly until the lesions have resolved. The mother is instructed to wash the area thoroughly after 4 h.

Dermatological conditions

The commonest dermatological condition affecting the vulvar area is napkin rash which may be exacerbated by infection with

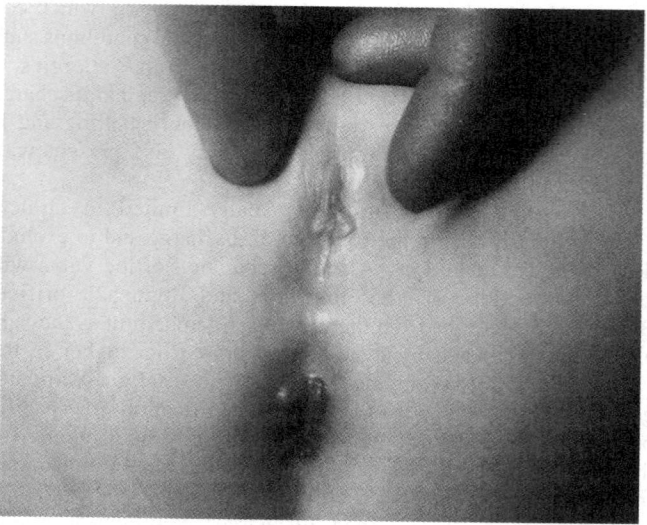

Fig. 18.1   Labial adhesions in a 3-year-old girl. Note the absence of anatomical structures beyond the vulva which is the feature which differentiates between this condition and vaginal agenesis.

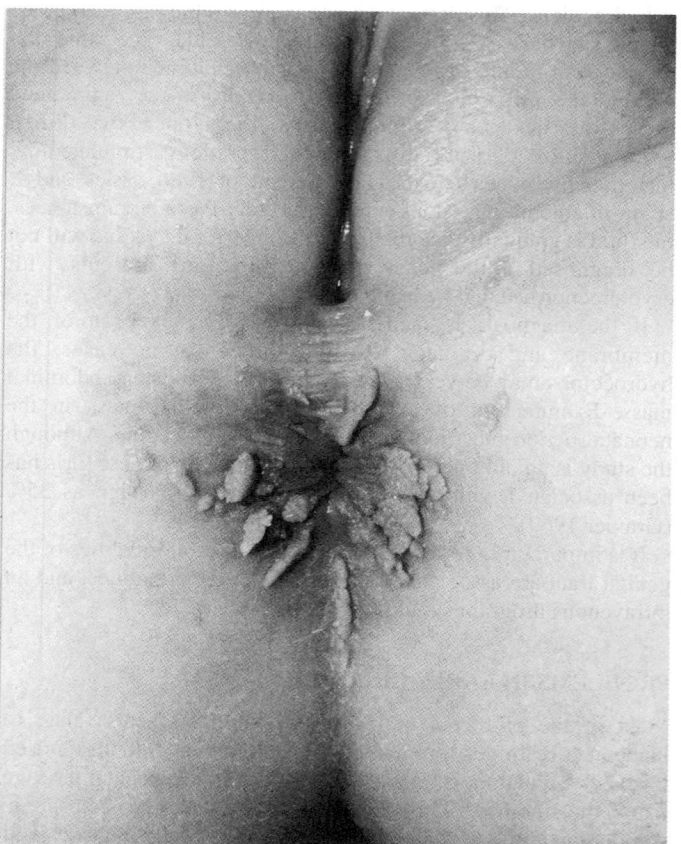

Fig. 18.2   Perianal warts in a prepubertal girl.

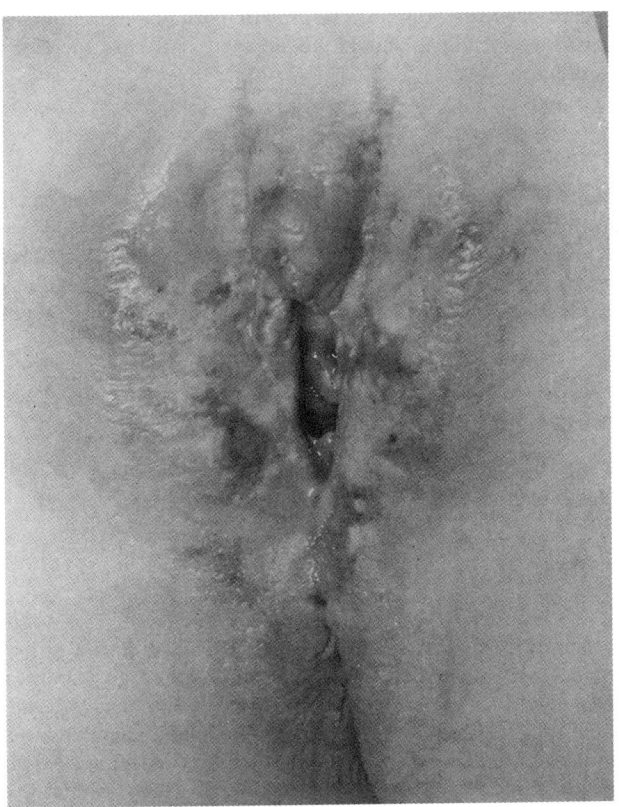

Fig. 18.3 Severe lichen sclerosis et atrophicus in a 9-year-old girl. Note the marked clitoral hypertrophy and the involvement of the perianal skin.

bacteria or Candida. Treatment involves instruction on hygiene and appropriate therapy for secondary infection. Thereafter, the use of a bland barrier cream such as E45 or zinc and castor oil is usually sufficient (see also Ch. 25).

Vulvar soreness may be secondary to any generalized dermatological condition such as eczema or psoriasis. Lichen sclerosis et atrophicus deserves a special mention (Fig. 18.3).

Lichen sclerosis et atrophicus. This first appears as discrete white papules which coalesce to form white plaques. Hemorrhagic areas, similar to bruising, may also be present. These are an integral part of the disorder and not secondary to trauma from scratching. The child presents with marked itching and vulvar soreness. Scratching and rubbing may result in excoriation, infection and fissuring. The diagnosis can usually be made on clinical examination, although biopsy may be required. Treatment in the first instance is with potent topical steroids such as Dermovate (clobetasol proprionate). Careful hygiene is also necessary and may be difficult to achieve because of the vulvar soreness. Unlike the postmenopausal condition, there is no risk of malignancy. The condition is usually self-limiting and resolves at or just after the menarche.

PROBLEMS OF PUBERTY

Puberty can be defined as the period of time when the child develops physically and mentally into adulthood. A wide variety of disorders may occur at this time; only the gynecological ones will be considered here.

Table 18.1 Stages of breast development (Tanner 1962)

Stage 1	Infantile breasts
Stage 2	Development of the breast bud
Stage 3	Enlargement of the breast and areola
	Breast develops rounded contour
Stage 4	Nipple and areola enlarge to produce secondary projection above contour of breast
Stage 5	Normal adult breast with rounded contours and assimilation of the nipple and areola into whole breast formation

The physical changes are usually an orderly sequence of events. The first event is development of the breast bud and appearance of pubic hair, followed by appearance of vaginal secretions, growth of the breast, appearance of axillary, hair and onset of menstruation. The process usually starts at around 9–10 years of age and is completed by the age of 16. Variations in the order may occur and it is important that the girl's overall development is considered (Chs 8 and 19).

Breast development usually begins with the development of the breast bud at around the age of 10 years and progresses as outlined in the classical descriptions by Tanner (1962) (Table 18.1). Pubic hair growth usually begins at about the same time as breast bud development.

The average age of the menarche in the UK is 12.8 years.

Precocious puberty

Precocious puberty is said to occur when the features of puberty appear in very young girls. Usually, menarche before the age of 10 years or development of secondary sex characteristics before 8 years are considered to be abnormal. Precocious puberty may be constitutional, neurological or gynecological. The constitutional and neurological causes are more common but will not be considered here (see Chs 8 and 14). The commonest gyneco-logical cause is a feminizing estrogen-secreting ovarian tumor, such as a thecoma or granulosa cell tumor. The inappropriate use of exogenous estrogens should also be considered, e.g. overuse of topical estrogen preparations or ingestion of the mother's oral contraceptive pills. Excess estrogen as a cause of precocious puberty usually has vaginal bleeding as the main feature, as opposed to breast and body hair development.

Diagnosis and treatment. Diagnosis is by pelvic ultrasound, as some of these tumors can be too small to palpate, and estimation of serum estrogen levels. It should be remembered that ovarian cysts may be secondary to ovarian stimulation from cerebral causes. Laparotomy is required as the lesions in the ovary may be too small to be readily identifiable through the laparoscope. Granulosa cell tumors can usually be recognized by their appearance, but if in doubt frozen section should be arranged. If a thecoma or granulosa cell tumor is present unilateral oophorectomy should be performed.

Girls in whom no cause can be identified should be treated with gonadotropin-releasing hormone (GnRH) analogues.

Amenorrhea

Amenorrhea is usually considered as primary amenorrhea (in a girl who has never menstruated) and secondary amenorrhea (in a girl/women who has not had a period for more than 6 months). The former is usually subdivided into those girls who have no evidence of sexual development and those with normal sexual development. It should be remembered, however, that this distinction is arbitrary and depends at which point in the girl's development the ovarian failure occurred. It is not unusual for women with Turner's syndrome to present at infertility clinics with regular, though often infrequent, periods, whereas girls with ovarian failure causing premature menopause prior to puberty, will present with failure of sexual development. Similarly, it is important to remember that pubertal development is a continuum and that cessation of development should also be investigated.

Primary amenorrhea with absence of secondary sex development

Absence of menstruation in the absence of normal secondary sex development should be investigated by the age of 14. The likely causes are shown in Table 18.2. Constitutional delay is characterized by delayed bone age and low gonadotropin and estrogen levels. There is frequently a family history. Chronic systemic disease, such as hypothyroidism, is not usually a diagnostic problem. Occasionally, primary amenorrhea may be the presenting complaint of disorders such as celiac disease.

Gonadal dysgenesis

This is usually due to a chromosomal abnormality the commonest being 45X (Turner's syndrome). The clinical features of short stature, web neck, shield chest with wide-spaced nipples and a wide carrying-angle are usually easily recognizable. Girls with mosaic Turner's syndrome may be more difficult to recognize and the condition should always be considered in girls with short stature. It is not unusual for the diagnosis not to be made until adolescence, when the girl presents with primary amenorrhea. Diagnosis is confirmed by chromosome analysis.

Treatment. This involves hormone replacement therapy given in such a way as to mimic natural hormone production to produce breast development and to induce cyclical withdrawal bleeding. Unless being delayed to allow treatment with growth hormone, estrogen replacement should begin around the age of 10 or 11, initially with low doses of ethinyl estradiol 0.01–0.02 mg daily. The dose is gradually increased over 18 months, initially to 0.05 mg daily, then to 0.10 mg daily. Intermittent treatment with estrogen/progestogen therapy, conveniently given in the form of a low-dose oral contraceptive pill or hormone replacement therapy, should be given and continued long term to prevent osteoporosis

Table 18.2 Causes of primary amenorrhea

Without sexual development
Constitutional delay
Chronic systemic disease
Gonadal dysgenesis
Hypothalamic/pituitary dysfunction
(Polycystic ovarian disease)

Normal development
Anatomical problems
  imperforate vagina
  absent vagina
  absent uterus
(Pregnancy)

and cardiovascular disease. If growth hormone is being used, estrogen replacement should be delayed until the increase in growth has ceased.

Hypothalamic/pituitary problems

Hypothalamic or pituitary causes for primary amenorrhea, such as craniopharyngiomas, Kallman's syndrome (p. 1031) or Laurence–Moon–Biedl syndrome (p. 1190), are usually diagnosed prior to puberty and therefore do not present as a diagnostic dilemma. Treatment is again with hormone replacement therapy as previously outlined.

Primary amenorrhea with normal sexual development

Primary amenorrhea with normal sexual development should be investigated by the age of 16. It is usually due to anatomical abnormalities.

Imperforate vagina

The commonest cause of absence of menstruation in a girl with normal development is cryptomenorrhea due to an *imperforate vagina* (Fig. 18.4) or, much less commonly, *absence of the vagina*. A careful history may reveal a history of cyclical lower abdominal pain. Not infrequently, the girl will have been admitted, often on more than one occasion, in recent months to the surgical wards with a provisional diagnosis of appendicitis. Retention of urine

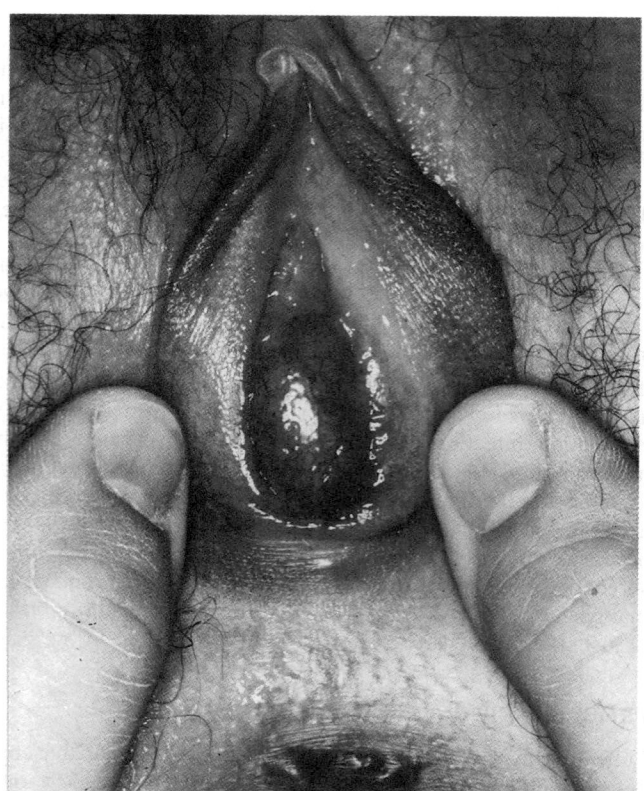

Fig. 18.4 Bulging membrane of hematocolpos.

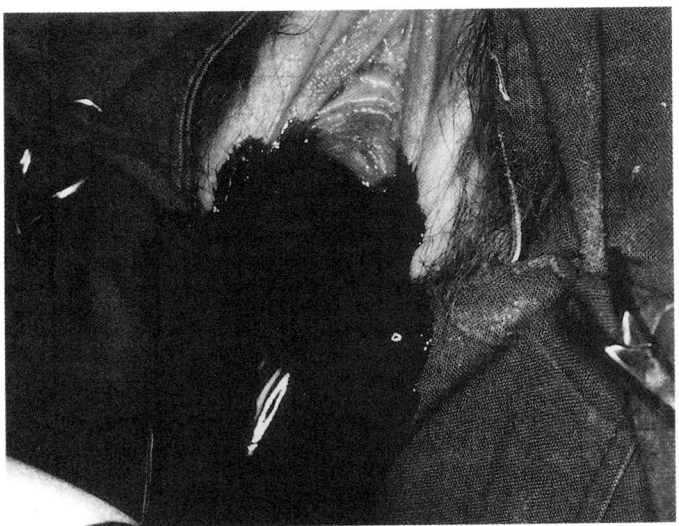

Fig. 18.5 Release of tarry material after incision of membrane in patient with hematocolpos.

may occur in serious cases owing to vaginal distention causing urethral blockage. General examination may show a lower abdominal mass arising out of the pelvis. The size of the mass is dependent on the duration of the cryptomenorrhea. Pelvic examination will show a distended blue-colored membrane on separating the labia. The diagnosis of hematocolpos may be confirmed by ultrasound scan. Treatment is with cruciate incision of the membrane under general anesthetic to release chocolate-colored tarry material (Fig. 18.5). The redundant membrane can then be excised. More complex causes of cryptomenorrhea will require more extensive investigation, including laparoscopy.

Absence of uterus

Other causes of primary amenorrhea with normal secondary sex characteristics include absence of the uterus and resistant ovary syndrome. *Absence of the uterus* may be the result of surgery or due to a congenital abnormality. Congenital absence of the uterus usually occurs in conjunction with congenital absence of the vagina owing to failure of development of the Müllerian duct system as in Rokitansky–Kuster–Hauser syndrome or complete androgen insensitivity syndrome (CAIS).

Complete androgen insensitivity syndrome

The condition results from the failure of the cells of the mesonephric duct and genital tubercle to respond to circulating androgens. Male genitalia, therefore, do not develop. At the same time, the paramesonephric ducts do respond to the Müllerian-inhibiting factor (MIF) produced by the testes and degenerate. This results in absence of the uterus, Fallopian tubes and upper two-thirds of the vagina. This is an X-linked disorder, and a history may be obtained of a sibling or an aunt similarly affected. Those affected are phenotypically female with female external genitalia and well-developed breasts with small nipples. They are, however, genetically male with a 46XY karyotype. Pelvic examination shows scanty pubic hair, an immature vulva, and a short blind vagina. The uterus is absent. Diagnosis is made by

chromosome analysis. Plasma testosterone levels are in the normal male range. Testes will be found in the abdomen, the inguinal canal or the vulva, and should be removed because of the risk of malignancy. The girl and her parents require appropriate support and counseling. Hormone replacement therapy as described elsewhere (p. 1033) will be required.

Pregnancy

Very occasionally, primary amenorrhea with normal secondary sex characteristics will be due to pregnancy.

PROBLEMS IN ADOLESCENCE

The main gynecological problems of the adolescent girl are those of menstruation – most commonly heavy or irregular periods, less commonly amenorrhea.

Dysfunctional uterine bleeding

Dysfunctional uterine bleeding presents as heavy periods which are often also irregular. Early menstrual cycles are usually anovulatory which result in overstimulation and proliferation of the endometrium from unopposed estrogen (Fig. 18.6). This thickened endometrium eventually breaks down to cause heavy irregular bleeding. The extent of the problem can be difficult to assess. It is difficult for a young girl unaccustomed to having periods to be able to say whether or not the bleeding is excessive.

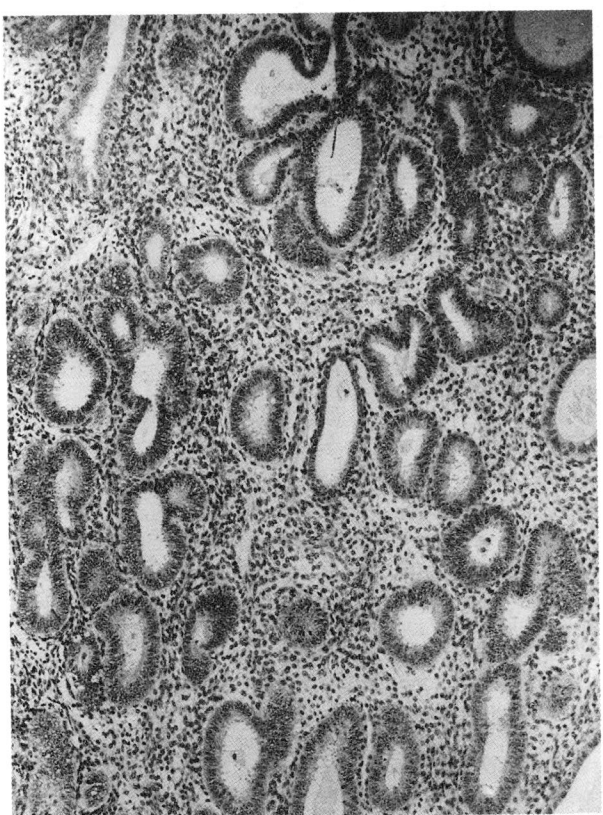

Fig. 18.6 Cystic appearance of endometrium from adolescent girl with hyperproliferation of the endometrium due to unopposed estrogen.

Her expectations and attitudes may well be significantly colored by those of her mother. An estimate of blood loss can be made by the number of pads and/or tampons required in a 24-h period, although this does depend on how fastidious the girl is about changing. Symptoms such as staining clothes, bedclothes or chairs are certainly indicative of excessive loss. In this age group, anemia is a not uncommon presentation of heavy periods. In the absence of such an obvious history, it is worth having her keep a diary of the frequency of her periods and the amount of protection she has to wear over a 2- to 3-month period. It may then be possible to reassure her – and her mother – that what she is experiencing is within normal limits. Treating her without establishing that her menstrual loss is excessive may lead to false expectations of the outcome of treatment and long-term gynecological problems.

Treatment. If her periods are regular, the simplest treatment is with prostaglandin synthetase inhibitors, such as mefenamic acid, 500 mg three times a day, perhaps in conjunction with a hemostatic agent such as ethamsylate, 500 mg four times a day, or tranexamic acid, 1–1.5 g three or four times a day. Although the prostaglandin synthetase inhibitors are primarily analgesics, they have the additional action of reducing menstrual flow. Both these medications need only be taken during the days of heavy menstrual flow. If the bleeding is irregular, hormone treatment will be required to regulate the cycle as well as reduce the flow. Norethisterone 5 mg three times a day, or dydrogesterone 5 mg twice a day, from day 15 to day 25 of the cycle (day 1 being the first day of menstruation) is usually satisfactory. One of the side effects of this treatment is weight gain, usually in the order or 3–6 kg. This should be mentioned before the onset of treatment, with reassurance that weight loss occurs quite quickly on cessation of therapy. The combined oral contraceptive pill is an alternative and is associated with less weight gain. Whatever treatment is used, it should be continued for 6–12 months, then stopped to ascertain whether or not the girl's cycle has become regular. Repeated courses may be given. If her periods do not improve while on therapy, an organic cause should be considered. These are rare in girls of this age group and do not need to be excluded at first presentation. Organic causes include pelvic inflammatory disease, endometriosis and genital tract tumors. Hematological disorders, such as von Willebrand's disease, presenting as heavy periods are uncommon but should be considered. The possibility of pregnancy must also be borne in mind.

Dysmenorrhea

This is also a common problem in adolescence. Classically, dysmenorrhea does not occur in the first few menstrual cycles as they are anovulatory which are purported to be painless. With the onset of ovulation, usually about 6 months after the menarche, dysmenorrhea may occur. The pain is usually spasmodic and colicky in nature. It may begin premenstrually and last until day 2 or 3 of the cycle. It affects the lower abdomen and back and occasionally radiates down the legs. In severe cases, the girl may also experience vomiting and diarrhea. In taking the history it is necessary to ascertain what medication, whether self-prescribed or medically prescribed, has been tried.

Treatment. In the first instance, treatment is with simple analgesics such as aspirin or codeine. If these are ineffective, the prostaglandin synthetase inhibitor group of analgesics should be used. The most commonly prescribed one is mefenamic acid,

250–500 mg three times a day. Girls should be instructed to start treatment with the onset of menstruation (or with the onset of pain if there is premenstrual dysmenorrhea) and to take it regularly during the days she is affected.

An alternative treatment, although not so satisfactory as it requires to be taken throughout the cycle, is dydrogesterone, 5 mg twice daily, or norethisterone, 5 mg three times daily from day 5 to day 25 of the cycle.

In severe cases when other therapy has failed, and particularly in girls who are losing time from school, the combined oral contraceptive pill may be used.

There is no place for dilation and curettage in the management of dysmenorrhea. It does not produce relief of symptoms and may result in cervical damage with consequent problems in adult life. Endometriosis is an unusual cause of dysmenorrhea in this age group but should be considered if there is no response to therapy. It can be excluded by a diagnostic laparoscopy.

Secondary amenorrhea

Secondary amenorrhea is said to occur if menstruation stops for more than 6 months (Table 18.3). The commonest cause is pregnancy. Pathological causes may be uterine, ovarian, pituitary or hypothalamic. Uterine causes are rare, particularly in this age group.

The causes of premature ovarian failure are listed in Table 18.4. Diagnosis is by hormone assay which shows low estrogen and elevated gonadotropin levels. Hormone replacement therapy is essential for these girls, not just for the psychological benefits of a monthly withdrawal bleed, but to prevent long-term problems with osteoporosis and cardiovascular disease.

Table 18.3 Causes of secondary amenorrhea

Physiological
Pregnancy

Pathological
Uterine
  absence
  Asherman's syndrome
Ovarian
  premature menopause
  polycystic ovarian disease
  hormone-secreting tumor
Hypothalamic/pituitary
  stress
  weight loss
  hypogonadotropic hypogonadism
  prolactinemia
  panhypopituitarism

Table 18.4 Causes of premature ovarian failure

Chromosomal, e.g. 45X

Autoimmune

Iatrogenic – surgery, radiotherapy, chemotherapy

Infection, e.g. mumps

Metabolic, e.g. galactosemia

Environmental

Idiopathic

Polycystic ovarian disease

This is responsible for 25% of cases of amenorrhea (Adams et al 1986). The etiology of the condition is unclear. The syndrome consists of amenorrhea or oligomenorrhea, obesity, hirsutism and reduced fertility. Not all patients manifest all symptoms. Diagnosis is confirmed by a raised LH : FSH ratio (greater than 3) and by an ultrasound examination which will show the ovaries to be larger than normal with increased dense stroma and a large number of small cysts arranged circumferentially (Fig. 18.7). The serum testosterone level may be mildly elevated.

Treatment. The mainstay of treatment must be the encouragement of weight loss. This reduces the peripheral metabolism of estrogen and circulating levels of LH (Bates & Whitworth 1982). Further treatment is with the combined oral contraceptive pill. Girls with polycystic ovarian disease should be reminded that the pill is merely masking the clinical features not curing the condition, and that the amenorrhea or oligomenorrhea is likely to recur when the pill is stopped. Girls in whom hirsutism is a major feature require careful investigation to exclude an adrenal lesion. In the absence of an adrenal lesion, cyproterone acetate (CPA) given in the reversed sequential regime is effective in limiting the hair growth in about three-quarters of the patients. Cyproterone acetate 50–100 mg is given from day 5 to day 15 of the cycle with ethinyl estradiol 0.30 mg daily (most conveniently in the form of the combined oral contraceptive pill). Girls on CPA therapy should have liver function tests assessed regularly.

Hypothalamic and pituitary lesions

These are the most common pathological causes of secondary amenorrhea. Secretion of gonadotropin-releasing factors from the hypothalamus is affected by emotional stress, such as examinations or problems at home, and by extreme weight loss in girls who have been on a crash diet or who are anorexic. Investigations in these girls are unlikely to reveal any abnormality. They can be reassured that their periods will resume when the stress is over or they have gained weight. Hypogonadotropic hypogonadism is a relatively common cause of amenorrhea and is associated with low levels of FSH, LH and estrogen. Treatment is by hormone replacement.

Pituitary disorders such as panhypopituitarism are extremely uncommon. Increased prolactin production is not an unusual cause of secondary amenorrhea in adults but not in adolescents. It is associated with galactorrhea and the presence of a pituitary microadenoma must be excluded.

GYNECOLOGICAL TUMORS

Gynecological tumors in childhood are fortunately rare, although their rarity may lead to a delay in diagnosis. The important ones to consider are ovarian tumors and the cervical/vaginal lesions.

Ovarian lesions

The commonest ovarian lesion is probably the *simple follicular cyst*. It is not understood why these lesions should arise in an ovary not being stimulated. Many of these are asymptomatic and may be found during ultrasound examination. The management should be as conservative as possible. Lesions smaller than 5 cm in diameter require no treatment and should only be followed with ultrasound examination. Larger cysts should be treated by aspiration either via ultrasound or laparoscopically with ultrasound follow-up. If surgery is required, care should be taken to conserve as much of the ovarian tissue as possible.

The commonest ovarian neoplasms in young girls are teratomas and dysgerminomas.

Teratomas are usually benign lesions that may be unilateral or bilateral. They derive from totipotential primordial germ cells and contain ectodermal, mesodermal and endodermal tissue in varying amounts, commonly with a preponderance of skin, sebum and hair (dermoid cysts). They usually present as asymptomatic abdominal masses, although abdominal pain may be the presenting symptom. Ultrasound examination confirms the presence of a multicystic tumor with mixed solid and cystic areas. X-ray examination may show areas of calcification or, less commonly, teeth-like structures. Treatment is by surgical removal with preservation of as much ovarian tissue as possible as the tumor is bilateral in approximately 10% of patients.

Dysgerminomas are malignant tumors though generally not of high malignant potential. They develop from the primordial germ cells. They are relatively more common in childhood than in adult life, 60% developing in the first two decades of life. Dysgerminomas present as a rapidly growing, often asymptomatic, abdominal mass. In advanced cases, ascites may be present.

Treatment depends on the degree of malignancy. In cases of obvious malignancy, with involvement of the opposite ovary, ascites and peritoneal involvement, total abdominal hysterectomy with bilateral salpingo-oophorectomy is required. The tumor is radiosensitive and postoperative irradiation may be required. In girls in whom the tumor is not so obviously malignant, unilateral oophorectomy may be sufficient with careful long-term follow-up.

Other ovarian tumors are less common in childhood.

Cervical/vaginal lesions

Cervical and vaginal tumors are the most important gynecological tumors of childhood. The commonest and most serious is *botryoid*

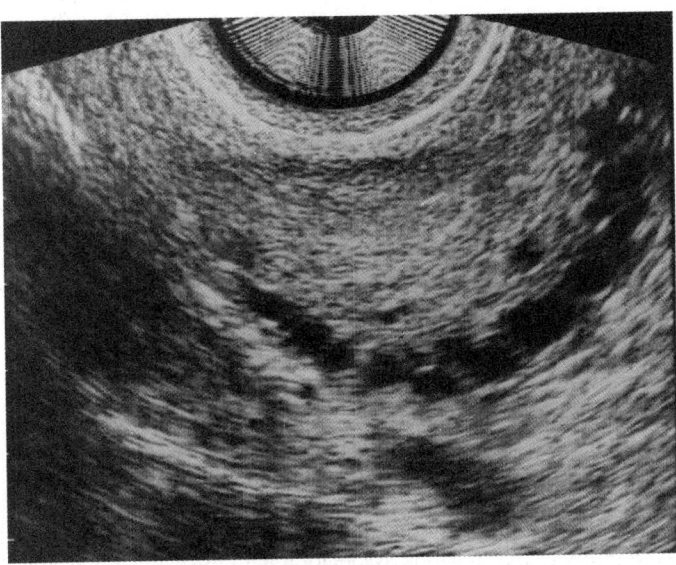

Fig. 18.7 Ultrasound appearance of polycystic ovaries showing the circumferential arrangement of small cysts.

sarcoma (*rhabdomyosarcoma*). This highly malignant tumor occurs most commonly in girls below the age of two, with 90% of the tumors occurring in girls below 5 years of age. It most commonly affects the vagina and, less commonly and usually in older girls and adolescents, the cervix. The tumor presents with bloodstained vaginal discharge or frank vaginal bleeding. On examination, a fleshy hemorrhagic lesion is seen which is classically described as 'grape-like', although it may also appear as a simple polyp. The tumor originates in the subepithelial layer of the cervical or vaginal epithelium and spreads widely within this layer, producing a classical polypoid appearance before invading the vaginal wall itself. In early stages, the tumor may not have a strikingly malignant appearance, leading to the diagnosis being missed. Later spread is via the lymphatics and bloodstream. Treatment is by combination chemotherapy over a period of 6 months, followed by extended hysterectomy and vaginectomy unless the response to chemotherapy has been dramatic when it should be continued for a further 6 months to a year (Bell et al 1986).

The other lesion of the vagina and cervix that deserves mention is *clear-cell adenocarcinoma*. This occurs in girls who were exposed to diethylstilbestrol (DES) in utero. DES was given to mothers for the treatment of threatened abortion and was more commonly used in the US than in Europe. Approximately two-thirds of girls exposed to DES in utero have a congenital abnormality of the cervix, including recessed areas around the cervix, pseudopolyp formation and hypertrophy of the endocervical tissue. Abnormalities of the vagina may also be seen, including incomplete septa, fibrous bands and vaginal adenosis. It has been estimated that the risk of these girls developing cancer is between 0.14 and 1.4 per 1000 (Herbst 1979). Girls exposed to DES in utero should be followed-up by colposcopy from their early teens. Treatment of clear-cell adenocarcinoma of the vagina is by extended hysterectomy and vaginectomy.

PREGNANCY IN TEENAGERS

The problems associated with teenage pregnancy are more social than medical. One UK survey of teenage mothers (Simms & Smith 1986) showed that four-fifths were from lower socioeconomic groups and that the incidence of smoking was twice that of their peers. As the pregnancies are usually unplanned and teenagers are often reluctant to acknowledge that they are pregnant, booking for antenatal care is usually late and clinic attendance sporadic.

Obstetric complications

Specific reported problems in teenagers are an increased incidence of pregnancy-induced hypertension (Konje et al 1992), premature labor (Osbourne 1981), low birth weight babies (Satin et al 1994) and anemia (Konje et al 1992, Khwaja et al 1986). All these complications are more common in women from the lower socioeconomic groups and most of them are also related to maternal smoking, making it difficult to identify the specific cause of the complication.

Contrary to the widely held view that young women have problems in labor because of their small pelvis, teenagers are at no greater risk of having a prolonged labor or delivery by Cesarean section (Satin et al 1994, Zhang & Chan 1991, Bradford & Giles

1989). There are no data to suggest a poor perinatal outcome for teenagers. A study from Hull (Konje at al 1992) showed no difference in birth weight or perinatal mortality in the teenage study group compared to controls.

A high percentage of teenage pregnancies end in abortion – the Hull study referred to above showed that 59.6% of pregnant teenagers had a termination of pregnancy. The social and educational background of the teenager (and her family) is a major factor, however. A study from Dundee (Smith 1993) showed that two-thirds of pregnancies in teenagers from affluent areas ended in abortion compared with a quarter of those from deprived areas.

Sexually transmitted diseases

Pregnancy is not the only unwanted outcome of early intercourse. An increased risk of sexually transmitted diseases, with subsequent risk to fertility, is a major problem. In the UK, as well as in the USA, adolescents account for 25% of sexually transmitted diseases seen in women. The organism causing most concern is *Chlamydia*, which is frequently asymptomatic but is associated with a high risk of tubal problems and consequent infertility.

Of even greater concern is the increasing number of teenagers presenting with *cervical intraepithelial neoplasia* (CIN), associated with an increase in the number of young women presenting with cervical cancer. The role of early intercourse and number of sexual partners in the development of cervical cancer is well recognized. Human papilloma virus types 16 and 18 has been implicated in the etiology of the disease, and it is essential that those involved in the sex education of teenagers make them aware of the correlation and of the importance of attending for cervical smears when they become sexually active.

CONTRACEPTION FOR TEENAGERS

The question of contraception for teenagers is a vexed one. The controversy that surrounded Mrs Victoria Gillick and the prescribing of contraception to girls under the age of 16 without parental consent revealed the depth of feeling on the matter within and outside the medical profession. While most doctors would probably agree that abstinence is ideal for young girls, in reality the choice for some girls is sexual intercourse with contraception or without it.

Methods of contraception

Barrier methods

Barrier methods such as the sheath or cap have much to recommend them. Not only are they an effective form of contraception if used correctly, they also protect against venereal diseases, cervical carcinoma and HIV infection. They have the big advantage of having no side effects. They are, however, unpopular with many teenagers. The use of the sheath requires the initiative to be taken by the male partner, or at least his agreement to use it, and he is usually less motivated to use contraception. The greater availability of the sheath in association with the campaign against AIDS may improve this, however, and increase the acceptability of the sheath.

The use by the girl of a vaginal cap or diaphragm requires having one fitted at a family planning clinic. In addition, the need to keep it hidden at home and the need to insert it prior to intercourse make it unsuitable for most teenagers.

Mechanical methods

Mechanical methods of contraception, such as the intrauterine contraceptive device, are not recommended for this age group, as they have a risk of causing pelvic inflammatory disease with resultant tubal infertility.

Hormonal methods

The oral contraceptive pill is probably the most widely used form of contraception. It does require medical supervision, but is often prescribed by the general practitioner thus avoiding visits to the family planning clinic, although many adolescents prefer the relative anonymity of the family planning clinic. In addition to its contraceptive effects, the pill has beneficial side effects. It may reduce menstrual flow, regulate menstrual periods and decrease dysmenorrhea. Some girls will present to their general practitioners with these symptoms in the hope that they will prescribe the pill and thus save them having to ask for contraceptive advice. The pill provides teenagers with continuous contraceptive cover, provided they take it regularly. As sexual intercourse in teenagers is likely to be sporadic and nonpremeditated, such continuous cover may be an advantage. By the same token, however, it may be argued that continuous hormone ingestion in a girl who is having intercourse infrequently is inadvisable. Numerous studies on the safety of the combined oral contraceptive pill in adolescents have been performed. An increased risk of breast cancer in later life as a result of oral contraceptive use during breast development has been suggested (Pike et al 1983). More recent studies have confirmed a slight increased risk (Wingo et al 1991, Bernstein et al 1990, Rookus & van Leeuwen 1994) especially if the combined oral contraceptive is taken for longer than 4 years prior to the age of 20. This risk, however, has to be balanced against the benefits mentioned above and the problems of an unplanned pregnancy.

An alternative form of oral contraceptive pill is the progestogen-only pill (mini-pill). This is not an advisable form of contraception for teenagers as it has to be taken regularly, preferably at the same time each day, and this is probably unrealistic. In addition, the progestogen-only pill may cause irregular periods, which many find unacceptable. For the same reason, the long-acting depot-progestogen is not advisable.

The ideal form of contraception for adolescents, therefore, is probably the sheath combined with the oral contraceptive (the so-called double Dutch method). The need for a realistic sex education and family planning program designed specifically for teenagers in which there is an opportunity for full discussion cannot be overstated.

REFERENCES

Adams J, Polson D W, Franks S 1986 Prevalence of polycystic ovaries in women with anovulation and idiopathic hirsutism. British Medical Journal 293: 355–359

Bates G W, Whitworth N S 1982 Effect of body weight reduction on plasma androgens in obese infertile women. Fertility and Sterility 38: 406–409

Bell J, Averette H, Davis J, Toledano S 1986 Genital rhabdomyosarcoma of the vagina or uterus. Cancer 37: 118–122

Bernstein L, Pike M C, Krailo M, Henderson B E 1990 Update of the Los Angeles Study of oral contraceptives and breast cancer. Royal Society of Medicine, London, pp 169–180

Bradford J A, Giles W B 1989 Teenage pregnancy in Western Sydney. Australia and New Zealand Journal of Obstetrics and Gynaecology 29: 1–4

David M, Forest M G 1984 Prenatal treatment of 21-hydroxylation of congenital adrenal hyperplasia resulting from 21-hydroxylase deficiency. Journal of Pediatrics 105: 799–803

Gravier L 1969 Hydrocolpos. Journal of Pediatric Surgery 4: 563–568

Herbst A L 1979 Current status of the DES problem. Obstetrical and Gynecological Survey 34: 844–850

Khwaja S S, Al-Sibai M H, Al-Suleiman A S, El-Zibdeh M Y 1986 Obstetric implications of pregnancy in adolescence. Acta Obstetrica Gynecologia Scandinavica 65: 57–61

Konje J C, Palmer A, Watson A, Hay D M, Imrie A 1992 Early teenage pregnancies in Hull. British Journal of Obstetrics and Gynaecology 99: 969–973

Landrum B, Ogburn P L, Feinberg S, Bendel R, Ferrara B, Johnson D A, Thompson T R 1986 Intrauterine aspiration of a large fetal ovarian cyst. Obstetrics and Gynecology 68: 11s–14s

Osbourne G K, Howat R C L, Jordan M M 1981 The obstetric outcome of teenage pregnancy. British Journal of Obstetrics and Gynaecology 88: 215–221

Pearce A N, Hart C A 1992 Vulvo-vaginitis: causes and management. Archives of Disease in Childhood 67: 509–512

Pike M C, Henderson B E, Krailo M D, Duke A, Roy S 1983 Breast cancer in young women and use of oral contraceptives: possible modifying effect of formulation and age at use. Lancet ii: 926–930

Purkiss S, Brereton R J, Wright V M 1988 Surgical emergencies after prenatal treatment for intra-abdominal abnormality. Lancet 1: 289–290

Rookus M S A, van Leeuwen F E 1994 Oral contraceptives and risk of breast cancer in women aged 20–54 years. Lancet 344: 844–851

Satin A J, Leveno K J, Sherman M L, Reedy N J, Lowe T W, McIntire D D 1994 Maternal youth and pregnancy outcomes: middle school versus high school groups compared with women beyond the teen years. American Journal of Obstetrics and Gynecology 171: 184–187

Simms M, Smith C 1986 Teenage mothers and their partners. Research report no 15. HMSO, London

Smith T 1993 Influence of socioeconomic factors on attaining targets for reducing teenage pregnancies. British Medical Journal 306: 1232–1235

Strachan T, Sinnott P J, Smeaton I, Dyer P A, Harris R 1987 Prenatal diagnosis of congenital adrenal hyperplasia. Lancet 2: 1272–1273

Tanner J M 1962 Growth at adolescence, 2nd edn. Blackwell Scientific Publications, Oxford

Widdowson D J, Pilling D W, Cook R C M 1988 Neonatal ovarian cysts: therapeutic dilemma. Archives of Disease in Childhood 63: 737–742

Wingo P A, Lee N C, Ory H W, Beral V, Peterson H B, Rhodes P 1991 Age-specific differences in the relationship between oral contraceptive use and breast cancer. Obstetrics and Gynecology 78: 161–170

Zhang B, Chan A 1991 Teenage pregnancy in South Australia, 1986–1988. Australia and New Zealand Journal of Obstetrics and Gynaecology 31: 291–298

19 Endocrine gland disorders and disorders of growth and puberty

Christopher J. H. Kelnar

Mechanisms of hormone action   996
History taking and examination   998
Endocrine tests   1000
Fetal endocrinology   1002
Fetal endocrine factors   1002
Ontogeny of fetal hormone secretion   1002
Long-term implications of fetal growth   1005
Placental hormone secretion   1005
Maternal disease and endocrine function   1005
Maternal drugs and endocrine function   1005
Control of onset of labor   1005
Neonatal endocrinology   1006
Growth assessment and disorders of growth   1011
The importance of growth assessment   1011
Growth hormone (GH) and growth   1012
Growth regulation   1014
The short or slowly growing child   1014
Investigation of poor growth   1018
Treatment of poor growth   1019
The tall or rapidly growing child   1020
Obesity and thinness   1021
Endocrinological aspects of puberty and adolescence   1023
The gonads   1023
Endocrine background to normal puberty   1024
Changes in fetus, infant and child and their relevance to the initiation of puberty   1024
Changes of body composition and metabolic signals for onset of puberty   1026
Abnormal puberty   1026
Precocious sexual maturation   1027
Delayed sexual maturation   1031
Other disorders related to female and male reproduction   1035
Amenorrhea   1035

Noonan's syndrome   1035
Klinefelter's syndrome (47 XXY)   1036
Gynecomastia   1036
Undescended testes   1037
The hypothalamo-pituitary unit   1037
Anterior pituitary hormones   1038
Posterior pituitary hormones   1039
Diseases of the hypothalamoneurohypophyseal unit   1039
Diseases of the adenohypophysis   1041
Other disorders   1043
The pineal gland   1043
The thymus   1044
The thyroid gland   1044
Hypofunction   1046
Hyperfunction   1050
Neoplasia   1052
Parathyroid glands and calcium metabolism   1053
Physiology of calcium homeostasis   1053
Calcium regulation in the fetus and neonate   1053
Disorders of calcium and bone metabolism   1055
Abnormal 1,25-dihydroxy vitamin D secretion or action   1055
Abnormal PTH secretion or action   1056
Abnormal calcitonin secretion   1057
Abnormalities of phosphate excretion   1058
Abnormalities of calcium excretion   1058
Practical differential diagnosis   1058
The adrenal glands   1059
The adrenal cortex   1059
The adrenal medulla   1069
Endocrine hypertension   1069
The pancreas and carbohydrate metabolism   1071
Pancreatic morphology   1071
Diabetes mellitus   1072
Hypoglycemia   1082
References   1084

MECHANISMS OF HORMONE ACTION

DEFINITION

Hormones are chemical substances secreted directly into the bloodstream which affect the specific functioning of a cell or system in some other part of the body. They are produced from endocrine glands. The integration of hormone activity is of vital importance for the maintenance of a stable and appropriate internal environment and for the response to external environmental changes. Few hormones have unique actions and few bodily processes are determined by one hormone.

TYPES OF HORMONE

Hormones can be divided into four distinct broad categories in terms of glands of origin, basic chemical nature, mode of synthesis, transport in the circulation, half-life, mode of action, metabolism and excretion. The properties of these groups, peptides, steroids, iodothyronines and catecholamines, are summarized in Table 19.1. Actions at cellular level are summarized in Figures 19.1 and 19.2.

ORGANIZATION OF THE ENDOCRINE SYSTEM

The biological effects of hormones are regulated within well-defined physiological limits by a complex system of stimulation, inhibition and feedback control – secretion, delivery to target cells, recognition by receptors, exertion of a specific biological action, appropriate degradation and feedback to secretory cells to inhibit further production. Control mechanisms are complex and

Table 19.1 Categories of hormone

	Peptides	Steroids	Iodothyronine	Catecholamines
Synthesis	From large precursors (prohormones) via enzymatic reactions	From common precursor (cholesterol) via enzymatic reactions	In thyroid gland from iodine and tyrosine via enzymatic reactions	In adrenal medulla and in sympathetic and central nervous tissues and chromaffin tissue from phenylalanine and tyrosine via enzymatic reactions
Storage (gland or origin)	High proportion	Very little	High proportion	Very little
Solubility	Aqueous	Lipid	?	?
Circulation	Unbound	Plasma protein bound	Plasma protein bound	Unbound
Half-life	Minutes	Hours	Days	? (short)
Periphery	Little transformation	Transformation ++ increasing biological activity	Little transformation	Little transformation
Action	Via specific plasma membrane receptors and cyclic AMP (cAMP)	Via binding to cytoplasmic receptors and stimulating nuclear messenger ribonucleic acid (mRNA) and protein synthesis	As steroids (no cytoplasmic receptor for T3)	Via alpha-, beta- and dopaminergic cell surface receptors

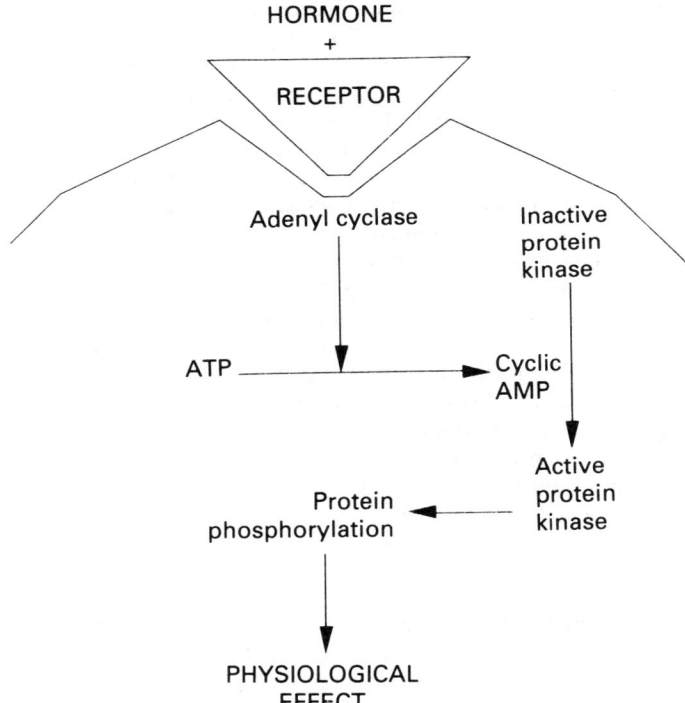

Fig. 19.1 Cellular mechanism of action of peptides.

may involve other hormones (facilitative, additive or antagonistic), neurotransmitters and metabolic substrates. The principles are summarized schematically in Figure 19.3.

Interrelationships between environment and endocrine and central nervous systems are close. Physiological states, such as sleep, are important in the hypothalamic control of growth and sex steroids modify behavior at puberty. The hypothalamus, situated between brain and pituitary gland, has an important integrative and regulatory role, exerting effects on the pituitary adenohypophysis via a series of small peptides secreted from the ventromedial nucleus near the median eminence. Their synthesis and release is determined by neurotransmitters such as dopamine, serotonin and noradrenaline, and others such as acetylcholine, melatonin and gamma-aminobutyric acid (GABA) may also be important. Some peptides have stimulatory and some inhibitory activity in terms of pituitary hormone secretion.

Neurosecretory cells producing neurotransmitters are in close anatomical relationship with hypothalamic secretory neurons whose axons anastomose with portal blood vessels traversing the pituitary stalk and transporting hypothalamic peptides to the pituitary. Blood-borne anterior pituitary hormones in turn control secretion by a number of glands – thyroid, adrenals and gonads – as well as physiological processes such as growth and lactation. The ontogeny of fetal pituitary hormone secretion and brain–hypothalamopituitary connections is discussed on pages 1002–1005. Other endocrine systems are independent of hypothalamopituitary axis control – serum calcium is the major controlling mechanism for parathyroid hormone (PTH) secretion as is plasma glucose for pancreatic insulin secretion.

Laboratory-based advances are making an important and relevant impact on the endocrine practice; protein chemistry is increasing understanding of how GH regulates growth, differentiation and metabolism; transmembrane signaling can now 'explain' such pediatric endocrine disorders as McCune–Albright syndrome, pseudohypoparathyroidism (PHP) type 1, acromegaly, and many thyroid, adrenocortical and ovarian granulosa cell tumors as disorders of heterotrimeric G proteins which are important for the GTP binding and hydrolysis that amplifies hormonal signals. Rapid molecular genetics advances are enabling recognition of the genetics and biochemistry of sex determination and new disease mechanisms – mosaicism in pseudoachondroplasia and McCune–Albright syndrome, placental mosaicism in some forms of IUGR; imprinting (parental origin effects) in Prader–Willi and Angelman syndromes, PHP, Beckwith–Wiedemann syndrome, and, possibly, Silver–Russell syndrome.

In addition, it is becoming recognized that fetal and childhood growth may have important implications, not only for the child but also for adult health and disease (see p. 1005).

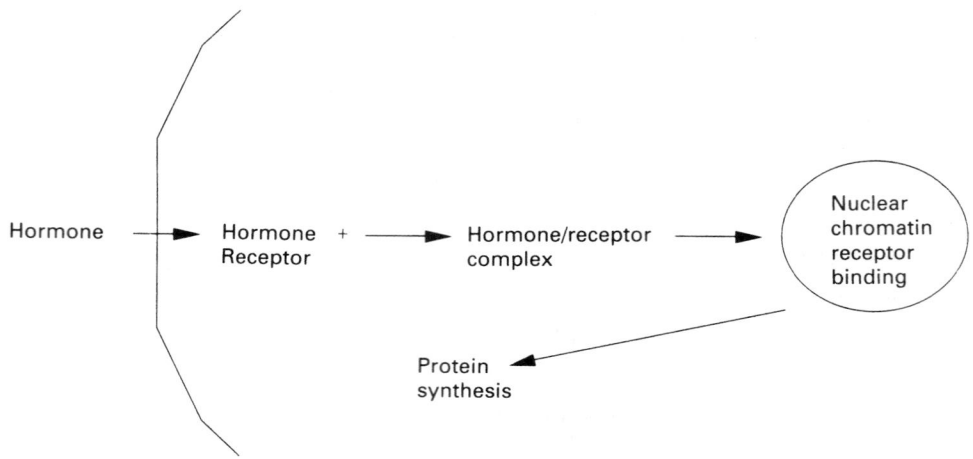

Fig. 19.2   Cellular mechanism of action of steroids.

HISTORY TAKING AND EXAMINATION

Clinical manifestations of endocrine disorders are diverse and subtle. A full history and comprehensive clinical examination can yield important clues.

FAMILY HISTORY

Some endocrine disorders are familial. Autosomal recessively inherited conditions include congenital adrenal hyperplasia. A history of unexplained neonatal deaths may be significant in this

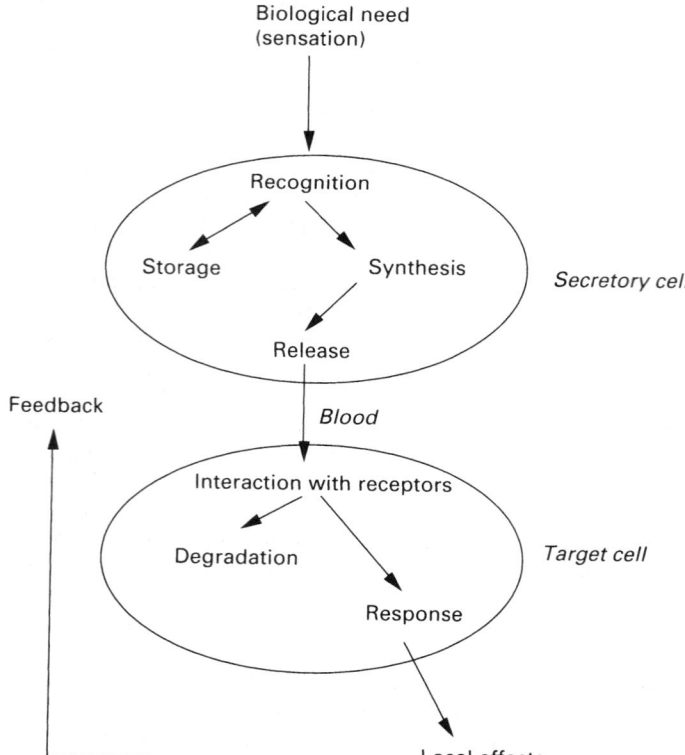

Fig. 19.3   Organization of the endocrine system.

context, particularly in parts of the world where neonatal pediatric services are poorly developed.

Inheritance in other conditions is less clear: the HLA identical sibling of a child with insulin-dependent diabetes mellitus has about a 90-fold increased risk of developing the disease before 15 years, yet less than 1% of genetically susceptible children will ever develop diabetes. Autoimmune processes are important in its pathogenesis and a family history of autoimmune disease (e.g. moniliasis, pernicious anemia, alopecia or vitiligo) should alert the clinician to disorders such as diabetes mellitus, Addison's disease, hypothyroidism or hypoparathyroidism. Growth hormone (GH) deficiency can run in families.

A family history of early or late puberty (ask about age of menarche in mother and older girl siblings; ask fathers whether they were growing fast after they left school and when they started shaving) is sometimes seen but there is considerable variation in the timing of puberty amongst normal family members.

Sometimes a child of normal stature is short for the parents (e.g. a girl with Turner's syndrome and tall parents). An unusually short parent can have an undiagnosed disorder (e.g. GH deficiency, skeletal dysplasia or pseudohypoparathyroidism (Fig. 19.4)) which the child has inherited.

PREGNANCY

Maternal illness during pregnancy may have significant effects on endocrine function in the fetus and neonate. Neonatal hyperthyroidism is seen in about 1.5% of infants born to mothers with Graves' disease. This relates to placental transfer of human thyroid-stimulating immunoglobulins. In the first trimester, 19-norprogestogens (e.g. norethisterone) for recurrent abortion are associated with masculinization of a female fetus. In the second or third trimesters, carbimazole and thiouracil are associated with neonatal goiter and hypothyroidism; chlorpropamide may cause neonatal hypoglycemia.

NEONATAL HISTORY

Breech delivery, micropenis, hypothermia and hypoglycemia are all commoner in infants with GH insufficiency or panhypopituitarism. Birth asphyxia may be associated with subsequent precocious puberty.

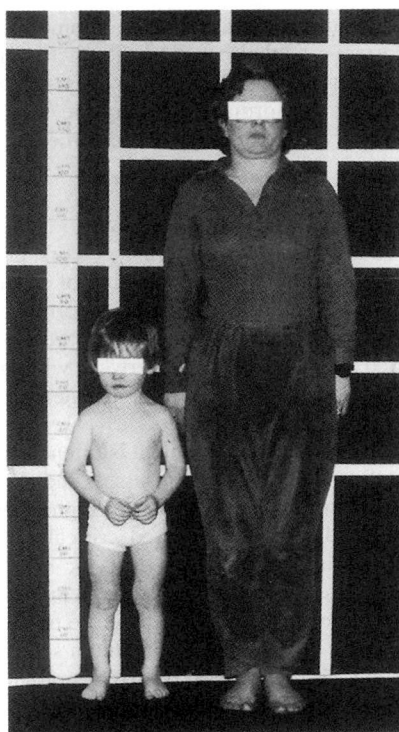

Fig. 19.4 Pseudohypoparathyroidism in mother and child (see also Fig. 19.7).

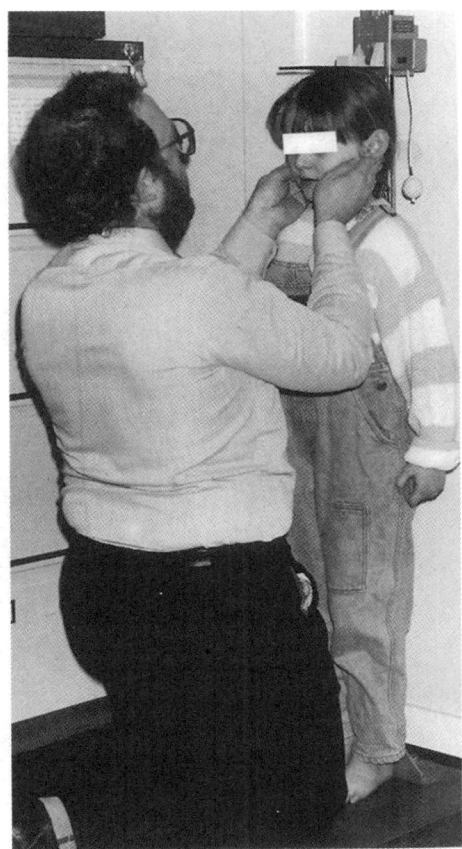

Fig. 19.5 Accurate measurement of height using a stadiometer.

Ambiguous genitalia suggest congenital adrenal hyperplasia (CAH, most commonly 21-hydroxylase deficiency in a genotypic female) or an androgen biosynthetic defect (in a phenotypic male). Severe vomiting, hyponatremic dehydration and excessive urinary sodium loss suggests a form of CAH, hypoplasia or pseudohypoaldosteronism (or renal disease). Hypertension can develop in the 11β-hydroxylase form of CAH.

Prolonged jaundice is a clue to congenital hypothyroidism. Other clinical signs may not be present until later. Even where screening programs are in operation, false negatives can occasionally occur.

PAST MEDICAL HISTORY

Very poor feeding in infancy may be associated with prolonged intrauterine growth retardation and later short stature. Recurrent hypoglycemia may be due to GH deficiency, panhypopituitarism or adrenal problems (e.g. Addison's disease). An insidious fall off in school performance is often a feature of acquired hypothyroidism.

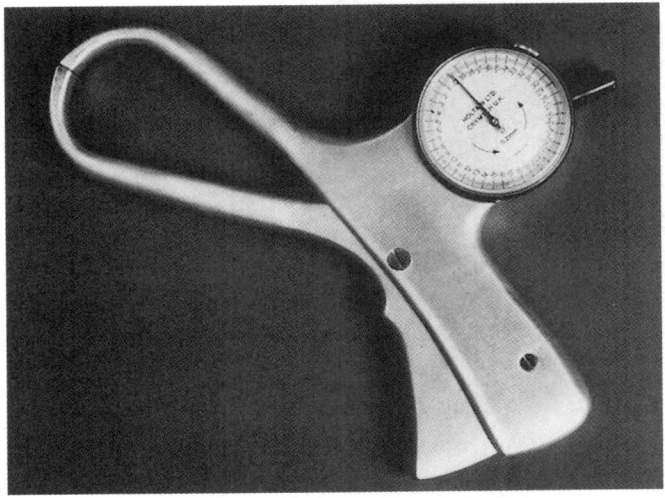

Fig. 19.6 Skinfold calipers.

CLINICAL EXAMINATION

Accurate height measurements (Fig. 19.5), repeated to determine growth velocity, are important in the diagnosis of endocrine (and many other) childhood disorders. Many cause slow growth (and, ultimately, short stature) and are associated with mild or moderate obesity (best assessed using skinfold calipers (Fig. 19.6) rather than weighing scales). In contrast, obesity due to an excessive food intake causes rapid growth and tall stature in childhood.

Endocrine causes of abnormally rapid growth in childhood include precocious puberty, thyrotoxicosis and gigantism.

Disproportionate stature (abnormal body proportions) is seen in long-standing panhypopituitarism, hypothyroidism and GH deficiency, skeletal dysplasias and some inborn metabolic errors. Short fourth and fifth metacarpal bones are characteristic of pseudohypoparathyroidism (Fig. 19.7) and Turner's syndrome.

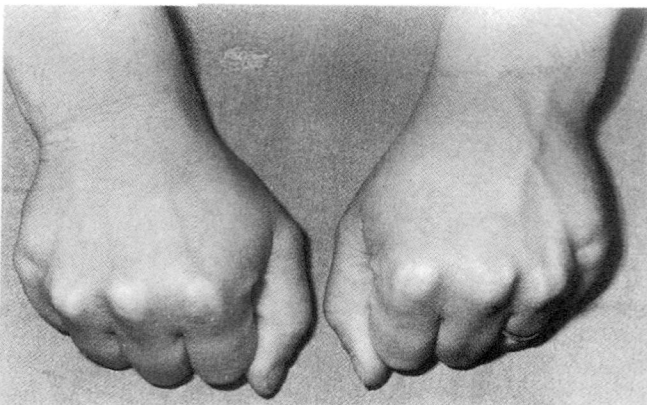

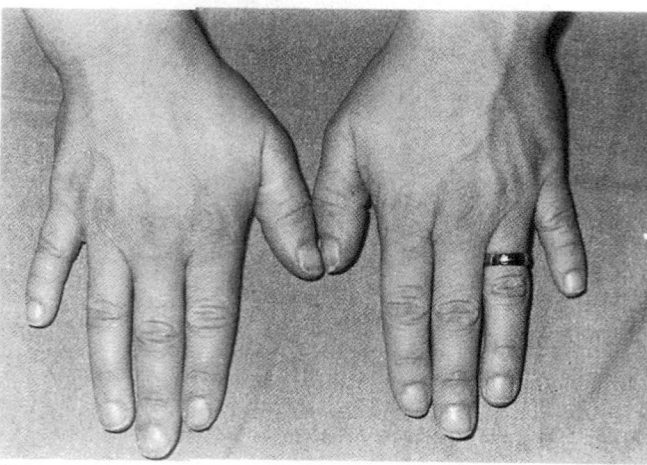

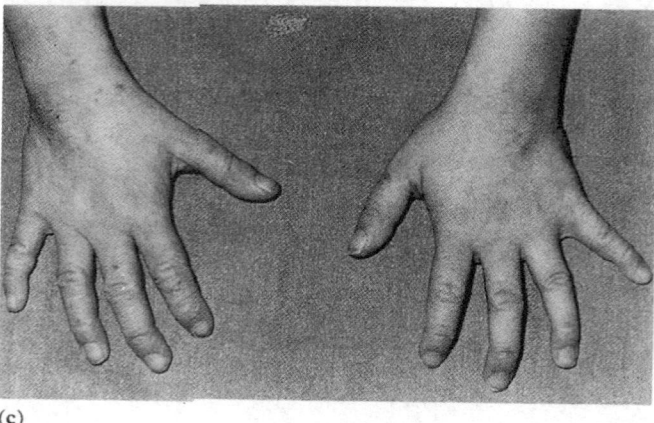

Fig. 19.7   Short 5th metacarpal in a mother (**a**, **b**) and child (**c**) with pseudohypoparathyroidism (see also Fig. 19.4).

Delayed puberty in girls may be due to Turner's syndrome. Primary amenorrhea may be associated with CAH, Turner's syndrome or rarer disorders of sexual differentiation.

Hirsutism may be due to CAH or Cushing's syndrome. The latter is often associated with temporarily rapid growth, truncal obesity, striae, and moon face. Secondary hypertension can be due to endocrine disease (usually adrenal cortical mineralocorticoid excess).

Fundal examination and visual fields assessment is vital in any child with abnormal growth or recurrent headache. Craniopharyngioma commonly presents in this way. Dysmorphic features (especially midline abnormalities) may be associated with hypothalamopituitary or other endocrine disorders.

ENDOCRINE TESTS

Diagnosis can often be suspected on the basis of history and clinical findings. In puberty, clinical staging of secondary sexual characteristics is an excellent 'bioassay' of hormone function. A girl of 14 years with stage 2 (Tanner 1962) breast development can be reassured that puberty is underway, without measuring estradiol or LH – indeed a 'random' clinic measurement would suggest the opposite (see below).

Nevertheless, biochemical assessment is often necessary, either to confirm or refute a diagnosis or to assess the appropriateness and effectiveness of treatment (Walker & Hughes 1995), but the information obtained must be assessed critically if misleading conclusions are not to be drawn.

Many hormones are secreted episodically in pulses or may vary diurnally. A single measurement may therefore be meaningless or misleading. Dynamic tests to assess maximum secretory capacity will give different normal values from physiological secretory profiles. Needless tests provide irrelevant information, waste laboratory time and resources and cause unnecessary discomfort to the child. Principles of tests and validation underlying diagnostic decisions are reviewed by Schönberg (1992).

BLOOD

A single, random blood test for hormone assay may give insufficient information. Dynamic tests requiring serial samples in children can be difficult or dangerous. There must be no errors in patient preparation (e.g. fasting), request forms, specimen collection, transport to and receipt by the laboratory, and reporting, communication and interpretation of results.

Stress from cannulation (or the thought of it) will affect levels of hormones such as cortisol, GH and prolactin (PRL). Baseline samples must be obtained before suppression or stimulation tests commence. A sample 30 min before baseline may help to quantify and reduce stress effects.

It may be necessary to measure simultaneously hormones at both ends of a feedback system – ACTH levels will be inappropriately high for the normal cortisol levels in untreated CAH; raised TSH levels with normal T4 levels indicate developing primary hypothyroidism.

Overnight fasting does not preclude day case tests if the family live nearby. Those traveling far are best admitted the previous evening. Fasting from midnight (water only allowed) is generally safe in the older child provided testing starts before 9 a.m. but is dangerous in a child with GH deficiency or panhypopituitarism. If this is suspected blood glucose levels should be checked at regular intervals overnight. Younger children are particularly vulnerable to fasting hypoglycemia (see p. 1082).

URINE

Urine sampling is atraumatic in children (less so in infants). 24-h collections can reflect overall production of (e.g.) steroids more accurately than isolated plasma samples but can be difficult to obtain, even in hospital. Expressing results per 24 h per gram excreted creatinine may not control for this (Vestergaard & Leverett 1958) and even distort results.

SALIVA

Many hormones (e.g. peptides) cannot be assayed in saliva but the technique is useful for steroids, e.g. cortisol, progesterone and testosterone (Butler et al 1989d) – concentrations are independent of flow rate and reflect free plasma levels (Riad-Fahmy et al 1982). Most children over about 6 years can produce saliva. Specimens can be collected easily and noninvasively, serially or during dynamic tests. Wash the mouth out with water and wait a few minutes before allowing saliva to dribble into a plain tube. Sialogogues (e.g. citric acid or a lemon sweet) may be helpful but are usually unnecessary.

ERRORS

Specimen collection, labeling, transport

Ensure that a sample of adequate volume is obtained in the correct tube at the appropriate time. Ensure, particularly during serial/dynamic tests that the collection time is marked on each container, that tubes are not muddled and that adequate, correct information is on the request form. Liaise with the laboratory beforehand if samples need special handling, e.g. ACTH assay samples into cooled lithium heparin tubes, centrifuged immediately at 4°C and plasma stored at 20°C until assay.

Reporting

Laboratory transcription errors can occur. Incorrect comments may be added about the normality or otherwise of a result if the child is of different age or sex from that recorded on the form (first names can be ambiguous), if a sample is thought to have been at a different time or is stimulated rather than basal. Reports may be delayed, lost or misfiled. Verbal reports may be misheard.

Interpreting results (Jeffcoate 1981, Fraser 1986, Fraser & Fogarty 1989)

Units can be misunderstood. The Système International has simplified and standardized the reporting of many hormones in molar amounts (SI units) but is still not used universally (e.g. USA). For a reference table for converting to and from SI units see Ranke (1992).

For larger polypeptides, including many hormones (whose structure cannot be physicochemically characterized), values are reported in terms of 'units' calibrated in terms of 'standards' derived from specific assays from material that may have different biological or immunological properties.

Laboratories sometimes report with spurious accuracy, e.g. to too many decimal places. Standard errors are seldom quoted and may be difficult to define as concentrations of many hormones are not normally distributed (Jeffcoate 1981) and skewed towards higher values. Log transformation often normalizes clinical, e.g. weight (Tanner 1951), and laboratory, e.g. urinary adrenal steroid metabolites (Kelnar 1985), data.

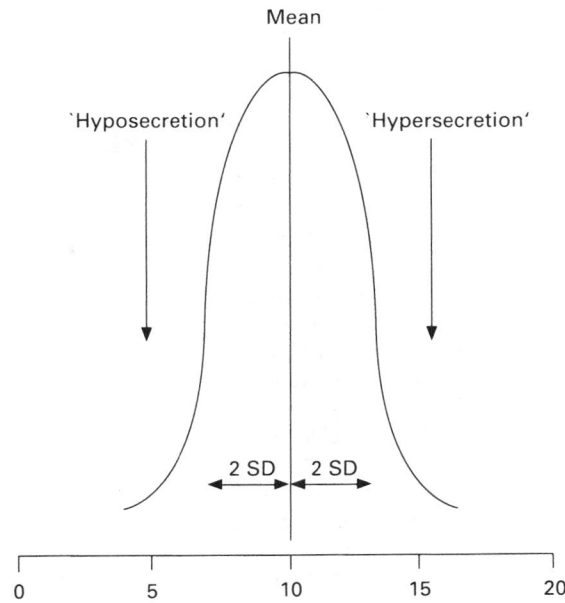

Fig. 19.8 Hypo- and hypersecretion – see text (after Jeffcoate 1981).

Hypersecretion is easier to diagnose than hyposecretion – a concentration half the mean of values in the normal population is more likely to fall within the 'normal range' than a concentration that is twice normal (Fig. 19.8) and it is more difficult analytically to measure low hormone levels.

This is important for screening tests (e.g. T4 or TSH for congenital hypothyroidism) or choosing particular assay techniques – TSH immunoradiometric assays (IRMA) give added precision at low levels compared to RIA (helpful in managing thyroxine replacement). LH and FSH IRMA and ultrasensitive immunofluorometric assays (IFA) are providing insights into the evolution of the hypothalamopituitary–gonadal axis during childhood and puberty control mechanisms for puberty (see pp. 1023–1026).

Prevalence of a condition is important in determining likely significance of an abnormal result in individual patients. Screening for congenital hypothyroidism (1 in 4000) with a TSH assay with 0.1% false positive rate will yield 4 out of 5 positive results in babies without the disease.

Quoted normal ranges may be based on an inappropriate 'normal' population (e.g. of adults) or taken over inappropriately from a laboratory using a different assay technique. Many clinicians underestimate the magnitude of change in laboratory values necessary before that change is significant in clinical terms – before two consecutive glycosylated hemoglobin results can be said to be significantly different a change of > 21% is likely to be required (Fogarty & Fraser 1989).

WHAT DO RESULTS MEAN?

Results are interpreted within pre-existing diagnostic frameworks which may be based on current concepts of disease classification rather than clear ideas of pathogenesis. Such preconceptions may lead to misinterpretation, e.g. the differential diagnosis of precocious puberty and the categorization of GH secretion into 'normal', 'partial deficiency' or 'deficiency'.

HORMONE ACTION AND MEASUREMENT

Many assays measure total hormone plasma levels of which only a small amount may be free, unbound and metabolically active. Direct measurement of the free, active hormone is of more value in diagnosis and treatment and abnormal hormone levels due to abnormalities of the binding protein can be more easily detected. It is invalid to extrapolate from isolated plasma samples to overall secretion or production rates. Circulating hormone levels may not reflect activity at tissue level. Many hormones have paracrine activity locally at tissue level and are not released in measurable quantities into the peripheral circulation.

Many laboratory assays are based on immunoassay techniques. These have, in many areas, replaced pre-existing bioassay (in vivo) techniques. One assay type is not intrinsically 'better' than another – which is preferable in particular circumstances will depend on the information sought.

What is measured in an immunoassay may not always have biological significance. For example, in mild acromegaly GH levels as measured by RIA may be very high, suggesting that GH molecular forms with low biological activity may be present.

CIRCULATING HORMONE LEVELS AND RECEPTORS

Endocrine disorders may not only result from hormone under- or overproduction but also from lack of tissue response to normal circulating concentrations. Receptor or postreceptor defects ('end-organ unresponsiveness') may be important, e.g. bone or renal unresponsiveness to PTH in pseudohypoparathyroidism, pseudohypoaldosteronism, partial insensitivity of androgen-dependent structures causing incomplete masculinization in some genotypic males or, as seems increasingly possible, in some children with 'idiopathic' growth failure.

Receptor assays, when available, may provide an indicator of biological activity. However, structural and functional properties of receptors may not be the same: in a given disorder they could be abnormal in number, function or both. In clinical practice, many defects must be inferred from finding functional inadequacy in clinical term with abnormally high circulating levels of the hormone(s) that stimulate that tissue activity.

LIAISON WITH LABORATORY STAFF, FAMILIARITY WITH TECHNIQUES

Pediatricians investigating potential endocrine disorders should establish good working relationships with their laboratory colleagues. In this way many potential pitfalls can be avoided. In addition, the clinician should try to become familiar with at least some basic principles of common and important assay techniques. Two-way interchange of information between clinician and laboratory staff increases knowledge and understanding in both and provides a more efficient service to patients.

FETAL ENDOCRINOLOGY

For recent detailed discussion, see Warshaw (1996) and Czernichow (1996).

FETAL ENDOCRINE FACTORS

Profound perinatal changes occur in many endocrine glands. Progress in understanding fetal endocrine functioning has come

Table 19.2 Factors reducing fetal growth

| Maternal illness during pregnancy |
| Chronic maternal disease |
| Maternal age (less than 20, over 35 years) |
| Increased parity |
| Maternal short stature |
| Ethnic group |
| Birthweight of other family members |
| Lower social class |
| Smoking |
| Poor nutrition |
| Alcohol |
| Poor weight gain |
| Multiple pregnancy |
| High altitude |
| Genetic factors |
| Fetal disease |
| Fetal abnormalities |

from increased access to wide ranges of abortus material from normal pregnancies, animal studies (which must be interpreted carefully in applying results to man), tissue culture experiments, advances in noninvasive (ultrasound) assessment of fetal growth and techniques such as fetoscopy.

Although fetal growth is ultimately controlled by genetic endowment, it is influenced by a number of fetal factors (including hormones and growth factors), uterine environment and other environmental factors. Control of fetal growth is by complex interaction between an evolving central nervous system, endocrine maturation, local tissue (paracrine) growth factors and placental and maternal hormone secretion – within environmental constraints which may impair fetal growth (Table 19.2).

Organogenesis occurs at a variety of times and tempos – organ embryogenesis and functional cell differentiation during the first trimester; rapid growth largely due to cell hyperplasia during the second; further functional maturation during the third. It is likely that endocrine factors, fetal, maternal and placental, are more involved with nonspecific growth stimulation or maturation (Milner & Hill 1989) and that specific stimuli to growth in individual cells and cell systems result from paracrine peptide growth factors derived locally. Measurable hormone levels in fetal circulation do not necessarily indicate a functional role at that time; target organs receptors may only appear later.

ONTOGENY OF FETAL HORMONE SECRETION

Anterior pituitary

The anterior pituitary is of ectodermal origin arising from Rathke's pouch, an evagination from the roof of the primitive buccal cavity appearing from about 3 weeks postconception. After 2 months, pouch anterior wall cells proliferate and differentiate to form the pituitary anterior lobe. Growth hormone (GH) is found in the fetal pituitary and circulation by 10 weeks gestation and levels are very high (greater than 200 mU/l) by mid-pregnancy.

In man, no anterior pituitary hormone crosses the placenta in physiologically significant amounts. Fetal growth continues relatively normally with absent GH secretion – anencephalics are only slightly small for gestational age (SGA) (Honnebier & Swaab 1973) as are children with severe growth hormone insufficiency. However, there is a small reduction in birth length for weight in babies with congenital GH deficiency (Gluckman et al 1992) although postnatal growth failure was more marked. GH receptors do not appear before the second trimester in man (not before birth in rat or sheep). In vitro, GH stimulates insulin-like growth factor 1 (IGF1) release from isolated fetal hepatocytes by 12 weeks' gestation (Strain et al 1987) but has no effect on fetal muscle growth. GH promotes β cell replication and insulin release in pancreatic islet cell cultures from 12- to 25-week fetuses (Sandler et al 1987) and any effects of GH in utero may be via insulin (see below).

PRL (198 amino acids structurally related to GH, molecular weight (MW) 22 500) is synthesized by the fetal anterior pituitary from about 7 weeks postmenstrual age (Siler-Khodr et al 1974) and the pituitary content increases subsequently (Aubert et al 1975). Fetal plasma levels rise during the third trimester to peak just before term. Cord blood levels are higher than maternal and normal in anencephalics (cf. GH). Its physiological role in man (other than in the initiation and maintenance of lactation in women) is unknown.

ACTH is present in fetal pituitary by 10 weeks and responsible for adrenal cortical steroidogenesis and growth.

LH and FSH may be present from as early as 5 weeks. At each stage, gonadotropin (GT) levels are higher in female than male fetuses. They are probably more important for later gonadal development than for early sexual differentiation.

Posterior pituitary

In the 6-week embryo, a downward extension of neural tissue from the floor of the diencephalon has formed the infundibulum. This gives rise to the stalk and neurohypophysis (posterior pituitary). From 12 weeks, nine amino acid peptides – vasopressin and oxytocin – are synthesized in and secreted from the supraoptic and paraventricular hypothalamic nuclei and transported via axons in the supraopticohypophyseal tract to capillaries drained by inferior hypophyseal veins. They have no known fetal function. Vasotocin seems to be concerned with water shifts across fetal membranes.

Thyroid

Fetal thyroid is active from mid-gestation and develops autonomously from the mother. Thyroxine (T4) is present at low but increasing levels from about 20 weeks but the more physiologically active metabolite triiodothyronine (T3) is present only in persisting low levels from about 30 weeks. Reverse T3 (rT3) levels are high due to active conversion from T4 in fetal liver, and placenta which also deiodinates T4 and T3 to inactive rT3 and T2 respectively.

T4, T3 and TSH were thought not to cross the placenta significantly. Thyroid hormones were also thought inessential for normal fetal somatic (and brain) growth (cf. other primate species). Recent research suggests that maternal–fetal transfer may protect the human fetus from adverse effects of fetal thyroid hormone deficiency to a limited extent and that thyroid hormones are important in human fetal development (Stein et al 1989, Calvo et al 1990) especially through regulation of gene expression for aspects of CNS development – neurogranin (RC3), tubulin (Stein et al 1989) and NGFI-A (Pipanon et al 1992). This has implications for limitations to effectiveness of screening programs in preventing adverse neurological sequelae in every case even with early thyroxine substitution (Grüters 1996).

Adrenal

During the second month adrenal cortical tissue differentiates into peripheral neocortex and active inner fetal zone. Rapid fetal zone hyperplasia and hypertrophy occurs (Idelman 1978) so that it makes up 85% of total adrenal size; it is the major site of dehydroepiandrosterone sulfate (DHAS) and 16-hydroxy DHAS production. As there is little fetal zone 3β-hydroxysteroid dehydrogenase (3βOHSD) activity, these compounds are produced in large quantities (equal to cortisol production) and placentally aromatized to estrogen, especially estriol. Fetal cortisol synthesis is maintained from placental progesterone and, possibly under the influence of progesterone, increased fetal zone 11β-hydroxylase and 21-hydroxylase activity leads to considerable cortisol production. Progesterone and PRL, as well as estrogens, are implicated in fetal 3βOHSD inhibition and thus fetal zone maintenance.

Fetal zone development and function is ACTH dependent. Fetal decapitation leads to adrenal atrophy, which is prevented by injection of ACTH. The anencephalic's fetal zone regresses during the second half of gestation causing no DHAS and pregnenolone secretion. Fetal adrenal atrophy occurs in pregnant women treated with high dose corticosteroids.

A high rate of DHAS secretion is an intrinsic property of human adrenocortical cells and ACTH is the only hormone required for its synthesis (Hornsby & Aldern 1984). In tissue culture, even fetal zone cells increase 3βOHSD activity in response to ACTH to levels of definitive zone cells (Simonian & Gill 1981) and distinction between zonae fasciculata and reticularis is lost (O'Hare et al 1980). ACTH stimulation increases intra-adrenal blood flow leading to enhanced zonae fasciculata and reticularis activity but has no effect on zona glomerulosa function (Vinson 1984). Zonal differences in blood flow may therefore have important consequences on zonal function – adrenarche (see p. 1026) may be a byproduct of the need of the inner cells of the fetal adrenal to respond to the hormonal milieu of pregnancy by developing an androgen (i.e. estrogen precursor) synthesizing zone (Anderson 1980).

It is speculated that fetal adrenal steroidogenic patterns, which could reflect placental and fetal growth (see below), might provide a link with the development of adult hypertension (Benediktsson et al 1993, Edwards et al 1993).

Within a few days of birth the fetal zone rapidly begins to atrophy. By 3 months the adrenal weight has halved and the weight at birth is not regained until puberty.

Gonads

Primitive gonads appears in the fourth week as a longitudinal ridge of proliferating celomic epithelium and underlying mesenchyme between mesonephros and dorsal mesentery.

Primordial germ cells appear in the yolk sac wall by 3 weeks and migrate towards and enter the ridges by 6 weeks, until when male and female human fetal gonads are morphologically identical. Primitive, undifferentiated gonads will develop in a female manner unless directed towards male differentiation by the presence of the sex-determining region of the Y chromosome – SRY (see below).

In females, proliferating epithelial cords surround primordial germ cells in the mesenchyme. These cords subsequently degenerate and are replaced by others which remain near the surface of the gland whilst the surface epithelium thickens. Germ cells develop into oogonia surrounded by follicular cells derived from surface epithelium.

From the third month, oogonia undergo meiosis to form primary oocytes which, by birth, have completed prophase of the first meiotic division and entered a resting stage. At sexual maturity, they complete the first meiotic division to form secondary oocytes which are extruded into the Fallopian tube at ovulation. Primary oocytes are surrounded by a layer of flat epithelial cells, later to form the granulosa cells – the complex is known as the primordial follicle. This is surrounded by a basal lamina and, externally, a layer of thecal cells. In the maturing follicle there is oocyte enlargement, granulosa cell proliferation and thecal differentiation into inner vascular and outer fibrous layers. Some 6–7 million oogonia are present by 6 months postconception but there are only 2–4 million primordial follicles at birth and less than half a million by menarche. Most follicles degenerate – only a few are lost by ovulation during reproductive life.

In males, presence of a Y chromosome carrying a testis-determining gene – sex-determining region of the Y chromosome (SRY) (Sinclair et al 1990, Hawkins 1993) – on its short arm and cell membrane histocompatibility (H-Y) antigen (Jost 1976), the primitive sex cords proliferate and differentiate to form testis cords. These become separated from surface epithelium by a layer of dense fibrous connective tissue (tunica albuginea) which, with the degeneration of the surface epithelium, forms the testis outer surface (capsule).

The testis cords differentiate to form the rete testis and straight and convoluted tubules. They remain solid until puberty when they develop a lumen and form seminiferous tubules. In the fetus they comprise primitive germ cells surrounded by supporting cells which will eventually develop into Sertoli (sustentacular) cells. Leydig (interstitial) cells develop from mesenchyme.

The major hormonal stimulus for fetal Leydig cells testosterone, and primitive seminiferous tubule, germ cell and Sertoli cell formation is placentally derived human chorionic gonadotropin (HCG). At this stage, there is little pituitary GT secretion – anencephalic male genital tract development is normal.

Before gonadal differentiation, Wolffian ducts have already developed (by 4 weeks). Müllerian ducts appear at about 7 weeks. In males, in the presence of a testis, degeneration of Müllerian structures occurs by 9 weeks under the influence of Müllerian inhibiting hormone (MIH), a high molecular weight glycoprotein secreted by the Sertoli cells (Josso & Picard 1986). MIH is a member of the transforming growth factor β (TGFβ) family (like the inhibins and activins). The human MIH gene has been cloned and mapped to the short arm of chromosome 19. There is a critical period during which Müllerian tissue is sensitive to inhibition by MIH – although MIH is now known to be produced by Sertoli

cells until puberty, no postnatal physiological effects have been identified.

Leydig cell testosterone secretion is responsible for persistence of the Wolffian ducts and their differentiation into epididymis, vas deferens, seminal vesicles and ejaculatory ducts. Male external genitalia are sensitive to dihydrotestosterone (DHT) rather than testosterone and the enzyme which converts the latter to the former, 5α-reductase, is present in high concentrations in these tissues. DHT is responsible for fusion of labia, growth of the phallus and formation of the scrotum.

In females, in the absence of Leydig cell testosterone secretion, Wolffian ducts virtually completely disappear. The Müllerian system, in the absence of Sertoli cell MIH secretion, differentiates into upper vagina, uterus and Fallopian tubes.

Parathyroid

The fetus accumulates calcium rapidly. Maternal PTH and 1,25-dihydroxycholecalciferol (1,25-DHCC) levels are high during pregnancy and there is active calcium (and phosphate) transfer to the fetus. 25-HCC crosses the placenta and preterm infants have lower levels than term infants, by when levels are comparable to those in the mother. PTH and 1,25-DHCC levels are low at birth but calcitonin levels are high. Calcitonin reduces fetal bone resorption; low PTH levels aid bone calcification.

Pancreas

Insulin is present in fetal pancreas by 8 weeks and plasma by 12 weeks and is an important anabolic factor with major, particularly last trimester, influence on somatic size and growth. Fetal hyperinsulinemia causes adiposity but has little effect on lean body mass (Naeye 1965); there is, however, a permissive effect on protein synthesis and hepatic glycogen deposition. Insulin does not cross the placenta in physiologically significant amounts. In normal pregnancy, fetal plasma glucose levels are modulated by maternal homeostatic mechanisms. The fetus of a poorly controlled diabetic mother has greatly increased adipose tissue stores, organomegaly and increased birth size. Other disorders associated with hyperinsulinism (e.g. nesidioblastosis and Beckwith–Wiedemann syndrome) are associated with fetal overgrowth. Insulin appears to have no direct action on release of IGF from human fetal connective tissue or hepatocytes in tissue culture and may act through stimulation of nutrient uptake and utilization (Milner & Hill 1989).

Glucagon is present in human fetal pancreatic tissue from 10 weeks and cannot cross the placenta. Its fetal metabolic role is still largely unknown but there is a high overall circulating insulin : glucagon ratio in the fetus, favoring anabolism (Aynsley-Green 1985).

Human pancreatic polypeptide (HPP) secreting cells are present in the pancreatic head by 18 weeks but sparse in the adult organ. HPP may have a role in liver glycogenolysis. The physiological role of pancreatic D (somatostatin-secreting) cells, present from 10 weeks, is unknown.

Growth factors

By the second trimester, insulin-like growth factors are present in many fetal tissues including liver, kidneys, gut, lung, cardiac and skeletal muscle, fetal zone adrenal, hemopoietic cells and dermis (Elgin et al 1987). They are regulated independently of GH and are important for fetal growth regulation. Both IGFI and IGFII are mitogenic and also cause tissue differentiation. IGFI is particularly important in muscle fiber, ovarian granulosa cells (causing LH receptor and sex steroid accumulation) and brain astrocyte differentiation. IGFII, like IGFI, increases extracellular connective tissue matrix synthesis, especially in chondrocytes. It synergizes with nerve growth factor in promoting neurite outgrowth from sensory and sympathetic ganglia (Milner & Hill 1989). Cellular growth is reviewed by Söder (1997).

Epidermal growth factor (EGF) (and its probable fetal form, transforming growth factor a (TGFα)) influences the growth, differentiation and function of epithelial cells, including lung and gut. It modulates trophoblast differentiation and function in tissue culture with release of human placental lactogen (HPL) and human chorionic gonadotropin (HCG) via placental receptors and may be important in fetal growth retardation (Lawrence & Warshaw 1989).

LONG-TERM IMPLICATIONS OF FETAL GROWTH

Most SGA babies are appropriately grown for their small parents, and maternal size, in particular, is an important determinant of birth weight. Some babies seem small because the expected date of delivery is incorrect. However, at any gestational age, babies can also be born small either because of (1) underlying pathology in the fetus (chromosomal or other genetic factors) or (2) intrauterine starvation due to abnormal placental function causing intrauterine growth retardation (IUGR). This uteroplacental insufficiency may relate to reduced maternal and placental perfusion and is associated with low PO_2, low pH and raised lactate levels in the fetus and neonate and redistribution of fetal blood flow from the thoracic aorta to the middle cerebral artery to protect, as far as possible, the growing and maturing fetal brain (Soothill & Holmes 1997a).

IUGR is now thought to be important not just in the short (e.g. neonatal hypoglycemia) or medium term (e.g. difficult feeding in infancy and poor growth) but because of possible long-term (adulthood) consequences. Epidemiological evidence suggests that small fetuses are more likely in adulthood to develop hypertension and other cardiovascular diseases and type 2 diabetes mellitus (Barker et al 1990, Barker 1992, Law et al 1993, Osmond et al 1993, Barker et al 1993) and that babies most at risk of subsequent hypertension are those born small with large placentae (Barker et al 1990). It is not yet clear how this relates to a pathophysiological classification of small babies nor whether, for example, 'normal' birth weight babies lighter than they should have been for their tall parents (and thus also starved in utero) are at risk.

Early nutrition is important for long-term outcomes, i.e. it has biological as well as nutritional effects. There is unequivocal evidence from animal experiments, human epidemiological studies and continuing long-term studies in the human, for nutritional imprinting (programming of function in later life – Lucas 1995). Early (fetal/neonatal) nutrition may be important for brain development, long-term cognitive function and IQ. An early brain 'insult' could lead to a 'good' or 'bad' outcome depending on nutritional state during the critical phase of tissue repair.

The management of the pregnancy with a growth retarded fetus is discussed in Soothill & Holmes (1997b).

PLACENTAL HORMONE SECRETION

The placenta is the source of a hormone structurally similar to pituitary GH (differing from pituitary GH by 13 amino acids), which is coded by a variant GH gene (human growth hormone V) inactive in the pituitary. Placental GH appears to be secreted into the maternal circulation in large amounts towards full term but has disappeared within 1 h of delivery (Frankenne et al 1988). Its role in fetal life is, at present, conjectural.

HPL is also structurally similar to GH (85% homology). HPL may be an important (necessary or permissive) fetal growth factor. By second trimester, levels are comparable to those promoting DNA synthesis and cellular anabolism in isolated human connective tissues and hepatocytes (Strain et al 1987). Actions on DNA synthesis are via paracrine IGF release. Specific HPL receptor binding sites are present in fetal liver and skeletal muscle in increasing numbers from 12 weeks (Hill et al 1988).

The placenta secretes HCG (structurally similar to thyrotropin and with significant thyroid-stimulating activity), which is more likely than fetal pituitary derived LH to be the important stimulus to fetal Leydig cell testosterone production.

MATERNAL DISEASE AND ENDOCRINE FUNCTION

Maternal thyrotoxicosis occurs in about 1 in 2000 pregnancies but hyperthyroid women seldom become pregnant unless treated and abortion commonly occurs. After the first trimester there is relative independence of fetal and maternal pituitary–thyroid axes. Iodine, antithyroid drugs and human thyroid-stimulating immunoglobulins (TSI) cross the placenta from mother to fetus. Neonatal thyrotoxicosis occurs in about 1.5% of infants born to mothers with Graves' disease (see later). The risk relates more to the presence of TSI than to disease activity and the disease may have been inactive for many years.

Hypocalcemia used to occur in full-term infants fed with high phosphate load cow's milk preparations. The same problem occurring in some babies on low phosphate milks suggests that maternal factors such as osteomalacia due to vitamin D deficiency (or rarer conditions such as pseudohypoparathyroidism with maternal hypocalcemia) may be important.

Fetal effects from poor maternal diabetic glycemic control are described above. Fetal hyperinsulinism causing neonatal hypoglycemia is seen there and in nesidioblastosis.

MATERNAL DRUGS AND ENDOCRINE FUNCTION

In the second and third trimesters, substances of MW < ~ 600 cross the placenta; this category includes most drugs, which are often more toxic to fetus than mother. Examples of drugs affecting endocrine function include iodides (cough mixtures, radiographic contrast media) which cause hypothyroidism with neonatal goiter, carbimazole and thiouracil (similar effects), and glucocorticoids.

CONTROL OF ONSET OF LABOR

In sheep there is evidence for the important role in parturition of the fetal adrenal. Increases in fetal cortical cell numbers, cortisol production and receptor sites with a fall in cortisol-binding globulin result in dramatic rises in free cortisol levels and placental enzyme induction, leading to a fall in progesterone and rise in estrogen levels. Arachidonic acid is released from the decidua and fetal membranes. Decreasing progesterone levels reduce inhibition of uterine epithelium prostaglandin (PG) secretion and the rise in $PGF_{2\alpha}$ initiates uterine contractions. Cortisol is important for pulmonary surfactant synthesis and fetal liver enzyme induction.

In the human, many events, particularly the role of PGs, may be comparable. That the hypothalamopituitary–adrenal axis is important is suggested by prolonged pregnancy in mothers with anencephalic fetuses. In anencephalic pregnancies unassociated with hydramnios there is inverse correlation between gestation length and size of fetal adrenals.

Other situations where fetal cortisol production is abnormal include congenital adrenal hypoplasia – the pregnancy may be prolonged – and unexplained preterm labor has been reported in fetal adrenal hyperplasia of unknown etiology. In contrast, in 21-hydroxylase deficiency (cortisol production often normal with high ACTH levels) gestation length appears normal.

Increased understanding of inhibiting and triggering mechanisms for labor is of potential practical relevance in prevention of preterm delivery and optimal management of labor.

NEONATAL ENDOCRINOLOGY

By late gestation, the fetus has developed significant endocrinological autonomy. Nevertheless, profound hormonal changes occur during and shortly after birth. This has implications for newborn screening: transient abnormalities may be misinterpreted as permanent, or vice versa.

Important endocrine disorders may present in the newborn. In this section, clinical and biochemical clues and general principles are discussed.

HYPOGLYCEMIA

Hypoglycemia is a common finding in the neonate. Fetal metabolism is essentially anabolic: enzymes concerned with formation of glycogen, fat and protein are increasingly active with advancing gestation in mammalian liver; glycogenolytic and gluconeogenic enzymes appear relatively inactive before birth. At delivery, transplacental glucose ceases. Full-term infants experience falls in blood glucose during the early hours after birth to about 2.5 mmol/l. Normal feeding is important for the subsequent rise in blood glucose levels as are hormonal changes stimulating liver glycogenolysis and gluconeogenesis and lipolysis. Glucagon levels rise, GH levels are high and there is a surge in TSH, T3 and T4 secretion.

Birth asphyxia is an important cause of neonatal hypoglycemia causing rapid depletion of glycogen stores. Glucose is the most important substrate for brain metabolism. The large neonatal brain : body mass ratio largely explains the increased susceptibility to hypoglycemia – prolonged or recurrent hypoglycemia is a preventable cause of long-term neurological damage and mental retardation.

Neonatal hypoglycemia may be an important clue to endocrine disorders such as nesidioblastosis or insulinoma, congenital hypopituitarism – panhypopituitarism or isolated ACTH or GH deficiency – and adrenal disease causing glucocorticoid deficiency (e.g. congenital adrenal hypoplasia, hyperplasia or following bilateral adrenal hemorrhage).

Hypoglycemia, at any age, is not a diagnosis in itself (see pp.

1082–1084). For reviews of neonatal hypoglycemia see Aynsley-Green & Soltesz (1992) and Cowett (1996).

MICROPENIS

Small penis and underdeveloped genitalia without hypospadias are characteristic findings in a male infant with pituitary disease – generalized, GT deficiency (Salisbury et al 1984) or GH deficiency – or rudimentary testes. The association with hypoglycemia is characteristic of hypothalamopituitary disorders; hypotonia and feeding difficulties suggest Prader–Willi syndrome. Other congenital abnormalities may suggest other syndromes in which hypogonadism is a feature.

AMBIGUOUS GENITALIA

The cause of ambiguity, and sex of the infant, cannot be identified by clinical examination alone (see Fig. 19.39); an urgent karyotype must be obtained. If both gonads are palpable in the labioscrotal folds the baby is likely to be a male with XY karyotype in whom there is a defect in testosterone biosynthesis or tissue insensitivity to androgen. If no gonads are palpable the most likely diagnosis is congenital adrenal hyperplasia (CAH); watch for possible salt loss in the commonest type (21-hydroxylase deficiency). Rarely hypertension will develop (11β-hydroxylase deficiency).

Fetal androgen deficiency in a male may result in appearances anywhere between severe hypospadias and 'normal female'. Exposure of a female fetus to androgen may result in appearances between clitoromegaly and 'normal male'. It is important, therefore, to try to classify disorders etiologically rather than descriptively.

Gender depends on a number of features which are normally self-consistent in any one individual: genetic sex – XX or XY; gonadal sex – presence of ovaries or testes; phenotypic sex – internal and external genital structures. Sex of rearing usually depends more on functional possibilities than on genetic or gonadal sex.

PROLONGED JAUNDICE

Primary hypothyroidism was a common cause of prolonged jaundice in the UK. Even now, no screening program is problem free (Grüters 1996) – check TSH levels again if there is clinical suspicion.

SALT WASTING

Vomiting, diarrhea and dehydration in the early days or weeks of life is seldom due to endocrine disease; sodium and water loss in the stool from gastroenteritis or vomiting associated with pyloric stenosis are much more common. Sodium loss in the urine is due to renal or adrenal disease. In renal disease, aldosterone levels will be high but they are generally low in adrenal disease (congenital adrenal hypoplasia (CAH) or corticosterone methyl oxidase deficiency (Veldhuis et al 1980)). In pseudohypoaldosteronism, aldosterone levels will be very high. If appropriate, prompt treatment is not given, symptoms can rapidly progress to vascular collapse with severe hyperkalemia and hyponatremia, hypoglycemia, metabolic acidosis, coma and death.

HYPOTHERMIA

Preterm babies are at particular risk of hypothermia. The SGA infant is at increased risk because of high surface area and lack of subcutaneous fat. Suspect hypothalamopituitary disease with persisting hypothermia, particularly in association with hypoglycemia or micropenis.

THE SMALL FOR GESTATIONAL AGE (SGA; LOW BIRTH LENGTH) BABY

Some SGA babies have grown slowly for much of pregnancy while others have done so only more recently. These situations can be distinguished by serial ultrasound measurements of biparietal diameter and lower thoracic circumference. The prognosis for growth and development varies with the time of onset of poor growth. Babies who have grown slowly before ~ 35 weeks are increasingly likely to be not only light but also short for dates at birth and to have a low head circumference. They characteristically feed extremely poorly in infancy and later may show characteristic dysmorphic features: body asymmetry, clinodactyly, triangular 'elfin' facies – the Silver–Russell syndrome – and present in childhood with short stature (see p. 1015).

Some SGA babies have specific reasons for slow intrauterine growth, e.g. congenital rubella, chromosome disorders or major congenital abnormalities. Suspect Turner's syndrome in an SGA female baby with peripheral edema.

UNDESCENDED TESTES

Cryptorchidism, in the context of otherwise normal external male genitalia, is much less common than normally retractile testes. Normal testes have usually descended by 36 weeks' gestation owing to the effects of GT-induced testosterone. They will not do so if there is GT deficiency, defective testicular testosterone production or anatomical impediment in the line of descent (much more commonly a unilateral problem). Bilateral cryptorchidism is thus usually due to an endocrine abnormality at pituitary or testicular level, or both. Karyotype and endocrine investigation should be undertaken before surgery is contemplated.

SCREENING

Few infants show diagnostic features of hypothyroidism at birth (see Grüters 1996 for a comprehensive review of screening, and page 1046). Screening programs in the USA and Europe have suggested an incidence of about 1 in 4000, double that expected from results of retrospective surveys.

Congenital hypothyroidism is an excellent disease to screen for – it is common, unreliably diagnosed clinically until too late, detectable with simple and cheap biochemical tests on small amounts of easily stored blood, and prompt and adequate treatment prevents significant neurodevelopmental deficit. It is generally thought that adequate treatment within 4 weeks leads to normal overall development but some studies suggest that subtle perceptual and hearing/speech deficits remain (Simons et al 1994, Grüters 1996). There are two alternative strategies for the screening program. If T4 alone is used, there is too much overlap between normal and hypothyroid values at the end of the first week. TSH must be measured in addition in those babies where the T4 is 'low'.

In many countries (including the UK) TSH is measured as the primary test; there is no overlap between normal and high levels, high levels are easier to interpret as abnormal (a level twice normal is less likely to fall within the 'normal range' – see p. 1046) and are easier to measure reliably. Hypothyroidism due to pituitary or hypothalamic disease is missed (TSH levels are low) but these babies usually have clinical features associated with other pituitary hormone deficiencies (e.g. micropenis, hypoglycemia) and thyroid function is usually sufficiently preserved to prevent neurological and intellectual problems even with later diagnosis.

Screening has shown transient abnormalities, previously unrecognized, to be almost as common in many countries. In particular, preterm infants may have temporary functional abnormalities and clear-cut diagnosis may be difficult. Any abnormal screening result must be confirmed by definitive tests before diagnosis and commitment to long-term therapy but the results should not be awaited before treatment is started.

It is possible to screen newborn babies for 21-hydroxylase deficiency using the 'Guthrie' test filter paper to detect raised 17OH progesterone levels (Pang et al 1977, Kelnar 1993b, Cheetham & Hughes 1996). The incidence is between 1 in 5000 and 1 in 23 000 (gene frequency in Europe and USA ~ 1 in 100). Boys do not have significant abnormalities at birth and there may be significant morbidity or even mortality if they present without warning with salt wasting. The non-salt-losing boy (around 50% in the UK) presents late with pseudoprecocious puberty, rapid growth and tall stature but a short final height prognosis. Despite severe consequences of late diagnosis, in the UK it is generally considered unnecessary (Virdi et al 1987) or 'uneconomical' to screen in the newborn even though this would only add a small additional unit cost in the screening laboratory already measuring TSH and phenylalanine (Wallace et al 1986, Hughes 1986).

Selective screening (of an 'at risk' population) has been suggested, and recently adopted in Italy (Cacciari et al 1986). In Hungary (Solyom & Hughes 1989), central laboratory measurement of 17OH progesterone concentrations in 'at risk' groups has led to earlier diagnosis, decreased mortality and yielded valuable clinical and epidemiological information in a country where blood steroid assays are not readily available.

DISORDERS OF SEXUAL DIFFERENTIATION (Savage 1989, Danon & Friedman 1996)

Normal fetal sexual differentiation is described earlier. It is increasingly possible to determine underlying pathophysiological processes which have led to inappropriate virilization or its inappropriate lack (Sultan et al 1996). Nevertheless descriptive terms are sometimes of value (if they are not used simply to hide ignorance).

Abnormal external genitalia may be found in many dysmorphic syndromes (Jones 1988). Specific disorders of fetal sexual differentiation have been descriptively categorized on the basis of gonadal (dys)morphology into the following three groups.

FEMALE PSEUDOHERMAPHRODITISM

This describes virilization of external genitalia with XX karyotype and normal ovaries and Müllerian structures. Important causes are summarized in Table 19.3. Virilization may be due to excessive fetal androgen production or exposure to increased transplacental androgen (maternal or iatrogenic). Some remain idiopathic.

Table 19.3 Causes of female pseudohermaphroditism

Virilization by:
1. Fetal androgens – congenital adrenal hyperplasia (21-hydroxylase, 11β-hydroxylase, 3β-hydroxysteroid dehydrogenase deficiencies)
2. Maternal androgen-secreting tumor
3. Iatrogenic (progestational abortifacients)
4. Miscellaneous (see text)
5. Idiopathic

Preterm female infants have underdeveloped labia mimicking 'clitoromegaly'. Clitoromegaly is found in some rare dysmorphic syndromes (e.g. Beckwith, Seckel and Zellweger).

Virilization by fetal androgens

Virilizing CAH

21-hydroxylase (P-450$_{c21}$) deficiency is the commonest cause of virilization in the genotypic female. The degree of intrauterine virilization may depend on the completeness of the block, but the degree of salt loss, when present, correlates poorly with the degree of virilization.

Some females have relatively normal looking genitalia at birth but in the majority there is clitoromegaly and variable labial fusion. There may be a urogenital sinus with common opening for urethra and vagina. In severely affected cases, appearances are 'normal male' with a 'penile' urethra but with no testes in the 'scrotum'. Ovarian and Müllerian development (upper vagina, cervix, uterus and Fallopian tubes) is normal. Most males appear normal at birth – the scrotum may occasionally appear pigmented and the penis large.

In 11β-hydroxylase (P-450$_{c11}$) deficiency, virilization is variable but seems more often severe enough for females to be brought up as males (Rosler & Leiberman 1984, Zachmann et al 1983). It is much less common than 21-hydroxylase deficiency but relatively common in the Middle East. Hypertension, which occurs in some, takes time to develop. Males appear normal at birth.

In contrast, in 3β-hydroxysteroid dehydrogenase deficiency (Bongiovanni 1962), ambiguous genitalia occur in either sex. Males are incompletely virilized (see below). Females are virilized by excessive production of the (weak) adrenal androgen dehydroepiandrosterone (DHA). There is usually severe associated salt wasting in early infancy.

Other causes of fetal androgen overproduction, for example adrenal adenoma or congenital nodular adrenal hyperplasia, seem excessively rare.

Transplacental virilization

Maternal androgens

Variable fetal virilization from maternal ovarian and adrenal tumors has been described.

Iatrogenic

During the 1950s recurrent spontaneous abortion was treated with natural (progesterone, 17-OH progesterone) and synthetic (medroxyprogesterone, norethynodrel) progestogens with androgenic properties resulting in significant virilization of female fetuses. Such treatment is now almost never used.

MALE PSEUDOHERMAPHRODITISM

This describes incomplete virilization of the external genitalia, XY karyotype and normally differentiated testes for one of three reasons (see Table 19.4): abnormality of MIH secretion or action, deficient fetal testosterone synthesis due to Leydig cell hypoplasia or an inborn metabolic error, or impaired peripheral androgen metabolism (Savage et al 1978). There is an association with other abnormalities in rare dysmorphic syndromes (e.g. Meckel, Opitz and Smith–Lemli–Opitz).

Persistent Müllerian structures

This is a rare familial condition. The original patient presented as a 'normal male' with an inguinal hernia, found at surgery to contain Müllerian structures (Fallopian tubes and uterus). External genitalia generally look normally male although cryptorchidism is common (Josso et al 1983).

Deficient fetal testosterone biosynthesis

Leydig cell hypoplasia

This is another rare disorder, probably autosomal recessive (but obviously male limited) with defective Leydig cell differentiation (Berthezene et al 1976) and testosterone response to HCG. Phenotype is female but Müllerian structures are absent because of normal Sertoli cell MIH production.

Inborn errors of testosterone biosynthesis (see Fig. 19.9)

These result in defective virilization of the male's internal and external genitalia. Adrenocortical steroid biosynthesis is affected when the defect is at an early stage in the pathway so that hypoglycemia and salt loss may occur. MIH synthesis is unaffected; Müllerian structures are absent.

Cholesterol desmolase deficiency ((P-450$_{scc}$) cholesterol side chain cleavage deficiency, lipoid adrenal hyperplasia)

This is due to deficiency of any of the microsomal enzymes 20α-hydroxylase, 20,22–desmolase (the rate-limiting step) or 22α-

Table 19.4 Causes of male pseudohermaphroditism

Impaired Leydig cell activity
  Leydig cell hypoplasia
  Inborn errors of testosterone biosynthesis (see Fig. 19.9)

Impaired peripheral tissue androgen metabolism
  5α-reductase deficiency
  Receptor defects
    Testicular feminization (complete)
    Testicular feminization (incomplete)
    Reifenstein's syndrome
    Infertile male syndrome
  Postreceptor defects

Abnormal secretion or action of MIH (persistent Müllerian duct syndrome)

Associated with dysmorphic syndromes (e.g. Opitz, Smith–Lemli–Opitz)

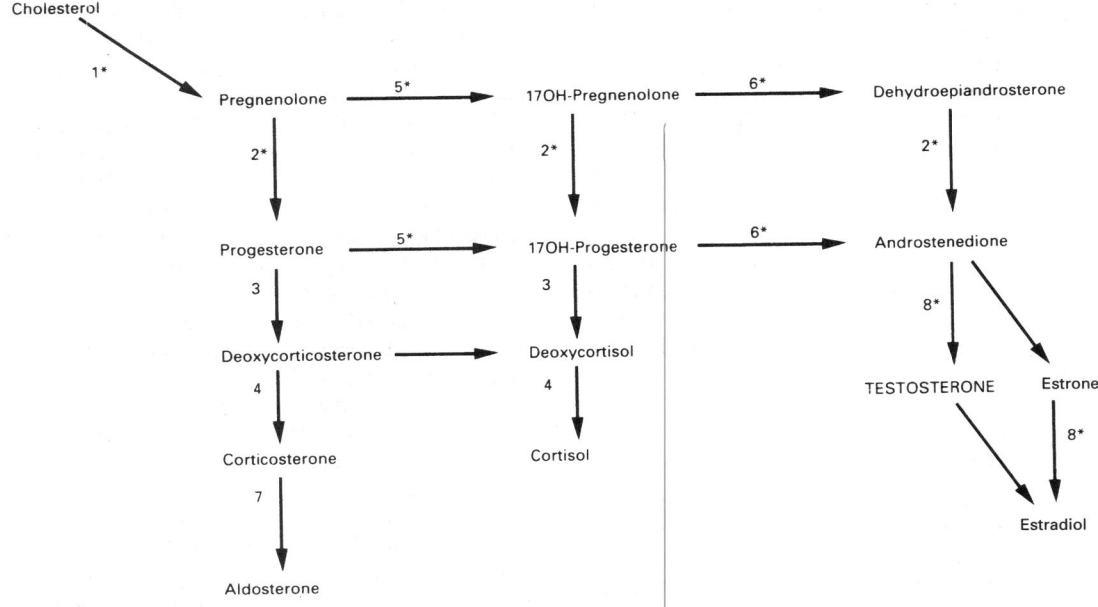

Fig. 19.9   Inborn errors of testosterone biosynthesis – marked with an asterisk (compare with Fig. 19.37). 1* – cholesterol side chain cleaving system (20α-hydroxylase, 20,22-desmolase, 22α-hydroxylase); 2* – 3β-hydroxysteroid dehydrogenase; 3 – 21-hydroxylase; 4 – 11β-hydroxylase; 5* – 17α-hydroxylase; 6* – 17,20-lyase (desmolase); 7 – 18-hydroxylase and 18-hydroxysteroid dehydrogenase; 8* – 17β-hydroxysteroid dehydrogenase.

hydroxylase converting cholesterol to pregnenolone, causing defective androgen, glucocorticoid (GC) and mineralocorticoid (MC) biosynthesis with cholesterol accumulation in the gland. The $P\text{-}450_{scc}$ gene is located in the q23 to q24 region of chromosome 15. In surviving cases, genitalia appear female and there is severe salt loss and hypoglycemia, often with fatal outcome – prompt treatment may be life saving.

3β-hydroxysteroid dehydrogenase deficiency (3β-HSD)

Two genes encode for 3β-HSD – type I (placental) and type II (adrenal and gonadal). Patients with classical 3β-HSD deficiency have type II gene point mutations. Genotypic males are incompletely (variably) virilized. Wolffian structures are normal. Salt loss and hypoglycemia are generally severe with high mortality.

17α-hydroxylase deficiency (P-450c17)

This results in GC and androgen deficiency (hypoglycemia and complete lack of virilization) plus mineralocorticoid excess due to ACTH drive (Fig. 19.9) resulting in hypokalemic alkalosis and hypertension (New 1970). At puberty there may be virilization with gynecomastia.

17,20-desmolase (P-450c17 17,20-lyase deficiency)

This is characterized by inadequate virilization and excessive urinary pregnanetriolone excretion (Zachmann et al 1972). Gluco- and mineralocorticoid pathways are intact. Nevertheless, a single gene encoding cytochrome P-450c17 controls both 17α-

hydroxylase and 17,20-desmolase activities – combined defects have been reported regardless of phenotype.

17β-hydroxysteroid dehydrogenase deficiency

There is defective conversion of androstenedione to testosterone and estrone to estradiol (Saez et al 1971). Adrenal steroidogenesis is normal. In most cases, male infants are sufficiently poorly virilized to be reared as females but there is significant virilization at puberty.

Impaired peripheral androgen metabolism (Danon & Friedman 1996)

There are three types, which collectively constitute the commonest group of male pseudohermaphrodite patients:

1. 5α-reductase deficiency
2. X-linked abnormalities of the androgen receptor (including complete or incomplete androgen insensitivity, and Reifenstein's and the infertile male syndromes)
3. postreceptor (receptor-positive) resistance (a similar clinical spectrum to 2 but normal receptor function).

5α-reductase deficiency

This is an autosomal recessive defect originally reported in a Dominican Republic inbred rural community (Imperato-McGinley et al 1974). The biochemical defect is in the conversion of testosterone to dihydrotestosterone (DHT) in the androgen target cell, characterized by a high plasma testosterone : DHT ratio (after HCG stimulation in prepuberty). Definitive diagnosis is by finding diminished 5α-reductase activity in genital skin fibroblast cultures. Two human cDNA clones for 5α-reductase have been isolated and the 5α-reductase 2 gene mapped to band 23 of the short arm of chromosome 2 (2p23).

Newborn external genitalia appear female (fetal DHT deficiency produces a very small phallus and perineal hypospadias) but the testosterone-dependent internal (Wolffian) genital structures develop normally with testes capable of spermatogenesis (Savage et al 1980).

At puberty considerable, but incomplete, virilization occurs spontaneously with male body habitus, psychosexual orientation and gender conversion. External genitalia remain small but large testosterone doses may produce cosmetic improvement (Price et al 1984). DHT therapy has proved disappointing.

Androgen receptor defects

These are either major structural abnormalities of the androgen receptor (AR) gene or point mutations altering either AR messenger RNA or single amino acids (Griffin 1992) resulting in a spectrum of appearance from 'female' (complete and incomplete testicular feminization) to 'male' (Reifenstein's syndrome and infertile male syndrome). The AR gene has been cloned and is located on the q11–12 region of the X chromosome. Mutations in exon 2 and 3 code for the DNA region have been identified in patients with 'receptor-positive' androgen insensitivity. However, most mutations are in exons 4–8 which code for the steroid-binding domain – 'receptor-negative' androgen insensitivity (French et al 1990).

Complete testicular feminization: patients generally present prepubertally with inguinal hernia(e) containing testes or after puberty with primary amenorrhea but normal breast development, scanty pubic and axillary hair, female body habitus and psychosexual orientation. There is a short blind-ending vagina as Müllerian structures have regressed. Gonads show Leydig cell hyperplasia with defective spermatogenesis and may undergo malignant change (Manuel et al 1976) if not removed. In incomplete testicular feminization there is more virilization with prepubertal clitoromegaly and variable labial fusion. There may be a mixture of virilization and feminization at puberty.

In *Reifenstein's syndrome* appearance is generally male but with severe (perineal) hypospadias. Virilization at puberty may be significant but still inadequate and associated with gynecomastia. There is male psychosexual orientation and infertility. In the infertile male syndrome there is a normal prepubertal male appearance although penis and testes may be rather small. Gynecomastia develops at puberty and there is oligospermia and infertility.

ABNORMAL GONADAL DIFFERENTIATION

This is a clinically heterogeneous group, including true hermaphroditism and syndromes of dysgenetic gonadal development. In most there is ambiguity of external genitalia in the newborn.

True hermaphroditism usually presents with abnormal external genitalia (e.g. phallus with urogenital sinus at the base). Testicular and ovarian tissue are present, more commonly as ovotestes than as separate gonads. The commonest karyotype is 46XX (58%); 10% are XY and the remainder mosaics, of which the commonest

is 46XX/46XY (13%). If the diagnosis is made neonatally, testicular tissue should be removed, and gender assignment should be female – there is good feminization at puberty with menstruation, and fertility is possible.

XX males usually present with hypogonadism as adults but genital ambiguity may occur (Rosler & Leiberman 1984). H-Y antigen is present (Kofman-Alfaro et al 1985).

Klinefelter's syndrome may be suspected in a neonate with hypospadias, small testes and extension of the scrotal skin on to the shaft of a small penis but is seldom diagnosed before the time of puberty (see p. 1036).

Mixed gonadal dysgenesis: generally there is a testis with Wolffian (and absent Müllerian) structures on one side, with streak gonad and Müllerian (but poorly developed Wolffian) development on the other. Karyotype is generally 46XY or 45XO/46XY mosaic, the latter associated with clinical features and the growth pattern of Turner's syndrome. Bilaterally dysgenetic testes are less common. In both groups there is a high risk of malignant change in the gonads (Savage et al 1986).

Turner's syndrome – see page 1032.

Pure gonadal dysgenesis seldom presents before puberty. There are normal female external genitalia but the karyotype may be 46XX or 46XY. Gonadal malignant change is common (Savage et al 1986).

Agonadism presents in a variety of clinical guises depending on the timing of testicular involution. There may be normal female appearances with absent Müllerian and Wolffian structures, micropenis with rudimentary testes or anorchia in an otherwise normal male.

CLINICAL MANAGEMENT

Initial assessment

Uncertainty as to the sex of their newborn baby is extremely distressing to parents. Emphasize that their baby's sex will be swiftly determined, the baby is either male or female (and not 'somewhere in between') and that the cause of the problem will be discovered. Birth should not be registered until sex of rearing is decided. Appearance of external genitalia is important in this decision – an adequately functional phallus cannot be created out of very little tissue – but is unhelpful in reaching an etiologic diagnosis.

Check the family history and for any hormone treatment during the pregnancy. Look for associated abnormalities or dysmorphic features. The most important aspect of clinical examination is for the presence of gonads – a clinical classification based on their number is useful for planning immediately relevant investigations (Savage 1989):

In *all* patients, an urgent karyotype is indicated.

If *no* gonads are palpable: the most likely diagnosis is the 21-hydroxylase deficiency in a genotypic female – salt loss may occur. Measurement of plasma 17OH progesterone will confirm the diagnosis; urinary pregnanetriol levels are high. 11-deoxycortisol levels are high in 11β-hydroxylase deficiency. Male pseudohermaphroditism with intra-abdominal testes is much less common and true hermaphroditism very rare.

If *one* gonad is palpable mixed gonadal dysgenesis (usually with XO/XY karyotype) is least uncommon. Pelvic ultrasound and genitogram, HCG test, gonadal biopsy and exploratory laparotomy may be necessary.

If *two* gonads are palpable, male pseudohermaphroditism is likely. An HCG test measuring testosterone, DHT, DHA and androstenedione will help distinguish 5α-reductase deficiency, testosterone biosynthetic disorders and androgen receptor or postreceptor defects. In vitro androgen binding studies and measurement of 5α-reductase activity in genital skin fibroblast cultures may be necessary. A genitogram may be helpful in imaging the internal genitalia and lower urinary tract.

MANAGEMENT: CHOICE OF GENDER/GENDER IDENTITY

Choice should be based on appearance of external genitalia and functional possibilities in the context of information (cytogenetic, biochemical and radiological) about the nature of the underlying defect and implications for pubertal development. The decision should be made jointly by parents (whose ethnic background may be important in determining their views), pediatric endocrinologist and surgeon. Karyotype is usually irrelevant. In cases where the phallus seems inadequate but there are pressures for male gender assignment, information about likely growth of the phallus in response to androgen can be predicted with depot testosterone (50 mg once monthly i.m. for 3 months).

It used to be thought that psychosexual orientation was dependent on sex of rearing (Money & Ehrhardt 1974) but, from observations in the 'natural history' of patients with 5α-reductase deficiency (Imperato-McGinley et al 1979a, Savage et al 1980) and those with 17β-hydroxysteroid dehydrogenase deficiency (Imperato-McGinley et al 1979b), this seems unlikely – the role of the fetal testis and androgens in 'imprinting' male gender identity seem more important.

Nevertheless, ideally, sex of rearing should be decided as early as possible and surgery carried out to achieve cosmetically acceptable external genitalia by 2 years. Sometimes, because of late presentation or late diagnosis in the older child, or if there is spontaneous 'inappropriate' feminization or virilization at puberty, gender reassignment is indicated. With expert psychiatric support and counseling this can be satisfactorily achieved but cultural considerations may again be important.

INCIDENCE OF TUMORS IN INTERSEX DISORDERS

Patients with a Y chromosome but androgen insensitivity or a disorder of gonadal differentiation are at increased risk of neoplasia in an intra-abdominal gonad by adolescence or early adulthood. The risk with scrotal gonads is probably much less, particularly with regular clinical and ultrasound follow-up.

Carcinoma in situ, benign hamartomas and seminomas (Manuel et al 1976) are reported in complete gonadal dysgenesis patients. In them, therefore, testes should be removed, but some argue that this should be done after spontaneous feminization has taken place at puberty. (In contrast, virilization at puberty will occur in incomplete testicular feminization (incomplete androgen insensitivity) or an androgen biosynthetic defect and the testes should be removed in childhood.)

Tumors are common in dysgenetic gonads. Benign gonadoblastomas may be endocrinologically functional and malignant seminomas, dysgerminomas, choriocarcinomas or yolk sac tumors are reported (Savage et al 1986). Unless there can be careful observation of scrotal gonads through childhood and puberty (with subsequent removal), they are best removed in childhood.

GROWTH ASSESSMENT AND DISORDERS OF GROWTH

For a comprehensive guide to the pathophysiology and treatment of growth disorders, see Kelnar et al (1997). Normal growth, including the growth curve, growth at puberty, measuring techniques, the interpretation of height and height velocity measurements and detailed discussion of the assessment of skeletal maturation, are included in Chapter 8. Hall et al (1989) is a useful reference manual of normal physical measurements and characteristics. The recent introduction in the UK of nine centile growth charts, based on a number of local growth surveys from various parts of the country in the 1980s (Freeman et al 1995), should help to facilitate the appropriate referral of children with growth disorders (Kelnar 1997).

THE IMPORTANCE OF GROWTH ASSESSMENT

Somatic growth is fundamental to childhood – a healthy, adequately nourished and emotionally secure child grows at a normal rate. Growth velocity remains one of the most useful indices of public health and economic well-being in both developing and socially heterogeneous developed countries (Floud et al 1990). Many hormones influence skeletal and somatic growth in childhood including GH, thyroxine, glucocorticoids, androgens and estrogens, insulin and polypeptide growth factors. Growth monitoring is important in the early detection of disease in children and of particular value in detecting a wide variety of endocrine abnormalities in which poor growth may be the earliest, or only, sign of a problem (Kelnar 1993a, 1995a, Buckler 1997, Stirling & Kelnar 1997). The value to the individual (as opposed to public health research) of growth screening has been questioned but overall benefit may be important and cost effective (Cernerud & Edding 1994).

Growth velocity represents the current dynamics of growth much better than does a single measurement of stature which merely reflects previous growth. A slowly growing child has a pathological disorder requiring diagnosis and, if possible, treatment. With conditions of recent onset, slow growth may not have occurred for sufficient time to cause short stature.

The ability to measure a child accurately and reproducibly is fundamental to growth assessment. Height measurements are often valueless or misleading because of inadequate apparatus and careless techniques. Measuring techniques eliminating postural drops and positional errors are readily learned (see Fig. 19.5 and Ch. 8).

Weight is a poor guide to obesity (see p. 1190) which is best assessed with skinfold calipers which measure directly the thickness of subcutaneous fat (Fig. 19.6). Slow growth with > 50th centile skinfold measurements is characteristic of an endocrine disorder in childhood. In severe GH insufficiency there is often a characteristic puckered or marbled appearance and texture to abdominal fat.

With accurate measurements, information on the normality of growth can be obtained over 3 months. Nevertheless seasonal growth variation can occur – not every child grows at a consistent rate month by month – and measurement over 1 year may be necessary before growth velocity can be clearly seen to be abnormal. In addition, normal growth may be cyclical (Butler et al 1989a) with the rate varying over 2–3 years. Rhythms of linear growth are reviewed by Wales & Gibson (1994) and Wales (1997) and the definition and pathogenesis of abnormal growth by Donaldson (1997).

Measurement of height velocity is an accurate, cheap and noninvasive way of assessing the appropriate dose of endocrine replacement therapy. This must be combined with a regular assessment of skeletal maturation (bone age). Otherwise, for example, rapid growth due to over-replacement with thyroxine in the management of acquired hypothyroidism may be taken as desirable 'catch-up' growth.

Knemometry is the technique of choice for studying short-term growth (Valk et al 1983, Hermanussen et al 1988a,b, Wales & Milner 1987, Ahmed et al 1995) as it allows precise, reproducible, noninvasive measurements of lower leg length in growing children, such that daily (or even within-day) and weekly fluctuations in leg length can be documented, e.g. during intercurrent illness or when daily (Wolthers & Pedersen 1990) or alternate-day (Wales & Milner 1988) steroids are administered therapeutically. Knemometry ignores spinal growth and may be influenced by the hydration of soft tissues overlying bone (Ahmed et al 1996b). It is only possible in neonates and children above about 4 years of age.

In certain circumstances, carefully chosen biochemical markers of growth may overcome some of these disadvantages. Biochemical markers are free from observer bias and their precision is independent of frequency of sampling. Bone alkaline phosphatase (BALP) is found in hypertropic chondrocytes of the epiphyseal growth plate, in matrix vesicles associated with bone mineralization and in mature osteoblasts. There is a close quantitative relationship between serial measurements of BALP and height velocity in short normal children undergoing GH treatment (Crofton et al 1995, 1996a).

Procollagen type I C-terminal propeptide (PICP) is released into the circulation by proliferating osteoblasts during collagen biosynthesis; the crosslinked telopeptide of type I collagen (ICTP) is released by collagen breakdown during bone modeling; procollagen type III N-terminal propeptide (P3NP) is released during soft tissue growth but is not present in bone (see Ch. 24). These markers are useful as early predictors of height velocity responses to growth-promoting therapies, and in evaluation of therapies with potentially adverse effects on growth – dexamethasone therapy in preterm neonates with bronchopulmonary dysplasia, and children receiving cytotoxic chemotherapy for leukemia and brain tumors (Crofton et al 1996b,c). Bone and cartilage growth and metabolism is reviewed by Horton (1997).

Skeletal maturation ('bone age') is computed from maturity of bones in radiographs of left hand and wrist by comparison with normal population standards. Bone age is that chronological age for which the maturity score is at the 50th centile. Whether 'delayed' or 'advanced', it is seldom helpful diagnostically. It estimates the percentage of completed growth more accurately than does chronological age and is useful in prediction of final height, assuming that the child and growth are normal and there are no significant bone abnormalities. This has implications not only for management of individual children but for interpretation of changes in height prognosis predicted following a treatment intervention in specific disorders. As with height measurements, bone age must be assessed accurately if it is not to be misleading

to the clinician. Practical auxology and skeletal maturation are reviewed by (Cox 1997a,b).

GROWTH HORMONE (GH) AND GROWTH

GH, a 191 amino acid anterior pituitary polypeptide, is secreted episodically throughout 24 h, but predominantly at night during slow wave sleep, during which there are usually three to five discrete pulses (Hunter & Rigal 1966, Finkelstein et al 1972), and is of cardinal importance in the control of growth. Release is mediated by the two hypothalamic peptides: GH-releasing hormone (GHRH) (Guillemin et al 1982, Rivier et al 1982, Frohman & Jansson 1986), which is stimulatory, and somatostatin, which is inhibitory. Dopaminergic, serotonergic and noradrenergic pathways impinge on the GH regulatory neuron system, but cholinergic neurotransmitter pathways seem particularly important in controlling GHRH and somatostatin release. Hippocampal impulses, perhaps sleep-related, are stimulatory whilst impulses from the amygdala may be either stimulatory or inhibitory. Somatostatin secretion is mediated via the hypothalamic ventromedial nucleus.

A number of drugs induce changes in GH secretion via specific neurotransmitter pathways: clonidine is stimulatory via α-adrenergic and diazepam via GABA pathways; bromocriptine, propranolol and cholinergic agents probably inhibit somatostatin release. This is relevant in understanding pharmacological stimulation tests and, potentially, for therapy to stimulate GH secretion.

GH-releasing hormone (GHRH) was first identified from the pancreas of a woman with Turner's syndrome who developed acromegaly which failed to resolve after transsphenoidal pituitary surgery. Full bioactivity resides in its first 29 amino acids. Recently, a long-recognized family of potent small synthetic GH-releasing peptides – GH-releasing hexapeptide (GHRP) and its analogues – have become important for their potential future therapeutic roles. GHRPs are active given by intravenous, subcutaneous, intranasal and oral routes releasing GH via a specific, nonopiate, non-GHRH pituitary receptor – GHRPs do not interact with GHRH and somatostatin (SRIH) receptors. The receptor is not species specific but is not yet cloned. An additional, hypothalamic, site of action is possible as they require intact GHRH secretion to be effective. Continuous GHRP administration leads to pulsatile GH release.

Analogues such as GHRP6 (hexarelin) and GHRP2 are currently under investigation as are nonpeptide orally active mimetics such as L-692,429. At equivalent (near-maximal) intravenous doses, hexarelin is a more potent GH secretagogue than GHRH but acts synergistically with GHRH when administered synchronously to healthy adult male volunteers (Massoud et al 1995). Intranasal hexarelin is also a potent GH secretagogue in prepubertal children with constitutional short stature (Laron et al 1995). GHRPs given intravenously and orally are currently under investigation in a variety of groups of short stature children. Their potent ability to stimulate GH synthesis and release plus their effectiveness when given orally make them potentially useful, both as diagnostic agents in the evaluation of pituitary disorders and as oral GH secretagogues in 'short normal' children and those in whom 'GH deficiency' is largely hypothalamic rather than pituitary in origin (e.g. post-radiotherapy). They are ineffective in children with organic pituitary disease. For a review see Rogol (1997).

The effective therapeutic use of GHRH itself, potentially a physiological way of treating GH deficiency when the pituitary is intact, has been hampered by the lack of a depot preparation. However, subcutaneous GHRH (given twice daily) has been shown to be effective at stimulating growth, e.g. in children with cranial-irradiation-induced GH deficiency (Ogilvy-Stewart et al 1997).

Yet other peptides are also important in the regulation of GH secretion: endorphins, neurotensin and vasoactive intestinal peptide (VIP) are stimulatory whilst substance P and central TRH pathways are inhibitory.

GH is unusual in being species specific. Two forms are present in man and it is secreted as an heterogeneous molecular species. The predominant, and presumably more bioactive, form is of MW 22 000 (22K). An approximately 20K form is present in smaller amounts. Structurally abnormal GH variants with varying bioactivity could be important in the etiology of growth failure in certain rare conditions but are unlikely to be common reasons for poor growth in the population as a whole.

GH is not inhibited by feedback from peripheral endocrine glands although thyroxine and glucocorticoids influence its secretion. Regulation is by GH itself (at hypothalamic and pituitary levels), peripheral GH-dependent growth factors (e.g. IGF1), GHRH and somatostatin and metabolic factors such as free fatty acids and glucose. The physiological role of GHRPs is still unclear. The integration of this control with physiological states – sleep, exercise, appetite and nutrition – is via the monoaminergic and peptide systems described above. GH neuroregulation in health and disease is reviewed by Dieguez et al (1988) and Robinson & Thomas (1997).

The plasma half-life of exogenously administered GH is 20–25 min; that of endogenous GH is thought to be similar or shorter although this remains controversial (Faria et al 1989, Hindmarsh et al 1989). GH affects linear growth directly by stimulating early epiphyseal growth plate precursor cell differentiation but it is uncertain whether it has anabolic effects that are independent of IGF1. Paracrine IGF1, produced locally in proliferating chondrocytes of the growth plate, is more important than liver-derived circulating IGF1 in stimulating epiphyseal cartilage growth (Underwood et al 1986).

In the interaction between GH and tissue growth, the GH receptor is of crucial importance (Waters et al 1990). The GH receptor was cloned from rabbit liver based on amino acid sequence data and from human liver by cross hybridization and consists of a 620 amino acid (AA) peptide situated astride the target cell membrane with a single transmembrane domain. The extracellular hormone-binding domain consists of approximately 245 AAs and there is a cytoplasmic region of 350 residues (Fig. 19.10) (Wood et al 1993).

85% of the cytoplasmic domain is unnecessary for signal transduction. Overall there is 24% homology with the PRL receptor – some sections are strikingly similar. Defects in the gene encoding the receptor have been identified in GH insensitivity syndrome (GHIS, Laron-type dwarfism) indicating that the receptor is required for normal growth. The extracellular component circulates as a high affinity GH-binding protein (GHBP). One molecule of GH binds to, and dimerizes, two molecules of receptor; thus there are two binding sites on the GH molecule with the second near the N terminus (Carter-Su et al 1993, Mullis 1997).

Receptor dimerization is the first step in the GH signaling pathway. A prediction of the model is that high levels of

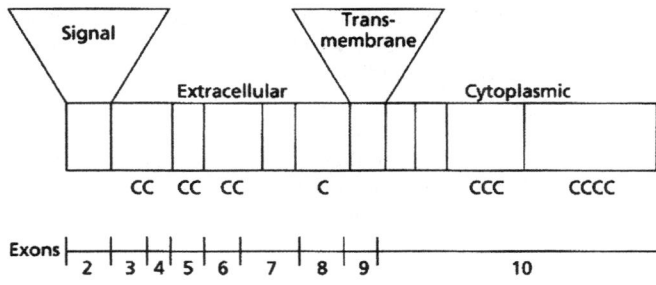

Fig. 19.10   The growth hormone receptor.

circulating GH, or GH with one abnormal binding site, should have antagonist rather than agonist activity. This is true of site 2 GH mutants although site 1 GH mutants show poor antagonism. GH to receptor concentrations of 1 : 1 show antagonism as predicted.

Laron dwarfism (Laron et al 1966, Laron 1993) is the classical form of GHIS resulting from molecular defects in the GH receptor caused by gene deletions or point mutations (Rosenfeld et al 1994, Amselem et al 1993). Recent evidence (Goddard et al 1995) that heterozygous expression of GH receptor mutations may be associated with growth failure, raises questions not only as to whether heterozygotic expression of Laron dwarfism results in a clinically important phenotype but also whether a significant minority of children with 'idiopathic short stature' could be heterozygous for mutations of the GH receptor (Rosenfeld 1995). This also has implications for investigation and diagnosis of short stature and GH 'deficiency'.

Current GH signal transduction models (Carter-Su et al 1993) involve activation by GH of a GH-receptor-associated tyrosine kinase (GHRTK), an important early (and perhaps initiating) step in signal transduction. Carter-Su et al (1993) have confirmed this by demonstrating that the GHRTK, which is stimulated by very low GH concentrations within less than 30 s of GH binding to the receptor, is likely to have a role in stimulation by GH of a variety of cellular responses including kinase activity and gene expression. In particular, GH stimulates tyrosyl phosphorylation and kinase activity of a GH-dependent GH-receptor-associated kinase JAK 2 (one of a family of Janus kinases). JAK 2 probably serves as a signaling molecule for multiple members of a cytokine/hematopoietin family which includes GH, PRL, erythropoietin, interleukin-3, etc. GHRTK functions both to activate other proteins by phosphorylation and to phosphorylate tyrosyl residues in itself and the GH receptor. These phosphorylated tyrosines may serve as docking sites for proteins in other signaling pathways. Such studies should lead to the identification of new cellular actions for GH.

GH receptors in sheep hepatocytes turn over rapidly (every 30–90 min); their number is regulated by, for example, nutritional factors and estrogens as well as GH itself (Gluckman et al 1990). It is likely that acuteness or chronicity of GH exposure profoundly influences GH receptor turnover rates. GHBP levels also vary diurnally and do not correlate with GH peaks. Human GHBP and GH receptor are encoded by a single species mRNA (Mullis et al 1995). Proteolysis is probably the major mechanism for GHBP production in man – GHBP blood levels probably do not represent GH receptor status in functional terms.

Thus to be biologically active, GH must bind to a transmembrane receptor, which must dimerize and activate an intracellular signal transduction pathway causing IGF1 synthesis and secretion. However, IGF1 which, in blood, is itself bound to members of a family of binding proteins (IGFBPs), must bind to the IGF1 receptor, in turn activating its own signal transduction pathways producing mitogenic and anabolic responses and tissue growth. The complexity of these pathways (together with the vagaries of GH assays and the pulsatile nature of GH release) help to explain the difficulties in measuring 'GH secretory ability' in many short stature children.

GROWTH REGULATION

Mechanisms by which physiological states, GH regulation and genetic determination of growth potential are integrated to achieve appropriate stature are largely unknown. Tanner has proposed (1963) that the CNS contains a 'sizostat' – the rate of synthesis or release of a specific molecule could decrease as maturity increases and another molecule could be synthesized in proportion to the amount of growth. A 'mismatch' would be sensed by the sizostat and growth adjusted accordingly. This concept, and 'catch-up' (Prader et al 1963) and 'catch-down' growth made it uncertain that exogenous hormone therapy in various categories of short children would necessarily increase final height significantly and this has, generally, been found to be the case in practice in recent years.

'Catch-up' growth, rather than CNS-dependent, could be intrinsic to the growth plate. Baron et al (1993) infused dexamethasone phosphate into one proximal tibial growth plate of 5-week-old rabbits over 4 weeks and inactive vehicle into the contralateral growth plate. Growth plate growth velocity was determined radiologically. Dexamethasone significantly decreased growth velocity in the growth plate compared to the contralateral control causing significant growth deficit. After the end of the infusion, growth velocity in the dexamethasone-treated growth plate rebounded above that of the control, ultimately correcting approximately half the deficit suggesting that 'catch-up' growth is, at least in part, intrinsic to the epiphyseal growth plate and cannot be explained by central mechanisms alone.

Mathematical models of human growth were descriptive (Stuetzle et al 1980) but models relating to possible underlying dynamics of hormonal (and other) control have since been proposed (Karlberg et al 1987). The 'infancy–childhood–puberty' model of growth suggests that the infancy component (which is a continuation of fetal growth) is primarily determined by nutritional factors, the childhood component by GH and the puberty component by sex steroids. The infancy component is initially rapid but decelerates as the influence of GH appears by the end of the first year. The effect of GH is sustained but in the absence of adequate sex steroid secretion the pubertal growth spurt is blunted or absent. The combined input of the three components results in the normal pattern of growth to final height. Such a model, simplistic if control mechanisms are seen as 'all or none' phenomena, does potentially enable effects of different insults which may affect growth and different treatment modalities to be studied more effectively.

Tall children secrete more GH than their short peers (Albertsson-Wikland et al 1983) and GH secretory pulse amplitude correlates with growth velocity although not very strongly. For detailed discussion of the endocrine control of growth see Robinson & Thomas (1997) and Holly (1997).

THE SHORT OR SLOWLY GROWING CHILD

The 'normality' of a child's height is determined by reference to growth charts showing population norms. Ideally each country and ethnic group should have its own growth standards. In practice, UK charts serve well even in developing countries and for ethnic minorities within the UK as differences in final stature reflect minor differences in growth velocity over the whole growing period. Recent introduction in the UK of nine centile growth charts, based on seven cross-sectional local growth surveys between 1978 and 1990 (Freeman et al 1995), should help to facilitate the appropriate referral of children with growth disorders following community height *screening*. The lowest centile is the 0.4 line – only 1 normal child in 250 will fall below that line which is a clear indicator for referral. The interval between each provided pair of centile lines is the same – two-thirds of a standard deviation. 2% of the normal population will have a height below the second centile. It is recommended that any children between the 2nd and 0.4 centiles are monitored to see whether their growth is normal. Versions are available for community and hospital use.

Revised charts based on the Tanner–Whitehouse growth standards (determined in a longitudinal study of South of England children in the 1960s) have recently been produced – the Buckler–Tanner 1995 longitudinal standards (Buckler & Tanner 1996). Height revision is adjusted to take account of the recent cross-sectional studies and of Buckler's longitudinal study of adolescent growth (Buckler 1990). For monitoring the growth pattern in an individual child such charts are preferable. 3% of normal children will, by definition, be below the third centile on a distance (height for age) chart yet a child with a growth disorder of recent onset will be of normal stature. Only serial measurements and calculation of growth velocity will distinguish normality from abnormality.

Parental genetic contributions reduce the population standard deviation of height by about 30%. 95% of the children of given parents will have a height prognosis within ± 8.5 cm of the mid-parental centile. Children also 'inherit' an environment from their parents. A child's shortness, whilst 'appropriate' for his short parents, may reflect poor nutrition or emotional deprivation continuing down the generations with no family member achieving his or her true genetic height potential. The mean height of children from social class IV and V families remains significantly less than that of those from social classes I and II in Britain in the 1980s as it did in the 1870s despite the secular trend to increasing height in both groups (Floud et al 1990).

The possibility of an unrecognized and untreated growth disorder in an unusually short parent must be excluded before attributing a child's shortness to constitutional reasons – pathology, e.g. GH deficiency, a skeletal dysplasia or pseudohypoparathyroidism, may also be genetically transmitted.

The differential diagnosis of short stature or slow growth is summarized in Table 19.5. Whatever their ultimate height prognosis many short children may suffer emotionally and underachieve. 'Western' society views tallness as a positive attribute and the social consequences of short stature are not dependent on the presence of underlying pathology, which must be sought if growth velocity is inadequate (Kelnar 1990). Without diagnostic clues from history or examination, the screening test for a child presenting with short stature is calculation of growth velocity.

Table 19.5   Differential diagnosis of short stature and slow growth

Short with currently normal growth velocity
Constitutional short stature, short normal parent(s)

Previous problem affecting growth, now cured or no longer operative
Prolonged intrauterine growth retardation – light for gestational age, low birth length and head circumference, difficult feeders in infancy, including Silver-Russell syndrome – triangular facies, clinodactyly, facial and limb length asymmetry
Congenital heart disease
Physiological growth delay (delayed bone age, normal height prognosis)

Growing slowly (whether already short or still of normal stature)
With increased skinfold thicknesses
Endocrine disease (e.g. panhypopituitarism, severe growth hormone insufficiency – idiopathic or secondary to tumor or irradiation, hypothyroidism, pseudohypoparathyroidism, Cushing's syndrome)
Disproportionate
Short limbs for spine (the dyschondroplasias) (e.g. achondroplasia, hypochondroplasia, multiple epiphyseal dysplasia)
Short limbs and spine (spine relatively shorter) (e.g. mucopolysaccharidoses, metatropic dwarfism)
Often without other obvious signs of disease (see text)
Chromosomal abnormalities (e.g. Turner's syndrome – other signs variable)
Unrecognized asthma (may be misdiagnosed)
Malabsorption due to celiac disease, ulcerative colitis, Crohn's disease (bowel habit may be normal)
Psychosocial deprivation
Malnutrition
Cardiovascular or renal disease

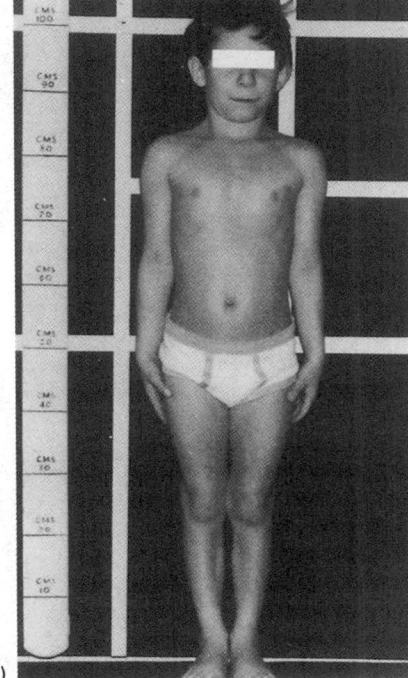

(a)

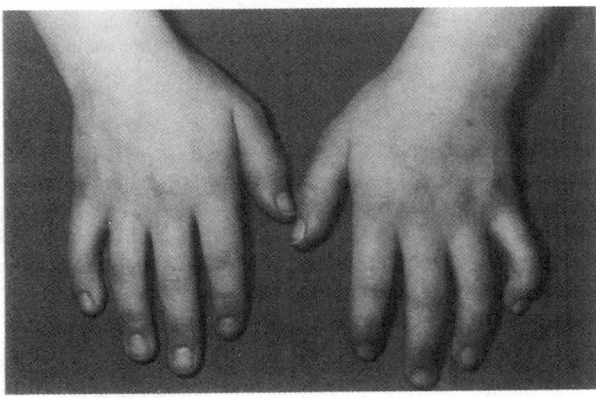

(b)

Fig. 19.11   A child with prolonged intrauterine growth retardation (Silver–Russell) syndrome presenting with short stature. Note the triangular facies, low-set ears, asymmetry (**a**) and clinodactyly (**b**).

A small child who is growing normally may have small parents (constitutional short stature but see above), growth (and likely maturational) delay, a previous period of poor growth (for example due to prolonged IUGR, e.g. Silver–Russell syndrome – see Fig. 19.11) or a combination of these factors.

The differential diagnosis of causes of slow growth, whatever the current height, is wide (see Table 19.5). Genetic and dysmorphic syndromes of short stature are reviewed by Rimoin & Borochowitz (1997).

Endocrine causes

Impaired GH secretion

A few children lack the gene for making GH (Illig et al 1971, Phillips et al 1986), demonstrate prenatal GH deficiency, respond to GH therapy with the major antibody response expected to a foreign protein and cannot be treated with any form of GH. Otherwise there is a wide spectrum of GH and IGF1 secretory ability (Albertsson-Wikland et al 1983), which, within the normal population, is likely to be largely genetically determined (see above). At one end of the spectrum are children, perhaps 1 in 4000 (Vimpani et al 1977), with severe GH insufficiency ('GH deficiency'). They grow slowly (Fig. 19.12) and demonstrate characteristic clinical features (truncal obesity with characteristic fat 'marbling' (Fig. 19.13), crowding of midfacial features with immature appearance and small genitalia with micropenis in boys) and show an inadequate (< 7 mU/l) response to a pharmacological stimulus to GH secretion.

There is a continuum from them through moderate GH insufficiency (so-called 'partial' GH deficiency with GH responses in the 7–15 mU/l range) and through short normal, averagely tall to tall normal individuals and those with gigantism (Fig. 19.14). The question as to whether GH therapy could increase the height of the normally growing short child is being actively investigated (Donaldson 1996, Hindmarsh & Brook 1996). Some short, slowly-growing children have what is considered to be an abnormal pattern of GH pulsatile release but normal GH responses to stimulation tests – 'neurosecretory dysfunction' (Spiliotis et al 1984). It is possible that genetic polymorphism for the GH or IGF1 receptor, IGF1 or IGFBP3, could also underlie the spectrum of height seen in a normal population. Heterozygosity for classical autosomal recessive disorders could, speculatively, explain growth abnormalities in many children with 'idiopathic' short stature (Rosenfeld 1995).

Severe GH insufficiency may be congenital, acquired, isolated or associated with other pituitary hormone deficiencies. Many children with 'idiopathic isolated GH deficiency' have a hypothalamic disorder of GHRH release, responding to a GHRH bolus by secreting GH normally (see below). In others, high resolution CT or MR scanning demonstrates abnormalities

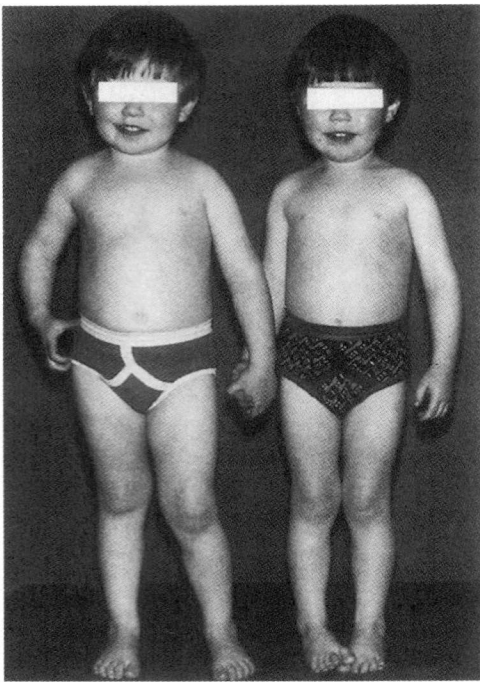

Fig. 19.12   A boy with severe GH insufficiency (right) who is shorter than his 2 years younger brother. Triceps and subscapular skinfold measurements were 97th centile.

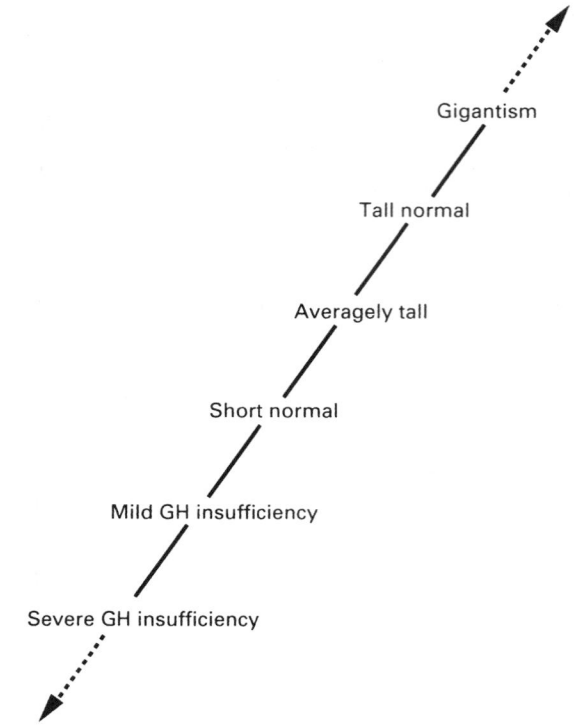

Fig. 19.14   The spectrum of growth hormone secretory ability.

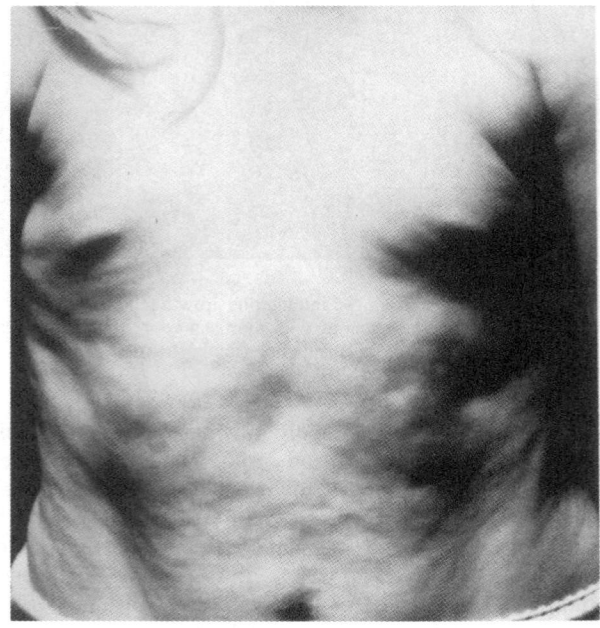

Fig. 19.13   Characteristic 'marbling' of fat in severe GH insufficiency.

ranging from absent septum pellucidum associated with other midline defects (septo-optic dysplasia) to pituitary hypoplasia.

Acquired GH 'deficiency' may result from intracranial tumor (e.g. craniopharyngioma) or from cranial irradiation for medulloblastoma or acute lymphoblastic leukemia (Ahmed et al 1986). The effects of chemotherapy on growth (and endocrine

function) are increasingly recognized (Wallace & Kelnar 1996a,b). Temporary GH deficiency is seen in children with psychosocial deprivation (see below) and occurs physiologically in late prepuberty and early male puberty. GH biosynthesis and release is also impaired in other conditions (e.g. primary hypothyroidism or celiac disease) – secretion normalizes with treatment of the underlying disorder.

Abnormalities of GH secretion and action are reviewed, respectively, by Heintze & Bercu (1997) and Rosenfeld (1997).

Hypothyroidism (see pp. 1048–1050)

Acquired primary hypothyroidism is usually autoimmune (Hashimoto's thyroiditis). Poor growth velocity and school performance often precede the well-known symptoms and signs by many months. Abnormal growth in thyroid disorders is reviewed by Grüters (1997).

Steroids (see also later)

Growth failure from glucocorticoids is usually iatrogenic (excessive medication) rather than due to pituitary-dependent Cushing's disease (excess ACTH secretion), adrenal tumor (benign or malignant) or ectopic tumor ACTH production, all rare in children. Alternate-day steroid regimes seem less growth suppressing. The effects of glucocorticoids on growth have been reviewed by Tönshoff et al (1996).

Disproportionate short stature

Most constitutional disorders of bone involve long bones and spine to a different extent leading to disproportionate short stature.

This may be obvious clinically when there is gross disproportion but may need to be specifically identified from sitting height measurements (subischial leg length equals standing height minus sitting height) and reference to standard charts.

The most important group of skeletal dysplasias affecting cartilage and/or bone growth and development are the osteochondrodysplasias. Those affecting tubular or spinal bone growth or both are known as chondrodystrophies. It is increasingly possible to classify skeletal dysplasias on a pathophysiological basis (Shohat & Rimoin 1996).

It is important to recognize disproportionate short stature so that accurate diagnosis can be made without unnecessary investigation. In general, biochemical investigation is unhelpful other than when a mucopolysaccharidosis or disorder of calcium metabolism is suspected and bone biopsy is rarely diagnostic. A full or selective skeletal survey generally yields most helpful diagnostic information and must be interpreted by a radiologist with particular expertise (Lachman 1997). Radiological atlases of skeletal dysplasias (e.g. Spranger et al 1974) are of great help. Even so, radiological changes in many conditions only become diagnostic in older children.

In general, specific therapy is unavailable (although there could be a response to GH therapy) but accurate diagnosis is necessary for genetic counseling and accurate prognosis. Limb lengthening orthopedic procedures are reviewed by Saleh (1997). Epiphyseal distal femur distraction in chondrodysplastic dogs results in damage to the epiphyseal growth plate and degenerative knee joint changes (Fjeld & Steen 1989).

Chromosomal abnormalities

Many chromosomal disorders are associated with poor growth and short stature (Rimoin & Borochowitz 1997). Absence, partial deletion or translocations of the X chromosome (Turner's syndrome and its mosaic forms – Fig. 19.15) are particularly so (see below). Turner's syndrome girls with tall parents may not become conspicuously short until puberty fails to start. Growth

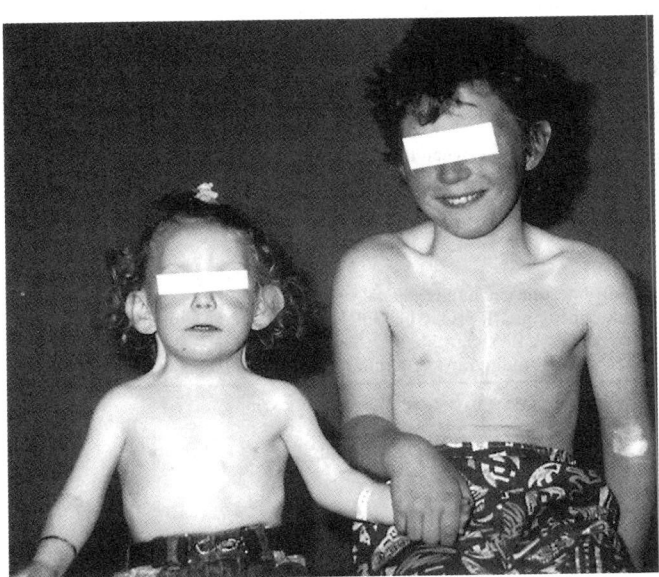

Fig. 19.15 Two unrelated girls with Turner's syndrome.

charts for Turner's syndrome (Lyon et al 1985b) and Down syndrome (Cronk et al 1988) are available.

Inheritance of two maternal alleles from the same parent (uniparental disomy), in this case on chromosome 7, may be a feature in some patients with severe IUGR (Silver–Russell syndrome or primordial dwarfism) (Schmitt et al 1995). There are several potentially relevant genes which map to the long arm of chromosome 7, e.g. those for IGFBP1, IGFBP3 and the EGF receptor. Whether any are influenced by the disomy, and thus involved in the pathogenesis of Silver–Russell syndrome remains to be determined.

Chronic disease

Differential diagnosis of the short but not fat child covers virtually the whole field of chronic disorders. Some may be suspected from history or clinical findings but poor growth is often the major diagnostic clue to psychosocial deprivation (see below), unrecognized or undertreated asthma, renal tubular acidosis and malabsorption syndromes such as celiac disease (Ashkenazi 1989) and chronic inflammatory bowel disease (Barton & Ferguson 1990, Kirschner 1990), Crohn's disease (Kanof et al 1988) or ulcerative colitis. Worldwide, protein/calorie deprivation is the commonest cause of growth failure; GH levels are high but peripheral growth factor synthesis and IGF1 levels are low. The effects on growth of gastrointestinal disorders are reviewed by Kirschner (1997). The effects of cardiac disease, neurological disorders and hemoglobinopathies are reviewed by Burns (1997), Minns (1997) and Wonke (1997) respectively.

Psychosocial deprivation

Psychosocial deprivation often causes poor growth, may mimic idiopathic hypopituitarism in terms of GH responses to conventional stimuli (Powell et al 1967a,b) and abnormal overnight GH secretory profiles may return to normal rapidly following admission to hospital (Stanhope et al 1988a, Skuse et al 1996). Any child growing poorly at home who thrives in hospital or when fostered (Fig. 19.16) should be suspected of being emotionally deprived. Accurately maintained growth data are increasingly accepted as evidence in British courts. Severe growth failure may result from Munchausen syndrome by proxy (Lyall et al 1992).

Laron dwarfism (Laron et al 1966, Laron 1993)

This is an autosomal recessively inherited syndrome associated with molecular defects in the GH receptor caused by gene deletions or point mutations (Rosenfeld et al 1994, Amselem et al 1993). These children, whose GH is active in in vitro GH receptor assays, characteristically demonstrate severe postnatal growth failure, secrete abundant GH (with normal or elevated serum levels) but have markedly reduced serum concentrations of IGF1 and IGFBP3 and do not respond to GH therapy. In clinical trials, some responded well to IGF1 therapy (Guevara-Aguirre et al 1995, Savage et al 1993) but its future availability is now in doubt. GH resistance is reviewed by Savage (1997).

Early cases demonstrated low serum GHBP concentrations indicating abnormalities of the extracellular domain of the GH receptor, i.e. circulating GHBP. Many may have deletions or point mutations of the GH receptor gene (nine coding regions (exons)

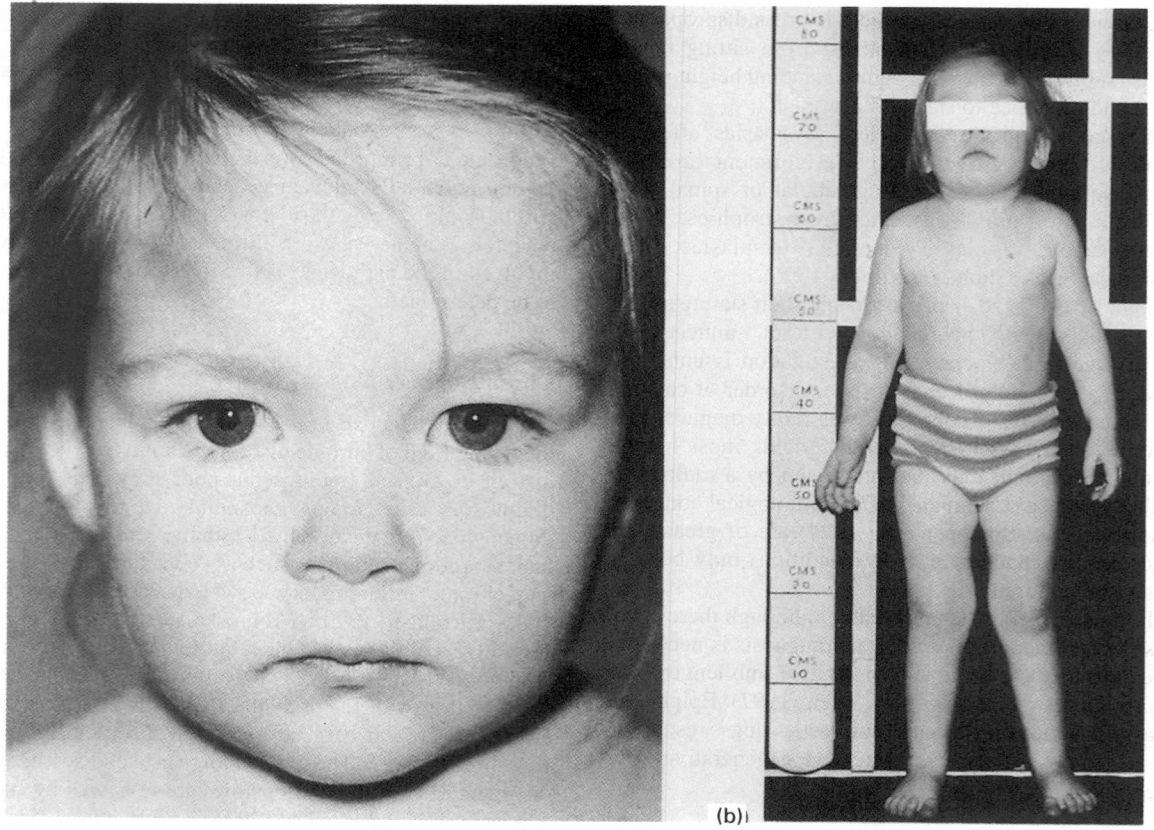

Fig. 19.16   An emotionally abused child (note the characteristic expression of 'frozen watchfulness'), photographed on the day of admission to hospital. In the ward environment she showed remarkable 'catch-up' growth and growth hormone secretion normalized. She has since been successfully adopted.

occupying an 87 kilobase segment of chromosome 5) coding for the GH-binding domain. However, it now seems that a minority of the several hundred cases identified worldwide have normal circulating GHBP levels suggesting a degree of heterozygosity and either defects in the portion of the extracellular domain of the GH receptor molecule needed for dimerization or intracellular defects affecting signal transduction (Buchanan et al 1991). There is now debate as to whether heterozygotic expression of Laron dwarfism results in a clinically important phenotype (Rosenfeld 1995).

INVESTIGATION OF POOR GROWTH

This is summarized in Table 19.6 and reviewed by Donaldson (1997). Random determination of serum GH levels is unhelpful – pulsatile release and short serum half-life often result in low levels in normal children. Establishing a reasonable assessment of GH secretory ability or a firm diagnosis of GH deficiency can be difficult (Rosenfeld 1995) because of the pulsatile, and predominantly nocturnal, nature of GH secretion, variability of GH assays (monoclonal, polyclonal, RIA, IRMA, which recognize different circulating forms of GH to varying extents) and the complexity of the control of GH secretion and the GH-IGF1–growth metabolic pathways.

All GH provocation tests may give false negative or positive responses. Screening tests are difficult to standardize and response

Table 19.6   Investigation of poor growth

Full medical and social history

Accurate measurement of the child and his parents

Thorough clinical examination (including measurement of blood pressure, fundi, visual fields)

Bone age

Karyotype (girls)

Specific investigation (when indicated)
    Hematological (e.g. Hb, FBC, ESR)
    Biochemical (e.g. Ca, PO_4, alkaline phosphatase, urea and electrolytes)
    Cardiac
    Respiratory
    Renal
    Gastrointestinal including jejunal biopsy
    Endocrine (e.g. T4, prolactin, GnRH, TRH tests, growth hormone provocation test*)
    Skeletal (e.g. radiograph of pituitary fossa, skeletal survey)

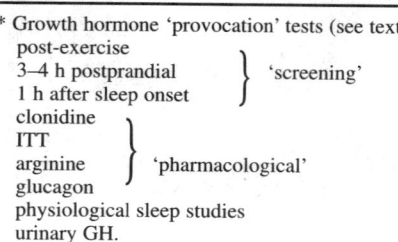

* Growth hormone 'provocation' tests (see text):
    post-exercise
    3–4 h postprandial   } 'screening'
    1 h after sleep onset
    clonidine
    ITT
    arginine   } 'pharmacological'
    glucagon
    physiological sleep studies
    urinary GH.

is variable. The insulin hypoglycemia (tolerance) test (ITT) remains the standard for confirming a diagnosis of severe GH insufficiency. Adequate (symptomatic) hypoglycemia must be obtained if results are to be meaningful (blood glucose < 2.2 mmol/l). Following adequate hypoglycemia, 85% of 'normal' children will produce a serum GH level of over 15 mU/l (usually after 30–60 min). In conjunction with an ITT, the GH response to GHRH is useful for determining whether 'GH insufficiency' is due to a pituitary defect or hypothalamic disorder of GHRH synthesis or release (Grossman et al 1983). In the latter case the GH response to GHRH will be normal indicating that pituitary somatotrophs are functional, e.g. in many children with 'isolated GH insufficiency' or 'GH insufficiency' secondary to cranial irradiation (Grossman et al 1984).

The role (and risks) of conventional GH stimulation tests have been reviewed by Ranke & Haber (1992), Shah et al (1992), Hindmarsh & Swift (1995) and Hindmarsh (1997). Tests of GH secretion must be performed only when indicated (and when other possible causes of poor growth have been considered). They should only be undertaken in specialist endocrine units experienced in their performance. An ITT is potentially dangerous and requires supervision by competent and experienced junior pediatric staff working from clear and understood protocols and guidelines. These should ensure that glucose and hydrocortisone are drawn up in readiness, and there is checking of insulin and glucose dosages, continual presence of a dedicated and experienced member of nursing staff for monitoring of blood glucose and conscious level, adequate and secure venous access established before insulin is administered and detailed instruction for management of hypoglycemia.

Some centers measure spontaneous nocturnal pulsatile GH release to provide greater insight into secretory control mechanisms (Adlard et al 1987, Hindmarsh et al 1987, Butler et al 1989c). Their relevance to short stature assessment or as a predictor of response to therapy remains controversial, though there may be a relationship between the amplitude of GH pulses and growth velocity. Such tests are impracticable for 'screening' large numbers of children.

Urinary GH measurement could become a useful, noninvasive, repeatable and cheap way of assessing physiological GH secretion (Albini et al 1988) but urinary GH levels vary considerably day by day, are approximately 1000-fold lower than in plasma and until recently, accuracy and reproducibility were poor (Girard et al 1990).

Measurements of serum IGF1 and IGFBP3 (and, perhaps, urinary GH) may be useful screening tests for identifying short children who need more complex investigations of GH secretory ability. Theoretical algorithms for the biochemical diagnosis of GH deficiency and insensitivity disorders have been proposed (e.g. Ranke 1994).

TREATMENT OF POOR GROWTH

Treatment aims to correct the underlying problem where possible (e.g. gluten-free diet in celiac disease, thyroxine in hypothyroidism) and can only maximize remaining growth potential. The sooner poor growth is recognized, its cause diagnosed and treated, the better the height prognosis. For a comprehensive review of the treatment of growth disorders see Kelnar et al (1997).

Growth hormone

Preparations

From 1958 to 1985, pituitary-derived GH was available in limited quantities for children with GH 'deficiency'. These preparations were withdrawn because some batches could have been contaminated with Creutzfeldt–Jacob disease (CJD) 'prion' and current purity could not be guaranteed. Biosynthetic GH, *E. coli* synthesized and produced by recombinant DNA technology, became available in the UK by late 1985. This was initially with an additional amino-terminal methionine (192 amino acids). Since December 1988, natural sequence 191 amino acid biosynthetic GH has been prescribable in the UK. This is physicochemically identical to natural human hormone. No brain tissue is involved in its production and its administration cannot transmit CJD.

Indications for use

Children with severe GH insufficiency (GH 'deficiency') and moderate GH insufficiency should be treated with GH, provided other causes of impaired GH secretion have been excluded. It is inappropriate to prescribe GH indiscriminately to short children (Stirling & Kelnar 1994, Hintz 1997, Guyda 1997): long-term studies are in progress (Cowell 1990, Ackland et al 1990, Donaldson 1996, Hindmarsh & Brook 1996). The improved psychological state resulting from knowledge that treatment is being given could itself have a growth-stimulating effect via hypothalamic pathways – children with psychosocial deprivation secrete more GH and grow better when in a normal emotional environment. However, placebo-controlled trials in our department have demonstrated no significant height velocity improvements on placebo over 1 year (and also no deleterious psychological effects) in short 'normal' children.

Although a social class-related and socially desirable attribute in 'developed societies', tall stature does not confer innate biological advantage in all societies. In disadvantaged environments (e.g. the Peruvian Andes), small mothers have more surviving offspring (Frisancho et al 1977); in an agricultural peasant economy, a small man is more efficient than a tall one, requiring to do less work to feed himself (Malcolm 1971, Stini 1972). Even if GH therapy increases the height of a normally growing short child, will taller stature in itself contribute to academic or material success or psychological contentment? Leaving aside methodological problems in assessing possible psychological disadvantage from short stature in childhood (Stabler 1997), it seems likely that there are genuine cultural differences in the psychological effects of short stature even between 'developed' countries (e.g. USA and UK) (Skuse et al 1994). For a discussion of the cultural, social and psychological background to the potential uses of GH in normal short children see Kelnar (1990).

GH therapy may be of particular benefit to children with Turner's syndrome (Ranke 1996, Ranke 1997) and could also benefit those with prolonged IUGR (who often remain short despite normal postnatal growth). The variable outcomes of studies of GH in IUGR probably reflect their heterogeneity of etiology of growth retardation (Albanese & Stanhope 1993, Czernichow 1996, Wollmann 1997). There is encouraging medium-term growth improvement in children with chronic renal failure treated with GH (Mehls 1997) and a product license for this use of GH is now available in a number of countries. Infants with chronic renal failure have also been found to benefit in the short term (Maxwell & Rees 1996).

GH is being evaluated in the treatment of some skeletal dysplasias (Hagenäs 1997). In these groups, surgical limb lengthening may be indicated once the postpubertal patient is able to decide whether he wishes to undergo these major and prolonged procedures (Saleh 1997).

Due to the shortage of available GH over many years, the dose used in severe GH insufficiency was the most 'cost effective' (in terms of increase in growth velocity achieved per unit GH given) rather than that which would maximally stimulate growth so that, even now, the optimal treatment regimen is not clearly established. A GH dose of 18–24 units/m^2/week divided into daily (bedtime) subcutaneous injections may be most effective. Higher doses are probably necessary during puberty. The role of short bursts of GH therapy in a variety of situations remains to be evaluated (Kelnar & Tanaka 1994). GH therapy in puberty has been reviewed by Shalet (1995).

GH antibodies could result in severe growth restriction in a previously normal child but antibodies of sufficient specificity and binding capacity to produce growth attenuation are rare. Potential metabolic side effects include glucose intolerance, hyperinsulinism, hyperlipidemia and hypertension. Psychological harm could result if expectations are not fulfilled. Leukemia may be more common in GH-deficient children treated with GH but there is no evidence causally linking GH treatment itself with leukemia. Adverse effects of GH therapy are reviewed by Saenger (1997).

GHRH therapy (Low et al 1988, Thorner et al 1988) may be appropriate in many 'GH insufficient' children when the problem is at hypothalamic, rather than pituitary, level but optimal treatment regimens are unclear (Smith & Brook 1988). Although it is possible that future growth-promoting treatment modalities could include intranasal GH (Hedin et al 1989), intranasal GHRH, depot (intramuscular) GHRH, and IGF1 in particular circumstances, with several of these preparations bioavailability, practical production difficulties and costs or possible side effects remain problematic. The most promising developments in the therapeutic application of growth-stimulating compounds seems currently to be in the use of GH-releasing peptides (see p. 1012) which may impinge significantly on the management of certain types of growth disorder in the future.

Anabolic steroids

Synthetic steroids with enhanced anabolic but little androgenic activity are valuable in growth delay, increasing (normal) slow growth in early male puberty (Stanhope et al 1988b) and in Turner's syndrome (see p. 1032). As with GH therapy, the decision to use these preparations should generally be the province of the specialist in growth disorders. Kelnar (1994) reviews their use in boys with constitutional delay of growth and puberty.

Emotional support

This is particularly important for short stature children and their families. Psychological measures for evaluating children with growth disorders are reviewed by Stabler (1997). Specific treatment may not be available, may be of unproven benefit or may start too late to achieve adequate stature. Any child

physically different from his or her peers will attract attention: short children have to cope with an identity which is determined primarily (and seen by others) in terms of their size (Skuse 1987). Growth-related changes in body shape and size are important determinants of perceived age and adult care-giving responses (Alley 1983). Short children must be treated appropriately for their chronological age, emotionally, intellectually and practically. Teasing, bullying and expectations based on physical size rather than on intrinsic abilities will cause immature behavior, underperformance at school and may impair growth further (Gordon et al 1982). They are likely to be aggressive to siblings and peers and more anxious and depressed than controls (Mussen & Jones 1957). Poor examination results cause the small school-leaver to have particular difficulties finding employment. The emotional and social consequences of short stature are not dependent on the presence of underlying pathology (Kelnar 1990). For a review see Skuse (1997).

THE TALL OR RAPIDLY GROWING CHILD (Table 19.7)

Tall stature presents less often than short: syndromes causing tallness are rare whereas poor growth is a common result of childhood disease, and childhood tallness, unless extreme, is socially advantageous. Nevertheless, a tall child is often taken for older and expectations may be greater than can be met. Clumsiness and gangliness may result from neurological immaturity for size.

Advanced skeletal maturation may be associated with tallness in childhood (and a normal growth velocity) but this rarely results in problems or medical help being sought (cf. growth delay).

Constitutional tall stature infrequently presents but tall mothers sometimes worry about their normal daughters' heights. In this situation, drug treatment – attempting to limit GH secretion whilst allowing normal sex steroid-mediated skeletal maturation (e.g. with bromocriptine (Schwartz et al 1987), somatostatin analogue (octreotide) or anticholinergic drugs such as pirenzepine (Hindmarsh & Brook 1995)) or rapidly advancing skeletal maturation (using sex steroids) – is unsatisfactory. Estrogen therapy causes an initial increase in growth velocity and potential side effects from the high doses necessary, both short term (headaches and nausea) and long term (diabetes mellitus, hyperlipidemia, hypertension, endometrial carcinoma, WHO 1985), limit its usefulness. It cannot be used much earlier than normal pubertal onset and treatment after the growth spurt is underway (early in female puberty) will have only a small effect on reducing final height. Medical management of tall stature is reviewed by Lamberts (1997).

When height prognosis remains unacceptably high to child and family, surgical epiphysiodesis, an established procedure for reducing moderate leg length discrepancy (Macnicol et al 1993, Alexeeff and Macnicol 1995) may be indicated. Surgical management of tall stature is reviewed by Macnicol (1997).

Tall stature syndromes

These are outlined in Table 19.7. Genetic and dysmorphic syndromes of tall stature are reviewed by Patton (1997). Gigantism due to excessive GH secretion is extremely rare in pediatric practice (cf. acromegaly after epiphysial closure).

Table 19.7   Differential diagnosis of tall stature or rapid growth

Tall with currently normal growth velocity
Constitutional tall stature (tall normal parent(s))
Previous rapid growth (usually due to overeating)
Physiological growth advance

Currently rapid growth (whether already tall or still of 'normal' stature)
Associated with precocious puberty
Idiopathic (physiological)
Pathological
   Intracranial space-occupying lesions
   Gonadal tumors
   Ectopic gonadotropin-producing tumor (e.g. hepatoblastoma)
   Adrenal
      Congenital adrenal hyperplasia (21-hydroxylase deficiency,
      11β-hydroxylase deficiency)
      Cushing's syndrome
      Neoplasia
   Estrogen ingestion (e.g. mother's oral contraceptives)
   Primary hypothyroidism
   Undefined mechanisms
      Birth asphyxia
      Mental retardation, including tuberous sclerosis
      Neurofibromatosis, McCune–Albright syndrome

Not associated with signs of puberty
Hyperthyroidism
Growth hormone excess (gigantism)

With obesity: currently excessive food intake

With dysmorphic features or disproportion
Marfan's syndrome
   Long, narrow limbs (dolichostenomelia)
   Arachnodactyly
   Scoliosis
   Aortic incompetence – dissecting aneurysm
   Myopia, retinal detachment, upward lens dislocation
   Autosomal dominant (often new mutation)

Homocystinuria
   Marfanoid body habitus
   Mental retardation
   Stiff joints with knock knee
   Downward lens subluxation
   Urine positive for homocystine
   Autosomal recessive

Congenital contractural arachnodactyly
   Kyphoscoliosis
   Joint contractures
   No ocular or CNS problems
   Autosomal dominant

Sotos' syndrome (cerebral gigantism)
   Large size at birth
   Hypertelorism, downslanting palpebral fissures, prominent forehead
   Large hands and feet
   Large male external genitalia
   Mental retardation ±, hypotonia, ataxia

Klinefelter's syndrome
   Disproportionately long legs
   Small firm testes
   Hypogonadism, infertility, with or without gynecomastia

Tallness and obesity

Tallness in childhood is commonly associated with food intake that is, or has been, excessive for growth and energy requirements. In wealthy societies, eating is a social as well as nutritional activity and moderate fatness in a baby may be seen as proof of mother love. Fat babies tend to be placid and little trouble. Once a child is overweight, calorie intake need not be excessive to maintain the situation. Continuing overeating causes rapid growth, skeletal maturational advance and early epiphyseal closure – adult height is not increased. If overeating stops but calorie reduction is insufficient to lose weight, growth velocity is normal but the child is tall and bone age remains advanced.

Rapid growth and precocious puberty

If nutrition has been normal, rapid growth is most commonly due to precocious puberty (see pp. 1027–1030). Final height may be significantly short (depending on etiology and duration) due to early epiphyseal closure.

Endocrine causes of rapid growth

These are either uncommon (thyrotoxicosis) or rare (gigantism, excess androgen secretion from an adrenal tumor).

OBESITY AND THINNESS

Malnutrition leading to obesity or thinness is discussed in Chapter 21. Discussion here is limited to some general comments and consideration of endocrine disorders which may be associated with each nutritional state.

Weight is a poor guide to nutrition – the interpretation of a high weight for a child's height as 'obesity' may be seriously misleading at times when growth and fatness are varying in opposite directions: a normal early pubertal boy is growing slowly but increasing body fat rapidly. Poor weight gain in a baby may be normal if the mother is tall and the father short as the maternal environment (in addition to genetic factors) is important in determining birthweight. In infancy weight gain largely reflects fluid flux; in the older child differences between normal and abnormal rates of weight gain are smaller than the reproducibility of weight measurements obtained some months apart even on sophisticated (and well-maintained and balanced) weighing scales.

The use of body mass index (BMI) – weight (kg)/height (m)^2 – provides a practical clinical tool for identification of adults with different degrees of obesity which carry particular adverse risks, for example hypertension, hypercholesterolemia and type 2 diabetes. However, use of a stable height as a basis for calculation, which is inapplicable to growing children, has limited its usefulness in pediatric practice. It can also underestimate the percentage of lean body mass by taking no account of variations in muscularity (Alemzadeh & Lifshitz 1996). At the least, age-related curves are necessary – UK pediatric standards have now been made available (Cole et al 1995) and show that BMI changes substantially in children, rising steeply in infancy, falling during preschool years and rising again into adulthood.

In normal and underweight individuals, between one-quarter and one-half of total body fat is subcutaneous – most excess fat in the obese is deposited there. Thus the adequacy, inadequacy or overadequacy of nutrition is best assessed from skinfold measurements using calipers (see Fig. 19.6) (Tanner & Whitehouse 1955) comparing results with available standards for age. Measurement of limb circumference assesses muscle and bone as well as fat. Measurements of triceps and subscapular skinfolds are representative of total body fat (Parizkova & Roth 1972) and show least between-observer error.

Care must be taken in interpretation: standards will depend on racial, maturational and genetic factors as well as age, and change as nutritional recommendations and feeding policies vary. British children were fatter in 1975 (Tanner & Whitehouse 1975) than 1962 (Tanner & Whitehouse 1962) but this trend may have been reversed more recently following Department of Health recommendations for infant feeding (DHSS 1974, 1980). Despite this, skinfold measurements provide quick, easy and reproducible estimates of nutritional state and are particularly useful in longitudinal assessment of an individual child.

OBESITY

Overeating is the commonest cause of childhood obesity. Energy intake surplus to requirements for growth, thermogenesis, basal metabolism and activity results in fat deposition (Fig. 19.17). It is likely that some, but not all, obese individuals eat, or have been eating, excessively. Nevertheless, observed variation between individuals in energy intake necessary to achieve normal fat deposition is likely to reflect genetic factors as well as differences in energy expenditure. Relative contributions of environmental and genetic factors remain poorly understood and certainly differ between different obese individuals.

It is no longer thought that there is a necessary progression from the fat infant to fat child with ultimate adult obesity and increased risk of hypertension, stroke, myocardial infarction or maturity-onset diabetes mellitus. The first year of life is not critical for determining adipocyte numbers which are related to the degree

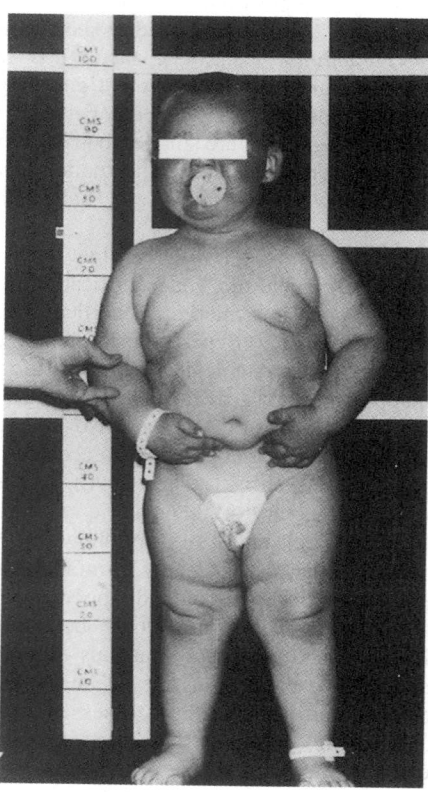

Fig. 19.17   Gross obesity in a toddler due to excessive food intake.

and duration of obesity rather than age at onset. Fat infants are two to three times likelier to become obese children than their normal peers but 80% will be of normal weight by primary school (Poskitt & Cole 1977).

Mild obesity seems unlikely to be associated with short- or long-term ill-health – the association with respiratory infection in infancy may not be very significant and social class factors may be linked. Advice about appropriate dieting should be given and will be successful only if child and whole family are motivated.

Height measurement is an important screening test. Overeating causes an increase in growth velocity and these children are generally tall for age with bone age advance. There is early epiphyseal closure and usually no final height increase. Some adolescent boys, in particular, may present with obesity, below average height and delayed puberty. Acceleration of height velocity is seen with rapid weight gain and strict dieting is associated with slowing of linear growth. Thus if overeating stops but there is insufficient reduction in calorie intake to lose weight, growth velocity may be normal but the child is tall and bone age remains advanced.

In contrast, virtually all endocrine and hypothalamic causes of obesity are associated with poor linear growth, short stature and bone age delay. Endocrine causes include excessive corticosteroid administration, GH insufficiency, hypopituitarism, hyper- or hypogonadotropic hypogonadism, hypothyroidism, pseudohypoparathyroidism and craniopharyngioma. Cushing's syndrome may initially cause rapid growth. Obesity also occurs with hyperinsulinism.

Hypothalamic damage from tumors, meningitis, encephalitis, radiotherapy or trauma may cause obesity. Possible mechanisms underlying the obesity include endocrine factors (hyperinsulinism – but this could be cause or effect, hyperprolactinemia, GH deficiency – but suppressed GH secretion may also be due to obesity) and nutritional and psychological factors (Didi et al 1995).

Hypothalamic syndromes associated with mental retardation and obesity include Laurence–Moon–Biedl and Prader–Willi. Craniopharyngioma may be associated with obesity after surgery or radiotherapy even if vision and activity are normal, food intake is appropriate and endocrine replacement therapy optimal. It seems likely that 'Fröhlich's syndrome' (one case of blindness, short stature, obesity and pubertal failure with a cyst in the region of the sella turcica) was due to craniopharyngioma.

The obesity of Down and other mental handicap syndromes may relate both to underlying genetic or metabolic abnormalities and physical inactivity – the latter is a major cause of obesity in physically handicapped children (e.g. spina bifida, muscular dystrophy).

Diagnosis of Prader–Willi syndrome (PWS – Prader et al 1956, Donaldson et al 1994a) is based on the characteristic history and clinical features (see Ch. 3). Diagnosis may often be made at birth from the association of characteristic facial features with history of poor fetal movements, hypotonia and poor feeding. Abnormalities of chromosome 15 were found in some (Leadbetter et al 1981) and molecular genetic techniques can now make the diagnosis more certain. Genomic imprinting (differential expression of genetic material depending on whether it originates from father or mother) occurs in the majority: if the 15q deletion (15q11q13) is paternally inherited, PWS results; when it is maternal, Angelman syndrome. 20–25% of PWS have normal chromosomes due to maternal uniparental 15 disomy (Webb 1994).

Endocrine features include hypogonadism (micropenis, hypoplastic scrotum and bilateral cryptorchidism in males), normal or increased GT secretion, poor secondary sexual development and delayed menarche, insulin resistance and diabetes mellitus, and growth failure. Energy requirements are abnormally low and appetite insatiable. Growth may be particularly poor when appetite is most successfully controlled and during adolescence. Scoliosis may impair spinal growth and, with gross obesity, predisposes to respiratory failure and death. GH therapy may have a place in stimulating growth in the older child and adolescent who is following a diet successfully.

'Simple' obesity (due to large appetite and excessive food intake) is associated with a number of minor (secondary) endocrine abnormalities. Increased adrenal androgen secretion for chronological (but not for bone) age could be a factor influencing the early onset of puberty in such children but increased GC metabolite excretion may reflect increased liver cortisol metabolism. There is frequently hyperinsulinemia, more marked in girls, older children and long-standing obesity, and unrelated to adipocyte size. It is thought to be related to both insulin resistance (with a fall in the concentration of adipocyte insulin receptors) and excessive CHO intake leading to a vicious cycle. A low calorie diet results in a rapid fall in insulin levels (before there are changes in weight, body fat mass or adipocyte size) with a rapid rise once dieting ceases, again preceding these other changes (Brook & Lloyd 1973). The risk of developing overt diabetes mellitus increases with age and the degree of obesity but is an uncommon complication.

THINNESS

Skinfold measurements, not weight, are best guides to thinness and undernutrition. A healthy child who is offered appetizing food in adequate amounts and variety in an emotionally supportive environment will eat enough to enable him to grow normally. This may be much less than mother (or granny) feels should be eaten. A thin child who is growing normally and not getting thinner should not be investigated or treated; one who is growing slowly or getting thinner needs investigation, diagnosis and treatment.

Recognizable syndromes (e.g. lipodystrophy, Marfan's syndrome) and malignancies are rare, but unrecognized organic disease (e.g. asthma, malabsorption due to celiac disease, ulcerative colitis or Crohn's disease), which may present with few overt signs, commonly causes poor growth and thinness. Calories may be too few (worldwide the most important cause of poor growth and thinness) but some children are on inadequate diets for ethnic or cultural reasons and some mothers are so concerned to prevent obesity that calorie intake is deficient. In the UK, emotional problems are common causes of thinness and poor growth. Anorexia nervosa may be life threatening in an adolescent. Nutrition and growth is reviewed by Ketelslegers (1997).

Acute malnutrition causes loss of fat and muscle; chronic malnutrition causes stunting but thinness may be masked by fat deposition (Cutting et al 1987, Raghupathy & Cutting 1997). Secondary endocrine responses to malnutrition result from the need to conserve the limited energy intake available. Cortisol, TSH, T3, GT and IGF1 levels are low.

IGF1 is controlled to a major extent by nutrition. In kwashiorkor and marasmus growth slows because of end-organ unresponsiveness to the action of GH – GH levels are high (Pimstone et al 1968) and IGF1 levels low.

Acute fasting in the human is associated with a reduction in GH receptor numbers and a low protein diet in the rat has the same effect. Receptor loss can be prevented with GH infusion suggesting that resistance is at the postreceptor level (Ketelslegers 1995). Amino acid deprivation has a direct effect on IGF1 gene expression. Protein restriction in very young rats leads to longer-term resistance to the growth-promoting effects of exogenous IGF1. Zinc deficiency in children is associated with reduced IGF1 levels (Ketelslegers 1995).

Anorexia nervosa patients (p. 1757) have normal cortisol production but decreased clearance rates due to low liver 11βOHSD activity. 5α-reductase levels are also reduced – this enzyme is also present in the liver. With gas liquid chromatography of urine, rises to normal in 5α androgen and GC metabolites are seen during recovery from cachexia in anorexia nervosa (Kelnar 1985). The secretory pattern of LH is immature and pubertal development either does not begin, halts (and may regress) or there is amenorrhea, depending on age at onset of anorexia and its degree. GH responses to stimulation are blunted. Estrogen deficiency is likely to reduce GH pulsatile release – induction of puberty with low dose gonadotropin releasing hormone (GnRH) causes marked changes in GH pulsatility (Stanhope et al 1985b) – and this may be an additional mechanism by which growth slows. Multicystic ovaries (a normal phase in ovarian maturation, see below) are seen during recovery (Treasure et al 1985). Vomiting, hypotension and cachexia may suggest Addison's disease but are generally much more severe in anorexia nervosa (although the vomiting may be concealed) – hirsutism may also occur in both.

The battle to get a healthy child to eat more than necessary is one parents are likely to lose and can produce emotional problems in both child and parents then or later. Reassurance that a thin child is healthy and growing normally will often, in itself, defuse an emotionally strained family situation. In other circumstances, treatment of the underlying cause of the thinness is necessary but may be easier with organic than emotional disorders.

ENDOCRINOLOGICAL ASPECTS OF PUBERTY AND ADOLESCENCE

THE GONADS

Ovaries and testes have two main functions: development and maintenance of secondary sexual characteristics and reproductive capability. Sex steroidogenic pathways in adrenals and gonads are identical – relative differences in types and quantities of individual androgens and estrogens reflect different enzymic activities.

PHYSIOLOGY

The ovary

Endocrine functions reside in ovarian follicles. Luteinizing hormone (LH) binds to theca cells to stimulate androstenedione and testosterone biosynthesis from cholesterol. These diffuse into granulosa cells which convert them to estrone (E1) and estradiol (E2) respectively (aromatization) under the influence of follicle-stimulating hormone (FSH). E1 and E2 interconversion also takes place in the granulosa cells. E1 is largely albumin bound; E2 is also bound to a specific globulin which also binds testosterone.

Estrogens stimulate secondary sex character development and, in the sexually mature, estrogens and progestogens ensure fertility by releasing ova and regulating the menstrual cycle. Estrogens are responsible for growth of vagina, uterus and fallopian tubes, and have a major role in the normal pubertal growth spurt and fusion of epiphyses at the end of puberty. They are metabolized in liver and excreted in urine.

The mechanism by which the dominant follicle suppresses others in both ovaries is unclear. Inhibin (McLachlan et al 1987, Ling et al 1986, Vale et al 1986) is found in follicular fluid, is thought to be secreted by granulosa cells and may have local effects as well as affecting feedback inhibition of FSH.

The testis

Both LH and FSH are required for spermatogenesis. FSH is necessary for initial establishment of mature germinal epithelium and initiation of spermatogenesis. LH effects are mediated through testosterone secretion by Leydig cells. Duration of spermatogenesis is approximately 74 days. Thus testosterone has both endocrine (secondary sexual characteristics and libido development) and paracrine effects (a permissive effect on spermatogenesis in the presence of FSH).

2% of testosterone in the mature male is in free active form, one-third is bound to a specific β-globulin – sex hormone-binding globulin (SHBG) and the remainder to albumin. In the target organs which require dihydrotestosterone (DHT) (scrotum, phallus, prostate), testosterone is converted to DHT by 5α reductase; in other tissues (e.g. bone, muscle, internal genitalia) testosterone acts directly.

Testosterone exerts negative feedback on LH secretion mainly at hypothalamic level but has little effect on FSH. However, FSH levels are high in the castrate. There is also a family of gonadal peptides which have inhibitory ('inhibin') (De Jong 1988, Ying 1988) and stimulatory ('activin') feedback effects at pituitary level and important gonadal (paracrine) effects. Modulation of FSH secretion at pituitary level is by mechanisms distinct from the GnRH receptor on the pituitary gonadotroph (Vale et al 1986). Inhibins are now known to be secreted in a variety of forms from the testis (Sertoli cells), placenta and ovary (granulosa cells).

The inhibins (A and B) are heterodimeric glycoproteins, consisting of two dissimilar subunits (Ling et al 1986), α and either βA (inhibin-A) or βB (inhibin-B), defined on the basis of the property of GT secretion, preferentially FSH, suppression (Burger & Igarashi 1988) and are similar to other glycoproteins such as TGFβ, erythroid differentiation factor and MIH. Activin consists of two inhibin β subunits.

Recent development of assays with sufficient sensitivity and specificity to distinguish different inhibin forms has led to important physiological insights. In women there is a characteristic pattern of changes in inhibin concentration during the menstrual cycle – inhibin-B is predominant during the follicular phase, inhibin-A during the luteal phase and early pregnancy (Groome et al 1994, Groome et al 1996, Illingworth et al 1996b). In men, there is no inhibin-A but inhibin-B concentrations reflect Sertoli cell function with an inverse relationship between FSH and inhibin-B suggesting a critical role for inhibin-B in regulation of FSH secretion (Illingworth et al 1996a). In both men and women, there are higher concentrations of the inactive inhibin precursor pro-αC than of the active dimer inhibin forms (Groome et al 1995). The inhibins may be important in normal puberty (see below).

Adrenals produce quantitatively more androgens than the testes and these are of importance in childhood in physiological and pathological situations (see pp. 1059–1061). In puberty and subsequently, the role of the testes is qualitatively paramount because testosterone is much more potent than androstenedione or dehydroepiandrosterone (DHA) – testicular failure causes hypogonadism despite normal adrenal function. Small quantities of estrogen are produced by normal testes by Sertoli cell aromatization of androgen. Testosterone is also metabolized to estrogen in some peripheral tissues (notably adipose cells) and the liver prior to urinary excretion.

ENDOCRINE BACKGROUND TO NORMAL PUBERTY

Physical changes of puberty are discussed elsewhere (see also Stirling & Kelnar 1992). Individual secondary sexual characteristics result from different hormonal events and must be assessed independently. Over the last century, children have tended to become taller and reach physical and sexual maturity earlier (Floud et al 1990). Although puberty timing and duration are very variable between individuals in the normal population, pubertal development is an harmonious process: marked discrepancies from the normal sequence of events (loss of 'consonance' – Bridges & Brook 1995) should lead to suspicion of pathology. In contrast, adolescence is sometimes far from harmonious – social pressures may be particularly marked in many who are sexually mature but still growing emotionally and intellectually (Hobsbawm 1994), and emotional problems may be seen in those whose timing of puberty is at either end of the normal spectrum.

CHANGES IN FETUS, INFANT AND CHILD AND THEIR RELEVANCE TO THE INITIATION OF PUBERTY

Fetal gonadotropin (GT) production occurs from the fifth week, rising until 20 weeks. Levels are higher in females perhaps because of feedback inhibition by fetal testosterone in males. Placental human chorionic gonadotropin (HCG) is secreted from implantation onwards and is the major stimulus for fetal Leydig cell testosterone and it seems unlikely that the fetal hypothalamopituitary–gonadal axis is fully functional by postpubertal standards. After delivery, a rise in GT levels persists for several months in both sexes. Total testosterone levels are high in males partly due to high SHBG levels (Forest et al 1973). During the first year, the axis becomes quiescent. There is little evidence for the existence of specific inhibitory hormones (see pineal gland, p. 1043) although CNS inhibitory influences could be important – precocious puberty is common following cranial irradiation for acute lymphoblastic leukemia (ALL).

Pulsatile GnRH secretion is of paramount importance in primate sexual maturation (Knobil 1980) but puberty initiation does not result from sudden hypothalamic GnRH activation – there is increasing biochemical and ultrasound evidence for activity well before the onset of clinical gonadarche. During childhood, there is gradual amplification of GnRH signals with pulses of low frequency and amplitude (Wu et al 1991) in the young child. From well before the clinical onset of puberty, around adrenarche, nocturnal pulsatile GnRH secretion is detectable with increasing pulse frequency (Wu et al 1989, 1990a) associated with multicystic prepubertal ovaries on ultrasound (Fig. 19.18). This normal stage of development (characterized by the presence of > 6 follicles of diameter > 4 mm) is associated with activation of the axis resulting in nocturnal pulsatile GnRH secretion (Boyar et al 1972) without (as yet) estrogen-mediated positive feedback (Stanhope et al 1985a).

Modulation of pituitary LH secretion resulting from increased GnRH pulse frequency is an important characteristic of transition between juvenile and peripubertal stages in man (Fig. 19.19) (Wu et al 1990a). Biochemical assessment in prepuberty has been helped by the development of sensitive LH radiometric assays (Butler et al 1987, 1988) although the bioactivity of what is measured is not beyond question. Using an ultrasensitive immunofluorometric assay (IFA), pulsatile LH and FSH fluctuations can be seen even in Kallmann's syndrome patients (Wu et al 1991, Brown et al 1996a, Wu et al 1996) but, in contrast to normal late prepubertal children, there is poor synchronization between LH and FSH pulses and absence of entrainment to sleep. A crucial condition for normal pubertal development may involve organization of neuronal circuits which not only maintain synchronized pulsatile GnRH release but enable their incorporation into the daily sleep–wake rhythm (Wu et al 1991, Wu et al 1996). It is likely that continuing pubertal transition to adult pituitary–gonadal function involves gradual further recruitment, organization and synchronization of GnRH neuronal discharge over an increasing proportion of the evening/night and resetting of gonadal negative feedback (Wu et al 1990b, 1991). Clinically, an early morning testosterone measurement is a useful predictor of the imminence of puberty (Wu et al 1993).

Recent data (Crofton et al 1997), using sensitive and specific assays to distinguish different inhibin forms, have shown that in normal boys testicular production of inhibin B increases as puberty progresses and that the initiation of puberty is accompanied by a dramatic switch from a positive to a negative relationship between inhibin B and FSH. Inhibin B may also be a more sensitive predictor than testosterone of clinical pubertal onset.

For normal ranges of ovarian and uterine size during childhood see Neu (1992). As puberty progresses, GnRH (and thus GT) pulse frequency remains at about 2 h (Jakacki et al 1982) but there is increasing amplitude and daytime as well as nocturnal pulses (Fig. 19.20). 24-h pulsatile release is necessary for full pubertal

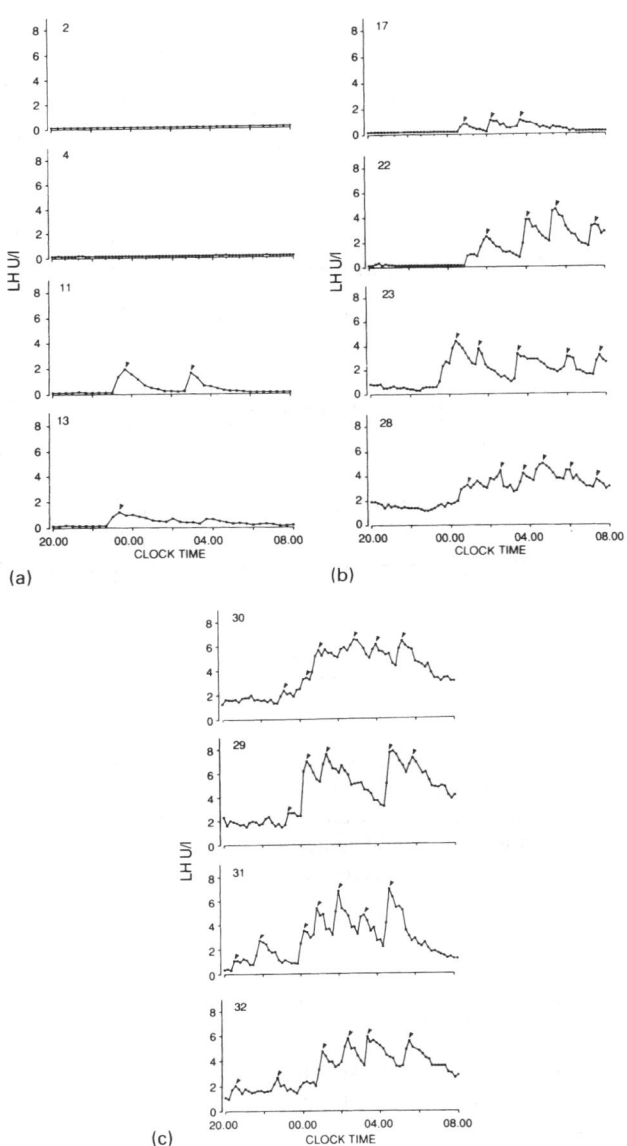

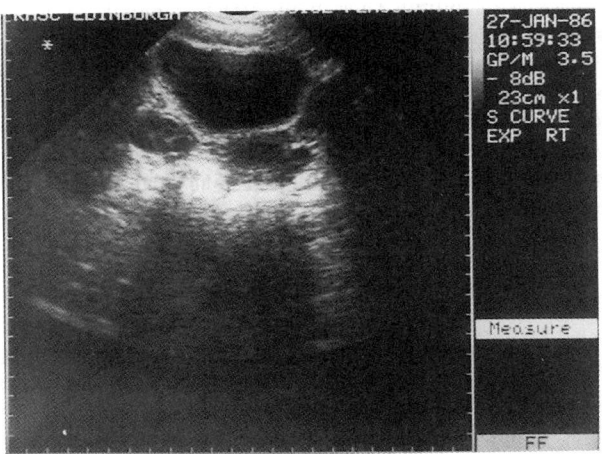

Fig. 19.18   The multicystic appearance of late prepubertal ovaries.

Fig. 19.19   Evolution of GT secretory profiles (1). Profiles of plasma LH between 20.00 and 08.00 h in (**a**) four young prepubertal subjects (G1 PH1 testicular volume ≤ 2 ml); arrowheads indicate a significant LH pulse; none of these patients progressed into puberty during the following 12 months; (**b**) four prepubertal subjects: two with G1 PH1 testicular volume ≤ 2 ml at time of study, but progression into puberty with testicular volume ≥ 4 ml within 12 months (subjects 15 and 19); two in earlier puberty at study (G1 PH1–2 testicular volume 3–4 ml); (**c**) four pubertal subjects (G2–3 PH1–3 testicular volume 6–10 ml). (From Wu et al 1990a.)

development, menarche and ovulation (Boyar et al 1972). In the follicular phase of the menstrual cycle, GnRH pulse frequency increases to approximately hourly and falls to 3-hourly in the luteal phase. Increasing sex steroid secretion resulting from increasing pulsatile GnRH secretion produces the physical changes of puberty and all pubertal events can be induced by pulsatile administration of exogenous GnRH (Brook et al 1987, Stanhope et al 1987a, Wu et al 1987) – even if this is a cumbersome way to do so in clinical practice.

Experiments in the rhesus monkey suggest the presence of an hypothalamic GnRH pulse generator but its site and nature are

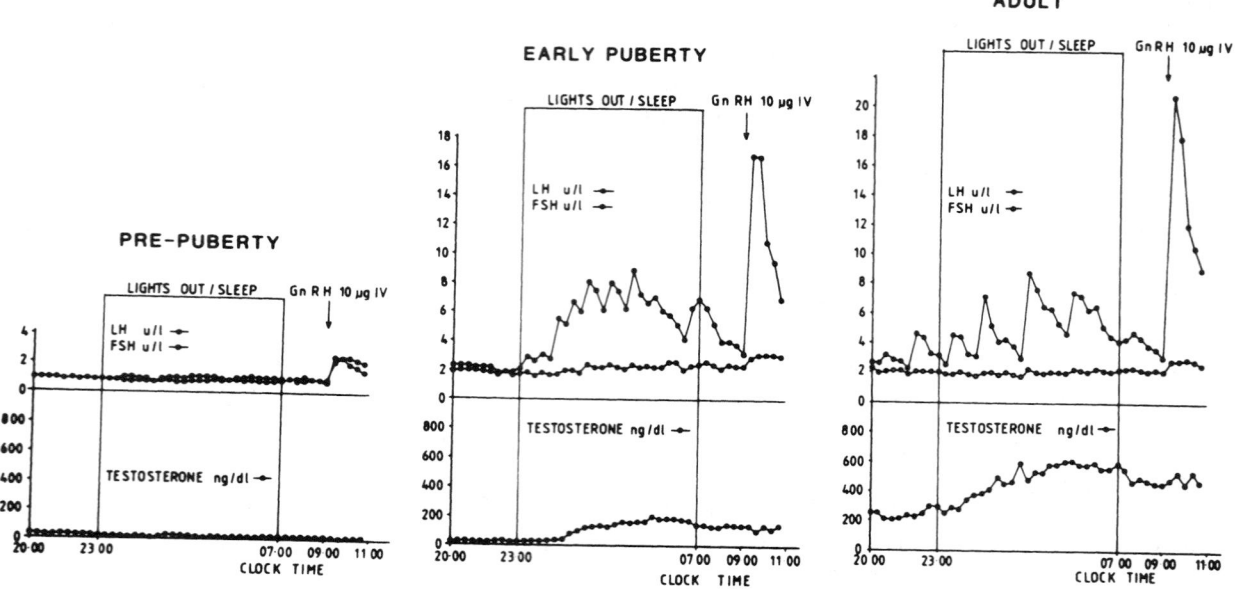

Fig. 19.20 Evolution of GT secretory profiles (2) and response to exogenous GnRH at different stages of pubertal development. (Data by courtesy of Dr F. C. W. Wu.)

unknown. A pulse of GnRH is associated with a burst of electrical activity and results in a pulse of LH secretion. There appears to be no other modulation of LH secretion but inhibins are important in FSH modulation and could underpin LH and FSH dissociation found in, for example, isolated premature thelarche.

ADRENARCHE AND GONADARCHE (see p. 1060)

CHANGES OF BODY COMPOSITION AND METABOLIC SIGNALS FOR ONSET OF PUBERTY

Although in pathological situations (e.g. anorexia nervosa, excessive exercise) nutritional factors are important for pubertal development and menarche, there is no evidence for the hypothesis (Frisch & Revelle 1970) that menarche depends on attainment of a critical weight for height. For a given bodyweight, the proportion of girls reaching menarche increases with age and the relative weight (weight as a percentage of standard weight) at 11 years explains less than 5% of variation in the age of menarche (Stark et al 1989). It is likely that in normally nourished populations genetic factors are of paramount importance for the timing of menarche – this is probably true of pubertal onset and events in general.

This does not mean that metabolic factors and signals are unimportant for pubertal development (Brown & Kelnar 1993, Brown et al 1996b,c). From rat, rhesus monkey and nonhuman primate experiments and circumstantial evidence in man, it is brain (rather than pituitary) maturation which is of primary importance for onset of puberty. Are there simply genetically determined biological clocks which, in the absence of pathological modulators, trigger puberty or could there be metabolic or other cues which signal into the CNS? In anorexia nervosa (p. 1757) or severe malnutrition (see p. 1191) there are low GT levels, menstruation ceases and puberty regresses as a way of conserving energy – the likely outcome of maintenance of

reproductive capacity in such circumstances would be disastrous for mother and fetus. Although anorexics who regain ~ 75% of ideal bodyweight resume menstrual cycling with normal pituitary responsiveness to GnRH (Warren et al 1975), leanness alone cannot account for the reproductive disturbances: sustained exercise (in female distance runners) affects GnRH pulse amplitude (Veldhuis et al 1985) and amenorrheic ballet dancers who stop training resume normal menstruation within a few months without detectable changes in bodyweight or composition suggesting that metabolic signals could be important in controlling reproductive function in these situations and, speculatively, in control of normal pubertal development.

There are pubertal increases in basal insulin levels in primates and man (Hindmarsh et al 1988, Dunger & Edge 1995) which may be secondary to changes in GH secretion, but insulin enhances basal and GnRH-stimulated GT release by pituitary cells in vitro and also affects brain neurotransmitter activity by regulating precursor availability. Thus both direct humoral stimuli and metabolic factors such as amino acids (AA) acting as neurotransmitter precursor substrates could influence the GnRH pulse generator. Combination CHO/AA infusions in monkeys produce dramatic increases in bioassayable plasma LH whereas CHO alone has no effect but much more work is needed before the role of metabolic factors in initiation of normal human puberty becomes clear.

ABNORMAL PUBERTY

As with other normally distributed characteristics (e.g. height or IQ) there is no absolute age at which pubertal timing becomes abnormal. Pubertal onset at an 'average' time does not necessarily exclude a pubertal disorder. The mean UK age of onset is such that 3% of boys or girls will have started puberty by 9 and 8 years and only 3% will have no pubertal signs by 13.8 and 13.4 years,

Table 19.8 A simplified classification of disorders of puberty (see text)

Precocious puberty
  Consonance:
    Idiopathic central precocious puberty
    Central precocious puberty due to, e.g.
      Intracranial tumors
      Cranial irradiation
      Raised intracranial pressure
  Gonadotropin-independent precocious puberty (GIPP, testotoxicosis)
  Loss of consonance (pseudopuberty)
    Isolated premature thelarche
    Thelarche variant
    Adrenal causes
      Premature pubarche
      Congenital adrenal hyperplasia
      Cushing's syndrome
      Adrenocortical tumors
    Gonadal causes
      Ovarian cysts
      Ovarian or testicular tumors
    Ingestion of sex steroid (accident or child abuse)
    Primary hypothyroidism
    McCune-Albright syndrome
    Extrapituitary tumors (e.g. hepatoblastoma)

Delayed puberty
  Consonance
    Constitutional delay of growth and puberty
    Chronic systemic disease
    Idiopathic hypogonadotropic hypogonadism
    Hypogonadotropic hypogonadism due to, e.g.
      Kallmann's syndrome
      Craniopharyngioma
      Cranial irradiation
    Panhypopituitarism
    Primary hypothyroidism
  Loss of consonance
    Turner's syndrome
    Ovarian agenesis with normal karyotype
    Polycystic ovaries
    Anorchia (primary or secondary to testicular irradiation)

respectively. A useful clinical rule is that puberty should be investigated if there is an abnormal sequence of pubertal changes (i.e. loss of 'consonance' – Bridges & Brook 1995), any abnormal sign or symptom of underlying pathology and if signs have or have not (respectively) appeared outwith the above age limits.

Children with precocious puberty may simply have early onset of normal (central) mechanisms (which may be idiopathic or secondary to underlying pathology) or may have an abnormal mechanism causing development (pseudopuberty) (Brown et al 1994). Children with no signs by 14 years may have delay in maturation (on a background of constitutional growth delay – see p. 1015) but may permanently lack ability to develop spontaneously. Investigations, potential outcomes and management are different in each situation and depend on not only presence or absence of underlying pathology but also emotional and psychological consequences. A clinical classification of disorders of puberty or its timing is given in Table 19.8.

PRECOCIOUS SEXUAL MATURATION

The concept of loss of consonance is particularly useful in the differential diagnosis of precocious puberty (Bridges et al 1994) but initiation of normal pubertal events can be due to underlying pathology and gonadotropin-independent precocious puberty (GIPP; an important cause of precocious puberty in boys) may be clinically identical to 'consonant' precocious puberty.

Pseudopuberty (loss of consonance)

Isolated premature thelarche

Breast development occurs in the absence of any other pubertal signs although vaginal bleeding may occur. Onset is usually in first year and uncommon after 2 years. There is usually cyclical waxing and waning of mild breast development (stage < B3) which may have persisted from postnatal breast enlargement (potentially in both sexes) due to maternal placental estrogen transfer. In contrast to true precocious puberty, pubic and axillary hair does not develop, growth velocity is normal for age and skeletal maturation is not advanced.

There is evidence for increased estrogen production, high basal and GnRH-stimulated FSH levels and pulsatile nocturnal GT, predominantly FSH, secretion (Stanhope et al 1986). Ultrasound may show several ovarian cysts whose size changes with breast size and moderate uterine enlargement.

A primary abnormality in GnRH pulse generation resulting predominantly in FSH secretion is unlikely as there is no response to GnRH analogues (see p. 1025). The activin/inhibin system (see p. 1025) may be important for pathogenesis – potentially exerting effects at both pituitary level, on FSH independently of the gonadotroph GnRH receptor (Vale et al 1986), and gonadal level by paracrine regulation.

There is waxing and waning of breast enlargement with gradual disappearance over months or years. Puberty generally takes place normally at appropriate age. Treatment consists of explanation and reassurance. Pelvic ultrasound and measurement of GTs basally and following a low dose (0.25 μg/kg i.v.) GnRH test may be helpful in doubtful cases. Occasionally, particularly in girls presenting after 2 years, there may be confusion with early true precocious puberty. An intermediate syndrome, 'thelarche variant', has been described (Bridges & Brook 1995) with GT independence and postulated ovarian lesion of folliculogenesis.

Adrenal causes

The normal rise in adrenal androgens in mid-childhood (adrenarche – see p. 1060) sometimes manifests with appearance of pubic (and less commonly axillary) hair – 'premature pubarche' – without breast development but with increased height velocity (Silverman et al 1952). Such children are particularly sensitive to adrenal androgens or at the upper end of a secretory spectrum. The timing of true pubertal onset is generally unaffected. In occasional children with true precocious puberty, pubic hair development may be the first sign. Other causes of adrenal androgen secretion must be considered in the differential diagnosis and excluded.

Congenital adrenal hyperplasia (CAH), specifically non-salt-losing 21-hydroxylase deficiency in boys, is the commonest cause of precocious pseudopuberty (see p. 1063). There is virilization in early childhood but testes classically remain prepubertal – adrenals are the androgen source. Occasionally ACTH-responsive adrenal rests will cause some testicular growth but significant enlargement signifies secondary central precocious puberty (Fig. 19.21) – a common consequence of GC therapy on the pre-existing advanced skeletal maturation. Mild or late-onset

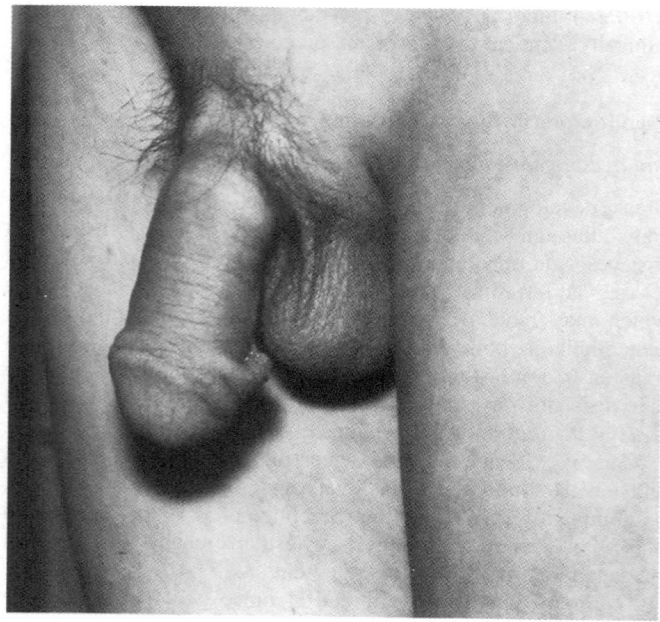

Fig. 19.21   True precocious puberty following glucocorticoid treatment of congenital adrenal hyperplasia. Note the testicular enlargement (same child as Fig. 19.40).

forms of 21-hydroxylase or 3β-hydroxysteroid dehydrogenase deficiencies may present with pubic hair growth in girls mimicking premature pubarche (Forest et al 1985, Temeck et al 1987).

Cushing's syndrome and adrenocortical tumors – see page 1069.

Gonadal causes

Testicular tumors are uncommon in children and (usually benign) Leydig cell androgen-secreting lesions are rare. Clinically, presentation may be with normal pubertal development but the affected testis is enlarged and the contralateral small and atrophic from suppression of the hypothalamopituitary–gonadal axis. Enlargement may be uniform or with a palpable nodule, causing confusion with enlargement due to ACTH-responsive adrenal rests in CAH. Rapid onset of true pubertal onset may follow surgical removal.

Ovarian tumors are also rare causes of precocious pseudopuberty, accounting for only around 1%. Least uncommon is the rare granulosa-theca cell tumor. Presentation is rarely before 4 years. Distinguishing features include early (in context of other pubertal signs) irregular vaginal bleeding or regular anovulatory cycles, marked areolar pigmentation and abdominal pain. A pelvic or abdominal mass is usually palpable. Although usually benign there are reports of significant mortality in children and adults.

Ovarian cysts are found in normal and precocious puberty. Multicystic appearances of late prepubertal and early pubertal ovaries are described above. Isolated follicular cysts may cause breast development, can be a feature of isolated premature thelarche and may regress spontaneously with conservative management (Brosnan 1985, Lyon et al 1985a, Stanhope & Brook 1985). Chronic estrogen secretion and large size may necessitate surgical removal. Polycystic ovaries may be common in puberty

and late prepuberty (Rao et al 1985) and can be associated with pubertal delay (Stanhope et al 1988d) – see page 1034.

Ingestion of sex steroid

Most commonly there is accidental ingestion of mother's contraceptive pills and estrogen will cause slight breast enlargement and, often, an estrogen withdrawal bleed. Contamination of animal feeds with estrogen has been implicated in isolated premature thelarche in Puerto Rico (Bongiovanni 1983).

Child abuse

Sex steroids may be administered deliberately and chronically as a form of child abuse (Munchausen syndrome by proxy – Meadow 1977, 1982). Sexual abuse (and pelvic neoplasia) must be excluded when vaginal bleeding is the presenting feature of precocious pseudopuberty. Factitious vaginal bleeding may be caused by presentation of mother's menstrual blood as though it came from the child. The laboratory can determine its origin.

Thyroid disease

Primary hypothyroidism may be associated both with delayed and precocious (Kendle 1905) puberty. Unusually (in the context of precocity) growth velocity will not have been rapid, stature may be short and bone age is characteristically delayed. It is usually seen in girls (in whom autoimmune hypothyroidism is commoner). Breast development is the main feature (sometimes with galactorrhea) but there is usually little (androgen dependent) pubic or axillary hair development. In boys (Laron et al 1970), enlarged testes consist of seminiferous tubules without Leydig cells, consistent with the postulated mechanisms (p. 1050). Pulsatile FSH release is common in primary hypothyroidism (Buchanan et al 1988) but only results in precocious pseudopuberty in a few. Follicular cysts are seen on ovarian ultrasound in association with FSH predominance and suppressed GH pulsatility during overnight sampling (Pringle et al 1988). The latter may contribute to slower height velocity.

The child may be clinically euthyroid at presentation in puberty with normally maintained TSH and thyroid hormone levels. The pituitary fossa may be enlarged (Fig. 19.22) (Van Wyk & Grumbach 1960) due to pituitary hyperplasia (Floyd et al 1984) – the pituitary gland shrinks rapidly on thyroxine therapy. Ultimately, secondary pituitary failure may result, with an empty but still enlarged fossa on CT or MRI scan. Menarche may occur early while growth is still accelerating (cf. normal puberty and central precocious puberty). Treatment is with thyroxine.

McCune–Albright syndrome

There is an association of hyperpigmented macules, precocious sexual development and thinning and sclerosis of bone with fractures in young children without systemic disease (McCune & Bruch 1937, Albright et al 1937b, Albright 1947b). The syndrome comprises macular brown skin hyperpigmentation with characteristic ragged edges, areas of rarefaction, commonly in long bones and elsewhere (polyostotic fibrous dysplasia – Fig. 19.23) and multiple endocrinopathies with glandular hyper-

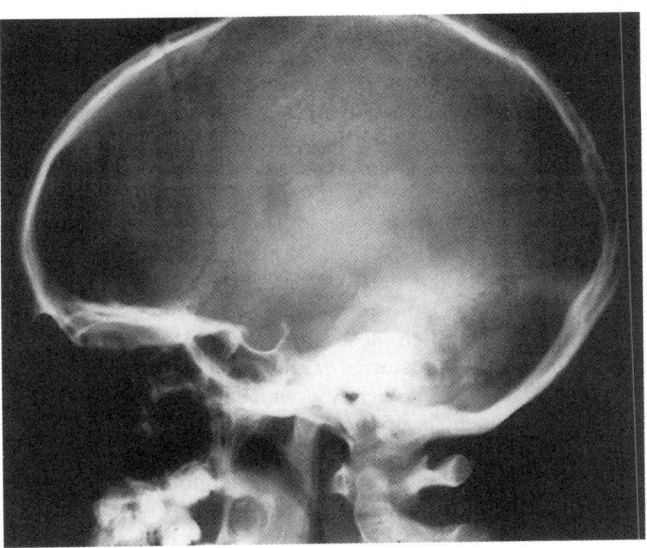

Fig. 19.22   Enlarged pituitary fossa due to pituitary (thyrotroph) hyperplasia in a child with primary hypothyroidism presenting with precocious puberty.

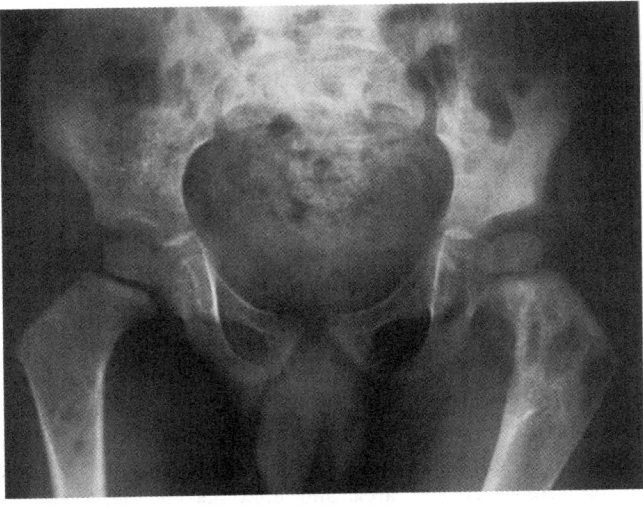

Fig. 19.23   Polyostotic fibrous dysplasia of bone in the McCune–Albright syndrome.

function (thyrotoxicosis with goiter, GH hypersecretion, Cushing's syndrome, hyperprolactinemia, hyperparathyroidism, precocious puberty and hyperphosphaturic rickets).

Endocrine hyperfunction is autonomous and not secondary to central tropic hormone stimulation. There are analogies with endocrinopathies in multiple endocrine neoplasia syndromes. They are due to an activating missense mutation in the gene encoding the Gsα subunit of the G protein that stimulates cyclic AMP formation (Mauras & Blizzard 1986, Shenker et al 1993a) (see p. 997). The mutation is variably expressed in different tissues consistent with a mosaic distribution of aberrant cells from a somatic cell mutation (Shenker et al 1993a).

Precocious puberty is the usual presentation, sometimes with early vaginal bleeding (cf. central precocious puberty). Bone lesions may not develop for many years and the skin pigmentation is inconstant. In girls, ovaries may be asymmetrically enlarged

(Foster et al 1986) by isolated follicular cysts. The GT response to exogenous GnRH is 'prepubertal' with absent GT pulsatility. As would be expected, suppression of puberty with GnRH agonists is ineffective. Cyproterone acetate or medroxyprogesterone are drugs of choice.

Extrapituitary tumors

These may cause precocious puberty as a result of the ectopic secretion of GT-like substances. Least uncommon are hepatoblastomas in boy and ovarian chorionepitheliomas and teratomas in girls; extrapituitary intracranial malignant teratoma and pineal choriocarcinoma have been reported. In boys testicular enlargement is rapid and vaginal bleeding often occurs early in girls.

Central precocious puberty

Normal activation of the hypothalamopituitary–gonadal axis may occur abnormally early secondary to an underlying disorder or idiopathically (Brown et al 1994). The pattern of secondary sexual characteristic development and endocrine findings are as in puberty developing at a more average time ('consonance') except that growth acceleration may occur relatively early in boys. This, plus more rapid epiphyseal maturation in boys in early puberty, may compromise final height more than expected in boys even with early presentation. In general early age at onset and short parents imply worse height prognosis but accurate individual prediction is difficult – predictive equations are most accurate for children of 'average' height developing normally at an 'average' time.

Mechanisms initiating normal pubertal development are still not clearly understood, perturbations in timing even less so. Central precocious puberty presents much more frequently in girls (female : male ratio of about 10 : 1) and in the majority (> 80%) of girls no sinister underlying cause is found. With high resolution neuroradiological scanning, hypothalamopituitary hamartomas have been reported (Cacciari et al 1983) but their incidence in the normal population at equivalent age is unclear. In boys, however, there is a high incidence of intracranial pathology, especially tumors such as teratomas, astrocytomas or gliomas causing pineal destruction (Kitay 1954) – neuroradiological investigation is necessary even without abnormal signs. The sex difference in incidence of idiopathic precocious puberty may relate to lower GT release thresholds to endogenous pulsatile GnRH in girls. GIPP (see below) may account for precocious puberty in a significant number of boys in whom normal central mechanisms had previously been implicated.

In girls, investigation is necessary to confirm the mechanism and to exclude an underlying cause. Ovarian ultrasound, which will show characteristic multicystic appearances (p. 1034), and a low dose (0.25 µg/kg i.v.) GnRH test (more practical than overnight GT profiling) will confirm central precocious puberty and exclude primary ovarian pathology. Neuroradiological investigation may be necessary (mandatory in boys). In addition to tumors, important central pathologies include CNS infection, raised intracranial pressure, trauma (during birth or childhood head injury) and previous cranial irradiation (Brauner & Rappaport 1985, Leiper et al 1987, Crowne et al 1992, Wallace 1996).

Silver–Russell syndrome (see p. 1015) (Russell 1954, Silver et al 1953)

Abnormalities of sexual development, including precocious puberty, can be associated with this prolonged IUGR syndrome (Silver 1964). Elevated urinary and serum GTs have been reported but the etiology is unclear.

Gonadotropin-independent precocious puberty (GIPP, testotoxicosis) (Rosenthal et al 1983)

Incidence, importance and classification are still controversial (Lee 1996) – characteristically there are normal somatic consequences (consonance) from abnormal mechanisms (pseudopuberty). Diagnostic criteria (Wierman et al 1985) are absent GT spontaneous pulsatility on bioassay and by RIA, poor but variable GT response to GnRH, no clinical response to GnRH analogue therapy and cyclical steroidogenesis. In reported studies there is a strong family history of precocious puberty but the etiology is unknown. Nearly all cases have been boys – girls may have the McCune–Albright syndrome (p. 1028). Maturation of testicular steroidogenesis and spermatogenesis is normal but GnRH/GT independent. An LH receptor mutation resulting in increased cAMP and autonomous Leydig cell activity has been found in some (Shenker et al 1993b). Treatment with medroxyprogesterone or ketoconazole (Holland et al 1985a,b) has been reported but in view of the latter's toxicity it cannot be generally recommended.

Investigation and diagnosis

In summary it is reasonable to investigate any girl < 8 and boy < 9 years with secondary sexual characteristics. Where a girl's development is harmonious and proceeds at a normal tempo (consonance) and clinical examination is normal, invasive investigation to exclude pathology is unnecessary, but basal TSH, estradiol and PRL measurement with skull X-ray, low dose GnRH test and pelvic ultrasound will give valuable information about mechanism and underlying pathology. Overnight profiling of GT secretion is essentially a research tool (Brown et al 1996a). If no underlying cause is found which itself requires treatment, the need to suppress GT secretion and further development is considered (see below). Adrenal or intracranial pathology must be actively sought in boys by steroid profiling and neuroradiological (CT or MRI) investigation. GIPP must be considered in boys, particularly if there is a family history of precocious puberty, as there is no response to GnRH analogue therapy.

Clinical consequences and management

Management of precocious pseudopuberty is of the underlying cause. In central precocious puberty, an underlying cause requires treatment and pubertal suppression may be necessary also. In idiopathic cases, suppression may be indicated on social and psychological (rather than medical) grounds (see below).

Treatment of central precocious puberty has traditionally been with progestogen-like drugs such as cyproterone acetate and medroxyprogesterone. Cyproterone has been widely used in the UK for many years and is generally effective and free from significant side effects in a dose of 75–100 mg/m^2/day given twice

daily. It has progestational, antiandrogenic, antigonadotropic and adrenal suppressive activities – the precise mechanism by which GT secretion is suppressed is unclear. It may predominantly directly inhibit ovarian steroidogenesis (Stanhope et al 1985a). Treatment is continued until such time as further pubertal progression is more appropriate – its actions reverse when treatment ceases.

Problems with cyproterone relate to adrenal suppression (Girard & Baumann 1975). Treated children must carry a steroid 'card' or talisman and need steroid cover during major stress, illness or surgery. Cortisol deficiency in other situations is uncommon unless high doses are used. Adults treated with cyproterone (for prostatic carcinoma) have altered lipid metabolism (Paisey et al 1986) which may be of concern if childhood treatment is prolonged. Taking the natural history of central precocious puberty into account, there is no evidence for improvement in height prognosis (Stanhope et al 1987b). Although cyproterone is still widely used, it has been replaced as treatment of choice by GnRH analogues (see below). It remains important for treatment of GIPP and is used by some to cover the initial (stimulatory) phase of GnRH analogue therapy (see below).

GnRH analogues are specific and effective in suppressing central precocious puberty (Crowley et al 1981). Although licensed in the UK for management of adults with prostatic carcinoma, the D-serine-6 analogue has been widely used in precocious puberty given intranasally (UK Collaborative Group 1988) although it is also effective subcutaneously. The D-tryptophan-6 analogue is effective given once monthly subcutaneously as a depot preparation (Roger et al 1984).

Although they act by desensitizing the pituitary to GnRH and inhibiting pulsatile GnRH secretion, analogues have an initial stimulatory effect (lasting several weeks) on sex steroid secretion. This is of most practical relevance in a girl sufficiently advanced for a menstrual bleed to occur. In this situation, particularly, additional treatment with cyproterone for the first 4 weeks of analogue therapy is appropriate. Height velocity may initially increase further due to the effect of sex steroids on spinal growth (Stanhope et al 1988c).

Effectiveness of therapy is best assessed by serial pelvic ultrasound in girls (assessing ovarian morphology and volume, uterine cross-sectional area and endometrial thickness), by clinical assessment of testicular volume in boys, plasma estradiol and testosterone measurements (respectively) and (if necessary) GT responsiveness to GnRH (0.25 μg/kg i.v.). There is no effect on the adrenal axis (cf. cyproterone) but (as with cyproterone) probably no effect on improving height prognosis. Slowing of epiphyseal maturation on treatment is mirrored by a slowing of height velocity (perhaps due to reduced GH pulsatile secretion secondary to sex steroid suppression – Stanhope et al 1988c). It is on this theoretical background that specific growth stimulation using GH therapy is being assessed. The effects of gonadal disorders on growth are reviewed by Ritzén (1997) and the treatment of growth problems associated with precocious puberty by DiMartino-Nardi (1997).

Ketoconazole (Sonino 1987), an antifungal agent and specific inhibitor of cytochrome P450-dependent enzymes and thus adrenal/gonadal steroidogenesis, has been used in precocious puberty (including GIPP – see above). Toxic side effects preclude its general use.

Whatever the therapy, secondary sexual development will seldom diminish significantly and families must be warned not to expect dramatic cosmetic improvement. GnRH analogues may allow further long-term progression of pubic and axillary hair. There is evidence in girls for reversibility of inhibition (Ward et al 1986) and for recovery of hypothalamopituitary–gonadal function and ovarian activity occurring from the pretreatment stage of puberty (Stirling et al 1989a,b). There is little experience of long-term outcomes of GnRH analogue therapy in boys – observed effects on inhibition of seminiferous tubule activity could impair subsequent fertility if irreversible.

Emotional problems are often considerable in these children who are already tall for age. They appear clumsy and, in association with precocious puberty, may be more aggressive with undesirable social consequences. They feel different because of both size and precocious development and are often ill-equipped to cope with psychological aspects of adolescence, particularly if parents and teachers are uncomprehending or embarrassed. Ultimate short stature, which may be severe, may be particularly emotionally disabling against this background.

The decision to treat idiopathic central precocious puberty depends on age at onset, rate of progression, level of emotional support provided by parents and other social and psychological factors. Menarche in primary school can cause additional psychological problems. In every case emotional support must be given.

DELAYED SEXUAL MATURATION

Late puberty, particularly when accompanied by short stature and delayed skeletal maturation, is the commonest reason for referral to a pediatric endocrinologist. This 'constitutional delay of growth and puberty' (CDGP) is seen more commonly in boys who are also more stressed by it as growth deceleration continues until puberty is well advanced. Pathological causes of late puberty are much commoner in girls (e.g. Turner's syndrome) – central causes are equally common in both sexes. A karyotype is an important early investigation in any slowly growing girl and mandatory if puberty is delayed even without any syndromic 'stigmata'. Virtually any chronic systemic disease may be associated with both growth retardation and pubertal delay (Preece et al 1986) (see below).

Constitutional delay of growth and puberty (CDGP)

This is the likely diagnosis in a healthy adolescent short for the family but not for pubertal stage and skeletal maturation, giving a normal height prognosis. There is often a family history of CDGP in parents or siblings but its presence does not make the diagnosis and absence does not exclude it. CDGP is commoner and often more stressful in boys. Emotional, psychological and social consequences may be severe despite absence of underlying pathology. Aspects of treatment which require consideration are puberty induction, growth stimulation and emotional support. Individual treatment modalities interact with each other in terms of their psychological and physical effects.

Chronic systemic disease

Chronic systemic disease may cause slowing of growth which may or may not be reversible and is often associated with subsequent maturational delay or pubertal failure. Anorexia nervosa results in secondary endocrine disturbances (see p. 1757)

whilst pubertal delay causes secondary psychological disturbances. A sympathetic child psychiatrist is helpful in providing evidence for underlying emotional disturbance and managing primary or secondary emotional problems.

Causes of growth and maturational delay or failure in these conditions may be explicable in nutritional, secondary hormonal, metabolic or therapeutic (e.g. glucocorticoid treatment) terms. However, in many conditions the etiology is both multifactorial and poorly understood (Preece et al 1986).

Malnutrition and weight loss

Undernutrition is the commonest worldwide cause of growth failure and pubertal delay and may occur in 'developed' countries, for example with inappropriate 'faddish' diets or emotional deprivation. Whatever the specific relevance of metabolic signals for the onset of puberty, it is likely that growth retardation and pubertal delay or failure are a secondary adaptation to the need to conserve energy and to prevent reproduction in suboptimal circumstances (see p. 1191).

Exercise

Intensive training sometimes leads to delayed sexual maturation.

Hypothalamopituitary disorders

Hypogonadotropic hypogonadism may cause pubertal delay, arrest or infertility depending on age at onset and severity. The cause is usually a hypothalamic disturbance in GnRH pulsatile release. Primary GT deficiency is usually associated with pituitary tumors (e.g. craniopharyngioma) and other pituitary hormone deficiencies. Cranial irradiation is associated with (hypothalamic) GT deficiency. Prolactinomas are rarely associated with delayed puberty – moderately elevated PRL levels are due to stress.

In contrast to CDGP, a child with hypogonadotropic hypogonadism is generally normal or tall for the family and bone age is arrested at around 13 'years' in the older child. A family history of delay with hypogonadism (cryptorchidism or micropenis) and anosmia suggests *Kallmann's syndrome* – inherited as an autosomal dominant with relative male limitation. Features may include color blindness, other midline craniofacial abnormalities, nerve deafness, mental retardation and renal anomalies. Differentiation from CDGP (Wu et al 1991, Brown et al 1996a) is generally possible at presentation.

Mental retardation syndromes associated with GT deficiency and obesity include Laurence–Moon–Biedl (with polydactyly and retinitis pigmentosa) and Prader–Willi (p. 60).

Hypothyroidism

Acquired hypothyroidism is often associated with pubertal delay but may cause precocious puberty (see p. 1050).

Gonadal

Disorders of ovarian function

These may relate to defective estrogen secretion or action (hypogonadism), androgen overproduction (hirsutism, amenorrhea or virilization), ovulatory failure (infertility) or menstrual abnormalities (amenorrhea and infertility).

Turner's syndrome (**TS**) (Ranke 1996, Ranke 1997). Primary gonadal dysgenesis is much commoner in girls because of the high incidence of Turner's syndrome (Turner 1938). Although diagnosis is usually possible well before the age when puberty should occur, even in those with no dysmorphic features, too many children are not measured regularly and accurately by primary carers so that presentation with delayed puberty is common. There is a poor correlation between physical manifestations (Figs 19.24 and 19.25) – neonatal lymphedema, broad ('shield') chest with widely spaced nipples, webbed neck, high arched palate, low posterior hair line, wide carrying angle, short fourth metacarpals and hypoplastic or malformed (spoon-shaped) nails (Fig. 19.26), cardiac and renal abnormalities – and the precise genetic abnormality.

1–2% of all conceptuses have TS but rates of early spontaneous miscarriage are very high so the birth prevalence is about 1 in 2500. About half have a single X chromosome and the remainder have one normal X and one abnormal because of partial deletions, ring formation or short or long arm isochromosomes (Palmer & Reichmann 1976). At least 10% have mosaicism (different proportions of abnormal cells in different tissues) and molecular analysis suggests that the proportion is much higher (Connor & Loughlin 1989). In children with mixed karyotypes, there is an equal abnormal genetic contribution from mother and father whereas in the 45X karyotype the missing chromosome is paternal in origin. The presence of Y chromosomal material can also be detected by karyotype and molecular genetic techniques (Pade 1994). If it is found, gonads should be removed to prevent possible malignant change (e.g. gonadoblastoma).

Genomic imprinting (differential expression of genetic material depending on whether it originates from father or mother) is important in several disorders (e.g. Prader–Willi/Angelman syndromes). It is important in determining some aspects of the TS phenotype (e.g. cardiac abnormalities, neck webbing) when the normal X chromosome is maternal in origin (Chu et al 1994).

The fetal ovary forms normally and germ cell numbers are normal until the end of the second trimester. These then decline to birth and subsequently at a variable but increased rate so that a 'menopause' occurs before puberty in the majority. However, 'streak' ovaries have been found in infancy with no increased incidence with age (Massarano et al 1986). Some will enter puberty spontaneously – this is commoner with 'mosaicism' (but see above).With partial deletions, long arm preservation may be important for ovarian function and short arm deletions are associated with the growth deficit.

There is defective end-organ responsiveness to growth factors at cartilage and collagen level and a spectrum of GH secretory insufficiency (Ross et al 1985). Intrauterine growth is poor,

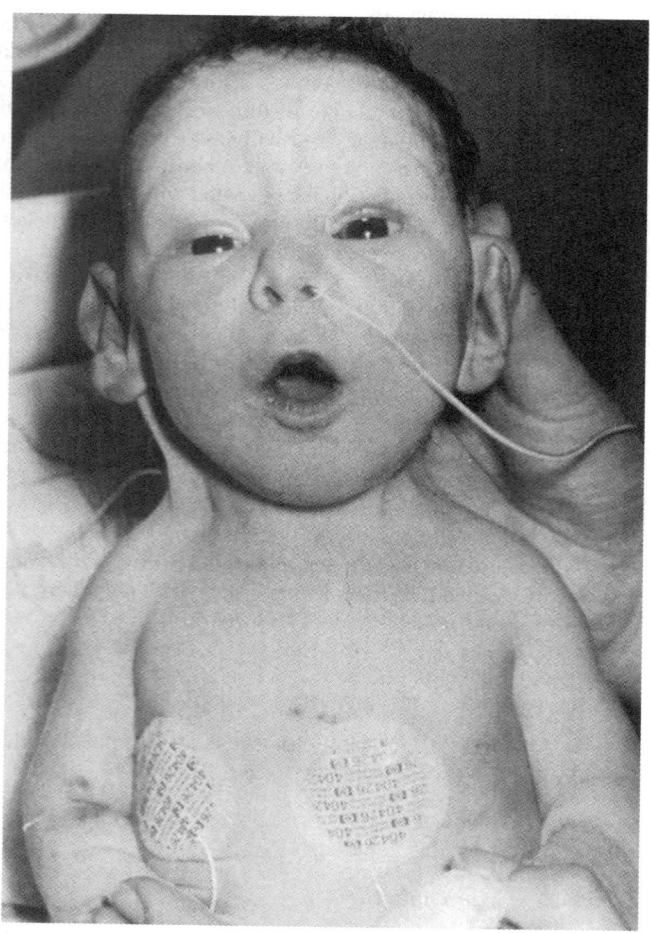
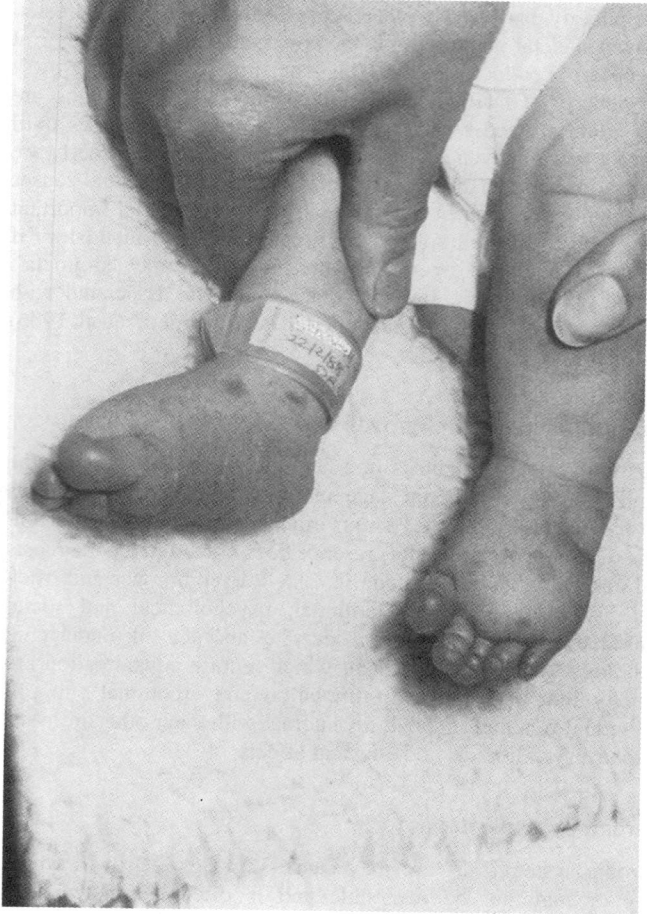

Fig. 19.24   Turner's syndrome diagnosed at birth – note the peripheral edema in a small for gestational age infant.

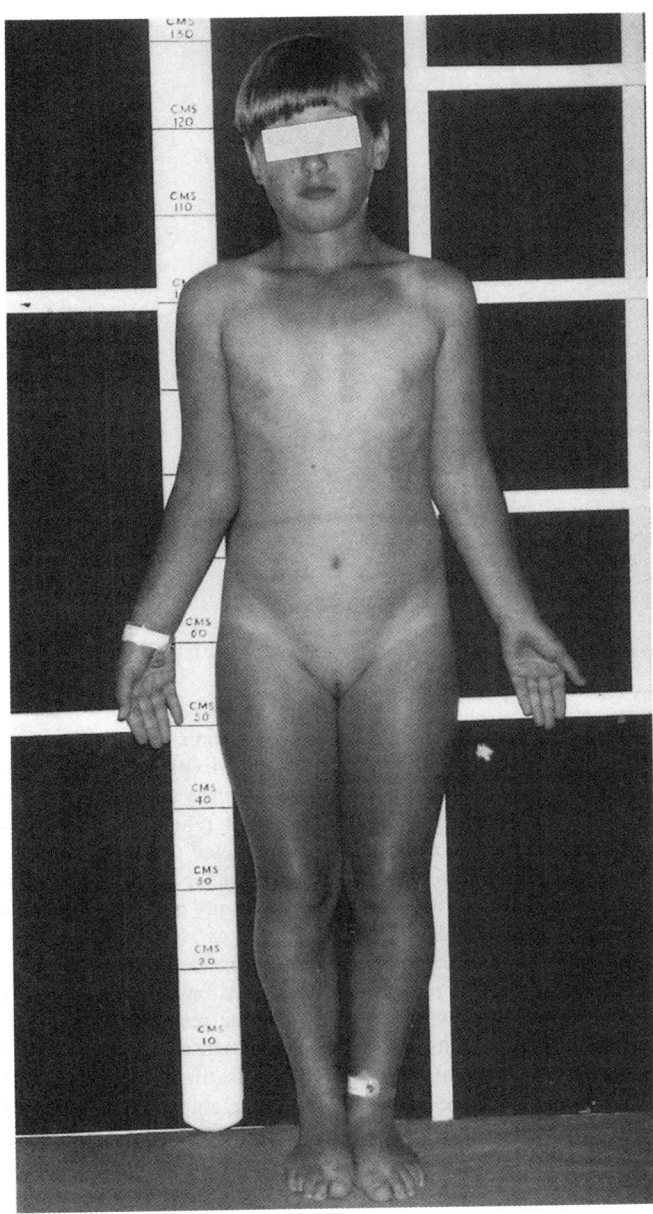

Fig. 19.25 Turner's syndrome presenting with pubertal delay in a 14-year-old girl.

syndrome-specific centiles necessitate a search for additional pathology (e.g. hypothyroidism or Crohn's disease).

Mean IQ is 95 and the majority have IQs within the normal range. Many have specific difficulties with visuospatial perception and full psychometric assessment will allow specific remedial help. Autoimmune disease is commoner in TS: autoimmune thyroiditis (Kelnar 1989) has an increasing risk with age and particularly by adolescence (Pai et al 1977). The frequency of antithyroid antibodies also increases with age (Germain & Plotnick 1986) as it does in the normal population – elevated antibody titers indicate the need for regular evaluation of thyroid function.

The nature of the dysplastic bone abnormality is unclear. However, bone mineralization is important in TS girls – it is uncertain whether absence of estrogen during early and mid-childhood compromises eventual acquisition of a healthy skeleton but GH therapy (see below) normalizes bone mineralization (Neely et al 1993).

Ideally estrogen replacement must be initiated to keep the TS girl in line with her peers and increased at a physiological rate. An appropriate regimen is described below. This produces good cosmetic breast appearances and allows normal psychological maturation. Oral estrogen enters the portal circulation and exposes the liver to high levels – transdermal natural estrogen patches will be preferable in the future. Estrogen replacement therapy is necessary at least until menopausal age and probably beyond. Ultra-low dose estrogen in early childhood (Ross et al 1986) cannot be recommended on present evidence (Rahim et al 1996). Delaying estrogen therapy beyond 11–13 years risks increased social isolation, stigmatization and psychological distress and reduced lifelong bone mineralization.

Growth-promoting therapy with GH with, or without, additional anabolic steroid (oxandrolone) has been widely studied in TS (e.g. Rosenfeld et al 1992, Chu et al 1997) but many questions remain unanswered. Current knowledge may be summarized as follows (Ranke 1996): pharmacological doses of GH produce a dose-related increase in height to socially acceptable levels in many TS girls; most gain is during the first 3 years of therapy; individual responses are variable and unpredictable; combining GH with oxandrolone increases the tempo of growth, thus shortening the duration of GH therapy to final height, and may contribute extra height gain – androgenic side effects of oxandrolone are dose related whereas the growth-promoting effect is not (Sobel 1968) and thus very low doses (0.0625 mg/kg daily) are optimal.

TS women are candidates for in vitro fertilization using donated ova (Navot et al 1986). In future, they, and perhaps women with acquired gonadal dysgenesis who have had abdominal irradiation in childhood (Critchley et al 1992), will be candidates for cryopreservation and ovarian autografts (Gosden et al 1994), although the latter group may have compromised uterine function.

Rarely ovarian agenesis occurs with a normal female karyotype. Stature is normal and there are no dysmorphic features. The presence of an XY cell line necessitates removal of dysgenetic gonads.

Disorders of testicular function

These are uncommon. Anorchia is usually detected prepubertally but may be secondary to testicular irradiation in the treatment of ALL or follow suboptimal management of testicular torsion.

growth velocity declines progressively after infancy and the pubertal growth spurt is absent. As the height relationship with parents is maintained (Brook et al 1974), TS girls with tall parents (or, more specifically, a tall parent from whom their normal X chromosome has been inherited (Chu et al 1994)) may not become conspicuously small until they fail to enter puberty when their normal peers are growing rapidly. Approximately 20 cm in height is lost compared to relevant population means – the mean adult UK height in TS is about 143.0 cm (Brook et al 1974, Lyon et al 1985b) although it may be a little more in 'mosaics' and when short arm material is present. Thus about 20% of TS girls will achieve a spontaneous final height above the 3rd centile for the normal population. Specific growth charts for Turner's syndrome are available (Lyon et al 1985b). Significant deviation from

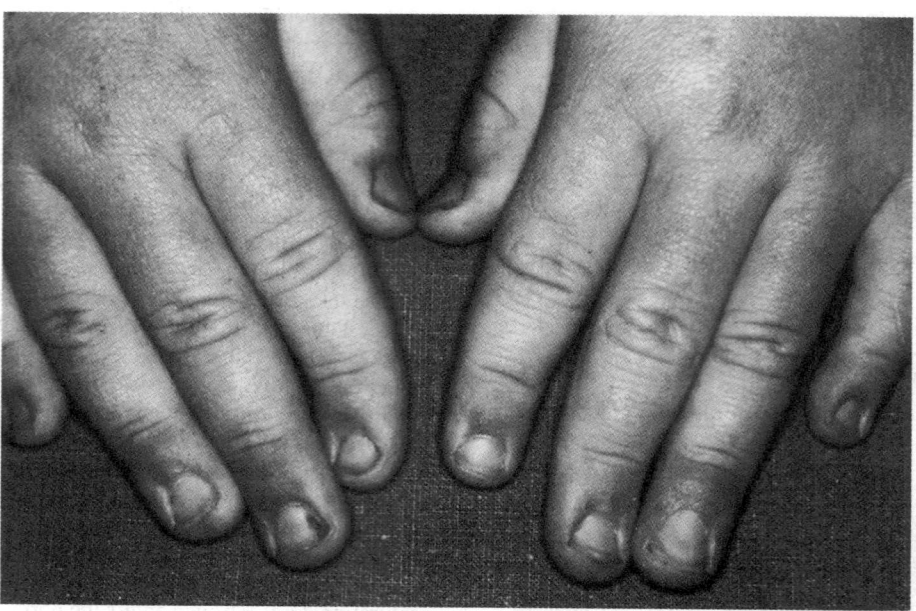

Fig. 19.26   The nails in Turner's syndrome (the same girl as in Fig. 19.25).

Polycystic ovarian syndrome

Menstrual disturbances in many adult women presenting with polycystic ovarian syndrome (hirsutism, obesity and menstrual irregularities) date from puberty and ultrasonic appearances (enlarged ovaries with many small circumferential cysts surrounding increased stromal tissue – Adams et al 1985) may be common in prepuberty and an important pathological cause of pubertal delay. The primary abnormality may be ovarian (Stanhope et al 1987c, 1988d) with secondarily raised LH levels, LH : FSH ratios and normal FSH levels.

Investigation

Distinguishing physiological from pathological delay may be impossible clinically. Assessment must include physical examination (nutritional state, fundal and visual field assessment) and calculation of height velocity. Loss of 'consonance' – tall stature for the family associated with pubertal delay and delayed bone age – is incompatible with CDGP and may be due to Klinefelter's syndrome, hypogonadism or GT deficiency; marked pubic or axillary hair growth in a girl with absent breast development suggests Turner's syndrome. The appropriateness or otherwise of height velocity can only be determined in the context of pubertal stage, e.g. growth should be accelerating in a girl with stage 2 breast development but slow growth is normal in a boy until 8–10 ml testicular volumes. Assessment of skeletal maturity may indicate likely delay before puberty starts spontaneously (if it will do so) but seldom distinguishes pathology from physiological delay.

Children with loss of consonance should be investigated at any age as should those with signs or symptoms attributable to an underlying pathological process. Where height and degree of skeletal maturational delay seem appropriate for the family in terms of final height prediction, delay is probably physiological. 3% of normal boys and girls will have no signs of puberty by 13.8

and 13.4 years respectively and it is reasonable to investigate those presenting after this. Even if delay is physiological it is unkind (in emotional and psychological terms) and inappropriate (in growth terms) to allow too much delay in relation to the child's peers, and pubertal induction may be indicated (Kelnar 1994).

Raised GT levels are diagnostic of primary gonadal failure but are not elevated before about 10 years. At any age, normal testes will respond to stimulation by LH (given as HCG) by secreting testosterone. In hypogonadotropic hypogonadism there is a presumed lack of LH receptors in the testis, basal and stimulated GT levels will be low and the testosterone response to HCG is absent. Pubertal imminence can be assessed by measuring nocturnal GTs (Brown et al 1996a) – pulsatile nocturnal GnRH release occurs well before clinically detectable signs – or more practically by measuring the GT response to a small (0.25 µg/kg/i.v.) dose of GnRH (see p. 1025). If puberty is imminent, LH responsiveness will exceed that of FSH and rise significantly. Where available, skilled ultrasound assessment is helpful in girls and noninvasive. An 8 a.m. plasma testosterone level may be a useful simple guide in boys (Wu et al 1993).

Raised basal PRL levels may be due to stress but are otherwise a sensitive indicator of the release of PRL following reduction in its dopaminergic inhibitory control secondary to hypothalamic lesions or those causing portal compression (e.g. craniopharyngioma, radiotherapy, histiocytosis X). Hyperprolactinemia (p. 1041) is itself a cause of delayed puberty. Prolactinomas are rare in children – PRL levels are generally very high (> 3000 mU/l). A significantly elevated PRL is a sensitive indicator of intracranial pathology as a cause of delayed puberty (see p. 1042) and an indication for neuroradiological investigation, which is important if an evolving endocrinopathy is suspected – hypogonadotropic hypogonadism may be the first sign of panhypopituitarism.

There is physiological blunting of GH secretion in late prepuberty in both sexes and in early male puberty so that, if pharmacological testing of GH secretion is deemed necessary and is to be interpreted correctly, sex steroid priming is necessary.

Stilbestrol is the drug of choice in both sexes but depot testosterone or oral estrogen may be used in boys and girls respectively.

If pathology is suspected, investigations should be carried out urgently (treatment of underlying pathology may be necessary) and puberty induced at normal time and tempo. Otherwise, although much can be learnt by several months' observation of growth and for early signs of puberty, the psychological pressures on some can be considerable (Kelnar 1990, 1994). The short, undeveloped and poorly qualified 16-year-old school leaver may find it particularly hard to obtain employment. It is inappropriate to induce puberty late to maximize prepubertal growth because continuing late prepubertal growth deceleration is leading to a lower point from which to accelerate and the magnitude of the pubertal growth spurt in a late developer is generally smaller (Prader 1975). It is also unkind to subject a child to unnecessary social and emotional pressures.

With optimal treatment, puberty can be started at an appropriate time and continued at a physiological tempo. In girls, too large a starting dose and too rapid escalation of estrogen therapy will reduce the magnitude of the growth spurt, produce cosmetically unattractive 'cylindrical' breasts and potential difficulties in important emotional and psychological aspects of adolescent development. A boy may have 2 years or more from early testicular enlargement until he notices height acceleration. Meanwhile his more average peers are both more developed and growing three- to fourfold faster. Stimulation of growth during early male puberty is thus of considerable potential psychological benefit (Kelnar 1990). Possible therapies (anabolic steroid, androgen or GH) are reviewed by Kelnar (1994).

Clinical consequences and management

Emotional and psychological consequences of delay are not dependent on the presence of underlying pathology – the commonest group, boys with CDGP, may suffer considerably yet are entirely normal. Where an underlying nonendocrine condition is responsible, diagnosis and optimal management may facilitate spontaneous development. When pubertal induction is necessary, it should closely mimic normal pubertal progression to optimize growth, cosmetic appearances and psychological maturation. Too rapid induction is deleterious and unnecessary if induction is not unduly delayed.

Puberty induction

Induction in girls is with estrogen whatever the precise nature of pubertal failure. An appropriate starting regimen is ethinylestradiol 1–2 µg orally daily, increasing to 10 µg over 18–24 months. At that dose, or before if breakthrough bleeding occurs, a progestogen (e.g. norethisterone 350 µg) should be added for 5 days every 4 weeks. Unopposed estrogenic endometrial stimulation otherwise increases risks of endometrial or breast carcinoma. Full secondary sexual development will generally occur with ethinylestradiol 20–30 µg – a low estrogen combined contraceptive pill may then be conveniently substituted. If hypogonadism is permanent, estrogen therapy must be maintained to enable sexual intercourse to be enjoyed without discomfort, prevent osteoporosis and, perhaps, early atherosclerosis. Transdermal natural estrogen, when available in low enough dosage for pubertal induction, will be preferable.

In boys, physiological sex steroid replacement is even more difficult. Conventionally, depot preparations of testosterone esters (e.g. Sustanon 50–100 mg i.m. once every 6 weeks increasing gradually over 2 years to 250 mg i.m. twice weekly) are used. Oral testosterone (undecanoate, TU) was considered too variably and excessively absorbed for pubertal induction but recent experience (Wu et al 1988, Butler et al 1992, Brown et al 1995) suggests that resulting high total testosterone levels reflect changes in SHBG on treatment, and that appropriate free (active) testosterone levels for pubertal induction are achievable with TU 40 mg on alternate days – TU may be the treatment of choice for the short, sexually immature adolescent boy where explanation and reassurance alone are not enough (Kelnar 1994, Bourguignon 1997). Long-term androgen replacement will probably be best given transdermally. Patches are now available in the UK and suitably low-dose regimens for pubertal induction need evaluation.

Human chorionic gonadotropin (HCG) therapy is an alternative in boys – in girls it may cause abdominal pain, ascites and hemorrhagic rupture of ovarian cysts. HCG (i.e. LH) is started alone (500 units i.m. weekly, increasing to 2000 units over 2 years) and then in combination with human menopausal gonadotropin (HMG, i.e. FSH) to induce spermatogenesis. Optimal fertility in both sexes requires eventual low dose pulsatile GnRH therapy.

The physician will need to assess carefully individual underlying psychological and social pressure before deciding on optimal management of CDGP which might comprise anabolic steroid (oxandrolone) or testosterone therapy (Kelnar 1994). Emotional support is always important whatever other treatment modalities are used but the morale boost from an increase in growth velocity in early male puberty is often dramatic, with improvement in school attendance and performance.

OTHER DISORDERS RELATED TO FEMALE AND MALE REPRODUCTION

AMENORRHEA (see Ch. 18)

Amenorrhea may be secondary (absent menstruation with previously normal menstrual history) – causes include pregnancy, anorexia nervosa, intense training or chronic underlying disease – or primary (menstrual bleeding has never occurred). Primary amenorrhea may be a consequence of abnormal GnRH pulsatile secretion or release – a middle stage between GnRH deficiency causing delayed or arrested puberty and infertility due to anovulatory cycles. Other important causes include primary ovarian failure (often in TS), gonadal dysgenesis with absent uterus (e.g. the XY girl – see p. 61) or imperforate hymen. Hypertension suggests 17α-hydroxylase deficiency (p. 1064).

NOONAN'S SYNDROME (Noonan & Ehmke 1963, Noonan 1968, Ranke 1997)

In this syndrome there is frequently variable hypogonadism associated with characteristic features such as pulmonary valvular stenosis, a broad forehead with hypertelorism, epicanthic folds, ptosis and downward slanting palpebral fissures, abnormal or low-set ears, neck webbing, low posterior hair line, shield chest or kyphoscoliosis (Fig. 19.27). However, as in TS, all these are inconstant. Cryptorchidism is found in about two-thirds of boys

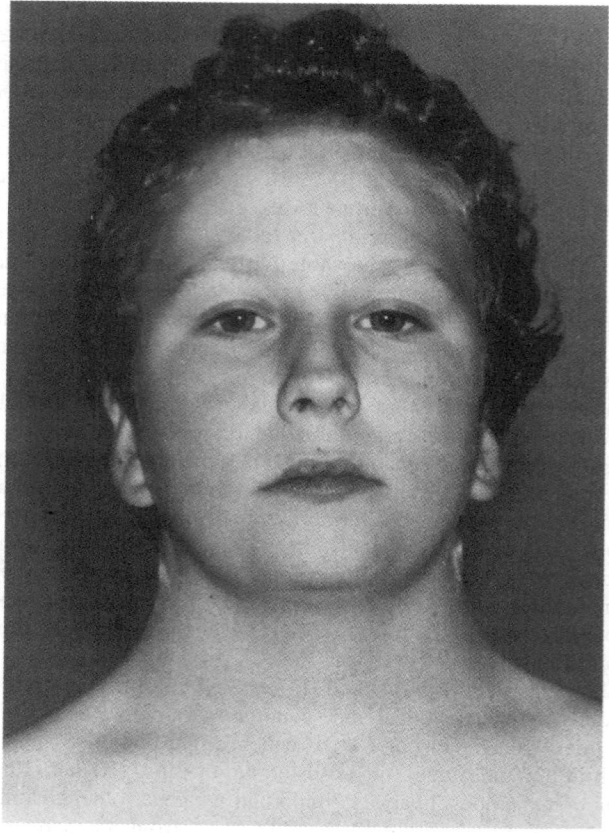

Fig. 19.27   Noonan's syndrome.

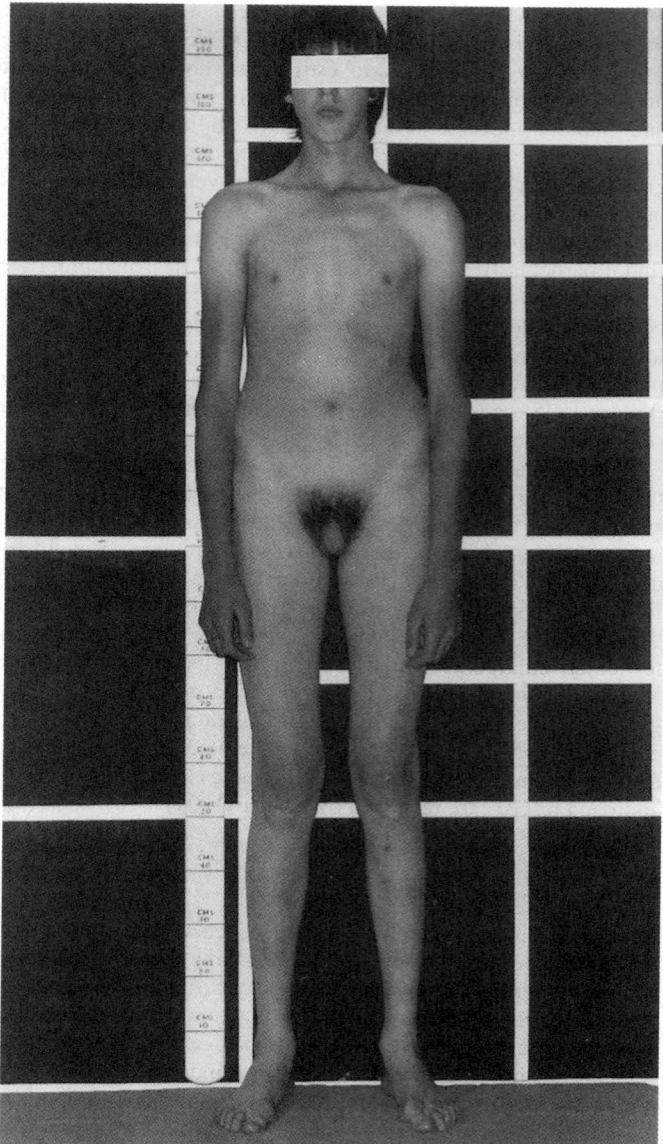

Fig. 19.28   Klinefelter's syndrome – note the disproportionately long legs in this 202-cm 18-year-old.

but sexual development generally occurs spontaneously but is delayed. Infertility is usual. In girls (whose karyotype is normal) puberty and menarche can be delayed (presentation may be with primary amenorrhea) but fertility seems common. There is an association with autoimmune thyroid disease. Mean final height is 165 cm and 152 cm in males and females respectively. GH treatment improves medium-term height velocity and theoretical adverse effects on cardiac ventricular wall thickness (potentially leading to hypertrophic obstructive cardiomyopathy) have not been seen (Cotterill et al 1996).

KLINEFELTER'S SYNDROME (47XXY) (Klinefelter et al 1942)

There is tall stature for the family with disproportionately long legs from childhood (Fig. 19.28) (Schibler et al 1974), small testes for apparent virilization (Fig. 19.29) and azoospermia. Presentation is usually with tall stature, hypogonadism (often with marked pubertal gynecomastia) or infertility. The incidence is about 1 in 500 to 1000 live births. Extremely tall ultimate height with increasingly disproportionately long legs relates to testosterone secretion inadequate for epiphysial closure at appropriate time or normal rapid late pubertal spinal growth – GH predominantly stimulates long bone growth. Spontaneous pulsatile GT secretion in pre- and peripubertal 47XXY boys may be normal (Butler et al 1989b) (cf. the usual GT elevation in adults). Pubertal onset is generally not delayed. Mean IQ is below

the population mean, but most are within the normal range. If the diagnosis is made sufficiently early, excessive stature can be prevented, or at least reduced, by high dose testosterone treatment or epiphysiodesis (see p. 1020).

GYNECOMASTIA (Braunstein 1996)

Hormonal effects on breast structures are complex (Anderson & Dewis 1989). In males androgens are important in inhibiting stimulatory estrogenic effects on breast tissue – breast development occurs in pubertal girls at estrogen levels comparable to those in adult males as also in androgen-insensitivity syndromes (see p. 991), where testosterone is inactive because of androgen receptor deficiency, at normal male estradiol levels.

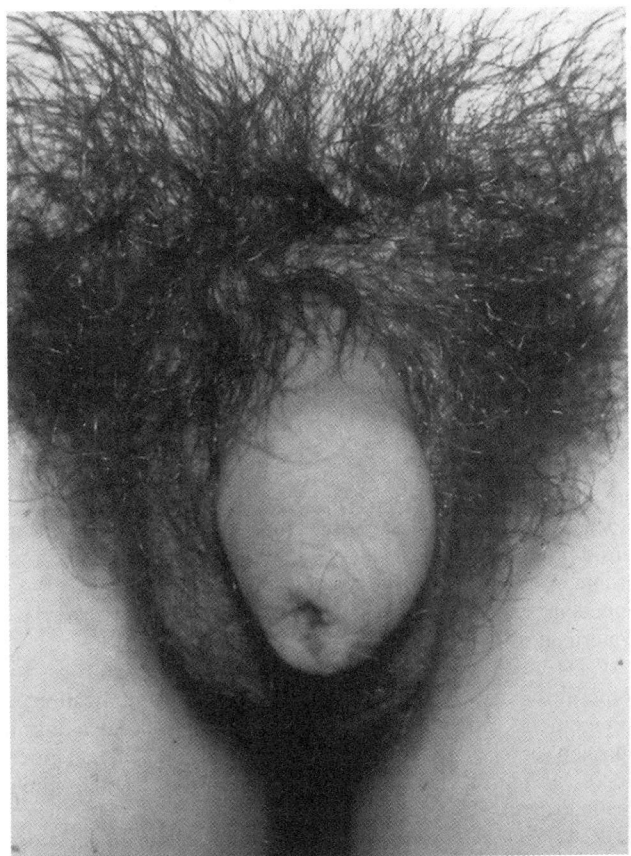

Fig. 19.29 Genitalia in Klinefelter's syndrome – note the small testes for the degree of virilization (the same subject as in Fig. 19.28).

Thus a degree of gynecomastia occurs in < 50% of normal boys during early to mid-puberty when estrogen levels are high in relation to androgens. It is usually mild resolving spontaneously within 12–18 months. Gynecomastia is a particular feature of Klinefelter's syndrome (see above). Gross pubertal gynecomastia, prepubertal gynecomastia or persistence in late puberty requires investigation.

Prepubertal gynecomastia may be unilateral or cause discomfort and is usually benign, self-limiting and idiopathic. Exposure to exogenous estrogen or endogenous production by adrenal, testicular or other tumors must be excluded and drugs such as digoxin, methyldopa, ketoconazole and cannabis and amphetamine abuse have been associated. Occasionally subareolar mastectomy is necessary if the condition is distressing and persistent.

UNDESCENDED TESTES

This common problem is considered elsewhere (see Ch. 31). Bilaterally undescended testes are much more likely to result from an underlying endocrine abnormality such as hypogonadotropic hypogonadism. All boys in this situation should be investigated (karyotype, GnRH and HCG tests) before surgery. Ensure that the testes are not simply retractile, i.e. can be manipulated into the scrotum and will descend (and stay in the scrotum) at puberty. In doubtful cases HCG (500 units daily i.m. for 1 week) will produce descent of retractile testes.

Scrotal testes are necessary functionally (testosterone biosynthesis, spermatogenesis) and cosmetically and because of the (difficult to quantify) risk of malignant change in functional intra-abdominal testes. A testis which is not in the scrotum by the middle years of childhood is unlikely to show adequate spermatogenesis. Although it may be undescended because it is intrinsically abnormal, orchidopexy should be carried out before school entry to optimize potential function and for psychological and cosmetic reasons. Functional but ectopic tissue which cannot be brought into the scrotum surgically is probably best removed unless it is easily accessible to clinical examination and follow-up can be assured. Nonfunctioning intra-abdominal testicular tissue is probably best left – it carries extremely low risk of malignant change and may be impossible to locate at laparotomy.

THE HYPOTHALAMO-PITUITARY UNIT

CONNECTIONS/ANATOMY/PHYSIOLOGY

Ontogeny of fetal hypothalamopituitary hormone biosynthesis is described on pages 1002–1003. By 15 weeks' gestation, the hypothalamus is anatomically mature and functionally active, and by 18 weeks' gestation, pituitary vascularization is complete. The hypothalamopituitary axis is functional by 20 weeks with development of the portal system.

Functional maturity is important for normal development of thyroid (secondary to TSH secretion), external genitalia in the male (GH and GTs) and adrenal (ACTH and related peptides).

The pituitary gland is situated within the pituitary fossa, directly below and in close relationship with the hypothalamus. Laterally are the cavernous sinuses, the internal carotid arteries, the 3rd, 4th and 6th cranial nerves and temporal lobes. Above lie arachnoid and subarachnoid spaces and above them the optic chiasma and hypothalamus.

The hypothalamus has afferent connections with frontal cortex, thalamus, amygdala, hippocampus and anterior thalamic (autonomic) nuclei and can integrate and respond to a wide range of physiological and behavioral inputs. Efferent pathways also connect with midbrain, pons, medulla, amygdala and hippocampus and there are specific pathways to adrenohypophysis via the portal system and to neurohypophysis via the supraopticohypophyseal tract.

Neuroendocrine control of hypothalamic secretion is by CNS neurotransmitters including dopamine, noradrenaline, serotonin, acetylcholine, gamma-aminobutyric acid (GABA), melatonin and histamine. Anterior pituitary hormone secretion is directly controlled by hypothalamic factors (regulatory peptides) which affect hormone synthesis and release (Table 19.9).

Table 19.9 Hypothalamic regulatory peptides and their properties

Regulatory peptide	Amino acids	Molecular weight
Growth hormone releasing hormone	40/44	4545/5040
Somatostatin (growth hormone release inhibiting hormone)	14	1638
Gonadotropin releasing hormone/ luteinizing hormone releasing hormone	10	1182
Thyrotropin releasing hormone	3	362
Corticotropin releasing hormone/factor	41	4758

ANTERIOR PITUITARY HORMONES

Corticotropin (ACTH)

ACTH is a single chain 39 amino acid polypeptide. The first 24 N-terminal amino acids are identical in most species and produce the biological (adrenocortical) activity. However, ACTH is one of a group of related pituitary peptides which originates from a common large molecular weight (31 000) glycosylated precursor molecule, pro-opiomelanocortin (POMC) (Mains et al 1977, Roberts & Herbert 1977). Glycosylation accounts for basophil staining of pituitary corticotrophs.

The bovine precursor protein (Fig. 19.30) consists of 265 amino acids encoding three peptides: ACTH, β-lipotropin (β-LPH) and a 105 amino acid N-terminal sequence N-POMC (Nakanishi et al 1979). Human N-POMC is a 76 amino acid peptide of molecular weight 11 200 (Seidah & Chretien 1981). All three POMC-derived peptides are found in the same secretory granules within the cell, are released concomitantly into the circulation in equal concentrations, become undetectable after hypophysectomy and their plasma concentrations rise after adrenalectomy. Secretion is stimulated by median eminence extracts containing CRF activity and suppressed by dexamethasone. Plasma concentrations of N-POMC and ACTH correlate closely, reflecting coordinated synthesis and secretion (Hope et al 1981).

No clearly defined physiological role for β-LPH and N-POMC has yet been identified although species similarity of the three POMC constituents makes such a role likely. Metencephalin (the first five residues of β-endorphin, β-LPH 61–65) has opiate agonist activity but no circadian secretory rhythm and may originate from the adrenal medulla rather than the pituitary.

Synthetic χ-3-MSH stimulates adrenocortical steroidogenesis and, in particular, cholesterol ester hydrolase (Pedersen et al 1980), and human N-POMC significantly potentiates ACTH-stimulated steroidogenesis in vitro using perfused isolated rat adrenocortical cells (Al-Dujaili et al 1981). Thus N-POMC or its derivatives could act as amplifiers of ACTH-induced steroidogenesis or regulators of adrenocortical cell growth.

There is no evidence linking POMC or any of its constituent fractions, other than ACTH, with adrenal androgen secretion. Nevertheless, there has been speculation that an ACTH biosynthetic precursor might be the prohormone of a specific adrenal androgen-stimulating hormone (Grumbach et al 1978) – see page 1059.

The principal modulator of ACTH secretion is CRF but vasopressin also has a stimulatory effect on ACTH secretion, directly and by potentiating the actions of CRF (Gillies & Grossman 1985). Neurotransmitter pathways important in ACTH secretion are α-adrenergic (perhaps most important), cholinergic, serotoninergic and histaminergic (all excitatory) and via GABA (inhibitory).

ACTH release is circadian resulting in the early morning peak of ACTH and cortisol in association with more frequent ACTH pulses (Krieger et al 1971). Factors modulating its secretion are cortisol (by negative feedback at hypothalamic (mainly) and pituitary levels via fast and slow feedback loops) and ACTH itself at pituitary level.

ACTH stimulates adrenal growth and cortisol synthesis and release. Plasma half-life is about 10 min. Mechanisms stimulating adrenocortical steroidogenesis are complex: ACTH binds to its adrenal cell membrane receptor, in the presence of calcium ions, to generate cyclic AMP; cyclic AMP activates, by phosphorylation, enzymes which stimulate hydrolysis of cholesterol esters (first steps in adrenal steroidogenesis). Rapid steroid production follows (see Fig. 19.37). There is also a slower, chronic effect on protein synthesis in the cytochrome P-450-dependent enzyme systems (11β-, 17α- and 21-hydroxylases) (Waterman & Simpson 1985).

ACTH acutely stimulates aldosterone release from zona glomerulosa cells – this has important practical implications for management of salt-losing CAH – and modulates adrenal androgen secretion (p. 1059). It stimulates amino acid and glucose uptake by muscle and lipolysis in adipose cells and inhibits thymic growth.

The 13 ACTH N-terminal amino acids are identical with α-MSH (see Fig. 19.37) and homologous with amino acids 7–13 of β-MSH. β-MSH is not present in the pituitary or circulation in man and may not exist in discrete form. The etiology of skin pigmentation in pathological states is unclear – ACTH itself is probably causative in some situations.

Somatotropin (GH) (see pp. 1012–1014)

Gonadotropins (GTs – LH, FSH)

LH and FSH are glycoproteins (MW 30 000, and 32 000 respectively), each with identical A but different B chains and possibly stored within the same secretory granules in pituitary gonadotrophs. Release is controlled by a single hypothalamic

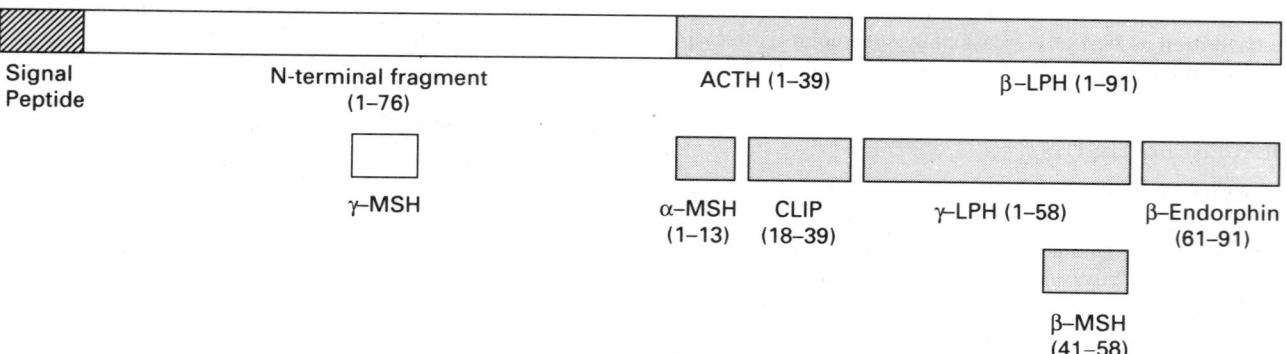

Fig. 19.30 Structure of bovine pro-opiomelanocortin (POMC) (after Nakanishi et al 1979) (the connecting peptide N-POMC 79–109 has been omitted).

hormone, GnRH (see Table 19.9). GnRH is released in a pulsatile manner. For puberty see pages 1024–1026.

In men, LH stimulates by testicular Leydig cell testosterone secretion and FSH stimulates spermatogenesis. In women, LH induces ovulation, maintains the corpus luteum and stimulates it to produce progesterone and estrogens. Ovarian follicles secrete estrogens in response to FSH and endometrial gland growth and secretion result from estrogen and progesterone secretion, respectively. In men, LH secretion is under negative feedback control from testosterone and FSH secretion is regulated by inhibin-B secreted by testicular Sertoli cells (Illingworth et al 1996a). In the female, estrogens exert either positive feedback at pituitary level (before ovulation) or negative feedback (at other times).

Prolactin (PRL)

PRL (198 amino acids, MW 22 500) is strikingly homologous with GH. Its major role is in initiation and maintenance of lactation. Its role in childhood, when levels are low and constant, is unknown although it rises in response to stress. There is no evidence that slight rises during normal puberty are important in its onset or control. Transiently high levels in neonates secondary to fetoplacental estrogen may cause galactorrhea ('witch's milk') from engorged breasts in either sex.

PRL is predominantly under inhibitory dopaminergic control and hyperprolactinemia is an important early nonspecific sign of neuroendocrine disturbance and intracranial pathology. A PRL-inhibiting factor (PIF) has been postulated but has not been characterized. GABA may also have some inhibitory effect but TRH and VIP are stimulatory.

Thyrotropin (TSH)

TSH is a glycoprotein, MW 26 600. It shares a common A chain with LH and FSH. TRH stimulates TSH synthesis and release which increases thyroid vascularity and stimulates follicular cell hypertrophy. TSH stimulates iodine uptake, organification, coupling of tyrosines and the synthesis and release of thyroxine (T4) and triiodothyronine (T3). Feedback inhibition is by T3, both directly and via deiodination of T4 within the pituitary. In man dopaminergic inhibition may occur at the level of the thyrotroph; the inhibitory role of somatostatin is unclear in normal physiology. Glucocorticoids inhibit TSH release at hypothalamic level.

After birth, there is a large rise in TSH release followed by a more gradual rise in circulating T4 and T3 levels. TSH levels return to normal by the end of the first week but thyroid hormone levels may be elevated for up to several weeks (p. 1046).

Melanocyte-stimulating hormones (α- and β-MSH)

See above under ACTH.

POSTERIOR PITUITARY HORMONES

Arginine vasopressin (antidiuretic hormone, AVP) and oxytocin

Vasopressin and oxytocin are 9 amino acid peptides differing from each other at two sites (amino acids 3 and 8). They are synthesized in the supraoptic (mainly vasopressin) and paraventricular (mainly oxytocin) hypothalamic neurons bound to proteins (neurophysins I and II) whose function is unknown. Both hormones reach the posterior pituitary, where they are stored in secretory granules, via the supraopticohypophyseal tract.

The principal stimulus to vasopressin (AVP) release is rising plasma osmolality but plasma volume and blood pressure may exert independent effects. Some physiological states (e.g. pain, stress, sleep) also stimulate vasopressin release. The most important physiological action is to cause water reabsorption by renal distal tubules and collecting ducts – water is reabsorbed in excess of sodium resulting in concentrated urine. Plasma osmolality is normally kept within the range 275–290 mosmol/kg throughout life. For a comprehensive review of the role of the neurohypophysis in water balance in health and disease see Perheentupa (1995) and Bode et al (1996). Tests of water regulation are reviewed by Czernichow (1992).

The principal stimulus to oxytocin release is suckling. Oxytocin stimulates the 'let-down' reflex during lactation and uterine contractility. It has weak antidiuretic activity. Except in pregnancy and the puerperium, its physiological role in man is unknown. Neither excess nor deficiency is associated with any syndrome in children (or adults).

DISEASES OF THE HYPOTHALAMONEUROHYPOPHYSEAL UNIT

Diabetes insipidus (DI)

Hypothalamic AVP deficiency leads to voiding of inappropriately large volumes of dilute urine (polyuria). If thirst sensation is normal, fluid lost is replaced and there is excessive drinking (polydipsia) to maintain normal plasma osmolality. Nocturia is invariable and may present as secondary enuresis in older children. If thirst recognition is defective (usually due to extensive hypothalamic damage to both AVP and thirst osmoreceptors) or there is no access to adequate or appropriate fluid (e.g. in neonate or infant), hypernatremic dehydration may result in fever, irritability vomiting and failure to thrive, and polyuria may be absent.

Polyuria and polydipsia may result from renal unresponsiveness to AVP (nephrogenic DI – see Ch. 17). Sometimes primary polydipsia ('compulsive water drinking') may develop in children (leading to secondary polyuria). Both these situations must be considered in the differential diagnosis as must other causes of polyuria (e.g. urinary tract infection, diabetes mellitus). Defects in AVP release are usually due to hypothalamic dysfunction – more than 75% of secretory capacity must be lost before symptoms develop. Removal of, or damage to, the neurohypophysis does not cause DI.

DI is rare in childhood – the incidence in Finland is 5 cases per million per year up to 14 years of age (Perheentupa 1995, Bode et al 1996). Causes are listed in Table 19.10.

Primary DI may be familial or sporadic and families with dominant or X-linked inheritance have been described (Forssman 1955). AVP deficiency is found in 25–50% of children with histiocytosis X and may precede other evidence of the disease by months or years (see Ch. 15). Other rare infiltrative causes include Hodgkin's disease, leukemias and sarcoidosis but transient DI is common after head injury and pituitary surgery. It may complicate severe neonatal infections and may be associated with autoimmune states with AVP antibodies (Scherbaum et al 1985).

Table 19.10 Causes of diabetes insipidus (data from Crawford & Bode 1975, Czernichow et al 1985, Niaudet et al 1985, Perheentupa 1995)

Hypothalamic tumor 38% – craniopharyngioma 23% (usually postoperative); germinoma 6.5%; optic neuroma rarely

Idiopathic 23% – autoimmune factors may be important

Congenital renal 23%

Histiocytosis X 8%

Cerebral malformations 3%

Primary polydipsia 3%

Traumatic 2%

Differential diagnosis of polyuria depends on history, examination and laboratory tests. Osmotic diuresis (e.g. due to salt or glucose) is readily excluded from the history and by testing the urine for glucose. Habitual polydipsia most often develops in response to fluids being offered to pacify a demanding infant or young child. Such primary polydipsia of 'psychogenic' origin is suggested by fluctuating symptoms, evidence of psychological difficulties in the child or family, and a refusal of water (as opposed to juice) if waking thirsty at night. A morning plasma osmolality in the normal range (cf. in DI) often contrasts with a low value in the evening.

History of head injury, meningitis or encephalitis should be sought. Poor growth suggests either inadequate appetite or food intake relating to the polydipsia or an associated anterior pituitary lesion with TSH, GH, GT or ACTH deficiencies. TSH or ACTH deficiency may temporarily conceal DI until thyroxine or cortisol replacement is given. Headaches, vomiting and visual disturbances indicate raised intracranial pressure secondary to tumor.

Synchronous measurements of plasma and urinary osmolality are valuable provided accurate assays are available. If not, plasma sodium (not specific gravity) should be substituted. Inappropriately low urinary osmolality with raised plasma osmolality confirms DI – charts aiding interpretation have been produced in children. To achieve this mismatch a water deprivation test may be necessary. Plasma AVP assays are increasingly available but their value in diagnosis of central DI in children is not established (high, diagnostic values are found in nephrogenic DI).

Water deprivation tests are potentially both dangerous and misleading if inadequately supervised and a strict protocol should be followed. Several protocols are available – Perheentupa (1995) is readily accessible. Specific additional endocrine and neuroradiological investigations may be necessary (Czernichow 1992).

Provision of adequate water with free access to solute-free fluid at all times is vitally important. Treatment with AVP has been much simplified by the availability of a synthetic AVP analogue 1-desamino-8D-arginine vasopressin (DDAVP, desmopressin) which has been administered intranasally. Convenience and simplicity of administration (the solution is blown into the nose via a soft plastic tube) outweigh problems such as variable therapeutic effect and duration of action (Robinson & Verbalis 1985). A reasonable starting dose is 0.25 µg (in neonates), 0.5–1.0 µg (infants) and 2.5 µg (children). Therapeutic effect is seen within 1 h. The 2- or 3-times-daily dose is adjusted to provide an antidiuretic effect for 8–12 h and may need increasing during rhinitis.

Special care must be taken with infants who do not have free access to water and children with an impaired sense of thirst. Water intoxication is a risk with overdosage or if water is given inappropriately. A talisman detailing the disease and its therapy should be carried or worn at all times. DDAVP, like other small peptides, is orally active and can now be given by mouth (initially 100 µg t.d.s.; maintenance 200–600 µg/day).

Poor control of DI is associated with nocturia, enuresis, irritability and poor behavior and school performance. Appetite and growth velocity may be poor. Polyuria may lead to secondary enuresis. If treatment is optimal, prognosis reflects the underlying condition in secondary DI; in treated primary DI growth and development should be normal.

DI, DIABETES MELLITUS, OPTIC ATROPHY, DEAFNESS SYNDROME ('DIDMOAD' SYNDROME, WOLFRAM SYNDROME) (see p. 1081)

Syndrome of inappropriate secretion of antidiuretic hormone (SIADH)

Causes are listed in Table 19.11. Excessive AVP secretion results in water retention, hypo-osmolality and dilutional hyponatremia. Inhibition of aldosterone with continuing AVP secretion leads to paradoxically high urinary sodium levels and concentrated urine. AVP levels may not be supranormal but are inappropriately high for the expanded extracellular volume and hypo-osmolality.

In pediatric practice, SIADH is usually seen either in neonates following birth asphyxia, hyaline membrane disease or intraventricular hemorrhage, or in older children in association

Table 19.11 Causes of inappropriate ADH secretion

CNS disease/disorder
  Meningitis/encephalitis
  Trauma
  Tumor
  Hemorrhage
  Hypoxia
  Ischemia
  Malformation
  Guillain-Barré syndrome
  Obstructed ventriculoatrial shunt

Lung disease
  Pneumonia
  Tuberculosis
  Pneumothorax*
  Asthma*
  Cystic fibrosis*
  Ventilation

Postoperative (including mitral valvotomy,* ductus arteriosus ligation*)

Drugs (e.g. analgesics, sedatives, anesthetics)

Malignancy

Trauma/burns

Endocrine/metabolic
  Hypothyroidism
  Adrenocortical failure
  Hypoglycemia

Idiopathic

* May be secondary to reduced left atrial filling.

with meningitis, encephalitis or CNS tumors. It occasionally complicates pneumonia or pulmonary tuberculosis, vincristine or cyclophosphamide therapy, and is a common, temporary (up to several days) complication of surgery requiring general anesthesia. It may be a particular problem in burns and trauma patients. SIADH may be iatrogenic, due to inappropriate intravenous fluid therapy.

The first signs and symptoms are often masked by, or taken as manifestations of, the underlying problem – anorexia, confusion, headaches, muscle weakness and cramps. Eventually, there is vomiting, convulsions or coma. There is no edema. Diagnosis depends on clinical suspicion and the biochemical findings described above.

Treatment is by water restriction to between 30 and 50% maintenance and sodium replacement to compensate for secondary sodium losses. Correction should be gradual (over several days). In situations where this cannot be achieved drug therapy may be indicated. Lithium and demethylchlortetracycline have serious side effects in children and should not be used. Frusemide (with slow infusion of hypertonic saline) may be indicated – AVP antidiuretic analogues which, it was hoped, would become the treatment of choice (Kinter et al 1985) have all had significant vasopressor activity (Hofbauer & Marr 1987).

DISEASES OF THE ADENOHYPOPHYSIS

GH insufficiency and excess (see pp. 1015, 1020)

ACTH excess

Hypercortisolism in children usually results from excessive GC medication. Endogenous adrenocortical overactivity is rare, whether due to adrenal tumor (benign or malignant), hyperplasia, ectopic tumor ACTH production or to pituitary-dependent ACTH secretion (Cushing's disease). Cushing's syndrome includes all pathological states secondary to excessive GC production (p. 1065). Cushing found a basophil pituitary adenoma in only six of his original 12 patients (Cushing 1932) – it is now thought that bilateral adrenal hyperplasia secondary to excessive ACTH secretion of pituitary origin is not a single entity and may be due to a variety of hypothalamic, pituitary or even CNS (neurotransmitter) abnormalities (Forest 1995a).

Classical clinical features of hypercortisolism (hypertension, striae, truncal obesity, moon face, osteoporosis) are less obvious in children than in adults. Growth failure is usually marked but there can be temporary adrenal androgen-mediated acceleration.

The (utopian) aim in treating Cushing's disease is to control cortisol overproduction (if appropriate by removing the source of ACTH hypersecretion) whilst avoiding permanent endocrine deficiencies and dependence on replacement therapy. In practice, treatment of Cushing's syndrome in children is still controversial given its poorly understood and diverse etiologic basis. Options include surgery to adrenals or pituitary, pituitary irradiation (conventional or with radioactive implants), or medical management with dopaminergic agents or serotonin antagonists.

ACTH deficiency

ACTH deficiency is usually associated with other anterior pituitary hormone deficiencies which may be congenital, idiopathic, due to brain malformations or pituitary hypoplasia or to tumors such as craniopharyngioma (especially following surgery and/or radiotherapy).

Isolated ACTH deficiency is rare, and may be congenital and have an unexplained association with primary hypothyroidism (Stephens et al 1985) – thyroxine therapy precipitates adrenal insufficiency by increasing cortisol clearance.

Congenital panhypopituitarism (see Fig. 19.31) is associated with severe neonatal hypoglycemia but isolated ACTH deficiency does not usually produce as severe adrenal hypofunction as in primary adrenal insufficiency. GC and adrenal androgen secretion are impaired; aldosterone secretion is normal. Collapse with salt loss may occur during severe intercurrent illness or general anesthesia. Treatment is with appropriate GC replacement.

TSH deficiency

Congenital hypothyroidism due to decreased TSH stimulation of thyroid hormone secretion may be due to abnormalities of hypothalamic or pituitary development, isolated TRH or TSH deficiency (familial or idiopathic) or panhypopituitarism. Congenital primary hypothyroidism is 15- to 30-fold commoner.

TSH deficiency may present in later childhood, usually in association with other anterior pituitary hormone deficiencies and secondary to tumors (especially craniopharyngioma), cranial irradiation or meningitis. Symptoms and signs due to associated deficiencies usually predominate.

Differential diagnosis of primary, secondary (pituitary) and tertiary (hypothalamic) hypothyroidism and management is discussed below.

Gonadotropin (GT) deficiency

Isolated GT deficiency may occur without underlying anatomical abnormality. Usually congenital abnormalities of brain development give rise to hypothalamic GnRH deficiency, either isolated (e.g. Kallmann's syndrome, p. 1031) or associated with other hypothalamic disturbances. GT deficiency may be associated with other pituitary hormone deficiencies in pituitary aplasia or hypoplasia, craniopharyngioma, etc.

Hyperprolactinemia

Moderately raised PRL levels are an early nonspecific sign of neuroendocrine disturbance and particularly of suprasellar or hypothalamic space-occupying lesions. Stress causes a rise in PRL levels and serial sampling at half-hourly intervals from an indwelling cannula may be necessary to distinguish the two. Very high levels result from PRL-secreting micro- or macroadenomas but these are extremely rare in children. They may cause delayed puberty (p. 1031). Raised PRL in association with raised GT (and especially FSH) levels cause precocious puberty in primary hypothyroidism (p. 1050).

Intracranial space-occupying lesions

These are the second commonest neoplasms in children (after leukemia) accounting for 20% of the total. Endocrine aspects are of practical importance in a variety of ways:

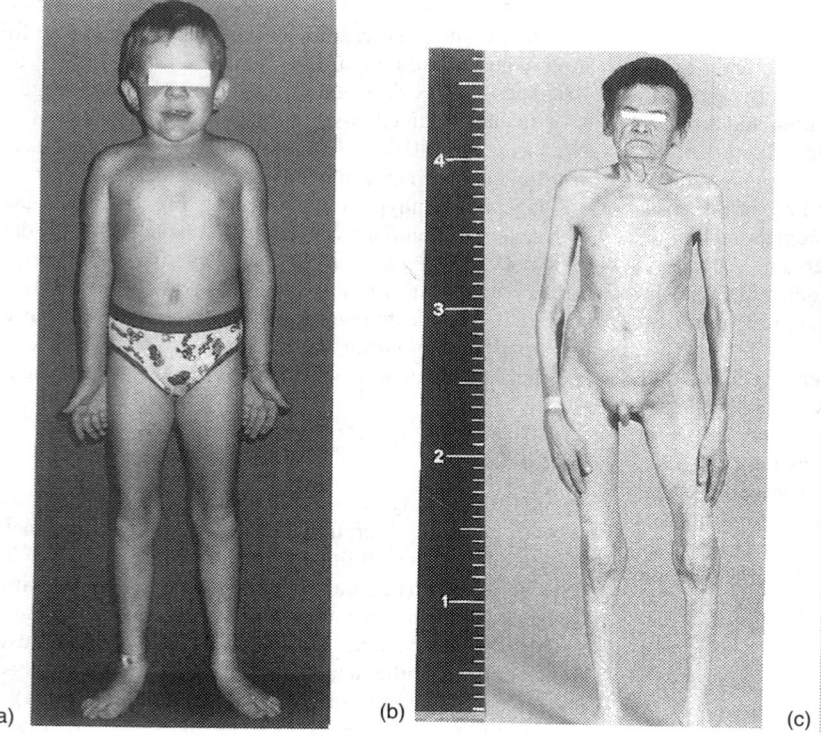
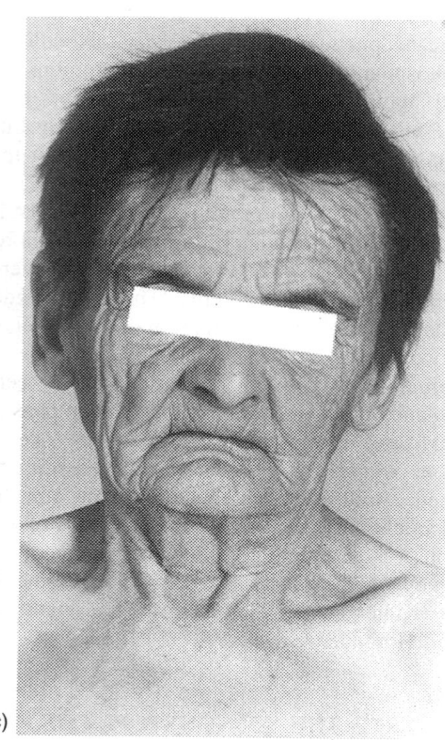

Fig. 19.31 Untreated panhypopituitarism (**a**) at age 11 years, (**b**) and (**c**) at age 71 years.

As 'early warning' signs of intracranial pathology

1. Moderately raised PRL levels in the absence of stress (see above).
2. Slow growth or signs of precocious or delayed puberty resulting from endocrine dysfunction may precede more specific clinical manifestations by many months.

In pre-, peri- and postoperative management

1. Hydrocortisone cover must be adequate for the stress of surgery, irradiation or radioactive implant.
2. Transient DI is common after surgery to the pituitary area but temporary inappropriate ADH secretion may occur (see p. 1040).

Permanent hormone replacement therapy after surgery and/or DXT

1. The need for therapy should be reassessed in terms of adeno- and neurohypophyseal function after these procedures – variable deficiencies of any or all hormones may be found. Long-term effects of irradiation on growth and endocrine function have become more obvious and important as survival following leukemia and brain tumors has improved. The hypothalamus is more susceptible than pituitary to damage. Spinal growth is impaired directly by spinal irradiation and GH deficiency (secondary to GHRH deficiency) is a virtually inevitable consequence of cranial irradiation in conventional (> 1800 cGy)

therapeutic dosage (Ahmed et al 1986). If a child has a good prognosis from the underlying condition 2 years from treatment, GH therapy is highly desirable. There is no evidence that GH is associated with reactivation of the primary lesion (Ogilvy-Stewart et al 1992). Other pituitary hormone deficiencies may also result from cranial DXT. Spinal irradiation may cause primary hypothyroidism or gonadal failure and chemotherapy may accentuate both problems. Growth and endocrine function following treatment of childhood malignant disease and the effects of chemotherapy are reviewed by Wallace (1996) and Wallace & Kelnar (1996a,b) respectively. Management of growth disorders secondary to treatment of childhood cancers is reviewed by Wallace & Kelnar (1997).

2. Some tumors are particularly associated with endocrine dysfunction. These include craniopharyngiomas, hypothalamic and optic nerve gliomas, third ventricular tumors and pituitary adenomas. Third ventricular tumors and hamartomas and other tumors of the pituitary stalk region may result in hypofunction, but may, like many pituitary adenomas, be functional. They seem commoner in boys and precocious puberty may be the earliest sign.

Craniopharyngioma

This is the commonest tumor affecting the hypothalamopituitary region in childhood and accounts for 8–13% of all intracranial tumors in those under 14 years of age. It results from embryonic, slowly growing remnants of Rathke's pouch and is initially suprasellar in origin. Expansion posterosuperiorly erodes the dorsum sellae causing hypothalamic and midbrain displacement. Nearly all contain areas of calcification but the tumors are usually cystic (containing cholesterol, cell debris and altered blood) with solid components (Kendall 1995).

Although benign, progressive local enlargement into important surrounding tissues, often late diagnosis (during the second decade of life) and difficulty of removal cause serious consequences. Regular growth assessment, clinical suspicion in a slowly growing child and fundal examination with recurrent headache or delayed puberty would all help reduce delay from first symptoms or signs to diagnosis which varies from 0.1 to 9 years (Lalu Keraly et al 1986). Obvious visual field defects, visual acuity impairment or neurological signs (cranial nerve palsies, optic atrophy, papilledema, effortless vomiting due to raised intracranial pressure) indicate a large tumor.

Plain lateral skull X-ray is often diagnostic revealing a mass containing calcification eroding the clinoid processes and an abnormally enlarged sella. CT or MRI scanning will confirm the diagnosis and determine any degree of suprasellar extension.

If the lesion is small (15% are still intrasellar at diagnosis) and adequate follow-up can be ensured with neuroradiological (CT or MRI) facilities, observation alone is justifiable (Lalu Keraly et al 1986). The endocrine situation is never improved by surgery or radiotherapy (usually it is made worse) and endocrine disturbance alone is not an indication for either form of treatment. When surgery is indicated, and it is urgent when there are visual or neurological disturbances, complete surgical excision without causing other damage is seldom possible because of the hardness of the tumor and its size (particularly if diagnosis is late). Subtotal excision is often inevitable whatever the preoperative intent and, although the tumors are not very radiosensitive, postoperative irradiation is thought to reduce recurrence risk.

Pre-, peri- and postoperative management and fluid balance must be meticulous. Pre-existing hormone deficiency should be corrected but hydrocortisone to cover the stress of the procedure must always be given even if ACTH reserve seems adequate. The need for long-term replacement therapies should be assessed several weeks postoperatively. DI may only become obvious after cortisol replacement. Occasional damage to the thirst center causes major management problems. In many cases, GH, thyroxine, hydrocortisone (certainly to cover stress and sometimes regularly), DDAVP and pubertal induction will be necessary. Despite appropriate hormone replacement, obesity can be a major long-term problem in many patients. The prognosis is improved with early diagnosis and careful initial management.

OTHER DISORDERS

Septo-optic dysplasia

This is a rare cause (Hoyt et al 1970) of disturbed hypothalamic function and resulting hypopituitarism (usually GT, GH and AVP deficiencies) usually presenting in infancy with hypothermia, hypoglycemia and blindness. CT or MRI scanning shows variable hypoplasia of the optic nerves, chiasma and hypothalamic infundibular region, often with absent septum pellucidum. Similar endocrine consequences are sometimes seen in other midline developmental abnormalities such as corpus callosum agenesis.

Empty sella syndrome

Pituitary hypoplasia is associated with a small fossa. The infundibulum and pituitary stalk are normal but the chiasmatic cistern may extend into the small sella and appear empty with the stalk outlined by CSF (Kendall 1995). Enlargement of the sella and pituitary has been found in some cases of primary hypothyroidism (Floyd et al 1984). Decreasing pituitary size on thyroxine replacement may give the appearance of an empty sella with the small pituitary gland situated posteroinferiorly within the enlarged fossa (Stanhope & Adlard 1987).

Diencephalic syndrome

This is usually due to an anteriorly growing hypothalamic glioma which presents in infancy or early childhood with excessive alertness and hyperexcitability, pallor, vomiting, gross wasting and failure to thrive. CSF protein levels are raised and tumor cells may be present. CT or MRI scanning will confirm the diagnosis.

Sotos' syndrome (cerebral gigantism) (Sotos et al 1964)

Birth weight and length are high reflecting rapid intrauterine growth. This continues until by middle childhood growth velocity is normal. As puberty occurs early, final stature is seldom excessive. Mental retardation is common but may be mild or absent. There are similarities with another tall stature syndrome, Beckwith–Wiedemann (p. 295) and excessive secretion of fetal growth factors could be etiologically important.

THE PINEAL GLAND

The pineal, like the hypothalamus, develops from the diencephalon. Ependymal cells and vascular mesenchyme from the anterior part of the diencephalic roof plate form the choroid plexus. Caudally, the roof plate of the diencephalon thickens, evaginates by about 7 weeks and forms an ultimately cone-shaped solid organ, the pineal, attached by a peduncle to the posterior border of the third ventricle. It lies in the quadrigeminal cistern between the superior colliculi covered by the splenium of the corpus callosum (Kendall 1995) and is innervated by postganglionic sympathetic superior cervical ganglionic nerve fibers. Pinealocytes form a mosaic pattern around capillaries, astrocytes and ganglion cells.

At one time thought to be the seat of the soul (Descartes), seen as guiding the cerebral hemispheres (Voltaire) or, more mundanely, being important in the control of the onset of human puberty (see p. 1023), the pineal role remains speculative. Pinealocytes convert tryptophan via serotonin to melatonin. It had been conjectured that endocrine pubertal events are inhibited prepubertally by melatonin, following reports that its concentration falls abruptly between pubertal stages G1 and G2 from age 11.5 to 14 years and that melatonin inhibits gonadal development in some males.

Other studies have demonstrated no inhibitory effect of melatonin on GT secretion. 24-h melatonin profiles are similar in prepuberty, puberty and adult males (low daytime levels, high nocturnal levels). Levels in precocious puberty are similar to those in normal puberty implying that melatonin has no major role in normal or precocious puberty, although blindness, which would upset the pineal circadian clock, is associated with early menarche (Zacharias & Wurtman 1964). Hypogonadal children with the Prader–Willi syndrome also have normal plasma melatonin rhythms and a study of urinary melatonin metabolite excretion during childhood and puberty found children to resemble adults with no marked changes of rhythm during puberty apart, surprisingly, from a rise in urinary 6-hydroxymelatonin excretion at the onset of breast development (Tanner stage 2) in girls.

Melatonin may have a role in inhibiting gonadal development – using a sensitive and specific assay, with frequent nighttime sampling, nocturnal melatonin levels decrease significantly with sexual maturation and age (Waldhauser et al 1984). However, the greatest fall in mean nocturnal melatonin levels was between prepubertal children under and over 7 years which does not support the hypothesis that it is that fall which triggers pubertal onset. There is evidence for a decline in the day to night increment of serum melatonin concentrations from infancy to childhood, that children with early puberty have lower melatonin day to night increments than age-matched controls, and that those with constitutionally delayed puberty show increments comparable to those of preschool children. This implies a relationship between maturation and the mechanisms controlling pineal gland secretion whether or not melatonin plays any significant role in the onset of puberty. For a review see Sizonenko & Lang (1988).

In pediatric practice, the pineal is important in two, sometimes related, contexts: rare pineal tumors and precocious puberty. Pineal tumors comprise < 1% of all intracranial tumors, are associated with precocious, delayed or absent puberty, but classically cause precocious puberty in boys. About half are radiosensitive germinomas; astrocytomas, gliomas, germ cell teratomas and carcinomas also occur. Pineal destruction is usually associated with precocious puberty (Kitay 1954). Germinomas sometimes secrete HCG and α-fetoprotein and secreting pineoblastomas and pineocytomas (pinealomas) occur.

Signs of raised intracranial pressure are common due to aqueduct compression. Visual loss, paresis of upward gaze and hypothalamic dysfunction (obesity, loss of temperature control, DI) may occur. Surgery is hazardous. Most pineal tumors recur after radiotherapy but germinomas are curable.

The pineal normally calcifies to varying extent with age. It is rarely seen radiographically before 6 years, is found in 2% by 8 years and 10% by 15 years (30% on CT scan). CT or MRI are indicated if calcification is seen on skull radiographs up to about 10 years (Kendall 1995) and in any boy with central precocious puberty (see p. 1029).

THE THYMUS

The thymus comprises cells of two origins. The epithelial component derives from 3rd and 4th pharyngeal pouches, the same embryological origin as the parathyroids. Thymic migration to the thorax from about 6 weeks is associated with parathyroid migration and branchial (pharyngeal) arch organization to form the aortic arch and other structures. Abnormal thymic stromal differentiation results in DiGeorge syndrome (p. 1252).

T lymphocyte progenitors travel from fetal liver and, postnatally, from bone marrow and undergo maturation within the thymus to form T lymphocytes – the lymphoid component. Thymic stromal cells manufacture humoral substances, thymosin and thymopoietin, thought to be important in this maturational process.

Thymus and other lymphoid tissues reach their greatest proportion of bodyweight at birth, and by puberty are nearly twice their size in the young adult (Scammon 1930). The decline to adult size is probably sex steroid mediated. Adrenalectomy delays involution and severe infection or stress hasten it.

Thymic tumors are rare, but may arise from either tissue component. There is an association with myasthenia gravis and tumors secreting an ACTH-like substance causing Cushing's syndrome are described.

THE THYROID GLAND

EMBRYOLOGY

The thyroid gland develops as an epithelial proliferation in the pharyngeal gut floor at 17 days between what will become the body and root of the tongue – the foramen cecum. It descends as a bilobed diverticulum in front of the pharyngeal gut, still connected to it by a canal – the thyroglossal duct. This normally disappears but cystic remnants may persist – a thyroglossal cyst. Migration continues in front of hyoid bone and laryngeal cartilages to the definitive position in front of the trachea by 7 weeks.

PHYSIOLOGY

By 30 min postdelivery, TSH levels surge, perhaps reacting to the cooler extrauterine environment. In response, within 28 h, total and free T3 and T4 levels rise – TBG levels do not change. High rT3 levels fall gradually over weeks. The importance of 'physiological neonatal hyperthyroidism' is not known, but animal data suggest a role in catecholamine-mediated brown fat and nonshivering thermogenesis.

Normal thyroid function is crucial in infancy and childhood because of its importance for normal somatic and brain growth and development. Thyroid hormone actions include protein synthesis, cholesterol turnover, water and ion transport and thermogenesis. There are direct and indirect (growth factor synthesis) effects on growth and CNS and skeletal development.

The thyroid concentrates iodide from blood (as do other tissues – salivary and mammary glands, placenta, uterus, stomach and small bowel) and (uniquely) combines it with tyrosine to form metabolically active derivatives. Endemic dietary iodine deficiency is the commonest cause of hypothyroidism and affects some 300 million people worldwide.

Steps in thyroid hormone biosynthesis are summarized in Figure 19.32. Inborn errors of each step are described and comprise about 10% of neonates with congenital nonendemic hypothyroidism. Transport of iodide into thyroid cells is rate limiting (Wolff 1983). Iodide oxidation (activation) is followed by peroxidase-catalyzed tyrosine iodination and iodotyrosine coupling to form T3 and T4. Thyroglobulin (TG), a high molecular weight iodinated glycoprotein, provides tyrosyl residues for iodotyrosine synthesis (any other physiological role is speculative) and reaches the circulation via thyroid lymphatics. Mono- and diiodotyrosine (MIT and DIT), T3 and T4 are stored as extracellular colloid. Thyroid hormone secretion involves formation of intracellular colloid droplets, fusion with lysosomes, proteolytic digestion and hydrolysis of thyroglobulin to form free MIT, DIT, T3 and T4. T3 and T4 are released into the circulation; MIT and DIT are deiodinated and free iodide is reutilized for hormone synthesis.

Physiological thyroid hormone action at cellular level is by binding to a specific nuclear plasma membrane and mitochondrial receptors. T3 binding to nuclear receptors seems most important.

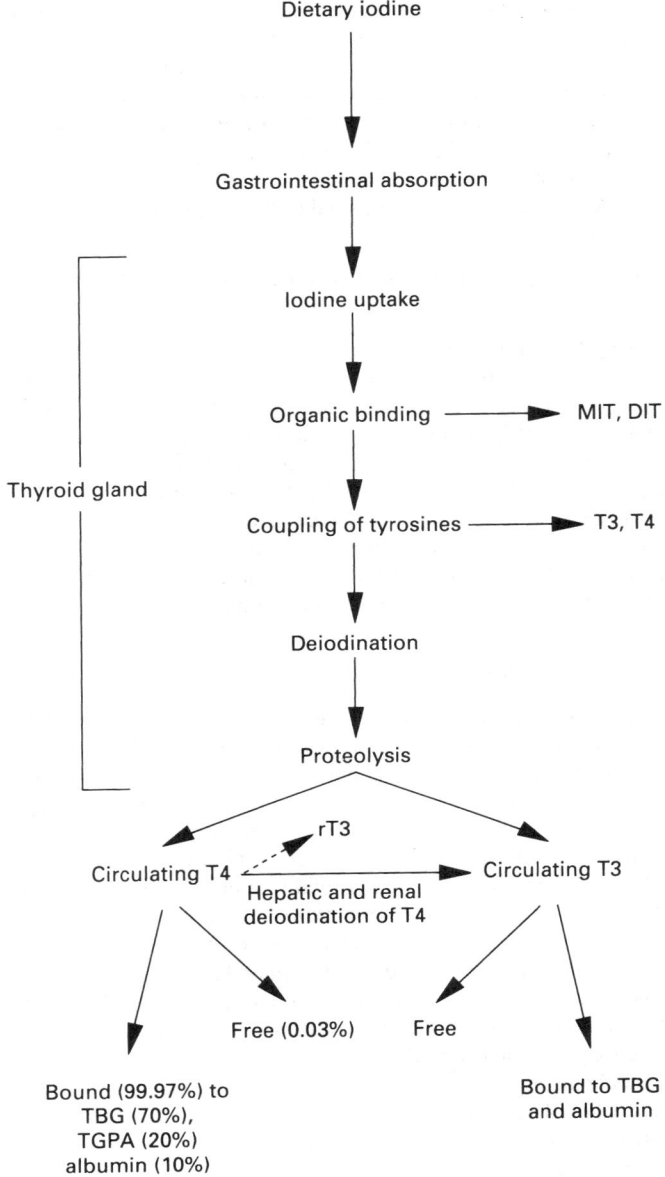

Fig. 19.32 Thyroid hormone biosynthesis.

REGULATION OF FUNCTION

Plasma iodide and circulating TSH levels regulate thyroid follicular cell function. Circulating FT4 exerts negative feedback on TSH release. 75–80% of circulating FT3 is produced by deiodination of T4 in peripheral tissues. The control mechanism for production of T3 in nonthyroidal tissue is poorly understood but during many disease states or fasting T4 conversion to T3 is reduced and (inactive) rT3 accumulates (Beckett & Seth 1989). T3 has three to four times the potency of T4 and binds to cell membrane receptor proteins with 10-fold greater affinity.

THYROID FUNCTION TESTS (TFTS)

Normal ranges for TFTs are age related and vary between laboratories. The most sensitive single test of primary thyroid

disease is plasma TSH immunoradiometric assay (IRMA). In primary hypothyroidism levels are raised; in hyperthyroidism (or overtreatment of hypothyroidism) levels are suppressed, usually to below the assay detection limit (< 0.1 mU/l). RIA TSH measurement will not reliably distinguish appropriate from excessive replacement.

Total T3 (TT3) and T4 (TT4) levels reflect TBG levels; free (active) hormone measurements (FT3, FT4) reflect functional thyroid status more accurately. T3 may be a more sensitive guide to developing thyrotoxicosis than T4 if TSH IRMA assays are unavailable, but diagnosis on clinical examination is seldom problematic.

Biochemical assessment strategies are reviewed by Vanderscheuren-Lodeweyckx (1992). It is good practice to measure TSH and FT4 simultaneously to assess the whole axis. TRH tests are useful in assessing hypothalamopituitary function: in hypothalamic or pituitary disease, basal TSH levels will be inappropriately low for the T4 levels; in pituitary disease, TSH levels will fail to rise in response to TRH (7 μg/kg i.v. over several minutes); in hypothalamic disease there is an exaggerated and delayed TSH response (60 min levels higher than at 20 min) as TSH must be synthesized before its release, but this is not always seen and can occur in normal children.

Most specific situations where nonthyroidal illness, pregnancy or drug treatment cause abnormal TFTs (e.g. malnutrition, anorexia nervosa) are uncommon in pediatric practice provided tests are not performed during severe intercurrent illness. During the acute phase of such illnesses (e.g. severe burns or trauma, diabetic ketoacidosis, liver or renal failure), TT3, TT4 and FT3 levels are often low; FT4 may be low or normal (depending on assay methodology (Beckett & Seth 1989); TSH may also be low or normal. During recovery, thyroid hormone levels gradually normalize, but persisting low levels, even with raised TSH levels, do not necessarily indicate hypothyroidism.

Drugs affecting TFTs include estrogens, salicylates, phenytoin, carbamazepine, glucocorticoids and propranolol. Iodide (in expectorants) can cause clinical, as well as biochemical, hypothyroidism.

Apparent thyroid disorders in euthyroid patients due to abnormal carrier proteins will not cause confusion if free hormone and IRMA TSH assays are available. Children with hereditary TBG deficiency (X-linked dominant inheritance, incidence 1 in 10 000, males : females 9 : 1) will have low TT4 and TT3 levels; high levels of TBG, and thus of TT4 and TT3, are seen during estrogen therapy. In both situations, FT4, FT3 and TSH levels are normal and the patient is clinically euthyroid.

Raised TSH levels with normal FT4 levels in treated hypothyroidism may indicate poor compliance (other than just before a clinic visit). TFTs must always be considered in the context of growth velocity and skeletal maturation and not in isolation (see earlier). Clinical examination alone for signs of hypothyroidism or thyrotoxicosis is a very insensitive guide.

FUNCTION IN PRETERM INFANTS

TT4 and FT4 levels increase with gestation – ~ 25% of preterm infants have low levels by term standards (50% at less than 30 weeks). FT4 levels are never as low as in congenital hypothyroidism. There is presumed hypothalamic immaturity: TSH levels may be normal or low; TSH and T4 levels rise normally following TRH. T4 levels correct spontaneously with maturation over 4–8 weeks, postnatal growth and development are normal and treatment is unnecessary.

There are babies (term or preterm), however, with significantly reduced FT4 levels (into the congenital hypothyroidism range). This seems much commoner in Europe than the USA (perhaps reflecting relative iodine availability). Prevalence in Belgium is 20% in the preterm and related to gestational length (Delange et al 1986). Cord blood T4 and TSH levels are normal for gestation – transient hypothyroidism develops during the first 2 weeks with important implications for screening. In many, thyroid function quickly normalizes; in others, recovery may take 1–2 months and treatment is necessary. Transient hypothyroidism may occur in preterm infants exposed in utero to maternal iodine-containing drugs or following injection of radiographic contrast agents.

Low T3 levels are commonly seen in preterm infants and may persist for 1–2 months. They are due to the lower T3 postnatal surge and reduced conversion of T4 to T3 in peripheral tissues resulting from, for example, birth asphyxia, hypoglycemia, hypocalcemia and relative malnutrition. FT4 and TSH levels are usually normal for gestational age and no treatment is necessary.

HYPOFUNCTION

Congenital

Thyroid dysgenesis

The commonest cause of congenital hypothyroidism is aplastic, hypoplastic or ectopic thyroid tissue – thyroid dysgenesis – occurring with consistent prevalence worldwide: 1 in 3500 to 4500 births. Females are twice as commonly affected but familial cases are rare – nearly all occur sporadically and idiopathically although there is increased incidence in Down syndrome babies and seasonal variation. In ~ 50% there is some functioning thyroid tissue resulting in a spectrum of severity of hypothyroidism. There is generally no relationship with maternal thyroid function, treatment with thyroxine or thyroid autoimmune status (see Grüters 1996). A role for immunoglobulins which block TSH-stimulated thyroid cell growth in vitro (Van der Gaag et al 1985) in pathogenesis remains speculative.

Dyshormonogenesis (inborn errors of thyroid hormone biosynthesis)

Autosomal recessively inherited defects in thyroid hormone biosynthesis are the second commonest causes of congenital hypothyroidism, accounting for about 10% of those identified on screening (i.e. about 1 in 40 000 births). Presence of a goiter at birth is strongly suggestive but goiter may not develop for months or years. There is a spectrum of hypofunction but it is generally less severe than in the dysgenetic group. Sex incidence is equal.

A defect may occur at any biosynthetic step (Fig. 19.32):

1. Decreased TSH responsiveness – very rare.
2. Decreased trapping of iodide: thyroid enlargement and reduced (or virtually absent) radioiodine (RAI) uptake by thyroid and tissues such as salivary glands and gastric mucosa.
3. Defective organification: peroxidase deficiency (defective oxidation of thyroidal iodide to reactive iodine). The association with high tone or complete nerve deafness (Pendred's syndrome, 2 per 100 000 children of school age) is not due to peroxidase deficiency – the precise etiology of the thyroid biosynthetic defect

(and deafness) is unknown. Together, these are the commonest dyshormonogenetic defects. In peroxidase deficiency (and most Pendred patients) there is a rapid fall in thyroid radioactivity with thiocyanate or perchlorate after radioiodine administration.

4. Defective iodotyrosine coupling or deiodination: nondeiodination of MIT and DIT leads to their leakage from the gland, urinary excretion and iodine loss.
5. Abnormal thyroglobulin synthesis, storage or release.

Hypothalamopituitary (tertiary/secondary) congenital hypothyroidism

Congenital hypothyroidism due to TRH or TSH deficiency may be familial or sporadic, isolated or associated with other hypothalamopituitary deficiencies and can be associated with anatomical defects (e.g. absent pituitary or sella turcica). Prevalence is about 1 in 100 000 births. Associated hypothyroidism will be missed by TSH screening. This is not critically important – there are often associated features (dysmorphism, micropenis, hypoglycemia) drawing attention to the differential diagnosis. Hypothyroidism is generally mild and treatment can be unnecessary for some months.

Clinical and laboratory features

During the early weeks of life, babies are usually asymptomatic and early clinical signs are nonspecific (Fig. 19.33): even in 'developed' countries only about 5% are diagnosed before the positive screening result and only ~ 50% can be diagnosed reliably before 3 months, by when subsequent neurodevelopmental problems are much more likely (Barnes 1985, Grüters 1996). No screening program is totally reliable – there must still be clinical suspicion in certain circumstances. Important features include: umbilical hernia, wide posterior fontanel or goiter at birth, a placid, sleepy, 'good' baby, poor feeding, constipation, hypothermia, peripheral cyanosis, edema, prolonged physiological jaundice. More specific features such as the coarse facies, large tongue, hoarse cry, dry skin and low hair line are late signs.

Biochemically, both dysgenetic and dyshormonogenetic groups have low T4 and high TSH levels after neonatal changes have settled. About 1 in 6 will have T4 levels in the lower part of the normal range.

Screening (see Grüters 1996)

Although clinical detection of congenital hypothyroidism is unreliable, no screening program is 100% specific and sensitive: there may be laboratory error, communication breakdown between laboratory and clinician and there is a minority of affected babies in whom the screening result will be normal. Up to 10% of babies with congenital hypothyroidism will not have grossly elevated screening TSH values. Where TSH is used for screening, hypothyroidism due to hypothalamic or pituitary disease will be missed; where T4 (followed by TSH for the lower range of T4 values) is used, a 10th centile or absolute T4 level of 130–140 nmol/l cut-off is used as < 20% of affected babies have low normal (90–140 nmol/l) T4 levels.

All abnormal or suspicious screening results must be confirmed before the infant is committed to long-term therapy but it is safer to start thyroxine whilst definitive results are awaited. If they are normal, full reassessment is necessary.

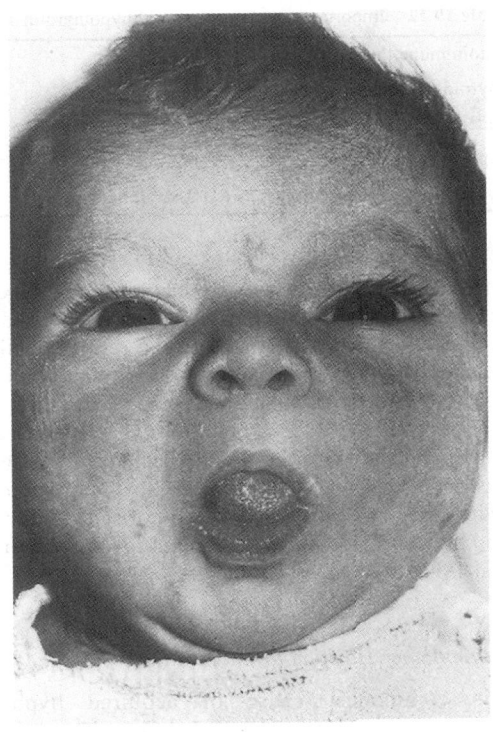

(a)

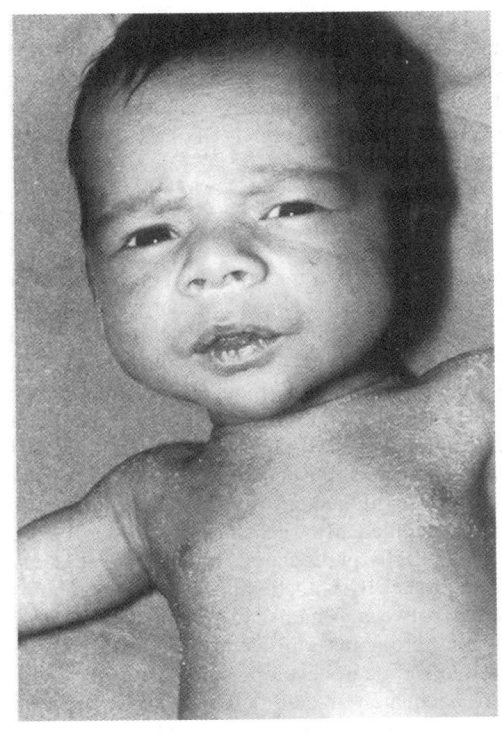

(b)

Fig. 19.33   Congenital hypothyroidism presenting (**a**) at 3 months in 1978 (prior to UK screening) and (**b**) at 10 days following a raised level of TSH screening (1983).

Scanning

Thyroid scans using ^{99m}Tc-pertechnetate or ^{123}I-labeled sodium iodide (the latter has the advantage of shorter half-life and better concentration in the thyroid (Walker & Hughes 1995)) are no longer routinely recommended in the newborn for detection and anatomical localization of functioning thyroid tissue and to exclude the commonest dyshormonogenetic defect (organification) (Grüters 1996). Results are unreliable, especially when tests are performed by inexperienced investigators, and misleading results can result from maternal blocking immunoglobulins or perinatal iodine contamination (Connors & Styne 1986). Ultrasound can reveal whether thyroid tissue is present in the normal position. If no gland is detectable with normal T3 but low T4 levels and measurable levels of thyroglobulin, an ectopic rest of thyroid tissue is likely.

Following ^{123}I-labeled sodium iodide scanning, most dyshormonogenetic defects (other than of iodide trapping) will show high or normal isotope uptake and normal thyroid position and anatomy. In the commonest defect (peroxidase deficiency) there is discharge of 60–70% of radioactive iodide within 1 h following perchlorate. If organification is normal, less than 5–10% is discharged within 1 h (Walker & Hughes 1995). Frequencies of different possible biosynthetic defects are unknown although molecular genetic studies have revealed mutations in the TPO and thyroglobulin genes in some familial cases (Bikker et al 1995).

Treatment

Once the diagnosis is suspected, treatment is urgent and should be started immediately blood has been taken for definitive testing without waiting for those results. Sodium-l-thyroxine (l-T4) is the treatment of choice as it is reliably absorbed and its peripheral endogenous conversion to T3 allows automatic 'fine tuning' of function. In infancy, T4 levels should be in the upper normal range and T3 levels normal. TSH levels must not be used as a guide to treatment efficacy in infancy – in > 50% the feedback set point is abnormal and TSH levels remain high in the presence of adequate replacement and normal T4 (Sato et al 1957).

Starting dose of l-T4 is 10–15 µg/kg orally once daily and is usually appropriate throughout infancy. A recent retrospective, nonrandomized study (Rovet & Ehrlich 1995) has shown higher full-scale and verbal IQ results at 7–8 years on this dose compared with lower doses, but the higher-dose group were also treated earlier. Prospective randomized studies are needed. Subsequently, the required daily dose is ~ 100 µg/m²/24 h. Overtreatment will cause symptoms and signs of thyrotoxicosis but clinical assessment alone only detects significant under- or over-replacement. Marginal over-replacement can generally be compensated for by endogenous deiodination but under-replacement may result in significant long-term neurological impairment.

Growth, TFTs, bone age maturation and clinical progress (including psychomotor development) should be checked regularly during the first year. Assessment should be at 1 month and then every 3 months. It is essential that parents know the importance of giving the l-T4 regularly and do not forget or stop treatment because baby seems normal.

By the third year of life, briefly interrupting medication will have no long-term effects on brain growth and development and is necessary to assess the need for permanent treatment. So as to minimize the time off treatment, T3 (with its shorter half-life) can be substituted for l-T4 therapy (100 μg l-T4 is equivalent to 20 μg T3) for 2 weeks, all treatment stopped for 7 days, thyroid function checked (and an isotope scan performed if indicated) and the previous l-T4 dose restarted immediately whilst results are awaited and assessed. Alternatively l-T4 can simply be discontinued for 2 weeks.

Outcome

'Not the magic wand of Prospero or the brave kiss of the daughter of Hippocrates ever effected such a change as that which we are now enabled to make in these unfortunate victims, doomed heretofore to live in hopeless imbecility, an unspeakable affliction to their parents and their relatives' – William Osler (1897) on the transforming effects of (recently introduced) thyroid replacement therapy. However, although gross physical manifestations of congenital hypothyroidism are abolished by treatment, significant neurodevelopmental and intellectual deficits remain unless treatment is started during the early weeks of life (Grüters 1996).

Delay beyond 3 months is particularly serious: in one study (Klein et al 1972) the mean IQ with treatment before 3 months was 89, 70 if started between 3 and 6 months and 54 after 6 months. With screening programs, sufficiently early diagnosis is almost always possible and neurodevelopmental prognosis good. At 2 years, children adequately treated before 4 weeks show no differences from controls on the Bayley mental development index, and at 3, 4 and 5 years in Stanford Binet IQ assessment, in contrast to those inadequately treated (New England Congenital Hypothyroidism Collaborative 1984). However, there may be subtle deficiencies in hearing/speech performance scales at 1 year and practical reasoning at 18 months and 3 years and, possibly, in motor and perceptual abilities, speech, behavior and personality.

It seems that a low T4 level (< 30–40 nmol/l) at diagnosis is associated with a deficit in mental development (Fuggle et al 1991). A recent comprehensive UK survey (Tillotson et al 1994) has demonstrated a discontinuous effect of severity of congenital hypothyroidism with a risk of a 10-point IQ deficit with initial thyroxine level of < 40 nmol/l. Lower social class (perhaps also associated with poorer compliance) accounted for another 10-point IQ decrement. Up to 10% needed special education (Simons et al 1994) in contrast to other studies (New England Congenital Hypothyroidism Collaborative 1990). Surprisingly, timing of onset of treatment did not seem important.

It is still controversial, therefore, how early treatment must be started to minimize problems and what the relevance of age of onset or severity of fetal hypothyroidism may be. Even if treatment is started within 10–14 days of birth, there is still likely to be a minority in whom long-term neurodevelopmental functioning is suboptimal.

Acquired

Hypothyroidism may develop, usually insidiously, at any age. Important causes are summarized in Table 19.12.

Endemic iodine deficiency

Worldwide, ~ 300 million people have endemic goiter. Simple iodine deficiency is generally responsible but genetic factors may predispose and environmental goitrogens (e.g. *Brassica* vegetables) potentiate the effects. Iodine deficiency leads to

Table 19.12   Important causes of acquired hypothyroidism in childhood

Autoimmune thyroiditis
Thyroid dysgenesis
Endemic iodine deficiency
Exposure to goitrogens
Hypothalamopituitary disease (TRH/TSH deficiency)

deficient thyroid hormone production, TSH hypersecretion and increased iodide trapping with goiter and raised T3 : T4 ratio. Such compensatory mechanisms can result in euthyroidism with goiter or varying degrees of goitrous hypothyroidism. In endemic areas < 8% of the population may be affected.

The problem is still common in some areas of Europe, Scandinavia and the Middle East including Switzerland, Finland, Austria, Germany, Italy, Spain, Greece, Lebanon and Iraq. In Switzerland and Finland iodination of salt is effectively reducing the prevalence – endemic cretinism is now uncommon (Delange et al 1986).

Autoimmune (Hashimoto) thyroiditis

This commonest cause of acquired hypothyroidism in nonendemic areas of iodine deficiency was described by Hashimoto (1912). Girls are much more commonly affected; a family history of thyroid disorders is found in about one-third.

The gland, infiltrated by lymphocytes and plasma cells (delayed hypersensitivity) with fibrosis and degeneration, is generally irregularly enlarged and firm. There is prominence of normal architecture but usually no nodules. Acinar regeneration can occur – growth immunoglobulins and TSH may be important for this (Toft 1989a). One or more of several possible types of circulating antithyroid antibodies are found in about 95% at presentation but such antibodies also occur in up to 20% of the 'normal' population (some of whom may eventually develop thyroiditis). The commonest antibodies are against thyroglobulin and microsomes but antiperoxidase, TSH-receptor blocking or stimulating, colloid and thyroid growth inhibiting or stimulating antibodies may occur. Antinuclear factor (ANF) is particularly likely to be positive in children.

Presentation may be with euthyroid goiter, goiter with hypothyroidism or in the context of pre-existing autoimmune disease. In < 10%, and particularly at adolescence, presentation may be with signs of thyrotoxicosis. Usually, however, onset is with insidious hypothyroidism – classical myxedema may not occur for many months (Fig. 19.34). School performance frequently deteriorates but can be attributed to other problems. Height velocity slows but this may not be recognized if children are not measured regularly – slow growth must be prolonged before a single measurement or simple observation detects conspicuous short stature.

In a still euthyroid child, diagnosis can be made on the basis of goiter, increased antithyroglobulin or antimicrosomal antibody titers, abnormal thyroid scan with positive perchlorate discharge test and biochemical signs of compensated hypothyroidism.

Associated multiple endocrine deficiency disease includes diabetes mellitus with or without adrenal insufficiency (Schmidt's syndrome), hypoparathyroidism, moniliasis, pernicious anemia and thrombocytopenia. < 30% of children with type 1 diabetes

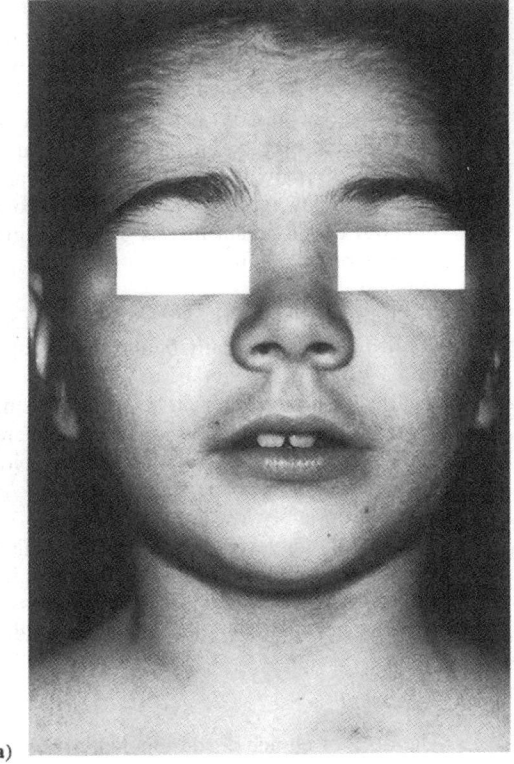
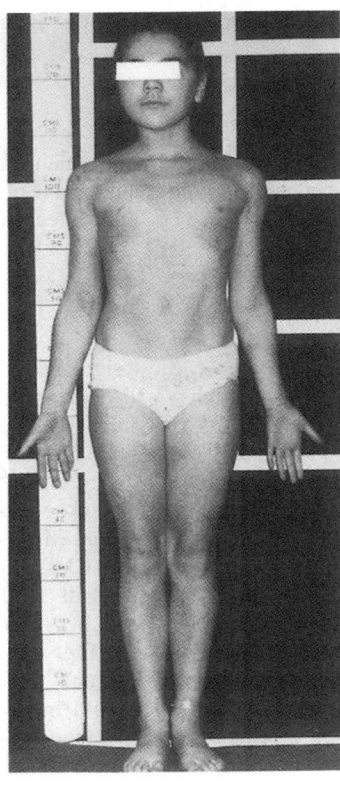

(a)   (b)

Fig. 19.34   The result of insidious development of hypothyroidism over several years.

mellitus will have detectable thyroid antibodies and 10% will have raised TSH levels. There is an association between autoimmune thyroid disease and a variety of cytogenetic disorders including Down, Turner's, Klinefelter's and Noonan's syndromes (Kelnar 1989). All children with diabetes mellitus and cytogenetic disorders should be screened regularly for thyroid disease.

There is usually progressive thyroid atrophy and treatment, once started, is generally lifelong. If there is initial hyperfunction, euthyroidism and eventual hypothyroidism will probably develop. Spontaneous remission is said to occur in < 30% of adolescents. Nodules in Hashimoto thyroiditis are due to lymphoid or thyroid hyperplasia and only rarely indicate malignancy.

Diffuse goiter in a euthyroid adolescent occurs commonly in nonendemic areas. Some have Hashimoto thyroiditis but in others aspiration biopsy shows a colloid goiter with no evidence of the characteristic lymphocytic infiltration and there may be autosomal dominant transmission. Although, in the medium term, the goiter usually regresses untreated, the common finding of thyroid-stimulating immunoglobulins (TSI), and the fact that a significant number of adults presenting with nodular goiters have a history of diffuse adolescent goiter, suggest that autoimmune mechanisms are important for pathogenesis.

Thyroid dysgenesis

Most inborn errors of biosynthesis present in the newborn or by infancy. However, if defects are mild and compensated, goiter develop slowly and hypothyroidism may not develop until childhood. There is increased incidence of thyroid dysgenesis in Down syndrome.

Ectopic and inadequately functional thyroid may present as an enlarging mass at the base of the tongue or along the course of the thyroglossal duct ('cryptothyroidism' – Little et al 1965). Removal of a 'thyroglossal cyst' may result in severe hypothyroidism if that is the only functional thyroid tissue present.

Thyroid destruction due to infiltration with cystine crystals may cause eventual hypothyroidism in children with cystinosis.

Exposure to goitrogens

Foods interfering with thyroid hormone biosynthesis include cabbage, cassava and soybeans. Ingestion of goitrogen in the context of a genetically predisposed population or iodine deficiency is more likely to result in frank hypothyroidism. Drugs acting similarly including iodide (in proprietary expectorants), perchlorate and thiocyanate, lithium, amiodarone, phenylbutazone, aminoglutethemide, aminosalicylic acid and the specifically antithyroid drugs, carbimazole and propylthiouracil.

Hypothalamopituitary-dependent hypothyroidism

Slowing of linear growth due to TSH or associated GH deficiency is the usual presentation with a history of head injury, cranial irradiation for leukemia or medulloblastoma, meningitis or granulomatous disease. Craniopharyngioma must be excluded. There may be associated neurological signs, and symptoms or signs relating to underlying disease, or hypothalamopituitary dysfunction. Latent hypothalamopituitary hypothyroidism may develop in 'isolated' GH deficiency treated with GH and may prevent growth acceleration. GH appears to inhibit the pituitary–thyroid axis in rats (Root et al 1986) but the mechanism in man is unknown.

Thyroid hormone unresponsiveness

Families with goiter and variable thyroid hormone unresponsiveness have been described with possible autosomal dominant or recessive inheritance (Refetoff 1982). The defect may be at receptor or postreceptor level.

Presentation and diagnosis

Slowing of height velocity is the earliest sign. Retrospectively, growth data (or holiday photographs) will help pinpoint age at onset. Skinfold measurements are usually increased and bone age delayed but both are common in many childhood endocrinopathies. Very delayed skeletal maturation (> 3 years over chronological age) is a particular feature. Muscle weakness is common on testing but is seldom a presenting complaint. Muscle atrophy, hypertrophy and dysfunction are described. Classical signs of myxedema (Toft 1989a) develop gradually with infiltration of many tissues (including skin) by mucopolysaccharides, hyaluronic acid and chondroitin sulfate (Fig. 19.34). Skin becomes yellow from high carotene levels and there may be tiredness (with poor school performance), cold intolerance and characteristically slow relaxation of tendon reflexes. Hypertrichosis with low hair line may occur (Stern & Kelnar 1985) as may hair loss with alopecia (Fig. 19.35).

Classically pubertal delay occurs, but a significant minority develop precocious puberty and this may occur whilst the child is still clinically euthyroid. A failing thyroid gland causes hypothalamic release of TRH; consequent high TSH levels initially maintain euthyroidism but TRH also stimulates PRL and GT (LH and FSH) causing ovarian estradiol secretion and breast development in girls and testicular (and sometimes penile)

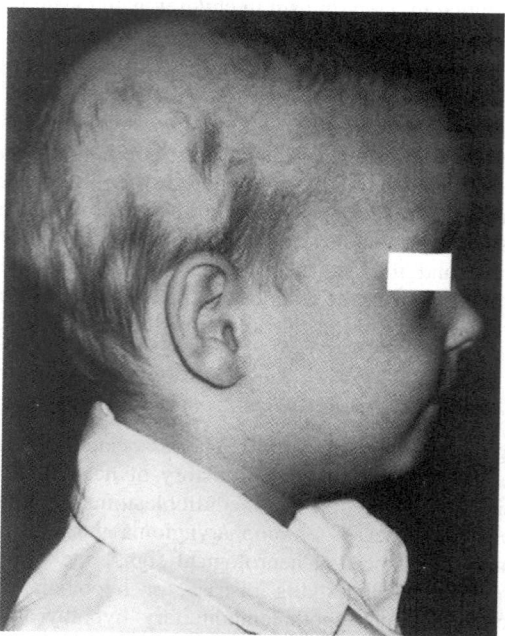

Fig. 19.35 Alopecia associated with autoimmune hypothyroidism.

enlargement in boys. PRL may cause inhibition of gonadal stimulation by LH but not FSH resulting in sustained gonadal stimulation (Castro-Magana et al 1988). A direct effect of TSH on the hCG receptor has also been described (Hidaka et al 1993).

Precocious puberty with bone age delay is pathognomonic. The sella turcica may be enlarged. Why a minority of children with acquired hypothyroidism develop sexual precocity rather than pubertal delay is unexplained. On thyroid replacement therapy pubertal development arrests and there may be some regression until puberty recommences at a time appropriate to bone age maturity.

Clinical diagnosis of acquired hypothyroidism must be confirmed biochemically before treatment is started. Low total or free T4 or T3 levels confirm hypothyroidism, raised TSH levels that the defect is at thyroid level. A goiter necessitates thyroid and other autoantibody measurement. If there is no goiter, or no evidence of autoimmune disease, thyroid scanning to exclude dysgenesis is valuable.

Inappropriately low (i.e. low or normal) TSH levels for low T3 or T4 levels suggest hypothalamic or pituitary disease. A TRH test may be helpful. With acquired TSH deficiency, pituitary function and neuroradiological tests are necessary to identify other pituitary hormone deficiencies and exclude a pituitary tumor.

Treatment

The drug of choice is sodium-1-thyroxine (l-T4) – usually ~ 100 $\mu g/m^2/24$ h once daily but precisely adjusted individually. Catch-up growth usually follows onset of treatment and height prognosis is favorable in comparison with most growth disorders. However, it is important to interpret height velocity on treatment in the context of accurate assessment of rate of bone age maturation. Inappropriately rapid skeletal maturation for height velocity indicates overtreatment and will result irretrievably in stunting due to early epiphyseal fusion. IRMA TSH levels are sensitive markers of over-replacement, under-replacement or noncompliance (except in hypothalamopituitary disease).

There is controversy about whether to treat euthyroid patients with compensated autoimmune hypothyroidism. Treatment does not alter the natural progression of the disease and chronic oversecretion of TRH/TSH is not generally associated with problems (although there are theoretical risks in children treated with radiotherapy for brain tumors), but enlarged pituitary fossa and secondary pituitary failure have been described. Often free T4 levels are low and if so, or growth velocity is slow, treatment should certainly start.

Outcome

Mental retardation does not occur in late-onset hypothyroidism. School performance and growth improve on appropriate replacement therapy. Final height is normal for the family.

HYPERFUNCTION (Dallas & Foley 1996)

Neonatal

Neonatal thyrotoxicosis is rare and usually due to transplacental passage of TSI from a mother with active or inactive Graves' disease or Hashimoto thyroiditis. High maternal antibody titers are strong predictors of neonatal disease in a clinically euthyroid mother whose disease has been inactive for many years. Only ~ 1.5% of mothers with thyrotoxicosis due to Graves' disease will have affected babies (Burrow 1974). Thyrotoxicosis is nevertheless rare in pregnancy – autoimmune disease tends to remit during pregnancy and anovulatory cycles are common in thyrotoxic women.

Goiter may be present at birth and an irritable infant rapidly develops tachycardia, dysrhythmias, flushing, hypertension and weight loss (until cardiac failure supervenes) despite ravenous hunger. There may be associated jaundice, hepatosplenomegaly and a bleeding tendency due to thrombocytopenia and low prothrombin levels. In some, symptoms and signs are delayed for 7–10 days either because of transplacental passage of maternal antithyroid drugs or postnatal T4 to T3 conversion.

Total and free T4 and T3 levels are high and TSH suppressed within a few days – cord blood levels may be normal. The half-life of TSI is 2–3 weeks and clinical resolution of the disorder mirrors their degradation – the condition is generally self-limiting over 4–12 weeks. In severely affected babies, mortality may be up to 25% due to cardiac arrhythmias or high output failure. Propranolol (1–2 mg/kg/24 h) with carbimazole (0.5–1 mg/kg/24 h) and Lugol's iodine (5% iodine, 10% potassium iodide, 8 mg t.d.s.) to inhibit thyroid hormone synthesis and secretion may be life saving. Satisfactory response is usually seen within 24–36 h. As thyrotoxicosis comes under control, iodine and propranolol can be gradually withdrawn and carbimazole gradually discontinued from about 6 weeks. Rarely, persisting hyperthyroidism suggests early-onset Graves' disease.

Graves' disease

In children, thyrotoxicosis is nearly always due to Graves' disease, is much rarer than hypothyroidism and rarer than in adults – only about 5% of patients with Graves' disease present in childhood or adolescence, usually in the second decade. It is three- to fivefold commoner in girls. As in Hashimoto thyroiditis, there is evidence of an autoimmune disorder on a background of genetic (HLA A1, B8, DR3) predisposition and positive family history of thyroid disease in ~ 60%.

The thyrotoxicosis is due to thyroid follicular cell TSH receptor IgG antibodies – thyroid-stimulating immunoglobulins (TSI) – which bind to the extracellular receptor domain stimulating thyroid hormone release analogously to TSH via the adenyl cyclase cAMP system (Toft 1989b). They do not cause the eye signs although these too are immunologically mediated. The TSH receptor is a 744 amino acid, single chain, polypeptide glycoprotein member of the guanine-nucleotide-binding (G) protein-coupled receptor family and represents the primary target antigen for autoantibodies mediating the hyperthyroidism and goiter of Graves' disease. Glycosylation is necessary for receptor expression and hormone–receptor interactions. The cDNA encoding the human TSH receptor has now been cloned and characterized (Nagayama & Rappoport 1992, Vassart & Dumont 1992).

Clinical features

The onset may be insidious and is usually well established before presentation to a physician. As in hypothyroidism, poor school performance may be marked, but usually from poor concentration, tiredness and behavior disturbances with temper tantrums and emotional lability. There is marked weight loss despite rapid growth and enormous appetite. The gland is usually diffusely enlarged and often with a bruit. Many systemic (tachycardia, tremor and sweating) and eye (staring due to lid retraction, wide palpebral aperture and lid lag) signs reflect sympathetic overactivity. Periorbital puffiness, exophthalmos, chemosis and squint due to infiltration of the orbit, lacrimal glands and ocular muscles occur less commonly and severely than in adults, but exophthalmos in particular may persist once euthyroidism is established. Pretibial myxedema characteristic of adults is rare in children.

Diagnosis

In children, a clinical diagnosis can usually be made confidently, but there must be biochemical confirmation and hyperthyroidism secondary to TSH hypersecretion must be excluded. Usually free and total T4 levels are high (occasionally they are normal but T3 levels are raised) and TSH is suppressed even using a sensitive (IRMA) assay. TSI are positive. Skeletal maturity is generally advanced disproportionately for the rapid growth.

Treatment

Treatment aims to reduce excessive thyroid hormone secretion and blunt the somatic consequences (largely mediated via β-adrenergic pathways). The former may be achieved with antithyroid drugs (e.g. carbimazole or propylthiouracil), surgery (subtotal thyroidectomy) or radioactive iodine (^{131}I). In childhood, in most centers, antithyroid drugs are the initial treatment of choice. These inhibit diiodotyrosine and iodothyronine formation and, to some extent, tyrosine iodination (Toft 1989b). Thyroid function normalizes by 3–4 weeks. The initial dose of carbimazole in childhood is 0.5 mg/kg/24 h and of propylthiouracil 5 mg/kg/24 h, both in three divided doses.

Skin rashes occur in ~ 2–3% on either drug, are usually transient and a change of therapy is not usually necessary, particularly if antihistamine is used symptomatically. More seriously, agranulocytosis may occur idiosyncratically, unpredicted from serial blood counts. Full recovery usually occurs on stopping treatment and the alternative can generally be substituted as cross-reactivity is rare. Progressive neutropenia can also occur and symptoms such as sore throat must be taken seriously and blood count checked regularly.

Once clinical and biochemical euthyroidism is achieved, it is probably beneficial (in terms of reducing both the goiter and necessity for frequent monitoring of thyroid function for developing hypothyroidism) to add l-thyroxine to an appropriate (usually half to one-third of initial dose) antithyroid medication. Combination therapy has also been reported to decrease production of TSI and the frequency of thyrotoxicosis recurrence in adults (Hashizume et al 1991).

Although antithyroid drugs do not alter the natural disease process, they do, in most children, allow maintenance of euthyroidism until spontaneous remission occurs (usually after about 2 years). Signs that this is not the case include persisting goiter and continuing presence of TSI. In any case there is a high relapse rate (50–70% within 2 years) (Toft 1989b).

Beta-blockers (e.g. propranolol) are valuable during the first 2–3 weeks of treatment in providing symptomatic relief of tachycardia, nervousness and tremor and can then be discontinued as the specific antithyroid drug becomes clinically effective.

Subtotal thyroidectomy is the treatment of choice in young adults in whom hyperthyroidism has returned after > 2 years of medical treatment or if compliance with treatment is poor – and, because of high relapse rates on medical treatment, is the primary treatment of choice in some centers with a surgeon experienced in thyroid surgery. Patients must be made euthyroid before surgery in which case morbidity and mortality are comparable to other major procedures. Specific complications include laryngeal nerve palsy (transient or permanent), transient hypocalcemia (~ 10%) and permanent hypoparathyroidism (~ 1%). 1 year postsurgery, 80% are euthyroid, 15% have permanent hypothyroidism (easily treated with thyroxine) and 5% are still thyrotoxic. Either thyrotoxicosis or hypothyroidism may develop many years after surgery in a previously euthyroid patient (Toft 1989b).

Radioactive iodine (^{131}I iodide) is the treatment of choice if judged by ease of administration, efficacy, short-term safety and cost (Hamburger 1985). UK use has traditionally been restricted to adults > 40 years because of fears (based on few data) that, if used in younger patients, leukemia or thyroid cancer could result – radiation is an important cause of thyroid cancer in children (Brill & Becker 1986) – or that risks of congenital malformations in subsequent pregnancies are increased. Use in UK pediatric practice has been restricted to poorly compliant adolescents who cannot be rendered euthyroid for surgery, but with increasing long-term experience (Farrar & Toft 1991) practice may change. There is a high incidence of hypothyroidism (25% in the first year, a subsequent annual rate of 24% and an incidence of 80% by 15 years post-treatment).

Hashimoto thyroiditis

About 5–10% of children, particularly adolescents, present with hyperthyroidism. Occasionally Graves' disease and Hashimoto thyroiditis coexist: there are clinical and laboratory features of the latter with TSI. Treatment is as for Graves' disease.

TSH hypersecretion

This is a rare cause of thyrotoxicosis, described either with a pituitary TSH-secreting tumor or a defect in TSH feedback inhibition by T3 causing goitrous hyperthyroidism associated with high TSH levels – an indication for neuroradiological evaluation.

Autonomous functioning nodules (Salas 1996)

These are uncommon in children and adolescents, usually occurring after ~ 35 years. Occasionally, single nodules of follicular adenoma (diameter > 3 mm) are found in association with thyrotoxicosis. Diagnosis is by isotope scanning. Carcinoma occurs in less than 1% of functional nodules (see below).

NEOPLASIA (Table 19.13) (Attie 1996)

A history of head and neck irradiation was common in children presenting with thyroid cancer. Palpable thyroid nodules must be taken seriously – the prevalence of malignancy in childhood thyroid nodules is currently ~ 15–20% which is about fourfold higher than in adults.

Table 19.13 Types of thyroid neoplasia

Follicular (epithelial) tumors
  Follicular adenoma
  Follicular carcinoma
  Papillary carcinoma
  Anaplastic carcinoma

Nonfollicular tumors
  Medullary carcinoma
  Lymphoma
  Teratoma
  Miscellaneous

Thyroid neoplasia may arise from follicular epithelium (follicular adenoma and carcinoma, papillary carcinoma, anaplastic carcinoma) or other tissue (medullary carcinoma, lymphoma, teratoma, metastatic tumor). More than 50% of solitary thyroid nodules in childhood are cystic lesions or benign adenomas. Hyperfunctioning adenomas are rare and 90% of malignant nodules consist of well-differentiated follicular carcinoma. In this group, prognosis is better than for rarer types.

Features suggestive of malignancy include history of head and neck irradiation, a hard or rapidly enlarging nodule, lymphadenopathy, hoarseness, dysphagia or metastases. Nodules in Hashimoto thyroiditis rarely represent carcinomatous change. In other situations, radioisotope and ultrasound scanning are valuable for differential diagnosis. Ultrasound identifies cystic lesions (usually benign); if iodide is concentrated by the nodule(s), carcinoma is rare. Small needle biopsy may aid further diagnosis of cystic lesions and distinguish benign from malignant lesions.

Treatment (where possible following needle biopsy histology) is surgical removal of the affected thyroid lobe and subsequent total thyroidectomy if frozen sections reveal malignancy. Radioiodine treatment postoperatively is reserved for metastatic disease or distant lymph node involvement. Prognosis is excellent even with metastatic well-differentiated follicular carcinoma. TSH must be fully suppressed chronically by adequate thyroxine therapy so as not to stimulate tumor growth or regrowth. Life expectancy is normal with follicular carcinoma but not with rarer carcinomas despite radical surgery, radiotherapy and chemotherapy.

An important rare thyroid carcinoma (medullary carcinoma, accounting for < 10% of thyroid carcinomas, Melvin 1986) arises from parafollicular (C) cells, nearly always secretes calcitonin and sometimes other hormones (e.g. ACTH, serotonin, prostaglandins). Although often sporadic, they are associated with syndromes involving tumors of neuroectodermal origin (multiple endocrine neoplasia – MEN) inherited autosomal dominantly. MEN type II (MEN II) comprises two syndromes with medullary thyroid carcinoma and pheochromocytoma: MEN IIa with hyperparathyroidism, MEN IIb with multiple mucosal neuromata (Voorhess 1996).

In a family with MEN II cases, molecular techniques, detecting the predisposing gene abnormality on chromosome 10, indicate whether a child (at 50% risk) has inherited the condition. The aggressive nature of the thyroid lesion, which may develop in childhood or adult life (usually before pheochromocytoma), has led to a search for markers of its presence whilst still microscopic. Calcitonin levels are usually normal at this stage but may rise significantly following pentagastrin infusion. Currently, annual stimulation tests provide the best monitor in affected children –

rising levels with time as well as raised absolute values may be suspicious (Telenius & Ponder 1993). Prophylactic thyroidectomy should be considered.

PARATHYROID GLANDS AND CALCIUM METABOLISM

There are two pairs of parathyroid glands, superior and inferior, although two, five or six glands may be present in normal individuals. Paradoxically, the inferior pair originates (at ~ 5 weeks) from 3rd pharyngeal pouch (endodermal) tissue, the superior pair from the 4th pouch. The inferior pair are pulled medially and caudally by the migrating thymus to the thyroid; the superior attach higher on its dorsal surface. There are two cell types: chief cells (secrete parathyroid hormone; PTH) and oxyphil cells (function unknown).

Although the major function is contributing to calcium and phosphate homeostasis by PTH production, its role in health and disease must be considered in conjunction with other hormones and metabolic factors.

PHYSIOLOGY OF CALCIUM HOMEOSTASIS

Calcium must be accumulated by a growing child – 99% of total body calcium is present in the skeleton. Nevertheless, as well as for bone mineralization, calcium is important for normal endocrine and neuromuscular function at plasma membrane level, enzymatic reactions and blood coagulation, so that the 1% in extra- and intracellular fluids must be closely regulated within narrow concentration limits. Thus homeostatic control mechanisms are inevitably complex. Serum calcium concentration is maintained within normal limits by the interaction of vitamin D, PTH and calcitonin acting at three target tissues: bone, kidneys and gastrointestinal tract. Unlike calcium, normal serum inorganic phosphate levels are age related during childhood (declining from high levels in infancy).

Calcium is present in serum in three fractions in dynamic equilibrium: 50% ionized (metabolically active), 40% protein bound (inactive), the remainder complexed to phosphate, citrate, etc. The proportion of ionized calcium is controlled by vitamin D, PTH and calcitonin but is affected by acid–base changes (acidosis increases and alkalosis decreases ionized calcium levels as hydrogen ions compete with calcium for albumin-binding sites). Vitamin D itself is biologically inactive and must be hydroxylated to active metabolite.

Total serum calcium is measured routinely – ionized levels may be measured directly using ion-selective electrodes. Indirect estimation of biologically active calcium using a formula may be misleading if serum protein concentrations are low. In hypoproteinemic states total calcium may be low but ionized calcium normal. Diet and diurnal variation will influence many indices of mineral and bone metabolism.

Although hypo- or hypercalcemia may be associated with disorders of vitamin D metabolism or parathyroid disease, nonendocrine disorders (e.g. chronic renal failure) may be etiologically important. Specific disorders of mineral and bone metabolism occur in infants, occasionally secondarily to maternal hyperparathyroidism.

Effects on growth of disorders of calcium and phosphate metabolism are reviewed by Kruse (1997). Peak bone mass accumulation and mineralization occurs during puberty, continues into early adult life and is influenced by genetic (racial) factors, body mass, adequate calcium intake during growth and physical activity. Vitamin D receptor genotypes may be diagnostically useful in selecting adults with osteoporosis at increased fracture risk (Spector et al 1995). Reduced peak bone mass occurs in GH deficiency, GT deficiency, male hypogonadism, Turner's syndrome and delayed puberty. Bone mass is also reduced by malnutrition, chronic illness and anorexia nervosa. Appropriate management of these conditions will reduce risks of clinically significant osteoporosis from middle-age. The subject is reviewed by Rahim et al (1996).

CALCIUM REGULATION IN THE FETUS AND NEONATE

Normal fetal bone mineralization requires considerable net calcium and phosphorus transfer from mother to fetus. There is active placental transport of calcium and some 80% of the total accumulates in the third trimester. Fetal blood total and ionized calcium levels exceed those in the mother by about 0.5 and 0.25 mmol/l respectively (Pitkin 1985) and absolute values have doubled from mid-gestation to a mean of 2.75 mmol/l at term.

PTH and calcitonin do not cross the placenta but it is not clear whether active vitamin D metabolites do. Both fetal kidney and placenta can synthesize the active metabolite 1,25-dihydroxy vitamin D. Although their importance compared with that of the maternal kidney is uncertain, it seems likely that that fetal 1,25-dihydroxy D is the major stimulus to placental calcium transfer, perhaps analogously to its effect on intestinal calcium absorption.

To accommodate fetal transfer, there is increased maternal intestinal calcium absorption – calcium loss to the fetus stimulates maternal PTH secretion and maternal 1,25-dihydroxy vitamin D levels are raised. In the fetus, conversely, PTH levels are suppressed and calcitonin levels high, encouraging bone mineralization.

At birth, cessation of transplacental calcium and these hormonal changes cause significant lowering of serum calcium. Lowest levels are reached, in the term neonate, between 24 and 48 h after birth; by 5 days rising PTH and falling calcitonin levels have established 'normal' serum calcium levels. Intestinal absorption of calcium and phosphate (very low in the fetus) is, suddenly, the sole mechanism and source – 1,25-dihydroxy vitamin D_3 secretion increases sharply.

As with other physiological changes from fetal to extrauterine life (e.g. circulatory, respiratory, bilirubin metabolism), these complex adaptations lead potentially to a variety of neonatal disorder, especially in the preterm.

Vitamin D

Vitamin D (calciferol) is a collective term for two steroid-related, cholesterol-derived, naturally occurring compounds, vitamin D_2 (ergocalciferol), derived from the plant sterol ergosterol, and vitamin D_3 (cholecalciferol), produced in skin by the effect of ultraviolet irradiation on a precursor (7-dehydrocholesterol) in the epidermal Malpighian layer (Fig. 19.36). In man D_2 and D_3 are equally active biologically. Serum D_3 levels are higher in summer than winter (reflecting differences in sunlight exposure). Pigmented skin synthesizes it less efficiently.

Plant and animal foods (e.g. fish, eggs, butter and margarine) are important sources of D_2 and D_3 respectively. Absorption is via

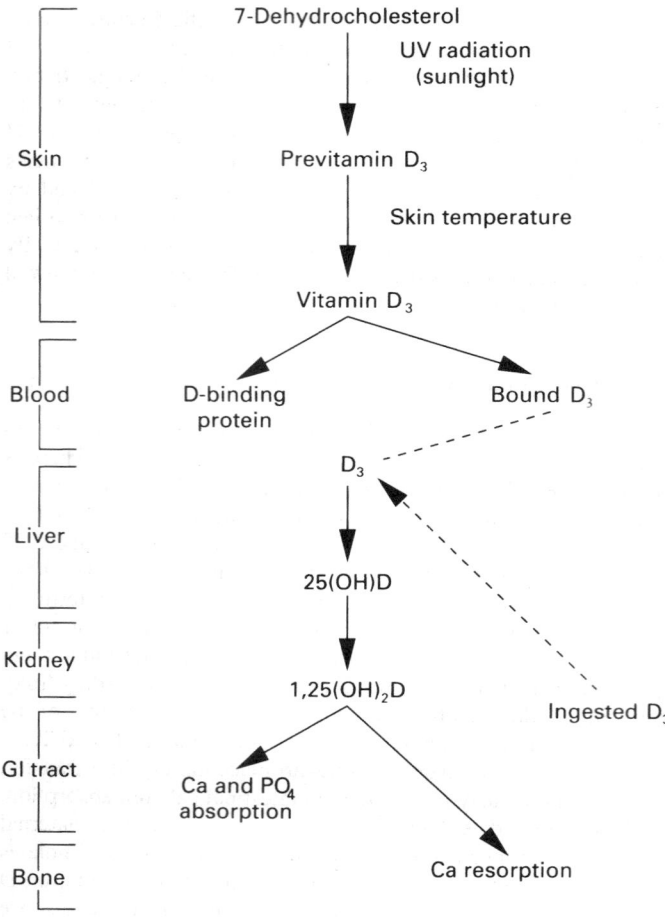

Fig. 19.36 Vitamin D metabolism and its regulation.

upper small intestine and lymphatic system in chylomicrons. Normal bile salt secretion is necessary – absorption is impaired by steatorrhea. In blood, ~ 98% is bound to a high MW liver-derived protein which also transports and binds active vitamin D metabolites and acts as a buffer against vitamin D toxicity.

The first step in vitamin D activation (Fig. 19.36) is 25-hydroxylation in liver microsomes but bowel and kidney may contribute. 25-hydroxy D is the major circulating metabolite but is metabolically inactive and converted in mitochondria of the proximal renal tubule to two major metabolites in proportions depending on physiological requirements: active 1,25-dihydroxy D and 24,25-dihydroxy D (some, but much less, biological activity). Other metabolites of uncertain pathophysiological significance and with varying biological activities can be formed. Placenta and bone can also hydroxylate at C 1.

1,25-dihydroxy D has major effects on intestinal villus and crypt cells, osteoblasts and osteoclasts and distal renal tubular cells. The net effect is to increase serum calcium and phosphate by stimulating intestinal absorption and mobilization from bone, and reducing renal excretion. Calcium mobilization from bone is also PTH dependent.

Average total serum concentrations of 1,25-dihydroxy D are 1000-fold lower than of 25-hydroxy D but there is only a 10-fold difference in relative concentrations of the free (metabolically active in the case of 1,25-dihydroxy D) components.

Parathyroid hormone (PTH)

PTH is an 84 amino acid peptide of MW 9500 (Keutmann et al 1978). 34 amino acids at the amino- (N-) terminal are essential for receptor binding and activation and thus biological activity. The PTH gene is close to the insulin gene on the short arm of chromosome 11. PTH is synthesized by parathyroid chief cells and cleaved from higher molecular weight biologically inactive precursors which are not released into the circulation. Both intact PTH and carboxy- (C-) terminal fragments are released into the circulation and the proportion of the latter is increased in primary hyperparathyroidism. Intact PTH is metabolized by liver (predominantly) and kidney and fragments returned to the circulation. Intact PTH and N-terminal fragments are cleared rapidly (< 10 min); C-terminal fragments (mainly metabolized by kidney) are cleared more slowly (2 h). Thus circulating PTH is a heterogeneous mixture of intact hormone together with N-terminal, C-terminal and intermediate fragments.

Serum calcium concentration is the major regulator of PTH synthesis and release. There is a greater response to evolving hypocalcemia than to falling levels within the normal range. Hypercalcemia suppresses PTH secretion. Catecholamines, vitamin D metabolites and cortisol increase PTH secretion but their physiological function is doubtful.

The major role of PTH is prevention of hypocalcemia by three main mechanisms: calcium resorption from bone, renal calcium reabsorption and, indirectly, increasing intestinal calcium absorption by stimulating renal 1,25-dihydroxy D synthesis.

In bone, it both regulates calcium movement between bone fluid surrounding surface and lacunar osteocytes and extracellular fluid, and influences remodeling. Osteoblasts (not osteoclasts) have PTH receptors and it is presumably release of an osteoblast factor which promotes osteoclast activation. A factor of MW 500–1000 has been postulated (McSheehy & Chambers 1986). PTH has several effects on renal tubules, acting distally to promote calcium and inhibit phosphate and bicarbonate reabsorption and proximally to stimulate hydroxylation at C1 to form 1,25-dihydroxy D.

Heterogeneity of circulating PTH forms (Berson & Yalow 1968) makes measurement difficult. There is cross-reactivity of RIAs against the intact molecule, the N- and C-terminal and the intermediate region. Because serum half-lives of intact PTH and N-terminal fragments are shorter than those of the C-terminal or intermediate fragments, the latter account for ~ 80% of immunoreactive material measured and better reflect PTH secretion rates. Except chronic renal failure (where C-terminal and intermediate fragments accumulate because of impaired glomerular filtration), assays specific for C-terminal or intermediate fragment PTH provide better discrimination between normal and raised PTH levels. Some PTH RIAs (and bioassays) are too insensitive to distinguish between normality and hyposecretion (Kruse 1995a).

There is diurnal circadian variation in serum PTH secretion – higher values in early morning. For correct interpretation, simultaneous serum calcium and phosphate concentrations should be measured. Renal phosphate reabsorption and urinary cyclic adenosine monophosphate (cAMP) may need assessment. The ratio of tubular maximal rate of phosphate reabsorption to glomerular filtration rate is calculated from simultaneous fasting serum and urinary phosphate and creatinine concentrations and reference to nomograms – ratios are high in hypoparathyroidism, low in hyperparathyroidism. cAMP is important in PTH release into the circulation in response to hypocalcemia; measurement is useful for indirectly assessing circulating active PTH, evaluating the renal response to exogenous PTH and distinguishing pseudohypo- from hypoparathyroidism.

Calcitonin

Calcitonin (Copp et al 1962) is synthesized in and secreted by thyroid parafollicular (C) cells of neuroectodermal origin. It is discussed here because of its importance in calcium metabolism.

As for insulin and PTH, the gene encoding calcitonin is on the short arm of chromosome 11 (Przepiorka et al 1984). Calcitonin is a 32 amino acid peptide, MW 3500, derived from a polypeptide precursor by loss of N- and C-terminal fragments. Species differences derive from mid-molecule amino acid sequences. The entire sequence is required for biological activity. Calcitonin-like bioactive material has been identified in thymus, lung, adrenal medulla, brain and parathyroid glands but none are major sources of circulating calcitonin.

As with PTH, serum calcium concentration is the major regulator of calcitonin secretion but with opposite effect: hypercalcemia stimulates and hypocalcemia suppresses calcitonin secretion. Gastrointestinal hormones such as gastrin, glucagon and cholecystokinin stimulate calcitonin secretion as do estrogens, β-adrenergic agonists and 1,25-dihydroxy D, but none seem physiologically important. Pentagastrin (a synthetic gastrin derivative) is used to stimulate calcitonin secretion in the diagnosis of medullary thyroid carcinoma.

More sensitive assays are helping to define calcitonin changes with age and deficiency states. In children, monomeric calcitonin (the major active circulating form) is present in very low concentrations (Kruse et al 1987) – levels are higher in infancy.

Like PTH, calcitonin influences serum calcium levels by action on bone, kidneys and bowel. It inhibits bone resorption by reducing osteoclast cytoplasmic motility. In kidney it binds to specific receptors to increase calcium, phosphate, magnesium, sodium and potassium excretion and stimulates 1-hydroxylation in the proximal tubule to produce 1,25-dihydroxy D (Jaeger et al 1986). This promotes intestinal calcium reabsorption indirectly but it may also have a direct, but inhibitory, effect.

The importance of calcitonin for the physiological regulation of calcium metabolism remains uncertain. Neither thyroidectomy nor calcitonin hypersecretion from medullary thyroid carcinoma affect serum calcium levels. Its major inhibitory effect on bone resorption is directly antagonistic to PTH and 1,25-dihydroxy D and its role in that context may be prevention of excessive resorption. It is secreted in response to eating calcium-rich food secondarily to secretion of various gastrointestinal and pancreatic hormones which it itself inhibits. The net effect is delayed calcium absorption which may be important in preventing postprandial hypercalcemia and hypercalciuria (Kruse 1995a).

A major physiological role may be in situations (fetal life, infancy, pregnancy and lactation) with extra needs for calcium and when calcitonin and 1,25-dihydroxy D levels are high – calcitonin may prevent unwanted bone resorption whilst allowing the stimulatory effect of vitamin D on intestinal calcium absorption.

DISORDERS OF CALCIUM AND BONE METABOLISM

Metabolic and hormonal interactions in many of these disorders are complex. Detailed pathophysiological information can be found in reviews by Kruse (1995b) and relevant chapters in Lifshitz (1996). Significant diagnostic pointers can be obtained from a full history (including family history) and specific abnormalities found on examination. To minimize effects of food and diurnal changes, blood is ideally taken in the fasting state in the morning and, when possible, without compression of the arm (venous stasis also influences calcium levels).

The important basic laboratory measurements are of serum calcium (Ca), phosphate (P) and alkaline phosphatase (ALP) which should be interpreted in the context of simultaneously estimated serum total protein and albumin, electrolytes, creatinine, magnesium and pH. Urine measurements (early morning or 24-h collections) of calcium, phosphate, creatinine and hydroxyproline (a measure of bone turnover) may be valuable. If significant abnormalities are found, more complex investigations can be instigated assessing aspects of parathyroid function, vitamin D metabolism and bone turnover as indicated – see Walker & Hughes (1995) and Kruse (1995b).

INFANCY

Important problems in infancy are (see also Ch. 5 and below):

1. hypocalcemia: early and late neonatal hypocalcemia
2. hypercalcemia
   a. idiopathic infantile hypercalcemia (see below)
   b. familial hypocalciuric hypercalcemia (see below)
   c. neonatal primary hyperparathyroidism
   d. hypervitaminosis D (see below)
   e. other associations: fat necrosis; phosphate deficiency
3. metabolic bone disease in the preterm infant.

ABNORMAL 1,25-DIHYDROXY VITAMIN D SECRETION OR ACTION

Increased intake (hypervitaminosis D)

Vitamin D intoxication usually results from excessive treatment of hypoparathyroidism, rickets, renal osteodystrophy, etc. with concentrated preparations – it is available in proprietary multivitamin preparations without prescription in many countries and may also be prescribed inappropriately. 'Stoss therapy' – administration of 600 000 units for the prevention of rickets – is not now used but was formerly a cause. Toxicity may persist for many weeks because of adipose tissue storage. Despite its potency, an advantage of the synthetic analogue of 1,25-dihydroxy D (1α-hydroxy D) is its short half-life with more rapid return to normocalcemia after inadvertent overdose.

Clinical signs reflect hypercalcemia from excessive intestinal calcium absorption and bone resorption. Initially, there is nausea and vomiting with anorexia, constipation and polyuria. Infants fail to thrive and become irritable. Ultimately, there may be nephrocalcinosis with renal insufficiency and ectopic calcification. Investigation confirms hypercalcemia with hypercalciuria; serum PTH will be suppressed – normal or elevated PTH with hypercalcemia indicate hyperparathyroidism.

Treatment is by withdrawing the vitamin D preparation and calcium supplements (if any), saline infusion and frusemide (to increase urinary calcium loss) and glucocorticoids (e.g. hydrocortisone 4 mg/kg/24 h 6-hourly) which gradually reduces intestinal calcium absorption.

Idiopathic hypercalcemia of infancy was thought to be due to excessive vitamin D administration. This is unlikely to be the case, although it remains a heterogeneous and poorly understood condition. The fall in incidence of the mild form (Lightwood & Stapelton 1953) observed in the UK preceded the reduction in vitamin D supplementation of artificial infant feeds. Incidence of the severe form (Martin et al 1984) often associated with mental retardation, cardiovascular abnormalities (supravalvar aortic stenosis or peripheral pulmonary stenosis) and facial and other dysmorphic features has not changed. The mild form is now rarely seen. The severe form may be due to a defect in calcitonin synthesis or release resulting from a neural crest developmental anomaly affecting face, heart and thyroid C-cell (calcitonin-producing) precursors (Culler et al 1985) which would explain the variable relationship between somatic developmental abnormalities and degree of calcium homeostatic disturbance (calcium levels may be normal).

Increased synthesis

Hypercalcemia from raised 1,25-dihydroxy D levels (with suppressed PTH) is seen in granulomatous disease (sarcoidosis, tuberculosis, etc.) due to conversion of 25-hydroxy D into the active metabolite by 1-hydroxylation in granulomatous cells. Similar findings in some patients with lymphoma are unusual – most patients with hypercalcemia due to malignant disease have low 1,25-dihydroxy D levels and reduced intestinal calcium absorption and other mechanisms are presumably involved.

Increased secretion and/or responsiveness (absorptive hypercalciuria)

This specific type of 'idiopathic' hypercalciuria is thought to be due to a primary abnormality of secretion of, or responsiveness to, 1,25-dihydroxy D. It may be transmitted autosomal dominantly and cause renal stones or hematuria. A form secondary to a renal tubular defect is also found (see renal hypercalciuria below) and may share a common pathogenesis.

Decreased formation or action (calciopenic rickets)

Rickets (Table 19.14) is caused by defective growth plate mineralization and may be due to decreased calcium and phosphate availability in extracellular fluid at those sites (deficiency or malabsorption of vitamin D, defective formation or action of 1,25-dihydroxy D – calciopenic rickets; increased renal

Table 19.14 Classification of rickets

'Classical': lack of sunshine, diet deficient in vitamin D	Immigrants (pigmented skin); during rapid growth (infancy/puberty)
Malabsorption	Celiac disease; giardiasis; hepatobiliary disease (biliary atresia/fistula; cirrhosis; neonatal hepatitis)
Hereditary renal (mainly tubular)	Hypophosphatemic; vitamin D dependency; fibrous dysplasia/neurofibromatosis (with hypophosphatemia); Fanconi's syndrome (including cystinosis, tyrosinemia, Lowe's syndrome, Wilson's disease); distal renal tubular acidosis
Acquired renal (mainly tubular)	Chronic renal failure (glomerular); hypophosphatemia; hypercalciuria

phosphate excretion or decreased intake – phosphopenic rickets). Phosphopenic rickets is usually due to renal phosphate loss (see below) but hypophosphatemia, commonly seen in low-birth-weight preterm infants, is due to inadequate phosphate intake – see also Chapters 5, 17 and 21.

ABNORMAL PTH SECRETION OR ACTION

Increased secretion (primary hyperparathyroidism)

Increased PTH secretion may be a normal physiological compensatory response to hypocalcemia (secondary hyperparathyroidism). Primary hyperparathyroidism is due to abnormally increased secretion of PTH, is rare in childhood and uncommon even by adolescence with an overall prevalence of 25 per 100 000.

The etiology is unknown but cases may be sporadic (nearly always associated with a solitary adenoma, rarely with carcinoma) or familial (usually due to hyperplasia of all four glands). Familial cases may be isolated (autosomal dominant and recessive forms are reported), associated with autosomal dominant multiple endocrine neoplasia syndromes (Telenius & Ponder 1993) (MEN I, in association with pancreatic tumors or gastrinoma and pituitary adenomas; MEN II, with medullary thyroid carcinoma and pheochromocytoma) or with autosomal dominant hypocalciuric hypercalcemia syndrome where there is defective renal calcium excretion (see below).

MEN I typically presents with clinical signs or symptoms in the middle decades of adult life but intractable peptic ulceration (Zollinger–Ellison syndrome due to a gastrin-secreting pancreatic tumor) is reported by adolescence and raised gastrin and calcium levels may be found in asymptomatic family members by then. Hypercalcemia occurs in about 97% and the serial fasting serum calcium measurement is a valuable screening test. In MEN IIa and IIb, calcitonin-secreting medullary thyroid carcinoma develops (see below).

The clinical spectrum of primary hyperparathyroidism ranges from asymptomatic to lethal. There may be fatigue, anorexia, constipation, polyuria, polydipsia, renal stones, bone pain and pathological fractures. Diagnosis depends on demonstration of inappropriately high PTH levels for hypercalcemia on three separate occasions. This is found otherwise only in familial hypocalciuric hypercalcemia (see below) where urinary calcium excretion is low for the hypercalcemia. Antibody against the C-terminal or intermediate PTH fragments is more sensitive to high PTH levels. Radiographically, there is usually generalized bone demineralization, osteolysis and subperiosteal bone resorption especially of the phalanges and, occasionally, cysts.

Once diagnosis is secure, surgical parathyroid exploration by an experienced surgeon is necessary. Preoperative localization of the responsible gland is unreliable (although ultrasound may detect enlargement < 1 cm) – hyperplasia of all four is common. In this situation total parathyroidectomy with autotransplantation of tissue into the forearm is the treatment of choice (Kruse 1995b). Other family members should be screened for hypercalcemia.

Decreased secretion (hypoparathyroidism – HP)

HP is much commoner than hypersecretion but less common than decreased peripheral hormone action ('end-organ resistance' due to receptor or postreceptor abnormalities – pseudohypoparathyroidism (PHP).

Cases may be sporadic or familial. Presentation may be in the neonate and may be transient, permanent (autosomal dominant, recessive, sex-linked recessive and sporadic forms have all been described), or part of the DiGeorge syndrome etc. – see Chapter 22. Postneonatal onset may be idiopathic or occur secondarily to neck surgery, irradiation, hemosiderosis, hypomagnesemia, etc.

A familial (autosomal recessive) form may be associated with autoimmune disease affecting other endocrine glands (especially Addison's disease) and mucocutaneous candidiasis (polyglandular autoimmune disease type 1). Presentation is with severe candidiasis (due to a defect in cellular immunity) followed, successively, by HP and Addison's disease (rarely before mid-childhood). Other autoimmune manifestations include alopecia, vitiligo, thyroiditis, chronic hepatitis and pernicious anemia. Parathyroid antibodies cause glandular destructions.

Clinical signs and symptoms of HP are from hypocalcemia due to decreased renal calcium reabsorption, bone resorption and, indirectly, decreased intestinal calcium absorption. Manifestations depend on age, severity and speed of onset and relate to the neuromuscular system (latent tetany – positive Chvostek and Trousseau signs; overt tetany – paresthesiae, muscle cramps, carpopedal spasm), brain (focal or grand mal convulsions, papilledema, basal ganglia calcification, eventual mental retardation), heart (prolonged Q–T interval), eyes (lenticular cataracts), ectodermal changes (dry skin, coarse hair, brittle nails, tooth enamel hypoplasia).

Treatment aims to correct hypocalcemia and prevent recurrence (treatment of associated problems may also be indicated). A vitamin D preparation is currently the long-term treatment of choice – PTH is expensive and must be given parenterally daily.

Acute hypocalcemia is treated with 10% calcium gluconate (9.4% calcium by weight) 1–2 ml/kg by slow i.v. injection repeated, as necessary, 6-hourly or carefully and slowly infused (in dilute form). Oral calcium supplements (e.g. calcium gluconate) and a vitamin D analogue (e.g. 1α-hydroxy D 25–50 ng/kg/24 h) should be started and serum and urinary calcium levels checked 3-monthly. Vitamin D will not correct renal calcium loss – although there is reduced urinary calcium excretion, there is relative hypercalciuria due to deficient (PTH-mediated) renal tubular calcium reabsorption and thus serum calcium levels should be maintained in low normal range to avoid nephrocalcinosis and renal stones. Treatment with a thiazide diuretic and sodium restriction may be necessary.

Decreased peripheral action (pseudohypoparathyroidism – PHP)

Uncommon causes of PTH-resistant HP include severe hypomagnesemia (which causes resistance to and decreased secretion of PTH) and calciopenic rickets (due to low 1,25-dihydroxy D levels). Receptor or postreceptor defects of response to PTH at the target organ (especially the renal tubule) are commoner, first described by Albright and termed pseudohypoparathyroidism (Albright et al 1942). This heterogeneous condition has been divided into several types:

Type 1 (originally described by Albright)

There is often symptomatic hypocalcemia in mid-childhood on a background of variable mental retardation and characteristic (but inconstant) somatic features ('Albright's hereditary osteody-strophy') including short stature, obesity, round face, short neck and marked metacarpal and metatarsal shortening (especially 4th and 5th – see Figs 19.4 and 19.7). There is no phosphaturic response to PTH administration and a blunted urinary cyclic AMP increase in comparison with both normals and patients with HP. This type has been further subdivided on the basis of decreased (Type 1a) or normal (Type 1b) amounts of a protein membrane component that couples the PTH receptor to the catalytic unit of the adenylate cyclase. The defect in Type 1b is unknown and somatic abnormalities are less common than in Type 1a.

Type 2

In this rarer form (Drezner et al 1973), the defect is thought to be due to an intracellular defect beyond cyclic AMP generation – cyclic AMP responses to PTH are normal but the phosphaturic response is defective.

These differences do not entirely explain the very variable clinical manifestations. Some patients with somatic features show no renal resistance to PTH – pseudopseudohypoparathyroidism (PPHP). In some families, PHP Type 1 and PPHP coexist and individuals may fluctuate between normo- and hypocalcemia (Barr et al 1994).

PTH activates the adenylate cyclase system via the 'G' protein, a heterotrimeric guanine nucleotide binding protein. The protein membrane component ('G' protein, formerly known as 'N' protein) may be deficient in PHP Type 1a/PPHP (Levine et al 1986). Mutations in the GNAS1 gene have been detected in kindreds with PHP (Ahmed et al 1996a).

The G protein family mediates numerous transmembrane hormone and sensory transduction processes in eukaryotic cells including LH, GH and TSH synthesis and release. Unsurprisingly, therefore, abnormalities of other peptide hormones, particularly thyroid and GT, have been described in these patients. It is likely that abnormalities of GH secretion also occur – the GRF/receptor complex on the somatotroph activates a similar coupling ('G') protein to stimulate adenylate cyclase and hence GH synthesis and release (Frohmann & Jansson 1986). Thus in PHP there could be a defect in GRF binding and/or activation of its regulatory protein similar to that postulated for the defect in PTH regulatory protein. Although these individuals are a heterogeneous group, they may grow better on GH treatment (Stirling et al 1991). Treatment of hypocalcemia in PHP is analogous to treatment in HP (see above).

ABNORMAL CALCITONIN SECRETION

Increased

Hypocalcemia is almost never a feature of calcitonin excess. High calcitonin levels are seen in medullary thyroid carcinoma (sporadic or in MEN II, see p. 1052) and a variety of nonthyroid tumors in adults but have not been described in children. Levels are high in the rare autosomal recessive condition pycnodysostosis and may be raised in pancreatitis. High levels, presumably due to a normal physiological response, are described in hypercalcemic states and renal insufficiency.

Decreased

A number of congenital and acquired hypocalcitoninemic conditions are described, including primary hypothyroidism or post-thyroidectomy, anticonvulsant treatment (phenytoin or primidone) and Williams syndrome. Hypercalcemia does not occur.

ABNORMALITIES OF PHOSPHATE EXCRETION

Increased

Phosphopenic rickets results from excessive urinary phosphate excretion with resulting hypophosphatemia (Table 19.14) and only rarely from inadequate intake (other than in the preterm infant (see above and Ch. 5). Familial forms of primary hypophosphatemia secondary to renal phosphate loss have been described including X-linked (dominant) hypophosphatemic rickets (Albright's vitamin D-resistant rickets – Albright et al 1937a) and autosomal dominant and recessive forms. Phosphopenic rickets is a feature of Fanconi's syndrome (sporadic or familial, idiopathic or secondary to a number of inborn metabolic errors), has been described in rare (usually benign mesenchymal) tumors and is a feature of distal renal tubular acidosis (sporadic and familial).

Decreased

Decreased renal phosphate excretion is important in the pathogenesis of renal osteodystrophy – other factors such as altered vitamin D metabolism become increasingly important as renal failure worsens. Tumor calcinosis (deposition of calcium phosphate around large joints due to increased phosphate reabsorption) is rarely seen outside Africa and may be familial or sporadic.

ABNORMALITIES OF CALCIUM EXCRETION

Increased

Hypercalciuria may be associated with hypercalcemia (e.g. vitamin D intoxication, primary hyperparathyroidism), normocalcemia (e.g. distal renal tubular acidosis, following corticosteroid, frusemide or immobilization) or may be 'idiopathic'. Absorptive (see above) and renal forms (renal hypercalciuria) of this last group occur but may share a common pathogenesis.

Decreased (familial hypocalciuric 'benign' hypercalcemia)

There are inappropriately raised (normal or high) PTH levels with hypercalcemia (see above). Inheritance is autosomal dominant. Hypercalcemia results from increased tubular calcium reabsorption, but there are no consequent symptoms of chronic hypercalcemia. There is a presumed abnormal set point for calcium-mediated PTH suppression but no abnormalities of vitamin D metabolism, calcitonin secretion or parathyroid histology have been found. Parathyroid surgery is ineffective and contraindicated.

PRACTICAL DIFFERENTIAL DIAGNOSIS (Kruse 1995c)

Rickets

Initial clinical assessment, characteristic radiographic changes and raised ALP, decreased P and normal (especially in phosphopenic rickets) or decreased Ca in serum usually make diagnosis straightforward. It is important to determine etiology (Table 19.14) and further tests will usually be necessary.

Normal PTH and cyclic AMP levels are characteristic of phosphopenic rickets (usually familial X-linked hypophosphatemic, but associated hypercalciuria suggests the rarer autosomal recessive type unless there is inadequate phosphate intake in, for example, the preterm infant). Tumor rickets should be considered in sporadic cases presenting in late childhood or adolescence. Renal function must be assessed to exclude primary renal causes such as chronic renal failure and Fanconi's syndrome (which may be secondary to other inborn metabolic errors) and is characterized by glycosuria and aminoaciduria.

Secondary hyperparathyroidism (i.e. secondary to calcium malabsorption) with raised PTH levels suggests calciopenic rickets, usually due to lack of vitamin D or impaired synthesis or action of the active metabolite 1,25-dihydroxy D. Further differential diagnosis necessitates measurement of individual vitamin D metabolites: low levels of 25-hydroxy D are found in all acquired forms (nutritional, liver disease, malabsorption, anticonvulsants). If 25-hydroxy D levels are normal, low 1,25-dihydroxy D levels indicate vitamin D-deficient rickets type 1 and high levels indicate end-organ resistance to its action (type 2).

Hypocalcemia

In the presence of normal total protein, albumin and magnesium levels and renal function, repeated fasting early morning hypocalcemia is interpreted in the context of serum phosphate levels. If these are high, HP or PHP are likely and can be differentiated on the basis of PTH and cyclic AMP measurements: in PHP, PTH levels are high and, in type 1 (the common form), there is blunted cyclic AMP response to PTH infusion; in HP, PTH levels are low and the cyclic AMP response is normal.

Low or normal serum phosphate levels suggests calciopenic rickets; elevated ALP and PTH levels will confirm the diagnosis which should be further elucidated as above.

Hypercalcemia

Confirmed raised fasting early morning hypercalcemia on at least three occasions with normal renal function and serum protein and albumin levels is uncommon in childhood. Raised or even detectable PTH levels in the presence of hypercalcemia are inappropriate and indicate primary hyperparathyroidism. MEN syndromes should be excluded and family members screened for hypercalcemia. Detectable PTH levels with hypercalcemia but hypocalciuria are characteristic of familial hypocalciuric hypercalcemia.

Suppressed PTH levels suggest vitamin D intoxication (most commonly), idiopathic infantile hypercalcemia, malignancy, sarcoidosis or Addison's disease.

HP from PHP

Hypomagnesemia, because of its dual effect on PTH secretion and resistance to PTH action, may produce features of both HP and PHP – serum magnesium must be checked in hypocalcemia. Somatic features of Albright's hereditary osteodystrophy (see above) and radiographic changes of hyperparathyroidism indicate PHP. In HP, PTH levels are inappropriately low for hypocalcemia; PTH levels are high in PHP. Deficient cyclic AMP generation after

PTH infusion is characteristic of PHP. Measurement of plasma cyclic AMP has replaced the older tests which measured urinary cyclic AMP excretion (Kruse & Kracht 1987, Stirling et al 1991b).

THE ADRENAL GLANDS

The adrenal glands are formed from mesodermal and ectodermal components which form cortex and medulla respectively. During the fifth week, mesothelial cells migrate and proliferate to form large acidophilic cells which constitute the fetal cortex. These become surrounded by smaller cells which later make up the definitive cortex. Meanwhile, sympathetic neural crest neuroblasts invade the medial aspect of the fetal cortex forming the adrenal medulla rather than nerve processes and known as chromaffin cells.

For ontogeny of fetal adrenal steroidogenesis, see page 1003. The neonatal adrenals are comparable in size to the kidneys. After birth, there is rapid atrophy of the fetal zone of the cortex and adrenal weight at birth is only regained by late puberty. The definitive cortex secretes glucocorticoids (GC) affecting carbohydrate metabolism, mineralocorticoids (MCA) affecting electrolyte balance and androgens (which are also estrogen precursors). The medulla secretes catecholamines (adrenaline and noradrenaline).

THE ADRENAL CORTEX

Morphology and steroidogenesis

The cortex comprises three histologically distinct zones but cells appear to migrate through them changing function as they do so. This has important implications for control of steroidogenesis. The outer (subcapsular) zone, the zona glomerulosa, consists of balls of small cells and overlies the radially arranged cord-like bundles of larger cells of the zona fasciculata. The innermost area, the zona reticularis, consists of a network of short cords with capillaries and only gradually becomes a distinct zone from ~ 6 years. Studies of adrenal histology at necropsy in children dying from accidents (Dhom 1973) demonstrate progressive subsequent reticularis development largely accounting for the pubertal adrenal size and weight spurt. In contrast, there is relatively little change in postnatal morphological glomerulosa and fasciculata appearances.

In tissue culture, fasciculata and reticularis cells differ functionally as well as histologically (O'Hare et al 1980) preferentially synthesizing GC (cortisol) and androgens respectively. Dehydroepiandrosterone (DHA) is a marker of zona reticularis function. Increasing production of androgens by reticularis from about 5 or 6 years and peaking around 12 or 13 years ('adrenarche' – Albright 1947a) is synchronous with morphological and functional reticularis development (Dhom 1973, Reiter et al 1977). Aldosterone, the main MC, is uniquely produced in the zona glomerulosa.

Since pioneering work in chemical characterization of adrenal steroids (Reichstein & Shoppee 1943) and excretion of 17 ketosteroids (Talbot et al 1943) in health and disease there has been enormous progress in measurement of individual plasma and urinary steroids. Plasma measurements reflect one moment in time, but many steroids are released episodically in relation to circadian rhythms and to environmental stimuli, often in sudden bursts at intervals.

Cortisol is secreted intermittently in response to pulsatile ACTH release. Most secretory activity occurs during sleep but there are, on average, about nine episodes of cortisol secretion through a 24-h period in adults under basal conditions (James et al 1978). The circadian diurnal cortisol rhythm results from maximal duration and number of ACTH secretory episodes between 3 a.m. and 8 a.m. Circadian cortisol rhythm is present by ~ 6 months (Onishi et al 1983) and is abolished in Cushing's syndrome.

ACTH binds to receptors on the adrenal cell membrane, activating adenylate cyclase (a calcium-dependent step); cyclic AMP activates enzymes (mainly intracellular protein kinases) which stimulate hydrolysis of cholesterol esters. Steroidogenesis is initiated in mitochondria by cholesterol binding to a C27 side chain cleavage enzyme which starts its stepwise conversion to pregnenolone, a necessary step in biosynthesis of all three groups of adrenal cortical hormones.

There are acute and chronic responses to ACTH in terms of GC biosynthesis. In contrast, the glomerulosa only seems to produce aldosterone acutely – chronic ACTH stimulation is not generally associated with sustained hyperaldosteronism. ACTH is probably the most, and perhaps only, important adrenal androgen modulator (see p. 1038). It is likely that changes in adrenal androgen production with age (cf. unchanging cortisol levels for surface area) result from ACTH-mediated intrinsic local vascular and morphological changes (Anderson 1980, Vinson 1984) rather than a specific, unidentified, pituitary adrenal androgen stimulating hormone.

Physiological ACTH levels regulate acute aldosterone fluctuations – ACTH is important in the pathogenesis of GC-suppressible hyperaldosteronism (Giebink et al 1973, New et al 1973). Although the primary control mechanism is the renin–angiotensin system, this ACTH role is important in managing salt-losing CAH.

GCs such as cortisol and corticosterone are fast feedback antagonists of ACTH secretion; other steroids (e.g. deoxycorticosterone (DOC), deoxycortisol (S) and synthetic GCs) show delayed feedback inhibition. The relative importance of these responses in normal physiological control of ACTH is unclear.

Simplified steroidogenic pathways are summarized in Figure 19.37. For the clinician, working knowledge of the pathways will aid understanding of physical and biochemical consequences of various types of congenital hyperplasia. Effects of adrenal disorders on growth are reviewed by Ritzén (1997).

Some 70% of circulating cortisol is bound to a 52 000 molecular weight α-2 globulin, transcortin (corticosteroid-binding globulin – CBG) and about 20% is albumin bound. Aldosterone, other GCs and precursors are less strongly bound to CBG and synthetic steroids only weakly. CBG is synthesized in liver; levels are increased by estrogen and decreased in cirrhosis. Binding sites are saturated when total plasma cortisol levels exceed about 600 nmol/l; at normal concentrations very little free cortisol is in plasma or excreted in urine. Urinary free cortisol is thus a sensitive screening test for Cushing's syndrome (p. 1065). Cortisol plasma half-life is 60–90 min; that of aldosterone is only ~ 20 min because proportionately much less is protein bound. Important adrenal androgens include DHA and its sulfated form (DHAS) which is also synthesized by the gland. DHAS half-life is 10–20 h; DHA secretion is episodic and concurrent with cortisol (Rosenfeld et al 1971). Aldosterone levels show marked circadian changes which follow cortisol but are significantly influenced by posture.

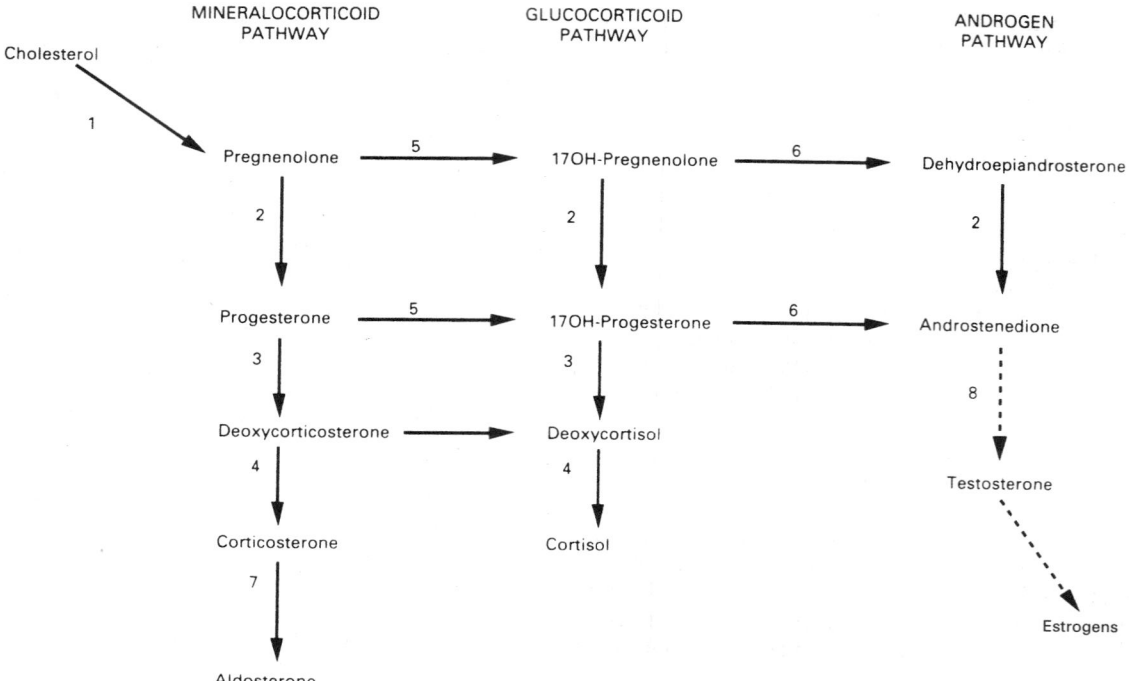

Fig. 19.37 Pathways of adrenal biosynthesis. 1-cholesterol side chain cleaving system (20α-hydroxylase, 20,22-desmolase, 22α-hydroxylase); 2–3β-hydroxysteroid dehydrogenase; 3–21-hydroxylase; 4–11β-hydroxylase; 5–17α-hydroxylase; 6–17,20-lyase; 7–18-hydroxylase and 18-hydroxysteroid dehydrogenase; 8–17β-hydroxysteroid dehydrogenase.

Normal values for individual steroids and urinary metabolites in infancy, childhood and puberty are now available (see Honour 1995, Honour et al 1991) based on cross-sectional and mixed longitudinal studies.

Urine sampling is atraumatic and 24-h collections are more likely than isolated plasma samples to reflect accurately overall steroid production. However, such collections may be difficult and unreliable in infants and young children. In general steroids are present in urine in about 1000 times their plasma concentrations. However, because of the complexity of metabolic pathways via which adrenal (and gonadal) steroids are excreted (and influences of disease or drugs) there can be uncertainty about clinical significance, relationship to gland of origin or even specific steroid from which they derive. Nevertheless, steroid profiles obtained by gas chromatography are valuable in complementing plasma steroid assays, e.g. studying normal children longitudinally to determine changes with age and the mechanism of adrenarche (Kelnar & Brook 1983, Kelnar 1985), detecting abnormal metabolites (e.g. secreted by tumors), metabolite ratios (e.g. in 5α-reductase deficiency), differential diagnosis of rarer or less clear-cut forms of CAH and differential diagnosis of salt-losing states in infancy due to aldosterone biosynthetic defects (Honour et al 1982).

Adrenarche

During the early months of life the fetal zone rapidly atrophies so that high fetal and neonatal DHAS levels (reflecting low 3β-hydroxysteroid dehydrogenase (3βOHSD) fetal zone activity) fall and remain low for ~ 6 years. During mid-childhood adrenal androgen secretion rises steeply ('adrenarche') (Fig. 19.38) – coincident with zona reticularis development.

Adrenarche is important because of (1) its role in precocious sexual (pubic and axillary) hair development in mid-childhood; (2) possible relevance to triggering normal puberty, although underlying mechanisms and relationship to subsequent rises in GT and gonadal steroids at clinical puberty onset ('gonadarche') are controversial; (3) potential etiologic relevance to concomitant steep rise in normal blood pressure (BP) centiles and the mid-childhood growth spurt.

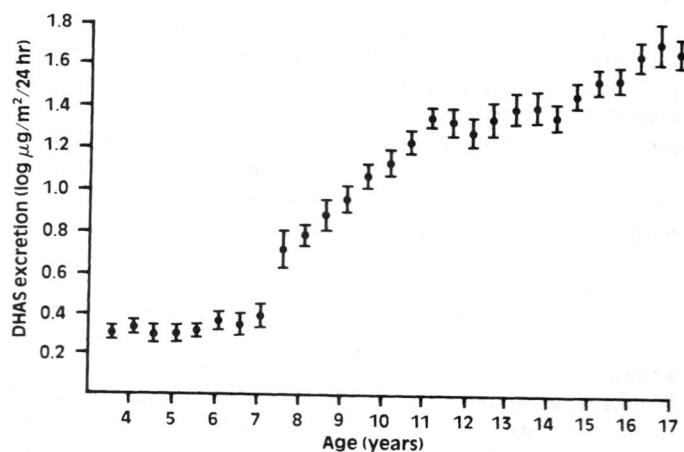

Fig. 19.38 Urinary excretion of dehydroepiandrosterone sulfate (DHAS) in childhood (from Kelnar 1985).

The adrenal androgen rise is not accompanied by significant increases in intermediate metabolites in cortisol or corticosterone biosynthesis when related to body surface area (Kelnar & Brook 1983). It is likely that this disassociation reflects changes in adrenal steroidogenesis with age in response to ACTH-mediated changes in adrenal blood flow and cell morphology (Kelnar & Brook 1983, Rich et al 1981, Schiebinger et al 1981, Hornsby & Aldern 1984) rather than a separate adrenal androgen stimulating hormone (Talbot et al 1951).

In some children, predominantly girls, the rise manifests as appearance of pubic, and sometimes axillary, hair ('premature pubarche' – Silverman et al 1952). These children probably represent one end of a spectrum of adrenal androgen secretion or perhaps of sensitivity to its action as plasma levels are not always high for age. It must be distinguished from nonclassical, late-onset (Forest et al 1985) or missed CAH and (rare) adrenal tumors (in which, in contrast, androgens are not dexamethasone-suppressible) as well as from true precocious puberty. In one clinic, a 30% incidence of nonclassical 21-hydroxylase deficiency was found in those presenting with premature pubarche (Temeck et al 1987). Although premature pubarche per se is probably physiological (puberty timing is normal or slightly early, Grumbach et al 1978), hirsutism or polycystic ovarian disease may develop at puberty – polycystic ovaries may be detected ultrasonically by pelvic ultrasound and androgen levels may remain high in adulthood (Forest 1995a).

The role of adrenarche in man remains controversial (Stirling & Kelnar 1990). It is difficult to extrapolate from pathological situations to normal gonadarche control. Adrenarche may be delayed in children with CDGP and isolated GH deficiency but not in hypergonadotropic hypogonadism (e.g. Turner's syndrome – Lee et al 1975). Children with Addison's disease enter puberty normally (Grumbach et al 1978) and in diabetic adolescents gonadarche may proceed normally despite delayed adrenarche. Children with congenital adrenal hypoplasia all have hypogonadotropic hypogonadism and do not enter puberty normally (Hay et al 1981). It is possible that adrenals may have a much earlier priming effect on gonadarche analogously to the situation in the rat (but rats do not have an adrenarche) but a causal role for adrenarche in gonadarche in man seems unlikely.

Adrenarche is coincident with the preadolescent fat spurt (Stolz & Stolz 1951, Tanner & Whitehouse 1975) and with the mid-childhood growth spurt (Tanner 1962, Molinari et al 1980). The latter could reflect a bone and muscle response to adrenal androgens, directly or indirectly by influencing GH secretion – androgens are important in determining the pulsatile nature of GH secretion in rats (Millard et al 1986) and at about 7 years a change in GH secretion with development of a dominant periodicity of ∼ 200 min is found in man (Hindmarsh & Brook 1995).

There is an apparent fall in 11β-hydroxylation during adrenarche (Kelnar & Brook 1983) and observed changes in steroidogenesis and their correlation with systolic BP in a group of normal boys followed longitudinally (Kelnar 1985) could implicate a role for adrenarche in the pathogenesis of essential hypertension in genetically susceptible individuals with other than low salt intakes. It is unlikely, however, that a primary abnormality in adrenal steroidogenesis is important in the generation of essential hypertension.

Adrenarche could simply be a byproduct of the need of inner fetal adrenal cells to respond to the hormonal milieu of pregnancy by developing an androgen (i.e. estrogen-precursor) synthesizing zone (Anderson 1980). Other than man, only the chimpanzee has adrenarche (Cutler et al 1978) which therefore occurs in two species which have the most prolonged interval between birth and puberty. Adrenarche may merely be revealed by such an interval. However, the more complex the organism the greater the advantage in prolonging the period between birth and reproductive activity to allow brain growth and childhood learning. If during that period androgens are required for continuing skeletal and muscular growth, this could be achieved by transferring androgen biosynthesis from gonad to adrenal – adrenarche (Tanner 1981).

Congenital adrenal hyperplasia (CAH)

CAH describes collectively a group of autosomal recessively inherited disorders of adrenal corticosteroid biosynthesis due to deficiency of one of five enzymes in the cholesterol to cortisol biosynthetic pathway – 21-hydroxylase (21OH, $P-450_{c21}$), 11β-hydroxylase (11βOH, $P-450_{c11}$), 3β-hydroxysteroid dehydrogenase (3βOHSD), 17α-hydroxylase (17αOH, $P-450_{c17}$) and cholesterol desmolase ($P-450_{scc}$) (see Fig. 19.37). Deficiencies of other enzymes such as 17,20-desmolase ($P-450_{c17}$ 17,20-lyase), 17β-hydroxysteroid dehydrogenase (17βOHSD) and 5α-reductase have effects limited to the adrenal androgen (and gonadal) biosynthetic pathway (p. 1060).

The steroidogenic block due to a specific enzyme deficiency will have potential clinical effects by two types of mechanism: (1) distal hormone deficiency and (2) the effect of ACTH drive, a compensatory response in CRF-ACTH release secondary to the defect in cortisol biosynthesis and reduced feedback inhibition of ACTH, leading to (a) proximal metabolite accumulation and (b) abnormal production of steroids whose biosynthesis is unaffected by the primary enzyme deficiency (Table 19.15).

Thus in the commonest form of CAH (21OH deficiency, $P-450_{c21}$ deficiency) there is, potentially, cortisol deficiency (in practice unstressed cortisol levels are normal as the enzyme deficiency is seldom complete), aldosterone deficiency and salt loss (when the defect is also present in the zona glomerulosa); plasma 17-hydroxyprogesterone (17OHP), and its principal urinary metabolite, pregnanetriol, levels are raised (and conveniently measured to confirm the diagnosis) and ACTH hypersecretion results in excess adrenal androgen and virilization (by birth in females, during early childhood in undiagnosed males).

Inappropriately raised plasma ACTH levels for plasma cortisol are pathognomonic of CAH – measuring cortisol alone is useless for diagnosis. Although the clinical picture may suggest the specific underlying enzyme defect, definitive diagnosis is dependent on detecting raised plasma levels of precursors by RIA or IRMA and characteristic urinary metabolite. Occasionally, measurement following ACTH stimulation may be necessary if the situation is not clear-cut. Pointers to the possibility of CAH include ambiguous genitalia in the newborn, vomiting with dehydration and urinary salt wasting during early days or weeks of life, collapse during stress (e.g. severe intercurrent illness or general anesthesia) at any age, hypertension, hirsutism or inappropriate virilization, primary amenorrhea, unexplained previous neonatal death (particularly if parents are consanguineous) and a family history of CAH.

For a comprehensive recent review of CAH, see New et al (1996b).

Table 19.15 Clinical and laboratory features in the commonest forms of congenital adrenal hyperplasia

Enzyme deficiency	Sexual ambiguity in newborn	Salt-wasting	Hypertension	Blood	Urine
21-hydroxylase (simple virilizing)	Female	–	–	17OHP ++ An ++ DHA n/+ Renin n/+	PT ++ Aldo n
21-hydroxylase (salt-wasting)	Female	+	–	17OHP ++ An ++ DHA n/+ Renin ++	PT ++ Aldo –
11β-hydroxylase	Female	–	+	17OHP + An ++ DHA + Renin – –	PT + THS ++ Aldo –
3β-hydroxysteroid dehydrogenase	Male and Female	+	–	17OHP n/+ An ++ DHA +++ Renin +	PT n/+ Aldo –

17OHP = 17 α-hydroxyprogesterone, An = δ-4-androstenedione, DHA = dehydroepiandrosterone, THS = tetrahydrodeoxycortisol, Aldo = aldosterone, PT = pregnanetriol
+++ = very high, ++ = high, + = moderately high, n = normal, – = low, – – = very low.

21-hydroxylase (21OH, P-450$_{c21}$) deficiency

This is by far the commonest form of CAH worldwide although there are considerable ethnic differences. The frequency of the homozygous state varies from 1 in 5000 (Europe) to 1 in 23 000 and is particularly common in Alaskan Eskimos (1 in 700). Nonclassical 21OH deficiency (see below) seems commoner and may affect 1 in 30 Jews of Eastern European (Ashkenazi) origin and 1 in 100 other whites (Speiser et al 1985).

Genetics. Molecular genetic techniques have localized two genes encoding the 21OH enzyme, CYP21B (active) and CYP21A (inactive), to the short arm of chromosome 6 either side of the genes for the fourth component of complement – there is close linkage with the HLA complex. Deletion of CYP21B is associated with severe, salt-wasting disease and the HLA B47, DR7 haplotype; deletion of CYP21A seems not to cause any hormonal abnormality (White et al 1985). Most affected individuals are compound heterozygotes (Cheetham & Hughes 1996). HLA associations with nonclassical 21OH deficiency vary between ethnic groups (Dupont et al 1977).

The presence of salt wasting in association with virilization was thought to breed true in affected families because of separate genetic regulatory control of glomerulosa and fasciculata – only salt wasters have an additional glomerulosa 21OH defect. Although there are separate control mechanisms for 21OH activity in these zones and simple virilizing and salt-wasting forms have different HLA associations, families who do not breed true are reported (Stoner et al 1986). Obligate heterozygote parents of salt-losing and simple virilizing patients show identical sodium, aldosterone and renin responses to a low sodium diet and some infants with aldosterone biosynthetic defects subsequently develop normal glomerulosa 21OH activity suggesting that other (non-HLA-linked) mechanisms are involved in enzyme expression (New et al 1996b).

The importance of these molecular genetic developments lies in the practical ability to confirm (pre- or postnatally) whether family members are affected or unaffected and in advancing understanding of pathogenesis. The genetics of 21OH deficiency is reviewed by Cheetham & Hughes (1996) and New et al (1996b).

Prenatal diagnosis of 21OH deficiency was first reported in 1965 (Jeffcoate et al 1965) on the basis of elevated 17-ketosteroids and pregnanetriol levels in amniotic fluid (i.e. dilute fetal urine) of an affected fetus. Raised 17OHP and andros-tenedione levels have since been found in many studies (e.g. Pang et al 1980) and HLA genotyping of amniotic cells was used in addition. Chorionic villus sampling, and molecular typing for restriction fragment length polymorphisms of the chromosome 6 loci, 21-hydroxylase gene and HLA, is now possible by 8–11 weeks' gestation and has replaced HLA genotyping of amniotic cells. Rapid early prenatal diagnosis by direct assay of specific mutations using DNA amplification by polymerase chain reaction (PCR) is now feasible (Owerbach et al 1992).

Antenatal diagnosis (AND) and treatment. Antenatal therapy with dexamethasone (which crosses the placenta) can be used (Evans et al 1985) (in a dose not exceeding 20 μg/kg/day of the prepregnancy weight in two to three divided doses) to suppress the excessive ACTH/androgen-induced virilization, and can be considered in managing a second affected female fetus. Although data from uncontrolled studies are now available concerning prenatal dexamethasone therapy (Pang et al 1992, Forest et al 1993, Mercado et al 1995) and reviewed in Kelnar (1993b), Cheetham & Hughes (1996) and Seckl and Miller (1996), the degree of benefit (reduced virilization) compared to potentially significant maternal side effects is unclear – possible long-term childhood side effects have not been studied. At present, therefore, there seems insufficient evidence regarding the safety of mother and fetus to recommend general dexamethasone use outwith controlled scientific studies. However, some consider it effective and safe and an algorithm for the prenatal management of the 'at risk' pregnancy has been published (New et al 1996b).

Heterozygote detection and neonatal screening. Stimulated 17OHP levels after ACTH will distinguish classical 21OH deficiency patients from heterozygotes for classical or nonclassical disease and from HLA-typed normal family members but HLA typing cannot be used on a population basis to detect heterozygosity (e.g. in the spouse of a potential carrier).

Newborn screening is highly desirable. Male infants (with normal genitalia) may give no warning of a salt-losing crisis with high morbidity and mortality. Females may be sufficiently virilized to be thought normal males leading to later gender reassignment or hysterectomy and sterility. Non-salt-losing males may be late diagnosed, by when secondary true precocious puberty and ultimate short stature may be inevitable. Classical 21OH deficiency is commoner than phenylketonuria and, in Europe, is nearly as common as congenital hypothyroidism. A reliable and cheap (in centers already providing a neonatal screening service) screening test is available (Pang et al 1977) using heel-prick capillary blood samples taken on to filter paper to measure 17OHP, easily done as part of the 'Guthrie test' procedure.

A Scottish pilot screening study demonstrated that large-scale (national) screening was feasible measuring 17OHP in neonatal blood spot samples using a nonextraction assay based on an iodinated steroid tracer (Wallace et al 1986). Only 30% of males were clinically suspected to have 21OHD before the positive screening result become available.

Significant mortality and serious physical and emotional morbidity consequent on late diagnosis has led to many screening programs worldwide, e.g. Italy, France, Japan, Ireland, New Zealand and a number of US States (Pang et al 1988). Experience from screening more than 1 million neonates in over 13 screening programs in six countries confirms that screening improves detection of salt-wasting newborns whose diagnosis is otherwise delayed or missed and in whom there is significant mortality and morbidity (Pang et al 1989). Morbidity in non-salt-losing males presenting in mid-childhood is also considerable.

In the UK it is generally considered unnecessary (Virdi et al 1987) or 'uneconomical' to screen the whole newborn population even though this would add only small additional unit cost in screening laboratories already measuring TSH and phenylalanine (Wallace et al 1986). There may be insufficient acknowledgment of considerable potential morbidity and concentration on mortality statistics. In one study (Donaldson et al 1994b) there was a 25% incidence of childhood learning difficulties in salt-losing patients. However, there are, to date, few published data on improvements in morbidity resulting from early detection and treatment.

Clinical presentation. Classical simple virilizing 21OH deficiency in a karyotypic female results in masculinization generally leading to ambiguous external genitalia recognized at birth (Fig. 19.39) but occasionally so severe that the infant is thought to be a normal male. Internal female structures including ovaries, Fallopian tubes and uterus are normal (there are no testes to elaborate MIH) but there is variable labioscrotal fold fusion with a urogenital sinus, genital pigmentation and clitoromegaly. Males usually appear normal at birth but present with penile enlargement, rapid growth (and tall stature) and advanced skeletal maturation (leading to eventual short stature) within a few years (Fig. 19.40). Finding small testes with clinical signs of precocious puberty suggests the adrenals as the androgen source but skeletal maturational advance can be so marked that true precocious puberty develops when treatment starts (see Fig. 19.21).

In the classical salt-wasting form (50–75%) there is an additional defect in mineralocorticoid biosynthesis with aldosterone deficiency due to an inability to convert progesterone to deoxycorticosterone in the glomerulosa. Presentation in both sexes is with severe renal wasting of sodium, dehydration and vomiting within a few days or weeks of birth – this should be foreseen as a possibility in a baby with ambiguous genitalia.

Nonclassical ('mild, late-onset') 21OH deficiency was

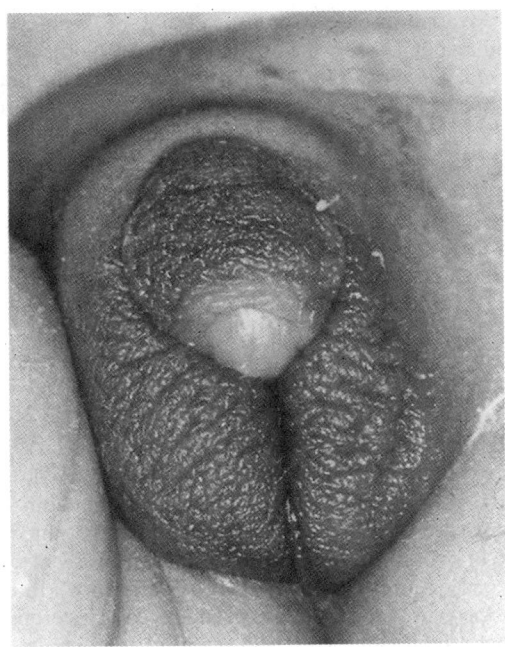

Fig. 19.39 Ambiguous genitalia in a 10-day-old genotypic female due to 21-hydroxylase deficiency.

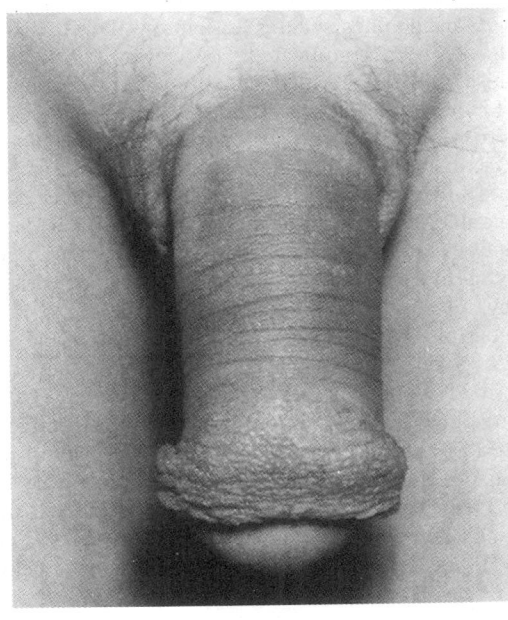

Fig. 19.40 Precocious pseudopuberty – a boy with non-salt-losing 21-hydroxylase deficiency at presentation at 5 years – testicular volume 2 ml (see also Fig. 19.21).

suspected in women presenting with hirsutism and infertility and family studies in classical 21OH deficiency characterized it (Rosenwaks et al 1979) as having different (and differing) HLA associations from classical forms but being also autosomal recessive. It may present as early as 6 months (Kohn et al 1982) or later with premature pubarche, rapid growth (and reduced height prognosis), acne, male-type baldness in the female, delayed menarche or secondary amenorrhea. There is an association with polcystic ovarian disease (Chrousos et al 1982) – infertility may result and respond to GC therapy (New et al 1996b).

Laboratory diagnosis. 17OHP measurement in the newborn is reliable for screening and diagnosis but false positives are reported in preterm or sick neonates. Plasma ACTH, androstenedione and urinary pregnanetriol levels will also be raised. In the salt-wasting form, there is urinary sodium loss (cf. the gut in gastroenteritis); aldosterone levels are low for the high renin levels (cf. renal disease). Clinical and laboratory features of this and the other least uncommon forms of CAH are summarized in Table 19.15. Management is discussed below.

11β-hydroxylase (11βOH, P-450$_{c11}$) deficiency

This accounts for some 5% of CAH. There is no HLA association (cf. 21OH deficiency). Clinical manifestations are, as predicted from biosynthetic pathways (Fig. 19.37), identical to 21OH deficiency from the virilizing point of view – in some affected individuals there is restriction of the defect to the glucocorticoid pathway. In over 50%, however, the glomerulosa is also affected but the consequences differ from 21OH deficiency (Table 19.15) because there is accumulation of deoxycorticosterone (DOC) which has significant MC (salt-retaining) properties and, in excess, causes hypertension. DOC may not be directly responsible for hypertension in all cases as some patients with 11βOH deficiency with raised DOC levels are normotensive and others are hypertensive with normal or only slightly raised DOC levels. Other DOC metabolites such as 18-hydroxy DOC (Rosler et al 1982) have been implicated. However fasciculata and glomerulosa 11βOH are undoubtedly under separate genetic control (Levine et al 1980).

18-hydroxylation (the next step in the aldosterone biosynthetic pathway) is a function of the same mitochondrial enzyme – a defect in 18-hydroxylase is often seen with 11βOH deficiency (Levine et al 1980, Yannagibashi et al 1986). Milder (late-onset) forms and even salt-wasting patients have been reported – clinically 11βOH deficiency is as heterogeneous as 21OH deficiency.

Hypertension, when present, is characteristic and may be extreme; hypokalemic alkalosis is common. Virilizing effects are as described under 21OH deficiency above. DOC and deoxycortisol (S) levels are raised, as are their respective urinary tetrahydro (TH) metabolites (THDOC and THS), and rise further following ACTH, but their proportional elevations vary between subjects. Prenatal diagnosis has been carried out (Rosler et al 1979) using a combination of amniotic fluid studies and maternal urinary THS measurement. Management is discussed below.

3β-hydroxysteroid dehydrogenase (3βOHSD) deficiency (Bongiovanni 1962)

This is also associated with ambiguous genitalia in newborns but the site of the block (Fig. 19.37) results in potential ambiguity both in genotypic males and females (Table 19.15): high levels of DHA and its peripheral conversion to potent androgens result in variable clitoromegaly in females but are insufficient to fully masculinize a male infant, resulting in variable hypospadias (often the severe perineoscrotal form) with palpable testes. The defect in MC biosynthesis usually causes severe salt wasting. Mild defects are important causes of hirsutism presenting in young adult women so that, as in 21OH deficiency, mild, late-onset forms are

apparently commoner than the classical severe type (Pang et al 1985). There is no HLA association and neither ethnic nor geographical clustering. Prenatal diagnosis is impossible because of low 3βOHSD fetal zone activity.

17α-hydroxylase (17αOH, P-450$_{c17}$) deficiency

Mineralocorticoid biosynthesis is intact (Fig. 19.37) and ACTH drive may result in neonatal hypertension and hypokalemic alkalosis. Deficient adrenal (and gonadal) sex steroid secretion means that karyotypic females usually present with failure of puberty and primary amenorrhea; males have ambiguous genitalia or virilize inadequately at puberty with gynecomastia. No HLA linkage has been demonstrated – the gene for 17αOH is on chromosome 10 (Chung et al 1987).

Cholesterol desmolase deficiency (P-450$_{scc}$, cholesterol side chain cleavage deficiency, lipoid adrenal hyperplasia)

This was originally described as lipoid adrenal hyperplasia because of adrenal accumulation of cholesterol. Pregnenolone is the precursor of all MCs, GCs and androgens (Fig. 19.37) and complete deficiency is presumably incompatible with life. In contrast to congenital adrenal hypoplasia (see below) gonadal steroids are also deficient. The P-450$_{scc}$ gene has been located in the q23 to q24 region of chromosome 15.

Management of CAH

The basic defect (in cortisol biosynthesis) has wide repercussions including survival itself, sexual differentiation, growth, pubertal development and adult sexual functioning. Management potentially involves sex assignment, hormone therapy, surgery and psychological and emotional support with attention to growth and puberty and not merely adrenal steroid levels (Cheetham & Hughes 1996).

Hormone replacement is aimed at appropriately suppressing excessive ACTH drive rather than simply replacing cortisol – cortisol levels are often normal in the unstressed situation. In a baby with salt loss, titration of the appropriate GC replacement dose (against ACTH, adrenal androgen or 17OHP levels) is misleading until there is sodium balance (evidenced by normal plasma renin and plasma and urinary sodium). In the older child also, raised ACTH levels may be due to inadequate MC replacement.

The normal cortisol production rate is lower than previously thought: approximately 6–7 mg/m²/day (Linder et al 1990, Kerrigan et al 1993). Appropriate GC replacement will allow normal growth, skeletal maturation and puberty – hydrocortisone (HC) 12–15 mg/m²/day in two to three divided doses is usually appropriate. However larger doses (< 20–25 mg/m²/day) may be necessary to suppress androgen levels (Sandrini et al 1993) and a combination regimen of physiological GC replacement with antiandrogens or aromatase inhibitors has been suggested (Cutler and Laue 1990).

To mimic normal diurnal rhythms, approximately two-thirds of the total HC dose is usually given first thing in the morning and the last dose at bedtime. In some it is necessary to give a longer-acting steroid (e.g. prednisone or dexamethasone) at bedtime if early morning ACTH and 17OHP levels are not to be too high – once-daily dexamethasone may be appropriate for adolescents and adults and may also improve ovarian function in women (Horrocks & London 1987).

The correct GC dose must be determined for each individual. Too low a dose will allow androgen-mediated excessively rapid growth, disproportionate bone age advance and eventual stunting. Too much will cause slowing of linear growth, delay (but not comparable delay) in bone maturation, also resulting ultimately in short stature. Swinging from one extreme to the other causes cumulative deficits in height prognosis.

Monitoring is by accurate growth and bone age assessment supplemented by home finger-prick blood spot 17OHP profiles four times daily approximately monthly. Abnormally rapid growth and bone age maturation is associated with nonsuppressed 17OHP levels (> 40 nmol/l), whereas GC over-replacement, evidenced by pathologically slow growth, is associated with levels < 10 nmol/l (Pincus et al 1993).

GC therapy must be increased two- to threefold during stress such as significant infection or general anesthesia which could otherwise precipitate hypoglycemia and collapse. The family should be provided with, and instructed in the use of, injectable hydrocortisone (phosphate) in case the child is vomiting or becomes rapidly ill at home. A Medicalert bracelet or talisman should be worn – as with other patients on steroid medication.

Mineralocorticoid (MC) replacement is necessary in salt-losing forms of CAH, given as the synthetic analogue 9α-fluorocortisol (fludrocortisone) 0.1–0.15 mg/m²/day in one or two daily doses. However, the salt-losing crisis cannot be treated with fludrocortisone (nor with hydrocortisone, which has limited MC activity) – emergency treatment with sodium replacement and i.v. normal or even hypertonic saline will be necessary as the total body sodium deficit is considerable. Once sodium balance is restored, fludrocortisone is introduced (and GC dose titration can begin) but oral sodium supplements (initially 2 mmol/kg/day) may also be required during infancy. Regular BP and urinary electrolyte measurements are sufficient check that MC replacement is appropriate. Renin and aldosterone clinic measurements may not be very meaningful. After infancy, children can adjust their salt intake and theoretically do not require long-term MC replacement. In practice, health and growth seem better if MC therapy is continued. The hypertension found in some forms of 11βOH and 17OH deficiencies responds to GC suppression of ACTH/MC overproduction.

Sex assignment seldom poses problems. In 21OH and 11βOH deficiencies karyotypic females with ambiguous genitalia should be reared as girls – internal sexual organs are normal female and with appropriate therapy there is about a 70% chance of fertility. Clitoral reduction is usually necessary for cosmetic reasons (see below). Assignment in rarer forms (3βOHSD, 17OH and cholesterol desmolase deficiencies) where males may be very poorly virilized depends on functional possibilities after potential reconstructive procedures (see p. 1796).

In virilized females, clitoral reduction is best undertaken before 6 months. The vascular and neural supply to the glans is maintained to aid later sexual functioning and pleasure. Labial separation, if necessary, may be carried out simultaneously. Vaginal reconstruction is best delayed until after puberty – often simple stretching will allow estrogen-mediated development at puberty obviating the need for major surgery. Early reconstruction is more commonly associated with discomfort at intercourse (Mulaikal et al 1987). Fertility prospects are good in males but only about 40% of affected women are fertile (Mulaikal et al 1987).

Emotional support is necessary for families of children with ambiguous genitalia particularly in the neonatal period and adolescence. Reports in the American literature of high rates of homosexuality in female CAH patients (Azziz et al 1986) may reflect inadequate vaginoplasty and difficult heterosexual relationships but effects of high androgen levels on the female fetal cerebral cortex could be important. Psychosexual outcomes in individuals treated prenatally will help to resolve the question but are not yet available.

Hyperadrenocorticism

Adrenal hypercorticism is commonly secondary to tropic hormone stimulation causing adrenal hyperplasia and hypersecretion and rarely primary (usually due to adrenal tumor). Clinical features are mimicked by (and in practice much more commonly due to) excessive GC administration (iatrogenic Cushing's syndrome – see below). Causes are listed in Table 19.16.

Cushing's syndrome (Cushing 1932)

Cushing's syndrome – disorders due to chronic excessive GC production – is uncommon in childhood – only 5–10% of reported cases – and rare in young children. It may be due to: (1) benign or malignant adrenal tumor (Lee et al 1984); (2) pituitary ACTH hypersecretion (Cushing's disease); (3) ACTH or CRF hypersecretion from malignant extrapituitary tumors (ectopic ACTH syndrome); (4) supraphysiological parenteral, oral or topical GC or ACTH therapy for other medical conditions – most frequently (Forest 1995a).

Clinical features are due to cortisol excess resulting in protein catabolism, increased carbohydrate production, fat accumulation and potassium wasting. In children, classical signs and symptoms (hypertension, truncal obesity, moon face, striae, proximal muscle weakness, osteoporosis, psychiatric symptoms) are usually less clear-cut than in adults and combined growth effects of hypercortisolism and excess adrenal androgen secretion may cause growth failure or temporarily rapid growth. The former is commoner, however, and hirsutism, progressive truncal obesity and growth failure (cf. obesity due to overeating) make up the most common presenting triad. Hypertension is usually only moderate and of multifactorial pathogenesis (Saruta et al 1986).

Table 19.16 Important causes of adrenocortical hyperfunction

Glucocorticoids	Iatrogenic (glucocorticoid therapy); Cushing's syndrome; carcinoma/adenoma; bilateral hyperplasia (Cushing's disease/pituitary tumor/ectopic ACTH-secreting tumor)
Mineralocorticoids	Primary hyperaldosteronism; Conn's syndrome (adenoma); Bartter's syndrome; congenital adrenal hyperplasia (17α-hydroxylase and 11β-hydroxylase deficiencies); deoxycorticosterone- (DOC) or corticosterone-secreting tumors
Sex steroids	*Androgens* Congenital adrenal hyperplasia (21-hydroxylase and 11β-hydroxylase deficiencies); 'premature' adrenarche (pubarche); virilizing carcinoma/adenoma *Estrogens* Feminizing carcinoma/adenoma

Iatrogenic disease must be specifically sought. ACTH is used to treat hypsarrhythmia and oral GC is used for a variety of chronic renal and connective tissue disorders (now less commonly for asthma). Large doses of inhaled steroids can be associated with significant adrenal suppression and growth failure (reviewed in Tönshoff et al 1996) as can topical steroids, depending on the extent of surface treated, frequency of application, potency of drug, use of occlusion and the age of patient (David 1989, Massarano et al 1993, Patel et al 1995). Infants, treated for seborrheic dermatitis/eczema, and adolescents are relatively sensitive to topical steroid side effects – an infant's (wet and occluded) napkin area has relative absorption 42-fold higher than the forearm; adolescents' increasing fat deposits and muscle mass inducing dermal remodeling makes them particularly susceptible to striae particularly around breasts and buttocks. If the hypothalamopituitary-adrenal axis is suppressed, treatment must be withdrawn gradually if acute adrenal insufficiency (see below) is not to be precipitated.

No single screening test is reliable in detecting Cushing's syndrome at an early stage or in differentiating it from exogenous obesity. A normal plasma cortisol diurnal rhythm, with normal urinary free cortisol levels and a normal short (overnight) dexamethasone suppression test (0.3 mg/m^2 orally at midnight measuring 8 a.m. plasma cortisol) will reasonably exclude the diagnosis. A 2-day low dose (6 mg/kg every 6 h) dexamethasone suppression test measuring plasma cortisol at 48 h, or urinary free cortisol corrected for creatinine, is necessary if results are equivocal.

Once the diagnosis is established, further differential diagnosis of the cause may also be difficult. Rapidly evolving symptoms, palpable abdominal mass and virilization at any age make adrenal carcinoma most likely and this is relatively common in infancy (Hayles et al 1966) but, generally, diagnosis depends on diagnostic imaging techniques (e.g. adrenal ultrasound, pituitary and adrenal CT scanning, adrenal iodocholesterol scintigraphy) and further dynamic hormone tests (e.g. response to metyrapone, high dose dexamethasone, CRF). Diagnostic algorithms are given and discussed by Forest (1995a) and Howlett & Besser (1989) – investigation should be carried out in specialist centers.

Treatment (Forest 1995a, Howlett & Besser 1989) depends on the cause and may be medical, surgical (to pituitary or adrenals), radiotherapy or radioactive implants. Medical treatment (e.g. with drugs blocking cortisol biosynthesis or GC antagonists) is of value in many patients prior to surgery, if inoperable lesions are found and in Cushing's disease. In virtually all situations treatment, however unsatisfactory, is urgent because of the progressive and severe natural course untreated.

Hyperaldosteronism

Primary mineralocorticoid (MC) hypersecretion is very rare in childhood and usually due to a zona glomerulosa adenoma (Conn's syndrome – Conn 1974) or bilateral hyperplasia. There is sodium retention and hypertension with hypokalemia, renin suppression and hyperaldosteronism which fails to suppress with dexamethasone. In addition to hypertension, there may be muscle weakness, polyuria and impaired growth. Treatment is medical (long-term spironolactone) in hyperplasia and surgical in adenoma.

Familial forms of hyperaldosteronism. Dexamethasone-suppressible hyperaldosteronism is clinically and biochemically indistinguishable from primary hyperaldosteronism but aldosterone levels suppress rapidly on dexamethasone administration. Hypertension can be controlled by GC therapy. Autosomal dominant inheritance (not HLA linked) has been proposed (New et al 1980). *Bartter's syndrome* (Bartter et al 1962) is discussed in Chapter 17. *Apparent mineralocorticoid excess (AME) syndrome* is often familial – aldosterone levels are low and there is no evidence for overproduction of other MCs. The pathogenesis is now known to be primary *11β-hydroxysteroid dehydrogenase* (11βOHSD) *deficiency* resulting in defective cortisol metabolism to cortisone. The resulting prolongation of cortisol half-life and bioactivity may result in sufficient MC activity to cause hypertension (Dimartino-Nardi et al 1987). Diagnosis depends on the finding of a raised (> 1) ratio of the main urinary metabolite of cortisol (tetrahydrocortisol, THF) to that of cortisone (THE) on gas chromatography, in association with low renin hypertension and normal or low aldosterone levels.

11βOHSD is a widely distributed enzyme which exists in two types – type II is found in the placenta and distal renal nephron, is NAD dependent and converts the (active) glucocorticoid cortisol (F) to (inactive) cortisone (E) (Fig. 19.41). The mineralocorticoid receptor (MR) has little affinity for E whereas aldosterone cannot be inactivated in this way and retains full access to the MR (New et al 1996a). Increased availability and binding of cortisol at the MR at the renal distal tubule is the currently accepted pathophysiological mechanism underlying AME (Stewart et al 1988).

11βOHSD may be of wider importance than simply in the etiology of AME. It is plentiful in the placenta and could be important in protecting the fetus from maternal cortisol. Epidemiological evidence suggests that small fetuses are more likely in adulthood to develop hypertension and other cardiovascular diseases and type 2 diabetes mellitus (Barker et al 1990, Barker 1992, Law et al 1993, Osmond et al 1993, Barker et al 1993). There is also epidemiological evidence that babies most at risk of subsequent hypertension are those born small with large placentae (Barker et al 1990). In rats, increased 11βOHSD activity is associated with increased fetal weight, decreased activity and large placentae. It is speculated that the growth-retarded human fetus has been exposed to excessive cortisol in utero due to relative placental 11βOHSD deficiency which could reflect placental and fetal growth and that this has long-lasting effects (e.g. adult hypertension) by imprinting via brain receptor or neurochemical mechanisms (Benediktsson et al 1993, Edwards et al 1993, Seckl 1993).

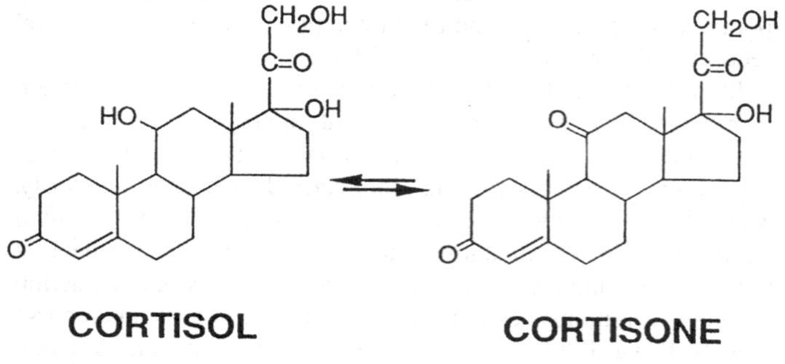

Fig. 19.41 Cortisol–cortisone interconversion (see text).

Secondary hyperaldosteronism may be due to various causes, most importantly renin-secreting tumors either of the juxtaglomerular apparatus or from ectopic sites such as pancreatic adenocarcinoma. Renin levels are very high.

Pseudohypoaldosteronism due to end-organ resistance to aldosterone is characterized by high levels of urinary aldosterone metabolites which distinguish it from 18-hydroxylase and dehydrogenase deficiencies. Clinical presentation is identical and it is discussed under sodium-losing states (see below).

Insufficiency

Adrenocortical hypofunction may result from primary adrenal disorders or may be secondary to hypothalamopituitary disorders (see p. 1046). Hypofunction may be complete or affect specific functions – GC, MC or androgen biosynthesis. Chronic conditions may present with dramatic symptoms relating to acute adrenal insufficiency ('Addisonian crisis') but may remain asymptomatic and diagnosis may be long delayed. Causes are listed in Table 19.17.

Congenital adrenal hypoplasia (Migeon & Lanes 1996)

After CAH, this is the commonest neonatal cause of adrenal hypofunction. Sporadic cases are associated with anencephaly or other congenital (e.g. renal and cardiac) malformations and maternal pre-eclampsia. Familial forms are sex-linked or autosomal recessive. Adrenocortical failure presents with adrenal hypoplasia or atrophy – combined adrenal autopsy weight < 1 g or < 1% of total bodyweight is characteristic. It is a rare cause of low maternal estriol levels during pregnancy.

Histological findings are heterogeneous but of three main types: (1) primary (cytomegalic) – a rare form in males, with poorly

Table 19.17 Important causes of adrenocortical hypofunction

Primary complete (glucocorticoids/mineralocorticoids/androgens)
   Congenital adrenal hypoplasia
   Lipoid adrenal hyperplasia (cholesterol desmolase deficiency)
   Addison's disease
   Adrenal apoplexy (Waterhouse–Friderichsen syndrome)
   Adrenal hemorrhage/cysts
   Adrenoleukodystrophy
   Autoimmune multiple endocrinopathy syndromes

Primary selective – glucocorticoids
   Congenital adrenal hyperplasia (21-hydroxylase, 17α-hydroxylase and 11β-hydroxylase deficiencies)
   Iatrogenic
   Hereditary unresponsiveness to ACTH

Primary selective – mineralocorticoids
   Pseudohypoaldosteronism
   Aldosterone biosynthetic defect (18-hydroxylase and 18-dehydrogenase deficiency)

Primary selective – androgens
   17,20-desmolase deficiency

Secondary
   Iatrogenic (glucocorticoid therapy)
   Hypothalamopituitary dysfunction
     Panhypopituitarism
     Isolated ACTH deficiency
     Craniopharyngioma
     Structural midline defects

differentiated cortex, disordered architecture and giant cells; (2) secondary (anencephalic) – the commonest in sporadic and familial cases – the fetal zone is reduced or absent but definitive cortex is well differentiated, mimicking the appearance in anencephalics; (3) miniature, comprising about one-third of cases – the glands are small but normally differentiated.

All three types occur sporadically. Two hereditary forms have been characterized: (1) autosomal recessive, usually associated with the miniature histological type; (2) X-linked, usually associated with the cytomegalic form and affecting boys. Pathogenesis is unclear but there is an association with hypogonadotropic hypogonadism (see under adrenarche) and with X-linked glycerol kinase deficiency.

In all types and forms, clinical presentation is within the first few hours or days of life with vomiting, diarrhea, apnea, hypoglycemia with convulsions, hyponatremic dehydration, hyperkalemia and metabolic acidosis. Plasma cortisol and aldosterone levels are very low with high renin. ACTH levels are very high (cf. adrenal failure secondary to pituitary disorders but not differentiating it from CAH). In karyotypic females it is indistinguishable from cholesterol desmolase deficiency (see p. 1064) but other forms of CAH can be identified as described above. Treatment is analogous to that of salt losing CAH (p. 1064). Prognosis was poor but is now much improved, particularly in those surviving the first few days.

Familial GC deficiency (hereditary unresponsiveness to ACTH) (Migeon et al 1968)

Onset is after the first year, sometimes with recurring hypoglycemia but often merely with a history of prostration during intrinsically mild intercurrent illness. There is hyperpigmentation and tall stature is common (Thistlethwaite et al 1975). Inheritance is probably autosomal recessive. Pathogenesis is unknown but may be degenerative – the glomerulosa is broad but fasciculata and reticularis are reduced to a fibrous band.

There is a selective defect in cortisol production with high ACTH levels. MC production is normal under basal conditions but may not remain so making the distinction from Addison's disease particularly difficult. Treatment is with GC which must be increased during severe intercurrent illness.

Addison's disease (Addison 1855)

This primary chronic form of adrenal insufficiency is rare in childhood affecting ~ 1 in 10 000. Hypoadrenalism much more commonly results from corticosteroid medication suppressing the pituitary–adrenal axis (see below). Variations in incidence – historically, geographically and in age of onset – probably represent changes in the epidemiology of the primary causes of adrenal damage and failure: until the 1950s, tuberculosis was overwhelmingly the commonest cause but 20 years later accounted for only about 1 in 5 UK cases.

The commonest cause is now autoimmune (AI) adrenal disease. As with other AI diseases there is a familial incidence and female preponderance. Adrenalitis is characterized by lymphocyte infiltration and adrenal microsomal and mitochondrial autoantibodies are found. The medulla is unaffected. There are associations with other AI conditions including hypothyroidism (Schmidt's syndrome – Carpenter et al 1964), hypoparathyroidism (in about 1 in 3 cases) and mucocutaneous candidiasis (Whitaker et al 1956), diabetes mellitus, cirrhosis and alopecia, but these can remain subclinical. Antibody titers are generally low, decrease further with age and do not correlate with the severity of the endocrinopathies. Cell-mediated (T lymphocyte) processes are more likely to be responsible for the adrenal cortical destruction. Familial (autosomal recessive) occurrence probably relates to the inheritance of the underlying tendency to AI disease – there is an association with HLA-A1, -A3 or -B8.

There is GC and MC deficiency which may not develop simultaneously. In childhood, presenting features are usually hypoglycemia, progressive lassitude and muscle weakness, gastrointestinal disturbances (including constipation or diarrhea, vomiting and abdominal pain), associated with mild hyperpigmentation (classically of buccal and vaginal mucosa, nipples and palmar creases and pressure areas – axillae and groin, due to pituitary β-lipotropin secretion). In practice, pigmentation may simply appear as excellent suntan or 'dirt' over extensor surfaces exposed to friction (e.g. knees, knuckles, elbows). For a comprehensive list of clinical and biological consequences of primary chronic adrenal insufficiency see Forest (1995b).

Major symptoms result from cortisol deficiency and consequent high plasma ACTH elevation. Glycogen stores are low – severe hypoglycemia may occur during fasting or intercurrent stress or illness. Hyponatremia results from aldosterone deficiency and reduced plasma volume induced vasopressin secretion causing water retention.

Characteristic laboratory findings are hyponatremia, hyperkalemia, raised urea, fasting hypoglycemia and anemia. Basal cortisol, aldosterone and adrenal androgen levels are commonly normal but with raised ACTH levels. Cortisol levels do not rise 60 or 120 min after a 'short' ACTH test (i.v. 1,24-ACTH 500 ng/1.73 m^2) (Dickstein et al 1991, Crowley et al 1993) – although the sensitivity of this test is still debatable (Crowley et al 1992, Patel et al 1995) – or after intramuscular ACTH 25 mg/m^2 (8-hourly for 3 days). Low T4 with raised TSH levels but often correct rapidly with GC treatment without thyroxine. Adrenal autoantibodies are characteristically present even before clinical onset and should lead to regular testing of adrenal function in patients with other AI disorders or siblings of affected individuals.

Acute 'Addisonian' crisis may occur as the presenting feature in a previously unsuspected case precipitated by intercurrent illness or stress. There is hypotension (otherwise uncommon in children with Addison's disease), dehydration, prostration and collapse, with hypoglycemia and the classical electrolyte disturbances described above, superimposed on symptoms and signs of the precipitating cause. Treatment with intravenous hydrocortisone and plasma or normal saline with 5 or 10% dextrose is urgent. Intravenous or intramuscular hydrocortisone must be continued whilst oral GC replacement is started. With adequate sodium replacement, MC treatment is not usually necessary acutely. After recovery, advice must be given about increasing GC dosage in appropriate circumstances (persistent vomiting requires hospitalization) and a Medicalert bracelet or talisman should be worn.

Long-term treatment is with oral hydrocortisone, usually 10–20 mg/m^2/24 h – the dose individually adjusted based on disappearance of symptoms, normal growth and skeletal maturation and normal diurnal ACTH levels. MC dosage (fludrocortisone 0.1–0.15 mg/m^2/24 h) is less critical provided it is adequate and assessed as in salt-losing CAH (p. 1064).

Treatment must be lifelong. Adrenal androgen therapy is unnecessary in childhood but a mild androgenic preparation may improve libido and pubic hair growth in adolescent and adult women. It is usually considered that puberty is normal in timing and progression (cf. congenital adrenal hypoplasia). Prognosis is normal in terms of health and life span presupposing optimal prevention and treatment of acute crises.

Sodium losing states

These may be due to renal disease (e.g. dysplasia, tubular disease, Bartter's syndrome, see Ch. 17, p. 946) or adrenal insufficiency. Adrenal urinary sodium wasting is characterized by hyperkalemia and due to defective aldosterone biosynthesis (congenital adrenal hypoplasia, salt-wasting forms of CAH – see above – or isolated aldosterone biosynthetic defects) or impaired action at the renal tubule (pseudohypoaldosteronism).

Isolated defects of aldosterone biosynthesis (Dillon 1995) may result from defective 18-hydroxylation (Degenhart et al 1966) or 18-dehydrogenation in conversion of corticosterone to aldosterone (see Fig. 19.37). Both are due to deficiency of corticosterone methyloxidase (CMO) which converts corticosterone to 18-hydroxycorticosterone – defective hydroxylation is known as CMO I, defective dehydrogenation as CMO II.

Inheritance is autosomal recessive. Presentation is with marked salt wasting, hyperkalemia and failure to thrive usually in early infancy. GC and androgen function are normal. Although, as in 21OH deficiency, there can be self-regulation of salt intake and proximal renal tubular maturation, the salt wasting tendency is lifelong and MC replacement should be for life.

Pseudohypoaldosteronism is due to a primary renal tubular sodium/potassium ATPase defect. Clinical presentation is identical to the 18-oxidation (CMO) defects (see above) but aldosterone is markedly elevated and MC therapy ineffective as the proximal renal tubule is unresponsive to its action. Treatment is with sodium supplements.

Adrenoleukodystropy (ALD)

Various uncommon associations between chronic adrenal insufficiency and progressive brain demyelinization are described with differing inheritance (see Migeon & Lanes 1996) but have in common the abnormal accumulation of saturated unbranched or monosaturated very long chain fatty acids owing to a defect in their catabolism. The ALD gene has been recently identified and maps to the long arm of the X chromosome (Xq28) (Mosser et al 1993). Adrenal insufficiency is secondary to cortical destruction; treatment is with GC and MC. The neurological disorder is progressive – these and related conditions (e.g. Zellweger syndrome) are further discussed in Chapter 14.

Other causes of acute adrenal insufficiency include adrenal destruction, e.g. hemorrhage due to birth trauma (see Ch. 5), and Waterhouse–Friderichsen syndrome (sepsis and collapse, often associated with meningococcemia).

Steroid withdrawal

Most commonly, adrenal crisis results from abrupt withdrawal of GC medication when the axis is suppressed from chronic GC administration (oral, inhaled or topical) or failure to increase GC during severe intercurrent illness or stress (see above). Alternate-day GC causes less hypothalamopituitary–adrenal axis suppression but the growth-sparing effects of such a regimen are less well documented. ACTH treatment is associated with more rapid current growth than is high dose GC, but this probably results from additional secondary adrenal androgen secretion and, if bone age advances disproportionately rapidly, ultimate stature may be just as impaired.

Tumors

Adrenal cortical tumors are rare in children. Virilizing tumors are relatively more common than feminizing or nonsecreting tumors and are usually carcinomas rather than adenomas. They are histologically identical to those causing Cushing's syndrome (p. 1065) but differ in secretory pattern and thus clinical manifestations. Predominantly androgen hypersecretion produces pseudoprecocious puberty (see p. 1063) – tall stature with growth acceleration and precocious pubic and axillary hair; in boys growth of the penis with prepubertal size testes, in girls clitoromegaly and labial enlargement. Treatment other than by surgical removal is disappointing and the prognosis often poor in any case.

THE ADRENAL MEDULLA

The medulla comprises cells of neuroectodermal origin which synthesize and secrete catecholamines, hormones containing a dihydroxylated phenolic ring. The most active compounds, adrenaline and noradrenaline, are both secreted by the medulla and noradrenaline is also produced in sympathetic ganglion cells.

Catecholamine biosynthesis

Catecholamines are synthesized (Fig. 19.42) from dietary tyrosine and tyrosine converted from phenylalanine by liver hydroxylation. Tyrosine is converted to dihydroxyphenylalanine (DOPA) in brain and sympathetic tissue as well as adrenal medulla, then to dihydroxyphenylethylamine (dopamine) and to noradrenaline and, only in the adrenal medulla and the organ of Zuckerkandl at the aortic bifurcation, to adrenaline. Catabolism and excretion (Fig. 19.42) is via vanillylmandelic acid (VMA), a urinary marker for catecholamine hypersecretion. Hypoglycemia, hypoxia, hypovolemia and exercise stimulate catecholamine release. Adrenaline has α- and β-adrenergic effects but noradrenaline is mainly α-adrenergic. Vasoconstriction is α receptor mediated; cardiac stimulation is via the β receptor. Dopaminergic effects also occur (Voorhess 1996).

Hypofunction

Adrenomedullary hypofuction is seldom important clinically. Adrenomedullary unresponsiveness is a rare cause of hypoglycemia in children but might be found less infrequently if catecholamines were measured more often during hypoglycemia. Sweating and pallor do not occur. The disorder may be of primarily hypothalamic origin as adrenocortical responsiveness may also be impaired and there is an association with perinatal problems.

In familial dysautonomia (Riley–Day syndrome), an autosomal recessive condition commonest in Ashkenazi Jews, there is disturbed autonomic function due to dopamine-β—hydroxylase deficiency resulting in impaired noradrenaline biosynthesis. Urinary VMA is decreased and urinary levels of homovanillic acid (HVA), a dopamine metabolite, are high. There is impaired swallowing in infancy with aspiration pneumonia, excessive sweating and salivation, defective lacrimation, labile BP, indifference to pain, loss of taste buds and corneal insensitivity and ulceration. Treatment is symptomatic and the majority die in childhood.

Hyperfunction

Catecholamine hypersecretion is usually associated with hypertension due to a neural crest catecholamine-secreting tumor – pheochromocytoma, neuroblastoma, ganglioblastoma or ganglioneuroma. It is discussed below.

ENDOCRINE HYPERTENSION

IMPORTANCE OF HYPERTENSION IN CHILDHOOD

The majority of children with higher than average blood pressure (BP) for age are part of a normal spectrum and those above the 95th centile will, in general, come within the category of essential hypertension although many will simply be obese (de Swiet & Dillon 1995). BP tracking occurs from an early age in normal children (de Swiet et al 1984) – there are steeper rises in normal levels from ~ 7 years of age. The pathogenesis of essential hypertension is poorly understood – primary endocrine abnormalities seem unlikely to be of paramount significance (but see p. 636). Until pathogenesis is clearer, preventive measures aimed at children in the upper BP centiles will remain controversial. Mass BP screening of children is probably unjustified (de Swiet et al 1989).

In contrast, children with sustained and very high BP are likely to have hypertension secondary to specific, and treatable, causes – overwhelmingly (~ 90%) renal disease (see Ch. 17). Diagnosis and treatment are urgent because, in this group, there is high morbidity and mortality from untreated hypertension. Too few ill children have BP measured. Regular measurements should be made in those with renal disease or diabetes and if previously high BP has been found (de Swiet et al 1989).

Endocrine hypertension usually results from corticosteroid excess (with low renin levels, cf. renal causes) or, less commonly, from catecholamine excess.

ENDOCRINE CAUSES OF HYPERTENSION

Corticosteroid excess

Congenital adrenal hyperplasia (CAH)

Some patients with 11βOH deficiency and all with 17αOH deficiency are hypertensive from ACTH-stimulated mineralocorticoid overproduction secondary to impaired cortisol biosynthesis. In both, excessive DOC levels are generally thought to be responsible for the hypertension (but see above). Appropriate GC treatment returns BP to normal.

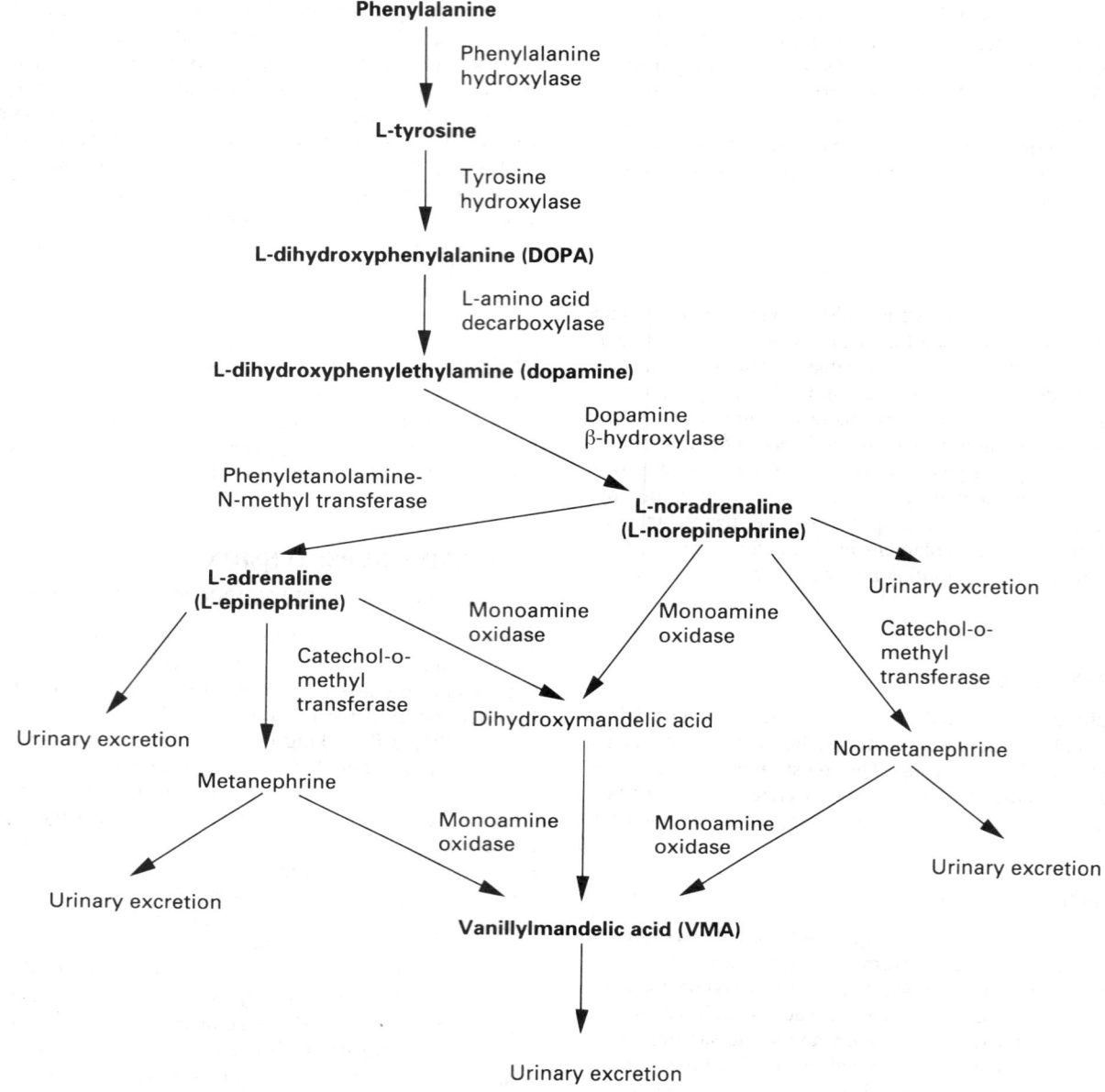

Fig. 19.42 Catecholamine biosynthesis and metabolism.

Primary and familial forms of hyperaldosteronism

Although these are rare conditions, their study has increased understanding of mechanisms which may have much wider significance.

Cushing's syndrome

Hypertension is common in children with Cushing's syndrome but BP may be only moderately elevated. Its etiology is multifactorial (Saruta et al 1986) including the significant mineralocorticoid effect of excessive cortisol secretion, increased renin substrate and, perhaps, increased vascular reactivity to vasoconstrictors.

Exogenous excessive administration of glucocorticoid is a much commoner cause of hypertension than any of the above.

Catecholamine excess

Pheochromocytomas are rare causes of secondary childhood hypertension which develop from chromaffin cells and can therefore arise from the sympathetic chain in the abdomen, the mediastinum or the neck; two-thirds are from the adrenal medulla. They are usually sporadic but may be familial or associated with MEN I and II (p. 1052) or neurofibromatosis. The tumors can be bilateral and multiple. In childhood, hypertension is nearly always sustained rather than paroxysmal and headaches, sweating, nausea and vomiting are common. There may be visual disturbances, abdominal pain, polydipsia and polyuria, convulsions and acrocyanosis.

Diagnosis depends on raised plasma catecholamine levels and increased urinary excretion of catecholamines and their metabolites (metanephrines, VMA and HVA). Repeated collections and estimations may be necessary. Localization of the tumor(s) may be possible by noninvasive techniques (ultrasound, CT scan, [131]I- or [23]I-metaiodobenzylguanidine (MIBG) scintigraphy).

If invasive techniques (e.g. arteriography or vena caval catecholamine sampling) are planned there must be full α- and β-sympathetic blockade, careful BP monitoring and drugs which will acutely lower BP immediately available. Blockade is necessary preoperatively to prevent severe hypertension, hypotension and dysrhythmias during definitive surgical removal. For full discussion of the pre- and perioperative management see Dillon (1995). Complete surgical removal results in BP normalization and, usually, 'cure' – only 5–10% are malignant. Analogous pharmacological blockade is necessary in children with hypertension associated with neuroblastoma.

THE PANCREAS AND CARBOHYDRATE METABOLISM

PANCREATIC MORPHOLOGY

The pancreas forms by proliferation of endodermal duodenal epithelium at the end of the fourth week of development as separate dorsal and ventral pancreatic buds. The ventral bud migrates posteriorly from a position close to the primitive liver bud and bile duct to lie in close contact with the dorsal bud. The duct systems and parenchyme subsequently fuse and the definitive (common) pancreatic duct is formed by the distal part of the dorsal and entire ventral duct. Failed fusion is a common normal variant. The pancreas is supplied by the splenic and superior mesenteric arteries and drained by the splenic and superior mesenteric veins into the portal vein. The islets of Langerhans, the pancreatic endocrine units, develop from the parenchymatous

pancreatic tissue during the third month, are scattered throughout the gland and secrete insulin by about 5 months. There is a rich blood supply to and rich sympathetic and parasympathetic (vagal) innervation in contact with the islet cells.

Exocrine pancreatic function is discussed in Chapter 11. The main endocrine secretions, insulin and glucagon, are intimately concerned in glucose homeostasis. Insulin is secreted from islet β cells, glucagon from α cells. There are also δ cells (thought to secrete somatostatin and perhaps gastrin) and a fourth cell type, F cells, which secrete pancreatic polypeptide (PP). The physiological importance of PP is unclear although it is secreted in response to food. Somatostatin's role in this context is in down-regulating the rate of entry of nutrients from the gut by delaying gastric emptying, decreasing duodenal motility, altering splanchnic blood flow, suppressing pancreatic exocrine and endocrine (insulin and glucagon) secretion and gastrin and secretin production from the gut. Thus integration of islet cell hormone and portal vein hormonal secretions is influenced by nutritional state, extrapancreatic hormones (especially gastrointestinal inhibitory polypeptide – GIP) and autonomic input.

INSULIN

Insulin is formed in β cells from a 9000 molecular weight precursor, proinsulin, itself derived from a larger polypeptide precursor, preproinsulin. Proinsulin is an 86 amino acid linear molecule with three peptide chains – A, B and (intermediate) C (Fig. 19.43). A and B peptides are joined by two disulfide bonds. C peptide is cleaved in the Golgi apparatus by proteolytic enzymes, leaving the covalently bonded A and B peptides (chains) – the definitive insulin molecule (MW 6000) (Fig. 19.43) – stored

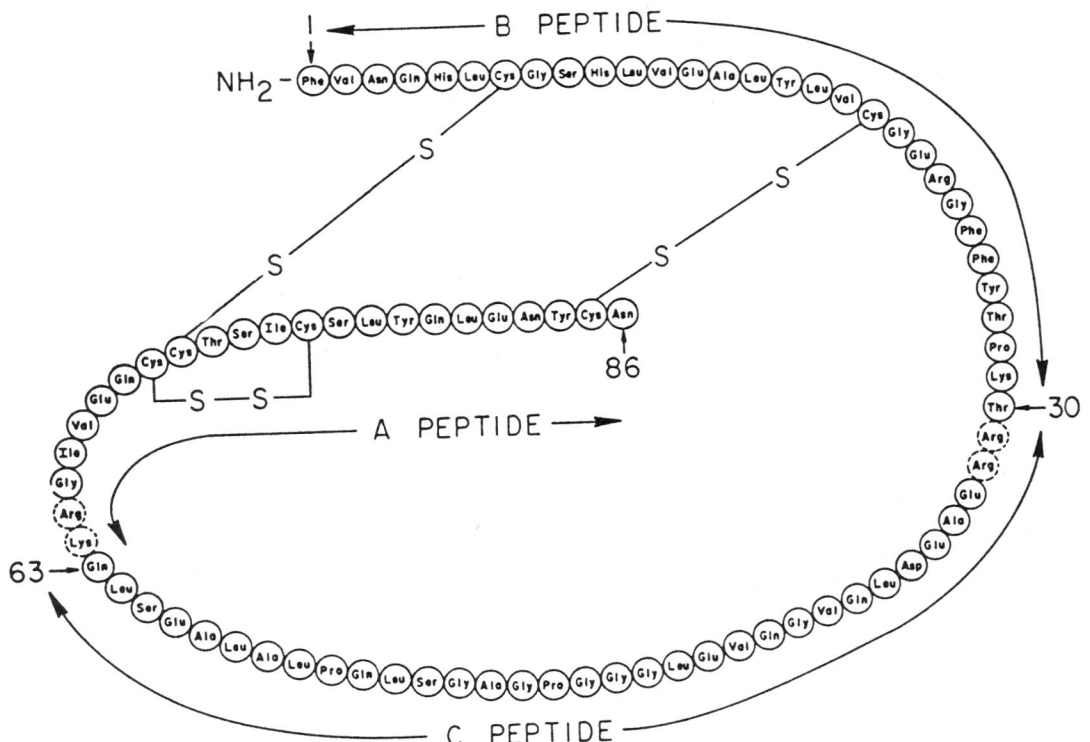

Fig. 19.43 Structure of proinsulin.

in cytoplasmic granules. Insulin and C peptide are thus present in granules in equimolar concentrations and expelled together into the draining capillary (emiocytosis). Circulating C peptide is a marker for endogenous insulin secretion, disappearing at the end of the 'honeymoon' period of diabetes mellitus (p. 1076).

Insulin is the major metabolic hormone. Factors modulating secretion include glucose, amino acids, glucagon, secretin, gastrin and GIP. During feeding, rising blood glucose and amino acid concentrations stimulate release – there are two phases in the response, a short-lived burst as preformed insulin is released and a slower and more sustained phase of de novo synthesis.

Insulin stimulates glucose uptake by muscle and fat cells, its conversion to glycogen and triglycerides and amino acid incorporation into muscle protein. Lipolysis, glycogenolysis, gluconeogenesis and muscle breakdown are inhibited and hepatic glycogen synthesis stimulated. The net effect is a fall in blood glucose associated with low circulating levels of free fatty acids, ketone bodies and branched chain amino acids. As plasma glucose levels fall below normal (e.g. during starvation), insulin secretion diminishes and secretion of glucagon and other hormones which increase blood glucose levels (catecholamines, GH, glucocorticoids) is stimulated ('counter-regulation') leading to stabilization of blood glucose levels. Insulin is mainly degraded in liver and kidney but also in pancreas and other tissues.

GLUCAGON

Glucagon is a single chain 29 amino acid polypeptide (MW 3485) secreted by islet α cells. Plasma levels increase during starvation – falling blood glucose levels are probably the major release stimulus but protein ingestion stimulates secretion through release of gut hormones such as pancreozymin. Anxiety and exercise increase secretion via sympathetic pathways. Somatostatin suppresses secretion.

Glucagon increases glucose levels by liver glycogenolysis and gluconeogenesis, stimulates fat cell lipolysis (increasing free fatty acids and ketones) and insulin, catecholamine, GH and calcitonin release. Circulatory half-life is only about 10 min – degradation is mainly in liver and kidney.

Integration

Interaction between insulin, glucagon and other counter-regulatory hormones is crucial in glucose and protein homeostasis, to provide sufficient and constant supply of glucose substrate to brain and for growth and energy requirements in infancy (Hawdon & Ward Platt 1995) and childhood (Stirling & Kelnar 1995a). Liver is particularly important for glucose homeostasis – liver gluconeogenesis, glycogen synthesis and glycogenolysis are summarized in Figure 19.44.

During *starvation*, two-thirds of daily glucose production is directly utilized by the brain as an energy source, insulin secretion falls and counter-regulation follows. This produces increased proteolysis, lipolysis, glycogenolysis and gluconeogenesis with reduced tissue glucose uptake resulting in increasing blood glucose levels. There are increased plasma fatty acids (used as an additional energy source), glycerol, ketone bodies and branched chain amino acids associated with high levels of glucagon, cortisol, GH and catecholamines and low or undetectable insulin levels (Fig. 19.45).

In the *fed* state, circulating glucose stimulates insulin secretion

and suppresses counter-regulation. Proteolysis, lipolysis, glycogenolysis and gluconeogenesis are suppressed, tissue glucose uptake increases and blood glucose levels fall (Fig. 19.45).

Understanding glucose homeostasis is necessary for rational differential diagnosis, investigation and treatment of hypoglycemia.

Surprisingly little is known about overnight blood glucose levels in normal children. Cyclical variation, periodicity 80–120 min, is described with a gradual fall until wakening with no evidence of a dawn blood glucose rise (Stirling et al 1991c). In some children levels fall to < 3 mmol/l. Maintenance of normoglycemia seems largely mediated through free fatty acid metabolism (with significant differences between 8 p.m. and 8 a.m. β-hydroxybutyrate levels) whereas lactate levels suggest that glycogen stores are relatively protected overnight but available for acute hypoglycemic crises (Stirling et al 1991c).

DIABETES MELLITUS

For detailed discussion of all aspects of childhood and adolescent diabetes, see Kelnar (1995a).

Historical introduction (Kelnar 1995c)

Diabetes mellitus was first mentioned (though not by name) in the 'Ebers' papyrus (about 1550 BC). 'Diabetes' (siphon or diuresis) was first used by the Turkish physician Aretaeos of Capadokia AD 130–200): 'Diabetes is an awkward affection melting down the flesh and limbs into the urine … patients never stop making water … life is short and painful … they are affected with nausea, restlessness and a burning thirst and at no distant term they expire.' The sweetness of diabetic urine ('mellitus' = sweet), first mentioned in sixth century AD Indian Vedic literature was rediscovered by Thomas Willis (1674). Matthew Dobson (1775) showed that the sweet taste was due to sugar and that serum also tasted sweet.

For 1500 years it was thought that the kidney's inability to retain water caused diabetes. Von Mering & Minkowski (1890) showed that total pancreatectomy in dogs resulted in diabetes mellitus and, within 10 years, islet function was becoming understood and fasting and dietary treatment introduced. The discovery of insulin by Banting & Best (1922) led to early development of insulin for treatment of human diabetes.

Recognition of the spectrum of diabetes and its manifestations led to a WHO classification: primary diabetes mellitus is insulin dependent (IDDM) – type 1, or non-insulin-dependent (NIDDM) – type 2, irrespective of age of onset. Definitions and classifications are discussed in Johnston (1995a). Diabetes is the commonest metabolic or endocrine disorder in children and adolescents and almost invariably type 1 (IDDM). Rarely, type 2 (NIDDM) may occur in this age group – maturity-onset type diabetes in the young (MODY). The discussion that follows relates to type 1 diabetes (IDDM). For MODY and transient neonatal diabetes see page 298.

Incidence and pathogenesis of type 1 diabetes mellitus
(Dorman et al 1995, Connor 1995, Foulis 1995, Mandrup-Poulsen & Nerup 1995)

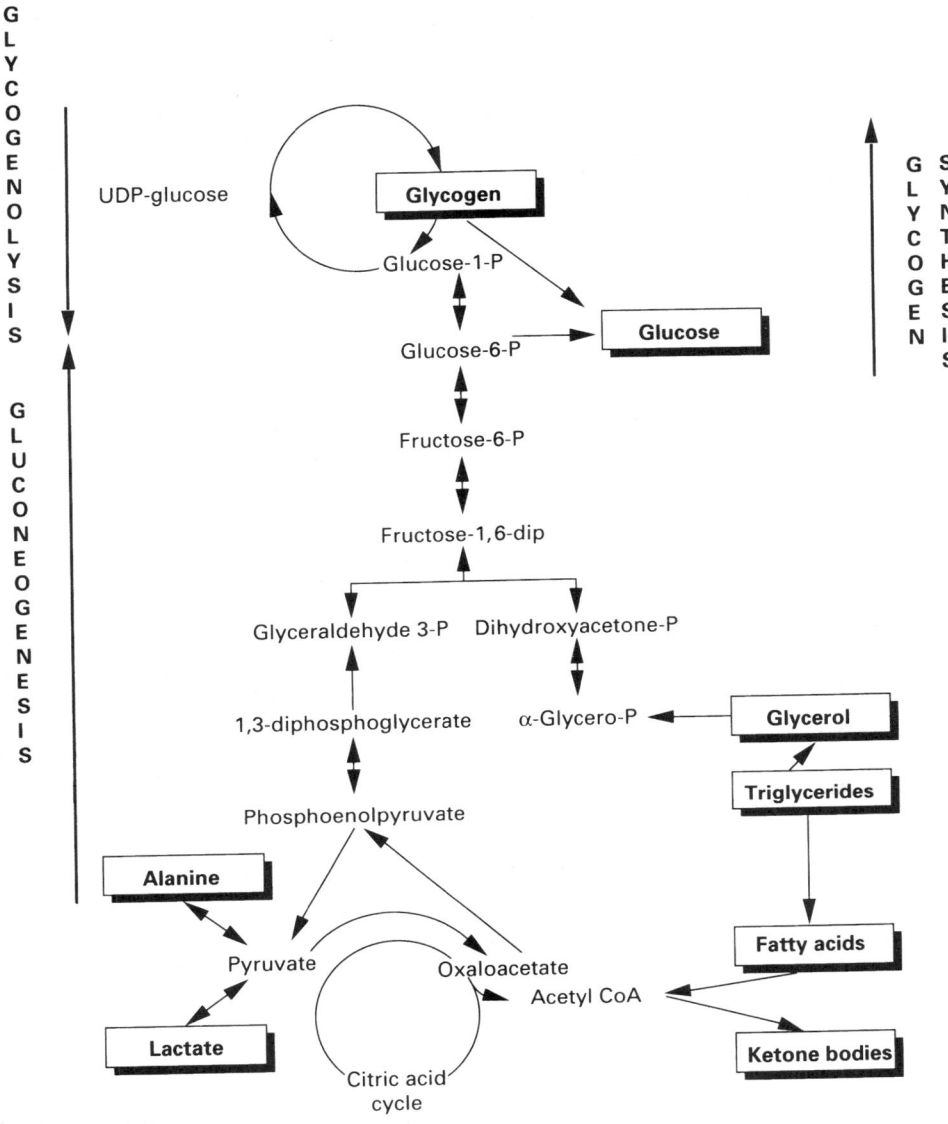

Fig. 19.44 Metabolic pathways of liver gluconeogenesis, glycogenolysis and glycogen synthesis.

Prevalence (sum of patients related to total age-related population) and incidence (age-related annual manifestations) data are available from many countries (for individual references see Dorman et al 1995). Both show wide variation and have yielded intriguing findings: annual incidence rates broadly increase with distance (north and south) from the equator both within Europe (3.7 per 100 000 in France, 38 per 100 000 in Finland) and within quite small distances within countries (about twofold higher in Scotland than England and higher in northern Scotland than south – Barclay et al 1988). Within individual areas, incidence is higher in whites than nonwhites, boys (M : F ratio about 1.1 : 1) and increases with age, peaking at adolescence. In many studies from geographically disparate countries an increasing incidence is reported.

Incidence and prevalence differences reflect the complex interaction of genetic and environmental factors (e.g. temperature, nutrition, viruses, chemical toxins) in the development of diabetes. Genetic factors are important (Dorman et al 1995,

Connor 1995): there is an increased incidence in parents and siblings of diabetics (Pincus & White 1933) – the risk to a sibling is 15- to 50-fold that in the normal population (Wagner et al 1942). Inheritance is likely to be polygenic or multifactorial rather than Mendelian (monogenic). Monozygotic twins are concordant for diabetes five times more frequently than dizygotic twins but the rate is much lower than in type 2 diabetes and a discordance rate of nearly 50% over a 30-year follow-up suggests the importance of environmental factors in clinical manifestation of the genetically determined predisposition.

There is strong association between developing diabetes and histocompatibility (HLA) markers and gene loci responsible for their synthesis on the short arm of chromosome 6 – loci DR3 and DR4 have particularly strong associations and increase the relative risk for developing diabetes between threefold (DR3) and 14-fold (DR3/DR4 heterozygosity). Molecular epidemiological studies have demonstrated that DNA sequences coding for the presence of an amino acid other than aspartic acid in the 57th

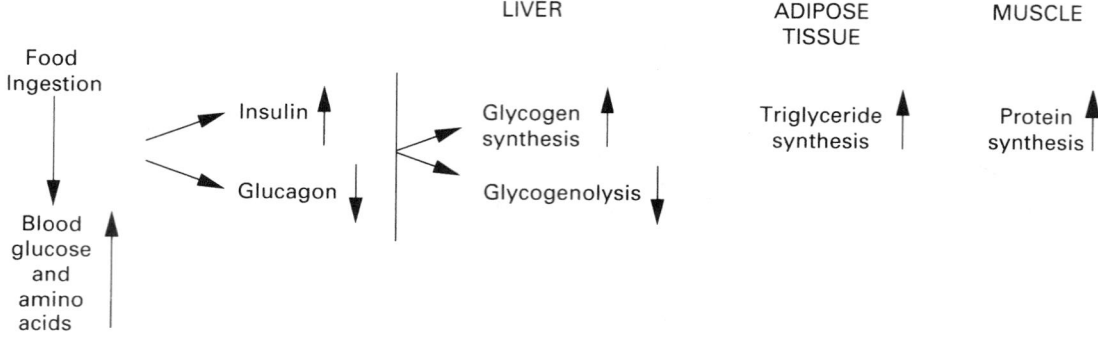

Effects: nitrogen sparing; triglycerides saved for future needs; low circulating levels of ketone bodies, free fatty acids and branched chain amino acids

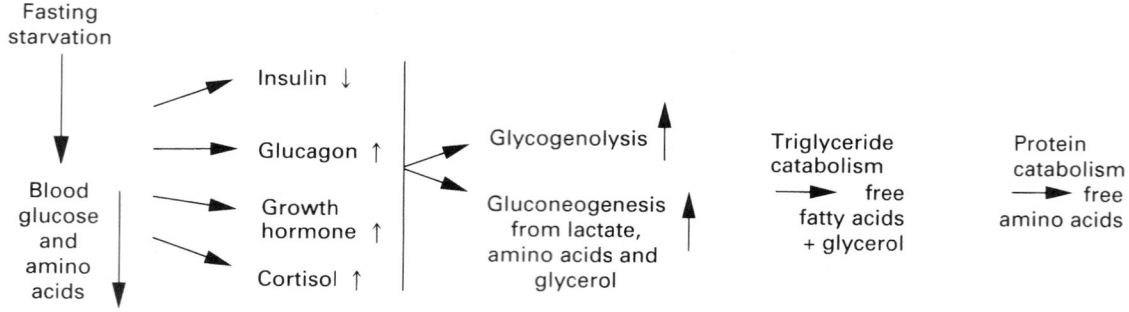

Effects: free fatty acids as energy source; ketone bodies generated from fatty acids; amino acids released by proteolysis as substrate for hepatic gluconeogenesis

Fig. 19.45 Metabolic and endocrine characteristics of fed and fasted states.

position of the DQB1 gene (non-ASP-57) is highly associated with IDDM susceptibility (much more strongly than for DR3/DR4) in most, but not all, racial or ethnic groups (Dorman et al 1995). The HLA identical sibling of a child with type 1 diabetes has about a 90-fold increased risk of developing the disease before 15 years. The risk is hardly increased at all if the sibling is HLA nonidentical. 90–98% of all type 1 diabetics express DR3 antigens, DR4 antigens or both, but less than 1% of healthy subjects with such markers will ever develop diabetes.

Environmental factors (Dorman et al 1995) are crucial for development of clinical diabetes in genetically predisposed individuals. Viruses can cause diabetes in animals; in humans there is seasonal variation of clinical onset in association with high viral prevalence (Gamble & Taylor 1969, Rayfield & Seto 1978) and a particular association with Coxsackie B4 (Banatvala et al 1985). However, it is known that β cell destruction, ultimately leading to decompensation and clinical onset of diabetes, has been occurring over many years. A virus or other 'insult' (early exposure to cow's milk protein, chemical toxin, food or cooking product or even stressful life events – reviewed by Bingley & Gale 1995, Dorman et al 1995) may, therefore, be responsible for triggering autoimmune (AI) β cell destruction in

genetically susceptible individuals. Relatively acute decompensation, up to many years later, leading to clinical presentation is often due to an intercurrent infection when insulin requirements rise and cannot, by then, be met.

Histopathological studies indicate that AI mechanisms are paramount in the pathogenesis of diabetes – reviewed by Foulis (1995), which has implications for its prevention or modification by immunosuppression (p. 1081). Development of complement-fixing ability by islet cell antibodies (ICA) seems to confer specific cytotoxic activity against the β cell (Bottazzo et al 1980) and continuing β cell destruction could occur by a cascade of AI mechanisms (involving B lymphocyte autoantibody production and cytotoxic T lymphocytes) in susceptible individuals (Bottazzo 1989). There is strong association between type 1 diabetes and other AI disease (e.g. thyroid, adrenal, parathyroid).

Clinical onset and diagnosis (Brink 1995)

Although, in retrospect, parents may feel their newly diagnosed diabetic child has not been 'right' for several months with poor appetite and malaise, the clinical onset in most children is usually relatively acute: increasing polyuria (due to osmotic glucose

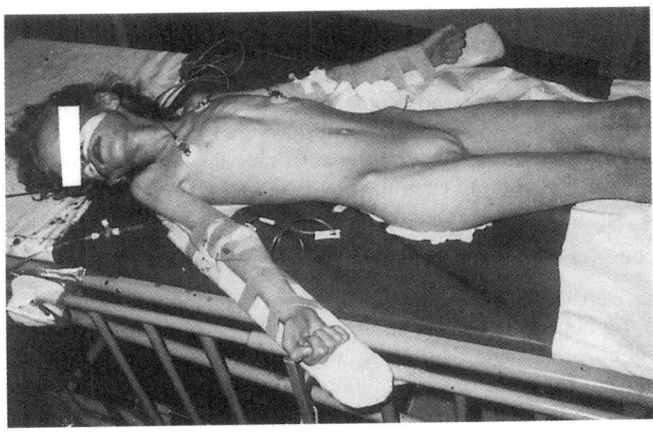

Fig. 19.46   A newly (and 'late') diagnosed diabetic with severe ketoacidosis and dehydration.

load), secondary polydipsia, weight loss, anorexia and fatigue develop over days or weeks. Some children present particularly acutely with rapid onset of ketoacidosis and coma. This may be commoner in DR3/DR4 heterozygotes (Knip et al 1986), DR3 patients presenting less acutely (Ludvigsson et al 1986). More acute onset is also reported in younger children (Jefferson et al 1985) perhaps because of lack of awareness by parents or health professionals, or pre-existing enuresis. The urine of any child with secondary enuresis should be tested for glucose.

Once suspected, diagnosis is not usually difficult. Too often there is delay because urine is not tested when a child presents with nonspecific symptoms – anorexia, vomiting, abdominal pain, 'pneumonia'. Finding glycosuria or hyperglycemia is an emergency – the child should preferably be seen the same day and certainly within 24 h and never simply referred by letter to an outpatient clinic. If diagnosis and treatment are not prompt, further catabolism may rapidly cause increasing ketosis and acidosis (Fig. 19.46) with coma and death. There is still significant morbidity and mortality in children who present with severe ketoacidosis and dehydration (Scibilia et al 1986) – children unconscious at presentation have a 12-fold increase in mortality compared to those not in coma (Tjima 1985).

Improvements in health education (of parents and professionals) and prompt access to a specialist pediatric unit will help reduce the incidence of severe ketoacidosis. Morbidity and mortality will be reduced if specific well-tried, well-understood and adequately supervised management guidelines are followed (see below).

Initial management of the child without ketoacidosis

Most children who have developed diabetes have only mild symptoms and are not ketoacidotic. Centers as disparate as Leicester, England (Hearnshaw 1985), and Tel Aviv, Israel (Laron et al 1982), with a network of primary carers (e.g. diabetes health visitors) successfully manage nearly all such children at home. Careful continuing assessment – frequent telephone contact and at least daily home visits – is necessary to prevent onset of ketoacidosis at home and to provide basic information (Brink 1995).

This approach is being increasingly adopted in many UK centers but may be inappropriate for socially deprived families or rural settings a long way from the hospital. Some parents are so

distressed at diagnosis that admission is desirable. Potential benefits of home management – greater acceptance by the family and a quick return to 'normal' family life – can also be achieved if the child's hospital admission is sensitively handled.

Several days in hospital may still be necessary for unhurried education in basic diabetic care of child and family. It is a mistake to try to impart too much early information – upset, anxious, grieving or frightened parents are not receptive learners. Simple practical information and instruction about insulin, injection techniques and dietetic principles are important with a positive emphasis that, provided simple guidelines are followed, the child will soon be feeling better than for some weeks and will be able to take part in all the activities he would wish. In some centers, before the child leaves hospital, hypoglycemia is induced in the parents' presence (morning insulin is given, breakfast omitted and the child exercised until symptoms occur) so that all can experience the symptoms for the first time in a controlled and supportive environment.

Recognition and treatment of ketoacidosis (Brink 1995)

A child with ketoacidosis and severe dehydration (Fig. 19.46) is dangerously ill and requires emergency treatment. Vomiting and abdominal pain with tenderness and guarding may mimic an acute abdomen whilst hyperventilation may be misdiagnosed as pneumonia. There may be circulatory collapse, oliguria and coma. Salicylate poisoning should be considered in differential diagnosis.

In known diabetics on insulin, ketoacidosis is usually precipitated by intercurrent infection, but may occur if too little insulin is given (perhaps because of fear of hypoglycemia), insulin is omitted altogether (e.g. by an emotionally disturbed adolescent) or with menstruation or severe emotional upset (Hinkle & Wolff 1952). In this group, particularly, there may not be pronounced hyperglycemia, particularly if insulin has been (correctly) continued or increased but vomiting has led to inadequate carbohydrate (CHO) intake. For this reason, urinary ketones should always be tested for by the established diabetic when there is significant hyperglycemia on home blood glucose testing (Bell & Hadden 1983) as metabolic decompensation may be more severe than realized.

The priority in management is appropriate volume repletion – rehydration is more crucial than insulin in the early stages. Initial fluid should be isotonic (0.9%, 150 mmol/l) saline, or plasma if there is circulatory collapse or unconsciousness – 20 ml/kg within the first 30–60 min. A rapid history, clinical examination and blood glucose (by indicator stick) will confirm the diagnosis and a sample for true blood glucose, urea and electrolytes, plasma osmolality and arterial blood gas estimation should be obtained as the infusion is set up. Full blood count, hematocrit, platelets and an infection screen (blood culture, urine microscopy and culture, viral cultures, swabs) should be obtained and ECG monitored.

Whilst hypernatremia is due to severe water loss (exceeding the sodium loss), hyponatremia is usually factitious and due to hyperlipidemia. Creatinine levels may be spuriously high owing to assay interference by acetoacetate, and the hematocrit may be falsely elevated by osmotic swelling of erythrocytes in the Coulter counter (Bock et al 1985).

Dehydration should be assessed clinically and, if possible, by weighing and comparing with average weights for age or previous records.

A short-acting *insulin* must be used and is best given as a continuous intravenous infusion by syringe pump at a rate of 0.05 units/kg/h, doubled if there is no response within 2 h (100 units of a short-acting insulin in 100 ml of normal saline produces a solution containing 1 unit/ml of insulin). This results in a smooth and steady fall in blood glucose.

Bicarbonate should be considered only with severe acidosis (pH < 7.0), circulatory collapse or respiratory depression and used only on advice of senior medical staff. In less severe ketoacidosis it increases risks of cerebral edema (due to the large sodium load) and hypokalemia (more rapid shift of potassium into cells) with increased morbidity. It must be infused slowly (over 30–60 min) and separately. The amount needed is derived from the formula:

$$\text{mmol bicarbonate (ml of 8.4\% NaHCO}_3\text{) required} = \text{wt (kg)} \times \text{base deficit (mmol/l)} \times 0.1$$

After 1 h, the saline infusion rate should be reduced. A simple, effective and safe regimen is to correct dehydration over 24 h:

$$\frac{\text{maintenance requirements} + \text{deficit}}{24} = \text{hourly infusion rate}$$

Once blood glucose levels are < 13 mmol/l, 0.45% saline/5% dextrose is substituted. Insulin solution should be renewed 6-hourly and the infusion rate adjusted to maintain blood glucose levels between 7 and 13 mmol/l.

Potassium 2–3 mmol/kg/h, but not exceeding 40 mmol/l concentration, should be started from the second hour if urine has been passed since admission without waiting for hypokalemia. If no urine is passed by 4 h, the child should be catheterized. Inappropriate ADH secretion may develop (low urine output, high urinary and falling plasma osmolalities) necessitating fluid restriction to prevent cerebral edema. Low plasma sodium levels may merely reflect hyperlipidemia (see above) – plasma osmolality is a better hydration guide.

All urine passed should be tested for glucose and ketones. A nasogastric tube should be passed and gastric losses included in an accurate fluid balance record. Blood glucose, gases, urea and electrolytes and osmolality should be checked at 2 and 5 h and thereafter as indicated with hourly indicator stick blood glucose monitoring. Antibiotics may be necessary if infection is suspected once bacteriology specimens are obtained.

From day 2 onwards (sometimes earlier) consider allowing oral fluids as tolerated and reduce fluid infusion rates accordingly. Solids are started as appetite recovers. Intravenous fluids should not be discontinued until the child is drinking and eating a light diet and urine is ketone free. If insulin infusion is stopped prematurely, ketonuria and anorexia will take longer to resolve and acidosis may persist. Subcutaneous short-acting insulin should be given as 1 unit/kg/24 h, 6- to 8-hourly for 24 h, with the first dose 30 min before the insulin infusion is stopped. Subsequently a twice-daily insulin regime is generally appropriate (see below). Potassium should be given orally (as KCl 1 mmol/kg/24 h) for 4 days. High quality, appropriately experienced nursing care is vital throughout (Mitchell et al 1995). After recovery, diabetes education begins.

Cerebral edema is the main cause of morbidity and mortality and single commonest cause of death in children with diabetes (Scibilia et al 1986) often developing several hours after treatment in a context of apparent biochemical and clinical improvement (Rosenbloom et al 1980). Over-rapid fluid replacement and insulin infusion and injudicious bicarbonate use

may well increase its likelihood, but the 'cause' is unknown and unlikely to be due solely to management factors – subclinical brain swelling may be common during even optimal treatment (Krane et al 1985) and seems generally not to be of long-term consequence. A nationwide study has commenced in the UK in 1995 under the auspices of the British Paediatric Association Surveillance Unit to examine possible etiologic factors.

Long-term management (Shield & Baum 1995)

Sir Derrick Dunlop opening a 1965 diabetes mellitus symposium in Edinburgh asked 'is the occurrence of these complications [retinopathy, nephropathy, neuropathy, coronary and peripheral angiopathy] to be regarded fatalistically as something inherent in the diabetic process … or can they be postponed by care and trouble directed to the control of the metabolic disturbance?'

It has taken nearly another 30 years to provide the answer. Perhaps observation of the effects of poor maternal diabetic control on her fetus should have alerted pediatricians earlier to likely long-term consequences of poor metabolic control and chronic hyperglycemia in childhood (Hepburn & Steel 1995), but there is now irrefutable epidemiological evidence (at least in those aged 13 years or over) from the American 10-year prospective Diabetes Control and Complications Trial (DCCT Research Group 1993) that if good long-term glycemic control is achieved, risks of microangiopathic complications (retinopathy, nephropathy and neuropathy) are greatly reduced. The question now is not 'why' or 'whether' to maintain good glycemic control but 'how'.

Other questions remain. Pediatricians seldom see complications silently bequeathed with their patients to adult diabetologists. What level of childhood or adolescent glycemic control constitutes 'good' or 'good enough' control? Is prevention of complications by establishment of good control in childhood and adolescence a realistic goal? How is it to be achieved in the context of normal physical and emotional growth and normal daily activities and family lifestyle? Will it be at expense of more hypoglycemia? If so, how frequent or severe must this be in children of different ages before it affects cognitive function long term? Does more education or new or improved skills in family or clinician necessarily produce better control? Risks for macrovascular disease seem unaffected by tight glycemic control. The St Vincent and ISPAD declarations (appendices in Kelnar 1995) seek to achieve maximum quality of life for patients with diabetes through efficient use of available resources. How is this to be attained with health care resources dwindling in many 'developed' countries, let alone in parts of the world (including even Eastern Europe) where insulin itself is unavailable?

Optimal control must be achieved in the context of normal family and school life and normal physical and emotional growth. Diabetes must not be ignored but should not need to preoccupy child or family. Education (instruction) attempts to achieve this through increased understanding of diabetes and self-confidence in management (Ingersoll & Golden 1995, La Greca & Skyler 1995). Motivation derives from encouragement and explanation, not coercion and arbitrary rules. Specific management aims and decisions will reflect the child's age, the family's diverse abilities, motivation and psychosocial backgrounds and personnel and resources available in hospital and community (Waine & Stavely 1995).

Achieving 'tight' glycemic control in the context of a 'normal' lifestyle may be difficult or impossible – in many children control is inadequate – but is helped by the multidisciplinary approach of the pediatric diabetes clinic (Johnston 1995b): doctors have specialist knowledge of pediatrics, growth and diabetes; there is a dietitian present; a child psychiatrist may sit in or be readily available. Family emotional problems may be precipitated by diabetes impacting on parents or other siblings; the child's and family's emotional responses to diabetes will themselves have major effects on glycemic control. Occasional omission of insulin, simulating hypoglycemia or making up test results is common and an understandable response in many situations either to gain reward or avoid reprimand (Tattersall & Walford 1985). This does not represent severe underlying psychopathology but should prompt a re-evaluation of management and a consistent parental and professional approach.

Liaison diabetes nurses are important assets to a clinic (Farquhar & Campbell 1980, McEvilly 1995) linking family, home, school, community and hospital in a way that other health professionals cannot. They provide specific support when the child first returns home after diagnosis and at times of crisis, visit schools to talk to teachers (Strang 1995), provide continuing support, advice and education, and report specific problems to the hospital-based team.

Specific attempts to increase the effectiveness of education in diabetes care may be beneficial in improving short- and perhaps long-term control (Bloomfield et al 1990). At the very least, a consistent approach by all members of the team will do much to create an environment in which the quality of control can improve.

Normoglycemia is dependent on appropriate balance between calorie (carbohydrate, fat and protein) intake necessary for normal growth and energy expenditure and insulin. Diverse uncontrollable or unpredictable factors affect glycemia, e.g. infection, a birthday party, attending the clinic, exams, GH, puberty, menstruation. Exercise has major effects and in children is variable and capricious (Greene & Thompson 1995).

Medical input provides a framework within which diabetes can be 'managed' – although many aspects of management remain controversial (Laron & Kalter-Leibovici 1995) – but living with diabetes may require support which can be derived from involvement with self-help organizations (Swift et al 1995).

Perioperative management of the diabetic child undergoing surgery is reviewed by Milaszkiewicz & Hall (1995).

Insulin regimens (Swift 1995)

The aim is to reproduce physiological insulin secretion – all currently practicable regimens do so relatively poorly. Only human or highly purified porcine insulins should be used to reduce lipoatrophy and insulin antibody formation. The regimen chosen must be individualized for child and family. Examples are shown in Figure 19.47. Human equivalents may be slightly quicker acting and can increase risks of nocturnal hypoglycemia from intermediate-acting insulin given before the evening meal, particularly in young children with early meal- and bedtimes. This may be overcome by moving the second injection of intermediate-acting insulin to bedtime or using a longer-acting insulin before the evening meal.

Most are potentially better controlled on two daily injections (a mixture of short-and intermediate-acting insulins) than one, but a single (before breakfast) injection may be satisfactory during the phase of partial recovery of endogenous insulin secretion (the 'honeymoon' period) and an acceptable compromise for longer in the toddler.

In some adolescents, flexibility of lifestyle can be achieved without loss of control by using a convenient pen injector giving small amounts of a short-acting insulin before the main meals (which can be varied in timing and quantity) and a long-acting (background) insulin at bedtime. In many countries (e.g. Scandinavia and Italy) this regimen is used even in young children. If premixed fixed mixtures are used in pens, potential flexibility (even compared to standard regimens) is lost but there is increased convenience compared to syringe and needle, welcomed by many children and their families, and no deterioration in control (Gall et al 1989). The number of insulin injections is less important for control than factors such as continuing support from the health care team, psychosocial factors (Belmonte et al 1988) or dedicated home blood glucose self-monitoring.

Usual insulin requirements are ~ 0.8 units/kg/day (less during the 'honeymoon'). On a twice-daily regimen, approximately two-thirds of the dose may be appropriate before breakfast with a ratio between short- and intermediate-acting insulins of between 1 : 2 and 1 : 3 often being satisfactory. Adjustments are ideally based on home blood glucose monitoring (Silink 1995) – with consistent abnormalities at a particular time of day the appropriate insulin is adjusted up or down by child or parent, if necessary after consultation by phone with a member of the diabetic team. Adjustment only every 3 months in clinic is unsatisfactory. Education and motivation are more important for good control than any specific insulin regimen (Hinde & Johnston 1986).

Subcutaneously injected insulin bioavailability is very variable (Swift 1995, Kurtz 1995, Danielsen et al 1995). Rates vary with injection site – fastest from the abdomen and slower from the thigh than the arm – and with exercise (see below) or if the site is rubbed after injection. If the same injection site is used repeatedly (because the injection becomes painless) lipohypertrophy (Fig. 19.48) is likely and insulin absorption extremely unpredictable. At least 30–45 min should elapse between morning injection and breakfast to avoid postprandial hyperglycemia (before adequate short-acting insulin absorption) and hypoglycemia before the midmorning snack (Kinmonth & Baum 1980). This is less crucial, but easier to achieve in practice, before the pre-supper injection.

Diet (Kinmonth et al 1989, Brenchley & Govindji 1995)

If it is to be acceptable to child and family and followed in practice, diet should be closely related to recommendations for nondiabetics, but is inevitably tempered by the family's eating habits which may fall short of that ideal. Rigid and dogmatic rules encourage noncompliance. Diets should give a 'stable' carbohydrate intake at regular intervals – breakfast, mid-morning snack, lunch, mid-afternoon snack, evening meal, bedtime snack. Dietary advice ('healthy eating' guidelines) have been produced by the British Diabetic Association (1992). A pediatric dietitian with an interest in diabetes is an important part of the management team.

The carbohydrate (CHO) exchange system (one exchange = 10 g CHO) has the virtue of dogmatic simplicity allowing a wide variety of foods to be eaten, but all nutrients can, of course, be converted directly or indirectly to glucose. The previously

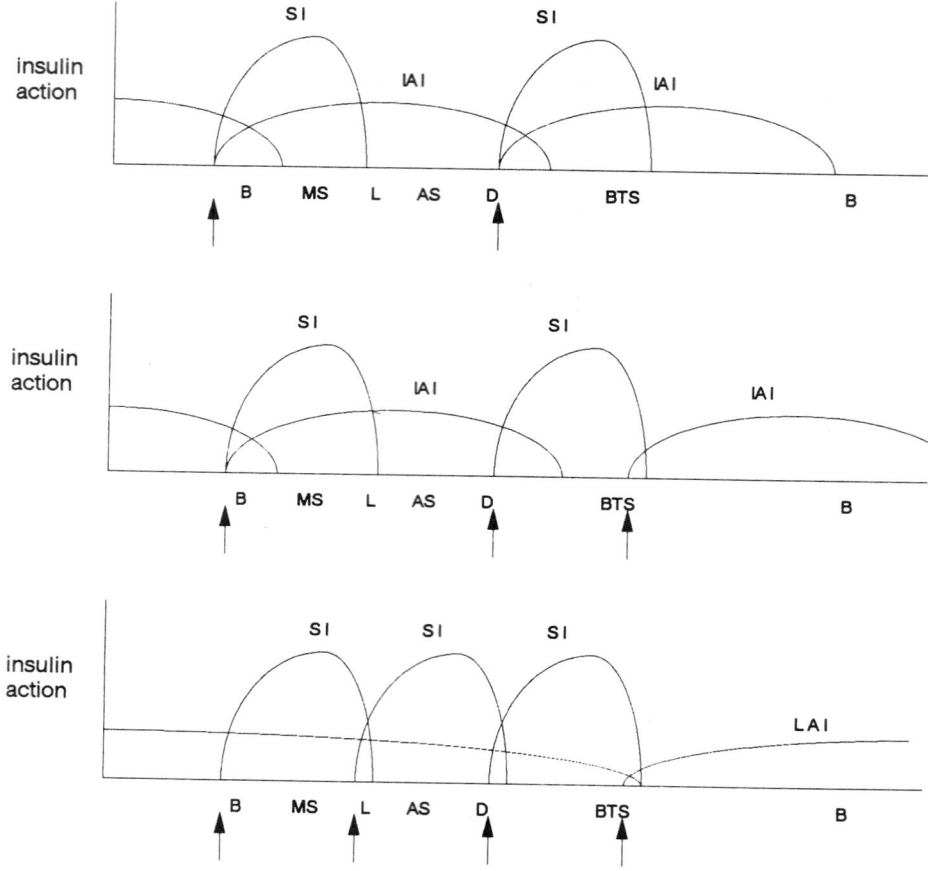

Fig. 19.47 Examples of insulin regimens: (**a**) two daily doses of short- and intermediate-acting insulins; (**b**) as (a) but the evening intermediate-acting insulin delayed until bedtime; (**c**) insulin pen regime – combination of preprandial short-acting insulin with long-acting insulin at bedtime. Key: B = breakfast; MS = midmorning snack; L = lunch; AS = afternoon snack; D = dinner (Scottish tea); BTS = bedtime snack; SI = short-acting insulin; IAI = intermediate-acting insulin; LAI = long-acting insulin; ↑ = insulin injection.

conventional guide to CHO intake (100 g per day for a 1-year-old plus an extra 10 g per day for each additional year of age) may need to be varied considerably to meet growth and energy requirements of the individual. The proportion of CHO should be high enough (40–50%) to enable fat intake to be reasonably low – less than 35% of calories should be from fat which should be polyunsaturated to reduce long-term risks of hyperlipidemia and cardiovascular disease.

CHO type remains important: concentrated, rapidly absorbed, sugary food taken in significant and regular amounts precludes stable glycemic control and should be confined to occasional treats before exercise, or at the end of a meal. Starchy, low fiber foods are acceptable, but starchy high fiber foods (Table 19.18) are best, because of their gradual absorption and metabolism. With education of the general population towards 'healthy eating' these foods are now more socially accepted and more easily obtainable cheaply.

Dietary management is therefore the 'art of the possible' and involves educating the whole family's eating habits. A sensible approach to 'treats', fast foods and reasonable flexibility over timing is more likely to lead to cooperation; psychological benefit in not being different from family and friends is likely to benefit lifestyle and control (Brenchley & Govindji 1995).

Exercise (Greene & Thompson 1995)

Regular exercise allows participation in peer group activities and improves self-confidence and physical fitness. Strenuous exercise usually results in rapid but unpredictable falls in blood glucose (increased insulin mobilization results from increased blood flow and muscular activity) but on a background of underinsulinization results in counter-regulation and hyperglycemia with ketosis.

Before unexpected activity, an extra 10–30 g CHO may be necessary depending on age, blood glucose level and intensity of exercise planned. Additional snacks may be necessary if exercise is prolonged and, if happening after school, reduction in pre-supper (Scottish 'tea') insulin may be necessary to allow for delayed hypoglycemia as muscle glycogen is replenished. On activity holidays it is often sensible to cut insulin by < 50% if severe hypoglycemia is not to result on the first day even with additional snacks.

Assessing control (Silink 1995)

Many diabetic children enjoy active and healthy lives but some are poorly controlled requiring frequent hospital admissions for ketoacidosis, hypoglycemia or stabilization. Poor control may

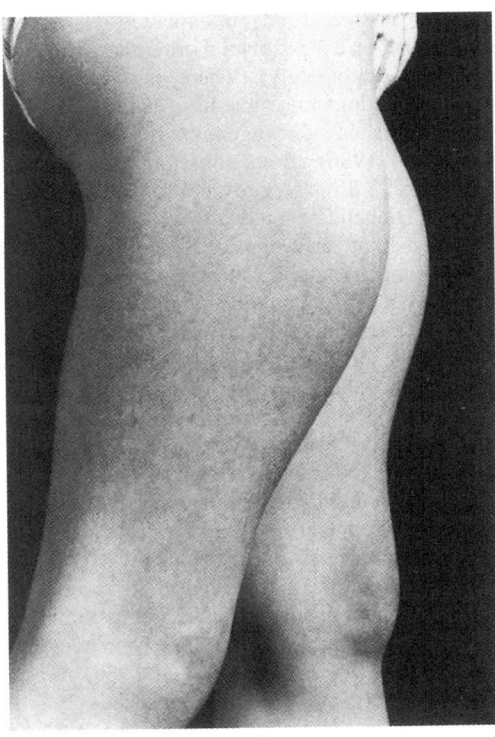

Fig. 19.48 Severe lipohypertrophy in a diabetic child on human insulin who was not adequately rotating the injection sites.

Table 19.18   Some high fiber foods

Wholemeal bread

Wholemeal spaghetti

Wholemeal cereals

Weetabix

Jacket potatoes

Ryvita

Oatcakes

Dried beans

Lentils

Fruits
   Apples
   Bananas
   Blackberries
   Pineapple
   Strawberries

Vegetables
   Brussels sprouts
   Cabbage
   Peas
   Sweetcorn

reflect unhappiness or instability in the family, particularly if there has never been emotional (cf. intellectual) acceptance of diabetes (Skuse 1995, Anderson 1995, Ingersoll & Golden 1995).

'Brittle' diabetes is almost invariable due to such problems – fruitless searches for underlying metabolic abnormalities are

counterproductive. Long-term poor control causes severe stunting of growth and pubertal development (Kelnar 1995b, Dunger 1995, 1997) and may be associated with 'Cushingoid' obesity and hepatomegaly (Mauriac's syndrome). Gross abnormalities are now seldom seen and assessment of physical and emotional growth and well-being while essential are, in themselves, insufficient – normal growth and no reported symptoms of hypo- or hyperglycemia may be found even when glycemic control is far from ideal.

Even young children find home blood glucose monitoring on capillary samples using indicator sticks acceptable. Urine tests give limited retrospective information about likely previous blood glucose levels (has the level been high enough to exceed the renal threshold for glucose since the bladder was last emptied?), do not warn of impending hypoglycemia, and are useless with normoglycemia the therapeutic goal. Even early morning glycosuria may be misleading, reflecting early morning hyperglycemia (excessive insulin the previous evening with counter-regulation, the Somogyi effect), too little insulin, or the 'dawn phenomenon' – decreased insulin sensitivity due to nocturnal GH peaks (Schmidt et al 1981, Dunger 1995, Dunger & Edge 1995).

Immediate knowledge of blood glucose level is only of practical benefit if child and parents understand its significance and relevance and are motivated to take appropriate action on the basis of consistent abnormalities. That home blood glucose monitoring does not, in itself, lead to better control (Hermansson et al 1986) is not surprising in this context. Blood tests done in rotation once or twice daily just before main meals and at bedtime, and occasionally 60–90 min after main meals, an acceptable regimen for many, will provide most information from fewest tests. Blood glucose estimation is of particular value during illness or symptoms that could relate to hypoglycemia. Nevertheless blood tests are uncomfortable and a chore. Education and motivation will reduce the number omitted, done inaccurately or results made up to 'keep the doctor happy'.

Hemoglobin forms a nonenzymatic link with glucose – percentage of glycosylated hemoglobin (HbA1c) is an objective measure of integrated glycemic control over the previous 6–8 weeks (Jovanovic & Peterson 1981, Silink 1995). Assessed in this way, the majority of diabetic children are less than ideally controlled and in some control is abysmal. Identifying this group is easier than improving the situation. There is doubt as to the appropriateness of some laboratory quoted normal ranges for HbA1c and the 'target range' may be lower than previously considered appropriate (DCCT Research Group 1993). This has implications for children, at greater risk of hypoglycemia and its consequences, when 'tight' glycemic control is the aim (see below). Finding high values is helpful when home monitoring results apparently indicate excellent control – either monitoring technique is faulty or there is deliberate manipulation due to emotional disturbance (Citrin et al 1980).

HbA1c estimation is much more valuable if the current result is available in clinic so that appropriate advice can be given. In some laboratories, assay techniques are available to provide such a service; in other circumstances, capillary blood samples on filter paper or in special containers can be obtained at home shortly before the next clinic visit and posted to the laboratory (Holman et al 1987, Petranyi et al 1986). Shorter-term indices of glycemic control, e.g. plasma proteins (Kennedy et al 1981) such as fructosamine, may be useful when assessing, for example, the efficacy of a specific therapeutic intervention.

Adolescence

Control may be particularly difficult to achieve in adolescents (Newton & Greene 1995): rapid growth necessitates a high calorie intake and must be paralleled by sufficient increases in insulin at that pubertal stage (Dunger & Edge 1995, Dunger 1995). Many adolescents are underinsulinized on conventional regimens. The role of insulin-like growth factors in the insulin resistance of puberty is reviewed by Dunger & Edge (1995). Menstruation may precipitate ketoacidosis; important examinations cause stress; emotional lability may cause rebelliousness against dietary restrictions, the need for monitoring control or insulin injections. Eating disorders (anorexia, bulimia) are common (Steel 1995). There is apprehension over desired independence, changing peer group activities and experiences, developing sexual relationships and, ultimately, career choices and learning to cope with an indifferent and ignorant public, employers and even 'friends'.

Psychological transition from childhood to adolescence and beyond (Skuse 1995, Anderson 1995) requires new approaches to motivation and education, flexible diet, insulin regimens and lifestyle. Although pen injector regimens give potential for maintaining or improving glycemic control in those motivated and well informed, such regimens can be disastrous in those who, even after many years, are unsure of the nature and consequences of what they eat or inject.

Special adolescent needs are often poorly met (Newton & Greene 1995). Specific adolescent clinics, jointly staffed by pediatricians and adult diabetologists with empathy for adolescents and their 'worldview' may be the ideal – a paternalistic approach is doomed to failure. Many adolescents appear to benefit from sharing experiences with others in a variety of contexts (Newton et al 1985, Thompson et al 1995).

Hypoglycemia (Gold & Frier 1995)

Parents, and many children, worry particularly about this and, especially, nocturnal hypoglycemia. It seems very common at home without need for hospital admission (Beaufrere et al 1986) and will become commoner with the quest for tighter control. The DCCT (DCCT Research Group 1993) reported a threefold increase in severe hypoglycemic episodes in the intensive treatment group – consequences for the child's developing immature brain require further elucidation.

There are few long-term neurophysiological and psychometric studies of effects of frequent mild hypoglycemia – children's hypoglycemic symptoms differ from adults' (McCrimmon et al 1995, Ross et al 1996a), as do their counter-regulatory responses which may also relate to prevailing glycemic control (Ross et al 1996b). Children diagnosed before 3 years have particular problems. This relates to the common occurrence of hypoglycemia in the young diabetic (the normal young child has a relative inability to maintain normoglycemia during periods of even 6–12 h without food – Kelnar 1976) and increased sensitivity to hypoglycemia of the still maturing brain. In a study of non-diabetic children, plasma glucose levels < 3 mmol/l occurred during sleep in 12% and plasma glucose levels immediately prior to wakening correlated significantly with age (Stirling et al 1991c,d).

Occasional mild hypoglycemia – a feeling of hunger with faintness, headache or belligerency if a meal is delayed – indicates tight control and seems harmless. Hypoglycemia is usually caused by delayed or missed food, unexpected (or unexpectedly strenuous) exercise or excess insulin administration (by mistake, or, more rarely, deliberately). There is particular risk after diagnosis when endogenous insulin secretion is temporarily partially re-established if exogenous insulin is not reduced (Fainmesser et al 1986). Both stress and early stages of an intercurrent viral illness can cause hypo- rather than hyperglycemia. Diabetics should always carry extra glucose or dextrose to be taken at early signs of hypoglycemia and followed by food. A semiconscious child who cannot coordinate swallowing a sweet drink should be given 'Hypostop' gel (rubbed into the gums or buccal mucosa and now available on prescription in the UK) or glucagon (1 mg i.m. or s.c.). Both should be kept at home for use by a relative in that eventuality and 'Hypostop', which should reduce the need for glucagon administration, can also be given readily by a schoolteacher. Both will improve neuroglycopenia and the conscious level sufficiently for oral CHO to be given. If it is not, glucose levels will fall again – a common problem with glucagon as it frequently induces vomiting.

With increasing use of human insulins, there have been anecdotal reports (Teuscher & Berger 1987, Berger et al 1989) of loss of hypoglycemia awareness in patients transferred from porcine or bovine insulins. Although there is no evidence that this is common (Berger 1987, Hepburn et al 1989) the problem is causing much anxiety and is being prospectively investigated (Fisher & Frier 1993).

Prolonged severe hypoglycemia resulting in cerebral edema is seen following deliberate and massive insulin overdose and in adolescents after significant alcohol intake and can cause death or permanent brain damage.

Complications

Complications are seldom seen before puberty even in long-standing diabetes. Sex steroid secretion could be important in their development and progression but pathogenesis is still poorly understood despite recent advances (Gregory & Taylor 1995, Becker et al 1995, Young 1995). Their relevance to the pediatrician is that – extrapolating from the results of the DCCT (DCCT Research Group 1993) – optimal childhood glycemic control is extremely important in prevention of microvascular disease and that very early changes can be detected by screening techniques (Clarke 1995).

The common association between diabetes and AI thyroid disease necessitates checking TSH levels routinely once yearly (and perhaps for other AI endocrine disorders also – MacCuish 1995) in all diabetic children. Microalbuminuria and retinopathy must be screened for and BP checked annually in all diabetics from puberty onward.

Microalbuminuria is a marker for early nephropathy in diabetic children (Davies et al 1985) and adults. Using the first morning urine sample (Cowell et al 1986) and relating concentration to creatinine is probably appropriate but its presence is likely to be related to such factors as acute glycemic control, posture, exercise, hydration and BP. It remains unclear how persistent and at what level it must be to cause concern or how justifiable is long-term antihypertensive therapy in a child with a raised diastolic BP and microalbuminuria.

Fluorescein angiography is said to detect retinal changes 4 years before direct ophthalmoscopy (Burger et al 1986) and all diabetics must have fundal examination by direct ophthalmoscopy through dilated pupils at least once yearly from adolescence.

Primary prevention (measures which will prevent or delay onset of a complication) and secondary prevention (interventions which halt or delay progression of an established complication) are reviewed by Young (1995).

The future

Much remains to be achieved – prognosis from childhood diabetes has remained gloomy in terms of complications and reduced life expectancy although it may be improving (Borch-Johnsen et al 1986). Of patients developing diabetes in childhood, half still died by the age of 50 years in the 1970s (Deckert et al 1978).

Current recognition of specific genetic, immune and metabolic markers is now allowing prediction of development of diabetes in high risk groups sufficiently early for intervention to prevent ongoing β cell destruction and prevent clinical disease (Bingley & Gale 1995). A variety of preventive strategies (e.g. with specific immunotherapy, oral insulin or nicotinamide) are currently in progress (Bingley & Gale 1995). Until now intervention has come too late – by clinical presentation more than 90% of β cell function is already destroyed. Nonspecific immunosuppressive therapy, with toxic drugs such as cyclosporine, prolongs the 'honeymoon' period, but no case of total remission or with normal glucose tolerance has been reported and renal toxicity is common. Nevertheless, less toxic immunosuppressive agents will be developed and may help make pancreatic, particularly islet cell, transplantation practical therapy (Sells & Brynger 1987, London et al 1995).

The epidemiological search for preventable environmental triggers for AI destruction and acute decompensation precipitating clinical onset continues (Diabetes Epidemiology Research International 1987, Dorman et al 1995).

Miniaturized portable 'closed loop' infusion pumps linked to glucose sensors are being developed and have exciting possibilities (Pickup 1995). The delivery of insulin more physiologically is an important goal (Danielsen et al 1995) but techniques such as implantation of an intraperitoneal pump to deliver insulin via portal vein to the liver without peripheral hyperglycemia are generally inappropriate. It is unclear whether even a 'desirable' childhood regimen combining nasal (bolus) and transdermal (basal) delivery (perhaps with a noninvasive glucose sensor) can be satisfactorily clinically and commercially developed in the foreseeable future (Danielsen et al 1995).

A promising and widely applicable approach is in modification of the molecular structure and formulation (e.g. preventing dimerization) of insulin which would alter timing of absorption from subcutaneous sites. Very rapidly absorbed insulin analogues could be administered subcutaneously with food (clinical trials in adult diabetics are in progress) or by other routes, such as intranasally (see above). There are obvious practical difficulties with the latter – absorption may be particularly erratic in children who have frequent upper respiratory infections and 'enhancers', which increase bioavailability, are associated with local irritation and polyp formation. Both altered structure and solubility of insulin could increase its immunogenicity and interfere with desired rapid and brief action (Van Haeften et al 1987). Insulin analogues with extended action – truly basal (background) insulins – are also being developed. With human (and porcine) insulins, antibodies are only very rarely of clinical importance.

Other diabetic syndromes in childhood (Batch & Werther 1995)

Maturity-onset diabetes in the young (MODY)

Presentation is usually in middle-aged adults but it is occasionally seen in children (MODY) with impaired glucose tolerance and insulin resistance usually associated with obesity. There may be a strong family history of type 2 diabetes. Treatment is with weight reduction. Insulin may be necessary but most children with impaired glucose tolerance will not develop diabetes and insulin should be reserved for those with fasting hyperglycemia or symptoms. Oral hypoglycemic agents should be avoided. There is no AI or HLA association. Other slow-onset forms with long remission periods (e.g. Mason-type) are probably closely related.

Secondary diabetes mellitus

Diabetes may occur with islet damage secondary to other factors, e.g. pancreatic exocrine disease in cystic fibrosis (Stutchfield et al 1988) and certain drug or poison ingestion, in association with genetic syndromes (e.g. Prader–Willi, DIDMOAD – see below) or with abnormalities of insulin or its receptors, and secondary to other endocrine disorders (e.g. Cushing's syndrome). There are no HLA or AI associations but an AI response to damaged pancreatic tissue may be a factor in the pathogenesis in cystic fibrosis (Stutchfield et al 1988).

DIDMOAD (diabetes insipidus, diabetes mellitus, optic atrophy and deafness) syndrome, Wolfram syndrome (Cremers et al 1977)

Optic atrophy (OA) and diabetes insipidus (DI) usually present on a background of established diabetes mellitus. The bilateral progressive OA is present in nearly all by young adulthood causing eventual blindness. DI occurs in about one-third and the (high tone) deafness is usually not severe. Inheritance is autosomal recessive.

Neonatal diabetes mellitus (Stirling & Kelnar 1995b)

This is a rare complication generally seen in SGA infants. Presentation is with rapid weight loss, severe dehydration, fever and vomiting without diarrhea. Thirst and polyuria are usually unnoticed. Babies appear pale and lively. Blood glucose is very high with glycosuria but only mild (if any) ketonuria and acidosis. There is extreme insulin sensitivity – treatment is with 0.01 unit/kg/h continuous infusion and normal saline initially. The condition is usually self-limiting, in which case ICA are absent, HLA alleles are not those which predispose to IDDM, and subcutaneous insulin can generally be stopped within weeks. Subsequent glucose tolerance is normal but there may be an increased risk of later diabetes. The cause is unknown but could relate to delayed β cell maturation (Pagliara et al 1973).

Occasionally permanent diabetes presents at this age (Hoffman et al 1980). Distinction from the transient form can only be made on follow-up but more 'typical' HLA alleles are generally present and other associated HLA-linked AI diseases (e.g. celiac disease) have been described.

A nationwide UK study under the auspices of the British Paediatric Association Surveillance Unit, to establish incidence rates for the transient and permanent forms and allow comparison of their clinical, physiological and genetic characteristics, is in progress.

HYPOGLYCEMIA

Hypoglycemia is a common, but often poorly investigated and managed, metabolic abnormality in infancy and childhood but not a diagnosis in itself. If prolonged or recurrent it can result in severe neuroglycopenia, potentially irreversible brain damage and long-term mental handicap particularly in the very young.

Blood glucose regulation and the metabolic consequences of starvation are discussed above (and see Figs 19.44 and 19.45) and by Aynsley-Green & Soltesz (1985), Lee & Leonard (1995), Hawdon & Ward Platt (1995), Stirling & Kelnar (1995a) and Dunger & Edge (1995).

Normal neonates and young children tolerate fasting less well than adults – blood glucose levels may start to fall after periods as short as 6–12 h which has implications for the preoperative management of children requiring surgery (Kelnar 1976). Reasons are unclear but use of stable (nonradioactive) isotopes should help to provide them. Glucose levels appear to fall in a cyclical fashion overnight in normal children, some falling into the 'hypoglycemic' range before compensation (Stirling et al 1991c,d).

The principal metabolic substrate for energy production in the fetus is glucose provided continuously via the placenta. After delivery the neonate must adapt to alternating periods of enteral milk feeding and starvation (p. 112). After the first 24 h normal babies fed on demand feed frequently (even twice an hour to begin with) taking small quantities with each feed. Until feeding is established, the neonate is dependent on glycogenolysis and gluconeogenesis to maintain normoglycemia. SGA babies (who have low liver glycogen stores but high glucose requirements) and those with sepsis or birth asphyxia are at particular risk of hypoglycemia (see also Ch. 5).

Neonatal symptoms are nonspecific and include 'jitteriness', hypotonia, feeding difficulties, pallor, apnea, tachypnea, convulsions and coma. In older children, symptoms and signs are attributable to neuroglycopenia (confused or bizarre behavior, bad temper, irritability, headache, visual disturbances, hunger, abdominal pain, convulsions, coma) or to counter-regulation (pallor, sweating, nausea, vomiting).

Blood glucose levels below which there is arbitrarily defined hypoglycemia (e.g. 2.2 mmol/l) are controversial – it is unclear whether 'low' but asymptomatic blood glucose levels cause short- or long-term problems in different age groups. There has been demonstration that levels below 2.6 mmol/l are associated with abnormal somatosensory and brain stem evoked potentials in asymptomatic infants (Koh et al 1988a) and further studies should provide information leading to definitions based on pathophysiological criteria (Koh et al 1988b). Prolonged or recurrent symptomatic hypoglycemia is undoubtedly associated with permanent neurological damage.

Etiology

There are many potential causes of hypoglycemia – the most important are classified by age at presentation in Table 19.19. Endocrine causes are discussed in the section relating to the relevant gland; causes of hyperinsulinism are discussed below.

Persistent neonatal hypoglycemia is usually due to

Table 19.19 Causes of hypoglycemia by age (after Aynsley-Green 1989)

Transient neonatal
Decreased glucose production
  Birth asphyxia
  Small for gestational age
  Sepsis
  Starvation
  Hypothermia

Hyperinsulinism
  Infant of diabetic mother
  Erythroblastosis
  Beckwith-Wiedemann (usually)
  Maternal glucose infusions
  Idiopathic

Persistent neonatal and infancy
Hyperinsulinism
  Nesidioblastosis
  Islet cell adenoma/hyperplasia/leucine sensitivity
  Beckwith-Wiedemann (sometimes)

Hormonal
  Growth hormone deficiency
  Hypopituitarism
  Glucocorticoid
    Congenital adrenal hyperplasia
    ACTH deficiency
    Glucagon deficiency
    Hypothyroidism (?)

Inborn errors of metabolism (enzyme deficiency – see Fig. 19.44)
  Glucose-6-phosphatase – glycogen storage disease (GSD) Type I*
  Amylo-1,6-glucosidase (GSD III)*
  Debrancher*
  Phosphorylase (GSD VI)*
  Phosphorylase kinase*
  Glycogen synthetase*
  Fructose-1, 6-diphosphatase*
  Phosphoenolpyruvate carboxykinase*
  Pyruvate carboxylase*
  Galactose-1-phosphate uridyl transferase (galactosemia)*
  β-oxidation defects*
  Fructose intolerance
  Maple syrup urine disease

Later childhood
Accelerated starvation

Hormonal
  As above
  Addison's disease
  Familial glucocorticoid deficiency

Enzyme deficiency
  Those marked* above
  Adrenomedullary hyporesponsiveness

Liver disease
  Fulminant hepatitis
  Reye's syndrome
  Jamaican vomiting sickness

Hyperinsulinism
  Insulin administration (including Munchausen by proxy syndrome)
  Oral hypoglycemics (including Munchausen by proxy syndrome)

Ingestion
  Alcohol
  Salicylates

hyperinsulinism, deficiency of a counter-regulatory hormone or of a gluconeogenic or glycogenolytic enzyme. Recent-onset recurring hypoglycemia is most commonly due to hyperinsulinism, 'accelerated starvation', defective hepatic gluconeogenesis or GH and/or glucocorticoid deficiency (Lee & Leonard 1995). Accidental or nonaccidental administration of hypoglycemic agents must be considered and hypoglycemia anticipated in any child who has ingested alcohol.

Differential diagnosis

History and examination may provide diagnostic clues, for example a family history of neonatal death or acidosis in an inherited metabolic disorder, short stature with micropenis in hypopituitarism, hepatomegaly in galactosemia or gluconeogenic or glycogenolytic disorders, macroglossia and transverse ear lobe creases in Beckwith–Wiedemann syndrome.

Essential diagnostic information is obtained from blood and urine samples taken *when there is hypoglycemia* and before treatment commences. Blood glucose, ketone bodies, lactate, free fatty acids, branched chain amino acids, insulin, GH, cortisol and catecholamines and urinary ketone bodies, catecholamine metabolites and reducing substances should ideally be measured. If sampling is difficult the most important assays are for blood glucose, plasma insulin and cortisol and urinary ketone bodies, and samples should be deep frozen for future analysis.

The metabolic consequences of starvation with counter-regulation are increased plasma fatty acids, glycerol, ketone bodies, and branched chain amino acids associated with high levels of cortisol, GH and catecholamines. Insulin levels will be low or undetectable. Significant ketosis excludes hyperinsulinism as the cause for hypoglycemia but 'ketotic hypoglycemia' is not a diagnosis in itself and requires further elucidation to find the cause. Important endocrine causes of ketotic hypoglycemia include deficiencies of counter-regulatory hormones (GH and ACTH deficiencies, CAH – especially during intercurrent stress or infection, Addison's disease, familial glucocorticoid deficiency and adrenomedullary unresponsiveness).

Hyperinsulinism results in hypoglycemia without ketonuria because insulin inhibits lipolysis. Plasma insulin levels may not be elevated but will be high for plasma glucose; plasma ketone bodies may be detectable but will be low for the glucose level.

Further differential diagnosis may necessitate 24-h metabolic profiles, calculation of the glucose infusion rate necessary to maintain normoglycemia, assessment of glycogen reserve by glucagon provocation tests and of gluconeogenesis.

After exclusion of other causes of ketotic hyperglycemia, there remains a group of children who regularly develop hypoglycemia during periods of fasting 'accelerated starvation'. Jewish children are absolved from fasting on Yom Kippur (Day of Atonement) until they are 'adult' (13 years). More severe hypoglycemia with convulsions may occur during intercurrent infection (particularly with vomiting), after pronounced physical activity or during preoperative starvation. There is often a history of difficult delivery or intrauterine growth retardation and the child (usually a boy) may be underweight. The hypoglycemic tendency is usually outgrown by later childhood. It is likely that they represent one end of a normal distribution of ability to maintain normoglycemia during fasting.

Defects in β oxidation of fatty acids (Turnbull et al 1988, Abdenur 1996) are increasingly recognized as important causes of hypoglycemia in previously 'idiopathic' groups. Ketone levels are low (cf. ketotic hypoglycemia including 'accelerated starvation'), plasma fatty acid levels are high (cf. hyperinsulinism). Medium-chain acyl CoA dehydrogenase (MCAD) deficiency may now be

specifically diagnosed by molecular genetic studies and by measuring urinary phenylpropionyl glycine levels, which are high following an oral phenylpropionic acid load owing to inability to convert phenylpropionic acid to hippuric acid, an essential step in fatty acid oxidation.

Endocrine pancreatic abnormalities causing hypoglycemia

These are almost always due to hyperinsulinism – glucagon deficiency seems very rare. Transient neonatal hypoglycemia due to hyperinsulinism is seen in the infant of a poorly controlled diabetic mother (fetal hyperinsulinism secondary to maternal hyperglycemia) and is found in erythroblastosis fetalis (cause unknown) and Beckwith–Wiedemann syndrome (see Ch. 5).

In a minority of infants of diabetic mothers hypoglycemia is delayed, but persisting neonatal hypoglycemia is usually associated with an underlying structural pancreatic abnormality. These conditions may not present until later in the first year, making hyperinsulinism the commonest cause of persistent hypoglycemia in infants below 1 year of age or even in childhood.

It is likely that the spectrum of histological findings, from discrete β cell adenoma(s) through diffuse β cell hyperplasia, microadenomatosis and nesidioblastosis to functional β cell disorder alone, and perhaps also 'leucine sensitive hypoglycemia', all result from the same pathological process, probably in the control of pancreatic endocrine secretion (Aynsley-Green & Soltesz 1985).

Nesidioblastosis

'Nesidioblastosis' ('germ islands') was first used to describe abnormal differentiation of isolated pancreatic islet cells from blastic duct cells, a process associated with severe hypoglycemia in infancy. Clinical and histological abnormalities are reviewed by Aynsley-Green et al (1981) and Polak & Bloom (1980), respectively.

The majority of infants present neonatally with symptoms (including convulsions) of intractable hypoglycemia. Occasionally presentation is later in the first 6 months. There may be a positive family history. They are obese, resembling the infant of the poorly controlled diabetic mother (hyperinsulinism is common to both). There may be a history of maternal glucose intolerance during previous pregnancies.

Diagnosis is dependent on demonstrating hyperinsulinemic hypoglycemia without significant ketosis. Very high glucose infusion rates (> 15 mg/kg/min) may be necessary to maintain normoglycemia – rates above 6–9 mg/kg/min are highly suggestive of hyperinsulinism. The demonstration, when hypoglycemic, of a glycemic response to glucagon, low branched chain amino acid levels, and insulin suppression following somatostatin infusion will confirm the diagnosis.

Priority is to correct hypoglycemia but this can be difficult because of the high glucose infusion rates necessary and technical problems with siting infusion lines. Glucagon (0.1 mg/kg) has only transient effects in mobilizing glucose from glycogen stores, but can be invaluable to cover resiting. Long-acting somatostatin analogues may aid longer-term maintenance of normoglycemia (Hindmarsh & Brook 1987, Kirk et al 1988) but GH (Hocking et al 1986) is as effective and has fewer potential side effects. Conventionally, medical treatment is with diazoxide (< 25 mg/kg/24 h), and its effect is potentiated by thiazide diuretics, but adequate control is seldom achieved without the need for continuing high rates of glucose infusion and side effects are common.

In these circumstances, surgery is urgently indicated. Preoperative imaging (ultrasound and CT scanning) may not discriminate between a diffuse process and a discrete lesion (and the biochemical consequences are identical). If a discrete adenoma is found it should be resected – this may be curative; if not, subtotal (95%) pancreatectomy (more effective than less radical removal) is performed. This may, commonly, result in 'cure' – normoglycemia without medical therapy, or normoglycemia on diazoxide – diabetes mellitus or still unstable glycemic control. In this last situation, or if the infant remains dependent on glucose infusion, total pancreatectomy is performed. Post-pancreatectomy diabetes (Greene et al 1984, Batch & Werther 1995) is generally easy to manage on small doses of insulin (e.g. once daily intermediate acting) because of associated α cell loss causing glucagon deficiency and altered CHO absorption secondary to pancreatic exocrine deficiency.

Maintenance of normoglycemia and early recourse to surgery prevent previously common permanent neurological damage and mental retardation.

REFERENCES

Abdenur J E 1996 Emergencies of inborn metabolic diseases. In: Lifshitz F (ed) Pediatric endocrinology. Marcel Dekker, New York, 791–808

Ackland F M, Jones J, Buckler J M H, Dunger D B, Rayner P H W, Preece M A 1990 Growth hormone treatment in non-growth hormone deficient children: effects of stopping treatment. Acta Paediatrica Scandinavica (suppl) 366: 32–37

Adams J, Polson D W, Abdulwahid et al 1985 Multifollicular ovaries; clinical and endocrine features and response to pulsatile gonadotrophin releasing hormone. Lancet ii: 1375–1378

Addison T 1855 On the constitutional and local effects of disease of the suprarenal capsule. Highley D, London

Adlard P, Buzi F, Jones J, Stanhope R, Preece M A 1987 Physiological growth hormone secretion during slow-wave sleep in short prepubertal children. Clinical Endocrinology 27: 355–361

Ahmed S R, Shalet S M, Beardwell C G 1986 The effects of cranial irradiation on growth hormone secretion. Acta Paediatrica Scandinavica 75: 255–260

Ahmed S F, Wallace W H B, Kelnar C J H 1995 Knemometry in childhood: a study to compare the precision of two different techniques. Annals of Human Biology 22: 247–252

Ahmed S F, Dixon P, Bonthron D T, Barr D G D, Kelnar C J H, Thakker R V 1996a Novel mutations in the GNAS1 gene as detected by single strand conformational polymorphism and direct DNA sequencing in a cohort of 13 kindreds with pseudohypoparathyroidism. Journal of Endocrinology 148 (suppl): 168

Ahmed S F, Wardhaugh B W, Duff J, Wallace W H B, Kelnar C J H 1996b The relationship between short term changes in weight and lower leg length in children and young adults. Annals of Human Biology 23: 159–162

Al-Dujaili E A S, Hope J, Estivariz F E, Lowry P J, Edwards C R W 1981 Circulating human pituitary pro-gamma-melanotropin enhances the adrenal response to ACTH. Nature 291: 156–159

Albanese A, Stanhope R 1993 Growth and metabolic data following growth hormone treatment of children with intrauterine growth retardation. Hormone Research 39: 8–12

Albertsson-Wikland K, Rosberg S, Isaksson O, Westphal O 1983 Secretory pattern of growth hormone in children of differing growth rates. Acta Endocrinologica 103 (suppl 256): 72

Albini C H, Quattrin T, Vandlen R L, MacGillivray M H 1988 Quantitation of urinary growth hormone in children with normal and abnormal growth. Pediatric Research 23: 89–92

Albright F 1947a Osteoporosis. Annals of Internal Medicine 27: 861–882

Albright F 1947b Polyostotic fibrous dysplasia: a defense of the entity. Journal of Clinical Endocrinology 7: 307–324

Albright F, Butler A M, Bloom E 1937a Rickets resistant to vitamin D therapy. American Journal of Diseases of Children 54: 529–544

Albright F, Butler A M, Hampton A O et al 1937b Syndrome characterised by osteitis fibrosa disseminata, areas of pigmentation and endocrine dysfunction with precocious puberty in females, report of five cases. New England Journal of Medicine 216: 727–746

Albright F, Burnett C H, Smith P H 1942 Pseudohypoparathyroidism: an example of 'Seabright-Bantam syndrome'. Endocrinology 30: 922–932

Alemzadeh R, Lifshitz F 1996 Childhood obesity. In: Lifshitz F (ed) Pediatric endocrinology. Marcel Dekker, New York, pp 753–774

Alexeeff M, Macnicol M F 1995 Epiphysiodesis in the management of limb length equality. Current Orthopaedics 9: 178–184

Amselem S, Duquesnoy P, Duriez B et al 1993 Spectrum of growth hormone receptor mutations and associated haplotypes in Laron syndrome. Human Molecular Genetics 2: 355–359

Anderson A B, Laurence K M, Turnbull A C 1969 The relationship in anencephaly between the size of the adrenal cortex and the length of gestation. Journal of Obstetrics and Gynaecology of the British Commonwealth 76: 196–199

Anderson B J 1995 Childhood and adolescent psychological development in relation to diabetes. In: Kelnar C J H (ed) Childhood and adolescent diabetes. Chapman & Hall, London, pp 107–119

Anderson D C 1980 The adrenal androgen-stimulating hormone does not exist. Lancet ii: 454–456

Anderson D C, Dewis P 1989 Gynaecomastia. Medicine International 64: 2647–2649

Ashkenazi A 1989 Occult celiac disease: a common cause of short stature. Growth, Genetics and Hormones 5(2): 1–3

Attie J N 1996 Carcinoma of the thyroid in children and adolescents. In: Lifshitz F (ed) Pediatric endocrinology. Marcel Dekker, New York, pp 423–432

Aubert M L, Grumbach M M, Kaplan S L 1975 The ontogenesis of human fetal hormones. III. Prolactin. Journal of Clinical Investigation 56: 155–164

Aynsley-Green A 1985 Metabolic and endocrine interrelations in the human fetus and neonate. American Journal of Clinical Nutrition 41: 399–417

Aynsley-Green A 1989 Hypoglycaemia. In: Brook C G D (ed) Clinical paediatric endocrinology 2nd edn. Blackwell Scientific Publications, Oxford, pp 618–637

Aynsley-Green A, Soltesz G 1985 Hypoglycaemia in infancy and childhood. Churchill Livingstone, Edinburgh

Aynsley-Green A, Soltesz G 1992 Disorders of blood glucose homeostasis in the neonate. In: Roberton N R C (ed) Textbook of neonatology, 2nd edn. Churchill Livingstone, Edinburgh, pp 777–797

Aynsley-Green A, Polak J M, Bloom S R 1981 Nesidioblastosis of the pancreas; definition of the syndrome and management of the severe neonatal hyperinsulinaemic hypoglycaemia. Archives of Disease in Childhood 56: 496–509

Azziz R, Mulaikal R M, Migeon C J, Jones H W, Rock J A 1986 Long term results of vaginal reconstruction in congenital adrenal hyperplasia (CAH). Fertility and Sterility 46 (suppl): 45 (A129)

Banatvala J E, Bryant J, Scherntaner G et al 1985 Coxsackie B, mumps, rubella and cytomegalovirus-specific IgM responses in patients with juvenile-onset insulin-dependent diabetes in Britain, Austria and Australia. Lancet i: 1409–1412

Banting F G, Best C H, Collip J B, Campbell W R, Fletcher A A 1922 Pancreatic extracts in the treatment of diabetes mellitus. Canadian Medical Association Journal 12: 141–146

Barclay R P C, Craig J O, Galloway C A S, Richardson J E, Shepherd R C, Smail P J 1988 The incidence of childhood diabetes in certain parts of Scotland. Scottish Medical Journal 33: 237–239

Barker D J P 1992 Fetal and infant origins of adult disease. BMJ Publishing Group, London

Barker D J P, Bull A R, Osmond C, Simmonds S J 1990 Fetal and placental size and risk of hypertension. British Medical Journal 301: 259–262

Barker D J P, Martyn C N, Osmond C, Hales C N, Fall C H D 1993 Growth in utero and serum cholesterol concentrations in adult life. British Medical Journal 307: 1524–1527

Barnes N D 1985 Screening for congenital hypothyroidism: the first decade. Archives of Disease in Childhood 60: 587–592

Baron J, Oerter K E, Yanovski J A, Novosad J A, Bacher J D, Cutler G B Jr 1993 Catch-up growth is intrinsic to the epiphyseal growth plate. Pediatric Research 33 (suppl): S41 A224

Barr D G D, Stirling H F, Darling J A B 1994 Evolution of pseudohypoparathyroidism: an informative family study. Archives of Disease in Childhood 70: 337–338

Barton J R, Ferguson A 1990 Clinical features, morbidity and mortality of Scottish children with inflammatory bowel disease. Quarterly Journal of Medicine 75: 423–439

Bartter F C, Pronove P, Gee J R et al 1962 Hyperplasia of the juxtaglomerular complex with hyperaldosteronism and hypokalaemic alkalosis. American Journal of Medicine 33: 811–828

Batch J A, Werther G A 1995 Unusual diabetes and diabetes in the context of other disorders. In: Kelnar C J H (ed) Childhood and adolescent diabetes. Chapman & Hall, London, pp 397–418

Beaufrere B, Giachino G, Francois R 1986 Treatment and prevention of hypoglycaemia. International Study Group of Diabetes in Children and Adolescents Bulletin 13: 25–26

Becker D J, Orchard T J, Lloyd C E 1995 Control and outcome: clinical and epidemiological aspects. In: Kelnar C J H (ed) Childhood and adolescent diabetes. Chapman & Hall, London, pp 519–538

Beckett G, Seth J 1989 Thyroid function tests. Medicine International 63: 2583–2587

Bell P M, Hadden D R 1983 Ketoacidosis without hyperglycaemia during self-monitoring of diabetes. Diabetes Care 6: 622–623

Belmonte M, Schiffrin A, Dufresne J 1988 Impact of SMBG on control of diabetes as measured by HbA1. Diabetes Care 11: 484–488

Benediktsson R, Lindsay R, Noble J, Seckl J R, Edwards C R W 1993 Glucocorticoid exposure in utero: a new model for adult hypertension. Lancet 341: 339–341

Berger M 1987 Human insulin: much ado about hypoglycaemic (un)awareness. Diabetologia 30: 829–833

Berger W G, Honneger B, Keller V, Jaeggi E 1989 Warning symptoms of hypoglycaemia during treatment with human and porcine insulin in diabetes mellitus. Lancet i: 1041–1044

Berson S A, Yalow R S 1968 Immunochemical heterogeneity of parathyroid hormone in plasma. Journal of Clinical Endocrinology and Metabolism 28: 1037–1047

Berthezene F, Forest M G, Grimaud J A, Claustrat B, Mornex R 1976 Leydig cell agenesis. New England Journal of Medicine 295: 969–972

Bikker H, Vulsma T, Baas F, de Vijlder J J M 1995 Identification of five novel inactivating mutations in the human thyroid peroxidase gene by denaturing gradient gel electrophoresis. Human Mutations 6: 9–16

Bingley P J, Gale E A M 1995 Prevention of IDDM. In: Kelnar C J H (ed) Childhood and adolescent diabetes. Chapman & Hall, London, pp 503–518

Bloomfield S, Calder J E, Chisolm V et al 1990 A project in diabetes education for children. Diabetic Medicine 7: 137–142

Bock H A, Flukiger R, Berger W 1985 Real and artefactual erythrocyte swelling in hyperglycaemia. Diabetologia 28: 335–338

Bode H H, Crawford J D, Danon M 1996 Disorders of anyidiuretic hormone homeostasis: diabetes insipidus and SIADH. In: Lifshitz F (ed) Pediatric endocrinology. Marcel Dekker, New York, pp 731–752

Bongiovanni A M 1962 The adrenogenital syndrome with deficiency of 3β-hydroxysteroid dehydrogenase. Journal of Clinical Investigation 41: 2086–2092

Bongiovanni A M 1983 An epidemic of premature thelarche in Puerto Rico. Journal of Pediatrics 103: 245–246

Borch-Johnsen K, Kreiner S, Deckert T 1986 Mortality of Type 1 (insulin-dependent) diabetes in Denmark: a study of relative mortality in 2930 Danish Type 1 diabetic patients diagnosed from 1933–1972. Diabetologia 29: 767–772

Bottazzo G F 1989 A biased attempt to reconstruct the pathogenic mechanisms leading to destructive endocrine autoimmunity. Acta Paediatrica Scandinavica (suppl) 356: 113–118

Bottazzo G F, Dean B M, Gorsuch A N, Cudworth A G, Doniach D 1980 Complement-fixing islet-cell antibodies in Type 1 diabetes: possible monitors of active beta cell damage. Lancet i: 668–672

Bourguignon J-P 1997 Treatment of constitutional delay of growth and puberty. In: Kelnar C J H, Stirling H F, Saenger P, Savage M O (eds) Growth disorders – pathophysiology and treatment. Chapman & Hall, London

Boyar R M, Finkelstein J, Roffwarg et al 1972 Synchronisation of augmented luteinising hormone secretion with sleep during puberty. New England Journal of Medicine 287: 582–586

Brauner R, Rappaport R 1985 Precocious puberty secondary to cranial irradiation for tumors distant from the hypothalamo-pituitary area. Hormone Research 22: 78–82

Braunstein G D 1996 Pubertal gynecomastia. In: Lifshitz F (ed) Pediatric endocrinology. Marcel Dekker, New York, pp 197–206

Brenchley S, Govindji A 1995 Dietary management of children with diabetes. In: Kelnar C J H (ed) Childhood and adolescent diabetes. Chapman & Hall, London, pp 271–281

Bridges N A 1995 Disorders of puberty. In: Brook C G D (ed) Clinical paediatric endocrinology, 3rd edn. Blackwell Scientific Publications, Oxford, pp 253–273

Bridges N A, Christopher J A, Hindmarsh P C, Brook C G D 1994 Sexual precocity: sex incidence and aetiology. Archives of Disease in Childhood 70: 116–118

Brill A B, Becker D V 1986 The safety of 131 I treatment of hyperthyroidism. In: Van Middlesworth L, Givens J R (eds) The thyroid gland; a practical clinical treatise. Year Book Publications, Chicago, pp 347–362

Brink S J 1995 Presentation and ketoacidosis. In: Kelnar C J H (ed) Childhood and adolescent diabetes. Chapman & Hall, London, pp 213–240

British Diabetic Association 1992 Dietary recommendations for people with diabetes: an update for the 1990s. Diabetic Medicine 9: 189–202

Brook C G D, Lloyd J K 1973 Adipose cell size and glucose tolerance in obese children. Archives of Disease in Childhood 48: 301–302

Brook C G D, Muerset G, Zachmann M et al 1974 Growth in children with 45XO Turner's syndrome. Archives of Disease in Childhood 49: 789–795

Brook C G D, Jacobs H S, Stanhope R, Adams J, Hindmarsh P C 1987 Pulsatility of reproductive hormones: applications to the understanding of puberty and the treatment of infertility. Baillière's Clinics in Endocrinology and Metabolism 1: 23–41

Brosnan P G 1985 Spontaneous resolution under ultrasonic observation of ovarian cysts causing precocious pseudopuberty in young girls. Pediatric Research 19: 182A

Brown D C, Kelnar C J H 1993 Metabolic signals for the initiation of puberty. Highlights 1(2): 4–5, Medicom Europe, The Netherlands

Brown D C, Stirling H F, Kelnar C J H 1994 Precocious puberty. Current Paediatrics 4: 184–188

Brown D C, Butler G E, Kelnar C J H, Wu F C W 1995 A double blind, placebo controlled study of the effects of low dose testosterone undecanoate on the growth of small for age, prepubertal boys. Archives of Disease in Childhood 73: 131–135

Brown D C, Kelnar C J H, Wu F C W 1996a Differentiation of normal male prepuberty and hypogonadotrophic hypogonadism using an ultrasensitive luteinizing hormone assay. Hormone Research 46: 83–87

Brown D C, Kelnar C J H, Wu F C W 1996b Energy metabolism during human male puberty I: changes in energy expenditure during the onset of puberty in boys. Annals of Human Biology 23: 273–279

Brown D C, Kelnar C J H, Wu F C W 1996c Energy metabolism during human male puberty II: use of testicular size in predictive equations for basal metabolic rate. Annals of Human Biology 23: 281–284

Buchanan C R, Stanhope R, Jones J, Adlard P, Preece M A 1988 Gonadotrophin, growth hormone and prolactin secretory dysfunction in primary hypothyroidism. Pediatric Research 23: A133

Buchanan C R, Maheshwari H G, Norman M R, Morrell D J, Preece M A 1991 Laron-type dwarfism with apparent normal high affinity serum growth hormone-binding protein. Clinical Endocrinology 35: 179–185

Buckler J M H 1990 A longitudinal study of adolescent growth. Springer Verlag, London

Buckler J M H 1997 Growth at adolescence. In: Kelnar C J H, Stirling H F, Saenger P, Savage M O (eds) Growth disorders – pathophysiology and treatment. Chapman & Hall, London

Buckler J M H, Tanner J M 1996 Buckler–Tanner (Tanner–Whitehouse revised) British longitudinal growth standards (1995). Castlemead Publications, Ware

Burger H G, Igarashi M 1988 Inhibin: definition and nomenclature, including related substances. Journal of Clinical Endocrinology and Metabolism 66: 885–886

Burger W, Hovener G, Dusterhus R, Hartmann R, Weber B 1986 Prevalence and development of retinopathy in children and adults with type 1 (insulin-dependent) diabetes mellitus. A longitudinal study. Diabetologia 29: 17–22

Burns J 1997 The effects on growth of cardiac disease. In: Kelnar C J H, Stirling H F, Saenger P, Savage M O (eds) Growth disorders – pathophysiology and treatment. Chapman & Hall, London

Butler G E, Sellar R E, Kelnar C J H, Wu F C W 1987 A sensitive immunoradiometric assay (RMA) for luteinising hormone (LH) in the assessment of prepubertal males with idiopathic hypogonadotrophic hypogonadism (IHH) and constitutional delayed puberty. Journal of Endocrinology 112 (suppl): A243

Butler G E, Kelnar C J H, Wu F C W 1988 Pituitary responsiveness in prepubertal and hypogonadotrophic hypogonadism is related to endogenous LHRH secretion. A study using a highly selective immunoradiometric assay. Journal of Endocrinology 117 (suppl): A277

Butler G E, McKie M, Ratcliffe S G 1989a An analysis of the phases of mid-childhood growth by synchronisation of the growth spurts. In: Tanner J M (ed) Auxology '88: perspectives in the science of growth and development. Smith-Gordon, London

Butler G E, Ratcliffe S G, Sellar R E, Kelnar C J H, Wu F C W 1989b Spontaneous pulsatile gonadotrophin secretion in pre- and peripubertal 47XXY boys. Journal of Endocrinology 121 (suppl): A160

Butler G E, Stirling H F, Wu F C W, Kelnar C J H 1989c Do growth hormone secretory patterns relate to growth velocity in both prepubertal and pubertal children? Hormone Research 31 (suppl): A109

Butler G E, Walker R F, Walker R V, Teague P, Riad-Fahmy D, Ratcliffe S G 1989d Salivary testosterone levels and the progress of puberty in the normal boy. Clinical Endocrinology 30: 587–596

Butler G E, Sellar R E, Walker R F, Hendry M, Kelnar C J H, Wu F C W 1992 Oral testosterone undecanoate in the management of delayed puberty in boys: pharmacokinetics and effects on sexual maturation and growth. Journal of Clinical Endocrinolgy and Metabolism 75: 37–44

Cacciari E, Frejauille E, Cicognani A et al 1983 How many cases of true precocious puberty in girls are idiopathic? Journal of Pediatrics 102: 357–360

Cacciari E, Balsamo A, Cassio A 1986 Neonatal screening programme for congenital adrenal hyperplasia in a homogeneous Caucasian population. Journal of Inherited Metabolic Disease 9 (suppl 1): 142–146

Cahill G F, Etzwiler L D, Freinkel N 1976 'Control' and diabetes. New England Journal of Medicine 294: 1004–1005

Calvo R, Obregon M J, Ruiz de Ona Escobar del Rey F, Morreale de Escobar G 1990 Congenital hypothyroidism as studied in rats. Crucial role of maternal thyroxine but not of 3,5,3'triiodothyronine in the protection of the fetal brain. Journal of Clinical Investigation 86: 889–899

Carpenter C C J, Soloman N, Silverberg S G et al 1964 Schmidt's syndrome (thyroid and adrenal insufficiency). A review of the literature and a report of fifteen new cases including ten instances of co-existent diabetes mellitus. Medicine 43: 153–180

Carter-Su C, Wang X, Campbell G S et al 1993 Molecular basis of growth hormone action. Pediatric Research 33 (suppl): S8 A34

Castro-Magana M, Angulo M, Canas A, Sharp A, Fuentes B 1988 Hypothalamo-pituitary–gonadal axis in boys with primary hypothyroidism and macroorchidism. Journal of Pediatrics 112: 397–402

Cernerud L, Edding E 1994 The value of measuring height and weight of schoolchildren. Paediatric and Perinatal Epidemiology 8: 365–372

Cheetham T M, Hughes I A 1996 Optimising the management of congenital adrenal hyperplasia. In: Kelnar C J H (ed) Paediatric endocrinology. Baillière's clinical paediatrics – international practice and research. Baillière Tindall, London, vol 4: 279–294

Chrousos G P, Loriaux D L, Mann D L, Cutler G B Jr 1982 Late onset 21–hydroxylase deficiency mimicking idiopathic hirsutism or polycystic ovarian disease: an allelic variant of congenital adrenal hyperplasia with a milder enzymatic deficiency. Annals of Internal Medicine 96: 143–148

Chu C E, Donaldson M D C, Kelnar C J H et al 1994 Possible role of imprinting in the Turner phenotype. Journal of Medical Genetics 31: 840–842

Chu C E, Paterson W F, Kelnar C J H, Smail P J, Greene S A, Donaldson M D C 1997 Variable effect of growth hormone on growth and final adult height in Scottish patients with Turner's syndrome. Acta Paediatrica 86: 160–164

Chung B C, Picado-Leonard J, Hanio M et al 1987 Cytochrome P450 c17: cloning of human adrenal and testis cDNA indicates the same gene is expressed in both tissues. Proceedings of the National Academy of Sciences USA 84: 407–411

Citrin W, Ellis G J, Skyler J S 1980 Glycosylated hemoglobin: a tool in identifying psychological problems. Diabetes Care 3: 563–564

Clarke B F 1995 Screening for complications in adolescence and beyond. In: Kelnar C J H (ed) Childhood and adolescent diabetes. Chapman & Hall, London, pp 539–552

Cohen H N, Paterson K R, Wallace A M, Beastall G H, Manderson W G, McCuish A C 1984 Dissociation of adrenarche and gonadarche in diabetes mellitus. Clinical Endocrinology 20: 717–724

Cole T J, Freeman J V, Preece M A 1995 Body mass index reference curves for the UK 1990. Archives of Disease in Childhood 73: 25–29

Conn J W 1974 Primary aldosteronism and primary reninism. Hospital Practice 9: 131–140

Connor J M 1995 Inheritance/genetics of childhood diabetes. In: Kelnar C J H (ed) Childhood and adolescent diabetes. Chapman & Hall, London, pp 161–168

Connor J M, Loughlin S A R 1989 Molecular genetics of Turner's syndrome. Acta Paediatrica Scandinavica (suppl) 356: 77–80

Connors M, Styne D 1986 Transient neonatal athyreosis resulting from thyrotropin binding inhibitory immunoglobulins. Pediatrics 78: 278–281

Copp D H, Cameron E C, Cheney B A, Davidson A G F, Henze K G 1962 Evidence for calcitonin – a new hormone from the parathyroid that lowers blood calcium. Endocrinology 70: 638–649

Cotterill A M, McKenna W J, Brady A F, Sharland M, Elsawi M, Yamada M, Camacho-Hübner C, Kelnar C J H, Dunger D B, Patton M A, Savage M O 1996 The short-term effects of growth hormone therapy on height velocity and cardiac ventricular wall thickness in children with Noonan syndrome Journal of Clinical Endocrinology and Metabolism 81: 2291–2297

Cowell C T in collaboration with the Australasian Paediatric Endocrine Group 1990 Effects of growth hormone in short, slowly growing children without growth hormone deficiency. Acta Paediatrica Scandinavica (suppl) 366: 29–30

Cowell C T, Rogers S, Silink M 1986 First morning urine albumin concentration is a good predictor of 24-hour urinary albumin excretion in children with type 1 (insulin-dependent) diabetes. Diabetologia 29: 97–99

Cowett R M 1996 Hypoglycaemia in the newborn. In: Lifshitz F (ed) Pediatric endocrinology. Marcel Dekker, New York, pp 677–692

Cox L 1997a Practical auxology. In: Kelnar C J H, Stirling H F, Saenger P, Savage M O (eds) Growth disorders – pathophysiology and treatment. Chapman & Hall, London

Cox L 1997b Skeletal maturation. In: Kelnar C J H, Stirling H F, Saenger P, Savage M O (eds) Growth disorders – pathophysiology and treatment. Chapman & Hall, London

Crawford J D, Bode H H 1975 Disorders of the posterior pituitary in children. In: Gardner L I (ed) Endocrine and genetic diseases of childhood and adolescence, 2nd edn. Saunders, Philadelphia, pp 126–158

Cremers C W, Wijdeveld P G, Pinckers A J 1977 Juvenile diabetes mellitus, optic atrophy, hearing loss, diabetes insipidus, atonia of the urinary tract and bladder, and other abnormalities (Wolfram syndrome). A review of 88 cases from the literature with personal observations on 3 new patients. Acta Paediatrica Scandinavica (suppl) 264: 1–16

Critchley H O D, Wallace W H B, Mamtora H, Higginson J, Shalet S M, Anderson D C 1992 Ovarian failure after whole abdominal radiotherapy – the potential for pregnancy. British Journal of Obstetrics and Gynaecology 99: 392–394

Crofton P M, Stirling H F, Kelnar C J H 1995 Bone alkaline phosphatase and height velocity in short normal children undergoing growth-promoting treatments: a longitudinal study. Clinical Chemistry 41 672–678

Crofton P M, Stirling H F, Schönau E, Kelnar C J H 1996a Bone alkaline phosphatase and collagen markers as early predictors of height velocity response to growth-promoting treatments in short normal children. Clinical Endocrinology 44: 385–394

Crofton P M, Stirling H F, Schönau E, Shrivastava A, Lyon A J, McIntosh N, Ahmed S F, Wallace W H B, Wade J C, Kelnar C J H 1996b Collagen markers and bone alkaline phosphatase as predictors of bone turnover and growth. In: Schönau E (ed) Paediatric osteology: new developments in diagnosis and therapy. Excerpta Medica International Congress Series, Elsevier Science, Amsterdam, pp 241–250

Crofton P M, Stirling H F, Schönau E, Shrivastava A, Lyon A J, McIntosh N, Ahmed S F, Wallace W H B, Wade J C, Kelnar C J H 1996c Biochemical markers of bone turnover. Hormone Research 45 (suppl 1): 55–58

Crofton P M, Illingworth P J, Groome N P, Stirling H F, Swanston I, Seth J, McNeilly A, Kelnar C J H 1997 Changes in dimeric inhibin A and B during normal early puberty in boys and girls. Clinical Endocrinology 46: 109–114

Cronk C E, Crocker A C, Pueschel S M et al 1988 Growth charts for children with Down's syndrome: 1 month to 18 years of age. Pediatrics 81: 102–110

Crowley S, Hindmarsh P, Honour J W, Brook C G D 1992 Failure of the short synacthen test to detect adrenal insufficiency in children on inhaled steroids. Journal of Endocrinology 132: 95

Crowley S, Hindmarsh P, Honour J W, Brook C G D 1993 Reproducibility of the cortisol response to stimulation with a low dose of ACTH (1–24): the effect of basal cortisol levels and comparison with low-dose and high-dose secretory dynamics. Journal of Endocrinology 136: 167–172

Crowley W F, Comite F, Vale W W, Rivier J, Loriaux D L, Cutler G B Jr 1981 Therapeutic use of pituitary desensitisation with a long-acting LHRH agonist: a potential new treatment for idiopathic precocious puberty. Journal of Clinical Endocrinology and Metabolism 52: 370–372

Crowne E C, Moore C, Wallace W H B, Morris-Jones P H, Shalet S M 1992 A novel variant of growth hormone insufficiency following low dose cranial irradiation. Clinical Endocrinology 36: 59–68

Culler F L, Jones K L, Deftos J J 1985 Impaired calcitonin secretion in patients with Williams syndrome. Journal of Pediatrics 107: 720–723

Cushing H 1932 Basophil adenomas of the pituitary body and their clinical manifastations (pituitary basophilism). Bulletin of the Johns Hopkins Hospital 50: 137–195

Cutler G B Jr, Laue L 1990 Congenital adrenal hyperplasia due to 21 hydroxylase deficiency. New England Journal of Medicine 323: 1806–1813

Cutler G B Jr, Glenn M, Bush M, Hodgen G D, Graham C E, Loriaux D L 1978 Adrenarche: a survey of rodents, domestic animals and primates. Endocrinology 103: 2112–2118

Cutting W A M, Elton R A, Campbell J L, Minton E J, Spreng J M 1987 Stunting in African children. Archives of Disease in Childhood 62: 508–509

Czernichow P 1992 Testing water regulation. In: Ranke M B (ed) Functional endocrinologic diagnostics in children and adolescents. J & J Verlag, Mannheim, pp 128–139

Czernichow P 1996 Pathophysiology and consequences of intrauterine growth retardation. In: Kelnar C J H (ed) Paediatric endocrinology. Baillière's clinical paediatrics – international practice and research. Baillière Tindall, London, vol 4: 245–258

Czernichow P, Pomerade R, Brauner R, Rappaport R 1985 Neurogenic diabetes insipidus in children. In: Czernichow P, Robinson A G (eds) Diabetes insipidus in man. Karger, Basel, pp 190–209

Dallas J D, Foley T P Jr 1996 Hyperthyroidism. In: Lifshitz F (ed) Pediatric endocrinology. Marcel Dekker, New York, pp 401–414

Danielsen G M, Drejer K, Langkjær, Plum A 1995 New routes and means of insulin delivery. In: Kelnar C J H (ed) Childhood and adolescent diabetes. Chapman & Hall, London, pp 571–584

Danon M, Friedman S C 1996 Ambiguous genitalia, micropenis, hypospadias and cryptorchidism. In: Lifshitz F (ed) Pediatric endocrinology. Marcel Dekker, New York, pp 281–304

David T J 1989 Short stature in children with atopic eczema. Acta Derm Venereol (suppl) 144: 41–44

Davies A G, Price D A, Postlethwaite R J, Addison G M, Burn J L, Fielding B A 1985 Renal function in diabetes mellitus. Archives of Disease in Childhood 60: 299–304

De Jong F H 1988 Inhibin. Physiological Reviews 68: 555–607

de Swiet M, Dillon M J 1989 Hypertension in children. British Medical Journal 299: 469–470

de Swiet M, Fayers P, Shinebourne E A 1984 Blood pressure in 4 and 5 year old children: the effects of environment and other factors in its measurement. The Brompton Study. Journal of Hypertension 2: 501–505

de Swiet M, Dillon M J, Littler W, O'Brien E, Padfield P L, Petrie J C 1989 Measurement of blood pressure in children. British Medical Journal 299: 497

Deckert T, Poulsen, J E, Larsen M 1978 Prognosis of diabetics with diabetes onset before the age of thirty-one. I Survival, causes of death and complications. II Factors influencing the prognosis. Diabetologia 14: 363–370, 371–377

Degenhart H J 1971 A study of the cholesterol splitting enzyme system in normal adrenal and in adrenal lipoid hyperplasia. Acta Paediatrica Scandinavica 60: 611

Degenhart H J, Frankena L, Visser H K A et al 1966 Further investigation of a new hereditary defect in the biosynthesis of aldosterone: evidence for a defect in 18–hydroxylation of corticosterone. Acta Physiologica Pharmacologica Neerlandica 14: 88–89

Delange F, Henderson P, Bourdoux P et al 1986 Regional variations of iodine nutrition and thyroid function during the neonatal period in Europe. Biology of the Neonate 49: 322–330

Department of Health and Social Security 1974 Present day practice in infant feeding. HMSO, London

Department of Health and Social Security 1980 Present day practice in infant feeding. HMSO, London

Dhom G 1973 The prepubertal and pubertal growth of the adrenal (adrenarche). Beitrage fur Pathologie 150: 357–377

Diabetes Control and Complications Trial Research Group 1993 The effect of intensive treatment of diabetes on the development and progression of long term complications in insulin-dependent diabetes mellitus. New England Journal of Medicine 329: 977–986

Diabetes Epidemiology Research International 1987 Preventing insulin dependent diabetes mellitus: the environmental challenge. British Medical Journal 295: 479–481

Dickstein G et al 1991 Adrenocorticotropin stimulation test: effects of basal cortisol level, time of day and suggested new sensitive low dose test. Journal of Clinical Endocrinology and Metabolism 72: 773–778

Didi M, Didcock E, Davies H A, Ogilvy-Stewart A L, Wales J K H, Shalet S M 1995 High incidence of obesity in young adults after treatment of acute lymphoblastic leukaemia in childhood. Journal of Pediatrics 127: 63–67

Dieguez C, Page M D, Scanlon M F 1988 Growth hormone neuroregulation and its alteration in disease states. Clinical Endocrinology 28: 109–143

Dillon M J 1995 Salt and water balance: sodium-losing states and endocrine hypertension. In: Brook C G D (ed) Clinical paediatric endocrinology, 3rd edn. Blackwell Scientific Publications, Oxford, pp 558–579

DiMartino-Nardi J 1997 Treatment of the growth disorders associated with precocious puberty. In: Kelnar C J H, Stirling H F, Saenger P, Savage M O (eds) Growth disorders – pathophysiology and treatment. Chapman & Hall, London

DiMartino-Nardi J, Stoner E, Martin K et al 1987 New findings in apparent mineralocorticoid excess. Clinical Endocrinology 27: 49–62

Donaldson M D C 1996 Jury still out on growth hormone for normal short stature and Turner's syndrome. Lancet 348: 3–4

Donaldson M D C 1997 Definition, pathogenesis and practical investigation of abnormal growth. In: Kelnar C J H, Stirling H F, Saenger P, Savage M O (eds) Growth disorders – pathophysiology and treatment. Chapman & Hall, London

Donaldson M D C, Savage D C L 1988 Testosterone therapy in boys with delayed puberty. Pediatric Research 23: 125 (A119)

Donaldson M D C, Chu C, Cooke A et al 1994a The Prader–Willi syndrome. Archives of Disease in Childhood 70: 58–63

Donaldson M D C, Thomas P H, Love J G, Murray G D, McNinch A W, Savage D C L 1994b Presentation, acute illness and learning difficulties in salt wasting 21-hydroxylase deficiency. Archives of Disease in Childhood 70: 214–218

Dorman J S, O'Leary L A, Koehler A N 1995 Epidemiology of childhood diabetes. In: Kelnar C J H (ed) Childhood and adolescent diabetes. Chapman & Hall, London, pp 139–160

Drezner M K, Neelon F A, Lebovitz H E 1973 Pseudohypoparathyroidism type II. A possible defect in the reception of the cyclic AMP signal. New England Journal of Medicine 289: 1056–1060

Dunger D B 1995 Endocrine evolution, growth and puberty in relation to diabetes. In: Kelnar C J H (ed) Childhood and adolescent diabetes. Chapman & Hall, London, pp 75–88

Dunger D B 1997 The effects on growth of diabetes mellitus. In: Kelnar C J H, Stirling H F, Saenger P, Savage M O (eds) Growth disorders – pathophysiology and treatment. Chapman & Hall, London

Dunger D B, Edge J A 1995 Glucose homeostasis in the normal adolescent. In: Kelnar C J H (ed) Childhood and adolescent diabetes. Chapman & Hall, London, pp 31–46

Dupont B, Oberfield S E, Smithwick E M, Lee T D, Levine L S 1977 Close genetic linkage between HLA and congenital adrenal hyperplasia (21-hydroxylase deficiency). Lancet ii: 1309–1311

Edwards C R W, Benediktsson R, Lindsay R, Seckl J R 1993 Dysfunction of the placental glucocorticoid barrier: link between fetal environment and adult hypertension. Lancet 341: 355–357

Eisenbarth G S 1986 Type 1 diabetes mellitus: a chronic autoimmune disease. New England Journal of Medicine 314: 1360–1368

Elgin R G, Busby W H, Clemmons D R 1987 An insulin-like growth factor (IGF) binding protein enhances the biologic response to IGF. Proceedings of the National Academy of Sciences USA 84: 3254–3258

Evans M I, Chrousos G P, Mann D W et al 1985 Pharmacologic suppression of the fetal adrenal in utero. Journal of the American Medical Association 253: 1015–1020

Fainmesser P, Laron Z, Feiman G, Flexer Z, Karp M 1986 The incidence of hypoglycaemia in newly diagnosed diabetic children during the first year of disease. International Study Group of Diabetes in Children and Adolescents Bulletin 13: 39–40

Faria A C, Veldhuis J D, Thorner M O, Vance M L 1989 Half-time of endogenous growth hormone disappearance in normal man after stimulation of growth hormone secretion by growth hormone-releasing hormone and suppression with somatostatin. Journal of Clinical Endocrinology and Metabolism 68: 535–541

Farquhar J W, Campbell M L 1980 Care of the diabetic child in the community. British Medical Journal 281: 1534–1537

Farrar J J, Toft A D 1991 Iodine-131 treatment of hyperthyroidism: current issues. Clinical Endocrinology (Copenhagen) 35: 207

Finkelstein J W, Roffwarg H P, Boyar R M et al 1972 Age-related change in the twenty four hour spontaneous secretion of growth hormone. Journal of Clinical Endocrinology and Metabolism 35: 665–670

Fisher B M, Frier B M 1993 Hypoglycaemia and human insulin. In: Frier B M, Fisher B M (eds) Hypoglycaemia and diabetes. Clinical and physiological aspects. Edward Arnold, London, pp 314–327

Fjeld T O, Steen H 1989 Limb lengthening by epiphyseal distraction in chondrodystrophic bone: an experimental study in the canine femur. Journal of Orthopaedic Research 7: 184–191

Floud R, Gregory A, Wachter K 1990 Height, health and history: nutritional status in the United Kingdom 1750–1980. Cambridge University Press, Cambridge

Floyd J L, Dorwart R H, Nelson M J, Mueller G L, Deyroede M 1984 Pituitary hyperplasia secondary to thyroid failure: CT appearance. American Journal of Neurological Radiology 5: 469–471

Fogarty Y, Fraser C G 1989 Problems of diabetics in prisons (letter). British Medical Journal 298: 521

Forest M G 1995a Adrenal steroid excess. In: Brook C G D (ed) Clinical paediatric endocrinology, 3rd edn. Blackwell Scientific Publications, Oxford, pp 499–535

Forest M G 1995b Adrenal steroid deficiency states. In: Brook C G D (ed) Clinical paediatric endocrinology, 3rd edn. Blackwell Scientific Publications, Oxford, pp 453–498

Forest M G, Cathiard A M, Bertrand J A 1973 Evidence of testicular activity in early infancy. Journal of Clinical Endocrinology and Metabolism 37: 148–151

Forest M G, Peretti de E, David M 1985 Late onset 21-hydroxylase deficiency (21-OHD) can be misdiagnosed as 'typical' premature pubarche (PP) in childhood. Pediatric Research 19: 624

Forest M G, David M, Morel Y 1993 Prenatal diagnosis and treatment of 21-hydroxylase deficiency. Journal of Steroid Biochemistry and Molecular Biology 45: 75–82

Forssman H 1955 Two different mutations on the X-chromosome causing diabetes insipidus. American Journal of Human Genetics 7: 21–25

Foster C M, Feuillan P, Padmanabhan V et al 1986 Ovarian function in girls with McCune Albright syndrome. Pediatric Research 20: 859–863

Foulis A K 1995 Pancreatic morphology/islet cell morphology. In: Kelnar C J H (ed) Childhood and adolescent diabetes. Chapman & Hall, London, pp 169–182

Frankenne F, Closset J, Gomez F, Scippo M L, Smal J, Hennen G 1988 The physiology of growth hormone in pregnant women and partial characterisation of the placental GH variant. Journal of Clinical Endocrinology and Metabolism 66: 1171–1180

Fraser C G 1986 Interpretation of clinical chemistry laboratory data. Blackwell Scientific Publications, Oxford

Fraser C G, Fogarty Y 1989 Interpreting laboratory results. British Medical Journal 298: 1659–1660

Freeman J V, Cole T J, Chinn S, Jones P R M, White E M, Preece M A 1995 Cross-sectional stature and weight reference curves for the UK 1990. Archives of Disease in Childhood 73: 17–24

French F S, Lubahn D B, Brown T R et al 1990 Molecular basis of androgen insensitivity. Recent Progress in Hormone Research 46: 1–42

Frisancho A R, Sanchez Z, Pollardel D, Yanez L 1977 Adaptive significance of small body size under poor socioeconomoic conditions in southern Peru. American Journal of Physical Anthropology 39: 255–262

Frisch R E, Revelle R 1970 Height and weight at menarche and a hypothesis of critical body weights and adolescent events. Science 169: 397–399

Frohman L A, Jansson J-O 1986 Growth hormone-releasing hormone. Endocrine Reviews 7: 223–253

Fuggle P W, Grant D B, Smith I, Murphy G 1991 Intelligence, motor skills and behaviour at 5 years in early treated congenital hypothyroidism. European Journal of Pediatrics 159: 570–574

Gall M-A, Mathiesen E R, Skott P et al 1989 Effect of multiple insulin injections with a pen injector on metabolic control and general well-being in IDDM. Diabetes Research 11: 97–101

Gamble D, Taylor K W 1969 Seasonal incidence of diabetes mellitus. British Medical Journal iii: 631–633

Germain E L, Plotnick L P 1986 Age related anti-thyroid antibodies and thyroid abnormalities in Turner syndrome. Acta Paediatrica Scandinavica 75: 750–755

Giebink G S, Gothin R W, Bighen E G, Katz F H 1973 A kindred with familial glucocorticoid-suppressible aldosteronism. Journal of Clinical Endocrinology and Metabolism 36: 715–723

Gillies G, Grossman A 1985 The CRFs and their control: chemistry, physiology and clinical implications. Clinical Endocrinology 14: 821–843

Girard J, Baumann J B 1975 Secondary adrenal insufficiency due to cyproterone acetate. Pediatric Research 9: 669

Girard J, Celniker A, Price D A, Tanaka T, Walker J, Welling K, Albertsson-

Wikland K 1990 Urinary measurement of growth hormone secretion. Acta Paediatrica Scandinavica (suppl) 366: 149–154

Gluckman P D, Breier B H, Sauerwein H 1990 Regulation of the cell surface growth hormone receptor. Acta Paediatrica Scandinavica (suppl) 366: 73–78

Gluckman P D, Gunn A J, Wray A et al 1992 Congenital idiopathic growth hormone deficiency associated with prenatal and early postnatal growth failure. Journal of Pediatrics 121: 920–923

Goddard A D, Covello R, Luoh S-M et al 1995 Mutations of the growth hormone receptor in children with idiopathic short stature. New England Journal of Medicine 333: 1093–1098

Gold A E, Frier B M 1995 Hypoglycaemia – practical and clinical implications. In: Kelnar C J H (ed) Childhood and adolescent diabetes. Chapman & Hall, London, pp 351–367

Gordon M, Crouthamel C, Post E M, Richman R A 1982 Psychosocial aspects of constitutional short stature: social competence, behaviour problems, self-esteem and family functioning. Journal of Paediatrics 101: 477–480

Gosden R G, Baird D T, Wade J C, Webb R 1994 Restoration of fertility to oophorectomized sheep by ovarian autografts stored at −196°C. Human Reproduction 9: 597–803

Greene S A, Thompson C 1995 Exercise. In: Kelnar C J H (ed) Childhood and adolescent diabetes. Chapman & Hall, London, pp 283–294

Greene S A, Aynsley-Green A, Soltesz G, Baum J D 1984 The management of secondary diabetes mellitus following total pancreatectomy in infancy. Archives of Disease in Childhood 59: 356–359

Gregory J W, Taylor R 1995 Biochemistry and intermediate metabolism. In: Kelnar C J H (ed) Childhood and adolescent diabetes. Chapman & Hall, London, pp 191–210

Griffin J E 1992 Androgen resistance – the clinical and molecular spectrum. New England Journal of Medicine 326: 611–618

Groome N P, Illingworth P J, O'Brien M et al 1994 Detection of dimeric inhibin throughout the human menstrual cycle by two-site enzyme immunoassay. Clinical Endocrinology 40: 717–723

Groome N P, Illingworth P J, O'Brien M, Priddle J, Weaver K, McNeilly A S 1995 Quantification of inhibin forms containing pro-aC in human serum by a new ultrasensitive ELISA. Journal of Clinical Endocrinology and Metabolism 80: 2926–2932

Groome N P, Illingworth P J, O'Brien M, Pai R, Rodger F E, Mather J P, McNeilly A S 1996 Measurement of dimeric inhibin-B throughout the human menstrual cycle. Journal of Clinical Endocrinology and Metabolism 81: 1401–1405

Grossman A, Wass J A H, Sueiras-Diaz et al 1983 Growth-hormone-releasing factor in growth hormone deficiency: demonstration of a hypothalamic defect in growth hormone release. Lancet ii: 137–138

Grossman A, Lytras N, Savage M O et al 1984 Growth hormone releasing factor: comparison of two analogues and demonstration of hypothalamic defect in growth hormone release after radiotherapy. British Medical Journal 288: 1785–1787

Grumbach M M 1997 Current controversies and future prospects. In: Kelnar C J H, Stirling H F, Saenger P, Savage M O (eds) Growth disorders – pathophysiology and treatment. Chapman & Hall, London

Grumbach M M, Richards G E, Conte F A, Kaplan S L 1978 Clinical disorders of adrenal function and puberty: an assessment of the role of the adrenal cortex in normal and abnormal puberty in man and evidence for an ACTH-like pituitary adrenal androgen stimulating hormone. In: James V H T, Serio M, Giusti G, Martini L (eds) The endocrine function of the human adrenal cortex. Academic Press, New York, pp 583–612

Grüters A 1996 Screening for congenital hypothyroidism – effectiveness and clinical outcome. In: Kelnar C J H (ed) Paediatric endocrinology. Baillière's clinical paediatrics – international practice and research. Baillière Tindall, London, vol 4: 259–276

Grüters A 1997 Thyroid disorders and abnormal growth. In: Kelnar C J H, Stirling H F, Saenger P, Savage M O (eds) Growth disorders – pathophysiology and treatment. Chapman & Hall, London

Guevara-Aguirre J, Vasconez O, Martinez V et al 1995 A randomized, double-blind, placebo-controlled trial on safety and efficacy of recombinant human insulin-like growth factor-1 in children with growth hormone receptor deficiency. Journal of Clinical Endocrinology and Metabolism 80: 1393–1398

Guillemin R, Brazeau P, Bolan P, Esch F, Ling N, Wehrenberg W B 1982 Growth hormone releasing factor from a human pancreatic tumour that caused acromegaly. Science 218: 585–587

Guyda H J 1997 Treatment of growth disorders – idiopathic short stature. In: Kelnar C J H, Stirling H F, Saenger P, Savage M O (eds) Growth disorders – pathophysiology and treatment. Chapman & Hall, London

Hagenäs L 1997 Treatment of skeletal dysplasias. In: Kelnar C J H, Stirling H F, Saenger P, Savage M O (eds) Growth disorders – pathophysiology and treatment. Chapman & Hall, London

Hall J G, Froster-Iskenius, Allanson J E 1989 Handbook of normal physical measurements. Oxford Medical Publications, Oxford

Hamburger J I 1985 Management of hyperthyroidism in children and adolescents. Journal of Clinical Endocrinology and Metabolism 60: 1019–1024

Hanssen K F, Dahl-Jørgensen K, Lauritzen T, Feldt-Rasmussen B, Brinchmann-Hansen O, Deckert T 1986 Diabetic control of microvascular complications: the near-normoglycaemic experience. Diabetologia 29: 677–684

Hashizume K, Icikawa K, Sakurai A et al 1991 Administration of thyroxine in treated Graves' disease. New England Journal of Medicine 324: 947

Hawdon J M, Ward Platt M P 1995 Glucose homeostasis in the normal fetus and infant. In: Kelnar C J H (ed) Childhood and adolescent diabetes. Chapman & Hall, London, pp 3–18

Hawkins J R 1993 The SRY gene. Trends in Endocrinology and Metabolism 4: 328–332

Hay I D, Smail P J, Forsyth C C 1981 Familial cytomegalic adrenocortical hypoplasia: an X-linked syndrome of pubertal failure. Archives of Disease in Childhood 56: 715–721

Hayles A B, Hahn J B Jr, Sprague R G et al 1966 Hormone-secreting tumors of the adrenal cortex in children. Pediatrics 37: 19–25

Hearnshaw J R 1985 Home treatment of diabetic children. 12th Congress of the International Diabetes Federation, Madrid, Spain

Hedin L, Diczfalusy M, Olsson B, Rosberg S, Pettersson A S, Albertsson-Wikland K 1989 Nasal delivery of human growth hormone: a new route of administration. Acta Paediatrica Scandinavica (suppl) 367: 158

Heintze H J, Bercu B 1997 Abnormalities of growth hormone secretion. In: Kelnar C J H, Stirling H F, Saenger P, Savage M O (eds) Growth disorders – pathophysiology and treatment. Chapman & Hall, London

Hepburn D A, Steel J M 1995 Maternal diabetes and the fetus. In: Kelnar C J H (ed) Childhood and adolescent diabetes. Chapman & Hall, London, pp 427–445

Hepburn D A, Eadington D W, Patrick A W, Colledge N R, Frier B M 1989 Symptomatic awareness of hypoglycaemia: does it change on transfer from animal to human insulin? Diabetic Medicine 6: 586–590

Hermansson G, Ludvigsson J, Larsson Y 1986 Home blood glucose monitoring in diabetic children and adolescents. A 3 year feasibility study. Acta Paediatrica Scandinavica 75: 98–105

Hermanussen M, Geiger-Benoit K, Burmeister J, Sippell W G 1988a Knemometry in childhood: accuracy and standardization of a new technique of lower leg measurement. Annals of Human Biology 15: 1–16

Hermanussen M, Geiger-Benoit K, Burmeister J, Sippell W G 1988b Periodical changes of short-term growth velocity (mini-growth spurts) in human growth. Annals of Human Biology 15: 103–111

Hidaka A, Minegishi T, Kohn L D 1993 Thyrotropin, like luteinizing hormone (LH) and chorionic gonadotropin (CG) increases cAMP and onositol phosphate levels in cells with recombinant human LH/CG receptor. Biochemical and Biophysical Research Communications 196: 187–195

Hill D J, Freemark M, Strain A J, Handwerger S, Milner R D G 1988 Placental lactogen and growth hormone receptors in human fetal tissues: relationship to human fetal hPL concentrations and fetal growth. Journal of Clinical Endocrinology and Metabolism 66: 1283–1290

Hinde F R J, Johnston D I 1986 Two or three insulin injections in adolescence? Archives of Disease in Childhood 61: 118–123

Hindmarsh P C 1997 Endocrine assessment. In: Kelnar C J H, Stirling H F, Saenger P, Savage M O (eds) Growth disorders – pathophysiology and treatment. Chapman & Hall, London

Hindmarsh P C, Brook C G D 1987 Short term management of an infant with nesidioblastosis using somatostatin analogue SMS 201-995. New England Journal of Medicine 316: 221–222

Hindmarsh P C, Brook C G D 1995 Normal growth and its endocrine control. In: Brook C G D (ed) Clinical paediatric endocrinology, 3rd edn. Blackwell Scientific Publications, Oxford 85–107

Hindmarsh P C, Brook C G D 1996 Final height of short normal children treated with growth hormone. Lancet 348: 13–16

Hindmarsh P C, Swift P G F 1995 An assessment of growth hormone provocation tests. Archives of Disease in Childhood 72: 362–367

Hindmarsh P C, Smith P J, Brook C G D, Matthews D R 1987 The relationship between height velocity and growth hormone secretion in short prepubertal children. Clinical Endocrinology 27: 581–591

Hindmarsh P C, Matthews D R, di Silvio L, Kurtz A B, Brook C G D 1988 Relation between height velocity and fasting insulin concentrations. Archives of Disease in Childhood 63: 665–666

Hindmarsh P C, Matthews D R, Brain C E et al 1989 The half-life of exogenous GH after suppression of endogenous GH secretion with somatostatin. Clinical Endocrinology 30: 443–450

Hinkle L E, Wolff S 1952 Summary of experimental evidence relating life stress to diabetes mellitus. Journal of Mount Sinai Hospital 19: 537–570

Hintz R L 1997 Treatment of growth disorders – growth hormone deficiency. In: Kelnar C J H, Stirling H F, Saenger P, Savage M O (eds) Growth disorders – pathophysiology and treatment. Chapman & Hall, London

Hobsbawm E 1994 Age of extremes – the short twentieth century 1914–1991. Michael Joseph, London, p 325

Hocking M D, Crase J, Rayner P H W 1986 Use of human growth hormone in treatment of nesidioblastosis in a neonate. Archives of Disease in Childhood 61: 706–707

Hofbauer K G, Marr S C 1987 Vasopressin antagonists: present and future. Kidney International 31: 521

Hoffman W H, Khoury C, Byrd H A 1980 Prevalence of permanent congenital diabetes mellitus. Diabetologia 19: 487–488

Holland F J, Fishman L, Bailey J D, Fazekas A T A 1985a Ketoconazole in the management of precocious puberty not responsive to LHRH-analogue therapy. New England Journal of Medicine 312: 1023–1028

Holland F J, Kirsch S E, Selby R 1985b Gonadotrophin-independent precocious puberty ('testotoxicosis'): influence of maturational status in response to ketoconazole. Journal of Clinical Endocrinology and Metabolism 64: 328–333

Holly J M P 1997 Endocrinology of growth – peripheral hormone action. In: Kelnar C J H, Stirling H F, Saenger P, Savage M O (eds) Growth disorders – pathophysiology and treatment. Chapman & Hall, London

Holm V A, Sulzbacher S, Pipes P L (eds) 1981 The Prader–Willi syndrome. University Park Press, Baltimore

Holman R R, Jelfs R, Causier P M, Moore J C, Turner R C 1987 Glycosylated haemoglobin measurement on blood samples taken by patients: an additional aid to assessing diabetic control. Diabetic Medicine 4: 71–73

Honnebier W J, Swaab D F 1973 The influence of anencephaly upon intrauterine growth of the fetus and placenta and upon gestation length. British Journal of Obstetrics and Gynaecology 80: 577–588

Honour J W 1995 The adrenal cortex. In: Brook C G D (ed) Clinical paediatric endocrinology, 3rd edn. Blackwell Scientific Publications, Oxford, pp 434–452

Honour J W, Dillon M J, Shackleton C H L 1982 Analysis of steroids in urine for differentiation of pseudohypoaldosteronism and aldosterone biosynthetic defect. Journal of Clinical Endocrinology and Metabolism 54: 325–331

Honour J W, Kelnar C J H, Brook C G D 1991 Urine adrenal steroid excretion rates in childhood reflect growth and activity of the adrenal cortex. Acta Endocrinologica 124: 219–224

Hope J, Ratter S J, Estivariz F E, McLoughlin L, Lowry P J 1981 Development of a radioimmunoassay for an amino-terminal peptide of pro-opiocortin containing the gamma-MSH region: measurement and characterization in human placenta. Clinical Endocrinology 15: 221–227

Hornsby P J, Aldern K A 1984 Steroidogenic enzyme activities in cultured human definitive zone adrenocortical cells: comparison with bovine adrenocortical cells and resultant differences in adrenal androgen synthesis. Journal of Clinical Endocrinology and Metabolism 58: 121–127

Horrocks P M, London D R 1987 Effects of long term dexamethasone treatment in adult patients with congenital adrenal hyperplasia. Clinical Endocrinology 27: 635–642

Horton W A 1997 Bone and cartilage growth and metabolism. In: Kelnar C J H, Stirling H F, Saenger P, Savage M O (eds) Growth disorders – pathophysiology and treatment. Chapman & Hall, London

Howlett T, Besser M 1989 Cushing's syndrome. Medicine International 63: 2605–2611

Hoyt W F, Kaplan S L, Grumbach M M, Glaser J S 1970 Septo-optic dysplasia and pituitary dwarfism. Lancet i: 893–894

Hughes I A 1986 Clinical aspects of congenital adrenal hyperplasia: early diagnosis and prognosis. Journal of Inherited Metabolic Disease 9 (suppl 1): 115–123

Hunter W M, Rigal W M 1966 The diurnal pattern of plasma growth hormone concentration in adults. Journal of Endocrinology 34: 147–153

Idelman S 1978 The structure of the mammalian adrenal cortex. In: Chester Jones I, Henderson I W (eds) General, comparative and clinical endocrinology of the adrenal cortex. Academic Press, London. vol 2: 1–199

Illig R, Prader A, Ferrandez A, Zachmann M 1971 Hereditary prenatal growth hormone deficiency with increased tendency to growth hormone antibody formation ('A type' isolated growth hormone deficiency). Acta Paediatrica Scandinavica 60: 607

Illingworth P J, Groome N P, Byrd W, Rainey W E, McNeilly A S, Mather J P, Bremner W J 1996 Inhibin-B: a potential candidate for the principal bioactive inhibin form in plasma in men. Journal of Clinical Endocrinology and Metabolism 81: 1321–1325

Illingworth P J, Groome N P, Duncan W C, Grant V, Tovanabutra S, Bairds D T, McNeilly A S 1996b Measurement of circulating inhibin forms during the establishment of pregnancy. Journal of Clinical Endocrinology and Metabolism 81: 1471–1475

Imperato-McGinley J, Guerrero L, Gautier T, Peterson R E 1974 Steroid 5-alpha-reductase deficiency in man: an inherited form of male pseudohermaphroditism. Science 186: 1213–1215

Imperato-McGinley J, Peterson R E, Gautier T, Sturla E 1979a Androgens and the evolution of gender identity among male pseudohermaphrodites with 5-alpha-reductase deficiency. New England Journal of Medicine 300: 1233–1237

Imperato-McGinley J, Peterson R E, Stoller R, Goodwin W E 1979b Male pseudohermaphroditism secondary to 17-beta-hydroxysteroid dehydrogenase deficiency – gender role change with puberty. Journal of Clinical Endocrinology and Metabolism 49: 291–295

Ingersoll G M, Golden M P 1995 The diabetic child in context: the family. In: Kelnar C J H (ed) Childhood and adolescent diabetes. Chapman & Hall, London, pp 449–456

Jaeger P, Jones W, Clemens T L, Hayslett J P 1986 Evidence that calcitonin stimulates 1,25-dihydroxyvitamin D production and intestinal absorption of calcium in vivo. Journal of Clinical Investigation: 78: 456–461

Jakacki R J, Kelch R P, Sauder S E et al 1982 Pulsatile secretion of luteinising hormone in children. Journal of Clinical Endocrinology and Metabolism 55: 453–458

James V H T, Tunbridge R D G, Wilson G A, Hutton J, Jacobs H S, Rippon A E 1978 Steroid profiling: a technique for exploring adrenocortical physiology. In: James V H T, Serio M, Giusti G, Martini L (eds) The endocrine function of the human adrenal cortex. Academic Press, London, pp 179–192

Jeffcoate S L 1981 Efficiency and effectiveness in the endocrine laboratory. Academic Press, London

Jeffcoate T N A, Fliegner J R H, Russell S H, Davis J C, Wade A P 1965 Diagnosis of the adrenogenital syndrome before birth. Lancet ii: 553–555

Jefferson I G, Smith M A, Baum J D 1985 Insulin dependent diabetes in under 5 year olds. Archives of Disease in Childhood 60: 1144–1148

Johnston D I 1995a Diabetes: definition and classifications. In: Kelnar C J H (ed) Childhood and adolescent diabetes. Chapman & Hall, London, pp 135–138

Johnston D I 1995b Children's diabetes clinics. In: Kelnar C J H (ed) Childhood and adolescent diabetes. Chapman & Hall, London, pp 323–330

Jones K L (ed) 1988 Smith's recognizable patterns of human malformation, 4th edn. Saunders, Philadelphia

Josso N, Picard J-Y 1986 The antimullerian hormone. Physiological Reviews 66: 1038–1090

Josso N, Fekete C, Cachin O, Nezelof C, Rappaport R 1983 Persistence of Mullerian ducts in male pseudohermaphroditism and its relationship to cryptorchidism. Clinical Endocrinology 19: 247–258

Jost A 1976 Hormonal and genetic factors affecting the development of the male genital system. Andrologia 8 (suppl 1): 17

Jovanovic L, Peterson C M 1981 The clinical utility of glycosylated hemoglobin. American Journal of Medicine 70: 331–338

Kanof M E, Lake A M, Bayless T M 1988 Decreased height velocity in children and adolescents before the diagnosis of Crohn's disease. Gastroenterology 95: 1523–1527

Karlberg J, Engstrom I, Karlberg P, Fryer J G 1987 Analysis of linear growth using a mathematical model. Acta Paediatrica Scandinavica 76: 478–488

Kelnar C J H 1976 Hypoglycaemia in children undergoing adentonsillectomy. British Medical Journal i: 751–752

Kelnar C J H 1985 Adrenal steroids in childhood. MD thesis, University of Cambridge

Kelnar C J H 1989 Thyroid disturbances in cytogenetic diseases. Developmental Medicine and Child Neurology 31: 400–404

Kelnar C J H 1990 Pride and prejudice – stature in perspective. Acta Paediatrica Scandinavica (suppl) 370: 5–15

Kelnar C J H 1993a Growth. Medicine International 21(6): 217–223

Kelnar C J H 1993b Congenital adrenal hyperplasia (CAH): the place of

prenatal treatment and neonatal screening. Early Human Development 35: 81–90

Kelnar C J H 1994 Does the short, sexually immature adolescent boy need treatment and what form should it take? Archives of Disease in Childhood 71: 285–287

Kelnar C J H (ed) 1995a Childhood and adolescent diabetes. Chapman & Hall, London

Kelnar C J H 1995b Normal childhood and pubertal growth and hormonal maturation. In: Kelnar C J H (ed) Childhood and adolescent diabetes. Chapman & Hall, London, pp 47–74

Kelnar C J H 1995c The historical background. In: Kelnar C J H (ed) Childhood and adolescent diabetes. Chapman & Hall, London, pp 123–133

Kelnar C J H 1997 Childhood growth: practice handbook. Medicom Excel, Kingston-on-Thames

Kelnar C J H, Brook C G D 1983 A mixed longitudinal study of adrenal steroid excretion in childhood and the mechanism of adrenarche. Clinical Endocrinology 19: 117–129

Kelnar C J H, Tanaka T 1994 Is there a place for short bursts of growth hormone treatment in short children without significant growth hormone deficiency? Acta Paediatrica 406 (suppl): 67–69

Kelnar C J H, Stirling H F, Saenger P, Savage M O (eds) 1997 Growth disorders – pathophysiology and treatment. Chapman & Hall, London

Kendall B E 1995 Neuroradiology. In: Brook C G D (ed) Clinical paediatric endocrinology, 3rd edn. Blackwell Scientific Publications, Oxford, pp 320–345

Kendle F W 1905 Case of precocious puberty in a female cretin. British Medical Journal 1: 246

Kennedy K, Mehl T D, Riley W J, Mezinole T J 1981 A non-enzymatically glycosylated serum protein in diabetes mellitus: an index of short term glycaemia. Diabetologia 21: 94–98

Kerrigan J R, Veldhuis J D, Leyo S A, Iranmesh A, Rogol A D 1993 Estimation of daily cortisol production and clearance rates in normal pubertal males by deconvolution analysis. Journal of Clinical Endocrinology and Metabolism 76: 1505–1510

Ketelslegers J M 1995 Presentation at the 34th Annual Meeting of the European Society for Paediatric Endocrinology, Edinburgh, June 25–28

Ketelslegers J M 1997 Nutrition and growth. In: Kelnar C J H, Stirling H F, Saenger P, Savage M O (eds) Growth disorders – pathophysiology and treatment. Chapman & Hall, London

Keutmann H T, Sauer R M, Hendy G N, O'Riordan J L H, Potts J T Jr 1978 Complete amino acid sequence of human parathyroid hormone. Biochemistry 17: 5723–5729

Kinmonth A-L, Magrath G, Reckless J P D et al 1989 Dietary recommendations for children and adolescents with diabetes. Diabetic Medicine 6: 537–547

Kinter L B, Dubb J, Huffman W et al 1985 Potential role of vasopressin antagonists in the treatment of water-retaining disorders. In Shrier R W (ed) Vasopressin. Raven Press, New York, pp 553–561

Kirk J M W, di Silvio L, Hindmarsh P C, Brook C G D 1988 Somatostatin analogue in short term management of hyperinsulinism. Archives of Disease in Childhood 63: 1493–1494

Kirschner B S 1990 Growth and development in chronic inflammatory bowel disease. Acta Paediatrica Scandinavica (suppl) 366: 98–104

Kirschner B S 1997 The effects on growth of gastrointestinal disorders. In: Kelnar C J H, Stirling H F, Saenger P, Savage M O (eds) Growth disorders – pathophysiology and treatment. Chapman & Hall, London

Kirtland J, Gurr M I 1979 Adipose tissue cellularity: a review. 2 The relationship between cellularity and obesity. International Journal of Obesity 3: 15–55

Kitay J I 1954 Pineal lesions and precocious puberty: a review. Journal of Clinical Endocrinology and Metabolism 14: 622–625

Klein A H, Meltzer S, Kenny F M 1972 Improved prognosis in congenital hypothyroidism treated before age 3 months. Journal of Pediatrics 81: 912–915

Klinefelter H F Jr, Reifenstein E C Jr, Albright F 1942 Syndrome characterised by gynaecomastia, aspermatogenesis without a-Leydigism and increased secretion of follicle-stimulating hormone. Journal of Clinical Endocrinology 2: 615

Knip M, Ilonen J, Mustonen A, Akerblom H K 1986 Evidence of an accelerated β-cell destruction in HLA-DW3/DW4 heterozygous children with type 1 (insulin-dependent) diabetes. Diabetalogia 29: 347–351

Knobil E 1980 The neuroendocrine control of the menstrual cycle. Recent Progress in Hormone Research 36: 53–88

Kofman-Alfaro S, Valdes E, Teran J et al 1985 Endocrine and immunogenetic evaluation of an XX male infant with perineoscrotal hypospadias. Acta Endocrinologica 108: 421–427

Koh T H H G, Aynsley-Green A, Tarbit M, Eyre J A1988a Neural dysfunction during hypoglycaemia in childhood. Archives of Disease in Childhood 63: 1353–1358

Koh T H H G, Eyre J A, Aynsley-Green A 1988b Neonatal hypoglycaemia – the controversy regarding definition. Archives of Disease in Childhood 63: 1386–1388

Kohn B, Levine L S, Pollack M S et al 1982 Late-onset steroid 21-hydroxylase deficiency: a variant of classical congenital adrenal hyperplasia. Journal of Clinical Endocrinology and Metabolism 55: 817–827

Krane E J, Rockoff M A, Wallman J K, Wolfsdorf J I 1985 Subclinical brain swelling in children during treatment of diabetic ketoacidosis. New England Journal of Medicine 312: 1147–1151

Kruse K 1995a Endocrine control of calcium and bone metabolism. In: Brook C G D (ed) Clinical paediatric endocrinology, 3rd edn. Blackwell Scientific Publications, Oxford, pp 713–734

Kruse K 1995b Disorders of calcium and bone metabolism. In: Brook C G D (ed) Clinical paediatric endocrinology, 3rd edn. Blackwell Scientific Publications, Oxford, pp 735–778

Kruse K 1995c Laboratory approach to the child with suspected disorders of calcium and bone metabolism. In: Brook C G D (ed) Clinical paediatric endocrinology, 3rd edn. Blackwell Scientific Publications, Oxford, pp 779–781

Kruse K 1997 The effects on growth of disorders of calcium and phosphate metabolism. In: Kelnar C J H, Stirling H F, Saenger P, Savage M O (eds) Growth disorders – pathophysiology and treatment. Chapman & Hall, London

Kruse K, Kracht U 1987 A simplified diagnostic test in hypoparathyroidism and pseudohypoparathyroidism type 1 with synthetic 1-38 fragment of human parathyroid hormone. European Journal of Paediatrics 147: 373–377

Kruse K, Suss A, Busse M, Schneider P 1987 Monomeric serum calcitonin and bone turnover during anticonvulsant treatment and in congenital hypothyroidism. Journal of Pediatrics 111: 57–63

Kurtz A B 1995 New insulins. In: Kelnar C J H (ed) Childhood and adolescent diabetes. Chapman & Hall, London, pp 565–570

La Greca A M, Skyler J S 1995 Psychological management of diabetes. In: Kelnar C J H (ed) Childhood and adolescent diabetes. Chapman & Hall, London, pp 295–310

Lachman 1997 Radiological assessment of the skeletal dysplasias. In: Kelnar C J H, Stirling H F, Saenger P, Savage M O (eds) Growth disorders – pathophysiology and treatment. Chapman & Hall, London

Lalu Keraly J, Aubier F, Derome P et al 1986 Evolution a moyen terme des craniopharyngiomes de l'enfant en fonction des choix therapeutiques initiaux. Archives of French Pediatrics 43: 593–599

Lamberts S W J 1997 Medical management of tall stature. In: Kelnar C J H, Stirling H F, Saenger P, Savage M O (eds) Growth disorders – pathophysiology and treatment. Chapman & Hall, London

Laron Z 1993 Laron syndrome: from description to therapy. Endocrinologist 3: 21–28

Laron Z, Hochman H 1971 Small testes in prepubertal boys with Klinefelter's syndrome. Journal of Clinical Endocrinology and Metabolism 32: 671–672

Laron Z, Kalter-Leibovici O 1995 Current controversies in the management of the diabetic child and adolescent. In: Kelnar C J H (ed) Childhood and adolescent diabetes. Chapman & Hall, London, pp 603–616

Laron Z, Pertzelan A, Mannheimer S 1966 Genetic pituitary dwarfism with high serum concentration of growth hormone. A new inborn error of metabolism? Israel Journal of Medical Sciences 2: 152–155

Laron Z, Karp M, Dolberg L 1970 Juvenile hypothyroidism with testicular enlargement. Acta Paediatrica Scandinavica 59: 317–322

Laron Z, Frankel J J, Amir S et al 1982 Long-term experience with a multidisciplinary, comprehensive ambulatory treatment scheme for diabetes mellitus in children. In: Laron Z, Galatzer A (eds) Psychological aspects of diabetes in children and adolescents. Pediatric and adolescent endocrinology vol 10. Karger, Basel, pp 182–186

Laron Z, Frenkel J, Silbergeld A 1995 Biochemical and growth promoting effects of a growth hormone releasing peptide – hexarelin – (HEX) in children. Hormone Research 44 (suppl 1): 20 (A76)

Larsson L I, Sundler F, Hakanson R 1975 Immunohistochemical localization of human pancreatic polypeptide (HPP) to a population of islet cells. Cell and Tissue Research 156: 167–171

Law C M, de Swiet M, Osmond C et al 1993 Initiation of hypertension in utero and its amplification throughout life. British Medical Journal 306: 24–27

Lawrence S, Warshaw J B 1989 Increased binding of epidermal growth factor to placental membranes in IUGR fetal rats. Pediatric Research 25: 214–218

Leadbetter D H, Riccardi V M, Airhart S D, Strobel R J, Keenan B S, Crawford J D 1981 Deletions of chromosome 15 as a cause of the Prader–Willi syndrome. New England Journal of Medicine 304: 325–329

Lee P A 1996 Disorders of puberty. In: Lifshitz F (ed) Pediatric endocrinology. Marcel Dekker, New York, pp 175–196

Lee P A, Kowarski A, Migeon C J, Blizzard R M 1975 Lack of correlation between gonadotrophin and adrenal androgen levels in agonadal children. Journal of Clinical Endocrinology and Metabolism 40: 664–669

Lee P D K, Winter R J, Green O C 1984 Virilizing adrenocortical tumours in childhood: eight cases and a review of the literature. Pediatrics 76: 437–444

Lee P J, Leonard J V 1995 Hypoglycaemia. In: Brook C G D (ed) Clinical paediatric endocrinolgy, 3rd edn. Blackwell Scientific Publications, Oxford, pp 677–693

Leiper A D, Stanhope R, Kitching P, Chessells J M 1987 Precocious and premature puberty associated with the treatment of acute lymphoblastic leukaemia. Archives of Disease in Childhood 62: 1107–1112

Levine L S, Rauh W, Gottesdiener K et al 1980 New studies of the 11β-hydroxylase and 18–hydroxylase enzymes in the hypertensive form of congenital adrenal hyperplasia. Journal of Clinical Endocrinology and Metabolism 50: 258–263

Levine M A, Jap T-S, Mauseth R S, Downs R W Jr, Spiegel A M 1986 Activity of the stimulating guanine nucleotide-binding regulatory ptotein in erythrocytes from patients with pseudohypoparathyroidism and pseudopseudohypoparathyroidism: biochemical, endocrine and genetic analysis of Albright's hereditary osteodystrophy in six kindreds. Journal of Clinical Endocrinology and Metabolism 62: 497–502

Lifshitz F (ed) 1996 Pediatric endocrinology. Marcel Dekker, New York

Lightwood R, Stapelton T 1953 Idiopathic hypercalcaemia in infants. Lancet ii: 255–256

Linder B L, Esteban N V, Yergey A L, Winterer J C, Loriaux D L, Cassoria F 1990 Cortisol production rate in childhood and adolescence. Journal of Pediatrics 117: 892–896

Ling N, Shao-Yao S Y, Ueno N et al 1986 Pituitary FSH is released by a heterodimer of the beta-subunits from the two forms of inhibin. Nature 321: 779–782

London N J M, Robertson G S M, Chadwick D, James R F L, Bell P R F 1995 Islet transplantation. In: Kelnar C J H (ed) Childhood and adolescent diabetes. Chapman & Hall, London, pp 595–602

Low L C K, Wang C, Cheung P T et al 1988 Long term pulsatile growth hormone (GH)-releasing hormone therapy in children with GH deficiency. Journal of Clinical Endocrinology and Metabolism 66: 611–617

Lucas A 1995 Presentation at the 34th Annual Meeting of the European Society for Paediatric Endocrinology, Edinburgh, June 25–28

Ludvigsson J, Samuelsson V, Beauforts C et al 1986 HLA-DR3 is associated with a more slowly progressive form of type 1 (insulin-dependent) diabetes. Diabetalogia 29: 207–210

Lyall E G H, Crofton P M, Stirling H F, Kelnar C J H 1992 Albuminuric growth failure. A case of Munchausen syndrome by proxy. Acta Paediatrica 81: 373–376

Lyon A J, DeBruyn R, Grant D B 1985a Transient sexual precocity and ovarian cysts. Archives of Disease in Childhood 60: 819–822

Lyon A J, Preece M A, Grant D B 1985b Growth curve for girls with Turner syndrome. Archives of Disease in Childhood 60: 932–935

McCrimmon R C, Gold A E, Deary I J, Kelnar C J H, Frier B M 1995 Symptoms of hypoglycaemia in children with IDDM. Diabetes Care 18: 858–861

MacCuish A C 1995 Childhood diabetes and other endocrine/autoimmune diseases. In: Kelnar C J H (ed) Childhood and adolescent diabetes. Chapman & Hall, London, pp 385–396

McCune D J, Bruch H 1937 Osteodystrophia fibrosa: report of a case in which the condition was combined with precocious puberty, pathological pigmentation of the skin and hyperthyroidism, with a review of the literature. American Journal of Diseases of Children 54: 806–848

McEvilly A 1995 Liaison nursing – the diabetic home care team. In: Kelnar C J H (ed) Childhood and adolescent diabetes. Chapman & Hall, London, pp 465–474

McGillivray B C 1989 Testicular differentiating factor current concepts. Growth, Genetics and Hormones 5(4): 1–3

McLachlan R I, Robertson D M, De Kretser D, Burger H G 1987 Inhibin – a non-steroidal regulator of pituitary follicle stimulating hormone. Baillière's Clinics in Endocrinology and Metabolism 1: 89–112

Macnicol M F 1997 Surgical management of tall stature. In: Kelnar C J H, Stirling H F, Saenger P, Savage M O (eds) Growth disorders – pathophysiology and treatment. Chapman & Hall, London

Macnicol M F, Krishnan J, Draper E R C 1993 Epiphysiodesis using a cannulated tube saw: comparison with the phemister technique. Journal of Paediatric Orthopaedics Part B 2: 70–74

McSheehy P M J, Chambers T J 1986 Osteoblast-like cells in the presence of parathyroid hormone release a soluble factor that stimulates osteoclastic bone resorption. Endocrinology 119: 1654–1659

Mains R E, Eipper B A, Ling N 1977 Common precursor to corticotrophins and endorphins. Proceedings of the National Academy of Sciences (USA) 74: 3014–3018

Malcolm L A 1971 Growth and development in New Guinea. Monograph no. 1: Institute of Human Biology, Madang

Mandrup-Poulsen T, Nerup J 1995 Pathogenesis of childhood diabetes. In: Kelnar C J H (ed) Childhood and adolescent diabetes. Chapman & Hall, London, pp 183–190

Manuel M, Katayama K P, Jones H W 1976 The age of occurrence of gonadal tumours in intersex patients with a Y chromosome. American Journal of Obstetrics and Gynecology 124: 293–300

Martin N D T, Snodgrass G J A I, Cohen R D 1984 Idiopathic infantile hypercalcaemia – a continuing enigma. Archives of Disease in Childhood 59: 605–613

Massarano A, Adams J, Preece M A, Brook C G D 1986 When do the ovaries in Turner syndrome fail? Presentation at British Society for Paediatric Endocrinology, Birmingham

Massarano A A, Hollis S, Devlin J, David T J 1993 Growth in atopic eczema. Archives of Disease in Childhood 68: 677–679

Massoud A F, Hindmarsh P C, Matthews D R, Pringle P J, Brook C G D 1995 The GHRP hexarelin is capable of releasing GH after two successive IV doses and acts synergistically with GHRH. Hormone Research 44 (suppl 1): 23 (A89)

Mauras N, Blizzard R M 1986 The McCune–Albright syndrome. In: Illig R, Visser H K A (eds) Paediatric endocrinology 1986. Acta Endocrinologica Copenhagen Supplementum 279: 207–217

Maxwell H, Rees L 1996 Recombinant human growth hormone treatment in infants with chronic renal failure. Archives of Disease in Childhood 74: 40–43

Meadow R 1977 Munchausen syndrome by proxy – the hinterland of child abuse. Lancet ii: 343–345

Meadow R 1982 Munchausen syndrome by proxy. Archives of Disease in Childhood 57: 92–98

Mehls O 1997 Renal disorders – management of associated growth disturbance. In: Kelnar C J H, Stirling H F, Saenger P, Savage M O (eds) Growth disorders – pathophysiology and treatment. Chapman & Hall, London

Melvin K E W 1986 Familial medullary carcinoma of the thyroid. In: Van Middlesworth L, Givens J R (eds) The thyroid gland, a practical clinical treatise. Year Book Publications, Chicago, pp 429–447

Mercado A B, Wilson R C, Cheng K C, Wei J-Q, New M I 1995 Prenatal treatment and diagnosis of congenital adrenal hyperplasia owing to steroid 21-hydroxylase deficiency. Journal of Clinical and Endocrinological Metabolism 80: 2014–2020

Migeon C J, Lanes R L 1996 Adrenal cortex: hypo-and hyperfunction. In: Lifshitz F (ed) Pediatric endocrinology. Marcel Dekker, New York, pp 321–346

Migeon C J, Kenny F M, Kowarski A et al 1968 The syndrome of congenital adrenal unresponsiveness to ACTH. Report of six cases. Pediatric Research 2: 501–513

Milaszkiewicz R M, Hall G M 1995 Peri-operative management of the diabetic child. In: Kelnar C J H (ed) Childhood and adolescent diabetes. Chapman & Hall, London, pp 345–350

Millard W J, Politch J A, Martin J B, Fox T 1986 Growth hormone secretory patterns in androgen resistant (testicular feminised) rats. Endocrinology 119: 2655–2660

Milner R D G, Hill D J 1989 Fetal growth signals. Archives of Disease in Childhood 64: 53–57

Minns R A 1997 The effects on growth of neurological disorders. In: Kelnar C J H, Stirling H F, Saenger P, Savage M O (eds) Growth disorders – pathophysiology and treatment. Chapman & Hall, London

Mitchell R M, Brown S C, Fallon, S, Smith L 1995 Hospital nursing care. In: Kelnar C J H (ed) Childhood and adolescent diabetes. Chapman & Hall, London, pp 331–344

Molinari L, Largo R H, Prader A 1980 Analysis of the growth spurt at age seven (mid-growth spurt). Helvetica Paediatrica Acta 35: 325–334

Money J, Ehrhardt A A 1974 Man and woman, boy and girl. The differentiation and dysmorphism of gender identity from conception to maturity. Johns Hopkins University Press, Baltimore

Mosser J, Douar A M, Sarde C-O et al 1993 Putative X-linked adrenoleukodystrophy gene shares unexpected homology with ABC transporters. Nature 361: 726–730

Mulaikal R M, Migeon C J, Rock J A 1987 Fertility rates in female patients with congenital adrenal hyperplasia due to 21-hydroxylase deficiency. New England Journal of Medicine 316: 178–182

Mullis P E 1997 Genetic control of growth. In: Kelnar C J H, Stirling H F, Saenger P, Savage M O (eds) Growth disorders – pathophysiology and treatment. Chapman & Hall, London

Mullis P E, Holl R W, Lund T, Brickell P M 1995 Regulation of growth hormone-binding protein production by r-hGH in a hepatoma cell line. Hormone Research 44 (suppl 1): 3 (A9)

Mussen P H, Jones M C 1957 Self-conceptions, motivations and interpersonal attitudes of late- and early-maturing boys. Child Development 28: 243–256

Naeye R L 1965 Infants of diabetic mothers: a quantitative morphologic study. Pediatrics 35: 980–988

Nagayama Y, Rappoport B 1992 The thyrotropin receptor 25 years after its discovery: new insight after its molecular cloning. Molecular Endocrinology 6: 145

Nakanishi S, Inove A, Kita T, Nakamura M, Chang A C Y, Cohen S M, Numa S 1979 Nucleotide sequence of cloned cDNA for bovine corticotrophin-—lipotropin precursor. Nature 278: 423–427

Navot D, Laufer N, Kopolovic J et al 1986 Artificially induced endometrial cycles and the establishment of pregnancies in the absence of ovaries. New England Journal of Medicine 314: 806–811

Neely E K, Marcus R, Rosenfeld R G, Bachrach L K 1993 Turner syndrome adolescents receiving growth hormone are not osteopenic. Journal of Clinical Endocrinology and Metabolism 76: 861–866

Neu A 1992 Sonographic size of endocrine tissue. In: Ranke M B (ed) Functional endocrinologic diagnostics in children and adolescents. J & J Verlag, Mannheim, pp 21–36

New England Congenital Hypothyroidism Collaborative 1984 Characteristics of infantile hypothyroidism discovered on neonatal screening. Journal of Pediatrics 104: 539–544

New England Congenital Hypothyroidism Collaborative 1990 Elementary school performance of children with congenital hypothyroidism. Journal of Pediatrics 116: 27–32

New M I 1970 Male pseudohermaphroditism due to 17-alpha hydroxylase deficiency. Journal of Clinical Investigation 49: 1930–1941

New M I, Speiser P W 1989 Congenital adrenal hyperplasia. In: Brook C G D (ed) Clinical paediatric endocrinology, 2nd edn. Blackwell Scientific Publications, Oxford, pp 441–462

New M I, Siegal E J, Peterson R E 1973 Dexamethasone suppressible hyperaldosteronism. Journal of Clinical Endocrinology and Metabolism 37: 93–100

New M I, Oberfield S E, Levine L S et al 1980 Demonstration of autosomal dominant transmission and absence of HLA linkage in dexamethasone suppressible hyperaldosteronism. Lancet i: 550–551

New M I, Crawford C, Virdis R 1996a Low-renin hypertension in childhood. In: Lifshitz F (ed) Pediatric endocrinology. Marcel Dekker, New York, pp 775–790

New M I, Ghizzoni L, Speiser P W 1996b Update on congenital hyperplasia. In: Lifshitz F (ed) Pediatric endocrinology. Marcel Dekker, New York, pp 305–320

Newborn Committee of the European Thyroid Association 1979 Neonatal screening for congenital hypothyroidism in Europe. Acta Endocrinologica 90 (suppl 223): 5–29

Newton R W, Greene S A 1995 Diabetes in the adolescent. In: Kelnar C J H (ed) Childhood and adolescent diabetes. Chapman & Hall, London, pp 367–374

Newton R W, Isles T, Farquhar J W 1985 The Firbush project – sharing a way of life. Diabetic Medicine 2: 217–224

Niaudet P, Dechaux M, Lercy D, Broyer M 1985 Nephrogenic diabetes insipidus in children. In: Czernichow P, Robinson A G (eds) Diabetes insipidus in man. Karger, Basel, pp 224–231

Noonan J A 1968 Hypertelorism with Turner phenotype. A new syndrome with associated congenital heart disease. American Journal of Diseases of Children 116: 373–380

Noonan J A, Ehmke D A 1963 Associated non-cardiac malformations in children with congenital heart disease. Journal of Pediatrics 63: 468–470

O'Hare M J, Nice E C, Neville A M 1980 Regulation of adrenal androgen secretion and sulfoconjugation in the adult human adrenal cortex: studies with primary monolayer cell cultures. In: Gennazani A R, Thijssen J H H, Siiteri P K (eds) Adrenal androgens. Raven Press, New York, pp 7–27

Ogilvy-Stewart A L, Ryder W D J, Guttameneni H R, Clayton P E, Shalet S M 1992 Growth hormone and tumour recurrence. British Medical Journal 304: 1601–1605

Ogilvy-Stewart A L, Stirling H F, Kelnar C J H, Savage M O, Dunger D B, Buckler J M H, Shalet S M 1997 Does growth-hormone releasing hormone (GHRH) promote growth in children with radiation-induced growth hormone deficiency? Clinical Endocrinology (in press)

Onishi S, Miyazawa G, Nishimura Y et al 1983 Postnatal development of circadian rhythm in serum cortisol levels in children. Pediatrics 72: 399–404

Osler W 1897 Sporadic cretinism in America. Transactions of the Congress of American Physicians and Surgeons 4: 169–206

Osmond C, Barker D J P, Winter P D, Fall C H D, Simmonds S J 1993 Early growth and death from cardiovascular disease in women. British Medical Journal 307: 1519–1524

Owerbach D, Ballard A-L, Draznin M B 1992 Salt-wasting congenital adrenal hyperplasia: detection and characterization of mutations in the steroid 21-hydroxylase gene, CYP21, using the polymerase chain reaction. Journal of Clinical and Endocrinological Metabolism 74: 553–558

Pade D C 1994 Y-chromosomal sequences in Turner's syndrome and risk of gonadoblastoma and virilisation. Lancet 343: 240–242

Pagliara A S, Karl I E, Kipnis D B 1973 Transient neonatal diabetes: delayed maturation of the pancreatic beta cell. Journal of Pediatrics 82: 97–101

Pai G S, Leach D C, Weiss L et al 1977 Thyroid abnormalities in 20 children with Turner syndrome. Journal of Pediatrics 91: 267–269

Paisey R B, Kadow C, Bolton C, Hartog M, Gingell J C 1986 Effects of cyproterone acetate and a long acting LHRH analogue on serum lipoproteins in patients with carcinoma of the prostate. Journal of the Royal Society of Medicine 79: 210–211

Palmer C G, Reichmann A 1976 Chromosomal and clinical findings in 110 females with Turner's syndrome. Human Genetics 35: 35–49

Pang S, Hotchkiss J, Drash A L, Levine L S, New M I 1977 Microfilter paper method for 17 alpha-hydroxy progesterone radioimmunoassay: its application for rapid screening for congenital adrenal hyperplasia. Journal of Clinical Endocrinology and Metabolism 45: 1003–1008

Pang S, Levine L S, Cederqvist L L et al 1980 Amniotic fluid concentrations of delta5 and delta4 steroids in fetuses with congenital adrenal hyperplasia due to 21-hydroxylase deficiency and in anencephalic fetuses. Journal of Clinical Endocrinology and Metabolism 51: 223–229

Pang S, Lerner A, Stoner E, Levine L S, Oberfield S E, New M I 1985 Late onset adrenal steroid 3βHSD deficiency: a cause of hirsutism in pubertal and postpubertal women. Journal of Clinical Endocrinology and Metabolism 60: 428–429

Pang S, Wallace A M, Hofman L, Dorche C, Lyon I C T, Fujeida K, Suwa S 1988 Worldwide experience in newborn screening for classical congenital adrenal hyperplasia due to 21-hydroxylase deficiency. Pediatrics 81: 866–874

Pang S, Dobbins R H, Kling S, Thuline H, Hofman L, Lyon I C T, Webster D R, Dorche C, Dhont J L, Wallace A M, Fujeida K, Suwa S 1989 Worldwide newborn screening update for classical congenital adrenal hyperplasia. In: Schmidt B J (ed) Current trends in infant screening. Elsevier Science Publishers, Amsterdam, pp 307–312

Pang S, Clark A T, Freeman L C et al 1992 Maternal side effects of prenatal dexamethasone therapy for fetal congenital adrenal hyperplasia. Journal of Clinical Endocrinology and Metabolism 75: 249–253

Parizkova J, Roth Z 1972 The assessment of depot fat in children from skinfold thickness measurements by Holtain (Tanner–Whitehouse) caliper. Human Biology 44: 613–620

Patel L, Clayton P E, Addison G M, Price D A, David T J 1995 Adrenal function following topical steroid treatment in children with atopic dermatitis. British Journal of Dermatology 132: 950–955

Patton M A 1997 Genetic and dysmorphic syndromes of tall stature. In: Kelnar C J H, Stirling H F, Saenger P, Savage M O (eds) Growth disorders – pathophysiology and treatment. Chapman & Hall, London

Pedersen R C, Brownie A C, Ling N 1980 Proadrenocorticotropin/endorphin-derived peptides: co-ordinate action on adrenal steroidogenesis. Science 308: 1044–1046

Perheentupa J 1995 The neurohypophysis and water regulation. In: Brook C G D (ed) Clinical paediatric endocrinology, 3rd edn. Blackwell Scientific Publications, Oxford, pp 560–615

Petranyi G, Patranyi M, Sharpe G R, Alberti K G M M 1986 Glycosylated haemoglobin measurements from filter paper blood spots using affinity chromatography. Diabetic Medicine 3: 386A

Phillips J A III, Ferrandez A, Frisch H, Illig R, Zuppinger K 1986 Defects of growth hormone genes – clinical syndromes. In: Raiti S, Tolinan R A (eds) Human growth hormone. Plenum, New York, pp 211–226

Pickup J C 1995 Biosensors and feedback-controlled systems. In: Kelnar C J H (ed) Childhood and adolescent diabetes. Chapman & Hall, London, pp 585–594

Pimstone B, Barberazat G, Hansen J, Murray P 1968 Studies on growth hormone secretion in protein–calorie malnutrition. American Journal of Clinical Nutrition 21: 482–487

Pincus D R, Kelnar C J H, Wallace A M 1993 17-hydroxyprogesterone rhythms and growth velocity in congenital adrenal hyperplasia. Journal of Paediatrics and Child Health 29: 302–304

Pincus G, White P 1933 On the inheritance of diabetes mellitus. 1 An analysis of 675 family histories. American Journal of Medical Science 186: 1–12

Pipanon C, Santos A, Perez-Castilloo A 1992 Thyroid hormone upregulates NGF1-A gene expression in rat brain development. Journal of Biological Chemistry 267: 21–23

Pitkin R M 1985 Calcium metabolism and pregnancy and the perinatal period: a review. American Journal of Obstetrics and Gynecology 151: 99–109

Polak J M, Bloom S R 1980 Decrease of somatostatin content in persistent neonatal hyperinsulinaemic hypoglycaemia. In: Adreani D, Lefebvre P J, Marks V (eds). Current views on hypoglycaemia and glucagon. Academic Press, London, pp 367–378

Poskitt E M E, Cole T J 1977 Do fat babies stay fat? British Medical Journal i: 7–9

Powell G F, Brasel A, Blizzard R M 1967a Emotional deprivation and growth retardation simulating idiopathic hypopituitarism. I. Clinical evaluation of the syndrome. New England Journal of Medicine 276: 1271–1278

Powell G F, Brasel, Raiti S, Blizzard R M 1967b Emotional deprivation and growth retardation simulating idiopathic hypopituitarism. II. Endocrinologic evaluation of the syndrome. New England Journal of Medicine 276: 1279–1283

Prader A 1975 Delayed adolescence. Clinics in Endocrinology and Metabolism 4: 143–155

Prader A, Labhart A, Willi H 1956 Ein Syndrom von Adipositas, Kleinwuchs, Kryptorchismus and Oligophrenie nach myatonieartigen Zustand im Neugeborenalter. Schweizer Medizinische Wochenschrift 86: 1260–1261

Prader A, Tanner J M, von Harnack G A 1963 Catch-up growth following illness or starvation. Journal of Pediatrics 62: 646–659

Preece M A, Law C M, Davies P S W 1986 The growth of children with chronic paediatric disease. In: Savage M O, Randall R A (eds) Growth disorders. Clinics in Endocrinology and Metabolism 15: 453–477

Price P, Wass J A H, Griffin J E et al 1984 High dose androgen therapy in male pseudohermaphroditism due to 5-alpha-reductase deficiency and disorders of the androgen receptor. Journal of Clinical Investigation 74: 1496–1508

Pringle P J, Stanhope R, Hindmarsh P C, Brook C G D 1988 Abnormal sexual development in primary hypothyroidism. Clinical Endocrinology 28: 479–486

Przepiorka D, Baylin A B, McBride O W, Testa J R, Bustros A, Nelkin B D 1984 The human calcitonin gene is located on the short arm of chromosome 11. Biochemical and Biophysical Research Communications 120: 493–499

Raghupathy P, Cutting W A M 1997 Growth failure in tropical and developing countries. In: Kelnar C J H, Stirling H F, Saenger P, Savage M O (eds) Growth disorders – pathophysiology and treatment. Chapman & Hall, London

Rahim A, Holmes S J, Shalet S M 1996 Bone mineralisation at puberty – clinical relevance for health and disease. In: Kelnar C J H (ed) Paediatric endocrinology. Baillière's clinical paediatrics – international practice and research. Baillière Tindall, London, vol 4: 349–364

Ranke M B 1992 Reference table for the conversion of current units to SI units. In Ranke M B (ed) Functional endocrinologic diagnostics in children and adolescents. J & J Verlag, Mannheim, pp 19–20

Ranke M B 1994 Growth hormone insufficiency: clinical features, diagnosis and therapy. In: DeGroot L (ed) Endocrinology, 3rd edn. W B Saunders, Philadelphia, pp 330–340

Ranke M B 1996 Optimising the management of Turner syndrome. In: Kelnar C J H (ed) Paediatric endocrinology. Baillière's clinical paediatrics – international practice and research. Baillière Tindall, London, vol 4: 295–308

Ranke M B 1997 Treatment of Turner and Noonan syndromes. In: Kelnar C J H, Stirling H F, Saenger P, Savage M O (eds) Growth disorders – pathophysiology and treatment. Chapman & Hall, London

Ranke M B, Haber P 1992 Growth hormone stimulation tests. In: Ranke M B (ed) Functional endocrinologic diagnostics in children and adolescents. J & J Verlag, Mannheim, pp 61–75

Rao J K, Chihal H J, Johnson C M 1985 Primary polycystic ovary syndrome in a premenarchel girl. Journal of Reproductive Medicine 3: 361–365

Rayfield E J, Seto Y 1978 Viruses and the pathogenesis of diabetes mellitus. Diabetes 27: 1126–1142

Refetoff S 1982 Syndromes of thyroid hormone resistance. American Journal of Physiology 243: E88–98

Reichstein T S, Shoppee C W 1943 Hormones of the adrenal cortex. Vitamins and Hormones 1: 345–413

Reiter E O, Fuldauer V G, Root A W 1977 Secretion of the adrenal androgen dehydroepiandrosterone sulfate during normal infancy, childhood and adolescence, in sick infants and in children with endocrinologic abnormalities. Journal of Pediatrics 90: 766–770

Riad-Fahmy D, Read G F, Walker R F, Griffiths K 1982 Steroids in saliva for assessing endocrine function. Endocrine Reviews 3: 367–395

Rich B H, Rosenfield R L, Lucky A W, Helke J C, Otto P 1981 Adrenarche: changing adrenal response to adrenocorticotrophin. Journal of Clinical Endocrinology and Metabolism 52: 1129–1136

Rimoin D L, Borochowitz Z 1997 Genetic and dysmorphic syndromes of short stature. In: Kelnar C J H, Stirling H F, Saenger P, Savage M O (eds) Growth disorders – pathophysiology and treatment. Chapman & Hall, London

Ritzén M 1997 Growth in adrenal and gonadal disorders. In: Kelnar C J H, Stirling H F, Saenger P, Savage M O (eds) Growth disorders – pathophysiology and treatment. Chapman & Hall, London

Rivier J, Speiss J, Thorner M, Vale W 1982 Characterisation of a growth hormone releasing factor from a human pancreatic islet cell tumour. Nature 300: 276–278

Roberts J L, Herbert E 1977 Characterization of a common precursor to corticotrophin and β-lipotrophin: cell-free synthesis of the precursor and identification of corticotrophin peptides in the molecule. Proceedings of the National Academy of Sciences (USA) 74: 4826–4830

Robinson A G, Verbalis J G 1985 Treatment of central diabetes insipidus. In: Czernichow P, Robinson A G (eds) Diabetes insipidus in man. Karger, Basel, pp 292–303

Robinson I A A F, Thomas G 1997 Endocrinology of growth – central control. In: Kelnar C J H, Stirling H F, Saenger P, Savage M O (eds) Growth disorders – pathophysiology and treatment. Chapman & Hall, London

Roger M, Chaussain J L, Raynaud F et al 1984 Treatment of male and female precocious puberty by monthly injections of a continuous release preparation of D-Trp6–LHRH. Pediatric Research 18: 120–129

Rogol A D 1997 Growth hormone releasing peptides. In: Kelnar C J H, Stirling H F, Saenger P, Savage M O (eds) Growth disorders – pathophysiology and treatment. Chapman & Hall, London

Root A W, Shulman D, Root J, Diamond F 1986 The inter-relationships of thyroid and growth hormones: effect of growth hormone releasing hormone in hypo- and hyperthyroid male rats. In: Illig R, Visser H K A (eds) Pediatric endocrinology 1986. Acta Endocrinologica Copenhagen Supplementum 279: 367–375

Rosenbloom A L, Riley W J, Weber F T, Malone J I, Donnelly W H 1980 Cerebral edema complicating diabetic ketoacidosis in childhood. Journal of Pediatrics 96: 357–361

Rosenfeld R G 1989 Update on growth hormone therapy for Turner's syndrome. Acta Paediatrica Scandinavica (suppl) 356: 103–108

Rosenfeld R G 1995 Broadening the growth hormone insensitivity syndrome. New England Journal of Medicine 333: 1145–1146

Rosenfeld R G 1997 Abnormalities of growth hormone action. In: Kelnar C J H, Stirling H F, Saenger P, Savage M O (eds) Growth disorders – pathophysiology and treatment. Chapman & Hall, London

Rosenfeld R G, Frane J, Attie K M et al 1992 Six year results of a randomized, prospective trial of human growth hormone and oxandrolone in Turner syndrome. Journal of Pediatrics 121: 49–55

Rosenfeld R G, Rosenbloom A L, Guevarra-Aguirre J 1994 Growth hormone (GH) insensitivity due to primary GH receptor deficiency. Endocrine Reviews 15: 369–390

Rosenfeld R S, Hellman L, Roffwarg H, Weitzman E D, Fukushima D J, Gallagher T F 1971 Dehydroisoandrosterone is secreted episodically and synchronously with cortisol by normal man. Journal of Clinical Endocrinology and Metabolism 33: 87–92

Rosenthal S N, Grumbach M M, Kaplan S L 1983 Gonadotrophin independent

sexual precocity with premature Leydig and germinal cell maturation (familial testotoxicosis): effects of a potent luteinising hormone-releasing factor agonist and medroxyprogesterone acetate therapy in four cases. Journal of Clinical Endocrinology and Metabolism 57: 571–579

Rosenwaks Z, Lee P A, Jones G S et al 1979 An attenuated form of congenital virilizing adrenal hyperplasia. Journal of Clinical Endocrinology and Metabolism 49: 335–339

Rosler A, Leiberman E 1984 Enzymatic defects of steroidogenesis: 11-beta hydroxylase deficiency congenital adrenal hyperplasia. In: New M I (ed) Adrenal disease in childhood. paediatric and adolescent endocrinology. Karger, Basel, vol 13: 47–71

Rosler A, Lieberman E, Rosenmann A, Ben-Veilio R, Weidenfeld J 1979 Prenatal diagnosis of 11β-hydroxylase deficiency congenital adrenal hyperplasia. Journal of Clinical Endocrinology and Metabolism 49: 546–551

Rosler A, Leiberman E, Sack J et al 1982 Clinical variability of congenital adrenal hyperplasia due to 11β-hydroxylase deficiency. Hormone Research 16: 133–141

Ross J L, Long L M, Loriaux D L, Cutler G B Jr 1985 Growth hormone secretory dynamics in Turner syndrome. Journal of Pediatrics 106: 202–206

Ross J L, Long L M, Skerda M et al 1986 Effect of low doses of estradiol on 6 month growth rates and predicted height in patients with Turner syndrome. Journal of Pediatrics 109: 950–953

Ross L A, McCrimmon R J, Kelnar C J H, Deary I J 1996a A comparison of hypoglycaemic symptoms reported by children with insulin dependent diabetes mellitus and those observed by their parents. Hormone Research 46 (supplement 2): A252

Ross L A, McCrimmon R J, Stephen R, Kelnar C J H, Frier B M 1996b Symptomatic and autonomic responses to acute hypoglycaemia in adolescents with insulin dependent diabetes mellitus (abstract) BDA Dublin March 1996

Rovet J, Ehrlich R M 1995 Longterm effects of l-thyroxine treatment for congenital hypothyroidism. Journal of Pediatrics 126: 380–386

Russell A 1954 A syndrome of 'intrauterine' dwarfism recognizable at birth with craniofacial dysostosis, disproportionately short arms and other anomalies (5 examples). Proceedings of the Royal Society of Medicine 47: 1040–1044

Saenger P 1997 Adverse effects of growth hormone therapy. In: Kelnar C J H, Stirling H F, Saenger P, Savage M O (eds) Growth disorders – pathophysiology and treatment. Chapman & Hall, London

Saez J M, de Peretti E, Morera A M, David M, Bertrand J 1971 Familial male pseudohermaphroditism with gynaecomastia due to testicular 17-ketosteroid reductase defect. 1 Studies in vitro. Journal of Clinical Endocrinology and Metabolism 32: 604–610

Salas M 1996 Thyroid nodules in children and adolescents. In: Lifshitz F (ed) Pediatric endocrinology. Marcel Dekker, New York, pp 415–422

Saleh 1997 Limb lengthening techniques. In: Kelnar C J H, Stirling H F, Saenger P, Savage M O (eds) Growth disorders – pathophysiology and treatment. Chapman & Hall, London

Salisbury D M, Leonard J V, Dezateux C A, Savage M O 1984 Micropenis: an important early sign of congenital hypopituitarism. British Medical Journal 288: 621–622

Sandler S, Andersson A, Korsgren O, Tollemar J, Petersson B, Groth C-G, Hellerstrom C 1987 Tissue culture of human fetal pancreas: growth hormone stimulates the formation and insulin production of islet-like cell clusters. Journal of Clinical Endocrinology and Metabolism 65: 1154–1158

Sandrini R, Jospe N, Migeon C J 1993 Temporal and individual variations in the dose of glucocorticoid used for the treatment of salt-losing congenital virilizing adrenal hyperplasia due to 21-hydroxylase deficiency. Acta Paediatrica 388 (suppl): 56–60

Saruta T, Suzuki H, Handa M et al 1986 Multiple factors contribute to the pathogenesis of hypertension in Cushing's syndrome. Journal of Clinical Endocrinology and Metabolism 62: 275–279

Sato T, Suzuke Y, Taetani T, Ishigura K, Nakajima H 1957 Age related change in the pituitary threshold for TSH release during thyroxine replacement therapy for cretinism. Journal of Clinical Endocrinology and Metabolism 44: 553–559

Savage M O 1989 Clinical aspects of intersex. In: Brook C G D (ed) Clinical paediatric endocrinology, 2nd edn. Blackwell Scientific Publications, Oxford, pp 38–54

Savage M O 1997 Treatment of growth hormone resistance. In: Kelnar C J H, Stirling H F, Saenger P, Savage M O (eds) Growth disorders – pathophysiology and treatment. Chapman & Hall, London

Savage M O, Chaussain J L, Evain D, Roger M, Canlorbe P, Job J C 1978 Endocrine studies in male pseudohermaphroditism in childhood and adolescence. Clinical Endocrinology 8: 219–231

Savage M O, Preece M A, Jeffcoate S L et al 1980 Familial male pseudohermaphroditism due to deficiency of 5-alpha-reductase. Clinical Endocrinology 12: 397–406

Savage M O, Lowe D G, Ransley P G et al 1986 Germ cell neoplasia in patients with abnormal sexual differentiation. Paediatric Research 20: 1183 (A131)

Savage M O, Wilton P, Ranke M B et al 1993 Therapeutic response to recombinant IGF1 in patients with growth hormone insensitivity syndrome (GHIS). Paediatric Research 33 (suppl): abstract 7

Scammon R E 1930 The measurement of the body in childhood. In: Harris J A, Jackson C M, Paterson D G, Scammon R E (eds) The measurement of man. University of Minnesota Press, Minnesota

Scherbaum W A, Bottazzo G F, Czernichow P et al 1985 Role of autoimmunity in central diabetes insipidus. In: Czernichow P, Robinson A G (eds) Diabetes insipidus in man. Karger, Basel, pp 232–239

Schibler D, Brook C G D, Kind H P et al 1974 Growth and body proportions in 54 boys and men with Klinefelter syndrome. Helvetica Paediatrica Acta 29: 325–333

Schiebinger R J, Albertson B D, Cassorla F G, Bowyer D W, Geelhoed G W, Cutler G B Jr, Loriaux D L 1981 The developmental changes in plasma adrenal androgens during infancy and adrenarche are associated with changing activities of adrenal microsomal 17-hydroxylase and 17,20 desmolase. Journal of Clinical Investigation 67: 1177–1182

Schmidt M I, Ndjii-Georgopoulos A, Rendell M et al 1981 The dawn phenomenon, an early morning glucose rise: implications for diabetic instability. Diabetes Care 4: 579–585

Schmitt S, Kotzot D, Lurie I W et al 1995 Uniparental disomy 7 in Silver–Russell syndrome and primordial growth retardation. Hormone Research 44 (suppl 1): 6 (A20)

Schönberg D 1992 Principles of hormone measurement and validation underlying diagnostic decisions. In: Ranke M B (ed) Functional endocrinologic diagnostics in children and adolescents. J & J Verlag, Mannheim, pp 1–18

Schwartz H P, Joss E, Zuppinger K 1987 Bromocriptine treatment in adolescent boys with familial tall stature. A pair-matched controlled study. Journal of Clinical Endocrinology and Metabolism 65: 136–140

Scibilia J, Finegold D, Dorman J, Becker D, Drash A 1986 Why do children with diabetes die? Acta Endocrinologica (Copenhagen) 113 (suppl 279): 326–333

Seckl J R 1993 11β-hydroxysteroid dehydrogenase isoforms and their implications for blood pressure regulation. European Journal of Clinical Investigation 23: 589–601

Seckl J R, Miller W L 1997 How safe is long-term prenatal glucocorticoid treatment. Journal of the American Medical Association 277: 1077–1079

Seidah N G, Chretien M 1981 Complete amino acid sequence of a human pituitary glycopeptide: an important maturation product of pro-opiomelanocortin. Proceedings of the National Academy of Sciences (USA) 78: 4236–4240

Sells R A, Brynger H 1987 Progress in pancreatic transplantation. Lancet i: 1024–1025

Shah A, Stanhope R, Matthew D 1992 Hazards of pharmacological tests of growth hormone secretion in childhood. British Medical Journal 304: 173–174

Shalet S M (ed) 1995 Growth hormone in puberty. Colwood House Medical Publications, Berkshire

Shenker A, Weinstein L S, Moran A et al 1993a Severe endocrine and non-endocrine manifestations of the McCune–Albright syndrome associated with activating mutations of stimulatory G protein Gs. Journal of Pediatrics 123: 509–518

Shenker A, Laue L, Kosugi S et al 1993b A constitutively activating mutation of the luteinizing hormone receptor in familial male precocious puberty. Nature 365: 652–654

Shield J P H, Baum J D 1995 long term management: scope and aims. In: Kelnar C J H (ed) Childhood and adolescent diabetes. Chapman & Hall, London, pp 241–252

Shohat M, Rimoin D L 1996 The skeletal dysplasias. In: Lifshitz F (ed) Pediatric endocrinology. Marcel Dekker, New York, pp 131–148

Siler-Khodr T M, Morgenstern L L, Greenwood F C 1974 Hormone synthesis and release from human fetal adenohypophysis in vitro. Journal of Clinical Endocrinology and Metabolism 39: 891–905

Silink M 1995 Testing for control – home and hospital. In: Kelnar C J H (ed) Childhood and adolescent diabetes. Chapman & Hall, London, pp 311–322

Silver H K 1964 Asymmetry, short stature and variations in sexual development: a syndrome of congenital malformations. American Journal of Diseases of Children 107: 495–515

Silver H K, Kiyasu W, George J, Daemer W C 1953 A syndrome of congenital hemihypertrophy, shortness of stature and elevated urinary gonadotrophins. Pediatrics 12: 368–375

Silverman S H, Migeon C, Rosenberg E, Wilkins L 1952 Precocious growth of sexual hair without other sexual development: 'premature pubarche', a constitutional variation of adolescence. Pediatrics 10: 426–432

Simonian M J, Gill G N 1981 Regulation of the fetal human adrenal cortex: effects of adrenocorticotropin on growth and function of monolayer cultures of fetal and definitive zone cells. Endocrinology 108: 1769–1779

Simons W F, Fuggle P W, Grant D B, Smith I 1994 Intellectual development at 10 years in early treated congenital hypothyroidism. Archives of Disease in Childhood 71: 232–234

Sinclair A H, Berta P, Palmer S et al 1990 A gene from the human sex-determining region encodes a protein with homology to a conserved DNA-binding motif. Nature 346: 240–244

Sizonenko P C, Lang U 1988 Melatonin and human reproductive function. In: Miles A, Philbrick D R S, Thompson C (eds) Melatonin – clinical perspectives. Oxford University Press, Oxford, pp 62–78

Skuse D H 1987 The psychological consequences of being small. Journal of Child Psychology and Psychiatry 28: 641–650

Skuse D H 1995 Developmental trends in coping in childhood and adolescence. In: Kelnar C J H (ed) Childhood and adolescent diabetes. Chapman & Hall, London, pp 89–106

Skuse D H 1997 Psychological disorders and management of the associated growth disturbance. In: Kelnar C J H, Stirling H F, Saenger P, Savage M O (eds) Growth disorders – pathophysiology and treatment. Chapman & Hall, London

Skuse D H, Gilmour J, Tian C S, Hindmarsh P C 1994 Psychosocial assessment of children with short stature: a preliminary report. Acta Paediatrica Scandinavica 406: 11–16

Skuse D, Albanese A, Stanhope R, Gilmour J, Voss L 1996 A new stress-related syndrome of growth failure and hyperphagia in children, associated with reversibility of growth hormone insufficiency. Lancet 348: 353–358

Smith P J, Brook C G D 1988 Growth hormone releasing hormone or growth hormone treatment in growth hormone insufficiency? Archives of Disease in Childhood 63: 629–634

Sobel E H 1968 Anabolic steroids. In: Astwood E V, Cassidy C E (eds) Clinical endocrinology II. Grune and Stratton, New York, pp 789–797

Söder O 1997 Cellular growth. In: Kelnar C J H, Stirling H F, Saenger P, Savage M O (eds) Growth disorders – pathophysiology and treatment. Chapman & Hall, London

Solyom J, Hughes I A 1989 Value of selective screening for congenital adrenal hyperplasia in Hungary. Archives of Disease in Childhood 64: 338–342

Sonino N 1987 The use of ketoconazole as an inhibitor of steroid production. New England Journal of Medicine 317: 812–818

Soothill P, Holmes R 1997a Fetal growth. In: Kelnar C J H, Stirling H F, Saenger P, Savage M O (eds) Growth disorders – pathophysiology and treatment. Chapman & Hall, London

Soothill P, Holmes R 1997b Pregnancy and the growth retarded fetus. In: Kelnar C J H, Stirling H F, Saenger P, Savage M O (eds) Growth disorders – pathophysiology and treatment. Chapman & Hall, London

Sotos J F, Dodge P R, Muirhead D et al 1964 Cerebral gigantism in childhood: a syndrome of excessively rapid growth with acromegalic features and non-progressive neurologic disorder. New England Journal of Medicine 271: 109–116

Spector T D, Keen R W, Arden N K et al 1995 Influence of vitamin D receptor genotype on bone mineral density in postmenopausal women: a twin study in Britain. British Medical Journal 310: 1357–1360

Speiser P W, Dupont B, Rubinstein P, Piazza A, Kastelan A, New M I 1985 High frequency of nonclassical steroid 21-hydroxylase deficiency. American Journal of Human Genetics 37: 650–667

Spiliotis B E, August G P, Hung W, Sonis W, Mendelson W, Bercu B B 1984 Growth hormone neurosecretory dysfunction. A treatable cause of short stature. Journal of the American Medical Association 251: 2223–2230

Spranger J W, Langer L O, Wiedemann H R 1974 Bone dysplasia: an atlas of constitutional disorders of skeletal development. Saunders, Philadelphia

Stabler B 1997 Psychological assessment. In: Kelnar C J H, Stirling H F, Saenger P, Savage M O (eds) Growth disorders – pathophysiology and treatment. Chapman & Hall, London

Stanhope R, Adlard P 1987 Empty sella syndrome. Developmental Medicine and Child Neurology 29: 397–399

Stanhope R, Brook C G D 1985 Precocious pseudopuberty and ovarian follicular cysts. American Journal of Diseases of Children 139: 222 (letter)

Stanhope R, Pringle P J, Adams J, Jeffcoate S L, Brook C G D 1985a Spontaneous gonadotrophin pulsatility and ovarian morphology in girls with central precocious puberty treated with cyproterone acetate. Clinical Endocrinology 23: 547–553

Stanhope R, Pringle P J, Brook C G D 1985b Alteration in the nocturnal pulsatile release of GH during the induction of puberty using low dose pulsatile LHRH: a case report. Clinical Endocrinology 22: 117–120

Stanhope R, Abdulwahid N A, Adams J, Brook C G D 1986 Studies of gonadotrophin pulsatility and pelvic ultrasound distinguish between isolated premature thelarche and central precocious puberty. European Journal of Paediatrics 145: 190–194

Stanhope R, Brook C G D, Pringle P J, Adams J, Jacobs H S 1987a Induction of puberty by pulsatile gonadotrophin-releasing hormone. Lancet ii: 552–555

Stanhope R, Huen K-F, Buzi F, Preece M A, Grant D B 1987b The effect of cyproterone acetate on the growth of children with central precocious puberty. European Journal of Pediatrics 146: 500–503

Stanhope R, Adams J, Pringle P J, Jacobs H S, Brook C G D 1987c The evolution of polycystic ovaries in a girl with hypogonadotrophic hypergonadism before puberty and during puberty induced with pulsatile gonadotrophin-releasing hormone. Fertility and Sterility 47: 872–875

Stanhope R, Adlard P, Hamill G, Jones J, Skuse D, Preece M A 1988a Physiological growth hormone secretion during the recovery from psychosocial dwarfism: a case report. Clinical Endocrinology 28: 335–340

Stanhope R, Buchanan C R, Fenn G C, Preece M A 1988b Double blind placebo controlled trial of oxandrolone in the treatment of boys with constitutional delay of growth and puberty. Archives of Disease in Childhood 63: 501–505

Stanhope R, Pringle P J, Brook C G D 1988c Growth, growth hormone and sex steroid secretion in central precocious puberty treated with GnRH analogue. Acta Paediatrica Scandinavica 77: 525–530

Stanhope R, Adams J, Brook C G D 1988d The evolution of polycystic ovaries in a girl with delayed menarche. Journal of Reproductive Medicine 33: 482–484

Stark O, Peckham C S, Moynihan C 1989 Weight and age at menarche. Archives of Disease in Childhood 64: 383–387

Steel J M 1995 Eating disorders. In: Kelnar C J H (ed) Childhood and adolescent diabetes. Chapman & Hall, London, pp 375–384

Stein A, Shanklin DR, Adams P M et al 1989 Thyroid hormone regulation of specific mRNAs in the developing brain. In: Delong G R, Robins J, Condliffe P G (eds) Iodine, pp 59–78

Stephens W P, Goddard K J, Laing I, Adams J E 1985 Isolated adrenocorticotrophin deficiency and empty sella associated with hypothyroidism. Clinical Endocrinology 22: 771–776

Stern S R, Kelnar C J H 1985 Hypertrichosis due to primary hypothyroidism. Archives of Disease in Childhood 60: 763–766

Stewart P M, Corrie J E T, Shackleton C H L, Edwards C R W 1988 Syndrome of apparent mineralocorticoid excess. a defect in the cortisol–cortisone shuttle. Journal of Clinical Investigation 82: 340–349

Stini W A 1972 Malnutrition, body size and proportion. Ecology of Food and Nutrition 1: 121

Stirling H F, Kelnar C J H 1990 Adrenarche. Growth Matters 1(4): 6–8

Stirling H F, Kelnar C J H 1992 Puberty. Current Paediatrics 2: 131–136

Stirling H F, Kelnar C J H 1994 Who needs growth hormone? Journal of the Royal Society of Medicine 87: 497–498

Stirling H F, Kelnar C J H 1995a Glucose homeostasis in the normal child. In: Kelnar C J H (ed) Childhood and adolescent diabetes. Chapman & Hall, London, pp 19–30

Stirling H F, Kelnar C J H 1995b Neonatal diabetes. In: Kelnar C J H (ed) Childhood and adolescent diabetes. Chapman & Hall, London, pp 419–426

Stirling H F, Kelnar C J H 1997 Postnatal, infantile and childhood growth. In: Kelnar C J H, Stirling H F, Saenger P, Savage M O (eds) Growth disorders – pathophysiology and treatment. Chapman & Hall, London

Stirling H F, Butler G E, Glasier A, Rodger M, Kelnar C J H, Wu F C W 1989a Hypothalamo-pituitary-ovarian function after D-ser LHRH agonist (buserelin) treatment for central precocious puberty. Journal of Endocrinology 121 (suppl): A153

Stirling H F, Kelnar C J H, Wu F C W 1989b What happens after treatment of precocious puberty? European Journal of Pediatrics 149: 150

Stirling H F, Barr D G D, Kelnar C J H 1991a Familial growth hormone releasing factor deficiency in pseudopseudohypoparathyroidism. Archives of Disease in Childhood 66: 533–535

Stirling H F, Darling J A B, Barr D G D 1991b Plasma cyclic AMP response to intravenous parathyroid hormone in pseudohypoparathyroidism. Acta Paediatrica Scandinavica 80: 333–338

Stirling H F, Darling J A B, Kelnar C J H 1991c What happens to children's blood glucose levels overnight? European Journal of Paediatrics 150: 75 (abstract)

Stirling H F, Darling J A B, Kelnar C J H 1991d Nocturnal glucose homeostasis in normal children. Hormone Research 35 (suppl 2): 54 (abstract 210)

Stolz H R, Stolz L M 1951 Somatic development of adolescent boys. A study of the growth of boys during the second decade of life. Macmillan, New York

Stoner E, DiMartino J, Kuhnle U, Levine L S, Oberfield S E, New M I 1986 Is salt-wasting in congenital adrenal hyperplasia genetic? Clinical Endocrinology 24: 9–20

Strain A J, Hill D J, Swenne I, Milner R D G 1987 The regulation of DNA synthesis in human fetal hepatocytes by placental lactogen, growth hormone and insulin-like growth factor 1/somatomedin C. Journal of Cell Physiology 132: 33–40

Strang S 1995 Childhood diabetes: the child at school. In: Kelnar C J H (ed) Childhood and adolescent diabetes. Chapman & Hall, London, pp 457–464

Stuetzle W, Gasser T H, Molinari L, Large R H, Prader A, Huber P J 1980 Shape-invariant modelling of human growth. Annals of Human Biology 7: 507–528

Stutchfield P R, O'Halloran S M, Smith C S, Woodrow J C, Bottazzo G F, Heaf D 1988 HLA type, islet cell antibodies and glucose intolerance in cystic fibrosis. Archives of Disease in Childhood 63: 1234–1239

Sultan C, Lobaccaro J M, Lumbroso S, Poujol N 1996 Disorders of sexual differentiation: recent molecular and clinical advances. In: Kelnar C J H (ed) Paediatric endocrinology. Baillière's clinical paediatrics – international practice and research. Baillière Tindall, London, vol 4: 221–244

Swift P G F 1995 Insulin: types and regimens. In: Kelnar C J H (ed) Childhood and adolescent diabetes. Chapman & Hall, London, pp 253–270

Swift P G F, North J, Redmond S 1995 Self-help in childhood diabetes. In: Kelnar C J H (ed) Childhood and adolescent diabetes. Chapman & Hall, London, pp 493–500

Talbot N B, Butler A M, Berman R H, Rodriguez P M, MacLachlan E A 1943 Excretion of 17 ketosteroids by normal and abnormal children. American Journal of Diseases of Children 65: 364–375

Talbot N B, Blodgett F M, Wood M S, Campbell A M, Christo E, Zygmuntowicz A S 1951 Concerning the probability that there are at least two adrenocorticotrophic hormones in the human. In: Mole J R (ed) Proceedings of the 2nd Clinical ACTH Conference. Blaiston, Philadelphia

Tanner J M 1951 Some notes on the reporting of growth data. Human Biology 23: 93–159

Tanner J M 1962 Growth at adolescence, 2nd edn. Blackwell Scientific Publications, Oxford

Tanner J M 1963 The regulation of human growth. Child Development 34: 817–847

Tanner J M 1981 Endocrinology of puberty. In: Brook C G D (ed) Clinical paediatric endocrinology. Blackwell Scientific Publications, Oxford, pp 207–223

Tanner J M, Whitehouse R H 1955 The Harpenden skinfold caliper. American Journal of Physical Anthropology 13: 743–746

Tanner J M, Whitehouse R H 1962 Standards for subcutaneous fat in British children. Percentiles for thickness of skinfolds over triceps and below scapula. British Medical Journal i: 346–350

Tanner J M, Whitehouse R H 1975 Revised standards for triceps and subscapular skinfolds for British children. Archives of Disease in Childhood 50: 142–145

Tattersall R B, Walford S 1985 Brittle diabetes in response to life stress: 'cheating and manipulation'. In: Pickup J C (ed) Brittle diabetes. Blackwell Scientific Publications, Oxford, pp 76–102

Telenius H, Ponder B A J 1993 Multiple endocrine neoplasia. Medicine International 21(6): 235–236

Temeck J W, Pang S, Nelson C, New M I 1987 Genetic defects of steroidogenesis in premature pubarche. Journal of Clinical Endocrinology and Metabolism 64: 609–617

Teuscher A, Berger W G 1987 Hypoglycaemia unawareness in patients transferred from beef/porcine insulin to human insulin. Lancet ii: 382–385

Thistlethwaite D, Darling J A B, Fraser R, Mason P A, Rees L H, Harkness R A 1975 Familial glucocorticoid deficiency. Studies of diagnosis and pathogenesis. Archives of Disease in Childhood 50: 291–297

Thompson C, Greene S A, Newton R W 1995 Camps for diabetic children and teenagers. In: Kelnar C J H (ed) Childhood and adolescent diabetes. Chapman & Hall, London, pp 483–492

Thorner M O 1995 Presentation at the 34th annual meeting of the European Society for Paediatric Endocrinology, Edinburgh, June 25–28

Thorner M O, Rogol A D, Blizzard R M et al 1988 Acceleration of growth rate in growth hormone-deficient children treated with human growth hormone-releasing hormone. Pediatric Research 24: 145–151

Tillotson S L, Fuggle P W, Smith I et al 1994 Relation between biochemical severity and intelligence in early treated congenital hypothyroidism: a threshold effect. British Medical Journal 309: 440–445

Tjima N 1985 Coma at the onset of young insulin-dependent diabetes in Japan: the result of a nationwide survey. Diabetes 34: 1241–1246

Toft A D 1989a Hypothyroidism. Medicine International 63: 2596–2600

Toft A D 1989b Hyperthyroidism. Medicine International 63: 2588–2595

Tönshoff B, Jux C, Mehls O 1996 Glucocorticoids and growth In: Kelnar C J H (ed) Paediatric endocrinology. Baillière's clinical paediatrics – international practice and research. Baillière Tindall, London, vol 4: 309–332

Treasure J L, Gordon P A L, King E A, Wheeler M, Russell G F M 1985 Cystic ovaries: a phase of anorexia nervosa. Lancet ii: 1379–1382

Turnbull D M, Shepherd I M, Aynsley-Green A 1988 Inherited defects of fatty acid oxidation. Biochemical Society Transactions 16: 424–427

Turner H H 1938 A syndrome of infantilism, congenital webbed neck and cubitus valgus. Endocrinology 23: 566–574

UK GnRH Analogue Collaborative Study Group 1988 Intranasal (D-ser6) GnRH analogue for the management of central precocious puberty. Pediatric Research 23: A134

Underwood L E, D'Ercole A J, Clemmons D R, Van Wyk J J 1986 Paracrine functions of somatomedins. In: Franchimont P (ed) Clinics in endocrinology and metabolism. 15: 58–77

Vale W, Rivier J, Vaughan J et al 1986 Purification and characterisation of an FSH releasing protein from porcine ovarian follicular fluid. Nature 321: 776–779

Valk I M, Langhout-Chabloz A M E, Smals A G H, Kloppenborg P W C, Cassorla F G, Schutte E A S T 1983 Accurate measurement of the lower leg length and ulnar length and its application in short term growth measurement. Growth 47: 53–66

Van der Gaag R D, Drexhage H A, Dussault J H 1985 Role of maternal immunoglobulins blocking TSH-induced thyroid growth in sporadic forms of congenital hypothyroidism. Lancet i: 246–250

Van Haeften T W, Heiling V J, Gerich J E 1987 Adverse effects of insulin antibodies on post-prandial plasma glucose and insulin profiles in diabetic patients without immune insulin resistance. Implications for intensive insulin regimes. Diabetes 36: 305–309

Van Wyk J J, Grumbach M M 1960 Syndrome of precocious menstruation and galactorrhea in juvenile hypothyroidism: an example of hormonal overlap in pituitary feedback. Journal of Pediatrics 57: 416–435

Vanderscheuren-Lodeweyckx M 1992 Thyroid function tests. In: Ranke M B (ed) Functional endocrinologic diagnostics in children and adolescents. J & J Verlag, Mannheim, pp 37–60

Vassart G, Dumont J E 1992 The thyrotropin receptor and the regulation of thyrocyte function and growth. Endocrine Reviews 13: 596

Veldhuis J D, Kulin H E, Santen R J, Wilson T E, Melby J C 1980 Inborn error in the terminal step of aldosterone biosynthesis. New England Journal of Medicine 303: 117–121

Veldhuis J D, Evans W S, Demers L M et al 1985 Altered neuroendocrine regulation of gonadotrophin secretion in women distance runners. Journal of Clinical Endocrinology and Metabolism 61: 557–563

Vestergaard P, Leverett R 1958 Constancy of urinary creatinine excretion. Journal of Laboratory and Clinical Medicine 51: 211–218

Vimpani G V, Vimpani A F, Lidgard G P et al 1977 Prevalence of severe growth hormone deficiency. British Medical Journal ii: 427–430

Vinson G P 1984 The antimatter of the adrenal cortex (abstract). 3rd joint meeting of the British Endocrine Societies, University of Edinburgh, 27–30 March

Virdi N K, Rayner P H W, Rudd B T, Green A 1987 Should we screen for congenital adrenal hyperplasia? A review of 117 cases. Archives of Disease in Childhood 62: 659–662

Von Mering J, Minkowski O 1890 Diabetes mellitus nach Pankreasextirpation. Archiv für Experimentalische Pathologie und Pharmacologie 26: 371–387

Voorhess M L 1996 Disorders of the adrenal medulla. In: Lifshitz F (ed) Pediatric endocrinology. Marcel Dekker, New York, pp 355–368

Wagner R, White P, Bogan I K 1942 Diabetic dwarfism. American Journal of Diseases of Children 63: 667–727

Waine C, Stavely E A 1995 Primary care and the community. In: Kelnar C J H (ed) Childhood and adolescent diabetes. Chapman & Hall, London, pp 475–482

Waldhauser W, Weiszenbacher G, Frisch H, Zeitlhuber U, Waldhauser M, Wurtman R J 1984 Fall in nocturnal serum melatonin during prepuberty and pubescence. Lancet i: 362–365

Wales J K H 1997 Rhythms of linear growth. In: Kelnar C J H, Stirling H F, Saenger P, Savage M O (eds) Growth disorders – pathophysiology and treatment. Chapman & Hall, London

Wales J K H, Gibson A T 1994 Short term growth: rhythms, chaos or noise? Archives of Disease in Childhood 71: 84–89

Wales J K H, Milner R D G 1987 Knemometry in the assessment of linear growth. Archives of Disease in Childhood 62: 166–171

Wales J K H, Milner R D G 1988 Variation in lower leg growth with alternate day steroid treatment. Archives of Disease in Childhood 63: 981–983

Walker J M, Hughes I A 1995 Tests in paediatric endocrinolgy. In: Brook C G D (ed) Clinical paediatric endocrinology, 3rd edn. Blackwell Scientific Publications, Oxford, pp 782–798

Wallace W H B 1996 Growth and endocrine function following treatment of childhood malignant disease. In: Plowman P N, Pinkerton C R (eds) Paediatric oncology: clinical practice and controversies. Chapman & Hall, London

Wallace W H B, Kelnar C J H 1996a The effect of chemotherapy in childhood on growth and endocrine function. In: Kelnar C J H (ed) Paediatric endocrinology. Baillière's clinical paediatrics – international practice and research. Baillière Tindall, London, vol 4: 333–348

Wallace W H B, Kelnar C J H 1996b The effect of chemotherapy in childhood on growth and endocrine function. Drug Safety: 325–332, Adis International, Auckland

Wallace W H B, Kelnar C J H 1997 The treatment of growth disorders in oncology patients. In: Kelnar C J H, Stirling H F, Saenger P, Savage M O (eds) Growth disorders – pathophysiology and treatment. Chapman & Hall, London

Wallace A M, Beastall G H, Cook B et al 1986 Neonatal screening for congenital adrenal hyperplasia: a programme based on a novel direct radioimmunoassay for 17-hydroxyprogesterone in blood spots. Journal of Endocrinology 108: 299–308

Walsh P C, Madden J D, Harrod M D et al 1974 Familial incomplete male pseudohermaphroditism type 2. New England Journal of Medicine 291: 944–949

Ward P S, Ward I, McNinch A W, Savage D C L 1986 Reversible inhibition of central precocious puberty with a long-acting GnRH analogue. Archives of Disease in Childhood 60: 872–874

Warren M P, Jewelewicz R, Dyrenfurth I, Ans R, Khalaf S, Vande Wiele R L 1975 The significance of weight loss in the evaluation of pituitary responsiveness to LH-RH in women with secondary amenorrhea. Journal of Clinical Endocrinology and Metabolism 40: 601–611

Warshaw J B 1996 Intrauterine growth retardation. In: Lifshitz F (ed) Pediatric Endocrinology. Marcel Dekker, New York, pp 95–102

Waterman M R, Simpson E R 1985 Regulation of the biosynthesis of cytochromes P-450 involved in steroid hormone synthesis. Molecular and Cellular Endocrinology 39: 81–89

Waters M J, Barnard R T, Lobie P E et al 1990 Growth hormone receptors – their structure, location and role. Acta Paediatrica Scandinavica (suppl) 366: 60–72

Webb T 1994 Genetic aspects of Prader–Willi syndrome. Growth Matters International 16 (June): 2–4

Weber B 1989 Pathophysiology of diabetes mellitus. In: Brook C G D (ed) Clinical paediatric endocrinology, 2nd edn. Blackwell Scientific Publications, Oxford, pp 555–598

Whitaker J, Landing B H, Esselborn V M et al 1956 The syndrome of familial juvenile hypoadrenocorticism, hypoparathyroidism and superficial moniliasis. Journal of Clinical Endocrinology and Metabolism 16: 1374–1387

White P C, Grossberger D, Onufer B J, New M I, Dupont B, Strominger J L 1985 Two genes encoding steroid 21-hydroxylase are located near the genes encoding the fourth component of complement in man. Proceedings of the National Academy of Sciences USA 82: 1089–1093

WHO Collaborative Study of Neoplasia and Steroid Contraceptives 1985 Invasive cervical cancer and combined oral contraceptives. British Medical Journal 290: 961–965

Wierman M E, Beardsworth D E, Mansfield J et al 1985 Puberty without gonadotrophins: a unique mechanism of sexual development. New England Journal of Medicine 312: 65–72

Wolff J 1983 Congenital goitre with defective iodine transport. Endocrine Reviews 4: 240–254

Wollmann H A 1997 Treatment of intrauterine growth retardation. In: Kelnar C J H, Stirling H F, Saenger P, Savage M O (eds) Growth disorders – pathophysiology and treatment. Chapman & Hall, London

Wolthers O D, Pedersen S 1990 Short term linear growth in asthmatic children during treatment with prednisolone. British Medical Journal 301: 145–148

Wonke B 1997 The effects on growth of the haemoglobinopathies. In: Kelnar C J H, Stirling H F, Saenger P, Savage M O (eds) Growth disorders – pathophysiology and treatment. Chapman & Hall, London

Wood W I 1993 Structure and functional analysis of the human growth hormone receptor. Pediatric Research 33 (suppl): S9 A35

Wu F C W, Feek C M, Glasier A 1987 Long-term pulsatile GnRH therapy in males with idiopathic hypogonadotrophic hypogonadism (IHH). Journal of Endocrinology 112 (suppl): A37

Wu F C W, Butler G E, Walker R F, Riad Fahmy D, Kelnar C J H 1988 Oral testosterone undecanoate in the induction of male puberty. Pediatric Research 24: 538 (A128)

Wu F C W, Borrow S M, Nicol K, Elton R, Hunter W M 1989 Ontogeny of pulsatile gonadotrophin secretion and pituitary responsiveness in male puberty in man – a mixed longitudinal and cross-sectional study. Journal of Endocrinology 123: 347–359

Wu F C W, Butler G E, Kelnar C J H, Sellar R E 1990a Patterns of pulsatile LH secretion before and during the onset of puberty in boys – a study using an immunoradiometric assay. Journal of Clinical Endocrinology and Metabolism 70: 629–637

Wu F C W, Butler G E, Kelnar C J H 1990b Pulsatile LH secretion during male puberty – a longitudinal study in patients with and without testosterone treatment for induction of sexual maturation. Journal of Endocrinology 124 (suppl): A182

Wu F C W, Butler G E, Kelnar C J H, Stirling H F, Huhtaniemi I 1991 Patterns of pulsatile luteinizing hormone and follicle stimulating hormone secretion in prepubertal (midchildhood) boys and girls and patients with idiopathic hypogonadotrophic hypogonadism (Kallmann's syndrome): a study using an ultrasensitive time-resolved immunofluorometric assay. Journal of Clinical Endocrinology and Metabolism 72: 1229–1237

Wu F C W, Butler G E, Brown D C, Stirling H F, Kelnar C J H 1993 Early morning testosterone is a useful predictor of the imminence of puberty. Journal of Clinical Endocrinology and Metabolism 76: 26–31

Wu F C W, Butler G E, Kelnar C J H, Huhtaniemi I, Veldhuis J D 1996 Ontogeny of pulsatile gonadotrophin releasing hormone (GnRH) secretion from midchildhood through puberty to adulthood in the human male: a study using deconvolution analyses and an ultrasensitive immunofluorometric assay. Journal of Clinical Endocrinology and Metabolism 81: 1798–1805

Yannagibashi K, Hanio M, Shively J E, Shen W H, Hall P E 1986 The synthesis of aldosterone by the adrenal cortex: two zones (fasciculata and glomerulosa) possess one enzyme for 11β, 18-hydroxylation and aldehyde synthesis. Journal of Biological Chemistry 261: 3556–3562

Ying S-Y 1988 Inhibins, activins, and follistatins: gonadal proteins modulating the secretion of follicle-stimulating hormone. Endocrine Reviews 9: 267–293

Young R J 1995 Prevention of complications. In: Kelnar C J H (ed) Childhood and adolescent diabetes. Chapman & Hall, London, pp 553–561

Zacharias L, Wurtman R 1964 Blindness: its relation to age of menarche. Obstetrics and Gynaecology 30: 507–509

Zachmann M, Vollmin J A, Hamilton W, Prader A 1972 Steroid 17,20 desmolase deficiency. Clinical Endocrinology 1: 369–385

Zachmann M, Tassinari D, Prader A 1983 Clinical and biochemical variability of congenital adrenal hyperplasia due to 11-beta-hydroxylase deficiency. A study of 25 patients. Journal of Clinical Endocrinology and Metabolism 56: 222–229

20 Inborn errors of metabolism

Chapter editor: N. R. M. Buist

Introduction   1099
N. R. M. Buist
Disorders of amino acid metabolism   1102
N. R. M. Buist   N. G. Kennaway   R. D. Steiner
Disorders of transport   1120
N. R. M. Buist   N. G. Kennaway   R. D. Steiner
**Disorders of mitochondrial energy generation
   1123**
N. R. M. Buist   N. G. Kennaway   R. D. Steiner
Disorders of carbohydrate metabolism   1131
J. Fernandes   N. R. M. Buist
Glycogen storage diseases   1135
J. Fernandes   N. R. M. Buist
**Disorders of purines, pyrimidines and DNA repair
   1140**
N. R. M. Buist   R. D. Steiner

The porphyrias   1142
R. Hume
Disorders of bilirubin and bile acid metabolism   1144
R. Hume
Disorders of metal metabolism   1145
N. R. M. Buist   R. D. Steiner
Disorders involving vitamins   1147
N. R. M. Buist   N. G. Kennaway   R. D. Steiner
Disorders of plasma lipids and lipoproteins   1148
R. J. West   N. R. M. Buist
Lysosomal storage disorders   1156
G. T. N. Besley   N. R. M. Buist
Disorders of peroxisomal function   1171
R. B. H. Schutgens   N. R. M. Buist
Inborn errors of plasma proteins   1174
N. R. M. Buist
References   1177

INTRODUCTION

References used in this chapter

Most journal articles have been eliminated; instead, we provide major textbooks and some resources that are available through electronic communication. These latter are updated every few months, are more comprehensive and should be more accessible to most readers than many of the arcane journals that are usually quoted.

The major reference is the three-volume textbook by Scriver et al (1995); it is the main resource for conditions discussed in this chapter unless otherwise indicated; the next edition will be available on CD-ROM. Four other review texts are by Holton (1994), Fernandes et al (1995), Blau & Blaskovics (1996) and Lyon, Adams & Kolodny (1996).

Radiological findings, particularly of brain MRI studies, are not extensively reviewed in this chapter; a good reference is Taybi & Lachman (1995). For laboratory techniques, Hommes (1993) is excellent.

In this chapter, a six-digit OMIM (On-line Mendelian Inheritance of Man) catalog number, if available, follows the first or main mention of each disorder (McKusick 1992); the OMIM is accessed through the Internet (*http: //www3.ncbi.nim.nih.gov/omim*).

Other useful contacts on the Internet include updated information on DNA based diagnoses and research laboratories (*http: //www.alces.med.umn.edu/vgc.html*) or through Genline (*http: //www.hslib.washington.edu/genline/index.html*).

Initial information for clinicians and for families is at *http: //hpb1.hwc.ca/healthnet.*

The Human Genome Organization can be contacted by fax on USA: (301)652–3368 and the Johns Hopkins University Genome Data Base by fax on USA: (410)614–0434.

HELIX maintains a register of DNA-based diagnoses and the laboratories that are capable of performing them (fax: USA: (206)528–2687).

An international metabolic bulletin board for any kind of inquiry is available by e-mail (*metab-l@rachael.franken.de*) or on the Internet as follows: *http; //frankende/users/daneel/c.renner/metab-l.html.*

Other resources include the Research Trust for Metabolic Diseases in Children (RTMDC), Crewe, UK (fax: UK: 1270–250244) and the National Organization for Rare Diseases (NORD), New Fairfield CT, USA (fax: USA: (203)746–8728).

GENETIC AND BIOCHEMICAL CONSIDERATIONS

The genome influences almost all disease. In the past 30 years, the boundaries between environmental, genetic and metabolic conditions, never very clear, have become increasingly obscure; the inclusion of some conditions in this chapter may seem arbitrary but the principles and the diagnostic approaches that apply to standard metabolic disorders also apply to an increasing array of other genetic disorders. Over 400 conditions are discussed in this chapter; others, such as the metabolic endocrinopathies (Ch. 19) and the metabolic defects of leukocytes (Ch. 15), are presented elsewhere. Some topics, such as the numerous defects of ion channeling and membrane dysfunction, are not included at all.

Sequencing of the human genome project is resulting in very rapid identification of gene location, gene function and gene families. Because the field is growing so fast, we have elected not to give gene locations, where known, in this chapter, although they can be of help in evaluating some patients.

Molecular techniques have shown that almost every human protein may be altered by mutations that can produce amino acid substitutions, deletions, duplications or other changes in the gene product that may be neutral or deleterious. Indeed, people may be heterozygous in 20% of their genes. It was long thought that analysis of DNA would explain many of the puzzling features of phenotype and genotype variation. In fact, it has rendered the field more complicated since even two siblings with the same genotype may show markedly different phenotypes; the mutant gene(s) do not work in isolation but only in the milieu of the rest of the genome.

For some conditions a single mutation is found in all or most cases. However, most single gene diseases for which DNA diagnosis is available can be caused by several mutations and for some, hundreds of allelic variants are known. At least 75 variants of α1-antitrypsin deficiency are distributed in about 10% of the population, yet only two appear to be deleterious. As many as 40% of females are heterozygous for different (and presumably mostly benign) mutations of the HGPRT locus; in a cohort of 24 cases of Lesch–Nyhan syndrome, at least 14 had different mutations of this gene. Such genetic heterogeneity is to be expected in most inborn errors of metabolism.

Some mutations are common in certain populations and rare in others but even the high incidences of Tay–Sachs, Gaucher disease and mild congenital adrenal hyperplasia in Ashkenazi Jews are caused by several different mutations, raising questions not only of founder effects but also of selective advantages. For diseases in this population contact the Internet at http://q.continuum.net/~wrosen/list.html. Even sickle cell anemia, long known to be due to a val→glu substitution in the β6 position, can be seen with other sickling hemoglobinopathies.

Allelic mutations may give rise to a spectrum of biochemical and clinical manifestations. Examples are vitamin B_6-dependent and non-dependent homocystinuria, both due to cystathionine synthase deficiency, or the hemolytic crises which occur in the presence of oxidant drugs with only certain mutants of glucose-6-phosphate dehydrogenase deficiency. Conversely, non-allelic mutations (involving different gene loci) may result in a similar biochemical and clinical picture as in the methylmalonic acidemias.

A gene product may be totally absent, as in analbuminemia, or it may be present in normal or reduced amounts as determined by enzymatic or immunological methods. If in normal amounts, the gene product may be functionally intact and detectable only by some abnormal physical property such as altered solubility or electrophoretic mobility or its function may be totally disrupted. If reduced, it may be from a decreased rate of synthesis, as in the thalassemias, or an increased rate of destruction, as in some forms of glucose-6-phosphate dehydrogenase deficiency.

Expression of an enzyme activity usually represents the sum of the effect of two alleles. In Figure 20.1, the contribution of each allele is indicated (0–50) and the total enzyme activity is shown as a percentage. The mother (I-2) is heterozygous for an allele producing a nonfunctional protein and I-1 is heterozygous for a minor mutant. Individuals like I-3, who is a compound heterozygote with 11% of residual function, might be totally asymptomatic, be mildly affected or may only exhibit problems when the enzyme is stressed. Such heterogeneity results in 0–100% of normal activity, giving rise to severe or mild cases of a disorder even within a single pedigree.

Methods to measure the biologic activity of a protein in vitro

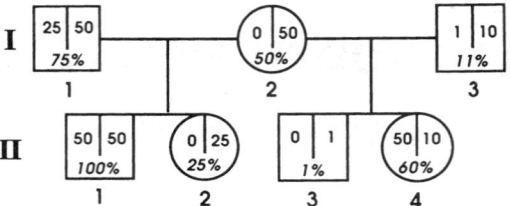

Fig. 20.1 Hypothetical pedigree showing the contribution of different mutant alleles to the total activity of an enzyme which is indicated as a percentage of the normal. Each normal allele contributes 50% of total normal function as seen in II-1. The index case II-3 has only 1% of normal activity. Case I-3 and even case II-2 might, under some circumstances, show evidence of the defect.

usually involve highly unphysiological conditions so that the results do not always reflect the in vivo activity. For example, most assays for lysosomal diseases use artificial substrates. Occasionally healthy people have no activity against an artificial substrate in vitro. Conversely, it is possible to have normal activity against an artificial substrate in vitro but no activity against the natural substrate in vivo. Enzyme assays usually use very high levels of substrate or cofactor and it is probable that some mutant enzymes can give normal activity under such conditions in vitro although not in vivo (abnormal K_m mutants). An example of this is seen in some vitamin-dependent diseases, when large doses of the vitamin cofactor improve the function of the enzyme.

The epitope of antibodies used in immunologic assays may not involve the active site of the enzyme; immunologic crossreactivity can therefore be present even though a mutant protein is functionally defective. Conversely a mutant protein can be functional but immunologically non-reactive.

Many enzymes have several distinct chemical forms in different tissues where different operating conditions may exist. Such *isoenzymes* may share some subunits but others are under separate genetic control. It is thus possible for a defect to occur in one tissue while normal activity is present in others. This must be remembered when leukocytes or cultured skin fibroblasts are used to diagnose an enzyme defect which is suspected to be present in other tissues. A further confounding fact is that some enzymes derive from a single gene but are matured to different forms in different tissues; an example is seen with an unusual form of acute intermittent porphyria in which the erythrocyte isoform is normal but the enzyme is deficient in the liver.

The potential metabolic consequences of an enzyme deficiency are illustrated in Figure 20.2. In phenylketonuria, for example, the metabolic derangements include inhibition of amino acid

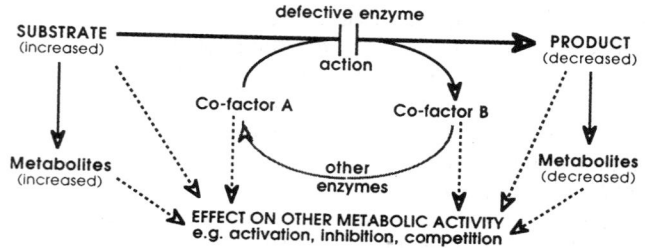

Fig. 20.2 Theoretical consequences of an enzyme deficiency.

transport into brain cells, diminished synthesis of myelin and the aromatic amines and inhibition of normal pyruvate metabolism, but it is not known how the brain damage is actually caused. Phenotypic variations even within a single family are presumed to be due to different environmental exposures or to inherited differences in the other metabolic steps which are affected by the biochemical upset. Genotype/phenotype correlations are proving to be very difficult to predict (Alper 1996).

Many metabolic disorders can be diagnosed by enzyme assay or by DNA analysis (Ch. 3) and more examples are constantly appearing. Each case needs to be considered separately, in view of the genetic heterogeneity between families. Thus when possible, the characteristics of the mutant enzyme or DNA abnormalities in the proband and the parents should be known before attempting prenatal diagnosis or carrier detection. Advances in DNA technology are leading to very rapid and accurate identification of both homozygotes and heterozygotes and will obviate the need for many of the methods currently in use.

Heterozygotes

Since heterozygotes should produce reduced amounts of the normal protein, most usually show a mild biochemical abnormality if a specific test can be devised. For example, carriers of maple syrup urine disease have normal plasma amino acid levels and cannot be detected by amino acid tolerance tests, but reduced enzyme activity can be shown in their leukocytes with sensitive techniques. On the other hand, 80% of carriers for phenylketonuria can be identified by the phenylalanine: tyrosine ratio in fasting plasma or a phenylalanine tolerance test.

Inheritance patterns

Most metabolic defects are recessively inherited. In this chapter, the genetics of each condition will not be discussed unless they vary from this pattern. With some unexpected exceptions, the OMIM catalog numbers indicate the inheritance pattern; 100000–199999 are autosomal dominant traits, 200000–299999 are autosomal recessives, 300000–399999 are X-linked, the 400000 and 500000 series are, respectively, Y-linked and mitochondrially inherited.

CLINICAL CONSIDERATIONS

Incidences

At least 1–2% of individuals have a pathogenic metabolic disorder of which most, such as hyperuricemia and the hyperlipidemias, are of little clinical importance in childhood. Almost all of the conditions in this chapter are rare (~1:100 000–1:250 000); many are extremely rare (10^{-6}–10^{-7})). However, if there are 1000 diseases each occurring only one in a million, 1 : 1000 people will have one of them and for *each* of these conditions, 1 : 500 is a carrier! This rarity constitutes a major diagnostic stumbling block for clinicians. Given these odds, the diagnosis of very rare disorders always raises the possibility of incest. Rough estimates of incidence are given for major disorders in italics in parentheses; there are huge regional variations.

Apart from gout and hyperlipidemia in adults, the commonest reasons for referral to our metabolic clinic in descending order are:

- suspected or confirmed lactic acidosis
- suspected or confirmed metabolic neurologic disorders
- metabolic bone diseases such as rickets (usually vitamin D resistant)
- abnormal results from newborn screening
- suspected or confirmed porphyria
- failure to thrive or to grow
- acute 'metabolic' crisis
- visceromegaly.

Clinical features

Metabolic disorders should always be considered when patients present with puzzling or unexplained problems whether of growth, development or of specific organ pathology. They can disrupt the function of any organ and may present at any age to specialists in any clinical discipline. It is therefore impossible to prepare a comprehensive guide to assist in recognizing all these disorders, but some of the more usual characteristics of metabolic disorders are displayed in Table 20.1.

Metabolic screening

Because of this diversity and the fact that the symptoms mimic nongenetic disorders, some kind of 'metabolic screen' is frequently done on blood or urine of potential cases in the hope that an abnormality may assist in the diagnosis. This screening is different from the newborn screen and varies in different centers but usually includes tests for sugars, mucopolysaccharides, amino acids and a variety of other compounds. Sometimes, organic acids and carnitine derivatives are included. It must always be remembered that these are only screening tests and that many disorders can not be detected by them. Nonetheless, examination of urine and possibly plasma or spinal fluid, for abnormal metabolites should be done in patients suspected of having a

Table 20.1 Some common presentations of metabolic diseases

Neonatal symptoms – see Ch. 5
CNS symptoms
    Developmental delay – static or progressive
    Movement or psychiatric disorder
    Seizures, neuropathy
    Cerebral palsy – athetoid, ataxic, spastic, hypotonic
Growth failure/failure to thrive
Episodic symptoms such as anorexia, vomiting, lethargy, coma
Gastrointestinal – anorexia, vomiting, diarrhea, malabsorption
Hepatocellular damage/visceromegaly
Renal dysfunction – Fanconi syndrome calculi
Ophthalmic – keratitis, cataracts, buphthalmos, retinopathy, optic atrophy
Auditory – nerve deafness
Muscular – cramps, myoglobinuria, weakness, wasting, loss of endurance
Cardiomyopathy
Osteodystrophies
Immune defects – leukocyte dysfunction
Dysmorphic features
Dermatologic – rashes, ulcers, cutis laxa
Metabolic acidosis, hypoglycemia

metabolic disease. In most centers, the cost of such testing is less than that of a CT scan.

Large-scale metabolic screening in retarded patients has led to the discovery of many new defects. Most are rare and the clinical variation even in diseases such as phenylketonuria can be considerable. When an unusual defect is associated with clinical symptoms it is tempting to assume that they are causally related. However, it is now clear that some are not consistently associated with clinical disease. Amino acid disorders once thought to cause retardation but now considered benign include cystathioninuria, methionine adenosyl transferase deficiency, some hyperlysinemias, saccharopinuria, α-ketoadipic aciduria, sarcosinemia, trimethylaminuria, hyperprolinemia, hydroxyprolinemia, histidinemia, carnosinemia, urocanic aciduria, β-aminoisobutyricaciduria and most group renal amino acidurias.

THERAPEUTIC CONSIDERATIONS

Roughly 12% of metabolic diseases are markedly ameliorated by therapy; in about 55%, treatment is clearly beneficial but in the remainder, treatment has little effect (Treacy et al, 1995). The only treatment for most enzyme defects is either to induce activity, as in the vitamin-responsive conditions, or to counteract the biochemical disturbance by diet or, occasionally, with drug therapy. There is no assurance, however, that correction of the biochemical defect will improve the symptoms since their basic cause is not usually known (Fig. 20.2). For example, in the Lesch–Nyhan syndrome, the blood urate is easily controlled with allopurinol, but the neurological symptoms are unchanged.

Parenteral administration of a protein requires that it must arrive at the site where it can function normally. For example, IgG deficiency can be treated by injections of gammaglobulin, but *secretory* IgA deficiency cannot. The half-life of many plasma proteins is so short that it is not feasible to replace them routinely by infusion of plasma. On the other hand, fresh plasma or plasma concentrate can be life saving, for example in hemophilia or hereditary angioneurotic edema.

Attempts to replace intracellular enzymes present formidable problems. In the first place, there must be adequate supplies of a stable, active product, which is nonallergenic. Secondly, the target cells must be able to take up the protein into the appropriate organelle, such as a lysosome, where it can function without being destroyed. Treatment of Hurler syndrome with infusions of fresh plasma is ineffective, which is not unexpected, but it is disappointing since cultured fibroblasts from Hurler and Hunter syndromes are mutually corrective in vitro. When some other lysosomal enzymes are infused, they are rapidly taken up by the liver, but not by the central nervous system. Infusion of genetically engineered human β glucosidase is dramatically effective in Gaucher disease but can cost more than £50 000/year. Similar therapy in Fabry disease lowers the abnormal plasma lipid and reduces symptoms. Experimental therapy with liposomes, fibroblasts, placental tissue and entrapment of the missing enzyme in red cell ghosts or polyethylene glycol are not promising. Bone marrow transplantation offers the possibility of 'cure' of lysosomal disorders not involving the brain, but is increasingly used in some that do involve the CNS. While some reports are encouraging, the long-term benefit is not known and its use in such cases should still be considered experimental. Liver transplantation for hepatocellular disorders, such as tyrosinemia type 1, α1-antitrypsin deficiency, ornithine transcarbamylase deficiency and Wilson disease amongst others, has been successful. Gene therapy for adenosine deaminase deficiency is currently under trial and seems promising but real gene therapy is still in the future.

DISORDERS OF AMINO ACID METABOLISM

GENERAL CONSIDERATIONS

The nutritional characteristics of proteins and amino acids are discussed in Chapter 21. Hydrolysis of protein to oligopeptides and free amino acids in the gut is controlled by enzymes which may be defective as a result of a hereditary disorder (Ch. 11).

Figure 20.3 shows the possible metabolic fate of plasma amino acids which normally are maintained within narrow limits, although they are also affected by nutrition, systemic diseases and hormones. Insulin and glucagon usually lower the plasma levels; conversely, many amino acids stimulate the release of insulin and other hormones. In obesity and early in fasting, the branched chain amino acids may be elevated. In starvation the essential

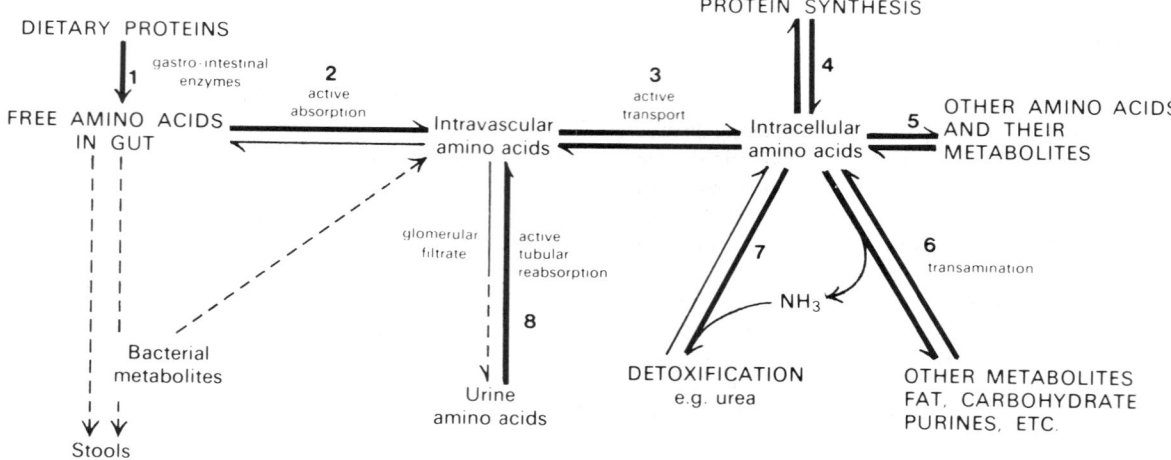

Fig. 20.3 Potential metabolic fate of amino acids. Numbers represent processes requiring active metabolism where congenital defects could occur. Dotted lines represent processes independent of metabolic activity.

amino acids are low and the non-essential amino acids may be elevated, although alanine, a major gluconeogenic substrate, is usually low. In sepsis, stress, renal failure and liver disease, there may be considerable changes, liver disease often causing marked elevation of methionine and tyrosine.

In Reye syndrome plasma levels of glutamine, alanine, proline, lysine, α-aminobutyric acid, methionine, leucine, isoleucine and taurine are markedly elevated. In early life, high protein intake and immature regulatory systems may cause major elevations of many amino acids. The level of free amino acids in intracellular fluid is about 10 times higher than in the plasma.

In PKU, the blood phenylalanine may be 20–60 times above normal. Conversely, a rise of alanine only 10–20% above normal may be the first indication of serious lactic acidosis or hyperammonemia. In some conditions, such as argininosuccinic aciduria and non-ketotic hyperglycinemia, the amino acid is excreted readily in the urine and blood levels may be only mildly abnormal, although in both these conditions the level is markedly increased in the cerebrospinal fluid.

The quantity of amino acids in urine can vary over 10-fold in normal people and depends greatly upon age and nutrition. The levels are higher in infants but the range is so wide that normal values are hard to establish; Table 37.2 is only a general guideline. Values expressed per unit volume are worthless and even when calculated per mg creatinine or per m², may be misleading. The predominant amino acids in urine (% of total amino acids in parentheses) are glycine (20–25%), taurine (5–15%), histidine (10–20%) and glutamine (7–10%). Normally, renal tubular reabsorption is nearly 100%, notable exceptions being histidine and glycine. In early infancy, many amino acids may be reabsorbed poorly, adult rates being reached by 3–6 months. Normal urine contains many metabolites arising from the diet, from drugs or from bacterial action in the gut; these compounds often pose diagnostic problems since many are detected on amino acid or organic acid analyses (Chalmers & Lawson 1982, Sweetman 1991).

The term *aminoaciduria* indicates that the urinary amino acids are greater than normal. This can be due to raised levels in the blood caused by a defect of amino acid catabolism which increases the filtered load. Conversely, renal aminoaciduria occurs when there is defective reabsorption by the renal tubular cells. Excess of a single amino acid may saturate the renal absorption mechanism for others which share the same transport site and thus cause a competitive aminoaciduria.

Routine newborn blood screening tests ('Guthrie test') are discussed in Chapter 5. Routine screening of urine reveals an amino acid disorder in about one in 6000 infants; other than PKU, the commonest are histidinemia (one in 20 000), cystinuria (one in 18 000) and Hartnup disease (one in 20 000). Detection of asymptomatic patients with mild variants of many other diseases is not infrequent. Such screening is usually done qualitatively. Quantitation by amino acid analysis, high pressure liquid or gas chromatography or other methods is essential to confirm most diagnoses and to monitor therapy. These methods require sophisticated interpretation since more than 200 compounds may be detected, even in normal urine, in a single analysis.

DISORDERS OF PHENYLALANINE METABOLISM (Fig. 20.4)

Several enzyme defects cause hyperphenylalaninemia; the most common involves phenylalanine hydroxylase (step 1), which causes the condition phenylketonuria (PKU). A bulletin board for both professionals and families is available on the Internet at *http://www.wolfenet.com/~kronwal*.

Phenylketonuria (PKU) (261600) (~1 : 10 000)

'Classic' untreated cases

With rare exceptions, the disease, when untreated, causes progressive brain damage, with a loss of 40–60 points in the IQ by 1 year. By then, microcephaly, eczematous or oily skin, hypertonicity, convulsions, dysphasia, hyperactivity with purposeless movements and an abnormal EEG are usual. In infants, vomiting may mimic pyloric stenosis. The skin and hair are often fair and the irides may be pale due to competitive inhibition of tyrosinase by phenylalanine. The plasma phenylalanine is over 1.2 mmol/l; when it exceeds 0.6–1.2 mmol/l, phenylalanine and its metabolites appear in the urine. Phenylacetic acid accounts for a subtle mousey, musty odor of these patients. The same smell is frequently encountered in incontinent patients and is due to bacterial degradation of phenylacetylglutamine, a major but unimportant constituent of normal urine.

Cerebral cortical atrophy is common; the cause of the brain damage is unknown but phenylalanine or its metabolites inhibit amino acid transport, protein and lipid synthesis and a number of metabolic pathways in the brain.

In the newborn

Phenylalanine is not detectably elevated in cord blood. It starts rising within 24 h of birth and reaches levels greater than 1.2 mmol/l within a few days. It is almost invariably 0.25 mmol/l or more within 48 hours if the baby receives adequate dietary protein although rare cases may be missed if tested before the third or fourth day. Newborn infants with PKU appear to be normal and abnormal metabolites may not be excreted in the urine for several weeks. Routine screening of newborn infants for metabolic diseases is discussed in Chapter 5. Urine pterin screening is discussed below.

In older patients who were treated in childhood

It is now clear that many older children develop learning and behavior problems if the diet is relaxed or stopped. These can reverse if the diet can be successfully reintroduced but this becomes extremely hard to do because of the restrictive and unpleasant nature of the available foods.

Changes in the brain MRI of older patients are usual with abnormal signal intensity in white matter. A severe and progressive neurodeterioration is being seen in a proportion of young adults most of whom were treated in childhood but often under the more relaxed guidelines of the 1960s and 1970s. It is not known if this will prove to be a common late complication or perhaps one which could be predicted by genotype. These emerging problems have lead to the philosophy of a 'diet for life', a sentence that is draconian and many find is untenable.

Intermediate forms of hyperphenylalaninemia

About 30–50% of untreated hyperphenylalaninemics have plasma phenylalanine levels between 0.2 and 1.3 mmol/l; phenylpyruvicaciduria is variable. Most represent less severe mutations of the

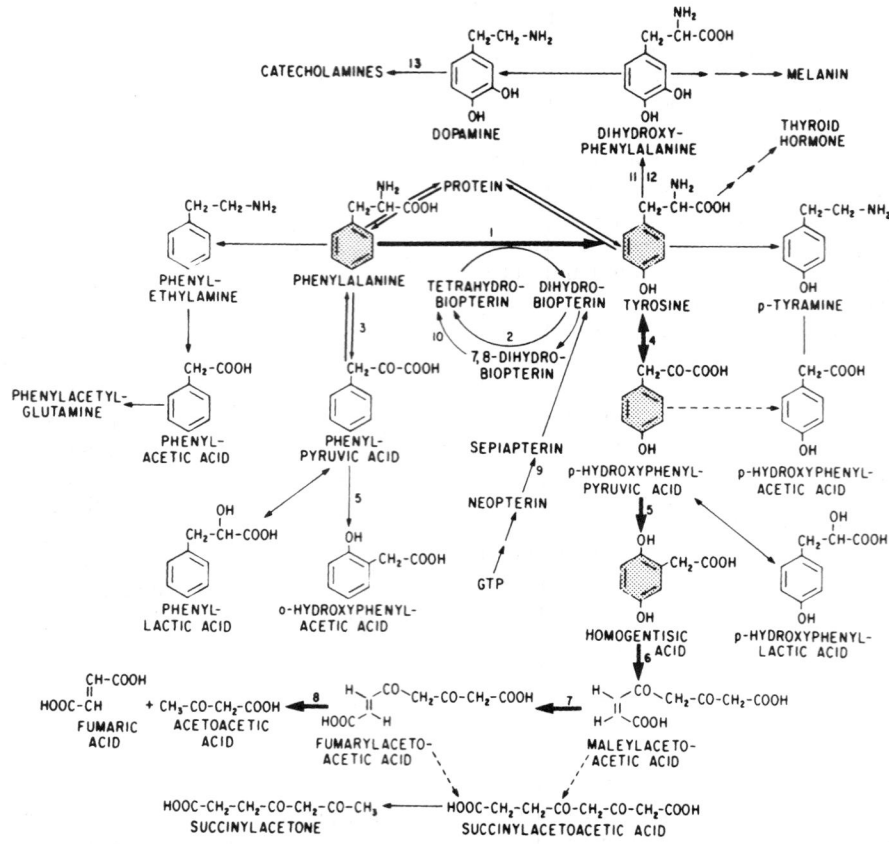

Fig. 20.4 Metabolism of phenylalanine and tyrosine. Numbers represent different genetic defects. 1, Phenylalanine hydroxylase (PKU and hyperphenylalaninemia); 2, dihydropteridine reductase (PKU, non-responsive to diet, malignant hyperphenylalaninemia); 3, phenylalanine aminotransferase (hyperphenylalaninemia); 4, tyrosine aminotransferase (tyrosinaemia, type II); 5, 4-hydroxyphenylpyruvate dioxygenase; 6, homogentisic oxidase (alcaptonuria); 7, maleylacetoacetate isomerase; 8, fumarylacetoacetase (tyrosinaemia, type I); 9, L-erythro-7,8-dihydrobiopterin synthetase (defective synthesis of biopterin); 10, dihydrofolate reductase; 11, tyrosinase (albinism); 12, tyrosine hydroxylase; 13, dopamine-{b}-hydroxylase (Riley–Day syndrome). Dotted arrows indicate non-enzymatic reactions.

hydroxylase although deficient phenylalanine transaminase might explain some cases. Brain damage is variable and depends on the chronic levels of phenylalanine and presumably individual susceptibility. However, phenylalanine can be very high in early life when the protein intake is relatively high and may remain elevated throughout life or may fall towards normal within a few months or years. Initially, such cases cannot be distinguished from the more severe cases and may be treated too vigorously. Heterozygotes for these traits may have normal results on carrier testing but DNA analysis is becoming a useful discriminant.

Transient hyperphenylalaninemia can occur during hyperalimentation and in the first 3 months of life, caused by delayed maturation of several enzymes; commonly associated with hypertyrosinemia, it appears to be benign.

Maternal hyperphenylalaninemia

Pregnancy in hyperphenylalaninemia poses a risk to the fetus which increases with higher blood levels of phenylalanine. However, as shown in Table 20.2, fetal damage may occur even at blood levels which, postnatally, are perfectly safe. In the past,

some women with intermediate forms of hyperphenylalaninemia were not retarded and were never diagnosed. Almost all such females are now normal and each year, more become adults. Most treated cases are still known but many of the milder cases have been lost to follow-up. All except the mildest cases are at increased risk of fetal damage during a pregnancy. This diagnosis should be considered in all cases of siblings with idiopathic mental retardation or microcephaly with growth delay. Children born to these mothers have elevated levels of phenylalanine in

Table 20.2 Maternal phenylalaninemia: risk of damage to fetus according to maternal phenylalanine level

	Blood phenylalanine (mmol/l)		
	>1.25	0.65–1.2	<0.625
Spontaneous abortion (%)	24	22	8
Mental retardation (%)	92	53	21
Microcephaly (%)	73	57	24
Congenital heart disease (%)	12	11	0
Low birthweight (%)	40	52	13

cord blood but the levels fall rapidly after birth and are normal within 24–48 hours of birth.

Frequent preventive counseling is essential for all these cases since the only effective treatment for the fetus is a phenylalanine-restricted diet *started before conception*. If it is started after conception, the outcome is not good. Management of adolescent females is controversial; some authorities suggest that all females should continue to take a phenylalanine-restricted formula throughout child-bearing years; others encourage sterilization. The blood phenylalanine should be maintained between 0.2 and 0.4 mmol/L through the use of elemental medical foods (p. 1119) which taste unpleasant and are poorly accepted. These cases are very difficult to manage and require intensive supervision and support, since a poorly managed diet can cause nutritional deficiencies or excesses which could also harm the fetus. Since these females are fertile, failure to control this problem could negate all the benefits of neonatal screening and could even result in an increase in the number of people with mental retardation.

Pregnancy does not appear to be a risk to the fetus in several other metabolic diseases including homocystinuria, argininosuccinic aciduria, isovalericacidemia, cystinosis, Hartnup disease, histidinemia, gyrate atrophy of the retina, galactosemia, several glycogen storage diseases, xanthinuria, Gaucher's disease, Wilson's disease and several of the porphyrias.

Diagnosis of hyperphenylalaninemia

Almost all cases are now detected by routine newborn screening (Ch. 3). At that stage, therapy is started to control the blood levels until the severity of the defect is known.

All new cases of persistent hyperphenylalaninemia should have urine and/or blood pterins fractionated and quantitated in order to differentiate the non-hydroxylase defects. In the pterin synthetic defects, a single dose of tetrahydrobiopterin 7.5–20 mg/kg p.o. usually causes a marked fall in the blood phenylalanine within 6 hours; in dihydropteridine reductase deficiency, its effect is minimal or transient and no change is seen in phenylalanine hydroxylase deficiency.

Overall, PKU occurs in about 1 in 10 000–20 000 white births but there is considerable geographic and ethnic variation. A number of RFLP haplotypes (see Ch. 3) and over 100 specific mutations occur with varying frequency in different populations. DNA methods are being used increasingly for prenatal diagnosis, genetic counseling and carrier detection and may become useful for prediction of long-term prognosis.

Heterozygotes may be detected by RFLP analysis or an oral phenylalanine tolerance test (100 mg/kg), blood levels at 1–4 hours being higher than controls. Also their fasting plasma phenylalanine:tyrosine ratio is usually greater than 1.2 : 1 although about 20% may give false results with one or both tests. Correlation of the phenylalanine:tyrosine ratio with the plasma phenylalanine is a better discriminant; pregnancy, oral contraceptives, obesity and some drugs can give false results.

Treatment

The level of phenylalanine at which brain damage can occur is not known, so most centers start treatment if the blood level exceeds 0.4–0.7 mmol/L. Elemental medical foods (Table 20.5), from which phenylalanine has been totally or partially removed, are mixed with ordinary infant formula or cow's milk or combined with a breast-feeding regime (without test-weighing) so that the total intake of phenylalanine is reduced sufficiently to maintain the blood level between 0.15 and 0.4 mmol/L. Weaning with low protein foods starts at the normal time but the special formula usually remains essential. After 2–3 years, a phenylalanine-free product remains the main source of protein and calories, but permits a larger selection of low protein foods to provide all the phenylalanine and a better variety of tastes and textures. Care must be taken to avoid the sweetener Aspartame (L-aspartylphenylalanine).

Treatment should be started as soon as possible without waiting for detailed genetic studies; if started in 2–3 weeks, the prognosis is excellent. If treatment is delayed by several weeks the outcome is more variable. Patients who are not treated until after 6 months show some improvement in IQ although they are likely to be brain damaged. Older patients usually show little change in IQ, but the diet may help to control behavior problems.

The diet should be continued as long as practical; most centers recommend life-long therapy with blood levels close to, or below, 0.6–0.8 mmol/L. By adolescence, the blood levels are usually 0.5–1.0 mmol/L or more and the restrictive diet is often the source of such great psychological turmoil in the family that it becomes too difficult to maintain. Even so, standard practice is that the formula should never be stopped, in view of the emerging risk of CNS deterioration and of the maternal PKU syndrome. If the diet is stopped after 5–7 years, structural brain damage does not seem to occur, but there is often some deterioration in IQ or in school performance and some children show minor neurological or behavioral problems. Phenylalanine restriction reverses these findings.

The phenylalanine requirement of these patients is highest (50–80 mg/kg/day for PKU) in the newborn period and gradually falls as growth slows. By 1 year it is around 20–40 mg/kg/day and by 2 years may be only 10–25 mg/kg/day. Infants with less severe enzyme deficiencies need considerably more phenylalanine since some is converted to tyrosine. Rarely, overtreatment can produce phenylalanine deficiency which causes failure to thrive, diarrhea, vomiting, eczema, napkin rash, radiological changes and, in the later stages, rising phenylalanine levels due to endogenous protein catabolism; permanent CNS damage or death may occur. During illness, plasma levels often rise rapidly due to endogenous protein catabolism. However, elevated phenylalanine is most commonly caused by too high an intake of the amino acid.

For these reasons, it is important to monitor the blood phenylalanine frequently, 2–3 times a week at the outset, reducing the frequency gradually as the management becomes clearer. By 1 year, once weekly assays may be sufficient. In some centers, the diet is stopped at 3 months for 2–4 days and daily tests are used to determine the severity of the defect. In severe cases, the phenylalanine rises over 1.2 mmol/L within 2–4 days; in milder cases it takes longer or may never reach this value. Regardless of the outcome of this challenge, the guidelines given above are still used to determine therapy.

'Malignant' hyperphenylalaninemia (<1 : 500 000)

About 1% of hyperphenylalaninemic cases have defects in one of the enzymes which regulate the cofactor tetrahydrobiopterin. The term 'malignant' implies that the standard diet therapy used for PKU does not arrest the development of seizures and progressive neurological deterioration which become evident within weeks or months of birth. Without treatment, most such cases die in the first decade. On normal diet, the blood phenylalanine is 0.27–3.5 mmol/L. *Dihydropteridine reductase* (261630) (step 2) is expressed in liver, cultured skin fibroblasts and other tissues, thus making enzymatic diagnosis possible. At least two enzyme *defects in biopterin synthesis* (261640) are also known (step 9). Tetrahydrobiopterin is also required for tyrosine and tryptophan hydroxylases. The neurological symptoms are thought to result from deficient synthesis of dopamine, serotonin and other neurotransmitters in the brain. Both temporary and partial forms have been described. Abnormal levels of biopterin due to a defect of *GTP cyclohydrolase* (128230) are reported in the CSF of adults with dominantly inherited dystonia due to *Segawa's disease* (128230).

Treatment of the biopterin synthetic defects may only require tetrahydrobiopterin (2.5–40 mg/kg/day) without dietary restriction or supplements. Dihydropteridine reductase deficiency may benefit from diet control and treatment with folinic acid (10–20 mg), L-dopa (10–95 mg/kg), 5-hydroxytryptophan (10 mg/kg), Carbidopa (5 mg/kg) or other methods to increase amine levels in the brain; Seligiline, a dopa decarboxylase inhibitor, has recently been reported to be beneficial. All these approaches are valuable but the long-term outlook is not yet clear.

DISORDERS OF TYROSINE METABOLISM (Fig. 20.4)

Several diseases cause high plasma levels of tyrosine (tyrosinemia) and excretion of tyrosine metabolites in the urine (tyrosyluria). These compounds reduce Benedict's solution and react with ferric chloride and nitrosonaphthol.

Tyrosyluria occurs in scurvy since step 5 is vitamin C dependent. It is also reported in rheumatoid arthritis, liver disease, thyrotoxicosis and megaloblastic anemia and occasionally in normal people where the cause is less well established. In malabsorption, such as cystic fibrosis, gut tyrosine is degraded by bacteria and tyrosyluria often occurs.

Neonatal hypertyrosinemia (276500)

In about 5% of prematures and some term newborns, gross tyrosinemia and tyrosyluria with secondary hyperphenylalaninemia may occur and last as long as 3 months. This is due to immaturity of liver enzymes, high protein intake or possibly suboptimal vitamin C intake of the mother and infant. These infants may show subtle learning defects in later childhood, but this is not certain. The biochemical defect is permanently reversed by lowering the protein intake to about 2.0–2.6 g/kg/day and giving 100 mg of vitamin C for several days.

Similar transient elevations of many of the plasma amino acids may occur in the newborn. They are usually associated with a high protein intake. Their long-term consequences are not known, but most are thought to be benign.

Tyrosinemia, type I (step 8) (276700) (~1 : 100 000)

Clinical features

Hepatocellular damage leading to cirrhosis and liver failure and renal tubular damage resulting in the Fanconi syndrome are the hallmarks of this condition, also referred to as hereditary tyrosinemia. Failure to thrive, rickets, thrombocytopenia and a profound clotting disorder, which may resist therapy with parenteral vitamin K, are frequent. Hypertrophic cardiomyopathy may occur. There is a severe form with rapid deterioration and death in the first weeks of life and milder cases who may survive until adult life; both may occur in the same family. In older cases hepatic carcinoma is very common. The disease occurs with increased frequency in Quebec and Scandinavia.

Diagnosis

Standard liver and kidney function tests are abnormal and the prothrombin time is markedly prolonged. The plasma tyrosine and methionine are usually, but not invariably, elevated. The serum α-fetoprotein is very high, there is generalized aminoaciduria and tyrosyluria and δ-aminolevulinic acid excretion is usually increased. Fumarylacetoacetate hydrolase activity is deficient in several tissues, which results in accumulation of powerful inhibitors of 4-hydroxyphenylpyruvate dioxygenase, δ-aminolevulinic acid dehydratase and methionine adenosyltransferase. This accounts for the abnormalities in these pathways and also forms the basis for a screening test from filter paper blood samples.

The disease should be considered in all infants and children with hepatocellular damage, especially if the family history is suggestive. Neonatal hepatitis, whether idiopathic or caused by viruses and the hepatitis of galactosemia or fructosemia may closely mimic the clinical and biochemical findings of this disease, since the blood tyrosine or methionine may be elevated by hepatocellular damage. The thrombocytopenia, profound clotting abnormality, elevated serum α-fetoprotein and urinary δ-aminolevulinic acid and the extent of the aminoacidemia and Fanconi syndrome may help to distinguish this disease. However, detection of *succinylacetone* by gas chromatography in fresh-frozen samples of urine is diagnostic since it is not excreted in other disorders. Confirmation by enzyme assay in cultured fibroblasts is feasible but false normals have been reported. A screening filter paper method to detect the enzyme and succinylacetone is highly effective and can even be used for confirmation. There are no unique histological characteristics, although hypertrophy of the islets of Langerhans is reported. Prenatal diagnosis by enzyme assay or finding succinylacetone in the amniotic fluid is possible.

Treatment consists of a low phenylalanine and tyrosine diet (300–500 mg/day; Table 20.5). This may produce considerable improvement in the clinical, biochemical and histological findings. Additional treatment for the Fanconi syndrome, such as 1,25-dihydroxyvitamin-D 3 or alkali and for the hepatocellular damage, such as vitamin K or dietary restriction of protein, may be required. A competitive inhibitor of pHPPA hydroxylase (step 5), known as NTBC, is extremely effective in reversing even severe liver damage and in reducing the level of succinylacetone to normal, but if liver damage is advanced liver transplantation is indicated and should be done as early as possible to prevent hepatic carcinoma; after transplantation, the patients still excrete succinylacetone, but appear to escape toxic damage to the transplanted liver. It is not known whether the drug can permanently prevent cancer.

Tyrosinemia, type II (step 4) (276600) (<1 : 500 000)

The Richner–Hanhart syndrome consists of corneal ulceration and unusual red, discrete raised hyperkeratotic lesions on the palms and soles together with hypertyrosinemia and tyrosyluria; about 60% have had developmental delay. Hepatic cytosol tyrosine aminotransferase activity is deficient. The eye and skin lesions are caused by tyrosine crystals and resist all conventional therapy but respond rapidly to tyrosine restriction. The relationship of the mental retardation to the metabolic defect is unclear but probably fortuitous.

Alkaptonuria (step 6) (203500) (<1 : 500 000)

A defect of homogentisic acid oxidase causes excretion of large quantities of homogentisic acid. Throughout life, homogentisic acid is deposited in cartilage where it polymerizes to a brown pigment and causes a characteristic degenerative arthritis and pigmentation of ears, nose and sclerae (ochronosis). High doses of vitamin C and a low tyrosine diet have been suggested, but their efficacy is unproven. Homogentisic acid turns brown on exposure to oxygen or alkali, reduces Benedict's reagent and Clinitest and turns ferric chloride a transient blue. The disease is often undetected in children unless discoloration of the napkin is noted.

Other disorders of tyrosine metabolism

A rarer form of tyrosinemia, *hawkinsinuria* (140350), is associated with severe metabolic acidosis and several unusual tyrosine metabolites in the urine, due to a partial abnormality of the *4-hydroxyphenylpyruvate dioxygenase* reaction (step 5) (276710). Other patients with deficient activity of this enzyme in liver, but without hawkinsinuria, have been reported; one had episodes of acute intermittent ataxia and drowsiness. *Tyrosinosis* (276800) is a term reserved for one patient described in 1932 who had myasthenia gravis and marked tyrosyluria of unknown etiology.

Congenital deficiency of *dopamine β-hydroxylase* (step 13) (223360) is associated with orthostatic hypotension, along with episodes of vomiting, coma, hypothermia and hypoglycemia; noradrenaline levels are greatly reduced (Biaggioni & Robertson 1987). A similar defect has also been shown in some cases of the *Riley–Day dysautonomia* syndrome (223900) (p. 1069) in which homovanillic acid levels are increased. Whether all such dysautonomic cases represent allelic disorders is not known

A defect of *L-aromatic amino acid decarboxylase* (107930) was found in twins with hypotonia, oculogyric crises, seizures and cerebral atrophy. L-dopa and 5-hydroxytryptophan were increased and several biogenic amines were decreased in plasma and CSF (Hyland & Clayton 1989).

A specific defect of *tyrosine hydroxylase* (191290) (Wevers et al 1996) is one cause of recessively inherited Segawa's disease in which there is diurnal dystonia and what seems to be developmental delay. Treatment with L-dopa and Carbidopa results in dramatic improvement. Other disorders affecting neurotransmitters are sure to be described as assays for these compounds in CSF become available.

Goiterous cretinism is discussed in Chapter 19.

Albinism (~1 : 10–20 000)

Albinism has been recognized since ancient times and occurs in most animals and all human races. Two major forms are recognized: oculocutaneous and ocular.

Piebald syndromes, in which there is a patchy depigmentation, often associated with deafness, include the Waardenburg syndrome, Woolf syndrome and heterocyclic irides and are not considered in the group. Hypopigmentation may be acquired in conditions such as malnutrition, PKU and Menkes' kinky hair syndrome.

Oculocutaneous albinism

Sixteen forms of oculocutaneous albinism are listed in OMIM and the molecular pathology is gradually becoming clearer. Different mutations of tyrosinase have no activity (*OCA1*) (203100) or some residual activity leading to yellow OCA1B (203320) and other variants (203200, 203280, 203290). Mutations of the P gene cause *OCA2* and the depigmentation of the Prader–Willi syndrome. Other syndromes include *Hermansky–Pudlak* (203300) and *Chediak–Higashi* (214500) and dominant albinoidism (103500, 126070).

The most severe albinism occurs in tyrosinase-negative patients, in whom the absence of pigment is complete and permanent. These patients have very pale hair and skin. They have no pigmented nevi or freckles and there is a greatly increased risk of skin neoplasia. The iris is always blue or gray, there is marked nystagmus and photophobia and most patients are legally blind. Lack of retinal pigment produces a red pupillary reflex. In OCA1B, the hair is yellow or reddish and the skin and hair may show slight pigmentation; in some forms, the hair is a metallic color, whereas others may have slight pigmentation in the skin, eyes and hair. OCA2 is milder and some pigmentation usually appears with age. Some types are more frequent in certain populations; in one type, the skin and irides have a reddish tinge but visual defects are not marked. Clinically these conditions are difficult to differentiate; electron microscopic or biochemical studies of hair roots or skin may be required. All of the above are autosomal recessive traits.

In the Hermansky–Pudlak syndrome, the albinism is very variable and may be confined to the eyes. Fibrotic lung disease, colitis, gum hypertrophy and cardiomyopathy may occur and a bleeding tendency, which may be mild or severe, is caused by a defect in platelet metabolism. Abnormal ceroid is present in the urine, leukocytes and bone marrow, similar to that seen in ceroid lipofuscinosis (p. 1171). In the Chediak–Higashi syndrome the albinism is less marked, the irides may be brown but the retina is depigmented and the hair has a metallic tinge. There are giant inclusions in the leukocyte lysosomes and leukotactic functions are defective, usually leading to marked susceptibility to infection and death in childhood. The black locks albinism and sensorineural deafness syndrome (*BADS*) and *Cross syndromes* (257800) include severe albinism and microphthalmia, cloudy corneas, cataracts or deafness and severe mental retardation, but are not considered as true albinism.

The incidence of both tyrosinase-positive and negative albinism is about 1 in 35 000, but in some genetic isolates the condition may be as common as 1 in 100. The other syndromes are less common.

Ocular albinism

In ocular albinism, the depigmentation is confined to the eyes and four syndromes are recognized. Two, Nettleship-Falls (*OA-I*) (300500) and albinism with sensorineural deafness (300700), are

X-linked. In the former, the hemizygous males have blue-green irides which may darken with age; nystagmus, strabismus and photophobia are severe and vision is usually markedly impaired. Rarely, heterozygous females are affected, presumably reflecting inactivation of the normal gene by lyonization of the X chromosome. In these rare females, the diagnosis can be confused with the autosomal recessive condition. The Forsius–Eriksson syndrome or Aland Island disease (*OA-II*) (300600), in which there is retinal depigmentation, is also X-linked. The condition can be associated with muscular dystrophy and adrenal hypoplasia in an X-microdeletion syndrome. Autosomal recessive ocular albinism (203310) and a dominantly inherited form with lentigines and deafness are also known.

Treatment

Albinos should avoid sunlight, both for their comfort and to diminish the risk of skin cancer. Sunscreen preparations with a sunscreen protection factor (SPF) of 25–50 are helpful; p-aminobenzoic acid, 5% in ethanol and titanium-based creams are cheap and quite effective. Tinted glasses, good ophthalmological supervision and regular examination of the skin for malignancies are required. Patients with the Hermansky–Pudlak syndrome should avoid aspirin-like drugs.

DISORDERS OF THE SULFUR-CONTAINING AMINO ACIDS (Fig. 20.5)

Methionine plays an important role in methylation reactions. Some is resynthesized from homocysteine by two separate

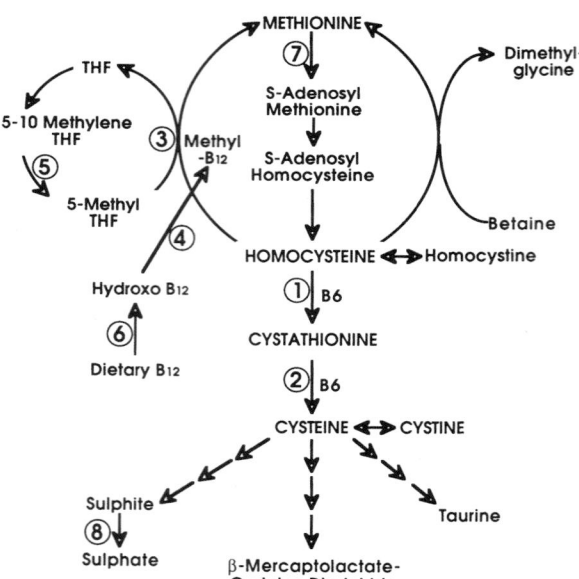

Fig. 20.5 Metabolism of the sulfur-containing amino acids. 1, Cystathionine synthase (homocystinuria); 2, cystathioninase (cystathioninuria); 3, 5-methyltetrahydrofolate-homocysteine methyl transferase; 4, cobalamin-activating system (homocystinuria and methylmalonic aciduria); 5, 5,10-methylenetetrahydrofolate reductase (homocystinuria); 6, gut absorption and reduction of vitamin B_{12} (homocystinuria and methylmalonic aciduria); 7, methionine adenosyltransferase (hypermethioninemia); 8, sulphite oxidase (sulfite oxidase deficiency). THF — tetrahydrofolic acid.

pathways, one of which interdigitates with folate metabolism and the 1-carbon pool. This uses one of only two known enzymes which require vitamin B_{12} as a cofactor, so that some defects of folate or vitamin B_{12} metabolism can cause accumulation of homocysteine. The disulfides, homocystine and cystine, are formed from two molecules of homocysteine and cysteine respectively. In proteins, two molecules of cysteine condense to form disulfide bonds which help to maintain the three-dimensional shape of the protein. Homocystine is not present in protein. Cystinuria and cystinosis are discussed on pages 1121 and 1123, respectively.

Breast milk contains taurine which is also present in high levels in muscle, leukocytes and other tissues; it is frequently excreted in large quantities as a result of liver disease, a high protein intake, leukemia or endogenous protein catabolism. No primary defect of taurine metabolism is known and its role in metabolism is unclear.

Homocystinuria

Homocystinuria can be caused either by defects in cystathionine synthase (step 1) or in the methionine recycling pathway (steps 3–5). Different mutations of cystathionine synthase result in varying response to pyridoxine both in vivo and in vitro but about half of such cases respond completely to this therapy due to its effect in stabilizing the mutant enzyme.

Cystathionine synthase deficiency (236200) (~1 : 250 000)

Clinical features

Infants usually appear normal but later, osteopenia with kyphoscoliosis, pectus excavatum or carinatum, genu valgum and pes cavus are common. The appearance may resemble Marfan's syndrome (Ch. 24) with arachnodactyly and long limbs. Often, however, the likeness is not striking and hypermobility of the joints is not marked; some patients may show few physical abnormalities. Dislocation (usually downward) of the lens develops and usually results in myopia and often in optic atrophy, glaucoma, cataract and retinal detachment. Commonly, the hair is fair and easily broken. The skin tends to become coarsened with telangiectasia and acne. Hepatomegaly is caused by fatty infiltration; standard liver function tests are usually normal. About 50% of these patients are developmentally delayed and those with normal intelligence often have psychiatric problems, which include nervousness, withdrawal and schizophrenic-like reactions.

There is a greatly increased tendency to develop intravascular thrombosis. Intermittent claudication, renal artery stenosis, coronary and carotid artery occlusions, portal vein thrombosis and pulmonary embolism have been reported. This disease should be considered in all patients with acute infantile hemiplegia. Cardiac arrhythmias are not uncommon. X-rays usually show a severe degree of osteopenia with some collapse of vertebral bodies. The physical deformities may become evident within a year. Around 1 in 200 persons is a heterozygote; recent studies suggest that minimal elevation of plasma homocystine in these cases may account for up to 10% of thromboembolic disease in adults.

Pregnancy in homocystinuric women is associated with an increased risk of miscarriage; surviving infants, at least in B_6-responsive cases, appear to be normal.

Diagnosis

The urine nitroprusside test is positive* unless the urine is very dilute; confirmation is by chromatography of the urine. Homocystine is barely detectable in normal plasma and, even in these patients, is only present in small amounts since it is rapidly cleared by the kidney.

The plasma methionine is elevated in cystathionine synthase deficiency but in methionine resynthetic defects, it is normal or low. A neonatal blood screening test is available for hypermethioninemia, but false-positive results can occur. Urinary methionine may be elevated but care must be taken to distinguish D-methionine which is contained in several infant formulae and which is absorbed from the gut and excreted unchanged in the urine. The urine test usually becomes positive within a few days of birth but may be delayed for up to 2 weeks. Carriers are best diagnosed by enzyme assay of cultured fibroblasts.

Histologically, the media of the major vessels is thin and many show evidence of thromboembolic disease. The cause of this is not known, but administration of methionine to animals causes arterial intimal damage and increased platelet adhesiveness. The zonular fibers of the lens show degenerative changes; the bones show no abnormalities to account for the osteoporosis, which may be due to disruption of the crosslinks in collagen by homocysteine.

Treatment

All patients should be treated initially with pyridoxine (100–500 mg/day) and folic acid (10–20 mg/day); if there is biochemical improvement, both vitamins should be continued for life. The aminoaciduria reappears promptly if the vitamins are stopped. In the event of pyridoxine nonresponsiveness, a higher dose of folic acid is administered together with a diet which provides only minimum requirements of methionine, 10–25 mg/kg for infants and possibly as low as 8–10 mg/kg for adults. All animal protein is withheld and protein is provided from a special formula (Table 20.5) and plant sources. Such a regimen is very hard to maintain. Betaine 6–30 g/day is used to recycle homocystine back to methionine and a supplementary source of methyl groups, such as choline (2–4 g/day), is probably advisable. Such treatment might prevent the development of complications but will not repair prior anatomic complications. Dipyridamole or low-dose aspirin should be used for anticoagulation. Oral contraceptives should be avoided in these women due to the increased risk of thrombosis.

Other causes of homocystinuria

$N^{5,10}$-methylenetetrahydrofolate reductase deficiency (step 5) (236250) (~1 : 500 000)

This is rare and these cases have none of the physical stigmata of cystathionine synthase deficiency. Some have had severe progressive neurological deterioration leading to early death; others have presented as teenagers or adults with slowly progressive deterioration or thromboembolic disease. Recurrent episodes of psychosis, proximal muscle weakness and seizures have also been reported. The variable clinical picture may reflect genetic heterogeneity or different thrombotic events in the brain. In contrast to most cystathionine synthase cases, the plasma methionine is low and urine homocystine, although elevated, may not be detected on a screening test. Homocystinuria due to a defect of the methyl transferase (step 3, Fig. 20.5) has also been reported. Therapy with folic acid (20 mg/day), B_{12} (1 mg/day) and betaine (6–30 g/day) should also be tried, as should extra methionine and L-carnitine.

Homocystinuria with methylmalonic aciduria (236270)

Several disorders of vitamin B_{12} metabolism cause either homocystinuria or methylmalonic aciduria or both (Table 20.7). In pernicious anemia, disorders of intrinsic factor synthesis, hereditary B_{12} malabsorption and transcobalamin II deficiency, megaloblastic anemia occurs and some degree of homocystinuria and methylmalonic acidemia can be expected. These disorders respond well to therapy with appropriate cobalamin derivatives (p. 1147).

Other disorders of sulfur amino acids

Cystathionine is found almost exclusively in nervous tissue where its function is unknown. Secondary cystathioninuria is found in liver disease and in some cases of primitive neuroblastoma when it can be used both as a diagnostic test and as a means of following the effect of treatment upon the malignancy. Cystathionine does not give a positive nitroprusside test; it is detected using an amino acid analyzer. Cystathioninase deficiency (step 2) (219500) is benign.

Transient neonatal hypermethioninemia occurs in a small number of infants, most of whom are on a high protein intake. Although there are no known toxic sequelae, modest protein restriction seems warranted in view of the toxic effects of methionine in laboratory animals. It is also frequent in tyrosinemia type I and in acute or chronic hepatocellular damage from any cause. D,L-methionine is added to some infant formulae and it is also given orally to treat napkin rash. Ingestion of this causes D-methioninuria since it is absorbed but not metabolized.

Persistent hypermethioninemia occurs in methionine adenosyl transferase deficiency (step 7) (250850), which appears to be benign. In another distinct syndrome, it is associated with developmental delay and a myopathy in which the creatine phosphokinase is markedly elevated. The basic defect is unknown; methionine restriction is warranted although its long-term effects are not known. Methionine malabsorption is discussed later (p. 1122).

Sulfite oxidase deficiency (step 8) (272300) is associated with dislocated lenses and progressive neurologic disease with spasticity, choreoathetosis and ataxia. Combined sulfite and xanthine oxidase deficiency, due to a defect in molybdenum metabolism, is discussed later (p. 1147). In neither instance is the nitroprusside test abnormal. β-Mercaptolactate-cysteine disulfiduria (249650) due to a sulfur transferase deficiency has also been reported in several patients, two of whom were retarded; one had dislocated lenses. The nitroprusside test is abnormal. No therapy was proposed.

---

* Cyanide-nitroprusside test. To 2.5 ml urine at pH 8, add 1.8 ml 5% sodium cyanide. Wait 15 min. Then add 0.5 ml 0.5% sodium ferricyanide. A pink color is given by disulfides such as cystine and homocystine and with generalized aminoaciduria. (A cystinuria test, Actessa, 23 Rue Mercier, Luxembourg, is also used.)

DISORDERS ASSOCIATED WITH HYPERAMMONEMIA (~1 : 25 000)

An average diet contains excess amino acids, the nitrogen of which is mostly excreted as urea. The enzymes of the urea cycle are active before birth. Steps 1–3 are mitochondrial so the full cycle requires the transport of ornithine into and the transport of citrulline out of the mitochondria. Arginine is an important regulator of the cycle since it induces N-acetylglutamate synthetase. N-acetylglutamate, in turn, activates carbamyl phosphate synthetase.

The urea cycle is only complete in the liver where urea is synthesized. Defects at all steps of the urea cycle have been described, the common feature of which is hyperammonemia. Some of the enzymes are present in other tissues where the enzymes must have other roles. In severe liver damage, hyperammonemia is sometimes found and may contribute to the cerebral symptoms of liver failure. It is also frequent in Reye's syndrome (p. 479), probably resulting from mitochondrial damage.

Clinical features

Patients with severe defects in the urea cycle often present in the newborn period with coma and acute metabolic crisis (Ch. 5). Postnatal catabolic events and protein intake contribute to the metabolic derangement. In infancy, the symptoms are commonly episodes of poor feeding, vomiting, failure to thrive, lethargy, irritability or other neurologic symptoms, all of which are aggravated by formula changes that increase protein intake and may be alleviated by reducing the protein content of the diet. Metabolic alkalosis is frequent.

In older children, with, presumably, less severe mutations, symptoms often develop for the first time during weaning and food intolerance or distaste for protein may be evident; most have failure to thrive, developmental or neurologic problems with seizures, migraine, ataxia and abnormal electroencephalogram. Even adults may present with new onset of hyperammonemic symptoms often induced by high-protein slimming diets. All such cases are at risk for acute metabolic decompensation which can be fatal during high protein intake or even minor catabolic events induced by intercurrent illnesses such as infections, dehydration or surgery.

Transient neonatal hyperammonemia

Hyperammonemia is sometimes seen in infants receiving intravenous alimentation. In these cases it may be due to an inappropriately high nitrogen intake. Other infants with profound, but transient hyperammonemia have mostly been preterm; respiratory distress is usual. There are signs of progressive neurologic damage with apnea, loss of reflexes and coma ensuing within 12–48 h of birth. Ammonia levels may be as high as 5 mmol/L. Liver function tests and amino acid studies may be normal. If the condition is treated early and vigorously the babies rapidly improve and the prognosis is excellent. In infants who recover, the protein tolerance becomes normal and liver enzyme assays show no abnormality. The cause is unknown but rapid protein catabolism, mitochondrial dysfunction or maternal carnitine deficiency may play a role.

Enzyme defects of the urea cycle (Fig. 20.6)

N-acetylglutamate synthetase deficiency (step 1) (237310) may be detectable in the first weeks of life but appears to be readily controlled by sodium benzoate. Arginine (1 mmol/kg/day) and carbamylglutamate (1.7 mmol/kg/day), which can substitute for acetylglutamate as an activator of carbamyl phosphate synthetase, were effective in controlling hyperammonemia at a protein intake of 2 g/kg/day. Acyl-CoA derivatives such as methylmalonyl-CoA, propionyl-CoA or valproic acid derivatives can inhibit N-acetylglutamate synthesis which explains the hyperammonemia that can occur in the 'ketotic hyperglycinemias' and valproic acid toxicity.

Carbamyl phosphate synthetase I is mitochondrial and provides carbamyl phosphate for the synthesis of urea. Deficiency (step 2) (237300), usually presents with severe neonatal hyperammonemia although others may present in infancy or childhood. Prenatal detection is possible. Carbamyl phosphate synthetase II is a separate enzyme in the cytoplasm and involved in the synthesis of pyrimidines.

Ornithine transcarbamylase deficiency (step 3) (311250) is an X-linked trait. Most affected males present as newborns in severe hyperammonemic crisis and most such cases die in spite of heroic efforts at treatment. 20–30% are less severely affected and some have normal mental development and almost normal tolerance for protein except during stress. Some female carriers are totally asymptomatic while others have mild aversion or intolerance to protein and some have recurrent hyperammonemic crises which can be fatal. Even during crises, plasma amino acids are not grossly distorted; citrulline is very low, ornithine is normal but glutamine, alanine and usually lysine are increased in blood and sometimes in urine; during stress, orotic acid is usually increased in the urine and serves to distinguish this disorder from Reye syndrome. L-citrulline (100–400 mg/kg) is added to the usual therapy.

Ornithine transcarbamylase can be assayed in liver or duodenal mucosa but not in fibroblasts. Enzyme activity from multiple liver biopsies from a single female carrier may vary widely, representing different degrees of inactivation of the mutant X chromosome in different areas. Most carriers can be detected by increased urine orotic acid from 0–8 and 8–16 hours after a provocative challenge of allopurinol (100 mg/kg p.o.) either alone or together with 1.0 g protein/kg or L-alanine 0.5 g/kg p.o. DNA

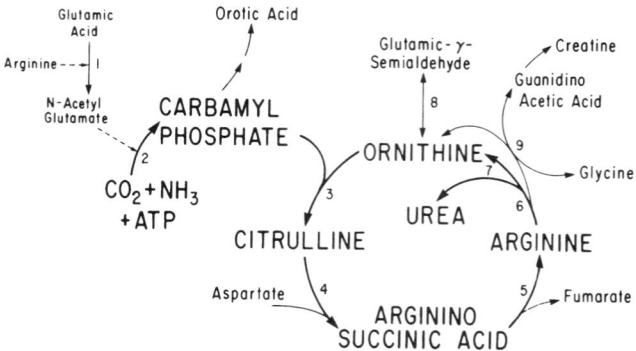

Fig. 20.6 The urea cycle. 1, N-acetylglutamate synthase; 2, carbamyl phosphate synthase; 3, ornithine transcarbamylase; 4, argininosuccinate synthase; 5, argininosuccinate lyase; 6, arginase; 7, ornithine uptake into mitochondria; 8, ornithine ketoacid aminotransferase.

analysis can now detect about 70% of gene carriers and, when possible, is best for prenatal diagnosis and carrier detection.

The clinical severity of *citrullinemia* (step 4) (215700) varies greatly, from death in the neonatal period to no symptoms at all, but most patients have been mentally retarded. Plasma and urine citrulline levels are markedly elevated, even between crises. The enzyme can be assayed in fibroblasts; prenatal diagnosis is possible. Some heterozygotes have elevated fasting plasma levels of citrulline.

Severe and mild cases of *argininosuccinic aciduria* (step 5) (207900) are known and almost all have been developmentally delayed. Trichorrhexis nodosa, an abnormal fragility of the hair, is found in some cases. The disease is easily diagnosed by chromatography of urinary amino acids since large amounts are excreted. Argininosuccinic acid is also found in the cerebrospinal fluid but is quite low in plasma. The enzyme defect can be shown in several tissues including red blood cells. Prenatal diagnosis is available. Large supplements of arginine (300–600 mg/kg/day) are added to the normal regime since urinary argininosuccinic acid provides a major pathway for waste nitrogen disposal.

Patients with *argininemia* (step 6) (207800) usually have increasingly severe pyramidal tract signs starting within the first 2 years of life. The plasma arginine is markedly raised. The urinary amino acid pattern may be similar to that seen in cystinuria, presumably caused by the high levels of arginine in the glomerular filtrate saturating the group reabsorptive site in the proximal renal tubules. Alternatively, urine amino acids may be normal or there may be a generalized aminoaciduria. Deficient arginase activity can be shown in the red blood cells of both patients and heterozygotes.

Hyperornithinemia (~1 : 500 000)

Hyperornithinemia with hyperammonemia and homocitrullinuria (*HHH syndrome*) (238970) is one of two distinct hyperornithinemic syndromes. Most reported patients have had developmental delay and older patients tend to have spasticity. Symptoms may develop at any age. Excretion of ornithine, polyamines, orotic acid and glutamine may be increased. The primary defect is in the mitochondrial uptake of ornithine (step 7). Large, bizarre mitochondria may be present in the liver. Oral ornithine supplements have been reported to be beneficial. Homocitrulline can also be formed during pasteurization of milk and, if ingested, is excreted in the urine.

Hyperornithinemia in the absence of hyperammonemia also occurs in *gyrate atrophy of the choroid and retina* (258870) which presents in adults without hyperammonemia but with a characteristic retinopathy, subcapsular cataract and progressive loss of peripheral vision leading to blindness by middle age. In children, small discrete circular patches of degeneration may be seen in the periphery of the retina; later these coalesce to form a characteristic lobular appearance which gives rise to the name. The electroretinogram, electro-oculogram and dark adaptation are abnormal. Plasma and CSF ornithine levels are markedly elevated. Ornithine ketoacid aminotransferase (step 8) is deficient in several tissues, including cultured skin fibroblasts. Heterozygotes may be detected by oral ornithine loading tests (100 mg/kg) or by enzyme assay. Abnormal inclusions have been reported in muscle and bizarre, elongated mitochondria are present in liver. Direct toxicity of ornithine, low proline or lysine or low creatine have all been suggested as a cause of the retinal damage.

Pharmacological doses of vitamin B_6, the cofactor of the mutant enzyme, improve the biochemical and ERG findings in some but not all cases. Severe, long-term arginine restriction improved visual function but such treatment is very hard to maintain. Oral creatine supplements (1–2 g/day) may improve muscle, but not retinal, function.

Secondary hyperammonemias

Other causes of hyperammonemia include the following:

Liver disease
Reye syndrome (p. 479)
Lactic acidosis (p. 1124)
The ketotic hyperglycinemias (p. 1116)
   Methylmalonic aciduria (p. 1117)
   Propionic aciduria (p. 1117)
   3-ketothiolase deficiency (p. 1118)
   3-hydroxy-3-methylglutaric aciduria (p. 1118)
Familial lysinuric protein intolerance (p. 1121)
Periodic lysinemia with hyperammonemia (p. 1113)
Neonatal glutaric aciduria type II (p. 308)
Defects of fatty acid oxidation
Valproic acid toxicity
Ureterostomy
Shock and after surgery

Diagnostic approaches

Assay of blood ammonia should be routine in any acutely sick child with neurologic findings; it is not so commonly done in patients with mild, episodic symptoms. Hyperammonemia may be present in the fasting state but is usually induced by a protein load. Great care must be taken in handling samples and in the assays – erroneously high values are common. When hyperammonemia is suspected, blood amino acids and urine organic acids should also be done routinely. Raised levels of glutamine and alanine are usual and should always suggest this possibility. In this group of disorders, blood urea and 24-h urinary urea excretion may be low or normal, suggesting that other systems for urea synthesis may exist. Patients with a defect at steps 3–6 of the urea cycle may exhibit orotic aciduria due to the diversion of carbamyl phosphate to the overproduction of pyrimidines.

Treatment

Every effort must be made to minimize catabolism for energy needs; (1 g of protein yields only 4 calories but 62 500 mg of nitrogen). Management of acute hyperammonemic crises includes the following steps:

1. maximal hydration p.o. or i.v. to enhance renal excretion
2. maximum tolerable nonprotein caloric intake p.o. or i.v. Dextrose 20–25%
3. sodium benzoate (250–500 mg/kg/day) and/or sodium phenylacetate or phenylbutyrate(250–500 mg/kg/day p.o. or i.v.) to trap ammonia in metabolites that are then excreted in the urine (Total 500 mg/kg/day)
4. gut sterilization with oral antibiotics and oral lactulose to reduce enterohepatic recirculation of nitrogen
5. anabolic steroid, aqueous testosterone (10–20 mg i.m.) for 1 or 2 days

6. L-arginine (300–400 mg/kg/day i.v. or p.o.) to enhance the urea cycle
7. L-carnitine (100 mg/kg/day) – mechanism of action is unclear
8. hemodialysis or peritoneal dialysis to remove ammonia; continuous extracorporeal hemodialysis is even better and can be continued for days if necessary
9. when blood glutamine or alanine are not elevated, citric acid cycle intermediates may be depleted and supplements of citric acid may be beneficial.

After the acute crisis, dietary protein is cautiously introduced starting at 0.5–0.75 g/kg/day. A mix of essential amino acids may be added. The protein intake is increased to the minimum daily requirement as tolerated. Chronic therapy with sodium benzoate (250 mg/kg/day), L-carnitine (50–100 mg/kg/day) and L-arginine (300–400 mg/kg/day) is usual. Although experimental, liver transplantation, if successful, should 'cure' the metabolic disease and prevent hyperammonemic brain damage but would not replace any functions of the mutant enzyme in the brain.

GLYCINE (Fig. 20.7)

Nonketotic hyperglycinemia (step 3) (238300, 238330) (~1 : 60–100 000)

Glycine enters into many biochemical pathways. Plasma glycine, along with other nonessential amino acids, may be elevated in protein malnutrition and plasma and urine glycine can be markedly elevated by valproate therapy. The term 'ketotic hyperglycinemia' has been discarded since most such patients have propionic acidemia or methylmalonic acidemia. Urinary glycine is very variable, even in normal people. Isolated hyperglycinuria is found in some iminoglycinuric carriers and in some patients with vitamin D-resistant rickets.

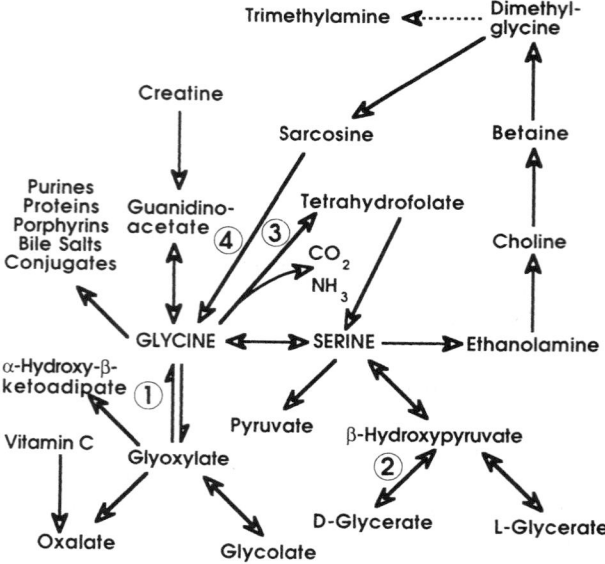

Fig. 20.7 Metabolite pathways of glycine. 1, Alanine:glyoxalate aminotransferase (peroxisomal) (type I hyperoxaluria); 2, D-glycerate dehydrogenase (type II hyperoxaluria); 3, glycine cleavage enzyme (non-ketotic hyperglycinemia); 4, sarcosine dehydrogenase (sarcosinemia).

Clinical features

Classically, nonketotic hyperglycinemia is associated with severe neurologic symptoms in the first days of life. Apnea, intractable seizures, spasticity, decerebrate rigidity and coma are usual and cause death in the neonatal period. Hiccuping occurs frequently and infants who survive have myoclonus, apathy, microcephaly, severe mental retardation and failure to thrive. The EEG may show hypsarrhythmia. Milder cases with less severe neurologic manifestations are known and there is a variant with late-onset spinocerebellar degeneration and relative preservation of cognitive functions.

Diagnosis

Plasma glycine is usually, but not invariably, elevated 10–200% above normal; the urine glycine is markedly elevated and in CSF, glycine is usually more than 10 times normal. Neutropenia and hyperammonemia may occur. Neither ketoacidosis nor organic aciduria is present. The symptoms are aggravated by valine. The diagnosis is made by quantitation of plasma, urine and CSF glycine; qualitative chromatography is unreliable. The plasma: CSF glycine ratio, normally about 30, is much reduced. The defect is in the glycine cleavage system which comprises four separate proteins; it is not expressed in fibroblasts.

Treatment

Glycine is a neurotransmitter in the spinal cord. Its action can be inhibited by strychnine and benzodiazepines which have been tried in some cases. Dextromethorphan and tryptophan have both been used with some apparent success. Sodium benzoate (250 mg/kg/day) or dialysis can remove large quantities of glycine from the body, but no therapy is known to prevent the cerebral damage.

Oxalosis (~1 : 500 000)

Calcium oxalate crystals are frequently seen in normal urine and calcium oxalate is the major constituent of about 70% of all kidney stones. In most of these cases, oxalate metabolism is normal. Oxalic acid used to be employed to commit suicide. Oxalosis is characterized by overproduction of oxalate. Type I oxalosis is due to a defect of *peroxisomal alanine glyoxylate aminotransferase* (259900): type II is caused by deficiency of *D-glycerate dehydrogenase* (step 2) (260000). The mechanism of increased synthesis of oxalate in type II oxalosis is not clear. Both defects can be shown in different tissues.

Clinical features

In both type I and type II oxalosis, renal oxalate stones develop and usually progress to nephrocalcinosis and renal failure. Symptoms may start in infancy, with death before the age of 10, although survival until the sixth decade is known. In type I, crystals of oxalate deposit in the kidney, muscle, heart, bone, bone marrow, joints and blood vessels.

Diagnosis

The diagnosis is made by finding characteristic birefringent crystals in the tissues and increased oxalate in the urine (normal adult <0.55 mmol (50 mg)/24 h). The two forms are distinguished by the excretion of large quantities of glyoxylate and glycollate in type I and L-glycerate in type II. Urinary oxalate is normal in heterozygotes, although rare families with dominantly transmitted hyperoxaluria are known. At postmortem, microscopic oxalate crystals can be seen in most tissues. A similar but lesser degree of tissue deposition of oxalate may also occur in some other types of renal failure.

Of the small amount of oxalate in normal urine, 30–50% is derived from ascorbic acid; the remainder comes either from the diet (10–40%) or from glycine (10–40%). Curiously, ingestion of large quantities of vitamin C usually barely increases the urinary oxalate because its catabolism is limited. However, in a few patients it results in marked oxaluria; these individuals are clearly at risk of renal calculus formation.

Hyperoxaluria with calculus formation may occur in patients with malabsorption, ileal resection or inflammatory bowel disease. In these cases, the oxalate is derived by gut bacteria from dietary precursors and glyoxylate and L-glycerate excretion are normal. Pyridoxine deficiency and ethylene glycol poisoning also cause oxaluria.

Treatment.

This includes alkalinization of the urine, dietary restriction of calcium and a large fluid intake to improve the urinary flow. Rhubarb, spinach, beets and cocoa are foods high in oxalate and should probably be avoided, particularly in patients with gastrointestinal hyperabsorption of oxalate. Only minimum daily requirements of vitamin C should be allowed. Some type I patients respond well to oral pyridoxine (200–500 mg/day), possibly by increasing conversion of glyoxylate to glycine. Transplanted kidneys are damaged by the continuing high levels of oxalate and this therapy is not effective unless oxalate overproduction can be prevented by drugs or by combined kidney and liver transplantation.

Other disorders of glycine metabolism

Trimethylaminuria (275700) is caused by malabsorption of choline and is recognized by the presence of an odor described as putrefying fish, although to us it is more like fresh cod. Most patients have been asymptomatic apart from the offensive odor which persists on the skin despite frequent washing. The amine arises from bacterial catabolism of dietary choline. In patients who feel a social stigma, a choline-reduced diet; intermittent courses of oral neomycin or metronidazole are very helpful and the use of phosphocellulose 10% applied as a deodorant in powder or wax is also advised.

D-glycericacidemia (238310) has presented with hypotonia, choreoathetosis, developmental delay, failure to thrive, recurrent infections, nonketotic hyperglycinemia and severe metabolic acidosis. The symptoms are aggravated by fructose. The relationship, if any, of this disorder to type II oxalosis is not clear. *Sarcosinemia* (step 4) (268900) is also reported; its role in the multiple acyl-CoA dehydrogenase deficiencies is discussed on page 1130.

LYSINE

Glutaric acidemia (type 1) (231670) (~1 : 250 000)

During the first months of life these infants appear to be normal until the onset of encephalopathy, which may be sudden or gradual. Macrocephaly, with dilated ventricles, seizures, dystonia and dyskinesia with progressive motor delay and fevers then develop, often exacerbated during infections; the development of a Reye's-like syndrome is probably caused by carnitine depletion. The urine usually, but not invariably, contains glutaric acid and 3-hydroxyglutaric acid and the diagnosis should always be considered in children with dystonic cerebral palsy. A low lysine diet improves the organic aciduria and riboflavin (200–300 mg/day) and L-carnitine (100–150 mg/kg/day) should be used but may not affect the outcome.

Other disorders of lysine metabolism

Mutations of a bifunctional enzyme, lysine ketoglutarate reductase and saccharopine dehydrogenase, may compromise either one or both functions; consequently, *hyperlysinemia* (238700) or *saccharopinuria* (268700) may occur together or separately. In α-aminoadipic aciduria (204750) the amino acid is increased in the blood and the urine and the keto acid in the urine. All these defects are now considered benign.

Lysine dehydrogenase deficiency is associated with neonatal hyperammonemia; plasma lysine and arginine and urinary lysine are increased. Protein restriction is warranted. The hyperammonemia may have been caused by inhibition of arginase by lysine.

Hydroxylysinemia (236900) has been found in several mentally retarded patients. The amino acid comes solely from collagen, where lysine is hydroxylated after incorporation into protocollagen. However, collagen metabolism was normal and the disorder was due to a defect in the metabolism of free hydroxylysine. A defect in lysine hydroxylation is found in Ehlers–Danlos syndrome type VI (225400). *Crotonic acidemia* with severe metabolic acidosis but without hypoglycemia has been reported; ketone bodies were increased. Lysine, palmitate and butyrate oxidation were impaired in leukocytes where crotonase activity was also reduced.

Secondary hyperlysinemia is usual in Reye's syndrome and in ornithine transcarbamylase deficiency. Pipecolic acid metabolism occurs in peroxisomes and is discussed on page 1173.

IMINO ACIDS

The imino acids are proline and hydroxyproline. Hydroxyproline is synthesized in situ from proline in precursor collagen molecules. In early infancy, both free proline and hydroxyproline are normally excreted; the latter is increased during growth and in diseases with increased collagen turnover such as rheumatoid arthritis, burns, rickets, scurvy, Marfan's syndrome and malignancy. After infancy, both are normally excreted only as small peptides. If hydroxyproline is excluded from the diet (no meat, fish, fowl, broth, gelatin or ice cream) total urinary hydroxyproline can be used as an index of endogenous collagen degradation. Plasma proline can be considerably elevated in renal failure or in certain mitochondrial disorders. *Iminoglycinuria* is discussed on page 1121.

Hyperprolinemia is found in proline oxidase (type I) (239500) and Δ1-pyrroline-5-carboxylate dehydrogenase (type II) (239510) deficiencies. Type I was reported in several kindreds with familial nephritis (Alport's syndrome) but the association is fortuitous. Type II has been found in several families, in some associated with mental retardation or seizures, in others with no symptoms. Plasma proline is high and the urine usually contains proline, hydroxyproline and glycine due to competitive inhibition of reabsorption by the renal tubules. In type II, Δ1-pyrroline-5-carboxylic acid is also excreted. Since the defects appear to be benign, treatment is unwarranted. Offspring of maternal hyperprolinemics have been normal.

After infancy hydroxyproline is barely detectable in plasma. Of the known cases of *hydroxyprolinemia* (237000), some were severely retarded while others were normal. No treatment was effective in lowering the plasma hydroxyproline and none is warranted.

Small quantities of several iminodipeptides, originating either from dietary or endogenous collagen, are excreted by normal people. Massive, generalized iminodipeptiduria occurs in *prolidase* deficiency (170100), an enzyme which normally degrades the dipeptides and returns them to the metabolic pool. Some patients are asymptomatic, others have developmental delay and often a chronic erythematous weeping dermatitis most marked on the hands, feet and face, splenomegaly with hypersplenism, recurrent infections and a collagen disorder similar to lathyrism. Therapy with vitamin C and Mn^{2+} has been tried but seems ineffective.

TRYPTOPHAN (Fig. 20.8)

1 mg of nicotinic acid is derived from 60 mg of tryptophan. This may seem trivial, but tryptophan deficiency and several disorders of tryptophan metabolism can cause pellagra. The incidence of these disorders is unknown because these compounds are not readily detected by most 'metabolic screening' tests. Pellagra-like symptoms may also occur in vitamin B_6 deficiency, secondary to prolonged treatment with isoniazid.

Dihydropteridine reductase deficiency (step 2, Fig. 20.4), one cause of PKU, also inhibits conversion of tryptophan to serotonin; this may be responsible for the mental symptoms seen in these patients.

Tryptophanemia (276100) due to tryptophan pyrrolase deficiency (step 2) is associated with pellagra-like symptoms, developmental delay and sometimes with ataxia and failure to thrive. Urine tryptophan is increased and excretion of its metabolites is reduced after a tryptophan load. Niacin should eliminate the symptoms of pellagra but may not affect the retardation.

Several other disorders, which may all represent aspects of the same metabolic defects, have been described. In all of them, nicotinic acid deficiency is to be expected and there is exaggerated excretion of various metabolites, either fasting or following an oral tryptophan load. *Kynureninase* deficiency (278600) is thought to be the basis of both xanthurenic aciduria and hydroxykynureninuria. The carcinoid syndrome, in which large amounts of dietary tryptophan are converted to serotonin and excreted as indole acetic acid, may also be associated rarely with pellagra-like symptoms.

Unabsorbed tryptophan is degraded by gut bacteria leading to absorption of indoles that are metabolized and/or conjugated by the liver and excreted in the urine as indican. This occurs in malabsorption and constipation, patients with transport disorders (p. 1120) such as Hartnup disease and the blue diaper (napkin) syndrome.

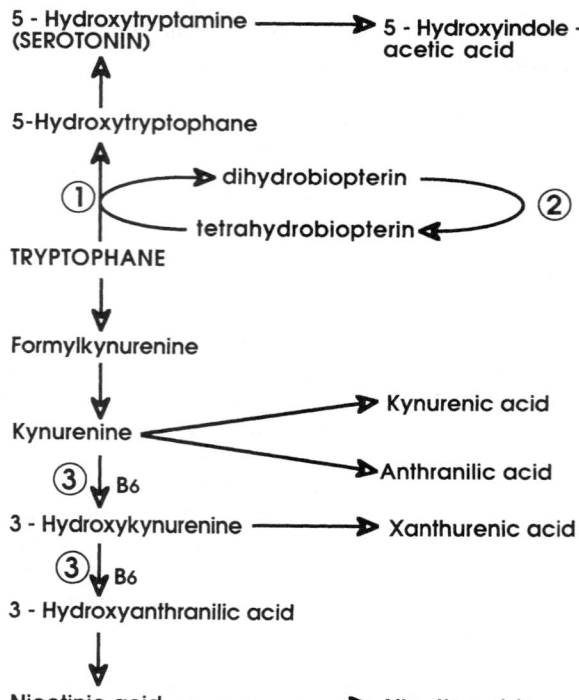

Fig. 20.8 Metabolism of tryptophan. 1, Tryptophan hydroxylase (tryptophanemia and tryptophanuria); 2, dihydropteridine reductase (atypical PKU); 3, kynureninase (xanthurenic aciduria and hydroxykynureninuria).

HISTIDINE

Histidine is normally excreted in large amounts. Its major metabolites in normal urine are 1- and 3-methylhistidine, anserine and carnosine; the range of normal values is very large. Carnosine (β-alanyl-histidine) is a normal constituent of muscle and brain and homocarnosine (γ-aminobutyrylhistidine) is found in CSF and brain. Anserine (β-alanyl-1-methylhistidine) is found in some mammals and birds. Small amounts of 3-methylhistidine are present in actin. Excretion of any or all of these compounds is increased by ingestion of flesh. On a meat-free diet, their excretion reflects endogenous muscle catabolism.

Histidinemia (1 : 20 000), caused by deficiency of histidase (235800), was thought to cause mental retardation and speech disorders. However, it is now clear from neonatal screening that this is not the case. Blood, urine and CSF histidine are increased and after some weeks imidazole derivatives are excreted. No treatment is indicated. Both paternal and maternal histidinemia appear to be benign.

Progressive neurological deterioration with spasticity and myoclonic seizures have been reported in several patients with *serum carnosinase* deficiency (212200), but others were clinically normal. Tissue and blood carnosine levels may be normal but urine contains about 0.5–1.0 mmol/g creatinine; anserine is also increased. Serum carnosinase activity is deficient but the tissue isozyme is normal. Elevated levels of homocarnosine (236130) in the CSF have been associated with progressive spastic paraplegia, developmental delay and retinal pigmentation; it is probably caused by a variant of serum carnosinase deficiency.

Excess histidine, carnosine, anserine and 1-methylhistidine have been found in the urine in several families with a form of cerebromacular degeneration. *Histidinuria* (235830) has been reported in a number of conditions including pregnancy. The mechanism is not clear.

Urocanic aciduria (276880) due to deficient hepatic urocanase activity has been described in several mentally retarded patients but also in some normal children. *Formiminoglutamic aciduria* (229100) is described under folic acid metabolism (p. 1147).

THE γ-GLUTAMYL CYCLE (Fig. 20.9) (~1 : 500 000)

This cycle involves both the synthesis of glutathione and the transmembrane uptake of amino acids; the former seems to be the main function since most patients with defects in the cycle do not have aminoaciduria. Defects of this cycle tend to be associated with hemolytic anemia, probably because of the reduced level of glutathione in erythrocytes. Conditions which predispose to hemolysis should be avoided; high-dose vitamin E therapy and other antioxidant approaches have been tried but they do not seem to be effective in increasing glutathione levels. Small amounts of glutathione can be found in the plasma and urine of normal people. Increased levels have been found in a few mildly retarded adults with *γ-glutamyl transpeptidase* deficiency (step 1) (231950) in cultured skin fibroblasts. No anemia or acidosis was noted and concentration of amino acids in serum and renal tubular reabsorption of most amino acids were normal. *γ-Glutamyl transferase* deficiency (step 2) has also been found in some patients with psychiatric disease but also in two normal siblings.

γ-Glutamylcysteine synthetase deficiency (step 4) (230450) is associated with developmental delay with spinocerebellar degeneration, peripheral neuropathy, hemolytic anemia and low erythrocyte glutathione levels. These patients had a generalized aminoaciduria which tends to confirm some role of the cycle in amino acid transport.

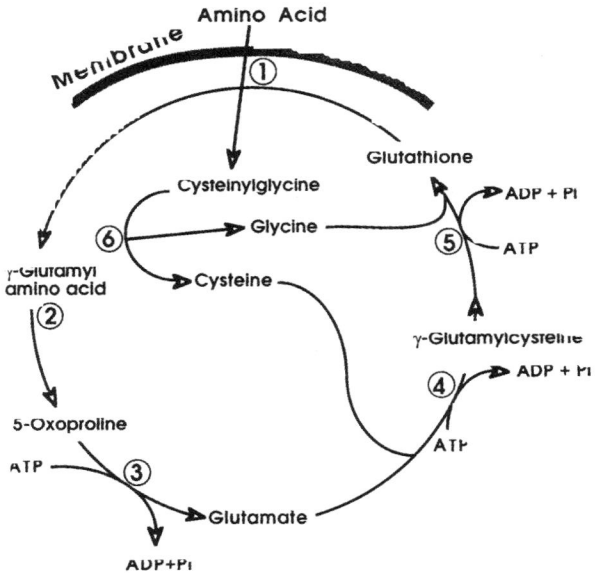

Fig. 20.9 The γ-glutamyl cycle. 1, Gamma-glutamyl transpeptidase; 2, γ-glutamyl cyclotransferase; 3, 5-oxoprolinase; 4, γ-glutamyl-cysteine synthase; 5, glutathione synthase; 6, peptidase.

Pyroglutamic aciduria (266130)

Defective function of two enzymes in this cycle cause the accumulation of large quantities of pyroglutamic acid which is excreted in the urine. Infants with severe *glutathione synthetase* deficiency (step 5) usually present in the newborn period with minimal neurological findings but with severe metabolic acidosis which may require 15–20 mEq/kg/day of sodium bicarbonate to correct. The acidosis tends to lessen and may disappear as the children grow. In addition there is severe hemolytic anemia, but it too diminishes as the children grow and disorders of phagocytosis can occur. These recur during times of metabolic stress and later, most but not all cases exhibit some neurological deterioration and developmental delay. Patients with less severe unstable mutants of glutathione synthetase (231900) usually have hemolytic anemia *without acidosis* since the labile enzyme is severely reduced only in the red blood cells where it cannot be replenished.

Oxoprolinase deficiency (step 3) (260005) does not cause metabolic acidosis, anemia or neurological deterioration and may be a benign condition. Excretion of pyroglutamic acid is much less than in glutathione synthetase deficiency. One woman with this defect had several children, all of whom had major congenital malformations.

ω-AMINO ACIDS*

The five ω-amino acids include β-alanine and β-aminoisobutyric acid (BAIB) which, along with taurine, are transported by a common system in the kidney. The ω-amino dipeptides carnosine and homocarnosine are discussed on page 1114. BAIB arises predominantly from thymine (the 'R' form); inherited defects in a catabolic enzyme cause excretion of large quantities of BAIB (100–300 mg/24 h) in 5–10% of whites and up to 95% of Orientals but this causes no disease. Increased DNA turnover from catabolism and in some malignancies also increases urinary R-BAIB.

Hyper-β-alaninemia (237400) occurs in deficiency of either dihydropyrimidine dehydrogenase or methylmalonate semialdehyde dehydrogenase deficiencies. It has also been seen with hypotonia and progressive neurological damage leading to death.

γ-Aminobutyric acid (GABA) decarboxylase deficiency in the brain is thought to be the cause of *pyridoxine-dependent convulsions* (266100) (p. 245); in this condition, GABA is low but glutamate is markedly elevated in the CSF. A different decarboxylase synthesizes GABA in other tissues, notably the kidneys; antibodies against this enzyme have been found in several conditions including some cases of diabetes and the stiff man syndrome in adults. *GABA transaminase* deficiency (137150) has been reported in siblings with severe psychomotor retardation, accelerated growth and early death. GABA and other ω-amino acids were elevated in the CSF. GABA metabolism is also altered in homocarnosinosis and succinic semialdehyde deficiencies.

Some cases of *glutamate dehydrogenase* deficiency (138130) have had progressive spinocerebellar degeneration not responsive to vitamin therapy. The Chinese restaurant syndrome is caused by monosodium glutamate which produces a burning sensation over

---

* The designation ω indicates that the amino group is the one farthest from the -COOH group.

the body and head; flushing and retrosternal pain may also occur. Monosodium glutamate has also been implicated as a possible cause of brain damage in infants; the mechanism, if any, is obscure.

Other amino acid disorders

Canavan's disease (Ch. 14) (271900) (<1 : 500 000), a disorder of developmental delay with spongy degeneration of the brain and macrocephaly, usually affecting Ashkenazi Jews, is due to a defect of aspartoacylase. N-acetylaspartic acid is excreted in the urine in large quantities. Enzyme and DNA testing is available but no treatment is known.

A myopathy associated with a defect of creatine synthesis has recently been reported.

DISORDERS OF BRANCHED CHAIN AMINO ACIDS (Fig. 20.10)

Mild *hyperleucine-isoleucinemia* (238340) due to a partial defect of their transaminase (step 1) (277100) and *hypervalinemia* (step 2) have both been found in rare infants with neurologic disease and vomiting, lethargy, failure to thrive and mental retardation.

Almost all of the branched chain disorders have been described with severe and lethal or mild or even asymptomatic variants.

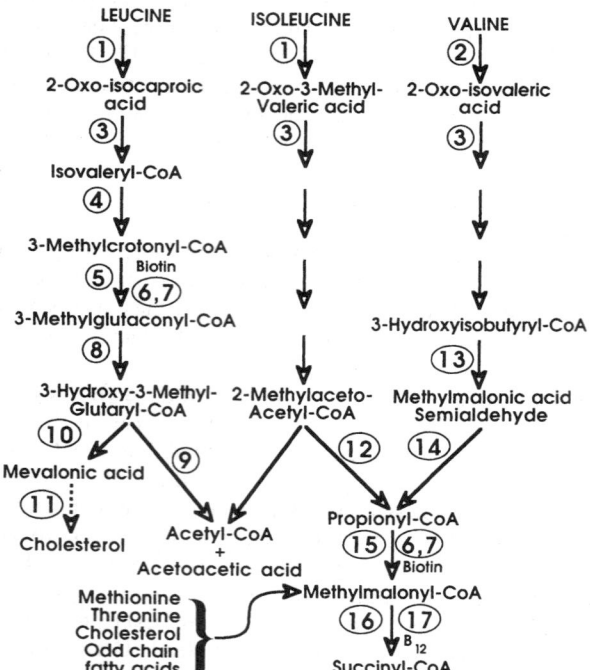

Fig. 20.10 Branched chain amino acid metabolism: numbers indicate known metabolic errors. 1, Leucine aminotransferase; 2, valine aminotransferase; 3, branched chain keto acid decarboxylase (Maple syrup urine disease); 4, isovaleryl-CoA dehydrogenase; 5, 3-methylcrotonyl-CoA carboxylase; 6, biotinidase; 7, holocarboxylase synthetase; 8, 3-methylglutaconyl-CoA hydrolase; 9, 3-hydroxy-3-methylglutaryl-CoA lyase; 10, 3-hydroxy-3-methylglutaryl-CoA reductase; 11, mevalonate kinase; 12, 2-methylacetoacetyl-CoA thiolase (β-ketothiolase); 13, 3-hydroxyisobutyryl-CoA deacylase; 14, methylmalonic semialdehyde dehydrogenase; 15, propionyl-CoA carboxylase; 16, methylmalonyl-CoA mutase; 17, cobalamin defects.

They usually present with metabolic acidosis and the excretion of characteristic organic acids (p. 1119) in the urine, some of which have distinctive odors. Most can be studied in cultured skin fibroblasts.

Maple syrup urine disease (step 3) (248600) (~1 : 250 000)

This condition is the exemplar of the inborn errors which cause metabolic acidosis. It affects the metabolism of leucine, isoleucine and valine, resulting in high levels in plasma, urine and CSF. Several variants are recognized, some with severe neonatal onset; others are less severe and some are intermittent, only precipitated by stress, intercurrent illness or a high protein diet. Another form responds to thiamine therapy. Mutations affecting the E_1, E_2 and E_3 components of the dehydrogenase complex are known.

Clinical features

The severe form presents in the first week of life with feeding and breathing difficulties and often a shrill cry. Severe neurological symptoms, vomiting, spasticity, convulsions, ketoacidosis and coma develop, progressing to death in a few weeks. A subtle sweet, malt-like odor is usually present and hypoglycemia may occur. If the disease is treated early, the prognosis can be excellent; untreated or poorly treated infants who survive are severely brain damaged. Organic acidemias should be suspected in any child becoming ill or acidotic within the first weeks of life.

In the milder forms, fluctuating levels of incoordination and lethargy are frequent and the metabolic abnormalities are always present (unless the patient is on a special diet) although the acidosis may be minimal. In the intermittent type, the patients may have some brain damage, but the biochemical abnormalities are only provoked by the stress conditions mentioned above; during such metabolic decompensation, the illness can be as severe as in the neonatal variety. Thiamin is required for the E_1 component of the decarboxylase and a thiamine-dependent form of the disease is recognized. Very mild variants can present as ketotic hypoglycemia (p. 1131).

Diagnosis

After birth, the amino acids rise rapidly and can be detected by a newborn blood screening test which is in wide, but not general use. Hypoglycemia, metabolic acidosis, increased anion gap or an abnormal dinitrophenylhydrazine test demands immediate amino acid chromatography which provides the diagnosis. High levels of the three branched chain amino acids and their keto acids are found, with leucine being most elevated and causing most of the symptoms. The defect can be found in white blood cells and cultured fibroblasts which can be used for all genetic testing.

Treatment

Strict dietary treatment, if started early, can prevent brain damage. In most cases the diet needs to be continued indefinitely since, if it is stopped, severe acidosis recurs within a few days. The diet is based on a mixture of synthetic amino acids in the approximate proportions of cow's milk, without the branched chain amino acids (Table 20.4). Small amounts of natural protein, providing 25–60 mg/kg/day of valine, isoleucine and leucine, are given to maintain normal blood levels. During periods of rapid growth, requirements for these amino acids may rise as high as 300 mg/kg/day. Mild cases require less aggressive protein restriction and have a proportionally better prognosis.

The dietary management is very difficult because each of the three amino acids must be individually adjusted, since excess of any one of them (especially leucine) may be toxic. Furthermore, deficiency of any one causes endogenous protein catabolism with a consequent *rise* in the plasma levels of all three. Unbalanced catabolism of only 20 g of the patient's own protein would release about 1.3 g (10 mmol) leucine which can rapidly cause a large elevation of the plasma levels. During any minor illness, the plasma levels may rise very rapidly to toxic levels. Dehydration must be avoided. Treatment with a glucose/insulin drip, anabolic steroids or dialysis may be helpful during acute crises. Thiamin (50–250 mg/day) should be given to all patients, since it may help to stabilize the mutant enzyme.

Leucine-induced hypoglycemia

Several amino acids stimulate the release of insulin without normally affecting blood glucose. Leucine, however, does lower the blood glucose by an unknown mechanism; occasionally this is excessive and symptomatic hypoglycemia is produced (Ch. 19); it is quite frequent in endogenous hyperinsulinism from any cause and can be seen at any age.

Methylmalonic acidemia (251000) (~1 : 250 000)

At least seven nonallelic conditions cause methylmalonic aciduria. Two, which tend to be severe, represent defects of the mutase apoenzyme with either no detectable activity (mut^0) or structurally altered enzyme with reduced activity (mut$^-$) in fibroblasts. Patients with these defects do not respond in vivo to high doses of cobalamin. Two result from deficient synthesis of the active cofactor, 5'-deoxyadenosyl-cobalamin (251000), one is due to deficient transferase activity (251120) and another to a defect in reduction of hydroxocobalamin or transport out of lysosomes. Homocystinuria occurs in the last two forms.

Clinical features

Severe cases present as newborns with marked and often lethal, metabolic acidosis (see below). Milder cases show intermittent symptoms of food refusal, vomiting, irritability, lethargy, hypotonia and failure to thrive, with a mild or compensated metabolic acidosis that may decompensate during illness; some cases are permanently asymptomatic. Untreated patients usually develop neurological damage with motor and mental retardation. Unusual but serious complications include renal damage with hypertension and uremia, cerebellar hemorrhage, basal ganglia infarcts and cardiomyopathy which may not be due to carnitine depletion and may not respond to it. Benign forms of the disease have been reported and temporary cases in infancy are also known.

Diagnosis and treatment

For general comments, see below. Hyperglycinemia and hyperammonemia are frequent and neutropenia may occur. Urine methylmalonic acid excretion may reach 5 g/day. A urine screening test is available. Tests for urinary ketones (e.g. Acetest) are often positive because of accumulation of the long chain ketones, butanone and hexanone.

Four of the variants respond clinically and biochemically to massive doses of vitamin B_{12} (1–2 mg day i.m.) and all cases should be given a trial of it. Other treatment is discussed on page 1119. The different types of disease can be identified in cultured skin fibroblasts.

Propionic acidemia (step 7) (232000, 232050) (~1 : 250 000)

This disorder results from a defect in the biotin requiring carboxylase, which converts propionyl-CoA to methylmalonyl-CoA. The symptoms and acidosis are identical to those of methylmalonic acidemia but propionic acid is elevated in serum and 3-hydroxypropionate, methylcitrate, tiglyl- and propionyl-glycines and long chain ketones are found in urine. Therapy (p. 1119) should include a trial of biotin (10–20 mg/day). In multiple carboxylase deficiency, propionic acid metabolism is also compromised, but the acidosis is usually mild.

Other disorders of branched chain amino acid catabolism

In *isovaleric acidemia* (step 4) (243500) (~1 : 250 000) symptoms are similar to methylmalonic aciduria except that a body odor of sweaty feet is characteristic. Glycine and certain other amino acids may be elevated in plasma. During remission, isovaleric acid levels may be near normal but excretion of isovalerylglycine is always high (up to 3 g/day). Treatment includes oral glycine up to 250 mg/kg/day and large doses of L-carnitine, in addition to the steps outlined on page 1119. *Jamaican vomiting sickness* is caused by eating unripe Ackee fruit which contains hypoglycin, and inhibits isovaleric acid metabolism causing hypoglycemia and ketoacidosis. Acute pancreatitis is a common complication.

3-Methylcrotonylglycinuria,* due to isolated deficiency of 3-methylcrotonyl-CoA carboxylase (step 5) (210200), is similar except that the urine smells similar to cats' urine. 3-Methylcrotonylglycine and 3-hydroxyisovaleric acid are excreted in large amounts in the urine but are not elevated in blood. A trial of biotin (10–20 mg/day) is indicated because most cases who excrete these metabolites have multiple carboxylase deficiency (p. 1254).

A defect of *3-methylglutaconyl-CoA hydratase* (step 8) (250950) causes excretion of 3-methylglutaconic acid and 3-methylglutaric acid. The usual symptoms are progressive neurological deterioration in infancy, *without obvious metabolic acidosis*. However, hypoglycemia, metabolic acidosis and cardiomyopathy have also been reported although these could have been due to carnitine depletion. Other patients with 3-methylglutaconic aciduria but normal enzyme studies have presented with various symptoms of neurological deterioration including choreoathetosis, spasticity, optic atrophy, tapetoretinal degeneration and nerve deafness. Metabolic acidosis may be absent or marked and most such cases die. Some cases are associated with defects of the respiratory chain but in most, the enzyme defect is not known.

Other reports involve *3-hydroxyisobutyryl-CoA deacylase* deficiency (277080) and *methylmalonic semialdehyde*

---

* Alternative nomenclature numbers carbon atoms sequentially starting with 1 for the carbon in -COOH. Thus 2 and 3 are equivalent to the Greek symbols α and β respectively.

dehydrogenase in different children with various problems including congenital abnormalities and failure to thrive; urinary organic acids provided the clue to the defects.

3-Hydroxy-3-methylglutaryl-CoA lyase, 3-ketothiolase and *2-methylacetoacetyl-CoA thiolase* deficiencies are discussed under defects of ketone utilization (p. 1130). *Mevalonic aciduria* (251170) is discussed on page 1156.

ORGANIC ACIDURIAS AND METABOLIC ACIDOSIS (Table 20.3)

There is a large group of disorders that are characterized by the excretion of either organic acids in abnormal quantities or of

Table 20.3 Disorders associated with metabolic acidosis and/or organic aciduria. The major metabolite excreted is indicated either by the name of the disorder or by the compounds in parentheses

Branched chain amino acid disorders
  Maple syrup urine disease (branched chain keto acids)
  Methylmalonic acidemia
  Propionic acid acidemia
  Isovaleric acidemia
  3-Methylcrotonylglycinuria
  3-Methylglutaconic aciduria
  3-Hydroxy-3-methylglutaryl-CoA lyase deficiency
  Mevalonic acidemia
  2-Methylacetoacetyl-CoA thiolase deficiency
  3-Ketothiolase deficiency (3-hydroxybutyrate)
  3-Hydroxyisobutyryl-CoA deacylase deficiency
  Methylmalonic semialdehyde dehydrogenase deficiency
  (3-hydroxypropionate)

Other disorders
  2-Ketoadipic aciduria
  Glutaric aciduria types I and II
  Crotonic acidemia
  Oxalosis types I and II (glycollate, L-glycerate)
  D-glyceric acidemia
  5-Oxoprolinuria
  Succinic semialdehyde dehydrogenase deficiency (4-hydroxybutyrate)
  Succinyl-CoA:3-ketoacid CoA transferase deficiency
  Threonine sensitive acidosis
  2-Hydroxyglutaric aciduria
  Barth syndrome (3-methylglutaconic acid)
  Fanconi syndrome
  The tyrosinemias (tyrosyluria) (succinyl acetone)
  Renal tubular acidosis
  Lactic/pyruvic acidosis
  Multiple carboxylase and biotinidase deficiencies
  Mitochondrial disorders
  Krebs cycle disorders
  Fructose 1,6-diphosphatase deficiency (lactate)
  Glycogen storage disease type 1
  Ketoacidosis as in diabetes mellitus
  Carnitine depletion
  Disorders of fatty acid catabolism
  Disorders of ketone body utilization

Other disorders in which pathologic organic aciduria can occur
  Urea cycle disorders (orotic acid)
  Canavan's disease-N-acetylaspartate
  Phenylketonuria

Other acquired causes of acidosis include:
  Poisoning: salicylate, methanol, benzyl alcohol, antifreeze, etc.
  Ethanol
  Starvation
  Dehydration
  Diarrhea
  Reye's syndrome

organic acids not normally found in urine. Most, but not all, are associated with metabolic acidosis which may be severe and fatal in the newborn period or may occur at any age thereafter. The acidosis may be persistent, with permanent abnormalities of acid–base balance and continuous excretion of abnormal metabolites, may be compensated or may be intermittent, usually being precipitated or aggravated by changes of diet or periods of stress such as infections, fever or surgery. These cases often die misdiagnosed as having respiratory distress and infection which, indeed, may coexist and aggravate the metabolic defect. These conditions are listed in Table 20.3. Not all metabolic acidoses are associated with pathological organic aciduria and some of the conditions can be very difficult to discriminate, clinically or biochemically, from the normal metabolic consequences of starvation or stress. Some of the conditions can be recognized by a characteristic odor of the body and urine but definitive identification usually requires organic acid analysis by gas-liquid chromatography (Chalmers & Lawson 1982, Sweetman 1991, Hommes 1993) with appropriate enzyme studies as confirmation.

Acidotic conditions not presented elsewhere include threonine-induced acidosis which occurred in a child with severe hypotonia, developmental delay, growth failure and recurrent attacks of ketoacidosis associated with hypoglycemia. Symptoms were not provoked by other amino acids; therapy with a low protein diet was beneficial. *Hyperthreoninemia* (273770) is a separate entity; it has been reported in a child with retardation and convulsions. In neither condition has the enzyme defect been localized.

D-2-hydroxyglutaric aciduria (600721) is associated with severe developmental delay and neurological abnormalities; no treatment seems to have been effective.

L-2-hydroxyglutaric aciduria (236792) is associated with progressive spongiform leukodystrophy, olivopontocerebellar abnormalities, mental delay and, in some cases, anemia and retinal dystrophy; it may be apparent in the newborn or later. The metabolic defect is not known.

Clinical features

In the severe cases, the metabolic acidosis causes air hunger, Kussmaul respiration and lethargy leading to coma; vomiting, failure to thrive, hepatomegaly and neurologic damage with seizures, spasticity, hypotonia and retardation are frequent. In milder cases the patients may only present during an acute exacerbation or may be detected as a result of a 'metabolic screen' performed for unexplained neurologic problems or an unexplained compensated metabolic acidosis in a child with no overt acidotic symptoms. Cases may present with chronic failure to thrive, chronic or acute neurologic problems, myopathy and even with cardiomyopathy. In some of the diseases, neutropenia and thrombocytopenia along with osteoporosis, mental retardation and seizures are seen.

Diagnosis

Unexpectedly severe acidosis, with or without ketosis, in any infant should suggest the possibility of one of these disorders. The blood pH may be normal or low, the PCO_2 is usually low and an anion gap* or base deficit is to be expected. In some disorders,

---

* Serum $(Na^+ + K^+) - (Cl^- + HCO_3^-)$ = anion gap (normal 12–18 mEq/l)

hypoglycemia is frequent and hyperammonemia or lactic acidosis reflect disturbed mitochondrial function. Hyperuricemia can be caused by inhibition of renal tubular secretion of uric acid by other organic acids. In the 'ketotic hyperglycinemia' syndromes (methylmalonic acidemia, propionic acidemia, isovaleric acidemia and 2-methyl-3-hydroxybutyric aciduria) the blood glycine is often raised; an elevated plasma glycine: alanine ratio is more consistent. The neutropenia and thrombocytopenia seem to be related to the glycine levels. In contrast, in lactic acidosis, hyperalaninemia reflects increased transamination of pyruvate.

The urine pH is low and the Acetest (Ames), Ketostix (Ames) or dinitrophenylhydrazine tests may be abnormal depending upon which metabolite is being excreted. Diagnosis can usually be made by identification of the organic acid pattern, or its glycine or carnitine conjugates, in blood or urine and can be confirmed by specific enzyme assay in tissues.

In milder cases, the diagnosis may be easily missed unless samples are obtained *during* an acidotic episode. Provocative tests with precursor amino acids have proved fatal and should rarely be used. *Blood and urine samples for metabolite identification should be taken from any child with unexplained acidosis.*

Gas chromatography with linked mass spectrometry of urine for organic acids is increasingly used as a screening test for the evaluation of unexplained clinical problems, particularly neurologic disorders. Some diseases, for example oxalosis, 3-methylglutaconyl-CoA hydratase deficiency or the glutaric acidurias, do not exhibit metabolic acidosis and the finding of unexpected poisoning, as with phenobarbital, or of novel iatrogenic substances such as benzyl alcohol or ethylene glycol may reveal an unexpected toxicological diagnosis.

A number of organic acids may occur in the urine of sick, ketotic or acidotic children, presumably reflecting secondary metabolic disturbances. Lactate can reflect poor tissue perfusion and the *dicarboxylic acids* adipic, suberic and sebacic acids, 3-hydroxyisobutyric acid, 2-methyl-3-hydroxybutyric acid and 3-hydroxyisovaleric acid, as well as the ketone bodies, can all accumulate when lipolysis is increased, making it difficult to distinguish between primary or secondary effects on fatty acid breakdown (p. 1128).

Treatment

The first priority is to supply sufficient alkali to counteract the acidosis. Unlike diabetic ketoacidosis, in which insulin results in rapid improvement of acid–base balance, the requirements for alkali may be enormous and permanent. Up to 200 mmol/day of sodium bicarbonate may be required in an infant. Since dehydration is associated with endogenous protein catabolism, it must be avoided; a urine output of 150–200 ml/kg/day or more, if tolerated, may help in the elimination of the metabolites.

Before the abnormal metabolites are identified, the patient should receive a low protein and low fat diet with as many calories as can be tolerated i.v. or p.o. If this aggravates a lactic acidosis, the defect may be in the pyruvate dehydrogenase complex (p. 1124). Once the abnormal metabolites are identified, their precursors are restricted in the diet to the limits of metabolic tolerance. Calories are then supplied from all other available sources. Thus in maple syrup urine disease, all three branched chain amino acids are restricted, whereas in isovaleric acidemia only leucine needs to be controlled. Before the diagnosis is established, large doses of vitamin B_{12} (1–2 mg), pyridoxine

(150–500 mg), thiamin (200–500 mg), folic acid (10–20 mg), biotin (10–20 mg), nicotinamide (100–500 mg) and riboflavin (100–500 mg) should be given in case the disorder is vitamin dependent (p. 1147). Once the definitive diagnosis is known, most of these can be stopped. Abnormal quantities of any CoA derivatives combine with carnitine to make acylcarnitine derivatives which are excreted. This frequently causes profound secondary carnitine depletion which in turn aggravates the metabolic acidosis and may add muscle weakness, hypoglycemia, hepatocellular damage and cardiomyopathy (p. 1129). Initial treatment should include L-carnitine (100 mg/kg/day or more) which should be continued indefinitely if subsequent studies indicate.

In extreme cases, hemo- or peritoneal dialysis or continuous extracorporeal hemoperfusion should be used and intramuscular testosterone propionate (12.5–25 mg for 1–2 days) or a glucose/insulin drip may help to reverse endogenous protein catabolism. Once the crisis is over, the diet is cautiously reintroduced over several days.

CONSTRUCTION OF AN AMINO ACID RESTRICTED DIET

Before constructing a metabolite-restricted diet, it is important to know:

- The normal amino acid and nutritional content of foods
- how much of the metabolites can be tolerated or manufactured by the body
- the minimum daily requirements for the nutrients in question
- the effects of deficiency of the nutrients upon other metabolites.

When such a diet is used, accurate, quantitative assays are essential to monitor the effects of therapy upon individual amino acids, trace elements and other nutrients and upon overall nitrogen balance and growth. Sometimes, daily assays are needed; qualititative assays are not adequate.

It might seem possible to provide protein as essential amino acids supplemented by a source of nitrogen such as glycine. In practice, such unphysiological mixtures do not work well and can be dangerous. Most diets are therefore based on the amino acid content of human or cow's milk (Table 20.4). There is a growing selection of elemental medical foods designed to treat different disorders. For example, products for maple syrup urine disease are based on a mixture of pure L-amino acids roughly in the proportions normally found in cow's milk, but without the branched chain amino acids. These are then provided, as tolerated, from a whole protein source such as any infant formula of known composition, so that their intake can be closely monitored. Manufacturers have up-to-date information on these and are very willing to give help in planning specific diets. Useful references include Schuett (1995), Evans et al (1994) and Dixon (1988).

As the child begins weaning, it is important to provide a variety of tastes and textures so that they learn normal feeding behavior. This is done using low protein foods, each containing similar quantities (e.g. 50 mg) or *equivalents* of the specified amino acid. The diet is then constructed so that the special formula provides most of the calories and protein requirements, whereas the additional equivalents provide texture, variety and the limiting nutrients. In most cases, this approach is reasonable but published figures for the amino acid content of foods are still scanty and those that are available are only average values; the composition of cow's milk can vary by 100% amongst different breeds and at different times of the year. In practice, the diet becomes largely vegetarian and similar to that used in renal failure, since greater variety can be achieved if low-protein compounds provide at least 50% of the limiting amino acids.

Daily requirements

The recommended daily intake of protein varies at different ages (see Table 21.5). The minimum requirements (Table 20.4) of amino acids have been estimated from very scanty data and clearly vary over time, during illness or if the diet is artificial and possibly deficient in other, still unknown, nutrients.

Deficiency of a single essential amino acid eventually results in failure to make new protein, increasing protein catabolism and metabolic bankruptcy. This leads to listlessness, eczema, anemia, fever, anorexia and vomiting and may progress to severe wasting, permanent brain damage and death. Deficiency of any one of the branched chain amino acids in a patient with maple syrup urine disease rapidly causes plasma elevations of all three amino acids, due to endogenous protein catabolism.

Table 20.4 Amino acid composition of human and cow's milk and a special formula for the treatment of maple syrup urine disease (MSUD)

	Human milk (mg/dl)	Cow's milk* (mg/dl)	MSUD† dried powder (g/100 g powder‡)	Approximate requirement of infants § (mg/kg/day)
L-alanine	35	120	0.45	
L-arginine	45	130	0.50	
L-aspartic acid	116	250	1.14	
L-cystine	22	30	0.25	
L-glutamic acid	230	800	2.09	
Glycine	0	70	0.6	
L-histidine	22	90	0.25	16–34
L-isoleucine	68	220	–	50–120
L-leucine	100	350	–	80–200
L-lysine	73	270	0.8	90–120
L-methionine	25	80	0.25	20–45
L-phenylalanine	48	170	0.55	25–90
L-proline	80	390	0.9	
L-serine	69	200	0.6	
Taurine	10	<1	–	
L-threonine	50	160	0.55	45–87
L-tyrosine	61	180	0.65	
L-tryptophan	18	50	0.20	15–40
L-valine	70	240	–	65–115
Carbohydrate	7 g	4.8 g	63.7	
Fat	3.8 g	3.8 g	20.1	

*Amino acid composition may vary widely amongst different breeds and in different countries.
†Or use a protein-free source of calories such as Hycal (Beecham), 80056 (Mead Johnson) or Caloreen (Scientific Hospital Supplies) and a source of pure amino acids such as MSUD-Aid (Scientific Hospital Supplies). See Table 20.5
‡Valine, isoleucine and leucine come from any regular infant formula of known composition as tolerated.
§These values have only been established in a few healthy babies over a short time.

Table 20.5 Some companies which produce special products for the treatment of inborn errors of metabolism

- Allen and Hanburys Ltd, Stockley Park West, Uxbridge, Middlesex UB11 1BT
- Carnation – now Clintec Nutrition Ltd, Shaftesbury Court, 18 Chalvery Park, Slough SL1 2ER
- Cow & Gate Nutricia Ltd, Newmarket Avenue, Whitehorse Business Park. Trowbridge, Wilts BA14 OXQ
- Farley Health Products Ltd, Torr Lane, Plymouth PL3 5UA
- G.F. Dietary Supplies Ltd – now Cow & Gate Nutricia as above
- ICI Ltd – now Zeneca Pharmaceuticals. Alderley House, Alderley Park, Macclesfield, Cheshire SK10 4TF
- Maizena Diat GmbH, Postfach 2760, W-7100 Heilbronn, FRG
- Mead Johnson Nutritionals, Bristol-Myers Pharmaceuticals, 141–149 Staines Road, Hounslow, Middlesex TW3 3JA
- Milupa Ltd, Milupa House, Uxbridge Road, Hillingdon, Uxbridge, Middlesex UB10 0NE
- Nestlé UK Ltd, St. Georges House, Park Lane, Croydon, Surrey CR9 1NR
- Procea, Alexandra Road, Dublin 1, Eire.
- Rite Diet, Welfare Foods – now Cow & Gate Nutricia as above
- Ross Laboratories – now Abbott Laboratories Ltd, Norden Road, Maidenhead, Berks SL6 4XE
- Scientific Hospital Supplies (UK) Ltd, 100 Wavertree Boulevard, Wavertree Technology Park, Liverpool L7 9PT
- Snowcrest Ltd, Unit 8–12, 1–7 Garman Road, Tottenham, London N17 0UN
- Ultrapharm Ltd, 23 New Street, Henley on Thames, Oxon RG9 2PB
- Welfare Foods Ltd, – now Cow & Gate Nutricia as above
- Wyeth Laboratories, Huntercombe Lane South, Maidenhead, Berks SL6 0PH

Minimum daily requirements for amino acids are about the same in children with disorders of amino acid metabolism as they are in normal children and are accepted as guidelines for the construction of a special diet. In certain circumstances the tolerance for amino acids may be less than the values given in Table 20.4. In disorders of the urea cycle, protein tolerance may be lower than 1 g/kg per 24 hours. In these cases supplementation with small quantities of essential amino acids or the keto acid analogs of amino acids which can be converted to amino acids in the body may be beneficial.

The composition of a number of infant formulae is given in Table 37.14 and European companies which manufacture special metabolic products are shown in Table 20.5.

DISORDERS OF TRANSPORT

AMINO ACIDS

In the kidney and gut, amino acids are actively transported across cell membranes in five major groups (Table 20.6). In addition, there are other separate, but probably minor, transport systems.

Disorders of both group-specific and individual amino acid transport systems exist. In tissues other than kidney and gut there are similar, but not identical active transport processes, but only in

Table 20.6 Group systems of amino acid transport in kidney and gut and their disorders

Group	Disorder
1. (a) Cystine, lysine, ornithine, arginine	Cystinuria type I, II and III
(b) Lysine, ornithine, arginine	Dibasic aminoaciduria
	(i) Familial protein intolerance
	(ii) Without protein intolerance
2. Glycine, proline, hydroxyproline	Iminoglycinuria
3. β-Amino acids, taurine	None known
4. Aspartic and glutamic acid	Dicarboxylic aminoaciduria
5. Neutral amino acids (e.g. glycine, alanine, valine, leucine, isoleucine, serine, threonine, cysteine, cystine, phenylalanine, tyrosine, methionine histidine, tryptophan	Hartnup disease

lysinuric protein intolerance is any other tissue known to be involved. Renal transport defects result in specific patterns of aminoaciduria, when, if anything, the plasma levels of the same amino acids are lower than normal. Plasma elevation of a single amino acid usually causes a single aminoaciduria, as in PKU, but a single amino acid may saturate the transport mechanism for all the other amino acids within the group causing a group aminoaciduria. For example, in hyperglycinemia, the imino acids (group 2) may be excreted.

Inherited defects of four group transport systems are known but they probably do not affect all cells. For example, the two types of iminoglycinuria imply that several genes must be required for amino acid transport in different tissues. *Dicarboxylic aminoaciduria* (222730) is also a benign trait. β-Amino acids and taurine are reabsorbed less efficiently than the α-amino acids but group amino aciduria with taurinuria is only reported in β-alaninemia. Heterozygotes for these disorders may show no abnormality in urine, as is seen in cystinuria type I, or a partial defect, as in cystinuria types II or III.

Cystinuria (220100) (~1 : 15 000) (see also Ch. 17)

There are at least three genetic abnormalities in the group transport of cystine and the basic amino acids (lysine, ornithine, arginine) in the kidney and gut. Urinary amino acid levels are similar in all three types of homozygotes and in compound heterozygotes, suggesting that the three forms are probably allelic. The condition is mainly important because cystine is very insoluble in normal urine and these patients tend to develop renal calculi at any age.

About 1–5% of patients with renal stones have cystinuria. Cystine crystals, which are flat and hexagonal, may be found in the urine. The diagnosis is based upon the nitroprusside test and amino acid chromatography. The aim of treatment is to keep urine cystine levels in the range of maximum solubility (approx. 0.1 mmol/mmol creatinine). It consists of maintaining a urine flow of 2–3 l/m² per 24 hours or more; 25% of the fluid intake should be taken during the night. Maximum alkalization of the urine to around pH 7.5 is important, since the solubility of cystine decreases markedly below that. L-penicillamine or mercaptopropionylglycine, which combine with cystine and render it more soluble, are both effective treatments. Captopril

produces a marked reduction in cystine and sodium restriction, possibly with added glutamine, may also be useful. The kidney stones can be totally dissolved by perfusing through a nephrostomy with THAM-E, an alkaline buffer, but they do not usually respond well to lithotripsy.

Heterozygotes for type I have no aminoaciduria, but carriers of types II and III have cystinuria and lysinuria of variable degree, sometimes sufficient to cause calculus formation. Heterozygotes for the three forms can be distinguished by differences of amino acid transport in biopsies from the gut and kidney. Excess cystine in the urine is seen in a number of conditions including argininemia, Fanconi's syndrome and in some organic acidemias. The incidence of heterozygous cystinuria in mental illness seems to be increased several-fold. There is also a report of progressive neurological deterioration and seizures with cystin-lysinuria and massive cadaverinuria (222350); intestinal uptake of amino acids appeared to be normal.

Isolated cystinuria, *isolated dibasic aminoaciduria* (lysine, ornithine, arginine) (222690) and *isolated lysinuria* (247950) have now been reported, showing that partial transport defects within the group can also occur. *Cystin-lysinuria* and recurrent pancreatitis (167800), both dominantly inherited, have been reported together in several families but the significance of the association, if any, is unclear.

Lysinuric protein intolerance (222700) (~1 : 500 000)

Clinical features

In this disorder, most common in Finland, symptoms of hyperammonemia become evident following weaning, when food intolerance, diarrhea, vomiting, hypotonia, hepatosplenomegaly, sparse hair, osteoporosis and marked failure to thrive develop. Interstitial pulmonary fibrosis is a late feature and may prove lethal. Mental development is usually normal.

Diagnosis

There is a defect in the renal and intestinal transport of lysine, arginine and ornithine, resulting in increased excretion in the urine and low levels in plasma. Cystine transport is normal. The hyperammonemia may be explained by deficient transport of urea cycle substrates into liver cells. In addition to other treatment for hyperammonemia, supplementation with citrulline (2–10 g/day) is very beneficial.

A dominantly inherited trait involving deficient renal and intestinal transport of the dibasic amino acids, but with no symptoms of hyperammonemia, is also known. Whether this is the heterozygous expression of the trait is unclear.

Iminoglycinuria (242600)

Free imino acids are normally present in urine in the first 6 months but they fall to very low levels thereafter. A defect of proline, hydroxyproline and glycine transport has been found in both retarded and normal people; it appears to be benign. Gastrointestinal transport may be either normal or defective. Hyperglycinuria is marked but renal absorption of the imino acids may only be slightly reduced. Urine glycine normally varies within wide limits and accounts for up to 25% of the amino acids in urine. It is commonly seen in iminoglycinuria heterozygotes but also occurs in the ketotic and nonketotic hyperglycinemias and in valproate therapy. Glycinuria with glucosuria can occur either alone or with vitamin D-resistant rickets, although the reason for this association is not known.

Hartnup disease (234500) (~1 : 20 000)

Hartnup disease is caused by defective transport in the kidney and usually the gut, of amino acids in group 5 (Table 20.6). The only constant feature is the characteristic aminoaciduria. The symptoms, if they occur, are those of pellagra which is due to tryptophan deficiency. They include photodermatitis, ataxia, psychiatric changes and mental deterioration, but these are usually intermittent and are only precipitated during protein deprivation or periods of stress. Symptoms usually lessen with age. Heterozygotes do not show aminoaciduria.

Urinary indoles arise in the gut from bacterial degradation of unabsorbed tryptophan. Malabsorption of tryptophan results in diminished nicotinic acid synthesis, so that patients on a high protein or niacin-supplemented diet are symptomless. Deficiency of the other amino acids causes no apparent problem. Treatment with oral nicotinic acid (25 mg/day) is effective.

Other amino acid transport defects

Methionine malabsorption (250900) in gut and kidney has been associated with mental retardation, convulsions, diarrhea and white hair. 2-hydroxybutyric acid produced by gut bacteria gave a peculiar, beery body odor that gives rise to the name oast-house syndrome.* Abnormal transport of several other amino acids may also occur. No treatment is known.

The *blue diaper* (*napkin*) *syndrome* (211000) is a rare isolated defect in gut absorption of tryptophan; gut bacteria degrade tryptophan to indoles which are then absorbed, metabolized in the liver and excreted in the urine. The defect may be associated with mental retardation, hypercalcemia and nephrocalcinosis. Urine from these patients intermittently contains the blue pigment indican. Gut sterilization, oral nicotinic acid and a low calcium diet might be indicated. Indoluria may occur in malabsorption, the blind loop syndrome, carcinoid and constipation.

Blue staining of the napkins can be produced by cuprammonium complexes from contact of the urine with brass. It can also be caused by pyocyanine produced by *Pseudomonas aeruginosa* which can be present in a reusable napkin, even after washing. Blue-green urine can also be produced by xanthurenic acid, methylene blue, amitriptyline, tolonium, methocarbamol and phenol poisoning.

A renal and intestinal deficiency causing *histidinuria* (235830) has been described.

Generalized aminoaciduria

More than 95–99% of filtered amino acids are normally actively reabsorbed by the proximal tubules. Renal aminoaciduria occurs if there is a detectable reduction in this value and accompanies renal tubular damage from any cause. A degree of generalized aminoaciduria is normal in the first 2–3 months of life, especially in prematurity, due to immaturity of the tubular transport systems. Many syndromes have been described in association with

aminoaciduria; in most of these the etiology of the disease and the relationship of the defect to the symptoms are unknown. Even in the presence of considerable tubular damage and 'generalized aminoaciduria', some amino acids may still be reabsorbed normally. Thus, there is no characteristic pattern of generalized aminoaciduria except that more than one of the major transport systems is involved. In the most severe forms, the urine has the chromatographic appearance of dilute plasma.

Recognition of aminoaciduria is not always easy. Amino acid concentrations in normal urine vary more than 10-fold so that quantitative results must be related to some relatively constant value such as age, weight, surface area or creatinine excretion and normal values vary so widely that they are rarely quoted. Tubular reabsorption rates are measured by comparing the clearance of each amino acid with the clearance of inulin or creatinine.*

Fanconi's syndrome†

The renal Fanconi syndrome is a generalized disturbance of renal tubular transport systems caused by a number of different conditions which may be hereditary or acquired. Reabsorption of glucose, electrolytes, bicarbonate, calcium, phosphate, amino acids, protein, uric acid and water are variably affected and H^+ excretion is compromised. This condition may occur at any age. The aminoaciduria causes no symptoms, but in the complete syndrome, polyuria, polydipsia, marked growth failure, anorexia, vomiting, rickets and renal tubular acidosis are marked and episodes of dehydration and electrolyte imbalance are frequent.

The most common hereditary cause is cystinosis; others include galactosemia, fructosemia, tyrosinemia, von Gierke's disease, cytochrome c oxidase deficiency, the Fanconi–Bickel syndrome (227810), Wilson's disease and Lowe's syndrome, most of which have prominent liver damage secondary to these recognizable conditions. The Busby and Luder–Sheldon (134600) syndromes are also hereditary but the underlying defect is not known. There is also an idiopathic group in which there is no recognizable underlying metabolic defect.

Acquired causes include shock, burns, heavy metals, lysol or salicylate poisoning, glue sniffing, hemoglobinopathies, degraded tetracycline, Sjögren's syndrome, hyperparathyroidism, nutritional rickets, scurvy, kwashiorkor, cirrhosis, potassium deficiency, myeloma or the nephrotic syndrome.

In all cases, therapy is directed to replacing the materials lost in the urine. Fluid, alkali and electrolytes are the most important but calcium, phosphate, vitamin D_3 and nutrition can also be critical. Carnitine (25–75 mg/kg/day) is also usually indicated.

Lowe's syndrome (309000) (~1 : 60–100 000)

This is an X-linked condition and is one cause of the Fanconi syndrome, associated with cataract, buphthalmos, marked hypotonia, frontal bossing and cryptorchidism and severe failure to thrive. Tendon reflexes are diminished or absent.

---

* An oast-house is where hops are prepared prior to making beer.

* Percent tubular reabsorption = creatinine clearance - amino acid clearance divided by the creatinine clearance and multiplied by 100.
† Fanconi and others all described a condition of generalized renal tubular dysfunction in which rickets, due to disturbed calcium and phosphorus metabolism, was a prominent feature: all their cases were probably cases of cystinosis and the terms are sometimes interchanged. The term 'renal Fanconi syndrome' should be used to describe any condition of generalized tubular dysfunction leading to the biochemical derangement described above.

Developmental delay is usually marked and many cases die in the first or second decade, although less severe cases are known. Osteoporosis from the Fanconi syndrome can be severe and, rarely, painful fibrous tumors develop. Electrolyte and mineral losses in the urine can be very high due to a transport defect in the kidney. The basic defect involves an inositol phosphatase but the mechanism of damage is unknown. Female carriers may have cataracts, be mentally retarded and have aminoaciduria, presumably due to variable inactivation of the X chromosome.

DEFECTS OF GLUCOSE TRANSPORTERS (Elsas & Longo 1995)

Two classes of these are known. Sodium/glucose cotransporters (SGLTs) concentrate glucose against a gradient. A defect of SGLT1 causes *glucose/galactose malabsorption* (231600) (Ch. 10) and abnormal SGLT2 may be the cause of benign renal glycosuria (233100).

There are several defects of facilitative glucose transport (GLUTs). GLUT 1 seems to be involved in defective *glucose transport into brain* (De Vivo et al 1995) which results in seizures, often unresponsive to regular anticonvulsants and hypoglycorrhachia with euglycemia. GLUT 7, in liver microsomes, may be involved in type IB glycogenosis. GLUT 2 is involved in pancreatic β-cell sensing and in peripheral tissues; predictably, these defects should cause diabetes. Other insulin resistance conditions like leprechaunism (246200) are associated with defects of insulin receptors.

LYSOSOMAL TRANSPORT DEFECTS

Cystinosis (219800) (~1 : 60 000)

This is not a group transport defect but a generalized disease in which there is intralysosomal storage of cystine in many tissues, secondary to deficient egress from the lysosomes. It is the most common cause of the Fanconi syndrome in childhood.

Clinical features

Children with infantile cystinosis present in the first year with tremendous water and salt craving, food refusal and failure to thrive, vomiting, lethargy, polyuria, irritability, anorexia and signs of progressive renal tubular and glomerular damage which can lead to death in the first decade. Growth failure is usually severe and rickets may be prominent. The skin is pale and the hair becomes blond due to inhibition of melanin formation; photophobia is common, probably due to a characteristic retinopathy combined with a crystal keratopathy. Progressive damage of the thyroid gland causes hypothyroidism and later, proximal myopathy and cerebral lesions may develop.

Milder variants present in childhood or adolescence (219900) with a slower progression of retinopathy and renal disease; there is also an adult form (219750) in which there is no renal damage, although cystine crystals are still present in the eye.

Diagnosis

The biochemical features of the severe form are those of the Fanconi syndrome with renal tubular acidosis, hypokalemia, hypouricemia, hypophosphatemia, glycosuria, proteinuria and aminoaciduria being prominent. Plasma amino acids, including cystine, are normal or low. The diagnosis may be confirmed by the demonstration of refractile corneal crystals seen on slit lamp examination (they can also be seen in bone marrow, lymph node, conjunctival or rectal biopsy) and by measurement of intracellular cystine levels in leukocytes or cultured skin fibroblasts (up to 100 times normal); levels in heterozygotes are 5–10 times normal. Microscopy shows severe damage of the proximal renal tubules. Cystinotic cells take up ^{35}S-cysteine at about twice the normal rate but accumulate the disulfide, cystine, in greatly increased amounts.

Treatment

There is no cure. Therapy is directed towards correction of the fluid and electrolyte imbalances, acidosis, rickets and hypothyroidism. Dietary restriction of cystine and methionine, along with penicillamine, have no effect. Cysteamine or phosphocysteamine are the drugs of choice since they deplete intracellular cystine; they must be given every 6 h and the dose monitored by regular assay of leukocyte cystine; these drugs delay or prevent tissue damage. Advanced renal failure is treated by renal transplantation; the transplanted kidneys do not express the cystinotic defect and have the same prognosis as kidneys transplanted for other reasons. The biochemical defect, however, continues in other tissues and long-term complications, including a myopathy and central nervous system damage, are now recognized.

OTHER DISORDERS OF TRANSPORT ACROSS CELL MEMBRANES

Other lysosomal defects include the CblF mutant of cobalamin metabolism (p. 1147) and Salla disease (p. 1169).

The transport of proteins into cells or organelles is performed by specific transport systems which require recognition sites on the proteins involved. Examples of such defects include α1-antitrypsin mutants which cannot exit from the Golgi in the liver and failure of enzyme uptake by lysosomes in I-cell disease, which are considered elsewhere. Selective *hypouricemia* (307830) is a benign condition caused by a disorder of urate reabsorption in proximal renal tubules and certain of the renal tubular acidosis syndromes are caused by transport defects for H^+ in the kidney. Mitochondrial uptake of ornithine is defective in the *HHH syndrome* (p. 1111).

At least two forms of *hypophosphatemic rickets* (p. 948) are associated with a renal and sometimes gut, defect of phosphate transport. One is inherited as an autosomal dominant trait (193100) in which the rickets can be cured with oral phosphate (2–3 g/day) alone. The other is an X-linked dominant trait (307800) in which vitamin D metabolism is also affected.

DISORDERS OF MITOCHONDRIAL ENERGY GENERATION

Mitochondria play a vital role in many pathways of intermediary metabolism, including the urea cycle and the catabolism of branched chain amino acids. The following section is confined to disorders of energy generation, involving either pyruvate, the citric acid cycle or the electron transport chain. Disorders of fatty acid and ketone metabolism are discussed on pages 1128 and 1130.

Defects of energy generation can be considered in five main categories:

1. defects of the pyruvate dehydrogenase complex (208800) which comprises five associated activities designated as E_1, E_2, E_3 (246900), an activating phosphatase and an inactivating kinase
2. defects of the gluconeogenic enzymes
3. defects of the citric acid cycle and related pathways
4. defects of the electron transport chain and ATP synthase
5. defects of fatty acid metabolism and ketone utilization (pp. 1128, 1130).

All of these defects are involved in the co-ordinated and tightly regulated production of ATP so it is not surprising that they share many characteristics although some disorders can be suspected on clinical grounds. All except group 5 characteristically exhibit *lactic acidosis* which is the hallmark of these disorders. Collectively, these are the most common conditions referred to most metabolic centers. Most are inherited in standard Mendelian ways but some of the electron transport chain defects are caused by mitochondrial DNA mutations which are maternally inherited.

DISORDERS OF PYRUVATE AND LACTATE METABOLISM (Fig. 20.11)

Pyruvate is the end-point of anaerobic glycolysis, the starting point of gluconeogenesis and an entry into aerobic metabolism in the citric acid cycle. Pyruvate is readily transaminated to alanine which, when even minimally elevated in blood or urine, may be the first clue to the diagnosis of lactic acidosis.

Pyruvate is converted to lactate by *lactic dehydrogenase* which comprises two subunits (H and M) in various tetrameric combinations in different tissues. Defects of both subunits have

been reported, the M form (150000) being associated with fatigue and myoglobinuria and the H form (150100) with a neurologic problem. A defect of a *lactate transporter* (245340) in muscle was benign.

Lactate arises in the body from normal anaerobic glycolysis. Under homeostatic conditions, it is in equilibrium with pyruvate with an L : P ratio of 15–25 : 1 which is determined by the NADH/NAD+ ratio (the redox state) in the cytosol. This ratio is usually increased in hypoperfusion and hypoxemia (as the H+ rises), defects of the respiratory chain and in some patients with pyruvate carboxylase deficiency; in pyruvate dehydrogenase deficiency, it is usually normal.

Venous lactate is normally <2 mmol/l. It can reach over 30 mmol/L with exercise and in anaerobic conditions such as hypoxemia or tissue hypoxia, as occurs in shock, and may take many hours to normalize after the stress is gone. Lactic acidosis without apparent hypoxemia is also seen in a number of conditions including diabetes mellitus, liver disease, prematurity, renal failure, malignancy, septicemia, dehydration, hypothermia, acute ethanol intoxication, methanol poisoning, mitochondrial damage and therapy with a number of drugs including phenformin and i.v. fructose. In these cases, the lactate is derived either from increased tissue production or decreased removal by the liver. Transient lactic acidosis may occur in small infants; it may last several months but seems to have a good prognosis.

Hereditary Lactic Acidosis (245400) (in aggregate perhaps as many as 1 : 1000)

Clinical features

Hereditary lactic acidosis, which can occur at any time from birth onward, may present with fulminating, rapidly fatal acidosis or

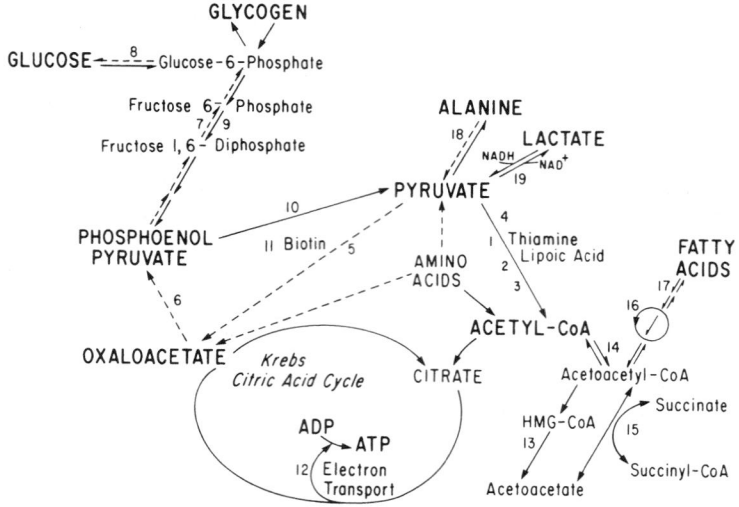

Fig. 20.11 Metabolic pathways involving lactate metabolism. Numbers indicate known metabolic defects. Dotted lines indicate gluconeogenic steps. 1, E_1 of pyruvate dehydrogenase (decarboxylase); 2, E_2 of pyruvate dehydrogense; 3, E_3 of pyruvate dehydrogenase; 4, pyruvate dehydrogenase phosphatase; 5, pyruvate carboxylase; 6, phosphoenolpyruvate carboxykinase; 7, fructose 1,6-diphosphatase; 8, glucose-6-phosphatase; 9, phosphofructokinase; 10, pyruvate kinase; 11, biotinidase and holocarboxylase synthase; 12, electron transport chain; 13, 3-hydroxy-3-methylglutaryl-CoA-lyase; 14, acetoacetyl-CoA thiolase; 15, succinyl-CoA:3-ketoacid-CoA transferase; 16, beta-oxidation spiral; 17, loporotein lipase; 18, alanine:pyruvate aminotransferase; 19, lactic dehydrogenase.

with milder attacks of metabolic acidosis which may develop spontaneously or be precipitated by illness or by changes in the normal diet. Between these attacks, some children exhibit continuous mild compensated metabolic acidosis with no changes in the blood pH; others have quite shortlived but severe episodes although they may be completely normal between attacks.

The spectrum of symptoms associated with lactic acidosis not obviously due to defects of the electron transport chain is wide and includes the following general categories:

1. Neonatal metabolic acidosis with a wide range of neurological symptoms including seizures, coma, hypotonia due either to neurologic damage or to myopathy, liver dysfunction, cardiomyopathy and the renal Fanconi syndrome.

2. Recurrent episodes of acidosis with failure to thrive.

3. Myopathy, generalized, peripheral or limb girdle, at any age from infancy to late adult life which can be stable or progressive.

4. Neurologic damage which may occur at any age and be chronic and stable or progressive, as is seen in Leigh syndrome (266150) (Ch. 14) which seems to be one of the responses of the CNS to energy deficiency associated with lactic acidosis, rather than the result of one specific enzyme defect.

5. Leigh syndrome and Alper's progressive poliodystrophy.

6. Cerebellar ataxia, which may be persistent or recurrent (208800).

7. Isolated cardiomyopathy (Kohlschutter & Hausdorf 1986).

Diagnosis

It is often very difficult to differentiate between a primary lactic acidosis which may be making a child ill and a secondary one in which the lactate is *because* the child is sick. It is essential to search for evidence of ischemic tissues (intracranial bleed? SGOT or LDH very high? etc.) since these can be the source of lactate for days. Several repeat estimations are needed to verify the situation but it must be remembered that even with profound enzyme defects, blood lactate can easily be normal at times and that it *may never rise high enough to alter the pH or the anion gap*. The clinical presentation and biochemical findings may provide a clue to the type of underlying defect but usually, even in patients with frank metabolic acidosis, an anion gap or even a compensated respiratory acidosis and an elevated serum lactate is only the first step in a very complicated metabolic evaluation. The detection of lactic acidemia should always lead to further diagnostic tests.

All patients in whom the blood or urine lactate or alanine are even marginally elevated should be investigated with repeated lactate determinations. Lactate should be assayed in arterial blood or in free-flowing venous blood to avoid the hypoxemic effects of stasis. The lactate in CSF is usually about 20% higher than in the blood; it increases after seizures, CNS infections or trauma and in metabolic diseases involving lactate production by the brain. Urine organic acids may be helpful in suggesting the site of the defect, but in many cases, these reflect only disturbed mitochondrial function and lactic acidosis can occur in several of the organic acid and fatty acid disorders.

Frequent pathologic findings in the brain include agenesis of the corpus callosum, cerebral atrophy, microcephaly and cystic lesions in the brainstem and basal ganglia.

Definitive diagnosis requires accurate enzyme analysis of liver, brain, muscle or other tissues. Some of the enzymes are expressed in leukocytes, platelets or fibroblasts and some exist in more than one form in different tissues. Laboratories that can assay some defects may be unable to test for others and often it is only possible to send fibroblasts or frozen tissues. Using the best methods available and with access to multiple, well-preserved tissues, a specific enzyme defect can only be shown in about 75% of patients.

In *D-lactic acidemia* (245450), there is no L-lactic acidosis and L-lactate metabolism should be normal. Profound D-lactic acidosis can be caused by abnormal proliferation of gut bacteria in the short bowel and blind loop syndromes and is a cause of intermittent neurologic symptoms. D-lactate is not detected by standard enzymatic methods which measure lactate so is one occult cause of a large anion gap.

Treatment

The first priority is to correct the metabolic acidosis; several hundred milliequivalents of bicarbonate per day may be required to combat the continuing production of lactate. Initially, treatment needs to be empiric; large doses of the vitamins involved in lactate metabolism should be tried, in case the defect is vitamin dependent (p. 1147), as follows: thiamin, up to 1000 mg; biotin, 10–20 mg; nicotinamide, 0.25–1.0 g; riboflavin, 0.2–1.0 g; pyridoxine, 100–250 mg; ubiquinone, 30–300 mg. Vitamins C and K can act as electron acceptors and doses of 0.5–2.0 g and 10–40 mg respectively should be considered. L-carnitine, 50–150 mg/kg, is also reasonable, at least until the defect is known. Starvation must be avoided and frequent feeding may be helpful. If hypoglycemia is evident, the defect is more likely to be in a gluconeogenic enzyme and a high carbohydrate diet should be tried. On the other hand, pyruvate dehydrogenase deficiency may be aggravated by carbohydrate and a glucose tolerance test can be disastrous.

Leigh syndrome (308930) and Alper syndrome (203700) (see Ch. 14)

In the past, these conditions have been attributed to one or another of the enzymes of pyruvate metabolism. It is now clear that they can be caused by any defect of energy generation that affects the brain. Common to both are the lactic acidosis and the neurodegenerative disease which may occur from infancy onwards. In the brainstem, the pathologic findings are reminiscent of thiamin deficiency but usually the lesions are more extensive, affecting the basal ganglia and then other areas. In both, the defects can usually be found in fibroblasts or other tissues but in about 30%, no defect is found, perhaps because the brain tissue is not available. Note that Leigh syndrome is accorded an X-linked OMIM number because some cases are due to defects of the E1α subunit of pyruvate dehydrogenase but at least as many cases are due to autosomal recessive or maternally inherited traits.

Pyruvate dehydrogenase deficiency (steps 1–4) (~1 : 100 000)

Defects of E_1 (312170, 179060), E_3 (246900), the phosphatase and possibly E_2 have been described. The most severe cases die in the first weeks or months with neurological deterioration. Optic atrophy, agenesis of the corpus callosum and mid-facial hypoplasia, reminiscent of the fetal alcohol syndrome, are frequent in this group. Most cases, however, present with the variable picture of Leigh syndrome. The mildest cases have normal development and intermittent ataxia, possibly with encephalopathic features which are induced or aggravated by carbohydrates and can be totally debilitating if not treated properly (208800).

The E_3 system is shared with the α-ketoglutarate and branched chain keto acid dehydrogenases, with corresponding amino acid and organic acid abnormalities. Antibodies against the E_2 component are found in primary biliary cirrhosis in adults. E_1α-subunit deficiency is X-linked but many such cases have been female, indicating the critical role of this enzyme in cerebral metabolism; the β-subunit is coded on autosomes.

Megadoses of thiamin (200–1000 mg/day) and lipoic acid (50–500 mg/day) should be tried, but are rarely effective. The ataxic cases can be dramatically helped with a ketogenic low carbohydrate diet (10–15% of total calories). Dichloroacetate activates this enzyme and is under trial at this time.

Disorders of gluconeogenesis

Pyruvate carboxylase deficiency (step 5) (266150) may be suspected if, in addition to the features presented above, there is recurrent hypoglycemia and ketoacidosis. In cases with total lack of the enzyme, there is hyperammonemia with elevated blood citrulline, lysine and proline; some cases have proximal renal tubular acidosis. Treatment, including biotin, seems ineffective but a high carbohydrate intake is advisable. In biotinidase and multiple carboxylase deficiencies, lactic acidosis can also develop, secondary to diminished pyruvate carboxylase activity.

Defects of either cytosolic (261680) or mitochondrial (261650) *phosphoenolpyruvate carboxykinase* (step 6) have been associated with severe hypoglycemia, hypotonia, hepatomegaly and failure to thrive; treatment has not been effective. *Fructose 1,6-diphosphatase* and *glucose-6-phosphatase* deficiencies can cause severe lactic acidosis and are discussed later.

Disorders of the citric acid cycle and related pathways

Deficiency of α-*ketoglutarate dehydrogenase* (203740) or *fumarase* (136850), both enzymes of the citric acid cycle, has been associated with lactic acidosis and neurological symptoms. Both can be suspected by the organic acid pattern in urine. Combined deficiency of *succinate dehydrogenase* and *aconitase* was associated with an abnormality of iron–sulfur proteins (251945).

DISORDERS OF THE ELECTRON TRANSPORT CHAIN

Four complexes, each comprising multiple polypeptide subunits, are assembled in the mitochondrial inner membrane and transfer electrons to molecular oxygen with the generation of a transmembrane proton gradient which drives the synthesis of ATP by ATP synthase (complex V). Most of the more than 70 polypeptides are coded on nuclear DNA and are transported into mitochondria where they are assembled in situ into the complexes together with the 13 coded on mitochondrial DNA (mtDNA). Defects of each complex have been reported and sometimes more than one is involved (Fig. 20.12). In some families the disorders are clearly inherited in classic autosomal recessive patterns. It is equally clear that clinically identical conditions can also be caused by defects of mitochondrial DNA. Techniques for defining this group of disorders and their molecular defects are gradually being developed.

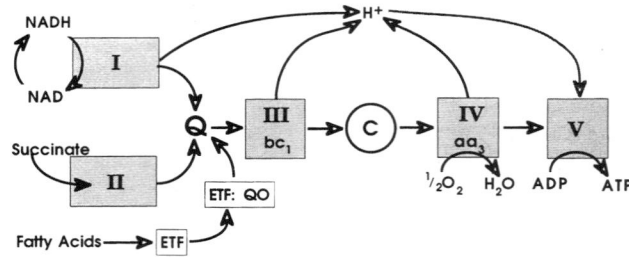

Fig. 20.12 The electron transport chain. I, Complex I, (NADH Co Q oxidoreductase); II, complex II, succinate Co Q oxidoreductase; III, complex III, ubiquinol cytochrome c reductase; IV, complex IV, cytochrome c oxidase; V, complex V, ATP synthase; Q, coenzyme Q; C, cytochrome c; ETF, electron transfer flavoprotein; ETF:QO, electron transfer flavoprotein oxidoreductase. Electrons generated by complexes I, III and IV create the proton gradient which drives ATP synthesis.

Mitochondrial genetics

All cells except erythrocytes contain thousands of mitochondria in numbers that reflect the metabolic and energy requirements of the tissues. The control of their replication is not well understood but they do proliferate in response to increased energy or other metabolic requirements. Mitochondria are all inherited from the mother (*maternal inheritance*); each possesses several copies of a distinct, circular 16.569 kb form of DNA which codes for two rRNAs, all the necessary tRNAs but only 13 polypeptides, all of which are components of the electron transport (respiratory) chain or ATP synthase. mtDNA exhibits a very high rate of spontaneous mutation which can readily be detected even in the healthy tissues of many young adults, with increasing quantities in older individuals. Some of these mutations occur with high frequency and may contribute to the normal decline of aerobic function with age. Mitochondrial proliferation can be seen in chronically hypoxemic tissues and defects of mtDNA are seen in affected parts of the brain in Alzheimer's, Huntington's and Parkinson's diseases but it is not clear which is primary or secondary.

During mitosis, mitochondria distribute randomly between the daughter cells so that if a mutation exists in some copies of the mtDNA (*heteroplasmy*) and there are no selective pressures, *replicative segregation* (presumed to be a random process akin to tossing a coin trillions of times) is likely to result in various mixtures (including *homoplasmy*) of the normal (wild) type and the mutated DNA in subsequent generations of cells. The proportions of these two populations determine the aerobic capacity of the cell and whether its functions will be compromised (*threshold effect*). This can result in very pleiotropic presentations involving different tissues within pedigrees (e.g. MERRF, MELAS or NARP); some of the mutations are expressed in tissue-specific forms. However, in Leber's optic atrophy the mutations are usually homoplasmic and in all tissues. Many benign polymorphisms are known and have been used to trace population migrations.

General clinical features of mitochondrial bioenergetic defects

All cells need to make energy and all, except RBC, rely on mitochondria to meet most of their ATP needs. This means that no organ or tissue escapes the risk of mitochondrial dysfunction, which can develop at any age. Even within a single family, there can be markedly different presentations; moreover, it is difficult or impossible to predict which of the complexes is involved without sophisticated biochemical studies since some of the disorders, such as the myopathies, can be due to defects of any, or all, of them.

Since most of the peptides of the electron transport chain are coded on autosomal genes, it follows that autosomal defects of these can cause similar problems to those produced by certain defects of mtDNA. While it is now possible to determine which of the complexes are involved in most patients, (e.g. complex I or IV deficiency causing *Leigh syndrome*), it is still rare that the precise genetic defect is identified (e.g. NARP mutation causing Leigh syndrome). The full spectrum of mitochondrial diseases is still emerging and it is not clear what determines the age of onset or the tissue susceptibility.

The commonest presentations in childhood are:

1. Neonatal. Profound lactic acidosis associated with severe neurologic damage, hypotonia with myopathy with or without ragged-red fibers* and quite often cardiomyopathy and evidence of involvement of other organs. Most of these cases die.

2. A severe infantile form similar to 1 above, with profound hypotonia and/or the *renal Fanconi syndrome*. Some of these cases are permanently affected but in others, the whole syndrome is *reversible* and by 1–3 years they are completely normal.

3. *Leigh* (308930) and *Alper* (203700) *syndromes* in which there is progressive neurological deterioration usually involving the brainstem and the basal ganglia together with myopathy.

4. A stable neurological syndrome in which there may be developmental delay, seizures or cerebral palsy with or without lactic acidosis.

5. Isolated myopathy with exercise intolerance and lactic acidosis, with or without chronic progressive external ophthalmoplegia (CPEO), occurring at any age (Table 20.7).

6. Isolated cardiomyopathy, occurring at any age.

7. The *Kearns–Sayre* syndrome.

8. Sudden severe but reversible organ failure; the liver is the most commonly affected.

There are many other presentations affecting adults; they are summarized below but the full spectrum is still emerging.

Maternally inherited mutations of mtDNA

Most of these syndromes involve point mutations in tRNA or protein coding regions and are encountered more frequently in adults. They include *Leber's hereditary optic neuropathy (LHON)* (308900, 535000) in which the symptoms usually develop in early adult life. The full-blown syndromes of *myoclonic epilepsy with ragged red fiber myopathy (MERRF)* (254775), *mitochondrial encephalopathy with lactic acidosis and stroke-like episodes (MELAS)* (251910) and *neuropathy, ataxia with retinitis pigmentosa (NARP)* are self-explanatory. However, they are very pleiotropic and many cases are oligosymptomatic with barely abnormal function of one or more tissues or organs; diabetes and

deafness are common in both kinds of pedigrees. In MELAS, the 'strokes' resemble transient ischemic episodes and the encephalopathy can include seizures and psychiatric or motor problems; the myopathy causes exercise intolerance and weakness. Excess mitochondria are seen in muscles and in the cerebral blood vessels. In the more aggressive forms of these syndromes, the encephalopathy and myopathy cause increasing debility and may be accompanied by other problems such as diabetes, deafness or pigmentary retinopathy. The NARP mutation is one cause of *Leigh syndrome*.

Other conditions include *type II diabetes with or without deafness* which is a combination of symptoms that is so frequent in older adults it is not clear how many such cases have one of these mutations. Rare cases of *chronic progressive external ophthalmoplegia (CPEO)* (251950, 258470) are maternally inherited and present in adolescence with ptosis and/or muscle weakness. *Aminoglycoside-induced deafness* (580000) and *familial nonsyndromic deafness* can also be maternally inherited.

It is critical to remember that these symptoms, often taken to be the manifestations of early aging and scattered randomly through a pedigree, seemingly unrelated to the problems in a child, can strongly suggest the possible etiology. A well-taken pedigree is tedious but often critical.

Spontaneous, sporadic errors in mtDNA

Most of these are major rearrangements (duplications or deletions) of several kb. They are almost always sporadic with little or no risk of recurrence in siblings or offspring.

The *Kearns–Sayre syndrome (KSS)* (530000) presents in childhood with growth failure, ophthalmoplegia, retinopathy and, variously, myopathy, encephalopathy, neuropathy, deafness, cardiac conduction defects, endocrinopathies and cerebellar damage with elevated CSF protein. Lactic acidosis is usual and should lead to referral to a center specializing in mitochondrial disorders.

Pearson's marrow/pancreas syndrome (260560) presents with early onset pancytopenic anemia, pancreatic dysfunction and lactic acidosis and a selection of involvement of other tissues.

A further syndrome which is not understood is sudden episodes of acute liver failure which is reversible and is associated most commonly with *depletion of hepatic mtDNA* (Wijburg et al 1995).

Mendelian inherited disorders of mtDNA

Mitochondrial myopathy with multiple deletions of mtDNA (160560) is dominantly inherited.

Mitochondrial neurogastrointestinal encephalopathy (MNGIE) (263080) causes myopathy, CPEO, leukodystrophy and chronic diarrhea with pseudo-obstruction which can be fatal; it can be sporadic or recessive. *Depletion of mtDNA* with loss of as much as 98% of the mtDNA usually affects only one tissue such as muscle, heart or kidney and is usually fatal before 1 year. Late onset cases are usually confined to muscle although recurrent episodes of liver failure have been reported. *Luft syndrome* (238800) is a hypermetabolic myopathy due to uncoupling of oxidative phosphorylation. *Myopathy with cytochrome oxidase deficiency* (220100) occurs in a fatal, infantile form and in a form which seems equally severe but is *reversible*. A defect of ion channeling at the mitochondrial membrane compromises mitochondrial function (314555) (Ruitenbeek et al 1995).

---

* This term denotes a histochemical staining characteristic which is caused by large subsarcolemmal accumulations of mitochondria. At one stage it was the main way that mitochondrial myopathies were diagnosed. While they are usually found in cases with mutations of mtDNA in a tRNA, their absence in no way excludes a disorder of mtDNA.

Mitochondrial myopathy and cardiomyopathy also occurs in Barth syndrome (p. 1156). Two siblings with Leigh syndrome had a defect of the flavoprotein subunit of complex II.

Investigations

The initial studies are outlined above; once a mitochondrial syndrome is suspected, the diagnostic approach varies depending on the facilities available. In some centers, it is possible to evaluate aerobic muscle function using exercise or other physiological approaches. P^{31}-NMR spectroscopy is being used to monitor energy generation in muscle but it is not widely available.

The detection of either lactic acidosis or ragged-red fiber myopathy leads to the complicated biochemical studies of the electron transport chain which are only available in a few centers. Defects of complex I (516000–516010, 252010), complex II, complex III (516020) and complex IV (cytochrome c oxidase) (220100) may exist alone or in any combination. In some cases, the defect may be expressed in fibroblasts or leukocytes but, frequently, a fresh sample of affected tissue such as muscle is required. Identification of the precise genetic defect requires sophisticated techniques only available in a few centers.

Treatment

Management of the lactic acidosis is discussed above. Some patients with complex I deficiency appear to respond to large doses of riboflavin or possibly nicotinamide. Vitamins C and K and ubiquinone (30–360 mg/day) should be tried in complex III deficiencies.

DISORDERS OF FATTY ACID METABOLISM (Fig. 20.13) (in aggregate ~1 : 10–20 000)

After birth, fatty acids are the major fuel for cardiac and skeletal muscle, both at rest and during aerobic exercise. Following release from circulating or stored triglycerides by lipoprotein lipase (step 1), free fatty acids are bound to albumin in the plasma. After diffusing across the cell membrane, the long chain fatty acids, primarily palmitic and oleic acids, are converted to fatty acyl-CoA esters by an acyl-CoA synthase (step 3). Neither this step nor the transport systems into mitochondria seem to be required for medium or short chain fatty acids but these are usually minor metabolic pathways.

Transport into mitochondria requires L-carnitine, which is both endogenously produced and also comes from animal sources in the diet. Carnitine palmitoyl transferase-1 (step 4) forms fatty acylcarnitine conjugates which are transported into the mitochondria by a translocase (step 5). Once inside the matrix, the reaction is reversed by CPT-2 and free carnitine and long chain fatty acyl-CoA are formed (step 6).

Fatty acid β-oxidation occurs in a repeating four-enzyme cycle, each 'spiral' of the cycle releasing one molecule of acetyl-CoA (steps 7–12). The first reaction is performed by very long chain or long chain ($C_{12–18}$), medium chain ($C_{6–12}$) or short chain ($C_{4–6}$) acyl-CoA dehydrogenases. These reactions provide reducing equivalents and are coupled directly through electron transfer flavoprotein (ETF) and ETF: CoQ oxidoreductase (ETF: QO) (steps 13–15) to coenzyme Q of the electron transport chain. Three further steps complete one cycle leaving a fatty acyl-CoA two carbons shorter for further β-oxidation. Fatty acid oxidation

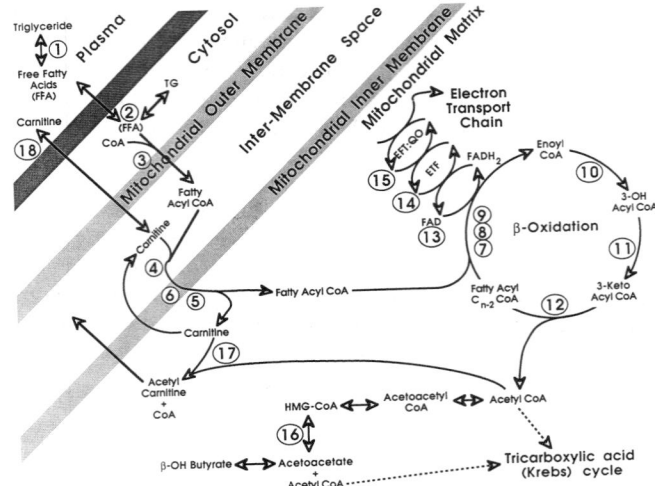

Fig. 20.13 Steps involved in fatty acid oxidation. 1, Lipoprotein lipase;* 2, fatty acid binding protein; 3, fatty acyl CoA synthase; 4, carnitine palmitoyl transferase I (CPT I);* 5, carnitine palmitoyl transferase II (CPT II);* 6, fatty acyl carnitine translocase;* 7, long chain acyl CoA dehydrogenase (LCAD);* 8, medium chain acyl CoA dehydrogenase (MCAD);* 9, short chain acyl CoA dehydrogenase (SCAD);* 10, enoyl-CoA hydratase; 11, 3-hydroxy acyl-CoA dehydrogenase;* 12, beta-ketothiolase; 13, flavin adenine dinucleotide (FAD);* 14, electron transfer flavoprotein (ETF);* 15, ETF: coenzyme Q oxidoreductase (ETF:QO);* 16, 3-hydroxy, 3-methylglutaryl CoA lyase (HMGCoA);* 17, carnitine acetyl transferase;* 18, carnitine transport.*
* Defects identified (see text).

in the liver produces the ketone bodies, acetoacetate and β-hydroxybutyrate, which, under homeostatic conditions, are recycled to fatty acids although they can be metabolized by the brain during prolonged fasting. In the liver, acetyl-CoA is used in the citric acid cycle, sparing glycogen and glucose depletion.

The transition from the continuous supply of glucose in fetal life to a mixed fuel system after birth requires efficient β-oxidation, which is not usually stressed by the normal, frequent feeding schedules of newborn infants. It is often only when the time between feeding increases, or during a catabolic illness, that symptoms develop in patients with defects of fatty acid oxidation. When β-oxidation is increased or disrupted, the dicarboxylic acids adipic (C_6), suberic (C_8) and sebacic (C_{10}) acids are produced by ω-oxidation of the excess intermediates. Thus they are seen in fasting and in ketoacidosis from any cause, as well as in the disorders of fatty acid catabolism or ketone utilization. In addition to carnitine deficiency, at least 12 defects in fatty acid oxidation have been identified. Their nomenclature is somewhat confusing since the clinical features and enzymology are still being defined. Collectively, they appear to be relatively common.

Clinical features

The clinical manifestations of disorders of fatty acid metabolism include episodes of lethargy with nausea and vomiting, hypoketotic hypoglycemia, progressive somnolence, hepatic encephalopathy indistinguishable from Reye's syndrome and sudden, unexpected death in infancy. Young children may have muscle weakness, hypotonia and developmental delay, exercise intolerance, muscle pain or cramps; in older patients, recurrent myoglobinuria may occur. Dysmorphic features and hypertrophic or dilated cardiomyopathy may occur in some of the disorders and CNS symptoms, when they occur, may be life threatening. Some patients may remain permanently asymptomatic. Severe and mild cases of many of these disorders are recognized.

Diagnosis

Hypoketotic hypoglycemia is discussed below. The majority of these cases are detected by studies of organic acids and carnitine status in patients with Reye's syndrome, myopathy, cardiomyopathy, unexplained liver disease or hypoglycemia. These patterns may be diagnostic at all times or only abnormal during metabolic stress. Plasma acyl-carnitine or acyl-glycine profiles by fast-atom bombardment/mass spectrometry often provide diagnostic patterns in these disorders. Histologically, microvesicular fat in the liver and myocytes are characteristic of carnitine depletion. Enzyme assays can usually be done on WBC or cultured skin fibroblasts.

Treatment

For those conditions which are treatable, avoidance of fasting and the ready provision of nonfat calories orally or parenterally if needed during stress are critical. L-Carnitine is indicated in all of these conditions in doses of 50–300 mg/kg/day and in depletion syndromes it is lifesaving. A lower fat diet is prudent and in the long chain disorders, MCT oil is a good source of calories. The tendency to develop symptoms falls with age as dependence on β-oxidation lessens.

Defects in the carnitine cycle

Carnitine derives partly from the diet and partly from endogenous synthesis. It can be depleted in liver or kidney disease, malnutrition and malabsorption. Low levels are usual in premature and neonatal infants and in pregnancy in which these lowered values are probably physiologically normal.

Marked depletion occurs either from interference with synthesis (e.g. methylene tetrahydrofolate reductase deficiency), renal loss (e.g. Fanconi's syndrome) or increased consumption (e.g. the organic acidemias or valproate therapy). The latter occurs because carnitine accepts any acyl-CoA ester and the resulting acylcarnitine, for example isovaleryl-carnitine, is then excreted. In removing the toxic acyl-CoA esters, more carnitine is lost. In addition, acylcarnitines inhibit the renal reabsorption of free carnitine, aggravating the depletion. In such cases, plasma and urine free carnitine levels are reduced but the acylcarnitine values are high so that the total may appear normal. In plasma, an acyl:free ratio above 0.5 warrants consideration of this mechanism.

No primary defect of carnitine synthesis is currently known. The term 'primary deficiency' is reserved for patients in whom there is a defect in the uptake of carnitine into cells. Such *carnitine transport defects* may be pancellular or tissue specific in myocytes (212160), renal tubular cells or, rarely, hepatocytes. Renal tubular losses (212140) produce very low plasma values and very high urine levels resulting in 'systemic deficiency', involving all tissues. Muscle depletion presents with hypotonia or weakness (see Table 20.7); cardiac depletion causes acute or chronic cardiomyopathy and hepatocellular depletion can cause hepatic steatosis or fulminant Reye's syndrome, any of which can

be precipitated during stress or minor starvation. In other cases, the plasma levels may be normal but the involved tissues are deficient. L-carnitine (25–350 mg/kg/day) should be used as replacement therapy; occasionally higher doses are warranted.

One idiopathic condition which seems not to be rare is the *Ruvalcalba–Myhre–Smith* syndrome (153480) in which low muscle carnitine tends to be associated with macrocephaly, hypotonia, cafe-au-lait spots that are frequent on the penis and poor development. In such depletion syndromes, nonspecific symptoms such as hypotonia, lassitude, anorexia and sleep disturbance often improve dramatically with oral L-carnitine therapy.

Carnitine palmitoyl transferase 1 deficiency (CPT-1) (255120) (steps 4 and 5) (~1 : 500 000) causes symptomatic fasting hypoketotic hypoglycemia and occasionally hepatocellular damage. The heart and muscle are rarely involved although plasma CPK can be high. The plasma carnitine is characteristically elevated.

In *CPT-2 deficiency* (255110) an infantile form presents with severe hypoglycemia, myopathy and cardiomyopathy leading to death. Plasma carnitine is low with elevated acylcarnitines. A milder form presents with lipid myopathy, recurrent rhabdomyolysis and myoglobinuria in young adults. *Carnitine/acylcarnitine translocase deficiency* (212138) is similar to infantile CPT-2 deficiency.

Medium chain acyl-CoA dehydrogenase deficiency (MCAD) (step 8) (201450) (1 : 10–20 000)

Clinical features

The most severe presentation (often an unusual G583A mutation) is of sudden death in the first days after birth. MCAD is also the cause of 1–3% of SIDS. Other common presentations include recurrent hypoglycemia, classically hypoketotic, often associated with hepatocellular dysfunction that can proceed to full-blown Reye's syndrome. Cardiomyopathy and/or signs of muscle carnitine depletion such as weakness or hypotonia are common and may be accompanied by fatigue or lethargy. As with all β-oxidation defects, these problems are produced or aggravated by poor nutrition or the stress of even a minor illness. It is important to note that many cases are never symptomatic, presumably because they never develop carnitine depletion together with sufficient stress; by mid-childhood, most of the risks are past.

Diagnosis

Characteristic medium chain fatty acyl–glycine and –carnitine conjugates are present in blood and urine (hexanoylglycine, suberylglycine and octanoylcarnitine); so far, phenylpropionylglycine has invariably been present. Using sophisticated technology, they can be detected on newborn filter paper samples as now employed in a few routine screening programs. 80–90% of cases are homozygous for the A985G mutation which can also be detected in filter paper samples.

Other defects of fatty acid oxidation

Long chain 3-hydroxyacyl-CoA dehydrogenase (LCHAD) is a component of a trifunctional enzyme that also comprises enoyl-CoA hydratase and CoA thiolase activities. Deficiency (step 11)

(143450, 600890) appears to be the second most common of these defects; long chain hydroxy acids are usually detectable. In it and in *long chain/very long chain acyl-CoA dehydrogenase deficiency* (*LCAD/VLCAD*) (step 7/11) (201460), the features are similar to, but more severe than MCAD. Older patients may develop late onset cardiomyopathy or myopathy with recurrent myoglobinuria and patients are generally carnitine deficient. Treatment with MCT oil is beneficial. Acute fatty liver of pregnancy or the 'HELP' syndrome occurs with some LCHAD affected fetuses.

Other defects include *short chain acyl-CoA dehydrogenase deficiency* (*SCAD*) (step 9) (201470), *short chain 3-hydroxyacyl-CoA dehydrogenase deficiency* (Bennett et al 1996) and *malonyl-CoA decarboxylase deficiency* (248360). These cases tend to have failure to thrive, recurrent vomiting with or without hypoglycemia and/or ketosis, hypotonia, marked developmental delay, seizures and early demise. The urine organic acid profiles tend to suggest the site of the defects but confirmation requires detailed studies in fibroblasts or other tissues. 3-hydroxy-3-methylglutaryl-CoA lyase deficiency (step 9, Fig. 20.13) (246450) is discussed on page 1118.

Glycerol derives from hydrolysis of fats and, reversibly, from glycolysis, making it available for gluconeogenesis. Isolated *glycerol kinase deficiency* (307030) causes recurrent attacks of a Reye-like syndrome with vomiting, acidemia, CNS depression and hypotonia which are precipitated by a high fat intake or fasting. Milder cases are found by chance with pseudohypertriglyceridemia on routine multichannel blood testing. It also can be part of an X chromosome microdeletion syndrome which includes Duchenne muscular dystrophy, retinopathy and adrenal hypoplasia which usually dominates the clinical picture; note that glycerol in urine may derive from body lotions or suppositories. Frequent high carbohydrate feeding with mild fat restriction is indicated. *Glycerol intolerance* is a different condition also causing recurrent hypoglycemia and Reye-like attacks.

Multiple acyl-CoA dehydrogenase deficiency (MAD) (Fig. 20.12)

This is actually a group of disorders at the level of entry of electrons into the electron transport chain from several amino acids as well as from numerous acyl-CoA dehydrogenases. Defects of transport, processing or binding of FAD, electron transfer flavoprotein (ETF) or the ETF: CoQ oxidoreductase (ETF: QO) are all possible. Three forms are generally recognized with clinical overlap between groups and genetic heterogeneity within each group.

The severe form (MAD:S), also called *glutaric aciduria type II* (231675, 231680), is usually lethal in the newborn period, secondary to profound acidosis, hypoglycemia, coma and multiple organ system involvement. A subgroup of these patients have dysmorphic facial and other features, characteristic subependymal brain cysts, dysmyelination of brain and polycystic kidneys. Milder cases have no dysmorphism but usually severe failure to thrive, hypotonia, cardiomyopathy and liver damage. An unusual 'acrid' odor and the 'sweaty feet' odor of isovaleric acid are often described. The biochemical profile in urine is generally diagnostic, with accumulations of ethylmalonic, glutaric, 2-hydroxyglutaric, adipic, suberic and sebacic acids, isovaleryl, isobutyryl- and 2-methylbutyryl-glycines and the amino acid sarcosine.

Milder, MAD:M patients, also called ethylmalonic-adipic aciduria (231680), may not even present until adulthood; they usually present similarly to other acyl-CoA dehydrogenase deficiency patients. The urine organic acid profile is simpler than in MAD: S, usually containing only ethylmalonic, adipic and methylsuccinic acids and hexanoyl and butyrylglycines. Dicarboxylic acids are abundant, giving rise to the original term *riboflavin-responsive dicarboxylic aciduria*.

Defects of both ETF and ETF: QO have been found in both forms of MAD. Generally, the severity of the enzyme deficiency correlates with the severity or type of disorder.

Some of these patients improve on riboflavin (100–300 mg/day); they may have a defect of cofactor binding.

DISORDERS OF KETONE METABOLISM (Figs 20.10 & 20.11)

Defects of ketone synthesis include *β-hydroxy-β-methyl glutaryl-CoA synthase* (HMG synthase) (142940) and *3-hydroxy-3-methylglutaryl-CoA lyase* deficiency (246450). They are associated with recurrent Reye's syndrome with stress-related episodes of vomiting, lethargy, severe *hypoketotic* hypoglycemia, metabolic acidosis and a characteristic pattern of urinary organic acids with elevated 3-hydroxy-3-methylglutaric, 3-methylglutaric, 3-methylglutaconic and 3-hydroxyisovaleric acidosis. This is the final enzyme of leucine degradation (step 9), but is also required for hepatic ketone body synthesis. Other patients with apparently similar biochemical findings have had normal enzyme activity. Growth failure, microcephaly, nerve deafness and basal ganglion lesions similar to Leigh syndrome were found in these cases. 3-hydroxy-3-methylglutaryl-CoA is also converted to mevalonic acid.

Defects of ketone utilization cause facile hyperketosis; they include *succinyl-CoA:3-ketoacid-CoA transferase* (245050) and several enzymes with *3-ketothiolase* activity. *2-Methylaceto-acetyl-CoA thiolase* deficiency (step 12) (203750) can present with severe neonatal acidosis, intermittent episodes of ketoacidosis with lethargy and coma or may be asymptomatic. Developmental delay may occur. Hypoglycemia, ketotic hyperglycinemia and hyperammonemia are reported. The urine contains 2-methyl-3-hydroxybutyric acid, other organic acids and butanone. Acetoacetic and β-hydroxybutyric acids can be greatly elevated and the disease may mimic salicylism. The enzyme defect can be shown in cultured skin fibroblasts. Deficiency of either of two other distinct 3-ketothiolases, *mitochondrial and cytosolic acetoacetyl-CoA thiolase*, both seem to be associated with progressive neurological deterioration, neuropathy and extrapyramidal movements. Lactic acidosis with abnormal lactate/pyruvate ratios and increased ketone body levels are usual. General treatment for these disorders is discussed on page 1125.

Diagnosis

These conditions are rare but definite causes of ketotic hypoglycemia. They are discussed below.

HYPOGLYCEMIA AND METABOLIC DISEASES

The half-life of metabolic fuels in the plasma is about 100 seconds. Great variations in the rate of glucose consumption must be balanced by intricate hormonal controls and the co-ordinated release of fuels from glycogen, fat or protein. Often, hepatomegaly or acidosis suggest a metabolic diagnosis but, for the most part, inborn errors causing hypoglycemia require extensive metabolic testing. Hyper- and hypoketosis are often not recognized because blood ketones must be quantitated at the same time as the glucose. In addition, free fatty acids, amino acids, carnitine and sometimes glycerol need to be measured *in samples obtained before any treatment has been given.* Urine for organic acids must also be obtained during the acute episode. Starvation/fasting stress tests can be used to create an acute episode but these should only be done in hospital with full emergency support available (Fernandes et al 1995, Ch. l, Scriver et al 1995, Ch. 5).

Hypoglycemia with ketosis and/or acidosis

Ketotic hypoglycemia occurs frequently in small undergrown infants and children. Most cases are due to poor growth, poor nutrition with inadequate and/or infrequent feeding. Lack of glycogen stores and of muscle protein for gluconeogenesis necessitate increased lipolysis. As a result, fatty acid intermediates and ketones readily accumulate in patterns that mimic hereditary defects of fuel homeostasis. In nutritional deprivation, plasma alanine and lactate are low and there is no response to an i.m. glucagon challenge. The metabolic diagnosis includes glycogen storage disorders and defects of ketone utilization, pyruvate, the citric acid cycle and organic acid metabolism.

Hypoketotic hypoglycemia

Hypoglycemia with inappropriately low levels of blood ketones suggests a defect of fatty acid oxidation or of ketone production; it is also typical in hyperinsulinism.

DISORDERS OF CARBOHYDRATE METABOLISM

Disorders of digestion and absorption are primarily addressed in Chapter 11. In the gut, hereditary defects of *lactase* (223000), *sucrose-isomaltase* (222900), *trehalase* and *glucose galactose absorption* (231600) are known.

In the kidneys, *renal glycosuria* (233100) is caused by a deficit in glucose absorption. *Pentosuria* (260800) is a benign condition, most common in Jewish people due to deficient L-xylulose reductase activity; xylulose is excreted in the urine where it reacts with Benedict's solution or Clinitest to give a false-positive test for glucose.

DEFECTS OF GLYCOLYSIS (Fig. 20.14)

In erythrocytes

Severe defects of glycolysis in erythrocytes are usually associated with hemolytic anemia (Ch. 15). Such conditions include defects of *glucose-6-phosphate dehydrogenase* (305900), *hexokinase* (235700) (step 2), *glucosephosphate isomerase* (172400) (step 4), *phosphofructokinase* (261670) (step 5), *aldolase* (103850), *triose phosphate isomerase* (*TPI*) (190450) (step 7), *phosphoglycerate kinase* (*PGK*) (311800) (step 9), *diphosphoglycerate mutase* (261670) (step 10), *pyruvate kinase* (266200) (step 12) and *lactate*

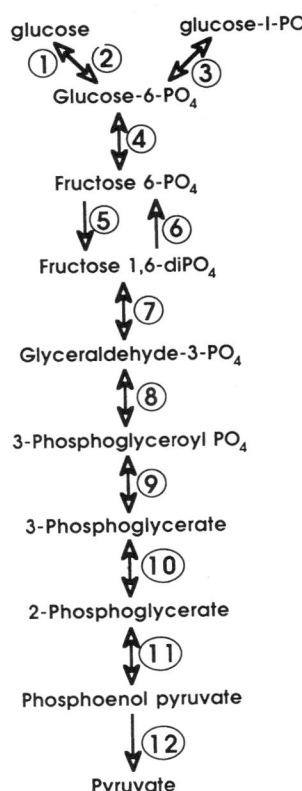

Fig. 20.14   The Embden–Meyerhof glycolytic pathway. 1, Glucose-6-phosphatase; 2, hexokinase; 3, phosphoglucomutase; 4, phosphohexose isomerase; 5, phosphofructokinase; 6, fructose-I, 6-bisphosphatase; 7, triose phosphate isomerase; 8, glyceraldehyde-3 phosphate dehydrogenase; 9, phosphoglycerate kinase; 10, phosphoglyceromutase; 11, enolase; 12, pyruvate kinase.

dehydrogenase. In contrast, deficiency of either *2,3-DPG mutase* (222800) or *diphosphoglycerate phosphatase* (171500) causes mild erythrocytosis. Hemolysis can also be caused by defects of the γ-glutamyl cycle (p. 1115) and certain steps in purine and pyrimidine metabolism (p. 1140) and *adenosine triphosphatase* (102800). Other red cell enzymopathies include defects of *6-phosphogluconate dehydrogenase* in the pentose monophosphate shunt and of *glutathione metabolism.* Finally, *cytochrome b_5 reductase* deficiency is often associated with methemoglobinemia and developmental delay.

In the nervous system

Several of these disorders also cause neurological or muscular disease. Severe TPI deficiency is associated with severe, progressive neurological disease with both upper and lower motor neuron damage; the intellect is relatively well preserved. There is also a tendency to sudden death and increased susceptibility to infection. Severe PGK deficiency can cause developmental delay and attacks of behavioral and emotional abnormalities, movement disorders including hemiplegia and even coma that develop during hemolytic crises. *Glutathione reductase* deficiency (138330) has also been reported to cause a variety of neurological abnormalities, including myelopathy. About 15% of cases with *cytochrome b_5 reductase* deficiency (250790) have severe progressive neurological deterioration with microcephaly, athetosis and hypertonia in addition to methemoglobinemia. In all of these disorders, management of these neurological symptoms is unsatisfactory but should include avoidance of oxidant drugs.

In muscle – the metabolic myopathies

There is a large and growing number of metabolic myopathies almost all of which involve energy metabolism. Since several are glycolytic disorders, the whole group are summarized here (Table 20.7).

Clinical features

The usual symptoms of these disorders are muscle weakness, lack of endurance and postexercise muscle pain or cramps; some are aggravated by fasting or a high fat diet. Muscle wasting, when present, is often due to disuse rather than to the intrinsic muscle disease. In glycolytic or fatty acid defects, excessive exercise leads to severe cramping and rhabdomyolysis with increased serum creatine phosphokinase levels with recurrent myoglobinuria leading to severe renal damage. These disorders tend to present only in adolescence or later. Curiously, the disorders of the electron transport chain, which may occur at any age, are rarely associated with myoglobinuria, perhaps because the dyspnea from lactic acidosis is so marked that exercise capacity is too limited to result in much muscle cell damage.

Nonspecific complaints of muscle weakness, lack of endurance or muscle cramps are very common and only 10–20% of such cases prove to have a real muscle disorder. Real cases are often not detected or evaluated for years or until a crisis such as rhabdomyolysis develops.

Diagnosis

Physiological measurements of muscle function are occasionally helpful and an ischemic exercise test is usually abnormal in the glycolytic defects. Muscle tissue, obtained by needle or open biopsy, should *not* be preserved in formalin but submitted fresh or flash frozen for histochemical examination which, when properly

Table 20.7 Metabolic disorders which cause myopathy

Glycogen storage diseases
  Acid maltase (II), debrancher (III), brancher (IV), phosphorylase (V) (Fig. 20.18)

Glycolytic defects
  Phosphofructokinase, phosphoglycerate kinase, phosphoglycerate mutase, glucosephosphate isomerase, lactate dehydrogenase, lactate transporter (Fig. 20.14)

Lipid catabolic defects
  Carnitine palmitoyl transferase, carnitine depletion, carnitine acetyl transferase, lipid storage myopathies, defects of β-oxidation (Fig. 20.13)

Purine disorders
  Myoadenylate deaminase (Fig. 20.20)

Mitochondrial defects
  Complexes I-V (Fig. 20.12), Lufts syndrome, malate–aspartate shuttle, calcium-ATPase, Krebs cycle defects, adenine nucleotide translocase, pyruvate dehydrogenase defects

Others
  Hypermethioninemia, periodic paralyses, malignant hyperthermia ion channelopathies

done, can indicate a number of enzymatic defects. Glycogen content is often increased in the glycogen storage diseases, the glycolytic defects and frequently in electron transport defects. The lipid content is usually increased in the lipid disorders but not in carnitine palmitoyl transferase deficiency. Mitochondrial disorders may exhibit ragged-red fibers and abnormal mitochondria on electron photomicrographs. Necrotic changes are usually only seen after severe exercise and sometimes the histology, including electron microscopy, is completely normal.

Intracellular levels of ATP, phosphocreatine and phosphate can be measured in vivo by ^{31}P-NMR spectroscopy and this is being used to detect defects of energy generation and to monitor the effects of treatment.

Treatment

This is usually restricted to limiting exercise which should stop before symptoms are provoked. Mild aerobic exercise can be encouraged but rigorous training is dangerous. In glycolytic and fatty acid disorders, 'carbo loading' may be useful and continuous intake of glucose during exercise is helpful; fasting and high-fat diets should be avoided, especially before exercise.

GALACTOSE

The main source of dietary galactose is lactose, the predominant carbohydrate in milk and most milk-based infant formulae, in which it provides a considerable amount of energy. Galactose is metabolized for energy, mainly in the liver. Other tissues such as erythrocytes can metabolize galactose too and can be used to evaluate galactose metabolism. The metabolic pathway of galactose is depicted in Figure 20.15.

Galactose-1-phosphate uridyltransferase deficiency (galactosemia) (step 2) (230400) (~1 : 60 000)

Clinical features

Babies with severe transferase deficiency become sick soon after beginning to ingest milk. The severity of the presentation depends on the quantity of milk ingested (breast milk contains more lactose than milk-based formulae) and any residual transferase activity of the liver. Severe cases mimic sepsis and many do develop Gram-negative or β-streptococcal sepsis presenting soon

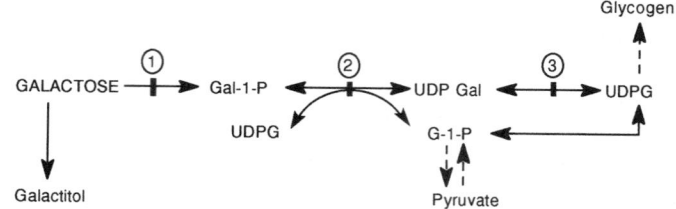

Galactose metabolism
- - - → metabolic pathway comprising several conversions
① galactokinase, ② galactose-1-phosphate uridyltransferase,
③ uridine diphosphate galactose 4'-epimerase
Abbreviations: see text

Fig. 20.15

after birth with vomiting, diarrhea, failure to thrive and persistent jaundice. Hepatosplenomegaly, progressive liver dysfunction with raised SGOT, hypoglycemia, anemia, purpura and deficient clotting factors and the biochemical findings of the renal Fanconi syndrome are typical. Cataracts may be evident at birth or appear soon after. Edema, ascites, malnutrition, cachexia and septicemia usually presage a fatal outcome from hepatic failure within a few weeks if the condition is not treated. Mental retardation and behavioral abnormalities develop if the disease has a more protracted course. With minimal enzyme activity, the course is less catastrophic, only causing failure to thrive and cataracts.

The acute abnormalities are rapidly corrected by complete elimination of galactose from the diet. However, long-term complications are frequent, regardless of how early or how well the infant is treated. Overall, there is a slight reduction in intelligence and visual perceptual skills; 50% have dyspraxic speech and hypergonadotropic hypogonadism with ovarian failure and often sterility occurs in approximately 80% of females. The causes of these late complications are unknown. Testicular function is unaffected.

Diagnosis

The simplest screening test is examination of the urine for reducing sugars (Clinitest) performed 24–36 hours *after* the start of lactose-containing feeds. Filter paper Guthrie tests for galactose, gal-1-P and the transferase (Beutler) test are in wide use (Ch. 5) but often these results are only available after symptoms have developed and when the diagnosis is suspected. Actually, gal-1-P is markedly elevated in cord blood so early detection in high-risk infants is feasible. Vomiting or changes to nonlactose formulae may obscure the diagnosis and blood transfusion or exchange transfusion negate the erythrocyte assays for gal-1-P and the enzyme. Any suspicious results are indications for initiating treatment, for identification of the reducing sugar by chromatography, for quantitative blood assays for galactose and gal-1-P and confirmatory enzyme assays on RBC or fibroblasts. Galactose tolerance tests should never be used.

The most obvious histological changes occur in the liver. There is fatty infiltration, fibrosis, bile duct proliferation and pseudoacinar arrangement of hepatic cells. The renal changes consist of widening of the proximal tubules and alterations of the tubular epithelium.

Transferase can be assayed in erythrocytes, cultured fibroblasts and chorionic villi. Many variants with lesser deficiencies of enzyme activity have been described; Duarte homozygotes and compound heterozygotes are about 1 : 3–5000. Most of these cases are asymptomatic

Variants (~1 : 4000)

Dozens of mutations are known; the commonest is the Duarte variant for which about 1 : 25 people are carriers who have about 75% of normal enzyme activity. Duarte homozygotes have about 50% and Duarte/classical compound heterozygotes about 10–25% activity (see Fig. 20.1). Such cases have elevated gal-1-P in cord blood and are often detected by routine newborn screening. If they drink milk, gal-1-P remains high for months but eventually falls to normal. There is no evidence that the gal-1-P is toxic in these cases or that there is any risk for any of the long- or short-term complications and opinion is sharply divided as to whether they

should be treated with galactose restriction or not. Some authorities require nonlactose formula for the first year; others allow partial breast-feeding but often prudence seems guided by medicolegal concerns.

Treatment

In infants with the full-blown disease, total elimination of dietary galactose corrects all of the acute problems within a few days and weight gain ensues. Residual liver damage is rare and sometimes the cataracts resolve.

Soy milks or synthetic formulae, which do not contain lactose, are used. Soy beans contain L-galactosides like raffinose and stachyose, which are not hydrolyzed in the small intestine; however, bacterial fermentation in the colon could release galactose, so these L-galactosides should be removed from the soy flour by dialysis.

Without question, the diet should be strictly followed for the first several years. It is less clear how important this is for older children; some authorities believe that the diet requires lifelong meticulous attention to detail. Many foods contain unlabeled lactose and even many fruits and vegetables contain galactose. With this approach, all foods, especially bread, sausage and candies of uncertain composition and medications which may contain lactose, must be rigidly excluded. Such diets are very restrictive and can lead to eating disorders and to serious parental anxiety. With the evidence that all these patients make significant quantities of galactose metabolites (see below), other authorities now believe that, after childhood, obsessive adherence is unnecessary and that small quantities of galactose are safe although deliberate and continuous exposure is clearly contraindicated. Adults can tolerate small quantities of galactose without acute symptoms or obvious biochemical abnormalities; the long-term safety of this is not known and some restrictions are clearly needed. Some children on a relaxed regime show deteriorating school performance and behavior problems but this may be due to suboptimal parenting as much as to galactose toxicity. Lifelong galactose restriction remains the standard of care.

Because cataracts may be present at birth, cord blood gal-1-P is markedly elevated and because it is also increased in the mother's blood, prenatal restriction of galactose has been advocated. However, this has no effect on the long-term outcome. Heterozygote offspring of properly treated homozygous mothers appear to be completely normal.

Self-intoxication

About 12–24 mg/kg/day galactose is synthesized by these patients (Berry et al 1995); it is essential for the synthesis of galacto-lipids and -proteins. Moreover, lactose is synthesized normally in the milk of a lactating mother. It is not surprising that, even with the use of strict galactose-free diets or parenteral nutrition, gal-1-P remains elevated in the blood. Galactose ingestion certainly raises the RBC gal-1-P and this test is still used to monitor diet compliance; in view of the dual sources, elevated values are often misinterpreted.

Galactitol from free galactose is the cause of the cataracts. The cause of the acute and the long-term complications is not known; they have been attributed to gal-1-P toxicity but, by inference from the variants, this seems unlikely. Perhaps they arise from excess or depleted metabolites in the tissues.

Other defects of galactose metabolism

Galactokinase deficiency (230200) (~1 : 150–250 000). As soon as galactose is consumed, it accumulates in the blood and urine; some is reduced to the polyol galactitol which causes cataracts because of osmotic swelling and disruption of lens fibers. Gal-1-P and UDP-galactose (UDP-gal) levels are normal and cataract is the only abnormality directly related to the enzyme defect. Fetuses from affected females may also develop cataracts, as may heterozygotes in later life. A galactose-free diet is indicated and should be continued for life. Early treatment prevents cataracts or arrests their further increase. A similar diet has been proposed for heterozygotes but no long-term studies have been reported. Prenatal diagnosis is possible.

Uridine diphosphate galactose-4-epimerase deficiency (230350) may be confined to the erythrocytes when it is completely symptomless and needs no treatment. Generalized epimerase deficiency is clinically similar to transferase deficiency and galactose, gal-1-P and UDP-gal increase after galactose consumption. Galactose elimination is followed by a drop of all three metabolites in the blood. UDP-gal is a critical substrate for the production of sphingolipids for the brain and an intake of 1.5–2 g galactose/day is necessary to meet the requirement of UDP-gal while simultaneously preventing gal-1-P accumulation.

The *Fanconi–Bickel* syndrome (227810) is associated with growth and developmental retardation, malabsorption, hepatomegaly, the renal Fanconi syndrome, sparse hair and lack of subcutaneous fat. Galactose accumulates if it is consumed but the galactose enzymatic cascade is normal. A transport defect is proposed.

FRUCTOSE (Fig. 20.16)

The main dietary sources of fructose are fruits, vegetables, potatoes, honey and all products which contain fructose or its disaccharide, sucrose. Another source is sorbitol which is used as a sweetener in diabetic foods.

Fructose-1-phosphate aldolase deficiency (hereditary fructose intolerance) (step 2) (229600) (~1 : 20 000–250 000)

There are three aldolase isozymes, A, B and C, each with specific properties and tissue localization. In this condition, aldolase B is deficient; it is localized in liver, intestine and kidneys and normally cleaves F-1-P and fructose-1,6-diphosphate (F-1,6-P) into two trioses. In fructosemia, F-1-P accumulates as soon as the patient ingests fructose; it is very toxic and it inhibits several enzymes of glycogenolysis and gluconeogenesis, causing rapid and profound hypoglycemia. Furthermore, ATP is not regenerated from ADP, which is degraded to AMP and then to uric acid.

Clinical features

Symptoms of intolerance develop as soon as fructose is ingested. This occurs usually after weaning, but sometimes much earlier, at the first introduction of fruit or when honey is misused as a pacifier. Acute symptoms are vomiting, sweating, trembling, lethargy, convulsions and other manifestations of hypoglycemia. The symptoms during chronic exposure to fructose are of progressive liver damage with anorexia, failure to thrive,

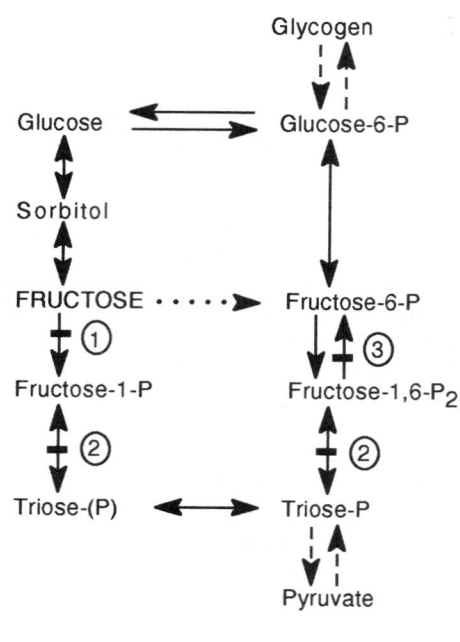

Fig. 20.16 The metabolism of fructose.

jaundice, hepatomegaly, splenomegaly, ascites, edema and hemorrhages. Aversion to sweets develops early in life and, by avoiding sweetened foods, most patients protect themselves from the toxic effects of fructose. Occasionally the condition is only diagnosed in adult life. Remarkably, the teeth remain free of caries.

Diagnosis

Fructosemia is easy to diagnose if the association of acute symptoms with fructose ingestion is recognized. Metabolic abnormalities include hypoglycemia, hypophosphatemia, hyperuricemia and hypermagnesemia along with all the manifestations of the Fanconi syndrome. The liver function tests are markedly abnormal and increased levels of some amino acids such as tyrosine and methionine are usual. Liver biopsy, during acute or chronic fructose ingestion, shows extensive abnormalities including focal areas of necrosis, fatty degeneration, proliferation of bile ducts, formation of pseudoacini and ultimately biliary cirrhosis.

The finding of a reducing sugar in urine is an important clue; it must be properly identified by sugar chromatography. When the diagnosis is in doubt, an intravenous (*not oral*) fructose tolerance test (200 mg/kg) is performed as soon as the child is reasonably stable. A positive test is signaled by a rise of nearly 50% in serum uric acid and a drop of 40–50% in the serum glucose and phosphate. In doubtful cases, DNA analysis or enzyme assay of a liver biopsy is required.

Treatment

A strict fructose-free diet can prevent or arrest all or most abnormalities and restore liver and kidney function to normal, except in cases of severe liver failure. The effects of the treatment are influenced by the age of the patient, the amount and duration of fructose ingestion and the residual aldolase B activity. Young infants are most susceptible to fructose toxicity. In older children, large amounts of fructose elicit acute symptoms; continued exposure to small amounts may cause growth retardation. Successful treatment requires knowledge of the varying composition of some nutrients, depending on their harvesting, cooking or storing (potatoes).

Fructose-1,6-diphosphatase deficiency (step 3) (229700)

This enzyme is one of the unidirectional enzymes in the pathway of gluconeogenesis and is also important for the conversion of fructose into glucose. Metabolic stress leads to hypoglycemia and increased protein and fat catabolism, resulting in the accumulation of lactate, pyruvate, alanine, ketone bodies and glycerol.

Clinical features

The symptoms of deficiency of this enzyme are similar to those of fructosemia or type 1 glycogen storage disease. They may develop in the neonatal period or later, provoked by insufficient food intake or by the inadvertent intake of fructose or sucrose. Fulminating lactic acidosis and hypoglycemia lead to hyperventilation, hypotonia, hepatomegaly, nausea, vomiting, lethargy and convulsions. Liver and kidney function may deteriorate and the course may be severe and rapidly fatal or episodic, being exacerbated during stresses.

Diagnosis

Hypoglycemia and lactic acidosis together with or without evidence of liver dysfunction demand metabolic studies. Precipitation of problems by fructose may be a clue and characteristically, glycerol and glycerol-3-phosphate accumulate during hypoglycemia and are excreted in the urine. These metabolites derive from excessive proteolysis and fatty acid oxidation which increase to compensate for the lack of glucose. The lactic acidosis can be profound and recalcitrant to therapy. Liver histology may show fatty degeneration and fibrosis and the renal Fanconi syndrome may be apparent. All these are reminiscent of type 1 glycogen storage disease. A fasting test might elicit the above symptoms. Fasting, fructose or glycerol stress tests are not without risk. Definitive diagnosis requires enzyme assay of leukocytes or liver tissue.

Treatment

Consists of frequent meals and the restriction of fructose, sucrose and sorbitol. Prolonged fasting must be avoided and early and aggressive treatment with glucose and bicarbonate intravenously may be necessary during infections.

Other disorders of fructose metabolism

In *fructokinase deficiency* (essential fructosuria) (step 1) (229800) (~1 : 150 000), fructose metabolism is blocked in the liver, intestine and kidney and fructose levels in blood and urine are increased if the patient consumes fructose. The condition is benign and treatment is not required. Fructose malabsorption is reasonably common associated with fermentative diarrhea following quite modest fructose ingestion.

A defect of *aldolase A* (103850) in fibroblasts is associated with nonspherocytic hemolytic anemia; some cases have had microcephaly and dysmorphic features.

GLYCOGEN STORAGE DISEASES (Fig. 20.17)

METABOLISM

Several inherited enzyme defects interfere with the degradation of glycogen and may raise the glycogen content of the organ in which the enzyme is normally localized. Glycogen is a giant polysaccharide in which glucose is stored in various organs, mainly the liver and the muscles. Ninety percent of the molecules are linked by α-1,4 bonds in straight chains; about 8% are α-1,6 bonds which form branching points. The usual glycogen concentration of the liver is < 5–7 g/100 g wet weight and in muscle < 2 g/100 g wet weight, these concentrations being influenced by factors such as the nutritional status, the pre- or postprandial condition of the patient and by hormonal stimuli.

Table 20.8 Glycogen storage diseases, classification

Type	Deficient enzyme	Tissue involved	Main clinical findings
IA	Glucose-6-phosphatase	Liver, kidney	Hepatomegaly, hypoglycemia, lactic acidosis
IB	Glucose-6-phosphatase-related transport	Liver, leukocytes	IB additional immunologic abnormalities
IC			
ID			IC, ID?
II	Acid α-glucosidase (lysosomal)	Generalized	Infant form: cardiorespiratory failure. Later forms: myopathy
III	Debranching enzyme	Liver, muscle, heart	Hepatomegaly, hypoglycemia, myopathy
IV	Branching enzyme	Liver	Hepatosplenomegaly, cirrhosis
V	Phosphorylase	Muscle	Myopathy, exercise intolerance
VI	Phosphorylase system	Liver (muscle)	Hepatomegaly (myopathy)
VII	Phosphofructokinase and other defects of glycolysis	Muscle (erythrocytes)	Myopathy, exercise intolerance (hemolysis)
O	Glycogen synthase	Liver	Hypoglycemia

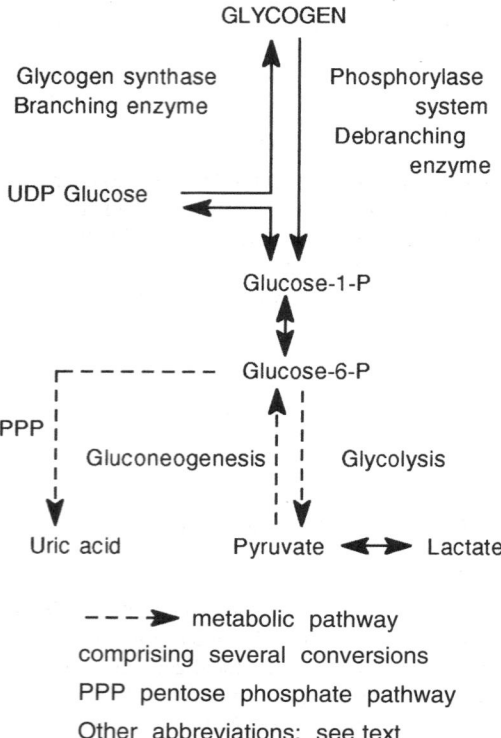

Fig. 20.17 Glycogen degradation and synthesis.

Therefore, quantitative glycogen analyses may not mean very much, even in the glycogen storage diseases (GSD).

In liver, the major function of glycogen is to provide reserve glucose for export to other organs, mainly the brain. In contrast, muscle glycogen is only used as a fuel for ATP synthesis during muscle contraction. It follows that GSD involving the liver is usually characterized by fasting hypoglycemia, whereas the muscle defects are characterized by myopathy (p. 1132).

Initially, phosphorylase cleaves glucose molecules from the α-1,4 linkages of the outer chains. Liver phosphorylase (enzyme VI) is different from muscle phosphorylase (enzyme V). It is activated by phosphorylase-β-kinase (not shown) which in turn is activated by a cyclic AMP-dependent protein kinase. The activation and inactivation of this cascade is mediated by hormones, mainly glucagon, insulin and adrenaline. The product of the phosphorylase reaction is not glucose but glucose-1-phosphate, which is converted to glucose-6-phosphate and subsequently dephosphorylated to glucose by glucose-6-phosphatase (enzyme I). Phosphorylase activity stops close to the branch points which are then degraded by debranching enzyme (enzyme III) so that more straight chains are available for further degradation by phosphorylase.

This main pathway of glycogen degradation by phosphorylation and dephosphorylation in the cytoplasm is different from that in the lysosomes. The significance of the latter pathway is apparent from consideration of Pompe's disease which results from deficiency of lysosomal α-1,4-glucosidase.

Two defects of glycogen synthesis are known, glycogen synthase deficiency and branching enzyme deficiency (enzyme IV). Although neither is really a glycogen storage disease, they are considered in the same group. Older numerical classifications are becoming outdated; specific enzyme nosology is preferable since different numbers have been assigned to the same enzyme defect.

Glucose-6-phosphatase deficiency (GSD type 1A: von Gierke's disease) (232200) (~1 : 150 000)

Clinical features

The most conspicuous clinical findings are a protruded abdomen because of marked hepatomegaly, hypotrophic muscles, truncal obesity, a rounded 'doll face' and short stature (Fig. 20.18). The liver may be enlarged at birth; its size increases gradually and may achieve a total height span of 15–20 cm. Initially, it is smooth with a normal consistency but by 10–20 years, it becomes firmer and nodular due to the development of adenomas; however, cirrhosis does not develop. There is no splenomegaly, but kidneys are moderately enlarged. Easy bruising and nose bleeds may be troublesome due to impaired platelet function. Linear growth is retarded but truncal obesity is obvious; both are improved by good treatment. Symptomatic hypoglycemia is frequent and occurs during the night or during even short periods of reduced caloric intake. Even minor delays or reduction of carbohydrate intake may provoke attacks which are always accompanied by lactic acidosis. Cerebral function is usually normal so long as recurrent hypoglycemic damage is prevented. When untreated, hyperuricemia frequently causes gout.

At present, there is controversy over whether abnormal function of the glucose-6-phosphatase system may be a cause of sudden death in infancy.

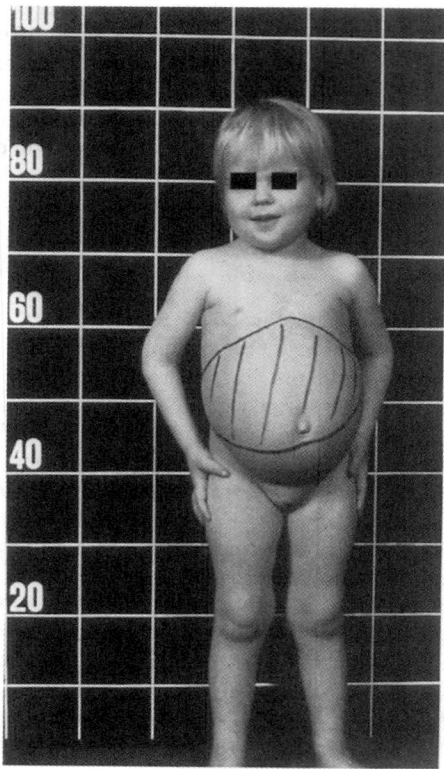

Fig. 20.18 The typical features of a patient with glucose-6-phosphatase deficiency.

With improved treatment, the life expectancy is much improved and some late-onset complications are emerging. Rarely, hepatic adenomas become malignant, hyperuricemia is now rare, but progressive focal glomerular sclerosis is a serious risk and can lead to renal failure. Anemia and osteopenia are also late-onset risks.

Metabolic derangements

Failure to dephosphorylate glucose-6-phosphate means that glucose production from both glycogenolysis and gluconeogenesis is blocked. However, the Embden–Meyerhof pathway (Fig. 20.14) is intact and during fasting is intensified under hormonal stimulation. This increases lactate production which is useful since lactate can serve as a fuel to the brain. However, chronic lactic acidemia is usual and probably contributes to the retarded growth and osteoporosis. Excess acetyl-CoA is also produced which is converted into fatty acids and cholesterol; this underlies the hyperlipidemia and hyperprebetalipoproteinemia of most of these patients. Some of the excess glucose-6-phosphate is channeled via the pentose phosphate shunt to urate, thus explaining the hyperuricemia, which can be severe.

Diagnosis

For a tentative diagnosis, an oral glucose tolerance test is the safest and most informative. During this test, the blood lactate *decreases* from an initially high level to (near) normal which is the opposite of the normal response. Assay of glucose-6-phosphatase activity in liver confirms the diagnosis and delineates the different forms of this syndrome. In the liver, fat accumulation often exceeds that of glycogen; this does not contradict the biochemical diagnosis. Antenatal diagnosis can only be done on fetal liver tissue or by DNA studies.

Treatment

Acute hypoglycemia should be treated with glucose 0.25 g/kg in 50–100 ml water by any means available; if needed, this should be followed by an intravenous drip providing twice the normal glucose requirement (see below). Lactic acidosis should be treated simultaneously by sodium bicarbonate although glucose administration suppresses lactate overproduction. Oral nutrition is reintroduced as soon as possible.

For maintenance, a high carbohydrate diet with 65–60% of the total energy as carbohydrates, 10% as protein and 20–25% as fat is used. Both lactose and sucrose should be restricted since neither galactose nor fructose can be converted to glucose because of the enzyme defect. Low-lactose, sucrose-free formulae are preferable if breast milk is not available. Maltose or dextrins are added to give a total 65% energy as carbohydrate. The feeding should be administered at 2–3 hours intervals around the clock before the age of 3 months, followed by a wider spacing from 3–6 months onwards. Gastric drip feeding at night is usually introduced as early as possible using carbohydrate derived from glucose, maltose or glucose polymers to provide a constant supply of carbohydrate at 7–9 mg/kg/min for infants, 5–6 mg/kg/min for 1–6-year-olds and 4 mg/kg/min for older children. This treatment improves the clinical condition, decreases the liver size, suppresses the bleeding tendency and promotes growth.

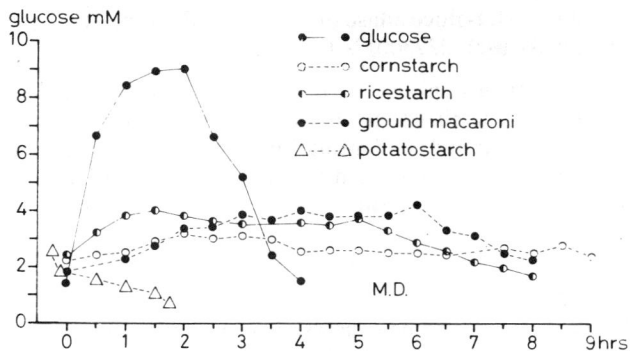

Fig. 20.19 Blood glucose curves of a patient with glucose-6-phosphatase deficiency after the ingestion of glucose or various uncooked starches, 2 g/kg bodyweight each.

Most older patients prefer to use uncooked cornstarch as a slow-release form of carbohydrate. It cannot be given by tube but can be given orally, between or together with meals and normalizes the blood sugar for several hours (Fig. 20.19); it is now considered a mainstay of therapy. It can be started when compliance issues are no longer a concern. Other raw starches from rice, wheat and tapioca are equally effective.

Even optimum treatment may not correct the hypoglycemia, lactic acidosis and hyperlipidemia completely and some patients continue to grow poorly. Captopril is being evaluated for treating the renal disease; osteoporosis requires a generous calcium and vitamin D intake and periodic assessment of bone density. Hyperuricemia is treated with allopurinol. Liver transplantation has been successful. Granulocyte/macrophage stimulating factor is used in type IB.

Glucose-6-phosphate translocase deficiencies (GSD types IB and IC)

These are defects of translocases located on the luminal wall of the endoplasmic reticulum which normally allow entry of glucose-6-phosphate (GSD type IB) (232220) and exit of phosphate (GSD type IC) (232240). Both defects render glucose-6-phosphatase functionally inactive. A defect of the glucose translocase has not yet been described.

The clinical and metabolic symptoms and treatment of GSD IB are not discernibly different from GSD IA except for a grave propensity to immunologic abnormalities.* There is neutropenia and defective neutrophil and monocyte function; bacterial infections are frequent and may be fatal. Inflammatory bowel disease akin to Crohn's disease and myelogenous leukemia are added complications. The prognosis of translocase 1 deficiency is much worse than that of glucose-6-phosphatase deficiency because of the increased risk of metabolic derangements due to the frequent infections.

Translocase 1 defect accounts for 12–15% of the total cases of glucose-6-phosphatase deficiency, whereas the translocase 2 defect is extremely rare.

---

* Other metabolic defects that affect leukocyte function include a severe form of glucose-6-phosphate dehydrogenase and myeloperoxidase deficiencies, two disorders of purine synthesis and two of the γ-glutamyl cycle and chronic granulomatous disease in which there is usually a defect of NADPH oxidase (see Ch. 22).

Lysosomal a-1,4-glucosidase deficiency (GSD type II: Pompe's disease) (232300) (~1 : 100 000)

Deficiency of this enzyme, also called acid maltase deficiency, leads to a generalized glycogen storage disease. There are infantile, juvenile and adult forms. This defect is not in the regular cascade of glycogenolysis and is not associated with defects of circulating fuels in the blood.

Clinical features

Infantile AMD or Pompe's disease is characterized by the rapid onset in the first months of life of profound muscle hypotonia, weakness, hyporeflexia, glossomegaly, massive cardiomyopathy without murmurs but no hepatomegaly except with cardiac failure. The infant is usually alert and the cerebral development is normal. The electrocardiogram shows a huge QRS complex, left or biventricular hypertrophy and shortened PR interval. The clinical course is downhill with cardiopulmonary failure or pneumonia leading to death in the first year.

Childhood or adult forms with onset in the second to fourth decades are less severe and progress more slowly. The heart is not affected but motor milestones are delayed and weakness develops of limb girdle and truncal muscles, mimicking other chronic myopathies. Involvement of respiratory muscles ultimately causes ventilatory insufficiency with death usually between the second and fourth decade.

Diagnosis

The enzyme can be assayed in leukocytes. In the infantile form, glycogen-laden lysosomes are present in all organs except the kidneys and the cerebral cortex, being particularly abundant in anterior horn cells and motor nuclei of the brainstem. In the adult disorder, glycogen storage is absent in heart, brain and liver and varies greatly in different muscles. A second enzyme, neutral maltase, is produced by the kidneys and is also present in the leukocytes and must be differentiated during enzyme analysis. Antenatal diagnosis is possible.

Treatment is only supportive.

Debranching enzyme deficiency (GSD type III; limit dextrinosis) (232400) (~1 : 5500 Sephardic Jews; otherwise rare)

During glycogenolysis, this enzyme normally prunes the α-1,6, linkage branch points as the straight, α-1,4 links are being broken down by phosphorylase. When this does not happen, glycogen degradation stops at the branch points, leaving 'limit dextrin'. This abnormal glycogen may behave as a foreign body and elicit high transaminase levels, recurrent jaundice, fibrosis and even cirrhosis. Gluconeogenesis, however, is unimpeded and this drains glucogenic amino acids from muscle protein, presumably contributing to poor growth and muscle wasting.

Clinical features

Two forms exist; one is confined to liver but the more common involves the muscles as well. In younger children the liver symptoms predominate and are very similar to glucose-6-phosphatase deficiency with severe hypoglycemia in the neonatal period or later or during decreased food intake or metabolic stress. The liver is markedly enlarged but the spleen and kidneys are not. Hypotonia, truncal obesity and a doll face develop and the patient may show retarded growth which gradually catches up later. Motor development is slow but mental development is usually normal. The liver has a normal consistency, but rarely cirrhosis may develop. Surprisingly, for unknown reasons, the liver size returns to normal at or before puberty.

In the myopathic form, which has probably been underdiagnosed in the past, there is increasing muscle weakness and a slowly progressive distal muscle wasting, sometimes starting in childhood, sometimes in adult life. It may be accompanied by cardiomyopathy with left ventricular hypertrophy and ECG abnormalities. These developments warrant close supervision of muscle function and regular ECG in all patients.

Diagnosis

Conspicuous findings during fasting are ketosis (not lactic acidosis), hyperlipidemia (mainly hypercholesterolemia) and hypoglycemia. An oral galactose tolerance test elicits a normal increase of blood glucose and an abnormal increase of blood lactate. A fasting glucagon test is characterized by an abnormally flat glucose response.

The liver pathology shows an increase of reticulin fibers between hepatocytes and of fibrous tissue in portal tracts. In the myopathic form, the muscles show myofibrillary destruction and degeneration of the neuromuscular junctions

Enzyme assay of blood cells or fibroblasts is diagnostic in the generalized disorder but for the isolated hepatic form, liver biopsy is required.

Treatment and prognosis

Treatment of the hepatic form is similar to that of GSD I except that restriction of galactose and fructose is not necessary as both can be converted normally into glucose. Although gastric drip feeding is not a prerequisite for glucose homeostasis at a later age, this treatment and extra protein are important for delaying or improving the myopathy. Thus, the diet for both forms of the disease should contain approximately 55–60% energy as carbohydrates, particularly starch, 15–20% energy as protein and 20–25% energy as fat, predominantly polyunsaturated. As for the prognosis, the late development of myopathy and cardiomyopathy remains a concern.

Branching enzyme deficiency (GSD type IV) (232500)

Clinical features

The main features of this disorder are marked hepatomegaly with progressive cirrhosis, splenomegaly, muscle hypotonia and weakness, hypo- or areflexia, retarded motor milestones, growth retardation and normal mental development. Death usually occurs in the first years of life. Rarely, milder variants with myopathy are observed in adults and cardiomyopathy with heart failure may be the only presentation. The metabolic derangements are hypoglycemia, usually mild, increased transaminases and decreased clotting factors.

Diagnosis

The enzyme defect causes insufficient ramification of the glycogen molecule and its prolonged inner and outer chains give it the appearance and properties of amylopectin. Apparently this abnormal glycogen is difficult to mobilize. It acts as a foreign body and glucose release from it is hampered. In contrast to the liver, muscle histology is usually normal in spite of absent enzyme activity in that tissue. The enzyme defect is expressed in all tissues and in fibroblasts; antenatal diagnosis is feasible.

Treatment

Treatment is symptomatic and consists of frequent high carbohydrate feedings and, eventually, gastric drip feeding. Liver transplantation has been successful.

Muscle phosphorylase deficiency (GSD type V; McArdle syndrome) (232600)

Clinical features

This disorder is characterized by increasing intolerance for strenuous exercise. During childhood no symptoms occur except easy fatiguability. In adults, strenuous muscle activity is accompanied by severe cramps and may be followed by myoglobinuria, which can precipitate anuria and renal failure. In middle life, the fatigue increases and muscle wasting and weakness predominate. The serum CPK may be permanently or intermittently elevated.

Diagnosis

Muscle exercise is normally accompanied by release of lactate and of inosine, hypoxanthine and ammonia through the purine nucleotide cycle (p. 1140). In myophosphorylase deficiency lactic acid production is blocked and release of the purine nucleotide cycle compounds is exaggerated. The ensuing myogenic hyperuricemia is one of the characteristic features of defects of muscle glycogenosis. The semi-ischemic exercise test gives abnormal results; it is carried out as follows. A blood pressure cuff is inflated above systolic pressure. A handgrip is formed and opened every second for 1 min. Prior to and for eight 1-min intervals after starting the exercise, venous blood is collected. Ammonia and hypoxanthine values rise abnormally but the normal increase in lactate is absent in this disorder and in other glycolytic defects in muscle, such as phosphofructokinase deficiency (see Table 20.8).

Phosphorylase activity must be assayed in muscle; liver phosphorylase is presumably normal, as is glucose homeostasis.

Treatment

Treatment is symptomatic and consists of the prevention of strenuous exercise. 'Carbo loading' and a high-protein diet are of some help and glucose should always be taken during exercise. Strenuous exercise is always a risk.

Liver phosphorylase (232700) and liver phosphorylase b kinase deficiencies (GSD type VI) (306000)

Phosphorylase b kinase is required to convert phosphorylase b (inactive) to the activated form and the kinase itself is regulated by another (cyclic AMP-dependent) kinase, the whole system being stimulated by hormones, particularly glucagon. The clinical heterogeneity of phosphorylase b kinase deficiency is due to the fact that it consists of four different subunits at least one of which is coded on the X chromosome. These two defects are discussed together because the clinical features and metabolic derangements are similar.

Clinical features

In early childhood, pronounced hepatomegaly, without splenomegaly and a protruded abdomen due to muscle hypotonia are the most striking features; the liver enlargement decreases slowly and usually disappears at puberty. Equally, the muscle hypotonia and weakness, which initially cause slow motor development, also tend to improve. Growth and puberty are often delayed. Mental development is normal. There are exceptions to this usually mild course, particularly in phosphorylase b kinase deficiency, of which many variants exist. Rare cases have had combinations of hepatic symptoms and myopathy (261750), fatal cardiomyopathy (261740) and even myopathy without hepatic symptoms.

Diagnosis

A tentative diagnosis is based on the pronounced hepatomegaly in contrast to the mild metabolic findings. Mild fasting hypoglycemia may develop; elevated serum transaminases, hypercholesterolemia and a marked tendency to fasting ketosis are evident at a young age, but normalize completely by puberty.

In the absence of galactosuria, an oral galactose test is abnormal as blood lactate increases excessively. Contrary to expectation, glucagon tests are not of much help as the increase of blood glucose is variable. Kinase defects can usually be detected in blood cells but assay of liver or muscle may be required in some cases.

Treatment

Treatment of this self-limiting disease is not necessary except for prevention of hypoglycemia which may require uncooked cornstarch. Use of polyunsaturated fat suppresses hypercholesterolemia.

Muscle phosphofructokinase deficiency (GSD type VII) (232800)

Clinical features

The three clinical and metabolic characteristics of this rare disorder are myopathy, increased hemolysis and gout. The myopathy is similar to GSD type V and manifests itself in childhood by weakness, limitation of vigorous activity and exercise-induced cramps, accompanied by myoglobinuria; CPK is often raised. As in muscle phosphorylase deficiency, there is no rise of venous lactate after exercise and ammonia, inosine, hypoxanthine and urate are produced in excess. Continued myogenic hyperuricemia explains the gout.

Different isoenzymes of phosphofructokinase exist in various tissues. The absence of the M-subunit in erythrocytes (261670) results in hemolytic anemia. In muscles, however, the block in glycolysis may be partly compensated by increased fatty acid oxidation.

Treatment

Provision of extra glucose does not bypass the enzyme defect and is therefore of no help. This is different from muscle phosphorylase deficiency in which glucose enters the glycolytic pathway 'downstream' from the enzyme defect. A high-protein diet and prevention of excessive activity are the only measures.

Glycogen synthase deficiency (240600)

Clinical features

This rare defect is usually grouped with the GSDs since it involves the same metabolic pathway. Failure to synthesize glycogen results in rapid and profound hyperglycemia after even quite modest meals. This is followed by a rapid and profound fall of the blood glucose when postprandial events normally turn to glycogenolysis to maintain blood glucose. Facile ketosis and postprandial hyperlactacidemia can be seen and bear superficial similarity to so-called ketotic hypoglycemia (p. 1131). The liver is not enlarged and its glycogen content is low. The enzyme defect can only be demonstrated in the liver or by DNA studies.

Treatment.

Consists of small, frequent protein-rich meals and regular cornstarch feeds to prevent hypoglycemia and ketosis.

DISORDERS OF PURINES, PYRIMIDINES AND DNA REPAIR

Metabolism of purines, two of the bases of DNA, involves an efficient salvage system and a complicated synthetic pathway normally regulated by feedback inhibition at step 1 (Fig. 20.20). On a purine-free diet, about 6–10 mg/kg is excreted per day as uric acid, the final degradation product. Uric acid is largely bound to albumin in the plasma; after glomerular filtration, it is reabsorbed and then re-excreted by the proximal renal tubules. Ingested purines are absorbed and mostly excreted.

Hypouricemia is seen in xanthinuria, molybdenum cofactor deficiency, in the Fanconi syndrome due to decreased renal tubular reabsorption and in a primary renal transport defect (307830) which results in uricosuria. There are no clinical consequences of the low purine levels.

HYPERURICEMIA

The solubility of uric acid in plasma is about 0.42 mmol/L (7.0 mg/dl). Values greater than this occur frequently, more often in adults, due to genetic or acquired problems of overproduction or underexcretion of uric acid.

Overproduction of purines occurs in glycogen storage disease type 1 (p. 1136) and in two defects of purine metabolism which are discussed below. The commonest cause is reduced renal fractional excretion of urate. Secondary hyperuricemia occurs in dehydration, renal failure, ethanol ingestion, during rapid tissue breakdown as in the early stages of chemotherapy and in

metabolic acidosis due to competitive inhibition of secretion in the renal tubules.

Hyperuricemia is frequently asymptomatic and its cause is often not sought. It frequently causes gout due to deposition in the tissues or urate lithiasis; both are common in adults but uncommon in children. Certainly, uric acid should be measured in patients with kidney stones, idiopathic renal disease, monoarticular arthropathy or tophi, but asymptomatic hyperuricemia in children should probably not be treated unless it exceeds about 0.5 mmol/L. Acute symptoms are treated with antiinflammatory drugs and colchicine; long-term, allopurinol is the drug of choice. Contrary to belief, ingestion of a purine (protein) rich diet is an uncommon cause of hyperuricemia.

Hypoxanthine-guanine phosphoribosyltransferase deficiency (step 8) (308000)

This defect is inherited as an X-linked recessive trait, partial deficiency is common and is the most frequent cause of gout in adults. Many different mutations have been described; more severe deficiency causes developmental delay without neurologic symptoms and even more marked deficiency is associated also with spasticity or cerebellar ataxia in about 20% of such cases. Complete deficiency causes the Lesch–Nyhan syndrome.

Lesch–Nyhan syndrome (1 : 150–200 000)

Clinical features

This condition is one of the cruelest inborn errors of metabolism. At birth, these infants appear normal but pink discoloration of the diapers (napkins) and urine due to excretion of large quantities of urates may be found. Within months, the children are noted to be irritable and sometimes hyperactive. By 1–2 years, choreoathetoid cerebral palsy is evident, the full spectrum of which is obvious by

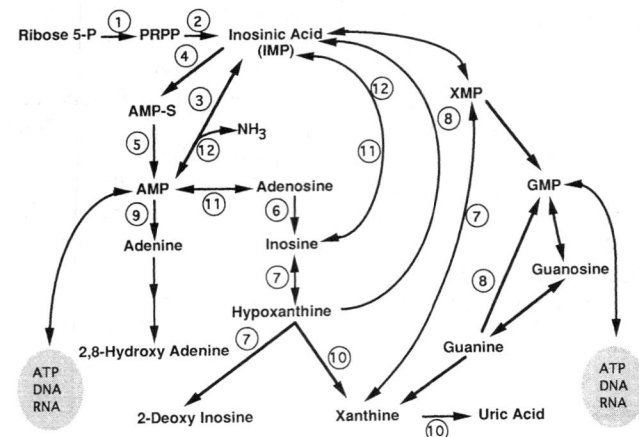

Fig. 20.20 The synthetic and salvage pathways of purine metabolism. 1, PRPP synthase; 2, multiple enzymes for purine synthesis; 3, AMP deaminase (myopathy); 4, adenylosuccinate synthase (AMP-S) (purine nucleotide cycle); 5, adenylosuccinase (autism); 6, adenosine deaminase (immune defect); 7, purine nucleoside phosphorylase (immune defect); 8, hypoxanthine guanine phosphoribosyltransferase (gout, kidney stones, ataxia, Lesch–Nyhan syndrome); 9, adenine phosphoribosyltransferase (kidney stones); 10, xanthine oxidase (kidney stones), 11, adenosine kinase (?malignant hyperthermia); 12, 5′-nucleotidase.

3–4 years. Speech is delayed and, when it occurs, is grossly dysarthric. Dystonic posturing accompanies almost any stimulation and compulsive self-destructive behavior is usual. This tends to take the form of finger or lip biting or hitting out at people or objects within reach, such that dental obturators or extraction may be necessary. Such children beg to be restrained with arm braces, gloves or straps and become anxious or even angry when these are removed. It is very difficult to assess intelligence in these patients, but the IQ is either normal or relatively well preserved. Orthopedic problems, arthropathy, obstructive nephropathy and large tophi develop in untreated cases.

Diagnosis

Diagnosis is made on clinical grounds and supported by the finding of hyperuricemia which may be only minimally elevated. It should be excluded in all male children with athetoid cerebral palsy. The enzyme defect can be identified in red blood cells, fibroblasts, amniocytes and chorionic villus samples.

Treatment

Allopurinol is used to control the blood urate, but increased xanthine production usually results in chronic nephrolithiasis and the drug has no effect on the neurologic disease. Many different sedatives, neuroleptics and other drugs have been tried to improve the emotional and neurological disorders, but they seem to be of little or no value. Extraordinary efforts are needed to provide a nurturing and educational milieu from which these children can benefit.

Other purine disorders causing nephrolithiasis

Increased activity of *PRPP-synthetase* (311850), an X-linked trait, results in urate overproduction and is one cause of neonatal diabetes (Von Muhlendahl & Herkenhoff 1995).

Xanthinuria (278300) is caused by a defect of xanthine oxidase (step 10), the ultimate step in purine degradation. There is hypouricemia and xanthine and hypoxanthine (oxypurines) are elevated in the urine. Xanthine is very insoluble and forms crystals and brownish, nonopaque stones. Occasionally xanthine stones are idiopathic and xanthinuria is a possible complication of allopurinol therapy. Treatment with alkali and a high fluid intake is indicated.

Adenine phosphoribosyl transferase deficiency (step 9) (102600) results in production of 2,8-dihydroxyadenine which is very insoluble, causing stones, sometimes even in neonates. Serum uric acid is normal. Characteristic yellow-brown, round crystals of the purine can be seen in the urine; however, it reacts chemically like uric acid from which it must be differentiated by special methods. A low purine diet is essential and allopurinol and renal transplantation are recommended. Alkalization of the urine is contraindicated.

Purine disorders causing immune problems

Adenosine deaminase deficiency (ADA) (step 6) (102700) and *purine nucleotide phosphorylase deficiency* (PNP) (step 7) (164050) both cause immune problems that are likely to be fatal in infancy although mild and asymptomatic variants are known. In ADA patients, both B and T cell functions are deficient leading to *severe combined immune deficiency* (Ch. 22), of which ADA is the

cause in about 50% of non-X-linked cases. In PNP deficiency, T cell function is depressed but B cell function may be normal, increased or decreased. In both, there are likely to be recurrent. severe, opportunistic infections with fungal and viral agents, diarrhea and failure to thrive being usual. In PNP, there is greatly increased susceptibility to viral infections and autoimmune problems; 50% have neurological problems with spastic diplegia or paralysis, ataxia, tremor and developmental delay being frequent. The thymus and other lymphoid tissues are greatly reduced in size.

Diagnosis

Lymphopenia is usual and the blood uric acid is extremely low. A filter paper screening test for ADA is available and cases of partial deficiency have been detected by this means. Immune testing is discussed elsewhere. Increased levels of this enzyme in red cells have been reported in a familial hemolytic anemia (102730).

Treatment

ADA is the first condition to be treated with patient cells reconstituted with wild-type (normal) DNA – true gene therapy. It is partially successful, but additional sources of the enzyme are also needed and the treatment costs over £20 000 every 2 weeks. For now, bone marrow transplantation seems more reasonable for both disorders.

Purine nucleotide cycle (steps 3–5)

The contribution of this system to muscle metabolism is not clear but, following exercise, inosine monophosphate and ammonia normally increase in muscle and blood due to the action of this cycle. *Myoadenylate deaminase* deficiency (254750) can be acquired (secondary to a large number of neuromuscular or rheumatologic disorders) or hereditary. It is often asymptomatic but can be associated with a spectrum of muscle symptoms occurring after exercise including cramps, fatigue and myalgia. Ammonia and inosine do not increase in blood after an ischemic exercise test, but elevation of CPK is noted in 50% of cases. The defect is found by immunohistochemistry in 1–2% of muscle biopsies. Muscle *adenylate kinase* deficiency (102990) may be one cause of malignant hyperthermia; hyperactivity of the enzyme can cause hemolytic anemia.

Adenylosuccinase deficiency (103050) has been found in some cases of autism; the significance of this is not yet clear.

DISORDERS OF PYRIMIDINES METABOLISM (Van Gennip 1996)

There are two isozymes of carbamyl phosphate synthase; one is mitochondrial and committed to the urea cycle, the other cytosolic and committed to synthesis of the pyrimidines, uridine and thymidine. In several urea cycle disorders, accumulation of carbamyl phosphate increases synthesis of pyrimidines. Four genetic defects of pyrimidine metabolism are known but are rarely detected.

Hereditary *orotic aciduria* (258900) is caused by a defect of uridine-5-monophosphate synthase which results in hypochromic, macrocytic or megaloblastic anemia that occurs in infancy or early childhood; later, orotic acid crystalluria can be so marked as to cause obstructive renal disease. Some patients have had problems with frequent infections and in vitro abnormalities of immune function have been reported. Lifelong treatment with uridine (50–150 mg/kg/day or more) improves the hematological abnormalities.

Pyrimidine 5-nucleotidase deficiency (266120) causes nonspherocytic hemolytic anemia. There is basophilic stippling of the erythrocytes which contain increased nucleotides. No effective treatment is known. Lead inhibits this enzyme, which explains the hemolytic anemia seen in lead poisoning.

Dihydropyrimidine dehydrogenase deficiency (274270) causes a spectrum of neurologic problems including seizures, psychomotor delay, microcephaly and autism. If given the antimetabolite 5-fluorouracil, asymptomatic patients can develop an acute neurotoxic syndrome which slowly resolves after the drug is stopped. Uracil and thymine levels are elevated in body fluids. *Dihydropyrimidinase* deficiency (222748) seems to cause similar problems.

DNA REPAIR

Several syndromes are associated with defects in DNA or RNA repair and more will undoubtedly be found. *Bloom's syndrome* (210900) is caused by defects in the BLM gene which belongs to the Rec Q helicase family. *Cockayne's syndrome* type A (216400) is associated with a defect of RNA polymerase II transcription and Type B is caused by a transcriptional regulator gene with homology to a yeast Snf2 protein. Seven genes have been found in *xeroderma pigmentosum* (16 entries in OMIM); they involve different functions of recognition (XP-A), unwinding (XP-B&D) and excision (XP-F&G) (Kraemer 1996). The gene involved in *ataxia-telangiectasia* (208900) has also been identified.

THE PORPHYRIAS

The porphyrias are a group of disorders in the pathway of heme biosynthesis which result in overproduction of porphyrins and porphyrin precursors. They have been classified as 'acute' (in which intermittent neurologic symptoms predominate) and 'nonacute' (in which photosensitivity is prominent) or as 'hepatic' or 'erythropoietic', depending on the major manifestations but are best classified according to the principal site of abnormal porphyrin biosynthesis (Table 20.9) (Kappas et al 1995).

The initial rate-limiting step is the formation of δ-aminolevulinic acid (ALA) from succinyl-CoA. Two molecules of ALA condense to form porphobilinogen, four molecules of which are converted into one of uroporphyrinogen. The basic tetrapyrrole ring structure is thus established and additional steps complete the synthesis of protoporphyrin. Finally, ferrochelatase (step 8) catalyzes the insertion of a molecule of iron into protoporphyrin IX to form heme. There are two naturally occurring isomers of the porphyrins, the I series and the III series, but only the III series act as precursors for heme synthesis (Table 20.9).

Heme normally exerts feedback inhibition of the rate limiting enzyme – ALA synthetase. When one of the enzymes is deficient, heme synthesis is reduced and loss of feedback control results in overproduction of precursors prior to the block, particularly when requirements for heme are increased. Excess uroporphyrinogens and coproporphyrinogens are then converted to uro- and coproporphyrins respectively and excreted in urine and feces.

Many drugs can induce synthesis of ALA synthetase thereby increasing production of porphyrins. The neurological features of acute attacks are thought to be partially related to increased levels of ALA and the photosensitivity occurs with excessive circulating porphyrins.

Table 20.9 The heme biosynthesis pathway with enumerated sites of partial enzyme deficiencies which are related to the clinical syndromes and abnormal sites of porphyrin production as follows: 1, aminolevulinic acid dehydratase (? sites); 2, porphobilinogen deaminase (liver); 3, uroporphyrinogen III synthetase (erythroid cells); 4, uroporphyrinogen decarboxylase (erythroid cells + liver) and porphyria cutanea tarda (liver); 5, coproporphyrinogen oxidase (liver); 6, ?coproporphyrinogen oxidase (? site); 7, protoporphyrinogen oxidase (liver); 8, ferrochelatase (erythroid cells + liver)

Disorder	Genetics	Pathway	Abnormal metabolites/enzymes		
			Urine	Stool	Blood
		Glycine + succinyl-CoA ↓ ALA synthetase	ALA	–	Proto
		δ-Aminolevulinic acid (ALA)			
ALA dehydratase porphyria	AR	①↓	ALA/PBG	–	Enzyme test
		Porphobilinogen			
Acute intermittent porphyria	AD	②↓	Uro I/Copro I	Copro I	Uro/Copro
		Hydroxymethylbilane			
Congenital erythropoietic porphyria	AR	③↳ **Uroporphyrin I**	Uro/7-Carbo P	IsoCopro	–
		Uroporphyrinogen III			
Porphyria cutanea tarda and hepatoerythropoietic porphyria	Variable AR	④↓	Uro/7-Carbo P	IsoCopro	Proto
		Coproporphyrinogen III			
Hereditary coproporphyria	AD	⑤↓	ALA/PBG Copro	Copro	–
		Harderoporphyrinogen			
Harderoporphyria	AR	⑥↓	ALA/PBG Copro	Copro	–
		Protoporphyrinogen IX			
Variegate porphyria	AD	⑦↓	ALA/PBG Copro	Copro/Proto	–
		Protoporphyrin IX			
Erythropoietic protoporphyria	AD	⑧↓	–	Proto	Proto
		Heme			

ACUTE PORPHYRIAS

Clinical features

The three major acute porphyrias are *acute intermittent porphyria* (*AIP*) (176000), the commonest type of acute porphyria in the UK (1:10–20 000), *variegate porphyria* (*VP*) (176200), which has an incidence of 3 : 1000 in Afrikaners, and *hereditary coproporphyria* (*HC*) (121300), which are all inherited as autosomal dominant traits. *Aminolevulinic dehydratase porphyria* (125270) is an autosomal recessive trait.

Over 80% of AIP patients are never symptomatic even after exposure to known precipitins. Most of the remainder develop an assortment of problems that include gastrointestinal symptoms, neuropsychiatric symptoms or cardiovascular problems. In perhaps 10%, the condition is fatal.

Gastrointestinal symptoms are the commonest presenting complaint. Generalized abdominal pain, which may be chronic or acute and may be colicky in nature, is usual but nausea, vomiting, constipation and ileus are common. Protracted vomiting can lead to dehydration and electrolyte disturbances which can also be due to inappropriate secretion of antidiuretic hormone.

Neurological abnormalities, particularly a peripheral neuropathy, are common during acute attacks with both motor and sensory nerves involved, usually symmetrically. Muscle weakness is common. Paresthesia, mainly involving hip and shoulder regions, may occur. Disorders of micturition, cranial nerve palsies with pseudobulbar palsy, respiratory paralysis and grand mal seizures may occur.

Psychiatric symptoms are frequent and chronic or acute depression, anxiety or even a frank psychosis can be the presenting feature. During acute attacks, almost any psychiatric symptom can occur with restlessness, confusion and disorientation being common.

The usual cardiovascular signs are tachycardia and systemic hypertension although postural hypotension commonly occurs and persists after other symptoms have settled.

Coproporphyria is similar but generally milder than AIP but photosensitivity is common in both HC and VP. Exposed parts of the body develop erythema, burning and itching and may produce eruptions with chronic hyperpigmentation and scarring.

Aminolevulinic dehydratase porphyria (125270) is rare with genetic heterogeneity; it may present even in the newborn period and is similar to the dominantly inherited disorders.

Other porphyrias include *Chester* porphyria (176010) and. *harderoporphyria* (121300) which seem to be associated with more than one enzyme defect.

Precipitating factors

Alcohol and a large number of drugs (Table 20.10) induce cytochrome P450, thereby creating the need for increased porphyrin synthesis. Sex steroids often precipitate attacks which explains the higher incidence of problems in females, with increasing frequency of attacks with oral contraceptives, prior to menstruation, in pregnancy or the puerperium. Stress, as with acute infections and reduced calorie intake, as in slimming diets or malnutrition, can cause attacks even before puberty.

Diagnosis and screening

The chronic and protean complaints strongly suggest psychosomatic disease. Moreover, the laboratory tests may only be abnormal transiently during acute attacks, some metabolites readily degrade if samples are improperly handled and the assays themselves are not easy to perform. Not surprisingly, the diagnosis is often overlooked, particularly given the high incidence of latent cases.

The clinical diagnosis of the type of porphyria depends on the presentation and the measurement of δ-aminolevulinic acid, porphobilinogen and porphyrins in urine; quantitative blood and fecal porphyrins are also needed. A simple screening test for porphobilinogenuria is the Watson–Schwartz reaction and urinary porphyrin may turn pink on exposure to sunlight. In acute intermittent porphyria, the urine metabolites are only raised during the acute phases of an attack; in HC and VP the urine and/or stool values are more consistently elevated but latent cases are easily missed. Nonetheless, blood relatives should be screened for *latent* disease and advised appropriately.

Several of these enzymes can be measured in peripheral blood cells. Erythrocyte porphobilinogen deaminase is used to detect AIP but there is an overlap between patients and controls and enzyme levels depend on red blood cell age and in rare families, the level is normal in RBC but deficient in the liver due to an unusual splicing mutation. Some laboratories assay coproporphyrinogen oxidase in RBC but since this is normally a mitochondrial enzyme, these results are doubted by many. Increasingly, these difficulties are being resolved by DNA analysis. Homozygous deficiency of several enzymes has been reported; not all such cases have severe disease.

Treatment of acute attacks

Precipitating factors should be identified and removed. Many drugs are listed as potentially unsafe, but each case responds differently (Table 20.10). Fluid and electrolyte imbalances require correction. A high-carbohydrate diet appears beneficial both in acute episodes and in their prevention; at least 300 g glucose per day p.o. or i.v. is recommended for adults. Chlorpromazine may alleviate anxiety, nausea and vomiting. Pain control usually requires aspirin and paracetamol, dihydrocodeine or morphine but many drugs can induce attacks. Convulsions can be treated with diazepam or sodium valproate and hypertension controlled with propanolol or captopril. Hematin (2–4 mg/kg q 12 h, i.v. for 10–14 days) is extremely useful in suppressing porphyrin synthesis but, if given too late, may only improve the biochemistry without improving the symptoms; experience with this treatment in children is limited. Respiratory paralysis is the commonest cause of death and assisted ventilation may be necessary. Physiotherapy should be instituted as soon as possible if neuropathy is present.

Table 20.10 Some of the drugs and toxins which may aggravate acute porphyrias. The list is not exhaustive

Barbiturates	Primidone
Chloroquine	Phenytoin
Ethanol	Estrogens
Erythromycin	Oral contraceptives
Griseofulvin	Sulfonamides
Ketamine	Trimethadione
Meprobamate	Theophylline
Pentazocine	Valproic acid

NONACUTE PORPHYRIAS

Erythropoietic protoporphyria (*EPP*) (177000) is relatively common, usually inherited as an autosomal dominant, rarely as a recessive. It is due to a deficiency of mitochondrial ferrochelatase in erythroid cells and also possibly in the liver. Protoporphyrin accumulates in red cells as well as in skin and liver. The excess protoporphyrin in skin produces photosensitization usually beginning in childhood with itching, burning and erythema but blistering is rare and there may be no visible skin signs in spite of symptoms. Early on, liver function tests are normal but later may show evidence of hepatic deterioration and cirrhosis may develop. Protoporphyrin is excreted in bile and gallstones pigmented with protoporphyrin can occur.

Congenital erythropoietic porphyria (*CEP*) (263700) is a rare autosomal recessive trait. Pink or red urine is often noted shortly after birth or during the first year of life. The increased level of porphyrins in the skin cause acute photosensitivity with burning or itching on exposure to sunlight followed by erythema, swelling and blister formation. Healing lesions may scar and hypertrichosis is common. Repeated eruptions of the same areas may produce extensive ulceration and mutilation. Accumulation of porphyrins in red blood cells causes them to fluoresce red under ultraviolet light while accumulation in bone and teeth produces discoloration and red fluorescence. Splenomegaly and hemolytic anemia are common. Life expectancy is shortened and many die before middle age. Uroporphyrinogen III cosynthase is absent in erythroid cells resulting in overproduction of uroporphyrinogen I. This is deposited in tissues and converted partly to uroporphyrin I which is excreted in urine and partly to coproporphyrinogen I and hence to coproporphyrin I which is excreted mainly in feces. Type III isomers are also elevated.

Hepatoerythropoietic porphyria (*HEP*) (176100) is a rare disorder due to homozygous uroporphyrinogen decarboxylase deficiency. It is similar to congenital erythropoietic porphyria causing a photosensitive skin eruption with erythema progressing to vesicles or even hemorrhagic bullae. Increased fragility of the skin is common and in less severe cases may be the only clinical sign. Hyperpigmentation and hirsutism are common.

Porphyria cutanea tarda (*PCT*) (176090, 176100) is the commonest nonacute porphyria and is also associated with reduced uroporphyrinogen decarboxylase. The hereditary form is dominantly inherited with enzyme activity about 50% in all tissues. Presentation is usually in childhood with mild to severe photosensitivity with blistering and scarring in exposed areas and often overt liver disease. Hyper- and hypopigmentation and hirsutism are common. *Toxic porphyria* is sporadic, occurring almost exclusively in adults and usually precipitated by alcohol, chloroquine, barbiturates, hemodialysis, estrogens or oral contraceptives. Clinically it is similar to the hereditary form of porphyria cutanea tarda but is thought to be due to a direct toxic effect on hepatic uroporphyrinogen decarboxylase. Hexachlorobenzene, used as a wheat dressing, caused an outbreak of several thousand cases in Turkey.

Treatment of the nonacute porphyrias

Precipitating agents should be avoided. Light exposure should be reduced as far as possible using long clothes and hats. Barrier creams with a high *spf* factor containing zinc or titanium oxide or hydroxyacetone cream may improve light tolerance and β-carotene may also improve light tolerance. Regular venesection is used in PCT, VP and HEP to reduce iron and porphyrin levels; in contrast, in CEP, blood transfusion benefits anemia and suppresses the patient's marrow so that porphyrin levels are reduced. Splenectomy, chelation therapy with charcoal, cholestyramine and chloroquine 125–500 mg/day have all produced encouraging results in different deficiencies. In severe cases, especially CEP, bone marrow transplantation should be considered.

DISORDERS OF BILIRUBIN AND BILE ACID METABOLISM

The pathophysiology and differential diagnosis of jaundice are discussed elsewhere (p. 216) and only those conditions with a genetic defect in bilirubin metabolism are considered here.

UNCONJUGATED HYPERBILIRUBINEMIA

The type I variant of the *Crigler–Najjar syndrome* (218800) is an autosomal recessive condition characterized by complete absence of UDP-bilirubin glucuronyl transferase. It presents in the neonatal period with severe unconjugated hyperbilirubinemia (360–850 μmol/L or 21–50 mg/dl) and, unless repeated exchange transfusions are performed and continuous phototherapy instituted, kernicterus rapidly develops. Death frequently occurs during the first year but rarely the onset of kernicterus may be delayed until after the late teens. Heterozygotes have normal serum bilirubin levels but may have impaired glucuronidation of other substrates. Diagnosis is based on the exclusion of other causes of hyperbilirubinemia, normal liver histology, lack of bilirubin conjugates and absent enzyme activity. Phenobarbitone is ineffective but regular phototherapy or plasmapheresis may help and liver transplantation should be curative.

The inheritance pattern of the type II variant (143500) is not clear; seemingly autosomal dominant, molecular studies suggest recessive inheritance with different mutations in the UGT1 gene. It is characterized by defective, but not absent, UDP bilirubin glucuronyl transferase activity. It presents with jaundice usually in the first year of life but this may be delayed until childhood or later. The serum bilirubin may be intermittently raised to 80–360 μmol/L (5–21 mg/dl) and falls with phenobarbitone treatment. Kernicterus is rare. Relatives may give a history of a similar pattern of jaundice.

Gilbert's syndrome (143500) (~1 : 1000) is characterized by a mild, chronic and variable unconjugated hyperbilirubinemia. It may represent more than one genetic defect (Bosma et al 1995) but the pathogenesis usually involves impaired uptake of bilirubin by liver, deficient UDP-bilirubin glucuronyl transferase activity and, in 50% of patients, slightly reduced erythrocyte survival time. Many cases are homozygous for an upstream mutation in the UDP1 gene; others may be heterozygotes for the Crigler–Najjar type 2 gene. Inheritance is usually autosomal dominant but autosomal recessive families are known; males are more commonly affected than females (Schmid 1995).

There is mild fluctuating jaundice (~50 μmol/L, 3 mg/dl) sometimes with upper abdominal discomfort, malaise and headache. Intercurrent infection, fasting, exertion and excessive alcohol intake may exacerbate the hyperbilirubinemia but intravenous nicotinic acid usually decreases it sharply. The condition often remains undiagnosed until adulthood. Hepatic morphology is normal and kernicterus does not occur. The disorder is benign but if skin pigmentation is distressing, phenobarbitone reduces the bilirubin level and may also give symptomatic relief.

PREDOMINANTLY CONJUGATED HYPERBILIRUBINEMIA

The *Dubin–Johnson syndrome* (237500) is caused by a basic defect in the transport of conjugated bilirubin and other low molecular weight anions from liver cells into bile.

Mild conjugated hyperbilirubinemia, 30–80 μmol/L (2–5 mg/dl) usually develops during adolescence but may be recognized in infancy; levels may reach as high as 340 μmol/L (20 mg/dl). At times, the stools may be acholic and the urine dark, the latter containing both bilirubin and urobilinogen. The patient may complain of generalized weakness, anorexia, nausea and of vague upper abdominal pain. The liver is enlarged in 50% of patients and may be tender. Infection, pregnancy or oral contraceptives may exacerbate jaundice.

Serum transaminases, alkaline phosphatase and bile salts are normal. Cholangiographic dye is not well concentrated. Bromsulphthalein secretion is characteristically deranged; retention in plasma is normal at 45 min. but is above normal at 90 min suggesting regurgitation of conjugated material from hepatocytes to plasma. Heterozygotes may show lesser abnormalities. Total urinary coproporphyrinogen is normal or slightly increased but the coproporphyrinogen I isomer is usually greater than 80% of the total. Characteristic coarse, blackish brown pigment, the nature of which is not understood, is present in the lysosomes of hepatocytes, particularly centrizonal areas. Hepatic structure is otherwise normal. Recent evidence suggests that the defect is a failure of localization of the multidrug resistance protein (MRP) to the canalicular membrane of hepatocytes. Phenobarbital has variable effects but may improve the symptoms in some patients.

Rotor disease (237450) is similar to the Dubin–Johnson syndrome in that the basic defect appears to be the transportation of conjugated bilirubin from hepatocytes into bile. The main difference is that, while the bromsulphthalein excretion is abnormal and shows a raised plasma value (greater than 25%) at 45 min, there is no secondary rise at 90 min. Total urinary coproporphyrinogens are markedly increased but the coproporphyrinogen I isomer is less than 80% of the total. Liver histology is normal with no pigmentation.

Benign recurrent cholestasis (243300) is another, similar, self-explanatory disorder. Malabsorption, steatorrhea and biliary cirrhosis can occur. Liver function tests are as expected with elevated bile acids in blood. Inheritance is autosomal recessive. No specific treatment is known. *Byler disease* (211600), which is usually fatal, is probably allelic.

DEFECTS IN BILE ACID METABOLISM

3β-hydroxysteroid-Δ5-oxidoreductase (231100), *3-oxo-Δ4-steroid-5β-reductase* and *3β-hydroxy-C27-steroid dehydrogenase/isomerase* deficiencies all cause severe 'neonatal hepatitis', marked cholestasis usually leading to cirrhosis and liver failure, the cause of which may be the abnormal bile acids. They cannot be readily differentiated from other causes of aggressive liver disease with biliary obstruction in infants, except by sophisticated mass spectroscopy techniques of serum bile acids. Such disorders may not be as uncommon as reports suggest since these methods are not readily available.

Early treatment with chenodeoxycholic, cholic and, in the latter, ursodeoxycholic acids may be very effective and can be continued for years. Liver transplantation is required in advanced cases.

In *cerebrotendinous xanthomatosis* (213700) (p. 1156) a defect of 27-hydroxylase leads to accumulation of cholestanol and cholesterol in tissues, especially in xanthomas, bile and brain, and to abnormal bile acid metabolism. The latter also occurs in several peroxisomal disorders in which there may also be liver damage.

DISORDERS OF METAL METABOLISM

Calcium and magnesium metabolism and the nutritional aspects of trace metals are discussed in Chapter 21.

COPPER

Copper is needed for normal function of cytochrome oxidase, tyrosinase, dopamine β-hydroxylase, lysyl oxidases and for the synthesis of hemoglobin. In serum, over 90% is bound to an α2-globulin, ceruloplasmin and most of the rest to albumin or to transcuprein. Within cells, copper is bound by a group of proteins called metallothioneins, but neither their role nor that of ceruloplasmin is clear. Copper deficiency compromises copper-dependent enzymes with, predictably, anemia, depigmentation, osteoporosis, fractures and disruption of collagen (Ch. 24). In several liver disorders, including Indian childhood cirrhosis, Alagille's syndrome and primary biliary cirrhosis, the copper content of the liver is very high; however, it is not clear if there is a causal relationship. Copper poisoning is said to be a frequent means of suicide in India.

Wilson's disease (277900) (~1 : 100 000)

This disorder, long an etiological mystery, has now been shown to be due to a defect of a P-type ATPase which is probably required for the normal extrusion of copper from cells. It probably has tissue specificity which may explain the limited tissue involvement.

Clinical features

Wilson's disease may present at any time from early childhood to the fifth decade. The two primary target organs are the liver and the nervous system. Liver disease usually becomes evident in the first or second decade. In early childhood, hepatosplenomegaly, jaundice and acute hepatitis or nodular cirrhosis of the liver are the most common findings. This disease should always be considered in such cases. Hemolysis is frequent.

After adolescence, the disease more commonly presents with progressive extrapyramidal signs, the most frequent of which include rigidity, dysarthria, dysphagia, drooling, intellectual deterioration and psychiatric disorders from mania to depression, paranoia or anxiety. Occasionally, flapping tremor, schizophrenic behavior or the renal Fanconi syndrome may be the presenting feature. A brown or green ring around the corneal limbus – the Kayser–Fleischer ring – is caused by copper deposited in Descemet's membrane, but is often not present in the first decade.

Diagnosis

Plasma copper and ceruloplasmin are almost invariably low and urine and liver copper levels are increased. However, the former can occur with liver damage from many causes and the urine copper varies widely in normal people. Some degree of Fanconi's syndrome is usual. Diagnostic tests which may be needed to establish the diagnosis include a penicillamine load, which causes a large increase in urine copper, assay of the hepatic copper content or rarely, ^{64}Cu isotope studies.

Slit lamp examination may be needed to see the Kayser–Fleischer rings. In the brain, there is gliosis in the basal ganglia, particularly the putamen. Carriers can be distinguished by linkage analysis or radioisotope studies.

Treatment

It is important to diagnose the disease early since treatment can prevent the onset of symptoms and results in striking clinical improvement. Oral D-penicillamine (0.2–2.0 g/day) is most frequently used; the drug should be continued for life. Possible adverse effects are pyridoxine deficiency, allergic reactions, nephrosis and bone marrow depression. Liver function should be monitored over the first 18 months of treatment. Triethylene tetramine 200–800 mg t.i.d. before meals is equally effective and a new drug, ammonium tetrathiomolybdate, is now under trial. Zinc reduces copper absorption and 100–150 mg/day can be given as zinc acetate. Liver transplantation is indicated for advanced liver disease and, if successful, reverses all the biochemical abnormalities.

Aceruloplasminemia (117700)

This is a newly described disorder due to mutations in the ceruloplasmin gene. Symptoms start in adults with extrapyramidal movement disorders, cerebellar ataxia and diabetes mellitus. Retinal and basal ganglia damage occur and excess iron deposits are seen in the liver, brain and pancreas. Plasma copper and ceruloplasmin are low; no specific treatment is known.

Menkes' kinky hair syndrome (309400) (~1 : 60–100 000)

The primary defect, long an enigma, is now known to be in a P-type ATPase needed to pump copper, and possibly other trace metals, out of cells. It has significant homology to the gene for Wilson's disease but is on the X chromosome

Clinical features

Drowsiness, lethargy, hypotonia, hypothermia and feeding difficulties are evident within a few days of birth. Severe developmental retardation becomes steadily more evident and seizures, variable muscle tone and immobility are frequent. The appearance is characteristic, with pudgy cheeks, a Cupid's bow upper lip and prominent eyebrows. The skin is soft and doughy and the hair soon becomes striking, being sparse, depigmented and coarse; it feels springy, like steel wool. Its appearance, reminiscent of spirochetes, is termed pili torti. X-rays show osteoporosis, flared metaphyses and fractures which may suggest battering; Wormian bones are usual. Arteries, ureters and the bladder are weakened and dilated. Heterozygotes may show some findings including kinky hair and developmental problems.

Death is commonly in the first decade. At autopsy, the brain is very small; focal cerebral and cerebellar degeneration are seen. Before birth, all tissues have access to transplacental copper and tissue levels are normal; later, however, levels are low in the blood and in all tissues except the gut and kidney, where copper is sequestered.

There are two allelic variants; one is a much milder form of the disease and the other is the *occipital horn syndrome* (304150), once considered as Ehlers–Danlos syndrome (type V) in which impaired function of lysyl oxidase leads to lax skin, arterial tortuosity and bony abnormalities at the lateral end of the clavicles and the occiput.

Treatment

Several different forms of oral or i.m. copper, the best of which is i.m. copper-histidinate, have been used to try and increase tissue levels. While blood levels increase, the neurologic damage rarely improves though seizures are much easier to control. Prenatal therapy with i.m. injections into the fetus has been tried but with only limited success.

IRON

The nutritional aspects of iron metabolism are discussed in Chapter 21. Absorbed iron is either released from the mucosal cells and bound to the β1-globulin transferrin in the plasma or is retained in the ferric form in the mucosal cells, bound to apoferritin, forming ferritin. The apoferritin:ferritin ratio regulates the absorption of iron which decreases as the mucosal ferritin increases. Much of this iron is subsequently lost through the sloughing of the mucosal cells into the gut lumen. Acute overload of the system results in release of free iron into the circulation, with devastating toxic effects.

In plasma, iron is bound either to transferrin, the major iron-binding protein in plasma, or to ferritin. After birth, the plasma iron-binding proteins are about 65% saturated with iron, this value falling to a norm of 20–30% as iron stores are used. The unsaturated iron-binding capacity of plasma is high in iron deficiency and low in overload or hemolytic states. An adult contains 3–4 g of iron, about 10–40% in stores, 40–60% in hemoglobin and 10–20% in myoglobin and tissue enzymes: a newborn infant contains about 250–400 mg.

In *atransferrinemia* (209300) the findings have included hypochromic anemia, resistant to all therapy, growth retardation and recurrent infections. Whether the deficiency is acquired or inherited is not clear. If the latter, the genetic mechanism is obscure because there are two separate loci which, together, code for over 20 different variants. Transferrin and iron may play a role in infection, unsaturated transferrin somehow having a protective function.

Hemosiderosis and hemochromatosis

One pint of blood contains ~200 mg of iron and *hemosiderosis* can result from repeated transfusions. Hemosiderosis can also occur in alcoholics or from dietary overload of iron, as seen in the Bantu in whom there may also be a genetic component. A high content of iron in the diet is the probable cause of Kashin–Bek disease which occurs in adolescents of short stature and consists of a symmetrical polyarthritis affecting the phalangeal joints particularly. Pulmonary hemosiderosis is discussed in Chapter 12.

Rare cases of idiopathic hepatic hemosiderosis or congenital iron overload are seen; some may have the Zellweger syndrome.

Primary hemochromatosis (bronzed diabetes) (235200) (said by some to occur in ~1 : 500) is associated with excessive iron absorption from the gut; the primary genetic defect is unknown. The symptoms do not develop until adulthood, when cirrhosis, arthropathy, skin pigmentation, hypogonadism, diabetes and cardiac failure become evident. The condition is inherited as a recessive trait, the gene being very tightly linked to the HL-A locus on chromosome 6. This can be used to identify patients in childhood. Heterozygotes are sometimes mildly affected. The serum ferritin is very high and hepatic iron increases steadily with age. Exfusion and desferrioxamine are used for treatment.

Neonatal hemochromatosis, one cause of neonatal giant cell hepatitis (231100), is a condition of unknown etiology. It is one cause of rapidly progressive and often fatal liver disease. There is cirrhosis, fatty infiltration and bile duct proliferation with hemosiderin deposits in the cells and in the pancreas, adrenals, thyroid and myocardium. It is unrelated to the disease discussed above. No specific therapy is known.

In *Hallervorden–Spatz* disease (234200) there are progressive extrapyramidal signs with dystonia, chorea, athetosis and developmental deterioration with death in the second decade. The basal ganglia show extensive iron deposits but the cause of this is totally unknown.

ZINC

Zinc forms an integral part of several enzymes and cofactors and is an essential element in cell growth. Hyperzincemia has been described in several members of a pedigree; the condition is benign and is probably due to an unusual zinc-binding protein in the plasma. *Acrodermatitis enteropathica* (201100) is discussed on page 1627. The primary defect is unknown. There may be several different causes of the syndrome; in all, there appears to be a defect in zinc metabolism or absorption. Plasma zinc levels are low and the symptoms respond completely to zinc sulfate (15–150 mg/day orally).

MOLYBDENUM

Molybdenum is incorporated in a cofactor required for xanthine oxidase, sulfite oxidase and aldehyde oxidase function. *Molybdenum cofactor* deficiency (252150) is associated with progressive neurological deterioration, seizures, dislocated lenses and early death. Serum uric acid is very low and the urine contains xanthine, sulfite and thiosulfate. The nitroprusside test is negative but a strip test (Merkoquant 10013 Sulfit test or Macherey-Nagel Quantofix SO_3) is available. No treatment is successful.

DISORDERS INVOLVING VITAMINS

Most vitamins are cofactors for enzymes and are involved in intermediary metabolism. Defective binding of cofactors can result in deficient activity or reduced stability of the protein. Increasing the level of a vitamin can sometimes improve the function of the mutant enzyme, resulting in a group of diseases that are *vitamin responsive* and which are not due to any defect in vitamin metabolism. Many vitamins in the diet are inactive precursors which undergo metabolic conversion before they are functional and defects in these processes also lead to vitamin-responsive conditions.

Most of the vitamin-responsive conditions are discussed elsewhere; they are summarized in this section.

FOLIC ACID

Folates are required for a number of one-carbon reactions related to DNA, RNA and amino acid synthesis. Four disorders of folate metabolism are recognized. *Congenital folate malabsorption* (229050) results in severe failure to thrive, megaloblastic anemia and neurologic dysfunction; most cases to date have been female. Serum folate is low and large doses of folate or folinic acid, orally or parenterally, are indicated. *Methylenetetrahydrofolate reductase* deficiency and the role of folate and vitamin B_{12} in methionine synthesis are discussed on page 1108. *Glutamate formininotransferase* deficiency (229100) has been reported with developmental delay and cerebral atrophy but is probably benign; FIGLU is excreted in large amounts. Folate-dependent *sarcosinemia* (268900) has been described and a syndrome of folinic acid-responsive seizures is associated with the presence of an unknown compound in CSF (Hyland et al 1995). Evidence for other disorders of folate metabolism, GTP-cyclohydrolase deficiency, 5-methyltetrahydrofolate homocysteine methyltransferase deficiency and dihydrofolate reductase deficiency is at present equivocal. Serum folate exists in several forms, all of which are included in normal folate assays. Deficiency of any one form may therefore not be apparent.

COBALAMIN: VITAMIN B_{12}

Ten disorders of vitamin B_{12} metabolism are known; three (defects of *intrinsic factor*, *ileal absorption* and *transcobalamin II* (275350)) affect the uptake and transport of cobalamin (cbl) (Table 20.11). In all of these, developmental delay and megaloblastic anemia are early features. *Transcobalamin I or III* deficiency is benign although serum B_{12} levels are low. Cobalamin is taken up by cells and undergoes a complicated metabolic fate involving both lysosomes and mitochondria. The cobalt is reduced and two cofactors, methyl B_{12} and 5'-deoxyadenosyl B_{12}, are formed; these are used in only two known reactions. The former interdigitates with folate in the recycling of

Table 20.11 Disorders of cobalamin metabolism

	Serum B_{12}	Anemia	H-cysuria	Me-maluria
Intrinsic factor absent or defective	Low	+	+	+
Defective ileal uptake	Low	+	+	+
TC I and III deficiency	Low	−	−	−
TC II deficiency	Normal	+	+	+
Cbl A and B	Normal	−	−	+
Cbl E and G	Normal	+	+	−
Cbl C, D and F	Normal	+	+	+

TC = transcobalamin; Cbl = cobalamin; Cbl A, etc. = cobalamin A mutant; H-cysuria = homocystinuria; Me-maluria = methylmalonic aciduria.

homocystine to methionine and the latter is required for catabolism of methylmalonyl-CoA. Two disorders, *cblA* (251100) and *cblB* (251110), affect the synthesis of adenosyl B_{12} causing methylmalonic aciduria (251100); two others (*cblE* (236270) and *cblG* (250940)) affect the synthesis of methyl B_{12}, causing failure to thrive, lethargy, megaloblastic anemia and homocystinuria and hypomethioninemia. Three other defects, *cblC* (277400), *D* (277400, 277410) and *F* (277380), affect the synthesis of both cofactors, thus producing both homocystinuria and methylmalonic aciduria. Lack of methyl B_{12} is thought to cause the megaloblastic anemia and most of the neurologic manifestations of pernicious anemia. All these disorders require sophisticated complementation studies in fibroblasts to differentiate between them. Therapy with B_{12} (1 mg/day i.m.) or the appropriate isoform is helpful in some of these conditions.

BIOTIN

Biotin is a cofactor for pyruvate, propionyl-CoA, 3-methylcrotonyl-CoA and acetyl-CoA carboxylases. All are activated by holocarboxylase synthetase which binds biotin to the enzymes. The biotin is subsequently removed by biotinidase and can then be reused.

Deficiency of both *holocarboxylase synthetase* (253270) and *biotinidase* (253260) (~1 : 60 000) is known. Both have been termed *multiple carboxylase* deficiency. The former usually presents in early infancy, the latter may not cause symptoms for months or years. In severe cases, symptoms include feeding difficulty, failure to thrive, hypotonia, ataxia, deafness, optic atrophy, seizures, lethargy, coma and developmental delay. When present, a rash, reminiscent of thrush or acrodermatitis and alopecia are characteristic and lactic acidosis, ketoacidosis, hyperammonemia and a characteristic organic aciduria are usual but not invariant. Definitive studies can be done in fibroblasts but a test for biotinidase is in wide use for newborn screening (Ch. 3), so that early recognition is now common. Treatment with biotin (10–20 mg/day or more) results in dramatic improvement.

OTHER DISORDERS INVOLVING VITAMINS

A familial defect in *retinol-binding protein* (180250) has resulted in reduced circulating levels of vitamin A and a tendency to keratomalacia in spite of good nutrition; supplements of the vitamin are indicated. Familial carotinemia is benign. *Thiamin-responsive conditions* include maple syrup urine disease, pyruvate dehydrogenase (E_1) deficiency and a rare disorder of megaloblastic or hypoplastic anemia, reminiscent of the Wiskott–Aldrich (301000) or the Wolfram (DIDMOAD) syndromes (222300) in which diabetes and deafness occur; thiamin corrects the anemia but not the deafness or the diabetes. At least one form of these syndromes is due to a defect of thiamin transport into affected cells. *Niacin* is effective in Hartnup disease and disorders of tryptophan degradation. It has also been used in idiopathic lactic acidosis and in some mitochondrial disorders. *Riboflavin* may be beneficial in these latter disorders, in glutaric acid type I and in several of the acyl-CoA dehydrogenase deficiencies. The *pyridoxine*-dependent conditions include B_6-dependent convulsions, B_6-responsive anemia, cystathionine synthase deficient homocystinuria, hyperoxaluria type 1, gyrate atrophy of the choroid and retina and xanthurenic aciduria. *Vitamin D*-dependent and resistant rickets are discussed in Chapter 21. A selective defect in *vitamin E* absorption (277460) leads to progressive spinocerebellar degeneration identical to that seen in abetalipoproteinemia; both respond to vitamin E therapy.

DISORDERS OF PLASMA LIPIDS AND LIPOPROTEINS

Basic biochemistry

Fatty acids are classified by chain length as *short* chain (2–6 carbon atoms), *medium* chain (8–10 carbon atoms) or *long* chain (> 12 carbon atoms) and also by the presence or absence of double bonds, those with two or more double bonds, such as linoleic acid, being termed *polyunsaturated*. Only a small proportion of the total plasma fatty acids exist in the free or nonesterified form (FFA or NEFA) which are transported by albumin; the majority are esterified with cholesterol forming cholesterol esters, with glycerol forming triglycerides or with phosphate base forming phospholipids. These three main lipid classes are all incorporated together with protein in four major lipoprotein fractions, each of which has a distinctive composition in respect both of the proportions of the individual lipids and protein and in respect of the type of proteins, called apoproteins, which are designated A, B, C or E according to their structure (Table 20.12).

Table 20.12 Nomenclature and composition of plasma lipoproteins

Nomenclature based on method of separation		Percentage composition					
Ultracentrifugation	Electrophoresis	Lipids			Protein		
		Cholesterol*	Triglyceride	Phospholipids	Protein	Apoproteins†	
						Major	Minor
Chylomicron	Chylomicron	3–7	80–95	3–6	1–2	apoA apoB apoC	apoE
Very low density lipoprotein (VLDL)	Prebetalipoprotein	20–30	45–65	15–20	6–10	apoC apoB	apoE
Low density lipoprotein (LDL)	Betalipoprotein	50–60	4–8	18–24	20–25	apoB	
High density lipoprotein (HDL)	Alphalipoprotein	18–25	2–7	26–32	40–50	apoA-1 apoA-2	apoC apoE

* Includes cholesterol esters (about 70% of total).
† Apoproteins A, C and E have a number of alleles designated apoA-1, etc.

Terms that are used to describe the lipoproteins reflect the different methods used for their separation. The terms β-, pre-β- and α-lipoproteins derive from electrophoretic separation. Ultracentrifugation gives rise to nomenclature based on the density of the lipoprotein and this is currently the preferred terminology. Low density lipoprotein (LDL) corresponds to β-lipoprotein, very low density (VLDL) to pre-β-lipoprotein and high density (HDL) to α-lipoprotein.

Metabolism

Much of the total body pool of triglyceride is derived from the diet. Dietary fat is hydrolyzed into free fatty acids in the small intestine and then re-esterified in the gut epithelium to triglycerides which, together with phospholipids, cholesterol, apoA-1 and apoB-48, are incorporated into chylomicrons. These then pass into the lymph where their surface proteins undergo changes, subsequently entering the general circulation. Once there, the chylomicrons acquire other apoproteins, mainly apoE and apoC, and the triglycerides are rapidly hydrolyzed by lipoprotein lipase; the fatty acids which are released are taken up by adipose tissue, muscle and other cells. After hydrolysis, the small particles remaining (remnants) transfer some of the apoA-1 and apoC to HDL and are finally taken up by apoE receptors in the liver (Fig. 20.21). Apoproteins are mainly formed in the liver and small intestine.

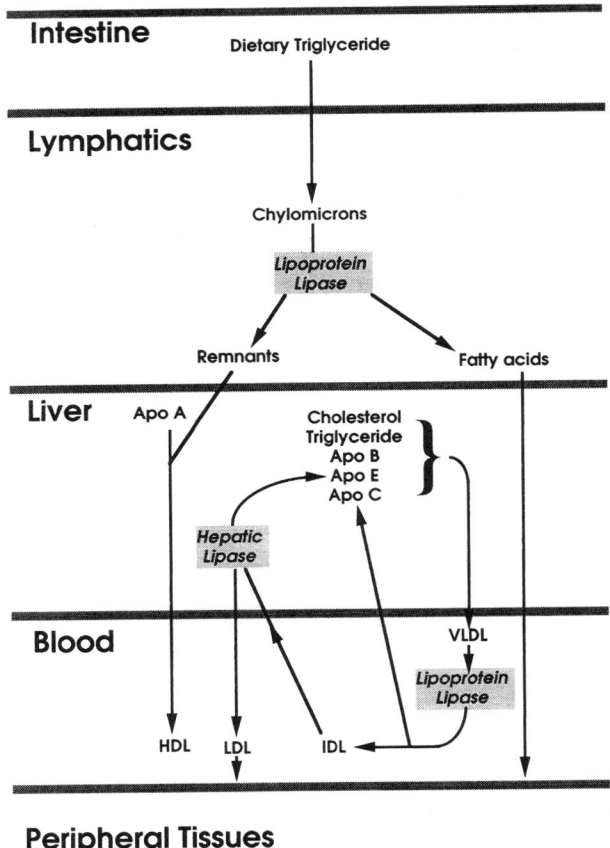

Fig. 20.21 Scheme showing main metabolic pathways of lipoprotein metabolism.

VLDL are formed in the liver from endogenously synthesized triglyceride, cholesterol and apoproteins B-100, C and E and are released into the circulation, where they too are hydrolyzed by lipoprotein lipase. The lipid-depleted particles that result (intermediate density lipoprotein, IDL) return to the liver and lose further triglyceride under the action of hepatic lipase, shedding all apoproteins with the exception of apoB-100. The molecule finally formed is LDL, which is then released into the plasma. LDL then binds to specific cell surface receptors, is internalized and subsequently degraded with release of the cholesterol. Some LDL is also probably taken into cells by bulk pinocytosis.

HDL derived from the liver contain mostly apoA-1, apoA-2 and apoE. Circulating HDL acts as a donor and acceptor of cholesterol and of apoproteins from chylomicrons, VLDL and IDL and is the site of cholesterol esterification by the enzyme lecithin-cholesterol acyl transferase (LCAT).

Normal values

A regular diet high in saturated fats tends to raise the plasma cholesterol, but the value changes little between the fasting and fed states. In contrast, triglyceride concentrations are raised for several hours after a meal and so should be measured in fasting samples. 'Normal' values are derived from epidemiological studies, most of which have been done in Western countries, many in the USA. Such results are not necessarily applicable in other societies around the world, plasma lipid levels being markedly affected by environmental factors, particularly diet. The data in Table 20.13 are based on the Bogalusa Heart Study in the USA. It must also be remembered that 'normal' values, defined by statistical analysis of values from population studies, may not indicate 'desirable' values in terms, for example, of the development of atherosclerosis.

Birth and the first year of life

Plasma lipid concentrations at birth are much lower than at any other age and proportionately more of the cholesterol is present in HDL than in later life. Lipid levels rise rapidly during the first week and more slowly until 4–6 months. Thereafter there is only a slight increase during the remainder of infancy. Nevertheless in individual children concentrations can fluctuate greatly and type of diet has considerable influence at this age.

Table 20.13 Fasting serum lipid concentrations in children from birth to 14 years (means, 5th and 95 centiles, mmol/l)

Age	TC	Tg	LDL-C	HDL-C
Birth	1.8 (1.1–2.6)	0.4 (0.1–0.9)	0.7 (0.4–1.3)	0.9 (0.3–1.5)
6 months	3.4 (2.3–4.9)	1.0 (0.6–1.9)	1.9 (1.0–2.8)	1.3 (0.6–2.2)
1 year	3.9 (2.5–4.9)	0.9 (0.5–1.8)	2.0 (1.2–3.1)	1.3 (0.6–2.2)
2–14 years	4.1 (3.1–5.4)	0.7 (0.4–1.4)	2.2 (1.5–3.3)	1.7 (0.8–2.6)

Data largely derived from Bogalusa Heart Study, USA (Berenson 1980). TC = total cholesterol; Tg = triglyceride; LDL-C = low density lipoprotein cholesterol; HDL-C = high density lipoprotein cholesterol. (1 mmol/l cholesterol ≡ 40 mg/dl.)

Later childhood

The values given in Table 20.13 agree relatively well with other North American studies although the cholesterol values are about 0.8 mmol/L lower than in European and Australian studies. Girls tend to have slightly higher cholesterol and triglyceride concentrations than boys, at least up to puberty. There are marked racial differences which emphasize the importance of allowing for genetic and environmental factors when making comparisons. Plasma cholesterol concentrations remain relatively constant until puberty when there is a fall which is more marked in boys. In individual children 'tracking' (that is, staying within the same centile grouping in relation to the peer group over the years) is obvious for plasma total and LDL cholesterol, with correlation coefficients around 0.6 over 6–8-year periods.

Calssification of disorders

These are classified according to the major lipoprotein fraction involved. Five main primary hyperlipoproteinemias (Table 20.14) are recognized but many of the conditions are ill defined, their primary etiology is unknown and their terminology is confusing. Many diseases result in secondary dyslipidemias (Table 20.15).

Table 20.14 Primary lipoprotein disease – classification and main features

Disorder	Lipoprotein class primarily affected	Plasma lipids involved	Basic defect	Genetics	Clinical features in childhood	Treatment
Hyperlipoproteinemias						
Familial hyperchylomicronemia (207750, 238600) type I	Chylomicrons	TG↑↑↑ Chol↑	a) Lack of lipoprotein lipase activity b) Mutation of Apo C-ll c) Lipoprotein lipase inhibitor	Recessive Rare	Eruptive xanthomata, abdominal pain, lipemia retinalis (may be none)	See text
Familial hypercholesterolemia (144400) type II A	LDL	Chol↑ TG	Deficiency of LDL receptors	Dominant ~1 : 500	Usually none in heterozygote; tendon and tuberous xanthomata in homozygote, See text.	See text
Familial dyslipoproteinemia, (Broad-beta disease) (107741) type III	IDL (normally not present)	TG↑ Chol↑	Mutation(s) of Apo-E having reduced binding to LDL receptors	Variable but common in adults	Rare in childhood; tuberous and palmar xanthomata	Reduce weight, clofibrate gemfibrozil
Prebetalipoproteinemia (144600) type IV	VLDL		Unknown	Dominant	Rare in childhood; no clinical features	Low CHO diet
Combined hyperlipidemia (144250) type IIB	LDL + VLDL	TGn-↑ Choln-↑	Unknown; probably several causes	Dominant	Rare in childhood; 1–2% of adults	Low-fat diet; drugs
Chylomicronemia with prebetalipoproteinemia type V (144650, 238400, 238500)	Chylomicrons + VLDL	TG↑↑	Unknown	Unclear ~1 : 500	Rare in childhood; eruptive xanthomata, abdominal pain, lipemia	Reduce weight. Moderate low fat and (HO diet)
Defective Apo B-100	LDL	Chol↑	Mutation(s) of Apo B	Dominant. ~1 : 500 adults	Rare but LDL cholesterol may be raised	As for type II
Hypolipoproteinemias						
Abetalipoproteinemia (200100)	LDL, VLDL, chylomicrons	Chol↓↓↓ TG↓↓	Defective synthesis of ApoB	Recessive	Fat malabsorption and acanthocytosis from birth; pigmentary retinopathy and ataxic neuropathy in later childhood	Low-fat diet; fat-soluble vitamins in large dosage
Familial hypobetalipoproteinemia (107730)	LDL	Chol↓ TG↓	Defective synthesis of ApoB	Dominant	May be none; malabsorption of fat; features of abetalipoproteinemia in homozygotes	Low-fat diet if malabsorption present
Familial alphalipoprotein deficiency (Tangier disease) (205400)	HDL	Chol↓ TG↑↑	Increased catabolism of HDL	Recessive	Large orange-yellow tonsils; hepatomegaly; later peripheral neuropathy and corneal opacity	None
Familial lecithin-cholesterol acyltransferase deficiency (LCAT) (245900)	HDL		Defective synthesis LCAT	Recessive	Corneal opacity; proteinuria, anemia	None
Fish eye disease (136120)	HDL		Defective synthesis β LCAT	Recessive	Corneal opacity	

While the primary conditions are genetically determined, some can be due to more than one genetic trait and others seem to be polygenic. Environmental factors play a large part in the expression of the clinical and biochemical manifestations of both primary and acquired disorders.

Classification of the primary hyperlipoproteinemias, based on electrophoresis, was agreed by the WHO, but the definition of type does not constitute a diagnosis; it merely describes an electrophoretic pattern. Understanding of the basic defects in these disorders is increasing rapidly and new disorders and new apoproteins, of unknown significance and function, are still being described. The genes for most of the apoproteins, LDL receptors and many of the enzymes are now known and it is likely that the WHO classification will be abandoned as understanding of the basic defects improves. Hyperlipoprotein type alone should not be used in deciding therapy.

Primary hypolipoproteinemias are rare.

PRIMARY DISORDERS OF LIPOPROTEINS

At least 1 : 100 children has a genetic predisposition to some form of hyperlipidemia but only familial hyperchylomicronemia (type I) and familial hyperbetaliproteinemia (type II) are likely to be encountered in children.

Familial hyperchylomicronemia (type I) (238600)

The three known causes are a primary defect of *lipoprotein lipase*, deficiency of the *activator* and *apoprotein C-II* deficiency (207750); all are rare. Defective clearance of lipoprotein triglyceride causes gross chylomicronemia which persists even in the fasting state. Heterozygotes have no clinical abnormalities but may show variable abnormalities of plasma lipoproteins. A further, dominantly inherited disorder due to a lipase inhibitor is also reported.

Clinical features

Although the enzyme lack is presumably present from birth, the clinical manifestations of eruptive xanthomata and/or attacks of abdominal pain due to recurrent pancreatitis do not usually occur until late infancy or childhood. Occasionally children are asymptomatic and the condition is detected by the chance finding of turbid plasma, hepatosplenomegaly or lipemia retinalis.

Diagnosis

The fasting plasma is grossly turbid and separates on standing at 4°C into a cream layer above a clear infranatant. Plasma triglycerides are very high (often 40–115 mmol/L or 3000–10 000 mg/dl) and cholesterol is also raised, although less markedly than the triglyceride; about 50% of the cholesterol is unesterified. Lipoprotein electrophoresis shows a heavy chylomicron band. Activity of lipoprotein lipase in plasma is often assayed after an i.v. dose of heparin; it does not increase in these conditions.

Treatment

Dietary fat must be severely restricted and the clinical response is usually excellent. Initially, a virtually fat-free diet (2–3 g day) is used and during attacks of abdominal pain, 'no fat' diets containing less than 1 g/day should be given. When the plasma is optically clear, fat intake can be increased but only to 5–10 g/day. Such diets are unpalatable and difficult to maintain. Atherosclerosis is not increased in later life so such severe restrictions may not be necessary for ever. Older children usually self-select a fat intake above which symptoms develop; it is unlikely to be more than 20 g/day. There is no evidence that the tolerance of fat increases with age. Medium chain triglycerides (MCT) enhance palatability of a low-fat diet and can be used for cooking and baking.

Familial hyperbetalipoproteinemia: familial hypercholesterolemia: FH: type II (144400)

The basic defect is an inherited deficiency or functional impairment of LDL receptors on cell surfaces. As a result LDL accumulates in the plasma and less cholesterol ester enters the cells. There is reduced feedback inhibition of cholesterol synthesis (HMG-CoA reductase) within the cell and circulating IDL is converted to LDL rather than binding to the receptors. The disorder is inherited in an autosomal dominant manner and is the most common primary hyperlipoproteinemia detectable in childhood with a frequency in the UK of around 1 : 500.

Clinical features

Heterozygous children are generally asymptomatic although some have corneal arcus or xanthomata. They are usually detected because of a family history of the disorder or the occurrence of early-onset coronary heart disease in a near relative. Fifty percent of males and 12% of females have an episode of cardiac ischemia before the age of 50 if untreated.

Homozygous children develop tendon and cutaneous xanthomata from early childhood, usually have evidence of aortic and coronary atheroma in late childhood and adolescence and rarely survive beyond the age of 25–30 years.

Diagnosis

The diagnosis is established by the demonstration of raised plasma LDL and hence of total plasma cholesterol (which is usually between 7 and 10 mmol/L; 270–400 mg/dl) but only after other causes of hyperbetalipoproteinemia have been excluded. Raised plasma cholesterol with normal triglycerides usually indicates an increase in LDL, but in some children the excess cholesterol may be in HDL and lipoprotein concentrations should always be measured. There is no absolute cut-off point for either total cholesterol or LDL above which the diagnosis can be established with certainty and difficulties arise in the interpretation of values in the 'borderline' range (6.5–7 mmol/L; 250–270 mg/dl). At least two estimations of plasma cholesterol and lipoprotein should be made before the diagnosis is established and treatment started. In homozygotes, plasma cholesterol is 18–25 mmo/l (700–1000 mg/dl). The measurement of LDL receptor function is not yet available for routine diagnosis.

Cord blood cholesterol cannot be used to make the diagnosis. However, if one parent is known to be a heterozygote and if LDL cholesterol is measured, the diagnosis can probably be made at this age. As treatment is not indicated in infancy and because plasma cholesterol may fluctuate markedly in early infancy, it is better to defer diagnostic tests until the child is weaned.

Routine screening for hypercholesterolemia

This has vociferous opponents and proponents. It has been tried using newborn filter paper samples but this seems inappropriate. Multiple battery blood tests (SMAC) inevitably provide cholesterol values even if they are unrequested and unwanted. Such results are different from values that are deliberately sought, which, when abnormal, presumably will occasion some planned therapeutic intervention. Practitioners must review these results and clarify their own policy. If, indeed, early treatment is beneficial, then the sooner the whole family starts, the better.

Treatment

It is accepted by most that lowering plasma cholesterol and LDL from an early age will prevent or delay the development of atherosclerosis. The goal is to achieve LDL cholesterol levels <110 mg/dl. A 'Step I' diet provides ~30% of calories as fat with roughly equal proportions of saturated, mono- and polyunsaturated fats and less than 100 mg cholesterol per 1000 calories. Step II diets reduce cholesterol to 66 mg/1000 calories and saturated fat to <7% of the fat. Saturated fat is considered deleterious but polyunsaturated fats and oils are not and can improve palatability and acceptance. With persistence, cholesterol may fall by ~20% but compliance is poor and diet is only effective in the long term in around 20%.

Ion exchange resins such as cholestyramine 12–20 g (up to 0.4 g/kg) or colestipol, which are nonabsorbable and bind bile salts in the gut, are currently the most effective form of treatment and lower plasma cholesterol levels by ~30–40%. Long-term compliance is better than for diet, but is still a major problem. Folic acid (5 mg/day) should be given with them and levels of other vitamins should be monitored in case they bind to the resin and are not absorbed. Other approaches, such as nicotinic acid, which is not often used in children and high-fiber diets are constantly appearing and may have some role.

Simvastatin and other HMG CoA reductase inhibitors have a marked effect in lowering plasma cholesterol and appear safe for long-term use in adults. In view of possible interference in steroid metabolism, they are not used in small children but in older children this is under study and seems encouraging.

Treatment of homozygotes is not satisfactory. Aggressive diet and drug therapy is required, xanthomata may regress, the onset of atherosclerosis may be retarded and there is some evidence that survival is prolonged but cholesterol levels seldom fall below 13 mmol/L (500 mg/dl). Treatment with regular plasmapheresis effectively lowers plasma cholesterol, but liver and/or heart transplantation are often required.

Other primary hyperlipoproteinemias

The main clinical features and treatment of the primary hyperlipoproteinemias are summarized in Table 20.14. *Defective apoB-100* (107730) and primary *hyperprebetalipoproteinemia* (*type IV*) (144600) are associated with elevated plasma cholesterol and LDL. *Familial combined hyperlipidemia* (*type II-b*) (144250) is associated with ischemic heart disease, obesity and diabetes, lipid levels are modestly high and *familial dysbetalipoproteinemia* (*type III*) (broad β) disease (107741) predominantly causes xanthomas and atherosclerosis. Though all are common in adults, they are rarely detected in children. They should not be diagnosed during childhood unless full clinical, biochemical and family studies have been carried out and the more common secondary causes of these patterns excluded. All are treated with diet modification of the whole family which may impact on children.

Lipoprotein(a) (Lp(a)) is another lipoprotein which is covalently linked to apolipoprotein B-100. Normal blood levels are around 1–>200 mg/dl, values being genetically determined, relatively static and high values strongly correlated to coronary heart disease in adults. The role of this protein in cholesterol-related coronary events in adults is being evaluated; it is structurally similar to plasminogen which might explain its thrombogenic and atherogenic properties.

The final story has not been written. Homozygous apoE (apo ε4) mutations are found in 2–3% of the population; they are associated with familial Alzheimer's disease but causal relations remain to be established.

Abeta- and hypobetalipoproteinemia

In abetalipoproteinemia (200100), the basic defect is a lack of apoB which is essential for the formation of LDL, VLDL and chylomicrons. These lipoproteins are absent from the plasma and HDL are reduced. Both apoB mRNA and immunoreactive apoB protein can be detected in hepatocytes and at least some cases are due to a defect of a microsomal triglyceride transfer protein.

Clinical features

The presenting features are usually those of fat malabsorption caused by the lack of chylomicron synthesis. This, together with acanthocytosis (spiky appearance) of the red cells, is present from birth. Malabsorption of vitamin K may cause a bleeding tendency; low levels of vitamin A are usually asymptomatic and clinical rickets is uncommon. Towards the end of the first decade pigmentary retinopathy and ataxia with peripheral neuropathy appear and are gradually progressive with crippling in early adult life. Cardiac arrhythmias may occur and have caused death. The neuro-ophthalmological features are the result of prolonged vitamin E deficiency.

Diagnosis

Very low plasma cholesterol concentrations, usually less than 1.3 mmol/L (50 mg/dl), together with failure of chylomicron formation after a fat meal and triglyceride levels below 0.2 mmol/L (15 mg/dl) suggest the diagnosis. Acanthocytosis of the red cells and failure of rouleaux formation (best seen in a fresh undiluted blood film) are always present but are not pathognomonic and the diagnosis must be confirmed by demonstrating the absence of LDL by electrophoretic and immunochemical methods. Intestinal biopsy shows normal villi with swollen epithelial cells laden with fat; similar appearances are found in primary hypobetalipoproteinemia.

Treatment

The malabsorption is controlled by a low-fat diet (5–20 g/day) which may achieve normal growth. Some polyunsaturated fat (e.g. corn oil 2–5 g/day) may be included. MCT should probably not be used since they may exacerbate the steatorrhea and possibly cause micronodular cirrhosis.

Supplementary fat-soluble vitamins should be given orally. Sufficient vitamin K to maintain a normal prothrombin time (usually 5–10 mg/day) and large doses of vitamin A (about 20 000 IU/day) to maintain normal plasma levels are required. Large doses of vitamin E (100 mg/kg/day) to correct red cell peroxide hemolysis (which is increased in vitamin E deficiency) should be given and will prevent the development or progression of the retinopathy and neuropathy. For vitamin D normal daily requirements appear adequate.

Primary hypobetalipoproteinemia (107730) is also due to defective synthesis of apoB. It is inherited as an autosomal dominant trait and is probably a structural or regulatory mutation of the apoB gene; there is some evidence of genetic heterogeneity. Total plasma and LDL cholesterol are about half the normal concentrations; many patients have no abnormalities while others may have some mild features of abetalipoproteinemia. Homozygous individuals have abetalipoproteinemia except they may not develop the most severe neuro-ophthalmological features. The two conditions can be differentiated by family studies. Hypobetalipoproteinemia occurs in some peroxisomal diseases.

In *chylomicron retention disease* (246700) apoB-100 is present in LDL but LDL levels are ~50% of normal. Symptoms are similar to the hypobetalipoproteinemias.

Familial alphalipoprotein deficiency: Tangier disease (205400)

Clinical features

The basic defect is unknown but loss of apoA results in virtual absence of plasma HDL. Cholesterol esters accumulate in all tissues of the body, especially the reticuloendothelial system. This results in grossly enlarged tonsils which have a peculiar and distinctive orange-yellow color. Lymphadenopathy and hepatosplenomegaly may occur; peripheral neuropathy of variable severity and sometimes relapsing in nature is common. Corneal opacities may develop in adult life. Premature atherosclerosis does not seem to occur. The tonsillar appearance is pathognomonic and even after tonsillectomy, the orange coloration may be seen in the pharyngeal lymphoid tissue.

The plasma is often turbid even when fasting, due to the increased concentration of VLDL. Plasma cholesterol is low and triglyceride levels high. No HDL can be visualized on electrophoresis, but ultracentrifugation and immunochemical studies are required to confirm the diagnosis. Heterozygotes are asymptomatic but have reduced HDL cholesterol, apoA-I and -II levels. There is no specific therapy.

Lecithin-cholesterol acyltransferase deficiency (LCAT) (245900)

This enzyme is synthesized in the liver; in the plasma it is associated with HDL where it transfers fatty acids from the phospholipid lecithin to HDL cholesterol, thus forming cholesterol esters.

Clinical features

The cardinal features are corneal opacity, proteinuria and mild normocytic, normochromic anemia with target cells. Moderate proteinuria may be the earliest finding and has been noted as early

as 4 years of age; in later life, red cells and casts may be found in the urine and ultimately renal failure can develop. Corneal opacity, most prominent in the periphery of the cornea, has been noted from puberty.

Diagnosis

Normally about two-thirds of the total plasma cholesterol is esterified; in LCAT deficiency this is reduced to about 10% or less. The diagnosis must be confirmed by enzyme estimation and liver disease, which can cause secondary LCAT deficiency, should be excluded.

Treatment

This is symptomatic. Diet seems to be unhelpful; chronic blood transfusion has been attempted Corneal grafting and renal transplantation for renal failure may be needed.

Fish eye disease (136120) is another rare disease characterized by striking corneal opacities but without anemia or renal abnormalities and is also associated with an LCAT abnormality. The β form of LCAT is present which has a substrate specificity restricted to free cholesterol in VLDL and LDL. Both the HDL and LDL are abnormal in composition with high triglyceride and low cholesterol ester.

SECONDARY DISORDERS

The cause of secondary hyperlipoproteinemia is usually obvious (Table 20.15) by the time the lipid abnormality is defined although it may be detected by routine screening so should lead to consideration of a secondary disorder. The lipid abnormality is seldom specific for a particular disorder; indeed, the pattern may differ in the same individual at different times. All secondary hyperlipoproteinemias tend to be reversed by the treatment of the basic disease process. Only rarely is treatment of the lipoprotein abnormality indicated for its own sake.

In poorly controlled diabetes mellitus the most usual lipoprotein abnormality is excess of VLDL, possibly with some excess of LDL, resulting in hypertriglyceridemia and some hypercholesterolemia. Massive hyperlipidemia causes falsely low plasma electrolyte values which may cause confusion in treating diabetic ketoacidosis. With treatment, the values usually return rapidly to normal.

In hypothyroidism, hypercholesterolemia due to excess LDL resulting from delayed catabolism is usual except in infants when the lipoproteins are often normal. Most cases of nephrotic syndrome have some form of hyperlipoproteinemia resulting from stimulation of hepatic protein synthesis caused by the continuing loss of albumin. There is a strong negative correlation between the plasma cholesterol and albumin levels. Increased plasma triglycerides are also common.

In the hepatic glycogenoses, hyperlipoproteinemia is common; its association with hepatomegaly without cirrhosis should always suggest the diagnosis. In type I, the predominant increase is in VLDL and in types III and V, the increase is mainly in LDL but the lipoprotein pattern cannot be used to differentiate these disorders. The plasma lipid patterns improve with good management of the glycogenosis.

Almost any type of lipoprotein pattern may occur in obstructive liver disease, unless the child is in terminal liver failure when lipoprotein levels are likely to be low. In intrahepatic biliary

Table 20.15   Secondary lipoprotein disorders – mechanisms and main features

Lipoprotein class primarily affected	Disease	Mechanisms	Clinical signs of lipoprotein defect	Management
Hyperlipoproteinemias Chylomicrons	Diabetes mellitus (rarely)	Defective lipoprotein lipase	Eruptive xanthomata, lipemia retinalis	Responds to diabetic (insulin) control
LDL (hypercholesterolemia)	Hypothyroidism	Delayed catabolism	Carotinemia, occasional tuberous xanthomata	Responds to thyroxine
	Nephrotic syndrome	Excess production	Probably none	Responds to correction of hypoalbuminemia
	Obstructive jaundice especially intrahepatic biliary atresia	Excess production especially of lipoprotein-X	Extensive skin xanthomata especially palms and soles if lipoprotein-X high	Ion exchange resin (e.g. cholestyramine)
	Hepatic glycogenosis types I & III	Uncertain	Usually none	Treatment by glycogenosis
IDL	Hypothyroidism (rarely)	? delayed catabolism	Xanthomata especially in palmar creases	Responds to thyroxine
VLDL (+ LDL) (hypertriglyceridemia and/or hypercholesterolemia)	Diabetes mellitus	Excess production + ? delayed clearance	Eruptive xanthomata, lipemia retinalis	Responds to diabetic (insulin) control
	Nephrotic syndrome	Excess production + ? delayed clearance	Probably none	Responds to correction of hypoalbuminemia
	Hepatic glycogenoses types I + VI	Excess production	Occasionally xanthomata	Treatment of glycogenosis
	Hypercalcemia	?	Probably none	May or may not respond to low-calcium diet
HDL	Obstructive jaundice (rarely)	Uncertain	None	
Hypolipoproteinemias Chylomicrons	Malabsorption of fat or malnutrition	Lack of triglyceride for chylomicron synthesis	None	
LDL	Malabsorption of fat	Uncertain	None	
	Hypothyroidism	Excess rate of catabolism	None	
	Hepatic failure	Defective synthesis	Occasionally acanthocytosis, indicates poor progress	
	Chronic anemia	Uncertain	None	
HDL	Obstructive jaundice and hepatic failure	Uncertain	None	
	Non-specific in many acute and chronic illnesses	Uncertain	None	

atresia, there is often accumulation of an abnormal lipoprotein termed lipoprotein X; this has a distinctive composition with a high proportion of unesterified cholesterol and of phospholipid in its molecule. Hypercholesterolemia may be gross but hyperphospholipidemia is even more marked. Extensive xanthomatosis may occur. Treatment by diet and drugs is often successful in alleviating this aspect.

The disorders commonly associated with reduced concentrations of plasma lipids and lipoproteins are given in Table 20.14. The hypolipoproteinemia itself does not give rise to clinical symptoms or signs and lipid levels revert to normal with correction of the underlying disease.

DISORDERS OF LIPID STORAGE

The lysosomal lipid storage disorders usually involve the storage of phospholipids or glycolipids; they are described later in this chapter. Only disorders involving storage of neutral lipids (triglyceride and cholesterol esters) are considered here.

Acid lipase (esterase) deficiency: Wolman's disease (278000)

This disorder is due to a deficiency of the lysosomal enzyme, acid esterase. Triglyceride and cholesterol ester accumulate within the cells in many tissues, especially the liver, spleen, intestinal mucosa and adrenal cortex.

Clinical features

Wolman's disease is variable and not necessarily related to the severity of the enzyme deficiency as measured by leukocyte enzyme assay. The acute infantile form usually presents in the first weeks of life with diarrhea, vomiting and failure to gain weight, with abdominal distention due to gross hepatosplenomegaly.

Neurological status is usually normal. Lymphocytes may contain vacuoles and large sudanophilic foamy cells are found in the bone marrow. Calcification of the adrenal glands may be visible radiologically. There is gross lipid deposition in histiocytes in the lamina propria of the small intestine. These infants usually deteriorate rapidly and die before the age of 1 year.

Hepatic cholesterol ester storage disease is a milder, allelic variant in which clinical manifestations occur later, are much less severe and may amount only to asymptomatic hepatosplenomegaly, although hypercholesterolemia and premature atherosclerosis are usual.

Diagnosis and treatment

Leukocyte enzyme assay can be used for diagnosis and carrier detection and prenatal diagnosis is possible in cultured fibroblasts. Treatment is symptomatic and consists of measures to alleviate the diarrhea and correct the secondary nutritional and electrolyte disturbances.

LIPODYSTROPHY

Generalized lipodystrophy (151660)

Total lack of adipose tissue may date from birth (congenital type) or be acquired in childhood, adolescence or adult life. Congenital total lipodystrophy is commonly familial and probably inherited as an autosomal recessive. The acquired type, also known as lipoatrophic diabetes, is usually sporadic and may follow an acute infection. The pathogenesis is unknown but excess circulating hypothalamic-releasing factors have been postulated.

Clinical features

In both sporadic and hereditary cases, the children tend to be tall for their family size, have advanced skeletal maturation, prominent muscles (due to an increase in muscle bulk as well as lack of overlying subcutaneous tissue) and enlargement of the penis or clitoris. They develop acanthosis nigricans, hirsutism and hepatomegaly and in later childhood or adolescence, a nonketotic insulin-resistant form of diabetes mellitus occurs. Some have associated renal, cardiac or neurological abnormalities; seizures and developmental delay may also occur. Metabolic abnormalities which vary with the stage of the disease include impaired carbohydrate tolerance and hyperinsulinemia usually progressing to overt diabetes mellitus. Hypertriglyceridemia is present in most patients. Levels of growth hormone, both resting and after stimulation, are low in spite of the increased height.

Treatment

Treatment designed to inhibit secretion of hypothalamic-releasing factors is currently under evaluation. At present management is symptomatic; children and their parents require considerable support to cope with the emotional consequences of the distressing clinical appearance.

Partial lipodystrophy

Clinical features

The classic form of partial lipodystrophy involves symmetrical

and expanding loss of subcutaneous fat from the face which may extend progressively to the arms, chest, abdomen and hips, but excludes the legs and lower trunk (Fig. 20.22). The process occurs relatively rapidly over a few months to 1–2 years. Girls are about four times more frequently affected than boys with the usual age of onset between 5 and 15 years. Abnormalities of glucose tolerance with insulin resistance are present in most patients and clinical diabetes eventually develops in about 20%.

Chronic glomerulonephritis develops at some stage in about 25% of cases. Low serum levels of the C3 component of complement, C3 splitting activity and activation of the alternate pathway are usually present, even in the absence of any clinical evidence of nephritis. The cause of the complement abnormalities and their significance in the pathogenesis of the lipodystrophy are obscure.

The prognosis should be guarded in view of the metabolic and immunological abnormalities and the possibility of later renal complications. Spontaneous recovery is documented but is extremely rare. For most children, however, the immediate problem is cosmetic which can cause severe emotional distress. Transplant of fat from nondystrophic areas are not effective in the long run and plastic surgery may be indicated.

Other forms of partial lipodystrophy are recognized and some children have patchy lipoatrophy that does not fit into a recognized type. A distinctive form in which the face is spared and the fat loss confined to the limbs and trunk has been described (151660). The onset is around puberty, girls are more commonly affected than boys, there is a strong familial tendency and the inheritance appears to be autosomal dominant. In addition to the

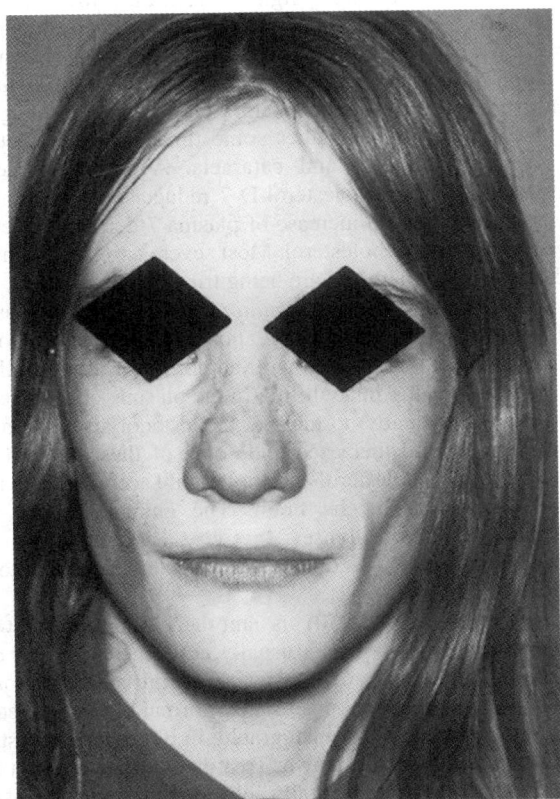

Fig. 20.22 A patient with lipodystrophy.

loss of fat, acanthosis nigricans, hypertrophy of the labia minora, diabetes mellitus and hyperlipidemia are common features. *Centrifugal lipodystrophy* is a progressive loss of subcutaneous fat occurring as a patch over the lower trunk. Most cases described have been in Japanese children but it has also been reported from the UK. In the *carbohydrate-deficent glycoprotein syndrome*, fat pads are usually present for the first 1–2 years over the buttocks and pudenda (p. 1174, Fig. 20.34).

DISORDERS OF CHOLESTEROL SYNTHESIS

Barth syndrome (302060) is an X-linked disorder in which symptoms develop in childhood. Cardiomyopathy with biventricular hypertrophy and systemic myopathy are associated with lipid deposition in the cells, there is severe neutropenia and often some growth failure. Plasma cholesterol and carnitine are modestly low and 3-methylglutaconic and 3-methylglutaric acids are elevated in the urine with some other less constant metabolites. The primary defect is not known but it may be in the 'mevalonic acid shunt' of cholesterol synthesis. Treatment includes carnitine and possibly extra cholesterol; cardiac transplantation may be needed.

Mevalonic aciduria (251170) is associated with severe failure to thrive, developmental delay, diarrhea, ataxia and recurrent fevers: 50% have splenomegaly, dysmorphic features and occasionally cataracts. Milder cases may only have ataxia and sparse neurological signs. Diagnosis is by urine organic acid analysis backed up with enzyme assay in leukocytes or fibroblasts. Treatment is empiric with cholesterol and ubiquinone being suggested.

Dysmorphic features, high forehead, low-set ears, micrognathia, syn- and/or polydactyly with microcephaly, cataracts, cleft palate and severe growth and developmental retardation are typical of the *Smith–Lemli–Opitz syndrome* (270400) (*1 : 40 000?*). Other malformations include congenital heart disease, genital anomalies some times with complete sex reversal (X/Y females) and cataracts. A defect of hepatic microsomal 7-dehydrocholesterol-D-7 reductase in the synthetic pathway causes marked increase of plasma 7-dehydrocholesterol and very low plasma cholesterol. Most severe cases die in infancy but cholesterol supplements are being tried.

In *cerebrotendinous xanthomatosis* (213700), progressive developmental delay, paralysis, ataxia and speech disorders develop in childhood or later and xanthomas on the Achilles or other tendons develop in adult life. In the plasma, cholesterol and triglycerides are usually normal but cholestanol and several bile acid metabolites are increased and some of these may also be detected in urine. Cholesterol and cholestanol accumulate in many tissues, particularly in the brain. The enzyme defect is in microsomal 26-hydrolyase activity. Treatment with chenodeoxycholic acid and HMG-CoA reductase inhibitors is beneficial.

Phytosterolemia (210250) is another disorder in which tendinous xanthomas develop, usually early in life. Some cases have chronic hemolytic anemia and premature atherosclerosis is usual. The serum cholesterol is usually normal but several sterols can be detected by gas chromatography in blood, urine or stools. The primary defect is not known. Treatment involves a diet from which plant sterols are totally eliminated and the use of cholestyramine.

Defects of steroid hormone synthesis are discussed in Chapter 19.

LYSOSOMAL STORAGE DISORDERS

LYSOSOMES

Lysosomes are organelles present in all cells except mature erythrocytes; they contain a large number of acid hydrolases which act as 'garbage disposal units' to degrade macromolecules within the cells. Intracellular materials destined for hydrolysis bind to receptors on the cell membrane forming vesicles which are coated with a specific protein, clathrin. These then fuse with an endosome formed from the Golgi creating a lysosome which has a very acidic interior. At the acid pH, the bound materials dissociate, making them available for hydrolysis. Once degraded, most monomeric units diffuse out of the lysosome to be recycled but some, such as cysteine and sialic acid (p. 1169), require specific transport proteins to facilitate their egress.

After transcription from RNA, all enzymes destined for lysosomes are glycosylated in the Golgi, receiving specific 'zip code' polymannose side chains which identify their destination and permit their uptake into lysosomes through specific mannose-6-phosphate receptors. The enzymes then dissociate from their receptors and act on macromolecules contained in mature lysosomes. Defective function of any one of the catalytic enzymes results in the intralysosomal accumulation (storage) of the undegraded substrates (Table 20.16).

General clinical features of lysosomal diseases

Storage diseases characteristically have three clinical phases. In the first, which may last from weeks to decades, clinical findings are absent or occult. In the second, the disorder becomes progressively symptomatic. In those diseases with nervous system involvement, increasing neurologic signs and slowing development lead to a third phase with increasing neurological or other organ decline. Prenatal onset can present as *nonimmune fetal hydrops* which may be caused by infiltration of the placenta with cells filled with storage material.

General diagnosis of lysosomal diseases

The first step is the recognition of symptoms suggesting one of these diseases. In conditions in which there is brain damage, there are predictable changes in the brain MRI. Coarsening of the facies associated with neurological deterioration, dysostosis and/or visceromegaly lead to the thought of a 'storage disease' and therefore to some sort of diagnostic algorithm.

Mucopolysaccharides and oligosaccharides can be screened, quantitated and identified in urine. There are specific enzyme assays for almost all the known disorders but some are only available in special research centers. Some assays can be done on serum, others require leukocytes or cultured skin fibroblasts – each laboratory has different protocols. Some of the assays require artificial substrates with fluorescent tags; others require natural substrates and all are performed under nonphysiologic conditions. Occasionally, normal people have low activity of one of the enzymes in vitro; it is assumed that their enzyme works normally against the natural substrates in vivo. Conversely, some affected individuals have normal activity in vitro but presumably, inadequate function in vivo. Except where indicated, all are recessively inherited and carrier identification is an important consideration. This is usually feasible but the possibility of partial defects and variants with 'normal' activity must always be remembered.

Table 20.16 Classification of the lysosomal storage diseases

Sphingolipidoses			Mucopolysaccharidoses		
GM$_1$-gangliosidosis	I,J,A*	β-Galactosidase	Hurler syndrome	I,J*	α-L-iduronidase
GM$_2$-gangliosidosis			MPS 1-H		
type B Tay–Sachs	I,J,A	Hexosaminidase A (α chain)	Scheie syndrome MPS I-S	J*	α-L-iduronidase
type O Sandhoff	I,J,A	Hexosaminidase A and B (β chain)	Hurler/Scheie MPS 1-H/S	J,A*	α-L-iduronidase
			Hunter syndrome MPS II	I,J,A*	Iduronate sulfatase
type AB	I	GM$_2$ activator	Sanfilippo syndrome		
Fabry disease	J → A	α-Galactosidase A	MPS III		
Metachromatic leukodystrophy	I,J,A	Arylsulfatase A	MPS IIIA	J*	Heparan-N-sulfatase
			MPS IIIB	J*	α-N-Acetyl-D-glucosaminidase
MLD with 'normal' enzyme	J	Arylsulfatase A activator protein?	MPS IIIC	J*	Acetyl-CoA;N-acetylglucosaminide transferase
Multiple sulfatase deficiency	I,J*	Multiple sulfatases	MPS IIID	J*	α-N-Acetyl-glucosamine-6-sulfate sulfatase
Krabbe disease	I,J,A	Galactosylceramide-β-galactosidase			
Gaucher disease	I,J,A	β-Glucosidase	Morquio syndrome (MPS IV)		
Niemann–Pick disease types A, B	I,J,A	Sphingomyelinase	MPS IV-A	J*	N-Acetyl-galactosamine-6 sulfatase
Niemann–Pick disease types C, D			MPS IV-B	J*	β-Galactosidase
(Sea-blue histiocyte syndrome)	J → A	? Defect in cholesterol esterification	Maroteaux–Lamy syndrome MPS VI	J,A*	Arylsulfatase B
			Sly syndrome MPS VII	I,J*	β-Glucuronidase
Farber syndrome	I	Acid ceramidase			
Glycoproteinoses			Other lysosomal disorders		
Aspartylglucosaminuria	J*	Aspartylglucosaminidase	Pompe syndrome (glycogenosis II)	I,J,A	α-D-glucosidase (acid maltase)
Fucosidosis	I,J*	α-Fucosidase			
α-Mannosidosis	I,J*	α-Mannosidase			
β-Mannosidosis	J*	β-Mannosidase			
Schindler disease	J*	α-N-Acetylgalactosaminidase			
Disorders involving sialic acid			Cystinosis	I,J,A	Cystine egress from lysosomes
Salla disease and infantile sialic acid storage disease	I,J*	Sialic acid egress from lysosomes	Cobalamin, Cbl F mutant	I	Vitamin B$_{12}$ egress from lysosomes
Sialidosis type I	J,A*	Neuraminidase			
Sialidosis type II	I,J*	Neuraminidase	Non-lysosomal disorders which may have Hurler phenotype		
(Mucolipidosis I)			Spinoepiphyseal dysplasia*	J*	Unknown
Galactosialidosis	I,J*	Neuraminidase and β-galactosidase	Geliophysic dwarfism*	I*	Unknown
			Winchester syndrome	I,J*	Unknown
Mucolipidosis IV	I*	not known	Kniest syndrome	J*	Unknown
Mucolipidoses					
Mucolipidosis II (I-cell disease)	I*	N-Acetyl-glucosamine-l-phosphotransferase			
Mucolipidosis III	J*	N-Acetyl-glucosamine-l-phosphotransferase			

* Conditions which usually have a 'Hurler-like' storage phenotype. I = infantile: symptoms or diagnosis usual within infancy; J = juvenile: symptoms or diagnosis usual within childhood; A = adolescents or adult: symptoms or diagnosis usually during or after adolescence.

In some centers, enzyme assays are the initial diagnostic tool, particularly when a specific condition is suspected. In others, particularly when the clinical diagnosis is obscure, electron microscopic study of fibroblasts from skin, conjunctival or rectal biopsy is used to search for the presence of lysosomal inclusions. This finding confirms the class of disorder and so leads to the appropriate analyses. The catalytic enzymes are linkage specific rather than substrate specific. Thus, α-L-iduronidase cleaves terminal α-L-iduronide from both dermatan sulfate and heparan sulfate which accounts for accumulation of both compounds in Hurler syndrome (Fig. 20.23).

In all patients who have or are thought to have one of these disorders, it is important to establish a long-term cell culture for genetic counseling and future prenatal testing and because a number of lysosomal enzyme defects await to be described.

All of these disorders, unless specified in the text, are amenable to prenatal diagnosis using chorionic villus samples or cultured amniotic cells.

General treatment of lysosomal diseases

Since there is no cure for any of these disorders, they are all considered here; any specific measures are discussed in the disease sections. For all the conditions with neurological deterioration, treatment is directed towards palliation and supportive measures such as physiotherapy and surgery to counteract orthopedic problems. Great care must be taken in those with spinal dysostosis since there is grave risk of cervical cord compression and atlanto-occipital dislocation. Extensive genetic counseling and family support measures are usually required.

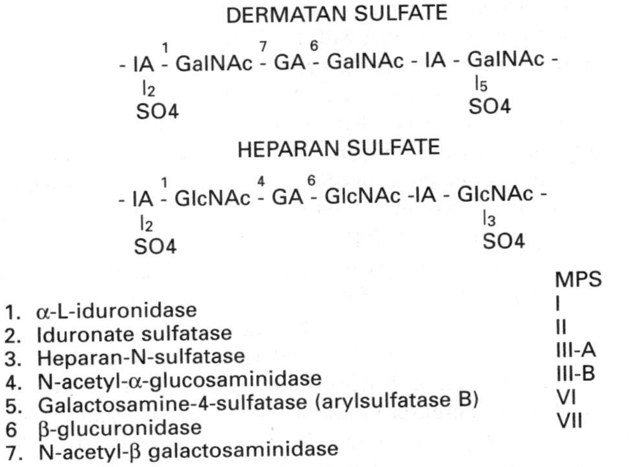

DERMATAN SULFATE

HEPARAN SULFATE

		MPS
1.	α-L-iduronidase	I
2.	Iduronate sulfatase	II
3.	Heparan-N-sulfatase	III-A
4.	N-acetyl-α-glucosaminidase	III-B
5.	Galactosamine-4-sulfatase (arylsulfatase B)	VI
6	β-glucuronidase	VII
7.	N-acetyl-β galactosaminidase	

Fig. 20.23 Portions of polysaccharide chains of dermatan and heparan sulfate and nature of the defects in the various mucopolysaccharidoses.

For Gaucher disease, purified or synthetic enzyme is now available and, though hideously expensive, is stunningly effective if properly used. These preparations must be given by regular infusion and are a prelude to true gene therapy.

In the interim, bone marrow transplantation is increasingly used in the hope that donor enzyme might be taken up by host cells and ameliorate or reverse the symptoms. For conditions in which the CNS is not involved, this approach seems logical. However, the procedure is also being done in patients with CNS involvement from lipidosis or mucopolysaccharidosis in which the results, though said to be encouraging, should still be considered experimental (Krivit et al 1995). It is not considered appropriate in Hunter or Sanfilippo syndromes.

THE MUCOPOLYSACCHARIDOSES (MPS)

Mucopolysaccharides (glycosaminoglycans) are complex macromolecules with a protein core to which are attached huge polysaccharide side chains. There are different repeating disaccharide units (e.g. iduronic acid and galactosamine in dermatan sulfate). In each species the uronic acids and hexosamines are variably sulfated (Fig. 20.23).

These disorders are the exemplar of the 'storage' diseases and in this section, reference is repeatedly made to 'Hurler' or 'storage' phenotypes. This is because these diseases call to mind certain physical and developmental characteristics that suggest, to an astute clinician, the possible diagnosis (Table 20.16). The phenotype is characterized by a progressive course after an earlier period of apparent normality, no exacerbations or remissions and multisystem involvement which may include characteristic facial and physical deformities, skeletal (dysostosis multiplex), ocular (corneal clouding and retinal degeneration), cardiac (valvular and myocardial), central nervous system (mental deterioration) and reticuloendothelial (hepatosplenomegaly and inclusion cells) manifestations. Spinal involvement leads to a very high risk of spinal cord compression and high cord paraplegia.

Radiographic features

The radiographic features of the Hurler-like phenotype are referred to as 'dysostosis multiplex'. A pattern of changes is seen and is best appreciated by a series of views, as seen in Figure 20.24 in an 18-month-old girl with I cell disease.

The earliest findings are in the spine where T12 and L1 start by showing a hooked vertebral body which progresses to a wedging with loss of anterior mass that results in a worsening gibbus. Eventually, many of the lumbar vertebrae show similar findings which are due to defective ossification of the anterior superior portion of the vertebral body. Striking thoracolumbar platyspondyly occurs in MPS IV.

There are obvious changes in the long bones, hands, ribs and clavicle; the basilar portions of the ilia are hypoplastic with flaring of the iliac wings. Dysplasia of the capital femoral epiphyses varies from severe in MPS VI to virtual absence in MPS I-S. Coxa valga and broad femoral necks are seen. Cardiomegaly is generalized and increased pulmonary markings occur after repeated respiratory infections. There is macrocephaly with decreased digital markings. Thickening of the calvarium is most apparent over the occiput. The sella becomes J- or shoe-shaped. The optic foramina are enlarged.

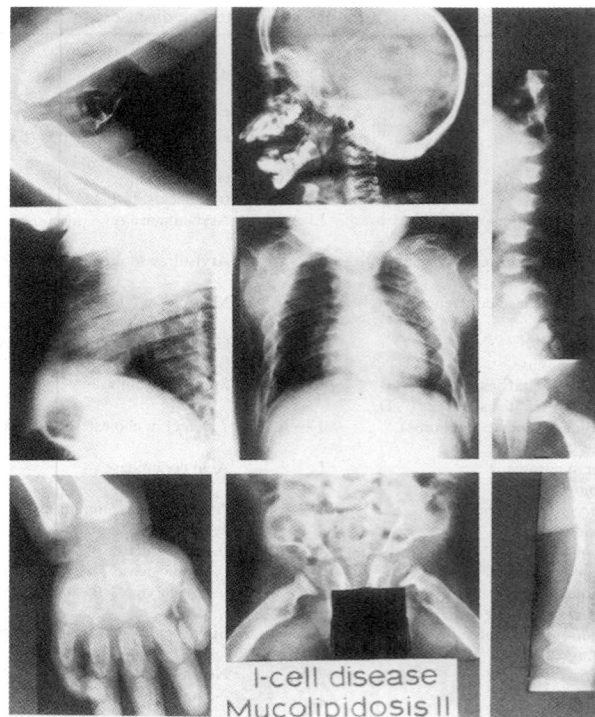

Fig. 20.24 Radiologic changes in lipidosis type II in an 18-month-old girl.

Mucopolysaccharidosis I (252800) (~1 : 80 000)

MPS I and Scheie's syndrome were originally thought to be different diseases; they are now known to be allelic variants of α-L-iduronidase deficiency. Genetic studies have both clarified and confused the picture, in that there are many mutations causing various degrees of residual function of the enzyme. There are therefore different phenotypes of MPS I as there are for almost all other metabolic disorders. For historic reasons, therefore, the terms 'Hurler's' (which denotes a severe condition with neurodegeneration) and 'Scheie's' (which is more indolent and involves the skeleton more than the brain) are retained in this chapter; intermediate forms are termed MPS I-H/S.

Clinical features

Hurler syndrome (MPS I-H) is the prototype of the MPSs. The disorder becomes clinically manifest between 6 and 18 months of age. At that age, affected infants are large with macrocephaly and by 18 months they demonstrate the full phenotype. This consists of hepatosplenomegaly, coarse facies with glossomegaly and grossly apparent corneal clouding, mild claw hand deformity (Fig. 20.25) with contractures at the elbow, shoulder, hips and knees, hirsutism and a lumbar gibbus, persistent mucoid rhinorrhea with recurrent respiratory and middle ear infections and umbilical and inguinal hernias. Thereafter, the course is one of unrelenting progression. By 18 months, mental development has slowed and plateaus between 2 and 4 years of age. Subsequent mental deterioration occurs. Valvular and myocardial accumulation of mucopolysaccharides leads to congestive heart failure, further complicated by recurrent pulmonary infections. These two

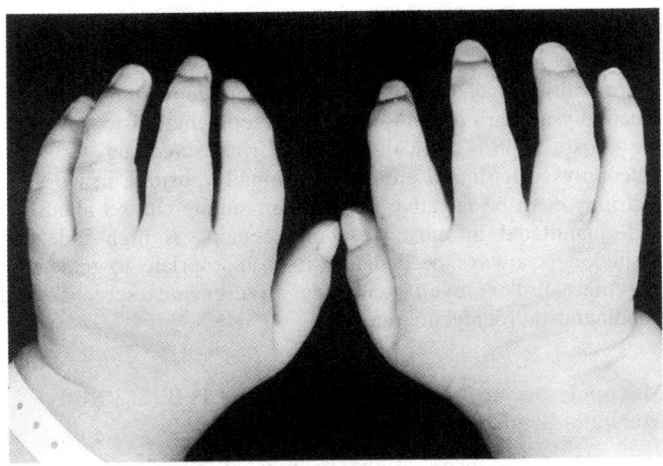

Fig. 20.25 Claw hand deformity in Hurler/Scheie mucopolysaccharidosis (21-year-old female).

complications lead ultimately to death between 6 and 10 years of age.

Although it can be severely crippling, *Scheie syndrome* (*MPS I-S*) is possibly the mildest of the MPSs, being compatible with normal intelligence and life expectancy. It becomes clinically apparent in early childhood with corneal clouding being the most common presenting complaint. Growth proceeds normally with minimal radiographic findings. Mild joint contractures occur but the hands suffer most with development of claw hand and further incapacity is often caused by a carpal tunnel syndrome. Compression of the cervical cord is always a risk. The corneal clouding becomes quite dense and vision is further compromised in later years by glaucoma and retinal degeneration. Cardiac abnormalities are apparent in early adulthood as valvular lesions and conduction defects, but progression of cardiac disease is slow.

The intermediate forms (*MPS I-H/S*) breed true in families, but there is striking interfamilial variability. Progression is slower but short stature, mild mental retardation and significant skeletal involvement are followed by death in the 20s or 30s from cardiopulmonary complications.

Diagnosis of MPS I

Any suggestion of a 'storage phenotype' should lead to a simple screening test, quantitation and identification of urine MPS. α-L-iduronidase deficiency can be shown in leukocytes or fibroblasts in serum or tissues. Determination of the severity and therefore the prognosis is made on clinical grounds sometimes aided by genotyping.

Under 6 months of age a Hurler-like phenotype is seen with generalized gangliosidosis, mannosidosis or mucolipidosis I or II. None of these four disorders is associated with mucopolysacchariduria and all are differentiated by specific enzyme assay. In early childhood Hurler's syndrome is quite similar clinically to MPS II, VI and VII. MPS IV, the Morquio syndrome, progresses to a more distinctive phenotype by 2–4 years of age. No corneal clouding occurs with MPS II and mental deterioration does not occur in MPS VI.

Intermediate forms are clinically similar to mucolipidosis III and mild forms of MPS II and MPS VI. Before other features of a mucopolysaccharidosis become apparent, the corneal clouding is reminiscent of an isolated corneal dystrophy.

Histologically, there is intralysosomal accumulation and storage of dermatan sulfate and heparan sulfate connective tissue cells in many tissues. Cornea, heart valve and cartilage are particularly rich in several mucopolysaccharides.

Affected fetuses that are aborted show widespread tissue accumulation of mucopolysaccharides. Affected newborns show no overt signs.

Treatment

As indicated above, supportive and symptomatic care requires aggressive effort and can only postpone the inevitable. Bone marrow transplantation is still controversial but is increasingly being used, particularly if it can be done before tissue damage is too far advanced. There are numerous reports of reversal of the findings, including clearing of the corneas and improvement of IQ, but bone deformity is not apparently easy to prevent.

Mucopolysaccharidosis II: Hunter syndrome (309900)

Hunter syndrome is differentiated from Hurler syndrome by its X-linked inheritance and absence of corneal clouding. The enzyme involved is iduronate sulfatase. Clinical variation depends upon allelic variation. The similarity of MPS I and II is readily apparent from Figure 20.23. Both result in similar accumulations of dermatan sulfate and heparan sulfate. The difference in the two disorders can be ascribed to the variation in sulfation of iduronate residues in different tissues. The lack of corneal clouding in MPS II reflects a low level of iduronate sulfation in normal corneal dermatan sulfate.

Clinical features

A severe form is most common and closely parallels Hurler syndrome clinically. Hunter syndrome becomes apparent 6 months to 1 year later and cases usually survive several years more. Characteristic differences include absence of corneal clouding and infiltration of the skin, producing a cobblestone appearance usually most apparent over the scapulae (peau d'orange).

The mild form of MPS II is similar to Scheie syndrome in that normal intelligence and life expectancy can be preserved. It differs in that mild dwarfism, skeletal contractures and deafness occur. The deafness is a neurosensory loss with a variable conductive component. The ocular complications of the Scheie syndrome do not occur. Management issues are the same as for MPS I. Behavior problems constitute a serious difficulty and should be dealt with early and sensitively.

Diagnosis

Diagnostic issues are the same as for Hurler syndrome.

Genetic issues

Because of X-linked inheritance, it is important that a specific diagnosis of Hunter syndrome be established. While the family history may strongly suggest the diagnosis, serum or cultured fibroblast studies with demonstration of iduronate sulfatase deficiency are required for confirmation.

Hunter syndrome presents the special problems inherent in severe X-linked recessive disorders. Severely affected males do not reproduce. Thus, one-third of the mutant genes are lost in each generation. The remaining two-thirds are carried by heterozygous females. One-third of all cases result from a new mutation. Thus, the birth of the first affected male in a family does not establish the mother as a carrier. If she has a second case, she might still represent a germ cell mutation. If an aunt and niece both bear an affected son, both establish themselves and their common first-degree female relative as carriers. These factors are important as, until recently, there has been no method to assure a female at risk that she is not a carrier. However, mutational analysis has been helpful and has shown that sporadic cases are rare. Accurate methods for prenatal diagnosis are available and should be offered to all families even when the risk of recurrence seems low.

Mucopolysaccharidosis IIIA (252900), IIIB (252920), IIIC (252930) and IIID (252940): Sanfilippo syndrome (~1 : 100 000)

Heparan sulfate is the mucopolysaccharide that accumulates and is excreted in Sanfilippo syndrome. A portion of the polysaccharide chain of heparan sulfate is shown in Figure 20.23. Two of the four linkages unique to this polymer are shown. Biochemical analysis has already established four enzymatic forms. Heparan N-sulfatase is the defect in MPS IIIA and α-N-acetyl-D-glucosaminidase in MPS IIIB. MPS IIIC is due to a defect of acetyl-CoA:N-acetyl-glucosaminide N-acetyl transferase and MPS IIID is due to defective function of N-acetyl-glucosamine-6-sulfate sulfatase. Two additional theoretical defects in α-glucosaminidase and α-glucosaminyl sulfatase have yet to be identified.

Type A seems to be more frequent than B. Types C and D have been described in only a few patients. Allelic forms of each enzymopathy should be expected but no good evidence for this currently exists.

Clinical features

In the early years, the children usually look normal but gradual coarsening of the facies is usual over the years. Early apparent normality soon changes to hyperactivity and aggressive behavior which represent the most difficult management problem for parents. Hearing may be compromised and speech is delayed even early on. Developmental retardation becomes obvious followed by plateauing and finally regression, usually apparent by 6 years of age. Physical health remains good through adolescence. This combination results in such serious behavioral problems that institutionalization or long-term custody is often needed. By this age, coarse hair is usual and corneal clouding may be found but only on careful slit lamp examination; hepatosplenomegaly is not present, joint contractures are minimal and facies are not obviously coarse. Radiologic changes are usually minimal or absent but may support the clinical impression; calvarial thickness over the occiput and ovoid vertebral bodies is usually present. Behavior modification, support of the family and appropriate use of local school facilities can allow the family to provide care within the home for many years. As the disorder progresses, patients may survive to adulthood but become totally incapacitated.

Diagnosis

The slow progression and the lack of obvious physical abnormalities make MPS III the most underdiagnosed of the mucopolysaccharidoses. A careful developmental history may be the most helpful clinical feature. Urine screening tests for mucopolysacchariduria are only marginally positive in MPS III and may even be negative but heparan sulfate can be identified and quantitated in most metabolic centers. A high index of suspicion is always needed and it is appropriate to undertake enzyme studies even with negative urine screens and nondiagnostic roentgenograms.

Mucopolysaccharidosis IVA (253000) and IVB (253010): Morquio–Brailsford syndrome (<1 : 250 000)

MPS IV shares many of the features of other mucopolysaccharidoses; keratan sulfate, which occurs in cornea, nucleus pulposus and cartilage, is the MPS that accumulates and is less readily detected by routine screening tests. The enzyme defect in MPS IVA is in N-acetyl-galactosamine-6-sulfatase. MPS IVB is due to a defect of β-galactosidase which is the same enzyme as is deficient in generalized gangliosidosis. It is an allelic mutant which retains activity against GM_1-ganglioside, but is deficient in activity towards keratan sulfate.

Clinical features

The clinical features are the same in both forms. Skeletal abnormalities predominate with dysplastic and dystrophic joint changes being prominent in weightbearing joints, whereas in the other forms of MPS the upper limbs are as severely involved as the lower.

Presentation is usually at 18–24 months because of gait problems from genu valgum and coxa valga, kyphosis and growth failure. The trunk and neck are obviously short and the facies are broad, but without the coarseness of MPS I or II. In the upper limbs, especially the hands, there is joint laxity rather than contractures. By 6 years, the cornea are cloudy, there is progressive spinal deformity with lumbar lordosis, dorsal kyphosis and a barrel-shaped chest (Figs 20.26 and 20.27). Contractures of the knees and hips produce a jockey-like stance and the fingers are short and hyperextensible with an ulnar deviation. Cardiac valvular lesions may occur. Intelligence is usually normal. An enamel dysplasia occurs that is not seen in other lysosomal storage diseases.

Survival well into adulthood is usual, females seeming to fare better than males. A common and critical problem is odontoid hypoplasia with subluxation of C-1 on C-2. Myelopathy may occur acutely or insidiously, being precipitated by even minor trauma. Mechanically induced pulmonary insufficiency and valvular heart disease are eventually fatal. Anesthetic risks are considerable in all MPSs, particularly if the neck is not fully protected, but the myelopathy should be treated early by surgical fusion of the spine and other orthopedic procedures may also be required. Bracing alone is rarely satisfactory.

Diagnosis

In early childhood MPS IV is similar to other MPSs, but the evolving skeletal features soon become distinctive. A number of

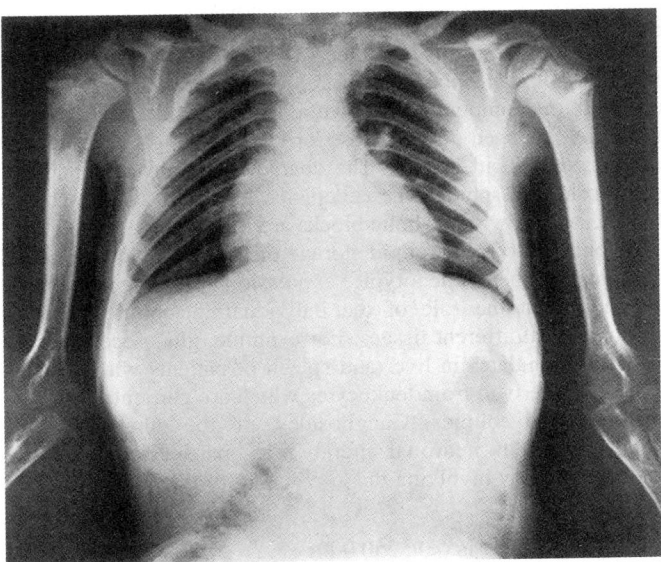

Fig. 20.26 Mucopolysaccharidosis IV. Crowding of ribs by dorsal kyphosis, imperfect modelling at shoulders and elbows.

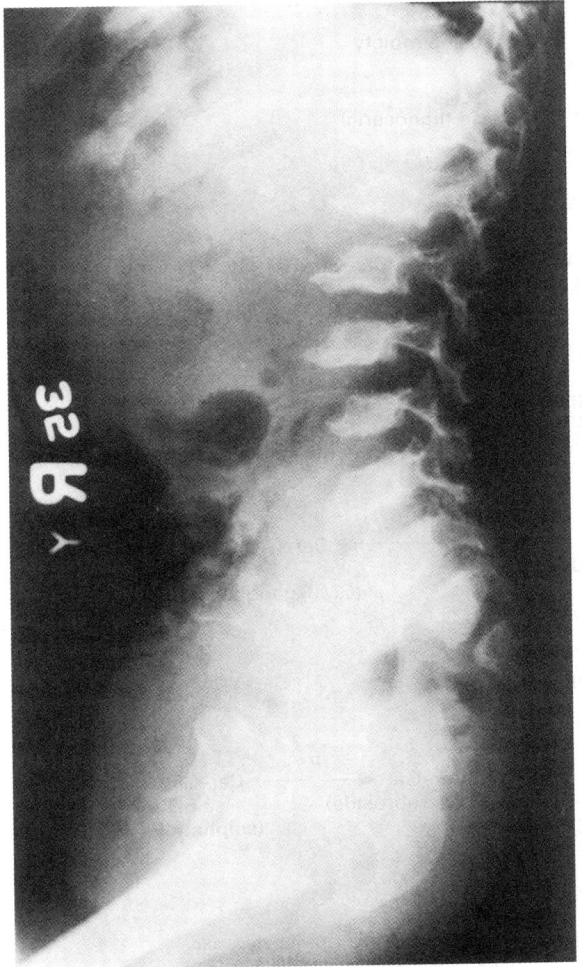

Fig. 20.27 Lateral view of the spine showing platyspondyly in mucopolysaccharidosis IV.

skeletal dysplasias with platyspondyly may resemble MPS IV; the spondyloepiphyseal dysplasias are easily confused, but corneal clouding and keratansulfaturia are absent. Specific enzymatic assays are required to confirm the diagnosis.

Mucopolysaccharidosis VI:* Maroteaux–Lamy syndrome (253200) (<1 : 250 000)

This disorder results from accumulation of dermatan sulfate secondary to a deficiency of arylsulfatase B (N-acetyl-galactosaminyl-4-sulfatase).

Clinical features

MPS VI resembles MPS I and II in physical features and multiple phenotypes but lacks mental deterioration. The severest form may even be apparent at birth but most classic cases have an onset around 1–2 years with survival to the late teens. Odontoid hypoplasia with myelopathy and increased intracranial pressure with optic atrophy and blindness are common; their occurrence is age dependent. Death is usually secondary to cardiopulmonary failure.

Intermediate cases are similar to mild MPS I and mucolipidosis III in severity, but lack the mild mental retardation of these two. The carpal tunnel syndrome and a severe claw hand deformity occur. As in mucolipidosis III, severe hip dysplasia produces pain and severely restricts activity. Valvular heart disease occurs but progression is slow.

The mild form of MPS VI is the least common. Mild dwarfism, joint contractures and valvular heart disease occur. Dense corneal clouding is often the presenting complaint.

Diagnosis

The physical and radiographic features with abnormal screening or identification of the type of mucopolysacchariduria establish the class of disease. In MPS VI, metachromatic inclusions in leukocytes are more striking than with any other form of MPS. Cornea, cartilage and heart valves are particularly rich in dermatan sulfate. Accumulation in these tissues accounts for the major pathology of MPS VI. Enzyme assays for arylsulfatase A or B both use the same substrate and require special techniques to differentiate the isoforms.

Mucopolysaccharidosis VII: Sly syndrome (253220) (?<1 : 500 000)

MPS VII is secondary to β-glucuronidase deficiency. β-Linked glucuronic acid occurs in dermatan sulfhate, heparan sulfate, hyaluronic acid and chondroitin sulfate. Deficiency of β-glucuronidase would be expected to result in widespread mucopolysaccharide accumulation. Among the patients described, mucopolysacchariduria has consisted of heparansulfaturia or dermatansulfaturia exclusively. This is consistent with the clinical heterogeneity seen.

* MPs V was originally the term for Scheie syndrome. It has now been dropped.

Clinical features

Severe cases present as fetal hydrops or in infancy with hepatomegaly and all the other findings of the Hurler phenotype of varying severity similar to that recognized in the other MPSs. Mild cases may not be overtly dysmorphic and may have few radiological findings and only minor developmental problems.

Diagnosis

The phenotype demonstrates typical features of a Hurler-like disorder. Mucopolysacchariduria may be minimal or not detected. The enzyme defect can be demonstrated in serum and in tissues.

THE SPHINGOLIPIDOSES

In sphingolipids, sphingosine is generally linked through its amino group to a variety of fatty acids containing 16–26 carbon atoms. These N-acylated sphingosines are called ceramide (Fig. 20.28). They form the basic building block for all the lipids that accumulate in the sphingolipidoses. More complex sphingolipids such as cerebrosides, sulfatides, sphingomyelin and gangliosides are formed by esterification through the hydroxyl group on the first carbon atom of ceramide. Glycosylation results in the formation of glycosphingolipids and when a terminal sialic acid is attached, the compound is known as a ganglioside. Sialic acid is generally attached to galactose or, in higher gangliosides, to another sialic acid residue. The degradative pathway for higher gangliosides to sphingosine is depicted in Figure 20.29 in which the sites of known metabolic blocks are indicated.

Although the sphingolipid storage diseases are closely related chemically, their phenotypic expression varies considerably depending on the role of the individual metabolites or their precursors in different tissues. For example, glucosecerebroside, which accumulates in liver and spleen of patients with Gaucher disease, is derived from leukocytes which are particularly rich in membrane glycolipids. Gangliosides, on the other hand, are concentrated in neuronal membranes, particularly at nerve endings, thereby involving the gray matter of the brain.

GM_1-gangliosidosis (<1 : 250 000)

Three types of GM_1-gangliosidosis have been described but most patients are of the infantile form (type I). All patients have the

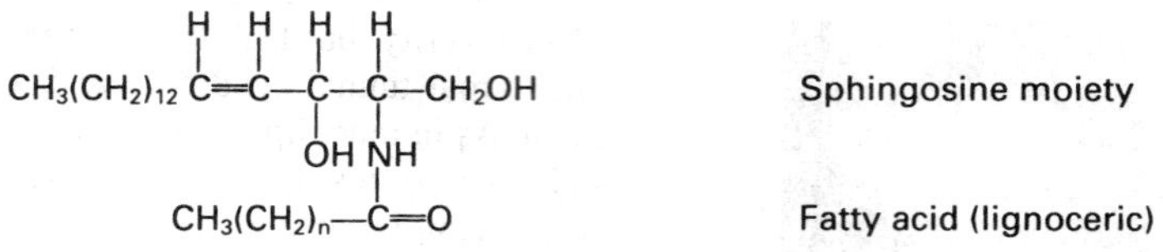

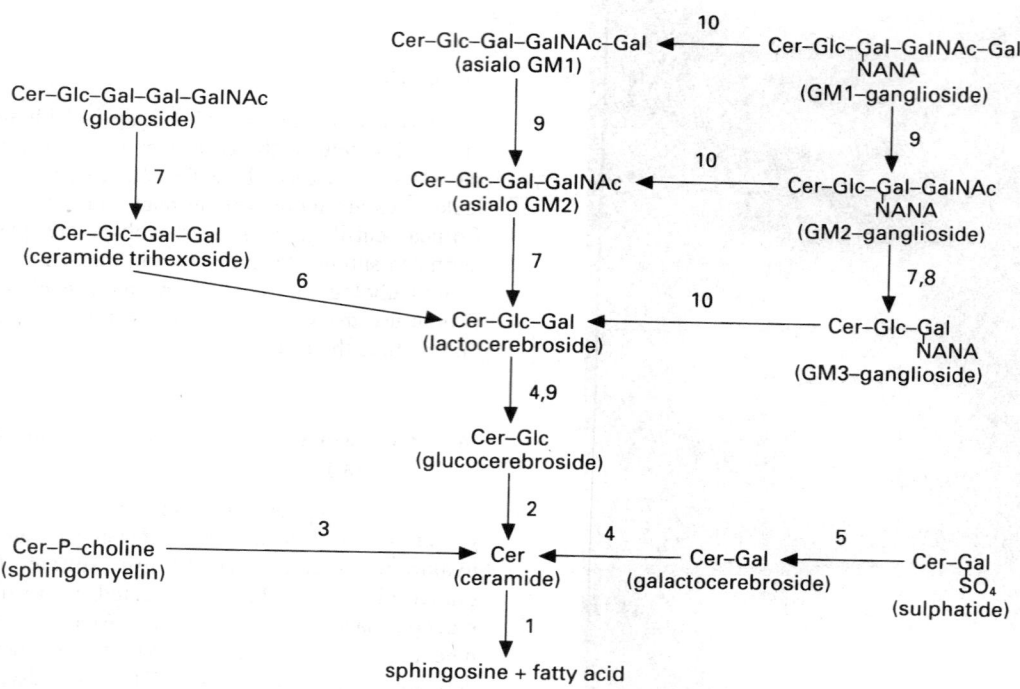

Fig. 20.28 Structure of a typical ceramide.

Fig. 20.29 Diagramatic representation of ganglioside and sphingolipid degradation, showing enzyme steps and metabolic blocks. 1, Ceramidase (Farber); 2, β-glucosidase (Gaucher); 3, sphingomylinase (Niemann–Pick); 4, galactocerebrosidase (Krabbe); 5, arylsulfatase A (metachromatic leucodystrophy); 6, α-galactosidase (Fabry); 7, Total hexosaminidase (Sandhoff); 8, Hexosaminidase A (Tay–Sachs); 9, β-galactosidase (GM_1-gangliosidosis); 10, α-neuraminidase (mucolipidosis I).

same enzyme deficiency as do patients with two unrelated conditions, Morquio type B (MPS IVB) and galactosialidosis.

Clinical features

Classic or *infantile* GM$_1$-gangliosidosis (230500) presents in the first months of life with psychomotor retardation, failure to thrive and severe developmental delay. The facies are coarse with frontal bossing and hypertrophy of the gums, similar to that seen in the mucopolysaccharidoses. About 50% have a macular cherry red spot similar to that in Tay–Sachs patients. Affected patients become blind and often exhibit an exaggerated startle response reflecting brainstem involvement. Hepatosplenomegaly is usual and peripheral edema and cardiomyopathy may develop. Skeletal changes, together with the radiological picture similar to that seen in the mucopolysaccharidoses, with beaking of the vertebrae and spatulate ribs, are prominent. By 1 year of age seizures are usual and continued deterioration results in neurorespiratory failure with death usual by 2 years of age.

Juvenile GM$_1$-gangliosidosis (type II) (230600) has a later onset and the course is slower. Skeletal changes, hepatomegaly and macular cherry red spots are usually absent. Slowing of normal development may be noticed around 1 year of age progressing to seizures, abnormal movements and progressive decline in function, leading to death between 3 and 10 years of age.

Adult GM$_1$-gangliosidosis (type III) (230650), with onset in the second or third decade, appears to be the least common variant but may be more frequent in Japan. Symptoms include slowly progressive dystonia, spinocerebellar degeneration and increasing cognitive deficits. It is important to note that none of the later onset forms of the disease is associated with dysmorphic features, visceromegaly, cherry red spots or seizures.

Diagnosis

β-galactosidase activity is deficient in all tissues. The assay is not reliable in plasma samples but lymphocytes often show a characteristic vacuolation. Because β-galactosidase deficiency is also found in Morquio type B and galactosialidosis (p. 1169), these conditions must be excluded on clinical and biochemical grounds. Some partially degraded keratan sulfate may be excreted but the levels are not as high as in Morquio disease. More often there is a characteristic oligosacchariduria which includes a specific octasaccharide; levels appear to correlate with the severity of the disease. At autopsy, many tissues contain large histiocytes ballooned with the storage material GM$_1$-ganglioside.

GM$_2$-gangliosidosis

GM$_2$-ganglioside is a complex glycolipid that contains a terminal *N*-acetyl-galactosamine which is hydrolyzed by a specific *N*-acetyl-galactosaminidase, in the presence of a substrate-binding activator protein. Because the enzyme also cleaves certain *N*-acetyl-glucosamine residues, it is generally referred to simply as *hexosaminidase*. The enzyme exists in two isoenzymic forms: hexosaminidase A contains α and β subunits whereas hexosaminidase B contains β subunits only. The two enzymes differ in their substrate specificities. The three major types of GM$_2$-gangliosidosis result from mutations affecting the α chain, the β chain or the activator protein. All result in the accumulation of GM$_2$-ganglioside in nervous tissue.

Tay–Sachs disease, GM$_2$-gangliosidosis B variant* (272800)

Clinical features

Infants appear to be normal for the first 4–6 months. Gradually it becomes obvious that development is slowing and soon stops. By 9–12 months, there is progressive neurological deterioration with loss of contact with the surroundings and feeding difficulties, seizures and a characteristic startle response to sharp sound. On ophthalmoscopy, a cherry red spot with a gray-white halo of lipid-laden cells can be seen in the macular region. By 18 months, the patients are unable to crawl or to sit unsupported. There is no visceromegaly but there is usually progressive enlargement of the head from the stored lipids in the brain. Patients often have fine facial features with pale skin and long eyelashes. During the second year, there are increasing numbers of seizures, patients become blind, progressively deaf and spastic and decerebrate rigidity sets in. Most patients die between 18 and 36 months of age.

Late-onset, juvenile Tay–Sachs disease usually presents between 2 and 10 years of age with ataxia, progressive spasticity, dementia and increasing seizures. The cherry red spot and loss of vision may be slow to develop. Most patients die in a vegetative state as teenagers.

Adult forms of the disease may start in childhood with subtle and variable symptoms leading to spinocerebellar degeneration and motor neuron disease with muscle weakness. Intellect and vision may not be affected, at least not initially. Such cases are often misdiagnosed as multiple sclerosis or other disorders and hexosaminidase should be assayed in all puzzling neurological cases.

The *GM$_2$-gangliosidosis B$_1$* variant (272800) is identical clinically to infantile Tay–Sachs. Hexosaminidase A activity is deficient in vivo but may appear normal when measured with the conventional assay (see diagnosis, below).

Other GM$_2$-gangliosidoses

Sandhoff disease – O variant (β subunit defect) (268800) is due to a mutation affecting the β chain of hexosaminidase. Since this subunit is common to both hexosaminidases A (αβ) and B (ββ), both major isozymes are deficient. As with the α chain defects, different mutations give rise to a variety of clinical phenotypes.

Infantile Sandhoff disease is clinically similar to infantile Tay–Sachs disease but with the combined enzyme deficiency, there is more extensive extraneural involvement with mild visceromegaly and occasional foamy histiocytes in bone marrow or vacuolated lymphocytes in peripheral blood. Minor bony changes may also be present. This condition is not specifically associated with Ashkenazi Jews.

Juvenile and adult forms are also identical to their counterparts of Tay–Sachs disease with delayed onset, slower progress and longer survival.

Activator deficiency, AB variant (272750) is clinically identical to Tay–Sachs disease except that hexosaminidase activities are *normal* when measured by conventional methods. At postmortem, the pathology is also identical. The defect is in a specific activator

---

* Tay–Sachs disease, also called type B on account of the retention of the B isozyme, is caused by a mutation in the α subunit of hexosaminidase A. Sandhoff disease type O is caused by a mutation of the β subunit of both hexosaminidase A and B. The nosology of this and other lysosomal diseases is confusing.

protein that facilitates the binding of GM$_2$-ganglioside to hexosaminidase A prior to degradation.

Diagnosis of the GM$_2$-gangliosidoses

Cherry red spots, once considered diagnostic of Tay–Sachs disease, are also present in other forms of GM$_2$-gangliosidosis and in GM$_1$-gangliosidosis, Niemann–Pick disease, Farber disease and sialidosis. Vacuolated lymphocytes are not present in Tay–Sachs but may be seen in Sandhoff. Urine oligosaccharides are normal in Tay–Sachs variants but in the Sandhoff disorders, a number of unusual oligosaccharides have been identified. The levels may correlate with the severity of the disease but the pattern may be difficult to interpret. Hexosaminidase activity can be measured in serum, leukocytes, tears, cultivated fibroblasts and a wide variety of other tissues.

Hexosaminidase A is heat labile and is assayed either as a percentage of the total activity (A + B) following thermal inactivation of the A component or by chromatographic or electrophoretic techniques. Reference laboratories provide sophisticated assays to identify unusual variants.

Sandhoff disease is characterized by profound deficiency of both the A and B activities with some apparent residual activity of A, due to an αα (S) isoform. In all the variant cases, the activities are more varied. Rarely, asymptomatic individuals with markedly reduced enzyme activities are detected.

Tay–Sachs disease occurs in about 1 : 3500 Ashkenazi Jews but only about 1 : 300 000 non-Ashkenazim. Since about 1 in 27 Ashkenazim is a heterozygote, widescale screening of serum hexosaminidase A is now common practice in selected populations. Pregnancy, hepatic disease and certain medications invalidate the serum assay in which case leukocytes are required for carrier detection.

Three mutations account for the majority of the Jewish cases. The reason for the high incidence of these and several other lysosomal diseases in Jews is not known but has raised issues of heterozygote advantage. DNA techniques have identified many other mutations and are sometimes used for genetic testing but it is unlikely that DNA methods will be routinely used to replace the standard tests which are more practical and cheaper. Assay of hexosaminidase activity in amniotic fluid, although reported, is not reliable for prenatal diagnosis of Tay–Sachs disease but may be useful in Sandhoff disease.

It should be noted that urinary hexosaminidase assays are sometimes used to assess renal damage due to rejection following transplantation.

Fabry disease, angiokeratoma corporis diffusum (301500) (~1 : 100 000)

Clinical features

Fabry disease with Hunter syndrome is one of the two X-linked lysosomal storage disorders. Patients usually first come to attention because of severe recurrent lancinating pain in the extremities. The cause often goes undiagnosed for years since there may be few, if any, obvious signs on examination. The pain may extend into the abdomen and is classically made worse by cold, heat or exercise; normal analgesics are of little benefit and sufferers may contemplate suicide to obtain relief. The pain is due to a neuritis caused by vasculitis of the vasa nervorum.

By adolescence characteristic angiokeratomata, which are clusters of dark, nonblanching, petechioid punctate lesions, are present usually in the 'bathing trunk' area but especially the umbilicus and scrotum. Angiokeratomata may also appear in other lysosomal storage diseases such as fucosidosis, β-mannosidosis, aspartylglucosaminuria, Schindler disease, β-galactosidase deficiency and sialidosis.

Ischemic heart disease, valvular damage and conduction defects are common in adults; although marked and progressive neurological involvement is rare, cerebrovascular problems may lead to a number of complications. Progressive renal damage is heralded by proteinuria and is a frequent cause of death. Abnormal eye findings include angioid streaks in the retina and characteristic whorl-like corneal opacities, which may be seen by slit lamp examination in most hemizygotes and in up to 70% of heterozygotes. Most carriers are asymptomatic, but females can be quite severely affected, presumably representing extreme forms of Lyonization. Most affected males die aged about 40 years, as a result of vascular disease, usually in renal failure.

A milder variant presents with isolated cardiomyopathy in mid-life.

Diagnosis

α-Galactosidase A is deficient and the major lipid which accumulates is ceramide trihexoside; the B isozyme is deficient in Schindler disease. In the urine, the lipid appears as characteristic 'Maltese crosses' and may be identified by thin layer chromatography. Heterozygotes usually have intermediate levels of enzyme activity, but DNA analyses are being increasingly used in family studies. The symptoms are caused by progressive accumulation of lipids in nerves and the vascular endothelium which increasingly compromises the blood supply to different organs.

Treatment

Analgesics and narcotics are usually needed for the pains. Phenytoin or carbamazepine is also useful. Renal transplantation is indicated for renal failure but lipid gradually accumulates in the transplanted organ. Therapy with enzyme replacement is now in trial.

The sulfatase deficiencies

There are several arylsulfatases designated as A, B and C. Arylsulfatase A is deficient in the metachromatic leukodystrophies; the B enzyme is deficient in Maroteaux–Lamy disease (MPS VI) and arylsulfatase C is involved in steroid sulfatase deficiency. All three, as well as iduronate sulfatase, heparan N-sulfatase and N-acetyl-galactosamine-6-sulfatase, are involved in multiple sulfatase deficiency.

Metachromatic leukodystrophy (~1 : 150 000)

This disease results from a defect in sulfatide degradation leading to accumulation of lipids which are deposited within neurons. Since sulfatide is a major constituent of myelin, progressive demyelination occurs, leading to a characteristic leukodystrophy. The most common presentation are late infantile and juvenile types.

Clinical features

In the late infantile type (250100), onset is usually between 1 and 2 years of age with learning difficulties and incoordination and gradually increasing signs of deteriorating psychomotor function with both cortical and cerebellar signs. Unexpectedly, the reflexes are diminished or absent indicating peripheral nerve involvement. Increasing speech difficulties with dysarthria, ataxia and optic atrophy accompany marked mental and motor regression and within a few years the children are decerebrate, rarely surviving beyond 8 years.

Most patients with the juvenile form (250100) present before 6 years, but onset may be delayed till puberty. Subtle behavioral difficulties and declining school performance accompany or precede increasing signs of cortical and cerebellar dysfunction. Clumsiness progresses to ataxia, spasticity and increasingly obvious deterioration. The course is quite variable but most patients succumb by about 20 years of age.

An adult onset (250100) is rare and may emerge at any age, starting with behavioral or personality changes which may include paranoia, dementia or psychosis. Neurodegenerative signs become progressively more obvious; once again, peripheral neuropathy results in absent reflexes. Most succumb after a prolonged course.

A defect of the *enzyme activator, saposin B* (249900), results in a disease that is clinically indistinguishable from the usual cases except that the activity of arylsulfatase A is totally normal in vitro. Such cases will be missed unless sulfatide-loading experiments are done in cultured fibroblasts.

Diagnosis

Imaging of the brain shows symmetrical attenuation of white matter most often in the parietal and occipital regions. Peripheral neuropathy causes decreased nerve conduction velocity, especially in late infantile and juvenile types and raised protein levels in cerebrospinal fluid.

Peripheral nerve biopsy shows segmental demyelination with metachromatic material within Schwann cells and histiocytes. Metachromatic granules may be seen within renal epithelial cells in freshly voided urine, but this is not constant and diagnosis requires enzyme assay of leukocytes or cultured fibroblasts.

Artificial substrates are usually used to measure the enzyme activity. Values less than 10% of control occur in all types of metachromatic leukodystrophy; however, 2.5% of people have 'pseudodeficiency' due to a mutant enzyme with in vitro activity up to ~20% of normal. These cases are best investigated by mutational analysis. Because real and pseudo-deficient genes can exist in the same family, prenatal diagnosis should always include a study of enzyme activity in the parents, as well as the proband. Chorionic villus tissue should be used with care due to the presence of high steroid sulfatase activity.

Treatment

In these diseases, treatment is symptomatic; bone marrow transplantation has its advocates who claim that the process can be stopped within a year and that it will then start to reverse.

Other sulfatase deficiencies

Multiple sulfatase deficiency (272200) involves many enzymes and is reminiscent of the mucopolysaccharidoses including coarse features, stiff joints, hepatosplenomegaly and short stature.

Arylsulfatase C (steroid sulfatase) (308100) (~1 : 5000 males) deficiency causes X-linked ichthyosis and reduced activity in the placenta often results in delayed onset of labor. The gene is located on the Xp22.3-pter region and escapes X-inactivation. A contiguous microdeletion can also involve the Kallman locus (308700). The ichthyosis responds quite well to topical 12% ammonium lactate.

Krabbe's disease (globoid cell leukodystrophy) (245200) (<1 : 250 000)

The basic defect is deficiency of galactosylceramide β-galactosidase (galactocerebrosidase). As a result, galactosylceramide, a major constituent of myelin and psychosine, which is neurotoxic, accumulate.

Clinical features

Most patients present between 3 and 6 months with pronounced irritability and increased sensitivity to stimulation. Progressive psychomotor retardation soon becomes obvious with increasing hyperactivity often accompanied by tonic spasms, scissoring of the lower limbs, flexion of the arms and neck spasms. Peripheral neuropathy is evidenced by diminished deep tendon reflexes. There is usually no retinal degeneration and even minimal cherry red spots are rare; however, optic atrophy leads to blindness. Seizures become more frequent and patients rapidly deteriorate, most dying before 2 years of age. There is no visceromegaly and the head is often small rather than large, as in other leukodystrophies.

Late infantile, juvenile and even adult forms are less common. The onset of symptoms is later, as the names imply; they are similar to the infantile form but with a more protracted course. The earlier the onset, the more aggressive is the neurological deterioration; later variants may present with loss of vision and hemiparesis.

Diagnosis

Leukodystrophy is apparent on CT scan or MRI and most patients have delayed nerve conduction velocity. CSF protein levels are usually raised in infants but may be normal in older patients. There is a general loss of white matter lipids and characteristic multinucleate globoid cells are seen concentrated within the perivascular regions of the white matter. These cells are probably derived from macrophages, stain positively with periodic acid-Schiff reagent and are strongly acid phosphatase positive. A natural substrate is required for the specific enzyme assay.

Gaucher's disease

Clinical features

This is the most prevalent lysosomal storage disease. Three main types are recognized; all have a marked deficiency of glucosylceramide β-glucosidase (glucocerebrosidase) activity and result in accumulation of glucosecerebroside.

Type 1, chronic nonneuronopathic type (230800) is most prevalent amongst Ashkenazi Jews with an estimated incidence between 1:600 and 1:2500. Symptoms may begin aggressively in infancy or the disease may be detected incidentally in a 70–80-year-old. The main presenting feature is hepatosplenomegaly, often with overt hypersplenism; the anemia and visceromegaly cause fatigue and the thrombocytopenia causes a bleeding diathesis. Marked bone marrow infiltration, most commonly in the femora, knees, pelvis and spine, leads to patches of osteopenia and osteonecrosis; avascular necrosis of the femoral head is common. Bone crises cause severe bone pain and can lead to considerable disability; they are often misdiagnosed as osteomyelitis and are caused by avascular necrosis, often in the extremities. A typical 'Erlenmeyer' flask deformity of the distal femur may result from expansion of the cortex. Rarely, pulmonary hypertension, infiltrative lung disease, portal hypertension and renal involvement are seen. There may be a yellow-brown pigmentation of the skin and patients appear to have a slightly increased risk of a malignancy. Most older patients have a normal life expectancy, but in younger patients, massive visceromegaly with pulmonary and hematological complications often prove fatal. Although these problems may be partly relieved by splenectomy, increased deposition of lipid in other sites may counteract this benefit and accelerate deposition of lipid in other tissues.

Type II, acute neuronopathic type (230900) presents in the first weeks or months of life; in the severest form it may lead to hydrops fetalis. Presenting features include hepatosplenomegaly and the neurological manifestations of brainstem involvement. Most patients exhibit strabismus, trismus and opisthotonus with retroflection of the head reminiscent of neonatal tetanus. There is increasing spasticity and gross failure to thrive with feeding and breathing difficulties. There is no cherry red spot but optic atrophy may be seen in some patients. Most patients die in their first or second year of life. This variant is panethnic; it is rare in North America but may be more frequent in the UK.

The *type III, subacute neuronopathic type* (231000) is sometimes called the Norrbottnian type after the region in Sweden where it is most prevalent. Onset is usually around 1 year but may vary between birth and 14 years. All cases have splenomegaly and most have hepatomegaly. Bone involvement is rare initially but may develop later. Neurological involvement seems minor but some patients develop seizures. The condition is probably a severe form of type I disease resulting from a different mutation. Survival is variable and tends to reflect the degree of involvement.

Diagnosis

All too often, the diagnosis is only suspected by finding large (20–100 μm) macrophage-like cells in the bone marrow and reticuloendothelial system. These cells stain weakly with periodic acid-Schiff reagent but strongly for tartrate-resistant acid phosphatase activity. The cytoplasm is heavily lipid laden and usually gives the appearance of crumpled tissue paper.

Acid phosphatase activity is often high in serum but this is *not* a satisfactory diagnostic test. Specific assay of β-glucosidase activity in leukocytes is diagnostic; there are five common mutations which are being increasingly used for carrier detection and prognosis.

Treatment

Recently, ceredase, β-glucosidase from placenta (a recombinant product is now available), has revolutionized this field. It is given intravenously every 1–4 weeks using protocols and dosage schedules that vary in different centers. After several months, depending on the accumulated load of lipid, the blood cell counts begin to rise and the viscera begin to shrink but bone lesions are very resistant to therapy. The drug is hideously expensive (>£50 000/year) and is therefore reserved for patients at high risk of complications; in severe cases, it is life saving but it has no effect on neurologic symptoms.

Niemann–Pick disease types A and B (<1:250 000)

The common feature of these disorders is accumulation of sphingomyelin. Types A and B are due to primary defects of sphingomyelinase but type C has emerged as a completely different entity although the name is retained.

Clinical features

Type A is an acute neuronopathic variant (257250); about 50% have a Jewish ancestry. Patients usually present in infancy with marked hepatosplenomegaly, failure to thrive and relentlessly progressive psychomotor regression. The skin may be discolored yellow-brown. About half the patients have a cherry red spot in the macula and there may be corneal and retinal opacification due to lipid deposits. There is widespread infiltration of foam cells in the lungs which produce fluffy deposits on X-ray. Most patients die in the first year or two of life.

Type B is a chronic nonneuronopathic variant (257200) with variable onset in childhood or adult life. All patients have marked hepatosplenomegaly usually with hypersplenism and studies for this may lead to the identification of foam cells or sea-blue histiocytes in the bone marrow. Patients may suffer general malaise and there may be a delay in sexual development. Lung infiltration may become prominent and lead to respiratory difficulties and cardiopulmonary failure but, unlike Gaucher's disease, there is generally no bone or neurologic involvement and cherry red spots are rarely found. In young cases, survival is variable but many older patients can have a relatively normal lifespan.

Diagnosis

Sphingomyelinase is markedly deficient in the A variant, especially in fibroblasts. Type B patients may have significant residual activities (up to 15% of control), especially in fibroblasts.

Treatment

Treatment is symptomatic; liver transplantation has been used in the severe non-neuropathic cases.

Niemann–Pick disease type C (257220) (~1:150 000)

Originally thought to be a form of type A, this is clearly a different disease. It is the commonest of the three and has several different names including juvenile dystonic lipidosis, neurovisceral storage disease with vertical supranuclear ophthalmoplegia and juvenile Niemann–Pick disease with sea-blue histiocytes. No primary defect has been identified.

Clinical features

Onset may vary from infancy to late adult life; neonatal hepatitis, sometimes with cholestasis, is often noted in the history and rare cases develop liver failure. Symptomatic patients have variable hepatosplenomegaly together with psychological and neurological symptoms which dominate the picture. The main finding is of dystonia with varying degrees of pyramidal or cerebellar signs. Supranuclear ophthalmoplegia with paralysis of upward gaze is almost invariable. As the disease progresses, bulbar palsy, mental regression and encephalopathy set in but the victims seem to maintain a cheerful demeanor though they do gradually lose contact with reality. There is generally no cherry red spot. Death occurs after 1–3 decades of deterioration. A former classification, *type D (Nova Scotian) variant* (257250), is now considered to be type C disease.

Diagnosis

This is often extremely delayed, many cases being diagnosed as multiple sclerosis, Leigh, Parkinson's or mitochondrial diseases although the ophthalmoplegia is highly suggestive. The marrow contains foam cells similar to those in types A and B and characteristic histiocytes that stain with an unusual sea-blue color which gives rise to one of the names. Similar foam cells and histiocytes may be found in some other conditions, including Wolman disease and cholesterol ester storage disease which also present with hepatosplenomegaly. These conditions are discussed on page 1154.

No primary defects have been identified in type C disease; sphingomyelinase activity is normal or partially reduced and the defect is in intracellular trafficking and esterification of cholesterol. Currently diagnosis rests on this and on characteristic filipin staining of intracellular cholesterol in cultured fibroblasts. Prenatal diagnosis is possible but tricky.

Farber disease (228000) (<1 : 500 000)

This rare condition has been divided into a number of clinical phenotypes. However, most patients present in the first months of life with joint deformities, subcutaneous nodules and laryngeal involvement. Joints become swollen and painful and contractures then develop. Subcutaneous nodules develop and increase in size and number as the disease progresses; they tend to concentrate around joints or at pressure points. Laryngeal involvement leads to a characteristic hoarseness and both breathing and feeding difficulties develop. In most patients, this, with lung infiltration, usually causes death in the first year or two. Most of the difficulties result from a granulomatous infiltration which causes thickening of cartilaginous tissue. A few patients have liver or spleen enlargement and a macular cherry red spot has occasionally been seen. Some cases have a neonatal onset and marked hepatosplenomegaly whereas others have had some neurological involvement and occasionally significant psychomotor regression.

Ceramidase deficiency can be found in leukocytes or cultured fibroblasts but this is a complex assay and not generally available. Ceramide levels are increased in the subcutaneous nodules.

THE GLYCOPROTEINOSES

Post-translational glycosylation of proteins occurs in the Golgi by linkage either to the hydroxyl group of serine or threonine (*O*-glycosylated) or to the free amino group of asparagine (*N*-glycosylated). The former are generally destined to be secretory glycoproteins whereas the latter, such as lysosomal enzymes, are usually intracellular. Defects in lysosomal degradation result in accumulation of oligosaccharides and glycoasparagines, mostly from incomplete degradation of *N*-glycosylated oligosaccharides. The structures of two typical oligosaccharide chains are shown in Figure 20.30.

Glycoproteinoses are rare disorders in which certain oligosaccharides and glycoasparagines accumulate and are excreted in excessive amounts in urine; some have ethnic predilections. The clinical presentation is often similar to a mild mucopolysaccharidosis but with no increased excretion of glycosaminoglycans. As with all lysosomal diseases, once the conditions manifest, they follow a steady downhill course. No specific treatment is known.

Aspartylglucosaminuria (208400) (<1 : 500 000)

Clinical features

Most cases originate from Finland, where a very consistent phenotype reminiscent of mucopolysaccharidosis is found. Patients usually present between 1 and 5 years of age with coarse features and loose, sagging skin, often with prominent acne. Angiokeratoma have been reported. Growth is usually poor, often with mild dysostosis multiplex. There is connective tissue involvement which leads to joint laxity. Progressive mental deterioration and bizarre behavioral changes become evident between 6 and 15 years with death 20–30 years later with pulmonary disease. About a third of patients have corneal opacities but there is generally no significant hepatosplenomegaly.

Diagnosis

Most patients have vacuolated lymphocytes and lymphopenia and increased levels of glycoasparagines are found in urine either on oligosaccharide or amino acid analysis. The deficient enzyme is aspartylglucosaminidase, which can be demonstrated in leukocytes, plasma or cultured fibroblasts.

Fucosidosis (230000) (<1 : 500 000)

Clinical features

Two major presentations are recognized: a severe form (type I) with onset between 3 and 18 months and type II with a less severe and more protracted course. The condition is rare, possibly being more frequent in southern Italy.

Both types are similar to the Hurler disease phenotype with skeletal abnormalities, coarse features, growth retardation, hepatosplenomegaly, cardiomegaly and mental retardation. Type I patients may never achieve their milestones and may never be able to sit unsupported. Type II patients have angiokeratomata identical to those seen in Fabry disease.

Diagnosis

Both types exhibit vacuolated lymphocytes and increased levels of Lewis A and B antigens in erythrocytes and saliva (these

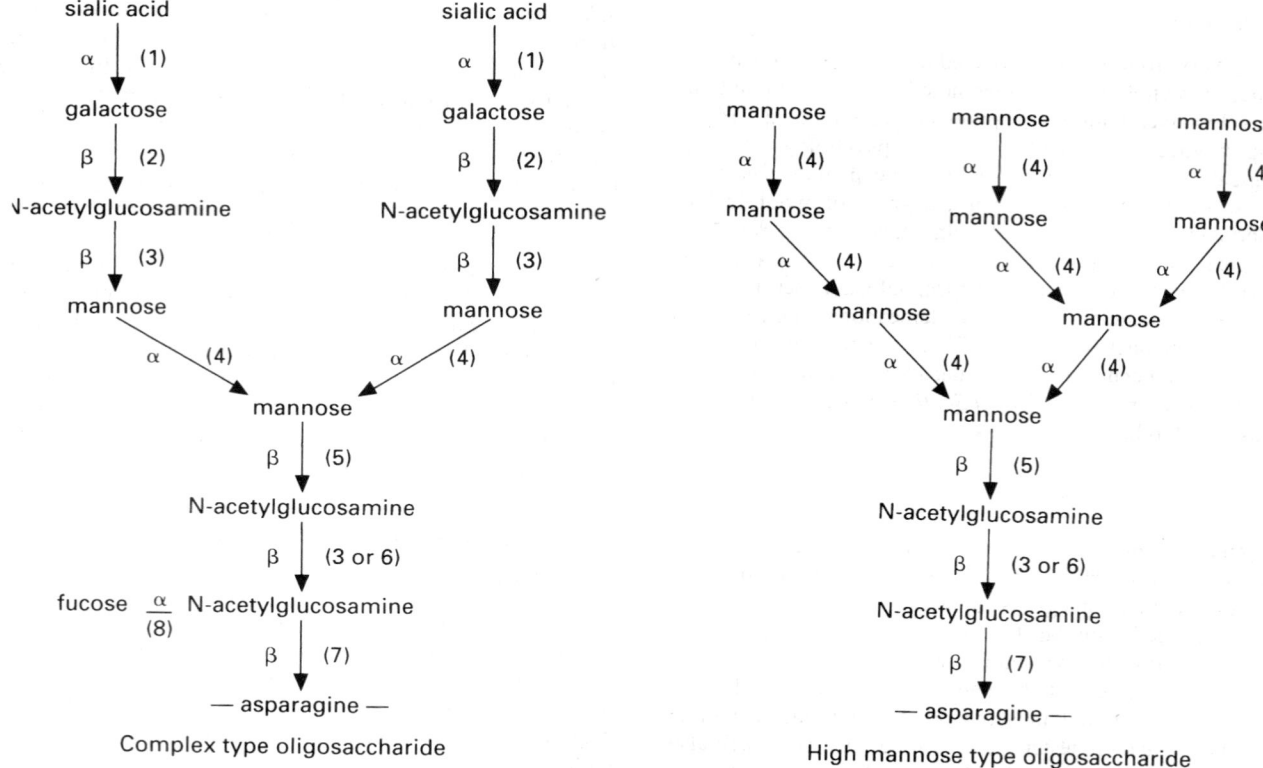

Fig. 20.30   Structures of two typical oligosaccharide chains as found on glycoproteins. Alpha and beta linkages are indicated and the specific degradative enzyme steps are numbered as follows: 1, α-neuraminidase; 2, β-galactosidase; 3, β-hexosaminidase; 4, α-mannosidase; 5, β-mannosidase; 6, endo-β-hexosaminidase; 7, aspartylglucosaminidase; 8, α-fucosidase.

antigens characteristically contain fucose linked (1–>4) to N-acetyl-glucosamine). Oligosaccharide analysis of urine is helpful. Deficient α-fucosidase activity in cells is diagnostic but activity in serum may not be diagnostic, since there is a polymorphism that gives low activity in some normal people.

Alpha-mannosidosis (248500) (<1 : 500 000)

Clinical features

Two phenotypes are described; both are rare. Type I presents between 3 and 12 months and type II between 1 and 4 years. The clinical features, however, are very similar and include mildly coarse Hurler-like facial appearance, marked mental retardation, recurrent infections, impaired speech, hearing loss, corneal clouding, hepatosplenomegaly and dysostosis multiplex. There may also be marked hyperplasia of the gingiva similar to that seen in I-cell disease.

Diagnosis

Vacuolated lymphocytes are generally present in peripheral blood and bone marrow. The urinary glycosaminoglycan pattern is normal but several mannose-rich oligosaccharides are found in urine. There is deficiency of a specific acid α-mannosidase; however, other acid (lysosomal) and neutral/intermediate (Golgi) α-mannosidase activities as well as any residual acid α-mannosidase activity in some patients could confuse the diagnosis.

Beta-mannosidosis (248510) (<1 : 500 000)

Clinical features

Severe cases have had seizures, quadriplegia and rapid decline to death. One case also had clinical and biochemical features of Sanfilippo's disease. Symptoms have included mental retardation, angiokeratoma, feeding difficulties, recurrent infections, speech difficulties and hearing loss.

Diagnosis

Vacuolated lymphocytes are not present and the major storage substance is an oligosaccharide which may co-chromatograph with lactose. Beta-mannosidase activity is markedly deficient in all tissues; prenatal diagnosis should be possible.

Schindler disease (104170) (<1 : 500 000)

Clinical features

This rare disorder is due to lack of N-acetyl-galactosaminidase (α-galactosidase B). Type I is an infantile onset neuroaxonal dystrophy with rapid deterioration starting about 1 year and leading to pancerebral damage, blindness and myoclonic seizures. There is no visceromegaly nor any peripheral storage cells. Type II develops later, even in mid-life. Angiokeratoma corporis diffusum, lymphedema and mild, progressive cerebral involvement are reported; inclusions may be seen in leukocytes and dystrophic axons are seen in rectal biopsies similar to those seen in Hallervorden–Spatz (234200) and Seitelberger (256600) diseases. Urinary oligosaccharides are abnormal. Enzyme assay is straightforward.

Sialidoses

The sialic acids are a family of compounds derived from neuraminic acid. Neuraminidase deficiency occurs in several forms; all are considered in this section even though the nomenclature suggests that they should be classified elsewhere.

Clinical features

In *type I* (256550), debilitating myoclonic seizures and sometimes movement disorders develop, usually in the second decade and are accompanied by progressive visual loss associated with cherry red spots at the macula. Nystagmus, ataxia and seizures may occur. The name cherry red spot-myoclonus syndrome is sometimes used. The intelligence is usually preserved until late and visceromegaly and bony abnormalities are mild or absent.

Type II (previously called mucolipidosis type I) is more severe and can present with fetal hydrops and neonatal ascites; others are detected in infancy. The phenotype is reminiscent of Hurler's syndrome with severe dysostosis, hepatosplenomegaly and developmental delay. Survival depends upon the severity of the symptoms.

Galactosialidosis (256540) is clinically very similar to type II sialidosis. There is an early infantile form with a Hurler-like phenotype and cherry red spots. Late infantile cases present with similar findings and mild developmental delay. Late juvenile cases are most common in Japan; symptoms develop more insidiously with survival into adult life.

Diagnosis

Vacuolated lymphocytes are rare in type I but present in type II. Vacuoles and lysosomal inclusions in other cells may be marked. The urine contains several sialylated oligosaccharides which can be detected by chromatography using a resorcinol reagent.

α-Neuraminidase activity is deficient in types I and II. The defect is best demonstrated in cultured fibroblasts. In galactosialidosis, there is a combined deficiency of neuraminidase and β-galactosidase activity which is due to lack of a specific intralysosomal protein that protects these enzymes from degradation. In all three disorders, foam cells may be seen in bone marrow.

Mucolipidosis IV (252650)

Clinical features

In this rare condition, there is prominent corneal clouding in early infancy and severe psychomotor retardation which becomes evident by 1–2 years of age. There is no facial dysmorphism, visceromegaly or skeletal changes; retinal degeneration is usual. Patients have lived until well into the third decade.

Diagnosis

There is no cellular metachromasia or mucopolysacchariduria although gangliosides and mucopolysaccharides accumulate in fibroblasts and inclusions can be seen in many tissues including conjunctiva. A proposed defect of ganglioside sialidase has not been confirmed

Infantile sialic acid storage disease (269920), Salla disease (268740) and sialuria (269920)

Clinical features

In contrast to the other lysosomal storage disorders, the first two conditions both result from defective sialic acid transport out of lysosomes; they are probably allelic. The *infantile* form is rare, presenting in the neonatal period with coarse 'storage' facial features, strabismus, hypotonia, hepatosplenomegaly, cardiomegaly and mental retardation. Some patients have had punctate calcification of the epiphyses similar to Zellweger syndrome. There is also marked hypopigmentation with pale wispy hair. Growth retardation is common but there may only be mild radiological abnormalities. There is generally no corneal clouding but optic atrophy is common. Marked failure to thrive leads to death in the first years of life.

In *Salla disease*, symptoms emerge in the first year or two of life, but most patients live for decades. Symptoms include ataxia, athetosis and pyramidal signs. Many patients are exotropic and later, most develop mild 'storage' facies. There is usually no corneal clouding and the fundi are normal. Speech is primitive and most patients have a very low IQ. Growth retardation is usual, but apart from a somewhat thickened calvarium, the radiological picture is usually normal.

Sialuria is a separate condition presenting with developmental delay, visceromegaly and coarse facies. There is massive excretion of free sialic acid in urine but no lysosomal storage. It is caused by overproduction of sialic acid due to a failure in negative feedback control on uridine diphosphate *N*-acetyl-glucosamine-2-epimerase.

Diagnosis

In the infantile disease there are prominent lysosomal vacuoles in lymphocytes and urinary free sialic acid levels are increased some 10-fold above normal in urine, leukocytes and fibroblasts. Glycosaminoglycan excretion is normal but abnormal urinary oligosaccharides can be seen using a resorcinol reagent. Patients with Salla disease have similar but less severe findings. In sialuria, the cells contain nonlysosomal sialic acid in the cytosol.

Prenatal diagnosis is possible and sialic acid is markedly raised in affected amniotic fluid in the infantile disease but not in Salla disease. Chorionic villous cells are vacuolated.

THE MUCOLIPIDOSES

Previously, four mucolipidoses were recognized. Types I and IV are now thought to be due to defects involving sialic acid metabolism and are discussed above.

The two remaining conditions are due to a defect of *N*-acetyl-glucosamine-1-phosphotransferase which normally attaches phosphate to a polymannose side chain on the precursor proenzymes in the Golgi. As a result the lysosomal 'zip code' is dysfunctional and several lysosomal enzymes that were destined for uptake into lysosomes are elevated in serum, their electrophoretic patterns are altered and multiple enzyme

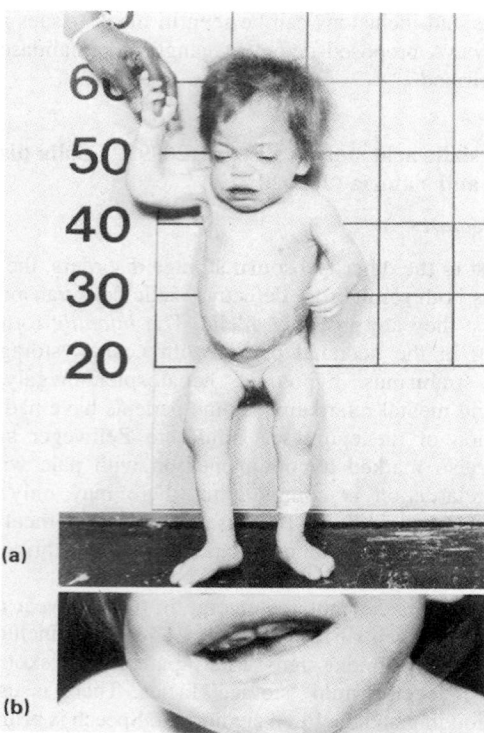

Fig. 20.31 Mucolipidosis II (I-cell disease) in an 18-month-old girl (**a**) Facies and habitus, (**b**) gum hypertrophy.

deficiencies inside the lysosomes account for a heterogeneous accumulation of storage material. The gross cytoplasmic inclusions seen in cultured fibroblasts gave rise to the name 'inclusion(I)-cell disease' (Fig. 20.31).

Mucolipidosis II: I-cell disease (252500) and mucolipidosis III (252600)

These two diseases were originally thought to be due to different enzyme defects. Complementation and molecular studies now show that they are allelic.

Clinical features

I-cell patients present with a severe Hurler-like phenotype (Fig. 20.31). Such features may be apparent in the newborn period but are always obvious by 9–12 months. The facies become ever more abnormal, the visceromegaly is obvious and the dysostosis is aggressive. The corneas are usually hazy, best seen by slit lamp examination. Striking gingival hyperplasia and thickened skin, mucoid rhinorrhea, severe joint contractures and claw hand are obvious. Radiologic findings are of a very severe Hurler osteodystrophy (Figs 20.24, 20.26 and 20.27). Death from cardiopulmonary disease usually occurs by 4–6 years of age. Diagnosis is discussed below.

Type III patients usually present by 3–4 years of age with stiffness in the hands and shoulders. Rheumatoid arthritis is often diagnosed but laboratory evidence of inflammatory disease is lacking. Thereafter, the disorder follows a slow, progressive course so that by 6–8 years of age these patients demonstrate short

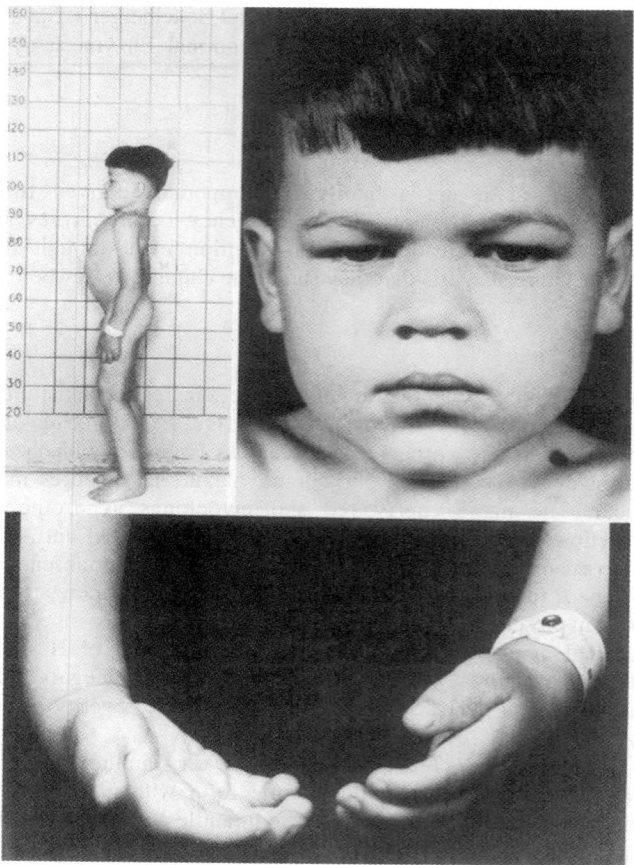

Fig. 20.32 Mucolipidosis III in an 11-year-old boy showing facies, dwarfed stature, barrel-shaped chest, lordosis and claw hands.

stature, mild coarsening of facies, joint contractures with claw hand deformity, fine corneal clouding located peripherally and demonstrable only by slit lamp examination and intelligence in the low normal to educably retarded range (Fig. 20.32). The radiographic features of mucolipidosis III are those of mild to moderate dysostosis multiplex. The most striking changes are in the hands, pelvis and spine.

By the late teens, severe joint contractures are present. Claw hand deformity, usually complicated by the carpal tunnel syndrome, and severe destructive hip changes both usually require surgery. Spinal fusion has been required to alleviate the pain and neurological problems. Aortic and mitral valve disease occur in all patients but cardiac failure has not been frequent. The disorder tends to stabilize in the 20s by which time patients have mild retardation and severe joint contractures as their major disabilities.

Diagnosis

As with other lysosomal diseases, the 'storage' phenotype should lead to an aggressive diagnostic algorithm of metabolite identification, enzyme analyses and possibly an electron microscopic examination for lysosomal inclusions. Type III takes much longer to recognize in view of the slow evolution. The differential diagnosis includes mild forms of mucopolysaccharidosis I, II, VI and VII, fucosidosis, aspartylglucosaminuria and rheumatoid arthritis.

In both conditions, the plasma hexosaminidase and arylsulfatase A are markedly elevated, often 5–20 times above normal. For I-cell disease, the striking clinical and radiographic changes and the massive increase of plasma hexosaminidase usually make the diagnosis easy. Assay of the specific transferase is required for genetic counseling and for prenatal diagnosis.

Ceroid lipofuscinosis, Batten, Spielmeyer–Vogt, Jansky–Bielschowski, Kufs diseases (CLN1–5) (204200, 204330) (~1 : 40 000)

In our clinic, this group of disorders is the most frequent of the nonethnic lysosomal diseases. At least five genes on different chromosomes account for infantile, late infantile, juvenile and adult forms. The infantile (CLN1) form is caused by a defect of palmitoyl protein thioesterase, an *extracellular* enzyme (1p32); a gene for the juvenile form has been identified (16p12.1). Lysosomal inclusions contain lipofuscin, a compound that is pigmented and contains degraded lipid, and dolichols. In some forms, the major protein component is subunit 9 of ATPase.

Clinical features

Infantile cases present with an early onset of seizures and deterioration. Juvenile cases usually present with subtle, slow but progressive behavioral and intellectual deterioration. Seizures soon develop accompanied by progressive neurologic decline that can take more than two decades before death. At some stage, there is a rapid loss of vision resulting in total blindness within a few months and a characteristic pigmentary retinopathy. The 'storage' phenotype does not occur and there is no visceromegaly or bone involvement. Kufs disease presents with myoclonic epilepsy and progressive ataxia, pyramidal signs and dementia in adults.

Diagnosis and treatment

The retinopathy is typical and the disease is confirmed by the presence of typical whorl-shaped or fingerprint inclusions in lysosomes visible in WBC, skin, rectum, conjunctival biopsies and many other tissues. These should be sought in any cases with unexplained neurological problems, particularly if they are progressive. Urinary dolichols may be raised and were formerly used for diagnosis. No treatment is proven effective but efforts are being made to try antioxidants.

DISORDERS OF PEROXISOMAL FUNCTION

PEROXISOMES

Peroxisomes are subcellular organelles which are present in all mammalian cells except mature erythrocytes. They lack DNA and glycoproteins. Their functions include the metabolism of hydrogen peroxide, the oxidation of D- and L-amino acids, urate, alcohols, polyamines and α-hydroxyacids, the biosynthesis of dolichols, cholesterol, bile acids and ether-phospholipids, including the plasmalogens, the β-oxidation of (very) long chain fatty acids, dicarboxylic acids, mono- and polyunsaturated fatty acids, prostaglandins, xenobiotics and, in humans, also in the degradation of L-pipecolic acid and phytanic acid. In man, alanine:glyoxylate aminotransferase (see oxalosis type I, p. 1112) is exclusively a peroxisomal enzyme.

The specific peroxisomal β-oxidation enzymes are acyl-CoA oxidase, the bifunctional protein with enoyl-CoA hydratase and L-3-hydroxyacyl-CoA dehydrogenase activities, and 3-oxoacyl-CoA thiolase. They accept fatty acids of a chain length of 12 carbons or more which are first activated to the corresponding acyl-CoA esters via a membrane-bound acyl-CoA synthetase. Another distinct peroxisomal synthetase activity catalyzes the activation of very long chain (>22 carbon) fatty acids. Peroxisomal β-oxidation is similar to the mitochondrial process but the first step only generates H_2O_2 and heat rather than ATP. The reason for the apparent duplication is unclear but it seems that peroxisomes can oxidize specific substrates that cannot be metabolized in mitochondria.

Unlike the lysosomal enzymes, the reason for sequestration of the disparate enzyme functions in peroxisomes is not clear. However, their functional significance, both in morphogenesis and in later life, is clear. A recent monograph (Roels et al 1995) includes 21 different inherited disorders of peroxisomal function many of which seem, at present, to be extremely rare. These can tentatively be classified into three groups (Table 20.17).

Diagnosis of peroxisomal disorders

These disorders represent a challenge to most clinicians and new defects are still being described. They should be considered in all of the following situations:

1. Neonatal dysmorphic syndromes with profound neurological findings.
2. Profound neurological findings in the newborn, particularly hypotonia, seizures and evidence of de- or hypomyelination, peripheral nerve damage without dysmorphic features.
3. Bleeding diathesis in the first 3 months.
4. Nerve deafness with any of the above findings.
5. Renal cysts in infants.
6. Addison's disease in infancy or in males at any age.
7. Late-onset neuropathy and/or myelopathy.
8. Retinitis pigmentosa, particularly with nerve deafness and/or neurological findings at any age.

The full spectrum of these disorders is becoming steadily more diverse and the symptoms tend to vary with the age at presentation. Clinicians should be familiar with Zellweger which is the florid, archetypic phenotype.

Screening tests for generalized peroxisomal dysfunction include plasma very long chain fatty acids (VLCFA), bile acids and, in some centers, RBC plasmalogens, phytanic acid and pipecolic acids but none is abnormal in all of the conditions. Extended tests are reviewed in Table 20.18; for the most part, these disorders are differentiated by extensive enzymatic testing in research laboratories Recently, nondysmorphic, nondeaf children with normal-appearing retinas but abnormal ERG have been reported; Usher's syndrome can be distinguished by the retinal findings and does not seem to involve peroxisomal dysfunction. Prenatal diagnosis is available for all of these disorders.

Therapy of peroxisomal diseases

With the exception of classic Refsum's disease, in which treatment is highly beneficial and X-linked ALD, reduction of

Table 20.17 Classification of peroxisomal disorders

Type	Enzyme defect
Impairment of a single peroxisomal function	
Adrenoleukodystrophy/adrenomyeloneuropathy (X-linked)	Peroxisomal very long chain fatty acyl-CoA synthetase
Acyl-CoA oxidase deficiency (pseudo-NALD)	Acyl-CoA oxidase
Bifunctional protein deficiency	Bifunctional protein
Thiolase deficiency (pseudo-Zellweger syndrome)	Peroxisomal thiolase
DHAP-acyltransferase deficiency	DHAP-acyltransferase
Bile acid defects	Tri(di)hydroxycoprostanoyl CoA synthase
Glutaryl-CoA oxidase deficiency	Glutaryl-CoA oxidase
Classic Refsum's disease	Phytanic acid oxidase
Hyperoxaluria type I	Alanine: glyoxylate aminotransferase
Acatalasemia	Catalase
Impairment of multiple peroxisomal functions	
Rhizomelic chondrodysplasia punctata	DHAP-acyltransferase, Acyl-DHAP synthase, phytanic acid oxidase
Zellweger-like syndrome	DHAP-acyltransferase, peroxisomal β-oxidation enzymes
General impairment of peroxisomal functions	
Cerebro-hepato-renal (Zellweger) syndrome	Generalized
Neonatal adrenoleukodystrophy	
Infantile Refsum's disease	
Hyperpipecolic acidemia	

Table 20.18 Diagnostically significant biochemical abnormalities in peroxisomal disorders

	ALD	Refsum's	RCDP	ZS/IRD/NALD	Pseudo-ZS
Number of peroxisomes reduced	−	−	−	++/+/+	−
Catalase in peroxisomes	+	+	+	−	+
Deficient synthesis and reduced tissue level of plasmalogens	−	−	++	++	−
Defective oxidation and accumulation of very long chain fatty acids	+	−	−	++	++
Deficient oxidation and accumulation of phytanic acid	−	++	++	+	−
Defects in bile acids biosynthesis and accumulation of bile acids	−	−	−	++	+
Defect in oxidation and accumulation of L-pipecolic acid	−	−	−	+	−

Abbreviations: ++ = substantial finding; + = less substantial finding; − = negative finding.

abnormal levels of metabolites in peroxisomal disorders does not appear to alter their clinical status. Bone marrow transplantation is now being evaluated in X-linked ALD; it appears to be beneficial.

DISORDERS WITH GENERAL LOSS OF PEROXISOMAL FUNCTIONS

In these disorders, there is defective assembly of peroxisomes so that only ghost (or empty) organelles containing no active enzymes are present.

Zellweger syndrome (214100) (? 1 : 50 000)

This is a classic example of a metabolic disease associated with characteristic dysmorphic features. There is some phenotypic variation, but the classic cases are remarkably similar. The facies (Fig. 20.33) show a high forehead, midfacial hypoplasia, small orbits, micrognathia, epicanthus, high arched palate, ear and neck abnormalities; these cases usually die in the first year of life. There is a typical pigmentary retinopathy, nerve deafness, severe weakness, hypotonia, hepatomegaly, cysts in the kidneys, neonatal seizures and the lack of psychomotor development.

Usually there are stippled calcifications of the patellae and often in other epiphyses. Patients with the milder forms survive the first years of life and may achieve some psychomotor development.

Pathological investigations show abnormalities in various organs, most notably in the brain where polymicrogyria and/or pachymicrogyria and deep parietal clefts are evident. Microscopic abnormalities represent specific dysontogenetic and degenerative abnormalities. Liver histology may reveal liver fibrosis, varying in severity depending upon the age of the patient, usually progressing into micronodular cirrhosis if the infant survives.

Neonatal adrenoleukodystrophy (202370) (<1 : 250 000)

These patients look similar to the Zellweger syndrome. It is, however, a separate disorder with a milder course and absence of renal cysts, cataracts or bony involvement and a somewhat longer survival, sometimes into adult life. Adrenal dysfunction is prominent. This condition is totally distinct from the X-linked disease; peroxisomes are absent or greatly diminished and plasmalogen, phytanic acid, pipecolic acid and bile acid metabolism are all abnormal. X-linked and neonatal ALD have never occurred in the same family. Biochemical abnormalities are summarized in Table 20.18.

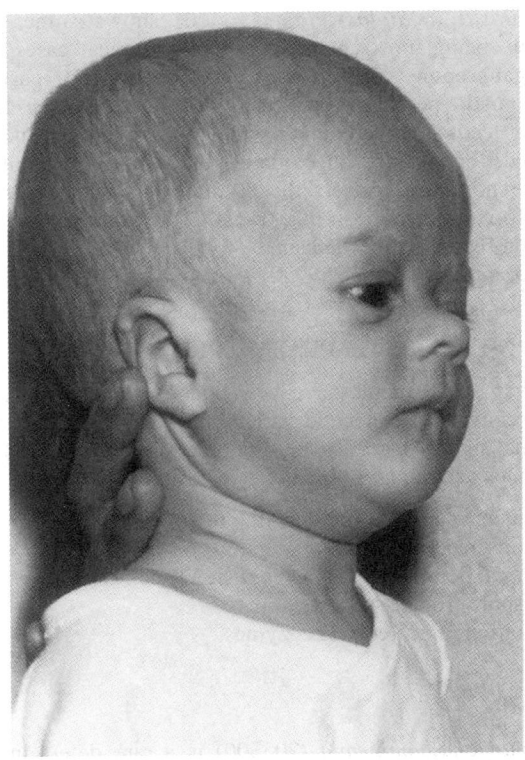

Fig. 20.33   An infant with the Zellweger syndrome (note the high forehead).

Infantile Refsum's disease (266510) (<1 : 50 000)

This is a milder allelic variant of the Zellweger syndrome. Patients have moderately dysmorphic features, midfacial hypoplasia, early hypotonia, marked sensorineural hearing loss, pigmentary retinopathy, an enlarged liver with impaired function and obvious psychomotor retardation. Some present with a bleeding diathesis in the first weeks of life. Chondrodysplasia punctata and renal cortical cysts are absent. Biochemical abnormalities are the same as in the Zellweger syndrome.

Hyperpipecolic acidemia (239400) (<1 : 500 000)

This may be a variant of the Zellweger syndrome with which both the phenotype and the biochemical findings share many similarities except that abnormal pipecolic acid levels may be the only biochemical abnormality detected in plasma.

PEROXISOMAL DISORDERS WITH LOSS OF MULTIPLE FUNCTIONS

Rhizomelic chondrodysplasia punctata (215100) (<1 : 250 000)

The phenotype clearly differs from Zellweger syndrome, but also shows some overlap. Patients have characteristic shortening of proximal limb segments, severely disturbed endochondrial bone formation and coronal clefts of vertebral bodies on lateral roentgenograms of the spine. Chondrodysplasia is more widespread than in Zellweger syndrome and most patients have cataracts and liver enlargement. Development is retarded and the infants fail to thrive. Survival can be up to 25 years.

Two enzymes of plasmalogen synthesis (DHAP acyltranferase and alkyl DHAP synthase) are defective in classic cases; variants may only show a defect of either one. There may be a defect in phytanic acid oxidation and peroxisomal 3-oxoacyl-CoA thiolase protein is in the unprocessed precursor form. The biochemical defects result in plasmalogen deficiency in tissues and in accumulation of phytanic acid in blood. VLCFA are normal.

In Conradi–Huenermann chondrodysplasia punctata, either autosomal dominant or X-linked recessive (118650, 302960), peroxisomal functions are usually normal. However, one nonrhizomelic type of chondrodysplasia can be associated with peroxisomal dysfunction.

Zellweger-like syndrome

Two patients were reported recently with a clinical presentation remarkably similar to the Zellweger syndrome, but showing abundant peroxisomes in liver. In both patients the three peroxisomal β-oxidation enzyme proteins were found to be absent as shown by immunoblotting. Moreover, DHAP acyltransferase activity was deficient in one of the patients. The biochemical basis for these multiple defects is not yet clear.

PEROXISOMAL DISORDERS INVOLVING ONLY ONE ENZYME

Adrenoleukodystrophy (ALD) (300100) (?1 : 150 000)

This X-linked disease, caused by a defect of 'ALD-protein', an ATP-binding membrane peroxisomal transporter which somehow affects VLCFA-CoA synthase, comes in several forms affecting two primary target organs: the adrenal glands and/or the CNS. The old name for this disease was Schilder disease. Neonatal adrenoleukodystrophy is considered above.

Clinical features

The most common form occurs in childhood with adrenal failure which is associated with progressive seizures, nystagmus, impaired hearing and neurological deterioration. Visual disturbances, deterioration in school achievement, behavior and/or memory are early features in this disorder. The disease is progressive, culminating within a few years in dementia, blindness, quadriplegia and death. Seizures are usually a late manifestation. By 10 years, the risk of developing the CNS damage declines markedly.

The second phenotype is termed *adrenomyeloneuropathy* which presents either with Addison's disease or with signs of myelopathy with progressive polyneuropathy and bladder dysfunction in the second or third decade of life; both may develop at about the same time. IQ and cerebral functions are remarkably preserved. Addison's disease may occur without any neurologic involvement and some 10% of males seem to escape altogether.

All these different phenotypes may occur within the same family. Furthermore, ~15% of adult female heterozygotes develop a chronic spinal cord disorder reminiscent of multiple sclerosis with which it is often confused even in males; some 50% have subtle signs of cord involvement.

Diagnosis

The differential diagnosis includes idiopathic Addison's disease, multiple sclerosis and spastic paraparesis and many of the neurodegenerative diseases. Serum and tissue levels of VLCFA (>22 carbon) are invariably elevated. They should be measured in all males of any age who develop Addison's disease. Typical pathological changes occur in the adrenal glands and in the cerebral white matter. DNA analysis may be valuable.

Treatment

Addison's disease is discussed on page 1069. Glyceryl trioleate (GTO) 1–2.5 g/kg/day lowers the VLCFA by about 50% but it has been supplanted by glyceryl trieruate (GTE) in a 4 : 1 mixture with GTO (popularly known as Lorenzo's oil). This lowers the plasma VLCFA close to normal; it can cause thrombocytopenia and presymptomatic use reduces the frequency and severity of neurologic disability. It is of no value in neurologically symptomatic ALD or in adrenomyeloneuropathy. Pentoxyphylline is under trial.

Bone marrow transplant is now being used experimentally. If done before the onset of CNS symptoms, it may have considerable protective effect; if postponed until after they develop, it is probably too late but even this is under study.

Other peroxisomal disorders with impairment of only one function

There are scattered reports of patients with an increasing array of rare defects of peroxisomal enzymes. Common to most of them has been a spectrum of severe neurologic disease including hypotonia, areflexia, feeding and developmental problems often with regression, severe nerve deafness, pigmentary retinopathy and seizures. Some have dysmorphic features suggesting a Zellweger phenotype; others have not been notably dysmorphic. Any combination of such features should occasion a 'peroxisomal screen' which includes blood for VLCFA, pipecolic and phytanic acids and possibly for abnormal bile acids.

Acyl-CoA oxidase deficient (pseudoneonatal ALD) (264470) infants are not dysmorphic but are profoundly delayed. A sensorineural hearing deficit and abnormal electroretinograms are characteristic. VLCFA are raised in blood and fibroblasts but levels of bile acids and ether-phospholipids (plasmalogens) are normal. *Bifunctional protein* deficiency (264470) differs mainly in that both plasma VLCFA and abnormal bile acids were increased. *Peroxisomal 3-oxoacyl-CoA thiolase deficiency (pseudo-Zellweger syndrome)* (261510) has been associated with all the physical features of Zellweger syndrome except that the liver contained abundant peroxisomes and deficiency of only a single enzyme. Isolated defects of either *alkyl DHAP synthase* or *dihydroxyacetone-phosphate acyltransferase* cause variant rhizomelic chondrodystrophy. Other peroxisomal defects have included *glutaryl-CoA oxidase* deficiency which caused failure to thrive that responded to riboflavin, and defects of *bile acid metabolism*.

Refsum's disease (phytanic acid storage disease) (266500) is asymptomatic in children. In adults the toxic accumulation of methylated branched chain fatty acid phytanic acid produces peripheral polyneuropathy, retinitis pigmentosa, cerebellar ataxia and nerve deafness. The CSF protein is elevated and cardiac conduction defects are common. The condition is caused by a defect in phytanic acid hydroxylase activity. Dietary restriction of plants (which contain phytanic acid) is beneficial.

Acatalasia (acatalasemia) (115500) shows some genetic variation, being most common in Japan. Typical cases present with gangrenous oral ulcerations but many cases are asymptomatic, perhaps protected by better oral hygiene. Lack of catalase leads to accumulation of toxic hydrogen peroxide, produced, for instance, in oxidative processes during infection. Catalase normally protects the erythrocytes against methemoglobin formation and also other cells against disturbances of the oxidation-reduction mechanism.

Hyperoxaluria type I (259900) – see oxalosis (p. 1112).

INBORN ERRORS OF PLASMA PROTEINS

Well over 100 proteins have been identified in plasma. Many exhibit considerable genetic variation which is usually without functional significance. The plasma proteins can be considered in five groups according to function:

1. maintenance of plasma oncotic pressure
2. clotting factors (Ch. 15)
3. humoral defense mechanisms (Ch. 22)
4. transport proteins
5. inhibition of proteolytic enzymes.

ALBUMIN

Congenital analbuminemia (205300) is a rare defect in which plasma albumin is missing and the substances in plasma which are normally bound to it, such as calcium, are lower than normal. However, the unbound (active) fractions of these compounds in the plasma are normal, so that mild edema may be the only finding. Heterozygotes have normal levels. Unless severe symptoms are present, no treatment is indicated. The reason for the lack of gross edema is unclear; it may be due to minor adjustments in the transcapillary hydrostatic pressure. Occasionally, electrophoretic variants of albumin are found in healthy people. Hypoalbuminemia due to malnutrition, hepatocellular disease and protein-losing enteropathy are discussed elsewhere.

TRANSPORT PROTEINS

Congenital deficiency of *thyroid-binding globulin* (314200) is usually inherited as an X-linked recessive trait; the T3 resin uptake is raised, plasma thyroxin levels are low, but the free thyroid hormone levels are within normal limits and the patients are euthyroid. These patients can cause confusion when found to have a low T4, for example on a newborn screening sample. *Transcortin deficiency* (122500) has also been reported.

Normal serum contains 0.3–2 g/l of *haptoglobin*, which binds to free hemoglobin in plasma. There are several common genetic variants (140100) and even total deficiency seems to be benign.

Carbohydrate-deficient glycoprotein (CDG) syndrome (212065) (?<1 : 250 000)

This is the term given to an emerging group of at least three subtypes in which the postribosomal addition of mannose side chains of a whole group of serum glycoproteins, most of which seem to have transport functions, including transferrin, thyroid-binding globulin and most other hormone transporters, and apoB

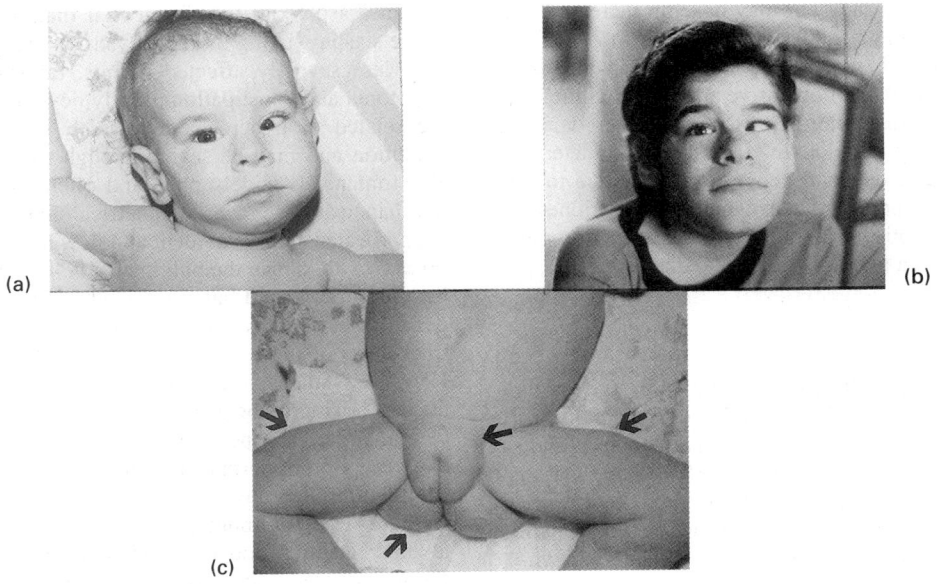

Fig. 20.34 The CDG sundrome: (**a**) Facies at 15 months. (**b**) Facies at 16 years. (**c**) Pelvic area at 18 months showing the fat pads.

lipoprotein are deficient. The side chains shown in Figure 20.30 are comparable, but different from those involved in this syndrome.

Clinical features

In this syndrome there is marked developmental delay, retinitis pigmentosa, characteristic dysmorphic features which include esotropia, inverted nipples and, in infancy, curious fat pads on the glutei, thighs, pudenda and upper arms (Fig. 20.34). Cardiomyopathy, peripheral neuropathy, moderate hepatomegaly with abnormal LFTs and myopathy are all common and hypogonadism seems universal. In type I, the commonest form, phosphomannomutase is deficient (Van Schaftingen & Jaeken 1995) and *N*-acetyl-glucoaminyltransferase II is low in type II. These defects involve the synthesis of the sialylated polymannose side chains in the Golgi.

Diagnosis and treatment

This can be suspected if the T4 is low and confirmed by electrophoresis of plasma transferrin which shows that the isoforms are hyposialated in a pattern similar to that seen in chronic alcoholism. No treatment is known.

C1-ESTERASE INHIBITOR DEFICIENCY (HEREDITARY ANGIONEUROTIC EDEMA) (106100)

At least 20 components of the complement system (Ch. 22) have been identified. Deficiency of C′1-esterase inhibitor causes hereditary angioneurotic edema, which is an autosomal dominant trait.

The disease presents with recurrent, acute, transient patches of edema in the skin, respiratory tract or gastrointestinal tract. Laryngeal edema is a common cause of death and acute intestinal edema causes attacks of abdominal pain, vomiting and diarrhea,

stimulating an acute surgical condition. In the skin, the patches are often preceded by tingling paresthesia. The edema may last for a few hours or several days. Symptoms, mainly vomiting and recurrent abdominal pain, can occur before puberty, but they are usually less severe than in adults. The symptoms are so varied and unpredictable that the sufferers are often considered neurotic – hence the name.

The anabolic steroid danazol (200–600 mg/day) is a very effective prophylactic, but will not abort an attack. Acute crises can be treated with infusions of fresh-frozen plasma or with intravenous ε-aminocaproic acid. Subcutaneous adrenaline (1 : 1000) may also be useful. Antihistamines and sedatives are recommended, although they do not directly affect the edema.

ALPHA-1-ANTITRYPSIN DEFICIENCY (107400) (≅1 : 3500)

α1-Antitrypsin is an α-1-globulin, one of a related family of antiproteases made in the liver. Over 75 variants are known, 90% of normal people being homozygous for the M form (Pi MM).* Most of the variants, designated by letters, are completely benign.

Clinical features

Homozygous Pi ZZ-deficient patients have 15–20% residual antitrypsin activity in plasma and almost all who smoke develop progressive panacinar emphysema in early middle life. In nonsmokers, emphysema occurs later or may never develop. Patients with the null or S phenotypes are at the same risk. There is an association between the Z genotype and cryptogenic cirrhosis and chronic active hepatitis in adults. There is no detectable lung damage through adolescence although there may be some association with reactive airway disease. Heterozygotes

---

* Pi – the designation of the α1-antitrypsin genotype Pi stands for protease inhibitor.

Pi MZ are usually asymptomatic but may have an increased risk of lung disease if they smoke heavily. About 10% of Pi ZZ infants develop neonatal cholestasis which may mimic biliary atresia or neonatal hepatitis. This may be progressive and fatal, but the liver function tests often return to normal. However, liver damage, including hepatoma, may develop in adolescence or later. As many as 30% of cases of neonatal hepatitis may be due to this disorder. Progressive glomerulotubular damage in the kidneys is also reported. A rare α_1-antitrypsin mutant possesses antithrombin III activity which causes a major hemorrhagic diathesis.

Diagnosis

Made by assay of α_1-antitrypsin activity in the blood, accompanied by electrophoretic identification of the genotype. A filter paper screening test is available. Liver biopsy shows characteristic intracellular accumulation of PAS-positive material which is the abnormal protein that is synthesized but not exported from the Golgi in the hepatocytes. Varying degrees of hepatitis and cirrhosis are also present, the cause of which is not known.

Treatment

Prevention of lung damage demands abstinence from smoking by the patient, the family and probably all close contacts; patients should avoid employment in polluted atmospheres. Purified antitrypsin is now available for treatment of adults with lung disease. Advanced liver damage is treated by liver transplantation which also normalizes the plasma α_1-antitrypsin values.

ALKALINE PHOSPHATASE

This term denotes a family of at least three genetically distinct enzymes which are normally bound to plasma membranes and accept a number of phosphocompounds, such as phosphoethanolamine, pyrophosphate and pyridoxal-5'-phosphate, as substrates. One isoenzyme is isolated to the intestine, a second to placenta. A third protein, which is present in most tissues and is called tissue nonspecific (TNSALP), undergoes post-translational modification in almost all tissues producing liver, kidney, bone, leukocyte, etc. isoenzymes which can be recognized electrophoretically. Alkaline phosphatase in plasma probably has no metabolic role; normally, in children, it derives largely from osteoblastic activity in bone, particularly during growth spurts. It can also reflect tissue damage in various organs, particularly the bile duct epithelium.

Hypophosphatasia

Clinical features

This condition is due to absence or defective function of tissue nonspecific alkaline phosphatase (TNSALP). Clinically, the most severely affected cases can be detected prenatally by X-ray and these infants usually die in the neonatal period (241500). The skull may be so soft as to seem like a bag of fluid and the skull bones may be almost invisible on X-ray. Shortening, bowing and rachitic changes of the bones are usual and undermineralization may seem reminiscent of osteogenesis imperfecta, although the radiologic features are distinct. Thoracic dystrophy causes severe

neonatal asphyxia; the differential diagnosis therefore includes Jeune's asphyxiating thoracic dystrophy (208500).

In less severely affected infants, failure to thrive, vomiting, hypotonia and constipation usually develop in the first year; they are related to hypercalcemia which is a usual feature of the condition and may be severe enough to cause nephrocalcinosis. The fontanel is widely open and often tense. The skull may be misshapen and the face asymmetrical. In the skull, osteoporosis or copperbeaten skull is evident and may be associated with delayed bone growth, hence the bulging of the fontanels. The sutures may be widely separated but permanent fusion may occur later. Bony deformities consist of shortening of long bones, bowing, thickening of the wrists, shortening of the digits, lordosis and a Harrison's sulcus; the metaphyses show characteristic translucencies arising in the growth plates. There may be premature loss of primary teeth, especially the incisors; there is no compensatory early eruption of permanent teeth.

Other children have little more than premature loss of primary teeth (241510) without periodontal disease, but with abnormal alveolar attrition and enlarged pulp chambers and root canals. Permanent teeth can also be involved. The disease may be first recognized in adults (146300). In such cases, osteoporosis and fractures are frequent, pseudofractures can be seen on X-ray and some have the deformities of previous 'rickets'. Dental abnormalities may be the only finding. It seems that some of the milder cases may represent manifesting heterozygotes.

Diagnosis

In the most severe cases, all TNSALP isozyme activities are virtually absent. In milder cases, the activity is present but diminished, a finding which becomes increasingly hard to evaluate in older cases since normal values are lower than in early childhood. Hypercalcemia is frequent in the infantile forms and can be life threatening when patients are immobilized, as for orthopedic treatment. The hypercalcemia develops from failure of synthesis of apatite crystals in bone; it can cause azotemia. Phosphoethanolamine is increased in the urine and pyridoxal-5'-phosphate is markedly increased in the blood. The latter test is less available but seems to be a better discriminant; both are most abnormal in the most severe cases.

Pseudohypophosphatasia was reported in a family with the findings of hypophosphatasia but normal enzyme levels. Low values for TNSALP may occur in a number of conditions including malnutrition, hypothyroidism, zinc deficiency and glucocorticoid therapy.

Treatment

There is no effective treatment; craniostenosis and limb deformity may require surgery. Prenatal diagnosis is tricky; ultrasound studies may help and analysis of TNSALP in an experienced laboratory is critical.

Hyperphosphatasia

The normal plasma alkaline phosphatase varies considerably throughout life; the normal ranges are not clearly defined. Elevated values derived from osteoblasts occur in any condition with increased bone turnover, such as rickets, fractures, osteogenic sarcoma, osteolytic malignancies or juvenile Paget's disease

(239100). The liver isozyme of ALP is increased whenever bile duct epithelium is damaged, as in obstructive jaundice.

Familial hyperphosphatasia (239000), usually involving liver ALP, is usually benign, but may be associated with bone disease and its association with mental retardation, seizures and neurologic damage is reported in several families (239300).

Transient hyperphosphatasemia of infancy is not uncommon; it involves the bone and liver forms and can occur following a minor viral prodrome and is often detected during routine blood tests. The plasma level can easily reach over 2000 IU/l but this only lasts for a few weeks. The etiology is unknown and no treatment is indicated (Wolf 1995).

CARBONIC ANHYDRASE II DEFICIENCY (259730)

This is a rare autosomal recessive trait which causes osteopetrosis, mixed proximal and distal renal tubular acidosis and developmental delay with cerebral calcifications; growth failure and dental malocclusion occur frequently.

The osteopetrosis in this condition is usually less severe than in the classic disorder and patients may be asymptomatic for months or years after birth but eventually fractures, failure to thrive or developmental delay bring the patient to attention.

Treatment for this disorder is symptomatic, whereas bone marrow transplantation is beneficial in 'classic', severe osteopetrosis. Prenatal diagnosis is not currently available.

AMYLOIDOSIS

Amyloidosis, which rarely occurs in children, is characterized by the extracellular deposition in different tissues of layers of amorphous, fibrillar material which is derived from one of several different proteins. Immunoglobulin-derived amyloid, usually monoclonal kappa or lambda light chains, usually signifies multiple myeloma. The commonest form of amyloid, which derives from an acute phase lipoprotein called amyloid A, is seen secondary to chronic inflammatory diseases such as tuberculosis, syphilis, leprosy, chronic sepsis, rheumatoid arthritis, ileitis, ulcerative colitis, diabetes and chronic drug abuse. Amyloid A also accumulates in familial Mediterranean fever (134610).

Hereditary amyloidosis

Over 25 varieties of hereditary amyloidosis are listed by McKusick (1992). Many are autosomal dominant traits involving specific mutations of transthyretin (prealbumin). Different forms have been described in different countries, leading to a tendency to a geographic nosology.

In the systemic disorders, familial amyloid polyneuropathy is usually prominent, but characteristic deposits may occur in other tissues leading to the carpal tunnel syndrome, leg ulcers, gastrointestinal dysfunction, a nephrotic syndrome and cardiomyopathy. Localized amyloid can occur in multiple endocrine adenomatosis type II as well as in the brain in Alzheimer's disease.

Most diagnostic tests depend on the property of amyloid to bind to various dyes. The intravenous Congo red test is positive if more than 80% of the dye is extracted from the serum in 1 hour. Values of 79–60% extraction are probably positive. A more certain way to establish the diagnosis is by biopsy of gingiva, rectal submucosa or an involved organ. This is positive in over 80% of cases; the tissue stains green with alkaline Congo red when examined under a polarizing microscope.

No treatment is proposed for the hereditary amyloidoses. The acquired forms may respond to vigorous therapy of the underlying condition.

REFERENCES

Alper J S 1996 Genetic complexity in single gene diseases. British Medical Journal 312: 196–197

Bennett M J, Weinberger M J, Kobori J A, Rinaldo P, Burlina A B 1996 Mitochondrial short-chain L-3–hydroxyacyl-coenzyme A dehydrogenase deficiency: a new defect of fatty acid oxidation. Pediatric Research 39: 185–188

Berenson G 1980 Cardiovascular risk factors in children. The early natural history of atherosclerosis and essential hypertension. Oxford University Press, New York, pp 151–159

Berry G T, Nissim I, Lin Z, Mazur A T, Gibson J B, Segal S 1995 Endogenous synthesis of galactose in normal men and patients with hereditary galactosaemia. Lancet 346: 1073–1074

Biaggioni I, Robertson D 1987 Endogenous restoration of noradrenalin by precursor therapy in dopamine-beta-hydroxylase deficiency. Lancet ii: 1170–1172

Blau N, Blaskovics M (eds) 1996 The physician's guide to the laboratory diagnosis of inherited metabolic diseases. Chapman & Hall, London

Bosma P J, Roy Chowdhury J, Bakker C et al. 1995 The genetic basis of the reduced expression of bilirubin UDP-glucuronyltransferase 1 in Gilbert's syndrome. New England Journal of Medicine 333: 1171–1175

Chalmers R A, Lawson A M (eds) 1982 Organic acids in man. Analytical chemistry, biochemistry and diagnosis of the organic acidurias. Cambridge University Press, Cambridge

DeVivo D C, Garcia-Alvarez M, Roner G, Trifiletti R 1995 Glucose transport protein deficiency: an emerging syndrome with therapeutic implications. International Pediatrics 10: 51–56

Dixon D E M 1988 Diets for sick children. Blackwell University Press, Oxford

Edwards M A, Grant S, Green A 1988 A practical approach to the investigation of amino acid disorders. Annual Review of Biochemistry 25: 129–141

Elsas L J, Longo N 1995 Glucose transporters: human disorders and insulin receptor regulation. International Pediatrics 10: 57–68

Evans J M, Prince A P, Huntington K L 1994 Phe-for-three. A tracking system for 1, 2 and 3 equivalents. Oregon Health Sciences University, Nutrition Dept., Portland, Oregon

Fernandes J, Saudubray J-M, van den Berghe G (eds) 1995 Inborn metabolic diseases: diagnosis and treatment, 2nd edn. Springer-Verlag, Berlin

Gieselmann V 1995 Lysosomal storage diseases. Biochimica et Biophysica Acta 172: 103–136

Holton J B (ed) 1994 The inherited metabolic diseases, 2nd edn. Churchill Livingstone, Edinburgh

Hommes F A (ed) 1993 Techniques in diagnostic human biochemical genetics. A laboratory manual. Wiley-Liss, New York

Hyland K, Clayton P T 1995 Aromatic L-aminoacid decarboxylase deficiency in twins. Proceedings of the Society for the Study of Inborn Errors of Metabolism, Munich, p 72

Hyland K, Buist N R.M, Powell B R et al 1995 Folinic acid responsive seizures: a new syndrome? Journal of Inherited Metabolic Disease 18:177–181

Kappas A et al 1995 The porphyrias. In: Scriver et al (eds) The metabolic bases of inherited disease. McGraw-Hill, New York, ch 66, p 2013–2160

Kohlschutter A, Hausdorf G 1986 Primary (genetic) cardiomyopathies in infancy. A survey of possible disorders and guidelines for diagnosis. European Journal of Pediatrics 145: 454–459

Kraemer K H 1996 Xeroderma pigmentosum knockouts. Lancet 347: 278–279

Krivit W, Lockman L A, Watkins P A, Hirsch J, Shapira E G 1995 The future for treatment by bone marrow transplantation for adrenoleukodystrophy, metachromatic leukodystrophy and Hurler syndrome. Journal of Inherited Metabolic Disease 18: 398–412

Lyon G, Adams R D, Kolodny E H 1996. Neurology of hereditary metabolic diseases of children. McGraw-Hill. New York

McKusick V A (ed) 1992 Mendelian inheritance in man, 10th edn. Johns Hopkins University Press, Baltimore

National Organization for Rare Diseases (NORD), PO Box 8923, New Fairfield, CT 06812–8923, USA (phone (203)746–6518, fax (203)746–8728)

Research Trust for Metabolic Diseases in Children (RTMDC), Golden Gates Lodge, Weston Rd, Crewe CW1 1XN, UK (phone (1270)250–221, fax (1270)250–244)

Roels F, De Bie S, Schutgens R B H et al (eds) 1995. Diagnosis of human peroxisomal disorders. Journal of Inherited Metabolic Disease (suppl 1) 18: 1–226

Ruitenbeek W, Huizing M, Thinnes F P, DePinto V, Wendel U, Trijbels J M F, van den Heuvel L P 1995 A novel cause of mitochondriopathies: a VDAC deficiency. Enzyme and Protein 48: 127

Schmid R 1995 Gilbert's syndrome – a legitimate genetic anomaly. New England Journal of Medicine 333: 1217–1218

Schuett V 1995 Low protein cookbook for PKU. Hemlock Printers, Burnaby, British Columbia, Canada

Scriver C R, Beaudet A L, Sly W S, Valle D (eds) 1995 The metabolic and molecular bases of inherited diease, 7th edn. McGraw-Hill, New York

Sweetman L 1991 Organic acid analysis. In: Hommes F A (ed) Techniques in diagnostic human biochemical genetics. Wiley-Liss, New York, pp 143–176

Taybi H, Lachman R 1995 Radiology of syndromes, metabolic disorders and skeletal dysplasias. C V Mosby, St Louis

Treacy E, Childs B, Scriver C R 1995 Response to treatment in hereditary metabolic disease. 1993 survey and 10-year comparison. American Journal of Human Genetics 56: 359–367

Van Gennip A H, Abeling N G G M, Vreken P, van Kuilenburg A B P 1996 Genetic metabolic disease of pyrimidine metabolism; implications for diagnosis and treatment. International Pediatrics (in press)

Van Schaftingen E, Jaeken J 1995 Phosphomannomutase deficiency is a cause of the carbohydrate-deficient glycoprotein syndrome type 1. FEBS Letters 377: 318–320

Von Muhlendal K E, Herkenhoff H 1995 The long term course of neonatal diabetes. New England Journal of Medicine 333: 704–708

Wevers R A, de Rijk-van Andel J F, Jansen M J T, Gabreels F J M, Ludecke B, Blau N, Bartholome K 1996 A new case of tyrosine hydroxylase deficiency. Journal of Inherited Metabolic Disease (in press)

Wijburg F A, van der Bogert C, Dingemans K P, Poulton J, Schotte HR, Bakker H D 1995 Liver disease in mitochondrial DNA depletion. Enzyme and Protein 48: 133–134

Wolf P L 1995 The significance of transient hyperphosphatasemia of infancy and childhood to the clinician and clinical pathologist. Archives of Pathology and Laboratory Medicine 119: 774–775

21 Nutrition

Chapter editor: L. T. Weaver

Introduction **1179**
L. T. Weaver
Nutritional requirements 1179
J. Reilly   C. A. Edwards
Nutritional assessment 1186
Anthropometric 1186
J. Reilly
Dietary 1187
B. Clark
Biochemical 1187
P. Robinson
Clinical 1188
L. T. Weaver
Normal diet 1188
B. Clark
Nutrition and disease 1190
Obesity 1190
J. Reilly
Failure to thrive 1191
L. T. Weaver
Protein–energy malnutrition 1191
B. A. Wharton   L. T. Weaver
Vitamin deficiencies 1194
D. Barltrop
Mineral deficiencies 1200
D. Barltrop
Inborn errors of metabolism 1203
P. Robinson   B. Clark
Inflammatory bowel disease 1206
T. J. Evans

Cystic fibrosis 1207
E. Buchanan   L. T. Weaver
Liver disease 1209
T. J. Evans
Diabetes mellitus 1209
A. Johnston
Congenital heart disease 1210
L. T. Weaver
Juvenile chronic arthritis 1210
L. T. Weaver
Renal disease 1211
K. Walker
Constipation 1211
L. T. Weaver
Short bowel syndrome 1211
L. T. Weaver
Food allergy and intolerance 1213
B. Clark
Enteropathies 1214
T. J. Evans
Gastroenteritis 1215
L. T. Weaver
Principles and practice of nutrition support 1215
Nutrition support team 1215
L. T. Weaver
Enteral nutrition 1217
B. Clark   L. T. Weaver
Parenteral nutrition 1219
J. W. L. Puntis
References and Bibliography 1226

INTRODUCTION

Nutrition is about maintenance of the *milieu interieur*. It is concerned with how food is used by the body and it touches upon gastroenterology, metabolism and endocrinology. In pediatrics, nutrition is inseparable from growth and development. The changing composition of the body of the infant and child is in part a reflection of what he or she eats.

Diets deficient in specific nutrients may cause specific diseases or syndromes (such as rickets, scurvy and kwashiorkor). Overeating causes obesity. Chronic disease is frequently associated with undernutrition and nutrient deficits. However, nutrient deficiencies lead to depletion of tissue stores, derangement of normal biochemistry and disordered tissue function before they are manifest as anatomic changes and may easily go unrecognized. Awareness of poor nutrition is critical to the effective management of many childhood diseases, particularly those that are chronic, and there is growing evidence that poor nutrition in early life may play a part in the genesis of a range of adult degenerative diseases (Barker 1992).

The emphasis of this chapter is on clinical nutrition. Nutrition is now a well-established subspecialty of pediatrics and research is rapidly extending and clarifying our understanding of the subject. We present here the core of clinical pediatric nutrition. The basic science of nutrition (composition of food, metabolic pathways, gastrointestinal physiology, body composition, etc.) is not covered here – several textbooks of human nutrition, listed at the end of the bibliography, deal comprehensively with these subjects.

Nutrition services should be provided by a nutrition team, composed of a pediatrician with expertise in nutrition, pediatric dietitians, nurse specialists and pharmacist, with the support of a pediatric surgeon, biochemist and bacteriologist, who work together in the clinic, ward and community to provide nutritional support for children.

NUTRITIONAL REQUIREMENTS

BACKGROUND AND DEFINITIONS

Figures for nutrient requirements set by expert committees emphasize the avoidance of nutrient *deficiency*. They do not concern themselves with the safety of excess intake (Tables 21.1 & 21.2).

Underlying the concept of requirement is the assumption that, for most nutrients, it is approximately normally distributed (Fig. 21.1) in any population. To determine requirements of nutrients that are sufficient to meet the needs of whole populations, they have been set 'high' in the distribution at approximately two standard deviations above the mean requirement (Fig. 21.1). With the exception of energy (excess energy intake leads to obesity) consumption of a nutrient in excess of requirements of this magnitude is not harmful and setting a high value as an RNI or RDA entails minimal risk for most nutrients.

In the UK the committee which recommended nutrient requirements most recently (DoH 1991) decided to use the term 'dietary reference values' rather than 'recommendations'. The basic approach to defining requirements remained the same, but the 1991 UK working party chose to set, where possible, up to three reference values for each nutrient, reflecting the range of nutrient requirements (low, medium and high) (Fig. 21.1) rather

Table 21.1   Definitions of nutrient requirements

- UK (1979) RDA (Recommended Daily Amount) 'The average amount of the nutrient which should be provided per head in a group of people if the needs of practically all members of the group are to be met.'

- USA (1980) RDA (Recommended Dietary Allowance) 'The level of intake of essential nutrients considered to be adequate to meet the known nutritional needs of practically all healthy persons.'

- Canada (1983) RNI (Recommended Nutrient Intake) 'The level of dietary intake thought to be sufficiently high to meet the requirements of almost all the individuals in a group; of necessity, the RNI exceeds the requirement of almost all individuals.'

In the UK the RDA has been superseded by several 'dietary reference values' (DoH 1991)

Table 21.2   Criteria used for setting nutrient requirements

- Amount taken by a group of people without deficiency developing
- Amount needed to cure deficiency
- Amount needed to maintain enzyme saturation
- Amount needed to maintain blood or tissue concentration
- Amount associated with an appropriate biological marker of adequacy

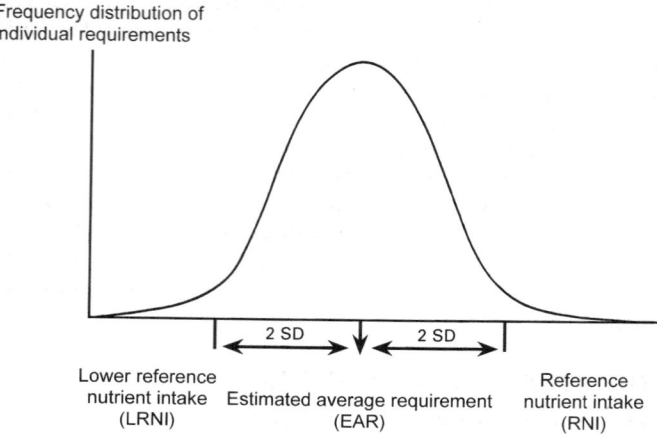

Fig. 21.1   Relation between various reference values for nutritional requirements. SD, standard deviation.

than just one reference value. These three values are now known collectively as 'dietary reference values' (DRVs) and are the 'estimated average requirement' (EAR), the mean requirement; 'reference nutrient intake' (RNI), the mean requirement plus two standard deviations; and 'lower reference nutrient intake' (LRNI), the mean requirement minus two standard deviations (Fig. 21.1). For some nutrients the 1991 UK report set a 'safe intake' if there were insufficient data upon which to set DRVs. This was judged to be an intake at which there was no risk of deficiency and below a level where there was a risk of adverse effects.

APPLICATIONS AND LIMITATIONS OF DIETARY REFERENCE VALUES

There are three main applications of DRVs.

1. To assess the adequacy of the dietary intake of individuals or groups. For example, if a hospital population of children consume a diet below the LRNI for a particular nutrient, their diet is probably deficient in that nutrient.

2. As a guide to prescribing or designing the diet of individuals or groups. The DRVs (often the EAR) can be a useful starting point in setting a diet prescription, in the absence of any other information on the requirements of the patient and DRVs are also used in the design of infant milk formulae.

3. Food labeling. A food might be described as containing x% of the EAR for iron, for example.

When applying DRVs their limitations must be borne in mind. In childhood estimates of requirement are usually based on limited data. They change over the years and DRVs should be regarded as best estimates at the time that they are set and they are often reviewed in the light of new information. For example, the 1979 UK estimates (DoH 1979) of energy requirements during infancy have subsequently been shown to be too high (Prentice et al 1988). In this chapter RNI is used in place of the formerly used RDA.

NUTRITIONAL REQUIREMENTS DURING INFANCY AND CHILDHOOD

Energy

Energy is required for physical activity, thermogenesis, tissue maintenance and growth. Dietary energy is consumed in the form of fat, protein and carbohydrate. Dietary protein does not simply build new tissue but is also oxidized to provide energy. In the UK and in most Western countries dietary surveys of children of school age show that they consume about 35–40% of dietary energy in the form of fat, 10–15% as protein and 40–50% as carbohydrate (DoH 1989). These figures are very similar to those of adults in the same countries and imply that the characteristic macronutrient composition of the diet is 'set' at a relatively young age. The main food sources of dietary fat are milk and milk products, fried foods and meat products (Table 21.6). In developing countries and in vegetarian children the contribution to energy intake of carbohydrate is much higher and the contribution of fat is generally much lower.

In infants and children the energy requirement is the amount of dietary energy needed to balance energy expended and energy deposited in new tissue (growth). Energy expenditure can be subdivided into basal (BMR) or resting metabolic rate (RMR,

50–60% of total energy expenditure (TEE) in most healthy children); energy expended on physical activity (30–40% of TEE in most healthy children) and thermogenesis (approximately 5–8% of total energy expenditure). BMR or RMR can be considered to be a 'maintenance' cost since it is the energy cost of biosynthesis, turnover, cellular ion pumps, physical work (respiratory and cardiac function). The energy expended on physical activity varies widely between children and is generally reduced when they are sick. The energy expended in thermogenesis is primarily the cost of digesting, absorbing and resynthesizing nutrients ('diet-induced thermogenesis'). Growth demands some energy expended on biosynthesis and the energy content of newly synthesized tissue. This represents up to about 35% of energy intake in rapidly growing infants, but falls for the rest of childhood (to about 1% of energy intake) because growth rate is so much slower thereafter.

The 1991 UK committee (DoH 1991) which set dietary requirements recommended an EAR for energy (Table 21.3) but no RNI or LRNI. In clinical or dietetic use the EAR can provide a basis for estimating the energy requirements of individual infants and children. Alternatively a more considered approach involves estimation of basal metabolic rate (Table 21.4) from equations based on age, weight and gender and multiplying this by a factor to take into account physical activity. In most children 1.5–2 times BMR will cover TEE. Estimation of minimum energy requirements using this approach, though better than depending on the EAR, can lead to large errors for individual children. However, although ideal, *measurement* of RMR and/or TEE is not usually a practical option in clinical practice and the former is therefore often the more widely used estimate.

In general dietary recommendations fall into two time frames; those for children under and over 5 years. The high demand for energy in the under-5s necessitates a more energy-dense diet with less complex carbohydrate and a greater proportion of energy from fat. Recommendations for children over 5 in general mirror those for adults based on a desire to encourage healthy eating habits in later life rather than specific needs for childhood.

Proteins and amino acids

Proteins are essential components of every living cell and subserve numerous biological functions. Dietary protein is essential to maintain nitrogen balance in the body and to provide sources of sulfur. Protein intake is particularly important in childhood where rapid growth requires amino acids to provide the building blocks for new muscle and other structural proteins. All amino acids provide nitrogen for synthesis of human proteins but some dietary amino acids are 'essential' as they cannot be synthesized de novo. Adequate intake of these essential amino acids is achievable only with a diet containing a wide variety of protein sources. Average requirements increase with age in absolute terms (EAR at 4 months is 10.6 g/day and at 18 years is 46.1 g/day) but decrease per kg body weight (EAR is 120 mg N/kg/day at 1 year and 96 mg N/Kg/day in adults; Table 21.5). If

Table 21.3 Estimated average requirements (EAR) for energy

Age	Boys		Girls	
	MJ/d	Kcal/d	MJ/d	Kcal/d
0–3 months	2.28	(545)	2.16	(515)
4–6 months	2.89	(690)	2.69	(645)
7–9 months	3.44	(825)	3.20	(765)
10–12 months	3.85	(920)	3.61	(865)
1–3 years	5.15	(1230)	4.86	(1165)
4–6 years	7.16	(1715)	6.46	(1545)
7–10 years	8.24	(1970)	7.28	(1740)
11–14 years	9.27	(2220)	7.92	(1845)
15–18 years	11.51	(2755)	8.83	(2110)

Adapted from DoH 1991

Table 21.4 Equations for predicting basal metabolic rate (MJ/d) from body weight (kg)

	Age (years)	Equation
Boys	0–3	0.255.w−0.226
	4–10	0.0949.w+2.070
	11–18	0.0732.w+2.720
Girls	0–3	0.255.w−0.214
	4–10	0.0941.w+2.09
	11–18	0.0510.w+3.12

Adapted from DoH 1991

Table 21.5 Estimated average requirements (EAR) and reference nutrient intakes (RNI) for protein and minerals in childhood

Age m=months y=years	Weight kg	Protein g/d		Calcium mg/d		Iron mg/d		Zinc mg/d		Magnesium mg/d		Iodine mg/d	Selenium mg/d
		EAR	RNI	EAR	RNI	EAR	RNI	EAR	RNI	EAR	RNI	RNI	RNI
0–3 m	5.9	–	12.5	400	525	1.3	1.7	3.3	4.0	40	55	50	10
4–6 m	7.7	10.6	12.7	400	525	3.3	4.3	3.3	4.0	50	60	60	13
7–9 m	8.9	11.0	13.7	400	525	6.0	7.8	3.8	5.0	60	75	60	10
10–12 m	9.8	11.2	14.9	400	525	6.0	7.8	3.8	5.0	60	80	60	10
1–3 y	12.6	11.7	14.5	275	350	5.3	6.9	3.8	5.0	65	85	70	15
4–6 y	17.8	14.8	19.7	350	450	4.7	6.1	5.0	6.5	90	120	100	20
7–10 y	28.3	22.8	28.3	425	550	6.7	8.7	5.4	7.0	150	200	110	30
Males													
11–14 y	43.1	33.8	42.1	750	1000	8.7	11.3	7.0	9.0	230	280	130	45
15–18 y	64.5	46.1	55.2	750	1000	8.7	11.3	7.3	9.5	250	300	140	70
Females													
11–14 y	43.8	33.1	41.2	625	800	11.4	14.8	7.0	9.0	230	280	130	45
15–18 y	55.5	37.1	45.4	625	800	11.4	14.8	5.5	7.0	250	300	140	60

Adapted from DoH 1991

Table 21.6 Sources of dietary protein, fat and carbohydrate

Nutrient	Main sources in UK diet	Alternative good sources
Protein	Meat and products, bread, cereal products, milk products, vegetables, fish *Milk, cereals, meat*	
Fat		
Saturated	Meat products, milk products, fat spreads, cakes, vegetables *Milk and milk products, cereals, meat, vegetables*	
PUFA n-3	Vegetables, meat products, cereal products, fat spreads, fish *Vegetables, cereal products, fish. meat, milk products*	Fish oils
PUFA n-6	Vegetables, cereal products, fat spreads, meat products *Vegetables, cereal products, fat spreads, meat products*	Vegetable oils
Mono-unsaturated	Meat products, cereal products, fat spreads, vegetables *Milk and milk products, meat products, cereal products, vegetables*	Olive oil
Trans	Fat spreads, cereal products, meat products *Cereals, cereal products, milk, meat fat spreads*	
Total	Meat products, fat spreads, milk products *Milk products, cereals, meat products and vegetables*	
Carbohydrate		
Starch	Cereals, wholemeal bread, potatoes *Cereals, vegetables*	
Sugars	Surcose, confectionary, beverages, milk products, cakes, biscuits *Beverages, milk and milk products, confectionary, cereals*	
Dietary fiber	Cereals (white bread, wholemeal bread, high fiber cereals), vegetables *Cereals, vegetables*	

In descending order of contribution to diet. Sources of nutrients for infants are shown in italics. From National Diet & Nutrition Survey 1990 and 1995, and Garrow & James 1993.

energy intake is below requirements protein stores will be used for energy, yielding approximately 17 kJ (4 kcal)/g. In the UK most diets contain protein well in excess of the daily requirements.

Fats

Fats are a major calorie source with an energy density of approximately 37 kJ (9 kcal)/g and they are also essential for the formation of membranes and neural tissue. Different types of fat play particular roles in the structure and function of cell membranes and neural tissue and the quality as well as the quantity, of fat intake is very important. Dietary fats (lipids) are mostly triglycerides containing a wide variety of fatty acids. Where a fatty acid is replaced with phosphate a phospholipid is produced and substitutions with other compounds produce other structural and functional lipids such as sphingolipids and glycolipids.

Fats from animal produce tend to contain saturated fatty acids with no double bonds and those from plants and fish tend to contain mono- or polyunsaturated fatty acids. This is not universally true: some plants, such as coconut, produce saturated fat. High saturated fat diets have been implicated in the development of coronary heart disease (CHD) in the adult whereas there is evidence that diets high in polyunsaturated or monounsaturated fats protect against CHD (DoH 1994a). To encourage good eating habits in adolescents and adults it is recommended that children over 5 years should adopt a diet with a similar fat content to that recommended for adults. Thus 10% of daily energy needs should be from saturated fat, 12% from monounsaturated fats, 6% from polyunsaturated, with a mixture of n-6 and n-3 fatty acids (with at least linoleic 1%, α-linolenic 0.2%) and transfatty acids 2%, giving a total fatty acid intake of 30% dietary energy or 33% including dietary glycerol. For children under 5 years a higher energy requirement makes these

recommendations unsuitable and a fat intake providing up to 50% of daily needs is recommended.

There are two essential fatty acids: linoleic (C18: 2 n-6) and α-linolenic (C18: 3 n-3) acid, which the human body cannot synthesize. These are precursors of phospholipids, prostaglandins, thromboxane, leukotrienes and arachidonic (AA), eicosapentanoic (EPA) and docosahexaenoic (DHA) acids. Young infants have limited ability to transform linolenic acid to DHA and linoleic to AA, which are both present in human milk. Many infant formulae do not contain DHA and the membrane phospholipids in the brain of infants whose intake of DHA is deficient have substituted saturated fatty acids for DHA. DHA is a major constituent of the developing brain and substitution by saturated fatty acids is likely to change the functional characteristics of the neural cells (Cockburn 1994).

Carbohydrates

Carbohydrates in the diet provide energy of approximately 17 kJ (4 kcal)/g and are also an important component of structural and functional glycoproteins and glycolipids. The variability of the bonds in oligosaccharides means that with five monosaccharides in a 13-residue oligosaccharide, 10^{24} combinations are possible making oligosaccharides ideal molecules for cell signals (Jackson 1990). Glucose is an essential fuel for the brain which cannot metabolize fat for energy. It can be synthesized by the liver from amino acids and propionic acid, but a minimum amount of dietary carbohydrate is necessary to inhibit ketosis and to allow complete oxidation of fat. In adults this is likely to be about 50 g/day (MacDonald 1987), a figure based on theoretical models, and the amounts needed in childhood are not known.

Carbohydrates can be divided into sugars (up to three residues), oligosaccharides (up to 10 residues) and complex carbohydrates (polysaccharides) on the basis of chain length. It is recommended that intake of extrinsic sugar is restricted to less than 10% of energy intake to prevent dental caries. There is very little evidence that excessive sugar intake plays a major role in the development of obesity. Indeed, diets high in sugar are often low in fat and in adults are associated with low BMI (Bolton-Smith & Woodward 1994).

Some oligosaccharides are undigestible in the human small intestine. These include fructo-oligosaccharides, stachyose and raftilose in beans. These pass to the colon where they are rapidly fermented to short chain fatty acids (SCFA) and gases and may produce flatulence if eaten in excess.

Complex carbohydrates include starch and dietary fiber. Starch is found in several forms in food, some of which are less digestible than others. Starch cooked under normal conditions can be rapidly or slowly digestible but is mostly digested and absorbed in the small intestine, whereas raw starches, as found in unripe bananas or raw potato and some processed starches (retrograded amylose) such as in some cornflakes or cooked cooled potatoes, may be resistant to human enzymes and pass into the colon undigested (Englyst et al 1992). These latter starches are called resistant starch. More starch may escape small intestinal digestion in young children than in adults and this will influence colonic function and the energy absorbed from food.

Dietary fiber has been defined as nonstarch polysaccharides and lignin although the debate on definition still continues (Southgate 1992). Dietary fiber polysaccharides are undigested in the small intestine and are fermented by the colonic microflora to SCFA and gases. These SCFA are rapidly absorbed resulting in an average energy value of 8.4 kJ (2 kcal)/g for dietary fiber. The calorific value of SCFA is closer to that of glucose, but many dietary fibers are poorly fermented and if dietary fiber escapes fermentation it can cause increased fecal output with increased loss of nitrogen and energy.

Because diets high in dietary fiber are less energy dense and more satiating than the converse, it is not recommended that young children consume high-fiber diets. Nevertheless dietary fiber plays an important part in normal large bowel function (see Constipation, pp. 461, 1211). There are anecdotal reports of overzealous mothers feeding young children high fiber, low fat diets with resultant growth failure (Wharton 1990) and vegan children are shorter than their peers (Sanders 1988). Older children, however, who do not need such an energy-dense diet, should be encouraged to eat foods rich in complex carbohydrates.

Vitamins and minerals

Vitamins are a group of naturally occurring organic nutrients that have little in common except their essentiality in the diet. They can be divided into water-soluble and fat-soluble vitamins. Water-soluble vitamins are easily absorbed, sometimes by active transport, and are not stored in the body to any great extent. Excessive intake normally results in excretion of the excess in the urine. Fat-soluble vitamins, on the other hand, are absorbed with fat and thus any factor reducing the amount of fat digested and/or absorbed will reduce their absorption. Fat-soluble vitamins are also stored in the body and thus deficiencies in the diet may take some time to affect nutritional status, but they are more likely to have toxic effects if eaten in excess.

Minerals are the inorganic elements (other than carbon, hydrogen and nitrogen) that are found in the body and which are essential constituents of diet. They include the 'trace elements' which are required in very small, but vital amounts. Minerals serve many different biological functions ranging from structural (calcium in bone), transport (iron in hemoglobin), energy metabolism (phosphorus in ATP), endocrine (iodine in thyroid), neurotransmission (magnesium) and enzyme action (molybdenum).

The dietary sources, function and requirements of vitamins and minerals are shown in Tables 21.7–21.12 and in Chapter 37. Deficiency diseases associated with these micronutrients are summarized in the sections on Nutrition and Disease.

Table 21.7 Dietary sources of vitamins

Vitamin	Food sources
Thiamin	Cereals: breakfast cereal, white bread, wholemeal bread Vegetables (potatoes), milk and meat products
Vitamin B_{12}	*Milk and milk products, meat and meat products, cereals.* (Alternative source, yeast extract for vegetarians.)
Folic acid	Vegetables, legumes, liver, meat products, eggs *Breakfast cereals, bread, vegetables, milk products*
Vitamin B_6	*Milk and milk products, vegetables, breakfast cereals.* (Alternative sources poultry, fish, eggs, nuts.)
Niacin	Meat and meat products, cereal products, bread, breakfast cereals, vegetables, milk and milk products
Riboflavin	Meat and meat products, cereal products, bread, breakfast cereals, vegetables, milk and milk products. *Cereals, milk*
Biotin	Liver, egg, cereals, yeast
Panthothenic acid	Widely distributed, meat, cereals, legumes
Vitamin C	Vegetables (potatoes), beverages (fruit juice), fruit and nuts. *Vegetables, beverages*
Vitamin A	Retinol: meat (liver, milk products, fat spreads. *Milk products, meat products, vegetables* β-carotene: vegetables, meat and meat products. *Vegetables*
Vitamin D	Fat spreads, cereal products, oily fish *Fat spreads, breakfast cereals, milk and milk products*
Vitamin E	Vegetable oils *Fat spreads, vegetables, meat and meat products, cereal products*
Vitamin K	Vegetables, margarines, but synthesized in colon

Sources of nutrients for infants are shown in italics
From National Diet and Nutrition Survey 1990, 1995a, and Garrow & James 1993

Table 21.8 Structure, function and mode of absorption of water-soluble vitamins

Vitamin	Chemical structure	Functions	Absorption
Thiamin	Pyrimidine ring joined to thiazole ring	Thiamin pyrophosphate coenzyme for many reactions in carbohydrate metabolism	Active transport or passive transport at concentration >1 μmol or 5 mg/day
Vit. B_{12}	Cobalamin, porphyrin-like ring containing cobalt; 5-deoxyadeno-sylcobalamin, methyl cobalamin, hydroxycobalamin	Cofactor for methionine synthetase, methylmalonyl-CoA mutase	Absorbed bound to various carrier proteins; R protein in stomach, IF protein in small intestine. Transcobalamin in basolateral membrane. 70% efficient
Folic acid	Folate, sustituted pteridine ring linked to p-aminobenzoic acid Exists as polyglutamated reduced or substituted forms of folic acid	Coenzyme for several reactions, transfer of single carbon units in reactions essential to metabolism of several amino acids and nucleic acid synthesis	Various dietary forms need to be hydrolyzed before absorption as monoglutamyl folate by active transport
Vit. B_6	Pyridoxine, pyridoxal, pyridoxamine, pyridoxine HCl	Pyridoxal phosphate coenzyme for reactions related to protein metabolism, amino transferase decarboxylase and for amine synthesis, e.g. 5HT, heme synthesis, glycogen metabolism, sphingolipid and niacin synthesis	Hydrolyzed and absorbed passively
Niacin	Nicotinamide	NAD, NADP for oxidoreductases	Absorbed as nicotinic acid, nicotinamide, NMM
Ribo-flavin	Isoalloxazine ring with ribityl side chain. Flavin mononucleotide, flavin adenosine dinucleotide	Flavoprotein enzymes in oxidative-reductive reactions, in metabolic pathways and cellular respiration	By sodium-dependent saturable proteins
Biotin	Imidazole ring fused to tetrahydrothiophene ring with valeric acid side chain	Cofactor for carboxylases in fatty acid synthesis, metabolism, gluconeogenesis, branched chain amino acid metabolism	Actively absorbed as free biotin in small intestine
Pantothenic acid	Dimethyl derivative of butyric acid linked to β-alanine	Constituent of CoA and esters essential for lipid and carbohydrate metabolism	Ingested as part of CoA released by intestinal phosphatase absorbed as pantnothenic acid
Vit. C	Ascorbic acid	Essential for hydroxylation of proline and lysine in collagen synthesis, needed for carnitine and noradrenaline synthesis	Active sodium-linked absorption

Table 21.9 Structure, function and mode of absorption of fat-soluble vitamins

Vitamin	Chemical structure	Functions	Absorption
Vit. A	Retinol, β-carotene, 6 β-carotene = 1 retinol equivalent	Cellular differentiation, vision, fetal development, immune system, spermatogenesis, appetite, hearing, growth	With fat 80% absorbed
Vit. D	Calciferol, ergocalciferol, cholecalciferol. Metabolized in skin, liver and kidneys to active forms	Essential for calcium absorption, regulates calcium metabolism, involved in immune system	With fat 80% absorbed
Vit. E	Tocopherols, tocotrienols; 8 naturally occurring forms	Antioxidant prevents lipid peroxidation	With fat absorption
Vit. K	2 metholnaphthoquinone rings, with side chains phylloquinone, menaquinone, menadione	Needed for gla-proteins. Catalyzes synthesis of prothrombin in liver for clotting factors VII, IX and X	With fat 50–80% absorbed

Table 21.10 Estimated average requirements (EAR) and reference nutrient intakes (RNI) for vitamins in childhood

Age m=months y=years	Weight kg	Thiamin mg/1000kcal		Riboflavin mg/d		Niacin mg equiv/ 1000kcal		B_6 μg/g protein		B_{12} μg/d		Folate μg/d		A* μg/d		C mg/d		D μg/d
		EAR	RNI	EAR	RNI	EAR	RNI	EAR	RNI	EAR	RNI	EAR	RNI	EAR	RNI	EAR	RNI	RNI
0–3 m	5.9	0.23	0.3	0.3	0.4	5.5	6.6	6	8	0.25	0.3	40	50	250	350	15	25	8.5
4–6 m	7.7	0.23	0.3	0.3	0.4	5.5	6.6	6	8	0.25	0.3	40	50	250	350	15	25	8.5
7–9 m	8.9	0.23	0.3	0.3	0.4	5.5	6.6	8	10	0.35	0.4	40	50	250	350	15	25	7
10–12 m	9.8	0.23	0.3	0.3	0.4	5.5	6.6	10	13	0.35	0.4	40	50	250	350	15	25	7
1–3 y	12.6	0.3	0.4	0.5	0.6	5.5	6.6	13	15	0.4	0.5	50	70	300	400	20	30	7
4–6 y	17.8	0.3	0.4	0.6	0.8	5.5	6.6	13	15	0.7	0.8	75	100	300	400	20	30	0
7–10 y	28.3	0.3	0.4	0.8	1.0	5.5	6.6	13	15	0.8	1.0	110	150	350	500	20	30	0
Males																		
11–14 y	43.1	0.3	0.4	1.0	1.2	5.5	6.6	13	15	1.0	1.2	150	200	400	600	22	35	0
15–18 y	64.5	0.3	0.4	1.0	1.3	5.5	6.6	13	15	1.25	1.5	150	200	500	700	25	40	0
Females																		
11–14 y	43.8	0.3	0.4	0.9	1.1	5.5	6.6	13	15	1.0	1.2	150	200	400	600	22	35	0
15–18 y	55.5	0.3	0.4	0.9	1.1	5.5	6.6	13	15	1.25	1.5	150	200	400	600	25	40	0

* μg retinol equivalents/d. From DoH 1991

Table 21.11 Dietary sources of minerals

Minerals	Food sources of major minerals	Alternative good sources
Iron	Cereal products (bread, breakfast cereals), meat/meat products, vegetables *Cereals, meat, vegetables*	
Calcium	Milk and milk products, cereal products *Milk, milk products, cereals*	
Phosphorus	*Milk and milk products, cereal products, meat*	
Potassium	*Milk and milk products, vegetables, cereal products*	
Copper	*Cereal products, meat and meat products, vegetables*	
Iodine	*Milk and milk products, cereal products*	Shellfish, legumes, cereals, liver, seafood, seaweeds, iodized salt
Zinc	Meat and meat products, milk	Cereals
Selenium	Cereals, meat, fish	Amount in foods depends on soil quality. Deficiency may occur where soil is poor
Magnesium	Cereals and green vegetables *Cereals, milk products*	
Chromium	Yeast, meat, cereals, legumes, nuts	

Sources of nutrients for infants are shown in italics.
From National Diet and Nutrition Survey 1990, 1995a, and Garrow & James 1993.

Table 21.12 Functions and mode of absorption of minerals

Mineral	Function	Absorption
Calcium	Bones, teeth, intracellular signal and messenger, neural signals, muscle contraction	Active transport stimulated by vitamin D. Bioavailability 20–30%. 60% from human milk, 40% from formula milk
Magnesium	Bones, nerve and muscles cofactor for DNA & RNA synthesis. Enzymes influence Ca^{2+} metabolism	Facilitated and passive absorption bioavailability low in meat and milk products
Phosphorus	Bones. Provides high energy bonds ATP, and used for phosphorylation for signaling activating enzymes and proteins in metabolism	Ubiquitous, 60% bioavailability
Sodium	Principal cation in ECF. Needed for general neural, muscle and membrane potentials	Passive and active absorption linked with glucose and amino acids
Potassium	Intracellular cation needed to maintain membrane potential, acid–base balance, Na/K+ ATPase pumps	90% bioavailability, excess not possible unless renal failure. Deficiency not diet related
Manganese	Many enzymes including pyruvate carboxylase, mitochondrial superoxide dismutase, phosphotransferases	Low bioavailability 10%
Chromium	Potentiates action of insulin	
Iodine	Thyroxine, triiodothyronine, maintenance of metabolic rate, cellular metabolism and integrity of connective tissue	Inorganic iodine well absorbed
Flourine	Not essential but protects against dental caries and aids bone remineralization	Passively absorbed
Arsenic	Methionine and polyamine metabolism	
Boron	Membrane signal transduction	
Bromine Lithium	} Can substitute for choride and iodide	
Nickel	Metabolism of branched chain amino acids and propionic acid	
Silicon	Cross-linking of glycoproteins and induction of calcification	
Vanadium	Regulation of phosphoryl transfer enzymes and receptor phosphorylation	
Chloride	Major electrolyte in ECF and in ICF	Passive absorption. Active absorption, dietary deficiency only been seen in infants fed formula containing less than 2 mmol
Iron	Hemoglobin, myoglobin, other iron-containing enzymes	Bioavailability 30% animal products, 10% plant products. 50% human milk absorption inhibited by tanins, phytate protein, Ca, Mn, Cu, Cd, Co. Enhanced by vit C, citric, lactic, malic and tartaric acid, fructose, sorbitol, alcohol, and amino acids
Zinc	Many enzyme systems in major metabolic pathways	Low bioavailability decreased by phytate, iron
Copper	Enzyme component cytochrome oxidase, superoxide dismutase, synthesis of neuroactive amines and peptides	Bioavailability 35–70%. 50% from infant formula
Selenium	Glutathione peroxidase protective against oxidative damage	
Molybdenum	Xanthine oxidase and other enzymes in metabolism of DNA and sulfites	80% bioavailability

NUTRITIONAL ASSESSMENT

Nutritional assessment is the evaluation of an individual's nutritional status and requirements. It is a means by which the undernourished (or overnourished) child can be identified, the nutritional effects of therapy and the efficacy of nutritional interventions monitored and the prevalence of under- or overnutrition in a group established. Nutritional assessment was used first in surveys of the nutritional status of populations, especially those in developing countries. More recently there has been a resurgence of interest in nutritional assessment in developed countries as a result of increasing awareness that malnutrition is common in hospital and community populations of children (Merritt & Suskind 1979, Parsons et al 1980, Listernick et al 1985, Moy et al 1990) and adults (McWhirter & Pennington 1994, Potter et al 1995) and the growing awareness of the clinical and functional consequences of malnutrition (Lennard-Jones 1992).

There are five principal approaches to nutritional assessment: anthropometric, dietary, biochemical, clinical and functional. Each evaluates a different aspect of nutritional status. While comprehensive assessment of nutritional status of patients requires adoption of all of these approaches, such a course of action is usually impractical and there is no agreed method of integrating the information derived from all of them to reach a judgment. Each will therefore be considered separately. All approaches have important limitations and there is still much debate over choice of methods, reference values and interpretation and reporting of measurements. These issues are summarized below under each heading. Functional assessment, the use of functional deficits (e.g. deficits in immune function or muscle function) to identify or measure undernutrition, is not discussed since it is so rarely used in children and is an approach that is still experimental. A fuller account of functional assessment is given in Gibson (1990). Assessment of growth is an integral part of the anthropometric assessment of nutritional status, but because growth assessment is dealt with in detail in Chapter 8 it will not be considered in depth here.

ANTHROPOMETRIC NUTRITIONAL ASSESSMENT

Anthropometry is the measurement of physical dimensions of the human body at different ages. Comparison with reference standards identifies abnormalities of growth that may result from nutrient deficiencies or excess. Anthropometric nutritional assessment is used to identify or quantify chronic or acute imbalance in intake/requirements of protein or (more commonly) energy. Imbalances of this kind alter the relative proportions of various tissues and/or disturb growth and measurement of 'indices' of these tissues forms the basis of nutritional anthropometry. Anthropometry is a reasonable guide to energy and protein status, in the sense that a disturbance in energy intake (for example) will usually result in a detectable anthropometric change, though these changes occur relatively slowly.

What should be measured?

A handful of simple anthropometric measurements are all that is necessary to carry out comprehensive nutritional anthropometry and these are often used to calculate 'derived indices' which are used to interpret the child's nutritional status. Three basic measurements (body height, weight and age) are recommended by the WHO (1983) and these are used to derive the following indices: height-for-age (low height-for-age, 'stunting', is an index of chronic undernutrition); weight-for-age; weight-for-height (low weight-for-height, 'wasting', is an index of acute undernutrition). A detailed description of how to perform these measurements is given in Gibson (1990).

The body mass index (BMI; weight (kg)/height (M)^2) is a simple and useful tool for assessing or monitoring overweight and underweight. The BMI is widely used in adults, but in children it has been restricted because the index is age dependent. There are now reference data for BMI from birth to adulthood for France (Rolland Cachera et al 1991), from the UK (Cole et al 1995) and the USA (Hammer et al 1991, Mast et al 1991). BMI can be expressed as standard deviation (SD) scores or as centiles.

In clinical practice in developed countries these anthropometric indices are useful but can be limited as, for instance, when a child has ascites, fluid retention or a large solid tumor. Such conditions can confound weight-based anthropometric indices and the most useful and widely used alternatives are mid upper arm circumference (MUAC – related to muscle mass and fat mass, an index of 'protein/energy' status), skinfold thickness (notably over the triceps, an index of fatness) and indices derived from these (arm muscle area or arm muscle circumference), which are more specific indices of muscle bulk and are particularly useful in measuring small changes (Gibson 1990, Potter et al 1995).

Analysis, presentation and interpretation of nutritional anthropometry

The purpose (application) of nutritional anthropometry defines how the data obtained are analyzed, presented and interpreted. If the purpose is to monitor changing nutritional status, for instance to evaluate the efficacy of supplementary feeding, the main outcome will be change in the parameter measured over time.

The other major purpose of nutritional anthropometry is screening, particularly for identification of patients that are undernourished (and who may need nutritional support) or overnourished (who need some other kind of dietary restriction). Screening of children in this way normally involves comparing the measured value of the index in question with the most appropriate set of reference values available and using 'cut-offs' to categorize them as undernourished (below the lower cut-off) or overnourished (above the upper cut-off). A wide variety of cutoffs and reference data sets are used and there is a distinct lack of uniformity in practice. Some of the anthropometric reference data used for this purpose are given in Table 21.13.

It is important to note that the cut-offs are usually fairly arbitrary and, since they involve 'slicing' off the bottom or top of the reference distribution, they inevitably include some healthy children (false positives). It is therefore more appropriate to think of anthropometric screening as a means of identifying children 'at risk' of malnutrition rather than 'malnourished'. If the purpose is not to identify individuals as under- or overnourished, but to establish the prevalence of under- or overnutrition in a population (for instance in hospital) the task is simplified since it becomes necessary only to show that the percentage of the sample above or below the cut-off is greater than expected (i.e. higher proportion than in the reference population).

When reporting and interpreting raw or derived anthropometric indices (e.g. BMI, weight-for-height, height-for-age) relative to a reference population there are three principal approaches:

Table 21.13 Anthropometric reference data for children from UK and USA

Index	Reference	Comments
Length	UK[a,b], USA[c]	
Height	UK[a,b], USA[c]	[c] Recommended by WHO
Weight	UK[a,b], USA[c]	
Body mass index	UK[d,e], France[f], USA[g,h]	
Weight-for-height	UK[i], USA[j]	[i] 4–12 yrs; [j]41–45 cm boys 49–137 cm girls [c] recommended by WHO
Mid arm circumference	USA[j]	
Triceps skinfold	UK[k,l], USA[j], Sweden[m]	[l]SD scores, [k]centiles, [m]to yr only
Subscapular skinfold	Sweden[m]	[m] to 3 yrs only

a   Tanner et al 1966
b   Freeman et al 1995
c   Hamill et al 1979
d   White et al 1995
e   Cole et al 1995
f   Rolland Cachera et al 1991
g   Mast et al 1991
h   Hammer et al 1991
i   Chinn et al 1992
j   Frisancho 1981
k   Davies et al 1993
l   Tanner & Whitehouse 1975
m   Karlberg et al 1968

classification with reference to centiles, use of percentage of reference median or use of standard deviation (SD) or 'Z' scores. While the first two approaches are most commonly used in clinical nutritional assessment, there is now a consensus that the third approach, the calculation of SD scores, is much more useful and should be adopted more widely. Detailed discussion and demonstration of this point is provided in Krick (1986) and Smith & Booth (1989).

Advantages and disadvantages of nutritional anthropometry

The main advantages are practical: the measurements described above are simple, noninvasive, inexpensive, portable and highly suitable for pediatric use in the ward, clinic or community. They are relatively specific indices of disturbance in energy balance, can be used to 'screen' patients, to monitor changes over time or to establish the prevalence of under- or overnutrition.

The practical disadvantages of nutritional anthropometry relate to the need for training in the methods, quality control (Gibson 1990) and the difficulty of accurately measuring small changes in nutritional status (for example, functional changes indicative of the development of malnutrition are often measurable before detection by anthropometry (Gibson 1990)). The statistical questions of sensitivity and specificity of nutritional anthropometry as a screening tool need to be considered carefully (Gibson 1990) and it should be noted that the validity of the indices is doubtful or limited in some cases (Davies 1994) and can be rendered invalid by disease states (e.g. alterations in fat distribution in cerebral palsy (Spender et al 1988)).

DIETARY NUTRITIONAL ASSESSMENT

Assessment of nutritional status based on dietary intake should take into account current and past food intake. Dietary assessments should be done by a pediatric dietitian who has the skills to ensure that all aspects of intake are considered, including assessment of the quantities of food eaten. Specific foods which appear to cause vomiting, diarrhea, malabsorption, etc. must also be identified and 'food' should not only refer to that taken at meals but also include snacks eaten.

Recording dietary intake can be done in a number of ways with the aim of measuring quality and quantity of food consumed and the macro- and micronutrients ingested. Food tables or computer programs are used to calculate intake of individual nutrients. Each dietary assessment method provides differing degrees of accuracy and the data obtained should always be interpreted with caution.

Weighed intakes should provide the most accurate record of food intake. However, the observer has to rely on the subject recording all food and drink taken (taking into account any wastage) and that the foods eaten reflect usual dietary habits rather than particular foods which are easy to weigh and record. Three-, 5- or 7-day food record diaries are used. The longer duration has the advantage of more clearly reflecting variations in food habits, but the disadvantage of the recording becoming onerous and thus more inaccurate. Alternatively a diet history, based on 'typical' or 'usual' food intake, can be recorded. Assessment of dietary intake based on a recall method is dependent on the parent and/or child remembering all food and drink taken during the previous 24 h and this being a typical day. A food frequency questionnaire presents the respondent with a list of foods that should be scored, in terms of the number of times that they are eaten each day, week or month.

All of these methods are adequate for the nutritional assessment of infants (excluding those who are exclusively breast-fed), since much food is provided by milk feeds and most mothers can readily provide a fairly accurate record of the number and volume of feeds and the amount of solids taken. The dietitian must include bottles taken during the night, as well as other fluids (types used, frequency and volumes taken). The accuracy of the history can often be verified by checking the number of tins of formula powder used each week. Intake of vitamin and mineral supplements can be calculated from how regularly they are taken and the type of preparation used.

Dietary assessment of an infant of less than 6 months should include assessment of the mother's nutritional status while pregnant and her lactational performance if she is breast-feeding. This may require weighing the infant before and after a feed (see Ch. 6).

BIOCHEMICAL NUTRITIONAL ASSESSMENT

Biochemical nutritional assessment requires measurement of nutrient concentrations in the blood, urine, other fluids or tissues. There is an optimal concentration of nutrients within the body, below and above which deficiency and toxicity can occur. However, circulating concentrations of nutrients are not an accurate measurement of tissue stores and reflect the immediate availability of particular nutrients. In the blood some nutrients are found 'free' (e.g. vitamin C), some 'bound' to carrier proteins (e.g. calcium, iron) and some as 'precursors' (e.g. β-carotene). Each nutrient has its own site of storage and function and it is not possible to make universal statements about biochemical nutritional assessment.

In pediatric practice, measurements of nutrient concentrations or biochemical markers of nutritional status and/or growth are made most commonly in the blood or urine. In certain nutritional deficiency or toxicity states and in some metabolic diseases, measurements of concentrations of particular nutrients in specific tissues should be made. It must be remembered that changes in circulating concentrations of many nutrients occur only when tissue stores have been depleted and normal blood concentrations do not necessarily indicate normal nutritional status.

The nutrients commonly measured in the blood are discussed here. Interpretation of the concentrations of those measured in other tissues will be found in relevant chapters.

Blood urea reflects not only renal function but also protein intake. It can be low in rapidly growing neonates and in children with hepatic failure. High blood urea can be a marker of the infant or toddler with a high cow's milk intake. Low serum albumin can be an early indicator of inadequate protein intake or excessive protein loss, because of its relatively short half-life as, for instance, in inflammatory bowel disease. Plasma amino acids measured quantitatively may show low glutamine. In the fasting state, hepatic uptake of alanine for gluconeogenesis causes blood levels of this amino acid to fall. In longer term protein deficiency levels of the essential amino acids will fall: first to do so are the branched chain amino acids leucine, isoleucine and valine. In patients on vegan diets or where severely reduced protein intake limits lysine availability for its synthesis, carnitine deficiency may develop. In these circumstances clinical effects are rare.

Alkaline phosphatase is a sensitive indicator of nutritional rickets and osteomalacia. Measurement of vitamin D level is not indicated in the presence of normal calcium and phosphate.

Prevalence studies have shown how difficult it is to make absolute definitions of iron deficiency. Hemoglobin and red cell indices may not fully reflect iron stores. Ferritin reflects total body iron stores but is also an acute phase protein and concentrations may be falsely high in acute infection. Serum iron, total iron-binding capacity (TIBC) and free erythrocyte protoporphyrin (FEP) may be measured: iron falls and TIBC and FEP rise in iron-deficiency anemia.

Deficiency of water-soluble vitamins is rare in the UK though it may develop rapidly in patients who are receiving inadequately supplemented intravenous fluids or total parenteral nutrition. None of these is widely routinely measured. Red cell transketolase activity gives an indirect indication of thiamin deficiency which can occur because of the demands of a high glucose intake for thiamin pyrophosphate cofactor. Deficiency of vitamin B_{12}, vitamin A or vitamin E develops late because of large tissue stores. Prothrombin time reflects vitamin K status if liver function is normal.

Circulating concentrations of trace elements (copper, zinc, selenium) decrease late in deficiency. Zinc or magnesium deficiency occurs in Crohn's disease and other causes of chronic diarrhea. Low glutathione peroxidase activity in red cells indirectly indicates selenium deficiency but a direct selenium assay may be preferable.

The section on Deficiency diseases (p. 1190) contains an account of the major features of macronutrient and micronutrient deficiencies.

CLINICAL NUTRITIONAL ASSESSMENT

Severe nutritional deprivation is easily detectable on clinical examination and can be confirmed by anthropometry. Clinical signs of 'pure' or single nutrient deficiencies rarely occur alone and subtle physical signs, such as glossitis or angular stomatitis, are relatively nonspecific. Physical examination should be interpreted in association with anthropometric, dietary and biochemical nutritional assessment.

The 'classic' physical signs of protein–energy malnutrition, vitamin and mineral deficiencies, including rickets and scurvy, are described in the section on Nutrition and Disease and in the relevant chapters of this book. It should be remembered, however, that physical signs are a late manifestation of nutrient deficiency, occurring after tissue stores have been depleted and adaptive changes have failed to maintain normal nutrient homeostasis and function.

NORMAL DIET

INFANCY (0–12 months)

Nutrition for the first year of life can be divided into two halves: birth to 6 months, when nutrition is essentially liquid and 6–12 months when reliance on fluids gradually diminishes as more solid foods are introduced to the diet.

0–6 months

Breast milk

The ideal feed for the human infant is human milk, a complex blend of nutrients and immunological and other bioactive substances which helps to confer protection on the infant from both bacterial and viral infections and assist in its adaptation to life outside the womb. The composition of human milk (see Ch. 6) changes both during the course of lactation and during a single feed. At the beginning of each feed, the fat content is low but gradually increases so that the most energy-dense milk is secreted at the end of the feed. The few contraindications to breast-feeding are for babies of mothers who have AIDS or HIV infection, infants who have galactosemia or congenital lactase deficiency and if certain drugs are being taken by the mother – the British National Formulary includes an up-to-date list of these.

Formula milk

Approved infant formulae provide a safe alternative to breast milk. They broadly resemble human milk in terms of their chemical composition but contain none of the enzymes, immunological or other bioactive substances found in human milk. The majority of formulae are based on cow's milk and comprise two groups: whey predominant and casein predominant. The former have a protein content based on demineralized whey with a whey : casein ratio similar to breast milk (60% whey:40% casein). Casein-predominant formulae have as their protein source skimmed cow's milk and a ratio of 80% casein:20% whey. Ideally infants should remain on the formula first used until the end of the first year of life but a follow-on formula may be used after the age of 6 months (Ch. 6).

A recent trend has been the use of formulae based on soy protein isolates. Although satisfactory growth has been achieved in babies fed these formulae, their nutritional composition is quite different from that of breast milk or milks based on modified cow's milk. Long-term studies on physical and neurological outcome of children taking these formulae have not been done and they should be used only when there is proven lactose or cow's milk protein intolerance (see Gastroenteritis pp. 1215, 1292) or for infants of vegetarian mothers who have elected not to breast-feed. The normal feeding of the newborn infant is considered in greater detail in Chapter 6.

6–12 months

Somewhere between 4 and 6 months of age, solids should be introduced into the diet because the infant's iron stores are becoming depleted, chewing needs to be developed and milk alone is insufficient to meet the growing nutritional requirements of the infant (DoH 1994).

Recommendations for weaning are that the infant, in addition to nonmilk diet, should continue to receive a minimum of 500–600 ml of breast or formula milk daily. Nonwheat cereals, fruit, vegetables and potatoes are all suitable first weaning foods. Between 6 and 9 months of age, meat, fish, all cereals, pulses, fish and eggs can be introduced. No salt should be added to home-prepared foods and only enough sugar used to make sour fruits palatable. Breast-fed and artificially fed infants consuming less than 500 ml formula feed daily should have supplements of vitamins A and D (DoH 1994b).

TODDLER

The feeding of the preschool child progresses through many skill-learning processes, from the semisolid/liquid diet of the weanling, through finger-feeding of bits of food which require chewing at around 1 year of age, to spoon-feeding by the age of 2 years, to mastering child-sized cutlery and adult-type food by the age of 5 years.

Nutritionally, the toddler diet bridges the gap between the energy-dense diet of the infant, which provides around 50% of energy from fat to that of the adult, where around 35% of energy should be derived from fat. Toddlers, however, have small stomach capacities and a balance must be struck between the gradual reduction of energy-dense fat-containing foods and the introduction of lower fat foods. Although surveys of nutritional intakes for this age group are sparse, recent studies have shown that the energy intake from fat declines in proportion to increasing age (National Diet & Nutrition Survey 1995a). The toddler should continue to consume around 500 ml of milk daily (or equivalent from other foods such as yogurt and cheese). Full fat milk should be used from 1–2 years of age. Thereafter, as long as growth and energy intake are satisfactory, semiskimmed milk can be given from the age of 2–5 years of age. After 2 years of age, other lower fat dairy products such as yogurt, spreads and cheese may be used. Many toddlers become fussy and difficult with meals and it may be more appropriate to follow a feeding regimen based on three small meals and three snacks daily. Care should be taken with fluids. Many toddlers begin to substitute easily assimilated liquids, particularly if given from bottles, for solid food which requires chewing and the use of cutlery. 'Bottle caries' is a result of continual ingestion of sweetened liquids from a teated bottle (National Diet & Nutrition Survey 1995b). After the first year, all drinks taken during the day should be given in a cup.

SCHOOL CHILD

After the age of 5 years, the diet can change towards that advised for adults (NACNE 1983, DoH 1992, Scottish Office 1993). Fiber intake should be increased, with generous consumption of fruits, vegetables and high-fiber cereals such as wholemeal bread, pasta and breakfast cereals. Efforts should be made to moderate saturated fat intake by the use of skimmed or semiskimmed milk, low fat or polyunsaturated spreads, low fat dairy products and eating fish, poultry and lean meats. The intake of nonmilk extrinsic sugars between meals should be avoided because of its association with dental caries. A reduction in energy intake from a lowering of fat intake should be compensated for by a commensurate increase in starch intake.

ADOLESCENT

Energy intake in adolescence should be a balance between the large demands needed to meet a peak growth velocity and that required for physical activity. The timing of the adolescent growth spurt varies between individuals so that nutrient requirements should be related to weight rather than age (WHO 1985). Weight gain in girls is mainly due to fat deposition whereas boys accumulate more muscle and skeletal tissue.

Many teenagers adopt a 'grazing' eating pattern, consuming snack foods and 'fast food' meals. Concern about body image may lead to abnormal eating and exercise patterns. In extreme cases anorexia nervosa and bulimia may result, but these disorders are primarily psychiatric rather than nutritional (Ch. 29).

A number of studies of teenage eating habits have shown that many children consume diets low in various nutrients, in particular iron, calcium, thiamin and riboflavin (Bull 1985, DoH 1989, Crawley 1993). The most comprehensive study of nutrient intakes of children aged 10–15 years based on 7-day weighed dietary records (DoH 1989) showed that, although weights and heights were within the normal ranges, on average children consumed 90% of EAR for energy. This may reflect the sedentary lifestyles of many children. Bread, milk, meat products, chips, cakes and puddings were the main sources of energy and around 75% of the children consumed about 38% of food energy as fat and 25% of this group took in excess of 40% of food energy from fat. Girls consumed less than the RNI for calcium, iron and riboflavin with one in three girls having iron intakes below the LRNI.

Many adolescents will experiment with different diets. Vegetarianism is increasing (Realit Survey Office 1993) and encompasses a range of dietary cultures (Table 21.14). 'Vegetarian' diets which include some animal foods such as milk, cheese or eggs usually achieve adequate nutrient intakes. Teenagers who elect to follow a vegan regimen should take supplements of vitamin B_{12}, calcium, vitamin D, iron and zinc. Avoidance of specific foods on religious or cult grounds may result in severe nutrient deficiencies unless the dietary regimen has been based on long established traditional practices.

Table 21.14 Types of vegetarian food regimens

Dietary regimen	Animal foods eaten	Animal foods avoided
'Semi-vegetarian'	White meat (chicken, turkey, fish), eggs, cheese	Red meat
Lacto-ovo-vegetarian	Eggs, milk, cheese	Meat, poultry, fish
Lacto-vegetarian	Milk	Meat, poultry, fish, eggs
Vegan	None	Meat, poultry, fish, eggs, cheese, milk

NUTRITION AND DISEASE

OBESITY

Obesity is a major pediatric health problem. Its prevalence is increasing steadily in children (Gortmaker et al 1987) and adults (Prentice & Jebb 1995) and there is evidence that children and adolescents of all ages are fatter than in the past (Lohman 1993).

There are many working definitions of pediatric obesity, but all include the idea that it is excess weight-for-height (e.g. BMI SD score >+2; weight-for-height >95th centile; weight more than 20% greater than median weight-for-height) or excess fat (e.g. body fat as % of bodyweight above an arbitrary threshold (Lohman 1993); triceps skinfold above a cut-off such as the 85th or 95th centile (Dietz 1993a)). The latter criteria, while more difficult to apply clinically, have the advantage of specifically distinguishing the child who is excessively fat from the child who has a particularly large fat-free ('lean body') mass. Dietz (1993b) estimated that up to 15% of children treated for obesity are not excessively fat, but simply have a large fat-free mass.

Despite the mystique surrounding obesity, the cause is well understood and quite simple. Obesity is a disorder of energy balance: *energy balance = (energy intake – energy expended)*. When energy intake exceeds energy expenditure (due to increased food intake and/or decreased energy expended on physical activity (Prentice & Jebb 1995)), the excess energy must be stored. It is important to note that excess energy is stored as both fat (adipose tissue) and fat-free tissue (muscle, connective tissue, etc.) and so obese children and adults have both a larger fat mass and a larger fat-free mass (lean body mass) than their nonobese peers (Forbes 1964). It is also important to note that once children (or adults) have become obese this expanded fat-free mass, together with the increased energy cost of most activities (energy cost of moving the extra body mass around), means that the energy requirements of the obese child are considerably higher than those of the nonobese child (and can be estimated using the approach outlined in the section on Nutritional Requirements). The obese patient tends to report a low energy intake, implying a low energy requirement and patients and their families often believe that the obese child has some defect in energy expenditure. This is rarely the case and most obese adolescents (Bandini et al 1990) and even young children (Maffeis et al 1994) substantially underreport their true dietary intake. One consequence of this is that self-reported dietary intakes from obese patients should not be used to estimate energy requirements or intakes in clinical practice, but can provide a crude estimate of eating habits (Dietz 1993b).

Clinical consequences of obesity

Obesity has important clinical consequences in childhood and adolescence. These include lowered fitness, increased blood pressure, increased total plasma cholesterol and decreased HDL concentration, polycystic ovarian disease (Dietz 1993a) and adverse psychological and socioeconomic consequences (Gortmaker 1993). In addition, obesity in childhood and adolescence has a strong tendency to persist or 'track' into adulthood. The relative risk of persistence into adulthood increases with age: obese 10–13-year-olds are 8–18 times more likely to become obese adults than their nonobese peers (Epstein 1993) and about 70% of children obese at this age will remain obese into adulthood. Relative risk is usually <4 in the prepubertal

child (Epstein 1993). Given the clinical consequences of obesity in childhood and adulthood, the high degree of resistance to treatment in adulthood and the phenomenon of 'tracking', the case for preventing or treating obesity in childhood and adolescence is strong.

Treatment of the obese child

Detailed discussions of therapeutic strategies for childhood obesity are provided elsewhere (Dietz 1993a,b, Epstein 1993). In summary, the focus of therapy is modest dietary restriction and 'healthy eating' (to reduce energy intake), usually with behavioral modification and parent training, often with an exercise prescription (to increase energy expenditure). One concern which is widely held is that diet restriction might compromise growth of the obese child, but evidence suggests that modest diet restriction does not compromise growth (Epstein et al 1993), though height and weight should of course be monitored during clinical intervention. As in adulthood, childhood obesity is often resistant to treatment and there is a need for more research in this area. Nevertheless, successful treatment can be achieved and can have both short- and long-term benefits (Epstein 1993).

Secondary obesity

A careful history and examination will usually readily differentiate between simple obesity and any underlying pathology which may be responsible (Table 21.15). The child with simple obesity often has relatively tall stature. In contrast, children with Cushing's syndrome and hypothyroidism have relatively short stature and growth failure. Hyperphagic dysmorphic syndromes include the Prader–Willi and Laurence–Moon–Biedl syndromes, but many other unclassified dysmorphic syndromes with mental handicap can be associated with voracious appetite. Some chromosomal abnormalities (Down and Klinefelter's syndromes) are associated with obesity. Obesity is a common long-term consequence of childhood acute lymphoblastic leukemia (Odame et al 1994) and is not uncommon in some neurologically impaired children who have limited mobility and activity, but good oral–motor function. In children with spastic cerebral palsy, excess weight gain adversely affects mobility and can present practical problems for the carer. Recurrent headaches with recent increases in severity and frequency may indicate a hypothalamic or pituitary tumor. Severe mood disturbance, unstable temperature, polyuria and polydypsia

Table 21.15 Causes of obesity

Functional	
Simple obesity	Excessive dietary intake
Lack of exercise/mobility (Spina bifida, muscular dystrophy)	
Organic	
Hypothalamic disturbance	Pituitary tumors
Hyperphagic syndromes	Prader–Willi syndrome
	Laurence–Moon–Biedl syndrome
Corticosteriod excess	Cushing's (iatrogenic, pituitary, adrenal)
Hypothyroidism	Thyroid failure
Chromosomal	Down syndrome
	Klinefelter's syndrome
Cerebral disease	Tumors, infection, hydrocephalus

and visual disturbance support this diagnosis. It is vital to identify causes of secondary obesity early. Management of secondary obesity obviously involves treatment of the underlying disease.

FAILURE TO THRIVE (see also Ch. 11)

Failure to thrive describes the infant or child who does not gain weight or height at the expected rate for his or her age. It is defined by reference to growth charts, on which serial measurements of weight and height have been recorded. When a child's weight remains below the 3rd centile and height above it, or crosses centiles downwards, a diagnosis of failure to thrive is made. Recently the use of a 'thrive index' to quantify the shift of weights across the centiles has been recommended to identify suboptimal weight gain (Wright et al 1994a). Failure to thrive may affect up to 10% of children at some time and there is an association with social deprivation (Wright et al 1994b).

The principal causes of failure to thrive in early life are listed in Table 21.16 and are discussed in greater detail in Chapter 11 and elsewhere (Frank & Zeisal 1988). Full assessment includes a family history of growth in weight and height, pregnancy and feeding, developmental progress, symptoms of gastrointestinal disease or metabolic disturbance and a social report (from health visitor or social worker). Physical examination should concentrate on ruling out organic causes, detecting dysmorphic features and signs of abuse, deprivation or neglect. Full dietary assessment should be made by a pediatric dietitian (see Dietary Assessment).

Failure to thrive in early life may be due to insufficient intake, excessive requirements or excessive losses of nutrients (Plate 21.1, Fig. 21.2, Table 21.16). The former is the most important and common cause. It is helpful to distinguish proportional (symmetric) from disproportionate (asymmetric) growth retardation: the former suggests a chronic, often intrauterine cause, while the latter (poor weight gain with preservation of length and head growth) suggests a peri- or postnatal cause.

Careful observation of the infant's feeding behavior and of mother's abilities to feed (test weighing the infant if breast-fed and supervision of formula preparation if bottle-fed) should be

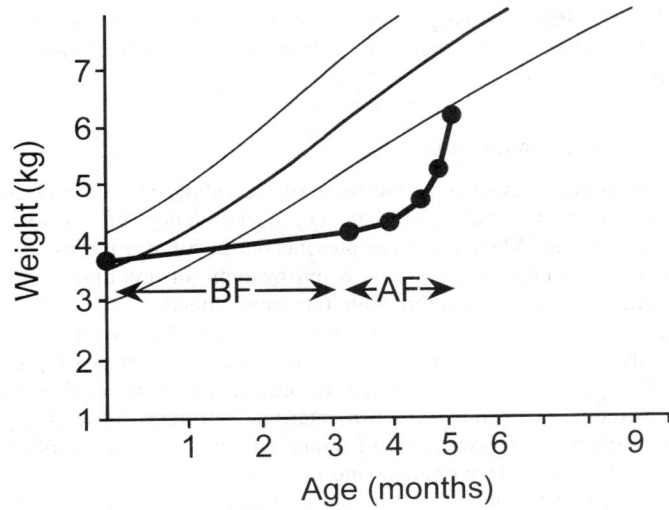

Fig. 21.2   Growth chart of infant with failure to thrive due to insufficent breast milk intake. BF, breast-fed; AF, artificial formula.

undertaken. This may require hospital admission, but separation of mother and baby should be avoided unless essential to determine accurate nutritional intake. Severe emotional deprivation may delay catch-up growth. Failure of adequate dietary intake to promote weight gain suggests underlying disease, such as renal failure, chronic infection (tuberculosis), etc. (Table 21.16).

In the toddler, it is important to rule out celiac disease (Ch. 11) and cystic fibrosis (Ch. 11). In the older child, inflammatory bowel disease (Ch. 11), chronic infection, including giardiasis, renal disease (urinary tract infection, renal tubular acidosis, chronic renal failure), immunodeficiency and chronic hepatic disease are other causes.

Nutritional management of failure to thrive will depend on the underlying cause. Nevertheless the 'final common pathway' of failure to thrive is nutrient deficiency in one form or another and dietary replenishment must be undertaken. This may involve increasing the energy density of feeds, their protein content or that of specific micronutrients. Enteral tube feeding may be required (see below) or in extreme cases, parenteral nutrition.

Nutritional requirements are based on the infant's size, gestation and clinical condition. Reference to appropriate centile charts for weight, length and head circumference and comparison of the infant's growth centiles with those of the parents are essential in making calculations of nutritional needs. These should be based on the infant or child's expected weight for age in order to provide adequate protein and calories for catch-up growth.

PROTEIN–ENERGY MALNUTRITION

Protein–energy malnutrition encompasses disease caused by a complex of dietary, infective and environmental factors. Milder degrees of deficiency result in failure to thrive with growth retardation (see above), while severe deficiencies cause the syndromes of nutritional marasmus and kwashiorkor. Globally malnutrition is one of the principal causes of childhood morbidity and mortality: more than 800 million children are malnourished with growth failure and it has been estimated that half of deaths under 5 years are due, in part, to undernutrition (Snyder & Merson

Table 21.16   Causes of failure to thrive in early life

Deficient intake	Increased metabolic demands
Maternal	*Infant*
Poor lactation	Congenital lung disease
Incorrectly prepared feeds	Congenital heart disease
Unusual milk or other feeds	Congenital liver disease
Inadequate care	Congenital infection
	Anemia
Infant	Inborn errors of metabolism
	Thyroid disease (hyper & hypo)
Prematurity	Cystic fibrosis
Small-for-gestational age	
Oropalatal abnormalities	**Excessive nutrient losses**
Neuromuscular disorders	
Intracranial disease	Gastroesophageal reflux
Genetic disorders	Pyloric stenosis
chromosomal	Necrotizing enterocolitis
dysmorphic	Gastroenteritis
skeletal	Protein-energy malnutrition
	Milk protein intolerance
	Lactose intolerance
	Persistent diarrhea
	Short bowel syndrome

1982). Protein–energy malnutrition often coexists with micronutrient deficiencies (see below) and diarrheal disease (Gracey 1996).

Nutritional marasmus

Nutritional marasmus is due primarily to eating very little of an otherwise well-balanced diet, i.e. a deficiency of all food components. When marasmus presents during infancy it is usually due to lactational failure, low birthweight or multiple birth, commonly in association with recurrent infection, particularly gastroenteritis. Later, it may indicate a local famine or social disruption. It often occurs in the overpopulated insanitary suburbs of large towns in developing countries. The combination of nutritional marasmus and gastroenteritis contributes substantially to the very high prevalence of infant and childhood malnutrition found in many developing countries (Wharton 1991).

Constant features of nutritional marasmus include low weight (<60% median weight-for-age) and wasting of muscles and subcutaneous fat (Fig. 21.3). Occasional features include vitamin deficiencies and infection. Weight-for-age is well below height-for-age, bone age is significantly retarded and the circumference of the chest shrinks to less than that of the head. Biochemical abnormalities are less common than in kwashiorkor: serum proteins are less depressed, plasma cholesterol is normal but fasting plasma concentrations of the free fatty acids and triglyceride are increased. Growth failure causes a low turnover of collagen and there is reduced urinary excretion of hydroxyproline. In contrast to kwashiorkor, loss of appetite is uncommon.

Treatment requires an ample supply of food over many weeks. Formulae composed of milk with added sugar and vegetable oils are used as a basis, together with locally available solid foods. An intake of at least 190 kcal (800 kJ)/kg per day should be achieved in the early days of treatment, increasing this if the child will take more. Children are usually ravenous so that enteral tube feeding is rarely necessary. A search for underlying infections, including HIV, should be made and treated accordingly.

Nutritional marasmus that begins during infancy has a relatively good prognosis when treated and only 1–2% of those sufficiently ill to be admitted to hospital will die. In those countries where it occurs in older children, mortality rate may be considerably higher (even higher than that of kwashiorkor) and recovery may take many months. Marasmus, which persists for many months during infancy, may lead to permanent stunting of stature, poor brain growth and compromised neurodevelopment (Galler & Ross 1993), but it is difficult to distinguish the effect of malnutrition alone since it has usually been accompanied by considerable social deprivation.

Kwashiorkor

Kwashiorkor is a weanling disease and its age of onset depends on the local pattern of breast-feeding, time of introduction of nonmilk diet and cessation of lactation. Almost all children in developing countries show some flattening of the growth curve at weaning, often associated with episodes of diarrhea and other infections (Fig. 21.4). The newly weaned child loses the supply of high-class animal protein from the mother and foods offered instead, such as sugar or banana, are not comparable in nutritional value. At the same time relative dietary protein deficiency occurs and total energy intake falls, because the child cannot eat a sufficient quantity of bulky weaning foods and because of anorexia due to protein deficiency. These changes in diet result in nutritional deficiencies and are accompanied by a substantial increased risk of enteric bacterial infection from contaminated milk or cereal gruels, leading to gastroenteritis and/or small bowel bacterial contamination. This situation has been described by Rowland (1986) as the 'weanling's dilemma' – is it better for the child to rely on a diminishing but clean supply of breast milk or should he try the more plentiful weaning diet with its risks of nutritional inadequacy and microbial contamination (Fig. 21.5)?

Clinical features (Fig. 21.6) can be divided into three groups:

1. *Constant*: edema: retardation in weight growth (even when there is edema) and in length, muscle wasting with some retention of subcutaneous fat, poor appetite, irritability and listlessness.

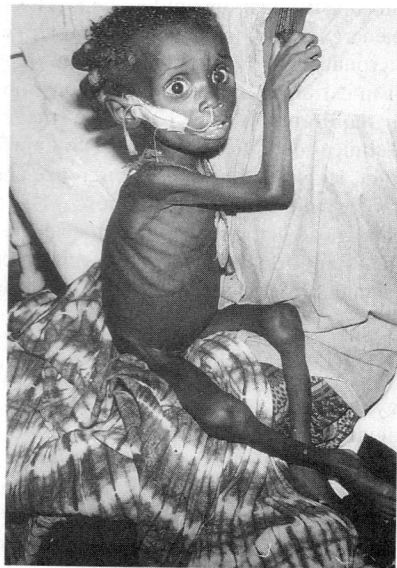

Fig. 21.3 Child with nutritional marasmus (with permission of Dr R G Whitehead).

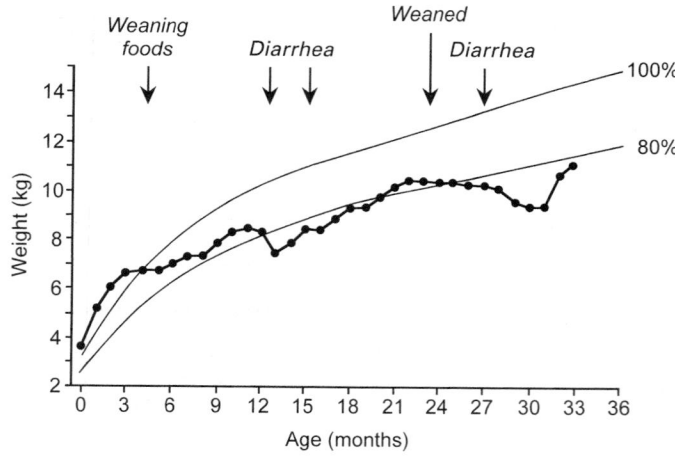

Fig. 21.4 Weight chart of infant with weaning diarrhea. Arrows indicate first introduction of weaning foods, episodes of acute diarrhea and cessation of breast-feeding. 100% and 80% weight-for-age reference standards are shown.

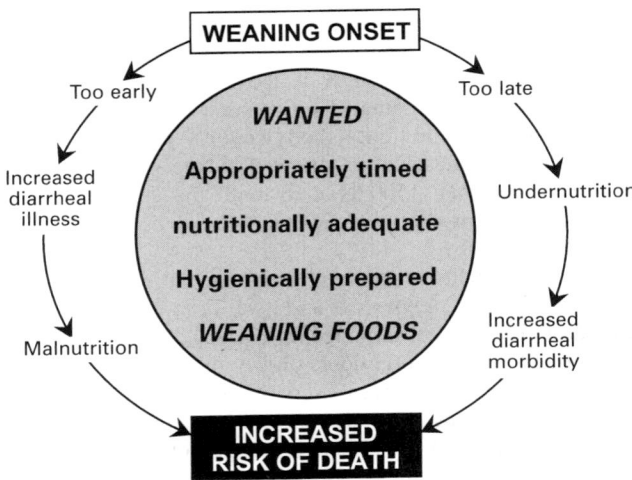

Fig. 21.5 The weanling's dilemma (adapted from Rowland 1986).

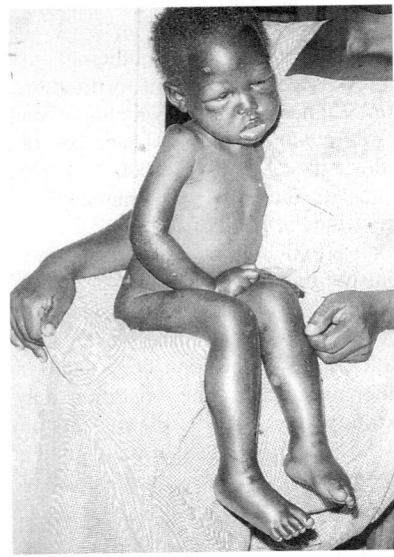

Fig. 21.6 Child with kwashiorkor (with permission of Dr R G Whitehead).

2. *Usual*: sparse, depigmented, friable hair, light-colored skin, moon face, moderate anemia and loose stools.
3. *Occasional*: 'flaky-paint' dermatitis, hepatomegaly, skin ulcers, fissures and blisters, associated vitamin deficiencies varying with the local dietary pattern and infection.

Pathologically, the main features of kwashiorkor are atrophy of the pancreas and small intestinal mucosa (Sullivan et al 1991) and a plethora of functional and biochemical abnormalities. The enteropathy and atrophic pancreas lead to malabsorption, steatorrhea, poor absorption and deficiencies of the fat-soluble vitamins. Small intestinal disaccharidase activity is depressed and the very ill child may also be intolerant of monosaccharides. Plasma protein concentrations are reduced. The plasma concentration of all substances normally carried by β-lipoprotein, such as cholesterol, triglyceride and the fat-soluble vitamins, is reduced too. The extracellular fluid is hypotonic and hypona-

tremia may occur as a result of overhydration rather than a total body deficit of sodium. Circulating cortisol concentrations are high, contributing to the fluid retention and hyponatremia. The protein deficiency results in hypoplasia of the bone marrow despite adequate amounts of erythropoietin.

Children with kwashiorkor often have associated infections. Those caused by Gram-negative bacteria are the most troublesome, presenting usually as gastroenteritis and septicemia, but sometimes as a urinary tract infection. Respiratory infection due mainly to Gram-positive organisms is common. Tuberculosis may be difficult to diagnose because of anergy induced by malnutrition. Measles is the most serious of the viral infections and abnormalities of cellular immunity have been demonstrated.

Nutritional treatment

Cow's milk is widely accepted as the most effective, economic and convenient basis of dietary therapy and lactose intolerance severe enough to warrant exclusion of milk is relatively uncommon. Sugar and vegetable oils are often added to increase the energy content of feeds and casein can be used in severe cases to augment the protein content. Partial digestion of cereal starches can reduce the viscosity of bulky feeds and thereby increase ingestibility and digestibility (Lancet 1991, Weaver et al 1995).

Dried skimmed milk is usually used as a base, but full-cream milk powder in any form is fully acceptable. Using these foods it is possible to formulate a diet which will provide 96–155 kcal (400–650 kJ), 2–4 g milk protein, 4–6 mmol potassium, 1–3 mmol magnesium and less than 2 mmol sodium/kg per day. Children with a reasonable appetite, normal body temperature and level of consciousness and with no serious infection can be treated outside hospital, but it is necessary to see the child at least once a week during the first month of treatment to assess progress.

In hospital, if the child is anorexic, has marked dyspnea or signs of heart failure, feeds should be given by nasogastric tube. In the second week solid foods are added to increase energy intake. Vitamin and mineral supplements are usually given: daily supplements of vitamin A (1500 µg retinol equivalents) and folic acid (1 mg) are recommended. If clinical signs of vitamin A deficiency are apparent, then more intensive therapy is required (see below). Zinc deficiency may delay recovery and should be reversed with 2 mg/kg of zinc per day.

During the treatment of children sufficiently ill to need admission to hospital, hypothermia, hypoglycemia, drowsiness and stupor, severe diarrhea, cardiac failure and infection may all occur. If all goes well the child begins to lose weight, from loss of edema, within the first 3 days after admission and continues to do so until the end of the first week, after which there should be a steady weight gain. If tube feeding has been necessary, it is usually possible during the second week to remove the tube and add solids to the child's milk diet. The recovery stage is used to educate the mother in the principles of child nutrition and welfare.

Mortality rate varies from 10% to 60%, averaging 15% in those sufficiently ill to be admitted to hospital. Some permanent defect in stature may occur if growth is arrested by malnutrition below the age of 2 years. Study of the effects of malnutrition on neurodevelopment suggests that mild retardation occurs in some malnourished children, reflecting as much the associated social deprivation as malnutrition itself (Grantham-McGregor et al 1991). The liver (Doherty et al 1992) and the exocrine pancreas (Sauniere & Sarles 1988) do not always show complete recovery of function and pancreatic endocrine function is slightly impaired. The appearance of the small intestinal mucosa some years after kwashiorkor is similar to that seen in the rest of the population.

Prevention of protein–energy malnutrition

Prevention of protein–energy malnutrition requires provision of a good supply of food and prompt treatment of gastroenteritis with oral rehydration therapy (Weaver 1994). Prolonged breast-feeding up to 2 years should be encouraged along with the use of locally available protein foods, either in their natural state (e.g. ground nuts, soya beans, etc.) or, as a temporary measure, the use of imported protein supplements such as dried skimmed milk. Early refeeding after episodes of diarrhea is recommended (Brown & MacLean 1984), as renourishment is as important as control of gastroenteritis in preventing undernutrition and reversing weight loss and growth failure (Briend 1990).

The pediatrician can also help in prevention by promoting health education, immunization programs, regular supervision of the child's growth and family planning. The best early indication that a child is at risk is poor growth. Supervision of a child's progress and recording growth at a child health clinic are important tools in the early detection of moderate deficiency, allowing advice and treatment to be given well before florid kwashiorkor occurs. Reviews of various aspects of protein-energy malnutrition in developing and industrialized countries are given in Haschke & Fjeld (1991) and Waterlow (1992). The management of the malnourished child with chronic diarrhea is summarized in Gastroenteritis (p. 1215).

VITAMIN DEFICIENCIES

The dietary sources, biological functions and requirements of vitamins are shown in Tables 21.7–21.10 and in Chapter 37.

Vitamin A deficiency

Xerophthalmia, due to vitamin A deficiency, is a major preventable cause of childhood blindness in many countries of the developing world. Infants born to mothers whose vitamin A nutritional status is low have low hepatic stores and receive breast milk containing reduced quantities of vitamin A. Weaning diets in these countries contain little preformed retinol from animal food and the child must rely on the presence in green and yellow vegetables of β-carotene which can be converted to retinol. Dietary intake may therefore be very low and during acute infections intestinal absorption of the vitamin is also depressed.

Vitamin A deficiency is usually extreme some time before ocular signs appear. In socially and economically susceptible populations, many children have minimal stores of vitamin A, even though there is no clinical evidence of deficiency. Xerosis of the conjunctiva occurs and Bitot's spots (triangular gray raised plaques on the temporal conjunctiva) appear first. The cornea becomes dry and hazy and, untreated, progresses to necrosis and scarring (keratomalacia), occasionally with perforation. Ocular changes are most common in schoolchildren, but the more severe corneal changes are seen in toddlers when there is also associated protein–energy malnutrition (see above).

Apart from the danger of permanent blindness, mortality rate is high in children with both protein-energy and vitamin A deficiency. Conjunctival abnormalities respond to 1–2 weeks'

treatment with oral vitamin A, 3000 μg daily. Treatment should be continued with 1500 μg daily (i.e. about 3–4 times RNI) for some months afterwards to replenish depleted stores. Corneal xerosis should be treated as an emergency. A water-miscible preparation of vitamin A (3000 μg/kg bodyweight) should be given immediately intramuscularly, followed by the same dose orally for 5 days and then 1500 μg daily until the eyes are normal. Associated protein–energy deficiency should be treated at the same time (see above).

Prevention includes vitamin supplementation of mothers, preferably before pregnancy and use of appropriate foods, particularly liver and unskimmed milk products where vitamin A is preformed. Massive oral doses of oily preparations of vitamin A (60 000 μg) may be given every 6 months or so with some success in preventing the appearance of eye signs. There is now evidence that vitamin A deficiency, though not severe enough to cause ocular abnormalities, is associated with a high infant mortality and intervention studies suggest that vitamin A supplementation in susceptible populations can reduce this (Sommer et al 1986, Keusch 1990), as well as morbidity from respiratory infections and diarrheal disease (Filteau & Tomkins 1995).

Vitamin A toxicity can follow injudicious use of vitamin preparations, excessive consumption of fortified breakfast cereals and the ingestion of polar bear liver (which may contain over 600 mg retinol/100 g). Acute poisoning has been described in an adult after a single dose of 100 mg (330 000 IU), characterized by drowsiness, headache, increased intracranial pressure, vomiting and subsequently desquamation of the skin.

Chronic vitamin A toxicity has been reported in childhood after the daily administration of 20 000 μg over a few weeks. It is characterized clinically by dry skin, hair loss, hepatosplenomegaly, headache, joint pains and muscular weakness. Osteoporosis, together with thickening of the long bone shafts and premature epiphyseal fusion, may occur. This condition may be confused with infantile cortical hyperostosis. Plasma vitamin A levels are markedly increased. The prognosis is usually good after vitamin A is withdrawn from the diet, though some deaths have occurred.

Vitamin D deficiency – rickets

Total vitamin D intake is represented by the sum of the intakes derived from ultraviolet irradiation of 7-dehydrocholesterol in skin secretions, ingestion of naturally occurring vitamin D in foodstuffs such as oily fish, eggs and margarine, ingestion of vitamin D-fortified foods including artificial milks, cereals and spreads (Table 21.7) and vitamin D-containing supplements such as multivitamin preparation recommended in the UK for infants and children aged 6 months to 5 years. Exposure of the face alone to sunlight has been calculated to yield 10 μg (400 IU) vitamin D per day, an amount close to the RNI for young children.

Inadequate intake, impaired absorption, defective metabolism of vitamin D and perturbations in the availability or retention of bone mineral substrates may all result in rickets, the features of which are shared with a number of other nonnutritional disorders that may be inherited or acquired (Ch. 20). Diminution of endogenous vitamin D production (through insufficient skin exposure) increases the need for an adequate exogenous source and potentiates the effects of dietary insufficiency.

Lack of vitamin D will impair bone formation and growth so that biochemical and radiological abnormalities may precede the clinical signs. The biochemical features reflect the action of vitamin D in the body and the compensatory changes which occur in a well-defined sequence (Marx 1989).

The absorption of calcium from the gut is impaired, leading to a decrease in plasma calcium concentration. As a result secretion of parathyroid hormone (PTH) is stimulated, leading to restoration of plasma calcium concentration to normal as a consequence of increased bone resorption. Increased PTH secretion, however, also affects renal tubular function so that aminoaciduria and phosphaturia leading to hypophosphatemia occur. Finally, in severe vitamin D depletion, the action of PTH on bone is itself impaired so that the plasma calcium concentration can no longer be sustained and hypocalcemia, which may be symptomatic, supervenes.

The clinical features of nutritional rickets vary with the age of onset. There is, however, an invariable impairment of linear growth and marked hypotonia associated with a protuberant abdomen. The onset of walking may be retarded. In infancy closure of the anterior fontanel is delayed and the bones of the calvarium are thin and soft (craniotabes) leading to a prominent forehead (frontal bossing). Swellings over the costochondral junctions give rise to the so-called 'rachitic rosary'. Deformity of the long bones is typically related to weight bearing and, in toddlers, comprises marked anterolateral bowing of the tibia at the junction of the lower and middle thirds together with an associated genu varum (bow leg) (Fig. 21.7). Marked swellings over the growing ends of the long bones, for example at the wrists, are evident, corresponding to the metaphyseal splaying observed radiologically. Enamel hypoplasia and delayed dental eruption occurs.

In long-standing cases, coxa vara, kyphoscoliosis, Harrison's sulci and pelvic deformities may occur (Fig. 21.8). By contrast, in late-onset rickets in adolescent Asian children, genu valgum (knock-knee) is more characteristic (Fig. 21.9). Rarely, nutritional rickets may present with features of hypocalcemia, namely stridor or seizures associated with positive Chvostek and Trousseau signs.

The most striking biochemical feature is a progressive increase in plasma alkaline phosphatase, presumably reflecting increasing, but ineffective, activity of the osteoblasts. Interpretation of plasma

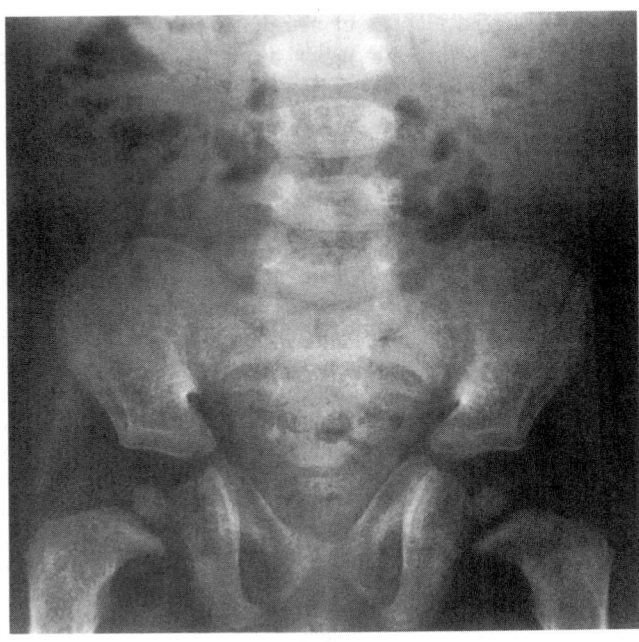

Fig. 21.8 Nutritional rickets. X-ray of 3-year-old girl showing triangular pelvic brim as a result of weight bearing causing acetabular protrusion.

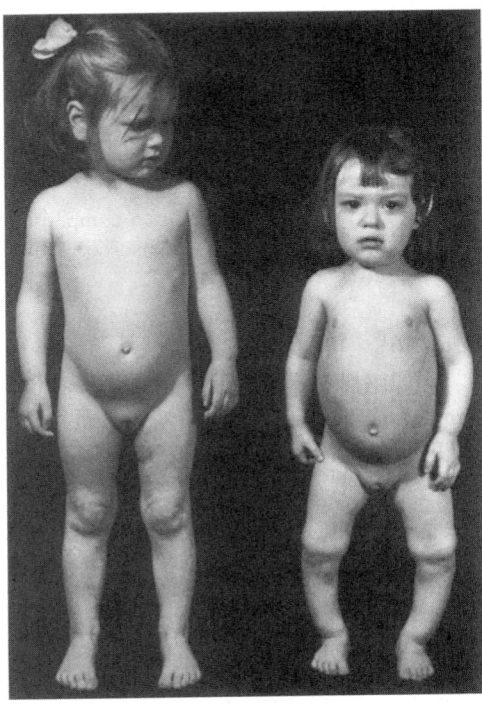

Fig. 21.7 Nutritional rickets. Dwarfing and bowing of legs in an affected girl (right) and a girl of the same age in good health (left).

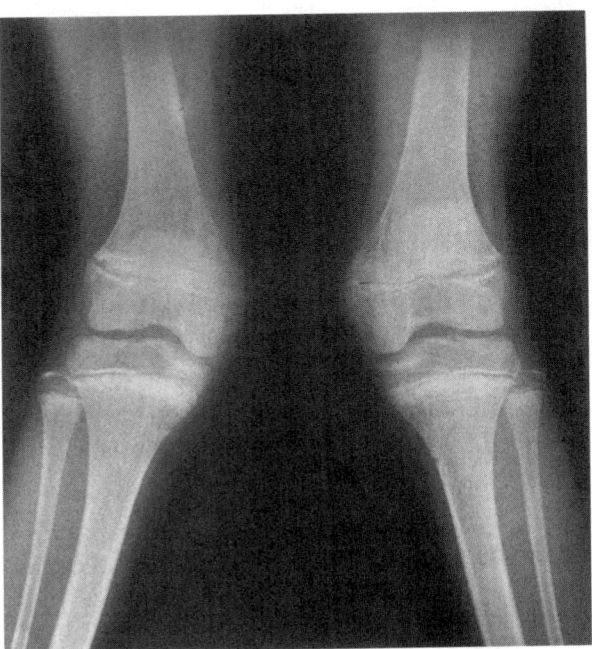

Fig. 21.9 X-ray of knees of adolescent Asian girl with rickets. Marked knock knee (genu valgum) with ill-defined transverse metaphyseal bands are seen.

alkaline phosphatase levels requires knowledge of the normal values encountered in various age groups and an awareness of the increased values which occur at times of rapid bone growth (Ch. 24). Confirmation of vitamin D deficiency can be made by measurement of plasma metabolite levels and a plasma 25(OH)D of less than 20 nmol/l supports the diagnosis. Paradoxically, plasma 1, 25(OH)2D values may be increased in vitamin D deficiency (Rosen & Chesney 1983).

The radiological features of nutritional rickets vary with the disease and the age of the patient (Figs 21.8 and 21.9). They include poor mineralization of both flat and long bones, delayed development of the epiphyses and marked changes in the metaphyses at the growing ends of the long bones in which concave, irregular margins are found together with a greater than normal diameter (cupping, fraying and splaying) (Fig. 21.10). In young children and infants, similar changes may be observed at the costochondral junctions. In advanced cases, the zone of provisional calcification is absent and both cortical greenstick fractures and radiolucent transverse bands (Looser's zones) may occur.

Nutritional rickets will respond to therapeutic doses of vitamin D in the range 25–125 µg (1000–5000 IU) daily. Biochemical improvement may be evident after a few days but radiological healing may not be recognized for 2–3 weeks. Careful biochemical monitoring of plasma phosphorus and calcium concentrations is required to insure that toxicity is avoided. This regime should be continued for at least 4–6 weeks until the plasma alkaline phosphatase values have decreased to within the normal range and a satisfactory radiological response has been obtained. Thereafter vitamin D intakes should be reduced to a maintenance level of 10 µg (400 IU) daily. Healing can be induced with the

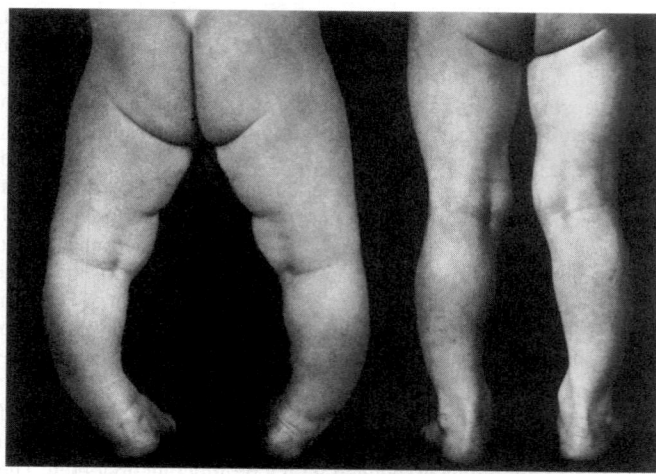

Fig. 21.11 Healing rickets. The legs shown severely bowed in a girl aged 2 years have straightened after 2 years' growth with adequate vitamin D intake.

vitamin D metabolites 25(OH)D and 1, 25(OH)2D, but they have no therapeutic advantage in this context. The resumption of normal bone growth and remodeling with vitamin therapy is usually sufficient to enable spontaneous resolution to occur, providing that there is sufficient residual growth potential (Fig. 21.11). An important corollary to treatment must be the provision of health education and dietary advice coupled with long-term follow-up to prevent recurrence. Identification of any child with nutritional rickets should lead to a search for other children at risk and review of existing prophylactic child health procedures in the community.

Malabsorption

Conditions associated with impaired gastrointestinal absorption of lipids will inevitably impair the absorption of the fat-soluble vitamins, including vitamin D. This may reflect the lack of factors required for the emulsification and digestion of fats in the gut lumen, for example in cystic fibrosis or obstructive jaundice, or alternatively any enteropathy in which mucosal function is impaired, as for example celiac disease (Ch. 11). Treatment requires an increased vitamin D intake to compensate for fecal losses and correction of the underlying disorder. Other causes of rickets are discussed in Chapter 19.

Vitamin D toxicity

Excessive intakes of vitamin D can result in toxicity and ultimately in death. The toxic dose is inversely proportional to the rate of administration so that when given for prolonged periods toxicity may be encountered with intakes of only 50 µg (2000 IU) per day. Clinically, toxicity is associated with anorexia, nausea, vomiting, constipation and failure to thrive. There is marked hypercalcemia and this may be associated with thirst and polyuria. In long-standing cases, metastatic calcification leading to nephrocalcinosis and renal failure may occur (Fig. 21.12). Radiologically, bone density is increased. Electrocardiographic changes, including an elevated S-T segment, may occur.

In addition to toxicity arising from the injudicious use of vitamin D preparations for prophylaxis, vitamin D-fortified milks and foods were thought to have been responsible for the

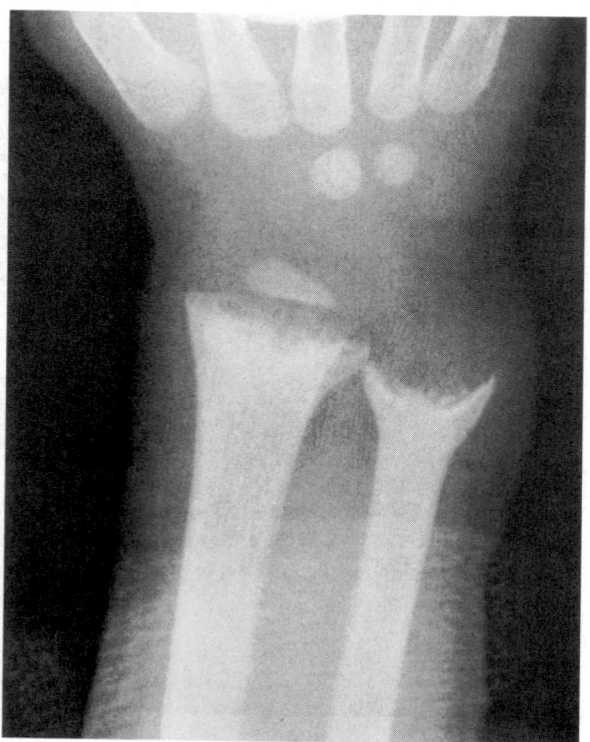

Fig. 21.10 Nutritional rickets. X-ray of wrist showing frayed radial and ulnar metaphyses with slight expansion.

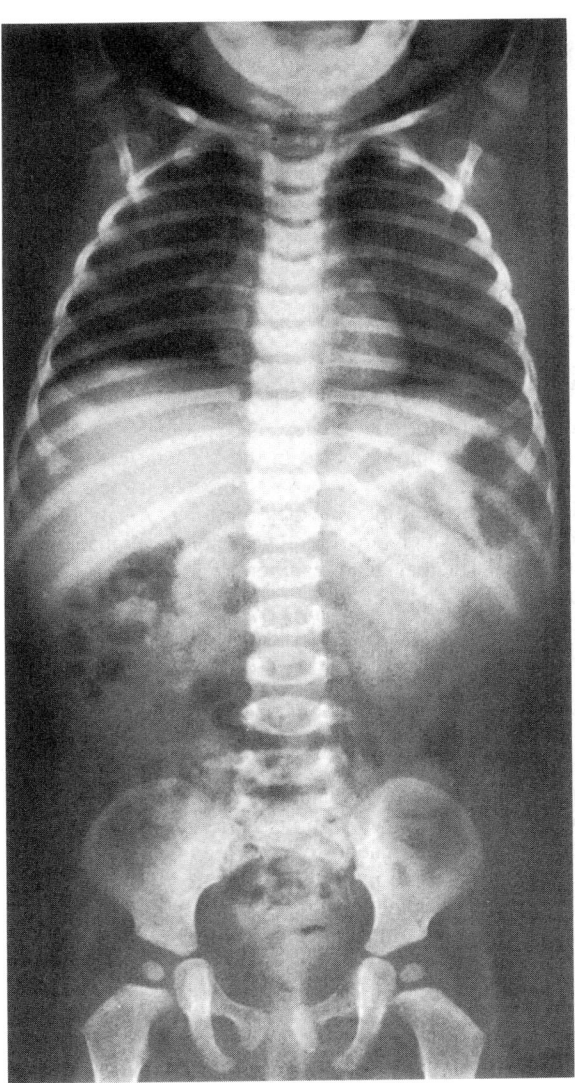

Fig. 21.12 Nephrocalcinosis. X-ray showing extensive bilateral renal calcification in a child with idiopathic hypercalcemia with increased density of spine, thorax and pelvis.

prevalence of idiopathic neonatal hypercalcemia (see Ch. 5). Reduction in the level of vitamin D fortification was associated with a marked decline in the incidence of hypercalcemia, but after a lag of several years, so that it remains uncertain whether there was a causal relationship. Conversely, therapeutic advantage is taken of the hypercalcemic effect of vitamin D in the treatment of vitamin D-resistant rickets, in which doses of the order of 1000 μg (40 000 IU) per day may be used with close supervision and monitoring. The more severe forms of the disorder, associated with an elfin-like facies, mental disorder and supravalvular aortic stenosis (Williams' syndrome), together with peripheral pulmonary aortic stenosis and abnormal dentition, continue to occur, suggesting a perinatal cause or metabolic disorder unrelated to exogenous vitamin D toxicity, but the etiology remains uncertain.

The immediate treatment of vitamin D toxicity requires the use of glucocorticoids, the provision of a low calcium diet and the withdrawal of all sources of exogenous vitamin D. The clinical features may, however, persist long after plasma calcium has returned to normal.

Vitamin K deficiency

The body's normal requirements for vitamin K are met by bacterial synthesis in the large intestine, but deficiency states can occur in the newborn before adequate colonic bacterial colonization has occurred, in malabsorption, in association with a biliary obstruction and after oral antibiotic therapy. Although the vitamin K content of human milk and cow's milk is low, it nevertheless appears to be sufficient for the dietary needs of most infants. It has been estimated that the infant probably requires only 5 μg vitamin K daily, although greater intakes are commonly recommended. The vitamin is involved with hepatic synthesis of the blood coagulation factors, II, VII, IX and X (Table 21.9) and deficiency therefore leads to hemorrhagic states (Ch. 15).

Hemorrhagic disease of the newborn (Ch. 5) occurs more commonly in breast-fed than formula-fed infants, presumably due to the lower content of vitamin K in human than artificial milks. Typically, gastrointestinal hemorrhage, or less frequently intracerebral hemorrhage or bleeding from the umbilical cord stump, occurs at about the third day of life, although presentation may be delayed until the age of 6 weeks or more. Blood loss may be severe and accompanied by shock. Treatment is by blood transfusion and parenteral administration of a water-soluble analog of vitamin K, such as phytomenadione 1 mg.

The disorder is attributed to an exaggeration of the normal diminution in plasma prothrombin content in young infants. Previously vitamin K was given to all infants at birth, but in the UK, owing to concerns about the relation between intramuscular injections and cancer in later life (Golding et al 1992) prophylaxis became restricted in some centers to infants who have been subjected to a traumatic or instrumental delivery. Present recommendations (Expert Committee 1992) are that multiple oral doses should be given to newborn babies, though nationally many other regimes are adopted (Rennie & Kelsall 1994). Infants of mothers receiving hydantoin anticonvulsants and those with prolonged cholestasis, biliary atresia, steatorrhea and parenteral nutrition should receive vitamin K supplementation. Excessive dosage of vitamin K and its synthetic analogs may lead to hyperbilirubinemia and kernicterus. Preterm or G6PD-deficient infants are predisposed to these complications.

Vitamin E deficiency

Vitamin E deficiency is uncommon and is largely restricted to preterm infants and children with malabsorption and steatorrhea. In the former the characteristic feature is a hemolytic anemia occurring at 4–6 weeks of age. The deficiency is enhanced in infants fed milks rich in linoleic acid since this results in a corresponding increase in the polyunsaturated fatty acid content of the erythrocyte membranes. Such erythrocytes are liable to hemolysis due to lipid peroxidation in their membranes by hydrogen peroxide and this forms the basis of a confirmatory laboratory test. A similar effect has been observed in infants fed milks rich in linoleic acid which contain supplementary iron, since this may also act as a lipid peroxidant. It follows that supplementary iron should be withheld from preterm infants unless they are fed milks with an appropriate vitamin E : linoleic acid ratio. In children with abetalipoproteinemia and less commonly with cystic fibrosis, a progressive neuropathy and retinopathy may occur in those with prolonged steatorrhea and fat malabsorption.

Vitamin B₁ (thiamin) deficiency – beri beri

The vitamin B_1 deficiency syndrome, infantile beri beri, is mainly confined to south east Asia and, like the adult form, is associated with a polished rice diet. Infantile beri beri occurs in breast-fed infants of thiamin-deficient mothers. Usually the mothers have no overt signs of deficiency. Probably, the fetus receives diminished amounts of vitamin from the deficient mother during prenatal life and postnatally the baby receives breast milk with a low thiamin content. A faulty maternal diet is therefore responsible, the low vitamin content usually being due to the use of oversoaked or overwashed polished rice.

Most commonly the deficiency presents as acute cardiac failure in a baby a few months old. Other forms of presentation, particularly in older infants, are changes in the cry, with hoarseness and eventual aphonia, or encephalopathy with apathy, drowsiness, convulsions, coma and death. The acute cardiac form with edema may be confused with kwashiorkor (see above), particularly if the child is drowsy, and children with kwashiorkor may have coexisting thiamin deficiency. Ethanol inhibits active transport of the vitamin and in adults thiamin deficiency is associated with alcoholism.

In the cardiac form, a diuresis within a few hours of giving parenteral thiamin hydrochloride – 25 mg i.v. or 100 mg i.m. – is diagnostic as well as therapeutic. This emergency treatment is followed by thiamin hydrochloride 25 mg i.m. daily for 3 days and then 10 mg orally b.d. The mother should be treated at the same time and should receive 10 mg orally b.d..

Vitamin B₂ (riboflavin) deficiency

Deficiency of riboflavin seldom occurs in isolation but is usually associated with other nutritional deficits. The clinical picture is both characteristic and relatively trivial. Features include an angular stomatitis, fissuring of the lips (cheilosis), nasolabial seborrhea and in some cases a painful magenta-colored tongue. Vascularization of the cornea from the periphery has been reported. Mouth lesions in childhood may become infected with monilia, giving rise to the appearance known as *perlèche*. Diagnosis of riboflavin deficiency may be confirmed by measurement of the increase in erythrocyte glutathione reductase activity after addition of flavine adenine dinucleotide. Treatment is with riboflavin 5–15 mg daily in divided doses.

Folic acid deficiency

Deficiency states are all characterized by megaloblastic anemia which, without laboratory tests, is indistinguishable from that of vitamin B_{12} deficiency (Ch. 15). Primary nutritional deficiencies are encountered most commonly in developing countries but folate deficiency may also occur as a secondary complication of increased requirements (in prematurity, malignant disease and its treatment, chronic hemolytic anemias), inadequate absorption in malabsorption syndromes, impaired utilization due to vitamin B_{12} deficiency and as a result of treatment with drugs such as methotrexate, trimethoprim and anticonvulsants. There is strong evidence that the incidence of recurrent and of first occurrence of neural tube defects is reduced after preconceptual treatment of the mother (MRC 1991, Czeizel & Dudas 1992) (Ch. 14). A number of inherited enzyme deficiencies may also impair folate metabolism (Rosenblatt 1989).

Hematological investigation in folate deficiency reveals a megaloblastic anemia, macrocytosis, leukopenia with increased segmentation of the nuclei of the polymorphonuclear cells and thrombocytopenia. Diagnosis is confirmed by assay of the red cell folate content. Treatment is with folic acid 1–5 mg daily with the exception of folic acid antagonist toxicity, in which parenteral folinic acid, the 5-formyl-tetrahydro derivative, is preferred.

Vitamin B₆ (pyridoxine) deficiency

Clinical pyridoxine deficiency is extremely rare. The best documented example occurred in the USA in infants fed with a milk formula which had been subjected to excessive heat sterilization, resulting in destruction of pyridoxal and pyridoxamine, which are more heat sensitive than pyridoxine itself. The principal features were epileptiform convulsions, abnormal EEG and abnormal tryptophan loading tests, all of which responded promptly to vitamin B_6 administration. A similar condition may occur in disorders of gamma-aminobutyric acid (GABA) metabolism.

Pyridoxine dependency should be considered in all persistent seizures in the newborn period in infants in whom hypoglycemia and hypocalcemia have been excluded and for which there is no adequate alternative explanation. Diagnosis and treatment are made by the intravenous administration of pyridoxine 100 mg, preferably with simultaneous monitoring of the EEG. Pyridoxine deficiency also occurs in children that are 'slow inactivators' of INAH, which is a potent antagonist of vitamin B_6, and following penicillamine and hydralazine therapy. Peripheral neuritis occurs in adults, but clinical features in children include weakness, depression, stomatitis, diarrhea and dermatitis.

Nicotinic acid (niacin) deficiency – pellagra

Deficiency of niacin gives rise to pellagra, which occurs principally in communities that subsist on maize. Isolated cases may occur in children treated with isoniazid, which competes with pyridoxal phosphate, in patients with malignant carcinoid tumors, which divert the metabolism of tryptophan to 5-hydroxytryptamine and as a complication of Hartnup disease secondary to impaired tryptophan transport.

Pellagra may occur in children receiving a maize diet. The nicotinic acid in maize is largely unavailable; tryptophan, which can be converted to nicotinic acid in the presence of vitamin B_6, is present in only small amounts and these deficiencies are made worse by machine milling.

The child is usually of school age, has a desquamating pigmented dermatitis affecting exposed areas of the skin, such as the extremities symmetrically, 'Casals necklace' on the neck and both cheeks. Pellagra occurs particularly in South Africa and is often associated with signs of protein deficiency. Dementia and diarrhea are less common than in adults. Pellagra is also seen in toddlers with kwashiorkor (see p. 1192). The skin lesions show the distribution of pellagra rather than the kwashiorkor distribution which is evenly spread over the trunk and proximal limbs and the children are edematous. Although nicotinamide 50 mg t.d.s. is required for the treatment of this disorder, treatment of the associated protein–energy deficiency which has resulted in the growth failure and low plasma albumin is important too.

Vitamin B$_{12}$ (cobalamin) deficiency

Nutritional deficiency of vitamin B$_{12}$ in infancy has been recognized increasingly in Europe reflecting recent maternal dietary trends (Scheenede et al 1994). It may be encountered in strict vegetarians, in infants born of vitamin B$_{12}$-deficient mothers, or as a result of prolonged feeding with either parenteral solutions or unfortified artificial milks based on soya bean isolates.

A congenital inability to absorb vitamin B$_{12}$ from the distal ileum may occur in the first 2 years of life owing to an inability to secrete intrinsic factor, associated with proteinuria and inherited as an autosomal recessive (Imerslund–Grasbeck syndrome). This occurs especially in Scandinavian Lapps and the North African Jewish population (Chanarin 1990). Preterm infants of less than 32–36 weeks' gestation are at risk of developing B$_{12}$ deficiencies as the transfer of maternal cobalamin occurs mainly in the third trimester (Bhatt 1990, Worthington-White et al 1994).

A specific deficiency of one of the transport globulins, transcobalamin II has been described and absent or poor synthesis of cobalamin-dependent enzymes has been reported. Examples of vitamin B$_{12}$ dependency have been reported due to defective synthesis of one or more of the B$_{12}$ coenzymes, methylcobalamin and 5-deoxyadenosyl cobalamin (Linnell & Bhatt 1995, Bhatt et al 1986), and in familial Addison's disease (Bhatt et al 1994).

In later childhood, true juvenile pernicious anemia may occur. This is an intrinsic factor deficiency associated with autoantibodies against the gasric parietal cells (Mirakian & Bottazzo 1994). Malabsorptive disease and resection of the terminal ileum may both interfere with absorption and lead to deficiency (see Short bowel syndrome). Absorption or metabolism may also be impaired by certain therapeutic agents including PAS, neomycin, nitrous oxide, anticonvulsants and the biguanides. Infestation with the fish tapeworm, *Diphyllobothrium latum*, may be associated with vitamin B$_{12}$ deficiency, apparently as a result of utilization of the vitamin by the parasite before absorption from the gut. Clinically the features of vitamin B$_{12}$ deficiency vary with the age of onset and the duration of the disorder; pallor, fatigue, glossitis or a smooth tongue may occur in the adult but splenomegaly and minimal jaundice are less frequent. Neurological complications due to myelopathy (subacute combined degeneration of the spinal cord) may occur with diminished tendon reflexes, loss of vibration sense, ataxia, and an extensor plantar response.

Hematological studies confirm the presence of a megaloblastic anemia, neutropenia with increased segmentation of the polymorphonuclear leukocytes, and thrombocytopenia, so that the picture is indistinguishable morphologically from that of folate deficiency. The plasma vitamin B$_{12}$ content is often below 100 pg/ml (normal, 180–950 pg/ml). The urine and/or plasma contains an excess of methylmalonic acid. A lack of intrinsic factor may be detected by means of the urinary excretion of [57]Co-labeled vitamin B$_{12}$ after oral administration (Schilling test). Impaired absorption results in poor recovery of the label in the urine when the vitamin is given alone, but normal values are obtained when it is given together with intrinsic factor. Failure of absorption may also occur if food cobalamin is not digested properly or the mucosal lysosomes trap the intrinsic factor or transcobalamin II bound cobalamin.

The treatment of vitamin B$_{12}$ deficiency depends on the cause, but all cases require the parenteral administration of the appropriate cobalamin. Simple nutritional deficiency and pernicious anemia respond to small doses of hydroxocobalamin (0.5 mg/day). Response is confirmed by a brisk reticulocytosis, increased circulating red cell mass and cessation of methylmalonic aciduria. After recovery, maintenance therapy with vitamin B$_{12}$ 0.5–1 mg every 2–3 months is required for life in the case of pernicious anemia and the congenital absorption defects, or until such time as the underlying cause has been corrected and/or central nervous system development is complete. Inherited cobalamin disorders (Cbl A–G and Mut^0/Mut$^-$) require more intensive treatment.

Pantothenic acid deficiency

Deficiency of pantothenic acid in man is unknown, as are its normal requirements. There are, therefore, no recommended advisable intakes or recognized deficiency syndromes.

Biotin deficiency

Experimental biotin deficiency in man results in lassitude, anorexia, paresthesiae, pale smooth tongue, anemia and hypercholesterolemia. There is desquamation of the skin. Among the few spontaneous cases of deficiency which have been reported is that of a boy with bulbar poliomyelitis who was fed a raw-egg-containing diet by gastric tube for 18 months. Several rare disorders of biotin metabolism including holocarboxylase and biotinidase deficiency have been described. In these conditions, treatment with oral biotin 10 mg/day is advocated.

Vitamin C (ascorbic acid) deficiency – scurvy

The clinical disorder associated with ascorbic acid is known as scurvy. Symptoms are rare in the first 6 months of life, but reach their peak at 8–9 months of age. Onset may be precipitated by acute infection. The earliest sign of deficiency is petechial hemorrhage in the skin and this may be perifolicular. Subsequently, impaired growth, irritability and unwillingness to be handled are common presenting features. Some degree of hematuria is invariably present. Pallor due to anemia is an inconstant feature. Capillary hemorrhage in relation to erupted teeth may occur and the teeth themselves can become loose. Subperiosteal bleeding at the distal end of the femur may lead to painful swellings of the lower limbs. The child may then adopt the 'frog position' with the thighs abducted and the knees flexed. Disinclination to move the lower limbs may be sufficiently marked to cause pseudoparalysis. Subluxation at the costochondral junctions may occur so that a sharp elevation is felt as the examiner's hand passes laterally from the sternum towards the osseous portion of the ribs. Sudden death has occurred in scorbutic adults.

Laboratory studies are of limited value in diagnosis. Anemia, which may be microcytic or megaloblastic, is an inconstant feature. Plasma concentration and the urinary excretion of ascorbic acid after an oral load are reduced but in practice do not differentiate well from asymptomatic normals with low intakes. Radiologically (Figs 21.13, 21.14) the long bones have a ground glass appearance due to atrophy of the trabeculae and there is thinning of the cortex. At the epiphyses this results in the so-called

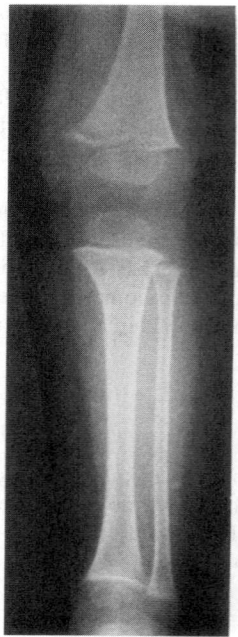 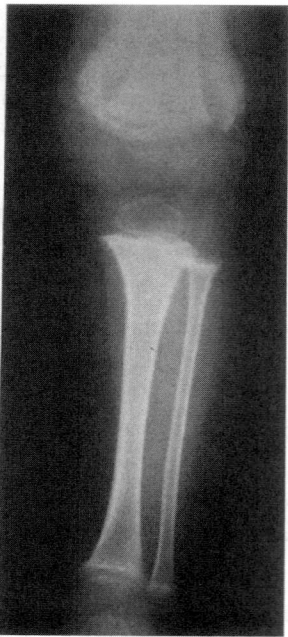

Fig. 21.13   Fig. 21.14

Fig. 21.13   Scurvy. X-ray of legs showing irregularly fragmented dense metaphyseal lines with proximal radiolucent bands and soft tissue swelling around the metaphyses from subperiosteal hemorrhage.
Fig. 21.14   Healing scurvy. X-ray of leg showing irregular dense bands across metaphyses, 'signet ring' epiphyseal centers with dense cortex and radiolucent center and copious callus formation in organizing subperiosteal hemorrhage round distal femoral shaft.

'pencil line', 'halo appearance' or 'ringing of the epiphysis'. A rarefied notch occurs at the lower end of the femur at the metaphysis, giving the 'corner sign'. Epiphyseal separation can occur. Although subperiosteal hemorrhage is not visible as such radiographically, periosteal elevation may be detected. Subsequently, the hemorrhage calcifies giving an appearance similar to the callus surrounding a fracture although it tends to be bilateral and symmetrical in distribution. Treatment is with ascorbic acid orally or parenterally, 300 mg daily.

MINERAL DEFICIENCIES

The dietary sources, biological functions and requirements of minerals are summarized in Tables 21.5, 21.11 and 21.12. Here the clinical features and treatment of the principal mineral deficiencies are outlined. The minerals that are generally regarded as electrolytes (sodium and potassium) and water are not discussed here.

Calcium

Dietary calcium is absorbed from the small bowel, principally in the duodenum. The availability of calcium may be diminished by other dietary components which bind calcium, such as phosphorus, phytate and oxalate. The nature and degree of absorption of other major nutrients, such as fat, carbohydrate and protein, may all modify absorption. Absorbed calcium is distributed through the metabolically exchangeable pool and thereafter is either deposited

in bone (accretion), excreted in the urine or back into the intestine (fecal endogenous excretion).

Nutritional calcium deficiency in childhood rarely occurs in isolation, so that there is limited information covering its sequelae. It has been suggested that deficient intake results in growth retardation, as it does in experimental animals (Nordin 1976). Juvenile osteoporosis has been reported in prepubertal children but does not seem to have a nutritional basis, although the affected children are in negative calcium balance. Impaired absorption of calcium in infancy has been attributed to interactions between dietary calcium and other components of infant milks, for example, the formation of calcium soaps with long chain saturated fatty acids in the intestinal lumen.

The homeostatic control of plasma calcium appears to respond effectively to wide ranges of calcium intake, partly by control of calcium-binding protein synthesis in the cells of the intestinal mucosa and partly by regulation of the accretion and resorption processes in bone. The most frequently reported disturbance of calcium homeostasis which was nutritionally induced was late neonatal hypocalcemia. This most commonly occurred in infants fed formulae based on unmodified cow's milk and was therefore unlikely to be due to deficient calcium intake but to other factors, such as a low dietary calcium/phosphorus ratio (see Ch. 5). Similarly, the disturbances of calcium metabolism associated with rickets and steatorrhea are usually related to vitamin D deficiency rather than to diminished intakes (see above), although rickets due to calcium deficiencies has been described. Marked depletion of body calcium occurs in protein–energy malnutrition but is complicated by several other mineral deficiencies.

Conversely, there is little evidence that excessive intakes of calcium will result in harm apart from the extreme situation of 'milk-alkali' syndrome which rarely occurs in childhood. The etiology of idiopathic hypercalcemia of infancy is unknown and juvenile osteopetrosis (Albers–Schönberg disease – Ch. 24) is an inherited disorder of bone metabolism rather than a nutritional problem. In both cases, however, calcium-restricted diets have been advocated. There is some evidence that individuals with a tendency to urolithiasis may be 'hyperabsorbers' of calcium, in spite of normal dietary intakes, leading to hypercalciuria.

Phosphorus

Phosphorus is contained in virtually all foodstuffs so that isolated deficiency states are virtually unknown. Prolonged treatment with the hydroxides of aluminum or magnesium is one of the few causes of phosphorus deficiency in the human and is due to binding with phosphorus in the intestinal lumen, thus rendering it unavailable for absorption. The effects of such induced phosphorus deficiencies are primarily skeletal, with the development of osteoporosis or rickets. By contrast, soft-tissue phosphate metabolism appears to be unimpaired. Advantage has been taken of the phosphate-binding properties of these agents in the management of hyperphosphatemic states.

Magnesium

Isolated magnesium deficiency of nutritional origin is rare although it is commonly encountered in protein–energy malnutrition and may occur in children receiving inappropriately constituted parenteral nutrition. Diminished absorption may occur after small bowel resection, in malabsorption syndromes, renal failure and hypothyroidism. A rare, selective inability to absorb magnesium, apparently inherited as an autosomal recessive, has been described. Interaction with other dietary compounds resulting in modified absorption can occur in a manner analogous to calcium. Thus, dietary phosphates and phytates are thought to diminish absorption and vitamin D, dietary protein and carbohydrates to increase absorption.

Excessive intakes of magnesium in children are likely to be iatrogenic, from the use of magnesium salts in therapy. Increased absorption from the gut has been described in primary hyperparathyroidism and hyperthyroidism. Clinical problems associated with hypomagnesemia are more likely to represent disorders of homeostasis than nutritional deprivation. In the newborn, hypomagnesemia may result in tetany and convulsions and is commonly associated with hypocalcemia. In these circumstances, administration of calcium may exacerbate the hypomagnesemia, whilst magnesium administration may restore both calcium and magnesium to normal values. Thus, the feeding of very low birthweight infants with a 'preterm' formula containing supplemental calcium and phosphorus has been shown to impair magnesium balance (Giles et al 1990).

Iron

Iron deficiency may result from insufficient dietary intake, impaired absorption or excessive losses. Blood loss most commonly occurs from the gastrointestinal tract and is an important cause of iron deficiency that is easily overlooked. Infestation with hookworm is probably the commonest single cause of severe iron deficiency in children worldwide (Ch. 23). Each of the numerous parasites in the bowel subsists on blood drawn from the host at the site of implantation at the rate of 0.2–0.3 ml/day. At least half the iron contained in this blood loss is excreted unabsorbed so that signs of deficiency rapidly appear. Chronic blood loss from the gut may complicate any ulcerative lesions in the intestinal tract and may also be a feature of hemorrhagic diatheses. Increased intestinal losses of iron occur in celiac disease due in part to increased shedding of mucosal cells from the intestinal epithelium. Some children have been reported to develop significant blood loss from the gut as a reaction to cow's milk protein (Ziegler et al 1990, Sullivan 1993). Chronic blood loss causing iron deficiency may also occur from the renal tract and from the nasopharynx. Less commonly, increased losses in the absence of bleeding may arise from the skin, for example in infantile eczema.

The clinical features of iron deficiency in childhood are almost all related to the concomitant anemia. Pallor is the most common feature and there may be splenomegaly. In extreme cases cardiac failure can occur. The laboratory findings are characteristic so that the red cells are hypochromic and microcytic. The serum iron, serum ferritin and the percentage transferrin saturation are reduced but the free erythrocyte protoporphyrin is increased. Many nonhematological sequelae have been attributed to iron deficiency, including diminished resistance to infection (Smith et al 1989) and poor neurocognitive development (Levitsky & Strupp 1993).

Another nonhematological problem attributed to iron deficiency in childhood is pica, the tendency to ingest nonfood materials. However, not all iron-deficient children manifest this practice and numerous other mineral and vitamin deficiencies have been implicated, together with emotional factors. The prevalence of pica in young children is high and inversely related to age so that it is more likely to represent a normal phenomenon of maturation than an elemental deficiency.

Iron overload

The chronic excessive ingestion of iron leading to iron overload is rare in childhood but may arise from foodstuffs and beverages contaminated at source or in preparation. Acute iron poisoning was formerly common in the UK but has diminished with replacement of ferrous sulfate by less readily ionized compounds as prophylactics in antenatal practice. Repeated blood transfusion for chronic hemolytic anemias such as thalassemia which, together with other advances in management, has greatly improved the prognosis for affected children, invariably results in siderosis with increased deposition of iron in the tissues (Barrett & Treleaven 1991, Rebulla & Modell 1991). The effects of transfusion siderosis can be mitigated by parenteral infusion of an iron-binding agent such as desferrioxamine. A number of rare metabolic disorders resulting in deposition of excessive tissue iron are known, for example, familial hemochromatosis in which reduction in tissue iron sources can be achieved by repeated phlebotomy. Iron overload and associated free radical damage has been reported in infants with rhesus hemolytic disease (Berger et al 1990).

Zinc

The clinical features of zinc deficiency in childhood include growth retardation, hypogonadism, hepatosplenomegaly and anemia. This syndrome has been described particularly in Egypt and Iran where zinc deficiency may have been due in part to impaired absorption as a result of interaction with other dietary components such as phosphates, phytates and calcium, rather than to low zinc intakes. Zinc deficiency may complicate the recovery of children with severe malnutrition (Golden & Golden 1981) and accompany chronic diarrheal disease (Roy et al 1990). Other associations with zinc deficiency have been described, including delayed wound healing, pica, diminished taste acuity (hypogeusia) and hyperkeratotic skin (Hambidge 1993). In severe deficiency states, supplements of 20–40 mg/day elemental zinc have been given, but in marginal deficiency doses of 0.2–0.4 mg/kg may be used.

Acrodermatitis enteropathica (Ch. 25) is a genetic defect that results in failure of zinc absorption and is not a 'nutritional' disorder. Zinc deficiency may produce an almost identical picture in newborn (Plate 21.2) and preterm infants. There is a dramatic response to zinc therapy in both cases.

Copper

Copper deficiency occurs principally in infancy, although it has been reported in children and young adults. Deficiency in normal infants is rare before the age of 5–6 months. It is encountered in protein–energy malnutrition (Lahrichi et al 1991), during prolonged parenteral feeding and as a complication of malabsorption. Deficiency of copper has been reported in prematurity and after prolonged total parenteral nutrition, when anemia, neutropenia, metaphyseal changes and periosteal reactions may occur.

The clinical manifestations of copper deficiency include hypochromic anemia which is unresponsive to iron and neutropenia. Skeletal changes, which are preceded by osteoporosis, include spontaneous fractures, epiphyseal separation and periosteal reactions suggestive of non-accidental injury or scurvy. There is decreased pigmentation of skin and hair and impaired growth. The neurological complications, degeneration of the internal elastic lamina of the great vessels and the growth of abnormal 'kinky' or 'steely' hair do not appear to have been described in pure nutritional deficiency. They may, however, be encountered together with mental retardation, seizures and instability of body temperature in the X-linked autosomal recessive disorder described by Menkes (Ch. 14). This condition is associated with impaired absorption of copper from the gut but is unresponsive to parenteral therapy.

Excessive intakes of copper are unlikely to occur apart from accidental contamination of foods or as a result of accidental poisoning. Abnormal retention of copper is encountered in hepatolenticular degeneration (Wilson's disease), in which deposition in the liver, basal ganglia and cornea lead to hepatic cirrhosis, tremor, personality changes and Kayser–Fleischer rings respectively (Ch. 14). Metabolic studies in this condition have suggested that copper retention is associated with diminished biliary excretion rather than excessive absorption. Now that the gene for Wilson's disease has been found (Petrukhin et al 1993) it will be possible to identify the affected siblings of patients with the disease and to offer appropriate genetic advice and treatment.

Fluoride

The importance of fluoride lies in its interaction with dental enamel, rendering the tooth less liable to caries. The mechanism is not understood, although diminished solubility and enhanced remineralization of the enamel have been suggested. The optimal concentration of fluoride in drinking water for communities which lack other dietary sources of fluoride is thought to be 1 p.p.m. (100 μg/dl) and there is evidence that this will reduce the incidence of caries by up to 50–60% in the permanent dentition and to a slightly lesser degree in the primary dentition.

Drinking waters containing fluoride in excess of 3 p.p.m. are associated with a tendency to increased fluorosis to a degree directly correlated to the water fluoride concentration. In severe cases, associated with fluoride contents of 10–14 p.p.m., permanent dentition becomes mottled with patches of chalky white and a secondary infiltration of yellow or brown staining. The integrity of the enamel is impaired so that pitting of the surface occurs. The osteosclerosis and exostoses of severe fluorosis are unlikely to be encountered in childhood.

Modification of water quality to provide optimal concentrations of fluoride can be successfully achieved by addition of fluoride salts or tertiary phosphates at source. Fluoridation of water supplies has encountered opposition in some communities so that other vehicles, such as table salt, toothpaste, milk, flour and cereals, have been used.

Iodine

The clinical disorder associated with iodine deficiency is described in Chapter 19. Excessive dietary intakes of iodine leading to impaired thyroid function and goiter have been described in communities with a high intake of foods of marine origin.

Chromium

It has been suggested that the impaired glucose tolerance found in children with protein–energy malnutrition may in some cases be related to chromium deficiency and enhanced glucose utilization after chromium therapy has been reported. A relationship between chromium deficiency and maturity-onset diabetes has also been described but there is no comparable evidence in juvenile diabetes. No recommendations for dietary allowances have been made although a tentative adequate intake in the range of 4–100 μg/day has been suggested (Mertz 1991).

Cobalt

The only known function of cobalt is as an essential component of the molecule of vitamin B_{12}. At present, no requirement for free cobalt in addition to that contained in the vitamin has been recognized so that no dietary allowances have been recommended.

Manganese

Although manganese is known to be essential for several animal species, its role in human metabolism remains uncertain. Deficiency in animals results in impaired growth, neonatal ataxia, chondrodystrophy and diminished fertility, but there is no evidence of the occurrence of related conditions in humans. Toxicity can occur in patients with impaired hepatic function receiving manganese in parenteral nutrition solutions (see below).

Molybdenum

The principal biological function of this element is as an essential component of the flavoprotein enzyme, xanthine oxidase, in addition to aldehyde oxidase and sulfite oxidase. Molybdenum deficiency has been described in man but little is known of its requirements. It is present in several foods and legumes; cereal grains, green leaf vegetables and offal are rich sources. Cow's milk contains approximately 7 μg/dl but the concentration varies according to the animal's diet. Human adult dietary intakes are of the order of 50 μg/day, but molybdenum contents of human milk and the dietary intake of children are unknown.

Selenium

Two disorders in man have been attributed to selenium deficiency: Keshan disease, an endemic cardiomyopathy principally affecting children in a defined zone extending from north eastern to south western China, and Kashin–Bek disease, an endemic osteoarthropathy also mainly affecting children in eastern Siberia and parts of China. Although both disorders have counterparts in animals and are reported to have responded to selenium prophylaxis, it is likely that other environmental factors are also involved.

Low selenium values have been reported in preterm infants receiving total parenteral nutrition but the significance of this finding has not been fully established. The nutritional requirements for selenium have not been defined with certainty, but intakes in the range of 10–40 μg/day in infancy have been estimated to be safe and adequate. Human milk contains selenium in the range 0.7–3.3 μg/dl but this may vary with geographical location. Excessive intakes of selenium from foodstuffs and water supplies in highly seleniferous areas have been associated with toxicity in local populations, with gastrointestinal disturbance, hair loss, nail changes and other symptoms (WHO 1987, Liton & Combs 1991).

INBORN ERRORS OF METABOLISM

The primary abnormality in an inborn error of metabolism is in the synthesis or regulation of a protein with important functional properties. This may result in an enzyme deficiency, alteration of the biological properties of a protein, abnormalities of transport mechanisms or alterations in the structure of subcellular organelles. In a typical enzyme defect, substrate accumulates, the normal product is depleted and an abnormal (toxic) metabolite results. For most inborn errors the genetic defect cannot be corrected, but an artificial diet may be used to alter the clinical expression of the disorder. Accumulation of essential precursors may be restricted and/or depleted products of synthesis may be replenished.

For all restricted diets it is absolutely essential that their overall nutritional adequacy is maintained. There must be adequate protein and energy, essential fatty acids and vitamin and mineral supplementation. As many 'natural' food sources as possible should be used. The child's biochemical status and growth must be monitored to ensure the therapeutic effectiveness and nutritional adequacy of the diet.

The principles of the dietary management of maple syrup urine disease, galactosemia, phenylketonuria, urea cycle disorders, organic acidemias, homocystinuria, fatty acid oxidation defects, glycogen storage diseases and hypercholesterolemia are summarized in Tables 21.17–21.25. Table 21.26 summarizes an emergency feeding regime that can be used when normal diet or prescribed feeds cannot be taken because of illness. Chapter 20 describes the management of inborn errors of metabolism in greater depth.

Table 21.17   Principles of dietary management of maple syrup urine disease (MSUD)

Metabolic defect	Principles of dietary management	Dietary modification	Prescribable products
A deficiency or reduced activity of the branch chain 2-ketoacid decarboxylase enzyme complex results in raised concentrations of the branched chain amino acids (BCAA) and their respective keto acids in plasma and urine	• To prevent accumulation of the BCAA: valine leucine and isoleucine • Aim for plasma concentration of: • leucine 100–700 µmol/l • valine 100–400 µmol/l • isoleucine 100–400 µmol/l • Usually plasma leucine concentrations are the most elevated • A few individuals have thiamine-responsive MSUD • Diet is lifelong	• Reduce intake of BCAA by restricted intake of protein-containing foods • Provide at least 120% of RNI of protein by use of AA mixtures free of BCAA • Provide the limited BCAA essential for growth from measured quantities of natural foods (amounts or exchanges of foods containing 50 mg of leucine). These are titrated with plasma leucine concentrations • Although these leucine-containing food exchanges will also contain valine and isoleucine, the dietary management based on the control of the plasma leucine may result in depletion of valine and/or isoleucine. Supplementation of the diet with one or both of these amino acids may be necessary • Energy requirements must be met by use of fats, sugars and low-protein prescribable foods • Poor appetite may necessitate use of NG feeds of BCAA-free AA supplement +/– energy source • Emergency feed regimen required for illness (see Table 21.26)	• Low BCAA infant formulae • Low-protein bread, biscuits, pastas, flour mixes • BCAA-free AA supplements • Vitamin and mineral supplements • Fat emulsion

Table 21.18   Principles of dietary management of galactosemia

Metabolic defect	Principles of dietary management	Dietary modification	Prescribable products
A deficiency or reduced activity of the red cell enzyme galactose-1-phosphate uridyl transferase which converts phosphorylated galactose, derived from hydrolysis of lactose, into glucose	• Maintain erythrocyte galactose-1-phosphate <0.57 µmol/g hemoglobin • Diet is lifelong • During pregnancy, the fetus of a heterozygote mother may benefit from maternal restriction of dietary galactose	• Exclude dietary lactose and galactose, i.e. avoid all milk-containing foods • Use a milk substitute based on soya or casein/whey hydrolysate • Liquid 'shop bought' soya milks are suitable for children >5 yrs of age • During the first year of life, exclude foods containing galactosides: offal, peas, beans, lentils, peanuts, chocolate, cocoa and coconut • Ensure adequate calcium and vit D intake • The CHO source in soya and whey/casein hydrolysates is frequently based on sucrose/glucose–care with dental and oral hygiene • Many medicines and artificial sweeteners contain lactose as a filler. These should always be checked before using or prescribing • Care with alcohol. Ethanol inhibits the elimination of galactose	• Low-lactose infant formulae based on whey/casein hydrolysates or soy protein isolates

Table 21.19   Principles of dietary management of phenylketonuria

Metabolic defect	Principles of dietary management	Dietary modification	Prescribable products
A deficiency or diminished activity of the enzyme phenylalanine hydroxylase which converts phenylanine (phe) to tyrosine This results in a raised concentration of phe and reduced concentration of tyrosine.	• Low phe diet to maintain plasma phe concentration 0–5 yrs 120–360 µmol/l 5–10 yrs 120–480 µmol/l >10 yrs 120–700 µmol/l Preconception and pregnancy 60–240 µmol/l (N phe = 60–100 µmol/l) • Maintain plasma tyrosine concentration within N range (40–100 µmol/l) • Discontinuation of diet no longer recommended	• Reduce dietary phe by restricted intake of protein-containing foods • Phe free amino acid (AA)/protein hydrolysate supplement with added tyrosine to provide protein in amounts: 0–2 yrs 3 gAA/kg/day >2 yrs 2 gAA/kg/day • Limited amount of phe, essential for growth, supplied from measured quantities of natural foods (exchanges of food containing 50 mg phe) such as potato, cereals. The number of food exchanges is titrated against plasma phe concentrations • Energy requirements must be met. Food sources are fats, sugar and low-protein prescribable foods • Natural foods allowed in low phe diet include fruits, most vegetables, fats, oils, sugars • L-tyrosine supplements if necessary	• Low phe infant formulae • Low-protein bread, pastas, biscuits and flour mixes • Phe free AA supplements • Low phe protein hydrolysate supplements • Fat emulsion • Vitamin and mineral supplements

Table 21.20   Principles of dietary management of urea cycle disorders

Metabolic defect	Principles of dietary management	Dietary modification	Prescribable products
Results in a deficiency or reduced activity of one of six enzymes involved in the urea cycle which converts waste nitrogen compounds derived from the degradation of protein foods into urea. Accumulation of nitrogen causes hyperammonemia and raised glutamine – both are neurotoxic	• Restriction of dietary protein to minimize accumulation of waste nitrogen. Supplement with L-arginine (except in the disorder arginase deficiency when accumulation of arginine results) • Provision of drug therapy to provide alternative pathways for the removal of waste nitrogen	See 'Organic acidemias' (Table 21.21) but none of the urea cycle defects have vitamin-responsive forms. If there is poor tolerance to dietary protein and growth is inadequate, supplements of essential amino acids may be used to 'top up' protein intake. Emergency feed regime required for illness (see Table 21.26)	• Low-protein biscuits, flours, pastas and flour mixes • Essential amino acids • Vitamin and mineral supplements • Fat emulsion • L-arginine

Table 21.21   Principles of dietary management of organic acidemias

Metabolic defect	Principles of dietary management	Dietary modification	Prescribable products
Isovalericacidemia (IVA) Methylmalonicacidemia (MMA) Propionicacidemia (PA) A defect in specific enzyme systems results in accumulation of organic acids derived from incomplete protein breakdown, e.g. methylmalonic acid in MMA. Excesses of these organic acids are found in plasma and urine. Plasma amino acid concentrations may be normal though glycine is elevated	• Reduction in total nitrogen intake but ensuring diet supplies sufficient protein, energy, vitamins and minerals for normal growth. Some centers advocate using amino acid supplements which are deficient in the individual precursor amino acids for the organic acidemia, i.e. the inefficient metabolism of valine, isoleucine, methionine and threonine contributes to a proportion of propionate production. These amino supplements can be used to 'top up' the natural protein food allowance if the child's tolerance to protein is very low and growth is poor. Children with IVA are usually more tolerant of protein than those with MMA and PPA • Adequate dietary energy, especially during illness is essential to prevent/minimize catabolism • Some individuals with MMA and PA have a vitamin-responsive form and administration of the respective cofactors, Vit B$_{12}$ for MMA and biotin for PA, may lessen the need for dietary restriction	• Initially reduce dietary protein intake to minimum amounts required for growth (WHO/FOA). If child remains well, gradually increase by increments of 0.2 g protein/kg/day until maximum tolerance is reached. More protein will be tolerated during periods of rapid/or catch-up growth. Dietary protein is measured by allowing a specific number of weighed portions of food which contain 1 g protein • Energy requirements must be met, usually by increased intake of CHO- and fat-containing foods • During illness/infection, protein should be discontinued for 24–48 hours but insure at least 100% EAR of energy is provided. After 48 hours, protein should be gradually reintroduced beginning with 0.5 g/kg/day and increasing by 0.2 g protein increments until tolerance level is reached. 100% EAR of energy must be continued. NG feeds may be necessary • Provide adequate amount of the appropriate vitamin precursor • Emergency feed regimen required for illness (see Table 21.26)	• Low-protein biscuits, flours, pastas and flour mixes • Amino acid mixtures free of the precursor amino acids – valine, threonine, methionine and isoleucine • Vitamin and mineral supplementation • Fat emulsion

Table 21.22 Principles of dietary management of homocystinuria

Metabolic defect	Principles of dietary management	Dietary modification	Prescribable products
Inherited as an autosomal recessive condition. A deficiency or reduced activity of the enzyme cystathionine β-synthase causes accumulation of homocystine and methionine in plasma and urine	• Low methionine diet to reduce/eliminate urinary excretion of homocysteine and derivatives and reduce plasma homocystine to <5 μmol/l • Approximately 40% of individuals with homocystinuria have a pyridoxine-responsive type • Diet is lifelong • Demands for folate are higher. Supplements of 10 mg folic acid daily should be given	• Reduce dietary methionine (meth) by restricted intake of protein foods • Meth-free amino acid supplement to provide 120–150% of RNI for protein • Limited amounts of meth, essential for growth, supplied from measured quantities of natural foods (exchanges of food containing 25 mg meth) such as potato, cereals. The number of food exchanges is titrated against plasma homocystine concentrations • Energy requirements must be met. Food sources are fats, sugar and low-protein prescribable foods • Natural foods allowed in the low meth diet include fruits, most vegetables, fats, oils and sugars • Betaine therapy may allow some relaxation of protein restriction	• Low meth infant formulae • Low-protein bread, pastas, biscuits and flour mixes • Meth-free amino acid supplements • Fat emulsion • Vitamin and mineral supplements (folic acid, vitamin B_6 (pyridoxine)

Table 21.23 Principles of dietary management of fatty acid oxidation defects

Metabolic defect	Principles of dietary management	Dietary modification	Prescribable products
Defects in the mitochondrial oxidative metabolism of fatty acids at any point from transport of long chain fatty acids across the mitochondrial outer and inner membranes to the later dehydrogenase steps of short chain fatty acids. Recognized disorders are deficiencies of carnitine palmitoyl transferases I and II, very long chain, long chain, medium chain, and short chain fatty acyl-CoA dehydrogenases, long chain hydroxyacyl-CoA dehydrogenase and a dienoyl-CoA reductase. They cause encephalopathy, hypoketotic hypoglycemia and an inappropriately high ratio of free fatty acids to ketones under fasting stress. Transferase deficiencies and the long chain defects may cause skeletal myopathy and cardiomyopathy. Broadly similar clinical presentation occurs with deficiency of electron transport flavoprotein (ETF) and electron transport lavoprotein-ubiquinone oxidoreductase (ETF-QO) causing glutaric aciduria type II. Hydroxymethylglutaryl CoA lyase is involved in the final step of synthesis of acetoacetate: deficiency also causes hypoketotic hypoglycemia	• Regular feeding and the avoidance of prolonged fasting • For some disorders, the use of fat supplements of shorter chain length to bypass the metabolic defect • Carnitine supplementation in cases of secondary deficiency • Glycine supplements in glutaric aciduria type II	• Avoid excessive carbohydrate to prevent iatrogenic obesity • For long chain fatty acid oxidation defects and hepatic carnitine transport defects CPT I and CPT II restriction of long chain (C18) fat and supplementation with medium chain fat (C8) may improve muscle strength and reduce hepatic steatosis. These supplements are contraindicated for medium chain and short chain effects • Use of an emergency regimen to provide an adequate carbohydrate source during intercurrent illness (Table 21.26)	• Glucose polymer • Medium chain triglyeride • Carnitine

Table 21.24 Principles of dietary management of glycogen storage diseases

Metabolic defect	Principles of dietary management	Dietary modification	Prescribable products
Type Ia, IaSP, Ib and Id (deficiency of glucose-6-phosphatase or its associated regulatory protein, phosphate transport protein or glucose transport protein). Severe hypoglycemia and lactic acidosis on fasting. Risk of hyperuricemia and hypercalciuria with stone formation. Severe growth failure with inadequate treatment. Longer term risk of renal hyperfusion syndrome and the development of hepatoma Type III (deficiency of debrancher enzyme, amylo-1,6-glucosidase) has less risk of hypoglycemia and of long-term growth failure. There may be skeletal myopathy in early childhood. There is risk of cardiomyopathy in later childhood, usually asymptomatic Type VI (deficiency of hepatic phosphorylase or of one of several phosphorylase kinases). Hypoglycemia is variable and often mild. The presenting feature may be hepatomegaly	• Maintain normoglycemia • Avoid oversupply of glucose causing large swings in blood glucose and paradoxical lactic acidosis. Ensure the nutritional adequacy of the diet as a whole: this can be overlooked in the efforts to avoid hypoglycemia • Prevent hypercholesterolemia and hypertriglyceridemia as a consequence of decreased lipolysis and increased synthesis. Prevent persistent acidosis which can cause rickets by leaching calcium from bone • Management principles for type III are similar to type I. Therapy need not be so aggressive as in type I as there is better tolerance of fasting and no fasting lactic acidosis • Type VI requires regular feeding or no treatment. Increased protein intake may be beneficial	• Frequent (2-hourly) formula feeding by day in very young infants. In older infants supplement formula and solids by giving glucose polymer drinks between meals. From preschool age onwards meals can be supplemented by uncooked cornstarch to provide a source of slowly absorbed carbohydrate (1–2 g/kg) • All children will require continuous gavage feeding overnight to provide glucose at the normal hepatic production rate (0.5 g/kg/h in infancy falling to 0.35 g/kg/h in older children). The continuous infusion must not be interrupted. Avoid rebound hypoglycemia at the end of the infusion period by giving cornstarch or a bolus of the infusate followed by breakfast • In type I restrict dietary fructose (and sucrose) and galactose as these cannot be converted to free glucose. Use a soya-based infant formula or a protein hydrolysate feed • Restriction of fructose or galactose is not necessary in type III • A high protein intake in type III promotes gluconoegenesis	• Low-lactose infant formula or enteral feeds based on whey/casein hydrolysates or soya protein • Cornstarch • Glucose polymers • Allopurinol for hyperuricemia • Calcium and vitamin D may be required for rickets

Table 21.25   Principles of dietary management of hypercholesterolemia

Lipid disorders & hyperlipidemias	Principles of dietary management	Dietary modification	Prescribable products
Polygenic hypercholesterolemia is the commonest abnormality of this group, followed by familial combined hyperlipidemia (type IIB – elevated triglycerides and cholesterol) and familial hypercholesterolemia (type IIA, FH). In homozygous FH total cholesterol levels usually exceed 16 mmol/l; in heterozygotes 8–12 mmol/l. Some heterozygotes may have values as low as 5 mmol/l in early life or as high as 15 mmol/l in adulthood. Homozygotes are very rare; heterozygotes are 1 in 500 of the population. All these predispose to earlier ischemic coronary artery disease. In familial hypertriglyceridemia (type IV) fasting triglycerides are greater than 2.2 mmol/l: risk of peripheral vascular disease is increased. In familial hyperchylomicronemia (type I) triglycerides are 35–100 mmol/l. There is hepatosplenomegaly and risk of recurrent pancreatitis	• For hypercholesterolemia: children over 2 years whose fasting total cholesterol exceeds 5.2 mmol/l should be treated. The aim is lowering of total cholesterol in all patients and to below 6.2 mmol/l in those with higher values at presentation • 'Step 1 diet.' Reduction of total fat intake to no more than 30% of total energy, and saturated fat to less than 10% of total energy without a rise (by substitution) of polyunsaturated fat to more than 10%. Cholesterol intake less than 300 mg/day • 'Step 2 diet.' Will be needed by most children whose total cholesterol level at presentation is >8 mmol/l. Saturated fat should be under 7% of total energy and cholesterol intake under 200 mg/day • For the others: moderate reduction in fat and total energy intake and avoidance of obesity will lower modestly raised triglycerides. The high values in type I require severe total fat restriction of 20–30 g/day or less	• Decreased intake of foods with high fat content. Avoid frying foods; grill instead • Use skimmed or semi skimmed milk and low-fat dairy products • Trim fat from meat products before cooking. Choose poultry (skin removed) and fish. • Restrict intake of high-cholesterol foods such as egg yolk and shellfish • Take care that total energy intake is adequate especially in the younger children who may not increase their unrefined carbohydrate adequately	• Fat-soluble vitamin supplements • Calcium supplements if the fat-reduced milk intake is low. • Folate supplements if bile salt sequestering agents are used • Specific drug therapy: in familial hypercholesterolemia the need for drug therapy is individual and should take into account the family history and other risk factors. In children over 10 years whose total cholesterol exceeds 6.2 mmol/l despite at least 6 months of adequate adherence to a 'Step 2 diet', consider: 1. Bile salt sequestering agents (cholestyramine, colestipol) 2. Fibric acid hypolipidemic drugs and HMG CoA lyase inhibitors have not been approved for use in children • Fish oil preparations and supplementary medium chain triglycerides for familial hyperchylomicronemia

Table 21.26   Emergency feeding regimen for children with inborn errors of metabolism

Age (years)	% CHO solution made from glucose polymer and oral rehydration solution*	Energy/100 ml kcals	Energy/100 ml kJ	Feed volume**
0–0.5	10	40	167	150–200 ml/kg
0.5–1.0	12	48	200	120–150 ml/kg
1–2	12	48	200	95 ml/kg
2–6	20***	80	334	1200–1500 ml/d
6–10	20***	80	334	1500–2000 ml/d
>10	20***	80	334	2000 ml/day

* If child has diarrhea, use oral rehydration solution in combination with glucose polymer. If no diarrhea, use glucose polymer alone.
** Emergency feeds should be administered at 2–3-hourly intervals over 24 hours.
*** A proprietary drink such as Lucozade may be more palatable for the older child.

INFLAMMATORY BOWEL DISEASE

At diagnosis around 75% of children with inflammatory bowel disease (IBD) have lost weight and as the disease progresses malnutrition becomes increasingly marked. The aim of nutritional management is to reverse nutrient deficiencies and growth failure and to provide a diet that will induce and maintain remission of disease.

Ulcerative colitis

Nutritional intervention has a limited role in the management of ulcerative colitis. Traditional wisdom suggests that during a relapse a low-lactose diet may improve diarrhea and colic and some patients are more comfortable on a low-residue diet, albeit at the risk of developing constipation. Parenteral nutrition (see p. 1219) may be used during a severe attack associated with toxic colonic dilatation, for pre- and postoperative nutrition and when the enteral route of nutrient delivery is not possible. There is no evidence that the colitis is improved, but overall nutritional status will benefit.

Dietary supplementation with fish oils rich in ω-3 polyunsaturated fatty acids (PUFA) has been claimed to reduce colonic inflammation in adults (Stenson et al 1992). The rationale is that ω-3 PUFA competes with ω-6 PUFA for δ-6 desaturase, which reduces the production of arachidonic acid from linoleic acid (an ω-6 PUFA) and consequently generates less potent precursors of proinflammatory leukotrienes. Their routine therapeutic use has not been established.

Crohn's disease

Anorexia, malabsorption, chronic inflammation, surgical resection and medical treatment may all result in malnutrition and growth failure in childhood Crohn's disease. There are sometimes specific nutrient deficiencies (iron, folate, vitamin B_{12}, zinc). Improving dietary intake by normal food or specially designed dietary supplements by the oral or nasogastric routes are important aspects of management of this chronic disorder. The aim of nutritional treatment is to restore normal nutritional status and growth using enteral or parenteral nutrition.

O'Morain and colleagues (1983) used an exclusively elemental diet for 6 weeks to induce clinical remission in predominantly small bowel Crohn's disease in children. Numerous subsequent studies (Seidman et al 1991) have shown an improvement equivalent in potency to a course of corticosteroids at inducing a remission of symptoms, enteric protein and lymphocyte loss and improvements in various clinical and laboratory test scores of disease activity. Whole liquid protein diets may be as effective as amino acid-based formulae, but this has not been shown in all comparative studies. Small bowel disease probably responds better than Crohn's colitis.

Children treated with elemental diets show improved growth in comparison with those treated with corticosteroids but may relapse earlier. Most pediatric gastroenterologists do not believe that specific foods induce a relapse and recommend rapid return of patients to a normal diet while encouraging a high energy and protein intake.

Elemental diets are unpalatable and hyperosmolar and are best given by nasogastric tubes, aiming at 75 to 80 kcal/kg ideal body weight per day with gradually increasing concentration, volumes and infusion rate over 3 to 7 days. Twelve-hour overnight infusion allows normal school attendance (see Enteral nutrition, p. 1217). The optimal duration of treatment is not established but 6 to 8 weeks usually induces remission. Why these diets reduce intestinal inflammation remains unclear but an adaptive response to bowel rest, immunological changes from decreased intraluminal antigens and nutritional improvement are possible factors.

Parenteral nutrition (PN), with its dangers, expense and limitation of patient activity, is only rarely required, as for example when intestinal obstruction or fistulae make the enteral route impossible or ineffective. Extensive small bowel resection resulting in dependency on total parenteral nutrition (TPN) is rare in childhood Crohn's disease. Management of the child on PN is outlined at the end of this chapter.

CYSTIC FIBROSIS

The nutritional management of cystic fibrosis (CF) aims to prevent malnutrition by anticipating and treating nutrient deficiencies that occur as a result of inadequate intake, malabsorption, chronic lung disease and other complications of the basic defect in transepithelial chloride transport (Table 21.27) (Chs 11, 12). There are several reasons why children with CF become malnourished: exocrine pancreatic insufficiency leading to malabsorption and increased nutrient losses, chronic lung disease leading to increased energy requirements (in excess of intake), small intestinal enteropathy and hepatobiliary disease (Table 21.28) (Shepherd et al 1991). Early diagnosis and prompt treatment, including a high-energy/high-fat diet, are associated with improved growth and outcome (Corey et al 1988, Dalzell et al 1992) and most children now survive well into adulthood.

Nutritional management

A dietitian should work with the pediatrician to make a careful

Table 21.28 Physiological disturbances leading to special nutritional requirements in cystic fibrosis

Pancreas and liver	Pancreatic insufficiency from birth resulting in diminished enzyme secretion with maldigestion of fat, complex carbohydrate and protein. Intraluminal sequestration of bile acids leading to reduction in bile salt pool and deficient solubilization of fat
Small intestine	Defect in active and passive absorption related to abnormalities of absorptive cell membrane structure and function
Energy metabolism	Increased energy expenditure related to basic defect and respiratory infection

assessment of nutritional status at diagnosis. A clinical nurse specialist can also provide invaluable support and advice to the family at home during this time (Nicholson 1992) and thereafter care should be the responsibility of a team that includes both. Although many infants are underweight at diagnosis, most achieve normal weight-for-age by 12 months (Weaver et al 1994). Clinical evaluation comprises measurement of bodyweight, length, head circumference, mid upper arm circumference and skinfold thicknesses, all of which should be plotted on appropriate centile charts. The chest should be X-rayed and blood taken for full blood count and film, baseline liver function tests and serum proteins. Nutritional assessment should include quantitative fat balance studies or, in centers where this is not possible, stool fat output can be assessed using the 'steatocrit' method or by fecal fat microscopy (Walters et al 1990). Stool chymotrypsin can be measured as an index of exocrine pancreatic function (Brown et al 1988). Vitamin and mineral deficiencies can occur early (Reardon et al 1984) and serum concentrations of the fat-soluble vitamins A, E and D should be measured at diagnosis and thereafter annually (see below). Trace elements are not routinely measured but this may be necessary in the severely malnourished child.

Milks for infants with CF

The choice of milk for the infant with CF depends on a number of factors, which include an understanding of the pathophysiology of exocrine pancreatic insufficiency (Green et al 1995). Breast-feeding has been widely advocated for the baby who is clinically well because human milk has an optimal essential amino acid and fatty acid content and the presence of taurine is particularly

Table 21.27 Principles of dietary management of cystic fibrosis

Aims of dietary management	Dietary modification	Prescribable products
• To achieve optimal nutritional status	• Aim to provide 100–150% of RNI for energy	• Energy supplement, e.g. Maxijul, Polycal, Caloreen
• To promote normal growth and development	• Use of dietary supplements if unable to achieve satisfactory growth on high-energy diet	• Protein-energy supplements, e.g. Fortisip, Fortimel, Ensure Plus, Entera, Fresubin
	• Use of nasogastric/gastrostomy feeds if above unsuccessful	• Enteral feeds, e.g. Nutrison Paediatric Standard, Nutrison Energy Plus, Elemental 028 Extra, Nutrison Standard, Pediasure, Ensure, Ensure Plus
	• Routine provision of fat-soluble vitamins A, D and E	
	• Use of pancreatic enzyme replacement therapy if indicated	

important because of its role in bile acid conjugation. In addition human milk contains a range of protective factors, trophic factors and digestive enzymes, including amylase and lipase, that may compensate for diminished pancreatic secretion.

However, human milk has a lower protein content than infant formulae and exclusive breast-feeding has been associated with failure to thrive and in a few cases with hypoproteinemia, edema, anemia and electrolyte depletion. In spite of these potential but rare problems, breast-feeding should be encouraged as long as adequate intake is ensured.

Infants with CF who are not breast-fed can thrive satisfactorily on normal infant formula (Holliday & Allen 1991) with adequate pancreatic enzyme replacement therapy (see below). If infants fail to gain weight satisfactorily, glucose polymers such as Maxijul (Scientific Hospital Supplies), Polycal (Cow & Gate-Nutricia) or Caloreen (Clintec) can be added to the feed. Glucose polymers have a low osmolality and are added in 1 g/100 ml increments to provide a total of 12 g carbohydrate/100 ml of feed. If further energy supplementation is required, long chain lipid emulsions, such as Calogen (SHS), can be added to provide a total of 5 g fat/100 ml feed. Duocal (SHS), a combined fat and carbohydrate supplement, may be used as an alternative energy supplement which can be added to infant formula. Many infants with CF consume large volumes of infant formula (150–200 ml/kg or more) (Holliday & Allen 1991), despite apparently adequate enzyme replacement.

Infants who require surgery for meconium ileus may develop a temporary disaccharide intolerance and protein hydrolysate milks such as Pregestimil (Bristol-Myers), Nutramigen (Bristol-Myers), Peptijunior (Cow & Gate-Nutricia) and Prejomin (Milupa) can be used (Farrell et al 1987). Pancreatic enzymes are still required with protein hydrolysate formulae, even though they contain a higher proportion of their fat as medium chain triglycerides. Occasionally a modular feed, such as comminuted chicken (Cow & Gate-Nutricia), with additional carbohydrate, fat, vitamins and minerals, may be necessary in infants who have undergone major surgery and fail to tolerate hydrolyzed protein formulae.

The infant with CF may become dissatisfied with breast milk or infant formula alone and solids should be introduced at 3 months of age to ensure an optimal intake of energy and protein. Parents are encouraged to give a normal to high fat intake to ensure adequate growth.

The child and adolescent

Elevated resting and total energy expenditure in children with CF (Girardet et al 1994) and excessive fecal losses require that total energy intake should be well above RNI. Despite improved pancreatic enzyme replacement therapy, fecal energy losses can be as high as 10–20% of energy intake (Murphy et al 1991). As the child gets older and pulmonary disease develops, with increasingly frequent episodes of infection, energy and protein requirements increase, but appetite declines in the face of anorexia, dyspnea and treatment. The older child may also become nitrogen depleted with muscle wasting and hypoalbuminemia because of excessive loss of protein in sputum and feces and on account of the chronic inflammatory response to lung disease.

In conjunction with pancreatic enzyme supplementation, RNI of energy and protein should be at least 150%, with fat representing around 40% of energy intake, to maintain positive nutrient balance (Morrison et al 1994). This can be achieved by adding high energy and/or protein supplements (glucose polymers and fat emulsions, such as Polycal and Calogen) to feeds or high energy and protein supplements (such as Fortisip) and in children whose requirements cannot be met by mouth, using nasogastric tube or gastrostomy feeding (see Enteral nutrition, p. 1218). Parenteral nutrition is sometimes indicated in severe undernutrition, as for instance after neonatal surgery and in preparation for heart–lung transplantation.

Pancreatic enzyme supplements

Neither pancreatin powders nor enteric-coated microsphere enzyme preparations are designed for administration with human milk. Pancreatin powders should be mixed with a little expressed breast milk and given at the beginning of each feed. Enzyme on the infant's lips may not only cause skin irritation, but also irritation of the mother's nipple. Enteric-coated preparations can be mixed either with expressed breast milk or formula or with fruit puree and given from a spoon. They should never be added to feeds. The advantage of the enteric-coated microspheres is that their enzyme contents are protected from hydrolysis in the stomach (Stead et al 1987). In older children enzyme supplementation should be 'titrated' against growth, nutritional status and stool fat or can be determined using fecal fat collection or other measures of fat balance (see above). There is no clear upper limit to the dose of enzymes, but caution has been aroused by reports of colonic strictures in association with high dose supplementation (Smyth et al 1994).

Vitamin, mineral and essential fatty acid supplements

Infants most at risk from fat-soluble vitamin deficiency are those with poorly controlled malabsorption, poor dietary compliance, liver disease, bowel resection or following late diagnosis. Bone demineralization can occur in children with CF but rickets is rarely seen, probably because dermal synthesis of vitamin D accounts for more than 80% of normal requirements. Vitamin E is a powerful antioxidant and hemolytic anemia has been reported in newly diagnosed infants. Clinically obvious vitamin K deficiency, presenting as hemorrhagic disease, is unusual in infants with CF and supplementation is not routinely undertaken unless there is evidence of liver disease (Scott-Jupp et al 1991).

Fat-soluble vitamins should be provided from time of diagnosis at levels of at least twice RNI: vitamin A 4000–8000 IU, vitamin D 400–800 IU and vitamin E 50–100 mg/day (Rayner 1991). Because there is no single vitamin preparation to provide all three vitamins in appropriate quantities, multivitamin preparations with additional vitamin E are usually prescribed. The water-soluble vitamins (B group and C) are not usually deficient but may be given as part of a multivitamin supplement.

Iron absorption is usually normal in infancy and iron supplements are not routinely prescribed in the first year. Low serum levels of trace elements, including selenium and zinc, have been reported (Walters et al 1990) and supplementation is not recommended routinely in early life, but may be necessary in childhood or adolescence.

Essential fatty acids are required for neurodevelopment and membrane synthesis and function and may be malabsorbed in the infant with steatorrhea, contributing to the enteropathy of CF (see above). Signs of essential fatty acid deficiency (desquamation, poor wound healing, thrombocytopenia) are rarely seen and supplementation beyond that recommended for inclusion in modern standard formulae is probably unnecessary in infancy.

Infants who have persistent diarrhea or fail to gain weight despite seemingly adequate diet and pancreatic enzyme supplementation should undergo jejunal biopsy to exclude celiac disease. This may occasionally also reveal partial or complete deficiency of lactase activity. Gastroesophageal reflux occurs more frequently in cystic fibrosis (Scott et al 1985). Treatment includes thickening of feeds, Gaviscon and sometimes cisapride.

LIVER DISEASE

Chronic liver disease leads to malnutrition from a combination of anorexia, metabolic disarray, diminished hepatic synthesis and fat malabsorption. Severe malnutrition (weight and/or height <2SD of mean) affects 50% of children with cirrhosis (Beath et al 1993). Improving nutrition not only improves quality of life, growth and development but also prognosis after hepatic transplantation (Moukarzel et al 1990, Charlton et al 1992). Anthropometric assessment must include measurement of skinfold thicknesses and mid upper arm circumference, as fluid retention (ascites and edema) and organomegaly make weight an unreliable index of growth (Sokol et al 1990) (see Nutritional assessment, p. 1186).

Appropriate early dietary advice may delay nutritional failure but aggressive intervention using nasogastric tube feeding is indicated when triceps skinfolds and mid arm circumference fall below the 10th centile (Chin et al 1992). Energy intake is increased by providing up to 6–8 g of fat and 15–20 g/kg of carbohydrate per day. A gradual increase in concentration and volume minimizes problems related to hyperosmolality (see Enteral nutrition, p. 1217).

Steatorrhea associated with reduced intraluminal duodenal bile concentration is improved by substituting 40–75% of dietary long chain triglyceride with medium chain triglyceride which is not dependent on micelle formation for absorption. At least 500 mg/kg per day of essential fatty acid is required to avoid deficiency.

Hepatic encephalopathy is usually a late event in chronic cholestatic liver disease and up to 4 g/kg per day of protein is required to avoid protein catabolism and more for growth. Vegetable protein is claimed to be less likely to produce hepatic encephalopathy than animal protein. Branched chain amino acids, which are metabolized in skeletal muscle, may be used as dietary supplements and in at least one report improved nutritional state, though not hepatic encephalopathy (Chin et al 1992).

Fat-soluble vitamin supplementation (vitamins A, D, E and K) is essential but there are unresolved problems relating to suitable preparations for young children. Up to 20 times normal daily oral intake may be required or use of special water-soluble preparations or parenteral therapy. Table 21.29 gives suggested doses and methods of monitoring. Hemorrhagic disease from vitamin K deficiency is life threatening and in severe cholestasis initial therapy should be parenteral. The vitamin K analog menadiol is water soluble but should not be used in jaundiced neonates or patients with G6PD deficiency or vitamin E deficiency. 25-hydroxycholecalciferol is better absorbed than ergocalciferol and is therefore preferred for this reason and not impaired hepatic hydroxylation. Water-soluble vitamin E (α-tocopherol PEG 100 succinate) is well absorbed and appears safe in the short term, but is not yet licenced for use in children.

Nutritional causes of liver disease are discussed in other chapters and include Indian childhood cirrhosis (copper), veno-occlusive disease (plant alkaloids) and parenteral nutrition-associated cholestasis.

DIABETES MELLITUS

The aims of dietary management are to optimize blood sugar concentrations (avoiding swings between hyper- and hypoglycemia), to ensure normal growth and development and to allow for variable exercise patterns, but without provoking obesity. It is the dietitian's role to teach the family how to establish sensible eating habits which take into account the need for strict glycemic control within the family's normal diet (Johnston & Maclean 1992). The diet should aim to minimize the development of complications such as microvascular and cardiovascular disease. A full account of the etiology and management of childhood diabetes mellitus is found in Chapter 19.

Nutritional requirements

Diabetic children have the same basic nutritional needs as nondiabetics. The eating plan may consist of a diet based on a 10 g carbohydrate exchange system, an unmeasured diet using 'healthy eating' or a plate model system. Fifty percent of dietary energy should be derived from carbohydrate (mainly fiber-rich polysaccharides), 35% from fat and 15% from protein (Nutrition Committee of BDA 1982, 1992). However, the distribution of energy between carbohydrate, fat and protein will differ according to age (Nutrition Committee of BDA 1989). Breast-fed infants will obtain approximately 55% energy from fat, 5% from protein and 40% from carbohydrate, whereas a 5-year-old may derive 35% energy from fat, 15% from protein and 50% from carbohydrate. The distribution of carbohydrate within the diet should balance the dose of injected insulin. A preprandial blood glucose concentration of 4–8 mmol/l is ideal. Meals should be consumed 30 minutes after insulin injection (unless blood sugar concentration is low).

Table 21.29 Fat-soluble vitamins used in the management of cholestatic liver disease

Vitamin	Daily dose (oral)	Plasma concentration	Assessment
K1(Phytomenadione)	5–10 mg		Prothrombin time
D (25-OH cholecalciferol)	5–7 µg/kg	25–30 ng/ml	Plasma Ca, P, Alk phosphatase X-ray metaphysis
A	5000–20 000 IU	400–500 µg/l (depends on plasma proteins/retinol binding globulin)	Dark adaptation
E	10–100 mg/kg	Vitamin E/Total lipid ratio >1.59 µmol/mmol	Peripheral nerve conduction, RBC hemolysis with peroxide

It is more practical, in most instances, to cover additional activity with extra carbohydrate because a child's energy expenditure is so variable, although insulin doses can be reduced before strenuous, prolonged exercise, particularly in older children. Extra carbohydrate given before exercise need not be in the form of sweets, but these may be favored by the child. The amount required will depend on the activity, the time of day in relation to insulin injections, the usual diet and the individual child. Blood sugar testing enables the family to gauge this.

Hypoglycemia

Families should know how to recognize and treat hypoglycemia. Low blood sugars are likely to occur during or after exercise, if insufficient carbohydrate is eaten or if there is a long delay between injection and eating. Glucose drinks such as Lucozade and glucose tablets (Dextroenergy) can be used to treat hypoglycemia; jam, honey or syrup can also be used. Hypostop (glucose gel) can be squirted into the mouth if the child is not conscious or is unco-operative. If hypoglycemia occurs just before a meal or snack then sufficient fast-acting carbohydrate should be given to alleviate symptoms and food given soon after. If the next food is not due for an hour or more it is important to use a back-up of slower-acting carbohydrate to prevent the blood sugar falling again. Regular episodes of hypoglycemia suggest that the eating plan and the dose or timing of insulin injections are out of balance and the regimen needs to be reviewed.

Infection

During periods of illness and infection children often do not want to eat. Blood sugar concentrations tend to be high and the insulin doses should be increased accordingly. Rapid-acting insulin may also be used through the day and carbohydrate intake needs to be adjusted according to the insulin dose. If the usual diet is refused it is not essential to replace all the carbohydrate, but realistically 70–80% of the usual intake should be the aim. Small frequent doses of rapidly absorbed carbohydrate, preferably as a liquid, are often best tolerated.

Dietary issues

Diabetic products are not recommended. They are often expensive, unpalatable, not always low in fat or calories and often contain the sugar substitute sorbitol which has a laxative effect. Low calorie drinks are an asset and other low sugar products marketed for the general population are useful. 'Sensible eating' should be advocated, without the inclusion of 'special foods'.

Toddlers and adolescents require special attention. The former can be faddy eaters and food refusal is common. Parents worry about maintaining good HbA1C levels with the accompanying risk of hypoglycemia. Force feeding is not recommended and the child's falling blood sugar concentration usually causes hunger and a desire to eat.

It is common for adolescents to snack and eat out in the evening and appropriate advice should be given. Advice about alcohol and its hypoglycemic effect will be necessary for most teenagers. Adolescent girls have a tendency to become obese and eating disorders may become a problem. Regular and continued dietetic advice is essential in order that the child's diet is appropriate for his or her continuing and changing nutritional needs.

CONGENITAL HEART DISEASE

Congenital heart disease (CHD), particularly complex anomalies and those associated with cyanosis and heart failure, can lead to failure to thrive. CHD may also, in some cases, be part of a syndrome including growth retardation and undernutrition, such as congenital rubella infection or fetal alcohol syndrome.

CHD leads to failure to thrive by a number of mechanisms: anorexia and dyspnea reduce food intake and the energy required for growth may not be met in the face of increased cardiac and respiratory work. Malabsorption may occur from vascular compromise of the gut and fluid restriction, because of heart failure, may lead to suboptimal milk intake. Overall increased resting energy consumption is probably the principal cause of growth failure in infants and children with CHD and they can become grossly underweight and continue to be so, in spite of apparently adequate intake, until the cardiac defect is corrected (Poskitt 1993).

Nutritional management must aim to provide at least 150 kcal/kg per day (often more) with the use of energy supplements to milk feeds and energy-rich foods to older children. Nasogastric feeding is often required (Barton et al 1994) (see Enteral nutrition, p. 1218).

JUVENILE CHRONIC ARTHRITIS

The etiology of nutritional impairment in juvenile chronic arthritis (JCA) is related to poor dietary intake, the disease itself and its treatment. Anorexia is not uncommon, mediated, it is thought, by high circulating levels of the cytokines IL-1 and TNF-α. Articular disease, particularly affecting the temporomandibular joint and the small joints of the hands, can make chewing and handling food difficult and painful. Corticosteroids and other anti-inflammatory drugs will also suppress appetite.

Nutritional impairment is most commonly protein–energy malnutrition, which occurs in 20–50% of children with JCA (Henderson & Lovell 1989), in addition to deficits in calcium, iron, zinc and selenium (Bacon et al 1990). These are reflected in decreased circulating concentrations of albumin and prealbumin, anemia and iron deficiency. Blood levels of IL-1 and TNF-α are often raised and IGF-1 is depressed. Growth hormone concentrations are usually normal.

Children with JCA are frequently underweight with decreased muscle mass, under height-for-age (with subnormal BMI and MUAC) and have decreased growth velocity. Growth failure is most common in systemic JCA, but can also affect children with polyarticular and pauciarticular disease.

The goals of nutritional treatment are to replete protein losses and stores by providing a protein and energy intake of up to 150% RNI and to reverse mineral and vitamin deficiencies. Elimination diets have been tried in the treatment of JCA because of the frequently reported aggravation of symptoms after the ingestion of certain foods (see Food allergies and intolerances, p. 1213) and up to 60% of children are treated with 'alternative (often vegetarian) diets': it is essential to ensure that their full nutrient requirements are met with these. There is also current interest in the possibility that polyunsaturated fatty acids (PUFAs) may have an anti-inflammatory effect in JCA. Arachidonic acid and eicosahexaenoic acid are precursors of prostaglandins and marine oils (rich in PUFAs) have been used to suppress inflammation (Cleland et al 1995). Whatever dietary intervention is used, growth and nutritional status should be monitored (see Nutritional assessment, p. 1186) with regular measure of weight, height, growth velocity, MUAC and serum albumin.

RENAL DISEASE

The kidney regulates the volume and composition of the extracellular fluid and in renal disease where there is a change in glomerular filtration rate, or tubular function, the homeostasis of this fluid composition becomes increasingly difficult to maintain. Complications of this metabolic derangement ensue, causing abnormalities in hematological, skeletal, endocrine, neurological and nutritional status. Chapter 17 includes a full account of the management of renal disease in children.

The dietary management of childhood renal disease is aimed at correcting the electrolyte and fluid imbalance, alleviating or preventing clinical problems such as metabolic bone disease and cardiac arrhythmias, avoiding catabolism and promoting optimal growth (Watson 1995). Choice of dietary prescription will depend on whether the disease is acute or chronic and the stage of the disease. Dialysis will also affect nutritional status and dietary modifications will be influenced by the length of time it is required and technique employed. Tables 21.30 and 21.31 summarize nutritional modifications recommended in the management of chronic and acute renal failure.

CONSTIPATION

The causes, investigation and treatment of constipation are dealt with in Chapter 11. The dietary management of constipation in childhood usually requires an increase in the consumption of dietary fiber and fluid. Medication that increases fecal bulk and stimulates the large bowel is often not enough alone to restore normal large bowel habit: hard dry stools require hydration to be passed easily and the colon functions best when it receives from the small intestine a significant amount of nonabsorbable polysaccharide (Weaver 1992).

The fiber content of the diet should therefore be increased. With the help of a dietitian, intake of high-fiber foods that the child likes (beans, raisins, fruit) should be maximized (Fulgoni & Mackay 1991). High fiber breakfast cereal, fruit, vegetables, whole grain products and wholemeal bread should become a major part of the diet of the whole family. Adequate fluid intake must be insured, as the effect of both dietary fiber and stool-bulking agents (such as lactulose) is to draw water into the large bowel and thereby soften the stool.

Recommendations for dietary fiber intake in childhood have not been clearly defined (see Nutritional requirements, p. 1183) but Table 21.32 provides a guide, based on a daily intake of fruit, vegetables and grains. Healthy intakes of dietary fiber should range from 8–10 g/day in children from 1 to 3 years to 14–16 g/day in those of 7–10 years.

SHORT BOWEL SYNDROME

Short bowel syndrome follows excision of a significant portion of the small intestine, leading to malabsorption, diarrhea and growth

Table 21.30 Principles of dietary management of chronic renal failure

Age (yrs)	Energy based on expected weight	Protein based on actual weight	Fluid	Other considerations
Conservative management and hemodialysis				
0–0.5	115–150 kcal/kg/d	2.1 g/kg/d		Phosphate: Dietary restriction usually necessary – aim for plasma phosphate 1.5–1.9 mmol/l
0.5–1.0	95–150 kcal/kg/d	1.5–2.0 g/kg/d	20 ml/day + urinary output	Potassium: Dietary restriction usually necessary – aim for plasma K 3.0–5.0 mmol/l
1.0–2.0	95–120 kcal/kg/d	1.0–1.8 g/kg/d		
>2.0	Minimum of EAR	1.0–1.5 g/kg		Vitamins: Water-soluble supplement only + vitamin D as 1-α-calciferol
Peritoneal dialysis				
0–0.5	115–150 kcal/kg/d	2.1–3.0 g/kg/d		Phosphate, potassium: As above but often less restriction is necessary
0.5–1.0	95–150 kcal/kg/d	2.0–3.0 g/kg/d	20 ml/day + urinary output + fluid loss in dialysate	Vitamins: as above
1.0–2.0	95–120 kcal/kg/d	2.0–3.0 g/kg/d		Monitor weight. Glucose is absorbed from the dialysate fluid and can contribute to energy intake. Protein can be lost in dialysate, extra dietary protein may be necessary
>2.0	Minimum of EAR	2.5 g/kg/d until puberty 2.0 g/kg/d during puberty 1.5 g/kg/d postpuberty		

Table 21.31 Principles of dietary management of acute renal failure in children not receiving dialysis

Age (yrs)	Energy based on expected weight	Protein based on actual weight	Fluid	Other considerations
0–2	95–150 kcal/kg/d	1.0–1.8 g/kg/d	20 ml/kg/day + previous day's urinary output	Potassium: may need restriction. Aim for plasma K 3.0–5.0 mmol/l
>2	Minimum of EAR	1.0 g/kg/d	20 ml/kg/day + previous day's urinary output	Restriction of phosphate and sodium may be necessary

Table 21.32 Guide to daily dietary fiber intake in childhood

Food	Serving size	1–3 years		4–6 years		7–10 years	
		Minimum recommended servings	Dietary fiber content	Minimum recommended servings	Dietary fiber content	Minimum recommended servings	Dietary fiber content
Fruit	$\frac{1}{2}$–1 (small)	2	2–4 g	2	2–4 g	2	2–4 g
Vegetables	$\frac{1}{4}$ cup	2	2 g	2.5	2.5 g	4	4 g
Grains	1 slice bread 1 cup dry cereal	2	4 g	4	8 g	4	8 g
Total			8–10 g		12.5–14.5 g		14–16 g

failure. Survival without parenteral nutrition is rare when less than 15 cm of small intestine remains after resection (Schwartz & Maeda 1985). Other factors which determine outcome are whether the jejunum or ileum was resected (the latter has greater powers of adaptation, the unique ability to absorb vitamin B_{12} and bile acids and has a longer transit time) and whether the ileocecal valve was preserved (Ch. 11).

Following extensive intestinal resection there is massive diarrhea which requires intravenous fluid and electrolytes. This usually lasts days and is associated with an increased transit rate and gastric hypersecretion (Hyman et al 1986). It is followed by a period of gradual intestinal adaptation when there is growth in length and diameter of the remaining bowel and mucosal hypertrophy (Ziegler 1986). Total parenteral nutrition (TPN) is required during this phase (Dorney et al 1985) (Table 21.33) (see below). Intestinal adaptation may continue for months, but maximal adaptation is usually achieved by 3 years of age in the infant who suffers neonatal intestinal resection.

Nutritional support

Enteral feeds should be introduced cautiously: while they may encourage mucosal growth and function they also stimulate

Table 21.33 Summary of management of short bowel syndrome

Phase I	Intravenous fluids and electrolytes
Phase II	Total parenteral nutrition
Phase III	Enteral feeds
	Elemental
	Lactose free
	High protein/low fat
	Fat- and water-soluble vitamins
	Supplement Ca^{++}, Mg^{++}, Zn^{++}, Fe^{++}
	Folate and vitamin B_{12}, especially if loss of ICV
	Restrict oxalates – risk of renal calculi
	Drugs H_2 antagonists
	Antimotility agents – loperamide
	Cholestyramine
	Somatostatin analogs
	Trophic agents Pectin
	Glutamine
	Short chain fatty acids
	Epidermal growth factor
	Home parenteral nutrition + ORS
	Surgical Antiperistaltic segments
	Colonic transposition
	Reconstruct ileocecal valve
	Recirculating loops
	Intestinal transplantation

intestinal and pancreaticobiliary secretion which, with gastric hypersecretion, rapid transit rate and loss of mucosal enterokinase, can contribute further to diarrhea. Therapies that may facilitate a trophic response of the mucosa include the use of pectin (to delay gastric emptying and intestinal transit and a substrate for production of SCFA), glutamine (preferential fuel for enterocytes) and SCFAs themselves (energy source that can be absorbed in the colon). However, none of these has been systematically demonstrated in human studies to be beneficial in children with short bowel syndrome (Booth 1994, Jenkins & Thompson 1994).

Feeds should be elemental, of high protein and low fat (composed of a protein hydrolysate and medium chain triglyceride) and lactose-free initially (Ch. 37). They should also contain adequate fat- and water-soluble vitamins and minerals, particularly calcium, magnesium, iron and zinc. Dietary oxalates should be restricted to reduce the risk of nephrolithiasis (Earnest et al 1974). As the child grows modular feeds may be used (see Enteral nutrition, p. 1217).

Weaning from PN to enteral feeding should be done gradually and methodically, changing one thing at a time (e.g. loperamide should not be stopped and cow's milk formula feeds introduced at the same time): the infant with short bowel syndrome is very susceptible to setbacks in growth and bowel habit. Close attention should be paid to weight gain, stool volume, nutritional status and fluid–electrolyte balance. Oral rehydration solutions can be used to replenish electrolytes lost in the stool.

Drugs and outcome

H_2-antagonists (cimetidine or ranitidine) and proton-pump inhibitors (omeprazole) may help to reduce gastric hypersecretion. Vitamin B_{12} supplements are necessary after terminal ileal resection. Antimotility agents such as loperamide may be effective, but should be used with care (Weaver et al 1984). Cholestyramine is indicated if there is evidence of bile acid diarrhea after ileal resection. Somatostatin analogs have been used in some intractable cases (Dharmasathaphorn et al 1982), but they require parenteral administration and have many unwanted effects on the endocrine system.

Properly managed, most infants climb back into the normal weight range by their third year, albeit on the lower centiles. They should be followed through childhood with particular attention to fat assimilation and vitamin B_{12} and fat-soluble vitamin status.

Failure to support infants with short bowel syndrome on enteral nutrition has led to attempts at surgical treatment aimed at slowing intestinal transit time or increasing absorptive surface area, by the reconstruction of the ileocecal valve, interposition of colon or antiperistaltic segments or recirculating loops (Thompson & Rikkers 1987). Small bowel transplantation offers hope to the infant who remains totally dependent on parenteral nutrition (Vanderhoof et al 1992).

FOOD ALLERGY AND INTOLERANCE

Food allergy and intolerance can be difficult to diagnose. Adverse reactions to foods are classified in four ways: allergies, defects in enzyme systems, psychological intolerances and pharmacological intolerances (RCP/BNF 1984). A fuller account of the immunological basis of food allergy may be found in Chapter 27 and of enzyme defects in Chapter 20. In general true allergic responses to foods are manifest as anaphylaxis, in the skin as eczema or urticaria and in the respiratory system as rhinitis and asthma. Food-intolerant reactions usually manifest themselves in the gastrointestinal system as protein enteropathies, failure to thrive, diarrhea and vomiting and in the central nervous system as migraine and possibly behavioral disorders (Minford et al 1982, RCP/BNF 1984, David 1993).

The dietary management of adverse reactions to food should be planned in a structured way based on clinical findings and must always be supervised by a clinician and a pediatric dietitian working as a team. No child should have foods excluded from his or her diet unless there is a clear indication for doing so and after the offending food(s) have been removed there has been a clear improvement in symptoms. It is also important to consider whether the child has severe enough symptoms to warrant dietary manipulation and to appreciate that any dietary change, if it is to be effective, requires compliance. The carer(s) of the child must be committed and fully understand the modifications to the dietary regimen advised. Noncompliance renders the diet or trial useless. Figure 21.15 outlines a guide to dietary exclusion choices.

Choice of diet

The initial choice of diet will depend on the severity of the symptoms, if the provoking foods have produced an immediate reaction and the age of the child. A food diary may help to identify offending foods but in practice it rarely adds to what can be elicited from a detailed dietary history.

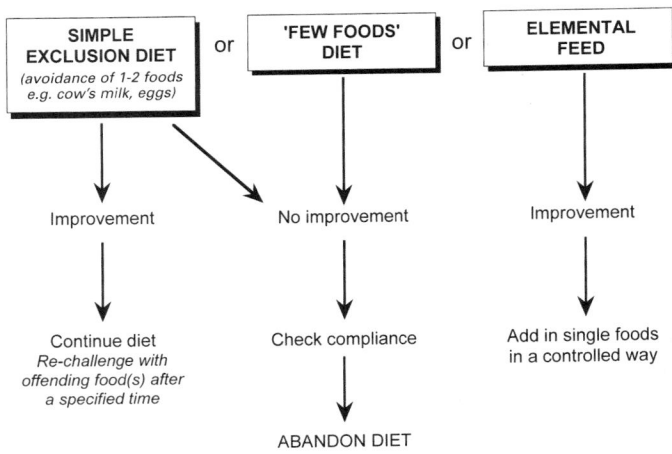

Fig. 21.15 Flow chart to plan dietary exclusion program.

Simple exclusion diet

If the reaction has been immediate and the provoking food is not a dietary staple it may be quite unimportant nutritionally. However, rapid-onset reactions can be life threatening and appropriate dietary advice should be given so that all likely sources of the food are avoided. This is particularly true of peanuts, which may be a 'hidden' constituent in ingredients labeled only as 'vegetable oils'. Parents need to be aware of this.

If the offending food is a dietary staple, such as wheat or milk, appropriate substitute foods must be used so that nutrient deficiencies are avoided. Practical dietary advice should be given with regard to how the food can be completely avoided and ways in which recipes and family meals can be adapted. It is not appropriate to simply prescribe a milk substitute for an infant who is already receiving solid foods. Dried milk powder is a common constituent of manufactured infant foods and milk-based foods such as butter, yogurt, ice cream and milk puddings are often part of the diet of infants and toddlers.

'Few foods diet'

When three or more foods have to be avoided, particularly those that are frequently eaten, such as cow's milk, eggs, wheat and soya, it is often easier to recommend foods that can be safely eaten rather than expect the carer(s) of the child to cope with complicated lists of ingredients which must be checked each time before a food is eaten. Usually the 'few foods diet' is based on one meat, one vegetable, one fruit, one carbohydrate and one fat. A milk substitute may also be allowed (Table 21.34). This diet is restrictive and monotonous and it takes a great deal of imagination to introduce variety within the allowed foods. Advice should be given for menu planning for meals, snacks and recipes using the allowed foods. These diets can be expensive and this aspect should be discussed with the family at the outset of treatment.

The 'few foods diet' should be given only for an agreed time, usually from 1–4 weeks. Thereafter single foods can be introduced every 2–5 days, the time interval determined by the child's history.

Elemental feeds

These should be reserved for children who have severe symptoms or who have not responded to the choices of diet summarized above, in spite of 100% compliance. Elemental or hypoallergenic formulae are unpalatable and often need to be administered via a nasogastric tube (see Enteral nutrition, p. 1217). It is essential that

Table 21.34 Example of a 'few foods' diet

Meat	Turkey or lamb
Vegetable	Cabbage or cauliflower
Starch	Rice or potato
Fruit	Apple or pear
Fats	Milk-free margarine, olive oil
Milk substitute	Casein or soya hydrolysate

A vitamin and calcium supplement will be required if a milk substitute is not taken. Ketovite tablets and Ketovite liquid are suitable vitamin supplements. Calcium gluconate is a suitable calcium supplement.

the required amount of these formulae is taken otherwise energy and other nutrient deficiencies can arise (Dorf 1989). The volume of feed expected to be consumed should be made clear to the older child and if this proves impossible a nasogastric tube should be passed or the feed discontinued.

Food challenges

Whatever the choice of diet, at some time foods that have been avoided should be reintroduced back into the child's diet in a controlled way. Food challenges can be open, blind or double blind. The risk of anaphylaxis should be assessed: infants are at particular risk and it may be necessary to admit the child to hospital for food challenge.

In whatever way the food challenge is given, it should replicate the way the food is generally taken. Initially very small quantities of the food are administered and the amounts slowly increased over a number of hours or days until a normal portion size is taken. If, however, hospital admission is necessary for the challenge, a very small amount of the food (e.g. 5 ml of cow's milk) can be given and the quantity increased every 15–60 minutes until a reasonable amount (such as 100 ml) is taken. However long the challenge takes, the child should always remain on the exclusion diet until it has been proven that the provoking food can be safely reintroduced.

ENTEROPATHIES

Dietary management may be specific, as in the exclusion of gluten in celiac disease (Ch. 11), or nonspecific, as in the management of the syndrome of protracted diarrhea/failure to thrive in infancy (see below). Severe malnutrition may necessitate the use of parenteral nutrition exclusively or in combination with enteral nutrients, followed by a gradual reintroduction of enteral feeds. In enteropathies with an associated secretory diarrhea, the intravenous route may be necessary to provide a substantial proportion of the water and electrolyte requirements. Table 21.35 lists the properties of an ideal diet for the management of enteropathies. No one feed has all of these attributes. Table 21.36 lists the dietary managements of the common childhood enteropathies and Table 37.14 (p. 1942) some of the formulae available. Certain basic physiological and pathophysiological principles guide the choice of formulae.

Protein

The rate of absorption of amino acids from a protein hydrolysate is greater than that from a mixture of free amino acids owing to an active carrier-mediated transport for oligopeptides and the

Table 21.35 Properties of ideal diet for management of enteropathies

1. Easily digested and absorbed
2. Low antigenicity
3. Low osmolality
4. Palatable
5. Liquid form available for tube feeding
6. Nutritionally complete
7. Modular (quantity of individual nutrients can be independently varied)
8. Simple feed preparation (parental use)

Table 21.36 Principles of dietary management of childhood enteropathies

Disease	Dietary management
Celiac disease	Wheat, barley, oats excluded
Cow's milk protein/soya enteropathy	Milk protein free (use protein hydrolysate or in refractory cases elemental diet)
Intestinal lymphangectasia (congenital or acquired)	Low fat (+/– MCT) – ensure adequate LCT to avoid EFA deficiency
Sucrase-isomaltase deficiency	Low sucrose diet
Hypolactasia	Low lactose (milk and most milk products)
Congenital glucose-galactose malabsorption	Exclude all carbohydrate other than fructose for infants (tolerance for other carbohydrate increases with age)
Abetalipoproteinemia	Low fat – avoid MCT if possible (vitamin E 100 mg/kg and large doses of vitamin A,D,K)

competitive inhibition of neutral amino acids. Amino acid solutions are of higher osmolality than whole protein or oligopeptide mixtures of equivalent nitrogen content so the latter are preferable if antigenicity is not a problem. Some food proteins may be tolerated better than others. Human milk protein is not usually available in large enough quantities to be a practical alternative for bottle-fed infants with a cow's milk protein enteropathy and there is a high degree of cross reactivity with protein in other ruminant milks and even some plant proteins such as soya. A chicken meat-based formula is sometimes better tolerated than casein hydrolysates in these infants (Larcher et al 1977).

Fat

Substitution of some dietary long chain triglyceride (LCT) with medium chain triglyceride (MCT) is commonly employed as MCT does not require bile acid micelle formation for absorption, is semi-independent of pancreatic lipase and is absorbed directly into the portal venous system, avoiding the enteric lymphatics. However, there are certain problems with MCT oils; they are unpalatable, hyperosmolar, laxative, have slightly fewer calories per gram than LCT, do not contain essential fatty acids and have a low flashpoint for cooking. A dietary MCT/LCT ratio of 60:40 is optimal in most situations.

Carbohydrate

Small intestinal brush border disaccharidase activity is commonly impaired in postinfective and immune-mediated enteropathies (see below). The β-galactosidase, lactase, is the first to be affected and the last to recover and lactose should be excluded from enteral feeds of infants with these disorders. The use of an oligosaccharide, of 15–20 glucose units length, is popular and justified by the relatively good survival of the enzyme for its hydrolysis, maltase-glucoamylase, in various enteropathies and its distribution throughout the small intestine. The disaccharidases are more maximally distributed in the proximal small intestine.

Apart from lactase activity, the rate-limiting step for carbohydrate absorption is the transport of monosaccharide into the enterocyte. The use of both the glucose-galactose and the fructose pathways has a theoretical advantage but in practice is not often beneficial. In congenital glucose-galactose malabsorption a fructose-based, glucose and galactose-free feed can be dramatically successful. Frequent testing of watery stools for unabsorbed carbohydrate following dietary changes (Kerry & Anderson 1964) is a useful guide to management. Practical aspects of the nutritional management of enteropathies are summarized in Enteral nutrition (p. 1217).

GASTROENTERITIS

The etiology, investigation and treatment of gastroenteritis are outlined in Chapter 23. The basis of treatment is rehydration and in most cases in the developed world, children return rapidly to normal diet with negligible adverse effect on nutritional status. In the developing world diarrheal disease is a major cause of growth faltering (Fig. 21.5) and, together with the undernutrition that follows, contributes to the high childhood mortality seen in the under-5s (see Protein–energy malnutrition, p. 1191).

The nutritional management of the infant and child with diarrheal disease aims to return the child to a normal diet as soon as possible and if there has been weight loss, to ensure that dietary intake meets requirements for catch-up growth. Present recommendations are that the breast-fed infant should continue on mother's milk during hydration whereas the formula-fed infant should receive oral rehydration fluid alone. When diarrhea stops the formula-fed infant should return relatively quickly to full-strength feeds (see Ch. 23) and the older child to solid diet. In the conditions discussed below dietary modifications are indicated.

Postenteritis syndrome

The infant or child that continues to have diarrhea after adequate rehydration and appropriate specific treatment, or who relapses after resumption of normal feeds or diet, is described as suffering from postenteritis syndrome. This is usually due to a persistent enteropathy of the small intestine and is usually manifest as lactose intolerance and/or milk protein intolerance.

Lactose intolerance

Because lactase (the enzyme responsible for hydrolyzing lactose, the principal carbohydrate in mammalian milks) resides at the tips of the villi, it is particularly vulnerable to damage by enterobacteria and viruses. Secondary lactase deficiency leads to lactose malabsorption with watery, frequent stools in which lactose and glucose (reducing substances) may be detected. Treatment of lactose intolerance requires a lactose-free diet. In the infant this may be achieved using a soya-based formula or a protein hydrolysate. Lactase deficiency can persist for weeks or months and a lactose-free diet should therefore be used for an appreciable duration (during which time the small intestinal mucosa heals) and then cow's milk or cow's milk-based formula reintroduced slowly.

Cow's milk protein intolerance

In some cases intolerance to dietary proteins can also coexist. This is thought to be due to a direct, toxic or immune-mediated reaction of food protein antigens with the intestinal mucosa (Ch. 27), and is manifest by persistent diarrhea, sometimes with blood in the stool. It may follow continued feeding with whole cow's milk or formula containing cow's milk or soya proteins. Treatment requires the use of a protein hydrolysate (see Enteral nutrition, p. 1217) such as Pregestimil (Mead Johnson), Prejomin (Milupa) or Peptijunior (Cow & Gate-Nutricia), which contain, instead of whole protein, peptides and amino acids. Such formulae should be used for several weeks until normal diet is cautiously resumed.

Persistent diarrhea

Persistent, intractable, chronic diarrhea of infancy is defined as diarrhea (more than two watery stools per day) for more than 2 weeks, with no gain in bodyweight. It may be caused by a range of congenital and acquired conditions (Rossi & Lebenthal 1984) (Ch. 11) and treatment consists primarily of nutritional support. Total parenteral nutrition (TPN) is usually required, following rehydration and restoration of electrolyte balance, while a diagnosis is made. It is advisable to continue with TPN until the infant's weight has returned to near normal growth centiles. Thereafter enteral nutrition may be used, depending upon the underlying diagnosis.

A detailed account of the nutritional management of persistent diarrhea in the developing world is outside the scope of this chapter. It is almost always associated with protein–energy malnutrition and treatment should aim to replenish lost weight and generate catch-up growth (see Protein–energy malnutrition, p. 1193). Nutritional treatment is often based on traditional or home available foods and undertaken outside hospital (Bhutta & Hendricks 1996). The single most effective strategy for preventing diarrhea in infancy remains breast-feeding. Cereal-based rehydration solutions may bridge the gap between rehydration and renourishment (Lancet 1992) and soft cereal or vegetable-based weaning foods are used, beginning with around 75 kcal/kg/day rising to 150 kcal/kg/day or more.

In idiopathic intractable diarrhea of infancy in the developed world, lactose-free protein hydrolysates are usually used in the first instance. These should be given in a volume and strength sufficient to meet both fluid requirements and energy and protein needs for growth (see Nutrition support, p. 1217). Human milk (Macfarlane & Miller 1984) and modular feeds (Lo & Walker 1984) have also been used and prognosis depends largely on early institution of nutritional support and the nature of the underlying disease.

PRINCIPLES AND PRACTICE OF NUTRITION SUPPORT

NUTRITION SUPPORT TEAM

There have been a number of surveys of the prevalence of undernutrition in hospitalized children. In an English children's hospital it was found that 16% of children were severely stunted, 14% were severely wasted and a further 20% were at risk of severe malnutrition if nutritionally stressed (Moy et al 1990). Comparable findings have been reported from Scotland (Hendrikse et al 1996), Canada (Merritt & Suskind 1979) and the USA (Parsons et al 1980). Poor nutrition is not only a consequence of specific diseases, as outlined above (Table 21.37),

Table 21.37 Diseases of childhood often associated with protein-energy malnutrition

Low birthweight
Short bowel syndrome
Cystic fibrosis
Mucosal disease of the gastrointestinal tract
   Celiac disease
   Recurrent gastroenteritis
   Milk protein enteropathy
   Soy protein enteropathy
   Tropical sprue
   Allergic gastroenteritis
   Persistent diarrhea
   Immune deficiency disorders
Chronic liver disease
Inflammatory bowel disease
Juvenile chronic arthritis
Chronic renal disease
Congenital heart disease
Burns and trauma
Anorexia nervosa
HIV infection and AIDS
Malignant disease

Table 21.38 Principal reasons why children become malnourished

Medical reasons
- Disease-related malabsorption
- Increased energy needs
- Altered taste perception
- Reduced ability to suck, chew or swallow
- Physical or mental disability

Hospital-specific factors
- Meals missed due to investigation or treatment
- Food served that takes no account of disability
- Lack of nursing supervision at meal times
- Reduced absorption following surgery

Social and psychological factors
- Poverty and disadvantage of family
- Chronic pain, depression or apathy

Table 21.39 Causes and effects of starvation or undernourishment

- Children are more vulnerable to malnutrition following trauma or major surgery and during infection
- Apathy and depression lead to loss of morale and will to recover
- Loss of muscle power (including respiratory and cardiac) occurs
- Impairment of immune response to infection occurs
- Recovery time is prolonged with need for high-dependency nursing care

but is also a feature of most chronic illnesses, follows major surgery and occurs when patients are unable to eat or make proper use of their diet (Lennard-Jones 1992). Children can also become malnourished for nonmedical reasons, such as inappropriate or missed hospital meals (Table 21.38).

There is a vicious cycle between chronic disease and malnutrition (Fig. 21.16) and undernutrition is associated with an increased risk of infection, poor muscle function (including cardiac and pulmonary muscle function), delayed mobility, retarded growth and prolonged admission to hospital (Table 21.39). It has been estimated that the cost of treatment of malnourished patients that develop complications in hospital is four times that of well-nourished patients that develop complications (Lennard-Jones 1992). Because of the recognition of the effects of undernutrition on health and recovery from illness, injury and operation, nutrition support has developed as an integral part of the care of sick children both in hospital and the community (Elia 1993).

As clinical nutritional care becomes more complex the skills required to deal with the details of assessment, prescription, administration and monitoring of treatment increasingly fall

outside the expertise of a single practitioner. Nutrition support should be provided by a team, led by a pediatrician trained and experienced in clinical nutrition, comprising dietitians, nutrition nurse specialists, a pharmacist in charge of the preparation and prescription of parenteral solutions, a biochemist responsible for monitoring biochemical outcome and a surgeon with experience of gastrostomies and insertion of intravenous long lines for parenteral nutrition (PN) (Puntis & Booth 1990). Introduction of nutrition teams is associated with a reduction of mechanical, metabolic and infection-related complications of TPN, shorter duration in hospital and decline in the cost of nutrition support (Lennard-Jones 1992).

Nutrition support may be provided either enterally or parenterally. Before starting nutrition support it is important to make a proper assessment of the patient's nutritional status and nutritional needs (see sections on Nutritional assessment (p. 1186) and Nutritional requirements (p. 1180)). The enteral

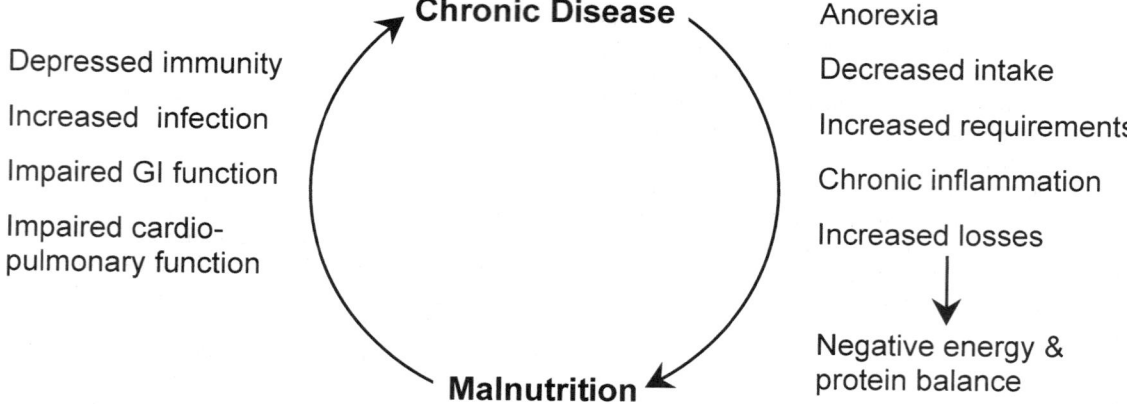

Fig. 21.16 Vicious cycle of chronic disease and malnutrition.

NUTRITIONAL ASSESSMENT

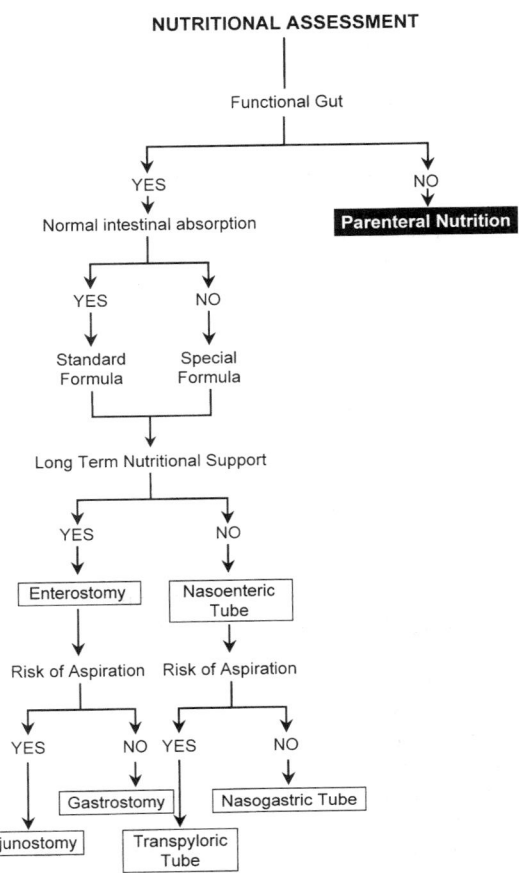

Fig. 21.17 Algorithm for choice of route for delivery of enteral feeds.

Table 21.40 Disease of children in which enteral nutrition may be indicated

Gastrointestinal disease
- Short bowel syndrome
- Inflammatory bowel disease
- Pseudo-obstruction
- Chronic liver disease
- Gastroesophageal reflux
- Glycogen storage disease types I and III
- Fatty acid oxidation defects

Neurological disease
- Coma and severe facial and head injury
- Severe mental retardation and cerebral plasy
- Dysphagia secondary to cranial nerve dysfunction, muscular dystrophy or myasthenia gravis

Malignant disease
- Obstructing disease
- Head and neck
- Esophagus
- Stomach
- Abnormality of deglutition following surgical intervention
- Gastrointestinal side-effects from chemotherapy and/or radiotherapy
- Terminal support care

Pulmonary disease
- Bronchopulmonary dysplasia
- Cystic fibrosis
- Chronic lung disease

Congenital anomalies
- Tracheoesophageal fistula
- Esophageal atresia
- Cleft palate
- Pierre Robin syndrome

Other
- Anorexia nervosa
- Cardiac cachexia
- Chronic renal disease
- Severe burns
- Severe sepsis
- Severe trauma

route should be used if the gastrointestinal tract is intact, accessible and functional. Parenteral nutrition should be reserved for conditions where enteral nutrition is not possible or suitable or nutrient requirements cannot be maintained via the gut alone (Fig. 21.17).

ENTERAL NUTRITION

The indications for enteral nutrition support, which include many of those discussed in the Nutrition and disease section, are listed in Table 21.40. Enteral feeding is a means by which nutrients can be delivered to the gastrointestinal tract by tube or enterostomy. This can be done in three different ways: continuously, as bolus feeds or as intermittent continuous feeds. The advantages and disadvantages of each are listed in Table 21.41.

Continuous feeding

The enteral feed is infused over a period of hours (usually from 8–24 h) using a feeding pump which regulates the volume administered. The feed is contained within a reservoir feeding bag or bottle which should be sterile prior to use and may contain enough volume of feed for 6 h. It is not advisable to have a larger volume in the reservoir because of the risk of bacterial multiplication (Anderton et al 1993).

With each change of reservoir, the position of the enteral feeding tube should be checked and feeds should not be infused continuously without supervision in case the tube becomes dislodged, causing feed to be infused into the lungs. The feed is administered via a giving set which connects the reservoir to the end of the feeding tube, the speed of administration being controlled by a predetermined hourly rate set on the pump.

Some feeds are not suitable for continuous infusion owing to the insolubility of certain ingredients. On standing, these gravitate to the bottom of the reservoir and will eventually block the enteral feeding tube. Continuous feeds have the advantage of allowing a reasonably high fluid intake with little gastric distention and aspiration.

Bolus feeding

Bolus feeding simulates the usual pattern of feeding, generating a gut hormone postprandial response that is greater than that when continuous feeds are given. Feeds can be given at various intervals from hourly to 4-hourly. Prior to each administration, the site of the feeding tube should be checked. The feed is usually administered via a syringe or funnel attached to the end of the feeding tube and is allowed to flow under the influence of gravity into the child's stomach. The disadvantage of bolus feeding is that a wider bore feeding tube is required. Delayed gastric emptying

Table 21.41 Advantages and disadvantages of enteral feeding methods

Feeding method	Advantages	Disadvantages
Continuous infusion	Larger volumes of feed can be administered Smaller bore tubes can be used Less gastric distention Less dumping so that feeds with higher nutrient densities can be given	Tube may become dislodged during feed administration with risk of aspiration Electric feeding pumps, reservoirs and giving sets are expensive Some feeds containing insoluble substances cannot be given
Bolus feeds	Mimics the gut hormonal responses of normal feeding Position of feeding tube can be checked prior to each feed Simple procedure: only a syringe required for feed to be administered Contact with child at each feed time	Gastric distention and vomiting A wider bore feeding tube may be required which may cause discomfort in nasopharynx if nasogastric feeding route used Dumping may be experienced especially if nutrient-dense feeds given Adequate fluid requirement may be difficult to achieve
Intermittent continuous feeds	Larger volumes can be tolerated Feeds containing insoluble substances can be administered Fine-bore tubes can be used The feeding tube position can be checked prior to each feed Nutrient-dense feeds can be administered	Requires a great deal of supervision Electric feeding pumps, reservoirs and giving sets are expensive

and vomiting are contraindications to bolus feeding and occasionally the dumping syndrome occurs.

Intermittent continuous feeding

This method combines the feeding techniques of bolus and continuous feeds. An electric feeding pump is used to infuse the feed at a predetermined rate over a period of 1 hour. The pump is switched off for a 1–3-hour period and then another infusion given over 1 hour. Although this involves greater commitment in time, it has the advantages of both methods without the disadvantages. The site of the feeding tube can be checked prior to each feed and aspiration, gastric distention and dumping are usually avoided. It is often possible to infuse feeds which contain insoluble products as the reservoir can be agitated prior to each administration.

Routes of delivery of feeds

Nasoenteral

Nasogastric tubes are easy to introduce and have fewer complications than nasojejunal tubes. Nasogastric tube feeding is also more 'physiological' in that the antimicrobial and digestive functions of the stomach are utilized, but gastroesophageal reflux and aspiration are more likely to occur. Nasojejunal tubes are used when these risks are high, such as in children with neuromuscular disease, severe neurological handicap and gastrointestinal motility disorders.

There is a wide range of enteral feeding tubes available of different lengths, widths and materials. For the majority of infants and children a tube of 56 cm is adequate. Larger children may need longer tubes which are usually 75 cm. Nasojejunal tubes are usually 109 cm long. The widths of the tubes are measured in French sizes; the narrowest is French size 4. Preterm infants and neonates most frequently manage with tubes of French size 4 or 5, older infants with French size 6 or 8, toddlers and older children with French size 8, 9 or 10 (external diameter 3.3 mm). In general the greater the volume and thickness of feed, the wider the bore of the tube required. Bolus feeds may take a long time to administer if the tube is very narrow, but with an infusion pump narrower

tubes can be used. As a general rule the tube with the smallest possible diameter that will not become occluded with feed should be used.

Tubes are made of polyvinylchloride (PVC), silicone or polyurethane. PVC tubes are relatively cheap but should be changed approximately every 10 days as plasticizers leach out on contact with gastric juices, resulting in them becoming hard and brittle. Silicone or polyurethane tubes are more inert and can remain in situ for many weeks or months depending on the manufacturer's specifications. They are, however, more expensive than the PVC tubes. Silicone and polyurethane tubes are very soft and pliable and require a guidewire so that they can be safely passed without twisting and kinking. Aspiration of these soft tubes should be done with a 50 ml syringe because smaller syringes will tend to collapse the tube when the gastric contents are being drawn up.

Enterostomies

Enterostomies offer a means of delivering enteral feeds directly into the stomach or jejunum, bypassing proximal mechanical, surgical or pathological obstructions. They are also preferred when pharyngeal discomfort is intolerable or the risk of aspiration is high. Percutaneous endoscopic gastrostomy is an increasingly popular technique of tube placement and the gastrostomy button is a useful innovation for long-term feeding. Flush with the skin, the button can be connected to a feeding tube at the child's convenience and avoids a long tube protruding from the abdomen. Many children who require long-term enteral nutrition have gastrostomies, including many who receive home enteral feeding (see below). For children with neurological handicaps, particularly those with difficulty swallowing, gastrostomies greatly facilitate both feeding and nursing. In some children a fundoplication may be necessary to control gastric regurgitation. The advantages and disadvantages of enterostomies are listed in Table 21.42.

Enteral feeding equipment and formulae

Feeding pumps

Continuous infusion of feeds may be delivered by simple gravity infusion using a roller clamp to control delivery rate or by an

Table 21.42 Advantages and disadvantages of enterostomies

Type	Advantages	Disadvantages
Gastrostomy	Stimulates normal feeding Intermittent bolus regimen Percutaneous endoscopic placement Conversion to transpyloric route	Aspiration Gastroesophageal reflux Dumping syndrome
Jejunostomy	Decreased risk of aspiration	General anesthesia Continuous infusion Tube occlusion Specialized formula

enteral feeding pump. The rate of infusion is difficult to control using the former and since infants and young children frequently require infusion of small precise volumes of feed, feeding pumps should always be used for pediatric enteral feeding. There are many different models available but it should be possible to adjust the flow rate of the pump to flow rates of 1 ml increments up to 50 ml/hour, 5 ml increments from 50–100 ml/hour, and 10 ml increments >100 ml/hour. Accuracy of the volume infused should be within +/–10%. All pumps run on mains power with the option of running for a limited period on rechargeable batteries.

Enteral feed reservoirs

Many enteral feeds are now available as ready-to-feed liquids which have been heat-treated and so are sterile. The majority are packed in glass or plastic bottles to which a compatible giving set can be attached if the feed is to be continually infused using a pump. Because the majority of children require a feed that has been 'tailor made' (in terms of volume and nutrient content), ready-to-feed liquids may have to be decanted into smaller more appropriate containers which contain a specified volume to be infused over a period not exceeding 6 hour. A range of feed reservoirs is available but the majority are only compatible with a certain feeding pump. Thus whenever an enteral feed system is chosen, the suitability of both pump and reservoir must be considered. A pump which is deemed satisfactory in terms of infusion rates, alarms and costs may not be appropriate for pediatric use if the smallest available reservoir is 1000 ml. Ideally pumps which have reservoirs in various sizes from 100 ml to 1000 ml are most acceptable for pediatric use.

The cost to health services of these items is increasing dramatically as more and more patients receive enteral nutritional support at home. Whenever a child is discharged on home enteral nutrition (see below), arrangements for the ongoing supply of these nonprescribable items must be clearly established.

Enteral feed formulae

There is an extensive range of enteral feeds available for adults. For children the range is smaller but growing (Table 37.16). There are feeds based on cow's milk for children with an intact and functional gastrointestinal tract and specialized formulae designed to meet the altered nutrient needs of children with specific clinical disorders. Home-prepared feeds and liquidized foods should never be used for enteral nutrition of children because of the risk of bacterial contamination, uncertain nutrient quality and the likelihood of the feeding tube becoming blocked with food particles (Dorf 1989). During the first year of life infants who require enteral feeding and have a normal functioning gastrointestinal tract and require no nutrient modification, should receive one of the standard infant formulae.

Home enteral nutrition

Home enteral feeding (HEF) should be considered when the sole reason for the child being in hospital is enteral nutritional support (Puntis & Holden 1991). It has been estimated that the expense and effort (of providing equipment, feeds and training) is justified by a minimum of 10 days of HEF (Moukarzel et al 1994). Children with chronic diseases, such as cystic fibrosis, neuromuscular disorders, malignant disease and renal failure, can greatly benefit from HEF: some have received it for more than 10 years and its use is growing (Holden et al 1991). Night-time HEF is preferred by many children, who are happy and able to pass their own nasogastric tubes. Children with enterostomies may also receive HEF.

PARENTERAL NUTRITION

Parenteral nutrition (PN) is a means by which nutrients are delivered to the patient via the vein. It may provide complete nutritional support – total parenteral nutrition (TPN) – or be combined with enteral feeding.

Indications for parenteral nutrition

The common indications for parenteral nutrition (PN) are shown in Table 21.43. Although sometimes a life-saving intervention, PN has been subjected to little in the way of controlled clinical trials and its precise benefits remain unclear. Intravenous feeding is both complex and expensive when compared with enteral nutrition and may be associated with serious complications. Recognition of these facts, together with growing evidence that nutrients in the bowel help maintain gastrointestinal structure and function (Booth 1994), has led to a reappraisal of the use of PN in some groups of patients, for example those receiving intensive

Table 21.43 Indications for parenteral nutrition

Neonates	
Absolute indications	Intestinal failure (e.g. functional immaturity, short bowel, pseudo-obstruction) Necrotizing enterocolitis
Relative indications	Respiratory failure Promotion of growth in preterm infants Possible prevention of necrotizing enterocolitis
Older infants and children	
Intestinal failure	Short bowel syndrome Protracted diarrhea Chronic pseudo-obstruction Postoperative gastrointestinal surgery Radiation/cytotoxic therapy (e.g. bone marrow transplant)
Exclusion of luminal nutrients	Crohn's disease Pancreatitis
Organ failure	Acute renal failure Acute liver failure
Hypercatabolism	Extensive burns Severe trauma

care. Whilst there can be little doubt that gastrointestinal 'failure' (from whatever cause) is an absolute indication for PN (Fig. 21.17), complete exclusion of luminal nutrients is frequently neither essential nor desirable. When planning nutritional intervention, therefore, it is important to bear in mind the maxim 'use the gastrointestinal tract if possible'. Total enteral nutrition may be feasible if a transpyloric or jejunostomy tube is used (Fig. 21.17). Even if only minimal volumes of enteral feed can be given in addition to PN, this will help prevent cholestasis by stimulating bile flow and pancreatic secretions, maintain splanchnic blood flow and provide nutrition to enterocytes.

Overall, the most frequent recipients of PN are preterm infants (Ch. 5), despite the fact that there are few data demonstrating benefit in terms of reduced morbidity and mortality. Surgical newborns comprise the next largest group and are fed parenterally usually because of gut failure following surgery for congenital or acquired gastrointestinal disease and PN has undoubtedly had a major impact on survival in children with short bowel syndrome (see above). Children undergoing gastrointestinal surgery, those with protracted diarrhea (see above) or severe dysmotility and others receiving intensive care, often with multiorgan failure, account for much of the remaining PN usage.

Nutrient requirements

Energy

The energy requirement for an individual patient must be determined to some extent by trial and error and recommendations are largely empirical. More precise measurements can be made using indirect calorimetry, but this approach is impractical for routine clinical use (see Nutritional assessment, p. 1187). Equations for calculating energy requirements, such as that produced by Schofield (Firouzbakhsh et al 1993), relate to normal, healthy children and take no account of the effect of disease processes. Infants need around 470 kJ/kg/day (112 kcal/kg/day) and this decreases to about 40% of this value in adult life. Approximately 20 kJ of energy is required for each gram of body tissue deposited, but in children recovering from severe malnutrition the energy cost may be twice this figure. When attempting to reverse long-term growth failure, therefore, caloric intake should be related to expected rather than actual weight. Children with severe burns are a group that requires a high energy intake and for whom predictions of energy needs have been attempted (Cunningham et al 1995).

Nitrogen

Nitrogen is supplied as a solution of synthetic crystalline essential and nonessential L-amino acids. In Vamin (Pharmacia and Upjohn), the proportions of amino acids are based on those found in egg protein. Egg was used as the reference protein since its balanced mixture of amino acids allows all the nitrogen to be used for protein synthesis. In children, histidine, proline, tyrosine, taurine, alanine and cystine/cysteine are required during infancy in addition to the eight amino acids regarded as essential in adults. Solutions which have been designed or modified to better suit the needs of the newborn infant (Ch. 5) include Vaminolact (Pharmacia and Upjohn), Primene (Clintec) and Aminoplasmal Ped (Braun). The ideal mix of amino acids for infants remains unknown (Mitton 1994), but for efficient utilization between 24 and 32 nonnitrogen calories should be given with each gram of amino acids.

Carbohydrate

Glucose is the carbohydrate of choice for PN because it is metabolized by all cells and is an essential nutrient for central nervous tissues, erythrocytes and the renal cortex. High infusion rates may lead to hyperglycemia, glycosuria and osmotic diuresis. Tolerance can usually be achieved by increasing intake over a number of days and should be monitored by BM stix and urine testing. Insulin infusion is rarely needed with the exception of the immature, very low birthweight infant (Binder et al 1989).

Fat

Lipid emulsions are nonirritant to veins, calorie dense and provide essential fatty acids. A dual energy system comprising both fat and glucose, rather than glucose alone, leads to improved protein synthesis, less water retention and less fatty infiltration of the liver. Intralipid (Pharmacia and Upjohn) is available as a 10%, 20% or 30% emulsion and is made from soybean oil emulsified with egg yolk phospholipid. It is composed entirely of long chain triglycerides (LCTs) and infusion gives rise to an increase in plasma cholesterol and phospholipid concentrations. Whilst there is no evidence that this is deleterious, the changes are much less marked with 20% than 10% emulsion. Lipofundin (Braun), in addition to LCTs, contains medium chain triglycerides (MCT) which have the theoretical advantage of more rapid clearance from the blood and more complete oxidation. There is relatively little experience with MCT emulsions in children receiving PN and their advantages over LCT preparations remain unclear.

Tolerance of lipid may be reduced in the preterm infant, particularly in those who are growth retarded. Plasma triglyceride should be monitored (usually kept below 2 mmol/l), particularly if higher than normal fat intakes are given. Lipid emulsions do not contain L-carnitine which enhances transfer of fatty acids across the inner mitochondrial membrane before oxidation. Although low plasma carnitine concentrations have been reported during PN there is no compelling evidence to support routine supplementation. Free fatty acids from metabolism of lipid emulsion in the newborn might theoretically displace bilirubin from albumin binding sites and increase the risk of kernicterus in a jaundiced baby. Recent evidence indicates that the risk is probably very low, but many still advocate withholding lipid if the unconjugated bilirubin is above 180 μmol/l. In the preterm infant with respiratory distress, lipid infusions can lead to a small reduction in arterial oxygen tension, possibly through vasoactive metabolites unblocking hypoxic vasoconstriction in the lung and effectively increasing ventilation perfusion mismatch. Lipid infusions and pulmonary function abnormalities have been reviewed by Stahl et al 1992.

Much has been written regarding the potential for lipid emulsion to compromise host defense against infection. Few studies have demonstrated a clinically significant effect, although lipid emulsion does appear to increase the risk of coagulase negative *staphylococcal* septicemia in preterm infants with indwelling central venous catheters. Unless there is overwhelming sepsis, the nutritional advantages of continuing lipid infusion outweigh the theoretical disadvantages (Palmblad 1991).

Calcium and phosphate

Bone mineralization is dependent upon adequate supply of calcium and phosphate. Metabolic bone disease in the preterm infant receiving PN appears to be related to insufficient mineral intake (Ch. 24). The limited solubilities of calcium and phosphate in PN solutions make it difficult to satisfy the relatively high requirements of these infants. In the preterm infant a calcium: phosphate ratio of 1.7 : 1 (ratio of retention in the fetus) in PN solution has been suggested as the ideal. The use of calcium glycerophosphate rather than the usual combination of calcium gluconate with monobasic and dibasic potassium phosphate allows higher concentrations of calcium and phosphate to be held in solution.

Vitamins and trace elements

The American Society for Clinical Nutrition (ASCN) reviewed the available data with regard to intake of vitamins and trace elements in infants and children receiving PN (Table 21.44) (Greene et al 1988). The optimal intake of vitamins and trace elements continues to be debated and the recommendations in the accompanying tables are therefore approximations. Although the current guidelines for Vitlipid N supply lower quantities of fat-soluble vitamins than the ASCN suggest, deficiencies seem to be rare in practice.

There is no ideal trace element solution for children over 10 kg. Additrace 0.2 ml/kg/day may be used, but since it contains no calcium and no phosphate, these should be closely monitored.

Table 21.44 Vitamin and trace element intakes recommended by the American Society of Clinical Nutrition (Greene et al 1988)

Vitamin	Term infants and children dose/day	Preterm infants dose/kg/day
Water soluble		
Ascorbic acid (mg)	80.0	25.00
Thiamin (mg)	1.2	0.35
Riboflavin (mg)	1.4	0.45
Niacin (mg)	17.0	5.00
Pyridoxine (mg)	1.0	0.30
Folate (µg)	140	40.00
Cyanocobalamin (µg)	1.0	0.30
Pantothenate (mg)	5.0	1.50
Biotin (µg)	20.0	6.00
Lipid soluble		
A (µg) *	700.0	500.0 (max. 700/day)
D (µg) *	10.0	4.0 (max. 10/day)
K (µg)	200.0	80.0 (max. 200/day)
E (mg) *	7.0	2.8 (max. 7/day)

* 700 µg retinol = 2300 IU; 10 µg vitamin D = 400 IU; 7 mg α-tocopherol = 7 IU

Element	Preterm infant µg/kg/day	Term infant µg/kg/day	Children µg/kg/day (max)
Zn	400	250 < 3 mo	50 (5000)
		100 > 3 mo	
Cu	20	20	20 (300)
Se	2.0	2.0	2.0 (30)
Cr	0.2	0.2	0.2 (5)
Mn	1.0	1.0	1.0 (50)
Mo	0.25	0.25	0.25 (5.0)
I	1.0	1.0	1.0 (1.0)

Table 21.45 Some of the consequences of trace element abnormalities described during parenteral nutrition

Trace element	Deficiency	Excess
Zinc	Perorifacial dermatitis Immune deficiency Diarrhea Growth failure	
Copper	Refractory hypochromic anemia Neutropenia Osteoporosis, subperiosteal hematoma Soft tissue calcification	
Selenium	Cardiomyopathy Skeletal myopathy, pain and tenderness Pseudoalbinism	
Chromium	Glucose intolerance Peripheral neuropathy Weight loss	Renal and hepatic impairment
Manganese	Lipid abnormalities Anemia	Liver toxicity Damage to basal ganglia
Molybdenum	Tachycardia Central scotomata Irritability Coma	
Aluminium*		Anemia Osteodystrophy Encephalopathy

* Contaminant of PN solution, not routinely added

Selenium is now given routinely and is included in Peditrace. Zinc requirements in the preterm infant are high and zinc deficiency sometimes occurs on current intakes of Peditrace, particularly in infants with gastrointestinal fluid losses. A low plasma alkaline phosphatase (a zinc-dependent enzyme) activity may be seen before the typical skin lesions of zinc deficiency manifest (Plate 21.2). Chromium added to long-term PN regimens has been associated with hepatic and renal impairment. There is probably sufficient chromium contaminating PN solutions for it to be unnecessary to make any specific addition; it is not included in Peditrace but is a component of Additrace. Consequences of some trace element abnormalities are shown in Table 21.45; trace element mixtures should be withheld in renal failure.

PN regimens

PN regimens for different age groups are shown in Tables 21.46–21.53. These may serve as a general guide as far as nutrient intake in different age groups is concerned, but do not take into account the influence of specific disease states on nutrient and energy requirements. The use of a portable computer assists in prescribing for children throughout the entire pediatric age range and allows flexibility when formulating individual prescriptions (Ball et al 1985). It is particularly helpful for children who are clinically unstable or who have abnormal fluid and electrolyte losses since macro- and micronutrient feed content can be adjusted largely independently of fluid intake. Thus, if a child is fluid restricted, it is possible to formulate a feed without compromising energy and nitrogen intake, as would happen if

Table 21.46 PN regimens for the newborn, 0–3 kg bodyweight. Regimens 1 to 3 are used for the first 3 days of parenteral nutrition, regimen 4 is used for day 4 and beyond

Regimen number	/kg/day	1	2	3	4
Amino acid	g	0.8	1.5	2.0	2.5
Carbohydrate	g	10	12	13	14
Fat	g	1	2	3	3.5
Sodium	mmol	3	3	3	3
Potassium	mmol	2.5	2.5	2.5	2.5
Calcium	mmol	1	1	1	1
Magnesium	mmol	0.2	0.2	0.2	0.2
Phosphate	mmol	0.4*	0.4*	0.4*	0.4*
Iron	µg	100	100	100	100
Solivito N	ml	1	1	1	1
Vitlipid N Infant	ml	1	1	1	1
Peditrace	ml	0.5	1	1	1

NB: The phosphate should be increased to 1 mmol/kg/day if the infant is preterm.
* When phosphate is added using Addiphos the sodium and potassium content of this product should be included in calculations, and if using sodium glycerophosphate injection, the sodium content should be included. Solivito N may be reconstituted with Vitlipid N Infant and 1 ml of the mixture used.

Table 21.47 PN regimens for patients over 1 month but under 10 kg body weight. Regimens 5 to 7 are used for the first 3 days of parenteral nutrition, regimen 8 is used for day 4 and beyond

Regimen number	/kg/day	5	6	7	8
Amino acid	g	1	1.5	2.0	2.5
Carbohydrate	g	10	12	13	14
Fat	g	1	2	2	3
Sodium	mmol	3	3	3	3
Potassium	mmol	2.5	2.5	2.5	2.5
Calcium	mmol	0.6	0.6	0.6	0.6
Magnesium	mmol	0.1	0.1	0.1	0.1
Phosphate	mmol	0.4*	0.4*	0.4*	0.4*
Iron	µg	100	100	100	100
Solivito N	ml	1	1	1	1
Vitlipid N Infant	ml	1	1	1	1
Peditrace	ml	1	1	1	1

* When phosphate is added using Addiphos the sodium and potassium content of this product should be included in calculations, and if using sodium glycerophosphate injection, the sodium content should be included. Solivito N may be reconstituted with Vitlipid N Infant and 1 ml of the mixture used.

Table 21.48 PN regimens for patients over 10 kg but under 15 kg body weight. Regimens 9 and 10 are used for the first 2 days of parenteral nutrition, regimen 11 is used for day 3 and beyond

Regimen number	/kg/day	9	10	11
Amino acid	g	1	1.5	2.0
Carbohydrate	g	5	8	10
Fat	g	1.5	2	2.5
Sodium	mmol	3	3	3
Potassium	mmol	2.5	2.5	2.5
Calcium	mmol	0.2	0.2	0.2
Magnesium	mmol	0.07	0.07	0.07
Phosphate	mmol	0.1*	0.1*	0.1*
Iron	µg	100	100	100
Solivito N	ml	1	1	1
Vitlipid N Infant	ml	1	1	1
Peditrace	ml	1	1	1

* When phosphate is added using Addiphos the sodium and potassium content of this product should be included in calculations, and if using sodium glycerophosphate injection, the sodium content should be included. Solivito N may be reconstituted with Vitlipid N Infant and 1 ml of the mixture used.

Table 21.49 PN regimens for patients over 15 kg but under 20 kg body weight. Regimens 12 and 13 are used for the first 2 days of parenteral nutrition, regimen 14 is used for day 3 and beyond

Regimen number	/kg/day	12	13	14
Amino acid	g	1	1.5	2.0
Carbohydrate	g	4	6	8
Fat	g	1.5	2	2
Sodium	mmol	3	3	3
Potassium	mmol	2	2	2
Calcium	mmol	0.2	0.2	0.2
Magnesium	mmol	0.07	0.07	0.07
Phosphate	mmol	0.1*	0.1*	0.1*
Additrace	ml	0.1	0.1	0.1
Solivito N	ml (total)	10	10	10
Vitlipid N Infant	ml (total)	10	10	10

* When phosphate is added using Addiphos the sodium and potassium content of this product should be included in calculations, and if using sodium glycerophosphate injection, the sodium content should be included. Solivito N may be reconstituted with Vitlipid N Infant and 10 ml of the mixture used.

Table 21.50 PN regimens for patients over 20 kg but under 30 kg body weight. Regimens 15 is used on day 1 of parenteral nutrition, regimen 16 is used for day 2 and beyond

Regimen number	/kg/day	15	16
Amino acid	g	1.5	2.0
Carbohydrate	g	4	8
Fat	g	1	2
Sodium	mmol	3	3
Potassium	mmol	2	2
Calcium	mmol	0.2	0.2
Magnesium	mmol	0.07	0.07
Phosphate	mmol	0.1*	0.1*
Additrace	ml	0.1**	0.1**
Solivito N	ml (total)	10	10
Vitlipid N Infant	ml (total)	10	10

* When phosphate is added using Addiphos the sodium and potassium content of this product should be included in calculations, and if using sodium glycerophosphate injection, the sodium content should be included. Solivito N may be reconstituted with Vitlipid N Infant and 10 ml of the mixture used.
** Additrace: Give 0.2 ml/kg up to 40 kg. When body weight exceeds 40 kg, the adult dose of 10 ml (total) may be given.

Table 21.51 PN regimens for patients over 30 kg. Regimen 17 is used on day 1 of parenteral nutrition, regimen 18 is used for day 2 and beyond

Regimen number	/kg/day	17	18
Amino acid	g	1	1.5
Carbohydrate	g	3	5
Fat	g	1	2
Sodium	mmol	3	3
Potassium	mmol	2	2
Calcium	mmol	0.2	0.2
Magnesium	mmol	0.07	0.07
Phosphate	mmol	0.1*	0.1*
Additrace	ml	0.1**	0.1**
Solivito N	ml (total)	10	10
Vitlipid N Adult	ml (total)	10	10

* When phosphate is added using Addiphos the sodium and potassium content of this product should be included in calculations, and if using sodium glycerophosphate injection, the sodium content should be included. Solivito N may be reconstituted with Vitlipid N Adult and 10 ml of the mixture used.
** Additrace: Give 0.1 ml/kg up to 40 kg. When body weight exceeds 40 kg, the adult dose of 10 ml (total) may be given.

Table 21.52 System for parenteral nutrition in infants using commercially available products (all values are quoted per kg body weight/24 hours)

Patient group	Day of PN	Post gestational age, days	Fluid ml	Vaminolact ml	Glucose 5% ml	Glucose 20% ml	Intralipid 20%* ml	Peditrace ml	Addiphos ml	Additional sodium mmol	Additional potassium mmol	Calcium mmol	Magnesium mmol	Iron µg
Preterm newborn	1	3	90	12	26	45	5	0.5	0.5	2.25	1.75	1	0.2	100
	1	4–5	120	12	66	35	5	0.5	0.5	2.25	1.75	1	0.2	100
	1	6+	150	12	106	25	5	0.5	0.5	2.25	1.75	1	0.2	100
	2	4–5	120	24	27	55	10	1	0.5	2.25	1.75	1	0.2	100
	2	6+	150	24	67	45	10	1	0.5	2.25	1.75	1	0.2	100
	3	5	120	32	11	60	15	1	0.5	2.25	1.75	1	0.2	100
	3	6+	150	32	51	50	15	1	0.5	2.25	1.75	1	0.2	100
	4+	6+	150	40	23	65	18	1	0.5	2.25	1.75	1	0.2	100
Term newborn < 1 mo	1	3	90	12	26	45	5	1	0.2	2.7	2.2	1	0.2	100
	1	4–5	120	12	66	35	5	1	0.2	2.7	2.2	1	0.2	100
	1	6+	150	12	106	25	5	1	0.5	2.7	2.2	1	0.2	100
	2	4–5	120	24	27	55	10	1	0.2	2.7	2.2	1	0.2	100
	2	6+	150	24	67	45	10	1	0.2	2.7	2.2	1	0.2	100
	3	5	120	32	11	60	15	1	0.2	2.7	2.2	1	0.2	100
	3	6+	150	32	51	50	15	1	0.2	2.7	2.2	1	0.2	100
	4+	6+	150	40	23	65	18	1	0.2	2.7	2.2	1	0.2	100
Infants > 1 month < 10 kg	1		150	15	61	35	5	1	0.2	2.7	2.2	0.6	0.1	100
	2		150	24	67	45	10	1	0.2	2.7	2.2	0.6	0.1	100
	3		150	24	41	55	10	1	0.2	2.7	2.2	0.6	0.1	100
	4+		150	40	26	65	15	1	0.2	2.7	2.2	0.6	0.1	100

* Vitamins to be added as in Tables 21.46–48.

Table 21.53 System for parenteral nutrition in children using commercially available products (all values are quoted per kg body weight/24 hours)

Patient group	Day of PN	Fluid ml	Vamin 9 glucose ml	Glucose 5% ml	Glucose 20% ml	Intralipid 20%* ml	Peditrace/ Additrace ml	Addiphos ml	Additional sodium mmol	Additional potassium mmol	Calcium mmol	Magnesium mmol	Iron µg
Children 10–15 kg	1	80	15	41	15	8	1.0P	0.05	2.2	2.1	0.2	0.07	100
	2	90	23	36	30	10	1.0P	0.05	1.8	2.0	0.2	0.07	100
	3	100	30	106	45	13	1.0P	0.05	1.4	1.8	0.2	0.07	100
Children 15–20 kg	1	75	15	51	0	8	0.1A	0.05	2.2	1.6	0.2	0.07	nil
	2	90	23	51	5	10	0.1A	0.05	1.8	1.5	0.2	0.07	nil
	3	90	30	33	17	10	0.1A	0.05	1.4	1.3	0.2	0.07	nil
Children 20–30 kg	1	60	23	29	3	5	0.1A	0.05	1.8	1.5	0.2	0.07	nil
	2	75	30	15	20	10	0.1A	0.05	1.4	1.3	0.2	0.07	nil
	3	75	30	15	20	10	0.1A	0.05	1.4	1.3	0.2	0.07	nil
Children >30 kg	1	50	15	35	0	5	0.1A**	0.05	2.2	1.6	0.2	0.07	nil
	2	60	23	18	9	10	0.1A**	0.05	1.8	1.5	0.2	0.07	nil
	3	60	23	18	9	10	0.1A**	0.05	1.8	1.5	0.2	0.07	nil

* Vitamins to be added as in Tables 21.49–51.
** Additrace: use 0.1 ml/kg up to 40 kg body weight. Above this, use adult dose of 10 ml total.
The sodium and potassium provided by Addiphos and Vamin 9 Glucose and the calcium and magnesium provided by Vamin 9 Glucose have been included in the above calculations.

only standard feeding solutions were available. The fluid and nutritional contribution from additional intravascular fluid infusions and partial enteral feeds can also be taken into account when prescribing PN. This should decrease wastage of PN solutions and help to maintain biochemical homeostasis. Additional advantages of computer-assisted prescribing include clearer communication between medical and pharmacy staff and an increased awareness of nutritional requirements.

Venous access

Peripheral PN

Short-term PN can be given using a standard peripheral venous cannula although overall dextrose concentration should be kept below 12.5%. Osmolality and titratable acidity of solutions, as well as particulate contamination and the type of material from which the cannula is made, are all known to affect the risk of phlebitis. Maintaining peripheral venous access becomes increasingly difficult with increasing duration of PN and interruptions to infusion can lead to suboptimal nutritional intake. Filtration of the amino acid–glucose solution through a 0.22 micron pore size in-line filter prolongs vein life. Recently filters with a 1.2 micron pore rating designed specifically for use with lipid emulsion have also become available. In general, the smallest possible intravenous cannula should be used and polyurethane is the preferred material since it causes less peripheral vein thrombophlebitis than Teflon. Patches supplying transdermal glyceryl trinitrate or nonsteroidal anti-inflammatory drugs applied adjacent to the cannula site reduce the incidence of thrombophlebitis in adult patients receiving peripheral PN but have not been evaluated in children.

Central venous catheterization

Central venous catheterization (CVC) provides reliable venous access and should be considered in any child who is likely to require PN for more than a week. Although there are a wide variety of external and totally implantable CVC devices, a single lumen cuffed catheter is the type most commonly used. The simplest method of access in infants is via 0.6 mm external diameter Silastic tubing such as the Vygon Epicutaneo-cava catheter. This is 30 cm in length, radiopaque and has a hub connection which locks on after insertion. The catheter can be inserted from almost any peripheral vein large enough to accommodate the 18G introducer needle, but temporal (preauricular) and antecubital veins are frequently employed. The tip should be placed just within the right atrium and the length of intravascular catheter required first estimated by measuring the distance from the right nipple to the site of insertion. The safe position of the catheter must be confirmed radiologically or by ultrasound since a number of potentially serious complications (usually related to extravasation) have been reported when the tip has not been ideally sited. These include subdural effusion of PN fluids following probable intracranial passage of a temporal vein catheter, chemical pneumonitis as a result of pulmonary artery catheterization and acute abdomen associated with inferior vena caval catheterization. If central venous access is undesirable or impossible, these very fine catheters perform well as a peripheral access device, functioning for a week or more (Childs et al 1995).

Alternatives to percutaneous fine Silastic catheter insertion include operative insertion from the internal jugular vein or a percutaneous infraclavicular subclavian vein approach using a Seldinger technique (Stringer 1995). These procedures should be carried out under general anesthesia and only by an experienced operator in order to minimize the risk of complications (Table 21.54). Additional access sites include femoral, axillary, facial, cephalic and azygos veins. In children who have required repeated chronic venous access complicated by infection or thrombosis, Doppler ultrasound scanning and venography may be necessary to identify remaining sites for catheter insertion.

Cuffed catheters are tunneled for some distance under the skin before entering the vein. Although this has not been shown to decrease the risk of catheter sepsis, the cuff becomes firmly fixed in place after a few weeks and minimizes the risk of accidental dislodgment. Most require a short general anesthetic for removal

when the cuff is dissected free via the exit site incision. In young children who may pull at their catheters, an interscapular exit site has been advocated. Totally implantable devices are used mainly for intermittent venous access and rarely for PN. They must be accessed using a side-fenestrated, noncoring Huber needle, their main advantage being the absence of an external component and the fact that swimming is permissible.

Catheter complications

Central venous catheter sepsis

This is the single most common serious complication associated with the use of CVCs and the reason why peripheral venous access is preferred by some units. The most common organism isolated is a coagulase-negative *Staphylococcus*, the usual route of access being via the catheter hub. Secondary CVC sepsis may result from bacteremia arising from focal infection elsewhere such as urinary tract or chest. Gram-negative organisms may come from the bowel, particularly if there has been previous gastrointestinal surgery. The incidence of reported CVC sepsis varies widely from just a few percent to over 40% of all catheters. Those interventions which are important in preventing sepsis are shown in Table 21.55 and the role of a nutrition nurse specialist has repeatedly been shown to be of the utmost importance.

In addition to sudden fever, infection may manifest non-specifically as vomiting, diarrhea, temperature instability, hyperglycemia or falling platelet count; Gram-negative infection can lead to rapid onset of circulatory collapse. When CVC sepsis is first suspected, blood cultures should be taken and treatment commenced with a combination of gentamicin and vancomycin to give broad-spectrum antibiotic cover given through the CVC. When possible, blood for bacterial culture should be taken both through the catheter and from a peripheral vein so that quantitative bacteriology can be performed on equal volumes of blood sampled. A 10-fold excess of colony-forming units comparing central with peripheral venous sample confirms catheter sepsis (Fan et al 1989). In the newborn, staining of through-catheter blood for bacteria using acridine orange provides a rapid and simple test for catheter infection which has a predictive value of around 90% (Rushforth et al 1993). This helps inform decisions with regard to catheter removal (only about 30% of suspected CVC sepsis is subsequently confirmed). The decision to leave a possibly infected catheter in situ will largely depend on how important it is to maintain central venous access; the threshold for removal will be much lower in a preterm infant approaching full enteral feeding than the child with short bowel syndrome or chronic protracted diarrhea. If, however, the patient becomes acutely unwell with hypotension, shock or evidence of septic emboli catheter removal

Table 21.54 Complications of central venous catheter insertion

Sepsis
Air embolism
Arterial puncture
Arrhythmias
Chylothorax
Hemothorax
Hydro(PNo)thorax
Pneumothorax
Hemo/hydropericardium
Malposition of catheter
Nerve injury
Central venous thrombosis
Thromboembolism
Extravasation from fractured catheter
Tricuspid valve damage
Catheter tethering

Table 21.55 Factors which may reduce the risk of central venous catheter sepsis

Insertion performed by limited number of experienced staff
Scrupulous aseptic technique
Catheter dedicated solely for parenteral nutrition
Minimum number of connections to catheter
Cleaning catheter hub with isopropyl alcohol
Nutrition nurse specialist
Nutrition care team

is mandatory. Continuing signs of sepsis or positive blood cultures despite appropriate antibiotic treatment are further indications for CVC removal, as is candidal infection since eradication is extremely unlikely. When signs of sepsis resolve with the CVC left in place, antibiotic treatment is usually continued for 10 days. Repeat blood cultures should be taken after 48 h of treatment and following completion of antibiotics.

Mechanical catheter problems

Catheters may block with blood, fibrin, fat, mineral deposits or a combination of these. Filling the catheter with urokinase, 90% alcohol or 1M hydrochloric acid and aspirating after 1 h can clear some occluded CVCs. Failing this, a 6-h infusion of urokinase (Haire & Lieberman 1991) or even a guidewire may successfully restore patency. Blockage of the 0.6 mm Silastic catheter sometimes occurs in the metal cylinder at the hub; this can be cut free whilst a new hub connection is established by inserting a 25G butterfly needle into the tubing rather than removing the catheter itself. Similarly, in larger cuffed catheters occlusion may be near the hub so that removing this and effecting a repair may salvage the catheter. Manufacturers of cuffed catheters supply kits which can also be used to repair splits in the external part of the catheter should this problem arise. When a cuffed CVC has to be removed, there is usually a fibrous capsule surrounding the catheter which can, with care, be exposed by the surgeon and used to thread a new catheter down the old track.

Rarely, a complete fracture of the intravascular catheter occurs on attempted removal. Application of radiopaque markers to the skin before X-ray helps localize the retained fragment which may be amenable to recovery via a cut-down. If the separated portion is inaccessible, retrieval may have to be transluminal with the help of a cardiologist using either a myocardial biopsy catheter or one with a snare attached. Neonatal Silastic catheters sometimes become tethered and can then be removed by gentle sustained traction over 24 hour achieved by stretching and taping the external catheter (Gladman et al 1990).

Infusing PN fluids

Although an all-in-one system (a single bag containing both amino acids/glucose and lipid emulsion) is commonly used in adult patients (Barnett et al 1995), a number of potential problems including the precipitation of calcium and phosphate in the aqueous phase have precluded its use in children. Amino acid/glucose and electrolytes are provided in one bag and lipid emulsion in another, the two being infused through a Y-connector. A volumetric pump should be used to deliver PN fluids; these are usually calibrated in ml/hour and use a peristaltic pumping mechanism which delivers volumes within an accuracy of ±5% (Auty 1992). For flow rates below 5 ml/hour either a syringe pump or a neonatal volumetric pump can be used.

Metabolic complications of PN

Some of the many reported metabolic complications of PN are listed in Table 21.56. Major unexpected biochemical disturbance simply as a result of PN is rare (Puntis et al 1993) and a suggested monitoring protocol is given in Table 21.57. One of the most common problems is cholestasis, the etiology of which is multifactorial. Lack of enteral feeding is one important and often

Table 21.56 Complications of parenteral nutrition

Phlebitis
Infection
Hypo- and hyperglycemia
Electrolyte disturbance
Fluid overload
Hypophosphatemia
Anemia
Thrombocyte and neutrophil dysfunction
Trace element deficiencies
Trace element excess
Vitamin deficiencies
Hyperammonemia
Essential fatty acid deficiency
Cholestasis and hepatic dysfunction
Metabolic acidosis
Hypercholesterolemia
Hypertriglyceridemia
Granulomatous pulmonary arteritis

Table 21.57 Monitoring protocol for parenteral nutrition

	Before PN	Daily	Twice weekly	Once weekly	Monthly	Six-monthly
Plasma						
Na	*		*			
K	*		*			
PO$_4$				*		
Bilirubin	*			*		
Ca				*		
ALP				*		
BM stix (glucose)		* week 1		*		
Cu, Zn, Se					*	
Cholesterol, triglycerides						*
FBC, PT/PTT ferritin						*
Al, Cr, Mn						*
Folate, Vitamins A, E, D, B$_1$, B$_2$ B$_6$, B$_{12}$						*
Urine						
Na	*		*			
K	*		*			
Glucose		*				
Other CXR Cardiac echo ECG						*

easily correctable contributory factor, although the child with short bowel may develop cholestasis and irreversible liver disease because of the inability to tolerate enteral feed necessary for stimulation of pancreaticobiliary secretions. Immaturity of bile salt secretion in the premature infant and recurrent sepsis are important additional factors. The complete or relative lack of taurine from amino acid solutions (because of its poor solubility) may contribute to cholestasis by disturbing the normal ratio of taurine and glycine conjugated bile salts. Manganese and aluminum from PN fluids are excreted in the bile and may add to hepatotoxicity when there is already cholestasis. Manganese accumulation can also lead to neurological impairment and the manganese content of Peditrace is now lower than in previous trace element formulations. Unmetabolized plant sterols from lipid emulsions have also been implicated in cholestatic liver disease during long-term PN, prompting calls for the development of phytosterol-free lipid preparations.

Recent deaths of patients both in the United States, attributable to calcium phosphate precipitation and in the United Kingdom, as a result of bacterial contamination of parenteral feeds, have emphasized the importance of quality control measures in relation to a PN service (Lattarulo 1995). Compounding of feeds should be performed aseptically in a laminar flow work station and subsequent additions to feed bags should not be made on the ward.

Long-term PN

Ethical dilemmas arise in relation to the care of children in whom there is little or no prospect of full enteral feeding becoming established at any time in the future, such as those with a congenital enteropathy. These issues should be discussed both with surgical colleagues and parents, although in practice this often has to take place following the process of investigation and diagnosis and after PN has already been initiated. The prognosis in short bowel syndrome has improved considerably over the past 20 years (Goulet et al 1991) and in some reported cases less than 20 cm of small bowel has ultimately sustained normal growth.

For any child receiving PN for more than a few weeks, cyclical nutrition should be considered. This involves a gradual decrease in the time over which the feed is given, so that eventually the PN can be infused overnight and the CVC left clamped for 12 hour during the day. Initially, blood glucose concentration should be monitored at the end of each period without intravenous fluids to detect hypoglycemia. The child is mobile during the day and can leave the ward or even visit home if otherwise stable. This helps encourage psychomotor development which is adversely affected by prolonged hospitalization. Oromotor skills should be promoted by use of comforters and, when possible, small amounts of enteral feed by mouth. The expert advice of a speech therapist should be sought at an early stage. Cyclical PN may help protect against cholestasis and hepatic dysfunction.

Other complications of long-term PN include a worryingly high incidence of major thromboembolic events affecting around 25% of children (Dollery 1996) and the possibility of granulomatous pulmonary arteritis and pulmonary hypertension (Puntis et al 1992). Effective preventive strategies for thromboembolism have not yet been evaluated and the potential risks and benefits of anticoagulation are unclear; in-line filtration of all PN fluids may reduce the risk of particulate-related pulmonary arteritis.

Home PN

For those children committed to long-term PN, home treatment is now an option (Bisset et al 1992). This has been facilitated by the development of the nutritional support industry and hospital outreach services which together provide the necessary organizational and support infrastructure. Home PN offers children who would otherwise become institutionalized the possibility of realizing growth and developmental potential, a good quality of life and a reduced risk of complications such as CVC sepsis. Suitable patients are those with long-term gastrointestinal failure who are medically stable and have adequate home circumstances. The carers must be highly motivated and capable of becoming expert in home therapy including sterile technique, setting up infusions, managing CVCs, setting pumps and recognizing and reacting appropriately to problems. The most frequent diagnoses in children receiving home PN are short bowel, severe dysmotility, congenital enteropathy and Crohn's disease. A recent British Paediatric Surveillance Unit survey identified 66 children on PN for longer than 6 months, of whom 34 were receiving home PN, while eight were regarded as unsuitable.

The nutrition nurse specialist plays a vital role in assessing suitability of families for home PN, training parents or carers and liaising with community staff such as general practitioner, health visitor and district nurse. Following discharge from hospital, the family have open access to the pediatric ward, keeping in regular touch through the nutrition nurse and outpatient visits. Children may be seen by a large number of different professionals and it is helpful for the parents to keep their own personal copies of medical records. These should include a list of contact numbers, written information to back up teaching sessions, equipment manuals, problem-solving advice and flow charts for biochemical monitoring. Equipment can be supplied by arrangement with one of the home care companies such as Fastnet or Caremark. Disposal of sharps and clinical waste needs to be arranged with the local authority and the electricity company should be appraised of the importance of maintaining supply. Additional support can be provided through the hospital social work department and the patient group PINNT, (Patients on Intravenous and Nasogastric Nutrition Therapy), which shares advice, produces a newsletter and organizes meetings for parents and families; children have their own section called Half-PINNT.

REFERENCES

Anderton A, Nwoguh C E, McKune L, Morrison L, Greig M, Clark B 1993 A comparative study of the numbers of bacteria present in enteral feeds prepared and administered in hospital and the home. Journal of Hospital Infection 23: 43–49

Auty B 1992 Advances in infusion pump design. In: Rennie M (ed) Intensive Care Britain 1991. Greycoat Publishing, London, pp 95–102

Bacon M C, White P H, Raiten D J et al 1990 Nutritional status and growth in juvenile rheumatoid arthritis. Seminars in Arthritis and Rheumatism 20: 97–106

Ball P A, Candy D C A, Puntis J W L, McNeish A 1985 Portable bedside microcomputer system for management of parenteral nutrition in all age groups. Archives of Disease in Childhood 60: 435–439

Bandini L G, Dale A S, Gyr H N, Dietz W F 1990 Validity of reported energy intake in obese and nonobese adolescents. American Journal of Clinical Nutrition 52: 421–425

Barnett M I, Cosslett A G 1995 Parenteral nutrition formulation. In: Payne-James J, Grimble G, Silk D (eds) Artificial nutrition support in clinical practice, Edward Arnold, London, pp 323–332

Barrett A J, Treleaven J 1991 Haematological diseases. In: Barltrop, D Brueton M J (eds) Paediatric therapeutics, principles and practice. Butterworth-Heinemann, London, pp 239–240

Barton J S, Hindmarsh P C, Scrimgeour C M, Rennie M J, Preece M A 1994 Energy expenditure in congenital heart disease. Archives of Disease in Childhood 74: 5–9

Beath S V, Booth I W, Kelly D A 1993 Nutritional support in liver disease. Archives of Disease in Childhood 69: 545–549

Binder N D, Raschko P K, Benda G I, Reynolds J W 1989 Insulin infusion with parenteral nutrition in extremely low birth weight infants with hyperglycaemia. Journal of Pediatrics 114: 272–280

Bisset W M, Stapleford P, Long S, Chamberlain A, Sokel B, Milla P J 1992 Home parenteral nutrition in chronic intestinal failure. Archives of Disease in Childhood 67: 109–114

Bhatt H R 1990 Urinary methylmalonic acid excretion in preterm infants. In: Cobalamin metabolism in health and disease. PhD Thesis, University of London

Bhatt H R, Linnell J C, Barltrop D 1986 Treatment of hydroxocobalamin-resistant methylmalonic acidaemia with adenosylcobalamin. Lancet 2: 465

Bhatt H R, Linnell J C, Barltrop D 1994 Deranged propionate metabolism in familial Addison's disease (isolated glucocorticoid deficiency). In: Bhatt H R, James V H T, Besser G M et al (eds) Advances in Thomas Addison's diseases. Journal of Endocrinology 1: 401–406

Bhutta Z A, Hendricks J 1996 Nutritional management of persistent diarrhea in childhood: a perspective from the developing world. Journal of Pediatric Gastroenterology and Nutrition 22: 17–37

Berger H M, Lindemann J H N, van Zoeren-Grobben D, Houdkamp E, Schrijver J, Kanhai H H 1990 Iron overload, free radical damage, and rhesus haemolytic disease. Lancet 335: 933–936

Bolton-Smith C, Woodward M 1994 Dietary composition and fat to sugar ratios in relation to obesity. International Journal of Obesity 18: 820–828

Booth I W 1994 Enteral nutrition as primary therapy in short bowel syndrome. Gut (suppl 1) 35: 569–72

Briend A I 1990 Is diarrhoea a major cause of malnutrition among the under fives in developing countries? A review of available evidence. European Journal of Clinical Nutrition 44: 611–628

Brown G A, Sule D, Williams J, Puntis J W L, Booth I W, McNeish A S 1988 Faecal chymotrypsin: a reliable index of exocrine pancreatic function. Archives of Disease in Childhood 63: 785–789

Brown K H, MacLean W C 1984 Nutritional management of acute diarrhea: an appraisal of alternatives. Pediatrics 73: 119–125

Bull N L 1985 Dietary habits of 15 to 25 year olds. Human Nutrition: Applied Nutrition 39A (Suppl 1): 1–68

Chanarin I 1990 Congenital cobalamin malabsorption. In: The megaloblastic anaemias, 3rd edn. Blackwell Scientific, London, p 126–127

Charlton C P J, Buchanan E, Holden C et al 1992 The use of enteral feeding in the dietary management of children with chronic liver disease. Archives of Disease in Childhood 67: 603–607

Childs A-M, Murdoch-Eaton D G, Standring P, Puntis J W L 1995 A prospective comparison of central and peripheral vein access for parenteral nutrition in the newborn. Clinical Nutrition 14: 303–305

Chin S E, Shepherd R W, Thomas B J et al 1992 Nutritional support in children with end stage liver disease: a randomised crossover trial of a branched chain amino acid supplement. American Journal of Clinical Nutrition 56: 158–163

Chinn S, Rona R J, Guildford M C, Hammond J 1992 Weight for height in children aged 4–12 years. European Journal of Clinical Nutrition 46: 489–500

Cleland L G, Hill C L, James M J 1995 Diet and arthritis. Baillière's Clinical Rheumatology 9: 771–785

Cockburn F 1994 Neonatal brain and dietary lipids. Archives of Disease in Childhood 70: F1–F2

Cole T F, Freeman J V, Preece M A 1995 Body mass index reference curves for the UK. Archives of Disease in Childhood 73: 25–29

Corey M, McLaughlin F J, Williams M, Levinson H 1988 A comparison of survival, growth and pulmonary function in patients with cystic fibrosis in Boston and Toronto. Journal of Clinical Epidemiology 41: 583–591

Crawley H F 1993 The energy, nutrient and food intakes of teenagers aged 16–17 years in Britain. British Journal of Nutrition 70: 15–26

Cunningham J J, Harmatz P R, Udall J N, Remensnyder J P 1995 Nutrition support during the acute care of moderately or severely burned pateints. In: Payne-James J, Grimble G, Silk D (eds) Artificial nutrition support in clinical practice. Edward Arnold, London, pp 459–468

Czeizel A E, Dudas I 1992 Prevention of the first occurrence of neural-tube defects by periconceptual vitamin supplementation. New England Journal of Medicine 327: 1832–1835

Dalzell A M, Shephers R W, Dean B, Cleghorn G Y, Holt T L, Francis P J 1992 Nutritional rehabilitation in cystic fibrosis: a 5 year follow-up study. Journal of Pediatric Gastroenterology and Nutrition 15: 141–145

Davies P S W 1994 Body composition assessment. Archives of Disease in Childhood 69: 337–338

Davies P S W, Day J M E, Cole T J 1993 Converting Tanner Whitehouse reference triceps and subscapular skinfold measurements to standard deviation scores. European Journal of Clinical Nutrition 47: 559–566

Department of Health 1979 Recommended daily amounts of food energy and nutrients for groups of people in the United Kingdom. Report on Health and Social Subjects No. 15. HMSO, London

Department of Health 1984 Diet and cardiovascular disease. Committee on Medical Aspects of Paediatric Policy. Report on Health and Social Subjects No. 28. HMSO, London

Department of Health 1988 Present day practice in infant feeding. Third report. Report on Health and Social Subjects No. 32. HMSO, London

Department of Health 1989 The diets of British schoolchildren. Reports on Health and Social Subjects No. 36 London, HMSO

Department of Health 1991 Dietary reference values for food energy and nutrients for the UK. Report on Health and Social Subjects No. 41. HMSO, London

Department of Health 1992 The health of the nation: strategy for health in England. HMSO, London

Department of Health 1994a Nutritional aspects of cardiovascular disease. HMSO, London

Department of Health 1994b Weaning and the weanling diet. Report on Health and Social Subjects No. 45. HMSO, London

Dharmasathaphorn K, Gorelick F S, Sherwin R S, Cataland S, Dobbins J W 1982 Somatostatin decreased diarrhea in patients with short bowel syndrome. Journal of Clinical Gastroenterology 4: 521–524

Dietz W H 1993a Childhood obesity. In: Suskind R M, Lewinter-Suskind L (eds) Textbook of pediatric nutrition, 2nd edn. Raven Press, New York

Dietz W H 1993b Therapeutic strategies in childhood obesity. Hormone Research 39 (Suppl 3): 86–90

Doherty J F, Adam E J, Griffin G E, Golden M H N 1992 Ultrasonographic assessment of the extent of hepatic steatosis in severe malnutrition. Archives of Disease in Childhood 67: 1348–1352

Dollery C M 1996 Pulmonary embolism in parenteral nutrition. Archives of Disease in Childhood 74: 95–98

Dorf A 1989 Tube feeding the young child: current practices and concerns of pediatric nutritionists. Journal of the American Dietetic Association 89: 1658–1660

Dorney S F A, Ament M E, Berquist W E, Vargas J H, Hassall E 1985 Improved survival in very short small bowel of infancy with use of long-term parenteral nutrition. Journal of Pediatrics 107: 521–525

Earnest D L, Johnson G, Williams H E, Admirand W H 1974 Hyperoxaluria in patients with ileal resection: an abnormality in dietary oxalate absorption. Gastroenterology 66: 1114–1122

Elia M 1993 Artificial nutritional support in clinical practice in Britain. Journal of the Royal College of Physicians 27: 8–15

Englyst H N, Kingman S M, Cummings J H 1992 Classification and measurement of nutritionally important starch fractions. European Journal of Clinical Nutrition 46: S33–S50

Epstein L H 1993 New developments in childhood obesity. In: Stunkard A J, Wadden T A (eds) Obesity: theory and therapy, 2nd edn. Raven Press, New York, pp 301–312

Epstein L H, Valsoski A, McCurley J 1993 Effect of weight loss by obese children on long term growth. American Journal of Diseases of Children 147: 1076–1080

Expert Committee 1992 Vitamin K prophylaxis. British Paediatric Association, London

Fan S T, Teoh-Chan C H, Lau K F 1989 Evaluation of central venous catheter sepsis by differential quantitative blood culture. European Journal of Microbiology and Infectious Disease 8: 142–144

Farrell P, Mischler E, Sonder S, Palta M 1987 Predigested formula for infants with cystic fibrosis. Journal of the American Dietetic Association 87: 1353–1356

Filteau S M, Tomkins A M 1995 Vitamin A supplementation in developing countries. Archives of Disease in Childhood 72: 106–109

Firouzbakhsh S, Mathis R K, Dorchester W L, Oseas R S, Groncy P K, Grant K E, Finklestein J Z 1993 Measured resting energy expenditure in children. Journal of Pediatric Gastroenterology and Nutrition 16: 136–142

Forbes G B 1964 Lean body mass and fat in obese children. Pediatrics 34: 308–314

Frank D A, Zeisel S H 1988 Failure to thrive. Pediatric Clinics of North America 35: 1181–1206

Freeman J V, Cole T J, Chinn S, Jones P R M, White E M, Price M A 1995 Cross-sectional stature and weight reference curves for the UK. Archives of Disease in Childhood 73: 17–24

Frisancho A R 1981 New norms of upper limb fat and muscle areas for assessment of nutritional status. American Journal of Clinical Nutrition 34: 2540–2545

Fulgoni V L, Mackay M A 1991 Total dietary fiber in children's diets. Annals of the New York Academy of Science 623: 369–379

Galler J R, Ross R N 1993 Malnutrition and mental development. In: Suskind R M, Lewinter-Suskind L (eds) Textbook of pediatric nutrition. Raven Press, New York, pp 173–179

Garrow J S, James W P T (eds) 1993 Human nutrition and dietetics, 9th edn. Churchill Livingstone, Edinburgh

Giles M M, Laing I A, Elton R A, Robins J B, Sanderson M, Hume R 1990 Magnesium in preterm infants: effect of calcium, magnesium and phosphorus and of postnatal and gestational age. Journal of Pediatrics 117: 147–154

Girardet J P, Tounian P, Sardet A, Veinberg F, Grimfield A, Tournier G, Fontaine J L 1994 Resting energy expenditure in infants with cystic fibrosis. Journal of Pediatric Gastroenterology and Nutrition 18: 214–219

Gladman G, Sinhq A, Shims D G, Chiswick M L 1990 *Staphylococcus epidermidis* and retention of neonatal percutaneous central venous catheters. Archives of Disease in Childhood 65: 234–235

Golden M H N, Golden B E 1981 Effect of zinc supplementation on the dietary intake, rate of weight gain, and energy cost of tissue deposition in children recovering from severe malnutrition. American Journal of Clinical Nutrition 34: 900–908

Golding J, Greenwood R, Bermingham K, Mott M 1992 Childhood cancer, intramuscular vitamin K, and pethidine given during labour. British Medical Journal 305: 341–346

Gortmaker S L 1993 Social and economic consequences of overweight in adolecence. New England Journal of Medicine 329: 1008–1012

Gortmaker S L, Dietz W H, Sobol A M, Wehler C A 1987 Increasing pediatric obesity in the United States. American Journal of Diseases of Children 141: 535–540

Goulet O J, Revillon Y, Jan D et al 1991 Neonatal short bowel syndrome. Journal of Pediatrics 119: 18–23

Gracey M 1996 Diarrhoea and malnutrition: a challenge to paediatricians. Journal of Pediatric Gastroenterology and Nutrition 22: 6–16

Grantham-McGregor S, Powell C A, Walker S P, Hines J H 1991 Nutritional supplementation, psychological stimulation and mental development of stunted children. Lancet 338: 1–5

Green M R, Buchanan E, Weaver L T 1995 Nutritional management of the infant with cystic fibrosis. Archives of Disease in Childhood 72: 452–456

Greene H L, Hambidge K M, Schanler R, Tsang R C 1988 Guidelines for the use of vitamins, trace elements, calcium, magnesium and phosphorus in infants and children receiving total parenteral nutrition: report of the Subcommittee on Pediatric Parenteral Nutrition Requirements from the Committee on Clinical Practice Issues of the American Society for Clinical Nutrition. American Journal of Clinical Nutrition 48: 1324–1342

Haire W D, Lieberman R P 1991 Thrombosed central venous catheters: restoring function with a 6 hour urokinase infusion after failure of bolus urokinase. Journal of Parenteral and Enteral Nutrition 16: 129–132

Hambidge M 1993 Trace element deficiencies in childhood. In: Suskind R M, Lewinter-Suskind L (eds) Textbook of pediatric nutrition. Raven Press, New York, pp 107–114

Hamill P V V, Drizd T A, Johnson C L J, Reed R B, Roche A F, Moore W 1979 Physical growth: National Center for Health Statistics percentiles. American Journal of Clinical Nutrition 32: 607–629

Hammer L D, Kraemer H C, Wilson D M, Ritter P L, Dornbusch S M 1991 Standardised percentile curves of BMI for children and adolescents. American Journal of Diseases of Children 145: 259–263

Haschke F, Fjeld C R 1991 Prevention and treatment of primary malnutrition in developing and industrialised countries. Acta Paediatrica Scandinavica (suppl 374)

Henderson C J, Lovell D J 1989 Assessment of protein-energy malnutrition in children and adolescents with juvenile rheumatoid arthritis. Arthritis Care Research 2: 108–113

Hendrikse W H, Reilly J J, Weaver L T 1997 Malnutrition in a children's hospital. Clinical Nutrition 16: 13–18

Holliday K, Allen J 1991 Growth of human milk-fed and formula-fed infants with cystic fibrosis. Journal of Pediatrics 118: 77–79

Holden C E, Puntis J W L, Charlton C P L, Booth I W 1991 Nasogastric feeding at home: acceptability and safety. Archives of Disease in Childhood 66: 148–151

Hyman P E, Everett S L, Harada T 1986 Gastric acid hypersecretion in short bowel syndrome in infants: association with extent of resection and enteral feeding. Journal of Pediatric Gastroenterology and Nutrition 5: 191–197

Jackson A A 1990 Sugars not for burning. In: Eastwood M, Edwards C, Parry D (eds) Human nutrition. Chapman and Hall, London

Jenkins A P, Thompson P P H 1994 Enteral nutrition and the small intestine. Gut 35: 1765–1769

Johnston A, Maclean M 1992 The team approach to practical management of childhood diabetes. European Journal of Clinical Nutrition 46 (Suppl 1): 547–550

Karlberg P, Ergstrom I, Lichtenstein H et al 1968 Physical growth during the first three years of life. Acta Paediatrica Scandinavica 187 (Suppl): 48–66

Kerry K R, Anderson C M 1964 A ward test for sugar in faeces. Lancet i: 981

Keusch G T 1990 Vitamin A supplements – too good not to be true. New England Journal of Medicine 323: 985–987

Krick J 1986 Using the Z score as a descriptor of discrete changes in growth. Nutrition Support Services 6: 14–21

Lahrichi M, Chabraoui L, Balafresj A, Baroudi A 1991 Zinc and copper concentration in Moroccan children with protein-energy malnutrition. In: Chandra R K (ed) Trace elements in nutrition of children II. Nestle Nutrition Workshop Series No. 23. Raven Press, New York, pp 176–178

Lancet 1991 Editorial: solving the weanling's dilemma: power flour to fuel the gruel. Lancet 338: 604–605

Lancet 1992 Editorial: cereal based oral rehydration solutions – bridging the gap between fluid and food. Lancet 339: 219–220

Larcher V F, Shepherd R, Francis E M, Harries J T 1977 Protracted diarrhoea in infancy. Analysis of 82 cases with particular reference to diagnosis and management. Archives of Disease in Childhood 52: 597–605

Lattarulo M 1995 Global quality assurance in parenteral nutrition. Clinical Nutrition 14: 61–63

Lennard-Jones J E (ed) 1992 A positive approach to nutrition as treatment. King's Fund Centre, London

Levitsky D A, Strupp B J 1993 The effects of iron deficiency, food additives and other nutrients on behavior. In: Suskind R M, Lewinter-Suskind L (eds) Textbook of pediatric nutrition. Raven Press New York, pp 107–114

Linnell J C, Bhatt H R 1995 Inborn errors of B12 metabolism and their management. In: Wickramasinghe S N (ed) Megaloblastic anaemia. Baillière's Clinical haematology. Baillière Tindall, London, vol 8, no 3: 567–601

Listernick R, Christoffel K, Pace J, Chiaramonte J 1985 Severe primary malnutrition in US children. American Journal of Diseases of Children 139: 1157–1160

Liton R E, Combs G F 1991 Selenium in pediatric nutrition. Pediatrics 87: 339–351

Lo C W, Walker W A 1983 Chronic protracted diarrhoea of infancy. A nutritional disease. Pediatrics 72: 786–800

Lohman T S 1993 Advances in body composition assessment. Monograph No. 3. Human Kinetics Publishers, Champaign, Illinois

MacDonald I 1987 Metabolic requirements for dietary carbohydrate. American Journal of Clinical Nutrition 45: 1193–1196

Macfarlane P I, Miller V 1984 Human milk in the management of protracted diarrhoea of infancy. Archives of Disease in Childhood 59: 260–265

Maffeis C, Schutz Y, Zaffanello M, Piccoli R, Pirelli L 1994 Elevated energy expenditure and reduced energy intake in obese children: paradox or poor dietary reliability in obesity. Journal of Pediatrics 124: 348–354

Marx S J 1989 Vitamin D and other calciferols. In: Scriver C R, Beaudet A L, Sly W S, Valle D (eds) The metabolic basis of inherited disease, vol II, 6th edn. McGraw-Hill, London, pp 2034–2035

Mast A, Gallal G E, Dietz W H 1991 Reference data for obesity, 85th and 95th percentiles for BMI and triceps skinfold thickness. American Journal of Clinical Nutrition 53: 839–846

McWhirter J P, Pennington C R 1994 Incidence and recognition of malnutrition in hospital. British Medical Journal 308: 945–948

Merritt R J, Suskind R M 1979 Nutritional survey of hospitalised patients. American Journal of Clinical Nutrition 32: 1320–1325

Mertz W 1991 General considerations regarding requirements and toxicology of trace elements. In: Chandra R K (ed) Trace elements in nutrition in children II. Nestle Nutrition Workshop Series No. 23. Raven Press, New York

Minford A M B, Macdonald A, Littlewood J M 1982 Food intolerance and food allergy in children: a review of 68 cases. Archives of Disease in Childhood 57: 742–747

Mirakian R, Bottazzo G P 1994 The autoimmune pathogenesis of chronic gastritis and pernicious anaemia. In: Bhatt H R, James V H T, Besser G M et al (eds) Advances in Thomas Addison's diseases. Journal of Endocrinology 2: 193–204

Mitton S G 1994 Amino acids and lipid in total parenteral nutrition for the newborn. Journal of Pediatric Gastroenterology and Nutrition 18: 25–31

Moukarzel A A, Najim J, Vargas J, McDiarmid S V, Busuhil R W, Ament M E 1990 Effect of nutritional status on outcome of orthoptic liver transplantation in pediatric patients. Transplant Proceedings 22: 1560–1563

Moukarzel A A, Reyer L, Ament M E 1994 Home enteral feeding in children. In: Baker S B, Baker R D, Davies A (eds) Pediatric enteral nutrition. Chapman and Hall, New York

Morrison J M, O'Rawe A, McCracken K J, Redmond A O B, Dodge J A 1994 Energy intakes and losses in cystic fibrosis. Journal of Human Nutrition and Dietetics 7: 39–46

Moy R J D, Smallman S, Booth I W 1990 Malnutrition in a UK children's hospital. Journal of Human Nutrition and Dietetics 3: 93–100

MRC Vitamin Study Research Group 1991 Prevention of neural-tube defects: results of the Medical Council vitamin study. Lancet 338: 131–137

Murphy J L, Wooton S A, Bond S A, Jackson A A 1991 Energy content of stools in normal healthy controls and patients with cystic fibrosis. Archives of Disease in Childhood 66: 495–500

National Advisory Committee on Nutrition Education (NACNE) 1983 Proposals for nutritional guidelines for health education in Britain. Health Education Council, London

National Diet and Nutrition Survey 1995a Children aged 1 1/2 to 4 1/2 years. Volume 1: report of the diet and nutrition survey. HMSO, London

National Diet and Nutrition Survey 1995b Children aged 1 1/2 to 4 1/2 years. Volume 2: Report of the dental survey. HMSO, London

Nicholson K 1992 The CF nurse specialist and neonatal screening: child care and research in East Anglia. In: David T J (ed) Role of the cystic fibrosis nurse specialist. Medicine Group, Abingdon, pp 32–38

Nordin B E C 1976 Nutritional considerations. In: Nordin B E C (ed) Calcium, phosphate and magnesium metabolism, clinical physiology and diagnostic procedures. Churchill Livingstone, Edinburgh, pp 19–23

Nutrition Sub-Committee of the Medical Advisory Committee of the British Diabetic Association 1982 Dietary recommendations for diabetics for the 1980's. Human Nutrition: Applied Nutrition 36A: 378–394

Nutrition Sub-Committee of the Professional Advisory Committee of the British Diabetic Association 1989 Dietary recommendations for children and adolescents with diabetes. Diabetic Medicine 6: 537–547

Nutrition Sub-Committee of the British Diabetic Association's Professional Advisory Committee 1992 Dietary recommendations for people with diabetes: an update for the 1990's. Diabetic Medicine 9: 189–202

O'Morain C A, Segal A W, Levi A J, Valman H B 1983 Elemental diet in acute Crohn's disease. Archives of Disease in Childhood 53: 44–47

O'Rawe A O, Dodge J A, Redmond A O B, McIntosh I, Brick D J H 1990 Gene/energy interaction in cystic fibrosis. Lancet 335: 552–553

Odame I, Reilly J J, Donaldson M, Gibson B E S 1994 Patterns of obesity in boys and girls after treatment for acute lymphoblastic leukaemia. Archives of Disease in Childhood 71: 147–149

OPCS 1990 The dietary and nutritional survey of British adults. HMSO, London

Palmblad J 1991 Intravenous lipid emulsions and host defence – a critical review. Clinical Nutrition 10: 303–308

Parsons M G, Francoeur T M, Howland P, Spengler R F, Pencharz P B 1980 The nutritional status of hospitalised children. American Journal of Clinical Nutrition 33: 1140–1146

Petrukhin K, Fisher S G, Pirastu M et al 1993 Mapping, cloning and genetic characterisation of the region containing the Wilson's disease gene. Nature Genetics 5: 338–343

Poskitt E M E 1993 Failure to thrive in congenital heart disease. Archives of Disease in Childhood 68: 158–160

Potter J, Klipstein K, Reilly J J, Roberts M A 1995 Nutritional status and clinical course of acute admissions to a geriatric unit. Age and Ageing 24: 131–136

Prentice A M, Jebb S A 1995 Obesity in Britain: gluttony or sloth. British Medical Journal 311: 437–439

Prentice A M, Lucas A, Vasquez-Velasquez L, Davies P S W, Whitehead R G 1988 Are current dietary guidelines in young children a prescription for overfeeding? Lancet ii: 1066–1069

Puntis J W L, Booth I W 1990 The place of the nutritional care team in paediatric practice. Intensive Therapy Clinical Monitoring 7: 132–136

Puntis J W L, Holden C E 1991 Home enteral feeding in paediatric practice. British Journal of Hospital Medicine 45: 104–107

Puntis J W L, Wilkins K M, Ball P A, Rushton D I, Booth I W 1992 Hazards of parenteral treatment: do particles count? Archives of Disease in Childhood 67: 1475–1477

Puntis J W L, Hall S K, Green A, Smith D E, Ball P A, Booth I W 1993 Biochemical stability during parenteral nutrition in children. Clinical Nutrition 12: 153–159

Rayner R M 1991 Fat soluble vitamins in cystic fibrosis. Proceedings of the Nutrition Society 51: 245–250

RCP/BNF 1984 Food intolerance and food aversion. A joint report of the Royal College of Physicians and the British Nutrition Foundation. Journal of the Royal College of Physicians of London 18: 83–123

Realit Survey Office 1993 The Realit Survey: changing attitudes to meat consumption. Realit Survey Office, Howard Way, Newport Pagnell, Bucks

Reardon M, Hammond K, Accurso F, Fisher C D, McCabe E R B, Cotton E K, Bowman C M 1984 Nutritional deficiencies exist before two months of age in some infants with cystic fibrosis identified by screening test. Journal of Pediatrics 105: 271–274

Rebulla P, Modell B 1991 Transfusion requirements and effects in patients with thalassaemia major. Lancet 337: 277–280

Recommended Dietary Allowances 1989, 10th edn. National Research Council, National Academy Press, Washington DC

Recommended Nutrient Intakes for Canadians 1983 Health and Welfare Canada Bureau of Nutritional Sciences, Health Protection Branch, Health and Welfare, Ottawa

Rennie J M, Kelsall A W R 1994 Vitamin K prophylaxis in the newborn. Archives of Disease in Childhood 70: 248–251

Rolland Cachera M F, Cole T J, Semple M, Tichet J, Rossignol C, Charraud A 1991 Body mass index variations: centiles from birth to 87 years. European Journal of Clinical Nutrition 45: 13–21

Rosen J F, Chesney R W 1983 Circulating calcitriol concentrations in health and disease. Journal of Pediatrics 103: 1–17

Rosenblatt D S 1989 Inherited disorders of folate transport and metabolism. In: Scriver C R, Beaudet A L, Sly W S, Valle D (eds) The metabolic basis of inherited disease, vol II, 6th edn. McGraw-Hill, London, pp 2049–2064

Rossi T M, Lebenthal E 1984 Pathogenic mechanisms of protracted diarrhea. Recent Advances in Pediatrics 31: 595–633

Rowland M G M 1986 The weanling's dilemma: are we making progress? Acta Paediatrica Scandinavica 323 (Suppl): 33–42

Roy S K, Haider R et al 1990 Persistent diarrhoea: clinical efficacy and nutrient absorption with a rice-based diet. Archives of Disease in Childhood 65: 294–297

Rushforth J A, Hoy C M, Kite P, Puntis J W L 1993 Rapid diagnosis of central venous catheter sepsis. Lancet 342: 402–403

Sanders T B 1988 Growth and development of British vegan children. American Journal of Clinical Nutrition 48: 822–825

Sauniere J P, Sarles H 1988 Endocrine pancreatic function in protein-calorie malnutrition in Dakar and Abidgan (West Africa). American Journal of Clinical Nutrition 44: 1233–1238

Scheenede J, Dagnelie P C, Refsum H, Ueland P M 1994 Nutritional cobalamin deficiency in infants. In: Bhatt H R, James V H T, Besser G M et al (eds) Advances in Thomas Addison's diseases. Journal of Endocrinology 1: 259–268

Schwartz M Z, Maeda K 1985 Short bowel syndrome in infants and children. Pediatric Clinics of North America 32: 1265–1279

Scott R B, O'Loughlin E B, Gall D G 1985 Gastro-esophageal reflux in cystic fibrosis. Journal of Pediatrics 106: 223–227

Scott-Jupp R, Lama M, Tanner M S 1991 Prevalence of liver disease in cystic fibrosis. Archives of Disease in Childhood 66: 698–701

Scottish Office 1993 Scotland's health, a challenge to us all. The Scottish diet. Scottish Office Home and Health Department, Edinburgh

Seidman E, LeLeikon N, Ament M et al 1991 Nutritional issues in pediatric inflammatory bowel disease. Journal of Pediatric Gastroenterology and Nutrition 12: 424–438

Shepherd R W, Cleghorn G, Ward L C, Wall C R, Holt T L 1991 Nutrition in cystic fibrosis. Nutrition Research Reviews 4: 57–67

Smith D E, Booth I W 1989 Nutritional assessment of children: guidelines on collecting and interpreting anthropometric data. Journal of Human Nutrition and Dietetics 2: 217–224

Smith I F, Taiwo O, Golden M H N 1989 Plant protein rehabilitation and iron supplementation of the protein-malnourished child. European Journal of Clinical Nutrition 43: 763–768

Smyth R L, Velzen D K, Smyth A R, Lloyd D A, Heaf D P 1994 Strictures in ascending colon in cystic fibrosis and high strength pancreatic enzymes. Lancet 343: 85–86

Snyder J O, Merson M H 1982 The magnitude of the global problem of acute diarrhoea. WHO Bulletin 60: 605–613

Sokol R J, Stall C 1990 Anthropometric evaluation of children with chronic liver disease. American Journal of Clinical Nutrition 52: 203–208

Sommer A, Djunaedi E, Leoden A A et al 1986 Impact of Vitamin A supplementation on childhood mortality: a randomised controlled community trial. Lancet i: 1169–1173

Southgate D A T 1992 The dietary fibre hypothesis: a historical perspective. In: Schweizer T F, Edwards C A (eds) Dietary fibre, a component of food. Springer Verlag, London, pp 3–20

Spender Q W, Cronk C E, Stallings V A 1988 Fat distribution in children with cerebral palsy. Annals of Human Biology 15: 191–196

Stahl G E, Spear M L, Hamosh M 1992 Lipid infusions and pulmonary function abnormalities. In: Polin R A, Fox W W (eds) Fetal and neonatal physiology. W B Saunders, Philadelphia, pp 346–353

Stead R J, Skypala I, Hodson M E, Batten J C 1987 Enteric coated microspheres of pancreatin in the treatment of cystic fibrosis: comparison with a standard enteric coated preparation. Thorax 42: 533–537

Stenson W F, Cort D, Rodgers J, Burakoff R, de Schryver-Kechkemeti K, Gramlich T L, Beeken W 1992 Dietary supplementation with fish oil in ulcerative colitis. Annals of Internal Medicine 116: 609–614

Stringer M D 1995 Vascular access. In: Spitz L, Coran A G (eds) Paediatric surgery. Chapman & Hall Medical, London. pp 25–37

Sullivan P B 1993 Cow's milk induced intestinal bleeding in infancy. Archives of Disease in Childhood 68: 240–245

Sullivan P B, Marsh M N, Mirakian R, Hill S M, Millar P J, Neale G 1991 Chronic diarrhea and malnutrition: histology of the small intestinal lesion. Journal of Pediatric Gastroenterology and Nutrition 12: 195–203

Tanner J M, Whitehouse R H 1975 Revised standards for triceps and subscapular skinfolds in British children. Archives of Disease in Childhood 50: 142–145

Tanner J M, Whitehouse R H, Takaishi M 1966 Standards from birth to maturity for height, weight, height velocity and weight velocity of British children, 1965. Archives of Disease in Childhood 41: 454–471 and 613–635

Thompson J S, Rikkers L F 1987 Surgical alternatives for the short bowel syndrome. American Journal of Gastroenterology 82: 97–106

Vanderhoof J A, Langnas A N, Pinch L W, Thompson J S, Kaufman S S 1992 Short bowel syndrome. Journal of Pediatric Gastroenterology and Nutrition 14: 359–370

Walters M P, Kelleher J, Gilbert J, Littlewood J M 1990 Clinical monitoring of steatorrhoea in cystic fibrosis. Archives of Disease in Childhood 65: 99–102

Watson A R 1995 Nutrition in renal disease. In: Davies D P (ed) Nutrition in child health. Royal College of Physicians, London, pp 133–142

Weaver L T (ed) 1992 Constipation: diagnosis and treatment. Seminars in Pediatric Gastroenterology and Nutrition 3: 1–14

Weaver L T 1994 Feeding the weanling in the developing world: problems and solutions. International Journal of Food Sciences and Nutrition 45: 127–134

Weaver L T, Richmond S W J, Nelson R 1984 Loperamide toxicity in severe protracted diarrhoea. Archives of Disease in Childhood 58: 569

Weaver L T, Green M R, Nicholson K et al 1994 Prognosis in cystic fibrosis

treated with continuous flucloxacillin from the neonatal period. Archives of Disease in Childhood 70: 84–89

Weaver L T, Dibba B, Sonko B, Bohane T D, Hoare S 1995 Measurement of starch digestion of naturally ^{13}C enriched foods, before and after partial digestion with amylase-rich flour, using a ^{13}C breath test. British Journal of Nutrition 74: 531–537

Wharton B A 1991 Protein energy malnutrition: problems and priorities. Acta Paediatrica Scandinavica 374 (Suppl): 5–14

Wharton B A 1990 Nutritional policy for children. In: Eastwood M A, Edwards C A, Parry D (eds) Human nutrition, a continuing debate. Chapman and Hall, London, pp 187–201

White E M, Wilson A C, Greene S A, McCowan C, Thomas G E, Cairns A Y, Rickets I W 1995 Body mass index centile charts to assess fatness of British children. Archives of Disease in Childhood 72: 38–4

World Health Organization 1983 Measuring change in nutritional status. World Health Organization, Geneva

World Health Organization 1985 Energy and protein requirements. Report of a joint FAO/WHO/UNU meeting. Technical report series 724. World Health Organization, Geneva

World Health Organization 1987 Selenium. Environmental Health Criteria 58. World Health Organization, Geneva

Worthington-White D A, Behnke M, Gross S 1994 Premature infants require additional folate and vitamin B12 to reduce the severity of the anaemia of prematuriy. American Journal of Clinical Nutrition 60 (6): 930–935

Wright C M, Matthews J N S, Waterston A, Aynsley-Green A 1994a What is a normal rate of weight gain in infancy? Pediatrics 83: 351–356

Wright C M, Waterston A, Aynsley-Green A 1994b Effect of deprivation on weight gain in infancy. Pediatrics 83: 357–359

Ziegler E E, Fomon S J, Nelson S E et al 1990 Cow milk feeding in infancy: further observations on blood loss from the gastrointestinal tract. Journal of Pediatrics 11: 611–618

Ziegler M M 1986 Short bowel syndrome in infancy: etiology and management. Clinics in Perinatology 13: 163–173

BIBLIOGRAPHY

Baker S B, Baker R O, Davis A 1994 Pediatric enteral nutrition. Chapman & Hall, New York

Barker D J P (ed) 1992 Fetal and infant origins of adult disease. BMJ Publishing, London

David T J (ed) 1993 Food and food additive intolerance in childhood. Blackwells, Oxford

Forman S J 1993 Nutrition of normal infants. C V Mosby, St Louis

Garrow J S, James W P T (eds) 1993 Human nutrition and dietetics. Churchill Livingstone, Edinburgh

Gibson R S 1990 Principles of nutritional assessment. Oxford University Press, Oxford

Gibson R S 1990 Nutritional assessment: a laboratory manual. Oxford University Press, Oxford

Hendricks K M, Walker W A 1990 Manual of pediatric nutrition. Decker, Philadelphia

Lebenthal E 1989 Textbook of gastroenterology and nutrition in infancy. Raven Press, New York

McLaren D S, Burman D, Belton N R, Williams A F (eds) 1991 Textbook of paediatric nutrition. Churchill Livingstone, Edinburgh

Paul A A, Southgate D A T 1991 The composition of foods, 5th edn. HMSO, London

Poskitt E M E 1988 Practical pediatric nutrition. Butterworths, London

Suskind R M, Lewinter-Suskind L 1993 Textbook of pediatric nutrition. Raven Press, New York

Taylor S, Goodison-McLaren S 1992 Nutritional support: a team approach. Wolfe, London

Waterlow J C 1992 Protein energy malnutrition. Edward Arnold, London

22 Immunodeficiency

E. G. Davies

Introduction   1231
The immune system   1231
Nonspecific immune mechanisms   1232
Specific immune mechanisms   1235
The development of the immune system   1240
Prenatal development   1240
The immune system in the newborn   1240
Postnatal development   1241
Immunodeficiency disorders: general principles
   1241
Classification and genetics   1241
Diagnosis of immunodeficiency   1243
Antenatal diagnosis   1248
Associations of immune deficiency   1248
Disorders of cell-mediated immunity: combined
   immunodeficiencies   1248
General features of severe combined
   immunodeficiency   1249
Types of severe combined and combined
   immunodeficiencies   1250
Combined immunodeficiency forming part of other
   syndromes   1252
DiGeorge anomaly   1252
Ataxia telangiectasia   1253
Other chromosomal breakage disorders   1253
Wiskott–Aldrich syndrome   1254
Other syndromes   1254

Defects of antibody production   1255
X-linked agammaglobulinemia   1255
Hyper IgM syndrome   1256
Common variable immunodeficiency   1256
Selective IgM deficiency   1258
IgG subclass deficiencies   1258
Disorders of phagocytic cells   1259
Neutropenia   1259
Defects of neutrophil killing   1259
Disorders of neutrophil chemotaxis   1260
Defects of mononuclear phagocytes   1262
Complement deficiency disorders   1262
Primary inherited deficiencies   1262
Secondary complement deficiencies   1263
Mannan-binding lectin deficiency   1263
Deficiencies of C3 receptors   1263
Secondary immunodeficiency   1263
Infection-induced immunodeficiency   1263
Immunodeficiency due to drugs and radiation   1265
Malnutrition   1265
Hyposplenism   1266
Treatment of immunodeficiency   1266
Supportive care   1266
Immunological intervention in neonates   1267
Replacement therapy for humoral deficiencies   1267
Replacement therapy for combined deficiencies   1268
References and Further Reading   1270

INTRODUCTION

The term 'immunity' is used to describe the state in which the immune system responds to a given antigenic challenge either in a useful (protective) sense or in a harmful way (allergy or hypersensitivity). The main role of the immune system is to repel invasion by microorganisms. Abnormalities in this system may result in an increased susceptibility to infection as well as other noninfective problems such as allergy and autoimmunity. Our increased understanding of the immune mechanisms used in handling microbes has led to a better understanding of both primary and secondary immunodeficiency (Steihm 1996). Conversely, much has been learned of the intricacies of immune function from studying patients with immunodeficiency.

THE IMMUNE SYSTEM

In addition to the immunological system, host defense against infection involves a whole variety of other important innate factors, such as the integrity of the skin, or the lack of receptors for microorganisms and their products. Though these will not be considered further in this chapter, their importance cannot be overemphasized.

The basis of the immune system lies in the cells which are derived from the pluripotent stem cells in the bone marrow. An important mechanism by which these cells signal to each other involves peptide messengers, or cytokines, which interact with specific receptors on their target cells.

Cells of the immune system

There are a large number of surface molecules present on all leukocytes and other cells of the immune system which are collectively known as leukocyte differentiation antigens. These can be identified by their reactivity with specific monoclonal antibodies. Monoclonal antibodies recognizing the same antigens are designated by CD (cluster designation or cluster of differentiation) numbers. Strictly speaking these designations apply to the group of antibodies of particular specificity but in common usage they have come to be used to designate the particular antigens recognized. Functional subsets of lymphocytes can be identified by the antigens on their surface. Other antigens can be used to classify cells according to their state of differentiation or activation. The more important surface antigens recognized by different CD antibodies are listed in Table 22.1. In many (but not all) cases the functional roles of these surface antigens have been established.

Table 22.1 Leukocyte antigens

Designation	Main cellular expression	Properties/Function
T cells		
CD1	Thymocytes. Langerhans cells	Unknown
CD2	Mature T cells	Sheep erythrocyte (E Rosette) receptor; LFA-3 ligand
CD3	Pan T cell marker	Part of T cell receptor complex
CD4	Helper/inducer T cells	MHC class II receptor; HIV receptor
CD5	Mature T cells. B cell subset (B1)	Unknown
CD8	Cytotoxic/suppressor T cells	MHC class I receptor
CD25	Activated T cells	IL-2 α receptor
CD28	T cells	CD80 receptor; T cell activation
CD38	Thymocytes Activated cells	Unknown
CD71	Activated T cells. Thymocytes	Transferrin receptor
B cells		
CD19	Pre B & B cells	Unknown
CD20	Pre B & B cells	Unknown
CD21	B cells	Complement receptor (CR) 2 EBV receptor
CD22	Pre B & B cells	Unknown
CD23	B cells	Low affinity IgE receptor
CD40	B cells	Ig isotype switching
Surface Immunoglobulin	B cells	Antigen receptor
Monocytes		
CD14	Monocytes	Receptor for Lipopolysaccharide
NK cells		
CD16	NK, monocytes	Fc γ receptor III
CD56	PMN, NK and some T cells	unknown
General		
CD11a	Leukocytes	cell adhesion ICAM-I receptor
11b	NK cells, MΦ, PMN	CR3
11c	NK cells, MΦ, PMN	CR4
CD15	PMN	Lewis X antigen
CD18	Leukocytes	β₂ integrin associated with CD11 antigens
CD34	BM Progenitor cells	L selectin ligand
CD35	Monocytes, PMN, B cells	CRI
CD43	All leukocytes	sialophorin
CD45	All leukocytes	Tyrosine phosphatase. T cell activation. Variable isoforms – see text
CD58	All leukocytes	LFA 3; CD2 ligand
CD80	Activated B & T mono	CD28 receptor
HLA Class I	All leukocytes	Antigen presentation
HLA Class II	B, monocytes, activated T cells	Antigen presentation

MΦ = macrophage; BM = bone marrow;
PMN = polymorphonuclear cells

Cytokines and receptors

Many aspects of immune responsiveness are dependent upon soluble protein messengers secreted either by leukocytes or by other organs such as the liver or vascular endothelium. These cytokines are involved in regulating afferent and efferent immune responses and direct effector mechanisms and act as growth factors. The more important cytokines and their main effects are listed in Table 22.2. It can be seen that many of these proteins have multiple and overlapping effects and that they are important in both the innate and specific adaptive immune systems.

Cytokines have their effect by interacting with their ligands (or receptors) present on the surface of the target cell population. Most receptors belong to a family of cytokine receptors which share important sequence homologies. In the case of receptors made up of more than one chain there is often one or more chains common to other receptors. An example is the γ chain of the IL-2 receptor which is shared with the receptors for IL-4, IL-6, IL-7, IL-9 and IL-15. Mutations in the gene for this chain result in X-linked severe combined immune deficiency (SCID) (see p. 1250).

Specific and nonspecific mechanisms

Figure 22.1 shows some of the specific and nonspecific components of the immune system. Non-antigen-specific immune mechanisms can be regarded as the less sophisticated, and phylogenetically more primitive, branch of the immune system. These include the polymorphonuclear and mononuclear phagocytes, as well as humoral factors such as those of the complement system.

The specific (or adaptive) immune system is distinguished by its ability to 'respond' to antigens in a way that potentiates the immune response. Such responses are then committed to 'immunological memory' resulting in more rapid and enhanced responses upon subsequent antigen exposure.

These two types of immune mechanism are far from independent, indeed, many specific immune mechanisms require the nonspecific elements as effectors. The functioning of the nonspecific system is often greatly potentiated by the influence of factors produced as part of the specific immune response.

Nonspecific immune mechanisms

Humoral

Complement. One of the most important humoral defense systems is the complement system. The central component in this system (Fig. 22.2) is C3b, the active product of cleavage of the C3 molecule. C3b bound to an antigen acts as a powerful opsonin by interacting with C3b receptors on neutrophils and monocytes. The splitting of C3 is achieved either by the classical (antibody-dependent) pathway, which requires specific antibody–antigen interaction, or by the alternative pathway, in which microbial products, such as polysaccharides and endotoxin, directly activate another cascade of reactions involving serum protein factors B and D to form an alternative C3 convertase which is stabilized by factor P (properdin).

The fixing of C3b to the surface of a microorganism becomes self-amplifying, since C3b itself forms a component of the enzyme responsible for C3 cleavage. This needs strict control, and there are a number of regulatory proteins involved.

The later complement components C5–C9 are used to produce a membrane-attack complex which can lyse cell membranes. This seems to be particularly important in the handling of systemic neisserial infections.

Table 22.2 Principal cytokines

Cytokine	Other (previous) names	Produced by	Main actions
IL-1		Monocytes	Proinflammatory; Fever; T cell activation
IL-2	T cell growth factor	T cells	T (mainly T_H1), NK cell activation/proliferation
IL-3	Multicolony stimulating factor	T cells	Proliferation of bone marrow progenitor cells
IL-4	B cell stimulating factor	T cells (T_H2)	T_H2 cell growth factor; B cell isotype switching especially to IgE
IL-5		T cells	T_H2 cytokine; activation and proliferation of eosinophils (and B cells)
IL-6		T, B cells monocytes	General cell growth and differentiation factor
IL-7	Lymphopoietin I	Bone marrow and thymic stroma	General cell growth factor
IL-8		T cells, monocytes, PMN	PMN activation, chemotaxis and adhesion
IL-9		T cells	T cell, mast cell growth and differentiation
IL-10	Cytokine synthesis inhibitory factor	T cells (T_H2) monocytes, mast cells	Inhibits T_H1 cytokine production
IL-11		Stromal cells	Growth factor similar in actions to IL-6
IL-12	NK stimulating factor	B cells, monocytes	Increases T and NK cell cytotoxicity; T_H1 growth and differentiation factor

Cytokine	Other (previous) names	Produced by	Main actions
IL-13		T cells (T_H2)	B cell isotype switching similar to IL-4
IL-14	High mol. wt. B cell growth factor	T, B cells	B cell growth and differentiation
IL-15		Stromal cells, monocytes	Similar actions to IL-2 (utilises same receptor)
IFN α and β		Leukocytes-α Fibroblasts-β	Antiviral, antiproliferative, Increased MHC expression, increased cytotoxic activity
IFNγ	Macrophage activating factor	T cells (T_H1) NK cells	Macrophage activation, increased MHC expression, T_H1 effects
TNF α	Cachectin	Monocytes	Proinflammatory
TNF β	Lymphotoxin	T cells	Proinflammatory
GM CSF		Leukocytes	Increased myelopoiesis, increased cytokine production by macrophages, proinflammatory
G CSF		Leukocytes	Increased granulopoiesis, activates PMN, reduces inflammatory cytokine production
M CSF		Monocytes, T, B cells	Increased monocyte growth and differentiation, increased cytokine production
TGF β		Platelets, Monocytes	Suppresses inflammation and cell proliferation

IL = Interleukin; IFN = Interferon; TNF = Tumor necrosis factor; CSF = Colony stimulating factor; GM = Granulocyte macrophage; G = Granulocyte; M = Monocyte; TGF = Transforming growth factor; PMN = Polymorphonuclear cells; T_H1/T_H2 = T helper cells

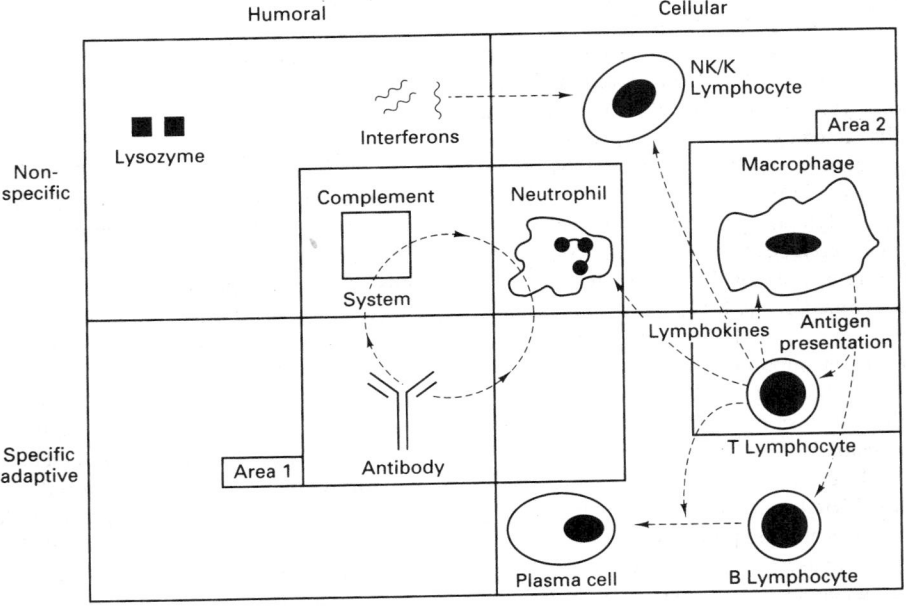

Fig. 22.1 Functional compartments of the immune system illustrating some of the more important interactions (dotted arrows). Area 1 mainly involved in handling pyogenic bacteria. Area 2 mainly involved with intracellular pathogens.

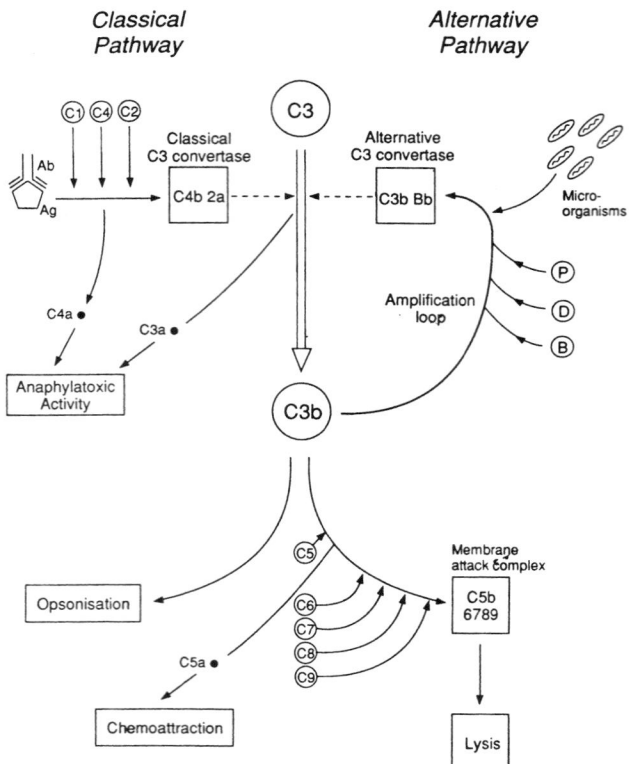

Fig. 22.2 The main features of the classical and alternative pathways of the complement system. Inactive cleavage and breakdown products are not shown.

As well as lysis and opsonization, the complement reactions generate a variety of pharmacologically and chemotactically active byproducts, such as the cleavage products C3a and C5a, for which there are cell surface receptors.

The major cell surface receptors for complement are the ligands for C3b and its derivatives and are responsible for the most important functions of the system. Complement receptor 1 (CR1 also designated CD35 – see Table 22.1) is widely distributed being found on neutrophils, monocytes, erythrocytes, B lymphocytes and glomerular epithelial cells. It recognizes C3b- and C4b- coated particles and facilitates phagocytosis. Its role on erythrocytes is important in clearing circulating immune complexes. CR2 (CD21) is found predominantly on B lymphocytes and recognizes C3d – the main C3b breakdown product. It is believed to play an important role in modulating activity of these cells. It is also the receptor for Epstein–Barr virus. CR3 (CD11b/CD18) is found on phagocytic cells and also on natural killer cells. It recognizes inactivated C3b (C3bi) and is important in phagocytosis. CR4 (CD11c/CD18) can bind C3bi but only weakly. CR3 and CR4 are both members of a family of adhesion molecules, the leukocyte β integrins. Intracellular adhesion is their more important function – see section on adhesion molecules.

Mannan-binding lectin (MBL) (Turner 1996). This fascinating protein, also known as mannan-binding protein (MBP), is the best known of a family of acute phase proteins known as *collectins* which possess both a collagenous region and a sugar-binding (lectin) site. These molecules are believed to form an important part of the innate immune system. MBL is a multimer of identical chains with mannose-binding moieties at the C terminal end. It

has some structural homology with the C1q component of the first complement component. When it reacts with mannose on the surface of microorganisms it opsonizes the organism partly by binding to a putative MBL receptor on phagocytic cells, but mainly by activating the classical complement pathway which it does in association with a serine protease MASP (MBL associated protein) which has structural homology with the other C1 components – C1r and C1s – to fix C4 and C2, resulting in the generation of classical C3 convertase (see Fig. 22.2). This can therefore be achieved in the absence of C1 and, more importantly, of antibody and as a consequence MBL is an important opsonin in the early stages of infection (before antibody production) and in young children (with immature ability to produce antibodies).

Other acute phase reactants. The serum levels of this diverse group of proteins rise rapidly at the onset of acute inflammatory responses. They include clotting factors, amyloid proteins and C-reactive protein (CRP). Their precise biological role is not well characterized. CRP has some immune modulating effects and can act as a nonspecific opsonin for bacterial phagocytosis.

Interferon. Alpha- and beta-interferons are families of proteins produced by virally infected cells. They have the ability to render other cells immune to virus infection (i.e. they produce an antiviral state). Interferons also have effects on some immune mechanisms, e.g. they increase natural killer cell activity; increase HLA class I antigen expression on cells, and decrease cell growth including that of tumor cells.

Gamma-interferon, though having some antiviral effect, is primarily a cytokine, whose chief function is concerned with modulating immune responses including the function of immune effector cells. Structurally, it is poorly related to alpha- and beta-interferons.

Iron-binding proteins. Many bacteria require iron for growth, and decreasing its availability is one mechanism of defense used by the host. An avid iron-binding protein, lactoferrin, present in human milk has the effect of reducing the growth of *E. coli*. The reduction of serum iron, which occurs during infections, increases the bacteriostatic effect of serum.

Lysozyme. This enzyme with antibacterial properties is found in neutrophil lysosomes and in body secretions including tears and saliva.

Cellular nonspecific immune mechanisms

Adhesion molecules. These molecules and their ligands facilitate the cell-to-cell association which is essential for normal immune and inflammatory responses. They are expressed on all cells of the immune system and on vascular endothelium. Their expression is tightly controlled being regulated during inflammatory responses by cytokines such as the interleukins, tumor necrosis factor α and interferon γ.

One group of adhesion molecules is the selectins. L selectin is constitutively expressed on neutrophils and monocytes and binds to its ligand, on the surface of vascular endothelium. E and P selectin expression on endothelial cells is induced during inflammation. These bind to ligands on leukocytes, an important one being a sialated carbohydrate called sialyl lewis x. Interaction between the selectins and their ligands results in the transient endothelial interactions of "rolling" and margination which occur early in inflammatory reactions. Subsequently, L selectin is shed by the cells and expression of more tightly adherent molecules is up-regulated.

The more firmly adhering molecules are a group called β$_2$ integrins. Their expression results in more firm adherence of neutrophils to endothelium and leads to their subsequent egress from the circulation. They also have a fundamental role in cell to cell interaction in the generation of immune responses and in effector cell functions such as cytotoxicity. The group comprises dimeric proteins with a common β subunit and variable α chain. They include molecules with some C3 receptor activity (see Table 22.3). Their expression is greatly up-regulated by the pro-inflammatory cytokines such as TNF-α or IL-1β.

Many other adhesion molecules are recognized as being important in allowing homing of recirculating cells to certain sites, for example the mucosal surfaces, and in cell to cell interactions.

Effector cells. Phagocytic cells include neutrophils and monocyte/macrophages. Phagocytosis of a bacterium by a neutrophil involves movement of the cell to the site of infection (chemotaxis). Products of the acute inflammatory response, including cleaved complement fragments (e.g. C5a), act as chemoattractants in this process. Chemotaxis is followed by adherence to the bacterium and ingestion (phagocytosis). This is facilitated by opsonization – the most important opsonic factors being IgG and complement (C3b) which bind to cell surface receptors Fcγ and CR1/3 respectively. Other opsonins include C-reactive protein, and soluble forms of the serum and tissue glycoprotein, fibronectin.

Following phagocytosis, there is rapid fusion of lysosomes with the phagocytic vacuole exposing the bacterium to lysosomal enzymes (e.g. myeloperoxidase) which are involved in killing and digestion. The process is accompanied by an oxidative metabolic burst which generates hydrogen peroxide as well as superoxide and hydroxyl radicals which aid bacterial killing.

Neutrophil numbers and function are generally enhanced by products of the inflammatory response, including cytokines and complement fragments.

Monocytes and macrophages can ingest and kill extracellular bacteria in a similar fashion to neutrophils but the process is slower and less efficient. However, they are very important in defenses against intracellular microorganisms, including bacteria such as *Mycobacterium tuberculosis* and *Listeria monocytogenes*. Such pathogens are either recognized via Fcγ or CR1/3 receptors following opsonization or microbial carbohydrate moieties such as mannose are recognized directly by the cell surface mannose/fucose receptor. They are also capable of cytotoxicity against infected host cells and malignant cells. The activity of macrophages is greatly enhanced by exposure to humoral substances (cytokines) produced by T lymphocytes as part of the specific cell-mediated immune response. One of the most important of these is gamma-interferon. Macrophages also produce cytokines which have effects on other aspects of immune/inflammatory responses, an example being tumor necrosis factor alpha (TNF-α).

Natural killer (NK) cells form part of the null (non-T, non-B cell) lymphoid population. They have the ability to recognize and kill tumor cells and virus-infected cells without prior sensitization. The precise mechanism of recognition is not known. They have surface receptors for the Fc part of IgG and, when 'armed' with specific IgG against a target cell antigen, can also kill by a process called antibody-dependent cellular cytotoxicity (ADCC). These cells are believed to have a role in the control of emerging malignant cells and in the early stages of intracellular infections, particularly viral infections.

Specific immune mechanisms

The essence of these responses is that antigen specifically stimulates T and B cells, expressing the relevant receptor specificities to trigger cell activation which leads to the generation of antigen specific effector immune mechanisms, e.g. antibody production or generation of specific cytotoxic T cells.

An important step in this process is the presentation of antigen to the T lymphocyte. This is performed mainly by specialized cells of the macrophage series called antigen presenting cells (APC) but also by B cells. These cells take up antigens, partially degrade them to small fragments (peptides) and then express them on the cell surface in association with the major histocompatibility complex (MHC) molecules (Klein et al 1993). The T cell receptor (TCR) will only recognize the peptide when it is presented in association with a self MHC molecule. Some MHC polymorphisms support better responses than others which goes some way to explaining genetic variability in immune responsiveness. Presentation of antigens to CD4 positive helper T cells is achieved in association with Class II MHC molecules (HLA-DR) while presentation to CD8 positive suppressor/cytotoxic cells is via the Class I (HLA-AB) molecules. Several other receptor ligand interactions between the APC and the T cell including adhesion molecule interactions are also important for maximising the stimulation of the latter.

The antigen is normally presented sitting in a groove in the MHC molecule where it can then interact with a complementary groove in the TCR (see Fig. 22.3) at the site is where the hyper-variable regions are expressed. Some antigens called

Table 22.3 Some important adhesion molecules in leukocyte/endothelial interaction

Molecule	Cellular expression	Ligand
L selectin (CD 62L)	PMN, monocytes	Uncertain ligand on vascular endothelium
E selectin (CD 62 E)	Endothelium, leukocytes	Sialyl lewis x on leukocytes
P selectin (CD 62 P)	Endothelium, leukocytes	Sialyl lewis x on leukocytes
Leukocyte function antigen I (LFA-1) - CD11a/CD18	Lymphocytes, monocytes	ICAM-1 on activated endothelium and leukocytes
Complement receptor 3 (CR3), MAC 1, CD11b/CD18	PMN, monocytes, NK cells	ICAM-1, C3bi
Complement receptor 4, P150/90 integrin, CD11c/CD18	Lymphocytes	ICAM-1, C3bi

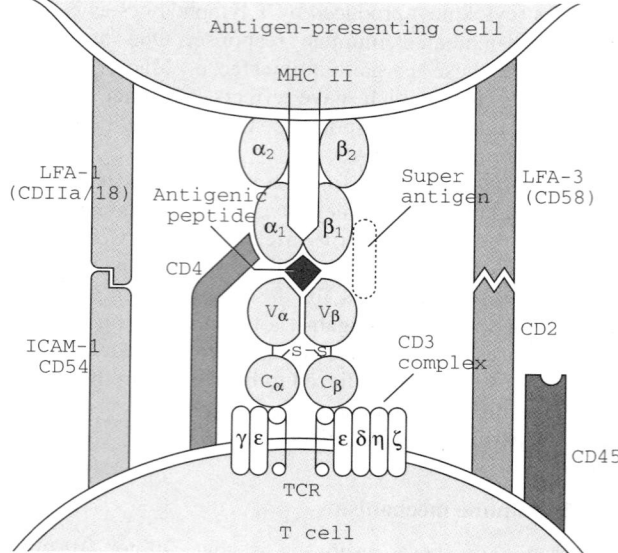

Fig. 22.3 Antigen presentation.

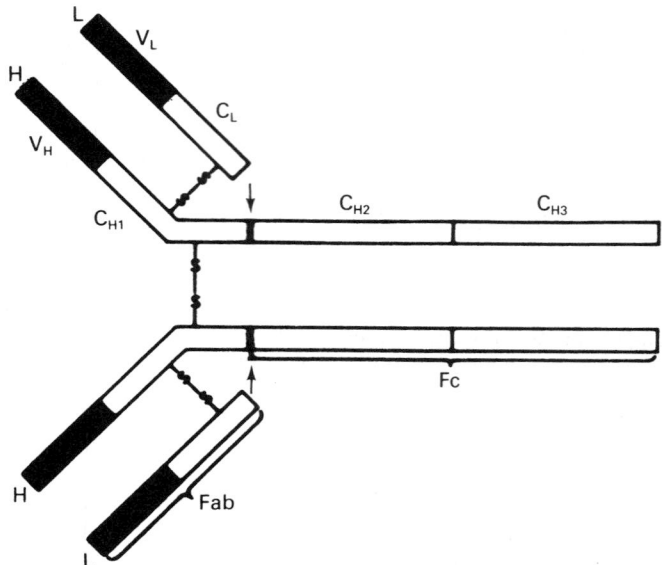

Fig. 22.4 Basic structure of an antibody molecule. Heavy (H) and light (L) chains comprise variable regions (V_H and V_L) – shown by solid bars – and constant regions (C_H and C_L) open bars. Constant region domains (CH_1, CH_2 and CH_3) are shown. Arrows indicate site of pepsin-mediated cleavage to give Fc and Fab fragments.

superantigens cross-link the presenting cell MHC molecule with other nonvariable parts of the TCR chains, resulting in stimulation of large numbers of T cells in an antigen nonspecific way. This is believed to be involved in the pathogenesis of some immune mediated diseases such as toxic shock syndrome and Kawasaki disease. Superantigens are usually microbial products such as exotoxins.

There are two arms of the specific immune system – antibody mediated and cell mediated.

Antibodies

These are immunoglobulins produced by B lymphocytes (and their derivative cells, plasma cells) in response to particular antigens. Antibodies produced against microbial antigens may follow exposure to the microbe or to a vaccine. Sometimes, specific antibodies may be present in the serum without prior exposure to the relevant antigen – so called 'natural' antibodies. These are produced as a result of cross-reactivity between antigens; particularly nonprotein (polysaccharide) antigens.

The basic structure of the immunoglobulin molecule is shown in Figure 22.4. The variable region is so called because of the great variability in amino acid sequence. This gives the antibody its particular (unique) specificity and makes its biochemical structure complementary to that of the relevant antigen. There are five main classes of immunoglobulin, each with its own structure and functions. Tables 22.4 and 22.5 show the main characteristics of these classes, and of the subclasses of IgG.

The immunoglobulin class is determined by the type of heavy chain present. During B cell development, rearrangement of the genes coding for the variable and constant parts of the immunoglobulin chain takes place (Fig. 22.5). One each out of the V, D and J heavy chain genes are 'moved' to lie adjacent to the relevant heavy chain constant region gene, so that transcription produces a single protein with a constant and a variable portion. Further rearrangement to bring a particular variable gene combination to lie adjacent to a different heavy chain constant

Table 22.4 Properties of serum immunoglobulins

	IgG	IgM	IgA	IgD	IgE
Heavy chain	γ	μ	α	δ	ε
Light chain	κ/λ	κ/λ	κ/λ	κ/λ	κ/λ
Mol wt ($\times 10^{-3}$)	150	900	160–320	180	200
Polymeric status	Monomer	Pentamer	Monomer or dimer*	Monomer	Monomer
Sedimentation coefficient (Svedberg units)	6.7	19	7	7	8
Mean adult serum concentration (g/l)	12	1.5	3	0.03	0.001
Biological half life (days)	23	5	7	2.8	2.3
Placental transfer	+	–	–	–	–

* Trimeric IgA may also occur. Secretory IgA is in dimeric form.

Table 22.5 Properties of IgG subclasses

	G1	G2	G3	G4
Mol wt ($\times 10^{-3}$)	150	150	165	150
% of total IgG (adults)	70	20	7	3
Biological half life (days)	23	23	9	23
Complement-fixing ability	++	+	++	–
Fc receptor binding				
Monocytes	++	+/–	++	+/–
Neutrophils	+	+	+	+
Lymphocytes	+	+/–	+	+/–

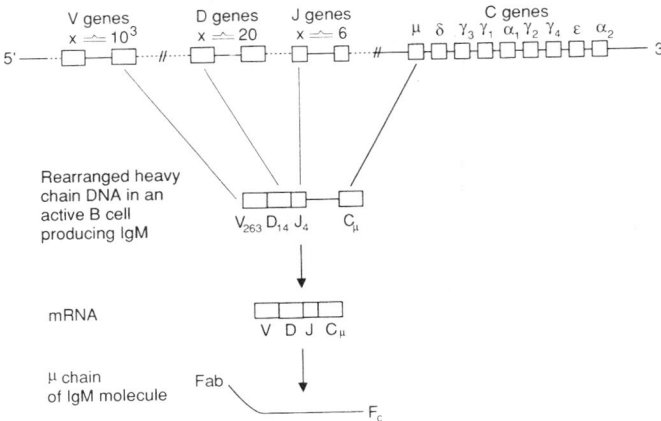

Germ Line DNA

Fig. 22.5 Immunoglobulin heavy chain gene arrangements on chromosome 14 in germ line configuration and showing an example of a rearrangement using V gene number 263, D_{14} and J_4 to produce a unique antigen binding site. In this example, the variable genes (V, D and J) have been combined with a μ constant region heavy chain gene (Cμ) to produce a complete μ chain of an IgM molecule.

region gene allows the B cell to switch production to another antibody class, but with the same specificity. The first heavy chain produced is always a μ chain and class switching occurs later to produce other immunoglobulin classes. The diversity of antibody specificities is created by the very large number of possible combinations of variable region genes which can be selected and is increased further by a very high mutation rate in V genes and the effect of the enzyme TdT (see p. 1238) occurring during the rearrangement process. A similar, but slightly less complex, process takes place with light chains, of which there are two types – kappa and lambda.

IgM. This is the first antibody class produced in primary immune responses. In response to most antigens, there is a subsequent switching to other classes but for some, e.g. responses to the lipopolysaccharides of Gram-negative bacilli, IgM remains the predominant class. Its large pentameric structure confines it mostly to the intravascular space where it is an excellent complement fixer.

IgG. This is the main class of antibody produced in secondary immune responses. Its functions include opsonization, complement fixation leading to C3 opsonization and complement mediated lysis, neutralization of toxins or viruses, and participation in antibody-dependent cellular cytotoxicity. Though there is considerable overlap, the four subclasses of IgG tend to have different functions. In adults, antibodies to bacterial polysaccharides are predominantly of IgG2 subclass, but in children significant amounts are found in the IgG1 subclass. Responses to protein antigens are mainly in the IgG1 and IgG3 subclasses. The role of IgG4 is, as yet, unclear.

IgA. This is the main antibody in secretions, where it is in the form of a dimeric molecule consisting of two IgA subunits joined by a J chain and associated with a protective secretory piece synthesized by epithelial cells. In addition to protecting mucus membranes and the gastrointestinal tract from infection, IgA may have a role in limiting food antigen uptake from the gut. Serum IgA is mainly in monomeric form, though dimeric and trimeric forms are also found.

IgD. This is mainly a surface molecule on the membrane of B cells. The small amounts found free in plasma are not thought to have any biological role. It has a role in regulating the differentiation and maturation of B cells.

IgE. Mast cells and basophils have receptors for the Fc part of this molecule. Antigen binding may trigger an immediate hypersensitivity response by causing degranulation of the cells. Such reactions are often harmful rather than beneficial, but may have a beneficial role in defenses against parasites.

Antibody production

Antibodies are produced by B (bone marrow derived) cells. Virgin B cells have membrane antibody which acts as a receptor for antigen (Fig. 22.6). B cells may be divided into two subsets on the basis of expression of the CD5 surface marker. B1 (CD5 +ve) cells predominate in fetal and neonatal circulations and produce a repertoire of antibodies against self antigens using a limited number of V region genes. They have an as yet poorly understood role in immune regulation and self tolerance. Their numbers may be raised in autoimmune disorders. B2 (CD5 –ve) cells are conventional B cells producing antibodies against foreign antigens.

The final stages of B cell differentiation require stimulation with the appropriate antigen leading ultimately (after final class switching) to maturation into plasma cells. The full process requires the cooperation of antigen-specific T helper (CD4 +ve) cells and is regulated by T suppressor (CD8 +ve) cells. Isotype switching from IgM production to the other antibody classes is critically dependent on T/B cell interaction via the CD40 antigen on B cells and its ligand expressed on activated T cells (antibodies to CD40 ligand have yet to be given a CD number). The responses to some antigens, e.g. bacterial polysaccharides, can result in limited antibody production without T cell help. There is no immunological memory generated in such responses.

Cell-mediated immunity

The T (thymus-derived) cell system is responsible for the predominant immune responses to intracellular microbes and, in addition, has regulating effects via cytokines and growth factors on many other aspects of the immune response.

T cells originate from bone marrow derived stem cells, but acquire their functional capabilities during a period of maturation in the thymus. Here the cells undergo a series of developmental stages including gene rearrangement to generate diversity in the variable domains of the T cell receptor. They also become educated with regard to self and nonself antigens. This education takes the form of both negative and positive selection. The former involves deletion of self-reactive clones, the latter selection of self reactive clones to develop a suppressor function against autoimmune reactions.

The T cell antigen receptor (TCR), though not an immunoglobulin molecule, has a similar arrangement of constant and variable parts and the generation of diversity is achieved along similar lines to the generation of antibody diversity. The TCR is a heterodimeric molecule with each chain having a constant and variable portion. The majority (> 90%) of mature circulating T cells express α and β chains and the minority γ and δ chains. The variable portions of the chains are made up by gene rearrangement

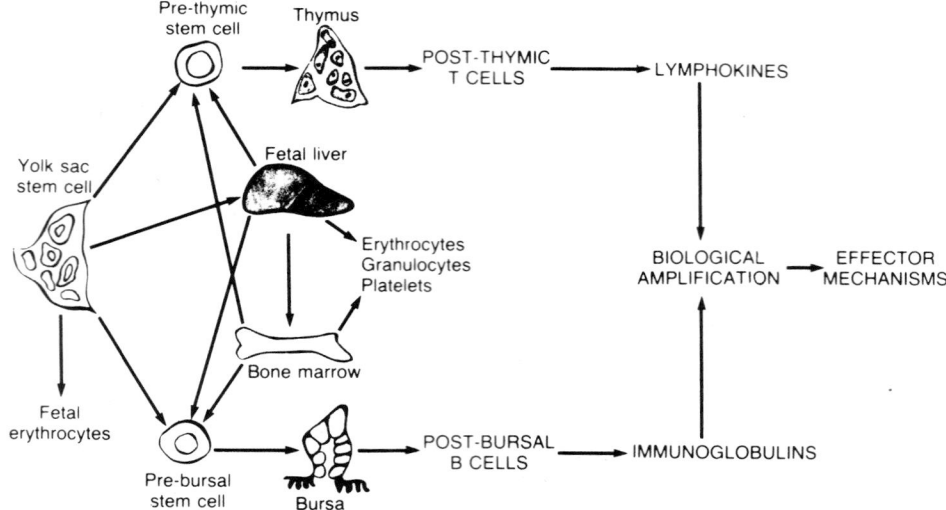

Fig. 22.6A T- and B-cell ontogeny in embryonic life. The yolk sac is the initial site of pre-T- and pre-B-cell production; later, the fetal liver produces these and, finally, the bone marrow, which becomes the permanent site of production. The 'bursa' is only found in avian species and its role in providing a site for maturation of pre-B-cells is fulfilled in mammals by the fetal liver and bone marrow. (Reproduced with permission from Steihm & Fulginiti 1980.)

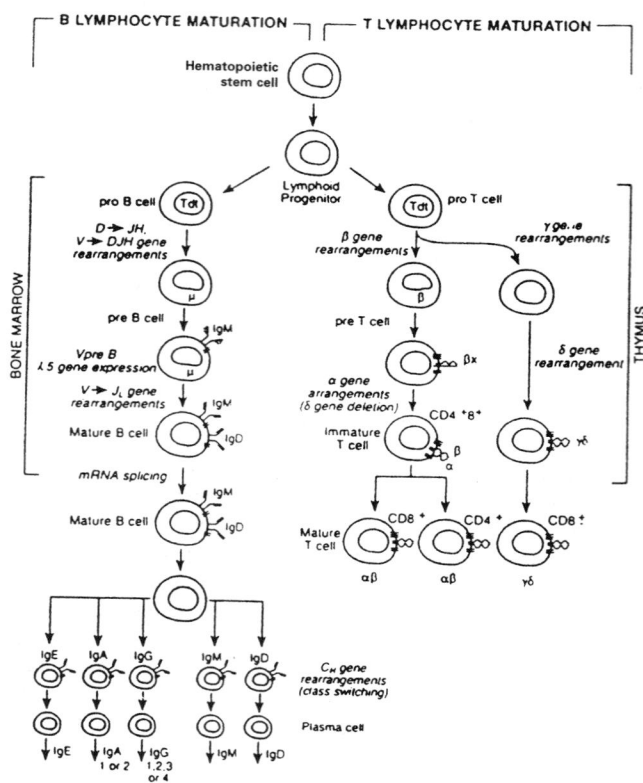

Fig. 22.6B Development of T and B lymphocytes. (Reproduced with permission from Rosen et al 1995.)

of a number of V, D and J genes (except γδ molecules which do not have J genes). This generates a large number of diverse receptors. Further diversity is added by the action of the enzyme terminal deoxynucleotidyltransferase (TdT) which inserts nucleotides in a random fashion at the N terminal end of each VDJ gene. Although this is wasteful in generating a lot of nonsense sequences it greatly increases diversity.

During thymic maturation T cells also acquire important functional surface molecules. CD3 is expressed on all T cells and is closely associated with the TCR (Fig. 22.3). Initially both CD4 and CD8 are expressed on the same cells, but by full maturation one or other molecule is expressed depending on the functional class of the cell. Most γδ T cells do not express CD4 or CD8. Their precise functional role is ill-understood.

The central cell in the immune response is the CD4 positive T helper cell (see Fig. 22.8). Once switched on by antigen presentation these cells develop in one of two ways – the T_{H1} route results in generation of IL-2 and interferon whose main role is in stimulating macrophage function and cell mediated immunity but also has effects on B cells including antibody class switching, particularly to IgG2. T_{H2} cells on the other hand produce predominantly IL-4 and IL-10 which promote antibody responses and class switching, particularly towards IgG1, IgG4 and IgE. Allergic responses and those against parasites are of T_{H2} type. Responses to an antigen may follow a T_{H1} or T_{H2} route depending on a complex set of circumstances. Once established these responses are self-amplifying in that production of interferon or IL-4 promotes T_{H1} and T_{H2} responses respectively and inhibits the other. There is much interest in learning more about these responses to allow therapeutic switching from T_{H2} to T_{H1} in allergic individuals.

The functions of T cells can be summarized as:

1. help and regulation of antibody production by B cells
2. lymphokine production which stimulates and regulates other nonspecific immune effector cells.
3. secretion of growth and differentiation factors, e.g. colony-stimulating factors, B cell growth factors.
4. T cell-mediated specific cytotoxicity, e.g. against virus-infected cells or against foreign tissues.

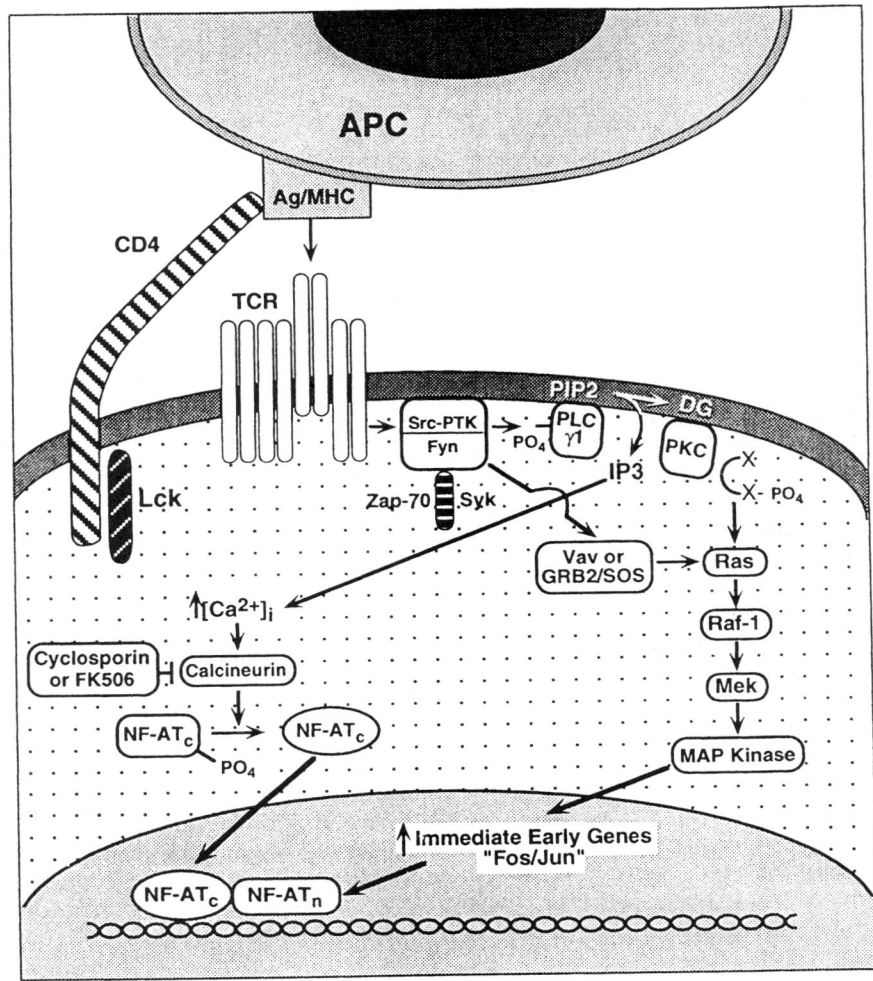

Fig. 22.7 Signaling pathways are induced following antigen-presenting cell/T-cell receptor interaction. APC = antigen-presenting cell; Ag-MHC = antigen/major histocompatibility class II interaction; Src-PTK = Src family protein tyrosine kinases; PIP2 = phosphatidyl-inositol bisphosphate; DG = diacylglycerol; PKC = protein kinase C; PLC-γl = phospholipase C-γl; IP3 = inositol trisphosphate; NF-AT = nuclear factor of activated T cells; n = nuclear; c = cytosolic. (Reproduced with permission from Steihm 1996.)

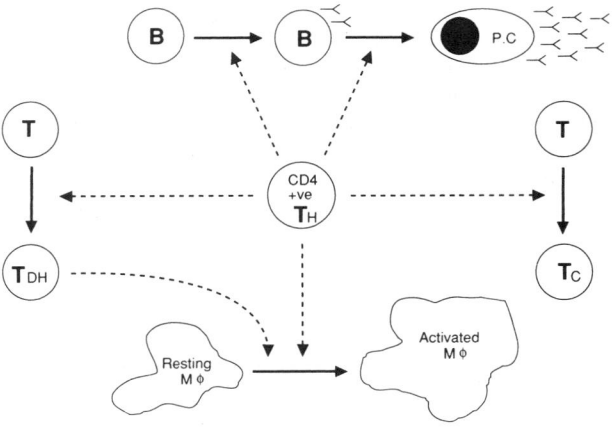

Fig. 22.8 Central role of CD4+ve T-helper (T$_H$) cell in immune responses. T$_C$ = cytotoxic T-cell; T$_{DH}$ = delayed hypersensitivity T-cell); M$_\Phi$ = macrophage; B = B-cell; PC = plasma cell.

Signal transduction

Once T and B cells have engaged antigen via their specific receptors they must activate to generate the next step in the immune response. This activation may take the form of increased transcription of the genes for surface receptors such as CD40 ligand and the IL-2 receptor on T cells, IL-2 production and preparation for cell division. The conveyance of the 'message' from the membrane receptors to the nucleus is called signal transduction (Fig. 22.7) and its study in recent years has revealed several inherited molecular defects resulting in failure of cell activation and thus immunodeficiency. Much is still to be learned about these processes. One of a number of pathways is described here.

Cross-linking of the TCR allows phosphorylation of the intracellular domains of the CD3ζ chain which contains a specific antigen recognition activation motif (ARAM) to bind to the tyrosine kinase ZAP-70 and trigger a cascade of reactions involving protein tyrosine kinases and lipid kinases resulting in a release of intracellular calcium. This is critical for the activation and translocation of nuclear messengers (transcription factors) such as NFAT (nuclear factor of activated T cells) which induce transcription of activation genes including the IL-2 gene.

In B cells a similar cascade occurs with transmembrane proteins Igα and Igβ possessing a similar ARAM motif to the CD3ζ chain of T cells. Full activation of T cells requires a number of signals apart from that via CD3 and the TCR. These come from CD28 engagement of its ligand CD80 on APC; LFA-1/ICAM interaction and the interaction of soluble IL-1 with its surface receptor.

THE DEVELOPMENT OF THE IMMUNE SYSTEM

Prenatal development

The ontogeny of the cellular components of the specific immune system is summarized in Figure 22.6A. T and B cell development commences very early in the gestation of the human fetus. Cells capable of responding in mixed lymphocyte culture or to the mitogen, phytohemagglutinin, and recognizable NK cells are present in the fetal liver from as early as 6 weeks. Precursors of T and B lymphocytes are identifiable from 7–8 weeks and the former start to colonize the rudimentary thymus from the 9th week. By the second trimester, fetal blood sampling reveals circulating lymphocytes with mature T cell surface antigens including the CD3, CD4 and CD8 markers. Surface B cell markers, including surface immunoglobulin, are also expressed at this stage. Absence of these markers can be used for the antenatal diagnosis of severe combined immunodeficiency by fetal blood sampling (see p. 1248).

Although the cellular elements of the specific immune system are present from early in gestation, their ability to respond to antigens, especially in terms of immunoglobulin production, is severely limited until the time of birth.

The nonspecific elements of the immune system also start developing early in fetal life. Neutrophil precursors can be identified in the yolk sac. Mature neutrophils appear in the circulation in the second trimester but remain present in low numbers until the onset of labor. C3 has been detected as early as 6 weeks of gestation. The serum levels of both C3 and of the other complement components, which are produced mainly by the fetal liver, rise slowly throughout fetal life.

The immune system in the newborn

'Physiological' immunodeficiency occurs in the newborn period due to an immaturity in function of the various elements of the immune system (Wilson 1986, Burgio et al 1987). This occurs in full-term as well as preterm infants, but is more exaggerated in the latter and is particularly prominent in sick or stressed preterm infants. It is responsible for the increased susceptibility to infection of the newborn, e.g. the susceptibility to overwhelming group B streptococcal sepsis, or to disseminated herpes simplex infection. Placentally transferred IgG partially offsets the deficiency. However, transfer of immunoglobulin (Fig. 22.9) is a late event in gestation, and so preterm infants have significantly reduced levels; those at the limits of viability (23–24 weeks) have extremely low levels. The protective effect of maternal immunoglobulin depends on the mother having IgG antibody to the appropriate antigens and, in the case of group B streptococcal sepsis, lack of maternal-type specific antibody to the relevant

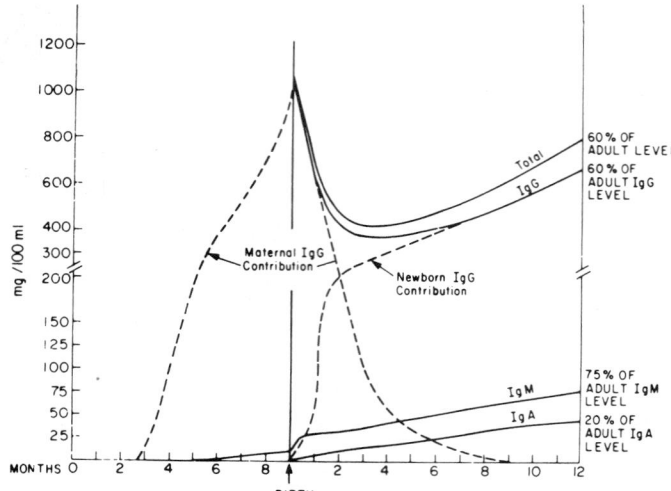

Fig. 22.9 Immunoglobulin levels in fetal life and in the first year postnatally. (Reproduced with permission from Miller & Steihm 1983.)

bacterial polysaccharides has been shown to be a major risk factor. The newborn does not itself produce very much immunoglobulin. Lymphoid cells, when cultured with B cell mitogens, produced a little IgM but no IgG or IgA (Table 22.6). These poor responses are a function of intrinsic B cell immaturity, poor helper and excessive suppressor T cell activity and probably also functional immaturity of the antigen presenting cells. A key factor in the failure of isotype switching is the diminished expression of CD40 ligand on neonatal T cells.

There are a number of differences in cell surface marker expression between neonatal and adult T cells. In addition to the reduced expression of CD40 ligand there is a high CD4 : CD8 ratio, a high expression of the thymocyte antigen CD38 and low numbers of cells expressing the γδ T cell receptor. There is also a high proportion of B cells expressing the CD5 antigen (B1 cells). These differences resolve over the early weeks of life as a result of antigen exposure. Neonates also differ from adults in the expression of CD45 isoforms on their T lymphocytes. They have usually less than 10% of the CD45RO (memory) form and predominant expression of the CD45RA (virgin, naive) form. These proportions gradually reverse during childhood. Exposure to intrauterine infection may alter these neonatal patterns towards a more mature picture.

Cell-mediated immune responses are poor at birth. Even though proliferative mitogen responses are normal, cytokine production (e.g. of gamma-interferon) is low. This may be particularly significant in the susceptibility to intracellular bacterial pathogens, such as *Listeria monocytogenes* or *Salmonella* species, since defenses to these pathogens rely heavily on cytokine-

Table 22.6 Protein A-induced plasma cell (PC) differentiation by newborn and adult lymphocytes (from Hayward & Lydyard 1979)

Source of lymphocytes	PC number/well × 10⁻³		
	IgM	IgG	IgA
Adult	8.1	1.3	1.3
Newborn	0.3	0	0

enhanced macrophage killing. Immaturity in these systems makes delayed hypersensitivity skin testing (as a test of immune competence) unreliable in this age group.

Nonspecific immune mechanisms are also immature at birth. Neutrophil bone marrow reserves are easily exhausted leading to neutropenia; chemotaxis and cell deformability are reduced (compared to values in adults or older children). Neutrophil bactericidal activity is also subnormal though to a lesser extent. In contrast to the situation at other ages, neutrophil numbers and function have a tendency to deteriorate in the presence of infection or other stress (Cairo 1989). Mononuclear phagocyte function and natural killer cell activity are also reduced in the neonate. Complement factor levels and function in a full-term infant are at approximately two-thirds of the adult level, and often below one-half in preterm babies. Alternative pathway factors are at relatively lower levels than classical pathway levels. The precise significance of these findings in predisposing to neonatal sepsis is not clear.

Low immunoglobulin and complement levels are directly proportional to gestational age, while immaturities in cellular function are relatively independent of this. Poor cellular function is more likely to be a feature in babies who have suffered intrauterine growth retardation. Such babies may be neutropenic and have subtly impaired cell-mediated immune functions. The latter have been demonstrated up to 5 years of age, though the clinical significance of such findings is unclear. The placental transfer of immunoglobulin in situations of severe intrauterine growth retardation is probably also compromised, though not all studies have confirmed this (Shapiro 1981).

Postnatal development

Following birth the neonate is exposed to a wide variety of antigenic stimuli, and this is the trigger for the next step in immunological maturation which proceeds regardless of the gestational age of the baby. Immunoglobulin production and the development of the ability to produce antibody responses commence soon after birth. Initially, mostly IgM is produced and there is a rapid rise in circulating IgM levels within days. Gradually, IgG responses develop and by 2 months of age infants are able to produce good IgG antibody responses to protein vaccines, such as tetanus toxoid. During this period, maternal IgG levels fall due to catabolism, and a physiological trough in IgG level occurs at 3–6 months of age before the infant's production picks up (Fig. 22.7). Thereafter the rate of maturation of levels varies for different isotypes. Adult levels of IgM are achieved by 4–5 years and of IgG by 7–8 years. Serum IgA levels (and secretory IgA) rise only very slowly, not achieving adult values until the teenage years.

The pattern of maturation of IgG subclass levels varies between subclasses. IgG2 shows a prolonged physiological trough compared to IgG1 and IgG3 (Fig. 22.10). Though antibody responses to most protein antigens mature early, responses to polysaccharide antigens do not. The latter parallels the development of IgG2 levels. In adults, most antipolysaccharide IgG antibody is found in the G2 subclass, while in children, a small (but probably important) part is found in the G1 subclass. These findings may explain the high degree of susceptibility to polysaccharide-encapsulated organisms, such as *Haemophilus influenzae* type B, shown by young children. They may also explain the lack of responsiveness of children under the age of 18–24 months to

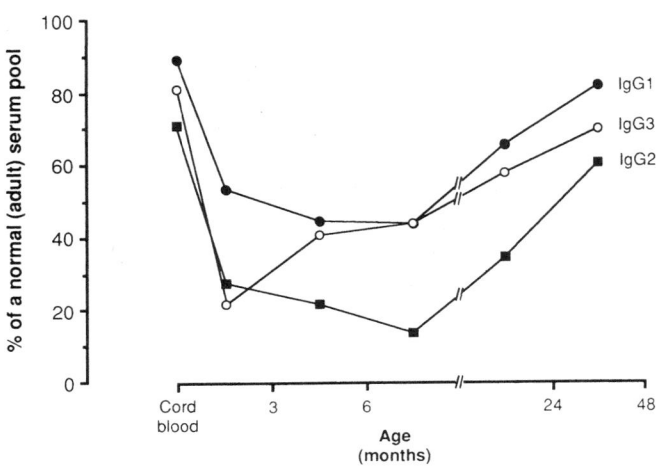

Fig. 22.10 Mean levels of IgG subclasses 1-3 in early life. Note the exaggerated fall and slow rise of IgG2 levels compared to IgG1 and IgG3. (Drawn from the data of Oxelius 1979.)

polysaccharide vaccines, such as pneumococcal or *Haemophilus* type b vaccines. Conjugation of the polysaccharide to a protein or peptide facilitates early responsiveness to both components as demonstrated by the high efficacy of Hib conjugate vaccine and the promising results with the new pneumococcal conjugate vaccines.

Maturation of cell-mediated immune mechanisms mostly occurs within the early weeks of life. Lymphokine production improves to levels comparable to those in adults. The differences in T cell numbers and CD4:8 ratios between children and adults, and the unreliable responses of children to delayed hypersensitivity skin test antigens, such as *Candida* antigen, does however suggest that maturation and development of the cell-mediated immune system continues through early childhood. Subtle immaturities in cell-mediated immunity probably account for the increased susceptibility of young children to tuberculosis, and of young infants to invasive salmonellosis and listeriosis.

IMMUNODEFICIENCY DISORDERS: GENERAL PRINCIPLES

Classification and genetics

Immunodeficiency may be due to a primary (usually inherited) defect or may be secondary (acquired). The WHO working party on immunodeficiency (1995) has attempted to classify the primary disorders, and the main categories are listed in Table 22.7. Figure 22.11 and Table 22.8 show the relative frequencies of the various disorders. The overall incidence of any significant immune deficiency disorder (excluding selective IgA deficiency) has been estimated at 1 in 10 000.

Many of the primary disorders have a genetic basis (Anon 1995, Buckley 1994, Fischer & Arnaiz-Villena 1995, Puck 1994). Identification of the responsible gene(s) has been achieved in a number of conditions, e.g. severe combined immunodeficiency due to adenosine deaminase deficiency and X-linked agammaglobulinemia. Chromosomal aberrations may be found in some immunodeficiency disorders. Deletions of heavy chain constant region genes have been described in a minority of patients with immunoglobulin class or subclass deficiencies, while deletions on chromosome 18 (in some cases of IgA deficiency) and on chromosome 22 (most cases of DiGeorge syndrome) have also been recorded. Immunodeficiency is often a feature of chromosomal breakage/repair disorders, such as ataxia telangiectasia.

Table 22.7A Combined or predominantly cell-mediated deficiencies (adapted from Rosen et al 1995)

Immunodeficiency	Defect	Inheritance
Autosomal recessive (Swiss type) SCID	Gene rearrangement (recombination activating genes)	AR
X-SCID	IL-2 receptor γ chain	XL
Adenosine deaminase deficiency	ADA de-oxy ATP accumulation	AR
Purine nucleoside phosphorylase deficiency	PNP de-oxy GTP accumulation	AR
Bare lymphocyte syndrome I	Defective Class I MHC expression	AR
Bare lymphocyte syndrome II	Defective Class II MHC expression	AR
Reticular dysgenesis	Unknown	AR
CD3 γ or ε deficiency	CD3 and TCR expression	AR
ZAP-70 (CD8) deficiency	ZAP-70 protein tyrosine kinase	AR

Table 22.7B Primary immunodeficiencies - predominantly antibody deficiency (adapted from Rosen et al 1995)

Immunodeficiency	Defect	Inheritance
X-linked agammaglobulinaemia	Btk protein	XL
X-linked Hyper IgM syndrome	gp 39 (CD40 ligand)	XL
Autosomal recessive Hyper IgM syndrome	Unknown	AR
Common variable immunodeficiency	Unknown–some closely linked to C4 gene	Varied (occasionally AR or AD)
Ig heavy chain deletions	Deletion at Ig heavy chain locus (14q32)	AR
Ig kappa chain deletion	Mutation in Ig κ chain locus (2p11)	AR
Selective IgA deficiency	Unknown–some closely linked to C4 gene	Varied (occasionally AR or AD)
IgG subclass deficiency (± IgA deficiency)	Unknown	?
Antibody deficiency with normal immunoglobulin levels	Unknown	?
Transient hypogammaglobulinemia of infancy	Unknown	?

Table 22.7C Defects of specific immunity associated with other major defects (adapted from Rosen et al 1995)

Immunodeficiency	Defect	Inheritance
Wiskott–Aldridge syndrome	WAS protein involved in cytoskeletal function	XL
Ataxia telangiectasia	ATM protein Cell cycle control	AR
DiGeorge anomaly	Developmental field defect. Chromosomal deletion (usually 22q11)	None
Cartilage hair hypoplasia	Unknown	AR
Immunodeficiency with partial albinism	Unknown	AR
Transcobalamin II deficiency	B₁₂ carrier protein	AR
Multiple co-carboxylase deficiency	Biotin metabolism	AR

Table 22.7D Defects of phagocytic function (adapted from Rosen et al 1995)

Immunodeficiency	Inheritance	Defect
X-linked chronic granulomatous disease (CGD)	XL	Killing gp91phox
Autosomal recessive CGD	AR	Killing gp22phox, gp47phox or gp67phox
Leukocyte adhesion deficiency Type I	AR	Chemotaxis & adherence β integrin (CD18)
Leukocyte adhesion deficiency Type II	AR	Chemotaxis & adherence Enzyme producing fucose residue needed for selectin ligand-sialyl lewis X
Chediak–Higashi syndrome	AR	Chemotaxis unknown molecular defect
Neutrophil G6PD deficiency	XL	Killing neutrophil G6PD
Myeloperoxidase deficiency	AR	Killing myeloperoxidase
Secondary granule deficiency	AR	Killing unknown molecular defect
Schwachman syndrome	AR	Chemotaxis unknown molecular defect
Papillion–Lèfevre syndrome	AR	Chemotaxis unknown molecular defect

Table 22.7E Other (less well characterized) immunodeficiency syndromes

Immunodeficiency	Defect	Inheritance
X-linked lymphoproliferative syndrome	Unknown Maps to Xq25	XL
Mucocutaneous candidiasis	Unknown – probably multiple types	?
Hyper IgE syndrome	Unknown	?AD

Table 22.7F Complement deficiencies (adapted from Rosen et al 1995)

Component	Inheritance	Main clinical associations
Clq	AR	SLE, MPGN, pyogenic infections
Clr*	AR	SLE
Cls*	AR	SLE
C4	AR	SLE
C2	AR	SLE, MPGN, HSP, pyogenic infections
C3	AR	Severe pyogenic infections
C5	AR	Neisserial infections, SLE
C6	AR	Neisserial infections, SLE
C7	AR	Neisserial infections, SLE
C8	AR	Neisserial infections, SLE
C9	AR	Neisserial infections (less marked than for C5–8 deficiency)
Factor D	?	Neisserial infections
Properdin	XL	Neisserial infections
C1 esterase inhibitor	AD	Hereditary angioedema
Factor H	AR	Pyogenic infections (less so than I deficiency), MPGN
Factor I	AR	Pyogenic infections

SLE = Systemic lupus erythematosus, MPGN = membrano-proliferative glomerulonephritis; HSP = Henoch Schönlein purpura. *NB* SLE is the most common immune complex disorder in complement deficiencies.
* Clr and Cls deficiency usually occur together.

Table 22.8 Incidence of some primary immunodeficiencies (from Hosking & Roberton 1983)

Immunodeficiency	Incidence
Severe combined immunodeficiency	1 in 66 000
DiGeorge syndrome	1 in 66 000
Common variable immunodeficiency	1 in 83 000
Chronic mucocutaneous candidiasis	1 in 103 000
Chronic granulomatous disease	1 in 181 000
Selective IgA deficiency	1 in 500
X-linked agammaglobulinemia	1 in 103 000

syndrome, the gene has yet to be identified but has been mapped to a particular location. Genetic diagnosis (including antenatal diagnosis) may involve a number of techniques including restriction fragment length polymorphism (RFLP) and single strand conformational polymorphism (SSCP) analysis.

The genetic basis of common variable immunodeficiency and IgA deficiency seems to be linked in that both conditions occur in the same families and are linked to a particular major histocompatibility complex haplotype which includes A1, B8, DR3. This haplotype is associated also with a tendency to autoimmune disorder which can occur in the same affected families. Within the complex the susceptibility to developing immune deficiency has been mapped as being very closely linked to one of the structural genes for the complement component C4. Deletions or duplications of the C4A gene may be found in these deficiency states.

Diagnosis of immunodeficiency

The diagnosis of an immunodeficiency disorder requires a careful history and clinical examination followed by the appropriate confirmatory laboratory tests (Wahn 1995). The first two are particularly important when deciding which children with recurrent minor infections should be investigated.

History

As in most pediatric histories, the pregnancy and birth history are important. Inquiry should be made about the possibility of congenital infection, premature delivery and intrauterine growth retardation, all of which can influence immunity in the early years of life.

In most cases, the presenting problem will be of an infective nature (Webster 1994). The age of onset of infections, their frequency and severity are all important considerations. Establishing the type of infecting organism can give clues to the presence and nature of an underlying immunodeficiency. Recurrent upper respiratory viral infections, however frequent, are not indicative of immune deficiency, unless associated with frequent 'bacterial' complications. Infections with common organisms may run an atypical course in that they are unusually severe, e.g. hemorrhagic chicken pox, or they fail to respond to standard treatments, e.g. a bacterial pneumonia which fails to respond to appropriate antibiotic therapy. Alternatively, infections may be caused by uncommon (atypical) organisms which are in themselves highly suggestive of immunodeficiency, e.g. *Pneumocystis carinii* pneumonia.

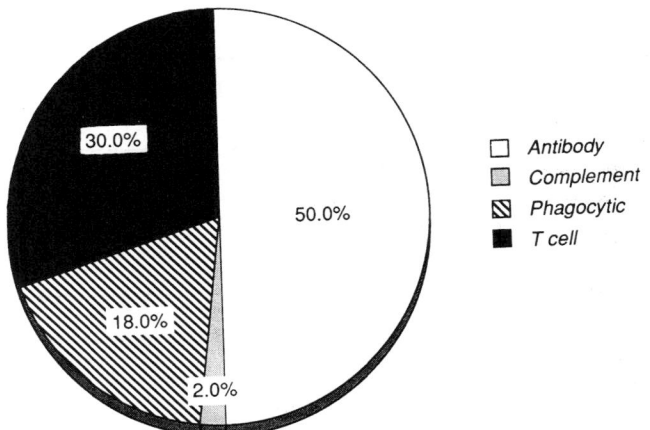

Fig. 22.11 Relative distribution of primary immunodeficiencies, based on combined experience from Japan, Switzerland and USA, excluding cases of asymptomatic selective IgA deficiency. T-cell deficiency group includes patients with combined cell-mediated and antibody deficiencies. (From Steihm 1996.)

The molecular basis of many of the primary ID disorders has been elucidated. Usually several different mutations in the relevant gene have been described. Occasionally mutations at certain points have been found associated with partial forms of the disease, presumably because of some residual function of the protein concerned. In other conditions, e.g. X-linked lymphoproliferative

The history should include inquiries about related problems which can be associated with immunodeficiency disorders. Failure to thrive is a common finding, and this may or may not be associated with diarrhea due to chronic or recurrent infection or noninfective enteropathy. Allergic/atopic problems are common and may be unusually severe. Autoimmune and malignant diseases, though not common, have an increased incidence (see p. 1248).

The family history will often be positive in primary immunodeficiency cases. Many of the major disorders show autosomal or X-linked inheritance. A history of consanguinity should be sought. Some tactful inquiries to ascertain whether the parents have any risk factors for infection with the human immunodeficiency virus should be made as infection with this virus is often a differential diagnosis. In some disorders, e.g. IgA deficiency, there may be a family history of collagen vascular or other immunopathological disease.

Examination

The general physical examination should look particularly for the presence of infection, such as candidiasis, or evidence of previous problems, such as failure to thrive, chronic lung disease, etc. The presence or absence of lymphoid tissue should be noted. In combined immunodeficiency, and in the more severe antibody deficiency states, there are usually no palpable lymph nodes and no visible tonsillar tissue.

In some diseases there may be specific physical signs, such as neurological signs and telangiectases in ataxia telangiectasia, skeletal and hair abnormalities in cartilage hair hypoplasia syndrome, or petechiae and eczema in Wiskott–Aldrich syndrome.

Radiological examination may be helpful. Anteroposterior and lateral chest views will show an absent thymic shadow in most young children with combined or T cell deficiencies. The lung fields may show evidence of chronic lung damage, such as bronchiectasis. The bones may show the skeletal dysplasia of Schwachman syndrome.

Laboratory investigations

The first problem that needs to be addressed is who to investigate. Table 22.9 gives some of the clinical indications for immune function testing. The second decision concerns the particular investigations needed. Clues from the clinical history may direct investigations toward particular branches of the immune system. Recurrent pyogenic infections, for example, would direct initial tests towards the antibody, complement and phagocyte systems

Table 22.9 When to investigate

1. Family history of immunodeficiency or other disorder

2. Single infection with an unusual/opportunistic organism

3. Single infection which is atypically severe or occurs at an atypical age

4. Recurrent minor bacterial infections, e.g. otitis media (> 2 per year*)

5. More than one episode of serious bacterial infection

6. Recurrent infections associated with severe allergy/autoimmune disorder

*in spite of appropriate management by an ENT surgeon

(Fig. 22.1). Table 22.10 shows how problems with different microorganisms tend to be associated with different types of immune defect, while Table 22.11 lists some of the more unusual infections which are suggestive of cell-mediated immune deficit, as in the acquired immunodeficiency syndrome. However, it should be emphasized that because of the multiple interactions and overlaps between the elements of the immune system, exceptions are common, e.g. *Pneumocystis carinii* infection can (rarely) complicate pure antibody deficiency syndromes.

The laboratory investigations available range from simple, widely available tests to complex assays available only in specialist centers (Pacheco & Shearer 1994, IUS/WHO Report 1988).

Blood picture. Much can be learnt from a careful examination of the blood film. A white cell count will detect neutropenic states,

Table 22.10 Association between infecting organisms and most likely type of immune defect

Organism causing problems	Most likely type of immune defect
Pneumococcus, *H. influenzae*	Antibody, Complement
Staphylococcus	Neutrophil, humoral
Meningococcus	Complement
Gram-negative bacilli	Neutrophil
Candida albicans	Cell-mediated, phagocytic†
Herpes viruses	Cell-mediated
Other viruses e.g. measles	Cell-mediated
Mycoplasmas	Antibody
Enteroviruses	Antibody, cell-mediated
Pneumocystis carinii	Cell-mediated
Mycobacteria	Cell-mediated
Salmonella	Cell-mediated
Giardia lamblia	Antibody

† Phagocytic = defects of neutrophil and monocyte function.

Table 22.11 Infections moderately predictive of cell-mediated immune defect (adapted from Jaffe et al 1983)

Protozoan/helminth
Cryptosporidiosis giving diarrhoea for more than 1 month
Pneumocystis carinii pneumonia
Strongyloides causing pneumonia, CNS or disseminated infection
Toxoplasma causing pneumonia or CNS infection

Fungal
Aspergillus – CNS or disseminated infection
Candida albicans – causing oesophagitis
Cryptococcus – pneumonia, CNS or disseminated infection

Bacterial
Atypical mycobacterial infection – disseminated

Viral
Measles – giant cell pneumonia without rash
Varicella zoster – disseminated zoster or hemorrhagic chicken-pox
Cytomegalovirus – pulmonary, gastrointestinal, renal or CNS infection
Herpes simplex – chronic mucocutaneous infection for more than 1 month
 Pulmonary gastrointestinal, or CNS infection
Papovavirus – progressive multifocal leukoencephalopathy

though in the condition of cyclical neutropenia a series of counts (twice weekly for a minimum of 4 weeks) is required. Lymphopenia is suggestive of severe combined immunodeficiency state – in one series (Hague et al 1994) the majority of cases had lymphocyte counts below $2.8 \times 10^9/l$. Eosinophilia is often found in T cell disorders. Abnormal white cell morphology is found in the Chediak–Higashi syndrome, and thrombocytopenia with abnormally small platelets is characteristic of Wiskott–Aldrich syndrome.

Bone marrow examination may be required and is almost always needed in cases with persistent neutropenia to determine whether the problem is one of production failure or excessive consumption and, if the former, to exclude conditions such as leukemia.

Histological tests. Histological examination is sometimes useful and may provide the only available information at postmortem examination if the possibility of immune deficiency is raised. Lymph nodes often show characteristic abnormalities in combined and in severe antibody deficiency disorders. The thymus will also be grossly abnormal in the former. Suction rectal biopsies can be used to demonstrate the absence of plasma cells in immunodeficiencies affecting B cell differentiation.

Tests of humoral immunity

Serum immunoglobulins. Circulating levels of the three main classes of immunoglobulin – IgG, IgM and IgA – are measured using automated methods such as nephelometry. Low levels may need confirmation by other techniques such as single radial diffusion. In very young children care must be taken to use the appropriate age related normal range and to allow for the effect of maternal transplacental IgG. Immunoglobulin deficiency may be due to failure of production or to excessive loss. In the latter, the serum albumin level may also be depressed. Normal or raised immunoglobulin levels do not exclude a significant antibody deficiency in the form of either IgG subclass deficiency or failure to produce 'functional' antibody.

IgG subclass estimations. These are measured in serum using specific monoclonal antisera usually in an ELISA. In standard assays, approximately 10% of normal individuals have undetectable levels of IgG4.

'Functional' antibody tests. Isohemagglutinins are naturally occurring IgM anti-blood-groups A and B antibodies which should appear (except in those with AB blood group) at around 6–9 months. In children older than this, measurement of the titer of these antibodies is a relatively simple test of functional IgM antibody.

Functional tests of IgG rely on the demonstration of antibody against an agent to which the child is known to have been exposed naturally or through vaccination. Tests are available for measurement of antibodies against tetanus toxoid, polio virus and the capsular polysaccharides of *Haemophilus influenzae* type B and some serotypes of pneumococcus. This can be done after primary or booster immunization. Polysaccharide vaccines such as pneumococcal vaccine are the most discriminating as they are the least immunogenic. However responses to these are unreliable in children of less than 2 years of age. Antibody titers against a panel of respiratory viruses can also be used to demonstrate the presence of functional antibody but negative tests are difficult to interpret because of lack of sensitivity. One sensitive test of 'in vivo'

antibody production is to use the harmless bacteriophage $\Phi X174$ injected intravenously. In addition to measuring IgM and IgG response (Pyun et al 1989), clearance of the bacteriophage (which is antibody dependent) can be followed. Patients with X-linked hypogammaglobulinemia fail to clear the virus for several weeks compared to a 3- to 4-day clearance time in normal individuals. Several other patterns of abnormal clearance caused by other immunodeficiency states have been found (Ochs et al 1971).

Immunoglobulins in other body fluids. Secretory IgA can be measured in saliva or tears by radial immunodiffusion. Since the concentration will be dependent on the flow rates, quantification should be related to albumin concentrations. A normal serum IgA with very low secretory levels suggests secretory piece deficiency but this is extremely rare. A small proportion of serum IgA deficient individuals have normal levels of secretory IgA.

Immunoglobulin and antibody levels can also be measured in cerebrospinal fluid, and this is used in the diagnosis of inflammatory or infective conditions affecting the central nervous system.

IgE. This is measured by radioimmunoassay. Its value in diagnosis of immunodeficiency is limited. One situation in which it is extremely useful is for the diagnosis of the hyper-IgE syndrome in which levels are usually at least 2000 U/l (Buckley & Sampson 1981). Undetectable levels of IgE are found in some cases of SCID, X-linked agammaglobulinemia and ataxia telangiectasia. In conditions with partial T cell deficiency, including Wiskott–Aldrich and DiGeorge syndromes, levels are moderately high, possibly due to disturbed regulation.

In vitro tests of immunoglobulin/antibody production. There are a variety of functional tests of immunoglobulin production. Culturing circulating lymphocytes with pokeweed mitogen leads to B cell activation and differentiation into plasma cells. There is polyclonal immunoglobulin production which can be measured in the supernatants. This test relies on T cell and antigen-presenting cell cooperation, and is thus a test of the whole cellular network involved in immunoglobulin production. Epstein–Barr virus is a B cell mitogen which will stimulate polyclonal immunoglobulin production in the absence of T cells. More subtle in vitro culturing methods can be used to look at specific antibody responses. This can be done using a variety of antigens, including tetanus toxoid and varicella-zoster virus.

Complement. Measurement of C3 and C4 levels is routinely available in many laboratories. A test for assessing functional activity of the whole complement pathway is called the total hemolytic complement or CH50 test. This involves using dilutions of serum as a complement source to lyse sheep erythrocytes which have been sensitized by antibody. Deficiency of any single component results in failure of lysis. If this occurs specific factor assays should be performed. Tests for the alternate pathway involve either measuring opsonization of particles, such as zymosan or yeasts (which activate the alternative pathway), or measuring complement component byproducts following alternative pathway activation. There are also assays for a number of the individual alternative pathway components. One practical consideration when investigating the complement system is that many of the components are labile, and so serum has to be separated and frozen at $-70°C$ within 2 hours of venesection.

Mannose-binding lectin. This can be measured in the serum by ELISA technique or deficiency can be inferred from finding one of the known mutations of the gene.

Tests of cell-mediated immunity

Lymphocyte numbers and subsets. Total T cell numbers and subsets are estimated using monoclonal antibodies (usually raised in mice) directed against surface antigens specific for the various human T cell populations (see Table 22.3). The cells are incubated with antibody and after washing, cells which have been labeled are identified by a second incubation with an anti-mouse immunoglobulin conjugated to an indicator molecule, e.g. a fluorescent marker such as fluorescein. Positive cells can be identified by UV microscopy or by an automated fluorescence activated cell scanner (FACS). The number of positive cells stained with a particular monoclonal can be expressed as a percentage of the total mononuclear cell population, as a derived (from the total lymphocyte count) absolute number of cells or as a ratio to other markers (e.g. CD4 : CD8 ratio). Care is needed in the interpretation of the results which will vary with age and with the state of general health at the time of testing. Around 60–80% of the circulating lymphocytes are T cells with roughly a 2 : 1 ratio of CD4 : CD8. Absolute CD4 counts at different ages are shown in Figure 22.12.

A modification of this method in which the second antibody is conjugated to an enzyme, such as alkaline phosphatase or peroxidase, can be used on slide preparations or even fixed histological sections – the cells being identified by the color change produced when the enzyme has reacted with its substrate.

B cell numbers can be measured using either the relevant monoclonal antibodies (CD19 or CD20) or an antihuman immuno-globulin antibody to identify the cell surface immunoglobulin molecules. In the latter fluorescein is usually tagged directly to the anti-immunoglobulin, making it a one-step reaction.

Tests of lymphocyte function: mitogen responses. Mitogens are substances which induce cells to proliferate. Measurement of the T cell mitogen response is a useful screening test for functional T cells. Plant lectin substances, phytohemagglutinin (PHA), concanavalin A and pokeweed mitogen are T cell mitogens. The last of these, as well as bacterial lipopolysaccharide and Epstein–Barr virus, are B cell mitogens and also induce immunoglobulin secretion (see above). After incubation with these substances, responses are measured by one of a number of methods – ^{3}H thymidine uptake as an index of DNA turnover, cytokine production (e.g. IL-2) as an index of cell activation or, in the case of B cell mitogens, immunoglobulin production in the culture supernatant.

Antigen specific tests. In vitro responses to antigens are more subtle tests of cellular immune function than those to mitogens. Cells are incubated with common antigens to which the individual has been exposed, e.g. candida antigen or tetanus toxoid and cell turnover or activation measured as above. Antibody production to specific antigens can also be performed in vitro and is a useful research technique.

Mixed lymphocyte culture reactivity is measured by the proliferative response of the patient's lymphoid cells to irradiated (stimulator) allogeneic lymphocytes.

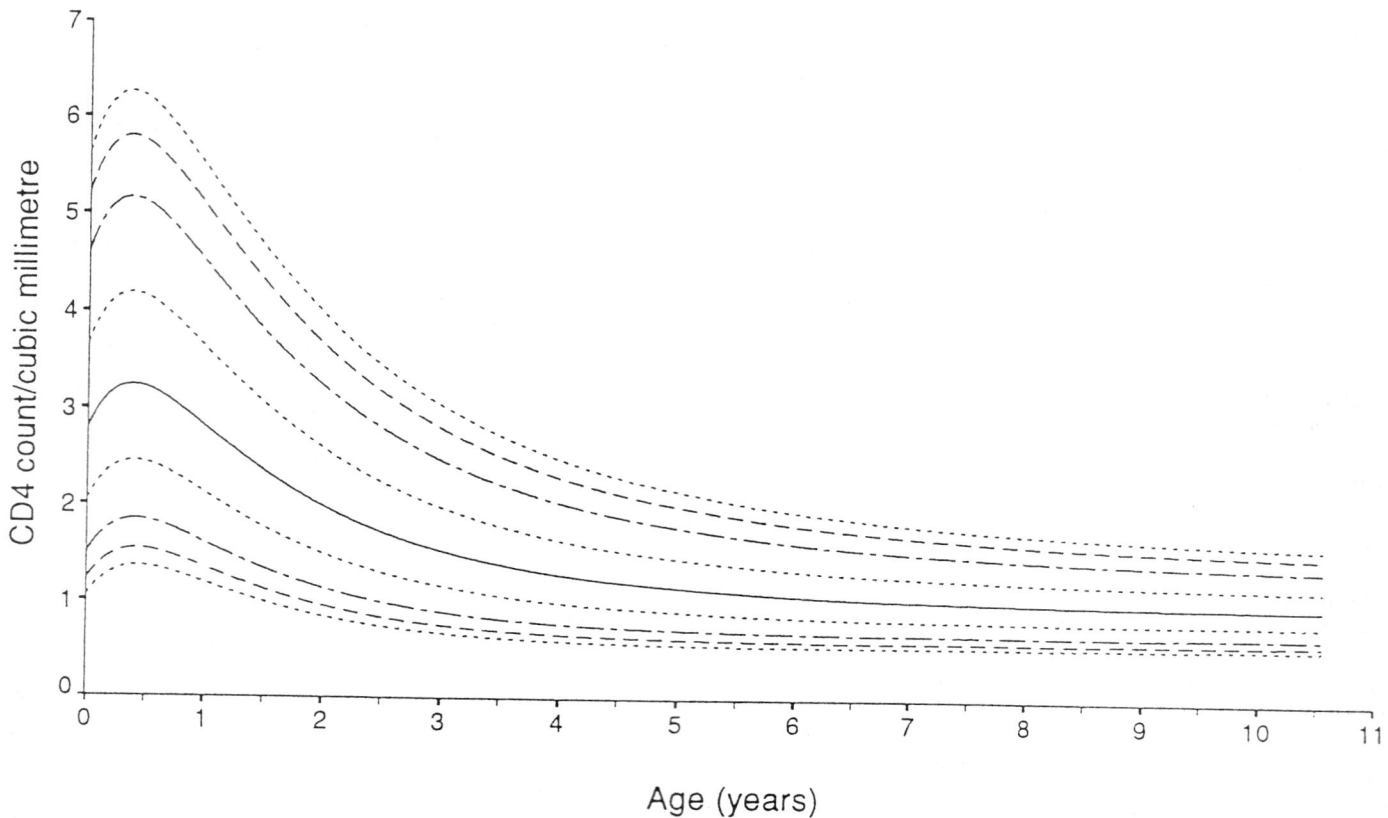

Fig. 22.12 CD4 lymphocyte counts in children by age: 3rd, 5th, 10th, 25th, 50th, 75th, 90th, 95th and 97th centiles. Created from data collected by the European Collaborative Study using the methods of Wade & Ades (1994).

Cytotoxicity assays look at T or NK cell cytotoxic function. In the most commonly used method, ^{51}Cr-EDTA-labeled 'target' cells are incubated with the lymphoid cells, and released ^{51}Cr is measured in the supernatant as an index of killing. Tumor cell lines can be used as targets for NK cell assay, whereas specific T cell cytotoxicity assays employ cell lines which express specific (most commonly viral) antigens.

In vivo tests of cell-mediated immunity. Delayed hypersensitivity skin tests can be performed using a number of common antigens, including those derived from candida, streptococcus and mumps as well as tetanus toxoid. Pre-prepared multiantigen kits are available for this purpose but are not recommended by all authorities (Rosen et al 1995). Positive responses make it quite unlikely that the patient has a major cell mediated immune deficiency. Children respond less reliably to these than adults and so negative results are less useful. Corticosteroid treatment can lead to false-negative results.

Neutrophil function tests. Chemotaxis. Neutrophil migration can be assessed by measuring the distance migrated through a millipore filter in a set time either by random movement or in response to a chemotactic stimulus. The test is affected by a number of unpredictable factors and even when strict controls are employed, the results can be difficult to interpret. Chemotaxis seems to vary greatly between individuals and with time in the same individual.

Phagocytosis. Phagocytic assays involve measurement of uptake of particles or microorganisms by direct microscopy, by scintillation counting (using radiolabeled organisms) or by FACS analysis (using fluorescent labeled organisms). The test can be used to assess opsonic activity of sera as well as the phagocytic function of the cell. Chemiluminescence can be used as an indirect measure of phagocytosis.

Chemiluminescence. The oxidative metabolic burst which neutrophils and monocytes undergo on phagocytosis results in the generation of photons (chemiluminescence) which can be measured (in a photomultiplier) in a quantitative way and used to assess neutrophil function.

Nitroblue tetrazolium (NBT) reduction. Nitroblue tetrazolium (NBT) is a dye taken up by phagocytes and reduced by the oxidative burst to a purple formazan deposit in the cells. After pretreatment of cells with the phorbol ester, phorbol myristate acetate (PMA), 98% or more of cells should reduce NBT. In chronic granulomatous disease (CGD), whichever stimulus is used, less than 1% of cells show NBT reduction. Approximately 50% of the cells from female carriers of the X-linked form show NBT reduction after PMA treatment. This test can be done rapidly on a microscope slide and is an excellent screening test for CGD and CGD carrier state (Fig. 22.13).

Bacterial killing tests. Neutrophils are allowed to ingest bacteria, e.g. staphylococci and then incubated at 37°C. After carefully washing the cells in antibiotic-containing medium, estimates of intracellular viable bacteria can be made by lysing the cells and culturing the lysate. A ratio of viable bacterial counts after 120 minutes compared to 20 minutes of incubation is calculated. This should be less than 0.2 in normal subjects. Ratios of up to 1.0 or even higher may be obtained in cells from patients with CGD or other bactericidal defects.

Enzyme assays. Killing defects not due to chronic granulomatous disease can be diagnosed by estimation of the specific granule enzymes including myeloperoxidase and glucose-6-phosphate dehydrogenase.

In vivo neutrophil function tests: Rebuck skin window. Creating a skin window by abrading the skin and covering it with a cover slip

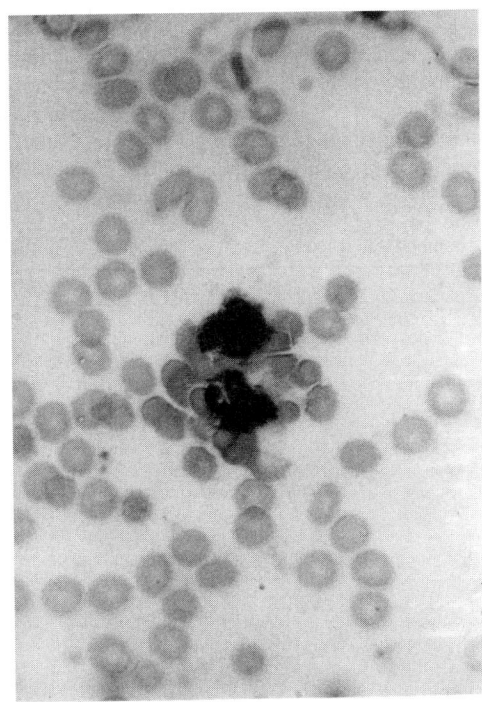 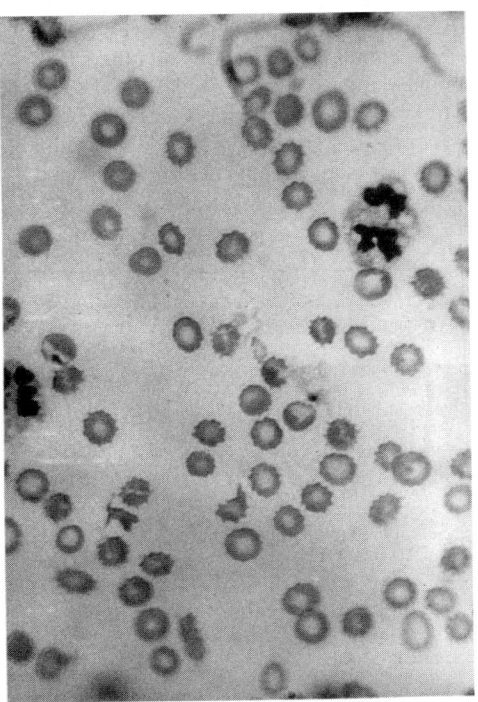

a   b

Fig. 22.13   Slide nitroblue tetrazolium (NBT) reduction test. (**a**) Normal subject. Neutrophils have taken up and reduced NBT to form a dense brown/black deposit. (**b**) Patient with chronic granulomatous disease. None of the cells have produced the deposit due to failure to reduce the NBT.

(to which neutrophils stick) allows in vivo assessment of neutrophil migration. This test is rarely used in clinical pediatric practice.

Antenatal diagnosis

The genetic basis for many of the primary immunodeficiency disorders has now been elucidated. This has greatly enhanced the ability to provide precise genetic counseling, carrier detection and antenatal diagnosis. The most used technique has employed informative restriction fragment length polymorphisms (RFLP) performed on first trimester chorionic villus samples. In the case of X-linked disorders, selective X chromosome inactivation studies can be performed, based on the fact that in some of the more severe X-linked immunodeficiencies female carriers show selective (100%) expression of the normal X chromosome in the affected cell series. This is in contrast to the usual finding of random expression of either X chromosome. This can be demonstrated by simultaneously utilizing markers which can distinguish maternal and paternal, as well as active and inactive, X chromosomes. This is of interest not only because of its usefulness for genetic counseling, but also because in complex immunodeficiencies, e.g. Wiskott–Aldrich syndrome, it has been used to identify which cell series are affected. Nongenetic tests are still used, e.g. the slide NBT test for detecting chronic granulomatous disease in affected fetuses and in female carriers. In those cases of severe combined immunodeficiency where the molecular basis has not been elucidated, second trimester fetal blood sampling can be used to detect absence or abnormalities of circulating T lymphocytes (Durandy et al 1982).

Associations of immune deficiency

Allergy and autoimmunity. Allergic diseases occur with increased frequency in patients with immune deficiency. Selective IgA deficiency is the most common association, but others include common variable immune deficiency and complement disorders.

Autoimmune disorders are also much more common than in the general population (Anon 1993). In the case of antibody, complement and phagocytic disorders, this might be explained by the poor handling and clearance of antigen and immune complexes. The gene(s), lying in the major histocompatibility complex, associated with IgA and common variable immune deficiencies are also associated with a susceptibility to various autoimmune disorders such as rheumatoid arthritis. In T cell disorders, defective regulation of the immune response is likely to be the cause. The fact that treatment of many of these disorders involves immunosuppression, makes the management particularly difficult.

Malignancy. Reports from the Immunodeficiency and Cancer Registry have confirmed that malignant disease occurs with higher frequency in primary immunodeficiency disorders (Spector et al 1978). Mostly lymphoid malignancies have occurred but, particularly in ataxia telangiectasia, carcinomas have also been reported (Table 22.12). Carriers of this condition may have an increased risk of developing breast cancer. Carcinomas also occur in selective IgA and common variable deficiencies, but this might be related to the relatively advanced age of the patients on the register with these conditions (Mueller & Pizzo 1995).

Defective immunological surveillance against cancer cells is one plausible explanation for these findings. Another possible mechanism is that the basic defect in the lymphoid cells which causes the immunodeficiency also has oncogenic potential. Certainly in ataxia telangiectasia the known DNA repair defect is likely to be important in this respect. The occurrence of lymphomas in secondary immune deficiency states, such as those induced by cyclosporine or by the human immunodeficiency virus (HIV), adds considerable weight to the immunological surveillance theory.

DISORDERS OF CELL-MEDIATED IMMUNITY: COMBINED IMMUNODEFICIENCIES

Failure of the normal development of T cells and cell-mediated immunity may result from primary abnormalities of thymic development or, more commonly, from intrinsic abnormalities in the T cell lineage affecting early pre-T cell development in the bone marrow. In the latter case the thymus also fails to develop,

Table 22.12 Incidence of malignancy in children with primary immunodeficiencies

Disease	Risk (%)	Main tumor type
X-linked agammaglobulinemia	6	Leukemia, NHL
Common variable immunodeficiency		
< 16 years at onset	2.5	NHL, gastric carcinoma
> 16 years at onset	8.5	
Selective IgA deficiency	?	NHL, gastric carcinoma
Severe combined immunodeficiency*	5	NHL
X-linked lymphoproliferative syndrome	24	NHL
Wiskott–Aldrich syndrome	>10	NHL, leukemia
Ataxia telangiectasia	>12	Leukemia, NHL carcinomas
Bloom syndrome	25	Leukemia, NHL carcinomas

Data from Immunodeficiency and Cancer Registry reported by Mueller & Pizzo, 1995
*very short latency period for development of malignancy compared to other disorders.
NHL = Non-Hodgkins lymphoma

and this is probably due to lack of inductive signals from the bone marrow.

Failure or abnormal regulation of T cell influences on B cell maturation and function means that in the more severe T cell deficiencies there is nearly always an accompanying deficiency in humoral responses resulting in a combined (cell-mediated and humoral) deficiency. The humoral element may range from subtle defects in antibody responses to complete hypogamma-globulinemia. In other combined immunodeficiencies the humoral component is due to a molecular defect which affects both T and B cells. Either way it is extremely unusual to find a significant pure T cell deficiency syndrome with preserved humoral immune function.

Combined immunodeficiency can result from a large number of disorders affecting T (±B) cells and showing X-linked or autosomal recessive inheritance. The molecular basis for many of these has been elucidated but many others remain uncharacterized. The term severe combined immunodeficiency (SCID) is used for the most severely affected cases. Typically such cases have profound T cell lymphopenia and panhypogamma-globulinemia and a very short life expectancy. However apparently less severe combined deficiencies can lead to equally devastating consequences. Furthermore with the recognition of attenuated ('leaky') forms of SCID (see below) it is clear that some infants with a SCID disorder may have a less severe phenotype. The distinction between SCID and CID is therefore rather arbitrary and, when known, it is best to use the name of the underlying molecular defect. The term SCID will be used here to describe the general features of the full blown syndrome described above.

General features of severe combined immunodeficiency

Full blown SCID

The particular features of individual disorders are discussed below. Some of the features of full blown SCID with early onset of problems and likelihood of being fatal at an early age are common to all the disorders and are considered here.

Clinical features. Affected babies appear well at birth and are normally grown. Problems usually start within the first few months of life. There are a number of different presentations. Chronic diarrhea and failure to thrive are amongst the commonest. This is often due to persistent and sometimes multiple gastrointestinal infection, and there is likely to be associated food intolerance. Persistent and extensive candidiasis also develops in many cases. Other presentations include severe bacterial infections, especially pneumonias, which may fail to respond to appropriate treatment, or atypical infections, e.g. caused by viruses or by *Pneumocystis carinii*. Presentation may sometimes follow vaccination with live vaccines, e.g. disseminated BCG infection or vaccine associated paralytic poliomyelitis. Vaccinia gangrenosum is fortunately no longer seen.

Since there is inability to reject foreign tissues, graft-versus-host disease (GVHD) can occur. Mild forms of this are seen if maternal engraftment has occurred following placental transfer of lymphocytes (in one series, this was found in 25% of cases). Even milder forms may occur through breast-feeding, although this is not a contraindication to breast-feeding. The GVHD in these cases typically causes a mild reticular skin rash with or without mildly deranged liver function tests. Its role in the gastrointestinal

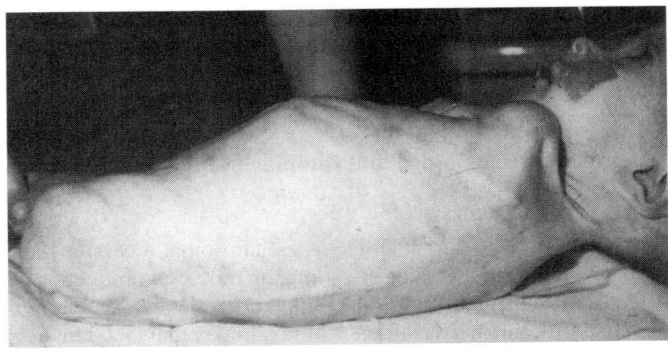

Fig. 22.14 Wasting in a child with severe combined immunodeficiency (SCID).

symptoms is not known. Fatal GVHD can follow transfusion with nonirradiated blood or with white cell or platelet concentrates.

Occasional cases of SCID have presented with a very similar clinical picture to severe Langerhans cell histiocytosis (Maarten-Egeler & D'Angio 1995, Pritchard et al 1994).

Examination may reveal a wasted child (Fig. 22.14) with evidence of candidiasis and other infections. However, in the early stages, the infant may appear well. There is no clinically detectable lymphoid tissue; and a thymic shadow is absent on chest X-ray. There may be hepatomegaly.

Investigations reveal lymphopenia, and lymphocytic markers show severely depleted T cell numbers. B cells are present, though nonfunctioning, in some cases (B cell SCID). Other cases have neither circulating T nor B cells. Occasional variants have odd patterns of immature T cell markers; in such cases maternal engraftment should be excluded. Mitogen responses, mixed lymphocyte reaction, in vitro antigen specific responses and delayed hypersensitivity skin testing to common antigens are all absent. Immunoglobulin estimations, depending on the age of the infant, show residual maternal IgG but typically very little or no IgM or IgA. Occasionally immunoglobulin, usually IgM, is produced but this is not functionally active.

In children who die, postmortem examination reveals severely depleted lymphoid tissue, with nodes and thymus showing no lymphoid cells and absent Hassall's corpuscles in the latter. Plasma cells are absent throughout the body.

Attenuated (leaky) severe combined immunodeficiency

In SCID a variety of different molecular defects can result in failure of development of T cells. Occasional cases of children with an attenuated phenotype have been found. It is believed that in these cases some T cells escape the block in differentiation and proceed to maturation. Circulating T cell numbers may be low or normal and mitogen responses may be present. Immunoglobulin may also be produced. However tests of antigen specific T cell proliferation and antibody production are defective and there is cutaneous anergy. Diagnosis may be difficult in these patients. In addition to the above test profile, patients can be shown to have a limited diversity of T cell receptor and immunoglobulin gene rearrangements. Screening of candidate genes for SCID may show the mutation.

It is possible that in these cases the mutation in the gene is in a position that allows some protein function to be expressed or possibly a second (correcting) mutation has occurred. It has been suggested that Omenn's syndrome (see below) is a form of leaky SCID.

Types of severe combined and combined immunodeficiencies

Reticular dysgenesis

In this variety of SCID, inherited as an autosomal recessive trait, there is severe leukopenia due to complete failure of production of all cells in the granulocyte and lymphoid series. Bone marrow examination confirms the absence of myeloid precursors. Platelets and red cells are formed normally. In some reports, leukopenia was not profound in all cases and erythrophagocytosis was noted. It is possible that in these cases maternal engraftment and GVHD had occurred. The absence of the nonspecific cellular elements of the immune system makes the immune deficiency even more severe than in other forms of SCID. Clinical presentation often occurs earlier, as does the inevitable fatal outcome if immune reconstitution cannot be achieved.

SCID with absent T and B cells (Swiss type agammaglobulinemia, autosomal recessive SCID)

In most or possibly all cases with this phenotype there is a defect in one of the genes controlling the gene rearrangements, recombination activating genes (RAG), necessary for the development of diversity in the antigen receptors on T and B cells.

γ Chain (of IL-2 receptor) deficiency (X-SCID)

Most X-linked cases of SCID have this disorder resulting from a mutation in the gene for the common γ chain of the IL-2, IL-4, IL-7, IL-9 and IL-15 receptors. Typically there is severe T lymphopenia with normal or high circulating numbers of (nonfunctional) B cells.

Defects of other cell surface molecules

Bare lymphocyte syndrome (Klein et al 1993). Defective expression of the Class I major histocompatibility complex antigens (HLA A, B and C) was the first form of this condition to be described. Subsequently, a second more common variety of defective MHC Class II (HLA DR) antigen expression with or without failure of Class I expression has been described. Both varieties are inherited in an autosomal recessive fashion. The failure to produce Class II antigens lies in the genes regulating their transcription. Since HLA antigens are of vital importance in lymphocyte function and interactions, their absence leads to a profound functional deficit. In contrast to other forms of SCID circulating T and B cell numbers are normal though the CD4 count is low in Class II and the CD8 count in Class I deficiency. Furthermore, lymph nodes are easily palpable and the thymus is of relatively normal size. Histological examination of lymph nodes shows poorly formed follicles, absent germinal centers and depleted T cell areas. Plasma cells are absent from all tissues. The thymus shows diminished Hassall's corpuscles. Mitogen responses are normal but antigen specific responses and delayed hypersensitivity tests are negative. There is panhypogamma-

globulinemia and it is not possible to induce B cell proliferation in vitro. Confirmation of the diagnosis depends on demonstration of the absence of the HLA antigens on the cells. Interestingly, two siblings have been described in whom absent HLA expression was not associated with clinical immune deficiency.

CD3 deficiency. Two genetic disorders have been described affecting the γ and ε chains of the T cell receptor. The expression of the receptor is reduced but not usually absent and may vary within the same affected family. Normal numbers of circulating T and B cells are found. The clinical consequences have yet to be fully described.

CD7 deficiency has been described. This molecule is thought to be important in early T cell development.

OKT4 deficiency is a defect in an epitope on the CD4 molecule recognized by a monoclonal antibody of that name. There is a mild immunodeficiency and a tendency to autoimmune disease.

Fas (CD95) deficiency. This is a cell surface molecule important in apoptosis. It is expressed on thymocytes and activated T cells. Three children described had a marked lymphoproliferative syndrome and two of them had autoimmune disease. CD4 cells are low but lymphocyte count is normal by virtue of a proliferation of CD4/CD8 double negative cells (Rieux-Laucat et al 1995).

Signal transduction defects

ZAP-70 defect (CD8 deficiency) (Elder et al 1995). Defective signal transduction in T cells results from this autosomal recessive condition. The defective kinase is important in T cell activation via the CD3/TCR complex. There is a marked effect on CD8 positive cell development. Though CD4 cells are present in normal numbers, they are nonfunctional.

JAK-3 defect. Mutations in the gene for this cytoplasmic kinase, named Janus (family) kinase, results in defective T cell activation and combined immunodeficiency.

Defects of cytokine production

Several defects have been described including IL-1, IL-2 and interferon γ deficiency which resulted in a spectrum of clinical problems including failure to thrive and a susceptibility to opportunistic infections. Humoral immunity is relatively preserved. A recently described defect in the gene for the interferon γ receptor led to a susceptibility to disseminated infection with atypical mycobacteria (Newport et al 1996).

Lymphocyte metabolism defects

Adenosine deaminase (ADA) deficiency (Hirschhorn et al 1979). This variety of SCID is due to a single gene defect which results in absence of the purine metabolic pathway enzyme, ADA. Though the enzyme is expressed widely throughout the body, the effects of the deficiency seem to be concentrated mainly in the lymphocytes, resulting in cell death. The exact mechanism by which this selective toxicity occurs is not fully elucidated and there are several theories. The most plausible is that there is accumulation of toxic deoxyadenosine triphosphate in lymphocytes due to the high activity of deoxyadenosine kinase. Skeletal abnormalities (cupping deformities of the ends of the ribs, as well as abnormalities of the transverse vertebral processes and the scapulae) are reported as occurring in up to 50% of cases and can be correlated with histological changes (Cederbaum et al 1976). Neurodevelopmental problems may also occur in some patients. Otherwise, the clinical and immunological features are similar to other SCID types. Partial forms of ADA deficiency can occur and are associated with a milder immunodeficiency or even normal immune function. Occasional cases of ADA deficiency have been described, where inexplicably, immune function is normal. The diagnosis is confirmed by assay of red cell ADA activity. First trimester antenatal diagnosis is possible.

Purine nucleoside phosphorylase (PNP) deficiency. Deficiency of another purine metabolic pathway enzyme, PNP, which results in combined immunodeficiency, is initially less severe than ADA deficiency though there is progression with age. It is an autosomal recessive condition the gene for which is found on chromosome 9. The toxic metabolite deoxyguanosine triphosphate accumulates in the cells resulting in lymphocytotoxicity.

The onset of symptoms is usually later than in ADA deficiency, and can be delayed for several years. Recurrent and severe infections, particularly with viruses and fungi, as well as a predisposition to GVHD following nonirradiated blood transfusion, suggest that the deficiency is predominantly of cell-mediated immunity. There is a marked tendency to autoimmune disease, especially hemolytic anemia which can progress to red cell aplasia. Skeletal abnormalities do not occur, but neurodevelopmental occurred in over half of the patients. Tests show a progressive fall in T cell numbers and function with time, poor in vitro mitogen responses and negative delayed hypersensitivity skin tests. Immunoglobulin levels and antibody responses are initially normal but in the late stages levels fall. Serum uric acid levels are low. The diagnosis is confirmed by demonstrating absent PNP activity in red cells or fibroblasts. Partial, asymptomatic, forms of the deficiency have not been reported.

Enzyme replacement therapy has not been used extensively but successful treatment has been achieved with bone marrow transplantation.

Poorly characterized defects

X-linked lymphoproliferative syndrome (Hereditary defective response to Epstein–Barr virus or Duncan's syndrome). An immunodeficiency specifically affecting the handling of Epstein–Barr (EB) virus was first recognized in the Duncan kindred (Purtilo et al 1975). It is inherited in an X-linked fashion, and affected boys are apparently normal until they meet the virus. Following infection, they develop profound secondary immune deficiency affecting T and NK cell function and antibody responses. Four clinical patterns, which are not mutually exclusive, have been described: severe infectious mononucleosis, malignant B cell lymphoma, aplastic anemia and panhypogammaglobulinemia. The prognosis is very poor with 75–85% mortality. Confirmation of the diagnosis involves demonstrating EB virus genome in lymphocytes by DNA hybridization, together with the immune defects outlined above and an abnormal serological response to the virus with absent antibody response to EB nuclear antigen (EBNA). The mothers of affected boys also have abnormal EB virus serology, with persisting very high titers against viral capsid antigen.

The responsible gene has been localized to Xq25 and using RFLP analysis it is possible to identify affected boys before they meet EB virus. In such circumstances administration of intravenous immunoglobulin on a regular basis as passive immunization against EB virus can be attempted though its efficacy is unproven. Correction of the disorder by bone marrow transplantation has been achieved.

Mucocutaneous candidiasis. This condition is characterized by chronic candidal infection of skin, nails and mucus membranes (Fig. 22.15). It is almost certainly made up of a heterogeneous group of conditions of varying severity and of varying inheritance. In some cases, there is an association with polyendocrinopathy including, in order of frequency, hypoparathyroidism, Addison's disease, pernicious anemia, hypothyroidism and diabetes mellitus. Iron deficiency exacerbates the condition. In severe cases, the skin lesions may be extremely disfiguring and distressing. Esophageal involvement can lead to dysphagia.

The underlying defect is poorly defined and may be variable. There is evidence of diminished T cell proliferation and cytokine production in response to candida antigens.

Treatment consists of correcting any associated deficiencies, and using systemic antifungal drugs. Oral ketoconazole has proved successful even in severe cases, but its potential toxicity and the emergence of drug resistance may be problematic. The

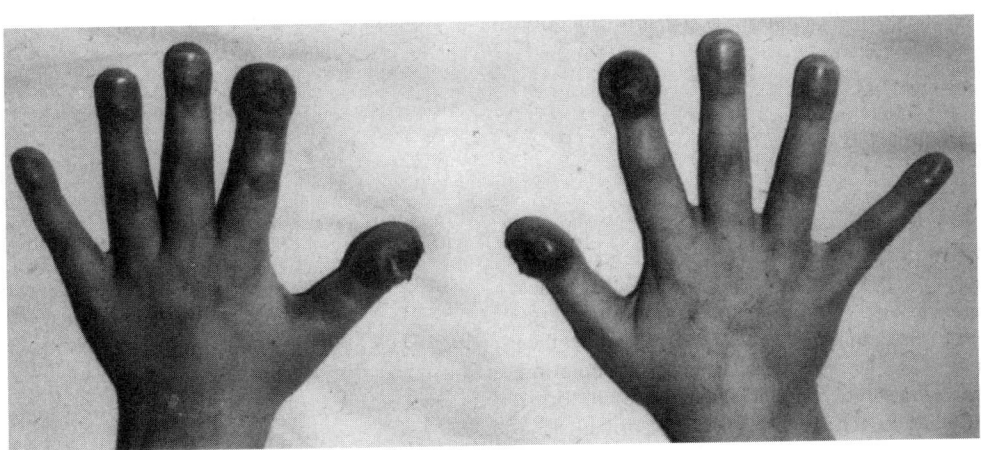

Fig. 22.15 Chronic mucocutaneous candidiasis.

newer agent itraconazole is promising in this respect. Immunological replacement therapy has met with some success in severe cases, and has included the use of transfer factor, thymic grafts and bone marrow transplantation.

Ommen's syndrome. The characteristic feature of this form of combined immunodeficiency is a severe immune dysregulation resulting in an infiltrative skin rash resembling seborrheic dermatitis (or sometimes with scaling and erythroderma), hepatomegaly and lymphadenopathy. Histologically there is a proliferation of CD8/CD4 double negative cells and histiocytes. There is marked eosinophilia, raised IgE levels and normal numbers of T and B cells. T cell mitogen proliferation is normal but antigen responses are poor.

It has been suggested that this is a form of 'leaky' SCID where the defect lies in the generation of the diversity of T and B cell receptors. The picture is caused by a relatively restricted number of clones of cells which escape the defect in differentiation and are then driven to proliferate by high cytokine levels of the T_{H2} variety.

Interferon γ may produce some clinical improvement but definitive treatment is with bone marrow transplantation.

Nezelof syndrome. Nezelof described a syndrome of T cell deficiency with normal immunoglobulin levels (Nezelof et al 1964). Subsequently, the term has been used to define combined deficiency states covering the whole range of severities in which, although one or more immunoglobulin classes (usually IgM) are preserved, antibody production is usually poor or absent. The term is probably best avoided.

Unknown defects

Idiopathic CD4 lymphocytopenia. A marked depression in the CD4 positive lymphocyte count characterizes this condition which is best regarded as a primary immunodeficiency disorder (Piketty et al 1994). Most reports have been on adult patients, but it can be seen in children. Strenuous efforts to look for a retroviral cause have proved negative and the epidemiology of the condition does not fit with a viral infection. Affected individuals are highly susceptible to opportunistic infections. Immunoglobulin levels and antibody responses are generally normal. The natural history of this recently described condition is not yet well understood. The CD4 cell count seems to remain stable for a prolonged period in most patients rather than progressively declining as in HIV infection. Prophylaxis against *Pneumocystis carinii* infection should be given.

COMBINED IMMUNODEFICIENCY FORMING PART OF OTHER SYNDROMES

DiGeorge anomaly

This condition results from abnormal embryological development of the third and fourth pharyngeal arch structures. Most cases (85–90%) are associated with a chromosomal deletion/microdeletion at 22q11 while the remainder are associated with other chromosomal anomalies. Together with other 22q deletion syndromes (velofaciocardiac or Shprintzen syndrome) it forms part of a group of disorders which have been described as a developmental field defect (Lammer & Opitz 1986). It is sporadic in occurrence, though familial cases, some associated with 22q

chromosomal deletions, have been reported. The syndrome is extremely heterogeneous and partial forms are more common than the full-blown condition. In its full-blown form, the syndrome comprises immunodeficiency, hypocalcemia (due to hypoparathyroidism), congenital heart defects and abnormal facies (low-set, abnormally formed ears, hypertelorism and antimongoloid slant, micrognathia, short philtrum to the upper lip and high arched palate; see Fig. 22.16). Many different heart defects have been described in the syndrome, including tetralogy of Fallot, and a number of other defects especially those involving the pulmonary artery and the aorta. Symptomatic hypocalcemia usually occurs within the first few days of life and may be poorly responsive to treatment.

Immune deficiency, resulting from failed thymic development, only occurs in 25% of cases. Particularly in partial forms of the condition, spontaneous improvement in immune function may occur with time. Affected children are excessively prone to candidiasis, recurrent pneumonias (typical and atypical), diarrhea and failure to thrive. Laboratory findings vary showing anything from severe T cell depletion with poor mitogen responses to relatively normal findings. Although previously considered a pure T cell defect, more recent studies have shown that antibody responses, particularly to polysaccharide antigens, are poor. Immunoglobulin levels are usually normal but hypogammaglobulinemia may develop. Chest X-ray shows lack of a thymic shadow.

In the full-blown form, the cardiac and metabolic problems are often the main prognostic determinants. Treatment of the immune

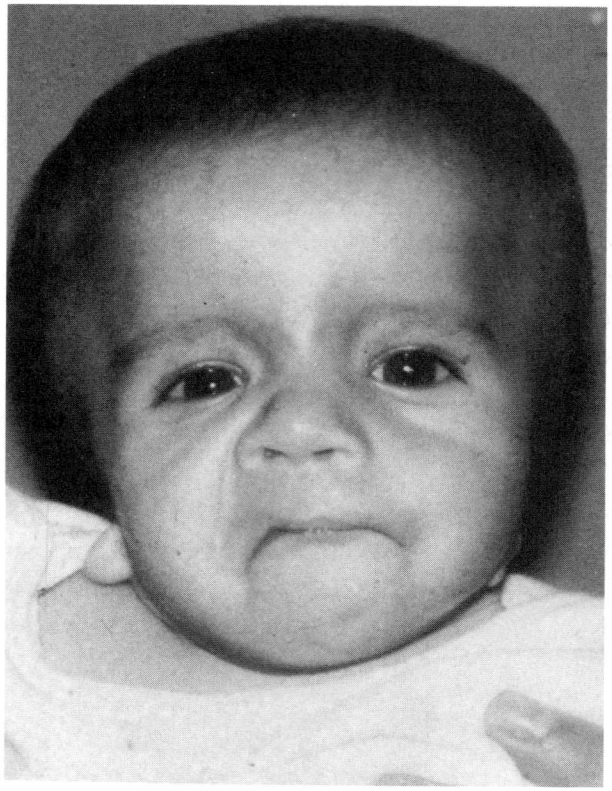

Fig. 22.16 Facies of a child with DiGeorge syndrome. (Courtesy of Professor C. B. S. Wood. Reproduced with permission of the family.)

deficiency has been successfully achieved using fetal thymus implants but bone marrow transplantation is the treatment of choice for severe cases. In less severe forms, expectant management should be pursued with avoidance of live vaccines, prophylactic antibiotics and intravenous immunoglobulin as required.

Ataxia telangiectasia

This multisystem autosomal recessive disorder is characterized by progressive neurological degeneration and telangiectases of conjunctivae and skin. Immunodeficiency is frequently, but not invariably, found in affected individuals. In addition, the condition is associated with a high incidence of malignant disease. No unifying hypothesis has been formulated to explain all these findings. The vast majority of cases show raised circulating α-fetoprotein levels, and all show a DNA-repair defect, with increased sensitivity of cells to radiation and mitomycin C treatment. Chromosomal breaks and translocations have a predilection for the sites of the T cell receptor and immunoglobulin heavy chain genes. The combination of immunodeficiency and DNA-repair defect is a likely explanation for the high incidence of malignancy. However, it is difficult to explain the other features on this basis. The situation is further complicated by experiments in which fibroblasts from different cases were fused and then checked for correction of the DNA repair defect. This showed that fusion of ataxia telangiectasia cells from some families could correct the defect in cells from others, suggesting a heterogeneity of the condition. At least six complementation groups were defined by this method (Jaspers et al 1984). Recently, the responsible gene (called ATM) has been identified at chromosome 11q22–23. It codes for an enzyme belonging to a family of phosphatidyl kinases involved in meiotic recombination and cell cycle control (Savitsky et al 1995). This single gene seems to be responsible for all of the disease complementation groups, a fact which has not yet been adequately explained.

The neurological symptoms are present uniformly. Ataxia and cerebellar signs usually appear in the second year, but may be delayed. Neurological degeneration progresses relentlessly, resulting in severe disability by late childhood. Mental function is usually preserved though retardation has been described. Telangiectases usually appear first on the bulbar conjunctivae (Fig. 22.17). The timing of their appearance is very variable and may be delayed until late childhood. It is unusual to see them before 4–5 years. Later they will appear elsewhere, particularly on the nose, the ears, and in the antecubital and popliteal fossae. Other cutaneous manifestations may include patches of hypo- or hyperpigmentation, cutaneous atrophy and atopic dermatitis. Gonadal atrophy occurs in both sexes, and growth failure is also prominent in the later stages. The immunodeficiency, which is present in 60–80% of cases, leads to frequent sinopulmonary infections which can progress to bronchiectasis. Impetigo and other skin infections are also common. Surprisingly, even though some cases have marked T cell abnormalities, infection with opportunistic pathogens is rare. On testing, the most common defects found are of immunoglobulins, where a number of patterns may occur. Deficiencies of IgE, IgA IgG2 and IgG4 are the most frequent findings (in up to 70% of cases). Antibody responses are poor particularly to polysaccharide antigens. T cell defects with T lymphopenia and depressed mitogen and antigen responses can be demonstrated in a lesser proportion of cases.

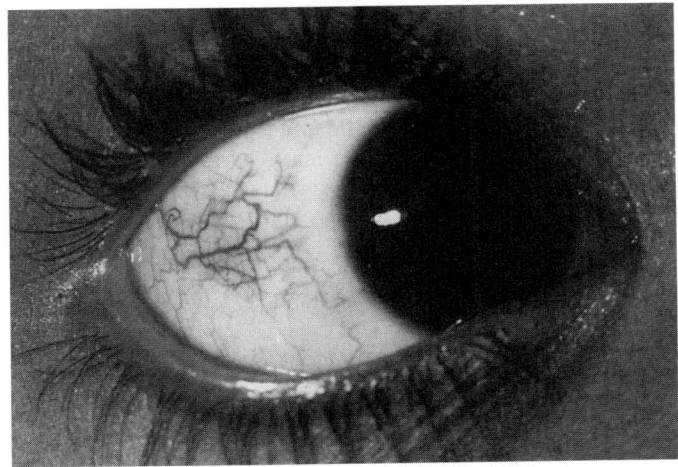

Fig. 22. 17 Ataxia telangiectasia.

Eosinophilia may be present. Chest X-ray usually shows an absent thymic shadow. Lymphoid and thymic tissue is hypoplastic, with absent Hassall's corpuscles in the latter.

Lymphoreticular malignancies and, in contrast to the findings in other immunodeficiencies, carcinomas occur with increased frequency in ataxia telangiectasia. The known radiosensitivity in the condition can complicate therapy for these diseases. Irrespective of the development of malignancy, survival beyond early adult life is unusual. It has been suggested that heterozygosity for the AT gene confers an increased risk of developing breast cancer.

Other chromosomal breakage syndromes

The rapid cell turnover and complex rearrangements of genetic material required in immune responses make this system very vulnerable to the effects of chromosomal instability and defective repair syndromes. Apart from ataxia telangiectasia there are several other disorders.

Bloom syndrome. Chromosome breaks and other aberrations are associated with severe growth failure in this syndrome which is an autosomal recessive disorder mapping to chromosome 11q23. Affected individuals may develop facial telangiectases and photosensitivity. Recurrent sinopulmonary pyogenic infections may occur and are associated with hypogammaglobulinemia affecting one or more immunoglobulin classes, most often IgM. T cell functional abnormalities are also found. The incidence of malignant disease is very high.

ICF syndrome (immunodeficiency, centromeric instability and facial anomalies syndrome) is an autosomal recessive disorder in which there are characteristic structural chromosomal abnormalities in chromosomes 1, 9 and 16 in lymphocytes. Other cells do not show these changes. Affected children develop severe recurrent infections predominantly bacterial and are found to have immunoglobulin deficiency with normal T and B cell numbers. The differential diagnosis is common variable immunodeficiency (CVID). Mental retardation may occur but there is no increased risk of malignancy.

Nijmegen breakage syndrome was described in Holland (Weemaes et al 1994) and involves neurological (microcephaly, mental retardation) and immunological features. Hypogamma-globulinemia and decreased T cell proliferative responses are found. Seemanova's syndrome is very similar but without mental retardation.

Fanconi's anemia. The main problem in this condition is usually of progressive bone marrow failure leading to pancytopenia. There may also be skeletal malformations. Immune deficiency can occur, and selective IgA deficiency and T cell abnormalities have been recorded.

In other chromosomal breakage disorders such as Xeroderma pigmentosa and Seckel syndrome immune deficiency may occur but is not a prominent feature.

Wiskott–Aldrich syndrome

Thrombocytopenia, eczema and immunodeficiency are found in this X-linked condition. There is a failure of the normal binding of actin bundles in the cytoskeleton resulting in lack of microvilli on lymphocyte surfaces. There is also instability in the expression of surface sialoglycoproteins notably sialophorin (CD43) but also the low affinity IgE receptor (CD23). Multiple lymphoid and hematological lines are affected. The gene has been identified and codes for a novel 501 amino acid protein called the Wiskott–Aldrich syndrome protein (WASP) whose precise function remains undetermined.

Clinical features. The classical features are thrombocytopenia, eczema and recurrent infections. The condition usually presents in the early months of life with bruising, petechiae and bleeding. There is however a variable range of clinical severities from mild thrombocytopenia alone to the full blown syndrome and this may depend on the position of the mutation in the gene. The thrombocytopenia and bleeding episodes may require platelet transfusions. An eczematous rash develops and after the first few months the child begins to have problems with infections – usually bacterial and/or viral infections of the upper and lower respiratory tract. There may also be infections with opportunistic pathogens, such as *Pneumocystis carinii*. Herpes viruses, including herpes simplex, are handled poorly and may cause severe disease. These infections invariably exacerbate the bleeding tendency, and early death may result from bleeding. With increasing age, bleeding problems may lessen only to be replaced by infective problems as the major cause of death. Immunization with polysaccharide and typhoid vaccines is ineffective and can cause severe, even fatal, reactions. In untransplanted children, the average age of death was $3^{1}/_{2}$ years. There is a high risk of lymphoid malignancy which often affects the central nervous system.

Laboratory tests. Blood count shows thrombocytopenia with abnormally small platelets. Electron microscopy shows 'bald' lymphocytes and platelets due to absence of microvilli. T cell lymphopenia and eosinophilia are common, and a Coombs-positive hemolytic anemia has been described. Serum immunoglobulins show a characteristic pattern with very low IgM, normal IgG (total and subclass) and markedly elevated IgA and IgE. FACS analysis shows low expression of CD43 on T cells. Antibody responses to polysaccharide antigens and isohemagglutinins are absent. There may be progressive lymphopenia affecting predominantly T cells numbers, with depressed responses to mitogens and antigens and negative delayed hypersensitivity skin tests.

Treatment. Acute bleeding episodes may be controlled by platelet transfusions (irradiated to prevent graft-versus-host disease). Splenectomy and systemic steroids should be avoided as they will increase the risk of infection. Topical steroids are required for the eczema. Intravenous immunoglobulin, with or without prophylactic antibiotics, reduces the bacterial sinopulmonary infections.

With only these supportive measures the prognosis is poor. Immunological and hematological reconstitution can be achieved by bone marrow transplantation though the results are less good than in SCID partly because of a high incidence of EB virus-driven lymphoproliferative disorders.

Other syndromes

Short-limbed dwarfism and immunodeficiency. Short-limbed dwarfism has been found to be associated with immunodeficiency which may be a combined deficiency or affect predominantly either T or B cell function. In its variant form – cartilage hair hypoplasia – the hair, including that of the eyebrows and eyelashes, is light-colored, fine and sparse, and lacks the normal central pigmented core. This variety is associated with a predominantly T cell defect and relatively normal B cell function. Characteristic radiological appearances of metaphyseal and spondyloepiphyseal dysplasia are found. The presence of immunodeficiency is variable and most children are not profoundly affected. However, they do seem excessively vulnerable to virus infections, particularly varicella, and in severe cases the full range of infections characteristic of T cell deficiency (e.g. *Pneumocystis carinii, Candida albicans*) can occur.

Immunodeficiency with multiple carboxylase deficiency. This autosomal recessive condition results in combined immunodeficiency of variable severity. Recurrent infections are associated with neurodevelopmental problems, alopecia, metabolic acidosis and marked susceptibility to chronic candidiasis. The syndrome is caused by dysfunction of a number of biotin-dependent carboxylase enzymes. The diagnosis is confirmed by the finding of lactic acidosis with elevation of specific organic acids in the urine. Treatment with pharmacological doses of biotin reverses the biochemical abnormalities with marked clinical improvement.

Griscelli syndrome (immunodeficiency with partial albinism). Children with this condition may resemble those with Chediak–Higashi syndrome, but the neutrophils lack the characteristic giant granules of the latter. There is a susceptibility to infection of all types and patients may develop a histiocytic proliferative disorder with hemophagocytosis. Decreased T, B and NK cell function has been found. Bone marrow transplantation corrects the immune problems.

Immunodeficiency associated with Down syndrome. Many children with Down syndrome suffer repeated sinopulmonary infections. They also have a tendency to develop chronic antigenemia following hepatitis B infection, and show an increased incidence of leukemia. Subtle defects affecting a number of aspects of immune function have been found. Neutrophils show relatively mild defects of chemotaxis and bacterial killing; T cells have impaired cytotoxic and cytokine-producing abilities; while antibody responses to certain antigens, including ΦX174 and influenza vaccine, are impaired.

DEFECTS OF ANTIBODY PRODUCTION

A number of primary immunodeficiency disorders result in failure of immunoglobulin production. This may take the form of a major deficiency affecting all immunoglobulin classes (panhypogammaglobulinemia) or there may be deficiencies affecting only some of the immunoglobulin classes or subclasses singly or in combinations. IgA deficiency is the commonest. In deficiencies affecting only one or a few classes or subclasses the defect is usually in the control of the immune response, but in a minority of cases gene deletions affecting the relevant immunoglobulin heavy chain constant region genes have been observed.

Since the control of antibody production lies with the T cells many of the antibody deficiency syndromes are strictly combined deficiencies but in practice they are classified according to the predominant problem.

X-linked agammaglobulinemia (XLA, Bruton's disease)

This X-linked condition is due to an intrinsic defect in the B cell line in which pre-B cells fail to differentiate into more mature B cells. The defective gene lying on the long arm of the X chromosome encodes a cytoplasmic enzyme, Bruton tyrosine kinase (Btk). Affected boys classically show a complete failure to produce immunoglobulins and antibody responses, but cell-mediated immunity is normal. Since the identification of the gene, boys with partial phenotypes have been found though it has been difficult to correlate phenotype with the multiple different mutations that have been found. Phenotypic variation has been described within the same family.

Clinical features. Typically, recurrent pyogenic infections commence in the latter half of the first year of life (when maternal IgG levels have declined). Sinopulmonary infections are most common, but gastroenteritis, pyoderma, arthritis, meningitis and osteomyelitis may be presenting features (Table 22.13). Despite these problems, the diagnosis is often made surprisingly late; in one series, the average age at diagnosis was $3\frac{1}{2}$ years without, and

$2\frac{1}{2}$ years with, a positive family history. The subsequent course may be complicated by such infections as giardiasis and chronic conjunctivitis caused by *Pseudomonas* species. Recovery from viral infections is normal with the notable exception of those caused by enteroviruses (especially echoviruses) which can cause a chronic meningoencephalitis or dermatomyositis like picture. Vaccine strain poliomyelitis can occur after live vaccination.

Hepatitis A is reported as running a severe course in these boys. Pathogens in which cell-mediated immunity is thought to be important are not usually a problem, though occasional cases of *Pneumocystis carinii* infection have been reported.

Other complications include a nonseptic arthritis affecting predominantly large joints. In some cases this has been shown to be due to mycoplasma infection. Neutropenia, alopecia totalis and amyloidosis are infrequent complications.

Laboratory findings. Once maternal IgG has declined, the usual pattern is one of absence or severe depletion of all serum immunoglobulin classes. It is not possible to demonstrate any antibody response to vaccines or to bacteriophage ΦX174. Circulating lymphocyte markers show a normal T cell pattern, but absence of B cells measured using surface immunoglobulin or CD19/20 markers. Bone marrow aspirate does, however, show pre-B cells (containing cytoplasmic μ chains). Lymph nodes show absent follicles and germinal centers. Plasma cells cannot be demonstrated in lymph nodes, bone marrow or suction rectal biopsy specimens. The recognition of partial phenotypes means that in the presence of any form of antibody deficiency in boys, particularly if circulating B cell numbers are low, the condition can only be fully excluded after examination of the Btk gene for mutations.

Foremost in the differential diagnosis of XLA is common variable immune deficiency. Table 22.14 lists some of the important differences between the two.

The mainstay of treatment is immunoglobulin replacement therapy (see p. 1267). In a large series reported in 1985 by Lederman & Winkelstein, there was a high incidence of chronic lung disease (75% of those over 20 years old) even with treatment and 17% of the patients had died with a mean age of 16.9 years

Table 22.13 Presenting features in 96 patients with X-linked agammaglobulinemia (from Lederman & Winkelstein 1985)

Presenting feature	%
Ear, nose and throat infections (otitis media)	75 (59)
Lower respiratory tract infections (pneumonia)	65 (56)
Gastrointestinal infections (diarrhea)	35 (32)
Pyoderma	28
Arthritis (septic)	20 (8)
CNS infections (meningitis)	16 (10)
Septicemia	10
Neutropenia	10
Positive family history	26
Others: Failure to thrive; fever of uncertain origin; complications of immunization; osteomyelitis and dermatomyositis.	<5% each

Diagnoses and figures in brackets indicate the predominant type of infection in each system and its overall incidence in the 96 patients.

Table 22.14 Comparison of X-linked agammaglobulinemia (XLA) and common variable hypogammaglobulinemia (CVH)

	XLA	CVH
Inheritance	X-linked	Mostly unknown (some may be AR or AD)
Age of onset	Infancy	Any age
Immunological defect	Antibody	Antibody +/– cell-mediated
Immunoglobulin classes	All decreased	One (usually IgM) or more often preserved
B cell numbers	Absent	Usually present
T cell numbers and function	Normal	Normal or decreased
Pyogenic infections	Yes	Yes
Opportunistic infections	Very rare	Yes
Autoimmune phenomena	Very rare	Yes
Chronic gastrointestinal problems	Rare	Common

(range 4–28). It is believed that these figures will be greatly improved following the introduction of intravenous immunoglobulin preparations in the last decade.

Hyper-IgM syndrome (CD40 ligand deficiency)

This condition is usually inherited as an X-linked trait, but autosomal recessive cases have been described. In the X-linked form the genetic defect lies in the gene for CD40 ligand, a glycopeptide expressed on activated T cells, which is necessary for immunoglobulin class switching by B cells. IgG and IgA deficiency are associated with serum IgM and IgD levels which are moderately or sometimes markedly elevated (Notarangelo et al 1992).

Usually, boys present a similar picture to XLA but with somewhat later onset. In contrast to XLA there is a susceptibility to opportunistic infections, especially *Pneumocystis carinii* pneumonia (Fig. 22.18) and cryptosporidium. This suggests that T cell function is subtly impaired but it is difficult to demonstrate this in the laboratory. Antibody activity can be shown in the IgM class. Autoimmune phenomena are relatively common and include hemolytic anemias, thrombocytopenia, hypothyroidism, arthritis and liver disorders. Neutropenia is particularly common affecting around 50% of cases and associated with recurrent or persistent oral ulceration. There is also an increased incidence of malignancy.

High doses of immunoglobulin replacement therapy are often required. With adequate replacement the rising IgM levels tend to stabilize. Prophylaxis against *Pneumocystis carinii* infection should be given. With the recognition of the high incidence of serious complications some authorities are recommending bone marrow transplantation for this condition.

Common variable immunodeficiency (CVID)

This category of immunodeficiency covers a heterogeneous group of disorders in which antibody deficiency is always present and there may be also a variable degree of cell-mediated immune defect (Cunningham Rundles 1989). Though the cell-mediated component may be significant, this condition is now classified by the World Health Organization Working Party as a condition predominantly of antibody deficiency. Inheritance of CVID does not usually follow a simple Mendelian pattern, although a minority of families do show autosomal recessive or dominant patterns. In other cases there are probably complex familial influences linked to the genes in the major histocompatibility complex (see section on genetics of immunodeficiency, p. 1241). Relatives of an affected person show an increased incidence of IgA deficiency or of autoimmune or other immunopathological disease. Chromosomal aberrations, such as breaks and centromeric instability, have been recorded in some patients suggesting some overlap with the ICF syndrome (see above).

Age of presentation appears to be very variable. Some cases present within the first few months of life and the defect is presumably present from birth. In others, onset may be at any later age (the peak being in the second to third decades) when the alternative names of 'late-onset' or 'acquired hypogammaglobulinemia' are given to this condition.

Pathogenesis. The existence of several patterns of immunological findings confirm the heterogenicity of the condition. These patterns include:

1. absence of B cells (± pre-B cell)
2. functionally deficient B cells which do not proliferate, differentiate or secrete immunoglobulin properly
3. apparently normal B cells, but T cell dysregulation usually with excessive T suppressor activity or, sometimes, with deficient T helper activity or antigen presenting cell dysfunction. In some patients there is a failure of T cells to produce B cell growth and differentiation factors, including interleukins 4 and 6, while in others poor IL-2 production has been found
4. occasional cases thought to be due to autoantibodies against T and B lymphocytes have been reported.

The majority of cases fall into the third category.

Clinical features. Most commonly it is the humoral immune deficiency which leads to clinical problems, with recurrent infections caused by pyogenic bacteria, especially pneumococci, *Haemophilus influenzae* and staphylococci. These usually affect the sinopulmonary system (upper and lower respiratory tract including middle ears and sinuses). Chronic lung damage leading to bronchiectasis is not uncommon if diagnosis is delayed or treatment inadequate. Mycoplasma and ureaplasma infections can be problematic, causing pneumonias, arthritis or genitourinary infections. Diarrhea and malabsorption are other presenting features most commonly caused by *Giardia lamblia*, with symptoms resolving after metronidazole treatment.

Sometimes in CVID the cell-mediated immune defect may cause problems leading to infections with *Pneumocystis carinii*, (Figs 22.18 and 22.19) viruses or *Candida*. Usually (but not always) in such cases, there are demonstrable T cell abnormalities.

Later complications of CVID include autoimmune diseases, which are either collagen type disorders such as systemic lupus erythematosus, or hematological diseases, including hemolytic anemia, thrombocytopenia or autoimmune neutropenia. Intestinal disorders include inflammatory bowel diseases, nodular lymphoid hyperplasia, malabsorptive syndromes and gastric carcinoma. Pernicious anemia and chronic active hepatitis have been described. Lymphoproliferation resulting in lymphadenopathy and splenomegaly is relatively common. Malignancy (either lymphoreticular or intestinal carcinoma) complicates CVID in 8% of cases.

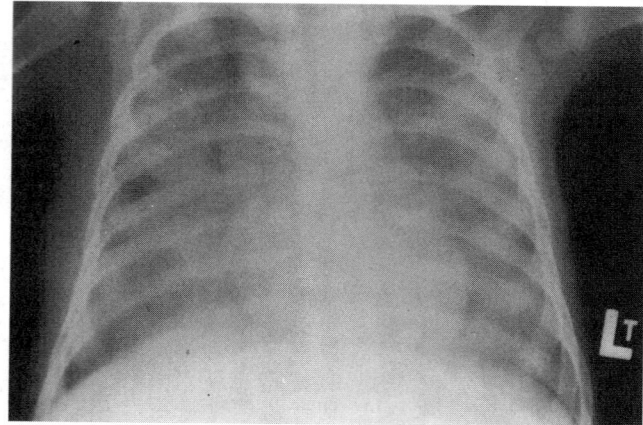

Fig. 22.18 Chest radiograph of a 6-month-old boy, presenting with *Pneumocystis carinii* pneumonia. The underlying immune deficiency was found to be immunoglobulin deficiency with hyper IgM syndrome.

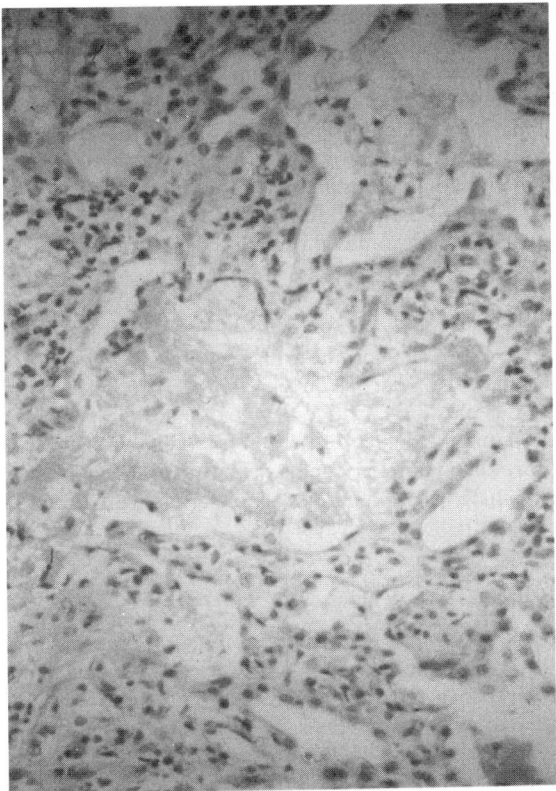

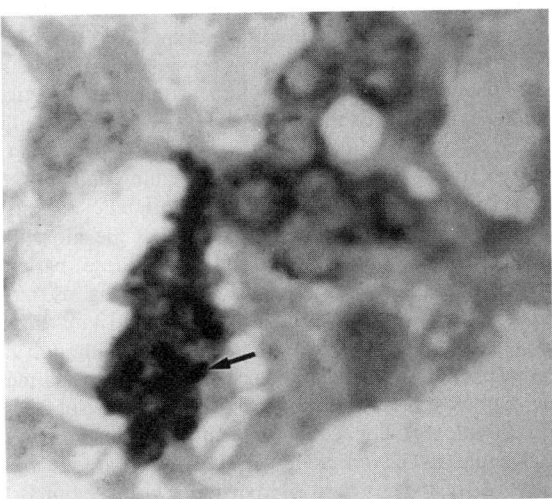

Fig. 22.19 Lung histology following open lung biopsy in the patient whose chest radiograph is shown in Figure 22.18.   (**a**) Hematoxylin and eosin stain showing marked inflammatory infiltrate. (**b**) Grocott methanamine stain showing pneumocystis organisms (arrowed).

Laboratory findings. Panhypogammaglobulinemia is found, with levels not usually as low as in X-linked agamma-globulinemia. Sometimes, IgM levels are preserved (including functional IgM antibody). B cells are usually present, but B cell function may be defective (see above). T cell numbers are low or normal, and subset and functional disturbances may be found in some cases. In those with the more severe defects of cell-mediated

immunity, mitogen responses and delayed hypersensitivity reactions may be depressed.

Treatment. The treatment of immunoglobulin deficiency is discussed below (p. 1267). Where significant cell-mediated immune dysfunction is also present, prophylaxis with co-trimoxazole and antifungals may also be required. Corticosteroids may be required for the autoimmune and lymphoproliferative complications but should be used as sparingly as possible. In selected patients with poor in vitro IL-2 production, treatment with polyethylene glycol conjugated IL-2 resulted in significant correction of cell mediated and humoral immune responses (Cunningham-Rundles et al 1995).

Hypogammaglobulinemia with growth hormone deficiency

In this very rare condition hypogammaglobulinemia with a clinical and immunological pattern identical or very similar to that found in X-linked agammaglobulinemia is associated with isolated growth hormone deficiency (Fleisher et al 1980). Genetic studies have not yet been completed but it has been suggested that there is a defect involving the Btk gene of XLA and an adjacent gene involved in regulation of growth hormone production.

Immunoglobulin deficiency with transcobalamin II deficiency

Hypogammaglobulinemia due to a failure of terminal (antigen driven) B cell differentiation can result from congenital absence of one of the vitamin B_{12} carrier proteins, transcobalamin II. There is associated pernicious anemia. Parenteral high dose vitamin B_{12} corrects the defect.

Selective IgA deficiency

This is by far the commonest primary immunodeficiency, with an incidence of between 1 in 500 and 1 in 700 of the population. The majority of affected individuals are asymptomatic. The precise abnormality has not been elucidated. Only a small minority of patients have deletions of the α chain genes. The rest have surface IgA positive B cells, indicating that at least some IgA molecules are being produced, but large scale production and export from the cells do not occur. There is evidence that this may be due to abnormal T cell regulation of immunoglobulin synthesis, and subtle T cell abnormalities, including defective interferon production, have been found in some cases. Most cases are sporadic, though Mendelian inheritance (dominant or recessive) can occur, sometimes associated with an 18q– chromosomal deletion. There is an increased incidence of common variable immune deficiency and of collagen vascular diseases in relatives of IgA-deficient individuals which maps to the major histocompatibility gene complex (see p. 1241 Genetics of immunodeficiency). Acquired (usually reversible) IgA deficiency can occur as a result of certain drug therapies including phenytoin, cyclosporine, penicillamine, sulfasalazine, sodium valproate and captopril. It has also been found in congenital infections and after hepatitis C infection.

Deficiency of serum IgA is nearly always associated with lack of secretory IgA. One family with secretory piece deficiency has been observed in which absent IgA in secretions occurred in the presence of normal serum IgA levels. A small proportion of serum IgA deficient individuals have normal levels of secretory IgA.

Clinical features. It is useful to divide IgA-deficient individuals into two groups. Complete IgA deficiency (levels less than 0.05 g/l) is usually lifelong, while partial deficiency (levels greater than 0.05 g/l but less than 2.5 SD below age-related mean level) is often found in young children. The latter corrects with time in most cases and therefore represents a delayed maturation of the immune system

Both types can be associated with IgG subclass deficiencies, most commonly IgG2 and/or IgG4 deficiency. These occur in approximately 15% of cases.

The reason why only a minority of affected individuals get symptoms is not clear – it seems to be irrespective of whether the deficiency is partial or complete. Indeed, frequency of infections is greater in the former though the latter, when symptomatic, may have more severe illness when infected. The presence of IgG subclass deficiency increases the likelihood and the severity of infective symptoms, but does not constitute the whole explanation. There is some evidence that asymptomatic individuals have increased levels of 7s (monomeric) IgM in their secretions. In at least a proportion of IgA-deficient adults immunization with oral cholera vaccine resulted in activation of IgG-producing intestinal cells.

Symptoms and complications.

1. Infective. Recurrent sinopulmonary infections are the commonest symptoms in young children. They are usually of a relatively minor, but persistent, nature and are frequently associated with asthma. Middle ear infections can be troublesome and severe pneumonias can occur. If repeated significant lower respiratory infections occur there is a risk of permanent lung damage. In most affected children, the frequency of infections diminishes with increasing age regardless of whether or not there is normalization of the IgA levels. Some remain symptomatic into adulthood. Gastrointestinal infections, especially those due to *Giardia lamblia*, are more common but a report of an increased incidence of urinary tract infections has not been confirmed.

2. Allergy and atopy. The incidence of IgA deficiency in children with allergic disease is of the order of 1 in 100 to 1 in 200. Atopic disease, such as asthma and eczema, as well as food allergic disease can occur. The probable mechanisms for this are discussed on page 1248.

3. Autoimmunity (Liblau & Bach 1992). There is a very strong correlation between autoimmune disease of all types and IgA deficiency. This is irrespective of whether individuals are symptomatic from the infection point of view. A prevalence of IgA deficiency of 4.6% in systemic lupus erythematosus, 3.4% in Still's disease and 2% in juvenile chronic arthritis has been reported.

Hematological, endocrine and other tissue-specific autoimmune disease have all been described. Autoantibodies (organ-specific and nonspecific) are often found in the absence of clinical disease. One particular autoantibody which may lead to problems is anti-IgA, which has been found in between 9 and 44% of IgA-deficient individuals. These antibodies can occasionally cause reactions after transfusion of blood, plasma or immunoglobulin preparations.

4. Gastrointestinal disease. An increased incidence of infection has been mentioned above. Celiac disease is frequently associated with IgA deficiency. Inflammatory bowel disease and nonceliac malabsorption syndromes have also been reported.

Treatment. Antibiotics, either commenced early in the course of each infection or used for long-term prophylaxis, are the mainstay of treatment for the infection problems. Immuno-globulin therapy is not usually indicated and may be dangerous if anti-IgA antibodies are present, since most of the immunoglobulin preparations contain small amounts of IgA. (For the same reason blood transfusion should be administered with care in individuals with known complete IgA deficiency.) If there is an accompanying demonstrable failure of antibody response to vaccine antigens with or without an IgG subclass deficiency, immunoglobulin therapy may be required, particularly if there is threatened lung damage. IgA depleted commercial preparations are available and should be used in this situation.

Selective IgM deficiency

A poorly defined syndrome with very low IgM levels (<0.2 g/l) but normal IgG and IgA levels has been reported (Inoue et al 1986). Surface IgM-positive B lymphocytes are present, and it is believed that the defect lies in T cell regulation of IgM secretion. T cell mediated immune functions, however, are normal. Affected patients have been reported as suffering from Gram-negative bacillary or meningococcal sepsis.

IgG subclass deficiencies

Partial or complete deficiencies of IgG subclasses may occur singly or in combination and may be associated with IgA deficiency. In a minority of cases, deletions on chromosome 14 corresponding to the relevant heavy chain constant region genes have been identified. In the remainder the genes are intact and there must be some regulatory problem. Occasionally IgG subclass deficiency progresses to the more profound deficiency of CVID. Less commonly an IgG subclass disturbance may be the only manifestation of one of the mild phenotypes of XLA. G2 and G4 deficiency are relatively common in ataxia telangiectasia and as a transient phenomenon after bone marrow transplantation for SCID.

Deficiency of any of the classes G1–G3 is associated with an increased susceptibility to infections, particularly of the respiratory tract with a risk of progressive lung damage. However there are many individuals with such deficiencies who remain perfectly healthy. It is generally agreed that the most important correlate with infection susceptibility in these patients is a deficiency in antibody responses to specific antigens particularly polysaccharides. G subclass disturbance may be a marker for such deficiencies rather than the primary problem although deficient functional antibody production is seen also in patients with normal subclass levels. The interpretation of subclass levels should therefore take account of antibody responses and the clinical context. G2 deficiency is the best characterized of the subclass disturbances and is particularly associated with a defective response to polysaccharide antigens. It is commonly associated with IgA and/or IgG4 deficiency. Like IgA, IgG2 levels rise slowly in childhood and in many young children transiently low levels are found representing a delay in maturation. Nevertheless such children may suffer frequent respiratory (especially ear) infections. The finding of isolated G4 deficiency is of unknown significance, since about one-fifth of the population have undetectable levels by standard assays. Cases of recurrent pulmonary infection where the only demonstrable deficiency was of IgG4 have been reported.

Diagnosis can be made by performing quantitative subclass assays and antibody assays (with or without immunization). The total IgG level is usually low in G1 deficiency but within the normal range for the other subclass deficiencies.

Treatment for symptomatic children involves prophylactic antibiotics such as co-trimoxazole or a macrolide which may only be needed over the autumn and winter months. Monitoring for hearing loss, for evidence of developing chronic lung problems and of growth are required. A minority of children with subclass deficiency and failure of antibody responses require intravenous immunoglobulin therapy.

Antibody deficiency with normal immunoglobulins

In patients with a clinical history suggestive of immunoglobulin deficiency but with normal or raised immunoglobulin levels, the possibility of functional antibody deficiency should be considered. This is the mechanism of the humoral immune deficiency in HIV infection, and also in some of the combined primary immuno-deficiency states. This pattern of deficiency is also found to a mild degree in Down syndrome and in splenectomized individuals. Most commonly, antibody responses to the polysaccharide antigens are affected, but defective responses to proteins, e.g. tetanus toxoid, can also be demonstrated.

Diagnosis is confirmed by the demonstration of a lack of specific antibody response following vaccination.

Transient hypogammaglobulinemia of infancy

This is thought to be a prolongation of the normal 'physiological' trough in IgG levels that occurs in infancy, IgA levels may also be low but there is usually preservation of the ability to produce functional antibodies, e.g. to blood group antigens, tetanus toxoid and Hib. The problem may be caused by a maturation defect in B cells. In some cases a transient T helper cell defect has been found. About 50% of cases have a family history of other types of immune deficiency. The condition usually resolves between 18 and 36 months, but in the meantime recurrent infections may occur. Management involves excluding the major primary immuno-deficiencies and minimizing morbidity if recurrent infections are occurring. Usually this can be achieved using prophylactic antibiotics and immunoglobulin therapy is rarely required.

Secondary immunoglobulin deficiency due to protein loss

Excessive loss of immunoglobulin occurs in protein-losing enteropathies and in nephrotic syndrome. IgG is the predominant class of immunoglobulin lost. Children become prone to pyogenic infections, especially invasive pneumococcal sepsis.

Intestinal lymphangiectasia can be one of the most severe of the protein-losing states. In children, it is usually a primary disorder which may be associated with lymphatic abnormalities in other organs. There is marked lymphopenia with diminished T cell mitogenic and antigenic responses and hypogammaglobulinemia particularly affecting IgG. In addition to bacterial sepsis, infections with T cell pathogens, e.g. *Pneumocystis carinii*, occasionally occur.

In myotonic dystrophy there is hypercatabolism of IgG resulting in low serum levels. It is unusual for this to be clinically significant.

DISORDERS OF PHAGOCYTIC CELLS

Neutropenia

This is most commonly secondary to a variety of disease processes or drug treatments. Usually, secondary neutropenia is caused by production failure in the bone narrow, but extensive consumption may be the cause as in some autoimmune diseases or overwhelming sepsis.

Congenital neutropenias (e.g. Kostman syndrome) are probably a heterogeneous group of conditions, usually inherited in autosomal recessive fashion, in which there is a maturation arrest in the neutrophil series (Kostman 1956).

In cyclical neutropenia, regular episodes of profound neutropenia may occur approximately every 3 weeks (range 13–35 days). During these episodes, infections and oral ulceration may occur and these clear after 3–4 days when the neutrophil count recovers. It may be inherited as a dominant trait. Immunoglobulin deficiency may be associated with congenital or cyclical neutropenias.

Neutrophil counts of less than $0.5 \times 10^9/l$ carry a major increased risk of infection, while counts below $0.2 \times 10^9/l$ are associated with a serious risk of septicemia (which may be fulminant due to Gram-negative organisms). Prophylaxis with antibiotics and antifungal agents may reduce the likelihood of these problems. Granulocyte colony stimulating factor (GCSF) has been shown to partly correct the deficiency in congenital agranulocytosis while in cyclical neutropenia it increases the frequency of the cycling resulting in shorter periods of neutropenia and thus less likelihood of infections. However prolonged usage of this growth factor may be complicated by an increased risk of the development of malignancy which is already higher than normal in these patients (Imashuku et al 1995). Bone marrow transplantation remains the definitive treatment for severe disorders of neutrophil production.

Defects of neutrophil killing

Chronic granulomatous disease (CGD)

This bacterial killing disorder is the best characterized of the inherited neutrophil defects. Affected individuals suffer from recurrent and chronic infections caused by bacteria and fungi. They develop widespread granulomatous lesions in lymph nodes, liver, spleen, lungs and skin. The originally described cases all died before reaching their teens, which led to the condition being named 'fatal granulomatous disease of childhood'. Since then, improved understanding and management of the condition have considerably reduced the early mortality, and the word, 'fatal', has been replaced by 'chronic' in the name.

Affected children have abnormalities of NADPH oxidase leading to failure of cells to generate superoxide, other reactive oxygen species and hydrogen peroxide in the phagolysosome after phagocytosis. The enzyme has four components, two subunits (91 kd and 22 kd) make up the cytochrome b558 component in the plasma membrane and two cytosolic components (67 kd and 47 kd). The commonest defect, accounting for around 60% of cases, lies in the gene for the 91 kd component called glycoprotein 91 phagocytic oxidase (gp91 phox). This is inherited as an X-linked recessive condition. Defects in the genes for the other three components account for the remaining cases and are inherited in an autosomal recessive fashion.

Children with CGD usually present in early life with suppurative infection involving the skin, lymph nodes and lungs (Mouy et al 1989). Other organs such as the liver can also be involved, and osteomyelitis is not infrequent. Hepatosplenomegaly is almost invariable even in the absence of frank infection in these organs. The liver cells are packed with amorphous material which presumably cannot be broken down because of the intracellular 'digestive' defect. Granulomata sitting in the intestinal wall, notably at the gastric outlet or in the renal pelvis or ureter occur leading to obstruction of those organs. These usually respond to steroid treatment which is given at the expense of further compromising immune defenses.

The types of organisms causing problems in this condition are shown in Table 22.15 and reflect the microbial species in which host handling is most dependent on intracellular oxidative pathways.

Diagnosis is made by demonstration of a neutrophil inability to reduce NBT, absence of the normal chemiluminescent response of neutrophils at phagocytosis, and severely impaired neutrophil killing.

Treatment of the condition is usually supportive, with good results from the use of long-term prophylactic antibiotics of which sulfamethoxazole/trimethoprim combinations have been used most extensively (Fischer et al 1993) (Table 22.16). However, although such management can achieve good results in many patients, a minority still develop severe problems often with fungal infections and in these individuals the prognosis is poor. Interferon γ therapy was found to reduce the incidence of infections in patients treated prophylactically and some authorities recommend its use in all patients. Others have suggested its use only as an interventional agent when problems develop. There is no correction of the defective oxidative burst by this treatment which must work by stimulating other less well defined protective mechanisms. Bone marrow transplantation offers a cure for the condition and has been successfully performed. The genes responsible for the disorder have been cloned and inserted into

Table 22.15 Microorganisms cultured from infection sites in chronic granulomatous disease patients (from Mouy et al 1989)

Microorganisms	Patients (n = 48)	Infectious episodes (n + 169)	Infections due to each organism
Staphylococcus aureus	25	53	31
Aspergillus sp.	19	24	16
Salmonella sp.	16	22	14
Serratia sp.	8	11	7
Escherichia coli	8	11	7
Mycobacteria	8	8	5
Staphylococcus epidermidis	7	10	6
Proteus sp.	6	7	4
Candida albicans	5	5	3
Klebsiella pneumoniae	4	4	2
Pseudomonas sp.	3	4	2
Enterobacter cloacae	2	5	3
Haemophilus influenzae	2	2	
Cephalosporium	1	1	
Pneumocystis carinii	1	1	
Campylobacter sp.	1		

Table 22.16 Morbidity rates in chronic granulomatous disease before and after starting antibiotic prophylaxis (from Mouy et al 1989)

Infection	Infections/year per patient		
	Patients without prophylaxis (n = 34)	Patients with prophylaxis (n = 34)	P
All infections	2.06	0.43	0.001*
Fungal infections	0.19	0.09	NS
Liver abscesses	0.15	0	0.01
Salmonella infections	0.14	0.01	0.02
Lymphadenitis	0.53	0.04	0.001

Prophylaxis consisted of sulfamethoxazole/trimethoprim plus ketoconazole 5 mg/kg per day for 3 weeks per month, 50 mg/kg per day of sulfamethoxazole, or a rotating regimen of sulfamethoxazole, oxacillin and pristinamycin. There were no differences between the regimens. Even though this is a retrospective uncontrolled study, it shows a highly significant advantage to using prophylaxis.
* Data analysed by paired Student-Fisher t test.
NS = No statistical difference.

cells in vitro with partial correction of the defect. Somatic gene therapy for patients is likely to follow.

Other neutrophil killing defects

Deficiencies of various enzymes which contribute to bacterial killing by neutrophils have been described. The clinical picture usually resembles chronic granulomatous disease, though usually in milder form. These conditions include: myeloperoxidase deficiency, glutathione synthetase and pyruvate kinase deficiency, and complete neutrophil glucose-6-phosphate dehydrogenase (G6PD) deficiency; (note: in the common red cell G6PD deficiency, there is sufficient enzyme present in the neutrophils for normal killing to occur). In transcobalamin II deficiency in addition to hypogammaglobulinemia, there is a neutrophil killing defect. Neutrophil secondary granule deficiency is an immune deficiency in which secondary (specific) granules, which contain lactoferrin and a vitamin B_{12}-binding protein are lacking. This results in defects of chemotaxis and neutrophil oxidative metabolism. Myeloperoxidase deficiency is relatively common with an incidence of 1 in 4000. Most affected individuals have only mild or no increased incidence of infections but a few suffer persistent problems with candida infection as myeloperoxidase seems to be important in the intracellular killing of this organism.

In most of these conditions, apart from G6PD deficiency, the NBT test will be normal and diagnosis is made by showing abnormal bacterial killing followed by specific biochemical assay. Myeloperoxidase in granules can be counted on automated blood counters.

Disorders of neutrophil chemotaxis

Several conditions are associated with defective neutrophil chemotaxis.

Leukocyte adhesion deficiency Type I

Deficiency of the 95 kd beta chain, common to the β_2 integrin family of cell surface adhesive molecules (see p. 1234 and

Table 22.3) leads to a profound immunodeficiency affecting the function of neutrophils, monocytes and certain lymphocytes, including T and NK cytotoxic cells (Crowley 1980). It is inherited as an autosomal recessive trait. In the phagocytic series, chemotaxis, adherence and phagocytosis are markedly depressed. There are a number of different mutations which can result in variable severity phenotypes depending on the number of surface molecules that can be expressed. It is interesting that although these molecules are involved in the lymphocyte interactions necessary for specific immune responses, there is no demonstrable defect in these. Even the impaired lymphocyte cytotoxicity in vitro is of uncertain clinical significance. The clinical pattern is almost entirely explicable on the basis of the phagocytic cell defect.

Individuals affected by the most severe phenotype (<1% expression) often present in the first weeks of life with delayed umbilical cord separation (the cord fails to shrink down and may not separate until 3–4 weeks of age). There is marked susceptibility to bacterial and fungal infections. The skin lesions may be necrotizing in nature and are characterized by a paucity of pus formation. Gingivitis is common. More deep seated infections are usually associated with the respiratory and gastrointestinal tracts.

Investigations invariably show a marked circulating neutrophilia (because of failure of the cells to migrate out of the circulation) and a profound neutrophil chemotactic defect. Diagnosis is confirmed by demonstrating the absence of the cell surface markers recognized by the anti-CD11/CD18 monoclonal antibodies.

In the severe form, early death from infection is the rule unless a successful bone marrow transplant can be performed. In the partial forms (2–10% expression) supportive and expectant management is pursued in the first instance.

Leukocyte adhesion deficiency (LAD) Type II

This recently described immunodeficiency results from failure to produce the fucose residues necessary for generating sialyl lewis x (CD15s) the ligand on neutrophils for the selectin molecules expressed on endothelial surfaces. There is a neutrophilia and neutrophil chemotaxis and migration from the circulation is severely impaired. There is no deficiency in specific immune responses. Patients suffer repeated bacterial infections and periodontal disease with a similar pattern to LAD I deficiency. The first two cases reported had mental retardation and abnormal facies (Etzioni et al 1992).

Hyper-IgE syndrome

Extreme elevation of the serum IgE level (up to 40 000 U/l or more) characterizes an immunodeficiency in which chronic dermatitis and repeated chest and skin infections occur (Buckley & Sampson 1981, Buckley 1994). Job's syndrome, so called because it was first described in fair-skinned red-headed girls, is characterized by eczema and recurrent staphylococcal infections (Davis 1966). It is almost certainly a milder variant of the hyper-IgE syndrome. Abscesses are said to be 'cold' with little surrounding inflammation but this is a relative description. The predominating organism causing these infections is *Staphylococcus aureus* and this can cause particularly serious chest disease with pneumatoceles and chronic lung damage. Other

bacteria, including streptococci and Gram-negative bacilli as well as fungi such as *Candida albicans*, can also be problematic. In addition to the high IgE level, there is a profound neutrophil chemotactic defect. The disorder is most likely due to a T cell immunoregulatory defect with imbalance of T_{H1}/T_{H2} responses resulting in a high IL 4 : γ-interferon ratio which drives B cells to IgE class switching during antibody responses. High titers of IgE antibody with specificity for *S. aureus*, *C. albicans* and tetanus toxoid are found. In a significant proportion of patients there is a failure of antibody responses to carbohydrate antigens which contributes to the susceptibility to infection. Defective T cell responses and cutaneous anergy have also been found in some patients. There is evidence that histamine released from mast cells by the IgE may mediate the chemotactic defect via histamine receptors on neutrophils. The gene for this disorder has not been identified. The mode of inheritance is thought to be autosomal dominant with incomplete penetrance.

The mainstay of treatment is long term antistaphylococcal antibiotic prophylaxis. Histamine 2 receptor blockers have been used though their value is disputed. γ interferon treatment has been tried in a few patients but although there was some lowering of the IgE levels, there was no apparent clinical benefit. Intravenous immunoglobulin therapy may be useful in those with a demonstrable antibody production deficit.

Schwachman syndrome

In this autosomal recessive syndrome, pancreatic insufficiency, short stature and skeletal abnormalities including metaphyseal dysostosis are associated with moderately severe variable neutropenia and a severe neutrophil chemotactic defect (Aggett et al 1979).

Chediak–Higashi syndrome

Neutrophils in this condition show giant cytoplasmic peroxidase positive granules. Affected patients have partial oculocutaneous albinism. They develop severe pyogenic infections and, later, a lymphoproliferative syndrome which may prove fatal. Neutrophil function, including chemotaxis and bactericidal activity, is depressed. There is also a profound defect in natural killer cell activity.

Papillon–Lefèvre syndrome

This recessively inherited condition is characterized by hyperkeratosis of the palms and soles, periodontal disease leading to early loss of teeth and a susceptibility to bacterial infection and pyoderma. There is markedly decreased expression of certain cell surface molecules including CD18, CD2 and CD45RO. Neutrophil chemotaxis is impaired.

Other causes of neutrophil chemotactic defect

Other poorly defined conditions have been described in which recurrent infections are associated with abnormal chemotaxis. In 'lazy leukocyte' syndrome, a chemotactic defect is believed to impair neutrophil mobilization from the bone marrow with resulting neutropenia. It is sometimes difficult to distinguish primary neutrophil chemotactic defects from secondary chemotactic defects which commonly occur as a result of severe illness.

Neutrophil chemotactic defects have also been found in association with metabolic defects, including glycogen storage disease type 1b, mannosidosis and diabetes mellitus.

Defects of mononuclear phagocytes

Abnormal monocytic function has been demonstrated in a number of immunodeficiency disorders affecting multiple cell series. These include chronic granulomatous disease, leukocyte adhesion deficiency syndromes, the bare lymphocyte syndrome (which despite its name also affects monocytes) and Wiskott–Aldrich syndrome. In cell-mediated immune deficiency states, lack of stimulatory cytokine production may lead to secondary subnormal macrophage function. A recently described syndrome in which there is a defect in the receptor for interferon γ results in severe disease due to disseminated atypical mycobacterial infection as a result of failure of upregulation of macrophage killing.

Defective monocyte function also plays a role in the immunodeficiency of immaturity in neonates, and in some secondary immunodeficiency states including those due to HIV infection and malignancy. In these circumstances there is a problem in handling intracellular pathogens such as mycobacteria and salmonella species. Additionally, since the most important antigen presenting cells are specialized macrophages, defects in this series can lead to poor specific immune responses.

Proliferative disorders of the monocytic series and immunodeficiency

These syndromes are summarized in Table 22.17. In Class I histiocytosis, immunological disturbance has been demonstrated but it is unclear whether this is primary or secondary (Pritchard et al 1994). In Class II histiocytosis, profound disturbance of immune function may be found but part of this may be secondary to the hypertriglyceridemia that occurs in these patients. This may be either a familial (autosomal recessive) condition (Ladish 1978) or infection (usually viral) driven. The latter often occurs in children with pre-existing immunopathological disease, suggesting that a subtle immune defect may be present before the onset of histiocytic proliferation (McClain 1988). Class III disorders are true malignancies of the monocyte series.

Table 22.17 Histiocytosis syndromes (from Writing Group of the Histiocyte Society 1987)

Class I	Langerhans cell histiocytosis (incorporates old histiocytosis X syndromes–eosinophilic granuloma, Hand–Schuller–Christian disease and Letterer–Siwe disease).
Class II	Histiocytosis of the mononuclear phagocytes other than Langerhans cells: –Familial hemophagocytic (or erythrophagocytic) lymphohistiocytosis (FHL or FEL) –Infection-associated hemophagocytic syndrome (virus-driven haemophagocytic lymphohistiocytosis)
Class III	Malignant histiocytic disorders hemophagocytic (or erythrophagocytic)

COMPLEMENT DEFICIENCY DISORDERS (Ross & Densen 1984)

Primary inherited deficiencies

The primary inherited deficiencies of complement components are listed in Table 22.7F. The defective genes responsible are inherited as autosomal codominants so that heterozygosity results in approximately half normal levels of the protein. A number of clinical patterns can occur depending upon which factor is deficient.

1. Autoimmune disease

Predisposition to autoimmune disease, particularly systemic lupus erythematosus and the other immune complex disorders, is a feature of most of the complement deficiency syndromes. Evidence, based on the finding that null alleles for a number of complement components (notably C2 and C4) occur with greater frequency in patients with autoimmune diseases such as SLE, suggests that heterozygosity for deficiency is also a risk factor. In general, the course of these diseases is similar to that in patients without complement deficiency. Some authorities would advocate regular screening for these diseases once the complement deficiency has been recognized.

2. Pyogenic infections

A predisposition to recurrent pyogenic infections is a feature of some complement deficiencies. The most severe of these is congenital C3 deficiency. Deficiency of the classical pathway components C1q and C2 and of factor D in the alternative pathway leads to these problems and the first two again carry a predisposition to autoimmune phenomena. Deficiencies of the alternative pathway control proteins, factors H or I lead to uncontrolled consumption of C3 resulting in increased susceptibility to pyogenic infections in factor I but, surprisingly, much less so in factor H deficiency.

3. Neisserial infections

Deficiency of one of the later complement components, C5–C9 (leading to failure of membrane lysis), or of properdin leads to a specific deficiency in handling neisserial species (N. meningitidis and N. gonorrhoeae) but not to a generalized increase in susceptibility to pyogenic infections. This is less of a problem in C9 deficiency where some lysis can still occur. Patients can suffer recurrent attacks of meningococcal septicemia/meningitis and severe invasive gonococcal disease. Deficiencies in factors 6–9 have been found more commonly in certain ethnic groups including middle eastern populations and in Japan (C9 deficiency in Japan affects up to 0.1% of the population). (Tedesco et al 1993). It has been argued that all cases of meningococcal infection should have complement assays performed in the convalescent phase, since incidences of deficiencies of up to 18% have been found after single episodes of infection. In the UK the figure would seem to be lower. After recurrent episodes the chances of finding a deficiency are high.

4. Hereditary angioedema

Deficiency of the control protein, C1 esterase inhibitor (C1INH), leads to spontaneous episodes of localized edema (angioedema) without urticaria. These occur spontaneously anywhere in the body but those affecting the upper airway are most serious and can be life threatening. Intra-abdominal swelling causes pain and can be misdiagnosed as a surgical condition. There is a high incidence of SLE and related diseases. Tests show persistently low C4 levels due to excessive consumption (which occurs even between attacks) and C1 INH assay shows one of two patterns – either very low levels of the protein or (in approximately 15%) a functionally defective protein. The condition is inherited as an autosomal dominant. Clinical problems do not usually commence until later childhood. Infusions of purified C1 INH are effective in terminating attacks. For prevention the treatment of choice is with one of the 'retarded' androgenic steroids, such as danazol, which raise functional C1 INH levels sufficiently to prevent attacks and are relatively free of virilizing side-effects. In post-pubertal girls, oral contraceptive preparations may be helpful prophylactically.

Secondary complement deficiencies

Many immunopathological diseases can result in excessive complement activation and consumption. In SLE and other immune complex diseases, low levels of C3 and the early classical pathway components can occur.

In acute nephritis, C3 levels are acutely depressed, while in membranoproliferative glomerulonephritis a more persistent depression of C3 levels occurs due to the presence of an autoantibody – C3 nephritic factor – directed against C3bBb, the alternative pathway C3 convertase. This autoantibody can also be associated with the condition partial lipodystrophy, with or without membranoproliferative glomerulonephritis. An increased susceptibility to pyogenic infections, occurs when C3 levels are reduced below approximately 10%.

Gram-negative sepsis, acute pancreatitis and acute vasculitis can all be associated with complement consumption. The first of these may be particularly important in neonatal sepsis, where complement levels are already low compared to those of older individuals.

Interaction of antibody and complement deficiencies

Deficiency of the early classical pathway complement components, has been shown to be associated with poor antibody responses, presumably because of some immunoregulatory role of the complement factors. Later components are not implicated.

Alternative pathway opsonization is less efficient in the absence of specific antibody to bacterial surfaces. There is evidence that antibody may 'neutralize' surface molecules, such as sialic acid, which otherwise inhibit alternative pathway activation.

Mannan-binding lectin (MBL) deficiency

Though not strictly a complement component, this deficiency is included here because this molecule interacts closely with the complement system. Low levels of MBL result from mutations in the gene which prevent correct association of the individual chains to form the multimeric molecular structure necessary for avid binding to mannose residues on the surface of microorganisms (Super et al 1989). These mutations are very common affecting 5–10% of Europeans and a higher proportion of certain African tribes. This condition was formerly known as

the yeast opsonization defect because of failure of serum from affected individuals to opsonize baker's yeast in a biological assay. In early childhood the deficiency often results in frequent infections while deficient adults are usually asymptomatic. MBL deficiency seems to be most important in the very early handling of microbial invasion and in the early years of life before the ability to make high affinity antibodies is fully developed (Turner 1996).

Deficiencies of C3 receptors

The distribution and function of cell surface receptors for C3b and its derivatives have been described on page 1234. Specific clinical syndromes have been attributed to deficiencies of some of these receptors. A dominantly inherited CR1 deficiency is associated with SLE and other immune complex disorders, presumably related to failure of the immune complex clearing function of this molecule.

Deficient expression of the CR3 receptor occurs as part of the leukocyte adhesion deficiency type I syndrome since it is a member of the β integrin family affected in this disorder (see p. 1260).

Management of complement deficiencies

Apart from C1 esterase inhibitor (see above) there are no specific preparations for replacement therapy. Fresh plasma infusions have been used prophylactically or can be reserved for the treatment of serious episodes of infection. Lifelong prophylactic penicillin and meningococcal vaccination are advised in the late complement deficiencies resulting in susceptibility to neisserial infections. Prophylactic co-trimoxazole can be used in deficiencies which result in an increased susceptibility to a wider range of organisms.

Clinical monitoring may allow earlier diagnosis and treatment of autoimmune disorders should they emerge.

SECONDARY IMMUNODEFICIENCY

Secondary deficiencies of immunity are relatively more common than primary disorders. They include natural immunosuppressive influences, e.g. viral infections, as well as iatrogenic causes. Table 22.18 shows the main causes of secondary immunodeficiency some of which, affecting specific immune parameters, have been discussed above in the relevant sections, e.g. protein-losing states leading to immunoglobulin deficiency and complement consumption states. The causes of more generalized, and sometimes less well-defined, secondary immunodeficiency are discussed here.

Infection-induced immunodeficiency

Infection with all types of microbial pathogens has been shown to depress immunity. These effects are most commonly seen after viral infection (Lamelin 1983) which is discussed below. However, chronic infection with other organisms have been well documented as producing similar effects, examples include the depressed antibody responses in malaria infected children which correlates with the parasite load; or the T cell depression that complicates advanced mycobacterial disease and which may be due to the effects of specific cell wall products.

Table 22.18   Some causes of secondary immunodeficiency

Drugs
Corticosteroids
Cytotoxic drugs
Specific immunosuppressives–e.g. cyclosporine A, anti-lymphocyte globulin
Miscellaneous–e.g. phenytoin

Radiation

Malnutrition

Protein-losing states
Nephrotic syndrome
Gastrointestinal disease (especially intestinal lymphangiectasia)
Burns

Excessive immunoglobulin catabolism
Myotonic dystrophy

Metabolic disturbance
Inherited   – galactosemia
             – glycogen storage disease
Acquired   – uremia
             – diabetes mellitus

Infections
Viruses   – human immunodeficiency virus
             – cytomegalovirus, Epstein–Barr virus
Bacteria   – overwhelming infections
Protozoa   – e.g. malaria

Immune complex disorders – e.g. systemic lupus erythematosus

Hyposplenism
Congenital asplenia
Sickle cell anemia
Splenectomy

Malignancy, esp. lymphoid

Histiocytic disorders
Langerhans cell histiocytosis
Hemophagocytic lymphohistiocytosis

Miscellaneous
Sarcoidosis
Surgery and anesthesia

Acute viral infection

Changes in circulating lymphocyte numbers associated with markedly reduced T cell responses and cutaneous anergy seem to be a 'normal' reaction to acute infection with a wide variety of common viral infections. This was first recognized in measles infection by Von Pirquet in 1908. It has also been shown to occur after live viral vaccines, including measles and oral polio. In some cases, it is due to direct infection of lymphocytes and/or macrophages. In others, there is an alteration in immunoregulation. The latter is most marked in acute infectious mononucleosis due to Epstein–Barr virus infection in which there is B and T cell proliferation and a reversal of the normal helper: suppressor T cell ratios. Influenza and measles virus infections have also been shown to have nonspecific depressive effects on neutrophil and monocyte function.

The clinical importance of these observations is not always certain. However, they are thought to be relevant to the very high incidence of secondary bacterial infection after measles and to the fatal downward spiral of infection and malnutrition that commonly complicates measles in the developing world.

Chronic viral infection

Congenital viral infection (and toxoplasmosis) result in an immune depression with specific failure of T cell reactivity, or tolerance, to the relevant agent and in some cases a more generalized depression of antibody responses and even hypogammaglobulinemia, sometimes of a pattern which mimics the hyper-IgM syndrome. Congenital cytomegalovirus and rubella infections can result in prolonged excretion of these viruses for several years. Other chronic viral infections, e.g. subacute sclerosing panencephalitis or persistent EB virus infection, are associated with an ill-defined immune suppression though this may be partly due to an element of preexisting immune incompetence. Hepatitis C virus infection has recently been shown to be associated with acquired IgA deficiency (Ilan et al 1993).

Human immunodeficiency virus (HIV) infection

HIV is 'par excellence' an example of a virus that produces profound immunodeficiency (McNamara 1989). The natural history, virology and epidemiology of this infection is dealt with in Chapter 23. This account will deal with the immunological effects of HIV infection and its consequences.

Immune deficiency caused by vertically acquired HIV infection is often the differential diagnosis of the primary immunodeficiency states presenting in early life. Affected children follow one of two courses, a rapid progression which results in the development of full blown AIDS symptoms, usually within the first year of life, or a more slowly progressive illness. The former may present with opportunistic infection such as *Pneumocystis carinii* pneumonia; severe failure to thrive; severe invasive bacterial disease or neurodevelopmental problems. The first three of these produce a clinical picture similar to children with SCID. Children with the slower progression picture may remain asymptomatic for a long period or may develop problems of relatively minor (non-AIDS defining) infections and thus mimic the clinical picture of children with less severe primary immune deficiencies such as the minor immunoglobulin disturbances. Lymphoid interstitial pneumonitis (LIP) (see Ch. 23), as a result of lymphocytic infiltration of the lungs producing nodular shadowing on the chest X ray, is a relatively frequent manifestation of HIV infection in children. If this is the first presenting illness, the clinical picture again raises the differential diagnosis of a primary immune deficiency with opportunistic lung infection.

HIV not only infects the CD4 +ve T cells but also cells of the macrophage/monocyte lineage, including those cells responsible for antigen presentation in immune responses. There is depression of both cell mediated and humoral immunity. The CD4 count in children correlates poorly with the degree of HIV induced immune suppression, and cannot be used as a guide for commencing prophylactic measures as is the case in infected adults. Normal ranges of CD4 counts at different ages have been devised (Fig. 22.12). A falling CD4 : CD8 ratio may be a better predictor of disease progression in young children, probably because of preservation of the CD4 count mitogen responses in children which are preserved until very late in the disease, whereas antigen specific T cell responses are depressed. Serum immunoglobulin measurements in most cases show a hypergammaglobulinemia which can become very marked. However, antibody responses are very poor particularly to polysaccharide antigens. IgG_2 subclass deficiency is sometimes seen and very occasionally hypogamma-globulinemia has been described.

The overall management of the HIV-infected child is discussed in Chapter 23. From the immunological point of view there are many strategies offering theoretical benefit but few that are of proven value. Intravenous immunoglobulin prophylaxis has been used against bacterial infections but in a large study (Spector et al 1994) was shown to give no additional benefit over that provided by prophylactic co-trimoxazole. Recombinant cytokines such as interferon γ are not useful prophylactically but may be useful as adjuvant therapy for specific infections. Recombinant hemo-poietic growth factors such as GCSF have been used to treat the myelosuppressive effects of some of the antiviral agents used.

Immunodeficiency due to drugs and radiation

Specific immunosuppressants

Antibodies to human lymphocytes (antilymphocyte globulin) or to specific T cell subsets are used therapeutically as immuno-suppressive agents. The former has been used to treat idiopathic aplastic anemia, and the latter for the prevention of graft-versus-host disease and graft rejection. They induce profound lympho-penia and depress primary antibody and delayed hypersensitivity responses.

Cyclosporine and tacrolimus are highly specific T cell immunosuppressants used in organ and bone marrow transplantation. They inhibit antigen processing as well as diminishing interleukin-1 and -2 production, and interleukin-2 receptor expression.

Corticosteroid drugs are less specific, but nevertheless potent, immunosuppressive drugs (Mukwaya 1988). The degree of immunosuppression induced is related to the dose, to the length of the treatment course and probably varies between individuals. Lymphopenia results from a diminution of recirculation of long-lived T cells. Cytotoxic function, mitogenic responses and delayed hypersensitivity responses are all depressed. With high-dose treatment for prolonged periods antibody responses, especially primary responses, also become impaired. Corti-costeroids also have effects on recirculating monocytes and polymorphs, and microbicidal ability is depressed.

Cytotoxic drugs used in the treatment of leukemia and solid tumors not surprisingly have major immunosuppressive side-effects. Cyclophosphamide has particular effects on B cell function and antibody production, but T lymphopenia (especially of CD4 cells) also occurs.

Azathioprine and 6-mercaptopurine also suppress antibody production, particularly primary responses. T cell functions including delayed hypersensitivity responses are also depressed.

Methotrexate has potent anti-inflammatory activity and may also suppress antibody responses in higher doses.

Radiation therapy, particularly total body or total lymphoid irradiation, has profound and long-lasting effects on cell-mediated immune function and on antibody responses.

The most severe immunosuppressed states occur during bone marrow transplantation for malignant disease. In these cases, a combination of radiotherapy and chemotherapy is often used.

Clinical effects. The immunosuppressed child will be susceptible to opportunistic infection, especially fungal infections and *Pneumocystis carinii* pneumonia (see Figs 22.18 and 22.19). After bone marrow transplant, there is a recognized pattern of

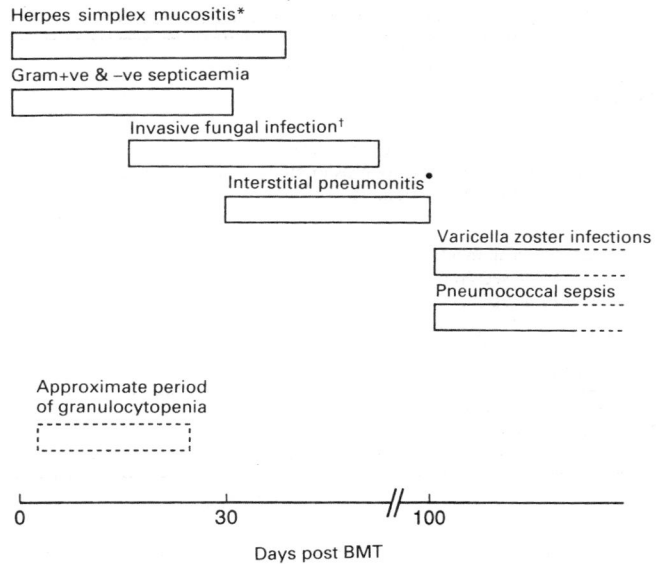

* Realighted infection

† Predominantly *Candida* and *Aspergillus* species

• Predominantly cytomegalovirus and *Pneumocystis carinii*

Fig. 22.20 Periods of maximal risk for various infectious complications after bone marrow transplantation with immunosuppression/marrow ablation. (Redrawn from Rogers 1985.)

susceptibility to different pathogens, depending on the elapsed time since the procedure (Fig. 22.20). In the absence of neutropenia, susceptibility to pyogenic infections is less of a problem. 'Live' vaccines should be avoided, as should contact with cases of measles and chicken pox. Post exposure prophylaxis should be given when inadvertent exposure to these viruses occurs. Co-trimoxazole is of benefit as prophylaxis against *Pneumocystis carinii* pneumonia.

Other drugs

A variety of miscellaneous drugs may cause immunosuppression as part of their side-effect profile. The effects of phenytoin and other agents on IgA production is discussed above (section on IgA deficiency).

Moderate or severe depression of neutrophil counts is a side-effect of a large number of drugs including antibiotics such as sulfonamides and flucloxacillin and results in a susceptibility to bacterial disease.

Malnutrition

This has potent effects on immunity. The most profound effects are seen in protein calorie deficiency (Table 22.19). There is increased susceptibility to tuberculosis, measles, *Pneumocystis carinii* as well as staphylococcal pneumonia, and Gram-negative sepsis.

Specific nutritional deficiencies can also affect immune function. Zinc deficiency has very specific effects on thymic function, with development of thymic atrophy, decreased levels of thymic hormones and T cell lymphopenia, anergy and impaired

Table 22.19 Main immunological effects of severe malnutrition

Cell-mediated immunity
T cell lymphopenia
Reduced CD4 cell numbers
Reduced CD4:CD8 ratio
Reduced delayed hypersensitivity responses
Reduced proliferative T cell responses to mitogens and antigens
Reduced lymphokine production

Antibody production
Polyclonal hypergammaglobulinemia
Decreased IgA in secretions
Increased serum IgE
Defective antibody responses
Reduced antibody affinity
Depressed function of antigen-presenting cells

Non-specific immune system
Depressed neutrophil bactericidal capability
Depressed levels of complement factors, especially C3

cytotoxic functions. Zinc deficiency may be secondary to nutritional problems or can occur as the primary defect in the autosomal recessive condition, acrodermatitis enteropathica in which specific zinc malabsorption occurs. Treatment with zinc supplements reverses most effects.

Iron deficiency, even without anemia, has subtle effects on T cell and phagocytic cell function. The clinical importance of this is not clear. Some studies have shown an increased frequency of infections which reverses with iron therapy, but others have not confirmed this.

Vitamin A deficiency is associated with depressed T cell and humoral responses. In populations at risk from malnutrition, vitamin A supplementation improves antibody responses to vaccines. In similar populations treatment with vitamin A during measles infection reduces mortality and has been shown to reverse some of the induced abnormalities in lymphocyte numbers and function.

Hyposplenism

Lack of splenic function occurs as a result of splenectomy, sickle cell disease and congenital asplenia. There is an increased risk of pyogenic infections, including pneumonia, septicemia and meningitis caused by pneumococcus and other polysaccharide encapsulated organisms (e.g. *Haemophilus influenzae* type b). The mechanism for this immune deficiency is not entirely clear – it would seem to be multifactorial. Immunoglobulin levels generally remain normal, though low serum IgM levels have been reported. Antibody responses to pneumococcal vaccine are impaired as are responses to protein antigens, but only if the latter are given intravenously. Defective alternative pathway complement activity was found in 10% of splenectomized and 16% of sickle cell patients. Deficiency of tuftsin – a tetrapeptide produced by the spleen which enhances phagocytosis – has been postulated as another contributory factor to immunodeficiency.

As pneumococcal infection is numerically the greatest risk, prophylaxis with penicillin is used. However, particularly in young children, awareness of the risks from other infections should be maintained. Vaccination with pneumococcal and *Haemophilus influenzae* type B vaccines may diminish the risk but do not remove the need to give penicillin. Immunization should be performed prior to elective splenectomy. New

conjugate pneumococcal vaccines may be particularly useful in this group of patients.

Sickle cell disease

Much, but not all, of the increased susceptibility to infection in sickle cell disease stems from the hyposplenism which develops. In addition, sickle cell patients have impaired reticuloendothelial clearing capacity (due to chronic hemolysis) and focal tissue ischemia (as a result of sickling). In addition to susceptibility to pneumococcus, these patients are also prone to Gram-negative sepsis, including salmonella osteomyelitis. The risk of these problems is less in the variant form, Hemoglobin SC disease, but is still higher than background so prophylactic measures (as discussed under hyposplenism) are still indicated.

Other causes of secondary immunodeficiency

A whole variety of other medical conditions lead to depressed immune function. Acquired metabolic problems, such as uremia and diabetes mellitus, have been shown to depress polymorph function (as do some primary inherited disorders, as discussed above – see p. 1262).

TREATMENT OF IMMUNODEFICIENCY

Supportive care

Children with immunodeficiency disorders will often require the full spectrum of pediatric care in their management. Particular attention needs to be paid to their nutritional status and to the management of dietary intolerances secondary to the gastrointestinal problems which frequently occur. Expert handling of the emotional needs of the family is also very important. Prevention and treatment of infections is the mainstay of supportive care.

Prevention of infection

Newborns suspected of having a severe immunodeficiency disorder should be protected using moderately strict isolation techniques, including limitation of the numbers of persons involved with care. Placement in sterile isolation facilities is fraught with difficulties and not of proven benefit, though this degree of isolation is usually initiated if and when bone marrow transplantation with immunosuppression is embarked upon (see below). Breast-feeding should be encouraged. Prophylactic nonabsorbable antifungals, e.g. nystatin, should be used in combined immunodeficiencies or phagocytic cell defects. Co-trimoxazole as prophylaxis against *Pneumocystis carinii* should be considered for defects involving cell-mediated immunity mechanisms (in newborns this treatment is delayed until at least 2 weeks of age or until physiological jaundice has subsided). Prophylactic co-trimoxazole may also be of benefit in reducing the incidence of pyogenic infections in phagocytic or humoral immune deficiencies. In conditions where the immune deficiency affects the handling of relatively few organisms, prophylaxis with a narrow spectrum antibiotic can be used, e.g. penicillin prophylaxis for the complement deficiencies which lead to predisposition only to neisserial infections.

Immunizations may be used judiciously if sufficient immune function is judged to be present to give an antibody response. 'Live' vaccines are contraindicated in combined immunodeficiencies and in the more severe antibody-deficiency states. In Wiskott–Aldrich syndrome, killed vaccines including polysaccharide and typhoid vaccines can cause severe reactions and are therefore contraindicated. Passive immunization is the basis of immunoglobulin replacement therapy (see below) and specific hyperimmune globulins are available for postexposure prophylaxis in patients with primary or secondary immunodeficiency exposed to chicken pox, hepatitis B or cytomegalovirus. For measles exposure standard immunoglobulin is used.

The prevention of complications of recurrent infections is obviously important. Evidence of middle ear disease which might lead to deafness should be sought and treated. Chronic lung disease leading to bronchiectasis is a serious complication, particularly of antibody deficiency states. Regular physiotherapy, with sputum cultures to direct appropriate antibiotic therapy and monitoring of pulmonary status are useful.

Treatment of infections

A policy of vigorous and early antimicrobial treatment of infections should be observed. Unusual etiologic agents may be responsible for infections, and broader spectrum antimicrobial cover may therefore be needed. In neutrophil disorders it is particularly important to cover *Pseudomonas* and other Gram-negative bacilli. Early treatment of an infection may be life saving, but its initiation should not detract from full attempts at identification of the causative agent. Invasive diagnostic procedures, such as bronchoalveolar lavage or, if this fails to produce a diagnosis, open lung biopsy, can be fully justified on the basis that they will facilitate precise and optimal therapy.

Antivirals such as the broad spectrum agent, ribavirin, and the anticytomegalovirus agent, gancyclovir, are particularly useful in the immunocompromised infant.

Blood product support

Blood product infusions may be necessary in some disorders. In combined deficiencies and in patients undergoing heavy immunosuppression (as for bone marrow transplantation), all such products except intravenous immunoglobulin may contain viable leukocytes and should be irradiated with 2000–3000 rad to prevent possible graft-versus-host disease. In those with no evidence of previous exposure to cytomegalovirus, blood products should be obtained from cytomegalovirus-antibody-negative donors.

Immunological intervention in neonates

The neonate, and particularly the sick premature neonate, must be regarded as severely immunocompromised, and the usual mechanisms for reducing the risk of cross-infection should be taken. The prophylactic use of intravenous immunoglobulin infusions to make up for the lack of maternally transferred IgG in premature infants has proved disappointing in that although some studies suggested benefit others have not and a recent meta-analysis concluded that there was no benefit (Lacy & Ohlsson 1995). The disparate results obtained may be due to the different spectra of organisms causing sepsis in the various studies and to the fact that commercial immunoglobulin preparations have been shown to vary considerably (from batch to batch and preparation to preparation) in the titers of antibody against relevant organisms. Few preparations have significant antibody against coagulase negative staphylococcus, the commonest cause of late onset neonatal sepsis. Future work in this field is likely to be directed to use of 'tailored' immunoglobulin preparations of known and appropriate antibody content (Fischer 1994). Such an approach has been successfully employed in studies of passive prophylaxis against *Respiratory syncytial virus* (RSV) infection in high risk infants (bronchopulmonary dysplasia and congenital cyanotic heart disease) using preparations with high titer anti-RSV content (Groothuis et al 1993).

Alternative preventative measures include active immunization of mothers and a vaccine against type III Group B streptococcus that has been shown to be immunogenic in pregnant women (Baker et al 1988). This approach may, in the future, produce a means by which the morbidity and mortality caused by this organism can be reduced in both mother and baby. This technique has the added advantage that it would help prevent early onset sepsis which is not amenable to passive prophylaxis. It would however be less beneficial for very low birthweight infants because of failure of placental antibody transfer. A similar strategy might be employed for the use of the RSV vaccines currently under development.

Immunological maneuvers may also be used in the treatment of established neonatal infections (Cairo 1989). Fresh blood transfusion (from donors known to have the relevant antibodies) as well as immunoglobulin infusion are beneficial in group B streptococcal sepsis. Exchange transfusion with fresh blood has the advantage that, in addition to supplying antibody, it replaces clotting factors, complement factors and polymorphs. The use of fibronectin or fibronectin-rich blood products (such as cryoprecipitate) to boost the depleted circulating levels of this protein in sick neonates has been advocated. The use of cytokines to boost immune responses is a theoretically attractive idea. Interleukin-2 and interferon γ are both poorly produced in the newborn, and experimental work suggests that the use of recombinant forms of these cytokines would boost cell-mediated immune function, especially macrophage-dependent mechanisms. However, they may have unpleasant side effects, and much work is needed to establish the precise role of these agents. Granulocyte colony stimulating factor (GCSF) is much better tolerated and has been shown to boost low neutrophil counts in neonates with proven or suspected sepsis though whether this has any beneficial effect on outcome remains to be established. In contrast to granulocyte macrophage colony stimulating factor, GCSF seems to have anti-inflammatory properties which makes it less likely to exacerbate lung damage in infected neonates.

Replacement therapy for humoral deficiencies

Immunoglobulin

This is the mainstay of treatment for the more severe antibody deficiency and combined immune deficiency states (Haeney 1994). Intravenous immunoglobulin (IVIG) preparations have superseded the use of intramuscular preparations, since they are more acceptable to the patients and their use enables higher and more reliable blood levels to be achieved.

Several IVIG preparations are licensed for use. They are all prepared by fractionation of human plasma followed by chemical or enzymatic treatment to reduce the tendency to aggregation. Although all donors are screened for blood borne viruses, a specific viral inactivation step must be involved in the preparatory process and regulatory bodies require proof that this will inactivate added virus. Inactivation steps used for different preparations include acidification, solvent/detergent treatment or pasteurization. Finally, the immunoglobulin is stabilized (at a concentration of approximately 5%) in a sugar or amino acid solution (maltose, sucrose or glycine). The preparations are almost entirely IgG with a fairly normal IgG subclass distribution but mostly with small amounts of IgA (which may cause problems; see below). One preparation not licensed in the UK contains significant amounts of both IgA and IgM. The current generation of products can be shown to have excellent preservation of antibody binding, Fc receptor binding and complement fixation functions.

IVIG replacement therapy is given in doses between 0.3 and 0.5 g/kg infused over 2–3 hours every 2–4 weeks. The exact dosage and frequency are very variable and are based on clinical response and trough IgG levels (the aim being to keep these well within the normal range). Home therapy with IVIG is becoming increasingly popular with families. This requires careful setting up and ongoing support. Though serious reactions are rare, families are taught simple resuscitation and are provided with adrenaline injections.

An alternative mode of immunoglobulin administration is via the subcutaneous route. This has mainly been used in adults where patient acceptability is high. It requires a more concentrated preparation (to reduce volume) and the infusions need to be given once or twice a week. Experience of using this route in children is increasing but the frequency of infusions is a drawback.

IVIG has also been successfully given directly into the cerebrospinal fluid in cases of chronic viral meningoencephalitis associated with immunoglobulin deficiency states.

Unwanted effects (Misbah & Chapel 1993). Immediate side-effects include reaction to the infusion and these are commoner than after intramuscular preparations. They include nausea, vomiting, flushing, rigors and occasionally hypotension. Generally they are not serious and can be avoided by slowing down the rate of infusion. The mechanism is probably complement activation by micro-aggregates in the preparations. More serious (anaphylactoid) reactions can occur in IgA deficiency due to anti-IgA antibodies (see IgA deficiency, p. 1258).

The risk of viral transmission is small, partly because of screening of donors, the viricidal steps in the preparation process and tight control by the regulatory authorities greatly reduce the risk of viral transmission by IVIG. Nevertheless, occasional instances of hepatitis C transmission have been reported. Monitoring of serum transaminases during therapy and testing for infection by polymerase chain reaction (antibody tests are of no use in most of these patients) are therefore advisable.

Plasma

Fresh plasma contains all the immunoglobulin classes as well as complement factors. It may be useful in boosting levels of these proteins during episodes of serious infection. However the risk of viral transmission is higher than for IVIG and this needs to be taken into consideration.

Replacement therapy for combined deficiencies

Replacement of thymus function

Fetal thymic grafts, grafts of thymic epithelium and thymic hormone therapy have been used for the treatment of a number of combined immunodeficiencies. Notable successes have been achieved in DiGeorge syndrome. No consistent success has been achieved in other conditions. Combined fetal thymus and fetal liver (as a source of stem cells) transplants have been used for severe combined immunodeficiency with some limited success. There are often major problems as a result of prolonged delay in immune reconstitution, severe infection and graft-versus-host disease. Lack of availability of fetal tissues and progress in bone marrow transplantation techniques have led to these methods being largely abandoned.

Bone marrow transplantation (BMT)

Virtually all of the primary immunodeficiency disorders which have a cellular basis are potentially correctable by bone marrow transplantation (Berthet et al 1994). The largest group of patients for whom this approach has been used were those with immediately life-threatening conditions, mainly SCID. In recent times with increasing understanding of the basis of the immunodeficiencies and improving techniques and results from BMT, a wider variety of conditions has been treated in this way (Table 22.20).

Early attempts at bone marrow transplantation using incompletely matched donors were largely unsuccessful. For a time, transplants were therefore restricted to those using HLA fully matched sibling donors. This meant that the approach was only available to the lucky few with matched sibling donors. Techniques were therefore developed to allow parent-to-child (one haplotype identical) grafts with T cell depletion to prevent graft-versus-host disease. These are called haploidentical or mismatched grafts and a large experience has been built up. There is also experience of the use of matched unrelated donors (MUD).

Table 22.20 Primary immunodeficiency disorders which have been treated with bone marrow transplantation

Lymphocyte disorders

Severe combined immunodeficiency
(including adenosine deaminase deficiency)
Wiskott–Aldrich syndrome
Ommen syndrome
Nezelof syndrome
Major histocompatibility antigen Class II deficiency
DiGeorge syndrome
Purine nucleoside phosphorylase deficiency
Cartilage hair hypoplasia syndrome
X-linked lymphoproliferative disease
Hyper IgM syndrome (CD40 ligand deficiency)
Mucocutaneous candidiasis
Immunodeficiency with partial albinism (Griscelli syndrome)

Phagocytic cell disorders

Chronic granulomatous disease
Leukocyte adhesion defect Type I
Congenital agranulocytosis
Chediak–Higashi syndrome
Familial hemophagocytic lymphohistiocytosis

Problems of bone marrow transplantation. The interrelationship between the three main complications of graft failure (rejection), graft-versus-host disease, and infection is shown in Figure 22.21. Complications are less troublesome after matched-related than after mismatched or matched unrelated transplantation.

Graft-versus-host disease (GVHD) can affect any organ in the body, but the three most commonly affected are skin, gut and liver. Severe acute inflammatory changes in these can be life threatening. The process itself causes further immunosuppression and bone marrow depression, the latter causing delay or failure of maturation of the graft which, in turn, increases the risk from infection. Prophylaxis against GVHD is usually employed with cyclosporine and/or methotrexate. Another approach to prophylaxis is to give the patient antibody of the CD11b/CD18 designation (against the leukocyte adhesion molecule LFA 1). Though this reduces GVHD it probably also increases the risk of infection. Treatment of GVHD involves the use of immunosuppressive drugs including high dose steroids which further increase the risk of infection. Intravenous immunoglobulin may be useful in GVHD as infection prophylaxis and possibly as an immune modulator.

Infection after transplantation is discussed above (see secondary immunodeficiencies and Fig. 22.20).

Matched related donor bone marrow transplantation. This usually will be from a sibling donor but in consanguineous relationships, other family members may be a full match.

For severe combined immunodeficiency, HLA-matched grafts are relatively straightforward. Prior immunosuppression ('conditioning') is not usually required or can be minimal. Graft-versus-host disease can occur but is usually mild and self-limiting and prophylaxis is not usually given. Full and long-lasting immune reconstitution is usually achieved though in some cases B cell engraftment and therefore reconstitution of humoral immunity does not occur necessitating continuing immunoglobulin therapy. In recent years, the success rate in the European experience has been of the order of 90% (Fischer et al 1990). Failures may be related to the pre-existing condition of the child, rather than the technique.

Matched transplants for other conditions (in which graft rejecting ability is present) have a lower success rate, at least in part because of the need to give immunosuppressive treatment,

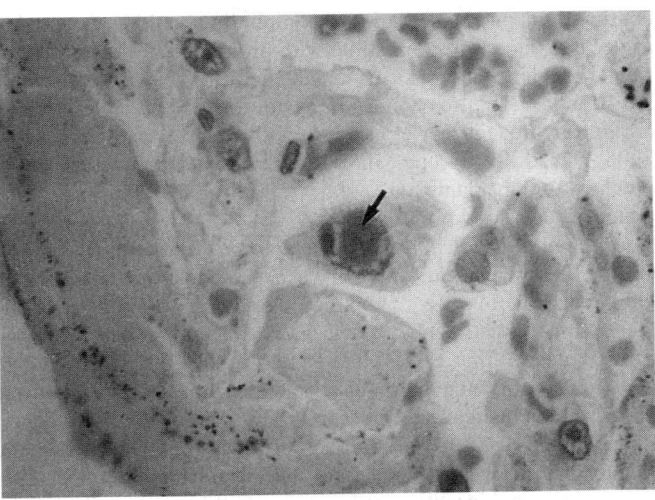
Fig. 22.22 Lung histology at postmortem from a bone marrow transplant recipient (adult) dying from cytomegalovirus (CMV) pneumonitis. Note the typical CMV nuclear inclusion (arrowed). (Courtesy of Dr Susan Dilly.)

with the consequent risks of infection. Nevertheless, encouraging results have been reported (Fischer et al 1994) with overall survival of 66% (81% in the period since 1985).

Mismatched bone marrow transplantation. By removing all T cell lineage cells (back to the prethymic stage) from harvested bone marrow, it is possible to prevent graft-versus-host disease even in an HLA-mismatched situation. Earlier grafts performed in this way utilized the differential binding of T cells to plant lectins, but these have now been largely superseded by T cell depletion techniques using monoclonal anti-T cell antibodies in a semiautomated system. The resulting T cell-depleted (but stem cell enriched) marrow will reconstitute T cell immunity by producing precursor T cells which are then 'educated' into a state of tolerance towards the foreign HLA haplotype in the new host. The fact that there is half matching of HLA antigen allows most immune functions to proceed normally.

However, successful mismatched BMT are not as easily achieved as matched ones. Even in SCID, the T cell-depleted bone marrow can be rejected (or fail to take), and to prevent this full conditioning therapy (marrow ablation) is often needed. Graft take is often slow, and achievement of full immune function will take months or even years. Not uncommonly, B cell function (antibody responses) never become fully reconstituted, and lifelong immunoglobulin therapy is still required. Failure to remove all the T cells can result in severe graft-versus-host disease (GVH) which may require the use of immunosuppressive drugs. On the other hand absolute deficiency of T cells inhibits graft take. The adding back of small numbers of T cells has been attempted to overcome this problem but it increases the risk of GVH. The prolonged period of immunoincompetence greatly increases the risk of opportunistic infections. In this group of transplants it has been shown that the use of high technology isolation facilities (such as laminar air flow) improves the outcome. Figure 22.21 summarizes the vicious cycle of problems that may occur. Despite these problems, refinements of the technique over recent years have resulted in continuing improvement in results, with most recent figures suggesting around 50% success rate. (Partial immune reconstitution with

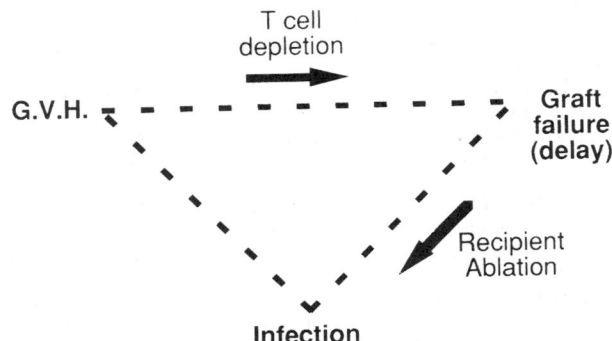
Fig. 22.21 Relationship between the three main complications of bone marrow transplantation. Maneuvers such as T cell depletion of the marrow reduce graft versus host (GVH) disease but increase the risk of graft failure; while marrow ablation of the recipient facilitates graft take but at the expense of an increased risk of infectious complications.

continuing dependence on immunoglobulin should be counted as a success, since it is compatible with prolonged life expectancy.)

The problems and risks of mismatched BMT have meant that it has been used less for non-SCID conditions. Nevertheless results are improving (Fischer et al 1994) with 47% survival in the post 1985 period in Europe. Interestingly, far better results were obtained in transplants for Leukocyte Adhesion Deficiency Type I than for other conditions.

Matched unrelated donor (MUD) bone marrow transplantation. For many years there have been 'banks' of tissue typed volunteer bone marrow donors in a number of countries allowing the option of using phenotypically matched unrelated donors. Early results in SCID suggested that the mismatched haploidentical donor approach was superior. However, with the increased sophistication of tissue typing techniques this may no longer be the case and the approach is increasingly being used and found to be at least as successful as the mismatched approach. There is considerable experience of this approach in the hematological field.

Transplantation technique. This is relatively straightforward for donor and recipient. Under general anesthesia marrow is harvested by multiple punctures along the posterior iliac crest. If it is to be given unfractionated it is passed through a coarse filter to remove bone particles, the nucleated cells are counted and if necessary the volume adjusted. T cell depletion if required is done under strict aseptic conditions (details of this are beyond the scope of this chapter). A relatively new approach which avoids the need for bone marrow harvest is the technique of peripheral stem cell harvest which is increasingly being used and is under evaluation.

Other replacement therapies

Enzyme replacement. Some immunological reconstitution of immunological function can be achieved by administering the deficient enzyme in adenosine deaminase deficiency. Purified bovine ADA is given in a conjugate with polyethylene glycol (PEG-ADA) by intramuscular injection. In full blown deficiency with SCID this treatment is unlikely to produce consistent clinical benefit, presumably because the lymphoid system has been too severely damaged by the time of birth and bone marrow transplantation remains the treatment of choice. However this form of treatment may be useful in partial forms of the condition and to temporarily improve immune function if somatic gene therapy is being attempted. It should not be used immediately prior to transplantation since the reconstituted immunity may make it more difficult to achieve engraftment.

Cytokines. Several cytokines and growth factors are available in recombinant synthetic form. Their widespread use in immunodeficiency disorders awaits evaluation. Gamma-interferon and interleukin-2 have been useful in improving cell-mediated immune function in deficiencies where their production was demonstrably absent (Cunningham-Rundles et al 1995). Growth factors such as granulocyte colony stimulating factor (G-CSF) or granulocyte-macrophage colony stimulating factor (GM-CSF) may be of benefit in phagocytic series defects. The use of γ interferon in chronic granulomatous disease has been discussed under the description of this disorder.

Somatic gene therapy. This has been attempted in adenosine deaminase deficiency using ADA transfected CD34 positive autologous cells. Some expression of the gene could be demonstrated but, to date, no consistent improvement in immunological or clinical parameters has been achieved. There is much work in this field and a number of other conditions for which such therapy might apply include chronic granulomatous disease and leukocyte adhesion deficiency type I (Thrasher & Kinnon 1995).

REFERENCES AND FURTHER READING

Aggett P J, Harries J T, Harvey B A M, Soothill J F 1979 An inherited disorder of neutrophil mobility in Schwachmann syndrome. Journal of Pediatrics 94: 391–394

Anon 1993 Primary immunodeficiency and autoimmune diseases in children: directions in defining the molecular basis. Symposium proceedings and festschrift in honour of Ralph J Wedgewood. Clinical Immunology and Immunopathology 67: S1–82

Anon 1995 Proceedings of the Jeffrey Modell immunodeficiency symposium. Advances in Primary Immunodeficiency Disease. Clinical Immunology and Immunopathology 76: S145–232

Baker C, Rench M A, Edwards M S, Carpenter R J, Hays B M, Kasper D L 1988 Immunisation of women with a polysaccharide vaccine of Group B Streptococcus. New England Journal of Medicine 319: 1180–1185

Berthet F, Le Deist F, Duliege A M, Griscelli C, Fischer A 1994 Clinical consequences and treatment of primary immunodeficiency syndromes characterized by functional T and B lymphocyte anomalies (combined immune deficiency). Pediatrics 93: 265–270

Buckley R H 1994 Breakthroughs in the understanding and therapy of primary immunodeficiency. Clinical Immunology 41: 665–690

Buckley R H, Sampson H A 1981 The hyperimmunoglobulinaemia E syndrome. In: Franklin E C (ed) Clinical immunology update. Elsevier North-Holland, New York, p 147–167

Burgio G R, Hanson L A, Ugazio A G (eds) 1987 Immunology of the neonate. Springer-Verlag, Berlin

Cairo M S 1989 Neonatal neutrophil host defence: prospects for immunologic enhancement during neonatal sepsis. American Journal of Diseases of Children 143: 40–46

Cederbaum S D, Kartila I, Runoin D L, Steihm E R 1976 The chondro-osseous dysplasia of adenosine deaminase deficiency with severe combined immunodeficiency. Journal of Pediatrics 89: 737–742

Crowley C A, Curnutte J T, Rosin R E et al 1980 An inherited abnormality of neutrophil adhesion: its genetic transmission and its association with a missing protein. New England Journal of Medicine 302: 1163–1168

Cunningham-Rundles C 1989 Clinical and immunologic analyses of 103 patients with common variable immunodeficiency. Journal of Clinical Immunology 9: 22–33

Cunningham-Rundles C, Kazbay K, Zhou Z, Mayer L 1995 Immunologic effects of low-dose polyethylene glycol-conjugated recombinant human interleukin-2 in common variable immunodeficiency. Journal of Interferon and Cytokine Research. 15: 269–276

Davis S D, Schaller J, Wedgwood R J 1966 Job's syndrome; recurrent 'cold' staphylococcal abscesses. Lancet i: 1013–1015

Durandy A, Dumez Y, Guy-Grand D, Oury C, Henrion R, Griscelli C 1982 Prenatal diagnosis of severe combined immunodeficiency. Journal of Pediatrics 101: 995–997

Elder M E, Hope T J, Parslow T G, Umetsu D T, Wara D W, Cowan M J 1995 Severe combined immunodeficiency with absence of peripheral blood CD8+ T cells due to ZAP-70 deficiency. Cellular Immunology 165: 110–117

Etzioni A, Frydman M, Pollack S, Avidor I, Phillips M L, Paulson J C, Gershoni-Baruck R 1992 Recurrent severe infections caused by a novel leucocyte adhesion deficiency. New England Journal of Medicine 327: 1789–1792

Fischer A, Arnaiz-Villena A 1995 Immunodeficiences of genetic origin. Immunology Today 16: 510–514

Fischer A, Landais P, Friedrich W 1990 European experience of bone marrow transplantation for severe combined immunodeficiency. Lancet 336: 850–854

Fischer A, Segal A W, Seger R, Weening R S 1993 The management of chronic granulomatous disease. European Journal of Pediatrics 152: 896–899

Fischer A, Landais P, Friedrich W et al 1994 Bone marrow transplantation (BMT) in Europe for primary immunodeficiencies other than severe combined immunodeficiency: A report from the European Group for BMT and the European Group for Immunodeficiency. Blood. 83: 1149–1154

Fischer G W 1994 Use of intravenous immune globulin in newborn infants. Clinical and Experimental Immunology 97 (Suppl 1) 73–77

Fleisher T A, White R M, Broder S et al 1980 X-linked hypogamma-globulinaemia and isolated growth hormone deficiency. New England Journal of Medicine 301: 1429–1434

Groothuis J R, Simoes E A F, Levin M J et al 1993 Prophylactic administration of respiratory syncytial virus immune globulin to high-risk infants and young children. New England Journal of Medicine. 329: 1524–1530

Haeney M 1994 Intravenous immune globulin in primary immunodeficiency. Clinical and Experimental Immunology 97 (Suppl 1): 11–15

Hague R A, Rassam S, Morgan G, Cant J 1994 Early diagnosis of severe combined immunodeficiency syndrome. Archives of Disease in Childhood 70: 260–263

Hayward A R, Lydyard P M 1979 B cell function in the newborn. Pediatrics 64: Supplement 758–764

Hirschhorn R, Vauter G F, Kirkpatrick J A Jr, Rosen F S 1979 Adenosine deaminase deficiency frequency and comparative pathology in autosomally recessive severe combined immunodeficiency. Clinical Immunology and Immunopathology 14: 107–120

Hosking C S, Roberton D M 1983 Epidemiology and treatment of hypo-gammaglobulinaemia. Birth Defects: Original Article Series 19: 223–227

Ilan Y, Shouval D, Ashur Y, Mains M, Naporstek 1993 IgA deficiency associated with chronic hepatitis C virus infection. Archives of Internal Medicine 153: 1588–1592

Imashuku S, Hibi S, Kataoka-Morimoto Y, Yoshihara T, Ikushima S, Morioka Y, Todo S 1995 Myelodysplasia and acute myeloid leukaemia in cases of aplastic anaemia and congenital neutropenia following G-CSF administration. British Journal of Haematology 89: 188–190

Inoue T, Okumura Y, Shirahama M, Ishihashi H, Kashiwagi S, Okubo H 1986 Selective partial IgM deficiency: functional assessment of T and B lymphocytes in vitro. Journal of Clinical Immunology 6: 130–135

IUS/WHO Report 1988 Laboratory investigations in clinical immunology: methods, pitfalls and clinical indications. Clinical and Experimental Immunology 74: 494–503

Jaspers N G, Painter R B, Patterson M C, Kidson C, Inoue T 1984 Complementation analysis of ataxia telangiectasia. In: Gatti R A, Swift M (eds) Ataxia telangiectasia: genetics, neuropathology and immunology of a degenerative disease of childhood. Alan R Liss, New York, p 147–154

Klein C, Lisowska-Grospierre B, LeDeist, F, Fischer A, Griscelli C 1993 Major histocompatibility complex class II deficiency: clinical manifestations, immunologic features, and outcome. Journal of Pediatrics 123: 921–928

Kostman R 1956 Infantile genetic agranulocytosis. Acta Paediatrica Scandinavica 45 (Suppl): 1–78

Lacy J B, Ohlsson A 1995 Administration of intravenous immunoglobulins for prophylaxis or treatment of infection in preterm infants: meta-analyses. Archives of Disease in Childhood 72: F151–F155

Ladish S, Holiman B, Poplack D G, Blaese R M 1978 Immunodeficiency in familial erythrophagocytic lymphohistiocytosis. Lancet i: 581–583

Lamelin J-P, Lenoir G M 1993 Immunodeficiency secondary to viral infection. In: Chandra R K (ed) Primary and secondary immunodeficiency disorders. Churchill Livingstone, Edinburgh, pp 204–218

Lammer E J, Opitz J M 1986 The DiGeorge anomaly as a developmental field defect. American Journal of Genetics 2 (Suppl): 113–127

Lederman H M, Winkelstein J A 1985 X-linked agammaglobulinaemia: an analysis of 96 patients. Medicine 64: 145–156

Liblau R S, Bach J F 1992 Selective IgA deficiency and autoimmunity. International Archives of Allergy and Immunology 99: 16–27

Lobato M N, Spira T J, Rogers M F 1995 CD4+ T lymphocytopenia in children: lack of evidence for a new acquired immunodeficiency syndrome agent. Pediatric Infectious Disease Journal 14: 527–535

Maarten-Egeler R, D'Angio G J 1995 Langerhans cell histiocytosis. Journal of Pediatrics 127: 1–11

McClain K, Gehrz R, Grierson H, Purtilo D, Flipovich A 1988 Virus associated histiocytic proliferations in children: frequent association with Epstein–Barr virus and congenital or acquired immunodeficiencies. American Journal of Pediatric Hematology Oncology 10: 196–205

McNamara J G 1989 Immunological abnormalities in infants infected with human immunodeficiency virus. Seminars in Perinatology 13: 35–43

Miller M E, Steihm E R 1983 Immunology and resistance to infection. In: Remington J S, Klein J O (eds) Infectious diseases of the fetus and newborn infant. Saunders, Philadelphia

Misbah S A, Chapel H M 1993 Adverse effects of intravenous immunoglobulin. Drug Safety 9: 254–262

Mouy R, Fischer A, Vilmer E, Seger R, Griscelli C 1989 Incidence, severity and prevention of infections in chronic granulomatous disease. Journal of Pediatrics 114: 555–560

Mueller B U, Pizzo P A 1995 Cancer in children with primary or secondary immunodeficiencies. Journal of Pediatrics 126: 1–10

Mukwaya G 1988 Immunosuppressive effects and infections associated with corticosteroid therapy. Pediatric Infectious Disease Journal 7: 499–504

Newport M J, Huxley C M, Huston S, Hawrylowicz C M, Oostra B A, Williamson R, Levin M 1996 A mutation in the interferon-gamma-receptor gene and susceptibility to mycobacterial infection. New England Journal of Medicine 335: 1941–1949

Nezelof C, Jammet M L, Lortholary P, Labrune B, Lamy M 1964 L'hypoplasie hereditaire du thymus. Sa place et sa responsabilité dans une observation d'aplasie lymphocytaire, normoplasmocytaire et normoglobulin émique du nourrisson. Archives Françaises de Pediatrie 21: 897–920

Notarangelo L D, Duse M, Ugazio A G 1992 Immunodeficiency with hyper IgM (HIM). Immunodeficiency Reviews 3: 101–122

Ochs H D, Davis S D, Wedgewood R J 1971 Immunologic responses to bacteriophage Φ-X174 in immunodeficiency diseases. Journal of Clinical Investigation 50: 2559

Oxelius V A 1979 IgG subclass levels in infancy and childhood. Acta Pediatrica Scandinavica 68: 23–27

Pacheco S E, Shearer W T 1994 Laboratory aspects of immunology. Pediatric Clinics of North America 41: 623–655

Papadatos C, Papalvangelou G J, Alexiou D, Mendis J 1970 Serum immunoglobulin G levels in small-for-dates newborn babies. Archives of Disease in Childhood 45: 570–572

Piketty C, Weiss L, Kazatchkine M 1994 Idiopathic CD4 lymphocytopenia. Presse Medicale 23: 1374–1375

Pritchard J, Beverley P C L, Chu A C, D'Angio G J, Davis I C, Malpas J S (eds) 1994 The proceedings of the Nikolas Symposia on the histiocytoses 1989–1993. British Journal of Cancer 70 (Suppl XXIII): S1–S72

Puck J M 1994 Molecular and genetic basis of X-linked immunodeficiency disorders. Journal of Clinical Immunology 14: 81–89

Purtilo D T, Cassel C K, Yang J P S, Harper R 1975 X-linked recessive progressive combined variable immunodeficiency (Duncan's disease). Lancet I: 935–940

Pyun K H, Ochs H D, Wedgewood R J, Yang X, Heller S R, Reimer C B 1989 Human antibody responses to bacteriophage ΦX174: sequential induction of IgM and IgG subclass antibody. Clinical Immunology and Immuno-pathology 51: 252–263

Rieux-Laucat F, Le Diest F, Hivroz C, Roberts I A, Debatin K M, Fischer A, de Villartay J P 1995 Mutations in Fas associated with human lymphoproliferative syndrome and autoimmunity. Science 268: 1347–1349

Rogers T R 1985 Prevention of infection in neutropenic bone marrow transplant patients. Antibiotics and Chemotherapy 33: 90–113

Rosen F S, Wedgewood R J, Eibl M 1986 Primary immunodeficiency diseases. Report of a World Health Organization Scientific Group. Clinical Immunology and Immunopathology 40: 166–196

Rosen F S, Wedgewood R J, Eibi M et al 1995 Primary immunodeficiency diseases. Report of a WHO Scientific Group. Clinical and Experimental Immunology 99 (Suppl 1): 1–24

Ross S C, Densen P 1984 Complement deficiency states and infection: epidemiology, pathogenesis and consequences of Neisserial infections in an immune deficiency. Medicine 63: 243–273

Savitsky K, Bar-Shira A, Gilad S, Rotman G et al 1995 A single ataxia telangiectasia gene with a product similar to PI-3 kinase. Science 268: 1749–1753

Shapiro R, Beatty D W, Woods D L, Malon A F 1981 Serum complement and immunoglobulin values in small for gestational age infants. Journal of Pediatrics 99: 139–142

Spector B D, Perry G S III, Kersey J H 1978 Genetically determined immunodeficiency disease (GDID) and malignancy: Report from the Immunodeficiency-Cancer Registry. Clinical Immunology and Immunopathology 11: 12–29

Spector S A, Gelber R D, McGrath N et al 1994 A controlled trial of intravenous immune globulin for the prevention of serious bacterial infections in children receiving zidovudine for advanced human immunodeficiency virus infection. Pediatric AIDS Clinical Trials Group. New England Journal of Medicine 331 : 1181–1187

Steihm E R 1996 Immunologic disorders in infants and children, 4th edn. Saunders, Philadelphia

Steihm E R, Fulginiti V 1980 Immunological disorders in infants and children, 2nd edn. Saunders, Philadelphia

Super M, Thiel S, Lu J, Levinsky R J, Turner M W 1989 Association of low levels of mannan binding protein with a common defect of opsonisation. Lancet ii: 1236–1239

Tedesco F, Nürnberger W, Perissutti S 1993 Inherited deficiencies of the terminal complement components. International Reviews of Immunology 10: 51–64

Thrasher A, Kinnon C 1995 Gene therapy for primary immunodeficiency. Gene Therapy 2: 601–602

Turner M W 1996 Mannose-binding lectin: the pluripotent molecule of the innate immune system. Immunology Today 17: 532–540

Wade A M, Ades A E 1994 Age related reference ranges: significance tests for models and confidence intervals for centiles. Statistics in Medicine 13: 2359–2367

Wahn U 1995 Evaluation of the child with suspected primary immunodeficiency. Pediatric Allergy and Immunology 6: 71–79

Webster A D 1994 Virus infections in primary immunodeficiency. Journal of Clinical Pathology 47: 965–967

Weemaes C M R, Smeets D F C M, Van der Burgt C J A M 1994 Nijmegen breakage syndrome: a progress report. International Journal of Radiation Biology 6 (Suppl): S185–S188

Wilson C B 1986 Immunological basis for increased susceptibility of the neonate to infection. Journal of Pediatrics 108: 1–12

Writing Group of the Histiocyte Society 1987 Histiocytosis syndromes in children. Lancet i: 208–209

23 Infections

Chapter editor: A. G. M. Campbell

Classification 1274
Mortality and morbidity in infectious disease 1275
A. Nicoll
Infection control in hospital: policies and procedures
  1281
A. G. M. Campbell
Clinical problems
The child with fever 1282
P. T. Rudd
The child with a rash 1284
P. T. Rudd
Vomiting 1285
P. T. Rudd
Diarrhea 1286
P. T. Rudd
Bacteremia and septicemia 1286
P. T. Rudd
Acute bacterial meningitis 1288
P. T. Rudd
Infantile gastroenteritis 1292
H. B. Wong
Bacterial infections 1297
The use of the bacteriology laboratory by the
  pediatrician 1297
T. M. S. Reid
Anthra 1300
A. G. M. Campbell
Bartonellosis 1300
G. C. Cook
Botulism 1301
A. P. Ball
Brucellosis: undulant fever 1302
P. D. Welsby
Cholera 1303
H. B. Wong
Diphtheria 1305
A. M. Geddes
Haemophilus influenzae 1307
P. T. Heath   E. R. Moxon
Leprosy 1309
G. C. Cook
Leptospirosis 1311
P. D. Welsby
Lyme disease 1312
D. Nathwani
Meningococcemia 1314
C. O'Reilly
Pertussis 1315
A. Nicoll
Plague 1318
G. C. Cook

Pneumococcus 1318
A. G. M. Campbell
Proteus 1320
C. O'Reilly
Pseudomonas 1320
G. Russell
Rat-bite fevers 1321
G. C. Cook
Relapsing fever 1322
G. C. Cook
Salmonellae 1323
J. B. S. Coulter
Shigella (bacillary dysentery) 1327
J. B. S. Coulter
Staphylococcus 1328
J. Main
Streptococcus 1330
J. Main
Tetanus 1333
A. M. Geddes
Tuberculosis 1334
J. B. S. Coulter
Diseases caused by environmental mycobacteria 1348
J. B. S. Coulter
Tularemia 1350
A. G. M. Campbell
Infections due to viruses and allied organisms 1351
D. Isaacs
HIV infection 1392
J. Y. Q. Mok
Treponematoses and sexually transmissible diseases 1398
A. McMillan   H. Young   C. Thompson
Protozoal infections 1445
Malaria 1445
M. Molyneux
Trypanosomiasis 1453
D. H. Smith
Leishmaniasis 1460
D. H. Smith
Toxoplasmosis 1464
J. Syme
Giardiasis 1466
A. G. M. Campbell
Amebic infections 1467
J. B. S. Coulter
Fungal infections 1470
J. Syme
Presumed infection: Kawasaki disease 1478
P. J. Smail
Helminth infection 1481
J. Goldsmid   M. A. Kibel   A. E. Mills
Flies, fleas, mites and lice 1513
J. Goldsmid   M. A. Kibel   A. E. Mills

Diseases transmitted by cats and dogs 1519
J. Goldsmid   M. A. Kibel   A. E. Mills
Poisonous animal bites and stings 1520
J. Goldsmid   M. A. Kibel   A. E. Mills

Principles of antimicrobial therapy 1526
T. M. S. Reid
References   1530

CLASSIFICATION

Table 23.1   A classification of infections according to the system principally involved

	Bacterial	Viral	Protozoal	Fungal	Helminthic
General	Streptococcal Staphylococcal Diphtheria Brucellosis Tetanus Botulism Meningococcemia Tularemia Plague Bartonellosis Tuberculosis Atypical mycobacteria Leprosy Sarcoidosis Leptospirosis Rat bite fever Relapsing fever Syphilis Yaws Pinta *Pseudomonas pyocyanea* Legionnaires' disease Cat-scratch disease	Measles Chickenpox Influenza Q fever Mumps Poliomyelitis Rabies Cytomegalovirus Infectious mononucleosis Roseola infantum Erythema infectiosum Arbovirus gp A (e.g. Chikungunya) Arbovirus gp B (e.g. yellow fever, dengue, etc.) Arbovirus group C (e.g. sandfly fever) Rickettsiae (e.g. typhus fever) Lassa fever Marburg virus disease	Malaria Toxoplasmosis Leishmaniasis Trypanosomiasis	Aspergillosis Blastomycosis	*Mansonella perstans* *Mansonella ozzardi* Schistosomiasis *Inermicapsifer* *Madagascariensis*
Alimentary	Typhoid Paratyphoid Other salmonellae Bacillary dysentery Cholera (Gastroenteritis) Staphylococcal (enterocolitis: toxins) Tuberculosis *E. coli*	Adenovirus (gastroenteritis) ECHO virus (gastroenteritis) Reovirus (gastroenteritis) Herpes simplex (ulcerative stomatitis) Coxsackie A (hand-foot-mouth disease) Cytomegalovirus (hepatic) Virus hepatitis A Virus hepatitis B Virus hepatitis C Arbovirus gp B (hepatic-yellow fever)	Amebiasis Acanthamebiasis Balantidiasis Giardiasis Leishmaniasis (visceral)	Moniliasis	Ascariasis *Enterobius vermicularis* Hookworm *Trichuris trichiura* *Strongyloides stercoralis* Trichinosis *Taenia saginata* *Taenia solium* *Hymenolepis nana, diminuta* *Dipylidium caninum* *Diphyllobothrium latum* Echinococcosis (hepatic) Schistosomiasis Liver flukes (hepatic) Intestinal fluke *Toxocara* *Oesophagostomum* sp. *Ternidens deminutus* Acanthocephala Capillariasis
Respiratory	Pertussis Pneumonia (pneumococcal: *H. influenzae*, group B streptococcal staphylococcal) Tuberculosis Atypical mycobacteria *Pseudomonas pyocyanea* (cystic fibrosis)	Measles Influenza Parainfluenza Respiratory syncytial virus Adenovirus Rhinovirus Psittacosis Ornithosis *Mycoplasma pneumoniae*	*Pneumocystis carinii*	Aspergillosis Blastomycosis Coccidioidomycosis Histoplasmosis Nocardiosis	Ascariasis Toxocara Echinococcosis Lung fluke (paragonimiasis) Strongyloides *Dirofilaria immitis*

Table 23.1 *Cont'd*

	Bacterial	Viral	Protozoal	Fungal	Helminthic
Neurological	Meningococcal *H. influenzae* Staphylococcal Pneumococcal Streptococcal Diphtheroids *E. coli* Proteus Pseudomonas *Listeria monocytogenes* Diphtheria Tuberculosis Botulism	Measles Herpes simplex, varicella-zoster Vaccinia Coxsackie A Coxsackie B ECHO virus Mumps Lymphocytic choriomeningitis Poliomyelitis Rabies (Guillain–Barré) (Infectious mononucleosis) Arbovirus gp A		Cryptococcosis (Torulosis)	Toxocara *Taenia solium* *Angiostrongylus cantonensis*
Skin and subcutaneous tissue	Erysipelas (streptococci) Impetigo (staphylococci) Rat bite fever Anthrax Bartonellosis Tuberculosis Leprosy Syphilis Yaws Pinta	Herpes simplex, zoster Varicella Smallpox Vaccinia Coxsackie A (hand-foot-mouth disease) Orf Molluscum contagiosum Rickettsiae (rickettsialpox)	Leishmaniasis (cutaneous)	Moniliasis Actinomycosis Aspergillosis Phycomycosis Sporotrichosis	Hookworm Dracunculosis Onchocerciasis Filaria, *Loa loa*, *Wuchereria bancrofti* Schistosomiasis Myiasis Strongyloides *A. braziliense* *A. caninum* Sparganosis
Genitourinary	Streptococci (*S. faecalis*) *E. coli* Proteus *Pseudomonas pyocyanea* Staphylococci Gonorrhea Tuberculosis	Herpetic vulvovaginitis (Lymphogranuloma venereum)			Schistosomiasis
Upper respiratory tract	Streptococcal Diphtheria *H. influenzae*	Adenovirus Coxsackie A (herpangina) Parainflueza Rhinovirus ECHO virus Reovirus		Rhinosporidioidosis	
Lymph glands and lymphatics	Diphtheria Plague Tuberculosis Atypical mycobacteria Sarcoidosis Cat-scratch disease	(Infectious mononucleosis) Rubella (Roseola infantum) (Lymphogranuloma venereum)	Toxoplasmosis Leishmaniasis (Splenomegaly) Trypanosomiasis		*Brugia malayi*
Blood (anemia)	Bartonellosis		Leishmaniasis Malaria		Toxocara Hookworm *Diphyllobothrium latum*
Ophthalmic and periorbital	Gonorrhea Tuberculosis	Adenovirus (conjunctivitis) TRIC virus (conjunctivitis) Trachoma Herpes simplex Acute hemorrhagic conjunctivitis	Trypanosomiasis (periorbital)		*Toxocara
Muscle		Coxsackie B (e.g. myocarditis Bornholm)	Trypanosomiasis		Trichinosis

MORTALITY AND MORBIDITY IN INFECTIOUS DISEASE

The global perspective

Worldwide, infections as a disease category are responsible for the majority of loss of life and good health in children. It is estimated that infectious diseases, in 1990, were responsible for 8.3 million of a total of 12.5 million deaths among a global child population (under 5 years of age) of 630 million (World Bank 1993). Most of these deaths occurred in developing countries where it is also estimated that five groups of infections: acute respiratory infections (ARIs), diarrheal diseases, congenital infections (principally human immunodeficiency virus type 1, HIV-1), malaria, measles and other vaccine-preventable diseases caused the death of more than 7 million children (Voelker 1995, Nicoll et al 1994, UNICEF 1996). In industrialized countries infections are responsible for proportionately fewer childhood deaths. However, they still caused an estimated 37 000 of a total of 214 000 annual deaths among 78 million children under 5 years old (World Bank 1993). Mortality statistics need to be supplemented by estimates of the burden of disability (morbidity) and to allow for the varying implications of the death of an individual at different ages. This can be done by use of disability adjusted life years (DALYs) (Murray 1994). Combining estimates of chronic disability and mortality statistics, this measure calculates the likely numbers of healthy years of life lost because of specific diseases and conditions, and, by 'weighting', an allowance is made for the different significance of ill health and mortality among infants, elderly persons and adults providing for dependents. Estimates of the burden of disease experienced (Table 23.2) further emphasize the importance of infectious disease in developing countries and the particular role in producing mortality in children under age 5

played by respiratory disease, diarrheal disease, five vaccine-preventable diseases (diphtheria, measles, pertussis, polio and tetanus), and in older children by tuberculosis and intestinal helminths (World Bank 1993).

The United Kingdom

Infections remain an important cause of death in children in the UK. Death registration data indicate that in 1993 infections were the main cause of death in 512 children, 244 infants and 268 older children (Table 23.3). The infant figure rises to 680 if sudden infant death syndrome is included.

Recent trends in a number of important infections are shown in Figures 23.1 to 23.7. The introduction of immunization against *Haemophilus influenzae* type b in 1992 led to a dramatic decline in invasive infections attributed to this organism (Fig. 23.1). Conversely it has led to heightened awareness of meningococcal infections (Fig. 23.2) as the most important single cause of septicemic infections and deaths in immunocompetent children (Public Health Laboratory Service 1995).

Immunization was highly effective in reducing the incidence of measles in the 1970s (Fig. 23.3a). However, measles vaccination only confers immunity in 90% of recipients and coverage is incomplete. Seroepidemiological investigations in the early 1990s indicated a growing number of susceptible (antibody negative) older children and hence an increasing risk of a substantial measles epidemic in school-age children, with an inevitable morbidity and mortality (Ramsay et al 1994, Gay & Miller 1995). An epidemic took place in Scotland in 1993/4 (Christie 1994) and to preempt further larger epidemics a UK-wide initiative immunized 8 million school children (90% of those eligible) in November 1994. Transmission of indigenous measles was almost entirely interrupted and confirmed notifications fell dramatically (Fig. 23.3b) and the risk of an epidemic was averted (CDSC 1995a).

Food poisoning has become one of the commonest notified infections in children. Sharply increasing trends in notified

Table 23.2 Estimated distribution of burden of disease (combined mortality and chronic morbidity) in children in developing countries – 1990

	Total DALYs lost (million)	
	Age under 5 years	Age 5–14 years
Perinatal conditions	13.5	Nil
Communicable disease	63.3	33.9
Congenital STDs (HIV and syphilis)	(2.0%)	(4.0%)
Diarrheal diseases	(32%)	(15%)
Tuberculosis	(1.0%)	(11%)
Other vaccine-preventable disease	(20%)	(18%)
Malaria	(8%)	(9%)
Intestinal helminths	Nil	(27%)
Respiratory infections	(35%)	(16%)
Noncommunicable disorder	20.8	16.9
Injuries	6.2	9.7
Total	103.7	60.5

Source: World Development Report 1993, World Bank 1993.

Table 23.3 Deaths due to infections in children aged 14 years and under; UK 1988–1993 (with rates per thousand births)

ICD code	Disease	1988	1989	1990	1991	1992	1993
001–009	Intestinal infectious disease	21	31	21	22	15	27
036	Meningococcal infection	117	134	121	120	100	115
038	Septicemia	16	42	32	28	20	30
030–041 (excluding 036 & 038)	Other bacterial disease*	147	184	169	159	140	155
045–079	Viral disease	61	46	37	38	20	31
001–139	All infectious and parasitic disease	235 (2.2)	273 (2.5)	246 (2.2)	228 (2.1)	192 (1.71)	252 (2.3)
320–322	Meningitis	62	70	65	69	58	54
466	Acute bronchitis and bronchiolitis	84	84	64	66	35	50
480–486	Pneumonia	195	159	149	150	92	156
–	Combined infections*	576 (5.6)	586 (5.4)	524 (4.8)	513 (4.7)	377 (3.4)	512 (4.5)
798.1	SIDS†	1566 (1.97)	1339 (1.69)	1226 (1.53)	1017 (1.23)	531 (0.64)	440 (0.57)
All causes	All causes‡	9696 (93.5)	1143 (84.4)	8793 (80.4)	8216 (75.2)	7180 (64.1)	7060 (63.0)
	Population denominators (100 thousands)	103.6	108.3	109.3	110.6	111.9	113.1

* Contains other totals not shown above.
† Rate in brackets is SIDS under 1 year per 1000 live births.
‡ All infectious and parasitic disease, plus meningitis, acute bronchitis and pneumonia. Excludes hepatitis not identifed as viral.
Source: OPCS, General Register Office Scotland, and Department of Health and Social Services, Northern Ireland.

numbers of cases of food poisoning in the 1980s and 1990s were mirrored by trends in national laboratory reporting of salmonellosis (Fig. 23.4). From 1986 to 1992 much of the increase was caused by *Campylobacter* spp. and one particular *Salmonella typhimurium*, phage type 4. Ensuing investigations implicated shell eggs and chicken meat as the main vehicles of *S. typhimurium* infection and led to specific legislation and public education to control the epidemic (PHLS 1989).

Diphtheria and poliomyelitis declined dramatically in the UK following the introduction of immunization in the 1940s (diphtheria – Fig. 23.5) and 1960s (poliomyelitis – Fig. 23.6). In contrast, control of another vaccine-preventable illness, tuberculosis, has been less successful with a rise in notifications during 1991–1993 especially among older children (Fig. 23.7).

Sexually transmitted diseases are now appreciated to be a substantial problem among adolescents. The highest incidences of gonorrhea and chlamydia seen among genitourinary medicine clinic attenders are in females aged 16–19 years (CDSC 1995b,c). Chlamydia is the more important because of its widespread distribution and serious sequelae of pelvic inflammatory disease, infertility and ectopic pregnancies. It is clear that the chlamydia infections seen in genitourinary medicine clinics are only a fraction of those prevalent in the teenage population.

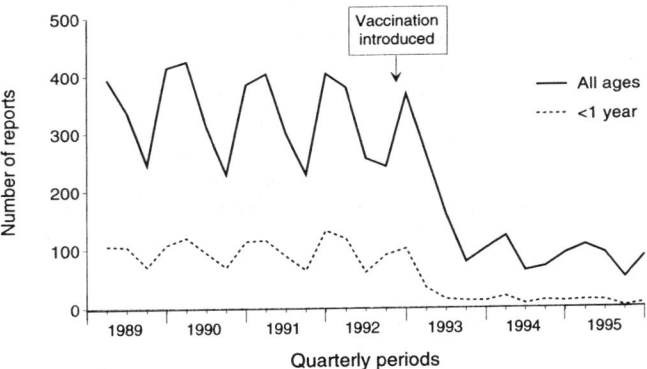

Fig. 23.1 Invasive *Haemophilus influenzae* b infections; UK 1989–1995 (1995 data are provisional). Source: PHLS/CDSC, SCIEH & DHSS (N. Ireland).

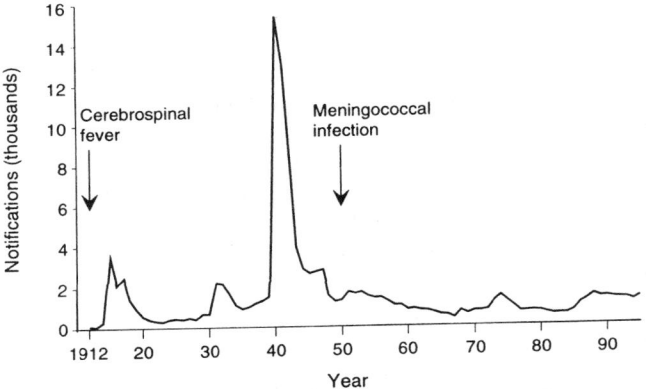

Fig. 23.2 Meningococcal infection notification; England, Wales and Northern Ireland 1912–1940, UK 1940–1995. Source: PHLS/CDSC, OPCS/ONS, GCIEH/GRS, DHSS (N. Ireland).

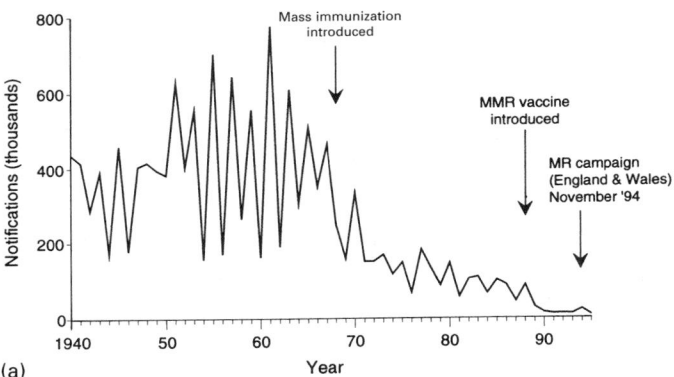

(a)

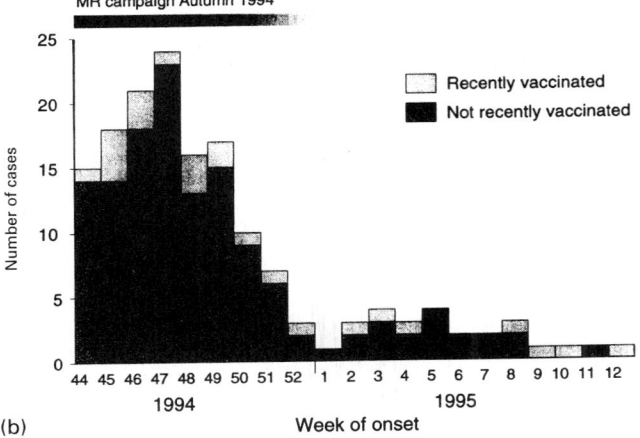

(b)

Fig. 23.3 (a) Measles notifications; UK 1940–1995. (b) Measles in England and Wales following the 1994 campaign: cases confirmed by salivary testing, by week of onset.

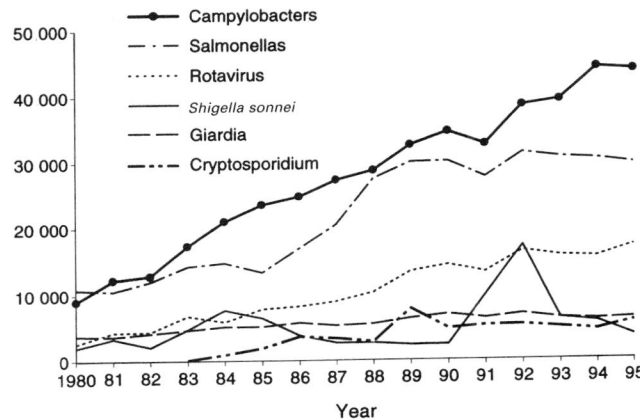

Fig. 23.4 Laboratory reports of selected gastrointestinal infections (adult and child data combined); England and Wales 1980–1995.

General practitioner (GP) reporting provides the least-selected surveillance data in the UK on the nature and burden of infectious disease in children in the community, particularly on conditions such as chickenpox or influenza unlikely to be investigated microbiologically or to lead to hospital admission. These data show that respiratory tract infections (mainly upper) account for

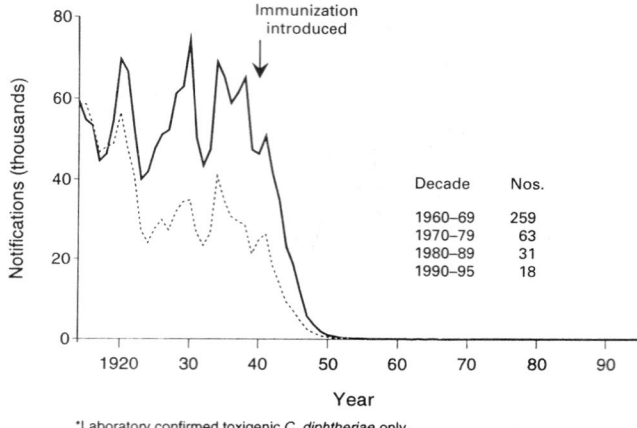

*Laboratory confirmed toxigenic *C. diphtheriae* only

Fig. 23.5 Diphtheria notifications; England and Wales 1914–1995. Source: OPCS/CNS, PHLS Diphtheria Reference Unit.

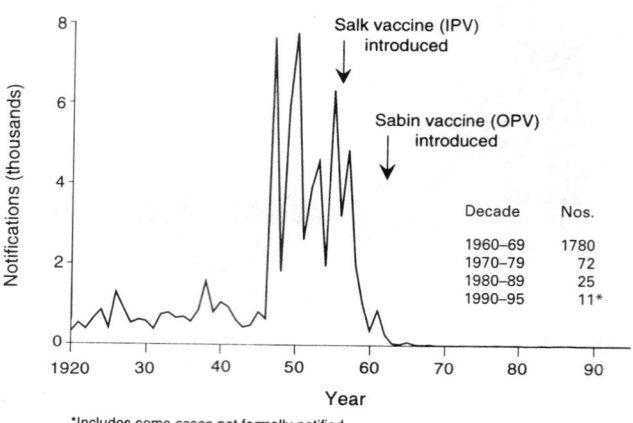

*Includes some cases not formally notified

Fig. 23.6 Poliomyelitis notifications; England and Wales 1920–1995. Source OPCS/ONS.

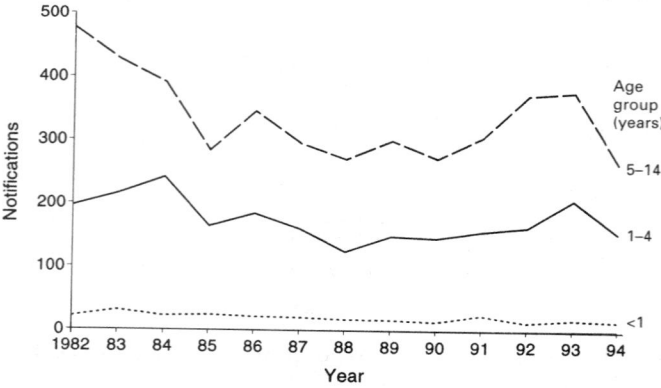

Fig. 23.7 Notifications of tuberculosis (all forms) in children; UK (Northern Ireland not included) 1982–1994.

over 80% of new GP consultations for infectious diseases in children (McCormick & Hall 1995).

The growing population of immunocompromised children, very low birth weight babies, children with congenital immuno-deficiencies, HIV infection and children on powerful immuno-compromising therapies represent an increasingly important source of deaths due to infections, often with organisms that are usually innocuous for immunocompetent children.

Emerging and re-emerging infections

In the 1960s and 1970s it was a medical commonplace that improving social conditions and medical treatments were leading to a relentless decline in the importance of infectious diseases. Emerging and re-emerging infections (WHO 1994), as well as some spectacular nosocomial outbreaks of legionnaires' disease and food poisoning in the UK (DoH 1988), have changed medical opinion and it is realized that infections remain important threats to the health of children and adults in every country. In 1995 the World Health Organization established a Division of Emerging Viral and Bacterial Disease Surveillance and Control and some countries and regional bodies (for example the European Union) are establishing or strengthening infrastructures to detect and respond to emerging or re-emerging infections. Some emerging infections are new or newly recognized pathogens (Table 23.4) examples being human immunodeficiency virus (HIV) and human herpes virus types 6 and 7 respectively. Others represent infections that have only recently come to affect humans in any numbers, such as Creutzfeldt–Jacob disease. Yet a third group are established infections whose incidence, pathogenicity or antimicrobial resistance has recently increased, for example dengue fever, invasive streptococci and multiply resistant *M. tuberculosis*. Of particular importance to children are HIV, diphtheria, pertussis, *E. coli* 0157 causing hemolytic-uremic syndrome, and STDs in adolescents. HIV in the 1990s in urban areas of sub-Saharan Africa is reversing earlier improvements in child survival (Nicoll et al 1994). The reasons for emergence and re-emergence are almost as varied as the organisms themselves (Table 23.5). Failure of public health programs can be an important cause. Diphtheria reappeared in the 1990s as an epidemic in Russia because of a collapse in vaccine production and the emergence of mistaken reasons among the public and professionals for refusing immunization. A similar phenomenon affecting pertussis occurred in the UK in the 1970s and 1980s from the mistaken impression that the vaccine was more dangerous than the disease (Begg & Nicoll 1994) (see p. 1315). Both *E. coli* 0157 and various salmonellas have been spread efficiently through industrialized production and distribution of foods (Gill et al 1983). An outbreak of hemolytic-uremic syndrome (HUS) due to contaminated commercial hamburgers occurred in the USA in 1993 (Bell et al 1994) and in 1995 an outbreak of gastrointestinal disease in children due to *S. agoma* in North London was traced to defective production in a factory in Israel. Changes in behavior can result in disease emergence. International trends towards earlier menarche and sexual debut are causing younger females to be exposed to STDs with a consequent rise in pelvic inflammatory disease, ectopic pregnancy and secondary infertility (Wasserheit 1994).

Effective interventions

In 1990 at a World Summit for Children government leaders including that of the UK, committed their administrations to 27 goals to improve the health and lives of children. Interventions designed to prevent or treat infections may be assessed by

Table 23.4 Diseases important to child and adolescent health: major etiologic agents identified since 1973

Year of report	Agent	Disease
1973	Rotavirus	Major cause of infantile diarrhea worldwide
1975	Parvovirus B19	Fifth disease; aplastic crisis in hemolytic anemia
1976	*Cryptosporidium parvum*	Acute enterocolitis
1977	Ebola virus	Ebola hemorrhagic fever
1977	*Legionella pneumophila*	Legionnaires' disease
1977	Hantaan virus	Hemorrhagic fever with renal syndrome (HFRS)
1977	Campylobacter sp.	Enteric pathogens distributed globally
1980	Human T cell lymphotropic virus-I (HTLV I)	T cell lymphoma – leukemia
1981	*Staphylococcus* toxin	Toxic shock syndrome associated with tampon use
1982	*Escherichia coli* 0157:H7	Hemorrhagic colitis; hemolytic-uremic syndrome
1982	HTLV II	Hairy cell leukemia
1982	*Borrelia burgdorferi*	Lyme disease
1983	Human immunodeficiency virus (HIV)	HIV disease including AIDS
1983	*Helicobacter pylori*	Peptic ulcers
1988	Human herpes virus-6 (HHV-6)	Roseola subitum and encephalitis
1989	*Ehrlichia chaffeensis*	Human ehrlichiosis
1989	Hepatitis C	Parenterally transmitted non-A, non-B hepatitis
1990	Human herpes virus-7 (HHV-7)	Roseola subitum and encephalitis
1991	Guanarito virus	Venezuelan hemorrhagic fever
1992	*Vibrio cholerae* 0139	New strain associated with epidemic cholera
1992	*Bartonella (=Rochalimaea) henselae*	Cat-scratch disease; bacillary angiomatosis
1993	Hantavirus isolates	Hantavirus pulmonary syndrome
1994	Sabiá virus	Brazilian hemorrhagic fever
1995	? Human herpes virus-8 (HHV-8)	? Kaposi's sarcoma
1996	Prion	New variant of Creutzfeldt–Jakob disease

Adapted from Satcher 1995

Table 23.5 Factors in infectious disease emergence and re-emergence relevant to child and adolescent health

Factor	Examples of specific factors	Examples of disease
Ecological changes (including those due to economic development and land use)	Agriculture: dams, changes in water ecosystems; deforestation/reforestation; flood/drought; famine; climate changes	Schistosomiasis (dams); Rift Valley fever (dams, irrigation); Argentine hemorrhagic fever (agriculture); Hantaan – Korean hemorrhagic fever (agriculture); hantavirus pulmonary syndrome, southwestern US, 1993 (weather anomalies)
Human demographics, behavior	Societal changes and events: population growth and migration (movement from rural areas to cities); war or civil conflict; urban decay; sexual behavior; intravenous drug use; preference for 'fast foods'; use of high-density facilities	Introduction of HIV; spread of dengue; spread of HIV and other sexually transmitted diseases, meningococcal disease, cholera, increases in food poisoning (*Salmonella enteritidis*)
International travel and commerce	Worldwide movement of goods and people; air travel	'Airport' malaria; dissemination of mosquito vectors; rat-borne hantaviruses; antibiotic-resistant gonorrhea; introduction of cholera into South America; dissemination of 0139 *V. cholerae*
Technology and industry	Globalization of food supplies; changes in food processing and packaging; organ or tissue transplantation; drugs causing immunosuppression; widespread use of antibiotics	Hemolytic-uremic syndrome (*E. coli* contamination of hamburger meat), *S. agoma* in kosher snacks; transfusion-associated hepatitis (hepatitis B,C), opportunistic infections in immunosuppressed patients, Creutzfeldt–Jakob disease from contaminated batches of human growth hormone (medical technology)
Microbial adaptation and change	Microbial evolution, response to selection in environment	Antibiotic-resistant bacteria (multiply resistant *M. tuberculosis*), 'antigenic drift' in influenza virus; zidovudine-resistant HIV
Breakdown in public health measures	Curtailment or reduction in prevention programs; inadequate sanitation and vector control measures, immunization myths	Whooping cough in the UK, resurgence of tuberculosis in the US; cholera in refugee camps in Africa; resurgence of diphtheria in the former Soviet Union

Adapted from Morse 1995.

measuring their resulting health gain as healthy years of life and comparing their costs relative to other interventions. Thus it is possible to come up with 'best buys' for countries and this has been undertaken for the developing world by the World Bank using the 'DALY' measure (Murray 1994). Interventions targeted against acute respiratory infections, diarrheal disease, malaria and the six vaccine-preventable diseases represent four of the six top interventions for health gain in children under age 5 and five out of six of those targeted at children aged 5–14 years (Bobadilla et al 1994) (Table 23.6). While new technologies and developments are necessary, greater health gains can come from the application of established interventions of proven effectiveness such as the

Table 23.6 Main cause of disease burden in children in demographically developing countries in 1990 and the cost-effectiveness of the interventions available for their control

Disease and injuries	Number of DALYs lost* millions (% total)	Main intervention	Cost-effectiveness ($ per DALY)
Respiratory infections	98 (14.8)†	Integrated management of the sick child	30–100
Perinatal morbidity and mortality	96 (14.6)	a. Prenatal and delivery care b. Family planning	30–100 20–150
Diarrheal disease	92 (14.0)	Integrated management of the sick child	30–100
Childhood cluster (diseases preventable through immunization)	65 (10.0)	Expanded Program on Immunization (EPI) EPI-plus†	12–30
Congenital malformation	35 (5.4)	Surgical operations	High (unknown)
Malaria	31 (4.7)	Integrated management of the sick child	30–100
Intestinal helminths	17 (2.5)	School health program	20–34
Protein–energy malnutrition	12 (1.8)	Integrated management of the sick child	30–100
Vitamin A deficiency	12 (1.8)	EPI-plus†	12–30
Iodine deficiency	9 (1.4)	Iodine supplementation	19–37
Subtotal	467 (71.0)	–	–
Total DALYs lost	660 (100)	–	–

* DALYs lost (for specific diseases and the total) are taken from the 1993 World Development Report (World Bank 1993).
† EPI-plus includes the six vaccines of the Expanded Program on Immunization (EPI), plus the vaccine against hepatitis B and vitamin A supplementation.

early detection and treatment of ARIs, and the use of oral rehydration therapy (ORT) for gastrointestinal infections (UNICEF 1996). Immunization represents a success story. Already by 1990 the Expanded Program of Immunization (EPI) reached a goal of immunizing 80% of children in most countries with an estimated benefit of 3 million lives saved in 1995. A particular priority has been polio immunization. The EPI, supported by Rotary International, had by 1995 eliminated wild polio from 145 countries, including all of the Americas (UNICEF 1996). However, the 80% target remains unachieved in sub-Saharan Africa where overall immunization rates are static. Because of economic or social reasons there are at least 40 countries where polio elimination looks difficult or impossible. This makes the goal of global polio elimination, and its prize of release of resources currently committed to polio immunization, look illusory (Hull et al 1994).

Surveillance to inform public health action

Given adequate resources, many infectious diseases can now be prevented or contained, but eradication of all infection-related morbidity and mortality is unachievable as many microorganisms have extensive animal and environmental reservoirs. Interventions can prevent infections or ameliorate the effects of disease. Knowledge as to which interventions are effective must be combined with timely surveillance data on the epidemiology of infection and susceptibility so as to allow rational decisions to be made on resource allocation for public health action. Routine data for surveillance of the commoner infectious diseases in the UK are derived from mortality statistics, disease notifications and laboratory reporting (Table 23.7). An infection may be made statutorily notifiable in the UK either because there is a need for rapid information for effective local control, or for the purpose of monitoring national immunization programs. Often taken for granted, these systems are the best in the world. Routine reporting

Table 23.7 Infectious disease morbidity and mortality: principal sources of data in the UK

Data source	Collected by	Type of information
Mortality data	OPCS, GRS, DHSS	Death entries from medical practitioners
Statutory notifications	OPCS, LAGs, SHHD, DH	Currently (1995) list of 39 IDs; selected because need for rapid local information for control, or to monitor national immunization program; clinical diagnoses
Laboratory reports	CDSC and SCIEH from PHLS and NHS laboratories	Wide range of microbiologically confirmed infections
General practitioners	RCGP from weekly returns from 40 practices	Wide range of infectious diseases presenting in general practice; clinical diagnoses
Computerized hospital discharge data	OPCS and SHHD, individual HAs and HBs	All diagnoses categorized by ICD code; combination of clinical and microbiological
Consultant pediatricians	Royal College of Paediatrics and Child Health Surveillance Unit	Changing 'menu' of rare infections and infection-related disorders; specified case definitions

CDSC = Communicable Disease Surveillance Centre; DHSS = Department of Health and Social Security, Northern Ireland; GRS = General Registrar's Office for Scotland; HA = health authority; HB = health board; ID = infectious disease; LGA = local government authority; OPCS = Office of Population Censuses and Surveys; PHLS = Public Health Laboratory Service; RCGP = Royal College of General Practitioners; SCIEH = Scottish Centre for Infection and Environmental Health; SHHD = Scottish Home and Health Department is supplemented by special surveillance systems for rare and/or more important infections such as HIV and congenital rubella syndrome. An example of this is active reporting by clinicians through the British Paediatric Association Surveillance Unit of the Royal College of Paediatrics and Child Health whereby researchers combine reports from RCPCH members with data from other systems to give optimal coverage. Surveillance of infectious disease mortality and morbidity in England and Wales is undertaken by the Office of Population, Censuses and Surveys (OPCS) and by the Communicable Disease Surveillance Centre (CDSC), the central epidemiological unit of the national Public Health Laboratory Service. CDSC and OPCS collaborate closely to obtain, analyze and interpret data from several sources which often overlap, but which are also complementary (Table 23.3). In Scotland most surveillance is coordinated by the Scottish Centre for Infection and Environmental Health. Public health policy is coordinated by national departments of health and enacted by local specialists in public health medicine.

ACKNOWLEDGMENTS

In the preparation of this section the assistance of the following is gratefully acknowledged: Office of Population Censuses and Surveys (now the Office for National Statistics); Registrar General's Office, Scotland; Department of Health, Northern Ireland; The Scottish Centre for Infection and Environmental Health, Glasgow; and the Public Health Laboratory Service Communicable Disease Surveillance Centre, Colindale.

INFECTION CONTROL IN HOSPITAL: POLICIES AND PROCEDURES

Infections make up the largest part of a family doctor's work with children and continue to be a major reason for admission to children's wards. Apart from these community-acquired infections, children are vulnerable to nosocomial infections especially in traditional open wards and modern intensive care units where a major infectious threat to patients is the increase in multiply resistant organisms. Outbreaks are usually related to failure in implementing infection control guidelines and often point to a breakdown in the discipline of rigorous handwashing (Table 23.8). Continuous education of the ICU staff appears to be at least as important as isolating patients (Garner & Hierholzer 1993).

Children are much more likely than adults to need isolation, a fact usually ignored in planning children's units. It has been suggested that separate rooms should be provided for all infants and young children especially in winter months when many respiratory infections are incubating on admission and as many as 25% of asymptomatic infants and toddlers may be shedding rotavirus, but few hospitals have enough single rooms or cubicles to accommodate these numbers and strictly conform to current isolation policies (Kim et al 1987). There is obviously a need for compromise. If possible infectious children should be nursed at home, and careful thought should be given to patient placement in hospital wards so that whatever isolation facilities are available, they are used appropriately. Single rooms are not popular with young children who feel lonely and abandoned but it is essential to protect those who are particularly vulnerable to nosocomially acquired airborne diseases, such as the immunocompromised or infants with symptomatic congenital heart disease. Single room

Table 23.8 Factors increasing or decreasing the threat of nosocomial infection

The threat	The defense
Crowded wards	Awareness of risk

Poor facilities for:
  Isolation
  Hygiene
	Effective infection control team (with administrative 'clout')

Inappropriate patient placement
Autoinfection
Cross-contamination
  Contacts
  Hands
  Environment
	Policies and procedures for:
	  Isolation
	  Handwashing
	  Aseptic techniques
	  Sterilization
	  Disinfection
	  Dosmestic cleaning

Impaired patient defenses
1. Local, e.g. skin breaks, invasive procedures
2. General
  Immunodeficiency
  Immunosuppression
	Waste disposal
	Antibiotic use

shortages can be eased by such measures as cohorting of the older children with respiratory infections and diarrheal diseases.

Two forms of isolation are practiced. First, children excreting transmissible organisms are isolated to prevent spread to contacts (standard or source isolation – 'barrier nursing'); and second, children who are at particularly high risk from infection are isolated to protect them from environmental pathogens (protective isolation – 'reversed barrier nursing').

For regularly revised and more comprehensive advice the reader is directed to official publications from departments of health and communicable disease centers (CDCs). For example, the CDC in Atlanta has recently revised its guidelines 'to meet the following objectives: (1) to be epidemiologically sound; (2) to recognize the importance of all body fluids, secretions and excretions in the transmission of nosocomial pathogens; (3) to contain adequate precautions for infections transmitted by the airborne, droplet and contact routes of transmission; (4) to be as simple and user friendly as possible; and, (5) to use new terms to avoid confusion with existing infection control and isolation systems.' (Garner 1996). The term 'Universal Precautions' has been replaced by 'Standard Precautions' which apply to blood, all body fluids, secretions and excretions, except sweat, whether or not they contain visible blood; nonintact skin, and mucous membranes. They are designed for all patients in hospital irrespective of infection status by reducing the risk of transmission of microorganisms from both recognized and unrecognized sources of infection. To further reduce the risk of transmission these Standard Precautions are reinforced by 'Transmission-based Precautions' either Airborne, Droplet or Contact in the case of patients with documented or suspected infection or colonized with highly transmissible or epidemiologically important organisms spread by airborne, e.g. varicella, measles, M. tuberculosis; or droplet transmission, e.g. invasive H. influenzae type b and N. meningitidis infection, pertussis, streptococcal (Lancefield Group A) infection, influenza, rubella, mumps; or direct contact with dry skin or indirect contact with contaminated surfaces, e.g. multiresistant staphylococci (MRSA) and Gram-negative organisms, Clostridium difficile, hepatitis A, gastroenteritic viruses, shigella and E. coli 0157.

Frequent and careful handwashing before and after each patient contact is the most important factor in preventing cross-infection. Gloves should be worn when touching blood, body fluids, secretions, excretions and contaminated items and changed before proceeding to another patient or handling noncontaminated items and environmental surfaces. Protective clothing – masks, eye protection, gowns – should be worn where appropriate when procedures or patient care activities are likely to generate splashes or sprays of blood, body fluids, secretions or excretions. Extreme care must be taken to prevent 'sharps' injuries when cleaning or disposing of instruments or used needles. Needles must never be resheathed after use and should be placed in puncture-resistant 'sharps bins'.

Where the risk of airborne transmission is high the patient should be isolated in a single room and with negative pressure ventilation. In the case of a patient with known or suspected pulmonary tuberculosis, measles or varicella infection, susceptible staff or visitors entering the room should wear a mask. Ideally only previously immune staff should nurse measles and varicella patients. Likewise for droplet infection, the patient should be nursed in a single room by staff wearing masks.

When there is a significant risk of direct or indirect contact transmission the patient should be isolated in a single room. Gloves and gown must be worn when entering the room and removed on leaving. Gloves should also be changed after handling infective material or sites which may harbor high concentrations of microorganisms. Hands must be washed whenever gloves or clothing are changed and care taken to avoid touching potentially contaminated items.

Each hospital or hospital group should have an efficient infection control team, a development shown to be effective in lowering hospital infection rates (Haley et al 1985). Inter alia, such a team will establish policies and procedures for infection prevention and control that are appropriate and feasible for local circumstances. These policies will address such issues as isolation, disinfection, sterilization, immunization (including staff protection), cleaning, waste disposal, staff education, etc. (Casewell 1989). Such a team may also exert some control or influence over the use of antimicrobial drugs and should be given considerable powers to require administrative action towards the eradication of infection hazards, e.g. the disposal of 'sharps' or infected waste. The key members of the infection control team are the Infection Control Officer, usually a microbiologist, and the Infection Control Nurse who can be particularly effective in initiating a quick response to outbreaks of infection, in continuing infection surveillance, and in staff education.

CLINICAL PROBLEMS

THE CHILD WITH FEVER

The most useful temperature measurement is the core or central temperature which has a normal range in young adults of 36.4–36.9°C, and fluctuation around these values of up to 0.4°C. Infants have a rectal temperature above 37°C which falls by about 0.8°C during sleep and rises before waking (Wailoo et al 1989). There is a circadian rhythm in childhood with the highest temperature at 6 p.m. The peripheral temperature is normally 0.5°C lower than that recorded centrally. The core temperature can be measured either rectally or orally using a mercury thermometer or electronic probe. The peripheral temperature is usually measured in the axilla using a thermometer. A number of disposable strip thermometers are available and should be used on the forehead. They are generally less accurate than the other methods described. Experiments on normal volunteers suggest that the most accurate recordings are made when a thermometer is left in the mouth for 3 min and readings taken for less than 2 min are inaccurate.

Although a central temperature reading is of value in the sick child, and measurement of the temperature difference between core and periphery is of particular value in the shocked patient, for most purposes a peripheral reading is adequate. Indeed in the inexperienced, measurement of both rectal and oral temperature carries considerable risk of injury from broken glass.

The commonest cause of fever in childhood is viral infection, usually resolving within a week of onset. Persistence of fever for longer demands thorough investigation; the term pyrexia or fever of unknown origin (PUO, FUO) is normally applied when fever has been present for 14 days.

FEVER IN THE NEWBORN (see pp. 145–150)

Fever during the neonatal period may be the presenting sign of bacterial infections. If investigation is delayed until other signs occur, such as lethargy, anorexia or apnea, infection may be far advanced before treatment is started. Features in the history suggesting such infection include prolonged rupture of membranes, chorioamnionitis, postpartum fever and spontaneous onset of preterm labor. Fever on the second and third day is characteristic of congenital bacterial infection. Acquired bacterial infection is not uncommon in preterm infants nursed in intensive care units and should be considered when fever occurs later in the neonatal period. However, both group B *Streptococcus* and *Listeria* meningitis tend to occur after the end of the first week of life. Sepsis may present with hypothermia or a normal body temperature during this period, probably because of insensitivity of the hypothalamic centers to pyrogens which would normally produce fever in the older child.

Viral infections, either congenital or acquired, may also be associated with fever. A careful history should be taken from the mother; primary herpes simplex infection during late pregnancy which carries a high risk of neonatal infection can easily be over looked. Enteroviral, or respiratory syncytial virus (RSV) infections with their seasonal distributions may present with fever.

The threshold for investigation of fever in the newborn is much lower than in the older child. Infections are characterized by a relative leukopenia (WBC $< 5 \times 10^9$/l) and raised band count ($>$ 20%). Normal investigations would include collection of blood cultures, cerebrospinal fluid and surface swabs, and where indicated tracheal aspirate and specimens for virology.

Dehydration fever has been described in large term infants. This diagnosis should only be made once there is certainty that the baby is not infected.

FEVER DURING INFANCY AND CHILDHOOD

The commonest cause of fever in this group is viral infection. Pyrexia tends to be shortlived and symptoms and signs are usually more generalized than those associated with bacterial infection. Thus typical signs of a viral upper respiratory tract infection include coryza, inflamed tympanic membranes, tonsillitis and fever. Bacterial tonsillitis and otitis media are difficult to differentiate from viral causes but a bacterial otitis media is more likely to be unilateral.

A good history and thorough examination are essential if a speedy diagnosis is to be achieved. Thus direct questions should be asked about the following:

1. previous immunizations
2. family members with fever
3. travel abroad
4. consumption of unpasteurized milk (to exclude listeriosis, brucellosis), or raw eggs (*Salmonella* sp.)
5. history of congenital heart disease
6. symptoms of this illness (abdominal pain, urinary frequency and dysuria)

7. signs noticed – rash, joint swelling.

Examination should take note of rash, lymphadenopathy, hepato- and splenomegaly, chest signs, heart murmurs, abdominal masses and tenderness. A rectal examination should be considered particularly when there is a history of abdominal pain associated with anorexia and a fever. The bones and joints should be assessed for swelling and tenderness.

When fever has been persistent – over a week for instance – and no cause has been found, serious consideration should be given to hospital admission to confirm pyrexia and to initiate investigations. The physical signs and investigations required to exclude conditions producing fever, or pyrexia of unknown origin (FUO, PUO), are given in Table 23.9.

However, certain basic investigations should be performed – of which urine and blood culture are the most useful.

Table 23.9   Causes of pyrexia of unknown origin

Disease	Signs	Investigations
Bacterial Brucellosis	Lymphadenopathy, splenomegaly	Antibody titers
Bacterial endocarditis	Murmur, splinter hemorrhages	Blood culture × 3, *Brucella, Coxiella* titers
Leptospirosis	Hematuria, jaundice conjunctivitis	Blood culture, serology
Osteomyelitis	Bone swelling, tenderness, redness, immobility	Blood culture × 3, bone aspirate culture, bone radioisotope scan
Pelvic abscess	Abdominal tenderness, tender mass rectally	Leukocytosis on FBC
Pyelonephritis	Loin tenderness	Urine microscopy and culture
Tuberculosis	Pneumonia, meningitis	Tuberculin test, culture gastric washings ± cerebrospinal fluid, chest X-ray
Typhoid fever	Abdominal tenderness, rose spots, splenomegaly	Blood culture
Septic arthritis	Swelling, tenderness, immobility at single joint	Joint aspirate culture
Psittacosis	Chest crackles, tachypnea	Chest X-ray, serology
Listeriosis	Arthritis, meningism	Blood culture, cerebrospinal fluid culture
Virus Cytomegalic inclusion disease	Lymphadenopathy, hepatosplenomegaly	Urine culture etc.
Human immunodeficiency virus	Lymphadenopathy, failure to thrive, chronic infection, e.g. candida	T4/T8 lymphocyte ratio, HIV antibody
Infectious mononucleosis	Tonsillitis, hepatosplenomegaly	Paul–Bunnell/ Monospot Epstein–Barr viral antibody
Hepatitis	Icterus, hepatomegaly	Hepatitis A antibody, Australia antigen
Parasite Malaria	Splenomegaly Hepatomegaly Encephalopathy	Thick or thin blood film
Toxoplasmosis	Cervical, supraclavicular lymphadenopathy	Smear from biopsy specimen, serology
Miscellaneous Crohn's disease	Abdominal tenderness and mass	Barium study of GI tract Exclude *Yersinia* and *Campylobacter* infection
Diabetes insipidus	Dehydration Polyuria, polydipsia	Dilute urine following water deprivation
Juvenile rheumatoid arthritis 1. Systemic	Fever characteristic Macular-papular rash, lethargy, arthritis, pericardial effusion	No diagnostic test
2. Monoarticular/ polyarticular	Fever not a consistent sign	
Kawasaki's disease	Cervical lymphadenopathy Bilateral conjunctival injection Red, fissured lips and tongue Macular-papular rash Swelling and desquamation of hands and feet	No diagnostic test Platelet count
Malignancy Leukemia Lymphoma Neuroblastoma	Includes anemia, lymphadenopathy, splenomegaly Abdominal mass, bone pain	Full blood count, blood film, lymph node biopsy Bone marrow trephine, VMA
Factitious fever (Munchausen by proxy)	Pyrexia only recorded by parent	None

FEVER IN THE IMMUNOSUPPRESSED

This requires urgent investigation in the neutropenic child. Blood cultures are frequently sterile in this group although endotoxin levels may be elevated. It has been suggested that it is endotoxin which is pyrogenic.

THE CHILD WITH A RASH

In some cases a rash will be diagnostic and in others the diagnosis will only be reached in conjunction with the history and appropriate investigations. Failure to recognize certain rashes could cost the life of a child, as in meningococcal infection or varicella in an immunocompromised child.

In establishing a diagnosis when an infectious cause is considered, certain information should be obtained by history as follows: prior infectious disease and or rashes; recent contact with infectious disease; prior immunization; foreign travel; prodromal illness; fever.

In the general examination note should be taken of the child's general state, the temperature, appearance of conjunctivae, ears and throat. Careful auscultation of the chest should be performed; all groups of lymph glands as well as liver and spleen should be examined.

Once this has been done interest should return to the rash which should be described carefully in its form (e.g. hemorrhagic, macular, papular):

1. macules – flat and impalpable
2. papules – circumscribed elevated lesions
3. vesicles – circumscribed, elevated, fluid filled and normally less than 0.5 cm in diameter
4. pustules – elevated lesions containing a purulent exudate
5. petechiae and other hemorrhagic spots – cannot be blanched by compression and may be flat or raised; the term purpura usually refers to the larger lesions with a diameter greater than 0.5 cm.

The distribution may be an important clue to certain infections. Consideration may need to be given as to whether the rash is itchy, e.g. are there signs of scratching?

RASHES IN THE NEWBORN

In this age group rashes are common. Neonatal urticaria or erythema toxicum is characterized by a mixture of erythematous macules, and white or yellow papules. These usually develop over the first few days and may persist until the end of the second week. Staphylococcal infection of the newborn may be difficult to distinguish from neonatal urticaria. Although erythematous lesions are seen pustules and vesicles predominate with staphylococcal infection. When there is uncertainty as to the diagnosis, a Gram stain of vesicle fluid should be performed. Plentiful polymorphs as well as Gram-positive cocci should be seen in the presence of staphylococcal infection; eosinophils predominate in neonatal urticaria.

Vesicles are also seen in neonatal varicella and herpes simplex infection. In the former a history of maternal varicella will be elicited; in the latter herpetic lesions of the genital tract are likely to be visible. The vesicles of herpes simplex tend to be larger and less opaque than those of staphylococcal infection. Urgent treatment is essential and diagnosis can be achieved by electron microscopy on vesicle fluid or by rapid viral identification tests.

Other rashes associated with infection may be petechial or purpuric as seen in congenital CMV or rubella as a result of thrombocytopenia and in most cases the rash is just one aspect of severe infection. Petechiae are also not uncommon in the newborn following birth asphyxia, phototherapy or in association with immune thrombocytopenia.

RASHES IN INFANCY AND CHILDHOOD

These will be described under descriptive headings.

Vesicular rashes

Varicella (see p. 1360)

Lesions normally appear without a prodromal illness, and progress rapidly (within a few hours) from papule to vesicles surrounded by an erythematous base. Crops of vesicles appear over 3 days, predominantly on the trunk and proximal limbs. Vesicles may also develop on mucous membranes.

Herpes zoster

Lesions similar to those seen in varicella infection may develop over specific dermatomes or cranial nerves. Although the immunosuppressed are at increased risk from zoster, this condition is also seen in normal children.

Herpes simplex type 1

Although infection is most commonly associated with gingivostomatitis during childhood, vesicles are seen on the skin in eczema herpeticum (Kaposi's varicelliform eruption). Pyrexia is followed by the appearance of crops of vesicles on the eczematous skin. Crops of lesions may occur over several days. Correct and rapid diagnosis is essential because untreated severe infection may be fatal.

Hand, foot and mouth

This is caused by Coxsackie virus type 16 and occurs in epidemics. It is associated with a papular-vesicular eruption of the mouth, hands, feet and buttocks.

Impetigo

This condition usually presents as a red macule and then becomes vesicular. The small vesicles burst to leave a honey-colored crust. Both streptococcal and staphylococcal impetigo occur commonly around the mouth but can occur elsewhere.

Molluscum contagiosum

This is caused by a pox virus. In this condition flesh-colored papules with a central dimple are seen. Although firm initially they become softer and more waxy with time. Lesions are 2–5 mm in size and may occur anywhere.

Dermatitis herpetiformis

This occurs in children from 8 years upwards who develop recurrent crops of pruritic papulovesicles over extensor surfaces including the elbows, buttocks and knees. Many of these children also have a gluten-sensitive enteropathy.

Maculopapular rashes

Measles

This is red in color and appears on the third day of illness, initially on the face and neck. The lesions tend to become confluent on the upper part of the body and remain more discrete lower down. The rash tends to fade after 2–3 days. The skin becomes brown and although desquamation occurs this is not seen on the hands and feet as in scarlet fever.

Rubella

This results in a pink rash which progresses caudally. The lesions are normally discrete and the rash develops more quickly and disappears earlier than in measles. Desquamation is not a characteristic.

Scarlet fever

The eruption is dark red and punctiform. The rash tends to be most prominent on the neck and in the major skinfolds. A distinctive feature is circumoral pallor as a result of the rash sparing the area around the mouth. As with measles, desquamation is seen but the hands and feet are involved. True scarlet fever is associated with inflammation of the tongue (white and red strawberry tongue). Scarlatina refers to the rash which may occur alone in milder streptococcal infection, and is often shortlived.

Kawasaki disease

Although several features are required for the diagnosis of this condition which is of unknown etiology the rash may be confused with that of scarlet fever. Discrete red maculopapules are seen on the feet, around the knees and in the axillary and inguinal skin creases. Desquamation of the hands and feet is a common feature (Plate 23.5).

Erythema infectiosum or Fifth disease

Infection caused by parvovirus is associated with a rash which develops in two stages. The cheeks appear red and flushed with circumoral pallor giving rise to a 'slapped cheek' appearance. A maculopapular rash then develops predominantly over the arms and legs which, as it fades, appears lace-like.

Roseola infantum

Recently attributed to a human herpes virus 6 this infection is characterized by a widespread rash seen in its most florid form on the trunk. The lesions tend to be discrete. As the rash appears the fever which is normally present over the previous 4 days effervesces.

Viral infections

Many viral infections, particularly those associated with the enteroviruses, may result in maculopapular rashes.

Petechial and purpuric rashes

Meningococcal infection

The first sign of meningococcal septicemia may be a petechial or purpuric rash anywhere on the body and often localized (Plate 23.2). On occasions these lesions may be preceded by or accompany a maculopapular rash (Plate 23.1). The petechiae will not blanch, and although it is conventional to make a microbiological diagnosis on blood culture, bacteria can also be isolated from these lesions.

Meningococcal petechiae can be confused with those seen on the face around the eyes following events that result in a transient rise in venous pressure such as vomiting. Rarely petechial rashes are associated with septicemia caused by other bacteria particularly Haemophilus influenzae.

Henoch–Schönlein purpura

This condition often follows an upper respiratory tract infection but no single infective agent has been implicated. Hemorrhagic macules and papules develop on buttocks and extensor surfaces of the limbs particularly the knees and ankles. The lesions come in crops and fade over a few days leaving a brown pigmentation.

Idiopathic thrombocytopenic purpura (ITP) and leukemia

A purpuric rash sometimes associated with frank bleeding is seen in this condition. Even postinfective cases are referred to as ITP and rubella infection is considered to be the commonest cause. Children with leukemia may present with a hemorrhagic rash as a result of thrombocytopenia but in addition, the pallor of severe anemia will usually be obvious.

VOMITING

Although the commonest cause of vomiting in childhood is gastrointestinal infection or food poisoning it may be a symptom of a large number of other conditions.

CAUSES OF VOMITING IN CHILDHOOD

Gastrointestinal infection and food poisoning

Bacterial (e.g. Salmonella sp. and staphylococcal enterotoxin)
Viral (e.g. rotavirus).

Infection elsewhere

Meningitis (bacterial or viral)
Encephalitis
Urinary tract infection
Pneumonia
Tonsillitis
Hepatitis
Pancreatitis.

Disease of the central nervous system

Meningitis and encephalitis
Migraine
Space-occupying lesion.

Metabolic disease

Diabetic ketoacidosis
Congenital adrenal hyperplasia
Chronic renal failure
Inherited metabolic disorders, e.g. urea cycle defects
Reye's syndrome.

Gastrointestinal disease

Neonatal intestinal obstruction; meconium ileus, Hirschsprung's disease, small bowel atresia
Volvulus
Pyloric stenosis
Reflux esophagitis
Acute appendicitis
Appendix abscess.

Others

Antibiotics and other drugs
Accidental poisoning
Toxic encephalopathy syndrome
Functional – recurrent, periodic.

The history and physical findings should indicate the cause of vomiting, e.g. fever and neck stiffness suggest meningitis; polydipsia and polyuria, diabetes mellitus. There is no place for antiemetic drugs in the treatment of vomiting. It is more important to establish a cause and treat the underlying condition, correcting dehydration and electrolyte imbalance if present.

DIARRHEA

Diarrhea is defined as the frequent passage of watery stools. What may be normal stool frequency for the young infant may be abnormal for an older child. Most cases of diarrhea result from gastrointestinal disease.

CAUSES OF DIARRHEA IN CHILDHOOD

Infection

Bacterial (*Salmonella* sp., *Shigella* sp., *Campylobacter jejuni*)
Viral (e.g. rotavirus, enteroviruses, Norwalk virus)
Protozoal (giardiasis)
Hemolytic-uremic syndrome
Staphylococcal toxic shock
Systemic infection – urinary tract infection, meningitis.

Malabsorption

Lactose intolerance
Cow's milk protein intolerance
Cystic fibrosis
Celiac disease
Shwachman syndrome.

Gastrointestinal disorders

Acute appendicitis
Appendix abscess
Ulcerative colitis
Crohn's disease.

Other causes

Toddler diarrhea
Kawasaki disease
Laxatives
Antibiotics.

Diarrhea of short duration and acute onset is more likely to be caused by infection. A long history might indicate conditions such as celiac disease, cystic fibrosis or inflammatory bowel disease. Enquiries should be made about the feeding history, the nature of the stools and presence of respiratory symptoms. Growth since birth should be recorded on a centile chart.

In children, particularly infants, dehydration may develop rapidly after onset of diarrhea. Because of this the physical examination should include an assessment of the degree of dehydration (Table 23.10). This allows an assessment of the severity of diarrhea and indicates the type and volume of rehydration fluid required. Further investigations such as measurement of plasma electrolytes may be important. When the history of diarrhea is less acute, further investigations to exclude conditions such as celiac disease should be performed.

BACTEREMIA AND SEPTICEMIA

BACTEREMIA

This is defined as the presence of bacteria in the bloodstream in the absence of systemic illness apart from fever. This should be distinguished from septicemia in which signs and symptoms of severe disease are present.

Transient bacteremia occurs in all subjects; vigorous tooth brushing may promote release of bacteria into the circulation but in the immunocompetent child these microorganisms quickly disappear without fever.

Bacteremia may accompany localized infection such as otitis media and pneumonia. A source of infection may not be identified in up to one-third of children under the age of 2 with *Streptococcus pneumoniae* bacteremia (McLellan & Giebink 1986). *Haemophilus influenzae* bacteremia is more likely to be associated with localized disease during infancy; other organisms include *Neisseria meningitidis* and *Salmonella* sp. Untreated occult bacteremia (with absence of localizing disease) caused by the pathogens described above appears to resolve in perhaps one-third of cases (Marshall et al 1979). A number of parameters have been examined to determine how predictive they are of bacteremia. There seems to be considerable variation between different studies but there is some agreement that a rectal temperature of less than 39°C is rarely associated with bacteremia. The probability of bacteremia in a child under the age of 2 with a temperature greater than 39°C is thought to be approximately 5% (McLellan & Giebink 1986). Of laboratory tests that have been evaluated – white blood count (WBC), erythrocyte sedimentation rate and C-reactive protein – the first appears to be the most useful. Bacteremia appears to be unusual

Table 23.10 Signs of different degrees of dehydration (from Nicoll & Rudd 1989, p. 59, reproduced with permission)

Sign	Less than 5% dehydration	More than 5% dehydration	More than 10% dehydration
Skin	Normal tension	Loss of turgor	Mottled, poor capillary return
Fontanel (if open)	Normal	Depressed	Deeply depressed
Eyes	Not sunken	Sunken, reduced intraocular pressure	Sunken, reduced intraocular pressure
Lips	Moist	Dry	Dry
Peripheral pulses	Normal	Normal	Poor volume and tachycardia
Blood pressure	Normal	Normal	Low
Behavior	Unchanged	Lethargic	Prostration, coma
Urine output	Still wetting nappies or urinating at usual frequency	Long periods between micturition	Anuric

Note: children with hypernatremic dehydration have a doughy feel to the skin and may not appear clinically as dehydrated.

with a total WBC between 5000 and 15 000/mm³ (Dagan et al 1985a). In meningococcemia at least, leucopenia is seen in fatal disease (Dashefsky et al 1983). The specificity of both an elevated and reduced WBC is low. Other work has suggested that the physician's general assessment of the child's condition is as important as any investigations.

When occult bacteremia is suspected, appropriate investigations should include blood and urine culture, and in spite of its limitations, a blood count. Because bacteremia, particularly in early infancy, may progress to meningitis and this diagnosis may be difficult on clinical grounds, a lumbar puncture should be considered. Although there is some concern that a lumbar puncture in a child with bacteremia may lead to meningitis there is no satisfactory evidence of this in the human subject. In one study there appeared to be a definite relationship between meningitis and recent lumbar puncture. However, the definition of meningitis was broad, and included children who may not have suffered from this condition. It is likely that of the two groups under comparison those children investigated by lumbar puncture were sicker than those who escaped this test (Teele et al 1981).

Treatment of the child with suspected bacteremia can be expectant; if antibiotics are not given when the child presents, careful observation should be performed looking for more specific evidence of bacterial infection – signs of meningococcemia for instance. If fever is still present when a positive isolation is made on blood culture, antibiotics should be given. Bactericidal antibiotics are recommended, directed towards the coliforms as well as *H. influenzae* and the pneumococcus in early infancy when an aminoglycoside and penicillin are indicated. In children over 3 months ampicillin is appropriate but account of culture results and susceptibility of bacteria isolated should be taken.

Fever in the immunosuppressed neutropenic child should lead to urgent investigation; and antibiotics should be started immediately. Studies indicate that pathogens are isolated in blood culture from less than a third of neutropenic children. Infection in these children may be caused by *Staphylococcus aureus, S. epidermidis* and *Pseudomonas aeruginosa* in addition to the pathogens affecting normal children. There may be local differences in the bacteria causing infection in the neutropenic child but a combination of an aminoglycoside and another agent effective against *P. aeruginosa* such as piperacillin is indicated. Antistaphylococcal agents may be required for children with indwelling cannulae who are susceptible to *S. epidermidis* infection.

SEPTICEMIA

Septicemia may follow untreated bacteremia and may develop rapidly in the immunocompromised child (e.g. the child with leukemia, nephrotic syndrome or sickle cell disease). Circulatory collapse from septic shock is a characteristic of infection with Gram-negative bacteria such as *P. aeruginosa, Escherichia coli* and *Klebsiella* sp., although similar events may be precipitated by *Staphylococcus aureus* infection.

The illness produced by Gram-negative septicemia is a result of endotoxemia. Endotoxins are lipopolysaccharides (LPS) found in the outer membrane of Gram-negative bacteria. They consist of a polysaccharide and a lipid, the latter mediating most of the biological effect of endotoxins. Endotoxins appear to activate complement, through both the classical pathway and alternative route. Activation of complement releases anaphylatoxins which have diverse effects in the body including vasodilation and chemotaxis of white blood cells. Other effects of endotoxin include the stimulation of prostaglandin production, and release of platelet activating factor (PAF) which causes platelet aggregation and secretion, degranulation of neutrophils, smooth muscle contraction, increased vascular permeability and hypotension (Morrison & Ryan 1987).

An early sign of septicemia may be a fever or even lowered body temperature. The child may develop rigors, hyperventilate and develop peripheral vasodilation. With release of anaphylatoxins hypotension occurs associated with a poor peripheral circulation. The cardiac output rises but cannot compensate for the fall in peripheral resistance caused by leakage of fluid from the circulation as a result of damage to capillary walls. With a fall in blood flow to the kidneys renal failure ensues. Characteristic skin lesions may develop in some forms of septicemia; petechiae or purpura with meningococcal infection; necrotic ulcerated lesions (ecthyma gangrenosum) with *Pseudomonas* sp. infections. Disseminated intravascular coagulation becomes evident with bleeding from venepuncture sites. Death occurs in a significant number of children with Gram-negative septicemia.

Early diagnosis is essential, and it should be recognized that certain children are at greater risk of such infection, e.g. the child who is neutropenic from immunosuppressive drugs or who has sickle cell disease. A careful history and examination should be performed to elucidate the origin of the infection; for instance the diagnosis of a pelvic abscess which would require urgent surgical drainage rather than medical treatment, or the recognition that an indwelling bladder catheter may be colonized with pathogens. It should also be recognized that a child with functional asplenia is at increased risk of pneumococcal or salmonella septicemia, and a child with nephrotic syndrome is at increased risk from pneumococcal or *H. influenzae* infection.

Investigations should include blood cultures. Measurements of endotoxin and tumor necrosis factor (TNF) which is released from macrophages during endotoxemia are not routinely available. Measurement of electrolytes, glucose and creatinine is important. Because of disseminated intravascular coagulation (DIC), platelet counts, clotting studies and fibrinogen degradation products should be measured.

Bactericidal antibiotics should be given once blood cultures have been taken. If the child develops endotoxemia in hospital, the selection of antibiotics may be dependent on bacterial cultures from surface swabs, or on the basis of recent infection among other hospitalized children. For Gram-negative septicemia an appropriate combination of antibiotics might be an aminoglycoside such as gentamicin (although care should be taken if renal function is impaired) and an antipseudomonal β-lactam penicillin – piperacillin or ticarcillin. Alternatively a third generation cephalosporin such as ceftazidime can be used. Unless staphylococcal infection has been excluded, an antistaphylococcal antibiotic should be given. Metronidazole for treatment of anerobic infection should be given when sepsis has risen from the abdomen. Children will require nursing in an intensive care unit, with careful monitoring of central venous pressure, pulmonary wedge pressure and urine output. Supportive treatment will require maintenance of an adequate circulating blood volume. Large volumes of plasma or blood are normally required but care has to be taken to prevent fluid overload with pulmonary edema. The β-adrenergic agent dopamine is of value for its positive inotropic effect on the myocardium, and for promoting renal perfusion. Treatment of DIC is symptomatic – heparin is of dubious value and if dosage is inappropriate may exacerbate disease. Transfusion of fresh frozen plasma and platelets may be required. Steroids may worsen the outcome. The prognosis for septicemia with DIC is grave.

TOXIC SHOCK SYNDROME (TSS)

This is caused by staphylococcal exotoxin and it was first described in five children and young adults (Todd et al 1978). It was characterized by an acute onset of high fever, with headache, confusion and rash. In addition sore throat, vomiting and diarrhea, oliguria and shock were normally seen. On examination, the patients appeared very ill and confused, with red conjunctivae, and a diffuse nonpruritic scarlatiniform rash most prominent on the trunk and extremities. Edema of the face and limbs was also seen, and episodes of severe and refractory hypotension were associated with reduced peripheral perfusion leading to ischemic changes in the tissues. Several children had an inflamed pharynx, and jaundice was common.

Laboratory investigation showed an increased number of immature neutrophils with toxic granulation. Thrombocytopenia was associated with disseminated intravascular coagulation. There was an elevation of bilirubin and glutamic-oxaloacetic transaminase levels. Microscopic hematuria was seen with increase in plasma creatinine.

In two patients localized infection was identified during the illness and *S. aureus* was isolated from swabs. Because of a similarity of this illness to other staphylococcal illness, scalded skin syndrome for example, attempts were made to identify a toxin from the *Staphylococcus* isolated from swabs of all the patients described. An epidermal toxin distinct from the exfoliation toxin associated with scalded skin syndrome was isolated although subsequent workers have been unable to identify this toxin from patients with TSS; the toxins that have been identified would not be expected to produce the type of systemic illness seen in this syndrome. It is of note that *S. aureus* could not be isolated from blood culture or CSF. In spite of intensive care and early treatment with antistaphylococcal antibiotics one patient died and another survivor had gangrene. As more cases were seen it was recognized that women using vaginal tampons were specially vulnerable to such infection. More recently *S. aureus* has been isolated from blood culture and *Streptococcus pyogenes* has been recognized as a cause of toxic shock.

HEMORRHAGIC SHOCK AND ENCEPHALOPATHY SYNDROME (HSE)

In 1983 Levin et al described what was thought to be a new syndrome. In just 1 year, 10 infants aged 3–8 months were admitted to the Hospital for Sick Children, Great Ormond Street, with similar symptoms and outcome – often fatal. A case history, said to be typical, described listlessness and two episodes of vomiting over 2 days. The child was found collapsed, fitting and breathing quickly. On admission to hospital he was pyrexial, and shocked with an unrecordable blood pressure. He then developed watery bloodstained diarrhea. Investigations showed features of disseminated intravascular coagulation. There was a severe metabolic acidosis, high plasma creatinine, bilirubin and transaminase enzymes. He was given positive pressure ventilation, plasma, dopamine and antibiotics as well as mannitol and dexamethasone for cerebral edema, but died from the effects of encephalopathy 36 h after admission. Only three out of ten infants in this series survived, all with severe neurological damage. Autopsy was similar in all cases with edema of the brain and swelling and degeneration of hepatocytes (rather than fatty change as seen in Reye's syndrome). Extensive biochemical and microbiological investigations were performed in most cases. Of note were a normal plasma ammonia (excluding Reye's syndrome) and negative culture for *S. aureus*. Bacterial pathogens were isolated from the sputum of three infants, and results of viral studies were unremarkable. The cause still remains unexplained. However, Bacon et al described a similar syndrome 4 years earlier – characterized by fever, shock, convulsions, diarrhea, liver failure and DIC (Bacon et al 1979). The age range of 3–8 months was the same as that in Levin's series. In Bacon's series of five infants there was one survivor. Autopsy revealed cerebral edema and hepatocyte degeneration. In spite of a comprehensive search for biochemical abnormalities and infective agents all results were negative. It was considered that the illness was caused by heatstroke; the oral or rectal temperatures of these infants were 39.9°C or more on admission and all had been swaddled in several layers of clothes or blankets. Although children with HSE had features of heatstroke only one of the 10 had been overwrapped.

ACUTE BACTERIAL MENINGITIS

Bacterial meningitis occurs at all ages, but is commonest in infancy. 80% of all meningitis occurs in childhood. Meningitis

Table 23.11 Reports of isolates in the cerebrospinal fluid to the Communicable Disease Surveillance Centre (CDSC) in 1990 and 1995 England and Wales (source: CDSC)

		Age groups			
	Year	1–11 months	1–4 years	5–9 years	10–14 years
Haemophilus influenzae	1990	214	247	19	1
	1995	9	9	1	2
Neisseria meningitidis	1990	211	220	58	43
	1995	98	92	31	17
Streptococcus pneumoniae	1990	79	51	9	7
	1995	57	24	6	4

may result in the death of a child within hours of the onset of the disease. Untreated it is usually fatal. During 1985 in England and Wales there were 64 deaths from meningitis in the first year of life; 33 from 1 to 4 years and 20 between 5 and 10.

During the neonatal period the main pathogens include the group B streptococcus, *Escherichia coli, Streptococcus pneumoniae* and less commonly *Haemophilus influenzae* and *Listeria monocytogenes*. Following this *S. pneumoniae* and *Neisseria meningitidis* predominate, the latter more common with increasing age. Voluntary reports of cerebrospinal fluid isolates to the Communicable Disease Surveillance Centre are shown in Table 23.11.

Meningitis may occur without warning in a perfectly normal infant or child but there are a number of circumstances in which there is increased risk of this disease. Of note is prematurity especially when associated with maternal chorioamnionitis, and in the term infant with spina bifida cystica.

Meningitis may be associated with septicemia particularly during the neonatal period. It may result from direct spread of middle ear infection and mastoiditis, frontal sinusitis, rupture of a cerebral abscess or compound fracture of the skull. It can occur as a result of an infected ventriculocardiac or ventriculoperitoneal shunt.

PATHOLOGY

The bacterial invasion of the cerebrospinal fluid is followed by an outpouring of polymorph leukocytes and fibrin. The meninges become inflamed, swollen and covered by fibrinopurulent exudate. The thickest exudate is usually at the base of the brain. In this situation it may temporarily obstruct the exit foramina of the fourth ventricle or the subarachnoid basal cisterns. This leads to obstruction of the cerebrospinal fluid circulation and hence to hydrocephalus particularly in young infants. The purulent exudate may also cover the spinal cord. If sufficiently thick, it may cause a spinal block and interfere with the free diffusion of drugs within the cerebrospinal fluid.

In some instances, particularly in pneumococcal meningitis, the exudate may be more profuse over the frontal lobes and vertex. Occasionally the pus may become encapsulated. In such cases cerebrospinal fluid may clear with therapy but if the patient dies thick fibrinopurulent exudate will be found over the vertex.

The ependymal lining of the cerebral ventricles may be the site of maximal inflammation (ventriculitis), particularly in infants with myelomeningocele. The ventricles not only enlarge, but may be divided into multiple loculi by the exudate. This renders antibiotic therapy or the later surgical treatment of the residual hydrocephalus more difficult. Not infrequently the ventricular cerebrospinal fluid may be normal even when the spinal CSF is purulent.

The cerebral vessels and cranial nerves may be involved in the purulent exudate at the base of the brain. Destruction of nerve fibres and thrombosis (septic or sterile) of the cerebral vessels can lead to permanent neurological damage.

Subdural effusions may develop over the vertex, particularly after *Haemophilus* meningitis. Such fluid may be clear and sterile or turbid and infected. Both types of effusion have a high protein content.

Early in the illness the brain is swollen and the ventricles are diminished in size. Later this cerebral edema disappears and the ventricles increase in size. In infants, manifest hydrocephalus frequently follows meningitis and is more frequent and severe in the youngest babies.

CLINICAL FEATURES

The fully developed clinical picture of acute meningitis in children is sufficiently characteristic to be recognized without difficulty. The diagnosis is more difficult in very young infants, and in the earliest stages of the disease in others.

In young infants the symptoms are often those of a generalized illness. They consist of irritability, refusal of feeds and vomiting. A vacant 'far away' look may be present and convulsions may occur. The cry may be high pitched and the fontanel tense and bulging. The infant looks ill and is usually fevered. The temperature need not be greatly elevated and rarely may be subnormal. Neck stiffness or a positive Kernig sign (see below) are often not present in the early stages of the illness in infants. They are late, not early diagnostic signs in infantile meningitis.

Older children will often complain of headache or pain at the back of the neck, nausea and photophobia. Projectile vomiting and fever are prominent features. Cranial nerve palsies, especially of the sixth nerve, may develop rapidly. The child resents being disturbed, lies with his face turned away from the light and is curled up as far as a stiff or retracted neck will allow. Later there is delirium or drowsiness which then proceeds to coma. Convulsions later in the disease are of ominous prognostic significance. Untreated, the illness tends to progress rapidly from early prodromal symptoms to convulsions, coma and death which, in fulminating cases, may all occur within a few hours, but more often take several days.

The physical signs of meningeal irritation are neck stiffness and a positive Kernig sign. Neck stiffness can be detected by placing a palm of the hand on the child's occiput while he is lying on his back. Any attempt at flexing the child's neck will result in the lifting of his whole trunk. The child himself is unwilling or unable to flex his neck and is unable to kiss his knees, or touch his toes without bending his knees. In advanced cases the head is held rigid and retracted. Kernig's sign is elicited with the child lying on his back. The hip and knee joints are bent to 90° and then an attempt is made to extend the knee fully. In normal children this is easily achieved but in the presence of meningitis there is considerable resistance, and long before the leg is fully extended the child complains of severe pain in the hamstrings and the small of the back. The hamstrings go into spasm and the leg cannot be straightened.

Papilledema is an uncommon late development and is not seen in infants with an open fontanel. The skull may give a 'crackpot sound' on tapping it with a finger, but this sign is difficult to interpret and it may occur in hydrocephalus and other conditions.

The choice of the appropriate antibiotic depends on the identity of the infecting organism. For this reason consideration should be given to associated clinical features which may indicate the likely organism. The age of the patient is important. Newborn infants are more likely to be infected by Gram-negative bacilli. If the mother had perinatal infection previous bacteriological evidence may be available to indicate the probable infecting organism. If the baby had myelomeningocele, organisms already obtained from an infected wound may provide a clue to the likely bacterial type of meningitis.

A petechial rash or more extensive purpura (Plate 23.2) almost certainly indicates meningococcal infection, in which case meningococci can be rapidly cultured from the blood. As lumbar puncture in this type of meningitis carries a risk of cerebellar coning with death in the unconscious child it may be considered unnecessary or unwise to carry out a diagnostic lumbar puncture. Otitis media or mastoiditis is likely to lead to pneumococcal meningitis. Infections produced by compound fracture of the skull or by surgical procedures are more likely to be due to staphylococci or pneumococci.

DIAGNOSIS

If meningitis is suspected the diagnosis should be confirmed by lumbar puncture and examination of cerebrospinal fluid (CSF). Although coning in childhood meningitis following lumbar puncture is very rare the risk is increased in the unconscious child who may show no evidence of the papilledema normally seen in the presence of longstanding increased intracranial pressure. It is acceptable to forego a lumbar puncture in a child suspected to have meningococcal meningitis by virtue of the characteristic purpuric or petechial lesions seen in this infection, but care should be taken not to confuse these with purpura seen on the face following vomiting or on the limbs produced by an attendant holding a struggling child during investigation. In this situation it is essential to obtain a blood culture, as is the case with all children undergoing lumbar puncture. Otherwise treatment of meningitis should not be started before CSF has been obtained.

Lumbar puncture should be performed in the 3rd to 4th lumbar space using a styleted needle; use of a needle alone has been associated with the development of implantation dermoid cysts. Although CSF pressure can be measured this technique is often very difficult in all but the unconscious child and should not be allowed to interfere with the collection of CSF. It is usual to collect a minimum of five drops into three bottles for use in the bacteriology laboratory as well as a small amount for protein and glucose analysis. When viral meningitis is suspected consider sending a specimen for viral studies.

Microscopy alone should indicate the presence of meningitis in the majority of cases. A Gram stain should be performed – a negative result may be seen early in the infection or where antibiotics have been given already. Interpretation of the cell count is perhaps most difficult in the newborn when increased numbers of leukocytes may be seen in CSF following intraventricular hemorrhage (IVH). Even in the absence of IVH, counts of up to 50 WBC/mm^3 may be seen in the absence of meningitis. In the presence of bacterial meningitis in childhood the CSF leukocyte count might be expected to range from 200 to 20 000/mm^3 (Smith et al 1973). However, positive cultures have been obtained from children with normal CSF microscopy. Because bacteremia may precede infection of the meninges it is likely that a lumbar puncture was performed in these cases prior to infection of the meninges. The physician may have to repeat the lumbar puncture if there has been deterioration in the condition of a child who shows the clinical signs of meningitis.

Although polymorphonuclear leukocytes predominate in the CSF of children with acute bacterial meningitis, lymphocytes may predominate in the newborn; indeed lymphocytosis is characteristic of *Listeria monocytogenes* meningitis. Lymphocytes may predominate in partially treated meningitis. In one series a lymphocytosis was seen in 14% of patients (both adults and children) and when the CSF leukocyte count was less than 1000, lymphocytes predominated in 32% (Powers 1985). Conversely in children with suspected aseptic meningitis 48 out of 230 had 71–87% polymorphs with leukocyte counts of 59–443/mm^3. Repeat lumbar puncture 6–8 h later showed a lower white count and fall in polymorph count (Feigin & Shackelford 1973). The characteristic CSF findings of tuberculous meningitis include an excess of polymorphs and lymphocytes. Polymorphs predominate in the CSF of children with amebic meningitis.

Although many clinicians assume that in the presence of a bloody tap the ratio of leukocytes to erythrocytes in CSF can be expected to correspond to that in the peripheral blood it has been shown that this is untrue. The white count in CSF was only 25% of that expected in neonates and 14% for older children (Osborne & Pizer 1981).

A specimen should be collected for plasma glucose prior to lumbar puncture when the CSF glucose should also be measured. In most cases of bacterial meningitis the glucose CSF/blood ratio is less than 0.5, but similar results are also seen in a small proportion of children with aseptic meningitis. A low CSF glucose is seen in tuberculous meningitis. Protein should also be measured – a value of more than 0.4 g/l is characteristic of septic and tuberculous meningitis.

Microscopy, culture, protein and glucose analysis are the essential investigations for suspected meningitis. Rapid identification of bacteria in CSF can be obtained by use of countercurrent immunoelectrophoresis or the more sensitive latex agglutination test. They have given disappointing results in cases of partially treated meningitis and are invariably negative in Gram stain negative but culture positive cases (Finlay et al 1995).

A number of other tests have been evaluated. A high lactate concentration in CSF may be a more sensitive means of distinguishing bacterial from aseptic meningitis than the blood/CSF glucose ratio. Evaluation of acute phase reactants suggests that the presence of C-reactive protein is a sensitive test for bacterial meningitis, detected in all 24 children with such infection (including two with CSF leukocyte counts of less than 50/mm^3) compared with two out of 32 with aseptic meningitis (Corrall et al 1981).

On occasions a presumed diagnosis of partially treated meningitis is made which fails to respond to what is thought to be appropriate antibiotic treatment. It is then important to consider antibiotic resistance, cerebral abscess, tuberculous or even amebic meningitis. Rarely a child with a cerebral tumor with ventricular extension may present with a cellular CSF response, increased protein and lowered glucose.

TREATMENT

There are several different antibiotic regimes known to be effective in treating *H. influenzae*, *Streptococcus pneumoniae* and *N. meningitidis* meningitis. The mortality of meningitis appears to be similar irrespective of the antibiotic used. Unfortunately there is a dearth of good long-term studies of morbidity and there remain a number of unanswered questions such as the value of steroids.

The antibiotic regime selected will depend on the age of the child. The treatment of neonatal meningitis, predominantly from group B *Streptococcus* and *E. coli* is discussed elsewhere. Cefotaxime is the treatment of choice for infection outside the neonatal period, except for Listeria meningitis when ampicillin is recommended. Cefotaxime has good CSF penetration and is effective against meningococcal, pneumococcal and the less common *H. influenzae* meningitis. Penicillin can be used for both meningococcal and pneumococcal disease but this antibiotic has relatively poor CSF penetration. Antibiotic regimes are listed in Table 23.12 (see also Ch. 38). Because meningococci are easily eradicated by antibiotics relatively short courses can be used; it is recommended that treatment is continued for 48 h after temperature returns to normal. Illness caused by *H. influenzae* and *S. pneumoniae* is slower to respond to treatment so that longer courses of antibiotics are often used; 10 days for the former and 10–14 days for the latter. However, 7-day treatment courses do not appear to be associated with an adverse outcome (Jadavji et al 1986). In uncomplicated cases there is no place for repeat lumbar puncture either during or at the completion of treatment to assess response to antibiotics. Treatment failure may be related to inappropriate antibiotics – susceptibility to the antibiotics used should be assessed by the laboratory early in the course of treatment although resistance is unlikely using the treatment regimes described. Persistence of fever associated with a bulging anterior fontanel may be caused by a subdural collection of pus. Surgical drainage of the smaller effusions is unnecessary. Although intrathecal antibiotics have been used, such treatment does not result in an improved prognosis, and death has been reported following inadvertent overdose. Evidence from a recent study suggested that dexamethasone treatment (0.15 mg/kg · dose^{-1} 6-hourly for 4 days) started immediately before antibiotics reduces the risk of sensorineural hearing loss in *H. influenzae* meningitis (Lebel et al 1988). Of note was the high rate of deafness in the control group. There is little evidence of benefit in other types of meningitis (Meningitis Working Party 1992).

Skilled nursing should be available and regular neurological observations performed. Although vomiting may be a presenting symptom of meningitis, dehydration is unusual and fluid overload associated with inappropriate ADH secretion is a more frequent occurrence. Plasma and urine electrolytes should be carefully monitored and fluids restricted until there are clear signs of recovery.

Anticonvulsants such as phenobarbitone and phenytoin should be used if fits occur. The unconscious child may need referral to a neurosurgeon for intracranial pressure measurement and treatment with mannitol and dexamethasone.

COMPLICATIONS

Incomplete notification of meningitis by clinicians makes assessment of mortality difficult but this is probably around 5%. Convulsions occur in 20–30% of children, in most within the first 48–72 h of hospitalization. Persistence of fits is associated with a poor prognosis. Subdural collections of fluid are common particularly during infancy. Presenting features include fever, irritability, vomiting and a bulging fontanel and rapidly enlarging head. A diagnosis may be made from abnormal transillumination of the head. In one series subdural fluid could be aspirated from nine out of 59 children with meningitis under the age of 2. All were less than a year old and as might be expected most were associated with *H. influenzae* infection. In only two infants were cultures positive. Persistent fever during treatment may also be

Table 23.12 Antibiotics used in treatment of childhood septic meningitis

Antibiotic(s)	Dosage	Advantages	Disadvantages	Reference
Benzyl penicillin	240 mg/kg/day × 6	*S. pneumoniae* and *N. meningitis* sensitive	Uncommon *S. pneumoniae* resistance	Standard combination against which newer antibiotics evaluated
Or ampicillin And	200 mg–400 mg/kg/day × 6		*H. influenzae* resistant in 15%	See references below
chloramphenicol	100 mg/kg/day × 4 75 mg/kg/day after 48 h	Extremely good CSF penetration Oral absorption good Inexpensive	Aplastic anemia in 1/50 000 courses Blood chloramphenicol levels should be estimated	
Cefotaxime	200 mg/kg/day × 4	Single agent Good CSF penetration		Odio et al 1986
Ceftazidime	150 mg/kg/day × 4	Single agent Good CSF penetration for Gram-negative enteric pathogens		Rodriguez et al 1986
Ceftriaxone	100 mg/kg/day × 1	Good CSF penetration Single daily dose	Diarrhea	Congeni et al 1986
Cefuroxime	225 mg/kg/day × 3	Single daily dose	Slow clearance of *H. influenzae* from CSF	Marks et al 1986

associated with thrombophlebitis and viral infection. Hydrocephalus may develop and is characterized by irritability, vomiting, a tense fontanel (if still patent) and rapidly enlarging head. Investigations such as ultrasound or CT scan may be required for diagnosis of both subdural collections and hydrocephalus.

The commonest long-term complication of meningitis is sensorineural deafness. All children should undergo audiological assessment after recovery from infection. A number of studies have shown either unilateral or bilateral hearing loss in about 10% of children. In one series deafness occurred in 31% of children following *S. pneumoniae*, 10% following *N. meningitidis* and 6% following *H. influenzae* meningitis. Bilateral hearing loss occurred in about half of the children (Dodge et al 1984). In a recent prospective study from the UK, permanent sensorineural deafness was seen in only 3/124 (2.4%). In a prospective study of children with *H. influenzae* meningitis, 28% had major handicaps: 10% deafness, 15% impaired speech, 10% mental retardation, 3–7% motor abnormality and 2–8% fits. The mean IQ of these children was 11 points less than the controls (Sell 1983). This group appears to have been a highly selected one. Other studies have been unable to determine a significant effect of illness on IQ.

There is little evidence that the duration of illness prior to hospital admission has any relationship to development of long-term sequelae. Focal neurological signs present on admission may be prognostic of a low intelligence quotient at follow-up.

MENINGOCOCCAL MENINGITIS

Caused by a Gram-negative diplococcus it is the commonest type of meningitis in children. Over recent years there has been an increased incidence with very high rates in certain areas.

In cases associated with meningococcemia the typical petechial or purpuric rash is seen often preceded or accompanied by a maculopapular erythematous eruption (Plate 23.1). The symptoms and signs of meningitis are as described above. Mortality is high in children with septicemia who should be nursed in units where intensive care can be provided.

The antibiotic of choice is cefotaxime given intravenously (see above). As with meningococcal septicemia it is recommended that antibiotics are given once a clinical diagnosis has been made rather than after investigation. Prophylaxis is discussed elsewhere (p. 1315).

HAEMOPHILUS INFLUENZAE MENINGITIS (Hib)

This is caused by a Gram-negative encapsulated rod; the same organism is isolated from children with acute epiglottitis. This infection has become uncommon in the UK since the introduction of *H. influenzae* vaccine in 1992. Cefotaxime is the treatment of choice, although chloramphenicol which has good CSF penetration can be used (see Table 23.12).

PNEUMOCOCCAL MENINGITIS

Infection caused by the Gram-positive coccus is seen throughout childhood. It is thought to have a higher mortality and complication rate than either meningococcal or *H. influenzae* meningitis. Children with functional asplenia are at increased risk. Recurrent episodes of pneumococcal meningitis should alert the pediatrician to the possibility of a communication such as a

congenital sinus into the subdural space. Chloramphenicol is the treatment of choice.

STAPHYLOCOCCAL MENINGITIS

This infection may occur in children with indwelling catheters connecting the cerebral ventricles and either atrium or peritoneum. Signs may be those of other forms of acute bacterial meningitis with fever, vomiting and neck stiffness, or may be more subtle with irritability and fever. Diagnosis is made following isolation of coagulase-negative *S. epidermidis* from the CSF obtained at lumbar or ventricular puncture. Although antibiotics such as cloxacillin and rifampicin may appear effective relapse is common unless the shunt is removed. Infection is also seen in children with meningomyelocele, and following compound skull fracture.

PREVENTION OF MENINGITIS

Meningitis is thought to occur following invasion of bacteria from the nasal passages into the meninges. During infancy it may also follow bacteremia. Children may become ill within a short time of colonization by pathogenic bacteria or may harbor organisms for a considerable period before infection develops.

When an index case presents, other family members may be at increased risk of infection. The risk is highest for meningococcal disease, lower for *H. influenzae* b infection and very low for pneumococcus.

Consequently chemoprophylaxis should be made available for all family members when meningococcal infection is seen. It is only necessary to give antibiotic to the family of *H. influenzae* cases when there are nonimmunized children under the age of 4 in close contact. The child with meningococcal disease should also be given prophylaxis because many of the antibiotics administered for the treatment of meningitis (apart from ceftriaxone) do not eradicate pathogens from the nasopharynx.

Rifampicin is at present the agent of choice for meningococcal prophylaxis (10 mg/kg per dose 12-hourly four times); *H. influenzae prophylaxis* is 20 mg/kg per dose given once daily for 4 days.

Immunization is available for community outbreaks of meningococcal disease of types A, C and W but because the B type (most common in the UK at present) is of low immunogenicity, a B vaccine has proved difficult to produce. The vaccine is quadrivalent and consists of the purified capsular polysaccharides, and is given subcutaneously as a 0.5 ml dose. The vaccine offers protection from the A serotype from the age of 3 months and C from 2 years.

A conjugate vaccine against *H. influenzae* b (Hib) is in routine use in the UK and is given as part of the primary course of immunization at 2, 3 and 4 months (see Ch. 7). Children with functional asplenia are at increased risk of pneumococcal septicemia, and should receive pneumococcal vaccine although it would appear that prophylaxis with penicillin has a more important role in prevention of infection.

INFANTILE GASTROENTERITIS

Infantile gastroenteritis is a distinct clinicopathological entity in which the most important problems are those of dehydration and electrolyte loss of a degree seldom encountered in adult patients.

The age of these patients renders them more prone to severe diarrhea accompanied by vomiting, further enhancing the fluid and electrolyte loss. Although the mortality rate has been reduced in the developed countries it is still considerable in the developing countries where poor hygienic conditions and malnutrition are both responsible for the higher morbidity and mortality rates. In developing countries about 5 million children below 5 years of age die from diarrhea annually (Grant 1988), while in the USA 500 children aged from 1 month to 4 years die annually from diarrhea (Ho et al 1988).

ETIOLOGY

Infective

The frequency of positive cultures for bacteria or viruses from the stools varies directly as the assiduity with which these organisms are looked for. Positive bacterial cultures vary from 4% to 62% (Connor & Barrett-Connor 1967). The most prevalent organisms are enteropathogenic *Escherichia coli* of various strains, *Shigella, Salmonella, Campylobacter* and *Yersinia. Staphylococcus, Bacillus proteus, Clostridium difficile* and *Pseudomonas* may overgrow gut organisms during massive antibiotic therapy especially in debilitated infants, and cause a fulminating enterocolitis. In this connection, thrush diarrhea can also occur owing to superinfection by *Candida albicans.* Intestinal parasites such as amebae, roundworms and hookworms, though rare in infancy, occasionally occur in tropical countries and can cause diarrhea. Food poisoning due to staphylococcal toxin and *Salmonella* organisms occasionally affects infants.

Escherichia coli are among the commonest bacteria found in the human colon. Morphologically they cannot be distinguished from salmonellae or other enterobacteria on a Gram-stained film but can be differentiated by biochemical characteristics. More than 300 strains can be identified on the basis of antigenic characteristics – somatic (O), flagellar (H) and capsular (K) antigens. Of the many known strains more than 17 are recognized as being potentially pathogenic. Of these 0 111, 0 114, 0 119, 0 125, 0 126, 0 127, 0 128, 0 142, 0 26 and 0 55 have been found to be the pathogens of gastroenteritis in infancy. In older children acute diarrhea has been associated with infection with types 0 127, 0 136, 0 44 and 0 144. Pathogenic *E. coli* can be cultured from at least 2% of children under the age of 5 years. In adult subjects outbreaks of diarrheal illness have been attributed to infection with type 0 111. All of these strains may be found in older subjects who are without evidence of disease (a carrier rate of 1–2% has been found) presumably because of immunity developed as a result of earlier contact.

It is probable that *E. coli* infection plays some part in the etiology of 'traveler's' diarrhea which so commonly attacks new arrivals, especially in tropical countries.

Gastroenteritis due to *E. coli* has been designated enteropathogenic *Escherichia coli* disease and the epidemiological preventive and therapeutic aspects of the subject have been reviewed by South (1971).

Since the description by Bishop et al (1973) of a form of reovirus, referred to as rotavirus (or orbivirus or duovirus), which could be detected by electron microscopy in the feces of infants and children with gastroenteritis, many workers have confirmed that it is the commonest type of virus associated with the disease all over the world. Other viruses which can cause gastroenteritis include the enteroviruses such as Coxsackie, poliovirus and ECHO, and also adenoviruses (Isaacs et al 1986).

Parenteral

The role of parenteral infections in the causation of diarrhea is difficult to prove but in the large numbers of patients in whom stool cultures are negative it is often assumed that symptoms are due to infections elsewhere. In these circumstances secondary changes in the bacterial flora, intestinal juices, gastric acid and digestive enzymes may occur and cause diarrhea.

Dietetic

Fully breast-fed infants are unlikely to suffer from gastroenteritis owing to the protective effect of breast milk against it. Dietary indiscretions may cause diarrhea in infants but seldom do they produce acute severe diarrhea. Cow's milk allergy, though uncommon, can cause diarrhea with abdominal colic and vomiting.

Miscellaneous

This group comprises some conditions not caused by infective organisms which are likely to present with recurrent bouts of diarrhea. Infantile Hirschsprung's disease sometimes presents with acute explosive bouts of diarrhea alternating with constipation, and death can result from these acute episodes. Infants with disaccharide intolerance and other malabsorptive states such as celiac disease, fibrocystic disease of the pancreas, acrodermatitis enteropathica and protein-losing gastroenteropathy often suffer from diarrhea.

PATHOLOGY

The important lesion is biochemical rather than histological. In fatal cases, autopsy may reveal nothing more than hyperemia of the submucosa of the intestines. The lymphoid tissues may be prominent and occasionally shallow ulcers may be seen. It is only in the pseudomembranous type of enterocolitis caused by staphylococci or *Pseudomonas* that large areas of the mucous membrane may be denuded and replaced by a pseudomembrane composed of bacteria, exudate and cellular debris. Generally, therefore, there is no correlation between the pathological lesions and the clinical state.

In infantile gastroenteritis, water and electrolytes are lost in the stools. On average, 50 mmol/l of sodium; 35 mmol/l of potassium and 45 mmol/l of chloride are found in stool water in infantile gastroenteritis. In all such stool analyses reported, the sum of the concentrations of sodium and potassium always considerably exceeded the concentration of chloride, and this is an indication of the loss of bicarbonate ion. This results in metabolic acidosis, a common accompaniment of moderate and severe gastroenteritis. Besides the loss of water and electrolytes in the stools, the loss is accentuated if there is vomiting, and further losses occur via sweating and pulmonary ventilation. Thus, infants can be moribund after 1 or 2 days of diarrhea or even within a few hours. Infants with a poor nutritional state will be less able to stand up to these water and electrolyte losses.

The metabolic acidosis (standard bicarbonate < 17 mmol/l) due to loss of bicarbonate is often made worse by poor renal function (reflected in raised blood urea) secondary to dehydration, and by the ketosis that results from inadequate food intake. This acidosis tends to cause a shift of calcium ions from bones to the extracellular fluid but the serum calcium tends to be within normal limits during the acute stage. However, with correction of the dehydration and acidosis, in some patients hypocalcemic tetany may ensue as extracellular calcium re-enters the bones.

In the acute stage of dehydration, owing to egress of potassium from the cells, serum potassium levels may be within normal limits despite potassium losses in the stools.

Generally, the loss of electrolytes parallels the loss of water, so that extracellular electrolyte estimations reveal that the dehydration is of the isotonic variety. However, when the loss of water exceeds that of sodium owing to the administration of fluids of high sodium content, *hypernatremic* dehydration with hypertonicity of the extracellular fluid may occur. Hypernatremia (i.e. serum sodium more than 160 mmol/l) may cause subdural effusions and abnormal neurological signs (p. 414). On the other hand, if too much water is administered without an equivalent amount of sodium, *hypotonic* dehydration then results. Dehydration and infection may predispose to thrombosis of the cerebral and renal veins.

Transferable resistance among *E. coli* may introduce a therapeutic problem where this organism is involved. Strains of organism resistant to antibiotics may transfer their resistance to other organisms which have not been exposed to antibiotic.

CLINICAL FEATURES

Gastroenteritis affects chiefly children under 2 years of age and tends to be more severe in infants under 6 months of age in whom about half of all cases occur.

The most important clinical features are those consequent on water and electrolyte disturbances. Attention should be paid to the history in regard to the loss by diarrhea and vomiting, the amount of fluid retained by the infant, the amount and color of urine passed, any fever, breathlessness or drowsiness, loss of consciousness or fits. The infant should be weighed, and if the weight just prior to diarrhea is known, the difference gives an indication of the amount of fluid lost. A full clinical examination should be carried out, particular note being taken of the signs of dehydration, such as dryness of the mucosa, depressed fontanel, sunken eyes, loss of skin turgor and deep acidotic breathing.

From the practical point of view it is useful to be able to assess clinically the degree of dehydration both from the point of view of treatment and prognosis. Each patient can be placed in one of three categories, designated as mild, moderate or severe dehydration, depending on the clinical criteria presented in Table 23.13.

Although there will be a certain amount of overlap in the assessment of particular patients, in practice it is not difficult to group them. Fever tends to be associated with dehydration.

Blood in the stools can be seen in any case of infective diarrhea, but often it merely stains the stools and it is not copious except in the dysenteries. Perianal excoriation is more likely to occur with longstanding diarrhea but the characteristic redness with whitish plaques of thrush with generalized wasting is typical of thrush diarrhea.

Hypernatremic dehydration may be suspected clinically if the infant shows no sign of circulatory collapse in spite of considerable fluid loss. This type of dehydration gives the

Table 23.13 Symptoms in gastroenteritis according to degree of severity

Symptom or sign	Degree of dehydration		
	Mild	Moderate	Severe
Fever	Mild or high	Mild or high	High
Oliguria	Nil	Present	Anuria
Fits	Nil	Nil	May be present
State of consciousness	Fully conscious	Drowsy	May be in coma
Acidosis	Nil	May be present	Usually present
Fontanel	Normal	Normal	Depressed
Eyes	Normal	Slightly sunken	Obviously sunken
Skin turgor	Normal	Slightly reduced	Markedly reduced
Skin color	Normal	Normal	Mottled, cold and clammy

subcutaneous tissues a doughy feel. In addition, neurological signs such as convulsions, impaired consciousness, neck rigidity and increased response to stimuli may be present.

Cerebral venous thrombosis may produce neurological signs such as convulsions and disturbance of consciousness, and renal venous thrombosis, albuminuria and palpability of the affected kidney.

DIAGNOSIS AND DIFFERENTIAL DIAGNOSIS

The diagnosis of infantile gastroenteritis rests on the history and clinical signs of dehydration, if any. It is usually straightforward, but there are certain conditions which produce the same history and clinical findings in which the diarrhea is symptomatic of some important basic lesions and in which it is vital to detect the original lesion with a view to instituting appropriate specific therapy. Such conditions include the following.

Intussusception

An infant may present initially with loose stools tinged with blood. In infants episodes of abdominal pain may be unrecognized. The appearance of the stools may be indistinguishable from that due to gastroenteritis. It is only later that the typical redcurrant jelly stools are passed. Failure to recognize intussusception in time while treating the baby mistakenly for gastroenteritis will jeopardize his chances of recovery. Only a minority of babies with intussusception present in this manner. Most show the classical features of intussusception (p. 1786). In some instances, infants develop intussusception as a complication of gastroenteritis.

Septic meningitis

Parenteral diarrhea due to septic meningitis may focus attention only on the diarrhea. Some such infants do not show any of the classical signs of meningitis or fits, and even the fontanel may not be bulging because of dehydration caused by the diarrhea. A persistent leukocytosis often with an increased number of platelets, continued fever, vomiting and diarrhea in spite of treatment for this should alert the attending pediatrician to the possibility of septic meningitis.

Hirschsprung's disease

Some infants with Hirschsprung's disease present with severe and recurrent enterocolitis, starting in the neonatal period. The infant becomes extremely dehydrated and toxic, and the mortality rate is about 80% if the condition is unrecognized and not properly treated. Between attacks there is usually constipation with abdominal distention. The cause of these episodes of diarrhea is unknown but may be related to the high intraluminal pressure proximal to the aganglionic segment, facilitating infection by bacteria and viruses. A rectal biopsy will establish the diagnosis, and colostomy will prevent further attacks.

Thrush diarrhea and other superinfections

This may occur in premature and feeble neonates who initially contract infantile gastroenteritis. Overenthusiastic use of antibiotics may favour excessive growth of the fungus *Candida albicans*. There is often perianal erythema and ulceration with the typical whitish monilial plaques. The whole gastrointestinal tract may be infected and the perianal skin secondarily infected by the fungus-laden stools. Recognition of the condition and the timely use of oral nystatin, 500 000 to 2 million units per 24 h, may save the infants's life.

Antibiotic usage may also result in overwhelming growth of resistant bacteria, particularly resistant staphylococci, in the alimentary tract with a resulting infective enterocolitis.

Ankylostomiasis

Normally, hookworm infestation is rare in infancy, but when it occurs it is usually severe. Hookworm infestation in the older child does not usually result in diarrhea but in the infant it leads to severe diarrhea with consequent anemia and dehydration. Failure to diagnose the condition in time results invariably in death.

Chronic refractory diarrhea

There is a group of chronic refractive diarrheas which include cow's milk intolerance, disaccharidase and monosaccharidase deficiency, immunodeficiency, short-gut syndrome, familial chloride diarrhea, vipomas, intestinal lymphangiectasia, acrodermatitis enteropathica and other malabsorptive states.

TREATMENT

Preventive

Prevention of infantile gastroenteritis can be achieved by paying close attention to hygienic measures in the preparation of feeds and maintaining a high standard of hygiene generally. In the hospital nursery, strict observance of measures to prevent cross-infection is necessary, because the disease, once it has occurred, can spread very rapidly. Strict isolation of cases and of contacts and barrier nursing are necessary in the ward. Breast-feeding is an important preventive measure. Oral vaccines against rotaviruses are now available and they are given in three doses. They are safe and effective (Griffiths et al 1995).

Parenteral fluid therapy (see also Ch. 10)

The treatment of the infant with gastroenteritis depends on the etiology, if known, and on the degree of dehydration. Patients with moderate and severe dehydration need parenteral fluids and hence must be hospitalized, while infants with mild dehydration may be treated at home or on a hospital outpatient basis.

Mild cases

The majority of infants with gastroenteritis suffer mild attacks. It is best to take such cases off milk and solids for 12–24 h. This period of 'starvation' will ensure some degree of rest for the intestines. In place of milk or solids, watery fluids are given in small amounts frequently, e.g. hourly feeds, and this will obviate vomiting. A total daily intake of at least 180 ml/kg will be required. 5% dextrose with 0.4% sodium chloride drinks have been used for many years with good results. Higher concentrations of dextrose should not be given as this may aggravate the diarrhea. After 12–24 h, when diarrhea is reduced, quarter-strength milk is given for 24 h, then half-strength and so on till gradually full-strength milk is taken without recurrence of the diarrhea. Solids can then be reintroduced at this stage.

Moderate or severe cases

When the dehydration is moderate or severe, the infant should be hospitalized as parenteral fluid therapy will be necessary. Fluids should be given intravenously, as fluids given by the subcutaneous route are absorbed erratically and too slowly for efficacious treatment. In infants, intravenous fluids can be given by scalp vein infusion or into a limb vein (pp. 1836–1838).

There are three main aspects of fluid therapy in infantile gastroenteritis, namely the type of repair fluid, the amount, and the rate at which it is administered. There are many regimes in use but there is little substantial difference between them. The following regime is simple and has been used for many years and found to be satisfactory. It is desirable, but not necessary, to have serum electrolyte estimations before starting off intravenous therapy.

First, the degree of dehydration is gauged from the history and clinical examination (using the criteria in Table 23.13), and the baby is weighed. If dehydration is very severe, with signs of peripheral vascular failure, it can be assumed that the infant has lost fluid equivalent to 10% of his bodyweight, with less severe dehydration 7–8%, and with moderate dehydration 5%. These assumptions are made because in most instances the weight of the baby just prior to the onset of the diarrhea is unknown so that the actual amount of fluid lost cannot be calculated. For example, if the baby weighs 10 kg and has moderate dehydration (i.e. 5% dehydration), the fluid lost is 5% of 10 kg = 500 ml. This amount must be replaced and is termed replacement fluid.

At the same time, the baby will have continued with normal fluid losses, and the amount necessary to replace these may be calculated as shown in Table 23.14.

This amount is termed maintenance fluid, and in our example above, the 10-kg baby (aged between 1 and 2 years) will need approximately 1000 ml. The total amount to be given intravenously over the first 24 h is the sum of the replacement and maintenance fluids, i.e. 500 + 1000 = 1500 ml. Half of this amount (i.e. 750 ml) is to be given in the first 8 h, and the other

Table 23.14 Approximate daily fluid requirements related to patient age

Age	Approximate daily fluid requirement
Up to 12 months	150 ml/kg body weight (70 ml/lb) up to a maximum of 1000 ml
1–2 years	100 ml/kg body weight (45 ml/lb)
2–4 years	90 ml/kg body weight (40 ml/lb)

half over the next 16 h. The rates at which these fluids are to be delivered will have to be adjusted so that these amounts will be administered in the stated times. Microdrip sets are readily available now and volumes delivered over a set period of time can be determined, preset as required beforehand and expressed as drops per minute. The continuing pathological fluid loss should be roughly assessed during the first 24 h, and this is added to the next 24 hours' therapy.

The next problem is the *type* of repair fluid to be used. For replacement therapy (i.e. over the first 8 h) half-strength isotonic saline containing 0.45% sodium chloride and 2.5% dextrose can be used. This solution contains 77 mmol/l of sodium and is a safe and effective replacement fluid for infantile gastroenteritis. Suitable maintenance fluids are quarter-strength isotonic saline containing 0.23% sodium chloride and 3.75% dextrose or one-fifth-strength isotonic saline containing 0.18% sodium chloride and 4.3% dextrose. In the example quoted above, 750 ml of half-strength isotonic saline solution would be given over the first 8 h and the other 750 ml of maintenance fluid (one-fifth or one-quarter strength) given over the next 16 h.

In addition to the fluid and electrolyte replacement therapy outline above, there are the problems of metabolic acidosis and potassium needs. In severe dehydration with marked acidosis, it is desirable to have the plasma bicarbonate estimated on admission so that the acidosis can be corrected with sodium bicarbonate solution. The deficit of bicarbonate in mmol/l can be calculated from the difference between the plasma bicarbonate in the patient and normal: the amount of sodium bicarbonate needed to correct the acidosis is calculated from the formula: 0.058 g of sodium bicarbonate per kg body weight would raise the plasma bicarbonate concentration approximately 1 mmol/l. Based on this, the amount necessary is given intravenously within the first 8-h period, and the volume given is subtracted from the volume calculated for replacement fluid. For example, if in the patient above the plasma bicarbonate is 10 mmol/l, the deficit is approximately 10 mmol/l (20 mmol/l–10 mmol/l). If 4.2% $NaHCO_3$ solution (one millequivalent or 0.84 g/2 ml) is used the volume needed to raise the plasma bicarbonate by 1 mmol/l is 1.4 ml/kg bodyweight. Therefore, the volume needed is $1.4 \times 10 \times 10 = 140$ ml, and the amount of replacement fluid to be given is modified to 750 ml – 140 ml = 610 ml. Alternatively, if base excess measurements are available the procedure described on page 421 can be used.

Although the serum potassium is usually within normal limits during the acute stage of dehydration, the total body potassium is reduced. After rehydration has been effected and urine passed, the serum potassium may fall. It is probably better not to give potassium at the beginning, but when urine is passed, potassium in the form of Darrow's solution can be given intravenously in a volume of approximately 100 ml/kg bodyweight, given over the first 24 h. When Darrow's solution is given the volume is subtracted likewise from the total volume of fluids to be given

over the first 24 h. Otherwise potassium can be given as indicated on page 411.

Although the above regimen is outlined in some detail, the amounts, rates and types of fluid recommended serve only as a working guide. The pediatrician cannot leave the patient totally to the care of the nursing staff with instructions as to amount and rates of fluid to be delivered within 24 h. He must reassess the infant time and time again especially during the critical first hours and be prepared to make changes in the intravenous fluid therapeutic regime as and when necessary to suit changing needs.

In moderate and severe cases no oral feeds should be given during the first 24 h since the fluid needs are being met intravenously. Another reason for omitting oral feeds is that these infants are often drowsy, and may be immobilized to some extent by restrainers because of the drip, so that if vomiting should occur, aspiration into the lungs is a distinct possibility.

Oral rehydration solutions (ORS)

Following experience in the use of ORS in the treatment of cholera, it was later found that mild and moderate degrees of dehydration in infantile diarrhea can be treated totally by oral dehydration therapy. The standard World Health Organization ORS enjoyed widespread use in developing countries and this confirmed the usefulness of ORS. However, the use of WHO ORS met with certain problems such as cost, inability to dilute the salts correctly, use of contaminated water, deterioration of the packet contents, etc. A cheaper and equally effective method of ORS using boiled rice water was advocated as an alternative (Wong 1981), and since then rice-based ORS have been shown to be sterile, cheap, effective and acceptable in developing countries (Mehta & Subramaniam 1986, Roesel & Schaffter 1989). It is considered that the use of ORS in infantile diarrhea may substantially reduce the large number of deaths in developing countries.

Antibiotics and chemotherapy

The place of antibiotics and chemotherapy in the treatment of infantile gastroenteritis is a matter of some controversy. Although most of the agglutinable *E. coli* isolated from cases of gastroenteritis are sensitive to a wide range of antibiotics there is little evidence that antibiotics benefit such cases and may merely lead to drug resistance which has already proved to be a problem in certain epidemics.

Likewise in cases of viral origin chemotherapy will be ineffective and may be harmful in producing superinfection. In general, antibiotics may be justified in the treatment of cholera, *Shigella* dysentery, some cases of *E. coli* diarrhea, *Clostridium difficile* diarrhea, *Salmonella* diarrhea with parenteral infection and a few other bacterial diarrheas.

Other symptomatic treatment

The use of the so-called absorbents such as kaolin and pectin in infantile gastroenteritis is of doubtful value and similarly opiates and allied drugs to reduce gastrointestinal mobility can be only symptomatic in their effect. They may, however, reduce the number of stools without affecting the primary lesion itself and may serve a purpose in allaying unnecessary worry on the part of parents of infants with mild gastroenteritis.

The treatment of parenteral diarrhea is, of course, the treatment of the primary disorder.

Management in recovery

After about 24 h, when the patient is seen to be fully conscious and dehydration and electrolyte deficits corrected, oral feeds can be offered. First bland fluids should be given and then milk formula in increasing concentrations as outlined for infants with mild gastroenteritis. When the infant is able to retain the oral feeds, and diarrhea is seen to be diminished or nonexistent, the intravenous drip can be removed. After this, in most instances, the infant will recover fully in 4 or 5 days. Occasionally, the severely dehydrated and acidotic infant, after correction of deficits, may exhibit signs of hypocalcemic tetany, when calcium gluconate injections may have to be given (5 ml/kg of 10% solution per 24 h in divided doses i.v.). In patients suffering from anemia and malnutrition at the same time blood or plasma transfusions may have to be given.

In a small minority of infants suffering from what is termed malignant or refractory diarrhea, the measures described above fail to stop the diarrhea, and fail to correct the fluid and electrolyte deficits. Even oral bland fluids result in a brisk and copious diarrhea, rapidly terminating in death. Under these circumstances, parenteral alimentation by the intravenous route (p. 1223) using synthetic amino acids, glucose and lipids (if available, and if not, plasma from blood donors after a fatty meal – postprandial plasma – will suffice), with vitamins and electrolytes will often give sufficient time for the intestinal epithelium to be repaired, so that oral feedings may then be tolerated. Though the central venous route with plastic catheters may be used for delivery of these parenteral foods, lack of suitable facilities may lead to secondary bacteremia and fungemia. Since scalp veins are freely available for intravenous feeding in infants, the use of scalp vein needles for peripheral delivery, with daily changes of veins, is equally effective.

PROGNOSIS

In severe epidemics the mortality may be as high as 50%. Early diagnosis and the effective control of fluid and electrolyte status are the primary factors in ensuring a satisfactory prognosis.

BACTERIAL INFECTIONS

THE USE OF THE BACTERIOLOGY LABORATORY BY THE PEDIATRICIAN

The diagnosis and treatment of infectious diseases are based on the detection and identification of the etiologic agent. The clinical microbiology laboratory specializes in the microscopic examination, isolation, identification and susceptibility testing of microorganisms. The quality of the specimen submitted will influence the number and type of the organisms isolated and, in turn, the clinical significance of the report. Equally, the request form which accompanies the specimen should provide the laboratory with sufficient clinical information for the paper processing of the specimen and interpretation of results. Thus, in addition to basic demographic data, information regarding the child's condition, antibiotic treatment and immune status is of great importance. Where unusual pathogens are suspected details of recent travel or potential exposure should also be included.

The safety of laboratory personnel is a major consideration in microbiology laboratories. Where there is a known or perceived high risk, the samples and request forms should be clearly marked 'Danger of Infection' by the sender and handled accordingly.

THE NATURE, COLLECTION AND TRANSPORTATION OF SPECIMENS FOR BACTERIAL EXAMINATION

Frequently, the laboratory receives inadequate amounts of sample for microscopic examination and the multiple cultures required to cover the range of potential pathogens.

The 'ideal' specimen is aseptically obtained fresh pus, fluid or tissue that is rapidly and safely transported to the laboratory. Swabs represent a convenient and economical method of specimen collection but they should not be sent if fluid or pus can be obtained. Certainly, swabs without a buffer-type nonnutritive transport medium (Stuart's or Amies) should not be used since they allow the specimen to dry out with resultant loss of microbial viability. This is particularly important where clinically significant bacteria are present in low numbers, or anaerobes are involved.

All specimens should be delivered to the laboratory as soon as possible. Where it is not possible for specimens to reach the laboratory timeously, they can be refrigerated, but it should be remembered that the result may not be optimal. *Neisseria* and anaerobic bacteria in particular may not survive refrigeration and these samples should be held at room temperature and processed as soon as possible.

BLOOD CULTURES

The detection of living microorganisms in the blood of a sick child has great diagnostic and prognostic importance. Blood should be obtained for culture from any child who has a fever ($\geq 38°C$) or hypothermia ($\leq 36°C$), leukocytosis or neutropenia (< 1000 polymorphs/ml) or any combination of the above. In addition, blood cultures are complementary to cultures of urine and cerebrospinal fluid and swabs from throat, umbilicus and ear in the investigation of neonates with suspected sepsis whose only clinical findings in addition to fever or hypothermia may be poor feeding and failure to thrive.

To detect bacteremia or fungemia at least one viable microorganism must be present in the sample of blood cultured. The volume cultured is relatively more important than the medium or atmosphere of incubation in the detection of sepsis. In infants and young children 1–5 ml per culture and in older children 10 ml per culture give optimal recovery (Szymczak et al 1979).

The number and timing of blood cultures should take into consideration the pathophysiology of bacteremia. Ideally blood should be obtained for culture during the hour before the spike since there is usually a lag of 1 h between the influx of bacteria and the onset of pyrexia. In practice, however, most samples are obtained after the fever. In children with unexplained fever two separate blood cultures initially, repeated 24–36 h later, give optimal recovery on culture.

When initial culturing is unsuccessful, blind repetition of cultures is expensive and often unhelpful. In these circumstances, discussion between microbiologist and clinician is strongly recommended.

A major problem in the interpretation of pediatric blood cultures is their contamination by skin microorganisms. To minimize this, the skin should always be cleansed with 70% isopropyl alcohol prior to venepuncture. Any blood culture isolate must be evaluated critically in relation to the clinical findings in the patient.

SPECIMENS FROM THE CENTRAL NERVOUS SYSTEM

Specimens of cerebrospinal fluid must be collected aseptically and submitted to the laboratory in sterile containers. The range of microbiological and immunological tests which can detect infectious agents in cerebrospinal fluid make it essential that an adequate volume of sample is received. When the volume collected is small, the microbiology laboratory may be compelled to centrifuge the whole sample and culture the deposit while referring the supernatant for serological study or biochemical analysis.

In the past the only technique for rapid detection of microbes was direct microscopy. This has now been supplemented by noncultural techniques such as antigen detection by latex agglutination in CSF or urine (concentrated) or more recently identification of organism-specific nucleic acid sequences by polymerase chain reaction (PCR) techniques. These are particularly useful in the diagnosis of meningitis where antibiotic therapy may have been commenced prior to hospital admission.

Where there is a brain abscess, pus should be aspirated and sent to the laboratory in a container which maintains the viability of any anaerobes present.

SPECIMENS FROM THE UPPER RESPIRATORY TRACT

In the case of the child with a sore throat it is not clinically possible to distinguish a self-limiting viral infection from a specific bacterial infection which requires antibiotic treatment. Diagnosis is best obtained by the laboratory. The diagnosis is made by isolating a putative pathogen from the mass of indigenous commensal respiratory tract flora. Even so the mere isolation of a potential pathogen should not necessarily be equated with pathogenicity since many of the organisms, e.g. β-hemolytic Lancefield group A streptococci, are frequently found in the carrier state. Consequently, pediatricians must make initial diagnostic decisions on clinical probabilities rather than proof and revise therapy later if necessary in the light of information received from the laboratories. A well-taken throat swab from both tonsillar areas and posterior pharynx is essential. In this instance a transport medium swab is not recommended as group A streptococci survive for days on albumin-coated or Dacron swabs and may be overgrown by normal flora if transport medium is used.

Cultures take at least 24 h to yield results. Recently, rapid (10–15 min) tests based on latex agglutination or enzyme-linked immunoassay for the detection of group A streptococcal antigen in throat swabs have offered a potential means of instituting early specific treatment and thereby minimizing morbidity (Kaplan 1988). The sensitivity and specificity of these assays compared to plate culture are 89–90% and 90–100% respectively. Thus caution must be observed if negative results are obtained where there is a high clinical index of suspicion and particularly if there is an increased incidence of acute streptococcal infection and its

complications such as rheumatic fever in the area (Kaplan & Hill 1987).

In acute epiglottitis, *H. influenzae* type b is invariably implicated but direct swabbing is contraindicated because the irritation may trigger complete respiratory obstruction and the isolation of *H. influenzae* may simply reflect local contamination. Blood cultures are the key to confirming the diagnosis.

Tracheostomy and endotracheal tubes compromise the defense mechanisms which protect the lower airways resulting in colonization within 24 h by Gram-negative organisms and potential pathogens from the environment regardless of the clinical status of the child. Interpretation of culture results requires careful correlation with clinical features.

Transtracheal aspiration provides a method for obtaining lower airway secretions free from contamination and may be particularly useful in cases of severe infection where noninvasive techniques have been unhelpful or obscure pathology is suspected.

Nasopharyngeal specimens are helpful in diagnosing pertussis and diphtheria and in identifying carriers of staphylococci or meningococci. The specimen of choice for the diagnosis of whooping cough is mucus from the posterior nasopharynx collected either by means of a flexible wire pernasal swab or suction catheter (Onorato & Wassilak 1987). Since *Bordetella pertussis* is particularly susceptible to drying it is advisable to employ transport medium. A rapid immunofluorescent test may give a presumptive diagnosis.

The diagnosis of thrush can be confirmed by finding numerous yeast cells on a direct smear of a visible white patch of exudate but not simply by culture of *Candida* from a mouth or throat swab since *Candida* is present in small numbers in the normal oral and pharyngeal flora.

Middle ear infection is one of the most frequent infections of infants and young children. To be sure of the causative agent tympanocentesis is required as cultures of throat and nasopharynx may be misleading.

SPECIMENS FROM THE LOWER RESPIRATORY TRACT

The significance of the results of sputum culture is largely dependent on the quality and source of the original sample and the organisms isolated. Some, such as *Mycobacterium tuberculosis*, are invariably pathogenic whereas others such as pneumococci may be part of the normal oropharyngeal flora and simply contaminants. Some contamination is virtually inevitable with expectorated sputum and nasopharyngeal aspirates. Previous antimicrobial administration will further complicate matters. Expectorated sputum from children receiving antimicrobial agents will commonly grow organisms resistant to the agent administered. This altered indigenous flora of the oropharynx invariably represents 'sputum superinfection' and not superinfection of the child. Ideally, specimens of expectorated sputum should be obtained with the help of the physiotherapist.

The diagnosis of the etiology of pneumonia in children is often difficult since positive cultures from blood or pleural fluid are obtained in only 10–20% cases. Other than by deep tracheal suction, adequate respiratory tract specimens are difficult to obtain from children.

Specimens obtained by invasive procedures such as bronchoscopy including aspirates, brushings and transbronchial biopsies may be particularly useful where mycobacteria, legionellae and other opportunistic pathogens are implicated in immunocompromised patients with severe infection.

URINE SPECIMENS

Nowhere is the collection, storage and transport of specimens more important than in the laboratory diagnosis of urinary tract infections. Urine is an excellent culture medium and contaminating perineal bacteria can multiply in specimens standing at room temperature, invalidating the results of both microscopy and culture. Specimens which cannot be handled immediately should be refrigerated and examined within 24 h or alternatively sample bottles containing boric acid should be used. The latter inhibits overgrowth of bacteria and preserves the pus cells for microscopic examination. Early morning specimens are ideal as overnight incubation in the bladder yields high bacterial counts.

It is imperative that the accompanying request form contains details of the clinical diagnosis, the method and time of collection and any current antimicrobial therapy.

Depending on the age and clinical condition of the child, urine specimens can be collected by clean-catch midstream urine technique, from an indwelling catheter, or urine bag specimen or preferably suprapubic aspiration in babies.

The clean-catch midstream specimen largely eliminates the risk of introducing infection but small numbers of urethral flora may be present.

When the child has an indwelling catheter, urine specimens should not be collected from the drainage bag. To ensure a fresh specimen of urine the tube of the drainage bag should be clamped, the sampling port or band cleaned with a medicated swab, and the urine sample aspirated with a needle and syringe.

Culture of bag urine specimens collected before a feed with the baby held in an upright position can help to eliminate a diagnosis of urinary infection but suprapubic aspiration is the preferred method for establishing an accurate diagnosis or clarifying equivocal bag specimen results.

Suprapubic bladder aspiration is particularly helpful in confirming infection in neonates and small children. The investigation is always diagnostic, any bacterial growth indicating bladder infection. However, screening of neonates for bacteriuria is not justified.

In the untreated child, whether symptomatic or asymptomatic, pure cultures of $> 10^5$ bacteria/ml are indicative of infection. Mixed growths imply contamination and a carefully collected repeat sample is indicated.

Urine microscopy should always be performed to establish the presence or absence of white cells (pyuria). The absence of pyuria does not preclude a diagnosis of infection. It should be remembered that the rate of white cell excretion is increased in pyrexial children and this may complicate the interpretation of a negative or equivocal culture result. Equally, white cells may appear in the urine as a result of local tissue inflammation, e.g. vulva, vagina or prepuce. A carefully collected repeat specimen will usually resolve this problem. Pyuria in the absence of a significant culture result should be investigated further. Repeated 'sterile pyuria' should raise the possibility of renal tuberculosis and a series of three consecutive early morning specimens of urine should be submitted.

The rapid chemical screening dipstick tests for urinary tract infection such as the leukocyte esterase test for pyuria and the nitrite test for bacteriuria currently lack sensitivity and specificity. None can supplant quantitative culture for confirmation and precise identification of the causative organisms and appropriate sensitivity testing where indicated.

Bacteriological quantitative dip slides consist of a flat paddle coated with selective and nonselective agar media, which is dipped into the urine, replaced in its container and incubated to give a rough quantitative estimate of the viable count.

SPECIMENS FROM THE INTESTINAL TRACT

The ideal specimen for the diagnosis of bacterial gastroenteritis is freshly passed feces. Specimens should be obtained as near to the acute onset of symptoms as possible and transported to the laboratory without undue delay. The yield of enteric bacterial pathogens from culture of feces is much greater than from rectal swabs which if used should be sent in transport medium.

While the immediate clinical concern in a child with acute diarrhea is appropriate rehydration, the identification of the infecting agent may provide invaluable information about possible clinical complications, infectivity, sources of infection, potential for spread to contacts, and the appropriateness of antibiotic therapy.

Given the frequency of mild gastrointestinal upset in children, attempts have been made to define clinical symptom complexes with a high predictive value for positive bacterial culture. The combination of watery stools, fever and blood (Kaplan et al 1980), and the sudden onset of frequent diarrhea without vomiting (De Witt et al 1985) have been positively associated.

With the ever increasing range of potential gastrointestinal pathogens it is important that any relevant clinical and epidemiological information is noted on the request form, e.g. recent antibiotic therapy, consumption of seafood meal, attendance at day nursery or contact with sick pet. This will ensure that the appropriate screening cultures are performed.

PROCEDURES FOR PROTOZOA AND HELMINTHS

The laboratory diagnosis of most protozoal and helminthic infections rests on the detection of the parasite or its cysts or ova in feces, urine (*Schistosoma haematobium*) or thick and thin blood films (malaria, babesiosis, trypanosomiasis and filariasis). Some filaria exhibit cyclical variation in parasitemia and hence blood for detection of *Wuchereria bancrofti* and *Loa loa* should be collected around midnight or noon respectively. Consultation with the laboratory to ensure appropriate specimens are submitted is essential.

SEXUALLY TRANSMITTED DISEASE

The isolation of a sexually transmitted disease pathogen from a child is presumed to be evidence of sexual abuse (Beck-Sague & Alexander 1987). The whole range of sexually transmitted diseases can be acquired and specimens (swabs in charcoal transport medium) should be taken from pharynx, rectum and vaginal introitus. It is important to warn the laboratory if sexual abuse is suspected as there will be a need to store any isolates for possible typing in the event of legal proceedings. If rapid antigen detection methods are used in such cases the results should be interpreted with extreme caution particularly where cultural confirmation is lacking.

SEROLOGICAL DIAGNOSIS

Immunological techniques are performed in the microbiology laboratory to measure the immune response to organisms particularly those for which isolation by culture is not possible, to establish or confirm a presumptive diagnosis, to assess the level of protective immunity whether naturally acquired or vaccine induced or to indicate the etiologic infective trigger of an ongoing immunological disease process, e.g. glomerulonephritis, reactive arthritis. The selection of the appropriate test and the timing of samples depend on the stage of the disease, the nature of the infectious agent and, in particular, the characteristics of the immunological response to that agent.

Serological diagnosis based on antibody detection is an indirect method of diagnosing an infection and as such cannot supplant isolation of the organism or direct antigen detection in tissues or fluid. Technical aspects regarding methodology and choice of test need not concern the pediatrician but the laboratory should be provided with adequate pertinent detail to enable the appropriate test to be performed. Thus, in the child suspected of having a recent infection, or the newborn with possible intrauterine infection, it is necessary to measure specifically the IgM antibody. Otherwise, it is essential to obtain an early acute or baseline serum sample and an appropriately timed convalescent sample in order to demonstrate a rising titer of IgG antibodies. As ever, the most efficient service will result from effective communication between the pediatricians and their laboratory counterparts.

MONITORING ANTIMICROBIAL THERAPY

Once the pediatrician has embarked on an antibiotic regimen, the microbiology laboratory can monitor the levels of the antimicrobial agent in blood and other body fluids to establish whether adequate therapeutic levels are being achieved or potentially toxic levels are present. This can be particularly important in neonates and young children where there can be wide individual variation in the levels resulting from standard dosage and there is a narrow margin between therapeutic and toxic levels. In addition, in the management of bacterial endocarditis, it is important to assess the bactericidal effect of the patient's serum against the offending organism.

ANTHRAX

HISTORY AND EPIDEMIOLOGY

Well known in antiquity, medical interest in anthrax waned after the development of successful vaccines and the arrival of penicillin but it remains a potential danger if the normal procedures of control are upset (Turnbull 1986). *Bacillus anthracis* was a candidate agent for biological warfare until the signing of the Biological Weapons Convention in 1972. A 1979 epidemic of human anthrax in the Russian city of Sverdlovsk, although attributed to tainted meat, raised suspicions of an accident at a biological warfare installation. Spores of *B. anthracis* persisted in the soil of the Scottish island of Gruinard for over 40 years after tests during World War II until decontamination in the mid-1980s. In the early 1980s a series of reports from Zimbabwe described a major epidemic resulting from breakdown of the livestock vaccination program during the insurgency. In developed countries a handful of cases occur each year in adults whose occupation involves the handling of infected animal products such as furs, hides, feeding stuffs and carcasses. It is rare in children.

CLINICAL MANIFESTATIONS

Cutaneous anthrax is the commonest presentation but infected spores can also enter the body by inhalation (*woolsorters' disease*) or by the ingestion of contaminated meat (*gastrointestinal anthrax*). Septicemia and hemorrhagic meningitis may occur as secondary manifestations.

For *cutaneous anthrax* the incubation period is 2–5 days but most cases develop within 48 h of exposure. At the site of cutaneous infection a papule develops which itches then vesicates containing clear serous or bloodstained fluid. The underlying tissue becomes swollen and edematous and secondary vesicles tend to form in the periphery of the primary lesion. The latter enlarges and the center becomes hemorrhagic and necrotic leaving a black eschar. Regional lymph nodes become involved. Constitutional symptoms in the form of malaise, pyrexia, headache and arthralgia are usual. The white cell count is raised.

Intestinal anthrax is particularly uncommon in children but a recent case in Iran demonstrates the importance of considering the diagnosis in endemic areas if gastrointestinal symptoms follow the ingestion of contaminated or uncooked meats (Alizad et al 1995).

DIAGNOSIS

1. Detection of *B. anthracis* by direct Gram-staining of fluid from a vesicle.
2. Fluorescent antibody identification of the organisms in vesicle fluid.
3. Fourfold or greater rise in antibody titer in paired sera by an ELISA test.

TREATMENT

Penicillin is the antibiotic of choice and is given parenterally for a 7-day course. Ciprofloxacin, erythromycin and chloramphenicol are also effective. Treatment for systemic anthrax should include not only vigorous antibiotic therapy (e.g. high dose i.v. penicillin), but the provision of the other supportive measures usually required for the critically ill child (LaForce 1994).

PREVENTION AND CONTROL

Protective clothing, good hygiene and programs of livestock vaccination are the most important elements in control. A cell-free vaccine is available for human use but is restricted to those persons at significant occupational risk and has not been licensed for use in children.

BARTONELLOSIS

Bartonellosis consists of a sandfly-borne infection, which is confined to South America and is endemic in some Andean valleys – in Peru, Ecuador, Columbia, Chile and Guatemala (Dooley 1980, Scott 1996). It is caused by *Bartonella bacilliformis*, a motile, flagellated Gram-negative coccobacillus (1–2 × 0.2–0.5 μm). Bartonella-like bacteria, which are also hemotropic, have been reported from Thailand, Pakistan, Sudan, Niger and eastern USA, but their relationship to *B. bacilliformis* is unclear. The acute febrile form of the disease is associated with severe hemolysis and a high mortality rate (Oroya fever); the chronic (benign) form presents with verrucous skin eruptions: *verruga peruana*. The disease has been known in Peru for many centuries, and the acute form produced a high mortality rate (> 7000) during construction of the Trans-Andean Railway between Lima and Oroya in the 1870s. In 1885, a Peruvian medical student Carrión inoculated himself with material from a verruca, developed Oroya fever and subsequently died; the causative organism was first demonstrated within erythrocytes by Barton in 1905. The sandfly vector *Lutzomyia verrucarum* (certain other species are also involved) was first incriminated by Townsend in 1912. The main reservoir lies in asymptomatic human cases; no animal reservoir has been demonstrated.

PATHOLOGY

After inoculation into the skin by the infected sandfly, *B. bacilliformis* proliferates in the vascular epithelium and subsequently invades erythrocytes (virtually all may be affected, containing up to 20 bacilli) in which rapid multiplication gives rise to hemolysis and hepatosplenic erythrophagocytosis (Benson et al 1986). The acute events subside as chronicity ensues; as bacilli decrease in number in peripheral erythrocytes they tend to assume coccoid features. During the chronic phase, cutaneous (Bhutto et al 1994) and noncutaneous verrucous lesions resembling pyogenic granulomata develop; the well-defined nonencapsulated nodules consist of prominent endothelial cells and an associated lymphohistiocytic inflammatory infiltrate. These highly vascular nodules are eventually replaced by fibrous tissue.

CLINICAL FEATURES

The incubation period is variable; in Oroya fever the mean is about 3 weeks and sometimes less (Scott 1996), and in those with skin lesions or positive blood cultures significantly longer. Oroya fever usually begins insidiously with headache, low grade intermittent fever and anorexia; however, an acute onset with a higher fever, profuse sweating and impaired consciousness also occurs. Bone, joint and muscle pains may be severe, together with anemia (occasionally accompanied by thrombocytopenia) and its sequelae. Pallor, jaundice, generalized lymphadenopathy, mild hepatosplenomegaly, and occasionally hemorrhagic manifestations may be apparent on physical examination. The reticulocyte count may approach 50%, and peripheral blood may contain nucleated cells; a polymorphonuclear leukocytosis is often present; CSF may show a pleocytosis with many intracellular organisms. The acute illness usually runs for 3–4 weeks although death may occur after 10 days; untreated a 10–40% mortality rate is likely – two-thirds of deaths result from infective complications. The most important is *Salmonella* sp. (usually *S. typhimurium*) infection (with its usual clinical manifestations) which occurs during convalescence from Oroya fever; this complication is present in 40–50% and results from interference with intracellular killing and reticuloendothelial blockade; untreated, a mortality rate of 90% is likely. Tuberculosis, brucellosis, bacterial pneumonias, malaria and *Entamoeba histolytica* infection are other associated infections.

Before the development of verrucous lesions, other clinical manifestations including phlebitis, parotitis, meningoencephalitis (which carries a high mortality rate), erythemas, myalgias and pruritus may occur in the partly immune host. The skin lesions appear on the extensor extremities, face, scalp, genitalia or in a generalized distribution at from one to several months later; soft, circular, erythematous (hemangioma-like) papules rapidly enlarge and reach a diameter varying from 3 to 5 mm (miliary) to several centimeters (nodular) – the latter may be tumor-like and sometimes ulcerate, bleed profusely after even mild trauma, and/or become secondarily infected. Similar lesions can develop throughout the gastrointestinal and genitourinary tracts. As the lesions heal, they flatten, become less erythematous and leave hypopigmented macules surrounded by a zone of hyperpigmentation. They should be differentiated from yaws, secondary syphilis, fibrosarcomas and angiomas.

DIAGNOSIS

Clinical diagnosis during the acute phase is confirmed by demonstrating intraerythrocytic bacteria in a Giemsa-stained thin peripheral blood film (Scott 1996); definitive diagnosis is dependent on isolation of *B. bacilliformis* from a blood culture using the appropriate media. In the chronic phase, the cutaneous lesions (in the presence of a consistent history) usually make the diagnosis straightforward; a Giemsa-stained skin biopsy provides confirmation (Recavarren & Lumbreras 1972). Asymptomatic carriers of *B. bacilliformis* can usually be identified by blood culture. Serological tests are of value in epidemiological studies.

TREATMENT

The chemotherapeutic agent of choice is chloramphenicol (which is also effective against *Salmonella* sp.) four times daily for 5 days (Scott 1996); penicillin, streptomycin, tetracyclines (contraindicated in young children) and co-trimoxazole are also effective. Defervescence usually takes 8–12 h. Blood transfusion and other supportive measures are necessary in the management of acute Oroya fever. Large chronic verrucous lesions do not usually require chemotherapy but excision is occasionally necessary. Recovery confers lasting immunity. Prevention depends on individual protection between dusk and dawn in endemic areas; vector control (*L. verrucarum* penetrates netting with < 8 meshes per cm) with DDT or another insecticide is effective. There is no vaccine.

BOTULISM

ETIOLOGY

Botulism, a rare systemic disease characterized by neurological paralysis, results from the effects of toxins, produced by an anaerobic sporing bacillus, *Clostridium botulinum*, on myoneural junctions in voluntary muscle. In older children this results from ingestion of preformed toxin in food. In infants, ingestion of spores is followed by colonization of the gut with vegetative organisms and subsequent elaboration and absorption of toxin (Wigginton & Thill 1993).

A number of types of *Cl. botulinum* are known to produce toxin, of which types A, B and E are associated with human disease. The organism is widespread in the inanimate environment and contamination of food by soils containing types A and B is usually responsible for human cases (Ball & Farrell 1979). Type E is found in freshwater or inshore marine environments and fish or marine mammals are the usual food vehicle (Ball et al 1979). The source of infant botulism is not clear but the use of wild honey as an infant milk sweetener has been implicated in some cases in the USA and most in Japan.

Botulinum toxin is produced only by vegetative organisms under anaerobic conditions. Thus, except in infants, ingestion of spore-contaminated fresh foods is quite safe. Problems arise in storage of inadequately preserved food. Canned or bottled foodstuffs, especially soil-contaminated vegetables, must be subjected to high temperatures to inactivate spores, and inadequate processing, whether by home bottlers or commercial canners, may risk toxin production in the food. This may also occur in smoked fish and continental sausage products. As type A and B strains are proteolytic and saccharolytic, spoiling of food and blowing of cans by gas production usually draws attention to the problem before ingestion. In addition, adequate cooking or reheating will render food safe as the toxin is inactivated at quite moderate temperatures. Botulism only results from cold or inadequately heated products and occasionally from raw products which have been left to decompose partially before ingestion, e.g. izushi – a Japanese fermented fish and rice product – or aged seal flipper, whale meat or salmon eggs eaten by Eskimos (Ball & Farrell 1979).

Once ingested, the highly potent, high molecular weight protein toxins circulate and then fix to unmyelinated cholinergic nerve fibrils proximal to the myoneural junction. The result is to block the quantal release of acetylcholine by interfering with normal calcium influx in response to depolarization. This effect is permanent and later recovery is associated with proliferative regeneration of motor endplates. Autonomic dysfunction may also be present.

CLINICAL FEATURES AND DIAGNOSIS

Botulism in older children presents with initial malaise, nausea, vomiting and dizziness followed after a variable period of hours (type E) to days (types A/B) by onset of paralysis. Early signs include ptosis, ophthalmoplegia with blurring of vision and diplopia, dysphagia and dysarthria followed in severe cases by systemic paralysis and resultant respiratory failure. Consciousness and sensation are unimpaired. Diagnosis is confirmed by detection of toxin in serum and demonstration of the organism and toxin in the ingested food if available. Electromyography may give confirmatory information.

Infant botulism can present as sudden infant death (cot death) syndrome but this is probably a rare occurrence (Byard et al 1992): it usually has an indolent onset following slow elaboration of toxin in the gut. The features include failure to suckle and swallow, generalized hypotonia, pooling of secretions in the hypopharynx and constipation. Sudden apnea may supervene. This syndrome must be differentiated from other causes of severe hypotonia of infancy. Examination of feces will yield both organism and toxin: toxin cannot usually be identified in serum. PCR may be of value in detecting toxin where animal inoculation proves negative.

TREATMENT

In older children rapid neutralization of circulating toxin by systemically administered specific polyvalent antitoxin is essential. Antitoxin has no effect on toxins bound to nervous tissue but should be given irrespective of its chronological relation to onset as toxins may circulate for many days and paralysis may slowly progress as a result. Those with respiratory failure will require ventilatory support in intensive care. No effective neuromuscular blockade antagonists are routinely available. Recovery may take many weeks.

Infants with botulism should also receive such therapy as appropriate. In addition, antitoxin can be given via a nasogastric tube in an attempt to neutralize toxin present in the gut. The use of penicillin to eradicate Cl. botulinum from the gut appears relatively ineffective and could possible exacerbate paralysis by causing increased toxin release from dying bacteria.

Although infant botulism usually occurs sporadically, food-borne disease in older children may cause family outbreaks possibly also involving visitors. All contacts should be traced as, in those who have shared the suspect food vehicle, induction of vomiting and use of purgatives to expel toxin from the gut may be justified. Where early signs of disease are present antitoxin should be administered urgently.

BRUCELLOSIS: UNDULANT FEVER

Brucellosis is usually caused by one of three organisms Brucella abortus, melitensis or suis. All three are primarily diseases of domesticated animals (cattle, goats and pigs, respectively). The clinical picture ranges from clinically asymptomatic infection via acute brucellosis (with septicemic manifestations) to chronic brucellosis (Young 1995).

EPIDEMIOLOGY

Human brucellosis is mostly a disease of those who come into contact with infected animals in rural areas. Spread of infection from animal to animal occurs readily and the resulting illness is often chronic with long-term excretion of the organism. Infection is transmitted to humans by infected milk or milk products and, less frequently, by direct contact or entry through skin. Person-to-person spread rarely occurs. Elimination of brucellosis in animal population (by vaccination or slaughter policies) will eliminate new infections in humans. World Health Organization sources estimate 500 000 cases worldwide each year (childhood infections accounting for less than 10% of cases). The low incidence in children in a milk-borne infection is unexpected and some have suggested that environmental exposure may be more relevant.

PATHOLOGY

Acute brucellosis is a septicemic illness with seeding of organisms in the body which may become apparent immediately or later after the systemic features have resolved. There is widespread reticuloendothelial system hyperplasia and focal manifestations may occur in many organs, particularly in the liver or spleen. Chronic brucellosis may follow acute brucellosis or begin insidiously. In chronic brucellosis the organisms usually remain intracellularly where they are relatively protected against host defenses and antibiotics.

B. melitensis often produces more invasive manifestations and debility than B. abortus, an important point to realize when generalizing about brucellosis.

CLINICAL FEATURES

The incubation period of acute brucellosis is from a few days to a month.

With acute brucellosis symptoms develop rapidly with high fever, rigors, arthralgia and profuse sweating: patients often feel much iller than signs suggest but recovery follows in most. Fever has no particular pattern. Weight loss and secondary anemia may develop. If the patient does not recover then a state of chronic brucellosis ensues with vague irritability, malaise, fatigue, musculoskeletal aches and pains, headaches and depression. Fever may be intermittent, occurring every few weeks – hence the name 'undulant fever'.

Although chronic brucellosis is rarely life threatening the morbidity may be significant.

With both acute and chronic brucellosis suggestive signs may be prominent or absent – constituting a pyrexia of unknown origin. There may be hepatomegaly, splenomegaly or lymph node enlargement. Particularly with *B. melitensis* infection lymph nodes may suppurate and osteomyelitis or arthritis may develop.

Other rare, but potentially life-threatening manifestations include meningitis, endocarditis, peritonitis and encephalitis.

DIAGNOSIS AND DIFFERENTIAL DIAGNOSIS

Clinical diagnosis may be easy in areas where animal infection is endemic. In nonendemic areas clinical diagnosis may be difficult unless it is realized that patients have visited endemic areas or ingested milk products from endemic areas.

In acute brucellosis blood cultures may be positive but the organisms are difficult to culture and cultures may take up to 2 weeks to become positive. Agglutination tests to detect IgM and IgG antibodies may be helpful but may be positive in asymptomatically infected patients in endemic areas. Nevertheless increasing titers are almost certainly diagnostic. Agglutination titers of greater than 1 : 160 in a patient with appropriate clinical features are very suggestive.

In chronic brucellosis blood cultures are rarely positive and bone marrow culture or, less often, liver or splenic biopsy culture may be necessary. If there is renal involvement urine cultures may be positive. Biopsy shows noncaseating granulomas.

If available, the presence of *Brucella*-specific IgM is diagnostic of acute brucellosis or of chronic brucellosis in an acute relapse, whilst *Brucella*-specific IgG indicates infection at some stage. Lymphocytosis with neutropenia may be found.

The differential diagnosis of acute brucellosis includes malaria, salmonellosis (including typhoid fever), tuberculosis, tularemia, rheumatic fever, infective endocarditis, Q fever, leptospirosis and noninfective conditions. If malaise and debility predominate, depression enters the differential diagnosis, as well as being a complication in its own right.

TREATMENT (Lubani et al 1989)

In acute brucellosis antibiotic treatment probably shortens the illness and reduces the risk of progression to chronic brucellosis. Opinions differ as to the optimal treatment: comparison of treatment results of *abortus* and *melitensis* infection are not necessarily valid. Most studies of children with brucellosis deal with children with *melitensis* infection. Regimens advocated include (either alone or in combination) co-trimoxazole, rifampicin or streptomycin. In chronic brucellosis suppression of intracellular infection may be attempted in the hope that the host's immunity will eventually eliminate or contain infection. Regimens advocated include protracted courses of the antibiotics used in acute brucellosis. Tetracyclines are useful but obviously cannot be used in children unless there is no alternative.

Antipyretics, analgesics and antidepressant treatment may be indicated. Vaccination of humans is not practicable – and would certainly make subsequent interpretation of serological tests very difficult.

CHOLERA

Pediatric cholera in many respects resembles cholera in adults and diarrhea in children due to other organisms, but often there are differences. For example, cholera in children is often more acute and severe with blunting of the sensorium and episodes of hypoglycemia. Cholera is caused by infection with the classical *Vibrio cholerae* or by its biotype El Tor strain of serotype 01. However, a new strain of serotype 0139 has caused severe outbreaks in South Asia and is termed the Bengal strain. Outbreaks occur as a result of ingestion of infected water due to poor sanitation and hygiene although occasionally they may occur as a result of ingestion of infected food.

ORGANISM AND PATHOPHYSIOLOGY

V. cholerae are Gram-negative curved rods measuring 1.5–3.0 μm × 0.5 μm. In culture, they may assume other forms such as spiral shapes. In hanging-drop preparations, they are highly motile. They possess somatic (O) antigens and flagellar (H) antigens. By the use of somatic (O) antisera, the serological strains such as Ogawa, Inaba and Hikojima can be distinguished one from the other.

The pathogenesis of diarrhea is mediated via the enterotoxin produced by the organisms. The enterotoxin consists of A and B subunits. There are five B subunits surrounding the single A subunit. The B subunits are responsible for the binding of the toxin to specific receptors on the cell membrane of the epithelium of the small intestine. Once binding has occurred, the A subunit breaks into two, the A_1 and the A_2 subunits, by the disruption of the disulfide bond. The A_1 subunit then activates the enzyme adenylate cyclase to produce cyclic adenosine monophosphate (cAMP) which then is responsible for the crypt epithelial cell pouring out excessive intestinal secretions, which accumulate in the intestinal lumen and are then expelled in the diarrheal stools.

The amount of electrolytes lost in stools of patients with adult cholera, cholera in children and infantile diarrhea due to other organisms is summarized in Table 23.15.

Table 23.15 Relative electrolyte constituents of stools

	Sodium	Potassium	Chloride	Bicarbonate
Cholera in adults	+++	+	+++	+++
Cholera in children	++	++	++	++
Noncholera infantile diarrhea	+	++	+	+

In pediatric cholera, stool sodium content is intermediate between that found in infantile diarrhea due to other organisms and adult cholera. Stool potassium is higher in pediatric cholera compared to adult cholera but similar to that in infantile diarrhea. Bicarbonate loss in stools in pediatric cholera is intermediate between that seen in adult cholera and infantile diarrhea. Generally, stool osmolarity in pediatric cholera is isotonic with plasma.

The organism is easily destroyed by the acidic gastric juice and most patients with cholera either show relative achlorhydria or are infected with large inocula of the organism. The enterotoxin also stimulates mucus production by goblet cells and this may prevent the organisms from reaching the crypt epithelium. Furthermore, the enterotoxin increases peristaltic activity and this itself clears the bowel of the toxin.

CLINICAL FEATURES

The textbook signs and symptoms of a child with cholera are usually those of severe dehydration with water and electrolyte loss. However, during an outbreak of cholera, it is important to realize that some children as well as adults may be totally asymptomatic or may suffer from mild or moderate diarrhea with minimal signs of dehydration. These milder cases are due to the factors described above (gastric acidity, dose of inoculum and other resistance factors, etc.). The stools of these mild cases should be examined for *V. cholerae* as they form a significant focus of dissemination of the organism. It has been estimated that in classical *V. cholerae* infection, the ratio of mild to severe cases is 1 to 1, while in an El Tor biotype outbreak, the ratio of mild to severe cases can be as high as 7 to 1.

Excluding these mild cases, the clinical features are those seen in any severe childhood diarrhea consequent on severe water and electrolyte loss (see p. 1294, Table 23.13).

In some cases there are differences in the mode of presentation in children compared to adults. Some of these differences are as follows:

1. *Fever.* In adults, there is usually hardly any rise in temperature but in children, fever is occasionally encountered.

2. *Alteration of consciousness.* In adults when drowsiness is present, they may be restless and on occasion are capable of talking almost in a rational manner. In other words, the altered consciousness is one of a detached mental state. This is due to the fact that adults with this degree of acute dehydration are still capable of maintaining cerebral circulation off and on. On the other hand, in children consciousness can be totally lost and they are unarousable.

3. *Convulsions.* It is rare to encounter fits in adults but this is not uncommon in the child with severe cholera. The cause of the fits is uncertain, although they have been attributed to hypoglycemia. Other signs and symptoms consequent on hypoglycemia may also be encountered.

4. *Hypoglycemia.* The blood glucose of all children with suspected cholera must be estimated as prolonged severe neuroglycopenia may cause death.

5. *Hypokalemia.* Just as hypoglycemia is commoner in pediatric cholera than in adult cholera, hypokalemia is also more common in children with cholera. This is due to the greater loss of potassium in the stools. Signs consequent on hypokalemia which should be looked for include paralytic ileus of the intestines, cardiac arrhythmias, electrocardiographic abnormalities such as depressed T waves and prominent U waves, and muscle weakness.

DIAGNOSIS

Diagnosis is confirmed by examining the stools under phase contrast or dark field microscopy. The latter is preferable and the vibrios are seen in large numbers and because of their motility, they give the typical appearance of shooting stars. Specific diagnosis can be made if specific antisera of the Ogawa and Inaba strains are added to the rapidly moving vibrios when they will totally cease their motility. Cultures can be obtained from stool samples or by rectal swabs and further confirmation of the diagnosis obtained.

MANAGEMENT

The initial treatment of a child with cholera is essentially the treatment of dehydration. In cases of mild dehydration oralyte solutions suffice. Oralyte solutions may have to be used in those with moderate dehydration in areas where intravenous therapy is not so readily available, but where pediatric intravenous therapy is readily available, intravenous fluid therapy is ideal. The type of fluid, amount and rate of flow of the intravenous fluid used are based on the usual principles which apply to any child with acute diarrhea with dehydration.

In general, those children with mild dehydration will have a 5% fluid deficit and may show tachycardia and slightly decreased skin turgor but with normal sensorium and blood pressure. Those with moderate dehydration may have a fluid deficit of up to 10% with markedly decreased skin turgor, tachycardia and hypotension but with an intact sensorium. Those with severe dehydration with fluid deficits of more than 10% will show all the above signs together with peripheral cyanosis, drowsiness or coma and absent peripheral pulses. Initially, fluids should be given to replace the fluid and electrolyte loss, followed by maintenance intravenous fluids, and then oralytes are given as the child improves.

Antibiotics can shorten the duration of diarrhea and in this way reduce fluid losses in cholera. Tetracycline is most commonly given in a dose of 50 mg/kg bodyweight per day in 6-hourly doses for 48 h. The first dose can be given 3 h after the onset of intravenous hydration. Other effective antimicrobials include ampicillin, trimethoprim, sulfamethoxazole, furazolidone and doxycycline. Electrolytes and blood sugar should be assessed at intervals to guide ongoing therapy. If hypoglycemia is present, an intravenous infusion of 3–4 ml/kg of 25% glucose is given immediately and glucose is added to the infusion fluid to provide 10 mg/kg of glucose.

Oral rehydration solutions (ORS) of various types are effective in rehydration of the cholera patient. The World Health Organization ORS consists of 90 mmol/l of sodium, 20 mmol/l of potassium, 80 mmol/l of chloride, 30 mmol/l of bicarbonate and 111 mmol/l of glucose. However, sucrose-based ORS as well as polysaccharide-based ORS are cheaper, more easily available and are just as effective (Wong 1981, Mehta & Subramanian 1986, Roesel & Schaffter 1989).

Prevention and containment of outbreaks are important methods of management of cholera. Effective sanitation and hygiene are prerequisites but in some developing countries these are still not available. During outbreaks, effective handwashing and boiling of all drinking water and ensuring that food is well cooked assist in prevention of spread. Identification of cases and carriers, their isolation and treatment are effective ways of preventing future outbreaks. Previous vaccines against cholera, both given parenterally and orally, have not been very safe nor effective. However, new safe and effective oral vaccines against the serotypes 01 and 0139 are now available (Coster et al 1995).

DIPHTHERIA

HISTORY AND INCIDENCE

Diphtheria is caused by *Corynebacterium diphtheriae*. It was first specifically defined by Klebs in 1881. The following year Löffler obtained the bacillus in pure culture and shortly afterwards its exotoxin was described; in 1894 von Behring developed an antiserum for treatment. In 1913 Schick described the skin test which distinguishes between immune and susceptible persons.

In developing countries diphtheria is still an important cause of illness and of death in children.

In developed countries diphtheria had almost been eliminated until the breakup of the former Soviet Union in the early 1990's. Since then significant outbreaks of diphtheria have occurred in Russia and other former Soviet Republics. Table 23.16 illustrates the dramatic fall in morbidity and mortality from diphtheria since routine immunization of children was introduced following the Second World War in England and Wales. Since 1980 only occasional cases have been diagnosed in the UK.

ETIOLOGY

C. diphtheriae is a Gram-positive, slender, sometimes curved or club-shaped organism. On direct smear from a suspected lesion it cannot be differentiated morphologically from harmless diphtheroid bacilli. Three strains can be differentiated: *gravis, intermedius* and *mitis*. It is readily destroyed by heat and by antiseptics, but may survive for several weeks in milk or water.

The diphtheria bacillus produces a powerful exotoxin which is responsible for the general symptoms and for the distant and often delayed damaging effect on the heart and peripheral nerves. Exotoxin production by the organism depends on the presence in the bacterium of a phage which carries the gene encoding for the toxin (tox+). *C. diphtheriae* strains are classified as toxigenic (pathogenic) or nontoxigenic (nonpathogenic) depending on whether or not they produce toxin. However, recent evidence suggests that conversion from nontoxigenic to toxigenic can occur by the acquisition of the appropriate phage. The toxin is destroyed by heat or light and in its freely circulating state it can be neutralized by antitoxin. Once it is fixed to the tissues, its effect cannot be modified by antitoxin.

EPIDEMIOLOGY: ACTIVE AND PASSIVE IMMUNITY

Diphtheria is spread by direct contact via the airborne route. The source of infection may be a patient suffering from diphtheria or a healthy carrier. The disease may spread rapidly among susceptible unimmunized child populations and can cause major epidemic outbreaks.

As long as most mothers had themselves suffered from diphtheria in childhood they transferred passive immunity to their infants. This persists for several months. In most advanced communities, however, babies born now do not have passive immunity, because their mothers have not had the disease. These infants can be successfully immunized (with diphtheria toxoid which is inactivated toxin) in the first few weeks of life and thus acquire active immunity. These procedures are usually carried out concurrently with immunization against whooping cough and tetanus ('DPT' – 0.5 ml at 4-week intervals for three injections for the primary course) with a booster dose at school entry. A further booster is given at the time of leaving school using the adult (low dose) vaccine (see Ch. 7). There are various other equally effective schemes.

PATHOLOGY

Diphtheria bacilli usually invade the pharynx and may spread from there to the nose, the palate or the larynx. These other sites may sometimes be the primary site of infection. Infection elsewhere in the body, such as in wounds or on the vulva, may also occur. Such infections might be primary or secondary to a throat lesion.

The bacteria multiply rapidly and elaborate the exotoxin, which inhibits the local inflammatory defense mechanisms and invades distant body tissues via the bloodstream. At the site of the invasion edema and hyperemia occur, with destruction of the superficial epithelium. The result is a 'washleather' membrane or 'pseudomembrane', consisting of necrotic tissue, fibrin, white cells and large numbers of bacteria. It becomes very adherent to underlying tissues and if separated, a raw, bleeding surface is exposed. The membrane may involve the fauces, the larynx or the nose. Laryngeal membrane may extend downwards to involve the trachea and bronchi, forming a cast of the bronchial tree. The regional lymph nodes become enlarged.

The distant effect of the exotoxin is mainly on the cardiac muscle which becomes flabby, with small hemorrhages scattered between the muscle bundles. The muscle becomes necrotic and is infiltrated with leukocytes. A myocarditis results.

The peripheral nerves are also affected by the toxin with destruction of the myelin sheath. The kidneys and liver can also be affected. Subject to survival none of these changes is likely to lead to permanent sequelae.

CLINICAL FEATURES

The incubation period of diphtheria is between 2 and 7 days. The illness may be so mild as to be overlooked (especially in partially immunized persons) or it may be fulminating, leading to death in a short time. Most commonly it is of insidious onset, with fever,

Table 23.16 Diphtheria – England and Wales

	Cases	Deaths
1920	69 481	5 648
1930	74 043	3 497
1940	44 281	2 480
1950	962	49
1960	49	5
1970	22	3
1980	5	0

malaise and headache. The commonest site of invasion is the throat (tonsillar or faucial diphtheria), but sore throat is not a conspicuous symptom. The fever does not usually rise as high as in streptococcal tonsillitis but may reach 39.5°C. Initially there is only mild edema and redness of the throat, but later individual spots appear on the tonsils which then coalesce to form a grayish membrane. By now the cervical glands enlarge and in highly virulent, massive infections these, together with edema of the subcutaneous tissues, produce the characteristic 'bullneck' appearance.

The throat lesion may be unilateral or of asymmetrical distribution. The membrane is difficult to separate from the underlying tissues. It may be noted on the tonsils, the uvula and the soft palate. Membrane in the nose will cause an offensive, thin, bloodstained nasal discharge. Difficulty with breathing and stridor will occur even without laryngeal involvement. There may also be difficulty in swallowing. Nasal regurgitation of food and a nasal voice indicate palatal paralysis, which is common. Meanwhile the child's general condition also deteriorates due to toxemia and myocardial involvement. The ECG may be abnormal, the changes reflecting myocarditis. There may be prolongation of the P–R interval, bradycardia or heart block. The blood pressure falls, the heart rate becomes irregular and the pulse is thready.

Death may occur at any stage from myocarditis, respiratory failure, or secondary bacterial infections such as bronchopneumonia.

The risk to life is even greater if the larynx is involved in the disease (laryngeal diphtheria). Membrane on the vocal cords will result in hoarseness, a brassy cough and variable degrees of respiratory obstruction, resulting in stridor (diphtheritic or membranous croup), subcostal, suprasternal and intrasternal recession, restlessness and cyanosis. The child is extremely anxious. He may die of suffocation unless his airway is kept open by laryngeal intubation or by tracheostomy.

Occasionally diphtheria only affects the nasal passages (nasal diphtheria). As this produces only a mild disease it may be overlooked, with considerable risk to contacts. There may be a serosanguineous nasal discharge. In other instances diphtheria may primarily or secondarily involve the skin (cutaneous diphtheria), vulva, eye or ear. If, at any site, a membrane is formed on a lesion, diphtheria should be suspected.

Lower motor neuron-type paralyses may affect any muscle or muscle group, and can cause paralytic squint, blurring of vision, diaphragmatic paralysis and weakness of legs and arms. These paralytic phenomena are usually late manifestations, coming several weeks after the primary infection. Palatal palsy often occurs in the third week of the illness, eye muscle paralysis in the fifth week, diaphragmatic involvement in the fifth to seventh weeks, and limb weakness up to 10 weeks. The child's sensorium may be disturbed with hallucinations and diminished consciousness.

DIAGNOSIS AND DIFFERENTIAL DIAGNOSIS

In countries in which diphtheria is still common, the diagnosis in most cases presents no difficulties. The isolation of the organism on culture should confirm the clinical suspicion, but while awaiting bacteriological confirmation there should be no delay in instituting therapy. Swabs should be taken from the lesions, preferably after removal of some of the membrane.

The diagnosis may readily be missed, especially in areas where

diphtheria is rare. Diphtheria should be considered in those cases in which the degree of a child's constitutional upset is greater than could be accounted for by the sore throat, pharyngeal exudate or the degree of the fever. Throat cultures should distinguish diphtheria from acute streptococcal tonsillitis, from less common Vincent's angina, or from croup of virus origin, which can also be mistaken for diphtheria. Infectious mononucleosis may present initially with a similar picture, but a negative throat swab, monocytosis (mononucleosis) in the peripheral blood and a positive 'Monospot' test should help to differentiate the two conditions. Recent travel from an area where diphtheria is known to occur may provide a clue to the diagnosis.

PROGNOSIS

Diphtheria caused by the *gravis* strain tends to be more severe than that due to other strains. Infants have a higher mortality than older children. Early diagnosis improves the outlook and the provision of facilities for dealing rapidly with laryngeal obstruction will reduce the risk of death.

TREATMENT

The essential part of treatment is the prompt administration of adequate doses of antitoxin, to neutralize the effect of circulating toxins before these become fixed to the tissues. It is best to give a single dose to prevent sensitization and anaphylactoid reactions. If given in sufficient dosage, a therapeutic level will persist for many days, until toxin production from the site of the lesion has ceased. Antibiotic therapy is of secondary importance. Most organisms are sensitive to penicillin, as well as to other agents including erythromycin. These should be given in adequate doses as soon as the diagnosis is made.

The dose of antitoxin depends on the degree of toxemia, on the site and extent of the diphtheritic membrane and on the duration of the illness. Thus it may vary from 10 000 units given intramuscularly in mild nasal diphtheria to up to 80 000 units given intravenously in cases of 'bullneck' diphtheria with severe toxic signs. The more extensive the membrane and the more toxic the patient the larger is the dose required. Laryngeal and late cases require a large dose. In urgent cases *intravenous* antitoxin is effective more rapidly and should be given slowly into the tubing of a 5% glucose intravenous drip.

As the antitoxin is a horse serum preparation a history should be obtained regarding any previous injections of horse serum and a test for sensitivity must be carried out before administering antitoxin. This consists of an intradermal injection of 0.1 ml of 1 : 1000 dilution of antitoxin in normal saline. A local reaction will be produced in 20 min in those who are hypersensitive. Even in the absence of a reaction a syringeful of 1 : 1000 adrenaline solution must be available before injecting the full dose. In case of a reaction the adrenaline solution should be given at once (up to 0.5 ml intramuscularly). Hydrocortisone, 100–200 mg intravenously should also be given. Large doses of antitoxin are not more dangerous than moderate doses.

If a child is shown to be hypersensitive, then a dilute and minute dose, 0.1 ml of 1 : 20 dilution, should be tried subcutaneously, followed with the same dose at a 1 : 10 dilution, then the same dose undiluted at 15- to 30-min intervals. Progressively increasing intramuscular injections (e.g. 0.3 ml, 0.5 ml, etc.) can then be given subject to no reaction until the full dose is reached.

The effectiveness of the antitoxin depends on the day of administration. If given on the first day of illness, the result will usually be full recovery.

Penicillin should be given in a single daily injection of a long-acting preparation (e.g. 600 000 units procaine penicillin) or in penicillin-allergic patients erythromycin orally, 40 mg/kg per day. Treatment is continued for 7 days.

In laryngeal obstruction tracheostomy is often necessary and may be life saving.

Treatment of the carrier state

The carrier state is not influenced by antitoxin therapy. Erythromycin should be given for 7 days. Post-treatment swabs should be taken to ensure eradication of the organisms.

Contacts

Close contacts (family and schoolfriends), even if fully immunized, should be given 7 days of erythromycin to prevent acquisition of the infecting organism and development of a carrier state. Unimmunized close contacts should also be immunized and observed closely for possible development of symptoms or signs suggestive of diphtheria – if these develop antitoxin should also be given.

HAEMOPHILUS INFLUENZAE

GENERAL FEATURES AND EPIDEMIOLOGY

Haemophilus influenzae was first reported by Pfeiffer in 1892, but the sensational claim that it was the primary cause of epidemic influenza proved fallacious. None the less, the bacterium has a wide spectrum of pathogenic capabilities. A small Gram-negative bacterium, it may be encapsulated or nonencapsulated (nontypable). Pittman (1931) described six antigenically distinct capsular types, designated a to f. The possession of the capsule is an important virulence determinant and it is *Haemophilus influenzae* of capsular serotype b (Hib) that stands out as the most virulent strain, responsible for the great majority of invasive *Haemophilus* infections. Prior to the widespread use of effective vaccines against Hib, it was the major cause of bacterial meningitis and the predominant cause of epiglottitis in young children. It was estimated to cause 1400 cases of invasive disease, including 900 cases of meningitis annually in UK children aged less than 5 years (Booy et al 1993). In addition to invasive life-threatening infections, *H. influenzae*, mostly capsule-deficient strains, is estimated to cause at least half a million cases of acute otitis media each year in the UK among children aged less than 10 years. Table 23.17 summarizes several characteristics relating to carriage and pathogenicity.

H. influenzae is among the bacteria normally found in the human pharynx and also colonizes the mucosae of the conjunctiva and genital tracts. Spread from one individual to another occurs by airborne droplets or by direct transfer of secretions. Exposure begins during or immediately after birth so that from infancy onwards, carriage of one or more strains for periods lasting from days to months is common. The presence of *H. influenzae* in cultures obtained from the upper (but not the lower) respiratory tract is therefore a common and normal finding. In about 3–5% of individuals, the organisms are encapsulated, most often with the

Table 23.17 Carriage and pathogenicity of *Haemophilus influenzae* (from Turk 1982)

Strains	Common upper respiratory tract carriage rates	Principal manifestation of pathogenicity
Nonencapsulated	50–80%	Exacerbations of chronic bronchitis, otitis media, sinusitis, conjunctivitis Bacteremic infections rare Patients commonly adults
Encapsulated, type b	2–4%	Meningitis, epiglottitis, pneumonia and empyema, septic arthritis, cellulitis, osteomyelitis, pericarditis, bacteremia Rarer manifestations include glossitis, tenosynovitis, peritonitis, endocarditis, ventriculitis associated with infected shunt tubing
Encapsulated, types a and c through f	1–2%	Rarely incriminated as pathogens

serotype b antigen (in an unvaccinated population). In general, carriers of *H. influenzae*, whether colonized with encapsulated or capsule-deficient organisms, remain healthy, but occasionally disease occurs. Two contrasting patterns of *H. influenzae* disease can be identified. The most serious in its consequences are invasive infections such as meningitis, septic arthritis, epiglottitis and cellulitis; these infections typically occur in young children, are associated with bacteremia and are caused by encapsulated type b strains. The second category includes less serious but numerically more common infections that occur as a result of contiguous spread of *H. influenzae* within the respiratory tract. *H. influenzae* is a common cause of otitis media (10–30% of bacteria isolated; Ruuskanen & Heikkinen 1994), sinusitis, conjunctivitis and lower respiratory tract infection. These infections are usually, but not invariably, caused by nontypable strains. These generalizations are not hard and fast; nontypable strains are a well-recognized cause of neonatal sepsis, including early-onset pneumonia and meningitis (Wallace et al 1983). They are a common cause of severe, acute lower respiratory tract infections (often accompanied by bacteremia) among young children living in the developing world (Shann et al 1984) and in one study were responsible for about 50% of all *H. influenzae* causing invasive disease in adults (Farley et al 1992). Outbreaks of an apparently new syndrome, Brazilian purpuric fever, have been described in which young children who present initially with a conjunctivitis develop a serious, potentially fatal form of septicemia which mimics meningococcemia but which is caused by *H. influenzae* biotype *aegyptius* (Brazilian Purpuric Fever Study Group 1987a,b).

PATHOGENESIS

The host and microbial determinants of colonization by *H. influenzae* are poorly understood. Infection is potentiated by viruses such as influenza in animal experiments. Adhesins facilitate attachment to mucus and to human epithelial cells and there are microbial factors which inhibit the normal ciliary function of respiratory tract epithelium. The primacy of type b capsule as a crucial factor in the pathogenesis of invasive disease has been well established. Lipopolysaccharide is also important in facilitating bloodstream survival and blood–brain barrier damage in experimental infections. In rat and primate models of *H. influenzae* type b meningitis, organisms were found to invade the submucosa of the nasopharynx and to reach the meninges as a result of bacteremia rather than by direct penetration of contiguous structures such as the cribriform plate or the inner ear. The occurrence of meningitis correlated strikingly with the duration and intensity of bacteremia; experimental manipulation of the host factors which decreased the efficiency of intravascular clearance (e.g. splenectomy) increased the incidence of meningitis (Moxon et al 1985).

IMMUNITY

Among the host factors governing susceptibility to invasive type b infection, the role of serum antibodies to polyribosyl-ribitol phosphate (PRP), the type b capsular antigen, has been shown to be critical (Robbins et al 1973). Serum anti-PRP antibodies in conjunction with complement-mediated bactericidal and opsonic activity mediate protective immunity against systemic infections in humans (Anderson et al 1972). The serum of newborns and young infants (up until about 3 months) generally have sufficient amounts of passively acquired antibody to afford protection. Thereafter, the natural decline of these maternally derived antibodies is followed by a period lasting until the age of 2–4 years when the levels of antibody are inadequate to provide protection. The delay in the acquisition of serum anti-PRP antibodies is characteristic of children less than 2 years and is a major reason for the high attack rates of *H. influenzae* b invasive disease in early infancy. Although some infants may be exposed to type b *H. influenzae* through nasopharyngeal carriage the antigenic stimulus for these antibodies may often be through exposure to different, commensal bacteria or ingested foods which immunize through their cross-reacting antigens (Bradshaw et al 1971). The role of local (mucosal) immunity and host defense against *H. influenzae* is poorly understood. In an infant rat colonization model anti-PRP antibodies given intranasally are able to prevent nasopharyngeal colonization by Hib. The same effect is seen when these antibodies are given intraperitoneally and a minimum effective serum level can be defined (Kauppi et al 1993). If it is assumed that anti-PRP antibodies function in a similar manner on the oropharyngeal mucosa of human children, both serum-derived IgG and locally produced IgA may reduce Hib carriage and thereby protect against invasive disease.

CLINICAL FEATURES

Meningitis is the most common, serious manifestation of invasive infection due to *H. influenzae* b. Antecedent symptoms of upper respiratory infection are common. The most common signs are fever and altered behavior – including poor feeding, vomiting, irritability and drowsiness. Thus, none of these clinical features distinguish the child with *H. influenzae* meningitis from several other infectious diseases or other forms of meningitis. In particular, young infants have few specific signs; nuchal rigidity and a bulging fontanel are typical but often absent early in the course of established meningeal infection. Seizures, cranial nerve involvement and coma may develop as the disease progresses and the effects of raised intracranial pressure, cerebral edema and vasculitis prevail. Subdural effusions are common but these very rarely require specific management and are usually sterile.

Overall mortality for *H. influenzae* meningitis is currently less than 5% in developed countries but significantly higher, ranging from 22–40% in the developing world. Sequelae occur in 15–30% of those who survive; the commonest complication is sensorineural deafness.

Acute respiratory obstruction caused by involvement of the supraglottic tissue by *H. influenzae* b is a potentially lethal disease of characteristically rapid onset. Typically, the child is aged 2–7 years and presents with sore throat, fever, dyspnea and dysphagia (causing pharyngeal pooling and then oral drooling of secretions). The child is restless and anxious and often adopts a characteristic posture in which the neck is extended and the chin is protruded in order to minimize airway obstruction. Abrupt deterioration leading to death within a few hours may occur if adequate treatment is not provided. The characteristic findings are supralaryngeal. The epiglottis is red and swollen and resembles a red cherry at the base of the tongue. Although an abrupt death is usually the result of acute airways obstruction, sudden collapse may result from less well-defined mechanisms associated with acute toxemia. It should be emphasized that examination of the pharynx and larynx of a child in whom acute epiglottitis is suspected should only be attempted under conditions in which the airway can be secured immediately, otherwise the examination may precipitate respiratory arrest.

Invasive disease due to non type-b encapsulated and nonencapsulated *H. influenzae* is rare but may present in a similar fashion. Presentation may also be similar in the rare group of children who develop invasive disease with Hib despite vaccination, 'vaccine failures'. In both groups predisposing host factors such as immunodeficiency are frequent and should be sought.

Confirmation of the clinical impression of invasive *H. influenzae* infection depends upon cultures of normally sterile fluids (e.g. CSF, blood, pleural or synovial fluid). Positive nasopharyngeal cultures are not helpful since carriage is common among healthy persons. Needle aspiration of the middle ear (tympanocentesis), maxillary sinus, the margins of an area of cellulitis or lung may occasionally prove helpful in selected cases, especially in a very sick child in whom no diagnosis has been established. Whenever practical, the results of Gram stain should be sought immediately; in about 70% of cases of meningitis, CSF smears show the typical pleomorphic, Gram-negative coccobacilli. Detection of capsular antigen in serum, CSF or concentrated urine by immunoassay (e.g. latex agglutination) may be useful, especially in children who have received prior antibiotic treatment. This test should be interpreted with caution, however, in those who have recently received Hib vaccine as a false positive result is possible.

TREATMENT

For many years, the treatment of choice for invasive *H. influenzae* b infections was chloramphenicol. However, increasing resistance to this agent together with the necessity of monitoring blood concentration has lead to treatment with parenteral, third generation cephalosporins. Commonly used agents which penetrate well into CSF include cefotaxime and ceftriaxone. There is no evidence however that third generation cephalosporins are superior as treatment when compared to the conventional regimens of ampicillin and chloramphenicol, or chloramphenicol alone, providing that the infection is caused by a susceptible organism.

The use of dexamethasone as adjunctive therapy in Hib meningitis can result in a reduction in sensorineural deafness (Schaad et al 1993). Early administration, close to or even prior to the first dose of antibiotic is preferable. Elective intubation and antibiotics are usually mandatory in cases of epiglottitis.

PREVENTION

Active immunization

A compelling body of evidence supports the case for active immunization against *H. influenzae* b. Predominant amongst these is its preeminence as a cause of childhood meningitis around the world. Relevant also is the increasing prevalence of type b strains resistant to antibiotics.

The first generation of vaccines against Hib consisted of the purified type b polysaccharide. A trial in 1974 in Finland demonstrated efficacy in children older than 18 months of age but not in younger infants, even when given two doses. No effect of the vaccine on nasopharyngeal carriage was observed (Peltola et al 1984). This led to the development of a second generation of vaccines in which the immunogenicity of PRP is enhanced by covalent linkage of the capsular polysaccharide or oligosaccharides to protein. Currently, four conjugates are licensed for use in infants. Although differences in the immunogenicity of these vaccines have been observed, all elicit significantly enhanced antibody responses when compared to PRP and, in contrast to the latter, are found to prime for a secondary antibody response. Large clinical trials have confirmed their efficacy in infancy (Booy et al 1994). An unexpected benefit has been a reduction in Hib colonization of the upper respiratory tract (Takala et al 1991), and this has contributed to the near elimination of Hib disease in countries where immunization has become routine (CDSC 1994).

Passive immunization

Individuals with congenital or acquired hypogammaglobulinemia are unduly susceptible to a variety of pathogens, among which infections due to *H. influenzae* are particularly frequent and troublesome. Replacement immunoglobulin therapy is the mainstay of treatment. A recent development is the use of a human globulin preparation, bacterial polysaccharide immune globulin (BPIG), prepared from donors actively immunized with Hib vaccine. It contains 10–60 times the anti-PRP antibodies available in conventional immune globulin. Its pharmacology and protective efficacy have been investigated in Apache Indian infants who have an exceptionally high incidence of type b infection occurring at an early age (Siber et al 1992). BPIG may have utility in the prevention of Hib infections in high-risk patients who cannot be immunized adequately with Hib conjugate vaccines.

Chemoprophylaxis

Young unimmunized children, especially aged less than 2 years in the same household, are likely to be at significantly increased risk of secondary invasive infections by *H. influenzae* b. In the prevaccine era secondary attack rates in household contacts were estimated to be 2–4% and in 'day-care centers' up to 1.3%. It has been suggested that antibiotic treatment of contacts of children with invasive *H. influenzae* could decrease this secondary attack rate. Susceptible individuals will be those less than 4 years of age who have not started or not completed a course of Hib conjugate vaccines. Rifampicin (20 mg/kg per dose, maximum dose 600 mg/day) given orally once daily for 4 days is effective in eradicating nasopharyngeal carriage. Treatment of household contacts (children and adults) where there are susceptible children (other than the index case) less than 4 years old should be considered as should treatment of such children in nurseries or playschool who are contacts of a case. The course of Hib vaccines should also be completed. None the less, several instances of apparent failure of rifampicin to prevent secondary cases have been reported, including cases in which the disease isolate was resistant to rifampicin. When a patient with *H. influenzae* b disease will return from the hospital to a household with a susceptible child, treatment of the patient with rifampicin 20 mg/kg once daily for 4 days is recommended prior to discharge in order to eradicate the carrier state and prevent secondary cases.

LEPROSY

Leprosy is a chronic bacterial infection caused by *Mycobacterium leprae*, which principally affects the cooler parts of the body – skin, upper respiratory tract, anterior segments of the eyes, the superficial sections of cutaneous nerves, and testes (Hastings 1985, Jopling & McDougall 1989). The current WHO estimate of prevalence of the disease is 15 million throughout the world; about 50% of those affected are in Africa or Asia. Since antiquity this disease has conveyed a serious social stigma; Judaic scripture recorded in the Old Testament probably included this infection amongst a group of diseases (*tsar-ath*, later translated to *lepra*) associated with uncleanliness. There is no doubt that leprosy was widespread in Europe, including the UK, in the Middle Ages; 11th century Crusaders returning from the Middle East suffered from the disease, Danish graveyards from the Middle Ages have yielded skulls with unmistakable evidence of lepromatous leprosy, and similar conclusive findings have also been documented in the skull of Robert the Bruce of Scotland.

MICROBIOLOGY AND PATHOLOGY

The acid-fast bacillus *M. leprae* ($0.3 \times 0.5 \times 4$–7 μm) was first visualized in 1873 by Hansen in Norway in fresh scrapings from the skin of an infected patient. The mouse foot pad and nine-banded armadillo (body temperature 32–35°C) are the sole experimental models for in vivo growth of *M. leprae*; limited evidence suggests that infection might be zoonotic in the armadillo. In vitro cultivation of the bacillus has not yet been achieved. The portal of entry for human infection is poorly worked out; nasal secretions are probably important; open ulcers also discharge a high concentration of bacilli, and breast milk from a lepromatous woman contains *M. leprae*. Ethnic factors are clearly important in predisposition; while lepromatous disease afflicts a mere 5–10% of Africans, up to 50% of some Asian populations may be affected. Male : female ratio is 2–3 : 1. Whereas underlying socioeconomic conditions are undoubtedly important background factors, the role of malnutrition as a predisposing factor to infection is unclear. The spectrum of disease – from tuberculoid to lepromatous (Table 23.18) – is governed by the ability of *M. leprae* to survive within the macrophage, and to elicit a delayed-type hypersensitivity reaction

Table 23.18   The clinical spectrum of leprosy

	Tuberculoid (TT)	Borderline tuberculoid (BT)	Borderline (dimorphous, intermediate) (BB)	Borderline lepromatous (BL)	Lepromatous (unusual in children) (LL)
Clinical	Single or several well-defined anesthetic areas; peripheral nerves thickened	Similar to TT; lesions more numerous and less distinct	Similar to BT; lesions more numerous, with satellites (unstable disease)	Similar to BB; some nerve damage	Multiple, symmetrical macular or papular nonanesthetic lesions No neutral lesions until late Leonine facies, testicular atrophy, etc. (late)
Histology	Epithelioid lymphocyte granulomas in nerves and skin; bacilli in nerves rare	Granulomas as in TT; nerves infiltrated, bacilli +	Epithelioid cells and histiocytic infiltrations; nerves similar to BT	Histiocytic infiltrations; lymphocytes +; nerves less infiltrated	Foamy histiocytes containing bacilli + Few lymphocytes Bacilli in nerves and perineurium ++
Density of bacteria in skin	–	±	+	++	+++
Lepromin reaction	+++	+	±	–	–

(cell-mediated immunity) (CMI). In lepromatous disease, CMI is markedly depressed and macrophages cannot clear dermal *M. leprae*; also, T lymphocyte numbers are decreased and lymphocyte–macrophage interaction seems deranged. In tuberculoid disease, a vigorous CMI response results in bacteriological recovery. In lepromatous disease, peripheral B lymphocytes are increased, and concentrations of serum immunoglobulins G, M and A are elevated; C-reactive and amyloid-related proteins may also be raised, together with autoantibodies to rheumatoid factor, thyroglobulin, ANF, etc. Histologically, many organs – nerves, lymph nodes, liver, spleen, upper respiratory tract, eyes and testes – exhibit evidence of cellular infiltration. Effect(s) of treatment on histological appearances have recently been addressed (Cree et al 1995).

CLINICAL FEATURES

The incubation period ranges from 2 to 20 years, but is usually in the 2–5 year spectrum. It is therefore unusual in young children (Sehgal & Chaudhry 1993, Dayal & Bharadwaj 1995). There are many clinical presentations. Owing to the long incubation period, it is unusual for manifestations to occur before late childhood or adulthood. The overt clinical lesions may be preceded by focal paresthesiae and/or pruritus. Clinical leprosy is usually described initially as being intermediate, and examination reveals a single macule or alternatively several poorly defined ones, which are either mildly hypopigmented or erythematous; skin smears either contain a few bacilli or are negative for *M. leprae*. Table 23.18 summarizes the clinical manifestations of fully developed disease. At the tuberculoid (TT) end of the spectrum, either a single or several randomly placed areas of hypopigmentation or erythema – with impaired sensation, sweating and hair loss – are usually present; thickened cutaneous nerves – ulnar, posterior tibial and greater auricular – are often palpated easily. At the lepromatous (LL) end of the spectrum, cutaneous manifestations are more overt and striking – they may be macular and/or nodular; pubic and axillary hair diminishes, the lateral parts of the eyebrows become thin, and later testicular atrophy, gynecomastia, and laryngeal and ophthalmic lesions (keratitis, conjunctival and

scleral changes) may occur. Dermatological lesions may be difficult to differentiate from those in many other diseases, including lupus erythematosus, onchocerciasis, leishmaniasis, psoriasis, etc.; other diseases producing a peripheral neuropathy should also be considered. Recent reports have focused on ocular (Nwosu & Nwosu 1994), oral (Scheepers et al 1993) and renal (Kirsztaju et al 1993) involvement. There are two major categories of inflammatory episode or clinical 'reaction':

1. *Reversal reaction* (CMI is enhanced) in which borderline (BB) lesions become erythematous and edematous and are often accompanied by an acute neuritis (the disease then moves towards TT and ultimately burns itself out leaving permanent residual deformities, e.g. a claw hand or dropped foot).

2. *Erythema nodosum leprosum* (ENL) (a local immune complex reaction) which occurs in lepromatous (LL) and borderline lepromatous (BL) cases, often several months after starting chemotherapy. There is a relatively sudden appearance of subcutaneous nodules which become erythematous and may ulcerate, these being accompanied by fever, arthropathy, iridocyclitis, synovitis and immune complex glomerulonephritis. Amyloidosis is a late sequel.

DIAGNOSIS

Diagnosis is essentially a clinical one (Nagaraju & Gupte 1994). However, histological confirmation by examination of a skin smear from the edge of a macule, plaque or nodule, an ear lobe or nasal mucosa is valuable (Table 23.18). The bacterial index (BI) reflects the density of *M. leprae* in tissue or smear, and the morphological index (MI) the percentage of solidly stained (this equates with viability) *M. leprae* using a standard procedure. Nonviable bacilli are irregular, granular or fragmented. The lepromin test (Table 23.18) is of limited value in diagnosis.

TREATMENT

The management of leprosy consists of (1) specific chemotherapy whilst active infection is present and (2) prevention. Later, correction of deformities and resultant disabilities becomes

Table 23.19   Single and multiple chemotherapeutic regimens for leprosy

Therapeutic agent*	Dose when used alone	Duration	Toxic effects
Single chemotherapeutic regimens			
1. Dapsone (4.4'-diaminodiphenylsulfone, DDS)	1.2 mg/kg daily or 2.4 mg/kg × 3 weekly	Continue for 18 months after activity is no longer detectable; for rest of life in LL	Allergy Desquamating dermatitis Anemia Hepatitis Peripheral neuropathy Psychosis
2. Rifampicin	Not recommended for use alone		
3. Clofazimine (Lamprene)	1.2–3.6 mg/kg daily		Hyperpigmentation Gastrointestinal disturbances Paralytic ileus

Multiple chemotherapeutic regimens
BB, BL and LL:
1. Dapsone: 1.2 mg/kg daily
2. Rifampicin: >35 kg 600 mg; <35 kg 450 mg; <20 kg 300 mg; <12kg 150 mg monthly (at least 2 years)
3. Clofazimine: 0.6 mg/kg daily together with 3.6 mg/kg monthly

BT and TT:
1. Dapsone: 1.2 mg/kg daily
2. Rifampicin >35 kg 600 mg; <35 kg 450 mg; <20 kg 300 mg; <12 kg 150 mg monthly (6 months)

* Prothionamide and ethionamide are alternative agents which are occasionally used.

important. This is usually undertaken on an outpatient basis; segregation of affected patients from those suffering from other infective diseases is not indicated. The first chemotherapeutic agent used successfully in leprosy was dapsone which was introduced in 1943; this is a bacteriostatic agent, but resistant strains of *M. leprae* are increasingly being encountered worldwide. Multiple chemotherapeutic regimens (Table 23.19) are now widely employed (Lancet 1988, Jakeman & Smith 1994, Kishore & Shetty 1995). Details of appropriate courses are summarized for the five major clinical varieties of the disease. Rifampicin is bactericidal; a similar action has also been demonstrated using clarithromycin and minocycline in lepromatous disease (Ji et al 1993). Clofazimine has anti-inflammatory in addition to antilepromatous properties and resistance to its action is rarely encountered; it is of value in the management of ENL reactions. Careful long-term follow-up is essential, and MI evaluations are of value in monitoring progress. In the management of leprosy reactions, special treatment is indicated. For reversal reactions (see above), analgesics and corticosteroids (e.g. prednisolone 2 mg/kg daily) are required when nerve involvement is severe. Physiotherapy is important. In ENL reactions, analgesics are also often required; thalidomide (daily) or corticosteroids (as for reversal reactions) are indicated rarely. The former agent should not be used in young children or pregnant women (or those who might become pregnant) owing to its teratogenic potential. In practice, however, LL is a very unusual event in childhood, and although ENL occasionally complicates BL this is a rarity. Corticosteroids are indicated for iridocyclitis in lepromatous disease. Management of longstanding complications is a long-term and complex problem. Further trauma must be minimized by using protective devices; eyes and limbs are important organs to protect. Evaluation by a surgeon with special expertise in dealing with deformities caused by *M. leprae* is important. When long-term management is started early, mutilation can be minimized if not prevented and prognosis should then be excellent. A vaccine is not available, but BCG vaccination has been shown to confer significant protection (Fine et al 1986, Baker et al 1993, Orega et al 1993).

LEPTOSPIROSIS

Leptospirosis is a worldwide zoonosis transmitted to humans by infected urine of a wide range of domestic and wild animals: often the causative spirochetes are excreted asymptomatically for long periods of time (Ferguson 1991, Farrer 1995).

Adults usually acquire infection because of occupational exposure: children may acquire infection by playing in areas contaminated with animal urine or by playing with the animals themselves.

PATHOLOGY

In Britain and America the common serotypes of the genus *Leptospira* include *L. icterohemorrhagica* (commonly acquired from rat's urine), *L. canicola* (commonly acquired from dog's urine), *L. pomona* (commonly acquired from pig's urine), *L. hebdomadis* and *L. ballum*. Correlation of named serotypes with specific syndromes is impossible because of the variability of illness produced by each serotype.

Leptospires gain entry to humans via ingestion, via mucous membranes, via skin abrasions or via the conjunctivae. After entry the organisms affect capillary epithelium and may cause capillary damage, hypoxia and hemorrhage into various organs. Liver damage may cause jaundice (although hemolysis may also play a part), renal damage may cause renal failure, central nervous system damage meningitis and encephalitis, and skeletal muscle involvement muscle pain. Blood clotting parameters are often not disordered enough to account for the hemorrhagic tendency. Illnesses may be biphasic with initial symptoms caused by leptospiremia and later symptoms by host immune responses.

CLINICAL FEATURES

The incubation period is probably from a few days to just under 3 weeks.

The clinical manifestations range through asymptomatic infection to multisystem disease. With clinical disease there is usually an abrupt onset of fever with several possible accompaniments:

1. muscular pains
2. marked constitutional upset and hemorrhagic manifestations
3. nephritic features usually without associated hypertension
4. jaundice with or without hemorrhages
5. jaundice with leukocytosis or a raised erythrocyte sedimentation rate (leukocytosis and a raised sedimentation rate are unusual in viral hepatitis)
6. meningitis with injected or hemorrhagic conjuctivae, or a lymphocytic meningitis with normal biochemical parameters: this syndrome is typically associated with *L. canicola* infection
7. persistent fever lasting up to 3 or 4 weeks, perhaps without other signs
8. jaundice with nephritis: Weil's syndrome, usually caused by *L. icterohemorrhagica* infection in which renal failure is a common cause of death (in contrast most patients with viral hepatitis have a low or normal urea and present with gradual-onset malaise and fever which usually remits once jaundice is apparent).

DIAGNOSIS AND DIFFERENTIAL

Blood cultures may be positive in early illness, but some *Leptospira* resist standard culture and the diagnosis has to be confirmed by dark ground microscopy or by serology. Usually reactive antibody becomes detectable after the first week of illness. Agglutination and complement fixation tests are often used. If there is a meningitic clinical picture the cerebrospinal fluid (CSF) is usually lymphocytic; the CSF biochemistry is often normal and CSF culture may be positive. Urine culture or dark ground microscopy may be positive once infection is established, and may remain positive for several weeks.

The differential diagnosis is very wide: if a zoonosis is suspected Q fever or brucellosis are major contenders.

TREATMENT

Eradication of noncommercial animals (such as rats) or reducing potential exposure to animal urine is ideal. *Leptospira* are sensitive to penicillin, tetracyclines (which are contraindicated in renal failure and which, depending on the severity of illness, are contraindicated in children) and erythromycin. Usually high doses are given for 10 days. Early treatment is essential as antibiotics will do little to alleviate the immune-mediated elements of the illness. Isolation of patients is unnecessary as person-to-person spread is unlikely. Despite serious dysfunction of infected organs in acute illness, recovery is usually complete in survivors.

LYME DISEASE

Lyme disease is a seasonal nonoccupational bacterial zoonosis which is distributed throughout the temperate zones of the world (Schmid 1985). It was first recognized in 1975 because of a geographic clustering of children with arthritis in Lyme, Connecticut (Steere et al 1977). It is now recognized that the causative agent is an arthropod-borne spirochete called *Borrelia burgdorferi* which is transmitted by the hard tick *Ixodes daminii* or related ixodid ticks depending on the geographical distribution (e.g. *Ixodes ricinus* is predominant in Europe (Muhlemann &

Wright 1987). The tick which has a wide range of hosts (deer, cattle, sheep, mice, squirrels, dogs) appears to prefer the white-footed mouse and white-tailed deer. Birds are now also recognized as reservoirs.

The illness is a multisystem disorder which consists of a prodromal febrile illness with the characteristic rash of erythema chronicum migrans (ECM) and associated symptoms. Without antibiotic treatment a substantial number of patients will go on to cardiac, neurological and rheumatological sequelae. However, progression from early to late stage is not inevitable, even in the absence of antibiotic treatment. 'Incomplete' cases with minimal or absent rash can occur, and patients may have aseptic meningitis, facial palsy, carditis or arthritis as the first sign of disease.

ETIOLOGY AND VECTOR

In 1982 a previously unrecognized spirochete was isolated from *I. daminii* ticks that had been collected from Shelter Island, New York. This discovery was followed in 1983 by the successful culture of the spirochete named *B. burgdorferi* from patients with Lyme disease (Steere et al 1983a).

The main vector species are *I. ricinus* in Europe and the *I. scapularis* group in North America (Anderson 1989). The life cycle of the tick consists of larval, nymphal and adult stages. The larvae and nymphs primarily feed on rodents such as the white-footed mouse, the natural reservoir for *I. daminii*. The adults usually feed on large mammals like deer, sheep and horses. Furthermore, the growth of the vector population is promoted by deer and fails to occur in their absence. The nymphal stage whose peak questing period is May through July is primarily responsible for transmission of disease. As these immature ticks feed aggressively on more animal species they facilitate rapid transmission of the organisms and often escape detection by the human host because they remain very small, even after a feed.

EPIDEMIOLOGY

Lyme disease is the most common vector-borne disease among children with more cases in children than adults. However, there is substantial regional variation in the incidence of Lyme disease although most cases appear to occur during the summer months. The estimated incidence in the USA in 1992 was 3.9 per 100 000 population with Connecticut having the highest incidence (53.6/100 000). These figures are undoubtedly underestimates as only a small proportion of cases are reported. In the UK, for example, the incidence of Lyme disease is not well documented although experience suggests that serious disease is not common. Children between the ages of 5 to 10 years appear to be at highest risk in endemic areas.

PATHOGENESIS

In early Lyme disease the spirochete is injected into the bloodstream or skin through tick saliva. It may also be deposited in fecal material on the skin, and from there the organism may invade the skin or blood. Following an incubation period of 3–32 days the organism migrates outwards in the skin to produce the classical immune-mediated lesion of ECM. It may also spread to the lymphatics or disseminate in the blood or organs such as the brain, heart or joints or to other sites to produce the secondary lesions of late-stage disease. The propensity to produce damage of a specific target organ appears to be determined by a number of factors including genospecies of *Borelia* isolate as well as host factors such as HLA phenotype. For Example, *B. afzelli* is more common in patients with mainly dermatological manifestations, whereas *B. garinii* is more often associated with neurological complications (Van Dam et al 1993). Furthermore, arthritis, which is a more common presentation of early or late Lyme in Europe as opposed to ECM in North America, is more commonly seen in patients with HLA-DR4 and -DR2 (Steere et al 1990). There is also some evidence that patients with severe and prolonged illness, especially neurological or joint disease, have an increased frequency of the B cell alloantigen HLA-DR2 (Steere et al 1979).

CLINICAL CHARACTERISTICS

Like other spirochetal infections the illness can occur in distinct stages which may overlap or occur alone without recalling earlier features.

Early manifestations (Steere et al 1983b)

Up to one-third of patients remember a tick bite which often leaves a nonspecific small red macule or papule. About 1 week later this area expands to the pathognomonic warm, painless, erythematous, annular lesion called ECM which reaches a maximum diameter of 15 cm (larger areas up to 70 cm have been reported) and usually has a bright red outer border. In the largest community-based prospective study reported in children, 89% of those studied presented with a single or multiple lesions of ECM (Shapiro & Gerber 1994).

This lesion, which resolves within 4 weeks without therapy, can occur at any site although the thigh, groin and axilla are particularly common. Concomitant signs and symptoms include high fever (particularly in children), malaise, regional lymphadenopathy, meningism, myalgia and migratory arthralgias. Most of the early clinical features are characteristically intermittent and fluctuating during a period of several weeks before spontaneous resolution occurs. About 10% of patients have features suggestive of anicteric hepatitis. Cellulitis secondary to an infected insect bite is a common misdiagnosis.

Two uncommon skin lesions, acrodermatitis chronica atrophicans and lymphadenosis benigna cutis, which are rare both in children and in North America, are regarded as specific late skin manifestations in Lyme disease (O'Neill & Wright 1988).

Late manifestations

These manifestations occur some weeks to months after the initial infection and the clinical features are dependent on the organ affected and the severity of damage.

In about 10–40% of patients, frank *neurological abnormalities* usually occur weeks to months after infection. The classical triad of early neurological disease includes a lymphocytic meningitis, cranial neuropathy, and radiculoneuritis. Neuroborreliosis in children most commonly presents as mild encephalopathy, lymphocytic meningitis and cranial neuropathy (Garcia-Monoco & Benach 1995). Radiculopathy, particularly in European children, and peripheral neuropathy both of which occur late in the disease are rare in children. Typically patients develop a fluctuating lymphocytic meningitis about 4 weeks after the onset of ECM often with superimposed cranial (especially facial) neuritis. Patients will have a CSF lymphocytic pleocytosis. Other less common neurological complications include ataxia, spastic paraparesis due to an acute myelitis, hemiparesis, optic neuritis, hydrocephalus, Guillain–Barré syndrome and a pseudotumor cerebri-like syndrome.

Cardiac disease, which is relatively uncommon in children, occurs roughly 5 weeks after the tick bite. The disease spectrum includes myopericarditis, cardiomegaly, left ventricular dysfunction and especially fluctuating degrees of atrioventricular block which may progress to complete heart block. The latter may require temporary pacing. The duration of cardiac involvement is usually brief (3 days to 6 weeks) and self-limiting. The clinical features show similarities to rheumatic fever although valvular involvement has not been reported.

Arthritis is a common late sequela of Lyme disease occurring in up to 60% of patients within a few weeks to 2 years after the onset of illness. 20–40% of patients do not remember having ECM. The spectrum of Lyme arthritis ranges from subjective joint pains which are often migratory, to intermittent attacks of arthritis to chronic erosive disease (10%) (Steere et al 1987). The commonest pattern of joint involvement is an acute asymmetric mono- or oligoarticular arthritis primarily affecting the large joints. Most commonly (> 90%) involved is the knee joint and the child typically presents with subacute effusion of the knee. The attacks of arthritis typically last for a few weeks to months and recur intermittently over several years. Fatigue is the commonest associated nonarticular symptom, whereas fever or other systemic symptoms are unusual.

Numerous other rare manifestations have been associated with Lyme disease. These include ophthalmic complications (conjunctivitis, episcleritis, photophobia, uveitis), hepatitis, hepatosplenomegaly and testicular swelling. There is no clear evidence that *B. burgdorferi* causes congenital disease, although the existence of this rare syndrome cannot be ruled out (Shapiro 1995). Furthermore, transmission of Lyme disease in breast milk has not been documented.

DIAGNOSIS

The diagnosis is not always easy, given that symptoms may be nonspecific, and serology may be misleading (Feder & Hunt 1995). The hallmark for confirming the diagnosis is to obtain appropriate fluid or tissue for culture. Such tests are unlikely to be of value in everyday clinical practice and future diagnostic tests such as polymerase chain reaction (PCR) have not yet been adequately tested. Therefore, serological tests which detect antibodies against *B. burgdorferi* are the most commonly used diagnostic tests. The most commonly used test which is now widely available as prepacked commercial kits is the enzyme-linked immunosorbent assay (ELISA). Unfortunately, this test yields many false positive reactions with other spirochetal infections, connective tissue diseases and certain viral infections (Shapiro 1995). There is also cross-reactivity with antigens of spirochetes belonging to the normal flora. The immunoblotting technique currently offers the best means of validating a positive or equivocal ELISA in a patient with a low likelihood of Lyme, although this test is not widely available and its proper interpretation is as yet unclear (Dressler et al 1993).

Currently the diagnosis of early Lyme disease, especially in the presence of skin lesions, is made on clinical and epidemiological grounds since serology (*B. burgdorferi* IgM) does not usually become positive until 3–6 weeks after the onset of the erythema migrans. Also, the antibody response may be aborted in patients with early Lyme who are treated promptly with an effective antimicrobial agent. The specific IgG antibody rises slowly and may not reach a level of diagnostic significance in early disease. It usually peaks months or years later, often when arthritis is present, and can persist for many years despite adequate treatment or cure. Furthermore, a substantial proportion of people who become infected by *B. burgdorferi* never have a clinical illness but have positive serology. Serological testing is not necessary for diagnosing typical ECM but is helpful in untreated atypical skin lesions, patients with acute meningitis, neuropathies and arthritis due to Lyme. The negative and positive predictive values of currently available serological tests are very much dependent on the pretest likelihood that a patient has Lyme disease. For example, a patient with ECM who lives in an endemic area has a very high probability of having Lyme even if the serological test is negative. Conversely, a patient with vague nonspecific symptoms with a positive test is unlikely to have Lyme despite positive serology. Therefore, serological tests should not be used on patients with nonspecific symptoms but clinicians should order serological tests for Lyme disease in selected groups such as those with clinical findings suggestive of Lyme or in highly prevalent areas so that the predictive value of the test is high (Shapiro 1995).

TREATMENT

Since no clinical trials of treatment have been performed in children the recommendations for treatment have been extrapolated from adult studies (Table 23.20). Lyme disease if treated early will respond well to antibiotic therapy, shortening the duration of illness and reducing the incidence of complications. The long-term prognosis for this group (Salazar et al 1993) as well as those treated for late Lyme disease is excellent (Szer et al 1991).

PREVENTION

Acquisition of Lyme borreliosis can be reduced by simple practical methods such as wearing long trousers, tucking trousers into socks, wearing boots, promptly removing any attached ticks and impregnating clothes with DEET or permethrin. A vaccine is currently under development.

MENINGOCOCCEMIA

Neisseria meningitidis, a Gram-negative diplococcus, is the most frequent cause of septicemia in the otherwise healthy child outside the neonatal period. The organism is carried in the nasopharynx of 2–5% of the population. All serogroups of *N. meningitidis* can cause septicemia.

In Western Europe the group B organism is still the most commonly isolated strain but is closely followed by group C organisms. *N. meningitidis* group A has been responsible for large epidemics. The antibiotic sensitivity of the organism is also changing. Sulfonamide resistance occurred in the 1960s and in the 1980s penicillin resistance was reported.

Children usually acquire the organism from a colonized adult. Acquisition is rare in infants under 3 months, probably due to the protection from maternal antibody. Not all nonimmune contacts become colonized and only a small number of colonized individuals develop invasive disease. The factors governing these

Table 23.20 The antibiotic therapy of Lyme disease

Skin
Children > 8 years: Tetracycline 40–50 mg/kg per day (max. 1 g) in divided doses p.o. for 10–30 days*
Children < 8 years: Phenoxymethyl penicillin 50 mg/kg per day in divided doses p.o. for 10 days; or erythromycin 30 mg/kg per day p.o. for 10–30 days for penicillin-allergic children

Neurological
Cefotaxime 100–200 mg/kg daily i.v. or i.m. for 14 days; or ceftriaxone 20–80 mg/kg daily†
Penicillin 300 mg/kg i.v. by continuous infusion or 6 divided doses daily for 14 days is now considered to be second line therapy

Cardiac
First degree atrioventricular block – oral regimens, as for skin infection
High degree atrioventricular block – penicillin G 300 mg/kg i.v., 6 divided doses daily for 14 days

Joint
Benzyl penicillin 300 mg/kg per day i.v. in divided doses for 14 days
Benzathine penicillin intramuscularly or ceftriaxone may also be used.
Aspirin or a nonsteroidal anti-inflammatory drug may be added

* Tetracyline is a drug of choice except in children < 8 years, because it is more effective than penicillin or erythromycin in preventing late sequelae (Steere et al 1983c).
† Cefotaxime or ceftriaxone have been found to be superior to penicillin in treating neurological complications, especially those that have failed to respond to penicillin (Pal et al 1988).

risks are poorly understood. Immune deficiency of properdin is known to increase the risk of infection and deficiencies of the terminal components of complement are associated with recurrent infections (Densen et al 1987).

The majority of people develop a bactericidal response to colonization. A concurrent viral upper respiratory tract infection predisposes to invasive disease by disrupting the mucosal barrier and possibly interfering with host defenses. Once the organism penetrates the mucosa it is carried by the leukocytes into the bloodstream and may cause clinical disease.

CLINICAL FINDINGS

Meningococcal septicemia may occur on its own in an acute, subacute or, rarely, chronic form.

Acute meningococcal septicemia may be very rapid in onset and rapidly fatal. In the younger child a rash, fever and malaise are the usual presenting complaints. The older child may complain of headache or abdominal pain. In the early stages fever, tachycardia and tachypnea may be present with the rash. This rash is often first found on the buttocks or abdomen and may be purpuric or morbilliform (Plate 23.1). Later signs of shock develop with poor peripheral perfusion, hypotension and oliguria. This is generally accompanied by an extensive purpuric rash and evidence of disseminated intravascular coagulopathy (DIC) (Plate 23.2). Hemorrhage into internal organs may occur. Classically this involves the adrenal glands in the Waterhouse–Friderichsen syndrome. DIC and circulatory failure due to endotoxic shock are the usual causes of death. In those who recover, skin necrosis or vascular occlusion may cause the loss of an extremity though most small lesions heal with minimal scarring.

The subacute form may present with a generalized petechial rash and progress to cause focal infection in the meninges, joints, heart or eye.

The chronic form of meningococcal sepsis is characterized by anorexia, weight loss, fever, arthralgia or arthritis and nonpurpuric skin rash. Erythema nodosum or bacterial endocarditis may occur.

Arthritis, pericarditis and pleural effusions may occur as autoimmune phenomena 5–10 days after the acute infection. This is due to immune complex formation and is self-limiting but a large pericardial effusion may cause cardiac tamponade.

In the differential diagnosis other bacterial and viral infections which cause purpura must be considered. Anaphylactoid purpura and idiopathic thrombocytopenic purpura may cause similar purpuric rashes. A morbilliform rash may be confused with a drug eruption or a number of viral infections including measles. Subacute or chronic meningococcemia presents a greater challenge. The differential diagnosis must include the many causes of arthritis and fever in children.

LABORATORY INVESTIGATION

The diagnosis is established by recovery of *N. meningitidis* from the blood, petechial lesions or the cerebrospinal fluid (CSF). The practice of giving penicillin before hospital admission has decreased successful culture of the organism. Meningococcal DNA may be detected by polymerase chain reaction (PCR) in blood and CSF. Serology may confirm the clinical diagnosis retrospectively. The complete blood count may show a polymorphonuclear leukocytosis or leukopenia in severe infection. Platelets are reduced in the presence of DIC when fragmentation of red blood cells may be seen on the blood film. On an appropriately stained blood film, Gram-negative diplococci may be identified.

TREATMENT

Penicillin is the preferred therapeutic agent unless there have been local reports of resistance. Cefotaxime is used in those with penicillin allergy and increasingly, as the antibiotic of first choice in suspected septicemia.

In shocked children vigorous resuscitation is undertaken. Large volumes of plasma and albumin may be required. Inotropic agents, dopamine and dobutamine, are useful if shock fails to respond to fluids alone. Artificial ventilation should not be postponed (Nadel et al 1995). New therapies which alter the immune response or inflammatory cascade are under investigation at present.

Prophylaxis against invasive disease should be given to the family and close contacts of the patient. The patient should receive similar therapy as penicillin does not eradicate the organism from the nasopharynx. Rifampicin in four doses has been shown to be effective in clearing the organism. A single injection of ceftriaxone or oral dose of ciprofloxacin are appropriate alternatives.

Polysaccharide vaccines are available for *N. meningitidis* groups A, C, Y and W but not for the more common group B. The immune response is poor in children under 2 years (Duerden 1988). Work is continuing on outer membrane antigens and conjugate vaccines. The mortality from acute meningococcemia remains high. Between 20% and 40% of those presenting with peripheral purpura and shock die, most within the first 12 hours. Those who present with a generalized morbilliform or petechial rash are more likely to develop meningitis but mortality is less than 10%. The outcome is related to the presence of shock and the state of consciousness of the child at the time of presentation.

PERTUSSIS

ETIOLOGY AND PATHOGENESIS

The causative organism *Bordetella pertussis* is a coccobacillus whose only natural host is man. Other microorganisms, *Bordetella parapertussis* and adenoviruses may cause a clinically similar condition but are only responsible for a minority of cases and rarely result in severe disease. *B. pertussis* is spread by aerosol or direct contact. Otherwise it is a relatively fragile organism that dies quickly outside of its host and is rarely transmitted through fomites.

Respiratory colonization takes place whereby the organisms attach and multiply on the cilia of the epithelium. The organism produces a number of biologically active molecules including a toxin. Some of these products determine attachment of the bacteria to the respiratory mucosa but the role of others is still unknown and the role of the toxin is uncertain beyond it producing the characteristic lymphocytosis. It seems unlikely that pertussis disease is only mediated through toxin production as acellular vaccines giving protection against toxin alone only confer limited protection (Miller 1995). The bacteria do not invade the body and symptoms are mediated through alteration in cell function rather than cell damage. Restoration depends on cell renewal not bacterial destruction. Infection can be well established before a clinical diagnosis can be made and so even though *B. pertussis* is vulnerable to antibiotics these will have little therapeutic value for the symptomatic child.

EPIDEMIOLOGY

Pertussis occurs worldwide with an estimated 60 million cases and 0.5–1 million deaths annually (Muller et al 1986). Where immunization is unavailable it is estimated that 80% of children are infected by age 5 and well over 90% by adulthood (Clarkson & Fine 1985). The disease can be acquired immediately after birth and in an unimmunized community its highest incidence is in the preschool years. However, it also occurs in adolescents and adults (Deville et al 1995, Wirsing von Konig et al 1995), increasingly so where successful immunization programs protect the younger children but give less protection to older individuals in whom induced protection declines with age (Jenkinson 1988, Ramsay et al 1993, Bass & Wittler 1994). A high herd immunity contributes to control (Nielsen & Larsen 1994). There is an unusual sex difference with pertussis being commoner and perhaps also more severe in girls. Because of diagnostic and other difficulties it is recognized that reported rates are a substantial underestimate of true incidence. The UK has one of the better surveillance systems but only 5–25% of cases are notified (Clarkson & Fine 1985). Under-reporting is common for the older age groups and the very young, partially because these are age-groups when the disease has more atypical presentations (Deville et al 1995, Wirsing von Konig et al 1995).

Epidemics used to occur once every 3–4 years in the UK (Fig. 23.8; Grenfell & Anderson 1989) and similar patterns have been reported in some other countries (Muller et al 1986). There was a substantial recrudescence of pertussis in the UK when immunization slumped in the mid-1970s (Joint Committee on Vaccination and Immunization 1981). 14 years had to elapse before immunization uptake recovered, during which time two substantial epidemics took place each producing cases estimated to be in excess of 400 000. By 1986 immunization had raised herd

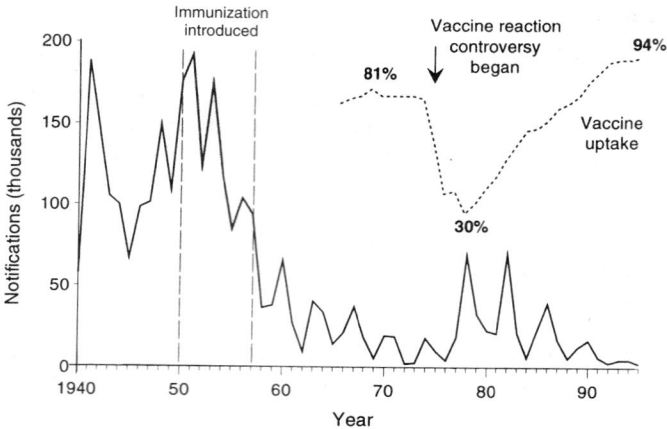

Fig. 23.8 Whooping cough notifications and vaccine uptake rate; UK 1940–1995.

immunity just enough to prevent the second half of the epidemic that began in 1985 and subsequent epidemics have been muted (Fig. 23.8). In the diverse and less densely populated US the epidemic pattern is less clear (CDC 1993a). It experienced a return of epidemic pertussis in the early 1990s and it has been suggested that this was because of an over-reliance on immunization in younger children without boosting in older individuals (Bass & Wittler 1994). Subsequent trial data suggests that the whole-cell vaccine used in the US may have lacked protective efficacy (Miller 1995).

Pertussis has high morbidity. In one study by the College of General Practitioners during the UK 1977–1979 epidemic 3% of all notified child cases were admitted to hospital whilst the proportion rose to 13% among infants. Deaths from whooping cough are uncommon in developed countries with widespread vaccination. 93 deaths from whooping cough were reported in the 15 years from 1974 to 1987 in England and Wales when the disease was widespread following the fall in immunization; subsequently in the 5 years from 1988 to 1993 there have been 9 deaths. However, these figures are likely to be an underestimate because of unrecognized pertussis deaths in the youngest infants which may appear as sudden infant death syndrome or deaths from respiratory infections (Southall et al 1988, Nicoll & Gardner 1988). An unusual epidemiological feature in the UK is that intervals between epidemics have not varied with levels of immunity. Despite a halving of the immunization rate after 1975 there was little if any change in the interepidemic interval (Fig. 23.8), suggesting that immunization is more successful in preventing disease than infection (Fine & Clarkson 1987).

NATURAL HISTORY

The incubation period ranges from 7 to 14 days (beyond 10 days is unusual). Once symptoms start the disease has customarily been divided into three phases. The first is the *catarrhal phase* when disease is essentially indistinguishable from a cough and cold, sometimes with a mild fever (never above 38°C). After 1 week to 10 days the cough worsens and the disease moves into the *paroxysmal phase* with bouts of coughing; the child's face becoming congested passing from red to blue during bouts. The classical whoop stems from the final desperate inspiration at the end of a bout of coughing. Equally commonly the bout may end with the child vomiting. The length and severity of this second phase is variable but can continue for 2 weeks without improvement. Finally if complications do not ensue the disease moves imperceptibly into the *convalescent phase* during which coughing slowly subsides over a period which can last for 3 months or more. In clinical practice the paroxysmal and convalescent phases are best considered as one and relapses back to paroxysmal coughing are common. It is not surprising that in some countries the disease is known as 'the cough of a hundred days'. The whole process is exhausting and extremely worrying for the family. The child will be scared and distressed during the illness and will often carry the memory into adulthood. Presentation of the disease can be atypical in adults (Deville et al 1995, Wirsing von Konig et al 1995) and young babies. In older patients the whoop may be absent. This is also the case in the youngest sufferers who may lack the strength to mount paroxysms. These are the patients most at risk and the disease can present as a serious respiratory infection or a cough proceeding to apneic attacks. Babies are especially vulnerable since protective antibodies acquired in childhood decline in adults and hence there is little passive protection of the newborn by maternal antibodies. Though there are mild cases at all ages truly asymptomatic infections are considered to be rare and chronic carriers do not exist. Immunized children can experience a typical disease though the clinical course is usually milder than in unimmunized individuals (Bortolussi et al 1995).

Complications are common, mostly resulting from the paroxysms. Pressure effects lead to venous congestion causing subconjunctival hemorrhages, skin petechiae, nose bleeds and hemoptysis. Intracranial hemorrhage is very rare but has been recorded. Raised intra-abdominal pressure may also enlarge a number of hernias. Respiratory complications frequently occur though rarely result in permanent lung damage in developed countries where antibiotics are available to treat secondary infections. However, children with an asthmatic tendency may have this revealed by their pertussis. Atelectasis is thought to be due to the inspiration of secretions during the 'whoop'; this in turn predisposes to secondary infection in the lungs. Such should be suspected in any infected child with a significant temperature. Most commonly it is due to otitis media or bronchopneumonia. Neurological sequelae are the most serious complications but are very rare. They are thought to occur through anoxia following apnea, though there may also be a direct toxin effect. They can manifest as loss of consciousness, convulsions or encephalopathy which when severe may lead to brain damage, handicap and death.

The child with pertussis is infectious from 2 weeks after infection and if untreated can remain so for up to 3 months, though this only applies to ≤ 5% of individuals after 5 weeks of starting the spasmodic phase (Madsen 1925). The disease is highly infectious and it can be expected that one child will infect 90% of nonimmune household child contacts.

DIAGNOSIS

Diagnosis is essentially clinical and once the paroxysmal phase has been reached the classical case is unmistakable even to those who have never experienced the disease before. The World Health Organization has suggested guidelines for diagnosis from which the following criteria have been adapted.

Whooping cough should be suspected whenever there is a history of severe cough lasting for 2 weeks or more. This *probable whooping cough* case should be notified and treated as whooping cough if *any* of the following exist:

1. prolonged coughing followed by a period of apnea and cyanosis, or in older children paroxysms of coughing followed by vomiting, or a typical breath intake and 'whoop', or subconjunctival hemorrhages
2. exposure of a suspect case in the previous 3 weeks
3. epidemic of whooping cough in the area
4. lymphocytosis of 15 000/mm^3 or more.

Simpler criteria based on a cough persisting more than 2 weeks have also been shown to be useful (Partriarca et al 1988).

A probable case is *confirmed* if there is laboratory evidence of *B. pertussis* from culture or immunofluorescence of nasopharyngeal secretions (Onorato & Wassilak 1987). The nasopharyngeal diagnosis is provided by a pernasal sample which requires a special cotton swab on a long flexible wand. This is inserted through a nostril into the postnasal space. It is an unpleasant procedure for the child, requiring gentle but firm positioning on a parent's lap. Such sampling will often trigger the paroxysmal cough the family has reported. The swab needs to be placed in a culture medium such as Stuarts, and, though storage overnight in a refrigerator is permissible, rapid transport to the laboratory for plating improves the chance of a positive result. Prior treatment with antibiotics will also reduce the chance of a successful culture. Once in the laboratory the sample will usually be subjected to fluorescent antibody study and/or culture techniques. These are highly specific but false negatives are commonly experienced with only 80% of suspected cases revealing positive results in the research laboratory whilst rates of 40–60% are more common in routine work. Immunofluorescence may detect dead organisms or miss a few live ones sufficient to give a positive culture. Hence a child with the disease may be positive on one test but negative on the other. Immunofluorescence is a rapid technique whilst culture requires 48–72 h. Polymerase chain reaction looks a promising tool and may be more sensitive than culture (He et al 1994) while serological testing can be performed in some laboratories but is essentially a research procedure.

TREATMENT

Once in the paroxysmal phase drug therapy makes little impact on the course of the illness. An antibiotic (erythromycin is highly effective) should always be given to render the sufferer noninfectious. This is normally achieved after 5 days of erythromycin; however, treatment is best continued for 2 weeks as a few individuals have been reported culture positive after only 1 week of antibiotics (Hoppe & Haug 1988). Managing the child with pertussis is mostly a nursing task either for the parents or professional staff. This is most critical in the small infant. Walker (1988) recommends five principles of care in these circumstances:

1. avoid provoking paroxysms of coughing
2. comforting during paroxysms
3. clearing away mucus and vomit during paroxysms to prevent inhalation
4. early recognition and treatment of complications
5. maintaining good hydration and reasonable nutrition.

The baby who is badly affected will need small frequent feeds. Experienced nurses used to give feeds at the end of coughing bouts when, presumably, secretions would have been cleared, but sometimes tube feeding is necessary. Being nursed in a sitting position seems to give some relief for the baby and it makes picking up and comforting easier during a coughing bout. Most cases will be managed at home. Parents need to be told about the natural history of the illness. After 5 days of treatment with an effective antibiotic there is no reason for isolating a child though most will not feel well enough to return to school for some time. Community child health or public health staff need to explain to schools that a treated child in the convalescent phase is noninfectious. Parents should be asked about other children who might have been exposed, particularly young babies, and appropriate action taken.

If spasms of coughing are frequent the child and the parents are soon exhausted. Young infants are commonly admitted during epidemics because the parents require a break from what is a most distressing illness. In hospital the child will need to be nursed in isolation until at least 5 days' treatment with erythromycin. If the child is in a cubicle baby alarms may be needed to alert the staff to paroxysms. The immunization status of nursing and medical staff who are immediately involved should be checked and rectified if deficient. Immunization in adults is both safe and effective. If staff develop a persistent cough this should be investigated.

PREVENTION AND CONTROL

Prophylaxis

Children suspected of being infected should be given a 2-week course of erythromycin to render them noninfectious. There is no strong evidence that such medication is effective in protecting an uninfected child; however, it would seem reasonable to give it, particularly if a baby has been exposed to infection.

Immunization (see pp. 341 to 345)

The fall in immunization in the UK and the consequences (Fig. 23.8) provided evidence of the effectiveness of immunization with a whole-cell preparation. That used in the UK is highly protective with estimates of its effectiveness ranging from 80–95% (Miller et al 1992). Efficacy is somewhat lower in epidemic years (Ramsay et al 1993). Protection wanes with years since immunization though a primary course with a whole-cell vaccine in the UK confers good protection to age 8 years (Jenkinson 1988, Ramsay et al 1993). The national schedule for the UK is for pertussis antigen to be given in combination with diphtheria and tetanus (DTP or the 'triple' vaccine) as three doses at the ages of 2, 3 and 4 months (DoH 1996). Children who missed out on protection as infants should also be immunized and may receive the single component vaccine. If the vaccine is given at other ages, intervals of 6–8 weeks are recommended between the first and second and second and third injections. Once the third birthday is reached the intervals can be reduced to 1 month. Boosting at older ages may need to be introduced in the UK to ensure adequate protection in adulthood (Miller 1995). Other immunization schedules may be appropriate in other circumstances, for example where pertussis mortality is high. The WHO schedule is for three doses at monthly intervals starting at 6 weeks of age.

If a child has an acute febrile illness immunization should be deferred for 1 week. Otherwise the *only* contraindication is a severe local or general reaction to a prior immunization including pertussis. Such reactions are defined as:

1. *Local*: an extensive area of redness and swelling which becomes indurated and involves part of the front and side surface of the thigh or a major part of the circumference of the upper arm.
2. *General*: any of: temperature over 39.5°C within 48 hours of immunization, anaphylaxis, bronchospasm, laryngeal edema, generalized collapse, prolonged unresponsiveness, convulsions or prolonged inconsolable screaming occurring within 72 h.

Many parents and professionals will have heard of other mythical contraindications concerning fits, asthma and other conditions (Begg & Nicoll 1994). These should not be allowed to deny children protection (Davies et al 1995, DoH 1996).

Mild reactions following pertussis immunization are relatively common, most often the child being mildly irritable and pyrexial. More severe reactions are rare and there is *no* evidence to support a causal relationship between the vaccine and irreversible neurological damage in the short or long term (Miller et al 1993).

A variety of acellular vaccines (vaccines not based on whole-cell preparations) have been developed and are in use in some countries (Cherry 1993, Miller 1995). They are less toxigenic than the whole-cell vaccines and may be more efficacious than some whole cell vaccines, for example that in use in the US (Edwards & Decker 1996). However, a combination of a variety of components is needed to achieve acceptable protection. A Swedish trial due to be completed in 1996 should reveal whether candidate acellular vaccines possess the same high efficacy (around 90%) as the whole-cell preparations currently in use in the UK (Miller 1995).

PLAGUE

A bacterial infection (primarily zoonotic) of man and animals, plague is caused by *Yersinia pestis* (an aerobic Gram-negative bacillus which is readily cultured in broth and agar media). Reservoirs of infection exist in sylvatic and urban rodents (especially *Rattus rattus* and *R. norvegicus*); it is transmitted amongst animals, and occasionally to man by the bite of an infected flea (Cook 1995). The bubonic variety is the most common and consists of acute regional lymphadenitis; pneumonic, septicemic and meningeal forms also exist. The disease is widely distributed, especially in tropical countries, and important foci are present in southeast Asia, Africa and South and North America (Craven et al 1993). Throughout history, this infection has caused devastating pandemics with high mortality rates; under these circumstances, in addition to flea-to-man spread, pneumonic man-to-man transmission has been important. The causative organism was identified (and cultured) by Yersin and Kitasato in Hong Kong in 1894.

CLINICAL FEATURES

The disease can afflict individuals of any age including infants (Kabra et al 1994). After an incubation period of 2–8 days, bacteria proliferate in the regional lymph node(s) nearest to the flea bite. A sudden onset of fever, headache and weakness precedes the appearance of an extremely tender bubo; the groin (most common), axilla or neck are most usually affected (Butler 1983, Florman et al 1986). Only rarely is there evidence of the bite and/or lymphangitis. Necrosis and hemorrhage into the bubo and ulceration may occur. Purpuric skin lesions resulting from vasculitis may also be present and these can become necrotic; they resemble the Schwartzmann reaction produced in rabbits by intradermal injection, and followed the next day by an intravenous injection, of endotoxin. Hepatosplenomegaly is often present. An intense intermittent bacteremia is common, and in a fulminant case death can follow as rapidly as 2–4 days after onset of symptoms. Hematogenous spread to the lungs can give rise to *pneumonic* plague (McClean 1995); this form is highly contagious (by airborne transmission). When septicemia is present in the absence of a bubo, the term *septicemic* plague has been used. *Meningitic* plague is less common and usually results following an interval after inadequate antibiotic treatment of the bubonic variety; primary infection of the meninges without an antecedent lymphadenitis is a far less frequent manifestation. Pharyngitis is a rare clinical presentation.

DIAGNOSIS

Bacteriological diagnosis is usually straightforward and is made by smear and culture (on blood and MacConkey agar plates) from a bubo aspirate obtained by inserting a needle attached to a 10-ml syringe containing 1 ml sterile saline and withdrawing several times until the saline is bloodstained. The polymorphonuclear leukocyte count is elevated (10–20×10^9/l); in children especially, a myelocytic leukemoid reaction (up to 100×10^9/l) may be present. Platelet count is normal or reduced, and disseminated intravascular coagulation is common. When acute- and convalescent-phase serum samples are available, a passive hemagglutination test is of value to confirm the diagnosis.

TREATMENT

Prompt antibiotic administration is essential; untreated (or when treatment is delayed) the mortality rate is > 50%. Streptomycin (15 mg/kg bodyweight twice daily for 10 days) is the antibiotic of choice; shorter courses can be associated with relapse. However, most patients are afebrile within 3 days. Tetracycline is an alternative agent, but this should be avoided in young children. Intravenous chloramphenicol (loading dose 25 mg/kg, followed by 15 mg/kg 6-hourly for 10 days) should be used when meningitis is present. When the bubo(s) becomes fluctuant during the first week of treatment, incision and drainage may be necessary; aspirated fluid should be cultured for evidence of superinfection with other bacteria. Plague (together with cholera and yellow fever) is a quarantinable disease and should be reported to the WHO. A formalin-killed vaccine is available for travelers to epidemic or hyperendemic areas, and individuals (including children) who live in close contact with rodents. Two injections separated by an interval of 1–3 months should be followed by booster doses at 6-monthly intervals. Vector control is essential for elimination of the disease (Kant & Nath 1994, Cook 1995).

PNEUMOCOCCUS

The pneumococcus (*Streptococcus pneumoniae*) is a common cause of serious disease in children, particularly otitis media (p.

1680), pneumonia (p. 565) and meningitis (p. 1288). It is also a frequent cause of occult bacteremia (Gray & Dillon 1989). *S. pneumoniae* are Gram-positive oval cocci, β-hemolytic on blood agar and occur in pairs or short chains. Pathogenic strains have a polysaccharide-containing capsule and produce smooth (S) colonies on culture; rough strains (R) are noncapsulated and nonpathogenic. 84 pneumococcal serotypes have been characterized but fewer than 10 are responsible for the great majority of infections in childhood.

EPIDEMIOLOGY

The pathogenicity of the pneumococcus is low and it may be recovered from the upper respiratory tract of up to 70% of healthy subjects. Most pneumococcal disease is probably spread by healthy carriers but patient-to-patient and patient-to-doctor transfer has been documented. Children under 2 years have the highest rate of carriage but why some children develop disease whereas others remain unaffected is unknown. In developing countries a high proportion of lower respiratory infection in young children is due to *S. pneumoniae*, and pneumococcal meningitis is associated with a high mortality (30–35%). Globally, *S. pneumoniae* is thought to cause over 1 million deaths in children under the age of 5 years (Obaro et al 1996). The 'pneumonia season' in late winter and early spring has been attributed to indoor crowding with more opportunities for cross-infection but more probably it is due to damage to respiratory mucosal defenses from virus infections.

From the nasopharynx pneumococci may reach the lungs or through impaired respiratory mucosa spread to the middle ear or meninges. Bacteremic spread to a variety of sites may occur, notably the joints (Earley et al 1988).

Antibiotics have reduced the severity of pneumococcal disease and case fatality rates but have had little influence on disease incidence. The effect on morbidity has been disappointing. Infants with pneumococcal meningitis remain at considerable risk from neurological sequelae and the pneumococcus is more likely to cause permanent deafness than either the meningococcus or *Haemophilus influenzae*. Recurrent pneumococcal meningitis is occasionally seen when CSF leakage complicates skull fracture. Children with an absent or nonfunctioning spleen or with other causes of an impaired immune response are at particular risk from serious infection.

DIAGNOSIS

In pneumococcal pneumonia there will be tachypnea with grunting, inspiratory retractions, nasal flaring and cyanosis but physical examination of the chest may be unhelpful and the radiological changes surprisingly few in the early stages of illness. Blood, CSF and urine cultures may be helpful in diagnosing pneumococcal disease particularly in preschool children. In bacteremic disease the white blood cell count is often elevated to over $20 \times 10^9/l$. Recovery of the pneumococcus from the upper respiratory tract is not always proof of causation because of the frequency of the carrier state. Rapid methods of pneumococcal capsular antigen detection (e.g. countercurrent immunoelectrophoresis, latex agglutination) in CSF, pleural fluid and serum may be useful for rapid diagnosis, especially in children who have received antibiotics prior to culture.

TREATMENT

A worrying trend is the increasing antimicrobial resistance among *S. pneumoniae* worldwide (Lister 1995). Susceptibility to penicillin (usually the drug of choice), cephalosporin and macrolide antimicrobials can no longer be assumed. Penicillin remains the drug of choice for most infections, but if resistant pneumococci are suspected, a third generation cephalosporin is the preferred initial treatment. Alternatively combination treatment such as ceftriaxone + vancomycin has been used successfully.

PREVENTION

Pneumococcal vaccine

A safe and effective 23-valent polysaccharide vaccine has been available for years but remains relatively little used, even where strongly recommended (Mayon-White 1996). Unfortunately the antibody response is not so reliable in young children, those with immunological impairment and those on treatment with immunosuppressive therapy. Antibody response is particularly poor in children under 2 years of age so that its potential for preventing pneumococcal meningitis is limited. A more immunogenic conjugate vaccine currently being developed should help to overcome this problem but its protective efficacy may be limited by the number of capsular antigens that can be included. The duration of protection with the current vaccine is unknown but antibody levels begin to decline after about 5 years and may decline more rapidly in asplenic patients and children with nephrotic disease.

At the present time, pneumococcal vaccine should be considered for the following children (DoH 1996): all those aged 2 years or older in whom pneumococcal infection is likely to be more common and/or dangerous:

- asplenia or severe dysfunction of the spleen, e.g. homozygous sickle cell disease and celiac syndrome
- chronic renal disease or nephrotic syndrome
- immunodeficiency or immunosuppression from disease or treatment (including HIV infection)
- chronic heart, lung or liver disease
- diabetes mellitus.

Note: Where possible, the vaccine should be given together with advice about the increased risk of pneumococcal infection, 4–6 weeks (but at least 2 weeks) *before* splenectomy and *before* courses of chemotherapy. If this is not possible, as for splenectomy following trauma, the vaccine should be given as soon as possible after recovery and before discharge from hospital. If not given before chemotherapy and/or radiotherapy its use should be delayed for at least 6 months after completion of treatment.

Chemoprophylaxis

An alternative for children with functional or anatomical asplenia, for those receiving immunosuppressive therapy, or for infants under 2 years is to give them continuous antibiotic prophylaxis, e.g. phenoxymethyl penicillin.

EDUCATION

Patients at risk (or their parents) need to be educated about the risks and the importance of seeking medical help at the onset of illness. A Medic Alert bracelet should be used. A patient card and information sheet for asplenic or hyposplenic patients is available from: Department of Health, PO Box 410, Wetherby LS23 7LL: Tel: 01937 845 381. Advice is also available from The Splenectomy Trust, Swinbrook Post Office, Swinbrook, Oxfordshire OX18 4EE.

PROTEUS

The proteus species are a large group of organisms occurring widely throughout nature. They are found in soil and compost and play an essential part in the decomposition of organic material. Proteus species are abundant in the colons of animals and man; hence large numbers are found in sewage.

The group consists of Gram-negative, non-lactose-fermenting, rod-shaped bacteria which readily grow on ordinary culture media. The commonest varieties causing disease in man are *Proteus mirabilis*, *Proteus vulgaris* and *Proteus penneri*. *Providentia stuartii* and *Morganella* are related organisms which may also infect man.

There are no specific disorders caused by these organisms but in common with other Gram-negative colonic bacteria, they cause urinary tract infection, neonatal sepsis and septicemia in immunocompromised individuals. *P. mirabilis* is the most virulent of the group, causing infection more often than all the others.

The urinary tract is the most common site of proteus infection. Prepubertal boys carry proteus at the urethral meatus and ascending infections occur.

Proteus mirabilis has a particular advantage as a urinary pathogen. It produces the enzyme urease in response to urea in the environment. Ammonia is released by splitting urea, increasing the urinary pH and enhancing the organism's ability to multiply. This sequence is facilitated by urinary stagnation and incomplete voiding (Senior 1987). It is therefore not surprising that urinary tract infection occurs readily where there is urinary tract obstruction. Alkalinization of the urine also favors the deposition of pyrophosphate stones in the kidney. These stones are particularly associated with recurrent proteus infection. In children with high urinary residues, release of ammonia by the organism may, rarely, lead to hyperammonemia with resulting central nervous system abnormalities (Kuntze et al 1985).

Other species are more often found as opportunistic infections. *Proteus vulgaris*, *Proteus penneri* and *Providentia stuartii* may be a problem where there is long-term urinary catheterization.

Outside the urinary tract, proteus infection occurs in the neonate causing Gram-negative septicemia and occasionally meningitis which may be complicated by cerebral abscesses (Smith & Mellor 1980). Postoperative infections may occur particularly after bowel surgery.

Diagnosis depends on recovering the organism from the site of infection. Proteus species, from any body fluid, are easy to culture in the laboratory, often outgrowing other pathogens.

Treatment is with broad spectrum antibiotics. In serious infection parenteral therapy with a third generation cephalosporin or a combination of ampicillin and an aminoglycoside may be used initially. In urinary tract infections in otherwise healthy children, trimethoprim or a cephalosporin may be used.

PSEUDOMONAS

Although most *Pseudomonas* spp. are of low pathogenicity, many can produce significant disease, particularly if tissue viability or defense mechanisms are impaired. They are resistant to many commonly used antibiotics, and rapidly acquire resistance.

PSEUDOMONAS AERUGINOSA

Ps. aeruginosa is a common contaminant of moist areas such as sink traps, water traps and ventilator and incubator humidification systems (Grundmann et al 1993, Gould 1987). For epidemiological purposes, typing of individual strains can be performed using various techniques including polymerase chain reaction (PCR) fingerprinting. *Ps. aeruginosa* classically infects wounds and burns, producing pyocyanin, a blue pigment which discolors pus. Best known to pediatricians as a cause of lung infection in cystic fibrosis, *Ps. aeruginosa* can infect virtually any part of the body; infection is particularly likely to occur in the presence of congenital or acquired immunodeficiency, neutropenia or white cell dysfunction, prematurity, malignant disease and its treatment, prolonged instrumentation of body cavities (e.g. tracheostomy, ventricular drainage, bladder catheterization, venous catheterization, peritoneal dialysis) and following puncture wounds.

Some of the more common infections are:

Septicemia. An important cause of septicemia in oncology and neonatal units, *Ps. aeruginosa* is seldom suspected as the infecting agent in children with no previous medical disorders, and antipseudomonal activity is not usually included in antibiotic protocols to cover presumed sepsis in such children. Even when appropriate antibiotic therapy is given, it has a high mortality (Rais-Bahrami et al 1990).

Meningitis. Seen mainly in premature babies and in patients with ventricular drainage catheters, this calls for immediate intravenous therapy with a suitable antibiotic, guided by the results of antibiotic sensitivities and, ideally, by the activity of the patient's own postantibiotic serum against the isolate.

Ear infection. *Ps. aeruginosa* is commonly cultured from chronically infected middle ears and mastoids, particularly in regular swimmers. Occasionally an aggressive and painful infection is produced which is difficult to eradicate and may require surgery.

Eye infections. Keratitis commonly follows trauma, especially from the use of contact lenses, but may also occur in association with immunosuppression and prematurity. The response to apparently appropriate systemic and topical antibiotic therapy is often disappointing and keratoplasty may be necessary. *Ps. aeruginosa* also causes orbital cellulitis,

Urinary tract infection. Urinary tract infection usually follows long-term catheterization, but also occurs when chronic infection has impaired local tissue viability. The organism is a common commensal under the prepuce, and this should be suspected as the source of unexpected *Pseudomonas* bacteriuria.

Peritonitis. Peritonitis following appendicitis, intestinal perforation or peritoneal dialysis may be caused by *Ps. aeruginosa*; failure to appreciate this possibility may result in inappropriate choice of antibiotics (Aronof et al 1987).

Pneumonia. Pneumonia caused by *Ps. aeruginosa* is common in cystic fibrosis, but also occurs in the presence of the predisposing factors already mentioned and following prolonged treatment of other bronchopulmonary infections.

Osteomyelitis. Pseudomonas infection should be considered in osteomyelitis which fails to respond to the usual antibiotic therapy directed against *S. aureus*. It is not always possible to isolate the organism from blood cultures, and antibiotic therapy may have to be broadened blindly.

Skin infections. Folliculitis occurs especially in users of whirlpool ('spa') baths. Skin infections are also seen where the skin of the foot has become macerated from prolonged immersion or the wearing of rubber footwear. Ecthyma gangrenosum, a more aggressive skin infection usually arising in children with one of the predisposing factors already mentioned, produces necrotic ulcerative lesions involving particularly the anogenital and axillary areas, and can be rapidly fatal (Boisseau et al 1992).

Management of *Ps. aeruginosa* infections (Tan 1995)

The choice of antibiotic therapy will depend mainly on the laboratory sensitivity of the isolate; many strains are sensitive to broad spectrum penicillins such as ticarcillin, aminoglycosides such as gentamicin, and 'third generation' cephalosporins such as ceftazidime, all of which must be given parenterally. Recently developed quinolines such as ciprofloxacin can be given orally, but resistant strains emerge with disappointing rapidity.

BURKHOLDERIA (PSEUDOMONAS) CEPACIA

Ps. cepacia, now classified as a *Burkholderia* species, has emerged as an important pulmonary pathogen in patients with cystic fibrosis. It has also been reported as a nosocomial infection in a wide variety of tissues, commonly in relation to contamination of sterile solutions including disinfectants. When contaminated solutions are used for skin cleaning prior to blood culture, an erroneous diagnosis of sepsis ('pseudosepticemia') may be made. It is, however, unwise to assume that *B. cepacia* isolates are invariably contaminants; it can be an aggressive pathogen producing bacteremia, endocarditis, meningitis and urinary tract infection (Goldmann & Klinger 1986).

B. cepacia is even more resistant to antibiotics than *Ps. aeruginosa* but may be sensitive to trimethoprim.

PSEUDOMONAS FLUORESCENS AND *PSEUDOMONAS PUTIDA*

These organisms occasionally cause infection, particularly in relation to hypothermia and following the administration of stored blood.

OTHER *PSEUDOMONAS* SPECIES

Numerous species of *Pseudomonas* (e.g. *Stenotrophomonas maltophilia*, *Ps. pickettii* and *Ps. stutzeri*) are recovered from time to time from clinical microbiology specimens, particularly from immunocompromised or otherwise vulnerable patients. *Ps. pickettii* has infected indwelling venous access devices.

Prevention of nosocomial pseudomonas infections

Environmental measures, such as heating sink traps, thoroughly drying (and preferably sterilizing) equipment after cleaning, and scrupulous attention to the manufacturer's instructions for the storage and use of antiseptic solutions are important in curtailing hospital epidemics. Every effort should be made to isolate (or not to admit) patients who are known to be carriers of *Pseudomonas* spp.

PSEUDOMONAS MALLEI

Ps. mallei causes glanders in horses, an occasional problem in the developing world with transmission from horses to man producing slowly progressive gangrenous nodules in the skin, respiratory mucosae and lungs. The organism is usually sensitive to tetracyclines, chloramphenicol and streptomycin.

PSEUDOMONAS PSEUDOMALLEI

Ps. pseudomallei causes melioidosis, spread mainly by rats and endemic in Southeast Asia. The illness typically includes pneumonia among its features, but may also present with multiple metastatic abscesses. Melioidosis has a high mortality, and although it responds better to intravenous ceftazidime than to conventional therapy with tetracyclines and chloramphenicol (White et al 1989), antibiotic resistance is an increasing problem (Yamamoto et al 1990, Sookpranee et al 1991).

RAT-BITE FEVERS

Two separate and distinct spirochetal infections which are characterized by a relapsing fever usually result from rat bites, and are prevalent in rat-infested communities (not necessarily in tropical countries) of low socioeconomic status (Ordog et al 1985, Cook 1996). *Spirillum* (sodoku or sokosha) has been reported worldwide, most often in Japan. *Actinobacillus muris* (formerly *Streptobacillus moniliformis*) (Haverhill fever) has been reported from Europe, the USA and elsewhere (Wullenweber 1995). Children living in poor socioeconomic conditions are especially vulnerable to rat bites; these can be inflicted during sleep.

SPIRILLUM MINUS

The causative organism of sodoku is a short Gram-negative spirochete (approximately 4 mm in length) which moves rapidly – rather like a vibrio; it is easily stained by Giemsa or methylene blue. Growth can be achieved in guinea pigs, mice and rats by intraperitoneal inoculation. Transmission is via the bite of an infected rat, cat, ferret or bandicoot which is usually a healthy carrier; food contaminated by infected rat urine can also produce infection. While rat bites produce sporadic cases, contaminated raw milk has occasionally been associated with epidemics. There may be local inflammation (occasionally with necrosis) and regional lymph gland involvement. In a fatal case, neuronal degeneration of the brain and degenerative changes in liver and kidneys have been demonstrated.

Incubation period varies from 5 to 30 (mean 8) days. Recurrent fevers at 5- to 10-day intervals with profuse sweating follow the bite which may already have healed or be necrotic and chancre-like but becomes inflamed in the presence of fever. Regional lymphadenopathy is usually present. A characteristic purplish, papular (sometimes nodular) exanthem or urticaria may be present especially on the chest and arms; muscle and joint pains (rarely with arthritis), hyperesthesia, and localized edema are additional signs. In a severe case, delirium (which results from meningoencephalitis) followed by coma ensues; other organ involvement includes endocarditis. The overall mortality rate is about 10%. Differential diagnosis is from the relapsing (see below) and trench fevers, other virus and rickettsial infections, plague and tularemia. In a tropical setting *Plasmodium* spp. infection is also an important possibility. Puffiness of the face may suggest acute nephritis. In children especially, persistent diarrhea and weight loss may be present.

Diagnosis is occasionally confirmed by detecting *S. minus* in a peripheral blood sample by dark ground illumination or Giemsa staining (this can only be demonstrated during a febrile episode); organisms are more likely to be present in exudate in proximity to the bite and in lymph node juice. Inoculation into mouse, rat, rabbit or monkey produces disease, and the organism can then be isolated. During paroxysms, there is usually a leukocytosis, and occasionally eosinophilia and anemia. CSF pressure may be raised. Treponemal serology (e.g. the Kahn test) is weakly positive; the Weil–Felix to proteus OXK strain is also positive. There is no specific serological test.

The usual chemotherapeutic agent is penicillin (Bhatt & Mirza 1992); streptomycin, erythromycin, chloramphenicol and the tetracyclines (contraindicated in young children) are also effective.

ACTINOBACILLUS MURIS

Haverhill fever is a more common cause than *S. minus* infection of a pyrexial illness following a rat bite or ingestion of *A. muris*. The causative organism is a commensal of the rat nasopharynx (Shanson et al 1983); it is a pleomorphic, slender, nonmotile, branching, filamentous organism $1–3 \times 0.3–0.4$ μm which forms chains of bacilli or coccoid bodies. Transmission can occur from raw milk contaminated by rat urine (Anderson & Thomas 1987); this route of infection has resulted in many epidemics. Pathologically, ulcerative endocarditis and subacute myocarditis have been reported; hepatomegaly may be present.

The incubation period is 1–22 (usually < 10) days during which gastroenteritis may be present. The wound usually heals rapidly and uneventfully (Fordham et al 1992). The fever, which is often relapsing and may continue untreated for many months, is accompanied by a generalized erythematous, morbilliform rash (most prominent on the hands and feet) often with a purpuric element, arthralgias, and a subsequent sore throat. Severe generalized muscular pain, extreme prostration and headache may also be present. Although in some cases the fever may subside spontaneously after 9–10 days, continuation with irregular relapses, accompanied by night sweats, can continue at variable intervals for weeks or months. A nonsuppurative shifting arthritis is common; infective endocarditis is an important complication. Untreated, the mortality rate is approximately 10%, usually from bacterial endocarditis and abscess (sometimes cerebral) formation. Coxsackie infections, meningococcal septicemia and erythema multiforme are some of the possible differential diagnoses.

Diagnosis is by isolation of *A. muris* from blood or pustules, using aerobic culture followed by subculture in a CO_2 atmosphere after 48 h. *A. muris* can be agglutinated by serum, and a fluorescent IgM antibody response to *Actinobacillus* sp. has been demonstrated. A polymorphonuclear leukocytosis and secondary anemia are frequently present.

Penicillin is usually effective (Rygg & Bruun 1992), and as with *S. minus* infection should be given as soon as possible after the rat bite. Some coccobacillary variants are resistant to penicillin;

streptomycin, erythromycin (Konstantopoulos et al 1992) or the cephalosporins are effective.

RELAPSING FEVER

Louse-borne and tick-borne relapsing fevers are usually caused by the blood spirochetes ($5–40$ μm $\times 0.5$ μm) *Borrelia recurrentis* and *B. duttoni*, respectively (Cook 1996); however, other species are also important in the etiology of the tick-borne variety. The tick-borne is usually milder than the louse-borne form. The diseases exist worldwide in both tropical (very high prevalence rates for the louse-borne variety have been reported in Ethiopia (Borgnolo et al 1993) and Sudan (de-Jong et al 1995)) and temperate climates, and cause an acute recurring febrile illness. High mortality rates (up to 70%) have been recorded with louse-borne relapsing fever when untreated. The term *relapsing fever* was introduced by Craigie in 1843 at Edinburgh, and the suggestion that arthropod-transmitted *Borrelia* were responsible was made by Flugge in 1891. The role of the tick was documented by Dutton and Todd in 1904. The sole reservoir for *B. recurrentis* is the human body louse; infection is acquired by crushing lice on the skin – this allows liberated spirochetes to penetrate at the site of a bite or alternatively via intact skin. People in crowded and unhygienic surroundings, e.g. migrant workers and their children, and soldiers during a war are especially vulnerable. *B. duttoni* and other species which cause tick-borne disease usually maintain reservoirs in various mammalian, reptile, or avian hosts while man is an accidental host. Transmission follows inoculation of infected saliva via a bite or through intact skin.

The pathophysiology is unclear. Although the clinical events (see below) seem to favor an endotoxin reaction, this has not been confirmed. Neither is the mechanism of the pathological changes understood. Splenomegaly is present in a severe infection; necrosis and hemorrhage into the white pulp, infarcts and occasionally rupture may result. Hepatic necrosis with hemorrhage (and liver failure), myocarditis (occasionally resulting in arrhythmias and sudden death), and cerebral edema (sometimes with hemorrhage) are other severe manifestations.

CLINICAL FEATURES

Clinically, the incubation period is 4–18 (mean 7) days and the illness begins with a sudden onset of fever, headache and fatigue; these symptoms increase in intensity over the first few days. Myalgias, arthralgias, anorexia, dry cough and abdominal pain may also be present. Conjunctival injection, a petechial rash – most marked on the trunk – and tender hepatosplenomegaly are frequently present; jaundice, generalized muscle weakness, spontaneous hemorrhages, disseminated intravascular coagulation, confusion and delirium, and neck stiffness may all be present. Untreated, the first attack in louse-borne relapsing fever usually lasts about 6 days and is followed by an afebrile period of around 9 days, and this is followed by a single relapse lasting about 2 days. In tick-borne relapsing fever, the first attack lasts about 3 days; an average of three but often more relapses (lasting 2 days each) then follow at about 7-day intervals.

DIAGNOSIS

Spirochetes can be demonstrated in a thin Giemsa-stained peripheral blood film. During a febrile episode, large numbers of spirochetes are present. Alternatively, dark ground illumination can be used. Spirochetes can be cultured in Kelly's broth medium (*B. recurrentis* is less easily grown). A spirochetemia can be produced in mice or rats after intraperitoneal inoculation. Serological tests have been used, but none is commercially available. Total white blood cell count is usually normal, but the platelet count is reduced. Liver function tests are often abnormal, and prothrombin time increased. Renal function tests are often mildly abnormal. C-reactive protein is elevated in the louse-borne variety; however, neither this nor tumor necrosis factor (TNF) or interleukin-6 are directly associated with the Jarisch–Herxheimer reaction (JHR) (see below) (Cuevas et al 1995).

TREATMENT

Erythromycin is usually effective (Butler 1985). Tetracycline is probably more effective but should not be administered to young children. In the tick-borne variety longer courses of antibiotic are often necessary to produce cure, e.g. in children, 125–250 mg erythromycin 6-hourly for 10 days. Penicillin has also been used, but clearance of spirochetes is slow and relapses frequent. In most patients with louse-borne, and in some with tick-borne relapsing fever, a JHR (2–3 h after treatment) is a common sequel (Warrell et al 1983). It is during this episode that spirochetes disappear from the peripheral blood and polymorphonuclear leukocyte and platelet counts decline; hyperpyrexia and hypotension are striking clinical features. As mortality is significantly related to JHR, and most relapses are both mild and easily treated, some physicians (Seboxa & Rahlenbeck 1995) favor low-dose penicillin in the initial management of this infection. Meptazinol is of value in diminishing these reactions (Teklu et al 1983). Following treatment, 95% of patients recover. The presence of a high spirochetosis, jaundice and hypotension (usually resulting from myocarditis) suggests a poor prognosis. Vector control and public health education are important in prevention; there are no vaccines.

SALMONELLAE

Salmonellae are motile, Gram-negative, non-spore-forming organisms. They can survive long periods in water, sewage, dried foodstuffs or in carcasses, and can withstand freezing. Their increasing prevalence in domestic animal produce, especially poultry and bovines, and their ability to develop resistance to antibiotics is a major health problem.

There are over 2000 serotypes of salmonellae. They can be divided into:

1. Those that cause *enteric fever* : *S. typhi* which is pathogenic only to man; *S. paratyphi A, S. schottmuelleri (S. paratyphi B), S. hirschfeldii (S. paratyphi C)* which are primarily but not exclusively pathogenic to man.

2. Those that cause *Salmonella* enteritis or salmonellosis; these salmonellae are primarily infectious to animals and may infect man, e.g. *S. typhimurium* and *S. enteritidis*. The infections are confined mainly to the bowel but they may result in septicemia or metastatic abscesses, particularly in young infants or old people and those immunosuppressed, especially in the case of *S. cholerae-suis* and *S. dublin*. *S. typhimurium* accounts for the majority of infections throughout the world. The term enteric fever includes typhoid and paratyphoid fever.

Two principal antigens, in the cell wall (O) and the flagellae (H), are used in the typing of *Salmonella*. A capsular polysaccharide antigen Vi is present in *S. typhi* and *S. paratyphi C*. It can block agglutination reactions with the underlying O antigen and so protect the bacillus from antibody.

SALMONELLOSIS

Salmonellosis is caused by nontyphoidal salmonellae. There has been a particularly dramatic increase in outbreaks of salmonellosis in Britain since 1980, and up to 80% of reported cases of food poisoning are due to *Salmonella*. These are associated with infections contracted abroad and infected food, e.g. poultry, bovine and pig produce and, to a lesser extent, milk and dairy produce. Intensive farming methods, especially of poultry, and the addition of antibiotics to feeds is a major cause. In Britain, many chickens and turkeys reaching retail shops are colonized by salmonellae.

Infection may occur from handling meat, directly or with utensils, or through improper cooking, especially when frozen meat has not been allowed to thaw fully. Infection, especially *S. enteritidis* which produces clinical disease in chickens, may pass to eggs from the ovary or oviduct of infected chickens, or through the shell if care is not taken when separating eggs from feces. *Salmonella* in eggs may resist boiling for 2–3 min, especially if the eggs have been stored in a refrigerator. Egg produce made from raw or improperly cooked eggs may be infected, e.g. homemade mayonnaise, egg powder, milkshakes and ice cream.

Spread between humans occurs from symptomatic or asymptomatic carriers who infect food, or less often by direct contact. A relatively large dose of *Salmonella* is required to cause infection and this usually results from bacterial multiplication in food. Intrafamilial spread and spread through institutions is common, and outbreaks at restaurants, parties and picnics are reported. Breast-feeding protects infants against infection, but occasionally a fully breast-fed infant may be infected by the mother.

In developing countries, where intensive rearing of food animals is not common, infection by chronic carriers and waterborne salmonellosis in sewage are more likely methods of spread.

Pathogenesis

The sites of invasion by salmonellae are usually the ileum and/or the colon. The bacilli can penetrate the mucosa to the lamina propria of the ileum without producing obvious damage to cells and invoke a mainly polymorph response (as opposed to *S. typhi* which produces a monocytic response). Infection of the ileum results in a watery diarrhea, secretory in nature. Less commonly, invasion of the colon may produce a dysentery-type illness.

Under certain conditions there may be bloodstream invasion, resulting in an enteric fever-type illness, septicemia, or localized foci of infection, such as meningitis, osteomyelitis, septic arthritis, pyelonephritis or endocarditis. Systemic infection is particularly associated with infants less than 1 year, malnourished infants, immunocompromised children, and conditions such as hypochlorhydria, hemolytic anemia, especially sickle cell disease, schistosomiasis and malignancy. A focal lesion, e.g. in bone, may manifest itself long after the enteritis has ceased.

In sickle cell disease, infarction of the gut may allow salmonellae access to the bloodstream from where they may invade infarcted areas of bone resulting in osteomyelitis. Also, the impaired opsonization and phagocytic activity in sickle cell disease may permit proliferation of bacteria which exacerbates the infection.

Subjects with schistosomiasis may harbor salmonellae, within the worm or perhaps the granuloma, which protects them from the body's immune system. There may be prolonged or intermittent fever with joint pains and malaise. Glomerulonephritis and an associated nephrotic syndrome may occur and are usually reversible with adequate chemotherapy, presuming there is no established glomerular disease (as occurs in *Schistosoma mansoni* infection). In *Schistosoma haematobium* infections there may be chronic *S. typhi* urinary excretion. Treatment should include appropriate chemotherapy for schistosomiasis and *Salmonella*.

Occasionally a cyst or infarcted area of the kidney or other organ may become a focus for chronic *Salmonella* infection.

Clinical features

The incubation period of *Salmonella* enteritis is 12–48 h. Symptoms in essentially healthy individuals include nausea, vomiting, abdominal pains and diarrhea. In mild cases there may only be diarrhea. The diarrhea may be secretory in nature with frequent high volume watery stools resulting in hypotonic dehydration. Alternatively, the presence of blood and mucus may indicate a colitis. Fever is common and occasionally there may be an enteric fever-type illness. A reactive arthritis may occur and is associated with HLA-B27 histocompatibility antigens. Symptoms usually settle after 5–7 days but loose stools may continue for several weeks.

In infants less than 1 year, especially neonates and infants less than 3 months of age, septicemia with metastatic infections is common. In a prospective study the incidence of *Salmonella* bacteremia was estimated to be 6% in children less than 1 year of age (Torrey et al 1986). In systemic salmonellosis, gastrointestinal symptoms may not be prominent and the infection may be diagnosed only by blood culture.

Serious consequences of blood invasion in young infants are meningitis, osteomyelitis and failure to thrive. In older infants, bacteremia is usually associated with fever or toxemia, but infants less than 3 months of age may be afebrile.

Diagnosis

Culture of *Salmonella* is more likely from feces than from a rectal swab. In suspected cases repeat culture may be necessary as excretion of the organisms may be intermittent. Leukocytes are often seen, and red blood cells and mucus may be present. In *Salmonella* colitis, proctoscopy or sigmoidoscopy may demonstrate a swollen edematous mucosa with mucus and areas of hemorrhage suggesting ulcerative colitis.

In invasive disease, blood, CSF, urine culture and culture of metastatic lesions such as bone will confirm the diagnosis. Blood culture is advised in infants < 3 months of age and immunosuppressed children with *Salmonella*-positive stools, irrespective of the presence or absence of symptoms of bacteremia. There may be a variable increase in blood neutrophils.

Management

In cases of secretory-type diarrhea with hyponatremia,

considerable volumes of normal and half-normal saline may be necessary to replace losses. In prolonged illness, with failure to thrive or in immunocompromised children, intravenous feeding should be considered before significant weight loss has occurred.

In healthy children, antibiotics usually do not alter the course of the disease and may result in prolongation of excretion of *Salmonella*. Resistance of *Salmonella* to antibiotics is related to their ability to acquire drug resistance from other bacteria in the gut through plasmids and transposons.

Indications for antibiotics in *Salmonella* enteritis include infants less than 3 months of age (particularly febrile infants and neonates), immunocompromised children, and systemic or metastatic disease (St Geme et al 1988).

A third generation cephalosporin, cefotaxime or ceftriaxone, or one of the fluoroquinolones, ciprofloxacin or norfloxacin should be given for 5–7 days (Gendrel et al 1993). Metastatic abscesses may require 4–6 weeks' treatment. The fluoroquinolones are not licensed for children but may be used on a compassionate basis (see section on typhoid fever). The advantage of fluoroquinolones is excellent efficacy particularly in eradicating intracellular infection, and both parenteral and oral administration, also eradication of intestinal carriage.

Persistent excretion of *Salmonella* may occur for weeks or some months, especially in young infants. No action is necessary, except for advice regarding hygiene, e.g. when changing nappies and the washing of hands of young children. No restriction of activities is necessary, if stools are normal.

TYPHOID FEVER

In England and Wales between 1981 and 1990 there were on average 168 cases of typhoid fever, 61 cases of paratyphoid A, and 40 cases of paratyphoid B per annum, the majority of which were contracted abroad, particularly in the Indian subcontinent (CDSC 1991). In many developing countries, where hygiene and sanitation are poor, typhoid fever is endemic and constitutes a major health problem (Edelman & Levine 1986). It is considered that up to 80% of infections are mild or subclinical and thus hospital statistics grossly underestimate the prevalence. It is mainly a disease of school-age children and young adults and when it occurs in young children the presentation is often atypical (Mahle & Levine 1993).

S. typhi only infects humans. Subjects are infectious during the acute phase of the disease and when chronic infection of the biliary system, especially the gallbladder, occurs persistent excretion of the bacteria in feces results. In subjects with structural abnormalities of the urinary tract such as those resulting from *Schistosoma haematobium* infection, there may be prolonged excretion of *S. typhi*.

Epidemiology

In technically advanced countries, typhoid fever is usually caused by contamination of food by a carrier. *S. typhi* can survive for long periods in food and can withstand freezing and drying. Outbreaks may occur from infected milk and ice cream, and in institutions a wide variety of foods have been infected when a carrier is involved with its preparation. Oysters and shellfish cultivated in contaminated sewage may be infected. In developing countries, flies and insects may transmit infection and a contaminated water supply may be the source of an outbreak. Contaminated ice may also be a cause. The infective dose is much smaller than in salmonellosis.

Pathogenesis and pathology

After ingestion, the bacilli invade mainly the upper bowel, with minimal inflammation, and pass to the local lymphatics where they are taken up by macrophages. Their easy access through the bowel is explained by *S. typhi's* ability to evade the killing properties of neutrophils. If the macrophages have not been sensitized by a previous infection they are unable to kill the bacteria, which are then transported within the macrophages to the thoracic duct and thus to the reticuloendothelial system where the uncontained bacilli proliferate in the bone marrow, lymphoid tissue, liver and spleen. At this stage, marrow and blood culture will be positive. The degree of infection depends on the dose and virulence of the organism, the protective effects of gastric juice, and the host's immune response.

Proliferation of bacilli, which is enhanced by bile, continues in the bile ducts and especially the gallbladder, from where large loads of bacteria pass into the gut and may be cultured from a duodenal aspirate. The organisms are taken up by macrophages in Peyer's patches, particularly those in the ileum. By now, the macrophages have been activated by sensitized lymphocytes and an inflammatory reaction takes place. This results in swelling, necrosis and ulceration of Peyer's patches which in most cases heal uneventfully. However, erosion of blood vessels may cause intestinal hemorrhage, and extension of the necrosis through the bowel wall may result in perforation. At this stage, which is usually 2–3 weeks after the initial infection, most of the bacteria are intracellular and so blood culture is less often positive, but continuous proliferation in the gallbladder results in shedding of large numbers of bacilli into the gut and stool culture becomes positive. Infection of urine reflects the bacteremia, and a quarter to one-third of subjects may excrete *S. typhi* during the illness.

Within the body, reaction to the infection continues. Many tissues are affected including the liver, spleen, kidney, heart and lungs. Typhoid nodules, which are foci of macrophages and lymphocytes, can be detected in a number of organs. Cloudy swelling of the liver and kidney occurs and the enlarged spleen is packed with proliferating cells in the sinusoids and pulp. Toxemia is the most likely cause of organ dysfunction as signs of inflammation are patchy and is also probably responsible for the mental confusion. Glomerulonephritis and renal failure may occur and are, in some cases, due to immune complex disease.

Rarely, local suppurative infections may develop in bone, joints, lung, kidney and the meninges. Osteomyelitis is commonly associated with sickle cell disease.

Clinical features

The incubation period is around 10–14 days and shorter in those receiving a high infecting dose of the organism. During the first week of illness there are vague influenza-like symptoms, viz. fever, malaise, aches and pains and headache. Persistence of fever for over a week should alert one to the diagnosis. At this stage, common symptoms are headache, drowsiness, anorexia, vomiting, abdominal pain, diarrhea and cough; constipation may be a symptom in older children. On examination the temperature is often 39–40°C and may have a 'swinging' septicemic pattern. Occasionally, the temperature may be normal in moribund

children and rise after resuscitation. Signs of toxemia and confusion are common. The respiration rate is often raised and nonlocalized rhonchi and rales may be heard in the chest. The pulse rate is raised and may be weak in late-diagnosed cases. A bradycardia relative to the level of temperature, common in adults, is usually not present in young children. Signs of heart failure may be present, especially if there is anemia and/or myocarditis. The abdomen is mild to moderately distended with vague nonlocalized tenderness. The spleen is enlarged in 20–30% of cases and the liver in a similar number of cases. Rates of hepatosplenomegaly vary geographically and according to the duration of the disease. Meningism may be detected. Rose spots which are pink macules and fade on pressure may be seen, especially on the trunk. *S. typhi* may be cultured from them. They may appear in successive crops lasting 2–3 days. They have rarely been reported in children with dark skin.

In uncomplicated cases, treatment results in symptomatic improvement within 2 days and the temperature is usually normal within the week. The physical signs resolve in 2–4 weeks but the child may not regain full strength for 1–2 months.

S. typhi infection during pregnancy may cause abortion. Though transplancental infection occurs perinatal infection is commonly due to infection during parturition (Reed & Klugman 1994).

In infants and young children, infection by *S. typhi* may present as a rapid septicemic-type illness with respiratory signs, seizures and meningism. Conversely, presentation may be milder in infants compared to older children (Mahle & Levine 1993).

In developing countries, the presence of nutritional anemia and malnutrition and diseases such as malaria, tuberculosis, sickle cell disease, schistosomiasis and leishmaniasis may complicate the picture. In these diseases, splenomegaly is a common feature. The tendency to anemia in typhoid, which is commonly due to marrow depression, may be exacerbated by the above diseases, and also by glucose-6-phosphate dehydrogenase deficiency and the thalassemias. The association between *Salmonella* infections and sickle cell disease and schistosomiasis is described in the section on salmonellosis.

Complications

Perforation of the gut is one of the major complications. It appears to be less common in young children. It is commonest in the second to third week of the illness but may occur at any time. If it is observed in hospital, it is often associated with sudden deterioration, hypotension, tachycardia and abdominal rigidity. Sometimes perforation is less dramatic and presents more as an ileus. Occasionally, air is detected under the diaphragm in a child who is not particularly sick. Presumably, the perforation, being small, has sealed off spontaneously. Intestinal hemorrhage may accompany or occur independently of perforation. Other complications include pneumonia, myocarditis, heart failure, glomerulonephritis, renal failure, hepatitis, focal or generalized central nervous system disorders and meningitis. The association between septic osteitis and sickle cell disease has already been mentioned.

Diagnosis

Blood culture is positive in 70–80% of cases in the first 7–10 days of the illness and in about half this number in the following 2–3 weeks and may still be positive after some weeks of illness. Culture of marrow is more often positive than blood, and both may remain positive despite previous or current antibiotic therapy. Early on, stool culture may be positive in 50% of cases and in over 70% later in the disease. Urine culture may be positive in 25–30% of cases. Thus, the combination of blood, stool and urine cultures should diagnose most untreated cases. Leukocytes, predominantly mononuclear, are usually detected in the stool and there is often some proteinuria.

The Widal test may be helpful but has its limitations. A high titer of O antibody (> 1 : 160) or fourfold rise in titer in a child in a nonendemic area who has not had a recent typhoid vaccination (within 1 year) is highly suggestive of typhoid fever. In endemic areas, H antibodies may be raised from previous infections and vaccination also results in a sustained raised H titer. Also, in endemic areas an anamnestic response of O antibody to nontyphoid illnesses may necessitate having a higher diagnostic level during the first week of illness. Conversely, O antibodies may fail to develop and, if present, fail to rise in confirmed typhoid fever. In tropical countries immunosuppression by malaria may be a factor. Persistence of Vi antibodies may be used as evidence of carrier status but they may be raised (> 1 : 5) in only 70% of cases. A number of rapid diagnostic tests including ELISA and antigen tests are being evaluated but none are sufficiently reliable as yet for routine service (Edelman & Levine 1986, Mandal 1994).

Anemia is common and the white cell count is usually within the normal range or depressed. In young infants there may be neutrophilia and also when there is a pyogenic abscess. There is usually a decrease in eosinophil count. Thrombocytopenia may occur. The serum bilirubin is usually normal unless there is a hemolytic anemia but serum transaminases are often raised. Hyponatremia is common.

Management

Correction and maintenance of fluid and electrolyte balance is important. Blood transfusion may be necessary. Care regarding overhydration is necessary in the presence of anemia, heart failure, nephritis and/or renal failure.

There is little to choose between chloramphenicol, co-trimoxazole (or trimethoprim), amoxycillin and furazolidone for treating typhoid fever when the organism is known to be sensitive. Chloramphenicol has a slightly higher chance of relapse, and does not treat the carrier state, but otherwise is a very effective and convenient drug, especially in developing countries, because of its low cost and good oral absorption. Chloramphenicol is given in a dose of 75 mg/kg/day. Therapy is continued for a minimum of 14 days; 21 days' duration significantly reduces the relapse rate.

Because of the emergence of multidrug-resistance to S. typhi alternative drugs need to be considered (Gupta 1994). Ceftriaxone 60–80 mg/kg once daily for 7–10 days or 3 days after defervescence is effective. Fluoroquinolones have the advantage of better tissue penetration, oral administration and eradication of the carrier stage. Ciprofloxacin 25 mg/kg/day intravenously followed by 30 mg/kg/day orally is given for 14 days. In mild cases a shorter duration (7–10 days) may be adequate (Hien et al 1995). The new fluoroquinolones, e.g. ciprofloxacin and ofloxacin are not licensed for children, owing to concerns regarding arthropathic effects on weightbearing joints in juvenile

animals. However, these fears appear unfounded (Kubin 1993). Fluoroquinolones may be given on a compassionate basis.

Corticosteroids may be beneficial in some cases. A controlled trial of dexamethazone in severely ill patients of 3 mg/kg followed by 1 mg/kg every 6 h for 48 h produced a significant reduction in mortality (Punjabi et al 1988). The general consensus is that perforation should receive operative management after full resuscitation with correction of electrolyte and fluid imbalance, and blood transfusion if necessary (Bitar & Tarpley 1985, Butler et al 1985). Procedures will vary according to circumstances and include local drainage only (in moribund patients), simple oversewing of the perforation, or resection, especially in those with multiple perforations. Additional antibiotics to cover Gram-negative organisms and anaerobes such as gentamicin and metronidazole should be given.

For clearance of infection, three consecutive stools should be cultured at weekly intervals after chemotherapy ceases. With adequate chemotherapy relapse is uncommon. Children may return to school when symptom-free; stools do not have to be culture-negative. Preschool children and children unable to practice normal hygiene may need to be excluded until clear of infection. Carriage of S. typhi for over 3 months indicates that the child may have become a chronic carrier but this is uncommon in children. It may be associated with defective cell-mediated immunity to Salmonella. Ciprofloxin or another fluoroquinolone should be given for relapse or chronic carriage.

Prognosis

In the preantibiotic era the mortality rate for typhoid fever for all ages was around 7–20% and in technically advanced countries is now < 0.5% (Butler et al 1985). In developing countries the overall mortality in children shows marked geographical variation. This may depend on age and stage of disease on admission, and management.

Prevention

Care should be taken in the handling of stools of infected children and attention paid to hygiene, particularly handwashing. Supervision of young and handicapped children is important.

There are two vaccines available for general use: parenteral Vi capsular polysaccharide and oral S. typhi Ty 21a vaccines. Whole cell heat-killed vaccine has been discontinued. A single dose of Vi polysaccharide vaccine is given by intramuscular or subcutaneous injection and side effects are usually only local and mild. There may be a suboptimal response in children under 18 months. A reinforcement dose is required every 3 years. The Ty 21a vaccine is given for three to four doses on alternate days. It is not recommended at present for children under 6 years. Reinforcement courses need to be given every year.

In developing countries there is potential for mass immunization of children with the Vi polysaccharide or Ty 21a vaccines (Ivanoff et al 1994).

PARATYPHOID FEVER

Paratyphoid fever is similar to typhoid fever but is usually milder, with a shorter period of fever, and a lower frequency of complications and mortality. The incubation period is often shorter and diarrhea is more common. However, in neonates and young infants complications and mortality may be high. It should be treated along the same lines as typhoid fever.

SHIGELLA (BACILLARY DYSENTERY)

The term *bacillary* (as opposed to amebic) *dysentery* is used to describe infections of the gut by shigellae otherwise known as shigellosis. The bacillus was first described by Shiga in Japan in 1898. The organism he described was *Sh. dysenteriae* type 1, previously known as the *Shiga bacillus*, and is the most virulent of all the shigellae.

Shigellae are nonmotile, Gram-negative, non-spore-forming rods. The genus *Shigella* is subdivided into four species: *Sh. dysenteriae* (12 serotypes, the most important is type 1 (*Shiga*)), *Sh. flexneri* (8 serotypes), *Sh. boydii* (18 serotypes) and *Sh. sonnei* (1 colicin type). Man and certain primates are the only hosts.

Although all four species may cause a wide spectrum of disease, generally *Sh. dysenteriae* is associated with severe, *Sh. sonnei* with mild and *Sh. flexneri* and *Sh. boydii* with intermediate severity. Host factors such as malnutrition and immunodeficiency may play a part and explain the vast difference in mortality between developing and technically advanced countries.

EPIDEMIOLOGY

Shigellae are important causes of diarrhea worldwide. They are transmitted by the fecal–oral route and are highly infectious. In Britain, *Sh. flexneri* and *Sh. sonnei* were of equal importance before the Second World War but since the 1940s *Sh. sonnei* is responsible for virtually all endemic infections. In the US, 60–80% of reported cases are due to *Sh. sonnei* and the remainder to *Sh. flexneri*. Of course, imported infections may be of any type. Since the 1920s, *Sh. dysenteriae* 1 infection has been uncommon in Europe and North America, but it still causes devastating epidemics in developing countries. Since 1968 there have been major epidemics of drug-resistant *Sh. dysenteriae* 1 in Central America, south Asia and central and southern Africa (WHO 1995a). In developing countries endemic disease is usually associated with *Sh. dysenteriae* and *Sh. flexneri* and is commonest during the hot humid and rainy seasons.

In industrialized countries, infection is commonest in preschool children, although less common in infants under 6 months of age. It is associated with poor hygiene and direct person-to-person spread. Outbreaks occur particularly in playgroups and nursery schools and also in institutions for the mentally handicapped of all ages. Outbreaks are commonest in late winter or early spring. In developing countries, in addition to the above, infection is associated with unprotected water and open latrines, and food- and waterborne transmission is common. Flies are also vehicles of transmission. Lack of soap and adequate water for washing after defecation are also factors. Breast-feeding has important protective factors against infection by shigellae.

Inoculi as small as 10–200 virulent organisms may be all that are required to cause disease. This explains the high infection rate through direct contact without the necessity for organisms to multiply in food, and contrasts with other bacteria such as salmonellae and *Escherichia coli* which are usually food-borne infections. Liquid stools contain large numbers of organisms and are highly infectious and may contaminate lavatory seats, lavatory and door handles, etc., and fingers. Shigellae can survive on fomites for long periods, and *Sh. sonnei* may survive on wooden lavatory seats for over 2 weeks.

PATHOGENESIS AND PATHOLOGY

Infection by *Shigella* produces a spectrum of disease varying from a mild catarrhal inflammation of the rectum and pelvic colon associated with *Sh. sonnei*, to widespread devastating necrosis of the entire mucosa of the colon, as occurs with some *Sh. dysenteriae* infections.

Shigellae can survive gastric secretions for up to 4 h. Once they have overcome the surface immune defences of the gut, they penetrate the epithelial cells and multiply in the submucosa and lamina propria of the colon and terminal ileum. The ability of cytotoxin to inhibit protein synthesis leads to cell destruction, resulting in mucosal inflammation and ulceration. The mucosa becomes swollen and covered in mucus and blood. In addition to blood, there is leakage of plasma proteins into the intestine. In severe cases, there may be widespread coagulation necrosis and destruction of the mucosa and, if the patient survives, there is often associated persistent colitis. Studies in experimental animals have shown that cytotoxin produced by *Shigella* binds to jejunal villus but not crypt cells, and inhibits villus cell sodium absorption which leads to fluid accumulation in the intestine (Keusch & Bennish 1989). This explains symptoms of watery diarrhea that occur in the initial stages of infection. In severe dysentery there is often a generalized systemic disturbance with neurological symptoms (described under Clinical Features). No toxin responsible for extraintestinal disease has been identified, apart from the Shiga toxin which is associated with the hemolytic-uremic syndrome. Bacteremia occurs but is uncommon.

In endemic areas the hemolytic-uremic syndrome (HUS) is a complication of *Sh. dysenteriae* 1, especially in young children, and is often associated with a leukemoid reaction. HUS usually occurs late in the course of the disease when active dysentery is resolving. Case fatality rates may be as high as 50%. There is structural and antigenic similarity between the Shiga toxin produced by *Sh. dysenteriae* and verotoxin produced by *E. coli* of 0157:H:2 (see section on hemolytic-uremic syndrome).

CLINICAL FEATURES

The incubation period is usually 1–3 days but may be up to 5–7 days in *Sh. dysenteriae* 1. The infection may be asymptomatic or associated with the passage of a few loose stools only, present as a secretory-type diarrhea, or dysentery of variable severity.

In the milder forms, as typified by *Sh. sonnei* or milder forms of *Sh. flexneri* infections, there are frequent loose stools for the first 24 h or so which subside over the next 1–2 days and the stools are usually normal within a week. There may be macroscopic blood and mucus. Abdominal pain may be a prominent feature and may simulate appendicitis or, in young infants, intussusception until the diarrhea becomes apparent. Young children may become dehydrated during the acute watery diarrheal period. Infection of the newborn and young infants is uncommon but mortality may be high (Huskins et al 1994). In the newborn it may be confused with necrotizing enterocolitis and perforation of the bowel has been described (Starke & Baker 1985).

Extraintestinal symptoms are an important feature of shigellosis especially during the initial period, and sometimes occur before the diarrhea. Convulsions are common in children less than 5 years of age. They are usually associated with a rapidly rising temperature. Other central nervous symptoms may occur including headache, confusion, hallucinations, lethargy and meningism. Toxic encephalopathy though uncommon may be fatal.

The etiology of these symptoms is not known. Release of a neurotoxin either from the bacillus or as a result of necrosis of bowel tissue would be a reasonable explanation but this is not proven. Bacteremia is uncommon but is more likely in malnourished infants who are dehydrated and are often afebrile with protracted diarrhea. It is associated with a high mortality. In developing countries measles is often complicated by *Shigella* dysentery. In HIV infected children *Shigella* may cause prolonged relapsing disease.

Other complications include rectal prolapse, reactive arthritis especially in HLA B27-positive children, rarely septic arthritis (Altman et al 1994) and myocarditis (Rubenstein et al 1993), infection of the vagina with bloody discharge, of the cornea, and urinary tract infection (Awadalla & Johny 1990). Infection of the cornea is presumably due to contact with infected fingers.

Sh. dysenteriae and *Sh. flexneri* infections may be relatively mild but in endemic areas, especially amongst populations with a high number of undernourished children, complications are common and are especially associated with *Sh. dysenteriae* 1. In addition to those described above they include severe hyponatremia, hypoglycemia, toxic megacolon, perforation, leukemoid reactions, disseminated intravascular coagulation and hemolytic-uremic syndrome (WHO 1995a). Protracted diarrhea often associated with tenesmus is a major nutritional problem, especially if complicated by protein-losing enteropathy.

DIAGNOSIS

If the patient presents with fever and diarrhea without macroscopic blood in the stools, the diagnosis of *Shigella* infection may be suggested by the presence of large numbers of leukocytes accompanied by red blood cells in the stool. The association of central nervous system symptoms such as convulsions, encephalopathy or meningism may also suggest the diagnosis. If blood and mucus are present, *Campylobacter jejuni* or *Salmonella* infection should also be considered. In tropical countries parasitic causes such as amebic dysentery, a heavy *Trichuris trichiura* infection, or *Schistosoma mansoni* may be responsible for bloodstained stools.

Shigella do not survive long if allowed to dry, or when exposed to sunlight, and thus stools for culture should be inoculated promptly into culture media or put in an appropriate transport medium.

MANAGEMENT

Dehydrated children, particularly young infants, will require correction of fluid and electrolyte balance, either orally or parenterally. Agents that suppress intestinal motility, such as diphenoxylate, loperamide and opium-containing preparations, are contraindicated as they may increase the severity of dysentery by delaying clearance of the organism.

Mild cases are self-limiting, last about a week and do not require chemotherapy. Severe cases with toxemia should be treated, especially in malnourished or young infants. The choice of agents depends on the sensitivity of the organism in the community. In some areas multiple antibiotic resistance is common. Suggested drugs are co-trimoxazole, ampicillin, pivmecillinam, ceftriaxone or nalidixic acid given for 5 days. Amoxicillin is not effective. For multidrug-resistant *Shigella*, one of the fluoroquinolones, e.g. ciprofloxacin, is presently the drug of choice. For discussion of use of fluoroquinolones in children see section on *Salmonella* (p. 1326).

In malnourished children nutritional support will be required and blood transfusion may be necessary.

PREVENTION

Children are most infectious during the acute phase of diarrhea. Occasionally they may excrete the organisms for some weeks. Chemotherapy decreases the duration of *Shigella* excretion and may be indicated in certain circumstances to reduce transmission. Hygiene, especially handwashing after defecation, is the main method of preventing transmission. Outbreaks in nursery schools and mental institutions are major problems. Rigorous attention to maintaining hygiene in lavatories, with adequate cleaning and disinfection, is required. Supervised washing of hands is essential. Management of outbreaks in Britain (Newman 1993) and developing countries (WHO 1995a) has been outlined.

Natural immunity to *Shigella* is serotype specific and thus an effective vaccine may need to be polyvalent. Oral live and parenteral vaccines have been developed which produce protection against some type-specific *Shigella* but as yet no effective vaccine is available (Dellert & Cohen 1994).

STAPHYLOCOCCUS

Staphylococci are Gram-positive cocci and include the coagulase-positive *Staphylococcus aureus* which is responsible for most of the clinical problems. Coagulase-negative staphylococci include *Staphylococcus saprophyticus*, a common cause of urinary tract infection and *Staphylococcus epidermidis*, a skin commensal, which has become an increasing problem particularly with the increasing use of intravascular devices.

STAPHYLOCOCCUS AUREUS

Staphylococci are relatively resistant to heat and drying enabling them to survive for some months on a variety of surfaces or in dust. Their pathogenicity depends on various cell wall components, enzymes and toxins. Catalase, coagulase, hyaluronidase, lipases and nucleases are cellular products with important enzymatic actions. The production of β-lactamases (penicillinases and cephalosporinases) is of particular clinical relevance as these enzymes effectively inactivate β-lactam antibiotics such as penicillin. Cephalosporins vary in their stability to β-lactamases but drugs such as flucloxacillin or clavulanate-potentiated amoxicillin remain useful. Staphylococci produce a variety of toxins with antimembrane actions. The scalded skin syndrome of infants, for example, appears to be caused by an 'exfoliative toxin'.

Asymptomatic carriage of *S. aureus* is common and the organisms can be found in the anterior nares and less often on the skin particularly on the perineum and axillae. This can be a particular problem in hospitals where staff can become carriers of resistant staphylococci and can have serious consequences in obstetric units, burns units and surgical wards; immuno-compromised patients on broad spectrum antibiotics are particularly at risk. Since the 1960s the emergence of methicillin-resistant strains of *S. aureus* (MRSA) has led to further problems and the more recent hospital outbreaks of epidemic MRSA (EMRSA) has necessitated stringent control measures. Patients, nursing and medical staff who are found to be EMRSA carriers require a decontamination program of daily baths for at least a week with an antiseptic detergent such as chlorhexidine, triclosan or povidone-iodine detergent solutions and the topical use of mupirocin (pseudomonic acid) applied three times daily for at least 5 days to the anterior nares. Frequently wards have to be closed for careful cleaning. Serious infection can occur with MRSA and strains are resistant to most antistaphylococcal agents with the exception of vancomycin.

Bacteremia and septicemia

Septicemia and bacteremia with *S. aureus* is generally associated with a focus of infection such as osteitis, pneumonia or a severe skin infection and can be associated with intravascular devices such as Hickman catheters, prosthetic heart valves and ventriculoatrial shunts used for treating hydrocephalus. Severe systemic upset is common with fever, anorexia and with prolonged illness weight loss and anemia can occur. Staphylococcal bacteremia can progress to endocarditis and risks of damage to previously normal heart valves. Toxic shock syndrome can follow infection with a strain of *S. aureus* which produces toxic shock syndrome toxin type 1 (TSST-I). This was particularly recognized with tampon usage but can occur with other foci of infection. Symptoms include fever, headache, diarrhea, myalgia and confusion. Clinical features include pyrexia, hypotension, a widespread erythematous rash, particularly on the hands and soles (which later desquamates) and mucosal involvement with conjunctivitis and red, inflamed lips. It is a multisystem disease with frequently renal impairment, hepatitis or thrombocytopenia.

Successful treatment depends on rapid institution of antistaphylococcal therapy after blood cultures have been taken and general supportive measures including surgical drainage or removal of tampon etc. as indicated (Table 23.21). Eradication of staphylococci from indwelling devices such as shunts is unlikely with antibiotic therapy alone and replacement of the infected device is usually required. If this is not possible then long-term therapy can be considered.

Staphylococci, particularly if hospital acquired, are generally penicillin resistant and suitable antimicrobial agents include flucloxacillin and fusidic acid. Erythromycin may be useful in combination with fusidic acid, particularly if there is a history of penicillin allergy. Aminoglycosides, such as gentamicin, have antistaphylococcal action and vancomycin is particularly useful where EMRSA infection occurs. 2 weeks of therapy is usually sufficient for uncomplicated bacteremia.

Skin infection

Intact skin is a powerful barrier against staphylococcal infection and most skin infection is fairly minor resulting in boils, pustules, furunculosis, carbuncles, styes, paronychia and impetigo. Topical therapy with mupirocin or fusidic acid ointment should suffice for the treatment of impetigo. Large abscess formation may require surgical drainage. Children who are prone to recurrent minor staphylococcal skin infections should be investigated for possible nasal carriage as they may benefit from a course of mupirocin applied to the anterior nares, and if necessary other family members may also be treated. Children with recurrent staphylococcal skin infection should be screened for metabolic abnormalities or phagocytic dysfunction.

Cellulitis, a more deep-seated, spreading infection of the skin is an indication for systemic antimicrobial therapy. Orbital cellulitis carries risks of cavernous sinus infection and should be treated promptly with high dose intravenous antibiotics.

The scalded skin syndrome is discussed on page 1635.

Gastrointestinal infection

Food poisoning

Foodstuffs such as cooked meat products, cream, custard and pastry can be a source of staphylococcal food poisoning. The

Table 23.21 Antimicrobial therapy for *Staphylococcus aureus* infection

Parenteral				
Flucloxacillin or cloxacillin	i.v. or i.m.	1 month to >12 years	12.5mg/kg	6-hourly
Fusidic acid	i.v. only	1 month–12 years >12 years	6–7 mg/kg 500 mg	8-hourly diethanolamine fusidate
Vancomycin (infusion over 60 min, monitor levels)	i.v. only	>1 month	15 mg/kg/day	
Oral				
Flucloxacillin		1 month–1 year 1–4 years 5–12 years >12 years	62.5 mg 125 mg 250 mg 500 mg	6-hourly 6-hourly 6-hourly 6-hourly
Fusidic acid		1 month–1 year 1–4 years 5–12 years >12 years	12.5 mg/kg 250 mg 250–500 mg* 500 mg*	8-hourly 8-hourly 8-hourly 8-hourly

* As sodium salt.

organism can often be isolated from the food handlers involved and often the food is found to have been undercooked and then refrigerated. Symptoms are caused by the enterotoxin (which is heat stable) occur 2–5 h after consumption and result in an acute onset of sweating, abdominal pain, diarrhea and vomiting. The symptoms rarely last longer than a few hours but occasionally supportive therapy with intravenous fluids is required. Antibiotics are not helpful.

Pneumonia, osteitis, meningitis

These staphylococcal infections are discussed on pages 281, 1292, 1589 respectively.

STAPHYLOCOCCUS EPIDERMIDIS

With the increasing use of invasive procedures, this skin commensal has become an important pathogen particularly in the neonate (p. 281) and in the presence of indwelling catheters and shunts. Children with ventriculoatrial shunts may have bacteremia and ventriculoperitoneal shunts can lead to peritonitis. In this situation eradication of infection with antimicrobial therapy may not be possible and relapse is common. Replacement of the infected device or catheter is therefore usually required.

Particularly in hospital-acquired infection, resistance to many antimicrobial agents is common. Resistance, however, to vancomycin is rare despite its widespread use in this setting. Rifampicin is another useful agent for this condition.

STREPTOCOCCUS

The large family of streptococci can be responsible for a variety of disease and sequelae. Streptococci are Gram-positive cocci which tend to form chains and are classified into three groups according to the degree of hemolysis when cultured on blood agar. *Streptococcus viridans* causes partial or 'alpha' hemolysis of the agar whereas *Streptococcus pyogenes* causes complete or 'beta' hemolysis and *Streptococcus faecalis* often produces no hemolytic effect and is therefore termed 'nonhemolytic' or 'γ-hemolytic' *Streptococcus*.

The β-hemolytic streptococci are responsible for most of the streptococcal disease in humans and streptococcal infections are among the most common bacterial infections of childhood. Streptococci belonging to the other two groups tend to be commensals of the pharynx or gastrointestinal tract and tend to be less virulent pathogens.

THE β-HEMOLYTIC STREPTOCOCCI

β-hemolytic streptococci can be further classified into Lancefield groups A to N depending on the serological characterization of the polysaccharide layer of the cell wall. Most human disease is caused by group A β-hemolytic streptococci and they can be further categorized by the protein make-up of the cell wall into various subtypes. Many subtypes produce similar infection and sequelae such as rheumatic fever but nephritis, for example, appears to be a specific complication of a group A type 12 infection.

β-hemolytic streptococci can produce disease by direct tissue invasion or by toxin production. Some strains have a hyaluronic acid capsule which is nonantigenic and has an inhibitory effect on phagocytosis. The cell wall is a complex structure built upon a peptidoglycan matrix. There are a variety of antigenic determinants including the protein M antigen which confers further resistance to phagocytosis. Streptococci lacking this antigen are generally avirulent. The T antigens are useful for epidemiological tracing. The polysaccharide layer determines the Lancefield group. Lipoteichoic acid is a further cell wall component which influences membrane affinity and adherence to epithelial cells. Virulence also depends on the production of toxins. Several strains can produce the erythrogenic toxin which causes the rash of scarlet fever. The two streptolysins O and S are responsible for the hemolytic action of streptococci and the estimation of the antistreptolysin O (or ASO) titer can be useful in diagnosing streptococcal infection. Persisting high ASO titers are seen, for example, in rheumatic fever. Other extracellular products which are possibly involved in spread of infection and the pyogenic process include DNAases, hyaluronidases and streptokinase. Streptokinase can be used therapeutically for thrombolysis.

Epidemiology

β-hemolytic streptococci are principally carried in the pharynx and asymptomatic carriage occurs in 15–20% of children. Infection is spread by direct contact or droplet spread and outbreaks may occur particularly in dormitory-type accommodation in winter months. Food- or waterborne outbreaks have been reported. In western Europe and USA the severity of streptococcal infection has decreased over this century. Scarlet fever, for example, which carried a high mortality rate is now much less of a problem and it may be that decreased virulence of the organism is as important a factor as increased host resistance with better nutrition and more widespread use of antibiotics. In many countries, however, streptococcal infection remains a significant cause of childhood morbidity and mortality.

Immunity

In view of the antigenic variety of the streptococcal strains repeated streptococcal infection is possible. A child who has suffered from scarlet fever and developed antibodies to the erythrogenic toxin should be protected against further attacks of the syndrome.

Clinical features

The usual focus for *S. pyogenes* infection is the throat and infection generally presents with symptoms and signs of acute tonsillitis. In children up to the age of 5 years the illness may be less specific. The incubation period is 2–4 days and the child usually complains of a sore throat and headache, is febrile and may have cervical lymphadenopathy. The pharynx may appear mildly inflamed or a more severe form of exudative pharyngitis may be present. Clinical discrimination from viral infection is not usually possible and uncomplicated carriage is always a possibility when streptococci are isolated from the throat swab. Classically after 10 days of illness a rise in the ASO titer will be apparent. Tonsillitis, otitis media, mastoiditis, sinusitis and the much rarer β-hemolytic streptococcal pneumonia, empyema, meningitis and septicemia are described elsewhere. Scarlet fever and erysipelas are unique to streptococcal infection.

Scarlet fever

Scarlet fever is caused by infection with an erythrogenic toxin-producing strain of group A β-hemolytic streptococci. The usual portal of entry is via the pharynx and the syndrome classically follows acute streptococcal tonsillitis. A mild form of pharyngitis may be present and the streptococci may gain access via broken skin following minor cuts, burns, surgical wounds or chickenpox infection.

Clinical features

The incubation period is usually 2–4 days and the illness may be of variable severity with sudden onset fever, headache, vomiting, sore throat and refusal to eat. In the past severe illness was more common and delirium a frequent feature. The erythematous rash appears some 2 or 3 days after the onset of illness and classically is first seen in the axillae and groins with blanching on pressure (Figs 23.9 and 23.10). Within 24 h the rash spreads to the trunk and limbs. The face may be flushed and circumoral pallor is a common feature. Pastia's sign – linear petechiae, seen in the flexures of the elbows – may be helpful diagnostically. After a week or so, desquamation usually occurs starting on the face, then the trunk and limbs. Initially the tongue appears swollen with a yellowish white coating and prominent papillae. This is known as

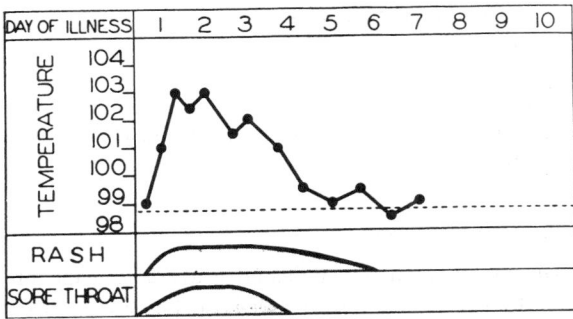

Fig. 23.10 The development of scarlet fever. (From Krugman & Ward 1968.)

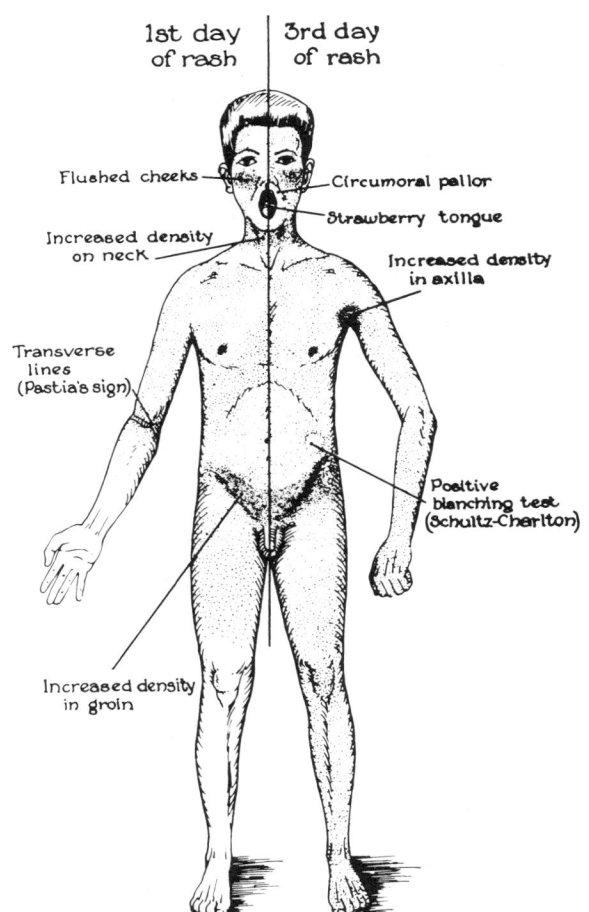

Fig. 23.9 The distribution and development of rash in scarlet fever. (From Krugman & Ward 1968.)

the white strawberry tongue which later becomes the red strawberry tongue as the coating disappears.

Untreated the illness runs its course within 10 days or less. A high fever and tachycardia are common.

Albuminuria is a common finding and a polymorphonuclear leukocytosis is usual.

Since the availability of antibiotic therapy serious complication are rare. Immediate complications include cervical lymphadenitis with more rarely abscess formation necessitating surgical drainage. Acute otitis media may develop and without treatment further complications including mastoiditis, meningitis or cerebral abscess may ensue. Involvement of the paranasal sinuses can lead to suppurative sinusitis. Other recognized local complications include peritonsillar cellulitis or abscess formation, laryngitis and retropharyngeal abscess.

Rarely bacteremic spread can lead to metastatic foci of infection and bronchopneumonia is a further complication which may lead to empyema or suppurative pericarditis.

2 or 3 weeks after the onset of illness the later complications include rheumatic fever, acute glomerulonephritis and erythema nodosum. Early antibiotic therapy should prevent such complications.

Differential diagnosis

Where acute tonsillitis is present the diagnosis is usually straightforward. With milder or subclinical pharyngitis the diagnosis may be less apparent and confused with other exanthemata. Measles is recognized by the prodromal catarrhal symptoms, diarrhea, conjunctivitis, the presence of Koplik spots and the different character and distribution of the rash. In rubella the contrasting severe rash with the mild illness and the presence of predominantly occipital cervical lymphadenopathy are distinguishing features. General lymphadenopathy with splenomegaly is often detectable in infectious mononucleosis; the blood film examination may reveal atypical mononuclear cells and the Monospot test is usually positive. Other viral exanthemata run a shorter course and have a leukopenia rather than polymorphonuclear leukocytosis.

Kawasaki's syndrome may be difficult to differentiate in the earlier stages of illness but the characteristic distribution of the rash and mucosal involvement are usually evident and classically desquamation starts periungually.

A similar rash may be seen as a result of infection with toxin-producing *S. aureus* but in the resulting syndrome of 'toxic shock' there is usually an obvious focus of staphylococcal infection and the rash tends to be more severe on the palms and soles.

Drug rashes particularly following antibiotic usage can be scarlatiniform (scarlet fever-like). The other features of disease are not usually present, however, and the rash fades with the cessation of therapy.

Prevention and treatment

The main aim of antimicrobial therapy is to eradicate the infection and thereby prevent the sequelae of local suppurative disease or later rheumatic fever and poststreptococcal glomerulonephritis (Table 23.22). Penicillin is the drug of choice for the treatment of β-hemolytic streptococcal infection. In severe cases intravenous or intramuscular administration may be required initially with benzyl penicillin. In milder cases oral phenoxymethyl penicillin for 10 days is usually sufficient. Erythromycin is a suitable alternative in cases of penicillin allergy. Ampicillin and amoxicillin should be avoided as if mistakenly given in infectious mononucleosis they can cause a severe rash and constitutional upset.

It is unusual to get multiple cases of scarlet fever in a family although uncomplicated streptococcal throat infection may develop in other children and this can be prevented by oral penicillin.

Erysipelas

Erysipelas is a skin infection caused by any of the group A β-hemolytic streptococci which can enter the skin through trivial wounds or abrasions. Children of all ages are susceptible and recurrent attacks often involving the same site can occur. Children with congenital lymphedema appear to be more at risk.

Clinical features

The illness may present with fever, malaise, vomiting and anorexia or the symptoms may be confined to the affected skin or occasionally the mucous membranes. A small erythematous patch may develop into a much larger area of affected skin which becomes red, hot, painful, indurated and well demarcated by a raised edge. In infants the periumbilical region is a common site whereas in older children the extremities or the face are sites of predilection and both cheeks may be involved in a butterfly type of distribution. Facial erysipelas must be differentiated from the violaceous cellulitis caused by *Haemophilus influenzae* infection or the slapped cheeks appearances seen with parvovirus infection. Resolution of erysipelas starts centrally and may be followed by desquamation.

Blood cultures are frequently negative but after 10 days of illness there may be a rise in the ASO titer.

Erysipelas responds quickly to penicillin or erythromycin. It may be difficult to differentiate erysipelas from other soft tissue infection such as cellulitis, the more deep-seated infection caused mainly by staphylococcal infection, and in cases where doubt exists antistaphylococcal antimicrobial therapy should also be prescribed, e.g. flucloxacillin.

Streptococcal pyoderma

Although most impetigenous lesions are caused by staphylococcal infection localized purulent streptococcal infection of the skin (streptococcal impetigo or pyoderma) may result from secondary infection of wounds or burns. In children particularly in the age range 2–5 years and living in tropical or subtropical climates it mainly involves the lower limbs and may follow intradermal inoculation of streptococci by minor trauma or insect bites. Multiple lesions are common and begin as small papules becoming vesicular with surrounding erythema. Pustule formation occurs and the lesions then enlarge and break down with formation of thick crusts. Systemic upset is not common but regional lymphadenitis is usually present. 10 days of penicillin therapy is advised although there appears much less risk of rheumatic fever with this type of infection.

Lymphangitis, characterized by red, linear streaks leading to the enlarged regional lymph nodes, may follow very minor skin infection or inoculation with streptococci. It may accompany cellulitis.

Streptococcus agalactiae

Streptococcus agalactiae is a β-hemolytic streptococcus belonging to Lancefield group B and may be pathogenic for the newborn infant who can become infected vertically at the time of birth or be horizontally infected in the nursery environment (p. 280).

Table 23.22 Antimicrobial therapy for *Streptococcus pyogenes* infection

Parenteral				
Benzyl penicillin	i.m.	1–12 months	15 mg/kg	6-hourly
		1–4 years	150 mg	6-hourly
		5–12 years	300–600 mg	6-hourly
		>12 years	600 mg – 1.2 g	6-hourly
	i.v.	All ages	25–50 mg/kg	4 to 6-hourly
Erythromycin	i.v. only	1 month–12 years	8–12 mg/kg	6-hourly
Oral				
Phenoxymethyl penicillin		<1 year	62.5 mg	6-hourly
		1–4 years	125 mg	6-hourly
		5–12 years	250 mg	6-hourly
		>12 years	500 mg	6-hourly
Erythromycin		1 month–1 year	125 mg	6-hourly
		2–8 years	250 mg	6-hourly
		>8 years	500 mg	6-hourly

α-HEMOLYTIC STREPTOCOCCI

α-hemolytic streptococci are generally oropharyngeal commensals and termed *S. viridans* and include *S. salivarius, S. milleri, S. mitior, S. sanguis* and *S. mutans* which appears to have a major role in the development of dental caries. Even minor dental procedures can be complicated by a transient bacteremia which is of no clinical consequence unless cardiac abnormality exists either in children who have suffered from rheumatic heart disease or who have congenital heart disease such as patent ductus arteriosus or bicuspid aortic valves. Infective endocarditis is a risk in such cases but regular penicillin prophylaxis in children who have suffered from rheumatic fever has practically eliminated the problem. In addition regular dental care with additional antibiotic cover is advised for children who have a history of rheumatic fever or congenital heart disease (p. 632). *S. pneumoniae* is a major cause of bacterial pneumonia (p. 565), otitis media (p. 1680) and meningitis (p. 1288). The polysaccharide capsule inhibits phagocytosis and is a major determinant of virulence. Children with sickle cell disease, previous splenectomy and agammaglobulinemia are particularly at risk and vaccination and penicillin prophylaxis should be considered.

NONHEMOLYTIC STREPTOCOCCI

The most important nonhemolytic streptococci are *S. faecalis* or enterococci as they are commensals of the intestinal tract. They can cause urinary tract infection particularly in cases of structural urinary tract abnormality or neurological dysfunction of the bladder such as in children with lumbar or sacral myelomeningocele. *S. faecalis* can also cause infective endocarditis. This group of organisms is generally penicillin resistant. Determination of the antibiotic sensitivity is important. In cases of endocarditis combinations of antimicrobial chemotherapy are advised such as the synergistic combination of amoxicillin and aminoglycoside such as gentamicin.

TETANUS

Tetanus is an often fatal disease which is still common in developing countries where it occurs in the newborn (see p. 285) and at any age thereafter but especially in schoolboys.

In England and Wales less than 12 cases are reported annually, few in children.

ETIOLOGY

Tetanus is due to infection by *Clostridium tetani*, which is a spore-bearing, anaerobic Gram-positive organism. The spores are resistant to heat and to many antiseptics. The organism produces a soluble exotoxin (tetanospasmin), which is neurotoxic and binds strongly to neural gangliosides. It usually enters the body through a wound, which is typically a puncture wound, but may be a crush injury or a burn. Nevertheless, any kind of wound can lead to tetanus, even one caused by a surgical operation. Occasionally, there is no history or sign of wound or injury. Tetanus in the newborn (p. 285) commonly results from the application of cow dung to the severed umbilical cord, a custom still existing in tropical countries.

EPIDEMIOLOGY AND PATHOGENESIS

The tetanus bacillus is a natural, harmless inhabitant of the intestinal tract of many animals and is commonly found in soil, particularly in rural areas. In a wound the bacillus is not invasive, but it produces tetanospasmin which has a strychnine-like action. It abolishes the synaptic inhibition between the neural end plates and the anterior horn cells in the spinal cord and the motor nuclei in the brain. Tetanospasmin is carried by retrograde axonal transport to the neuroaxis from where it passes to other neurons, especially the presynaptic inhibitory cells. Once it has reached central nervous tissue, the toxin is not accessible to neutralization but, as in diphtheria, it can be inhibited by antitoxin while it is still in the bloodstream.

PREVENTION

Active immunization of all susceptible persons of any age is the method of choice. The tetanus toxoid (inactivated toxin) is usually incorporated into a triple antigen against diphtheria, whooping cough and tetanus (DPT) but may be given separately. A primary course of immunization consisting of three injections at monthly intervals any time from about 6 weeks of age onwards is a sound assurance against contracting tetanus provided that a booster dose is given 3 years later (or at school entry). A further dose is recommended for those aged 15–19 or before leaving school. A booster dose should be given where there has been any injury which might result in the introduction of tetanus bacilli or spores into the body. In contaminated wounds and those involving penetrating injuries or necrotic tissue human tetanus immunoglobulin should also be administered intramuscularly especially if there is uncertainty about the immunization status of the child or the child has not been immunized. Serum antitoxin levels of 0.01 units/ml or over are thought to be protective.

CLINICAL FEATURES

The incubation period of tetanus varies between 1 and 20 days, but it is usually between 5 and 14 days, depending on the inoculating dose, the nature of the injury and the immunity state of the patient.

The symptoms begin with progressive, intermittent, painful stiffness of the muscles, particularly those of the jaws. This feature can give the appearance of the sardonic grin (risus sardonicus). These painful spasms increase in strength and frequency. They can be precipitated by noise, by light or by touch. Occasionally only muscles near the site of injury may be involved particularly in partially immunized subjects. Commonly the spasms are generalized, all muscle groups being involved. As the extensor muscles of the neck and trunk are more powerful than the flexors, head retraction and opisthotonos are striking features. The jaws are clenched (lockjaw, trismus), the arms and legs are outstretched and exhibit clonic spasms, and the hands are clenched. The abdominal wall may exhibit board-like rigidity, which may be mistaken for an acute perforation of a viscus.

The spasms are brief to begin with, interspersed with periods of complete relaxation, but they increase progressively in duration and frequency and may cause very severe pain. They may be so severe as to result in spontaneous tearing of or bleeding into muscles, or compression fracture of the spine. In spite of the severity of the paroxysms the patient remains afebrile and fully conscious. Involvement of the bladder sphincters may cause retention. There may be asphyxia and cyanosis due to spasms of the glottis and the respiratory muscles. Inability to get rid of respiratory secretions may lead to bronchopneumonia. This, or cardiac failure or complete exhaustion, may be the cause of death. The shorter the time between the wound and the onset of symptoms, the more severe is the disease. Death, if it occurs, usually does so within 10 days of the onset of symptoms. In those who recover the spasms tend to continue for several weeks with diminishing force and frequency.

Neonatal tetanus often presents with generalized disease within 2 weeks of birth and has a high mortality.

DIAGNOSIS AND DIFFERENTIAL DIAGNOSIS

Diagnosis must rest on clinical grounds and is not usually difficult. The spasms are different from those of epilepsy and there is no loss of consciousness. In meningitis there is high fever and the cerebrospinal fluid is abnormal. In tetanus the CSF is normal and this feature also distinguishes tetanus from rabies, apart from the history of an animal bite and the absence of trismus in rabies. Neonatal tetany is unassociated with abnormal serum calcium and phosphate levels. Hysteria and certain drugs, e.g. metoclopramide, can mimic tetanus.

TREATMENT

The patient is best nursed in a special care unit. Subdued light, silence and adequate sedation are essential. All nursing procedures or laboratory tests should be preceded by adequate sedation to prevent or minimize further muscle spasms. There is a choice of several sedative drugs. Diazepam is the drug of first choice and is given in increasing dosage until muscle spasm is controlled. The advice of an anesthetist should be sought especially if diazepam fails to produce the desired effect. The patient may have to be paralyzed to control spasms in severe cases and assisted ventilation commenced.

Adequate food and fluid intake is given by indwelling nasogastric tube.

Specific treatment

Tetanus antitoxin is given to neutralize circulating toxin. It has no influence on toxin already combined with the cells in the central nervous system. Human tetanus immune globulin should be used whenever possible (and always in developed countries) because this avoids the serious risk of hypersensitivity reaction which exists if horse or other animal antitoxin is used. Human tetanus immune globulin must only be given intramuscularly, in a single dose of 3000 units. Only if human immune globulin is not available should antitoxin derived from the horse be used. The dose is 100 000 units, half of it given intravenously, half of it intramuscularly, in a single dose, but preliminary testing for sensitivity to horse serum should be carried out as for diphtheria antitoxin (p. 1306).

Penicillin should be given intravenously.

Concurrent with this treatment active immunization with toxoid is begun and must be followed by a second injection 4–6 weeks later, to prevent relapse as tetanus does not confer immunity against recurrence of infection.

Debridement must be carried out according to the nature of the wound, but should not be started until some hours after the intramuscular administration of the immune globulin, which in such cases should also be infiltrated locally around the wound.

PROGNOSIS

The prognosis of tetanus is still serious in spite of the best treatment, but if a patient survives for 10 days, he is most likely to recover completely.

TUBERCULOSIS

In technically advanced countries morbidity and mortality from tuberculosis have declined progressively over the decades. This is associated with improved living conditions and medical care, particularly case finding and chemotherapy. However, it is still an important problem, especially in immigrant and minority groups. In some developing countries the case rate has hardly changed and any decline is offset by an increase in population.

The majority of children infected by *Mycobacterium tuberculosis* are asymptomatic. However, in a small number, especially young children, the disease is serious or fatal, cf. meningitis or miliary disease, and survivors may be left with sequelae such as cerebral palsy, mental retardation, bone and joint disease.

BACTERIOLOGY

The 'tubercle bacillus' was first described by Robert Koch in 1882 and is now called *Mycobacterium tuberculosis*. However, the identification of the transmissible nature of tuberculosis is attributed to Jean Antoine Villemin in 1865. Mycobacteria derive their name from their mold-like appearance on culture. One of their unique characteristics is a highly complex lipid-rich cell wall which protects the bacillus from digestion by the lysosomal enzymes of macrophages and which, when stained, resists decolorization by acid alcohol. Like *M. Leprae*, and different from other mycobacteria, *M. tuberculosis* is an obligate parasite with total dependence on the living host.

The two major species of mycobacteria infecting man are *M. tuberculosis* and *M. bovis*. *M. tuberculosis*, the classic human variety, has an Asian variant originating in the Madras area of south India but is also found in other parts of India, southeast Asia and Africa. It differs from the classical type in having low virulence for the guinea pig and is susceptible to hydrogen peroxide (Grange 1988). Another variant, *M. africanum*, was isolated from man in equatorial Africa and has properties intermediate between the classical and bovine types. *M. bovis* differs from the other types in its resistance to pyrazinamide. The identification of these variants of the classical variety is of mainly epidemiological importance.

M. tuberculosis is aerophilic but *M. bovis* is microaerophilic (prefers reduced oxygen tension). Within the host, mycobacteria may lie dormant for many years.

M. tuberculosis is cultured on Lowenstein–Jensen medium and is slow growing, taking an average time of 21 days, and occasionally 1–2 months or longer. Growth of *M. tuberculosis* may be detected in 7–10 days using the Bactec radiometric or the Roche biphasic systems.

There are two major methods for direct identification in specimens: Ziehl–Neelsen stain and fluorescence microscopy. For fluorescence microscopy the specimen is stained with auramine–rhodamine. The latter is more rapid, more sensitive, and less likely to yield false positive results than the Ziehl–Neelsen method.

A number of serological tests have been developed using purified protein derivatives of *M. tuberculosis* by ELISA or solid-phase radioimmunoassays. However, many lack sensitivity and specificity especially for culture-negative cases and thus are not used for routine laboratory diagnosis (Wilkins 1994). Gene probes can provide a rapid identification of mycobacteria once they have grown on culture. Polymerase chain reaction (PCR) is a sensitive test for the diagnosis of tuberculosis. It can be applied to gastric aspirates, bronchial washings and specimens obtained from nonrespiratory disease (Delacourt et al 1995). It can differentiate between *M. tuberculosis* and environmental mycobacteria and provides a rapid diagnosis. DNA fingerprinting is a valuable tool in studying transmission of tuberculosis.

EPIDEMIOLOGY

In studies of tuberculosis, differentiation has to be made between tuberculous infection (as evidenced by a positive tuberculin test) and disease. In tuberculous disease there is clinical, radiological or bacteriological evidence of infection. In Britain, subjects who are tuberculin positive without demonstration of disease are not notified as tuberculosis. The great majority of infected people remain asymptomatic. In England and Wales in 1949–1950, a national survey showed that nearly half of 14-year-old children were tuberculin positive. Today, less than 1% of 11- to 13-year-old children are tuberculin positive at routine school examination.

Three-quarters of tuberculosis cases occur in developing countries where 0.2–1% of the population are expectorating the tubercle bacillus. A rise in case rates in adults and children has been observed in countries with a high prevalence of HIV infection. Estimates predict a marked rise in southeast Asia and particularly sub-Saharan Africa by the year 2000 (Dolin et al 1994).

In technically advanced countries where the prevalence of smear-positive cases is small, the infection rate in children will be low and the majority of adults with tuberculosis will have endogenous reactivation. Conversely, in developing countries, the high prevalence of smear-positive cases will result in a significant proportion of children and young adults developing primary tuberculosis, and exogenous reinfection in older adults will be common. However, despite the high prevalence of infection in these countries, up to 50% of 15-year-old adolescents may be tuberculin negative and thus prone to primary tuberculosis.

National surveys in England and Wales for the periods 1978–9, 1983, 1988 and 1993 found 747 (estimate based on 6 months' survey), 452, 294 and 389 newly notified children under 15 years, respectively (Medical Research Council Cardiothoracic Epidemiology Group 1994). The annual rate of notifications of tuberculosis in children increased from 3.1 to 3.9 per 100 000 between 1988 and 1993 (J. M. Watson, personal communication). In 1993, rates (per 100 000) for children of Pakistani/Bangladeshi (36) and Indian (26) ethnic origin were higher than black Caribbean (6), other ethnic minorities (12) and white groups (2). Since 1988 there has been a rise in notifications in other ethnic minority groups.

The decline in the incidence of tuberculosis began in Europe before the introduction of BCG and chemotherapy. In the decade 1979–88 there was an average reduction in notification rates in England of 7.2% per year. However, since 1988 there has been no further decrease and notifications in some areas have shown an increase (Darbyshire 1995). Responsible factors include recent immigration, socioeconomic factors and homelessness. There has also been a rise in notifications in parts of Europe and the US. Factors associated with the rise in notifications in the US since 1987 include HIV infection, homelessness, immigration and decline in resources for tuberculosis control. The increase is focal, mainly confined to inner cities and 80% of childhood cases are in minority groups. Multidrug resistance is a major problem. However, with increased support for tuberculosis control the rise in cases has reversed in 1993–94 (CDC 1995a).

The vast majority of cases of tuberculosis are caused by *Mycobacterium tuberculosis*. *Mycobacterium bovis*, which was an important cause of tuberculosis of the gastrointestinal tract, lymph nodes and bones, has virtually disappeared from technically advanced countries through eradication of tuberculosis in cattle and pasteurization of milk. In Britain, before 1950, *M. bovis* was the cause of 33% of childhood and 10% of adult extrapulmonary disease. It is also considered to be an uncommon cause of tuberculosis in developing countries, except in communities where large amounts of raw milk are consumed, e.g. in cattle-herding tribes. In Britain it is still isolated from reactivated lesions in approximately 1% of adults (O'Reilly & Daborn 1995). *M. bovis* is resistant to pyrazinamide.

PATHOLOGY

The pathology has been described by Miller (1982). The first response to the presence of the tubercle bacilli at the point of entry and in the regional nodes is a serous exudate. Soon neutrophils accumulate followed by macrophages. The macrophages ingest the bacilli. Some may be transformed into epithelioid cells which contain more effective digestive enzymes in their lysosomes. Fusion of either the macrophages or epithelioid cells forms the characteristic multinucleate giant cells. Death of the cells in the center of the tubercle (granuloma) results in the appearance of caseation necrosis. Lymphocytes form a zone around the tubercle and are particularly apparent during the second month of infection which coincides with the development of tuberculin sensitivity. Healing takes place with the deposition of collagen fibrils by fibroblasts which wall off the caseous area from healthy tissue. After 12 months or more calcification may be seen which remains for years but may be completely reabsorbed. It usually has a stippled appearance. Alternatively, healing may not occur or the tubercle containing dormant bacilli may reactivate after months or years. Extensive necrosis with caseation and liquefaction may develop. Liquefaction allows bacilli to survive, inhibits macrophage and lymphocyte function because of oxygen lack, and prevents drug penetration. Activity and healing of the lesion may occur concurrently.

IMMUNOLOGY

The main defense against infection by the tubercle bacillus is cell mediated. The role of B cells is unclear.

Tubercle bacilli are readily ingested but are not killed by macrophages in which they multiply. Toxic substances and other properties in the lipid-thick cell wall protect the bacillus against lysosomal enzymes. CD4 T lymphocytes (T helper cells) when sensitized by tubercle bacilli produce cytokines which activate macrophages and CD8 cytotoxic cells. Cytotoxic cells lyse cells containing mycobacteria and enable macrophages to kill their ingested bacilli. The positive effect of T helper cells may be countered by suppressor T lymphocytes. In advanced disease or in the presence of a large bacterial load these suppressor effects may predominate, which may explain the anergy commonly seen in these children.

Defense against tuberculosis can be described as two components: one where cell-mediated immunity (CMI) controls the infection by activating macrophages which enables them to kill ingested mycobacteria; the other is delayed type hypersensitivity (DTH) which when the bacillary antigens reach high levels results in caseous necrosis of host tissues (Dannenberg 1989). DTH is responsible for the tissue damage and caseation necrosis which is characteristic of postprimary tuberculous disease. There is no correlation between the degree of hypersensitivity and resistance to tuberculosis. The balance between hypersensitivity and resistance will influence the manifestation of tuberculosis, i.e. the former will be associated with clinical and radiological signs of the disease whereas with the latter there will be a paucity of signs. Subsets of T helper cells include Th_1, Th_2 and Th_0. Th_1 produces IL-2 and gamma interferon (IFN-γ) which activates CMI and controls infection. Th_2 produces IL-2, IL-5 and IL-6 amongst other interleukins. The combined effect of Th_1 and Th_2 makes cells very sensitive to TNF resulting in necrosis and cavity formation.

A number of factors influence the outcome of the immune response, including the number of inhaled bacilli, their virulence and the immune response by the host. These are affected by secondary factors which may affect the immune system, e.g. age of the patient, infections such as measles, malnutrition, malignancy and immunodeficiency states such as HIV infection, or immunosuppressive therapy.

PATHOGENESIS

The first infection by tubercle bacillus occurs most commonly by inhalation through the lungs, less often by ingestion through the alimentary tract (tonsils and ileum), and rarely by infection of an open wound on the skin. Infection of the mouth, skin and eyes may result from exposure to a dental surgeon with pulmonary tuberculosis. Enlargement of the regional lymph nodes occurs which provides an indication of the site of primary focus.

Primary infection

The primary focus or site of entry in the lung is usually single and situated just under the pleura (*Ghon focus*) in a well-ventilated part of the lung. Because there is no acquired immunity the bacilli multiply at the primary focus and in the regional lymph nodes. The primary focus and nodes form the primary complex. In most cases there is hematogenous and lymphatic dissemination throughout the body and to other parts of the lungs. Certain organs favor survival of the bacilli and these may later be affected by disease, e.g. apical and subapical regions of the lungs (*Simon focus*), where there is a higher oxygen tension, renal parenchyma, epiphyseal lines of bones, cerebral cortex and regional nodes. At about 4–8 weeks acquired immunity develops, which coincides with sensitivity to tuberculoprotein, and this usually contains the infection. Multiplication of bacilli ceases and, in the great

majority of cases, they either die or remain dormant indefinitely within the healing tubercle or macrophages. The tubercles, especially those which are large and are situated in the apical and subapical regions of the lungs, may become active again (reactivate) at any time during the person's life if the balance between the organism and the host defense is upset.

In children, the primary focus in the lung is usually small or invisible on chest X-ray, but the regional nodes are enlarged and prominent. In contrast, regional nodes are usually not prominent in primary infection in adults.

The initial infection is usually asymptomatic. Occasionally a short period of fever and malaise may have been noted. Erythema nodosum may appear within a few weeks of the primary infection and coincide with tuberculin conversion. It is an allergic hypersensitivity reaction which may be associated with high levels of circulating immune complexes. Phlyctenular conjunctivitis is another, though rare, manifestation of hypersensitivity.

If the infecting load of bacilli is large or the host defense inadequate there may be (Fig. 23.11):

1. extension of the lung focus
2. softening of the regional nodes
3. extension of foci in other parts of the body
4. hematogenous spread due to erosion of a blood vessel with dissemination of bacilli throughout the body (miliary tuberculosis), or chronic low-grade dissemination (cryptogenic tuberculosis).

In a newly infected person the risk of developing tuberculous disease is highest in the first 2 years following a primary infection (especially in the first year), and diminishing thereafter. The risk is more in infants and young children and those with malnutrition or immunosuppression. Pulmonary disease, miliary tuberculosis and meningitis are usually manifest within 1 year of infection, especially in young children, whereas bone disease presents later (within 3 years), and renal disease usually much later (over 5–7 years).

Postprimary tuberculosis

Postprimary tuberculosis is characterized by strong resistance which keeps the disease localized to the affected organ, also an active hypersensitivity state which results in extensive tissue destruction and necrosis. The tubercle bacillus may have reached this area through blood spread following primary infection or via the airways in exogenous reinfection. For the latter, as the apices are not well ventilated, multiple exposure will usually be necessary (Smith & Wiegeshaus 1989). It affects particularly the apical regions of the lungs where the oxygen tension is higher. There is widespread caseation necrosis, liquefaction with cavity formation and healing by fibrosis.

Postprimary tuberculosis can develop from endogenous reactivation of a primary lesion, exogenous reinfection or both. Though sometimes termed 'adult'-type pulmonary tuberculosis, it may be seen in children (Miller 1982).

TUBERCULIN SENSITIVITY

The intradermal tuberculin test using old tuberculin was described by Charles Mantoux in 1908. A positive response results in induration within 72 h associated with migration of activated

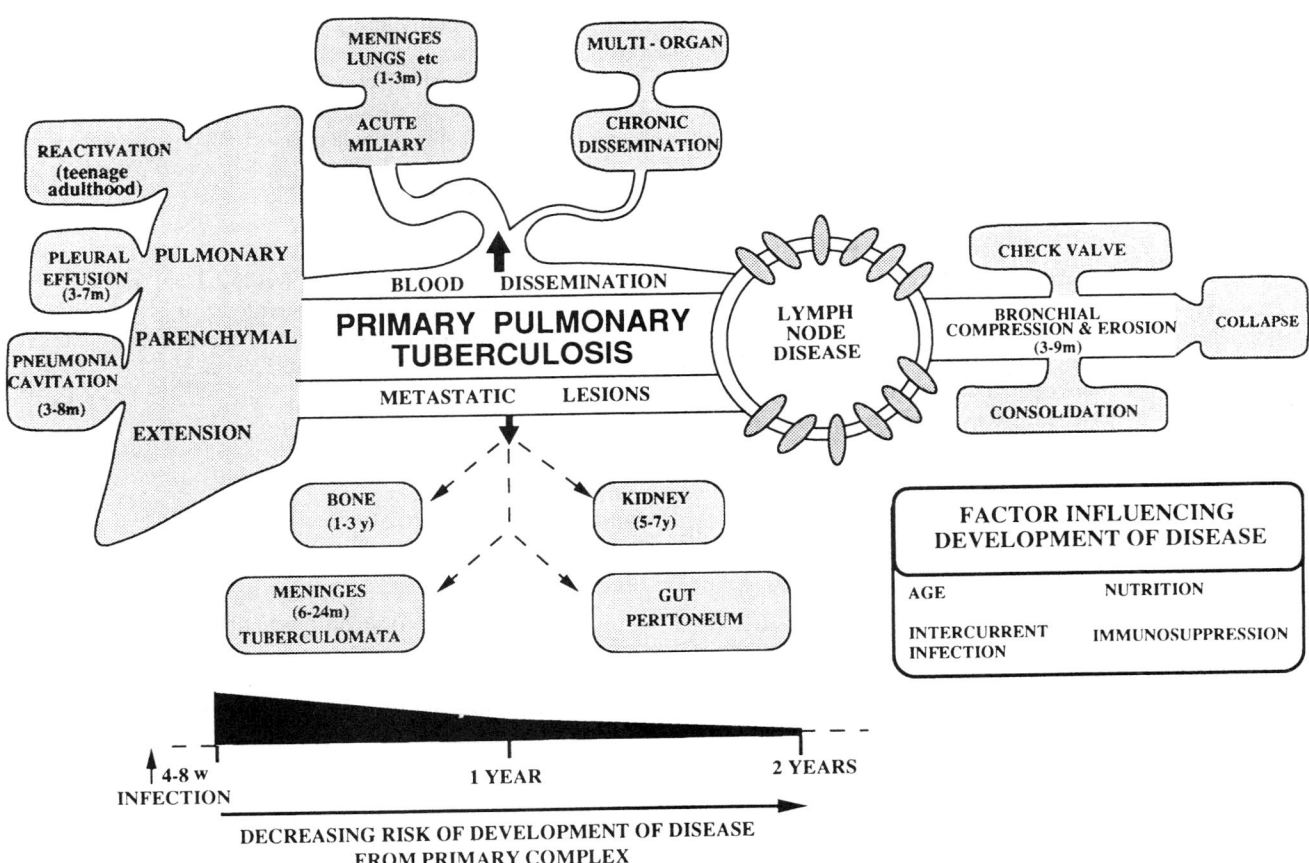

Fig. 23.11 Complications of primary pulmonary tuberculosis. Approximate interval between establishment of primary complex and development of complications in parentheses.

lymphocytes and macrophages to the site of injection. It has been suggested that the dermal swelling is caused by at least two different immunological reactions: the listeria-type reaction, which is associated with protective immunity and is enhanced by BCG, and the Koch-type reaction with necrosis, which does not indicate immunity and is not enhanced by BCG (Lancet 1984).

Two antigen preparations are used: old tuberculin (OT) is a liquid preparation of an extract of dead bacilli and is now mainly used for multiple-puncture skin tests; and purified protein derivative (PPD-S) which is more easily standardized. Different strengths are available: 1 TU/0.1 ml (1 : 10 000 solution), 5 TU/0.1 ml (1 : 5000 solution), 10 TU/0.1 ml (1 : 1000 solution) and 100 TU/0.1 ml (1 : 100 solution). The addition of Tween 80 to PPD reduces the adsorption to the walls of the syringe and multiplies the strengths by a factor of 4–5. Thus, 1 TU with Tween 80 is approximately equivalent to 5 TU without it (Miller 1982). For surveys, 2 TU of PPD with Tween 80 is commonly used. In clinical practice, 10 TU PPD in 0.1 ml solution is given, except where tuberculosis is strongly suspected in which case a weaker dose, 1 TU, is given initially as the former may result in painful necrosis with ulceration. In phlyctenular conjunctivitis or tuberculosis of the eye 1 TU is used initially as a stronger solution may result in a severe eye reaction. In the US and some other countries 5 TU PPD-S is the standard dose. 100 TU is rarely used as it may give a false positive response, more likely to be due to environmental mycobacteria.

Technique of tuberculin test

If necessary, the skin may be cleaned with spirit and allowed to dry. The injection is given *intradermally* into the upper third of the flexor surface of the forearm with a 1.0 ml syringe and a small needle (short bevel gauge 25–27) producing a wheal of at least 5 mm. The result should be read at 48–72 h, but a valid result may be obtained at up to 96 h. In strongly tuberculin-positive subjects, a wheal may appear within 24 h. A positive result consists of induration of at least 6 mm diameter measured transversely. Only the area of induration, not the erythema, should be measured. Rarely, lymphangitis or a systemic reaction may develop following the tuberculin test. If necrosis and ulceration develop local hydrocortisone ointment may relieve the discomfort.

Interpretation

In older children and adults, a wheal of 5 mm or less is regarded as negative, 6–9 mm likely to be associated with infection by environmental mycobacteria, and 10 mm or more is indicative of infection by *M. tuberculosis*, unless the person has received BCG. *In infants and young children with clinical evidence suggestive of tuberculosis, those with malnutrition or immunosuppression or in close contact with a case, an intermediate reaction of 6–9 mm should be considered positive.* After BCG the Mantoux response is usually less than 10–15 mm or Heaf grade 1–2. A Mantoux reaction ≥ 15 mm is suggestive of sensitivity to *M. tuberculosis* in any child.

A negative or weak response in the presence of tuberculosis may occur in the following conditions: 6–10 weeks after infection, but before tuberculin sensitivity has developed, malnutrition, miliary or overwhelming tuberculosis, nonrespiratory disease, especially tuberculous meningitis, tuberculosis in infants less than 6 weeks of age, recent viral infections such as measles and glandular fever, or whooping cough, recent immunization (within 6 weeks) against measles, mumps or rubella (MMR), immunosuppressive diseases including HIV, malignancy, and other debilitating diseases, and current treatment with immunosuppressive agents (including corticosteroids). In developing countries, the tuberculin test is often negative in children with tuberculosis, probably owing to the presence of malnutrition and current infections.

In malnourished children the use of the accelerated BCG test may be of value (see under BCG).

When the tuberculin test is negative in children with tuberculosis due to malnutrition, overwhelming infection or other causes, if it is repeated some months later when the general condition of the patient has improved, it will usually be positive. However, there are a small proportion of children with culture-proven tuberculosis (perhaps 5%) who are consistently negative, despite the absence of adverse factors such as malnutrition, overwhelming tuberculosis or other infections (Steiner et al 1980). In children infected by *M. tuberculosis* (and those given BCG) tuberculin sensitivity may revert to negative over some years, particularly those in whom there was not a strong initial reaction or who have had prompt treatment. This does not necessarily imply that they are not protected from reinfection. Repeated administration of tuberculin may enhance tuberculin sensitivity (booster phenomenon).

Multiple puncture techniques

Multiple puncture tests such as the Heaf test are used to screen large numbers of children. Other tests include the Tine and Imotest. The Heaf test is the most reliable, but all doubtful reactions following multiple puncture techniques should be confirmed by a Mantoux test.

The Heaf gun has six needles arranged in a circle which puncture the skin through a strong solution of PPD (100 000 units/ml). The needles are set at 2 mm for children 2 years and over, and at 1 mm for those younger. Disposable heads or units are now used which dispenses with the need for sterilization. The result may be read at any time from 3 to 10 days after the puncture, and is graded as follows: grade 1, at least four small indurated papules; grade 2, an indurated ring formed by confluent papules; grade 3, a disc of induration; grade 4, induration over 10 mm. Grade 1 is interpreted as unlikely to be associated with *M. tuberculosis* infection, grades 3–4 strongly suggest tuberculous infection and grade 2 is indeterminate. A grade 2 Heaf response is approximately equivalent to that of a positive Mantoux test of 5–14 mm using 10 TU and grade 3 or 4 to a Mantoux response ≥ 15 mm.

BCG VACCINATION

BCG vaccine is an attenuated bovine strain of mycobacteria introduced by Calmette and Guérin in France in 1921 and originally given orally. It was first used in Sweden in 1927 and in England in 1948.

After intradermal injection of BCG, there is dissemination of small numbers of bacilli to internal organs, particularly the liver and lungs where granulomata develop. BCG sensitizes individuals so that when they are infected by *M. tuberculosis* multiplication of bacteria is curtailed and a granuloma develops quickly which walls off the infection. Systemic hematogenous dissemination is reduced, as also is secondary infection of the lung either from local extension of lesions or seeding from the blood. BCG vaccination does not prevent tuberculous infection; it particularly reduces the chances of miliary spread and meningitis (and death), and, to a lesser extent, pulmonary disease.

Indications

In Britain BCG vaccination is recommended for the following groups (DoH 1996):

1. Schoolchildren between the ages of 10 and 14 years
2. Newly born babies, children or adults where the parents or the individuals themselves request BCG vaccination
3. Health service staff who may have contact with infectious patients or their specimens (it is particularly important to test and immunize staff working in maternity and pediatric departments in which the patients are likely to be immunocompromised, e.g. transplant, oncology and HIV units)
4. Veterinary and other staff who handle animal species known to be susceptible to tuberculosis, e.g. simians
5. Staff of prisons, old people's homes, refugee hostels and hostels for the homeless
6. Contacts of cases known to be suffering from active pulmonary tuberculosis (see Prevention and contact tracing, and Management during pregnancy and of the newborn')
7. Immigrants from countries with a high prevalence of tuberculosis, their children and infants wherever born
8. Those intending to stay in Asia, Africa, Central or South America for more than 1 month.

Mass campaigns

In countries with a high prevalence of tuberculosis, BCG is given at birth or in early infancy and may be repeated at school entry and school leaving. In countries such as the UK where there is a low prevalence of tuberculosis, it is given at 10–14 years. With the decreasing risk of tuberculosis and, thus, low cost-effectiveness, the BCG Schools Programme in Britain is under regular review.

Contraindications

Contraindications to BCG vaccination include patients with immunosuppressive disorders, malignancy and those receiving corticosteroids or immunosuppressive treatment, and generalized infective conditions. If eczema exists vaccination should be given in an area free from skin lesions. An interval of 3 weeks should be allowed between administration of BCG vaccine and other live vaccines, with the exception of oral polio vaccine. BCG vaccination is not given to tuberculin-positive subjects including those Heaf grade 2 or more.

The recommendations for BCG vaccination of infants born to mothers infected by human immunodeficiency virus (HIV) varies according to the prevalence of tuberculosis. BCG is contraindicated in HIV-infected infants, whether they are symptomatic or not. In countries where both HIV infection and tuberculosis are endemic, routine immunization of newborns is still recommended.

Technique

BCG is given to subjects whose Mantoux is less than 6 mm or who are Heaf grade 0 or 1. In persons with a BCG scar of at least 3–4 mm, even though the tuberculin test is negative, revaccination is unnecessary. Newborns and infants up to the age of 3 months do not require a prevaccination tuberculin test. In developing countries, a prevaccination tuberculin test is not usually given at any age.

The vaccination is given by *intradermal* injection, usually into the left upper arm at the insertion of the deltoid muscle; 0.1 ml is given with a 1 ml syringe and a gauge 25–27 needle (as per Mantoux test). It is advised that newborn infants are given 0.05 ml because of the increased chance of local lymphadenopathy. Older infants may be given 0.1 ml. Proper technique is essential. The needle should be inserted for about 2 mm and a wheal of at least 5–7 mm produced. If resistance is not felt during injecting, the needle has been inserted too far (or the fluid has leaked externally) and it should be withdrawn. Injecting the vaccine subcutaneously may result in an abscess or large ulcer. BCG vaccination may also be given by the percutaneous multiple puncture technique using a modified Heaf gun (18–20 needles). It is more convenient and easier for newborn infants. A specific vaccine for percutaneous BCG should be used. A scar is detected less often than with the intradermal method but there are similar rates of conversion (Cundall et al 1988). Jet injectors are not advised because of the likelihood of mechanical fault. Normally a small papule develops at the site of vaccination within 2–6 weeks. Sometimes it may ulcerate and discharge but it usually heals after about 2–3 months, leaving a small scar (for management see Complications).

Accelerated BCG reaction

If BCG vaccination is given to subjects infected by tuberculosis or who have received BCG previously, an accelerated reaction may result; a papule appears within 24–48 h, a pustule by 5–7 days, and a scab by 2 weeks. In malnourished children with tuberculosis, the Mantoux test is often negative but there may be an accelerated reaction to BCG. A papule of 5 mm or more appearing by the third day is regarded as positive. BCG is considered to be equivalent to 20–50 TU PPD and in India is used as a diagnostic test for tuberculosis, particularly in malnourished children.

Complications

Adverse reactions to BCG over 1% usually indicate incorrect dosage or bad technique. The commonest complication is abscess formation and the development of a large ulcer. Swelling of local lymph nodes with or without sinus formation is more likely in young infants. These complications usually result from an inadvertent subcutaneous injection. Excess volume of vaccine or the use of a vaccine with a higher potency may also be responsible. Outbreaks of lymphadenitis have been associated with certain manufacturers' preparations, e.g. the Pasteur strain (WHO 1989). Both *Staphylococcus aureus* and/or the BCG mycobacterium may be cultured from the lesion.

Nonfluctuant enlarged nodes should be left untreated. Abscesses should be aspirated. If repeated aspiration of fluctuant nodes does not result in resolution they may be excised. Discharging ulcers should be cleaned with an antiseptic two or three times a day, left uncovered as much as possible, and, when necessary, a nonadherent dressing should be used. For ulcers that do not respond to these methods, isoniazid 6 mg/kg/day for 6 weeks usually results in healing. Hypertrophic or keloid scars may develop at the site of vaccination especially if given at sites other than insertion of the deltoid. Excision is not always successful. Local injection of triamcinolone at monthly intervals for three to four doses may result in atrophy.

Other rare complications of BCG vaccination include anaphylactic reactions, satellite lesions, bone lesions, meningitis or overwhelming infection. The latter usually occurs in immunodeficient infants (Casanova et al 1995). Risk of complications in infants of HIV-infected mothers given BCG in the neonatal period is small; rarely disseminated BCG may occur (O'Brien et al 1995). Focal lesions such as osteitis may occur in apparently immunocompetent infants and in some cases have been associated with increased potency of the vaccine. This complication has been reported particularly from Sweden and Finland (WHO 1989, Kroger et al 1995). Osteitis may develop some years after vaccination. In HIV-infected infants, enlarged lymph nodes with sinus formation may develop months after the vaccination has apparently healed, coinciding with the onset of immunosuppression.

Efficacy

The effectiveness of BCG in preventing tuberculosis, particularly miliary spread and meningitis, has been demonstrated in a number of prospective trials and case-control studies (WHO 1989). It also provides some protection against leprosy and Buruli ulcer. Protection is greatest within a few years after neonatal BCG vaccination and persists for up to 10 years. However, the results of studies vary between different communities and are influenced by factors such as the prevalence of and exposure to tuberculosis, distance from the equator, the prevalence of environmental mycobacteria, the administration and potency of the vaccine, and the age and nutritional status of the subjects (Fine 1995).

British school children vaccinated at around 13 years have demonstrated a consistent level of protection of about 75% persisting for 15 years (Sutherland & Springett 1987). Other studies, notably a trial in the Chingleput area (50 km from Madras, India), have not demonstrated any protection against tuberculosis. The reasons for failure in this trial have been debated. Children less than 1 month of age were not included in the trial and the trial was not designed to detect tuberculosis in children. The prevalence of environmental mycobacteria is high in that area and immunity produced by these mycobacteria may not be enhanced by BCG vaccination. A similar reason is given for failure of BCG in Georgia, USA.

Two controlled trials of BCG in the newborn, one in North American Indians living in Saskatchewan, the other in Chicago, have shown 75–80% protection rate, and some case-control studies have also demonstrated considerable protection

(Rodrigues & Smith 1990, Colditz et al 1995). BCG given a few months after birth may result in a better immunological response and have a lower complication rate.

In the northern hemisphere BCG continues to provide substantial protection against tuberculosis overall and up to 80% for disseminated disease (Romanus et al 1992). Some reasons for failure in warm climates are outlined above.

Tuberculin sensitivity after BCG vaccination

When the technique and potency of vaccine is adequate, most vaccinated infants will have a scar and over 90% will be tuberculin positive. Tuberculin sensitivity (usually Heaf grade 1–2) will remain in most children for at least 5–12 years (Ormerod & Garnett 1992, Teale et al 1992). However, some infants with a scar may be tuberculin negative and some of those with no scar may be tuberculin positive. Preterm infants and those with severe intrauterine growth retardation may have a reduced response to BCG vaccination, possibly due to impaired cell-mediated immunity. Scars are less likely to persist in infants vaccinated in the neonatal period.

In developing countries tuberculin sensitivity may wane considerably over the years. Most older children will be tuberculin negative or have low sensitivity (Eason 1987). In children vaccinated with BCG a Mantoux reaction ≥ 10–15 mm or Heaf grade 3–4 should be interpreted as likely infection by *M. tuberculosis*. Repeat BCG vaccination is associated with larger tuberculin reactions.

New vaccines

Vaccines are required which are more effective in preventing exogenous reinfection and in persons already infected by environmental mycobacteria or in those who have received the conventional BCG. Preliminary studies of administration of *M. vaccae* to adults on chemotherapy for tuberculosis have demonstrated improved outcome (Stanford & Stanford 1996).

PREVENTION AND CONTACT TRACING

In Britain today, the majority of children in whom tuberculosis is diagnosed are detected through contact tracing of smear-positive cases of tuberculosis. Children with primary tuberculosis and subjects with nonrespiratory tuberculosis are rarely infectious. Smear-positive adults who receive drug regimens which include rifampicin usually have a negative sputum culture within 2 weeks.

Procedures for control and prevention of tuberculosis in Britain have been outlined (British Thoracic Society 1994). When a case of tuberculosis is diagnosed, household contacts should be screened. Children and young adults should have a tuberculin test and, when positive, a chest X-ray. Older adults and those who have received BCG vaccination should have a chest X-ray. If the tuberculin test is negative, it should be repeated after 6 weeks as the first test may have been done too early in the course of infection. Tuberculin-negative subjects should be offered BCG. Tuberculin-positive subjects with a normal chest X-ray should be given prophylaxis (see below).

In the majority of cases of tuberculosis in young children, the source of infection is in the home. For older children it may be necessary to search outside the home, e.g. staff at school, a swimming pool attendant or a youth leader. In tuberculosis of the face or gums, the possibility of infection by a dentist should be considered.

Chemoprophylaxis and follow-up of contacts

Chemoprophylaxis is indicated for tuberculin-positive children (Heaf grades 2–4) with a normal chest X-ray, who have not had BCG, and in those who seroconvert. It should be considered in those with grade 3–4 who have received BCG.

Tuberculin-negative children under 2 years of age in close contact with tuberculosis should also be given chemoprophylaxis followed by BCG. Follow-up chest X-rays should be done at 3 and 12 months.

For chemoprophylaxis isoniazid (INH) 6 mg/kg/day should be given for 6 months or INH plus rifampicin (RIF) for 3 months. In young infants exposed to smear-positive patients, or in contacts at any age when the source is suspected to harbor INH-resistant *M. tuberculosis*, rifampicin may be added to INH and the combination given for 4–6 months. If INH resistance is confirmed RIF alone can be given for 6–9 months (Swanson & Starke 1995).

Schools BCG Programme

Children with a definite BCG scar do not require a Heaf test.

Children with Heaf grade 0 and 1 are given BCG; no action is required for those with grade 2; for Heaf grade 3–4 with normal chest X-rays, chemoprophylaxis is recommended for those with a history of contact with tuberculosis or residence in a high prevalence area within the preceding 2 years, and should be considered for others in high-risk groups.

CLINICAL FORMS OF TUBERCULOSIS

The commonest presentation of tuberculosis is respiratory disease followed by involvement of lymph nodes. However, unless the culture of lymph node tissue is obtained infection by environmental mycobacteria cannot be differentiated from that by *M. tuberculosis*. In the 1988 survey of childhood tuberculosis in England and Wales nonrespiratory lesions were present in approximately one-third of children some of whom also had a respiratory lesion (Table 23.23). In developing countries, where the diagnosis is often late, nonrespiratory disease is common with or without respiratory disease. It is important to remember that tuberculosis can infect virtually any part of the body.

Figure 23.11 shows an outline and a time scale of some of the complications of primary pulmonary tuberculosis.

Intrathoracic tuberculosis

The distribution of respiratory and nonrespiratory disease seen in children in England and Wales in 1988 is shown in Table 23.23.

Primary pulmonary tuberculosis

The primary complex consists of a focal lesion usually 1–2 cm in diameter which may be found in any part of the lung, and enlarged hilar nodes or, in heavier infections, the paratracheal nodes (Figs 23.12 and 23.13). Lymph node enlargement is particularly prominent in infants and young children. It is usually asymptomatic and discovered during contact tracing or a routine tuberculin test. Often the primary focus has resolved or is not

Table 23.23 Clinical presentation of tuberculosis in children in England and Wales for 1988

Respiratory disease*	n = 213	%	Nonrespiratory disease*	n = 101	%
Pulmonary	166	78	Peripheral lymph nodes	61	60
Intrathoracic lymph nodes	55	26	Central nervous system	15	15
Pleural	12	6	Miliary	7	7
			Abdominal	7	7
			Bone and joint	6	6
			Other†	13	13

* 20 children had both respiratory and nonrespiratory disease.
† Other includes: genitourinary (3), pericarditis (1), abscesses (2).
Source: Medical Research Council Cardiothoracic Epidemiology Group 1994.

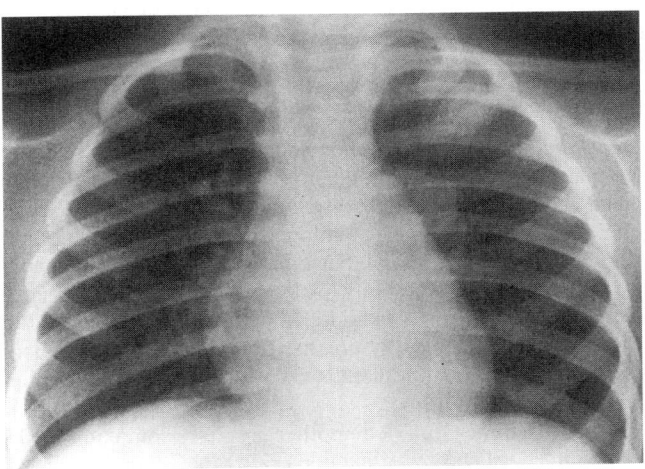

Fig. 23.12 Primary tuberculosis in a 2-year-old child. Primary focus in the left upper lobe with enlarged regional nodes.

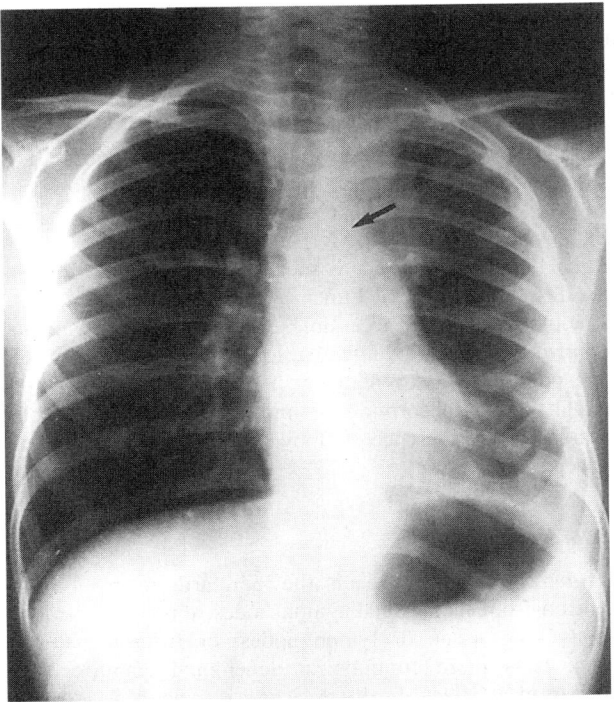

Fig. 23.13 A 10-year-old boy with primary tuberculosis. There is consolidation of the left upper lobe, displacement of the lower trachea and left main bronchus by enlarged nodes (→) and a pleural effusion.

visible and the diagnosis is based on the enlarged regional nodes. Calcification of the focus and, more often, the nodes may occur after about 12 months, generally within 2–3 years of the infection, and remains an indication of previous infection. Calcification usually indicates healing of the tuberculous process, but healing and progression of the disease may continue concurrently. In many cases the calcium slowly resolves leaving clear lung fields, which explains the common situation in adults where the tuberculin test is positive and the chest X-ray normal.

In older children and adolescents, the lung component is more prominent and commonly presents as an enlarging upper lobe infiltrate and cavitation, usually without lymph node enlargement, and indistinguishable from postprimary tuberculosis. Pleural effusion is commoner at this age (Fig. 23.13).

Progressive primary tuberculosis

Progressive primary tuberculosis may result from extension of the pulmonary focus or softening of regional lymph nodes. Extension of the pulmonary focus may cause bronchopneumonia or rupture into the pleura resulting in *pleural effusion. Tuberculous empyema* may result from rupture of caseous material into the pleural space. It may be complicated by pneumothorax (pyopneumothorax). Evacuation of caseous material into a bronchus may result in the appearance of a cavity. Cavities in primary pulmonary tuberculosis are not uncommon in malnourished and debilitated infants.

Complications from enlargement or softening of regional nodes are more common. The bronchus can be compressed externally; more likely, the wall is eroded and caseous material either partly or completely blocks the lumen (endobronchial tuberculosis); or rupture of the wall results in bronchopneumonia. Partial obstruction may result in a ball valve effect with lobar emphysema. This is often transient, because either the bronchus blocks completely or the material is coughed up with clearing of the obstruction (Miller 1984). More commonly, there is *segmental* collapse with or without consolidation. Rupture of caseous material into the bronchus may result in a predominantly allergic response with exudation, or, if there are a large number of bacteria present, a progressive tuberculous bronchopneumonia. The former may be associated with marked changes on chest X-ray but which clear spontaneously, whereas the latter, which is more often seen in debilitated children, may prove fatal if not treated.

Rarely, a caseous node may rupture into the trachea, resulting in bilateral obstructive emphysema or asphyxia, into the esophagus resulting in a fistula or the development of an esophageal pouch, or into the pericardium. Other complications from enlarged nodes include superior vena cava obstruction, and recurrent laryngeal or phrenic nerve compression.

There may be nonspecific symptoms of irregular fever, anorexia, weight loss and, in severe or longstanding cases, the child may be marasmic. Compression of the bronchi may result in a spasmodic cough simulating whooping cough. When there is obstructive emphysema the symptoms may be mistaken for asthma, though clinical examination will usually demonstrate signs of mediastinal shift. In longstanding cases, the child may present with clubbing of the fingers and bronchiectasis.

Postprimary pulmonary tuberculosis

The pathogenesis of postprimary pulmonary tuberculosis has been described earlier. The infection is usually in the upper lobes or the superior segments of the lower lobes, and is confined to the lungs with no hematogenous spread. In many cases it results from reactivation of a former primary lesion and, though usually associated with adults, may be seen in children and adolescents. Evidence of a previous primary pulmonary complex may be detected (Miller 1984). Common symptoms include a productive cough, especially in the morning, and there may be hemoptysis, fever, night sweats, malaise and weight loss.

Chest X-ray may show a variety of lesions including nodular or patchy shadows, cavities and various stages of healing with fibrosis and calcification. Both lungs may be affected and there may be a pleural effusion.

Diagnosis

The diagnosis of *primary tuberculosis* is based on a positive tuberculin test and enlarged nodes on chest X-ray with or without a pulmonary infiltrate. Enlarged lymph nodes may not be easily demonstrated; a lateral chest X-ray may be helpful. Persistent pulmonary infiltrate(s) in the presence of a positive tuberculin test is highly suggestive of tuberculosis.

In *progressive primary tuberculosis* the chest X-ray usually shows enlarged nodes with opacities more often in the middle or lower lobes, due to collapse and/or consolidation. In progressive pneumonia, cavities may be seen. In debilitated children, the tuberculin test may be negative. This is a common problem in developing countries where in the absence of facilities for mycobacterial culture the diagnosis is often based on the response to a trial of chemotherapy.

In young children specimens for microscopy and culture are usually obtained from gastric aspirates or less commonly laryngeal swabs. In older children sputum may be available from expectoration or sputum induction (Shata et al 1996) or, if bronchoscopy is required, from an aspirate or a biopsy. Mycobacteria may be cultured from gastric aspirate of patients with regional intrathoracic nodes without a radiologically detectable pulmonary lesion or rarely those with normal chest X-ray. Also, lymph nodes may be detected on CT scan in children with normal chest X-rays (Delacourt et al 1993). Gastric aspiration is performed in the morning in a fasting child usually on three consecutive mornings. The specimen must be *immediately* examined by fluorescent microscopy or Ziehl–Neelsen stain, and cultured. Gastric aspirates are seldom positive on direct smear but *M. tuberculosis* may be cultured in about one-third of children and two-thirds of infants (Vallejo et al 1994).

A *pleural effusion* is due to an allergic response to the mycobacteria and thus the tuberculin test is usually strongly positive. If large, or required for diagnostic purposes, it should be aspirated. The fluid is usually clear straw colored but may be opalescent if there is a high cell count. Lymphocytes will be seen on microscopy, but early in the disease neutrophils may also be present. The protein content will be raised, > 40 g/l, and the glucose low, < 1.7 mmol/l. Mycobacteria are often not detected on direct smear but in about half the cases they may be cultured, especially if a large volume of fluid is centrifuged. Mycobacteria are more likely to be cultured from an empyema. Pleural biopsy may also be taken for histology.

The blood count usually shows a normal white cell count. There may be an increase in pale-staining monocytes. A raised ESR is associated with activity of the disease but otherwise has no diagnostic value.

Management

Uncomplicated primary infection usually heals without treatment. The main purpose of chemotherapy is to prevent hematogenous spread and progression of disease which is more likely in young, debilitated or malnourished children. Segmental collapse may occur despite chemotherapy, but tuberculous bronchopneumonia or pleural effusion is usually prevented. Radiological changes resolve slowly and 50% of children may still have evidence of the primary complex after 18 months. Lymph nodes may enlarge during chemotherapy but there is usually no necessity to prolong therapy because of this.

Standard three-drug chemotherapy is isoniazid (INH), rifampicin (RIF) and pyrazinamide (PZA) for 2 months followed by INH and RIF for 4 months. If PZA is not given INH + RIF should be given for 9 months. For alternative regimens see section on Chemotherapy. For hilar lymphadenopathy alone a three-drug regimen followed by INH + RIF for just 2 months or two drugs INH + RIF for 6 months is adequate (WHO 1993, American Thoracic Society 1994).

Bronchial obstruction. Incomplete bronchial obstruction with air trapping and the development of *obstructive emphysema* may respond to corticosteroids (see Management). However, the transient nature of this lesion should be remembered, i.e. it may resolve or the bronchus may become completely obstructed. Complete obstruction will result in absorption collapse, and bronchoscopy should be performed to exclude other pathology, such as foreign body, and to suck out as much of the caseous material in the bronchial lumen as possible. Unfortunately, the obstruction may not be accessible, especially in young infants.

Pleural effusion. The infective load in pleural effusion is low and responds quickly to treatment. The addition of corticosteroids may enhance the absorption of fluid and help to prevent pleural adhesions. In the presence of empyema, surgical drainage may be required.

Pericarditis

M. tuberculosis may reach the pericardium by lymphatic extension from mediastinal lymph nodes, direct extension from caseous lung tissue or lymph nodes, or from hematogenous spread. It is more common in developing countries (Hugo-Hamman et al 1994). In dry pericarditis, a loud pericardial rub may be heard. Occasionally, there is a large effusion which may cause tamponade. An effusion will be detected by echocardiography. Pericardial aspirate is often bloodstained, and polymorphonuclear leukocytes may be seen in the early stages after which lymphocytes predominate. *M. tuberculosis* may be cultured in over half the cases. Diagnosis may also be made by culture and histology of a pericardial biopsy. Constrictive pericarditis may follow in spite of treatment.

Standard antituberculous treatment is given. Open drainage may prevent subsequent requirement for pericardial aspiration. Corticosteroids, may enhance the rate of improvement, reduce the requirement for aspiration and may possibly reduce the need for pericardiectomy (Strang et al 1987, Strang et al 1988).

Extrathoracic tuberculosis

Nonrespiratory tuberculosis usually results from hematogenous spread and arises from extension of a primary focus or extension of a regional node. It is less common than pulmonary disease. Virtually any organ may be affected and particularly in developing countries where nonrespiratory disease is still relatively common tuberculosis should be remembered in *any* unusual lesion where the diagnosis is not known. Some of the common types are described below. Tuberculosis may also affect the larynx, middle ear and mastoid bones. Virtually any part of the eye may be infected and tuberculosis should be remembered as a cause of an orbital mass. Tuberculosis of the skin may result from primary inoculation, from hematogenous dissemination, or from a cold abscess in an underlying structure.

Lymph node tuberculosis

Superficial lymph node tuberculosis commonly occurs in the cervical or supraclavicular, and, less often, the axillary or inguinal regions. As in primary tuberculosis of the lungs, the regional nodes enlarge in response to a focus. Less commonly, enlargement of a number of superficial lymph nodes results from hematogenous spread, especially during chronic disseminated tuberculosis. The focus may be the tonsils, gums, lungs, or elsewhere. In cervical adenitis the commonest focus is the upper lung fields. Enlarged axillary or inguinal nodes may be due to infection of the skin. In Britain, in the majority of cases of white children with histological evidence of mycobacterial infection of the cervical glands, it is associated with environmental mycobacteria such as *M. avium-intracellulare*. *M. tuberculosis is* commoner in immigrant children.

Initially the nodes are discrete, mobile and nontender later becoming matted together. The primary node is the largest with those draining it being progressively smaller. Without treatment, softening of nodes usually develops within 6 months of infection, and nodes may discharge forming a sinus or track along the fascial planes. Swelling and softening may occur in up to a third of patients during treatment or even years after the node is calcified and apparently healed. This phenomenon may be due to hypersensitivity to tuberculoprotein released at intervals from the lesion and does not necessarily indicate active infection.

The tuberculin test is usually positive and a chest X-ray should be taken to exclude pulmonary tuberculosis. Calcification within the node may be detected radiologically. Fine needle aspiration for smear and culture or biopsy will usually confirm the diagnosis. All specimens either from biopsy or aspiration should be cultured as it is important to know whether the infection is caused by *M. tuberculosis* or environmental mycobacteria. However, culture may be positive in only two-thirds of cases. The main differential

diagnosis is from a cervical pyogenic abscess. Local viral or streptococcal infection of the tonsils may cause enlargement of existing tuberculous nodes. Other differential diagnoses include glandular fever, HIV infection, cat-scratch disease, actinomycosis, malignancy or an infected branchial or thyroglossal cyst.

Treatment with standard chemotherapy is adequate (Jawahar et al 1990). If softening of the node occurs, it may be aspirated. If excision is necessary the primary node should be removed intact, or if not feasible as much of the caseous material as possible (Miller 1982). It is important to remember that cold abscesses are frequently of the 'collar stud' variety and that adequate drainage of the abscess in the deep fascia is necessary.

Miliary (disseminated) tuberculosis

Hematogenous dissemination of small numbers of bacilli probably occurs in the majority of children with primary uncomplicated tuberculosis. In developing countries a liver biopsy for an unconnected disease may show tuberculous granulomata in children not known to have had tuberculosis. These rarely become symptomatic. Erosion of a pulmonary vessel with massive hematogenous spread is referred to as acute miliary tuberculosis and if untreated is usually rapidly fatal. It may be found at autopsy without being evident on chest X-ray. A more chronic form, cryptogenic disseminated, also occurs. In both forms disease may develop in virtually any organ of the body.

Acute miliary tuberculosis. Acute miliary tuberculosis is commonest in young children and usually occurs within a year of the primary infection. The most important complication is meningitis. The onset is usually insidious. Presenting signs include pyrexia, dyspnea, anemia, hepatosplenomegaly and lymphadenopathy (Hussey et al 1991). Anorexia and weight loss are common and variable degrees of malnutrition will be evident depending on the length of the illness. The lungs show a 'snowstorm' picture on chest X-ray. Rarely respiratory failure with adult respiratory distress syndrome may develop (Monier et al 1992). Choroid tubercles are pathognomonic of the disease. Cutaneous lesions include macules, papules, purpura and papulonecrotic tuberculides.

Except in the early stages the diagnosis will usually be evident from a chest X-ray (snowstorm appearance). There may also be lobar infiltrates and hilar lymphadenopathy. The tuberculin test may be weak or negative in the early stages or if the child has severe debility. A lumbar puncture is essential in all cases to exclude meningitis. Bacteriological confirmation will be obtained in the majority of children particularly from culture of gastric contents, and also CSF and urine. In difficult cases the diagnosis is sometimes made on liver, lung or marrow biopsy.

The differential diagnosis is wide depending on the geographical situation. The lung disease may simulate histiocytosis X, cystic fibrosis or idiopathic pulmonary hemosiderosis, and the systemic disease typhoid fever, systemic leishmaniasis, leukemia, collagen diseases and chronic malaria.

Acute miliary disease usually responds promptly to chemotherapy. Most deaths are related to meningitis and/or late diagnosis. A short course of corticosteroids will speed the resolution of symptoms, especially if there is alveolar capillary block. Standard chemotherapy is adequate. Prolonged (9 months) therapy may be required in complicated cases or meningitis.

Chronic disseminated (cryptic) tuberculosis. In chronic disseminated tuberculosis, small numbers of bacilli seed the bloodstream at intervals and produce metastatic foci in organs throughout the body. Apart from the lung lesions, there is usually generalized lymphadenopathy and often hepatosplenomegaly, and involvement of the pleural, pericardial and peritoneal cavities, bones and kidneys may occur. There may be multiple bone involvement with dactylitis or involvement of the skin with papulonecrotic tuberculides. In some cases the chest X-ray is normal and the primary site is unknown. A variety of hematological abnormalities may be seen, e.g. pancytopenia, or leukemoid reactions, which suggest leukemia or a lymphoma. The tuberculin test may be negative. Bone marrow biopsy may show necrotic foci with little cellular reaction but teeming with mycobacteria.

Treatment is similar to that of acute miliary disease. Corticosteroids may be of benefit in debilitated children.

Tuberculosis of the central nervous system

Tuberculosis of the central nervous system may have a variety of manifestations. There may be generalized inflammation affecting brain and spinal cord; less commonly, single or multiple tuberculomata enlarge and present as an intracranial space-occupying lesion or rarely tuberculous disease may be confined to the spine.

Tuberculous meningitis. Tuberculous meningitis is commonest in children under 5 years of age, often occurring within 6 months and usually within 2 years of primary infection, but it may occur at any age. It results from rupture of one or more tubercles (Rich focus) into the subarachnoid space. The tubercle(s) is commonly situated in the subcortex of the brain, and less often in the meninges or spinal cord. Characteristically the severe inflammatory response results in a thick gelatinous exudate and adhesions around the base of the brain with hydrocephalus and spinal block. Involvement of cranial nerves may result in single or multiple palsies. Arteritis may cause thrombosis and infarction of nervous tissue with permanent damage. Occasionally there is little exudate and the illness is termed *serous meningitis*. Spontaneous recovery without treatment has been described in some of the latter cases.

Symptoms develop over some weeks and may be grouped into stages which give a guide to prognosis. Initially, the symptoms are nonspecific and include irritability, malaise, anorexia, vomiting, constipation and low grade fever. Unless the child is a contact of tuberculosis or there is a high index of suspicion, the diagnosis is rarely made at this stage. Within a few weeks specific features in addition to the above become apparent: there is headache, disorientation, meningism, focal neurological signs, such as cranial nerve palsy, hemiplegia or visual defect, and seizures may develop. In young infants the fontanel may be distended. In older infants a 'cracked pot' sound may indicate separation of the cranial sutures due to raised intracranial pressure. Fundoscopy may demonstrate choroid tubercles, especially when there is miliary disease, papilledema or the development of optic atrophy. The third and often terminal stage is manifest by coma, a posture of decerebrate rigidity, dilated pupils, and the child is usually wasted.

Diagnosis. The diagnosis is based on CSF findings in association with a positive tuberculin test. There may be radiological evidence of pulmonary disease, or disease elsewhere in the body. The tuberculin test is positive in most cases but may be negative, especially in the advanced stages when there is wasting. The latter situation is particularly common in developing countries. The differential diagnosis includes viral and partially treated pyogenic meningitis, cerebral abscess, subdural empyema, fungal infections, e.g. *Cryptococcus neoformans*, and unusual causes such as sarcoidosis, Lyme disease, leptospirosis, collagen diseases and malignancy.

The CSF is clear, unless there is a high cell count, when it may appear turbid. The cell count is usually less than 500/mm^3 and mainly lymphocytic, except in the very early stages when polymorphoneutrophils may predominate. Polymorphoneutrophils may also increase after chemotherapy has started. The protein rises to between 0.8 and 4 g/l and in spinal block may be well over 10 g/l and the CSF xanthochromic. The glucose is usually low. However, it should be remembered that the first lumbar puncture may be normal, that the cell count, protein and glucose levels may fluctuate from day to day, and that the cell count and protein may be lower in ventricular than in spinal fluid (Donald et al 1991). The chance of detecting tubercle bacilli microscopically is higher if a large amount of CSF is obtained and centrifuged; the success rate claimed varies from 30% to 90% depending on the care and time taken in examining the fluid. A CT scan will be abnormal in 75–100% of cases, usually there is hydrocephalus, also parenchymal disease and basilar meningitis may be detected. If raised intracranial pressure is suspected, the CSF should be taken off slowly with a fine needle or from the ventricles. The CSF should always be cultured for mycobacteria, but is positive in less than half the cases. It may be possible to detect tubercle bacilli after chemotherapy has commenced. Occasionally, tuberculous meningitis may be complicated by pyogenic meningitis. A number of methods have been developed to detect antigen from, and antibody to, *M. tuberculosis* in the CSF but none are commercially available and so are not used in routine diagnosis. PCR shows the most promise in the rapid diagnosis of tuberculous meningitis (Mancao et al 1994).

Spinal tuberculosis. Spinal tuberculosis is usually secondary to downward extension of the tuberculous process and occurs during treatment of tuberculous meningitis. There is pain and stiffness in the spine at the level of the lesion and symptoms are related to involvement of the spine or nerve roots. The CSF protein is high and there is evidence of a spinal block which can be confirmed by a myelogram.

Rarely, diffuse tuberculous spinal subarachnoiditis may occur as a result of extension of a primary focus in the spine. It presents as a subacute, transverse or ascending myelitis with upper and lower motor neuron signs and may be mistaken for other causes of cord compression and polyneuritis.

Tuberculoma. A tuberculoma is a tuberculous focus which enlarges within brain tissue without rupturing. It may be single or multiple. It may give rise to signs of raised intracranial pressure or a hemiplegia, or cranial nerve palsy if in the brainstem. A skull X-ray may show calcification. CT scan usually shows a hypodense mass and ring enhancement with contrast. MRI scan may be more useful in detecting tuberculomata, infarcts and spinal lesions. Tuberculomata may expand weeks to months after commencing treatment for pulmonary tuberculosis and result in raised intracranial pressure sometimes requiring surgical decompression (Teoh et al 1987). This phenomenon may be a hypersensitivity response to release of tuberculoprotein and other antigens following destruction of the mycobacteria.

Management. The key to success in treating tuberculous meningitis is early diagnosis and immediate treatment. If there is doubt as to whether the child has a partially treated meningitis or other causes, antituberculous chemotherapy should be commenced, along with conventional antimicrobials for bacterial meningitis, if necessary.

Optimal chemotherapy is the use of a combination of drugs with good penetration into the CSF and low toxicity. Standard chemotherapy is isoniazid (10 mg/kg) and rifampicin (15–20 mg/kg) which are given for 9 months, with the addition of pyrazinamide (35 mg/kg) for the first 2 months of treatment. A 6-month course may be adequate in most cases (Jacobs et al 1992). If drug resistance is suspected ethambutol (or streptomycin) should be added. Drugs cross the blood–brain barrier more readily in the first 2–3 months of the disease when the meninges are inflamed.

Isoniazid and pyrazinamide, achieve high levels in the CSF even when meninges are not inflamed. Ethionamide has adequate, rifampicin and ethambutol moderate to poor, and streptomycin poor penetration across the meninges (Donald & Seifart 1989, Humphries 1992, Ellard et al 1993). Ethionamide is useful for isoniazid-resistant *M. tuberculosis*. In children who are vomiting, isoniazid, rifampicin and streptomycin can be given parenterally and other drugs by nasogastric tube. Controlled trials on the value of corticosteroids in tuberculous meningitis are few but have demonstrated benefit especially in stage II and III disease (Girgis et al 1991, Humphries 1992). The rationale is based on their ability to reduce the inflammatory exudate and thus prevent the development of adhesions which result in internal hydrocephalus and basilar arachnoiditis. Dexamethasone 0.6 mg/kg/day may be given for 2–3 weeks then tailed off over 2–3 months.

Serial CT scans should be performed to detect cerebral edema and the presence or development of hydrocephalus. In the presence of cerebral edema, controlled ventilation with monitoring of intracranial pressure may be indicated. Hydrocephalus is common and is not always clinically evident. If it is symptomatic, it may be treated by a ventriculoperitoneal shunt. In the initial stages before the drugs have controlled the infection the shunt may be exteriorized.

Spinal arachnoiditis with a CSF block may develop during treatment. If not improved by corticosteroids, release of pressure by surgery may be necessary.

Tuberculomata are treated on similar lines to meningitis. Most of the small and medium-sized lesions resolve completely with chemotherapy. Large lesions and those not responding to chemotherapy may require excision. Enlargement may occur during treatment of pulmonary or tuberculous meningitis, with the development of raised intracranial pressure or localizing signs such as cranial nerve palsy. It may settle without a change of treatment. Corticosteroids should be tried and, failing this, a ventriculoperitoneal shunt may be necessary. Prolongation of antituberculous therapy is advised.

Prognosis. The prognosis for meningitis is related to age of the child (young children have worse prognosis) and the stage of the disease at which therapy is commenced. The stages have been classified as follows:

Stage I: Consciousness undisturbed; no, or only mild and focal, neurological signs.
Stage II: Consciousness disturbed, but patient not comatose or delirious. Mild or moderate neurological signs, such as paraparesis, hemiparesis, and cranial nerve palsies, may be present.
Stage III: Patient comatose or delirious with mild, moderate or severe neurological signs.

In a study of 199 children in Hong Kong complete recovery occurred as follows: stage I 96%, stage II 78% and stage III 21%. 17% of children in stage III died as opposed to 1% in stage II (Humphries et al 1990). Resolution of neurological disability may continue for many months after commencement of therapy.

Abdominal tuberculosis

Abdominal tuberculosis usually results from swallowed sputum or *M. bovis*-infected milk; it may be associated with extension from thoracic nodes, hematogenous dissemination, and after the menarche may be an extension of pelvic tuberculosis. The primary focus is usually in the terminal ileum. Symptoms of disease in children are generally due to enlargement or softening of regional mesenteric nodes, and/or involvement of the peritoneum. In adults with cavitatory pulmonary disease, there may be a chronic enteritis and fistulo-in-ano resembling Crohn's disease or other inflammatory bowel disease.

Common symptoms are abdominal pain, fever, weight loss and abdominal swelling or there may be symptoms of intestinal obstruction. Enlarged mesenteric lymph nodes or a mass associated with adhesions of the omentum and intestines may be palpated, usually on the right side of the abdomen.

Peritonitis may be the dominant condition and is often unassociated with demonstrable pulmonary disease. It may result from extension of a mesenteric node or hematogenous spread. In the latter situation, rarely there may be a polyserositis with involvement of the pleura and pericardium. The ascitic fluid has a predominance of lymphocytes, and a protein concentration above 25 g/l (usually lower than in a tuberculous pleural exudate). Mycobacteria are not often identified and the culture may be positive in only a quarter of cases.

Diagnosis is made on the basis of a positive tuberculin test, peritoneal aspiration and bacteriological and histological examination of specimens obtained by laparoscopy, endoscopy, or at laparotomy. Ultrasonography and CT scan are useful for diagnosis and guidance for needle aspiration. Calcification may be detected on abdominal X-ray.

Treatment is by standard chemotherapy.

Tuberculosis of bones and joints

Tuberculosis of bones and joints results from hematogenous spread usually affecting a single or a few joints within 6–36 months of primary infection. The spine is affected in over half the cases, followed by the knee, hip and ankle. In chronic disseminated tuberculosis, multiple large or small joints may be affected with or without associated abscesses or there may be dactylitis of one or both hands. Sometimes punched out cystic lesions are seen with few inflammatory changes affecting surrounding tissue. Lesions confined to the skull may resemble eosinophilic granuloma of bone, or, if associated with miliary disease, the Letterer–Siwe form of histiocytosis X.

Infection usually starts in the well-vascularized metaphyses near the epiphyseal line of long bones, or, less commonly, in the synovium of the joint. Typically there is minimal periosteal reaction or new bone formation. Progression of the disease may result in destruction of the joint, and/or abscess or sinus formation. The cold abscess may track a considerable distance from the primary focus. For example, a cold abscess from the cervical vertebrae may present as a retropharyngeal mass or, from the lumbar vertebrae, as a psoas abscess in the groin.

Treatment is by standard 6-month chemotherapy. However, if evacuation of necrotic sequestrum and abscesses is not adequate, which might prevent drug penetration, a longer course (9–12 months) may be necessary (Dutt et al 1986, Starke & Correa 1995). Ambulatory chemotherapy without surgery has been found the most satisfactory treatment for spinal disease in developing countries. Acute cord compression may respond to chemotherapy alone, but if the necessary technical expertise is available, early spinal decompression is the treatment of choice. A bone graft in cases of extensive destruction of vertebrae or weightbearing bones, such as the neck of the femur, may be necessary.

Genitourinary tuberculosis

Tuberculosis of the kidneys is uncommon in children as it usually presents 5–7 years or more after the primary infection although it may occur sooner. The first symptom is dysuria and typically there is a sterile pyuria with or without red cells. There may not be any symptoms and even in advanced disease there may be very few leukocytes in the urine. Culture of urine for mycobacteria is usually positive.

Glomerulonephritis with immune complex disease complicating miliary tuberculosis has been described, and may be found to be more common if actively sought (Shribman et al 1983).

Tuberculous epididymitis is seen in young boys and epididymo-orchitis in older boys (Miller 1982). The development of a cold abscess may be the first manifestation of disease. In girls, tuberculosis of the uterus or Fallopian tubes occurs after the onset of puberty and may be complicated by peritonitis.

Tuberculosis of the kidneys and genital tracts should be treated by standard chemotherapy.

Management during pregnancy and of the newborn

Active tuberculosis during pregnancy is associated with infection of the placenta in approximately half the cases; congenital tuberculosis is rare. The main considerations are of the mother during pregnancy and management of the infant at birth. Situations that may arise include a tuberculin-positive woman with a normal chest X-ray, radiologically inactive disease with negative sputum cultures, or active disease.

The only commonly used drug absolutely contraindicated during pregnancy is streptomycin because of its ototoxic effect on the fetus. Isoniazid and rifampicin are given for 6 months and pyrazinamide is added during the first 2 months of treatment. Pyridoxine supplements should be given with INH because of increased requirements during pregnancy.

At birth if the mother has completed treatment or has inactive disease the infant is given BCG. If she has active disease and/or is receiving treatment the infant is given isoniazid 6 mg/kg per day for 3–6 months and is then given a tuberculin test and chest X-ray. If these are negative, isoniazid may be stopped (presuming the mother is not infectious) and BCG given. Where it is doubtful that the mother will comply with treatment, as in developing countries, BCG may be given at birth and the infant also given isoniazid for 3–6 months. The extent to which isoniazid may interfere with BCG vaccination is not clear but is probably small (Lancet 1990a). It is not necessary to use isoniazid-resistant BCG.

If the tuberculin test is positive (> 5 mm), full investigation for tuberculosis should be undertaken. If no clinical or bacteriological evidence of disease is detected INH + RIF should be given for 3–4 months, or INH alone for a total of 9–12 months. If disease is detected full treatment as for congenital infection should be given.

Where possible, the mother should not be separated from her child and should continue breast-feeding. Small amounts of antituberculous drugs are excreted in breast milk, but they are not harmful to the infant.

Perinatal tuberculosis

Congenital tuberculosis is rare although at least 300 cases have been reported (Nemir & O'Hare 1985, Rosenfeld et al 1993, Cantwell et al 1994). Whether the infection is contracted before birth or in the neonatal period is probably only of epidemiological significance. There are three possible routes for congenital infection:

1. transplacental, when the primary infection will be in the liver, or it may possibly bypass the liver through the ductus venosus and be detected in the lungs
2. aspiration of infected amniotic fluid or infected material in the genital tract when the lungs will be infected
3. ingestion, when presumably the liver will be infected.

Symptoms of congenital infection may occur from birth up to 2 months of age with the majority presenting within 2–5 weeks. In neonatal infection onset of symptoms is later (1–2 months). Common clinical features are respiratory distress, fever, hepatosplenomegaly, lymphadenopathy, poor feeding, and failure to thrive; there may also be skin lesions, ear discharge, jaundice and, in late-diagnosed cases, meningitis. The tuberculin test is usually negative but may become positive 6 weeks or more after birth. Chest X-ray may show bronchopneumonia, sometimes resembling staphylococcal pneumonia, or miliary changes but may not be abnormal in the early stages. Mycobacteria are often isolated from gastric aspirates and the diagnosis has also been made on CSF, or liver, lung or lymph node biopsy. The mortality is high in overwhelming or late-diagnosed cases and preterm infants. Also, other bacterial or viral infections may be superimposed.

Treatment is with standard chemotherapy. If drug resistance is suspected, ethambutol or streptomycin should be added.

HIV infection

Few cases of coinfection with HIV and tuberculosis have so far been reported in industrialized countries (Gutman et al 1994). Dual infection is commoner in children in HIV endemic areas of sub-Saharan Africa. In Lusaka, Zambia, up to 70% of children with tuberculosis may be HIV seropositive (Luo et al 1994). However, the epidemiology and disease spectrum of tuberculosis in HIV-infected children is not yet clear. HIV seropositivity in infants with tuberculosis may be due to maternal antibodies and in older children in endemic areas it reflects the high level of perinatal HIV infection and HIV/tuberculosis coinfection in the community. In developing countries lymphadenopathy, miliary disease and wasting are common in dually infected children and there may be a poor response to antituberculous chemotherapy.

There is limited experience on treatment, and at present standard chemotherapy of 9 months' duration is advised. In some cases lifelong prophylaxis with INH may be necessary. In HIV-endemic areas, streptomycin should be avoided because of risks from unsterilized needles (WHO 1993). Thiacetazone may cause severe skin reactions in HIV-infected children and should be replaced by ethambutol.

Chemotherapy

6 months' short-course therapy is now standard for pulmonary and most extrapulmonary disease (British Thoracic Society 1998). There are still differences of opinion regarding dosage of drugs especially INH, and the management of meningitis, bone or joint disease, HIV infection and drug resistance. In developing countries, the main constraint is the cost of drugs, especially rifampicin, which is essential for short-course regimens. The use of cheaper drugs may be a false economy, particularly in areas with a high incidence of drug resistance, as the longer the period of treatment, the more the chance of noncompliance. The duration of therapy need not exceed 1 year, except in unusual circumstances such as drug resistance or noncompliance. Intermittent therapy is useful where compliance may be in doubt and is cheaper, although probably only of practical value in areas where supervision is possible. Drugs are usually given thrice-weekly. Directly observed therapy (DOT) is very successful in overcoming poor compliance.

Different drugs are effective (in order of efficacy) in:

1. killing actively dividing bacilli, e.g. in open cavities: INH, RIF and SM
2. killing dormant, intermittently or nondividing bacilli, e.g. in closed caseous lesions: RIF, INH; or within macrophages: PZA, RIF, INH
3. suppressing drug-resistant mutants: INH, RIF.

Pyrazinamide is particularly active against bacteria inhibited by an acid environment (e.g. within macrophages and in areas of acute inflammation). Killing actively dividing bacilli and clearing the sputum of *live* infective bacilli can be accomplished rapidly but for *cure* or 'sterilization' a prolonged course of treatment is necessary to eradicate dormant and intracellular bacilli. Failure to do this may result in relapse. Mycobacteria may survive for years in a dormant state when metabolism is inhibited by low oxygen tension or low pH.

The most commonly used drugs are bactericidal, e.g. INH (the most potent), RIF, PZA, SM. Isoniazid can kill up to 90% of the bacillary population during the first few days of chemotherapy. Bacteriostatic drugs may be used along with bactericidal drugs to prevent emergence of resistance to the bactericidal drugs, e.g. ethambutol (bactericidal in large doses), thiacetazone, PAS and ethionamide.

The *standard regime* is INH + RIF + PZA for 6 months stopping PZA after 2 months, or INH + RIF for 9 months. The three-drug course is used for all types of tuberculosis. A longer duration of 9–12 months is advised for some types of disease as indicated in the respective sections. Other schedules are shown in Table 23.24. Ethambutol is not advised for children under 6 years because of the possibility of optic neuritis, the symptoms of which they would be unable to report. However, it may have to be used in drug resistance. With a dose of 15 mg/kg it is unlikely that problems should arise (Swanson & Starke 1995). Visual testing should be undertaken where possible. In Table 23.25 the drug dosage and common side effects are shown. The recommended daily dose of isoniazid is 6 mg/kg except for tuberculous

Table 23.24 Drug regimens

Regimen	Duration
Standard daily	
HRZ(E)†: 2 months, then HR: 4 months	6 months
HR: 9 months	9 months
HRZ: 2 months, then HR: 2 months	4 months*
Intermittent thrice weekly	
HRZ: 2 months, then HR thrice weekly: 4 months	6 months
Alternative less potent daily	
HRZ: 2 months, then HE: 6 months	8 months
HRZ: 2 months, then HT: 6 months	8 months

H = isoniazid, R = rifampicin, Z = pyrazinamide, E = ethambutol, T = thiacetazone
† Add E if drug resistance suspected.
* For hilar lymphadenopathy alone.

meningitis when the dose should be 10 mg/kg. There are a large number of reported adverse reactions to tuberculosis chemotherapy (Reed & Blumer 1983). They occur in 1–2% of patients and some of the commoner ones are shown in Table 23.25. They are uncommon in children and are usually apparent within 6–8 weeks of starting treatment. Peripheral neuropathy as a complication of isoniazid is rare in children. Slow acetylators are at increased risk. Pyridoxine will prevent it, but is necessary only if high doses of isoniazid are given. Pyridoxine 10 mg is indicated for children on meat- or milk-deficient diets, breast-feeding infants, malnourished children, and during pregnancy. Higher doses may interfere with the activity of isoniazid.

The main complication is hepatic toxicity. Transient elevation of transaminases occurs in 7–17% of children taking isoniazid which is dose related and is increased if rifampicin is also given. There are case reports of hepatocellular toxicity and death from isoniazid therapy in children (Reed & Blumer 1983). Unless there is pre-existing liver disease or high doses of these drugs are administered, e.g. in meningitis, there is no need to monitor serum transaminases. Parents should be asked to report persistent nausea, vomiting, malaise and especially jaundice. Children who are rapid acetylators do not have an increased risk of hepatitis when exposed to isoniazid.

Cutaneous reactions if mild may not require cessation of treatment, but generalized hypersensitivity will. If toxicity occurs all drugs should be stopped and reintroduced sequentially in the order isoniazid, rifampicin and pyrazinamide in a small dose (approximately a quarter of the full dose) the first day increasing to full dose over the next 2–3 days (Ormerod et al 1996).

The value of corticosteroids is their ability to reduce the host's inflammatory response if it is contributing to tissue damage or impairing function. Their use is discussed in the respective sections, and may be indicated in the following conditions: meningitis, spinal block, obstruction of bronchi by lymph nodes, miliary disease with alveolar capillary block, pleural effusion and pericarditis (Alzeer & FitzGerald 1993). Prednisolone 1–2 mg/kg/day is given for 2 weeks and gradually tailed off over 2–3 months.

In children, knowledge of drug resistance is usually obtained from culture and sensitivity of the contact. If drug resistance is suspected, four bactericidal drugs, e.g. INH, RIF, PZA and ethambutol (EMB) or streptomycin, should be given. If possible streptomycin should be avoided because of the trauma of daily injections. For INH resistance RIF, PZA and EMB are given for a 6- to 9-month course. For multiple drug resistance, e.g. to INH,

Table 23.25   Recommended drugs

Drug	Daily dose			Thrice weekly dose			Side effects
	Children	Adolescents		Children	Adolescents		
		<50 kg	>50 kg		<50 kg	>50kg	
Isoniazid (INH)	6 mg/kg p.o., i.m. 10 mg/kg (meningitis)	300 mg	300 mg	10 mg/kg (max. 900 mg)	10 mg/kg	Max. 900 mg	Hepatic enzyme elevation, hepatitis, peripheral neuropathy, hypersensitivity
Rifampicin (RIF)	10 mg/kg p.o., i.v. 15–20 mg (meningitis)	450 mg	600 mg	15 mg/kg (max. 600 mg)	15 mg/kg	Max. 900 mg	Orange discoloration of secretions and urine (also contact lens), nausea, vomiting, hepatitis, febrile reactions, thrombocytopenia
Pyrazinamide (PZA)	30–35 mg/kg p.o.	1.5 g	2.0 g	50 mg/kg	2.0 g	2.5 g	Hepatotoxicity, Hyperuricemia, arthralgia, gastrointestinal upset, skin rash
Ethambutol (EMB)	15–20 mg/kg	15 mg/kg (max. 2.5 g)	15 mg/kg (max. 2.5 g)	30 mg/kg	30 mg/kg	Max. 2.5 g	Optic neuritis, skin rash
Streptomycin (SM)	15–20 mg/kg i.m.	750 mg	1.0 g	15–20 mg/kg	750 mg	1.0 g	Ototoxicity, nephrotoxicity
Thiacetazone	4 mg/kg p.o.	150 mg	150 mg	Not recommended	Not recommended	Not recommended	Gastrointestinal disturbance, vertigo, visual disturbance, hepatitis, agranulocytosis, exfoliative dermatitis in HIV infection
Ethionamide	15–20 mg/kg p.o. (divided doses)	750 mg	1.0 g	Not recommended	Not recommended	Not recommended	Gastrointestinal disturbance, hepatotoxicity, allergic reactions

* In young children give no more than 15 mg/kg throughout.

RIF and SM, four or more drugs should be given for 12–24 months (Swanson & Starke 1995). Depending on sensitivities, PZA and EMB are given with two or more second line drugs, e.g. ethionamide, ciprofloxacin, cycloserine or parenterally administered drugs, e.g. kanamycin, amikacin or capreomycin. DOT should be considered.

The patients should be seen monthly for the first 2–3 months to make sure of compliance and to monitor any problems with the drugs. Chest X-ray should be repeated at 1–2 months, at the end of therapy and 3 or more months thereafter. Resolution of pulmonary infiltrates may take over a year and lymphadenopathy (intra- or extrathoracic) 2–3 years. If adequate chemotherapy has been given, there is no need to prolong treatment; if relapse occurs or the patient stops treatment for a period, the same standard drug regimen should be given, preferably for 9 months' duration. If in doubt about activity of a pulmonary lesion, gastric aspirates may be obtained for microscopy and culture. Chest X-rays should be repeated every 6–12 months after cessation of therapy until stable.

Children with primary tuberculosis are rarely infectious and sputum is usually noninfectious after 2–3 weeks of chemotherapy and so they may return to school after this period.

DISEASES CAUSED BY ENVIRONMENTAL MYCOBACTERIA

Mycobacteria may be divided into those associated with tuberculosis and leprosy and those causing disease associated with the environment, referred to as nontuberculous, or atypical, mycobacteria (Table 23.26). The former (including M. leprae) are highly infectious and are passed from person to person.

Environmental mycobacteria of which there are over 50 species exist principally as harmless saprophytes in water, soil and vegetation, and also as pathogens in animals such as birds, reptiles

Table 23.26   Mycobacteria and disease in humans

Pathogen	Disease
M. tuberculosis	
M. bovis (including BCG)	Tuberculosis
M. africanum	
M. leprae	Leprosy
Slow-growing potential pathogens	
M. avium*	
M. intracellulare*	
M. scrofulaceum*	
M. kansasii*	
M. malmoense*	
M. marinum	Swimming pool granuloma
M. ulcerans	Buruli ulcer
M. xenopi	
M. szulgai	
M. semiae	
M. gordonae	
M. haemophilum	
Rapidly growing potential pathogens	
M. fortuitum*	Soft tissue abscess, wound infection
M. chelonei*	and otolaryngeal infection
M. abscessus	

* Associated with cervical adenitis in children.
M. avium, M. intracellulare and M. scrofulaceum are sometimes termed the MAIS complex; and M. avium and M. intracellulare as MAC.

and fish. Person-to-person transmission is extremely rare. Environmental mycobacteria generally prefer warm climates and the geographical distribution of the different species is quite variable. Water (fresh or salt) is probably a major vector, e.g. drinking, washing or aquatic sports, or by inhalation of aerosols (Grange 1988). The main portals of entry are probably through the skin or mucosa, and by inhalation or ingestion.

DIAGNOSIS

Environmental mycobacteria may be detected as commensals in sputum or gastric aspirates, swabs from wounds or abscesses, or in inadequately sterilized sputum pots. More definite proof of their pathogenicity is obtained when they are derived from a closed lesion, e.g. by aspiration or resection or the same strain of mycobacteria is repeatedly isolated. Differentiation between mycobacteria is by their cultural characteristics also by PCR. Histologically, it is usually not possible to clearly differentiate lesions from the granulomata of tuberculosis, although nontuberculous infection is more likely to show 'nonspecific' inflammation with less prominent caseation. Variable numbers of acid-fast bacilli may be seen.

There may be a moderate reaction to the Mantoux test (PPD-S): 5–15 mm, less or no reaction. Differential intradermal tests with antigens prepared from specific environmental mycobacteria, e.g. *M. avium*, *M. intracellulare*, *M. malmoense*, *M. scrofulaceum* or *M. kansasii* are more likely to produce a larger reaction than that with PPD-S. However, if the antigen is not specific for the infecting organism the reaction may be small or nil. Repeat differential testing some months later may be of value as the PPD-S reaction may be relatively smaller.

The commonest clinical problem due to infection by environmental mycobacteria in children is cervical adenitis. Other conditions include cutaneous infections, rarely pulmonary or otolaryngeal disease, osteitis, disseminated disease and meningitis (Lincoln & Gilbert 1972, Starke 1992, Wolinsky 1992). In adults infection of pre-existing pulmonary disease (including cystic fibrosis) is the commonest association.

LYMPHADENITIS

There appears to be a relative if not an absolute increase in incidence in areas of the world where tuberculosis is now uncommon which may be partly due to decline in neonatal BCG vaccination (Romanus et al 1995). It usually presents in children between 1 and 5 years. The submandibular group of nodes is most often infected; other nodes in the neck include the tonsillar, preauricular and anterior cervical groups. They are usually unilateral. Outside the neck, infection of axillary, inguinal and epitrochlear nodes has been described. The area of entry is rarely identified, although occasionally a lesion on the tonsil or buccal mucosa is seen. Enlargement of preauricular nodes suggests that the eye might be a portal of entry in some cases. Enlargement of nodes is fairly rapid over some months, the overlying skin becoming erythematous prior to discharge of the abscess but is not usually warm unless secondarily infected. It is commonly mistaken for a pyogenic cervical abscess. A sinus may develop and later calcification may occur. Some nodes probably settle spontaneously. Infection by environmental mycobacteria should be considered when a submandibular or preauricular node enlarges in a young child from a background of low tuberculous endemicity in the presence of a normal chest X-ray and a negative or low grade sensitivity to PPD.

The treatment of choice is excision biopsy of the primary group of involved nodes (Schaad et al 1979, Wolinsky 1995). A fluctuant abscess may be aspirated for diagnosis, but if possible aspiration should be avoided. Often the lesion is incised when mistaken for a cervical abscess, or it has discharged spontaneously. In these circumstances as much necrotic material as possible should be removed and later, if necessary, the primary node excised.

Chemotherapy is not usually indicated as the disease is local and the usual mycobacteria causing disease, e.g. MAC and *M. malmoense* are commonly resistant to standard chemotherapy. However, if surgery is difficult, e.g. involvement of the parotid gland or closeness of the lesion to the facial nerve, incision and drainage or needle aspiration together with antimycobacterial drug therapy should be considered. Suggested drugs are clarithromycin or azithromycin plus one of the following: ethambutol, rifabutin or ciprofloxacin for 6 months (Berger et al 1996). Recurrence or disease in another site sometimes occurs and should be treated as usual.

OTOLARYNGEAL DISEASE

Chronic infection of the middle ear associated with tympanotomy tubes (Franklin et al 1994) and chronic mastoiditis (Nylen et al 1994) due to colonization by, particularly, rapidly growing mycobacteria, e.g. *M. abscessus* and *M. chelonei*, has been described. Debridement with removal of all diseased tissue and in the case of chronic mastoiditis securing maximum ventilation of the cavity is essential. Chemotherapy with appropriate drugs is given for 6 months. Treatment for *M. abscessus* and *M. chelonei* includes parenteral therapy with amikacin and cefoxitin or imipenem for a few weeks followed by oral clarithromycin and or ciprofloxacin depending on sensitivities (Wolinsky 1992, Starke & Correa 1995).

SOFT TISSUE INFECTION

The most common soft tissue infections are 'swimming pool granuloma' and 'fish tank granuloma', both caused by *M. marinum*. Local abscesses may follow infection by *M. fortuitum* or *M. chelonei* at injection sites, trauma or surgery, and often present 3–4 weeks after infection although the incubation period may be much longer in deep infections. Buruli ulcer (*M. ulcerans*) occurs in tropical countries. Regional nodes are not usually enlarged. Mycobacteria can usually be detected in the lesions. Management comprises debridement of diseased tissue with chemotherapy reserved for extensive or deep-seated disease.

'Swimming pool granuloma' commonly affects children bathing in infected water on areas of abrasion such as the knees or elbows. Papules which may ulcerate appear on the affected areas; scab formation follows. Spontaneous healing occurs within a few months. If drug therapy is required a single agent such as co-trimoxazole, clarithromycin or ciprofloxacin, or for more severe infections, rifampicin plus ethambutol are given for 3–6 months.

Buruli ulcer derives its name from a district in northern Uganda and is known as Bairnsdale ulcer in Australia where the causative agent (*M. ulcerans*) was originally identified. It occurs in localized areas in a number of tropical rain forest areas around swamps and river banks. It starts as a subcutaneous nodule, often on a leg or arm, ulcerates and gradually progresses to a large ulcer with deep undermined edges. Satellite nodules or ulcers may be present. Treatment requires wide excision, cleansing with antiseptic such as 0.5% silver nitrate, and immediate skin grafting. Application of heat to maintain the temperature of the ulcer above 40°C which inhibits growth of *M. ulcerans* may be successful (Goutzamanis & Gilbert 1995). Chemotherapy is not generally rewarding, but may be tried along with surgery to assist healing. Suggested drugs are clofazimine or rifampicin. BCG may give some protection.

PULMONARY DISEASE

Pulmonary disease due to environmental mycobacteria is rare in immunocompetent children. It presents similarly to pulmonary tuberculosis: primary complex, bronchial obstruction, bronchopneumonia or primary progressive disease. The majority of cases are caused by MAC, less often by *M. kansasii* and, in some cases, by other mycobacteria such as *M. fortuitum*. Obstruction of a bronchus should be resected either at bronchoscopy or thoracotomy. Prolonged drug therapy is usually given as per disseminated disease.

DISSEMINATED AND EXTRAPULMONARY DISEASE

Disseminated disease is usually associated with severe immunological defects, especially AIDS. When bone disease occurs, it is usually disseminated osteomyelitis, but rarely, multifocal osteomyelitis without an apparent underlying immunodeficiency is seen. Infection of the meninges may also occur. A familial disease has been described associated with disseminated environmental mycobacterial or salmonella infections probably due to macrophage dysfunction and responding to gamma interferon (Levin et al 1995).

In HIV infection, disseminated infection is usually seen in older children with a low CD4 count and advanced disease. MAC are the commonest mycobacteria. Trials are in progress regarding optimal chemotherapy. A suggested regimen is clarithromycin or azithromycin and ethambutol plus one or more of the following clofazimine, rifabutin, rifampicin, ciprofloxacin or amikacin (Starke & Correa 1995).

Rifabutin has been suggested for prophylaxis for MAC in children with low CD4 counts. The benefit has to be considered against cost, side effects and development of rifampicin-resistant strains of mycobacteria including *M. tuberculosis* (Starke & Correa 1995).

DRUG THERAPY

Drugs appropriate for environmental mycobacteria are outlined in Table 23.27. In vitro drug sensitivities may not predict clinical response as minimal inhibitory concentrations are not known for many environmental mycobacteria. Duration of treatment and synergy between drug combination are important factors. In general neither isoniazid or pyrazinamide are useful for environmental mycobacteria. Experience with many of the newer drugs is limited in children and it is important to be aware of side effects particularly when used in combination, e.g. plasma levels of rifabutin may be increased by clarithromycin and fluconazole with a risk of uveitis.

Table 23.27 Suggested drugs for environmental mycobacteria

Organism	Drugs
M. avium-intracellulare *M. scrofulaceum* *M. malmoense*	Clar (or Azith), Emb, Cpfx, Clof, Rif/Rifb, Amik
M. kansasii	Rif, Emb, Cpfx, Clar
M. marinum	Rif, Emb, Clar, TMP-SMZ, Cpfx
M. fortuitum *M. chelonei* *M. abscessus*	Amik, Cef, Clof, Clar, Cpfx Ipm

Amik = amikacin, Azith = azithromycin, Clar = clarithromycin, Cef = cefoxitin, Clof = clofazimine, Cpfx = ciprofloxacin, Emb = ethambutol, Ipm = imipenem, Rif = rifampicin, Rifb = rifabutin, TMP-SMZ = trimethoprim-sulfamethoxazole

TULAREMIA

ETIOLOGY

This disease derives its name from Tulare, a county in California, where it was first discovered amongst ground squirrels by McCoy in 1911. It is caused by a small Gram-negative coccobacillus *Francisella tularensis* which commonly causes disease in wild animals such as rabbits, hares, squirrels, foxes, rats and deer. Domestic animals like sheep, cattle and cats, blood-sucking arthropods (e.g. ticks, mosquitoes) that bite these animals and water contaminated by infected animals also act as sources of human disease.

EPIDEMIOLOGY

Human infection occurs as a result of a bite or scratch by an infected animal, or by infected arthropod vectors, like fleas, ticks, lice or bedbugs. Human case-to-case contact has not been documented, though care must be taken in dressing discharging wounds. Tularemia is extremely infectious for laboratory workers, who must take exceptional care in the handling of infected material or cultures. The disease is common in North America where in some areas the incidence is 30–40 times that of Lyme disease (CDC 1993b). It is also relatively common in parts of northern Europe, Russia and in Japan, but rare in the rest of Europe.

PATHOLOGY

There is a local lesion at the site of inoculation and disseminated lesions in many parts of the body. The local lesion may be a papule or abscess with regional lymph node enlargement. The disseminated lesions occur in the lungs, the liver and spleen, in the bone marrow and many other sites. They resemble the lesions of miliary tuberculosis, but the center of the lesions consists of polymorph leukocytes and hence may be purulent.

CLINICAL FEATURES

The incubation period ranges from 1 to 21 days but most cases occur 3–5 days after exposure. The severity of the disease is variable with children usually showing more constitutional upset than adults. The onset may be abrupt with high fever, headache, vomiting and rigors. A number of tularemic syndromes have been described of which the commonest is the *ulceroglandular syndrome* characterized by a primary painful maculopapular lesion at the point of skin entry with subsequent ulceration and slow healing. This is associated with painful, acutely inflamed regional lymph nodes which may ulcerate and proceed to abscess formation. Other forms of the disease include *glandular* tularemia, *pneumonic* tularemia which seems to be increasing in incidence and a *typhoidal* form with high fever and hepatosplenomegaly (Jacobs et al 1985).

DIAGNOSIS

The circumstances of the disease onset, especially a history of bite or scratch, should readily suggest the diagnosis in endemic areas. Confirmation is obtained by culturing the organism from infected sites on special media or guinea pig inoculation. A fourfold or greater rise in serum agglutination titer to *F. tularensis* is evident after the second week of illness.

There is a significant risk to laboratory personnel when performing cultures so the laboratory should be informed if tularemia is suspected. The differential diagnosis includes a number of causes of prolonged fever including brucellosis, disseminated tuberculosis, salmonellosis (especially typhoid) and septicemias of all kinds.

TREATMENT

Gentamicin administered two to three times daily is the antibiotic of choice. There seems to be no advantage in giving more than a 7-day course (Cross et al 1995).

PREVENTION

In endemic areas, opportunities for arthropod bites should be minimized by the wearing of protective clothing and regular tick inspections. Prevention also involves avoidance of contact with infected or potentially infected animals and insect vectors and the boiling of water from springs and streams.

In the US, a live attenuated vaccine is available for those repeatedly exposed to the organism such as laboratory technicians (American Academy of Pediatrics 1994).

INFECTIONS DUE TO VIRUSES AND ALLIED ORGANISMS

THE USE OF THE VIROLOGICAL LABORATORY BY THE CLINICIAN

Over the last few decades a widespread and rapid advance in our knowledge of viruses has taken place. Rapid diagnosis of many viral infections is now the rule rather than the exception (Burgner et al 1996).

The usefulness of the virologist to the clinician is often limited by lack of knowledge of the most appropriate specimens to submit to the laboratory. All too often the wrong specimens are sent, they are sent in bacteriology transport media or virological studies are only considered at a late stage in a difficult case, by which time virus isolation may be impossible and the opportunity to perform serological tests, designed to demonstrate a rising antibody titer,

irretrievably lost. It is essential that the virologist is given a full clinical account of difficult cases, which are best discussed in person or by phone. Determined efforts are also needed to ensure that convalescent samples of serum are sent at the appropriate time.

A significant clinical example of the above can be found in the case of presumed paralytic poliomyelitis occurring in a fully immunized child. In general, poliomyelitis immunization is highly successful and, if full clinical details and the immunization history are given to the virologist, he will at once suspect that the 'poliomyelitis-like' illness in question could have resulted from infection by an ECHO virus or Coxsackie virus. Armed with this information he will then suggest sending stool samples as well as CSF and will know the appropriate tissue cultures to use for isolation of the virus and will appreciate that suckling mice should be inoculated to exclude Coxsackie infection. In several instances, where poliomyelitis immunization might have appeared to have failed, the virologist has been able to exonerate the immunization program.

THE NATURE, COLLECTION AND TRANSPORTATION OF SPECIMENS FOR VIROLOGICAL EXAMINATION

Blood specimens

A high proportion of virus diagnoses are made by serology. Even in those cases where a virus is isolated, the significance of the isolation is greatly enhanced where serological tests demonstrate a rising antibody titer to the agent in question. An acute sample of clotted blood should be removed *as early as possible* in the illness and a convalescent sample sent 2–3 weeks later. Ideally at least 2 ml should be obtained though lesser quantities have often to suffice in the case of infants. Provided the blood samples arrive in the laboratory within a day they will withstand cool atmospheric conditions; on no account should such specimens undergo freezing as this will provoke lysis of the erythrocytes. In the laboratory serum will be separated from the clot and stored at −20°C pending examination. IgM assays are available to diagnose some virus infections on a single sample. In most cases, however, acute and convalescent sera are necessary to look for a rise in IgG antibodies. Infants under 6 months mount a relatively poor IgG response, and viral detection isolation or an IgM response (if the assay is available) are the best ways to make a viral diagnosis.

As a general rule blood is not a suitable medium from which to isolate viruses and blood viral culture is not a procedure that is routinely used.

Specimens from the upper respiratory tract

Nasal swabs may be taken for isolation of respiratory viruses but throat swabs have a more universal application. The latter should be taken in a vigorous manner in order to ensure that mucus and cellular material is wiped from the pharynx. In older children throat garglings can be obtained. Nasopharyngeal aspirates are particularly useful in the isolation of respiratory syncytial virus and other respiratory viruses. Viruses which can be isolated from saliva include mumps, herpes simplex and cytomegalovirus.

After the collection of any specimen by swabbing, the swab should be immersed in the virus transport medium (VTM) supplied. Normally this will be contained in a small sterile bottle and after immersion the wooden shaft of the swab should be broken level with the neck of the container. The bottle cap should then be firmly replaced and the fluid gently agitated. Nasopharyngeal aspirates need not have VTM added unless there is a long transit time.

If the time interval between the collection of the specimen and delivery to the laboratory is under 2 h ordinary room temperature is unlikely to produce significant loss in viability of the virus. For periods exceeding 2 h but less than 24 h specimens should be retained at + 4°C and transported in water-ice in a vacuum flask. Where greater delay is involved the specimen should be surrounded by solid CO_2 and packed in an insulated container. A notable exception to the above recommendations is any specimen suspected of containing respiratory syncytial virus; such specimens should not be frozen, but transported to the laboratory as soon as possible.

Specimens from the lower respiratory tract

As a general rule viral specimens are not taken from the lower respiratory tract. However, the agents of psittacosis, Q fever and *Mycoplasma pneumoniae* may be recovered from specimens of sputum, and rhinoviruses have been grown from sputum.

Specimens from the intestinal tract

Examination of feces by electron microscopy and culture can produce a rich harvest of viruses. It is particularly important to culture stools in the cases of suspected viral meningitis or encephalitis. Often the infectivity is high and virus may persist within the specimen for over 24 h. As a result fecal samples often withstand transport by mail. Rectal swabs are less suitable but may be employed where feces are not immediately available and urgent study of the case is desirable.

Storage and transportation at room temperature is satisfactory providing the time interval does not exceed 24 h.

Specimens from the central nervous system

A sample of CSF, approximately 1 ml in volume, should be submitted from cases of suspected viral infection of the CNS. It should be aseptically collected and placed in a sterile container without the addition of transport medium. Rapid transportation to the laboratory is desirable but where the delay exceeds a few hours the specimen should be placed in a thermos flask surrounded by water-ice. Further delay will necessitate the employment of solid CO_2 during transit (see above: respiratory specimens).

In certain forms of encephalitis a brain biopsy may be taken for detailed virological study. It is essential that such specimens reach the laboratory as soon as possible but, in view of the fact that the method of transportation may vary depending on the nature of the studies to be made, the virologist should be consulted in each individual case.

Specimens from the skin

Successful virus isolation is most likely to arise from samples of vesicle fluid but viruses may also be grown from, or seen in, pustular fluid, scabs and carefully taken scrapings from macules or papules. Fluid material should be collected from vesicles and pustules by puncturing their surface with a fine, sterile capillary

tube. Scabs or crusts are removed by fine forceps and placed in a small sterile bottle. Scrapings from any lesion are carefully smeared on to scrupulously clean microscope slides.

Skin specimens will usually be examined for poxviruses and in this case transportation can be made under normal atmospheric conditions. The material should be packed with care to prevent breakage, and contamination of the outside of the package avoided.

Urine specimens

Specimens of urine, preferably midstream, must be fresh and sent to the laboratory without delay. The specimen (approximately 10 ml in volume) should be collected in a screw-capped glass container and if delay in transportation exceeds a few hours, the container should be kept in contact with water-ice during transit.

Other specimens

On occasion it may be desirable to submit specimens for examination from suspected viral lesions of the eye and genital tract. Virus isolation has also proved possible from mesenteric and other lymph glands as well as from serous exudates, such as ascites or pericardial fluid. The methods of collection and transportation are broadly as outlined above but a more detailed account is given in the appropriate section of the text.

Finally reference should be made to the obtaining of specimens at autopsy for virological examination. These require to be collected with scrupulous care so that contamination of the organs does not arise from instruments and other contacts. Each specimen should be collected with separate sterile instruments and careful labeling is essential. Contamination by fixatives such as formalin must be avoided.

THE PRACTICAL APPLICATION OF THE LABORATORY DIAGNOSIS OF VIRAL INFECTIONS

At the present time, when specific chemotherapy and specific preventive measures are not available for many viral infections, detailed laboratory investigation may provide no immediate benefit to the affected patient. However, the widespread use of such investigations (Table 23.28) has immeasurably increased our knowledge of the role of viruses in producing disease; this is particularly seen in the studies of various disease syndromes involving the respiratory tract and the central nervous system.

There are various situations in which laboratory diagnosis of viral infections is particularly valuable:

1. Rapid diagnosis of respiratory syncytial virus (RSV) infection is not only useful for clinical management, e.g. decisions on antibiotic use, but also for decisions about isolation of infected babies to prevent hospital-acquired infections.
2. Rapid diagnosis of HSV encephalitis can help rationalize the use of antivirals, e.g. acyclovir.
3. Rapid diagnosis of measles and VZV can help make decisions about the use of passive or active immunization to protect high-risk immunocompromised children who have been exposed.
4. Viral diagnosis can be important for epidemiological reasons, e.g. the example used previously of paralytic illness due to poliomyelitis or other enteroviruses.

Table 23.28 Some laboratory techniques used in viral diagnosis

Direct microscopy	Electron microscopy
	Fluorescent antibody methods
	Presence of inclusion bodies
Virus isolation	Tissue culture
	Fertile hen's eggs
	Laboratory animals
Serological	Complement fixation
	Hemagglutination inhibition
	Neutralization
	Enzyme-linked immunosorbent assay
	Radioimmunoassay
Antigen detection	Immunfluorescence
	Enzyme-linked immunosorbent assay
Genome detection	Polymerase chain reaction

THE EXANTHEMATA

MEASLES (MORBILLI AND RUBEOLA)

Measles is a viral disease of high infectivity which presents with an acute catarrhal illness, fever, characteristic Koplik's spots on the buccal mucous membranes followed by a distinctive maculopapular rash. There is a high incidence of serious complications of the respiratory and nervous systems. In large cities and towns, measles is most likely to occur in infants and preschool children, but in rural and less crowded urban areas the principal incidence is between the ages of 5 and 10 years. Measles is extremely rare under 3–4 months of age, because of protective maternal antibody, but authenticated cases have occurred.

In some countries measles outbreaks have shown a characteristic biennial periodicity but such a pattern is by no means universal and the introduction of active immunization has altered the natural epidemiology of the disease.

Mortality

In developing countries, where malnutrition is common, measles may have a mortality as high as 25% and produce serious complications (Aaby et al 1986). Children are at increased risk of dying for a year after their measles due to impaired cellular immunity. Measles can cause devastating outbreaks when the virus is introduced into the relatively virgin soil of remote islands. Although the morbidity and mortality are lower in highly immunized industrialized countries, outbreaks can still occur if a population of unimmunized children, usually preschool, is allowed to develop (National Vaccine Advisory Committee 1991). In more exposed communities, measles is now comparatively mild and its morbidity and mortality lower, although several deaths still occur each year in the UK. Unimmunized children who contract measles are at particular risk when in remission from acute leukemia or other conditions in which immunity is compromised.

Etiology

Measles virus is usually transmitted by droplet infection from the respiratory tract of a case before, or close to, the onset of the rash. Entry probably occurs through the respiratory tract but infection through the intact conjunctiva has been postulated. The measles virus is approximately 140 nm in diameter and morphologically

resembles the parainfluenza viruses. It is an RNA virus. No antigenic variation has been described. An attack is usually followed by lifelong immunity and there is little or no authenticated evidence of second attacks of measles except in individuals with severe immunological defects. Subclinical infection can probably occur but is rare.

Clinical features

Measles has an incubation period of 8–14 days. A mild illness may occur at the time of infection but most cases develop a prodromal illness some 3–5 days before the eruptive stage. The main features of this illness are pronounced catarrh, characterized by a constantly running nose, conjunctivitis and a harsh dry cough. Fever and irritability are usually present and there may be a fleeting scarlatiniform or morbilliform rash. Koplik's spots, the most pathognomonic sign of measles, appear during this stage and are seen as small, grayish white lesions on the buccal mucosa close to the posterior molar teeth; they are usually quite numerous but may be scanty or occasionally cover the entire lining of the cheek. They can be difficult to demonstrate and the angle of the inspecting light is critical; having faded, they are replaced by a dry, matte appearance on the mucosa which has a ground-glass-like surface.

The true rash of measles (Fig. 23.14) starts behind the ears and along the hair line. Fever, which will have lessened at the end of

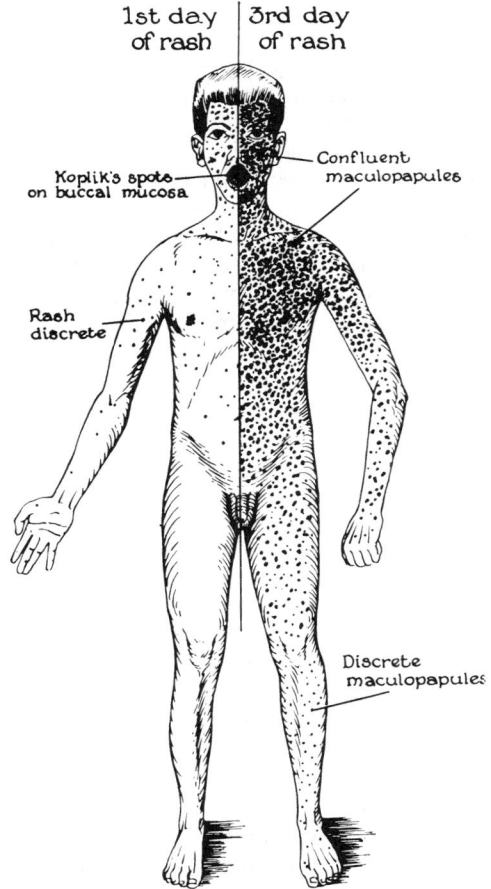

Fig. 23.14 The distribution and development of rash in measles. (From Krugman & Ward 1968.)

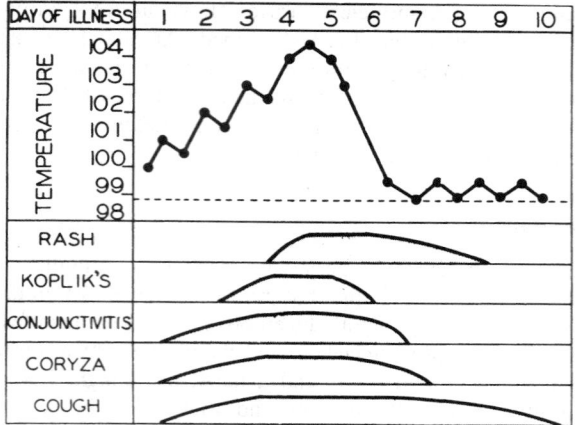

Fig. 23.15 The development of measles. (From Krugman & Ward 1968.)

the prodromal period, may now rise again to 39–40°C (Fig. 23.15), and the eruption spreads rapidly to involve the face. The lesions are maculopapular in character and of a dusky hue. Over the next 2 days the eruption spreads downwards and becomes generalized; marked confluence of the spots develops and this gives a blotchy appearance.

The extent and severity of the rash show wide variation. In some, especially the younger cases, the eruption may be unusually sparse and modification by maternal antibody has been suggested. There is frequently some degree of hemorrhage or diapedesis into the rash giving it a purpuric quality and subsequent skin staining. This should not be confused with the rare and usually fatal hemorrhagic measles in which extensive bleeding occurs into the skin and from the mucous membranes.

Fading of the rash can be surprisingly rapid but it usually disappears quite slowly beginning to fade on the third day in the order of appearance; the rash may be largely gone from the face and upper trunk by the fourth day though persisting on the lower extremities. After a further 3–4 days a brownish staining appears, probably due to capillary hemorrhage and on occasions this staining can be very intense. In severe cases a fine desquamation may occur at the site of the rash but this does not usually involve the hands and feet like scarlet fever.

Complications

Respiratory

Measles virus always attacks the respiratory tract causing some degree of laryngotracheobronchitis. An element of bronchitis is universal and can be severe extending even to bronchiolitis; the latter can be complicated by acute mediastinal emphysema. Croup may be prominent. Viral damage may denude the respiratory tract of its protective lining and allow the aspiration of bacteria. Bronchopneumonia may result and the severity will depend on the nature of the aspirated material. Staphylococcal pneumonia can be life threatening.

In a few instances measles virus involvement of the respiratory tract may spread to the lung parenchyma giving rise to the condition known as giant cell pneumonia. This complication may be prolonged, is often fatal and the illness may be accompanied by little or no rash. It is usually found in association with underlying disease such as immune deficiency, leukemia, cystic fibrosis or Letterer–Siwe disease, particularly when there is impaired T cell function. In view of its atypical nature, this illness is often undiagnosed during life and the true diagnosis is made as a result of the autopsy findings.

Ophthalmic

Some degree of conjunctivitis and keratitis occurs in every case of measles. It is typically nonpurulent and nonfollicular and can be characterized by Koplik's spots. When pseudomembranes or corneal ulcers occur they are the result of secondary bacterial infection. Optic neuritis and retinitis are associated with measles encephalitis.

Ear

Involvement of the middle ear used to be commonplace and could result in suppurative otitis media, chronic perforation or mastoiditis. The lessening severity of measles and prompt antibiotic treatment has reduced the incidence of these complications to a low level.

Gastrointestinal tract

Severe oral inflammation due to secondary infection by bacteria, *Treponema vincenti*, or thrush can occur but cancrum oris is only likely to be seen where malnutrition is rife. Cancrum oris is a gangrenous form of stomatitis which commences with a dusky red spot on the inside and outside of the cheek. This rapidly spreads to form a sloughing gangrene of the gums and jaws and in extreme cases teeth may be shed. The breath develops a peculiarly foul odor and death can supervene.

Gastroenteritis is common in measles in nonindustrialized countries and can be prolonged; it probably results from direct viral involvement of the gut with or without superinfection with organisms such as *Cryptosporidium*. Appendicitis can occur in measles though abdominal pain is more commonly due to associated mesenteric adenitis.

Enlargement of the spleen is more frequently encountered in measles than is generally realized.

Central nervous system

Measles, with its pronounced constitutional upset and high fever, is often complicated by febrile convulsions (1 in 10 000). These are most commonly encountered at the start of the eruptive stage and either settle spontaneously or in response to simple sedation; they should not be assumed to be indicative of encephalitis.

True postinfectious encephalomyelitis occurs in from 1 in 1000 to 1 in 5000 cases of measles and has a mortality of about 10% and leaves about 15% with neurological residua. It normally presents after 7–14 days, when the rash is subsiding, but can commence earlier in the disease and rarely even before the rash. Drowsiness, fits, a recrudescence of fever, focal neurological signs and progressive coma suggest that severe cerebral involvement is occurring. In some cases the process may arrest at this juncture and be followed by rapid improvement; in others there is a steady deterioration and death. Between these extremes there are patients in whom recovery is slow and permanent cerebral damage likely.

Rarely *subacute sclerosing panencephalitis* (see p. 794) may complicate measles infection, though not apparently measles immunization. In SSPE, measles virus becomes latent in the cerebrum following primary infection and is then reactivated, usually 5–10 years later, by some unknown stimulus. An alternative hypothesis suggests that a partially immune individual, is reinfected by measles which then provokes this unique form of encephalitis. It is commoner in children whose primary measles occurs before 1 year of age.

Others

Uncomplicated measles tends to produce a leukopenia and significant thrombocytopenia is occasionally encountered. Epistaxis is a common and occasionally troublesome feature.

Lastly, there is a traditional belief that measles may activate, or predispose to, tuberculosis. This association now seems less common but authenticated examples still occur. Diagnostic difficulty is provided by the fact that measles may suppress the Mantoux reaction for several weeks.

Diagnosis

Provided the medical attendant is consulted at its inception, measles can be diagnosed on clinical grounds with a fair degree of accuracy. Difficulties can arise when an opinion is required later in the disease.

Measles virus can be isolated in primary tissue cultures of human kidney, human amnion or monkey kidney and several other tissue culture systems have been used. The growth rate of measles virus in tissue culture is relatively slow and serological tests will often yield a positive result before the virus has been isolated and identified. Immunofluorescence can be used to detect measles virus antigen in respiratory secretions if rapid diagnosis is needed.

During the late prodromal stage of the illness virus can be recovered from the nasopharynx, urine, conjunctival secretions and blood. By the second day of the rash, virus isolation becomes more difficult, though the urine may continue to contain virus for a further 2 days.

Neutralizing, complement-fixing and hemagglutination-inhibiting antibodies to measles develop during the illness and appropriate serological tests can confirm their presence. The demonstration of a significant rise (fourfold or greater) in antibody titer to measles virus confirms the clinical diagnosis. The hemagglutination-inhibition and complement-fixation tests are usually employed on account of the ease and rapidity with which they can be performed.

In subacute sclerosing panencephalitis (SSPE) measles antibody in high titer is demonstrable in the serum many years after a typical attack of measles. Antibody may also be detected in the cerebrospinal fluid and the ratio of this antibody to that in the serum may be of diagnostic significance. In SSPE the ratio of antibody in the serum to antibody in the CSF may be of the order of 50 : 1 and even lower ratios have been described. Brain biopsy can confirm the diagnosis of SSPE where facilities for electron microscopy and immunofluorescence are available.

Differential diagnosis

Kawasaki disease (p. 1478) can cause a morbilliform rash with fever, conjunctivitis and lymphadenopathy and can be quite difficult to distinguish clinically from measles. The milder illness of rubella with its pinker rash and selective involvement of the suboccipital glands is usually distinguishable. The rash of infectious mononucleosis can cause confusion but its other clinical and laboratory features usually lead to the correct interpretation. Enteroviral infections associated with a rash are usually more transient and lack the catarrhal involvement. Influenza virus infections, both A and B, can occasionally cause a morbilliform rash with respiratory symptoms and fever. In roseola infantum, the rash is just like measles, but as it appears the fever falls and the child is well, in contrast to measles. Scarlet fever and drug eruptions have readily distinguishing features.

Treatment

Amongst the earliest complications that may require treatment are croup and febrile convulsions. These are managed symptomatically (see Chs 12 and 14).

Secondary bacterial infection, superimposed on viral damage to the respiratory tract, will require treatment. Staphylococcal pneumonia is the most feared complication, and if bacterial pneumonia is suspected antistaphylococcal antibiotics should be used. Prophylactic antibiotics are unnecessary.

Mastoiditis should not occur if adequate treatment of otitis media is given early, but if it does occur surgical drainage is required. Any sign of secondary infection of the conjunctivae should be treated with appropriate antibiotics and chloramphenicol eye ointment smeared on to the lids often proves efficacious.

It is rare for gastroenteritis to be so severe as to cause fluid and electrolyte depletion but where this occurs appropriate measures require to be taken (see p. 1295). True appendicitis can present in the course of measles.

Postinfectious encephalitis (see p. 695) requires intensive supportive treatment. Convulsions, which may be a particularly troublesome feature, should be treated with anticonvulsants. The use of corticosteroids remains controversial, but many clinicians feel such therapy warrants trial in severe cases whose progress is unsatisfactory.

Preventive measures

Quarantine

In view of the high infectivity of this disease and since the maximum infectivity is before the rash appears, quarantine measures are frequently ineffective. However, any child who is suffering from a severe debilitating disease should be protected from exposure wherever possible.

Passive immunization

Passive immunization against measles has been an established procedure for many years and has proved highly effective. Normal human immunoglobulin (gamma globulin) is used (0–2 ml/kg i.m. for normal children, 0.5 ml/kg for immunocompromised children, maximum dose 15 ml). The use of passive immunization is particularly important when immunocompromised children, in whom active immunization is contraindicated, become exposed to measles.

Active immunization

In the early years of measles vaccines, an inactivated measles vaccine was used which not only failed to protect against infection but resulted in the children developing severe, atypical illness with giant cell pneumonitis when exposed to wild-type virus.

Live, attenuated measles vaccines are highly protective and have very few side effects. Where they have been used to immunize whole populations acute measles, encephalitis and subacute sclerosing panencephalitis have virtually disappeared. In countries where immunization rates are relatively low, there are many cases of acute encephalitis with several children each year dying or handicapped as a result (Noah 1984). Measles vaccine is readily inhibited by maternal antibody and may be ineffective if given before 1 year of age. If it is wished to protect a child exposed to measles who has no contraindications to immunization and is over 1 year old, then measles vaccine is preferable to passive immunization. Many countries now give measles vaccine in conjunction with mumps and rubella vaccines (MMR) in the second year of life (Peltola et al 1986), and a second dose may be given at school entry or at 12–14 years old. The only contraindication to measles vaccine is immune deficiency (including high dose but not low dose steroids). Anaphylactic egg allergy is no longer considered to be a contraindication (Aickin et al 1994). HIV infection is not a contraindication and on the contrary, as they are at high risk from wild-type measles virus, every attempt should be made to immunize HIV positive children against measles, whether or not they have symptomatic HIV infection.

RUBELLA (GERMAN MEASLES)

Rubella has been recognized as a distinct clinical entity for some time. Some of the original accounts of the disease emanated from Germany and because of this and a certain similarity to measles, the name of German measles became a popular, if ill-conceived, descriptive title. The disease has no relationship to measles. In its postnatally acquired form rubella is characterized by its mild nature and relative freedom from complications.

Etiology

Rubella virus was first cultured and identified as recently as 1962. Since then it has proved possible to grow it quite readily on suitable tissue cultures, a factor that has considerably enhanced our knowledge of the disease.

Incidence

The true incidence of rubella is difficult to assess as infection is subclinical in a sizable proportion of cases; even the clinical illness itself has no pathognomonic features and this point is well substantiated in surveys of rubella antibody levels where the results show a poor correlation with the history of previously suspected infection. By early adult life as many as 90% of city dwellers may show serological evidence of previous rubella but the figure can be much lower in rural communities. Rubella is less common in preschool children than, for example, measles and in one survey less than 10% of children under 2 years showed evidence of previous infection, though this figure had risen to 25% between the ages of 2 and 5 years. By 12 years of age 80% showed evidence of antibody suggesting that the bulk of infection occurs between 6 and 12 years of age.

Clinical features

Rubella has an incubation period of 14–21 days with an average of 17 days. In children it is rare to have a significant prodromal illness and the first indication of rubella infection is the appearance of a rash over the face (Fig. 23.16). This soon spreads to cover the trunk and later the limbs. The basic lesions are fine, pink macules which, originally discrete, can soon coalesce over the face and trunk. The rash usually disappears within 2–3 days but may persist for as long as 5 days. Occasionally it has a duration measured in hours and in this instance can be readily missed. A biphasic type of rash, with complete regression in between, has been described and a small area of the eruption may persist on the medial aspect of the thighs after the main rash has subsided. Small purpuric spots sometimes appear on the soft palate but have no diagnostic significance as other infections are associated with a similar enanthem.

Lymph node enlargement is an important feature of the disease. It may appear as much as a week before the rash, though usually just before, and may persist for some time after the eruption has faded. The cervical, postauricular and suboccipital glands are most commonly involved, can be tender and are sometimes unassociated with any rash.

In adolescents and adults, especially female, prodromal symptoms are more likely and include malaise, headache, stickiness of the eyes, conjunctivitis and fever. In children the

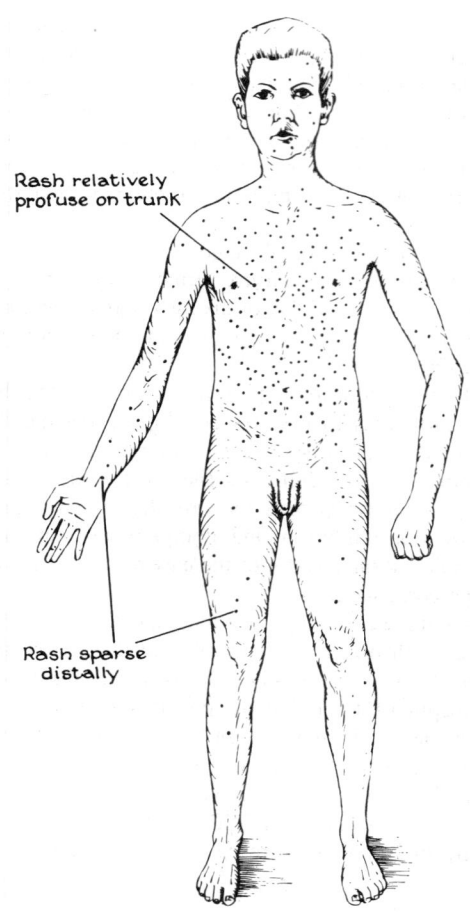

Rash relatively profuse on trunk

Rash sparse distally

Fig. 23.16   The distribution and development of rash in rubella. (From Krugman & Ward 1968.)

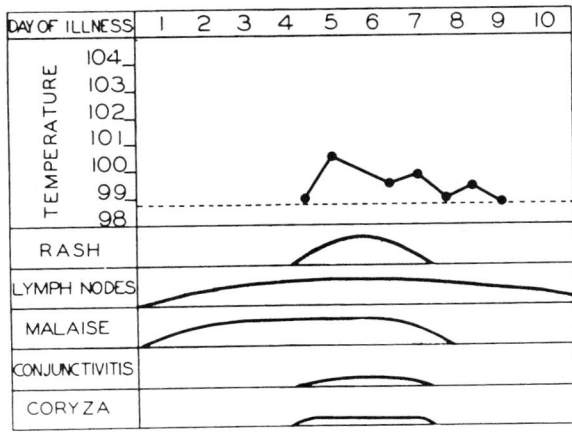

Fig. 23.17 The development of rubella. (From Krugman & Ward 1968.)

temperature rarely rises above 37.1–37.4°C but can attain 39.5–40.0°C in adults (Fig. 23.17).

Complications

In general complications are unusual though a higher incidence is encountered in certain epidemics and some seem age dependent.

Polyarthritis may be a sequel of rubella. It usually commences when the rash has subsided, is more common after florid eruptions and occurs in adults, especially women, rather than in children. The small joints of the hands and the wrist joints are most often involved but the large joints can also be attacked. The condition usually resolves within 2 weeks.

Postinfectious encephalitis, myelitis and polyradiculitis may follow an attack of rubella and have a similar pathology to these syndromes when they occur after other infections. However, in rubella they appear to have a better prognosis.

Thrombocytopenia is quite common in the course of the illness and may become clinically manifest as purpura. Epistaxis, hematuria and melena can also develop. Some cases of so-called idiopathic thrombocytopenic purpura can be shown by laboratory tests to have resulted from subclinical rubella infection. Leukopenia is frequently found at the height of the illness and there may be an increase in plasma or Turk cells.

Diagnosis

Owing to the lack of pathognomonic features, one cannot rely on a clinical diagnosis of rubella and, whenever confirmation is important, laboratory tests (in the form of appropriate serological studies) should be used.

A serological diagnosis depends on the demonstration of a significant rise in antibody titer (fourfold or greater) when a sample of serum collected at the onset of the illness, and a further sample taken 2–3 weeks later, are compared.

Antibodies to rubella virus may be detected by hemagglutination-inhibition (HI), neutralization, complement-fixation or radial hemolysis test. Nowadays, the HI test is generally preferred, owing to its reliability and the ease with which it can be performed.

Following infection both neutralizing and HI antibodies persist, at a variable titer, for a long time whereas complement-fixing antibodies disappear more rapidly.

Virus may be recovered with relative ease from the nasopharynx during the last week of the incubation period and for up to 2 weeks thereafter. It is less readily isolated from the urine and blood. However, many laboratories do not offer viral culture for rubella.

Differential diagnosis

Rubella may be confused with many common exanthemata and other skin eruptions. Differentiation from measles, glandular fever and drug eruptions does not present great difficulty but scarlet fever can cause confusion. Enteroviral infections accompanied by a rash, especially those associated with ECHO virus infection, provide the greatest diagnostic challenge. The presence of the herald patch, the distribution over the trunk and the complete well-being of the patient help to distinguish pityriasis rosea.

Resort to laboratory tests is always desirable when doubt exists in regard to a suspicious rash in a pregnant woman or her contacts.

Treatment

There is no specific treatment for rubella. A rapid recovery is to be expected. Prodromal symptoms rarely cause trouble but analgesics may be needed when polyarthritis occurs. Neurological complications are managed along the usual lines for such conditions.

Prevention

As a general rule preventive measures are unnecessary in view of the mild nature of the disease. However, the situation is quite different in the case of women in early pregnancy and attempts to prevent rubella have traditionally been made by the intramuscular injection of normal human immunoglobulin. Evaluation of this procedure has proved difficult but cases of rubella, confirmed by laboratory tests, have occurred despite this use of immuno-globulin. Attenuated live rubella vaccines are now widely used and in general stimulate reasonable antibody levels. Opinions differ as to how they are best employed. Some recommend they are given to girls around puberty and nonimmune pregnant women postpartum (selective immunization) while others believe children of both sexes should be given the vaccine in early childhood, usually in conjunction with measles and mumps vaccine as MMR, in an attempt to reduce the pool of infection in the community (universal immunization). Although terminations of pregnancy are frequently performed on pregnant women who have been inadvertently immunized there have been no cases of congenital rubella syndrome caused by the vaccine.

Congenital rubella (p. 286)

Congenital rubella may occur when a nonimmune mother acquires rubella in early pregnancy. The possibility of fetal involvement seems to persist up to the 16th week and possibly longer, though during this period the overall risk steadily diminishes. In the very early weeks of the pregnancy spontaneous abortion may occur but thereafter survival of the fetus is probable.

In general the earlier the mother contracts rubella the greater the risk of fetal involvement and the greater the risk that such involvement will be severe. Proven rubella infection before 13 weeks' gestation is an indication for termination of the pregnancy. Between 13 and 16 weeks deafness may result from congenital infection but not usually the full congenital rubella syndrome. After 16 weeks the risk is very low.

Congenital rubella syndrome can very rarely occur following reinfection with rubella virus in a woman previously shown to be immune (Best et al 1989).

Diagnosis by laboratory tests

It is desirable to confirm a clinical diagnosis of congenital rubella and attempts should be made to isolate the virus; this may be recovered from the nasopharynx, urine, CSF and many other tissues of the body. An infant with this condition will continue to shed virus for weeks or even months though this usually shows a quantitative reduction with increasing age.

The serum of an infant with congenital rubella contains both IgM and IgG antibodies against rubella. Serological testing of healthy infants may also demonstrate the presence of antibody, but in them this is entirely of the IgG variety having been transplacentally acquired from the mother. After some months maternal IgG antibody disappears from the serum of healthy infants but quite high levels of IgM antibody may persist in those with congenital rubella.

ERYTHEMA INFECTIOSUM (FIFTH DISEASE, SLAPPED CHEEK DISEASE)

This disease may occur at any time of year, but outbreaks in primary school children are classically in the winter and spring. Joint involvement may occur. Children with shortened red cell survival can develop profound anemia (aplastic crises). Infection during pregnancy can lead to hydrops fetalis.

Etiology

Erythema infectiosum is caused by parvovirus B19 (human parvovirus), a small, single-stranded DNA virus (Anderson et al 1983). Spread is by droplet infection, although as the virus can be seen in plasma during infections it could be transmitted by blood products. Erythrocyte precursors are particularly susceptible to the virus causing a mild fall in hemoglobin (of about 1 g/dl) in normal individuals but profound anemia in those whose red cell survival is already shortened.

Clinical features

B19 infection may be asymptomatic or may cause a mild febrile illness with rash (Anderson L J 1987). In children the first sign of infection is usually marked erythema of the cheeks or slapped cheek appearance often with relative circumoral pallor (Fig. 23.18). In volunteer studies, however, there is an initial febrile episode with headache, chills, myalgia and malaise associated with viremia and the rash appears about 7 days later (Fig. 23.19). 1 to 4 days after the slapped cheeks an itchy, erythematous, maculopapular rash develops on the trunk and limbs. As the rash on the limbs clears it leaves a lacy, reticular pattern. The rash may fluctuate over the next 1–3 weeks and a hot bath, for example, may lead to recrudescence of an evanescent rash.

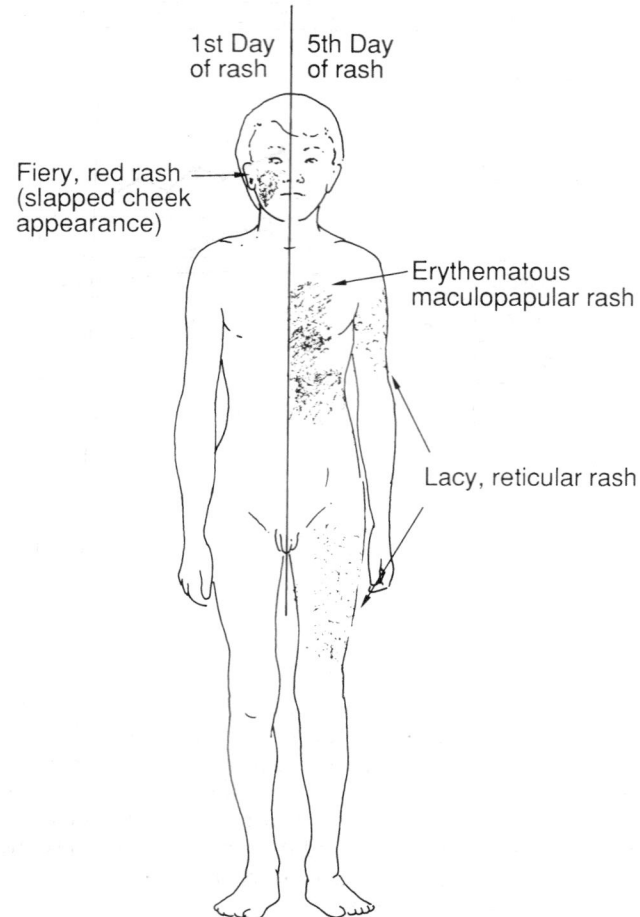

Fig. 23.18   The distribution and development of rash in erythema infectiosum (fifth disease).

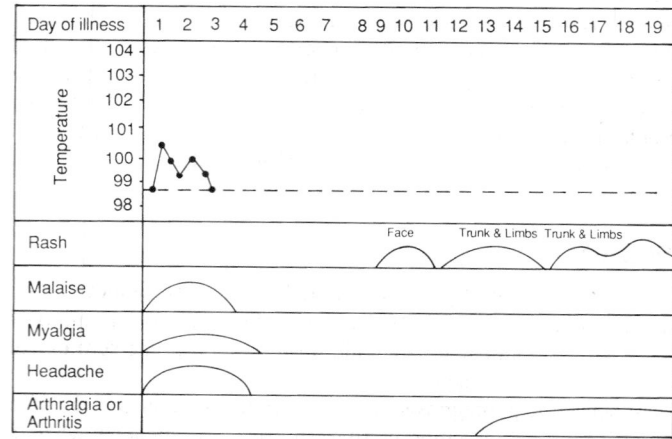

Fig. 23.19   The development of erythema infectiosum (fifth disease).

Complications

Arthritis or arthralgia is more common in adults, but certainly can occur in children. It usually appears 1–6 days after the rash but there may be no history of rash at all. Arthritis is characteristically transient and asymmetrical, affecting wrists, knees, ankles, elbows and fingers, though it may persist for weeks or even months.

Children with a shortened red cell survival, such as those with sickle cell anemia, thalassemia major, hereditary spherocytosis or other hemolytic anemias, may have severe aplastic crises with hemoglobin levels falling as low as 1–2 g/dl and no reticulocytes.

Children with malignancy, particularly acute leukemia, may develop prolonged anemia from chronic parvovirus B19 infection (Kurtzman et al 1988).

Infection during pregnancy can result in hydrops fetalis due to fetal anemia, which may be fatal, but no congenital syndrome has been described in babies of infected mothers who delivered at term (Anand et al 1987).

Encephalitis with or without neurological sequelae has rarely been reported after clinical erythema infectiosum, but as this was prior to the identification of the causative agent it is not certain that this is a true complication of B19 infection.

Diagnosis

Erythema infectiosum may closely mimic rubella, and the two diseases can circulate concurrently. The slapped cheek appearance with circumoral pallor can be mistaken for scarlet fever.

The diagnosis can be made serologically by demonstrating parvovirus B19-specific IgM on an acute serum sample, although it is always better to get a paired sample in case there is a late rise in antibody. The virus can be detected by electron microscopy in the plasma of patients with aplastic crises. This is particularly important in patients with sickle cell disease in whom severe anemia might be due to sequestration or pneumococcal sepsis. DNA probes and PCR have been used to detect the viral genome in stillbirths with hydrops fetalis and to demonstrate persisting antigen in children with leukemia and chronic anemia.

Treatment

There is no specific treatment. Isolation of patients is unnecessary since they are no longer infectious when the rash appears.

Arthritis may require salicylates or nonsteroidal anti-inflammatory agents. Children with aplastic crises may require blood transfusion until the red cell aplasia resolves spontaneously after 1–2 weeks.

ROSEOLA INFANTUM (SIXTH DISEASE, EXANTHEM SUBITUM, THREE DAY FEVER)

Roseola infantum is a common disease of infancy, characterized by fever and the appearance of an erythematous maculopapular rash as the fever defervesces. It may be confused with measles clinically. It is generally benign.

Etiology

A viral cause has long been postulated, since roseola was transmitted to a 6-month-old boy by injecting him with serum from a child with pre-eruptive roseola. There is good evidence that human herpesvirus 6 (HHV-6) is the main causative agent (Yamanishi et al 1988, Jones & Isaacs 1996). Seroconversion has been demonstrated in infants in association with clinical roseola, with modest rises in IgG but no IgM response, and the virus has

been cultured from lymphocytes of affected children. Human herpesvirus 7 is responsible for most clinical cases of roseola infantum which are HHV-6 negative (Torigoe et al 1995).

Clinical features

The illness starts abruptly with fever, and some anorexia and irritability although in general the child appears relatively well. Mild cough, coryza, diarrhea and vomiting rarely occur. The pyrexia of 38.9–40.6°C persists for 3–5 days, then falls precipitately as the rash appears (Fig. 23.20). The rash is erythematous, with discrete macular or maculopapular lesions, and starts on the trunk and neck, sometimes spreading to the face and limbs. It lasts 1–2 days. Cervical lymphadenopathy is common and may sometimes be prominent: the suboccipital, posterior cervical and posterior auricular nodes are most commonly involved. There is no characteristic enanthem, although there may be pharyngitis, small exudative follicular tonsillar lesions, or small ulcers on the soft palate, tonsils and uvula.

For the first day or two of fever the white count is often elevated with a neutrophil leukocytosis, but then may fall as low as 3 × 10⁹/l predominantly lymphocytes with an absolute neutropenia.

Complications

Convulsions may occur in association with roseola. These are usually febrile convulsions but encephalitis has rarely been described, sometimes with severe residua such as hemiparesis or mental retardation. Rarely thrombocytopenic purpura may occur following roseola (Jones & Isaacs 1996).

Diagnosis

The diagnosis of roseola infantum is primarily clinical, although the diagnosis can now be confirmed serologically. The characteristic fever chart and discrete rash that does not become confluent distinguish roseola from other childhood exanthemata including measles. The rash may be confused with a drug rash if antibiotics have been given and a vaccine reaction may cause confusion if the illness comes on soon after immunization.

Treatment

There is no specific treatment. Antipyretics may lessen the risk of convulsions, but if these occur, encephalitis should be considered and the child treated appropriately.

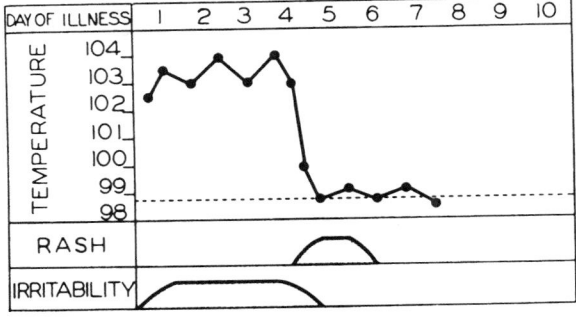

Fig. 23.20 The development of exanthem subitum. (From Krugman & Ward 1968.)

HERPESVIRUSES

CHICKENPOX (VARICELLA)

Chickenpox is a common and highly infectious disease caused by varicella-zoster virus (VZV), also known as human herpesvirus 3 (HHV-3). In general it is a benign condition and has a virtually worldwide distribution. However, chickenpox is not endemic in some isolated areas and if introduced to such a community a more serious disease may occur. It can also prove fatal in neonates and sometimes in adults and can be fatal when contracted by a patient on immunosuppressive drugs. To some extent varicella had a reflected importance due to a clinical similarity to smallpox.

Immunity following chickenpox is usually lifelong and second primary attacks are rare. Like all herpesviruses, however, the virus can remain latent and recur years later in the form of zoster (shingles).

Etiology

Chickenpox is transmitted from person to person by direct contact, droplet or airborne spread; infection can also arise through articles recently contaminated by an infected person. Infectivity is maximal during the prodromal period and has completely waned by the time the eruption becomes crusted.

The causative agent, varicella-zoster virus, is a DNA virus. The virus particle is surrounded by a membrane and the approximate diameter of the capsid is 100 nm; it is readily seen under the electron microscope.

Clinical features

Chickenpox is predominantly a disease of childhood and usually occurs between 2 and 8 years of age. Cases may occur in infancy. Peripartum intrauterine infection can lead to varicella neonatorum (see below) which, untreated, has a mortality up to 20%. Postnatal infection can cause classical chickenpox of a lesser severity occurring only in babies whose mothers have not had chickenpox.

Following an incubation period of 14–21 days, usually around 16 days, the disease starts with mild malaise and fever (Fig. 23.21). In children prodromal symptoms may be absent and the illness begins with a rash. Older children and adults have more definite prodromata and symptoms include malaise, fever, headache, sore throat and backache.

The rash (Fig. 23.22) commences as a crop of macules, which within hours pass through a papular stage to become vesicular; the

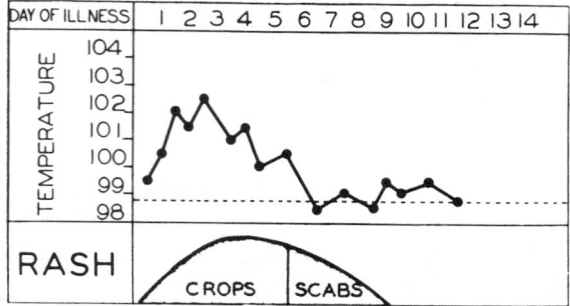

Fig. 23.21   The development of chickenpox. (From Krugman & Ward 1968.)

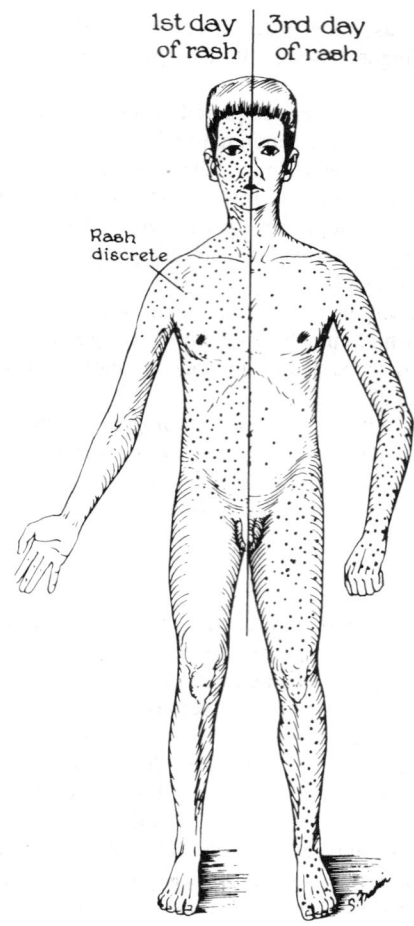

Fig. 23.22   The distribution of rash in chickenpox. (From Krugman & Ward 1968.)

vesicles persist for 3–4 days, becoming pustular and finally forming a crust. The spots are superficial and the vesicles may be round, oval, elliptical or irregular in shape; they are often surrounded by a red areola.

Evolution of the rash occurs by a series of crops, and lesions at different stages may be seen. The trunk is principally involved but spots also appear over the face, scalp and the proximal parts of the limbs. Lesions tend to be more abundant on covered rather than exposed parts of the body.

In mild cases the entire eruption may consist of a few spots; less often, the rash is almost generalized, extending to the distal parts of the limbs including the soles and palms. By the time of vesiculation there is often an intense pruritus. In some patients crusts can be very tenacious and 2–3 weeks may elapse before their separation is complete.

An enanthem is usually found and presents as vesiculation over the palate, tongue or buccal mucous membranes; the conjunctivae and vagina may be similarly affected.

Hemorrhagic chickenpox

In this there is usually a marked constitutional disturbance and high fever. Extensive bleeding into the vesicles develops and the lesions become black; areas of ecchymosis can appear on otherwise uninvolved skin. Bleeding may occur from mucous membranes and present as hematuria or melena. Both children and adults may contract this form of chickenpox and it has been particularly reported in patients receiving corticosteroids or cytotoxic drugs suggesting the importance of cell-mediated immunity as well as antibody in recovery from infection. It can be associated with profound thrombocytopenia (purpura fulminans) and is often fatal.

Varicella gangrenosa

This form of the disease usually results from severe secondary bacterial infection (usually due to group A streptococci) of the vesicles which may extend down to muscle. These lesions are slow to heal and can leave considerable scarring. Occasionally this form of varicella appears to start ab initio before any apparent secondary infection.

Varicella neonatorum

If the maternal rash appears less than 7 days before delivery or up to 2 days after delivery there is a risk that the baby will receive a large inoculum of virus without maternal antibody. Such babies are at very high risk of disseminated disease with death from pneumonitis, and should be protected at birth by giving zoster immune globulin (ZIG) (Hanngren et al 1985, Paryani & Arvin 1986). Since this does not always protect them, early treatment with acycloguanosine (acyclovir) is advisable if symptoms develop. Babies whose mother's rash develops 7 days or more before or 3 days or more after delivery are at low risk. Postnatally acquired chickenpox is nearly always mild although if the mother has not had chickenpox the use of ZIG should be considered for a neonate exposed to the virus.

Varicella bullosa

Bullous varicella may occur in children, the lesions developing into large bullae with a positive Nikolsky sign. It is due to superinfection with a toxin-producing *Staphylococcus aureus*, and the prognosis is excellent. Treatment is with antistaphylococcal antibiotics.

Complications

Sepsis

Secondary skin infection is the commonest complication. Abscesses may form locally or in regional lymph nodes. Cellulitis, erysipelas and scarlet fever can also develop. Bacteremic spread may give rise to pneumonia, osteomyelitis and septic arthritis. Common infecting organisms include group A streptococci and *Staphylococcus aureus*.

Neurological

Postinfectious encephalitis can occur and usually starts as the rash reaches maturity. The most common manifestation is a pure cerebellar ataxia with an excellent prognosis. Complete recovery is virtually invariable, usually rapidly, though may rarely take some weeks. Acute disseminated encephalomyelitis (ADEM) is a more sinister but rarer form of post-varicella encephalitis with cerebral demyelination giving rise to long tract signs, cranial nerve lesions, convulsions, etc. Examination of the CSF may show a mild lymphocytic pleocytosis and slight elevation of the protein content. About 10% of cases of Reye's syndrome occur secondary to chickenpox. Transverse myelitis, acute infantile hemiplegia and Guillain–Barré syndrome have been described complicating varicella.

Pneumonitis

Pneumonitis is usually seen in adults and immunocompromised children (and varicella neonatorum) and may present with acute respiratory distress or hemoptysis; diffuse nodular infiltration is seen on X-ray of the chest. The diagnosis is often obscure until the typical exanthem develops. Some cases die and, in those who recover, miliary calcification may be seen in the lung fields some years later.

In normal children, pneumonia complicating chickenpox is most likely to be bacterial, due to *S. pneumoniae*, group A streptococcus or occasionally *S. aureus*.

Others

Myocarditis, pericarditis, endocarditis, hepatitis and glomerulonephritis have rarely been reported. Appendicitis may also occur and can present before the eruptive phase; this sometimes leads to cross-infection in pediatric surgical wards. Keratitis and conjunctivitis are rare and usually benign. Arthritis may mimic septic arthritis but the latter should always be excluded by examination of the joint fluid because septic arthritis can complicate chickenpox. If ampicillin is prescribed a drug eruption may occur as with EBV infection, probably as a result of drug–hapten interaction.

Congenital varicella

If the mother contracts chickenpox in the first trimester there is about a 2% risk of the baby developing congenital varicella syndrome with cicatricial scarring of the limbs, cortical atrophy, hypoplasia of limbs, digital defects, retinitis or cataracts.

Diagnosis

The clinical course of varicella and the nature of the rash are usually typical and a firm clinical diagnosis can be made. Rapid diagnosis can be by electron microscopy or by immunofluorescence.

Varicella-zoster virus can be isolated from vesicle fluid collected during the first 3 or 4 days of the rash. For growth of the virus it is usual to employ cultures of human fibroblast cells.

Complement-fixing antibody develops during an infection and a retrospective diagnosis can be made if a significant rise in antibody titer has occurred during the illness. It is necessary to test two sera – an acute sample collected within a day or two of the onset of the illness and a convalescent sample collected 2 or 3 weeks later.

High complement-fixing antibody titers to varicella-zoster virus are usually present in the serum of patients suffering from herpes zoster.

Differential diagnosis

Chickenpox can be confused with impetigo, scabies, dermatitis herpetiformis, eczema herpeticum or vaccinatum and erythema multiforme. In most of these the absence of the typical, centripetal distribution and cropping of varicella helps in the differentiation.

Treatment

General

No treatment is usually required and bed rest is probably unnecessary except in ill patients. Simple analgesics will control prodromal symptoms where these are troublesome. Aspirin should not be given because of the risk of Reye's syndrome. Calamine lotion will normally soothe pruritus; if not, an antihistamine should be tried. If the enanthem is unusually severe careful oral toilet is needed and lesions on the conjunctiva should be protected from secondary infection. Treatment with acyclovir is indicated if infection develops in immunosuppressed cases, and in any patient with severe disease.

Sepsis

In convalescence simple antiseptics should control superficial skin infection. More severe sepsis will require appropriate antibacterial chemotherapy which should be guided by swabbing of the affected lesions and by cultures of the blood and of any pus. Flucloxacillin will adequately treat hemolytic streptococcal infection or staphylococcal infection until culture results are available.

Encephalitis

No specific treatment is available for the neurological complications and the usual supportive measures will be employed. Some clinicians favor the use of corticosteroids in severe cases despite the unhappy association of chickenpox with these drugs. It is argued that the encephalitis is of allergic origin and that by this stage of the illness there is sufficient antibody response to prevent further dissemination of the virus. In practice no serious untoward effects have been reported where steroids have been used in this condition although it is difficult to assess how much this therapy contributes to any recovery. Similarly the role of acyclovir in treating varicella encephalitis is unclear.

Others

Cases of severe varicella pneumonitis and profound thrombocytopenia have also been treated with acyclovir and corticosteroid drugs but an accurate evaluation of their benefit is impossible. Appendicitis should be treated surgically.

Prevention

The infectivity of chickenpox is such that the strictest isolation measures may fail to prevent its spread. As a result quarantine measures are of little value and it can be argued that it is preferable to contract the disease when a child as it will probably run a benign course – in contrast to the potentially more serious form in the adult.

An exception must be made in the case of patients who are receiving corticosteroid drugs or cytotoxic drugs. In this instance every effort should be made to prevent exposure to chickenpox and herpes zoster for reasons already described. If such exposure should occur then hyperimmune chickenpox gamma globulin (zoster immune globulin, ZIG) has been shown to modify severity even if it does not always prevent the disease, and should be given. The use of ZIG in neonates has already been discussed.

HERPES ZOSTER (ZOSTER: SHINGLES)

The clinical relationship between chickenpox and herpes zoster has long been recognized. The virus causing the two syndromes is identical, and is referred to as the varicella-zoster virus. Nonimmune persons may develop chickenpox when exposed to herpes zoster but the converse rarely occurs. The inoculation of children with virus obtained from zoster patients has resulted in clinical chickenpox which has then spread to other children as chickenpox.

Following an attack of varicella, the virus survives in a latent form in the sensory root ganglia of the cord and brain; a situation with similarities to latent infection by herpes simplex virus. After an interval of many years, but sometimes earlier, the virus becomes activated by local precipitating factors or by some depression of protective immunological mechanisms. Virus then spreads along the sensory root in question; adjacent motor areas of the cord, or other parts of the cerebrum, may become involved. A degree of systemic spread can also occur which provokes a modified form of chickenpox called zoster varicellosa; such modification may result from the antigenic stimulus provided by the reactivated virus, and the very high antibody levels found early on in the course of herpes zoster support this impression.

Patients who develop zoster are usually elderly but the disease does occur in children and younger adults. In young children, pain is much less marked than in adults, and zoster is not suggestive of immune deficiency or malignancy. There is often a history of maternal varicella during pregnancy or early neonatal varicella: it is thought that varicella at a time of relatively poor immunity is more likely to result in childhood zoster. In a few instances, primary infection by the varicella-zoster virus appears to provoke zoster rather than chickenpox; the explanation is not known. On occasion zoster may also occur simultaneously with a primary attack of chickenpox.

For reasons alluded to above, zoster is seen quite frequently in persons suffering from leukemia or other malignant disease and can follow radiotherapy.

Clinical features

Zoster may start with constitutional disturbance or progressive pain over a particular dermatome, although in children zoster may be pain free. Clusters of macules and papules appear on the skin overlying the dermatome, rarely crossing the midline. These soon vesiculate and the vesicles formed may be larger than in chickenpox and tend to coalesce. Extensive crusting follows which slowly separates to expose a raw, ulcerated area. This will bleed readily and is liable to secondary infection. Healing is slow and after months or years, vitiligo may develop and the involved skin is often anesthetic. Enlargement of the regional lymph nodes is very common.

Acute pain tends to subside as crusting sets in but extreme irritation and neuralgia may persist for months and even years (postherpetic neuralgia). In children the illness tends to be much milder, pain is mild or absent and recovery is considerably quicker.

In hospitals, one tends to find selected examples of zoster but more representative surveys show that thoracic segments are most commonly involved. However, zoster of the trigeminal nerve, and usually of the supraophthalmic division, is the commonest variety seen in hospital.

Geniculate herpes is of special interest and is frequently misdiagnosed; in this form of zoster, vesicles appear on the meatus and pinna of the ear. Pain may be experienced in the throat, in or behind the ear and taste may be lost over the anterior two-thirds of the tongue. Facial paralysis, sometimes permanent, may result. This condition is sometimes referred to as the *Ramsay Hunt* syndrome. A modified generalized rash over the trunk and face is seen in many cases provided examination is sufficiently diligent. Other features include involvement of the adjacent motor root with resultant paralysis which can be permanent, and meningitis, encephalitis or myelitis can be encountered.

Occasionally zoster occurs without any accompanying rash, the so-called zoster sine herpete.

Diagnosis

Prior to the appearance of the skin eruption diagnosis is difficult in children, in whom zoster is rather unexpected. Diagnoses such as pleurisy or fibrositis may be made but the difficulties are quickly resolved when the classical rash, along the line of a nerve, makes its appearance. Laboratory tests are referred to in the section on chickenpox.

Treatment

The illness is usually mild in children and simple analgesics such as paracetamol will usually control pain. Relief may follow the application of a dusting powder of zinc oxide or the use of cold sprays.

Supraophthalmic zoster requires special care. It is advisable to dilate the pupil with atropine and any break in the cornea may require treatment with topical antibiotics to prevent secondary bacterial infection. Topical idoxuridine is effective against ophthalmic VZV. The help of a qualified ophthalmologist is advisable.

In some instances, particularly severe zoster may show a dramatic response to treatment by corticosteroid drugs. However, their general use is not advised and they are best avoided in zoster affecting the eye and wherever any underlying immunological defect may be present. Acyclovir or vidarabine is only needed for immunocompromised children or those with severe zoster.

Prognosis

This is usually good in children. Postherpetic neuralgia is uncommon but may persist for a long time. Certain paralyses can prove permanent and impairment of vision has followed supraophthalmic zoster. Such complications are more commonly found in adult cases.

HERPES SIMPLEX (see also pp. 1435–1442)

Primary infection by *Herpesvirus hominis* (herpes simplex virus)

usually occurs in early childhood and is generally subclinical. However, in a small percentage of children it may produce a variable clinical illness, the main features of which include localized vesiculation on some part of the body and a sharp constitutional reaction. Some children avoid infection altogether and may reach adolescence or adult life with no immunity to this virus. This is more likely to occur when they have been brought up in rural, as opposed to urban, areas and, as with many other viral infections, an attack in adult life can often be more severe.

An interesting feature of this virus is its ability to persist in a latent form once the primary infection, whether clinical or subclinical, has subsided (Lancet 1989a). In some people the virus becomes reactivated by certain nonspecific stimuli at various times in their lives and the resultant clinical manifestations tend to differ from those seen with primary infection.

Etiology

Herpes simplex virus (HSV) is a DNA virus surrounded by a membrane and is approximately 150–180 nm in diameter. There are two strains, HSV types 1 and 2. HSV type 2 primarily infects the genital tracts of adults, and infection in the pregnant woman near term can result in serious infection in the newborn infant. HSV type 1 is primarily oral, although type 2 can cause oral disease and type 1 can infect the genitalia.

Clinical features: primary herpes

A variety of different syndromes may result from primary infection by HSV and are now described in detail.

Acute herpetic gingivostomatitis (ulcerative stomatitis)

This, the commonest manifestation, commences with a sharp constitutional reaction with high fever, malaise, anorexia and irritability. The patient, usually a young child, has difficulty feeding due to pain in the mouth. Inspection, often hampered by severe discomfort, reveals marked swelling and inflammation of the gums which may bleed at the merest touch. Deeper inspection will reveal the typical shallow ulcers, white in color, on such sites as the tongue, palate, gums, buccal mucosa and tonsils. In mild cases the ulcers are few; in more severe examples there may be a contiguous sheet of ulcers involving all the sites mentioned. Saliva tends to flow from the mouth and satellite lesions form down the chin or cheek where the child dribbles. Regional lymph nodes in the neck enlarge and fever will persist for several days. Mild cases subside rapidly but the worst may take up to 2 weeks before the local lesions disappear. Younger children may implant the virus on to other sites such as the sucked finger or perineal region, where vesiculation will develop.

Perineal herpes (acute herpetic vulvovaginitis)

This is a less common primary manifestation though it may be underdiagnosed in view of confusion with severe napkin and other eruptions in the same area. It is diagnosed far more often in girls, though primary perineal herpes sometimes occurs in boys. Some degree of constitutional upset will again herald the infection, to be followed by painful vesiculation over the perineum which may extend into the vagina in girls. Lesions close to the external urethral orifice may cause difficulties with micturition and regional adenitis may develop. The lesions usually subside without scarring despite the likelihood of secondary infection. Reactivation occurs over the buttocks, thighs or perineum.

Traumatic herpetic infection

The intact skin appears relatively resistant to this virus but primary infection may arise over the site of abrasions and burns. An interesting variety is the herpetic whitlow of the finger which is sometimes seen in nurses who contract the infection by virus entering such lesions as needle puncture wounds or the abrasions that can result from opening glass phials – lesions that are common on the nurse's hand. Here again there may be a marked constitutional upset and regional lymphadenitis.

Acute herpetic keratoconjunctivitis

Primary herpetic infection of the eye is a serious presentation of this infection though relatively rare. Only one eye is normally involved and cases present with constitutional upset and pain. Marked reddening and edema appear on the affected conjunctiva, the cornea becomes hazy and the eye will usually close. Vesicles appear around the lids and a purulent discharge often occurs. So long as the infection remains superficial the condition will usually subside without complications in 10–14 days. Deeper involvement may give rise to keratitis disciformis, hypopyon keratitis or iridocyclitis, all of which may be followed by scarring; however, these are more commonly encountered in recurrent herpetic infection.

Kaposi's varicelliform eruption (KVE) or eczema herpeticum

Children with eczema are prone to superinfection of the involved skin by a number of organisms including herpes simplex virus. The disease starts with a particularly sharp constitutional upset and vesicles then appear on the skin and are most intense at the eczematous areas. An experienced observer may readily recognize the condition; more often the true diagnosis is unappreciated and extensive secondary infection accompanied by a marked serosanguineous discharge will develop. Further crops of vesicles may appear and the child's condition deteriorate further. The most severe cases may be fatal without acyclovir therapy; in the remainder there is a slow recovery over a period of 3–4 weeks.

Primary herpetic meningoencephalitis

Previously considered an infrequent infection, modern virological techniques have shown that herpetic meningoencephalitis is more common than was believed. The signs of central nervous system involvement may appear shortly after a primary lesion at some other site but there is usually no clinical evidence to indicate the basic etiologic agent (Whitley 1988). Cases may present as mild forms of aseptic meningitis or as a rapidly fatal form of encephalitis principally involving the temporal lobes. Confusion with a brain abscess or tumor may arise and in those who recover severe cerebral damage may persist. Neonatal herpes encephalitis classically presents with facial twitching and focal fits at 7–28 days, and there is rarely a history of skin lesions or maternal herpes.

Generalized herpetic infection (see p. 287)

This form is normally confined to the newborn and occurs in infants with no protective maternal antibody. The source of the infection is usually the mother or rarely an attendant in the nursery or a relative. The condition presents with fever, hepatosplenomegaly and deepening jaundice, the infant becoming progressively weaker with vomiting and anorexia. The outcome is usually fatal and the diagnosis made at autopsy when typical inclusion bodies are found in the affected viscera. Visible involvement of the skin and mucous membranes is absent in most cases.

Neonatal infection

Skin, eye or mouth lesions may not precede the development of generalized or CNS herpes infection. Nevertheless there is a very high risk of progression from such isolated lesions, about 70% without treatment. Any vesicular lesion in a neonate should be treated as an emergency, and urgent electron microscopy or immunofluorescence obtained on the vesicle fluid, and treatment started.

Clinical features: recurrent herpes

Exacerbations of latent herpes simplex virus infection may be provoked by a variety of nonspecific stimuli which include upper respiratory infections, any febrile illness, gastrointestinal upsets, overexposure to sunlight and emotional upsets. Drugs and certain foods have also been incriminated.

Whatever the excitant, recurrent herpes present as a crop of tiny vesicles which are sometimes painful and after a few days will dry up to form a scab. They may erupt on almost any part of the skin or on the mucous membranes of the mouth, conjunctivae or genitalia. The most usual site is on the skin around the nose and mouth. Exacerbations tend to recur at the same site in any particular individual. Recurrent herpes gives rise to little or no constitutional upset or fever but the excitant, such as lobar pneumonia, may do so.

Diagnosis

The clinical features are often diagnostic in themselves but resort to laboratory aid is of help in certain instances. The procedures available are:

1. growth of the virus in tissue culture
2. demonstration under the electron microscope of herpesvirus particles in material taken from a lesion
3. demonstration of viral antigens in the material by a fluorescent antibody technique
4. antibody estimations on acute and convalescent serum samples to show specific IgM or a significant rise in IgG during a suspected primary infection
5. histological evidence of intranuclear inclusions and giant cells.

Primary herpes

The oral lesions of primary herpetic gingivostomatitis may be confused with a variety of conditions such as thrush, tonsillitis, Vincent's stomatitis, agranulocytosis and leukemia. Careful clinical and laboratory studies readily differentiate most of these but herpangina, due to infection by Coxsackie viruses group A, can cause genuine confusion; however, gingivitis does not normally accompany herpangina, but is common in herpetic infections. Virus studies may be needed in difficult cases. Herpetic vulvovaginitis is readily confused with ammoniacal dermatitis which has been secondarily infected. Impetigo of the vulva is usually accompanied by involvement elsewhere. Kaposi's varicelliform eruption may be confused with severely infected eczema, with eczema vaccinatum and occasionally with varicella. Herpetic meningoencephalitis is difficult to diagnose on clinical grounds; usually, virological studies are required to make a conclusive diagnosis.

Recurrent herpes

Recurrent herpes produces a fairly precise diagnostic picture but, on occasion, can resemble herpes zoster. The absence of pain, lack of a definable, neurological distribution and differing nature of the vesicles should differentiate these conditions.

Treatment

As a rule primary herpetic infections do not require other than supportive treatment. Severe examples of gingivostomatitis may have feeding difficulties due to pain, and careful coaxing will be needed to ensure adequate hydration; cleansing of the mouth is also difficult on account of this pain. Irritating acidic fluids should be avoided and diet restricted to cold, bland drinks during the most acute phase. Superinfection by *Candida* may occur but this usually responds to treatment by the local application of nystatin suspension; secondary bacterial infection rarely warrants any antibiotic therapy though this may be required in herpetic vulvovaginitis. Eye involvement is best managed by an experienced ophthalmologist.

Herpetic infections are amongst the few viral diseases in which highly successful treatment by antiviral agents has been reported; topical 5-iodo-2-deoxyuridine (IDU) or acyclovir are effective in herpetic eye infections. Acyclovir is the treatment of choice for herpes simplex encephalitis, for KVE and for any herpetic skin lesion in a neonate (Arvin et al 1987, Whitley 1988).

CYTOMEGALOVIRUS INFECTIONS

Prior to 1950 cytomegalic inclusion disease (CID) was recognized as a fatal disease of infancy in which the diagnosis was invariably made at autopsy. A viral cause was always suspected and the discovery of large intranuclear inclusions in epithelial cells from stained urinary deposits lent support to this hypothesis. Subsequently the responsible virus was successfully grown in tissue cultures and the knowledge of cytomegalovirus (CMV) infections has greatly expanded in recent years. CMV is a DNA virus of the herpesvirus group and electron microscopic studies show it to be structurally similar to *Herpesvirus hominis*.

Types

There are three main clinical syndromes produced by CMV. Firstly, infection in the newborn, usually acquired congenitally, results in the established picture of cytomegalic inclusion disease. Secondly, an illness may be produced in older children and adults which has similar clinical features to infectious mononucleosis. Lastly, there is increasing evidence of opportunistic infection by CMV in immunocompromised patients who have recently

undergone open heart surgery or have had organ transplantation performed; it is postulated in these instances that the virus is transmitted through blood transfusion or that a latent infection becomes reactivated. Concurrent immunosuppressive therapy used in this field of surgery is an obvious factor of importance in disseminating the infection further, regardless of the mode of entry. A whole new spectrum of diseases caused by CMV has been described in AIDS patients.

It is also relevant to comment on the frequency with which healthy individuals may be found with antibodies to CMV in their blood or occasionally have the virus isolated from their urine, indicating that widespread subclinical infection by this agent occurs.

Clinical features

Cytomegalic inclusion disease of infants is described in the chapter relating to neonatal infection (see p. 287).

In older children and adults CMV infection may present with fever, cough, headaches and pains which are usually situated in the back and limbs. The clinical picture is one of infectious mononucleosis, with lymphadenopathy, hepatosplenomegaly and sometimes jaundice. Examination of the peripheral blood reveals the presence of atypical lymphocytes, and there is a varying degree of derangement in liver function tests. Hemolytic anemia can occur, and cold agglutinins, cryoglobulins and antinuclear factor may be present. Ampicillin may cause a rash as in EBV infection. The suspected diagnosis is usually glandular fever, but this is not supported by the heterophile antibody test and a significant rise in titer of complement-fixing antibodies to CMV together with the possible isolation of this virus from the urine substantiates the true diagnosis. CMV may produce a pneumonitis but this is usually seen in neonates or children suffering from underlying diseases such as chronic hepatic disorders, leukemia and other malignancies (Grundy et al 1987).

A febrile illness with features suggesting infectious mononucleosis may also be encountered in patients who have recently undergone open heart surgery or organ transplantation and investigation of obscure postoperative illness in such cases should include the possibility of CMV infection. In patients with immune deficiency, particularly AIDS patients, CMV may cause pneumonitis, hepatitis, severe retinitis and colitis. It is a frequent cause of death due to hepatitis or pneumonitis in liver transplant patients and of graft rejection in renal transplant patients. The virus is usually acquired from the donor organ or blood products, although reactivation of latent host CMV may also occur.

Laboratory diagnosis

Histological lesions due to CMV infection are characterized by large cells containing intranuclear and cytoplasmic inclusion bodies; the inclusion-containing cells may be widely disseminated.

A clinical diagnosis may be confirmed by:

1. the presence of typical histological lesions in a biopsy specimen, e.g. liver
2. typical inclusion bodies in cell deposits of fresh urine
3. isolation of the virus
4. demonstration of a significant rise in antibody titer during the illness.

Rapid viral diagnosis using DNA probes or by early immunofluorescence testing of tissue cultures (so-called shell viral cultures) is increasingly available, and particularly useful for immunocompromised patients.

With improved virological techniques, efforts should always be made to grow CMV when cytomegalic inclusion disease is considered to be present. Suitable specimens are fresh urine samples and saliva swabs but these specimens must be delivered to the laboratory with minimum delay as the virus easily loses its infectivity. Isolation of the agent is usually carried out in tissue cultures of human fibroblasts.

Differential diagnosis

Cytomegalic inclusion disease requires to be differentiated from other congenital infections such as rubella, syphilis, toxoplasmosis, disseminated herpes simplex and sepsis of the newborn. CMV infections acquired in later life may mimic a variety of febrile states but infectious mononucleosis is the most likely condition to cause confusion; where jaundice occurs infectious hepatitis, serum hepatitis and leptospirosis require exclusion.

Prevention

Blood products from CMV antibody-negative donors should always be given to preterm neonates and immunocompromised patients, particularly post-transplant or HIV-infected patients. Alternatively, as the virus is cell associated, filtration or freezing of the donor blood to remove white cells also reduces the risk of acquired CMV infection.

Passive immunoprophylaxis of transplant patients with immunoglobulin is partially successful in reducing the risk of CMV infection. Seropositive CMV patients may reactivate when immunosuppressed, and interferon but not acyclovir reduces this risk.

Treatment

Ganciclovir, a derivative of acyclovir, has been successfully used to treat immunocompromised patients with CMV retinitis, enteritis and pneumonitis (Meyers 1988). In adult patients, 70–80% cease excretion of CMV within a week, with the exception of marrow transplant patients with CMV pneumonitis of whom somewhat fewer respond. However, relapse occurs in about half when ganciclovir is stopped, it causes significant marrow suppression, the drug is incorporated into the host genome, and there is little experience with children.

Foscarnet causes less marrow suppression although transient renal impairment may occur. There are few controlled data on its use in CMV infections.

Prognosis

Congenital CMV infection has a variable outcome (see p. 287). Normal individuals who contract CMV infection rarely suffer any sequelae, but in immunocompromised patients blindness due to retinitis, graft rejection and death from pneumonitis, hepatitis and disseminated infection may occur.

EPSTEIN–BARR VIRUS

Epstein–Barr virus (EBV) is the cause of infectious mononucleosis or glandular fever, a disease primarily of older children, adolescents and young adults. An almost identical syndrome can be caused by CMV and *Toxoplasma gondii* as well as EBV. An anginose form of glandular fever primarily affecting the tonsils is increasingly being recognized in younger children under 5 years of age (Krabbe et al 1981). EBV has a worldwide distribution and like the other herpesviruses can persist in a latent state and reactivate. It is potentially oncogenic and has been linked with nasopharyngeal carcinoma, Burkitt's lymphoma and other lymphomas, particularly in immunocompromised patients (Allday & Crawford 1988).

Etiology and epidemiology

Primary infection of the lymphoid tissue of the nasopharynx may be asymptomatic or may lead to symptomatic infection of lymph nodes. Transmission is by the respiratory route and the virus is of low infectivity, usually requiring intimate oral contact. The 'kissing disease' refers to its spread among adolescents and young adults by this route. Epidemics are unusual. The virus persists in the nasopharynx (Lung et al 1985) and the uterine cervix (Sixbey et al 1986). The virus primarily infects B lymphocytes but the atypical mononuclear cells seen in the blood film are activated T lymphocytes.

Clinical features

The anginose form of glandular fever is characterized by fever and sore throat with moderate or marked cervical lymphadenopathy. The tonsils are red and inflamed and there is often white exudative folliculitis. Other lymph nodes and spleen are rarely enlarged and the clinical picture is not readily distinguishable from acute tonsillitis.

Glandular fever usually starts insidiously with malaise, anorexia and fever. Usually sore throat is a prominent symptom. Occasionally the patient merely has malaise and fever for 1–3 weeks with chills and sweats (febrile form of infectious mononucleosis) and presents with pyrexia of unknown origin. Generally, however, there is marked enlargement of posterior and anterior cervical lymph nodes, and the suboccipital, postauricular, axillary, epitrochlear and inguinal nodes may also be enlarged (glandular form). The tonsils may be inflamed with exudate and rarely this can be sufficient to impair swallowing and even breathing. Splenomegaly is usual and hepatomegaly may also be present, sometimes with jaundice.

Skin eruptions occur in about 10–15% of cases. The commonest is a widespread maculopapular rash but morbilliform, scarlatiniform, purpuric and urticarial rashes may occur. Ampicillin causes a particularly florid, confluent maculopapular rash in EBV infection, and this ampicillin rash may also be seen though less commonly in conjunction with other herpesvirus infections such as CMV and chickenpox.

In Duncan's syndrome, or X-linked lymphoproliferative disease, affected males are unable to control EBV infection and develop generalized lymphadenopathy and hepatosplenomegaly which persists and is rapidly fatal. These patients usually have persistently high levels of IgG antibodies to the viral capsid antigen (VCA).

EBV may be responsible for the lymphoid interstitial pneumonitis that can occur in children with HIV infection, since the EBV genome has been demonstrated in lung biopsy specimens from these patients. It can also cause CNS and other lymphomas in patients with HIV infection.

Complications

Threatened obstruction of the airway may occur in the severe anginose variety especially when there is secondary edema in the neck. Neurological complications include aseptic meningitis, cranial nerve palsies (including Bell's palsy), encephalomyelitis, transverse myelitis and Guillain–Barré syndrome. Cardiac involvement may present as myocarditis or as transient arrhythmias. Other complications include pneumonitis, orchitis, rupture of the spleen, hemolytic anemia, thrombocytopenic purpura and various ocular manifestations; hepatic involvement has been referred to previously. A prolonged illness with fatigue and relapses over many months has occasionally been described in children, in association with raised EBV antibodies (Lancet 1985, 1986a). Chronic EBV infection is not a common cause of the 'chronic fatigue syndrome' or myalgic encephalopathy (ME).

EBV is thought to be the cause of Burkitt's lymphoma and of nasopharyngeal carcinoma, in both of which tumors the EBV genome can consistently be demonstrated.

Diagnosis

Five main points arise in the diagnosis of glandular fever – a suggestive clinical picture, typical changes in the peripheral blood, a positive heterophile antibody test, IgM antibody to EB virus, and certain nonspecific changes in other laboratory tests.

Blood changes

Most important is the presence of large atypical mononuclear cells which have an irregular nucleus, whose cytoplasm contains vacuoles and in which characteristic pale staining of the cellular cytoplasm is found. Often there is a leukocytosis of $10–20 \times 10^9$ cells/l and sometimes the predominant cells are initially polymorphonuclear. However, atypical monocytes and lymphocytes soon appear, or may be present from the outset, and these can represent from 5–50% of the total leukocyte count. Other changes in the blood include occasional cases where there is a leukopenia and rare instances of profound thrombocytopenia and transient autoimmune hemolytic anemia.

Heterophile antibody test (Paul–Bunnell reaction)

Frequently sheep red cell agglutinins (heterophile antibodies) develop by the second week of infectious mononucleosis but occasionally the appearance of these agglutinins may be delayed for 2 or 3 weeks, so an early negative test should be repeated.

Sheep red cell agglutinins are not specific for infectious mononucleosis and may occur in other conditions. However, by means of absorption tests using guinea pig kidney and ox erythrocytes the specificity of the test may be increased; the following are the salient features:

1. Antibodies present in infectious mononucleosis are not absorbed by guinea pig kidney but are absorbed by ox erythrocytes.
2. Antibodies found in normal serum are not absorbed by ox erythrocytes but they are absorbed by guinea pig kidney.
3. Antibodies found in serum sickness are absorbed by both guinea pig kidney and ox erythrocytes.

Agglutinins to horse erythrocytes may also be present in the serum of a patient suffering from infectious mononucleosis and in many laboratories a test based on the agglutination of horse erythrocytes is in use. This is the basis of the rapid slide test, the 'Monospot' test. This test may sometimes be negative early in the disease and if EBV is suspected should be repeated. The test is unreliable under 5 years of age owing to false negative results.

EB virus antibody tests

The presence of specific EB IgM antibody indicates a recent or current infection, whereas the presence of IgG antibodies to the viral capsid antigen (VCA) or nuclear antigen (EBNA) merely indicate an infection with EB virus some time in the past. Only a small proportion of affected patients show a rise in IgG to VCA so the IgM test is preferred to show acute infection.

Nonspecific laboratory tests

In well over half the cases, some derangement of liver function tests will be found. Most often there is mild or moderate rise in the serum alanine aminotransferase (AAT) or glutamic pyruvate transaminase (SGPT) level but the alkaline phosphatase and serum bilirubin levels may also rise. Usually these changes are transient but in cases with clinical evidence of hepatic involvement the derangement in liver function tests is more marked.

On occasion a false positive Wassermann reaction occurs in infectious mononucleosis and high antistreptolysin 'O' titers may be found; the latter probably arise from an anamnestic reaction.

Differential diagnosis

Infectious mononucleosis may be diagnosed too readily. Young children with mild fever and lymph node enlargement in the neck are more likely to have a respiratory viral infection.

Cases that present with fever and little else may be confused with influenza, brucellosis or typhoid; those with a sore throat need to be differentiated from streptococcal tonsillitis, Vincent's stomatitis, diphtheria, agranulocytosis and leukemia. Glandular enlargement may be mistaken for toxoplasmosis, cytomegalovirus infection or reticulosis, and the icteric form of the disease has to be distinguished from infectious hepatitis, leptospirosis and, occasionally, from obstructive liver disease.

The skin eruption of glandular fever has produced confusion with measles, rubella, secondary syphilis and drug rashes.

In all the above situations careful attention to the five main diagnostic criteria will confirm or refute a suspected diagnosis of infectious mononucleosis.

Treatment

There is no specific treatment. Acyclovir has virtually no activity against EBV. The disease tends to be mild in children but simple analgesics may be required to ease pain and gargles to soothe the sore throat. There is increasing evidence that antibiotics can do more harm than good as toxic skin eruptions appear to follow their use and ampicillin is especially incriminated in this direction.

However, in cases where significant secondary infection is fully substantiated antibiotics may need to be employed. Corticosteroids can have a dramatic symptomatic effect but should be strictly reserved for those cases where edema of the airway is severe or used in cases where life-threatening complications such as thrombocytopenic purpura or severe neurological involvement are encountered.

Prognosis

The prognosis is good and children recover more quickly than adults though some cases run a protracted course and patients may take months to recover their full health. Death is rare and usually results from rupture of the spleen or severe neurological involvement. Recurrences in the immediate convalescent phase can occur but are usually shortlived.

VIRAL AND ALLIED INFECTIONS OF THE RESPIRATORY TRACT

Infections of the respiratory tract are frequent and ubiquitous. They are the most common cause of illness in almost any age group and have a predilection for the extremes of life. Agents that are capable of attacking one part or another of the respiratory tract include viruses, rickettsiae, mycoplasmas and fungi.

Respiratory infection frequently results from a combination of different organisms because, once the initial assault has damaged the defensive mechanisms within the air passages, secondary infection is readily superimposed. This often renders it difficult to deduce the primary cause. Nevertheless detailed studies on the etiology of acute respiratory tract infection indicate that 85% of such disease may be initiated by a virus.

In the ensuing account a description is given of the various viruses, and allied organisms, which play a significant role in the production of infective respiratory disease.

INFLUENZA

Influenza is an acute infectious disease of variable severity with an emphasis on general illness rather than on symptoms arising from the respiratory tract. It tends to occur in pandemic form every few years. In most instances the disease is a benign condition but may have a devastating effect when it attacks immunosuppressed patients or those with chronic cardiorespiratory disease, when there is a high mortality.

Etiology

Influenza may result from infection by three myxoviruses, types A, B or C, collectively known as orthomyxoviruses. Infection by type C is relatively uncommon, results in mild or inapparent illness and does not produce epidemics. Type B virus produces more significant illness followed by reasonably effective immunity. Outbreaks or small epidemics may occur, especially in schoolchildren, but are often of a localized nature. Some variation in antigenicity of type B virus occurs and outbreaks appear sporadically at intervals of 3–6 years.

Most clinical, virological and epidemiological interest is focused upon type A viruses as these produce the most noteworthy outbreaks or epidemics and, when major new variants emerge, pandemics. Pandemics have usually been identified by titles

which reflect the suspected geographical origin as indicated by titles such as 'Asian flu' or 'Hong Kong flu'. The World Health Organization has devised a more definitive classification of influenza viruses which reflects the nature of mutation more precisely (WHO 1980).

Structurally, influenza viruses comprise a central core of ribonucleoprotein with a covering envelope. From this envelope spikes containing hemagglutinins project and between these spikes the mushroom-shaped protrusions composed of neuraminidase.

Each basic type of influenza (A, B or C) has its own distinctive ribonucleoprotein consisting of the S or soluble antigen. Protein antigens on the viral surface are related to hemagglutinins (the H antigens) and to neuraminidases (the N antigens). In the case of type A viruses minor changes may occur year by year producing what is known as antigenic drift. However, at intervals usually exceeding a decade, major changes take place producing antigenic shift. The virtually new type A virus which emerges has thus acquired the potential to produce a pandemic.

Strain designation of influenza viruses is, therefore, based on the following points:

1. identification of the S antigen – that is whether virus is type A, B or C
2. the host origin – when isolated initially from man no specific identification is recorded but, if from an animal source, a suitable suffix is appended
3. the geographical origin
4. the strain number and the subtype of the hemagglutinin and neuraminidase identified
5. the year of isolation.

Without an appreciation of the relatively complex antigenic structure and its variation, an understanding of the epidemiology of influenza is difficult (Lancet 1986b). Furthermore, effective vaccination will require the use of vaccines whose antigenic components accurately reflect the strain of influenza virus prevalent at the time of use.

Epidemiology

Man is the principal reservoir of infection and the disease is transmitted by direct contact, through droplet infection and by articles that have been freshly soiled with discharges from the nose or throat of infected persons. Infectivity appears to persist for 4–5 days after the clinical onset of the disease. Occasional cases originate from animals, e.g. pigs. In view of the high infectivity of influenza and the rapidity of modern travel an epidemic can soon develop pandemic proportions.

Pathogenesis

Influenza infection causes necrosis of ciliated respiratory epithelium and this commences in the nose and spreads downwards to the trachea and bronchi. Edema and leukocyte infiltration follow causing pharyngitis, tracheitis and bronchitis; in severe cases considerable exudation of blood and edema fluid may occur and enter the alveoli with resultant pneumonia.

Primary respiratory damage from influenza virus may in itself produce a severe illness but secondary bacterial infection is more often the cause of fatal pneumonia; organisms such as *Staphylococcus aureus* and *Klebsiella pneumoniae* are particularly dangerous in this context.

Clinical features

The incubation period of influenza is short and ranges from 1 to 3 days. In children over 5 years of age there is a sudden onset of fever, headache and shivering, with pains in the limbs and back. Anorexia, listlessness and malaise may also be experienced and in some instances, particularly in children, nausea and vomiting may be unduly pronounced. Abdominal pain ('gastric flu') can be a prominent symptom. A dry, painful cough, discomfort in the throat, hoarseness and nasal discharge are usual.

The temperature may reach 39–40°C, but apart from signs of pharyngitis, objective physical findings are few and in uncomplicated cases clinical and radiographic examination of the chest is usually clear. Leukopenia will be found in uncomplicated cases and the ESR becomes moderately elevated.

The illness usually runs a short course and is followed by rapid improvement. Some patients experience a period of mental and physical lethargy in convalescence but seriously complicated cases are rarely seen outwith epidemics.

In younger children and infants influenza A typically causes high fever (over 39.5°C) and upper respiratory tract infection with coryza, cough, irritability and pharyngitis. Otitis media, laryngotracheitis, bronchitis, bronchiolitis indistinguishable from that due to RSV, and pneumonia may all occur. Vomiting and diarrhea are frequent in infants. Febrile convulsions are frequent, as are fleeting erythematous rashes, which can be morbilliform. The risk of severe lower respiratory tract involvement is greater in immunocompromised children.

In neonates the picture is nonspecific with apneic episodes, lethargy, poor feeding and impaired circulation. Outbreaks may occur in neonatal units.

Diagnosis

At epidemic times a clinical diagnosis of influenza has a high likelihood of being correct but such a diagnosis in a sporadic case can often be incorrect. Other respiratory viral infections and some quite unconnected diseases may present with a similar clinical picture and a specific diagnosis can only be based on definitive laboratory tests.

Virological confirmation of influenza can be established by serological studies or by demonstrating the presence of influenza virus. The latter can be isolated from pharyngeal swabs, nasal swabs or throat washing during the acute stage of the illness and can be grown in the amniotic cavity of chick embryos or in tissue cultures. Influenza may be isolated in monkey kidney tissue cultures. During epidemics immunofluorescence, using an antiserum to the epidemic strain to test nasopharyngeal secretions, can be used for rapid diagnosis. Complement-fixation, neutralization and hemagglutination-inhibition tests are available for the serological study of antibody responses to infection with influenza. In all these tests it is desirable to show a significant (fourfold or greater) rise in antibody titer during the illness.

Complications

Viral complications such as myocarditis, polyneuritis, encephalitis and psychosis are rarely seen in childhood cases. Secondary bacterial infection of the respiratory tract is more likely, and pneumonia, otitis media and purulent sinusitis may occur. Death can result from severe overwhelming infection by influenza virus itself though a fatal outcome is more likely to result from secondary bacterial infection. Acute myositis may be severe, particularly affecting the calves, with a raised serum CPK. Reye's syndrome has sometimes followed influenza B infection.

Treatment

In mild cases this is essentially symptomatic. Bed rest is advisable and pain will be eased by simple analgesics such as aspirin or paracetamol; troublesome cough should respond to codeine or similar preparations. Bacterial complications may require antibiotic treatment and wherever possible this should be guided by appropriate laboratory studies. Amantadine and rimantadine have been successfully used to treat immunocompromised patients with severe infection, and nebulized ribavirin may be of some benefit.

Prophylaxis

The extreme infectivity of influenza renders such measures as isolation and quarantine virtually ineffective. There is evidence that killed virus vaccine can significantly reduce the incidence of influenza though the sudden emergence of a fresh A mutant may render it impossible to produce the specific vaccine in time to influence an outbreak. Encouraging accounts of the use of amantadine in the prophylaxis of this disease have been reported and, more recently, live virus vaccines have become available, but their exact value has still to be established. So far they are not recommended for use in children.

PARAINFLUENZA VIRUS INFECTIONS

The parainfluenza viruses are members of the *Paramyxovirus* group. They have some properties in which they differ from the influenza viruses and they appear more closely related to the agents of mumps and Newcastle disease. They are approximately 150–220 nm in diameter, and contain RNA.

Four antigenic varieties, called 1, 2, 3 and 4, are recognized though type 4 has an undetermined role in the production of disease in humans. Types 1, 2 and 3 have frequently been isolated from cases of acute laryngotracheobronchitis (croup), bronchitis, bronchiolitis and pneumonia occurring in infants and children; less often they have been isolated from cases of rhinitis and pharyngitis. They are undoubtedly the commonest cause of acute laryngotracheobronchitis in which other viruses, such as influenza A and ECHO virus type 11, play a lesser role.

Serological studies indicate that infection, especially with type 3, is a common event in preschool children. Type 3 infection is endemic and occurs at any time of the year. Type 1 infection tends to occur in summer or autumn outbreaks every second year while type 2 outbreaks are less predictable.

Laboratory diagnosis

Parainfluenza viruses can be isolated from nasal and pharyngeal swabs. The viruses are relatively labile so these swabs should be placed in virus transport medium and delivered to the laboratory with minimum delay. Antigen detection by immunofluorescence or ELISA is increasingly available. Serological diagnosis is rarely helpful, other than in epidemiological studies, because of heterotypic antibody rises among the three types and related viruses particularly mumps.

RESPIRATORY SYNCYTIAL VIRUS INFECTIONS

Respiratory syncytial virus (RSV), first identified in 1956, is now recognized to be amongst the most important agents causing respiratory infection in infants and young children worldwide. RSV is an RNA paramyxovirus. The virus grows well in many tissue cultures. In contrast to members of the *Myxovirus* group, to which it shows some resemblance, RSV has no hemagglutinins so does not cause hemagglutination, but produces a fusion protein which causes in vitro and in vivo fusion of cells to form syncytia. Only two antigenic strains of RSV have been described.

Clinical features

RSV has been found in association with several clinical syndromes including mild upper respiratory tract infection, croup, bronchitis, bronchiolitis and pneumonia. Its principal association is with acute bronchiolitis in infants below 1 year of age. Epidemics of RSV infection occur annually in late autumn and winter in temperate climates. Outbreaks are mainly found in urban communities. In tropical climates there is not such a clear-cut annual epidemic. Nosocomial infections can be a major problem in hospitals.

Bronchiolitis is described elsewhere (p. 564) and although infection by influenza viruses, parainfluenza viruses, mycoplasmas, adenoviruses and rhinoviruses may produce a similar picture, few clinical respiratory syndromes have so close an etiologic association as bronchiolitis and RSV infection.

Neither maternal nor acquired antibody protect against RSV, so RSV can infect neonates. Reinfections throughout childhood are common, but successively milder. Toddler-age children may develop bronchitis or pneumonia, school-age children more commonly develop otitis media while adults get a severe cold with sore throat.

Laboratory diagnosis

The ideal specimen is a nasopharyngeal aspirate of mucus. Rapid viral diagnosis by immunofluorescence (or ELISA) has greatly aided the management of infants with bronchiolitis. The virus can be isolated successfully in various tissue culture systems, but as it is relatively unstable it is recommended that the specimen should be inoculated directly into the cultures without previous freezing. If the specimen has to be stored for a few hours it should be kept in virus transport medium at 4°C.

Serology can be used in children over 6 months of age, usually by complement-fixation test on paired sera. Under this age there is often no IgG response.

Treatment

Nebulized ribavirin may be indicated in proven severe RSV infection in infants at high risk, particularly those with pre-existing cardiopulmonary disease or immune deficiency (MacDonald et al 1982, Hall et al 1986, Isaacs et al 1988).

ADENOVIRUSES

The first isolation of an adenovirus took place in 1953 from fragmented human adenoids grown in tissue culture, hence the name. Subsequently a number of different strains, chiefly types 1, 2, 5 and 6, were isolated from cultures of tonsils and adenoids. Outbreaks due to these agents have been encountered in children at boarding schools, at summer camps and amongst those attending communal swimming pools; outbreaks in adults are mainly found in military recruits. The nature of the clinical illness produced shows considerable variation and overlap but some relatively specific syndromes are included (Ruuskanen et al 1985).

Adenoviruses are DNA viruses. They are relatively stable to changes in temperature and pH. They are widespread in nature and have been isolated from monkeys, pigs, dogs, birds and cattle, as well as from man. They may persist for weeks or even months in the upper respiratory tract.

Clinical features

Adenovirus infections are principally diseases of childhood, occurring mostly in children under the age of 5. Furthermore, certain adenovirus types show a pronounced age association.

Amongst syndromes recognized to be associated with adenoviral infection are the following.

Acute febrile pharyngitis

This syndrome has a high endemic rate in infants and young children and mainly results from infection by types 1, 2 and 5. It can also occur in epidemic form when type 3 is usually involved.

Pharyngoconjunctival fever (PCF)

Most commonly associated with infection by type 3, and less frequently with types 7A and 14, this syndrome can also follow infection by types 1, 2, 5 and 6. Epidemics occur in children, some of which have been associated with swimming pool infection. Symptoms of the syndrome include sore throat, headache, myalgia, eye discomfort, abdominal pain and stiffness in the back. Examination of the throat often reveals a degree of pharyngitis, and follicular conjunctivitis, unilateral or bilateral, may be seen.

Acute respiratory disease (ARD)

Uncommon in children, ARD is usually found in military recruits. It is most commonly due to infection by types 4 and 7; less often by types 3 and 14. The main clinical features include pharyngitis, cough, hoarseness and chest pain.

Viral pneumonia in infants

Adenoviruses may cause severe pneumonia and outbreaks have been reported in hospital nurseries and fatalities have resulted. Types 3, 7 and 21 have caused the most severe cases. Infection may disseminate (see below) or may result in bronchiolitis obliterans, bronchiectasis and unilateral hyperlucent lung.

Ocular syndromes

Two specific ocular syndromes are associated with adenovirus infection. The first is called *epidemic keratoconjunctivitis* and is associated with type 8 infection; the second, *follicular conjunctivitis*, usually results from infection by type 3 and may expand into the fuller syndrome of pharyngoconjunctival fever.

Disseminated disease

Adenovirus types 7 and 21 are particularly prone to cause pneumonia and disseminate to involve the liver (hepatitis), heart (myocarditis or pericarditis) and CNS (meningitis or encephalitis). This is more likely in immunocompromised patients.

Gastroenteritis

Noncultivable enteric adenoviruses (types 40 and 41), seen on electron microscopy of feces, have been associated with gastroenteritis (Brandt et al 1985).

Laboratory diagnosis

Adenoviruses can be grown in a wide range of tissue cultures. These viruses are relatively stable and can readily be isolated from throat swabs and feces. In respiratory disease the specimen should consist of a pharyngeal swab, sent to the laboratory in virus transport media. Cytopathic effect may be slow to appear, so cultures should be incubated for at least 3 weeks before being regarded as negative.

Serological evidence of infection can be determined by examination of acute and convalescent samples of serum for complement-fixing antibodies to adenoviruses. Antigen detection by ELISA is possible in some laboratories (Ruuskanen et al 1985).

Treatment

There have been anecdotal reports of successful treatment of adenovirus pneumonia with nebulized ribavirin (Buchdal et al 1985).

MUMPS (EPIDEMIC PAROTITIS)

To mump is an old English word meaning to mope. Mumps is an acute infectious disease characterized by nonsuppurative enlargement of the salivary glands, particularly the parotids. It results from infection by mumps virus, one of the myxoviruses, and is associated with an unusually diverse range of complications. Infection may be inapparent in as many as 30% of cases and the illness may present with a complication and no history of preceding salivary gland involvement.

Epidemiology and etiology

It is an endemic disease of urban communities which occasionally occurs in epidemic proportions especially in certain closed communities. Spread is by droplet infection or from recently contaminated articles and close contact is required. The quite high incidence in adults bears witness to the comparatively low infectivity of the disease, though when mumps is introduced into a virgin community, a serious and widespread outbreak may follow.

The responsible agent is an RNA virus approximately 150 nm in diameter although considerable variation in size can occur. Man appears to be the only reservoir and the portal of entry is through the mouth or nose. Infectivity may extend from several days before the illness to several days after the first sign of salivary gland involvement. Virus has been isolated from the blood in the prodromal stage and from the urine up to 14 days after the commencement of clinical illness. It is not clear whether spread to the salivary glands occurs locally or through the bloodstream.

Clinical features

The main incidence occurs between 5 and 15 years of age and is relatively uncommon in younger children and in adults over 30 years.

The incubation period is between 14 and 21 days and the illness may commence with malaise, fever, headache and anorexia; these prodromal symptoms may be absent. Salivary gland involvement commences 1–2 days later and the parotid glands are the most frequently affected. Pain develops around the ear and a swelling appears which extends forwards from the lobe of the ear, downwards over the angle of the jaw and backwards behind the pinna, which is usually pushed outwards. The swelling may be so trivial as to escape casual inspection or be very marked and exquisitely tender. Often only one parotid is involved initially followed in 75% of cases of swelling of the other parotid 1–5 days later. Less often simultaneous and synchronous swelling of both parotids occurs.

Submandibular salivary gland involvement can easily be overlooked as the soft tissues under the jaw readily absorb such swelling, unless it is particularly marked, and it is often the concomitant swelling of the parotids that directs attention to it. Sublingual involvement is much less common but is extremely painful and can be seen readily beneath the upturned tongue.

In addition to salivary gland involvement, the orifice of Stensen's duct may be swollen and the mouth rather dry. Fever is present in the majority of cases, may reach 40°C and persist for up to a week; in fact, cases without salivary gland involvement may present as examples of unexplained fever and recover without the true diagnosis being appreciated, though in others the later development of a typical pattern of complications may indicate mumps to be the cause.

There may be some degree of leukopenia in mumps though certain complications, such as meningitis and pancreatitis, may provoke a leukocytosis.

Complications

Complications are common and varied.

Central nervous system

Aseptic meningitis is the commonest complication and may present before, coincidentally with, or after the illness. The CSF will show a lymphocytic pleocytosis and the count may exceed 1000 cells/μl. The protein content may be moderately raised and the glucose level is usually normal. However, the latter is occasionally decreased in mumps meningitis and where no salivary gland enlargement occurs to indicate the diagnosis, confusion with tuberculous meningitis has occurred. Other less common complications include postinfectious encephalitis, myelitis and polyradiculitis. Although usually unilateral, bilateral nerve deafness, often complete, can also occur as may transient facial paralysis. The virus is easily isolated from the CSF of patients with mumps meningitis which is generally benign. The postinfectious encephalitis is, however, more severe; although complete recovery is usual, neurological sequelae and even death may occur. Virus can be grown from the CSF and an immune-mediated mechanism is likely.

Orchitis

This may occur in 20% of postpubertal males and in younger children can occasionally occur in an undescended testicle. The involvement is usually unilateral but even after severe orchitis sterility is rare, and cases with orchitis should be firmly reassured of the good prognosis.

Pancreatitis

A significant degree of pancreatitis is rare and this complication is overdiagnosed. Salivary gland enlargement by itself raises the serum amylase level but when the pancreas is significantly involved intense pain will occur with rigidity of the abdominal wall and there is often a marked leukocytosis.

Other complications

These include oophoritis, mastitis, bartholinitis, myocarditis, hepatitis, thyroiditis and thrombocytopenic purpura. An occasional case of diabetes mellitus has also been reported following mumps.

Laboratory diagnosis

Viral confirmation of mumps depends on isolation of the virus or the demonstration of a significant rise in antibody titer during the illness.

Mumps virus can be cultured from saliva swabs and urine during the acute illness and from the CSF in cases complicated by meningitis.

Serological tests are readily available to demonstrate a significant rise in antibody titer during the illness and the complement-fixation test is most commonly employed. In this test two specific antigens, soluble (S) and viral (V), are often used. In general, antibody to S antigen rises earlier in the illness than antibody to V antigen, but whereas S antibody may only persist for a few months the V antibody is present for a very long period. Hemagglutination-inhibition and virus neutralization tests are also of help where available.

Differential diagnosis

In children the differential diagnosis is more limited than in adults as in the latter one may encounter more diseases that involve the salivary glands. Conditions that cause lymph node enlargement produce most confusion but careful clinical examination should resolve the difficulty. Pyogenic submandibular abscesses and glandular fever can prove more perplexing and in these instances the blood picture and serum amylase estimations can be helpful. Suppurative parotitis may be considered where there is overlying inflammation and where pus can be expressed from the appropriate salivary duct. Recurrent parotitis is quite common in children. It is not due to repeated attacks of mumps. Sometimes an underlying allergic disorder, sialectasis or duct calculi may be found. Other conditions which may require exclusion are tumors, Mikulicz's syndrome, uveoparotid fever in sarcoidosis, HIV infection, tuberculosis and dental conditions.

Treatment

There is no specific treatment. Pain may be relieved by simple analgesics and the application of heat to the glands can prove soothing. The mouth should be kept clean and a fluid diet is needed until swelling subsides. Neurological complications are managed along customary lines though the diagnostic lumbar puncture in mumps meningitis often produces dramatic relief of headache. In orchitis the testes should be supported and ice bags may ease the discomfort; there is no evidence that corticosteroid drugs, stilbestrol or incision of the tunica albuginea significantly alter the course of this complication.

Prognosis

This is generally good and a fatal outcome exceedingly rare, although permanent brain damage and deafness have been described. Sterility is most unlikely and one attack of mumps appears to provide lifelong immunity.

Prevention

Injections of human antimumps immunoglobulin have been used prophylactically and appear beneficial if given sufficiently early in the incubation period. Live vaccines are safe and produce a good antibody response with long immunity though the duration has not been fully substantiated. They can be used to immunize contacts, and are incorporated into the mumps–measles–rubella (MMR) vaccine for routine immunization in many countries.

COXSACKIE AND ECHO VIRUS INFECTIONS

Respiratory illness in association with these enteroviruses is usually of a mild character.

Certain *Coxsackie viruses* produce specific respiratory syndromes; some group A serotypes are identified as the cause of *herpangina* and certain group B viruses are the agents responsible for pleurodynia (Bornholm disease). Agents from both groups of Coxsackie viruses have been found in association with mild febrile respiratory disease and one strain, Coxsackie A 21 (Coe virus), has been recovered with particular frequency from outbreaks in young servicemen.

ECHO viruses are not usually regarded as respiratory pathogens but they have been found in the throat or feces during upper respiratory disease. Amongst serotypes isolated in these circumstances are ECHO viruses types 6, 11, 19 and 20.

The laboratory diagnosis of infections due to Coxsackie and ECHO viruses is described in the section specifically devoted to these agents.

RHINOVIRUS INFECTIONS

Rhinoviruses are the main cause of the common cold. There are many serologically distinct types. They belong to the large group of picornaviruses, meaning small RNA viruses, but unlike Coxsackie and ECHO viruses they are acid labile at pH 3.

The common cold is probably the most ubiquitous infection in man and the illness tends to be more severe in children than in adults with an acute catarrhal inflammation involving the nose, nasopharynx and accessory sinuses. The onset is usually abrupt and is accompanied by a copious watery discharge which may later turn mucopurulent even in the absence of bacterial superinfection. Little or no fever occurs and constitutional symptoms are mild.

Apart from their ability to produce the common cold, rhinoviruses have been found in association with acute wheezing episodes in children and with pneumonia.

Laboratory diagnosis

Nasopharyngeal aspirates in virus transport medium, nose swab or throat swab collected during the acute stage of the respiratory illness should be sent to the laboratory for the isolation of rhinoviruses. Serology is generally unhelpful. ELISA and PCR for rhinovirus have been developed but are not widely available.

CORONAVIRUSES

Human coronaviruses (HCV) are probably almost as frequent a cause of colds and acute upper respiratory tract infections as rhinovirus infections (McIntosh 1985). Coronaviruses have also been associated with wheeze and pneumonia (Isaacs et al 1983). The exact frequency of HCV infections has been difficult to ascertain because coronaviruses are difficult to grow and can often only be isolated in tracheal organ cultures. The diagnosis can be made by ELISA on respiratory secretions or serologically by detecting antibody to one of the two main serotypes, 229E and 0043. PCR is not widely available.

REOVIRUS INFECTIONS

In 1954 a new group of respiratory-entero or reovirus agents was recognized. It had originally been thought to belong to the ECHO virus group. Since then three distinct types (1, 2 and 3) have been serologically differentiated though they share a common complement-fixing antigen.

Following these preliminary investigations reoviruses have been isolated from many different animal hosts in widely separated areas. These viruses have also been recovered from rectal and throat swabs taken from children suffering from mild respiratory disease, diarrhea, and occasionally fatal pneumonia.

The exact role of reoviruses in producing human disease is largely undetermined. However, the family Reoviridae also includes the agents named rotaviruses which are associated with gastroenteritis, especially in children (see p. 1293).

Laboratory diagnosis

Reoviruses can be isolated from pharyngeal swabs and nasal secretions but they are more commonly recovered from feces.

Acute and convalescent samples of serum are required for hemagglutination-inhibiting antibody titer estimations; a fourfold, or greater, rise in titer during the illness is evidence of infection with a reovirus.

Rotaviruses are difficult to culture and diagnosis depends on electron microscopic examination or ELISA tests on feces.

PSITTACOSIS

Psittacosis is a zoonosis contracted from birds or objects they have contaminated. It was originally considered that infection could only result from birds of the psittacine group (psittacosis) but it is now appreciated that infection may arise from many other birds, both wild and domesticated (ornithosis) and animals such as sheep and goats (Macfarlane & Macrae 1983).

Chlamydia psittaci, the causative organism, belongs to the genus *Chlamydia*. This genus appears to occupy an intermediate position between viruses and rickettsiae. The organisms are obligate intracellular parasites which show sensitivity to certain antibiotics.

Clinical features

The presentation is usually with high fever, chills, headache, myalgia, chest pain, anorexia and fatigue. A dry cough may become productive and fine rales are heard. The pulse may be relatively slow. There may be no history of bird or animal contact, but contact with a sick bird is suggestive. Chest radiography may show perihilar infiltrates, atelectasis or even consolidation. Children and adolescents seem less susceptible to psittacosis than adults (Nagington 1984). However, this may merely reflect the fact that less specific illness is produced in the young and the diagnosis may therefore be overlooked.

Laboratory diagnosis

A clinical diagnosis of psittacosis can be confirmed by serological tests or by isolation of the causative agent. The estimation of complement-fixing antibodies in acute and convalescent samples of serum is a reliable and popular test, which avoids the hazards involved in the isolation of a highly infectious agent. The acute sample of serum should be collected as early in the illness as possible and a convalescent sample may be taken about 2 weeks after the onset of the illness; it is often worthwhile examining a third sample of serum obtained after a further 2 weeks. A fourfold, or greater, rise in antibody titer during the illness is indicative of infection with a member of the psittacosis–lymphogranuloma venereum group of agents.

The psittacosis agent can be isolated from blood in the early stages of the illness and later from pleural fluid and infected tissues. In the case of respiratory illness it is usual to send sputum or throat washings to the laboratory. Positive results may be available within a few days but it is frequently necessary to passage the material.

Prognosis

Spontaneous recovery is to be expected but where the diagnosis is confirmed during the clinical illness tetracycline (except in children less than 8 years old) or erythromycin should be given, as this may reduce symptoms and hasten convalescence.

CHLAMYDIA PNEUMONIAE

Chlamydia pneumoniae, previously called the TWAR agent (from Taiwan-associated respiratory agent) is closely related to *Chlamydia psittaci*, and cross-reacts with it in complement-fixation serological tests (Grayston et al 1986). As the serological assays for *C. pneumoniae* are not widely available this organism may be responsible for reported cases of person-to-person spread of psittacosis and cases with no history of bird or animal contact. During mass chest X-ray screening in Finland a number of young adults were identified with a single patch of pneumonic consolidation. They mostly had mild respiratory symptoms with dry cough, and were found to have antibodies to *C. pneumoniae*. Serological surveys suggest it is a not uncommon cause of pneumonia in children, particularly in developing countries. Treatment is as for psittacosis.

CHLAMYDIA TRACHOMATIS

Chlamydia trachomatis, acquired by passage through an infected birth canal, can cause a pneumonitis usually at 3–11 weeks of age (Rettig 1986). There may be a history of maternal vaginal discharge and the infant may have had conjunctivitis (see p. 1430). The infant is afebrile with a characteristic staccato cough. There are often rales and rhonchi on auscultation. About half the infants have otitis media with a pearly white tympanic membrane. The radiographic appearance is of diffuse pulmonary infiltrates with peribronchial thickening and focal consolidation. Definitive diagnosis is by culturing *Chlamydia trachomatis* or detecting antigen in a nasopharyngeal aspirate or conjunctival swab, or by detecting specific IgM by immunofluorescence. Presumptive evidence can be obtained by demonstrating characteristic inclusions on conjunctival scrapings if there is active conjunctivitis. Treatment is with erythromycin 40 mg/kg/day 6-hourly for 14 days but there may be chronic pulmonary sequelae. The parents should also be treated.

MYCOPLASMA PNEUMONIAE

For many years a distinct clinical entity known as *primary atypical pneumonia* was recognized but an exact basis could not be demonstrated. A specific viral causation was always suspected, and following Eaton's studies on this syndrome, a causative filterable agent (subsequently referred to as Eaton's agent) appeared to have been found. Later work has shown that *Mycoplasma pneumoniae*, a pleuropneumonia-like organism (PPLO) belonging to the distinctive genus of mycoplasmas, and not a virus, is responsible for some cases of primary atypical pneumonia.

Clinical features (see p. 569)

Mycoplasma pneumoniae may give rise to inapparent infection, mild upper respiratory tract infection, bronchitis, bronchiolitis, bronchopneumonia and bullous myringitis both in adults and children; furthermore, some childhood infections occur in epidemic form. *Mycoplasma pneumoniae* may have an etiologic role in some cases of Stevens–Johnson syndrome and can also cause myocarditis, pericarditis, arthritis and encephalitis. When it causes pneumonia, the radiological appearance may be of bilateral, diffuse reticular infiltrates or of consolidation including lobar consolidation (Sabato et al 1984).

Laboratory diagnosis

The isolation of *Mycoplasma pneumoniae* can now be undertaken by many laboratories but the agent grows slowly and often the results of serological tests are available before the isolation and identity of the mycoplasma has been established. The agent can be isolated from sputum, throat washings or pharyngeal swabs.

For serological studies, acute and convalescent samples of serum should be collected. Various serological tests are available but the complement-fixation test appears popular and reliable. A single high titer of IgG antibodies to *Mycoplasma pneumoniae* on an acute serum sample may also be helpful since there is often a fairly long history before presentation.

Cold agglutinins are present in the serum in many cases and, although their detection is not specific for *Mycoplasma* infection, may be useful in acute management.

Treatment

Mycoplasma pneumoniae displays sensitivity to certain antibiotics, particularly tetracycline (25–50 mg/kg/day) and erythromycin (30–50 mg/kg/day), and where a diagnosis is made during the active stage of illness, treatment by one of these drugs should be employed. Erythromycin is preferable in children under 9 years old in view of the potential toxicity of tetracycline.

Q FEVER (QUERY FEVER)

This disease results from infection by *Rickettsia burnetii* (*Coxiella burnetii*) and usually presents as an influenza-like illness with fever and headache, often followed by an atypical pneumonic illness. Unlike other rickettsial infections, Q fever is unaccompanied by a rash.

Rickettsia burnetii is an obligate intracellular parasite which is highly pleomorphic and contains both RNA and DNA. It is more resistant to chemical and physical agents than other pathogenic rickettsiae and is relatively sensitive to certain antibiotics.

The natural reservoir of *R. burnetii* is animals such as cattle, sheep and goats, as well as certain ticks, and the latter are probably involved in animal-to-animal spread. Infection in humans may arise from the handling of infected meat and placentae, the inhalation of infected dust in farmyards and from the consumption of infected raw milk. Cases are most likely to be found in farm workers, slaughtermen and shepherds; however, where milk is the vehicle of transmission, the disease may occur without any apparent occupational link and involve children.

Clinical features

Q fever is less commonly diagnosed in children than in adults because the illness produced in younger age groups is less severe and less intensively studied.

There is usually an incubation period of 2–3 weeks and the illness starts abruptly with fever, rigors, headache, malaise and weakness. In some instances the illness may terminate in approximately 1 week without any further progression but in most diagnosed cases the patient goes on to develop a cough and chest pain. Physical signs may be absent or minimal, though chest X-ray shows pneumonitis.

Severe cases may have symptoms for up to 3 weeks and radiological abnormalities can take a similar period to resolve. The surveying of contacts shows that inapparent infection can also occur. Occasionally Q fever presents with meningoencephalitis and in such instances diagnosis can be difficult.

Complications

The main complication is Q fever, or rickettsial, endocarditis (Tobin et al 1982). To date this has only been seen in persons with pre-existing valvular disease of the heart and the clinical presentation is one of subacute bacterial endocarditis in which repeated blood cultures prove negative. Granulomatous hepatitis and bone granulomas have been described.

Laboratory diagnosis

Rickettsia burnetii can be isolated in laboratory animals or fertile hen's eggs. However, owing to its high infectivity, serological tests are preferably employed to confirm a clinical diagnosis and a complement-fixation test or immunofluorescence is used on acute and convalescent sera.

Treatment

Prodromal symptoms require symptomatic treatment. Once the diagnosis is made tetracycline (25 mg/kg/day) should be given in standard dosage for 2 weeks. Chloramphenicol is the drug of choice in young children. Therapy should not be withheld where the diagnosis is retrospective and the patient has recovered; it is important to ensure eradication of the infection and avoid the possibility of chronicity. Endocarditis has a grave prognosis.

VIRUS INFECTIONS OF THE CENTRAL NERVOUS SYSTEM

The viruses that may occasionally result in devastating neurological damage are more usually associated with a benign clinical illness or even subclinical infection. The reasons for this selective vulnerability remain unexplained but older theories of specific neurotropism have been largely disproved; in fact only a few viral agents such as rabies appear to have a particular predilection to attack the nervous system.

Viral infection of the nervous system may be established beyond question by the demonstration of specific viruses in neural tissue or in the cerebrospinal fluid (Grandien & Olding-Stenkvist 1984). However, in certain instances of suspected viral infection no such proof has been forthcoming and in these instances it is postulated that an autoimmune or other immunological process takes place within the nervous system.

Against some of these diseases, such as poliomyelitis and rabies, immunization procedures are available and antiviral chemotherapy may have some part to play in the treatment of herpes simplex and certain types of encephalitis. In the main, however, treatment is symptomatic.

VIRUS MENINGITIS (ASEPTIC MENINGITIS, LYMPHOCYTIC MENINGITIS)

Meningitis may follow infection by a wide variety of viruses. Most frequently Coxsackie and ECHO viruses are involved, but cases may also arise following infection by the viruses of mumps, measles, lymphocytic choriomeningitis, herpes simplex, poliomyelitis, varicella-zoster and the *Arbovirus* (*Togavirus*) group.

The prognosis of uncomplicated viral meningitis is good and the pleocytosis stimulated in the CSF is usually, but not exclusively, lymphocytic in character. In fact, the terms viral and lymphocytic meningitis may be used synonymously but the latter term lacks strict accuracy as the pleocytosis may be entirely polymorphonuclear in the earliest days of attack. Perhaps benign, acute aseptic meningitis is a preferable descriptive title since certain nonviral infections, such as leptospirosis, can cause a similar picture in the spinal fluid. Enteroviral meningitis commonly occurs in the summer and autumn months in temperate climates but no such seasonal variation is seen in the tropics.

Clinical features

Viral meningitis is most commonly encountered in children up to the age of 10 years although a sizable proportion of cases is also encountered in adolescents and young adults. There is quite a marked male preponderance in early childhood cases. The clinical picture of viral meningitis may be variable. Where infection is due to such agents as mumps or measles, the well-defined stigmata of these diseases may suggest the actual virus responsible. However, in many instances there is no pathognomonic clinical picture that permits the exact viral cause to be deduced. Certain enteroviral infections may produce a rash but these are rarely so characteristic as to be diagnostic and detailed virological studies are required to elucidate the responsible agent.

In general, there is an introductory illness of short duration and symptoms and signs of meningitis may follow immediately. In some, a short period of apparent recovery intervenes between the prodromal illness and nervous system involvement – a situation rather like the minor and major illness seen in poliomyelitis. The actual symptoms and signs simulate those of any other type of infective meningitis but are usually less pronounced. The progressive coma and marked toxicity of bacterial meningitis are usually absent and, in the average case, the full clinical picture together with analysis of the CSF permits broad division of the case into a bacterial or aseptic group, most of the latter being the result of viral infection.

The blood count is usually normal though an early leukocytosis or leukopenia may be noted. The cerebrospinal fluid will usually be clear with a moderate increase in lymphocytes. The glucose level will be within normal limits with the exception of aseptic meningitis following mumps in which there may be some degree of hypoglycorrhachia. The protein content is modestly increased but rarely exceeds 100 mg/100 ml (1 g/l) of CSF.

Differential diagnosis

Although the epidemiological background and clinical features may suggest a likely etiologic cause, a definitive diagnosis is dependent on detailed laboratory studies. Confusion can arise from leptospiral meningitis, cryptococcal infection, partially treated bacterial meningitis and tuberculous meningitis. Less often noninfectious conditions such as sarcoidosis, leukemia and other forms of malignant disease can produce CSF findings that are confusing.

Laboratory diagnosis

Virus may be isolated from throat swabs, feces, CSF or urine and the specimens should be inoculated into appropriate tissue cultures and, where indicated, into suckling mice. As the yield from CSF is low in viral meningitis it is particularly important to send a stool and throat swab for virus isolation. Acute and convalescent samples of serum, preferably collected 3 weeks apart, should be tested for appropriate antibodies, but enteroviral serology is not very satisfactory and virus isolation is preferable.

Treatment

There is no specific treatment. Bed rest is desirable until symptoms and fever have settled as hasty mobilization may provoke paralytic disease in certain enteroviral infections. Where the clinical picture is unclear and bacterial infection is the possible cause of the presenting syndrome, empirical antibiotic treatment is justified until the situation becomes clarified by laboratory studies or further developments.

VIRAL ENCEPHALITIDES

See page 693.

POSTINFECTIOUS MYELITIS

Some degree of myelitis may often be found in association with postinfectious encephalitis but on occasion may present as an isolated clinical syndrome (Boos & Esiri 1986). It is rare and there is usually a latent interval between the initiating infection and the development of spinal cord involvement. Age distribution tends to follow the same pattern as postinfectious encephalitis, though in the case of rubella the age tends to be higher. The pathological changes are those associated with postinfectious neurological involvement and direct viral invasion of the cord seems rare except in infections due to polioviruses and enteroviruses. In one study of 911 cases of measles associated with neurological complications 877 showed encephalitis, 24 myelitis and 10 polyradiculitis; a similar distribution can be found for the neurological complications of rubella and chickenpox. Most recorded cases have followed specific exanthemata and the association seems well substantiated by the circumstantial evidence. Occasional reports of myelitis in association with other viral infections are difficult to evaluate as these reports often involve single cases and the association may have been fortuitous; nevertheless, there are good reasons to believe that other agents could play a role in this condition.

The prognosis is difficult to evaluate. Those developing ascending paralysis have a poorer outlook and most of the reported deaths are associated with this picture. Others may be left with permanent spastic paraplegia but those presenting with transverse myelitis often make an unexpectedly rapid and full recovery. The main differential diagnoses are Guillain–Barré syndrome and space-occupying or vascular lesions of the spinal cord.

POSTINFECTIOUS POLYNEURITIS (POSTINFECTIOUS POLYRADICULITIS, LANDRY–GUILLAIN–BARRÉ SYNDROME)

See page 725.

LABORATORY TESTS APPLICABLE TO ENCEPHALITIS, MYELITIS AND POLYNEURITIS

A postmortem examination may confirm a clinical diagnosis of encephalitis but during life the specific type can only be established by isolation and identification of the virus or by serological examination. Several viruses have been associated with encephalitis and consideration requires to be given to geographical and epidemiological factors in determining the possible causative agents.

Brain biopsy material may prove suitable for examination and this is well established in the case of herpes simplex encephalitis (Whitley 1988). It may also be of value in some types of arbovirus infection and in the subacute sclerosing panencephalitis associated with measles (p. 794). Cerebrospinal fluid should certainly be submitted for culture as such agents as enteroviruses and mumps virus may be cultured. Acute and convalescent serum samples should always be collected and tested for a significant rise in antibody titer; guidance will often be available from the associated clinical illness as to which antigens the serum should be tested against. PCR or CSF is increasingly available for a range of different viruses.

LYMPHOCYTIC CHORIOMENINGITIS

The agent, first recognized in 1934, was entitled lymphocytic choriomeningitis (LCM) virus. This virus is now classified as a member of the Arenavirus group. It occurs in mice.

Sporadic cases and small outbreaks of aseptic meningitis in man due to LCM have been reported in Europe and America in circumscribed areas where infected mouse colonies have been shown to exist (Biggar et al 1975). Although originally suspected to be a common cause of aseptic meningitis, it is now known to have a very small role except in areas of endemic infection in mice.

Clinical features

The incubation period of LCM lies between 7 and 14 days. Any age group may contract the disease if contact with the relevant infected mouse colonies occurs. The clinical picture and the abnormalities in the CSF are identical with those found in other types of viral meningitis and etiologic diagnosis can only be made by laboratory studies. LCM can also cause mild respiratory illness and, rarely, pneumonia. Orchitis, myopericarditis, arthritis or alopecia may rarely occur. The prognosis is usually excellent though an occasional fatality has been reported in infants. No specific treatment is indicated though control of infected mouse colonies should be undertaken by expert rodent exterminators.

Laboratory diagnosis

The lymphocytic choriomeningitis virus can be isolated from blood in the initial febrile phase of the illness, and from the CSF after the onset of meningitis. The virus can be propagated in young mice and in various tissue cultures.

Complement-fixing and neutralizing antibodies appear in the patient's serum following infection and a serological diagnosis can be made by demonstrating a significant rise in antibody titer during the illness. The antibodies tend to be produced rather late in the illness; as a result the convalescent serum sample for complement-fixing antibodies should be collected about the third week of the illness and that for neutralizing antibodies about 6 weeks after the onset of the disease.

RABIES (HYDROPHOBIA)

Rabies, the most feared of all zoonoses, has been a recognized disease of man since early times (Fishbein & Robinson 1993). Spread to man may occur from a wide variety of warm blooded animals which demonstrate variable susceptibility. Although this susceptibility is extremely high in such animals as foxes, jackals and wolves, it is only moderate in others including the dog. However, as man has a closer association with domestic animals, such as the dog, they provide a greater risk to him. In any particular geographical area enzootic or epizootic infection may predominate in only one or two species of wild animal; in Central and South America the dominant animal is the vampire bat, in Russia the wolf, in North America the skunk, and in Europe the fox.

Certain areas of the world are currently free of rabies including Australia, New Zealand, certain Pacific islands, parts of Scandinavia and Great Britain. In an attempt to retain this position the movement of animals is governed by strict regulations including compulsory quarantine of animals, but such measures can be severely stretched. Enzootic rabies was eradicated from Great Britain in 1922 but fears exist that the current epizootic amongst foxes in Europe, which has spread rapidly westwards over recent years, may result in the reintroduction of rabies.

Casual contact with a rabid animal should not produce infection in man as this will usually only follow a specific bite. However, infection can follow the licking of abraded skin or mucosae by an infected animal. It is also suggested that airborne infection from bats to man can occur within caves where such animals are roosting. In most instances suspicion will arise that the animal concerned is rabid especially where the furious form of the disease occurs. Should the less dramatic, dumb form occur, however, the true nature of the illness is not so readily suspected.

Clinical features

The incubation period may be as short as 10 days or as prolonged as 7 years but is usually between 1 and 3 months. Wounds on the hands, forearm and neck are especially dangerous and in them, or where there is extensive biting at any site, the incubation period may be shortened. Age may also be a factor and cases in young children tend to have a shorter incubation period.

The onset of clinical illness is heralded by a prodromal period which may last from 2 to 7 days. Indefinite sensory changes may be experienced at the site of the bite together with such nonspecific features as slight fever, headache, malaise, nausea and sore throat. Paresis and paralysis then develop and the muscles of deglutition go into spasm at any attempt to swallow (hence the term hydrophobia). Increasing depression and anxiety become apparent and the patient may become very withdrawn.

The disease may now enter a stage of excitement (furious rabies) with alternating manic activity and calm. The patient will remain lucid but fearful and the spasms in the throat become more violent. Cranial nerve palsies may develop and generalized convulsions become frequent. Death follows in virtually every case from either cardiac or respiratory arrest. Less often the picture is not so florid and a progressive ascending paralysis occurs giving rise to the so-called dumb form of the disease.

Clinical diagnosis

A classical case, following a significant bite, provides a clearly recognizable clinical picture. Otherwise, forms of viral encephalitis, bulbar poliomyelitis, hysteria and tetanus may produce similar features and cause diagnostic confusion. Encephalitis following antirabies vaccination with the old vaccines can occur and produce a similar picture to that of rabies itself, although this has not been recorded following the human diploid cell vaccine.

Laboratory diagnosis

Rabies virus is probably not a single antigenic species and four rabies-related viruses are recognized. These agents have a marked predilection for nervous tissue but multiply in other organs such as the salivary glands. Within the nervous system the main pathological process is an encephalomyelitis leading to the development of inclusion bodies particularly within the hippocampus. These inclusions are known as Negri bodies.

During life the laboratory diagnosis of rabies depends on testing such specimens as saliva, cerebrospinal fluid and conjunctival secretions by animal inoculation and immunofluorescent techniques. The rapidly fatal outcome, and the confusion which serum or vaccine can introduce, may render serological tests unhelpful.

After death, specimens of brain tissue should be inoculated intracerebrally into mice. The specimens should also be subjected to rabies immunofluorescent tests and examined for Negri bodies. These tests should yield results within 1–2 days. However, if they are inconclusive the results of mouse inoculation must be awaited, and it may take up to 3 weeks to declare this test negative.

Treatment

The treatment of clinical rabies is largely symptomatic but intensive supportive therapy including artificial ventilation has been employed and at least two cases of proven rabies have survived following such measures. Appropriate steps must be taken to avoid possible spread to the attendants and to the immediate environment.

Postexposure prophylaxis

Local treatment of the wound. This can prove highly beneficial and should not be overlooked or delayed. Ideally wounds should be thoroughly cleansed using a 20% soap solution and, after washing any residual soap away with water, a 0.1% quaternary ammonium compound such as cetrimide should be applied. Alternatives include 40–70% alcohol or tincture and aqueous solutions of iodine. Should none of these agents be immediately available, extensive cleansing with clean water should be used as early as possible and the chemical agents employed when practicable. Primary suturing of the wounds should be avoided and human rabies immunoglobulin (HRIG) may be infiltrated into the tissue beneath the wound. If there is any suspicion of exposure to tetanus, appropriate prophylaxis against this disease should be instituted.

Special systemic treatment. The aim of prophylaxis by vaccination is to induce a rapid antibody response which may prevent clinical disease developing, and is safe and highly effective. Several vaccines are available for postexposure treatment and the site and frequency of injections will depend on the vaccine used. If the human diploid cell vaccine is used, vaccination should commence as soon as possible after the incident and injections should be given by deep subcutaneous or intramuscular injection on days 0, 3, 7, 14, and 28. As antibodies do not develop for some days human rabies immunoglobulin may be given intramuscularly as well as infiltrating the wound

(Bahmanyar et al 1976) of those not previously immunized. Treatment may be discontinued if the suspected dog or cat remains healthy after observation for 5 days; other animals may require longer periods of observation.

Pre-exposure prophylaxis. Prophylaxis by the human diploid cell rabies vaccine may be used for those at high risk of contracting rabies, e.g. laboratory staff or veterinary staff in endemic areas (Anderson et al 1980). Immunization is not routinely recommended for those visiting endemic areas.

SLOW VIRUS DISEASES

Slow virus diseases, transmissible diseases with an incubation period of some years, were described in animals long before man. In 1976 Gajdusek was awarded the Nobel Prize for his classic description of the CNS degenerative disease, kuru, which affects the Fore people in New Guinea as a 'slow virus' disease. A number of other viruses have now been implicated as falling into the general realm of slow virus diseases (Adams & Bell 1976). Of these, infection with human immunodeficiency virus (p. 1392) is surely the best studied.

Subacute sclerosing panencephalitis (SSPE)

There is now overwhelming evidence that this progressive CNS degenerative disorder is caused by measles virus. It is suspected that the disease reflects an abnormal immunological response to persisting measles virus or measles virus antigen. Children with SSPE make antibodies to most measles antigens but do not make antibodies to the matrix (M) protein. Whether this is important in permitting the virus to become latent is not known. Children with SSPE have high titers of antibody to measles virus by complement-fixation test in both serum and CSF. The clinical features of SSPE are described elsewhere (p. 794). Measles vaccination of a population leads to a decreased incidence of SSPE.

Rubella panencephalitis

Progressive panencephalitis may complicate both stable congenital and acquired rubella infections. The disease somewhat resembles SSPE but in active rubella encephalitis there is detectable virus in the CSF, together with a pleocytosis and elevated protein. Rubella antibodies are present in both blood and CSF. The pathological picture is variable but usually one of a chronic meningoencephalitis with focal areas of degenerative vascular change.

Children present between 8 and 12 years of age with mental decline followed some months to years later by myoclonic jerks, chorea, ataxia, nystagmus and spasticity. The course is slower than SSPE and patients may survive 10 or more years.

Progressive multifocal leukoencephalopathy

This disease is a demyelinating disease caused by infection of astrocytes and oligodendrocytes with one of two papovaviruses, namely JC virus and simian virus 40 (SV40). The commoner of the two to cause disease, JC, is named after the initials of the first affected patient, a 38-year-old man with Hodgkin's disease who developed PML, and should not be confused with Creutzfeldt–Jakob disease. All cases have been in patients who are immunosuppressed, e.g. postrenal transplant, have a malignant lymphoproliferative disorder or have a chronic disease such as tuberculosis or sarcoidosis. All areas of the brain and spinal cord may be affected. The usual presentation is early dementia with confusion, impaired cerebration and labile affect. There is often focal weakness progressing to hemiparesis and later bilateral long tract signs. Blindness, aphasia and ataxia are usual with death occurring in less than 6 months.

Subacute spongiform encephalopathies (kuru, Creutzfeldt–Jakob disease)

The subacute spongiform encephalopathies of man, kuru and Creutzfeldt–Jakob disease, closely resemble two animal diseases, scrapie and transmissible mink encephalopathy. Progressive degeneration of neurons with demyelination and gliosis of gray matter cause a spongiform appearance of the brain. The incubation period is up to 20 years. In kuru the cerebellum is most affected, and the disease is characterized by a progressive ataxia with a shivering tremor (the word 'kuru' means shivering). It was acquired by the women and children of the Fore tribe in New Guinea who ate the brains of dead kinsfolk.

Creutzfeldt–Jakob disease (CJD) is a progressive dementia with varying neurological features. Myoclonus, ataxic tremor, spasticity and parkinsonian features have all been described. CJD is sometimes familial. Cases have occurred in children who received human growth hormone from human pituitary extracts unwittingly infected with the agent and through brain and eye surgery. These two diseases are currently thought to be due to *prions*, transmissible proteins.

INFECTIONS DUE TO ENTEROVIRUSES

POLIOMYELITIS (INFANTILE PARALYSIS, ACUTE ANTERIOR POLIOMYELITIS)

Poliomyelitis is amongst the most feared of the communicable diseases. Documentation over the last century has recorded many epidemics of variable severity with sporadic cases being reported at interepidemic periods. Furthermore, there are historical references which show that poliomyelitis has been a disease of man for many centuries though these indicate that it has become more virulent since the late 19th century.

Modern epidemiological and virological surveys show that in the great majority of infected persons poliomyelitis is a harmless subclinical event; nevertheless, severe epidemics can arise with remarkable rapidity and the mortality and morbidity that result demonstrate that the fear in which the disease is held is well founded.

Epidemiology

Man appears to be the main reservoir of polioviruses in nature and their proven presence in sewage, flies and food is probably of minor importance. In temperate climates epidemics occur in summer months. Poliomyelitis has shown a change in its epidemiological pattern; the large epidemics of the early 1950s were associated with a higher attack rate in older children and in young adults. The clinical severity showed a parallel rise and these severe epidemics occurred in countries with a high standard of living; a possible explanation put forward for this change was that improved hygienic standards led to a diminished rate of subclinical infection in infancy. In view of this it became a matter of great urgency to provide effective immunization against poliomyelitis and it was fortuitous that developments in this field were so timely. The Expanded Program of Immunization of the World Health Organization has led to a steady decline in the world incidence of poliomyelitis since 1973, and the total eradication of poliomyelitis from the Americas has been one of the major health achievements of the 20th century (Patriarca et al 1993).

Etiology

There are three strains, polioviruses types 1, 2 and 3, which show little antigenic overlap. They are particularly small having a diameter of 25 nm and contain RNA. Poliovirus type 1 has been associated with most of the major epidemics and shows the greatest propensity to cause paralytic forms of the disease, whereas type 2 causes sporadic cases or small outbreaks with a low incidence of paralysis; type 3 occupies an intermediate position. Certain factors appear to influence the virulence of polioviruses in the human host. Clinical severity is increased by age and pregnancy. Excessive muscular activity in a recently infected person makes a paralytic form of the disease more probable as do certain intramuscular injections into the limbs and other minor, traumatic procedures. Tonsillectomy, especially where recent, predisposes to bulbar poliomyelitis and corticosteroid drugs can have an adverse effect. Antibody is clearly important as there is a higher incidence in patients with antibody deficiency.

The disease is spread by direct contact with infected persons through pharyngeal secretions and feces. Infectivity is probably maximal early on and oral–oral spread may be more common than fecal–oral spread. Rarely paralytic poliomyelitis may result from oral vaccine strains which revert to virulence.

Pathogenesis and pathology

Polioviruses enter the body via the oral route and multiply in the tonsillopharyngeal tissues and in the intestinal wall. From the former they pass to regional lymph nodes and infectivity of the pharyngeal secretions disappears rapidly; from the latter, viruses also pass to the appropriate regional lymph nodes but in this case there is continued excretion into the bowel. This is shown by the ease with which polioviruses can be isolated from the feces for weeks and sometimes months.

The viruses probably pass to the bloodstream from the infected lymph nodes and can be isolated from the blood on occasion. The mode of passage thereafter to the nervous system is not fully understood.

In man the pathological lesions in the central nervous system are mainly found in the anterior horns of the spinal cord but the posterior horns and intermediate columns may be involved. The essential lesion is neuronal damage and though some neurons will die others may recover. Meningitis occurs and in some cases there is an extensive encephalitis involving motor cells in the medulla and pons, the vestibular nuclei and the motor and premotor areas of the cerebral cortex. Sometimes the lesions are concentrated in the medulla with little damage at lower levels in the cord.

Clinical features

Poliomyelitis is highly infectious and has an incubation period of 1–3 weeks. Paralytic disease virtually only occurs in unimmunized children or adults, as the virus still circulates in the community. In countries where vaccination is not performed and where low economic standards obtain, poliomyelitis is still primarily a disease of infants and young children. Most persons infected will have an inapparent illness which can only be demonstrated by retrospective serological surveys or by examination of contacts in the course of an actual epidemic.

The minor illness

Persons infected by polioviruses may respond with a mild, insignificant illness whose features may include fever, anorexia, headache, lassitude and gastroenteritic symptoms. The title of 'abortive poliomyelitis' was sometimes used to describe this condition which is now more commonly referred to as the minor illness.

The major illness (nonparalytic or preparalytic poliomyelitis)

The major illness may immediately follow the minor or there may be a short gap of apparent recovery. Occasionally the minor illness does not occur.

In the preparalytic stage of the major illness, the symptoms simulate those of aseptic meningitis. The patient will experience headache, vomiting, malaise and fever. Later, pain and stiffness may be felt in the neck and back. Nuchal rigidity and a positive Kernig's sign are usually elicited on examination. Patients may also complain of an aching pain and spasm in the limbs but this is rarely as marked a feature as older accounts of the disease suggest.

A lumbar puncture performed at this time will normally demonstrate a mild CSF pleocytosis (either polymorphonuclear or lymphocytic) and slight to moderate elevation of the protein content.

A variable percentage of cases presenting with this picture will gradually improve over the ensuing 7–10 days and thereafter make an uninterrupted recovery (nonparalytic poliomyelitis). Others, unfortunately, proceed to paralysis. Most paralytic cases pass through the preparalytic stage outlined above; the paralysis starting some 2–3 days later. Occasionally, paralysis comes on earlier or the preparalytic stage is absent.

Paralytic poliomyelitis

Spinal paralysis. The cervical and lumbar segments of the cord are most frequently involved and patchy, asymmetrical paralysis in the limbs results. This may be trivial and can be confined to part of one muscle group when it is easily overlooked. Unilateral involvement of the dorsiflexors of the feet, of the quadriceps or of the deltoids is a common finding. The paralysis is of lower motor neuron type.

Spinal respiratory paralysis. This form is usually associated with rapid, severe limb paralysis, and neuronal damage may then extend through the central part of the cord. Paralysis of the abdominal muscles may show itself by weakness in the cough though lower intercostal involvement may be symptomless to the patient at rest and only evident to the examiner. Eventually such signs as tachypnea, tachycardia, cyanosis, a rising blood pressure and mental confusion will become apparent. In some instances the signs of increasing ventilatory failure are difficult to distinguish from those of bulbar involvement or encephalitis and these conditions can be simultaneously present.

Bulbar poliomyelitis. This form may be seen with unusual frequency in some epidemics and can be associated with recent tonsillectomy. Difficulty in swallowing is the cardinal sign and the subject is unable to clear mucus and saliva from the throat. There is a reluctance on the part of the patient to breathe deeply in case secretions become aspirated into the lung. Such symptoms arise from pharyngeal involvement and further spread may occur manifesting itself in weakness of the flexors of the neck, facial paralysis, external ocular palsies and, occasionally, true laryngeal paralysis. Extension to the respiratory center, with totally irregular breathing and periods of apnea, has a grave prognosis and involvement of the circulatory center will result in circulatory collapse and an irregular, rapid pulse. Involvement of these vital centers is usually fatal.

Laboratory diagnosis

Isolation of the poliovirus from the patient is the method of choice. Polioviruses grow well in a variety of tissue cultures and providing specimens are collected early in the illness successful virus isolation is not difficult. Virus may be recovered from throat swabs during the early stages of the illness and from the feces for several weeks after the onset. Cerebrospinal fluid should be cultured for polioviruses but unlike Coxsackie and ECHO viruses, these are found infrequently.

Acute and convalescent samples of serum should be obtained and tested for a significant rise in antibody titer during the illness; tests for both complement-fixing and neutralizing antibodies are available.

Differential diagnosis

Nonparalytic poliomyelitis cannot be differentiated on clinical grounds from other conditions causing the syndrome of aseptic meningitis. Paralytic poliomyelitis may be confused with a variety of disorders including acute polyneuritis (both of infective and toxic types), acute porphyria, localized paralysis following specific infections such as mumps or infectious mononucleosis, paralytic episodes in sickle cell disease, myasthenia gravis and familial periodic paralysis.

Particular forms of poliomyelitis can be specially confusing, such as isolated facial paralysis which may mimic Bell's palsy and bulbar paralysis which can be mistaken for tetanus. Pseudo-paralysis may be found in acute rheumatism, osteomyelitis, fractures, scurvy, congenital syphilis and hysteria.

Emphasis must also be laid on the fact that a true poliomyelitis-like illness can follow infection by other enteroviruses such as Coxsackie virus A7, ECHO virus type 3 and others. Wherever possible the diagnosis of any case of clinical poliomyelitis should be supported by virus isolation and positive serological tests.

Complications, course and prognosis

Nonparalytic poliomyelitis

There are no complications of nonparalytic forms of polio-myelitis. However, unsuspected paralysis may be detected in cases of this type once they become mobilized and this is particularly seen in the back muscles, the strength of which is difficult to assess whilst the patient remains in bed.

Spinal paralytic poliomyelitis

Some recovery may occur in the first 4 weeks following paralysis. Improvement thereafter is much slower. In those muscles where the neuronal supply has been severely affected, permanent paralysis with extremely rapid wasting will result.

Spinal respiratory paralysis

At the height of the illness in this group various cardiac irregularities and even cardiac failure may be encountered and this may be a secondary effect from the respiratory complications or a direct effect of the virus on the myocardium.

Major complications include pneumonia, hypertension, urinary retention and constipation. Renal calculi are not uncommon.

Bulbar poliomyelitis

This form of poliomyelitis is of great seriousness if it spreads to the vital centers in the medulla. However, in those cases without involvement of these centers there is remarkably full and quite rapid recovery of the cranial nerves. Involvement of the diaphragm may be permanent.

Late effects (post-polio syndrome)

People with paralytic polio may develop new symptoms many years later, characterized by pain in muscles, weakness, fasciculation, breathlessness and problems with speech and swallowing. The mechanism is unknown (Dalakas et al 1986).

Treatment

Spinal paralysis

The mainstay of therapy is physiotherapy, emphasizing passive movement and hydrotherapy if available. Paralytic limbs should be supported and splinting may prevent contractures.

Patients may remain fecal excretors of poliovirus for several weeks and isolation procedures must be used.

In children lack of growth in severely paralyzed limbs may lead to significant shortening, and skilled orthopedic advice is needed in such instances.

Spinal respiratory paralysis

Ventilatory support may be required and a constant watch for the incipient onset of respiratory insufficiency must be maintained; if these difficulties are diagnosed late, hypoxia may increase neuronal damage. Where respiratory paralysis is marked ventilation is best achieved by the use of intermittent positive pressure ventilation combined with tracheostomy.

Bulbar poliomyelitis

The milder examples of this condition, where the major defect is inability to swallow, can often be managed conservatively with nasogastric tube feeding and suction of secretions. These patients often do well and undergo spontaneous recovery in 2–3 weeks. More severe cases require tracheostomy. Even in these severe cases the prognosis is good and the tracheostomy can often be closed within a few weeks.

Prevention

Virtually all cases of paralytic poliomyelitis occur in children who have not been immunized. Poliomyelitis outbreaks are unlikely to occur in a community where there is a high level of protection by immunization and where that level is maintained. Active immunization can be produced by either killed virus vaccines (Salk type) or live attenuated virus vaccines (Sabin type). The former require to be given by injection and the latter by the oral route. A full primary course of either type involves three doses with periodic boosting thereafter to maintain protection. In general, Sabin-type vaccines result in higher humoral antibody levels, are easy and painless to administer and also produce local immunity in the gut. Children with immune deficiency are at increased risk of paralytic polio and must be immunized with the killed vaccine. Children with HIV infection can receive either live or killed vaccines, but if there is a relative at home with AIDS who might be infected by the vaccine virus, Salk (killed) vaccine should be given.

COXSACKIE AND ECHO VIRUS INFECTIONS

The *Coxsackie* and ECHO viruses, together with the *polioviruses* are called enteroviruses and are classified with rhinoviruses into a larger group known as the *picornaviruses* (pico = small, RNA viruses). The agents in this group have a similarity in size, a similar nucleic acid core (RNA) and other common physical and chemical properties. Clinical and epidemiological studies show that the Coxsackie and ECHO viruses are widely distributed in man and can cause a considerable variety of clinical syndromes (Dagan et al 1985b). However, they have not demonstrated the same propensity to produce such large and serious epidemics as polioviruses.

COXSACKIE VIRUS INFECTIONS

The existence of this group of viruses became apparent in 1948 when unidentifiable, filterable agents were isolated from the feces of two children in whom a clinical diagnosis of paralytic poliomyelitis had been suspected. These children resided in Coxsackie in New York State and the large group of similar viruses subsequently identified has been named after this town. At the present time there are approximately 30 different varieties of Coxsackie viruses and these have been classified into two groups, known as A and B. 24 of the strains have been allocated to group A and the remaining 6 to group B.

Some, but not all, viruses of the Coxsackie groups may be grown on suitable tissue cultures but all produce a characteristic histopathological effect when injected into suckling mice.

Coxsackie group A virus diseases

Relationship of group A viruses to disease

Viruses of this group may be isolated from a variable percentage of healthy individuals; as a result their isolation from a sick patient must not necessarily be construed as a diagnostic event.

Herpangina

This is one of the most clearly defined clinical syndromes caused by infection with Coxsackie A viruses. It is most commonly seen in infants and children, though can occur in adults. The onset is characterized by fever, anorexia and pain in the throat; other features include headache, abdominal pain and myalgia. Infection will normally derive from another human and the agent may be transmitted from nasal secretions as well as from the feces. The incubation period lies between 3 and 5 days and fecal infectivity may last for several weeks.

Local examination of the mouth will usually reveal hyperemia of the pharynx, and characteristic papulovesicular lesions, approximately 1–2 mm in diameter and surrounded by an erythematous ring, will be seen. Most commonly the lesions are present over the tonsillar pillars, soft palate and uvula though on occasion the tongue may be involved. It is rare to find more than five to six lesions and these soon enlarge and form shallow ulcers. The illness will usually subside within a week and few complications are found in children. Second attacks may result from infection by different antigenic strains. In a classical case the clinical picture is highly suggestive, but laboratory studies are required for full confirmation and at least nine different group A viruses are known to produce this syndrome.

Central nervous system involvement

Aseptic meningitis is the most common clinical manifestation and may result from infection by several different Coxsackie A virus strains. As with other types of viral meningitis young children are most likely to be involved and a rather higher incidence is encountered in male children. There is usually no characteristic clinical picture that differentiates this from other causes of viral meningitis although in a few instances one of the more specific syndromes associated with group A infection may be simultaneously present. On occasion this group may also be associated with paralytic disease that is clinically indistinguishable from poliomyelitis; Coxsackie virus A7 is the most frequently implicated but other strains such as A9 have also been involved. Severe and fatal encephalitis has been described in only a small number of cases of Coxsackie A virus infection.

Hand, foot and mouth disease

In 1957 there was a small epidemic in Toronto of an illness which had certain characteristic features. These included the presence of vesicular lesions in the mouth as well as on the hands and feet. Virological studies on these cases indicated infection with Coxsackie virus A16 and in the ensuing years several similar outbreaks, including some from Britain, were reported. In the majority, Coxsackie virus A16 was once again the responsible virus though in some instances types A5 and A10 were responsible.

This illness presents with little or no constitutional upset. In babies, reluctance to feed may be an early sign and in older children a reluctance to eat. Examination of the mouth often shows some mild ulceration over the tongue and further examination indicates the pearly white vesicles, sometimes surrounded by a red halo, on the extremities. The lesions are mainly found over the ventral surface of the fingers and toes and have a characteristic distribution along the sides of the feet. Some cases also show a maculopapular rash over the buttocks which may extend on to the thighs mimicking Henoch–Schönlein purpura. Fever may occur but it is rarely marked and there is little associated lymphadenopathy.

A fully developed case is extraordinarily characteristic and once seen is readily recognized thereafter. The mouth lesions can be confused with herpetic gingivostomatitis and herpangina as the peripheral lesions are painless, and may be overlooked. An occasional case has been confused with scabies.

Outbreaks of this syndrome are usually small and tend to occur in the summer months. Subclinical infection of family contacts can be demonstrated by the isolation of viruses from them and the prognosis is excellent.

Miscellaneous Coxsackie A virus infections

Coxsackie A viruses have been isolated from children suffering from a febrile illness with a rash, from cases of pharyngitis and from cases of benign pericarditis. They have also been associated with mild undifferentiated respiratory tract infection, especially Coxsackie A21 virus (previously known as Coe virus), with acute febrile lymphadenitis, gastroenteritis, tracheobronchitis and pleurodynia.

Laboratory diagnosis

The isolation of Coxsackie group A viruses is not difficult provided suitable specimens are sent to the laboratory. Suitable specimens include vesicle fluid, throat swabs, feces and CSF, depending on the clinical syndrome under investigation. Serological tests on acute and convalescent serum samples can be carried out but owing to the large number of serotypes this is not a practical procedure unless an agent has been isolated. The Coxsackie virus complement-fixation test frequently employed cross-reacts with all enteroviruses and is not very sensitive. PCR is available in a small number of laboratories.

Coxsackie group B virus diseases

Bornholm disease or epidemic pleurodynia

This disease, first recognized clinically over a century ago, is now known to result from infection with certain group B Coxsackie viruses. Children and young adults are usually involved and more severe cases occur in the latter.

After an incubation period of 2–4 days, the illness commences in a nonspecific manner with fever, malaise and headache. However, the characteristic pain will soon follow and is principally experienced over the lower chest and may be associated with acute dyspnea. A clinical diagnosis of pleurisy may be made though no friction rub is audible and X-ray of the chest is clear. Pain may also be felt lower down the trunk and this may spread over the abdomen and simulate an acute surgical condition. Palpation over the affected muscles may reveal exquisite tenderness and this can have a band-like distribution suggestive of a neurological disorder or shingles.

In many instances the illness subsides within a few days but it may run a relapsing course and last for as long as 3–4 weeks. Several members of a family may be attacked in quick succession and show a wide variation in the severity.

Bornholm disease requires to be differentiated from pleurisy and pneumonia. Acute appendicitis and cholecystitis have been mimicked by an abdominal presentation but milder varieties, without significant pain, can be confused with influenza. In general, there is no significant leukocytosis and this may be helpful in the differentiation of pyogenic infection.

Outbreaks are small and often confined to family units. However, an epidemic can be more widespread and in these instances the correct clinical diagnosis may be made with reasonable accuracy. Nevertheless, full confirmation requires detailed virological assessment.

Central nervous system involvement

The etiologic role of the group B viruses in *aseptic meningitis* is fully established and all six types have been incriminated in this illness. The age incidence appears similar to that encountered in aseptic meningitis due to other viruses as indicated on page 1375. Clinical differentiation from other possible causes is impossible though pleurodynia is an occasional accompaniment. Severe and fatal encephalitis has been described in only a small number of cases as has mild paralytic disease.

Cardiac involvement

The clinical syndrome of *acute myocarditis* in infants and children has been variously described as idiopathic, isolated, Fiedler's or interstitial myocarditis. However, in the light of present knowledge, it has proved possible to make a definitive, causative diagnosis in an increasing proportion of such illness and the role of Coxsackie B viruses, and to a lesser degree some group A agents, has become firmly established.

Coxsackie B myocarditis of infancy

Coxsackie viruses B1–5 have been incriminated in this disorder though types B3 and B4 have been implicated most frequently (Kaplan et al 1983). The illness usually commences within the first 2 weeks of life though older babies have been involved. Most neonatal cases are probably caused by vertical spread from an infected mother, and a maternal history of respiratory or gastrointestinal illness is common. Nursery outbreaks can also occur.

Clinical features. (see p. 630). The onset is always sudden. Presenting symptoms include feeding difficulties, lethargy, fever, cyanosis, respiratory distress and shock. Cardiomegaly, tachycardia, hepatomegaly and electrocardiographic changes soon appear. Involvement may not be confined to the cardiovascular system. In up to one-third of cases central nervous signs such as convulsions, neck stiffness, coma and CSF disturbances are encountered.

The prognosis is poor and up to 75% of cases die in spite of intensive therapy. At autopsy an intense inflammatory infiltration and necrosis is found in the myocardium and changes may also be found in the liver, pancreas, suprarenal glands, bone marrow and central nervous system.

Differential diagnosis. Myocarditis is a difficult entity to diagnose in a neonate. Most cases are initially considered to be some form of acute respiratory disorder (e.g. respiratory distress syndrome), other overwhelming infections or congenital heart disease.

Treatment. Infants with this condition require to be intensively nursed in hospital; oxygen, diuretics and digitalization may be required, although the heart is often very sensitive to digoxin and low doses may be needed.

Pericarditis and myocarditis due to Coxsackie B viruses in older children

Acute pericarditis in older children and adults is a syndrome where the causative role of Coxsackie B viruses (types B1–5) is well established. Less often, myocarditis may also occur in these age groups but, unlike infection in neonates, the prognosis is generally good. Clinical recovery is quite rapid and although the electrocardiographic changes can take some months to resolve, recovery seems complete and there is little evidence of any permanent cardiac damage. Rare cases of myocarditis are fulminant and fatal.

Miscellaneous Coxsackie B virus infections

Amongst other disorders found in association with group B viruses are mild respiratory tract illness, febrile illness with an exanthem and orchitis. They are also reputed to cause endocardial fibroelastosis, the infection of the fetus occurring in utero.

Laboratory diagnosis

The six types of Coxsackie group B viruses can be readily isolated in the laboratory either in tissue cultures or suckling mice. Virus can be grown from throat swabs, feces, CSF and in some cases from other organs, e.g. myocardium and testis. Acute and convalescent samples of serum should be sent to the laboratory so that, if present, a significant rise in antibody titer during the illness can be shown. Serological tests may be of special value if a Coxsackie group B virus has been isolated as in this instance the sera need only be tested for an antibody rise against this specific isolate. In all cases it is advisable to try to isolate a virus from the patient as early in the illness as possible. PCR is available in some laboratories.

ECHO VIRUS INFECTIONS

Agents of this group are so named after the initial letters of their original name, enteric cytopathogenic human orphan viruses. There are some 30 distinctive serotypes and their association with aseptic meningitis, encephalitis and paralytic diseases is well documented. They may also cause respiratory tract infections, gastroenteritis, myocarditis and exanthemata of a rather nonspecific character. Subclinical infection with this group is common but clinical examples may present sporadically or in moderate-sized epidemics.

A number of different types of ECHO viruses have been associated with each of the various clinical syndromes that this group may cause and most types have been found in association with more than one syndrome. A few of the identified types have not, as yet, been found in association with obvious disease. In general infection by this group of agents is relatively benign and, except in neonates, few fatalities have been described. They spread in a fashion similar to polioviruses and Coxsackie viruses.

Clinical syndromes

The most commonly associated disease is *aseptic meningitis*; this may be found sporadically or in epidemics. A considerable number of different ECHO virus types may be found in association with this syndrome but the age incidence once again follows the pattern found with infection by other viruses and this is referred to in greater detail on page 1375. In general the prognosis is good and in many instances the cases are clinically indistinguishable from those produced by other viral infections. However, in some there is a rash and where this is seen in a reasonable proportion of cases in any outbreak of aseptic meningitis, it often indicates that an ECHO virus is responsible.

Sporadic cases of *poliomyelitis-like illness* with paralysis have been reported in which evidence of ECHO virus infection has been established; the involvement has usually been slight but instances of permanent residual paralysis are recorded. Cases of *encephalitis* due to ECHO viruses have also been reported and a fatal outcome has occasionally resulted. Children with antibody deficiency can get chronic ECHO virus infection of the brain and/or muscle.

Mild upper respiratory illness has been found in association with a few ECHO viruses, particularly types 11, 19 and 20. These agents may also cause gastroenteritis in infants and young children; fecal samples cultured from such cases have produced evidence of infection by ECHO viruses 5, 11, 14, 18, 19 and 20.

ECHO viruses have been isolated in association with sporadic cases of pleurodynia, pericarditis and myocarditis. However, as these agents may be cultured from many otherwise healthy people their etiologic relationship should not necessarily be assumed.

Where rashes occur as a result of ECHO virus infection they tend to be of a fine maculopapular character, have a widespread distribution and fade rapidly. Generally there is no classical distribution or typical enanthem, although lesions may be papular, arranged in lines and located peripherally, the so-called papular acrolocated syndrome (PALS).

Neonatal ECHO virus infection can cause disseminated infection with massive hepatic necrosis, disseminated intravascular coagulation, bleeding and usually death (Modlin 1986). Such severe cases are almost always acquired vertically and a maternal history of peripartum illness is usual. Although nursery outbreaks may occur most horizontal cases are relatively mild, although meningitis and myocarditis are well described (Jenista et al 1984).

Laboratory diagnosis

The ECHO viruses can be readily isolated in various tissue culture systems. Specimens usually required by the laboratory are CSF, throat swabs and feces depending on the clinical manifestations of the illness. Serological tests on acute and convalescent serum samples can be carried out to show a significant rise in antibody titer during the illness, but owing to the large number of different types of ECHO viruses it is usually not a practical procedure unless an agent has been isolated and identified. Some ECHO viruses cause hemagglutination, so in these cases hemagglutination-inhibiting antibodies can be estimated; otherwise it is usual to test for a rise in neutralizing antibody titer.

VIRUSES AND THE GASTROINTESTINAL TRACT

Many viral agents may inhabit the intestinal tract without producing obvious clinical illness. As a result when such agents are cultured in the presence of gastrointestinal symptoms, their etiologic role is difficult to establish. Nevertheless epidemiological studies in the recent past seemed to indicate that some agents, such as certain ECHO viruses, may be involved in outbreaks of diarrhea in infants. The picture has, however, changed in the last few years as a wide variety of new viral agents has been discovered by electron microscopy of feces. Notable amongst these are *rotaviruses* and *Norwalk-like viruses*.

GASTROENTERITIS

Amongst viral agents which are found in association with gastroenteritis are rotaviruses, Norwalk-like viruses, caliciviruses, coronaviruses, astroviruses, adenoviruses, stool parvoviruses and enteroviruses. The role of rotaviruses and Norwalk virus is more clearly established, but the other viruses can cause limited outbreaks of infantile diarrhea.

Rotaviruses were initially found on electron microscopy of duodenal biopsies taken from children with diarrhea in Australia in 1973. Since then these agents have been found to be common worldwide and their presence may be detected by a variety of methods. Several different human types have been identified as well as many animal varieties. Species specificity appears incomplete.

Between 1 and 7 days after infection, but usually within 2 days, the affected child starts to vomit and develops a low grade fever. Watery diarrhea soon follows and, although mucus may be seen in the stools, blood is rarely present. The vomiting stops after 1–2 days but diarrhea persists even if intravenous fluids are started with no oral intake. Nonspecific respiratory symptoms may occur and, although the illness terminates in about 5–7 days, virus may be found in the stool for up to 10 days.

The peak age of attack is between 6 and 24 months of age, mainly from 9 to 12 months; there is a slight male preponderance. Asymptomatic cases will often be found in older members of the household. Neonatal infection occurs and has been associated with a clinical picture resembling necrotizing enterocolitis. However, neonatal infection is often subclinical, perhaps due to the presence of maternal antibody. It is suggested that breast-feeding can be protective.

Up to 50% of hospitalized cases of infantile gastroenteritis, and a somewhat lower proportion of community cases are caused by rotaviruses (Isaacs et al 1986). Transmission is by the fecal–oral route and, in temperate climates, it is mainly a winter disease although cases can occur throughout the year. Serological surveys show that up to 90% of children aged 3 years or over possess antibody to rotaviruses and surveys in the adult population show figures of up to 70%.

Treatment of gastroenteritis due to rotavirus infection is along standard lines (see p. 1295). Fatalities are rare in industrialized countries and usually in otherwise debilitated children. A variety of complications has been found but the role of rotaviruses in their production is not firmly established.

The *Norwalk virus*, which was first discovered in 1972, and other similar agents since, is also known to produce gastroenteritis. Outbreaks have usually occurred in older children with secondary cases in adults, some involving schoolchildren and their teachers. These agents, first discovered in America and certain Far Eastern countries, are now found on a worldwide basis. After an incubation period of some 2 days the illness starts with nausea and vomiting. Diarrhea, abdominal cramps and fever follow in about half of those involved but symptoms usually abate within a day or so. Treatment is purely symptomatic.

Enteric adenoviruses are the second most important cause of viral diarrhea of infancy, in terms of hospitalization, and often cause prolonged diarrhea with or without vomiting. Astroviruses rarely result in hospital admission, but can cause winter vomiting and may cause rare outbreaks in hospitals.

INTUSSUSCEPTION

The etiology of this condition, which involves the invagination of a portion of the intestine into an adjacent portion, is not fully understood, but in some instances association with a recent infective illness appears to be present. Further investigation of this possible association in recent times has revealed evidence of infection of the intestinal tract by *adenoviruses* and this association appears to be encountered more often than one would expect to occur by chance. Furthermore, adenoviruses have been isolated from regional lymph glands in children found to be suffering from mesenteric adenitis and, as this condition is considered to be associated with the development of intussusception, the possible etiologic role seems strengthened.

OTHER CONDITIONS

Attempts to establish an association between viral infection and appendicitis have not proved very rewarding. Pancreatitis is a recognized complication of mumps and has occasionally been found in association with infection by Coxsackie viruses.

LABORATORY DIAGNOSIS

Various viruses have been associated with diseases of the gastrointestinal tract but the isolation of agents from clinically fit children is not infrequent, so caution must be used before incriminating a virus as the cause of a disease.

In general, it is probably worthwhile examining feces from outbreaks of gastroenteritis, by culture and electron microscopy, for the presence of viruses if no other cause has been found. Some laboratories prefer ELISA testing for rotavirus, but this is restrictive and will not diagnose other viruses. The most common viruses isolated are members of the picornavirus group.

OCULAR VIRAL DISEASES

It is now recognized that viral chlamydial infections of the eye constitute a larger proportion of ocular disease than was formerly appreciated. In part this stems from the enormous advances in viral technology but many ocular diseases are now recognized to have a viral basis because chemotherapy has cleared secondary bacterial infection and revealed the true, underlying viral pathogenesis.

In most instances viral infection of the eye presents as part of a systemic infection which may manifest itself by direct tissue invasion or indirectly through neural involvement, as in the viral encephalitides. However, some viral infections seem to involve the eye selectively, and those include *certain adenoviral infections, trachoma, inclusion conjunctivitis* and *acute hemorrhagic conjunctivitis*.

ADENOVIRUS INFECTIONS OF THE EYE

Two main ocular syndromes are associated with adenovirus infection – *pharyngoconjunctival fever* and *epidemic kerato-conjunctivitis*.

Pharyngoconjunctival fever

This condition may result from infection by several types of adenoviruses though type 3 is most commonly implicated. Clinically it may present as a follicular conjunctivitis, often with associated fever and pharyngitis, producing the recognized clinical entity of pharyngoconjunctival fever. The virus may infect one or both eyes causing an acute conjunctivitis with follicular hypertrophy and mild preauricular lymphadenopathy. A mild transient keratitis sometimes develops.

Children are most often affected and cases may occur sporadically or in epidemics, sometimes associated with swimming pools.

Epidemic keratoconjunctivitis

This disease presents as an acute keratoconjunctivitis with follicular hypertrophy of the conjunctiva and marked preauricular lymphadenopathy. A distinctive keratitis then develops and about a third of the cases have pseudomembranes.

Large epidemics may occur and adults are involved rather than children. Infection is usually due to adenovirus type 8 and spread may occur through ocular instruments, infected eyedroppers and contaminated solutions used in hospitals, first aid stations and surgeries. Complete recovery usually occurs but permanent impairment of vision can occasionally result.

Laboratory diagnosis

Ocular infection with an adenovirus can be confirmed by culturing the virus. Swabs or scrapings in virus transport medium should be sent to the laboratory for virus isolation. The adenoviruses are not difficult to propagate.

TRACHOMA AND INCLUSION CONJUNCTIVITIS (see pp. 283, 1430)

Agents of the genus *Chlamydia* are organisms with properties that are intermediate between viruses and bacteria, and they show sensitivity to certain antibiotics. *Chlamydia trachomatis* is the cause of trachoma, inclusion conjunctivitis, afebrile pneumonitis and lymphogranuloma venereum.

Trachoma

Trachoma is a specific form of keratoconjunctivitis which first involves the upper tarsal follicles. Later upper limbal changes appear followed by pannus formation and the development of Herbert's peripheral pits. The disease is mainly encountered in tropical areas where water is scarce. In such areas there is often a very high incidence. Permanent scarring and blindness may occur especially where adequate facilities for treatment are not available.

Infection occurs at an early age but the mode of transmission is still far from clear; all ages are affected but the disease is especially common in children and is often associated with secondary infection. Theories to explain the spread have included person-to-person contact, infection through fomites and dissemination by flies.

Treatment

Among drugs which may be used are sulfonamides, tetracycline and, less often, erythromycin. Opinions differ as to the efficacy and mode of treatment. However, where topical therapy is conscientiously applied over a period of several weeks, or even months, a good response can be anticipated. Some advocate supplementation by oral therapy.

Inclusion conjunctivitis

This condition is caused by certain strains of *Chlamydia trachomatis* which may reside in the genital tract and produce cervicitis or urethritis. There is a danger of spread to infants, resulting in inclusion blennorrhea, during their passage through the birth canal. Older children and adults may contract inclusion conjunctivitis from swimming pools which have been contaminated by urine or by discharge from the genital tract.

Treatment of inclusion conjunctivitis is also by sulfonamides or topical broad spectrum antibiotics. However, the response is quicker than in trachoma and treatment need not be so prolonged. The prognosis is also better and permanent scarring does not occur. Neonates with inclusion conjunctivitis should be treated with oral erythromycin 40 mg/kg/day 6-hourly for 14 days because of the risk of progression to afebrile pneumonitis.

Laboratory diagnosis

The agents are situated in the epithelial cells of the conjunctiva, and for successful culture epithelial scrapings or eye swabs in special transport medium should be sent to the laboratory. Cultural methods consist of inoculation of suitable tissue cultures and then after incubation, examination under the microscope for typical inclusion bodies. Direct microscopy on Giemsa-stained smears may reveal typical inclusions. ELISA antigen-detection tests and PCR which avoid the need for culture and give a rapid diagnosis are increasingly being used.

ACUTE HEMORRHAGIC CONJUNCTIVITIS (APOLLO 11 DISEASE)

This condition was recognized as a clinical entity in 1969 at the same time as the Apollo 11 moon landing, and a virus, now classified as enterovirus type 70, has been isolated from the conjunctiva of affected patients. Extensive outbreaks have been reported from Africa, Pakistan, India and South America. The disease appears to have an incubation period of about 24 h and to be highly contagious in unhygienic and crowded conditions. The infection is of sudden onset with swelling, congestion, watering and pain in the eye. The most characteristic sign is subconjunctival hemorrhage of varying intensity, which may sometimes be accompanied by corneal keratitis. The disease is not influenced by antibiotics and symptoms usually subside within 1–2 weeks.

Laboratory diagnosis

Conjunctival scrapings or swabs should be sent to the laboratory where suitable tissue cultures can be used to isolate the causative agent.

VIRAL INFECTION OF THE LIVER

Acute inflammation of the liver may be caused by a number of viruses including hepatitis viruses A to F, cytomegalovirus, adenoviruses, picornaviruses, herpes simplex virus, EB virus and the viruses of diseases such as yellow fever and rubella (Lancet 1990b).

VIRUS A HEPATITIS OR INFECTIOUS HEPATITIS (EPIDEMIC HEPATITIS, EPIDEMIC JAUNDICE OR CATARRHAL JAUNDICE)

This disease has an incubation period of 15–50 days (average 30 days) and is mainly found in young children. It is also quite common in older children and young adults but the attack rate declines with increasing age though a higher proportion of severe and complicated cases may be found in these older age groups. Pregnant women may contract a particularly severe form.

The distribution of infectious hepatitis is worldwide and epidemic periodicity varies greatly in different communities. Experimental studies indicate that the responsible agent, hepatitis A virus, is present in both blood and feces at the peak of the illness and persists in the feces for a relatively short time. Susceptible human volunteers have been fed filtered fecal extracts and virus could be found in the feces of those who developed jaundice from 14 to 26 days before the onset of icterus and for over a week thereafter. Furthermore, although at least two-thirds of the recipients displayed no clinical evidence of hepatitis, subclinical evidence of infection was found on serial examination by appropriate liver function tests. This indicates a ratio of 1 : 2 for clinical, as opposed to subclinical, infection and this impression is further substantiated by epidemiological studies in naturally occurring epidemics.

Although infectious hepatitis is mainly transmitted by the fecal–oral route through contamination of food and water, transmission may also occur from blood, urine, nasopharyngeal secretions and saliva. Large epidemics usually occur in institutions and closed communities and, in some of these, infection of a communal water supply has been responsible. Prevention of waterborne outbreaks of this type is difficult though carefully controlled superchlorination may be effective. Outbreaks have also followed the ingestion of raw oysters and raw clams infected by sewage. Infection may also result from the use of imperfectly sterilized instruments, syringes and needles which have been contaminated by infected blood or blood products.

The diagnosis, differential diagnosis and detailed treatment of infectious hepatitis are referred to elsewhere (p. 476). Complement-fixation tests, immune-adherence hemagglutination, ELISA and radioimmunoassay can be used to detect specific IgM and IgG antibody to HAV; the presence of specific IgM antibody indicates a recent infection with hepatitis A virus. In the majority of childhood cases the illness is mild and treatment need not extend beyond simple bed rest and a moderate period of convalescence.

Mortality amongst otherwise healthy, well-nourished individuals is as low as 0.1–0.2% but can rise to 2 or 3% in those poorly nourished. Death may either be early from fulminating hepatitis leading to acute hepatocellular failure or occur considerably later from chronic liver damage.

Prevention

Killed vaccines are now available and are safe and effective (Goilav et al 1995), and indicated for older children and adults at long-term risk. Human normal immunoglobulin is effective prophylaxis and should be given to adult and child contacts of index cases and to people traveling to areas with poor sanitation for short periods.

HEPATITIS B (SERUM HEPATITIS, AUSTRALIAN ANTIGEN-POSITIVE HEPATITIS)

Hepatitis B is enormously important for a number of reasons: some 200 million worldwide carry hepatitis B virus, which is one of the most important causes of liver cirrhosis and hepatoma, the incidence of these being greatly increased in chronic carriers. Because of both vertical and horizontal transmission of the hepatitis B virus (HBV) infection is endemic in some parts of the world, notably the Far East where carriage rates may exceed 15%. About half of all carriers will die liver-related deaths.

The incubation period is 60–160 days, much longer than hepatitis A. Virus antigen can be detected in the blood up to 3 months before jaundice occurs and often for many years after clinical recovery. The virus is mainly transmitted via infected blood, and is highly infectious, far more so than human immunodeficiency virus. Infected blood transfusions, needle sharing by intravenous drug abusers, tattooing and ritual scarification are all well-documented means of spread. The virus can be sexually transmitted and the incidence is high in many homosexual communities. Vertical spread is common and is thought to be mainly peripartum rather than transplacental, thus being largely preventable by intervention immediately after birth. Most vertically infected babies become chronic carriers. The virus is also found in breast milk, although breast-feeding has not been shown to be a clear risk factor for transmission. Clinical features of hepatitis B infection are discussed elsewhere (p. 476).

Etiology

In 1965 geneticists investigating inherited variations in human plasma proteins discovered an unusual protein antigen in the serum of an Australian aborigine. This antigen, originally called Australia antigen (Au), subsequently serum hepatitis antigen (SH) and now hepatitis B surface antigen (HBs), was found to be associated with hepatitis of long incubation. On electron microscopy of serum three particles are identifiable. Dane particles, 42 nm in diameter, are complete virus comprising an inner core containing double-stranded HBV DNA within a core antigen (HBc) and surrounded by an outer coat of surface antigen (HBs). A further antigen, the e antigen, a component of the inner core, may also be seen (see Fig. 23.23). The detection of e antigen in the absence of e antibody correlates with high infectivity. Subjects may be either:

1. HBs antigen positive, with no e antigen or e antibody detected. These will be mainly chronic carriers.
2. HBe antigen positive, but e antibody negative. Usually also HBs positive. Suggests recent active infection and highly infectious.
3. HBe antibody positive. Recovery phase, much less infectious.

Tests commonly used to detect the presence of HBV antigens and antibodies include hemagglutination tests and ELISA tests, which are often used to screen sera for surface antigen (HBs), and radioimmunoassays which are more sensitive.

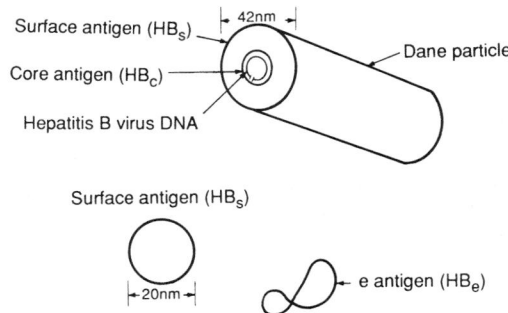

Fig. 23.23 Diagrammatic representation of electron microscopic appearance of hepatitis B virus.

Detection of HBs antibody indicates either recovery from acute HBV infection or a response to immunization. Presence of HBc IgM antibody indicates acute HBV infection, while HBc IgG antibody is detected following infection but not immunization (which uses HBs).

Prevention

In many countries blood or blood product donations are routinely screened for surface antigen (HBs) and antenatal screening of all pregnant women or those from high-risk groups allows intervention to prevent vertical transmission. Great care should be taken handling blood and excreta from HBV-positive patients because of the high infectivity, although any person doing so should be immunized.

Passive immunization with specific immunoglobulin is given for accidental contamination with infected blood, e.g. in the laboratory or from a syringe and needle from a drug abuser. It is also given to babies of infected mothers as soon as possible after birth.

Hepatitis B vaccines are now widely available. The early vaccine, still much used, is purified from human plasma of HBV carriers and inactivated so that there is no risk of transmission of HIV or other viruses. Recombinant DNA techniques have been used to insert the gene for HBs into yeast particles and yeast HBs vaccines are also available (Zuckerman 1985). All health care personnel likely to come into contact with HBV-positive patients, i.e. doctors, dentists, nurses, midwives, students, laboratory staff, etc. should receive a course of three doses of the vaccine.

Babies of mothers who are in the above risk groups 1 (HBs positive) and 2 (HBe antigen positive) are at high risk of becoming chronic carriers without intervention (Zuckerman 1984). Indeed this will be the case in up to 90% of babies of HBe antigen-positive mothers. Such babies should receive both passive HBV-specific immunoglobulin and be actively immunized with HBV vaccine (Beasley et al 1983). Babies of mothers in group 3 (HBe antibody positive) are at lower risk but may rarely develop acute hepatitis, and there is a risk of later horizontal transmission from the mother or an infected sibling. They should therefore be immunized and many would feel they should also receive specific immunoglobulin.

Many countries are now advocating universal neonatal hepatitis B immunization.

Treatment

Interferon alpha has been shown to have some antiviral effect in chronic carriers and its clinical evaluation is continuing (Alexander & Williams 1986).

HEPATITIS C (TRANSFUSION-ASSOCIATED NON-A, NON-B HEPATITIS)

It has been long known that hepatitis could be transmitted by blood transfusion in the absence of hepatitis B virus, and the condition was previously called non-A, non-B hepatitis. The great majority of transfusion-associated hepatitis in which hepatitis B has been excluded are now known to be caused by hepatitis C virus, a flavivirus.

The structure of hepatitis C (HCV) was determined by molecular biology techniques in 1988, yet the virus is extremely difficult to grow. Serological tests have been developed to screen blood products, and PCR testing for the presence of viral nucleic acid is widely available (van der Poel et al 1994).

Hepatitis C virus has an incubation period of around 30–60 days. Transmission is mainly via blood transfusion or by needle sharing between intravenous drug abusers. Screening of donated blood for the presence of hepatitis C antibodies has greatly reduced the risk from blood transfusion. HCV is more resistant to inactivation than HBV or HIV, and blood products such as intravenous immunoglobulin have occasionally transmitted HCV despite viral inactivation steps (Lever et al 1984).

Vertical transmission from mother to fetus occurs in about 10% of pregnancies, and is thought to occur antenatally or perinatally. HCV is not detectable, even by PCR, in breast milk, although it is found in saliva.

A high proportion of those infected with HCV become chronic carriers and may progress to cirrhosis. Interferon alpha therapy is effective in reducing viral replication in around 40% of chronic carriers, though half of these responders will relapse when interferon is stopped.

DELTA AGENT (HEPATITIS D)

The delta agent is a defective RNA virus which requires HBV for its own synthesis. This is one of the most important examples of viral coinfection described. The delta agent was detected by immunofluorescence studies of liver cell nuclei of chronic HBV carriers. Delta antigen and antibody are detected by radioimmunoassay or ELISA and have never been demonstrated other than in association with HBV. The delta agent is most prevalent in intravenous drug abusers in Italy and the Mediterranean but has been detected worldwide. It appears to be a risk factor for acute hepatitis in drug abusers. About half of HBs-positive hemophiliacs in America and Italy have antidelta antibodies.

HEPATITIS E (ENTERIC NON-A, NON-B HEPATITIS)

Hepatitis E is the enterically transmitted form of non-A, non-B hepatitis and is transmitted by the fecal–oral route. It is of major importance in developing countries as a cause of hepatitis due to waterborne epidemics, which mainly affect young adults, but rarely children. It causes a high mortality, sometimes as high as 40%, in pregnant women. The viral genome has been cloned and sequenced, and serological tests are available.

HEPATITIS F

This is an as yet putative virus thought to cause hepatitis by the parenteral route, as some such cases are negative for all currently known hepatitis viruses (Lancet 1990b).

HEPATITIS – THE ROLE OF OTHER VIRUSES

Despite the ubiquity and prevalence of infectious and serum hepatitis, other viral infections may involve the liver.

Cytomegalovirus is known to attack the liver in 85% of newborn infants suffering from cytomegalic inclusion disease; the same virus may also cause hepatitis when older children or adults contract the acquired form of the infection. *Infectious mononucleosis*, due to EBV, is frequently accompanied by some degree of liver involvement; most often this will reveal itself as a mild derangement of liver function tests though some cases will manifest obvious jaundice. Infection by *arboviruses* may be accompanied by a similar picture, though amongst these yellow fever produces a more specific and severe form of hepatitis.

Herpes simplex virus infections of the newborn are serious and usually fatal, one pathological feature being an extensive hepatic necrosis. Neonatal echovirus hepatitis is often fulminant.

Lastly, there are instances where transient liver involvement has been found in a variety of viral infections including some due to ECHO viruses types 4 and 9, Coxsackie viruses, adenoviruses and lymphocytic choriomeningitis virus. In most the involvement has been extremely mild with full recovery, though in some severe hepatitis may occur.

MISCELLANEOUS INFECTIONS

ORF (CONTAGIOUS PUSTULAR DERMATITIS OF SHEEP, CONTAGIOUS ECTHYMA OF SHEEP)

This is a common and widespread viral infection of sheep and to a lesser extent of goats. In general infection is from animal to animal but virus can persist in the soil of affected pastures for several months. Lambs are most commonly involved and they develop a papulovesicular eruption on the mouth, lips and non-hair-bearing areas of the skin. Transmission to man is relatively rare and the main incidence occurs in springtime. The infection is most commonly encountered in shepherds, farm and abattoir workers. However, children can be infected owing to their liking for handling young lambs.

Orf virus is included amongst the poxviruses and has certain similarities to the virus of molluscum contagiosum. It can be grown with difficulty on tissue culture but is usually identified by electron microscopy. Scrapings from the base of the bullae are to be preferred to vesicle fluid in these studies.

Clinical features

Lesions, which are usually but not exclusively single, most commonly appear on the hand or forearm. Initially there is an area of infiltration presenting as brawny edema but this soon develops into a flaccid bulla. However, on puncture a rather clear serosanguineous fluid is obtained. There is little or no constitutional upset but the progression of the lesion is slow and may take 6–8 weeks before it finally heals. No specific treatment is available or required in view of the benign nature of the condition but it is wise to protect the lesion with dressings to counteract the possibility of secondary infection.

MOLLUSCUM CONTAGIOSUM (see p. 1633, Plate 25.11)

This viral disease is seen in children more often than in adults. The responsible agent is a DNA virus belonging to the pox group but serologically unrelated to vaccinia or variola; it is readily identified by electron microscopy of the curettings from a lesion or on the histological appearances of a biopsy. Transmission is by close contact but infectivity is low.

Clinical features

Molluscum contagiosum is unassociated with any constitutional upset and presents as a chronic viral infection of the epidermis. Lesions, which may be multiple, take the form of pinkish white or flesh-colored, dome-shaped nodules between 2 and 8 mm in diameter and some show a central depression or umbilication. They may appear on the face, arms, legs, buttocks, scalp or genitalia but sparing of the palms of the hands and the soles of the feet is a characteristic feature. Occasionally the margins of the eyelids are involved and chronic follicular conjunctivitis can supervene (Plate 25.11). HIV infection may be associated with disseminated molluscum.

Treatment

The disease is benign and self-limiting. Treatment is advised only to prevent spread by autoinoculation or to others. Treatment is simple and consists of the removal of the lesions with a sharp curette. Other methods include electro- or cryocautery. The lesions will usually heal without scarring and recurrence is rare.

LASSA FEVER

Lassa fever was first reported from Lassa in Nigeria in 1969. The Lassa virus shows some morphological and antigenic similarities to lymphocytic choriomeningitis virus. It is one of the arenaviruses and it is widely distributed throughout West Africa. It is one of five African viruses (yellow fever, Lassa, Ebola, Marburg and Congo-Crimean) that cause hemorrhagic fever (see p. 1389). The natural host is the rat *Mastomys natalensis*.

The virus is transmitted from person to person by close contact. It causes a diffuse serositis, hemorrhage and shock and is often fatal. Intravenous ribavirin reduces mortality from Lassa fever and is the treatment of choice (McCormick et al 1986). Additional treatment involves the use of plasma from a convalesced patient. For the adult 250–500 ml are used. Stocks of this are held in Nigeria, Sierra Leone, the London School of Hygiene and Tropical Medicine and the Communicable Disease Center, Atlanta, Georgia, USA. Strict isolation of patients is mandatory.

MARBURG VIRUS DISEASE (GREEN MONKEY DISEASE, VERVET MONKEY DISEASE, JO'BURG VIRUS DISEASE)

Marburg virus disease was first recognized in Germany in 1967 in personnel who had handled a consignment of African green monkeys (*Cercopithecus aethiops*) from Uganda. Outbreaks have occurred in Sudan and Zaire (Bowen et al 1977). The Marburg virus is long, rod shaped (rhabdovirus-like) and does not appear to possess antigenic affinity with other known viruses. Although the Marburg outbreak appeared to follow contact with African green monkeys no similar infections have been recognized as a result of other contacts with these monkeys and such monkeys suffer 100% mortality if experimentally infected. Thus the natural host or possible vectors are unknown.

The disease is highly infectious and carries a high mortality: 7 of the 31 Marburg cases died. Secondary cases appear to have a better prognosis than primary cases. There is as yet no protective vaccine. Strict isolation and barrier nursing of patients is necessary.

EBOLA VIRUS DISEASE

This disease is clinically indistinct from Marburg virus disease. The virus is morphologically identical to the Marburg virus, but antigenically distinct. The disease has been found in the Sudan and Zaire (Baron et al 1983, McCormick et al 1983).

INFECTIONS DUE TO ARBOVIRUSES (TOGAVIRUSES)

The principal feature linking the viruses of this group is the fact that all are arthropod borne (hence the name) and well over 200 such agents have been recognized. Most viruses in this group are natural parasites of animals or birds and multiply in their arthropod vectors, the latter being unharmed in the process. Infection in the human may take several forms; most commonly encephalitis of varying severity results, but other diseases produced include yellow fever, dengue and sandfly fever. Arboviruses may also result in mild influenza-like illness. Children are particularly susceptible to this group of diseases.

ARBOVIRUSES GROUP A

Some 20 arboviruses are included in this group of which the best known are the viruses of eastern and western equine encephalitis; these present in humans as aseptic meningitis or meningoencephalitis of varying severity. Children tend to be more seriously affected and death may result. Those who survive the illness may have permanent mental retardation, deafness, epilepsy and paralysis. Mortality may vary with age and the responsible virus; on average 5% of patients may die but this can be considerably higher following infection by certain agents of the group, reaching 74% in eastern equine encephalitis.

Other viruses of this group produce a mild dengue-like illness and most have their animal reservoir in wild or domestic birds. Their arthropod vectors are culicine and anophiline mosquitoes.

ARBOVIRUSES GROUP B

This, a larger group, can be divided into (1) *mosquito-borne* and (2) *tick-borne* sections. The best known disease associated with the former is yellow fever; the latter are mainly associated with a variety of encephalitic illness.

Yellow fever (yellow jack)

Mosquito-borne, this disease has been a recognized clinical entity for over 300 years and in 1881 Carlos Finlay suggested that *Aedes aegypti* spread the infection. This theory was substantiated by the classical studies of Walter Reed and his colleagues working in Cuba (Monath 1984). Yellow fever occurs in parts of Africa, South America and Central America but not Asia. The last cases of infection within Britain occurred in the latter part of the 19th century when ships arrived carrying infected *Aedes aegypti*.

Disease may vary from a mild fever to a fulminant hepatitis with jaundice, hepatic necrosis, hemorrhage and shock. In the jungle it is predominantly an adult disease. Where infection occurs in an urban community all ages and both sexes are equally affected.

There is no specific treatment.

Elimination of the responsible vector is of prime importance and infection has been eradicated from certain areas where this has been diligently performed. Vaccination with the 17 D attenuated strain of virus is compulsory for travel to endemic areas and immunity will usually last for up to 6 years. Complications of immunization are confined to an occasional case of benign encephalitis, usually encountered in young infants, and the vaccine is not recommended under 9 months of age if exposure to mosquitoes can be avoided.

Dengue fever (breakbone fever)

Mosquito-borne like yellow fever, this disease is caused by a virus from group B and the same vector, *Aedes aegypti*, is involved. The disease is widespread and is mainly found in warm areas, amongst which are Australia, Greece, Japan, India, Malaysia and Hawaii. So far, four antigenic varieties, known as types 1, 2, 3 and 4 have been described (Halstead 1980).

Clinical features

There is an incubation period of 5–9 days. The illness starts with high fever, malaise, headache, pain in the eyes, backache and excruciatingly painful limbs. Between the third and fifth days a maculopapular, scarlatiniform, or petechial rash appears and lasts up to 4 days; following this there is a rapid recovery. Occasionally, however, particularly in children the disease progresses to a severe hemorrhagic form, dengue hemorrhagic shock syndrome (DHSS), which may be fatal (see Hemorrhagic Fevers below). It is thought that DHSS follows prior sensitization with a different strain of dengue virus, and is an example of antibody-mediated enhancement of disease.

Control

Eradication of the vector is desirable. Dengue viruses are poor antigens and this has frustrated efforts to produce effective vaccines.

HEMORRHAGIC FEVERS

A number of virus infections may occur in a hemorrhagic form, e.g. Lassa fever, yellow fever and measles. The arboviruses, particularly the Chikungunya (group A) and dengue (group B) viruses, are also prone to cause hemorrhagic disease. Hemorrhagic fever due to the mosquito-borne Chikungunya virus has been reported in Africa, India and Thailand. In southeast Asia hemorrhagic fever due to dengue virus is transmitted by the bite of the *Aedes aegypti* mosquito which is common in urban areas.

The hemorrhagic fevers affect mainly children in these countries, and patients develop fever, erythematous or petechial rashes, hepatosplenomegaly and bleeding which may be mild or severe. The majority of the patients recover but a certain number develop shock and die. Thrombocytopenia is common. In fatal cases there are gross effusions into the serous cavities, petechial hemorrhages on the surface of organs and bronchopneumonia. Treatment is symptomatic, and in shocked cases intravenous plasma together with the usual measures for collapsed patients should be administered.

Hemorrhagic fever with renal syndrome

This name is used for several similar conditions including Korean hemorrhagic fever and nephropathica epidemica occurring in Scandinavia, central Europe, Russia, China, Japan and Korea (WHO 1983). At least two viruses, Hantaan (Hantavirus) and Puumala, transmitted by arboviruses from rodents, are implicated. The clinical manifestations are of fever, shock, massive proteinuria followed by acute renal failure, and thrombocytopenia and bleeding with bruising, hematuria, hematemesis and melena. With supportive treatment the mortality is low.

TICK-BORNE ARBOVIRUS INFECTIONS

These including louping ill (a disease of sheep in Scotland and northern England; rarely aseptic meningitis can occur if man is infected by an infected tick), Russian spring–summer encephalitis (western and eastern forms), Omsk hemorrhagic fever and Kyasanur Forest fever. Illness associated with this group may range from aseptic meningitis to severe and even fatal encephalitis though the prognosis is better than with infection by group A strains. On occasion paralytic disease simulating poliomyelitis can occur and Omsk fever is usually characterized by bronchopneumonia and hemorrhage from various orifices.

ARBOVIRUSES GROUP C AND UNCLASSIFIED ARBOVIRUSES

Group C, comprising seven viruses, are responsible for influenza-like illness in parts of South America. Amongst the unclassified infections, sandfly fever is perhaps the best documented illness.

Sandfly fever (phlebotomus fever, pappataci fever)

This illness results from infection by one of the unclassified arboviruses. It is relatively common in countries bordering the Mediterranean and occurs in parts of Africa, Russia, India and China. The responsible vector *Phlebotomus papatasi*, often called sandfly, is extremely small and may pass through mosquito nets. Infection in these sandflies may be a permanent feature owing to transovarian infection and no definite animal reservoir is known. Several different strains of virus have been isolated with established immunological variation.

Clinical features

The incubation period is 3–7 days. Onset is sudden and rigors may occur. Headache, pain behind the eyes, muscular aching and fever are typical features. Occasionally photophobia, neck and back stiffness occur and mimic meningitis. After 3 or 4 days there is an abrupt termination by crisis. Severe apprehension often accompanies this illness and acute depression may follow an attack for a short time; leukopenia is a common accompaniment. A clinical diagnosis is readily made in endemic areas or during an outbreak.

There is no specific treatment and the prognosis is good. Control is confined to attempts at eradication of the vector in its breeding grounds.

RICKETTSIAL INFECTIONS

Rickettsial infection in man produces a number of different diseases, spread over a wide geographical area. The resultant illnesses have certain basic similarities and all but one are characterized by some form of skin eruption. Definitive clinical diagnosis can be difficult and confirmatory laboratory tests are desirable. A simple classification of rickettsial infection is shown in Table 23.29.

Rickettsiae have biophysical properties which place them in an intermediate position between viruses and bacteria and are small coccobacilli, usually less than half a micrometer in diameter, with rigid cell walls. They contain both RNA and DNA but are obligate intracellular parasites and are sensitive to certain antibiotics.

Table 23.29   Rickettsial diseases: causal agents, vectors, reservoirs and differential Weil–Felix reactions

	Disease	Causal rickettsiae	Principal vectors	Animal reservoir	Geographic occurrence
Typhus	Epidemic (louse-borne typhus)	*R. prowazekii*	Lice	Man	Worldwide
	Brill–Zinsser disease	*R. prowazekii*	–	Man	Worldwide
	Endemic murine (flea-borne) typhus	*R. mooseri*	Fleas	Rats	Worldwide
	Scrub typhus (mite-borne) (Tsutsugamushi fever)	*R. tsutsugamushi*	Mites	Small rodents	Japan, Southeast Asia, Pacific
Spotted fevers	Rocky Mountain spotted fever	*R. rickettsii*	Ticks	Small rodents	East and west USA
	Mediterranean fever (fièvre boutonneuse)	*R. conori*	Ticks	Small rodents and dogs	Mediterranean, Caspian and Black Sea, Africa, Southeast Asia
Rickettsial pox		*R. akari*	Mites	House mice	USA, Russia, Korea
Q fever	Query fever	*R. burnetii*	Occasionally ticks	Cattle Sheep Goats Bandicoots	Worldwide

LABORATORY TESTS

Procedures to isolate the causative organisms exist but should only be undertaken by a laboratory well equipped to deal with the risks involved. In view of the hazards involved in isolation, serological methods of diagnosis are usually employed.

The Weil–Felix agglutination reaction has been used for several years; this depends on the fact that patients with certain rickettsial infections develop agglutinins in their serum during the illness which agglutinate some strains of proteus organisms, namely OX 19, OX 2 and OXK. If possible paired sera should be examined in the Weil–Felix test but agglutinins may appear as early as the fifth or sixth day after the onset of the fever and usually reach a peak during the second or third week.

TYPHUS FEVER (EPIDEMIC LOUSE-BORNE TYPHUS FEVER)

Historical writings suggest that typhus fever (classical or historic typhus) has been a scourge of humanity for many centuries. Typhus fever and war are inextricably linked. Although the responsible agent may be endemic in many parts of Europe, serious epidemics only arise during times of war or in their aftermath, due entirely to the increased infestation by lice that occurs in these periods. Epidemics occur chiefly in winter when persons are crowded together for warmth and shelter, enhancing chances of spread of the louse. Following the 1914–1918 war it was estimated that 30 million cases of typhus occurred in Russia alone and some 10% of these probably died. In the 1970s large epidemics occurred in central Africa (Ruanda-Burundi).

The responsible organism is *Rickettsia prowazekii* and transmission is by the body louse *Pediculus corporis* or the head louse *P. capitis*. The lice become infected by biting a human who is carrying the specific rickettsiae in the blood. Spread of the infection thereafter results from the infected feces of the lice rather than by an actual bite and the irritation set up on the human body by the infestation results in the organisms being scratched into the skin; infection may also result from the inhalation of louse feces in dust. At times fleas may act as a vector and also convey the infection through their feces.

Clinical features

The incubation period lies between 6 and 15 days. There are three main clinical phases – prodromal, invasive and eruptive.

Prodromal symptoms, which are not always present, comprise mild headache, lassitude, weakness and pyrexia. The invasive stage is characterized by a sharp rise in temperature, severe headache and generalized aching. Rigors may occur and the fever may reach 40.0–41.0°C. The pulse is rapid, the blood pressure reduced and a variable degree of prostration develops. A wide variety of additional symptoms and signs may be encountered including suffusion of the conjunctivae, facial flushing, photophobia, deafness, tinnitus, vertigo and cough.

The characteristic rash arises about the fifth day of illness and the initial lesions, comprising pinkish red macules, appear on the trunk and soon spread to the limbs. Most cases show sparing of the face, palms and soles. In mild cases the rash may develop no further but in the more severely ill the eruption becomes hemorrhagic or even purpuric. During this eruptive phase the mental state becomes dulled; stupor, delirium and coma may follow. Hypotension also becomes more intense and oliguria with azotemia is common. Severe cases will die between the 9th and 18th day of illness; those who recover slowly improve after 2 weeks, the mental recovery being more rapid than the physical. Typhus is usually accompanied by a leukopenia and normochromic anemia.

Complications

Bronchopneumonia, otitis media, skin sepsis, arterial thrombosis and gangrene are all encountered. Less often there may be areas of skin necrosis and secondary infection of the salivary glands. Prolonged hypotension has a grave prognosis.

Differential diagnosis

Typhus may be readily considered and diagnosed at epidemic times but sporadic cases can cause considerable confusion. Amongst diseases that may require differentiation are other rickettsial infections, typhoid fever, measles, malaria and meningococcal septicemia.

Treatment

In children 75–100 mg/kg/day of chloramphenicol or 50 mg/kg/day of tetracycline is used and treatment should continue until the temperature has settled for 48 h. Antibiotics should be reinstituted if there is clinical relapse.

Careful nursing and general supportive measures are required. A high protein diet is desirable and transfusion of blood or plasma may be needed. Electrolyte imbalance can readily occur and requires appropriate correction. Oxygen may be given for pulmonary complications and digoxin for cardiac failure.

Prognosis

The disease is rarely fatal in children, but about 10% of young adults and 60–70% of people over 50 may die.

Control

Killed vaccines prevent mortality though not necessarily infection. Scrupulous hygiene is desirable and insecticides should be used to eliminate lice: DDT, lindane and malathion have proved effective.

BRILL–ZINSSER DISEASE (RECRUDESCENT TYPHUS)

This condition represents a recrudescence of epidemic louse-borne typhus which occurs years after the primary attack. It is usually mild and the illness is drastically modified; skin rashes are usually absent and the prognosis is good. In view of its atypical clinical nature and the fact that a case may arise when no other typhus infection is occurring, diagnosis is difficult. Less marked reaction in the laboratory tests can also be misleading. However, if a diagnosis is made, treatment is along the lines employed for epidemic typhus. The real danger of Brill–Zinsser disease is to the community. If epidemiological factors are favorable, especially if the environment is heavily louse infested, an epidemic could arise from such a case.

MURINE TYPHUS (ENDEMIC FLEA-BORNE TYPHUS FEVER)

This disease is clinically similar to classical epidemic typhus but is milder and has a much lower fatality rate (2%); the management and treatment are also similar. The responsible agent is named *Rickettsia mooseri* and it is usually spread to man from its animal host by the rat flea (*Xenopsylla cheopis*).

Widely distributed throughout the world, the disease appears to be on the decline probably owing to stricter control of rats. It is commoner in summer when rats are more numerous and has a higher infection rate amongst persons in the food trade where rats may abound. Unlike lice which die from *Rickettsia prowazekii*, the rat flea is not killed by the multiplication of *R. mooseri* in its tissue. Control depends on flea eradication and extermination of rats.

SCRUB TYPHUS (TSUTSUGAMUSHI FEVER)

This disease, known by many different names according to the locality where it occurs, is transmitted to man by the bite of the larvae of different species of chiggerlike mites; best known of these are *Trombicula akamushi* and *T. deliniensis*. The responsible agent is known as *Rickettsia tsutsugamushi* and the cycle of infection involves chiggermite and various wild rodents. Clinical features are again like those of other rickettsial infections though fairly mild. A diagnostic finding in some is a small necrotic ulcer or eschar where the responsible mite has attached itself to the skin and introduced the infection. The disease occurs in the southwest Pacific and southeast Asia between Japan, the Solomon Islands and Pakistan.

Treatment is with chloramphenicol or tetracycline and the mortality is under 5%. Elimination of the disease is difficult and mite-infested areas are best avoided. Alternatively protective clothing, treated with a mite repellent, should be used. Vaccines have not proved effective in this condition.

ROCKY MOUNTAIN SPOTTED FEVER

This disease results from infection by *Rickettsia rickettsii* which is transmitted to man through a variety of ticks which are both the vector and the common reservoir for the responsible agent. Some rodents, dogs and sheep also act as additional but less prolific reservoirs. The clinical course has many similarities to classical typhus but the incubation period is often shorter (2–5 days in severe cases). Furthermore, the rash is usually more pronounced and frankly petechial. It can also be more widespread and may take some time to subside.

Complications, differential diagnosis and laboratory findings are also similar to epidemic typhus as is the treatment and management. Reported mortality rates have varied between 3% and 90% with an average, for all ages, of 20%. Despite its name this disease is now much more common in the eastern than the western US. In the western US adult males are most frequently attacked whereas in the east children are most commonly affected.

Control is difficult owing to the disseminated nature of the vector in the wild and where possible it is best to avoid tick-infested areas or to ensure that adequate protective clothing is worn.

TICK TYPHUS FEVERS (FIÈVRE BOUTONNEUSE)

There are three tick-borne spotted fevers caused by rickettsiae which share the same group-specific antigen as *Rickettsia rickettsii*, the cause of Rocky Mountain spotted fever, but have distinct type-specific antigens.

Rickettsia conorii causes fièvre boutonneuse which is also called Mediterranean fever along the Mediterranean, Black and Caspian sea littorals; called Kenyan tick typhus and South African tickbite fever; and called Indian tick typhus in southeast Asia. *Rickettsia australis* causes Queensland tick typhus in eastern Australia. *Rickettsia sibirica* causes Siberian tick typhus which occurs throughout central Asia.

The main animal reservoir is dogs. These tick typhus fevers are clinically similar. A small indurated lesion, the tache noire, develops at the site of the tick bite, and central necrosis gives way to eschar formation. There is regional lymphadenopathy. The tick typhus fevers are much milder than Rocky Mountain spotted fever, with a mortality under 1%. Antibiotic treatment is as for the latter disease.

RICKETTSIALPOX

Due to *Rickettsia akari*, this disease is usually transmitted to man by a mite and the house mouse is the main animal reservoir. Epidemics tend to occur where mice and mites are found together primarily in urban populations worldwide.

The illness is comparatively mild. The incubation period is 10–21 days. Fever is usual and a mild rash develops, most closely resembling adult chickenpox. Death is extremely rare. Tetracycline is the drug of choice.

Q FEVER (QUERY FEVER)

Q fever, caused by *Rickettsia burnetii*, has clinical features quite unlike those of other rickettsial infections. The features are often those of respiratory or influenza-like illness with no rash (see p. 1374). Endocarditis can occur and children may present with fever of unknown origin.

HIV INFECTION

EPIDEMIOLOGY

The first cases of pediatric acquired immune-deficiency syndrome (AIDS) were reported in 1982, in children of intravenous drug-using or promiscuous mothers, and in infants who had received infected blood transfusions. Between 75 and 80% of children with AIDS have acquired the infection from the mother, across the placenta, during the intrapartum period, from breast milk or close mother–child contact. The majority of children have been infected in the intrapartum period (European Collaborative Study 1994b).

Infection can also result from receiving infected blood or blood products, and rarely, because of sexual abuse. No case of pediatric AIDS has been transmitted through social and family contact, nor in the school or daycare setting.

ETIOLOGY AND PATHOGENESIS

In 1983, the causative agent for AIDS was isolated and is currently known as the human immunodeficiency virus (HIV).

Infection occurs when the HIV envelope protein, gp120, binds on

Infection occurs when the HIV envelope protein, gp120, binds on to the CD4 receptor on the cell surface. The viral membrane fuses with the cell membrane, and viral core material enters the host cell. The genetic material, encoded in RNA, is converted to DNA by reverse transcriptase and this DNA 'provirus' is integrated into the host genome. Therefore infection is lifelong although the integrated virus may remain latent. The viral DNA directs the production of new viral RNA and viral proteins, which migrate to the periphery, combine and form new virus particles which bud from the cell membrane.

The distribution of HIV-infected cells in the body is determined by cells which bear the CD4 antigen. These include the CD4+ lymphocytes, monocytes, macrophages, certain antigen-presenting cells in lymph nodes and skin, as well as a minority of B lymphocytes. Neuroglial cells and chromaffin cells in the gastrointestinal tract can be infected by HIV in vitro although CD4 cannot be detected directly in these cells.

Infected cells form syncytia, or are cleared by the immune system. Free viral gp120 may circulate in the blood and bind to CD4 receptors of uninfected cells, rendering them susceptible to destruction by the immune system although the cells themselves are not infected by the virus. Antibodies directed against gp120 and other HIV proteins may also activate complement, and lead to destruction of cells.

LABORATORY DIAGNOSIS

Humoral responses to HIV can be measured by various antibody assays. Antibodies to core (p24) and envelope (gp120) proteins can be detected 6 weeks to 3 months following infection. For screening, enzyme-linked immunoassays (ELISA) are commonly used because of ease of administration. A positive result can be confirmed with a different ELISA technique, such as antiglobulin assay and a competitive binding technique. Western blot analysis of serum samples can be used for specific antibody responses.

In the adult, a positive antibody test is a sensitive and specific indicator of HIV infection. The presence of transplacentally acquired maternal HIV antibody in a newborn limits the usefulness of antibody testing as a criterion for infection. Maternal antibodies clear at around 12–18 months of age. The European Collaborative Study (1988) reported some children with clinical features of HIV infection but no HIV antibody response because of B cell dysfunction.

HIV antigen can be detected, either soon after infection or in the late stages of the disease. The test is rendered more sensitive after acid dissociation of immune complexes. While a positive antigen test confirms infection, a negative test does not necessarily exclude it, as antigen is infrequently detected in symptom-free antibody-positive individuals. With disease progression, antigen reappears and is correlated with the loss of antibody to core protein.

HIV can be cultured from peripheral blood lymphocytes. The technique involves co-culturing the patient's cells with donor cells prestimulated with phytohemagglutinin, and assaying supernatants for the presence of p24 antigen or reverse transcriptase activity. A new, sensitive method for detecting HIV is the polymerase chain reaction (PCR) technique to amplify HIV-DNA or RNA sequences. The amplified product can be visualized in agarose or acrylamide gel, or detected with radiolabeled probes.

LABORATORY EVALUATION OF IMMUNE COMPETENCE

A full blood count with differential allows assessment of absolute numbers of lymphocytes. The blood film may reveal atypical lymphocytes at the time of seroconversion. Total T and B lymphocyte numbers can be determined, along with T lymphocyte subsets. Although lymphopenia (< 1000 cells/ml) is rarely seen until end-stage disease, CD4+ cells are often decreased in numbers. The ratio of CD4/CD8 cells is less than 1.0 with progression of disease (European Collaborative Study 1991).

Cell-mediated immunity is assessed by mitogen stimulation of lymphocytes, and the response may remain normal for prolonged periods until end-stage disease, when most infected children lose proliferative responses to tetanus and diphtheria toxoids (Borkowsky et al 1992).

Abnormalities in B cell function usually precede T cell abnormality and include polyclonal hypergammaglobulinemia or hypogammaglobulinemia. Hypergammaglobulinemia is an early and reliable marker of infection, and is seen in about 50% of infected children at 4 months and in more than 75% by 9 months of age (European Collaborative Study 1991).

Thrombocytopenia is seen at various stages of HIV infection, although the actual mechanism is not known. Sequential platelet counts show that counts can drop to less than $100 \times 10^9/l$, and recover with no specific therapy.

Figure 23.24 shows the relationship between laboratory tests and clinical progression of disease.

CLINICAL FEATURES

The incubation period is variable, ranging from approximately 6 months to several years. The clinical spectrum ranges from asymptomatic carriers to those with terminal AIDS. Infected infants rarely present with AIDS in the neonatal period although HIV-related symptoms and signs may appear during the first year of life, at a median age of 5 months. It is estimated that about 20% of infants develop the more severe infantile form of the disease, with 10% dying before 1 year of age. In contrast, HIV progresses less rapidly in the majority of infected infants, with 75% surviving at 5 years (European Collaborative Study 1991, 1994a).

The new classification for HIV infection in children less than 13 years of age, according to the Centers for Disease Control (1994), considers the clinical status as well as immune function, and is shown in Tables 23.30 and 23.31. In developing countries, the lack of laboratory facilities makes it difficult to diagnose opportunistic infection, neurological and pulmonary complications. Therefore the World Health Organization (WHO Global Program on AIDS 1989) proposed a clinical case definition for AIDS in adults and children where diagnostic resources are limited. Signs and symptoms, shown in Table 23.32, are easily identified by clinicians. This definition has been found to have a specificity of almost 90% and a sensitivity of 40%.

INFECTIOUS COMPLICATIONS

Recurrent bacterial infections occur commonly, despite hypergammaglobulinemia. Organisms implicated are *Streptococcus pneumoniae, Haemophilus influenzae, Salmonella* species, *Escherichia coli, Staphylococcus aureus* and *Pseudomonas* species. Clinical manifestations include respiratory sepsis,

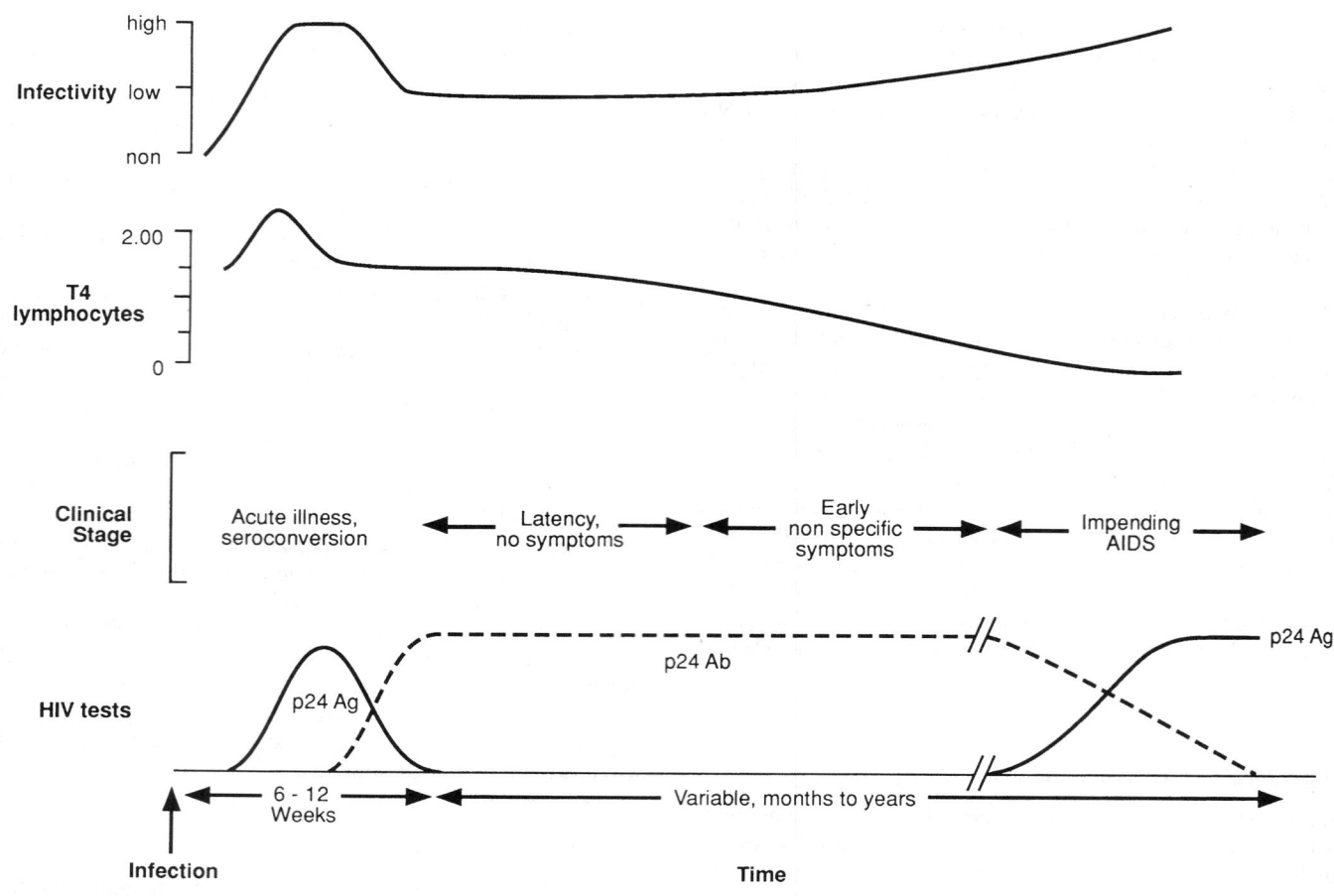

Fig. 23.24   The clinical progression of HIV infection.

Table 23.30   1994 Revised classification system for pediatric HIV infection*

Immunological categories†	Clinical categories (signs and symptoms)			
	N: none	A: mild	B: moderate	C: severe
1. No evidence of immune suppression	N1	A1	B1	C1
2. Moderate immune suppression	N2	A2	B2	C2
3. Severe immune suppression	N3	A3	B3	C3

* Centers for Disease Control 1994.
† Based on age-specific CD4+ lymphocyte count or CD4% of total lymphocytes.

meningitis, cellulitis, osteomyelitis, gastrointestinal as well as urinary infections.

With immune deficiency, opportunistic infections occur with *Pneumocystis carinii*, cytomegalovirus, varicella-zoster virus, *Herpes simplex, Candida albicans, Toxoplasma gondii* and atypical mycobacteria.

NONINFECTIOUS COMPLICATIONS

Neurological disease

Encephalopathy presents as delay or regression in developmental milestones or cognitive function (Epstein et al 1986). Progressive symmetrical motor deficits include gait disturbances, abnormal tone and pathologic reflexes. Seizures may occur. Serial head measurements show acquired microcephaly, and computerized tomography reveals cerebral atrophy with calcification of the basal ganglia. Early demyelination of cerebral white matter may be seen with magnetic radioimaging. Even with clinical evidence of neurological disease, the cerebrospinal fluid may be normal or show mild pleocytosis with elevated protein. Postmortem examination of brain tissue reveals cerebral atrophy and infiltration with inflammatory cells, microglial nodules and perivascular calcification. HIV viral particles, antigen and DNA sequences have been found in brain tissue and cerebrospinal fluid.

Gastrointestinal symptoms

HIV-enteropathy or infection of the gut leads to debilitating symptoms which ultimately result in the child failing to thrive. Symptoms include anorexia, nausea, abdominal discomfort and diarrhea, which may be intractable. A wasting syndrome is seen in advanced disease, and is an AIDS-defining condition.

Table 23.31 Clinical categories for pediatric HIV infection (adapted from Centers for Disease Control 1994)

Children are placed in four mutually exclusive clinical categories based on clinical signs, symptoms and diagnoses, which have been designed to provide prognostic value

Category N: Not symptomatic. No signs or symptoms considered to be the result of HIV infection, or has only one condition listed in Category A

Category A: Mildly symptomatic. Two or more of the following – lymphadenopathy, hepatomegaly, splenomegaly, dermatitis, parotitis, recurrent or persistent upper respiratory infections

Category B: Moderately symptomatic. Commonly encountered conditions include: anemia (< 8 g/dl), neutropenia (< 1000/mm^3), thrombocytopenia (< 100 000/mm^3) persisting > 30 days; single episodes of bacterial sepsis, meningitis or pneumonia; oropharyngeal candidiasis persisting > 2 months; cardiomyopathy; CMV infection before 1 month of age; intractable diarrhea; hepatitis; recurrent herpes simplex (HSV) stomatitis; systemic HSV infection before 1 month of age; herpes zoster involving > 1 dermatome; lymphoid interstitial pneumonia; nephropathy; fever > 1 month; toxoplasmosis after 1 month of age; disseminated varicella

Category C: Severely symptomatic. AIDS-defining conditions include: recurrent serious bacterial infections; disseminated candidiasis; extrapulmonary cryptococcosis; cryptosporidiosis or isosporiasis with diarrhea > 1 month; CMV disease after 1 month of age; encephalopathy; persistent HSV infection after 1 month of age; lymphoma; disseminated *Mycobacterium tuberculosis* or atypical mycobacteria; *Pneumocystis carinii* pneumonia; progressive multifocal leukoencephalopathy; recurrent salmonella (nontyphoid) septicemia; cerebral toxoplasmosis after 1 month of age; wasting syndrome in the absence of concurrent disease

Table 23.32 WHO modified definition for pediatric AIDS (1989)

Major signs
Weight loss or failure to thrive
Chronic diarrhea > 1 month
Prolonged fever > 1 month
Severe or repeated pneumonia

Minor signs
Generalized lymphadenopathy
Oropharyngeal candidiasis
Repeated common infections
Generalized pruritic dermatitis
Confirmed maternal HIV infection

Note: pediatric AIDS is suspected when at least two major signs are associated with at least two minor signs, in the absence of known causes of immune deficiency.

Lymphoid hyperplasia syndrome

Lymphoid interstitial pneumonitis (LIP)

This presents insidiously with dyspnea on exertion, with a chronic nonproductive cough. The chest X-ray shows diffuse reticulonodular shadowing, which persists despite appropriate antimicrobial therapy. Auscultatory findings are minimal. The condition progresses, resulting in hypoxia and finger clubbing. Other causes of interstitial infiltrates should be excluded, such as tuberculosis or infection with *P. carinii* and cytomegalovirus.

No pathogens have been identified in lung biopsy tissues from children with lymphoid interstitial pneumonitis, although the role of Epstein–Barr virus in pathogenesis is debated. HIV-RNA has been found, suggesting that the pneumonitis may be a direct result of HIV infection. Children with LIP seldom develop opportunistic infections, and the overall prognosis is better.

Polyglandular enlargement

Some children with lymphoid interstitial pneumonitis have recurrent attacks of parotitis, resulting in parotid gland enlargement. There may also be paratracheal or perihilar lymphadenopathy. Foci of lymphoid infiltrates have been reported in spleen, liver, gastrointestinal tract, skeletal muscle, adrenal medulla and epicardium (Joshi et al 1987). The nature of the lymphoid proliferation is not clear, nor is it known if this lymphoproliferative disorder is a precursor of lymphoma.

CUTANEOUS MANIFESTATIONS

Hair and skin texture

The majority of children with HIV infection are reported to have 'dry flaky skin' and 'wispy hair'. Alopecia is not uncommon as the disease progresses, probably secondary to malnutrition or recurrent infections.

Bacterial infections

Severe and recurrent bacterial infections result from the underlying defective humoral immunity. Staphylococcal skin lesions are the most frequent, and present as persistent folliculitis, cellulitis, impetigo and skin abscesses.

Fungal infections

Infection with C. *albicans* presents in atypical or severe forms because of immune suppression. Persistent mucocutaneous candidiasis occurring without prior use of antibiotics is often the first sign of HIV infection. It recurs when therapy is stopped and may involve the esophagus and larynx.

Viral infections

An early manifestation of immune compromise is *molluscum contagiosum*, which can affect the face. Dermatological conditions tend to occur when CD4+ lymphocytes fall below 1000 cells/mm^3. With increasing immune deficiency, *herpes simplex* virus type 1 infection presents with severe perioral ulcers. Lesions can become chronic, despite therapy with acyclovir. Herpes varicella-zoster infection can be disseminated and persistent, requiring several courses of acyclovir.

Rashes

Almost all children with symptomatic HIV infection have rashes at some stage of the illness. Atopic dermatitis, 'eczematous rashes', diffuse erythematous flushes and urticarial reactions have been described. Drug eruptions are common following therapy with ampicillin or co-trimoxazole. Skin changes compatible with acrodermatitis enteropathica, scurvy and zinc deficiency follow chronic diarrhea.

Neoplasia

Kaposi's sarcoma, frequently seen in adults with AIDS, has been described in less than 10% of children. Those who do present have an aggressive and fulminant form which rarely manifests as skin lesions, although large tumors are often found in lungs, liver, lymph nodes and intestine.

OTHER FEATURES

Hematological abnormalities which have been reported include microcytic anemia, immune thrombocytopenia and atypical lymphocytosis in the early stages of infection. Anemia is seen in end-stage disease, along with lymphopenia.

Other conditions thought to be caused by HIV include cardiopathy, nephropathy, neuropathy and hepatitis.

DIFFERENTIAL DIAGNOSIS

Primary and secondary causes of immune deficiency which must be excluded include agammaglobulinemia and hypogammaglobu-linemia, severe combined T and B cell immunodeficiencies, DiGeorge syndrome, ataxia telangiectasia, Wiskott–Aldrich syndrome, adenosine deaminase deficiency, purine nucleoside phosphorylase deficiency, severe malnutrition, immuno-suppression and congenital infections.

A careful history should elicit risk factors in the child or mother, time of onset of symptoms and the presence of significant opportunistic infections. Examination may reveal evidence of dysmorphism or neurological defects. Initial screening tests should include lymphocyte subsets and quantitative immuno-globulin measurement. Polyclonal hypergammaglobulinemia is rare in other immunodeficiencies, and in the presence of CD4+ lymphopenia should lead to the presumptive diagnosis of HIV infection especially if risk factors are documented.

MANAGEMENT

GENERAL SUPPORTIVE CARE

A major concern amongst medical, nursing and ancillary staff is the transmission of HIV. The risks are minimal in the work environment, especially if care is taken to avoid accidental inoculation injuries and mucocutaneous blood contamination. Studies of close family and household contacts of patients with AIDS have failed to demonstrate horizontal transmission, except when stringent precautions have not been adopted when dealing with large quantities of blood or feces (Friedland & Klein 1987).

A thorough assessment of the home and the parents' ability to care for the infected child is necessary. Families need counseling to cope with the stigma and stresses produced by living with AIDS. Financial problems arise either because the families usually come from areas of multiple deprivation or because of parental ill health. If both parents are infected, alternative care for the child may have to be sought. When considering care or education for the infected child, decisions should be individually tailored. Amongst issues to be considered are the health and development of the child, such as the presence of oozing skin lesions, bleeding disorders, transmissible diseases and socialization skills. All child care staff should follow universal guidelines for handling spillages of blood and body fluids, including the routine use of gloves and a dilute bleach solution for disinfection.

IMMUNIZATION

Live virus vaccines can cause serious adverse side effects when administered to immunocompromised individuals. Retrospective review of case records of HIV-infected children revealed no cases of atypical measles, paralytic poliomyelitis or aseptic meningitis following receipt of measles, mumps, rubella or polio vaccines. With the exception of BCG, it is probably safe to give live vaccines to HIV-positive individuals, with or without symptoms of the disease (Tarantola & Mann 1987). Vaccination should be offered prior to the onset of immune deficiency. However, vaccine efficacy may be reduced compared to that of immunocompetent children, and should therefore be monitored. The use of hyperimmune immunoglobulin should be considered for HIV-infected children, following exposure to measles or chickenpox.

Because oral polio vaccine virus may be excreted for prolonged periods from individuals with immune dysfunction, the clinician may choose to use inactivated polio vaccine especially if there are other HIV-infected members in the household.

There are no contraindications to the use of inactivated vaccines such as diphtheria, tetanus and pertussis vaccines. The theoretical risk of accelerating HIV infection by immunization has not been supported by clinical information that is available, and the risks are insignificant when compared to antigenic stimulation provided by endemic infectious diseases.

BACTERIAL INFECTIONS

Despite raised gamma globulin levels, HIV-infected children are functionally hypogammaglobulinemic. Prompt treatment of infections should be started with broad spectrum antibiotics until results of sensitivities are available. Prophylactic co-trimoxazole may be used. A double-blind, placebo-controlled study has shown that, compared to albumin, regular infusions of immunoglobulin (400 mg every 4 weeks) reduced the frequency of bacterial and viral infections in children with CD4+ counts in excess of 200 cells/mm³ (Mofenson et al 1992).

Infection with *Mycobacterium tuberculosis* requires prolonged therapy with antituberculous agents. No effective agent exists against *Mycobacterium avium-intracellulare* which presents as a disseminated infection in terminally ill children.

VIRAL INFECTIONS

Regular intravenous immunoglobulin therapy offers some passive protection against common viruses. Following known exposure to measles or chickenpox, hyperimmune immunoglobulin should be given as soon as possible. In an immunocompromised child, measles and varicella can run atypical courses. Fatal measles pneumonia has been documented in the absence of an identifiable rash. Infection with varicella can lead to pneumonitis, encephalitis or chronic cutaneous varicella-zoster. Therapy with acyclovir should be started promptly, to avoid onset of complications, and prolonged treatment may be necessary.

Many children with HIV infection are asymptomatic carriers of cytomegalovirus. With onset of immune deficiency, disseminated CMV infection occurs. Ganciclovir and trisodium phosphonoformate (Foscarnet) have reported efficacy in adults but experience with children is limited.

FUNGAL INFECTION

Topical nystatin or miconazole should be used for candidal infection of the mouth and nappy area. With esophageal candida, intravenous fluconazole, clotrimazole or ketoconazole may be more effective. Cases which are refractory to therapy might require therapy with amphotericin B or flucytosine. Candidiasis is likely to recur unless maintenance treatment is initiated.

Pneumocystis carinii is the major opportunistic pathogen in children with AIDS, although diagnostic difficulties arise when a child is unable to cooperate in methods to induce sputum production. Bronchoalveolar lavage and examination of the washings improves diagnostic acumen, along with newer methods such as detection of *P. carinii* antigen in respiratory tract secretions, using monoclonal antibodies. Treatment may have to be empirical, with high-dose co-trimoxazole. Side effects include hypersensitivity to the sulfonamide component, and myelosuppression. Intravenous pentamidine has been used, but toxic effects on the liver, kidneys and adrenals have led to aerosolized delivery as the method of choice in adults. Following one attack of *P. carinii* pneumonia, prophylaxis with co-trimoxazole or inhaled pentamidine must be instituted. Prophylaxis is also recommended for all infants born to HIV-infected women until it is established that the infant is not infected with HIV. For infected children, prophylaxis is recommended when the CD4+ lymphocyte count falls below the age-appropriate cut-off (Centers for Disease Control 1995b).

PROTOZOAL INFECTION

Infestation of the gastrointestinal tract with *Cryptosporidium* leads to diarrhea refractory to treatment. An empirical course of metronidazole might be helpful in eradicating *Giardia lamblia*. *Isospora belli* has been isolated, which responds to treatment with co-trimoxazole. Infection of the central nervous system with *Toxoplasma gondii* merits therapy with sulfadiazine and pyrimethamine.

NUTRITION

Nutritional assessment should be performed early, by a dietitian. With progression of disease, nutritional intervention is essential. Oral and esophageal candidiasis will result in a poor intake, requiring nasogastric or nasoduodenal continuous or overnight feeding. If malabsorption has been excluded, gastrostomy feeding can result in good weight gain. Parenteral nutrition may be the only option in some children. Care must be taken when indwelling catheters are used in an immunocompromised child.

Microbiological investigations may be unhelpful, and some children have persistent diarrhea despite parenteral feeding. A regimen of oral gentamicin and cholestyramine has been suggested, while others have tried zidovudine, on the basis that the diarrhea and wasting result from a direct infection of the gut with HIV.

RESPIRATORY DISEASE

Acute respiratory failure is caused by infection of the lungs with *P. carinii*, CMV, *C. albicans* or bacterial pathogens. Antimicrobial therapy alone may be insufficient, and some children require respiratory support. The prognosis for children who require mechanical ventilation is poor, and the justification for resorting to such action must be questioned.

Although children with lymphoid interstitial pneumonitis have a lower mortality, morbidity is considerable. Chronic hypoxemia results in restricted exercise tolerance and home oxygen therapy may be required. Repeated episodes of acute respiratory infections warrant several courses of antibiotics. Corticosteroids have been used with good results, although this is potentially hazardous in a child with poor immune function. Zidovudine therapy may produce favorable results.

NEUROLOGICAL DISEASE

Apart from infectious complications, the central nervous system is susceptible to primary lymphoma and cerebrovascular accidents as well as demyelination. With impaired brain growth, loss of cognitive function and motor milestones, the child suffers multiple handicaps. The encephalopathy can be static or progressive, and may be accompanied by seizures.

Significant improvement in clinical signs and neurodevelopmental scores have resulted when zidovudine was administered to children with neurological involvement (Pizzo et al 1988). However, the long-term effects are as yet unknown, and it may only delay the onset of physical and mental handicap. In such cases, physiotherapy, occupational therapy, speech therapy and special educational services will be required along with the medical input.

HIV-ASSOCIATED THROMBOCYTOPENIA

Thrombocytopenia may be the presenting feature of HIV infection. It is indistinguishable from idiopathic immune thrombocytopenia, and may not require active intervention. When the platelet count drops to less than $20 \times 10^9/l$ spontaneous bruising and bleeding occurs. Corticosteroids and splenectomy might result in a raised platelet count, but are not without dangers in an immune-compromised child. Although controlled studies are lacking, a safer alternative may be provided by high-dose intravenous immunoglobulin (0.4–1.0 g/kg/day over 2–5 days). The total dose depends on the response to the initial dose, and maintenance treatment may be required.

Zidovudine can increase the count in those individuals with previously low levels, probably owing to an antiviral effect.

ANTIRETROVIRAL THERAPY

The first available antiretroviral drug was zidovudine (AZT) with activity against reverse transcriptase. However, longer term studies in adults showed that the benefits of monotherapy were short-lived, owing mainly to the emergence of resistant strains of HIV. Many of the therapeutic advances since 1996 have focussed on treatments using a combination of two or more drugs. The availability of protease inhibitors (ritonavir, nelfinavir), non-nucleoside reverse transcriptase inhibitors (nevirapine) as well as a wider range of reverse transcriptase inhibitors (didanosine, zalcitabine) and newer drugs (lamivudine, stavudine) have also opened up exciting prospects in the treatment of HIV infection. Debates continue as to when to start treatment, especially in a child who is asymptomatic (Pizzo & Wilfert 1994). New research on viral dynamics and pathogenesis shows the very high viral loads which can exist in apparently well individuals with HIV infection, and advocates of early intervention argue that in most infectious diseases, treatment is started as soon as infection is diagnosed. Against this, is the fact that many long-term survivors do so without therapeutic intervention, and the drugs available have appreciable toxicity.

At present, antiretroviral therapy is recommended in the following circumstances:

- an AIDS-defining illness
- CD4 count very low for age or falling rapidly
- failure to thrive
- persistent HIV-related symptoms
- rising viral load.

Quantitative measures of viral activity (viral load) are now used to guide decisions to start as well as change therapy. In theory, more than 200 combinations of drugs are now possible; but few are licenced for use in children. Many formulations are also unpalatable or unsuitable for young children. The future direction for anti-HIV therapy is likely to follow the models developed for childhood leukemia, using relatively toxic drugs to halt viral replication to prevent disease progression. This can only be achieved with multi-center collaboration, such as the Pediatric European Network for Treatment in AIDS (PENTA) and the AIDS Clinical Trials Group in the US (ACTG).

IMMUNOLOGICAL RECONSTITUTION

Agents like interferon α and γ, interleukin-2 and tumor necrosis factor suppress HIV replication and may have a place when combined with antiretroviral therapy. In adults, passive neutralization of antigenemia has been described, using plasma rich in p24 antibody. This form of therapy has few side effects, and merits further evaluation in children.

International collaboration is the way forward to evaluate all forms of therapy, as few centers have large enough numbers of infected children to conduct meaningful trials.

PROGNOSIS

HIV infection in children has been shown to be compatible with long-term survival (Tovo et al 1992, European Collaborative Study 1994a, Italian Register 1994). Although infants who develop an opportunistic infection in the first year of life have the poorest prognosis, with few surviving beyond 2 years of age, the median survival for the remaining children is 10 years. In developing countries, common causes of death include protracted diarrhea with wasting, pneumonia and measles. Table 23.31 outlines the prognostic value of some clinical signs.

PREVENTION

With the routine screening of blood, treatment of blood products and self-deferral of donors, the number of transfusion-associated cases will diminish. There will, however, be an increase in the number of children infected by vertical transmission, whose mothers have acquired the infection heterosexually. The present challenge is therefore to limit the current spread of HIV by sexual transmission. Vertical transmission can be reduced by the use of zidovudine in the antenatal, intrapartum and postnatal period, although the longer-term effects of zidovudine on the fetus and newborn are unknown (Connor et al 1994). While no effective vaccine or cure exists, an intensive educational approach is important, which should include information on the modes of transmission of HIV. For the pediatrician, this means educating schoolchildren and teenagers, as well as women of childbearing age, about good hygiene standards, avoidance of intravenous drug use and safer sexual practices.

TREPONEMATOSES AND SEXUALLY TRANSMISSIBLE DISEASES

In sexually transmissible disease (STD) the pediatric interest arises for a number of reasons. The need for prevention and protection in children necessitates an unambiguous commitment to education in the difficult and controversial field of sexual behaviour. Sexual abuse of children is being increasingly revealed as a serious medicosocial problem (Lancet 1987a); this will need understanding of the approach and procedures necessary to detect or exclude sexually transmitted infection. In STD infection of one parent is likely to lead to infection of the other and in the case of pregnancy vertical transmission to the fetus or neonate may take place. Specific treatment will have to take into account the sensitivity of the organism to antibiotic or chemotherapy prevailing in the locality and in the control of STD the tracing of contacts is essential. In endemic treponematoses, however, it is not sexual transmission which is the method of spread but close contact among children and others with skin lesions in an infectious stage.

PREVENTION

The need for primary prevention, always important, has been sharpened in recent times and becomes more pressing for everyone responsible for the education of the young as human immunodeficiency virus (HIV) infection and the acquired immune-deficiency syndrome (AIDS) have spread inexorably since first recognized in 1981. In STD secondary prevention has an important role and this will require insight by the young person of the possible risks of sexual behavior and a willingness to seek help when needed. It will need readily available medical facilities for diagnosis and specific treatment as well as those for counseling and the tracing and treatment of contacts.

Worldwide, wherever AIDS is found, the causative agent, the human immunodeficiency virus (HIV) is spread only in the same ways – through penetrative sexual intercourse, blood transfer and from infected mother to infant. There is now increasing evidence that other STDs, particularly those like syphilis, chancroid and genital herpes, that cause genital ulceration, may increase the likelihood of the spread of HIV. For the reasons stated, because effective vaccines have not yet been created and because there is not yet a fully effective drug for treatment, sex education and information programs are critical to AIDS prevention and STD control. The short-term actions, often strident in their urgency, have to be replaced by education programs which will last and which will be brought into the schools (Director of the World Health Organization Global Programme on AIDS 1988).

In relation to the transmission of STD it is appropriate here to refer to the evidence that psychosexual development in both sexes is determined by nutrition. In developed countries sexual maturity in girls, for example, occurs at an earlier age than in the developing countries as a result of good nutrition. Intellectual maturity, upon which her capacity to cope with her sexuality depends, is, however, more dependent upon chronological age and comes later. The social consequences of lowering the age of puberty are profound:

earlier sexual activity requires access to sex education. Rights to health education, including sex education, can be claimed from the European Convention of Human Rights. Judgments of the European Court of Human Rights have made these obligations clear as well as the bounds that may be set in this subject. The principles characterizing a 'democratic society', which are relevant to discussion on education and have been outlined in the European Court of Human Rights (ECHR) at Strasbourg, emphasize the value of 'freedom of expression'. The importance of pluralism, tolerance and broadmindedness is again and again emphasized as well as the balance which must be achieved to secure the fair and proper treatment of minorities. None the less, teaching materials should not contain sentences or paragraphs that young people, at a critical stage of their development, could interpret as encouragement to indulge in precocious activities harmful for them, or even to commit criminal offences (for further discussion see Robertson et al 1989, pp. 56–58).

SUMMARY OF CLINICAL AND LABORATORY PROCEDURES FOR THE DETECTION OR EXCLUSION OF STD

The clinician, when considering the possibility of a sexually transmitted disease in a patient, will find it useful to follow the summary of the clinical procedures (detailed more fully in the text) necessary to detect or exclude such infection and to consider a number of other important issues as listed below.

EARLY STAGE SYPHILIS

Detect or exclude syphilis. If detected give specific treatment for patient and trace contacts.

1. Clinical inspection: surface lesions of early syphilis, e.g. chancre, condylomata lata.
2. Microscopy (serum obtained from depth of mucocutaneous surface lesions): detection of *T. pallidum:* dark ground illumination, monoclonal antibody immunofluorescence.
3. Serological tests: e.g. venereal disease research laboratory (VDRL) test and *Treponema pallidum* hemagglutination assay (TPHA) (confirmation if necessary by the fluorescent treponemal antibody-absorbed (FTA-ABS) test at 0, 30 and 90 days); trace particularly *contacts* of primary and secondary syphilis.

GONORRHOEA

Detect or exclude: if infected give specific treatment and trace contacts.
Bacteriological diagnosis:

1. Gram-stained film.
2. Selective medium, direct plating, when immediate incubation available, or use transport (e.g. Amies) (serogroup/serovar analysis in medicolegal cases).
3. *N gonorrhoeae:* test all for β-lactamase production, chromosomally mediated resistance.
4. Sites examined (number of occasions): heterosexual male – urethra ($\times$ 1); throat ($\times$ 2) if indicated; homosexual male – urethra ($\times$ 1); anorectum ($\times$ 2); throat always ($\times$ 2); female – urethra ($\times$ 2); cervix ($\times$ 2); throat ($\times$ 2) if indicated. (Indications for throat culture: history, if *N. gonorrhoeae* is detected in any site or if patient is a contact of *N. gonorrhoeae* case.)

OTHER STD

Detect or exclude; specific treatment for affected patient; trace contacts. Some other issues to consider at this stage:

1. By inspection: *Phthirus pubis, Sarcoptes scabiei* (or characteristic lesions), molluscum contagiosum, human papillomavirus (HPV) or herpes simplex virus (HSV) lesions.
2. Heterosexual male: nongonococcal urethritis (NGU) and recurrences (common).
3. Homosexual male: positive HBsAg, HIV, enteric infection (possibly common).
4. Female: cervical cytopathology (annual smears/colposcopy when indicated); pelvic inflammatory disease (PID); *Trichomonas vaginalis:* (diagnosis by microscopy of wet vaginal film); *Candida*: (diagnosis by microscopy of Gram-stained film); *Chlamydia*: 0.2 M sucrose phosphate (2SP) transport medium (see later), smear fixed in acetone for immunofluorescence test; 'anaerobic vaginal infection' (Amies) (pH > 4.5; amines released by potassium hydroxide solution (10%).

OTHER MEDICAL CONDITIONS

History:

Hepatitis B (see pp. 476, 1386)
Allergy to drugs
Recent or present antibiotic or chemotherapy (if any)
Drug misuse/addiction (especially i.v. and sharing of needles)
Contraception/pregnancy
Glycosuria (diabetes important cause of balanitis).

SOCIAL ASPECTS

Nonjudgmental attitude in staff.
Conciliation important.
Avoid making situation worse.
Right of patient to truth.
Confidentiality strict, information within STD department.
Medicolegal (sexual abuse, marital issues).
Trace contacts: persuasion: no threats, no coercion, legal or otherwise.

HIV INFECTION AND AIDS

HIV antibody test requires the following:

Pretest counseling
Consent
Informing of results
Learning to live
Partners, consideration of
Prevention; unambiguous counseling
Infection control (HIV, HBV, *M. tuberculosis*)
Safer sex, information on
STD, exclusion or detection of other
Link with other support services
Follow-up
Tests predictive of AIDS

SUMMARY OF AIMS

Organismal diagnosis first; specific treatment afterwards.
Contact tracing (source and secondary contact) after diagnosis; priority related to seriousness.
Epidemiological treatment.
Prevention: counseling and risk reduction.

OTHER GROUPS (SPECIAL CONSIDERATIONS)

PREGNANT FEMALE

Treponema pallidum can be transmitted transplacentally long after a woman has ceased to be infectious sexually. Early diagnosis and treatment with penicillin is essential to prevent spread to or to cure fetus (crystalline benzyl pencillin, procaine penicillin).

Neisseria gonorrhoeae – cervical infection, with spread to the fetus during passage down birth canal to cause conjunctivitis of newborn (benzyl penicillin, or ampicillin for mother).

Chlamydia trachomatis – cervical infection, treat with erythromycin.

Herpes simplex virus – see text for discussion on prevention in newborn.

Hepatitis B virus – babies of HBeAg positive mothers: give to newborn 0.5 ml HBIG at delivery within 48 h, and vaccinate at 0, 1 and 6 months.

Human papillomavirus: genital warts – commonly increase in size and spread during pregnancy; recede during puerperium. Laryngeal papillomas rare in neonate/children.

Human immunodeficiency viruses: intrauterine and postnatal transmission.

NEONATE

Congenital syphilis is rare in areas where antibiotics are easy to obtain: 'early' form and 'late' form.
Conjunctivitis of newborn:

N. gonorrhoeae (see p. 283)

Chlamydia trachomatis spread to fetus during delivery to cause conjunctivitis and sometimes pneumonitis (erythromycin ethylsuccinate 50 mg/kg/day orally and topical tetracycline for 3 weeks for affected infant).

Hepatitis B: HBIG/vaccine.

Herpes simplex virus – acyclovir treatment if any lesions seen.

Human immunodeficiency viruses: acquired immune-deficiency syndrome.

THE PREPUBERTAL CHILD

When sexual abuse of prepubertal children is suspected screening for sexually transmissible disease forms an important part of medical investigation. Firstly it allows treatment of what otherwise might be an undetected and damaging infection. Secondly the presence of an STD, particularly early stage syphilis and gonorrhea, may be supportive evidence that sexual abuse has occurred and in the case of gonorrhea serotyping of the organism may allow it to be matched with a supposed assailant. Furthermore STD including HIV infection may be an important factor to consider when compensation for criminal injury is being assessed (Criminal Justice Act 1988, UK legislation).

The circumstances of the examination of young children are important. At all times a sympathetic and understanding approach is required in the management of these children and repeated examinations by different doctors are to be avoided. When possible a single detailed examination should be performed in the presence of both a police surgeon and pediatrician, with the child sedated if necessary. A general physical examination which will include throat, eyes, ears, chest and abdomen should precede the examination of genitalia and anus. Time should be given to set the child at ease, so that examination of the genitalia and anus is seen as a routine part of the procedure (DHSS 1988). Evidence of trauma can be sought and satisfactory specimens obtained for the detection of STD; follow-up examinations for the exclusion of STD are not avoidable.

In the case of children suspected of having been sexually abused or proved to have been so abused the clinician should be aware of the importance of the multidisciplinary process and ensure that medical confidentiality does not work against the protection of the child.

Diagnosis of STD (for further detail see summary of clinical laboratory procedures for the detection or exclusion of STD, above) in prepubertal children.

1. Direct plating on selective media for *Neisseria gonorrhoeae*: pharynx, anorectum, urethra and vagina. Obtaining specimens may be facilitated by gentle insertion of an auriscope or a suitable nasal speculum (e.g. Killian's Nasal Speculum 2–2 $\frac{1}{2}$, Downs Surgical plc, Church Path, Mitcham, Surrey CR4 3UE, England); a swab is then passed along the speculum to sample the vaginal contents. Taking the anorectal specimen may be facilitated by the gentle use of a child's proctoscope.
2. Collection in 2SP (0.2 M sucrose phosphate transport medium) for isolation of *Chlamydia trachomatis*:* pharynx, rectum, urethra and vagina.
3. Collection on a swab placed in Amies' transport medium for anaerobes, *Trichomonas vaginalis*: vagina.
4. Note any anogenital discharge and exclude presence of foreign body in vagina or rectum.
5. In the presence of genital/oral vesicular lesions collect vesicular fluid or scrapings from roof or base of vesicle in virus transport medium for herpes simplex virus.*
6. Serological tests for syphilis (e.g. VDRL and TPHA) and hepatitis B (e.g. HBsAg and antibody).
7. Store serum (for retrospective anti-HIV testing if necessary).

Specific consent from person with legal responsibility for the child for testing is necessary.

THE TREPONEMATOSES

AETIOLOGY

Treponema pallidum is the causative organism of syphilis and the other treponematoses, yaws and pinta. Because of their very close genetic homology the treponemes of syphilis (including endemic syphilis) and yaws are designated as subspecies of *T. pallidum* (Penn & Pritchard 1990):

---

*If delay more than 3 h store at − 70°C.

1. *Treponema pallidum* subspecies *pallidum* (causative organism of syphilis, worldwide in distribution): sexually transmitted and congenital infection
2. *Treponema pallidum* subspecies *pertenue* (causative of yaws, endemic in some warmer countries): not sexually transmitted, spread mostly by skin lesion to skin contact in childhood
3. *Treponema pallidum* subspecies *endemicum* (causative organism of endemic syphilis, e.g. *bejel* of seminomads of Arabian peninsula and sub-Saharan Africa): spread by skin contact etc.
4. *Treponema carateum* (causative organism of pinta, found in scattered foci in northern South America or Mexico): direct skin to skin contact.

As these pathogenic treponemes cannot be cultured in vitro, *T. pallidum* is grown in vivo in the testes of rabbits to produce antigen for diagnostic tests and for research purposes. *T. pallidum* is a delicate tightly coiled spiraled filament 6–10 μm by 0.1–0.18 μm in diameter and is often referred to as a 'spirochete'. It is feebly refractile and too narrow to be seen well by ordinary light microscopy. Dark ground illumination has been the technique normally used to detect this organism in the lesions of early syphilis since its demonstration as the cause of syphilis by Schaudinn and Hoffman in 1905. Immunofluorescent techniques can now be used to demonstrate the organism in tissue and body fluids.

SYPHILIS

Transmission

Syphilis is spread principally by sexual intercourse but it may be transmitted congenitally, that is to say transplacentally to the fetus in utero by the infected mother (see p. 1404). Although congenital syphilis in children is rare in many parts of Europe, and most doctors will never have seen a case, it is important to continue universal antenatal screening for syphilis (Nicoll & Moisley 1994).

Transfusion-acquired syphilis is now rare. Nevertheless screening for syphilis in all units of donated blood intended for immediate transfusion should remain national policy (Schryver & Meheus 1990). When infected blood is stored at 4°C in citrate anticoagulant, infectivity is lost between 96 and 120 h. The actual survival times may depend on the number of treponemenes present in donor blood (van der Sluis et al 1985). The risk of accidental syphilis is highest where fresh heparinized blood is used as in exchange transfusion in neonates (Risseeuw-Appel & Kothe 1983).

Pathogenesis and immunology

The pathogenesis of syphilis reflects invasive properties of *T. pallidum*, but the actual mechanism of tissue invasion is unknown. It is likely that the highly motile spirochetes leave the circulation by invading the junctions between endothelial cells (Thomas et al 1988). Syphilis can be considered as a generalized infection of vascular tissues since, within lesions in each stage, treponemes localize primarily in vascular areas. Capillary destruction inhibits blood supply leading to necrosis and ulceration, characteristics of syphilis pathology (Quist et al 1983). *T. pallidum* has a remarkable ability to evade the humoral and cellular responses

that it elicits in infected hosts. T cell-mediated delayed-type hypersensitivity is the predominant mechanism for clearing tissues of infecting organisms in the primary lesions of syphilis (Sell & Hsu 1993). The dermal inflammatory infiltrate in primary and secondary syphilis is composed mainly of lymphocytes and plasma cells: in primary lesions CD4-positive cells predominate (Engelkens et al 1993). Genital ulceration due to syphilis increases the risk of acquiring HIV (Stamm et al 1988).

Human immunodeficiency virus infection may have a profound influence upon the natural history of syphilis and be associated with unusual presentations of this disease (Rufli 1989, Musher et al 1990).

Acquired syphilis

General description

Syphilis is systemic from the onset and produces short symptomatic and prolonged asymptomatic stages. In the early infectious stage of the disease lesions, containing many treponemes, occur on the moist mucocutaneous parts of the body, particularly the genitalia, and enable transmission to occur by sexual intercourse. Even if untreated these lesions tend to heal but may recur during the first 2–4 years, after which the disease becomes latent or hidden. The latent form or the noninfectious late stage of the disease may persist for decades without producing obvious clinical changes, but a proportion of patients will unpredictably develop active involvement of the cardiovascular system (about 10%), the central nervous system (about 10%), or localized gummatous destructive lesions which can affect the musculoskeletal system (about 10%), the viscera and mucous membranes (about 15%) (Fig. 23.25).

If treated in the early stage clinical cure can be achieved by penicillin treatment and with certain other antibiotics. In the late stages curative effects are often spectacular in some forms of neurosyphilis and in gummatous syphilis. In cardiovascular forms of the disease the effects of antibiotic therapy are not easy to define.

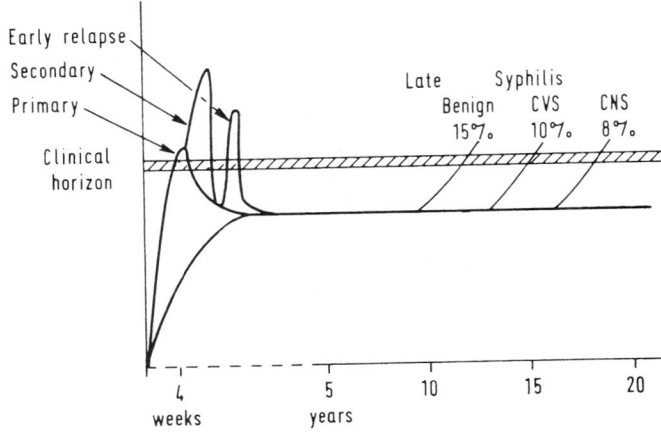

Fig. 23.25 Simplified diagrammatic representation of the course of untreated syphilis from the times of infection. The early stages, whether primary, secondary or early relapse or latent syphilis, are indicated together with the subsequent development of late stage effects, whether late benign or gummatous, cardiovascular, central nervous system or late stage latent syphilis. The percentage of effects may vary in different populations. (Modified from Robertson et al 1989.)

There are a number of reports, mainly from the USA, to suggest that in HIV-infected patients, syphilis runs a more severe course and lesions may be more aggressive in both early and late stage disease; neurological complications of secondary syphilis occur more frequently and at an earlier stage and may increase the risk of treatment failure (Musher et al 1990, Goldmeier & Hay 1993, Malone et al 1995).

Congenital infection

See page 1411.

Laboratory diagnosis of syphilis

In syphilis a clinical diagnosis must be confirmed in the laboratory either by:

1. demonstrating *T. pallidum* in the serous exudate obtained from the depth of early lesions
2. demonstrating specific antibodies in the serum.

For a detailed review of the value and limitations of screening tests and diagnostic strategies as well as an outline of new technological approaches see Young (1992).

Demonstration of T. pallidum *in primary and secondary lesions*

Dark ground microscopy. After cleansing the surfaces of the primary or secondary lesions with a swab soaked in physiological saline, serum is obtained from the depth of the lesion by gentle squeezing and examined by dark ground microscopy using the oil immersion objective. *T. pallidum* is recognized by its slender structure, characteristic slow movements and angulation. If the initial test is negative the procedure should be repeated daily for at least 3 days: antibiotics should be withheld during this period although co-trimoxazole orally may be used to reduce local sepsis. Many commensal treponemes occur in the mouth and therefore dark ground illumination is not suitable for examining oral lesions. Organisms are not easily found in skin lesions of secondary syphilis except those in moist skin areas.

Fluorescence microscopy. Direct fluorescent-antibody staining for *T. pallidum* (DFA-Tp) overcomes the problem of examining potentially infectious material. A smear of the material to be tested is made on a glass slide, dried and fixed (5 min immersion in acetone) prior to sending to the laboratory. When a monoclonal antibody-staining reagent is used the DFA-Tp test has similar sensitivity to dark ground microscopy but greater potential specificity (Romanowski et al 1987).

The Centers for Disease Control (CDC), Atlanta, recommend that when clinical findings suggest syphilis, but serological tests are negative, biopsy tissue should be examined by DFA-Tp or silver staining (MMWR 1989).

Demonstration of antibodies in the serum

During treponemal infection, whether in syphilis or in the endemic treponemal diseases such as yaws or pinta, a variety of antibodies are produced. These can be classified into nonspecific antitreponemal antibodies and antibodies specific for pathogenic treponemes.

After infection, the first humoral immune response is the production of antibodies of the IgM class. Specific anti-*T.*

pallidum IgM is detectable during the second week of infection but disappears usually within 3–9 months of the beginning of treatment in cases of early syphilis or within 1–1.5 years after treatment of late disease.

Production of IgG begins around the fourth week after infection and usually reaches much higher titers than those for IgM. IgG secretion may be continued by memory cell clones long after elimination of the antigen thus accounting for the persistence of reactivity in sensitive tests such as the *Treponema pallidum* hemagglutination assay (TPHA) and the fluorescent treponemal antibody-absorbed (FTA-ABS) test.

Tests to detect nonspecific treponemal antibodies

Cardiolipin antigen tests

Cardiolipin is widespread in nature and the lipids of *T. pallidum* include cardiolipin as do mammalian mitochondria. Cardiolipin tests now use defined antigens comprising cardiolipin mixed with lecithin and cholesterol to provide optimum reactivity.

There are a wide range of cardiolipin antigen tests available (Young & Penn 1990) but the most widely used are the Venereal Disease Research Laboratory (VDRL) carbon antigen test in the UK and the Rapid Plasma Reagin RPR test in the USA. Both tests are suitable for routine screening as they are cheap, simple to perform (can test serum or plasma), can be read by eye, and are quantifiable yielding a titer by end-point doubling dilution of the patient's serum. They usually become positive 10–14 days after the appearance of the chancre, the titer gradually increasing. After treatment the titer tends to diminish and the test becomes negative. In late or latent syphilis the cardiolipin antigen tests are often negative.

One of the most serious, and often underestimated, disadvantages of these tests is the prozone phenomenon, i.e. the occurrence of false negative reactions resulting from inhibition of agglutination by excess antibody in the serum (Young 1992). In the US, false negative serological tests due to the prozone phenomenon have been reported in women who gave birth to infants with congenital infection. This is unlikely to occur in Europe as the VDRL is not recommended as a single screening test.

In syphilis, the antibody is now generally considered to be directed against cardiolipin present in treponemes, i.e. it is antibody against a nonspecific antigen shared by treponemes and mammalian tissues. However, the serum of patients with an acute febrile infectious disease, or an autoimmune disorder, may give a positive cardiolipin antigen test but negative specific treponemal antigen tests in the absence of past or present treponemal infection. This is widely referred to as a 'biological false positive reaction' or BFP but the term 'nontreponemal cardiolipin antibody response' is more accurate. Other tests are required to distinguish between positive cardiolipin tests resulting from treponemal infection and those due to other causes (Robertson et al 1989).

Tests to detect antibodies specific for pathogenic treponemes

The antigen used in these tests is derived from Nichols strain of *T. pallidum* which is maintained in rabbits by intratesticular inoculation and weekly passage. Tests using pathogenic *T. pallidum* antigen tend to remain positive for a very long time after treatment and can be used to confirm the treponemal nature of a positive cardiolipin antigen test result or as a sensitive screen for all stages of infection. The main treponemal tests are:

The Fluorescent Treponemal Antibody Absorbed (FTA-ABS) Test

The FTA-ABS is an indirect immunofluorescence test which makes it unsuitable for routine screening but it is currently the standard confirmatory test. It becomes reactive around the third week of infection and in primary infection has a sensitivity ranging from 86 to 100%. It is positive in all secondary cases and 96–100% of late stage infections. Reactivity persists after adequate therapy although the test may occasionally become nonreactive if treatment is given early in the disease. Although the FTA-ABS is considered to be a very specific test it is not endowed with the high level of specificity usually accorded. The reputation for high specificity stems from the fact that it is applied to sera that have been preselected thus increasing considerably the probability that they contain antitreponemal antibodies. The specificity of the FTA-ABS test is not absolute, however, and varies from 92 to 99% (Hunter et al 1986). The total prevalence of false reactivity is around 1% in normal persons, but higher rates have been reported in hospital patients (Luger 1988). Reactivity only in the FTA-ABS test must be treated with caution: in one study 43% of patients with Lyme disease were reactive in this test (Carlsson et al 1991). More widespread use of *T. pallidum* antigen tests for screening also suggests that the FTA-ABS may be marginally less sensitive in detecting antibody in infections treated many years previously.

The T. pallidum *Hemagglutination Assay (TPHA)*

The TPHA is a hemagglutination assay in which sheep erythrocytes coated with an extract of *T. pallidum* are agglutinated by antibody from serum of patients with syphilis. Components of Reiter treponemes, rabbit testis and erythrocyte membranes are used to absorb test sera in order to eliminate hemagglutination due to antibody against any of these agents. TPHA reactivity may be detectable around the fourth week of infection. The sensitivity in untreated primary infection ranges from 64–87%. The TPHA titer tends to be low in primary syphilis (80–320) but rises sharply in the secondary stage reaching 5120 or greater. The titer declines during the latent stage but invariably remains positive, often a low titer (80–1280). Titers may decline after therapy but, with the exception of patients coinfected with HIV, the test almost always remains positive (Lukehart 1991).

According to Luger (1988) the TPHA, with an overall margin of error in the range of 0.07% false positive reactions and 0.008% false negative reactions, is the most sensitive and specific method for detecting antibodies to *T. pallidum*. When false negative reactions occur they are usually associated with early primary infection and this is the main reason why the TPHA has not been widely used as a single screening test in laboratories serving STD clinics.

Enzyme Immunoassay (EIA)

EIA is a relatively simple serological technique with the additional advantage of automation and electronic reporting. The majority of EIAs are noncompetitive – patients' serum is allowed to react with antigen coated on the surface of small plastic beads or on the inside surface of plastic tubes or wells in a microhemagglutination plate. Specific antibodies binding to the antigen are then quantitated by means of anti-immunoglobulin conjugated to an enzyme such as alkaline phosphatase or horseradish peroxidase. By use of appropriate enzyme substrates, color changes, which increase in intensity as the degree of specific antibody increases, can be measured spectrophotometrically allowing objective interpretation of the results. In contrast, in competitive EIAs a known positive serum competes with the patient's serum for binding sites on the antigen – a positive result is indicated by a decrease in the optical density of the test specimen relative to the control. Competitive EIAs are theoretically more sensitive in early primary infection. In general, the performance of EIAs using treponemal antigens, is similar to that of the TPHA. Recombinant antigen-based tests are already available although the most appropriate cocktail of recombinant antigens remains to be defined.

Serological tests in clinical practice

Since syphilis can be acquired concomitantly with any other STD those at risk should be screened to exclude syphilis. As congenital infection is preventable by appropriate treatment during pregnancy and the costs of congenital syphilis are so high it was calculated in 1983 that screening may be cost beneficial when the prevalence of maternal infection is as low as 0.005% (Stray-Pedersen 1983). Although the role of antenatal screening has been questioned more recently (Holland & O'Mahony 1989) the overwhelming body of opinion is that routine antenatal screening for syphilis is not only cost effective but is a valuable public health measure that must continue, even in countries where the disease has a relatively low prevalence (Pritchard & Hudson 1989, Clay 1989).

Screening with a combination of VDRL and TPHA tests

When used together, the VDRL and TPHA tests provide a highly efficient screen for the detection or exclusion of treponemal infection. The VDRL test is more sensitive than the TPHA in the detection of very early syphilis while the TPHA is more sensitive in the detection of latent and late stage infection (Young et al 1974).

Although the VDRL carbon antigen and TPHA tests can be performed without inactivation, heating patients' serum at 56°C for 30 min is recommended: this not only decreases the incidence of nonspecific agglutination but also destroys HIV or at least renders the levels noninfective.

The VDRL test usually becomes positive 10–14 days after the appearance of the chancre or approximately 3–5 weeks after acquiring the infection. It is positive in approximately 75% of cases of primary syphilis. After the secondary stage the VDRL titer declines and eventually becomes negative in approximately 30% of untreated latent and late cases. The VDRL test also tends to become negative after treatment, particularly in early syphilis.

The TPHA test

Patients' serum is screened at a final dilution of 1 in 80: if any hemagglutination is noted the test is repeated with a series of twofold dilutions from 1 in 80 to 1 in 5120. The reciprocal of the final serum dilution resulting in marked hemagglutination is termed the titer. TPHA titers are reported as positive-80, positive-160, etc. Each specimen is also tested against control cells (no antigen) at a serum dilution of 1 in 80: if the control cells agglutinate the serum is reported as 'nonspecific – agglutination test invalid'.

The TPHA may be negative in early primary syphilis but usually becomes positive at low titer (80–320) towards the end of the primary stage. The TPHA titer may give some indication of the duration of the infection. Titers rise sharply during the secondary stage and commonly reach 5120 or greater. The TPHA titer declines during the latent stage but invariably remains positive at low titer (80–640).

The only stage of syphilis likely to escape detection by screening with a combination of VDRL and TPHA tests is early primary syphilis, although repeated tests over a 3-month period will detect such an infection.

EIA

EIA used as a single screening test offers comparable performance to the VDRL/TPHA combination but has the additional advantage of an objective reading, automation and electronic report generation. There is no evidence to suggest that, in the case of primary syphilis, screening for antitreponemal IgG by EIA is significantly less sensitive than the combination of VDRL and TPHA tests (Young et al 1992). Provided that clinicians are aware of the 'seronegative window' that may exist for 1–2 weeks during the early primary infection, maintain a high index of clinical suspicion and have the facility to request additional tests (e.g. specific IgM or FTA-ABS) in cases of suspect primary infection, then detection of early infection will not be compromised by using antitreponemal IgG EIA as a single screening test.

Activity of infection and response to treatment

Cardiolipin antigen tests. Because there is no microbiological 'test of cure' patients treated for syphilis are conventionally followed using quantitative nontreponemal tests such as the VDRL. All cardiolipin antigen tests tend to become negative after treatment particularly in early syphilis. Patients with early syphilis should be followed clinically and serologically until they are free of clinical disease and seronegative in nontreponemal tests or have achieved a stable very low titer (Lukehart 1991). Serial quantitative tests should be carried out for up to 2 years following treatment for early acquired syphilis and for up to 5 years in late stage infection. The VDRL titer should become negative within 1–2 years of effective treatment for early syphilis. Seroreversal is governed by a range of factors and will take longer in the case of high initial titers, longer-duration infections, and repeat infections. As seroreversal does not always occur and may take many months when it does occur the rate of decline in titer is often more useful. In primary and secondary syphilis the titer should decrease fourfold by 3–6 months and eightfold at 6–12 months (Brown et al 1985, Romanowski et al 1987). In early latent infection a fourfold response may take up to 12 months. After adequate treatment of late infection the VDRL test may remain reactive (titer ≤ 8) for many years. In monitoring efficacy of treatment it is important to use the same type of cardiolipin test as the end-point titer may vary between tests: a twofold difference in titer is not considered significant but a fourfold difference is.

Quantitative VDRL testing is to some extent useful in assessing treatment status as titers ≥ 16 are rarely found in adequately treated infections (Luger 1988).

Detection of antitreponemal IgM. The presence of antitreponemal IgM in the sera of neonates and adults is an indication of the persistence of treponemal antigen within the body. In theory, tests to detect specific IgM should provide a more direct indication of treatment status and response to therapy. The variety of methods available for detecting antitreponemal IgM have been reviewed elsewhere (Young & Penn 1990): many of these methods are not available commercially and are technically unsuitable for routine use. In general, the titers of specific IgM decline after adequate treatment of early syphilis and reactivity ceases within 3–9 months; reactivity may be found from 1–1.5 years after treatment of late disease (Luger 1988). The detection of IgM by a commercially available EIA for antitreponemal IgM (Captia Syphilis M) was not recommended as a replacement for the VDRL test to monitor patients treated for syphilis (Ijsselmuiden et al 1989).

Detection of specific antitreponemal IgM, in patients without a history of recent treatment, suggests active disease and the need for chemotherapy. The simple Captia Syphilis M test is as sensitive as the technically complex 'gold standard' 19S(IgM) FTA-ABS test in early infection (Ijsselmuiden et al 1989, Lefevre et al 1990). Previous exposure to antibiotics combined with the general decrease in the spectrum and strength of antibody response which occurs with increased duration of infection may contribute to poor sensitivity in late infection. A reactive antitreponemal IgM test in a patient with positive serological tests supports the need for treatment. However, untreated or inadequately treated infection, particularly beyond the primary stages, as well as reinfections, cannot be excluded reliably on the basis of a nonreactive result. When considering treatments due consideration must be given to clinical findings, the history of the patient, and quantitative VDRL and TPHA tests.

Congenital syphilis

There remains a considerable risk for congenital infection in many developing countries. The diagnosis of congenital syphilis can present a considerable problem since it depends mainly on the results of serological tests and also because most infected neonates are asymptomatic at birth. Early stage congenital syphilis is a rarity in the UK and there are few up-to-date serological data available. During the 1980s there was a steady increase in the number of cases of congenital syphilis occurring in certain areas of the US which stimulated extensive interest in the diagnosis of congenital infection. In 1988 the surveillance case definition changed in the US which resulted in more reported cases (approximately 4000 in 1990) but thereafter the numbers began to decrease and fell to around 3000 cases in 1993 (Stoll 1994). The 1988 surveillance case definition was broad and covered any infant whose mother had untreated or inadequately treated syphilis at delivery. Confirmed cases were restricted to infants in whom *T. pallidum* was identified by dark ground microscopy, fluorescent antibody or other specific stains in placenta, umbilical cord or autopsy material.

The US surveillance definition is highly sensitive but lacks specificity and will include noninfected infants. A major clinical and laboratory dilemma is to determine which asymptomatic or at-risk neonate is infected and therefore requires evaluation and treatment. As the standard serological tests for syphilis depend on responses involving IgG and IgM antibodies their interpretation is extremely difficult; the IgG found in the serum of neonates is largely passively acquired through the placenta and does not represent the infant's own response. Lower titers in neonates when compared to their mothers are, however, suggestive of passively transferred antibody but serial testing is required. In the absence of infection passively transferred antibody detected by the VDRL, TPHA or EIA test for antitreponemal IgG will decrease and the tests will usually become negative in approximately 3–6 months. Whereas a rising or higher titer in the neonate than in the mother is suggestive of infection, the detection of specific antitreponemal IgM in the infant's serum provides more direct support for congenital infection. The simple to perform Captia Syphilis M test is as sensitive as the 19S(IgM) FTA-ABS test in cases of clinically diagnosed congenital infection (Schmitz et al 1994, Stoll et al 1993). Because an IgM response may take some time to develop, a negative IgM test result does not exclude congenital infection and it is important to follow up the infant with repeat IgM testing. Apart from specific antitreponemal IgM, infected infants tend to have raised total IgM (usually in the range of 1–4 g/l compared with < 0.7 g/l in noninfected neonates) which returns to normal after treatment (Borobio et al 1980).

Data on specific antitreponemal IgM in late stage congenital infection are inadequate. In late stage infection, either treated or untreated, test results tend to fluctuate over a period of months or years. The VDRL test often remains positive at low titer in association with a low TPHA titer and positive FTA-ABS test.

Newer technologies such as immunoblotting (to detect antibodies to the KDal antigen in particular) and PCR show promise and in future may play a major role on the detection of congenital infection. However, the major goal in congenital infection is prevention through good prenatal care and serological testing.

Diagnosis of neurosyphilis

The use of cerebrospinal fluid (CSF) for routine screening tests in patients in whom there is no clinical suspicion of syphilis is unjustified; a negative TPHA test (or an EIA using treponemal antigen) on the blood will virtually exclude active neurosyphilis and is a better screen for the detection of all forms of late syphilis (Lancet 1977). Neurosyphilis is also most improbable at serum or CSF titers below 320 (Luger et al 1988).

In the case of early syphilis it is traditional policy to carry out a lumbar puncture 12 months after treatment as part of the test of cure. In the case of patients with syphilis of uncertain duration or in the late symptomatic or late latent stage, CSF examination is an essential part of the investigation necessary before treatment. CSF examination prior to treatment has been recommended for all patients who are HIV-positive (Lukehart et al 1988). When there is evidence of clinical relapse or a fourfold rise is noted in the titer of the serological tests in the follow-up of a patient, CSF examination is necessary (Catterall 1977).

Examination of the cerebrospinal fluid

Investigation of the CSF should include:

1. serological tests (VDRL, TPHA or FTA-ABS)

2. a total white cell (normally less than 3 leukocytes/mm³, 3 × 10⁶/l) and differential count
3. estimation of total protein, IgG, IgM and albumin.

Whereas a reactive CSF VDRL test is highly specific for neurosyphilis it lacks sensitivity and 25–50% of patients with neurosyphilis will give a negative CSF VDRL test result. In contrast tests such as the TPHA and FTA-ABS are highly sensitive and while a negative result on the CSF excludes neurosyphilis a positive reaction, particularly at low titer, could be due to the permeability of the blood–CSF barrier.

Serological tests and estimation of IgG and albumin should be performed in parallel on serum.

Blood-CSF barrier function and the TPHA index

Conventional criteria such as raised CSF cell count and increased total protein may give evidence of an inflammatory response in the CNS but these examinations are not specific for neurosyphilis: these parameters are even less specific indicators of neurosyphilis in HIV-infected patients as 40–60% of such patients without syphilis have abnormalities of CSF protein or cell counts (Hollander 1988). In addition normal cell counts and total protein values do not exclude absolutely involvement of the CNS.

Quantitative TPHA tests on CSF combined with albumin, IgG, and IgM estimations are helpful in suggesting synthesis of *T. pallidum*-specific IgG and in excluding errors that may arise from disturbed function of the blood–CSF barrier. Details of the various methods and expected values are reviewed elsewhere – for details see Young (1992). The TPHA index (CSF TPHA titer/albumin quotient) is one of the most reliable indicators: neurosyphilis is most probable at a TPHA index above 70 and is strongly suggested at values above 500. The TPHA index has also provided support for the diagnosis of neurosyphilis in HIV-infected patients (Tomberlin et al 1994).

Acquired syphilis: clinical features

Early Stage

Primary syphilis. Following a period of about 3 weeks (range 10–90 days), the primary lesion or chancre develops at the site of inoculation of *T. pallidum*. The initial lesion noted in primary syphilis is a single dull red papule which becomes an ulcer, well demarcated from the surrounding tissue, with a smooth, flat, dull red surface, which may be covered by a thin yellow or brown crust. Characteristically the ulcer is painless, not tender and on pressure serous fluid, but no blood, exudes from the lesion. Induration of the ulcer is often marked giving it a cartilaginous consistency. Occasionally there may be considerable edema of the adjacent tissues.

In the male the chancre may be found on any part of the external genitalia, especially in the coronal sulcus, on the inner surface of the prepuce, on the glans or on the shaft of the penis. Rarely an intraurethral chancre may occur. In male passive homosexuals the chancre may be found at the anal margin or less frequently in the rectum. Chancres may also occur in the lips, buccal cavity, tongue, tonsil and pharynx, particularly in homosexual patients. Lesions of the tonsil and pharynx may be painful.

Chancres may occur on the labium majus (Fig. 23.26), labium minus, fourchette, clitoris or cervix. Lesions of the cervix usually

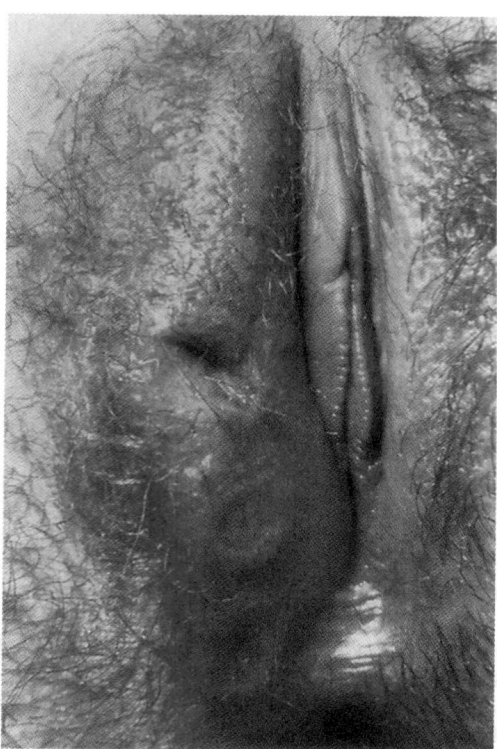

Fig. 23.26 Primary chancres of right labium majus. Lesions are indurated; edema of the adjacent labial tissues is conspicuous.

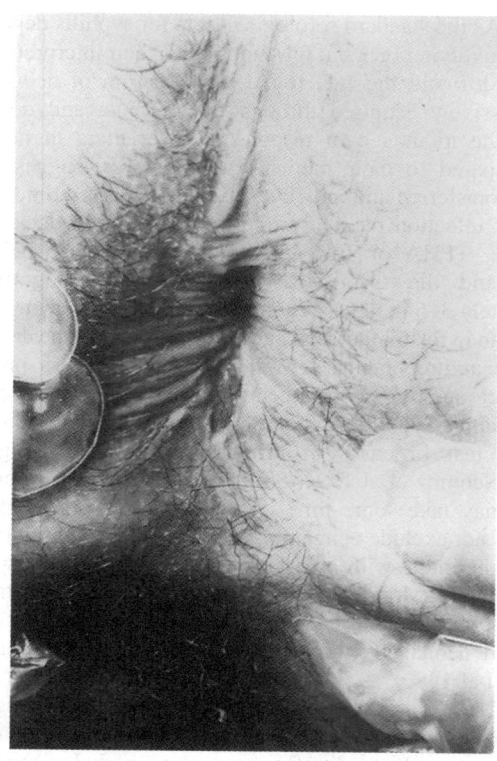

Fig. 23.27 Anal fissure in homosexual male. Serous fluid obtained from fissure showed numerous *Treponema pallidum* on dark ground microscopy.

produce no symptoms and as the lymph drains to the iliac nodes, these may be found to be enlarged on abdominal examination. Extragenital chancres are uncommon.

Many lesions of primary syphilis are atypical and in the anal region, primary lesions may resemble slightly indurated anal fissures (Fig. 23.27).

Within a few days of the appearance of the chancre there is usually regional lymph node enlargement; the enlarged lymph nodes are typically discrete, rubbery and painless. Without treatment, the primary lesion heals within 3–8 weeks, leaving a thin atrophic scar.

Secondary syphilis. Signs of secondary syphilis usually appear 7–10 weeks after infection or 6–8 weeks after the appearance of the primary lesion, which may still be present and unnoticed by the patient, in about third of patients with early secondary syphilis.

Symptoms. The patient often feels generally unwell, with mild fever, malaise, headache and anorexia. He may complain of a non-itchy skin rash, patchy loss of hair, hoarseness, swollen lymph nodes, bone pain and, rarely, deafness or other evidence of neural damage.

Signs. (a) Skin lesions (syphilides). Skin lesions are seen in over 80% of patients with secondary syphilis. Mucocutaneous lesions, particularly, contain many treponemes and are infectious. Skin eruptions are often polymorphic – several types of eruption appear simultaneously – during the course of secondary syphilis and, although early skin lesions are usually symmetrically distributed, later lesions are not always in this pattern. Just over 40% of patients with secondary syphilis complain of pruritus. Histological appearances are not always classical but more

variable and in at least 25% of biopsies plasma cells are either inconspicuous or absent.

Macular syphilide (roseola): these lesions are usually the earliest to appear, but are often overlooked, being faintly colored. The individual macules are rose pink in color, about 1 cm in diameter, discrete and with indistinct margins.

Papular and papulosquamous syphilide: these are the commonest lesions to be detected in secondary syphilis. Papules are dull red lesions, variable in size, distributed symmetrically – during the early stages of secondary syphilis – over the body, and especially prominent on flexor aspects. They are firm to touch and initially have a shiny surface. Later, as the papule ages, scaling is noted on the surface. When scaling papules predominate in the eruption, the term papulosquamous syphilide is applied.

Although papules may be found anywhere on the body, the following sites require special mention:

1. Face: this is often affected, papules being especially prominent in the nasolabial folds and on the chin. Occasionally a group of papules may be noted on the forehead just below, and parallel to, the hairline, sometimes described as '*corona veneris*'.

2. Scalp: when a hair follicle is involved in the inflammatory changes in the skin, hair growth is arrested and shedding of the contained hair occurs. Hair loss in secondary syphilis is characteristically irregular, the scalp having a 'moth-eaten' appearance (syphilitic alopecia). Occasionally, as a nonspecific reaction to a systemic disease, there may be a more diffuse hair loss (*telogen effluvium*) after recovery from the secondary stage.

3. Palms and soles (palmar and plantar syphilide): papular lesions on these sites do not project much above the surface of the

skin, but appear as firm lesions, dull red in color, associated with thickening and scaling (Fig. 23.28). A collar of scales may often surround individual lesions.

4. External genitalia: on moist areas such as the vulva and perianal region, papules may become hypertrophied, forming broad-based, flat-topped, moist, wart-like lesions called condylomata lata (Fig. 23.29). The surface is often eroded and the exudate from the erosion contains large numbers of *T. pallidum*. Commonly papules encircle the free margin of the prepuce, and, as a result of moisture, trauma and secondary infection, deep painful fissures develop. Papulosquamous lesions are often found on the shaft of the penis and on the scrotum.

In the later stages of secondary syphilis, papules become fewer in number and asymmetrical in distribution. Occasionally, a large papule may be found, surrounded by smaller satellite lesions – corymbose syphilide. Nail growth may be affected, particularly in the late secondary stage. The nail loses its luster, becomes brittle and may be shed.

Pustular syphilide: rarely papules become pustular due to necrosis of the upper dermis and epidermis as a result of occlusion of the lumen of blood vessels. Multiple pustular lesions are very seldom found in western countries (Miller 1974).

With the exception of pustular syphilide, the skin lesions of secondary syphilis heal without leaving scars. Areas of faint pigmentation may persist for months. Occasionally, depigmentation of the skin of the neck may be noted, particularly in dark-haired women – *leucoderma colli*. This residual depigmentation lasts for life.

(b) Lesions of the mucous membranes. These are found in about 30% of patients with secondary syphilis. The characteristic lesion is the so-called 'mucous patch' which appears at the same time as the skin rash. The mucosal lesions appear as round or oval gray areas surrounded by a narrow zone of erythema. Shedding of the gray necrotic membrane reveals superficial ulceration and if several patches coalesce, a 'snail-track ulcer' (Fig. 23.30) may result. Mucosal lesions are generally painless and resolve within a few weeks, or, less commonly, within a few days. Various sites may be involved in secondary syphilis, viz. tonsils, cheeks, palate and lips, tongue, larynx (produces hoarseness), nasal mucosa and mucous membranes of the genitalia (patches may be found on the glans penis, subpreputial surface of the prepuce, vulva, fourchette and cervix).

(c) Lymph node enlargement. Generalized lymph node enlargement is found in at least 60% of cases of secondary syphilis. Cervical, suboccipital, axillary, epitrochlear and inguinal nodes are often palpably enlarged. The lymph nodes are discrete with a rubbery consistency and are not tender. Not uncommonly, the spleen is enlarged in secondary syphilis. Histologically there is follicular hyperplasia with fibrosing endarteritis and periarteritis. Treponemes are rarely found in affected lymph nodes.

(d) Periostitis. Bone pain may occasionally be the presenting feature of the disease Periostitis is usually a localized process most commonly affecting the anterior tibia. Localized bone pain, especially at night, relieved by movement and exacerbated by immobilization is the chief symptom and localized tenderness may be noted on examination. Radiological examination usually reveals no abnormalities although osteolytic foci and periostitis may be seen. Bone scanning using technetium-99 may show areas of increased bone uptake; the superficial bones, including the

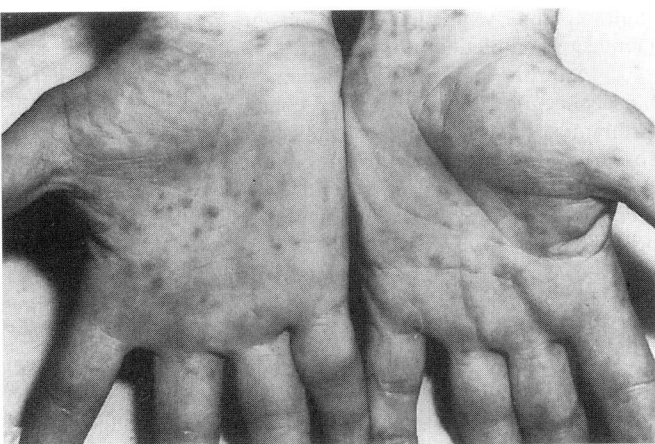

Fig. 23.28 Papulosquamous syphilide of the palms (early stage syphilis).

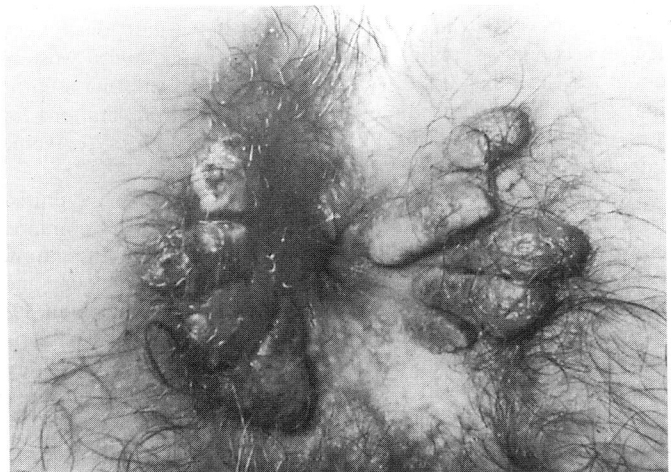

Fig. 23.29 Perianal condylomata lata of early stage syphilis in a homosexual male.

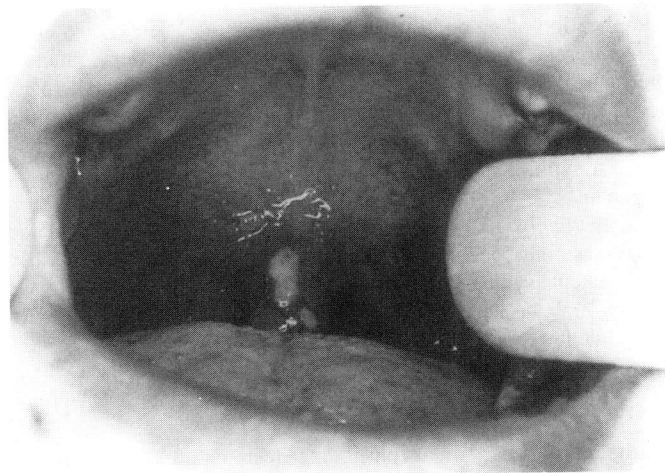

Fig. 23.30 Mucous patch of the uvula in early stage syphilis in a heterosexual male.

skull, are chiefly affected. These changes resolve within about 9 months of completion of therapy.

(e) Arthritis and bursitis. Painless effusion into joints and bursae occurs rarely during the course of secondary syphilis. Arthralgia, however, either localized or generalized, is more common, affecting at least 6% of patients.

(f) Hepatitis. Rarely, jaundice may be associated with secondary syphilis. The serum alkaline phosphatase – of hepatic origin – is often disproportionately elevated in comparison with only a moderate elevation in the case of alanine aminotrasferase. Usually within 6 weeks of treatment the plasma enzyme activities revert to normal.

(g) Glomerulonephritis and the nephrotic syndrome. Patients with secondary syphilis frequently have mild albuminuria, possibly as the result of immune complexes trapped by the glomeruli and setting up an inflammatory reaction there. Such changes are usually mild and transient, but rarely a membranous glomerulonephritis results, being manifest as the nephrotic syndrome. If untreated, the nephrotic syndrome appears to resolve spontaneously.

(h) Iridocyclitis and choroidoretinitis. Iritis, usually discovered late in secondary syphilis, is now a rare complication in western countries (less than 1% of cases). Uveitis and choroidoretinitis may be precipitated by the use of corticosteroid preparations for some other complication (e.g. glomerulonephritis) or for some intercurrent illness.

(i) Neurological abnormalities in secondary syphilis. Headache, especially noticeable in the morning, is a common complaint and probably reflects meningeal inflammation. Although transitory abnormalities of the white cell count and protein content in the cerebrospinal fluid occur in only about 5% of patients with secondary syphilis, frank meningoencephalitis may rarely be encountered. Peripheral neuritis may be a rare complication. Perceptive nerve deafness with or without vestibular dysfunction is another uncommon complication. It is usually associated with tinnitus and the CSF tends to show some abnormality. Improvement, both subjective and objective, occurs following antibiotic treatment. Although pure tone, speech and impedance audiometry are usually normal in patients with early syphilis, brainstem electrical response audiometry often indicates subclinical brainstem disease (Rosenhall & Roupe 1981).

(j) Parotitis. Unilateral parotitis has been described as a complication of secondary syphilis (Hira & Hira 1984).

Differential diagnosis of secondary syphilis. The appearance of the rash of secondary syphilis is variable and as a result many dermatological conditions have to be considered in the differential diagnosis; the problem is generally resolved by the serological tests for syphilis and by the generally rapid response to antibiotic treatment.

Early latent syphilis. The lesions of early syphilis may heal and the disease may become latent. During this stage, known as early stage latent syphilis, recurrence of infectious mucocutaneous lesions may be seen. Latency may, however, persist, and early stage latent syphilis is arbitrarily taken to last for 2 years.

Late stage

In the early years of syphilis the lesions already described (chancre, mucous patch, condyloma latum) are infectious and there is evidence of a recurrent spirochetemia and recurring mucocutaneous lesions. In pregnant women infection of the fetus in utero is inevitable in early untreated syphilis. Syphilis then enters a subclinical stage of latency, in which the only readily detectable evidence of infection is serological and this latency may persist for years or even for life. Transmission of the disease by sexual intercourse does not occur although in the case of pregnancy the woman can infect her fetus long after she has ceased to be infectious sexually. Further activity of the disease may, at any time during latency, cause profound effects and lead to death as long as three decades or more after infection. The main forms of late stage acquired syphilis are more appropriately discussed in a general text (Robertson et al 1989).

Treatment of syphilis: general considerations

Among the kaleidoscopic changes in medical practice since 1946 when penicillin first became easy to obtain, the effect of this antibiotic in microbial disease has nowhere been more spectacular than in syphilis where it continues to be the antibiotic of first choice for the treatment of all stages of the disease. The persisting susceptibility of *Treponema pallidum* to penicillin over an extensive period of time suggests that these organisms, in distinction from many other pathogens, do not have the genetic capacity to develop resistance to this antibiotic.

Penicillin is only effective against actively growing bacteria, the optimum effect being achieved when there is unhindered and rapid multiplication. It follows that penicillin will be most effective against the treponeme during early syphilis where there is rapid multiplication of the organism. Treponemes, like other bacteria, can exist in a resting phase when there is minimal cell wall synthesis and when penicillin effects are minimal.

In the case of rapidly growing bacteria, such as gonococci, the organism will be particularly sensitive to the action of penicillin many times over a 24-h period. In organisms with a longer generation time these phases of optimal sensitivity are correspondingly less frequent; for example, as in the case of *Treponema pallidum*. It is, therefore, an important determinant for therapeutic success to ensure that effective plasma concentrations are maintained over an adequate time.

T. pallidum is one of the most penicillin-sensitive microorganisms known. For penicillin to be effective in the therapy of syphilis, however, two requirements are believed to be essential: a minimal benzyl penicillin concentration of 0.018 mg (30 IU)/l of serum, which gives several times the serum and tissue levels needed to kill *T. pallidum*, should be maintained for at least 7–10 days in early syphilis; penicillin-free or subtreponemicidal intervals during treatment should not exceed 24 h.

Healing of lesions occurs rapidly and treponemes disappear from early stage lesions; biological cure, that is total eradication of treponemes, is difficult to prove, however, as *T. pallidum* cannot be cultured in vitro. In patients, however, the passage of time has given confidence that individuals treated for early syphilis will not suffer ill effects due to late syphilis provided that they have had a course of penicillin which gives adequate blood levels over a sufficient length of time.

Clinical and serological follow-up after treatment has always been maintained as important in clinical practice and there are occasional reports of failure after a generally acceptable course of penicillin (Giles & Lawrence 1979).

The finding of treponemes, apparently avirulent and incapable of causing further clinical disease, persisting after treatment of late syphilis, does not alter the fact that the treatment of early syphilis produces a clinical cure and prevents the emergence of late effects and that it is only in early syphilis with moist lesions that transmission can occur by sexual contact.

There are a multiplicity of empirically developed treatment plans but in spite of these variations in the case of long-acting penicillins results have been good. Imperfections in the understanding of penicillin effects in late and latent syphilis and more particularly in the long-term value of alternative antibiotics leave some questions unanswered.

Long-acting forms of penicillin diminish the need for repeated injections and consist of procaine penicillin, an equimolecular compound of penicillin and procaine; benethamine penicillin; and benzathine penicillin; with these relatively low concentrations are produced for periods respectively of 24 h, 5 days or for some weeks.

Guidelines in treatment

Guidelines established by a group of experts and the staff of the Centers for Disease Control (CDC), US Public Health Service, form a valuable source of guidance when considering therapy. In keeping with practice in the UK, the authors tend to place less reliance on single-dose schemes than is given in current recommendations in the USA. In all cases regular clinical and serological follow-up is advised following treatment.

CDC guidelines (1993c) suggest that primary and secondary syphilis in children should be treated with a single intramuscular injection of benzathine penicillin in a dosage of 50 000 units/kg up to the adult dose of 2.4×10^6 units (equivalent to 1.4 g of benzyl penicillin). For late latent syphilis, or syphilis of unknown duration, benzathine penicillin should be given for three total doses (total 150 000 units/kg up to the adult dose of 7.2 million units).

Doses for young persons over 50 kg bodyweight or past puberty for treatment of early syphilis (primary, secondary, latent syphilis of less than 1 year's duration) are given in Table 23.33. In early latent syphilis it is difficult to obtain direct information regarding the duration of the disease and it is advisable in cases of doubt to examine the CSF, because when it is abnormal a diagnosis of asymptomatic neurosyphilis can be made and adequate treatment ensured.

Doses are given in Table 23.34 for treatment of early syphilis (young persons over 50 kg bodyweight or past puberty) who are hypersensitive to penicillin. These antibiotics appear to be effective but results have been evaluated less fully than in the case of penicillin therapy. Clinical and serological follow-up are therefore very important. It should be noted that doxycyline or tetracycline should not be used in children under the age of 12 years.

Treatment of syphilis of more than 1 year's duration (latent syphilis of indeterminate or more than 1 year's duration, cardiovascular or late benign syphilis) except neurosyphilis is given in Table 23.35. Optimal treatment schedules for syphilis of greater than 1 year's duration are less well established than those for early syphilis. Cerebrospinal fluid (CSF) examinations are mandatory in suspected symptomatic neurosyphilis and desirable in other patients with syphilis of greater than 1 year's duration.

Alternative antibiotics and the doses given for those who are hypersensitive to penicillin are given in Table 23.36. Cerebrospinal fluid examinations and follow-up are important in

Table 23.33 Treatment of primary, secondary, latent syphilis of less than 1 year's duration in young persons over 50 kg or past puberty

Antibiotic	Route	Daily dose	Approximate benzyl penicillin equivalent		Number of doses
Benzathine penicillin	i.m.	1.8 g	1.4 g	2.4×10^6 i.u.	Single dose
Procaine penicillin	i.m.	900 mg	550 mg	0.9×10^6 i.u.	One daily for 10 days (seronegative primary syphilis)
Procaine penicillin	i.m.	1.2 g	730 mg	1.2×10^6 i.u.	One daily for 14 days (seropositive primary or secondary)

i.u. = international units

Table 23.34 Treatment of early syphilis in young persons over 50 kg bodyweight or past puberty who are hypersensitive to penicillin. Results have been evaluated less fully than in the case of penicillin; clinical and serological follow-up are therefore very important

Antibiotic	Route	Daily dose	Number of divided doses	Number of days treatment
Tetracycline hydrochloride*	Oral	2 g	4	15
Oxytetracycline*	Oral	2 g	4	15
Doxycycline*	Oral	200 mg	2	14
Erythromycin	Oral	2 g	4	15

* Not to be used for children under 12 years of age.

Table 23.35 Treatment of syphilis of more than 1 year's duration (latent syphilis of indeterminate or more than 1 year's duration, cardiovascular or late benign syphilis) except neurosyphilis; doses are given for young persons over 50 kg bodyweight or past puberty

Antibiotic	Route	Daily dose	Approximate benzyl penicillin equivalent		Number of doses
Benzathine penicillin	i.m.	1.8 g	1.4 g	2.4×10^6 i.u.	Once weekly for 3 successive weeks
Procaine penicillin	i.m.	900 mg	550 mg	0.9×10^6 i.u.	Once daily for 14 days
Procaine penicillin	i.m.	1.2 g*	730 mg	1.2×10^6 i.u.	Once daily for 14 days

i.u. = international units
* Dose for much heavier patients.

Table 23.36   Treatment of syphilis of more than 1 year's duration (latent syphilis of indeterminate or more than 1 year's duration, cardiovascular or late benign syphilis) except neurosyphilis, in those hypersensitive to penicillin; doses are given for young persons over 50 kg bodyweight or past puberty. Results have been evaluated less fully than in the case of penicillin

Antibiotic	Route	Daily dose	Number of divided doses	Number of days treatment
Tetracycline hydrochloride	Oral	2 g	4	30
Oxytetracycline	Oral	2 g	4	30
Erythromycin	Oral	2 g	4	30
Doxycycline	Oral	200 mg	2	30

patients being treated with these regimens as their efficacy in the long term is not yet clear.

Neurosyphilis. Early diagnosis and the rapid institution of treatment are of prime importance in neurosyphilis. Results of treatment depend to a very great extent upon how much irreversible damage to the central nervous system has occurred before treatment has begun and it is clear that any patient should be seen as a matter of urgency. CDC guidelines (1993c) recommend the use of 12–24 million units of benzyl penicillin daily given as 2.4 million units every 4 hours for 10–14 days. An alternative regimen is 2.4 million units procaine penicillin given daily by intramuscular injection plus probenecid 500 mg orally four times per day, both for 10–14 days. Patients with a history of penicillin hypersensitivity should be treated with penicillin, after desensitization.

Syphilis in pregnancy and the care of the fetus. In localities where the number of reported cases of transplacental (congenital) syphilis are more than very rare the antenatal care and the regular serological testing of pregnant women is a matter of major importance and will enable the eradication of congenital syphilis. Penicillin is recommended for pregnant women in dosage appropriate for the stage of syphilis.

Alternative antibiotic therapy in pregnant women with a history of hypersensitivity to penicillin. In the case of syphilis in the pregnant woman who gives a history of hypersensitivity to penicillin, treatment is problematic since tetracyclines are not used. Treatment with erythromycin may control the infection in the gravid patient but it may fail to prevent or cure the infection in her fetus. The infection in the fetus might or might not be seriously damaging and would be treatable effectively with penicillin at birth although damage already sustained would not necessarily be reversed.

Treatment of syphilis in HIV-infected individuals. Although HIV-infected patients with early syphilis are at increased risk of neurological disease, the use of the above treatment regimens are likely to be curative (CDC 1993c). In individuals with latent syphilis, irrespective of duration, examination of the CSF should be routine. Careful follow-up is essential and patients should be evaluated clinically and serologically at 1 month and at 2,3,6,9 and 12 months after treatment.

Follow-up after treatment

The CDC (1993c) guidelines advise that quantitative nontreponemal tests (e.g. VDRL) should be taken 3,6 and 12 months after treatment. A detailed discussion of the serological responses to treatment is given above. If disease is of more than 1 year's duration serological tests for syphilis should be repeated 24 months afterwards. Follow-up is especially important in patients treated with antibiotics other than penicillin. CSF is examined at the last follow-up after treatment with alternative antibiotics. In patients with neurosyphilis a follow-up after treatment is advised with periodic quantitative cardiolipin tests (e.g. VDRL), clinical evaluation and repeat CSF examinations, for at least 3 years (CDC 1993c). A life-time follow-up is, however, generally recommended.

In the case of early syphilis a 2-year follow-up is maintained where possible.

In the case of cardiovascular syphilis follow-up by a cardiologist is advisable and in neurosyphilis a life-time follow-up is best.

Retreatment

Reinfection with syphilis is a possibility particularly in the promiscuous who have casual relationships and where contacts may fear or neglect to surface for medical help. A CSF examination should be carried out before retreatment unless reinfection and a diagnosis of early syphilis is clearly established.

Retreatment should be considered under the following circumstances (CDC 1993c):

1. if clinical signs or symptoms persist or recur
2. if there is a fourfold increase in the titer of a nontreponemal test
3. if an initially high titer nontreponemal test fails to show a fourfold decrease in titer within 1 year.

When a patient is retreated one retreatment course is indicated and the course used will be that recommended for syphilis of more than 1 year's duration.

Treatment on epidemiological grounds

Patients who have clearly been exposed to infectious syphilis and who are not likely to cease sexual intercourse for 3 months, or to attend for surveillance, should be considered on epidemiological grounds for treatment and followed up; the regimen advised is that for early syphilis. It is our practice to treat couples such as husband and wife simultaneously if possible, if one partner develops early syphilis. Every effort is made, however, to establish a diagnosis beforehand in such cases.

In the case of early stage syphilis immediate treatment for the infected person or 'epidemiologic' treatment for potentially infected contacts will interrupt a possible chain of infection. The CDC (1993c) guidelines recommend that those exposed to infectious syphilis within the preceding 3 months and those who, on epidemiological grounds, are at high risk for early syphilis should be treated as for early.

Jarisch-Herxheimer Reaction (JHR)

This reaction is a complication that usually follows within a day of the initial treatment of a number of organismal diseases, including syphilis, and it is characterized by fever and an aggravation of existing lesions together with their attendant symptoms and signs. The salient features are as follows:

1. Prodromal phase with aches and pains.
2. A rise and then a fall in body temperature: the rise is accompanied by a chill and the fall by sweating. Defervescence lasts up to 12 h.
3. Aggravation of pre-existing lesions and their attendant symptoms and signs, e.g. flaring of the rash in syphilis or more seriously exacerbation in deafness in labyrinthitis.
4. Characteristic physiological changes, which include early vasoconstriction, hyperventilation and a rise in blood pressure and cardiac output, and later a fall in blood pressure associated with a low peripheral resistance.

CONGENITAL SYPHILIS

Congenital syphilis is an uncommon disease in the UK; in England during the 12 months ending in December 1992 only one case was reported. Antenatal examination routinely includes serological tests for syphilis and this screening, together with adequate treatment of infected mothers, accounts for the low incidence of the disease in this country. In Africa and South America, congenital syphilis is still common although where yaws is endemic an immune effect may modify the consequences of syphilis in the adult females and its transmissibility to the fetus. It can be prevented in utero by treatment of the infected woman with penicillin during early pregnancy or cured later in pregnancy; its occurrence in a community is an indicator of defective antenatal care and the result of insufficient primary medical care.

Transmission of infection

Although it had long been considered that involvement of the fetus did not occur before the fourth month of gestation, studies have clearly demonstrated that infection may occur within 10 weeks of conception. Any infection before 20 weeks' gestation will not stimulate immune mechanisms because the fetal immune system is not as yet well developed and thus no histological evidence of fetal reaction to infection will be seen. The theory that the cytotrophoblastic layer (Langhan's layer) of the early placenta protects, until its disappearance at 18–20 weeks' gestation, against transmission of the organism from the maternal to the fetal circulation has now been discounted. Electron microscopic studies have shown that this layer of cells does not completely atrophy.

Infection of the fetus is more likely to occur when the mother's infection is in the early stage, as at this time considerable numbers of organisms are present in the circulation. During the first year of infection in an untreated woman there is an 80–90% chance that the infection will be transmitted to the fetus. The probability of fetal infection declines rapidly after the second year of infection in the mother and becomes rare after the fourth year. In general, the greater the duration of syphilis in the mother, the less chance there is of the fetus being affected.

In preantibiotic days it was common for a mother of a child with congenital syphilis to give a history of previous miscarriages succeeded by a premature stillbirth, then a stillbirth at term, and later an apparently healthy child at birth. The widespread use of antibiotics for concomitant infection has completely altered this pattern of events, and such an obstetrical record is now virtually unknown.

Although uncommon, a woman with late syphilis, however, may give birth to a child with syphilis, although the child of a previous pregnancy had been apparently healthy. This may be explained by the speculation that there is an intermittent release of treponemes from lymphoid tissue into the circulation in late syphilis. Should such an event occur the fetus may become infected.

If mothers with early stage syphilis are not treated, 25–30% of fetuses die in utero, 25–30% die after birth, and of the infected survivors 40% develop late symptomatic syphilis.

Clinical features

The manifestations of congenital syphilis may conveniently be divided into two stages, early and late; the end of the second year of life is the arbitrary point of division between the two stages. Fuller details of the clinical features of congenital syphilis may be found in Nabarro's book (Nabarro 1954) as well as by reference to individual papers quoted.

Early congenital syphilis

When congenital syphilis was common it was rare to find acute signs of syphilis in the newborn and in cases that occurred, death usually followed within a few days. Infants were often born prematurely or, if full term, were often of low birthweight. The skin was wrinkled and there was a bullous skin rash (syphilitic pemphigus), particularly on the soles and palms. The clear or purulent fluid from the bullae contained large numbers of *T. pallidum* and was highly infectious. Other skin lesions, most often maculopapules, were usually present and were found around the body orifices. Rhinitis produced a mucoid or mucopurulent nasal discharge, and a hoarse cry resulted from laryngitis.

Abdominal distention was common, and hepatic and splenic enlargement almost invariably found. Hemorrhagic manifestations occasionally occurred. This has been shown to have been due to thrombocytopenia and macroglobulinemia. The majority of infants infected with syphilis appear healthy at birth as the characteristic clinical features do not develop until between 2 and 12 weeks. After a period of normal development, the child fails to thrive and the clinical picture of congenital syphilis becomes apparent.

It is convenient to describe the manifestations according to the particular part of the body affected.

Cutaneous manifestations. Skin rashes of varied character are found in 70–90% of infants with congenital syphilis. The rash is symmetrical in distribution and erythematous macular, papular and papulosquamous lesions may exist together in different parts of the body. On the face the eruption is particularly prominent around the mouth. Where the skin is moist, for example on the buttocks and external genitalia, the rash appears eczematous. In these sites hypertrophic lesions resembling condylomata lata may appear, usually as a manifestation of a recurrence following resolution of the initial rash. Deep fissures develop round the body orifices, and healing of these lesions leaves characteristic scars (rhagades).

The skin of the palms and soles may show peeling. In severe cases, the hair becomes scanty and brittle and involvement of the nails leads to shedding, and replacement by narrow, atrophic nails.

In addition to the eruptions described, the skin may show wrinkling from weight loss and there is café au lait pigmentation.

If an infant is not treated, or is inadequately treated, the skin lesions usually heal within a year, but there may be recurrences during the second year. Recurrent lesions usually differ from those seen in the original rash and include condylomata lata.

Mucosal lesions. Clinical evidence of rhinitis is found in 70–80% of infected infants. There is nasal obstruction and a mucoid nasal discharge which becomes mucopurulent and occasionally bloodstained (syphilitic snuffles). Numerous treponemes may be demonstrated in the discharge which is highly infectious. Arrested development of nasal structures, and continued pressure changes within the nose as a result of obstruction, lead to deformities of the nose (saddle nose).

Mucous patches resembling those seen in secondary acquired syphilis may occur in the mouth and pharynx. Laryngitis produces a hoarse or aphonic cry.

Lymphadenitis and splenic enlargement. Although not a constant accompaniment of early congenital syphilis, moderate generalized enlargement of the lymph nodes is common. The spleen is enlarged in at least 60% of infected infants.

Bone and joint manifestations. Bone disease, diagnosed by clinical or radiological examination, or both, occurs in at least 85% of infected infants under the age of 1 year. In only about 40% of cases is there clinical evidence of bone involvement. Bones are usually affected symmetrically, but one side may be more involved than the other. The child cries when adjacent joints are passively moved and he rarely moves affected limbs (Parrot's pseudoparalysis).

Radiological examination of infected infants under the age of 12 months, who have no clinical evidence of bone involvement, demonstrates abnormalities in at least 75% of cases. Multiple long bone involvement is most commonly found, the metaphyses being particularly affected. Variable degrees of calcification at the growing ends of the bone result in a variety of radiological changes (Hira et al 1985). Most commonly there is an irregular (saw tooth) dense zone of calcification overlying an osteoporotic area at the metaphysis. Peripheral osteoporosis of the metaphysis is less often observed, as is the appearance of dense bands sandwiching such zones.

Irregular patchy areas of loss of bone density are commonly found in both metaphyses and diaphyses. A characteristic sign is loss of density of the upper medial aspect of the tibiae (Wimberger's sign). In severe cases there may be a fracture at the site of bone destruction in the metaphysis, with impaction or displacement of the epiphysis.

Periostitis appears radiologically either as a single layer or as multiple layers of new bone formation along the cortex of the shaft of the bone; it is common in early congenital syphilis particularly amongst children aged 4 weeks and over (Hira et al 1985). Although any long bone may be affected, the distal femur and radius and the proximal tibia and humerus are the most often involved. The changes described are not specific for syphilis, similar radiological findings being encountered in rubella, cytomegalovirus infection, rickets and hemolytic disease of the newborn. Occasionally in early congenital syphilis lens-shaped areas known as Parrot's nodes appear around the anterior fontanel on the frontal and parietal bones. These nodes are probably due to

periostitis. Usually the changes described resolve within the second 6 months of life, but periostitis persists and may become more pronounced.

During the later stages of early congenital syphilis, dactylitis, manifest clinically as painless, spindle-shaped swelling of the fingers, may occur in a small number of cases (less than 5%). Radiographic examination shows that up to 25% of all infected children under the age of 2 years have dactylitis.

Hepatic and pancreatic involvement. The liver is almost invariably enlarged, usually in association with the spleen, in congenital syphilis appearing in the neonatal period and in at least 60% of older infants. Jaundice is an uncommon feature, but its presence in the neonate should alert the physician practicing in areas where syphilis is common to the possibility that syphilis may be the cause of the jaundice.

Although not clinically apparent, pancreatitis is a common finding at autopsy of infants dying of congenital syphilis in the neonatal period.

Renal involvement. The nephrotic syndrome may rarely be associated with early congenital syphilis, and is thought to be the result of deposition of soluble complexes of treponemal antigen and antitreponemal antibody in the glomeruli. Acute nephritis is a rarity.

Bronchopulmonary involvement. In the aborted fetus and stillborn infant the lungs are always affected, as bronchi and lung parenchyma have developed abnormally.

Neurological involvement. Although meningitis is common in early congenital syphilis, particularly during the exanthem stage, clinical signs relating to the nervous system are uncommon. Epileptiform seizures, irritability and bulging of the anterior fontanel may occur. There may be focal changes in the cerebral tissue due to thrombotic occlusion of blood vessels affected by a panarteritis. These cerebral lesions may produce hemiplegia, monoplegia and cranial nerve palsies.

In about a third of infants under the age of 12 months, the cerebrospinal fluid is abnormal with respect to cell content and protein levels, and gives positive results when examined by the serological tests for syphilis.

Ocular manifestations. Iritis is rare in early congenital syphilis. Choroidoretinitis is considerably more common during the first year of life. Examination with ophthalmoscope shows small spots of pigment surrounded by yellow areas (salt and pepper fundus). If untreated the inflammatory process progresses and if the macular or optic disc regions are involved, blindness may result.

Hematological abnormalities. Anemia of varying severity occurs in at least 20% of infants with congenital syphilis. Normocytic, normochromic anemia reflects depression of hematopoiesis in the bone marrow as a result of the chronic infection. Increased hemolysis probably plays a small part in the development of the anemia. Secondary iron deficiency produces a microcytic, hypochromic anemia. Occasionally a leukoerythroblastic anemia occurs.

Thrombocytopenia, associated with a bleeding disorder during the first few weeks of life, has been described. Macroglobulinemia may be associated with the bleeding diathesis.

In early congenital syphilis, the white cell count is usually elevated, with lymphocytosis.

Late congenital syphilis

Infected and untreated children are said to have entered the late stage of syphilis after their second birthday. In at least 60% of affected children there are no clinical signs of the disease, the only abnormal finding being positive serological tests, that is latent congenital syphilis.

Interstitial keratitis. This is the most common clinical manifestation of late congenital syphilis, occurring in about 40% of affected children. Interstitial keratitis appears to be the result of immunological reaction in the cornea to the treponeme, penicillin treatment having no influence on the course of this manifestation. In most cases this develops between the ages of 6 and 14 years, but it may occur earlier or very much later (even over the age of 30 years). Although commencing in one eye, both become involved in more than 90% of cases; the second eye shows features of the condition a few days to several months after the first. The patient complains of pain in the affected eye, photophobia with excessive lacrimation and dimness of vision. A diffuse haziness near the center of the cornea of one eye is the earliest clinical sign, but within a few weeks the whole cornea becomes opaque. This is usually associated with circumcorneal sclerotic congestion.

Examination by slit lamp microscopy shows that these corneal changes are attributable to blood vessels extending into the cornea from the sclera, and to exudation of cells from these vessels.

The condition gradually improves over a period of 12–18 months, leaving a variable degree of corneal damage which may lead to blindness or be only detectable by slit lamp examination. This latter investigation may show empty blood vessels (ghost vessels) within the cornea of patients who have had interstitial keratitis earlier in life, but have had no apparent residual scarring.

After resolution of the initial episode of interstitial keratitis, 20–30% of patients suffer a relapse of this condition.

Bone lesions. The essential bone lesion in late congenital syphilis is hyperplastic osteoperiostitis, a process which may be diffuse, resulting in sclerosis of bone, or localized (periosteal node or gumma). Gumma formation may lead to necrosis of underlying cortex with softening of the bone. The tibias are most commonly affected by these changes.

Usually bone lesions develop between the fifth and 20th year of life, when the patient complains of pain in the affected bone. Palpation may reveal nodules on the anterior surface of the bone, and rarely ulceration may be observed where a gumma has involved skin and bone. In older children, thickening of the anterior surface of the tibia may result in forward bowing of that bone (saber tibia).

Painless gummatous lesions may be found on the hard and soft palates or in the pharynx. These are often extensive, with considerable necrosis of tissue. Perforation of the palate, absence of the uvula and scarring about the oropharynx may be the result.

Destructive gummatous lesions of the nasal septum may cause perforation of the septum with or without deformity of the lower part of the nose.

Joint lesions. The commonest type of joint lesion (Clutton's joints), seen in about 20% of untreated children, is bilateral effusion into the knee joints. This condition, like interstitial keratitis, is unaffected by antibiotic treatment, and appears to be an immunological reaction to *T. pallidum*. Less commonly, other joints are similarly affected. Although most frequently occurring in children between the ages of 5 and 10 years, joint involvement may be seen at any age from 3 years to the mid-20s.

The onset of the arthritis starts acutely often with a history of antecedent trauma. Although most commonly painless, the affected joints may be acutely painful, particularly at the onset. Radiological examination reveals no specific changes in the joint.

There is gradual resolution of the arthritis over many months, with recovery of full function.

Neurosyphilis. In about 20% of infected children over the age of 1 year neurosyphilis is latent or hidden and diagnosis depends upon the detection of abnormalities in the cerebrospinal fluid. As a late result of the meningitis of early stage congenital syphilis, epileptiform seizures, mental deficiency and cranial nerve palsies may be found in children over the age of 2 years. Parenchymatous involvement produces two main clinical conditions, juvenile general paralysis of the insane and tabes dorsalis.

Juvenile general paralysis of the insane (juvenile GPI). This occurs in about 1% of affected children appearing about the age of 10 years, but occasionally much earlier, or much later as in middle age. The sexes are affected equally (in contrast to the GPI of acquired syphilis in which males are more often affected than females). There is usually a gradual onset of symptoms, the child becoming dull, irritable, apathetic and forgetful. Later, delusions, usually paranoid in type, occur and speech becomes disturbed. The voice is monotonous, articulation becomes stumbling and tremulous and speech is eventually lost. There is generally tremor of the lips, hands and legs. Handwriting becomes indistinct. Epileptiform seizures are common at a late stage of the disease.

Pupillary abnormalities are seen in over 90% of cases; the pupils are of the Argyll Robertson type or immobile and dilated. Optic atrophy occurs in between 10% and 35% of cases.

Other physical findings resemble those found in general paralysis of acquired syphilis.

Juvenile tabes. This is much rarer than general paralysis. The onset of the condition is generally between the ages of 10 and 17 years. Failing vision and paresthesiae are the most common symptoms; lightning pains and ataxia are rare. Later in the course of the disease headaches, photophobia and diplopia occur frequently. Sphincter disturbances are uncommon although enuresis may be found. Clinical examination may detect nystagmus, pupillary abnormalities, optic atrophy, and absent or diminished tendon reflexes. Trophic disturbances are rare and it is unusual to find evidence of loss of cutaneous sensation.

Ear disease. The middle ear may be affected by a painless otolabyrinthitis, showing as a slight purulent aural discharge. Conduction deafness may result without treatment. The deafness of congenital syphilis, however, is predominantly sensory.

In sections of the temporal bone of individuals with longstanding sensorineural deafness which has resulted from congenital syphilis, there is patchy osteitis with inflammation of all three layers of the otic capsule. Hydrops of the cochlear duct, saccule and utricle occurs and there is degeneration of the organ of Corti with loss of cochlear neurons. Similar changes may affect the sensory epithelium or neurons of the vestibular system.

Even after what has been considered adequate penicillin treatment, treponemes have been demonstrated in endochondral bone, a dense structure into which antibiotics do not readily diffuse.

Subjective hearing impairment is commonly a late manifestation often not occurring until adult life, although it can occur in childhood. In addition the patient may not be seen first till middle age, when the diagnosis of congenital syphilis may not come readily to mind unless there are other stigmata of the disease.

Vestibular disease is frequent in patients with congenital syphilis, the symptoms, which include dizziness, unsteadiness of gait and paroxysmal vertigo, usually beginning with the onset of deafness.

Audiograms show a variety of patterns. The most common (35%) is high tone loss, followed by a flat audiogram (25% of cases) and low tone loss (15% of cases). There is progressive deterioration of deafness although spontaneous fluctuation may occur. The most severe difficulty is in discrimination of speech. It is usually an isolated finding, bilateral, although one side is often more severely affected than the other. There are usually no abnormalities in the cerebrospinal fluid.

Skin lesions. Gummata similar to those occurring in late acquired syphilis may be found.

Cardiovascular lesions. Myocarditis may be found in children dying of congenital syphilis, but aortitis is exceedingly rare.

Liver disease. Gummata of the liver are rarely found.

Paroxysmal cold hemoglobinuria. This rare condition occurring in less than 1% of patients with late congenital syphilis, may be seen also in acquired syphilis. Large quantities of hemoglobin are excreted in the urine after exposure to cold. Shivering or a rigor heralds the attack and this is rapidly followed by fever, headache and pains in the back or limbs. A generalized urticarial rash may also develop. Within the next few hours the urine becomes dark brown in color and contains hemoglobin and methemoglobin but few red blood cells. In most cases, the clinical features described resolve within several hours, but occasionally mild jaundice may develop and persist for some days. This condition is liable to recur periodically when the patient is exposed to cold of varying severity.

Cold hemolysins are found in the blood, and demonstrated by the Donath–Landsteiner test. The basis of this test is the ability of the hemolysin to unite with red cells when the blood is chilled; when the blood is then warmed to 37°C, these sensitized cells are lysed in the presence of complement.

Stigmata of congenital syphilis

Lesions of early and late congenital syphilis may heal leaving scars and deformities characteristic of the disease. Such scarring and deformities constitute the stigmata of congenital syphilis, but only in some 40% of patients do they occur.

Stigmata of early lesions

Facial appearance. The 'saddle nose' deformity may result from rhinitis. The palate may appear high arched as a result of underdevelopment of the maxilla.

Teeth. The tooth germs of deciduous teeth are fully differentiated by the 10th week of gestation before tissue reaction to treponemes appears to occur; hence these teeth are usually unaffected. Teeth which develop later may, however, be affected. Two groups of teeth bear the brunt, the upper central incisors and the first molars.

Typically the affected upper incisor is smaller than normal, and darker in color and peg-like, instead of being flat, with the sides converging to the cutting edge which classically has a notched center (Fig. 23.31), the so-called Hutchinson's incisor. Affected incisors do not always show this typical appearance but may often be thickened anteroposteriorly, with rounding of the incisal

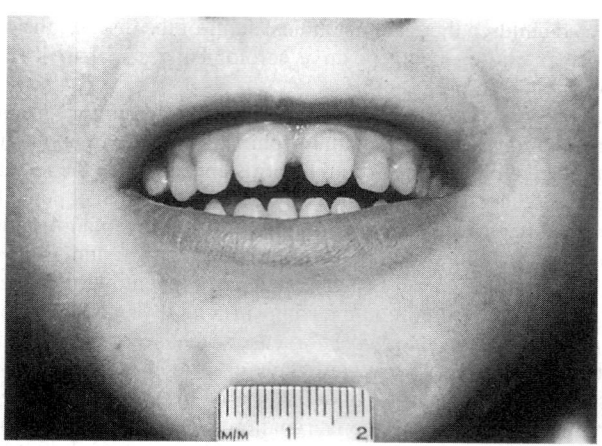

Fig. 23.31 Hutchinson's incisors; one of the classical stigmata of congenital syphilis. Note the peg-like appearance with convergence towards the cutting edge, which classically has a notched center. Affected incisors do not always have this typical appearance (see text).

angles; they may have a shallow depression on the incisal edge rather than a notch.

The typically affected molar, Moon's molar, shows a constricted occlusal surface and rounded angles. The cuspules of the molar are poorly developed and appear crowded together. Such teeth are prone to dental caries and as a result are lost early.

In one series, in 45% of patients with congenital syphilis the upper central incisors were affected, and in about 20% the first molars were involved. The incidence of dental changes is high in patients who also develop interstitial keratitis.

Rhagades. The deep cutaneous lesions around the orifices of the body heal producing scars radiating from the orifice known as rhagades.

Nails. Atrophy and deformity of the nails may be seen in adult life as a result of nail bed inflammation in infancy.

Choroidal scarring. Healing of choroidoretinitis produces white scarred areas surrounded by pigmentation on the retina.

Stigmata of late lesions

Corneal lesions. Opacities of the cornea and ghost vessels observed on slit lamp examination are the result of interstitial keratitis.

Bone lesions. Saber tibia resulting from osteoperiostitis may be observed, as may the scars of destructive lesions of the oropharyngeal and nasal regions. Broadening of the skull may result from osteoperiostitis of the frontal and parietal bones.

Optic atrophy. This may occur as a single entity without iridoplegia (e.g. Argyll Robertson pupils).

Nerve deafness.

Diagnosis of congenital syphilis

The serological diagnosis of congenital syphilis is described above.

In western industrialised countries, the discovery of positive serological tests in an otherwise healthy person often raises the question as to whether syphilis has been acquired before birth or later. This problem is difficult as stigmata appear to be rare now. A family history may be misleading. Patients should, however, be carefully examined for the presence of obvious stigmata and slit lamp microscopy of the cornea should be included in the investigation to search for ghost vessels, as a trace of previous interstitial keratitis. Nerve deafness may be obvious or, if mild, demonstrable by audiography. In doubtful cases, serological examination of parents or brothers and sisters may be helpful, and, to avoid serious social upset, consultation and collaboration with the general practitioner is advised.

Treatment of congenital syphilis

Early congenital syphilis

Although infants with massive infection may still die in the neonatal period, the majority will be cured by adequate penicillin treatment. Stigmata, particularly dental, will, however, be detectable. Prior to instituting treatment, the CSF should be examined to detect neurological involvement. Benzyl penicillin in an intramuscular dose of 30 mg (50 000 IU)/kg should be given daily in two divided doses. Alternatively, procaine penicillin 50 mg (approximately equivalent to 30 mg or 50 000 IU benzyl penicillin)/kg/day may be used. Treatment should be continued for at least 10 days, and preferably longer if the CSF is abnormal. Further details on prevention, treatment and the problem when erythromycin has been used for treatment of the pregnant woman with syphilis are discussed elsewhere (p. 1410).

After the neonatal period the dose should be the same dosage used for neonatal congenital syphilis. For larger children the total dose need not exceed the dosage advised in adult syphilis for more than 1 year's duration. If hypersensitive to penicillin, erythromycin may be used. Tetracycline or oxytetracycline should not be used in children under 12 years of age.

Late congenital syphilis

The dosage of procaine penicillin required for the treatment of late congenital syphilis is similar to that used in the therapy of late acquired syphilis. Treatment, however, does not prevent the development or course of interstitial keratitis, hydrarthrosis and neural deafness.

Management of interstitial keratitis. Patients with interstitial keratitis should be managed in hospital, in consultation with an ophthalmologist. Topically applied corticosteroids rapidly suppress the inflammatory reaction in the cornea and anterior uveal tract, and their use, until spontaneous cure occurs, has revolutionized the management of this condition. Although the infiltration of the cornea by inflammatory cells resolves, scarring from previous episodes of keratitis is not affected.

Betamethasone eyedrops, BPC 0.1%, instilled into the affected eye(s) every 1–2 h is a useful preparation. Treatment should be continued until the corneal inflammatory infiltrate has cleared, and visual acuity is restored to the patient's normal level. Slit lamp examination is essential before steroid treatment is discontinued, as mild degrees of keratitis may not be apparent otherwise. Regular examination is required after cessation of treatment, as corneal scarring may result from continuing mild inflammation.

During steroid treatment, mydriatics such as atropine eyedrops BPC 1% may be useful adjuvants by reducing ciliary muscle tension.

Corneal grafting may be required in patients with corneal scarring acquired during attacks of interstitial keratitis.

Hydrarthrosis (Clutton's joints). This is a self-limiting disorder, and does not require any specific therapy.

Nerve deafness. Despite previous treatment of congenital syphilis with what has been regarded as adequate doses of penicillin, progressive neural deafness may develop at any age, but most commonly in the adult of middle age. This may be the result of failure of the drug to reach adequate concentrations in the perilymph or endolymph.

The use of benzyl penicillin in a dosage of 300 mg (500 000 IU) given by intramuscular injection every 6 h for 17 days, together with probenecid in a dose of 1 g 6-hourly by mouth has been advocated. During the first week of treatment, 30 mg of prednisone is given orally, the dose thereafter being reduced to 25 mg daily for 3 weeks. As a response to treatment is seen within the first month, treatment may be discontinued if there has been no improvement at that time. When the response has been satisfactory, steroids may be continued for 3–6 months in gradually diminishing doses. A further course of penicillin is then given. Occasionally patients have required maintenance treatment with low doses of steroids to abolish vertigo and maintain hearing. In advanced cases where there has been considerable tissue damage, however, no response to medical treatment occurs.

Ampicillin in a dosage of 1.5 g 6-hourly for 4 weeks, together with prednisolone 30 mg daily for 10 days, tailing off over the succeeding 10 days, has been used in the management of this condition.

Audiometry may give useful information regarding response to treatment. The value of treatment has not been fully assessed. In some cases, the disease process may be arrested, but in others improvement in hearing may only be temporary.

ENDEMIC TREPONEMATOSES

The treponematoses of man have developed in differing geographical and epidemiological situations as parasite and host and have evolved a modus vivendi. The nonvenereal diseases tend to exist among primitive peoples in rural communities, where transmission occurs by skin contact in childhood with other younger or older children who, themselves, have relapsing crops of infective skin lesions. If infected in childhood susceptibility to venereal syphilis later as adults is diminished.

In the world maps provided the geographical distribution of the endemic treponematoses in the early 1950s (Fig. 23.32) is contrasted with that of the 1980s (Fig. 23.33).

Syphilis, on the other hand, probably evolved as a venereal disease in those who, as a result of social and climatic change, began to wear clothes and, apart from sexual contact, tended to live more separate existences. The survival and transmission of the treponeme under these circumstances became possible only when susceptible adults, escaping yaws in childhood, became infected by contact with genital lesions at sexual intercourse.

Pinta (Synonyms: in Mexico, *mal de pinto*; in Colombia and Venezuela, *carate*; and in Chile and Peru, *azul*)

This is a disease of remote rural communities, affecting the skin (blue-stain disease) and it is the least damaging of the human treponematoses. The causative organism is *Treponema carateum*, the most attenuated of the pathogenic treponemes. Pinta used to be prevalent in semiarid regions of Brazil, Colombia, Cuba, southern Mexico and Venezuela with scattered foci in Central and South

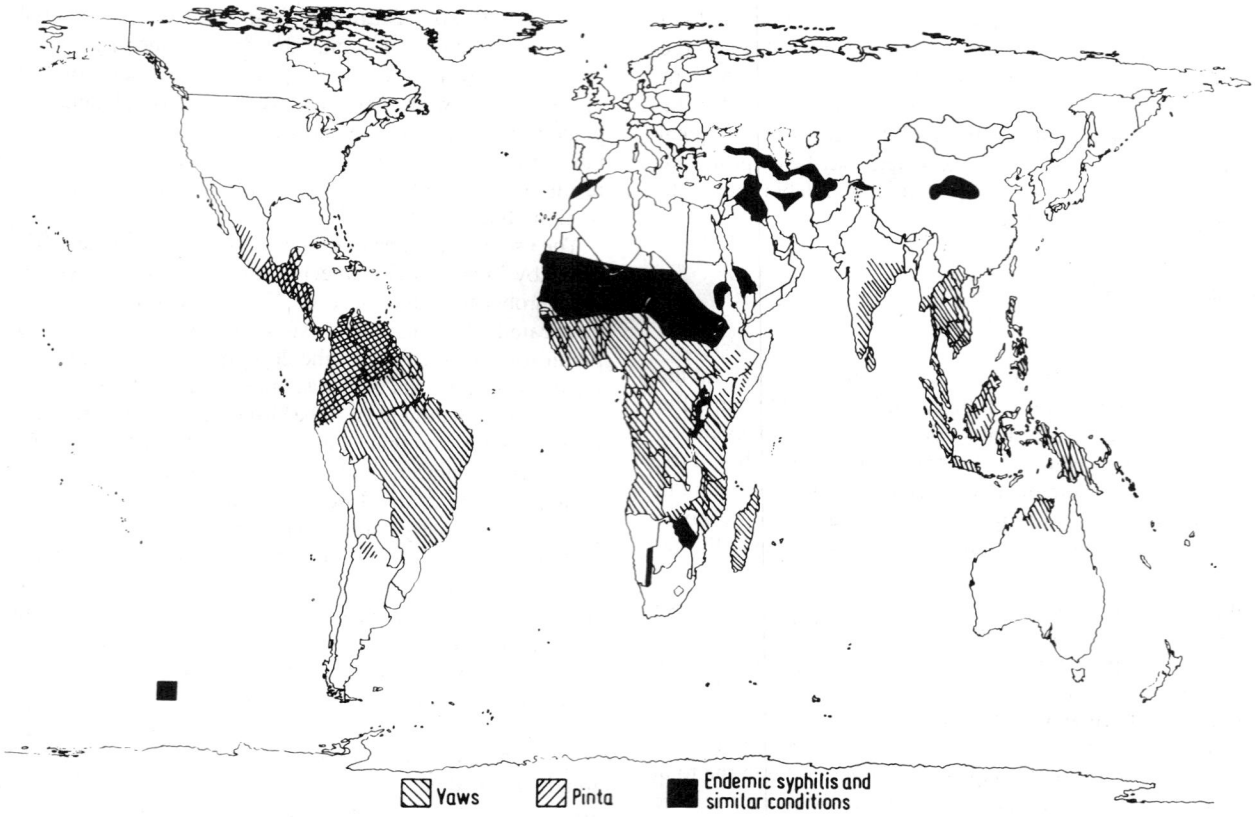

Fig. 23.32   Geographical distribution of the endemic treponematoses in the early 1950s – World Map, Arno Peters projection; data from WHO Chronicle, 1982.

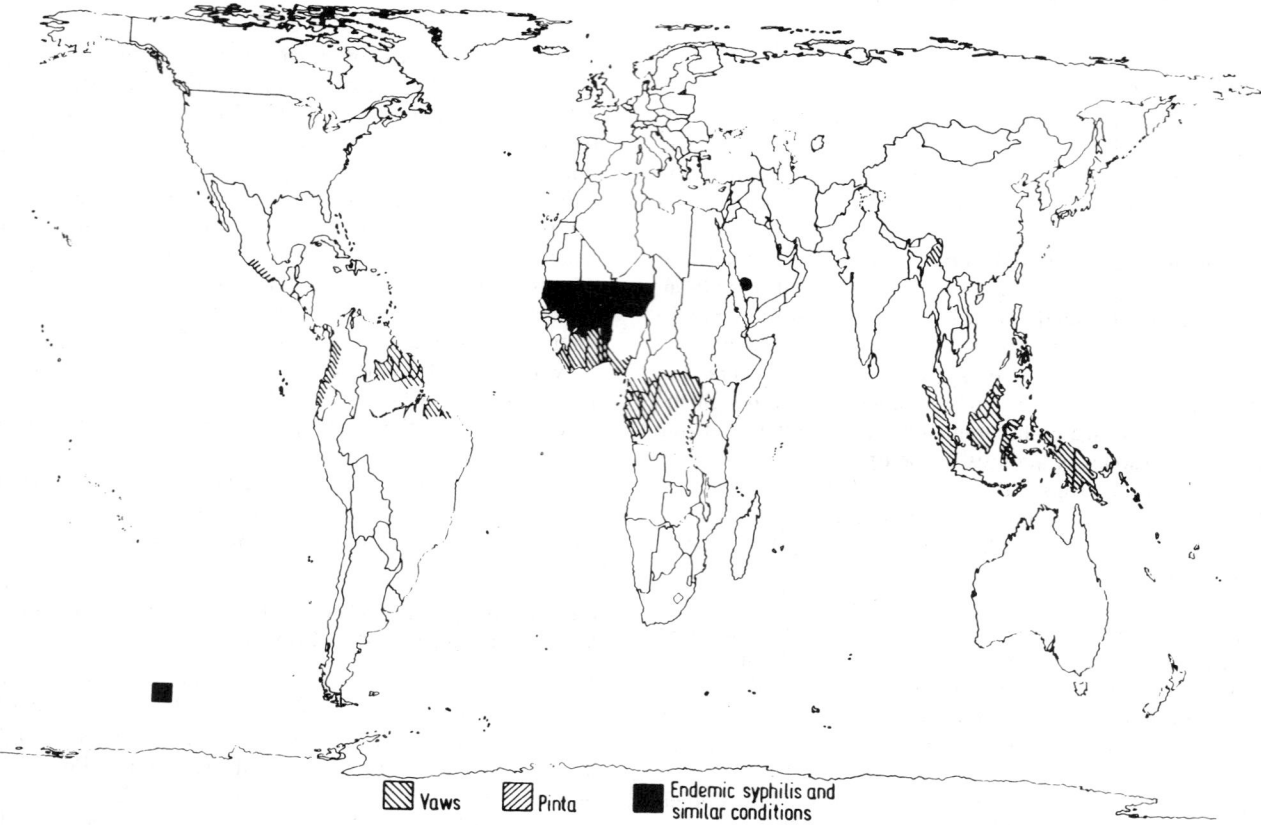

Fig. 23.33   Geographical distribution of the endemic treponematoses in the early 1980s – World Map, Arno Peters projection; data from WHO Chronicle, 1982.

American countries and the Caribbean islands; today only scattered foci remain in northern South America and Mexico. It differs from yaws and endemic syphilis in that it affects children and adults of all ages. Throughout its course the disease is confined to the skin, where pigmented and achromic lesions may remain infective for years, permitting spread by direct skin-to-skin contact.

Clinical features

The primary or initial lesion develops usually after 2–3 weeks, often on an uncovered part of the body as a lenticular and slightly scaly papule which enlarges to form a plaque; mostly the initial lesion is to be found on the legs, the dorsum of the foot, the forearm or the back of the hands. At first pink in color in fair skins it becomes pigmented or hypochromic to a variable degree as it enlarges; lymph nodes draining the area enlarge. After 2 months or up to 1 year later, secondary lesions develop, some on occasions appearing on the same site as the initial lesion. At first erythematous and afterwards copper colored these 'pintids' become pigmented to a varying degree, changing slowly from a copper color to lead gray and slate blue as a result of photosensitization and areas of erythema, hypopigmentation and leukoderma develop. The polychromic lesions become keratotic.

In late stage pinta residual areas of hyperchromia and achromia develop in isolated patches to form multicolored lesions; the depigmentation process occurs at different rates even within the same lesion. No disability or complication other than leukoderma occurs.

The causative organism, *T. carateum*, is detected by dark ground illumination microscopy in serum obtained from the base of a lesion after abrading the surface; although numerous in early stage lesions treponemes persist through to the late dyschromic stage.

Yaws (Synonyms: *pain* in French; *framboesia* in German, Dutch; *bouba* in Portuguese; *buba* in Kiswahili)

Yaws has shown the greatest changes in regional prevalence since the mass treatment campaigns of the 1950s. In South America only scattered foci of active yaws persist; Brazil and Surinam are almost yaws free and in Colombia, Ecuador, French Guiana and Guyana only a few dozen or a hundred cases are reported annually. In southeast Asia yaws still exists in Indonesia and Papua New Guinea.

Africa remains the part of the world mostly affected although where there is improved rural medical care and improved standards of living, as in the Ivory Coast and Nigeria, the numbers of clinical cases are declining. In Ghana, however, resurgence of yaws occurred following cessation of active yaws surveillance; the numbers of reported cases of infectious yaws increased 21-fold between 1969 and 1976.

In a WHO survey in the Central African Republic, Congo and Gabon, clinical yaws was detected in over 20% of the pygmy population and positive serological tests in 80%. Out of a total pygmy population of between 100 000 and 200 000 two major groups have undergone less assimilation than the others – the Binga of the tropical rain forests to the west of the Ubangi River and the Mbuti, several hundred miles to the east in the Ituri Forest. In a survey (486 examined) of the former group in 1978–1979, in the dry season, a time when these nomadic forest people were accessible, it was found that there were clinical signs of yaws in

50% and serological tests (VDRL and TPHA) were positive in 86% of the children and 95% of the adults. In the case of neighbouring nonpygmy peasant cultivators clinical evidence of yaws was also common (30%) and 78% of the children and 98% of the adults had positive serological tests (Widy-Wirski et al 1980). Eradication campaigns had clearly not reached such isolated populations and total mass treatment (see Antibiotics in treatment and control in endemic treponematoses, p. 1419) would be the appropriate medical strategy. To achieve success, however, anthropological understanding would be essential as the forest pygmies have no formal social structure and organization and small bands constantly change in size and composition throughout the year.

Clinical features

Yaws is a contact disease of childhood, caused by *Treponema pertenue* and is characterized by crops of highly infectious and relapsing skin lesions in the first 5 or 6 years of the natural course of the infection. The classification and nomenclature for the lesions of yaws were established in an illustrated monograph of the World Health Organization (Hackett 1957) and the bone lesions were discussed more fully by Hackett (1951). A classification of lesions and the degrees of infectiousness of such lesions, based on Perine et al (1984), is summarized in Table 23.37.

The most characteristic lesion in early yaws is the papilloma (Fig. 23.34) and in the exudate of all early lesions, which may be macular, maculopapular or papular, treponemes are numerous. The early papule enlarges to form a papillomatous lesion bearing some resemblance to a raspberry (a synonym is framboesia). There may also be adenitis. After 2–6 months the initial lesion heals, often without scarring. Further papillomata often in crops develop most often around the body orifices, near the nose, mouth, anus and vulva. A change in climate may influence the number and morphology of yaws lesions: in the dry season lesions tend to be fewer in number and macular in form and papillomata tend to be more concentrated in moist areas of the skin such as the axilla (Fig. 23.35) and anal cleft. Hyperkeratotic lesions occur on the soles of the feet and palms of the hands. On the feet plaques develop which are painful and walking becomes difficult (crab yaws).

A periostitis may affect long bones or cause a polydactylitis affecting the phalanges and metacarpals (Fig. 23.36). An osteitis of the nasal processes of the maxilla produces paranasal swellings (goundou) and is common in Africa. The tibia may become saber shaped. Nocturnal bone pain and tenderness of the tibial shaft are common in early yaws.

Ganglions, particularly at the wrist, and hydrarthrosis can also occur in early yaws. There is also an early latent stage which may be interrupted by relapses of active early lesions.

Late lesions (Table 23.37) develop 5 or more years after the infection and the characteristic late lesion is a destructive ulcer, which may involve skin, subcutaneous tissue, the mucosae and the bones and joints. Deep destructive lesions are typified by the hideous mutilation of the central part of the face (*rhinopharyngitis mutilans*) called gangosa in which there is destruction of cartilage and bone structures of the septum, palate and posterior part of the pharynx. It is probable, however, that there is no bone lesion that occurs in yaws that does not also occur in syphilis (Hackett 1951).

There is no certain evidence of transplacental or congenital infection in yaws. Serologically it cannot be distinguished from syphilis.

Table 23.37 Classification of yaws lesions (Hackett 1951, 1957, Perine 1984)

Yaws lesions	Examples	'Infectiousness' (+ to +++)
Early stage cutaneous (often pruritic, tendency to cropping, often polymorphous, modified by climate, if lesions moist then infectious)		
Initial lesion	Papule, papilloma	+++
Papillomata	Papilloma, some serpiginous, some ulcerated	+++
Macules		++
Micropapules, papules		+++
Squamous macules		+
Squamous micropapules, papules		++
Polymorphous or mixed		++
Plaques		+
Nodules	Front of knees	+
Hyperkeratosis	Palmar, plantar (as in crab yaws – painful)	–
Early stage bone		
Osteoperiostitis	Polydactylitis tibia	–
	Goundou (osteitis of nasal processes of maxilla)	–
Early stage joint	Ganglion, hydrarthrosis	–
Late stage cutaneous		
Hyperkeratosis	Palmar, plantar	–
Ulcer with characteristic tissue destruction (gummatous)		–
Late stage bone		
Gummatous osteoperiostitis	Saber tibia	–
	monodactylitis	
	Gangosa	
Late stage joint	Ganglion	–
	Hydrarthrosis	–
	Bursitis	–
	Juxta-articular nodes	–

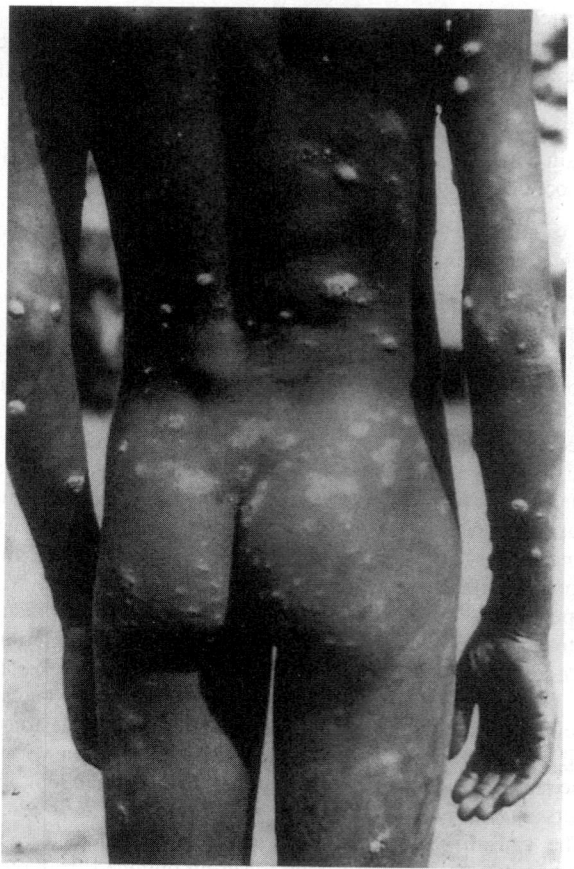

Fig. 23.34 Back of patient showing papillomata and papules of yaws. Over the inner surface of the buttocks are papular lesions and on the posterior surface of the upper limbs are macular lesions. On the back are acuminate micropapules. The association of macular and maculopapular lesions with papillomata is frequent in the early stages of the disease. (Courtesy of Professor H. M. Gilles.)

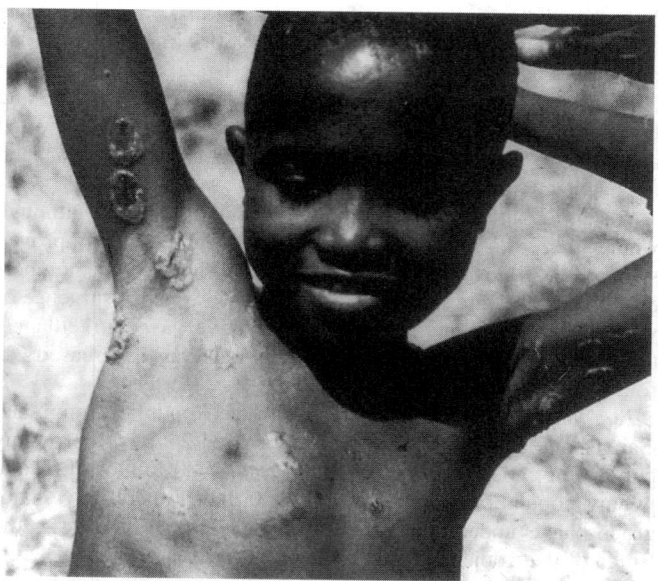

Fig. 23.35 Circinate early papules in yaws. (Courtesy of Professor H. M. Gilles.)

Endemic syphilis (Synonyms: *bejel* in Arabic; *njovera*, *dichuchwa* in Zimbabwe; Endemic Syphilis in Bosnia; Extinct Forms of Disease: *sibbens* in Scotland, *radesyge* in Norvway and *skerljevo*, of the Croation Coast, Yugoslavia)

Endemic syphilis is prevalent today primarily among the seminomads in the Arabian peninsula and along the southern border of the Sahara desert. A recent survey found thousands of cases of early endemic syphilis in Mali, Mauretania, Niger and Upper Volta; in sub-Saharan Africa the disease may be a greater problem today than it was formerly. It used to be found also in scattered foci in central Asia, Australia and India but these have been eliminated by the mass penicillin treatment campaigns of the 1950s.

The infection may be spread in the early stage through the use of recently contaminated drinking vessels, by direct skin-to-skin contact, or by the fingers contaminated with saliva and mucus

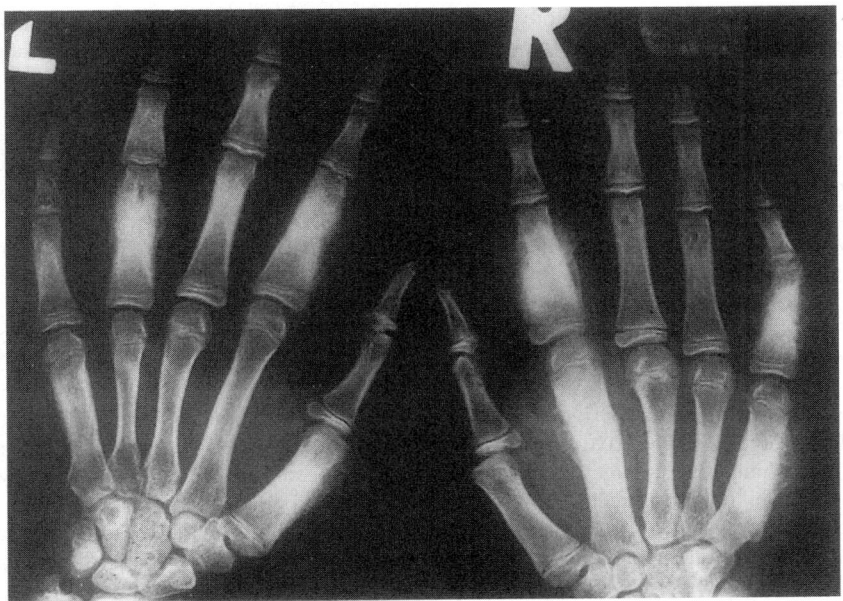

Fig. 23.36 X-ray showing osteoperiostitis of early yaws in a boy aged 12 years with polydactylitis and circinate early stage lesions in the axilla.

from infective lesions containing treponemes (Perine et al 1984).

In Arabia endemic syphilis, known as bejel, presents in its early stage and generally in children aged 2–15 years with a mucocutaneous eruption and exuberant papules predominantly around the genitalia and anus. Mucous papules or shallow ulcerations (mucous patches) appear on the lips, in the mouth and in the fauces. Symptoms such as hoarseness, dysphagia or dyspnea have been attributed to extension of the mucous patches to the larynx. Condylomata may be seen in the moist areas of the skin. Periostitis also occurs.

Late lesions are granulomatous and destructive and the nose and its bony structure, the oral cavity and the hard palate and larynx are favourite sites. Destructive skin ulcers, plantar keratosis, juxta-articular nodes and depigmented lesions are common late manifestations.

Control of endemic treponematoses

Although the treatment of whole communities with long-acting penicillin preparations for the control of endemic treponematosis of childhood was followed initially by a remarkable regression of the community disease, early clinical yaws has not been eliminated in large endemic areas where transmission continues and periodic focal outbreaks tend to occur. Without renewed control programs gains made by mass treatment campaigns of the 1950s and afterwards may be lost, particularly for yaws in some African countries (Perine et al 1984).

In the 1950s, on the basis of pilot studies in yaws in Haiti, endemic syphilis in Yugoslavia and pinta in Mexico, mass treatment campaigns with penicillin were undertaken in 46 countries in the context of the World Health Organization Treponematoses Campaign. Up till 1970 some 160 million people had been examined and in 50 million clinical cases, latent cases and contacts treatment had been given. In western Samoa, for example, the prevalence of clinically active yaws was about 11% in 1955 with about 3% with infectious lesions. On resurvey of the population after mass treatment a year later clinically active yaws was found in only 0.06% and infectious cases in 0.02%. In Yugoslavia the careful campaign, follow-up and progressive environmental changes reduced the rate of endemic syphilis to nil and results of surveys in 1968–1970 confirmed that eradication had been achieved (Arslanagic et al 1989).

Clinical surveys for active yaws may be conducted without any sophisticated laboratory test but surveys for latent disease require serological tests. The original indices were clinical and the detection of cases of active yaws is likely to continue to be the mainstay of surveillance and most appropriate for economic and logistic reasons. Age-specific seroreactor rates are, however, useful to define areas as hyperendemic, mesoendemic and hypoendemic and in surveys after mass treatment such profiles demonstrate the age at which infections are occurring.

The socioeconomic status of a large segment of the populations in the rural areas of West Africa has either not improved or has actually regressed in the last decade. In these areas, patients with reported yaws infection now number tens of thousands, but epidemiological estimates place the true incidence as four times higher. In areas of increasing prevalence, atypical early yaws lesions may be underdiagnosed owing to the inexperience of clinicians unfamiliar with the manifestations of the disease.

Antibiotics in treatment and control in endemic treponematoses

Benzathine benzyl penicillin (available as Extencilline, Specia, Paris) has been recommended by a recent WHO Expert Committee on Venereal Diseases and is preferred to other forms of penicillin for the treatment of treponemal diseases. Since a single deep intramuscular injection of benzathine benzyl penicillin 1.8 g (approximately equivalent to 1.4 g or 2.4×10^6 IU benzyl penicillin) in a healthy ambulant adult produces a penicillinemia above the treponemicidal level for more than 3 weeks, this dose is effective not only for curing treponemal diseases but also for providing protection against reinfection during this period.

Currently schedules for the endemic treponematoses (not including venereal syphilis) are: a single intramuscular injection of 460 mg benzathine benzyl penicillin (approximately equivalent to 360 mg or 600 000 IU of benzyl penicillin) for patients and contacts aged under 10 years; and 918 mg benzathine benzyl penicillin (approximately equivalent to 720 mg or 1.2×10^6 IU benzyl penicillin) for those over 10 years (Perine et al 1984).

The extent of treatment given to a community, village or other group living close to one another is based on the prevalence of clinically active yaws in the community. World Health Organization treatment policies recommend for hyperendemic areas (approximate prevalence of clinically active yaws in the community of over 10%) benzathine benzyl penicillin treatment to the entire population, viz. total mass treatment (TMT); for mesoendemic areas (approximate prevalence of clinically active yaws in the community of 5–10%) treatment with benzathine benzyl penicillin in all active cases, all children under 15 years of age, and obvious contacts of infectious patients, viz. juvenile mass treatment (JMT); and for hypoendemic areas (approximate prevalence of clinically active yaws in the community under 5%) treatment with benzathine benzyl penicillin in all active cases and all household or other obvious contacts. In isolated and remote villages TMT may be appropriate even if the prevalence of active yaws is less than 10% (Perine et al 1984).

Penicillin treatment always carries the risk of serious side effects including fatal anaphylaxis. During the initial mass treatment campaigns when almost all are receiving penicillin for the first time risks are very low but those undertaking such campaigns should be prepared to treat penicillin reactions. Alternatives to penicillin have been suggested; children between 8 and 15 years may be given erythromycin 250 mg orally four times per day for 15 days. Although tetracycline is generally not advised in children under the age of 12, Perine et al (1984) have suggested that in those between 8 and 15 years of age who are allergic to penicillin a dose of 250 mg four times per day for 15 days is acceptable in mass campaigns. In children under the age of 8 years only erythromycin in doses appropriate to their bodyweight (8–12 mg/kg) may be used and tetracycline must not be given. Tetracycline is not recommended in pregnancy.

Adults who have acquired yaws in childhood may be seen in the clinics of western countries, when the results of serological tests will not differentiate from syphilis; in such cases, treatment appropriate for syphilis is advised.

GONORRHEA

Gonorrhea, an infection of the mucosal surfaces of the genitourinary tract with the bacterium *Neisseria gonorrhoeae*, is mainly transmitted by sexual intercourse. In men the infection is associated with an acute purulent urethritis in approximately 90% of cases, but the organisms may spread also to the epididymis and the prostate. In women the urethra and cervix are infected in 65–75% and 85–90% of cases respectively and the rectal mucosa in 25–50%. Occasionally (about 10%) infection extends from the cervix to the endometrium and Fallopian tubes. Infection of the fauces may occur in both sexes (5–35%); eye infections are seen rarely in adults. In homosexual men, who act as passive partners in anal intercourse, rectal infections also occur.

In children before the age of puberty gonorrhea is commoner in girls than boys and those affected are usually in a low socioeconomic group. In girls the infection may follow contamination but sexual abuse is a frequent mode of transmission causing vulvovaginitis or a rectal infection. In boys the source of gonorrhea may be homosexual contact with older men. In the US, the routine surveillance of pediatric gonococcal infection has been suggested as a useful tool for monitoring the occurrence of child sex abuse (Desenclos et al 1992).

In the neonate gonococcal conjunctivitis (ophthalmia neonatorum), acquired during birth, is potentially blinding and requires urgent treatment. In localities where gonorrhea is common, primary care for all difficult to secure and antenatal care inadequate, then active consideration of prophylaxis for gonococcal infections in the newborn will be required, particularly gonococcal conjunctivitis.

In a small percentage of untreated cases, systemic spread gives rise to an entity known as disseminated gonococcal infection, characterized clinically by arthritis with or without skin lesions.

ETIOLOGY

The causative organism, *Neisseria gonorrhoeae*, exists as small Gram-negative cocci, kidney shaped and arranged in pairs (diplococci) with the long axes in parallel and the opposed surfaces slightly concave; the organisms are typically intracellular, are delicate and have exacting nutritional and environmental requirements. Media containing blood or serum, a temperature of 36–37°C and a moist atmosphere, enriched with 10% carbon dioxide must be provided to ensure growth. The organism is liable to die if separated from its host and is also readily killed by drying, soap and water, and many other cleansing or antiseptic agents.

Gonococci in pus appear in specific clusters in which they are surrounded by organelles and granules derived from the host cells in which they multiplied. These clusters are called infectious units in which the cocci are probably protected against humoral defense mechanisms. Serum antibody to gonococci can be detected within a few days of infection but such antibodies are not protective with regard to mucosal reinfection.

TRANSMISSION OF INFECTION

Owing to the poor viability of the gonococcus away from the mucosal surfaces of the host, gonorrhea is ordinarily acquired by sexual intercourse with an infected person. Gonorrhea is highly infective and the risk for a female having intercourse with an infected male is between 60% and 90%; for a male the risk with an infected female is 20–50%. The gonococcus can be transmitted to the pharynx by orogenital contact; infection in this anatomical site is usually without symptoms.

The incubation period in the male tends to be about 3–5 days (range 2–10 days). In the female a precise incubation period is difficult to determine since approximately 70% or more of infections may cause no symptoms. Such asymptomatic infections make it possible for individuals to remain as sources of infection within the community whilst at risk themselves of developing pelvic inflammatory disease or disseminated infection: the risk of developing these sequelae are generally given as 10% and 1% respectively.

In young children under the age of puberty vulvovaginitis is caused more commonly by organisms other than *N. gonorrhoeae*. Although gonococcal vulvovaginitis can result from accidental contamination of the child with discharge when sleeping with an infected parent, sexual abuse may be the more likely mode of spread and involve more than one child in the family. In the sexual abuse of boys the source of gonorrhea may be homosexual contact with older males. Pharyngeal gonorrhea, usually asymptomatic, may be the only anatomical site of infection in sexually abused children.

During birth, a baby passing through an infected cervix may acquire gonococcal conjunctivitis of the newborn (ophthalmia neonatorum). Gonococcal conjunctivitis in older children and in adults is usually acquired by contact with fingers and/or moist towels contaminated with fresh pus.

PATHOLOGY

Infection involves the columnar epithelium of the urethra and paraurethral ducts and glands of both sexes, the greater vestibular glands (Bartholin's), the cervix, the conjunctiva and the rectum. Infection may also be established in the soft stratified squamous epithelium of the vagina of young girls; involvement of this type of epithelium in other parts of the body such as the skin of the glans penis, cornea and mouth is extremely rare.

Inflammation induced by infection by *N. gonorrhoeae* of the mucosal surfaces may be mild or acute with the production of pus. A chronic inflammatory process of mucous membranes may have serious sequelae causing pelvic inflammatory disease, infertility, or an increased risk of ectopic pregnancy. In the male urethritis sometimes involving the deeper tissues may lead to urethral stricture and abscess formation.

EPIDEMIOLOGY

Since man is the only natural host for *N. gonorrhoeae* the epidemiological factors that are important in gonococcal infection relate to human behavioral factors as much as to properties of the organism. Gonorrhea is common in developed as well as developing countries. On a global scale there are in the region of 200 million cases per year. In developed countries there has been a decrease in the incidence of gonorrhea during the late 1980s and early 1990s, partly due to changes in sexual behavior in response to the HIV epidemic. In England and Wales the incidence of gonorrhea fell from 231 to 43 cases/100 000 in men and from 132 to 22 cases/100 000 in women between 1981 and 1993 (CDSC 1995b). In developing countries the prevalence of gonorrhea remains much higher and in women attending prenatal clinics is generally between 10 and 15%, indicating an important risk of postpartum salpingitis and transmission of the infection to the eyes of the newborn (Meheus & Schryver 1991). Prostitution probably plays an important part in the spread of infection in developing countries. Modern travel enables the rapid spread of antibiotic-resistant strains.

It is a disturbing fact that worldwide many millions of children 'live rough' in the streets and are frequently forced into prostitution by economic necessity; such 'street kids' also share 'comfort' sex with friends. In such situations special methods of help can be devised (World AIDS 1989). The only discoverable

indicator of sexual abuse in prepubertal children may be the isolation of a sexually transmitted infection such as gonorrhea. In England in 1990 there were 16 reported cases of prepubertal gonorrhea (Estreich & Forster 1992) while 5% of 183 children under 16 years of age attending a genitourinary medicine clinic in Leicester, England, between 1990 and 1992 had gonorrhea (Young & Keane 1992). In the US between 1980 and 1985 the incidence of gonococcal infection in children aged 0–9 years was 6.5 cases/100 000. In developing countries levels are much higher: in one report in 1980 from a Nigerian STD clinic 35% of female patients with gonorrhea were girls under 12 with vulvovaginitis (Richens 1994)

Epidemiology of antibiotic resistance

Antibiotic resistance in the gonococcus results from mutations in chromosomal genes and/or from resistance genes located on plasmids.

Chromosomally mediated resistant *N. gonorrhoeae* (CMRNG)

Fully sensitive wild strains of gonococci have penicillin minimum inhibitory concentrations (MICs) of less than 0.06 mg/l. Mutations at a series of loci on the chromosome result in small additive increases in penicillin resistance resulting in isolates with penicillin MICs of 1 mg/l or greater, levels at which currently recommended doses of penicillin become ineffective. These levels of resistance are over 100 times greater than those which prevailed when penicillin therapy was introduced in the 1950s.

As these mutations exert their effect by altering the permeability of the gonococcal cell envelope, isolates with clinically significant levels of resistance to penicillin are likely to be relatively resistant to a range of antibiotics such as erythromycin, tetracycline and chloramphenicol. Resistance to tetracycline and chloramphenicol is controlled by specific loci as well as the nonspecific loci.

CMRNG have an MIC to penicillin of ≥ 1.0 mg/l at which point clinical cure using recommended antibiotic dosages begins to lose efficacy. In the UK the level of CMRNG is generally low (2–5%) but in parts of Africa and Southeast Asia more than half of the strains may be CMRNG.

Recently chromosomally mediated ciprofloxacin-resistant isolates with MICs ≥ 16 mg/l have been imported to the UK (Birley et al 1994, Thompson et al 1995). In Japan, where fluoroquinolones have been widely used as first-line therapy for gonorrhea for several years the decrease in the susceptibility of gonococci to quinolones has been so rapid that fluoroquinolone resistance in gonorrhea may be a new worldwide problem complicating the treatment of gonococcal infections (Tanaka et al 1994). Between 1989 and 1994 more than half of the ciprofloxacin-resistant isolates referred to the Gonococcal Reference Unit at Bristol, England, also showed plasmid-mediated resistance to penicillin (CDSC 1995b)

Plasmid-mediated resistance

Plasmids are small circular pieces of DNA that can replicate within a bacterial cell independently of the chromosome. Gonococci totally resistant to penicillin owing to a plasmid coding for a β-lactamase (penicillinase) enzyme (PPNG) were first reported in 1976 while isolates with high level plasmid-mediated tetracycline resistance (TRNG) were reported in the US in 1985 (Heritage & Hawkey 1988).

PPNG: A total of six β-lactamase plasmids have been described in *N. gonorrhoeae* (Sarafian et al 1991): these are the 3.2 megadalton (MDa) plasmid originally associated with Africa; the 4.4 MDa plasmid originally associated with Asia; the 2.9 MDa 'Rio' plasmid; the 3.05 MDa 'Toronto'; the 4.0 MDa 'Nimes'; and the 6.0 MDa 'New Zealand' plasmids. In Europe and North America the 3.2 and 4.4 MDa plasmids account for most of the PPNG with a few infections due to strains containing the other plasmids (Sarafian et al 1991, Young & Moyes 1996a). Many PPNG strains also posess a 24.5 MDa plasmid that promotes transfer of plasmid DNA and can thus spread resistance to sensitive strains in mixed infections.

TRNG: TRNG have high levels of resistance to tetracycline (MIC ≥ 16 mg/l) mediated by the *tet*M gene which is located on a 25.2 MDa plasmid that can also promote the transfer of plasmid DNA.

PPNG/TRNG: There has been a decrease in the number of PPNG strains without resistance to other antibiotics but an increase in TRNG and in gonococci with plasmid-mediated resistance to both penicillin and tetracycline (PPNG/TRNG) (CDSC 1995b).

The prevalence of PPNG and TRNG shows marked geographical variation. In Scotland during 1994, 3.4% of strains were PPNG, 1% TRNG and 1% PPNG/TRNG (Young & Moyes, 1996a); in one London clinic 12.5% of isolates were PPNG and 3% PPNG/TRNG (Lewis et al 1995a); and in Jamaica between 1990 and 1991 11% were PPNG, 22% TRNG and 47% PPNG/TRNG (Knapp et al 1995).

The majority of antibiotic-resistant isolates found in the UK are imported so early diagnosis, effective therapy (which depends on appropriate antibiotic susceptibility surveillance) and intensive contact tracing are vitally important to control the level of resistant strains and prevent them becoming endemic.

Epidemiological typing of gonococci

Typing of gonococci is important in epidemiological studies and has shown correlations between isolates and sexual orientation, antibiotic resistance, site of infection, presence of symptoms, dissemination of infection, and geographical origin. Typing is useful in recognizing multiple infection and differentiating between reinfection and treatment failure and is also useful in medicolegal cases (Bygdeman 1987). The various phenotypic systems have been reviewed elsewhere (Sarafian & Knapp 1989). The most widely used typing system determines serovars (serovariants) based on the reactivity of a gonococcal isolate with a panel of monoclonal antibodies reactive with protein I, the major outer membrane protein of *N. gonorrhoeae* which exists in two forms termed IA and IB: there are 24 IA and 32 IB serovars. Serovar typing is often combined with auxotyping (a system based on the nutritional requirements of gonococci) to increase the discrimination between isolates. For example in Scotland, during 1994 seven different IA and 13 different IB serovars were found compared with 14 IA and 34 IA serovar/auxotype combinations – certain combinations were associated with homosexually acquired infection while others were found in distinct geographical areas (Young & Moyes, 1996a). The

combination of serovar, auxotype and plasmid profile is particularly useful in monitoring PPNG and supports the epidemiological data which suggest that the majority of isolates are imported into the UK. Molecular biological typing techniques such as polymerase chain reaction (PCR) amplification of the protein I gene and restriction fragment length polymorphism of chromosomal DNA are currently being developed and evaluated.

DIAGNOSIS OF GONORRHEA: LABORATORY AND CLINICAL PROCEDURES

Microbiological tests are mandatory in making a diagnosis of gonorrhea. Because of the short incubation period and high infectivity, rapid diagnosis followed by immediate treatment and contact tracing are important in the control of infection within the community.

Neisseria gonorrhoeae is a very fastidious organism and very careful techniques are necessary for the collection of specimens and their transport to the laboratory for culture and investigation. Ideally the patient is seen at a clinic with an adjacent or closely sited laboratory. Under these conditions the majority of infected patients (about 90–95% of males and 50–60% of females) can receive appropriate effective treatment on the first attendance after examination of Gram-stained smears. In parallel with the decrease in gonococcal infection during the late 1980s and early 1990s some centers have reported a decrease in the sensitivity of Gram staining in detecting gonorrhea in women (Lewis et al 1995b). Cultural diagnosis of additional cases and confirmation of smear-positive cases can be made within 24–72 h.

Specimens required for bacteriological examination

Microscopy

This enables a presumptive diagnosis to be made in the clinic so that appropriate treatment can be given immediately. Immediate treatment facilitates the prevention of spread of infection and progression of the disease to its more serious sequelae, particularly in those patients likely to default.

A smear of secretion or discharge is prepared, dried, fixed by gentle heating and Gram stained by standard bacteriological technique (Collee et al 1989) but 0.1% neutral red is the preferred counterstain. The stained and dried slide is examined under a 2 mm oil immersion objective lens.

Specimens from males

In males, material for examination is obtained by inserting a sterile bacteriological loop into the everted urethral meatus and gently scraping the walls of the terminal part of the urethra. A loopful or less of the exudate obtained may be examined by microscopy of a Gram-stained smear and by culture. If anal intercourse is acknowledged or suspected a cotton wool tipped applicator stick should be passed gently and blindly into the anal canal to a distance of 5 cm; a proctoscope should be passed and if mucopus is seen it may be examined microscopically and by culture. If there has been orogenital contact with a person who may possibly have been infected, material should be obtained for culture from the tonsillar crypts or bed and pharynx.

Specimens from females

In female patients specimens for cultural investigation should be taken from the urethra (traditionally specimens are taken from the urethra after massaging from above downwards to expel any discharge from the para-urethral glands), external cervical os and cervical canal, rectum and throat. If pus is expressed from the orifice(s) of the ducts of the greater vestibular glands, this should be similarly examined. Smears should be taken from the urethra and endocervix for microscopic examination after Gram staining.

In prepubertal children vaginal cultures may be obtained uncontaminated by organisms at the introitus by gentle insertion of an auriscope or a suitable nasal speculum (e.g. Killian's Nasal Speculum 2–21/2″, Downs Surgical plc, Church Path, Mitcham, Surrey CR4 3UE, England); a swab is then passed along the speculum to sample the vaginal contents. Anorectal and pharyngeal cultures should also be taken.

Tests in disseminated gonococcal infection

When disseminated gonococcal infection (DGI) is suspected the routine tests described and several blood cultures should be taken before commencing therapy. It is most important to inform the laboratory that DGI is a possible diagnosis. Fluid obtained by aspiration of a joint effusion should be similarly investigated. Although patients with suspected DGI may have no genital symptoms it is important to take anogenital (and pharyngeal) cultures as these are most likely to yield gonococci.

Importance of culture site and number of diagnostic tests

Repeated testing of multiple sites is necessary since not all infections in women will be detected on first attendance. The efficiency of detecting gonorrhea varies depending on factors such as the culture medium used. Ordinarily in the female two consecutive culture tests will be taken from the endocervix (and if possible the urethra), cervix and anorectum.

A 'high vaginal swab' in the adult female is totally inadequate for diagnosing or excluding gonorrhea. Rectal cultures are important in the female and particularly so in screening for infection and assessing effectiveness of treatment.

If pharyngeal or anorectal infection is suspected two consecutive tests are advised in this site. Heterosexual men and women with pharyngeal gonorrhea require higher penicillin dosage than those with uncomplicated infection. In all patients it is important to know which sites are infected in order that all infected sites can be sampled to assess the efficacy of treatment.

Culture

Immediate diagnosis must be supplemented as well as confirmed by culture if the maximum number of positive results is to be obtained. Cultures are obligatory in the diagnosis of rectal, oral, disseminated and asymptomatic infections in both sexes, and are also essential in order to determine antibiotic sensitivities, to type the infecting strain, and to assess treatment efficiency. Cultures are advisable when medicolegal issues require special consideration.

Culture media

The vast majority of laboratories now use some form of selective media containing vancomycin or lincomycin to inhibit Gram-positive organisms, colistin to inhibit Gram-negatives, trimethoprim to prevent overgrowth by swarming *Proteus spp.*, and amphotericin or nystatin to inhibit yeasts. There are many variations of media in use but media that contain lincomycin rather than vancomycin are preferred as they are less inhibitory to certain strains of gonococci (Young & Moyes 1996b).

Transport and culture systems

As the gonococccus is very susceptible to drying dry swabs should never be used. Best results are achieved by direct plating. Culture plates, preferably warmed beforehand to 37°C, are inoculated directly with patients' secretions and immediately incubated at 36–37°C in a moist atmosphere containing 5–10% carbon dioxide.

When direct plating and immediate incubation are impracticable transport media should be used. Amies' medium is more effective than Stuart's at maintaining gonococcal viability (Human & Jones 1986) and should be used more widely. Nutrient transport and culture systems are expensive, do not perform well in a clinical setting (Genzmer et al 1984) and seem to offer little advantage when the transit time is about 3–4 h. In situations where transport is a problem the new tests to detect gonococcal nucleic acid (see below) should be used.

Identification

After 24 h of incubation, plates are examined and any colonies suspected as being gonococcal are tested by the cytochrome oxidase test. In negative cultures incubation is continued for 48 h and the plate re-examined before the culture can be reported as negative. Bacteriological techniques include examination of a Gram-stained smear from a colony. Oxidase-positive Gram-negative diplococci growing on selective media inoculated from a genital site have a very high probability (> 99%) of being gonococci and this level of identification is sufficient for developing countries where resources are limited.

A definitive diagnosis has traditionally been made by carbohydrate utilization tests. In the rapid carbohydrate utilization test (RCUT) preformed enzyme is measured by adding a suspension of the overnight growth of the suspect organism to a buffered, nonnutrient solution containing the sugar to be tested and a pH indicator (Young et al 1976). Apart from rapidity, this enables identification of other neisseriae and confirmation of *N. gonorrhoeae* to be made within 24–72 h of seeing the patient. The Phadebact Monoclonal GC test® based on two pools of monoclonal antibodies against protein I provides a rapid and reliable confirmation of *N. gonorrhoeae* while at the same time differentiating the isolate into serogroup IA or IB but it does not identify nongonococcal neisseriae. A combination of biochemical (RCUT) and immunological (Phadebact Monoclonal GC test) provides a highly reliable identification. There are a variety of commercial identification systems based on enzyme profiles determined by chromogenic substrates. Whilst these may be attractive to units dealing with small numbers of gonococci such tests are not absolutely reliable and the identification should be confirmed by another method, or preferably, the isolate forwarded to a reference laboratory, particularly if there are any medicolegal implications. Accurate identification is essential – *N. cinerea* in particular can cause problems and has been misdiagnosed as gonococcal infection in a child (Dossett et al 1985).

Antibiotic sensitivity tests

Once the gonococcus has been fully identified, antibiotic sensitivity tests are carried out. Since the majority of patients with gonococcal infection will have been treated on the basis of a positive smear, antibiotic susceptibility tests are only of help in the initial management of smear-negative cases or if the patient has been diagnosed and treated outwith a special clinic. Nevertheless, susceptibility testing is important, in identifying resistant isolates, for epidemiological purposes, and in planning rational therapy for use in the geographical area concerned.

Susceptibility testing can be performed by disk or, more accurately, by agar dilution methods and should be capable of identifying PPNG and TRNG as well as the various forms of chromosomal resistance described above.

Normally gonococci are defined as susceptible (> 95% efficacy), intermediate (> 90% efficacy), or resistant (< 85–90% efficacy) based on predictive values for clinical cure using recommended dosages for uncomplicated urogenital infection (Jones et al 1989, Ringertz et al 1991 CDC 1990). With regard to penicillin: susceptible equates to an MIC of ≤ 0.06 mg/l; intermediate 0.12–1.0 mg/l; and resistant > 1.0 mg/l. Standardization of susceptibility testing is important both for an accurate result in the case of the individual patient and to allow valid monitoring of temporal and geographical resistance trends.

Detection of nucleic acid

Although this new molecular approach requires more widespread evaluation it is likely that reliable noncultural detection of genital gonococcal infection can be achieved with commercial test kits to detect gonococcal ribosomal RNA in a chemiluminescent reaction (Hale et al 1993), and DNA by PCR or the ligase chain reaction (LCR) (Quinn 1994). In a preliminary evaluation LCR also performed well on urine specimens (Smith et al 1995), and since this approach has also been shown to give good results with chlamydia, it may provide a simple noninvasive screen for gonococcal and chlamydial infection in women.

CLINICAL FEATURES

The clinical features of gonorrhea reflect the inflammatory changes induced by infection of mucosal surfaces by *Neisseria gonorrhoeae*; in some cases the inflammation may be so mild that the patient is unaware of being infected. A chronic inflammatory process of mucous membranes may have serious sequelae, however, particularly in women in whom infertility or an increased risk of ectopic pregnancy may result. An infrequent but serious complication is systemic dissemination of the organism.

Clinical features in infants and children under the age of puberty

Purulent conjunctivitis of the newborn (gonococcal conjunctivitis of the newborn)

The chief cause of a purulent conjunctivitis of the newborn (in the past generally referred to as 'ophthalmia neonatorum') in developed countries before the antibiotic era was *N. gonorrhoeae*, but now in such parts of the world it is more commonly caused by other organisms including *Chlamydia trachomatis*.

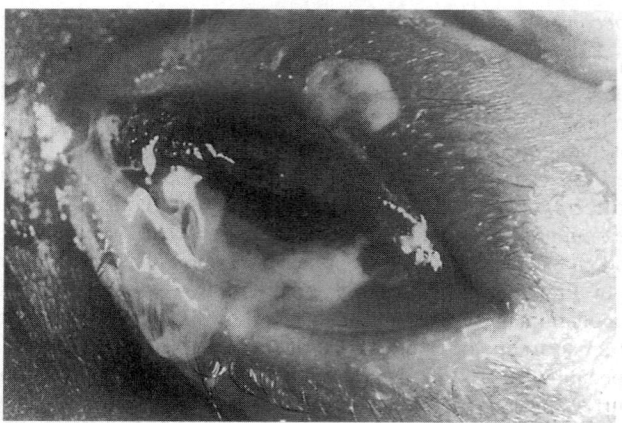

Fig. 23.37 The eye of a newborn infant with gonococcal conjunctivitis. The inflamed conjunctiva is infiltrated and swollen, so that it extrudes beyond the lid margin when the lower lid is pulled down. In such cases it is difficult to examine the cornea, which is hidden by inflamed conjunctiva and discharge. (From World Health Organization 1986a, with permission.)

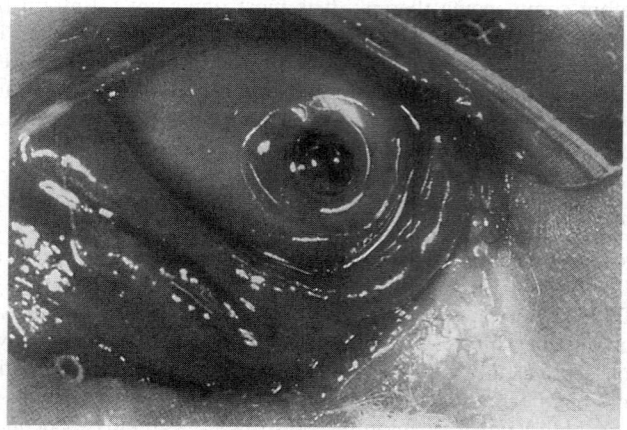

Fig. 23.38 Untreated gonococcal conjunctivitis in a 3-week-old infant. The cornea is opaque and a peripheral ulcer has developed which has perforated the cornea. The iris can be seen forming a plug at the base of the ulcer. (From World Health Organization 1986a, with permission.)

Gonococcal conjunctivitis (Fig. 23.37) generally manifests itself within 1–13 days after birth, usually by the third day. Commencing with hyperemia and shedding of tears, a mucopurulent, sometimes bloodstained, discharge appears about a day later. The eyelids swell and profuse pus collects often under pressure in the conjunctival sac. The palpebral and bulbar conjunctiva become edematous. If untreated, corneal involvement first shows as a hazy grayish appearance due to a diffuse epithelial edema. Opacities appear near the border of the cornea and sclera. Ulceration of the center of the cornea (Fig. 23.38) may develop and proceed to perforation of the eyeball with loss of vision. If untreated, gonococcal infection of the newborn may be associated with extraocular manifestations such as arthritis and septicemia (WHO 1986a).

Acute vulvovaginitis in children

The parents usually notice discharge on the child's underwear and on examination a purulent vaginal discharge, with reddening and edema of the vulva, may be found. It is usually accompanied by a gonococcal urethritis. Pelvic inflammatory disease may be seen in 60% of female children with gonorrhea.

Oropharyngeal and rectal infection

Workers in the USA have described the occurrence of gonorrhea in these sites in a number of children from lower socioeconomic groups (Nelson et al 1976) and victims of sexual abuse. Mostly infections of the pharynx and anorectum are asymptomatic.

Clinical features in the adolescent male (uncomplicated gonococcal infection)

Urethral infection

The patient complains of urethral discharge and an often mild dysuria in about 90% of cases. If infection has spread proximally to the posterior urethra there may be symptoms of frequency of micturition, urgency and painful erections. Clinical examination may reveal a reddened urethral meatus with a purulent or mucopurulent discharge. Inguinal lymph nodes may be enlarged on both sides. Examination of the urine by the two glass test will show pus in the first glass if the anterior urethra is mainly affected, or in both glasses if the posterior urethra and/or bladder is involved. Threads (cellular casts from mucus-secreting submucosal glands) may be found in the urine. A considerable number (possibly as many as 15% in some localities) of males with urethral gonorrhea have few symptoms if any (Neilsen et al 1975).

Postgonococcal urethritis may occur in at least 20% of cases of adequately treated gonorrhea in males.

Oropharyngeal infection

Infection of the pharynx by the gonococcus may produce symptoms in only about 20% of cases, when there may be sore throat, perhaps with referred pain in the ear. Clinical examination may reveal no abnormalities, or a mild pharyngitis or tonsillitis.

Anorectal infection

Infection in this site in the male is invariably the result of a homosexual act. The majority of patients (more than two-thirds) with anorectal gonorrhea have no symptoms of infection. In other there may be a history of pruritus and mucoid or mucopurulent anal discharge, anal pain, bleeding and tenesmus.

Proctoscopic examination may show a normal appearance, or there may be either patchy or generalized erythema of the rectal mucosa with mucopus in the lumen of the anal canal and rectum. The histology is that of a nonspecific proctitis.

Local complications of untreated anorectal infection include perianal and ischiorectal abscesses and anal fistulae.

Local complications of gonorrhea in the male

Inflammation and abscess formation may occur in the parafrenal glands (Tyson's glands). As the gonococcus tends not to attack the squamous epithelium of the gland penis balanitis is uncommon.

Inflammation may also affect and cause abscesses in the paraurethral glands on either side of the urethral meatus. When medical help is delayed periurethral cellulitis may develop. Although rare in developed countries urethral strictures and fistulae as late complications are common in tropical countries.

Abscess affecting the bulbourethral glands (Cowper's glands) is uncommon in countries with good medical services. The patient complains of fever, throbbing pain in the perineum, painful defecation and frequency of micturition. Reflex spasm of the sphincter urethra may produce acute retention of urine. An abscess, which is usually unilateral, may point in the perineum.

Epididymitis is usually unilateral, when the patient complains of a painful swollen testis. On examination there may be erythema of the scrotum on the affected side; the epididymis is enlarged and tender; and there is often a secondary hydrocele. Inflammation of the testis itself is rare.

Infection of the median raphe of the penis is rare but when it occurs a bead of pus may be expressed from a duct opening on to the skin on the ventral surface of the penis.

Clinical features in the adolescent female (uncomplicated gonococcal infection)

In most cases females with gonorrhea (70% or more) have few, if any, symptoms. They may occasionally complain of vaginal discharge, but this may be attributable to concomitant vaginitis caused by *Trichomonas vaginalis*. Uncommonly, inflammation of the trigone of the bladder produces urinary frequency. The sites infected in the uncomplicated cases are: cervix 85–90%, urethra 65–75%, rectum 25–50%, oropharynx 5–15%. The affected cervix may appear normal on inspection, or there may be signs of inflammation with mucopus exuding from the external os. There may be no clinical evidence of urethritis but occasionally pus may be expressed from the orifice. Rectal gonorrhea in the female, as in the male, usually produces few symptoms. Oropharyngeal gonorrhea in the female results from fellatio and the features are similar to those in the male.

Local complications of gonorrhea in the female

Inflammation and abscess formation may affect the paraurethral glands including those lying externally on either side of the external meatus (Skene's glands), as well as greater vestibular glands (bartholinitis and Bartholin's abscess). The glands may be involved on one or both sides. There may be few symptoms of bartholinitis but, in the routine examination, on compressing the gland, pus may be expressed from the orifice of the duct. When an abscess forms, the patient may complain of pain in the vulva, and examination reveals a tender cystic swelling of the posterior half of the labium majus, the skin of which may be reddened. In less acute and partially treated cases a chronic inflammation may result, causing palpable thickening of the glands.

Acute pelvic inflammatory disease (PID)

The symptoms of acute PID usually occur during or shortly after menstruation or in the puerperium.

The patient complains usually of lower abdominal pain, often exacerbated by movement of the psoas muscle, fever, rigors, malaise, anorexia and vomiting. With the increased use of the laparoscope, it has become apparent that whilst abdominal pain is the most reliable symptom, it may be minimal in at least 5% of cases. Pyrexia (temperature of 38°C or greater) may be found in only about two-thirds of women with acute PID, and more commonly in cases due to *N. gonorrhoeae*.

There is usually tenderness and a variable degree of muscular guarding over the lower abdomen. Pain is elicited by moving the cervix during bimanual examination. Palpation of the uterus and tubes is usually impossible on account of tenderness and guarding.

In about half the cases of acute PID, the white cell count is elevated. The erythrocyte sedimentation rate is raised in about 75% of cases, especially when the salpingitis is associated with gonorrhea.

Paralytic ileus presenting with abdominal distention and vomiting may occur in 1% of cases. In such cases fluid levels are noted on the plain X-ray film of the abdomen, taken with the patient in an upright position.

Chronic pelvic inflammatory disease

Chronic PID may be asymptomatic and undiscovered until the patient is investigated for infertility. Symptoms, when they occur, consist of intermittent lower abdominal pain or discomfort, discomfort in the groins, backache, malaise and frequent heavy menstrual periods. The tubes may not be palpable, or they may be irregularly thickened; the uterus may be retroverted and fixed.

For a fuller discussion on the subject of pelvic inflammatory disease and its treatment the reader is referred to a general text (Robertson et al 1989).

Gonococcal conjunctivitis

This is rare except in the newborn and presents as a purulent conjunctivitis affecting one or both eyes. If untreated, keratitis or panophthalmitis with blindness may result.

Disseminated gonococcal infection, involving both sexes

This uncommon complication, occurring in less than 1% of cases, is usually seen in women and in homosexual males in whom the infection has been asymptomatic and untreated (Graber et al 1960). Dissemination may occur from any infected site and more often during or just after menstruation and in pregnancy.

The clinical manifestations of disseminated gonococcal infection usually take the form of fever, rash and arthralgia or arthritis. The spectrum of clinical features of this complication is fairly broad but two forms possibly represent successive stages of the disease.

In the initial bacteremic stage or form, symptoms are usually of short duration, the patient complaining of fever, rigors, joint pains and perhaps a skin rash. There are characteristic skin lesions and polyarticular arthritis involving usually the knees, wrists, small joints of the hands, ankles and elbows, without sufficient joint effusion present to allow aspiration. If obtained, the fluid from joints is sterile on culture but blood cultures are often positive for *N. gonorrhoeae* if taken within 2 days of onset of the illness. There may be a tenosynovitis.

In the second form, involvement of one joint is usual, a considerable effusion is present and *N. gonorrhoeae* may be recoverable from the synovial fluid, which contains many polymorphonuclear neutrophil leukocytes. This form, sometimes called the 'septic joint stage', occurs usually after symptoms have been present for at least 4 days. A large joint, especially of the upper limb, tends to be affected, e.g. shoulder or elbow. The sternoclavicular or temporomandibular joint may also be affected. Systemic features are usually milder than in the bacteremic form, skin lesions are seldom found and blood cultures are usually negative for *N. gonorrhoeae*.

Intermediate stages of the disease may be seen and in the 'septic joint stage', if untreated, the articular surfaces of the joint may be destroyed and fibrous or bony ankylosis may follow.

The skin lesions in disseminated gonococcal infection

These are usually associated with constitutional disturbance, including fever and polyarthritis. There are essentially two types of skin lesion:

1. hemorrhagic lesions
2. vesiculopapular lesions on an erythematous base.

Both types of lesion begin as erythematous macules but in the hemorrhagic type the lesions become purpuric, especially on the palms and soles. In the second type lesions become papular and progress through vesicles to pustules.

The lesions of a disseminated gonococcal infection are clinically and histologically similar to those seen in meningococcal septicemia.

Meningitis, endocarditis and pericarditis

Meningitis is an uncommon manifestation of disseminated gonococcal infection and is usually found associated with arthritis and dermatitis. Gonococcal endocarditis is also a rare but often lethal complication.

Hepatitis

Hepatitis may occur following the bacteremia of disseminated gonococcal infection.

Perihepatitis

In both gonococcal and chlamydial infection in women acute perihepatitis usually occurs in association with pelvic inflammatory disease. This complication is very rarely found in men. The patient complains of pain in the right hypochondrium and sometimes in the right shoulder from irritation of the right side of the diaphragm.

TREATMENT OF GONORRHEA

Since its introduction into medical practice in 1944, penicillin has been widely and successfully used in the treatment of gonorrhea and, more recently, semisynthetic penicillins and other antimicrobial agents have been added to the therapeutic armamentarium. Although the proportion of strains with reduced sensitivity to penicillin has been rising slowly since the 1960s, the problem of resistance to penicillin has become more ominous with the discovery of β-lactamase-producing strains. The development of chromosomal-mediated resistance to a variety of antibiotics may cause difficulties in treatment in some areas of the world.

Principles of treatment

The aim of treatment is to eradicate the organism from the body as quickly as possible. Ideally the treatment used should be based on the pattern of sensitivity to antibiotic and chemotherapeutic agents observed amongst the strains of the organism in the population served. Regimens of treatment should be constantly reviewed, account being taken of the results of continuous monitoring of isolates for the emergence of drug resistance.

A course of treatment with almost any antimicrobial drug to which the organism is sensitive will cure the majority of patients with gonorrhea. Patient compliance, however, is often unsatisfactory and tablets may be inadvisably shared with a consort.

For these reasons a single large dose of antibiotic, given under supervision either orally or parenterally, is preferred as treatment of uncomplicated infection. In most cases blood and tissue concentrations of drug reach a high level and are maintained for sufficient time to eradicate the organism. Oral administration of antibiotics is preferred to intramuscular injections which are not only painful but more liable to cause hypersensitivity reactions. Single dose therapy has not proved satisfactory, however, in the treatment of oropharyngeal, or complicated gonococcal infections.

As concurrent chlamydial infection is common, it is recommended that all treatment for gonococcal infection should be accompanied by effective antichlamydial therapy (CDC 1993c).

Treatment schedules

Uncomplicated infections

With N. gonorrhoeae (not β-lactamase-producing strains, viz. non-PPNG). Regimens for single dose treatment currently used in the treatment of uncomplicated gonorrhea in adults together with suggested dosage for children are given in Table 23.38. In children the dosage should be given according to weight until 50 kg or puberty is reached.

With high level plasmid-mediated tetracycline-resistant N. gonorrhoeae (TRNG). As none of the regimens described in Table 23.38 are based on tetracyclines any should be suitable for treating infection with TRNG. However, as TRNG strains often show plasmid-mediated penicillin resistance the regimens described below for PPNG are preferred.

With β-lactamase-producing N. gonorrhoeae (PPNG). Some antimicrobial agents, available for the treatment of PPNG infections, are indicated in Table 23.38. The following groups of patients with uncomplicated genital infection should be treated with one of these:

1. if their infection is known to be caused by PPNG
2. if they are the sexual partners of such patients
3. if individuals have acquired their infection in areas of the world where the prevalence of PPNG is known or suspected to be high.

With chromosomally mediated resistant N. gonorrhoeae (CMRNG). Patients (adults or those over 50 kg weight or after puberty) who fail with standard treatments or who are infected with penicillin-resistant strains that do not produce β-lactamase (CMRNG) may be treated with ciprofloxacin 500 mg orally or ceftriaxone 125 mg intramuscularly (CDC 1993c).

With the high in vitro resistance of gonococcal strains isolated in Bangkok to a number of antimicrobials (penicillin, tetracycline, erythromycin, trimethoprim/sulfamethoxazole, kanamycin, spectinomycin, chloramphenicol) it has been considered that the adaptation of the gonococcus to antimicrobial selective pressures may mean that single drug treatments of the condition are no longer appropriate and 'combination therapies' need to be evaluated to delay further antimicrobial resistance.

The regimen spectinomycin 2.0 g and cefuroxime 1.5 g intramuscularly plus probenecid was suggested for Bangkok and where such trends may be found in other countries (Brown et al 1982).

Table 23.38 Suggested dosage regimens for the treatment of uncomplicated gonococcal infection

Antibiotic	Single dosage for adults or adolescents	Suggested dosage in children	
		Neonate 0–4 weeks	4 weeks–12 years
Ampicillin*	2 g oral		
Amoxicillin*	2 g oral		
Co-amoxiclav*† (amoxicillin 250 mg + clavulanic acid 125 mg)	8 tablets		
Ciprofloxacin†‡	500 mg oral	NOT SUITABLE FOR CHILDREN OR GROWING ADOLESCENTS	
Ceftriaxone†‡	125 mg i.m.	25–50 mg/kg i.v./i.m. as single dose†	125 mg i.m. as a single dose†
Cefixime†‡	400 mg oral		
Ofloxacin†‡	400 mg oral	NOT SUITABLE FOR CHILDREN OR GROWING ADOLESCENTS	
Spectinomycin†‡	2 g i.m.	NOT RECOMMENDED IN BABIES	40 mg/kg (max. 2 g) i.m. as single dose in children over 2 years†

* With 1 g probenicid orally.
† Recommended by CDC.
‡ Suitable for PPNG strains.

Oropharyngeal and rectal gonorrhea

Early single dose treatments for uncomplicated genital gonorrhea in adults were generally considered to be less effective in the treatment of oropharyngeal infection in both sexes and in rectal infection in the male. Infection in these sites usually can be eliminated by a course of antibiotics given by mouth; ampicillin (250 mg) may be given four times daily for 5–7 days. The single dose regimens of ceftriaxone, cefixime, ciprofloxacin and ofloxacin (Table 23.38) are effective in rectal infection.

Pharyngeal infection, including PPNG can be treated with either a single dose of ceftriaxone 125 mg intramuscularly or ciprofloxacin 500 mg orally (CDC 1993c).

Complicated gonorrhea

Any complications, if severe, may require parenteral therapy initially (see Table 23.39). This should be continued for at least 24 hours after the start of clinical improvement, when oral therapy may be substituted, to complete 7 days of treatment:

cefixime 400 mg orally twice daily, or

ciprofloxacin 500 mg orally twice daily.

Epididymitis. Epididymitis necessitates rest, scrotal support and an antibiotic which will eradicate both gonococcal and chlamydial infection (CDC 1993c): ceftriaxone 250 mg i.m. stat. *and* doxycycline 100 mg orally twice daily for 10 days. If severe and the organism is penicillin sensitive, then parenteral benzyl penicillin may be used (see Table 23.39).

Bartholinitis and abscess. The patient may need admission to hospital if the inflammation is severe and she should be treated with benzyl penicillin in the dosage given in Table 23.39. In less severe cases there is usually a response to a course of oral antibiotics. If an abscess persists, this is best treated by aspiration during antimicrobial therapy or by marsupialization if this fails.

Pelvic inflammatory disease including salpingitis. Reference has already been made to pelvic inflammatory disease (p. 1425). For a fuller discussion of this subject and its treatment the reader is referred to a general text (Robertson et al 1989).

Disseminated gonococcal infection (DGI) with or without arthritis and/or skin lesions. The patient should be admitted to hospital, the affected joint(s) rested in a position of function and treatment with parenteral benzyl penicillin 600 mg (1 million units) 6-hourly instituted. Usually the condition of the patient improves within 48 h and oral treatment may be substituted and continued for 10–14 days. In such cases the gonococci have been found to be very sensitive to penicillin.

For the treatment of disseminated gonococcal infection due to β-lactamase-producing *N. gonorrhoeae* (PPNG), or for treatment of infection in those allergic to penicillin, a number of alternative treatments are available (see Table 23.39).

Endocarditis and meningitis

In the preantibiotic era 4–10% of all cases of endocarditis were due to *Neisseria gonorrhoeae* and in one series of 38 cases encountered over a 12-year period 10 (26%) infections were due to this organism. Since deterioration may occur rapidly in endocarditis despite apparently appropriate antibiotic treatment, and delay in valve replacement therapy may prove fatal, it is strongly recommended that such patients should be referred early for expert management by a cardiologist and a cardiac surgeon (Working Party of British Society for Antimicrobial Chemotherapy 1985).

Treatment with 1–2 g ceftriaxone i.v. every 12 hours is recommended, and should be continued for at least 4 weeks in endocarditis, and 2 weeks in meningitis.

Treatment of pregnant women with gonorrhea

Care is needed in giving any drug in pregnancy. Penicillin is considered generally safe, and benzyl penicillin given intramuscularly in a dose of 1 million units 6-hourly for 12 doses is effective. Erythromycin is also considered to be safe although cure rates may be low, say 70%, and absorption uncertain; a dose of 500 mg erythromycin base 6-hourly orally for 7 days is an alternative in patients hypersensitive to penicillin.

Cerftriaxone 125 mg (for adults) intramuscularly as a single dose will be necessary for PPNG infections. Pregnant women who are allergic to penicillin or cephalosporins should be treated with spectinomycin 2.0 g intramuscularly as a single dose and be given erythromycin (base) 500 mg by mouth four times daily for 7 days (CDC 1993c).

Table 23.39 Suggested dosage regimens for the treatment of complicated gonococcal infection

Antibiotic	Dosage for adults or adolescents	Suggested dosage in children	
		Neonate 0–4 weeks	4 weeks–12 years
Benzyl penicillin	600 mg i.v./i.m. 6-hourly	30 mg/kg daily in four divided doses	10–20 mg/kg daily in four divided doses
Ceftriaxone*†	1 g i.v./i.m. daily	25–50 mg/kg/day i.v./i.m. in a single daily dose for 7 days (10–14 days in meningitis)*	
Cefotaxime*†	1 g i.v. 8-hourly	25 mg/kg i.v./i.m. every 12 hours for 7 days (10–14 days in meningitis)*	
Ceftizoxime	1 g i.v. 8-hourly		
Spectinomycin*†	2 g i.m. 12-hourly	NOT RECOMMENDED FOR TREATMENT OF COMPLICATED INFECTION	

* Recommended by CDC.
† Suitable for PPNG strains.

Gonococcal conjunctivitis of the newborn (ophthalmia neonatorum)

Combined local and parenteral therapy is necessary.

1. Local: frequent, repeated instillations of sterile normal saline into affected eye. Topical antibiotic treatment may produce sensitisation reactions and should on this account be avoided.
2. Parenteral: benzyl penicillin should be given in a dosage of 30 mg/kg bodyweight per day in two or three divided doses by intramuscular injection until cure is obtained, generally within a week.
3. Ceftriaxone 25–50 mg/kg i.v. or i.m. as a single dose (not greater than 125 mg) (CDC 1993c).

In developing countries where hospital facilities are limited, kanamycin given as a single intramuscular injection of 75 mg or 150 mg given with gentamicin eye ointment (1% w/v) applied every 30 min for the first 10 h and then four times per day (Fransen et al 1984) for 3 days is effective in treating infection with PPNG and non-PPNG. Possible ototoxicity of kanamycin, however, must be taken into account.

Both parents must be examined and treated appropriately.

Also see section on chlamydial infection (p. 1430).

PROPHYLAXIS

Systematic detection and treatment of mothers infected with gonorrhea is a goal not attainable in many areas of the world and prophylactic measures to the newborn child are the only means of reducing the incidence of this potentially blinding disease. Although none of the presently recommended approaches for prophylaxis against gonococcal or chlamydial neonatal conjunctivitis (ophthalmia neonatorum) is completely satisfactory tetracycline hydrochloride (1%) eye ointment appears to be effective when applied after careful cleaning of the baby's eyes after birth. It should be instilled into the conjunctival sac of all neonates as soon as possible after birth. Erythromycin 0.5% ophthalmic ointment – not widely available – is an alternative. Conjunctival sac instillation of 1% silver nitrate (CDC 1993c) has been used for more than a century (Carl Siegmund Credé, Leipzig, published his method in 1881). The latter frequently causes a chemical conjunctivitis and will not protect against chlamydial infection. In areas of the world where gonococcal infections are very uncommon prophylaxis has been replaced by good primary care systems, good antenatal care and in the neonate early diagnosis and specific therapy. The *prophylaxis of gonococcal conjunctivitis* should not be abandoned prematurely (WHO 1986a). A recent report (Isenberg et al 1995) suggests that a 2.5% ophthalmic solution of povidone-iodine as prophylaxis against ophthalmia neonatorum is not only more effective than treatment with silver nitrate or erythromycin but is cheaper and less toxic.

TESTS OF CURE IN GONORRHEA

After treatment every patient should be carefully examined to ensure that the infection has been cured. Culture is necessary in men when urethritis persists, or in those treated for an asymptomatic infection. In women at least two consecutive tests of cure by culture of the urethra, cervix and rectum should be carried out.

TREATMENT WHEN DIAGNOSIS OF GONORRHEA IS SUSPECTED ON EPIDEMIOLOGICAL GROUNDS

Accurate diagnosis and treatment is the approach of choice when adequate facilities exist. Treatment before diagnosis is not desirable as a routine even in contacts, except when there are special problems. For example a female contact of a known case of gonorrhea may be treated if she is unlikely to reattend. In such a case a form of treatment known to produce high cure rates in that locality (say of 95%) may be justified. In the case of contacts of patients with an infection due to PPNG then treatment with spectinomycin or cephalosporin is justified. Follow-up is important.

CHLAMYDIAL INFECTIONS

Although the etiology of nonspecific genital infections, particularly nonspecific urethritis in men, is not wholly resolved chlamydial infection plays an important part. From the pediatric point of view *Chlamydia* is the main agent to consider and the possible roles of *Ureaplasma urealyticum* and *Mycoplasma* spp. remain controversial (Robertson et al 1989).

CHLAMYDIA

Organisms belonging to the genus *Chlamydia* are the cause of ocular, genital and systemic diseases in man. Three species are recognized, viz. *Chlamydia trachomatis, Chlamydia psittaci* and *Chlamydia pneumoniae* (previously known as TWAR *Chlamydia*). These are obligate intracellular parasites which cannot by themselves synthesise the high energy compounds adenosine triphosphate (ATP) and guanosine triphosphate (GTP) and multiply by binary fission. Now regarded as Gram-negative bacteria, *Chlamydia* contain DNA and RNA, possess enzymes, contain cell wall material, have a developmental cycle and share common antigens. *C. trachomatis* forms glycogen-containing inclusions that can be stained with iodine. DNA homology within *C. trachomatis* strains lies between 96% and 100% (Kingsbury & Weiss 1968, Becker 1978) and supports their classification as a single species. In so far as sexually transmitted diseases are concerned, *C. trachomatis* is the most important of the three species. Of the three biovars of this species known, one is found as a latent infection in mice and two which concern man have no animal reservoir, viz. *C. trachomatis* biovar *trachoma* and *C. trachomatis* biovar *lymphogranuloma*.

All chlamydiae, unique among prokaryotic cells, undergo a developmental cycle in the cytoplasm of eukaryotic cells (Ward 1983) and the tendency of these to produce persistent infection is characteristic.

Pathology of chlamydial infection

In conjunctivitis due to chlamydiae the formation of a follicle commonly occurs, but this is a tissue reaction to irritation and is not specific. In trachoma, cellular inclusions were first described in 1907 by Halberstaedter & von Prowazek. In histological sections of cervical mucosa similar inclusions appear as cytoplasmic vacuoles when examined by light microscopy and are most easily seen in columnar endocervical cells. The vacuoles may occupy nearly the entire volume of the cell and, on electron microscopy, are seen to contain numerous small spherical bodies about 1 μm in diameter; these represent infectious elementary bodies, noninfectious reticulate bodies and transitional stages. The pathology of the urethra and conjunctiva is not easy to study as biopsy is not justified; urethral follicles, however, have been seen with the operating microscope in some men with *Chlamydia*-positive NGU. Changes are not necessarily attributable wholly to chlamydiae as other organisms commonly colonize the cervix. Neutrophil polymorphonuclear leukocytes are dominant in the early stages of eye infections and are similarly found in urethritis and cervicitis.

Laboratory diagnosis

Because chlamydiae are obligate intracellular organisms, diagnostic culture techniques require viable cells in which to replicate. Alternative nonculture diagnostic techniques have therefore been developed, but none of these are without their individual problems, and there is as yet no ideal test. Current methods for the laboratory diagnosis of chlamydial infection are reviewed by Taylor-Robinson & Thomas (1991) and summarized below:

1. Detection of inclusion bodies by direct microscopy is too insensitive to be of practical value.

2. Detection of *Chlamydia* antigen by immunocytochemical methods. Monoclonal antibodies have been used in fluorescent antibody and ELISA methods for the detection of chlamydial antigens in conjunctival, urethral and endocervical material (Taylor et al 1984, Thomas et al 1984, Pugh et al 1985). The major advantages of immunocytochemical methods over culture are that they are simpler, quicker and a little more sensitive. Problems of transport are also circumvented. A disadvantage is that nonviable organisms are likely to be detected.

3. Culture. Isolation of *C. trachomatis* on McCoy cells, irradiated or otherwise treated to stop their replication, is a sensitive method, whereas the isolation in the yolk sac of an egg is insensitive and prone to contamination. As irradiation is inconvenient for some laboratories alternative methods of comparable sensitivity have been described, e.g. treatment of cells with the nucleoside analogue 5-iodo-2-deoxyuridine (IDU) or with the fungal metabolite cytochalasin B. Culture methods depend on viable organisms reaching the laboratory and are not suitable for clinicians for whom rapid transport of specimens to the laboratory is a problem. It should be noted that culture of *C. psittaci* should not knowingly be attempted if the laboratory is not equipped for the culture of microorganisms defined as being of category B1.

4. Ligase chain reaction. This in vitro nucleic acid amplification technique is currently being developed for the diagnosis of chlamydial infections, but is not yet widely available (Schachter et al 1994).

5. Serology. Information on antibody responses during chlamydial infections is based largely on microimmuno-fluorescence (micro-IF) tests. Only a few laboratories, however, offer this test at present. The more widely available serological tests are not type specific, and cross-reaction between *C. trachomatis* and *C. pneumoniae* makes the results difficult to interpret. A fourfold rise in titer or conversion from seronegative to seropositive correlates well with the isolation of *C. trachomatis*, but this does not provide rapid diagnosis. In the neonate, passive transfer of maternal IgG antibody makes this test unreliable and diagnosis should be based on the detection of IgM.

Disease due to *C. trachomatis* biovar *trachoma* (tropical trachoma, serovars A, B, Ba and C)

In hyperendemic tropical trachoma, due to biovar trachoma (serovars A, B. Ba and C), the organisms are spread by eye-to-eye transmission particularly in unhygienic conditions, affecting about 500×10^6 people and causing blindness in some 2×10^6. *Chlamydia* require rapid transmission in moist conditions and hyperendemic trachoma occurs in conditions of 'ocular promiscuity' – that is to say in conditions that favour the frequent, unrestricted and indiscriminate mixing of ocular contacts or of ocular discharges.

Disease due to *C. trachomatis* biovar *trachoma* (ocular or genital infections, serovars D, E, F, G, H, I and K)

The ocular or genital infections of western countries, on the other hand, tend to occur when there is frequent mixing of genital contacts or discharges with occasional transfer to the eye. These chlamydial infections, due to serovars D-K, are predominantly genital, i.e. nongonococcal urethritis (NGU) in men, or endocervical infection in women (Robertson et al 1989) and the incidence of both adult chlamydial conjunctivitis and conjunctivitis of the newborn, with or without involvement of other sites, e.g. nasopharynx, are dependent upon the incidence of genital infections in the adult population and, in the case of infants, in their mothers.

Although mainly genital, either alone or with *N. gonorrhoeae* in women, these organisms can cause pelvic inflammatory disease and sometimes perihepatitis in the form of the Fitz-Hugh and Curtis syndrome (Robertson et al 1989). In the latter syndrome the combination of right upper quadrant abdominal pain and perihepatitis occurs in association with genital tract infection.

There is evidence which suggests that chlamydiae may be a cause of peripheral and axial forms of human arthritis either in association with lymphogranuloma venereum or as a reactive arthritis, as in Reiter's disease.

In the sexually active adolescent, the manifestations of genital infection are similar to the adult. Pediatric infections due to *C. trachomatis* are largely confined to the neonate and young baby as a result of vertical transmission from an infected mother. The estimated attack rate is 60–70%

Infections in the newborn due to *Chlamydia trachomatis*

Conjunctivitis

Conjunctivitis is the most obvious clinical form of neonatal chlamydial infection since contamination can occur from the mother's infected cervical excretions during birth or by shedding of *Chlamydia* in inflammatory discharges from an infected eye in the newborn.

The increase in incidence of NGU in men and the increasing isolation rate of certain serotypes of *C. trachomatis* in some 40% or more in this condition is likely to be associated with a large number of women acting as carriers. As chlamydial infection can be asymptomatic in men with minimal signs of urethritis, and is ordinarily so in women, conjunctival infections of the newborn are to be expected.

There are difficulties in assessing the true incidence of chlamydial conjunctivitis because babies are rarely in hospital for the full incubation period of the order of 3–13 days or longer, but it has been estimated to be as high as 50% of babies born to infected mothers. In the case of gonococcal conjunctivitis diagnosis is usually made 24–48 h after birth.

Clinical features. The infection usually presents as a mucopurulent conjunctivitis (Fig. 23.39) which may vary from mild to severe within the incubation period already stated. The discharge may be only scanty and not obviously purulent but it is sometimes more copious and frankly purulent, or on occasions bloodstained. On examination the palpebral conjunctiva shows mild to severe inflammation and papillary hyperplasia. In its more severe form there is also edema of the eyelids and palpebral conjunctiva particularly of the lower lid. Signs may be minimal and inflammatory reaction apparently transitory but in some cases conjunctival scarring develops.

In the absence of specific treatment, the course is usually benign, but may be protracted. The sight is not usually compromised although micropannus and conjunctival scarring may be found on long-term follow-up.

Diagnosis. The discharge should be wiped gently away from the surface of the eyelids with a swab and the lower lids everted. A cotton wool swab should be passed gently but firmly along the lower and upper palpebral conjunctiva and then agitated gently in 2SP transport medium;* excess fluid is removed by rotating the swab while gently pressing against the inside of the container. The sample should reach the laboratory within 2 h or be stored at a temperature of – 70°C until cultured.

Similar samples are taken from the posterior pharyngeal wall, particularly in older children and on follow-up.

The earlier the provisional diagnosis the earlier the full investigation and treatment, not only of the baby but also of the mother who is at risk of pelvic inflammatory disease and of the sexual partner.

In the investigation of neonatal conjunctivitis the following are essential steps:

1. Microscopy of Gram-stained smear from the palpebral conjunctiva for Gram-negative diplococci (*N. gonorrhoeae*)
2. Direct inoculation of selective medium with material from the palpebral conjunctiva to detect or exclude *N. gonorrhoeae*
3. Swab from palpebral conjunctiva placed in 2SP or other chlamydial transport medium for the isolation of *C. trachomatis*
4. Swab taken in Amies' transport medium for isolation of other bacterial pathogens
5. Pelvic examination of the mother to exclude *N. gonorrhoeae*, *C. trachomatis* and other pathogens
6. Examination of sexual partner of the mother.

Treatment. Once *N. gonorrhoeae* has been excluded it is justifiable to treat a mild neonatal conjunctivitis with a 0.5% (w/v) solution of neomycin prescribed as single dose sterile eye drops ('Minims' Neomycin sulfate, Smith and Nephew Pharmaceutical Ltd., 20 units in each single dose), instilled into the eye every 4 h. Neomycin is effective against most isolates of staphylococci and some strains of *Proteus vulgaris* and *Pseudomonas aeruginosa*. It

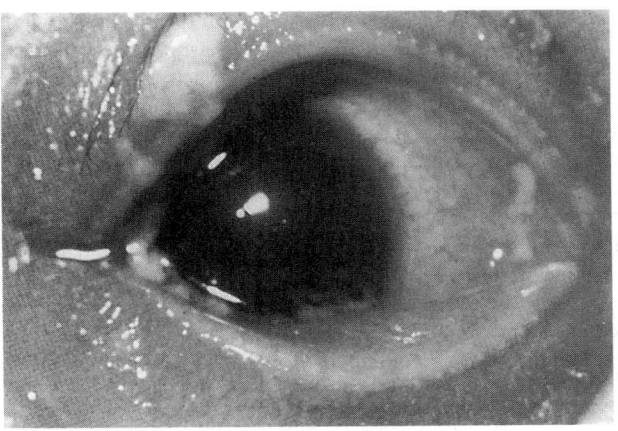

Fig. 23.39 Chlamydial conjunctivitis in a newborn infant. (From World Health Organization 1986a, with permission.)

has no action against fungi, viruses or intracellular *Chlamydia*. If the conjunctivitis is marked and does not respond to neomycin then isolation of *Chlamydia* should be attempted and if this organism is *discovered, or suspected*, systemic treatment with erythromycin should be commenced.

Infants with chlamydial infections frequently have concurrent pharyngeal infection which is likely to persist after topical chemotherapy alone with eye ointments and may be a focus for reinfection of the eye. In addition the eye infection may be associated with concurrent or subsequent pneumonia and otitis media and even myocarditis.

There is therefore a very strong case for systemic treatment of all infants with chlamydial conjunctivitis and erythromycin ethylsuccinate given in divided doses to a total of 40–50 mg/kg bodyweight per day for 2–3 weeks is reliable. There appears to be no advantage in giving systemic and topical treatment simultaneously.

Pneumonia

Spread of the organism from the nasopharynx to the lower respiratory tract can result in pneumonitis, with an estimated incidence of 11–20% of babies born to infected mothers. Onset of pneumonitis occurs later than that of conjunctivitis, usually between 3 and 11 weeks, with gradual development of a 'staccato' cough, partial nasal obstruction and tachypnea. Typically, the baby is afebrile and not systemically unwell. Chest signs may be minimal compared with the diffuse bilateral interstitial opacities and hyperinflation seen on chest X-ray.

The chest X-ray appearances, the presence of circulating IgM antichlamydial antibodies and demonstration of *C. trachomatis* in concurrent conjunctivitis or from the nasopharynx are all supportive evidence for the diagnosis of chlamydial pneumonitis. The presence of other respiratory tract pathogens (e.g. respiratory syncytial virus) must be excluded.

Treatment with erythromycin ethylsuccinate 25 mg/kg twice daily for 3 weeks produces a rapid response and chronic chlamydial pneumonia or recurring infection has not yet been shown to occur.

As with conjunctivitis, examination of the mother for evidence of chlamydial infection is mandatory.

---

* '2SP' is 2.4 ml of a sucrose phosphate solution, i.e. 0.2 M sucrose in 0.02 M phosphate buffer pH 7.2 with 50 µg/ml of streptomycin, 100 µg vancomycin, and, except for 2SP to be used for conjunctival specimens, 25 units/ml of nystatin. Specimens may be stored at – 70°C before culture (Gordon et al 1969).

Other mucosal surfaces in the newborn have been shown to be colonized by *C. trachomatis*, namely nasopharynx, rectum and vagina. It is difficult to be certain whether the isolation of *Chlamydia* from the nasopharynx of infants represents an 'established infection' or pathological condition of the pharynx rather than contamination by tears. The infection is usually light in terms of numbers of infectious units and is often clinically inapparent and without sequelae but it can persist for as long as 866 days in the absence of chemotherapy (Bell et al 1992). Otitis media has been described in infants infected with *C. trachomatis* but the exact role of the organism in the pathogenesis of otitis media remains controversial (Mardh et al 1989, pp. 221–232). Rectal and vaginal infections do not appear to have clinical significance.

Infections in the adolescent male

Chlamydial infection in men causes up to 50% of cases of nongonococcal urethritis, and may be asymptomatic in up to 25% of patients. In untreated infections epididymo-orchitis may develop as a complication. A reactive arthritis (Reiter's syndrome) may develop in 1% of men with a chlamydial infection.

Clinical features. The majority of men will notice a urethral discharge, which may vary from clear to grossly purulent, and may often be associated with dysuria, although not usually frequency of micturition.

Diagnosis. The presence of 10 or more polymorphonuclear lymphocytes in at least five fields on microscopy of a Gram-stained urethral smear at times 100 magnification, in the absence of gonorrhea is diagnostic of nongonococcal (nonspecific) urethritis. Specific chlamydial testing is required to establish *C. trachomatis* as the pathogen, and one of the diagnostic techniques described above should be used, according to local availability. Traditionally, a fine-tipped cotton swab is used to sample the urethral epithelium, requiring to be inserted 2–3 cm proximally to ensure adequate sampling. As this is an uncomfortable procedure, recent studies have been evaluating the use of first void urine as an alternative sampling site, with varied results (Chernesky et al 1990, Leonardi et al 1992 Chernesky et al 1994).

Treatment. Oral treatment with a tetracycline preparation or erythromycin for a minimum of 7 days is recommended. Oxytetracycline 250 mg four times daily for 7 days has shown to be effective (Robertson et al 1989) and is inexpensive, although the frequent dosage may result in problems with compliance with some individuals. A new azalide, azithromycin as a single 1 g dose is effective for uncomplicated chlamydial infections and although relatively expensive, has the advantage of allowing supervized therapy. For epididymo-orchitis, doxycycline 100 mg once or twice daily for 14 days is often used for its better tissue penetration.

It is mandatory in the management of chlamydial infections that all sexual partners are sought and screened for infection to eliminate the possibility of reinfection from an untreated consort.

Infections in the adolescent female

Endocervical infections in women are predominantly (70%) asymptomatic and may persist untreated for years. Ascending infection can cause endometritis and salpingitis (often known as pelvic inflammatory disease, of which chlamydial infections are the cause in up to 60% of cases (Taylor-Robinson 1994)) and occasionally perihepatitis, and chronic infection with fibrosis is now recognized as the commonest cause of tubal infertility. Other sequelae of chronic infection and tubal scarring are ectopic pregnancy and chronic pelvic pain. These complications use considerable resources for investigation and management, and early detection and treatment is therefore important in preventing future morbidity.

Clinical features. Although mainly asymptomatic, the commonest symptoms produced by chlamydial infection are a purulent vaginal discharge, irregular vaginal bleeding and pelvic pain. Infection of the urethra is less common, but can occur in isolation or in conjunction with endocervical infection, and may cause dysuria.

Diagnosis. Diagnosis depends on the detection of *C. trachomatis* by one of the methods outlined above. Specimens are taken with a cotton-tipped swab from the endocervix by rotating it gently within the entrance to the os and then placing in transport medium or on to a slide for immunofluorescent staining. Urethral swabs are taken using a fine-tipped cotton swab.

Treatment. The same treatment regimens as given above for men are effective. Where there is any risk of pregnancy, erythromycin is advocated (500 mg twice daily for 7 days) as tetracyclines are contraindicated in pregnancy. There are no data on the safety of azithromycin in pregnancy and it should be avoided in such cases. In cases of pelvic inflammatory disease, anaerobic infection may also be present and concurrent treatment with doxycycline 100 mg twice daily and metronidazole 400 mg thrice daily for 14 days is recommended. The sexual partners should always be screened and treated to prevent reinfection from an untreated consort.

Pregnancy

Chlamydial infection during pregnancy is important to recognize in order to prevent vertical transmission to the baby during birth via an infected cervix, with the consequences outlined above. However, chlamydial infection in pregnancy has also been demonstrated to be associated with chorioamnionitis and premature delivery, and postabortal and postpartum endometritis (Smith & Taylor-Robinson 1993).

Disease due to *C. trachomatis* biovar *LGV* (lymphogranuloma venereum, serovars L-1, L-2 and L-3)

Biovar *LGV* is sexually transmitted (serovars L-1, L-2 and L-3) and in contrast to biovar *trachoma*, which is pathogenic to the squamocolumnar cells of mucous membrane, it causes primarily a disease of the lymphatic tissue, involving characteristically the lymph nodes of the genitoanal region.

Psittacosis (p. 1373)

C. psittaci causes a disease (psittacosis) in parrots and certain other birds. In man the disease may arise when infected dust or droplets are inhaled: illness ranges from an 'influenza-like' syndrome to a severe illness with delirium and pneumonia.

Atypical pneumonia due to *Chlamydia pneumoniae* (TWAR Agent)

There has been recent interest in the group of chlamydiae called TWAR agents, now known as *C. pneumoniae*, and antichlamydial

IgG antibodies are found in 25–45% of healthy adults. These infections are a common cause of community-acquired pneumonia, may occur endemically and affect children and adults alike.

Symptoms of cough, sore throat and fever may accompany an elevated ESR, normal white blood cell count and chest X-ray abnormality: often a single lesion, normally in one of the lower lobes. Mild asymptomatic infections occur, but in debilitated patients the infection can be severe and even fatal.

Diagnosis is difficult as *C. pneumoniae* is difficult to culture. Serological studies using the genus-specific complement-fixation test are not sensitive enough and require to be confirmed by a micro-IF test. However, in primary *C. pneumoniae* infections, the IgG micro-IF test can take several weeks to demonstrate a response. An IgM antibody titer may be demonstrated in 70% of cases of primary infection but not in recurrences.

Treatment by tetracycline is recommended, but satisfactory results have been obtained from treatment of chlamydial pneumonia by a 2-week course of erythromycin (Mardh et al 1989) or a 3-day course of azithromycin.

CANDIDOSIS

Candidosis (synonyms: candidiasis, thrush) is a convenient generic term for infections caused by yeasts, acting as opportunistic pathogens in individuals whose host defenses are impaired.

ETIOLOGY

Pathogenic yeast cells are typical of aerobic eukaryotes possessing intracellular organelles including mitochondria and ribosomes and a double-membraned nucleus containing chromosomes. Taxonomically the yeasts have been mostly assigned to a single genus *Candida*, but molecular studies show that this 'genus' should be regarded as an artificial one comprised of nonsexually reproducing forms of members of a variety of other genera some of which have now been identified (Riggsby 1985). The most important member of the group, *Candida albicans*, is capable of causing the very common superficial infections of the mouth and vagina as well as widespread or more deep-seated disease, viz. systemic candidosis, an important hazard in modern medical procedures such as transplantation surgery, intravenous hyperalimentation and immunosuppressive surgery as well as in the emergent epidemic retrovirus infection with human immunodeficiency viruses (HIV) leading to the acquired immune-deficiency syndrome (AIDS).

The formation of germ tubes is accepted as a reliable property for identifying *Candida albicans* and is used in medical laboratories because of its rapidity. The germ tube of *C. albicans* is a thin filamentous outgrowth from the cell without a constriction at its point of origin. Presumptive identifications based on the formation of germ tubes are 95–100% accurate when compared with stricter taxonomic methods (Kreger-van Rij 1984).

In the vagina in those with vaginitis *C. albicans* comprises a very high proportion of isolates (70–90%). *Torulopsis glabrata* (synonymous with *C. glabrata*) is less frequently found in those with vaginitis (6%) than in those without (17%).

Adherence of microorganisms to epithelial cells is a critical step in the colonization of mucosal surfaces and their subsequent capacity to cause disease. Hyphal production in candidosis in vivo is not necessarily indicative of tissue invasion and the case for the connection of yeast-to-mycelium conversion to pathogenicity remains a matter for debate.

Conditions which favor transition from saprophyte to pathogen and are relevant to vaginal candidosis particularly include pregnancy, diabetes mellitus, damage or maceration of the tissue, the use of immunosuppressive drugs, possibly also the oral contraceptive – particularly estrogenic rather than progestagenic preparations – and oral antibiotics (Ridley 1988).

In those infected with HIV and in AIDS, there is profound damage to the cell-mediated branch of the immune system and, although it is oropharyngeal candidosis spreading to cause esophageal erosions that is most often seen, disseminated candidosis occurs rarely (Ebbesen et al 1984).

PATHOLOGY

In the mouth at least, in acute and chronic candidosis there is invasion of the epithelium by hyphae, which grow downwards in more or less straight lines without respect for epithelial boundaries.

CLINICAL FEATURES OF CANDIDOSIS

Candidosis of the female genitalia

Vulvar pruritus which may vary from slight to intolerable is the cardinal symptom of candidosis. Burning is a common complaint, particularly upon micturition and dyspareunia, especially in the nulliparous, may be severe enough to make intercourse intolerable. Vulvar edema is more common in vaginal candidosis in pregnancy.

Erythema of the vulva is the commonest sign of candidosis and tends to be limited to the mucocutaneous surfaces between the labia minora but may extend more widely. The vagina is abnormally reddened in about 20% of cases. If adherent patches or plaques of 'thrush' or pseudomembrane are removed the vaginal skin underneath appears erythematous and superficial ulceration with bleeding may be seen.

In contrast, primary cutaneous candidosis involves the outer parts of the labia majora and the genitocrural fold and not infrequently the mons veneris, the perianal region and inner thighs. Vulvar lesions tend to be reddened and moist with defined scalloped edges.

T. vaginalis or *N. gonorhoeae* may coexist with the yeast infection and on occasions all three organisms are found together.

Candidosis of the glans penis and prepuce

Characteristic symptoms of soreness and itching of the penis, accompanied sometimes by a discharge from under the prepuce, are seen in candidosis of the penis where there may be a balanoposthitis with superficial erosions.

Neonatal candidosis

Candidosis in the newborn may involve the umbilicus, mouth and napkin areas. The maternal vagina is only one source as colonization may involve also the mouth and bowel. Attendants and environmental sources may also contribute to transmission.

Pharyngeal and esophageal candidosis in AIDS

This usually manifests itself as dysphagia and retrosternal discomfort in patients who also have oral involvement with *Candida*.

DIAGNOSIS

Microscopy

Direct microscopy, to detect yeast cells or hyphae, is an essential as an 'on-the-spot' procedure in the diagnosis of candidosis of the vagina and of the glans penis. Material is emulsified in 20% potassium hydroxide in water or dimethyl sulfoxide. Alternatively the smear is dried in air, fixed by heat and then Gram stained; all yeasts, like all fungi, are Gram-positive and detected using the oil immersion ($\times$ 100) objective.

Culture

The swab of vaginal discharge, obtained from the vaginal fornices, may be sent to the laboratory in Amies transport medium. It is plated on malt agar and the yeast isolated and tested with horse serum for germ tube formation (see Etiology). The isolate found to be germ tube positive is considered to be *Candida albicans*; germ tube negative isolates are sent to specialist mycology units for identification. In deep-seated lesions identification to species level is desirable.

TREATMENT

Preparations widely used in the topical treatment of candidosis include the polyene antibiotics nystatin and amphotericin B and the imidazoles, clotrimazole and miconozole. Fluconazole, a triazole antifungal agent (see reviews in Fromtling 1987), is available for vaginal and oropharyngeal candidosis but in children under 16 years of age it is *not* recommended owing to lack of clinical data in this group; it should not be used in pregnancy or in those at risk of pregnancy.

For life-threatening systemic candidosis 5-fluorocytosine and amphotericin B are available for parenteral use.

The polyene antifungal antibiotics

The polyene antibiotics nystatin and amphotericin B are effective antifungal agents that act by increasing the permeability of the fungal membrane, causing a leakage of intracellular solutes and cell death. Nystatin is prescribed as vaginal tablets, each containing 100 000 units, with instructions to insert one at night for 14 nights continuing during menstruation. The patient should wash her hands and vulva before bedtime, lie down on the bed and gently insert the tablet into the upper third of the vagina. It should be explained that the nystatin is itself yellow in colour and that the appearance of a yellow discharge is not a cause for worry. Nystatin cream (100 units/g) may be applied to the skin on the vulva and, if required, to the adjacent skin. Should relapse occur the administration of oral nystatin (500 000 units four times a day for 1 week) together with local treatment and the use of nystatin cream in the male partner is justified.

Amphotericin B

Amphotericin B, a polyene derived from *Streptomyces nuclosus*,

may be also used topically as a 3% cream (Fungilin, Squibb); it is very toxic if used parenterally and liable to cause renal damage.

The antifungal imidazoles

The antifungal activity of the antifungal imidazoles differs from that of the polyenes in that the imidazoles have a very broad spectrum of activity affecting many filamentous fungi and dermatophytes as well as yeasts.

Clotrimazole (Canesten, Bayer) is supplied as a 1% cream for topical use and as 100 mg vaginal pessaries: One 100 mg vaginal tablet inserted every night for 6 nights is an effective alternative to nystatin and more pleasant to use; a shorter course of one 200 mg vaginal tablet inserted for three consecutive nights may be sufficient in the uncomplicated case, and the insertion of a single 500 mg vaginal tablet at night may also suffice. Sometimes (1% cases) vaginal applications of clotrimazole may cause burning sensation.

Miconazole nitrate (Daktarin, Dermonistat) is supplied as a 2% cream for topical use, as a 2% intravaginal cream (GynoDaktarin, Monistat) and as vaginal pessaries, each containing 100 mg.

Econazole (Ecostatin, Squibb) is another effective antifungal imidazole. It is supplied as pessaries containing econazole nitrate 150 mg and a cream, 1% econazole nitrate.

TRICHOMONIASIS

This common condition in women is caused by *Trichomonas vaginalis*, a flagellate protozoan which can infect the vagina, urethra, bladder, paraurethral ducts and ducts of the greater vestibular glands. It is usually sexually transmitted with an incubation period of 4–28 days (Robertson et al 1989).

CLINICAL FEATURES

Women. Many individuals are asymptomatic, and in others the clinical features may be those of vaginal discharge or manifestations of vulvovaginitis: dysuria, vulval discomfort. On examination, the commonest sign is an abnormal vaginal discharge, classically frothy yellow in 10–30% but it may vary widely in consistency. There is often an associated vaginitis, and occasionally a marked vulvitis may be present.

Men. Infections in men are commonly asymptomatic (90%), but may produce symptoms suggestive of urethritis.

Neonate. Vertical transmission may result in a vulvovaginitis although this is rare (Al-Salihi et al 1974).

Prepubertal Infection. In girls this may produce a vulvovaginitis, and acquisition of the organism as a result of sexual abuse should be considered.

DIAGNOSIS

Both direct microscopy and culture of patients' secretions are used for the diagnosis of trichomoniasis. In men, isolation of trichomonads from the urethra, prostatic secretions and centrifuged deposit of urine may be attempted, but are often unsuccessful. The organism can be found in vaginal secretions from the posterior fornix in women.

Microscopy. Examination of a freshly prepared saline mount of secretions by phase contrast microscopy will identify the typical oval shape (slightly smaller than an epithelial cell) with its rapidly moving flagella in 50% cases. Examination of stained films (as in

Papanicolaou smears) is insensitive, and prone to error due to the presence of artefacts.

Culture. A variety of liquid media have been used (Feinberg and Whittington's, Diamond's) but no one medium has been consistently superior.

TREATMENT

Metronidazole is effective treatment for most cases of trichomoniasis, although occasional treatment failures have been reported (Robertson et al 1989). In adolescents, a single oral dose of 2.0 g is as effective as 200 mg three times daily for 7 days, usually produces fewer gastrointestinal side effects, is less expensive and has better patient compliance.

In children, the dosage regimens are as follows:

1–3 years: 50 mg thrice daily
3–7 years: 100 mg twice daily
7–10 years: 100 mg thrice daily

for a total of 7 days.

There is inadequate evidence for the safety of metronidazole in pregnancy and during lactation, and it should therefore be used with caution. It is advisable to defer use in pregnancy until after the 16th week of gestation, and to strictly advise against concurrent alcohol ingestion.

In the treatment of sexually active women, it is advocated that the male partner be also treated empirically as the insensitivity of the diagnostic tests in men make it difficult to exclude the presence of infection. This will prevent reinfection.

BACTERIAL VAGINOSIS

This syndrome is a common cause of vaginal discharge and/or offensive vaginal odour, and although it is not sexually transmitted the incidence increases with sexual activity. Recent reports suggest it may have a role in adverse pregnancy outcome. For a detailed review, see Eschenbach 1993.

ETIOLOGY

The presence of large numbers of *Gardnerella vaginalis*, anaerobic Gram-negative rods, anaerobic Gram-positive cocci, genital mycoplasmas and probably *Mobiluncus* spp., with a reduction in vaginal *Lactobacillus* is associated with the syndrome. These organisms coat the surface of vaginal epithelial cells giving a characteristic appearance known as 'clue cells' (Gardner & Dukes 1955) and also produce amines, the commonest being putrescine and cadaverine, responsible for the 'fishy' smell. In bacterial vaginosis, the vaginal pH is high, and the addition of alkaline prostatic fluid in semen will allow release of these amines, thus exacerbating the odor.

CLINICAL FEATURES

Characteristically an offensive ('fishy') vaginal odor often worse post-coitally, which may be associated with a milky vaginal discharge. Direct inspection will often reveal a thin whitish-gray discharge coating the inner labia and introitus, and on speculum examination of the upper vagina, an homogeneous milky discharge is evident. There is no inflammatory component to the syndrome.

DIAGNOSIS

The diagnosis is made on the basis of a combination of several clinical and microbiological features:

1. the characteristic smell noted by the patient, and the presence of the typical vaginal discharge
2. vaginal pH > 4.5
3. positive 'whiff' test: characteristic smell produced by the release of amines when potassium hydroxide is added to the vaginal secretions on the posterior blade of the speculum once withdrawn from the vagina
4. presence of 'clue cells' on microscopy of vaginal secretions.

Culture of *G. vaginalis* alone is not sufficient to make the diagnosis.

TREATMENT

Oral metronidazole 500 mg twice daily for 7 days is effective treatment, although the relapse rate is high (up to 50% within 6 months). Alternative effective therapies include single-dose metronidazole 2 g orally, 2% clindamycin vaginal cream once daily for 7 days, 0.75% metronidazole vaginal gel twice daily for 5 days, oral clindamycin 300 mg twice daily for 7 days (Joesoef & Schmid 1995). There is no evidence that treating the sexual partner prevents relapse.

PREGNANCY

As in other sexually active women, bacterial vaginosis is common during pregnancy – 12% (Hay et al 1994) to 32.5% (McGregor et al 1995). It has recently been recognized that the organisms commonly associated with bacterial vaginosis are also commonly found in the amniotic fluid of women with clinical chorioamnionitis, and that pregnant women with bacterial vaginosis have an increased risk of mid-trimester miscarriage, preterm premature rupture of membranes and preterm birth. Treatment trials are currently underway to assess whether treatment of bacterial vaginosis during pregnancy will reduce the incidence of adverse pregnancy outcome, and preliminary reports suggest that this may be so (McGregor et al 1995). One study shows that bacterial vaginosis does not develop after the first trimester and suggests that any treatment should be initiated before the start of the mid-trimester (Hay et al 1994). However, data are insufficient as yet to enable any firm recommendations to be made regarding the treatment of bacterial vaginosis in asymptomatic pregnant women.

HERPES SIMPLEX INFECTION

HERPES SIMPLEX

Herpes simplex is an acute infectious disease, characterized by a sometimes recurring vesicular eruption, occurring anywhere on the skin, but most often on or near the lips or the genitals. Sometimes the infection involves the eye to cause a conjunctivitis with or without corneal involvement. The causative virus, herpes simplex virus (HSV), can be divided into two types on the basis of certain antigenic, biochemical and biological differences. Type 1 HSV (HSV-1) is usually isolated from lesions round the mouth or eye and transmitted by the direct contact of kissing, or by droplet in cases or from carriers; type 2 HSV (HSV-2) is responsible for the majority of genital tract infections and spread is by direct contact during sexual intercourse. The very common nature of inapparent infections, whether of HSV-1 or HSV-2, is becoming better appreciated.

HERPES SIMPLEX VIRUS (HSV) (SYNONYM: HUMAN ALPHA-HERPESVIRUS)

Herpes simplex virus is a member of the subfamily Alpha-herpesviridae which is characterized by the capacity to cause rapid spread of infection in cell culture resulting in mass destruction of susceptible cells. The mature herpes virion contains a core enclosing viral DNA in the form of a torus (Roizman & Batterson 1985). With restriction endonuclease it is possible to fingerprint HSV types. Its mode of transmission is mainly by contact of oral or genital mucosal surfaces.

NATURAL HISTORY OF HERPES SIMPLEX

In most virus infections affecting humans the virus rapidly establishes itself in susceptible cells, is replicated and after a few days it and its progeny are eliminated by host-mediated immunity. In a number of viruses, however, and in particular in herpes simplex virus and varicella-zoster virus, an elegant stratagem has been evolved by which, in spite of immunity, the virus can persist in the host for life and also provide for its spread to other hosts. To understand the natural history of HSV infection it is necessary first to define and name the various events in infection. The definitions given below are based on those of Wildy and his Cambridge colleagues (1982) but modified to take into account suggestions made by Rawls (1985); clinical and virological features in herpes genitalis at various stages in its natural history are represented diagrammatically in Figure 23.40.

1. *Primary infection.* This is an infection which may be asymptomatic, remain localized or become generalized in an individual who has not been previously infected with either type of HSV as shown by a lack of antibodies to herpes viruses.

2. *Initial infection.* This denotes the first infection of a virus type. It may be a *primary infection* in those without serological evidence of a previous herpetic infection or *nonprimary* in those with evidence of previous infection. Clinically primary and nonprimary initial infections may be indistinguishable on physical examination.

3. *Latency.* There is apparent recovery but some virus remains dormant in nervous tissue, particularly in certain sensory ganglion cells; this is latency (latent means hidden).

4. *Reactivation.* Virus may be reawakened spontaneously, or as a result of external stimuli so that infective virus may once again be found.

5. *Recurrence.* The reactivated virus may on occasion initiate a peripheral lesion in the dermatome relating to the sensory ganglion. The lesion is referred to as a *recurrent lesion* and the phenomenon is *recurrence*. Wildy et al (1982) used the term 'recrudescence' to describe this phenomenon but since the term 'recurrence' is deeply embedded in the literature it is used instead (Rawls 1985).

6. *Axonal transport.* The whole phenomenon requires translation of the virus from the periphery to the sensory ganglion and back again by way of, it is believed, the cytoplasm within the axon. The rate of translocation from the skin to the ganglion lies within the range of 2–10 mm/h.

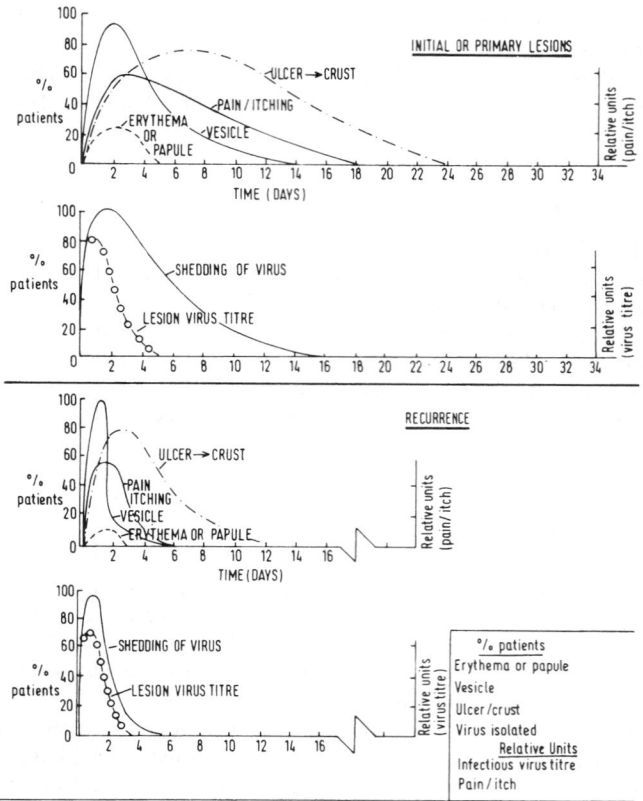

Fig. 23.40 Diagrammatic representation of surface clinical and virological features in herpes genitalis at various stages in its natural history. The patterns evolve during the approximate times shown and latency is indicated by the horizontal axis (sketches based on Wildy et al 1982, Spruance et al 1977, Rawls 1985, and other sources – see text). (Courtesy of Professor J. C. Southam.)

7. *Asymptomatic virus shedding.* Sometimes the virus evidently reactivates and passes to a peripheral site but fails to cause a noticeable lesion, although it probably multiplies and can be isolated. The term *asymptomatic virus shedding* (Rawls 1985) is used in this situation to distinguish this event from *recurrence*.

The cell bodies of the sensory neurons are situated in the dorsal root ganglia and the axons of these cells pass to the dorsal columns of the spinal cord and peripherally to the skin. Each dorsal root ganglion innervates an area of skin, called the dermatome. The ganglion cell, the sensory nerve and the skin it innervates occupy the area of operation of both herpes simplex virus and varicella-zoster virus and is conveniently called the *neurodermatome*.

Herpes simplex is the commonest virus infection encountered in humans and as a successful parasitic agent herpesvirus has few equals. It is able to infect generally without causing serious disease, it is readily transmitted from person to person and can persist in its host.

Notwithstanding the wide variation in the severity of clinical disease in *primary infection* the majority appears to be asymptomatic. The severity of signs and symptoms in primary infection appears to be age related; usually asymptomatic infections occur in the 2–3-year age group and symptomatic infections in the adolescent or young adult. In the majority of cases of clinically apparent disease the lesions are localized to the site of inoculation, the sensory neurons innervating that site, and the lymphatics draining it. Spread to contiguous areas or transfer to more distant sites by autoinoculation can also occur. Although primary infections can occur at any site, the lesions are characteristically vesicles affecting the mucosa and/or adjacent skin of the mouth or genitals which evolve rapidly into grayish or yellowish painful shallow ulcers.

Asymptomatic virus shedding occurs in between 1% and 5% of adults in their oral secretions. In the case of genital secretions this depends upon age and sexual behaviour and may vary between 0.5% and 7.0%. Asymptomatic virus shedding is thus a substantial source of virus.

The majority of the adult population, including women of childbearing age, particularly in the lower socioeconomic groups, carry neutralizing antibody to HSV. This antibody is transferred across the placenta and confers passive immunity to the newborn child, but antibody will have disappeared by the age of 6–8 months when a primary infection can then occur in the nonimmune infant. The commonest time at which the infection is acquired, particularly in lower socioeconomic groups, is between 2 and 3 years of age. Primary infections at this age are HSV-1 infections and the vast majority are subclinical; in an important early study, only between 1% and 11% of children showed some manifestation clinically, usually of stomatitis. Following primary infection antibody appears and usually remains at a constant level for a prolonged period, although it may decline until reinfection or reactivation may bring about an increase and stabilization of the titer. As the amounts of virus antigen produced may influence the magnitude of response, in many recurrent infections where virus replication is limited little or no increase in virus antibody may be observed.

DISTRIBUTION OF HERPESVIRUS TYPES

HSV-1 may occasionally be recovered from saliva, tears and the genital tract between attacks and regularly from lesions during attacks. In the case of HSV-2, as well as in HSV-1, asymptomatic carriers probably constitute the principal source of infection and the virus may be isolated from genital sites (cervix in the female or from the urethra in the male). Transmission is more likely when there is a lesion producing a high titer of virus. In the sexually active age groups spread occurs by sexual intercourse, kissing or direct or indirect orogenital contact.

In the case of genital lesions HSV-1 is less commonly found than HSV-2. In higher socioeconomic groups high proportions (40–90%) of young adults may have no antibody to either HSV-1 or HSV-2 whereas the corresponding figure in lower groups is only 20%. HSV-1 is associated with the mouth and stomatitis but genital infection with HSV-1 is likely to occur particularly in populations where 30% of young adults (15–24 years) are without antibody to HSV (Smith et al 1967). Orogenital contact or contact of the genitals with saliva-contaminated fingers may be the means of transmitting the virus.

The prevalence of Herpes simplex virus type 2 antibody varies throughout the world, ranging between 8% in Japan to up to 40% in Afro-Americans in the USA (Dwyer & Cunningham 1993).

Complement-fixing antibody can be detected before neutralizing antibody and conversion from absence of antibody to its presence in serum will signify a primary infection, which can occur in the genital area with either type 1 or type 2.

Using the restriction endonuclease patterns of HSV DNA to 'fingerprint' the virus isolates on the basis of the presence or absence of known cleavage sites it has been possible to begin to study the spread of the agent in the community (Buchman et al 1978). The possibility of transmission of HSV-1 within a nursery for the newborn has been confirmed (Linnemann et al 1978). Restriction endonuclease analysis for epidemiological tracing of HSV-1 is useful but because there is only a small number of variable cleavage sites in the HSV-2 genome caution is needed in the extrapolation of the results of HSV-2 analysis to establish proof of the source of an infection.

IMMUNITY IN HSV INFECTION

Herpes simplex virus persists throughout the life of the individual infected and achieves this by mechanisms which enable it to avoid host responses, viz. the ability of the virus to pass from cell to cell by a fusion process circumventing the need to emerge into the extracellular environment; to secure latent infection of a neuronal cell, by a mechanism as yet not precisely known; and to evade natural defense systems of the host, i.e. macrophages, natural killer cells and interferon.

Following infection there are both humoral and cell-mediated immune responses lasting many years.

Primary infection yields a rise in antibody with titers reaching a peak in about 4–6 weeks and remaining stable afterwards. Virus-specific IgM antibodies are produced in the early stages and persist for 6–8 weeks.

In individuals with pre-existing antibodies recurrence is not associated with a marked change in antibody titer.

In the newborn passively transferred maternal antibodies are often present but are gradually lost during the first 6 months of life.

PATHOLOGY

The basic lesion is one of localized necrosis. The nuclei of affected cells become swollen and the chromatin marginated. A dense basophilic mass fills the whole nucleus and later retracts from the nuclear margin. Finally an eosinophilic intranuclear inclusion appears (the Lipschutz or Cowdry type A inclusion); all stages may be found in any one section. The lesions of the skin and mucous membrane are characterized by intraepidermal vesicle formation followed by ulceration, crusting and usually rapid healing.

In severe disseminated infections visceral lesions consist of parenchymal lesions of coagulative necrosis with specific intranuclear changes. In the liver and adrenals, the areas of focal necrosis can be seen with the naked eye. In early encephalitis, necrosis is a marked feature and in the adult form, there is asymmetrical softening with numerous hemorrhages on the surface of affected areas. The temporal lobes and the posterior orbital gyri are most commonly affected.

CLINICAL FEATURES

The very common nature of inapparent infections, whether by HSV type 1 or 2, is becoming better appreciated with increasing availability and improvement of isolation techniques. When apparent the prepatent or incubation period of HSV-1 or HSV-2 infections lies between 3 and 9 days.

Primary herpetic gingivostomatitis

Primary herpetic gingivostomatitis is the commonest clinical manifestation of primary infection of HSV-1 in children between 1 and 5 years of age. The stomatitis begins with fever, malaise, restlessness and excessive dribbling. Drinking and eating are very painful and the breath is foul. Vesicles containing high titers of virus appear as white plaques on the tongue, pharynx, palate and buccal mucosa. The plaques are followed by ulcers with a yellowing pseudomembrane. Regional lymph nodes are enlarged and tender.

An identical clinical picture (Figs 23.41 and 23.42) may be seen in adolescents and young adults who escaped infection in childhood but acquired the infection by kissing. Primary infections, including ocular, in adolescence are becoming more common in developed countries, so more severe clinical forms of the disease will be seen more often in this age group. Virus shedding continues for 14–21 days on average after the appearance of lesions caused by a primary infection.

Primary herpes genitalis

Signs and symptoms of primary genital herpes tend to be more severe in women than in men and are usually those of vulvovaginitis accompanied by systemic symptoms of fever and malaise; local pain and dysuria can be severe. Difficulty in starting micturition or retention may be the presenting clinical feature. White plaques are present on the red swollen mucosae of the vulva, cervix and occasionally in the vagina (4%); scattered vesicles are seen on the labia (Fig. 23.43) and these may extend to involve the perianal skin and the skin of the thigh. The regional lymphatic glands are enlarged and tender and there may be a vaginal discharge. Healing tends to take place over a period of 1 or 2 weeks, but new lesions sometimes continue to develop over a period of 6 weeks.

In primary cervicitis there may be only swelling and redness of the mucosa but sometimes there is a necrotic ulceration and friability of the cervix which bleeds easily. The range of clinical effects is wide and asymptomatic cases are common.

Primary infection with systemic dissemination of HSV appears to be rare in immunocompetent adults but fulminating systemic HSV infection in pregnant women during the last trimester, although rare also, is a recognized and important clinical entity with a high mortality in both mother and fetus (Robertson et al 1989).

Early diagnosis is very important and the characteristic primary lesions, viz. vesicles or painful ulcers of the vulva with or without involvement of the cervix or of the mouth and pharynx, are seen in the majority. It should be emphasized, however, that the patient may not give a spontaneous history of either genital or throat lesions owing to the predominant systemic symptoms, particularly of fever and vomiting.

In primary herpes genitalis in the male the lesions can involve the glans or coronal sulcus and, if severe, there may be a phimosis with accumulation of secondarily infected exudate and occasionally a resulting necrotizing balanitis. In the homosexual the anorectum may be involved and show vesicles and/or

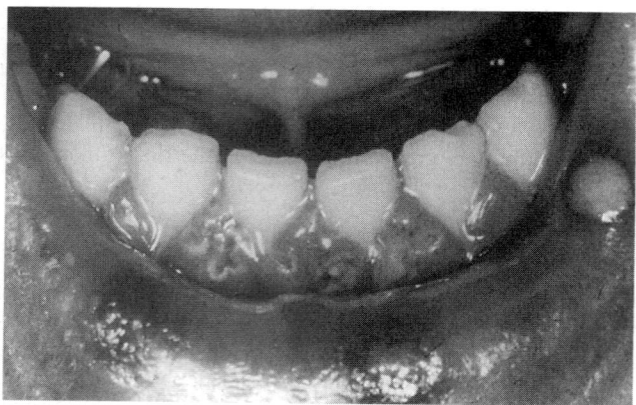

Fig. 23.41 Primary herpetic gingivostomatitis. (Courtesy of Professor J. C. Southam.)

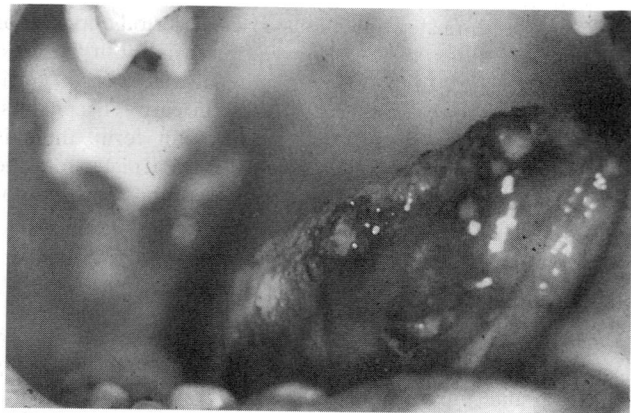

Fig. 23.42 Primary herpetic glossitis.

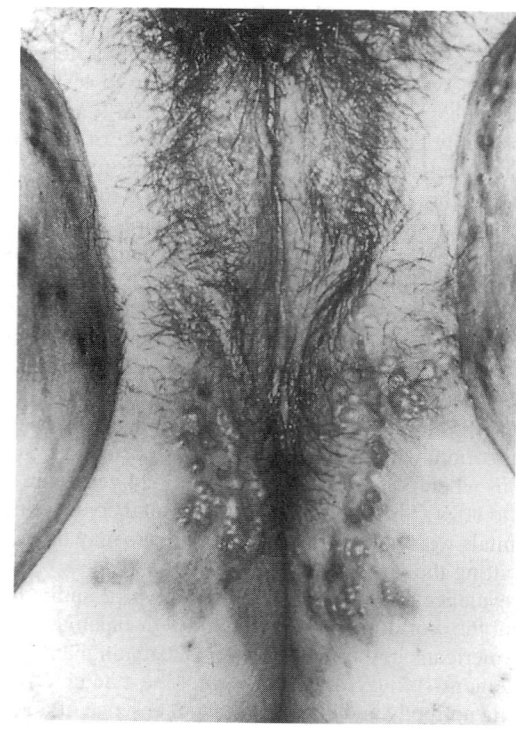

Fig. 23.43 Primary herpes simplex of the vulva.

ulceration. Anorectal pain, constipation, tenesmus, anal pruritus, difficulty in starting micturition, paresthesia in the sacral area, pain in the back of the thigh, fever and enlargement of the inguinal lymph nodes are characteristic symptoms. Herpesvirus may be acquired at other sites by contact. Other forms of herpes simplex include keratoconjunctivitis and eczema herpeticum, where infection has become superimposed on eczematous skin (Kaposi's varicelliform eruption).

The significance of the immune responses becomes clinically evident in a variety of immunodeficiency states in which HSV infection or reactivation may lead to severe local or general disease, e.g. malnutrition, Wiskott-Aldrich syndrome, lymphoma, immunosuppresive therapy in renal transplantation and in the acquired immune-deficiency syndrome (AIDS).

Complicated primary herpes genitalis

Aseptic meningitis

Fever, severe headache, malaise, photophobia, neck rigidity and the presence of Kernig's or Brudzinski's sign indicate meningeal involvement. There is a lymphocyte pleocytosis (5–1000/mm³) in the CSF which diminishes spontaneously. This complication may occur within 6–12 days of onset in 36% of women and 13% of men (Corey et al 1983).

Sacral autonomic dysfunction

Sacral anesthesia, urinary retention requiring intermittent catheterization and constipation may occur. The patient may complain of numbness and tingling in the buttocks or of perineal pain and there may be a decrease in perception of fine touch. Urinary retention and constipation may follow. In men impotence is associated with decrease in the bulbocavernosus reflex.

Extragenital lesions

Extragenital herpetic lesions may occur nearby particularly in the buttocks, groin or thighs. Any site may be involved including the finger and conjunctivitis may also occur.

Esophagitis

Primary herpetic esophagitis may be encountered as a rarity in the apparently immunocompetent adult without accompanying lesions of the lip or gingivostomatitis. In HIV infection this form of HSV infection may be severe.

Dissemination

In the rare disseminated infections in adults, HSV type 2 can be isolated from vesicular or pustular lesions that may appear anywhere on the body. In such cases HSV meningitis or encephalitis does not necessarily occur.

RECURRENCE AND RECURRENT LESIONS IN HSV INFECTION

After the primary or initial infection, whether obvious or inapparent, there may be no further clinical manifestations throughout life. Certain febrile illnesses, such as malaria and pneumonia, provoke attacks in those in whom the disease is latent.

Exposure to sunlight, menstruation or emotional stress may have a similar effect.

In the commonest form of herpes of the face, lips or genitals, itching or burning precedes by an hour or two the development of small, closely grouped vesicles on a sometimes slightly raised erythematous base. Ordinarily healing is complete within a week or 10 days. The shallow ulcers which develop may be very painful. Recurrent ulcers tend to be in the same region but not precisely on the same site.

Recurrent lesions in genital sites are not as frequent in HSV-1 infections as in those of HSV-2; this could be due to relative inefficiency of HSV-1 in establishing a latent infection of the sensory nerve cells in the sacral ganglia. After a primary genital herpes simplex due to HSV-1 recurrent episodes were reported in 55% of patients compared with 88% of patients with primary genital herpes simplex due to HSV-2 (Corey et al 1983).

COMPLICATIONS AND SEQUELAE

In the eye, repeated attacks of ulceration may result in corneal opacity. Transmission to the fetus and newborn may have serious implications, which are discussed later.

DIAGNOSIS

In herpes simplex involving the genitals, it is essential to exclude other sexually transmitted diseases, particularly syphilis, gonorrhea and chlamydia infection, which may have been acquired concurrently.

Cells from lesions may contain characteristic intranuclear inclusions. Multinucleated giant cells can also be found in scrapings as for example in cervical smears. Virus particles may be also found in lesion material by electron microscopy but the different herpesviruses cannot be distinguished by microscopy alone. Viral antigens are detectable in cells using immunofluorescence or enzyme-linked immune techniques. In the case of vesicular lesions diagnosis by tissue culture of lesion material is more sensitive as infectious virus is usually present. In later ulcers or in crusted lesions where the virus cannot be isolated the diagnosis can be better made by the detection of antigen (Rawls 1985).

Isolations by tissue culture are best made from vesicular fluid when present and/or exudate. Cellular debris is gently scraped from the lesions with a cotton wool applicator. The specimen obtained is then agitated in a bijou bottle containing virus transport medium (VTM) (Collee et al 1989).

Virus isolates may be characterized in the laboratory by antigenic, biological or biochemical typing by various methods:

1. Cytopathic effect (CPE) in tissue culture cells.
2. Immunofluorescent antibody test: fluorescein-conjugated monoclonal antibodies which are type specific are now available.
3. Restriction-endonuclease analysis: HSV-1 and HSV-2 can be separated unambiguously by restriction endonuclease analysis and the endonuclease Hpal shows the distinction most clearly (Lonsdale 1979).

Serological testing

Blood samples should be taken on first attendance and again after 10–14 days for a complement-fixation test to determine whether the lesion is due to a primary or a recurrent infection. Serological tests are now available in some large centers which use type-specific antibody to glycoprotein G, and are useful in differentiating the patient's serological response to HSV-1 and HSV-2.

TREATMENT

Acyclovir

In 1978 the discovery of a new compound with both remarkably good antiviral activity and extremely low toxicity to the host cell – 9-(2-hydroxyethoxymethyl)guanine – heralded a new era in the chemotherapy of HSV infections. This compound, now known as acyclovir, has proved to be a highly potent inhibitor of HSV-1, HSV-2 and varicella-zoster and has extremely low toxicity for the normal host cells.

The high potency and selectivity of acyclovir for herpes simplex viruses can be understood on the basis of a number of differences between cellular and HSV-specified enzymes. Firstly, whereas the HSV-specified thymidine kinase phosphorylates acyclovir to a monophosphate, cellular thymidine kinase does not. The acyclovir monophosphate is subsequently converted to acyclovir triphosphate by cellular enzymes which persists in HSV-infected cells. The acyclovir triphosphate is a more potent inhibitor of the viral DNA polymerases than of the cellular polymerases.

Acyclovir is normally given orally, but in those unable to swallow, the intravenous route may be used. The drug has the potential to crystallize out in the kidney tubules; therefore patients should be hydrated and the acyclovir administered by slow intravenous infusion over approximately 1 h to avoid this problem. In those with impaired renal function the dosage of acyclovir should also be reduced.

Reduced sensitivity to acyclovir in herpes simplex virus

Resistance to acyclovir has been shown experimentally to arise by mutations in the gene of the virus-specified enzymes and DNA polymerase. Three cases have been described in immuno-compromised patients on courses of intravenous acyclovir therapy (Crumpacker et al 1982, Burns et al 1982). Although 'wild' HSV has not been shown to be resistant, Field & Wildy (1982) considered that extreme caution should be applied to the widespread prophylactic use of acyclovir, especially at low dosage to avoid possible promotion of resistance. However, a large study of immunocompetent patients on long-term suppressive therapy found no evidence of viral resistance (Baker 1994).

Acyclovir formulations available

Acyclovir for oral use. Acyclovir is available as a pale blue shield-shaped tablet impressed with ZOVIRAX and containing 200 mg acyclovir; a suspension – one 5 ml spoonful equivalent to one Zovirax tablet – may be used as an alternative. The standard dose in adults is 200 mg five times daily at approximately 4-h intervals, omitting the night-time dose. Administration should commence as early as possible during the prodromal period or when the lesions first appear. It is contraindicated in patients known to be hypersensitive to acyclovir.

In children under the age of 2 years, half the adult dose is advised; children over 2 years may be given the adult dose.

In patients with severe renal impairment (creatinine clearance less than 10 ml/min), a dose of 200 mg every 12 h is recommended. In pregnancy caution should be exercised in prescribing but for further details about the use of acyclovir in pregnancy, see below.

Acyclovir does not seem to decrease the likelihood of subsequent recurrences when used to treat patients either during a primary attack or a recurrence. If given continuously in adults for a period of 12 months it seems to be effective in reducing the frequency of recurrences but costs are high (Baker 1994); in the seriously affected or in the immunocompromised, however, acyclovir treatment is very effective (see paragraph below).

Acyclovir for skin use. Acyclovir 5% w/w in a white aqueous cream base is available as Zovirax Cream (2.0 g or 10.0 g tube) for the treatment of herpes simplex of the skin (this preparation is NOT for eye use), including recurrences of genital and labial herpes. The cream is applied five times daily at approximately 4-h intervals and this treatment should be continued for 5 days. If healing is not complete treatment may be continued for a further 5 days. Therapy should begin as early as possible after awareness of the lesion and preferably in the prodromal period. Patient-initiated therapy with the skin cream is effective therapy when treatment is used early.

Acyclovir for eye use. Acyclovir 3% w/v in a white soft paraffin base is available for ophthalmic use as Zovirax Ophthalmic Ointment (4.5 g tubes). A 1 cm ribbon of ointment should be placed inside the lower conjunctival sac five times daily at approximately 4-hourly intervals. Treatment should continue for at least 5 days after healing is complete. The acyclovir eye ointment is superior to other antiviral agents for the eye.

Acyclovir for intravenous infusion. Acyclovir for intravenous use is available in vials containing 250 mg sterile acyclovir as the freeze-dried sodium salt (Zovirax IV, Wellcome). It is indicated in HSV infections in immunocompromised patients and is given by slow intravenous infusion of 5 mg/kg over 1 h every 8 h in patients with normal renal function. In children (3 months–12 years) the dose 250 mg/m^2 is given similarly and doubled in the immunocompromised and in herpes simplex encephalitis. Suggested dosages are shown in Table 23.40. 5 days treatment is usually adequate. Reconstituted Zovirax IV has a pH of about 11 and should not be given by mouth. Severe inflammation sometimes leading to ulceration may occur if infused accidentally into the tissues extravascularly.

Other antiviral agents have recently been introduced:

Famciclovir (**SmithKline Beecham**). This oral preparation is converted in vivo into penciclovir, which in turn within virus infected cells is converted into penciclovir triphosphate which

Table 23.40 Dosage of acyclovir (Zovirax) in herpes simplex infections in children. Suggested dose is given as single dose in this table

Route	Acyclovir single dose in children			Times daily
	0–4 weeks	4 weeks–2 years	Over 2 years	
Oral*	–	100 mg	200 mg	5
i.v.†	10 mg/kg	5 mg/kg	5 mg/kg	3

* Available as tablets (200 mg) or as a suspension (200 mg/5 ml).
† Available as 250 mg vial of the sodium salt acyclovir for reconstitution and given over 1 h.

inhibits viral DNA replication. Famciclovir has a much longer half-life than acyclovir, and as a result need only be given three times a day for acute herpetic infections, at a dose of 250 mg. There are at present no preparations for topical or intravenous use. It has been shown to be successful in the management of acute genital herpes and its efficacy in the suppression of recurrent disease is currently being studied. There is no information about its safety in pregnancy, and as acyclovir has not been shown to have any adverse effects, it is recommended that acyclovir be used should an antiviral be needed in pregnancy.

Valaciclovir **(Wellcome).** This is the L-valine ester of acyclovir, and in man is rapidly and almost completely converted to acyclovir. It is currently only licensed for use in the management of herpes zoster and genital herpes simplex virus infections but may in the future be available for herpes simplex infections.

HERPES SIMPLEX VIRUS IN NEONATAL INFECTIONS AND ENCEPHALITIS

The very serious and often fatal infections with HSV are rare and occur as neonatal infections, acquired before or at birth, as sporadic encephalitis, acquired later in life, or as disseminated herpes simplex in the immunologically deficient. HSV is a rare cause of the aseptic meningitis syndrome.

HERPES SIMPLEX VIRUS IN THE IMMUNOCOMPROMISED

Acyclovir has given new hope for immunocompromised patients in whom relatively simple local herpes simplex recurrence can otherwise develop into disseminated and sometimes life-threatening conditions. Such patients may be immunosuppressed by drugs or radiation given as therapy for malignancy or to prevent graft rejection; or they may have impaired immune response, inborn, due to malignancy or seen in AIDS.

VERTICAL TRANSMISSION OF HSV TO NEONATE FROM MOTHER AT THE TIME OF DELIVERY

The importance of transmission by sexual intercourse and timing is illustrated by the case cited by Hanshaw & Dudgeon (1978). The report describes the exposure of a wife, 1 week before delivery, to her husband, who had an episode of penile herpes genitalis in a recurrent form at the time of intercourse. His wife had a primary genital herpes lesion at the time of delivery and the infant, born by Cesarean section 6 h after rupture of the membranes, contracted a disseminated infection and died at 8 days of age. The risk of neonatal infection is highest in infants born vaginally to women with a primary genital HSV infection at term when about half will be infected. Primary genital infections in late pregnancy are more likely to be clinically apparent with a serious outcome for mother and fetus than nonprimary infections. The risk of development of neonatal infection is determined by the level of maternal antibody transmitted to the neonate, duration of ruptured membranes (longer than 6 hours), and damage to neonatal skin, e.g. by scalp electrode (Dwyer & Cunningham 1993).

In recurrent genital herpes simplex, in contrast, in neonates exposed to the virus at the time of vaginal delivery the risk of infection is low. In the USA Prober et al (1987) reported that in pregnant women with a history of recurrent herpes (HSV-2) the theoretical maximal infection rate was 8% for vaginally delivered infants. His work suggested that the presence of neutralizing antibody contributed to the low infection rate.

Estimates of incidence of neonatal herpes in the US vary between 1 in 1500 and 1 in 2000 (Dwyer & Cunningham 1993), with a frequency greater in the lower socioeconomic groups. In some countries or social groups, a major source of virus to the infant is the mother's genital tract at the time of delivery and more than 80% of HSV isolated from the newborn belongs to type 2, the common form of genital herpesvirus. In the UK, in Manchester, however, in the period 1969–1973, the incidence of neonatal herpes was thought to be 1 in 30 000 live births; in one-third of the cases infection was acquired from a person other than the mother and in these cases HSV-1 predominated (Tobin 1975). Over an 18-month period from July 1986 the British Paediatric Surveillance Unit, under an active surveillance scheme, reported 20 cases of confirmed neonatal herpes simplex (Hall & Glickman 1988). The rarity of recognized infection makes it difficult to formulate preventive measures. In Canada severe neonatal herpes is estimated to be 1 per million.

It has been suggested that if viral cultures are taken from the vulva and cervix in women with suspected herpes genitalis in late pregnancy and Cesarean section carried out if HSV is cultured near the time of delivery the risk of neonatal infection can be avoided and indeed this procedure is recommended by the American Academy of Pediatrics Committee on Fetus and Newborn (1994). In some 70% of cases of neonatal herpes, however, the mother has had no signs or symptoms of the infection at the time of delivery and the shedding of virus during pregnancy but without manifest disease is known to occur.

In a study by Prober et al (1988) of 6904 women at the time of delivery HSV-2 was recovered in 14 (0.2%). 12 (86%) of the HSV-2-positive women had serological evidence of previous infection with HSV-2 and none of their infants contracted neonatal herpes. One of the two infants born to women with serological evidence of a primary HSV infection at the time of delivery contracted neonatal herpes. These findings showed that most infants at risk of exposure to HSV at delivery will not be identified if concern about asymptomatic shedding of virus and surveillance by culture is limited to women with a history of genital herpes infection. Most neonatal exposure to asymptomatic HSV infection at delivery is not predictable or preventable.

The advice now given is that all pregnant women, regardless of their history of genital herpes, be assessed for genital herpes at time of their admission in labour – history, current symptoms and signs of external genital lesions and questions should be asked about any sexual contacts with persons with genital herpes. If lesions consistent with genital herpes simplex are noted Cesarean section should be performed before rupture of the membranes. When vulval lesions are present the vagina and cervix should be examined with a speculum (Kelly 1988). Any suspicious lesion should be noted and scrapings sent by prior arrangement to the virologist for immunofluorescence testing. The use of acyclovir in pregnancy is under study, and Burroughs Wellcome keep the 'Acyclovir in pregnancy registry' which so far has noted no increase in the incidence of congenital abnormalities or spontaneous abortions in those women given acyclovir compared with the general population. However, the numbers are still too small to allow reliable conclusions about the safety of acyclovir in the treatment of pregnant women (Andrews et al 1992) and it is recommended that the Centers for Disease Control Sexually

Transmitted Disease Treatment Guidelines 1993c be followed: 'In the presence of life threatening maternal Herpes simplex virus infections (eg disseminated infection that includes encephalitis, pneumonitis, and/or hepatitis), acyclovir administered intravenously is probably of value. Among pregnant women without life threatening disease, systemic acyclovir treatment should not be used for recurrent genital herpes episodes or as suppressive therapy to prevent reactivation near term.' In an uncomplicated primary infection during pregnancy, the role of antiviral therapy is uncertain but may be of benefit in preventing transmission.

The infant may acquire the infection after delivery from maternal herpes or herpes infection in one of the medical or nursing attendants. Men with herpes genitalis should be told of the dangers of communicating HSV particularly when untreated lesions are present and advised against intercourse with women who are pregnant.

Infants exposed to viral shedding during labour should have specimens taken for HSV isolation from the eyes, nasopharynx, umbilicus and any abrasions or puncture sites acquired at delivery. Intravenous acyclovir should be given to the infant in primary infection in the mother if any of the infant's cultures yield HSV or if the infant's condition shows cause for concern. Careful follow-up is very desirable to assess the effect of therapy (Kelly 1988).

Uncertainties remain as the majority of infants born per vagina to mothers with overt disease do not become clinically ill. In theory hyperimmune anti-HSV-2 gamma globulin given to the neonate would be expected to be useful in preventing involvement of an infant delivered vaginally in a woman with genital HSV-2 infection. Acyclovir, however, might well become a more acceptable line of approach in such situations. Physicians who care for the newborn should consider neonatal herpes in the differential diagnosis when infants become ill during the first weeks of life regardless of the presence or absence of identifiable risk factors (Prober et al 1988).

In the case of patients who become clinically very ill during the last trimester of pregnancy with a primary HSV infection with actual or suspected dissemination acyclovir offers an important advance in treatment. In such cases early diagnosis and early institution of treatment is important; mouth, throat, vulva, vagina and cervix should be carefully examined for characteristic vesicular or ulcerative lesions. Virological diagnosis by electron microscopy of the roof, base or fluid of any vesicle can be made rapidly but the clinical appearance may be sufficiently characteristic.

Infection in the neonate can produce a wide spectrum of clinical effects from subclinical to disseminated forms or to those localized to the central nervous system, the eye or mouth. Increased application of virus isolation methods has shown that the incidence of subclinical infection is commoner than the serious clinical forms.

Neonatal HSV infection and its management is discussed on page 287. The serious problems of sporadic HSV encephalitis are referred to in Robertson et al (1989).

ASEPTIC MENINGITIS

In the aseptic (or abacterial) meningitis syndrome characterized by fever, signs of meningeal irritation, an increased leukocyte count in the CSF, but no signs of frank encephalitis, HSV is a very rare cause among the wide array of other viruses which have been implicated in the etiology of a varying minority of cases.

PAPILLOMAVIRUS INFECTION AND GENITAL WARTS

Not only are genital warts due to human papillomavirus unsightly but their persistence and inconstant response to treatment give rise to anxiety and introspection in the patient as well as the added burden of multiple attendances. Their high prevalence, high infectivity, long prepatent period (average 3 months, range 2 weeks to 8 months) and often poor response to treatment all make effective control by therapy and contact tracing possible only to a limited extent. Until quite recently genital warts have been regarded virtually as wholly benign growths which regress spontaneously, but human papillomaviruses may not be solely causes of benign tumors of skin and mucosa, but in the longer term and possibly in association with herpesvirus-type 2 and/or other cofactors, such as cigarette smoking, may play a part in the etiology of cancer particularly of the cervix uteri. The case against papillomaviruses in regard to cancer of the cervix is, however, not yet proven.

In children anogenital warts appear to be more commonly reported. They cannot, however, be regarded as a definite indicator of sexual abuse but the possibility of this has to be considered by the clinician – see Anogenital warts in prepubertal children, below.

ETIOLOGY

Since papillomaviruses cannot be propagated in vitro and the quantities of viral material in anogenital lesions were so low, their characterization directly from such material was not possible. Molecular cloning of wart virus DNA in bacterial plasmids or in bacteriophage lambda has now, however, enabled the preparation of quantities sufficient to develop a classification of the papillomaviruses from lesions in a variety of anatomical sites (Lancet 1983).

At the present time classification of HPV into separate types is based on nucleic acid hybridization studies; a virus is considered to be a separate type if such DNA studies reveal less than 50% homology with known virus types (Pfister 1984).

On the basis of these nucleic acid studies, more than 60 types have been reported of which at least seven are most commonly associated with mucosal lesions including those of the urogenital tract, viz. the common types HPV-6, 11, 16, 18 and the less common HPV-31, 33 and 35.

Skin warts appear to be acquired from environmental sources, but genital warts are acquired mainly by sexual intercourse. The prepatent period varies between 3 weeks and 8 months with an average of about 3 months. Genital warts in one sexual partner will also be found in the other in about 65% of cases. Vulvar and penile warts are more clearly associated with transmission by sexual intercourse, while anal warts are less certainly associated with anal intercourse so their origin remains speculative.

HISTOLOGY

Hyperkeratosis is not a feature of a condyloma acuminatum of the genital area where the stratum corneum consists as a rule of only one or two layers of parakeratotic cells. In these warts acanthosis combined with extensive papillomatosis results in layers of the wart that consist entirely of sheets of hyperplastic keratinocytes showing multiple mitotic figures. As the condylomata age hyperkeratosis may develop.

CLINICAL FEATURES

Genital lesions

Various clinical types of wart can be distinguished. In men the fleshy hyperplastic warts (condyloma acuminatum), either one or many, occur most often on the glans penis and on the inner lining of the prepuce. The appearance depends upon the location, although moisture and accompanying inflammation may enhance the size and tendency to coalesce. Those in the terminal urethra have a bright red color in particular. Hyperplastic genital warts in the female are commonly seen on the vulva and may extend to the adjacent skin (Fig. 23.44).

In children anogenital warts are being more commonly reported possibly associated with increasing incidence of the disease in the adult population (23 126 cases in 1975 and 90 891 in 1992 recorded by UK departments of genitourinary medicine – PHLS Communicable Disease Surveillance Centre 1993). Clinically they resemble those seen in adults (Rock et al 1986). Their discovery is an indication for taking tests to exclude other sexually transmissible disease (see Fig. 23.45), but genital warts are not a definite indicator of sexual abuse – see Anogenital warts in prepubertal children, below.

Cervical warts

HPV infection of the cervix frequently does not produce lesions that are recognizable by naked eye inspection. McCance et al (1983) have found HPV-6 DNA by these techniques in over half of histologically proved cases of cervical intraepithelial neoplastic lesions. Different types (e.g. 6, 11, 16 of 18) may also be involved.

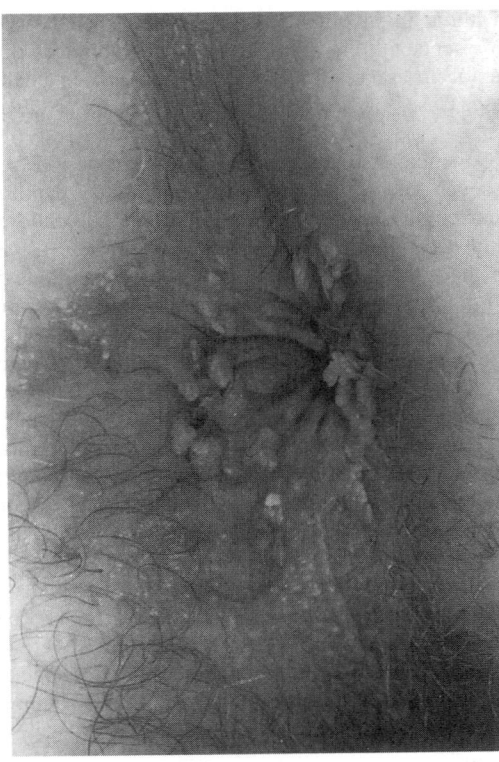

Fig. 23.45 Perianal warts and nearby a moist papule due to early stage syphilis in male aged 15 years; *Treponema pallidum* were numerous in serum obtained from the depth of the moist papule. Infection acquired homosexually.

Sessile warts of the genitalia

Sessile warts, resembling plane warts on the not-genital skin, tend to be seen on the shaft of the penis and although often multiple they do not coalesce. Sessile warts do not seem to occur on the vulva.

Oral papilloma

Mouth lesions (lips, tongue, cheek, gingiva, hard palate, floor of mouth) may occasionally occur after orogenital contact with an infected partner.

Laryngeal papillomata

Papillomata of the larynx may very rarely appear within the first 6 months of life in babies born to mothers with genital warts at the time of delivery. Hybridization analyses have shown that the papillomaviruses found in laryngeal papillomata are the same as the papillomaviruses found to infect the genital tract. In juvenile-onset disease intrapartum infection is most likely to be the method of transmission of the disease, so Cesarean delivery, prior to the rupture of the membranes, would be expected to provide a high degree of protection against infection. The relative rarity of transmission, however, is to be weighed against the risks of Cesarean section.

In juvenile-onset disease (viz. onset of the disease before 16 years) hoarseness is the first symptom in 90% of cases. The larynx is the most common primary site but papillomata can occur in the

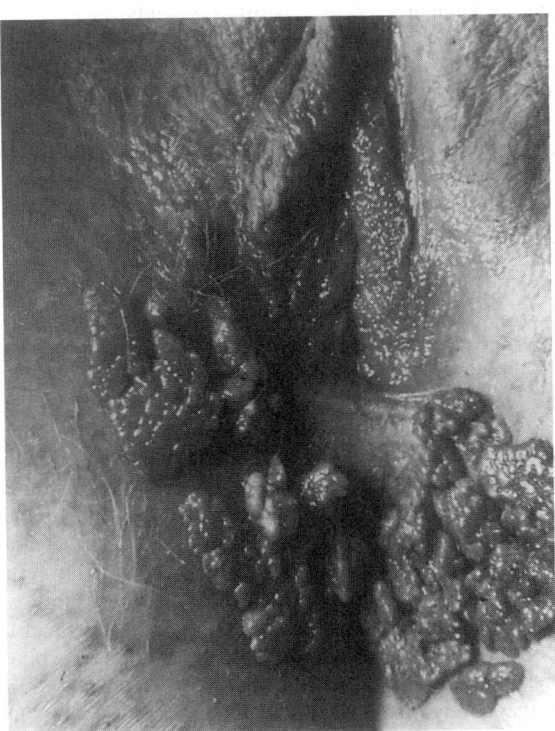

Fig. 23.44 Multiple hyperplastic condylomata acuminata of the vulva and perianal skin (genital warts).

trachea without involvement of the larynx. The laryngotracheal location presents a threat to the airway and respiratory distress or stridor can occur as a result. Persistent recurrence is a hallmark of the disease. Cases of adult-onset disease can be as severe as in juveniles.

In the Copenhagen district during the 4-year period from 1980 to 1983 seven new cases of juvenile laryngeal papillomatosis (JLP) occurred; in an at-risk population of 300 000 children under 14 years of age this gave an incidence of 0.6 per 10^5 (Bomholt 1988). In the total population of 1 740 000 inhabitants 53 were operated upon for laryngeal papilloma – arising *before* puberty – during the 4-year study, giving a prevalence of 0.8 per 10^5.

Juvenile laryngeal papillomatosis has, in areas with good specialist surgical facilities, mostly a good prognosis, i.e. short duration, low morbidity and no mortality unless malignant change occurs. Treatment has been by microsurgical removal but currently vaporization by means of carbon dioxide laser technique has been developed. Regression before puberty does not ensure recovery and more than half the adult patients in the Copenhagen study experienced recurrences between 6 and 22 years after puberty (median 21 years). Since in both pregnancy and at puberty itself JLP may subside it has been postulated that the condition may be subject to hormonal influence. Severe diffuse papillomatosis involving the bronchi may be associated with malignancy and is itself a serious prognostic sign (Bomholt 1988).

ANOGENITAL WARTS IN PREPUBERTAL CHILDREN

Although anogenital warts in prepubertal children cannot be regarded as a definite indication of sexual abuse, it is a possibility that requires to be taken into account by the clinician. These warts are often caused by the same HPV types – 6 and 11 – that cause condylomata acuminata in adults, but the source of infection is often in doubt.

The transplacental transmission of HPV is suggested by the finding of HPV DNA in the cord blood of infants born to mothers with known HPV infection (Tseng et al 1992). Perinatal transmission of these viral types from an infected mother must also be a possibility. HPV DNA has been detected in scrapings from the oral mucosa, nasopharynx and genitalia of neonates born to mothers with anogenital warts or CIN (Sedlacek et al 1989, Smith et al 1991). Although some studies (Rock et al 1986) have suggested that anogenital HPV infections in young children are most likely to have been acquired sexually, others consider vertical transmission to be the most important means by which they are infected, particularly if the child is under the age of 3 years (Cohen et al 1990, Handley et al 1993).

Cutaneous HPV-2 is sometimes found in anogenital warts of children especially when aged 3 years and over (Obalek et al 1990), and this may reflect transmission of the virus from, say, the hands of the child or parent.

DIAGNOSIS

Identification of the virus in the lesion is as yet seldom undertaken except for research purposes and diagnosis is based on recognizing genital warts clinically. In young persons in the case of cervical infection, colposcopy is indicated if cervical cytopathology smears show abnormalities.

Skin lesions of secondary syphilis, viz. condylomata lata and papular skin eruptions, require to be differentiated by dark field microscopy for *T. pallidum* and serological tests for syphilis. Lesions of molluscum contagiosum (see p. 1633) are commonly found on the genitalia of young adults where they may have been acquired through sexual contact; the differentiation from warts may require the use of a magnifying lens.

TREATMENT

General considerations

Although anogenital condylomata acuminata tend to regress spontaneously treatment is important as, in the case of moist hyperplastic warts, spread is sometimes rapid and sepsis can be troublesome. The exclusion, detection and, if required, treatment of other sexually transmissible infections in the affected individual and the sexual contact(s) are essential first steps (Robertson et al 1989). Although there are a wide range of procedures available there is no certain once-only treatment for warts.

Before local treatment of genital warts is started it is important to attend to any other local infection, whether sexually transmitted or not, as warts tend to spread more readily in inflamed skin. Any cause of vaginitis or discharge must be discovered and eradicated.

Papillomavirus is frequently present in clinically and histologically normal skin adjacent to the condylomata acuminata. Latent HPV may be responsible for recurrences so commonly observed following all forms of therapy (Ferenczy et al 1985).

Podophyllin

Podophyllin, an ethanol extract of rhizome and roots of the plant *Podophyllum*, often produces spectacular initial effects particularly when applied to hyperplastic condylomata acuminata of the genital skin. This extract contains, among other compounds, podophyllotoxin, the main active agent. The latter acts in a manner similar to colchicine and binds specifically at the same (or greatly overlapping) site to tubulin, a component protein of microtubules but in contrast to colchicine, this binding is reversible. The disintegration of chromatin and arrest of mitosis produced by podophyllin and colchicine are explained by the disassembly of microtubules produced by these compounds.

Clinical effects

Condylomata acuminata rapidly and occasionally permanently undergo involution after one or two treatments with a 25% suspension of podophyllum resin (podophyllin) in liquid petrolatum (liquid paraffin) or in 95% alcohol (see review in von Krogh 1981). Painful local inflammatory reactions are sometimes a problem and washing off medication 3–24 h after application and protection of the surrounding epithelial surfaces with inert pastes, creams or ointments is advocated. It is generally recommended that 1 week should elapse between applications. Condylomata acuminata show first blanching (4–8 h) and later a drying effect when the pink or red moist warts appear white, gray and dry; in some cases there is dark brown discoloration. In 4–24 h the condylomata decrease in size and in 48 h there is sometimes complete involution. Failures occur in chronic perianal condylomata where penetration was prevented by the dry keratinized surface.

Unwanted effects

Unwanted local effects of podophyllin, even with the washing of the preparation after an interval, vary from local itching, burning, tenderness and erythema to pain, swelling and minor erosions.

Podophyllin should not be used aggressively and in quantities beyond that now recommended (Stoehr et al 1978). In children great caution is required in its use.

The present authors recommend dispensing about 0.5 ml quantities to be used for once-only applications given by trained personnel within the clinic; the use of single containers for repeated applications in the clinics is condemned as it may bring risks of cross-infection. Ordinarily, a few warts should be treated at a time, the adjacent skin being protected by yellow or white soft paraffin (BNF), powder or both. It is good practice to treat, with due regard to any local reaction produced, at frequent intervals (every 3–7 days) with small amounts of 25% podophyllin in liquid paraffin or methylated spirit (not more than 0.3 ml at a time). In the case of the preparation in spirit time should be given to allow drying. The patient should be instructed to wash off the podophyllin after an interval of about 6 h.

An ethanolic solution of purified podophyllotoxin (0.5% w/v), the active substance in podophyllin resin, is now available (Warticon, Cph; Condyline, Gist-brocades) its use in children is not advised by the manufacturers.

Electrocautery

Electrocautery with a 1% solution of lignocaine is used as a local anesthetic and the wart removed with the cautery. The aim should be to coagulate the wart down to the basement membrane and cause minimal damage to surrounding skin. In the case of intrameatal warts, lignocaine gel (20 mg/ml) may be instilled into the terminal urethra and the wart cauterized after 5–10 min. Occasionally removal of warts by diathermy or cautery will require general anesthesia and circumcision is sometimes required, particularly when there is phimosis.

Scissor excision

Under general anesthesia the wart-bearing area, in the case of intra-anal warts in particular, is infiltrated with saline adrenaline solution (1 : 300 000). The warts are then removed with scissors by cutting at the base of the wart from back to front so that exudate and blood do not obscure progress.

Cryotherapy

The application of liquid nitrogen (boiling point − 195.8°C) to discrete warts is sometimes effective. The aim should be to freeze the wart until a halo of frozen skin is just visible at the base. A cotton tipped applicator can be immersed in a vacuum flask of liquid nitrogen and then applied to the wart, exposed and immobilized by stretching the skin between the fingers.

PROGNOSIS AND CONTACT TRACING

Whenever possible it is important to ensure that each sexual partner is examined. Although treatment of warts is far from satisfactory it is important to examine the patient to exclude other sexually transmitted diseases and to relieve anxieties by explanations. In the case of the female contact a cervical smear should be taken for exfoliative cytology examination and an explanation given about the importance of a lifetime follow-up.

MALIGNANT TRANSFORMATION OF ANAL AND GENITAL CONDYLOMATA ACUMINATA

Condylomata acuminata, cervical koilocytosis and respiratory papillomatosis appear all to be linked in that HPV-6 and HPS-11 are the commonest types seen. Malignant conversion is a rarity but in respiratory papillomatosis X-irradiation of recurrent laryngeal or tracheal papillomatosis has been followed by carcinoma after intervals between 5 and 40 years.

The incidence of anal carcinoma in homosexual men in the USA is increasing and probably reflects the high prevalence of HIV infection and its attendant immunosuppression.

PROTOZOAL INFECTIONS

MALARIA

Malaria is a disease of humans caused by infection with one or more of four species of protozoa of the genus *Plasmodium (P. falciparum, P. vivax, P. malariae* and *P. ovale)*. It is usually acquired through the bite of an infected female *Anopheles* mosquito, although it may also follow the transfer of infected blood as in blood transfusion, or transplacentally or by the use of contaminated syringes. Worldwide some 45 *Anopheles* species effectively transmit malaria, although the identity, behavior and importance of local vectors varies widely with geographic location. The most effective vector is probably *A. gambiae* – a mosquito that is widely distributed in tropical Africa. *P. falciparum* is the most pathogenic of the malaria parasites and infections with it must always be regarded as serious and potentially life threatening. The other three species tend to cause less serious illness, although on occasion a lethal nephrosis may complicate *P. malariae* infections.

THE PARASITE LIFE CYCLE

Malaria parasites undergo a complex stage of asexual development in the human host and a stage of sexual development (sporogony) which occurs partly in man and partly in the mosquito vector (Garnham 1988).

Asexual development in man

This begins with the introduction of infective forms (sporozoites) in mosquito saliva during the biting act. Sporozoites circulate for less than 60 min, eventually gaining access to parenchymal liver cells either directly or after passage through Küpffer cells. The invasion process may entail specific ligand/receptor interaction. Once within the hepatocyte, the sporozoite initiates the exoerythrocytic (EE) phase of asexual development during which it grows and undergoes repeated nuclear fission (schizogony) – eventually producing a cyst-like schizont filled with daughter parasites (merozoites). This phase usually proceeds without interruption and both the time taken to schizont maturity and the number of merozoites produced varies with the identity of the plasmodial species involved. *P. falciparum* completes its EE development fastest (about 5 days) and produces most merozoites per schizont (about 30 000). The other species are slower and less prolific, the respective values for *P. malariae*, for example, being about 15 days and about 15 000 merozoites. In two parasite species, *P. vivax* and *P. ovale*, some sporozoites initiate this uninterrupted EE stage of development but some do not. These latter on entering hepatocytes produce small unicellular forms (hypnozoites) which persist without development for periods varying from several weeks to many months. Eventually the hypnozoites, activated by mechanisms as yet not known, resume growth and proceed to schizont maturation and merozoite liberation. Hypnozoites are currently widely believed to give rise to the relapsing parasitemias which characterize *P. ovale* and, particularly, *P. vivax* infections and which can occur even after drug treatment has effectively eliminated erythrocytic parasites. Hypnozoites do not develop in infections with *P. falciparum* and *P. malariae* and in these species recrudescence of parasitemia is generally considered to be due to persistent erythrocytic infection.

Merozoites liberated from EE schizonts are short lived and must find and enter a red blood cell within a few minutes. Within the erythrocyte each grows rapidly through ring form and uninucleate trophozoite stages eventually to form a schizont containing merozoites. On schizont rupture, the merozoites enter the bloodstream, attach to and penetrate fresh erythrocytes and again begin the cycle of erythrocytic asexual development. Attachment and penetration by merozoites are complex operations which appear to require specific ligand/receptor interaction. Erythrocyte invasion by *P. vivax* appears to require a ligand that is associated with Duffy blood group antigens, while attachment of *P. falciparum* merozoites to red cells requires one associated with sialic acid on the erythrocyte membrane. Age of the red cell also influences invasion by merozoites; *P. vivax* preferentially invades reticulocytes – a feature which tends to limit the density of parasitemia attained by this species.

The duration of the erythrocytic phase of asexual development and the merozoite yield per schizont vary with the plasmodial species. *P. malariae* has the longest cycle (72 h, i.e. quartan periodicity); the remaining species have cycles of about 48 h duration (i.e. tertian periodicity). *P. falciparum* has the greatest capacity to replicate and the merozoite yield of its schizonts is in the range 8–32. For the others the yields are 8–24 for *P. vivax*, 4–16 for *P. ovale* and 8 for *P. malariae*. The ability of *P. falciparum* to replicate rapidly in both the hepatic and erythrocytic phases of development partly accounts for the severity of the illness this species causes.

The time taken for parasites to become detectable in the peripheral blood following sporozoite inoculation is termed the prepatent period, while the time from infection to the onset of symptoms is termed the incubation period. While the two periods may be of equal duration, more usually the incubation period is about 2 days longer.

Late in its asexual erythrocytic cycle *P. falciparum* withdraws from the peripheral circulation and sequesters in deep vasculature. The phenomenon, which contributes importantly to the serious pathological effects that this *Plasmodium* causes, is effected by the binding of receptors on the surface of red cells infected with nearly mature parasites to ligands exposed on the surface of the endothelial cells lining deep blood vessels. Sequestration does not occur in the course of infections with the other plasmodial species that infect man.

Sexual development

In the course of blood stage schizogony in the human host some merozoites differentiate, by mechanisms which are not yet understood, to give rise to male and female sexual forms (gametocytes). When mature, gametocytes circulate in the blood but do not undergo further development unless they are ingested by an anopheline mosquito during feeding. Once in the midgut of the mosquito, the female (macrogametocyte) escapes from the enclosing erythrocytic membrane and becomes a macrogamete. The male (microgametocyte) undergoes a process of exflagellation during which eight slender, uninucleate filaments (microgametes) are extruded and break free. Each microgamete seeks a macrogamete and, if successful, penetrates and fertilizes it. The two nuclei fuse and a zygote is formed. This is probably the only point in the life history of the parasite that genetic recombination occurs. The diploid zygote then undergoes meiosis and, as an ookinete, migrates to penetrate the epithelium of the mosquito midgut wall where it comes to rest on the external surface. There it rounds up, becomes an oocyst and begins a series of nuclear divisions. Oocyst maturity is reached after a period which is dependent on the identity of the plasmodial species and the ambient temperature to which the mosquito is exposed but which may be 1–4 weeks or longer. At maturity the oocyst is filled with as many as 10 000 daughter parasites (sporozoites), each some 10–15 mm long and feebly motile. The sporozoites escape at oocyst rupture and travel in the hemocelomic fluid to the salivary glands where they accumulate in the acinal cells to be discharged with saliva when next the mosquito feeds.

Infected humans constitute the only known source of mosquito infection for *P. falciparum*, *P. vivax* and *P. ovale*. For *P. malariae* some apes and monkeys may constitute reservoirs of infection in addition to humans.

EPIDEMIOLOGY

Despite widespread operations promoted by the World Health Organization between 1955 and 1975 with the aim of achieving global eradication, malaria remains probably the most prevalent important communicable disease throughout much of the tropical and subtropical world. It is estimated that more than 2500 million persons live at risk of contracting the infection and that many – 200 million in sub-Saharan Africa alone – remain chronically and persistently infected (WHO 1985, 1987). New cases are thought to exceed 100 million per year and, while no reliable data are available on overall morbidity and mortality, it is believed that in Africa alone mortality exceeds 1 million per annum. Over the past 15–20 years *P. falciparum* parasites have become resistant to chloroquine and other currently available antimalarial drugs. This development has greatly complicated the treatment and management of acute falciparum infections and has jeopardized effective chemoprophylaxis by drugs that are inexpensive and of proven low toxicity. As a result travelers to endemic areas are at higher risk of contracting infections than perhaps at any time since the end of World War II, with the consequence that malaria must be considered as a possible diagnosis in all instances of illness – especially febrile illness – presenting in residents of temperate climate countries who have recently visited endemic areas.

Many factors influence the epidemiology of malaria. Atmospheric temperature is important. For successful development in the mosquito vector *P. vivax* requires a sustained temperature of at least 16°C, while *P. falciparum* requires one of 20°C. The geographic limits of *P. vivax* transmission are thus more widely set than those of *P. falciparum*. Other factors relate to the identity and biology of the *Plasmodium*, the identity and behavior of the vector, the social and economic customs of human populations and the topography and climate of the region. It follows, therefore, that the epidemiological pattern of the infection is not uniform but varies considerably between and within countries.

Where transmission occurs the measurement of endemicity has in the past relied on establishment of spleen rates and parasite rates in children aged 2–9 years. Thus categories classified as hypo-, meso-, hyper- and holoendemic were characterized by both spleen and parasite rates of < 10%, 11–50%, constantly > 50% and constantly > 75% respectively. In hyperendemic areas spleens in adults were frequently enlarged; in holoendemic areas they were not.

However, the widespread use of antimalarial drugs in areas where malaria is endemic has adversely affected these classical indices of endemicity and they are today less useful than formerly. This change has prompted the use of seroepidemiological techniques in the identification of malaria transmission and the measurement of its intensity. These techniques detect and quantify specific malaria antibody in serum and establish age-specific profiles for prevalence and titer. Briefly, profiles which show little change with age denote low transmission while profiles showing values which rise rapidly with age denote high transmission (Molineaux 1988).

Epidemiologically malaria presents in two extremes, one of which is stable and shows little change from one year to another and the other which is unstable and may fluctuate violently in intensity at regular or irregular intervals. Stable malaria is most in evidence in areas where transmission rates are high; it is characterized by rates of mortality and morbidity which are high in infants and young children and which fall to low, even negligible, levels as age advances and effective immunity is acquired. Unstable malaria occurs where transmission rates remain low for periods of several years then suddenly increase greatly for climatic or other reasons; it is characterized by the occurrence of epidemics in which morbidity and mortality are conspicuous at all ages. Acquired immunity is not a feature of unstable malaria, save possibly at the end of a protracted epidemic period. Between the extremes of stability and instability, a range of intermediate epidemiological presentation occurs.

IMMUNITY

Malarial immunity may be innate, i.e. genetically determined, or acquired. Innate immunity may be due to the lack of ligands on the erythrocyte surface which bind to specific receptors on the merozoite surface at an essential stage in the invasion process, or to the presence of abnormal intramembranous erythrocytic components which inhibit but do not totally prevent growth of the parasite within the red cell. An example of the former is the freedom from *P. vivax* infection that is apparent in persons whose erythrocytes lack Duffy blood group antigens, while an example of the latter is the partial protection and survival advantage towards *P. falciparum* infections that heterozygosity for the sickle cell gene confers (Miller 1988).

Acquired immunity may be passive or active. Passive immunity due to the transplacental transfer of specific IgG malarial antibodies from mother to fetus probably accounts, at least in part, for the relative resistance to malaria that infants born in highly endemic areas show over the first few months of life. Acquired active immunity develops slowly in response to infection with malaria (McGregor & Wilson 1988). The first evidence is an ability to restrict the clinical effects of infection despite the persistence of high density parasitemia. This 'clinical' immunity is usually discernible in young children in highly endemic areas around the third to fourth year of life. Later an ability to restrict parasite density develops and slowly strengthens throughout later childhood and adolescence to reach maximum expression in adult life. When fully developed, malarial immunity is species, strain and stage specific.

Acquired active immunity entails the collaboration of different cell populations, notably T cells, B cells and macrophages, during which specific and nonspecific humoral factors are elaborated which restrict parasite growth and replication (Allison 1988). Knowledge as to how this complex response is assembled and controlled remains incomplete. T cells play a central role and their recognition of and response to defined malarial antigens are probably controlled by immune response (Ir) genes. Sensitized T cells respond to antigen by replication and the secretion of lymphokines which promote further T cell replication and diversification, induce replication of B cells with antibody production and activate macrophages.

Specific malarial antibodies belong to the immunoglobulin classes G, M and A. They function in agglutinating parasites and parasitized cells, in inhibiting interactions between host cell surface ligands and parasite receptors, by mediating cellular cytotoxicity and phagocytosis and by inhibiting sequestration of mature asexual erythrocytic forms of *P. falciparum* in deep vasculature. Antibodies do not kill parasites directly through the activation of complement. Natural malaria infection induces synthesis of a wide range of antibodies directed against specific parasite antigens. Thus antibodies with specificity for the antigens of sporozoites, EE forms, asexual blood stages and sexual stages can be detected and titrated in the sera of residents of endemic areas.

The killing of parasites is probably mainly carried out by activated macrophages and cytotoxic T cells, involves release from the host cells of toxic oxygen derivatives and occurs principally in spleen and liver. However, other killing mechanisms exist. Gamma-interferon released by sensitized T cells has been observed to kill EE stages in hepatic cells, while tumor necrosis factor (TNF) liberated from macrophages stimulated with endotoxin has been reported to inhibit replication of both EE and erythrocytic stages of the parasite.

PATHOLOGY

The pathogenic sequences which develop in malaria are attributable to events which arise during the asexual erythrocytic stage of development of the parasite in man.

Anemia is common and is due partly to the rhythmic invasion and destruction of erythrocytes by parasites and partly to additional mechanisms, such as dyserythropoiesis and immune hemolysis following sensitization of nonparasitized red cells (Weatherall 1988). Bone marrow changes in dyserythropoiesis include erythroblast multinuclearity, karyorrhexis, incomplete and unequal nuclear division and cytoplasmic bridging. The marrow may contain large amounts of stainable iron and show evidence of phagocytosis of defective red cell precursors by macrophages.

Whether these changes are initiated by toxic substances liberated by the parasite or represent the nonspecific effects of macrophages rendered hyperactive by parasite antigens remains to be ascertained. The sensitization of uninfected red cells occurs commonly in malaria, often involves C3 and/or IgG and can be detected by the direct antiglobulin test (DAT) using specific antisera. DAT positivity of red cells, which is frequent in patients with falciparum malaria, has been found to be associated with enhanced blood destruction, but the association appears to be relatively uncommon (Weatherall 1988).

A characteristic feature of *P. falciparum* infections is the collection ('sequestration') of large numbers of late-stage parasites in the venules and capillaries of a variety of organs (Boonpucknavig & Boonpucknavig 1988). This results from the ability of this parasite, in the later stages of its development in the red cell, to induce changes in the erythrocyte surface causing it to adhere to endothelial cells. Sequestration is believed to be the mechanism underlying some of the clinical complications of *P. falciparum* infection, including the coma and convulsions of cerebral malaria. It is not known how sequestration may lead to tissue dysfunction: one possibility is that the huge number of actively metabolizing parasites consume oxygen and glucose at the expense of neighboring tissue, or produce toxic metabolites, including lactate, that may affect cellular function. Another possibility is that sequestration stimulates the release of host transmitters, such as nitric oxide, that may have a local effect on blood flow or on the conduction of nerve impulses. Host cytokines, too, are released and these may make endothelial cells more adhesive for the surface of parasitized red cells, thus augmenting sequestration (Clark 1987).

Enlargement of the spleen and liver is common in acute and chronic infections and, on section, both organs are dark from the accumulation of malarial pigment (hemozoin). Evidence of phagocytosis of parasites, parasitized cells and hemozoin is usually present in the splenic pulp and in the sinusoidal macrophages and Küpffer cells of the liver.

In *P. falciparum* infections an acute diffuse glomerulonephritis may occur in which deposits of immunoglobulins, complement and malarial antigens are detectable in the mesangium and capillary loops. The condition is usually transient and resolves with appropriate antimalarial treatment. In *P. malariae* infections, however, a much more progressive and frequently lethal nephropathy may develop, again with evidence of antigen/antibody deposition. In children these lesions may progress despite antimalarial treatment to total glomerular sclerosis with secondary tubular atrophy. Clinically, the manifestations of a nephrotic syndrome develop with severe generalized edema and ascites accompanied by heavy proteinuria and hypoalbuminemia.

During pregnancy, *P. falciparum* may attain very high densities in the maternal placental blood and cause damage to the syncytiotrophoblast. Placental infection is associated with reduced infant birthweight and, in endemic areas, the association is most marked in first pregnancies. Occasionally, parasites cross the placenta giving rise to congenital infection in the infant at or soon after birth.

Thrombocytopenia commonly occurs in *P. falciparum* infections for reasons that remain poorly understood. It usually occurs independently of changes in other measures of coagulation (prothrombin time, partial thromboplastin time) or to plasma fibrinogen concentrations and is usually unaccompanied by

bleeding. Spontaneous bleeding may occur associated with disseminated intravascular coagulation (DIC), but this appears to be an uncommon event (Harinasuta & Bunnag 1988).

PROPHYLAXIS

In recent years the development and spread of drug-resistant *P. falciparum* parasites together with increasing evidence that some antimalarial drugs are associated, albeit rarely, with serious side effects have gravely compromised chemoprophylaxis. While *P. ovale* and *P. malariae* have shown no changes in drug susceptibility, *P. falciparum* parasites resistant to chloroquine and sometimes to a range of other drugs as well have developed and are now present in many endemic countries. In southeast Asia resistance of *P. vivax* to chloroquine has also been reported. The overall effectiveness of chemoprophylaxis, therefore, can no longer be guaranteed. When Fansidar (pyrimethamine–sulfadoxine) has been used as a weekly prophylactic drug, episodes of Stevens–Johnson syndrome and toxic epidermal necrolysis have occasionally occurred, some with fatal outcome. Maloprim (pyrimethamine–dapsone) has been associated with agranulocytosis and amodiaquine with neutropenia and hepatocellular dysfunction (Cook 1988).

These events have emphasized the need to limit contact between humans and mosquitoes as much as possible and advice to parents to this effect should be given. Protective measures include the wearing of clothing which effectively covers the arms and legs and the careful application of insect repellents (dimethylphthalate (DMP) or dimethyl-m-toluamide (DEET)) to exposed skin areas over periods of mosquito activity, the screening of houses, the use of knock-down insecticides in bedrooms before retiring, and sleeping under mosquito nets impregnated with permethrin.

When contemplating the need for chemoprophylaxis in particular instances, the physician should ascertain the risk to which the child is or will be exposed, the duration of exposure, the presence or absence of drug-resistant malaria in the area of residence and possible drug toxicity. Useful information on disease incidence and drug resistance in the malarious countries of the world is to be found in the periodic reviews published by the World Health Organization in its Weekly Epidemiological Record.

Children are highly susceptible to malaria, particularly *P. falciparum* infections, and the need for chemoprophylaxis must be seriously considered when they visit malarious areas. When the visit is short term, e.g. 1–2 months, and the risk of infection very low, chemoprophylaxis may be deemed unnecessary. In this event, however, the parents should be advised that the risk of infection does exist and that any illness, febrile or not, which occurs abroad should be properly investigated to exclude malaria as a diagnosis, and any illness developing within 6 months of return from abroad should be reported to a physician as should details of the visit made. For children visiting or residing in areas where the risk of infection is other than very low, chemoprophylaxis should be prescribed.

Suggested chemoprophylactic regimens (Bradley & Warhurst 1995) are as follows:

1. Where only *P. vivax* malaria exists, prophylaxis should be by chloroquine proportional to an adult dose of 300 mg (two tablets) once weekly or by proguanil (Paludrine) proportional to an adult dose of 200 mg (two tablets) daily (see Table 23.41).

Table 23.41 Age-related dosage of antimalarial drugs for chemoprophylaxis in children

Age	Fraction of adult dose
<6 weeks	$^1/_8$
6 weeks–1 year	$^1/_4$
1–5 years	$^1/_2$
5–12 years	$^3/_4$
>12 years	Adult dose

2. Where *P. falciparum* exists and is sensitive to chloroquine, chemoprophylaxis is as in 1 above.

3. Where chloroquine-resistant *P. falciparum* exists, chemoprophylaxis should be by mefloquine proportional to an adult dose of 250 mg taken once weekly; this is not advised for young children, for whom chloroquine plus proguanil should be used (doses as in 1 above).

4. Where chloroquine-resistant *P. falciparum* exists but where regimen 3 above is apparently ineffective, as is sometimes the case in southeast Asia, the choice of a prophylactic antimalarial can be a difficult problem. Local advice should be sought. For visits confined to cities, it may be best to take no drug prophylaxis. For visits to high-risk areas, options include Maloprim proportionate to an adult dose of one tablet (pyrimethamine 12.5 mg; dapsone 100 mg) once weekly plus chloroquine proportionate to an adult dose of 300 mg once weekly. (Maloprim should not be given to infants less than 6 weeks of age because of immaturity of several enzyme systems.) Doxycycline 100 mg daily, which is a useful prophylaxis for adults, is not suitable for children.

Chemoprophylaxis should be started 1 week before residence in an endemic area (to permit detection of early signs of idiosyncrasy or side effects) and continued for 4 weeks after return. Parents should be advised to ensure that physicians attending illness in children after return from endemic areas are aware of the need to exclude a diagnosis of malaria. Similarly, parents who live in endemic areas and are visited from time to time by children being educated in nonendemic areas should ensure that guardians and school authorities are alerted to the need to exclude malaria as a diagnosis in any illness developing in the repatriated child.

Chemoprophylaxis of indigenous children in endemic areas

Currently studies are in progress to assess the benefits and disadvantages of mass chemoprophylaxis administered to indigenous children in endemic areas. At the present time the balance of opinion seems to favor a view that large-scale continuous prophylaxis is not to be recommended, the main reason being that it is economically and logistically almost impossible to achieve. Other theoretical but unproven disadvantages of mass chemoprophylaxis include interference with the development of acquired immunity, enhancement of the development and spread of drug resistance and risk of toxicity from long-term drug usage. Chemotherapy at the individual level, however, remains a matter for parental decision taken in the light of experienced medical advice. Continuous chemoprophylaxis is indicated in children who are homozygous for the sickle cell gene, because malaria may precipitate a crisis. There is no evidence yet

(1997) that chemoprophylaxis against malaria improves life expectancy in children with HIV infection or AIDS.

Vaccination

While much interest attaches to the development of malaria vaccines, a safe and effective one is not yet available. Trials of two *P. falciparum* antisporozoite vaccines employing the immunodominant circumsporozoite epitope NANP have been made in human volunteers. In both instances protection appeared to be conferred in some, but not all, instances. A vaccine (SPf66) comprising antigens from both the sporozoite and asexual blood stages of the same parasite has also been tested in human volunteers. Field trials of SPf66 have given conflicting results: a 31% reduction in episodes of uncomplicated *P. falciparum* malaria was achieved in a study involving 600 Tanzanian children aged 1–5 years (Alonso et al 1994), but the vaccine failed to afford any protection in Gambian children who were aged 6–12 months at the time of the first dose (D'Alessandro et al 1995). These initial vaccines must be regarded as prototypes and improved, more effective, formulations are to be expected (Hockmeyer & Ballou 1988).

CLINICAL FEATURES

The manifestations of malaria in an individual are determined by the infecting species of *Plasmodium* and the resistance or immunity of the host.

Each of the four species of parasite causing human malaria may produce a febrile illness with nonspecific symptoms including anorexia, malaise, headache, chills, rigors, sweating, irritability and failure to eat and drink (Chongsuphajaisiddhi 1988). Symptoms begin about 10 days after the infective mosquito bite, but longer incubation periods are common, and sometimes the first symptoms are not experienced until months or years after exposure. Vomiting and cough are both common, but not severe, early symptoms; diarrhea is unusual. Febrile convulsions commonly complicate sudden rises of temperature. The pattern of fever is irregular at first; the classical periodicity appears only if the illness is protracted and untreated, when *P. malariae* may cause quartan fever (72 h between spikes), *P. vivax* and *P. ovale* tertian fever (48-h intervals) and *P. falciparum* subtertian fever (less than 48-h intervals). The liver and spleen may become palpable during the first few days of fever; the spleen may become very large after repeated or untreated infections.

Anemia develops, its degree being greatest in those with the heaviest or most protracted infections. Minor abnormalities of hepatic enzymes may be found, but jaundice is unusual except in complicated falciparum malaria.

The most important distinction between species in their clinical effects is in the capacity of *P. falciparum* to cause, in susceptible individuals, a rapidly progressive severe or complicated disease, which may be fatal. Most of the estimated 1–2.5 million deaths from malaria every year (Stürchler 1989) are due to *P. falciparum* infections in young children living in endemic areas.

In endemic areas the patient's first encounter with *P. falciparum* may be in utero. Parasitemia is common in pregnant women, and both placenta and cord blood may contain parasites at the time of delivery. Babies born to infected primigravid mothers may have a low birthweight but are otherwise unaffected. Parasitemia usually clears rapidly in the newborn, who remains relatively resistant to falciparum malaria for the first few months of life. Occasionally the newborn goes on to develop congenital malaria, features of which may include fever, failure to feed, anemia, jaundice and hepatosplenomegaly: congenital malaria is rare in endemic areas. Severe disease begins to affect children in endemic areas after the first few months of life, and for the next few years. During this time the majority of children are increasingly able to tolerate parasitemia with few or no symptoms, and malaria-related mortality decreases later in childhood.

In areas where there is little or no malaria transmission, children are susceptible to infection and severe disease at any age, and congenital malaria is sometimes seen (Quinn et al 1982).

Acute *P. falciparum* infections

Falciparum malaria usually presents as a febrile illness similar to that caused by other species of malaria. In a proportion of patients, however, complications develop which may threaten life. The most important manifestations of severe malaria in children are altered consciousness, labored breathing (due to acidosis) and severe anemia. These features may occur singly or in any combination (Marsh et al 1995). Hypoglycemia may accompany any of the above syndromes and is associated with increased mortality, especially when the hypoglycemia is profound. Some of the organ complications of falciparum malaria which are common in nonimmune adults are uncommon in children. Renal failure, pulmonary edema and disseminated intravascular coagulation are less likely to develop in children, and are not present in most of those who die of falciparum malaria.

Cerebral malaria (CM)

When impaired consciousness in a child with falciparum malaria cannot be explained by the presence of hypoglycemia or a transient postictal state, and no other causative disease is present, the term 'cerebral malaria' is used.

Clinical measurements of the depth of coma are helpful in defining severity (Molyneux et al 1989).

CM develops rapidly. In the majority of children febrile symptoms precede coma by 2 days or less; in some the interval is only a few hours. Most patients have been feverish, irritable, listless and unable to eat or drink prior to losing consciousness. Convulsions are common and sometimes herald the onset of coma. In CM there is no postictal recovery of consciousness as occurs after a febrile convulsion. Other symptoms that may precede coma include vomiting and cough; minor looseness of stool may occur, but severe diarrhea is unusual.

The rectal temperature may exceed 40°C, and is usually sustained during the first day or two of treatment. Occasionally a patient with CM may be afebrile when first examined, and rarely may remain so throughout the illness. Tachycardia is appropriate to the degree of fever, and the systolic blood pressure is normal in most patients. Dehydration is not clinically obvious, but vigorous fluid therapy in some patients leads to correction of acidosis and to improved tissue perfusion, suggesting that hypovolemia is commonly important. Respiration is rapid; in some patients breathing is stertorous, in others deep suggesting acidosis. About 5% of children with CM are jaundiced. The heart and lungs are normal on examination. The abdomen is soft; the liver may be moderately enlarged and the spleen may be palpable. In a minority of children with CM a shock-like state, with hypotension, cold peripheries and a wide core-to-skin temperature difference, may develop. Anemia is clinically apparent in some patients, and may develop during the course of illness in others.

The most striking clinical features are neurological. By definition the patient is unconscious and cannot be roused. Coma may be profound, the child being unable to withdraw from or localize a painful stimulus, and unable to moan or cry in response to pain. With less severe neurological impairment, motor and vocal responses to pain are retained but the patient is unable to watch or recognize familiar people. Corneal and pupillary reflexes are usually intact, but brainstem reflexes may be lost in the most severely ill. Retinal hemorrhages are common. Other retinal features include intraretinal edema, macular edema, exudates and occasionally papilledema. In some patients the motor picture suggests decerebration or decortication, with symmetrical rigidity or posturing of limbs, which may be sustained or repetitive. It is not uncommon for such patients to be opisthotonic (see Fig. 23.46). Focal asymmetrical twitching movements of the face or of a limb may be witnessed, sometimes but not invariably proceeding to a generalized convulsion. These events are not associated with extremes of fever and cannot be regarded as febrile convulsions. The plantar reflexes may be symmetrically abnormal. Abdominal reflexes are almost invariably absent.

The peripheral blood film reveals ring stages of *P. falciparum*. Occasionally parasites may be scanty, and rarely absent, in the blood film of a child with CM, perhaps as a result of the sequestration of mature parasites; parasitemia is usually revealed with repeated examination at intervals of a few hours. More commonly parasitemia is heavy: it is not uncommon for up to 20% of red cells to be parasitized, and in some patients the figure exceeds 50%. The packed cell volume may be normal or may be reduced; it invariably falls further. Life-threatening anemia may

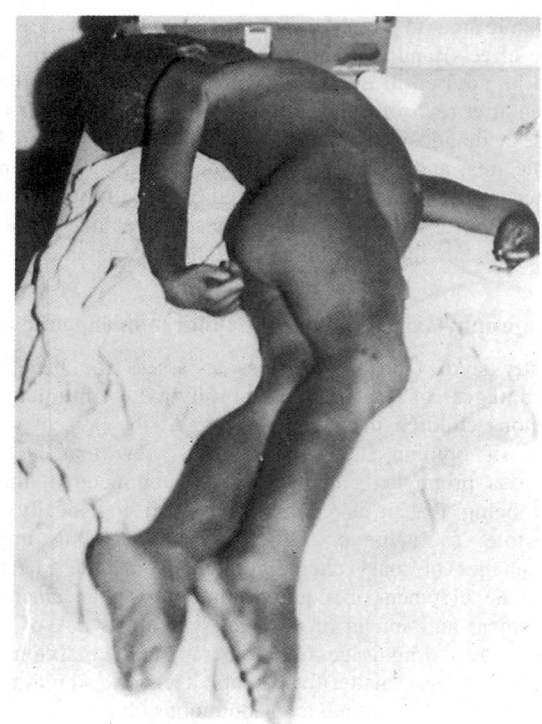

Fig. 23.46   Child with cerebral malaria showing opisthotonos.

develop rapidly in patients with hyperparasitemia. Commonly the fall in hematocrit exceeds what would be predicted from the level of parasitemia. In the severely ill, red cells containing late trophozoite and schizont stages of the parasite, normally sequestered in deep capillary beds, may appear in the peripheral blood. The peripheral white cell count is normal in the majority of patients but may be elevated in the very ill. The most severely affected patients are acidotic. There are minor abnormalities of hepatic enzymes, and the plasma creatinine may be mildly elevated. Plasma sodium, potassium, chloride, phosphate and calcium concentrations may show mild abnormalities but are commonly normal. Plasma and cerebrospinal fluid lactate levels are abnormally raised in some patients, commonly in association with hypoglycemia. Cerebrospinal fluid opening pressure is raised in most patients, and probably fluctuates over time. The mean and distribution of opening pressures were similar in a series of patients with fatal and those with nonfatal cerebral malaria, and the pathogenetic importance of raised intracranial pressure remains uncertain. The cerebrospinal fluid is clear with normal cell counts and protein concentration.

A significant proportion of patients with CM are hypoglycemic when first admitted to hospital (White et al 1987, Taylor et al 1988). These patients do not differ from others in their duration of illness, fasting or coma, or by any distinctive physical signs, but they tend to be younger and are more likely to be profoundly unconscious, to exhibit motor abnormalities and to have elevated levels of lactate and alanine in the plasma.

Even with optimal treatment the mortality among children admitted to hospital with CM is 10–20%. The cause of death is not known, and in most cases cannot be attributed to renal, cardiac, pulmonary or hematological complications of malaria. Presenting features associated with an increased risk of death in children with CM include profound coma, age under 3 years, hypoglycemia, witnessed convulsions, motor abnormalities (hypertonicity, posturing), extreme hyperparasitemia (> 20% of red cells parasitized), acidosis, lactic acidemia and leukocytosis (> 15×10^9 white blood cells/l) (Molyneux et al 1989).

In patients who survive CM, the duration of coma after the start of treatment ranges from a few hours to several days, the average duration being about 30 h. The change from deep coma to full consciousness may be dramatically rapid, and usually occurs before the temperature has fallen to normal and before parasitemia has cleared. The great majority of children who survive CM make a full neurological recovery; 5–10% of patients, however, suffer neurological sequelae, including hemiparesis, spasticity and cerebellar defects, from which a gradual recovery is made in some patients over the subsequent months. Risk factors for the development of sequelae are the same as those associated with mortality. It is not yet known whether minor defects of motor or cognitive function may persist in some children recovering from cerebral malaria.

Anemia

Anemia is a component of most episodes of malarial illness. In areas endemic for *P. falciparum* severe anemia (hemoglobin concentration < 5 g/dl) is an important clinical consequence of acute or recurrent malaria.

The history of fever and associated symptoms may be similar to that of any malarial illness, but it is common for a child to present without such symptoms, or for anemia to be identified when a child is examined for an unrelated complaint. Some children with severe malarial anemia develop respiratory distress, which is usually due to acidosis resulting from impaired tissue perfusion and oxygenation.

Peripheral blood films reveal parasitemia and a normochromic normocytic or, in chronic infections, hypochromic anemia. The reticulocyte count is inappropriately low. Unconjugated bilirubin may be increased in the plasma, free hemoglobin may be present in plasma and urine, and the plasma haptoglobin concentration is usually decreased or absent in the acute stage of the illness. The bone marrow shows normoblastic erythropoiesis with minimal dyserythropoiesis and increased myeloid precursors (Weatherall 1988). Unless other diseases are present, serum and red cell folate values are normal. Serum iron may be normal or moderately reduced, but there is usually normal or increased stainable iron in the bone marrow.

After the start of treatment for acute malaria, the hemoglobin level falls further in proportion to, or in excess of, the degree of parasitemia. In endemic areas many children have a positive direct antiglobulin test. Reticulocytosis begins within a few days, and the hemoglobin level rises rapidly in convalescence.

In endemic areas anemia is a common presenting sign in children who have *P. falciparum* parasitemia but no recent history of febrile illness. The role of malaria in the pathogenesis of the anemia is suggested by rapid improvement after antimalarial chemotherapy. In these patients the bone marrow may show severe dyserythropoiesis.

Other manifestations

P. malariae nephrotic syndrome

P. malariae infection if recurrent or prolonged may be complicated by a nephrotic syndrome characterized by nonselective proteinuria, unresponsiveness to steroid or cytotoxic treatment and relentless progression. Immunofluorescent studies suggest that the renal damage is due to the deposition of immune complexes on the glomerular basement membrane. Treatment with antimalarial drugs does not reverse the renal disease.

Hyperreactive malarial splenomegaly

Some children with protracted or frequent *P. falciparum* infection develop hyperreactive malarial splenomegaly, a condition in which massive enlargement of the spleen is accompanied by raised serum IgM, high titers of antimalarial antibody, and hepatic sinusoidal lymphocytosis. Splenomegaly resolves slowly with prolonged antimalarial treatment.

DIAGNOSIS AND DIFFERENTIAL DIAGNOSIS

Delayed diagnosis of *P. falciparum* malaria can have tragic consequences. In endemic areas all fevers must be regarded as malarial until proved otherwise or treated. In nonendemic areas a history of travel should alert the physician to the possibility of malaria, even if travel was many months or years ago. Malaria should be considered in the differential diagnosis of all fevers accompanied by cerebral complications, acidosis or anemia, and in patients with fever who develop acute renal failure, disseminated intravascular coagulation, pulmonary edema or hypoglycemia.

The diagnosis of malaria depends on finding the parasite in the peripheral blood. Thick smears stained with Field's or Giemsa stain, and thin films stained with Leishman's or Giemsa stain, allow identification of the species and density of malaria parasitemia. There have been occasional well-authenticated reports of fatal falciparum malaria in which blood films were repeatedly negative during life; treatment should therefore not be withheld from a patient with an illness suggestive of malaria even if films are negative. In such patients blood films should be repeated at intervals during treatment, when parasitemia may be revealed. Serological methods of identifying malarial infection are valueless for individuals in endemic areas, and of limited use to the clinician seeing patients elsewhere. Serology identifies past or current infection, and may help towards diagnosis in a patient with recurrent fever in a nonendemic area in whom parasitemia cannot be found on repeated testing. Antigen-detecting test-strips and DNA probes can identify parasitemia; the use of these methods for clinical and epidemiological purposes is likely to increase.

TREATMENT

Malaria due to *P. falciparum* differs from disease due to other plasmodial species in two important respects: *P. falciparum* may cause severe and complicated disease, and the parasite may be resistant to chloroquine. In the patient with falciparum malaria treatment must therefore be undertaken urgently; complications must be foreseen, recognized and treated; and the antimalarial drugs must be chosen with care.

Drug treatment of the acute attack

The correct drug, dosage and route are important. In general, antimalarial drugs should be given by mouth unless the patient is too ill to swallow. Chloroquine is a safe and effective drug for sensitive parasites, and is the treatment of choice for nonfalciparum malaria.

For severe or complicated falciparum malaria quinine is the drug of choice. Appropriate schedules for treatment are given in Table 23.42. In areas where *P. falciparum* is known to be partially quinine resistant, an additional drug may be given concurrently with quinine as soon as oral treatment is possible. The choice of additional drug should be guided by drug sensitivities of parasites in the area where the infection was contracted – options include pyrimethamine–sulfadoxine (Fansidar) in a single dose, equivalent to an adult dose of three tablets (see Table 23.41), or, in children over 10 years of age, tetracycline 250 mg 6-hourly for 5 days.

Both chloroquine and quinine may cause severe hypotension if given by rapid intravenous injection, but do not have this effect if infused slowly (over 3 or more hours). Parenteral quinine is known to stimulate the secretion of insulin from the pancreatic beta cells, but hypoglycemia in children being treated for malaria is usually due to the disease rather than to drug therapy (Taylor et al 1988). If intramuscular quinine is used in the treatment of a comatose child, supplementary glucose must be given or the blood glucose level checked frequently.

Oral drugs should replace parenteral as soon as a patient can take them.

Other measures

Hypoglycemia. This complication should be suspected in any child with impaired consciousness, convulsions, or acidosis, whether at the time of admission or during the course of treatment. Glucose should be administered as 25% or 50% solution by slow intravenous injection (0.5 g/kg) and the blood glucose concentration must be measured again at hourly intervals until the patient's condition improves.

Convulsions. Hypoglycemia and hyperpyrexia should be corrected. Prolonged seizures should be treated with the optimal available drug regimen – drugs which may be used include lorazepam, diazepam, paraldehyde, phenytoin or phenobarbitone, using drugs in sequence if convulsions prove refractory.

Acidosis. Deep or labored breathing due to acidosis is a common presentation of severe malaria in children. Possible

Table 23.42 Drug treatment of acute malaria. In this table the first regimen listed in each section is the treatment of choice

Diagnosis	If patient can take oral drugs	If patient unable to take oral drugs
Malaria due to *P. vivax, ovale, malariae,* and uncomplicated CQ-sensitive falciparum malaria	Oral CQ: 10 mg/kg first dose then 5 mg/kg after 6, 24 and 48 h	CQ: 10 mg/kg over 8 h in saline or 5% dextrose; then 5 mg/kg by similar infusions × 3 (total 25 mg/kg in 32 h)
	Or: AQ, same doses	*Or*: CQ i.m. or s.c. 2.5 mg/kg 4-hourly to 10 doses. Substitute oral CQ when possible
Uncomplicated falciparum malaria of doubtful CQ sensitivity	S/P single dose (S: 25 mg/kg, P: 1.25 mg/kg) *Or*: oral AQ as above *Or*: oral MQ 15 mg/kg first dose, then 10 mg/kg after 8 h	As for complicated falciparum malaria
Severe or complicated falciparum malaria	QN: i.v., first dose* 16.7 mg/kg over 4 h in 5% dextrose, then 8.3 mg/kg over 2–4 h each, 8-hourly, until oral drug can be taken (viz. quinine 8.3 mg/kg 8-hourly) to complete 7-day course *Or*: QN i.m. 8.3 mg/kg 8-hourly as solution containing 60 mg/ml. Give supplementary glucose. Substitute oral quinine as soon as possible, 8.3 mg/kg 8-hourly to complete 7-day course *Or*: quinidine i.v. 7.5 mg/kg 8-hourly, each dose over 4 h in 5% dextrose, until oral treatment can be taken; this may be QN 8.3 mg/kg 8-hourly or quinidine 7.5 mg/kg 8-hourly. Total course 7 days	

* The first dose of i.v. quinine should be reduced to 8.3 mg/kg if the patient has received any quinine or mefloquine in the two preceding days.
CQ = chloroquine; AQ = amodiaquine; QN = quinine; MQ = mefloquine; S/P = sulfonamide–pyrimethamine combination, e.g. Fansidar. All doses of CQ, QN and quinidine refer to base, not salt (8.3 mg quinine base = 10 mg quinine dihydrochloride).

contributory causes are dehydration, severe anemia, shock, repeated convulsions and hypoglycemia, all of which should be looked for and corrected in the acidotic child (see below under Anemia).

Hyperpyrexia (rectal temperature > 39°C) should be corrected by administration of oral or rectal paracetamol (15 mg/kg 4- to 6-hourly).

Severe anemia. Because of the increasing risk of transmission of human immunodeficiency virus by blood in parts of the world where malaria is endemic, blood transfusion should only be given if life-threatening anemia is present or can be predicted on the basis of the hematocrit and level of parasitemia on admission. Recent studies suggest that blood transfusion is particularly important for the child with severe anemia and respiratory distress (Lackritz et al 1992). Most children with severe malarial anemia who are breathless have acidosis rather than heart failure, and may be in urgent need of fluid volume replacement (M. C. English, personal communication).

Exchange transfusion has been advocated and successfully used for patients with hyperparasitemia, but no controlled trials have been done to prove the superiority of this measure.

Fluid therapy must be sufficient to correct hypovolemia, acidosis and oliguria. Pulmonary edema is rare in children with malaria, but the usual precautions are needed to avoid overhydration. Acute tubular necrosis is uncommon as a complication of falciparum malaria in children, but if it occurs peritoneal or hemodialysis may be required.

Antibiotics. Unresponsive fever or a shock state in falciparum malaria may be due to a complicating septicemia requiring treatment with an appropriate or broad spectrum antibiotic. It may be impossible to distinguish clinically between pneumonia and severe malaria with acidosis, in a child with fever and respiratory distress. The clinical setting and radiological features may help, but in some cases it is necessary to treat for both conditions.

There is no place for heparin, dexamethasone or dextran in the treatment of cerebral malaria (WHO 1986b).

Primaquine

P. vivax and *P. ovale* malaria (unless acquired congenitally or by blood transfusion) may relapse if treatment does not include a drug to eliminate hepatic hypnozoites. Primaquine (0.25 mg/kg daily for 2 weeks) will achieve this, but is not worth giving in areas where reinfection is inevitable, and it should not be given to children under the age of 5 years. Primaquine causes severe hemolysis in patients with glucose-6-phosphate dehydrogenase deficiency; the red cell concentration of this enzyme should therefore be measured before the drug is given; if low, an alternative method of radical cure is weekly chloroquine for 6 months in prophylactic doses. Primaquine need not be given after malaria due to *P. falciparum* or *P. malariae*. Primaquine has the additional action of killing gametocytes of all species of malaria parasites; it therefore reduces transmission and is sometimes used for this purpose in areas of moderate endemicity.

MALARIA CONTROL

Since the epidemiology of malaria varies greatly between and even within countries, control measures which are effective in one area may prove ineffective in another. It is important, therefore, that national control programs be designed having regard to local epidemiological, social and economic circumstances. Vector control by residual insecticides remains valid in many countries despite the acquisition of resistance by mosquitoes in some areas. Its cost however restricts its use.

The mainstay of malaria control in areas of intense transmission is the prompt recognition and treatment of both mild and severe disease at all levels of the health service. This requires appropriate diagnostic policies (often including presumptive diagnosis of fever as malarial) and treatment schedules (depending on availability and competent use of effective, safe and affordable drugs).

Alternative strategies that are suitable for implementation in primary health care programs are being assessed. These include administration of antimalarial drugs for treatment or prevention by village health workers, environmental management to restrict mosquito breeding, the use of mosquito repellents and the use of mosquito (bed) nets impregnated with pyrethroid insecticides. The latter measure has proved highly efficacious in a community research context (Alonso et al 1991), and effective (but less so) in an ongoing community program in The Gambia (d'Allessandro et al 1995), but the sustainability of this method in other settings remains uncertain.

The success of any method or combination of methods of control is likely to be materially influenced by the degree to which the causes and consequences of malaria are appreciated by populations and by the willingness of communities to participate in, and even finance, specific operations (WHO 1986b).

TRYPANOSOMIASIS

AFRICAN TRYPANOSOMIASIS: SLEEPING SICKNESS

Human African trypanosomiasis (HAT) is caused by two morphologically identical 'subspecies' of *Trypanosoma brucei* which cause sleeping sickness or African trypanosomiasis in man and are transmitted by the bite of the tsetse fly. Sleeping sickness is widely distributed in 36 countries in sub-Saharan Africa as far south as a latitude of 20°. The number of new cases reported annually to WHO, 20 000–50 000, underestimates the actual numbers substantially. *T. b. gambiense* occurs in west and central Africa and is slow in onset and progress while the more acute *T. b. rhodesiense* disease is distributed in east and southeast Africa. Infection is often more common in adults but where transmission is peridomestic any age group may be affected. In *T. b. rhodesiense* infections the progress of diseases to meningoencephalitis may be more rapid in childhood.

1. *Trypanosoma brucei brucei.* Parasite mainly of wild and domestic two-toed ungulates not usually infective to man. Morphologically identical to *T. b. gambiense* and to *T. b. rhodesiense.*

2. *Trypanosoma brucei gambiense.* Parasite of the insidious form of sleeping sickness (Gambian or *T. b. gambiense* sleeping sickness). Infected humans can provide long-term sources of infection for the tsetse and the disease may be largely an anthroponosis.

3. *Trypanosoma brucei rhodesiense.* Parasite of the acute form of sleeping sickness with an abrupt onset often lethal to the patient within a few months (Rhodesian or *T. b. rhodesiense* sleeping sickness). This form of the disease is a true zoonosis: humans are infected by tsetse that acquired their infection from wild ungulates.

Life cycle

The parasite exists only as a *trypomastigote* in the blood of the mammalian host but *gut trypomastigotes, epimastigotes* with the kinetoplast anterior to the nucleus and *metacyclic trypomastigotes* are seen in the vector. The continual movement of the trypomastigote (Fig. 23.47) is activated by a flagellum and the fold of membrane which is lifted up by the motion of the flagellum – the 'undulating membrane'. In the insect vector stumpy blood forms ingested with the blood meal transform into slender midgut forms of trypomastigotes which appear eventually to reach the peritrophic space. From there they penetrate the semisolid peritrophic membrane at its origin, move to the hypopharynx in the proboscis and then reach the salivary glands. In the salivary gland epimastigotes are formed (Fig. 23.47) which transform to the infective metacyclic trypomastigote.

In the vertebrate host the three 'subspecies' of *T. brucei* group are found in the form of trypomastigotes. After inoculation the metacyclic trypomastigotes, on reaching the subcutaneous tissue, are converted into long slender forms. Blood forms are polymorphic comprising slender and stumpy forms.

T. b. brucei, which is not infective to humans, cannot be distinguished morphologically from *T. b. rhodesiense* and *T. b. gambiense*. However, biochemical techniques including DNA analysis and isoenzyme characterization have shown the diversity of *T. brucei* populations and increased understanding of the epidemiology. *T. b. rhodesiense* comprises two distinct zymodemes; the 'Zambezi' group in southern Africa and the 'Busoga' group in east Africa associated with more acute severe disease. *T. b. gambiense* is less variable with no animal reservoir whilst the 'bouafle' group also occurring in west and central Africa also occurs in wild and domestic animals (Godfrey et al 1990, Stevens & Godfrey 1992).

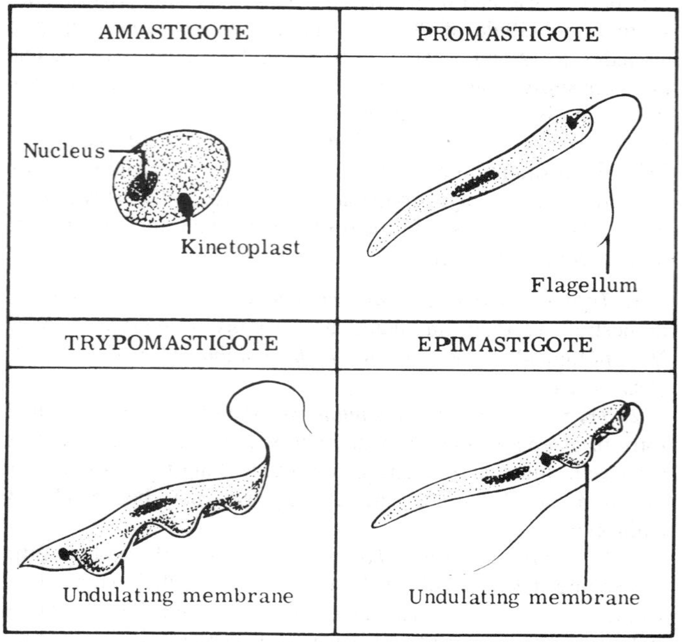

Fig. 23.47 Morphological forms produced by the genera *Trypanosoma* and *Leishmania*. (From Hoare & Wallace 1966.)

Epidemiology

It is probable that all infections with human infective African trypanosomes proceed to sleeping sickness, which, if untreated is invariably fatal. Recent evidence suggests that African trypanosomiasis is increasing as a human health problem. Substantial epidemics have recently occurred in Uganda, Mozambique, Angola and Zaire.

T. b. gambiense (Gambian sleeping sickness)

The spread of *T. b. gambiense* is restricted to west and central Africa and is transmitted by 'palpalis group' tsetse which inhabit dense vegetation along rivers and in forests. The most common vectors, *Glossina palpalis, G. tachinoides* and *G. fuscipes*, tend to attack man, bovids and aquatic reptiles but *G. palpalis* will feed preferentially on man where man–fly contact is intense, near riverine vegetation at water collecting points and river crossings, where people concentrate. In *T. b. gambiense* the man–fly–man cycle of transmission may maintain the disease in the absence of an animal reservoir but it is now clear that human infective parasites occur in both wild and domestic animals especially in west African foci although their epidemiological significance remains uncertain. *T. b. gambiense* frequently persists in foci (foyers) where transmission is maintained at high levels.

Without continued surveillance and control efforts the prevalence can rise to high levels in human populations as is presently occurring in Zaire and Angola.

T. b. rhodesiense (Rhodesian sleeping sickness)

In *T. b. rhodesiense* sleeping sickness 'morsitans group' tsetse are involved, especially *G. morsitans, G. pallidipes* and *G. swynnertoni* whose habitats are in the low woodland and thickets of the east African savanna and lake shores. Throughout much of the geographical range of *T. b. rhodesiense*, infection is sporadic and occurs in individuals coming into contact with savanna species of tsetse flies. Under these conditions infection is clearly zoonotic, from wild animal reservoirs of infection. Intrusion by man into the enzootic cycle of *T. b. rhodesiense* is typified in Tanzania, in the Kahama and Tabora districts for example, by the activities of game hunters, fishermen and more particularly honey gatherers whose travel brings them into contact with *G. morsitans*. This tsetse species exists among game including bushbuck and other potential mammalian reservoirs. In Kenya the focus in the Llambwe valley is maintained by *G. pallidipes* and wild animal reservoirs but in epidemics domestic cattle provide a domestic animal reservoir and permit increased human transmission.

In southeast Uganda and western Kenya *T. b. rhodesiense* was predominantly transmitted by *G. pallidipes* with an animal reservoir especially in the bushbuck (*Tragelaphus scriptus*) with sporadic human infection in adult males, notably fishermen who came into close fly contact in lacustrine situations. However, more recently, large epidemics have occurred in western Kenya and especially Busoga in southeastern Uganda with infections occurring in both sexes and all age groups. The vector is *G. f. fuscipes*, a palpalis group tsetse which invaded *Lantana camora* thickets close to human habitation with consequent epidemics of up to 8000 infections a year.

Transplacental infections with *T. b. rhodesiense* and *T. b. gambiense* are known but often unrecognized. In congenital infection, trypomastigotes have been found in the blood film from an infant with meningoencephalitis during the first week of life.

As well as population movements leading to local spread of the disease, trypanosomiasis as an imported disease has increased as a result of tourism. Tourists are more likely to become infected with game-associated *T. b. rhodesiense* than with *T. b. gambiense*.

Pathogenesis and pathology

In both *T. b. gambiense* and *T. b. rhodesiense* infections the pathological processes are similar but vary in intensity. Metacyclic trypomastigotes introduced with the tsetse saliva into the subcutaneous tissue change into slender blood forms and multiply locally with the formation of the trypanosomal chancre, with edema and an infiltrate of polymorphonuclear leukocytes, lymphocytes and plasma cells. Between the fifth and 12th day after infection parasitemia occurs and continues in waves. *T. brucei*, including its subspecies, attempts to evade immune response in its host by altering its surface antigens every 5–6 days. The infection consists of a series of waves of parasitemia, each one differing antigenically. The antigens consist of two classes, the variable antigen (VSG – variant surface glycoprotein) contributed by the outer coat of the trypomastigote and the stable core antigens. The succession of variable antigens induces a profuse production of IgM antibody which reaches high levels in the serum and, when the central nervous system is involved, the cerebrospinal fluid. This response leads to the high IgM levels exploited for diagnostic purposes.

Hyperplasia of the reticuloendothelial system with lymph node and spleen enlargement occurs as a response to antigenic stimulation together with phagocytosis by macrophages. Later lymph nodes become atrophic and fibrotic and there is evidence of immunosuppression. Expressions of cell-mediated immunity, induction of cell-mediated immunity and expression of humoral immunity have been shown to be impaired in *T. b. gambiense* infections in man (Greenwood & Whittle 1980). In *T. b. rhodesiense* trypanosomiasis a hemolytic anemia may develop and thrombocytopenia can be marked in *T. b. rhodesiense* infections, which may proceed to disseminated intravascular coagulation. Major damage due to immune complexes (type III hypersensitivity) may explain less common lesions of the kidney, lungs, liver and heart.

Parasites subsequently invade the central nervous system from the choroid plexus leading to the characteristic meningoencephalitis. Involvement of the central nervous system, indicated by abnormalities of the cerebrospinal fluid, mark the onset of the second stage of the disease. There is widespread vasculitis and predominantly lymphocytic meningoencephalitis with focal accentuation. Cell aggregates are seen more frequently at the mouth of the sulci and typical 'morular' cells (Mott cells) are found but may be few. Perivascular infiltrates are striking especially in the subcortical white matter, the caudate nucleus, thalamus and putamen but seldom in the globus pallidus. The midbrain, pons and medulla oblongata are substantially affected. The white matter of the brainstem is characterized by small foci of perivascular demyelination and diffuse gliosis. The cerebrospinal fluid in the late stage contains trypanosomes, mononuclear cells most of which are lymphocytes and elevated protein levels. IgM is probably produced locally in the central nervous system and plasma cells and the morular cells of Mott play an important part in its production releasing free IgM into the CSF.

Clinical features

The trypanosomal chancre

The primary lesion (trypanosomal chancre) develops as a painful erythematous and edematous swelling at the site of the infecting bite appearing within 2 or 3 days and healing with residual scarring in 2–3 weeks. It occurs in *T. b. rhodesiense* infection but only exceptionally in *T. b. gambiense*. Skin vesicles and ulceration may develop. The lesion subsides over 2 or 3 weeks often leaving hyper- or hypopigmented lesions. As the chancre develops the regional lymph glands become enlarged and tender.

The hemolymphatic stage

The parasitemic phase occurs 5–12 days after the bite and the waves of irregular remittent fever, more severe in *T. b. rhodesiense* infections than in *T. b. gambiense*, occur in association with the waves of parasitemia. In *T. b. gambiense* the hemolymphatic stage may be mild, subclinical or asymptomatic. The febrile episodes, sometimes associated with rigors, are accompanied by malaise, headache, muscular tenderness, joint aches, weight loss, generalized lymphadenopathy and sometimes an annular erythematous rash (circinate erythema) visible particularly in the fair skinned. The rash is usually on the trunk but may appear on the face and limbs; individual patches may be 10–15 cm or more across and fade without desquamation. A generalized lymphadenopathy develops especially in *T. b. gambiense*; the soft adenopathy in the posterior cervical triangle, known as Winterbottom's sign, occurring particularly in *T. b. gambiense* develops probably as a sequel to an infected bite by *G. palpalis* as bites of this species of tsetse tend to be on the head.

Edema may affect the ankles or feet and puffiness of the face produce a dull expressionless facies. Irritability, insomnia, sense deceptions and confusion may occur even in the early stage. The spleen and liver may enlarge. The serum albumin is low and bilirubin levels may be raised as well as a slight rise in transaminases. Tachycardia is usual and myocarditis with arrhythmias or cardiac failure, pleural or pericardial effusions occur especially in *T. b. rhodesiense* and may cause mortality during the hemolymphatic stage. Anemia with a normocytic normochromic picture and hemolytic in nature is also more frequent in *T. b. rhodesiense* as well as severe thrombocytopenia and a hemorrhagic coagulopathy.

Meningoencephalitic stage

Meningoencephalitis is an inevitable consequence of human African trypanosomiasis. In *T. b. gambiense* it tends to occur late in the course after months or years while in *T. b. rhodesiense* it occurs early, often during the febrile illness and progresses rapidly to a fatal outcome. As the central nervous system becomes involved a wide variety of neurological signs can occur. Changes in behavior and sleep disorders occur before other evidence of meningoencephalitis. Diurnal and inappropriate somnolence with insomnia and agitation at night are common and patients lose interest in themselves and their surroundings. They become apathetic, lacking in attention and may exhibit trance-like states. Behavior becomes inappropriate, aggressive or overtly paranoid. There is weakness, lassitude, unsteadiness of gait, expressionless facies, slurred speech, tremors of the limbs and progressive emaciation, nutritional deficiencies and intercurrent infections.

Hyperreflexia and delayed deep hyperalgesia occur. As the disease progresses focal epileptic attacks, profound ataxia, choreoathetosis and psychotic changes may be followed by somnolence, deepening coma and death.

Diagnosis

The clinical diagnosis of African trypanosomiasis is often difficult. The presence of a chancre is almost pathognomonic, the hemolymphatic stage must be differentiated from a wide range of febrile illness including malaria and the meningoencephalitis differentiated from other causes of meningitis and encephalitis as well as psychiatric illness. HIV/AIDS and associated cryptococcal and tubercular meningitis present particular diagnostic difficulty. A parasitic diagnosis must be attempted in all suspected of trypanosomiasis. Routine laboratory tests show a normal total white cell count, raised ESR, anemia, thrombocytopenia, low serum albumin and elevated serum IgM.

Parasitological diagnosis

In the early stages of the disease the recognition of trypomastigotes in the blood is usually simple, particularly in *T. b. rhodesiense* infections, as the concentration of trypanosomes is high. Organisms are readily recognized by single or repeated microscopic examination of fresh aspirates of lymph nodes (especially in *T. b. gambiense*) or trypanosomal chancres (in *T. b. rhodesiense*) and thick blood films stained with Field's stain or Giemsa and sometimes in wet blood films. Microscopy of blood films is less reliable in *T. b. gambiense*; repeated examination of blood films and concentration techniques are more often required. Trypanosomes may also be identified in cerebrospinal fluid, various effusions and marrow smears.

Concentration methods in common use include microhematocrit centrifugation and microscopic examination of the area above the buffy coat. Multiple hematocrit tubes increase the sensitivity and recently the quantitative buffy coat technique (QBC®) a modification of the hematocrit method where motile trypanosomes are stained with fluorescent acridine orange and examined by fluorescent microscopy has proved a very sensitive and rapidly performed test (Bailey & Smith 1992).

The miniature anion exchange centrifugation technique MAEC (Lumsden et al 1979) involves passing a sample of blood through an ion exchange column using a DEAE-cellulose anion exchange column, in which red cells are held back and trypanosomes pass through into a collecting tube which is centrifuged and examined for motile trypanosomes. This is a sensitive technique but technically difficult especially under field conditions. Inoculation of blood, aspirates from lymph node or trypanosome chancre into laboratory rodents is valuable in *T. b. rhodesiense* infections but less so for *T. b. gambiense*.

Once trypanosomiasis is diagnosed or suspected the CSF must be examined, preferably within 15 min of lumbar puncture. Increase in cell count (more than 5 cells/mm^3), protein elevation, CSF IgM or trypomastigotes in the centrifuged deposit indicate CNS involvement.

Immunodiagnosis

Immunodiagnostic tests utilized in human African trypanosomiasis include IFAT, ELISA, CFT and IgM estimation. IFAT, in particular, has been found of value in epidemiological investigation and screening of populations and suspects. They provide only presumptive evidence of infection. More recently an agglutination test, the card agglutination test for trypanosomiasis (CATT), has been developed for the diagnosis of *T. b. gambiense*. This relies on a the presence of common antigens (LiTat 1.3) not present in all foci of *T. b. gambiense*. The test provides a rapid field test for preliminary screening of populations in endemic areas. With all existing serological techniques problems with sensitivity and specificity require that a parasitic diagnosis should be established prior to treatment. Antigen detection techniques are also being developed.

Treatment

Although it is important to initiate treatment as soon as possible after reaching a parasitological diagnosis and to avoid unnecessary delays resulting from multiple investigations, particularly in extremely virulent *T. b. rhodesiense* infections, it is advisable in view of the possibilities of immunosuppression in the disease to exclude other intercurrent infections. Patients should be nursed as inpatients and attention given to correction of nutritional disturbance or intercurrent infection.

Examination of the cerebrospinal fluid is mandatory and the results allow the separation of early from late cases. An increase in cells above 5/mm^3, elevation of protein or the presence of trypanosomes indicate late-stage meningoencephalitis regardless of the clinical features. Prior to lumbar puncture suramin is useful in clearing the parasitemia.

Treatment of hemolymphatic trypanosomiasis

In the treatment of the early case suramin (Bayer 205, Germanin) is effective in both *T. b. rhodesiense* and *T. b. gambiense* disease and will rapidly clear the parasitemia in both early and late sleeping sickness. Pentamidine is also effective in *T. b. gambiense* but not in *T. b. rhodesiense*. Neither suramin or pentamidine are effective in meningoencephalitis.

Suramin. Suramin is a whitish powder freely soluble in water. It is best shaken on to the surface of the sterile distilled water and allowed to dissolve to produce a 10% w/v solution. The usual dose is 20 mg/kg bodyweight with a maximum single dose of 1.0 g. The drug is given intravenously. Five doses on days 1, 3, 7, 14 and 21 are advised although, because about 1 person in 20 000 appears to have an idiosyncrasy, a test dose of one-fifth of the desired dose is given initially.

Pentamidine. Pentamidine, an aromatic diamidine, is available as the isethionate (Pentamidine) and as the methanesulfonate (Lomidine). Pentamidine, a white powder, is made up freshly as a 10% solution in water. It tends to dissolve slowly and it is important to ensure that every particle is in solution before use. 'Lomidine' comes already prepared as a 4% solution of the base. Both preparations are administered intramuscularly. The dosage is 3–4 mg/kg bodyweight, calculated on the pentamidine base. Injections are given daily or on alternate days for 7–10 days. Side effects including faintness due to hypotension and vomiting and abdominal pain may occur within the first half hour. Peripheral neuritis is a rare complication and severe hypoglycemic reactions occur during the course of treatment. Adrenaline and glucose should be available when treatment with pentamidine is given.

Meningoencephalitic trypanosomiasis

Melarsoprol. Melarsoprol (Mel B, Arsobal) is a compound of the trivalent arsenical melarsen oxide and dimercaprol (BAL). It enters the cerebrospinal fluid and, prior to the development of DFMO, was the only drug which offered a chance of cure in *T. b. rhodesiense* infection in which involvement of the central nervous system had occurred. Melarsoprol is presented as a 3.6% solution in propylene glycol and *must* be given intravenously since the propylene glycol is highly irritant. The maximum dosage is 3.6 mg/kg bodyweight (WHO 1986d).

A variety of treatment schedules have been developed based on clinical experience and without the benefit of pharmacokinetic information. In *T. b. rhodesiense* infection melarsoprol is given in 3-day courses each course separated by 1 week for three or four courses, giving a total of 35–37.5 ml melarsoprol. A widely used schedule (Table 23.43) starts with low doses and rises throughout the four courses of treatment. Based on experience in Kenya and Uganda this schedule appears to be less toxic than regimes starting with larger dosage and given over three courses, especially in advanced, late-stage disease.

In west Africa a variety of other regimes have been developed either providing a rising dosage in each successive course or starting with a dose of 5 ml daily for 3 days and varying the number of courses according to the degree of meningoencephalitis as determined by the CSF cell count.

All syringes and needles must be sterilized dry: thrombophlebitis is a frequent complication of treatment and the technique of injection must be impeccable as the smallest leak will result in a severe local reaction at the site of injection. The most severe complication is a *reactive arsenical encephalopathy* (RAE) developing usually after the third injection or at the beginning of the second course. The onset is usually sudden with neurological deterioration, confusion, convulsions and coma. It occurs more commonly in severe meningoencephalitis. RAE occurs in up to 5% of patients treated with melarsoprol and is fatal in 50%. In *T. b. gambiense* prophylactic prednisolone significantly reduces the incidence of RAE (Pepin et al 1994, 1995). Occasionally the encephalopathy may be hemorrhagic due to intolerance rather than reactive with an immunopathological basis (Robertson 1963a,b). Other toxicity includes agranulocytosis, aplastic

anemia, thrombocytopenia and peripheral neuropathy. Jaundice, diarrhea, conjunctival infection, pyrexia, edema of the lips, pruritus, arthralgia, renal and hepatic damage and an erythematous papular rash have also been recorded.

During therapy there is generally a striking improvement in the mental and physical condition of patients with sleeping sickness but unwanted effects are common. In parasitemic patients if melarsoprol is given as initial treatment a febrile reaction with or without rigor, a Jarisch–Herxheimer-like reaction, occurs after the first injection and subsides usually within 12 h.

Difluoromethyl-ornithine (DFMO). The ornithine decarboxylase inhibitor difluoromethyl-ornithine (DFMO, Eflornithine Ornidyl) has recently been introduced. Initially used in the treatment of arsenic-refractory *T. b. gambiense* it has also been used in both early and late stage *T. b. gambiense* with encouraging results but treatment remains very expensive. DFMO is less effective in *T. b. rhodesiense*. Trials of combined therapy with DFMO and suramin are currently being carried out. The dose advocated is 100 mg/kg 6-hourly for 14 days. Nifurtimox (see Chagas' disease) has also been used in the treatment of arsenic-refractory *T. b. gambiense*.

Follow-up and relapse

After treatment patients should be followed for 2 years to identify relapse. Ideally follow-up should initially be at 3 months and then 6-monthly. Relapse may be difficult to identify clinically and presents as a chronic meningoencephalitis without a peripheral parasitemia. Follow-up should include lumbar puncture to identify rising levels of pleocytosis or protein estimations. Relapse following treatment with suramin or pentamidine should be with melarsoprol. Ornidyl (DFMO) is valuable in the treatment of relapse after melarsoprol therapy.

Control of sleeping sickness

Sleeping sickness caused by *T. b. rhodesiense* is usually detected at fixed medical units in rural areas with patients presenting with the obvious symptoms associated with early parasitemias (passive surveillance). In *T. b. gambiense* the clinical symptoms tend to be few and mild in the early stage and active search for infected individuals is necessary (active surveillance). In the event of epidemics active surveillance has also been used in *T. b. rhodesiense*. The aim is to identify infected individuals through mass screening as early in the course of infection as possible. Blood film examination is effective in *T. b. rhodesiense* but in *T. b. gambiense* gland aspiration and CATT tests are frequently used for initial population screening. Surveillance programs require adequate laboratory resources.

In *T. b. gambiense* areas pentamidine has been used in the past as a chemoprophylactic although its role has never been clearly demonstrated and the risk of masking infections is substantial.

Historically trypanosomiasis control involved destruction of tsetse habitats and animal reservoirs, human resettlement and extensive ground and aerial spraying with insecticides. In recent years control efforts are attempting to integrate into primary care systems with emphasis on community education and participation. However, this is resource intensive and requires technical and logistic support. Trypanosomiasis is associated with economic decline, deteriorating health services and civil

Table 23.43 Treatment schedule for late stage. *T. b. rhodesiense* (dosage for 50 kg adult)

Day	Drug	Volume (ml)	mg/kg
1	Suramin	2.5	5
3	Suramin	5.0	10
5	Suramin	10.0	20
7	Melarsoprol	0.5	0.36
8	Melarsoprol	1.0	0.72
9	Melarsoprol	1.5	1.1
16	Melarsoprol	2.0	1.4
17	Melarsoprol	2.5	1.8
18	Melarsoprol	3.0	2.2
25	Melarsoprol	3.0	2.2
26	Melarsoprol	4.0	2.9
27	Melarsoprol	5.0	3.6
34	Melarsoprol	5.0	3.6
35	Melarsoprol	5.0	3.6
36	Melarsoprol	5.0	3.6

disturbance; in many endemic foci control efforts have declined substantially and, as a result, disease endemicity has deteriorated as was the situation in Uganda and is currently occurring in Zaire and Angola. The costs of surveillance, diagnosis and treatment are substantial and inevitably require external support. New, less toxic drugs are urgently required to limit the substantial morbidity and mortality of trypanosomiasis as well as the toxicity and difficulty of administration of existing chemotherapy.

The most favored method of tsetse control in many areas is still ground spraying with insecticides. Aerial spraying has been applied effectively against *G. morsitans* in Botswana and against *G. palpalis*, *G. tachinoides* and *G. morsitans* in Nigeria. More recently insecticide-impregnated (and/or odor-baited) traps and targets have been used in vector control programs. Attractant traps (such as the pyramidal trap) have been deployed over large areas and have brought about a reduction in fly populations without the environmental problems associated with ground spraying or aerial application of insecticides.

AMERICAN TRYPANOSOMIASIS: CHAGAS' DISEASE

The discovery of *Trypanosoma cruzi*, of the disease it causes in man and of its vector, by Carlos Chagas, were first detailed in April 1909 to the National Academy of Medicine in Rio de Janeiro by Oswaldo Cruz. Chagas unraveled the biology of the flagellate and the vector, a blood-sucking triatomine bug; he found the parasite first in domestic animals and finally in the blood of a sick child (Lewinsohn 1979). Estimates of the public health importance indicate that some 65 million are at risk in Latin America, some 20 million may be infected and 2 million have chronic Chagas' disease. Although the initial *T. cruzi* infection is usually benign and asymptomatic and the mortality resulting from the early acute disease is low, the public health and socioeconomic importance of the chronic stages of the disease are substantial.

Life cycle of *Trypanosoma cruzi*

The organism occurs in three distinct forms: amastigotes, epimastigotes and trypomastigotes (Fig. 23.47). The *amastigote* is 2–4 μm in diameter and occurs intracellularly in 'pseudocysts' in the tissues of the mammalian host. The *trypomastigote*, about 20 μm long, tends to be crescent shaped, has a prominent kinetoplast and is found in mammalian blood. *Epimastigotes*, with the kinetoplast anterior to the nucleus, are found in the digestive tract of the triatomine bug. After ingestion by the vector, trypomastigotes change into and multiply as epimastigotes and in the succeeding 2–4 weeks develop into metacyclic trypomastigotes in the rectal ampulla of the bug. Infective forms, excreted with the feces, enter through an abrasion in the skin or through an intact mucous membrane such as the conjunctiva. Within 1–2 weeks trypomastigotes enter and circulate in the bloodstream. After an undetermined period the trypomastigote invades tissue cells, preferentially muscle and glial cells of the host, and is transformed into the amastigote which multiplies within a pseudocyst in the infected cell.

Epidemiology

T. cruzi occurs in more than 100 mammalian species. The most frequent wild hosts are rodents and small marsupials (e.g. opossum, *Didelphis*). *T. cruzi* does not infect birds or reptiles.

Many triatomine bugs are sylvatic and maintain infection among reservoir hosts. Three species have adapted to human dwellings: *Rhodnius prolixus*, *Triatoma infestans* and *Panstrongylus megistus*. Transmission between man, domestic animals and these domestic bugs provides the majority of human infections and accounts for the public health importance of Chagas' disease. Infection rates among bugs are often high and household populations may reach hundreds or thousands. High infection rates (40–50% or higher in some localities) in the exposed populations are due to factors which encourage triatomine bug infestation such as poor housing, thatched roofs and lack of wall resurfacing. Most transmission occurs in rural populations but transmission in periurban areas is increasing.

The risk of acquiring Chagas' disease by blood transfusion has increased in recent years and serological tests have been widely adopted to detect Chagas' disease in donors. Seropositive blood is ideally discarded but the addition of 0.5% gentian violet (at 1 : 4000) to stored blood will eliminate the organism within 24 h. Contaminative transmission for example in the laboratory is also well recognized and transmission via transplant surgery is now well documented.

The rapid urbanization occurring throughout much of South America by those from rural endemic areas has increased the frequency of transfusion-transmitted Chagas' disease from infected donors and increased the risks of transmission in periurban situations from importation of vector triatomines. The increasing frequency of international travel and emigration from tropical countries has resulted in Chagas' disease being more frequently identified in developed countries.

Congenital disease is an important public health problem in rural areas of endemic transmission. It is associated with severe disease in early infancy including abortion, prematurity, and stillbirth.

Pathogenesis and pathology

The *acute phase* may be asymptomatic or subclinical in two-thirds to half of infected infants and children. Within a few hours some will develop a chagoma at the site of inoculation of metacyclic trypomastigotes. This frequently develops around the eye. There is edema and a local inflammatory reaction which may persist for a few days or be prolonged for months. *T. cruzi* preferentially parasitizes histiocytes, neuroglia, smooth muscle and cardiac muscle cells and skeletal muscle cells. In those dying with cardiac disease in acute Chagas' disease there is infiltration of mononuclear cells, variable degenerative processes in the myocardial fibers and the development of pseudocysts containing amastigotes. The intensity of inflammation shows wide variation and is not related to the number of amastigotes present.

In the *chronic phase* Chagas' cardiomyopathy is characterized by the presence of fibrous tissue, degenerating myocardial fibers and infiltrates of mononuclear cells. Fibrous plates in the subendocardium may produce mural thrombi. Hypertrophy of the heart muscle and dilation of the cavities are found and there is thinning of the ventricular wall. This leads to the formation of aneurysms which develop usually at the apex of the left ventricle, less frequently in both ventricles and rarely at the apex of the right ventricle. At autopsy, in 1700 cases. Köberle (1974) found cardiopathy in 90%, megacolon in 20%, megaesophagus in 18%, bronchiectasis in 7% and other mega formation in 5% respectively. He ascribed these changes in hollow muscular organs to a reduction in the number of ganglion cells.

As a result of immune mechanisms induced by the parasite the infection is controlled at subpatent levels. The immune response may be responsible also for tissue damage in chronic Chagas' disease and parasite-modified host cells can be killed in vivo, releasing self components which are themselves immunogenic. Although a wide variety of cells can be destroyed, neurons are especially vulnerable because the cells are not regenerated. Events occurring in the acute phase may also initiate the chronic phase which itself can be exaggerated by secondary autoimmune mechanisms (Lancet 1980). Among other unexplained problems is the disparate distribution of Chagas' disease syndromes in man, megacolon, megaesophagus and other mega conditions being highly prevalent in certain areas such as southern Brazil, but reported less frequently in Chile and Argentina and almost totally absent in countries such as Venezuela.

Clinical features

Acute Chagas' disease

The chagoma. Although the acute illness occurs as such (see below), the acute phase can be totally asymptomatic and go unrecognized in approximately two-thirds of affected infants and children. Shortly after penetration of the connective tissue of the host the parasites elicit a local inflammatory reaction with marked edema at the site of the portal of entry (chagoma). The skin over the chagoma becomes hard and may desquamate. In most cases this occurs within the region of the eye or within the conjunctival sac and is accompanied by a hard nonpitting edema of both eyelids and chemosis on the affected side (Romana's sign). Local areas of hard edema may develop elsewhere.

The acute illness. After 1 or 2 weeks a febrile reaction develops with the temperature rarely exceeding 40°C. The acute phase lasts for 1–3 months, following an incubation period of 1–3 weeks and usually occurs in the first decade of life. Lymphadenopathy and moderate hepatosplenomegaly are observed; vomiting, diarrhea and meningoencephalitis may follow. Myocardial involvement varies widely in severity and may even be clinically silent. Tachycardia, dysrhythmias and cardiomegaly are encountered with electrocardiographic changes. Cardiac failure may follow with death from myocarditis, arrhythmia or meningoencephalitis, particularly in the very young. A leukocytosis and lymphocytosis accompany the parasitemia.

The majority survive and the disease may persist as a latent (hidden) infection with a low-level parasitemia. This latent phase may persist for the life of the patient.

Chronic Chagas' disease

Chronic Chagas' disease affects some 15% of those infected and occurs generally between the ages of 15 and 50 years. It is characterized by the reappearance of clinical disease perhaps 10–20 years after infection. The pancarditis becomes more severe. There may be very marked thinning of the muscle wall especially in the apical region, mural thrombi and the development of biventricular, congestive cardiomyopathy. The other main clinical feature is the development of cardiac rhythm disturbances. Complete right bundle branch block with left bundle hemi-block is characteristic. AV block, extrasystoles and Stokes–Adams attacks are common. There is electrocardiographic evidence of

myocardial damage. The predominant causes of death are heart failure, embolic phenomena and cardiac arrest.

Dysfunction of hollow organs develops owing to inflammatory changes and destruction of parasympathetic ganglion cells in muscle. Disturbances of esophageal peristalsis and the development of eventual megaesophagus give rise to the characteristic symptom of inability to swallow dry food without drinking, parotid gland hypertrophy and recurrent lung infections. When the lower bowel is affected the first symptom is constipation which may be prolonged for months. Megacolon is also associated with fecolith formation and sigmoid volvulus and can reach enormous dimensions; megatrachea, megacystis and megaureter can also occur.

Involvement of the central nervous system with parasites in glial tissue and focal decrease in neurons in the cerebellum and elsewhere have been found (Tafuri 1979) and may account for a variety of signs such as agitation, irritability and insomnia which occur in Chagas' disease. A peripheral neuropathy has also been described.

Congenital Chagas' disease

Congenital infection with *T. cruzi* probably occurs in between 2 and 10% of maternal infections. Infection is associated with abortion, stillbirth and death in early infancy in a high proportion. Clinical features include cardiac, megaesophagus, pneumonitis and meningoencephalitis. Transmission is also thought to occur through breast milk.

Diagnosis

Parasitic diagnosis

Specific diagnosis, made by the demonstration of *Trypanosoma cruzi* in the peripheral blood is easy in the early acute illness. In Romanowsky-stained thick or thin films the parasite appears as a C- or S-shaped trypomastigote with a prominent kinetoplast.

Culture requires the use of Nicolle–Novy–MacNeal (NNN) medium with an overlay of Locke's solution. Although useful in the laboratory the medium cannot be autoclaved and contamination is a problem in the field.

Xenodiagnosis is a method for detecting subpatent parasitemia in chronic infections by allowing triatomine bugs to feed on the individual patient: it is preferable to animal inoculation which is unreliable. Unfed third instar *Dipetalogaster maximus* have replaced *Triatoma infestans* as a xenodiagnostic agent in the University of Brasilia. Examination of the bugs for gut infection is made after 20–40 days. To avoid direct contact with patients, triatomine bugs may be allowed to feed through a membrane from a fresh blood sample contained in a warmed (37°C) capsule.

Serological diagnosis

The commonly used serological tests for Chagas' disease are the complement-fixation test, IFAT and an indirect hemagglutination test. Enzyme-linked immunosorbent assay (ELISA) may supplement other techniques. Whilst existing serodiagnostic tests are sensitive, poor specificity is more important. False positive tests occur with parasitic infections and autoimmune disorders.

Treatment

Chemotherapy in Chagas' disease is uncertain and unreliable. Two drugs have been widely used: nifurtimox (Lampit) a nitrofurfurylidine compound 8 mg/kg bodyweight daily for 60–90 days and benzidazole (Rochagan) 6 mg/kg bodyweight daily for 30 or 60 days. The later drug is now the drug of choice. Treatment is of value in shortening the course of the acute illness and preventing complications and deaths from myocarditis and meningoencephalitis. Both drugs affect bloodstream trypomastigotes and may render the patient aparasitemic although cure, both in the acute and chronic stages, is far from sure. In congenital infection the effect of chemotherapy is uncertain. If any success is to be achieved, patients require to be treated for prolonged periods. Side effects can be severe (weight loss, polyneuropathy and psychoses) especially during the last 40 days. Hypersensitivity reactions (dermatitis, anaphylaxis and jaundice) also occur and gastrointestinal symptoms may be severe. Results of clinical trials have been difficult to assess and results vary both geographically and according to the stage of the infection. The suppressive action of nifurtimox has been clearer in some areas than in others and the results better in Argentina than in Brazil. There is no evidence that antiparasitic treatment in the chronic stages of Chagas' disease provides any benefit.

Heart failure may respond poorly to digitalis. Sensitivity to digitalis is common and β-adrenergic blockers are contraindicated. Pacemakers are now commonly implanted for heart block.

Control

The socioeconomic cost of South American trypanosomiasis although unquantified is substantial, whether measured in terms of years of productive life lost or cost of medical care including pacemaker implantation and corrective surgery.

The control of South American trypanosomiasis is based on efforts to control transmission. This requires the widespread use of vector control in endemic rural and periurban populations in domestic situations and the prevention of transfusion and organ transplant transmission.

In recent years control programs have been effective in countries in the southern cone of South America (Argentina, Brazil, Bolivia, Chile, Paraguay and Uruguay) which have led to a reduction in transmission with notable success in Brazil, Argentina and Venezuela. Following seroprevalence surveys, insecticides are used as sprays, paints and fumigant canisters. Housing improvements, health education and community involvement help to promote sustainability. House improvements include the use of bricks and roofing tiles and replastering internal walls.

Programs to control blood transfusion transmission are based on serological testing and usually combine serological tests for HIV and hepatitis B as well as T. cruzi. In some circumstances the high prevalence of seropositivity requires that seropositive blood has to be used and in these circumstances the addition of gentian violet 24 h before use appears effective and safe.

Gentian violet added routinely to banked blood at a concentration of 1 : 4000 has proved effective in preventing transmission of T. cruzi. Neither effective antiparasitic chemotherapy or vaccines have been developed.

LEISHMANIASIS

Leishmaniasis is a group of diseases caused by infection with protozoan parasites of the genus Leishmania, which in the vertebrate host, including man, are intracellular (the amastigote) in cells of the reticuloendothelial system. Infection in man ranges from a self-limiting cutaneous lesion to potentially fatal visceral leishmaniasis. All forms are transmitted by sandflies (genera Phlebotomus and Lutzomyia). In the insect vector, the amastigote transforms to a flagellated extracellular parasite, the promastigote. Most forms of leishmaniasis are zoonoses with rodent or canine reservoirs of infection.

Apart from minor variations in size of amastigotes, leishmania infecting man are morphologically similar regardless of the type of clinical infection. However, in recent years the development of biochemical techniques defining isoenzyme patterns, DNA and serological characterization as well as cultural characteristics has allowed a clearer understanding of the species and complexes of Leishmania and their relationship to human clinical infection. In addition differences in the development of Leishmania in vector species have identified two subgenera of importance in human leishmaniasis (Lainson & Shaw 1987): Leishmania which develop in the midgut and foregut of the vector (suprapylaria) – Leishmania subgenus Leishmania (L. donovani, L. mexicana, L. tropica and L. major) and Leishmania which also develop in the hind gut with subsequent migration to the foregut (peripylaria) – Leishmania subgenus Viannia (L. braziliensis complex).

The important leishmania affecting man (Table 23.44) include parasites causing visceral leishmaniasis and cutaneous leishmaniasis and those restricted to Central and South America causing mucocutaneous leishmaniasis.

Life cycle of leishmania in the vector

Leishmania are transmitted by sandflies of the genus Phlebotomus in the Old World and Lutzomyia in the New World. Sandflies take in blood from a minute hemorrhage made in the skin by their mouthparts. The aflagellate stage (amastigotes), taken in the blood meal, divide at least once before changing into the motile flagellate stage (promastigotes). In the peripylaria, hindgut forms are retained but parasites also migrate to the midgut and foregut and transmission is by bite. In the suprapylaria hindgut development is lost and parasites are restricted to the foregut with transmission again by bite. The speed of development of leishmania in the sandfly varies from a possible 4 days to more than 14 (Lainson & Shaw 1979). Sandfly populations show substantial fluctuations and transmission is often seasonal.

Life cycle in the vertebrate host

The intracellular stage in the vertebrate host is a small uninucleate ovoid body (2–5 μm long and 1–2 μm wide) containing a kinetoplast with a flagellar remnant and known as the amastigote (also referred to as the Leishman–Donovan body). The amastigote multiplies repeatedly by binary fission eventually destroying the host cell, e.g. macrophage. Stained with Romanowsky stains such as Leishman or Giemsa the cytoplasm of the amastigote appears blue, the nucleus pink or violet and the kinetoplast bright red. In cutaneous leishmaniasis the amastigote may be found in the skin or, in visceral disease, more diffusely in the internal organs in the reticuloendothelial system.

Table 23.44 Summary of human leishmaniasis

Parasite	Geographical distribution	Animal reservoir	Disease
Visceral leishmaniasis (*Leishmania donovani* complex)			
L. donovani	India, Bangladesh, China	None	VL PKDL
	Kenya	(Dog)	VL PKDL
	Sudan and Ethiopia	Rodents	VL (CL) (MCL)
L. infantum	Mediterranean littoral, Central Asia, China	Canine sp.	VL (CL) VL CL
L. chagasi	Central and South America	Canine sp.	VL
Old World cutaneous leishmaniasis			
L. tropica	Middle East to India	(Dog)	CL (dry), LR
L. aethiopica	Ethiopia and Kenya	Rock hyrax	CL DCL
L. major	Africa, Middle East and Asia	Rodents	CL (wet)
American cutaneous leishmaniasis (*Leishmania mexicana* complex)			
L. mexicana	Mexico, Belize, Guatemala	Forest rodents	CL (DCL) Chiclero's ulcer
L. amazonensis	Brazil–Amazon basin	Forest rodents	CL DCL
American mucocutaneous leishmaniasis (*Leishmania braziliensis* complex)			
L. braziliensis	Brazil, Amazon forest, Peru, Ecuador, Bolivia, Venezuela, Colombia, Paraguay	Uncertain, forest animals	CL and MCL
L. guyanensis	North Amazon, Guyana	Sloth, lesser anteater	CL MCL
L. panamensis	Panama, Costa Rica	Sloth	CL (MCL)
L. peruviana	Western Andes	(Dog)	CL (Uta)

VL = visceral leishmaniasis; CL = cutaneous leishmaniasis; MCL = mucocutaneous leishmaniasis; DCL = diffuse cutaneous leishmaniasis; LR = leishmania recidivans; PKDL = post-kala-azar dermal leishmaniasis

Parasitic diagnosis of leishmaniasis

Whenever possible a specific parasitic diagnosis should be made in all forms of leishmaniasis. Parasites may be detected in needle aspirates, smears and biopsy. The morphology of the leishmania amastigote is similar regardless of the species. Smears are fixed in methanol and stained with a Romanowsky stain such as Giemsa or Leishman. Leishmania although intracellular are commonly seen lying free on smear preparations. They contain a central nucleus and a kinetoplast. Culture of leishmania can be attempted using NNN medium or Schneider's medium. Cultures must be maintained free of bacterial contamination. Some *Leishmania* species grow poorly in culture and culture characteristics have been used to differentiate *L. braziliensis* which is slow growing from *L. mexicana*.

More sophisticated techniques have now been developed for the taxonomic identification of leishmanias. They include isoenzyme profiles, DNA characterization, PCR, monoclonal antibody techniques and serotyping. Such techniques are, however, complex and not generally available for clinical investigation (Chance 1985).

VISCERAL LEISHMANIASIS (kala azar)

Visceral leishmaniasis is caused by leishmania of the *L. donovani* complex and characterized by fever, splenomegaly and anemia. It has become evident that less than 1 in 5–10 infections lead to clinical disease; the remainder have subclinical or asymptomatic infection and develop immunity to subsequent infection.

L. donovani is endemic and epidemic in northeastern India and Bangladesh predominantly in young adults and children. Epidemics tend to occur every 10–15 years. Infection is confined to man and no animal reservoirs have been identified. The vector, *P. argentipes*, is peridomestic and readily feeds on man, thus predisposing to human epidemics. Similar parasites are found in east African foci of disease. In Sudan, rodents are reservoirs of infection whilst in Kenya clear evidence of an animal reservoir is lacking. The disease is widespread and focally endemic and epidemic, predominantly in children and occurs especially in association with population movements and land development.

L. infantum is widely distributed through the Mediterranean littoral, southern Europe, the Middle East, southern regions of the former USSR and China. In endemic areas children under 5 are predominantly affected although in visitors infection may occur at any age and especially in the immunosuppressed. The domestic dog is an important reservoir host and in addition wild canine species and foxes also act as reservoirs.

L. chagasi in South and Central America resembles *L. infantum* clinically and epidemiologically. Children are predominantly affected and both domestic and wild canine species and foxes are reservoir hosts. Infection occurs in Amazonian Brazil where it is hyperendemic in eastern Brazil, Bolivia, Paraguay, Argentina, Colombia and Venezuela.

Clinical features

The clinical features of visceral leishmaniasis are similar throughout the geographical range of the *Leishmania donovani* complex. A small cutaneous lesion may occur at the site of inoculation (a leishmanioma), weeks after infection but is rarely observed clinically. The incubation period is variable but usually 4–6 months after which the characteristic triad of fever, splenomegaly and anemia develop. Amastigote-laden macrophages are found in liver, spleen, bone marrow, lymphatic tissue and under certain circumstances in the skin. The disease has a variable course ranging from an acute febrile infection with anemia, pancytopenia and splenomegaly to a protracted illness slowly progressing over 2 or more years with severe anemia and massive splenomegaly. *L. infantum* infections are usually more acute than infection with *L. donovani* but even in the latter, acute forms are seen especially in children. In southern Europe simple cutaneous leishmaniasis occurs in adults due to *L. infantum*.

Fever is frequent, commonly remittent or intermittent, and may show a characteristic double diurnal periodicity. Patients often remain active despite high fever. Especially in chronic cases patients may be afebrile for prolonged periods. In the most acute form fever is usually high and associated with prostration and toxemia and minimal splenomegaly.

The spleen progressively enlarges usually associated with hepatomegaly. In more chronic infections the spleen is grossly enlarged often to the iliac fossa and is smooth and hard. A generalized lymphadenopathy is common in some geographical foci and may occur in the absence of hepatosplenomegaly or other features of visceral leishmaniasis. A more localized lymphadenopathy may also occur notably in the cervical region.

Well-established cases are characterized by pallor and in India especially, develop an earthy gray color with areas of hyperpigmentation (kala azar). In Africa a diminution in skin pigmentation is more typical. In chronic forms there is progressive wasting, nutritional skin changes and hair changes similar to those observed in kwashiorkor.

Anemia and pancytopenia are invariable and secondary infections common, related to the immunosuppression and neutropenia. Bacterial infections commonly occurring in the course of visceral leishmaniasis include pneumonia, bronchitis, gastroenteritis, meningitis and tuberculosis, and such infective episodes commonly bring patients to health facilities.

Episodes of diarrhea are common and may be due either to secondary infection or submucosal infiltration with leishmania-laden macrophages. Deterioration of anemia and pancytopenia are associated with episodes of secondary infection. Dependent edema and ascites are common but jaundice is unusual. Hemorrhagic features are common, especially recurrent epistaxis and major or fatal hemorrhagic episodes occur.

Laboratory findings

The hematological features of visceral leishmaniasis are usually characteristic. There is a moderate to severe normocytic, normochromic anemia with hemoglobin levels of 6–8 g/dl accompanied by a pancytopenia and neutropenia. Lymphocytes are usually in the normal range and circulating eosinophils reduced or absent from the peripheral blood. There is a moderate thrombocytopenia, commonly $80–100 \times 10^9/1$. The serum albumin is reduced and there is a substantial elevation of immunoglobulins, almost all of which is polyclonal IgG.

Immunodiagnostic tests of value in the investigation of VL include IFAT, ELISA and CFT. ELISA techniques in particular are both highly specific and sensitive. High titers are associated with active disease and fall slowly after treatment. Recently the direct agglutination test, DAT, has been introduced for field diagnosis.

The leishmanin skin test (a test of delayed hypersensitivity using leishmanial antigen) is invariably negative in active disease but becomes positive after effective treatment.

Parasitic diagnosis

Parasites are demonstrated in smears stained with Giemsa from material aspirated from bone marrow or splenic aspiration. Splenic aspiration is a more sensitive technique and reasonably safe if performed carefully in the absence of disturbed hemostasis or thrombocytopenia. Culture in NNN media improves the sensitivity of direct smear examination. Marrow aspiration is preferable to spleen puncture especially in children, acute illness or in the presence of thrombocytopenia or disturbed hemostasis. Leishmania may also be identified in lymph node and buffy coat examination and liver biopsy.

Visceral leishmaniasis and acquired immune-deficiency syndrome

In the last decade visceral leishmaniasis has been increasingly recognized as an important infection in HIV infection in Europe as a result of reactivation of *L. infantum* in emerging AIDS infections. This has caused an increase in the incidence of visceral infections in adults in southern Europe. The presentation may be with fever, splenomegaly and anemia but may be atypical with pulmonary and skin lesions and leishmanial serology frequently negative.

Differential diagnosis

Visceral leishmaniasis should be considered in the differential diagnosis of both short-term and long-term fever accompanied by hepatosplenomegaly and anemia especially when there is a history of residence in an endemic area. Malaria, especially *P. malariae* infection, is particularly important but typhoid, brucellosis, relapsing fever and tuberculosis (which may coexist with visceral leishmaniasis) may simulate leishmaniasis. Splenomegaly must be differentiated from schistosomiasis, tropical splenomegaly syndrome, reticulosis or leukemia in particular. In the immunocompromised, especially in AIDS, visceral leishmaniasis may present as a fulminant infection without characteristic splenomegaly.

Treatment

Pentavalent antimonial compounds are the treatment of choice in visceral leishmaniasis. Two preparations are in common use, sodium stibogluconate containing 100 mg antimony (Sb) per ml (Pentostam) and methylglutamine antimoniate containing 85 mg Sb per ml (Glucantime).

Pentavalent antimony compounds

Sodium stibogluconate is administered by daily intravenous or intramuscular injection. The dose is 10–20 mg/kg Sb per day for 20–30 days. Children require relatively higher dosage (20 mg/kg per day), when calculated on bodyweight. Clearance is rapid with almost 90% excreted in the urine within 8 h. Caution is therefore required in the presence of reduced renal function. Cardiotoxicity, notably prolonged Q–T interval and dysrhythmias, is rare at standard dosage but increases at higher dosage regimes used to treat antimony-resistant patients. Anaphylactic shock is rare following administration. Caution is also required in the presence of pneumonia, intercurrent viral infections, myocarditis, renal or hepatic disease. Sodium stibogluconate has been used in pregnancy without untoward effects on the fetus.

Aminosidine (an aminoglycoside) is also effective in the treatment of visceral leishmaniasis. It is administered intravenously or by intramuscular injection at a dose of 14 mg/kg daily for 3–4 weeks. More recently liposomal amphotericin B (Ambisome) has proved effective with low toxicity but is expensive (Bryceson 1996).

Supportive and symptomatic treatment is important with attention to infection, nutritional status and vitamin deficiencies. Intercurrent infections must be sought and appropriately treated. Management of anemia and hemorrhage includes vitamin K, and blood transfusion in acute hemorrhage but is seldom required otherwise.

Response to treatment

In the first week of treatment fever usually subsides and patients feel better. Hematological improvement with rising Hb and total white cell count improve in 2–4 weeks while the splenomegaly reduces more gradually over subsequent weeks or months. Patients should be followed up for at least 1 year to detect relapse.

Relapse and nonresponsiveness

A proportion of treated patients relapse, usually within 6 months. Relapse is more frequent if initial therapy is inadequate, and after repeated relapse patients may become resistant to antimony treatment. Treatment of relapse is initially with further courses of sodium stibogluconate at 20 mg/kg for 60 days. Subsequently in nonresponsive patients, pentamidine may be effective or the more recently developed regimens with aminosidine, amphotericin B and liposomal amphotericin (Ambisome).

Post-kala azar dermal leishmaniasis

Post-kala azar dermal leishmaniasis (PKDL) is most commonly seen in Indian visceral leishmaniasis (20%) and less often in African infections (1–5%). Following treatment of visceral disease cutaneous lesions develop with symmetrical depigmented lesions especially on exposed surfaces. Lesions progress to become papular or nodular and mucosal surfaces may be involved with abundant leishmania (*L. donovani*) in lesions. Treatment with pentavalent antimonial compounds is effective although lesions also heal spontaneously.

CUTANEOUS LEISHMANIASIS

Various leishmania typically produce a localized cutaneous lesion which heals spontaneously with residual scarring in 6 months to 2 years. Lesions start as a small raised nodule surrounded by a zone of erythema often with fine papery desquamation. The lesion grows slowly and central shallow ulceration may occur. Lesions remain raised above the level of normal skin; ulcers are shallow and do not have undermined edges. Lesions continue to progress for 6–24 months followed by healing eventually leaving a slightly depressed papery scar. Local satellite lesions may develop and,

especially in some forms, a local lymphadenitis. Lesions may be single or multiple and are more common on the face, hands, feet or limbs.

Cutaneous leishmaniasis occurs in the Middle East, Afghanistan, the Mediterranean littoral, Sudan and sub-Saharan Africa due to *L. tropica* and *L. major*. In endemic areas clinical infection is observed mainly in children. In Central and South America cutaneous leishmaniasis is caused by *L. mexicana* and *L. braziliensis*.

L. tropica (urban cutaneous with a human reservoir) tends to cause single lesions lasting for 1–2 years. Local tissue reaction is mild and lesions may not ulcerate. Parasites are plentiful especially early in the evolution of the lesion.

L. major (rural leishmaniasis with a rodent reservoir) tends to cause larger, often multiple lesions with more tissue reaction and ulceration.

L. mexicana in Central and South America (with a reservoir in forest rodents) causes ulcerating lesions especially affecting the pinna of the ear in forest workers, notably chicleros (chewing gum collectors), and *L. braziliensis* (with a reservoir in domestic animals and forest rodents) which causes cutaneous lesions and which progresses to mucocutaneous leishmaniasis (espundia).

Diffuse cutaneous leishmaniasis

In the Ethiopian highlands and western Kenya, *L. aethiopica* (with a reservoir in hyraxes) causes initial skin lesions similar to *L. tropica*. In approximately 1 in 10 000 infections leishmania then disseminate widely throughout the skin with an absence of cell-mediated immunity (negative leishmanin skin test). Lesions are widespread, often symmetrical especially on exposed surfaces. Similar syndromes occur in Central and South America associated with *L. mexicana* and *L. amazonensis*. DCL resembles lepromatous leprosy. It is chronic and resistant to antimony treatment but may respond to prolonged treatment with pentamidine.

Leishmania recidivans

This is an unusual form of cutaneous leishmaniasis found in the Middle East, in areas of *L. tropica*, and causing a chronic skin lesion which heals but then progressively spreads. The appearances are similar to lupus vulgaris. Leishmania amastigotes are difficult to find but the leishmanin skin test is strongly positive.

Mucocutaneous leishmaniasis

The *L. braziliensis* complex is characterized by single often self-healing primary lesions of the skin with subsequent late metastatic spread to the oronasopharynx (espundia). The nasal septum is commonly an early involved site. Granulomatous lesions develop with necrosis and destruction of cartilage and soft tissue. Secondary infection is common and contributes to tissue destruction. Lesions extend to involve the nose, mouth, tongue and soft palate leading to gross deformation. Granulomatous destruction proceeds to involve the pharynx, larynx and trachea. Sepsis and mutilation cause considerable morbidity and malnutrition and death from aspiration and respiratory infection may follow.

Diagnosis of cutaneous leishmaniasis

Parasitic diagnosis should be attempted in suspect lesions but the frequency with which parasites are found varies with the parasite species and the stage of the lesion. Parasites are more numerous in early lesions and especially in *L. tropica* and DCL. Techniques include aspiration or slit smear preparation from the raised margins of a lesion or a punch biopsy. In the latter, impression smears should be prepared before fixation of tissue. Culture on NNN should be attempted when facilities are available.

The leishmanin skin test becomes positive during the course of infection and remains positive thereafter. It is of little value in endemic areas as a high proportion of inhabitants are positive but may be helpful in travelers. It is negative in DCL and strongly positive in *Leishmania recidivans*. Serodiagnostic tests are also of limited value (IFAT and ELISA) especially in endemic areas. In *L. braziliensis*, IFAT is of some value in the diagnosis and follow-up of mucocutaneous disease.

Treatment

Many cutaneous leishmaniasis lesions can be left to heal spontaneously without specific treatment. Local treatment including cleansing and antibiotics to control secondary infection and covering to prevent secondary contact lesions is all that is required. Local infiltration with antimonials is widely used and local paromomycin creams are being evaluated. Specific treatment with systemic pentavalent antimonials is indicated for multiple lesions and lesions associated with tissue damage or potential metastatic spread.

In *L. braziliensis* areas where mucocutaneous leishmaniasis occurs, all leishmanial lesions must be treated with prolonged systemic pentavalent antimonials as for visceral leishmaniasis in an attempt to prevent metastatic spread. Established mucocutaneous disease requires 6–8 weeks of systemic pentavalent antimony or prolonged amphotericin.

Diffuse cutaneous leishmaniasis is resistant to pentavalent antimonials but may respond either to combinations of aminosidine and antimonials or to prolonged courses of pentamidine.

Control of leishmaniasis

When the disease is restricted in its reservoir to man (anthroponosis) effective control can be achieved by medical surveillance of the population at risk and where the vector is peridomestic as in Indian visceral leishmaniasis, by destruction of the domestic sandfly vector by insecticide spraying of houses. If the reservoir host and the sandfly vector can be discovered, as in central Asia, the simultaneous use of rodenticide and insecticide in gerbil burrows have reduced markedly the incidence of *L. major* infection: similarly, control of stray dog populations and residual insecticide spraying have reduced *L. infantum* infection in many areas. In the vast forested areas of the Americas cutaneous and mucocutaneous leishmaniasis remains a problem largely unsolved; the use of insecticides in tropical rain forests is scarcely practicable and the destruction of the extensive reservoir of infected wild animals equally impossible. Deliberate infection with a live vaccine of *L. major* has been practiced with some success in the former USSR and Israel and appears to protect against either *L. major* or *L. tropica*.

TOXOPLASMOSIS

Toxoplasmosis is of importance in pediatrics as a congenital infection, producing an acute and often severe illness in the newborn, or a less severe acute febrile illness in later childhood.

Congenital infection may produce major damage to the central nervous system, including the eye.

ETIOLOGY

The causative organism, *Toxoplasma gondii*, is, in its free active state, a small crescentic protozoon, which is a strict intracellular parasite multiplying only within the cytoplasm of the nucleated host by binary fission or, probably more frequently, by internal budding (endodyogeny). The active form, responsible for acute infection, stimulates an immunological response by the host. At the same time, cyst forms of the parasite develop in any tissue, but chiefly in nervous tissue or striated muscle, and may persist for the life of the host.

PATHOGENESIS

Toxoplasma gondii infects virtually all species of mammals, and several species of birds. In man, the incidence of infection measured by serological methods varies from 5% to 9%, being most prevalent in tropical and subtropical climates. In Great Britain, children under the age of 5 years are seldom infected, while 25–50% of adults show evidence of past or present infection.

While transplacental infection is responsible for congenital toxoplasmosis, the mode of transmission of the protozoon under other circumstances is not known. Among mechanisms suggested are transmission from the oropharynx in the saliva, supported by the high incidence of cervical lymph gland involvement in acquired infections, and ingestion of the cysts in raw or undercooked meat. Cat feces is also suspected as a major source of infection of humans with *T. gondii*, because of persistence of oocysts in that species. Domestic animals are commonly infected, and cysts may be found in feces, urine and oral secretions, while infection can be transmitted to cats by transmission within the egg of the cat roundworm *Toxocara cati*.

Congenital infection in man (p. 288)

It is believed that infection of the fetus by *Toxoplasma gondii* occurs during a primary maternal infection, usually symptomless, or accompanied by mild fever and malaise. Parasites form small focal lesions in the placenta, proliferate and are released as active forms into the fetal bloodstream.

It is generally accepted that women who bear a congenitally infected child do not have infected children in subsequent pregnancies, probably owing to persistence of immunity after the primary infection. Exceptions to this rule occur and it is suggested that the persistence of *Toxoplasma gondii* as cysts in the myometrium with liberation of active forms during pregnancy is one of the main infectious causes of repeated abortion in women. The low antibody titers in some women with affected fetuses suggest incomplete immunological response. Good results, in terms of successful pregnancies, are claimed for treatment of the mothers with pyrimethamine and sulfonamides during pregnancy.

Infection of the fetus with virulent strains early in pregnancy will, it is thought, produce fetal death and abortion; still later, severe fetal damage or stillbirth; and later still in a liveborn infant with stigmata of congenital toxoplasmosis, including neurological and visceral manifestations. The French Ministry of Health advocates screening of pregnant women for acquisition of toxoplasmosis. Congenital infection does not always cause disease, however. In a study among Parisian women, serological evidence of infection was present in 20 of the infants born to 47 women who developed primary toxoplasma infection during pregnancy, as detected by conversion from seronegative to seropositive with rising antibody titers. Of the 20 infected infants 7 at most had signs of disease at birth (Desmonts et al 1985). By ultrasound studies of the fetal brain, fetal blood sampling and amniocentesis it was reported that 6% of fetuses were affected if mother converted from seronegative to seropositive. Further features of congenital toxoplasmosis are described on page 288.

Acquired infection in man

Lymph node involvement is the most common feature of acquired toxoplasmosis in man. However, chorioretinitis, though usually congenital, may be due to acquired toxoplasmosis. Lesions of the lungs, skeletal muscle, myocardium and, recently, the liver have been recorded in acquired toxoplasmosis in man. Meningoencephalitis has long been considered as a possible result of acquired toxoplasma infection, although few cases have been recognized.

Acquired toxoplasmosis has increasingly become recognized as an opportunistic infection complicating acquired immune-deficiency syndrome; Holliman (1988) reports 140 cases responding to a variable extent to treatment with pyrimethamine and sulfadiazine.

CLINICAL FEATURES

Congenital toxoplasmosis

The clinical features of congenital toxoplasmosis in the newborn infant are described on page 288. The most common single presenting feature is chorioretinitis and both eyes are involved in 40% of cases. Severe infection early in fetal life may result in serious central nervous manifestations at birth or in early infancy with signs of meningoencephalitis, hydrocephalus and cranial nerve palsies but convulsions may occur at this stage, or up to 18 years of age. In the intervening period, congenital toxoplasmosis may present as mental retardation. Calcified lesions may be radiologically demonstrable as a curvilinear streak in the line of a lateral ventricle or, in the case of lesions in deeper layers, as small irregular foci of calcification.

Acquired toxoplasmosis

Acquired infection with *Toxoplasma gondii* is uncommon in Britain in children under 5 years, but in a recent survey of 51 patients with acquired toxoplasmic lymphadenopathy 28 (55%) were aged 3–15 years. Serological surveys suggest a peak acquisition of infection in early and mid-teens.

The commonest manifestation is lymphadenopathy, particularly of cervical nodes, which may be accompanied by no ill health, or may be accompanied by fever and prostration, and resemble severe infectious mononucleosis. Hepatosplenomegaly may

occur. Lymphocytosis may be found. A common symptom associated with acquired toxoplasmic lymphadenopathy is muscle pain, due, it is believed and occasionally confirmed, to infection of voluntary muscle. Cardiac arrhythmias occurring during acquired infection are probably due to lesions in the region of the conducting system, while the occurrence of cardiac failure due to toxoplasma infection of the mycocardium is conjectural. Recently, it was confirmed that acute hepatitis could be caused by acquired toxoplasmosis. Pneumonitis is a rare feature. In a review of acquired toxoplasmosis in children in Galway the frequency of this condition in childhood was emphasized, the authors finding 1 case in every 2000 new pediatric patients, a higher incidence than that of brucellosis (McNicholl & Flynn 1978). The clinical manifestations described included chorioretinitis, hepatitis, myocarditis, encephalitis, myositis and arthritis.

DIAGNOSIS AND DIFFERENTIAL DIAGNOSIS

Congenital toxoplasmosis should be considered a possible cause of generalized lymphadenopathy, hepatosplenomegaly, thrombocytopenia or severe and otherwise unexplained jaundice in the newborn. Cytomegalic inclusion disease, congenital rubella, neonatal hepatitis, rhesus incompatibility and congenital syphilis would also be considered. In later infancy and childhood congenital toxoplasmosis enters into the differential diagnosis of hydrocephalus and of fits. Congenital toxoplasmosis should be considered as a possible cause of chorioretinitis whatever the stage of development of the lesions or age of the patient. It is believed that 25–35% of chorioretinitis is due to toxoplasma infection. Chorioretinitis could also be due to congenital rubella.

Acquired toxoplasmosis should be considered in any case of unexplained lymphadenopathy, particularly when maximal in, or confined to, the cervical region whether or not it is accompanied by pyrexia. Lymph node enlargement in acquired toxoplasmosis may persist for several months, leading to the consideration of Hodgkin's disease and allied conditions and tuberculous lymphadenopathy in the differential diagnosis.

Laboratory diagnosis

Laboratory aids to the diagnosis include isolation of the organism, serology, skin testing and histology.

Culture of *Toxoplasma gondii* from lymph node biopsy material or, less often, from other tissue fluids is possible although generally less widely used than serological methods. The organism can be cultured in suitable laboratory animals, particularly mice, embryonated eggs and tissue cultures. The most reliable of these procedures is that of intraperitoneal inoculation of mice.

A number of serological methods are available, the most commonly used being the *cytoplasm modifying* or *dye test* which depends upon the inhibition by antibody-containing serum of methylene blue staining of laboratory cultures of *Toxoplasma gondii*. Dye test antibody titers rise rapidly to a maximum 3–6 weeks after infection and then gradually decline over the course of many years. Interpretation of dye test titers as indicating past or present infection may therefore be difficult, since asymptomatic infection is so common in the community. Equally, passive transfer of maternal antibody may complicate the diagnosis of congenital toxoplasmosis in the newborn. However, the half-life of passively transferred antibody is approximately 3 weeks, so a repeated estimation of dye test titer after 3–4 weeks will be informative. If the newborn is infected, the antibody titer will rise. Actively produced antibody is in part IgM, while passively transferred antibody contains little or no IgM – a further aid to interpretation of antibody titers. During the first 5 years of life asymptomatic infection appears to be uncommon, and a raised and especially a rising antibody titer in this age group should be regarded as probably indicating recently acquired infection. Generally, apart from the neonatal period, a dye test titer of 1 : 16 or higher indicates past or present infection, while in Britain, dye test titers of over 1 : 250 are found in only 0.2% of clinically normal persons.

While the dye test for *Toxoplasma* antibody remains the 'gold standard' for diagnosis, the need for the use of live organisms, fresh frozen human plasma or antibody-free serum creates disadvantages. A number of other serological tests have been assessed and several are in use. The latex agglutination test, while technically reasonably simple, gives a 1–2% false positive rate. The ELISA test for IgM antibodies and the latex test are widely used for screening purposes, while a direct agglutination test using formalin-treated *T. gondii* is extensively employed in France. The laboratory diagnosis is well reviewed in the Journal of Clinical Pathology (1989).

Dermal hypersensitivity to injection of a suspension of killed *Toxoplasma* is indicated by a delayed tuberculin-type response. There is good correlation between a positive skin test and a positive dye test titer of 1 : 8 or more. The test may be negative in very recent infections and is used chiefly in epidemiological surveys in man. Histological examination of biopsy material is of value, limited chiefly by the availability of suitable material. Cysts can be identified readily, but vegetative forms are recognized with difficulty.

TREATMENT AND PROGNOSIS

Antibiotics, other than spiramycin, have proved to be of little value in the treatment of toxoplasmosis. Sulfonamides have proved disappointing and sulfones too toxic in the doses required. The most effective form of chemotherapy is a combination of pyrimethamine, 1 mg/kg bodyweight per day and sulfadiazine 100 mg/kg bodyweight per day, for a total duration of 10–21 days. The hematological toxic effects of pyrimethamine, due to its antifolic acid action, can be prevented or reversed by folinic acid. Spiramycin, though less toxic than the pyrimethamine and sulfadiazine combination, is clearly less effective. An alternative is the use of a combination of trimethoprim and a sulfonamide, e.g. co-trimoxazole.

The major indication for the use of pyrimethamine and sulfadiazine is the presence of active *Toxoplasma gondii* infection, particularly when it is confirmed or strongly suspected in the newborn. Treatment may also be indicated in active ocular infection; concurrent administration of prednisolone is believed to assist in preventing spread of existing lesions of the choroid retina.

The prognosis of congenital toxoplasmosis varies greatly with the severity and timing of fetal infection and the distribution of the lesions. In acquired toxoplasmosis the prognosis is almost uniformly good.

GIARDIASIS

Giardia lamblia is a relatively common parasitic cause of diarrhea in children. The active form or trophozoite is a pear-shaped flagellated protozoan measuring about 9–21 μm in length and 5–15 μ in width. Variations in the organism have been identified in different isolates, e.g. in the DNA-binding patterns or surface antigens. These differences together with a number of nonimmune and immune host factors may partly explain the great variation in the severity and duration of giardiasis (Pickering & Engelkirk 1988).

Epidemiology and pathogenesis

Giardiasis is encountered worldwide but often comes to public attention in developed countries only when outbreaks are reported in travelers returning from parts of the world where the disease is particularly prevalent. The infestation commonly involves the duodenum and upper small intestine. Giardia is excreted usually in cyst form in the stools and infection may occur directly through hand-to-mouth transfer or indirectly from the ingestion of contaminated water or food. Most epidemics result from contaminated water. Epidemics from person-to-person transmission are particularly likely to occur in institutions for the mentally handicapped and among children in day-care centers. Children with immunodeficiency or who are immunodepressed from disease or treatment are particularly vulnerable to giardiasis.

Infection is endemic in Britain and principally involves children aged 5–10 years. There is a potential reservoir of infection in domestic pets (Winsland et al 1989). In many infected children the protozoon is a commensal but microscopic studies of material obtained by small intestinal biopsy have demonstrated a variety of lesions associated with intestinal giardiasis such as edema, round cell infiltration of the lamina propria and focal acute inflammation of the crypt epithelium.

Clinical features

After an incubation period of 1–2 weeks, a variety of clinical manifestations may occur. Children may excrete *Giardia* cysts yet be completely asymptomatic; they may have brief episodes of acute explosive infectious diarrhea, or they may have chronic debilitating diarrhea with failure to thrive. Commonly an episode of giardiasis is relatively short with or without low grade fever, nausea, anorexia, abdominal distention and flatulence. The stools are watery and foul smelling. In some children, particularly if debilitated, the diarrhea is more protracted with general malaise, abdominal cramps and weight loss. The stools may become greasy and foul smelling suggesting significant malabsorption. Giardiasis is relatively common in cystic fibrosis and will contribute to the malabsorption of fat and fat-soluble vitamins (Roberts et al 1988). Chronic giardiasis may interfere with the absorption of drugs and at times may account for a lack of clinical response to drugs such as antibiotics.

Diagnosis and differential diagnosis

Giardiasis should be suspected in infants and children suffering from chronic or recurrent diarrhea and from recurrent abdominal pain when associated with malaise and poor general health.

The trophozoite is readily recognizable on simple wet film microscopy of a suspension of fresh stool, but because intermittent excretion of the organism occurs, several stool specimens from different days may be necessary. Specimens should be examined within an hour of being passed. If this is not possible they should be transmitted to the laboratory in a preservative (e.g. polyvinyl alcohol or 10% formalin), but it is best to check with the local laboratory before dispatch. Some laboratories base their diagnosis on cyst identification, especially on specimens received late or from a distance. Examination of duodenal or jejunal aspirate or biopsy material is more reliable and should be carried out in cases where stool specimens are negative in spite of a convincing history. False negative results are common, possibly produced by altered morphology or by the temporary disappearance of the parasite after the use of various medications such as antibiotics, antacids or antidiarrheal drugs. As far as possible oral drugs should be withheld for 72 h prior to the collection of stool specimens.

Countercurrent immunoelectrophoresis (CIE) and enzyme-linked immunosorbent assay (ELISA) are available as complementary techniques to microscopic diagnosis. The ELISA appears to be more sensitive for *G. lamblia* than stool microscopy. It is a useful test in assessing and controlling community outbreaks and for confirming clinical diagnoses (Addiss et al 1991).

Treatment

Only symptomatic infections should be treated as the benefits and risks of treating asymptomatic carriers have not been established. Indeed healthy day-care children with asymptomatic infection show no disadvantage. (Ish-Horowicz et al 1989). The generally accepted treatment of symptomatic intestinal giardiasis is the oral administration of metronidazole (15–20 mg/kg/day) three times daily for 1 week.

An alternative, indeed more effective, drug is *mepacrine* given in a dose of 50 mg twice daily for children aged 1–5 years and 100 mg twice daily for those aged 5–10 years. Unfortunately its use in children is limited by a bitter taste and a tendency to induce vomiting. *Tinidazole* similar to metronidazole has a longer plasma half-life and can be given as a single dose. In the US *furazolidone* is more popular with children as it is the only drug available in liquid suspension. A dose of 6 mg/kg/day is divided into four doses.

Control measures

In nurseries and child care centers personal hygiene should be emphasized. Handwashing by staff and children should be stressed particularly after toileting and handling soiled napkins. In outbreaks, efforts would be made to identify and treat all symptomatic children, family members and staff who are infected with *Giardia*. Persons with diarrhea should be excluded until asymptomatic, but treating asymptomatic carriers has not proved effective in controlling outbreaks.

Prognosis

The prognosis is excellent except in immunocompromised children where relapse is common and treatment may need to be continued for prolonged periods. At the same time attention must be paid to adequate nutrition and the treatment of concurrent infections.

AMEBIC INFECTIONS

Amebae are characterized by two forms, the motile feeding trophozoite and the cyst. The cyst has a rigid wall resistant to environmental conditions which allows it to survive for variable periods without feeding. The major ameba of importance to man is *Entamoeba histolytica* which is anaerobic and an obligate parasite of the gut. It has to be differentiated from other nonpathogenic gut amebae, e.g. *E. coli* and *E. hartmanni*. There are a number of free-living aerobic amebae which are found in the soil and feed on bacteria in muddy water. In dry conditions the cysts may be dispersed by wind. Two species that are pathogenic to man and may cause meningoencephalitis are *Naegleria fowleri* and the opportunist *Acanthamoeba culbertsoni*.

AMEBIASIS

Amebiasis is caused by *E. histolytica* and is transmitted by the fecal–oral route. Sewage contamination of water supplies, infection by food handlers and direct fecal contact from person to person, as may occur in mental institutions, have been identified as sources of infection. Transmission by sexual contact, especially among homosexuals, also occurs. It is worldwide in distribution with a high prevalence in tropical countries where hygiene is poor.

There are two groups of *E. histolytica*, pathogenic and nonpathogenic (Reed 1992). Only the pathogenic strains are able to invade tissue and produce disease. The two groups are morphologically identical but cultured pathogenic and nonpathogenic strains can be distinguished by a number of processes, viz. isoenzyme or zymodeme patterns, monoclonal antibodies and gene probes. Pathogenic amebae engage in active erythrophagocytosis, but nonpathogenic strains ingest few red blood cells. Infection by nonpathogenic strains is always, and by pathogenic strains is often, asymptomatic.

Why pathogenic strains are activated to invade is not known. Malnutrition, pregnancy, ulcerative colitis, immunosuppression, corticosteroids, and intercurrent infection by bacteria or parasites may be precipitating factors. Ulcerative colitis should not be treated with corticosteroids until amebiasis has been excluded.

The majority of amebae detected in carriers in nonendemic areas are noninvasive. The incidence of disease does not necessarily correlate with prevalence of infection. Invasive disease is reported, particularly from southeast Asia, Natal (South Africa), the west coast of Africa, Mexico and parts of South America. In the US, infection is associated especially with children of Hispanic origin.

Perinatal transmission occurs and there have been reports of amebic liver abscess presenting within the neonatal period.

Pathogenesis and pathology

Infection occurs from ingestion of cysts which on digestion release trophozoites. The trophozoites feed on bacteria and fecal matter in the cecum and further down the colon. When they reach areas where the feces are more solid they encyst and the cysts are passed in the stool. Trophozoites may be detected in the stool if there is no intestinal hurry, but the presence of either trophozoites or cysts is not necessarily indicative of invasive disease. However, the presence of hematophagous trophozoites (containing ingested red blood cells) is usually suggestive of invasion. Invasion is accomplished by lytic enzymes secreted by the trophozoites which result in tissue necrosis and erosion of blood vessels but with a surprising lack of inflammatory response. Initial lesions are small superficial erosions. With progression they penetrate the muscularis mucosae and may expand to produce flask-shaped ulcers. Further extension may result in intestinal perforation but more commonly the parasite is carried to the liver in the portal vein and rarely to other organs such as the lung, heart or brain. The colonic lesions may vary from small pinhead erosions confined to the cecum and rectosigmoid to extensive, deep, confluent ulcers extending throughout the colon. It is probable that the majority of amebae reaching the liver do not cause detectable disease. Possibly, an area of tissue necrosis is necessary for the disease to be established. Similarly to the bowel, liver abscess is characterized by localized necrosis without much inflammatory response unless there is secondary infection.

Clinical features

The major organs affected in invasive amebic disease are the colon, the liver and adjacent organs, such as the right lung, pericardium and rarely the skin or eye.

Intestinal amebiasis

Intestinal amebiasis has a wide spectrum of severity. It may occur within a few weeks of infection or be delayed several months. There may be mild intermittent diarrhea with blood and mucus accompanying the fecal material usually with no systemic upset or fever. Severe fulminating dysentery is associated with watery, bloodstained, mucoid stools resulting in dehydration, electrolyte disturbance and toxemia. Abdominal pain, tenesmus and tenderness may be present. Perforation, which is often multiple with slow leakage, and peritonitis may occur. Other complications include hemorrhage, ameboma, stricture, intussusception and rectal prolapse. Chronic or relapsing dysentery may occur unless the initial attack has been managed by adequate chemotherapy and nutritional support.

Enlargement of the liver may occur without evidence of an abscess, presumably the result of toxic products transported in the portal vein from the diseased bowel.

Liver abscess and related disorders

Liver abscesses may be single or multiple and more often involve the right lobe. Multiple abscesses are common in young children (Fig. 23.48). The liver is tender and, if the abscess is situated anteriorly, a mass is commonly visible (Fig. 23.49). There is nearly always fever and usually anemia, leukocytosis and raised ESR. Jaundice is infrequent and serum transaminases are usually not raised. There is a history of previous, or evidence of concomitant, dysentery in only half the cases. In over two-thirds of cases elevation and immobility of the right diaphragm produces corresponding signs in the right lung.

Complications of amebic liver abscess include secondary bacterial infection, extension or rupture into the peritoneal cavity, the pleural cavity and/or the lung. Involvement of the left lobe of the liver may result in a pericardial effusion or rupture into the pericardium. Rarely, there may be extension to abdominal organs including the stomach, gut or kidneys. Blood-borne spread may result in a brain or lung abscess.

Skin

Cutaneous amebiasis may be associated with rupture of a liver abscess, colostomy stomata or a laparotomy incision. In infants, amebic abscess of the perineum may result from direct contact with infected feces (Fig. 23.50).

Diagnosis

The diagnosis of amebic dysentery is based on the finding of motile, hematophagous *E. histolytica* trophozoites in feces. Red cells, bacteria but few leukocytes are usually present. Examination

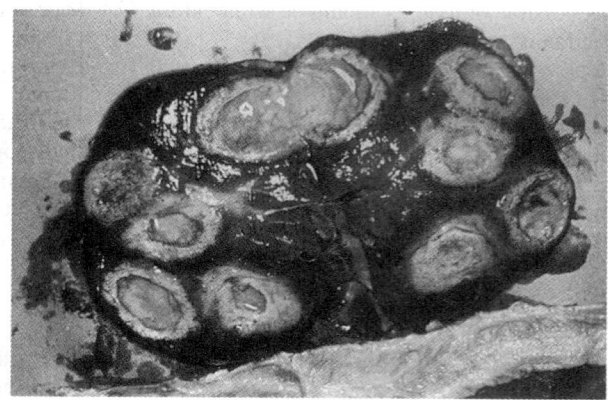

Fig. 23.48 Typical multiple amebic abscesses in the liver of an infant aged 8 months.

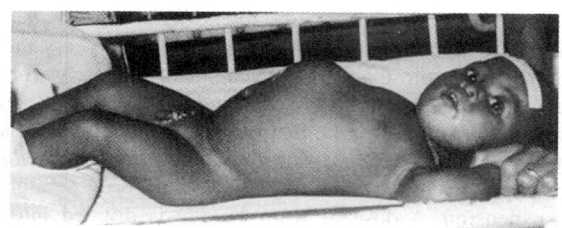

Fig. 23.49 An African infant of 10 months with a large amebic liver abscess presenting as a fluctuant mass in the epigastrium.

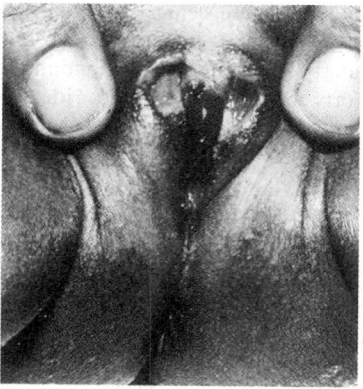

Fig. 23.50 Cutaneous amebiasis involving the vulva in an infant aged 5 months.

of a freshly passed warm stool is important because, when the stool cools, the amebae stop moving and release the contained red cells in their vacuoles. Three or more stool examinations may be necessary and both direct and concentrated methods should be used. Proctoscopy or sigmoidoscopy may demonstrate amebic ulcers which are usually shallow, covered with a yellowish-gray exudate and contain numerous hematophagous trophozoites. The intervening mucosa is often relatively normal in appearance. Antibody titers may be raised and in endemic areas are diagnostic in young children, but their presence in older children does not distinguish between past and current infection.

The definite diagnosis of amebic liver abscess is made by aspiration of bacteriologically sterile pus. The pus is usually gray-yellow at the first aspiration and only at subsequent aspirations takes on the pink or red-brown 'anchovy' color. Amebae are seldom detected in necrotic material from the center of the abscess but are more common in the walls of the cavity and thus are more likely to be detected in the last portions of the aspirate.

In most cases an ultrasound scan can localize and delineate the size of the abscess cavity. More than 95% of abscesses may be detected by CT scan. Differential diagnosis includes pyogenic abscess and hydatid disease. X-ray and screening may demonstrate a raised diaphragm with reduced movement and there may be an effusion or other signs of inflammation at the lung base. Usually there is a leukocytosis and a raised ESR. Antibody titers are usually high and may be detected in serum in over 95% of cases. A number of different methods are used including indirect hemagglutination, agar gel diffusion, fluorescent antibody test, counterimmunoelectrophoresis and ELISA. ELISA has high sensitivity and specificity and usually becomes negative 6–12 months after response to treatment whereas indirect hemagglutination titers may remain raised for many years. For reasons unknown, infection is only detected in the stool in about one-third of cases, and usually only cysts are present.

Management

Chemotherapy of invasive amebiasis must include drugs which can eliminate amebae both from the lumen of the bowel and the tissues. Metronidazole and tinidazole achieve both but are less effective as lumenal amebicides.

For asymptomatic patients and following invasive disease the lumenal amebicide diloxanide furoate 20 mg/kg/day in three divided doses for 10 days, is the treatment of choice. In endemic areas older asymptomatic children are usually not treated as reinfection is so common.

In symptomatic intestinal disease metronidazole or tinidazole is recommended. Metronidazole 35–50 mg/kg/day in three divided doses orally is given for 5–10 days depending on the severity of the infection. Side effects such as nausea and a metallic taste in the mouth may make compliance difficult. Alternatively, oral tinidazole 50–60 mg/kg is given as a single dose for 5 days. Both drugs may also be given intravenously. In severe colitis, correction of fluid and electrolyte imbalance is important, and gastric suction is necessary when there is ileus. Blood transfusion may be required. Broad spectrum antibiotics may be necessary if septicemia or other infection is suspected. Perforation of the bowel with leakage into the peritoneum may require surgery.

For liver abscess, metronidazole or tinidazole is effective and is given in doses similar to intestinal disease. In difficult cases, chloroquine 10 mg/kg/day in two divided doses may be added and given for 3 weeks. The second-line drugs dehydroemetine and emetine are rarely required and limited by adverse effects. Diloxanide furoate should be given to eradicate the bowel infection.

Indications for aspiration of the abscess include: suspected pyogenic abscess (particularly when there are multiple lesions), a palpable mass, a markedly raised diaphragm, failure of symptoms to remit after 72 h of drug therapy, and abscess in the left lobe. Aspiration, by relieving the pressure within the liver tissues, allows better drug penetration of the abscess. Surgical evacuation may be necessary for multiple or inaccessible abscesses, or when secondary infection has occurred. For needle aspiration, a wide-bore needle with a three-way tap should be used and the abscess cavity evacuated fully. Aspiration is usually through the right chest wall at the point of maximum tenderness, or through the abdomen if the abscess is superficial. Aspiration should be guided by ultrasound scan. Repeat aspiration may be necessary.

Resolution of the abscess cavity may take many months. Follow-up should be made to ensure complete eradication of infection otherwise relapse may occur.

NAEGLERIA AND ACANTHAMOEBA

Two distinct types of meningoencephalitis are caused by free-living amebae: primary amebic meningoencephalitis by *Naegleria fowleri* and granulomatous amebic encephalitis, usually by *Acanthamoeba culbertsoni* (Simon & Wilson 1986, Ma et al 1990). Acanthamoeba infections of the cornea particularly associated with contact lenses are an increasing problem.

Primary amebic meningoencephalitis

This is an acute necrotizing meningoencephalitis where *N. fowleri* gains access to the nasal cavities and results in direct invasion of the nervous system through the olfactory apparatus. There is usually a history of swimming under water or diving in warm fresh water or hot springs. In Nigeria there are reports of infection from cysts, transmitted in dust, colonizing the nasal cavities of children (Lawande 1980). The cerebrospinal fluid (CSF) has changes similar to bacterial meningitis, viz. a predominant neutrophil count, often accompanied by red cells, a raised protein (usually > 1 g/l) and low glucose concentration. Careful search for trophozoites should be undertaken on fresh CSF. Nasal secretions or washings should also be examined for amebae.

The course of the disease is usually rapidly fulminating within 3–6 days. Intravenous and intraventricular (through a reservoir) amphotericin is the main treatment. In addition miconazole is usually given by the intravenous and intrathecal route and rifampicin orally. Duration of therapy is 8–10 days.

Granulomatous amebic encephalitis

This is a slowly progressive disease occurring in immuno-suppressed individuals. Infection by acanthamebae may result from swallowing or inhaling cysts, or by direct skin or corneal contact. The CSF shows a lymphocytosis, a raised protein and low or normal glucose. Acanthamoeba may be detected in histological specimens. Serology may also be of value.

Severe brain damage may have occurred by the time diagnosis is made. Suggested drugs for treatment include polymyxin B, pentamidine isethionate and sulfadiazine.

Acanthamoeba keratitis

Most cases of acanthamoeba keratitis are associated with use of contact lenses owing to a combination of abrasions of the cornea and contamination of the lens from washing in homemade solutions, especially fresh or tap water.

Treatment is difficult and often involves keratoplasty. Local application of 0.1% propamidine isethionate solution, 0.15% dibromopropamidine ointment and neomycin have been used. Local 1% clotrimazole may also be of value. Corticosteroids are required to control inflammation. Only fresh, sterile, commercial solutions should be used to clean contact lens.

BALANTIDIASIS

Balantidium coli is a parasite of pigs which may colonize the colon of man producing a disease similar to *E. histolytica* but extracolonic disease does not occur. Treatment is with metronidazole or tetracycline for 8–10 days.

FUNGAL INFECTIONS

Infections due to the fungi known as dermatophytes are described in Chapter 25. Other fungus infections in infancy and childhood fall into two main groups:

1. *Superficial infections* with *Candida* species, thriving on intact surfaces, seldom invading deeper structures and in general, responding to topical treatment. *Sporotrichosis* is a fungal infection which usually involves the skin primarily and can occur in childhood.
2. Infections known as the *deep mycoses* caused by fungi which enter the body, usually via the respiratory and alimentary tracts and which may spread to other organs. Such infections are actinomycosis, aspergillosis, blastomycosis, coccidioidomycosis, cryptococcosis, histoplasmosis and nocardiosis. Treatment is generally by the use of systemic antibiotics, in most instances amphotericin B or ketoconazole (Table 23.45). To prevent repetition, details of dose, administration and toxic effects of amphotericin B and of other systemic antifungal agents are described at the end of the section.

Systemic fungal infections have assumed increasing importance in immunosuppressed children including the very low birthweight infant, those undergoing treatment by radiation and cytotoxic drugs and those suffering from acquired immune-deficiency syndrome.

MONILIASIS (CANDIDOSIS, CANDIDIASIS)

AETIOLOGY

Candida species have a worldwide distribution. They grow in the form of budding ovoid yeast cells and as nonbranching filaments or hyphae. Both yeasts and hyphal forms are Gram positive. In humans, the fungus commonly exists as a saprophytic yeast form in body cavities or clefts, and less often in intact skin and can be isolated in healthy persons from the oral cavity (30%), gastrointestinal tract (38%) and vagina (59%). Under certain environmental conditions the organism can assume a pathogenic

mycelial form. At least seven *Candida* species have been recognized as pathogenic in man; by far the most important is *Candida albicans*.

Candida albicans is commonly pathogenic in the newborn, but in older children, as in adults, lesions due to *C. albicans* infection are associated with certain predisposing factors, including antibiotic or corticosteroid therapy and pre-existing diseases, particularly those involving the reticuloendothelial system.

The source of *C. albicans* infection in the newborn is most commonly the vagina of the mother, demonstrated by the strong relationship between the frequency of isolation of the fungus from mothers and the incidence of subsequent infection in their infants. The role of cross-infection is much less important than was once believed. The readiness with which oral moniliasis develops in otherwise healthy newborns appears to be due not only to the large size of inoculum but also to deficient humoral factors. Serum anticandidal activity in newborns is low, with titers in the region of 1 : 128, compared with levels rising to 1 : 4000 in adults.

Antibiotics do not enhance the growth of *C. albicans* in vitro and may act by suppression of gut flora, some of which produce anticandidal components. Similarly corticosteroids have no in vitro effect, and may predispose to *C. albicans* infection by impairing the host's local or humoral resistance to infection. Certain diseases, particularly diabetes mellitus, acute and chronic leukemia, myeloma and Hodgkin's disease are known to predispose to moniliasis. *C. albicans* infection is associated with deficiency of thymus-mediated ('T-cell') immunity, e.g. in the DiGeorge syndrome, and the association in a newborn of severe moniliasis and intractable hypocalcemia should raise the suspicion of this diagnosis. Intractable *C. albicans* infection is also a common complication of hypoparathyroidism. The frequency of superficial monilial infection in patients with diabetes mellitus has been attributed to high free glucose levels in the skin. In diseases of the reticuloendothelial system, low levels of serum anticandidal activity have been described.

The lesions of moniliasis follow rapid proliferation of the pathogenic mycelial form. In the commonest form, oral moniliasis, the lesions are superficial plaques, but appearances vary with the site of the infection.

CLINICAL FEATURES

Superficial moniliasis

In *oral moniliasis* (thrush) in the newborn the typical lesions are gray-white plaques, on a background of inflamed mucosa. They are pliable and adherent and if scraped off, leave a raw red base. Lesions are commonly found on the buccal mucosa, tongue and gums but may extend to the pharynx, esophagus and trachea. In many infants there are associated scaly macular or vesicular erythematous perianal lesions with clearly defined margins. Oral moniliasis, by causing pain and discomfort may hinder feeding, and, in a small proportion, extension to the esophagus may occur with consequent refusal to feed and vomiting. Pulmonary infection rarely follows oral moniliasis in newborns but may occur as a complication of the infection in older children. Premature infants are particularly liable to thrush.

Chronic superficial infections may occur in older children. Diffuse *Cutaneous C. albicans infection* of the skin has been reported in some children suffering from acrodermatitis enteropathica, in which an erythematous papulovesicular or

Table 23.45 Systemic fungus infections

Disease	Causative organism	Geographical distribution	Predominant clinical features	Treatment
Actinomycosis	*Actinomyces israelii*	Worldwide	Abscesses and sinuses in face and neck, lungs, abdomen	Benzyl penicillin*
Aspergillosis	*Aspergillus* species	Worldwide	Granulomata of lungs, skin or generalized	Nystastin aerosol*, i.v. amphotericin B* or oral ketoconazole or itraconazole
North American blastomycosis	*Blastomyces dermatitidis*	North America	Granulomata of lungs or generalized	i.v. amphotericin B* or oral itraconazole
South American blastomycosis	*Blastomyces brasiliensis*	South America	Ulcerating granulomata of oropharynx, lungs or generalized	i.v. amphotericin B* or oral itraconazole
Coccidioido-mycosis (San Joaquin Valley fever)	*Coccidioides immitis*	North and South America	Influenza-like illness. Progressive pulmonary or central nervous system infection in minority	i.v. amphotericin B* or 5-fluorocytosine* or i.v. miconazole* or oral itraconazole
Cryptococcosis (torulosis)	*Cryptococcus neoformans*	Worldwide	Chiefly central nervous system infection, meningoencephalitis, or focal lesion	i.v. amphotericin B* or oral itraconazole
Histoplasmosis	*Histoplasma capsulatum*	Central USA	Granulomata in lungs, or in miliary distribution	i.v. amphotericin B* or oral itraconazole
Moniliasis	*Candida* sp., usually *albicans*	Worldwide	Usually superficial infection. Systemic resembles septicemic illness	i.v. amphotericin B* or 5-fluorocytosine* or oral itraconazole
Nocardiosis	*Nocardia asteroides* or *brasiliensis*	Worldwide	Pulmonary suppuration, occasionally central nervous system infection	Sulfonamides*
Phycomycosis (mucormycosis)	*Phycomycetes*	Africa and Indonesia	Indurated subcutaneous swelling – neck, shoulder, upper arm, thighs, buttocks. Painless, nonulcerating tumor mass. General health good. Self-limiting. Diagnosis by biopsy	Potassium iodide 30 mg/kg/day for 4–6 weeks
Rhinosporidiosis	*Rhinosporidium seeberi*	India and Ceylon	Polypoid tumors of mucous membrane – nose, nasopharynx, conjunctival sac. Gelatinous lesions, bleeding easily. Diagnosis by microscopic examination of crushed fragments of polyp. Pulmonary and nasopalatal types with tissue destruction may occur in patients subject to severe metabolic disturbance	Surgical removal
Sporotrichosis	*Sporotichum schenckii*	Worldwide	Subcutaneous nodule (usually on hands or feet) which enlarges and adheres to skin and breaks down to form chronic ulcer. Satellite nodules develop by lymphatic spread. Usually localized but may be widely disseminated. Diagnosis by culture of exudate or scrapings or antibody tests. Extracutaneous forms involving muscles, lungs, eyes, CNS, urinary tract and widely disseminated may occur	For lymphangitic form, potassium iodide, 30 mg/kg/day up to maximum tolerance. For disseminated form i.v. amphotericin B or oral itraconazole

* See also Chapter 38.

pustular rash around body orifices is associated with paronychia, alopecia, diarrhea and retardation of growth. A familial incidence has been described, and the prognosis is poor. *Candida* has been isolated from the skin or alimentary tract in 55% of such children. The response to antifungal therapy is poor.

Deeper moniliasis

Monilial infection of deeper tissues and organs occurs rarely in otherwise healthy patients. Oral or *esophageal moniliasis* may be complicated by extension of infection to the *intestine*, typically with symptoms of diarrhea, abdominal pain and pruritus ani. The child may present with a celiac-like syndrome. In *pulmonary moniliasis* the symptoms of fever and productive cough sometimes with hemoptysis are nonspecific. On radiological examination, patchy consolidation is seen, and cavitation may occur with infections of sufficient duration. Pulmonary moniliasis should not be diagnosed too readily on the evidence of culture of *Candida* from sputum, since the organism may be isolated in a proportion of healthy individuals, or particularly from hospital patients.

Disseminated monilial infection, although very uncommon in infancy and childhood, is thought to be increasing in frequency and has been reported in debilitated infants and children, particularly those treated with antibiotics or corticosteroids or with diseases of the reticuloendothelial system, and in patients requiring prolonged intravenous therapy. Several *Candida* species have been isolated from such patients, whose clinical features are those of septicemia. Disseminated moniliasis, which can be confirmed by blood culture, should be suspected when a septicemic illness supervenes in debilitated infants or children in the course of antibacterial antibiotic therapy, especially in the presence of a portal of entry of the organism such as an indwelling intravenous cannula.

The isolation of *Candida* from a specimen of urine obtained by suprapubic aspiration is highly suggestive of disseminated infection. The appearance of papular lesions of skin containing *Candida* has been noted in preterm infants under such circumstances. Disseminated moniliasis also raises the possibility of hypogammaglobulinemia.

Monilial endocarditis, though rare, has been reported in childhood. Previously damaged heart valves are the site of localization of infection in a patient with disseminated *Candida* infection.

DIAGNOSIS AND DIFFERENTIAL DIAGNOSIS

Oral thrush can usually be diagnosed on observation of the typical lesion which may be confused with deposits of milk. The latter can be scraped off without effort, revealing a normal mucosal surface. Monilial napkin rash may be confused with ammoniacal dermatitis, and, although it is common for the two lesions to coexist, the sharply demarcated edges of the former and its association with oral thrush should suggest the diagnosis. Confirmation of superficial moniliasis is readily made by the finding of typical mycelia on microscopic examination and by culture of the organism from swabs from superficial lesions. Fecal material can be examined in the form of smears either stained with Gram stain or as wet films with 10% sodium hydroxide. Yeast cells are not significant as they occur in 15% of normal children but hyphal forms occur only with invasion of mucous membranes and their presence can therefore be taken as indication of enteric candidiasis.

The clinical and radiological features of pulmonary moniliasis can be confused with a number of subacute and chronic bacterial infections of the lungs. The presence of characteristic predisposing circumstances should suggest the diagnosis, especially if pulmonary cavitation is present. Laboratory confirmation is best made by repeated sputum culture or, preferably, by culture of tracheal or bronchial aspirate.

In disseminated moniliasis, the organism can be isolated by blood or urine culture.

TREATMENT AND PROGNOSIS

Oral moniliasis is best treated by local application of antifungal agents. Preparations in common use are suspensions of nystatin (100 000 units/ml) and miconazole (2% in a gel). Gentian violet (1% aqueous solution) is by far the cheapest but it is messy, may produce excoriation of buccal mucosa, and generally fails to eradicate the fungus from the lower alimentary tract and is now little used in western countries. Nystatin and miconazole are probably equally effective. Nystatin is given in a dose of 1.0–2.0 ml dropped in the oral cavity 4 to 6-hourly for 7–10 days while miconazole gel is given as 5.0 ml, two to four times each day. Apparent failure of such treatments is seldom, if ever, due to the presence of antibiotic-resistant species of *C. albicans*. While resistance to nystatin and amphotericin B by *Candida* species other than *C. albicans* can readily be induced in vitro, only a minor degree of diminished antibiotic sensitivity can be induced in *C. albicans*. A dose of 1 ml of nystatin by oral instillation 6-hourly may be inadequate; higher and more frequent doses should be employed if the infection appears to be unresponsive. In perianal forms of moniliasis of skin or nails, topical nystatin (100 000 units/g of ointment) or miconazole are effective. Oral therapy with either antibiotic is effective in monilial enteritis.

In the treatment of moniliasis of deeper structures and organs, oral nystatin therapy is not recommended, since absorption from the gastrointestinal tract is poor. Oral ketoconazole may be effective. In pulmonary moniliasis, nystatin may be administered by aerosol, e.g. 500 000 units in 15 ml distilled water. In systemic moniliasis and monilial endocarditis and probably in pulmonary moniliasis the most effective treatment is the intravenous administration of amphotericin B, 1 mg/kg per day (p. 1478). Recent reports have indicated that the liposomal amphotericin B (AmBisome) treatment is less toxic and at least equally effective. Flucytosine (p. 1478) has the advantages over amphotericin B of oral administration and lower toxicity. Many strains of *C. albicans* are resistant, however, and the drug cannot be administered parenterally to those patients too ill to take it by mouth. It should be reserved for those patients in whom amphotericin B has proved to be too toxic.

The prognosis of superficial moniliasis is excellent; that of monilial enteritis has to be guarded. Disseminated moniliasis carries a poor prognosis, largely related to the nature of the predisposing conditions. Meningeal moniliasis, however, may run a surprisingly mild course.

SPOROTRICHOSIS

ETIOLOGY

Sporotrichum schenckii is a fungus which thrives on living and dead vegetation. Disease usually follows inoculation of the pathogen into the skin but it can be acquired by ingestion or inhalation. Most of the reported cases in children have come from North America.

CLINICAL FEATURES

Child patients have been aged from 3 years upwards. The initial lesion is an ulcer of the skin with nodular changes in the course of its lymphatic drainage and regional lymphadenopathy. The face and limbs tend to be involved. There is often some degree of erythema and tenderness adjacent to the primary ulcer. There is little constitutional upset. Rarely, extracutaneous sporotrichosis involving the lung has been reported. A disseminated, extracutaneous form may follow the development of a primary focus, especially in children with immunological suppression.

DIAGNOSIS AND DIFFERENTIAL DIAGNOSIS

Diagnosis is made by culturing *S. schenckii* from the primary lesion. Aspiration of subcutaneous nodules has also revealed the organism. Agglutination and complement fixation tests are also available. The differential diagnosis is from coccidioidomycosis, blastomycosis, histoplasmosis, tuberculosis, leishmaniasis, syphilis, anthrax, tularemia and cat scratch disease.

TREATMENT

Iodides are specific for the lymphangitic form. Potassium iodide is given in the form of the concentrated solution starting with 1–5 drops (50 mg/drop) three times per day according to age and increasing over 10 days to 10–40 drops three times per day. Treatment should be continued for a minimum of 4–6 weeks after healing of the lesion. Amphotericin B should be used in the treatment of the disseminated form. *S. schenckii is* sensitive in vitro to imidazoles.

ACTINOMYCOSIS

ETIOLOGY

Actinomycosis, affecting humans and certain animals, is a disease of worldwide distribution caused by the Gram-positive anaerobic branching filamentous actinomycete *Actinomyces israelii*, which also occurs as a saprophyte on mucous surfaces, especially in the oropharynx, and in the gastrointestinal tract.

PATHOGENESIS

Actinomyces israelii on invading the tissues produces a characteristic granulomatous suppurative lesion. The lesions commonly occur in the cervicofacial region, the abdomen and the lungs. Trauma, such as dental extraction or fractures predispose to infection in the cervicofacial region, probably by providing devitalized tissue suitable for anaerobic growth. Infection produces dense cellular infiltration, with abscess and sinus formation. On examination, actinomycotic 'sulfur' granules are seen in infected tissue. Similar lesions occur in the lungs, which are probably infected by aspiration from the oropharynx. Histologically, the granules consist of mycelial filaments. The organism can infect the apparently healthy gastrointestinal tract, usually the cecum or appendix, with later spread to other tissues on draining of sinuses to the surface.

CLINICAL FEATURES

The disease in uncommon, particularly in children, although a small series has been reported (Drake & Holt 1976). Actinomycosis of the cervicofacial region is the commonest form and is seen as a brawny swelling in the region of the mandible, with later, the formation of one or more sinuses over the mandibular region. Less often the tongue, pharynx or bone may be infected. Regional lymph glands are seldom involved.

Infection of the lungs by *Actinomyces israelii* produces subacute or chronic pulmonary disease, with multiple abscess formation and progressive lung destruction. Lesions are commonly found in the lung bases, while spread to pleura and thoracic wall may occur. Fever, cough and the production of purulent sputum with hemoptysis are common symptoms. Consolidation and multiple small abscess cavities are seen on radiological examination.

In abdominal actinomycosis, the common presenting feature is an abdominal mass, which progresses to fluctuation and possible sinus formation.

DIAGNOSIS AND DIFFERENTIAL DIAGNOSIS

Actinomycosis of the cervicofacial area is suspected from the typical lesion, and confirmed by histological examination and by culture of the actinomycete. It must be distinguished from other indolent suppurative infections of the area, including chronic pyogenic osteitis, and tuberculosis. Pulmonary actinomycosis may closely resemble other subacute or chronic lung infections, including bronchiectasis and pulmonary tuberculosis. Repeated culture of sputum or bronchial aspirate and histological examination will confirm the diagnosis.

The mass typical of abdominal actinomycosis may mimic an appendix abscess, abdominal tuberculosis or carcinoma of the intestine. Laparotomy with examination of the pus obtained may be necessary to establish the diagnosis.

Infection with the fungus *Nocardia asteroides* produces clinical features similar to actinomycosis. Differentiation, chiefly by cultural methods, is of importance since the sensitivity of the two fungi to antibiotics differs greatly.

Serological methods are unreliable in the diagnosis of actinomycosis, probably owing to the existence of several serotypes of *Actinomyces israelii*.

TREATMENT AND PROGNOSIS

Actinomyces israelii is sensitive in vitro to benzyl penicillin, streptomycin and isoniazid. Benzyl penicillin is the antibiotic of choice; most strains are inhibited by concentrations of 0.01–0.5 units/ml although occasional strains show degrees of resistance. In 1952, Garrod showed that the minimal concentration of benzyl penicillin required to kill whole colonies of the fungus was five times higher than for ground up colonies. Benzyl penicillin should therefore be given in a high dose 1–6 million units daily, by intramuscular injection and treatment must be prolonged, if necessary, for 6–8 months. *Actinomyces israelii* is not sensitive in vitro or in vivo to the polyene antifungal antibiotics. Antibiotic therapy must often be complemented by surgical drainage of actinomycotic pus. Ciprofloxacin may be effective in cases recalcitrant to penicillin (Macfarlane et al 1993).

The prognosis, owing to modern treatment, is good although pulmonary actinomycosis in particular may require prolonged and energetic treatment.

ASPERGILLOSIS

ETIOLOGY

Aspergillosis is a fungus infection of worldwide distribution affecting several mammalian species and birds. The causative organism of human infection is usually *Aspergillus fumigatus*, although *A. flavus, A. versicolor, A. nidulans, A. oryzae, A. glaucus* and *A. sydiovii* have also been proved to be pathogenic in man. These organisms are found widely in nature and are common laboratory contaminants. Aspergillosis is frequently acquired by workers in areas of high contamination, particularly stables, barns, flour mills and aviaries.

PATHOGENESIS

Aspergillosis may occur in previously healthy children, but more often occurs in the presence of debilitating disease or as a complication of corticosteriod or antibiotic therapy (Walmsley et al 1993). Pulmonary aspergillosis is the commonest form of the disease, and usually complicates pre-existing diseases such as pulmonary tuberculosis, pneumonia, bronchiectasis, and especially cystic fibrosis. In the respiratory tract *Aspergillus* species proliferate in the bronchial tree, or produce diffuse pulmonary infiltration. Local lung necrosis may occur, with dense surrounding inflammatory and granulation tissue – an aspergilloma.

Disseminated aspergillosis, involving virtually all or any organs, has a strong association with severe debilitating and usually malignant disease, particularly carcinoma, leukemia and lymphoma and with corticosteroid and antibacterial therapy.

CLINICAL FEATURES

The clinical features of pulmonary aspergillosis may resemble bronchitis or diffuse pneumonitis. The most common form, the bronchopulmonary aspergilloma, is localized in bronchial or lung tissue. The area of lung affected may be the site of bronchiectasis or tuberculosis. Recurrent hemoptysis is frequent, and on radiological examination the diagnosis is suggested by the presence of a cavitated lesion with a solid center, especially if there exists a crescent of air between the solid center and the wall of the cavity, and if the center is mobile.

The clinical features of disseminated aspergillosis resemble those of septicemia and vary with the organs involved.

DIAGNOSIS

Confirmation of diagnosis depends on culture of *A. fumigatus* or other pathogenic *Aspergillus* species, from blood or sputum. The possibility of laboratory contamination by the fungus makes repeated examination advisable. Histological examination of biopsy material and demonstration of characteristic hyphal elements provides valuable confirmation. Hildick-Smith et al (1964) provide comprehensive reviews of the pathogenesis, clinical features and management of aspergillosis.

TREATMENT AND PROGNOSIS

Antibacterial drugs are of little value in the management of aspergillosis. Pulmonary aspergillosis is best managed by surgical removal of localized lesions, combined with administration of antifungal antibiotics. Nystatin, too toxic for systemic administration, may be given in aerosol suspension, and amphotericin B by aerosol or, preferably, by the intravenous route for 1–3 months (p. 1478). Oral itraconazole is a less toxic alternative. The prognosis of pulmonary aspergillosis has been considerably improved by such therapy. Natamycin in a 2.5% solution may be given by aerosol. *Aspergillus* is sensitive in vitro to clotrimazole, but the drug appears to be too toxic for systemic administration.

Systemic aspergillosis carries a poor prognosis, in part due to the serious nature of the debilitating condition often present. The intravenous administration of amphotericin B is the treatment of choice.

BLASTOMYCOSIS

ETIOLOGY

Infections caused by *Blastomyces dermatitidis* are titled North American blastomycosis, while *Blastomyces brasiliensis* causes South American blastomycosis.

PATHOGENESIS

North American blastomycosis is endemic in the southern, southeastern and mid-western areas of the United States. Infection arising in other countries has not been reported. It is uncommon in children.

The organism can be isolated from the soil and from domestic animals. The portal of entry in humans is not known with certainty, but inhalation from the oropharynx is probable.

South American blastomycosis is contracted only in South America, the probable portal of entry being the oral cavity. As with its northern counterpart, children are seldom infected.

CLINICAL FEATURES

Both forms of blastomycosis are characterized by the formation of granulomatous lesions. In many patients the disease process is chronic and progressive.

North American blastomycosis most commonly involves the respiratory tract, resulting in clinical and radiological features resembling those of pulmonary tuberculosis. Erythema nodosum may be observed. A disseminated form of the disease is common, and may involve the skin, bones, central nervous system and the genitourinary system, producing granulomatous lesions which, in the skin, take the form of papulopustular nodules, which later enlarge and ulcerate.

South American blastomycosis most commonly produces ulcerating lesions of the oral mucosa which extend locally and by lymphatics. Subsequent dissemination to other tissues and organs may follow.

DIAGNOSIS AND DIFFERENTIAL DIAGNOSIS

Blastomycosis, although uncommon in children, should be suspected in patients from endemic areas, with superficial granulomatous and ulcerating lesions, especially if there is evidence of infection of other organs. In the differential diagnosis of either form of blastomycosis, tuberculosis and coccidioidomycosis should be considered since both may produce similar skin lesions and run an equally chronic and progressive course.

The diagnosis is best confirmed by culture of the fungus responsible and by histological examination of superficial lesions.

Immunological tests are of some value in North American blastomycosis. Skin tests using an antigen derived from *B. dermatitidis* yield a delayed tuberculin-type response, the value of which is reduced by cross-reactions with *Histoplasma capsulatum*.

TREATMENT AND PROGNOSIS

The prognosis of North American blastomycosis is extremely variable, but poor in the disseminated form, while disseminated South American blastomycosis is, if untreated, a progressively fatal disease. For both forms of blastomycosis, the intravenous administration of amphotericin B (p. 1478) is the treatment of choice, with oral itraconazole as a less toxic alternative.

COCCIDIOIDOMYCOSIS

ETIOLOGY

Coccidioidomycosis is most common in specific endemic areas of North and South America, especially in California and Argentina, but isolated cases have been described in other continents. It is caused by infection with the fungus *Coccidioides immitis* found as a saprophyte in mycelial form in the soil of endemic areas. Children and adults are affected alike.

PATHOGENESIS

Clinical studies of US Army personnel training in endemic areas have clarified the pathogenesis and clinical features of coccidioidomycosis. The incidence of infection in endemic areas may be as high as 90% and primary infection can take place at all ages. Nonwhites are more commonly affected.

Primary infection follows inhalation of spores of the fungus, which form, in lung or bronchial tissue, spherules which undergo protoplasmic division to form endospores which, in turn, are liberated into the tissues involved. The initial infection usually causes no symptoms or may result in a transient febrile illness arising 10–18 days after infection. In the majority, the disease progresses no further, but in a small proportion, estimated at 5%, postprimary pulmonary infection may follow, with pulmonary fibrosis, hilar lymphadenopathy and, in a few, lung cavitation.

In a very small minority of those primarily infected, disseminated coccidioidomycosis ensues, with the development of granulomatous lesions in skin or bone. Single or multiple cold abscess formation with sinus formation is frequently observed in the disseminated form of the disease, which may pursue a fulminating, subacute or chronic course.

CLINICAL FEATURES

Smith (1955) studied a group of patients developing *primary coccidioidal infection* (incubation period 1–3 weeks) in an endemic area. Only 40% showed any clinical features of infection, chiefly a transient febrile illness, and in some, cough, chest pain, malaise and headache. Erythema nodosum was noted in 25% arising 6–16 days after the onset of symptoms. Signs of pulmonary infection varied from nonexisting or minimal to severe, with pneumonic consolidation, fever and production of purulent sputum.

Postprimary or *progressive coccidioidomycosis* (coccidioidal granuloma) represents dissemination of the disease in certain individuals. Pulmonary involvement produces fever, cough, purulent sputum and, if the pleural cavity is involved, pleuritic pain, but the disease may run a more subacute or chronic course. Secondary skin lesions may appear as large subcutaneous abscesses or bones may be involved. Meningitis and miliary dissemination are serious secondary forms. The rate of progress and the organs involved in disseminated coccidioidomycosis vary greatly and so, therefore, does the clinical picture.

DIAGNOSIS AND DIFFERENTIAL DIAGNOSIS

Coccidioidomycosis should be suspected in children in or from endemic areas, especially nonwhites, who develop an acute febrile illness. Primary coccidioidomycosis, with erythema nodosum, and especially with clinical features of primary pulmonary infection, is readily confused with primary tuberculosis, while postprimary pulmonary disease resembles postprimary tuberculosis.

The diagnosis may be confirmed by culture of the fungus if sputum is available but generally depends upon immunological methods. A positive tuberculin-type test to coccidioidin, an antigen preparation of the fungus, develops within 21 days of infection. The finding of a positive reaction to coccidioidin strongly suggests present or past infection, although cross-reactions with histoplasmosis and blastomycosis do occur. A positive precipitin-fixation test is suggestive of recent infection. The complement-fixation test titer may be raised to titers of 1 : 16 or more, most often in disseminated coccidioidomycosis.

TREATMENT AND PROGNOSIS (Graybill 1993)

Primary coccidioidomycosis seldom requires more than symptomatic treatment. Amphotericin B, the most effective drug, should in view of its toxicity be reserved for severe primary or postprimary pulmonary disease. Intravenous amphotericin B therapy is, however, essential in disseminated coccidioidomycosis and, where there is infection of the central nervous system, may be given by intrathecal injection. Until recently the only alternative form of therapy was intravenous miconazole but oral itraconazole has been shown to be of value and of relatively low toxicity.

The prognosis of primary coccidioidomycosis is excellent, while that of postprimary pulmonary disease is good. Disseminated coccidioidomycosis carries a poor prognosis, especially with meningeal infection, unless treated vigorously and at an early stage.

CRYPTOCOCCOSIS (TORULOSIS)

ETIOLOGY

Cryptococcosis is an uncommon infection in man, caused by one species of fungus, *Cryptococcus neoformans*, formerly named *Torula histolytica*; the disease was previously known as torulosis or European blastomycosis. The organism possesses a capsule and elaborates a toxic polysaccharide product. It occurs widely throughout the world, being isolated from air, soil, milk, fruit and from healthy individuals. Diseases of the reticuloendothelial system and corticosteroid therapy are important predisposing factors, probably by interference with immunological mechanisms. Cryptococcosis is more common in adults than in children, but can occur at any age.

PATHOGENESIS

The portal of entry of *Cryptococcus neoformans* to the body is uncertain but infection probably follows inhalation of the fungus, although ingestion or direct inoculation are possible.

Tissues infected with *C. neoformans* show surprisingly little inflammatory and cellular response, and the immunological response of the body to infection is difficult to detect. The typical lesion produced is a cluster of encapsulated budding cells, loosely contained within a scanty framework of connective tissue. The fungal mass may excite the formation of granulation tissue but does not caseate. Masses of gelatinous material thus formed produce clinical features chiefly by compression. Any tissue may be involved, the central nervous system most frequently, producing meningoencephalitis or a localized cryptococcal granuloma. In a review of 220 published cases, only 19 were free of central nervous system involvement (Carton 1952). Cryptococcal meningitis is the most common type of meningitis due to fungal infection.

Pulmonary cryptococcosis, an uncommon form of the disease, may accompany meningeal infection or occur alone. There may be diffuse infiltration of peribronchial or miliary distribution, or solitary lesions.

In 15% of patients with cryptococcosis, usually in the disseminated form, skin and mucosal lesions occur. Bone and joints may be infected by dissemination of the fungus.

CLINICAL FEATURES

The most common clinical features of cryptococcosis in children or adults are those produced by central nervous system involvement. The disease may be of acute onset, with symptoms and signs of meningoencephalitis, or subacute with more gradually developing signs of meningeal irritation. In a proportion of patients enlarging cryptococcal lesions within the brain or spinal cord result in symptoms and signs of an expanding tumor of the central nervous system.

Pulmonary cryptococcosis may cause no symptoms, or may be accompanied by fever and a productive cough. Chest X-ray examination may show diffuse peribronchial or miliary-type infiltration or solitary masses.

The skin and mucosal lesions of cryptococcosis are protean, and may resemble acne, or present as abscesses, ulcers, granulomata or plaques. The most common lesion of the skin consists of circular erythematous papules exuding pus from the center.

DIAGNOSIS AND DIFFERENTIAL DIAGNOSIS

The diagnosis of cryptococcal meningoencephalitis may not be suspected until cerebrospinal fluid shows on microscopy the typical capsulated organism, which may be observed more readily by staining with Indian ink, or fluorescent antibody. By this observation, the condition may be differentiated from acute bacterial, tuberculous or viral meningitis or meningoencephalitis. The symptoms and signs are due to an enlarging cryptococcal mass in the brain or spinal cord and closely resemble those due to cysts or tumors, and again differentiation will depend chiefly upon the finding of C. neoformans in the cerebrospinal fluid or, more probably, upon examination of tissue removed at operation.

The organism may be isolated from the sputum in pulmonary cryptococcosis or from skin lesions.

Immunological and skin sensitivity tests are of little value.

PROGNOSIS AND TREATMENT

The prognosis of disseminated cryptococcosis, particularly with central nervous system involvement, is poor. No effective treatment existed before the introduction of amphotericin B in 1957. The antibiotic should be given intravenously in the maximum tolerated dose, until clinical and cerebrospinal fluid observations cease to indicate active infection. Intrathecal therapy is indicated in the gravely ill child, or in the case of failure of intravenous alone. An alternative is oral administration of flucytosine or itraconazole (p. 1478).

HISTOPLASMOSIS

ETIOLOGY

Histoplasmosis, thought at one time to be a protozoal infection, is caused by the fungus *Histoplasma capsulatum*, isolated from air, silos, bird and bat guano, and from soil especially that contaminated by chicken excreta. It is most commonly encountered in the east central area of the US, but cases have been reported from all continents. It occurs at all ages, but the disseminated form is most commonly encountered below the age of 2 years. A variant of histoplasmosis due to infection with *Histoplasma duboisii* has been described in Africa.

PATHOGENESIS

The clinical manifestations with *H. capsulatum* mostly result from the formation of granulomatous lesions. The fungus has a strong predilection for reticuloendothelial tissue. Histologically the lesions of histoplasmosis resemble tuberculous infection.

In the great majority of children, infection with the fungus is a brief, self-limiting disease with a focal pulmonary granuloma and hilar lymphadenopathy. Further progress of the infection within the lungs may result in a state of chronic pulmonary infection. In a very small number of patients, usually infants, the disseminated form of the disease occurs, with granulomata in many organs, particularly lungs, suparenal glands, liver, spleen and lymph nodes. Less often the brain, kidneys and intestine and occasionally the heart may be infected. Cutaneous or mucosal granulomata are often present in the disseminated stage of the disease.

CLINICAL FEATURES

The clinical manifestations of infection with *H. capsulatum* are well reviewed by Sweaney (1960) and Butler (1994). The *acute primary infection* resembles primary pulmonary tuberculosis in many respects. It is estimated that 65–75% of those infected develop no clinical disease, while the remainder experience an influenza-like illness, excepting 0.1–0.2% who progress to the generalized disseminated form. In the acute pulmonary infection, symptoms, if they occur, are malaise, fever, cough or chest pain. Chest X-ray reveals minimal changes or diffuse nodular densities with hilar lymphadenopathy. In the majority of patients healing ensues, and, in endemic areas, the finding of nontuberculous pulmonary calcification is commonly associated with a positive histoplasmin skin test. A chronic pulmonary form, with lung consolidation and cavitation is described, most commonly in middle-aged males. Cases have also been reported with abdominal pain and vomiting and in certain areas of America up to 10% of appendices removed under age 16 years showed evidence of histoplasmosis. In a review of symptomatic histoplasmosis in 32 children, 29 had clinical or radiological evidence, or both, of lung involvement. Chronic fever, peripheral lymphadenopathy and enlargement of liver and/or spleen were common findings, while four children had erythema nodosum. The histoplasmin skin test was positive in all (Kakos & Kilman 1973).

The *disseminated form* in children resembles in its clinical features acute miliary tuberculosis, with fever, cachexia and enlargement of liver, spleen and lymph nodes. Disseminated histoplasmosis has been reported in six children receiving chemotherapy for acute lymphoblastic leukemia; in all fever was present and in five, enlargement of liver and spleen. Cutaneous or mucosal granulomata should suggest the possibility of disseminated histoplasmosis, especially in endemic areas.

DIAGNOSIS AND DIFFERENTIAL DIAGNOSIS

Positive confirmation of histoplasmosis depends on isolation of the fungus. Identification is helped by the use of fluorescent antibody techniques.

A tuberculin-type response to the intradermal injection of histoplasmin, an antigenic preparation of the fungus, is of help in diagnosis and in epidemiological studies, but cross-reactions occur with *Coccidioides immitis* and *Blastomyces dermatitidis*. A positive complement-fixation titer is most often found in severe, chronic or disseminated histoplasmosis. Gram stain and culture of bone marrow may be very helpful in disseminated histoplasmosis.

Histoplasmosis should be suspected in endemic areas, and should be distinguished from primary pulmonary, miliary and postprimary tuberculosis, chiefly by the absence of laboratory confirmation of tuberculosis and by a positive histoplasmin test, or raised complement-fixation titer.

TREATMENT

The prognosis of primary pulmonary histoplasmosis is very good and no antifungal therapy is indicated. For other forms, however, the prognosis is guarded, while for the disseminated form of the disease, it is poor especially in infancy. In such patients good results have followed intravenous amphotericin B therapy, continued for periods of up to 30 days, and more recently from oral itraconazole.

NOCARDIOSIS

ETIOLOGY

Nocardiosis is caused by the fungi *Nocardia asteroides* and *Nocardia brasiliensis*, members of the order Actinomycetales. It is a fungus of worldwide distribution, isolated from soil and from mucous surfaces, especially in the respiratory tract. Infection can occur at any age, but the disease is more common in adults than in children although it may occur in children suffering from leukemia (particularly where immunosuppressive drugs are being used), diabetes mellitus and other debilitating conditions.

PATHOGENESIS

The characteristic lesion of nocardiosis is abscess formation, usually multiple, with central necrosis but little surrounding fibrous tissue reaction. Giant cells are uncommon, and the organism may be organized readily if it exists as beaded branching filaments. However, in its bacillary form it is morphologically indistinguishable from *Mycobacterium tuberculosis*, another member of the order Actinomycetales. Lesions are most commonly found in the lungs, but a disseminated form occurs in 30% of patients, involving the skin, kidneys and adrenals. In 5%

of patients, nocardial infection involves the central nervous system, either as diffuse meningitis or as localized abscess formation.

CLINICAL FEATURES

Pulmonary infection is found in 75% of patients with nocardiosis, alone or in association with disseminated infection, and may produce no symptoms. In other patients, malaise, cough, fever and dyspnea may develop. Hemoptysis is an uncommon symptom. Involvement of the central nervous system may result in the clinical features of meningoencephalitis, or, if the lesion is a single abscess, of a localized intracranial or intraspinous tumor.

DIAGNOSIS AND DIFFERENTIAL DIAGNOSIS

Nocardiosis produces no typical symptoms and signs. The pulmonary form may readily be confused with other suppurative conditions of the lung. Radiological examination of the chest provides no characteristic signs, the most common being patchy infiltration, possibly with cavitation. Diagnosis therefore depends upon isolation of the organism which may be distinguished with difficulty from *M. tuberculosis*.

The difficulty of producing suitable antigens has limited the value of dermal sensitivity testing.

TREATMENT AND PROGNOSIS

Prior to the advent of the sulfonamides, nocardial infection was usually fatal, and at present the outlook is poor, partly because of the nature of the predisposing conditions and partly because of delay in diagnosis.

The treatment of choice is prolonged administration of sulfonamides. Treatment may be necessary for several months, and may be combined with surgical treatment, for example lobectomy. It is recommended that sulfonamides be given in a dose adequate to maintain a blood level of not less than 10 mg/100 ml.

Treatment with antibiotics, including benzyl penicillin and chloramphenicol, has been reported to be successful on occasions and, as indicated by sensitivity of the organism in vitro, may be given in addition to sulfonamides.

MADURA FOOT

Two types of fungi, from the actinomycetes on the one hand and maduromycoses on the other, may cause a chronic infection of the foot. Subcutaneous nodules develop and may arrest at that stage or go on to form abscesses which spread to involve a progressively wider area. Ultimately, in progressive cases, the feet (and hands or other areas) show multiple sinuses discharging pus. Spontaneous healing of one sinus may be followed by development of another. There is little pain or constitutional upset.

Diagnosis is based on examination of the pus. Surgery is of benefit in early cases.

ANTIFUNGAL CHEMOTHERAPY (Warnock 1989, Ruhnke & Trautman 1994)

The majority of systemic fungal infections can be successfully treated by the use of intravenous amphotericin B. Nystatin and amphotericin B are similar in chemical structure and belong to the group of polyene antibiotics. They are macrolides with four to seven conjugated double bonds on the lactone ring. Nystatin is a tetrene, with four such bonds, and amphotericin B a heptene with seven. While both antibiotics can equally readily be employed in the treatment of superficial infections, especially moniliasis, the high degree of toxicity of nystatin precludes its systemic administration.

AMPHOTERICIN

Amphotericin B is active in vitro against a wide range of fungi, with minimum inhibitory concentrations ranging from 0.04 μg/ml for *H. capsulatum* to 1.9 μg/ml for *C. albicans*. It is poorly absorbed when given by mouth, and since its action is uncertain when given by intramuscular injection the intravenous route is preferred. Amphotericin B is slowly excreted by the kidneys over several days; accumulation of the drug is therefore probable.

Amphotericin should be given by continuous intravenous infusion over a 6-h period, dissolved in 5% dextrose, in an initial dose of 0.25 mg/kg bodyweight per day. Too rapid infusion may lead to convulsions and cardiac arrhythmias. The solution should be agitated frequently to avoid precipitation of the antibiotic. The dose should be gradually increased to an average daily dose of 1.0 mg/kg bodyweight per day, and should never exceed 1.5 mg/kg bodyweight per day. For intrathecal administration, doses of 0.1–0.5 or even 1.0 mg have been given in children, according to weight and tolerance of the drug.

The duration of parenteral amphotericin B therapy is dictated by the rate of disappearance of clinical and laboratory signs of fungus infection, but is usually 1–3 months.

Toxic effects are very common during parenteral amphotericin B therapy. Milder toxic effects include fever, rigors, anorexia and vomiting. The most important toxic effect is that of renal damage. The blood urea concentration should be measured frequently during treatment and, should it be elevated, treatment should be discontinued until the level has fallen to normal, when treatment can be commenced at a lower dose. Cardiac irregularities, even arrest may occur. Bone marrow depression and liver damage may occur. Liposomal amphotericin B (Ambisome) appears to be better tolerated and less toxic when given in a dose up to 1.0 mg/kg/day.

FLUCYTOSINE

Flucytosine (5-fluorocytosine) is a fluorinated pyrimidine thought to act by replacing uracil in the RNA of yeasts. It is well absorbed from the gut and against susceptible strains is effective in a dose of 150–200 mg/kg bodyweight per day. Unfortunately, its activity is confined to *Candida albicans* and *Cryptococcus neoformans* and many strains of even these organisms are resistant. Flucytosine is much less toxic than amphotericin B although marrow depression, jaundice, and bowel perforation have been reported. Its limited range of antifungal activity probably confines its role to that of a less toxic alternative to amphotericin B in infection by susceptible fungi.

IMIDAZOLES

Miconazole and econazole are marketed in various topical formulations while one, miconazole, is available in the UK for oral and parenteral administration. They appear to act by inhibition of peroxidative enzymes, allowing a cytotoxic intracellular accumulation of peroxides.

Absorption of miconazole from the gastrointestinal tract is poor so that miconazole tablets are most effective in eradication of susceptible fungi from the gut.

The imidazoles are active against a wide range of filamentous organisms and yeasts and are particularly useful for topical application in dermatophytic infections and in oral and cutaneous moniliasis. Intravenous miconazole should be considered in patients unable to tolerate amphotericin B and as an alternative to the latter drug in systemic infections with monilia resistant to fluocytosine.

Recommended dosage for oral moniliasis is 5 ml of miconazole gel (20%) two to four times per day. For systemic infections, an ampoule containing 200 mg of miconazole should be diluted with 5% dextrose or physiological saline solution and administered by slow intravenous infusion three times daily. In children, the total daily dose is of the order of 40 mg/kg bodyweight, no single infusion to exceed 15 mg/kg bodyweight.

Toxic effects are in general less frequent and less severe than those encountered with amphotericin B therapy. They include gastrointestinal, mental and liver enzyme disturbances. The poor water solubility of miconazole necessitates the use of a lipophilic solvent causing major problems with venous irritation and occlusion.

Ketoconazole, a systemically active imidazole, shows promise in the treatment of systemic fungal infections and is a less toxic alternative to amphotericin B. Its use has been reported in systemic candidosis, coccidioidomycosis and histoplasmosis. An appropriate dose is 3 mg/kg daily orally for a child and 200–400 mg once daily for an adult. Treatment should be maintained for 10 days in the case of oral thrush and for at least 1 month in the case of systemic infections.

TRIZOLES

This, the most recently introduced class of antifungal drugs, includes two drugs of potential value, fluconazole and itraconazole, of which the latter has wider application. The trizoles have a similar mechanism of action to miconazole. Both drugs are of low toxicity but as both are metabolized by the liver they should be used with caution where there is a possibility of hepatic dysfunction. Fluconazole is poorly absorbed from the intestinal tract and its intravenous use has been confined to systemic candidosis and cryptococcosis. Itraconazole is well absorbed by mouth and has been shown to be effective in systemic candidosis, cryptococcosis, aspergillosis, histoplasmosis, blastomycosis, coccidioidomycosis and sporotrichosis. Treatment should not be continued beyond 30 days.

For further information on antifungal agents, the reader should consult the reviews by Dismukes (1988), Graybill (1988), van't Wout (1988), Walsh & Pizzo (1988) and Davey (1990).

PRESUMED INFECTION

KAWASAKI DISEASE

Kawasaki disease (mucocutaneous lymph node syndrome) is a multisystem disorder which presents as a febrile illness in prepubertal children, particularly the under-5s. Up to 20% of patients develop coronary artery aneurysms which can lead to fatal infarction or long-term morbidity. Early recognition and treatment of the disease prevents these complications. The disease was described by Kawasaki in Japan in the 1960s and first reported in English literature in 1974. It was subsequently reported from many other countries. It is probably not a new disease for the infantile form of polyarteritis nodosa, first described in the 19th century, is very similar clinically and identical pathologically. It does, however, seem to have become much more prevalent in the last 30 years.

MAJOR CLINICAL FEATURES (see Table 23.46)

In the absence of a definitive laboratory test the diagnosis of Kawasaki disease is made by careful clinical assessment of a constellation of progressive clinical features and associated nonspecific laboratory findings. With experience a probable diagnosis can often be made in the first few days of illness, peripheral desquamation and thrombocytosis in the second or third week being particularly helpful confirmatory features (Hicks & Melish 1986).

Fever

This is an essential criterion. Fever is usually abrupt in onset, high (40°C) and swinging, lasting from 5 to 30 days. It is unresponsive to antibiotics but responds in 2–3 days to aspirin or gamma globulin.

Conjunctivitis

This is nonpurulent and without corneal ulceration. It persists throughout the acute phase of the illness, and is often accompanied by a mild uveitis detectable by slit lamp examination.

Oral changes

These appear within a day or two of fever. The oropharynx is diffusely reddened without ulceration or membrane. The lips are swollen, red and cracked. The tongue is also diffusely red with prominent papillae (strawberry tongue) (Plates 23.3 and 23.4).

Changes of the extremities

Erythema of the palms and soles and nonpitting edema of the hands and feet appear early. In the second or third week

Table 23.46 Diagnostic criteria for Kawasaki disease

Fever
Conjunctivitis
Oral changes
Changes of the extremities
Polymorphous rash
Cervical lymphadenopathy (present in only 50%)

Five of six features should be present including fever.

desquamation of the skin of hands and feet occur, characteristically starting at the finger tips followed by toe tips (Plate 23.5).

Polymorphous rash

This appears soon after the onset of fever and fades within a week (Plate 23.6). It is usually macular, sometime maculopapular and may be scarlatiniform, morbilliform or urticarial or shows the appearance of erythema multiforme or marginatum. Vesicles are rare. The rash may be confined to the napkin area in infants or is particularly intense in the perianal area where desquamation may occur.

Cervical lymphadenopathy

Unlike other major criteria which occur in most cases this feature is only found in 50%, usually as a single cervical node 1.5 cm or larger in diameter. Diffuse lymphadenopathy suggests other diagnoses such as infectious mononucleosis.

Incomplete forms

Incomplete forms of Kawasaki disease may occur, particularly in infants under 6 months of age, the group in which cardiovascular complications are commoner.

Progression and severity

The acute febrile phase of the illness usually lasts up to 10 days (prolonged fever being a bad prognostic sign) and is followed by a subacute phase up to 30 days when cardiovascular complications may present, with full recovery by 8 weeks. Many cases admitted to hospital are severely ill and require intensive care but the clinical spectrum is wide and mild cases may go unrecognized in the community.

ASSOCIATED FEATURES

Arthritis, particularly affecting the knees, hips, elbows and fingers, is a common association. It usually resolves in the acute phase but may persist for several months. Irritability and mood swings are almost universal and aseptic meningitis is common. Diarrhea and abdominal pain are frequent. The latter may indicate hydrops of the gallbladder which occurs in up to 15% of cases, is self-limiting, and can be monitored by ultrasound. Mild hepatitis with transient elevation of hepatic enzymes is often seen with occasionally more prolonged hepatitis or obstructive jaundice.

Cardiovascular complications including pericarditis, myocarditis and coronary artery aneurysm are described in Chapter 13.

Aneurysms can occur in other arteries. They may be silent but occasionally result in peripheral gangrene, especially in infants, or cerebral infarction. Other less common complications include pneumonitis, sterile otitis media, myositis and pancreatitis.

DIFFERENTIAL DIAGNOSIS

Kawasaki disease has to be differentiated from a number of similar infectious and noninfectious conditions, particularly the febrile exanthemata. These include streptococcal scarlet fever, staphylococcal toxic shock syndrome, staphylococcal scalded skin syndrome, Stevens–Johnson syndrome (erythema multiforme major), measles, Reiter's syndrome and in endemic areas, Rocky Mountain spotted fever (tick typhus) or leptospirosis. Other similar presentations include infectious mononucleosis and juvenile chronic arthritis.

LABORATORY TESTS

Simple laboratory tests may help to support the clinical diagnosis. The white blood count is usually elevated in the first week (to $20–30 \times 10^6$/ml) with a neutrophilia. Later a lymphocytosis is seen. A mild normochromic, normocytic anemia is common with the nadir at the end of the second week. The platelet count, normal in the first week, almost always rises in the second or third week. Acute phase reactants such as ESR and C-reactive protein are usually elevated. A platelet count higher than 1000×10^6/ml or ESR over 100 are quoted by some authorities as bad prognostic signs. Sterile pyuria (probably from meatal ulcer or urethritis) is a frequent finding as is proteinuria.

EPIDEMIOLOGY

Kawasaki disease probably only occurs in prepubertal children. Isolated reports of cases in teenagers or young adults most likely represent toxic shock syndrome or infectious mononucleosis. The median age at presentation is 24 months (12 months in Japan) with 80% of cases aged less than 5 years. Boys outnumber girls by 1.5 : 1 and may have a higher rate of complications. A recurrent episode may occur in 1% of cases.

National surveys in Japan have shown an incidence varying between 15 and 100 cases annually per 100 000 children under the age of 5 years with major national epidemics on a 2- to 4-year cycle. In North America where more cases are seen in the early spring, overall incidence is much lower but approaching 20 per 100 000 children under 5 in epidemic years (Shulman et al 1995).

Direct person-to-person spread has not been described but in Japan in epidemic years the second case rate in siblings of affected children is significantly higher than in the general population. Some surveys have shown increased rate in upper and middle income families. Mortality was reported as 2–3% in the 1960s and 1970s. In most areas it is now less than 0.5%. This may relate to better recognition but early treatment undoubtedly also plays a role.

ETIOLOGY AND PATHOGENESIS

There is general agreement that the disease must be regarded as an infection but no single agent has yet been confirmed in spite of an enormous number of suggested candidates. These have included *Streptococcus sanguis, Coxiella burnetti, Rickettsia,* and, lately, *Staphylococcus aureus* toxin or parvovirus B19 (Leung et al 1993, Nigro et al 1994). The possible roles of house dust mite antigen or of *Proprionobacterium acnes* carried by a mite vector have not been confirmed.

There has on the other hand been considerable progress in elucidating the immunological changes involved in a disease which is in association with a diffuse vasculitis of small and medium blood vessels. There is an acute rise and convalescent fall in all classes of immunoglobulin including IgE. Rheumatoid factor, antinuclear factor and anti-DNA antibodies are negative but immune complexes have been demonstrated by multiple

assays including a factor that induces aggregation and serotonin release in normal platelets. Other factors related to platelet aggregation are increased including thromboxane A2 and betathromboglobulin. Cellular immune imbalance includes a reduction of suppressor cytotoxic T cells (CD8+), increased activated helper T cells (CD4+), and monocytes and polyclonal B cell activation accompanied by high levels of interleukin-1, tumor necrosis factor and interferon gamma. The acute T cell and B cell changes are reduced by treatment with gamma globulin. Antineutrophil cytoplasmic antibodies and antiendothelial antibodies have also been demonstrated.

TREATMENT

See Chapter 13, page 633.

Aspirin

Aspirin, with its anti-inflammatory action and activity against platelet aggregation, has long been the mainstay of therapy in Kawasaki disease. This is now the main indication for aspirin in childhood, since its widespread use as an antipyretic was implicated in the etiology of Reye's syndrome. High dose treatment (100 mg/kg/day in four divided doses) is recommended for the first 14 days or until fever remits. Some authorities suggest monitoring serum salicylate levels and liver enzymes to ensure adequate treatment and avoid drug toxicity. Treatment should be started as early as possible, as soon as there is a strong suspicion of the diagnosis. Meanwhile active monitoring is continued for alternative diagnoses, particularly treatable ones such as streptococcal or staphylococcal disease, and for cardiac complications including the use of two-dimensional echocardiography.

During the recovery phase aspirin is continued at 3–5 mg/kg per day as a single dose until repeat assessment at 6–8 weeks confirms the absence of cardiac involvement.

Intravenous gamma globulin

Controlled trials from the US and Japan of high dose intravenous gamma globulin treatment in the acute phase of the illness have shown a significantly lower subsequent incidence of coronary artery aneurysms. A single infusion of 2000 mg/kg over 12 hours of intravenous gamma globulin is recommended in addition to high dose aspirin whenever Kawasaki disease is diagnosed in the first 10 days of the illness (Shulman et al 1995). Side effects such as chills, fever, headache or backache can be relieved by slowing or interrupting the infusion. True anaphylaxis is rare. Because of passively transferred measles antibody following such treatment, primary measles–mumps–rubella vaccination may need to be delayed for 12 months thereafter. The mechanism of action of intravenous gamma globulin in Kawasaki disease is unknown. It may act by downregulating cytokine production.

Gamma globulin is an expensive treatment. If cost is a factor alternatives are to use dipyridamole (see below) in addition to aspirin or to reserve treatment for cases with established cardiac disease or high cardiac risk factors such as age less than 1 year.

Dipyridamole

This inhibitor of platelet aggregation can be used at a dose of 3–5 mg/kg/day in divided doses as an alternative to gamma globulin in the acute phase, or instead of aspirin in the recovery phase during epidemics of influenza or varicella to prevent the remote possibility of Reye's syndrome.

Steroids

Steroids have no place in the routine management of Kawasaki disease having been shown in several Japanese studies to increase the frequency of coronary artery aneurysms. The only indication is for high dose pulse therapy combined with heparinization in the rare complication of peripheral gangrene.

SUMMARY

Kawasaki disease is an acute self-limiting multisystem vasculitis of childhood almost certainly caused by an infectious trigger. Though no single agent has yet been discovered there have been many advances in assessment, understanding and management of the condition. It is to be hoped that ongoing study of the immunological derangement may produce a quick and reliable laboratory test to help in the diagnosis and assessment of the condition in its early stages to facilitate more effective treatment and limit the severity, particularly of the cardiovascular complications.

HELMINTH INFECTION

Helminth or worm infections are worldwide although in warmer, moister areas, especially where standards of hygiene are low, the range of species and prevalence tends to be greater. In such parts, multiple infections are also often the rule. Because children tend to live more closely with nature and with their pets, many helminth infections are commoner in children than in adults.

The following is a list of the estimated prevalence of various worm infections in man, worldwide. The medical relevance of these figures indicates that a vast health problem exists.

Intestinal, liver and lung flukes	33 million infections
Schistosomes	200 million infections
Taenia spp.	42 million infections
Hymenolepis nana	20 million infections
Ascaris lumbricoides	1000 million infections
Hookworm	800 million infections
Trichuris trichiura	500 million infections
Enterobius vermicularis	209 million infections
Strongyloides stercoralis	35 million infections
Trichinella spiralis	28 million infections
Filariasis	280 million infections

Many such tentative prevalence figures are undoubtedly underestimates and thus, referring to the trematodes alone, Rim et al (1994) have concluded that there are more of these helminths infecting humans than any other group of animal parasites, with over 100 species of trematode infecting humans, mostly acquired from poorly prepared or cooked food.

Helminth infections are by no means confined to tropical or developing countries and the increase in travel and of refugee movements in recent years has led to an increasing awareness in the industrialized world of the dangers of imported diseases (Goldsmid 1988).

Helminth infections differ in most cases from those caused by viruses, bacteria or protozoa in that the clinical effects exhibited by the host are mostly related to the worm load carried, and the latter in turn is usually related to the degree of infection. The controversy regarding the possible adverse effects of helminth infections on cognitive function and learning or educational ability remains unresolved, but the concept may well be valid (Nokes & Bundy 1994).

The common parasitic helminths infecting humans include the Nematoda (roundworms) and Platyhelminthes (flatworms) which comprises the Trematoda (flukes) and Cestoda (tapeworms). Less commonly humans may be infected with such worms as the Acanthocephala (thorny headed worms) (Goldsmid 1988).

The control of human helminth infections usually depends on a detailed knowledge of the epidemiology and life cycles of the species concerned – the aim being to break the cycle. The following principles are utilized either alone or in combination, depending upon the species:

1. treatment of infected individuals
2. control of animal reservoirs where such exist
3. hygiene, which includes education and provision of adequate and *acceptable* toilet facilities
4. vector control where applicable
5. the wearing of shoes where infection occurs from the soil through the skin
6. instruction in food preparation and cooking
7. immunization – a field which continues to be of great interest.

Of all the above, the most important method of control of human helminthiases remains improved personal hygiene.

NEMATODES (ROUNDWORMS)

The nematodes or roundworms are nonsegmented worms, round in transverse section with separate sexes. They possess both gut and body cavity (pseudocele). Roundworms especially important to humans include amongst others: *Ascaris lumbricoides, Toxocara canis, Enterobius vermicularis, Ancylostoma duodenale, Necator americanus, Trichuris trichiura, Strongyloides stercoralis, Angiostrongylus cantonensis, Oesophagostomum* spp., *Ternidens deminutus, Trichinella spiralis, Capillaria* spp., *Dracunculus medinensis, Onchocerca volvulus, Loa loa, Wuchereria bancrofti, Mansonella perstans, Mansonella ozzardi* and *Brugia malayi*.

ASCARIASIS

The intestinal roundworm *Ascaris lumbricoides* is cosmopolitan although variable in its distribution, thriving in a moist climate, be it temperate or tropical and especially under conditions of overcrowding. The adult ascarids, male and female, live in the lumen of the small intestine, maintaining only an intermittent attachment to the mucosa. The gravid female lays an average of 200 000 eggs each day. Newly excreted eggs may remain dormant for a long period; if conditions are suitable they develop into an infective stage in about 2 weeks, in which condition they can remain viable for months or years until ingested (Janssens 1985). The hosts of these worms are humans, although cases of human infection with *Ascaris suum*, the pig ascarid, are also on record. The life cycle of *A. lumbricoides* is depicted in Figure 23.51.

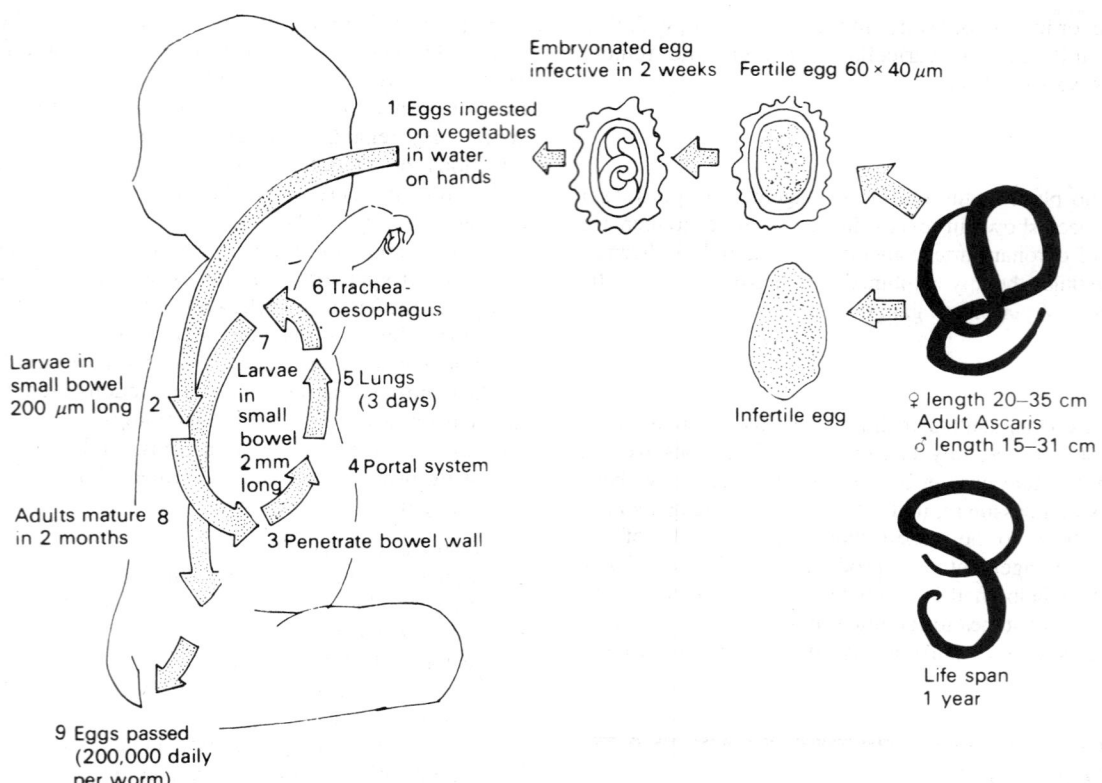

Fig. 23.51 Character and life cycle of *Ascaris lumbricoides*.

Clinical features

In fully 80% of cases the only manifestation of ascariasis in the human is the asymptomatic passage of eggs and adult worms in the stool. Symptoms, when they do occur, are related to three phases of the ascarid's life cycle:

1. invasion of larvae
2. presence of a large adult worm load
3. migration of adult worms from their normal habitat.

To this one may add symptoms associated with the development of true allergy to the ascarid (Lancet 1989c).

Ascariasis is potentially serious and may contribute a significant proportion of abdominal emergencies in children (Crompton 1985).

Larval pneumonitis

The initial migration of larvae through the intestinal wall and by way of the portal circulation to the lungs may, in the case of heavy infection, or if there have been repeated reinfections, cause a characteristic and often seasonal clinical picture (Pawlowski 1987a). The patient develops a dry spasmodic cough with intermittent wheezing and breathlessness, transient rhonchi and crepitations in the lung fields; rarely, hemoptysis occurs. There may be malaise with fever as high as 40°C, discomfort over the liver, and urticarial rashes. Radiological examination of the chest reveals diffuse mottled opacities, peribronchial infiltration or areas of pneumonitis. Marked eosinophilia is present. Symptoms and signs subside after 2 or 3 weeks and the eosinophilia generally

diminishes to 3–5% of the total white cell count. Chronic lung disease occasionally results from repeated larval onslaughts. Severe pulmonary infiltration with asthma, eosinophilia and raised IgE levels can result in children infected with *A. suum* which may or may not become patent.

Worm load

Although some features of intestinal ascariasis are of an allergic or reflux nature, in the healthy child on a normal diet it is unlikely that the presence of a few ascarids will cause any significant disturbance (Pawlowski 1987a). A large worm load will, however, drain off a considerable proportion of a child's nutritional intake and *Ascaris* infection in children can be associated with impaired lactose digestion and absorption (Crompton 1985). Cases of heavy infection are usually seen in underprivileged communities where nutrition is already inadequate. The combination of malnutrition, vitamin and iron deficiency and the almost invariable presence of intestinal parasites of other types, make the part played by ascarids difficult to assess. However, studies in Columbia have shown steatorrhea and d-xylose malabsorption associated with heavy loads of *Ascaris* which improved after deworming. These children are ill, stunted and marasmic, with abdominal distention. Colicky abdominal pain is frequent. There may be low grade fever and a mass of worms can often be palpated abdominally. Toxins from ascarids may play a part in producing the chronic illness.

Intestinal complications associated with a heavy worm burden are frequently seen in hyperendemic areas (Crompton 1988). A

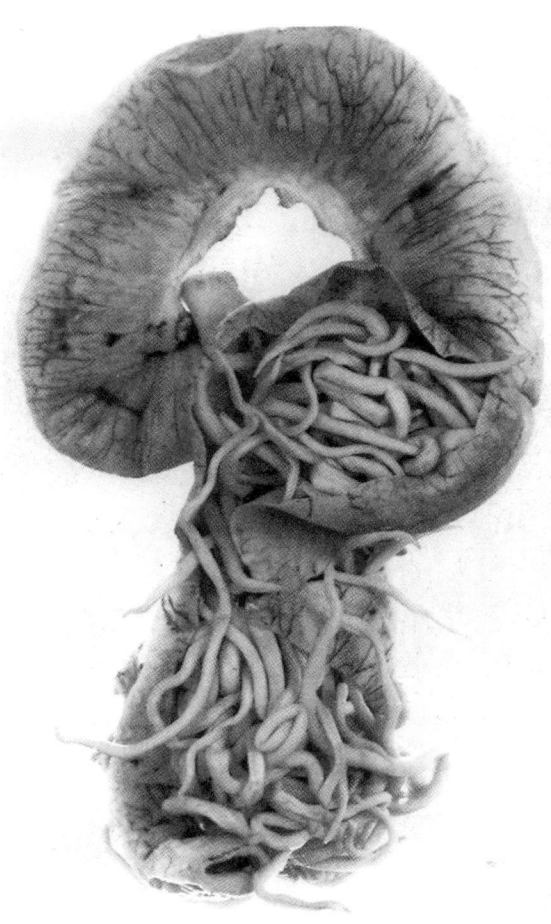

Fig. 23.52 Intestinal obstruction by *Ascaris lumbricoides* in a 14-year-old boy.

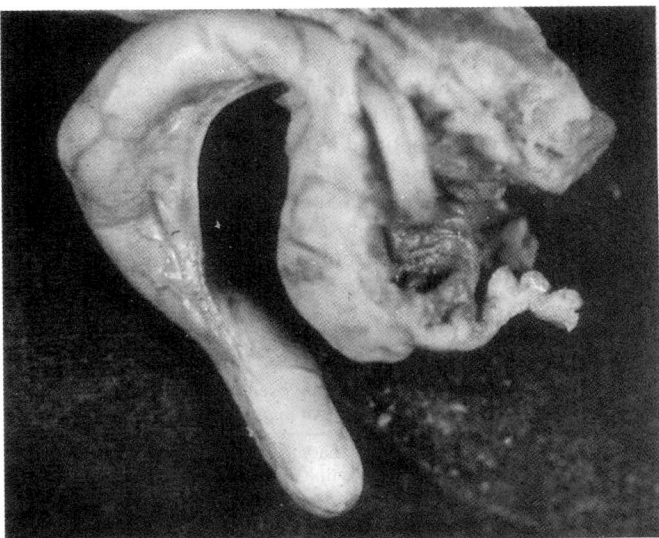

Fig. 23.53 Adult *Ascaris* in appendix.

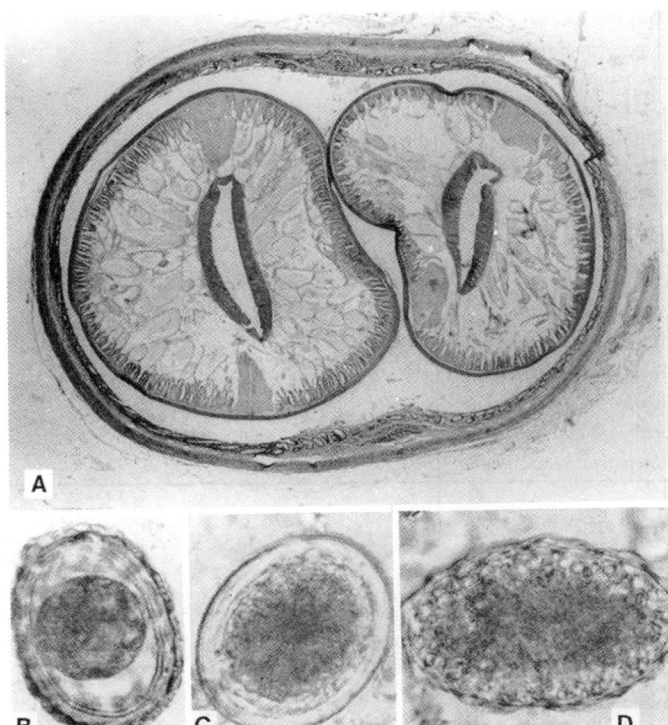

Fig. 23.54 (a) Pair of *Ascaris* in appendix (approx. ×10). (b) Fertilized egg of *Ascaris lumbricoides* (approx. ×600). (c) Decorticated fertilized egg of *A. lumbricoides* (approx. ×600). (d) Unfertilized egg of *A. lumbricoides* (approx. ×600).

bolus of worms (usually both dead and living) may impact, particularly near the ileocecal junction (Fig. 23.52). A mass of ascarids may also precipitate temporary obstruction from spasm, cause inflammatory reactions and adhesions, or lead to volvulus or intussusception.

Migration of adult worms

Under certain circumstances, particularly with high fever, gastrointestinal upset or ineffectual anthelmintic therapy (e.g. the use of tetrachlorethylene for a concomitant hookworm infection), an ascarid will migrate from its normal habitat in the bowel and be vomited, or wriggle unaided, up the esophagus and emerge through the nose. Lodgment in the appendix (Figs 23.53 and 23.54) or Meckel's diverticulum can result in obstruction and perforation. The common bile duct may be blocked by a roundworm, leading to severe upper abdominal pain, vomiting, tenderness and enlargement of the liver, a palpable gallbladder, and jaundice. Pancreatitis is a further complication. Other manifestations of the migrating ascarid include intestinal perforation with peritonitis, chronic peritonitis due to the presence of eggs, soft tissue or liver abscess, laryngeal impaction and even the passage of a worm per urethram. Ascarids also have a special propensity to congregate at the scene of incidental catastrophe –

penetrating perforations, suture lines and into drainage or suction tubes.

The development of roundworm sensitivity can produce a variety of allergic manifestations – nasal, pulmonary, dermal, or gastrointestinal (Pawlowski 1987a).

Diagnosis

Larval pneumonitis (Löffler's syndrome) is generally suspected by the presence of eosinophilia, but other parasites can produce this syndrome (Table 23.47), and proof of diagnosis can only be obtained if a larva is identified in the sputum (Fig. 23.55). Adult worms may later be passed in the stool or seen on radiological examination (Figs 23.56 and 23.57) of the abdomen using barium. Diagnosis, however, rests almost wholly on finding eggs in the stools (Fig. 23.54b, c, d), except in the event of early infection or a population of purely male worms. Serological and intracutaneous tests are available but as yet are of little practical value.

Table 23.47 Worms and fly larvae giving rise to pulmonary infiltrations, visceral larva migrans and cutaneous larva migrans

	Pulmonary infiltration with eosinophilia	Visceral larva migrans	Cutaneous larva migrans
Ancylostoma braziliense			×
Ancylostoma caninum			×
Ancylostoma duodenale	Rare		
Angiostrongylus cantonensis		×	
Anisakis species		×	
Ascaris lumbricoides	×	Rare	
Ascaris suum	×	×	
Capillaria hepatica		×	
Dirofilaria species	×	×	
Fly larvae			
Dermatobia species		×	
Gasterophilus species			×
Hypoderma species			×
Gnathostoma species		×	×
Necator americanus	Rare		'Ground itch'
Schistosoma species			'Swimmer's itch'
Strongyloides stercoralis	×	Rare	'Ground itch'
Toxocara canis	×	×	
Toxocara cati	Uncertain	Uncertain	
Uncinaria stenocephala			×

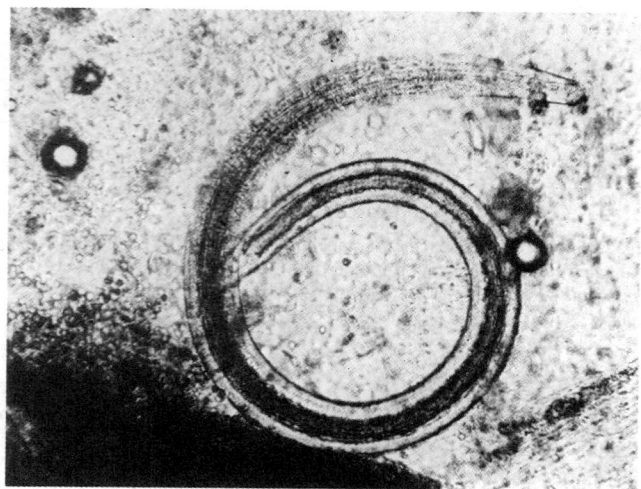

Fig. 23.55 *Ascaris* larva in sputum.

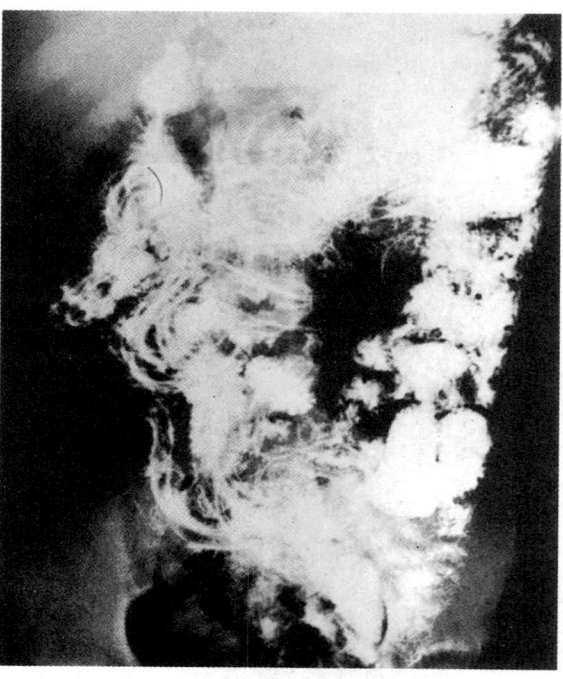

Fig. 23.56 *Ascaris lumbricoides*. Barium follow through showing infestation in small bowel with worms coated with barium.

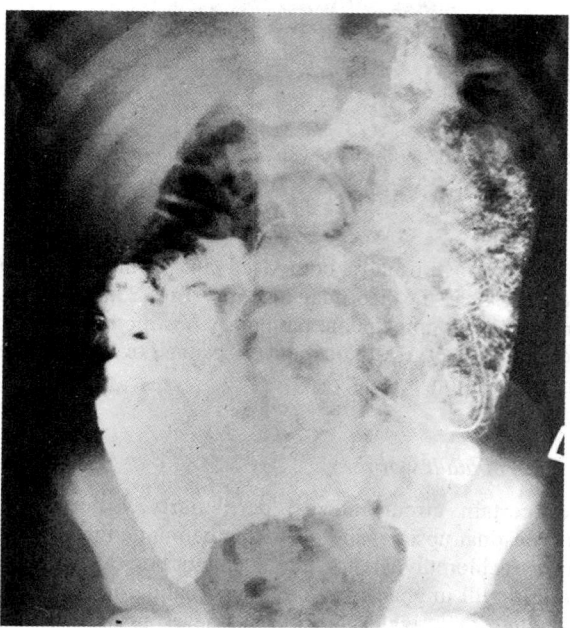

Fig. 23.57 *Ascaris lumbricoides*. Barium follow through showing infestation in jejunum with worms as tubular opacities having ingested barium.

Treatment

No treatment is known to remove migrating larvae although some have claimed success using piperazine or pyrantel and the pneumonitis responds dramatically to prednisone (Pawlowski 1987a). A safe and effective treatment for established ascariasis is piperazine. Syrup is best and is given before the evening meal in a dosage of 75 mg/kg bodyweight to a maximum of 4 g. If the bowels have not acted by the following morning a mild laxative is administered. The dose is repeated on the second evening. Worms are narcotized and eliminated by normal peristalsis. Nausea, vomiting, transient neurological disturbance and EEG changes have been reported when the drug is given in excessive doses. Piperazine is contraindicated in the presence of liver and renal disease and where there is a history of neurological disease (Janssens 1985).

Two anthelmintics highly effective in ascariasis and with minimal side effects are pyrantel embonate/pamoate (Combantrin) (10 mg/kg) and mebendazole (Vermox) (100 mg twice a day for 3 days). Levamisole (Ketrax) 50–100 mg is also effective. Newer anthelmintics include flubendazole (200 mg twice in one day) and albendazole 400 mg as a single dose (Janssens 1985, Pawlowski 1987a, Schneider et al 1990). Albendazole in particular is a very valuable, broad spectrum anthelmintic with a wide activity against intestinal nematode species. It is generally well tolerated at doses recommended for these helminths and has, in fact, been designated as a 'WHO essential agent'. Thiabendazole (50 mg/kg) although effective, is better avoided owing to its side effects (James & Gilles 1985).

Prevention of ascariasis depends on the sanitary disposal of feces, on preventing contamination of drinking water and raw vegetables, and on education in hygiene.

TOXOCARA CANIS AND VISCERAL LARVA MIGRANS

Toxocara canis is a close relative of *Ascaris*. Its natural hosts are the young dog and the fox, in which it undergoes a cycle essentially similar to *Ascaris* in humans (Fig. 23.58). The cycle in dogs is complicated by the development of immunity with expulsion of adult worms by the animals at about 6 months of age. In pregnant bitches, however, this immunity is lost and dormant larvae in the tissues are reactivated or reinfection occurs, resulting in the puppies being infected in utero and being born with worms. Children ingest infective eggs from dirt contaminated with dog feces or directly from the animals themselves, especially young puppies or lactating bitches (Gillespie 1988). The larvae, after penetrating the intestinal wall, are incapable of completing their pulmonary migration in an unnatural host and wander aimlessly never to find their intestinal habitat. They pass through, or become encysted in liver, lungs, kidneys, heart, muscle, brain or eye, causing an intense local response from the tissue.

Clinical features

The child (most commonly 1–5 years of age) shows marked failure to thrive associated with pica (90% of cases), anemia (Hb below 9 g/dl in 45%), fever (80%) and enlargement of liver (65%) and spleen (45%). There is cough (80%), bronchospasm and wheezing (63%) (Gillespie 1988). A single organ may bear the brunt of the infection so that pulmonary symptoms, or neurological abnormalities due to brain involvement (convulsions, disturbances of consciousness, hemiparesis) may predominate. Intense and persistent eosinophilia lasting months or years and reaching levels as high as $80 \times 10^9/l$ is characteristic and may be the only abnormality found. Serum globulin levels are raised, particularly IgM, IgG and IgE, and elevated titers of anti-A and anti-B isoagglutinins have been described in 39% of cases.

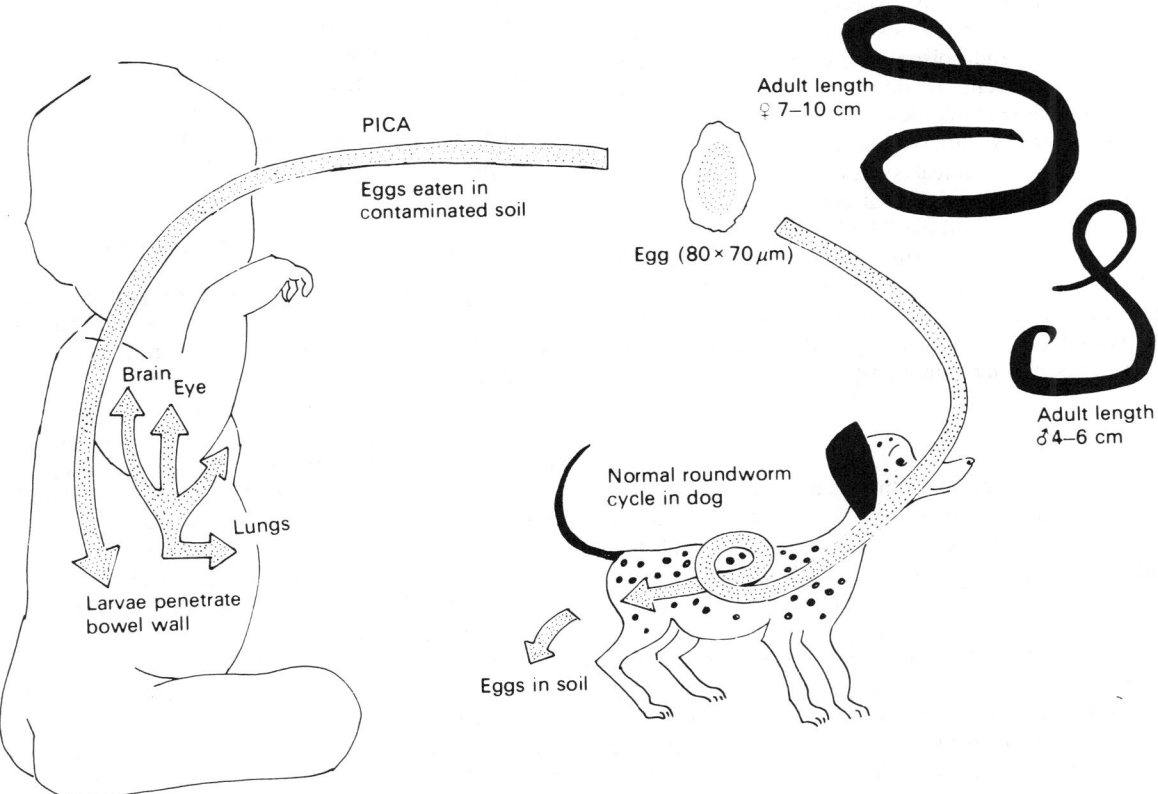

Fig. 23.58 Character and life cycle of *Toxocara canis*.

Transient chest shadows are recorded in about 50% of cases and the CSF may show an eosinophilia where the CNS is involved. The infection usually runs a chronic, benign course of 18 months or so and generally the prognosis is good, although deaths have been reported.

Ocular manifestations of toxocariasis may be the only evidence of the disease. The age of maximal ocular involvement is higher than that of systemic involvement, the average age being about 7–8 years. Loss of sight in the affected eye generally results, and usually only one eye is involved. A diagnosis of ocular toxocariasis should be considered when there is inflammatory detachment of the retina or retinitis of the posterior pole in a child, especially in one with geophagic habits, who has contact with young dogs. The diagnosis can be confused with retinoblastoma and this may lead to the unnecessary surgical removal of an eye in a child with ocular toxocariasis.

It appears, therefore, that there are two toxocaral syndromes in humans:

1. larvae in the eye presenting as granulomatous pseudotumors of the retina
2. generalized toxocariasis with numerous larvae in the liver and other organs and associated with fever and eosinophilia.

Because ocular lesions are seldom found in the generalized forms, and because ocular disease is almost entirely confined to children, it has been postulated that ocular toxocariasis could be the manifestation of congenital infection of the child from an infected mother in a similar fashion to the transplacental infection of puppies. This hypothesis, if true, would have important implications for expectant mothers. Similarly contact with cats or cat litter might entail risk of fetus-damaging infection due to toxocariasis from *T. cati* as well as toxoplasmosis.

It has been suggested that the eosinophilia so often seen in children suffering from lead poisoning resulting from pica may well be due to concurrent *Toxocara* infection. Physicians managing children with lead intoxication should be aware of this possibility and treat the toxocariasis concurrently.

Undoubtedly, a similar clinical syndrome can be caused in children by filarial parasites of animal origin and by larvae of other types (Gillespie 1988) (Table 23.47). Thus it still remains unclear whether *Toxocara cati* (the cat roundworm) can be responsible for systemic larva migrans and warnings have been sounded that another dog ascarid, *Toxascaris leonina*, previously thought to be noninfective to humans, should be considered as a potential cause of visceral larva migrans.

Diagnosis

Acquisition of a puppy in the preceding year has proved to be a good suggestive indicator of *Toxocara* infection in symptomatic patients (Gillespie 1988). The diagnosis can only be established with certainty, however, by a biopsy (generally of the liver) or, undesirably and rather drastically, after enucleation of the eye. Skin tests and serological tests are available and in the past, the indirect fluorescent antibody test has been the most widely used. This test has been improved by using frozen sections of adult worms, refined antigen bound to sepharose beads or larval secretory antigen. The *Toxocara* ELISA test appears to be gaining popularity and is considered by many to be the serological test of choice with a 78% sensitivity and a 92% specificity, while an antigen-detecting ELISA is being developed (Gillespie 1988).

It is worth noting that 2–7% or more of symptomless adults and up to 23% of children with no symptoms may have detectable *Toxocara* antibodies (Gillespie 1988, Milstein & Goldsmid 1995).

Treatment

Diethylcarbamazine (Hetrazan, Banocide) (5–10 mg/kg per day for 7 days) is reportedly effective but several courses may be necessary. An alternative regime is up to 6 mg/kg in divided doses for 3 weeks (Gillespie 1988). Repeated courses may be necessary and if respiratory distress or myocardial involvement develop, corticosteroids may be life saving.

Thiabendazole (Mintezol) at a dose of 50 mg/kg for 3–5 days or 25 mg/kg for 1–4 weeks has also been recommended. It is especially useful for early ocular cases where diethylcarbamazine should not be used, as the cellular response it elicits could aggravate visual problems. Corticosteroids are also useful in controlling ocular lesions. Albendazole (50 mg/kg) for 3 days has shown promise and flubendazole has also proved encouraging (Rochette 1985).

Prevention

While the dangers of infection from pets cannot be overstressed, this is a very emotive issue. It might be worth quoting Hungerford (1977) who stated: 'In our stress distorted society, pets ... may be the critical factor in maintaining or restoring mental health or happiness to an only child, or to a psychotic, mentally distraught or lonely child or adult.'

The answer, therefore, is not destruction of pets, but regular and routine deworming of dogs, especially puppies and pregnant bitches, with mebendazole, fenbendazole, piperazine or pyrantel pamoate. Also important is education to impress upon children and expectant mothers the need to wash after handling their pets and not to allow dogs to lick them on the face. Dogs and cats should also be prevented from defecating where children play (sandpits etc.).

ENTEROBIUS VERMICULARIS (OXYURIASIS)

Enterobius vermicularis (threadworm, pinworm, seatworm) is a common parasite throughout the world but, unlike most nematodes, it is more prolific in temperate and cold climates. The incidence is highest in school children from 5 to 9 years with another peak at 30–49 years (Pawlowski 1987b). Boys and girls are equally affected. Enterobiasis is particularly common in highly populated districts, institutional groups, and among members of the same family. Incidences as high as 40–50% have been reported in London children and in institutions such as mental hospitals, prevalence may reach 90–100%. The absence of a prolonged developmental stage outside humans (Fig. 23.59) favors reinfection and transmission from child to child. Hands are contaminated by scratching the perianal area where eggs are deposited, and by contact with soiled underclothing, nightclothing or bedding. Infection is also acquired by inhalation of egg-containing dust which may be disseminated from bedclothing by shaking, or movements of the sleeper. At room temperature eggs survive for 2–3 weeks. Furthermore, retroinfection may occur when the eggs hatch on the perianal area and larvae find their way back through the anus into the intestinal tract.

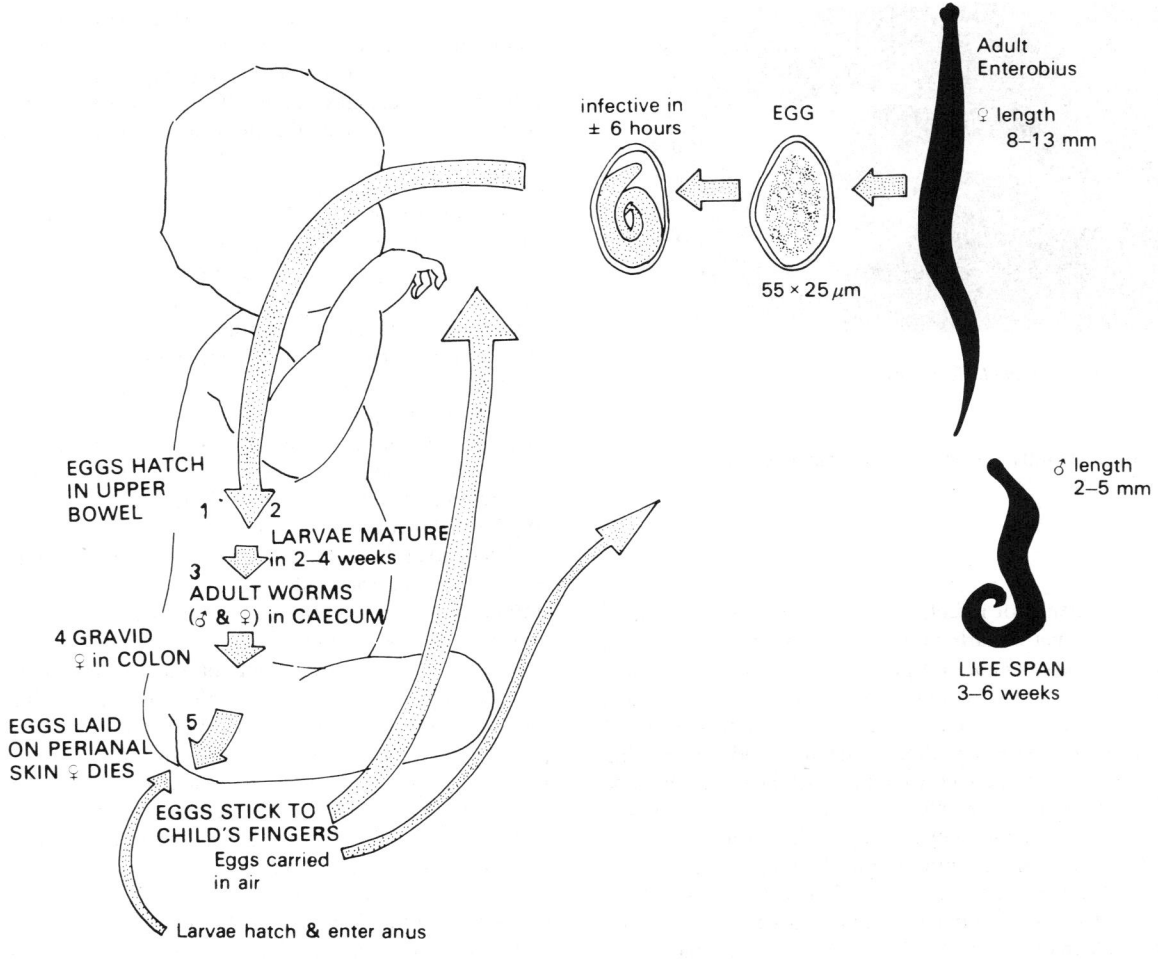

Fig. 23.59 Character and life cycle of *Enterobius vermicularis*.

The usual habitat of the threadworm of both sexes is the cecum and adjacent appendix, lower ileum, and colon. The worms are free in the intestinal lumen or lie with their heads attached to the mucosa. The gravid females migrate to the lower colon and rectum and crawl through the anus to deposit thousands of sticky eggs on the anal verge and perineum at night, usually dying thereafter. It is worth emphasizing that dogs and cats play no part in the transmission of enterobiasis to humans (Janssens 1985).

Clinical features

Threadworm infection generally causes no symptoms whatsoever. The most common manifestation is pruritus of the perineal areas due to migration of the worms and the presence of eggs. Restless sleep, nightmares, teeth grinding, and perhaps bed-wetting may result. In up to 20% of girls, vulval irritation and vaginal discharge are caused by threadworms and can persist for years (Janssens 1985) and night crying may be due to a threadworm in the vaginal introitus. Excoriation and pyogenic infection can follow from constant scratching.

It is most unlikely that threadworms play any significant part in causing the variety of symptoms commonly attributed to them. For example, threadworms are no commoner in children with recurrent abdominal pain than in those without pain. Similarly, threadworms are found as often in normal appendices as in appendices showing acute or chronic inflammation (Fig. 23.60), so that they are not considered to play any material role in the production of appendicitis, although appendiceal blockage resulting in a simulated chronic appendicitis may occur at times (Pawlowski 1987b). Nail biting, nose picking, masturbation, convulsions, hyperkinesis and other behavior disturbances are also often erroneously ascribed to these parasites.

Very heavy infections can, however, result in catarrhal inflammation of the bowel from the attachment and irritation of worms, resulting in gastrointestinal disturbance. Intestinal obstruction has even been reported. Rarely, heavy infections have led to invasion of the bowel and appendiceal walls, peritoneum or viscera by larvae and immature worms. In their external migration gravid threadworms may occasionally crawl up the vagina into the uterus and Fallopian tubes or into the urethra and bladder depositing eggs in these sites with resulting, low grade salpingitis; cystitis or urethritis, and cases are on record of worms penetrating the intestinal wall, probably through a pre-existing mucosal breach, to reach the peritoneal cavity.

Enterobiasis may be associated with infection by the protozoan flagellate, *Dientamoeba fragilis* which is believed to be transmitted within the egg of the threadworm and may be a cause of diarrhea (Mills & Goldsmid 1995).

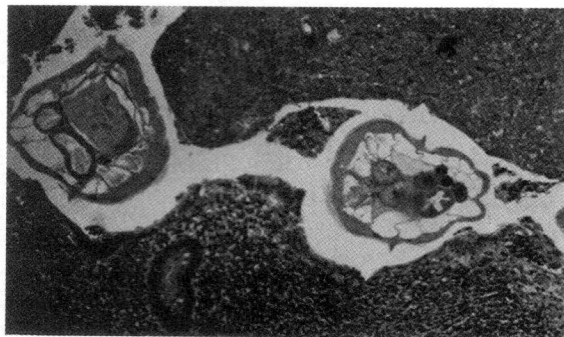

Fig. 23.60 *Enterobius vermicularis* in appendix.

Eosinophilia is usually absent in enterobiasis but may occur in up to 12% of cases.

Diagnosis

Often the first evidence of infection is the discovery of the adult worms in the feces, particularly after enemas, or on the perineum. Worms may be clearly visible on proctoscopy. The most widely used and effective method of obtaining eggs from the perianal region is the adhesive cellulose tape method. The adhesive side of a piece of transparent tape is applied to the anus and surrounding skin – either directly or wrapped round a test tube – and the tape then transferred adhesive side down to a glass slide. The adhering eggs are clearly visible under a microscope (Fig. 23.61a). The test must be performed in the morning before bathing or defecation, and in view of the irregular migrations of gravid worms at least three examinations should be made on consecutive days. Eggs are found in the stools in only 5–10% of cases, but five perianal swabs reveal eggs in 97% of infections.

Treatment

A wide range of effective drugs are available for the elimination of threadworms. The drugs of choice at present are mebendazole

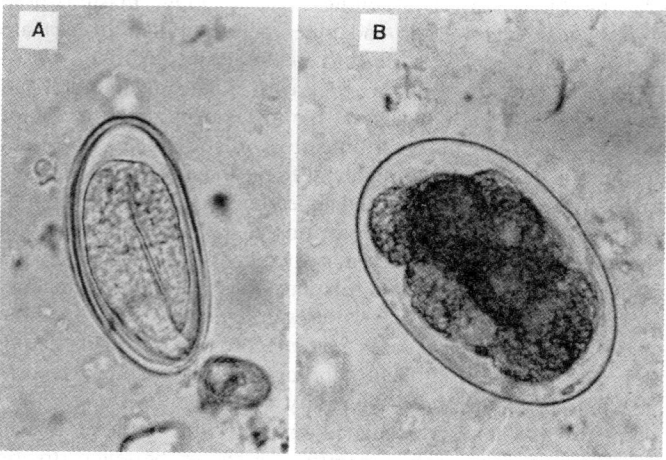

Fig. 23.61 (a) Fully developed egg of *Enterobius vermicularis* (approx. ×600). (b) Hookworm egg (approx. ×600).

(Vermox) and pyrantel embonate/pamoate (Combantrin, Antiminth). Mebendazole is given in a single dose of 100 mg (1 tablet) stat. which is recorded as giving a cure rate of about 95% with no or very few side effects (Janssens 1985), but some authorities advise that the drug should not be used in children under 2 years of age. Albendazole is also reported as being effective (Marty & Andersen 1995).

Pyrantel is also very effective as a single dose treatment, giving cure rates of over 90% at doses of 10 mg/kg. Side effects are usually mild (e.g. nausea and vomiting) and uncommon – about 3% of cases (James & Gilles 1985, Janssens 1985).

Other treatments for enterobiasis include pyrvinium pamoate (Vanquin, Povan) which is effective as a single dose of 5 mg/kg. With this drug, however, the stools and sometimes the teeth are stained red and parents should be warned of this and also of the fact that clothing and sheets may also be stained. Bilious vomiting may occur in some cases. Piperazine citrate (Antepar) is no longer recommended owing to low efficacy and the prolonged course required (Pawlowski 1987b).

Thiabendazole (Mintezol) (50 mg/kg in two divided doses) is also efficacious but side effects are common and often very unpleasant making the recommendation of the drug for enterobiasis inadvisable.

In general terms, treatment for most cases of threadworm is unnecessary, especially as reinfection of children is almost inevitable. However, if for clinical reasons or to satisfy distressed parents treatment is deemed necessary, then whichever drug is used, the whole family must be treated and a second course should be given after 3 weeks. Intractable family infections can be controlled by the treatment of all family members with 100 mg mebendazole a week for 12 weeks.

Prevention of recurrence is extremely difficult, particularly in crowded communities and in humid temperate climates, which facilitate prolonged survival of eggs. Personal cleanliness is essential and this includes cutting of finger nails, regular washing of hands before meals and after using the toilet, washing the anal area on rising, and regular changing of underclothing and bed linen.

HOOKWORM (ANCYLOSTOMIASIS)

Ancylostoma duodenale (Old World hookworm) and *Necator americanus* (tropical hookworm) are morphological variants, tropical hookworm being rather smaller with many differences of fine morphology.

Hookworm occurs in most tropical and subtropical areas of the world, with *Ancylostoma duodenale* distributed mainly around the Mediterranean littoral and *Necator americanus* in south and central Africa and southern America. Both species are, however, widely distributed today in Asia as well as in most other tropical countries. In southeast Asia and Brazil, *A. ceylanicum* infections of humans occur as well and *A. malayanum* is yet another species from humans (Janssens 1985). Hookworm is one of the world's chief causes of anemia.

Ancylostoma braziliense, one cause of cutaneous larva migrans (Table 23.47) and a natural parasite of dogs and cats, is widely distributed throughout tropical and subtropical areas, while the common dog hookworm *Ancylostoma caninum* is also widely distributed, and *Uncinaria stenocephala* infects dogs in temperate regions. These latter two species can also cause cutaneous larva migrans in humans and it is claimed that in northern Queensland

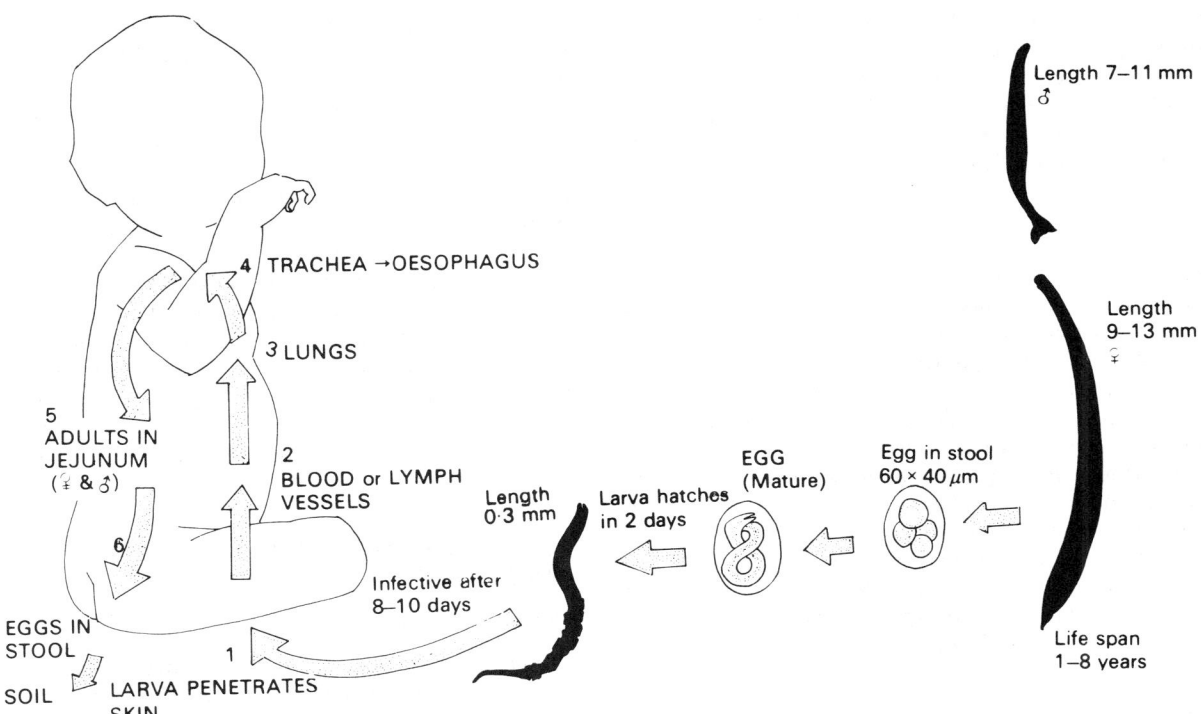

Fig. 23.62 Character and life cycle of hookworm.

in Australia, *A. caninum* may be a cause of eosinophilic gastroenteritis in humans as discussed by Smyth (1995).

The excreted egg, in favorable damp, shady conditions, hatches on the soil in about 2 days, releasing a rhabditiform larva which develops 8–10 days after hatching into the infective (filariform) larva. This larva penetrates the skin of the host in the case of *N. americanus*, although *A. duodenale* is believed also to enter via the oral route, with fecally contaminated food and water and may infect by the transmammary and transplacental routes from infected mother to child (Crompton 1989). The life cycle in humans from larval penetration to oviposition lasts about 5 weeks (Fig. 23.62). The adult worm may survive within its host for 7 years or longer.

The adult worms are attached to the wall of the jejunum, or, less commonly, the duodenum, by the buccal capsules, sucking blood from their hosts. Each worm may suck up to 0.5 ml of blood per day; thus heavy worm loads may result in a loss of 100–150 ml/day. Significant damage is therefore produced by hookworms, but clinical manifestations depend on the host's general resistance, on the worm load, and on the child's dietary intake and iron reserves.

Clinical features

Larval invasion

Penetration of the skin, usually of the feet or buttocks, by the filariform larvae may produce within minutes a series of wheals which soon develop into an itchy, papular and vesicular eruption ('ground itch'). The rash may become ulcerative or pustular, but generally subsides within 10 days and the larvae do not wander within the skin as in the case of cutaneous larva migrans (see below).

Migration through the lungs

After penetration of the skin, larvae reach the small intestine via the heart and lungs as in ascariasis.

Respiratory symptoms are unusual in children except in the case of heavy or repeated infections, particularly of *N. americanus*, when there may be cough, sore throat, bloody sputum and pulmonary changes on X-ray (Table 23.47).

Adult worms in the intestine

A distinction should be made between hookworm infection (where patients carry a subclinical worm load) and hookworm disease which results from heavy worm loads and inadequate diet. Where heavy infections occur symptoms develop in 2–7 weeks after initial infection and consist of abdominal discomfort especially after meals, anorexia and sometimes nausea and vomiting. There may be intermittent diarrhea, general debility and undue tiredness. Once the adult worms are well established there is little disturbance to the child provided that the intake of iron, vitamins and protein keeps pace with the chronic blood loss produced by the parasites. When diet is inadequate and worm load heavy, severe hookworm disease results, characterized by profound iron deficiency anemia, hypoalbuminemic edema, cardiac failure and even death. It has been estimated that 100 worms will cause a daily loss of 4 mg of iron. A balanced diet easily compensates for this loss, but iron deficiency soon develops on a marginal dietary intake. Children with heavy hookworm infections are stunted, marasmic and anemic; the skin is dry and the face puffy. All aspects of development are retarded. An important concomitant which makes hookworm infection much more serious is sickle cell anemia.

A marked eosinophilia (40%) is characteristic of early hookworm infection. It reaches maximum intensity at about 3 months after initial infection and then diminishes gradually to levels of 5–20% (Migasena & Gilles 1987). A partially effective protective immunity seems to develop in hookworm infection (Behnke 1987, Pritchard 1995).

Diagnosis

This depends on finding the eggs (Fig. 23.61b) in the feces and an egg count should be performed if a causal relationship with a concomitant iron deficiency anemia is to be established. An egg count greater than 2000 eggs/g of feces is generally considered to be of clinical significance.

In old stool specimens rhabditiform larvae are occasionally found and can be separated from those of *Strongyloides* by the short buccal chamber and larger genital primordium of the latter.

Eggs similar to those of hookworms can be recovered from humans infected with *Trichostrongylus* spp. and *Ternidens deminutus*. The eggs of the former species are more pointed than those of hookworm and the eggs of *T. deminutus* are significantly larger than those of the hookworm species. These infections can be treated as for hookworm (Goldsmid 1991).

Treatment

Albendazole is reported to be effective against the migrating larval stages of the human hookworms, *A. duodenale* and *N. americanus* (Reynolds 1996). The avermectins (Ivermectin) have shown promise against all stages of hookworm development, including migrating larvae (Janssens 1985). Children with severe anemia, malnutrition, infection or heavy worm load should receive preliminary supportive treatment in the form of blood transfusion, high calorie and protein diet, vitamins and iron therapy before definitive treatment of the worms. Highly effective anthelmintics for hookworm infection include pyrantel embonate/pamoate (Combantrin) (10 mg/kg) which is effective for *A. duodenale* given in a single dose regimen, but which for *N. americanus* needs to be given as a multiple dose treatment. Phenylene diisothiocyanate (Jonit) (adult dose: 100 mg every 12 hours × 3) is reported to be equally effective against both *A. duodenale* and *N. americanus*. Mebendazole (Vermox) gives excellent cure rates for both species of hookworm at a dose of 100 mg twice a day for 3 days – and with no side effects.

Albendazole and flubendazole at a single dose of 400 mg have both proved highly effective against a wide range of intestinal helminths including hookworm (Janssens 1985) and albendazole is reported to have ovicidal activity against hookworm, ascariasis and trichuriasis, making it especially valuable in integrated control programs for these infections (Reynolds 1996).

Well-tried treatments include bephenium hydroxynaphthoate and tetrachlorethylene. Bephenium hydroxynaphthoate (Alcopar) has proved highly successful against hookworm, but rather less so in *N. americanus* than in *A. duodenale*. The recommended dose is 2.5 g for children under 2 years, or 10 kg in weight, and 5.0 g in ages and weights above these figures. The drug should be taken when the stomach is empty and at least 1 h before food. The bitter taste can be masked by giving it in a sweet liquid. A second dose is only given if eggs continue to be passed. Side effects are uncommon but include nausea and vomiting. In *N. americanus* the older treatment, tetrachlorethylene (TCE), is stated to be more effective. The dose is 0.1 ml/kg, with a maximum single dose of 5 ml. The dose can be repeated for up to three successive days. It should probably not, however, be given to very small, severely ill children, and is contraindicated in cases of liver disease. It is important to note here, however, that TCE must not be used for *Necator* when a concomitant *Ascaris* infection is present as it often results in the ascarids migrating up the bile duct and causing obstructive jaundice. In these cases, the ascarids must be treated before TCE is administered.

The preventive aspects of hookworm are complex and include education of the public into the mode of spread of the disease, provision and proper usage of latrines, improvement of diet, and, where the incidence is high, mass population treatment. The wearing of shoes will also help to prevent infection. Interest is continuing regarding the possibility of vaccination against hookworm infection (Hotez et al 1987, Crompton 1989, Pritchard 1995).

CUTANEOUS LARVA MIGRANS (CREEPING ERUPTION, SAND WORM)

Clinical features

The larvae of the dog hookworms *A. braziliense*, *A. caninum* and *U. stenocephala*, together with certain other parasites (Table 23.47), produce in humans a skin eruption which differs from that caused by 'human' hookworms. The larva, after penetrating the epidermis, is unable to enter the blood or lymph streams and instead burrows just below the corium, traveling up to an inch a day. Papules mark the site of entry and advancing end of the larva and the tunneling causes linear, slightly elevated erythematous and serpigenous areas which itch intensely (Fig. 23.63). Vesicles may form along the course of the tunnels and scaling develops as the lesions age. The most common sites in children are the buttocks and the dorsa of the feet, but any area can be affected. The eruption generally disappears after 1–2 months, but may present for 6 months or longer.

Treatment

The time-honored treatment for cutaneous larva migrans is freezing of the area with ethyl chloride or similar refrigerant sprays. This is both extremely painful and ineffective. The larvae

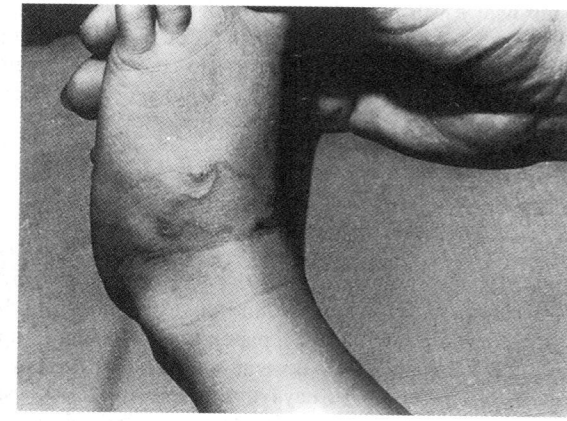

Fig. 23.63 Cutaneous larva migrans.

may be eliminated by a course of diethylcarbamazine (Hetrazan, Banocide) (5 mg/kg per day for 7 days), or thiabendazole (Mintezol) (50 mg/kg in two divided doses twice daily for 3 days, the treatment being repeated at weekly intervals if necessary). Best cure rates, however, are achieved with topical thiabendazole which can easily be made from the oral preparation if not commercially available.

TRICHURIS TRICHIURA (TRICHOCEPHALIASIS, WHIPWORM)

The whipworm, so called for its thin anterior lash-like end (Fig. 23.64), is widely distributed, being most common in hot, damp environs. The adult nematode frequents the cecum but can occur in the appendix, colon or terminal ileum, its thin anterior extremity threaded or embedded in the mucosa (Fig. 23.65a). Children usually acquire whipworm by sucking fingers or objects contaminated with fecal-polluted soil containing infective eggs, but contaminated vegetables and fly-borne contamination are also important means of spread. Trichuriasis is by no means confined to the tropics (Cooper & Bundy 1987) and may prove troublesome in mental institutions at times.

T. vulpis, the dog whipworm, may occasionally infect humans (Milstein & Goldsmid 1995).

Clinical features

Whipworm infection is often asymptomatic but should not be underrated as a pathogen in humans (Cooper & Bundy 1987).

Heavy worm loads may be responsible for intestinal symptoms, usually abdominal pain, which is most marked in the right iliac fossa, bloody diarrhea, tenesmus, and sometimes mild pyrexia. Appendicitis may also result. Excessive loads can lead to marked anemia, weight loss, and a picture closely resembling hookworm disease or amebic colitis. Clubbing of the fingers and toes is often seen in these children and is reversed with eradication of the infection. Rectal prolapse is a well-recognized complication. Trichuriasis often causes insidious disease and is frequently associated with growth retardation in children (Cooper & Bundy 1988).

Diagnosis

This is readily accomplished by finding the characteristic eggs (Fig. 23.65b) in the stools. These eggs under suitable conditions in damp soil require about 3 weeks to mature to the infective stage. A barium enema may assist in diagnosis (Fig. 23.66).

Treatment

The drug of choice remains the very safe mebendazole (Vermox) which should be administered at a dose of 100 mg twice a day for 3 days (Janssens 1985). If the child is suffering from diarrhea, the diarrhea should be controlled before the mebendazole is administered, in order to achieve maximal efficiency. Difetarsone (Bemarsal) has been reported to be most useful in the treatment of whipworm – 2 g daily in divided doses for 10 days are given in adults. Oxantel pamoate is also reported to be effective at a dose

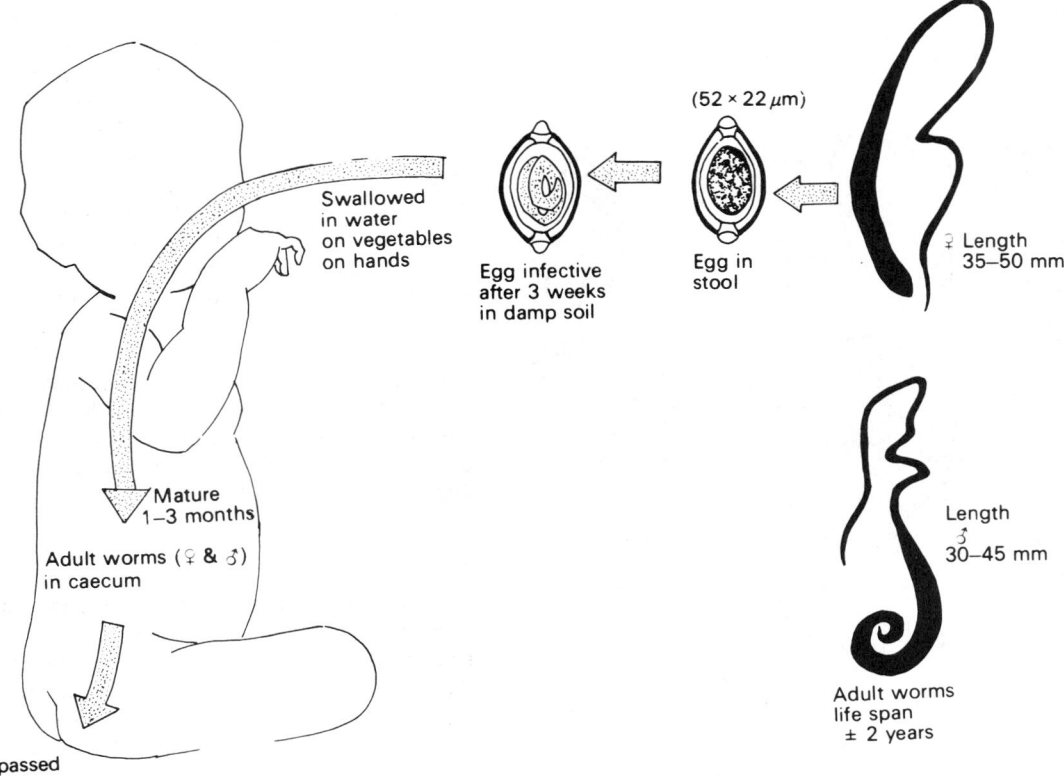

Fig. 23.64 Character and life cycle of *Trichuris trichiura*.

of 15 mg/kg bodyweight (Janssens 1985). Albendazole (600–800 mg for 2–3 days) is a most promising treatment if available (Gustafsson et al 1987).

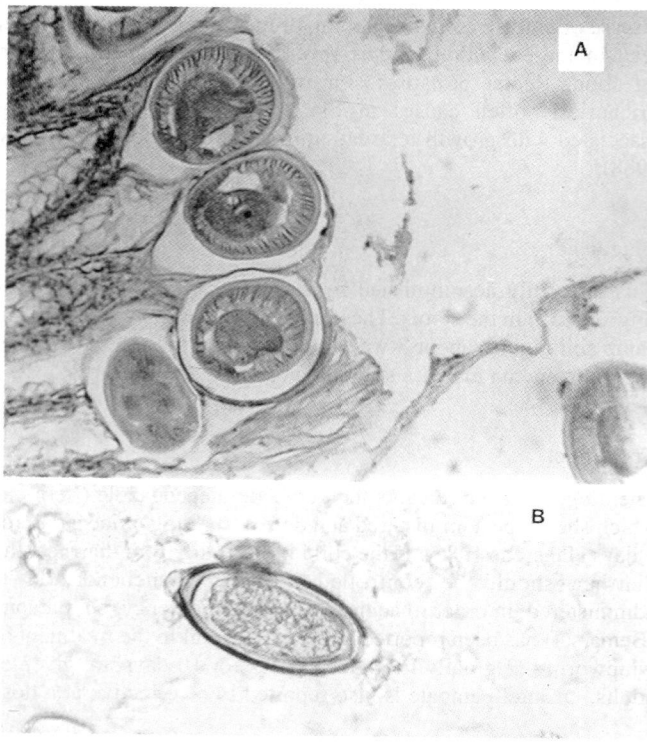

Fig. 23.65 (a) Histological section of *Trichuris trichiura* showing body of worm in lumen of cecum and proboscis threaded into the mucosa (approx. ×250). (b) Egg of *Trichuris trichiura* (approx. ×600).

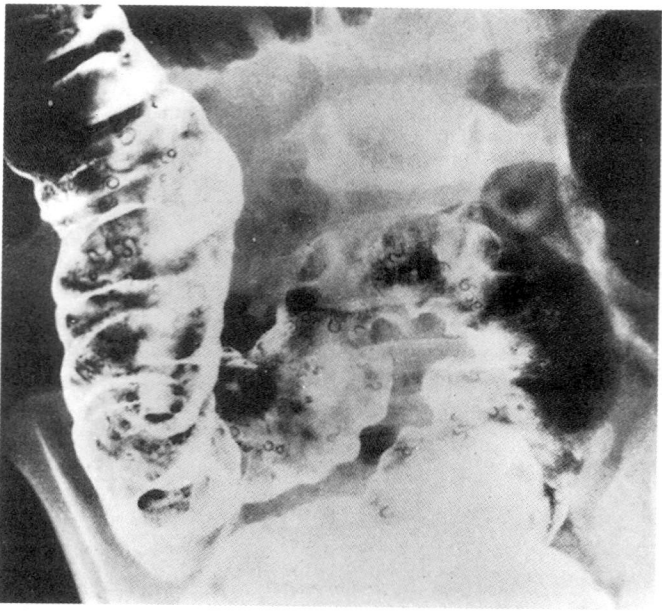

Fig. 23.66 *Trichuris trichiura*. Double contrast barium enema examination showing infestation and numerous small circular or sigmoid defects in barium coating of colon.

STRONGYLOIDES STERCORALIS (STRONGYLOIDIASIS)

Strongyloides stercoralis (sometimes termed 'threadworm' in the American literature) is a facultative parasite with a human cycle closely resembling hookworm, except that internal autoinfection is common and a free-living cycle can occur if external conditions are favorable (Fig. 23.67). Strongyloidiasis is essentially an affliction of tropical or semitropical climates but its sporadic occurrence in temperate zones is recognized. The minute adult worms are to be found in the crypts of Lieberkuhn's glands in the upper part of the small intestine, where they burrow in mucosa.

In central Africa, *Strongyloides fülleborni* is often found in humans and a similar species is reported to cause 'swollen belly syndrome' in infants about 6 weeks of age in Papua New Guinea (Ashford & Barnish 1987). The species in Papua New Guinea has been designated as *Strongyloides fülleborni kellyi* and infants can become infected in the first days of life, with children as young as 18 days of age being found to have patent infections – possibly owing to transmammary infection, as may also occur with *S. fülleborni* in Africa (Ashford et al 1992).

Clinical features

Skin penetration by filariform larvae may be accompanied by a transient prickling sensation, but following heavy infection there is a pruritic petechial rash with local edema. Autoinfection also frequently occurs, especially in immunodeficient patients or patients on immunosuppressant drugs or corticosteroids, larvae in the feces entering the skin in the perianal region. This gives rise to an often recurring eruption resembling cutaneous larva migrans (termed *larva currens*) but of shorter duration. Larvae may also re-enter through the anus. Generalized urticaria is sometimes seen as a result of hypersensitivity. Eosinophilia is common. Clinical manifestations of pulmonary migration of larvae are infrequent, but respiratory symptoms can occur and, rarely, chronic lung disease develops due to misguided larvae maturing within the lung.

In chronic strongyloidiasis the presence of the adult worms in the intestine is often asymptomatic (Genta 1986). A heavy worm load causes epigastric pain, episodes of acute appendicitis (Marty & Andersen 1995) bowel upset often with bloody diarrhea, iron deficiency anemia, and debility. Infection can last for 20 years or more owing to constant internal and external autoinfection (Oliver et al 1990). In immunocompromised patients, fatal autoinfection can occur, but it is noteworthy that despite the AIDS epidemic in central Africa, *S. stercoralis* has not proved an important opportunistic pathogen (Genta 1986, Goldsmid 1991). *Strongyloides* hyperinfection syndrome carries a high mortality and may be complicated by Gram-negative bacteremia in both immunocompromised and noncompromised individuals (Smallman et al 1986, Pagliuca et al 1988).

Diagnosis

Considerable eosinophilia is usual and can be an important diagnostic indicator in some circumstances (Oliver et al 1990). Diagnosis of *S. stercoralis* is established by demonstrating rhabditiform larvae (Fig. 23.68a) in fresh stools (repeat examinations may be necessary) or duodenal fluid. A most useful method for diagnosing *Strongyloides stercoralis*, giardiasis, and other upper intestinal parasites is duodenal drainage or the use of the duodenal capsule (Enterotest), of which a special pediatric size is available. The capsule, containing a length of thread and 3-

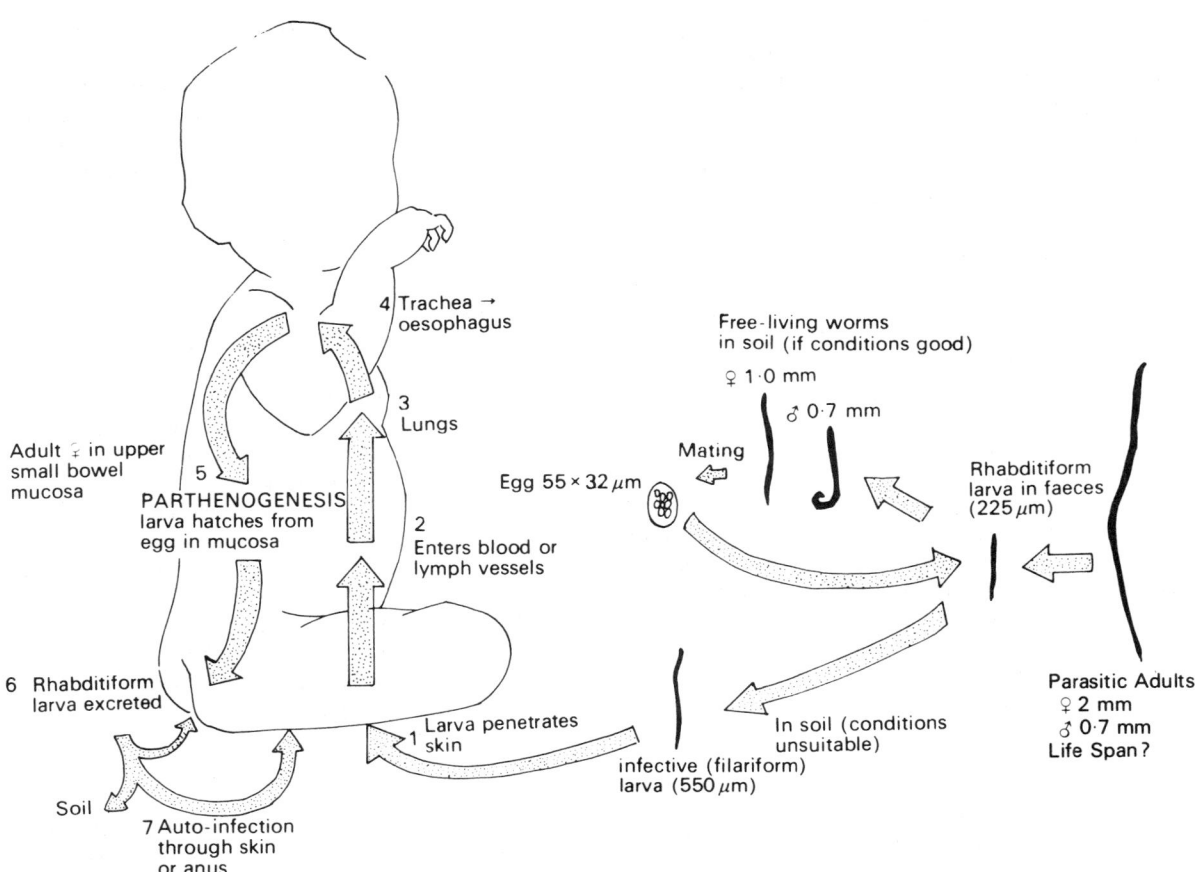

Fig. 23.67 Character and life cycle of *Strongyloides stercoralis*.

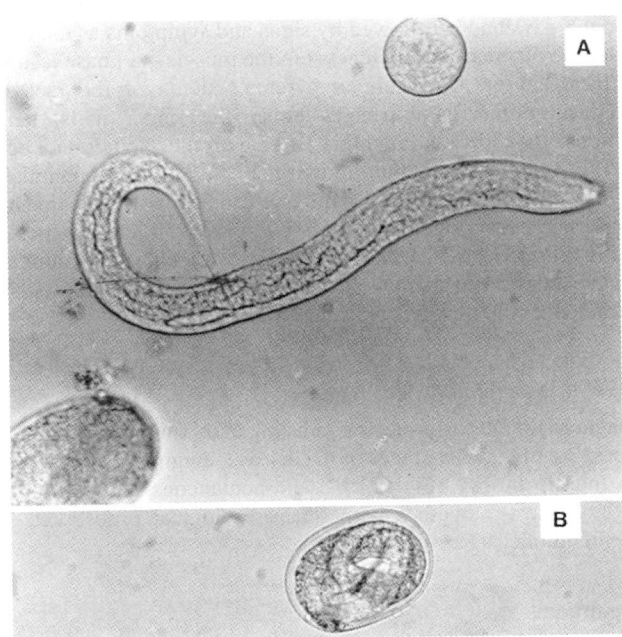

ply nylon yarn, is swallowed while the protruding free end of thread is held at the mouth. The yarn within the capsule plays out, and within 3–4 h the line has almost invariably extended to the duodenum or jejunum. The gelatin capsule dissolves. The nylon yarn is then pulled back through the mouth and the adhering mucus examined for parasites.

In *S. fülleborni* infections, fully embryonated eggs (Fig. 23.68b) are passed in the feces. These are small, being about 50 × 36 μm in size and fully developed at time of passage (Goldsmid 1991).

Treatment

Because of the dangers of autoinfection, strongyloidiasis must always be treated when diagnosed.

The treatment of choice for strongyloidiasis remains thiabendazole (Mintezol) which is effective (50 mg/kg divided into two doses and given morning and evening up to a total of 3 g daily max.). It may, however, have most unpleasant side effects. Ivermectin appears promising but requires further evaluation (Genta 1986) and albendazole is reported to be an effective treatment at a dose of 400 mg given on three consecutive days (Reynolds 1996).

ANGIOSTRONGYLIASIS

Angiostrongylus cantonensis is a natural parasite in the lungs of rats over a wide area of the world, with human infection being

Fig. 23.68 (a) Rhabditiform larva of *Strongyloides stercoralis*. Note short buccal cavity and large genital primordium. Also in the field, an *Entamoeba* cyst and a hookworm egg (approx. ×600). (b) Egg of *Strongyloides fülleborni*. Note its small size. It contains a fully developed, motile larva when passed (approx. ×600).

recorded from Indonesia, Papua New Guinea, northern Australia, Africa, the Pacific, Asia, Cuba and Puerto Rico. The intermediate hosts are snails (such as the giant African land snail *Achatina fulica*) and slugs which are eaten by the rodents. Humans become infected by eating certain edible snails or by accidental ingestion of small infected slugs on food plants or ingestion of paratenic (or 'carrier') hosts such as edible crustacea (Cross 1987).

In humans, larvae migrate to the brain causing a condition known as eosinophilic meningitis, with neck stiffness, photophobia, pyrexia, decreased consciousness and vomiting.

The diagnosis in endemic areas can be suspected when large numbers of eosinophils are found in the CSF in patients with a history of eating snails or perhaps crustacea. Occasionally adults or larvae of *A. cantonensis* may also be detected. A blood eosinophilia may also be present.

No effective treatment is known and may in any case be inadvisable as dead worms cause more clinical problems than live ones.

Other forms of angiostrongyliasis include an abdominal form caused by *A. costaricensis* in several Latin American countries. This species causes intestinal and liver lesions similar to those caused by *Toxocara*. It is usually diagnosed at surgery and has an epidemiology similar to *A. cantonensis* (Morera 1987).

HELMINTHOMA

The nodular worms belong to the genera *Oesophagostomum*, naturally occurring in simian and ruminant hosts, and the false hookworm, *Ternidens deminutus*, a natural parasite of nonhuman primates, are known in central Africa to cause human disease characterized by tumor-like granulomatous reactions in the wall of the colon (Polderman & Blotkamp 1995). Eggs of these species are hookworm-like but larger in size (Goldsmid 1991).

The drug treatment of choice for the expulsion of the adult worm would appear to be mebendazole (Vermox) (100 mg twice a day for 3 days) and albendazole is promising (Goldsmid 1991, Polderman & Blotkamp 1995).

ANISAKIASIS (ANISAKIDOSIS)

This parasitic infection of humans is caused by the larval stages of some 30 genera of anisakid nematodes, of which the commonest are *Anisakis*, *Contracaecum* and *Terranova* (Marty & Andersen 1995). These helminths are intestinal parasites of a range of fish-eating vertebrates, including dolphins, and the larval stages of the worm are found in intermediate hosts such as small fish (e.g. mackerel, herring, salmon), squid or octopus (Bier et al 1987, Oshima 1987). Humans become infected when they eat raw or undercooked fish.

The ingested worms live in the human gastrointestinal tract or penetrate the tissues, giving rise to abscesses or eosinophilic granulomata.

Clinically the infection may be asymptomatic or mild with nausea, vomiting, epigastric pain and often an eosinophilia which may reach 41%. Death, although rare, may result from peritonitis following perforation of the gut (Bier et al 1987).

While the infection has for many years been recognized in Japan, an increase has been noted in the USA owing to better diagnostic techniques (Oshima 1987).

Diagnosis is established at laparotomy, by X-ray, or most reliably, by endoscopy. Serological tests for diagnosis include the radioallergosorbent test (RAST) and counterimmunoelectrophoresis.

The most effective treatment, where possible, is removal of worms from the stomach by endoscopy and prevention is best achieved by removal of worms from fish prior to eating and by thorough cooking of fish. No effective anthelmintic treatment is presently available (Bier et al 1987).

TRICHINOSIS

The genus *Trichinella* contains at least four species of which the best known is *Trichinella spiralis* (Flockhart 1986). *Trichinella spiralis* has a cosmopolitan distribution and the worm is usually transmitted to humans by inadequately cooked, infected pig meat, although outbreaks from other meat sources (e.g. horse meat) are recognized (Anonymous 1986, Campbell 1988), so that the disease may occur in outbreaks (Fig. 23.69). Trichinosis due to *T. spiralis* is rare in communities which shun pork and in those with vigilant agricultural control but human disease, especially with other species (e.g. *T. pseudospiralis*, *T. nelsoni* or *T. nativa*) may be associated with other species of animal. The nematode, of which the adult worm is microscopic in size, naturally infects humans, pigs and rats, as well as other animals. Porcine infection usually results from the ingestion of either infected rats or garbage containing uncooked pork meat.

Clinical features

Human trichinosis is frequently mild or symptomless. Although symptoms may occur as early as 24 h following a pork meal, it is usually during the incubation period of 5–7 days or longer (Kociecka 1987b) in which the ingested larvae mature into adults, that a clinical picture resembling food poisoning develops – nausea, vomiting, diarrhea, and abdominal pain. This phase lasts about 5 days and is followed by signs and symptoms as the larvae enter the bloodstream and encyst in the muscle – a phase lasting a further 2–3 weeks. There is pyrexia, edema of the face and eyelids, splinter hemorrhages under the finger nails, tender lymphadenopathy, and myalgia, often extreme. Cough may occur and in severe cases the illness may suggest encephalitis or myocarditis. Marked eosinophilia is usual. Final encystment of the larvae occurs only in voluntary muscles particularly those of the diaphragm, throat, chest wall, extrinsic ocular apparatus and tongue, and patients may die of toxemia or myocarditis. The encysted larvae may live for many years.

Diagnosis

Diagnosis in the early stages can be made by finding worms in the feces, but in the later stages of the disease, diagnosis is established by muscle biopsy (Fig. 23.70). Intracutaneous and fluorescent antibody tests, together with other serological procedures, are useful adjuncts (Kociecka 1987b).

Treatment

There is evidence that thiabendazole (Mintezol) (50 mg/kg per day in two doses for 2–7 days) rapidly kills off migrating larvae and relieves the symptoms. If taken early, the drug also kills larvae in the bowel but is not lethal to the adult worms. Corticosteroids, previously recommended for the treatment of

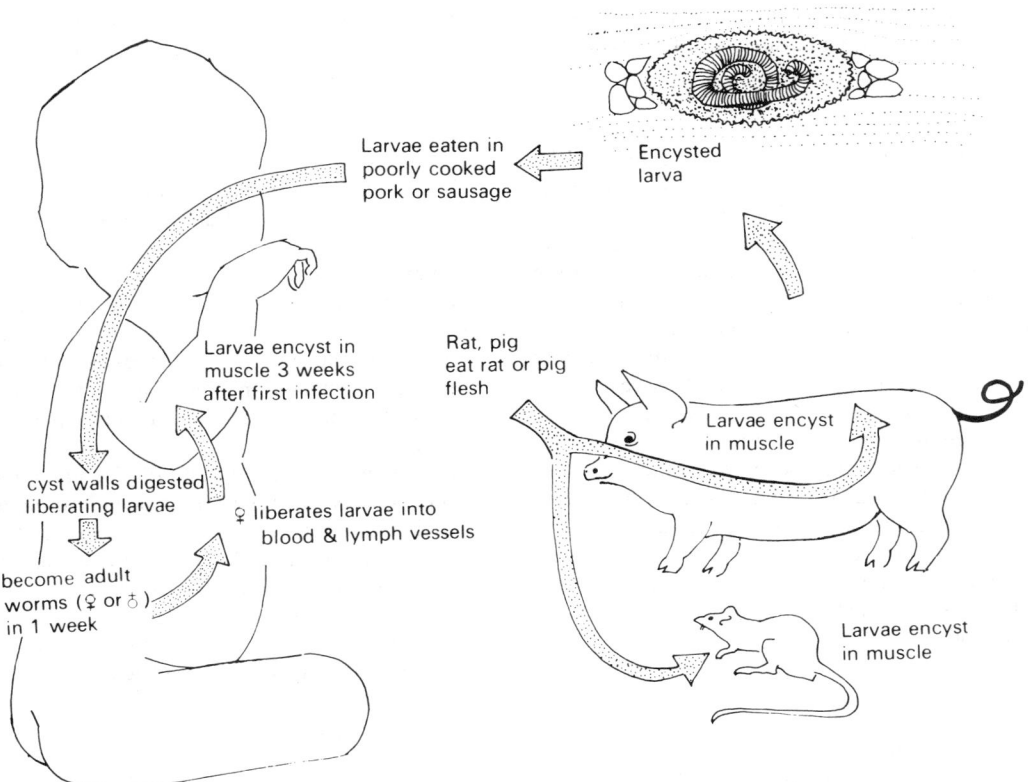

Fig. 23.69   Character and life cycle of *Trichinella spiralis*.

trichinosis, should be restricted to critically ill cases, and then only used in conjunction with anthelminthics. Other drugs found to be of value, especially during the intestinal phase of trichinosis, include mebendazole and pyrantel (Kociecka 1987b).

CAPILLARIA PHILIPPINENSIS (CAPILLARIASIS)

It has long been known that the nematode *Capillaria hepatica* can cause a visceral larva migrans-like syndrome in people who have eaten meat (e.g. infected liver) or sand containing the eggs of the worm. These children exhibit such symptoms as fever, eosinophilia, abdominal pain and hepatomegaly, with large numbers of typical eggs being found in the liver on histological examination.

Another species of the genus, *C. philippinensis*, has also been

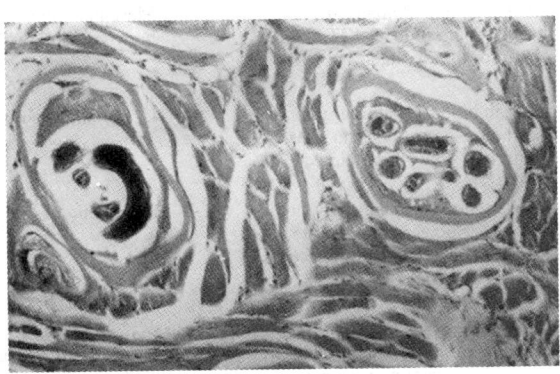

Fig. 23.70   Tongue biopsy showing *Trichinella spiralis*.

shown to be an important cause of epidemic diarrhea in humans. Clinical features in these cases include abdominal pain, malabsorption and diarrhea which is often severe and not uncommonly fatal (35%) without medical care (Cross & Basaca-Sevilla 1987).

C. philippinensis is a parasite of the small intestine and it is believed to be a zoonotic infection but the life cycle has not been elucidated for certain. Humans become infected by ingestion of eggs or infected raw fish, the usual intermediate host, and loads within the host may increase as a result of autoinfection (Marty & Andersen 1995).

C. aerophila is a zoonotic species found in the lungs of cats, and occasional human infections have been recorded (Marty & Andersen 1995).

Diagnosis of capillariasis is based upon histology or finding eggs and larvae in feces. These eggs are like those of *Trichuris*, but the polar plugs are inset and the shells are striated or pitted. *Capillaria hepatica* eggs can be found as spurious 'transit eggs' in feces of patients who have recently eaten infected liver (Goldsmid 1995).

Treatment for capillariasis is thiabendazole (Mintezol) 25 mg/kg per day for 30 days or longer. Side effects and relapses are, however, common (Cross & Basaca-Sevilla 1987). Mebendazole and albendazole are also reported to be effective for the treatment of capillariasis (Marty & Andersen 1995).

DRACUNCULOSIS (DRACONTIASIS)

Despite its bizarre mode of propagation, the guinea worm (*Dracunculus medinensis*) is widely distributed in equatorial Africa, the Middle East and India. However, with new international efforts to improve drinking water supplies, dracontiasis eradication may well be feasible (Muller 1985).

Clinical features

Children from the age of 2 years upwards may be infected by drinking water containing *Cyclops*, a tiny crustacean which is infected with the larvae of *Dracunculus*. During the asymptomatic incubation period, lasting approximately 1 year, the guinea worm matures in retroperitoneal tissues. The male, after having fertilized the female, apparently dies. The gravid female, often over 100 cm in length by 1.5 mm in width, then migrates through the subcutaneous tissues to distal parts of the extremities, usually the lower limb, to form a large pruritic papule. This vesiculates and then bursts leaving a shallow ulcer. On immersion in water the worm's uterus prolapses through the ulcer releasing myriads of larvae. Occasionally adult worms may develop in ectopic sites.

Papule formation may be associated with a marked allergic reaction (vomiting, diarrhea, urticaria and bronchospasm).

Secondary infection of sinuses, subcutaneous cysts, sterile abscesses, and perarticular fibrosis with joint deformity are recognized complications. Calcified worms may be discovered on radiological examination.

Treatment

The ancient technique of repeatedly stimulating the parturient worm with cold water, grasping the uterus which then protrudes, and then cautiously winding the worm round a stick an inch or two per day is still used. However, drug treatments recommended for dracontiasis include the use of niridazole (Ambilhar) (25 mg/kg daily in two divided doses for 7–10 days) and thiabendazole (Mintezol) which has also been reported to be effective at a total dose of 25 mg/kg orally daily for 3 days.

Metronidazole (Flagyl) is also claimed to be highly effective at an oral dose of 25 mg/kg (max. 750 mg/day) daily in three doses for 10 days (Gustafsson et al 1987).

FILARIASIS

Filariasis has been ranked by the World Health Organization as number two on the list of diseases causing disabling conditions in humans.

Humans are the primary hosts to several species of filariae, the adult worms living in the tissues. The adult female worms produce eggs which hatch to release prelarval microfilariae. These are ingested by an appropriate blood-sucking arthropod vector in which they undergo metamorphosis to form infective larvae. Important characteristics of the principal human filariae are shown in Table 23.48.

During the early stages of all filarial infections moderate to high eosinophilia is usual, but this gradually diminishes in those who have been infected for long periods. Apart from *Onchocerca volvulus* where microfilariae are found in skin snips, parasitological diagnosis is best achieved by using stained blood films or concentration techniques applied to peripheral blood. However, very promising and effective serological tests for the detection of circulating filarial antigen have been developed.

Onchocerca volvulus

Onchocerciasis is a filarial disease which is transmitted to humans by bites from black flies of the genus *Simulium*. It is characterized by subcutaneous nodules containing adult worms of *O. volvulus*, by skin eruptions due to microfilariae and by serious eye disease. The condition is only seen in central Africa and in Central and parts of South America (Table 23.48) especially along the banks of fast flowing rivers in which the flies breed.

Table 23.48 Types of filaria worms responsible for human disease

Type and distribution	Insect vector	Important features of microfilaria	Human adult worm location
Onchocerca volvulus, west, central and east Africa, Guatemala, Mexico, and Surinam	*Simulium* black flies	Do not occur in blood, but in skin as unsheathed intradermal microfilariae (microfilariae may penetrate eye)	Subcutaneous tissue
Mansonella perstans, tropical and subtropical areas mainly of Africa and South America	*Culicoides* midges	Occur in blood. Nonperiodic. Unsheathed. Nuclear column extends into tip of thick, blunt tail	Mesentric perirenal and retroperitoneal tissues
Mansonella ozzardi, South America	*Culicoides* midges	Occur in blood. Nonperiodic. Nuclear column does NOT extend into tip of thin, pointed tail	Mesentery and serous body cavities
Wuchereria bancrofti, tropical and subtropical areas throughout the world	Many mosquitoes belonging to the genera *Culex, Aedes, Anopheles,* and *Mansonia*	Occur in blood. Nocturnal periodic. Sheathed. Nuclear column does NOT extend into tip of thin pointed tail	Lymphatic tissue
Brugia malayi, East Indies and Southern Asia	Many mosquitoes belonging to the genera *Mansonia, Culex,* and *Anopheles*	Occur in blood. Nocturnal periodic. Sheathed. Nuclear column extends into tip of tail with single spaced nuclei in terminal bulb and subterminal swelling	Lymphatic tissue
Loa loa, West and Central Africa	*Chrysops* flies	Occur in blood. Diurnal periodic. Sheathed. Nuclear column extends into tip of thick blunt tail	Subcutaneous tissue

Clinical features

Adolescents are most commonly affected but children down to 1 year of age may be afflicted.

Signs of disease begin to appear in 4–18 months and the commonest manifestation is the *Onchocerca* nodule. These subcutaneous fibrous nodules (onchocercomata), containing one or more adult worms in each, vary from a few millimeters to about 3 cm in diameter and become fully developed within a year of exposure. In Africa they tend to occur most commonly in the pelvic region especially over the hips and on the buttocks, while in America the head is more usually involved. Nodules do not generally give rise to much discomfort, but at times they may be painful, and secondary infection with abscess formation can occur. The number and size of nodules increase with intensity of the infection (Fig. 23.71).

Typical skin lesions (onchodermatitis) consist of an intensely itchy papular dermatitis with edema in the early stages progressing to lichenification and atrophy ('lizard skin'). Large numbers of microfilariae are present in the skin and involvement may be generalized or limited to one area of the body. Transient urticaria is often the only skin manifestation, and indeed the condition may be entirely asymptomatic despite the presence of microfilariae in the skin. General well-being is seldom disturbed.

Ocular lesions (river blindness) due to microfilariae penetrating the eyes represent the most serious feature of onchocerciasis and are a frequent cause of blindness in endemic areas. They occur especially when the disease is present in the upper half of the body and are commoner in America. Children rarely show advanced ocular lesions, but hyperemia of the conjunctiva and nummular keratitis may be seen on occasions in older children. Any part of the eye can be involved.

Diagnosis

Diagnosis is best established by demonstrating microfilariae in skin snips and the adult worms on nodule biopsy (Fig. 23.71). Intradermal and complement-fixation tests are also available in onchocerciasis. Microfilariae are not uncommonly found in urine.

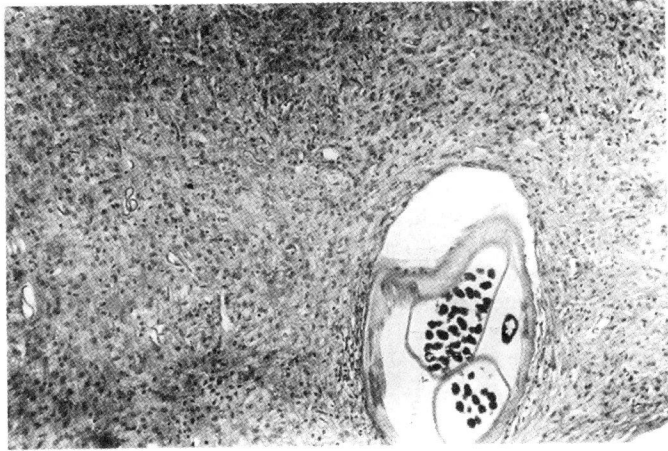

Fig. 23.71 Section of skin nodule caused by *Onchocerca volvulus*. Note section of adult worm and numerous microfilariae migrating through the skin.

Treatment

Excision of nodules is recommended prior to chemotherapy, especially those near the eyes because of the danger of ocular involvement. Microfilariae are killed by diethylcarbamazine but the drug causes a temporary exacerbation of skin and eye lesions, tenderness of nodules, and enlargement of regional lymph glands. This reaction forms the basis for the Mazzoti test – a useful diagnostic procedure. Diethylcarbamazine should, therefore, be given in small doses initially (0.5 mg/kg three times daily) gradually increasing to 2 mg/kg (max. 150 mg/day) three times daily for 2–3 weeks. Severe reactions can be controlled with corticosteroids. Suramin (Antrypol) is lethal to the adult worms. A course consists of 6 doses of 20 mg/kg intravenously at intervals of 7 days. Regular urine tests should be made as the drug is nephrotoxic. Ivermectin is now accepted as the treatment of choice for onchocerciasis at a single dose of 200 µg/kg for both adults and children (Cupp 1992, Whitworth 1992, Chodakewitz 1995). Its use for mass treatment has given hope for the effective control of this disease. Amocarzine and albendazole are also being evaluated for efficacy in the treatment of onchocerciasis (Marty & Andersen 1995).

Vector control would require the simultaneous application of control measures (spraying with appropriate insecticides) over whole river systems.

Loa loa

Microfilariae of the worm *Loa loa* are transmitted to humans by flies of the genus *Chrysops*, which, in turn, are infected by sucking human blood containing microfilariae. These are present in blood during the daytime, thus corresponding with the diurnal biting habits of most *Chrysops*. The disease is endemic in western and central Africa. Adult worms live in the subcutaneous tissues, the male being some 3 cm and the female 6 cm in length. They may remain viable for as long as 30 years.

Clinical features

Symptoms of loiasis are trivial. The most characteristic manifestation is a recurrent, painless, puffy, pink, swelling, often referred to as a calabar, or fugitive, swelling. This lesion marks the journey of the adult worm in the subcutis. It develops over a period of 3–4 h and may acquire a diameter of 10 cm or more, before subsiding in a few days. The upper extremities and eyelids are most often involved and on occasions the thin worm may be seen rapidly traversing the bulbar conjunctiva and sometimes accompanied by periorbital edema. The appearance of the calabar swelling is frequently associated with fever and malaise. Eosinophilia is present.

Some patients remain afilaremic, no microfilariae being found in the peripheral blood despite intensive investigation (Pinder 1988).

Treatment

Diethylcarbamazine is a highly effective remedy in loiasis. The recommended dose is 0.5 mg/kg three times daily for 2 days, and if no unfavorable reactions follow, the dose is increased to 3 mg/kg three times a day for a further 3 weeks. Mebendazole and ivermectin appear less effective (Pinder 1988).

Wuchereria bancrofti and Brugia malayi

Infections by *Wuchereria bancrofti*, *Brugia malayi* and *B. timori* (termed 'lymphatic filariasis') occur in the tropics and in some semitropical areas, being transmitted by various species of mosquito. The adult female and male worms (some 85 mm and 40 mm in length respectively) attain maturity in the lymphatic system about 1 year following entry to the body, after which time the nocturnal periodic microfilariae are demonstrable in peripheral blood between 10 p.m. and 2 a.m. (Fig. 23.72). Some Pacific strains of *W. bancrofti* are nonperiodic.

Clinical features

First infection may occur in children but the full clinical picture may take many years to develop. As with other filarial diseases, the early phases may be entirely asymptomatic or associated with florid allergic manifestations. The commonest manifestations of the mature filariae are acute and recurring lymphangitis. The affected lymph node together with its afferent vessel, usually in the groin, are painful and tender. The lymphatic vessel becomes palpable and cord-like and is associated with a linear red streak in the overlying skin. This stage is often accompanied by pyrexia, malaise, nausea, and headache. The attacks, which subside after several days, have a variable periodicity of weeks or months, gradually becoming less severe, often with persistence of residual subcutaneous swelling. Recurrent funiculitis may occur and involvement of intra-abdominal lymph nodes may give rise to the clinical picture of peritonitis. Chylous ascites, chyluria, varicose groin nodes, hydrocele and elephantiasis are classical end results but as they arise from chronicity over many years, emphasis on this aspect is out of place in a pediatric context. Nevertheless, early manifestations of chronic disease may sometimes appear in the late years of childhood.

Work by Hightower et al (1993) has suggested that children born to mothers infected with *W. bancrofti* are more susceptible to infection than those born to uninfected mothers.

Tropical eosinophilia syndrome. In some patients, an abnormal response to *W. bancrofti* infections results in a clinical picture reflecting a specific allergic sensitization to filarial antigens – a condition known as tropical pulmonary eosinophilia or tropical eosinophilia syndrome. These patients present with cough, asthma-like symptoms, respiratory distress and eosinophil counts of 3000/mm³ or greater. X-ray of the lungs usually shows extensive changes. An interesting feature of this syndrome is that patients do not develop a filaremia – hence the name of 'occult filariasis'.

A similar condition can be caused by infection with *Brugia malayi* and perhaps by infection with nonhuman filariae.

Diagnosis

The clinical diagnosis based on symptoms can now be greatly aided by ultrasonography and lymphoscintigraphy.

The recovery of typical sheathed microfilariae (Fig. 23.72) in midnight blood slides and occasionally in urine will establish the diagnosis. Concentration techniques may need to be used to recover microfilariae from the blood.

In the case of tropical pulmonary eosinophilia, diagnosis is made clinically and confirmed by serology or rapid response to diethylcarbamazine (Partono 1985).

It is worth noting that visitors to endemic areas who contract lymphatic filariasis often do not develop a microfilaremia, which can make parasitological confirmation of the infection impossible. Thus the development of an EIA test (TropBio, Australia) to detect circulating filarial antigen has provided a major breakthrough in the diagnosis of lymphatic filariasis, the test for *W. bancrofti* being highly specific and very sensitive.

Treatment

Diethylcarbamazine rapidly removes circulating microfilariae but large doses are required to kill adult worms. The initial dosage should be 0.5–1.0 mg/kg in divided doses daily for 3 days, followed by 2.0 mg/kg three times daily for a further 2–3 weeks (Gustafsson et al 1987). There is often an acute exacerbation during therapy, for which antihistamines should be given. Ivermectin which has significantly fewer side effects than diethylcarbamazine is also very effective in the treatment of lymphatic filariasis, but may not be readily available. It kills microfilariae but not adult worms and the single oral dose of 200 µg/kg should be repeated at yearly intervals. Ottesen et al (1990) concluded that a single oral dose of ivermectin was a favorable method for controlling lymphatic filariasis and the review by Chodakewitz (1995) has confirmed its value against *W. bancrofti*.

The use of yearly or 6-monthly doses of ivermectin or the regular use of salt fortified with diethylcarbamazine has proved invaluable in the control of lymphatic filariasis in endemic regions.

Mansonella perstans and Mansonella ozzardi

Mansonella perstans has had many recent changes in name (Muller 1987) and is widely distributed in those tropical and subtropical areas which favor the habitat of the vector. The microfilariae (Fig. 23.73) are transmitted by *Culicoides* midges from person to person, and the adult worms develop in the mesentery, perinephric and retroperitoneal tissues where they may survive for many years. The females measure 75 mm and the males 45 mm in length (Table 23.48).

Clinical features

This form of filariasis was long held to be harmless, but it is now known that symptoms can be associated with infection, particularly in people visiting from nonendemic regions. Infection

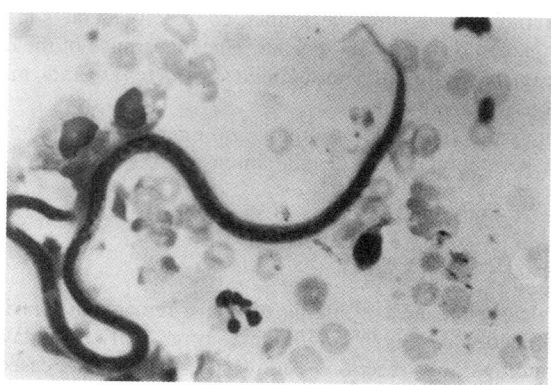

Fig. 23.72 *Wuchereria bancrofti* in peripheral blood.

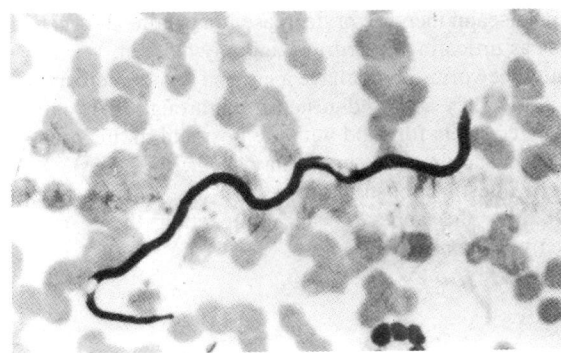

Fig. 23.73   *Mansonella perstans* in peripheral blood.

with these helminths may result in lethargy, arthralgia, urticaria and headache. Less frequently calabar-like swellings around the eye ('bung eye'), and pericardial or pleural effusions occur. Among indigenous inhabitants of endemic areas *M. perstans* is often asymptomatic.

The prepatent period from exposure to the appearance of nonperiodic microfilariae in the blood is unknown.

Diethylcarbamazine is ineffective in treatment of the disease, but trichlorophone has been used with success in an adult dose of 10 mg/kg given every 2 weeks with a total of four doses. The judicious use of corticosteroids is valuable in severe cases. Mebendazole or a combination of mebendazole (Vermox) and levamisole (Ketrax) have proved effective.

In rain forest areas of central Africa, a related species, *M. streptocerca*, infects humans. Microfilariae of this species are unsheathed and have a curled tail with nuclei extending to the tip. The adult and microfilariae of this species are found in skin and diagnosis is by skin snips as for *Onchocerca*. Symptoms include a dermatitis, with macules and papules. Infection is more common in older people than in children.

Mansonella ozzardi in South America is a species with many clinical similarities to *M. perstans*. In the past it too has been considered a commensal, but studies have suggested that this parasite may also not be as harmless as is often believed (Table 23.48).

Dirofilaria immitis

The dog heartworm is a common filarial nematode infecting dogs in most tropical regions of the world including parts of the USA and northern Australia. It is transmitted by mosquitoes.

Occasional human cases are diagnosed during serological surveys or on biopsy for investigations of pulmonary 'coin' lesions found on X-ray (Smyth 1995). Cases of pleural effusion, intraocular infection and eosinophilic meningitis are also caused by *D. immitis* in humans. Most cases of dirofilariasis are recorded in adults, but clinical infections are seen at times in children and Hungerford (1977) believes that dirofilariasis is much commoner in Australia than at present believed.

As *D. immitis* infection in humans does not usually exhibit a filaremia, diagnosis is usually made on biopsy of a lung lesion, on removal of a worm from the eye, by skin tests or such serological tests as the indirect fluorescent antibody test.

Other species of *Dirofilaria* are also recorded from humans, usually from subcutaneous tissue or from the conjunctival sac.

CESTODES (TAPEWORMS)

The cestodes are platyhelminths, which are dorsoventrally flattened, have no gut or body cavity and are hermaphroditic. Adult tapeworms have a characteristic morphology with a scolex armed with suckers and sometimes hooks, an unsegmented neck region and a long segmented strobila.

Life cycles are complex, with the adult tapeworms living in the gastrointestinal tract of the vertebrate definitive hosts and with larval stages occurring in a range of vertebrate or invertebrate intermediate host species. Larval forms vary from the free-living ciliated coracidium larva and worm-like procercoid and plerocercoid (sparganum) larvae of the pseudophyllidean tapeworms (e.g. *Diphyllobothrium latum*) to the cysticercoid, cysticercus (bladderworm) or hydatid larvae of the cyclophyllidean tapeworms.

Humans can become infected with a range of cestode species and mostly harbor the adult tapeworm although human infection with larval cestodes includes sparganosis (*Spirometra* sp.), cysticercosis (*Taenia solium*) and hydatidosis (*Echinococcus granulosus*).

The cestodes relevant to humans are *Taenia saginata, Taenia solium, Hymenolepis nana, Hymenolepis diminuta, Dipylidium caninum, Diphyllobothrium latum, Echinococcus* spp. and *Inermicapsifer madagascariensis*.

TAENIASIS

Taeniasis is caused by infection with adult *Taenia saginata* or *T. solium* (Table 23.49). In both these infections, the adult tapeworm is found in the intestinal tract of humans – the only definitive host. The intermediate hosts harboring the larval stage (cysticercus) of the tapeworm are cattle in *T. saginata* (the beef tapeworm) and usually pigs in *T. solium* (the pork tapeworm). However, in the case of *T. solium*, in addition to pigs, a wide range of mammals, including humans, can harbor the cysticerci.

It has been suggested that in the Asia-Pacific region, other but as yet incompletely defined, species of *Taenia* may infect humans (Ito 1992, McManus & Bowles 1994). One such species found in Indonesia, Taiwan and Korea, morphologically resembles *T. saginata* but is acquired from pork and has been named *T. asiatica* (Marty & Andersen 1995).

Infection with adult *Taenia* results from ingestion of infected meat and as such is not common in very young children.

Taenia saginata (the beef tapeworm)

The beef tapeworm is cosmopolitan, occurring in almost all countries where beef is eaten. It is especially common where local

Table 23.49   Characteristics of *Taenia saginata* and *Taenia solium*

	Taenia saginata	*Taenia solium*
Parasite		
Scolex	4 suckers only	Crown of hooklets and 4 suckers
Length	5–20 m	3–15 m
Lateral branches of uterus	15 or more	8–13
Intermediate host	Cattle	Pig, but occasionally man
Final host	Man	Man

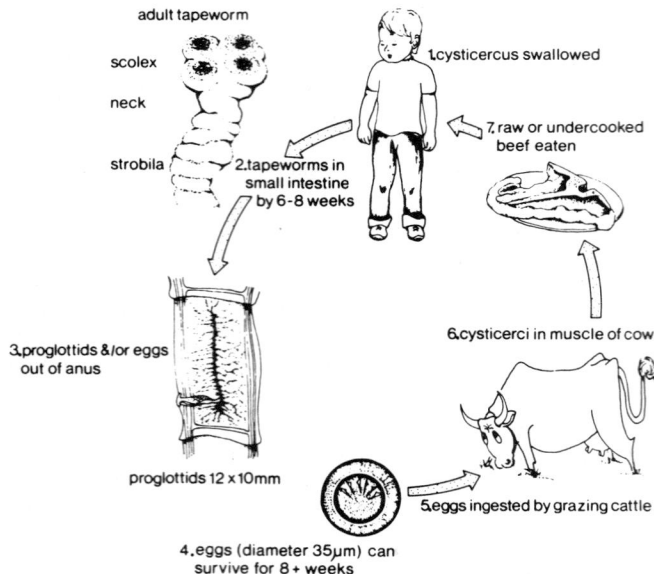

Fig. 23.74 Life cycle of *Taenia saginata*.

eating habits favor the consumption of raw or undercooked beef. The cysticerci in the beef can even survive salting and a moderate degree of drying.

The adult worm is harbored in the human intestine with the scolex, which has four suckers but no hooks, attached to the mucosa of the small intestine. The adult tapeworm may reach 20–25 m in length and gravid proglottids (or segments), their uteri packed with eggs (often in excess of 40 000 eggs per segment) break from the strobila singly or in chains of 2–5 segments, and either migrate actively out of the anus or pass out passively with the feces.

The proglottids crawl about on the ground releasing eggs which are also liberated when the proglottid dies and disintegrates on pasture land. Eggs lying on the grass are ingested by grazing cattle (Fig. 23.74). The oncosphere (hexacanth) larva is released in the intestine, penetrates the intestinal wall using its six hooklets and is carried via the bloodstream to the heart and voluntary muscles, especially the tongue, shoulder and masseter muscles. Here it loses its hooklets, develops an inverted scolex with suckers but no hooks and changes into a bladderworm (or cysticercus) larva, termed *Cysticercus bovis*, over about 3 months. These cysticerci are about 8 × 5 mm in size and meat infected with them is commonly termed 'measly' owing to its spotted appearance.

When ingested the cysticercus evaginates the scolex and elongates into the adult stage. Humans eating such 'measly' beef raw or undercooked thus become infected with adult tapeworm. Gravid segments are shed about 3 months after infection.

Epidemics of 'measles' in cattle have not uncommonly resulted from cattle grazed on pastures fertilized with untreated effluent from sewage outlets. Such cattle become infective in about 3 months after ingestion of eggs.

Clinical features

In most cases infection with *T. saginata* is quite symptomless, the only feature being the intermittent passing of segments. In 5–50% of cases, eosinophilia may occur while abdominal pain, weight loss, malaise, an increase or decrease in appetite and such allergic features as urticaria and pruritus ani may be seen.

Adult tapeworms do not have a gut and do not feed on the tissue of the host. They absorb digested food through their cuticles and thus they compete for food with the host and in this process food deprivation and digestive upset may occur.

Rarely intestinal obstruction results and at times proglottids wander into the appendix and, impacting there, may cause obstructive appendicitis.

Diagnosis

Diagnosis is generally made when proglottids are seen in the stool. These can readily be identified by pressing them between two glass microslides and counting the number of uterine branches on each side of the central stem. In *T. saginata* there are usually 15 or more primary uterine branches on each side.

In the cases where proglottids cannot be found, eggs (Fig. 23.75a and b) may be detected in the feces or on anal tapes as used for *Enterobius*, a process which is more effective for recovery of *T. saginata* eggs than stool examination. Eggs of *T. saginata* and *T. solium* are identical.

Treatment

The treatment of choice for *T. saginata* infection is now praziquantel as a single oral dose of 10–20 mg/kg (Schneider et al 1990). Niclosamide (Yomesan) is also effective, being usually given without purgation at a dose of 0.5 g (1 tablet) which should be chewed before swallowing. A repeat dose is given after 1 h and the worm is passed in a partially digested state. Treatment can be followed, if desired, by a saline purge after 2 h.

Treated patients should be rechecked 3 months after treatment to assess cure. With modern anthelmintics it is not feasible to examine post-treatment stools for the scolex.

Prevention of *T. saginata* infection depends upon avoidance of consumption of raw or undercooked beef and hygienic disposal of human feces to prevent infection of cattle. Freezing of meat (− 10°C for 10 days) is also reported to be effective in killing cysticerci.

Taenia solium (the pork tapeworm)

T. solium is widely distributed, but less so than the beef tapeworm. It is common, however, in Africa, Asia, Latin America and parts of eastern Europe.

The life cycle of *T. solium* (Fig. 23.76) is similar to that of *T. saginata* but with some very important differences. In both

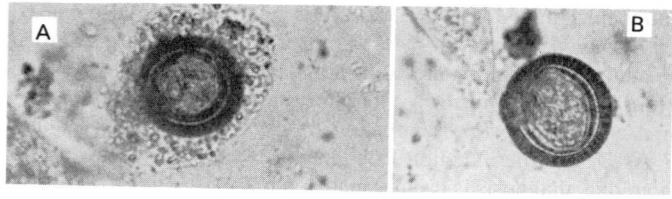

Fig. 23.75 (a) Complete egg of *Taenia* sp., the embryophore being surrounded by the remains of the vitelline cell. (b) Other egg has lost all traces of the vitelline cell and consists only of the oncosphere larva surrounded by its thick, striated embryophore (approx. ×600).

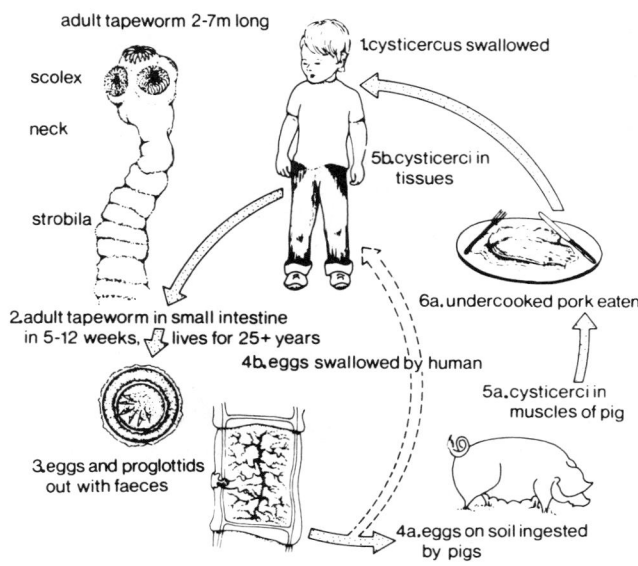

Fig. 23.76 Life cycle of *Taenia solium*.

adult tapeworm 2-7m long

scolex

neck

strobila

1.cysticercus swallowed

5b.cysticerci in tissues

6a.undercooked pork eaten

5a.cysticerci in muscles of pig

2.adult tapeworm in small intestine in 5-12 weeks, lives for 25+ years

4b.eggs swallowed by human

3.eggs and proglottids out with faeces

4a.eggs on soil ingested by pigs

species humans comprise the only definitive host and may harbor one or more tapeworms. In *T. solium* infections humans become infected with the adult tapeworm after eating raw or undercooked 'measly' pork containing cysticerci. The range of intermediate hosts of *T. solium* is wider than that of *T. saginata* and besides pigs, can include the domestic dog. In fact, in areas where dogs form a significant part of human diet, they may serve as an important source of human *T. solium* infection. Humans too can become infected with cysticerci of *T. solium* (known as *Cysticercus cellulosae*) after ingestion of eggs – a condition termed cysticercosis.

The adult *T. solium* is, on average, a little shorter than *T. saginata*, reaching about 15 m in length. The scolex has both suckers and a double row of hooks. The cysticerci of both species are essentially similar, but again the invaginated scolex of *C. cellulosae* has hooks which are absent in *C. bovis*.

Clinical features

Taeniasis. Infection with the adult *T. solium* is much the same as with the adult *T. saginata* except that proglottids of the pork tapeworm are less mobile than those of the beef tapeworm and so such features as appendiceal blockage are rarer. Most cases are asymptomatic, but diarrhea and constipation have been recorded and a moderate eosinophilia may develop.

Cysticercosis. The greatest danger in infection with *T. solium* is the danger to others of infection with eggs via food or water (heteroinfection) and the danger to the patients themselves of autoinfection by external means (hand-to-mouth transfer of eggs) or internal means (vomiting up and reswallowing of proglottids).

The clinical effects of cysticercosis are essentially dependent upon the number and sites of the cysticerci. Cysticerci can develop almost anywhere in the body – beneath the skin (subcutaneous cysticercosis); in the myocardium; in the muscles; within the eye or in the brain (cerebral cysticercosis). If within the ventricles of the brain the cysticerci can become greatly enlarged resulting in a racemose cyst.

Usually cysticerci do not cause clinical symptoms until they

die, swell and calcify – a process which occurs about 3 years or longer after infection. Whether or not they cause symptoms is also dependent upon their site. In the muscles, heart or beneath the skin they are relatively benign but within the eye they can cause retinal detachment, loss of vision and even blindness, while if sited in the brain they may result in neurological disorders, personality changes or jacksonian-type epileptic convulsions. Cerebral cysticercosis is a not uncommon cause of epilepsy among Africans in southern Africa and although more common in adults, it has even been recorded in children as young as 3 years of age (McKelvie & Goldsmid 1988). Death can follow hydrocephalus resulting from blockage of the ventricular spaces.

Diagnosis

Taeniasis. Diagnosis of infection with adult *T. solium* is established by the finding of eggs (indistinguishable from those of *T. saginata*) in feces (Fig. 23.75) or by the passing of typical gravid proglottids. The proglottids of *T. solium* have less than 13 lateral uterine branches on each side and so can be differentiated from those of *T. saginata* although some degree of overlap may occur. (*Note*: gloves must be worn when examining proglottids for counting of the uterine branches as eggs of *T. solium* are infective to humans.)

Cysticercosis. Cysticercosis can be diagnosed by palpation and biopsy of cysticerci if accessible and their microscopic examination after squashing between two glass microslides (Fig. 23.77a) or after histological sectioning (Fig. 23.77b).

In patients in whom cysticercosis is clinically suspected confirmation can sometimes be obtained by radiology, where calcified cysticerci are visible as millet seed-shaped shadows in the muscles (Fig. 23.78b), or small spotted areas on skull X-ray (Fig. 23.78a). X-rays are also useful in differentiating cerebral cysticercosis from CNS infection due to *Angiostrongylus*, *Gnathostoma* and *Paragonimus* (Jaroonvesama 1988).

Eosinophils can at times be found in the CSF of patients with cerebral cysticercosis. About 25% of patients with cerebral cysticercosis will be found to harbor adult *T. solium* in their intestines or have a history of such infection.

Serological tests for blood or CSF are available for the diagnosis of cysticercosis – these include solid-phase radioimmunoassay and ELISA tests (Tillez-Giron et al 1987, Jaroonvesama 1988). In addition, standard ELISA and DOT ELISA tests have been developed to detect cysticercal antigen in CSF.

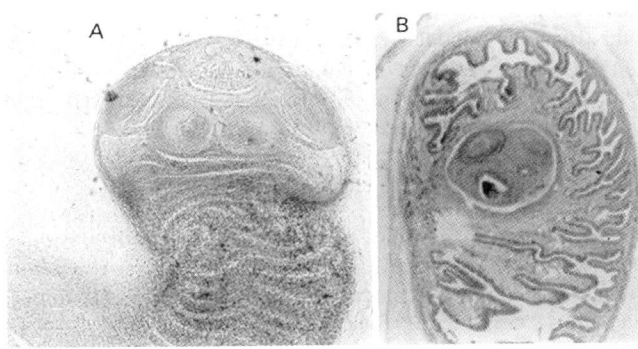

Fig. 23.77 (**a**) Squash preparation of *Cysticercus cellulosae* (approx. ×35). (**b**) Histological section of *Cysticercus cellulosae* in heart section through scolex region (approx. ×35).

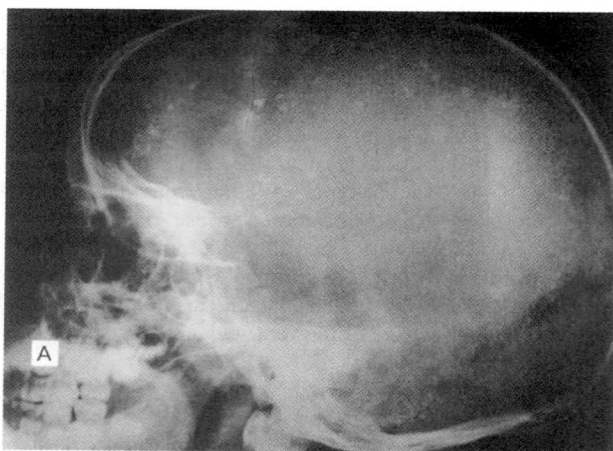
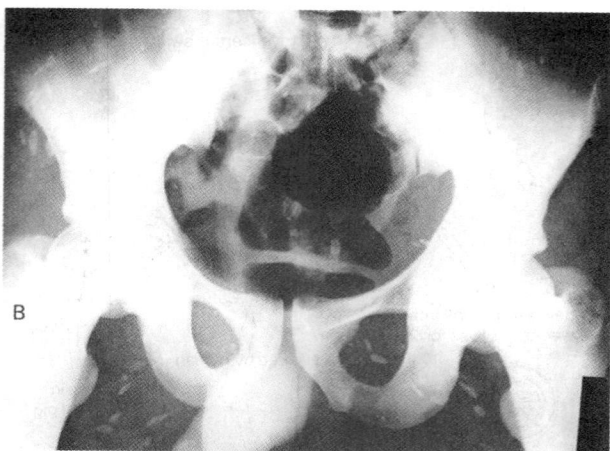

Fig. 23.78   (a) Cerebral cysticercosis. (b) Calcified cysticerci visible in the muscles in X-ray of pelvis.

CT scans are of great value, not only for the diagnosis of cerebral cysticercosis, but also for an assessment of the length of infection and for post-treatment progress evaluation (Camargo & Marshall 1987, Jaroonvesama 1988).

Treatment

Treatment for *T. solium* is similar to that for *T. saginata* with praziquantel or niclosamide (Yomesan) being the drugs of choice (Kociecka 1987a). Mepacrine or similar drugs which tend to cause nausea and vomiting should be avoided because of the danger or regurgitation of proglottids into the stomach and reswallowing them.

Cysticercosis. Recent studies have shown that praziquantel at a dose of 50 mg/kg in three divided doses for 14 days is effective for the treatment of cysticercosis (James & Gilles 1985, Kammerer 1985, Gustafsson et al 1987, Schneider et al 1990). The simultaneous administration of steroids may help reduce inflammatory complications which can follow the death of the cysticerci after anthelmintic treatment (Marty & Andersen 1995).

Surgical removal of cysticerci is seldom feasible, especially if the cysticerci are numerous and deep seated.

Anticonvulsants to control fits, steroids to control raised intracranial pressure and occasionally surgery to control hydrocephalus may be required for controlling the fits in cerebral cysticercosis. Praziquantel is frequently associated with side effects in neurocysticercosis and its use is not universally accepted in this situation (Moodley & Moosa 1989, Schneider et al 1990).

Prevention of *T. solium* infection and cysticercosis is essentially the same as for *T. saginata*. Cysticerci can be destroyed during cooking by heating the meat to 50°C.

Hymenolepis spp.

Two species of this genus of tapeworm infect man, *Hymenolepis nana* (the dwarf tapeworm) and *H. diminuta* (the rat tapeworm). These are small tapeworms, reaching only 40 mm in length for *H. nana* and 40 cm in length for *H. diminuta*.

Hymenolepis nana

H. nana is harbored in the small intestine of the human host and the gravid proglottids disintegrate in the gut so that eggs pass out in the feces. When an egg is ingested by another person, it releases an oncosphere into the small intestine, and this burrows into a villus, forming a cysticercoid. It develops here before leaving the villus after about 14 days to grow into an adult tapeworm in the intestinal lumen (Fig. 23.79).

Because of its direct person-to-person mode of transmission, *H. nana* is a common tapeworm in Third World countries and tends to be commoner in children than in adults. In fact, Goldsmid et al (1976) recorded 18.7% of children infected with *H. nana* in a survey in Zimbabwe as opposed to only 3.8% of adults infected.

Diagnosis is based upon the recovery of characteristic *H. nana* eggs (Fig. 23.79) and the treatment of choice is praziquantel or niclosamide as for taeniasis (James & Gilles 1985). Praziquantel at a dose of 25 mg/kg has a cure rate of 98.5% and no side effects have been claimed by Schenone (1980).

Hymenolepis diminuta

The rat tapeworm, *H. diminuta*, is common in many parts of the world in rats and mice. Its intermediate hosts are fleas and flour beetles. Children may become infected when they accidentally swallow the intermediate host – often with insect-infested meal or flour.

Diagnosis of *H. diminuta* infection is based upon finding the eggs in feces. These eggs differ from those of *H. nana* in being larger, rounder, lemon yellow in color, and having a striated shell and no polar filaments.

Treatment is as for *H. nana*.

Neither *H. nana* nor *H. diminuta* cause serious clinical effects, but abdominal pain, diarrhea, loss of appetite and eosinophilia may occur when loads are heavy. One problem with *H. nana* is a build-up of worm load as a result of external autoinfection by ingestion of eggs.

Dipylidium caninum

This tapeworm is worldwide, commonly infecting both dogs and cats. The intermediate hosts are fleas, such as the common dog and cat fleas (Fig. 23.80a) which contain the cysticercoids and infection of the final host occurs when the flea is swallowed.

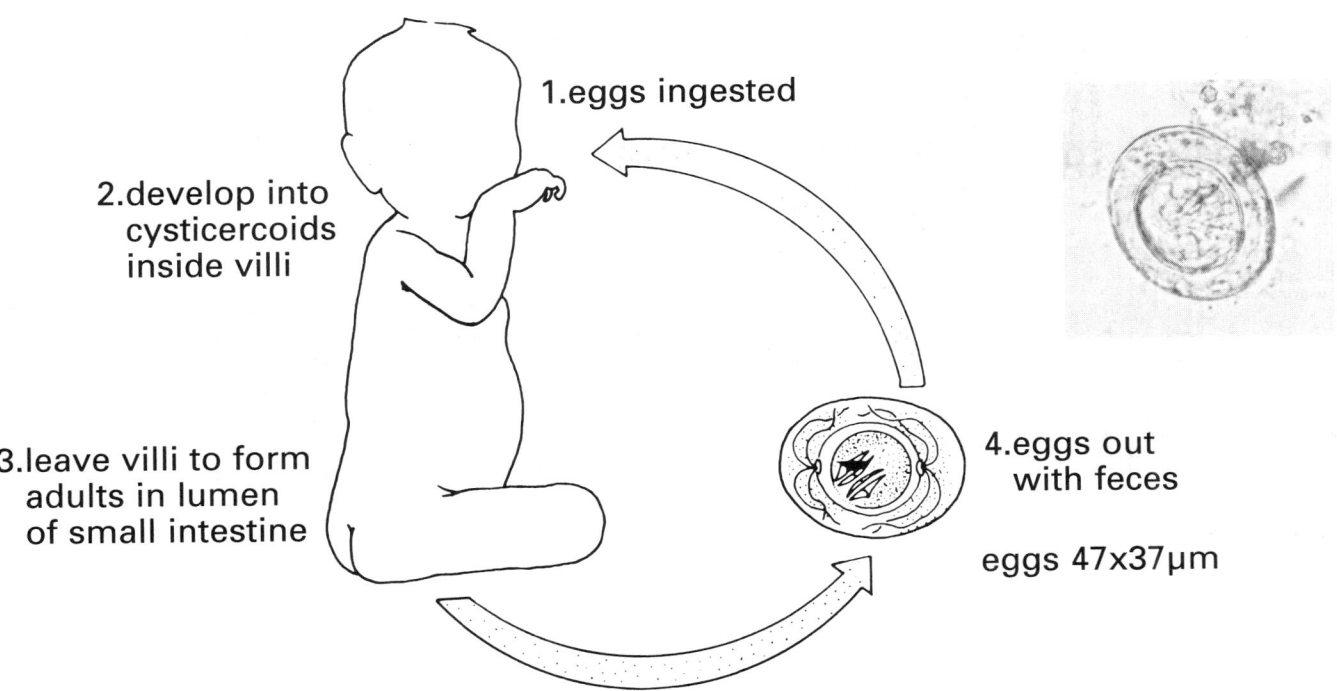

1.eggs ingested

2.develop into cysticercoids inside villi

3.leave villi to form adults in lumen of small intestine

4.eggs out with feces

eggs 47x37μm

Fig. 23.79 Life cycle of *Hymenolepis nana*. Egg inset (approx. ×600).

Children can become infected when they accidentally swallow a flea or when they are licked on the mouth by a dog which has been 'fleaing' itself and has cysticercoids on the tongue.

It is a relatively small tapeworm (20 cm long) and usually causes little discomfort, although at times diarrhea, fever, restlessness and even convulsions have been recorded.

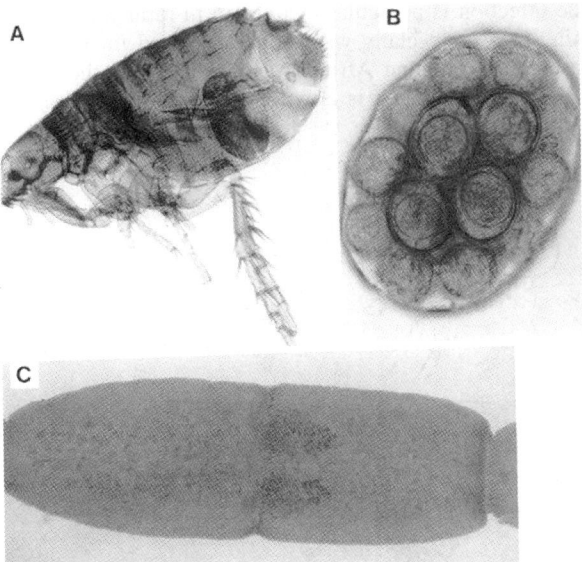

Fig. 23.80 (a) *Ctenocephalides* sp. – dog flea intermediate host of *Dipylidium caninum* (approx. ×50). (b) Egg capsule of *Dipylidium caninum* (approx. ×600). (c) Stained gravid proglottid of *Dipylidium caninum*. Note characteristic double set of reproductive organs and twin genital pores (approx. ×20).

Diagnosis is made when actively motile proglottids with two genital pores (Fig. 23.80c) are found by the mother on nappies or when typical egg capsules (Fig. 23.80b) are found in the feces on microscopic examination.

Yomesan is reported to be effective in treatment although in some cases repeated treatments with this drug have failed.

Diphyllobothrium latum

The fish tapeworm is one of the largest of the parasites of humans, the adult worm reaching 20 m or more. It is a common tapeworm of a variety of fish-eating mammals, including dogs and cats, in Scandinavia, the Baltic, South America, the Great Lakes of North America, parts of the Middle and Far East and Indonesia, while occasional cases are encountered in other parts such as Labrador and Australia (Kociecka 1987a, Marty & Andersen 1995).

The scolex of this species has sucking grooves and eggs are shed from the gravid proglottids to pass out with the feces.

When the eggs fall into water, a ciliated coracidium larva develops and is released through the operculum into the water. It swims around and is ingested by the microscopic crustacean, *Cyclops*, in which a procercoid larva is formed. When the *Cyclops* is eaten by a fish, the procercoid changes into a plerocercoid (sparganum) larva in the muscles of the fish. Finally the life cycle is completed when the fish is eaten by the mammalian definitive host (Fig. 23.81), which may include humans.

Clinical effects of infection include, in heavy loads, diarrhea, abdominal pain, generalized weakness (Kociecka 1987a) and occasionally intestinal obstruction. *D. latum* is also recorded in Finland, as causing a megaloblastic (macrocytic) anemia in susceptible patients who have a genetic predisposition and who are on a diet deficient in vitamin B_{12}, by competition with the host for this vitamin – especially when the worm is attached high up in

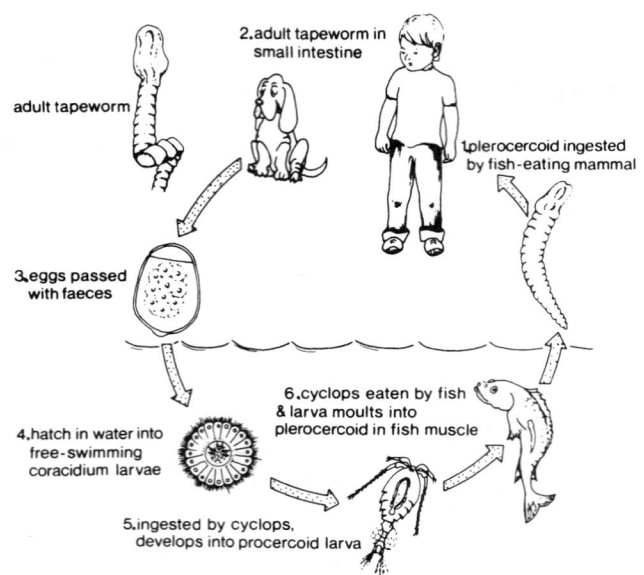

Fig. 23.81   Life cycle of *Diphyllobothrium latum*.

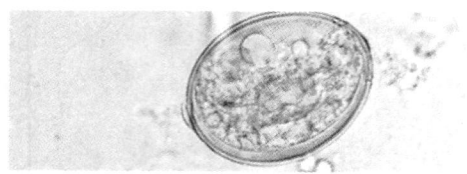

Fig. 23.82   Operculate egg of *Diphyllobothrium latum* (approx. ×600).

the small intestine. Eosinophilia is not usually a feature of infection.

Diagnosis is based upon the finding of the typical operculate eggs in the feces (Fig. 23.82). Proglottids passed in the feces can be recognized by their centrally situated uterus and genital pore.

Treatments recommended are praziquantel or niclosamide (Yomesan). Whichever anthelmintic is used, concurrent vitamin B$_{12}$ should also be given if the patient is anemic.

A common source of human infection is the eating of raw or smoked fish, so cooking of fish is an important factor in preventing infection of humans. Freezing fish (− 10°C for 15 min) is also effective in killing plerocercoids.

The plerocercoids of certain species belonging to the related genus, *Spirometra*, the adults of which inhabit the intestines of dogs, can infect humans causing a condition called sparganosis. These elongated plerocercoid (sparganum) larvae can infect

humans after ingestion of infected frogs, or *Cyclops* with water (East Africa, North America) or by application of infected frog flesh to skin ulcers or eye wounds as poultices. Plerocercoids in the frog muscle migrate into the human flesh where they settle – a condition occurring in southeast Asia.

These spargana can encyst in any tissues. Perhaps the commonest manifestations are nodules about 2 cm in size under the skin with painful surrounding edema. They can be detected radiologically as elongated shadows and can usually be removed surgically if accessible. One species of sparganum can bud and proliferate so spreading through the tissues.

ECHINOCOCCOSIS (HYDATID DISEASE)

Echinococcosis (hydatid disease) in humans is caused by the larval stage of *Echinococcus granulosus* and to a much lesser extent by *E. multilocularis*, *E. oligarthrus* or *E. vogeli*.

The life cycle of *E. granulosus* is shown in Figure 23.83. The small adult tapeworms (Fig. 23.84a) live in the intestine of the dog and related canids. After ingestion of the eggs by the intermediate hosts, which are usually sheep, the larval tapeworms develop into hydatid cysts in the viscera. Humans also become infected when they ingest the tapeworm eggs, and children are particularly susceptible because of their often intimate contact with dogs. They may pick up eggs contaminating the animal's coat or from the dog's tongue after licking.

The infection is particularly common in rural sheep and cattle farming areas, especially where dogs are used for herding. It is widespread throughout Africa, Australasia, Asia, the Near East and South America and is also found in the Mediterranean, the

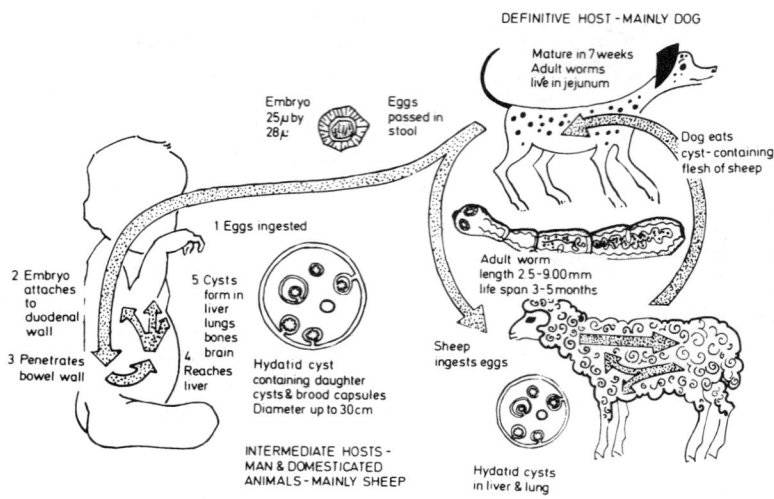

Fig. 23.83   Character and life cycle of *Echinococcus granulosus*.

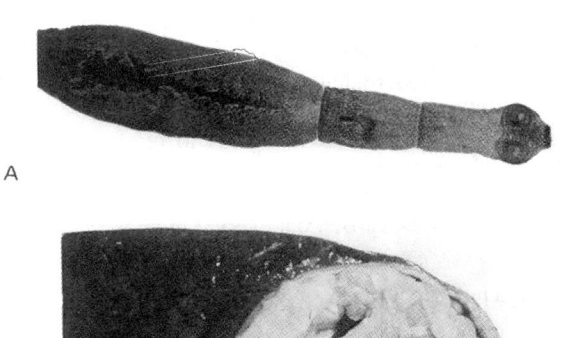

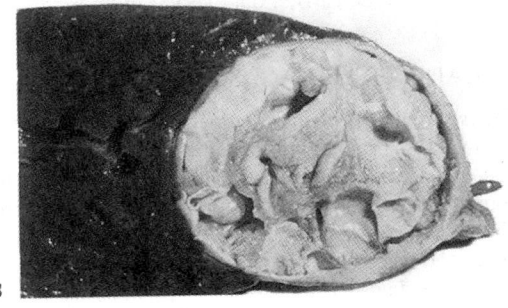

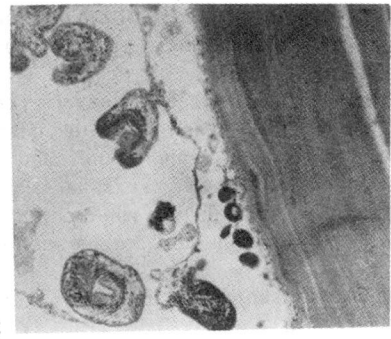

Fig. 23.84   (**a**) Adult *E. granulosus*. Note scolex and proglottids (approx. ×12). (**b**) Hydatid cyst in human liver. (**c**) Histological appearance of the wall of a pulmonary hydatid cyst.

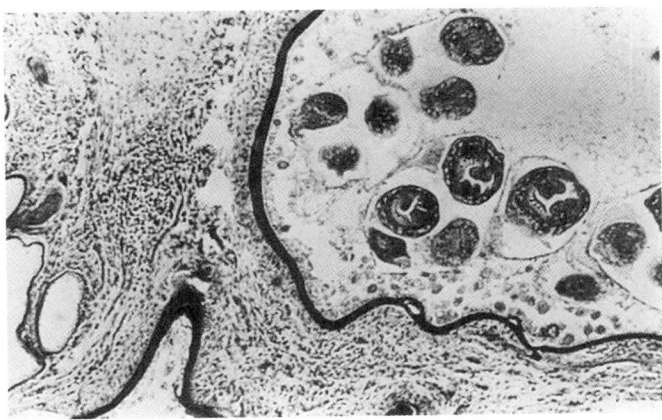

Fig. 23.85   Liver section showing cyst of *E. multilocularis*. Note protoscolices (approx. ×120).

USA and the UK (McManus & Smyth 1986, Goldsmid 1988). *E. multilocularis* is widespread in the northern hemisphere, with human cases being common in parts of the former USSR, China, northern Japan, Alaska and central Europe including possible spread into eastern Germany (McManus & Smyth 1986, Craig et al 1991, Lucius et al 1995). Cycles involving wild animals are also found in certain parts of the world.

In hydatidosis due to *E. multilocularis*, wolves, coyotes and foxes are the definitive hosts, and small field rodents serve as the natural intermediate hosts. Urban cycles involving the domestic cat and house mouse have been demonstrated.

The incidence of echinococcosis is decreasing in some areas owing to regular anthelmintic treatment of dogs and strict controls prohibiting the feeding of offal to dogs (Goldsmid & Pickmere 1987) and global control has been mooted (Gemmell et al 1987).

Clinical features

Because development of cysts is slow, an infection acquired in childhood may only become clinically evident in adulthood, but manifestations of the disease in children are by no means uncommon. It has, in fact, been widely believed in the past that most hydatids detected in adults were acquired in childhood. Studies in Australia, however, have indicated clearly that adults

are susceptible to infection and that the latent period between infection and diagnosis is, in many cases; only a few years.

The most frequent sites for cysts are the liver (Fig. 23.84b) and lungs (Fig. 23.84c). Spleen, peritoneum, kidneys, bone, orbital fossae, brain, heart and reproductive organs may also be invaded. In children, lung disease is reported to be the commonest form. Cysts sited in parenchymatous organs are large unilocular, well-circumscribed, fluid-filled structures in *E. granulosus* infections.

In bone, the parasite ramifies along bony canals, eroding bone and later involving the medullary cavity to form a large osseous cyst which often results in spontaneous fracture. The much rarer *E. multilocularis* infection may produce complex, multilocular alveolar cysts with a gelatinous matrix (Fig. 23.85). Alveolar hydatid disease has a 93% mortality within 10 years of diagnosis (Gemmell et al 1987).

Many cases of hydatid disease are silent. When symptoms occur they are usually those of a slow-growing tumor with pressure on, or blockage to the affected organ. Thus, recurrent pyrexia, paroxysmal cough, chest pain, hemoptysis and even expectoration of cyst fluid and membrane (should rupture occur into a bronchus) may occur as manifestations of pulmonary hydatidosis. Abdominal pain, vomiting, hepatomegaly and obstructive jaundice may indicate liver involvement. Intracranial localization produces symptoms and signs indistinguishable from those of a tumor – epilepsy, personality change, intellectual deterioration, signs of raised intracranial pressure or neurological abnormalities. Orbital cysts produce proptosis.

Sensitivity to cyst contents, resulting from slow leak of fluid, may develop with resulting allergic symptoms, notably urticaria. Severe anaphylaxis has been reported following rupture of a cyst, and secondary metastatic cysts may develop in other parts of the body following such rupture.

Diagnosis

Diagnosis depends initially upon clinical awareness of the condition – especially in patients from endemic areas. A moderate eosinophilia is almost invariably present in childhood cases, except during febrile illnesses.

Often an X-ray provides the first indication of hydatid disease especially in thoracic cases (Fig. 23.86). Ultrasound or CT scanning may be required to demonstrate the cystic nature of the

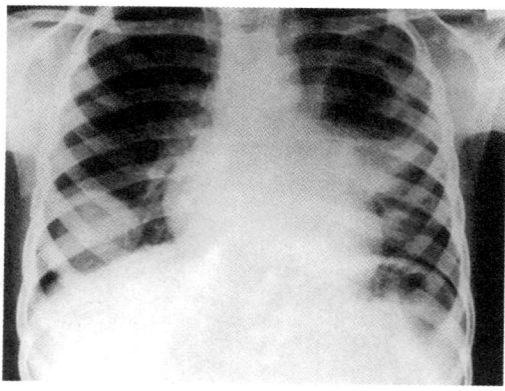

Fig. 23.86 Hydatid cysts in lung. Noncalcified cyst in right lung. Cyst in left lung has ruptured into a bronchus and contains fluid and air.

lesion. Serological tests such as the complement-fixation test, the indirect fluorescent antibody test and the hemagglutination test may be helpful. A skin test (the Casoni test) is available but gives variable results and should perhaps only be used where other serological tests are unavailable. Other serological tests include the hydatid ELISA test and the improved immunoelectrophoresis, Arc 5 test. The latter is considered by many to be the only reliably specific serological test available for hydatidosis although false positives have been reported for this test in patients with certain types of tumors. The double diffusion Arc 5 test is reported to be even better.

It is worth remembering that pulmonary hydatids appear less serologically active than cysts in other parts of the body, and that after surgical removal of hydatid cysts, antibodies may remain in low titers for a while, but that sooner or later they disappear completely.

At times a cyst in the lung may rupture and diagnosis can then be made by finding hydatid sand or hooklets in the sputum. The latter are easily detected by using a standard Ziehl–Neelsen or auramine stain with UV microscopy as they are intensely acid fast.

If hydatid cysts are suspected, aspiration must *not* be attempted because of the danger of anaphylaxis and metastatic spread.

If children vomit what appears to be hydatid cysts, care should be taken to confirm their nature microscopically by the presence or absence of a germinal membrane as gel cysts, closely resembling small hydatids, can easily mislead the unwary. These gel cysts are not uncommonly vomited after ingestion of commercial fruit gels containing carrageenan by children up to 2 years.

Treatment

Treatment is surgical if cysts are accessible, but due precautions must be observed to prevent release of hydatid fluid and to sterilize cysts prior to removal, using formalin or 0.5–1% sodium hypochlorite (EUSOL).

Results of chemotherapy for hydatid cysts using mebendazole have been disappointing, but albendazole can be used for treatment of inoperable hydatids at a dose of 10 mg/kg daily for 8 weeks (McManus & Smyth 1986, Schneider et al 1990).

Prevention

While highly successful control programs have resulted in decreases in the prevalence of hydatid disease in Tasmania and New Zealand, elsewhere the disease remains common and may even be spreading (McManus & Smyth 1986, Gemmell et al 1987, Goldsmid 1988).

Dogs should not be allowed access to offal to limit canine infection, and regular treatment with an effective teniafuge such as praziquantel (Droncit) is indicated. In endemic areas deworming should be carried out every 2 months.

INERMICAPSIFER MADAGASCARIENSIS

I. madagascariensis is primarily a parasite of rodents with various arthropod vectors probably involved as intermediate hosts. Human infection, however, is common, especially in Africa, and it has been sporadically reported also from tropical and subtropical areas throughout the world, particularly Cuba where the parasite was introduced and has dispensed with its rodent reservoir.

This cestode has a rounded scolex containing four unarmed suckers and ranges up to 42 cm in length. The small, actively motile proglottids are shed in the stool and have the appearance of rice grains; they contain characteristic parenchmyatous egg capsules (Fig. 23.87).

I. madagascariensis most frequently involves children between the ages of 1 and 5 years, and while the infection is usually asymptomatic, anorexia, asthenia, anemia and abdominal pain have occasionally been attributed to it. It has been found to be the most common tapeworm affecting white children in Zimbabwe and more cases in African children are coming to light as awareness increases.

Niclosamide (Yomesan) is the treatment of choice – 1 tablet (0.5 g) repeated in 1 h.

TREMATODES (FLUKES)

Trematodes are parasitic helminths belonging to the class Platyhelminthes (flat worms). Trematodes are dorsoventrally flattened worms which have a gut, no body cavity and possess a dorsal and ventral sucker. Most are hermaphrodite, except the schistosomes. The flukes have a complex life cycle involving

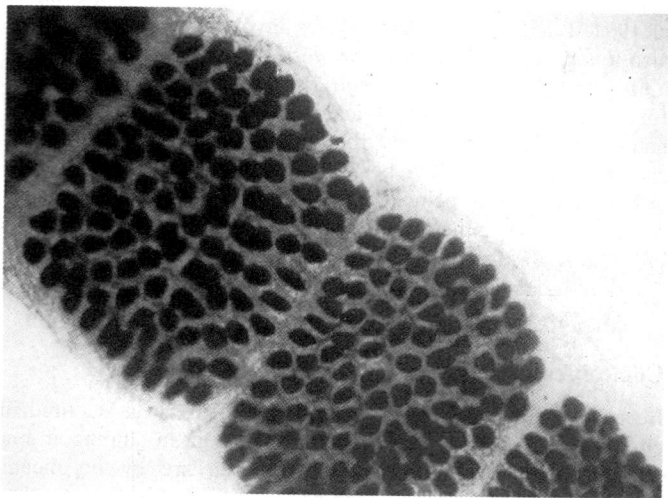

Fig. 23.87 Gravid proglottids of *Inermicapsifer madagascariensis* to show masses of parenchymatous egg capsules in each segment (approx. ×50).

Table 23.50 Main snail hosts involved in important trematode life cycles

Trematode	Genera of snails
S. haematobium S. intercalatum }	Bulinus and Physopis
S. mansoni	Biomphalaria
S. japonicum	Oncomelania
F. hepatica F. gigantica }	Lymnaea
Fasciolopsis buski	Polypylis, Planorbis (Hippeutis), Trochorbis
O. sinensis	Bithynia (Bulimus), Parafossarulus, Alocima
O. felineus	Bithynia
P. westermani	Semisulcospira (Melania), Thiara, Oncomelania
M. yokogawai	Semisulcospira
H. heterophyes {	Pironella (in Egypt) Cerithidea (in China and Japan)

various species of snail as intermediate hosts (Table 23.50). Trematodes infecting humans include blood flukes (*Schistosoma*), liver flukes (*Fasciola, Opisthorchis*), intestinal flukes (*Fasciolopsis, Heterophyes, Metagonimus*) and lung flukes (*Paragonimus*).

BLOOD FLUKE INFECTION (SCHISTOSOMIASIS OR BILHARZIASIS)

Adult blood flukes live in the veins of the final host. There are three main species which infect humans – *Schistosoma japonicum, S. mansoni* and *S. haematobium*. *S. japonicum* is a zoonotic species found in the Far East. It frequents the superior mesenteric veins of humans and causes a more virulent and rapidly progressive illness than the other species, involving mainly the small and large intestine and liver. *S. mansoni* occurs in Africa, the Caribbean and South America, the worms living in the inferior mesenteric veins with resultant damage to the colon and liver. *S. haematobium* is found in the veins of the vesical plexus of humans throughout much of Africa, the Middle East and parts of India. In this infection, the disease predominantly affects the urinary tract.

The geographical distribution of the main schistosome species is shown in Table 23.51. Other blood flukes less commonly recorded in humans include *S. intercalatum* (in Zaire), *S. bovis* (in North Africa and Iraq) and *S. mattheei* (in southern Africa). The latter two are zoonotic species of cattle and sheep. In southeast Asia, *S. mekongi* is found.

The life cycle of the human blood flukes is shown in Figure 23.88.

Pathogenesis and clinical features

Humans are usually infected by direct penetration of the cercariae through intact skin. The pathological changes in schistosomiasis are produced by cercariae, schistosomulae, adult worms and eggs – by their physical presence or by virtue of metabolic products. The severity of the disease depends primarily upon the number of parasites that can gain entry to the body and mature.

Despite the wealth of knowledge that has been accumulated regarding the pathophysiology of schistosomiasis, the extent of ill health and mortality caused by this disease is still debatable (Mahmoud 1987).

Table 23.51 Geographic distribution of schistosomiasis (after Warren & Mahmoud)

Species	Distribution				
	Africa	Middle East	Asia	South America	Caribbean
S. mansoni	Egypt Libya Sudan South of the Sahara Malagasy Republic	Yemen* Aden* Saudi Arabia*		Brazil Surinam Venezuela	Puerto Rico Dominican Republic* Guadeloupe Martinique St Lucia
S. japonicum				Malaysia* China Japan Philippines Sulawesi* Thailand* Laos* Kampuchea* Vietnam	
S. haematobium	Widespread including Malagasy Republic and Mauritius‡	Lebanon Iran* Turkey Iraq Jordan Yemen Israel Saudi Arabia	India†		

* Very small focal areas.
† Focal distribution.
‡ Limited foci have been reported in Portugal in the past.

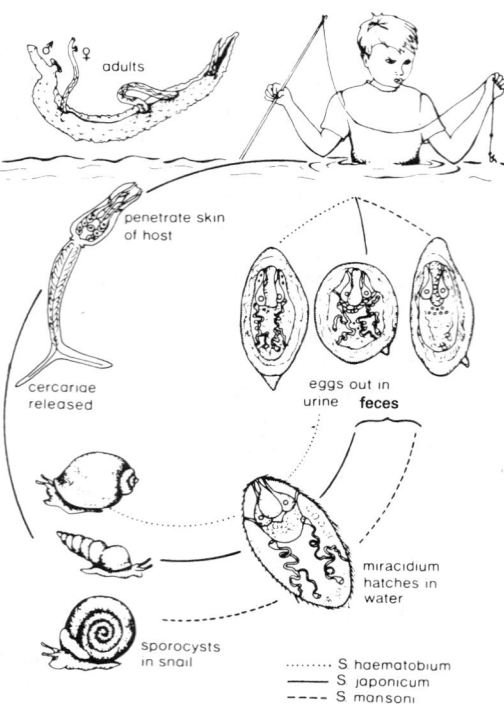

Fig. 23.88   Life cycle of schistosomes

While in many areas, large sections of the population harbor the parasites, it is certain that many individuals come to terms with the disease and suffer virtually no morbidity owing to a complex interplay of factors such as immunological tolerance, worm load, and rate of reinfection. The role of protective immunity in schistosomiasis continues to be a subject of debate (Woolhouse 1993). Increased prevalence and intensity of infection in childhood lends credence at least to some protective immunity playing a part (Lancet 1987b). The immunity involved in schistosomiasis is complex (Woolhouse 1993), being described as concomitant immunity, whereby the adult worms are not affected by the hosts' immune responses to the infection although newly invading cercariae are destroyed (Hagan & Williams 1993, Terry 1994, Butterworth 1994, Greyseels 1994).

The later stages of schistosomiasis generally take many years to develop so that the spectrum of clinical disease in children is narrowed. Nevertheless, such late manifestations as portal hypertension, calcification of the bladder and even vesical carcinoma are by no means rare in adolescents living in hyperendemic areas. A further difference in the disease as it affects children compared with adults is related to the caliber of blood vessels. Because of the smaller and more tenuous venous plexuses and collaterals, schistosomes are less able to migrate in sites far removed from their normal habitat, as they do in older persons. The relative lack of immunity in young patients renders them more liable to severe systemic disturbance during the early stages of the disease. Determinants of infection in human communities are complex (Anderson R M 1987).

Clinical features can be related to the phase of parasitic invasion, and symptomatology is generally, but not always, proportionate to worm load. The pathogenesis of schistosomiasis is complex but it is essentially an immunological disease (Colley 1987, Warren 1987, Wyler 1992).

Penetration of cercariae

At the time of penetration, within a few hours to a few days of exposure, a dermatitis termed swimmer's or Kabure itch may develop and last for 2–3 days. The condition is commoner in nonindigenous inhabitants. It can also be caused by avian or mammalian schistosomes in countries where human schistosomiasis is unknown. For example it is quite common in Australia where it is sometimes termed 'pelican itch'. These latter cercariae, however, die while attempting to penetrate the skin. A prickly sensation is followed by intense itching and an urticarial, papular or occasionally vesicular rash appears, lasting from a few hours to several days.

Migratory/toxemic stage: the Katayama syndrome

Having passed through the skin, the cercariae lose their tails and the resulting schistosomulae enter the lymphatics, pass to the veins and travel to the heart and hence to the lungs to circulate freely in the systemic circulation. Many die, but those that gain access to the portal system reach the liver where they mature into adult male and female worms. Rarely, worms mature in other ectopic sites such as veins of the brain and spinal cord. Coupling takes place in the liver and the male transports the female against the flow of blood to their sites of predilection where egg laying begins. The prepatent period in schistosomiasis (i.e. from infection to egg laying) is normally about 5–9 weeks (Sturrock 1987).

During the migratory stage of the life cycle with a crescendo just prior to egg laying, the patient may develop an illness known as the Katayama syndrome due to antigenic challenge by the parasitic metabolites in the nonimmune host. Malaise, pyrexia, liver tenderness and splenomegaly, occur. Eosinophilia is constant. Urticaria, joint and muscle pains, cough, abdominal discomfort and diarrhea may also occur. Encephalopathy, myocarditis and anaphylactoid purpura are reported complications (Marty & Andersen 1995).

Katayama syndrome is commonest in *S. japonicum* infections but also occurs in schistosomiasis mansoni when a previously uninfected individual is exposed to a heavy invasion by cercariae.

Early egg laying stage

Many eggs laid by female worms in the submucosal venules of the intestine or bladder pass through the tissues and are discharged in the feces (*S. japonicum* and *S. mansoni*) or urine (*S. haematobium*). This early egg laying stage may be associated with dysenteric symptoms or with dysuria, frequency and terminal hematuria.

Late egg laying stage – pathology of chronic schistosomiasis

Initially eggs pass through the tissues relatively easily but as infection progresses marked tissue reaction occurs. As a result of this eggs can no longer pass through the tissues so readily and many are swept back by the flow of blood to be deposited elsewhere.

The morbidity of chronic schistosomiasis is complex and is mainly related to the presence of eggs (Phillips & Lammie 1986) which initially stimulate a granulomatous reaction characterized by a pseudotubercle, rich in eosinophils (Fig. 23.89a). This is

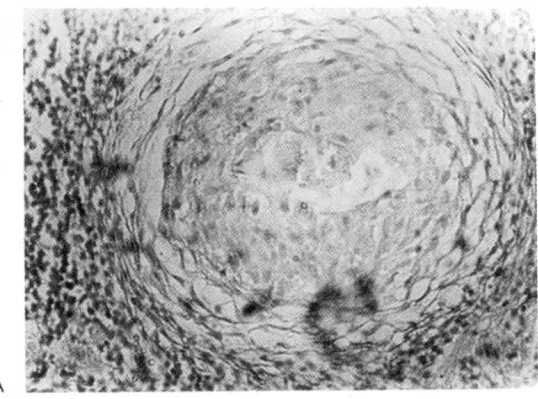

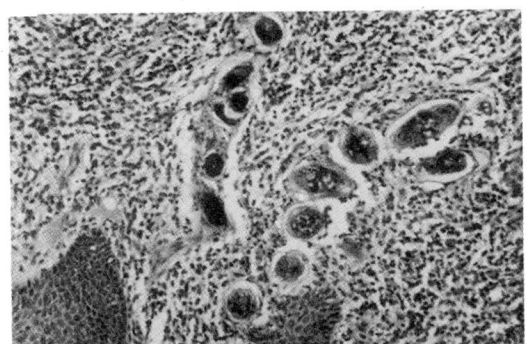

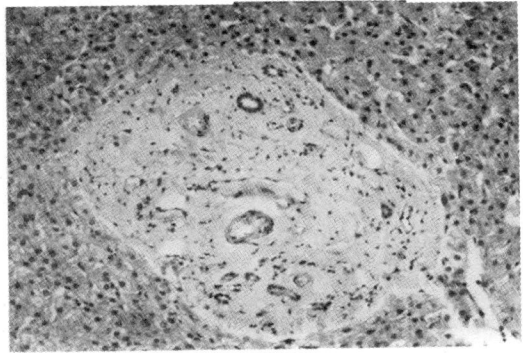

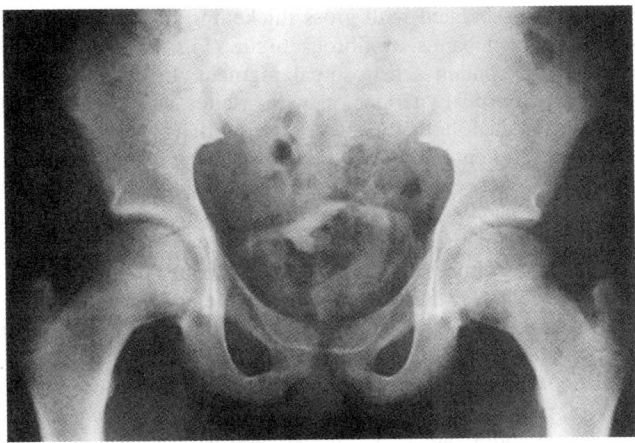

Fig. 23.90 X-ray showing bladder calcification due to schistosomiasis in a 10-year-old girl.

Fig. 23.89 (a) Schistosomal pseudotubercle. (b) Bilharzioma. (c) Liver biopsy showing collagenized periportal thickening due to schistosomiasis.

followed by degeneration and calcification of the eggs with much reactive fibrosis. The principal pathological effects are as follows:

Genitourinary system. S. haematobium is the principal cause. The early bladder lesions usually occur on the trigone where deposition of phosphates round the egg deposits imparts a velvety appearance termed 'sandy patches'. Subsequent mucosal proliferation may produce multiple papillomata before ulceration, calcification (Fig. 23.90) and fibrosis lead to diminished bladder capacity. A similar process may involve the ureters, especially at their lower ends, leading to ureteric stricture and consequent hydronephrosis. This complication can also occur from vesical reflux in the absence of overt ureteric involvement. Vesical or ureteric calculi may occur. An important long-term complication is the predisposition of the bladder affected by schistosomiasis to

develop carcinoma, usually of squamous cell type. The pathogenesis of such bladder carcinoma in *S. haematobium* infection is complex and has still not been fully elucidated. While this is naturally commonest in adults, it is not unknown in adolescents. Genital lesions are usually diagnosed after puberty. These include epididymo-orchitis (often with associated secondary hydrocele) salpingo-oophoritis and chronic cervicitis. Large schistosomal granulomata (bilharziomas) consisting of masses of eggs enveloped in granulation tissue (Fig. 23.89b) may involve the skin of the perineum and vulva. The lesions have a warty papillomatous appearance and when situated at the urethral meatus such a lesion is indistinguishable from a caruncle. Cutaneous schistosomiasis may rarely involve other parts of the body, and bilharzial granuloma of the conjunctiva has even been described in children.

An extended bacteremia with *Salmonella typhi* or *S. paratyphi* can occur – including a prolonged urinary carrier state – in concurrent *S. haematobium* infections.

Bacteriuria is generally considered to be commoner in patients with *S. haematobium* than in uninfected controls.

Intestinal tract. Involvement of small bowel is usually only seen in *S. japonicum* infection but schistosomiasis of the colon may be due to both *S. japonicum* and *S. mansoni*. Eggs of *S. haematobium* may also be encountered in rectal snips taken from the lower part of the rectum. Mucosal involvement of the bowel gives rise to a similar appearance to that seen in the bladder with a velvety roughening of the mucosa. This may be associated with dysentery in the early egg laying phase of the disease, especially with *S. japonicum* infection. Gross lesions of the bowel are rare, but on occasions papillomata, granulomata, ulcers, stricture and fistulae occur. The appendix is frequently involved and signs of chronic appendicitis are common, although acute obstructive appendicitis consequent upon fibrosis, is a rare complication.

Liver. Hepatic fibrosis may result from the presence of eggs of *S. mansoni* or *S. japonicum* with formation of granulomata and healing by fibrosis leading to thick tracts of periportal fibrous tissue traversing the liver in different directions. This 'pipe stem' fibrosis (Symmers' liver) gives the surface of the liver an irregular bosselated contour due to tethering of the capsule. In the later stage eggs are scanty and may even be absent from biopsy material in which the essential features are of preserved liver architecture associated with gross thickening of the portal tracts by collagenized bands of fibrous tissue (Fig. 23.89c). Kupffer cells usually contain schistosomal pigment. Liver involvement can lead to portal hypertension with ascites and splenomegaly which is occasionally massive ('Egyptian splenomegaly'). Anemia is frequent and may be due to chronic hemorrhage from varices or to associated 'hypersplenism'. There is usually only mild impairment of liver function and thus the results of portal systemic shunting procedures usually give good results in selected cases. Splenectomy combined with lienorenal anastomosis is a helpful procedure if there is associated hypersplenism.

A relationship has been postulated between schistosome infection and carcinoma of the liver.

Cardiopulmonary systems. Lung involvement is usually the result of pulmonary embolization by eggs of *S. haematobium*. Though generally rare it is reported with some frequency from Egypt. Two forms of lung disease occur:

1. A bronchopulmonary form characterized by parenchymal egg granulomata. Chronic bronchitis and bronchiectasis may result.
2. A cardiovascular form which is due to occlusion of pulmonary arterioles by obliterative endarteritis resulting in Ayerza's syndrome with cor pulmonale.

Nervous system. Eggs may lodge in any part of the central nervous system generally seeded there by gravid females ectopically situated in nearby veins. Migrating schistosomulae may also be arrested in the nervous system if treatment is administered during the early migratory phase of the disease. However, neurological complications are unusual in schistosomiasis, cerebral involvement being best known with *S. japonicum* and spinal cord lesions with *S. mansoni* and *S. haematobium*.

It has been claimed that school performance can be adversely affected by chronic schistosomiasis.

In patients infected with *S. mansoni*, glomerulonephritis has been reported due to the deposition of immune complexes (IgM and IgG) in the kidney.

Laboratory diagnosis

Confirmation of the diagnosis of active schistosomiasis can only be obtained by finding typical viable eggs (Fig. 23.91a, b and c). Eggs can be recovered by examination of urinary deposit (*S. haematobium*) or from stool (all other species) by direct smear (including a Kato smear), sedimentation or water centrifugation (Peters & Kazura 1987). Flotation techniques are not satisfactory and formol ether concentration kills the eggs with the result that no report can be made on egg viability as judged by miracidial activity or flame cell activity. Confirmation of viability of the egg is important to differentiate active disease from past infection.

Egg recovery is not easy and as many as 20% of infected persons may not pass eggs. Repeated examination of stool and urine specimens, the latter collected at midday, is essential. If urine or stools fail to reveal eggs, a rectal snip may prove rewarding in *S. japonicum*, *S. mansoni* and *S. haematobium* infections. In fact a single rectal snip gives more positives than three urines and stools. Cystoscopy may be indicated where urinary symptoms are present, the cystoscopic picture depending on the worm load.

A type I response skin test and various serological tests (CFT, indirect fluorescent antibody test, indirect hemagglutination test, etc.) are available. These indicate present or past infection, and

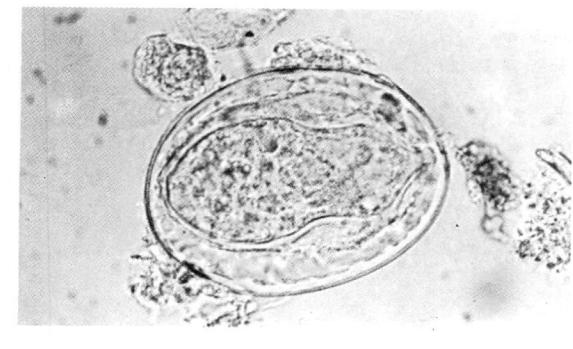

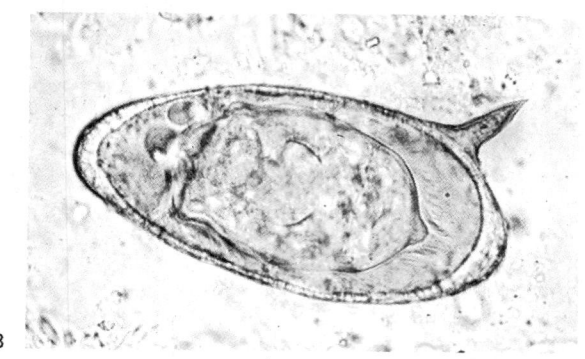

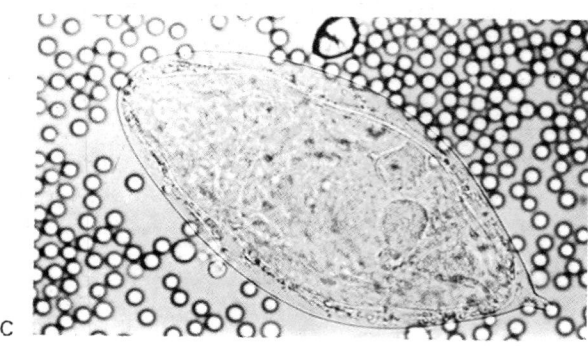

Fig. 23.91 (**a**) Egg of *Schistosoma japonicum* (approx. ×600). (**b**) Egg of *Schistosoma mansoni* (approx. ×600). (**c**) Egg of *Schistosoma haematobium* (approx. ×1000).

therefore a positive result with these tests is not, in itself, an indication for treatment. However, these tests often provide good negative screens to exclude a diagnosis of schistosomiasis.

Treatment

The treatment of choice for all forms of schistosomiasis, and the only effective and safe treatment for *S. japonicum* infections, is praziquantel (Biltricide) (James & Gilles 1985, Webster 1987). This drug is designated as a 'WHO essential agent', being extremely safe and highly effective when given as a single dose of 40 mg/kg for *S. haematobium* and *S. mansoni* and at a dose of 60 mg/kg divided into two doses and given in a single day for *S. japonicum* (Gustafsson et al 1987).

Other treatments for schistosomiasis include hycanthone (Etrenol), mostly used against *S. haematobium* and given as a single intramuscular injection of 2.5–3.5 mg/kg. This drug can be hepatotoxic and deaths following its use are on record. Metrifonate (Bilarcil) is an organophosphorus compound, achieving a cure of about 60% in cases of infection with *S. haematobium*. It is not used for other species of schistosome. The dosage used for children is 7.5 mg/kg per fortnight for a total of three doses. Although side effects are minimal, some have been recorded. The drug does depress cholinesterase levels and caution is needed in cases where patients may require some form of surgery necessitating the use of the muscle relaxant, suxamethonium. Oxamniquine (Mansil) is only effective against *S. mansoni* infections. The dose regime is 20–30 mg/kg given as a single or divided doses over 1–2 days after food (Schneider et al 1990). High cure rates and few side effects are recorded (James & Gilles 1985). This drug is useful for treating children orally at a rate of 800 mg/m³ body surface area per day in divided doses for 2 days. Antischistosome drugs such as the antimonials and niridazole (Ambilhar) have been superseded by the newer, more effective and safer compounds.

Prevention

Attempts to control schistosomiasis are complex and generally employ a two-pronged attack on the life cycle of the fluke. The first is aimed at eliminating the snail population. Planned water systems for irrigation, which give a flow rate too high for survival of snails, is an ideal, but not always feasible method. Nontoxic molluscicides such as Frescon or Bayluscide have been found effective.

The experimental introduction of snail-eating predators and parasites has not proved to have any long-term effect.

The second approach to control is aimed at preventing pollution of waterways by human excreta and involves public health education combined with provision of adequate and effective toilet facilities. In some control projects, mass treatment of infected humans has been used in conjunction with snail control. However these aspects of prevention are ineffective in the case of *S. japonicum* which is extensively propagated by rodents. In *S. japonicum*, cercariae can be prevented from penetrating the skin by using topical applications of niclosamide or niclosamide-impregnated leggings.

Current research is aimed at the development of vaccines and chemoprophylactic methods and the results to date appear to be encouraging, but debatable in application (James & Sher 1986, Butterworth 1987, Butterworth et al 1987).

OTHER TREMATODES

The life cycles of these flukes involve snail hosts (Fig. 23.92).

LIFE CYCLES OF LIVER, INTESTINAL AND LUNG FLUKES

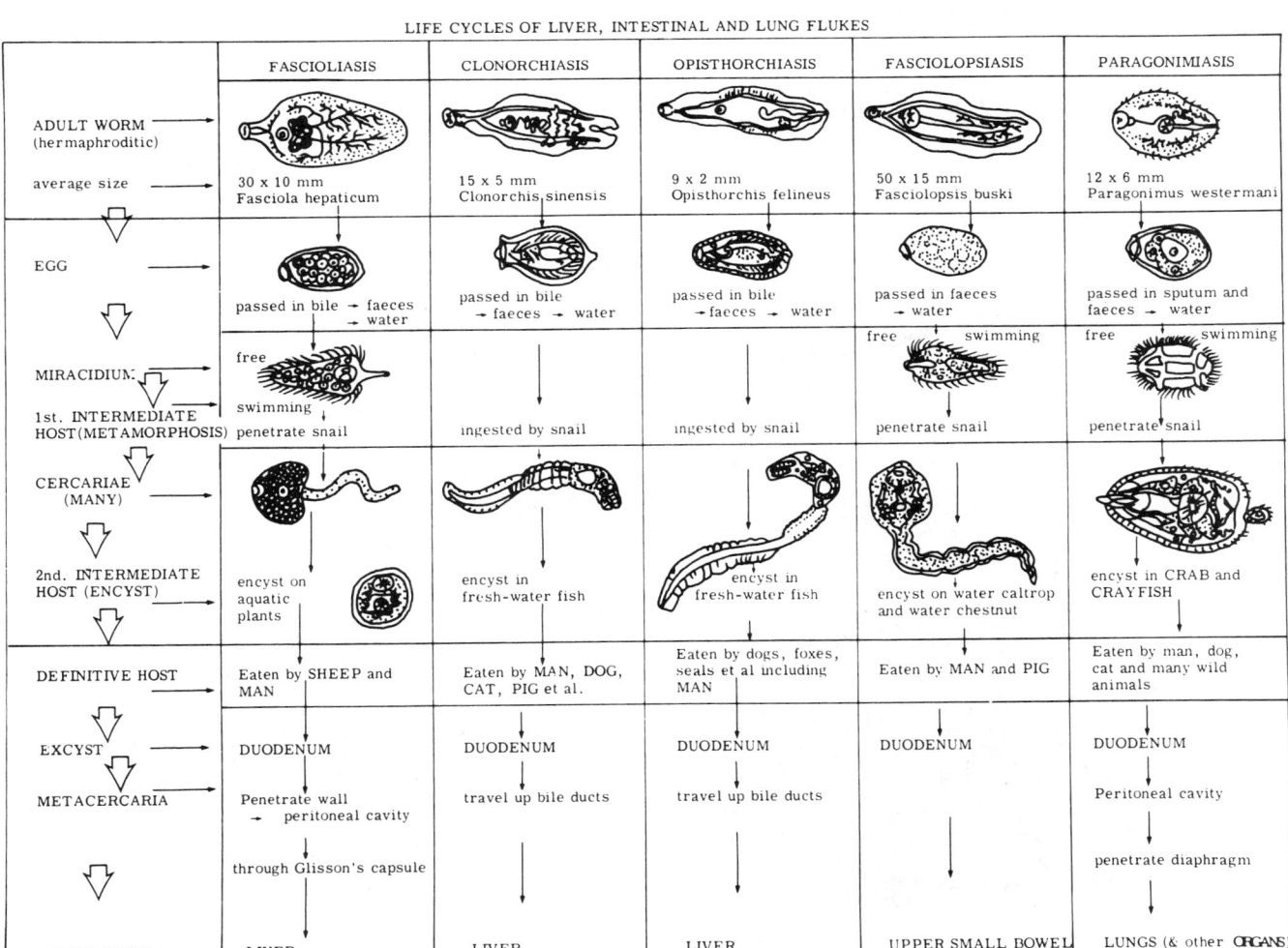

	FASCIOLIASIS	CLONORCHIASIS	OPISTHORCHIASIS	FASCIOLOPSIASIS	PARAGONIMIASIS
ADULT WORM (hermaphroditic) average size	30 x 10 mm Fasciola hepaticum	15 x 5 mm Clonorchis sinensis	9 x 2 mm Opisthorchis felineus	50 x 15 mm Fasciolopsis buski	12 x 6 mm Paragonimus westermani
EGG	passed in bile → faeces → water	passed in bile → faeces → water	passed in bile → faeces → water	passed in faeces → water	passed in sputum and faeces → water
MIRACIDIUM 1st. INTERMEDIATE HOST (METAMORPHOSIS)	free swimming penetrate snail	ingested by snail	ingested by snail	free swimming penetrate snail	free swimming penetrate snail
CERCARIAE (MANY) 2nd. INTERMEDIATE HOST (ENCYST)	encyst on aquatic plants	encyst in fresh-water fish	encyst in fresh-water fish	encyst on water caltrop and water chestnut	encyst in CRAB and CRAYFISH
DEFINITIVE HOST	Eaten by SHEEP and MAN	Eaten by MAN, DOG, CAT, PIG et al.	Eaten by dogs, foxes, seals et al including MAN	Eaten by MAN and PIG	Eaten by man, dog, cat and many wild animals
EXCYST METACERCARIA	DUODENUM Penetrate wall → peritoneal cavity through Glisson's capsule	DUODENUM travel up bile ducts	DUODENUM travel up bile ducts	DUODENUM	DUODENUM Peritoneal cavity penetrate diaphragm
ADULT WORM	LIVER	LIVER	LIVER	UPPER SMALL BOWEL	LUNGS (& other ORGANS)

Fig. 23.92 Life cycles of liver, intestinal and lung flukes.

Liver fluke infection

The main trematode infections of the liver are fascioliasis, caused by the cattle and sheep liver flukes *Fasciola hepatica* (temperate regions) and *F. gigantica* (tropical Africa, Asia and Hawaii); clonorchiasis caused by *Opisthorchis* (*Clonorchis*) *sinensis* in the Far East; and opisthorchiasis, caused by *Opisthorchis felineus* in parts of Europe and Asia or *O. viverrini* in Thailand.

Clinical features

Infection with these flukes results when the metacercariae are ingested with aquatic plants (*Fasciola*) such as watercress to which the encysted metacercariae are attached, or in undercooked fish (*Opisthorchis*).

Symptoms of liver fluke infection depend largely upon the worm load and mild infections are often asymptomatic. Heavier infections tend to produce a triphasic response with an initial phase of invasion being accompanied by irregular fever and eosinophilia. Diarrhea and urticaria are common and there may be tender hepatomegaly. This phase lasts for about 4 weeks and is followed by an asymptomatic latent period usually lasting several months before the stage of obstructive jaundice occurs. Rarely the parasites of *F. hepatica* may settle in ectopic sites such as the pharynx and mature there with resulting local reaction. Pharyngeal fascioliasis is known in the Middle East as *halzoun*. Individual worms may migrate into the liver parenchyma resulting in liver abscess formation. Eosinophilia is often present and the ESR is usually raised.

In Thailand cholangiocarcinoma has been found to be associated with infection by *O. viverrini* (Haswell-Elkins et al 1992).

Local prevalences are often dependent upon social customs and dietary habits and epidemic outbreaks of fascioliasis have been recorded (Gillett 1985, Haswell-Elkins et al 1992).

Diagnosis

The diagnosis is usually based upon the finding of typical operculate eggs in the feces (Figs 23.92 and 23.93) although in some infected patients stools are consistently negative for eggs. The finding of eggs of *Fasciola* in the feces must be regarded with

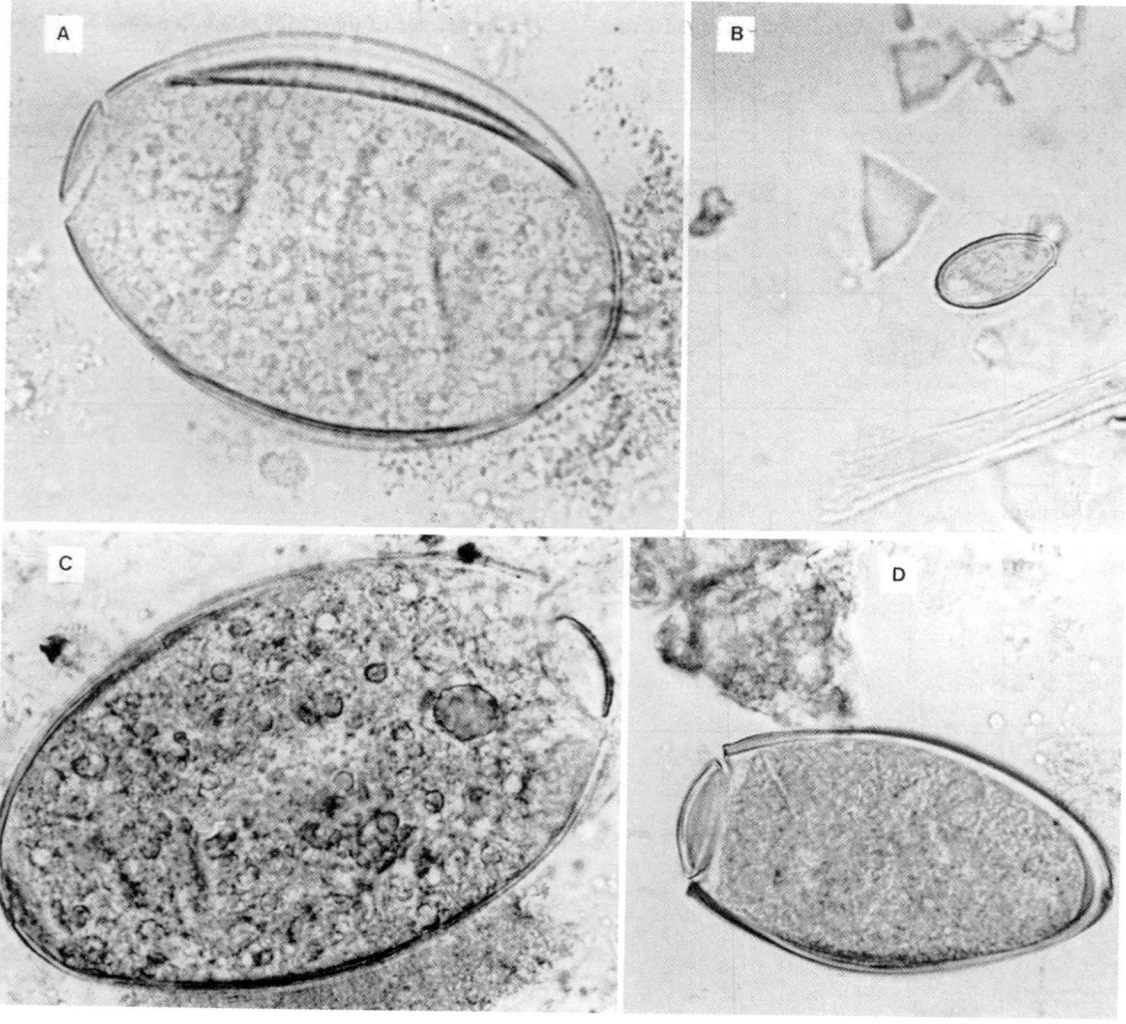

Fig. 23.93 Eggs of (**a**) *Fasciola hepatica* – ruptured to demonstrate operculum (approx. ×600); (**b**) *Opisthorchis sinensis* (approx. ×600); (**c**) *Fasciolopsis buski* – ruptured to demonstrate operculum (approx. ×600); (**d**) *Paragonimus westermani* (approx. ×600).

caution as persons eating infected cattle or sheep liver can pass 'transit eggs' and this condition of spurious infection or false fascioliasis must be distinguished from true fascioliasis by the examination of repeat stool specimens (Goldsmid 1995).

Treatment

On the whole, treatment of liver fluke infection remains unsatisfactory. For fascioliasis, Bithionol 50 mg/kg orally in divided doses on alternate days for 2–3 weeks is the drug of choice, although chloroquine and dehydroemetine have also been used. Drug treatment of choice for clonorchiasis and opisthorchiasis is praziquantel 25 mg/kg t.d.s. for 1–2 days (James & Gilles 1985, Gustafsson et al 1987) although Hetol (1:4 bistrichloromethyl bensol) has also been shown to be promising.

Intestinal fluke infection

Many species of fluke infect the human intestinal tract (Harinasuta et al 1987) including the large intestinal fluke *Fasciolopsis buski* in parts of southeast Asia, the small intestinal fluke *Heterophyes heterophyes* in the Nile Delta and the Far East, and *Metagonimus yokogawai* in the Far East and eastern Europe.

Infection with these flukes results from ingesting metacercariae with aquatic vegetation (*F. buski*) or with raw or undercooked fish (*H. heterophyes* and *M. yokogawai*). As in the case of liver fluke infection, a local high prevalence may be caused by local eating habits (Gillett 1985).

Symptoms of intestinal fluke infection may vary from a mild inflammatory reaction at the site of worm attachment in the small intestine to ulceration or abscess formation in the bowel wall, associated with severe bloody diarrhea.

Infections due to *F. buski* may result in vague abdominal symptoms, ascites and edema, probably as a result of protein-losing enteropathy and toxemia (Harinasuta et al 1987). An eosinophilia may be present, and iron deficiency anemia is common in fasciolopsiasis.

Diagnosis

As in liver fluke infection, diagnosis is made by finding typical operculate eggs in the feces of infected patients (Figs 23.92 and 23.93).

Treatment

Intestinal fluke infections, especially that due to *F. buski*, can be treated with praziquantel in a dose of 25 mg/kg 8-hourly for 1 day (Gustafsson et al 1987, Schneider et al 1990). Niclosamide (Yomesan) can also be used (James & Gilles 1985), while tetrachlorethylene has been described as an effective and cheap anthelmintic (Marty & Andersen 1995).

Lung fluke infection

Human lung fluke infection is caused by eleven species of the genus *Paragonimus*. In the Far East the species involved is *P. westermani* while in central and west Africa (and probably South Africa) the species is *P. africanus* or *P. uterobilateralis*. In the Western Hemisphere, *P. mexicanus* and *P. kellicotti* are the commoner species (Marty & Andersen 1995).

Infection occurs with the ingestion of the metacercariae in crabs and crayfish. Again local high prevalences are largely dependent upon dietary habits and culinary practices of preparing and cooking the crustacean intermediate hosts (Gillett 1985). However, an interesting epidemic is on record which resulted from the use of crab juice as an antipyretic for children suffering from measles.

Symptoms of lung fluke infection are often suggestive of pulmonary tuberculosis, which may also often be present concurrently. The onset is insidious with cough and chest pain. Hemoptysis is usual, with copious blood-tinged sputum containing many eggs. Bronchiectasis and pulmonary fibrosis are late results and finger clubbing is often present. An eosinophilia may occur and variable symptoms may result from flukes developing in ectopic sites, e.g. epilepsy, transverse myelitis and skin ulceration.

Diagnosis

The characteristic asymmetrical operculate eggs of *Paragonimus* may be recovered in sputum or feces (Figs 23.92 and 23.93). An intradermal test is available. Sputum should also be examined for tuberculosis in proven cases of paragonimiasis.

Treatment

The drugs of choice are Bithionol (or Bitin) at a dose of 30–40 mg/kg in divided doses given orally every other day for 10–15 days, or the newer derivative of Bithionol, Bitin-S, given at a dosage regimen of 10–20 mg/kg every other day for 10–15 days. Praziquantel is also effective (James & Gilles 1985, Gustafsson et al 1987, Schneider et al 1990).

Side effects include diarrhea, nausea, vomiting and abdominal pain, but these are mild and soon subside.

ACANTHOCEPHALA

This group of helminths, the thorny-headed worms are intestinal parasites of rats throughout the world. They are characterized by having a proboscis covered with rows of recurved hooklets and have as their intermediate hosts insects such as cockroaches. The only species recorded from humans are *Moniliformis moniliformis* and *Macracanthorhynchus hirudinaceus*.

Humans, especially children, are occasionally infected after accidental ingestion of the intermediate host.

The worms live in the small intestine and diagnosis is made by passing of the adult worms or the finding of eggs in the feces. Spurious transit eggs can be passed by humans after eating of rodents as food.

Pyrantel pamoate and thiabendazole appear to be ineffectual, and mebendazole (Vermox) is the drug of choice, being given at a dose of 100 mg (1 tablet) twice a day for 3 days.

FLIES, FLEAS, MITES AND LICE

MYIASIS

Given access, a number of fly larvae may penetrate the skin of children or enter wound tissue as is discussed in detail in a review of myiasis by Hall & Wall (1995).

The tumbu, or putsi fly, *Cordylobia anthropophaga*, of tropical and subtropical Africa is but one of a large variety of flies capable of causing myiasis, which is the infestation of viable tissue by dipterous larvae or 'maggots'. Foci of infection with this species have recently been recorded in northern Europe (Goldsmid 1988). The large pale brown tumbu deposits her eggs on shady soil contaminated with urine, or damp clothing, where they hatch to release larvae in about 3 days. Laundry placed out to dry is an ideal site for oviposition, especially if laid out on grass or on the ground and for this reason thorough ironing of clothes on all surfaces is desirable in endemic areas. The larvae penetrate intact skin where they grow rapidly, and unless removed, abandon the host in about 8 days to pupate.

The cutaneous lesions, which may be single or multiple, can occur on any part of the skin, particularly the waist area, back (Fig. 23.94a) and feet. The characteristic lesion is a tender, large, furuncular swelling with a central pore (Fig. 23.94b). Following application of petroleum jelly, the pore widens revealing movement of the posterior spiracles. The tough larva, about 0.5–1.0 cm in length, may then be squeezed out or grasped with forceps and extracted. Secondary infection of these lesions is rare.

In South America the eggs and larvae of the tropical warble fly *Dermatobia hominis* may be transferred to the human skin by flies, mosquitoes or ticks and produce similar papular lesions.

Cutaneous myiasis is being increasingly recognized as an imported infection in many nontropical areas (Goldsmid 1988). The maggot can be gently squeezed out of the lesion or treated by covering the lesion with a thick layer of Vaseline which causes it to leave the skin.

In areas of the world where sheep are farmed, the sheep nasal bot fly, *Oestrus ovis*, has been at times recorded as causing ophthalmo-myiasis – a self-limiting but extremely painful condition.

Other larvae (e.g. those of *Gasterophilus*) may produce itching skin lesions related to the wanderings of the larvae or tender short-lived subcutaneous cystic swellings. *G. intestinalis* can cause intestinal myiasis.

Maggots in wounds tend to be related to the amount of necrotic tissue and their control to the maintenance of adequate wound toilet.

Myiasis may occur rarely in mucous membrane-lined orifices such as the mouth, anus and vagina and in the eye. One species *Auchmeromyia luteola* lives in cracks and crevices of floor in Africa, coming out at night to suck blood from the sleeping human host.

TUNGIASIS

Tungiasis is infection with the jigger (or chigoe) flea, *Tunga penetrans*. This flea, originally endemic to South America, has spread to central Africa and parts of India.

The young adult fleas live in soil or in the dust and cracks of earth floors of houses. After mating, the female flea penetrates the skin of the host (rodents, dogs, cats or humans). Here she develops in the epidermis under the stratum corneum, her abdomen swelling tremendously with developing eggs. The lesion starts as a small black spot in the skin but then becomes inflamed and erythematous, developing into a pustule which may crust over or even form a suppurating ulcer if secondarily infected by bacteria. Lesions mostly occur on the feet, especially under the toe nails or between the toes (Fig. 23.95a). Itching, pain and even regional lymphadenopathy are common.

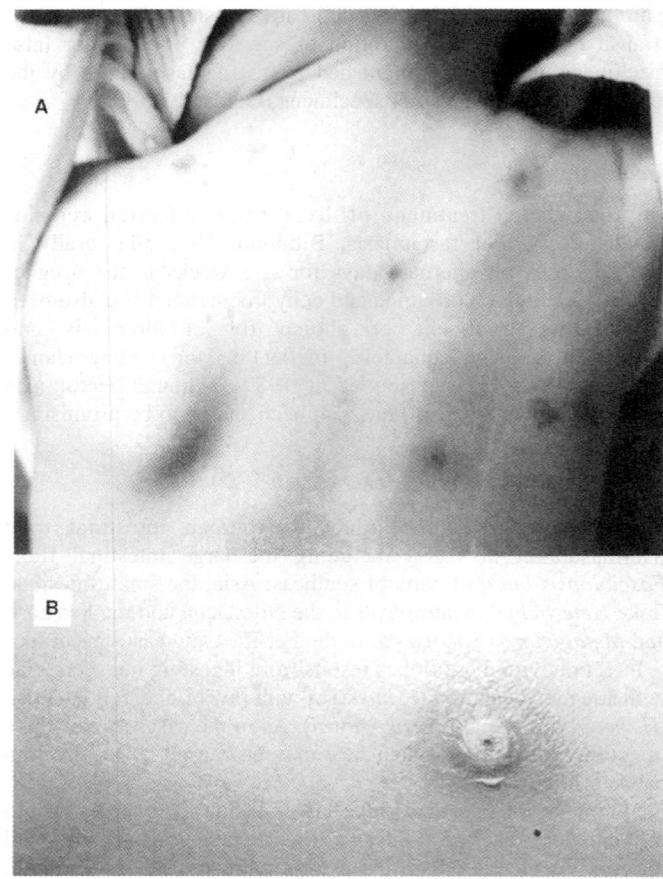

Fig. 23.94 (a) Child with multiple putsi lesions on back. (b) Lesion due to *Cordylobia anthropophaga* on leg to show characteristic appearance.

Eggs are expelled by the female flea, fall to the ground and form free-living larvae and pupae in the soil.

Diagnosis is made by finding the flea in the lesion (Fig. 23.95b) and carefully removing it. In unsuspected cases, diagnosis may be made after biopsy of the lesion and finding the fragmented flea in the lesion.

Treatment consists of a careful removal of the flea without rupturing it, using a sterile needle, followed by a cleaning of the wound with chloroform and a careful curetting of the affected area.

DEMODICIDOSIS

The hair follicle mite, *Demodex folliculorum* (Fig. 23.96a) is one of the commonest parasites of the human skin, with infection rates of 25% or higher.

Human infection is probably acquired by direct person-to-person contact – often at a very young age (e.g. sucking babies infected from their mother). Human infection with other species of *Demodex* from animals has not been ruled out.

The mites live in the pilosebaceous glands and hair follicles especially of the face, scalp, external ear and breast. They are common in the eyelids and mites can often be found clinging to removed eyelashes.

Clinically the condition may be asymptomatic or infected hair follicles may result in the formation of 'blackheads' with crops of

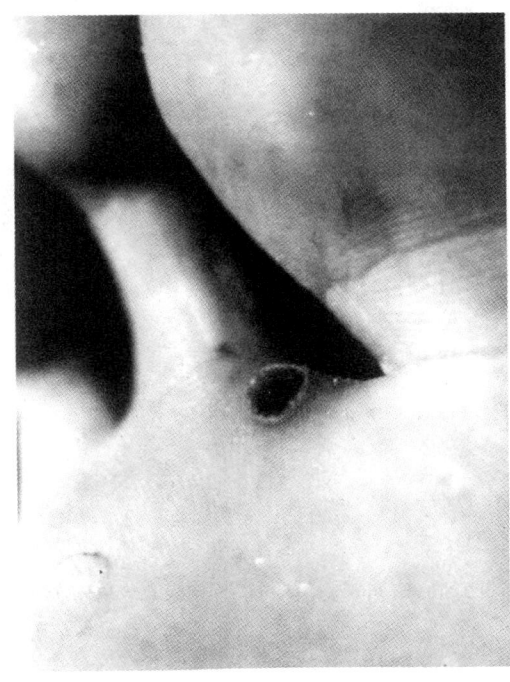

A

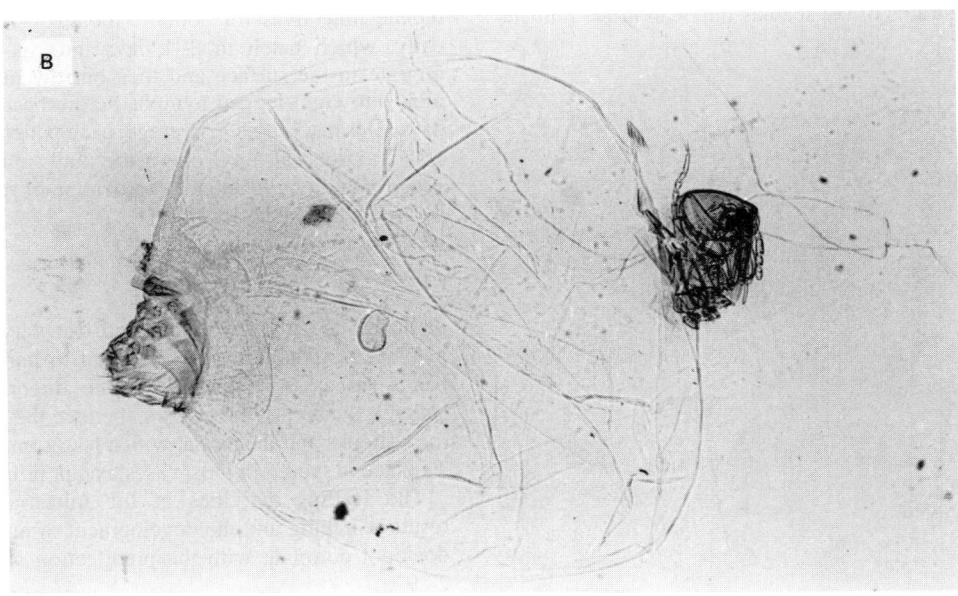

B

Fig. 23.95 (**a**) Lesion due to jigger flea (*Tunga penetrans*) (courtesy of Dr K. Ott). (**b**) Gravid female *Tunga penetrans* – note grossly swollen abdomen (approx. ×35).

red papules appearing often on the forehead. In heavy infestations, or in sensitized patients, dermatitis may follow, with scaling of the skin. Papulonodular demodicidosis may be associated with acquired immune-deficiency syndrome in the form of a papulonodular rash of acute onset, usually localized to the head and neck (Dominey et al 1989).

Diagnosis is established by finding the mites, often in seropurulent fluid expressed from the lesions, or in biopsied specimens of skin in which mites can be found (Fig. 23.96b).

Treatment consists of good hygiene, soap and water together with sulfur ointment or gamma-benzene hexachloride (lindane) if necessary.

SCABIES (see p. 1638)

Scabies is a disease caused by the mite *Sarcoptes scabiei* (Fig. 23.97b). It is worldwide, being especially common in the underdeveloped areas of the world and in countries with a low standard of living. Scabies appears to sweep the world in cyclical pandemics (Christopherson 1986, Goldsmid 1988). It afflicts both

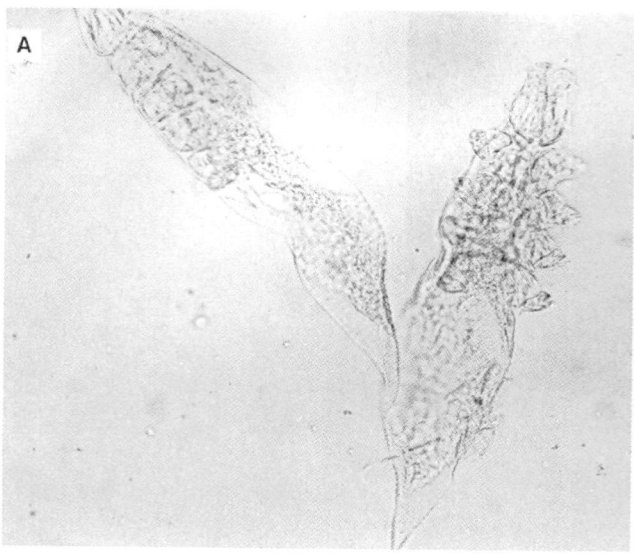
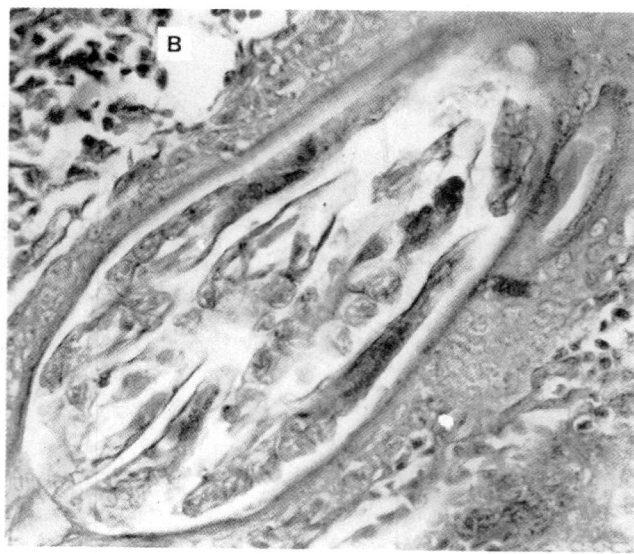

Fig. 23.96 (a) *Demodex folliculorum* (approx. 300). (b) Histological section showing *D. folliculorum* mite in hair follicle (approx. ×300).

rich and poor alike and is commoner in children. Most cases of human scabies are contracted from other infected humans, but occasionally animal strains of the scabies mite can infect humans (Alexander 1984).

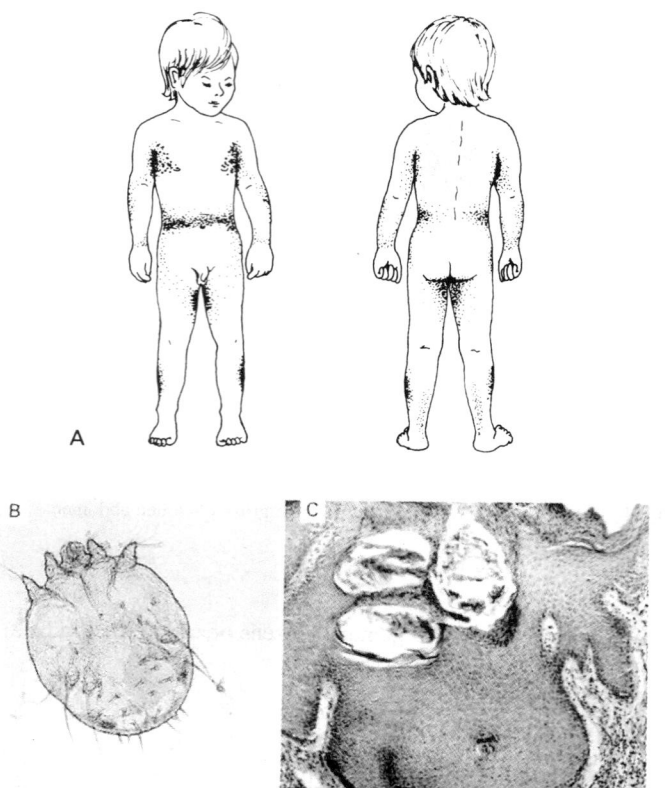

Fig. 23.97 (a) The distribution of the rash in scabies. (b) Adult *Sarcoptes scabei* (approx. ×100). (c) Histological section of skin in scabies showing tunnels (approx. ×300).

The gravid female mites burrow into the horny layers of the skin, forming tunnels (Fig. 23.97c) in which the eggs are laid. The female mite lives for about 1 month, laying two to three eggs daily, which hatch in 3–4 days into six-legged larvae. These migrate to the surface and then burrow into the skin again and molt into eight-legged nymphs before becoming adults about 10 days after hatching. On average, each patient is infested with only 10–12 mites at any one time and much of the observed symptomatology is due to sensitization of the host to the mite and its products (Robinson 1985).

CLINICAL FEATURES

Although the main sites infested can vary with the age of the patient, the commonest sites found to harbor mites include the hands (especially the sides of the fingers and the interdigital spaces), the wrists, the elbows, the feet, the penis and the scrotum, the buttocks and the axilla, with a lesser involvement of the body. The face is spared in most cases except in infants (Burgess 1994).

The feeding activities of the mites and host sensitization result in itching and the development of an extensive rash which does not correlate with the predilection sites of the mites (Fig. 23.97a).

The characteristic lesions of scabies are the burrows in the skin, but there may also be pruritic papules, vesicles and pustules. Often there is eczematization and crusting of the lesions, especially when they are secondarily infected by bacteria. Scabies lesions can provide an entry site for infection with Group A β-hemolytic streptococci and thus glomerulonephritis may follow scabies (Burgess 1994).

Scabies may present in variable forms. Thus in the 'clean' and in patients on corticosteroids, scabies may present with minimal signs and symptoms. In young children, vesicles rather than tunnels are often the rule, while in some patients, the disease occurs in the nodular form. In mentally handicapped patients, debilitated patients and the immunosuppressed, crusted or 'Norwegian scabies' is sometimes seen. Here the infestation is highly contagious and large numbers of mites can be found.

A common feature of scabies is the characteristic nocturnal itching, especially when the patient is warm in bed.

The infestation is transmitted by direct contact, including sexual contact. Fomites such as clothing and blankets generally play no part in the transmission of scabies.

DIAGNOSIS

Scabies is usually diagnosed clinically and should be a considered diagnosis for any patient presenting with an itchy rash covering the whole body but sparing the face. In fact scabies should be the first disease to be *excluded* in any patient presenting with such a rash (Commens 1994). Confirmation by the finding of mites is often difficult, even extensive lesions being associated with very few mites. Mites can sometimes be found in the tunnels after careful removal of the horny layers of skin over the tunnel entrance and the extraction of the shiny white glistening mite with a pin and examination under a microscope. An improved method of obtaining mites is to scrape a suspect lesion and then float the mite out using mineral oil.

TREATMENT

Treatment traditionally begins with a hot bath and a brisk scrub with a soft brush, but this is unnecessary or even inadvisable. Treatment of scabies involves the widespread application over the body of such topical preparations as benzyl benzoate (Ascabiol), gamma-benzene hexachloride (Lorexane, lindane) or crotamiton (Eurax). Of these, benzyl benzoate is the classic treatment but its application causes an unpleasant stinging if used in full strength (25%). In children it should be diluted to half strength, and in infants to quarter strength. Monosulfiram and crotamiton are possibly less effective but the latter is believed to be especially useful as it is said to have some antipruritic activity. Monosulfiram is sometimes used for treating scabies in children. Gamma-benzene hexachloride 1% has in the past proved to be cheap and effective (Burgess 1994).

The newer synthetic pyrethroids are also effective (Burgess 1994, Commens 1994). Resistance to both lindane and the pyrethroids (including permethrin) has been recorded and the problem of resistance as opposed to incomplete treatment is discussed in the review of scabies by Burgess (1994).

For adequate treatment and control, *all members of the family must be treated whether or not they exhibit symptoms,* or relapses and treatment failure will result. In conditions of overcrowding and poor hygiene, the regular use of Tetmosol soap prevents reinfection.

Overtreatment resulting from a temporary persistence of symptoms due to sensitization and the development of a 'parasitophobia' must be resisted at all costs.

It is worth noting that many animal parasitic mites (e.g. *Dermanyssus* and *Ornithonyssus* from rodents or birds and mange mites from dogs and cats) as well as many free-living and nonparasitic mites can attack humans and cause an extensive rash with a severe dermatitis and an itchy allergic reaction resulting in the formation of papules, vesicles and skin blotches. This condition can be very distressing and infestation usually derives from pets, animals nesting in roofs, straw and other packing materials (Goldsmid 1985).

The use of ivermectin, once established for human mite infestations, may prove suitable for the treatment of scabies but toxicity may prove a problem (Burgess 1994).

LOUSE INFESTATION

Humans can become infested with three types of lice – the head louse (*Pediculus humanus capitis*; Fig. 23.98), its morphologically identical, but behaviorally different variant, the body louse (*P. h. corporis*) and the crab or pubic louse, which forms a distinct species, *Pthirus pubis*. All three types are confined to humans worldwide and tend to be more prevalent in areas with poor living standards (Burgess 1995).

PEDICULUS HUMANUS CAPITIS (THE HEAD LOUSE)

P. h. capitis is worldwide in distribution but tends to be commoner in colder countries. Its incidence is subject to unpredictable

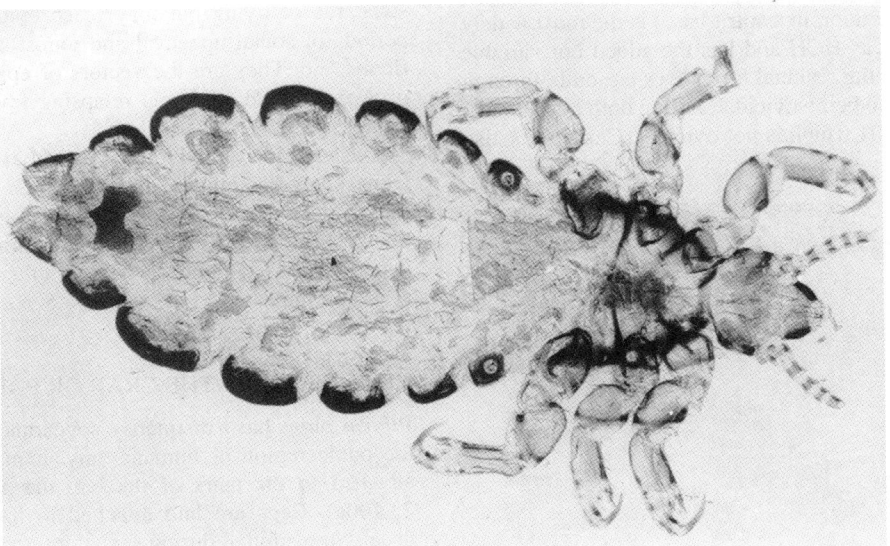

Fig. 23.98 Photomicrograph of adult *Pediculus humanus capitis* – the head louse (approx. ×50).

increases and decreases and with sporadic extensive pandemics. Prevalence figures vary from country to country and from year to year but vary from low percentage prevalences to prevalences of 60% or more amongst schoolchildren (Robinson 1985, Burgess 1995).

Head lice tend to be confined to the scalp, but are occasionally found on other hairy parts of the body. The insects live close to the scalp and feed on blood which they obtain with their sucking mouthparts. After mating, the female louse lays 6–8 eggs every 24 h. These eggs ('nits') (Fig. 23.99) are glued tightly to the hairs close to the scalp and hatch in about 7 days into a nymph which feeds and passes through three nymphal instars before becoming adult in 10–11 days (Burgess 1995).

Head louse infestation may be asymptomatic or, in heavily infested cases, may be manifested by scalp pruritus, loss of sleep, mild pyrexia and, with secondary bacterial infection, by cervical gland enlargement.

Pediculosis capitis is found in people of all age groups, but is commoner in children especially those aged 3–13 years, being maximal at 6–9 years. Although not directly correlated to hair length, head lice are commoner in girls than in boys. Both rich and poor alike are afflicted, but infestation is more frequently but not exclusively encountered in low socioeconomic areas than in higher class environments.

While transmission is mostly by direct contact and is thus facilitated by overcrowding, many studies have suggested strongly that transmission can occur through shared headgear, hat and coat hooks, combs and brushes.

Head lice can only be controlled by regular inspection and treatment of infected cases *and all their family members*, whether or not lice or nits can be found in the latter.

In the past, DDT has been used for treatment, but its toxicity and resistance in the lice led to its replacement by gamma-benzene hexachloride (γ-BHC, γ-HCH; Quellada, Lorexane). However, resistance is being recorded to HCH and this, plus its toxicity, has resulted in its being considered obsolete in many parts of the world (Robinson 1985, Meinking & Taplin 1990, Vander Steichele et al 1995). It is being replaced by safer preparations such as carbaryl, malathion (Maldison, Prioderm) and the synthetic pyrethroids such as permethrin (Nix). Of these, malathion (a 0.5% preparation in a spirit base) is the most widely used. It is twice as safe as HCH and has the added but variable advantage of possibly being residual for at least a month, through bonding to the hair, and in being ovicidal, killing both lice and nits – a feature absent in HCH which is not ovicidal. Carbaryl is also said to be ovicidal but Burgess (1991) has challenged this concept of an inherent ovicidal efficacy for malathion and carbaryl. Pyrethrins (Paralice) especially those in a mousse formulation (e.g. Banlice) may also be effectively used to treat head lice (Burgess 1995) with the third generation synthetic pyrethroids such as permethrin (Nix) proving the most promising (Meinking & Taplin 1990, Vander Steichele et al 1995). All these preparations are toxic to some extent and care should thus be exercised in their use, with particular care being taken to avoid accidental ingestion or contact with eyes. Both shampoos and lotions are available but lotions are far superior (Goldsmid 1989, Goldsmid et al 1989, Burgess 1995). Developing resistance to headlouse preparations may prove a problem, albeit a sometimes controversial one (Burgess 1995, Burgess et al 1995).

Nits, although killed by malathion and carbaryl, remain tightly attached to the hairs and may have to be combed out with special fine toothed 'nit combs', although with ovicidal compounds this exercise is not necessary in louse treatment or control.

In the control of head lice, sterilization of clothing, bedding, combs, etc. is unnecessary as insecticide treatment of the hair will provide sufficient protection from reinvasion by the short-lived lice that have strayed from the head.

In community control programs, antilouse preparations should be changed on a regular basis to prevent the emergence of resistance.

PEDICULUS HUMANUS CORPORIS (THE BODY LOUSE)

Pediculus humanus corporis is identical to the head louse in appearance but differs in that it lives on the clothing and only visits the skin to suck blood. The eggs are glued to the clothing, especially the seams, and hatch in about 1 week to nymphs, which like those of the head louse, develop into adults in 7–10 days.

Body lice cause pediculosis corporis which may be characterized by the presence of feeding punctures appearing as small papules which, in sensitized patients, may become swollen, pigmented and hardened, a condition formerly known as vagabond's disease or *morbus errorum*.

Body lice are more limited to areas of overcrowding and poorer standards of living but may reach epidemic proportions during periods of social upheaval and unrest such as war, earthquakes, floods, etc. They are the vectors of epidemic typhus (*Rickettsia prowazekii*) and epidemic relapsing fever (*Borrelia recurrentis*) (Burgess 1995).

Transmission of body lice is directly from person to person and from shared clothing and blankets. Control is with 0.5% malathion lotion or 5% carbaryl dust and treatment of clothing, blankets, etc. with methyl bromide fumigation, washing in hot water at 60°C or higher by heating in a domestic tumble drier for at least 5 min.

PTHIRUS PUBIS (THE CRAB OR PUBIC LOUSE)

Pthirus pubis has a distinctive appearance and is usually found in the pubic region of humans only. It may also be found tightly attached to the hairs of the leg, the axilla or the beard (Fig. 23.100a). Eggs are laid attached to hairs (Fig. 23.100b). It is usually transmitted during sexual intercourse and because of this, it is mostly found infesting adults. However, children can harbor the lice and even young children may become infected from

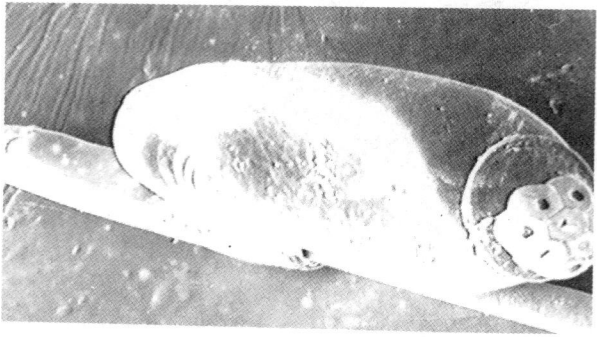

Fig. 23.99 Scanning electron micrograph of egg ('nit') of the head louse attached to a hair (approx. ×80).

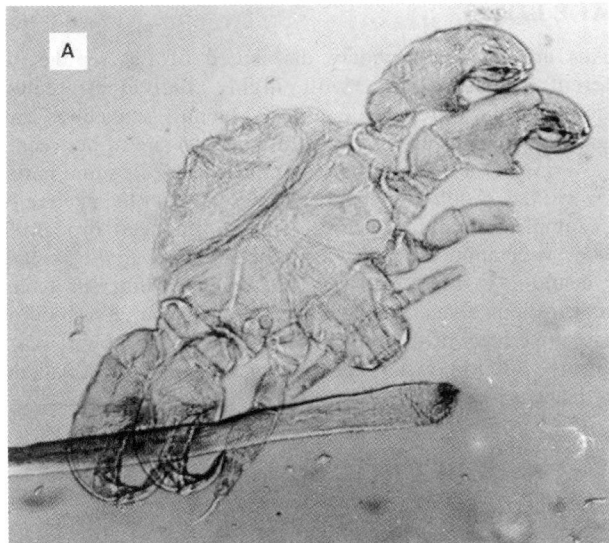

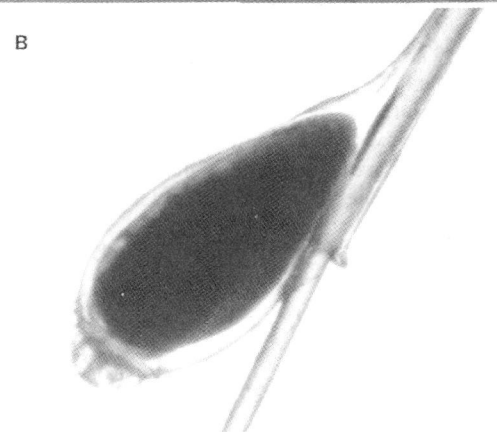

Fig. 23.100 (a) Photomicrograph of nymph of *Pth. pubis* tightly attached to hair (approx. ×100). (b) Egg of crab louse (*Pth. pubis*) attached to hair (approx. ×60).

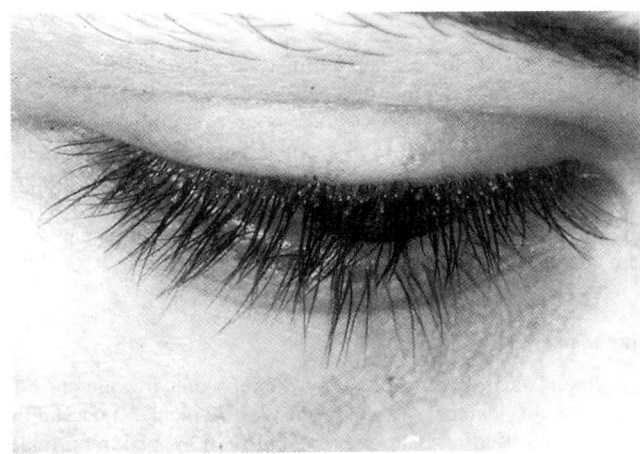

Fig. 23.101 Eggs of pubic louse on eyelashes.

heavily infested parents. Thus toddlers are at times found to have phthiriasis, the lice being found attached to the eyelashes and even the hair of the forehead. The lice can survive for 9–44 h off the host and infestation from clothing and toilet seats is thus feasible, although unlikely.

Again, heavy infestations may result in itching and rarely, *maculae cerulae* or bluish spots due to repeated biting may be found.

Treatment is similar to that for head lice, namely the use of insecticides such as gamma-benzene hexachloride (lindane) as a lotion, shampoo or 2% powder. This insecticide is toxic and treatment needs to be repeated as it is not ovicidal. 0.5% malathion or carbaryl are safer and, being ovicidal, are more effective, but spirit base preparations should not be used. Pyrethroids are also effective and are widely used.

When on the eyelashes (Fig. 23.101) *Pth. pubis* should be dealt with by removal of individual lice or by treating each egg individually with a paint brush dipped in an ovicidal insecticide. Alternatively, the thick application of Vaseline twice daily for 8 days may be effective (Burgess 1995). Laundering of clothing, sheets, etc. in hot water is advisable to prevent spread.

DISEASES TRANSMITTED BY DOGS AND CATS

These are summarized in Table 23.52.

CAT-SCRATCH DISEASE

First described in 1950, cat-scratch is a relatively benign, widely encountered infection characterized by malaise, low-grade fever and lymphadenopathy. It usually resolves spontaneously in a few weeks. Rarely, complications can occur such as encephalitis, follicular conjunctivitis and neuroretinitis (Margileth 1993). Contact with cats followed by skin lesions associated with a scratch or bite are found in the majority of cases. There may be a maculopapular rash. Chronic lymphadenitis may occur with the cervical lymph nodes frequently involved. Systemic symptoms are unusual.

Table 23.52 Diseases transmitted from dogs and cats

Dogs	Cats
Rabies (p. 1376)	Rabies (p. 1376)
Ringworm (p. 1636)	Cat-scratch fever (*Bartonella henselae*)
Scabies (pp. 1515, 1638)	Ringworm (p. 1636)
Echinococcus granulosus infection (p. 1504)	Scabies (pp. 1515, 1638)
Toxocara canis infection (larva migrans) (p. 1485)	*Toxocara cati* (larva migrans) (p. 1486)
Leptospirosis (p. 1311)	Pasteurellosis (*Pasteurella multocida*)
Canicola fever (*Leptospira canicola*) (p. 1311)	Cutaneous larva migrans (p. 1490)
Leishmaniasis (p. 1460)	Toxoplasmosis (p. 1464)
Dipylidium caninum (p. 1502)	
Cutaneous larva migrans (p. 1490)	
Dirofilaria immitis (p. 1499)	
Capnocytophaga canimorsus (DF-2)	

Etiology

A causative agent for cat-scratch disease was identified in 1988 and classified as a member of a new genus named *Afipia* – Gram-negative, motile, oxidase-positive, nonfermenting bacilli. Only one species *Afipia felis* is associated with cats (Brenner et al 1991). The bacterium *Bartonella* (formerly *Rochalimaea*) *henselae*, which is morphologically similar to *A. felis*, may be more important in etiology, but the proportion of cases caused by each agent is unknown (Adal et al 1994).

Diagnosis

The diagnosis is confirmed if the history of cat contact and a primary skin lesion is associated with typical silver-staining bacteria identified on histopathological sections of lymph nodes, skin or eye lesions. A skin test for scratch disease is available, but this is being superseded by serology using an indirect fluorescent antibody test for *B. henselae* which is said to be more sensitive.

Treatment

As most patients with this disease are not ill and spontaneous recovery is common, treatment is usually symptomatic. Antibiotics should be reserved for patients with severe disease. The most commonly used antibiotics are not effective and a recent review indicated that only four antimicrobial drugs are useful, with the oral drugs in decreasing order of efficacy being rifampicin (87%), ciprofloxacin (84%) and trimethoprim-sulfamethoxazole (58%). Intramuscular gentamicin was 73% effective (Margileth 1992).

Cat-scratch encephalopathy

CNS complications may develop from a few days to some weeks after the first evidence of illness, usually a mildly tender lymphadenopathy. Fever is not characteristic and may occur in only 50% of cases. Convulsions of varying severity will also affect about 50% of the children with encephalopathy, and they may remain lethargic or even comatose for several weeks. In the recovery phase, 'transient combative behavior' seems to be a characteristic feature of this particular type of encephalopathy. Changes in the CSF are neither consistent nor characteristic and peripheral blood counts are not helpful. In addition to the control of convulsions and supportive measures, the most important aspect of this encephalopathy is to establish the diagnosis and differentiate it from other causes of encephalopathy as quickly as possible to avoid extensive and invasive investigations. The prognosis is excellent with no evidence of lasting neurological impairment (Carithers & Margileth 1991).

POISONOUS ANIMAL BITES AND STINGS

In a recent overview of poisonous animal bites and stings published by the World Health Organization, it was stated that in excess of 100 000 deaths result worldwide each year from bites by snakes, stings from scorpions and from anaphylactic reactions to insect stings (WHO 1995b).

SNAKE BITES

Snakes are the most widely distributed of the reptiles, and different species, often with highly individual features, predominate in different countries. Overall, snakebites cause thousands of deaths each year, with a fatality rate of between 1.5 and 3% (WHO 1995b). Environmental change in some parts of the world has resulted in changes in the pattern of snakebite – as for example in parts of Africa, where prolonged drought has reduced vegetation cover, favoring the spread of *Echis ocellatus*, and resulting in more bites (WHO 1995b). Clinicians have to concern themselves primarily with the characteristics and venomous effects of the poisonous snakes in their own area. Of the nearly 3000 known varieties only some 300 are of medical significance.

ADDER BITES (EUROPE)

There is only one poisonous species in Britain, the common viper or adder (*Viper berus*), and its bite seldom causes death in an adult, although young children very occasionally die as a result. The fully grown adder may be 50–60 cm in length and is recognized by the dark zigzag band which runs along the center of the back, although rarely the snake may appear uniformly black. It is a shy creature, living in clearings, the edges of woods, moors and low lying damp ground, and normally disappears quickly on the approach of people. It is only likely to bite if disturbed unexpectedly.

Clinical features

When the amount of venom injected is small, as is usual in a defensive bite, there may be few signs or symptoms, but fear often causes transient pallor, sweating or vomiting. With moderate poisoning there may be local swelling increasing over 1 or 2 days to involve the whole limb. This swelling resolves within a few weeks. In more serious cases, a burning pain is experienced at the place bitten, usually an extremity. Vomiting may begin within a few minutes of the bite (often accompanied by diarrhea) and may continue for up to 48 h. Shock is likely with weakness, sweating, thirst, coldness, absent pulse, hypotension, drowsiness and occasionally loss of consciousness. Swelling of the face, lips and tongue may occur, Soon hemorrhagic discoloration and swelling appear and may gradually extend up the limb. Bleeding may occur from gums, wound and infection sites. With recovery, discoloration slowly changes from blue to green and finally to yellow before disappearing. The child generally recovers quickly from the initial collapse but in severe poisoning there may be persistent or recurrent hypotension. Full recovery may take 1–6 weeks.

In hospital, blood pressure should be monitored hourly, and bleeding time should be recorded; the white cell count (raised), serum creatine phosphokinase (may be raised), serum bicarbonate (may be low) and ECG should be determined twice daily.

Treatment

When a child is bitten by a snake, the reptile should be killed for identification, if this can be done without risk of further bites. The bite should not be incised but merely covered with a clean handkerchief or cloth. The patient should be kept quiet and the limb maintained at rest by splinting, helping to retard absorption of venom. The child and his parents should be reassured about the expected outcome and taken to hospital as quickly as possible. On admission to hospital paracetamol may be given for the pain, chlorpromazine if required for vomiting and an antihistamine drug for the swelling. The blood pressure should be recorded hourly and repeated observations made for any bleeding tendency, leukocytosis or electrocardiographic changes. Antibiotics and tetanus antitoxin are not required routinely. Antivenom (two ampoules) should be given if there is evidence of systemic poisoning especially hypotension, bleeding or ECG changes. It should be given diluted with isotonic saline, by slow intravenous infusion, over a period of 30–60 min with adrenaline ready in case of need. The antivenom is produced in Zagreb and can be obtained in Britain from Regent Laboratories Ltd., London NW10 6PN. Before antivenom arrives or if a history of allergy contraindicates its use, blood transfusion may help to combat collapse.

TROPICAL AND SUBTROPICAL SNAKES

Morbidity and mortality from snake bites are highest in those areas where snakes have adapted to farm, plantation and village life and live in close proximity to large human populations. Examples are the Indian cobra, krait and Russell's viper in southeast Asia, and some pit vipers in Latin America.

Land snakes may be classified according to the presence or absence of poisonous injecting fangs, and their position when present in the snake's mouth (Table 23.53). Sea snakes, of which there are some 50 varieties, have characteristic flattened tails and short front fangs.

Although the Elapidae include many highly venomous varieties, these usually retreat when approached by humans and are generally nonaggressive unless cornered or molested. The large family of Colubridae contains only a few snakes of medical significance and these are rarely the cause of bites in humans. The Viperidae, on the other hand, are broad sluggish snakes which hold their ground and may easily be trodden on (puff adder) or touched, on or in the ground or among rocks (rattlesnake, burrowing adder, berg adder). These snakes, despite their sluggishness, strike with great rapidity and power, virtually stabbing their victim with frontally situated large fangs which are swung forward during the strike.

Many nonvenomous snakes are capable of inflicting bites which are liable to become infected, sometimes with exotic bacteria, such as *Arizona* species.

Snake venoms broadly correspond with the families shown in the table. They are complex mixtures of toxins and enzymes and effects depend upon which of these predominate. Viper (and some cobra) venoms are mainly cytotoxic. Elapid venoms produce neurotoxic effects, as do varieties of tropical rattlesnake (*Crotolinea*). The Australian tiger snake has a complex venom with at least three distinct neurotoxins. The venoms can also cause hemolysis, hemorrhage and coagulation disturbances.

Colubrid (boomslang) venoms are hematoxic and anticoagulant, while hydrophiid (sea snake) venoms are mainly myotoxic. Nephrotoxic properties have also been demonstrated in puff adder, sea snake and rattlesnake venoms.

Children are particularly at risk in areas where snakes are common because of their love of outdoor pursuits, together with their curiosity and carelessness. However, it is important to realize

Table 23.53 Classification of snakes

Group of snake	Features of groups	Common examples and habitat	Principal action of venom
Viperidae	Mobile front fangs	Viperinae Puff adder, widespread in Africa Gaboon viper, central and southern Africa Berg adder, southern Africa Russell's viper, Asia and Indonesia Saw-scaled viper, India, Iraq, North Africa European viper (adder), Europe, Asia, Japan Crotalinae (pit vipers) Cottonmouth mocassin, southeastern United States Fer-de-lance, Mexico and South America Jaracara, South America Rattlesnakes, Mexico, southern and western United States Taiwan Habu, southeastern China	Cytotoxic (tropical rattlesnakes and Berg adder are mainly neurotoxic)
Elapidae	Fixed front fangs	Cobras, widespread in Africa and Asia Mambas, east, central and southern Africa Rinkhals, southern Africa Indian krait, India, Burma, Malaya, Indonesia Tiger snake, Australia Death adder, Australia and New Guinea Coral snake, southern United States	Neurotoxic (king cobra also has cytotoxic effect)
Colubridae	Back fangs	Boomslang Herald snake } widespread in Africa Vine snake	Hematoxic
Hydrophidae (sea snakes)	Short fixed front fangs	Beaked sea snake and many other species, mainly in Pacific. A few varieties in Indian Ocean	Myotoxic
Nonvenomous	Fangless	House snake } Grass snake } cosmopolitan Python, Africa, Asia	Nil

that the majority of bites from snakes are not caused by venomous species. In these circumstances two distinct puncture marks are not seen and the bites are irregular and lacerated to a greater or lesser degree, with little local swelling or pain. Even venomous species do not always inflict clinically significant envenomation as the bite may be deflected by clothing or the venom stores of the snake depleted. When envenomation has occurred, symptoms tend to be more severe in children because of their smaller size relative to the volume of injected venom.

Despite popular belief, signs of systemic envenomation in even the most poisonous snake bites seldom occur before 30 min. The earliest features are often those due to fright – shock, pallor, sweating, vomiting, weak pulse and faintness. Severe pain and swelling at the site of the bite, with rapidly spreading edema, are the first signs in most viperine and some cobra bites. Later large blisters may form around the bite and painful lymphadenopathy develops. Sometimes there is extensive bruising in superficial and deeper tissues. Within 5 or 6 h the whole limb may be tensely swollen. There is thus a profound local cytotoxic effect and subsequent systemic disturbance is largely due to this tissue damage rather than to circulating venom. Necrosis of superficial or deep tissues may be seen. 'The intravascular clotting–fibrinolysis syndrome', with resultant hemolytic anemia, hemorrhagic manifestations and hemoglobinuric nephrosis, can complicate the bite.

In heavy envenomation, especially by puff adders and Gaboon vipers, bloody saliva may be expectorated, and sudden death may follow due to circulatory collapse. Notable exceptions in this family of snakes are the hemorrhagic reactions seen in bites from saw-scaled and Russell's vipers and the neurotoxic effects occurring in tropical rattlesnake and berg adder bites.

Elapid bites cause much less local reaction, but have profound systemic effects which are predominantly neurotoxic. The first symptoms are ptosis, rapidly followed by strabismus, slurred speech and dysphagia, with drooling saliva. There is confusion and hypersensitivity to tactile stimuli. If untreated, respiratory paralysis may result in death within 15 h. In survivors there are no neurological sequelae. In the case of mamba bites, the first systemic symptoms are combined with a sensation of tightness and pain across the chest. Violent abdominal pain sometimes occurs after krait and coral snakebites. Local blistering may be seen after envenomation by some cobras and a burning sensation at the site is often described. Local pain after snake bites is, however, extremely variable. Hematuria and hemoglobinuria may occur as may hemorrhage or menorrhagia.

Some elapids, for example the spitting cobra, or rinkhals, of southern Africa, are able to eject venom with considerable force and accuracy at the victim's head. Should this enter the eyes, a very severe keratoconjunctivitis is produced which may lead to blindness.

The boomslang is the only venomous snake in the large family of Colubridae which is a significant hazard to humans. Fortunately bites from this species are rare usually occurring in those handling or working with snakes. There is little or no local reaction apart from mild burning pain but severe headache about 1 h after the bite is a regular and unexplained phenomenon. Colubrid venoms contain mainly fibrinolysins and hemorrhagins which result in severe, systemic defibrination and generalized hemorrhage, widespread cutaneous bruising especially at sites of trauma, and free bleeding from fang punctures. There may be massive intestinal, urinary tract or intracranial hemorrhage

leading to death. As mentioned earlier, the venom of certain vipers and also some elapids (such as the Papuan black snake) produces similar hemorrhagic effects.

Sea snakes do not attack in water if unmolested. Most bites result from handling the snake when caught in fishing nets. The bite shows no local reaction and in most sea snake bites no envenomation occurs (Heatwole 1987). Initial symptoms, due to a myotoxin, are seen after a latent period of 30–120 min. There is muscular pain, stiffness and trismus followed by ptosis and progressive weakness which may threaten respiratory function. Myoglobinuria, renal tubular necrosis and acute renal failure may ensue.

Treatment

The only effective treatment for a case of envenomation by a poisonous snake is the administration of antivenom, preferably intravenously. The use of antivenom, especially polyvalent antivenom, carries a substantial risk of anaphylaxis and serum sickness because of its foreign protein content, but there is no doubt that the benefits of antivenom treatment far outweigh the risks (WHO 1995b). Its administration in every case of snake bite is, however, dangerous, wasteful and unnecessary. As only a minority of bites are due to poisonous snakes, it is obviously of paramount importance, as an initial step, to identify the snake accurately, or at least to decide into which group it falls. Much can be deduced from the color and shape of the snake, manner and circumstances of striking, the situation of the bite and presence or absence of fang marks. For instance, the puff adder, responsible for 95% of poisonous snake bites in Africa, is encountered on paths or in grassy terrain, and almost always strikes at the feet or ankles. On the other hand, cobras often attack when they are surprised near outbuildings or chicken runs. They rear up prior to striking and bites are frequently inflicted above the knees or even on the trunk or upper limbs.

As many victims of snake bites are not within easy access of clinic or hospital, it is most important to lay down firm and easily understood guidelines which can be applied to a layman on the spot:

1. *Symptoms* developing within the first half hour of a bite are almost always due to fear and its effects – and not to envenomation. The patient should be calmed and reassured, and encouraged to lie down quietly so as not to disseminate the poison by restless body movements. The affected limb should be kept horizontal at this stage and gently splinted to avoid movement. A mild analgesic (paracetamol) should be given and a placebo injection of saline has been found of value in older patients to allay anxiety.

2. *Bites* from nonvenomous snakes should be thoroughly cleansed with a dilute antiseptic solution, any loose teeth removed, and a light dressing applied. Tetanus toxoid (or antitetanus serum if applicable) should be administered within 24 h to all cases of snake bite and broad spectrum antibiotics should be given at the first indication of possible infection.

3. *Signs of significant envenomation* generally develop from half to 2 h after the bite. These may be local in the case of viperine bites, with swelling and pain, or systemic in the case of elapid and some other snakes, with varying manifestations, as noted earlier. They call for urgent administration of antivenom: get the patient to a hospital or a trained person to the patient, so that it can be

given intravenously. If this is not possible, the antivenom should be administered intramuscularly (see below). Premedication with parenteral antihistamine and low dose subcutaneous adrenaline (0.003–0.007 mg/kg) prior to administration of antivenom will prevent anaphylaxis. This should be followed by a 5-day course of prophylactic oral corticosteroids to avoid delayed serum sickness. (Sutherland 1992a, Tibballs 1994)

4. *Tourniquets:* under no circumstances should a tourniquet be applied in the case of viper or colubrid bites. The local effects and subsequent complications are aggravated by compression. However, where highly venomous snakes with pronounced systemic effects are incriminated (e.g. cobras, mambas, crotalids and sea snakes), and especially if there are already signs of systemic toxicity, a tourniquet should be applied to the affected limb above the bite to prevent further absorption. It should be broad and tightly applied to constrict arteries and veins. The tourniquet should be completely released for 90 s every 15 min, and finally removed after 1 h. The time of initial application should be clearly marked on the patient. There is no place for the application of a tourniquet more than 1 h after a bite or if antivenom has been given. Australian experience with elapid bites has much to recommend it. Thus it has been found that for this group, venom movement can be effectively delayed for long periods by the application of a firm crepe bandage to the length of the bitten limb combined with immobilization by a splint. It is worth noting here that this 'pressure immobilization' method may be used for all snake bites and some other types of bites or stings such as those from bees, wasps, or ants in sensitive subjects, and funnel-web spider bites (Sutherland 1992a). However, exceptions when the method should *not* be applied include ant, bee and wasp stings in normal, nonsensitive subjects, red-back spider bites and jelly-fish stings (Sutherland 1992a).

5. *Suction:* suction apparatus is available in many commercial snake bite kits, and if used immediately may be of help in withdrawing venom from fang punctures. Suction by mouth, however, entails a definite risk of absorption of venom through the oral or intestinal mucous membranes. In general, suction is not recommended for snakebite (WHO 1995b).

6. *Incision:* most authorities now condemn the use of deep incisions over fang marks as a first aid measure. Superficial incisions, if made within minutes of the bite, may be of possible benefit in enhancing removal of venom, when coupled with efficient suction but again, in general, its use is not recommended (WHO 1995b).

7. *Other local measures*, such as freezing, injection of antivenom, EDTA or other agents into the bite and application of permanganate crystals to incised wounds, have no place in the management of snake bites, and can only serve to aggravate tissue damage.

Antivenom

Some 30 centers in different countries manufacture antivenom appropriate to local varieties. Polyvalent antisera generally cover most bites encountered, but in the case of certain snakes (e.g. boomslang) monospecific antisera are required. Antivenom is preferably given intravenously but the intramuscular route may be necessary when a doctor is not available. If more than 2 h have elapsed since the bite, the allergic status of the patient should be tested with a small intradermal test dose. A positive skin test constitutes a relative contraindication to its use, but this must be

assessed according to the clinical condition of the patient. Adrenaline should always be at hand to combat possible anaphylaxis. It is advisable to give a corticosteroid, such as hydrocortisone, prior to antivenom as this tends to modify serum reactions as well as having anti-inflammatory and antihypotensive effects.

Once a decision to administer antivenom has been reached, it must be given in adequate dosage, especially in the case of children and thus it must be emphasized that the dosage for children is the same as that for adults (WHO 1995b). Antivenom is undoubtedly best given in an intravenous drip, diluted in about four times its volume of normal saline over a period of half an hour. A recommended initial intravenous dose is 40 ml. This should be repeated every 4 h if clinical response is not satisfactory and if necessary up to 200 ml should be given within the first 24 h. When large doses are used, steroids should be continued to modify possible serum sickness reactions. With the use of i.v. antivenom administration, the incidence of anaphylactoid reactions does increase, but these reactions respond quickly to prompt adrenaline injection. If a doctor is not available, the usual dose that can be tolerated intramuscularly is about 20 ml.

In the case of ophthalmia due to a spitting cobra, the affected eye should be well washed with water or other bland fluid before diluted antivenom is instilled.

ELISA kits, suitable for field use, are available in some areas such as Australia for detection and species identification in snakebite washings, blood or urine (CSL Diagnostics, Australia).

Further supportive care

Unless it has been shown with the passage of some hours that the bite is trivial all cases of poisonous snake bite require admission to hospital.

If severe bulbar or respiratory paralysis have developed, airway suction, oxygen and assisted respiration with or without tracheostomy are indicated.

Management of acute renal failure should be anticipated by adequate intravenous replacement, careful monitoring of input and output, urinalysis and measurement of plasma urea and electrolytes.

Hemorrhagic manifestations require careful appraisal with a coagulation profile as hemorrhagins (Russell's viper), fibrinolysins (boomslang) or intravascular clotting (puff adder) can be responsible. Intravenous vitamin K, blood transfusion, fresh plasma, or fibrinogen, low molecular weight dextran, heparin or ε-aminocaproic acid may be required according to circumstances.

In the event of severe local swelling, the limb should be kept elevated. Bullae should not be burst as this increases the likelihood of infection. Skin or fascial release to ease jeopardized circulation, debridement of necrotic tissue, and subsequent grafting or amputation are not uncommonly required, especially in untreated puff adder bites.

In an interesting analysis of deaths from snake bites Sutherland (1978) has emphasized that snake bite deaths result from:

1. victims not being observed for an adequate period – suspected snake bite victims should be observed for at least 12–24 h after the bite
2. antivenom being withheld despite clear indication of systemic envenomation

3. giving the wrong antivenom – often more than once
4. giving too little of the correct antivenom or not giving more antivenom if signs and symptoms reoccur.

Prevention

1. Treat all snakes with respect.
2. Endeavor to know the snakes in your area.
3. Watch out in summer months particularly after first rains. Be careful when walking at night; use a torch.
4. Wear boots and leggings or at least shoes and socks when walking in the bush (80% of human snake bites are on the legs and 55% on the ankle and foot).
5. Avoid thickly bushed country, long grass, etc.
6. Do not panic and run away when confronted by a snake; movement will attract attention whereas the snake is likely to move off if you keep still.
7. Keep an appropriate anti-snakebite kit with you.

It has also been found important in Australia to emphasize the need to believe a child who claims to have been bitten by a snake (Sutherland 1979).

INSECTS, SPIDERS, TICKS, BEETLES, SCORPIONS, CENTIPEDES AND CATERPILLARS

HYMENOPTERA STINGS

All stinging insects, such as bees, wasps, hornets and ants, are included in the order Hymenoptera. Bee venom contains many toxic fractions, the most important being mellitin which alters capillary permeability, causes local pain, hemolyzes red cells, and lowers blood pressure. The venom also contains antigenic components which are capable of invoking an allergic response in the form of hypersensitivity in a significant proportion of the population if subjected to a subsequent challenge. Cross-antigenicity may occur between wasp and bee stings.

In Australia serious clinical problems are becoming more common owing to severe allergy to jumper ant (*Myrmecia pilosula*) and bull ant (*Myrmecia pyriformis*) bites and stings.

The management of insect stings has been well reviewed by Reisman (1994). In general terms, uncomplicated stings require no treatment, apart from mild analgesics. Bee sting barbs should be carefully removed with a flat blade, taking care not to express further venom, which will happen if the sting is grasped with forceps. It has been claimed that meat tenderizer, available in most kitchens, applied in a dilute solution (a quarter teaspoon mixed with 1 teaspoon of water), rubbed into the sting relieves all pain within seconds. In sensitive individuals, however, even a single sting may result in acute anaphylactic shock with urticaria, hypotension, tachycardia and sweating, glottic edema, or bronchospasm. Prompt treatment is vital. Adrenaline is indicated, either by injection or inhalation. Inhalation of an adrenaline aerosol (Medihaler EPI, Riker) from a pressurized can similar to that used for asthma, is more rapid than administering an injection. Five inhalations of this aerosol are equivalent in effect to 0.5 ml of injected 1 : 1000 adrenaline. People who are known to be allergic to bee or wasp stings should always carry such a can. An appropriate dose of an antihistamine is then given parenterally. In the case of laryngeal edema, hydrocortisone should also be injected intravenously. Tracheostomy may be life saving in the event of severe edema of the glottis.

Skin tests to detect hypersensitivity to Hymenoptera stings are unreliable. However, children who are known to react in a hypersensitive manner should undergo desensitization with a carefully planned immunization schedule, using polyvalent Hymenoptera antigen. Immunotherapy may become more reliable with the development and use of pure venom immunization and phospholipase A, when and if it becomes available. However, children appear to exhibit considerably less frequent severe side effects to stings than adults. Accordingly Valentine et al (1990) conclude that immunotherapy is unnecessary for most children allergic to insect stings.

Bee venoms also possess hemolytic properties and multiple stings, usually in excess of 100, may result in significant hemolysis with acute anemia and subsequent renal failure. Cases of massive bee stings should be admitted to hospital and carefully observed for early signs of these complications, where prompt treatment can be instituted and renal failure minimized to ensuring a high urine output. Biphasic renal failure has been known to occur with early renal failure due to hemolysis and a second episode of azotemia about 10 days later, corresponding with a depressed serum complement C3 level and nephritic changes on renal biopsy – a phenomenon probably representing a serum sickness reaction caused by a large volume of foreign protein.

Studies in Australia have shown that 'Stingose' (an aqueous solution of 20% aluminum sulfate and 1.1% surfactant) is an effective, wide-acting first aid treatment to counteract the venoms of insects, marine invertebrates and plants when applied topically soon after the bite or sting.

The application of ice packs to insect stings (and platypus stings in Australia) will help to relieve local pain (Sutherland 1992b).

SPIDER BITES

Only a small fraction of the several hundred genera of spiders contain poisonous species and Alexander (1984) has discussed these in detail. The most important medically are *Latrodectus* and *Loxosceles* with *Latrodectus mactans* (the black widow spider) and *L. geometricus* (the brown widow spider) being the commonest species, being widely distributed throughout the warmer areas of the world. The former is known locally as the button spider in South Africa and the red back spider in Australia.

Only the aggressive females are hazardous to humans. They have black or dark velvety globular bodies about 15 mm in length with orange-red markings often in the shape of an hourglass on the ventral surface of the abdomen. They tend to spin their webs in dark places, such as under lavatory seats, hence the number of bites which occur on the buttocks or genitalia. *Latrodectus* venoms possess neurotoxic properties and cause stimulation of neuromuscular junctions. Following a bite from *Latrodectus*, there is a very variable local reaction. Signs of systemic envenomation occur between 20 and 200 min later. There is often a regional lymphadenopathy within 30 min of the bite, followed by severe muscular pains involving the limbs and trunk with tightness around the chest and abdominal rigidity which may mimic an acute abdomen. Hyperreflexia is often present. Death is rare, even in untreated cases, but when it occurs, is usually due to respiratory or cardiac failure. Treatment is aimed at relieving muscular spasm. Calcium gluconate 10% (5–10 ml by slow i.v. injection) is effective in depressing the excited neuromuscular junctions. However, specific *Latrodectus* antivenom is available in most endemic areas, and in cases of severe envenomation it should be given intravenously (5 ml) and if necessary repeated. If the victim shows only a mild local reaction and no systemic effects are detectable after 24 h then antivenom should not be given (Sutherland 1978). The possibility of adverse serum reactions although uncommon should be borne in mind and adrenaline and corticosteroids should always be at hand.

The genus *Loxosceles* includes many long-legged spiders occurring throughout Latin America as well as in focal areas elsewhere. The venom is cytotoxic and a bite is accompanied by severe local pain rapidly followed by marked edema, which may progress to necrosis. Treatment is aimed at controlling the local reaction. Parenteral antihistamines have been shown to decrease both the pain and the swelling.

In the Sydney region of Australia, the Sydney funnel web spider, *Atrax robustus*, is the cause of a number of serious spider bites each year. This is a large aggressive spider which rears up before attacking when disturbed. It has a complex venom and with multiple bites being the rule, considerable pain and panic ensue. In cases where systemic envenomation develops, airway obstruction may occur due to muscle spasm, excessive salivation, and vomiting. Loss of consciousness may occur and death can result from respiratory failure.

In management of bites from this spider, atropine and diazepam have proved useful, but repeated doses may have to be given. Encouraging results have been obtained in the development of a funnel web spider venom antagonist.

Bites of the white-tailed spider, *Lampona cylindrata*, are being increasingly recognized in Australia as causing chronic nonhealing skin ulcers (Sutherland 1982).

TICK BITES: TICK PARALYSIS

Ticks are the vectors of a number of human diseases in both tropical and temperate regions. These include the tick bite fevers, certain arbovirus diseases and Lyme disease due to *Borrelia burgdorferi* (Piesman 1987). However, as well as this role in the transmission of infectious diseases, dealt with elsewhere, tick bites may have other unpleasant effects.

Engorging ticks should be encouraged to detach themselves, by applying a lubricant such as liquid paraffin, before gently extracting them. They should never be hastily pulled off, as the tick's mouthparts may be retained in the skin. This may subsequently give rise to a granuloma composed of a dense dermal granulomatous reaction associated with overlying pseudoepitheliomatous hyperplasia, which on occasions may be so marked in biopsy material that it can lead the unwary pathologist to an erroneous diagnosis of squamous carcinoma. On other occasions, the bite may lead to ulceration which is slow to heal. It remains covered by a necrotic, black eschar which takes many days to separate.

Certain ticks of the genera *Ixodes, Dermacentor, Haemaphysalis, Rhipicephalus* and *Hyalomma* produce a neurotoxin in their saliva which may cause 'tick paralysis'. The condition is commoner in children than in adults and particularly tends to afflict girls, probably because their longer hair hides the tick engorging on the scalp or neck, often with little or no local discomfort. A period of irritability occurs several days after the tick has been present. This is followed by ascending symmetrical flaccid paralysis. Initially there is difficulty in walking and standing (Alexander 1984). Within a day or two, paralysis spreads up from the legs to involve the trunk, arms and neck. Bulbar involvement

causes dysphagia, slurring of speech and may result in death from respiratory failure. A local paralysis of the face, for example, may result when the tick is attached to the eardrum. Sensory changes are minimal although there may be paresthesia in the paralyzed limbs. The cerebrospinal fluid remains normal. Mortality may reach 11%, although death is uncommon if the engorging tick is removed (Sutherland 1978). Tick paralysis should be considered in the differential diagnosis of Guillain–Barré syndrome and it can mimic poliomyelitis (Alexander 1984). Rapid and complete recovery usually attends the removal of the offending tick, although sometimes neuroparalysis may become transiently worse after removal of the tick. In Australia a canine antitick antivenom has been used in children with promising results.

Tick bites can also cause a severe life-threatening anaphylactic reaction in sensitized patients.

BEETLES

Two large families of beetles, found in many parts of the world, produce urticating toxins. These are the Staphylinidae (rove beetles) and the Meloidae (blister beetles).

In Africa, and parts of Asia, America and Europe, rove beetle dermatitis due to the genus *Paederus* poses a difficult problem. When the tiny beetles are brushed off the skin, or crushed, an irritant toxic principle, pederin, is released. This causes blistering 1–2 days later. The blisters vesicate in 2–8 days and have a tendency to spread as a result of the release of fluid. Thereafter, the lesions flatten and dry out with subsequent peeling. On occasions the blistering is accompanied by systemic symptoms, with headache, fever, myalgia and arthralgia. A severe conjunctivitis, commonly known as 'Nairobi eye' results if pederin comes into contact with the eyes.

Several genera of Meloidae, including *Lytta* ('Spanish fly'), produce a vesicant, cantharidin, which is falsely credited with aphrodisiac properties, but which is toxic if ingested.

Treatment of dermatitis due to rove or blister beetles relies on the topical application of compresses, such as magnesium sulfate, and eye lesions should be bathed with isotonic saline (Alexander 1984).

The condition termed 'Christmas eye' in Australia is as yet of undetermined origin. It may prove to be due to an orthopteran of some type, but a blister beetle seems more likely.

SCORPION STINGS

Scorpions have a single caudally placed sting with which they can inject venom. Some varieties, such as the genus *Parabuthus*, are dangerous especially to young children. Serious stings are characterized by hypersensitivity and severe pain at the site of the sting, paresthesia and myalgia in the affected limb, quickly followed by generalized weakness, muscle spasm, epigastric pain, excessive salivation and rhinorrhea, excitement, coma, convulsions and respiratory failure, often fatal. Less venomous varieties, or stings in older subjects, result in only local pain and swelling, sometimes with lymphangitis. Nausea, vomiting and headache may also occur, and pancreatitis is a reported complication.

Treatment

In India, it has been noted that scorpion sting in children can have a high mortality rate unless adequate symptomatic and specific therapy are given. Prompt application of a tourniquet will slow the spread of venom. Ice packs applied to the sting site may help to reduce pain and limit local circulation. Scorpion antivenom is available and can be life saving in severe envenomation; 10 ml should be given intramuscularly, as soon as possible, keeping adrenaline and corticosteroids on hand in case of anaphylaxis. When antivenom is not available, general supportive treatment is needed and subcutaneous atropine and intravenous calcium gluconate have been reported to be effective. The need for assisted respiration must be anticipated. In milder stings, immersion of the affected part in very hot water alleviates the pain, but injection of a local anesthetic into the site may be required.

CENTIPEDES

Bites from centipedes can cause considerable pain and swelling, and sometimes local ulceration and spreading lymphangitis result.

CATERPILLARS (LEPIDOPTERISM)

The fine, spiny, venom-containing hairs of some species of caterpillar induce a very painful urticarial or vesicular dermatitis. This may be acquired by actual contact with the larva or from hairs blown in the wind. Where caterpillars are very prolific, severe symptoms may occasionally be induced in children, with extensive rashes, fever, vomiting and even paralysis. Hairs are best removed by applying adhesive tape to the site. Immersion in a very hot bath is soothing, and analgesics may be required. There is little evidence for the development of an allergic response from repeated exposure. Shock syndrome can follow stings from caterpillars of *Megalopyge* and can be treated with subcutaneous 1 : 1000 adrenaline solution twice a day if necessary (Alexander 1984).

STINGS FROM VENOMOUS MARINE ANIMALS

Stings from venomous marine animals can be a major health problem in many parts of the world, including Australia, Papua New Guinea, Southeast Asia, Asia and the Far East, the Mediterranean, North and Latin America, the Caribbean and even Russia. As might be expected, the problem is greatest in tropical waters and its magnitude can be gauged by figures from Australia where, over the summer months of 1990–1991, more that 18 000 people were treated for marine stings (Fenner et al 1995) while in the USA, in Chesapeake Bay alone, about 500 000 jellyfish envenomations occur each year (Fischer 1995).

Although mostly seasonal, the problem of marine stings in the waters of northern Australia is so significant that it often precludes swimming during the summer months, except in areas protected by special nets – termed 'stinger enclosures'.

Overall, the most common cause of jellyfish stings is coelenterates of the genus *Physalia*, the common blue bottle or Portuguese man-of-war. Stings from these animals occur in the water or on the beach and, especially with the short-tentacled species, can be painful for up to an hour or so, but are not usually life threatening (Sutherland 1992b). Stings from the multiple-tentacled species, however, can be severe and rare fatalities are on record (Sutherland 1992b, Fenner et al 1995).

The so-called 'nematocyst dermatitis' from the blue bottle jellyfish is often exacerbated by the tentacles sticking to the skin, with subsequent discharge of the nematocysts causing ongoing pain and discomfort.

Treatment of blue bottle stings consists of gentle washing off of the attached tentacles with water (not vinegar) and then covering the affected area with a plastic bag containing ice and water to alleviate the pain (Sutherland 1992b).

By contrast, stings due to the seawasp or box jellyfish (*Chironex* spp.) are excruciatingly painful and are associated with a significant mortality. Thus stings by this species in northern Australia have resulted in over 300 cases between 1984 and 1994, with in excess of 80 deaths being recorded from these stings this century in Australia – often only minutes after the sting has occurred in the water (Sutherland 1982, Pearn 1995).

The bodies of people stung by this jellyfish are often covered with long red wheals which, if the victim survives, can result in permanent scarring (Sutherland 1992b). Reactions to the sting can, however, in some cases be delayed for some time (Fenner et al 1995). The toxin of this species has three modes of action – it damages the skin, attacks the red blood cells and, most importantly, can affect the heart and respiration (Sutherland 1982, Pearn 1995).

The treatment for *Chironex* stings is the immediate application of vinegar by pouring it liberally over the affected area to prevent further nematocyst discharge. In severe cases, CPR can be life saving (Pearn 1995) and the use of a specific *Chironex fleckeri* antivenom produced by the Commonwealth Serum Laboratories in Melbourne, Australia is beneficial. The recommended dosage should not be reduced for children (Fenner et al 1995).

It is worth reiterating that vinegar is essential to inhibit the discharge of further nematocysts but will not reduce pain and, paradoxically, may initially increase pain. Compression-immobilization bandaging may be helpful (Beadnell et al 1992).

In Australia, a third type of jellyfish sting is the so-called 'Irukandji sting' which is caused by a minute carybdeid jellyfish (*Carukia barnesi*) and which can result in severe joint pains, low back pain, trunk pain, headache, shivering, sweating, hypotension and cardiac involvement (Sutherland 1982, Pearn 1995). Stings usually occur in the water in the afternoon and the jellyfish, being so small, is often not seen.

Treatment for the pain in Irukandji syndrome involves the use of ice packs, and 20 mg i.v. frusemide proved beneficial in one case (Fenner et al 1995). Again the application of vinegar will help prevent further envenomation from undischarged nematocysts (Pearn 1995).

Other jellyfish known to cause stinging of humans include the large carybdeids ('firejellies') in Tomoya or Morbakka stings; the 'hairjelly' or 'sea blubber', *Cyanea*, and *Pelagia noctiluca*, the 'mauve blubber' (Sutherland 1992b, Pearn 1995).

There are, of course, a large number of other potentially dangerous marine animals, including stingrays, the blue ringed octopus, sea urchins, starfish, stonefish and lion fish amongst others. The management of such a diverse range of envenomations is obviously beyond the scope of this chapter, but the topic has been well reviewed by Auerbach (1991) and Pearn (1995).

PRINCIPLES OF ANTIMICROBIAL THERAPY

Of all drugs in the therapeutic armamentarium, few can have had a greater impact than the antimicrobials. The confidence with which the pediatrician may now approach a seriously ill child, affected by almost any infection, is a tribute to their potency and potential. In developed countries few children will pass through childhood without receiving antimicrobial treatment at some stage. Therapeutic successes far outweigh failures, just as beneficial results outweigh harmful effects. As drugs they are held in high medical and public esteem, but this will be maintained only if they are used rationally, through knowledge of the advantages and disadvantages of the many varieties now available. The following general principles are relevant to the use of antimicrobial agents in the treatment and prophylaxis of infection.

CLINICAL DECISION MAKING

When faced with a seriously ill child, the pediatrician will often consider infection in the differential diagnosis. Knowing that rapid deterioration can occur, especially in neonates, empirical antimicrobial therapy will need to be given before information is to hand from bacterial, viral and fungal investigations. Appropriate samples should be taken before beginning chemotherapy to establish the microbial cause of infection but this should not delay treatment. This applies particularly to children less than 1 year of age where the early signs of serious infection are often nonspecific. Where life-threatening infection is present as in meningococcal meningitis/septicemia prompt administration of penicillin by the primary care physician may be life saving. This will not necessarily vitiate later confirmation of the precise microbial diagnosis as polysaccharide meningococcal antigen may be detected immunologically and the polymerase chain reaction (PCR) technique can be used to detect bacterial DNA in the CSF.

When infection is suspected the pediatrician should be in contact with the microbiologist who will be aware of the unique local bacterial ecology and can give invaluable advice.

SITE OF ANTIMICROBIAL ACTION

The site and mode of action determine whether an antimicrobial drug is microbicidal or simply inhibits pathogen replication. When the patient's defense mechanisms are intact this distinction has little clinical relevance as these defense mechanisms will eliminate nonreplicating organisms. However, the selection of cidal or static agents is of great importance when treating infections in immunocompromised patients particularly those with moderate or severe neutropenia or patients with infective endocarditis when bactericidal agents are essential.

There are six principle sites of action for antimicrobials:

1. Cell wall: penicillins, cephalosporins and vancomycin.
2. Cell membrane: polymyxins (colistin) and nystatin.
3. Metabolic processes: sulfonamides and trimethoprim prevent synthesis of folic acid and folinic acid respectively preventing the synthesis of purines required for DNA.
4. Protein synthesis: chloramphenicol acts at the ribosome level; tetracycline confuses transfer RNA and amino acid sequences; lincomycin, erythromycin, fusidic acid and aminoglycosides, e.g. gentamicin and tobramycin, act on protein synthesis.
5. RNA synthesis: rifampicin inhibits.
6. DNA synthesis: nalidixic acid, quinolones, e.g. ciprofloxacin and metronidazole, interfere with DNA synthesis.

PHARMACOKINETICS

The pediatrician must be aware of the pharmacological properties of the drugs available so that the antimicrobial agent chosen will achieve adequate concentration at the site of infection.

Once in the blood, antibiotics vary in their distribution to tissues and body fluids and in their renal handling owing to differences in binding to plasma proteins. There is a reversible equilibrium between bound and unbound drug, but it may be only the unbound portion that is free to diffuse out of the circulation. The size of the molecule, its lipid solubility, the degree of protein binding and the route of elimination determine the penetration of the drug to the site of infection. Lipophilic compounds such as ciprofloxacin penetrate bronchial mucosa and secretions better than β-lactams.

Antibacterial drugs also vary widely in their ability to pass into body fluids other than urine. For example, chloramphenicol levels in the CSF are usually 40–80% of the prevailing blood levels. On the other hand, only traces of the penicillins reach the CSF from the blood if the meninges are healthy; though much larger amounts go through and much higher CSF levels are achieved when the meninges are inflamed, and high concentrations can be achieved by direct intrathecal or intraventricular injection.

The appropriate route of administration will depend on the pharmacokinetics of the drug, the severity of infection and the maturity and clinical state of the child. Antimicrobials given *orally* are absorbed in the stomach and small bowel. Absorption of acid-labile β-lactams can be increased by using enteric-coated formulations which delay drug release until after the stomach or by giving an inactive pro-drug which on hydrolysis with gastric acid releases the active form. With the exception of doxycycline and itraconazole most drugs are best absorbed on an empty stomach.

Parenteral antimicrobial therapy is recommended:

- when speedy delivery of an effective drug concentration at the site of infection is required in a seriously ill patient
- when oral administration is contraindicated by vomiting, ileus or gastrointestinal surgery
- when using aminoglycoside or glycopeptide agents which are not absorbed from the gut.

Topical antimicrobials are only used to treat:

- superficial skin infections
- mucosal candidiasis
- superficial eye and ear infection.

DOSAGE

The dose of antimicrobial agent to be used is based on the pharmacokinetic profile of the drug and the susceptibility of the infecting organism. Where possible, efforts should be made to increase patient compliance by reducing the frequency of drug administration.

The killing effect of aminoglycosides and quinolones is concentration dependent – the higher the concentration the more rapid the bactericidal effect – but is limited by potential toxicity. By contrast, β-lactams (penicillins, cephalosporins) are most effective when the drug concentration is maintained in excess of the minimal inhibitory concentration (MIC) of the infecting organism. This is often best achieved by continuous infusion.

The relationship between the therapeutic concentration of a drug and its toxic concentration is known as the therapeutic index. This is high for penicillins and cephalosporins but much lower in the case of aminoglycosides and amphotericin B where the dose must be calculated using a mg/kg schedule and toxicity monitored clinically and biochemically during treatment. Therapeutic drug monitoring is essential during treatment with these antimicrobials to ensure therapeutic concentrations are attained and toxic levels avoided. This is particularly important in patients with impaired renal function.

The potential benefits of the treatment prescribed are balanced against the toxicity related to the individual patients. In the preterm and newborn infant, liver enzyme immaturity and reduced renal clearance of drugs must be taken into account. On occasion, the pediatrician may be faced with a child with an infection associated with an inborn error of metabolism which may affect the choice of drug. For example, a sulfonamide would produce severe intravascular hemolysis in a child with glucose-6-phosphate dehydrogenase deficiency.

DURATION OF TREATMENT

The duration of treatment depends on the type of infection, the site involved and the response. In uncomplicated infection 5–7 days' treatment will often be more than sufficient but in meningitis particularly due to *Haemophilus influenzae*, osteomyelitis and infection in immunocompromised patients where penetration to the site involved is difficult or the adjuvant effect of the host's immune system is lacking longer courses of treatment are required. While clinical trial evidence has established that 4–6 weeks' treatment for infective endocarditis and 6 months for pulmonary tuberculosis are effective, in many infections the optimal duration of treatment is yet to be defined. In serious infection treatment will often be commenced with parenteral agents followed by a switch to oral therapy after a few days when the patient is clinically stable and apyrexial.

It is reasonable to expect the pediatrician to have some idea of the relative cost of the antimicrobials that are available. If the drugs are of equal efficacy then it is only sensible to use a cheaper one. Many hospitals have a drug and therapeutics committee made up of clinicians, microbiologists and pharmacists who produce a local formulary and policies recommending a limited number of antimicrobials which can be used in routine practice and the most appropriate therapy for specific infections – including dosage and duration.

ANTIMICROBIAL COMBINATIONS

There are three possible results of combining two antimicrobials, namely addition (2 + 2 = 4), synergy (2 + 2 = 5) or antagonism (2 + 2 = 3). These effects can be demonstrated in vitro in the laboratory but clinical demonstration of synergy and antagonism is difficult because of many interacting variables. A possible outcome of a bactericidal/bacteriostatic combination is antagonism.

There are, however, a number of valid reasons for combining antimicrobials, namely:

1. To broaden the antibacterial spectrum particularly if the causal organism is unknown and the initial clinical response is poor.

2. For mixed infections where no single agent is sufficient, e.g. in peritonitis secondary to a perforated viscus where a mixture of aerobic and anaerobic organisms is involved.

3. To produce synergy where the inhibitory effect of the combination is greater than the sum achieved by the individual components, e.g. penicillin and gentamicin in treatment of enterococcal endocarditis, amphotericin B and flucytosine in the treatment of cryptococcal meningitis.

4. To prevent emergence of resistant organisms, e.g. using a combination of three antimicrobials in the treatment of *Mycobacterium tuberculosis* infection minimizes the possibility of drug-resistant strains emerging causing clinical relapse.

5. For unknown causal organisms, e.g. in pyogenic meningitis or septicemia where there are a number of possible causes.

β-lactamase blocking agents have been introduced such as clavulanic acid, sulbactam and tazobactam. These β-lactamase inhibitors are themselves relatively inactive β-lactam antibiotics but are used in combination with susceptible β-lactams (penicillins and cephalosporins) to enhance their spectrum of activity and clinical usefulness.

PROPHYLAXIS AGAINST INFECTION

The possible benefits of using prophylactic antimicrobials have to be balanced against the risks of encouraging the emergence of resistant strains or superinfection with organisms such as *Candida albicans* or *Clostridium difficile* which may become 'opportunist' pathogens particularly if the patient is debilitated or immunologically deficient. Despite this, well-designed, double-blind, controlled trials have shown the advantages of prophylaxis in some surgical procedures and medical conditions where the risk of infection and the sensitivity of the likely organisms is predictable and the consequences of sepsis are serious.

SURGICAL PROPHYLAXIS

It is now established that prophylaxis for selected surgical procedures reduces postoperative infection and is cost effective – colorectal surgery, vascular, neurosurgical and prosthetic implant procedures are examples. The choice of antimicrobial must be appropriate for the contamination that is likely to occur. Thus in colorectal surgery prophylaxis directed against Gram-negative aerobic (broad spectrum cephalosporin or gentamicin) and anaerobic organisms (metronidazole) is appropriate. High doses and short courses are the rule, given intravenously with the premedication or at induction of anesthesia. Single dosing may suffice, otherwise it is seldom necessary to administer antimicrobials for longer than 12–24 h.

MEDICAL PROPHYLAXIS

There are certain situations in which single-dose or short-course prophylaxis is of value:

1. to prevent meningococcal infection in close contacts of patients with meningitis – rifampicin, ceftriaxone
2. to prevent streptococcal/enterococcal bacteremia and infective endocarditis in patients with congenital or rheumatic heart disease or other cardiac conditions – amoxicillin

3. to prevent pertussis or diphtheria infection in exposed unimmunized infants under 1 year of age – erythromycin
4. to prevent tetanus or gas gangrene in an open injury – penicillin.

Long-term 'prophylaxis' is used:
1. to prevent pneumococcal infection following splenectomy or in patients with asplenia, hyposplenism or sickle cell disease – penicillin
2. to prevent recurrence of rheumatic fever – penicillin
3. to prevent renal scarring resulting from recurrent urinary tract infection
4. to prevent infection in immunodeficient patients, e.g. co-trimoxazole for *Pneumocystis carinii*.

ANTIBIOTIC RESISTANCE

Resistance to currently available antimicrobial drugs continues to increase worldwide posing major therapeutic problems.

Mechanisms of resistance:

- The target site for the antibiotic may be lacking or bypassed, i.e. the resistance is intrinsic.
- The antibiotic fails to reach its target site as a result of impaired permeability. In Gram-positive organisms the antibiotic enters the cell by passive diffusion while in Gram-negatives entry is facilitated by protein channels known as porins. Any alteration in the configuration of these porins may affect drug penetration.
- Enzyme inactivation – plasmid or chromosomally mediated β-lactamase enzymes located extracellularly in Gram-positive bacteria or in the periplasmic space of the Gram-negative cell wall can destroy the activity of β-lactam antibiotics (penicillins and cephalosporins).

Extended spectrum β-lactamases have recently been described in Gram-negative organisms such as *Klebsiella*, *Enterobacter* and *Serratia* which render these strains resistant to nearly all established broad spectrum penicillins and cephalosporins.

- Substrate competition – absence or alteration in the penicillin-binding proteins which are the receptor sites for β-lactam antibiotics can result in antibiotic resistance.
- Efflux resistance – tetracycline, macrolides and norfloxacin can be extruded from the cell by an energy-dependent mechanism.

Antibiotic resistance which is genetically acquired can be transferred from one organism to another by transduction, transformation or most importantly by conjugation in which plasmid DNA coding for resistance is transferred, e.g. ampicillin resistance in *Haemophilus influenzae*.

When resistant strains of bacteria are produced by chromosome mutation in the antibiotic-rich environment of hospitals they have a decided selection advantage over their sensitive counterparts. These strains which may show multiple resistance are often involved in outbreaks of cross-infection. When this occurs the use of certain antibiotics may need to be restricted to allow time for the offending plasmids to be lost. There is a need for continuous vigilance and regular monitoring of sensitivity/resistance patterns to prevent the emergence and spread of these strains within hospitals. Patients colonized or infected with these organisms must be isolated.

Changes in antibiotic resistance of many common pathogens which were previously predictably sensitive have necessitated additional sensitivity testing in the microbiology laboratory and major changes in prescribing practice and the management of infection worldwide, e.g. the emergence of penicillin-resistant strains of *S. pneumoniae* demands that pneumococcal meningitis should now be treated with cefotaxime or ceftriaxone pending confirmation of antibiotic sensitivity.

LABORATORY INVESTIGATION – SENSITIVITY AND RESISTANCE

Standardized laboratory antibiotic sensitivity testing distinguishes between bacteria which are susceptible to drug concentrations that are attainable in patients (sensitive) and those which are not (resistant). While such testing can predict bacteriological outcome it cannot predict clinical outcome. Thus intracellular pathogens such as salmonellae which appear sensitive in vitro to a wide range of antibiotics are only eliminated effectively in practice by those such as the quinolones which are concentrated intracellularly. Treatment guidelines should therefore be based on good clinical trial data.

Sometimes it is desirable not just to classify an organism as sensitive or resistant but to determine more precisely the smallest drug concentration that will inhibit or kill it – the minimal inhibitory concentration (MIC) or minimal bactericidal concentration (MBC). Since MIC and MBC values are expressed in numbers (e.g. 0.5 µg/ml or mg/l) they appear more accurate than they are; with some organisms and some antibiotics in particular, they are markedly dependent on inoculum size and precise techniques used. By testing large numbers of strains of a particular organism it is possible to determine the MIC_{90} for a given antibiotic against that species, i.e. the concentration that will inhibit 90% of strains, as a general guide to the selection of suitable treatment. Some organisms are inhibited but not killed by usually bactericidal antibiotics; such tolerance results in a wide difference between the MIC and the MBC. This phenomenon may have important clinical implications, e.g. in the treatment of endocarditis.

MONITORING ANTIMICROBIAL THERAPY

Most antibacterial treatment can be carried out satisfactorily without any monitoring of the levels achieved in blood and other body fluids. This is because, by the time that an antibacterial drug is on the market, the ranges of levels to be expected following recommended dosage schedules have been reliably established. Monitoring may be required, however, when there is wide individual variation in the levels resulting from a standard dose, e.g. in neonates, to determine either that the patient is having enough of the drug for a therapeutic effect to be likely, or that he is not having too much and therefore exposed to unnecessary toxicity. This is true, for example, of gentamicin and related drugs, and for them there is the additional complication of a narrow margin between dosage which is adequate and that which may give toxic levels. For these and many other antibacterial drugs, impaired renal function is one of the most important factors that may invalidate deductions based on results obtained in healthy volunteers, so that it is necessary to check the levels actually achieved in the patient to avoid toxic levels.

Serum levels assayed in the laboratory measure total antimicrobial (protein bound and free) and, provided the MIC for the causal organism is also measured in the presence of serum, it is only necessary to reach this level at the site of infection to achieve a good clinical response. In heart valve infections and other sites where penetration is poor, much higher levels must be aimed for (always within the limits of toxicity). In such cases it may be useful to measure the inhibitory or bactericidal power of the patient's serum against his causal organism. These are termed minimum inhibitory and minimum bactericidal dilutions (MID, MBD) and a four- to eight-fold ratio is aimed for.

ANTIVIRAL DRUGS (see Davey 1990)

Much painstaking research is now yielding the reward of a cohort of antiviral agents which are not unacceptably toxic to the patient despite the viral dependence on host cell metabolic function. They act by arresting or modifying different stages of the viral replicative cycle without destroying the host cell. Interferons have in addition the ability to modulate the immune system. Amantadine and rimantadine interrupt attachment and intracellular coating of influenza A virus but the largest group of antiviral agents are purine or pyrimidine nucleoside analogues which interfere with the biosynthesis of viral nucleic acid – idoxuridine, acyclovir, ganciclovir, ribavirin, vidarabine and zidovudine. Phosphonoformate (foscarnet) is a pyrophosphate analog that inhibits the DNA polymerase of herpes viruses.

As for antibacterial drugs, the same general priciples apply. Pediatricians must consider the spectrum required on a 'best guess' basis or from laboratory data; potential toxicity; cost; dose; route of administration; trial results; special effects; and availability.

Early and accurate diagnosis is important so that treatment can begin before tissue damage is irreversible. For example, amantadine or rimantadine will only be of value if the diagnosis is established as influenza A infection. Hitting the target proteins will only be possible if the viral genes are expressed. During the latent phase of infection, the targets are not revealed and therapy will fail.

The efficacy of antiviral therapy can be monitored by measuring the levels of marker proteins, e.g. p24 protein of HIV, or the viral load by quantitative PCR (polymerase chain reaction) techniques.

Resistance to antiviral drugs is becoming more important clinically. It occurs following treatment with acyclovir for herpes simplex virus, ganciclovir for cytomegalovirus and prolonged therapy with zidovudine for HIV. Combinations of antivirals are increasingly being used to diminish the emergence of resistant mutants and to reduce the toxicity associated with many of the current antiviral agents.

ANTIFUNGAL DRUGS (see Davey 1990)

Deep-seated mycoses are assuming greater importance year by year, especially in patients with underlying disease and immunocompromised hosts. Factors responsible for this new challenge are:

1. use of broad spectrum antibacterials
2. use of long-term catheters and implanted prostheses
3. improvements in neonatal care
4. aggressive anticancer chemotherapy
5. more immunocompromised patients, e.g. AIDS and postsurgical.

If the underlying condition can be ameliorated or the source of infection, e.g. long-term catheter, removed the chances of a successful clinical outcome following antifungal therapy are greatly increased.

The range of antifungal agents is increasing. They differ in mode of action. Griseofulvin inhibits the formation of cellular microtubules, the polyenes (nystatin, amphotericin) act on the sterol content of the cell membrane causing increased permeability and disruption of the cytoplasm, flucytosine is a synthetic pyrimidine analogue which inhibits protein synthesis, and the imidazoles (clotrimazole, miconazole and ketoconazole) and newer triazoles (fluconazole and itraconazole) inhibit ergosterol biosynthesis.

Antifungal susceptibility testing is becoming more readily available and reliable. It can be particularly helpful in detecting the development of resistance during therapy with potential clinical relapse or treatment failure. *Candida albicans* resistance to fluconazole is growing together with an increase in infections due to intrinsically fluconazole-resistant species such as *Candida krusei*.

Amphotericin B treatment is associated with significant toxicity – fever, hypotension and renal impairment with tubular damage. The risk of renal impairment may be reduced by

- giving an initial test dose of 1 mg and increasing to an optimum over 3–5 days
- using one of the new lipid formulations of the drug – AmBisome (liposome), Amphocil (colloidal dispersion) or Abelcet (lipid complex)
- combining amphotericin B and flucytosine – the dose can be lowered and the efficacy of both drugs improved.

Flucytosine is the only drug for which monitoring of serum levels is clinically useful particularly in patients with renal failure – levels in excess of 80 mg/l are associated with marrow toxicity.

Prophylactic use of antifungal agents – oral amphotericin B, nystatin, fluconazole or itraconazole is now being increasingly used to prevent local and systemic infection in immuno-compromised patients.

REFERENCES

Aaby P, Bukh J, Hoff G et al 1986 High measles mortality in infancy related to intensity of exposure. Journal of Pediatrics 109: 40–44
Adal K A, Cockerell C J, Petri W A Jr 1994 Cat scratch disease, bacillary angiomatosis, and other infections due to *Rochalimaea*. New England Journal of Medicine 330: 1509–1515
Adams D H, Bell T M 1976 Slow viruses. Addison-Wesley, London
Addiss D G, Mathews H M, Stewart J M et al 1991 Evaluation of a commercially available enzyme-linked immunosorbent assay for *Giardia lamblia* antigen in stool. Journal of Clinical Microbiology 29(6): 1137–1142
Aickin R, Hill D, Kemp A 1994 Measles immunization in children with allergy to egg. British Medical Journal 309: 223–225
Al-Salihi F, Curran J, Wang J 1974 Neonatal *Trichomonas vaginalis*: report of three cases and review of the literature. Pediatrics 53: 196–200
Alexander G, Williams R 1986 Antiviral treatment in chronic infection with hepatitis B virus. British Medical Journal 292: 915–917

Alexander J O'D 1984 Arthropods and human skin. Springer, Berlin

Alizad A, Ayoub E M, Makki N 1995 Intestinal anthrax in a two-year-old child. Pediatric Infectious Disease Journal 14(5): 394–395

Allday M J, Crawford D H 1988 Role of epithelium in EBV persistence and pathogenesis of B-cell tumours. Lancet 1: 855–857

Allison A C 1988 The role of cell-mediated immune responses in protection against plasmodia and in the pathogenesis of malaria. In: Wernsdorfer W H, McGregor I A (eds) Malaria: the principles and practice of malariology. Churchill Livingstone, Edinburgh, vol I, pp 501–513

Alonso P L, Lindsay S W, Armstrong J R M, Conteh M et al 1991 The effect of insecticide-treated bed nets on mortality of Gambian children. Lancet 337: 1499–1502

Alonso P L, Smith T, Armstrong-Schellenberg J R M A et al 1994 Randomized trial of efficacy of SPf66 vaccine against Plasmodium falciparum malaria in children in Southern Tanzania. Lancet 344: 175–1181

Altman R L, Li K I, Van Horn KG et al 1994 Hip joint infection caused by Shigella sonnei in a one-year old boy. Pediatric Infectious Disease Journal 13: 1156–1158

Alzeer A H, FitzGerald J M 1993 Corticosteroids and tuberculosis: risk and use as adjunct therapy. Tubercle and Lung Disease 74: 6–11

American Academy of Pediatrics 1994 Report of the Committee on Infectious Diseases. American Academy of Pediatrics, Elk Grove Village, Illinois

American Thoracic Society 1994 Treatment of tuberculosis and tuberculosis infection in adults and children. American Journal of Respiratory and Critical Care Medicine 149: 1359–1374

Anand A, Gray E S, Brown T et al 1987 Human parvovirus infection in pregnancy and hydrops fetalis. New England Journal of Medicine 316: 183–186

Anderson D, Thomas T J 1987 Septic arthritis due to Streptobacillus moniliformis. Arthritis and Rheumatism 30: 229–230

Anderson J F 1989 Epizootiology of Borrelia in Ixodes tick vectors and reservoir hosts. Reviews of Infectious Diseases 11(suppl 6): S1451–S1459

Anderson L J 1987 Role of parvovirus B 19 in human disease. Pediatric Infectious Disease Journal 6: 711–718

Anderson R M 1987 Determinants of infection in human schistosomiasis. In: Mahmoud A A F (ed) Baillière's clinical tropical medicine and communicable diseases. Baillière Tindall, London, pp 279–300

Anderson L J, Sikes R K, Langkop C W et al 1980 Postexposure trial of human diploid cell strain rabies vaccine. Journal of Infectious Diseases 142: 133–138

Anderson M J, Jones S E, Fischer-Hoch S P et al 1983 Human parvovirus, the cause of erythema infectiosum (fifth disease). Lancet 1: 1378

Anderson P, Johnston R, Smith D H 1972 Human serum activities against Haemophilus influenzae type b. Journal of Clinical Investigation 51: 31–38

Andrews E B, Yankaskas B C, Cordero J F et al 1992 The Acyclovir in Pregnancy Registry Advisory Committee: acyclovir in pregnancy registry: six years experience. Obstetrics and Gynecology 79: 7–13

Anonymous 1986 Trichinosis outbreak associated with horsemeat. Parasitology Today 2: 295

Aronof S C, Olson M M, Gauderer M W L, Jacobs M R, Blumer J L, Izant R J 1987 Pseudomonas aeruginosa as a primary pathogen in children with bacterial peritonitis. Journal of Pediatric Surgery 22: 861–864

Arslanagic N, Bokonjic M, Macanovic K 1989 Eradication of endemic syphilis in Bosnia. Genitourinary Medicine 65: 4–7

Arvin A M, Johnson R T, Whitley R T et al 1987 Consensus management of the patient with herpes simplex encephalitis. Pediatric Infectious Disease Journal 6: 2–5

Ashford R W, Barnish G 1987 Strongyloidiasis in Papua New Guinea. In: Pawlowski Z S (ed) Baillière's clinical tropical medicine and communicable diseases. Baillière Tindall, London, vol 2.3, pp 765–773

Ashford R W, Barnish G, Viney M E 1992 Strongyloides fuelleborni: infection and disease in Papua New Guinea. Parasitology Today 8: 314–318

Auerbach P S 1991 Marine envenomation. New England Journal of Medicine 325: 486–493

Awadalla N B, Johny M 1990 Urinary tract infection caused by Shigella sonnei: a case report. Annals of Tropical Paediatrics 10: 309–311

Bacon C, Scott D, Jones P 1979 Heatstroke in well wrapped infants. Lancet 1: 422–425

Bahmanyar M, Fayaz A, Nour-Salehi S 1976 et al Successful protection of humans exposed to rabies infection: postexposure treatment with the new diploid cell rabies vaccine and antirabies serum. Journal of the American Medical Association 236: 2751–2754

Bailey J W, Smith D H 1992 The use of the acridine orange QBC (R) technique in the diagnosis of African trypanosomiasis. Transactions of the Royal Society of Tropical Medicine and Hygiene 86: 630

Baker D A 1994 Long-term suppressive therapy with acyclovir for recurrent genital herpes. Journal of International Medical Research 22 (suppl 1): 24A–31A

Baker D M, Nguyen Van Tam J S, Smith S J 1993 Protective efficacy of BCG vaccine against leprosy in southern Malawi. Epidemiology and Infection 111: 21–25

Ball A P, Farrell I D 1979 Problems in human botulism. Journal of Infection 1: 121–125

Ball A P, Hopkinson R B, Farrell I D 1979 Human botulism caused by Clostridium botulinum Type E: the Birmingham outbreak. Quarterly Journal of Medicine 48: 473–491

Baron R C, McCormick J B, Zubeir O A 1983 Ebola virus disease in Southern Sudan: hospital dissemination and intrafamilial spread. Bulletin of the World Health Organization 61: 997–1003

Bass J A W, Wittler R R 1994 Return of epidemic pertussis in the United States. Pediatric Infectious Disease Journal 13: 343–345

Beadnell C E, Rider T A, Williamson J A, Fenner P J 1992 Management of a major box jellyfish sting. Medical Journal of Australia 156: 655–658

Beasley R P, Hwang L-Y, Lee G C-Y et al 1983 Prevention of perinatally transmitted hepatitis B virus infections with hepatitis B immune globulin and hepatitis B vaccine. Lancet 2: 1099–1102

Beck-Sague C, Alexander E R 1987 Sexually-transmitted diseases in children and adolescents. Infectious Disease Clinics of North America 1: 277–304

Becker Y 1978 The chlamydia: molecular biology of procaryotic obligate parasites of eucaryotes. Microbiological Reviews 42: 274–306

Begg N, Nicoll A 1994 Myths in medicine. British Medical Journal 309: 1073–1075

Behnke J M 1987 Do hookworms elicit protective immunity in man? Parasitology Today 3: 200–206

Bell B P, Goldoft M, Griffin P M et al 1994 A multistate outbreak of E. coli 0157: H7–associated bloody diarrhea and hemolytic uremic syndrome from hamburgers. Journal of the American Medical Association 272: 1349–1353

Bell T A, Stamm W E, Wang S P et al 1992 Chronic Chlamydia trachomatis infections in children. Journal of the American Medical Association 267: 400–402

Benson L A, Kar S, McLaughlin G, Ihler G M 1986 Entry of Bartonella bacilliformis into erythrocytes. Infection and Immunity 54: 347–353

Berger P, Pfyffer G E, Nadal D 1996 Treatment of non-tuberculous mycobacterial lymphadenitis with clarithromycin plus rifabutin. Journal of Pediatrics 128: 383–386

Best J E, Banatvala J E, Morgan-Capner P, Miller E 1989 Fetal infection after maternal re-infection with rubella: criterion for defining re-infection. British Medical Journal 299: 773–775

Bhatt K M, Mirza N B 1992 Rat bite fever: a case report of a Kenyan. East African Medical Journal 69: 542–543

Bhutto A M, Nonaka S, Hashiguchi Y, Gomez E A 1994 Histopathological and electron microscopic features of skin lesions in a patient with bartonellosis (verruga peruana). Journal of Dermatology 21: 178–184

Bier J W, Deardorff T L, Jackson G J, Raybourne R B 1987 Human anisakiasis. In: Pawlowski Z S (ed) Baillière's clinical tropical medicine and communicable diseases. Baillière Tindall, London, vol 2.3, pp 723–733

Biggar R J, Woodall J P, Walter P D et al 1975 Lymphocytic choriomeningitis outbreak associated with pet hamsters: fifty-seven cases from New York State. Journal of the American Medical Association 232: 494–498

Birley H, McDonald P, Carey P, Fletcher J 1994 High level ciprofloxacin resistance in Neisseria gonorrhoeae. Genitourinary Medicine 70: 292–293

Bishop R F, Davidson G P, Holmes I H, Ruck B J 1973 Virus particles in epithelial cells of duodenal mucosa from children with acute non-bacterial gastroenteritis. Lancet 2: 1281–1283

Bitar R, Tarpley J 1985 Intestinal perforation in typhoid fever: a historical and state of- the-art review. Reviews of Infectious Diseases 7: 257–271

Bobadilla J-L, Cowley P, Musgrove P, Saxenian H 1994 Design, content and financing of an essential national package of health services. In: Murray C J L, Lopez A D (eds) Global comparative assessments in the health sector. World Health Organization, Geneva, pp 171–192

Boisseau A M, Sarlangue J, Perel Y et al 1992 Perineal ecthyma-gangrenosum in infancy and early childhood: septicaemic and non-septicaemic forms. Journal of the American Academy of Dermatology 27: 415–418

Bomholt A 1988 Juvenile laryngeal papillomatosis: an epidemiological study from the Copenhagen region. Acta Oto-Laryngologica 105: 367–371

Boonpucknavig V, Boonpucknavig S 1988 The histopathology of malaria. In: Wernsdorfer W H, McGregor I A (eds) Malaria. The principles and practice of malariology. Churchill Livingstone, Edinburgh, vol I, pp 673–734

Boos J, Esiri M E 1986 Viral encephalitis. Blackwell, Oxford

Booy R, Hodgson S A, Slack M P E et al 1993 Invasive *Haemophilus-influenzae*-type-b disease in the Oxford region (1985–91). Archives of Disease in Childhood 69: 225–228

Booy R, Hodgson S, Carpenter L et al 1994 Efficacy of *Haemophilus-influenzae* type b conjugate vaccine PRP-T. Lancet 344: 362–366

Borgnolo G, Denku B, Chiabrera F, Hailu B 1993 Louse-borne relapsing fever in Ethiopian children: a clinical study. Annals of Tropical Paediatrics 13: 165–171

Borkowsky W, Rigaud M, Krasinski K et al 1992 Cell mediated and humoral immune responses in children infected with human-immunodeficiency-virus during the first four years of life. Journal of Pediatrics 120: 371–375

Borobio M V, Nogales M C, Palomares J C 1980 Value of serological diagnosis in congenital syphilis: report of nine cases. British Journal of Venereal Diseases 56: 377–380

Bortolussi R, Miller B, Ledwith M, Halperin S 1995 Clinical course of pertussis in immunized children. Pediatric Infectious Disease Journal 14: 870–874

Bowen E T W, Platt G S, Lloyd G et al 1977 Viral-haemorrhagic-fever in southern Sudan and northern Zaire. Lancet 1: 571–573

Bradley D J, Warhurst D C 1995 Malaria prophylaxis: guidelines for travellers from Britain. British Medical Journal 310: 709–714

Bradshaw M W, Schneerson R, Parke J C et al 1971 Bacterial antigens cross-reactive with the capsular polysaccharide of *Haemophilus influenzae* type b. Lancet i: 1095–1096

Brandt C D, Kim H W, Rodriguez W J et al 1985 Adenoviruses and pediatric gastroenteritis. Journal of Infectious Diseases 151: 437–443

Brazilian Purpuric Fever Study Group 1987a *Haemophilus aegyptius* bacteraemia in Brazilian purpuric fever. Lancet ii: 761–763

Brazilian Purpuric Fever Study Group 1987b Brazilian purpuric-fever: epidemic purpura fulminans associated with antecedent purulent conjunctivitis. Lancet ii: 757–761

Brenner D J, Hollis D G, Moss C W, English C K et al 1991 Proposal of *Afipia* gen. nov., with *Afipia felis* sp. nov. (formerly cat scratch disease bacillus), *Afipia clevelandensis* sp. nov. (formerly the Cleveland Clinic Foundation strain), *Afipia broomeae* sp. nov., and three unnamed genospecies. Journal of Clinical Microbiology 29: 2450–2460

British Thoracic Society: Joint Tuberculosis Committee 1998 Chemotherapy and management of tuberculosis in the United Kingdom. Thorax (in press)

British Thoracic Society: Joint Tuberculosis Committee 1994 Control and prevention of tuberculosis in the United Kingdom: code of practice 1994. Thorax 49: 1193–1200

Brown S, Warrnissorm T, Biddle J, Panikabutra K, Traisupa A 1982 Antimicrobial resistance of *Neisseria gonorrhoeae* in Bangkok: is single drug treatment passé? Lancet ii: 1366–1368

Brown S T, Zaidi A, Larsen S A, Reynolds G H 1985 Serological response to syphilis treatment. A new analysis of old data. Journal of the American Medical Association 253: 1296–1299

Brunell P A, Bass J W, Daum R S et al 1985 Prevention of hepatitis B infections. Pediatrics 75: 362–364

Bryceson A D M 1996 Leishmaniasis. In: Weatherall D J, Ledingham J G G, Warrell D A (eds) Oxford textbook of medicine. Oxford Medical Publications, Oxford, vol 1, pp 899–907

Buchdal R M, Taylor P, Warner J O 1985 Nebulised ribavarin for adenovirus pneumonia. Lancet 2: 1070–1071

Buchman T G, Roizman B, Adams G, Stover B H 1978 Restriction endonuclease fingerprinting of herpes simplex virus DNA: a novel epidemiological tool applied to a nosocomial outbreak. Journal of Infectious Diseases 138: 488–498

Burgess I 1991 Malathion lotions for head lice – a less reliable treatment than commonly believed. Pharmaceutical Journal (Nov 9): 630–632

Burgess I 1994 *Sarcoptes scabiei* and scabies. Advances in Parasitology 33: 235–292

Burgess I 1995 Human lice. Advances in Parasitology 36: 271–342

Burgess I, Peock S, Brown C M, Kaufman J 1995 Headlice resistant to pyrethroid insecticides in Britain. British Medical Journal 311: 752

Burgner D, Isaacs D, Givney R 1996 New microbiological diagnostic techniques. Journal of Paediatrics and Child Health 32: 83–85

Burns W H, Saral R, Santos G W et al 1982 Isolation and characterisation of resistant herpes simplex virus after acyclovir therapy. Lancet i: 421–423

Butler J C 1994 Histoplasmosis during childhood. Southern Medical Journal 87: 476–480

Butler T 1983 Plague and other yersinia infections. Plenum, New York, pp 220

Butler T 1985 Relapsing fever: new lessons about antibiotic action. Annals of Internal Medicine 102: 397–399

Butler T, Knight J, Nath S K et al 1985 Typhoid fever complicated by intestinal perforations; a persisting fatal disease requiring surgical management. Review of Infectious Diseases 7: 244–256

Butterworth A E 1987 Potential for vaccines against human schistosomes. In: Mahmoud A A F (ed) Baillière's clinical tropical medicine and communicable diseases. Baillière Tindall, London, vol 2.2, pp 465–483

Butterworth A E 1994 Human immunity to schistosomiasis: some questions. Parasitology Today 10: 378–380

Butterworth A E, Wilkins H A, Capron A, Sher A 1987 The control of schistosomiasis – is a vaccine necessary? Parasitology Today 3: 1–3

Byard R W, Moore L, Bourne A J et al 1992 *Clostridium botulinum* and sudden-infant-death-syndrome: a 10 year prospective study. Journal of Paediatrics and Child Health 28: 156–157

Bygdeman S M 1987 Polyclonal and monoclonal antibodies applied to the epidemiology of gonococcal infection. In: Young H, McMillan A (eds) Immunological diagnosis of sexually transmitted diseases. Marcel Dekker, New York, pp 117–165

Camargo C A, Marshall W H 1987 Radiological diagnosis of cysticercosis. Parasitology Today 3: 30–31

Campbell W C 1988 Trichinosis revisited – another look at modes of transmission. Parasitology Today 4: 83–86

Cantwell M F, Shehab Z M, Costello A M et al 1994 Brief report: congenital tuberculosis. New England Journal of Medicine 330: 1051–1054

Carithers H A, Margileth A M 1991 Cat scratch disease: acute encephalopathy and other neurologic manifestations. American Journal of Diseases of Children 145: 98–101

Carlsson B, Hanson H S, Wasserman J, Brauner A 1991 Evaluation of the fluorescent treponemal antibody-absorption (FTA-Abs) test specificity. Acta Dermato-Venereologica 71: 306–311

Carton C A 1952 Treatment of central nervous system cryptococcosis: a review and report of four cases treated with actidione. Annals of Internal Medicine 37: 123

Casanova J-L, Jovanguy E, Lamhamedi S et al 1995 Immunological conditions of children with BCG disseminated infection. Lancet ii: 581

Casewell M 1989 Control of hospital infection: enhancing present arrangements. British Medical Journal 298: 203–204

Catterall R D 1977 Neurosyphilis. British Journal of Hospital Medicine 17: 585–604

Centers for Disease Control and Prevention (CDC) 1990 Disc diffusion antimicrobial susceptibility testing of *Neisseria gonorrhoeae*. Morbidity and Mortality Weekly Report 39: 167–169

Centers for Disease Control and Prevention (CDC) 1993a Resurgence of pertussis – United States. Morbidity and Mortality Weekly Report 42: 952, 959–953, 960

Centers for Disease Control and Prevention (CDC) 1993b Cases of selected notifiable diseases, United States. Morbidity and Mortality Weekly Report 42: 955–958

Centers for Disease Control and Prevention (CDC) 1993c STD treatment guidelines. Morbidity and Mortality Weekly Report 42: RR–14

Centers for Disease Control and Prevention (CDC) 1994 Revised classification system for human immunodeficiency virus infection in children less than 13 years of age. Morbidity and Mortality Weekly Report 43: RR 12: 1–10

Centers for Disease Control and Prevention (CDC) 1995a Tuberculosis morbidity – United States 1994. Morbidity and Mortality Weekly Report 44: 387–395

Centers for Disease Control and Prevention (CDC) 1995b Revised guidelines for prophylaxis against pneumocystis carinii pneumonia for children infected with or perinatally exposed to human immunodeficiency virus. Morbidity and Mortality Weekly Report 44: RR 4: 1–11

Chance M L 1985 The biochemical and immunological taxonomy of leishmania. In: Chang K P, Bray R S (eds) Human parasitic diseases, Vol. 1 Leishmaniasis. Elsevier, Amsterdam, pp 93–110

Chernesky M, Castriciano S, Sellors J et al 1990 Detection of *Chlamydia trachomatis* antigens in urine as an alternative to swabs and cultures. Journal of Infectious Diseases 161: 124–126

Chernesky M, Lee H, Schachter J et al 1994 Diagnosis of a *Chlamydia trachomatis* urethral infection in symptomatic and asymptomatic men by testing first-void urine in a ligase chain reaction assay. Journal of Infectious Diseases 170: 1308–1311

Cherry J 1993 Acellular pertussis vaccines – a solution to the pertussis problem. Journal of Infectious Diseases 168: 21–24

Chodakewitz J 1995 Ivermectin and lymphatic filariasis: a clinical update. Parasitology Today 11: 233–235

Chongsuphajaisiddhi T 1988 Malaria in pediatric practice. In: Wernsdorfer W, McGregor I A (eds) Malaria. The principles and practice of malariology. Churchill Livingstone, Edinburgh, vol I, pp 889–902

Christie P 1994 Measles in Scotland. Communicable Diseases and Environmental Health in Scotland 28(41): 3–8

Christopherson J 1986 Epidemiology of scabies. Parasitology Today 2: 247–248

Clark I A 1987 Monokines and lymphokines in malarial pathology. Annals of Tropical Medicine and Parasitology 81: 577–585

Clarkson J A, Fine P E M 1985 The efficiency of measles and pertussis notification in England and Wales. International Journal of Epidemiology 14: 153–168

Clay J C 1989 Antenatal screening for syphilis. British Medical Journal 299: 409–410

Cohen B A, Honig P, Androphy E 1990 Anogenital warts in children: clinical and virologic evaluation for sexual abuse. Archives of Dermatology 126: 1575–1580

Colditz G A, Berkey C S, Mosteller F et al 1995 The efficacy of Bacillus Calmette–Guérin vaccination of newborns and infants in the prevention of tuberculosis: meta-analyses of the published literature. Pediatrics 96: 29–35

Collee J G, Duguid J P, Fraser A G, Marmion B P 1989 Mackie and McCartney practical medical microbiology, 13th edn. Churchill Livingstone, Edinburgh, p 872

Colley D G 1987 Dynamics of the human immune response to schistosomes. In: Mahmoud A A F (ed) Baillière's clinical tropical medicine and communicable diseases. Baillière Tindall, London, vol 2.2, pp 315–332

Commens C A 1994 We can get rid of scabies: new treatment available soon. Medical Journal of Australia 160: 317–318

Communicable Disease Surveillance Centre (CDSC) 1991 Enteric fever in England and Wales 1981–90. CDR Review 16: 71

Communicable Disease Surveillance Centre (CDSC) 1994 Invasive Haemophilus influenzae infections: changing patterns. CDR Review 4(48): 227

Communicable Disease Surveillance Centre (CDSC) 1995a The national measles and rubella campaign – one year on. CDR Review 5: 237

Communicable Disease Surveillance Centre (CDSC) 1995b Sexually transmitted diseases, quarterly report: gonorrhoea in England and Wales. CDR Review 5: 61–64

Communicable Disease Surveillance Centre (CDSC) 1995c Sexually transmitted diseases, quarterly report: genital infection with Chlamydia trachomatis. CDR Review 5: 122–123

Congeni B L, Bradley J, Hammerschlag M R 1986 Safety and efficiency of once daily ceftriaxone for the treatment of bacterial meningitis. Pediatric Infectious Disease Journal 5: 293–297

Connor E, Sperling R S, Gelber R et al 1994 Reduction of maternal–infant transmission of HIV type 1 with zidovudine treatment. New England Journal of Medicine 331: 1173–1180

Connor J D, Barrett-Connor E 1967 Infectious diarrhoea. Pediatric Clinics of North America 14: 197–221

Cook G C 1988 Prevention and treatment of malaria. Lancet 1: 32–37

Cook G C 1995 Plague: past and future implications for India. Public Health 109: 7–11

Cook G C 1996 Other spirochaetal diseases. In: Cook G C (ed) Manson's tropical diseases. W B Saunders, London, pp 951–962

Cooper E S, Bundy D 1987 Trichuriasis. In: Pawlowski Z S (ed) Baillière's clinical tropical medicine and communicable diseases. Baillière Tindall, London, vol 2.3, pp 629–643

Cooper E S, Bundy D 1988 Trichuris is not trivial. Parasitology Today 4: 301–306

Corey L, Adams H C, Brown Z A, Holmes K K 1983 Genital herpes simplex infections: clinical manifestations, cause and complications. Annals of Internal Medicine 98: 958–972

Corrall C J, Pepple J M, Moxon E R, Hughes W T 1981 C-reactive protein in spinal fluid of children with meningitis. Journal of Pediatrics 99: 365–369

Coster T S, Killen K P, Waldor M K et al 1995 Safety, immunogenicity and efficacy of live attenuated vibrio cholerae 0139 vaccine prototype. Lancet 345: 949–950

Craig P S, Desham L, Zhaoxun D 1991 Hydatid disease in China. Parasitology Today 7: 46–50

Craven R B, Maupin G O, Beard M L et al 1993 Reported cases of human plague infections in the United States, 1970–1991. Journal of Medical Entomology 30: 758–761

Cree I A, Coghill G, Subedi A M et al 1995 Effects of treatment on histopathology of leprosy. Journal of Clinical Pathology 48: 304–307

Crompton D 1985 Chronic ascariasis and malnutrition. Parasitology Today 1: 47–52

Crompton D 1988 The prevalence of ascariasis. Parasitology Today 4: 162–165

Crompton D H 1989 Hookworm disease: current status and new directions. Parasitology Today 5: 1–2

Cross J H 1987 Public health importance of Angiostrongylus cantonensis and its relatives. Parasitology Today 3: 367–369

Cross J H, Basaca-Sevilla V 1987 Intestinal capillariasis. In: Pawlowski Z S (ed) Baillière's clinical tropical medicine and communicable diseases. Baillière Tindall, London, vol 2.3, pp 735–744

Cross J T, Schutze G E, Jacobs R F 1995 The treatment of tularemia with gentamicin in pediatric patients. Pediatric Infectious Disease Journal 14(2): 151–152

Crumpacker C S, Schnipper L E, Marlowe S I et al 1982 Resistance to antiviral drugs of herpes simplex virus isolated from a patient treated with acyclovir. New England Journal of Medicine 306: 343–346

Cuevas L E, Borgnolo G, Hailu B et al 1995 Tumour necrosis factor, interleukin-6 and C-reactive protein in patients with louse-borne relapsing fever in Ethiopia. Annals of Tropical Medicine and Parasitology 89: 49–54

Cundall D B, Ashelford D J, Pearson S B 1988 BCG immunisation by percutaneous multiple puncture. British Medical Journal 297: 1173–1174

Cupp E W 1992 Treatment of onchocerciasis with ivermectin in Central America. Parasitology Today 8: 212–214

D'Alessandro U, Leach A, Drakely C J, Bennett S et al 1995 Efficacy trial of malaria vaccine SPf66 in Gambian infants. Lancet 346: 462–467

Dagan R, Powell K R, Hall C B, Menegus M A 1985a Identification of infants unlikely to have serious bacterial infection although hospitalized for suspected sepsis. Journal of Pediatrics 107: 855–860

Dagan R, Jenista J A, Prather S L et al 1985b Viremia in hospitalized children with enterovirus infections. Journal of Pediatrics 106: 397–401

Dalakas M C, Elder G, Hallet M et al 1986 A long-term follow up study of patients with post-poliomyelitis neuromuscular symptoms. New England Journal of Medicine 314: 959–963

Dannenberg A M 1989 Immune mechanism in the pathogenesis of pulmonary tuberculosis. Reviews of Infectious Diseases ii(suppl 2): 369–378

Darbyshire J H 1995 Tuberculosis: old reasons for a new increase? British Medical Journal 310: 954–955

Dashefsky B, Teele D W, Klein J O 1983 Unsuspected meningococcemia. Journal of Pediatrics 102: 69–72

Davey P G 1990 New antiviral drugs and antifungal drugs. British Medical Journal 300: 793–798

Davies E G, Elliman D, Hart C A H, Nicoll A, Rudd P T 1995 British Paediatric Association manual of childhood infections. Saunders, London

Dayal R, Bharadwaj V P 1995 Prevention and early detection of leprosy in children. Journal of Tropical Paediatrics 41: 132–138

De Witt T G, Humphrey K F, McCarthy P 1985 Clinical predictors of acute bacterial diarrhoea in young children. Pediatrics 76: 551–556

de-Jong J, Wilkinson R J, Schaeffers P et al 1995 Louse-borne relapsing fever in southern Sudan. Transactions of the Royal Society of Tropical Medicine and Hygiene 89: 621

Delacourt C, Mani T M, Bonnerot V et al 1993 Computed tomography with normal chest radiograph in tuberculous infection. Archives of Disease in Childhood 69: 430–432

Delacourt C, Poveda J-D, Chureau C et al 1995 Use of polymerase chain reaction for improved diagnosis of tuberculosis in children. Journal of Pediatrics 126: 703–709

Dellert S F, Cohen M B 1994 Diarrhoeal disease: established pathogens, new pathogens and progress in vaccine development. Gastroenterology Clinics of North America 23: 637–654

Densen P, Weiler J M, McLeod-Griffiss J, Hoffman L G 1987 Familial properdin deficiency and fatal meningococcemia. New England Journal of Medicine 316: 922–926

Department of Health (DoH) 1988 Public health in England: the report of the committee of enquiry into the future development of the public health function. HMSO, London

Department of Health (DoH) 1996 Immunization against infectious disease. HMSO, London

Department of Health and Social Security (DHSS) 1988 Diagnosis of child sexual abuse: guidance for doctors. HMSO, London

Desenclos J C, Garrity D, Wroten J 1992 Pediatric gonococcal infection, Florida, 1984 to 1988. American Journal of Public Health 82: 426–428

Desmonts G, Forrester F, Thuliez P H 1985 Prenatal diagnosis of congenital toxoplasmosis. Lancet i: 85

Deville J G, Cherry J D, Christenson P D et al 1995 Frequency of unrecognized *Bordetella pertussis* infections in adults. Clinical Infectious Diseases 21: 639–642

Dismukes W E Azole antifungal drugs: old and new. Annals of Internal Medicine 1988 109(3): 177–179

Dodge P R, Davis H, Feigin R et al 1984 Prospective evaluation of hearing impairment as a sequela of acute bacterial meningitis. New England Journal of Medicine 311: 869–874

Dolin P J, Raviglione M C, Kochi A 1994 Global tuberculosis incidence and mortality during 1990–2000. Bulletin of the World Health Organization 72: 213–220

Dominey A, Rosen T, Tschen J 1989 Papulonodular demodicidosis associated with acquired immunodeficiency syndrome. Journal of the American Academy of Dermatology 20: 197–201

Donald P R, Seifart H I 1989 Cerebrospinal fluid concentrations of ethionamide in children with tuberculous meningitis. Journal of Pediatrics 115: 483–486

Donald P R, Schoeman J F, Cotton M F, Van Zyl L E 1991 Cerebrospinal fluid investigations in tuberculous meningitis. Annals of Tropical Paediatrics 11: 241–246

Dooley J R 1980 Haemotropic bacteria in man. Lancet ii: 1237–1239

Dossett J H, Appelbaum P C, Knapp J S, Totten P A 1985 Proctitis associated with *Neisseria cinerea* misidentified as *Neisseria gonorrhoeae* in a child. Journal of Clinical Microbiology 21: 575–577

Drake D P, Holt R J 1976 Childhood actinomycosis: report of three recent cases. Archives of Disease in Childhood 51: 979–981

Dressler F, Whalen J A, Reinhardt B N, Steere A C 1993 Western blotting in the serodiagnosis of Lyme disease. Journal of Infectious Diseases 167: 392–400

Dutt A K, Moers D, Stead W W 1986 Short course chemotherapy for extrapulmonary tuberculosis. Annals of Internal Medicine 104: 7–12

Dwyer D E, Cunningham A L 1993 Herpes simplex virus in pregnancy. Baillière's Clinical Obstetrics and Gynaecology 7: 75–105

Earley A, Richman S, Ansell B M 1988 Pneumococcal arthritis mimicking juvenile chronic arthritis. Archives of Disease in Childhood 63: 1089–1090

Eason R J 1987 Tuberculin sensitivity. Annals of Tropical Paediatrics 7: 87–90

Ebbesen P, Biggar R J, Melbye M (eds) 1984 AIDS: a basic guide for clinicians. Munksgaard, Copenhagen, p 93

Edelman R, Levine M M 1986 Summary of an international workshop on typhoid fever. Reviews of Infectious Diseases 8: 329–349

Edwards K M, Decker M D 1996 Acellular pertussis vaccines for infants. New England Journal of Medicine 334: 391–392

Ellard G A, Humphries M J, Allen B W 1993 Cerebrospinal fluid drug concentrations and the treatment of tuberculous meningitis. American Review of Respiratory Disease 148: 650–655

Engelkens H J, ten Kate F J, Judanarso J et al 1993 The localisation of treponemes and characterisation of the inflammatory infiltrate in skin biopsies from patients with primary or secondary syphilis, or early infectious yaws. Genitourinary Medicine 69: 102–107

Epstein L G, Sharer L R, Oleske J M et al 1986 Neurologic manifestations of human immunodeficiency virus in children. Pediatrics 78: 678–687

Eschenbach D A 1993 Bacterial vaginosis. American Journal of Obstetrics and Gynecology 169(2): 441–445

Estreich S, Forster G E 1992 Sexually transmitted diseases in children: introduction. Genitourinary Medicine 68: 2–8

European Collaborative Study 1988 Mother-to-child transmission of HIV infection. Lancet ii: 1039–1042

European Collaborative Study 1991 Children born to women with HIV-1 infection: natural history and risk of transmission. Lancet 337: 253–260

European Collaborative Study 1994a Natural history of vertically acquired human immunodeficiency virus-1 infection. Pediatrics 94: 815–819

European Collaborative Study 1994b Perinatal findings in children born to HIV infected mothers. British Journal of Obstetrics and Gynaecology 101: 136–141

Farley M M, Stephens D S, Harvey R C et al, and the CDC Meningitis Surveillance Group 1992 Incidence and clinical characteristics of invasive *Haemophilus influenzae* disease in adults. Journal of Infectious Diseases 165(suppl 1): S42–S43

Farrer W E 1995 *Leptospira* species (leptospirosis). In: Mandell G L, Bennet J E, Dolon R (eds) Principles and practice of infectious disease. Churchill Livingstone, Edinburgh, pp 2137–2141

Feder H M, Hunt M S 1995 Pitfalls in the diagnosis and treatment of Lyme disease in children. Journal of the American Medical Association 274: 66–68

Feigin R D, Shackelford P G 1973 Value of repeat lumbar puncture in differential diagnosis of meningitis. New England Journal of Medicine 289: 571–573

Fenner P, Williamson J, Burnett J 1995 Some Australian and international marine envenomation reports.

Ferenczy A, Mitao M, Nagai N et al 1985 Latent papillomavirus and recurring genital warts. New England Journal of Medicine 313: 784–788

Ferguson I R 1991 Leptospirosis update. British Medical Journal 302: 128–129

Field H J, Wildy P 1982 Clinical response of herpes simplex virus to acyclovir. Lancet i: 1125

Fine P E M 1995 Variation in protection by BCG: implications of and for heterologous immunity. Lancet ii: 1339–1345

Fine P E M, Clarkson J A 1987 Reflections on the efficacy of pertussis vaccines. Reviews of Infectious Disease 9: 866

Fine P E M, Ponnighaus J M, Maine N et al 1986 Protective efficacy of BCG against leprosy in northern Malawi. Lancet ii: 499–502

Finlay F O, Witherow A, Rudd P T 1995 Latex agglutination testing in bacterial meningitis. Archives of Disease in Childhood 73: 160–161

Fischer P R 1995 The danger of marine envenomations. Travel Medicine Adviser Update 5: 32–33

Fishbein D B, Robinson L E 1993 Rabies. New England Journal of Medicine 329: 1632–1638

Flockhart H A 1986 *Trichinella* speciation. Parasitology Today 2: 1–2

Florman A L, Spencer R R, Sheward S 1986 Multiple lung cavities in a 12-year-old girl with bubonic plague, sepsis and secondary pneumonia. American Journal of Medicine 80: 1191–1195

Fordham J N, McKay-Ferguson E, Davies A, Blyth A 1992 Rat bite fever without the bite. Annals of Rheumatic Diseases 51: 411–412

Franklin D J, Starke J R, Brady M T et al 1994 Chronic otitis media after tympanotomy tube placement caused by *Mycobacterium abscessus*: a new clinical entity. American Journal of Otology 15: 313–320

Fransen L, Nsanze H, D'Costa L et al 1984 Single dose kanamycin therapy of gonococcal ophthalmia neonatorum. Lancet ii: 1234–1236

Friedland G H, Klein R S 1987 Transmission of the human immunodeficiency virus. New England Journal of Medicine 317: 1125–1135

Fromtling R A (ed) 1987 Recent trends in the discovery, development and evaluation of antifungal agents. J R Prous Science Publishers, SA, pp 125–139

Garcia-Monoco J C, Benach J I 1995 Lyme neuroborreliosis. Annals of Neurology 37: 691–702

Gardner H L, Dukes C D 1955 *Haemophilus vaginalis* vaginitis. American Journal of Obstetrics and Gynecology 69: 962–976

Garner J S 1996 Special report: guidelines for isolation precautions in hospitals. Infection Control and Hospital Epidemiology 17(1): 54–80

Garner J S, Hierholzer W J 1993 Controversies in isolation policies and practices. In: Wenzel R P (ed) Prevention and control of nosocomial infections. Williams & Wilkins, Baltimore

Garnham P C C 1988 Malaria parasites of man: life cycles and morphology (excluding ultrastructure). In: Wernsdorfer W H, McGregor I A (eds) Malaria. The principles and practice of malariology. Churchill Livingstone, Edinburgh, vol I, pp 61–96

Gay N, Miller E 1995 Was a measles epidemic imminent? CDR Review 5: R204–R207

Gemmell M A, Lawson J R, Roberts M G 1987 Towards global control of cystic and alveolar hydatid disease. Parasitology Today 3: 144–151

Gendrel D, Raymond J, Legall M A, Bergeret M, Badoual J 1993 Use of perfloxacin after failure of initial treatment in children with severe salmonellosis. European Journal of Clinical Microbiology and Infectious Diseases 12: 209–211

Genta R M 1986 *Strongyloides stercoralis*: immunobiological considerations on an unusual worm. Parasitology Today 2: 241–246

Genzmer U, Naumann P, Nemes G 1984 Usefulness of commercial culture media for gonococcal diagnosis in general practice: comparative study of various test systems. Hautarzt 35: 517–521

Giles A J H, Lawrence A G 1979 Treatment failure with penicillin in early syphilis. British Journal of Venereal Diseases 55: 62–64

Gill O N, Sockett P N, Bartlett C L R et al 1983 Outbreak of *Salmonella napoli* caused by contaminated chocolate bars. Lancet 2: 544–547

Gillespie S H 1988 The epidemiology of *Toxocara canis*. Parasitology Today 4: 180–182

Gillett J D 1985 The behaviour of *Homo sapiens*, the forgotten factor in the transmission of tropical disease. Transactions of the Royal Society of Tropical Medicine and Hygiene 79: 12–20

Girgis N I, Farid Z, Kilpatrick M E, Sultan Y, Mikhail I A 1991 Dexamethasone adjunctive treatment for tuberculous meningitis. Pediatric Infectious Disease Journal 10: 179–183

Godfrey D G, Baker R D, Rickman L R, Mehlitz D 1990 The distribution, relationship and identification of enzymic variants within the subgenus *Trypanozoon*. Advances in Parasitology 29: 1–74

Goilav C, Zuckerman J, Lafrenz M et al 1995 Immunogenicity and safety of a new activated hepatitis A vaccine in a comparative study. Journal of Medical Virology 46: 287–292

Goldmann D A, Klinger J D 1986 *Pseudomonas cepacia*: biology, mechanisms of virulence, epidemiology. Journal of Pediatrics 108: 806–812

Goldmeier D, Hay P 1993 A review and update on adult syphilis with particular reference to its treatment. International Journal of STD and AIDS 4: 70–82

Goldsmid J M 1985 Unusual arthropod ectoparasitic infestations of man. Australian Family Physician 14: 386–388

Goldsmid J M 1988 The deadly legacy. University of NSW Press, Sydney

Goldsmid J M 1989 The treatment and control of head lice: a review. Australian Journal of Pharmacy 70: 1021–1024

Goldsmid J M 1991 The African hookworm problem: an overview. In: Macpherson C, Craig P (eds) Parasitic helminths and zoonoses in Africa. Unwin & Hyman, London

Goldsmid J M 1995 More than meets the eye: artefacts and pseudoparasites in faeces. Australian Microbiologist 16: 87–89

Goldsmid J M, Pickmere J 1987 Hydatid eradication in Tasmania – point of no return? Australian Family Physician 16: 1672–1674

Goldsmid J M, Rogers S, Parsons G S, Chambers P G 1976 The intestinal protozoa and helminths infecting Africans in the Gatooma region of Rhodesia. Central African Journal of Medicine 22: 91–95

Goldsmid J M, Langley J, Naylor P, Bashford P 1989 Further studies on head lice and their control in Tasmania. Australian Family Physician 18: 253–255

Gordon F B, Harper I A, Quan A L, Treharne J D, Dwyer R St C, Garland J A 1969 Detection of Chlamydia (Bedsonia) in certain infections of man. 1 Laboratory procedures: Comparison of yolk sac and cell culture for detection and isolation. Journal of Infectious Diseases 120: 451–462

Gould I M 1987 *Pseudomonas aeruginosa*: its clinical importance. Intensive and Critical Care Digest 6: 9–11

Goutzamanis J J, Gilbert G L 1995 *Mycobacterium ulcerans* infection in Australian children: report of eight cases and review. Clinical Infectious Disease 21: 1186–1192

Graber W K, Sanford J P, Ziff M 1960 Sex incidence of gonococcal arthritis. Arthritis and Rheumatism 3: 309–313

Grandien M, Olding-Stenkvist E 1984 Rapid diagnosis of viral infections in the central nervous system. Scandinavian Journal of Infectious Diseases 16: 1–8

Grange J M 1988 Mycobacteria and human disease. Edward Arnold, London

Grant J P 1988 The state of the world's children. Oxford University Press, Oxford

Gray B M, Dillon H C 1989 Natural history of pneumococcal infections. Pediatric Infectious Disease Journal 8(1) (suppl): S23–S25

Graybill J R 1988 The long and the short of antifungal therapy. Infectious Disease Clinics of North America 2(4): 805–825

Graybill J R 1993 Treatment of coccidioidomycosis. Current Topics in Medical Mycology 5: 151–179

Grayston J T, Kuo C-C, Wang S-P, Altman J 1986 A new *Chlamydia psittaci* strain, TWAR, isolated in acute respiratory infections. New England Journal of Medicine 315: 161–168

Greenwood B M, Whittle H C 1980 The pathogenesis of sleeping sickness. Transactions of the Royal Society of Tropical Medicine and Hygiene 74: 716–725

Grenfell B T, Anderson R M 1989 Pertussis in England & Wales: an investigation of transmission dynamics and control by mass. Proceedings of the Royal Society 236: 213–250

Greyseels B 1994 Human resistance to schistosome infections. Parasitology Today 10: 380–384

Griffiths R I, Anderson G F, Powe N R et al 1995 Economic impact of immunizing against rotavirus gastroenteritis: evidence from a clinical trial. Archives of Pediatrics and Adolescent Medicine 149: 407–414

Grundmann H, Kropec A, Hartung D et al 1993 *Pseudomonas aeruginosa* in a neonatal intensive care unit: reservoirs and ecology of the nosocomial pathogen. Journal of Infectious Diseases 168: 943–947

Grundy J E, Shanley J D, Griffith P D 1987 Is cytomegalovirus interstitial pneumonitis in transplant recipients an immunopathological condition? Lancet 2: 996–999

Gupta A 1994 Multidrug-resistant typhoid fever in children: epidemiology and the therapeutic approach. Pediatric Infectious Disease Journal 13: 134–140

Gustafsson L L, Beerman B, Abdi Y A 1987 Handbook of drugs for tropical parasitic infections. Taylor and Francis, London

Gutman L T, Moye J, Zimmer B, Tian C 1994 Tuberculosis in human immunodeficiency virus exposed or infected United States children. Pediatric Infectious Disease Journal 13: 963–968

Hackett C J 1951 Bone lesions of yaws in Uganda. Blackwell Scientific Publications, Oxford

Hackett C J 1957 An international nomenclature of yaws lesions. World Health Organization, Geneva

Hagan P, Williams H A 1993 Concomitant immunity in schistosomiasis. Parasitology Today 9: 1–6

Hale Y M, Melton M E, Lewis J S, Willis D E 1993 Evaluation of the PACE 2 *Neisseria gonorrhoeae* assay by three public health laboratories. Journal of Clinical Microbiology 31: 451–453

Haley R W, Culver D H, White J W et al 1985 The efficacy of infection surveillance and control programs in preventing nosocomial infection in US hospitals. American Journal of Epidemiology 121: 181–205

Hall C B, Powell K R, McDonald N E et al 1986 Respiratory syncytial virus infection in children with compromised immune function. New England Journal of Medicine 315: 77–80

Hall M, Wall R 1995 Myiasis of humans and domestic animals. Advances in Parasitology 35: 257–334

Hall S M, Glickman M 1988 The British Paediatric Surveillance Unit. Archives of Disease in Childhood 63: 344–346

Halstead S B 1980 Dengue haemorrhagic fever: a public health problem and a field for research. Bulletin of the World Health Organization 58: 1

Handley J, Dinsmore W, Maw R 1993 Anogenital warts in prepubertal children; sexual abuse or not? International Journal of STD and AIDS 4: 271–279

Hanngren K, Grandien M, Granstrom G 1985 Effect of zoster immunoglobulin for varicella prophylaxis in the newborn. Scandinavian Journal of Infectious Diseases 17: 343–347

Hanshaw J B, Dudgeon J A 1978 Viral diseases of the fetus and newborn. In: Schaffer A J, Markowitz M (eds) Major problems in clinical pediatrics. Saunders, Philadelphia, pp 153–181

Harinasuta T, Bunnag D 1988 The clinical features of malaria. In: Wernsdorfer W H, McGregor I A (eds) Malaria. The principles and practice of malariology. Churchill Livingstone, Edinburgh, vol I, pp 709–734

Harinasuta T, Bunnag D, Radomyos P 1987 Intestinal flukes. In: Pawlowski Z S (ed) Baillière's clinical tropical medicine and communicable disease. Baillière Tindall, London, vol 2.3, pp 695–721

Hastings R C 1985 Leprosy. Churchill Livingstone, Edinburgh, p 331

Haswell-Elkins M R, Sithithaworn P, Elkins D 1992 *Opisthorchis viverrini* and cholangiocarcinoma in northwest Thailand. Parasitology Today 8: 86–89

Hay P E, Morgan D J, Ison C A et al 1994 A longitudinal study of bacterial vaginosis during pregnancy. British Journal of Obstetrics and Gynaecology 101: 1048–1053

He Q, Mertsola J, Soini H, Viljanen M K 1994 Sensitive and specific polymerase chain reaction assays for detection of *Bordetella pertussis* in nasopharyngeal specimens. Journal of Pediatrics 124: 421–426

Heatwole H 1987 Seasnakes. University of NSW Press, Sydney

Heritage J, Hawkey P M 1988 Tetracycline-resistant *Neisseria gonorrhoeae*. Journal of Antimicrobial Chemotherapy 22: 575–579

Hicks R V, Melish M E 1986 Kawasaki syndrome. Pediatric Clinics of North America 33: 1151–1175

Hien T T, Bethell D B, Hoa N T T et al 1995 Short course of cefloxacin for treatment of multidrug-resistant typhoid. Clinical Infectious Disease 20: 917–923

Hightower A W, Lamine P J, Eberhard M C 1993 Maternal filarial infections – a persistent risk factor for microfilaraemia in offspring? Parasitology Today 9: 418–429

Hildick-Smith G, Blank H, Sarkany I 1964 Fungus diseases and their treatment. Little Brown, Boston, p 334

Hira S K, Hira R S 1984 Parotitis with secondary syphilis. A case report. British Journal of Venereal Diseases 60: 121–122

Hira S K, Bhat G J, Patel J B et al 1985 Early congenital syphilis: clinico-radiologic features in 202 patients. Sexually Transmitted Diseases 12: 177–183

Ho M S, Glass R I, Pinsky P F et al 1988 Diarrhoeal deaths in American children. Journal of the American Medical Association 260: 3281–3285

Hoare C A, Wallace F G 1966 Developmental stages of trypanosomatid flagellates: a new terminology. Nature 212: 1385–1386

Hockmeyer W T, Ballou W P 1988 Sporozoite immunity and vaccine development. Progress in Allergy 41: 1–14

Holland E F, O'Mahony C P 1989 Is it time to review antenatal screening for syphilis? British Journal of Obstetrics and Gynaecology 96: 1005–1006

Hollander H 1988 Cerebrospinal fluid normalities and abnormalities in individuals infected with human immunodeficiency virus. Journal of Infectious Diseases 158: 855–858

Holliman R E 1988 Toxoplasmosis and the acquired immune-deficiency syndrome. Journal of Infection 16: 121–128

Hoppe J E, Haug A 1988 Treatment and prevention of pertussis by antimicrobial agents (Part II). Infection 16: 148–152

Hotez P J, Le Trang N, Cerami A 1987 Hookworm antigens: a potential for vaccination. Parasitology Today 3: 247–249

Hugo-Hamman C T, Scher H, De Moor M M A 1994 Tuberculous pericarditis in children: a review of 44 cases. Pediatric Infectious Disease Journal 13: 13–18

Hull H F, Ward N A, Hull B F et al 1994 Paralytic poliomyelitis: seasoned strategies, disappearing disease. Lancet 343: 1331–1337

Human R P, Jones G A 1986 Survival of bacteria in swab transport packs. Medical Laboratory Sciences 43: 14–18

Humphries M 1992 The management of tuberculous meningitis. Thorax 47: 577–581

Humphries M J, Teoh R, Lau J, Gabriel M 1990 Factors of prognostic significance in Chinese children with tuberculous meningitis. Tubercle 71: 161–168

Hungerford T G 1977 Hazards from domestic pets. Australian Family Physician 6: 1503–1507

Hunter E F, Russell H, Farshy C E et al 1986 Evaluation of sera from patients with Lyme disease in the fluorescent treponemal antibody-absorption test for syphilis. Sexually Transmitted Diseases 13: 232–236

Huskins W C, Griffiths J K, Faruque A S G, Bennish M L 1994 Shigellosis in neonates and young infants. Journal of Pediatrics 125: 14–22

Hussey G, Chisholm T, Kibel M 1991 Miliary tuberculosis in children: a review of 94 cases. Pediatric Infectious Disease Journal 10: 832–836

Ijsselmuiden O E, van der Sluis J J, Mulder A et al 1989 An IgM capture enzyme linked immunosorbent assay to detect IgM antibodies to treponemes in patients with syphilis. Genitourinary Medicine 65: 79–83

Isaacs D, Flowers D, Clarke J R et al 1983 Epidemiology of coronavirus respiratory infections. Archives of Disease in Childhood 58: 500–503

Isaacs D, Day D, Crook S 1986 Childhood gastroenteritis: a population study. British Medical Journal 293: 545–546

Isaacs D, Moxon E R, Harvey D et al 1988 Ribavirin in respiratory syncytial virus infection. Archives of Disease in Childhood 63: 986–990

Isenberg S J, Apt L, Wood M 1995 A controlled trial of povidone-iodine as prophylaxis against ophthalmia neonatorum. New England Journal of Medicine 332: 562–566

Ish-Horowicz M, Korman S H, Shapiro M et al 1989 Asymptomatic giardiasis in children. Pediatric Infectious Disease Journal 8: 773–779

Italian Register for HIV Infection in Children 1994 Features of children perinatally infected with HIV-1 surviving longer than 5 years. Lancet 343: 191–195

Ito A 1992 Cysticercosis in the Asian-Pacific regions. Parasitology Today 8: 182–183

Ivanoff B, Levine M M, Lambert P H 1994 Vaccination against typhoid fever: present status. Bulletin of the World Health Organization 72: 957–971

Jacobs R F, Condrey Y M, Yamauchi T 1985 Tularemia in adults and children: a changing presentation. Pediatrics 76: 818–822

Jacobs R F, Sunakorn P, Chotpitayasunonah T, Pope S, Kelleher K 1992 Intensive short course chemotherapy for tuberculous meningitis. Pediatric Infectious Disease Journal 11: 194–198

Jadavji T, Biggar W D, Gold R, Prober C G 1986 Sequelae of acute bacterial meningitis in children treated for seven days. Pediatrics 78: 21–25

Jakeman P, Smith W C 1994 Evaluation of a multidrug therapy programme of leprosy control. Leprosy Review 65: 289–296

James S L, Gilles H M 1985 Human antiparasitic drugs. Wiley, Chichester

James S L, Sher A 1986 Prospects for a non-living vaccine against schistosomiasis. Parasitology Today 2: 134–137

Janssens P G 1985 Chemotherapy of gastrointestinal nematodiasis in man. In: Vanden Bossche H, Thienpont D, Janssens P G (eds) Chemotherapy of gastrointestinal helminths. Springer, Berlin, pp 183–406

Jaroonvesama N 1988 Differential diagnosis of eosinophilic meningitis. Parasitology Today 4: 262–266

Jawahar M S, Sivasubramanian S, Vijayan V K et al 1990 Short course therapy for tuberculous lymphadenitis in children. British Medical Journal 301: 359–362

Jenista J A, Powell K L, Menegus M A 1984 Epidemiology of neonatal enterovirus infection. Journal of Pediatrics 104: 685–690

Jenkinson D 1988 Duration of effectiveness of pertussis vaccine: evidence from a 10 year community study. British Medical Journal 296: 612–614

Ji B, Jamet P, Perani E G et al 1993 Powerful bactericidal activities of clarithromycin and minocycline against Mycobacterium leprae in lepromatous leprosy. Journal of Infectious Disease 168: 188–190

Joesoef M R, Schmid G P 1995 Bacterial vaginosis: review of treatment options and potential clinical indications for therapy. Clinical Infectious Disease 20(suppl 1): S72–S79

Joint Committee on Vaccination and Immunization 1981 The whooping cough epidemic 1977–79. In: Whooping cough: Report from the Committee on Safety of Medicines and the Joint Committee on Vaccination and Immunization. HMSO, London, pp 170–184

Jones C A, Isaacs D 1996 Human herpesvirus-6 infection. Archives of Disease in Childhood 74: 98–100

Jones R N, Gavan T L, Thornsberry C et al 1989 Standardization of disc diffusion and agar dilution susceptibility tests for Neisseria gonorrhoeae: interpretative criteria and quality control guidelines for ceftriaxone, penicillin, spectinomycin and tetracycline. Journal of Clinical Microbiology 27: 2758–2766

Jopling W H, McDougall A C 1989 Handbook of leprosy. Heinemann, Oxford, p 180

Joshi V V, Kauffman S, Oleske J M et al 1987 Polyclonal polymorphic B-cell lymphoproliferative disorder with prominent pulmonary involvement in children with acquired immune deficiency syndrome. Cancer 59: 1455–1462

Journal of Clinical Pathology 1989 Annotation. Diagnosis of toxoplasmosis. Journal of Clinical Pathology 42: 191

Kabra S K, Jain Y, Seth V 1994 Plague – clinical features and management. Indian Journal of Paediatrics 61: 619–623

Kakos G S, Kilman J W 1973 Symptomatic histoplasmosis in children. Annals of Thoracic Surgery 15: 622

Kammerer W S 1985 Chemotherapy of tapeworm infections in man. In: Vanden Bossche H, Thienpont D, Janssens P G (eds) Chemotherapy of gastrointestinal helminths. Springer, Berlin

Kant S, Nath L M 1994 Control and presentation of human plague. Indian Journal of Paediatrics 61: 629–633

Kaplan E L 1988 The rapid identification of Group A beta-haemolytic streptococci in the upper respiratory tract. Pediatric Clinics of North America 35(3): 535–542

Kaplan E L, Hill H R 1987 Return of rheumatic fever: consequences, implications and needs. Journal of Pediatrics 111: 244–246

Kaplan M H, Klein S W, McPhee J, Harper R G 1983 Group B coxsackie virus infections in infants younger than three months of age: a serious childhood illness. Reviews of Infectious Diseases 5: 1019–1032

Kauppi M, Saarinen L, Kayhty H 1993 Anti-capsular polysaccharide antibodies reduce nasopharyngeal colonization by Haemophilus influenzae type b in infant rats. Journal of Infectious Diseases 167(2): 365–371

Kelly J 1988 Genital herpes during pregnancy: routine virological screening is futile. British Medical Journal 297: 1146–1147

Keusch G T, Bennish M L 1989 Shigellosis: recent progress, persisting problems and research issues. Pediatric Infectious Disease Journal 8: 713–719

Kim M-H M, Mindorff C, Patrick M L et al 1987 Isolation usage in a pediatric hospital. Infection Control 8: 195–199

Kingsbury D T, Weiss E 1968 Lack of deoxyribonucleic acid homology between species of the genus Chlamydia. Journal of Bacteriology 96: 1421–1423

Kirsztaju G M, Nishida S K, Silva M D et al 1993 Renal abnormalities in leprosy. Nephron 65: 381–384

Kishore B N, Shetty J N 1995 Bacterial clearance with WHO-recommended multidrug regimen for multibacillary leprosy. Indian Journal of Leprosy 67: 301–308

Knapp J S, Brathwaite A R, Hinds A et al 1995 Plasmid-mediated antimicrobial resistance in Neisseria gonorrhoeae in Kingston, Jamaica 1990–1991. Sexually Transmitted Diseases 22: 155–159

Köberle F 1974 Pathogenesis of Chagas' disease. In: Elliott K, O'Connor M, Wolstenholme G E W (eds) Trypanosomiasis and leishmaniasis. Ciba foundation Symposium 20 (new series). Elsevier, Excerpta Medica, North Holland, Amsterdam, pp 137–152

Kociecka W 1987a Intestinal cestodiasis. In: Pawlowski Z S (ed) Baillière's clinical tropical medicine and communicable diseases. Baillière Tindall, London, vol 2.3, pp 677–694

Kociecka W 1987b Intestinal trichinellosis. In: Pawlowski Z S (ed) Baillière's clinical tropical medicine and communicable diseases. Baillière Tindall, London, vol 2.3, pp 755–763

Konstantopoulos K, Skarpas P, Hitjazis F et al 1992 Rat bite fever in a Greek child. Scandinavian Journal of Infectious Diseases 24: 531–533

Koplan J P, Benfari Ferraro M J, Fineberg H V, Rosenberg M L 1980 Value of stool cultures. Lancet ii: 413–416

Krabbe S, Hesse J, Uldall P 1981 Primary Epstein–Barr virus infection in early childhood. Archives of Disease in Childhood 56: 49–52

Kreger-van Rij N J W (ed) 1984 The yeasts: a taxonomic study. Elsevier, Amsterdam

Kroger L, Korppi M, Brander E et al 1995 Osteitis caused by Bacille Calmette–Guérin vaccination: a retrospective analysis of 222 cases. Journal of Infectious Diseases 172: 574–576

Krugman S, Ward R 1968 Infectious diseases of children. Mosby, St Louis

Krugman S, Ward R 1996 Infectious diseases of children. C V Mosby, St Louis

Kubin R 1993 Safety and efficacy of ciprofloxacin in paediatric patients – review. Infection 21: 413–421

Kuntze J R, Weinberg A C, Ahlering T E 1985 Hyperammonaemic coma due to proteus infection. Journal of Urology 134: 972–973

Kurtzman G J, Cohen B, Meyers P et al 1988 Persistent B19 parvovirus infection as a cause of severe chronic anaemia in children with ALL. Lancet 2: 1159–1162

Lackritz E M, Campbell C C, Ruebush T K II et al 1992 Effect of blood transfusion on survival among children in a Kenya hospital. Lancet 340: 524–528

LaForce F M 1994 Anthrax. Clinical Infectious Diseases 19: 1009–1014

Lainson R, Shaw J J 1979 The role of animals in the epidemiology of South American leishmaniasis. In: Lumsden W H R, Evans D A (eds) The biology of the Kinetoplastida. Academic Press, London, vol 2, pp 1–116

Lainson R, Shaw J J 1987 Evolution classification and geographical distribution. In: Peters W, Killick-Kendrick R (eds) The leishmaniases in biology and medicine, biology and epidemiology. Academic Press, London, vol 1, pp 1–20

Lancet Editorial 1977 Routine tests for syphilis on cerebrospinal fluid. Lancet ii: 340–341

Lancet Editorial 1980 Chagas' disease: potential for immunoprophylaxis. Lancet i: 466

Lancet Editorial 1983 Human papillomaviruses and neoplasia. Lancet ii: 435–436

Lancet Editorial 1984 New tuberculins. Lancet i: 199–200

Lancet Editorial 1985 EBV and persistent malaise. Lancet i: 1017–1018

Lancet Editorial 1986a Enervating illness and Epstein–Barr virus. Lancet ii: 141–142

Lancet Editorial 1986b Reinfection with influenza. Lancet 372: 374

Lancet Editorial 1987a Ill-treatment of children. Lancet i: 367–368

Lancet Editorial 1987b Immunity to schistosomiasis. Lancet i: 1015–1016

Lancet Editorial 1988 Chemotherapy of leprosy. Lancet ii: 487–488

Lancet Editorial 1989a Herpes simplex virus latency. Lancet i: 194–195

Lancet Editorial 1989b Will the real hepatitis C stand up. Lancet ii: 307–308

Lancet Editorial 1989c Ascariasis. Lancet i: 997–998

Lancet Editorial 1990a Perinatal prophylaxis of tuberculosis. Lancet ii: 1479–1480

Lancet Editorial 1990b The A to F of viral hepatitis. Lancet 336: 1158–1160

Lawande R V 1980 The seasonal incidence of primary amoebic meningoencephalitis in northern Nigeria. Transactions of the Royal Society of Tropical Medicine and Hygiene 74: 141–142

Lebel M H, Freij B J, Syrogiannopoulos G A 1988 Dexamethasone therapy for bacterial meningitis: results of two double-blind, placebo controlled trials. New England Journal of Medicine 319: 964–971

Lefevre J C, Bertrand M A, Bauriaud R 1990 Evaluation of the Captia enzyme immunoassays for detection of immunoglobulins G and M to Treponema pallidum in syphilis. Journal of Clinical Microbiology 28: 1704–1707

Leonardi G P, Seitz M, Edstrom R et al 1992 Evaluation of three immunoassays for detection of Chlamydia trachomatis in urine specimens from asymptomatic males. Journal of Clinical Microbiology 30: 2793–2796

Leung D Y M, Meissner H C, Fulton D R et al 1993 Toxic shock syndrome-toxin secreting Staphylococcus aureus in Kawasaki syndrome. Lancet 342: 1385–1388

Lever A M L, Webster A D B, Brown D, Thomas H C 1984 Non-A, non-B hepatitis occurring in agammaglobulinaemic patients after intravenous immunoglobulin. Lancet 2: 1062–1064

Levin M, Kay J D S, Gould J D et al 1983 Haemorrhagic shock and encephalopathy: a new syndrome with a high mortality in children. Lancet ii: 64–67

Levin M, Newport M J, D'Souza S et al 1995 Familial disseminated atypical mycobacterial infection in childhood: a human mycobacterial susceptibility gene? Lancet i: 79–83

Lewinsohn R 1979 The discovery of Trypanosoma cruzi and of American trypanosomiasis. Transactions of the Royal Society of Tropical Medicine and Hygiene 73: 513–523

Lewis D A, Ison C A, Livermore D M et al 1995a A one-year survey of Neisseria gonorrhoeae isolated from patients attending an east London genitourinary medicine clinic: antibiotic susceptibility patterns and patients' characteristics. Genitourinary Medicine 71: 13–17

Lewis D A, Forster G E, Goh B T 1995b The falling accuracy of microscopy in the diagnosis of gonorrhoea – a cause for concern? Genitourinary Medicine 71: 136

Lewis L L, Taber L H, Baughn R E1990 Evaluation of immunoglobulin M western blot analysis in the diagnosis of congenital syphilis. Journal of Clinical Microbiology 28: 296–302

Lincoln E M, Gilbert L A 1972 Disease in children due to mycobacteria other than Mycobacterium tuberculosis. American Review of Respiratory Disease 105: 685–714

Linnemann C C, Light I J, Buchman T G et al 1978 Transmission of herpes simplex virus Type 1 in a nursery for the newborn. Identification of viral isolates by DNA 'fingerprinting'. Lancet i: 964–969

Lister P D 1995 Multiply-resistant pneumococcus: therapeutic problems in the management of serious infections. European Journal of Clinical Microbiology and Infectious Diseases 14(suppl 1): 18–25

Lonsdale D M 1979 A rapid technique for distinguishing herpes-simplex virus Type 1 from Type 2 by restriction-enzyme technology. Lancet i: 849–852

Lubani M M, Dudin K I, Sharda D C et al 1989 A multicenter therapeutic study of 1100 children with brucellosis. Pediatric Infectious Disease Journal 8: 75–78

Lucius R, Frosch M, Kern P 1995 Alveolar echinococcosis: immunogenics and epidemiology. Parasitology Today 11: 4–5

Luger A F H 1988 Serological diagnosis of syphilis: current methods. In: Young H, McMillan A (eds) Immunological diagnosis of sexually transmitted diseases. Marcel Dekker, New York, pp 249–274

Luger A, Marhold I, Schmidt B L 1988 Laboratory support in the diagnosis of neurosyphilis. WHO/VDT/RES/88.379. World Health Organization, Geneva

Lukehart S A 1991 Serologic testing after therapy for syphilis: is there a test for cure? Annals of Internal Medicine 114: 1057–1058

Lukehart S A, Hook E W, Baker-Zander S A et al 1988 Invasion of the central nervous system by Treponema pallidum: implications for diagnosis and treatment. Annals of Internal Medicine 109: 855–862

Lumsden W H R, Kimber C D, Evans D A, Doig S J 1979 Trypanosoma brucei: miniature anion-exchange centrifugation technique for detection of low parasitaemias: adaptation for field use. Transactions of the Royal Society of Tropical Medicine and Hygiene 73: 312–317

Lung M L, Lam W-K, So S Y et al 1985 Evidence that respiratory tract is major reservoir for Epstein–Barr virus. Lancet 1: 889–892

Luo C, Chintu C, Bhat G et al 1994 Human immunodeficiency virus type-1 infection in Zambian children with tuberculosis: changing seroprevalence and evaluation of a thiacetazone-free regimen. Tubercle and Lung Disease 75: 110–115

Ma P, Visvesvara G S, Martinez A J et al 1990 Naegleria and Acanthamoeba infections: review. Review of Infectious Diseases 12: 490–513

McCance D J, Walker P G, Dyson J L et al 1983 Presence of human papillomavirus DNA sequences in cervical intraepithelial neoplasia. British Medical Journal 287: 784–788

McClean K L 1995 An outbreak of plague in northwestern province, Zambia. Clinical Infectious Diseases 21: 650–652

McCormick A, Hall S 1995 Infectious disease in childhood. In: Botting B (ed) Office of Population Censuses and Surveys: the health of our children. (Decennial Supplement) Series DS, No 11. HMSO, London, pp 168–176

McCormick J B, Bauer S P, Elliott L H et al 1983 Biologic differences between strains of Ebola virus from Zaire and Sudan. Journal of Infectious Diseases 147: 264–267

McCormick J B, King I J, Webb P A et al 1986 Lassa fever. Effective therapy with ribavirin. New England Journal of Medicine 314: 20–26

MacDonald N E, Hall C B, Suffin S C et al 1982 Respiratory syncytial virus infection in infants with congenital heart disease. New England Journal of Medicine 307: 397–400

Macfarlane J T, Macrae A D 1983 Psittacosis. British Medical Bulletin 39: 163–167

Macfarlane D J, Tucker L G, Kemp R J et al 1993 Treatment of recalcitrant actinomycosis with ciprofloxacin. Journal of Infection 27: 177–180

McGregor I A, Wilson R J M 1988 Specific immunity acquired in man. In: Wernsdorfer W H, McGregor I A (eds) Malaria. The principles and practice of malariology. Churchill Livingstone, Edinburgh, vol I, pp 559–619

McGregor J A, French J I, Parker R et al 1995 Prevention of premature birth by screening and treatment for common genital tract infections: results of a prospective controlled evaluation. American Journal of Obstetrics and Gynecology 173: 157–167

McIntosh K 1985 Coronavirus. In: Mandell G L, Douglas R G Jr, Bennett J E (eds) Principles and practice of infectious diseases. John Wiley, New York

McKelvie P, Goldsmid J M 1988 Childhood central nervous system cysticercosis in Australia. Medical Journal of Australia 149: 42–44

McLellan D, Giebink G S 1986 Perspectives on occult bacteremia in children. Journal of Pediatrics 109: 1–8

McManus D P, Smyth J D 1986 Hydatidosis: changing concepts in epidemiology and speciation. Parasitology Today 2: 163–167

McManus D P, Bowles J 1994 Asian (Taiwan) *Taenia*: species or strain? Parasitology Today 10: 273–275

McNicholl B, Flynn J 1978 Acquired toxoplasmosis in children. Archives of Disease in Childhood 53: 414–416

Madsen T 1925 Whooping cough. Its bacteriology, diagnosis, prevention and treatment. Boston Medical and Surgical Journal 192: 50

Mahle W T, Levine M M 1993 *Salmonella typhi* infection in children younger than five years of age. Pediatric Infectious Disease Journal 12: 627–631

Mahmoud A A F 1987 Baillière's clinical tropical medicine and communicable diseases: schistosomiasis. Baillière Tindall, London, vol 2(2)

Malone J L, Wallace M R, Hendrick B B et al 1995 Syphilis and neurosyphilis in a human immunodeficiency virus type-1 seropositive population: evidence for frequent serologic relapse after therapy. American Journal of Medicine 99: 55–63

Mancao M Y, Nolte F S, Nahmias A J, Jarvis W R 1994 Use of polymerase chain reaction for diagnosis of tuberculous meningitis. Pediatric Infectious Disease Journal 13: 154–156

Mandal B K 1994 *Salmonella typhi* and other salmonellas. Gut 35: 726–728

Mardh P-A, Paavonen J, Puolakkainen M 1989 Chlamydia. Plenum Medical Book Company, New York, pp 277–281

Margileth A M 1992 Antibiotic therapy for cat-scratch disease: clinical study of therapeutic outcome in 268 patients and a review of the literature. Pediatric Infectious Disease Journal 11: 474–478

Margileth A M 1993 Cat scratch disease. Advances in Pediatric Infectious Diseases 8: 1–21

Marks W A, Stutman H R, Marks M I et al 1986 Cefuroxime versus ampicillin plus chloramphenicol in childhood bacterial meningitis: a multicenter randomized controlled trial. Journal of Pediatrics 109: 123–130

Marsh K, Foster D, Waruiru C, Mwangi I et al 1995 Indicators of life-threatening malaria in African children. New England Journal of Medicine 332: 1399–1404

Marshall R, Teele D W, Klein J O 1979 Unsuspected bacteremia due to *Haemophilus influenzae*: outcome in children not initially admitted to hospital. Journal of Pediatrics 95: 690–695

Marty A M, Andersen E M 1995 Helminthology. In: Doerr W S, Siefert G (eds) Tropical pathology. Springer, Berlin, vol 8, pp 801–982

Mayon-White R T 1996 Pneumococcal vaccine. Journal of Medical Microbiology 44: 397–398

Medical Research Council Cardiothoracic Epidemiology Group 1994 Tuberculosis in children: a national survey of notifications in England and Wales in 1988. Archives of Disease in Childhood 70: 497–500

Meheus A, Schryver A D 1991 Sexually transmitted diseases in the Third World. In: Harris J R W, Forster S M (eds) Recent advances in sexually transmitted diseases and AIDS. Churchill Livingstone, Edinburgh, pp 201–217

Mehta M N, Subramanian S 1986 Comparison of rice water, rice electrolyte solution and glucose electrolyte solution in the management of infantile diarrhoea. Lancet 1: 843–845

Meinking T L, Taplin D 1990 Advances in pediculosis, scabies and other mite infestations. Advances in Dermatology 5: 131–152

Meningitis Working Party British Paediatric Immunology and Infectious Diseases Group 1992 Should we use dexamethasone in meningitis? Archives of Disease in Childhood 67: 1398–1401

Meyers J D 1988 Management of cytomegalovirus infection. American Journal of Medicine 85(suppl 2A): 102–106

Migasena S, Gilles H M 1987 Hookworm infection. In: Pawlowski Z S (ed) Baillière's clinical tropical medicine and communicable diseases. Baillière Tindall, London, vol 2.3, pp 617–627

Miller E 1995 Acellular pertussis vaccines. Archives of Disease in Childhood 73: 390–391

Miller F J W 1982 Tuberculosis in children. Churchill Livingstone, Edinburgh

Miller F J W 1984 The natural history of primary tuberculosis. WHO/TB/84.144. World Health Organization, Geneva

Miller L H 1988 Genetically determined human resistance factors. In: Wernsdorfer W H, McGregor I A (eds) Malaria. The principles and practice of malariology. Churchill Livingstone, Edinburgh, vol I, pp 487–500

Miller R L 1974 Pustular secondary syphilis. British Journal of Venereal Diseases 50: 459–462

Miller D, Madge M, Diamond J et al 1993 Pertussis immunisation and acute neurological illnesses in children. British Medical Journal 307: 1171–1176

Miller E, Vurdien J E, White J M 1992 The epidemiology of pertussis in England and Wales. CDR Review 2: R152–R154

Mills A, Goldsmid J M 1995 Intestinal protozoa. In: Doerr W S, Siefert G (eds) Tropical pathology. Springer, Berlin, vol 8, pp 477–556

Milstein T, Goldsmid J M 1995 The presence of *Giardia* and other zoonotic parasites of urban dogs in Hobart, Tasmania. Australian Veterinary Journal 72: 154–155

Modlin J F 1986 Perinatal echovirus infection: insights from a literature review of 61 cases of serious infection and 16 outbreaks in nurseries. Reviews of Infectious Diseases 8: 918–926

Mofenson L M, Moye J Jr, Bethel J et al 1992 Prophylactic intravenous immunoglobulin in HIV-infected children with CD4+ counts of 0.20 × 10⁹/L or more. Effect on viral, opportunistic and bacterial infections. Journal of the American Medical Association 268: 483–488

Molineaux L 1988 The epidemiology of human malaria as an explanation of its distribution, including some implications for its control. In: Wernsdorfer W H, McGregor I A (eds) Malaria. The principles and practice of malariology. Churchill Livingstone, Edinburgh, vol II, pp 913–998

Molyneux M E, Taylor T E, Wirima J J, Borgstein A 1989 Clinical features and prognostic indicators in pediatric cerebral malaria: a study of 131 comatose Malawian children. Quarterly Journal of Medicine 71: 441–459

Monath T P 1984 Yellow fever. In: Warren K A, Mahmoud A A (eds) Tropical and geographical medicine. McGraw Hill, New York

Monier B, Fauroux B, Chevalier J Y 1992 Miliary tuberculosis with acute respiratory failure and histiocyte hemophagocytosis. Successful treatment with extracorporeal lung support and epipodophyllotoxin VP 16-213. Acta Paediatrica 81: 725–727

Moodley M, Moosa A 1989 Treatment of neurocysticercosis: is praziquantel the new hope. Lancet 1: 262

Morera P 1987 Abdominal angiostrongyliasis: intestinal helminthic infections. In: Pawlowski Z S (ed) Baillière's clinical tropical medicine and communicable diseases. Baillière Tindall, London, vol 2.3, pp 747–753

Morrison D C, Ryan J L 1987 Endotoxins and disease mechanisms. Annual Review of Medicine 38: 417–432

Morse S S 1995 Factors in the emergence of infectious diseases. Emerging Infectious Diseases 1: 7–15

Mortality and Morbidity Weekly Reports (MMWR) 1989 Recommendations for diagnosing and treating syphilis in HIV-infected patients. Archives of Dermatology 125: 15–16

Moxon E R, Zwahlen A, Rubin L B 1985 Pathogenesis of *Haemophilus influenzae* meningitis: use of a rat model for studying microbial determinants of virulence. In: Sande M, Smith A, Root R (eds) Bacterial meningitis. Churchill Livingstone, Edinburgh, pp 23–36

Muhlemann M F, Wright D J M 1987 Emerging pattern of Lyme disease in the United Kingdom and Irish Republic. Lancet 1: 260–263

Muller A S, Leeuwenburg J, Pratt D S 1986 Pertussis: epidemiology and control. Bulletin of the World Health Organization 64: 321

Muller R 1985 Guineaworm eradication – the end of another disease? Parasitology Today 1: 39

Muller R 1987 *Dipetalonema* by any other name. Parasitology Today 3: 358

Murray C J L 1994 Quantifying the burden of disease: the technical basis for disability-adjusted life years. In: Murray C J L, Lopez A D (eds) Global comparative assessments in the health sector. WHO, Geneva, pp 3–19

Musher D M, Hamill R J, Baughn R E 1990 Effect of human immunodeficiency virus (HIV) infection on the course of syphilis and on the response to treatment. Annals of Internal Medicine 113: 872–881

Nabarro D 1954 Congenital syphilis. Edward Arnold, London

Nadel S, Levin M, Habibi P 1995 Meningococcal disease. Wiley, Chichester, pp 208–243

Nagaraju B, Gupte M D 1994 Diagnostic problems of early leprosy in field studies. Indian Journal of Leprosy 66: 463–472

Nagington J 1984 Psittacosis/ornithosis in Cambridgeshire 1975–1983. Journal of Hygiene (Cambridge) 92: 9–19

National Vaccine Advisory Committee 1991 The measles epidemic: the problems barriers and recommendations. Journal of the American Medical Association 266: 1547–1552

Neilsen R, Sondergaard J, Ullman S 1975 Asymptomatic male and female gonorrhoea. Acta Dermato-Venereologica (Stockholm) 55: 499–501

Nelson J D, Mohs E, Dajani A S, Plotkin S A 1976 Gonorrhea in preschool and school-aged children. Report of the Prepubertal Gonorrhea Cooperative Study Group. Journal of the American Medical Association 236: 1359–1364

Nemir R L, O'Hare D 1985 Congenital tuberculosis. American Journal of Diseases of Children 139: 284–287

Newman C P S 1993 Surveillance and control of *Shigella sonnei* infection. CDR Review 3(5): R63–R70

Nicoll A, Gardner A 1988 Whooping cough and unrecognized postperinatal mortality. Archives of Disease in Childhood 63: 41–47

Nicoll A, Moisley C 1994 Antenatal screening for syphilis. British Medical Journal 308: 1253–1254

Nicoll A, Rudd P 1989 British Paediatric Association manual on infections and immunizations in children. Oxford University Press, Oxford

Nicoll A, Timaeus I, Kigadye R-M et al 1994 The impact of HIV-1 infection on mortality in children under five years of age in sub-Saharan Africa: a demographic and epidemiological analysis. AIDS 8: 995–1005

Nielsen A, Larsen S O 1994 Epidemiology of pertussis in Denmark: the impact of herd immunity. International Journal of Epidemiology 23: 1300–1308

Nigro G, Zerbini M, Krzysztofiak A, Gentilomi G et al 1994 Active or recent parvovirus B 19 in children with Kawasaki disease. Lancet 343: 1260–1261

Noah N D 1984 What can we do about measles? British Medical Journal 289: 1476

Nokes C, Bundy D P 1994 Does helminth infection affect mental processing and educational achievement? Parasitology Today 10: 14–18

Nwosu S N, Nwosu M C 1994 Ocular findings in leprosy patients in Nigeria. East African Medical Journal 71: 441–444

Nylen O, Alestig K, Fasth A 1994 Infections of the ear with non-tuberculous mycobacteria in three children. Pediatric Infectious Disease Journal 13: 653–656

O'Brien K L, Ruff A J, Louis M A et al 1995 Bacillus Calmette–Guérin complications in children born to HIV-1 infected women with a review of the literature. Pediatrics 95: 414–418

O'Neill P M, Wright D J M 1988 Lyme disease. British Journal of Hospital Medicine 40: 284–289

O'Reilly L M, Daborn C J 1995 The epidemiology of *Mycobacterium bovis* infections in animals and man: a review. Tubercle and Lung Disease 76(suppl 1): 1–46

Obalek S, Jablonska S, Faure M, Wakzak L, Orth G 1990 Condylomata acuminata in children: frequent association with human papilloma viruses responsible for cutaneous warts. Journal of the American Academy of Dermatology 23: 205–213

Obaro S K, Monteil M A, Henderson D C 1996 The pneumococcal problem. British Medical Journal 312: 1521–1525

Odio C M, Faingezicht I, Salas J L et al 1986 Cefotaxime vs conventional therapy for the treatment of bacterial meningitis of infants and children. Pediatric Infectious Disease Journal 5: 402–407

Oliver N W, Rowbottom D J, Sexton P et al 1990 Chronic strongyloidiasis in Tasmanian veterans – clinical diagnosis by use of a screening index. Australian and New Zealand Journal of Medicine 19: 458–462

Onorato I M, Wassilak S G F 1987 Laboratory diagnosis of pertussis – the state of the art. Pediatric Infectious Disease Journal 6: 145–151

Ordog G J, Balasubramanium S, Wasserberger J 1985 Rat bites: fifty cases. Annals of Emergency Medicine 14: 126–130

Orega P A, Fine P E, Lucas S B et al 1993 Case-control study of BCG vaccination as a risk factor for leprosy and tuberculosis in western Kenya. International Journal of Leprosy and other Mycobacterial Diseases 61: 542–549

Ormerod L P, Garnett J M 1992 Tuberculin skin reactivity four years after neonatal BCG vaccination. Archives of Disease in Childhood 67: 530–531

Ormerod L P, Skinner C, Wales J 1996 Hepatotoxicity of antituberculosis drugs. Thorax 51: 111–113

Osborne J P, Pizer B 1981 Effect on the white cell count of contaminating cerebrospinal fluid with blood. Archives of Disease in Childhood 56: 400–401

Oshima T 1987 Anisakis – is the Sushi Bar guilty? Parasitology Today 3: 44–48

Ottesen E A, Vijayasekaran V, Kumaraswami V et al 1990 A controlled trial of ivermectin and diethylcarbamazine in lymphatic filariasis. New England Journal of Medicine 322: 1113–1117

Pagliuca A, Layton D, Allen S, Mufti G 1988 Hyperinfection with strongyloides after treatment for adult T-cell leukaemia–lymphoma in an African immigrant. British Medical Journal 297: 1456–1457

Pal G A, Baker J T, Wright D J M 1988 Penicillin resistant borrelia encephalitis responding to cefotaxime. Lancet i: 50–51

Partono F 1985 Diagnosis and treatment of lymphatic filariasis. Parasitology Today 1: 52–57

Paryani S G, Arvin A M 1986 Intrauterine infection with varicella-zoster virus after maternal varicella. New England Journal of Medicine 314: 1542–1546

Patriarca P A, Biellik R J, Sanden G et al 1988 Sensitivity and specificity of clinical case definitions for pertussis. American Journal of Public Health 78: 833–836

Patriarca P A, Foege W H, Swartz T A 1993 Progress in polio eradication. Lancet 342: 1461–1464

Pawlowski Z S 1987a Ascariasis. In: Pawlowski Z S (ed) Baillière's clinical tropical medicine and communicable diseases. Baillière Tindall, London, vol 2.3, pp 595–615

Pawlowski Z S 1987b Enterobiasis. In: Pawlowski Z S (ed) Baillière's clinical tropical medicine and communicable diseases. Baillière Tindall, London, vol 2.3, pp 667–676

Pearn J 1995 The sea, stingers, and surgeons: the surgeon's role in prevention, first aid and management of marine envenomations. Journal of Pediatric Surgery 30: 105–110

Peltola H, Kayhty H, Virtanen M et al 1984 Prevention of *Haemophilus influenzae* type b bacteremic infections with the capsular polysaccharide vaccine. New England Journal of Medicine 310: 1561–1566

Peltola H, Karanko V, Kurti T et al 1986 Rapid effect on endemic measles, mumps, and rubella of nationwide vaccination programme. Lancet 1: 137–139

Penn C W, Pritchard D G 1990 The spirochaetes. In: Parker M T, Duerden B I (eds) Topley and Wilson's principles of bacteriology, virology and immunity. Edward Arnold, London, pp 603–628

Pepin J, Milord F, Khonde A N et al 1994 Gambian trypanosomiasis: frequency of and risk factors, failure of melarsoprol therapy. Transactions of the Royal Society of Tropical Medicine and Hygiene 88: 447–452

Pepin J, Milord F, Khonde A N et al 1995 Risk factors for encephalopathy and mortality during melarsoprol treatment of *Trypanosoma brucei* gambiense sleeping sickness. Transactions of the Royal Society of Tropical Medicine and Hygiene 89(1): 92–97

Perine P L, Hopkins D R, Niemel P L A et a 1984 Handbook of endemic treponematosis. World Health Organization, Geneva

Peters P A S, Kazura J W 1987 Update on diagnostic methods for schistosomiasis. In: Mahmoud A A F (ed) Baillière's clinical tropical medicine and communicable diseases. Baillière Tindall, London, vol 2.2, pp 419–433

Pfister H 1984 Biology and chemistry of papillomaviruses. Review of Physiology, Biochemistry and Pharmacology 9: 111–181

Phillips S M, Lammie P J 1986 Immunopathology of granuloma formation and fibrosis in schistosomiasis. Parasitology Today 3: 296–302

Pickering L K, Engelkirk P G 1988 *Giardia lamblia*. Pediatric Clinics of North America 35: 565–577

Piesman J 1987 Emerging tick-borne diseases in temperate climates. Parasitology Today 3: 197–199

Pinder M 1988 *Loa loa* – a neglected filaria. Parasitology Today 4: 279–284

Pizzo P A, Wilfert C M 1994 Antiretroviral therapy for infection due to human immunodeficiency virus in children. Pediatric AIDS and HIV Infection 5(5): 273–295

Pizzo P A, Eddy J, Falloon J et al 1988 Effect of continuous intravenous infusion of zidovudine (AZT) in children with symptomatic HIV infection. New England Journal of Medicine 319: 889–896

Polderman A M, Blotkamp J 1995 *Oesophagostomum* infections in humans. Parasitology Today 11: 451–456

Powers W J 1985 Cerebrospinal fluid lymphocytosis in acute bacterial meningitis. American Journal of Medicine 79: 216–220

Pritchard D I 1995 The survival strategies of hookworms. Parasitology Today 11: 255–259

Pritchard R C, Hudson B J 1989 Antenatal screening for syphilis. Medical Journal of Australia 151: 363–364

Prober C G, Wayne M, Sullender W M et al 1987 Low risk of herpes simplex virus infections in neonates exposed to the virus at the time of vaginal delivery to mothers with recurrent genital herpes simplex virus infections. New England Journal of Medicine 316: 240–244

Prober C G, Hensleigh P A, Boucher F D et al 1988 Use of routine viral cultures at delivery to identify neonates exposed to herpes simplex virus. New England Journal of Medicine 318: 887–891

Public Health Laboratory Service 1989 Salmonella in eggs: PHLS evidence to agriculture committee. PHLS Microbiology Digest 6(1): 1–9

Public Health Laboratory Service: Meningococcal Infections Working Party and Public Health Medicine Environmental Group 1995 Control of meningococcal disease: guidance for consultants in communicable disease control. CDR Review 5: R189–R195

Pugh S F, Slack R C B, Caul E D et al 1985 Enzyme amplified immunoassay: a novel technique applied to direct detection of Chlamydia trachomatis in clinical specimens. Journal of Clinical Pathology 38: 1139–1141

Punjabi N H, Hoffman S L, Edman D C et al 1988 Treatment of severe typhoid fever in children with high dose dexamethasone. Pediatric Infectious Disease Journal 7: 598–600

Quinn T C 1994 Recent advances in diagnosis of sexually transmitted diseases. Sexually Transmitted Diseases 21: S19–S27

Quinn T C, Jacobs R F, Mertz G J et al 1982 Congenital malaria: a report of four cases and a review. Journal of Pediatrics 101: 229–232

Quist E E, Repesh L A, Zeleznikar R, Fitzgerald T J 1983 Interaction of Treponema pallidum with isolated rabbit capillary tissues. British Journal of Venereal Diseases 59: 11–20

Rais-Bahrami K, Platt P, Naqvi M 1990 Neonatal pseudomonas sepsis: even early diagnosis is too late. Clinical Pediatrics 29: 244

Ramsay M E B, Farrington C P, Miller E 1993 Age-specific efficacy of pertussis vaccine during epidemic and non-epidemic periods. Epidemiology and Infection 111: 41–48

Ramsay M, Gay N, Miller E et al 1994 The epidemiology of measles in England and Wales: rationale for the 1994 national vaccination campaign. CDR Review 4: R141–R146

Rawls W E 1985 Herpes simplex virus. In: Fields B N (ed) Virology. Raven Press, New York, pp 527–561

Recavarren S, Lumbreras H 1972 Pathogenesis of the verruga of Carrion's disease: ultrastructural studies. American Journal of Pathology 66: 461–470

Reed M D, Blumer J L 1983 Clinical pharmacology of antitubercular drugs. Pediatric Clinics of North America 30: 177–193

Reed S L 1992 Amebiasis: an update. Clinical Infectious Diseases 14: 385–393

Reed R P, Klugman K P 1994 Neonatal typhoid fever. Pediatric Infectious Disease Journal 13: 774–777

Reisman R E 1994 Insect stings. New England Journal of Medicine 331: 523–527

Rettig P J 1986 Infections due to Chlamydia trachomatis from infancy to adolescence. Pediatric Infectious Disease Journal 5: 449–457

Reynolds J E F (ed) 1996 Martindale, the extra pharmacopoeia. The Pharmaceutical Press, London

Richens J 1994 Sexually transmitted diseases in children in developing countries. Genitourinary Medicine 70: 278–283

Ridley C M 1988 The vulva. Churchill Livingstone, Edinburgh, pp 88

Riggsby W S 1985 Some recent developments in the molecular biology of medically important Candida. Microbiological Sciences 2(9): 257–263

Rim H-J, Forag H F, Sormani S, Cross J H 1994 Food-borne trematodes: ignored or emerging. Parasitology Today 10: 207–209

Ringertz S, Rylander M, Kronvall G 1991 Disc diffusion method for susceptibility testing of Neisseria gonorrhoeae. Journal of Clinical Microbiology 29: 1604–1609

Risseeuw-Appel I M, Kothe F C 1983 Transfusion syphilis: a case report. Sexually Transmitted Diseases 10: 200–201

Robbins J B, Schneerson R, Argaman M et al 1973 Haemophilus influenzae type b: disease and immunity in humans. Annals of Internal Medicine 78: 259–269

Roberts D M, Craft C, Mather F J et al 1988 Prevalence of giardiasis in patients with cystic fibrosis. Journal of Pediatrics 112: 555–559

Robertson D H H 1963a The treatment of sleeping sickness (mainly due to

Trypanosoma rhodesiense) with melarsoprol: I Reactions observed during treatment. Transactions of the Royal Society of Tropical Medicine and Hygiene 57: 122–133

Robertson D H H 1963b A trial of Mel W in the treatment of Trypanosoma rhodesiense sleeping sickness. Transactions of the Royal Society of Tropical Medicine and Hygiene 57: 274–289

Robertson D H H, McMillan A, Young H 1989 Clinical practice in sexually transmissible diseases. Churchill Livingstone, Edinburgh

Robinson J 1985 Fight the mite, ditch the itch. Parasitology Today 1: 140–142

Rochette F 1985 Chemotherapy of gastrointestinal nematodiasis in carnivores. In: Vanden Bossche H, Thienpont D, Janssens P G (eds) Chemotherapy of gastrointestinal helminths. Springer, Berlin, pp 487–504

Rock B, Naghashfar Z, Barnett N et al 1986 Genital tract papilloma virus infection in children. Archives of Dermatology 122: 1129–1132

Rodrigues L C, Smith P G 1990 Tuberculosis in developing countries and methods for its control. Transactions of the Royal Society of Tropical Medicine and Hygiene 84: 739–744

Rodriguez W J, Puig J R, Khan W N et al 1986 Ceftazidime vs standard therapy for pediatric meningitis: therapeutic, pharmacologic and epidemiologic observations. Pediatric Infectious Disease Journal 5: 408–415

Roesel C, Schaffter T 1989 Rice water/salt solution for diarrhoea. Lancet i: 620–621

Roizman B, Batterson W 1985 Herpesviruses and their replication. In: Fields B N (ed) Virology. Raven Press, New York, pp 497–526

Romanowski B, Sutherland R, Fick G H et al 1987 Serologic response to treatment of infectious syphilis. Annals of Internal Medicine 114: 1005–1009

Romanus V, Svensson A, Hallander H O 1992 The impact of changing BCG coverage on tuberculosis incidence in Swedish born children between 1969 and 1989. Tubercle and Lung Disease 73: 150–161

Romanus V, Hallander H O, Wahten P et al 1995 Atypical mycobacteria in extrapulmonary disease among children. Incidence in Sweden from 1969 to 1990 related to changing BCG vaccination coverage. Tubercle and Lung Disease 76: 300–310

Rosenfeld E A, Hageman J R, Yogev R 1993 Tuberculosis in infancy in the 1990's. Pediatric Clinics of North America 40: 1087–1103

Rosenhall U, Roupe G 1981 Auditory brain-stem responses in syphilis. British Journal of Venereal Diseases 57: 241–245

Rubenstein J S, Noah Z L, Zales V R, Shulman S T 1993 Acute myocarditis associated with Shigella sonnei gastroenteritis. Journal of Pediatrics 122: 82–84

Rufli T 1989 Syphilis and HIV infection. Dermatologica 179: 113–117

Ruhnke M, Trautman M 1994 Editorial: Recent trends in antimycotic therapy. Infection 22: 117 (also see related articles)

Ruuskanen O, Heikkinen T 1994 Otitis media: etiology and diagnosis. Pediatric Infectious Disease Journal 13: S23–S26

Ruuskanen O, Muerman O, Sarkinnen J 1985 Adenoviral diseases in children: a study of 105 hospital cases. Pediatrics 76: 79–83

Rygg M, Bruun C F 1992 Rat bite fever (Streptobacillus moniliformis) with septicaemia in a child. Scandinavian Journal of Infectious Diseases 24: 535–540

Sabato A-R, Martin A J, Marmion B P et al 1984 Mycoplasma pneumoniae: acute illness, antibiotics and subsequent lung function. Archives of Disease in Childhood 59: 1034–1037

St Geme J W, Hodes H L, Marcy S M et al 1988 Consensus management of Salmonella infection in the first year of life. Pediatric Infectious Disease Journal 7: 615–621

Salazar J C, Gerber M A, Goff C W 1993 Long term outcome of Lyme disease in children given early treatment. Journal of Pediatrics 122: 591–593

Sanchez P J, Wendel G D, Grimprel E et al 1993 Evaluation of molecular methodologies and rabbit infectivity testing for the diagnosis of congenital syphilis and neonatal central nervous system invasion by Treponema pallidum. Journal of Infectious Diseases 167: 148–157

Sarafian S K, Knapp J S 1989 Molecular epidemiology of gonorrhoea. Clinical Microbiology Reviews 2: S49–S55

Sarafian S K, Chu M L, Kojima H M et al 1991 Distribution of the 3.05-Mdal 'Toronto' beta-lactamase plasmid among penicillinase-producing isolates of Neisseria gonorrhoeae in the Far East. Sexually Transmitted Diseases 18: 201–204

Satcher D 1995 Emerging infections: getting ahead of the curve. Emerging Infectious Diseases 1: 1–6

Schaad U B, Votteler T P, McCracken G H, Nelson J D 1979 Management of atypical mycobacterial lymphadenitis in childhood: a review based on 380 cases. Journal of Pediatrics 95: 356–360

Schaad U, Lips U, Gnehm H et al 1993 Dexamethasone therapy for bacterial meningitis. Lancet 342: 457–461

Schachter J, Stamm W E, Quinn T C et al 1994 Ligase chain reaction to detect *Chlamydia trachomatis* infection of the cervix. Journal of Clinical Microbiology 32: 2440–2443

Scheepers A, Lemmer J, Lownie J F 1993 Oral manifestations of leprosy. Leprosy Review 64: 37–43

Schenone H 1980 Praziquantel in the treatment of *Hymenolepis nana* infections in children. American Journal of Tropical Medicine and Hygiene 19: 320–321

Schmid G P 1985 The global distribution of Lyme disease. Reviews of Infectious Diseases 7: 41–50

Schmitz J L, Gertis K S, Mauney C et al 1994 Laboratory diagnosis of congenital syphilis by immunoglobulin M (IgM) and IgA immunoblotting. Clinical and Diagnostic Laboratory Immunology 1: 32–37

Schneider J, Hughes J, Henderson A 1990 Infectious diseases: prophylaxis and chemotherapy. Appleton & Lange, Australia

Schryver A De, Meheus A 1990 Syphilis and blood transfusion: a global perspective. Transfusion 30: 844–847

Scott G 1996 Bartonellosis. In: Cook G C (ed) Manson's tropical diseases. W B Saunders, London, pp 892–898

Seboxa T, Rahlenbeck S I 1995 Treatment of louse-borne relapsing fever with low dose penicillin or tetracycline: a clinical trial. Scandinavian Journal of Infectious Diseases 27: 29–31

Sedlacek T V, Lindheim S, Eder C et al 1989 Mechanism for human papilloma virus transmission at birth. American Journal of Obstetrics and Gynecology 161: 55–59

Sehgal V N, Chaudhry A K 1993 Leprosy in children: a prospective study. International Journal of Dermatology 32: 194–197

Sell S H 1983 Long term sequelae of bacterial meningitis in children. Pediatric Infectious Disease Journal 2: 90–93

Sell S, Hsu P L 1993 Delayed hypersensitivity, immune deviation, antigen processing and T-cell subset selection in syphilis pathogenesis and vaccine design. Immunology Today 14: 576–582

Senior B W 1987 *Proteus morgani* is less frequently associated with urinary tract infection than *Proteus mirabilis* – an explanation. Journal of Medical Microbiology 16: 317–322

Shann F, Gratten M, Germer S et al 1984 Aetiology of pneumonia in children in Goroka hospital, Papua, New Guinea. Lancet 2: 537–541

Shanson D G, Gazzard B G, Midgley J et al 1983 *Streptobacillus moniliformis* isolated in blood from four cases of Haverhill fever: first outbreak in Britain. Lancet ii: 92–94

Shapiro E D 1995 Lyme disease in children. American Journal of Medicine 98(suppl 4A): 69S–73S

Shapiro E D, Gerber M A 1994 Lyme Disease in Children Study Group: Lyme disease in children. Sixth International Conference on Lyme Borreliosis, Bologna, Italy

Shata A M A, Coulter J B S, Parry C M et al 1996 Sputum induction for the diagnosis of tuberculosis. Archives of Disease in Childhood 74: 535–536

Shribman J H, Eastwood J B, Uff J 1983 Immune complex nephritis complicating miliary tuberculosis. British Medical Journal 287: 1593–1594

Shulman S T, De Inocencio J, Hirsch R 1995 Kawasaki disease. Pediatric Clinics of North America 42(5): 1205–1222

Siber G R, Thompson C, Reid G R et al 1992 Evaluation of bacterial polysaccharide immune globulin for the treatment or prevention of *Haemophilus influenzae* type b and pneumococcal disease. Journal of Infectious Diseases 165 (suppl 1): S129–S133

Simon M W, Wilson H D 1986 The amoebic meningoencephalitides. Pediatric Infectious Disease Journal 5: 562–569

Sixbey J W, Lemon S M, Pagano J S 1986 A second site for Epstein–Barr virus shedding: the uterine cervix. Lancet 2: 1122–1124

Smallman L A, Young J A, Shortland-Webb W R et al 1986 *Strongyloides stercoralis* hyper-infestation syndrome with *Escherichia coli* meningitis: report of two cases. Journal of Clinical Pathology 39: 366–370

Smith C E 1955 Coccidioidomycosis. Pediatric Clinics of North America 2: 109–125

Smith D H, Ingram D L, Smith A L 1973 Diagnosis and treatment. Bacterial meningitis. A symposium. Pediatrics 52: 586–600

Smith D W, Wiegeshaus E H 1989 What animal models can teach us about the pathogenesis of tuberculosis in humans. Reviews of Infectious Diseases II(suppl 2): 385–393

Smith E M, Johnson S R, Cripe T P et al 1991 Perinatal vertical transmission of human papilloma virus and subsequent development of respiratory tract papillomatosis. Annals of Otology and Rhinology 100: 479–493

Smith I W, Peutherer J F, McCallum F O 1967 The incidence of herpesvirus hominis antibody in the population. Journal of Hygiene (Cambridge) 65: 395–408

Smith J R, Taylor-Robinson D 1993 Infection due to *Chlamydia trachomatis* in pregnancy and the newborn. Baillière's Clinical Obstetrics and Gynaecology 7: 237–255

Smith K R, Ching S F, Lee H et al 1995 Evaluation of ligase chain reaction for use with urine for identification of *Neisseria gonorrhoeae* in females attending a sexually transmitted disease clinic. Journal of Clinical Microbiology 33: 455–457

Smith M L, Mellor D 1980 *Proteus mirabilis* meningitis and cerebral abscess in the newborn period. Archives of Disease in Childhood 55: 308–310

Smyth J D 1995 Rare, new and emerging helminth zoonoses. Advances in Pathology 36: 1–47

Sookpranee T, Sookpranee M, Mellencamp M A, Preheim L C 1991 *Pseudomonas pseudomallei*, a common pathogen in Thailand that is resistant to the bactericidal effects of many antibiotics. Antimicrobial Agents and Chemotherapy 35: 484–489

South M A 1971 Enteropathic *Escherichia coli* disease: new developments and perspectives. Journal of Pediatrics 79: 1

Southall D P, Thomas M G, Lambert H P 1988 Severe hypoxaemia in pertussis. Archives of Disease in Childhood 63: 598

Spruance S L, Overall J C Jr, Kern E R et al 1977 The natural history of recurrent herpes simplex labialis. New England Journal of Medicine 297: 69–74

Stamm W E, Handsfield H H, Rompalo A M et al 1988 The association between genital ulcer disease and acquisition of HIV infection in homosexual men. Journal of the American Medical Association 260: 1429–1433

Stanford J L, Stanford C A 1996 Immunotherapy for tuberculosis with *M. vaccae*. Journal of Medical Microbiology 44: 1–34

Starke J R 1992 Nontuberculous mycobacterial infections in children. Advances in Pediatric Infectious Diseases 7: 123–159

Starke J R, Baker C J 1985 Neonatal shigellosis with bowel perforation. Pediatric Infectious Disease Journal 4: 405–407

Starke J R, Correa A G 1995 Management of mycobacterial infection and disease in children. Pediatric Infectious Disease Journal 14: 455–470

Steere A C, Hardin J A, Malawista S E 1977 Erythema chronicum migrans and Lyme arthritis. Cryoimmunoglobulins and clinical activity of skin and joints. Science 196: 1121

Steere A C, Gibofsky A, Patarroyo M E et al 1979 Chronic Lyme arthritis. Annals of Internal Medicine 90: 896–901

Steere A C, Grodzicki R L, Lornblatt A N et al 1983a The spirochaetal etiology of Lyme disease. New England Journal of Medicine 308: 733–739

Steere A C, Bartenhagen N H, Craft J E et al 1983b The early clinical manifestations of Lyme disease. Annals of Internal Medicine 99: 76–82

Steere A C, Hutchinson D J, Rahn D W et al 1983c Treatment of the early manifestations of Lyme disease. Annals of Internal Medicine 99: 22

Steere A C, Schoen R T, Taylor E 1987 The clinical evolution of Lyme arthritis. Annals of Internal Medicine 107: 725–731

Steere A C, Dwyer E, Winchester R 1990 Association of chronic Lyme arthritis with HLA-DR4 and HLA-DR2 alleles. New England Journal of Medicine 323: 219–223

Steiner P, Rao M, Victoria M S, Jabbar H, Steiner M 1980 Persistently negative tuberculin reactions. American Journal of Diseases of Children 134: 747–750

Stevens J R, Godfrey D G 1992 Numerical taxonomy of Trypanozoon based on polymorphisms in a reduced range of enzymes. Parasitology 104: 75–86

Stoehr G P, Peterson A L, Taylor W J 1978 Systemic complications of local podophyllin therapy. Annals of Internal Medicine 89: 362–363

Stoll B J 1993 Congenital syphilis: evaluation and management of neonates born to mothers with reactive serological tests for syphilis. Pediatric Infectious Disease Journal 13: 845–853

Stoll B J 1994 Congenital syphilis: evaluation and management of neonates born to mothers with reactive serologic tests for syphilis. Pediatric Infectious Disease Journal 13(9): 845–853

Stoll B J, Lee F K, Larsen S et al 1993 Clinical and serologic evaluation of neonates for congenital syphilis: a continuing diagnostic dilemma. Journal of Infectious Diseases 167: 1093–1099

Strang J I G, Kakaza H H S, Gibson D G et al 1987 Controlled trial of prednisolone as adjuvant in treatment of tuberculous constrictive pericarditis in Transkei. Lancet ii: 1418–1422

Strang J I G, Kakaza H H S, Gibson D G et al 1988 Controlled clinical trial of complete open surgical drainage and of prednisolone in treatment of tuberculous pericardial effusion in Transkei. Lancet ii: 759–764

Stray-Pedersen B 1983 Economic evaluation of maternal screening to prevent congenital syphilis. Sexually Transmitted Diseases 14: 167–172

Stürchler D 1989 How much malaria is there worldwide? Parasitology Today 5: 39–40

Sturrock R F 1987 Biology and ecology of human schistosomes. In: Mahmoud A A F (ed) Baillière's clinical tropical medicine and communicable diseases. Baillière Tindall, London, vol. 2.2, pp 249–266

Sutherland S 1978 Venomous bites and stings. Medicine Australia 6: 402–412

Sutherland S 1979 First aid for snakebite in Australia. CSL, Parville

Sutherland S 1982 Venomous creatures of Australia. Oxford University Press, Melbourne, p 127

Sutherland S 1992a Antivenom use in Australia. Medical Journal of Australia 157: 734–739

Sutherland S 1992b Poisonous Australian animals. Hyland House, Victoria, p 64

Sutherland I, Springett V H 1987 Effectiveness of BCG vaccination in England and Wales in 1983. Tubercle 68: 81–92

Swanson D S, Starke J R 1995 Drug-resistant tuberculosis in pediatrics. Pediatric Clinics of North America 42: 553–581

Sweaney H C 1960 Histoplasmosis. Thomas, Springfield

Szer I S, Taylor E, Steere A C 1991 The long term course of Lyme arthritis in children. New England Journal of Medicine 325: 159–163

Szymczak E G, Barr J T, Durbin W A, Goldman D A 1979 Evaluation of blood culture procedures in a pediatric hospital. Journal of Clinical Microbiology 9: 88–92

Tafuri W L 1979 Pathogenesis of *Trypanosoma cruzi* infections. In: Lumsden W H R, Evans D A (eds) Biology of Kinetoplastida. Academic Press, London, vol 2, pp 548–618

Takala A K, Eskola J, Leinonen M 1991 Reduction of oropharyngeal carriage of *Haemophilus influenzae* type b (Hib) in children immunized with an Hib conjugate vaccine. Journal of Infectious Diseases 164: 982–986

Talio M, Zapata A G, McGreevy P B, Marsden P 1991 Strickland Hunter's tropical medicine. Saunders, Philadelphia, pp 628–637

Tan J S 1995 Anti-pseudomonal penicillins. Medical Clinics of North America 79(4): 679–693

Tanaka M, Kumazawa J, Matsumoto T, Kobayashi I 1994 High prevalence of *Neisseria gonorrhoeae* strains with reduced susceptibility to fluoroquinolones in Japan. Genitourinary Medicine 70: 90–93

Tarantola D, Mann J M 1987 Acquired immunodeficiency syndrome and expanded programmes on immunization. Special programme on AIDS. World Health Organization, Geneva

Taylor H R, Agarwala N, Johnson S L 1984 Detection of experimental *Chlamydia trachomatis* eye infection in conjunctival smears and in tissue culture by use of fluorescein-conjugated monoclonal antibody. Journal of Clinical Microbiology 20: 391–395

Taylor T E, Molyneux M E, Wirima J J et al 1988 Blood glucose levels in Malawian children before and during the administration of intravenous quinine for severe falciparum malaria. New England Journal of Medicine 319: 1040–1047

Taylor-Robinson D 1994 *Chlamydia trachomatis* and sexually transmitted disease. British Medical Journal 308: 150–151

Taylor-Robinson D, Thomas B J 1991 Laboratory techniques for the diagnosis of chlamydial infection. Genitourinary Medicine 67: 256–266

Teale C, Cundall D B, Pearson S B 1992 Heaf status 12 years after BCG vaccination. Tubercle and Lung Disease 73: 210–212

Teele D W, Dashefsky B, Rakusan T, Klein J O 1981 Meningitis after lumbar puncture in children with bacteremia. New England Journal of Medicine 305: 1079–1081

Teklu B, Habte-Michael A, Warrell D A et al 1983 Meptazinol diminishes the Jarisch–Herxheimer reaction of relapsing fever. Lancet i: 835–839

Teoh R, Humphries M J, O'Mahony G 1987 Symptomatic intracranial tuberculoma developing during treatment of tuberculosis: a report of 10 patients and review of the literature. Quarterly Journal of Medicine, New Series 63: 449–460

Terry R J 1994 Concomitant immunity in schistosomiasis. Parasitology Today 10: 377–378

Thomas B J, Evans R T, Hawkins D A, Taylor-Robinson D 1984 Sensitivity of detecting *Chlamydia trachomatis* elementary bodies in smears by use of a fluorescein labelled monoclonal antibody: comparison with conventional chlamydial isolation. Journal of Clinical Pathology 37: 812–816

Thomas D D, Navab M, Haake D A et al 1988 *Treponema pallidum* invades intercellular junctions of endothelial cell monolayers. Proceedings of the National Academy of Sciences 85: 3608–3612

Thompson C, Young H, Moyes A 1995 Ciprofloxacin resistant *Neisseria gonorrhoeae*. Genitourinary Medicine 71: 412–413

Tibballs J 1994 Premedication for snake antivenom. Medical Journal of Australia 160: 4–7

Tillez-Giron E, Ramos M C, Dufour I 1987 Detection of *Cysticercus cellulosae* antigens in cerebrospinal fluid by DOT enzyme-linked immunosorbent assay (DOT-ELISA) and standard ELISA. American Journal of Tropical Medicine and Hygiene 37: 169–173

Tobin J O H 1975 Herpesvirus hominis infection in pregnancy. Proceedings of the Royal Society of Medicine 68: 371–374

Tobin M H, Cahill N, Gearty G et al 1982 Q fever endocarditis. American Journal of Medicine 72: 396–400

Todd J, Fishaut M, Kapral K, Welch T 1978 Toxic shock syndrome associated with phage-group-1 staphylococci. Lancet 2: 1116–1118

Tomberlin M G, Holtom P D, Owens J L, Larsen R A 1994 Evaluation of neurosyphilis in human immunodeficiency virus-infected individuals. Clinical Infectious Diseases 18: 288–294

Torigoe S, Kumamoto T, Koide W et al 1995 Clinical manifestations associated with human herpesvirus 7 infection. Archives of Disease in Childhood 72: 518–519

Torrey S, Fleisher G, Jaffe D 1986 Incidence of *Salmonella* bacteraemia in infants with *Salmonella* gastroenteritis. Journal of Pediatrics 108: 718–721

Tovo P A, de Martino M, Gabiano C et al 1992 Prognostic factors and survival in children with perinatal HIV-1 infection. Lancet 339: 1249–1253

Tseng C J, Lin C Y, Wang R L et al 1992 Possible transplacental transmission of human papilloma viruses. American Journal of Obstetrics and Gynecology 166: 35–40

Turk D C 1982 Clinical importance of *Haemophilus influenzae* – 1981. In: Sell S H, Wright P F (eds) *Haemophilus influenzae* epidemiology, immunology and prevention of disease. Elsevier, New York, pp 3–9

Turnbull P C B 1986 Thoroughly modern anthrax. Abstracts on Hygiene and Communicable Disease 61(9): R1–R13

United Nations Children's Emergency Fund 1996 The state of the world's children 1996. Oxford University Press, Oxford

Valentine M D, Schuberth K C, Kagey-Sobotka A et al 1990 The value of immunotherapy with venom in children with allergy to insect stings. New England Journal of Medicine 323: 1601–1603

Vallejo J G, Ong L T, Starke J R 1994 Clinical features, diagnosis and treatment of tuberculosis in infants. Pediatrics 84: 1–7

Van Dam A P, Kuiper H, Vos K et al 1993 Different genospecies of *B. burgdorferi* are associated with distinct clinical manifestations of Lyme borreliosis. Clinical Infectious Diseases 17: 708–717

van der Poel C L, Cuypers H T, Reesink H W 1994 Hepatitis C virus six years on. Lancet 344: 1475–1478

van der Sluis J J, ten Kate F J, Vuzevski V D 1985 Transfusion syphilis – survival of *Treponema pallidum* in stored donor blood: II Dose dependence of experimentally determined survival times. Vox Sanguinis 49: 390–399

van't Wout J W 1988 Developments in treatment with new antifungal drugs. Mycoses 31: 59

Vander Steichele R H, Dezeure E M, Bogaert M G 1995 Systematic review of clinical efficacy of topical treatments for head lice. British Medical Journal 311: 604–608

Voelker R 1995 Achieving global child health goals. Journal of the American Medical Association 274: 103–106

von Krogh G 1981 Podophyllotoxin for condylomata acuminata eradication. Clinical and experimental comparative studies on *Podophyllum lignans*, colchicine and 5-fluorouracil. Acta Dermato-Venereologica (Stockholm) Supplementum 98

Wailoo M P, Petersen S A, Whittaker H, Goodenough P 1989 Sleeping body temperatures in 3–4 month old infants. Archives of Disease in Childhood 64: 596–599

Walker E 1988 Clinical aspects of pertussis. In: Wardlaw A C, Parton R (eds) Pathogenesis and immunity in pertussis. John Wiley, London, pp 273–282

Wallace R J, Baker C J, Quinones F J et al 1983 Non-typable *Haemophilus influenzae* (Biotype 4) as a neonatal, maternal and genital pathogen. Review of Infectious Diseases 5: 123–136

Walmsley S, Devi S, King S et al 1993 Invasive *Aspergillus* infections in a pediatric hospital: a ten year review. Pediatric Infectious Disease Journal 12: 673–682

Walsh T J, Pizzo A 1988 Treatment of systemic fungal infections. Recent advances and current problems. European Journal of Clinical Microbiology and Infectious Diseases (August): 460

Ward M F 1983 Chlamydial classification, development and structure. British Medical Bulletin 39: 109–115

Warnock D W 1989 Antifungal drugs. Current Opinion in Infectious Diseases 2: 362–366

Warrell D A, Perine P L, Krause D W et al 1983 Pathophysiology and immunology of the Jarisch–Herxheimer-like reaction in louse-borne relapsing fever: comparison of tetracycline and slow-release penicillin. Journal of Infectious Diseases 147: 898–909

Warren K S 1987 Determinants of disease in human schistosomiasis. In: Mahmoud A A F (ed) Baillière's clinical tropical medicine and communicable diseases. Baillière Tindall, London, vol 2.2, pp 301–313

Warren K S, Mahmoud A A F 1975 Algorithms in the diagnosis and management of exotic diseases: I Schistosomiasis. Journal of Infectious Diseases 131: 614–620

Wasserheit J N 1994 Effect of changes in human ecology and behaviour on patterns of sexually transmitted diseases, including immunodeficiency virus infection. Proceedings of the National Academy of Sciences 91: 2430–2435

Weatherall D J 1988 The anaemia of malaria. In: Wernsdorfer W H, McGregor I A (eds). The principles and practice of malariology. Churchill Livingstone, Edinburgh, vol 1, pp 735–751

Webster L T 1987 Update on chemotherapy of schistosomiasis. In: Mahmoud A A F (ed) Baillière's clinical tropical medicine and communicable diseases. Baillière Tindall, London, vol 2.2, pp 435–447

White N J, Miller K D, Marsh K et al 1987 Hypoglycaemia in African children with severe malaria. Lancet 1: 708–711

White N J, Dance D A B, Chaowagul W et al 1989 Halving the mortality of severe melioidosis by ceftazidime. Lancet 2: 697–701

Whitley R J 1988 Herpes simplex virus infections of the central nervous system. A review. American Journal of Medicine 85(suppl 2A): 61–67

Whitworth J 1992 Treatment of onchocerciasis with ivermectin in Sierra Leone. Parasitology Today 8: 138–140

Widy-Wirski R, D'Costa J, Meheus J 1980 Prevalance du pian chez les pygmees en Centrafrique. Annales de la Societe Belge de Medecine Tropicale (Bruxelles) 60: 61–67

Wigginton J M, Thill P 1993 Infant botulism: a review of the literature. Clinical Pediatrics 32: 669–674

Wildy P, Field H J, Nash A A 1982 Classical herpes latency revisited. In: Mahy B W J, Minson A C, Darby G K (eds) Virus persistence. Cambridge University Press, Cambridge, pp 133–167

Wilkins E G L 1994 The serodiagnosis of tuberculosis. In: Davies P D O (ed) Clinical tuberculosis. Chapman and Hall, London, 367–380

Winsland J K D, Nimmo S, Butcher P D et al 1989 Prevalence of giardia in dogs and cats in the United Kingdom: survey of an Essex veterinary clinic. Transactions of the Royal Society of Tropical Medicine and Hygiene 83(6): 791–792

Wirsing von Konig C H, Postels-Multani S, Bock H L, Schmitt H J 1995 Pertussis in adults: frequency of transmission after household exposure. Lancet 346: 1326–1329

Wolinsky E 1992 Mycobacterial diseases other than tuberculosis. Clinical Infectious Diseases 15: 1–12

Wolinsky E 1995 Mycobacterial lymphadenitis in children: a prospective study of 105 non-tuberculous cases with long-term follow-up. Clinical Infectious Diseases 20: 954–963

Wong H B 1981 Rice water in treatment of infantile gastroenteritis. Lancet 2: 102–103

Woolhouse M E J 1993 International Conference on schistosomiasis. Parasitology Today 9: 235–236

Working Party of British Society for Antimicrobial Chemotherapy 1985 Antibiotic treatment of streptococcal and staphylococcal endocarditis. Lancet ii: 815–817

World AIDS 1989 Children need knowledge too. The Panos Institute, 8 Alfred Place, London, p 9

World Bank 1993 Investing in health, World Development Report. Oxford University Press, Oxford

World Health Organization 1980 Memorandum: a revision of the system of nomenclature for influenza viruses. Bulletin of the World Health Organization 58(4): 585–591

World Health Organization 1983 Haemorrhagic fever with renal syndrome. Bulletin of the World Health Organization 61: 269–275

World Health Organization 1985 Tropical diseases research(TDR) 7th Programme Report. World Health Organization, Geneva

World Health Organization 1986a Conjunctivitis of the newborn: prevention and treatment at the primary health care level. World Health Organization, Geneva

World Health Organization 1986b Severe and complicated malaria. Report of an informal technical meeting in Geneva, 1985. Transactions of the Royal Society of Tropical Medicine and Hygiene 80(suppl): 1–50

World Health Organization 1986c Technical Report Series No 735: malaria. World Health Organization, Geneva

World Health Organization 1986d Epidemiology and control of African trypanosomiasis. Technical Report Series No 739. World Health Organization, Geneva

World Health Organization 1987 World malaria situation 1985. World Health Statistics Quarterly 40: 142–170

World Health Organization 1989 Quality control of BCG vaccines by the World Health Organization: a review of factors that may influence vaccine effectiveness and safety. WHO/EPI/GEN/89.3. World Health Organization, Geneva

World Health Organization 1993 Treatment of tuberculosis: guidelines for national programmes. World Health Organization, Geneva

World Health Organization 1994 Global surveillance programme for recognition and response to emerging diseases 1994–95. World Health Organization, Geneva

World Health Organization 1995a Guidelines for the control of epidemics due to Shigella dysenteriae. CDR/95.4. World Health Organization, Geneva

World Health Organization 1995b Poisonous animal bites and stings. WHO Weekly Epidemiological Record 44: 315–316

World Health Organization Global Program on AIDS 1989 Report of the meeting of the technical working group on HIV/AIDS in childhood. WHO/GPA/SF1/89.2AF. World Health Organization, Geneva

World Health Organization Scientific Group 1982 Endemic treponematoses making a comeback. WHO Chronicle 36(2): 77–78

Wullenweber M 1995 Streptobacillus moniliformis – a zoonotic pathogen. Taxonomic considerations, host species, diagnosis, therapy, geographical distribution. Laboratory Animals 29: 1–15

Wyler D J 1992 Why does liver fibrosis occur in schistosomiasis? Parasitology Today 8: 277–279

Yamamoto T, Naigowit P, Dejsirilert S et al 1990 In vitro susceptibilities of Pseudomonas pseudomallei to 27 antimicrobial agents. Antimicrobial Agents and Chemotherapy 34: 2027–2029

Yamanishi K, Okuno T, Shiraki K et al 1988 Identification of human herpesvirus-6 as a causal agent for exanthem subitum. Lancet i: 1065–1067

Young E J 1995 Brucella species. In: Mandell G L, Bennet J E, Dolon R (eds) Principles and practice of infectious diseases. Churchill Livingstone, Edinburgh, pp 2053–2060

Young H 1992 Syphilis: new diagnostic directions. International Journal of STD and AIDS 3: 391–413

Young H, Moyes A 1996a Gonococcal infections in Scotland 1994. Scottish Centre for Infection and Environmental Health Weekly Report 30(96/01): 2–5

Young H, Moyes A 1996b An evaluation of pre-poured selective media for the isolation of Neisseria gonorrhoeae. Journal of Medical Microbiology 44: 253–260

Young H, Henrichsen C, Robertson D H H 1974 Treponema pallidum haemagglutination test as a screening procedure for the diagnosis of syphilis. British Journal of Venereal Diseases 50: 341–346

Young H, Paterson I C, McDonald D R 1976 Rapid carbohydrate utilisation test for the identification of Neisseria gonorrhoeae. British Journal of Venereal Diseases 52: 172–175

Young H, Moyes A, McMillan A, Robertson D H H 1989 Screening for treponemal infection by a new enzyme immuno assay. Genitourinary Medicine 65: 72–78

Young H, Moyes A, McMillan A, Paterson J 1992 Enzyme immunoassay for anti-treponemal IgG: screening or confirmatory test? Journal of Clinical Pathology 45: 37–41

Young H, Penn C W 1990 Syphilis, yaws and pinta. In: Smith G R, Easmon C S F (eds) Topley and Wilson's principles of bacteriology, virology and immunology. Edward Arnold, Kent, pp 588–604

Young S M, Keane F E A 1992 Children seen by Leicester genitourinary medicine physicians 1988–1990. Genitourinary Medicine 68: 423

Zuckerman A J 1984 Perinatal transmission of hepatitis B. Archives of Disease in Childhood 59: 1007–1009

Zuckerman A J 1985 New hepatitis B vaccines. British Medical Journal 290: 492–496

24 Disorders of bone, joints and connective tissue

D. G. D. Barr   P. M. Crofton   K. M. Goel

DISORDERS OF BONE, CARTILAGE AND
   COLLAGEN   1544
Congenital limb malformations of variable
   distribution   1545
Congenital limb malformations affecting the upper
   limbs predominantly   1548
Congenital limb malformations affecting the lower
   limbs predominantly   1549
Structural defects of thorax and spine   1556
Structural defects of skull and facial bones   1558
Specific skeletal dysplasias (the
   osteochondrodysplasias)   1565
Skeletal defects associated with major disorders in
   other organs and tissues   1586
Infection in bone and joint   1589
The osteochondroses   1593
DISORDERS OF JOINTS AND CONNECTIVE
   TISSUE   1596
Acute rheumatic fever   1596

Juvenile chronic arthritis (JCA)   1600
Ankylosing spondylitis   1605
Systemic lupus erythematosus (SLE)   1605
Neonatal lupus erythematosus   1606
Dermatomyositis–polymyositis   1606
Progressive systemic sclerosis or scleroderma   1608
Mixed connective tissue disease   1609
Vasculitic syndromes   1609
Arthropathy in cystic fibrosis of pancreas   1611
Arthropathy in inflammatory bowel disease   1611
Psoriatic arthritis   1611
Reiter's syndrome   1611
Behçet's syndrome   1611
Lyme arthritis   1611
Viral arthritis   1612
Hypermobility syndrome (including Ehlers–Danlos syndrome)
   1612
Limb pains of childhood with no organic disease   1612
References and Bibliography   1613

DISORDERS OF BONE, CARTILAGE AND COLLAGEN

Congenital and acquired disorders of the musculoskeletal system are an important cause of handicap in children.

Limb defects and deformities cause increasing functional disability for the developing infant. Early energetic physiotherapy, corrective splinting, and close supervision to determine defects which require early reconstructive surgery will enable adjustments to take place with growth. Thus, the early diagnosis and effective management of relatively common disorders such as club foot and congenital dislocation of the hip will greatly improve the prospects of a good functional result.

Similarly, structural defects of the spine and thorax, such as scoliosis, require early recognition, regular assessment and timely intervention to prevent or mitigate the effects of progressive deformity on growth, posture, and the dynamics of breathing.

Malformations of the craniofacial structures, in addition to their cosmetic impact, are often associated with significant disorders in, for example, intellect, vision, hearing, speech, airway, palate and dentition. Early diagnosis and management of any coexistent problems will help to minimize the child's disability. The prospects for corrective surgery to skull and face have improved with advances in surgical techniques in specialized centers.

The inherited skeletal dysplasias, individually rare, are collectively quite common. The biochemical basis and molecular genetics of these disorders are increasingly being identified (p. 1566, Table 24.4). In the absence of an etiologic diagnosis, the clinical, radiological and genetic diagnosis should be as precise as possible, both in order to assess the child's prognosis and for counseling the family.

Infection of bone and joint presents a considerable threat to life with a high risk of residual orthopedic disability in survivors, and the osteochondroses remain conditions of uncertain etiology and unpredictable course.

In assessing the child with musculoskeletal disorder, coexistent abnormalities must be carefully sought, complications anticipated and the effects on growth and development monitored. Many of these disorders are at the interface of pediatrics, genetics and orthopedics, and the child and family require a multidisciplinary approach and, often, protracted follow-up.

This account is arranged under the following headings:

1. Congenital limb malformations of variable distribution.
2. Congenital limb malformations affecting the upper limbs predominantly.
3. Congenital limb malformations affecting the lower limbs predominantly.
4. Structural defects of thorax and spine.
5. Structural defects of skull and facial bones.
6. Specific skeletal dysplasias.
7. Infection in bone.
8. The osteochondroses.

Endocrine and metabolic disease affecting bone are covered in Chapters 19 and 20 respectively, and tumors of bone are reviewed in Chapter 16.

CONGENITAL LIMB MALFORMATIONS OF VARIABLE DISTRIBUTION

Clinical terminology for these defects tends to be imprecise. The anatomical classification of O'Rahilly (1969), covering both upper and lower limbs, defines four major groups of limb defects, with further subdivision of the longitudinal defects according to whether the preaxial or postaxial side of the limb is affected (Fig. 24.1). A comprehensive nomenclature for congenital limb deficiencies has been proposed (Developmental Medicine and Child Neurology 1975).

HAND MALFORMATIONS

For hand malformations, Temtamy & McKusick (1969) give a primary morphological classification with seven main categories (absence deformities, brachydactyly, syndactyly, polydactyly, contracture deformity, symphalangism, and malformations with ring constrictions). Further anatomic subdivision is possible in most cases. Each main category can also be further divided according to the presence or absence of malformation in other organs and the pattern of inheritance in the family (Table 24.1).

PHOCOMELIA, AMELIA, HEMIMELIA

These defects are defined in Figure 24.1. In the classical form of phocomelia (literally seal-limb) the hand or foot is attached to the trunk; this appearance may be due to a variety of underlying anatomic defects. Upper and/or lower limbs may be affected. Amelia indicates complete absence of a limb, or, rarely, of all four limbs (amelia totalis). Various forms of hemimelia are described. In thalidomide cases the radius and radial side of the hand are most specifically defective. Conditions known as radius aplasia, radius hypoplasia, or congenital absence of the radius may also be defined in terms of hemimelia. Other descriptive terms such as ectromelia and peromelia are used for a variety of reduction defects and 'amputation' is used to indicate any absence of a distal part through developmental failure. Most of the terms, therefore, require further qualification if a precise meaning is to be conveyed. 'Intrauterine amputation' should be confined to the rare occasion in which it can be shown that there has been mechanical severance of a formed limb. Some amputations appear to be related to congenital constriction bands (see below).

Treatment

A long range plan of orthopedic management should be explained to the parents. In the first year, severe deformities may require vigorous physiotherapy with splinting and corrective plaster casts to avoid contractures. Enough time out of corrective devices must be allowed to encourage use of the part. Minor surgery may be indicated, such as excision of the rudimentary floating thumb associated with radial aplasia. A prosthesis may be fitted after secure sitting balance has been achieved. A passive device assists prehension movements and crawling, gives better balance and may allow the child to feel more 'whole'. At 2–3 years the child, successful with a passive device, may be considered for a voluntary opening appliance, when a period of special training is necessary. When significant deformity is increasing in spite of conservative measures, soft tissue procedures or arthroplasty may be required to achieve realignment. At 4–5 years, when considerable growth has occurred and cooperation is more predictable, major reconstructive surgery may be appropriate.

Genetic counseling

For the large majority of congenital limb defects the recurrence risk for siblings is negligible. For a minority this risk may be high (roughly 1 in 10) or very high (between 1 in 4 and 1 in 2). Similar malformations may have different recurrence risks in different families. Within any one family the same gene may produce different malformations so that firm prediction of future defects cannot be made from knowledge of existing ones.

CONGENITAL HEMIHYPERTROPHY

Asymmetrical overgrowth of unknown etiology may involve the whole of one side of the body or be limited in extent (e.g. predominant enlargement of the leg) (Fig. 24.2). The tissues are structurally and functionally normal. There may be associated defects such as mental retardation, hypertrophy of ipsilateral paired internal organs, and, rarely, an association with Wilms' tumor or adrenal carcinoma. With short stature, elevated gonadotropins, and anomalous sexual development the condition is described as Silver–Russell syndrome (p. 1015). The abnormality may be evident at birth, become more marked with growth, and accentuate at puberty. Congenital hypertrophy has to be differentiated from regional overgrowth due to neurofibromatosis, hemangiomas or lymphangiomas.

CONGENITAL HEMIATROPHY

Unilateral growth failure usually presents as an orthopedic problem due to short, slim, but otherwise normal limbs. An elevated shoe on the dwarfed side is required and later tibial

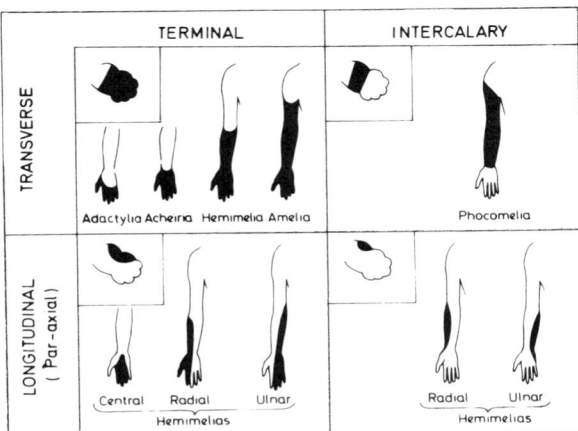

Fig. 24.1 Anatomical classification of limb defects. Note: (a) dark areas represent missing portions; (b) insets represent the four major types of limb deficiency as seen in upper limb of human embryo aged 6 postovulatory weeks; (c) 'hemimelia' is a primary description for three different types of defect and requires further qualification; (d) an analogous description applies to the lower limbs. (After O'Rahilly 1969.)

Table 24.1   Classification of hand defects (after Temtamy & McKusick 1969)

Categories	As an isolated malformation	Inheritance	As part of a syndrome
Category I – absence deformities			
Terminal transverse defects	Aphalangia, adactylia, acheiria amelia, transverse hemimelia acheiropody (Brazilian type)	Sporadic Mostly sporadic Recessive	Aglossia – adactylia Ankyloglossum superius syndrome With micrognathism (Hanhart) With skull, scalp defects
Radial defects	Terminal or intercalary radial hemimelias of various degrees (phocomelia was also included in this group)	Mostly sporadic	Acrofacial dysostosis Fanconi panmyelophthisis Radius-platelet hypoplasia With craniosynostosis In trisomy 17/18 Absent thumb with ring D2 chromosome With congenital heart lesion (Holt–Oram) Thalidomide syndrome
Ulnar defects	Terminal or intercalary ulnar hemimelias	No genetic pattern	Cornelia de Lange syndrome Weyers oligodactyly syndrome
Split hand, split foot defects	Central longitudinal terminal hemimelia (lobster-claw) Deficiency of radial rays with no cleft (monodactylic type)	Some sporadic, some dominant	With cleft lip and palate With anodontia With mandibulofacial dysostosis With perceptive deafness With anonychia With congenital nystagmus, fundal changes and cataracts
Category II – bradydactyly			With absent pectoralis major (Poland)
Type A	Middle phalanges: A_1 all digits, A_2 index and 2nd toe, A_3 5th finger		Mongolism (type A_3 brachydactyly) Sorsby syndrome (type B) — type D Heart–hand syndrome of Tabatznick Rubinstein syndrome
Type B	All digits, middle and terminal phalanges		
Type C	Middle and proximal phalanges fingers 2 and 3	Dominant	Turner's syndrome Albright hereditary osteodystrophy
Type D	Terminal phalanges short and broad in great toes and thumbs ('stub thumbs')		Silver–Russell syndrome — type E Biemond syndrome 1
Type E	Shortened metacarpals and metatarsals		With renal and other anomalies
Category III – syndactyly			
Type I	Fingers 3 and 4 ± toes 2 and 3		type I Apert II Vogt
Type II	Fingers 3 and 4 + polydactyly Toes 4 and 5 + polydactyly		Acrocephalosyndactyly
Type III	Fingers 4 and 5, feet unaffected	Dominant	III IV Waardenburg V Pfeiffer
Type IV	Complete bilateral + 6 digits and 6 metacarpals (Haas type)		
Type V	With metacarpal and metatarsal fusion		Oculodentodigital dysplasia
Category IV – polydactyly			
Postaxial	Type A – well-formed extra digit articulating	Dominant with marked penetrance	Ellis–van Creveld Infantile thoracic dystrophy (Jeune)
	Type B – poorly formed digit or skin tag	Complex genetic pattern	Laurence–Moon–Biedl Biemond syndrome II D1 trisomy With mental retardation (Oliver) With median cleft upper lip With hydrocephalus, polycystic kidneys
Preaxial	Thumb (mostly unilateral) Triphalangeal thumb	Sporadic	
	Triphalangeal thumb with tibial defect + preaxial polydactyly of toes	Dominant	Acrocephalopoly syndactyly (Carpenter)
	Thumb replaced by 1 or 2 triphalangeal digits Polysyndactyly		Polysyndactyly with peculiar skull shape Orofacial digital syndrome – type II (Mohr)
Category V – contracture deformities			
	Camptodactyly	Dominant	Craniocarpotarsal dystrophy – 'whistling face' syndrome Camptodactyly, pectus carinatum, ptosis, hypogonadism and multiple osteochrondritis dissecans
Category VI – symphalangism			
	Proximal Distal	Dominant	Diastrophic dysplasia Along with brachydactyly type A, C, E

Miscellaneous hand malformations are associated with a variety of other inherited syndromes such as: microphthalmos, anophthalmos; orofacial digital (OFD) syndrome type I (Gorlin); focal dermal hypoplasia (FDH); syndrome of cleft lip palate, popliteal pterygium, digital and genital anomalies; achondrogenesis, and the syndrome of complex brachydactyly with aplasia of the fibula.

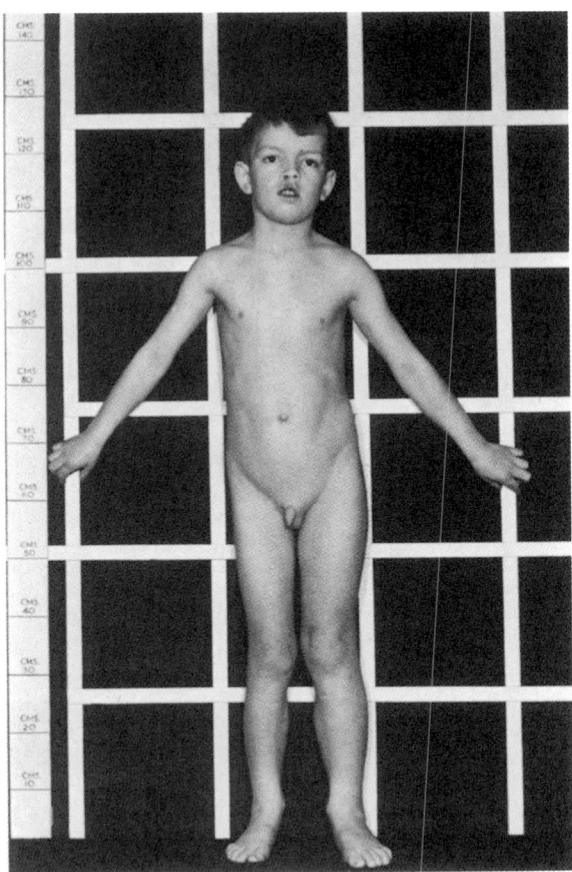

Fig. 24.2   Hemihypertrophy.

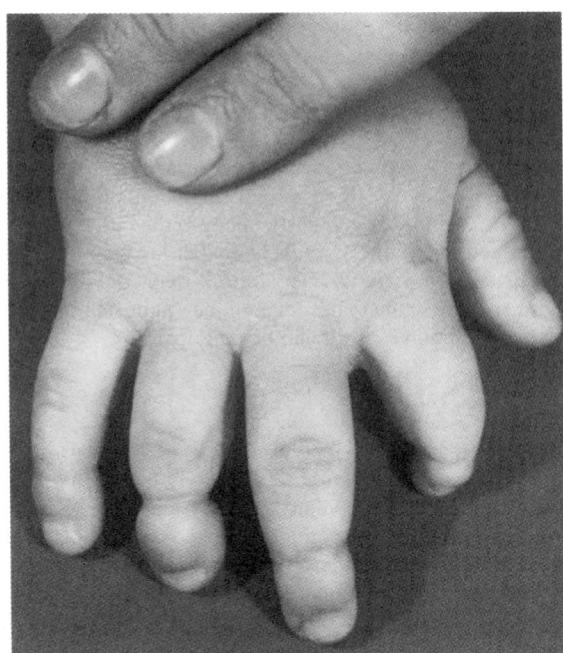

Fig. 24.3   Constriction bands.

SYNDACTYLY

Fusion of digits (Fig. 24.4) varies from a cutaneous web to synostosis and is somewhat more common in the foot than the hand. Various forms of hand syndactyly are described, all inherited as autosomal dominant, and some as components of

lengthening, or epiphyseal arrest on the normal side, may be indicated to equalize final leg lengths. This condition is of unknown etiology and has to be differentiated from wasting secondary to neuromuscular disease.

CONGENITAL CONSTRICTION BANDS

Ring-like constriction may affect any part of a limb (Fig. 24.3) with the legs more commonly involved than the arms. The constrictions may be single or multiple, shallow (affecting skin and subcutaneous tissue) or deep (through to bone). Distal parts may be swollen or edematous. Severely affected hands or feet may show syndactyly or terminal transverse defects. Superficial grooves require no treatment, deeper bands are divided and excised by Z-plasty.

SYMPHALANGISM

Ankylosis across interphalangeal joints occurs as a failure of segmentation of the primitive bony anlage. Before fusion, the bones appear separate on X-ray. Proximal and distal forms are described most commonly in both hands with resultant brachydactyly. Coalition of joints in the feet may coexist. There is stiffness, immobility and impaired function in the affected parts which may be amenable to surgery. Symphalangism is inherited as a dominant and may be part of a syndrome (Table 24.1).

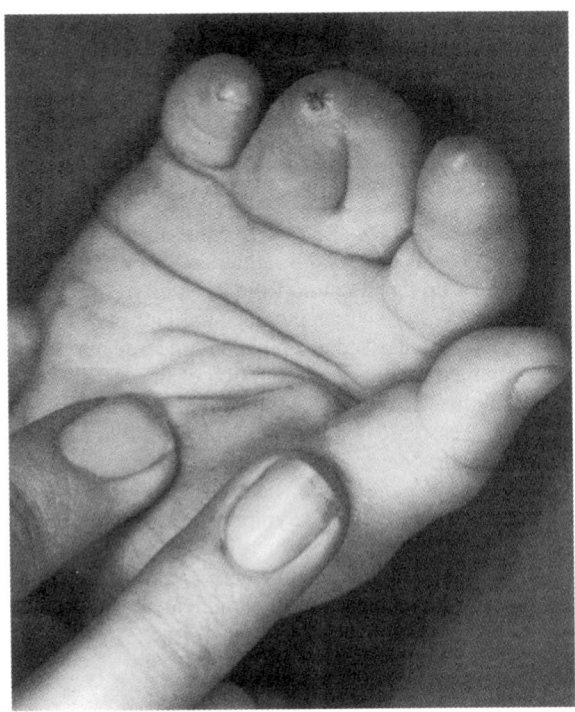

Fig. 24.4   Syndactyly (secondary to constriction bands).

syndromes (Table 24.1). From a surgical point of view, fusion of digits can be separated into two types:

1. those in which the digits are otherwise normal
2. those in which there are associated skeletal abnormalities.

In the first type separation with skin grafting is carried out at about 4 years of age. Where a long finger is being distorted by attachment to a short finger, early operation is indicated.

In the second type the small webbed hand is the most common, and is usually unilateral. Separation may be requested for cosmetic reasons but should not be undertaken unless a satisfactory functional result can be anticipated.

POLYDACTYLY

Extra digits on hands or feet vary from a fleshy protrusion to partial or complete duplication. Polydactyly has been extensively subdivided and may be associated with a wide range of syndromes (Table 24.1). Small fleshy digital nubbins or flail digits should be excised within the first few months for cosmetic reasons, to avoid interference with the application of splints, and to provide a smooth stump for a later prosthesis. If the supernumerary digit is more firmly fixed with tendons and joints, removal should be delayed until the parts have grown to allow adequate dissection and careful reconstruction of capsules and ligaments, avoiding injury to remaining growth centers and malalignment of remaining digits.

BRACHYDACTYLY

Short fingers or toes may be due to reduced metacarpal length, absence or abnormal segmentation of phalanges, or bony ankylosis. Several types are described which may occur in association with other defects (Table 24.1). Occasionally, surgery may lessen the disability, for example by removal of nonfunctional digits.

CONGENITAL LIMB MALFORMATIONS AFFECTING THE UPPER LIMBS PREDOMINANTLY

MADELUNG'S DEFORMITY

This involves a characteristic wrist deformity with posterior bowing of the lower end of the radius and a prominence of the head of the ulna on the dorsum of the wrist giving an appearance of subluxation. X-ray features include shortening of the radius, a triangular-shaped distal radial epiphysis underdeveloped on the ulnar side, and a triangular configuration of the carpal bones with the lunate at the apex (Fig. 24.5). The condition is frequently bilateral, has been more commonly reported in females, and may show a dominant mode of inheritance. The defect is probably one part of the more generalized disorder of dyschondrosteosis (Leri–Weill disease) (p. 1581). Symptoms of joint pain are liable to occur at adolescence and may be related to the growth spurt. If deformity is severe or symptoms of pain and weakened grasp are marked, corrective osteotomy may be indicated.

RADIOULNAR SYNOSTOSIS (Fig. 24.6)

This is usually proximal in site and associated with poorly developed pronator and supinator muscles. It is often bilateral,

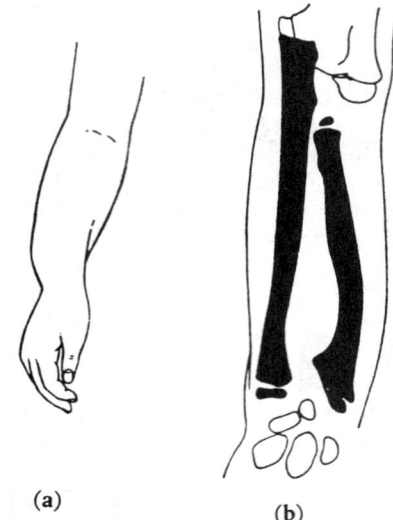

(a)   (b)

Fig. 24.5 Madelung's deformity: (**a**) characteristic wrist deformity caused by dislocation of the inferior ulnocarpal joint; (**b**) premature fusion of the lower end of the radius with a disproportionately long ulna. (From Wynne-Davies 1973, with permission.)

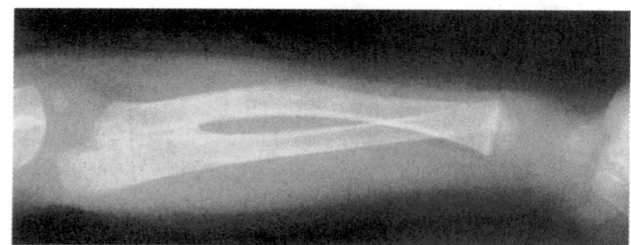

Fig. 24.6 Radioulnar synostosis.

may show a familial incidence, and has been frequently encountered in XXXY chromosome aberrations. Impaired forearm rotation may be partly corrected by resection of the synostosis.

SPRENGEL'S SHOULDER

On one side the scapula is fixed in an abnormally high position due to failure of descent during fetal development (Fig. 24.7). It may be attached to the cervical spine by a fibrous or bony connection, and the shoulder girdle muscles may be hypoplastic. There is limitation of shoulder abduction, and occasionally signs of brachial plexus compression. There may be other malformations such as cervical ribs, hemivertebrae, Klippel–Feil syndrome, and scoliosis. Physiotherapy is indicated to achieve maximum mobility. If there is significant functional or cosmetic disability, surgical procedures are available to release and refixate the scapula and this is best undertaken between 4 and 7 years of age.

CLINODACTYLY

Bony irregularity or defects in tendon and joint formation cause lateral, medial or flexion deformity of one or more fingers, often with associated brachydactyly. The little finger is most commonly

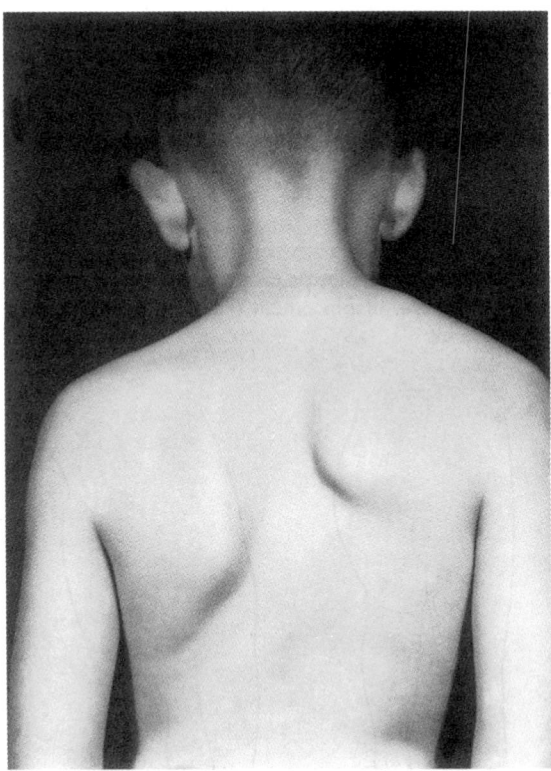

Fig. 24.7   Sprengel's shoulder.

affected. The disorder shows dominant inheritance. In severe cases, hand surgery involving osteotomies and soft tissue release may be indicated to improve function.

CAMPTODACTYLY

This is one form of congenital contracture of the hand affecting the fingers, particularly the fifth, seen more commonly in girls and with a tendency to increasing deformity at adolescence. It is usually bilateral. It may be sporadic or autosomal dominant and may be part of a syndrome (Table 24.1). There appears to be a web contracture of the skin with underlying tight fibrous bands. Corrective splinting before the age of 2 may correct and improve the condition, and release of the sublimis may assist correction in the younger child.

CONGENITAL TRIGGER FINGER

This is one of the commonest hand disorders in children. There is a fixed flexion deformity of the terminal interphalangeal joint, usually in the thumb and frequently bilateral. Painless loss of passive extension of the interphalangeal joint is demonstrated. Of those presenting in the first year of life, about one-third resolve spontaneously. If the condition persists, incision of the stenosed tendon sheath may allow free mobility and prevent contractures.

OTHER CONGENITAL FLEXION CONTRACTURES

Volar skin webs over the metacarpophalangeal and interphalangeal joints limit finger flexion and may be associated with defective finger extensors. Flexion deformities of the hands are a common feature in trisomy 17/18. Congenital shortness of deep flexor tendons has been described as a dominant inheritance. Soft tissue contractures are a major secondary problem in congenital deformities such as radius aplasia (radial club hand).

CONGENITAL LIMB MALFORMATIONS AFFECTING THE LOWER LIMBS PREDOMINANTLY

CONGENITAL PSEUDARTHROSIS AND TIBIAL BOWING

Congenital posterior bowing of the tibia, often with associated talipes calcaneovalgus, has a good prognosis with a tendency to correction with growth. There is no liability to fracture or pseudarthrosis. Congenital anterior bowing is evident at birth and tends to fracture or form pseudarthrosis with the start of weightbearing. Fibrous dysplasia may be evident at birth as a cystic area at the junction of the lower and middle thirds of the tibia. Fracture and pseudarthrosis may occur in the second or third year of life. The disorder may be dominant in association with neurofibromatosis. The prognosis for bone union is good. In congenital pseudarthrosis of the tibia (Fig. 24.8) there is a major defect at birth, with fracture, fibrous defect in tibia and fibula, sclerotic bone and absent medullary canal. Neurofibromatosis is the usual cause and other neurocutaneous stigmata may develop. Excision and bone grafting with internal fixation is recommended but the prognosis is poor with frequent refractures.

CONGENITAL DISLOCATION OF THE HIP

Types

An early developmental defect causing marked structural change in the acetabulum and upper femur with dislocation of the hip joint has been named 'teratologic' dislocation. The acetabulum is small and shallow, the femoral head distorted and the neck shortened with lack of normal anteversion. The capsule is thickened and adherent and reduction of the dislocation difficult

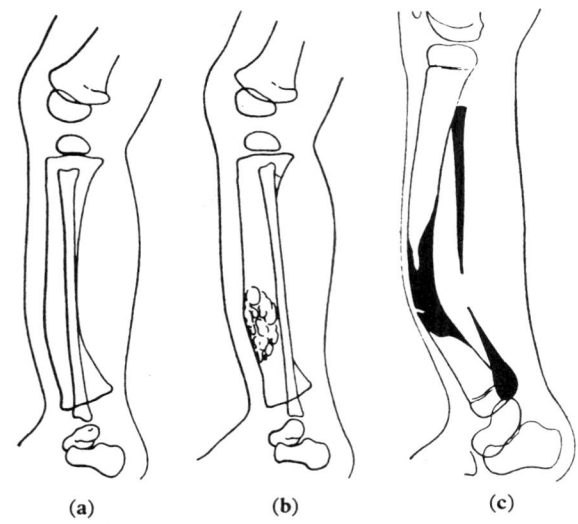

Fig. 24.8   Tibia: (**a**) congenital anterior bowing which may fracture in early infancy; (**b**) fibrous dysplasia – may fracture in early infancy but bone union is not difficult; (**c**) congenital pseudarthrosis with partial absence of fibula – bone union difficult. (From Wynne-Davies 1973, with permission.)

or impossible. This is often part of a generalized disorder such as arthrogryposis multiplex congenita, and a similar picture is commonly seen in myelomeningocele. Comparable changes may occur after some years in children with untreated simple or 'typical' congenital dislocation of the hip (see below).

These advanced disorders have to be differentiated from the much commoner dislocation unassociated with gross structural pathology in the joint. This type is also present at birth when the femoral head may lie outwith the acetabulum (dislocated hip) or may be induced by manipulation to ride over the posterior lip of the acetabulum (dislocatable, unstable or lax hip). There is abnormal laxity of the joint capsule and elongation of the ligamentum teres. The osseous roof of the acetabulum may be shallow, but the cartilaginous cup is intact and provides a normal socket. The femur is often excessively anteverted.

Etiology

Genetic factors operate to some extent in the common type of dislocation but the inheritance is complex. The risk to first degree relatives of female patients is about 1 in 15 for females, and 1 in 100 for males. For first degree relatives of male patients the risks are thought to be appreciably higher. Mechanical factors may be important, as shown by the increased incidence in babies who have been born in the breech position. The incidence is the same in infants born by cesarean section, which supports the belief that the normal birth process does not contribute to the dislocation. Undue ligamentous laxity has been attributed to exposure of the fetus to high concentrations of the normal fibrous tissue softening hormones of the mother.

Incidence

The generally accepted incidence of persistently dislocated hip is of the order of 1.25 per 1000. A higher incidence (4 per 1000) is found in the immediate newborn period with a subsequent fall due to spontaneous recovery (see below). Girls are affected some six times more frequently than boys, and the left hip more than the right for reasons unknown. A low incidence in babies of low birthweight may be due to their premature delivery excluding them from the joint-relaxing effects of maternal hormones in the last few weeks of pregnancy. Regional differences in incidence may be explained partly by varying criteria of diagnosis but there appear to be areas of high incidence (e.g. northern Italy). People of Negro race and those accustomed to carrying their infants astride the mother's back have a lower incidence. In some series a seasonal variation with increased incidence during the winter months has been described.

Diagnosis

The diagnosis of congenital dislocation of the hip is made by routine physical examination of the newborn, as described on page 110. In most series reporting the follow-up of neonatal screening for congenital dislocation of the hip, occasional cases appear to be missed. These may be failures of the initial examination technique or possibly represent genuine late-occurring dislocation. The need for repeated hip examination, e.g. at infant welfare clinics, until a child is walking normally is evident. Increased vigilance is required where there is a positive family history of dislocated hip.

Beyond 2 or 3 months of age the characteristic instability of the joint may be lost and there is more likely to be limited abduction of the hip and asymmetrical skin folds.

Persistent dislocation (missed diagnosis or failure of splinting) and late onset subluxations are associated with permanent dysplastic changes at the hip. An unstable waddling gait and a positive Trendelenburg test (Fig. 24.9) are evident.

The place of radiology in the diagnosis of congenital dislocation of the hip is controversial. Our current practice is to obtain a single anteroposterior radiograph of the pelvis with the legs parallel. Lateral displacement (see Fig. 24.10) is suggestive of an unstable hip.

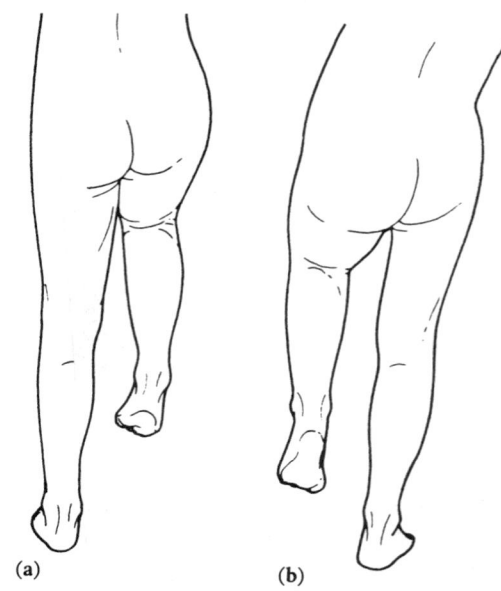

(a)   (b)

Fig. 24.9 Trendelenburg's test. Bearing weight on the normal left leg causes the pelvis to tilt up with elevation of the opposite buttock. Standing on the right leg with unstable hip causes the pelvis to tilt down, the buttock falls, and a compensatory scoliosis develops. (From Hendrickse et al 1991, with permission.)

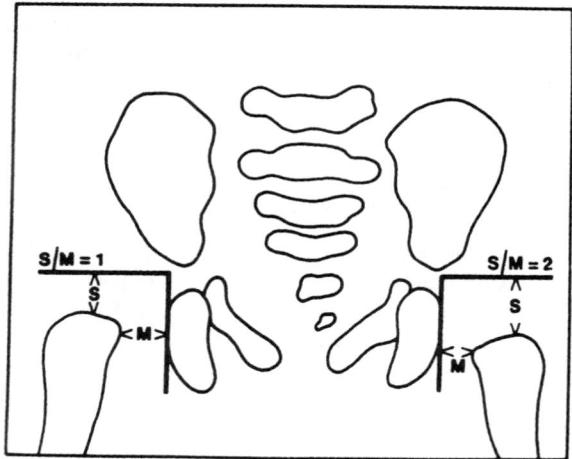

Fig. 24.10 Method of measuring radiographs. The medial gap (M) and superior gap (S) are measured in millimeters. In the stable hip the ratio S/M = 2. Progressive instability produces a ratio that approximates to 1. (From Macnicol 1990, with permission.)

Ultrasound examination of the hip has proved to be a valid alternative and has the advantage of showing the cartilaginous areas of the joint and revealing dynamic instability during manipulation of the hip. Ultrasound is also useful to monitor the quality of reduction and degree of stability on treatment.

Treatment

The treatment of teratologic dislocation (see above) is usually by skeletal traction followed by open reduction. In simple (typical) dislocation, the diagnosis should be made in the newborn period (see p. 110) and treatment started at once. In this the hips are held in at least 90° of flexion and in 60° abduction which should be achieved without force. If this degree of hip abduction is not possible an adductor tenotomy should be considered. Various splints are available to maintain the required position and the Malmö design is illustrated in Figure 24.11. This is a malleable plastic-covered splint which can be bent to fit the baby and to retain the hip joints in the required degree of abduction. The lower struts of the splint should be wide enough to allow the thighs to move forward through an arc of 30° from the fully abducted position. The baby must not be taken out of the splint. Care of pressure areas should be ensured, and the splint readjusted at regular outpatient attendances at 1 or 2 week intervals. The splint should be retained for 8–12 weeks, with regular reexaminations thereafter till 6 months of age. Follow-up is advised at 1 year and until the child is seen to be walking normally and is known to have radiologically normal hip joints. The Pavlik harness can be used in cases where there is limitation of abduction of the hip at birth or where an abduction splint is poorly tolerated (Fig. 24.12). Because of flexibility of freedom of movement it may be preferred in all cases from birth.

Hips which are clearly unstable (dislocatable), but not frankly dislocated are usually splinted for about 8 weeks, but examination at 2-weekly intervals may show spontaneous recovery and allow early relaxation of splinting. Where there is a family history of congenital dislocation an early X-ray is justified. If there is doubt about the stability of the joint, splinting should be continued longer. Dislocated hips which cannot be reduced in a splint, or hips which dislocate on mobilization usually have an inverted limbus which will be seen in arthrography. Successful reduction follows excision of the limbus. Persistent anteversion may correct with weightbearing or may require derotation osteotomy.

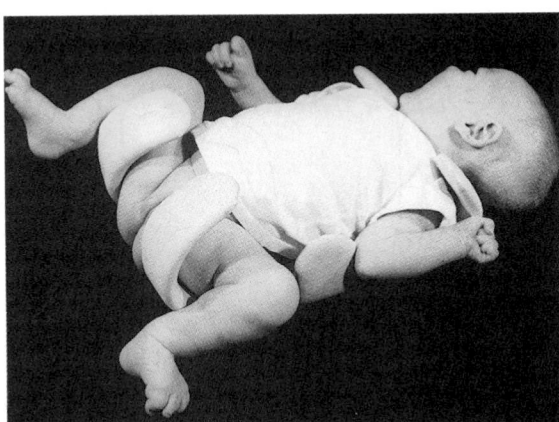

Fig. 24.11   Malmö splint for congenital dislocation of the hip.

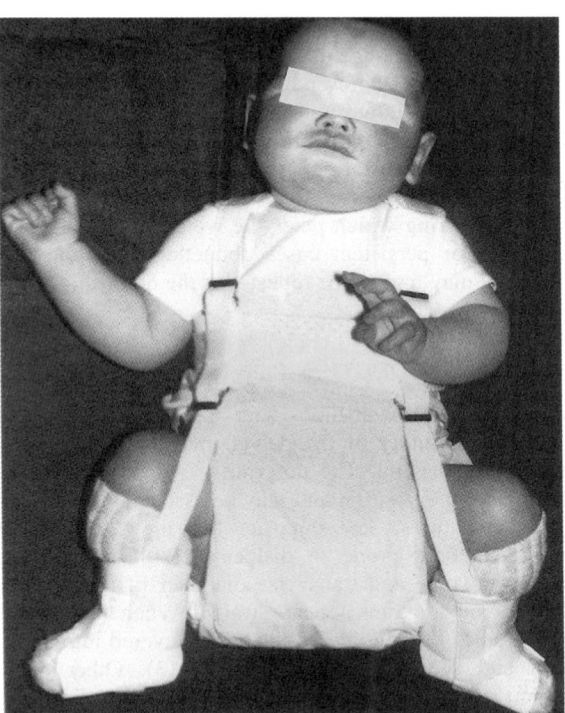

Fig. 24.12   Pavlik harness for congenital dislocation of the hip.

The treatment of teratologic dislocation, the missed or the neglected simple dislocation, presents considerable problems in management. The femoral head has a relatively fixed displacement laterally and superiorly and abduction is limited with adductor contracture. The head of the femur has to be brought down by a period of traction, then relocated by gradual abduction with subsequent immobilization in a hip spica. Adductor tenotomy may be required to aid reduction. The plaster cast is maintained for about 6 months. Reduction of the dislocation may fail due, for example, to distortions of the joint capsule, an inverted limbus, or accumulation of aberrant fibrofatty tissue within the socket. These may be evident in an arthrogram and are an indication for open reduction. In late untreated dislocation conservative treatment is inadequate and surgical correction is necessary.

Avascular necrosis of the femoral head due to a splint which is too tight, allowing little movement of the joint, may complicate congenital dislocation, and forced manipulations of the joint must be avoided. Late presenting congenital dislocation of the hip is associated with a high incidence of premature osteoarthritis.

Handicap due to congenital dislocation of the hip is preventable by early diagnosis and treatment based on thorough and meticulous routine examination of all infants in the newborn period and throughout early infancy.

CONGENITAL COXA VARA

Varus deformity of the hip with decrease in the angle between neck and shaft occurs as a localized abnormality (congenital, infantile, or developmental coxa vara), or as part of a generalized bone dysplasia (e.g. achondroplasia, Morquio's disease). These conditions should be differentiated from coxa vara secondary to acquired lesions such as avascular necrosis, osteomyelitis, or severe rickets. The congenital form may not be noted until the child walks. The picture resembles that of untreated dislocation of the hips with a waddling gait and exaggerated lumbar lordosis, particularly when the coxa vara is bilateral. The varus deformity increases with weightbearing and early treatment in mild cases is directed at relieving pressure on the proximal femur by a caliper with an ischial ring which takes the weight off the hip joint. In more severe or persistent cases abduction osteotomy will be required and may have to be repeated if the deformity recurs.

CONGENITAL ABDUCTION CONTRACTURE OF THE HIP

Asymmetry of the lower limbs with apparent shortening on one side (due to obliquity of the pelvis) may be due to abduction contracture of the hip. The deformity is apparently caused by faulty intrauterine position and may be associated with torticollis or foot deformities. The opposite hip may show adduction contracture and is prone to dislocate. With the affected hip abducted the spine and transverse diameter of the pelvis are at right angles and the trunk appears straight. When the affected limb is brought in to the midline, the pelvis is levered into an oblique position and scoliosis results (Fig. 24.13). Other causes of congenital pelvic obliquity such as vertebral anomalies should be excluded and the condition differentiated from congenital dislocation of the hip by manipulative tests (see above) and by radiographic examination.

Passive stretching exercises are begun as soon as the diagnosis is made. With the baby on his face the affected hip is extended in a posterior direction, followed by adduction of the hip with internal rotation (Fig. 24.14). Correction is usually possible within

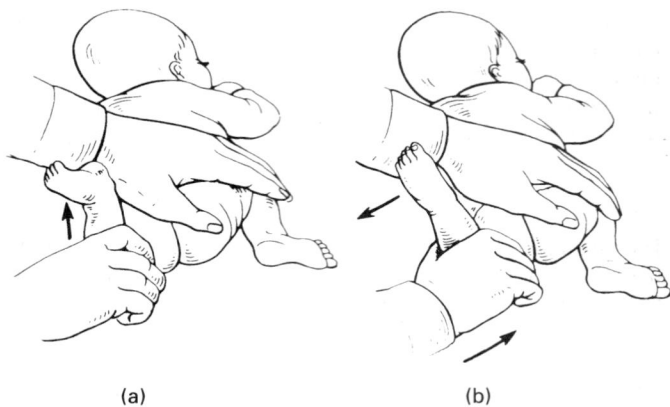

(a)

(b)

Fig. 24.14 Passive stretching exercises for congenital abduction contracture of the hip: (**a**) maximally extend the affected hip by lifting the thigh towards the ceiling; (**b**) adduct the thigh and internally rotate hips. Perform exercise 20 times, 4 to 6 times per day. (Redrawn from Tachdjian 1967.)

a few months, but severe contractures may require more intensive physiotherapy followed by some weeks of fixation in a bilateral hip spica.

FEMORAL TORSION

At birth, the femoral head is normally anterior to the mediolateral plane of the femoral shaft making an angle of about 40°. With growth and development the hips take up a more extended position, and the ligaments and capsule mold the bone, reducing the angle finally to about 12°. Diminished anterior positioning of the femoral head is associated with excessive tightening in the anterior ligaments of the hip joint which restricts external rotation and causes internal femoral torsion (anteversion). On standing erect the patellas are turned in towards the midline and the child has a toe-in gait. This appearance has to be differentiated from inturning due to tibial torsion or metatarsus varus. The femoral torsion is aggravated by the common sitting posture of these children (Fig. 24.15) and may be helped by insisting on a cross-legged position with exercises consisting of downward pressure on the knees to externally rotate the hips. Femoral anteversion may lead to an increased incidence of degenerative arthritis of hip

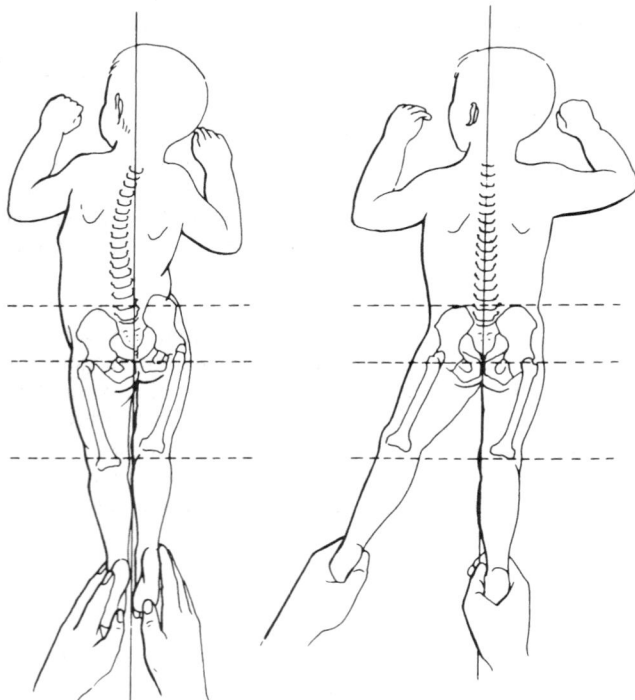

Fig. 24.13 Congenital abduction contracture of the hip. (Redrawn from Tachdjian 1967.)

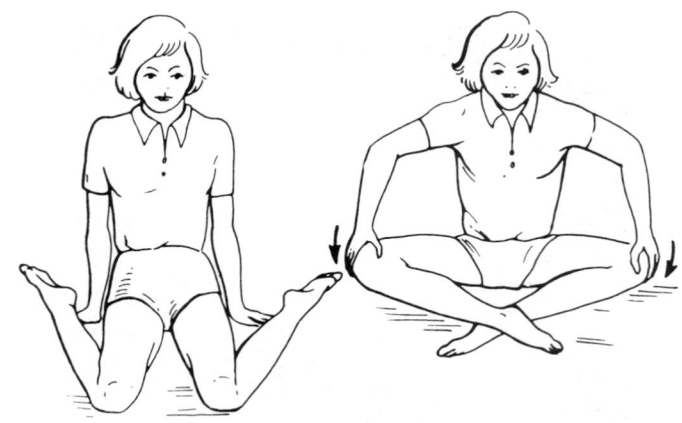

Fig. 24.15 Sitting posture in femoral torsion and corrective cross-legged position. (Redrawn from Connolly et al 1970.)

and knee joints, which emphasizes the need for early recognition and corrective physiotherapy.

GENU VALGUM (KNOCK-KNEE)

The knees are deviated medially so that with the child standing erect, there is a wide space between the medial malleoli (Fig. 24.16b). The ligaments of the knee joint, and often other joints, are abnormally lax and a degree of flat foot may coexist. The deformity is relatively common in the preschool child and mild cases often correct spontaneously. In one study about 20% of infants aged $3-3\frac{1}{2}$ years had a knock-knee of 5 cm or more and in only 2% of children was this degree of valgus evident at 7 years. Underlying pathology (such as rickets, epiphyseal dysplasia, or epiphyseal damage from trauma or infection) should be sought: if the intermalleolar distance with the child lying flat is greater than 9 cm; if the knock-knee is of unequal amount in the two legs; if the child is of short stature; or if there is a family history of bone deformity. Foot pronation is treated as outlined below. In severe and resistant deformities, operative correction may become necessary and may involve osteotomy or medial epiphyseal arrest.

GENU VARUM (BOW LEGS)

Prenatal bowing of the lower extremities is considered to be due to abnormal intrauterine posture. Single or multiple sites may be affected producing, for example, upper tibial angulation or more generalized bow leg deformity. The site of angulation may show internal cortical thickening on the concave aspect of the bone and the overlying skin may show dimpling. Gradual regression takes place in the years after birth but more severe deformities may persist into adult life. Manipulations, corrective plaster casts, and eventually osteotomies may then be necessary. Congenital bowing of the long bones is part of the syndrome of camptomelic dysplasia (p. 1572).

In the first few years of life a degree of bowing involving femora and tibia may be considered physiological (Fig. 24.16a). It may be associated with internal rotation of the tibia and a tendency to pigeon toe. Spontaneous correction usually occurs.

Genu varum in older children may be secondary to the various forms of rickets, osteogenesis imperfecta, chondrodysplasias, or infantile tibia vara (Blount's disease).

Correction of the deformities may be assisted by strong shoes with arch support and an outer sole wedge, and for more severe bow leg in young children the Denis Browne night shoe splint. In older children with severe deformity consideration may have to be given to corrective osteotomy below the tibial tubercle, or epiphyseal stapling at 8–10 years, before fusion of the growth plate occurs.

GENU RECURVATUM

Hyperextension at the knee with a tendency to backward dislocation may be evident at birth and may be associated with congenital hip dislocation or talipes equinovarus. In older children, genu recurvatum may occur with ligamentous laxity or secondary to neuromuscular disorders (e.g. poliomyelitis, cerebral palsy), or after damage to the tibial tubercle or anterior parts of the epiphyses at the knee (e.g. trauma, infection).

In the congenital form, early passive flexion at the knee is advised with care to ensure that movements are in the correct plane of the joint. Thereafter serial plasters are applied with increasing degrees of flexion, and finally bivalved casts with further physiotherapy. The aim is to promote shortening of the posterior part of the capsule. A brace to prevent recurrence of hyperextension may be required when weightbearing is commenced. With severe and resistant deformities, operative reduction may be indicated. Postparalytic deformities or those associated with irregular premature epiphyseal closure may require osteotomy, or sometimes epiphyseal arrest or stapling procedures. The mild deformity of ligamentous laxity may be improved by appropriate physiotherapy.

PATELLAR INSTABILITY

Congenital fixed dislocation of the patella is associated with quadriceps contracture, valgus knee deformity and external tibial rotation. It may be part of a generalized skeletal dysplasia.

In older children with habitual dislocation from various causes, the patella pulls over the lateral femoral condyle each time the knee is flexed, and activities are severely restricted.

Surgical release, realignment and fixation is usually indicated in these groups.

Recurrent patellar dislocation may also develop in adolescents with episodes of pain and the knee 'giving way'. There is often evidence of generalized joint laxity. As the condition usually improves with time, conservative treatment is indicated, with physiotherapy and a stabilizing orthosis if necessary.

NAIL PATELLA–(ILIAC HORN) SYNDROME

This consists of nail dystrophy (especially the thumb), hypoplastic patella, radial head dislocation, and in about one-third of cases pelvic abnormalities. The latter include flaring of the iliac crests and horn-like projections from the posterolateral surface of the iliac crest which are visible or palpable. The disorder is transmitted as an autosomal dominant. No specific treatment is indicated.

Ocular abnormalities including ptosis, strabismus, glaucoma and microcornea occur and in about half the patients there is proteinuria and a significant risk of progressive glomerulonephritis leading to renal failure (Ch. 17).

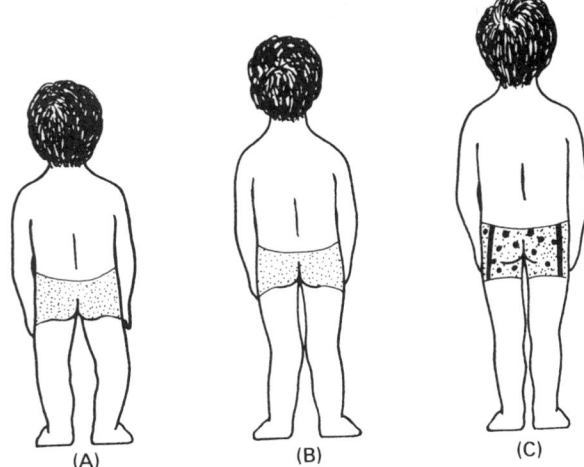

Fig. 24.16 Normal variation of stance with age: (**a**) genu varum, 18 months; (**b**) genu valgum, 3 years; (**c**) legs straight, 6 years.

POPLITEAL PTERYGIUM SYNDROME

There is a web in the popliteal fossa varying from a dense fibrous cord (which may contain the tibial nerve) to a prominent fold running the length of the limb. The toenails may be dysplastic, and associated defects are cleft palate with or without cleft lip, and salivary pits in the lower lip. The syndrome is inherited, usually as an autosomal dominant; intelligence is normal, but there is a wide range of other possible associated malformations.

TIBIAL TORSION

Internal tibial torsion is one of the causes of 'toeing-in' or 'pigeon toe'. Congenital internal tibial torsion is associated with genu varum, infantile tibia vara and talipes equinovarus. There is frequently limitation of rotation in the hip joint. Acquired torsion may develop in neuromuscular disorders. Passive stretching exercises for the hip and foot are recommended and shoes with arch support and outer sole wedges. In severe cases corrective plaster casts or the Denis Browne shoe splint may be used and in a few resistant cases osteotomy may be required.

Less commonly, external tibial torsion occurs and this may be associated with knock-knees. This deformity will usually respond to arch supports and inner heel wedges.

INFANTILE TIBIA VARA (BLOUNT'S DISEASE, OSTEOCHONDROSIS TIBIAE)

Marked internal rotation of the tibia with acute medial angulation may occur progressively with growth in a child who had 'physiological' bow legs. The upper tibial growth plate develops beaking on the medial side and later the tibial epiphysis is markedly distorted with changes ascribed to 'osteochondrosis'. The use of a Denis Browne night splint may prevent progression in the early stages but with established deformity realignment osteotomy may be required or more radical surgery on the tibial plateau.

TALIPES EQUINOVARUS (CLUB FOOT)

This relatively common deformity consists of fixed plantar flexion (equinus), inversion of the heel hindfoot and forefoot (varus), and adduction of the forefoot (Fig. 24.17), and in some the talus is small and underdeveloped. It may be associated with internal rotation of the tibia and muscle contractures or atrophy.

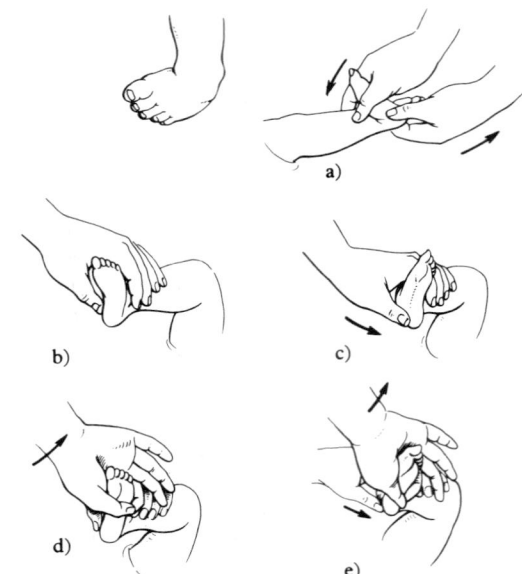

Fig. 24.17 Talipes equinovarus (top left) and corrective manipulation: (**a**) manipulation of foot out of equinus; (**b**) and (**c**) manipulation of foot out of varus; (**d**) manipulation of forefoot into abduction; (**e**) twisting of forefoot into eversion. (Redrawn from Tachdjian 1967.)

The congenital form has an incidence of about 1 per 1000 births, is commoner in males (2 : 1) and is bilateral in some 50% of cases. Familial cases are described which may be accounted for by an autosomal dominant with partial penetrance and a recurrence risk of about 10% for siblings.

Secondary clubfoot is seen with neuromuscular disorders, as in myelomeningocele, poliomyelitis, or cerebral palsy.

Manipulation of the foot should begin as soon as possible (Fig. 24.17) and the mother instructed in this. Correction must be gentle but repeated several times a day while position is maintained by adhesive strapping changed weekly and applied as in Figure 24.18. The treatment is continued to 3 months when, if the position is satisfactory, Denis Browne lace up boots with crossbar splint are used to age 1 year. Conservative treatment alone is likely to be adequate in only 30–50% of cases, and there is an increasing acceptance of the need to obtain the benefits of surgery early. If correction is unsatisfactory at 3 months, soft tissue release

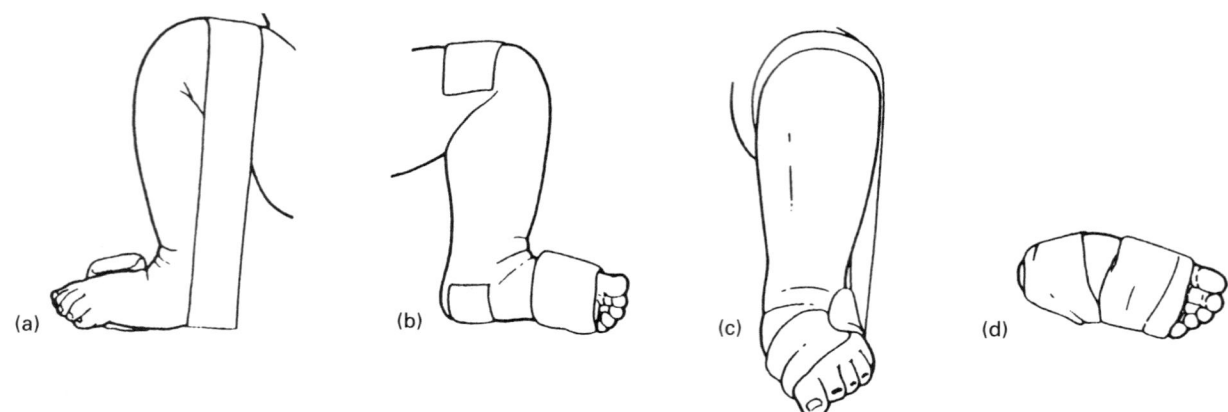

Fig. 24.18 Adhesive strapping for talipes equinovarus: (**a**) heel to lateral aspect of knee; (**b**) pad forefoot; (**c**) forefoot to lateral knee; (**d**) sole of foot. (From Hendrickse et al 1991, with permission.)

may be indicated with elongation of the tendo Achilles, posterior capsulotomy, and division of tight tendons such as tibialis posterior, flexor hallucis longus or flexor digitorum longus. Plaster of Paris fixation is maintained for a further 3 months, then Denis Browne boots used, with follow-up, till walking. Strong leather shoes with straight last and outer heel and sole wedges should be prescribed. The deformity may relapse in later childhood due to muscular imbalance between anterior tibial and peroneal group of muscles, or to shortening in the tendo Achilles in which case tendon transfer or lengthening operations may be indicated. In resistant club foot various forms of soft tissue release or tendon transplantation may allow correction and in later years severe or neglected cases may require osteotomies or arthrodeses to achieve a stable foot.

TALIPES CALCANEOVALGUS

In this less common variety of clubfoot, the foot is dorsiflexed and everted with soft tissue contractures over the dorsum of the foot. It may be evident in the newborn due to abnormal intrauterine position or it may be a persistent deformity due to neuromuscular imbalance as in spina bifida. Gentle passive stretching should be performed regularly but if the deformity is severe or persistent, Denis Browne splints or serial plaster casts may be required to achieve overcorrection into an equinovarus position. Later, when the child begins to walk, a pronated foot may persist, requiring appropriate treatment (see below).

PES PLANUS (FLAT, PRONATED OR VALGUS FOOT)

Types

Some degree of foot pronation is physiological in the early months of weightbearing. Persistent or excessive flattening of the medial longitudinal arch is most commonly due to lax ligaments with undue mobility at the midtarsal and subtalar joints. The heel is everted in valgus with diversion of the Achilles tendon, and the forefoot is commonly turned outwards (Fig. 24.19). There is often associated laxity at the knee with genu valgum. Some correction

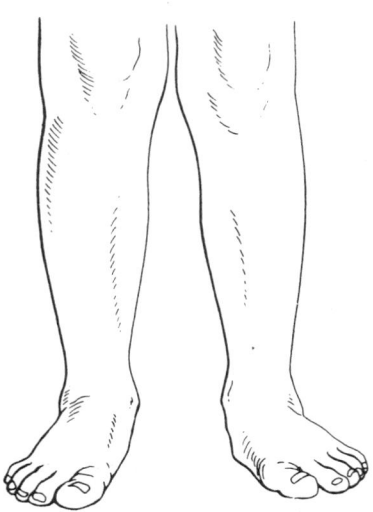

Fig. 24.19 Pes planus.

of this type of pes planus deformity is possible by pushing up on the arch of the foot or by having the child stand on tiptoe. In some older children, the arch appears normal when the foot is plantar flexed but with dorsiflexion an abnormally tight Achilles tendon fixes the os calcis. This results in undue leverage and movement in the tarsal joints with collapse of the longitudinal arch.

A painful persistent flatfoot with rigidity or hypermobility requires investigation. A fixed pes planus is seen when abnormal bars of bone, cartilage, or fibrous tissue cause fusion and rigidity of the subtalar or calcaneonavicular joints ('tarsal coalition'). Another rare form of fixed flat foot is caused by talonavicular dislocation with the talus taking up a vertical position ('congenital vertical talus'). The head of the bone presents a prominence on the sole of the foot and there is a rounded ('rocker-bottom') deformity. This latter disturbance may also be caused by faulty forceful manipulation of a talipes equinovarus club foot. Pathological flat foot may also be associated with neurological disorders such as cerebral palsy, spinal dysraphism and poliomyelitis.

The child with pes planus may avoid active games, show undue fatigability, or complain of sore legs. Tarsal coalition tends to present in later childhood with pain and limited exercise tolerance.

Management

Mild pes planus in young children usually improves with time: when flat feet are pain free, mobile and without evidence of bony or neurological abnormality treatment is hardly ever required. The foot may be strengthened by encouragement to walk barefoot and to walk on the outer aspect of the foot as a specific exercise. Shoes, when worn, should be strong and give good support to the foot. In severe early deformities a Denis Browne bar bent to turn the foot into inversion will stimulate arch development as the child kicks. In older children inversion exercises should be continued along with foot grasping exercises (i.e. lifting objects with the feet). Postural correction can be provided by a strong leather shoe with an inner heel wedge and an extension of the heel-piece anteriorly on the medial side. If a tendency to pigeon toe is aggravated by this, an outer sole wedge can be added. A tight Achilles tendon may be stretched by appropriate exercises. Surgical removal of a bony bridge may be indicated in tarsal coalition or open reduction and fixation of talonavicular dislocation in congenital vertical talus. In persistent severe pes planus a stable foot may be achieved by triple arthrodesis, which is performed when skeletal maturity is well advanced, preferably over 15 years of age.

METATARSUS VARUS AND HALLUX VALGUS

Medial deviation of the forefoot (Fig. 24.20) is often seen in the normal newborn as an extension of the intrauterine posture and this is likely to correct spontaneously. If the varus cannot be passively corrected, true deformity exists. Gentle stretching should be commenced in the neonatal period holding the heel in a neutral position. Later a Denis Browne bar may be fitted between the shoes to ensure that the feet are rotated outwards. Alternatively, serial plaster casts can be applied and if internal tibial torsion (p. 1554) coexists, the casts may be extended above the knee. Care should be taken to avoid producing valgus of the

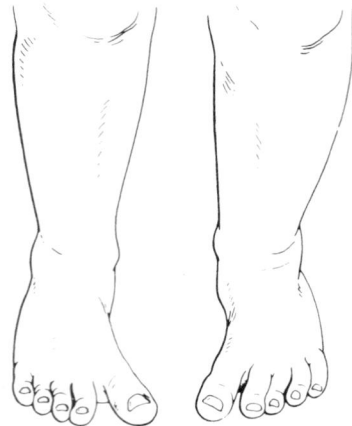

Fig. 24.20   Metatarsus varus.

heel. In the older child with an advanced deformity, metatarsal osteotomies and soft tissue release procedures may be necessary.

In metatarsus varus primus, only the first metatarsal is deviated. Treatment is as described above. This deformity tends to be overlooked and may lead to secondary deformity in later life as the great toe is pushed laterally producing a hallux valgus. Up to 20° valgus at the first metatarsopharyngeal joint is within normal limits but requires observation. Once the valgus angle is greater than 25°, progressive deformity is very likely and surgical correction of the hallux valgus deformity should be considered.

PES CAVUS (CLAW FOOT)

The foot is high-arched with the metatarsal heads pushed down, clawing of the toes, and often a degree of calcaneovarus (Fig. 24.21). The common idiopathic form may show a familial incidence with dominant inheritance. A cavus deformity due to muscular imbalance affecting intrinsic, peroneal, tibial, or Achilles tendon muscles is seen in neurological disorders such as spina bifida, poliomyelitis, Friedreich's ataxia, muscular dystrophy, peroneal muscular atrophy and some forms of cerebral palsy.

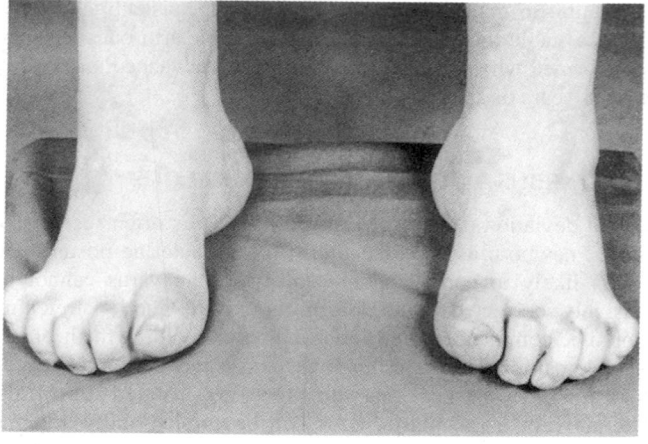

Fig. 24.21   Pes cavus with clawing of toes.

Conservative management includes exercises to increase the strength of intrinsic muscles and metatarsal pads to relieve pressure on the metatarsal heads. Surgical procedures may be directed at correction of the clawing, the cavus, or the varus deformity. Tendon transplant and plantar fascia release may be necessary and in older children osteotomies of tarsus, metatarsus and os calcis, or a triple arthrodesis may eventually be required.

STRUCTURAL DEFECTS OF THORAX AND SPINE

FUNNEL CHEST (PECTUS EXCAVATUM)

Depression of the sternum, often familial, is seldom evident at birth but appears worse in later childhood with decreased anteroposterior diameter of the chest, thoracolumbar kyphosis and rounded shoulders. There may be psychological effects. Impaired cardiorespiratory function is unlikely. A disfiguring defect in the young child may be treated by division of the xiphoid process and retrosternal ligament before fixed deformity has developed. In more advanced deformities, resection of costal cartilages and osteotomy at the point of angulation may be necessary.

PIGEON CHEST (PECTUS CARINATUM)

A prominent anterior projection of the sternum occurs with increased anteroposterior diameter of the chest. The deformity may cause psychological disturbance but probably no functional impairment. The cosmetic disability may lessen as breasts and pectoral muscles develop. In severe cases, resection of xiphoid and the angulated costal cartilages may be indicated.

SPLIT STERNUM

This varies from a notched xiphoid to a total cleft with absent sternum. Major defects frequently have associated anomalies such as abdominal wall defect, lung herniation, or ectopia cordis. In the latter malformation, the heart presents through the lower sternum or epigastrium either exposed completely or covered by skin and sometimes an intact pericardium. Often serious cardiac defects exist. Prognosis depends on the degree of cardiac displacement and severity of any associated congenital heart lesion. Thoracoplasty procedures may be attempted for large sternal defects.

CONGENITAL PSEUDARTHROSIS OF THE CLAVICLE

This is a rare defect, usually of the right clavicle, presenting as a painless swelling due to proliferating fibrous tissue. X-ray shows the bony defect and lack of callus formation. It has to be differentiated from clavicular fracture and craniocleidodysostosis. Surgery involves excision of fibrous tissue, bone grafting, and intramedullary pin fixation.

KLIPPEL–FEIL SYNDROME

There is a variable degree and extent of fusion in the cervical spine involving the vertebral bodies, lateral masses, joints and posterior arches, and sometimes an associated cervical spina bifida. The neck is short with restricted movements, webbing of soft tissues, low hair line and sometimes torticollis. Neurological involvement may occur due to cord or root compression. Malformations such as thoracic hemivertebrae, fused ribs or Sprengel's deformity may coexist. Profound deafness, micrognathia, cleft palate, Moebius' syndrome, syringomyelia, platybasia and congenital heart disease are other reported associations. Physiotherapy to obtain and maintain maximum mobility should be started as early as possible. Webbing and muscle contractures may be released surgically. An elevated scapula may be lowered and resection of upper ribs has been described.

CERVICAL RIBS

These are usually discovered incidentally at X-ray, are rarely symptomatic in children and require no treatment. In a few cases there may be signs of pressure on the subclavian artery, brachial plexus, or sympathetic nerves. Similar features can be produced by pressure from the anterior scalene muscle in the absence of cervical rib.

OCULOAURICULOVERTEBRAL DYSPLASIA (GOLDENHAR'S SYNDROME)

The vertebral anomalies in this disorder include synostoses, spina bifida, hemivertebrae, and cuneiform vertebrae. (See page 1564.)

DIASTEMATOMYELIA

This consists of a midline septum of fibrous tissue, cartilage, and bone which divides the neural canal and splits the spinal cord longitudinally. It is most common in lower thoracic and lumbar regions, and may be suspected in a child with neurological deficits such as lower limb pareses and bladder and bowel dysfunction (Ch. 14).

SPINA BIFIDA

Posterior defect occurs with failure of fusion of the vertebral arches. The milder forms (spina bifida occulta) may be indicated by an overlying skin defect. Larger spina bifidas may be associated with herniation of the meninges and cord to give a myelocele or meningomyelocele. An anterolateral defect can occur with failure of union of the vertebral body with the lateral masses. Herniation gives an anterior meningocele. Anterior spinal anomalies may be associated with a persistent neuroenteric communication (neuroenteric cyst). For management and neurological aspects of spina bifida see Chapter 14.

SACRAL AGENESIS

Aplasia of terminal spinal segments varies in extent. Severe cases with iliac bones approximating in the midline show flattened buttocks with dimples lateral to a short intergluteal fold. Rectal and X-ray examination confirms the defect. Associated congenital dislocation of the hips, talipes, and neurological deficit affecting bladder, bowel and lower limbs usually occurs. Visceral anomalies exist in about one-third of cases. This defect is rare but occurs with increased frequency in infants of diabetic mothers. Treatment is supportive with physiotherapy, orthopedic surgery and prostheses as necessary, and management of the neurological complications.

SPONDYLOLYSIS, SPONDYLOLISTHESIS

Spondylolysis is a congenital and probably inherited defect in the isthmus of a vertebral arch, particularly the fifth lumbar. It may be associated with spina bifida and other bony abnormalities of the lumbar spine and is usually asymptomatic. In some physically active adolescents a defect of the pars interarticularis appears to occur as a stress fracture and presents as low back pain or an instability syndrome. Anterior displacement of the affected vertebra and the vertebral column above it is referred to as spondylolisthesis. In addition to congenital dysplasia and trauma, causes include degenerative osteoarthritis and underlying bone pathology (infection, metastases, metabolic bone disease, etc.). Back pain, sciatica, and an increasing lumbar lordosis may develop. When displacement is marked or progressive, particularly if associated with neurological features, spinal fusion affords stability and relief of symptoms.

CONGENITAL HEMIVERTEBRAE

These arise through underdevelopment of one of the paired chondrification centers. Single or multiple vertebrae may be affected. Scoliosis is likely. In the thorax absence or fusion of ribs or lung hypoplasia, and in the lumbar region renal anomalies may coexist. Congenital heart disease and spinal dysraphism are known associations. When many spinal segments are involved, significant shortening of the trunk with dwarfing occurs. There is not usually any neurological involvement but a posteriorly placed hemivertebra can cause a severe kyphotic deformity with cord compression.

SCOLIOSIS

Postural scoliosis

This is usually mild and easily corrected with no rotation or fixed anatomical changes. It is most common in the lumbar spine as compensation for a short leg and disappears with the child sitting or with a corrective block under the foot. This curve is not progressive and does not in itself require treatment.

Structural scoliosis

In this the lateral curve is accompanied by vertebral rotation which is clinically apparent (Fig. 24.22). Idiopathic structural scoliosis is a condition diagnosed by exclusion of causes of secondary scoliosis (see below) which may prove difficult. Truly idiopathic scoliosis is classified into three groups according to the age of onset: infantile from 0 to 3 years, juvenile from 4 to 9 years, and adolescent from 10 to 15 years.

Infantile scoliosis is commoner in Europe than North America and is more common in males. The curve is usually in the thoracic region and convex to the left in over 80% of cases. It is frequently associated with plagiocephaly. Scoliosis should be considered if a newborn fails to show lateral trunk curvature equally to both sides on stimulation of the flank. Later the parents may notice the

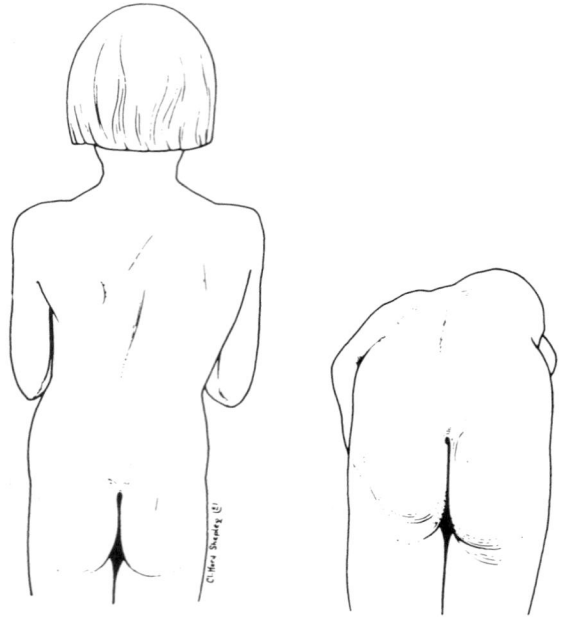

Fig. 24.22 Structural scoliosis with vertebral rotation shown by rib hump on bending forward. (From Wynne-Davies 1968.)

infant's asymmetrical posture, and permanent skin folds may develop over the concave side of the chest. Anteroposterior X-rays of the spine with the shoulders and pelvis forced laterally show limited movement of the scoliotic area towards the convex side. A scoliosis splint for correcting the spinal bend has been recommended, along with corrective movements and in advancing cases, spinal fusion at an age (over 10 years) when spinal growth is diminishing. Spontaneous resolution of the scoliosis by 1 year of age is thought to occur in over 50% of cases. The juvenile group is quantitatively the smallest and appears to have some characteristics of both infantile and adolescent forms.

The adolescent type is usually in a girl and it does not disappear spontaneously. The majority are midthoracic with 90% convex to the right. There is a distinct tendency to progression, especially if associated with compensatory curves. Asking the patient to touch the toes accentuates the asymmetry (Fig. 24.22). Daily stretching exercises and a restraining device such as the Milwaukee brace may prevent progression. X-rays are taken every 3–6 months and if an increasing fixed deformity develops, serial plaster casts, halopelvic traction, fixation rods or spinal fusion should be considered.

In severe kyphoscoliosis, chest movements may be so restricted as to cause alveolar hypoventilation. Pulmonary fibrosis and hypertension leading to cor pulmonale rarely occurs in childhood but this potential complication further emphasizes the need for early and effective orthopedic management.

Secondary scoliosis

Lateral curvature of the spine occurs with spinal vertebral anomalies (e.g. hemivertebrae), or with other defects such as Sprengel's shoulder or shortening of a lower limb due to, for example, femur hypoplasia. It is also seen secondary to disorders such as Marfan's syndrome, postparalytic poliomyelitis, muscular dystrophy, neurofibromatosis, and familial dysautonomia and is

described in Fallot's tetralogy. Kyphoscoliosis may be a prominent feature of Friedreich's ataxia.

KYPHOSIS

Primary kyphosis

A primary form with congenitally defective anterior spinal segments has been described. Physiotherapy and a corrective brace may help but there is a tendency to progression, especially at adolescence, when posterior spinal fusion may be necessary to avoid further deformity.

Secondary kyphosis

Posterior angulation of the spine is seen secondary to a wide range of disorders including Hurler's syndrome, Morquio's disease, hypothyroidism, rickets, Scheuermann's disease, and tuberculosis of the spine. It can be a major deformity in spina bifida with myelomeningocele.

STRUCTURAL DEFECTS OF SKULL AND FACIAL BONES (see Ch. 14)

ANENCEPHALY

The cranial vault is absent in anencephaly where there is aplasia of the forebrain and midbrain. Spina bifida and absent spinal vertebrae may coexist.

MICROCEPHALY

A small cranial vault of approximately normal contour is seen in microcephaly associated with hypoplasia of the brain. Premature synostosis may occur. Secondary forms are also seen after intrauterine brain damage as in maternal rubella, maternal hyperphenylalaninemia or exposure to X-irradiation.

A rare familial (autosomal recessive) form with severe mental retardation occurs in which the dome of the cranial vault is somewhat pointed when viewed from the front and in which the forehead slopes backwards.

MEGALOENCEPHALY (MACROCEPHALY)

In this the cranial vault is enlarged without increased intracranial pressure. A large brain with an overgrowth of glial cells is present. Mental retardation and seizures are frequent.

ANTERIOR FONTANEL BONES

These arise from a center of ossification within the fontanel and may be present at birth or appear later. They are a normal variant and do not interfere with skull growth but should be recognized as causes of apparent smallness or early closure of the fontanel. They are analogous to wormian bones arising within a suture.

PARIETAL FORAMINA

Bone defects which may be readily palpable can occur in the superior posterior angles of the parietal bones. They may show a familial incidence, and are of benign significance, but should be differentiated from other causes of bony defect such as meningoencephalocele, neoplasms, eosinophilic granuloma, myelomatosis or reticulosis.

LACUNAR SKULL

This congenital anomaly of the cranial vault (especially frontal and parietal regions) consists of multiple areas of deep circumscribed rarefaction (lacunae) with dense intervening bone. There may be associated malformation in the central nervous system, especially myelomeningocele with subsequent hydrocephalus. Lacunar skull has to be differentiated from the 'digital impressions' or 'beaten bronze' appearance which occurs secondary to increased intracranial pressure. Lacunar skull is usually recognized earlier and the lacunae are more clearly circumscribed.

PLATYBASIA

Flattening of the skull base is diagnosed radiologically by measuring the angle between the sphenoid and the clivus of the occipital bone, which is normally less than 145°. This condition is usually of no clinical significance and should be differentiated from basilar impression. It may occur secondarily to nursing infants in the upright position but in such cases tends to improve spontaneously as the child grows.

BASILAR IMPRESSION

Upward displacement of the bony margins of the foramen magnum (basilar, condylar, and squamous occipital bones) occurs as a congenital malformation and is frequently associated with fusion of the upper cervical vertebrae and occiput (occipitalization of the atlas). Rarely, an acquired type is seen with gross bony softening in rickets or osteomalacia. Neurological sequelae include compression of cerebellum and brainstem and obstruction of cerebrospinal fluid with acute hydrocephalus and sudden rise in intracranial pressure. This is likely to require neurosurgical intervention.

PREMATURE CRANIOSYNOSTOSIS (CRANIOSTENOSIS, STENOCEPHALY)

Early fusion of single or multiple cranial sutures may be congenital (e.g. as part of inherited syndromes), or acquired after metabolic disorders such as hypophosphatasia, rickets, or idiopathic hypercalcemia. The mechanism of craniosynostosis is not clear but clinical evidence of craniostenosis with increased intracranial pressure and exophthalmos may antedate radiographic evidence of synostosis, suggesting that the primary defect is a resistance to expansion of the intrasutural preosseous membrane. Bony closure of the suture line may be present at birth or develop many months later.

Generalized craniosynostosis affecting all suture lines produces a microcephalic type of deformity which is associated with mental retardation, increased intracranial pressure and other neurological sequelae (Figs 24.23 and 24.24).

Localized forms of craniosynostosis produce an asymmetrical skull and only a short segment of suture need be fused to produce deformity. These forms may also be complicated by signs of increased intracranial pressure and this is especially liable to occur in oxycephaly (see below). Localized craniosynostoses

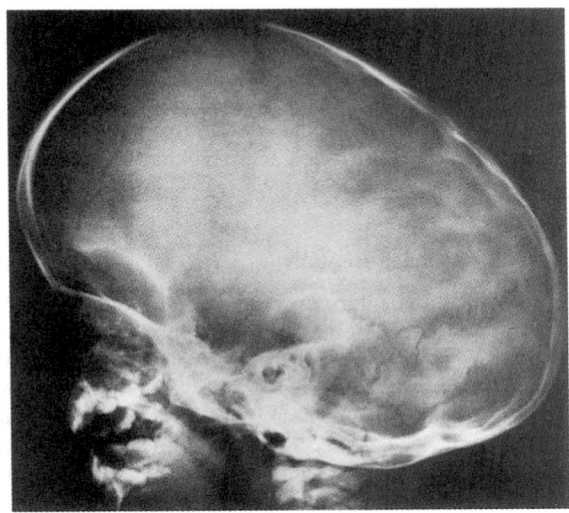

Fig. 24.23 Craniostenosis. Lateral film of skull showing scaphocephaly from sagittal suture stenosis.

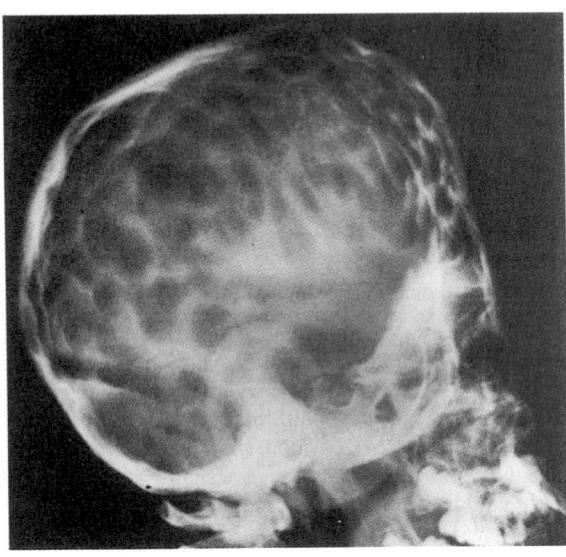

Fig. 24.24 Craniostenosis. Lateral view of skull showing oxycephaly with maximal growth towards bregma. Stenosis of coronal, sagittal and lambdoidal sutures. Beaten copper appearance.

should be differentiated from asymmetrical skull due to the effects of gravity when head posture is relatively fixed. Such flattening is seen, for example, in the small premature infant, the immobile mental defective, or the infant fixed in the splint. This postural effect is aggravated if the skull is abnormally soft as in osteogenesis imperfecta, rickets, or hypophosphatasia.

The uncomplicated forms of craniosynostosis are usually nonfamilial, but a dominant pattern has also been observed.

Plagiocephaly

Unilateral synostosis affecting a coronal (and occasionally lambdoidal) suture may be evident as a visible or palpable bony ridge. Flattening of the forehead and elevation of the orbit on the affected side result, with relative frontal prominence on the other side. This type of synostosis in severe form is rare. However, a minor degree of plagiocephalic asymmetry is common in early infancy, tends to improve with time and is of no significance. Plagiocephaly may be an isolated deformity or may coexist with other 'skew' abnormalities such as thoracic asymmetry, scoliosis and pelvic obliquity.

Scaphocephaly, dolichocephaly

Fusion in the sagittal suture prevents lateral growth of the skull and abnormal expansion occurs superiorly and in the anteroposterior axis (Fig. 24.23). The midline ridge gives a resemblance to an inverted keel. The occipitofrontal circumference may be above normal. Isolated sagittal suture closure is mainly a cosmetic problem and increased intracranial pressure is very unlikely. Scaphocephaly may be seen as one manifestation of Hurler's syndrome.

Brachycephaly

Synostosis in both coronal sutures produces anteroposterior shortening of the skull, with abnormally increased growth laterally and superiorly (Fig. 24.24). The occipitofrontal circumference is reduced and the anterior fontanel usually small. The face appears flat and broad, the eyes prominent and rather wide set. Up to 50% of cases of bicoronal synostosis may have associated defects such as mental defect, cerebral anomalies, cleft palate, or syndactyly and polydactyly. Brachycephaly is a common feature of Down syndrome.

Acrocephaly, turricephaly, oxycephaly

This deformity arises from synostosis in the coronal, sagittal, and to a lesser extent lambdoidal sutures. Anteroposterior and lateral growth is inhibited and compensatory upward growth occurs. The increased vaulting of the skull may assume a pointed form (oxycephaly; Fig. 24.24) or more rounded form (acrocephaly, turricephaly; Fig. 24.25). The orbits are shallow giving a tendency to exophthalmos. Increased intracranial pressure is especially prone to occur with convulsions, brain damage and optic atrophy. The association with hand and foot malformations is defined below.

Trigonocephaly

This deformity is characterized by a wedge-shaped skull coming to a point anteriorly where the metopic suture is ridged and commonly, but not necessarily, fused. There is orbital hypotelorism and a small anterior fossa. Hypoplasia of the forebrain may coexist, especially where there are other associated defects such as arrhinencephaly, microcephaly, or aplasia of the premaxilla. It has been suggested that barbiturates administered to the mother during early pregnancy may predispose to this anomaly.

Fusion of the metopic suture

The frontal bones are normally in close proximity at birth and have fused solidly across the midline by 2 years. Early synostosis produces a central ridge of the forehead which may be a cosmetic disability. Metopic fusion may be part of trigonocephaly but is not the sole cause of this abnormality.

ACROCEPHALOSYNDACTYLY

This combination of defects may take a variety of forms.

Apert's syndrome (type I)

In this there is acrocephaly and the middle third of the face is underdeveloped with a small nose, hypertelorism (telecanthus), shallow orbits with proptosis and strabismus. The jaw is relatively prominent and the palate frequently abnormal with a high arch and a midline furrow or posterior cleft. The syndactyly is severe with complete fusion of all five digits or the second to fifth digits of the hands and feet (Fig. 24.25). An association with other skeletal defects, congenital heart disease, anal atresia and other malformations is described. Most cases show subnormal intelligence. Inheritance appears to be dominant but the majority of cases are sporadic due to new mutation. The defect is in fibroblast growth factor receptor 2 (see Table 24.4 below).

Vogt cephalodactyly (type II)

Here the features of Apert's syndrome (but with less severe hand syndactyly) are combined with the facies of Crouzon's syndrome (see below). Inheritance is unknown.

Type III

This is characterized by mild acrocephaly, skull asymmetry, and soft tissue syndactyly of second and third fingers and third and fourth toes.

Waardenburg type (type IV)

This includes acrocephaly and plagiocephaly with an abnormal facies showing asymmetrical orbits, strabismus, and a long narrow nose. Brachydactyly and slight soft tissue syndactyly occur with some instances of bifid terminal phalanges and absent

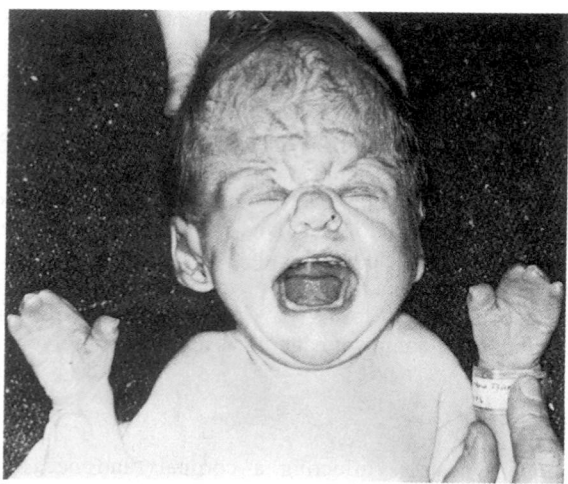

Fig. 24.25 Apert's syndrome (acrocephalosyndactyly).

first metatarsal. This disorder has been traced through six generations.

Pfeiffer type (type V)

This is characterized by acrocephaly, mild syndactyly but markedly broadened and shortened thumbs and toes (Fig. 24.26) and autosomal dominant transmission. The Jackson–Weiss syndrome, first described in a large Amish kindred, resembles Pfeiffer's syndrome with midfacial hypoplasia, craniosynostosis, and foot abnormalities but without thumb defects. Mutations in both fibroblast growth factor receptors 1 and 2 have been described (see Table 24.4 below).

ACROCEPHALOPOLYSYNDACTYLY

This is differentiated from the acrocephalosyndactylies by the additional feature of polydactyly. In the Carpenter syndrome there is brachydactyly and syndactyly in the hands, preaxial polydactyly and syndactyly in the feet, a tendency to mental retardation and a recessive inheritance.

CRANIOFACIAL DYSOSTOSIS (CROUZON'S SYNDROME)

The coronal, sagittal and lambdoidal sutures all fuse prematurely but at a variable rate and the skull may be scaphocephalic or, more commonly, brachycephalic with frontal prominence and a degree of towering. X-ray also reveals prominent convolutional markings, a small anterior fossa, and sometimes widening of the pituitary fossa. The facial features are typical consisting of hypertelorism, exophthalmos with shallow orbits, hypoplastic maxilla, a beaked parrot-nose, rather low-set ears, short upper lip and relative prognathism (Fig. 24.27). Nystagmus, external strabismus and optic atrophy are common. The palate is short and high-arched, teeth may be absent, defective, crowded and maloccluded.

Increased intracranial pressure, mental retardation, progressive exophthalmos and visual loss are liable to occur. Management is

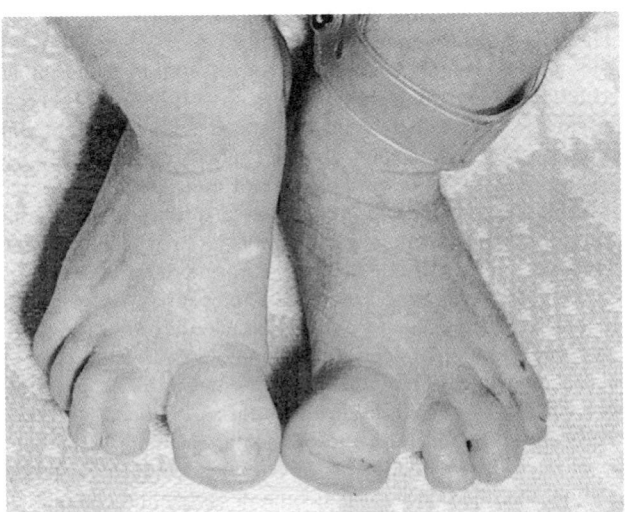

Fig. 24.26 Broad toes with webbing in Pfeiffer's type of acrocephaly syndactyly.

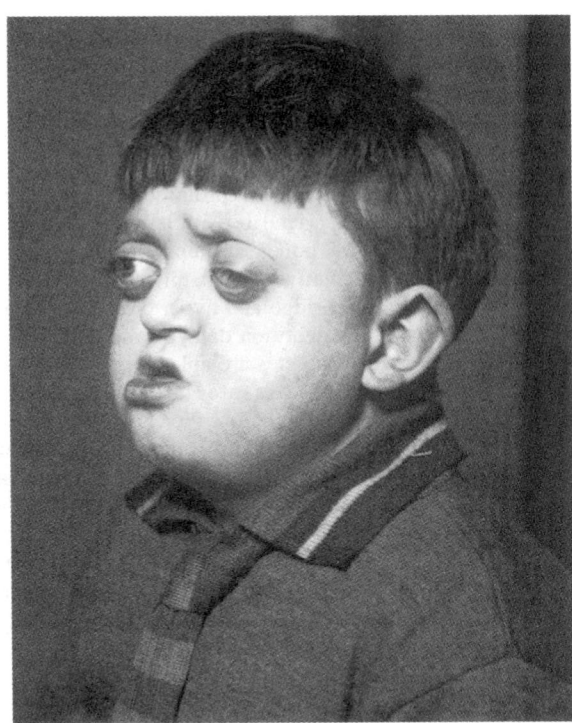

Fig. 24.27 Crouzon's syndrome.

discussed below. Inheritance is dominant although a proportion of cases appear sporadic. The mutation is in fibroblast growth factor receptor 2 (see Table 24.4 below).

MANAGEMENT OF CRANIOSYNOSTOSIS

Increased intracranial pressure should be suspected in a child with an abnormal skull who shows manifestations such as irritability, convulsions, vomiting, developmental retardation, headache or visual impairment. There may be exophthalmos, papilledema (rare in early infancy), or optic atrophy. A ridge of bone may be palpable along the suture line, and on X-ray the suture is closed and parasutural bone abnormally dense. This situation is a clear indication for craniotomy. Neurosurgery should also be considered for progressive exophthalmos and if there is X-ray evidence of increased pressure ('beaten bronze' appearance) in the absence of other signs and symptoms of craniostenosis. Craniotomy is also advised in 'high risk' situations such as bilateral coronal synostoses (especially if other sutures are also involved) and especially if significant cranial abnormality is obvious from birth. Such surgery is customarily undertaken in the first 3 months of life. Contraindications to operation include the presence of severe mental defect and serious brain or other malformations.

The object of surgery is to recreate the sutures and take steps by interposing an inert material such as polyethylene sheeting to prevent them from reuniting.

Cosmetic surgery (e.g. in uncomplicated sagittal synostosis) should be agreed to only if parents are very anxious to have something done, where there is appreciable disfigurement, and where a high standard of surgical and postoperative care can be offered. Considerable advances in the surgery of facial abnormality (e.g. Crouzon's syndrome) have been made in specialized centers.

CLEIDOCRANIAL DYSPLASIA

There is delayed closure of the fontanels and sutures giving a skull with increased transverse diameter, prominent frontal regions separated by a gutter, and parietal bossing. Wormian bones are frequently seen. The facial bones are underdeveloped with a hypoplastic maxilla and relative prognathism, and there is a depressed, broadened nasal bridge and hypertelorism. The palate may be high-arched and the dentition delayed and defective with marked malocclusion. The clavicles are aplastic, especially at the outer end so that the shoulders are narrow, drooped and hypermobile and can be folded in across the chest (Fig. 24.28).

The neck appears relatively long. This is a generalized disorder and other skeletal manifestations may include aplasia or hypoplasia of the pubic bones with pubic diastasis and coxa vara. The second metacarpals tend to be elongated and terminal phalanges blunted. A degree of short stature is common but intelligence is usually normal. The condition is an autosomal dominant and sporadic cases are considered new mutations. Dental and orthopedic treatment may be necessary.

OCULOMANDIBULODYSCEPHALY WITH HYPOTRICHOSIS (HALLERMANN–STREIFF SYNDROME)

Microphthalmia, bilateral congenital cataracts and other eye defects occur in association with hypomandibulosis and a long tapering beak-like nose giving a parrot-like facies. The skull may be small and show brachycephaly with frontal bossing, open fontanel and gaping sutures. Hypotrichosis may be generalized but especially affects the scalp along the suture lines. There may be areas of cutaneous atrophy and a variety of dental anomalies. Other bony defects (spina bifida, syndactyly, scoliosis), deafness and urogenital anomalies have been reported. The patients are

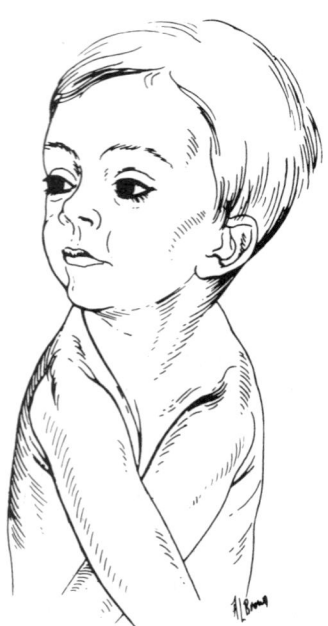

Fig. 24.28 Cleidocranial dysplasia.

underheight but mostly of normal intelligence. The genetics are uncertain; most cases appear to be sporadic.

HYPERTELORISM (TELECANTHUS, GREIG'S SYNDROME)

Wide separation of the eyes occurs due to underdevelopment of the greater wings and relative overgrowth of the lesser wings of the sphenoid. Standard measurements of the outer orbital and inner canthal distances are available (p. 22). There is no premature synostosis. Strabismus is common and binocular vision may be impaired. High-arched palate, cleft lip and palate, hypoplastic maxilla and hearing defect may exist.

The isolated form of this defect is rare, may be dominant, and may be associated with mental defect.

Hypertelorism may occur as part of a syndrome as in acrocephalosyndactyly, Crouzon's syndrome, craniocleidodysostosis, Waardenburg syndrome, midfacial cleft syndrome, and in some sex chromosome anomalies. Hypertelorism has to be differentiated from separation of the eyes due, for example, to frontal meningocele, facial cleft, or expansion of maxillary marrow in Cooley's anemia.

HYPOTELORISM

Abnormal approximation of the eyes is seen in trigonocephaly, the oculodentodigital syndrome, and in variants of the cyclops malformation (cebocephaly, arrhinencephaly). With severe defects which are not fatal there is a high incidence of mental defect, epilepsy, and hydrocephalus.

PIERRE ROBIN SYNDROME (MICROGNATHIA, GLOSSOPTOSIS AND CLEFT PALATE)

Clinical features

The mandible is hypoplastic producing a 'shrew-like' facies (Fig. 24.29) and reducing the size of the buccal cavity. The tongue, which is poorly anchored, is displaced backwards and downwards (glossoptosis). The palate is high-arched or, more commonly, shows a postalveolar cleft through which the tongue may prolapse. There is no associated cleft lip.

The clinical features are due to respiratory (pharyngeal) obstruction and interference with swallowing. Increased respiratory efforts are evident from birth with head retraction, inspiratory obstruction and stridor, subcostal and intercostal recession and a tendency to cyanotic attacks. Distress is aggravated by nursing in the supine position or by feeding. Respiratory difficulty may be relatively mild in the first week of life and worsen thereafter. Attempts at normal infant feeding lead to choking and regurgitation with failure to thrive or weight loss so that an advanced state of emaciation may develop. Death may occur from asphyxia or aspiration pneumonia.

Associated defects are not uncommon. Cardiac murmurs or other evidence of congenital heart disease have been reported in 10–25% of cases and a degree of mental retardation (including cases of microcephaly and hydrocephalus) in some 25%. The eyes may show microphthalmos, glaucoma or congenital cataract and, less commonly, there may be low set or deformed ears and deafness. A variety of skeletal malformations is described including congenital dislocation of the hip, club foot, syndactyly,

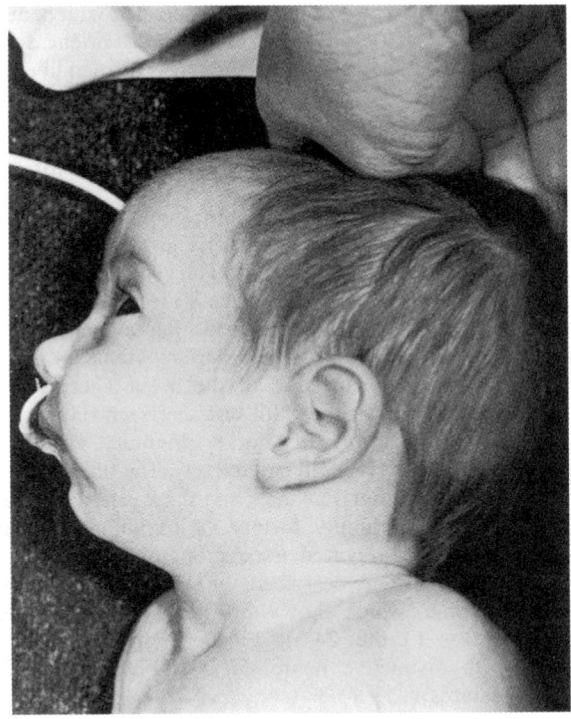

Fig. 24.29 Pierre Robin syndrome.

terminal transverse defects, and achondroplasia. Surviving infants usually show good jaw growth so that a normal profile is attained by 4–6 years, but the children tend to have mouth breathing, 'adenoidal' facies and recurrent middle-ear infections.

Treatment

Successful management lies firstly in early recognition. Nursing in the prone position with the chest and shoulders supported allows the tongue to fall forward. Tube feeding is usually necessary and a large nasopharyngeal tube may prevent the tongue falling back and occluding the oro- and nasopharynx. The use of an angulated teat may allow the infant to suck in the prone position. With good nursing technique, surgical intervention can usually be avoided. Various forms of tongue fixation have been recommended including stitching the tongue to the alveolar margin or attaching it to the anterior floor of the mouth, and these may be useful as temporary expedients. If serious respiratory obstruction persists, tracheostomy should be performed. Gastrostomy may be helpful if vomiting and malnutrition persist. The cleft palate is managed with an orthodontic plate and later surgical repair.

MANDIBULOFACIAL DYSOSTOSIS (TREACHER COLLINS', FRANCESCHETTI–KLEIN SYNDROMES)

In its complete form, there is a characteristic facies with marked hypoplasia of the mandible and malar bones, often a high-arched or cleft palate and dental malocclusion (Table 24.2). The palpebral fissures show antimongoloid obliquity, and often coloboma in the outer lower eyelids. The ears show deformed pinnae or microtia with absent external auditory canal, and deafness is present in about one-third of cases. Ear tags and fistulae are also common. Associated malformations, including congenital heart disease, mental defect and other skeletal malformations, may occur. Minor variants of the syndrome are seen. It appears that the disorder is inherited as an autosomal dominant with incomplete penetrance and variable expressivity.

Table 24.2 Differential diagnosis of three facial syndromes – oculoauriculovertebral dysplasia (Goldenhar's syndrome), mandibulofacial dysostosis (Treacher Collins syndrome) and hemifacial microsomia (from Gorlin & Pindborg 1964)

Sign	Oculoauriculovertebral dysplasia	Mandibulofacial dysostosis	Hemifacial microsomia
Epibulbar dermoids	++++	0	0
Upper-lid coloboma	+++	0	0
Lower-lid coloboma	0 → +	++++	0
Antimongoloid lid obliquity	+ → ++	++++	0 → +
Iris and/or choroid coloboma	+	+	+
Microphthalmia	+	+	+
Frontal bossing	++	0	0
Malar and/or maxillary hypoplasia	+ → ++	++++	+ → ++
Unilateral facial hypoplasia	+++	0	++++
Vertebral anomalies	++++	0	0
Microtia	+++	++++	+++
Deficiency of external auditory meatus	+ → ++	++++	+++
Supernumerary ear tags	++++	++ → +++	++
Antetragal pits	++	+++	++
Macrostomia	+++	+	+++
Aplasia of mandibular ramus and condyle	++	0	++++
Malocclusion	++	+++	++
Pulmonary agenesis	0	0	++
'Hair tongue'	0	+ → ++	0
Mental retardation	+	++	0

One form known as maxillofacial dysostosis consists of malar hypoplasia, overdeveloped lower jaw and open bite and antimongoloid obliquity of the eyes without colobomas. It is also dominantly inherited.

HEMIFACIAL MICROSOMIA (UNILATERAL FACIAL AGENESIS, OTOMANDIBULAR DYSOSTOSIS)

This is a unilateral disturbance with microtia, undeveloped mandible and tendency to macrostomia (Table 24.2). The ear defect varies from complete aplasia to a distorted pinna. The auditory canal is often absent. Flattening of the face on the affected side is due to aplasia of the mandibular ramus and condyle and some deficiency in the maxillary and malar bones (Fig. 24.30a). The muscles of mastication and facial expression may be hypoplastic. There may be macrostomia, or apparent macrostomia due to the hypoplastic cheek. Ipsilateral pulmonary agenesis has occurred in a few cases. No hereditary pattern has been defined.

OCULOAURICULOVERTEBRAL SYNDROME (GOLDENHAR'S SYNDROME)

In addition to the vertebral anomalies (p. 1557), there are eye defects including epibulbar dermoids (Fig. 24.30b), unilateral coloboma and occasionally microphthalmia, cataract or atrophy of the iris (Table 24.2). The ears show bilateral appendages, and pretragal fistulae; occasionally microtia, absent external auditory canal and deafness are present. The facies is characteristic with frontal bossing, hypomandibulosis, and sometimes poorly developed nostrils giving a 'parrot-like' appearance. Various inherited patterns are described.

Goldenhar's syndrome is sometimes associated with hemifacial microsomia (Fig. 24.30a), of which it may be a variant, and both of these conditions show some resemblance to mandibulofacial dysostosis. The differential features are indicated in Table 24.2.

OROFACIAL–DIGITAL DYSOSTOSIS (OFD SYNDROME)

The mouth shows hyperplasia of the frenum and a midline pseudocleft of the upper lip. There are lateral and other palatal clefts and the tongue shows an irregular margin, clefts, and frequently a small hamartoma. The teeth are malpositioned and the mandible hypoplastic. The face shows lateral displacement of the canthi giving apparent hypertelorism (telecanthus), and hypoplasia of the alar cartilages of the nose. There is frontal bossing. Abnormalities of the skull base are seen on X-ray. The hair is sparse. Malformed digits include clinodactyly, camptodactyly, syndactyly, and polydactyly. The tubular bones of the hands and feet are short and thick and show patchy rarefaction. Mental defect and a family history of trembling involuntary movements have been reported associations.

Two distinct entities are described, OFD type I and OFD type II (Mohr's syndrome) which shows different genetic patterns and clinical features (Table 24.3). Further variants have been described with distinctive neurological (OFD III) or skeletal (OFD IV) features.

OCULODENTODIGITAL SYNDROME

Microphthalmos, abnormalities of the iris, and sometimes glaucoma are associated with enamel hypoplasia of the teeth and limb defects including camptodactyly, syndactyly, and hypoplasia of middle phalanges in the toes. The facies is characterized by small eyes with medial epicanthus, ocular hypotelorism and a thin nose with underdeveloped alae. The condition may be an autosomal dominant.

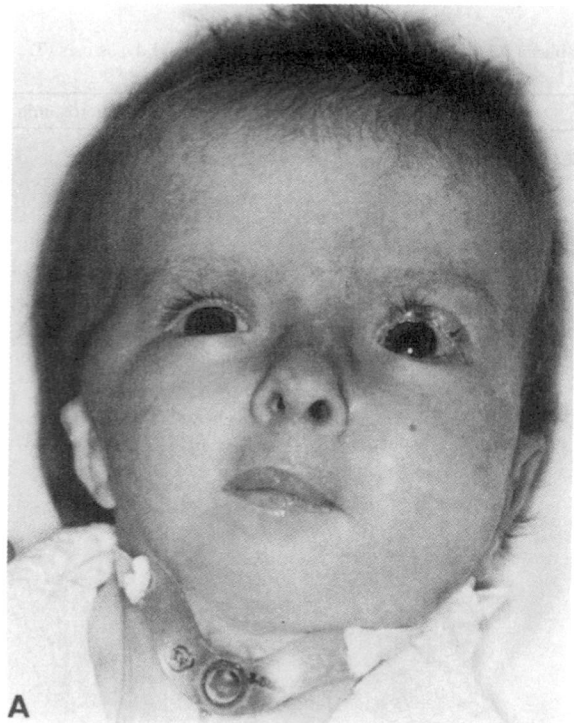

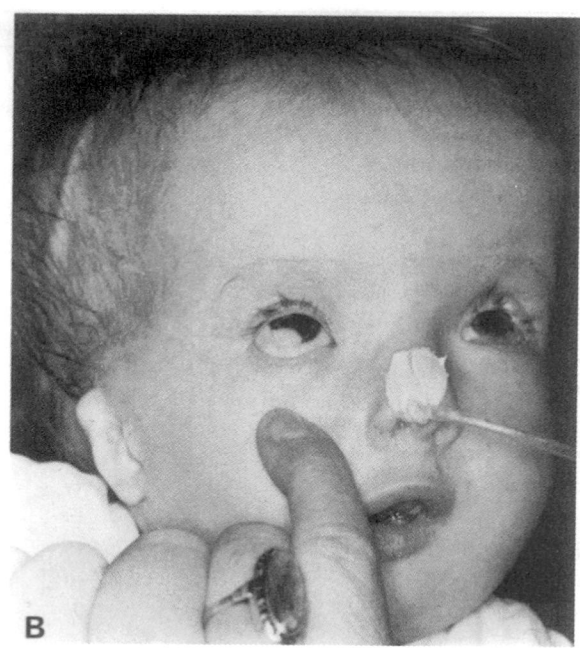

Fig. 24.30 Goldenhar's syndrome (oculoauriculovertebral dysplasia) showing (**A**) hemifacial microsomia and (**B**) epibulbar dermoid.

Table 24.3 Differences between OFD I and OFD II (Mohr's syndrome) (from Rimoin & Edgerton 1967)

	OFD I	OFD II (Mohr's syndrome)
Inheritance	X-linked dominant	Autosomal recessive
Sex distribution	Only female subjects	Male and female subjects
Alveolar ridge	Thick bands	Normal or flaring
Dentition	Lateral incisors absent	Normal or absent central incisors
Nose	Alar hypoplasia	Broad, bifid tip
Mandible	Hypoplasia of ramus of mandible	Hypoplasia of body of mandible
Hair	Coarse and thin	Normal
Skin	Granular or papular lesions	Normal
Digits	Polysyndactyly not present bilaterally	Bilateral polysyndactyly of halluces
Skeleton	Irregular reticular areas of the short tubular bones	Metaphyseal irregularity and flaring
Hearing	Normal	Conductive hearing defect

FAMILIAL FIBROUS DYSPLASIA OF THE JAWS (CHERUBISM)

This is characterized by maxillary and gross mandibular swelling with replacement of bone by fibrous tissue. The infant is normal at birth and facial swelling appears characteristically in the second year. The lower eyelids are pulled down by the swelling to reveal a band of sclera, dentition is disrupted, and submandibular lymph nodes may be enlarged. X-ray shows irregular rarefaction. The maxillary sinuses may be obliterated. The swelling increases for the first 2 years and shows a tendency to regress at puberty. There is no associated mortality and no specific treatment. Sporadic cases and a familial incidence have been described. The syndrome has to be differentiated from Caffey's disease and infection or tumor in the jaw or facial bones.

MANAGEMENT OF FACIAL AND ASSOCIATED DEFECTS

This should involve a multidisciplinary approach including the family doctor, pediatrician, child psychiatrist, speech therapist, hearing aid center, special school facilities and various surgical subspecialties as required. Dermoids, or auricular appendages may require to be removed. Disordered dentition or cleft palate will require orthodontic care and surgical repair. Reconstructive operations for external ear deformity are available. Macrostomia may be improved by Z-plasty and eyelid deformity corrected by skin flap insertions. Epicanthic folds and broadened nasal bridge may be reduced. Soft tissue aplasia may be built up with fat grafts and severe hypoplasias of the middle third of the face, mandible, or orbital regions may be built up by bone grafts. With these procedures, considerable cosmetic and functional improvements may be achieved and psychological disturbance minimized. The recommended age is 4–5 years. In hypertelorism, operative reduction of the interocular distance is possible. In all defects, however, the magnitude of the operation, its risks and the need for prolonged supervision should be balanced against the likely cosmetic and psychological benefits, and embarked on only after careful assessment of the child and his family, taking their attitudes and aspirations into account.

SPECIFIC SKELETAL DYSPLASIAS (THE OSTEOCHONDRODYSPLASIAS)

The osteochondrodysplasias (or simply chondrodysplasias) are a group of disorders in which there is an intrinsic abnormality of cartilage and/or bone growth and development. A large number of such entities exist and a comprehensive classification has been proposed (International Working Group 1992). Descriptions of the more common types follow.

Clinically, the disorder may be evident as disproportion or deformity in the newborn. Some of these neonatal presentations are likely to be lethal (stillborn, neonatal death or death in infancy); some are compatible with survival and show the features of disproportionate short stature in the older child.

A variety of milder skeletal dysplasias tend to be delayed in presentation. Some will present as short stature, some with locomotor disability or orthopedic deformity.

Diagnosis is based on careful clinical examination and radiological skeletal survey. In all cases, including the newborn, biochemical screening should be carried out to avoid missing renal, vitamin D or parathyroid related bone disease or hypophosphatasia. In patients with suggestive features, specific tests may be required to diagnose inborn errors of metabolism such as the mucopolysaccharidoses.

Much new information has come to light in recent years concerning the genetic and molecular defects underlying many skeletal dysplasias (Table 24.4). This, in turn, has led to a deeper understanding of many of the pathophysiological processes governing the structure and development of collagen, bone and cartilage. In some cases, clear patterns are emerging concerning the relationship between genotype and clinical phenotype, whereas in others the situation is more complex. As our knowledge increases, this may lead to the rational design of new therapies for some of these distressing conditions.

COLLAGEN

Collagen forms the most abundant protein family in the body and is responsible for many of the structural, tensile and load-bearing properties of the tissues in which it is found. More than 16 different types of collagen have been described, coded for by more than 28 genes. Type I forms by far the largest proportion of collagen in the body and is ubiquitously distributed, being the major protein in bone, skin, ligament, sclera, cornea and blood vessels. Types V and VI are also widely distributed, although in much smaller amounts. Type III collagen is found in most tissues except bone and cartilage, whereas types II, IX, X and XI are restricted largely to cartilage and the vitreous of the eye. Type IV

Table 24.4 Mode of inheritance and genetic defect in selected skeletal dysplasias

Skeletal dysplasia	Inheritance	Genetic defect	Reference
Collagen defects			
Stickler's syndrome	AD	Mutations in COL2A1, e.g. premature stop codon: reduced production of type II collagen or truncated protein	Byers 1994b
Stickler's syndrome – no eye involvement	AD	Type XI collagen mutations	Vikkula et al 1995
Kniest syndrome	AD	Mutations in COL2A1	Tilstra & Byers 1994 Spranger et al 1994
Achondrogenesis type II	AD	Point mutations in COL2A1 resulting in Gly substitutions at N-terminal end of triple helix	Spranger et al 1994 Bonaventure et al 1995
Hypochondrogenesis	AD	Point mutations affecting Gly in the triple helix	Horton et al 1992 Bogaert et al 1992 Bonaventure et al 1995
Spondyloepiphyseal dysplasia congenita	AD	Mutations in COL2A1	Tilstra & Byers 1994
Metaphyseal chondrodysplasia type Schmid	AD	Mutations in COL10A1, affecting molecular assembly or resulting in a truncated protein	Warman et al 1993 McIntosh et al 1995
Defects in non-collagen proteins in cartilage			
Pseudoachondroplasia	AD	Mutations in one region of cartilage oligomeric matrix protein, disrupting pentameric structure (allelic with some forms of multiple epiphyseal dysplasia)	Hecht et al 1995 Briggs et al 1995
Multiple epiphyseal dysplasia (some forms)	AD	Mutations in one region of cartilage oligomeric matrix protein, disrupting pentameric structure (allelic with pseudoachondroplasia)	Briggs et al 1995
Fibroblast growth factor receptor defects			
Achondroplasia	AD	Mutation affecting transmembrane domain of fibroblast growth factor receptor 3	Shiang et al 1994
Hypochondroplasia	AD	Mutation affecting intracellular tyrosine kinase domain a of fibroblast growth factor receptor 3	Bellus et al 1995
Thanatophoric dysplasia	AD	Mutation affecting intracellular tyrosine kinase domain b of fibroblast growth factor receptor 3	Tavormina et al 1995
Apert's syndrome	AD	Mutations in fibroblast growth factor receptor 2	Muenke & Schell 1995
Pfeiffer's syndrome	AD	Mutations in fibroblast growth factor receptors 1 and 2	Muenke & Schell 1995
Crouzon's syndrome	AD	Mutations in fibroblast growth factor receptor 2	Muenke & Schell 1995
Jackson–Weiss syndrome	AD	Mutations in fibroblast growth factor receptor 2	Muenke & Schell 1995
Miscellaneous defects			
Diastrophic dysplasia	AR	Mutation in sulfate transporter gene	Hastbacka et al 1994
Camptomelic dysplasia	AD	Mutations in SOX9 (SRY-related) gene	Foster et al 1994 Wagner et al 1994
Metaphyseal chondrodysplasia type Jansen	AD	Mutation in parathyroid hormone–parathyroid hormone-related peptide receptor gene	Schipani et al 1995
Osteopetrosis	AR	Mutations in carbonic anhydrase II gene	Ohlsson et al 1980 Hu et al 1992 Hu et al 1994
Marfan's syndrome	AD	Mutations in fibrillin-1 gene (many)	Dietz et al 1991 Njibroek et al 1995

AD = autosomal dominant; AR = autosomal recessive
Nomenclature: COL2A1 refers to the gene coding for the α 1 chain of type II collagen.

collagen is a structural component of basement membranes. The structures of the collagens reflect their functions. For example, the fibrillar collagens (types I, II, III, V and XI) are either homo- or heterotrimers that contain long stretches of triple helix, conveying great tensile strength. The triple helix requires repeated sequences of Gly-X-Y in each polypeptide chain, where X and Y can be any amino acid except tryptophan and cysteine. Glycine is essential at every third position to allow proper folding of the triple helix.

Collagen biosynthesis is complex, involving both intracellular and extracellular events. Post-translational modifications include hydroxylation of proline and lysine residues, glycosylation of hydroxylysine residues and triple helix formation. After secretion of fibrillar procollagen from the cell, the bulky N- and C-terminal propeptides are removed to leave a molecule that is almost entirely triple helix, with small peptide extensions at the N- and C-terminals. The collagen molecules then aggregate in a quarter-staggered array to form fibrils. Fibril formation and diameter are thought to be controlled by interactions with other collagens, proteoglycans or other glycoproteins. During collagen maturation, chemical crosslinks are gradually formed between adjacent fibrils, of which the best characterized are the pyridinoline and deoxypyridinoline crosslinks formed between hydroxylysine and lysine residues. These crosslinks stabilize the mature collagen and augment tensile strength.

Any mutation that changes the primary sequence of the amino acids, especially if it affects a glycine residue in the triple helix, thereby preventing proper folding, may have profound clinical effects. Such mutations may slow down translation, result in increased hydroxylation and glycosylation, prevent collagen secretion, and/or enhance degradation of the defective protein. Defects in processing, such as lysyl hydroxylation, may reduce the ability of collagen to form crosslinks and hence diminish tensile strength. Mutations affecting the N- or C-terminal procollagen cleavage sites may prevent these large globular structures from being detached, thereby disrupting fibril formation.

A large number of mutations have been described which, depending on the type of collagen affected, their site and nature, may lead to a variety of clinical consequences. For example, mutations in type I collagen generally result in osteogenesis imperfecta (see below). Several different chondrodysplasia phenotypes arise from mutations in type II collagen (Table 24.4). Type III collagen mutations result in the severe type IV form of Ehlers–Danlos syndrome (Byers 1994a; see p. 1612). Other forms of Ehlers–Danlos syndrome result from failure of crosslinking owing to a defect in the lysyl hydroxylase gene (type VI) or mutations affecting the N-proteinase cleavage site (type VIIA) or the N-proteinase enzyme itself (types VIIB and C). Type IV collagen mutations affect basement membranes and result in Alport's syndrome (Byers 1995; see p. 965). Mutations in type VII collagen, which forms anchoring fibrils in skin and mucosa, result in dystrophic epidermolysis bullosa (Tilstra & Byers 1994; see p. 1621).

Recently, biochemical markers have become available that reflect some of the processes involved in the biosynthesis and maturation of collagen. For example, the C-terminal propeptide of type I collagen quantitatively reflects the amount of type I collagen synthesized and secreted by the cell and can now be readily measured in plasma (Risteli & Risteli 1993). In children, most derives from bone, although there is some contribution from other tissues. Urinary hydroxyproline has been used as a measure of collagen degradation but it has limited value, owing to interference by dietary collagen and extensive hepatic metabolism. However, the newer urinary markers, pyridinoline and deoxypyridinoline, reflect the degradation of mature crosslinked collagen, are not affected by diet, have no significant metabolism and are excreted quantitatively in urine (Seibel et al 1992). Neither of the pyridinium compounds is specific for collagen type, but deoxypyridinoline is almost completely specific for bone-derived collagen. At present, there is no simple plasma-based biochemical assay that reflects type II collagen synthesis in cartilage, or type X collagen synthesis in the hypertrophic chondrocytes of the growth plate.

CARTILAGE

Cartilage has many functions, including cushioning of the joint and elongation of bone at the epiphyseal growth plate. It is a complex and highly metabolically active tissue that shares many of its macromolecules with the vitreous humor of the eye, thereby explaining the link between joint disease, growth abnormalities and ocular problems. Many proteins contribute to the structure and development of cartilage. Its principal collagen is type II but it also contains type XI and nonfibrillar type IX collagen containing a chondroitin sulfate moiety. Fibrils are composed of a mixture of type II and XI collagens, overlaid with type IX. Type II collagen mutations may result in several phenotypes, depending on their nature and location: glycine substitutions towards the N-terminal of the triple helical domain tend to result in more severe phenotypes such as achondrogenesis type II (Bonaventure et al 1995), but such predictions are not entirely reliable. Type X collagen is nonfibrillar and confined to the hypertrophic chondrocytes of the growth plate. Important noncollagenous macromolecules in cartilage include chondroitin sulfate proteoglycan, hyaluronic acid, link protein and cartilage oligomeric matrix protein.

GROWTH FACTORS

A variety of growth factors are also involved in the development of bone and cartilage. Some of the most important are the fibroblast growth factors, which regulate cell proliferation, differentiation and migration in many different tissues. Their actions are mediated via receptors that contain a ligand-binding domain, a transmembrane domain and two intracellular tyrosine kinase domains involved in signaling. Mutations in fibroblast growth factor receptor 3 all cause abnormal endochondral bone formation, affecting the growth of the cartilaginous growth plate of the long bones and the base of the skull. Whether the resulting phenotype is achondroplasia, hypochondroplasia or thanatophoric dysplasia depends on which receptor domain is affected (Muenke & Schell 1995; Table 24.4). On the other hand, mutations in fibroblast growth factor receptors 1 and 2 result in poor ossification of the flat bones of the skull, giving rise to the craniosynostosis syndromes: Apert, Pfeiffer, Jackson–Weiss and Crouzon (Muenke & Schell 1995; Table 24.4). Identical mutations have been described which in some individuals give rise to Crouzon's syndrome and in others to Pfeiffer's syndrome; the mechanism for this is unknown.

OSTEOGENESIS IMPERFECTA (FRAGILITAS OSSIUM)

Pathogenesis

Osteogenesis imperfecta (OI) is a clinically and genetically heterogeneous group of inherited disorders, associated with mutations in the genes encoding the chains of type I collagen. A large number of such mutations have now been described, with overlapping clinical effects depending on the site of the mutation and the secondary consequences on other matrix components. At present, the Sillence classification provides the best prediction of the natural history of these disorders, although in time biochemical and genetic studies may supersede or complement this classification. In general, mutations that result in reduced synthesis, stability or secretion of type I procollagen, but normal structure of the reduced amount of type I collagen that is incorporated into fibrils are associated with the milder phenotypes. By contrast, mutations that produce an abnormal procollagen structure frequently result in an overmodified protein that is secreted poorly (causing intracellular accumulation) and that causes fibril disruption: such mutations are associated with more severe or lethal phenotypes (Brenner et al 1989, Mörike et al 1992). Mutations towards the C-terminal end of the triple helix are usually more severe than those at the N-terminal, although there may be functional domains that disrupt this relationship.

A secondary consequence of some mutations may be that the defective type I collagen may not form proper quarter-staggered fibrillar arrays, leading to reduced apatite crystal size (Vetter et al 1991a) and poor mineralization. Any mutation that results in a reduced collagen content in bone frequently results in secondary changes in the noncollagenous proteins such as osteocalcin, osteonectin and bone sialoprotein (Castells et al 1986, Vetter et al 1991b).

Osteogenesis imperfecta (OI) type I

This is the mildest and commonest form of OI, with an autosomal dominant inheritance. Most of these individuals have a mutation in one of their COL1A1 alleles (see footnote to Table 24.4 for collagen gene nomenclature) that results in defective production of type I procollagen, for example m-RNA splicing defects, premature stop codons and mutations resulting in an unstable protein product. In each case, the other COL1A1 allele produces normal proα1(I) chains that associate with normal proα2(I) chains to form normal procollagen but in reduced amounts. Point mutations affecting nonglycine residues in the triple helix, or a few glycine substitutions near the N-terminal end of the triple helix also tend to result in the mild type I OI (Byers 1995).

Fractures are rare at birth (about 10% of cases); the disorder usually first manifests in the toddler or older child where the picture is dominated by pathological fractures, particularly in the lower extremities. The vertebrae may show osteoporosis and collapse with spinal deformity. Some improvement in bone fragility may occur after puberty.

Other manifestations include hypotonia and hypermobile joints which may dislocate, hernias, and thin atrophic skin. The conjunctival sclera is thin and transparent with blue discoloration due to choroid pigment showing through. In affected patients opacities in the cornea or lens may also occur. Blue sclerotics are common in the families of affected patients and some two-thirds of these relatives have fragile bones. Deafness due to otosclerosis is a common but not invariable feature. Thus about one-third of patients are deaf by 40 years, and half by 60 years of age. Aortic regurgitation and mitral valve prolapse may occur.

The teeth may be normal (OI type IA) or show dentinogenesis imperfecta with teeth which are translucent (opalescent) or discolored bluish-gray or yellow. Patients with defective dentin (OI type IB) show more severe bone disease with increased fractures and deformity.

Radiologically, the bone cortex is thin and the bones have a 'ground glass' appearance with lack of normal trabeculation. The vertebrae are shallow and biconcave with wide intervertebral spaces. The skull vault is poorly ossified with wide sutures and wormian bones (Fig. 24.31). Callus develops well but is not replaced by normal bone. Unfractured bones are thin and poorly calcified, very slender and bent. Fractures may show nonunion and develop pseudarthrosis, and occasionally there is

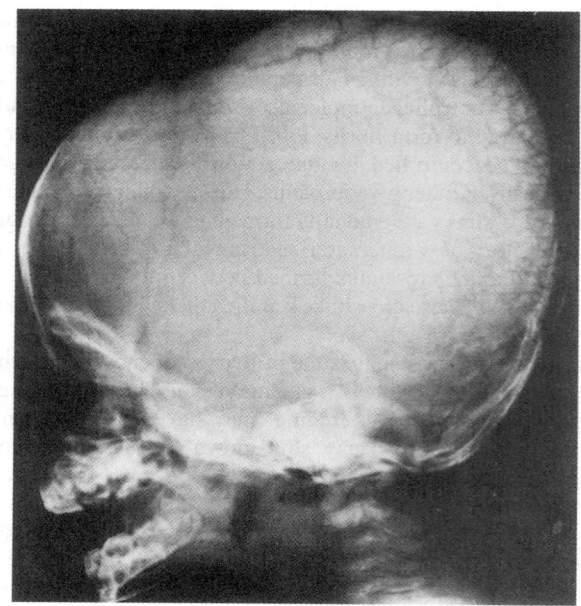

Fig. 24.31 Osteogenesis imperfecta. Skull with mosaic pattern of vault from deficient ossification; also generalized osteoporosis.

overabundant (hyperplastic) callus formation which causes a brawny swelling of the affected limb.

Concentrations of procollagen type I C-terminal propeptide in plasma have been found to be markedly reduced in this disorder compared to age-matched controls and unaffected family members, providing useful supportive evidence in its diagnosis (Brenner et al 1993, Minisola et al 1994). Urinary type I crosslinked telopeptide is usually increased in type I OI (Brenner et al 1994).

Osteogenesis imperfecta (OI) type II

Almost all cases of this lethal perinatal form are associated with a new dominant mutation. In the few families in whom there is recurrence (about 6% risk overall), this is due to parental mosaicism for the mutation which becomes lethal in the heterozygous infant. The type I collagen mutations that give rise to OI type II are very diverse: point mutations affecting glycine in the triple helical domain, multiple exon rearrangements, exon-skipping mutations, small deletions in the triple helix of either chain, and mutations in the C-terminal propeptide that interfere with molecular assembly have all been described (Byers 1995). Nearly all infants with OI type II are heterozygous for the mutation involved, but occasionally compound heterozygotes or homozygotes are found.

There is poor fetal ossification and multiple intrauterine fractures with distortion of long bones, spine and thorax giving stunting and deformity (Figs 24.32 and 24.33). The skull is soft with wide sutures. The skin is thin and fragile and the joints hyperextensible.

Radiologically, various subgroups have been identified. In type IIa, the long bones are broad and crumpled and the ribs broad with continuous beading. In type IIb, the long bones are similar but the ribs have discontinuous or no beading. In type IIc, the long bones are thin and fractured, and the ribs slender and beaded.

Pseudarthrosis of the tibia or other bones may be seen. Multiple islands of bone are evident in the skull vault.

A distinction has to be made from the severe form of congenital hypophosphatasia (see p. 1176).

Osteogenesis imperfecta (OI) type III

Inheritance in this disorder is most commonly autosomal dominant, usually as a result of a new mutation, but autosomal recessive inheritance has also been well documented. Autosomal dominant mutations include specific glycine substitutions in the triple helical domain of either the proα1 or the proα2 chains of type I collagen, resulting in less efficient secretion of unstable and overmodified molecules. A single autosomal recessive mutation has been identified in which a small deletion in both COL1A2 alleles caused a frameshift, resulting in an altered sequence of amino acids downstream of the mutation. This prevented proα2 chains from being incorporated into the procollagen molecule, which was composed of overmodified proα1 homotrimers instead of the normal heterotrimers (Byers 1995). In addition to these mutations affecting type I collagen, other so far uncharacterized mutations may also give rise to the OI type III phenotype.

Although clinically heterogeneous, multiple fractures tend to occur in the newborn and through infancy. Severe progressive osteopenia with kyphosis, chest and limb deformity, short stature and complicating bronchopneumonias lead to death from cardiorespiratory failure by the third or fourth decade. Although the sclera may be bluish early on, the appearance becomes normal with age. Deafness is not a usual feature.

Procollagen type I C-terminal propeptide concentrations in plasma are frequently reduced in type III OI, although not to the same extent as in type I OI (Brenner et al 1993). Urinary excretion of type I collagen crosslinked N-telopeptide is markedly increased and may help to support the diagnosis (Brenner et al 1994).

Osteogenesis imperfecta (OI) type IV

Type IV OI is inherited in an autosomal dominant fashion, and occurs both in sporadic and familial forms. Considerable intrafamilial variation in the clinical phenotype may be found. Linkage studies indicate that the mutation is usually in the COL1A2 gene, although in some cases the COL1A1 gene has been implicated. Mutations described include point mutations and a small deletion in the triple helical domain, resulting in overmodification, increased degradation and reduced secretion of the abnormal molecules (Byers 1995).

This form has white sclera, although a bluish tinge is usual at birth. The bone disease is similar to the usual dominant OI type I with osteopenia and fractures at a variable age from birth onwards and a tendency to remission in adolescence. Bowing of long bones and short stature results, but the bone disease is not so severe as in types II and III. Hearing is intact but some patients have opalescent dentin.

Procollagen type I C-terminal propeptide concentrations in plasma are moderately reduced in type IV OI (Brenner et al 1993). Urinary excretion of type I collagen crosslinked N-telopeptide is usually increased (Brenner et al 1994).

Treatment

Supportive management involves measures to reduce fractures and the resulting deformity. The young baby should be protected

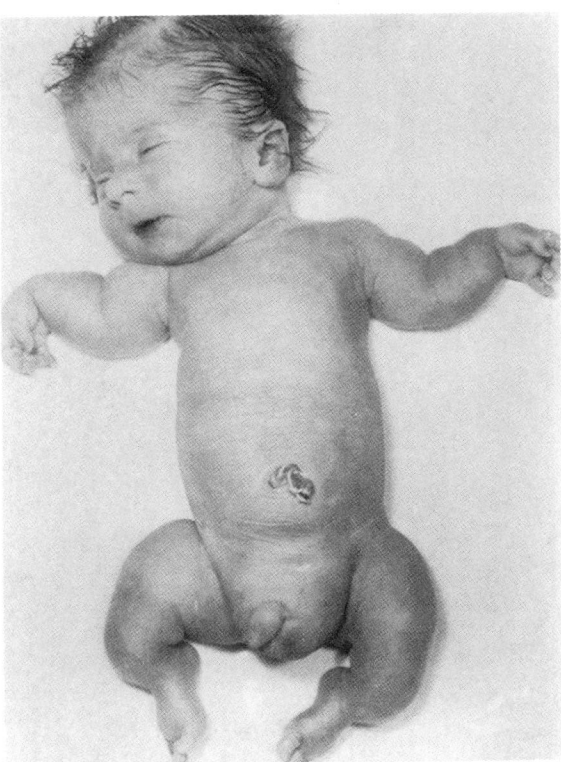

Fig. 24.32   Osteogenesis imperfecta type II.

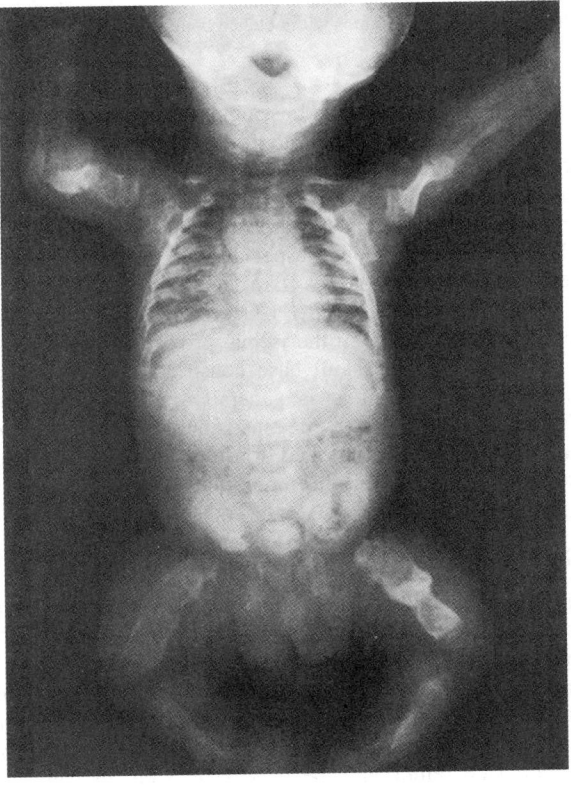

Fig. 24.33   Osteogenesis imperfecta type II. Newborn infant with multiple deformities of limbs and thoracic cage from fractures in varying stages of healing; generalized osteoporosis.

from trauma. Fractures are treated by standard orthopedic techniques but immobilization should be minimized and early ambulation with a protective (weightbearing) brace is preferable. With multiple fractures and deformity, osteotomies and intramedullary rods may help to preserve straight limbs. These patients are not unintelligent and can often adapt to a considerable degree of physical handicap. No specific therapy is known to be of benefit.

THANATOPHORIC DYSPLASIA

This is a lethal condition (thanatophoric = leading to death), distinguished from classical achondroplasia. It is the commonest type of fatal micromelic dwarfism.

A single sporadic point mutation in the intracellular tyrosine kinase domain b of fibroblast factor receptor 3 gives rise to one form of this lethal autosomal dominant disorder, which is associated with severe cloverleaf skull but straight, relatively long femurs (Tavormina et al 1995). Other point mutations in the extracellular domain of the protein are associated with curved, short femurs with or without cloverleaf skull.

The clinical appearance is characteristic (Fig. 24.34). Total body length ranges from 35 to 47 cm, the limbs are short, extended and abducted with excessive skin folds, the thorax is constricted and the abdomen protuberant. The head is disproportionately large with

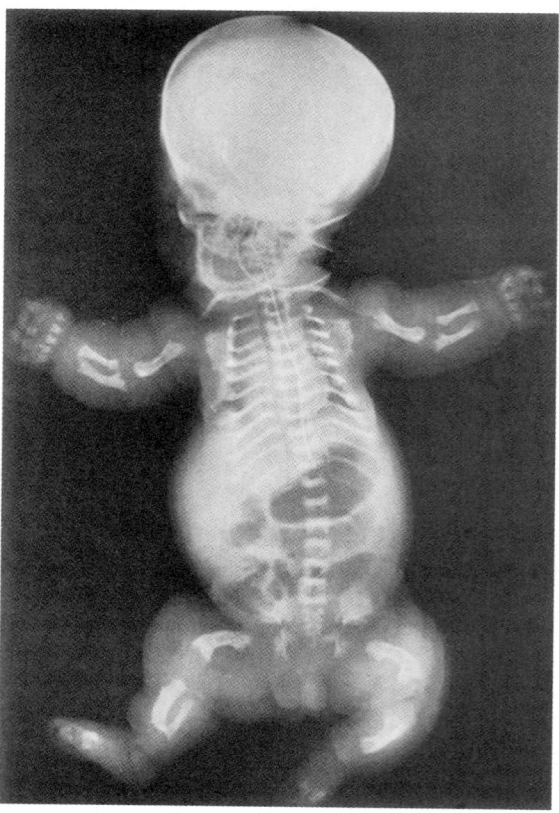

Fig. 24.35 Thanatophoric dysplasia. Skeletal survey of newborn infant with extremely short ribs, narrow vertebral bodies, tiny sciatic notches in flared iliac bones, and shortened limbs with notched bone ends.

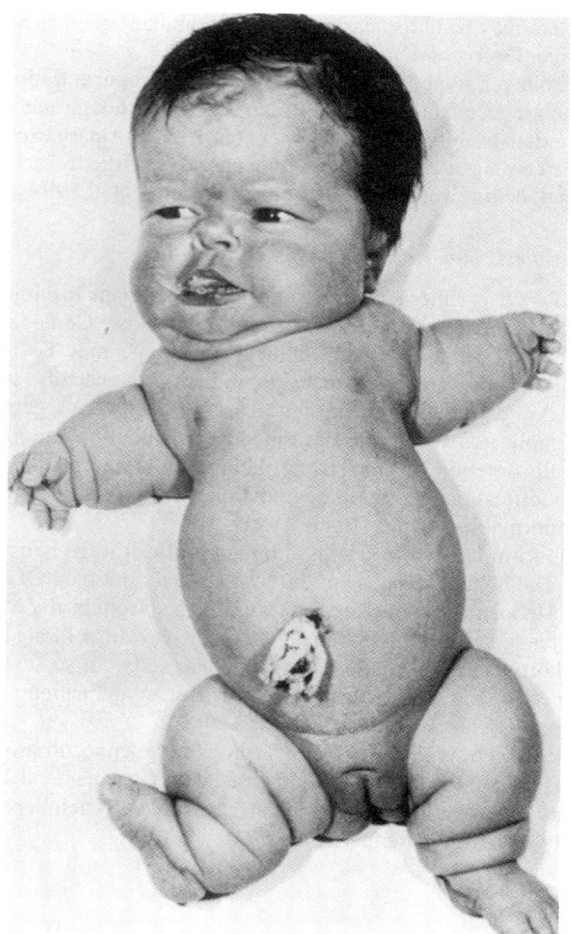

Fig. 24.34 Thanatophoric dysplasia.

a depressed nasal root, frontal bossing and enlarged fontanels, and may be hydrocephalic. Radiologically (Fig. 24.35) there are distinctive features, including extreme platyspondyly with an intravertebral disc space three or four times the depth of the vertebral body. The iliac bones are small and square with a small sciatic notch. The long bones, especially the femora, are short and bowed with flared metaphyses (like 'telephone receivers'), but in one variety the femora are relatively straight. Spike-like projections may be seen in the ischia, proximal femur and tibia. The ribs are short, the skull base constricted and the foramen magnum small. The infant is generally hypotonic and severe respiratory distress leads to death, usually within a few days. Occasional cases have survived for months or years. Prenatal diagnosis by ultrasound has been reported.

ACHONDROGENESIS AND HYPOCHONDROGENESIS

In these rare conditions, dwarfism and micromelia are extreme (Figs 24.36a and b). The head appears relatively large, the neck scarcely evident and the abdomen swollen. There is usually hydramnios, premature delivery and stillbirth. The radiological signs are unique with parts of the vertebral column and pelvic bones entirely unossified. The ribs are short and the limb bones very short (the femur may be only 2 or 3 cm in length) with 'cupped' and expanded metaphyses. Some cases have shown additional features of intrauterine fractures and gross distortion of the long bones and pelvis.

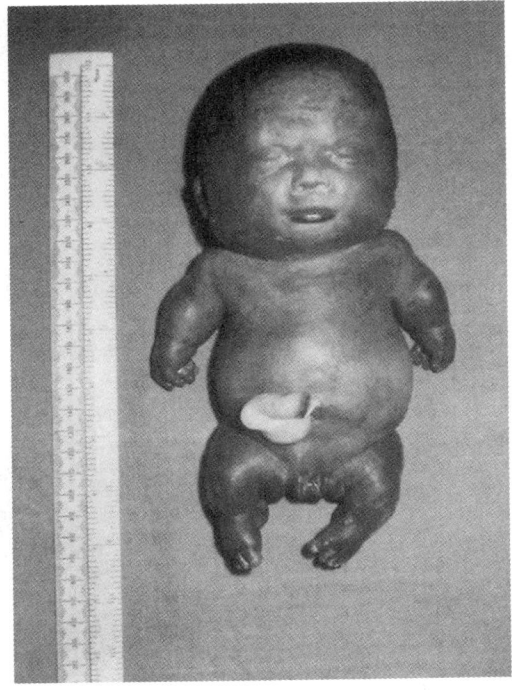
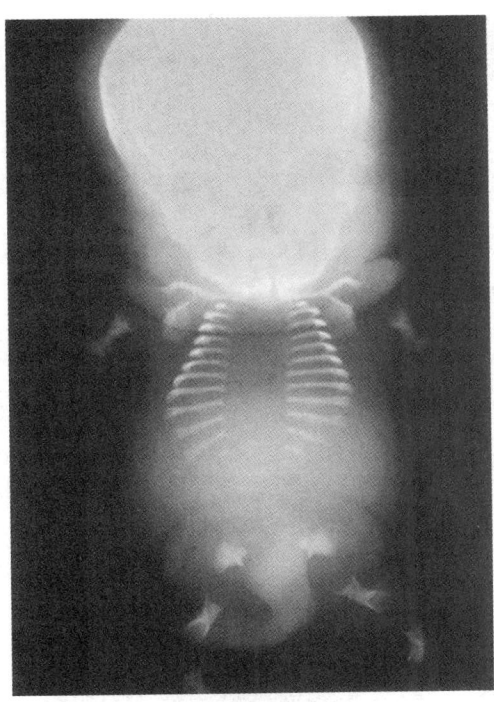

(a)

(b)

Fig. 24.36 Achondrogenesis: (**a**) phenotypic appearance with extreme micromelia in a stillborn achondrogenesis; (**b**) achondrogenesis type IB with absent spinal ossification.

Achondrogenesis types IA (Parenti–Fraccaro) and IB (Langer–Saldino), which is also designated type II, have been differentiated on phenotypic and radiographic features, but considerable heterogeneity seems to occur.

In hypochondrogenesis the clinical and radiological features are similar to those of achondrogenesis II, but the phenotype is less severe. Ossification of the lower thoracic and upper lumbar spine is seen but with severe hypoplasia in the cervical region and sacrum.

Achondrogenesis type II arises from new autosomal dominant point mutations in the COL2A1 gene that result in glycine substitutions at the N-terminal end of the triple helical domain (Bonaventure et al 1995). The amount of type II collagen in cartilage is reduced or has an abnormal structure. Occasional recurrence within families appears to arise from parental mosaicism for a dominant mutation, rather than autosomal recessive inheritance. Other mutations in the COL2A1 gene result in hypochondrogenesis (Horton et al 1992, Bogaert et al 1992, Bonaventure et al 1995).

HOMOZYGOUS ACHONDROPLASIA

This condition is the result of conception by parents of whom both have classical achondroplasia (see below). The skull is large with a depressed nasal bridge, there are short limbs with redundant skin folds, the chest is small and death tends to occur within the first few weeks of life. Radiologically the dysplasia is more severe than in achondroplasia but less severe than in thanatophoric dysplasia.

SHORT RIB–POLYDACTYLY (SRP) SYNDROMES

These autosomal recessive conditions are characterized by a tiny chest with pulmonary hypoplasia leading to death in respiratory failure.

In the Saldino–Noonan (SRP 1) syndrome there is postaxial polydactyly, a hypoplastic pelvis, dysplastic long bones and a high incidence of rectal and urogenital anomalies.

In the Majewski syndrome (SRP 2) there is pre- and postaxial polydactyly, relatively normal pelvic and long bone radiology, and a high incidence of cleft lip and palate, defects in the heart and other internal organs.

Differentiation is from other disorders with thoracic dystrophy, notably Jeune's (p. 1576) and the Ellis–van Creveld (p. 1575) syndromes.

Prenatal diagnosis of the SRP syndromes has been described.

CHONDRODYSPLASIA PUNCTATA (CHONDRODYSTROPHIA CALCIFICANS CONGENITA, STIPPLED EPIPHYSES, CONRADI'S DISEASE)

This disorder is characterized pathologically and radiologically by punctate mineralization in the epiphyses and also the joint capsules, trachea, larynx, hyoid, and vertebral discs. The calcification appears to occur in areas of mucoid degeneration in cartilage. Clinically (Fig. 24.37) there may be a peculiar facies with saddle nose, frontal bossing, hypertelorism, mongoloid slant to the eyes, high-arch palate, short neck, flexion contractures at the hips, knees and elbows, foot deformities, cataracts and dystrophic changes in hair and skin. Psychomotor retardation and failure to thrive may be prominent features and intercurrent infection the likely mode of death. Associated defects have included congenital heart disease, renal anomalies, cleft palate, and polydactyly.

The disorder has been classified into two main types. The rhizomelic type is usually lethal, often within the first year of life,

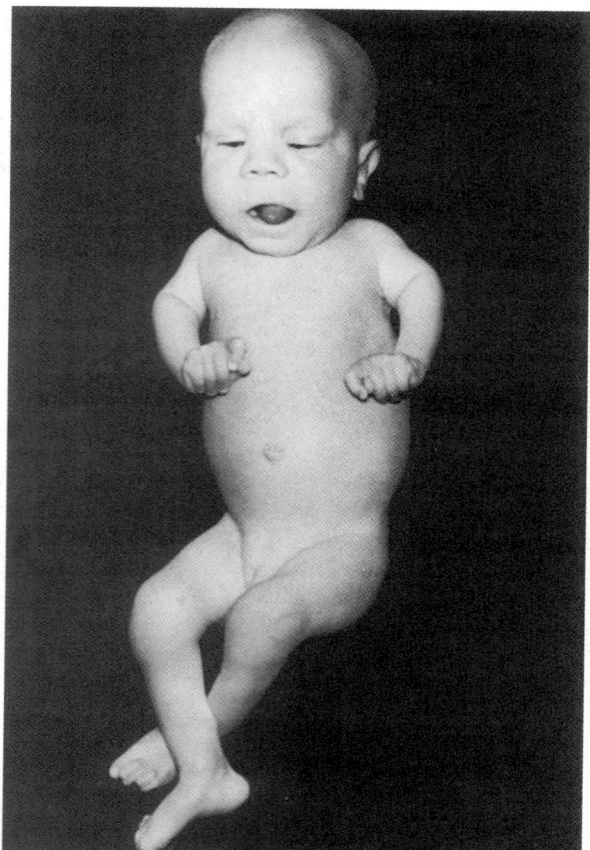

Fig. 24.37 Chondrodysplasia punctata (rhizomelic type).

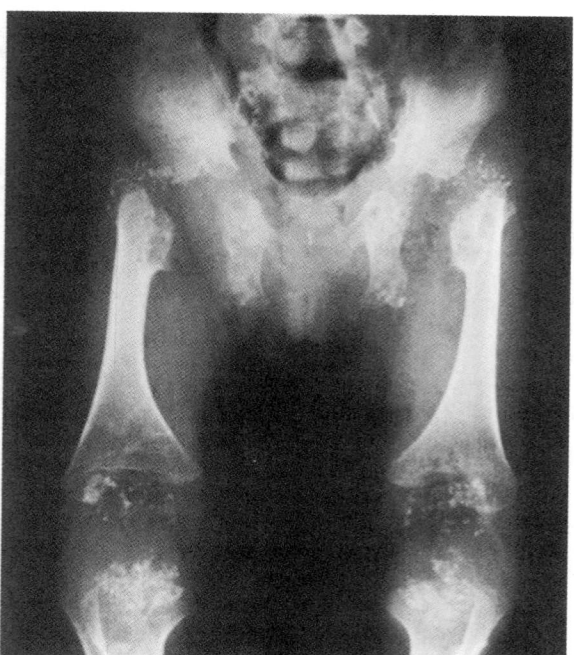

Fig. 24.38 Chondrodysplasia punctata (chondrodystrophia calcificans congenita). Extensive stippled calcification of articular cartilage at knees, hips and sacroiliac joints. Long bones short with flared and notched ends.

and inherited as an autosomal recessive. There is severe symmetrical rhizomelia with marked shortening of the humerus and femur and abundant punctate calcification around the epiphyses with coarse irregularity of the metaphyses (Fig. 24.38). Histologically there is severe disorganization of endochondral ossification. In this type there tends to be microcephaly, severe psychomotor retardation and a high incidence of cataracts. Deficient activity of peroxisomal enzymes has been demonstrated.

The other form, known as the Conradi–Hunermann type, is milder and an autosomal dominant. Cataracts and mental retardation are relatively rare and the prognosis for survival after the neonatal period is said to be good. Radiologically the limb bones are slightly shortened with mildly expanded metaphyses. The distribution of lesions is frequently asymmetrical. The calcifications are mainly paravertebral and there may be congenital hemivertebrae and scoliosis. Histologically, endochondral bone is normal or only mildly affected. In survivors, improvement in skeletal growth and joint mobility may occur and epiphyseal stippling becomes less obvious and eventually disappears.

CAMPTOMELIC DYSPLASIA

This autosomal dominant disorder has been linked to a defect in the SOX9 gene (Foster et al 1994, Wagner et al 1994). SOX9 is expressed in fetal testis and bone and encodes a transcription factor structurally related to the testis-determining factor, SRY. This may explain the combination of severe skeletal abnormalities and frequent sex reversal of chromosomal males to phenotypic females in this disorder.

There is striking deformity with anterior angulation of femora and tibiae and associated cutaneous dimples. There may be mild bowing of the forearms, bilateral talipes equinovarus and dislocation of the hips. The facies is peculiar with flattening, micrognathia and often a cleft palate. On X-ray there is evidence of prenatal bowing of the legs, with angulation in the midfemur and lower tibia with a hypoplastic fibula (Fig. 24.39). Other skeletal defects include a narrow thorax, scoliosis, hypoplasia of scapulae, various vertebrae and parts of the pelvis.

The infant tends to be stillborn or to show severe hypotonia, respiratory distress and early neonatal death. Rarely, survival has occurred with moderation of the bony deformities. Prenatal diagnosis by ultrasound has been reported.

ACHONDROPLASIA

The gene defect in this autosomal dominant disorder has been located on the transmembrane domain of fibroblast growth factor receptor 3 (Shiang et al 1994). This receptor mediates a variety of effects on cell growth and differentiation and is highly expressed in the growth plate. Unusually, more than 90% of achondroplasia patients have the same glycine to arginine substitution, mostly arising as new mutations (Muenke & Schell 1995). Such homogeneity makes DNA diagnosis a simple procedure.

In this disorder endochondral bone formation is defective with failure of proliferation of cartilage so that the cartilage columns of the growth plate are poorly developed. Membranous bone formation and articular cartilage are normal. Epiphyseal centers

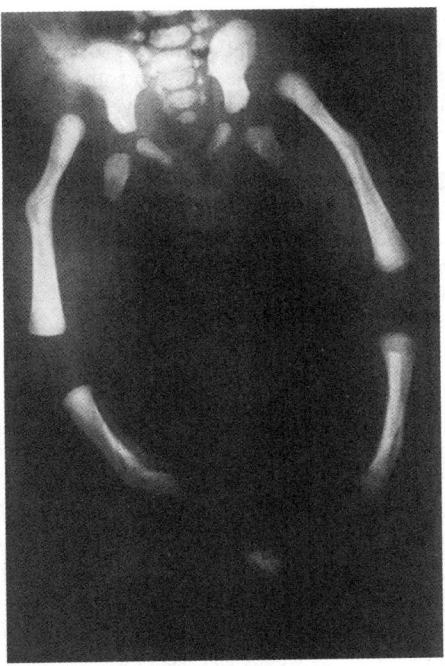

Fig. 24.39 Camptomelic dysplasia showing prenatal bowing of the legs with angulation of femur and tibia and a hypoplastic fibula.

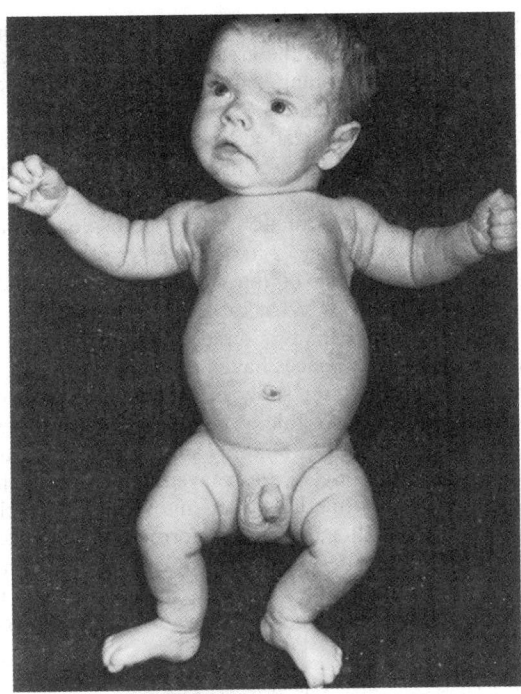

Fig. 24.40 Infant achondroplasia.

are less affected than the growth plates but may be small, delayed, and irregular with lateral expansion which contributes to the splaying of the growing end of the bone. Being developed in cartilage, the base of the skull is poorly formed whereas the vault of the skull (developed in membrane) is capable of full growth.

Clinical features

Clinically the condition is recognizable at birth. The infant is dwarfed; the limbs are shortened and as the shortening is primarily bony, there are rolls of soft tissue and transverse skin creases (Fig. 24.40). The limbs are also bowed and the bone ends

are bulbous. The feet and hands are short and broad. The fingers are all similar in length and lack full adduction giving the typical trident hand deformity. Secondary to the poor development of the base of the skull, the cranium enlarges, and with this disproportion between skull base and vault the head appears large. There is frontal bossing, the face is small with a depressed nasal bridge and the jaw is relatively prominent. The infant is mildly hypotonic and early motor progress is often slow.

The older child has, in addition to these early features, a characteristic erect posture with lumbar lordosis, mild thoracolumbar kyphosis and protuberant abdomen (Fig. 24.41). The legs are bowed with internal tibial torsion and the gait

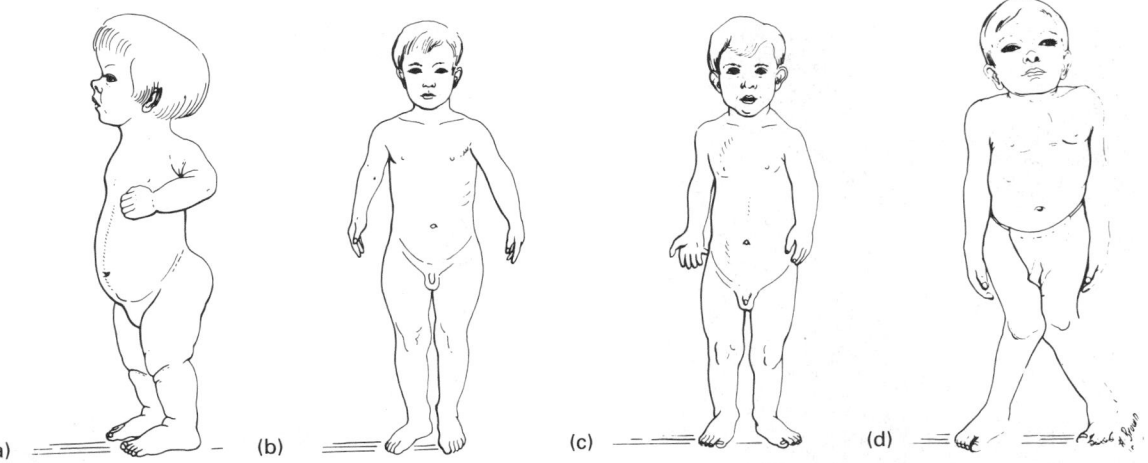

Fig. 24.41 (a) Achondroplasia. (b) Hypochondroplasia. (c) Ellis–van Creveld syndrome. (d) Morquio's disease. Note: (a) large cranium, abnormal facies, broad trident hand, lumbar lordosis, short limbs – especially proximally; (b) craniofacial structures relatively normal, hands small – not trident, short limbs – especially proximal; (c) craniofacial structures normal, narrow thorax, polydactyly, short limbs – especially distal; (d) skull and face little affected, short neck, deformed chest, short trunk, relatively long limbs, genu valgum.

waddling. The midpoint of the body lies above the umbilicus, the fingers do not reach beyond the greater trochanter. Intelligence is usually within the normal range but mental changes may develop with neurological complications (see below).

The neurological complications of achondroplasia are quite frequent and serious. A degree of hydrocephalus is often present. The hydrocephalus is usually communicating in type but is commonly related to obstruction of cerebrospinal fluid flow secondary to lack of space in the posterior fossa, basilar impression, and narrowing of the foramen magnum and upper cervical vertebrae. Narrow vertebral arches and interpedunculate spaces may cause cord compression leading to paraplegia.

No biochemical disturbances have been reported.

X-rays in achondroplasia show certain typical features. The long bones are short and thick (Figs 24.42 and 24.43). The proximal bones (humeri and femora) are more affected than the distal bones. The metaphyses are splayed and have a central V-shaped notch which forms a 'socket' into which the epiphyses protrude (so-called 'ball and socket' deformity). The metacarpals, metatarsals and phalanges appear short and stubby. The skull shows underdevelopment of the cartilaginous base with a small foramen magnum (Fig. 24.44). The vault appears large with

frontal bossing. The midface is hypoplastic and the jaw disproportionately large giving a degree of prognathism. The thorax appears long and narrow and the ribs short. The interpeduncular spaces narrow from above downwards (opposite

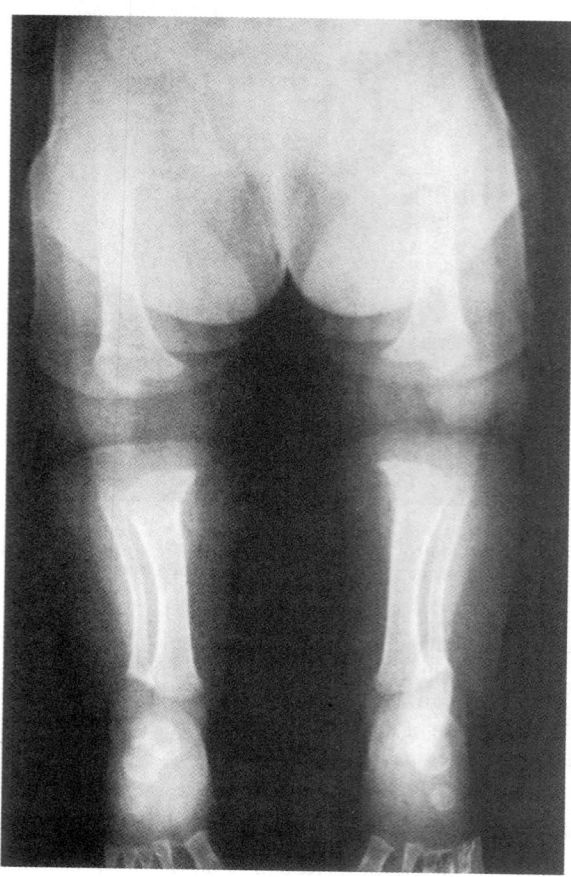

Fig. 24.43 Achondroplasia. Lower limbs showing shortening of long bones, more marked in proximal limb segments, and expanded ends with characteristic notching of femora at knees.

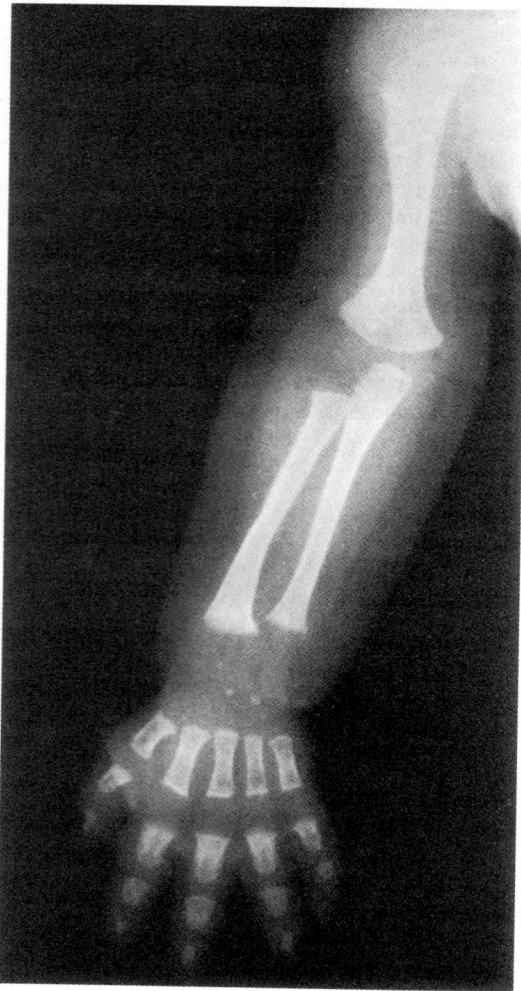

Fig. 24.42 Achondroplasia. Short humerus with broad ends; proximal limb segment shorter than distal; broad hand with relatively short bones.

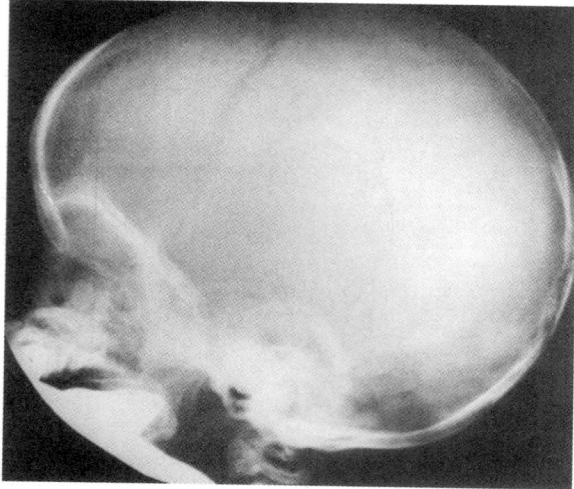

Fig. 24.44 Achondroplasia. Skull with short base producing domed vault with prominent forehead.

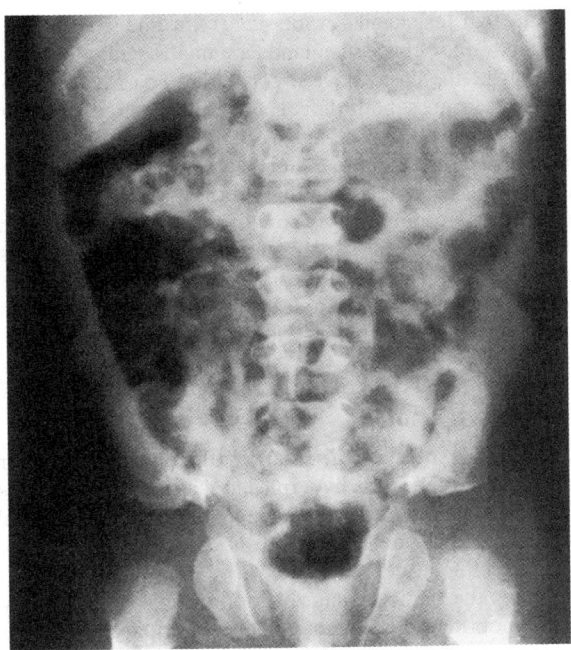

Fig. 24.45 Achondroplasia. Pelvis showing flared ilia with narrow sciatic notches and expanded proximal ends of femora. Spine shows interpedicular distances narrowing caudally in lumbar region.

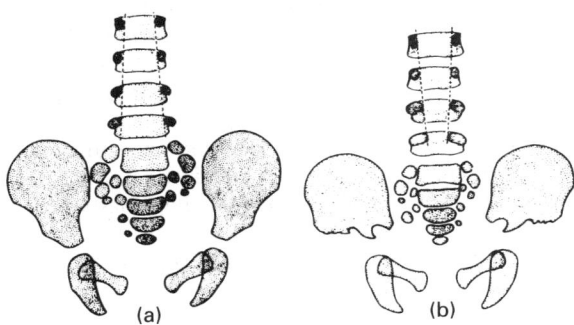

Fig. 24.46 Radiological appearance of pelvis and lumbar vertebrae in achondroplasia: (**a**) normal; (**b**) achondroplasia. (From Kaufmann 1964.)

of normal), particularly at the fifth lumbar vertebra, and there is some tapering of the pedicles (Figs 24.45 and 24.46). The vertebral bodies are small, cuboidal and irregular anteriorly, with beaking of lumbar 1 or 2. The posterior aspect of the vertebral bodies tends to be concave and the spinal canal narrowed. The pelvis shows a narrow sacrum which articulates low on the ilia. The iliac wings are small, the acetabular roof almost horizontal, and the sciatic notch narrow (Fig. 24.45). The pelvic inlet is wider than its depth ('champagne glass' appearance) (Fig. 24.46).

Prognosis

Contrary to older reports in which there had been confusion with the lethal forms of short-limbed dwarfism, the newborn achondroplast has a good life expectation, and in later years has good general health, is physically active, and fertile. The deformities do not increase after puberty but final adult height is

less than $4\frac{1}{2}$ feet (137 cm). There is no particular tendency to osteoarthritis but intervertebral disc degeneration and herniation are liable to occur.

Treatment

No treatment for achondroplasia is available. Hydrocephalus may require shunting, and extensive laminectomy may be necessary in cases complicated by transverse myelopathy due to lumbar canal stenosis. The place of leg lengthening operations remains controversial.

Children with achondroplasia may respond to recombinant growth hormone treatment with increased growth velocity, but this is at the cost of worsening disproportion (Bridges & Brook 1994), and there remains uncertainty about ultimate improvement in final height.

HYPOCHONDROPLASIA

The gene defect in this disorder has been located on the intracellular tyrosine kinase domain a of fibroblast growth factor receptor 3 (Bellus et al 1995), and is inherited in an autosomal dominant fashion. Most, but not all, patients share the same mutation. Since this relatively mild disorder is difficult to diagnose both clinically and radiologically, DNA testing for this common mutation should be of great value.

This disorder differs from classical achondroplasia in that growth retardation is less well marked and there is a relatively normal skull and facies (Fig. 24.41b). Sufficient positive radiological features are present to suggest the diagnosis. The cranium may be somewhat enlarged but without much basal maldevelopment and the face may be relatively small but without prognathism. The femur and humerus are most noticeably shortened and thickened with some metaphyseal flaring. The peripheral bones are also thick and small so that the hands are short, but not trident. The pelvis has well developed iliac wings, a somewhat reduced sacroiliac notch and horizontal acetabular roof. The spine shows less narrowing of the interpeduncular spaces than in achondroplasia and tapering of the pedicles is not seen. The vertebrae are reduced in anteroposterior diameter but of normal height.

Children with hypochondroplasia have a variable response to recombinant growth hormone, with some having a good response and others having no benefit (Bridges & Brook 1994). The greatest benefit may be gained by starting treatment in puberty. Orthopedic leg lengthening is an alternative treatment option that may be considered.

ELLIS–VAN CREVELD SYNDROME (CHONDROECTODERMAL DYSPLASIA)

This is a complex dysplasia in which skeletal defects are associated with ectodermal anomalies affecting hair, teeth and nails and, commonly, a mesodermal defect in the form of congenital heart disease. The condition is autosomal recessive, uncommon except among a certain Amish community in Pennsylvania. The growth plate cartilage appears deficient in cells with poorly organized columns.

Shortening of the long bones is most marked distal to the elbow and knee, which is the reverse of achondroplasia. Polydactyly of fingers and sometimes toes is a regular feature. The thorax is small and narrow. Dwarfism is moderate to severe (Fig. 24. 41c; Figs 24.47a and b). Craniofacial structures are normal. X-rays show the radius, ulna, tibia and fibula to be very short and widened at the ends. The changes in the proximal tibia are especially typical with a widened metaphysis showing an irregular ridged margin and a small medially placed epiphysis. There is a tendency to genu valgum. The hands and feet have prominent defects. The shortening is progressively more severe towards the distal bones so that the terminal phalanges are extremely hypoplastic. Epiphyses may be 'cone-shaped'. Carpal and tarsal bones may be fused into solid masses. The metacarpal of the extra digit tends to be fused with the adjacent fifth metacarpal.

The bones of the skull, vertebrae and pelvis are normal.

Teeth may be present at birth but dentition is generally delayed. The teeth tend to be small and conical and irregularly spaced giving rise to malocclusion. The mouth may show a short upper lip bound down to the underlying alveolar margin, accessory frenula and alveolar ridge defects. The nails are hypoplastic or

absent, the hair (especially of the scalp) fine and sparse. The skin, sweat glands and sebaceous glands are unaffected.

One-half of the cases have a congenital heart defect which is usually an atrial septal defect of either ostium primum or secundum type. About one-half of patients die in infancy from cardiac or respiratory disease. Survivors are not usually mentally subnormal and achieve a final height of 3–5 feet (107–152 cm). Surgery for the polydactyly or genu valgum will improve function. Regular dental supervision and treatment is necessary. Repair of the congenital heart lesion should be considered.

Prenatal diagnosis has been described.

ASPHYXIATING THORACIC DYSTROPHY (JEUNE'S SYNDROME)

This chondrodysplasia particularly affects the costochondral junction where there is hyperplastic cartilage which ossifies poorly. An autosomal recessive gene appears to be responsible.

Stillbirth or early neonatal death is associated with the small thorax and pulmonary hypoplasia.

In infancy the clinical picture is dominated by the narrow and rather immobile thorax with episodes of extreme respiratory distress often precipitated by respiratory infection. Death in respiratory failure may occur in the first year of life but if it does not, thereafter relative growth of the thorax occurs and respiratory problems remit. The patients are underheight with a variable degree of shortening of limbs and fingers and occasional polydactyly. Extension at the elbow may be limited. Hereditary nephritis leading to death in childhood has occurred with a variety of renal cystic dysplasias. Hypoplasia of the lungs and of the hepatic duct, pancreatic insufficiency with malabsorption, and retinal degeneration have also been reported.

X-rays show a small thorax with short horizontally placed ribs which have broad irregular anterior ends (Fig. 24.48). This is associated with pelvic changes, including hypoplastic iliac bones with a hook-shaped sciatic notch and sometimes a hook-shaped projection at the lateral margin of the acetabulum. The shortened

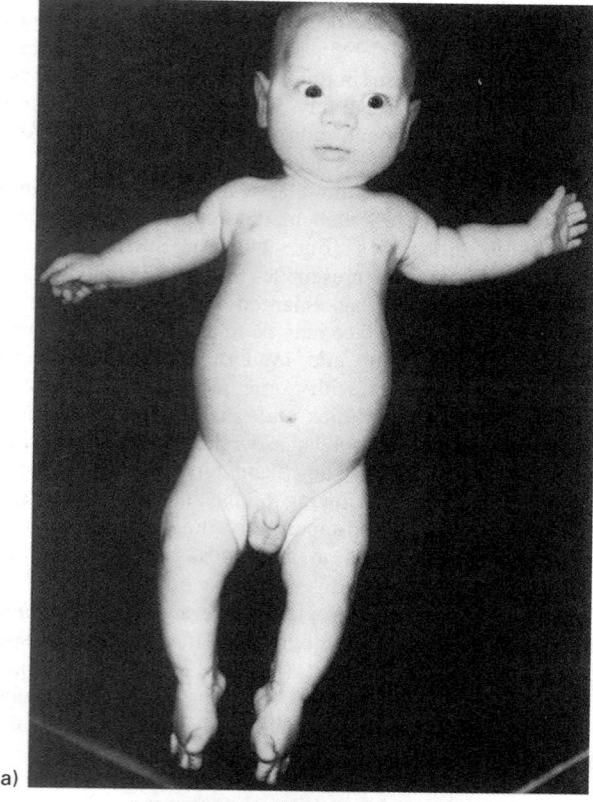

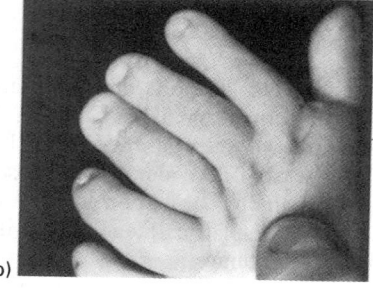

Fig. 24.47 Ellis–van Creveld syndrome: (**a**) dwarfism and short limbs; (**b**) polydactyly and hypoplasia of nails.

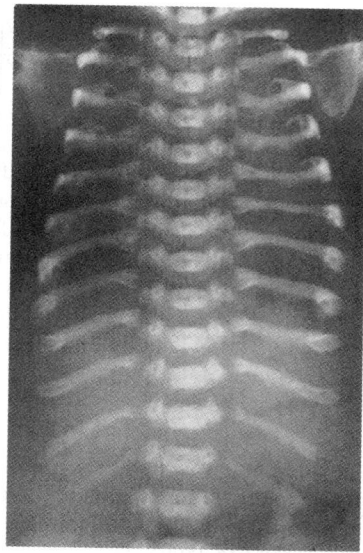

Fig. 24.48 Severe asphyxiating thoracic dystrophy, lethal in the newborn, showing extremely short ribs.

limb bones show variable irregularity of metaphyses and epiphyses. The hands have broad short metacarpals and proximal phalanges with small hypoplastic terminal phalanges, and the epiphyses may be 'cone-shaped'. The skull, face and spine are radiologically normal.

The differential diagnosis includes other bone dysplasias associated with a small thorax (e.g. thanatophoric, diastrophic, and metatropic dysplasia) and, particularly in the presence of polydactyly, the Ellis–van Creveld syndrome. The latter condition, however, also shows nail hypoplasia, upper lip malformations, dental anomalies and often congenital heart disease.

In the severely affected fetus, prenatal diagnosis by ultrasound may be possible.

DIASTROPHIC DYSPLASIA

These misshapen children (diastrophic = twisted or crooked) (Fig. 24.49) are differentiated from achondroplastics. Diastrophic dysplasia has been linked to a mutation in the sulfate transporter gene, leading to reduced activity of the protein (Hastbacka et al 1994). Only cartilage and bone are affected since the reduced activity is sufficient for the other tissues in which the gene is expressed, but insufficient for chondrocytes which have a high sulfate requirement.

The condition appears to be autosomal recessive. The growth retardation is present in infancy and is associated with marked

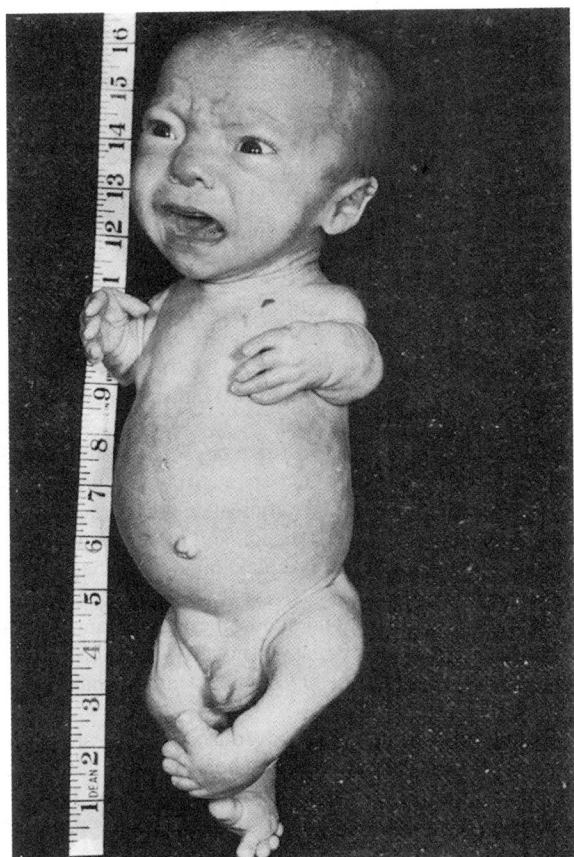

Fig. 24.49 Diastrophic dysplasia.

talipes equinovarus and limitation and contracture of other joints. Later, dislocations in the hip or knee and the development of (kypho)scoliosis lead to further deformity. There may be a superficial resemblance to arthrogryposis. The long bones are shortened with flared metaphyses and irregular epiphyses. The thumb is displaced proximally and the first metacarpal especially hypoplastic. The external ear shows deformity with soft cystic masses which develop into hypertrophied cartilage. Cleft palate occurs in one-fourth of cases. The skull and intelligence are normal. The orthopedic deformities are particularly resistant to correction. Prenatal diagnosis by ultrasound has been described.

METATROPIC DYSPLASIA

This disorder is characterized by variation in the clinical picture with age (metatropic = variable). At first the patients superficially resemble achondroplasia with limbs which are short for the trunk; later the proportions reverse with predominant shortening of the trunk more resembling Morquio's disease. Metatropic dysplasia is believed to be autosomal recessive but genetic and phenotypic variants have been described. In early infancy the limb shortening is associated with reduced length of the long bones and expanded metaphyses. There is limited joint movement. The hands are comparatively normal and the skull and face unaffected. The trunk at this stage may appear long and thin with a narrow chest and short ribs. There may be a caudal appendage. A degree of kyphoscoliosis may be evident but in spite of early spinal involvement body length at this stage may be within the normal range. As the years pass, however, shortening and deformity of the trunk with kyphoscoliosis and sternal protrusion dominate the clinical picture, producing an appearance comparable to Morquio's disease. The limb bones are radiologically abnormal at birth with defective remodeling and expanded epiphyses; the head of the femur is especially deformed with hypertrophy of the trochanters, and the pelvis has small iliac wings and a displaced acetabular roof. The spine shows markedly reduced height of the vertebral bodies with intervertebral disc spaces which may be two or three times wider than the vertebrae. Later the spine shows progressive kyphoscoliosis and wedge deformity of the lumbar vertebrae.

The spinal deformity in this disease is exceptionally severe requiring early and constant supervision.

KNIEST SYNDROME

This disorder resembles metatropic dysplasia (see above) and has been designated 'metatropic dwarfism type II'. Kniest syndrome is an autosomal dominant disorder that has been linked with a number of mutations in the COL2A1 (α1 chain of type II collagen) gene (Tilstra & Byers 1994, Spranger et al 1994). Short stature, a broad thorax, kyphoscoliosis and progressive limitation of joints are associated with craniofacial dysmorphism including macrocephaly, a flattened profile and cleft palate. Associated problems include severe myopia, retinal detachment and deafness. Radiologically, there is osteoporosis, platyspondyly with anterior wedging and coronal clefts in the vertebrae, hypoplastic iliac bones and slim long bones with bulky expanded metaphyses (dumbbell shape). The upper femoral epiphyses are particularly delayed and may never ossify. There appears to be a similar but distinct entity which is autosomal recessive, lethal in the newborn and designated 'Kniest-like dysplasia'.

THE METAPHYSEAL CHONDRODYSPLASIAS (METAPHYSEAL DYSOSTOSES)

These disorders are characterized by splayed irregular metaphyses and radiotranslucent areas of deficient ossification giving a rachitic-like appearance at the end of the long bones (Figs 24.50, 24.51 and 24.52). The epiphyseal contour is usually normal and

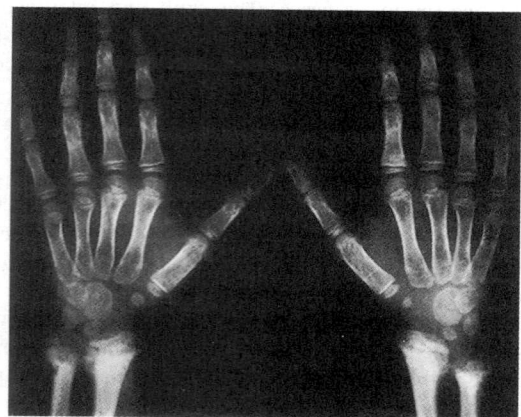

Fig. 24.50 Metaphyseal chondrodysplasia. Rachitic-like appearance with severe deformities at hands and wrists resembling renal osteodystrophy or hypophosphatasia but blood chemistry normal.

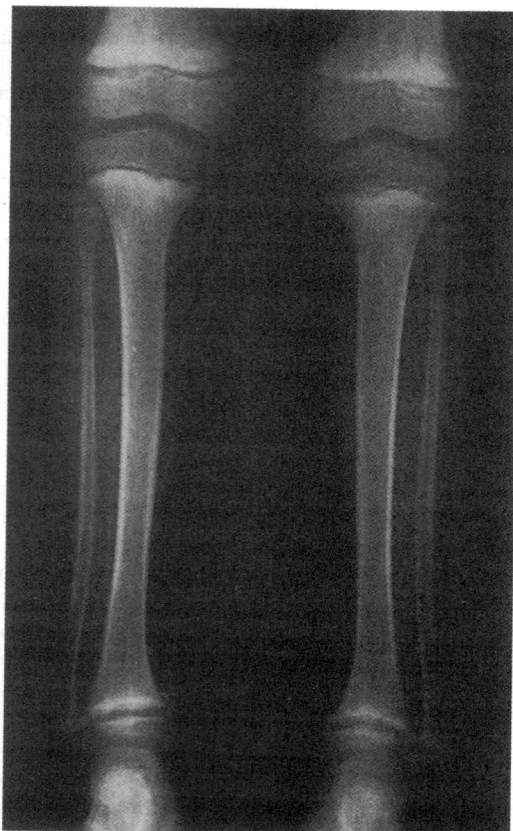

Fig. 24.51 Metaphyseal chondrodysplasia. Rachitic-like appearance showing irregularly frayed and expanded metaphyses at knees and ankles in girl of 5 with normal blood chemistry.

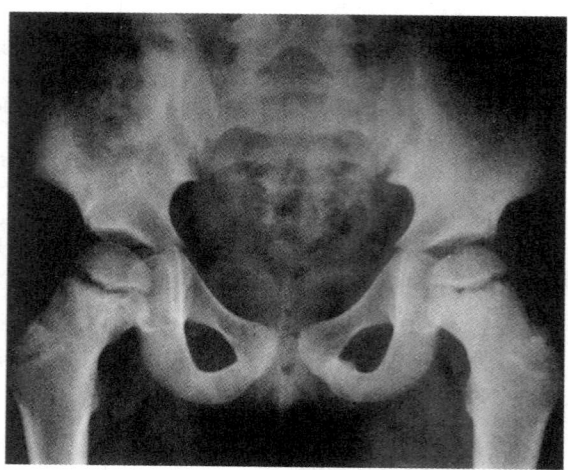

Fig. 24.52 Metaphyseal chondrodysplasia (dysostosis). Irregular defects in both femoral necks in girl with changes confined to hips.

the round bones of the wrists and ankles unaffected. The blood chemistry is normal. Clinically, some forms show only moderate short stature, others may show noticeably short or bowed limbs, swellings at the ends of long bones, flexion contractures, exaggerated lumbar lordosis, a waddling gait, or more severe dwarfism. The condition may mimic vitamin D-resistant rickets or bear a superficial resemblance to achondroplasia.

Some forms have a curious combination of extraskeletal manifestations with variable immunological deficiencies, malabsorption, and ectodermal abnormalities.

Metaphyseal chondrodysplasia type Jansen produces a phenotype that mimics hyperparathyroidism. It has been associated with a defect in the gene for the receptor that binds both parathyroid hormone and parathyroid hormone-related peptide, resulting in a permanently activated receptor (Schipani et al 1995). Its inheritance is autosomal dominant.

Metaphyseal chondrodysplasia type Schmid is an autosomal dominant disorder associated with mutations affecting the C-terminal noncollagenous domain of type X collagen, interfering with molecular assembly or producing a truncated protein (Warman et al 1993, McIntosh et al 1995). This explains the histological growth plate abnormalities and modest short stature observed in this disorder.

In cartilage–hair hypoplasia (metaphyseal chondrodysplasia type McKusick), scalp hair is fair, sparse, fine and brittle and the eyebrows and eyelashes may be deficient. Hirschsprung's disease, malabsorption syndrome, neutropenia, and increased virulence of certain virus infections, notably chickenpox have been noted in some patients.

In the Shwachman–Diamond syndrome there is an association of metaphyseal chondrodysplasia (notably of the hips) with exocrine pancreatic insufficiency, neutropenia or pancytopenia, and dwarfism.

A form of metaphyseal chondrodysplasia causing short-limbed dwarfism and associated with hereditary lymphopenia, hypogammaglobulinemia (particularly IgA and IgM), and ectodermal dysplasias affecting hair, eyebrows and skin has been described.

The main types of metaphyseal chondrodysplasia are summarized in Table 24.5. Other rare recessive forms include a

Table 24.5   The main groups of metaphyseal chondrodysplasias (after Shmerling et al 1969)

Type	Mode of transmission	Dwarfism	Bone lesions			
			Localization	Severity	Hips (coxa vara)	Vertebrae
Jansen	AD	++	Generalized	+++	+	+
Kozlowski	?	+	Generalized (epimetaphyseal)	++	−	−
Schmid	AD	+	Generalized	+	+	+
Spahr	AR	+	Generalized	+	−	−
Maroteaux	AR	+	Knees	(+)	−	−
McKusick, (cartilage – hair hypoplasia)	AR	++	Knees mainly	+	−	−
Shwachman	AR	++	Generalized including ribs	++	++	+

AR = autosomal recessive; AD = autosomal dominant.

congenital lethal type, a distinctive radiological type, and cases associated with retinitis pigmentosa, mental deficiency and deafness, optic atrophy and skin atrophy, and spastic paraplegia with plaque-like skin lesions. A dominant form associated with maxillary hypoplasia and brachydactyly has also been described.

SPONDYLOEPIPHYSEAL DYSPLASIAS

The chondrodysplasia in this group of diseases selectively affects the vertebrae, the carpal and tarsal bones, the epiphyses of the long bones and occasionally the adjacent metaphyses. These sites are affected to a variable degree so that some forms are mainly epiphyseal, some epiphysometaphyseal, and some characterized by platyspondyly (see below and Table 24.6).

Multiple epiphyseal dysplasia (MED) is one of the commoner skeletal dysplasias. Some forms of this autosomal dominant disorder have been linked to mutations in the same region of the cartilage oligomeric matrix protein gene that is affected in

Table 24.6   Spondyloepiphyseal dysplasia (SED) (after Maroteaux 1969)

Group	Sites of involvement	Clinical nomenclature	Dwarfism	Short limbs	Short trunk	X-ray	Mode of transmission
Multiple epiphyseal	Long and short tubular bones	Classical type of multiple epiphyseal dysplasia	+ or ++	++ Distal	+	Small irregular epiphyses. Prone to hip arthritis	AD and AR forms
	Spine and proximal long bones		+ or ++	+	++	Vertebral plates irregular ± wedging. Irregular proximal epiphyses of femur and humerus. Prone to hip arthritis	AD and AR forms
	Limited to specific sites	Brailsford's peripheral dystosis; Thiemann's disease	0	0 or +	0	Irregular epiphyses of hands and feet ± metaphyseal defect of phalanges. Some forms localized to hips or elbows	?
With generalized platyspondyly	Spine ± upper femoral epiphyses	SED tarda	+ late	0	++	Platyspondyly, small pelvis. Irregular, deformed femoral head	X-linked recessive
	Spine + proximal epiphyses ± peripheral epiphyses	SED congenita	+++	+	+++	At birth, platyspondyly with ovoid vertebral bodies, retarded pelvic ossification, proximal femur and humerus very deformed	AD
	Spine + generalized epiphyses	Morquio and similar syndromes*	+++	++	+++	Flattened vertebrae with anterior hypoplasia and posterior displacement of D12. L1. Coxa valga, protrusio acetabuli. Conical metacarpal ends. Irregular epiphyses	AR
Epiphysometaphyseal	With minor spinal changes†	Pseudoachondroplastic type	+++	++	+ or ++	Irregular metaphyses of long bones, epiphyses small and deformed. Vertebral bodies biconvex with anterior projection but not flattened	AD and AR forms
	Without spinal changes	Leri's pleonosteosis	0	0 or + distal	0	Irregular metaphyses in hands and feet. Joint contractures	AD

* Morquio-like syndromes have been described such as pseudo-Morquio's disease and the spondylometaphyseal dystosis of Kozlowski which vary from Morquio's in some clinical, radiological, and biochemical features and probably in mode of inheritance.
† A further heterogeneous group of epiphysometaphyseal dysplasias with severe spinal changes is also suggested. Dwarfism with micromelia and a short trunk occurs with a variable radiological appearance in the spine and long bones (see Maroteaux 1969).
AR = autosomal recessive; AD = autosomal dominant.

pseudoachondroplasia (Briggs et al 1995). The two disorders therefore appear to be allelic.

The child is likely to present with stiffness in the hips, limited exercise tolerance and/or a degree of short stature. Craniofacial appearance and intelligence are normal. The hands may be broad with stubby digits. The radiological changes in the femoral head simulate Perthes disease and the diagnosis of MED should be considered in all patients with apparently bilateral Perthes, particularly if 'familial' (Fig. 24.53). Lesser epiphyseal changes are usually seen elsewhere, e.g. hands, feet, and shoulders. MED is very heterogeneous with severe (Fairbank) and relatively mild (Ribbing) types. A form with myopia and conductive deafness has also been described. Degenerative osteoarthritis can be crippling and replacement of the femoral head by hip prosthesis may become necessary in adult life.

The form known as spondyloepiphyseal dysplasia congenita is an autosomal dominant disorder that has been linked to several mutations in the COL2A1 (α1 chain of type II collagen) gene (Tilstra & Byers 1994, Spranger et al 1994). It is evident at birth (see Table 24.6) and is characterized by short-limbed dwarfism and delayed ossifications, especially in the pelvis and proximal femora, along with flattened vertebral bodies. Facial dysmorphism is seen with hypertelorism, upward slanting palpebral fissures, cleft or high-arch palate, a short neck, and a tendency to prominent eyes, severe myopia, cataracts and retinal detachment. Later there may be hypotonia with delayed motor milestones, a waddling gait, pectus carinatum, kyphoscoliosis, knock-knee and flexion contractures of the hip (Fig. 24.54).

In other forms of spondyloepiphyseal dysplasia, growth usually appears normal in the first year of life and the disease becomes apparent in the second year with stunting which may eventually be very severe. Some varieties, however, show little or no dwarfism and present with orthopedic complaints such as abnormal gait, limited joint mobility, or shortening of the extremities. The craniofacial appearance is normal. A classification based on sites of involvement (Table 24.6) includes Morquio's disease, which is the prototype of these disorders, and this disease is described further in the section on

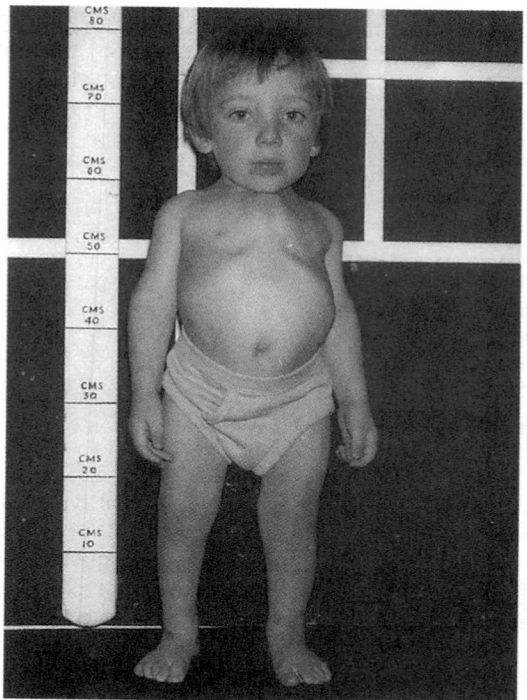

Fig. 24.54 Disproportionate short stature and rib cage deformity in spondyloepiphyseal dysplasia congenita.

mucopolysaccharidoses (p. 1158). The table excludes other mucopolysaccharidoses and certain disorders such as the metaphyseal chondrodysplasias, Conradi's disease, diastrophic and metatropic dysplasia which have distinctive features.

The classification is tentative and overlap between groups may occur so that, for example, the epiphyseal dysplasias may show some metaphyseal change.

Pseudoachondroplasia is an autosomal dominant disorder in which there is severe dwarfing with the limbs more affected than the axial skeleton. It has been linked to mutations in one region of the gene encoding cartilage oligomeric matrix protein, presumably disrupting its normal pentamer structure (Hecht et al 1995, Briggs et al 1995). It appears to be allelic with some forms of multiple epiphyseal dysplasia.

Stickler's syndrome is an autosomal dominant disorder characterized by early degenerative joint disease, mild skeletal epiphyseal dysplasia and ocular problems. In some cases there is cleft palate which may be coupled with Pierre Robin anomaly, or hearing loss. Many families have mutations in the COL2A1 gene, including premature termination codons, resulting in either reduced production of type II collagen or a truncated protein that may affect the structure of the cartilage matrix (Byers 1994b, Spranger et al 1994). Mutations in type XI collagen may give rise to a form of Stickler's syndrome without eye involvement (Vikkula et al 1995).

MESOMELIC DYSPLASIA

In this group of conditions there is disproportionate shortening in the middle segments (forearms, shanks) of the extremities (mesomelic brachymelia).

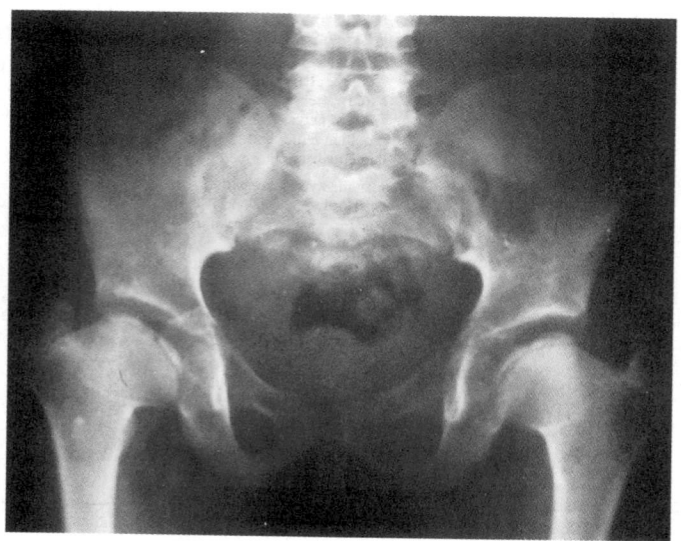

Fig. 24.53 Radiological changes in the femoral heads in multiple epiphyseal dysplasia (MED).

Certain rare and severe forms may be evident at birth. Langer's dwarfism shows a relatively normal trunk, severe mesomelia with particular hypoplasia of ulna, fibula and mandible and a probable autosomal recessive inheritance. In Nievergelt's mesomelic syndrome, the forearms and legs are about one-third the length of the arms and thighs at birth, there are flexion deformities of the elbows and fingers, severe clubfoot, a rhomboidal shape to the tibia and fibula on X-rays, and an autosomal dominant mode of inheritance. Robinow's syndrome shows clinical features at birth with saddle-nose, prominent forehead, hypertelorism along with moderate mesomelic dwarfism and later dental malalignment. There may be a superficial resemblance to achondroplasia but the hands, pelvis and spine are normal. It is considered an autosomal dominant.

In dyschondrosteosis, changes are relatively mild and present in later childhood. Also referred to as Leri–Weill disease, there are short forearms with bilateral Madelung's deformity (p. 1548), mesomelic shortening of the lower extremities, inconstant changes in metacarpals and metatarsals and moderate short stature (Fig. 24.55). It is probably inherited as an autosomal dominant.

SKULL AND LONG BONE DYSPLASIAS AND HYPEROSTOSES

Craniotubular dysplasias

Gorlin et al (1969) have categorized a number of genetically determined disorders which have in common cranial dysplasia and modeling defects of the tubular bones (Table 24.7).

Craniotubular hyperostoses

The same authors bring together a second group of conditions with the distinctive feature of hyperostoses of cranial and tubular bones, with bony overgrowth rather than defective modeling (Table 24.8).

ALBERS-SCHÖNBERG DISEASE (OSTEOPETROSIS, MARBLE BONES DISEASE)

This disorder occurs in several forms, one severe and recessive, one relatively benign and dominant, and one autosomal recessive

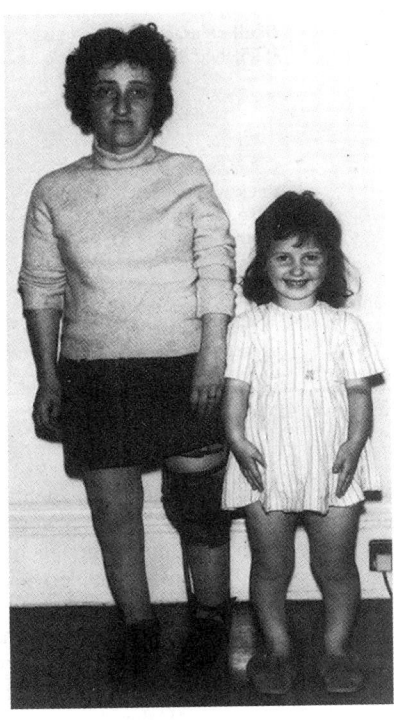

Fig. 24.55   Mesomelic dysplasia (dyschondrosteosis) in mother (with old poliomyelitis of leg) and child who presented with short stature and Madelung's deformity of the wrist.

Table 24.7   Genetic craniotubular dysplasias (after Gorlin et al 1969)

Type	Skull	Spine	Femur	Hand	Clinical	Genetics
Pyle's disease	Frontal bulge, little or no hyperostosis of vaults, obtuse mandibular angle	May show slight flattening	'Abrupt' metaphyseal flare	Marked metaphyseal flare	Muscle weakness, joint pains, genu valgum	AR
Craniometaphyseal dysplasia, dominant form	Fronto-occipital hyperostosis or sclerosis	Normal	'Soft' metaphyseal flare (club shape)	Mild metaphyseal flare	Broad nasal bridge, hypertelorism, nasal obstruction, cranial nerve palsies, deafness	AD
Craniometaphyseal dysplasia, recessive form	Massive sclerosis and hyperostosis of cranial vault and mandible	Normal	'Soft' metaphyseal flare (club shape)	Mild metaphyseal flare	As above but with more severe involvement of skull, nose and cranial nerves	AR
Craniodiaphyseal dysplasia	Massive sclerosis and hyperostosis of cranial vault and mandible	Normal	Widened diaphyses (cylindrical shape)	Diaphyseal widening	Severe facial and cranial distortion with bony thickening and nasal obstruction, mental defect, fits, deafness, visual loss, stunting and delayed sexual maturation	AD
Frontometaphyseal dysplasia	Extreme frontal bulge, negligible hyperostosis of vault, mandible hypoplastic and dysplastic	Normal	Moderate metaphyseal flare of distal onset	Moderate metaphyseal flare Subluxation of small joints	Marked supraorbital ridge, hirsutism, deafness and various long bone changes	X-linked dominant
Dysosteosclerosis	Moderate sclerosis of cranial vault, mild frontal hyperostosis	Platyspondyly and sclerosis	Very wide translucent metaphyses Sclerosis of epiphyses and diaphyses	Marked metaphyseal flare Epiphyseal sclerosis	Short stature with limbs more shortened than trunk. Narrow chest. Tendency to fracture. Cranial nerve palsies	AR

AR = autosomal recessive; AD = autosomal dominant.

Table 24.8 Genetic craniotubular hyperostoses (after Gorlin et al 1969)

Type	Skull	Tubular bones	Clinical	Genetics
Van Buchem	Calvaria thick, base dense. Mandibular enlargement	Thickened diaphyses, cortical hyperostosis (endosteal) with medullary constriction	Broad prominent mandible. Facial palsy, optic atrophy, deafness. Raised alkaline phosphatase	AR
Sclerosteosis	Skull enlarged. Calvaria grossly thickened. Skull base thick	Increased density, lack of diaphyseal modeling	Steep, high forehead, hypertelorism, broad nasal root. Broad, square prognathic jaw. May have syndactyly. Deafness, facial palsy	AR
Congenital hyperphosphatasia	Calvaria irregular and thick without sclerosis (also platyspondyly and protrusio acetabuli)	Expansion, hyperostosis of diaphyses. Bowing	Fever, bone pain, fractures, shedding of teeth. Stunting, blue sclera, tight skin, deafness. Raised alkaline phosphatase	AR
Camurati-Engelmann	Mild to moderate sclerosis of base and vault, especially anterior two-thirds	Diaphyseal hyperostosis, both endosteal and periosteal. Cortex may be lamellated. Metaphyses spared	At 3–5 years, painful limbs, muscle hypoplasia and abnormal gait	AR

AR = autosomal recessive; AD = autosomal dominant.

form associated with renal tubular acidosis, mental retardation, and carbonic anhydrase II deficiency.

Experiments on gene knock-out animal models have suggested that mutations in several genes that govern osteoclast development and function have the potential to produce an osteopetrosis phenotype. These include macrophage colony-stimulating factor 1 which acts at several stages during macrophage and osteoclast development (Yoshida et al 1990); C-fos which is required for normal development of osteoclast progenitors (Johnson et al 1992); and c-src which is necessary for the development of ruffled borders in the osteoclast, where bone resorption is initiated (Soriano et al 1991). Whether mutations in any of these genes also give rise to the human forms of osteopetrosis remains to be established. However, mutations in the carbonic anhydrase II gene, necessary for osteoclast action, have been shown to be associated with some human cases of osteopetrosis, mostly in kindreds of Arabic and Caribbean Hispanic origin (Ohlsson et al 1980, Hu et al 1992, Hu et al 1994).

Pathology

There is a persistence of primary calcified cartilaginous matrix with an apparent failure of resorption by osteoclasts. Remodeling of bone is defective and cortical compact bone is poorly differentiated as the marrow space fails to form. The entire skeleton is sclerotic to a greater or lesser extent. The tubular bones are widened, dense and fragile. Hemopoiesis is impaired.

Clinical features

Congenital form

The autosomal recessive congenital form is severe, presents in early infancy, and has been recognized radiographically in utero. The infant may be stillborn or may die within a few months with failure to thrive, severe anemia, hemorrhage, or intercurrent infection. Clinical manifestations include generalized lymphadenopathy and enlargement of the liver and spleen. There is a pancytopenia and evidence of a hemolytic process, sometimes with visible jaundice. Immature myeloid cells may appear in the peripheral blood. The bone foramina carrying the cranial nerves fail to enlarge with growth so that progressive compression and destruction of nerves occurs. Thus, loss of vision due to optic atrophy, deafness, extraocular palsies, facial and other paralyses may develop. A progressive hydrocephalus may occur and chronic subdural hematomas are recorded. Older children surviving the severe form of the disease may be mentally retarded and stunted. Serum calcium, phosphorus and alkaline phosphatase are not consistently abnormal but calcium balance has been found to be strongly positive. X-rays of the long bones show typical 'clubbed' metaphyses due to lack of modeling. The bones are dense with a poorly defined cortex and, in severe cases, an obliterated medulla (Fig. 24.56). The epiphyses are sclerotic but normally formed. In older children the metaphyses may show transverse bands of osteosclerosis as though activity of the disease has fluctuated over the years. The base of the skull is particularly dense, the vault appears less so. The pituitary fossa is small and the posterior clinoids clubbed. The sinuses are poorly aerated, the facial bones dense. Fractures are frequent and are often transverse. Callus forms normally and healing is not delayed. Rickets has occurred as a complication in some young infants. Teeth are often severely carious. Treatment for the severe 'malignant' form of osteopetrosis includes blood transfusion for anemia, antibiotics for infection, and standard orthopedic treatment for fractures. Optic nerve decompression may save sight if optic atrophy is developing.

Bone marrow transplantation has been undertaken with dramatic resolution of bone lesions and hematological features. Transient hypercalcemia is described after engraftment. Pre-existing neurological deficits are likely to persist.

Splenectomy has been performed on the basis that the hemolytic process is due to hypersplenism, with apparent benefit in some cases. Corticosteroids have controlled the anemia and thrombocytopenia in some patients but have been of no obvious benefit in others. A low calcium diet, if necessary supplemented with cellulose phosphate to inhibit calcium absorption, has led to

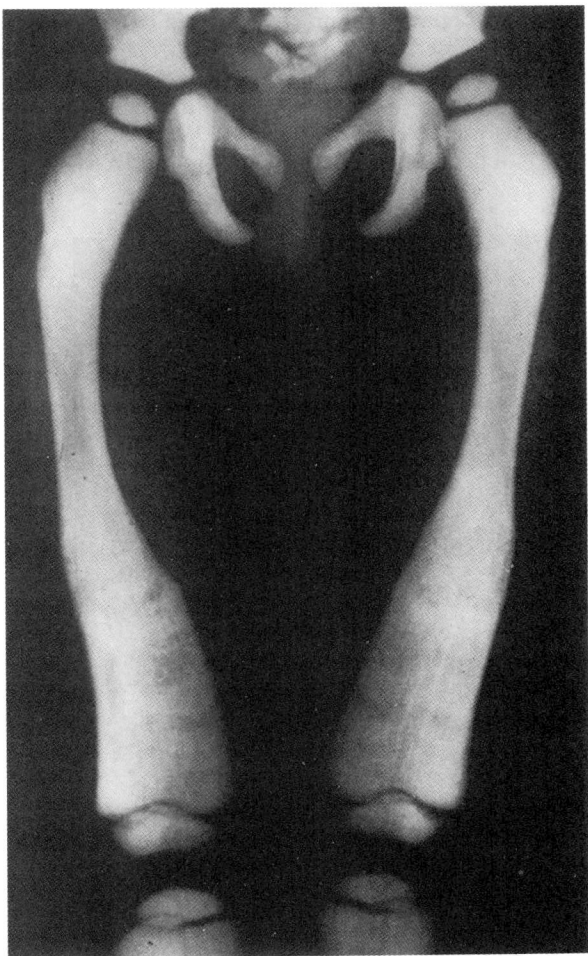

Fig. 24.56 Albers–Schönberg disease (osteopetrosis). Lower limbs showing imperfect modeling and greatly increased density with poorly developed trabecular pattern and no cortical definition.

demineralization of bone and prevented progression of the disease. High dose calcitriol promotes bone resorption, and can lead to clinical improvement.

Until the basic pathogenesis of the disorder is more fully understood, all of these various forms of treatment may reasonably be considered.

Tarda form

This is a relatively benign autosomal dominant form of osteopetrosis. It often presents as a pathological fracture, osteomyelitis or an unexplained anemia and may not be diagnosed until later childhood or adult life. The skeleton is generally osteosclerotic. All the long bones are dense but may show less clubbed metaphyses than in the congenita form. The patient may succumb to the hematological complications after many years, or there may be an entirely benign course with a normal life span.

Prolonged vitamin D overdosage, idiopathic hypercalcemia and fluoride poisoning may cause osteoscleroses, but other features of these conditions such as systemic effects, hypercalcemia and ectopic calcification will differentiate them.

Treatment of the tarda form is symptomatic.

PYKNODYSOSTOSIS

This disorder shows some resemblance to Albers-Schönberg disease. Clinically there is short stature, an undue tendency to fracture and a number of dysplastic stigmata including delayed closure of the sutures, facial hypoplasia, narrow palate, failure of angulation of the mandible and irregular or delayed dentition. The lateral end of the clavicle may be poorly formed and with the large fontanels may simulate craniocleidodysostosis. The terminal phalanges are typically atrophic.

On X-ray there is generalized osteosclerosis. It is differentiated from Albers-Schönberg by the absence of cranial nerve involvement or hematological complications and by the presence of the dysplastic features noted above. The disease appears to be autosomal recessive.

A number of affected cases have been mentally retarded.

INFANTILE CORTICAL HYPEROSTOSIS (CAFFEY'S DISEASE)

Pathology

In the early stage there is a swollen, mucoid and highly active cellular periosteum. This intraperiosteal inflammatory reaction extends into neighboring tissues. The elements are at first poorly differentiated and the lesion may resemble an osteosarcoma. Later, the reactive periosteum becomes enclosed in fibrous tissue. Periosteal new bone is laid down and in the healing phase is gradually resorbed from the endosteal surface, the bone becoming remodeled to a normal contour. The marrow is unaffected. The arterioles have been described as showing intimal proliferation and it has been postulated that vascular obliteration may be the primary lesion. A raised platelet count has been noted in some cases and vascular thromboses due to thrombocythemia suggested as a cause of the hyperostoses. There is no reported biochemical disturbance apart from an elevated alkaline phosphatase.

Cortical hyperostosis may affect the flat bones, particularly the mandible, but also the scapulae, ilium, and frontal and parietal regions of the skull. Scapular involvement is usually unilateral. Rib lesions have sometimes been associated with pleural effusion. In the extremities the forearms, especially the ulnae, are commonly involved but any tubular bones except the phalanges may show changes. Hyperostosis is confined to the diaphysis; the metaphysis and epiphysis are normal. The spine and the round bones are not affected.

Clinical features

This disorder of unknown etiology occurs in the first few months of life and is characterized by systemic disturbance and an acute inflammatory reaction in the periosteum. Most cases are sporadic with both sexes equally involved but a familial incidence compatible with dominant inheritance has been recorded. Bone changes have been recognized in utero but generally some weeks elapse before signs and symptoms develop (average 9 weeks). The onset is said never to be delayed beyond 5 months. A triad of irritability, soft tissue swellings and cortical thickening of the underlying bone is typical. The nonspecific signs of irritability, fever, pallor and a raised erythrocyte sedimentation rate are associated with soft tissue swellings which are tender, brawny and deep sited. The overlying skin is not reddened or hot. The distribution of lesions is one of the most diagnostic features with the mandibles (Fig. 24.57a), the clavicles, and in the extremities the ulnae being most frequently involved. Less commonly the scapulae (Fig. 24.57b), ilium, frontal and parietal bones and other tubular bones may be involved. Pseudoparalysis of a limb may occur. The soft tissue swellings appear before any radiological abnormalities appear and subside while X-ray changes persist (Figs 24.58 and 24.59).

The course of the disease varies from weeks to months. In some cases it remains localized (e.g. to the jaw), in others there is widespread or progressive involvement and unpredictable remissions and relapses occur. Disseminated disease with severe constitutional upset may be fatal, perhaps due to intercurrent infection in the debilitated infant. Prolonged disease causes failure to thrive, delayed development and motor handicap. The hyperostosis usually resolves some 3–12 months after signs of activity (swellings, fever, etc.) have subsided. A chronic form

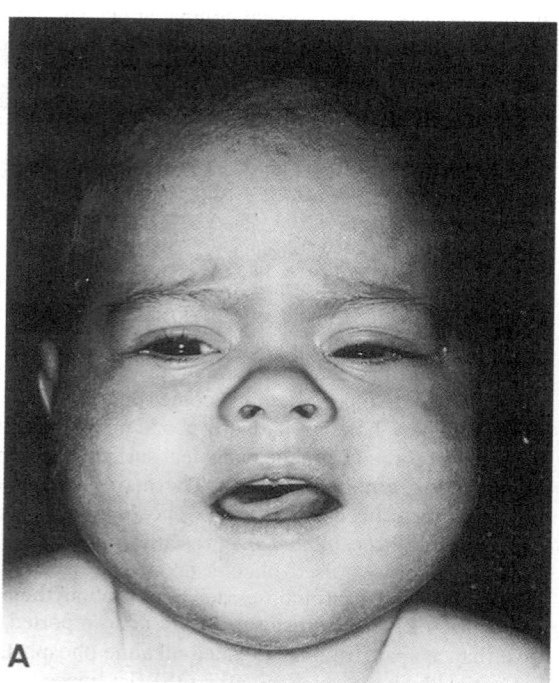
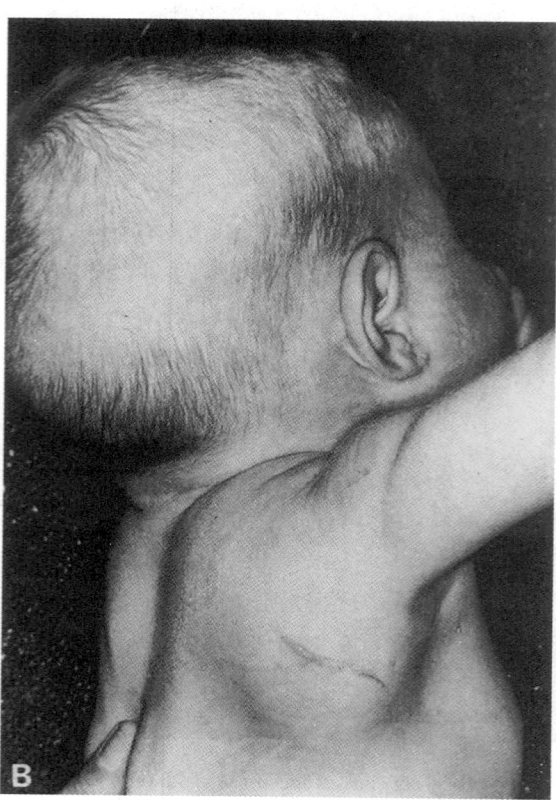

Fig. 24.57 Infantile cortical hyperostosis (Caffey's disease) showing: (**a**) mandibular swelling; and (**b**) scapular swelling (operation scar over scapula where incision carried out on account of mistaken diagnosis of osteomyelitis).

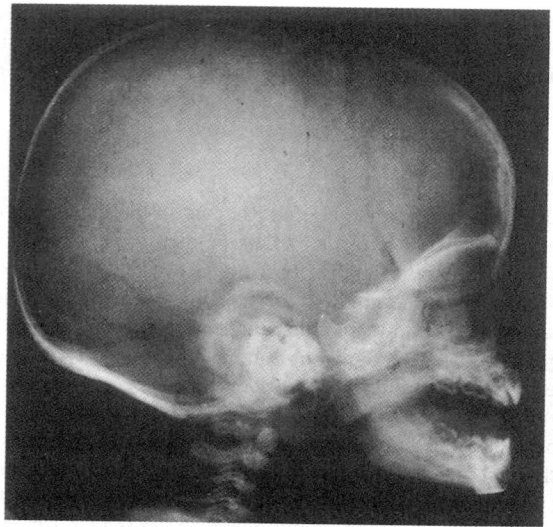
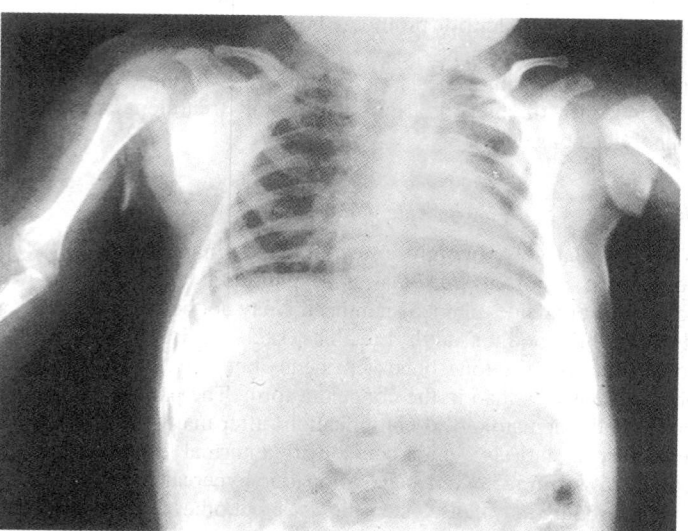

(a)

(b)

Fig. 24.58 Infantile cortical hyperostosis (Caffey's disease): (**a**) skull showing thickening of mandible; (**b**) chest film showing excessive new bone round right scapula and minimal changes in right clavicle and left lower ribs.

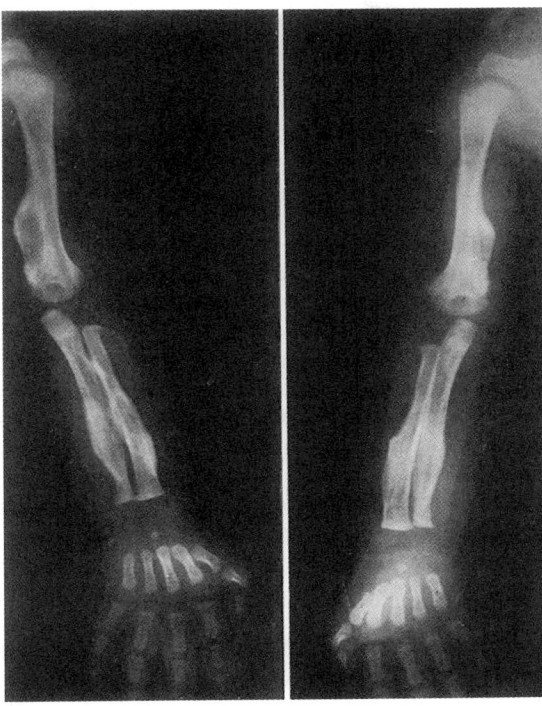

Fig. 24.59 Infantile cortical hyperostosis. Upper limbs showing extensive irregular new bone formation along shafts of long bones sparing metaphyses.

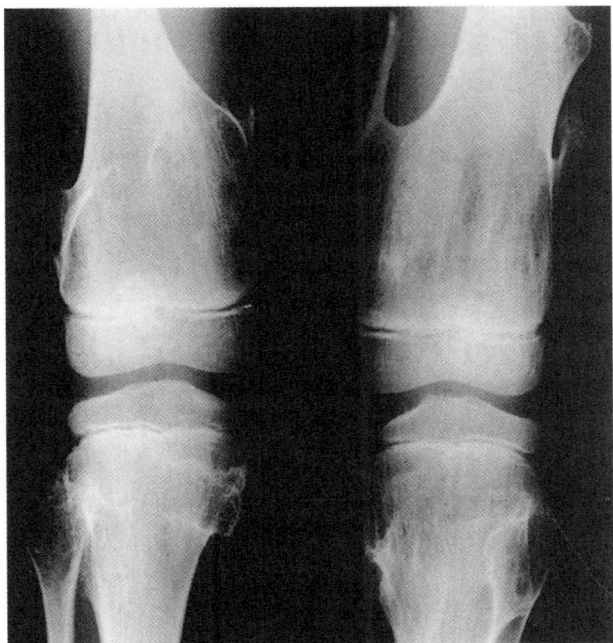

Fig. 24.60 Diaphyseal aclasis with multiple spurs of bone in metaphyseal regions of femora and tibia.

going on for years has been described and residual orthopedic deformity has occurred, e.g. when a bony bridge forms between the radius and ulna.

Treatment

Corticosteroids are highly effective in controlling the systemic disturbance. In ill children and those with widespread disease, oral prednisolone 1–2 mg/kg per day is recommended for 1–2 weeks with gradual reduction in dosage thereafter to minimize 'rebound' reactions with a fresh flare up in the disease.

MELORHEOSTOSIS

This rare condition of unknown etiology shows cortical hyperostosis in a characteristic distribution limited to one side of a long bone of one extremity (resembling wax flowing down a candle). The cortical proliferation tends to show a 'flowing' progression from shoulder to fingers or pelvis to toes. The child presents with pain, swelling or limitation of movement in the affected part but general health is unimpaired. Young infants have not been affected. Rarely, an association with localized scleroderma has been described.

MULTIPLE EXOSTOSES (DIAPHYSEAL ACLASIS)

Single or multiple spurs of bone develop at the growing ends of long bones (Fig. 24.60). The lesion appears to be an osteochondroma in the metaphyseal region but with increase in length of the bone it may appear more diaphyseal and the tip of the bony spur comes to point away from the epiphysis. The condition is frequently familial and inherited as an autosomal

dominant. It may be recognized in infancy as a superficial swelling or swellings attached to bone but more commonly presents in an older child as a swelling adjacent to a joint, particularly knee, ankle or wrist. Movements may be impaired. The flat bones of pelvis and scapula may be affected and rarely the spine, but the skull is spared. There may be unequal growth in the different bones of the extremities. Total height may be normal or decreased. Enlargement of exostoses and new outgrowths occur with some remission at puberty. A few cases have been described as undergoing sarcomatous change in adult life. Rarely, peripheral nerve involvement or spinal cord compression may cause neurological complications.

Deformities due to inequalities in growth may require corrective osteotomy. Exostoses causing pressure effects, pain, or impaired joint mobility should be removed and any which are growing fast should be excised due to the risk of chondrosarcomatous degeneration.

MULTIPLE ENCHONDROMATOSIS (OLLIER'S DISEASE)

The ends of the long bones are widened by a mass of hypertrophied cartilage which may derive from a nest of cartilage cells from the growth plate persisting in the bony cortex. A familial tendency is rare. The disease may be recognized in infancy but more commonly at age 2–10 years. It may present as bony swellings (Fig. 24.61) or as an orthopedic complaint due, for example, to shortening of a limb, joint limitation, or rarely a pathological fracture. Some degree of dwarfing is common in cases with disseminated lesions. On X-ray there may be atrophy of bony cortex, cystic translucencies and areas of striate sclerosis (Figs 24.62a and b). Adjacent epiphyses may be irregular and poorly developed and affected bones shortened and deformed. Lesions may be limited to the hands and feet, and may tend to

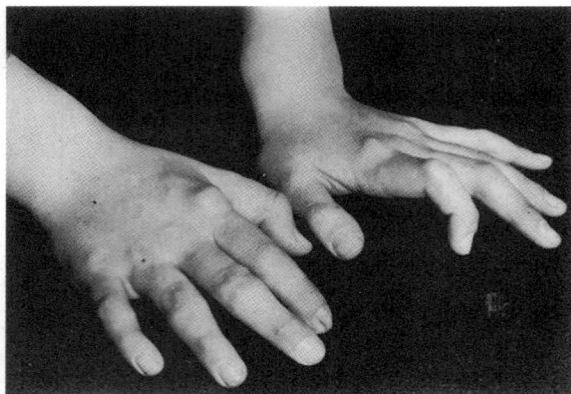

Fig. 24.61 Multiple enchondromata.

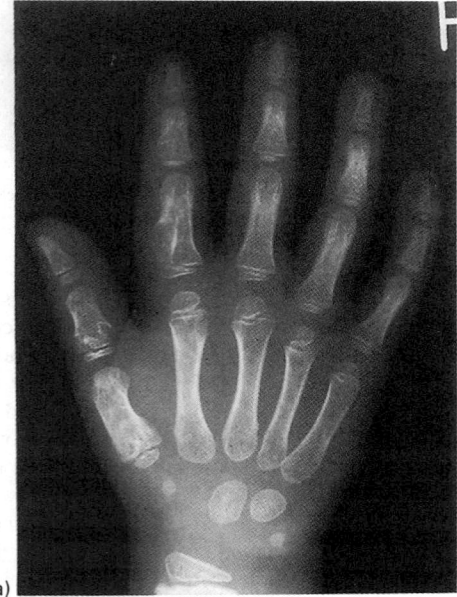

(a)

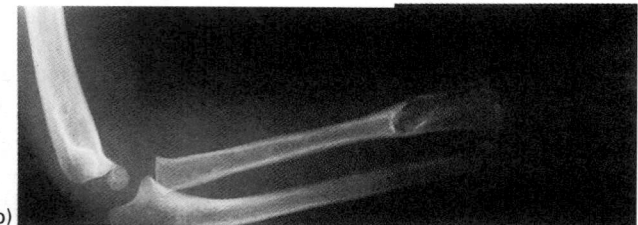

(b)

Fig. 24.62 Multiple cystic translucencies and striate sclerosis in multiple enchondromatosis: (a) hand; (b) forearm.

show a unilateral distribution, or a patchy distribution throughout the skeleton. The vertebrae and skull base are not involved. Development of lesions tends to remit as growth as a whole slows down and enchondromata ultimately ossify. An isolated lesion may simulate bone tumor but malignant change probably occurs rarely. Chondromas of the short bones with multiple hemangiomas and a tendency to develop malignant solid tumors in other organs is known as Maffucci's syndrome. An association with ovarian juvenile granulosa cell tumor has been reported.

Orthopedic procedures may be indicated to equalize leg lengths or to match discrepancies in length of paired bones in the forearm or lower leg. Fractures heal normally. Excision of enchondromas should be carried out when there is any sudden or rapid increase in size.

FIBRODYSPLASIA OSSIFICANS CONGENITA (MYOSITIS OSSIFICANS)

Fibrodysplasia ossificans is now the preferred name for this disease in which the fibrous tissue of fasciae, aponeuroses, ligaments, tendons and muscles is involved in a process of edematous swelling and proliferation of connective tissue with areas of calcification and ectopic bone formation. The etiology is unknown but an incidence in families, including twins, has been described. An autosomal dominant with variable expression appears responsible but about 90% of cases appear as fresh mutations (particularly with older fathers). No biochemical disturbance has been described.

Clinical features

Clinical features may develop at any age from birth to adulthood, but generally occur before the sixth year. Soft tissue swellings which may be painful and hot to touch develop over the course of a few days associated with some generalized upset such as irritability, anorexia and fever. Most often the lesions arise in the neck and occiput, back, shoulders, and proximal parts of the limbs. The hands, forearms and lower legs are usually spared. The skin over the lumps may break down and exude cheese-like material. After some weeks, the lesions become indurated and after some months calcification with areas of ossification appears. Biopsy reveals edema and connective tissue proliferation, osteoid and bone, but no inflammatory reaction. The appearance may simulate sarcoma. The disease relapses and remits but ultimately the child is encased in a rigid sheet which fixes his posture and embarrasses cardiorespiratory function. With early onset of severe disease, death occurs by the age of 15 years in most cases.

The majority of patients have associated minor congenital malformations and some of these, particularly short (often monophalangic) hallux, are common in otherwise unaffected relatives. The short great toe may be associated with synostosis, there may be a short thumb or other short phalanges, clinodactyly of the fifth finger, polydactyly, or shortening of the femoral neck. Deformities of ears, absence of teeth, and spina bifida have also occurred.

Treatment

Analgesics and possibly corticosteroids may provide symptomatic relief during relapse but have no certain effect on the progression of the disease. Bisphosphonates may inhibit the ectopic calcification, but have a detrimental effect on normal skeletal development.

SKELETAL DEFECTS ASSOCIATED WITH MAJOR DISORDERS IN OTHER ORGANS AND TISSUES

ARTHROGRYPOSIS MULTIPLEX CONGENITA

This is a descriptive term for a syndrome involving multiple persistent joint contractures which may arise from a number of pathological processes.

The condition is rare, nearly always sporadic, and the etiology is unknown. A slight male preponderance has been reported.

Pathology

The disorder can be classified into myopathic and neuropathic forms but mixed pathology may occur. The form associated with hypoplastic musculature (amyoplasia congenita) appears to arise from a developmental defect in fetal muscle. There are atrophic muscle fibers, fibrosis and fatty infiltration. The neuropathic form shows denervation atrophy of muscle. Anterior horn cells are degenerative. Corticospinal tract and, rarely, cerebral lesions may also be evident. Intrauterine compression of the fetus may contribute to the deformity but does not appear to be an underlying cause.

Clinical features

Clinically the baby shows various fixed postural deformities of all or some of the limbs (Fig. 24.63). The shoulders tend to be internally rotated, the forearms pronated often with radial head dislocation, and the wrists and fingers flexed. The hips are usually flexed and dislocated with the thighs approximated to the lower abdominal wall: the knees are hyperextended and may be dislocated so that the feet may touch the chest. Talipes is common.

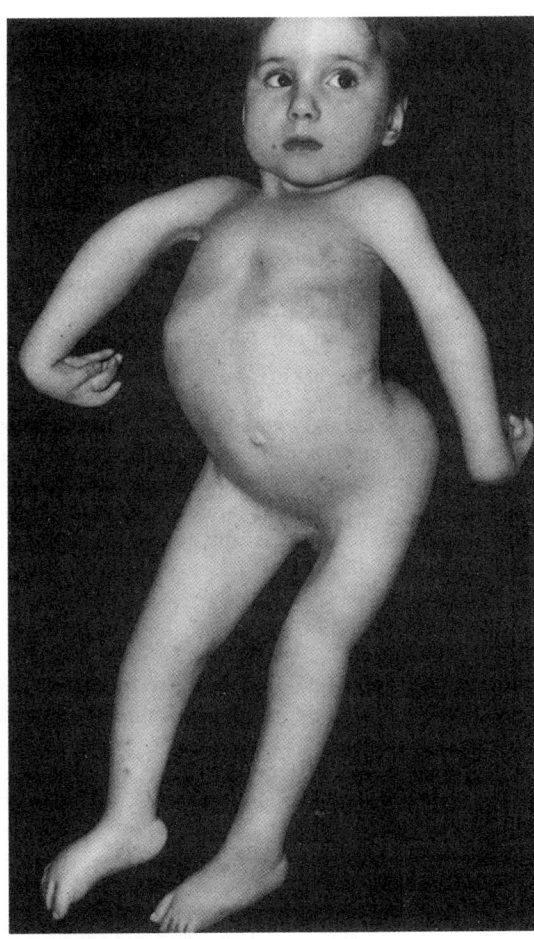

Fig. 24.63 Arthrogryposis.

Due to their abnormal position and fixity, limbs may be fractured at birth, e.g. if an attempt is made to bring down an extended leg. The extremities appear small with wasted, hypotonic muscles and absent reflexes. Some joints look large and fusiform. Contracture is often in fixed flexion with webbing of soft tissue but hyperextension at the knees is usual. In spite of the rigidity of the joints some degree of passive movement is usually possible. The skin and subcutaneous tissues may be thickened, there is loss of normal skin creases and abnormal folds may appear (e.g. over the front of the knee). The joint capsules are thick and inelastic, and an incomplete fibrous ankylosis of the joints is apparent. Congenital dislocations of the hip and knee and club feet are relatively common.

Radiologically, soft tissue views show defective muscle in overabundant fat. Patellar ossification is frequently absent and other ossification centers may be dysplastic. With immobility, bony atrophy tends to develop. Fractures may occur later as well as at birth.

Associated malformations may include scoliosis, thoracic deformity, arachnodactyly, absent sacrum or fibula, premature craniosynostosis, cleft palate, congenital heart disease and genitourinary abnormalities. These children are not usually mentally retarded.

Treatment

Treatment is primarily by passive stretching which must be started immediately. Later, active physiotherapy and occupational therapy are promoted. Splints are used to hold the corrections achieved; traction and soft tissue and bone surgery may be indicated. Part of the aim is to prevent the further handicap of increasing contractures and deformities as the child grows. The lower limbs have to be aligned and stable for weightbearing and the hands and arms as mobile as possible for manipulative skills. A comprehensive approach to the care of these severely handicapped children and their families is required, with due attention to their psychological, educational, and social needs.

MARFAN'S SYNDROME

Marfan's syndrome is caused by mutations in the gene encoding fibrillin 1 (Dietz et al 1991), an important structural component of microfibrils in the lens of the eye, in elastic tissues such as aorta and blood vessels, and also in skin, tendon, bone, muscle, lung and kidney. These microfibrils are important as a structural matrix in their own right, as a scaffolding upon which elastin is subsequently deposited and as a link between elastin and other matrix structures. The wide distribution of the tissues containing fibrillin 1 explains the multiorgan manifestations of Marfan's syndrome. Inheritance is autosomal dominant with high penetrance: about 20–40% of cases arise from new mutations. A large number of different mutations have been described, including missense mutations, insertions, deletions and premature stop codons (Nijbroek et al 1995, Tilstra & Byers 1994).

The disorder occurs with a frequency of around 1 per 10 000 individuals and is characterized by wide clinical variability both within and between families, presumably related to the large number of mutations that have been described. However, no clear pattern has so far emerged to link genotype to phenotype. Diagnosis is largely clinical and relies on a combination of major and minor manifestations involving the musculoskeletal,

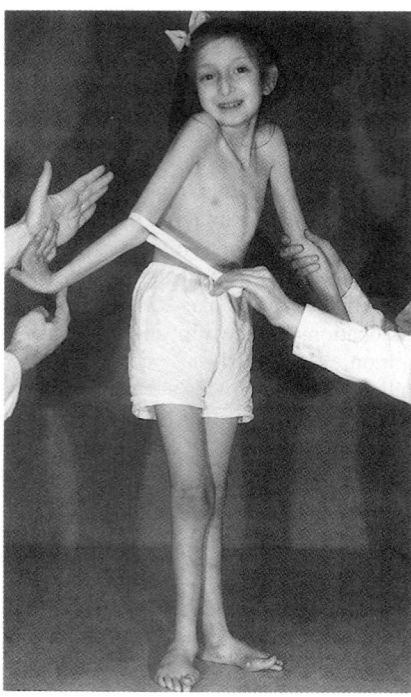

Fig. 24.64   Marfan's syndrome. Long limbs, chest deformity and hyperextensibility of the joints.

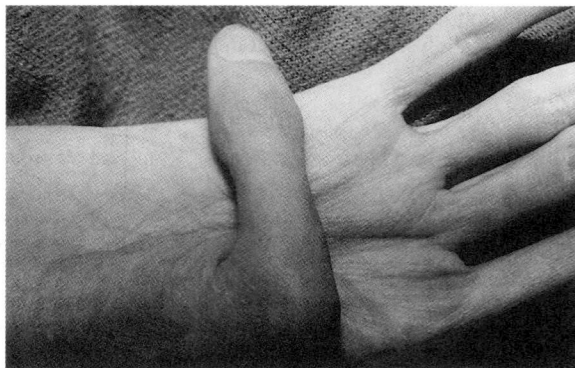

Fig. 24.65   Steinberg's sign in Marfan's syndrome.

cardiovascular, ocular and other systems. Major manifestations include aortic root dilation, mitral valve prolapse, ectopia lentis and the characteristic 'marfanoid' habitus (see Fig. 24.64). Minor manifestations include myopia, spontaneous retinal detachment, glaucoma, spontaneous pneumothorax, emphysema, pulmonary cysts, cutaneous striae distensae, inguinal, femoral and incisional hernias and high-pitched voice. To establish the diagnosis without a family history, a major manifestation from at least two of the three systems is required, plus at least one further minor manifestation. If there is a family history, a single major manifestation from one of the three systems plus two minor manifestations will suffice. Confirmation of the diagnosis may be possible using panels of DNA tests (Nijbroek et al 1995), but will be unnecessary in many instances.

Clinical features

The phenotype described as arachnodactyly involves a tendency to tall stature with abnormally long thin limbs (Fig. 24.64). Span (distance between finger tips with arms outstretched to the side) is greater than height. The distance from the pubis to the soles of the feet greatly exceeds the distance of the pubis from the top of the skull (normal upper to lower segment ratio is 0.93 after maturity is reached and in adult Marfan's syndrome it is 0.85). In the limbs the abnormal lengthening becomes greater as one progresses distally from the shoulders to the fingers or from the hips to the toes. The length of the middle finger usually exceeds 1.5 times the length of its metacarpal. When the thumb is enclosed in the closed fist it protrudes beyond the medial border of the hand (Steinberg thumb sign; Fig. 24.65). This is not pathognomonic but is a virtually constant feature of Marfan's syndrome. There may be clinodactyly of the fifth finger. An elongated great toe is especially characteristic. Many cases have a final height greater than 6 feet (183 cm) but this diagnosis should be suspected in someone whose height is not excessive but whose extremities are disproportionately long. The skull may be dolichocephalic with a long narrow base, the forehead high and full, and the palate narrow and high-arched. Teeth may be noticeably long. The chest may show a funnel-breast or pigeon-breast deformity. Kyphosis and scoliosis occur and are related to ligamentous laxity (see below) (see Fig. 24.65 for finger/palm length).

There is a tendency to generalized hypotonicity of muscles, laxity and hyperextensibility of joints. Pes planus, genu recurvatum, habitual dislocations, and 'double jointedness' are common. An association with arthrogryposis and congenital dislocation of the hip has been recorded.

Infantile Marfan's syndrome is a term used to describe a severe phenotype recognizable in early life and including facial dysmorphism with deep set eyes, ectopia lentis, high-arched palate, chest deformity, arachnodactyly, flexion contractures, pes planus, aortic dilation and multivalvular involvement.

Radiologically the distal limb bones are long and slender but the architecture and mineralization appear normal. Skeletal maturation is normal or somewhat advanced. The iliac wings are large. The vertebral bodies are normal or slightly increased in height.

Kyphoscoliosis is common and an occasional association with hemivertebrae, vertebral fusions or spina bifida is recorded. The skeletal changes have been attributed to generalized endochondral hyperplasia. Some of the clinical features of Marfan's syndrome may resemble homocystinuria (see pp. 1108, 1673) in which a definitive biochemical diagnosis is possible.

Management

Chest deformity is common but is mainly of cosmetic significance and surgical correction is rarely indicated. Scoliosis may appear in early childhood or at adolescence and a progressive curve will require bracing or surgical fixation.

Physiotherapy is valuable in improving muscle tone and power, and orthopedic procedures may be required to stabilize hypermobile joints.

Regular eye examination should be carried out to assess ocular complications including lens dislocation, myopia, retinal detachment, glaucoma, iritis and loss of visual acuity (see also Ch. 26).

The cardiovascular complications are serious and life-threatening as they are responsible for a median age of death in the mid-40s.

Multivalvular incompetence in childhood, mitral valve prolapse, pulmonary artery enlargement, progressive dilation of the aortic root and branches, and aortic dissection should be anticipated. Regular (annual) echocardiogram surveillance is recommended.

Long term treatment with beta-blockers (e.g. propanolol) is advocated to reduce the progression of aortic dilation but clear benefit has not been proven by controlled trials. Surgical treatment for valvular disease and aortic graft repair may be required.

Long term support with multidisciplinary involvement is indicated for Marfan patients and their families.

CONGENITAL CONTRACTURAL ARACHNODACTYLY

This inherited connective tissue disorder is similar to, but distinct from, Marfan's syndrome. The genetic defect is in a different fibrillin gene locus (FBN2) located in chromosome 5 (Tilstra & Byers 1994). The cardinal features are arachnodactyly along with congenital joint contractures (Fig. 24.66), deformed ears with crumpled antihelix and kyphoscoliosis. Those with severe spinal deformity tend to show progression of contractures with increasing disability, whereas those with mild kyphoscoliosis may show improvement in the contractures with time.

The prognosis for life is relatively favorable in comparison with Marfan's syndrome, with no propensity to ocular or cardiovascular complications.

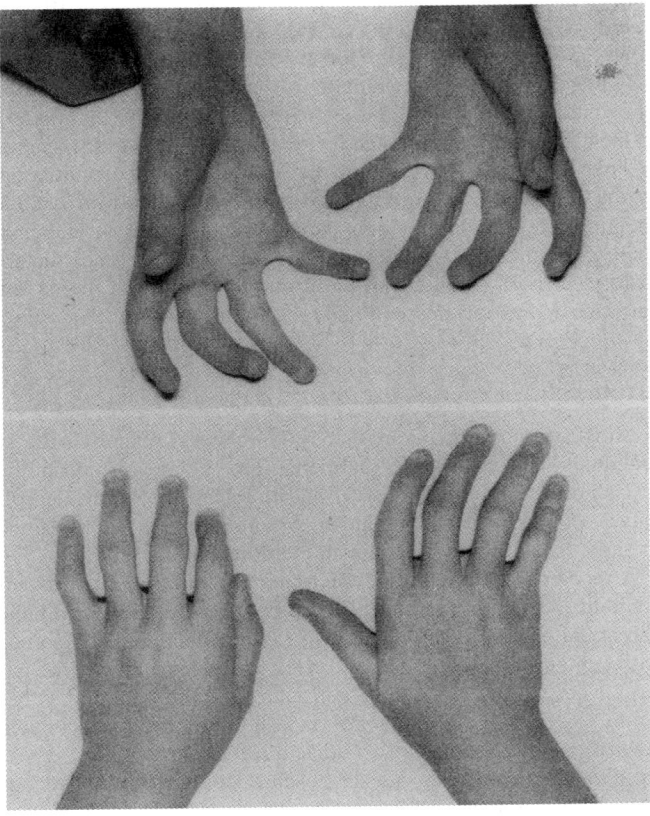

Fig. 24.66 Long tapering fingers and joint contractures in congenital contractural arachnodactyly.

The disease is inherited as an autosomal dominant with considerable variation in expressivity.

POLYOSTOTIC FIBROUS DYSPLASIA (McCUNE–ALBRIGHT SYNDROME)

Pathology

In this condition normal bone is in part replaced by fibrous tissue with islands of cartilage and trabeculae of poorly calcified immature bone. There is shortening, deformity and widening of long bones (especially the femur) with areas of rarefaction. There may be patchy sclerosis, cystic areas, and fractures. In severe cases the pelvis, facial bones, skull and vertebrae may show lesions with swelling and deformity. These may encroach on bony foramina.

Clinical features

This syndrome consists of irregular patchy brown pigmentation of the skin which is often unilateral, precocious puberty (especially in females) (p. 1028) and bone dysplasia (see Fig. 19.23). It is caused by an activating mutation in Gs, the protein that transduces the signal of many 7-transmembrane domain receptors, including the gonadotrophin receptor (Weinstein et al 1991).

Ossification is advanced and early closure of the epiphyses will lead to stunting. The bone dysplasia may show an irregular distribution throughout the skeleton but tends to be unilateral or to affect one side more than the other.

Cranial nerve compression by lesions adjacent to skull foramina may cause optic atrophy or deafness. Callus forms adequately and fractures heal well but angulations occurring at these sites tend to increase deformity. With widespread involvement the possibilities of corrective orthopedic procedures are slight.

Fibrous dysplasia of bone is also seen in a localized form unassociated with the other features of the McCune–Albright syndrome and presents as localized swelling, pain, or pathological fracture of a limb.

INFECTION IN BONE AND JOINT

OSTEITIS (OSTEOMYELITIS)

Acute osteitis

This is usually pyogenic and arises by hematogenous spread from a distant focus which may be clinically inapparent. Direct spread of infection to bone may occur from a penetrating wound, especially with a retained foreign body, or after an open fracture.

Chronic osteitis

This arises after failed or inadequate treatment of an acute osteitis, in patients with diminished body defenses, or from infection with organisms of relatively low virulence.

Septic arthritis

This may complicate bacteremia from a pre-existing source of infection, or may arise by direct spread to the joint from an adjacent focus of osteitis.

Pathology

In previously healthy children, the commonest organisms causing osteitis remain *Staphylococcus pyogenes* (approximately 70% of cases), group A and group B streptococci, *Haemophilus influenzae*, *Staphylococcus epidermidis* and *Streptococcus pneumoniae*. In infants, enteric and other Gram-negative bacteria are more often responsible and in the neonate, group B hemolytic streptococci have become increasingly important. *Salmonella* osteitis is a recognized complication of sickle-cell anemia and *Candida* infection of bone and joint can occur after prolonged intravenous alimentation. Other rare mycotic infections such as histoplasmosis, coccidioidomycosis, actinomycosis, and blastomycosis have to be considered, along with tuberculosis and syphilis, in the differential diagnosis of chronic pyogenic osteitis.

In acute pyogenic osteitis, an abscess first forms in the metaphysis where the vascular loops terminate. From this primary focus, spread may occur (Fig. 24.67) through the cortex to form a subperiosteal abscess, or into the medullary cavity. Where the metaphysis is intracapsular, as in the hip, pus may rupture into the joint to give a septic arthritis. Spread directly through the center of ossification to the articular cartilage is uncommon but may occur in young infants where vascular connections through the growth plate still exist. Although usually in the metaphysis of a long bone, any bone may be affected by osteitis including the craniofacial bones, ribs, scapula, sternum, pelvic bones, tarsus, and vertebral bodies. Multiple foci of bone infection are not uncommon, especially in infants.

In chronic osteitis, the separated periosteum lays down a cuff of new bone (involucrum) around the infected shaft. Areas of devitalized old cortical bone (sequestra) form, fragments may detach, and be extruded through the involucrum towards the surface along with pus in a chronic discharging sinus.

Brodie's abscess is a primary subacute pyogenic osteitis which occurs as a sharply localized metaphyseal focus of infection of low virulence with relatively mild symptoms and an extended time course.

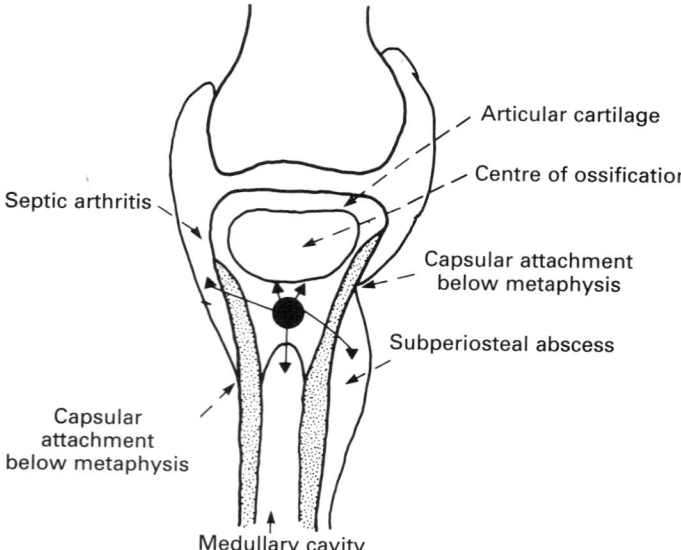

Fig. 24.67 Possible routes of spread of infection from primary metaphyseal focus in head of tibia to subperiosteum (subperiosteal abscess), knee joint (septic arthritis), medullary cavity or articular cartilage.

Garré's diffuse sclerosing osteitis is another form of low-grade infection which appears to be confined to the cortex, producing thickening with little evidence of bone destruction.

Clinical features

The onset of osteitis is usually sudden although there may have been a preceding boil or septic infection, particularly of the skin. There is acute and usually severe local tenderness at the site of infection. Untreated, swelling and erythema develop in the affected area. Movement of an affected limb is severely restricted and handling resented. There is malaise, anorexia, headache and pyrexia. The polymorph count usually reaches 20 000/mm³ (20 × 10⁹/l) or above. Serological tests (e.g. antistaphylococcal titer) may give an indication of the responsible pathogen.

With the early use of antibiotics, a practice so prevalent on empirical grounds, the classical clinical picture of osteomyelitis is often modified. The infection may be eradicated without its nature being appreciated or the acute phase may subside quickly to be replaced by a much more chronic and insidious disease. Low grade intermittent pain and swelling may involve the ends of long bones including metacarpals, and joints may be involved. There may be little systemic upset.

Diagnosis and differential diagnosis

Blood culture should be carried out before treatment and is positive in about 50% of acute untreated cases. Radiological examination in the acute phase of the disease shows no bony change but after 5 days or so in young children and up to 10 days in older children rarefaction occurs at the site of the lesion. Later, bone destruction is likely to become more evident and sequestra may form (Fig. 24.68). A technetium bone scan may reveal an area of osteitis before this becomes evident radiologically (Fig. 24.69). In the more chronic attenuated form of the disease, a cyst-like area or areas (Brodie's abscess) may be evident on first examination. In the acute form the differential diagnosis is likely to include rheumatic fever (flitting joint pain), trauma (history), leukemia (pallor, anemia and hepatosplenomegaly), scurvy (age, dietary history, X-ray). In the chronic form dysplasias of bone and cartilage and neoplasms will need to be considered.

Treatment

A satisfactory outcome in osteitis is closely related to early diagnosis and effective treatment. The extent of antibiotic resistance among staphylococci and the deep seated, walled-off nature of the infection create a special problem in antibiotic therapy. Isolation of the organism by blood culture will help.

A bactericidal antibiotic such as a penicillinase-resistant penicillin (e.g. flucloxacillin) should be given frequently in large parenteral dosage (e.g. 200 mg/kg per day) and can be combined with gentamicin (20 mg/kg per day) or ampicillin (200 mg/kg per day) to cover the possibility of nonstaphylococcal infection. Other antibiotics giving good bone concentration are clindamycin (20–40 mg/kg per day) or fusidic acid (20 mg/kg per day). These are given in three doses per day, each dose by slow intravenous infusion over 6 h.

If a non-penicillinase-producing staphylococcus is isolated a change to benzyl penicillin (penicillin G) may be considered using

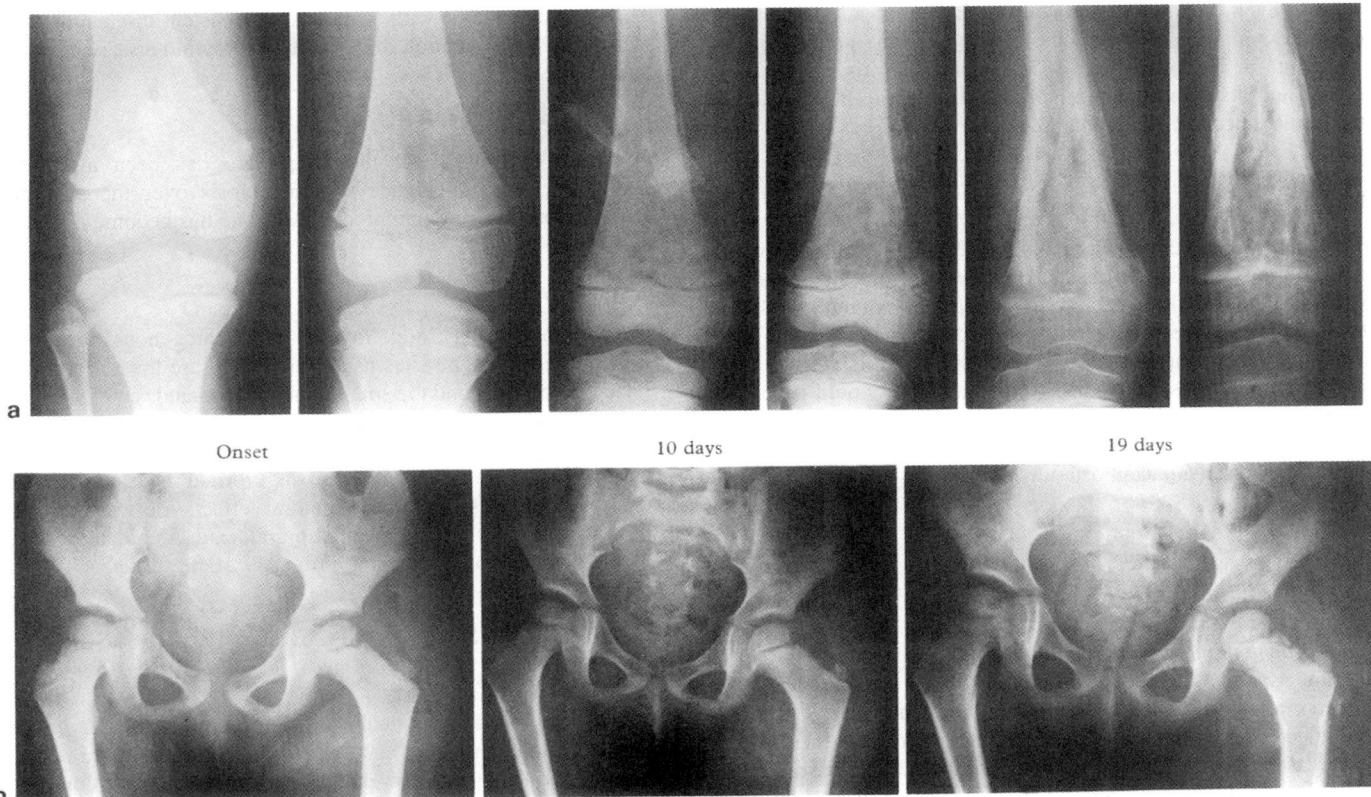

Onset   10 days   19 days

Fig. 24.68   Osteitis: (**a**) of the lower end of the right femur progressing to sequestrum formation; (**b**) of the head of the left femur (soft tissue swelling before bony lesion evident).

50 000 IU (30 mg)/kg per dose by slow intravenous infusion every 4 h.

Intravenous therapy should be used initially and oral therapy should not be considered until at least 7 days of parenteral therapy has been given. Therapy should be continued for at least 6 weeks and for 2 weeks after local and constitutional signs of infection have subsided.

In early cases most would allow 24–48 h to pass to assess

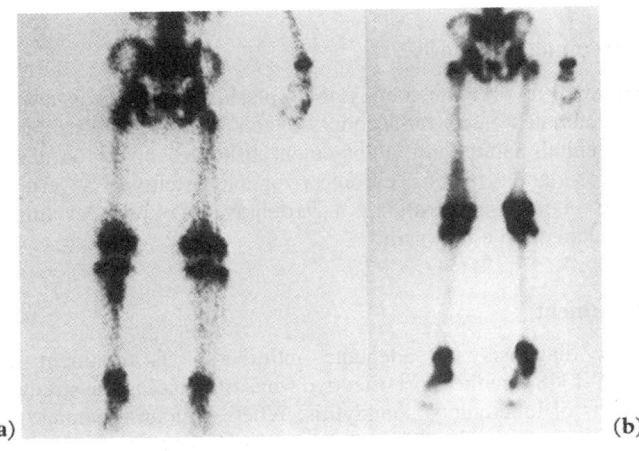

(a)   (b)

Fig. 24.69   Bone scans in osteitis: (**a**) acute osteitis of upper end of right tibia; (**b**) reactivation of old osteitis of lower end of right femur 3 years after onset of original infection.

response before instituting surgical drainage but delay in presentation, doubt as to the stage of the illness, or continuing toxicity with local signs of abscess formation indicate the need for incision of the periosteum to relieve any pus under tension. More extensive drilling of bone or opening the metaphysis for debridement and drainage is also advocated but the need for this formal decompression of bone has been questioned on the grounds that natural drainage of a metaphyseal abscess will be adequate.

In chronic osteitis 6–12 months of systemic antibiotic may be needed and surgery is essential to remove sequestra and other devitalized tissue.

SEPTIC ARTHRITIS

The majority of cases of septic arthritis are under 3 years of age with a significant proportion in the neonatal period. Single or multiple joints may be affected with the main sites in the large joints of the hip, knee, ankle, shoulder, and elbow. Pyoarthrosis may be an isolated lesion or occur as a complication of an adjacent osteitis. The common organisms are *Staphylococcus pyogenes*, Gram-negative enteric bacteria, and *Haemophilus influenzae*; less commonly, streptococci, pneumococci, gonococci, meningococci, and salmonellae may be involved.

Clinical features

The onset is usually sudden and the child is pyrexial and ill. The infant will resent handling and show rigid guarding of the affected limb. The joint is swollen, tender, and hot to touch with intense pain on even the slightest movement. By contrast, in osteitis the tenderness may be maximal on pressure over the metaphysis, and the joint can be gently moved. In septic arthritis of the hip, a flexed and abducted posture is adopted. Edema may spread into the inner aspect of the thigh and genital region.

Diagnosis

The total white cell count may be elevated or may be within normal limits; the ESR is raised to a variable extent. Blood cultures should be done in all suspected cases. Aspiration of the joint should be undertaken urgently to confirm the diagnosis and identify the organism. The aspirate is turbid with 100 000 cells/mm³ or more, mainly polymorphs: immediate Gram staining should be carried out and cultures set up. Radiologically, widening of the joint space may be evident, along with periarticular swelling, and in some cases signs of an adjacent osteomyelitis.

Treatment

In septic arthritis the same antibiotic therapy as for osteitis is required, with a minimum duration of 3 weeks. Under the age of 2 years *Haemophilus influenzae* is relatively common and the initial therapy should include ampicillin or chloramphenicol. Good concentrations of antibiotic can be obtained in synovial fluid and the injection of antibiotic directly into the joint is unnecessary.

Pus under tension within a joint rapidly leads to dissolution of articular cartilage and the epiphysis may undergo avascular necrosis. Repeated daily aspiration through a wide-bore needle is required in accessible joints, and if there is no reduction in volume of aspirate after 3 or 4 days, arthrotomy should be considered. In the hip joint, open surgical drainage from the outset is more likely to be successful.

Immobilization by splinting in the position of function, or traction may be needed and it is especially important to keep a severely affected femoral head positioned in the joint to avoid disabling shortening.

In the recovery stage, physiotherapy is required to prevent contractures and renew muscle. All cases should be followed up for residual disability (see below).

COMPLICATIONS OF OSTEITIS AND SEPTIC ARTHRITIS

In the acute phase of these illnesses, metastatic foci of infection may occur, particularly in other bones and joints. When osteitis has caused extensive destruction of the bony cortex, pathological fracture may occur. Acute osteomyelitis may be complicated by pyoarthrosis, particularly in infancy and in those sites where the metaphysis is within the joint capsule. In septic arthritis with damage to articular cartilage, dislocation of the joint can occur, sometimes with great rapidity. Shortening of a limb, or local overgrowth of bone due to hyperemia, may lead to inequality of limb size and disturbance of gait which may be revealed only when an infant learns to walk. An incidence of 30% sequelae after sepsis in weightbearing joints has been reported and emphasizes the importance of long term follow-up. Flexion contractures and impaired joint mobility require active physiotherapy and may need orthopedic correction.

In vertebral osteitis, paravertebral abscess, epidural abscess with cord compression, and pyogenic meningitis may develop.

In chronic osteitis with sequestra, a persistent discharging sinus with poor health, anemia, and eventually amyloid disease can occur.

TUBERCULOSIS OF BONE

In some countries, e.g. the UK, there has been a dramatic reduction in the incidence of tuberculosis over the past three decades and tuberculous infection of bone has become a rarity.

Pathology

Tubercle bacilli may lodge in bone by hematogenous spread from a primary focus. The sites usually involved are the vertebrae, the head of the femur and the small bones of the hands and feet. Single foci are usual but multiple foci are not uncommon. The lesions consist of granulation tissue with absorption of bone or caries, or assume a caseating type with necrosis. Normal bone architecture is destroyed with significant structural effects on weightbearing bones such as the vertebrae and femoral head. A cold abscess may form within the bone tracking ultimately to the surface.

TUBERCULOSIS OF THE SPINE (POTT'S DISEASE)

Clinical features

The onset is usually gradual with dull local pain in the affected vertebra. Local swelling and destruction of the vertebra result in pressure on the spinal nerves with referred pain. Most commonly the lower thoracic, followed by the lumbar and then cervical regions are involved. The child holds the back rigid and walks stiffly. Vertical jarring of the back and bending forward will aggravate his symptoms. He may become reluctant to walk or stand, preferring to be in the face down position. With cervical involvement head movement becomes restricted by pain. With collapse of the vertebra kyphosis and scoliosis may develop and if the upper part of the spine is affected paraplegia may result. Pus from a cold abscess may track down the psoas or lumbar muscles to form psoas (Fig. 24.70) or lumbar abscesses which may present in the groin or may rupture into the pleural cavity; in the cervical region an abscess is likely to point into the pharynx as a retropharyngeal abscess. Radiological examination shows rarefaction and destruction of the affected bone.

Differential diagnosis

This will involve the spondylar dysplasias which can usually be differentiated easily on account of their widespread distribution, congenital nature and involvement of other bones; structural scoliosis and kyphosis; chronic pyogenic osteitis of a vertebra; bone neoplasms involving a vertebra; or intrathecal tumors producing nerve root pain.

Treatment

Early diagnosis and adequate antituberculous treatment (pp. 1347–1348) are the most effective ways of avoiding the structural effects of tuberculous spondylitis. Where structural damage and nerve pressure effects have occurred, prolonged rest and spinal traction are likely to be required with surgical removal of diseased bone and, in a few cases, bone grafting as possible additional measures.

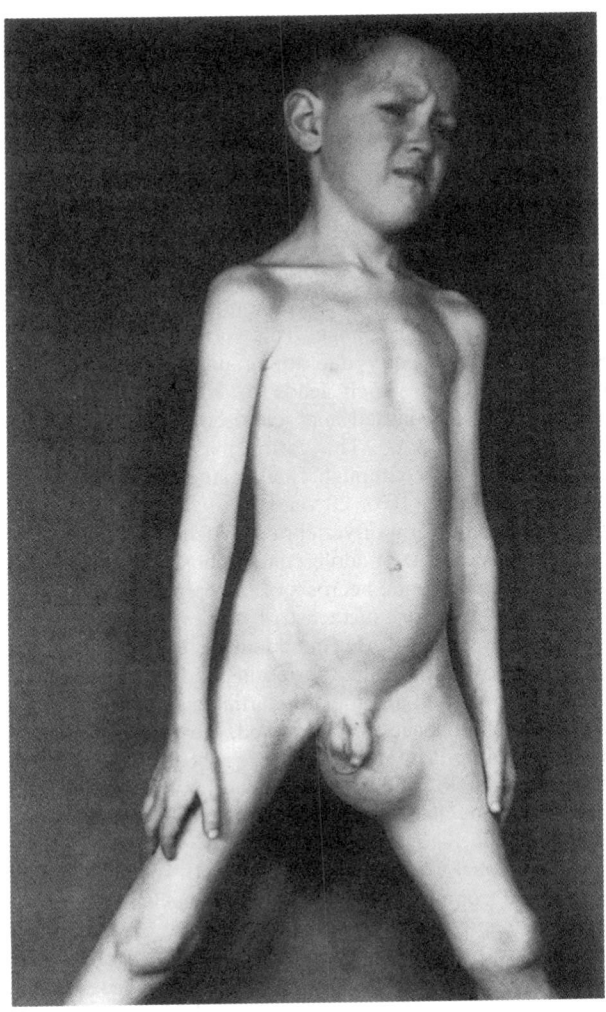

Fig. 24.70 Tuberculous abscess draining from tuberculous lesion of spine.

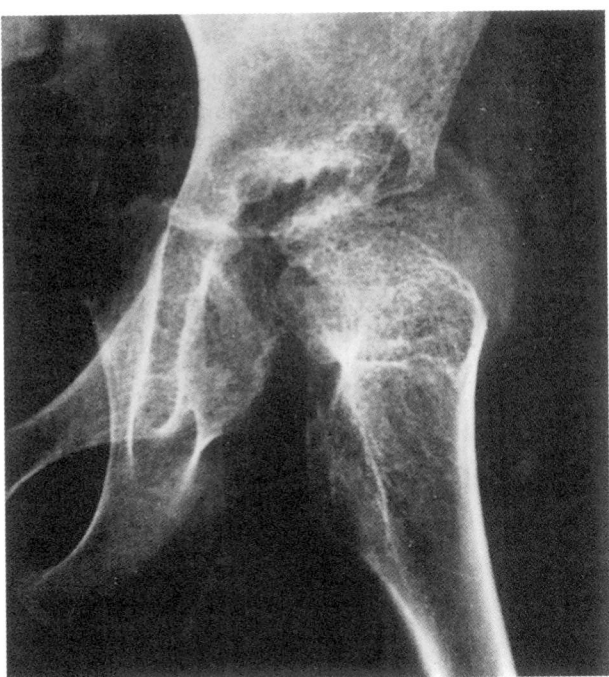

Fig. 24.71 Tuberculosis of hip joint. Left hip joint showing destruction of femoral head and acetabulum with commencing calcification within an abscess on lateral aspect of joint.

In more advanced cases antituberculous treatment will need to be combined with prolonged rest of the joint combined with traction.

TUBERCULOUS DACTYLITIS

This tends to occur in the preschool age group and is more likely to be multiple, involving fingers and metacarpals or toes and metatarsals. Spindle-shaped swelling is often the first sign (Fig. 24.72). This becomes indurated and may be reddened with limitation of finger movement but little pain may be experienced. Radiologically, rarefaction and cystic-like change may be seen in affected bones with involvement of the medullary canal and thinning and distention of the cortex.

In early cases antituberculous treatment and rest of the affected part are likely to be effective but in late cases permanent deformity may result.

Dactylitis, part of a periostitis, can also occur as an early manifestation of congenital syphilis.

THE OSTEOCHONDROSES

These disorders involve focal ischemic aseptic necrosis at a center of ossification in the growing bone. The process occurs at certain specific sites and in any affected child is usually localized to that one site.

The etiology is uncertain but a primary vascular disturbance which may be precipitated by trauma is postulated. Some may be related to a traction lesion at the insertion of a powerful muscle (tibial tubercle and os calcis), others may be a compression lesion (hip, navicular).

TUBERCULOSIS OF THE HIP

Clinical features

Symptoms are usually of gradual and intermittent onset. A limp develops on account of ill-defined pain which often becomes referred to the knee or inner side of the thigh. Symptoms may be worse in the morning or after exertion. On examination an early sign is limitation of rotation in the joint and as destruction of the head of the femur progresses the hip joint becomes maintained in a position of flexion, adduction and internal rotation. An abscess may form in the head of the femur, spread to the hip joint and point, usually anteriorly. Radiological examination shows rarefaction and then destruction of the head of the femur (Fig. 24.71). Untreated the disease is a chronic one with progressive destruction of the femoral head and then the hip joint over a period of years. Recovery is usually associated with ankylosis of the joint.

Treatment

With prompt diagnosis early tuberculous changes may be reversed by adequate antituberculous treatment (pp. 1347–1348) and rest.

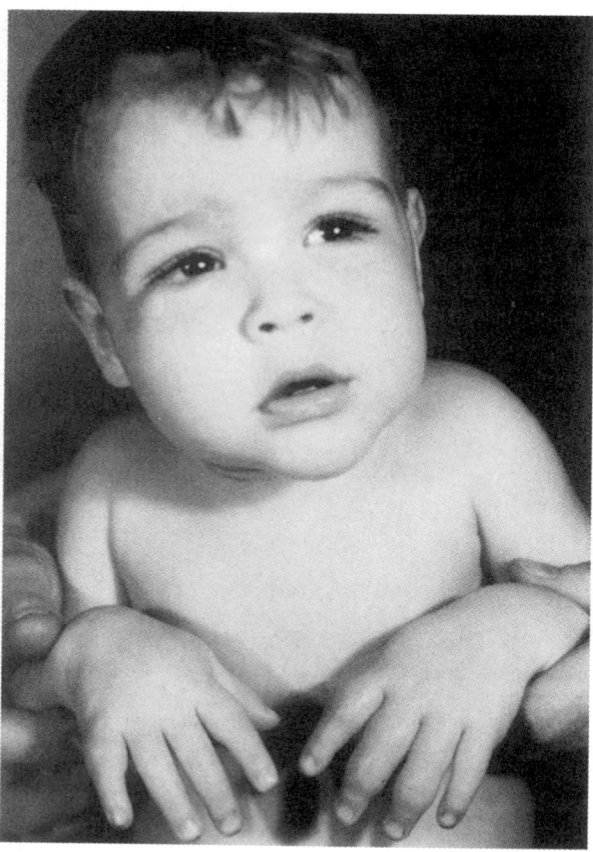

Fig. 24.72   Tuberculous dactylitis.

PATHOLOGY

There is perivascular edema and thickening of soft tissues, impaired blood supply, and cell degeneration. These changes lead to necrosis with loss of structure, particularly under mechanical stress such as weightbearing. With repair there is new growth of capillaries from the periphery into the mesenchyme of the lesion, leading to differentiation of cells and reconstitution of tissues.

The process of necrosis and repair may occur over many years. The end result is dependent on the amount of destruction and structural deformity which impairs growth and function of the affected part and predisposes to premature degenerative change.

Scheuermann's disease of the spine and Osgood–Schlatter disease of the tibial tubercle are sometimes referred to as pseudo-osteochondroses on the grounds that they have a different pathogenesis, but both are included in this account.

CLINICAL FEATURES

Osteochondroses may be asymptomatic or cause localized pain which can be severe, constant, or intermittent and aggravated by exercise. Depending on the site there may be localized swelling (e.g. over the tibial tubercle), functional impairment such as limp (proximal femoral epiphysis), or deformity with, for example, kyphosis (vertebral bodies) or bow legs (proximal tibial epiphyses).

Constitutional upset is uncommon and mild.

Radiologically there is focal irregularity in bone density progressing to fragmentation and deformity. Particular care

should be taken to avoid diagnosing ischemic necrosis on radiological evidence alone as irregular mineralization may be a normal feature of growing bone at these sites.

The differential diagnosis is from local infective, traumatic, or neoplastic disease of bone and rheumatoid disorders.

Spine (Calvé's disease, Scheuermann's disease)

The 'infantile' form of vertebral osteochondrosis described by Calvé appears as a single flattened vertebra in a child of 2–15 years. The lesion may be asymptomatic or associated with backache and postural change. This form of vertebra plana is thought to be frequently due to an unsuspected eosinophilic granuloma of bone which leads to ischemic necrosis. The vertebral body is collapsed and sclerosed but the intervertebral spaces are little affected. This lesion may develop rapidly and healing is very slow although final restitution of the vertebral body may occur after 10 or 20 years.

The 'adolescent' form of vertebral osteochondrosis is known as Scheuermann's disease or adolescent kyphosis. The original view that this was an ischemic necrosis of the epiphyseal plates on the superior and inferior surfaces of the vertebral body was contradicted by Schmorl. He found that there was prolapse of the nucleus pulposus into the vertebral bodies, probably after mechanical stress had disrupted the articular cartilaginous plates. The intervertebral spaces are narrowed, the vertebra compressed and wedged anteriorly giving rise to kyphosis. Several adjacent vertebrae in the lower thoracic, upper lumbar region may be affected. The nuclear herniations (Schmorl's nodes) may be demonstrable on X-ray tomography.

The child, usually a boy, presents at age 10–15 years with dorsal kyphosis and compensatory lumbar lordosis. Pain is frequently absent. The spinal deformity may advance or remain static. Treatment is directed at improving posture by physiotherapy supplemented by a corrective brace in some instances. In a few cases progression is such that posterior spinal fusion is justified.

Femoral head (Perthes disease)

Perthes disease (Legg–Calvé–Perthes, coxa plana) is ischemic necrosis of the femoral head affecting the epiphysis and sometimes an area of adjacent metaphysis. The articular and epiphyseal cartilages are swollen but not eroded. The destructive process can continue for 1 or 2 years and may lead to flattening and shrinking of the ossification center and widening of the femoral neck. Repair by ossification of fibrous tissue takes place over a further $2–3\frac{1}{2}$ years. An incidence of one in 2000 has been suggested, with a 3% recurrence risk for siblings but no clear pattern of inheritance. The disease is most often isolated but has been described in association with a wide range of other disorders including congenital dislocation of the hip, achondroplasia, the mucopolysaccharidoses, and rickets.

It presents in the age group 2–10 years (peak 4–6 years), is some four times more common in boys, and in about 10% of cases is bilateral. Clinically, there is a lurching gait with a limp. Pain may be mild or severe, localized to the hip joint or referred to the thigh or knee. There is protective spasm with limitation of hip movements especially abduction and internal rotation. The signs and symptoms are of very variable duration – from days to months – and correlate poorly with the progression of the disease as judged by X-ray.

X-rays should be taken anteroposterior with the feet pointing forward and in a lateral projection with the hips in the 'frog' position. There is first widening of the joint space between the femoral head and acetabulum due to edema of the soft tissues. In the ossification center there may be slight sclerosis, then early irregularity (Fig. 24.73), or fragmentation. With advancing necrosis the epiphysis becomes grossly irregular and a destructive cystic area may appear in the metaphysis. Where less than half of the epiphysis is involved the prognosis is good, especially under the age of 4 years. Where more than half the epiphysis is affected there is usually metaphyseal damage and the prognosis is less favorable, especially in girls who tend to present with severe changes. With healing, anatomical deformities of the femoral head and neck become more apparent. The recalcified femoral head may be large and flat (coxa magna) (Fig. 24.74), the femoral neck short and broad. The acetabulum remolds to accommodate the deformed femur and in adult life premature degenerative osteoarthritis is seen. Premature closure of the growth plate with shortening of the limb may occur.

Perthes disease is a self-limiting disorder which progresses through stages of destruction and repair. Initially, pain and muscle spasm require relief by recumbency, traction and physiotherapy. The femoral head has then to be protected from undue mechanical stress and attempts made to contain the head within the acetabulum.

In those patients under 4 years with less than half the epiphysis involved, symptomatic treatment only is required. Where more than half the epiphysis is involved relative mobility in a patten-ended ischial weight-bearing caliper is employed or ambulation is allowed in Petrie long leg casts with the hips held abducted and medially rotated. In the latter group a few patients may benefit from varus rotation femoral osteotomy, with full mobilization after 6–8 weeks in plaster.

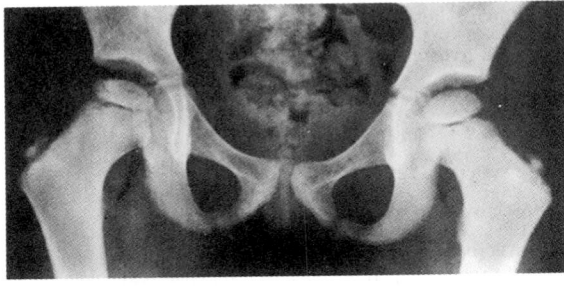

Fig. 24.73 Perthes disease. Right femoral head shows slight flattening, slight increase in density with commencing fragmentation indicating early stage in child of 3 years.

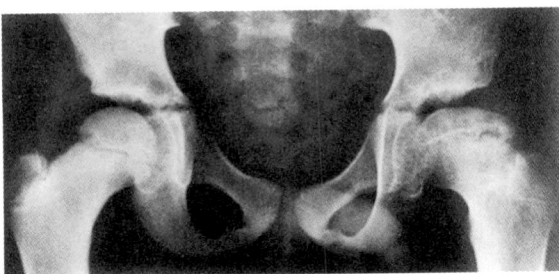

Fig. 24.74 Perthes disease. Left femoral head showing residual widening of femoral neck and flattening of head on healing.

Regular re-examination of the hip and X-rays at about 3-monthly intervals are used to follow progress. Late arthritis has been reported in one-third to one-half of cases, irrespective of treatment. Continuing physiotherapy is essential to avoid contractures and prevent disuse atrophy. Surgical procedures to assist revascularization of the Perthes are of unproven value.

Tibial tubercle (Osgood–Schlatter disease)

This typically presents at puberty, most often in boys, as a painful swelling over the tibial tubercle and patellar tendon, with limp or restricted gait. In some cases avulsion of the infrapatellar tendon occurs. X-ray shows fragmentation and irregularity of outline of the tubercle with soft tissue swelling. Treatment is by immobilization for 6–8 weeks in a plaster cast with gradual return to activity over the next 2 months.

Tarsal navicular (Köhler's disease)

Köhler's disease is most common in boys between the ages of 3 and 8 years and is often bilateral. There may be limp, local pain, swelling and tenderness and symptoms aggravated by walking. X-ray shows sclerosis and irregular rarefaction with flattening of the navicular. Treatment may require a 6–8 week period of plaster cast support and immobilization. Healing generally takes place spontaneously and is radiologically evident over the course of 2–3 years.

Os calcis (Sever's disease)

Osteochondrosis of the posterior epiphysis of the os calcis is known as Sever's disease. It may cause a painful heel and awkward gait in adolescents. X-ray shows irregularity and sclerosis of the apophysis and swelling of overlying soft tissues. Symptomatic relief can usually be achieved by fitting a raised heel, but a walking plaster for 6 weeks may be necessary. Healing eventually takes place without complication.

Metatarsal (Freiberg's disease)

Osteochondrosis of the epiphysis at the head of the second metatarsal is Freiberg's disease. It tends to develop in adolescence with local pain and tenderness which is aggravated by manipulating the metatarsal head. Pressure on the affected area is relieved by a metatarsal arch support and healing is usually complete.

OTHER SITES FOR OSTEOCHONDROSIS

There are many other bones which have been described as foci of osteochondrosis. These include the proximal tibial epiphysis (Blount's disease – see p. 1554), the carpal lunate, lower ulna, humerus, distal tibia, patella, femoral trochanters, symphysis pubis and iliac crest.

OSTEOCHONDRITIS DISSECANS

This disorder is analogous to the osteochondroses in that it is also an area of focal ischemic necrosis in bone. It is probably traumatic in origin and occurs in adolescents and young adults, predominantly males. The focus of necrosis is limited to a marginal defect at the edge of bone which is subchondral in relation to a freely articulating joint. The overlying layers of epiphyseal and articular cartilage are not grossly affected but may become cracked or defective and allow extrusion of the necrotic bone fragment to give a loose body in the joint. The femoral condyle is most often involved and about one-third of cases are bilateral. Other sites are the hip, capitellum of the humerus, and talus.

The condition presents as arthralgia and sometimes effusion, instability or locking of the joint.

X-rays reveal a crater of necrosis which may be cup-shaped with a sclerotic margin. The enclosed fragment shows a variable detachment and may finally be lying loose in the joint cavity.

Treatment for the early lesion is by plaster cast support for 3–4 months to avoid weightbearing stress during the phase of repair. If healing does not progress, operative fixation of a partially detached fragment or removal of a loose body may be indicated.

SLIPPED UPPER FEMORAL EPIPHYSIS (ADOLESCENT COXA VARA)

This disorder is also described as adolescent coxa vara (cf. congenital and infantile coxa vara, p. 1551). It is somewhat commoner in males (ratio 3 : 2), and has been associated with obesity and hypogenitalia, and multiple epiphyseal dysplasia (Table 24.6). There is gradual slippage of the capital femoral epiphysis and about 20% are bilateral. The presenting symptom is frequently pain in the knee so that hip disease is not suspected. There is a limp and swelling and limitation of movement of the hip joint will develop. Sometimes the slip occurs suddenly after a twisting injury and there is acute pain and inability to move the leg which is held in external rotation. The upper femoral epiphysis is apparently displaced posteriorly and inferiorly but this is due to the remainder of the bone moving upward and anteriorly relative to it with resultant anterior angulation of the neck of the femur (Fig. 24.75). The defect is best seen on a lateral X-ray. Complications include premature fusion of the epiphysis, avascular necrosis of the slipped head and necrosis of the articular cartilage.

Rarely, if the slip is acute, reduction by gentle manipulation and pinning is possible. With gradual slipping, reduction is

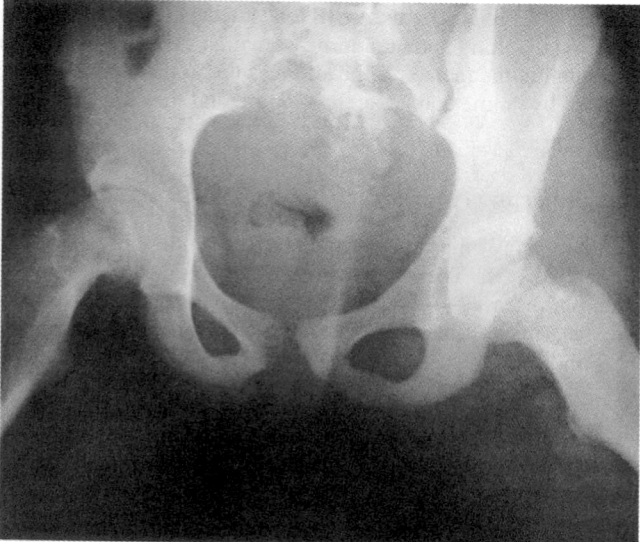

Fig. 24.75 Slipped left upper femoral epiphysis.

contraindicated because of compromise of the blood supply to the femoral head, and the head should be pinned in situ. If the condition is chronic a subtrochanteric osteotomy can be carried out to realign the femoral head with the acetabulum.

DISORDERS OF JOINTS AND CONNECTIVE TISSUE

With the new information available on the structure and biosynthesis of collagen it has become possible to explain a number of genetic diseases on the basis of molecular defects in collagen biosynthesis. Acquired diseases involving collagen are important in medicine but knowledge of how they alter collagen synthesis or metabolism is still fragmentary. At present, there are a number of diseases which can be classed as collagen diseases, and others which are best classed as collagen diseases until they are fully understood. In the following account, only inflammatory diseases of connective tissue of significance to pediatrics (Table 24.9) will be discussed, in order of clinical importance.

ACUTE RHEUMATIC FEVER

Over the past few decades, major changes have occurred in the epidemiology of acute rheumatic fever (ARF) resulting in a

Table 24.9 Connective tissue diseases in children

Acute rheumatic fever

Juvenile chronic arthritis
  a. Systemic onset
  b. Polyarticular onset
  c. Pauciarticular onset

Ankylosing spondylitis

Systemic lupus erythematosus

Neonatal lupus erythematosus

Dermatomyositis–polymyositis

Progressive systemic sclerosis or scleroderma

Mixed connective tissue disease

Vasculitic syndromes
  a. Henoch–Schönlein purpura (anaphylactoid purpura)
  b. Polyarteritis
  c. Mucocutaneous lymph node syndrome (Kawasaki's disease)
  d. Wegener's granulomatosis
  e. Aortic arch arteritis (Takayasu's disease)
  f. Giant cell arteritis

Arthropathy in cystic fibrosis of pancreas

Arthropathy in inflammatory bowel disease

Psoriatic arthritis

Reiter's syndrome

Behçet syndrome

Lyme arthritis

Viral arthritis

Hypermobility syndrome

Limb pains of childhood with no organic cause

decline of the disease in Europe and developed countries. The reasons for this decrease in incidence and severity are not clear but may be related to better standards of living with a decrease in overcrowding, and perhaps from easier access to medical care. Moreover, pathogenic streptococci are less prevalent since the introduction of penicillin. The recent resurgence of the disease in the USA remains unexplained (Congeni et al 1987, British Medical Journal 1988).

ARF remains the leading cause of acquired heart disease in developing countries and it is the commonest cause of cardiovascular death in the first five decades of life.

ETIOLOGIC FACTORS

Acute rheumatic fever is perhaps unique among the connective tissue disorders in that there is a clear and constant association between the disease and a specific pathogenic organism – the Lancefield group A β-hemolytic streptococcus. A high titer of the most commonly measured antistreptolysin-O (ASO) in the blood is so regularly a feature of this disease as to be almost diagnostic. It is generally agreed that in the rheumatic fever group as a whole, ASO antibody titers are higher and last longer than in uncomplicated streptococcal infections. Only a small proportion of children infected with β-hemolytic streptococci develop acute rheumatic fever although a wide range of serological subtypes of Lancefield group A streptococci may be responsible for the disease.

The incidence of ARF in any outbreak of acute streptococcal infection is low in contrast to the high incidence of recurrence in known rheumatic subjects who develop further streptococcal infection – a point of preventive importance. Outbreaks of ARF amongst young people living together at close quarters occur 2–3 weeks after the peak of acute streptococcal infection and there is often a clear history of preceding streptococcal infection. It is more prevalent in some families than one would expect from the random incidence of streptococcal infection and HLA B17 occurs with undue frequency in patients with rheumatic fever.

The incidence of ARF and chorea in childhood shows marked variation with age. ARF is very rare below the age of 5 years and even rarer below 3 years. The peak incidence of first attacks is highest between the ages of 10 and 14 years with a brisk fall over the next decade. First attacks of ARF after the age of 30 years are rare but do occur. The sex incidence of ARF shows a slight preponderance of females. In girls approaching puberty there is an inexplicable predominance of chorea. In countries where ARF and rheumatic chorea are prevalent, a late rise in the incidence of chorea may be seen in young pregnant women.

CLINICAL MANIFESTATIONS

There are five major clinical features of the clinical complex of ARF, namely polyarthritis, carditis, erythema marginatum, subcutaneous nodules and chorea. To these may be added a few nonspecific clinical features which occur frequently in rheumatic fever, but because they also often occur in numerous other diseases, their diagnostic value is limited. Their usefulness is in supporting the diagnosis of rheumatic fever when only a single major manifestation is present.

The diagnosis of acute rheumatic fever should be made by using the revised Jones criteria (1984). This requires two major or one major and two minor criteria plus evidence of streptococcal

Table 24.10 Jones criteria (revised) for guidance in the diagnosis of rheumatic fever

Major manifestations	Minor manifestations	Supporting evidence of streptococcal infection
Carditis Polyarthritis Chorea Erythema marginatum Subcutaneous nodules	*Clinical* Previous rheumatic fever or rheumatic heart disease Arthralgia Fever *Laboratory* Acute phase reactants Erythrocyte sedimentation rate C-reactive protein Leucocytosis Prolonged P–R interval	Increased titer of anti-streptococcal antibodies. Positive throat culture for Group A streptococcus. Recent scarlet fever

infection from a throat swab or streptococcal antibodies (Table 24.10).

Polyarthritis

The polyarthritis of ARF is characteristically both flitting and fleeting – a fact that has led to semantic confusion in some textbooks. In older children and young adults the arthritis tends to be more acute with more obvious signs of joint involvement. The joints may be swollen, red and exquisitely tender. At the other end of the scale, there may be vague joint pains (without redness or swelling) which move from joint to joint within hours or a few days. The joints involved are almost always the larger joints – the knee, ankle, wrist, elbow and shoulder in that order of frequency – and the smaller joints of the hands and feet are hardly ever affected. The spine is unaffected by this disease.

Carditis (see also p. 628)

Acute rheumatic fever accounts for a considerable amount of chronic cardiac disease in adult life. Stenosis and/or incompetence of the mitral and/or the aortic valves have been a major concern of physicians since before the invention of the stethoscope. During the acute phase of the disease there is often an endocarditis, myocarditis, and pericarditis, the latter often being identified on an echocardiogram. In mild cases no demonstrable cardiac involvement may be present. On a pathological basis, the diagnosis of ARF implies the likely existence of carditis with possible chronic valvular damage even if the clinical signs are not detectable.

The presence of a cardiac murmur and/or of cardiac enlargement may be the first indications of carditis. Knowledge that a new murmur has developed or that a murmur has changed in character has more significance than the mere hearing of a soft systolic murmur, but information on the cardiac signs prior to the current illness is often not available or accurate. Cardiac enlargement is likely to be a more important indicator of acute disease.

A soft systolic murmur may be the first sign of carditis but such murmurs are so common in children as to be of limited diagnostic value. A soft mid-diastolic murmur at the apex is more significant and usually indicates myocarditis. Presystolic and aortic diastolic murmurs are rarer but of greater significance. When acute rheumatic fever was more prevalent in the UK, 50% of children developed murmurs in the first attack (75% in the first week of the illness).

Tachycardia is another important sign of carditis, especially if the pulse rate is taken when the child is asleep and there is little difference between waking and sleeping heart rates. Bradycardia due to partial heart block may occur and is also common in patients on corticosteroid therapy. Arrhythmia may be due to atrial fibrillation or extrasystoles. An electrocardiogram (ECG) is necessary for differentiation.

A prolonged PR interval on the ECG to more than 0.18 s indicates delayed conduction. A pericardial friction rub indicates severe cardiac involvement. An unequivocal sign of cardiac involvement is cardiac failure and overwhelming rheumatic infection may present as congestive cardiac failure without polyarthritis. Cardiac failure is likely to be associated with orthopnea, gallop rhythm, hepatomegaly, edema and ascites. Under the age of 5 years, carditis predominates and joint symptoms are mild. In the developing countries gross rheumatic heart disease may present in the school-age child without previous history of acute rheumatic fever.

Subcutaneous nodules

These are characteristic bilateral firm nodules varying in diameter from a few millimeters to a centimeter. They occur mainly over the bony prominences and over tendons. The skin is freely mobile over them and they are nontender. Nodules occur in both juvenile chronic arthritis and rheumatic fever although they are infrequent in both. If present in acute rheumatic fever, the cardiac involvement is usually severe. They are best demonstrated by fully flexing the joint and stretching the skin over the extensor surface. Blanching occurs over nodules. Nodules may continue to appear during salicylate therapy (Fig. 24.76).

Erythema marginatum (erythema circinatum or erythema centrifugatum)

This occurs only occasionally in acute rheumatic fever and when present is virtually diagnostic consisting of erythematous rings of

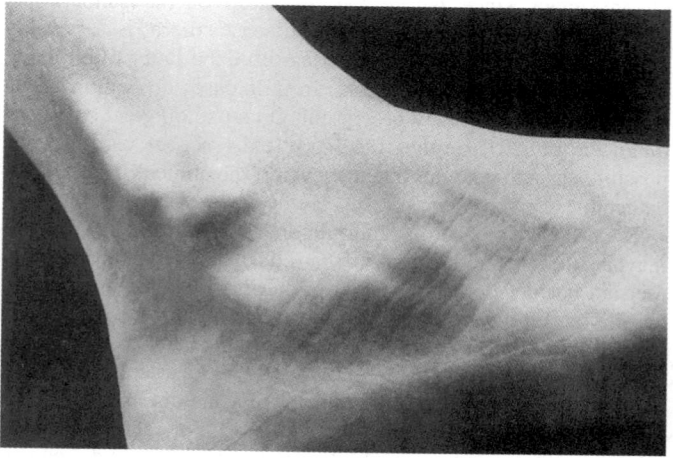

Fig. 24.76 Subcutaneous nodules on ankle in a child with acute rheumatic fever.

1–2 inches or more in diameter with large pale centers of normal skin. The rash occurs mostly on the trunk and limbs. The lesions frequently coalesce forming irregular circinate patterns which vary in shape and site from hour to hour. The changing pattern of the rash may be demonstrated by outlining its edge and observing the changes in outline and site in an hour or so.

Rheumatic chorea

Rheumatic chorea or Sydenham's chorea is a major manifestation of acute rheumatic fever and differs in many ways from other forms of chorea. Chorea is an involuntary movement resulting from disorder of the extrapyramidal system. It is without any implication as to etiology.

The onset of rheumatic chorea is usually insidious and at first may appear to be an emotional disorder associated with clumsiness. The disease may at times remain mild and undiagnosed recovering spontaneously. The fully developed picture is readily recognized but more easily demonstrated than described. There are irregular, nonrepetitive fidgeting or jerking movements of the limbs which are either generalized or focal. There is also a characteristic grimacing of the face. The movements invariably affect function, are exaggerated by emotional stress and disappear in sleep. The child tends to drop things; to spill from a cup; dressing, particularly fastening and unfastening of buttons, becomes difficult or impossible; handwriting deteriorates; speech is commonly slurred and sometimes the child finds speech so difficult that he gives up the attempt and appears mute. There is almost invariably an alteration of temperament with a characteristic lability of emotion, the child laughing and crying without apparent reason. The disease may progress to become so severe as to be seriously incapacitating and the movements may be so gross as to require a padded cot. Sometimes the weakness of voluntary movement is such as to create an impression of paralysis with only minimal choreic movements in the fingers being apparent (chorea mollis). Not uncommonly, chorea appears to be confined largely to one side of the body (hemichorea) but close observation will usually reveal some choreic movements on the other side as well.

On examination a marked fluctuation in muscle tone is common and best felt by asking the patient to squeeze the examiner's hand. When the arms and hands are extended there is a characteristic deformity in which the wrist is acutely flexed and the fingers extended at both the interphalangeal and the metacarpophalangeal joints, the so-called 'dinner fork' deformity. When the tongue is extruded it is rapidly withdrawn to prevent being bitten by the involuntary jaw movements. The knee jerk is either of the 'pendulum' type or, more commonly, is sustained or 'hung up'. The movements differ from multiple habit spasms in which each movement, taken individually, resembles a normal movement but is abnormal in its course and repetition. In chorea the movements are bizarre. Huntington's chorea is unlikely to cause diagnostic difficulties because typically the onset is later in life and there may be a strong family history. It may present in childhood but muscle rigidity is more prominent and the progressive nature of the disease soon becomes apparent.

There are some significant differences between chorea and the other major manifestations of acute rheumatic fever which are worthy of note. The most striking difference is the frequency with which it is the only overt manifestation. Carditis, nodules, and erythema marginatum may be found but the combination of chorea and arthritis is very rare. Chorea is much more commonly seen in girls, particularly in the age group 11–15 years.

When chorea occurs without complications, there are none of the associated clinical findings such as tachycardia, a raised ESR, or even a raised ASO titer. There is a marked tendency to relapse in chorea which (contrary to the experience with the relapsing arthritis of acute rheumatic fever) does not seem to carry with it an increasing tendency to carditis. Nevertheless, patients with frequent relapses of chorea over several years without any other rheumatic manifestation may finally develop severe rheumatic carditis with rheumatic nodules and signs of congestive failure.

Sydenham's chorea needs little treatment apart from rest and quiet. Haloperidol has been used with possible benefit and the use of tetrabenazine may shorten the duration of chorea. If the involuntary movements are very severe or the condition shows a relapsing course, treatment with steroids may be tried. Prophylactic penicillin is required as for rheumatic fever.

LABORATORY FINDINGS

It is vital to realize that rheumatic fever is a clinical diagnosis, with investigations playing only a secondary role.

The ESR is usually considerably raised in active rheumatic fever and is a useful index of progress. The ESR is usually normal when congestive cardiac failure is present but other acute phase reactants such as the C-reactive protein remain raised despite cardiac failure. An elevated ASO titer is an essential criterion for diagnosis. It is always over 200 Todd units/ml and is usually much higher, remaining elevated for weeks or months. More direct evidence of streptococcal infection may be found by culture of a throat swab. Although the onset of infection usually precedes the rheumatic process by some 2 or 3 weeks, the β-hemolytic streptococcal infection may still be present and identified by throat swab provided that antibiotics have not been given.

Anemia is a common feature of a prolonged rheumatic process and a polymorphonuclear leukocytosis is usual at the onset. A polymorphonuclear exudate into the joints during the acute phase of rheumatic arthritis can be demonstrated, but aspiration of the joint in acute rheumatic fever is not justifiable.

A chest X-ray and echocardiography may reveal cardiac enlargement due to congestive cardiac failure or pericarditis with effusion. It is also useful for comparison if cardiac involvement is suspected later. All children with suspected rheumatic fever should also have an ECG for evidence of carditis. The earliest feature of myocarditis is prolongation of the PR interval to greater than 0.18 s but flattened T waves, a prolonged QT interval and rhythm disturbances can also occur.

DIFFERENTIAL DIAGNOSIS

The differential diagnosis of ARF depends largely upon its mode of presentation. Polyarthritis must be distinguished from the arthritis of juvenile chronic arthritis, Henoch–Schönlein disease and serum sickness. Other causes of arthritis such as pyogenic infection (osteitis and septic arthritis) and gout are unlikely to cause difficulty. Subacute rheumatism with carditis but little or no joint involvement is more likely to be confused with other cardiac conditions such as a viral myocarditis, tuberculous pericarditis or acute myocarditis with cardiac failure. Subclinical ARF is probably quite common. Vague illness, associated with aches and pains, pallor and tachycardia, should always be investigated and if

the diagnosis of rheumatic fever is confirmed, prophylactic penicillin should be instituted to prevent further attacks and possibly crippling heart disease.

TREATMENT

Bed rest

A child with ARF will need no urging to remain in bed; the pain is acute and the child has no inclination to move. The child with severe cardiac insufficiency may sit gasping in bed or in a chair. Apart from these two extremes, the question of bed rest poses problems, especially since the administration of adequate doses of salicylate speedily banishes the joint pain. It is traditional to urge that the child with ARF be kept in bed until all clinical signs of disease activity have ceased (normal temperature and pulse rate). Awaiting a normal ESR may mean confining a child to bed for months. There is no evidence that such prolonged bed rest is beneficial and there is evidence that it is harmful psychologically and physically. Once the initial acute phase of the illness is over, exercise within tolerance is beneficial even if the heart is affected.

Antibiotic therapy

Eradication of the streptococcus is an essential part of treatment. Benzyl penicillin should be instituted without delay since a substantial proportion of children with ARF are shown to have β-hemolytic streptococci in their throats at the time of diagnosis. The offending organism may be deeply embedded in infected tonsils and eradication may require high concentrations. It is therefore desirable to begin treatment with high doses of benzyl penicillin intravenously (by indwelling cannula). A suitable dosage is 250 000 units 6-hourly for 3 days followed by oral phenoxymethyl penicillin 250 mg 6-hourly for a further 10 days. Thereafter a prophylactic regime takes over.

Antirheumatic drugs

Salicylates

Acetylsalicylic acid (ASA) (aspirin) gives rapid symptomatic relief of ARF (particularly arthralgia) but is not curative. A starting dose of 80–100 mg/kg per day is regulated by measurement of the plasma salicylate, 2 mmol/l (25–30 mg/dl) (children vary considerably in their reaction to salicylates and manifestations of intoxication with over breathing may occur even with apparently acceptable plasma levels). The pyrexia of ARF usually settles within 12 hours of starting ASA. The optimal duration for salicylate therapy is a matter of personal opinion. Some continue until all signs of activity have disappeared, others use salicylate only to alleviate symptoms. The author's personal practice is to prescribe full doses of aspirin for 6 weeks.

Corticosteroids

Corticosteroids are best reserved for those patients with moderate to severe carditis or cardiac failure; they are much more potent than salicylates in suppressing acute exudative inflammation. There is no evidence that cardiac damage is prevented or minimized by steroids, even if used early in the course of the disease.

There is immediate improvement in arthritis, nodules and in returning the ESR to normal. The 'rebound phenomenon' which occurred after treatment with corticosteroids, with the return of arthritis and/or carditis, often with alarming acuteness, is reduced by suitably tapering treatment. Side-effects are common and related to both dose and duration of therapy. Nevertheless, the immediacy of the effect has so impressed clinicians that whenever acute rheumatic fever is seen at its most severe (and that implies cardiac or pericardial involvement) steroids are advocated, but there is little evidence that the ultimate prognosis is influenced. Full tapered dosage of steroid is given, e.g. 60 mg prednisolone per day for 10 days, reducing to 40 mg then 20 mg and then 10 mg every successive 10 days until a maintenance dose of 5 mg daily is reached, when the problem of when to stop treatment has to be faced. Many centers use salicylate in full doses at the same time and continue this beyond the course of steroid therapy in the hope of avoiding a rebound. Others begin salicylate therapy when the maintenance dose of glucocorticosteroids begins.

PROPHYLAXIS

The prevention of rheumatic fever depends upon the prevention of β-hemolytic streptococcal infection. This is not practicable for children in general but is crucial for the child with a previous history of ARF. Benzathine penicillin 1.2 megaunits intramuscularly once monthly, or oral phenoxymethyl penicillin 125 mg twice daily, or, for those allergic to penicillin, sulfadimidine (0.5–1.0 g twice daily) give suitable prophylaxis until the age of 25 at least. It is difficult for a teenager who has not been ill for many years, and for his parents, to understand the continuing need to take a tablet twice a day but the importance must be emphasized.

COURSE AND PROGNOSIS

An average attack of rheumatic fever usually lasts for about 6 weeks. About 50% of patients escape lasting cardiac involvement in their first attack. Early cardiac enlargement lasting for a few days is quite common. Repeated attacks tend to mimic each other so that if there is no carditis in the first attack it is unlikely that there will be carditis in the second and subsequent attacks. Cardiac involvement is much more likely in children under the age of 12 years and unlikely in adults over the age of 25 years. Prognosis is worse where presystolic or aortic systolic murmurs develop or where there is progressive cardiac enlargement, nodules or pericarditis.

JUVENILE CHRONIC ARTHRITIS (JCA)

The clinical picture of chronic polyarthritis with lymphade-nopathy, splenomegaly, a rash and pericarditis was first described in Britain by George Frederic Still (1897). Since then, the term 'Still's disease' has been used to encompass the whole spectrum of rheumatoid arthritis in children. Recently the term juvenile chronic arthritis (JCA) has been accepted. This is still a generic descriptive term with considerable heterogeneity. The criteria for diagnosis are shown together with the subgrouping in Table 24.11.

SYSTEMIC ONSET JCA

The most common age of onset of the disease is under 5 years, but

Table 24.11   Criteria for diagnosis of juvenile chronic arthritis

Onset – under 16 years
Duration – minimum of 3 months
Classification by onset
Systemic onset
Polyarticular onset
Pauciarticular onset (4 or fewer joints)

it can occur throughout childhood. Boys are affected as frequently as girls. The children are toxic and irritable usually with swinging fever. Splenomegaly and general lymphadenopathy are almost invariably present but arthritis may often be delayed for weeks or even months. These children have a daily rise in temperature, to in the range of 39.5–40.5°C. Daily intermittent fever may be the only symptom present initially, but a large number of children in this subtype have a typical maculopapular rash of coppery red color (Fig. 24.77). It is usually nonpruritic and most florid where the skin has been rubbed from the pressure of underclothing (Köbner's phenomenon). The rash is best seen just after the child has had a hot bath or at the height of the temperature.

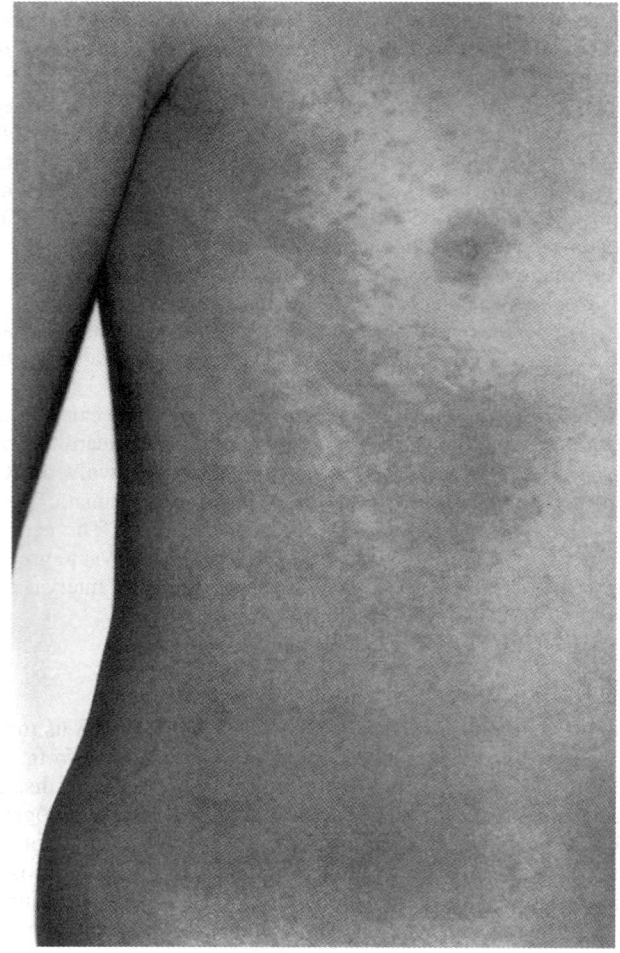

Fig. 24.77   Rheumatoid rash in a child with systemic onset type juvenile chronic arthritis.

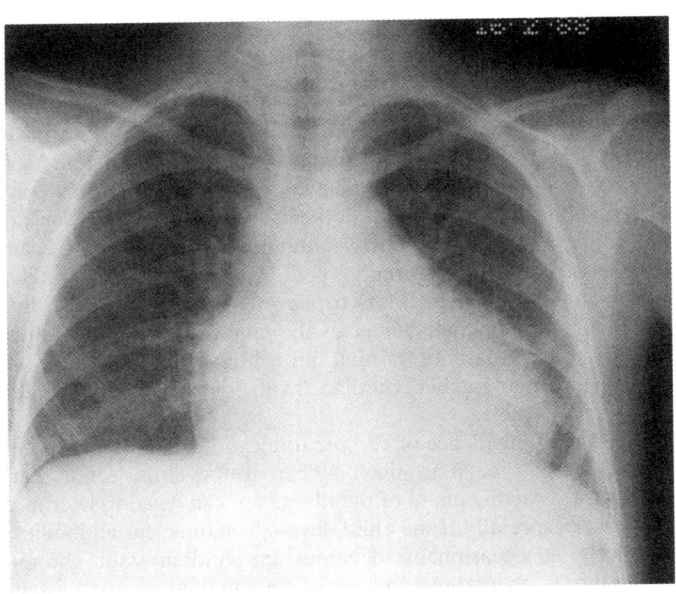

Fig. 24.78 Myopericarditis leading to congestive cardiac failure in a child aged 8 years with systemic onset type juvenile chronic arthritis.

Pericarditis may occur but is usually benign, asymptomatic and demonstrable at an early stage by echocardiography. Rarely, myocarditis can occur and may lead to congestive cardiac failure (Fig. 24.78). Endocarditis is not a feature of JCA. Hepatitis is an uncommon manifestation during the systemic phase.

Laboratory findings

There is no definitive diagnostic test for juvenile chronic arthritis. Laboratory findings in systemic onset JCA are nonspecific. The WBC count is high (about 25 000/mm³) and there is a neutrophil leukocytosis. The platelet count may also be high with counts around 750 000/mm³. Anemia is also present in the acute phase but it resolves as the disease activity is brought under control. The ESR is usually markedly raised, as are other acute phase reactants (CRP). Rheumatoid factor is almost always absent in the serum and to find antinuclear antibody in this subtype is rare. The immunoglobulins (IgG, IgA, and IgM) are frequently raised.

Differential diagnosis

Systemic onset JCA must be distinguished from fever of unknown origin, a viral infection, bacterial, rickettsial and *Mycoplasma pneumoniae* infections. The presence of splenomegaly, hepatomegaly, generalized lymphadenopathy and fever raises the possibility of leukemia and systemic lupus erythematosus. When rheumatic fever was common in children, it was the most difficult differential diagnosis. Diagnosis of the systemic subtype is based on the clinical findings with the exclusion of infection and neoplastic disorders and it may take several weeks before the correct diagnosis is made.

POLYARTICULAR ONSET JCA

In this subtype, involvement of five or more joints must be present for diagnosis. The commonest joints involved are the

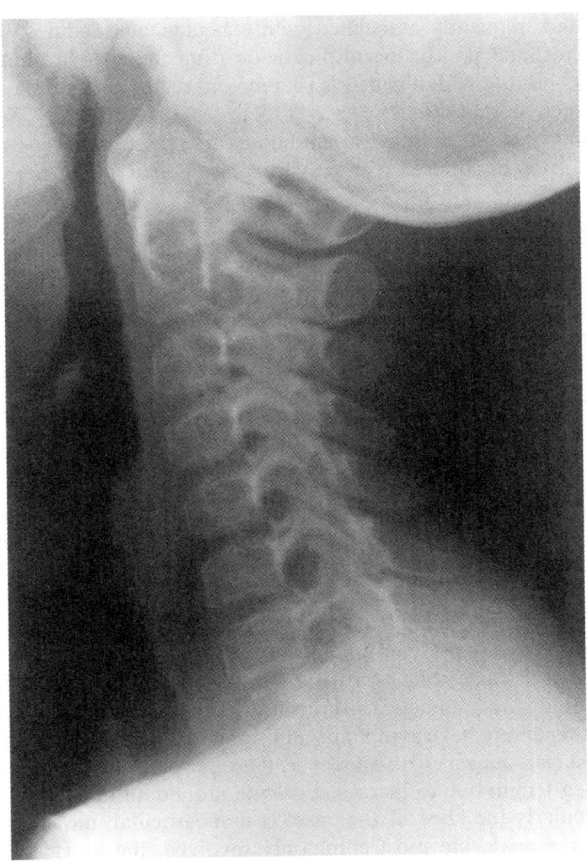

Fig. 24.79 Cervical spine showing apophyseal and disc changes at the C2/3 level in a child with polyarticular onset type juvenile chronic arthritis.

knees, wrists, ankles, metacarpophalangeal joints, proximal interphalangeal joints and metatarsophalangeal joints. Joint involvement is usually symmetrical. In addition to the joint synovitis, tenosynovitis may also be present. The cervical spine is also involved at an early stage, with limitation of movement and pain in the back of the neck so that torticollis can be a presenting feature (Fig. 24.79). Temporomandibular joint involvement is usually bilateral and failure of development of the jaw may lead to micrognathia. If the elbow joint is affected it occurs early, while hip and shoulder joint involvement is uncommon within the first year of onset of the disease. A low-grade fever is usually present but the marked spiking temperature seen in the systemic onset type is absent. Lymphadenopathy, though not necessarily generalized, and splenomegaly may also be present.

Laboratory findings

Children with polyarticular onset are divided into two groups: those negative for rheumatoid factor (seronegative group), and a smaller number (10%) who are positive (seropositive group). Clinically, rheumatoid factor positive polyarticular onset JCA is the subtype of JCA most similar to adult onset rheumatoid arthritis. The main reason for dividing them into two groups is because of the difference in prognosis. Patients with a positive rheumatoid factor are usually girls over 10 years of age and are more likely to develop destructive joint disease, particularly in the hip and frequently associated with subcutaneous nodules. They also respond poorly to antirheumatic drug therapy. In contrast, most children with a negative rheumatoid factor will not develop destructive joint disease.

On the whole, antinuclear antibodies are present in a very small proportion of children with polyarticular onset JCA.

Differential diagnosis

The early diagnosis of polyarticular onset may be as difficult as in systemic onset type JCA. Differential diagnosis includes connective tissue diseases, especially systemic lupus erythematosus (SLE) and mixed connective tissue disease (MCTD) (p. 1609).

PAUCIARTICULAR ONSET JCA

Nearly 50% of the children present with arthritis where one to four joints are involved. Monoarticular arthritis is included within the pauciarticular onset subgroup of JCA as the majority will develop a pauciarticular pattern within weeks to months and usually within 1 year of the onset of the disease. When persistent monoarthritis is present, it is most often in a knee.

When a single joint is involved it must be differentiated from infections or traumatic arthritis. Children with pauciarticular arthritis do not have symptoms and signs of a systemic or chronic illness and appear well. However, there may be a discrepancy in the leg length due to increased growth around an inflamed joint, particularly the knee. If the onset is monoarticular, the knee and then the ankle are most commonly involved, the wrist and the elbows and hips less frequently. Involvement of the small joints of the hands and feet, the cervical spine or the jaw is much less common in pauciarticular arthritis than in the polyarticular onset type.

There are two subgroups to pauciarticular JCA. The largest subgroup consists of children in whom the disease starts at an early age and the majority are girls. In this subgroup, children rarely have progressive joint disease but the development of iridocyclitis (uveitis) may be a serious problem. Antinuclear antibodies (ANA) are found in the majority, with close correlation with the presence of iridocyclitis. Children who are negative for ANA may not escape iridocyclitis but are at less risk. Rheumatoid factor is negative and HLA B27 is not present in these patients.

In the second subgroup, the majority are boys and joint disease usually begins about the age of 9 years. There is a tendency for this group to have predominantly lower limb arthritis involving the large rather than the small joints particularly the hips, knees and ankles. These children are usually positive for HLA B27 and negative for ANA. A significant number eventually develop ankylosing spondylitis. If uveitis develops it is usually acute and symptomatic.

Some patients with pauciarticular JCA do not fall into either of the above categories and may be separated into two additional groups by the number of joints that become involved during long-term follow-up. In some children, the total number of joints involved will never exceed four even after years of disease, and the arthritis is relatively benign. This group has been labeled as persistent pauciarticular JCA. Finally, some children have a pauciarticular onset, but proceed to a polyarticular course. The total number of joints involved increases with time so that after 6 months at least five joints may be affected. This type occurs less frequently than the persistent pauciarticular type.

COURSE AND PROGNOSIS OF JCA

Rheumatoid arthritis is a chronic systemic disease with a markedly fluctuating course. The arthritis tends to remit and relapse and with each exacerbation the ultimate deformity becomes worse. The disease seems to be self-limiting in that activity of the disease finally ceases. In some children this may occur within a few months or years resulting in little or no deformity, in others the course is more prolonged and a greater degree of articular deformity, possibly permanent, is likely. Fortunately, incapacity due to severe joint deformity and ankylosis is rare. Involvement of the temporomandibular joints may lead to failure of normal growth and be the cause of permanent micrognathia. Cardiac involvement seldom leads to permanent sequelae.

The overall incidence of chronic iridocyclitis is 10% but in the pauciarticular type it is much higher. Iridocyclitis is not seen during the systemic phase of the illness but can develop later in a few cases especially if the child develops antinuclear antibodies. Similarly, it occasionally develops in children with chronic polyarthritis. Symptoms and signs are minimal so routine slit lamp examination is mandatory in every child with juvenile chronic arthritis. Posterior synechiae form in the majority and chronic inflammation may eventually lead to band keratopathy, cataracts and secondary glaucoma (Fig. 24.80).

Apart from direct orthopedic effects, complications are rare except for those resulting from prolonged corticosteroid therapy.

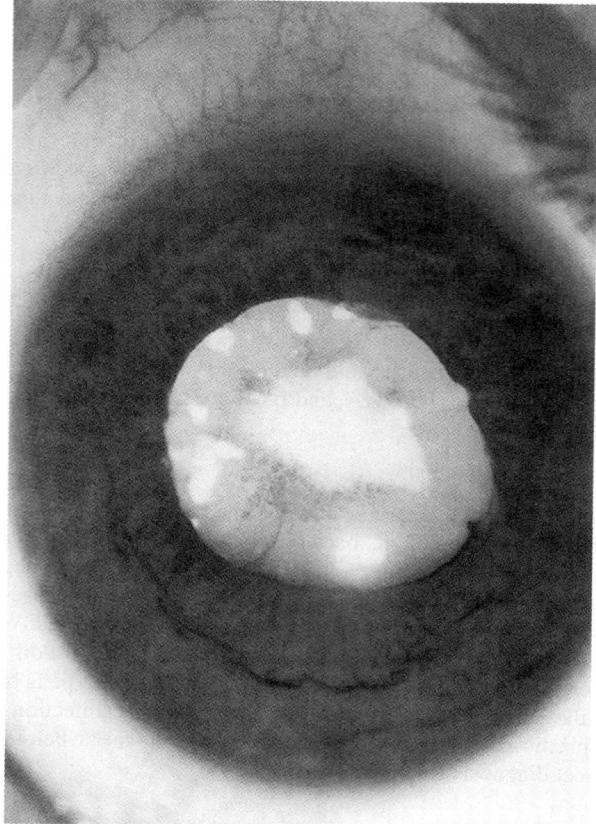

Fig. 24.80 Eye involvement in a child with pauciarticular onset type juvenile chronic arthritis showing synechiae, irregular pupil and complicated cataract as a result of prolonged chronic iridocyclitis.

Amyloid disease is a rare but potentially fatal complication. Abdominal pain, with progressive enlargement of the liver and spleen, diarrhea and the development of albuminuria are likely warning signs. The diagnosis of amyloidosis is confirmed by rectal or renal biopsy. Cytotoxic therapy such as chlorambucil has been used in amyloidosis with some success. There is an increased risk of mortality in juvenile chronic arthritis which is related to infection within the first 5 years of onset and later to amyloidosis.

TREATMENT

The treatment program of JCA consists of antirheumatic drugs, patient and family education, physiotherapy, occupational therapy, family support and orthopedic surgery.

Rest

A child with JCA should have an adequate period of rest in bed during the night and also some rest during the day, but complete bed rest is advised only for those children who are severely ill.

Antirheumatic drugs

The main aim of treatment of JCA is to relieve pain by using a relatively nontoxic drug. Some children have only mild symptoms and do not require drug treatment, only reassurance, supervision and physiotherapy. Others have intermittent problems that can be solved by the use of simple analgesics taken on demand. Still others will require regular treatment with antirheumatic drug(s) and sometimes a combination of antirheumatic drugs.

First line drugs

Nonsteroidal anti-inflammatory drugs (NSAIDs) are the mainstay of treatment of rheumatic diseases. NSAIDs are used initially for the acute flare up of rheumatic disease and later for long-term maintenance therapy. Since the variation in response to NSAIDs is greater between patients than between drugs, it is simply a matter of trial and error to find the one which suits a particular child. It is wise to start treatment with a low toxicity NSAID and if there is no response to try stronger and potentially more toxic ones. A 2-week trial is probably adequate to judge the efficacy of any single drug. Of the various NSAIDs, only those which are currently available for use in children will be discussed.

Acetyl salicylic acid (aspirin) is the oldest NSAID and remains the drug of first choice. Children tolerate aspirin well but should be observed closely for evidence of salicylism. In the young preschool child toxicity may occur even on low dosage and with low plasma levels. Unlike adults, children – particularly the very young – may not be aware of tinnitus or decreased auditory function. Other toxic manifestations are nausea, vomiting and gastrointestinal bleeding. The incidence and severity of gastric irritation can be decreased by ensuring that the prescribed aspirin or buffered aspirin disintegrates and dissolves properly. Should gastric symptoms still occur, enteric coated aspirin should be prescribed. 50% of children with JCA have high AST levels when their serum salicylate levels go above 35 mg/dl but this 'biochemical hepatitis' promptly disappears when aspirin is discontinued. The hepatic toxicity appears to be dose related and does not lead to chronic liver damage. Aspirin should be given with caution to children who have a history of chronic asthma,

sensitivity reaction to drugs, or other allergies. The dose of aspirin is 80–100 mg/kg daily and one should monitor the plasma salicylate level midway between doses (therapeutic range 25–30 mg/dl or about 2 mmol/l).

Propionic acids. This heterogeneous group have similar pharmacological and similar but fewer side-effects.

Ibuprofen. Ibuprofen has proved to be an effective anti-inflammatory agent and is well tolerated by the gastrointestinal tract. The toxicity seems to be low. The daily recommended dosage is 20 mg/kg in divided doses although, at the clinician's discretion, larger doses (40 mg/kg daily in divided doses) have been tolerated. Ibuprofen should be given with caution to patients with any form of bronchospasm and should be avoided in all patients allergic to aspirin or similar drugs. It is not recommended for children weighing less than 7 kg.

Naproxen. This drug is well tolerated in children and the biological half-life of 13 h makes it suitable for twice daily dosing. 15 mg/kg given in two divided doses produces very few side-effects.

Acetic acids. Indomethacin should be used cautiously in children. Side-effects include vomiting, abdominal pain, gastrointestinal bleeding, headaches, dizziness, confusion, vertigo and skin rashes. The side-effects related to the central nervous system are dose related. A single dose at night is often helpful in relieving early morning stiffness. The total daily dose should not exceed 2.5 mg/kg.

Full salicylate, ibuprofen or naproxen dosage by day and indomethacin by night is a satisfactory combination.

Tolmetin sodium. Tolmetin sodium is a new NSAID, and is effective for those who find aspirin and other NSAIDs difficult to tolerate. The side-effects are not clinically significant. In children under 2 years of age, safety and effectiveness have not been established. Therapy is started at 20–25 mg/kg daily in three or four divided doses and daily maintenance doses range from 15 to 30 mg/kg. Doses higher than 30 mg/kg are not recommended.

Phenylbutazone and oxyphenbutazone. These are the oldest and most potent NSAIDs but are potentially the most toxic, with a moderately high incidence of bone marrow suppression. They have a place in the treatment of juvenile ankylosing spondylitis and perhaps also in those children who respond to no other antirheumatic drugs. The daily dose is 5–10 mg/kg.

Second-line drugs

If a child continues to show evidence of active and progressively destructive joint disease in spite of an adequate trial of first line drugs, one needs to consider disease modifying drugs such as gold salts, penicillamine, hydroxychloroquine or salazopyrine.

Chrysotherapy. Although gold therapy in children is mentioned in scattered reports, most major contributions to our understanding of chrysotherapy relate to adults. Patients who respond to gold tend also to respond to penicillamine and vice versa. Maximal effects develop only after 4–6 months.

Hall & Ansell (1977) studied 41 children with seronegative juvenile arthritis treated with gold or penicillamine. They found the drugs to be equally effective in controlling disease activity and probably equally toxic in the doses employed. Toxic and allergic side-effects such as nephropathy with proteinuria, skin rashes and bone marrow suppression are common; the nephropathy is rarely permanent. A full blood count including platelets and urinalysis are needed at least once a month and parents should be asked to report any untoward side-effects immediately. Test doses of 0.25, 0.5 and 0.75 mg/kg are given intramuscularly at weekly intervals before continuing with 1 mg/kg intramuscularly once a week for 6 months. If effective, the treatment should not be interrupted but should be continued on an indefinite basis with a reduction in dosage (giving the same amount per injection but less frequently, such as every 2, 3 or 4 weeks). Remission is not an indication for cessation of therapy. The newer oral gold preparation, auranofin, has obviated the need for weekly intramuscular injections but Athreya & Cassidy (1991) reported that auranofin, although seemingly effective if used early in mild to moderate disease, provided long-term control for only a small percentage of children with JCA.

Penicillamine. Like gold, penicillamine has no immediate effect and begins to work only after several weeks. Because of its side-effects, it should be reserved for those children who cannot be managed with NSAIDs. Full blood and platelet counts are mandatory at 2-week intervals for the first 6 months and monthly thereafter. Urine is checked for presence of protein and red cells monthly throughout treatment. Any increase in dose should be considered only after results of blood and urine tests have been checked. Three successive falls in platelet or neutrophil counts, even within the normal range, must be taken as a signal for dose reduction or withdrawal. Proteinuria may persist for months without increasing above 1+ on stick testing. It should be quantified and if it does not increase above 2 g/24 h, penicillamine may be continued. A reduction in dose is sometimes followed by diminution in protein loss.

The starting dose is 50 mg daily, increasing by 50 mg at intervals of not less than 4 weeks up to 450 mg daily to children under 20 kg body weight and up to 600 mg above this, though maintenance doses of less than 375 mg are often adequate. Children tolerate penicillamine at least as well as adults but require equally close surveillance.

Hydroxychloroquine. Because of the risk of eye complications such as keratopathy and retinopathy, hydroxychloroquine should only be used when eye monitoring is available. The dose of 5–7 mg/kg daily of hydroxychloroquine will not be associated with the development of serious side-effects. After 6 months, if there has been no effect, it should be stopped. If there has been a considerable improvement, the dose of hydroxychloroquine should be reduced to an alternate day regimen and should not be used for more than a maximum of 2 years in any one course.

Sulfasalazine. Ansell et al (1991) found sulfasalazine in a dose of 40 mg/kg/day is ineffective in children with JCA with the possible exception of older onset pauciarticular arthritis, which is often associated with HLA B27 positive antigen and which tends to spread to more than four joints.

Third-line drugs

Steroids. There is general agreement that steroids do not alter the long-term course of rheumatoid arthritis or prevent permanent joint damage. Because of very significant side-effects they should only be used in the following situations:

1. acute systemic involvement
2. severe inflammatory joint disease refractory to other drugs
3. chronic uveitis unresponsive to local steroid therapy.

Prednisolone 1 mg/kg is started on alternate days to minimize both adrenal suppression and growth retardation. If necessary it can be increased and once the disease activity is controlled, the dose should be gradually decreased, aiming at keeping the disease activity just suppressed. NSAIDs should be considered in addition, especially on the 'nonsteroid day'.

ACTH has been used instead of oral steroids, as growth retardation is less, but repeated injections may distress a child.

Immunosuppressant therapy. The use of cytotoxic immunosuppressants in the treatment of JCA is based on the assumption that the disease is an immune disorder and that any observed effects of therapy are related to induced alterations of immune mechanisms. Their efficacy should be weighed against their serious side-effects. Methotrexate (MTX) is given at a starting dose of 5 mg/m^2/week orally, increasing to 10 mg/m^2/week at 1–2 month intervals to achieve maximal efficacy. A daily supplement of 1 mg of folic acid or 5 mg once a week 3 days after MTX dose is useful in lessening MTX toxicity. Liver function tests (AST, ALT and albumin levels) should be monitored every 4–8 weeks.

Splints

Joints may need to be splinted to prevent deformities. Rest splints on wrists, knees and ankles worn at night avoid the development of flexion deformities which, if untreated, may progress to contractures. Work splints protect joints in use and provide some relief of symptoms particularly during school lessons when there is movement of the neck and wrists.

Physiotherapy

A physiotherapist should be involved in treating a child with JCA and should plan an exercise program tailored to the child's needs. The purpose of the exercise program is to maintain joint motion and muscle strength. Hydrotherapy may allow easier movement of painful joints – a hot water bath is a useful substitute (Fig. 24.81). All joints must be moved as fully as possible every day. Cycling and swimming are the best activities for children with arthritis. Competitive sports such as running, football and hockey are not advised while the disease is active.

Occupational therapy

The role of the occupational therapist is to keep the child as independent as possible. Mildly affected children can enjoy normal activity for most of the time but others may have problems with everyday activities such as dressing, washing, eating, toileting and getting in and out of bed. The occupational therapist can assess any difficulties and teach the child techniques to make these activities easier, e.g. by using specially designed cutlery at meals.

Surgery

Most cases of JCA do not require surgery but the child with severe arthritis may present serious difficulties for the anesthetist because of an inability to extend the neck or open the mouth. Synovectomy is useful when overgrowth of the epiphysis or metaphyses is occurring. The most common sites are the knee and elbow. The synovium regrows within 6 months. Soft tissue release is occasionally required for progressive hip disease associated with flexion deformity. It allows the deformities to be corrected and provides additional time for growth. Whether it avoids ultimate joint replacement or merely delays it is uncertain. Total

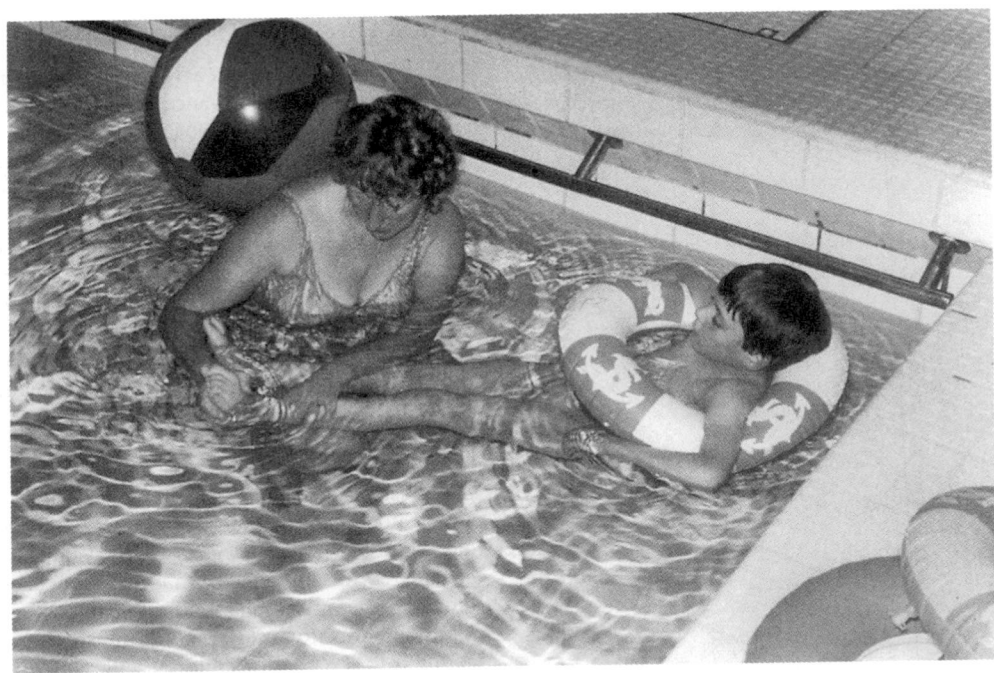

Fig. 24.81 Exercises in the hydrotherapy pool.

hip or knee replacement (arthroplasty) may be required for severe functional impairment and pain. Every attempt should be made to delay surgery until growth has ceased. Most surgeons now favor uncemented prostheses in both children and adolescents.

Local corticosteroid injections

Intra-articular corticosteroid injections may be useful for regaining function of the knee, elbow and the shoulder joints in pauciarticular JCA. Triamcinolone hexacetonide in the dosage of 20 mg for an elbow and 40 mg for a knee is recommended. If improvement does not occur, the injection should not be repeated. Should improvement last for some months followed by a relapse, it is reasonable to consider a further local steroid injection after approximately 6 months.

ANKYLOSING SPONDYLITIS

Ankylosing spondylitis is rarer in childhood than rheumatoid arthritis but has been described in children as young as 5 years of age. The classic presenting features of stiffness and backache in the lumbosacral region may also occur in childhood. In children and adolescents the presentation may, however, be as an asymmetrical polyarthritis in the large joints such as the hips and knees, and sometimes may be preceded by attacks of iritis, episcleritis and scleritis. The laboratory findings are not particularly helpful as IgM and IgG, rheumatoid factors, antinuclear antibodies and anti-DNA antibodies tend to be normal but these patients almost always possess tissue antigen W27.

SYSTEMIC LUPUS ERYTHEMATOSUS (SLE)

SLE is a multisystem disease with multiple and complex manifestations. The disease in children is more severe than in adults and previously often had a fatal outcome. The use of corticosteroids and immunosuppressive drugs has improved the outlook for children with SLE. The age of onset is between 11 and 15 years of age though the occasional case presents at even less than 1 year. It is more common in girls than in boys.

ETIOLOGY

The etiology is unknown but immunological mechanisms play a vital role in pathogenesis. The hallmark of this disorder is the presence of antibodies directed against a wide variety of nuclear, cytoplasmic and serum proteins. Drug-related lupus (identical to idiopathic lupus) may arise after administration of drugs such as hydralazine, procainamide, isoniazid, para-aminosalicylic acid and various anticonvulsants, especially phenytoin. It is sometimes difficult to discriminate between idiopathic and drug-related lupus.

CLINICAL MANIFESTATIONS

The clinical symptomatology may be variable and unpredictable with any number of organ systems eventually becoming involved. The disease is either acute or subacute and hardly ever chronic. The erythematous rash with its 'butterfly' distribution on the cheeks and bridge of the nose is characteristic and is present in one-third of children at presentation. (Fig. 24.82) but is often subtle and easily missed. Another characteristic skin eruption is a maculopapular erythema of the hands and feet, especially on the soles and around the nail beds. In addition various other skin manifestations may occur such as nonspecific erythemata, purpura, telangiectasia, urticaria, abnormal pigmentation, Raynaud's phenomenon and alopecia. Many children have a history of photosensitivity. There may be anemia with evidence of hemolysis, thrombocytopenia and leukopenia. Renal involvement manifested by red cells, white cells, protein and casts in the urine

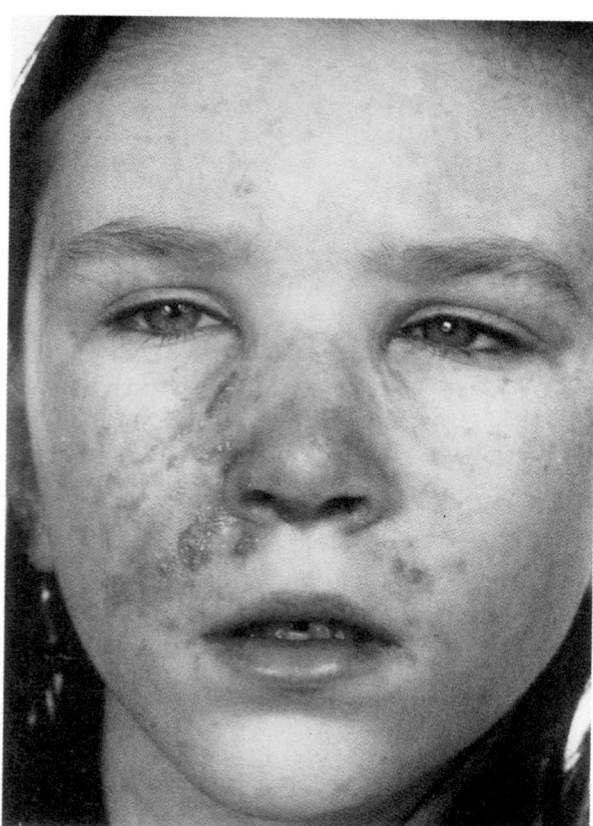

Fig. 24.82 Erythematous butterfly rash in a 10-year-old girl with systemic lupus erythematosus.

may progress to significant renal damage associated with azotemia and hypertension. This is the usual cause of death in SLE. Even where there is no clinical evidence of nephritis the characteristic histological picture may be present on renal biopsy. Joint involvement is common and varies from pain to a deforming arthritis closely resembling that of rheumatoid arthritis. In the chronic state, erosion of cartilage is in favor of JCA, even in the presence of antinuclear antibodies, while the presence of glomerulonephritis is likely to indicate SLE. Cardiac involvement may occur as myocarditis, endocarditis and pericarditis. Pleurisy with a serous effusion may also occur. Serositis may also involve the pericardium and peritoneum. Manifestations of central nervous system involvement include convulsions and mental confusion and various localizing manifestations due to focal vascular lesions. Enlargement of the liver and spleen and generalized lymphadenopathy may be present. Vascular occlusions may occur with bizarre consequences such as constrictive loss of visual fields, aseptic bone necrosis and gangrene of the fingers and toes. There may be a rapidly progressive retinopathy and extensive retinal hemorrhages, exudation and papilledema.

Sjögren's syndrome (sicca syndrome of dry mouth and dry eyes) is a connective tissue disorder which has elevated ANA and other autoantibodies. It is not uncommon and is usually benign and requires no special treatment. Symptomatic relief of dry eyes with artificial tears or of the dry mouth (xerostomia) by sucking lemon drops may be helpful.

LABORATORY FINDINGS

SLE is associated with an assortment of autoantibodies. The most important and striking advance in our understanding of this disease was the demonstration of the LE cell, used in diagnosis (but the LE cell test is now superseded). Anti-double strand DNA (dsDNA) is considered the most specific antibody for lupus, while anti-single strand DNA (ssDNA) is relatively nonspecific and commonly found in many rheumatic syndromes. The presence of anti-double stranded DNA is often coincident with evidence of serum complement (C3, C4) consumption and indicates renal disease. Anemia is present in most patients but only a fraction have positive Coombs' tests. Lymphopenia is possibly one of the most common manifestations of SLE and thrombocytopenia may be seen.

TREATMENT

Corticosteroids can be given in high dosage (1–2 mg/kg per day) either alone or in conjunction with azathioprine (2–5 mg/kg per day) or other immunosuppressants. Cyclophosphamide should be considered for any child with biopsy-proven diffuse proliferative glomerulonephritis and active nephritis. Intravenous 'pulse' methylprednisolone (30 mg/kg up to 1 g) is another useful addition to the care of children with SLE. It is effective for the control of both renal and extrarenal disease flares. Unfortunately its beneficial effects are often transient, and its use may be associated with severe toxicity.

PROGNOSIS

The course of SLE in childhood is highly variable and unpredictable. Prognosis relates closely to renal involvement (Ansell 1980). Fish et al (1977) have suggested that children and adolescents with lupus nephritis might have a better prognosis than adults.

NEONATAL LUPUS ERYTHEMATOSUS

Neonatal lupus erythematosus is rare and is characterized by cutaneous and/or cardiac abnormalities. Babies with neonatal lupus are born to mothers who have symptoms of a connective tissue disease and have circulating anti-Ro antibodies. Neonates with lupus erythematosus usually have a positive antinuclear antibody test and are also anti-Ro positive.

The cutaneous lesions may be confused initially with seborrheic dermatitis but the lesions are photosensitive. Even without treatment the cutaneous lesions will disappear spontaneously within 4–6 months after birth (Lee et al 1983). Cardiac abnormalities are usually permanent and characterized by conduction abnormalities, usually congenital complete heart block (Ch. 13). Cardiac and cutaneous abnormalities usually occur separately but patients have been reported with both abnormalities. Neonates with the lupus syndrome may also have a Coombs' positive anemia, hepatosplenomegaly, thrombocytopenia and/or leukopenia. As in the cutaneous disease, these hematological abnormalities should disappear spontaneously by the age of 4–6 months.

DERMATOMYOSITIS–POLYMYOSITIS

Approximately 5% of patients with connective tissue disease attending a pediatric rheumatology clinic will have dermatomyositis. Polymyositis is characterized by predominantly proximal muscle weakness but without any evidence of skin involvement. In dermatomyositis the muscle involvement is clinically and histologically indistinguishable from that of polymyositis but there is also a rash involving the face and extremities.

The clinical and histological features are different in childhood from dermatomyositis seen in adults. In children dermatomyositis is not associated with underlying malignancy. There is usually both skin involvement with subcutaneous induration and muscle weakness of all four limbs, together with general misery and constitutional upset.

The onset is usually insidious with facial erythema, muscle weakness and fatigue, and general constitutional upset, but occasionally the onset is acute. It may occur at any age from the second year into adolescence. A heliotrope color of the eyelids and periorbital skin is quite characteristic of this disorder and periorbital edema is also common (Fig. 24.83). Patches of erythema occur particularly over the extensor surfaces of the fingers, elbows and knees and later become atrophic, wrinkled, shiny and bluish in appearance. Often there is an associated low grade fever. The weakened muscles become stiff and tender on movement, sometimes leading to a mistaken diagnosis of JCA. Calcinosis of the affected areas is common in childhood and readily demonstrated by X-ray. The course is usually slow and insidious over many years. Contractures are common, requiring orthopedic management, and a varying degree of physical

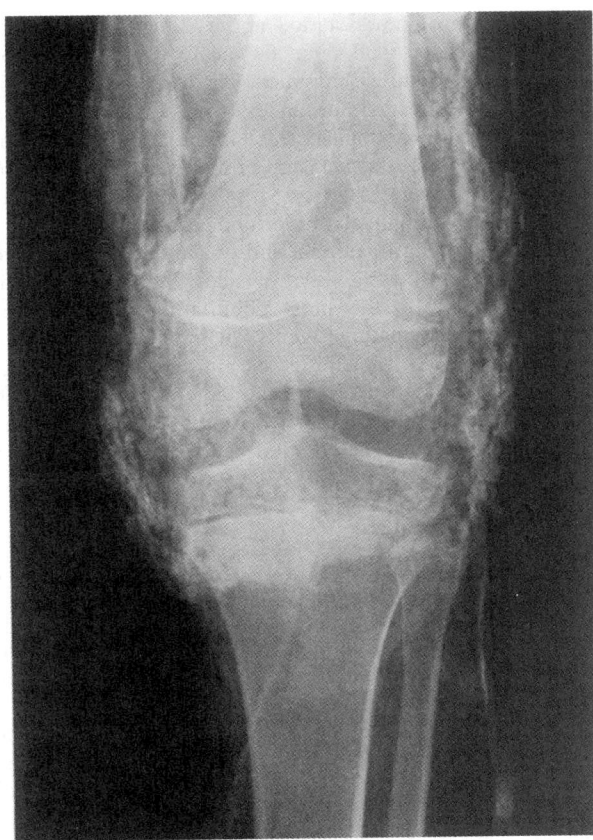

Fig. 24.84 Extensive soft tissue calcification at the knee joint in a 12-year-old child with dermatomyositis.

incapacity may result. Nevertheless, the ultimate prognosis seems to be better in childhood than in adults and this may be associated with a higher incidence of calcinosis (Fig. 24.84) (Goel & King 1986).

LABORATORY FINDINGS

The diagnosis is based on the clinical features of symmetrical muscle weakness and the typical cutaneous manifestations and may be confirmed by elevation of the serum muscle enzymes and/or a muscle biopsy showing inflammatory myositis. The ESR is often raised. Of the serum muscle enzymes the creatine kinase (CK) is often two to threefold above normal but is a nonspecific criterion for diagnosis. A normal level may simply mean that the patient is already so wasted that the CK may not rise even in an exacerbation of the disease. Electromyography (EMG) may demonstrate a myopathic/neuropathic pattern and this finding is helpful in supporting the diagnosis of inflammatory muscle disease. Muscle biopsies often show a characteristic vasculitis with accompanying degeneration of muscle fibers. 10–40% of biopsies have been reported as normal even in patients with clear-cut active disease.

TREATMENT

In long-term management, physiotherapy and orthopedic assistance are essential as contractures must be prevented or

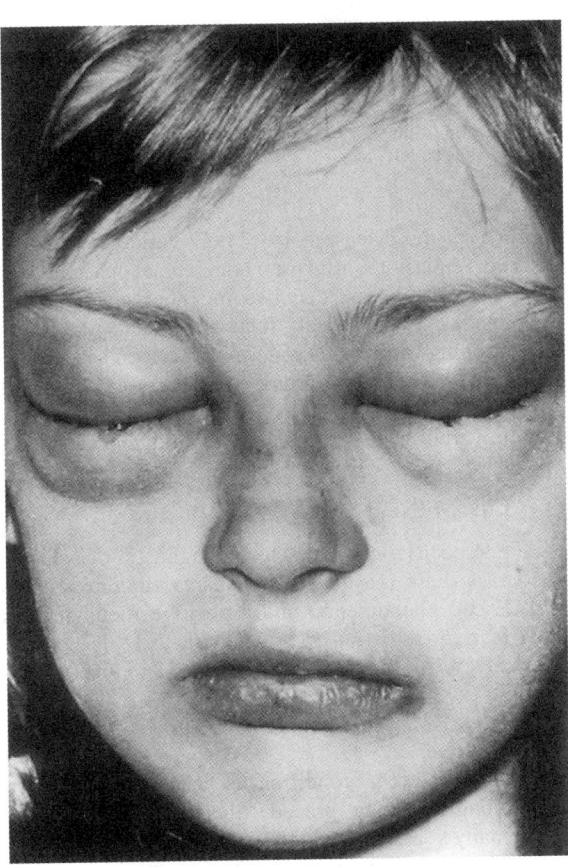

Fig. 24.83 Periorbital edema and erythema in a 10-year-old girl with dermatomyositis.

corrected. Prednisolone is started at 1.5–2 mg/kg per day as a single morning dose, and once the acute phase is controlled reduced to an alternate day regimen. The response to steroids is slow with improvement of the skin lesions, a diminution in muscle pain and tenderness, and an increase in muscle strength. Serum creatine kinase is a useful measure of disease activity and of its control by treatment. Cytotoxic drugs such as methotrexate, cyclosporine, cyclophosphamide and azathioprine may be valuable in improving functional ability and decreasing the total steroid requirement but the risks of side-effects limit their use. Calcification may be the most debilitating consequence of dermatomyositis. Chelating agents such as ethane hydroxy-diphosphate (EHDP) are ineffective in either controlling or preventing calcification. However the large, painful or unsightly lumps of calcinosis may be removed surgically. The deep tissue infections which occur usually require both surgical drainage and antibiotics.

PROGRESSIVE SYSTEMIC SCLEROSIS OR SCLERODERMA

The term progressive systemic sclerosis is nowadays preferred, indicating the important and often lethal nature of the systemic manifestations of this disorder. The skin manifestations are still striking and the disease may be neither systemic nor progressive. This disease is exceptionally rare in childhood. Patches of skin become edematous and then atrophic and inelastic, becoming adherent to the underlying tissues. The consequent atrophy and tightening of the skin gives the characteristic appearance of a pinched nose and pursed lips. The hands become shiny with tapered finger ends and restricted movement, producing claw-like deformities which may also affect the feet. This indirect involvement of the joints may be complicated by a true arthritis, particularly of the knees, ankles, metacarpophalangeal and interphalangeal joints. Ulceration of the affected skin may occur, as may calcification of the underlying tissues. The underlying muscles may atrophy and fibrose, leading to permanent contractures. Raynaud's phenomenon is common and narrowing of the radial artery may be demonstrable on angiography. The well-known gastrointestinal system involvement with esophageal fibrosis and dysphagia is less common in childhood but incoordination of esophageal peristalsis may cause dysphagia and consequent anorexia and is demonstrable on barium meal examination. A similar disorder may occur in the small bowel and lead to serious bacterial overgrowth with deconjugation of bile salts and resultant steatorrhea. This is much the same as the 'blind loop syndrome' but is better termed the 'small bowel contamination syndrome'. Malabsorption and persistent intractable diarrhea may be a consequence. Long-term antibiotic therapy beginning with co-trimoxazole is often quite dramatically effective. There may also be protein loss with severe hypoproteinemia and generalized edema. Intravenous salt-poor albumin and diuretics may be necessary to control this aspect of the condition. A falling hemoglobin may require blood transfusion in spite of the addition of iron, folic acid and vitamin B_{12}. Pulmonary fibrosis and renal involvement may occur.

Linear scleroderma is a strange condition in which half the body is affected while the other half remains untouched (Fig. 24.85). With growth there is an increasing disparity in bone length and girth, with consequent deformity and disability.

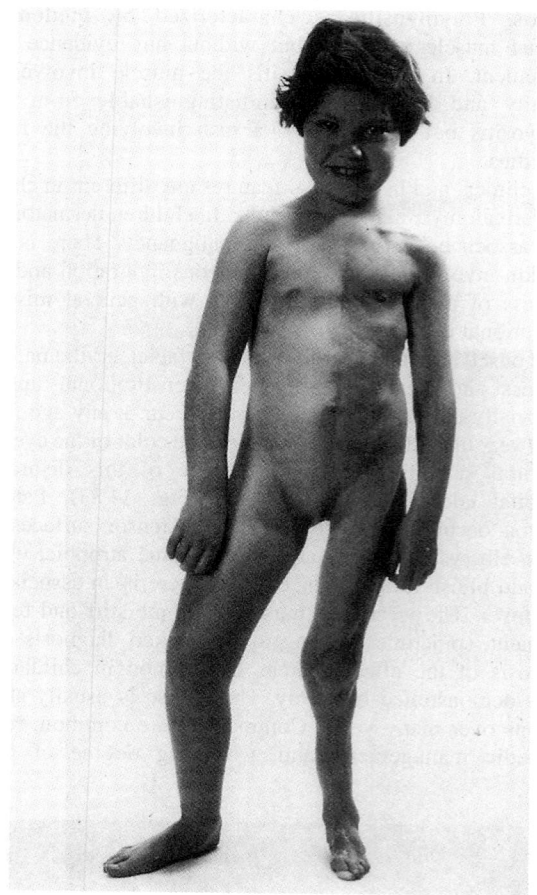

Fig. 24.85 A case of linear scleroderma showing gross hemiatrophy of trunk and limbs of the left side.

The course of the disease is extremely variable, with frequent relapses and remissions affecting both cutaneous and systemic manifestations. The disease may become quiescent and regress, or become progressive and rapidly fatal as in adults. An apparently slowly developing form of scleroderma described largely in adults and called the CREST syndrome may be found in children. CREST is an acronym for calcinosis, Raynaud's phenomenon, esophageal dysfunction, sclerodactyly and telangiectasia.

LABORATORY FINDINGS

There are no specific laboratory tests diagnostic of scleroderma. In some cases there may be antinuclear antibodies and even a positive LE cell phenomenon and a positive rheumatoid factor. The ESR is frequently raised and where there is considerable muscle involvement, the transaminases are also raised.

DIAGNOSIS

The characteristic skin condition is usually not difficult to diagnose though it may precede the clinically recognizable disease by many years. Occasionally the involvement of the joints may be such as to suggest juvenile chronic arthritis and synovial biopsy may be necessary to make the diagnosis clear, and skin and muscle biopsy may be necessary to differentiate dermatomyositis.

TREATMENT

No treatment at the present time is of any certain value. It is important to provide physical and occupational therapeutic measures to maintain good position and function of the joints and to maintain muscle strength. Corticosteroid therapy does not seem to alter the progression of the disease. Immunosuppressive agents and penicillamine have been reported to be of benefit to some patients, but both these forms of therapy should still be considered as experimental.

MIXED CONNECTIVE TISSUE DISEASE

Mixed connective tissue disease (MCTD) is a distinct syndrome in which patients have antibody to ribonucleoprotein (RNP) antigen, high titers of speckled fluorescent antinuclear antibody, and overlapping clinical features suggestive of systemic lupus erythematosus, scleroderma, dermatomyositis and rheumatoid arthritis. Significant renal and cardiac involvement appears to be more common in children than in adults. The disease evolves over months to years and only frequent determination of ANA and anti-RNP antibody titers with atypical rheumatological syndromes will allow earlier identification of MCTD. Children with MCTD may be less responsive to corticosteroids than adults, with consequently a poorer prognosis.

VASCULITIC SYNDROMES

HENOCH–SCHÖNLEIN PURPURA (ANAPHYLACTOID PURPURA)

This is a systemic vasculitis of unknown etiology involving skin, joints and some viscera. Schönlein associated the purpura and arthritis, and Henoch the purpura and gastrointestinal involvement. The syndrome may also include urticaria and not infrequently focal proliferative glomerulonephritis. A previous history of an upper respiratory tract infection is not unusual but such infections are commonplace among children. The disease is commonest among preschool children, affecting boys more often than girls, but a wide range of age groups may be affected including the first year of life.

Pathology

HSP is rarely fatal and pathological studies are largely confined to skin and renal biopsies. The basic lesion is a diffuse angiitis with perivascular exudates of leukocytes and leukocyte-platelet thrombi as seen in lupus erythematosus. The renal lesion is dealt with elsewhere (Ch. 17).

Clinical picture

The characteristic onset is a symptomless purpuric eruption confined largely to the extensor surfaces of the lower limbs, including the buttocks (Fig. 24.86). The trunk may also be affected and occasionally in the very young, the face. The eruption begins as a raised urticarial rash rapidly becoming purpuric without losing its urticarial character. Such a rash is virtually diagnostic of HSP. The lesions tend to fade through the typical brown-yellow discoloration of hemorrhage in the skin. Joint involvement is not always present and is usually transient but

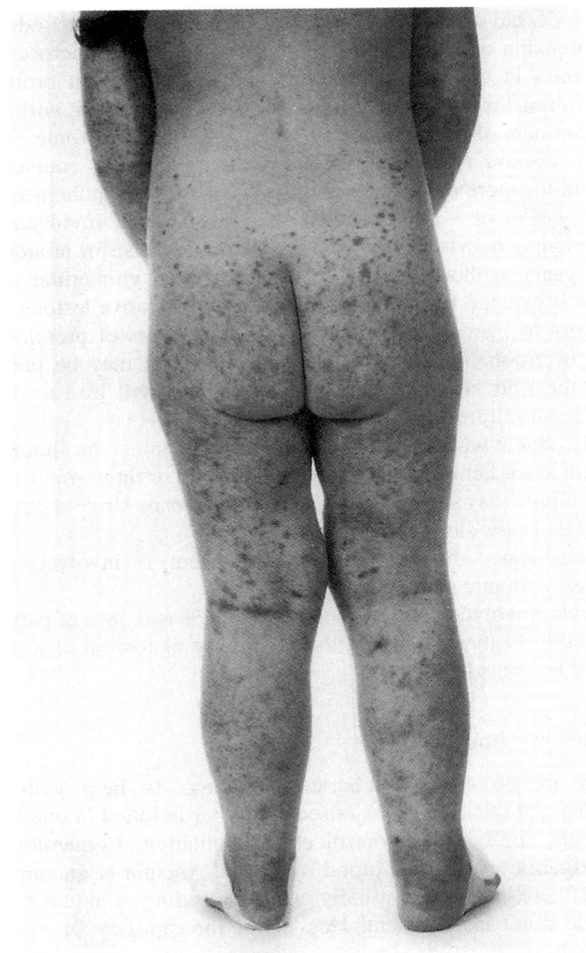

Fig. 24.86 Purpuric rash on buttocks in a child with Henoch–Schönlein purpura.

without the obvious migratory or 'flitting' character of the arthritis of acute rheumatic fever. Joint involvement may be confined to tenderness and pain on movement or associated with distinct swelling and intra-articular exudate.

Gastrointestinal involvement is often common and distressing. Hemorrhage into the gut wall produces intermittent or persistent colicky pain, occasionally vomiting, and less commonly melena. Where there is no frank blood in the stools, occult blood is usually present. It is not infrequent for the pain to be so severe as to suggest an acute abdominal emergency and this may lead to unnecessary laparotomy. Nevertheless, intussusception can occur and in this case surgery may be life saving. The differential diagnosis of intussusception may be very difficult. General abdominal tenderness usually makes palpation difficult and the continual complaints of abdominal pain may lull the medical attendants into a sense of false security. A plain X-ray film of the abdomen interpreted by a skilled pediatric radiologist is often the deciding factor and in all cases of doubt a pediatric surgeon should be consulted.

Renal involvement is more common than usually recognized and may occur in 25–50% of patients. It is usually asymptomatic in contradistinction to the acute glomerulonephritis of streptococcal origin. The patient presents without edema, hypertension or oliguria and the hematuria is often microscopic. Azotemia is unusual as are alterations in the serum proteins. Continuing renal involvement may be associated with the development of hypertension or of the nephrotic syndrome.

The disease runs a variable and often relapsing course but seldom for more than a year and many cases remit spontaneously by 6 weeks or so. In patients with overt renal involvement, microscopic hematuria and proteinuria may persist for months or even years. Although recovery from the focal glomerular renal lesion is usual, a few cases with diffuse proliferative lesions may progress to irreversible renal damage after years of proteinuria. Very occasionally, diffuse glomerular nephritis may be present from the start and an inexorable progression will lead to death from renal failure within a matter of months.

Any patient with unexplained abdominal or joint pain should be examined for hemorrhagic spots, as even two or three small spots on an elbow may suggest the definitive diagnosis. Urine should be tested daily for albumin and blood.

Occasionally the central nervous system is involved with pareses, epileptic seizures or coma.

Scrotal involvement occurs in between 2% and 38% of patients with HSP. In these children, the possibility of torsion of a testis should be considered.

Laboratory findings

There are no specific laboratory findings to help with the diagnosis of this disease. A raised ASO titer is found in one-third of cases, similar to a control child population. Hematological investigation excludes a blood dyscrasia. Anemia is uncommon unless there has been unusually profuse bleeding or in cases with chronic renal involvement. Hess's test for capillary fragility is negative.

Treatment

There is no specific therapy but symptomatic treatment may be of great benefit. If a streptococcal infection is detected, penicillin should be given. While purpura persists it may be wise to confine the child to bed as it is the general clinical impression that the purpura becomes worse if the child is allowed to run about. Frank hematuria and a raised ESR may also be indications for bed rest. Arthritic pain responds very promptly to oral NSAIDs which should be limited to the time required for symptomatic relief. The abdominal pain may be the most difficult and distressing feature of the disease and these children are, moreover, very prone to show a continued depression that causes their parents considerable anxiety. While a simple analgesic such as paracetamol may be of some value, severe cases will only respond to oral pethidine with considerable benefit, and with improvement in temperament of the patient. Occasionally, abdominal pain may be so gross and prolonged as to defy even large doses of morphine or heroin. In such a situation, prednisolone treatment may resolve this feature (and this feature only) of HSP. Such therapy should be of short duration and will not affect the nephritis.

POLYARTERITIS

Polyarteritis may be subdivided into at least five entities: infantile polyarteritis, polyarteritis of older children, polyarteritis associated with hepatitis B antigen, cutaneous polyarteritis and mucocutaneous lymph node syndrome (Kawasaki's disease).

Infantile polyarteritis

This affects mainly children under 12 months of age and is very rare. The coronary arteries are the primary sites involved. Respiratory symptoms and a morbilliform rash are common, and the course tends to be brief and downhill. Diagnosis is usually made at postmortem examination.

Polyarteritis of older children

This resembles the adult form of the disease. Fever is present in almost all cases as are irritability, weight loss and lethargy. Skin rashes of different kinds have been described – none being diagnostic. Significant arteritis involving the kidneys, heart, CNS and gastrointestinal tract result in clinical manifestations related to these organs. The pathology in children is similar to that in adults with polymorphonuclear infiltration and necrosis occurring mainly in small and medium sized muscular arteries, involving all layers of the vessel. Elevated ASO titers suggest a possible pathogenetic role for previous streptococcal infection. The prognosis is poor but may be improved with steroids and/or cyclophosphamide.

Polyarteritis associated with hepatitis B antigen

HBsAg immunoglobulin complexes have been shown in the serum of a small group of patients with biopsy-proved polyarteritis. These patients have evidence of mild hepatic damage. No children have yet been described with this type of polyarteritis.

Cutaneous polyarteritis

This primarily affects the skin in children and presents with crops of small, painful nodules. Fever and arthralgia are common features. Skin necrosis and ulcerations are frequent. Most patients respond to a low dose of steroids.

Mucocutaneous lymph node syndrome (Kawasaki's disease)

Kawasaki's disease has many similarities to infantile polyarteritis and is discussed elsewhere (Ch. 23).

WEGENER'S GRANULOMATOSIS

Wegener's granulomatosis is rare and is characterized by a necrotizing granulomatous vasculitis of the upper and lower respiratory tract in association with focal necrotizing glomerulonephritis. Diagnosis is based on biopsy. Therapy with steroids does not prolong life but immunosuppressive therapy has proved effective.

AORTIC ARCH ARTERITIS OR TAKAYASU'S DISEASE

This syndrome may be a variety of polyarteritis. It is classically a disease of the aortic arch and its major arteries. It is a slowly progressive panarteritis with marked dilation of the aorta and resultant aortic regurgitation together with occlusion of major vessels causing a weakening and finally abolition of the radial pulses at the wrist, from which it also receives the name 'pulseless disease'. A relative pulselessness of the upper limbs may be demonstrated by a significantly higher blood pressure in the legs than in the arms. Occlusion of the renal arteries may cause renal ischemia and hypertension while, rarely, decreased blood flow in the cerebral vasculature may produce central nervous system manifestations. Fever, constitutional symptoms and occasionally arthralgia may mimic rheumatic fever. The ESR is usually raised. Cineangiography provides the diagnosis. There is no specific therapy although corticosteroids have been used with apparent effect.

GIANT CELL ARTERITIS

Giant cell arteritis is primarily a disease of older adults. It would appear that only one child with giant cell arteritis has been reported (McEnery 1977).

ARTHROPATHY IN CYSTIC FIBROSIS OF PANCREAS

Due to the increasing life expectancy of patients with cystic fibrosis, age-related complications have now begun to appear. An arthropathy may be associated with cystic fibrosis mainly in three ways:

1. episodic arthritis, a specific complication
2. hypertrophic pulmonary osteoarthropathy (HPOA) as in any other chronic respiratory disease
3. coincidental, such as juvenile chronic arthritis (McGuire et al 1982).

EPISODIC ARTHRITIS IN CYSTIC FIBROSIS

The onset is usually sudden with one or more acutely inflamed joints, the most commonly affected being the knees and ankles. The patient is otherwise well and there is no temporal relationship between the appearance of joint lesions and respiratory disease. The X-ray may show an effusion, but erosive changes do not occur. Usually the symptoms and signs disappear either spontaneously or with the aid of NSAIDs.

HYPERTROPHIC PULMONARY OSTEOARTHROPATHY

Patients with hypertrophic pulmonary osteoarthropathy (HPOA) may present with joint effusions, tenderness and swelling of limbs, usually the legs, or the X-ray changes may be clinically silent. The periosteal changes in long bones can be seen using conventional radiology or isotope bone scanning. The bone and joint symptoms in HPOA relapse with acute pulmonary deterioration.

ARTHROPATHY IN INFLAMMATORY BOWEL DISEASE

Arthritis is the commonest extraintestinal manifestation of inflammatory bowel disease. The reported incidence varies from 5% to 25%, and the incidence is generally somewhat higher in ulcerative colitis than in Crohn's disease. It predominantly affects the large joints, especially the knees and ankles, but involvement of the spine (spondylitis) has been reported. The etiology of the joint manifestations remains unknown as does the etiology of the bowel disease. The onset of arthritis usually follows bowel symptoms by months or years but in some patients arthritic symptoms develop at the same time, while occasionally the arthritis is the first manifestation. In general, the episodes of arthritis occur when the underlying bowel disease is active. The prognosis for ultimate joint function is excellent.

PSORIATIC ARTHRITIS

Juvenile psoriatic arthritis may precede, be coincident with or follow psoriasis. Rheumatoid factor is absent from the serum. Psoriatic arthritis is rare in childhood and is more common in girls than in boys. Asymmetrical polyarthritis, frequently involving the distal interphalangeal joints, is the most frequent pattern. Pauciarticular large joint involvement is seen in some patients, and a minority have sacroiliitis and spondylitis. The major difference between JCA and psoriatic arthritis is the paucity of systemic manifestations including fever, generalized lymphadenopathy, hepatosplenomegaly or heart and lung involvement. There is an increased incidence of HLA B17 in psoriasis with peripheral arthritis and some increase in HLA B27 in the spondylitis group.

REITER'S SYNDROME

Reiter's syndrome, with the typical triad of urethritis, arthritis and conjunctivitis, is rare in childhood. The most common cause in childhood is an infective diarrhea due to *Shigella*, *Salmonella* or other enteric pathogens. The lower limb joints are usually involved, the knee being the most commonly involved joint followed by the ankle. Swelling of single toes or fingers has been noted. Systemic symptoms are not prominent although low grade fever and malaise may be present. Diagnosis of Reiter's syndrome is primarily clinical. Rheumatoid factor and antinuclear factor are absent but there is an association with HLA B27 in these patients. The prognosis is usually good with gradual amelioration of signs and symptoms. However, in some patients the arthritis can be very severe and persistent and may go on to a spondylitis indistinguishable from ankylosing spondylitis.

BEHÇET'S SYNDROME

This rare syndrome is characterized by recurrent oral and genital ulceration and eye inflammation. In addition, other associated clinical features are arthritis, fever and, less commonly, gastrointestinal and cardiovascular involvement and neurologic abnormalities. Laboratory findings are not diagnostic. There is no generally effective treatment although some children may benefit from high dose corticosteroids.

LYME ARTHRITIS

'Lyme arthritis' was identified in 1977 and is transmitted by the deer tick, *Ixodes dammini* (p. 1312). In 1982 it was discovered that the infectious agent is a spirochete (*Borrelia burgdorferi*). The clinical syndrome consists of a prodromal febrile illness with a characteristic rash, erythema chronicum migrans and cardiac, neurologic and articular manifestations. Arthritis may be the initial manifestation of Lyme disease, usually with pauciarticular-type joint involvement. The joints predominantly involved are knees, elbows, wrists, ankles and hips (Eichenfield et al 1986).

Lyme arthritis may be confused with septic arthritis, especially as the synovial fluid leukocyte counts can be very high, and usually show a neutrophilic preponderance. Lyme arthritis should be ruled out in patients with episodic, self-limiting attacks of arthritis even in the absence of the typical rash. The borrelia specific antibody indicative of Lyme disease can be measured in the immunofluorescent assay test: a significant titer is 1 : 256. The finding of an elevated titer in association with clinical manifestations is considered diagnostic. Lyme disease can benefit from antibiotic therapy such as high dose penicillin intravenously for 10 days. If antibiotics fail, synovectomy is curative (see p. 1314).

VIRAL ARTHRITIS

Virus infections commonly cause generalized musculoskeletal pain and stiffness but localized joint symptoms are uncommon and usually acute and self-limited. Thus, the main point of interest is in recognizing the viral arthropathy and excluding it from JCA and acute rheumatic fever. Arthralgia is relatively common but actual arthritis is rare, particularly in children. Viral infections that may be associated include rubella, both natural and vaccine induced, mumps, chickenpox, glandular fever, cytomegalovirus, hepatitis B, adenovirus (type 7), influenza and arboviruses. The arthropathy is usually polyarticular, transient, nonrecurring and resolves spontaneously.

HYPERMOBILITY SYNDROME (INCLUDING EHLERS–DANLOS SYNDROME)

Generalized joint laxity is a feature of the hereditary connective tissue disorders such as Marfan's syndrome, the Ehlers–Danlos syndrome (see below) and osteogenesis imperfecta. A subject is considered hypermobile if he can perform two of the following three maneuvers: passive opposition of both thumbs to the volar aspect of the forearms (Fig. 24.87); passive hyperextension of the fingers so that they lie parallel to the extensor aspect of both forearms; and active hyperextension of both elbows beyond 180°. Hypermobility is relatively common in the general population. The term 'hypermobility syndrome' has been coined to define a clinical situation in which there is generalized joint laxity

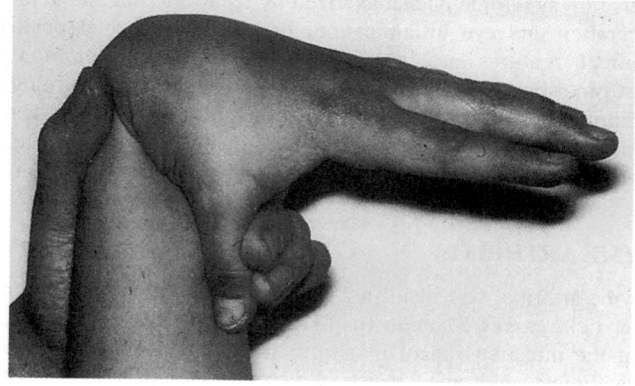

Fig. 24.87 Passive opposition of the thumb to the flexor aspect of the forearm in a girl of 8 years who presented with pain in the knees: hypermobility syndrome.

associated with musculoskeletal complaints without cutaneous or internal signs of connective tissue disease in otherwise normal subjects. In young children this syndrome is observed equally in both sexes but towards puberty it predominates in girls. The knees are the most frequent sites of complaint but occasionally the ankles may also be affected. The discomfort usually comes after exercise and the whole clinical picture is consistent with an episode of traumatic synovitis. There is a strong familial tendency to this syndrome and the diagnosis is therefore essentially clinical combined with an awareness of family history. The management is mainly reassurance as to the absence of serious disease, and activity which precipitates symptoms should be avoided if possible. Most young subjects will grow out of their complaints altogether.

EHLERS–DANLOS SYNDROME

The Ehlers–Danlos syndrome comprises a heterogeneous group of connective tissue disorders, clinically characterized by skin fragility and hyperextensibility, and joint hypermobility. More than 10 types have been defined on the basis of clinical and biochemical features: for many of these, the molecular defect has been defined (Table 24.12).

Types I and III are the commonest and are inherited in an autosomal dominant fashion. They are associated with marked joint hypermobility but are distinguished by the extent and severity of skin involvement.

In types I and II, scarring has a characteristic distribution on elbows, knees, shins, forehead and under the chin, which is more severe in type I than type II. Scarring is not a feature of type III. Electron microscope studies have demonstrated abnormalities in collagen fibrils in the dermis, but the primary defects are unknown.

Most of the Ehlers–Danlos syndrome types are relatively benign with the exception of type IV, in which arterial or bowel rupture leads to shortened life expectancy. Diagnosis is largely based on the clinical features. Because of the severe complications in type IV, its diagnosis should be confirmed by measuring type III collagen in skin. Type VI may be confirmed by the demonstration of a markedly increased deoxypyridinoline to pyridinoline ratio in urine, arising from a reduced number of hydroxylated lysyl residues and altered crosslink formation (Pasquali et al 1994). This constitutes a relatively simple biochemical test for this disorder. Type IX is confirmed by the finding of low plasma copper and ceruloplasmin concentrations.

There is no specific treatment for any of these disorders, but prompt recognition of the major complications of type IV Ehlers–Danlos syndrome may be life-saving.

LIMB PAINS OF CHILDHOOD WITH NO ORGANIC DISEASE

So-called 'limb pains' or 'growing pains' are more common in childhood than all the other rheumatic diseases put together.

Growth in children involves two phases – 'shooting up' and 'filling out'. A limb may show bony growth followed by (not accompanied by) muscle growth. It may be that in such a shooting up phase, extra strain is put upon the muscle, which tires easily and gives pain towards the end of the day or during the night when relaxation is incomplete (Craig J O 1989 personal communication). A history of rheumatic disorders is commoner in the

Table 24.12   Clinical features, mode of inheritance and molecular defect in Ehlers–Danlos syndrome (from Byers 1994b, with permission)

Type	Clinical features	Inheritance	Molecular defect
I Gravis	Soft, velvety, hyperextensible skin; easy bruising; cigarette paper scars; hypermobile joints; varicose veins; prematurity	AD	Not known
II Mitis	Similar to Type I, but less severe	AD (AR, rare)	Not known COL1A2 null alleles
III Familial hypermobility	Soft skin, no scarring, marked large and small joint hypermobility	AD	Not known
IV Arterial	Thin, translucent skin with visible veins; marked bruising; skin and joints have normal extensibility; arterial bowel and uterine rupture	AD	Mutations in COL3A1 gene that alter Type III collagen synthesis, secretion and structure
V X-linked	Similar to Type II	XLR	Not known
VI Ocular	Soft, velvety, hyperextensible skin; hypermobile joints, scoliosis; ocular fragility and keratoconus	AR	Mutations in lysyl hydroxylase gene, leading to enzyme deficiency
VII A and B Arthrochalasis multiplex congenita	Congenital hip dislocation; joint hypermobility; soft skin with normal scarring	AD	COL1A1 exon 6 skipping mutation that deletes N-proteinase cleavage site
VII C Dermatosparaxis	Very soft, fragile, bruisable skin; marked joint hypermobility	AR	Procollagen N-proteinase cleavage site
VIII Periodontal	Generalized periodontitis; skin similar to Type II	AD	Not known
IX X-linked cutis laxa; occipital horn syndrome	Soft, extensible, lax skin; bladder diverticulae and rupture; short arms, limited pronation and supination, broad clavicles, occipital horns	XLR	Abnormal intracellular copper utilization (probably allelic to Menkes' syndrome) leading to decrease in copper-dependent lysyl oxidase
X Fibronectin defect	Similar to type II	AR	Defect in fibronectin (uncharacterized)

AD, autosomal dominant; AR, autosomal recessive, XLR, X-linked recessive.

families of children with limb pains than in controls, therefore parents often become worried and feel their child suffers from rheumatic diseases. In two-thirds of affected children limb pains occur during the daytime or evening. In the remainder the pains are predominantly nocturnal, and can wake the child and may be severe enough to cause crying. The age group mainly affected is 9–12 years, and girls more than boys. The children site pain between joints, suggesting that the pain is muscular. Most children like to have the area gently rubbed by a parent, which effectively excludes acute rheumatism. With reassurance based on discussions, it should be possible to convince parents that their child does not suffer from a rheumatic disorder. Occasionally, children have psychosomatic musculoskeletal pain and these should have a full psychological evaluation. They should respond well to treatment directed toward decreasing pain and restoring function.

REFERENCES AND BIBLIOGRAPHY

Ansell B M 1972 Hypermobility of joints. Modern trends in orthopaedics. Butterworths, London, p 25

Ansell B M, Bywaters E G L 1959 Prognosis in Still's disease. Bulletin on the Rheumatic Diseases 9: 189

Ansell B M, Hall M A, Loftus J K et al 1991 A multicentre pilot study of sulphasalazine in juvenile chronic arthritis. Clinical and Experimental Rheumatology 9: 201–203

Athreya B H, Cassidy J T 1991 Current status of the medical treatment of children with juvenile rheumatoid arthritis. Rheumatic Disease Clinics of North America 17(4): 877

Ayoub E M, Schiebler G L 1986 Acute rheumatic fever. In: Kelly V C (ed) Practice of pediatrics. Harper & Row, New York, Vol 8

Beighton P H, Horan F T 1970 Dominant inheritance in familial generalised articular hypermobility. Journal of Bone and Joint Surgery 52B: 145–147

Bellus G A, McIntosh I, Smith E A et al 1995 A recurrent mutation in the tyrosine kinase domain of fibroblast growth factor receptor 3 causes hypochondroplasia. Nature Genetics 10: 357–359

Bogaert R, Tiller G E, Weis M A, Gruber H E, Rimoin D L, Cohn D H, Eyre D R 1992 An amino acid substitution (Gly853→Glu) in the collagen alpha 1 (II) chain produces hypochondrogenesis. Journal of Biological Chemistry 267: 22522–22526

Bonaventure J, Cohen-Solal L, Ritvaniemi P et al 1995 Substitution of aspartic acid for glycine at position 310 in type II collagen produces achondrogenesis II, and substitution of serine at position 805 produces hypochondrogenesis: analysis of genotype–phenotype relationships. Biochemical Journal 307: 823–830

Brenner R E, Vetter U, Nerlich A, Wörsdorfer O, Teller W M 1989 Osteogenesis imperfecta: insufficient collagen synthesis in early childhood as evidenced by analysis of compact bone and fibroblast cultures. European Journal of Clinical Investigation 19: 159–166

Brenner R E, Schiller B, Vetter U, Ittner J, Teller W M 1993 Serum concentrations of procollagen I C-terminal propeptide, osteocalcin and insulin-like growth factor-I in patients with non-lethal osteogenesis imperfecta. Acta Paediatrica 82: 764–767

Brenner R E, Vetter U, Bollen A-M, Mörike M, Eyre D R 1994 Bone resorption assessed by immunoassay of urinary cross-linked collagen peptides in patients with osteogenesis imperfecta. Journal of Bone and Mineral Research 9: 993–997

Bridges N A, Brook C G D 1994 Progress report: growth hormone in skeletal dysplasia. Hormone Research 42: 231–234

Briggs M D, Hoffman S M, King L M et al 1995 Pseudoachondroplasia and multiple epiphyseal dysplasia due to mutations in the cartilage oligomeric matrix protein gene. Nature Genetics 10: 330–336

British Medical Journal 1988 Transatlantic warning bells sound on rheumatic fever 296: 1215

Byers P H 1994a Ehlers–Danlos syndrome: recent advances and current understanding of the clinical and genetic heterogeneity. Journal of Investigative Dermatology 103: 47S–52S

Byers P H 1994b Molecular genetics of chondrodysplasias, including clues to development, structure, and function. Current Opinion in Rheumatology 6: 345–350

Byers P H 1995 Disorders of collagen biosynthesis and structure. In: Scriver C R, Baudet A L, Sly W S, Valle D (eds) The metabolic and molecular bases of inherited disease, 7th edn. McGraw-Hill, New York, p 4029

Castells S, Yasumura S, Fusi M A, Colbert C, Bachtell R S, Smith S 1986 Plasma osteocalcin levels in patients with osteogenesis imperfecta. Journal of Pediatrics 109: 88–91

Congeni B, Rizzo C, Congeni J, Sreenivasan V V 1987 Outbreak of acute rheumatic fever in north-east Ohio. Journal of Pediatrics 3: 176–179

Connolly J, Regen E, Hillman J W 1970 Pigeon-toes and flat feet. Pediatric Clinics of North America 17: 291

Developmental Medicine and Child Neurology 1975 The proposed international terminology for the classification of congenital limb deficiencies. Supplement 34, Vol 17

Dietz H C, Cutting G R, Pyeritz R E et al 1991 Marfan syndrome caused by a recurrent de novo missense mutation in the fibrillin gene. Nature 352: 337–339

Eichenfield A H, Goldsmith D P, Benach J L, Ross A H, Loeb F X, Doughty R A, Athreya B H 1986 Childhood Lyme arthritis: experience in an endemic area. Journal of Pediatrics 109: 753–758

Fish A J, Blau E B, Westberg N G et al 1977 Systemic lupus erythematosus within the first two decades of life. American Journal of Medicine 62: 99

Foster J W, Dominguez-Steglich M A, Guioli S et al 1994 Camptomelic dysplasia and autosomal sex reversal caused by mutations in an SRY-related gene. Nature 372: 525–530

Friere-Maia N 1969 Congenital skeletal limb deficiencies – a general view. In: Birth defects. Original Article Series, Vol 5, No 3. March of Dimes: The National Foundation

Goel K M, King M 1986 Dermatomyositis – polymyositis. Scottish Medical Journal 31: 15–19

Gorlin R T, Pindborg T T 1964 Syndromes of the head and neck. McGraw-Hill, New York

Gorlin R J, Spranger J, Koszalka M F 1969 Genetic craniotubular bone dysplasias and hyperostoses. A critical analysis. In: Birth defects. Original Article Series, Vol 5, No 4, p 79. March of Dimes: The National Foundation

Hall M A, Ansell B M 1977 A comparative study of gold and penicillamine in the management of seronegative juvenile chronic polyarthritis. Paper presented at 14th International Congress of Rheumatology, San Francisco, Programme Abstract No 164

Hastbacka J, de la Chapelle A, Mahtani M M et al 1994 The diastrophic dysplasia gene encodes a novel sulfate transporter: positional cloning by fine-structure linkage disequilibrium mapping. Cell 78: 1073–1087

Hecht J T, Nelson L D, Crowder E et al 1995 Mutations in exon 17B of cartilage oligomeric matrix protein (COMP) cause pseudoachondroplasia. Nature Genetics 10: 325–329

Hendrickse R G, Barr D G D, Mathews T S 1991 Paediatrics in the tropics. Blackwell Scientific, Oxford

Horton W A, Machado M A, Ellard J et al 1992 Characterization of a type II collagen gene (COL2A1) mutation identified in cultured chondrocytes from human hypochondrogenesis. Proceedings of the National Academy of Sciences of the United States of America 89: 4583–4587

Hu P Y, Roth D E, Skaggs L A, Venta P J, Tashian R E, Guibaud P, Sly W S 1992 A splice junction mutation in intron 2 of the carbonic anhydrase II gene of osteopetrosis patients from Arabic countries. Human Mutation 1: 288–292

Hu P Y, Ernst A R, Sly W S, Venta P J, Skaggs L A, Tashian R E 1994 Carbonic anhydrase II deficiency: single-base deletion in exon 7 is the predominant mutation in Caribbean Hispanic patients. American Journal of Human Genetics 54: 602–608

International Working Group on Constitutional Diseases of Bone 1992 International classification of osteochondrodysplasias. European Journal of Pediatrics 151: 407–415

Johnson R S, Spiegelman B M, Papaioannou V 1992 Pleiotropic effects of a null mutation in the c-fos proto-oncogene. Cell 71: 577–586

Jones Criteria 1984 Ad hoc committee to revise the Jones criteria (modified). Council on Rheumatic Fever and Congenital Heart Disease of the American Heart Association. Jones criteria (revised) for guidance in the diagnosis of rheumatic fever. Circulation 69: 204A–208A

Jones K L 1988 Smith's recognisable patterns of human malformation, 4th edn. W B Saunders, Philadelphia

Kaplan E L 1978 Acute rheumatic fever. Pediatric Clinics of North America 25: 817–829

Kaufmann H J 1964 In: Rontgenologische am Becken im Sauglings und Kindesalter bei Angeborenen Skelleter-krankungen und Chromosomalen Aberrationen. Georg Thieme Verlag, Stuttgart

Lamy M, Maroteaux P 1960 Le nanisme diastrophique. Presse Medicale 68: 1977

Lee L A, Bias W B, Arnett F C et al 1983 Immunogenetics of the neonatal lupus syndrome. Annals of Internal Medicine 99: 592–596

McEnery G 1977 Giant cell arteritis with gangrene in a child. Archives of Disease in Childhood 52: 733–735

McIntosh I, Abbott M H, Francomano C A 1995 Concentration of mutations causing Schmid metaphyseal chondrodysplasia in the C-terminal noncollagenous domain of type X collagen. Human Mutation 5: 121–125

Macnicol M F 1990 Results of a 25-year screening programme for neonatal hip instability. Journal of Bone and Joint Surgery 72B: 1057–1060

Maroteaux P 1969 Spondyloepiphyseal dysplasias and metatropic dwarfism. In: Birth defects. Original Article Series, Vol 5, No 4, p 35. March of Dimes: The National Foundation

Minisola S, Piccioni A L, Rosso R et al 1994 Reduced serum levels of carboxy-terminal propeptide of human type I procollagen in a family with type I-A osteogenesis imperfecta. Metabolism (Clinical and Experimental) 43: 1261–1265

Mörike M, Brenner R E, Bushart G B, Teller W M, Vetter U 1992 Collagen metabolism in cultured osteoblasts from osteogenesis imperfecta patients. Biochemical Journal 286: 73–77

Muenke M, Schell U 1995 Fibroblast-growth-factor receptor mutations in human skeletal disorders. Trends in Genetics 11: 308–313

Nijbroek G, Sood S, McIntosh I et al 1995 Fifteen novel FBN1 mutations causing Marfan syndrome detected by heteroduplex analysis of genomic amplicons. American Journal of Human Genetics 57: 8–21

Ohlsson A, Stark G, Sakati N 1980 Marble brain disease: recessive osteopetrosis, renal tubular acidosis and cerebral calcification in three Saudi Arabian families. Developmental Medicine and Child Neurology 22: 72–84

O'Rahilly R 1969 The nomenclature and classification of limb anomalies. In: Birth defects. Original Article Series, Vol 5, No 3, p 14. March of Dimes: The National Foundation

Pasquali M, Dembure P P, Still M J, Elsas L J 1994 Urinary pyridinium cross-links: a noninvasive diagnostic test for Ehlers–Danlos syndrome type VI. New England Journal of Medicine 331: 132–133

Rimoin D L, Edgerton M T 1967 Genetic and clinical heterogeneity in the oral–facial–digital syndromes. Journal of Pediatrics 71: 94–102

Risteli L, Risteli J 1993 Biochemical markers of bone metabolism. Annals of Medicine 25: 385–393

Russell A S, Sturge R A, Smith M A 1971 Serum transaminase during salicylate therapy. British Medical Journal 2: 428–429

Schipani E, Kruse K, Juppner H 1995 A constitutively active mutant PTH-PTHrP receptor in Jansen-type metaphyseal chondrodysplasia. Science 268: 98–100

Seibel M J, Robins S P, Bilezikian J P 1992 Urinary pyridinium crosslinks of collagen. Specific markers of bone resorption in metabolic bone disease. Trends in Endocrinology and Metabolism 3: 263–270

Shiang R, Thompson L M, Zhu Y-Z et al 1994 Mutations in the transmembrane domain of FGFR3 cause the most common genetic form of dwarfism, achondroplasia. Cell 78: 335–342

Shmerling D H, Prader A, Hitzing W H, Giedion A, Hadorn B, Kuhni M 1969 The syndrome of exocrine pancreatic insufficiency, neutropenia, metaphyseal dysostosis and dwarfism. Helvetica Paediatrica Acta 24 (fasc 6): 547

Soriano P, Montgomery C, Geske R, Bradley A 1991 Targeted disruption of the c-src proto-oncogene leads to osteopetrosis in mice. Cell 64: 693–702

Spranger J, Winterpacht A, Zabel B 1994 The type II collagenopathies: a spectrum of chondrodysplasias. European Journal of Pediatrics 153: 56–65

Still G F 1897 On a form of chronic joint disease in children. Medico-Chirurgical Transactions 80: 47

Tachdjian M O 1967 Diagnosis and treatment of congenital deformities of the musculoskeletal system in the newborn and the infant. Pediatric Clinics of North America 14: 307

Tavormina P L, Shiang R, Thompson L M et al 1995 Thanatophoric dysplasia (types I and II) caused by distinct mutations in fibroblast growth factor receptor 3. Nature Genetics 9: 321–328

Temtamy S, McKusick V A 1969 Synopsis of hand malformations with particular emphasis on genetic factors. In: Birth defects. Original Article Series, Vol 5, No 3, p 125. March of Dimes: The National Foundation

Tilstra D J, Byers P H 1994 Molecular basis of hereditary disorders of connective tissue. Annual Review of Medicine 45: 149–163

Vetter U, Eanes E D, Kopp J B, Termine J D, Gehron Robey P 1991a Changes in apatite crystal size in bones of patients with osteogenesis imperfecta. Calcified Tissue International 49: 248–250

Vetter U, Fisher L W, Mintz K P et al 1991b Osteogenesis imperfecta: changes in noncollagenous proteins in bone. Journal of Bone and Mineral Research 6: 501–505

Vikkula M, Mariman E C, Lui V C et al 1995 Autosomal dominant and recessive osteochondrodysplasias associated with the COL11A2 locus. Cell 80: 431–437

Wagner T, Wirth J, Meyer J et al 1994 Autosomal sex reversal and camptomelic dysplasia are caused by mutations in and around the SRY-related SOX9. Cell 79: 1111–1120

Warman M L, Abbott M, Apte S S et al 1993 A type X collagen mutation causes Schmid metaphyseal chondrodysplasia. Nature Genetics 5: 79–82

Weinstein L S, Shenker A, Gejman P N, Merino M J, Friedman E, Spiro A M 1991 Activating mutations of the stimulating G protein in the McCune–Albright syndrome. New England Journal of Medicine 325: 1688–1695

Wynne-Davies R 1968 Familial (idiopathic) scoliosis. Journal of Bone and Joint Surgery 50B: 24

Wynne-Davies R 1973 Heritable disorders in orthopaedic practice. Blackwell, Edinburgh

Yoshida H, Hayashi S-I, Kunisada T et al 1990 The murine mutation osteopetrosis is in the coding region of the macrophage colony stimulating factor gene. Nature (London) 345: 442–443

25 Diseases of the skin

Maureen Rogers   Ross St C. Barnetson

Introduction   1616
Management of a skin problem in a child   1616
Treatment of skin diseases   1617
Nevi and other developmental defects   1617
Melanocytic nevi   1617
Epidermal nevi   1618
Vascular nevi   1618
Congenital aplasia cutis   1620
Hereditary diseases   1620
The ichthyoses   1620
Epidermolysis bullosa   1621
Ectodermal dysplasias   1624
Tuberous sclerosis (epiloia)   1625
Incontinentia pigmenti   1626
Acrodermatitis enteropathica and nutritional zinc
    deficiency   1627
Neurofibromatosis   1628
Psoriasis   1628
Hereditary photosensitive disorders   1629
Infections and infestations of the skin   1631
Virus infections   1631

Bacterial infections   1634
Fungal infections   1636
Ectoparasitic infestations   1638
Hypersensitivity disease (and those diseases clinically related)
    1639
Type I hypersensitivity: anaphylactic hypersensitivity   1639
Type II hypersensitivity: cytotoxic/cytolytic hypersensitivity   1639
Type III hypersensitivity: immune complex-mediated
    hypersensitivity   1640
Type IV hypersensitivity: delayed type hypersensitivity   1641
Eczema and dermatitis   1642
Connective tissue diseases   1644
Lupus erythematosus (LE)   1644
Dermatomyositis   1644
Scleroderma   1644
Idiopathic photosensitivity eruptions   1645
Skin diseases of the neonate   1645
Neoplastic diseases   1646
Langerhans' cell histiocytosis (histiocytosis X)   1647
References   1648

INTRODUCTION

The skin comprises roughly 15% of the bodyweight. It is a complex organ which undergoes constant repair. Its main functions are:

1. barrier to loss of fluid and electrolytes
2. barrier to external injurious agents
3. protection against ultraviolet light
4. protection against bacteria and fungi
5. regulation of body temperature
6. as a sensory organ
7. synthesis of vitamin D.

To perform these functions, the skin requires a complicated structure. It consists of three layers:

1. epidermis, derived from ectoderm
2. dermis, derived from mesoderm
3. subcutis, derived from mesoderm.

The main function of the epidermis is to act as a barrier. The main barrier to fluid and electrolyte loss and to external injurious agents is the horny layer on the external surface of the epidermis: this is formed from flattened *keratinocytes* which originate from the basal layer of the epidermis and progress towards the exterior. *Melanocytes* are also found in the basal layer, and are differentiated from keratinocytes by darkly staining nuclei and clear cytoplasm: their main function is protection against ultraviolet radiation by distributing melanin throughout the basal layer. The amount of melanin determines the racial color. A third type of cell is the

Langerhans cell, found in the midepidermis which has been shown to be a dendritic antigen-presenting cell, and plays an important role in allergic contact eczema and forms part of the immune defense in the skin. A fourth cell has recently been described, the *Merkel cell*: the exact function of this cell has not been determined, but the present evidence suggests a sensory role.

The dermis is composed of collagen, elastin and reticulin within a matrix of ground substance. Blood vessels, sensory and autonomic nerves and nerve endings, hair follicles (pilosebaceous units) and sweat glands traverse the dermis. Temperature regulation is mainly effected by shunting of blood between the superficial and deep arteriolar and venular plexuses, modified by the glomus apparatus between the two plexuses which are under autonomic control. Secondary temperature regulation, which is particularly important where the ambient temperature exceeds 37°C, depends on evaporation from the eccrine sweat glands which are under adrenergic control.

The subcutis consists mainly of adipose tissue, whose main function is insulation of the body. In sites such as the sole of the foot, fibrous bands within the subcutis have a buffering and protective effect.

The skin appendages such as hair and nails are largely vestigial in the human; loss of either does not constitute any threat to the survival of the individual.

MANAGEMENT OF A SKIN PROBLEM IN A CHILD

It is important to take a detailed history either from the child or from the parents. History taking is similar to that in internal medicine, though the emphasis is different. Of particular importance are the following:

1. *family history* – many skin diseases are hereditary
2. *past history of the skin disease* – conditions such as psoriasis and atopic eczema tend to be intermittent
3. *general health* – some diseases (e.g. connective tissue diseases) are multiorgan problems
4. *previous treatment* – both oral and topical: treatment may have modified the clinical picture (for better or for worse).

Examination of the child

The child should be undressed completely to allow full assessment of the condition. A general medical examination should also be performed. If a rash is present, note should be taken of the following points: (1) color, nature and distribution; (2) relationship of the rash to skin appendages, such as hair follicles and sweat ducts; (3) mucous membranes: some skin diseases have a banal appearance in the skin, but a characteristic appearance in mucous membranes, e.g. lichen planus, congenital syphilis; (4) examination of the hair and nails, as changes may give a clue as to the diagnosis.

TREATMENT OF SKIN DISEASES

As the skin is so accessible, it is sensible where possible to treat skin diseases with topical preparations. It is also important to introduce the active agent (e.g. steroid, antibiotic) in a suitable form or vehicle:

1. *Lotions* (solutions) are very useful for exudative rashes as 'wet dressings', where ointments and creams would 'float off', e.g. potassium permanganate.
2. *Shake lotions* (solution + 15–30% powder), e.g. calamine lotion.
3. *Creams* (oil–water emulsion). Bases such as cetomacrogol or aqueous cream are very acceptable to the patient, e.g. topical steroid creams.
4. *Ointments* such as petrolatum have a greasy base. They are useful for dry skin conditions, such as atopic eczema, e.g. steroid and antibiotic ointments.
5. *Gels* (semicolloids in alcohol base, which dry on the skin). Useful for scalp conditions.
6. *Pastes* (ointments + 15–30% powder). Used on linen dressings, e.g. tar paste.
7. *Powders*, e.g. antifungal foot powders, miticides.

NEVI AND OTHER DEVELOPMENTAL DEFECTS

MELANOCYTIC NEVI

Congenital melanocytic nevi (CMN) (Plate 25.1 and Fig. 25.1)

These occur in approximately 1.5% of the population. They are arbitrarily classified as large (greater than 20 cm), medium (1.5–20 cm) and small (less than 1.5 cm) sized on the basis of the maximum diameter as measured in infancy. They occur at birth as raised, verrucose or lobulated nodules or plaques of varying shades of brown to black, sometimes with blue or pink components. They have an irregular margin and often long dark hairs and may become increasingly lobulated and hairy with time. Giant sized lesions may produce considerable redundancy of skin and often occur in a 'garment' distribution on the trunk and

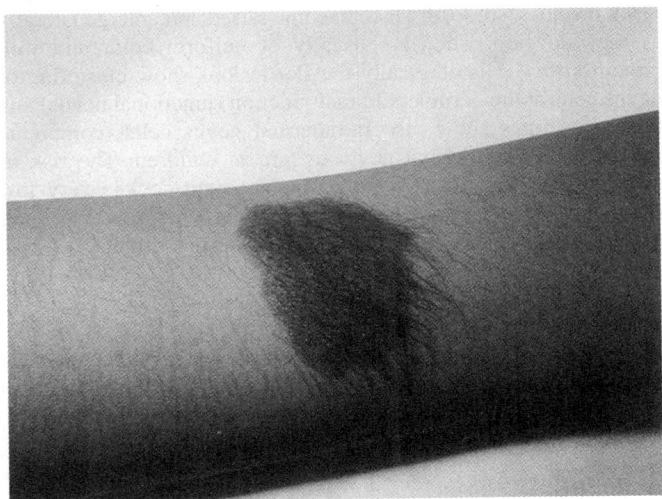

Fig. 25.1   Congenital melanocytic nevus.

adjacent limbs. The very small CMN may be only slightly raised and of a fairly uniform color. In patients with multiple large nevi an eruption of smaller ones may occur over the first year of life. Once established, the nevi increase in size in proportion to the patient's growth. CMN over the head and neck may rarely be associated with leptomeningeal melanocytosis and those over the spinal column with spinal dysraphism.

Considerable controversy exists regarding the risk of development of malignant melanoma in these lesions and hence the approach to management (Jacobs et al 1984). Malignancy can arise from the dermal as well as the junctional component of CMN. The incidence of malignancy in large nevi has varied from 2% to 31% in different series but most studies have been retrospective and biased. A long-term prospective study based on the Danish birth register is probably the most reliable and a lifetime risk of 4.6% is calculated from it (Lorentzen et al 1977). Malignant change in large CMN can occur in childhood (Kaplan 1974). Melanoma also occurs in medium sized and small CMN (Illig et al 1985, Rhodes et al 1982) but the exact incidence for small lesions is not known, though it is definitely lower than for large nevi. The development of malignancy in small lesions is always postpubertal.

While small lesions, in which the risk is low, can be easily excised, removal of large lesions in which the risk is much more significant is more difficult and with giant lesions may be impossible. In all cases the risk must be weighed against possible functional impairment and the morbidity of multiple operations. Many surgical procedures are available and are chosen singly or in combination, depending on the site and extent of the lesions. These include excision with direct closure, with or without prior use of tissue expansion techniques, advancement, rotation, transposition and distant flaps and skin grafting. Dermabrasion and laser therapy may improve the appearance of the nevus by removal of superficial pigment cells but the bulk of the lesion remains and the malignancy risk is not substantially reduced.

Acquired melanocytic nevi (AMN)

These nevi usually first appear after the age of 1 year and increase in number throughout childhood. They commence as brown or black macules, some of which become raised and enlarge laterally as they develop. They are usually of uniform color and well circumscribed. Histologically the flat lesions show clustering of nevus cells at the dermoepidermal junction (junctional nevus) and the raised ones show also intradermal nevus cells (compound nevus). Pure intradermal nevi are rare in children. The risk of melanoma arising from acquired melanocytic nevi is very low (less than 0.1%) and does not occur in childhood so their prophylactic removal in young patients is not justified.

Halo nevi (Fig. 25.2)

A depigmented halo may occur around the lesion. The nevus may appear inflamed and often disappears leaving a white spot which may eventually repigment. This is a completely benign change.

Dysplastic or atypical nevi

Dysplastic or atypical nevi are a subtype of acquired melanocytic nevi with characteristic clinicopathological features. They are a marker for the development of malignant melanoma, occurring in over 90% of patients with familial melanoma and over 10% of those with sporadic melanoma. They are commonly found contiguous with malignant melanomas on histopathology of the latter. These nevi differ from more typical AMNs by being larger (more than 5 mm diameter), having irregular and indistinct margins and irregular tan brown coloration, often with an erythematous component. They are predominantly macular, sometimes with a central elevated portion. They may appear in childhood as small typical appearing nevi which after puberty develop the atypical features. In adolescence and early adult life new atypical lesions may appear de novo. Characteristic dysplastic nevi may appear on the scalp in childhood. The final confirmation is based on the finding of some or all of a constellation of histopathological features of which the most important are nuclear atypia and a lymphocytic infiltrate.

Patients with multiple dysplastic nevi should be observed frequently and monitored with serial photography. Any mole showing significant alteration should be immediately removed. Family members should be checked for the presence of dysplastic nevi or melanoma.

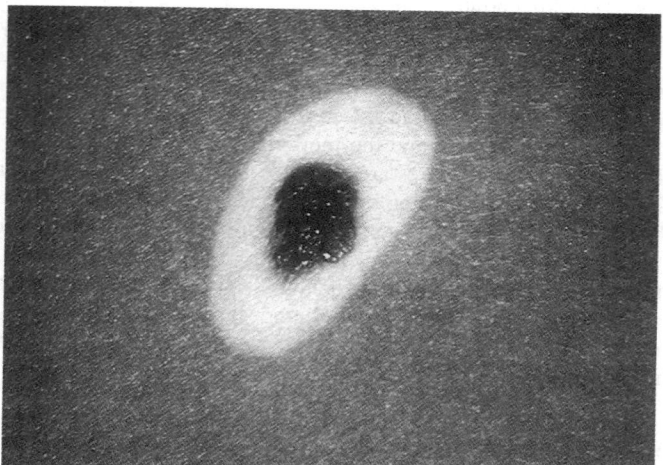

Fig. 25.2   Halo nevus.

EPIDERMAL NEVI

Epidermal nevi arise from the basal layer of the embryonic epidermis which gives rise to skin appendages and keratinocytes. These nevi have been conventionally classified according to the tissue of origin (keratinocytic, sebaceous and follicular) but the use of the general term 'epidermal nevus' is preferred (Solomon & Esterly 1975).

Epidermal nevi can involve any area of skin and may be present at birth (particularly those on the head) or appear in the first few years of life (or exceptionally later). They may simply grow with the patient or can extend well beyond their original distribution over months or years. Extension occurs less often with nevi on the head and with nevi present at birth, whatever their location.

On the scalp and face the nevi have a yellowish color due to prominent sebaceous glands and present as a hairless, often linear plaque, usually flat in infancy and childhood and becoming verrucose at puberty. Lesions elsewhere are usually dark brown but occasionally are paler than the normal skin. They occur as single or multiple warty plaques or lines often arranged in a linear or swirled pattern. They may be subtle or grossly verrucose. Small papillomas and comedo-like structures may occur. Some lesions are inflammatory, clinically and histologically resembling psoriasis. Epidermal nevi are rarely complicated in adult life by basal cell or squamous cell carcinoma.

It is now clear that the linear and swirled patterns taken by epidermal nevi follow the lines of Blaschko, which define the tracks of clones of genetically identical cells, and that all epidermal nevi can be explained on the basis of genetic mosaicism (Happle 1991) with each type of nevus representing the cutaneous manifestation of a different mosaic phenotype. In most patients the nevus is the only detectable manifestation but in some patients there are associated abnormalities in other organ systems, particularly skeletal, neurological and ocular (Solomon & Esterly 1975, Rogers et al 1989). This association has been called the 'epidermal nevus syndrome' (Happle 1991, Rogers 1992). Skeletal abnormalities occur particularly with nevi of keratinocytic type on the limbs, and neurological and ocular abnormalities with nevi of sebaceous type on the head. The major clinical neurological features are seizures, developmental delay and hemiparesis. All patients with epidermal nevi should have a careful physical examination at presentation. Patients with nevi on the head who present in infancy and are normal on initial examination should be followed for several years. Most centers embark on imaging studies only in patients with clinical abnormalities.

Therapy of these lesions is difficult. Topical retinoic acid may temporarily flatten very thick areas. There are a few reports of improvement of gross lesions with oral retinoids but the effect depends on continued use of the drug. Recurrence is almost invariable following diathermy and cryotherapy. Both CO_2 and argon laser have been used, in some cases with good results though these may be temporary. Excision is appropriate for small and linear lesions and for irritating or cosmetically troubling areas of more widespread nevi.

VASCULAR NEVI

These can be divided into hemangiomas, which are proliferative vascular tumors, and vascular malformations which represent fixed collections of dilated abnormal vessels (Enjolras & Mulliken 1993).

Hemangiomas (Plate 25.2)

Hemangiomas are usually not present at birth, undergo a fast growth phase and then, over a long period, tend to spontaneous resolution. It is now clear that hemangiomas, whether superficially or deeply located in the skin, have the same structure, being composed, in the early stage, of proliferating masses of endothelial cells with occasional lumina and later, as they resolve, of large endothelial lined spaces. The terms capillary, cavernous and capillary–cavernous are misleading and should be abandoned in favor of the simple term hemangioma.

Clinical features

Superficial hemangiomas are usually not present at birth but appear in the first weeks of life as an area of pallor followed by a telangiectatic patch. They then grow rapidly into a lobulated, well-demarcated, bright red tumor. Rapid growth continues over the first 6 months; the growth rate then slows and further growth after 10 months is unusual. After a stationary phase signs of involution appear with the appearance of gray areas which enlarge and coalesce. The tumor becomes softer and less bulky and then disappears in 90% of cases by 9 years of age.

Deeper hemangiomas may occur alone or beneath a superficial lesion. They also usually appear after birth and undergo a growth phase which however may be less striking than that of the more superficial lesions. The overlying skin is normal or bluish in color. As they resolve they soften and shrink and complete disappearance occurs in many cases: occasionally some redundant tissue remains in the place of large lesions. Apparent deep hemangiomas which show no sign of resolution are now recognized as vascular malformations, usually of venous type, and are not hemangiomas at all.

Complications

Ulceration may occur during the rapid growth phase of superficial hemangiomas. If secondary infection is controlled the ulcers usually heal in a few weeks but some scarring is inevitable. Ulceration of lesions on eyelids, lips or ala nasae can lead to full thickness tissue loss. Scarring following ulceration of lesions on or near the eyelids can result in a cicatricial ectropion and alopecia may be permanent after scalp ulceration.

Hemangiomas may encroach on vital structures. A hemangioma closing the eye for as little as 4 weeks in infancy can produce amblyopia. However, even without occluding the pupil an eyelid lesion, by pressing on the eye and producing a refractive error, can lead to failure of development of binocular vision and partial amblyopia. Large hemangiomas around the mouth may interfere with feeding and one blocking both nares can lead to respiratory difficulties while the child is being fed. A large deep hemangioma around the neck may displace the pharynx or trachea; the upper respiratory tract may also be directly involved with the hemangioma. The possibility of laryngeal involvement should be considered whenever there is a fast growing extensive lower face or neck hemangioma, particularly when there is accompanying intraoral involvement, and a lateral airways X-ray should be arranged. If there is stridor, an urgent laryngoscopy is mandatory. Even when traumatized, uncomplicated hemangiomas rarely bleed significantly.

Management

Simple observation and reassurance while awaiting natural resolution is the ideal approach for most hemangiomas. Serial photography and showing photographs of other resolving lesions are encouraging. Indications for active intervention are: an alarming growth rate; threatening ulceration in areas where serious complications could ensue; interference with vital structures; and severe bleeding. Oral corticosteroids will slow the growth of potentially dangerous or cosmetically serious lesions. A useful regime is prednisolone 2 mg/kg per day for 2 weeks, 1 mg/kg for a further 2 weeks, and 0.5 mg/kg for the last 2 weeks. Repeated courses should be avoided wherever possible. Intralesional steroids may shrink localized hemangiomas which fail to respond to steroids, and interferon-α has been effective in some life-threatening cases. Cosmetic surgical procedures can improve the appearance when loose tissue remains. Laser therapy has a place for upper respiratory tract lesions and as an adjunct or alternative to surgery in some complicated lesions.

Kasabach–Merritt syndrome (hemangioma–hemorrhage syndrome) (Plate 25.3)

This is the rare association of thrombocytopenia with vascular tumors. In children these are usually either large, deep hemangiomas, especially on limbs and around limb girdles, or diffuse hemangiomatosis. Thrombocytopenia is caused by entrapment of platelets within the lesions and is sometimes followed by disseminated intravascular coagulation (DIC). At first there may be bleeding into the hemangioma, which rapidly enlarges: widespread life-threatening hemorrhage may follow. When bleeding is confined to the hemangiomas the approach should be conservative; in severe cases high dose systemic corticosteroids are indicated together with resuscitation, transfusion, and management of the DIC.

Diffuse infantile hemangiomatosis

This is a condition with multiple small hemangiomas in a widespread distribution. A benign form has lesions limited to the skin but a potentially serious systemic form may occur with lesions in many organs, particularly liver, gastrointestinal tract, lungs and central nervous system with or, rarely, without cutaneous lesions. All patients with multiple cutaneous lesions should be carefully assessed with full blood count, chest X-ray, and examination for cardiac failure due to arteriovenous shunts and for bleeding from the gastrointestinal tract. Ultrasound or abdominal CT scan should be performed to exclude hepatic involvement and other organs may need to be further investigated. Angiography and technetium-labeled red blood cell scans can delineate further the extent of internal involvement (Esterly et al 1984). With severe systemic involvement high dose corticosteroids are required along with management of cardiac failure and other complications, and active surgical intervention may be necessary in selected cases.

Vascular malformations

Vascular malformations are structural abnormalities and as such are present at birth, grow in proportion to the patient's growth and have no tendency at all to resolution. They can be further divided according to their vessel of origin into capillary, arterial, venous and lymphatic types and mixed entities with more than one vessel type may occur.

Capillary malformation (port-wine stain, nevus flammeus)

This is a vascular malformation composed of dilated mature capillaries. It is present at birth and shows no involution. Lesions may be unilateral or, less often, bilateral, and occur anywhere on the body, though they are most commonly found on the face. They are deep pink in infancy becoming later more purple. After puberty they may become raised and nodular. Until recently only cosmetic cover could be offered but good results are now being achieved with the pulsed dye laser.

Sturge–Weber syndrome

This is the association of a facial capillary malformation and a vascular malformation of the ipsilateral meninges and cerebral cortex. The cutaneous lesion always involves the skin in the distribution of the first division of the trigeminal nerve (Enjolras et al 1985). The neurological manifestations of the syndrome include convulsions, hemiparesis and mental retardation. When the facial lesion involves the skin innervated by both the first and second divisions of the trigeminal nerve, congenital glaucoma may occur; this does not occur when only one division is involved (Stevenson et al 1974).

Patients presenting with a capillary malformation in the appropriate distribution should have early neurological and ophthalmological consultation and continued close follow-up. A CT scan may demonstrate the intracranial malformations in the first few months of life. Parallel streaks of calcification may be demonstrated radiologically after about 2 years of age.

Vascular malformations with limb hypertrophy

The eponyms Klippel–Trenaunay and Parkes–Weber syndromes refer to cutaneous vascular malformations associated with overgrowth of a limb, with soft tissue hypertrophy and/or bony hypertrophy. The cutaneous nevus is of capillary or capillary–lymphatic type and may or may not exactly overlie the area of tissue hypertrophy. Arteriovenous shunts can occur and deeper lymphatic and venous elements may be present. These are mixed vascular malformations and are best described by their component parts rather than using the eponyms. Treatment is generally unsatisfactory with few cases being amenable to surgical correction. Compression bandaging may help to some extent with the increased girth of a limb.

CONGENITAL APLASIA CUTIS

Aplasia cutis congenita (ACC) is a congenital absence of skin, usually localized but sometimes occurring as multiple lesions in a widespread distribution. The commonest form involves a localized oval, stellate or linear area at or near the midline of the scalp which presents as an ulcerated area which crusts, and finally after some months heals with a scar which is usually atrophic but is occasionally hypertrophic. There is permanent alopecia at the site. Rarely the lesion is already scarred at birth. The defect may involve not only skin but also subcutaneous fat and even bone.

The bony defect will eventually heal but until it does there is a risk of meningitis. Deep aplasia may erode large vessels producing serious hemorrhage. A skull X-ray should be performed in all cases unless the lesion is obviously very superficial. Early management of scalp ACC is conservative with protection of the area and early treatment of secondary infection. Very deep lesions, however, may require skin and/or bone grafting. In later life scalp reduction techniques can be used to deal with the area of alopecia.

After the scalp the next commonest site is the lower limbs. When multiple lesions occur their distribution is often strikingly symmetrical and they may be covered with a shiny transparent membrane rather than being open erosions. Cases with extensive truncal and limb ACC are often associated with a fetus papyraceus at delivery, indicating the death of a twin early in the second trimester.

ACC-like lesions can occur on the lower limbs of patients with several types of epidermolysis bullosa probably resulting from intrauterine mechanical trauma. ACC may occur in a number of syndromes including trisomy 13, 4p– syndrome, 46XY gonadal dysgenesis and the Johanson–Blizzard syndrome. It may also be associated with a number of morphological abnormalities, particularly those involving the limbs.

HEREDITARY DISEASES

THE ICHTHYOSES

These are a group of inherited conditions with dry thickened skin of varying severity. The major ichthyoses comprise:

1. ichthyosis vulgaris (IV) – autosomal dominant
2. recessive X-linked ichthyosis (RXLI) – sex-linked recessive
3. lamellar ichthyosis (LI) – autosomal recessive
4. congenital ichthyosiform erythroderma (CIE) autosomal recessive (Plate 25.4)
5. bullous ichthyosis (BI) – autosomal dominant.

The histopathological and clinical features of the major ichthyoses are listed in Table 25.1. They are lifelong disorders with little tendency to spontaneous improvement. The pathogenesis is unclear in most cases but several facts are known. IV and RXLI show a delayed shedding of stratum corneum cells. In RXLI there is a virtual absence of the enzyme steroid sulfatase from most tissues. In CIE there is an increased epidermal turnover and an abnormal stratum corneum lipid profile. In BI there is epidermal hyperproliferation and abnormal keratinization.

Management

Simple emollients such as wool fat ointment and cetomacrogol aqueous cream may be adequate in IV. Keratolytics containing urea, propylene glycol or α-hydroxy acids may be more effective and useful in IV and RXLI but they may sting on fissured skin. The more severe ichthyoses often show little improvement with these topical agents. Oral retinoids may be very helpful in CIE but their effectiveness must always be weighed against their potential side-effects, especially skeletal abnormalities and teratogenicity. In BI their usefulness is limited by their tendency to increase skin fragility. Detection and treatment of secondary bacterial infection is important in BI and topical disinfectants may reduce bacterial colonization and malodor.

Table 25.1 Classification and features of the major ichthyoses

	Onset	Clinical features	Complications and associations	Histopathology
Ichthyosis vulgaris	After birth but within the first year of life	Fine pale branny scales especially on extensor surfaces of limbs. Wide sparing of flexures of limbs. Trunk less severely involved. Face usually spared. Hyperlinear palms	Rarely corneal dystrophy, keratosis pilaris, atopy	Thickened stratum corneum. Reduced or absent granular layer
Recessive X-linked ichthyosis	Appears within the first 3 months of life. Sometimes congenital with a thin shiny covering membrane	Large dark adherent scales mainly on extensor surfaces of limbs. Scaling encroaches on limb flexures and axillae with narrow sparing. Trunk is diffusely involved. Sides of face often involved. Usually severe involvement of neck and thick scalp scaling. Palms and soles are uninvolved	Frequent corneal dystrophy (also in carriers). Cryptorchidism. Steroid sulfatase deficiency in most tissues including the amnion (which is derived from fetus). This placental steroid sulfatase deficiency may result in a failure of spontaneous onset of labour	Thick stratum corneum. Normal or thick granular layer. May be slight thickening of whole epidermis
Lamellar ichthyosis	Usually at birth as 'collodion baby'	Large dark plate-like scales. Mild to moderate erythroderma. The whole body surface is involved, including palms and soles	Ectropion. Blockage of external auditory meati with scale resulting in hearing loss. Block of nares with scale. Pyrexia from sweat duct obstruction. Failure to thrive. Alopecia	Very thick stratum corneum. Epidermis of normal or slightly increased thickness
Congenital ichthyosiform erythroderma	Usually at birth as 'collodion baby'	Fine white scale in most areas, sometimes larger and darker on lower legs. Mild to very severe generalized erythroderma. Whole body surface is involved including palms and soles	Similar to those of lamellar ichthyosis but of lesser extent	Moderately thick stratum corneum with some parakeratosis. Marked epidermal thickening
Bullous ichthyosis (epidermolytic hyperkeratosis)	At birth with erythroderma and widespread blistering. After a few days the redness subsides and over early months the blistering tendency reduces	Thick dark warty scales from time to time to leave denuded areas with a red base. Blistering is rare after 1 year. The condition may be localized to extensor surfaces but is usually widespread although the face is usually spared. Palm and sole involvement is variable	Bacterial superinfection is a recurrent problem. Heavy bacterial colonization is inevitable. Maceration and offensive odor are major problems	Very thick stratum corneum, thick granular layer with increased numbers of large abnormal keratohyaline granules. Vacuolation of cells in granular and upper spinous layers and loss of cell boundaries. Marked epidermal thickening. Chronic inflammatory infiltrate in dermis

Collodion baby (Plate 25.5)

This is a descriptive term for the child who is encased at birth in a shiny tight membrane resembling collodion or plastic skin, producing ectropion and eclabium and fissuring. The skin peels off in days or weeks. This may be a presentation of various conditions, particularly CIE, Netherton's syndrome and chondrodysplasia punctata. Rarely the membrane peels off to leave normal skin: this condition is called lamellar exfoliation of the newborn. Collodion babies show temperature instability and excessive fluid loss. Corneal exposure may result if the eyes are not covered and the eclabium may necessitate squeeze bottle, tube or dropper feeding. As the fissures appear, secondary infection becomes a risk. The child should be nursed in a humidicrib with minimum handling. Emollients are best avoided in the early stages.

Harlequin fetus

This may represent a phenotype of several disorders, all recessively inherited. Various abnormalities of keratinization and epidermal lipid metabolism have been demonstrated. At birth the child is covered in large dark plates of scale with severe ectropion and eclabium, deformed ears and claw hands and feet. Most die as neonates but the few who have survived have had a severe ichthyosiform erythroderma. (Note – this is different from the harlequin color change.)

Ichthyosis as part of other syndromes

Some of the syndromes of which ichthyosis is a part are listed in Table 25.2.

EPIDERMOLYSIS BULLOSA

This is a group of diseases characterized by trauma-induced blistering of skin and mucosae. There are over 15 types now identified, separated on the basis of inheritance, clinical features

Table 25.2 Syndromes associated with ichthyosis

Syndrome	Type of ichthyosis	Other major features
Chondrodysplasia punctata	Onset may be as 'collodion baby'. Initially occurs as a diffuse redness and scaling. Later occurs in a whorled patchy distribution	Epiphyseal dysplasia, cataracts, follicular atrophoderma
Sjögren–Larsson syndrome	Generalized ichthyosis at birth. Later large dark scales most prominent in flexures	Mental retardation, spasticity
Chanarin–Dorfman syndrome (neutral lipid storage disease with ichthyosis)	Ichthyosis simulating mild to moderate congenital ichthyosiform erythroderma	Lipid vacuoles in almost all cells. Normal serum lipids. Cataracts, deafness, developmental delay
Refsum's syndrome	Delayed onset of ichthyosis of mild form, simulating ichthyosis vulgaris	Failure to degrade phytanic acid. Retinitis pigmentosa, peripheral neuropathy, cerebellar ataxia
Netherton's syndrome	Erythroderma at birth. Late development of circinate migratory scaly, lesions (ichthyosis linearis circumflexa) in widespread distribution. Some cases simulate congenital ichthyosiform erythroderma	Alopecia due to hair shaft abnormalities, especially trichorrhexis invaginata, atopic diathesis, developmental delay, generalized aminoaciduria

and electron microscopic (EM) identification of the cleavage plane of the blister. The split may be within the epidermis (epidermolytic), at the dermoepidermal junction in the lamina lucida (lucidolytic, junctional; Plate 25.6 and Fig. 25.3) or in the upper dermis (dermolytic; Plate 25.7). A classification is given in Table 25.3 and the clinical features and complications are outlined in Table 25.4.

Blisters are clear or filled with serosanguinous material depending on their level. They may rupture or spontaneously subside. Secondary bacterial infection is common. Milia are small retention cysts resulting from a split through pilosebaceous or sweat ducts: these eventually extrude. Permanent scarring is mainly a feature of the dermolytic types and varies from mild, with minor cosmetic significance, to severe, with gross deformity and functional disability. Strictures can occur with scarring of mucosal lesions, leading to such complications as visual impairment, nasal obstruction, dysphagia, reflux and malabsorption and urinary obstruction and its sequelae.

Anemia is an important complication of the severe form and results from a combination of blood loss, malnutrition and chronic infection. Hypoproteinemia is caused by constant loss of protein in blister fluid, malabsorption and malnutrition. Severe failure to thrive is a feature of the serious cases. Management involves a multidisciplinary approach.

A firm diagnosis should always be established as soon as possible by EM examination of a new blister. This enables a prognosis to be given and a management plan to be established for present and future.

In mild epidermolytic and dominant dystrophic cases advice is required regarding avoidance of trauma, a reduction of friction, appropriate clothing and footwear. New blisters should be pricked to drain them but not deroofed and various dressings of nonstick material are appropriate. Secondary bacterial infection is treated with topical or oral antibiotics.

In the severe forms with extensive neonatal blistering the infant should initially be nursed naked in a humidicrib lying on nonadherent material with barrier nursing to prevent infection. Blisters should be drained and antibacterial creams such as silver sulfadiazine applied to large erosions. Vaseline gauze or nonadherent plastic dressings should be used as required, secured with tubular gauze or by other means but never taped to the skin

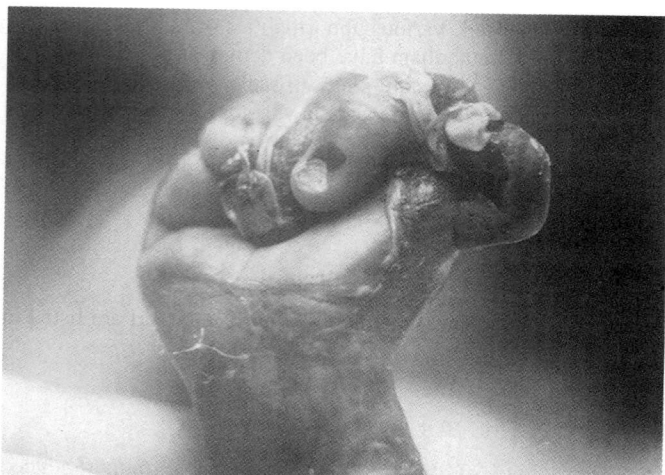

Fig. 25.3 Junctional epidermolysis bullosa.

Table 25.3 Classification of major types of hereditary epidermolysis bullosa

	Inheritance
EPIDERMOLYTIC	
Epidermolysis bullosa simplex (EBS)	
Generalized EBS (Koebner)	Autosomal dominant
Localized EBS (Weber Cockayne)	Autosomal dominant
Herpetiform EBS (Dowling Meara)	Autosomal dominant
LUCIDOLYTIC	
Junctional epidermolysis bullosa (JEB)	
Generalized severe (Herlitz)	Autosomal recessive
Generalized atrophic benign	Autosomal recessive
Localized	Autosomal recessive
DERMOLYTIC	
Dystrophic epidermolysis bullosa (DEB)	
Dominant DEB	
Hyperplastic (Cockayne Touraine)	Autosomal dominant
Albopapuloid (Pasini)	Autosomal dominant
Recessive DEB (Hallopeau Siemens)	Autosomal recessive

Table 25.4a   Epidermolytic epidermolysis bullosa – epidermolysis bullosa simplex (EBS)

	Generalized EBS	Localized EBS	Herpetiform EBS
Onset	Birth or early infancy	Usually early childhood; sometimes later, even in adult life	Birth
Skin	Blistering which may be widespread but especially in areas of trauma, hands, feet, knees and elbows. Worse with increase in temperature. No scarring	Blisters on hands and feet. Worse with increase in temperature. Hyperhidrosis of feet. No scarring	Widespread blistering at birth. Transient milia develop later groups of blisters, in anular and arcuate configurations, on proximal limbs and trunk. Large blisters on hands and feet. Palmoplantar keratoderma. May improve with increase in temperature. No scarring
Mucosae	Occasional involvement of oral mucosa, particularly in early infancy	Normal	Involves oral and sometimes esophageal and laryngeal mucosae especially in infancy
Teeth	Normal	Normal	Often normal. Occasionally natal teeth, hypodontia
Nails	Normal	Normal	Often dystrophic, may be lost
Prognosis	Continues through life. Normal life span	Continues through life. Normal life span	May improve considerably in late childhood

Table 25.4b   Lucidolytic epidermolysis bullosa – junctional epidermolysis bullosa (JEB)

	Generalized severe JEB	Generalized atrophic benign JEB	Localized JEB
Onset	Birth	Birth	Birth
Skin	Severe widespread blistering from birth, with relative sparing of hands and feet apart from around nails. Slow healing areas of exuberant granulation tissue especially on face. Healing without scarring. May be some atrophy	Generalized blistering. Slow healing areas of granulation tissue. No scarring	Blisters localized to hands and feet and sometimes pretibial area
Mucosae	Often involves nasal, oral, esophageal and anal mucosae. May involve other parts of respiratory, urogenital and gastrointestinal tracts and conjunctivae. Urethral stenosis, tracheal and laryngeal obstruction may occur	Involves nasal, oral and anal mucosae. Other mucosae less often affected	Moderate involvement of nasal and oral mucosae
Teeth	Severely dysplastic	Dysplastic	Dysplastic
Nails	Dystrophic, repeatedly lost, sometimes permanently	Dystrophic, often lost	Dystrophic, often lost
Other	Secondary infection, anemia, growth retardation. Pyloric atresia. Hydronephrosis	Postlesional hyperpigmentation. Alopecia following blistering of scalp and pubic area	
Prognosis	Death in early weeks is common. Survival to adolescence rare	Decreased blistering in adolescence. Life span not shortened	Normal life span

with adhesive. A squeeze bottle or dropper should be used for feeding when there is severe oral ulceration. A nasogastric tube should never be passed. Tourniquets, adhesive urine collection bags, name tags and pacifiers should all be avoided. The parents should be encouraged to hold the child but the need for extreme gentleness in handling must be both explained and demonstrated.

Later, the child with severe involvement should be dressed in soft loose clothing without elastic. He should sleep on a sheepskin or waterbed, and have padded swings and walkers provided and be encouraged in suitable activities such as swimming, exercise programs and interesting sedentary pursuits. Teeth are cleaned with a sponge or water jet 'toothbrush'. The child should be fed small portions of soft or blended food. The adequacy and balance of the diet must be constantly assessed. Regular assessment of growth parameters, blood count and protein levels should be made and a constant watch kept for secondary infection.

Severe complications may require the involvement of plastic surgeons, urologists, nephrologists, orthopedic surgeons, ophthalmologists, ear, nose and throat specialists, physiotherapists, occupational therapists, nutritionists, manufacturers of customized footwear, psychiatrists and other professionals.

Where possible, one physician should coordinate the entire management program to provide stability and continuity. The family should be directed towards support organizations, which can offer practical advice, emotional support and companionship. Finally, genetic counseling of the parents and later the patient should be arranged at an appropriate time.

Table 25.4c Dermolytic epidermolysis bullosa – dystrophic epidermolysis bullosa (DEB)

	Dominant DEB, Hyperplastic or Cockayne Touraine	Dominant DEB, Albopapuloid or Pasini	Recessive DEB or Hallopeau Siemens
Onset	Infancy or early childhood	Birth	Birth
Skin	Blisters especially on hands feet, knees and elbows. Heal with milia and scars which may be hypertrophic. Areas of hyperkeratosis may occur	Large blisters on trunk and extremities in infancy. Later more acral. Scar leaving white papules and plaques	Severe widespread blistering at birth, producing large erosions which heal with milia and scars. Later blistering, especially acral and over bony prominences. Repeated blistering and scarring can provide syndactyly of fingers, toes and club-like deformities of hands and feet with several digits encased together in a scar
Mucosae	Occasional mild oral involvement	Occasional mild oral involvement	Severe involvement of oral and anal mucosa. Esophageal blistering leads to scarring with obstruction and disordered motility. Laryngeal and tracheal involvement may threaten airway. Urethral stenosis may produce urinary retention
Teeth	Normal	Normal	Dysplastic
Nails	Dystrophic, thick, may be lost	Dystrophic. Toenails often lost	Dystrophic, often lost
Other	Keratitis. Squamous cell carcinoma in scars	Keratitis. Squamous cell carcinoma in scars	Severe flexion contractures, infection, anemia, severe growth retardation, eye involvement with keratitis and symblepharon. Hydronephrosis, hearing loss from stricture of external auditory meatus. Carcinoma in scars
Prognosis	Lifelong disorder	Less generalized with age	Significant shortening of life span in severe cases.

ECTODERMAL DYSPLASIAS (Fig. 25.4)

The ectodermal dysplasias are a heterogeneous group of inherited conditions with a primary defect in one or more of teeth, nails, hair or sweat gland function in addition to another abnormality in a tissue of ectodermal origin, including eyes, ears, oral and nasal mucosa, melanocytes and central nervous system. A detailed classification of these syndromes has been produced (Freire-Maia & Pinheiro 1984).

The major features of some of the more important ectodermal dysplasias are documented in Table 25.5.

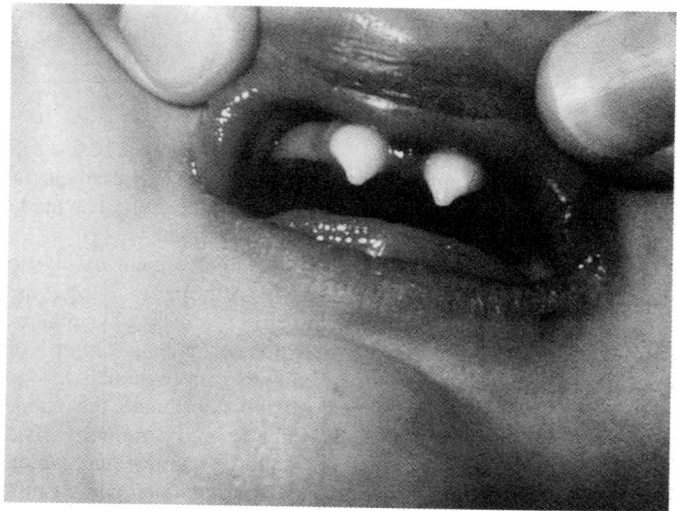

Fig. 25.4 Ectodermal dysplasia.

Management

As these are disorders manifesting very diverse features, a multidisciplinary approach is essential.

If the scalp hair is very sparse the cosmetic benefit of a good wig may be invaluable. Primary and secondary dentitions can be assessed with dental X-rays in infancy in conjunction with a pediatric dentist experienced in these conditions. Early use of prostheses may prevent development of some of the structural facial abnormalities. Newer techniques include osseous implants into which prosthetic teeth can be fitted.

Mechanical files are available to shorten and flatten thickened nails and some patients with nail dystrophies may require special footwear. Antibiotics may be required for acute paronychia. If hypohidrosis is extreme hyperthermia may result and may be severe and life threatening. Advice regarding activities, clothing, methods of cooling and even relocation to a cooler climate may be required.

Atopic eczema often accompanies hypohidrotic ectodermal dysplasia and will require the usual treatment. Many patients have dry skin and require emollients, and keratolytics may improve palmoplantar keratoderma.

All patients with eye abnormalities should be managed in conjunction with an ophthalmologist. Artificial tears are essential for dry eyes to prevent corneal damage. Reconstructive procedures will be required for atresia of nasolacrimal ducts and canaliculi. Severe respiratory infections complicate some of these syndromes and need antibiotics, physiotherapy and regular pediatric follow-up. Surgical therapy may be required for cleft lip and palate, urethral stenosis, vaginal adhesions, mucosal and cutaneous malignancy, syndactyly and other structural abnormalities. Regular follow-up for the development of malignancy in mucosal leukoplakia and atrophic skin and for blood dyscrasias in dyskeratosis congenita is essential.

Table 25.5a   The ectodermal dysplasias

	1. Hypohidrotic ectodermal dysplasia (Christ Siemens Touraine syndrome)	2. Autosomal recessive hypohidrotic dysplasia	3. Hidrotic ectodermal dysplasia	4. Dyskeratosis congenita
Inheritance	X-linked recessive	Autosomal recessive	Autosomal dominant	X-linked recessive, autosomal dominant, autosomal recessive
Hair	Hypotrichosis of scalp, body hair, eyebrows and lashes. Beard normal. Hair fine and fair	Hypotrichosis. Fair hair with hair shaft abnormalities	Hypotrichosis. Hair fine and dry	Normal or sparse. Premature canities.
Teeth	Hypodontia. Conical teeth	Hypodontia. Conical teeth	May be normal. Hypodontia, caries, widespaced teeth	Malalignment. Early caries.
Nails	Often normal. Sometimes fragile and occasionally dystrophic or absent	Often normal. Sometimes dystrophic	Thick, striated, discolored. Paronychia and nail loss. Rarely thin and brittle	Dystrophic from age 5–10. May be shed or reduced to horny plugs. Paronychia
Sweating	Hypohidrosis often with hyperthermia	Hypohidrosis with hyperthermia	Normal	Palmoplantar hyperhidrosis. May be reduced sweating elsewhere
Skin	Smooth and dry, loss of dermatoglyphics, wrinkled and hyperpigmented around eyes, atopic dermatitis	Thin, smooth and dry. Wrinkled around eyes	Thick over finger joints, knees and elbows. Palmoplantar keratoderma	Atrophy, telangiectasia, reticulate pigmentation, palmoplantar keratoderma with blistering. Carcinoma may develop in atrophic skin
Eyes	Hypoplasia of nasolacrimal duct, decreased lacrimal gland secretion, dry eyes, photophobia and corneal opacities	Hypoplasia of nasolacrimal duct, decreased lacrimal gland secretion	Usually normal. Occasionally premature cataracts	Erosions on tarsal conjunctiva producing scarring with block of lacrimal puncta
Facies	Variable. Thick lips, saddle nose, frontal bossing, maxillary hypoplasia. Occasionally abnormal ears	Thick lips. Saddle nose, frontal bossing, maxillary hypoplasia. Protruberant ears	Normal	Normal
Mucosae	Poor development of mucous glands in gastrointestinal and respiratory tracts. Atrophic rhinitis, thick nasal secretion, recurrent chest infections, dysphagia. Dry mouth	Chronic rhinitis, respiratory infections	Normal	Leukoplakia of oral and anogenital mucosae. May be mucosal involvement throughout gastrointestinal and urogenital tract. Urethral stenosis. Carcinoma in affected mucosae
Miscellaneous	Absent or supernumerary nipples. Absent breast tissue in carriers. Asthma	Brachydactyly	Tufting of terminal phalanges with finger clubbing. Thickening of skull bones	Blood dyscrasias, including myeloid aplasia and pancytopenia

Genetic counseling is important in this group of hereditary diseases. In many countries, including the UK and USA, there are ectodermal dysplasia societies for education about, stimulation of research into and more importantly, support of patients with these distressing conditions.

TUBEROUS SCLEROSIS (EPILOIA)

This is a neurocutaneous disorder with autosomal dominant inheritance (though a high rate of spontaneous mutation occurs). Epilepsy occurs in 80% and mental retardation in 70%. Other systemic abnormalities include retinal phacomata and a variety of hamartomata in renal tract, heart and other organs.

Dermatological features (Figs 25.5 and 25.6)

The most pathognomonic features are angiofibromas (adenoma sebaceum), periungual fibromas, shagreen patches and ash leaf macules. The angiofibromas appear as 1–4 mm bright red papules in a centrofacial distribution. Sometimes they coalesce to form cauliflower-like masses. Their onset is usually between the ages of 3 and 10 years and they may become more extensive at puberty.

Numbers vary from few to several hundred. Periungual fibromas appear around puberty as firm smooth flesh-colored papules in a periungual or subungual location. The shagreen patch is a connective tissue nevus comprising an accumulation of collagen as an irregularly thickened yellow-white plaque, usually in the lumbosacral area. It develops between the ages of 2 and 5 years. Ash leaf macules are depigmented macules, usually 1–3 cm in diameter but occasionally much larger. They are usually oval in shape, with a minority truly ash leaf shaped. They may be present at birth or appear during the first year. Large numbers may be present. Café au lait patches are no more common in tuberous sclerosis than in the general population (Bell & MacDonald 1985).

Other dermatological features include fibromatous plaques on brow or scalp, intraoral fibromas, multiple fibroepithelial polyps around the neck and in the axillae and a variety of other depigmented lesions including numerous guttate macules and large dermatomal lesions. Poliosis and canities may also occur.

Patients who present with these characteristic skin signs should be referred for neurological assessment, skull X-ray and computerized axial tomography to demonstrate any intracranial lesions.

Table 25.5b The ectodermal dysplasias

	5. Pachyonychia congenita	6. Rapp Hodgkin's syndrome	7. EEC syndrome (ectrodactyly ectodermal dysplasia and clefting)	8. AEC syndrome (ankyloblepharon ectodermal dysplasia and clefting) (Hay–Wells' syndrome)
Inheritance	Autosomal dominant	?Autosomal dominant	Autosomal dominant	Autosomal dominant
Hair	Occasional hypotrichosis	Sparse, coarse and stiff with hair shaft abnormalities	Sparse wiry hair	Severe hypotrichosis
Teeth	Natal teeth; early caries	Hypodontia, abnormally shaped teeth. Early caries	Hypodontia, abnormally shaped teeth	Variable hypodontia, abnormal shape, delayed eruption
Nails	Very thick and wedge shaped, marked subungual hyperkeratosis. Paronychia and nail shedding	Small and dysplastic	Thin, pitted and striated	Severe dystrophy. Short due to absence of distal nail plate
Sweating	Palmoplantar hyperhidrosis	Hypohidrosis	Occasional hypohidrosis	Variable hypohidrosis
Skin	Palmoplantar keratoderma, keratosis pilaris of limbs, buttocks, epidermoid cysts	Dry and coarse. Thick over elbows and knees. Reduced dermatoglyphics	Dry and thin. Palmoplantar keratoderma	Large weeping areas at birth, later dry and scaly. May be recurrent scalp crusting. Palmoplantar keratoderma
Eyes	Corneal dyskeratosis	Atresia of lacrimal puncta producing epiphora, corneal opacities	Nasolacrimal duct stenosis, dacryocystitis, corneal scarring	Ankyloblepharon filiforme adnatum, nasolacrimal duct atresia
Facies	Normal	Cleft lip, hypoplastic maxilla. Microstomia. Prominent malformed ears	Cleft lip	Cleft lip often, microstomia, broad nasal bridge, sunken maxilla, abnormal pinnae
Mucosae	Leukoplakia of tongue, oral, nasopharyngeal, and anogenital mucosae and larynx. May be complicated by carcinoma	Chronic rhinitis	Hoarseness due to abnormality of laryngeal mucosa	Filamentous bands in vagina, anal fissure
Miscellaneous		Short stature. Cleft palate. Syndactyly	Cleft palate. Ectrodactyly (split hands and feet). Syndactyly	Cleft palate. Syndactyly

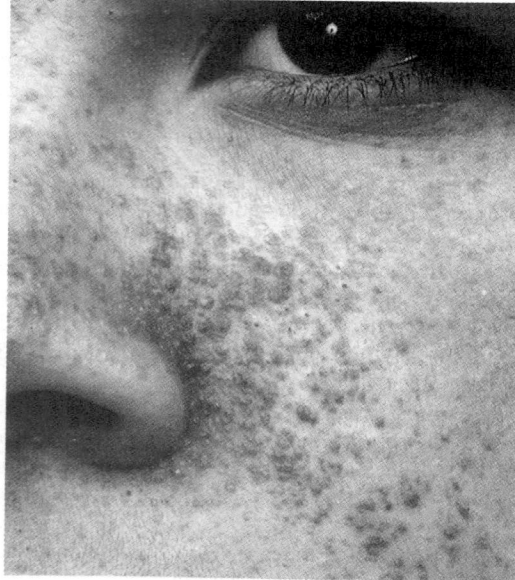

Fig. 25.5 Adenoma sebaceum: tuberous sclerosis.

Fig. 25.6 Ash leaf patch: tuberous sclerosis.

INCONTINENTIA PIGMENTI (Plate 25.8 and Fig. 25.7)

This is a multisystem disorder believed to be inherited as an X-linked dominant trait and is usually lethal in males. Neurological abnormalities occur in about 30% of cases and include epilepsy, mental retardation and spastic diplegia and tetraplegia. Ocular abnormalities are seen in 30% and include strabismus, cataracts, retinal vascular proliferation and retinal detachment. Almost 70% of patients have dental abnormalities with partial anodontia and peg-shaped or conical teeth. A variety of skeletal abnormalities

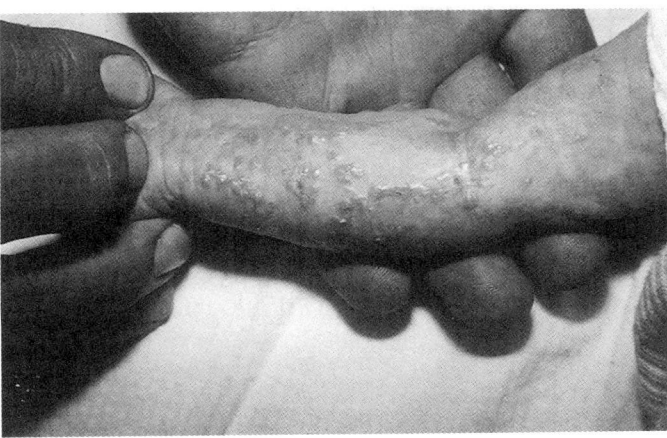

Fig. 25.7 Incontinentia pigmenti: vesicular stage.

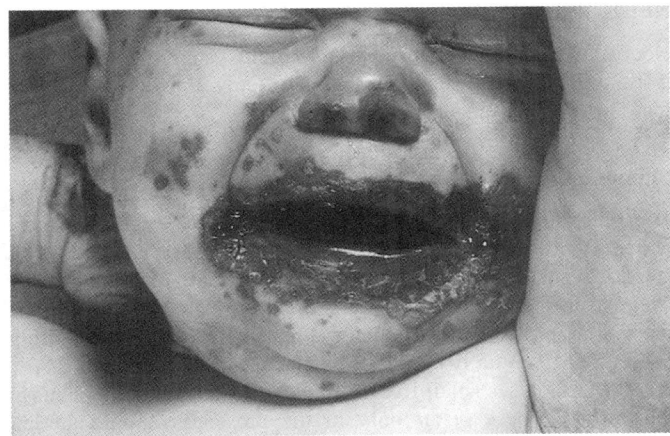

Fig. 25.8 Acrodermatitis enteropathica: mouth.

including limb reduction defects occur, and rarely cardiac abnormalities are seen.

Cutaneous lesions

There are four cutaneous stages of the disease which may follow each other in an orderly progression; however, there may be overlap, particularly in the earlier stages. Stage one comprises linear groups of vesicles which appear mainly on the limbs at birth or in the first days of life: they are accompanied by a peripheral blood eosinophilia and clear spontaneously over several weeks. Stage two is the verrucose stage with linear warty lesions appearing between 1 and 4 months of age: they occur particularly on the limbs, especially on dorsa of hands and feet, and resolve spontaneously after weeks or months. Stage three comprises streaks and whorls and splattered patterns of macular hyperpigmentation which appear on both limbs and trunk at 12–24 months of age. Lesions persist till early adult life. Stage four has been recently described: linear hypopigmented streaks with alopecia occur particularly on the lower legs, and these lesions are permanent.

Other dermatological features of incontinentia pigmenti are cicatricial alopecia and nail dystrophy.

ACRODERMATITIS ENTEROPATHICA AND NUTRITIONAL ZINC DEFICIENCY

Acrodermatitis enteropathica is an autosomal recessive condition in which there is a defective absorption of zinc, possibly due to the absence of a specific carrier protein. An identical condition occurs in infants with nutritional zinc deficiency. This may occur as a result of prematurity with low zinc stores, particularly in bottle-fed babies (as there is a lower bioavailability of zinc in bovine milk as compared to breast milk), or as a result of low breast milk zinc. Zinc deficiency also occurs in acquired immunodeficiency disease, cystic fibrosis and other causes of malabsorption and in infants on parenteral nutrition solutions not containing adequate zinc.

Clinical features

The onset in the primary form occurs usually when the child is weaned or in the first few weeks of life in a bottle-fed infant. In

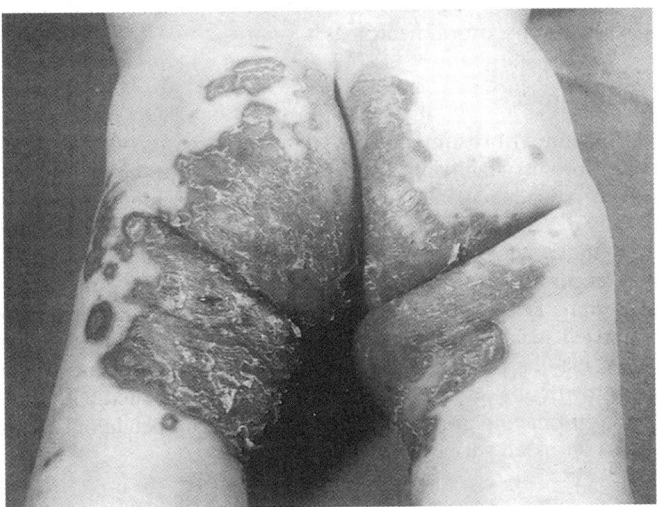

Fig. 25.9 Acrodermatitis enteropathica: buttocks.

the children with nutritional zinc deficiency the onset is usually at the time of the first growth spurt. Erythematous and crusted, sometimes vesicular and pustular lesions appear in an acral distribution particularly around nose, mouth and eyes (Fig. 25.8) and sometimes on tips of digits and the paronychial areas. An anogenital rash (Fig. 25.9) is also common and psoriasiform lesions may occur on knees and elbows and occasionally elsewhere. Secondary bacterial and candidal infection is common. In the primary form mucosal involvement with glossitis, cheilitis and conjunctivitis may occur, a nail dystrophy is usual, and alopecia and diarrhea may occur.

The diagnosis is confirmed by finding a low serum zinc (<50 μg/dl).

Management

All features of the condition respond rapidly to the administration of high doses of oral zinc as either zinc gluconate or zinc sulfate. This is required lifelong in the primary form but only for a few weeks in the secondary variety.

NEUROFIBROMATOSIS

Neurofibromatosis is a very variable multisystem disorder which is described in detail in Chapter 14. Only the dermatological features will be considered here.

Pigmented lesions

The café au lait macule is the most common of these: most patients with neurofibromatosis have at least six macules of at least 1.5 cm in maximum diameter. They are usually oval or irregular in shape and most are 2–5 cm long. Some lesions may be present at birth and they increase in size and number during childhood. Eventually hundreds of macules may be present.

In 20% of cases small freckle-like pigmented macules occur in the axillae. These occur only in the presence of café au lait macules and the combination is of great diagnostic significance. Similar small pigmented macules may occur in a widespread distribution, especially in patients with large numbers of café au lait spots. Larger pigmented patches 10 cm or more in diameter may overlie plexiform neuromas.

Neurofibromas

Molluscum fibrosum is the name given to a cutaneous neurofibroma which appears as a soft pink or skin-colored tumor, sessile or pedunculated and characteristically indentable. These usually develop after puberty. Their distribution is widespread and up to thousands of tumors half to several centimeters in diameter may occur. Small firmer discrete nodules occur along the course of peripheral nerves. The plexiform neuroma is a larger diffuse elongated neurofibroma along the course of a peripheral nerve. These may be present at birth or develop later. There may be an overgrowth of skin and subcutaneous tissue associated with these lesions producing gross disfigurement as a giant pendulous tumor with a wrinkled surface.

PSORIASIS

Psoriasis is probably an autosomal dominant condition with variable penetrance. It appears by the age of 15 years in 30% of patients. Children may present with typical adult large erythematous plaques, with a thick silvery white scale, predominantly on the knees, elbows, buttocks and scalp but usually the plaques are smaller and with a finer scale. A common presentation is acute guttate psoriasis with the eruption of small papules in a widespread distribution, often following an intercurrent illness, particularly a streptococcal throat infection. A micropapular form of psoriasis occurs particularly in dark-skinned children with 1–2 mm papules most marked on the extensor aspects of the limbs. These lesions are usually skin colored until scratching demonstrates the white scale.

The face and intertriginous sites, such as retroauricular areas, axillae, groin, genital and perianal area, are commonly affected in children. Children presenting with vulvitis, balanitis and perianal itching may be found to have psoriasis. In these areas the typical scale is absent and the condition presents as a glazed erythema often with fissuring. Generalized pustular psoriasis is rare in children and has an explosive onset with sheets of pustules on a background of bright erythema accompanied by severe systemic toxicity. It may be the first presentation of psoriasis and settle spontaneously in a few weeks leaving normal skin. It often recurs

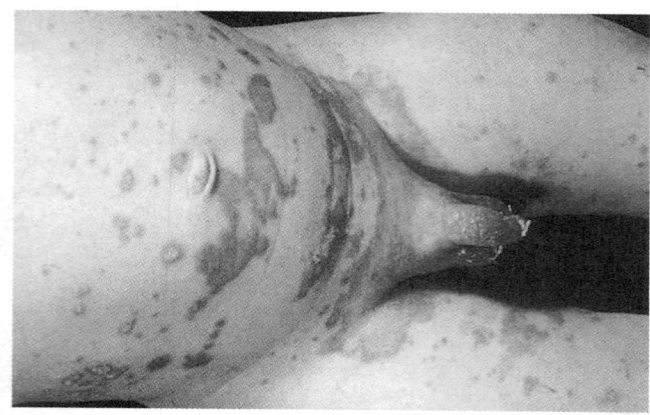

Fig. 25.10 Napkin psoriasis.

and usually more typical psoriasis eventually supervenes. Pustular psoriasis of the palms and soles is also very rare in children. Acropustulosis, a glazed erythema studded with pustules followed by thick scaling and fissuring, involving one or more digits, is an occasional childhood presentation. Nail involvement is usually absent or minimal with minor pitting, and psoriatic arthropathy is extremely uncommon in children.

Controversy exists over whether or not the condition called 'napkin psoriasis' or 'sebopsoriasis' (Fig. 25.10) is in fact a form of psoriasis. It occurs in the first 3 months of life with a nonspecific napkin dermatitis suddenly becoming more severe and extensive with bright, well-demarcated erythema involving most of the napkin area including the folds. Lesions resembling typical psoriasis then erupt elsewhere, usually first on face and scalp, then neck fold and axillae and finally trunk and limbs. In the scalp the lesions may appear similar to seborrhea. Evidence for this representing a form of psoriasis rather than dermatitis comes from the work of Andersen & Thomsen (1971) who found a family history of psoriasis in 26% of patients compared with 4.9% of controls, and of Neville & Finn (1975) who, on review of these patients at 5–13 years, found psoriasis in 17% with the expected rate being 0.4%.

In any child with a difficult napkin dermatitis responding poorly to conventional measures psoriasis should be considered, particularly if the lesions have well-defined margins and remain fairly fixed in position.

Management

Many therapies used in adults are inappropriate in children, including oral retinoids, psoralens and UVA light (PUVA), retinoid–PUVA combinations, cytotoxics, intralesional steroids and prolonged UVB therapy. As a general rule, psoriasis in children is better treated with tars than topical corticosteroids. They are often more effective, are safer for long-term use, and rebound on their cessation is less of a problem. Tars may be irritant in infants, as they may be at any age when applied to the face or intertriginous areas. A useful preparation for guttate or small plaque psoriasis is 4% liquor picis carbonis (LPC) and 4% salicylic acid in an aqueous cream base applied twice a day. A half-strength preparation may be tolerated on the face and in the flexures but if not 1% hydrocortisone cream can be used. If there is evidence of a recent streptococcal infection an oral course of penicillin should be given. For large plaque psoriasis in older children the adult regimes of various tars (dithranol 0.1–0.2%, crude coal tar 1–4%) combined with measured graduated UVB exposure are usually tolerated.

Scalp psoriasis usually responds well to the nightly application of an ointment containing 3% LPC, 3% sulfur and 3% salicylic acid; a tar shampoo can be used for maintenance.

Patients with generalized pustular psoriasis require hospitalization and close monitoring of fluid and electrolyte balance and evidence of infection. Wet compresses give symptomatic relief while awaiting spontaneous recovery. Tars are contraindicated and topical steroids must be used very cautiously due to the risk of considerable absorption. Palmoplantar pustulosis and acropustulosis usually respond slowly to tar preparations. Napkin psoriasis often clears quickly with hydrocortisone and anticandidal agents for the flexural areas and a weak corticosteroid elsewhere.

It is essential for the parents, and the child if old enough, to appreciate that psoriasis is a capricious recurrent disease which will require varying treatments depending on the site, nature and severity of the condition at different stages. Long-term follow-up, preferably with the same practitioner, is important.

HEREDITARY PHOTOSENSITIVE DISORDERS

Photosensitivity is the cardinal feature of most of the porphyrias (p. 1142) and occurs in other metabolic diseases including phenylketonuria (p. 1103) and Hartnup disease (p. 1122).

Severe photosensitivity occurs in oculocutaneous albinism and in xeroderma pigmentosum, and photosensitivity is an important feature, particularly in the early years, in Bloom's syndrome and Cockayne's syndrome and in some cases of the Rothmund–Thomson syndrome.

Oculocutaneous albinism

The term oculocutaneous albinism (OCA) refers to a group of autosomal recessive conditions with an absence or severe reduction in the pigmentation of skin, hair and eyes. In ocular albinism only ocular pigmentation is defective. In OCA melanocytes are present but are functionally abnormal with a variety of defects leading to decreased or absent production of melanin. The clinical and laboratory findings in the main forms of OCA are documented in Table 25.6.

Patients with severe OCA are unable to live a normal life due to their extreme photosensitivity and visual deficit. These patients should be managed in conjunction with an ophthalmologist who will arrange appropriate facilities and aids for the visual handicap. The child should be directed towards hobbies, sports and other activities which are performed indoors, and there should be early counseling regarding appropriate future careers. When outside, covering clothing, hats and broad spectrum sunscreens will be necessary. Patients should be examined regularly for the development of solar-induced premalignant and malignant lesions to which they are significantly more likely due to the lack of protective cutaneous pigmentation.

Table 25.6 Classification of reduced pigment disorders

	Tyrosinase negative albinism	Tyrosinase positive albinism	Yellow mutant albinism	Chédiak–Higashi syndrome	Hermansky–Pudlak syndrome	Cross syndrome
Skin pigmentation	Nil	Much reduced	Reduced	Much reduced	Reduced	Reduced
Development of pigmented nevi and freckles	Absent	Present and may be numerous	Present	Present	Present	Present
Hair colour	White	Blonde to light brown	Yellow or yellow-brown	Blonde, light brown or steely gray	Red to red-brown	White or blonde
Eye colour	Blue-gray. No visible pigment	Blue-gray early, darken with age	Blue-gray early, darken with age	Blue to brown	Blue to brown	Blue-grey
Nystagmus	Very severe	Moderate to severe	Mild to moderate	Absent or mild	Mild to moderate	Severe
Visual acuity	Most are legally blind	Severely reduced early. Some improvement with age	Severely reduced early. Some improvement with age	Normal to moderately reduced	Moderately reduced	Normal to mildly reduced
Other features				Increased susceptibility to infection due to neutrophil phagocytic defect. Risk of lymphoreticular malignancy	Abnormality of platelet function	Mental retardation
Pigment produced on incubation of hair bulbs in tyrosine	No pigment produced	Pigment produced	No pigment produced (some pigment produced if cysteine added)	Pigment produced	Pigment produced	Pigment produced
Hair bulb melanosomes (electron microscopic study)	Stages 1 and 2 are present	Up to early stage 3 are present	Up to stage 3 present	Stages 1 to 4. Some are giant-sized	Up to stage 3	Up to stage 3

Xeroderma pigmentosum (XP) (Plate 25.9)

This is a group of autosomal recessive conditions with a defect in the capacity to repair ultraviolet radiation (UVR)-damaged deoxyribonucleic acid (DNA). In 80% of cases there is a defect in the initiation of DNA repair and nine genetically separate forms have been demonstrated. In the remaining 20% (XP variants) there is a defect in the S phase of DNA replication following UVR exposure.

In XP the skin is usually normal at birth and the first lesions appear on exposed areas between the age of 6 and 24 months. The earliest lesions are small and large pigmented macules. Later telangiectases and small angiomas appear, and finally white atrophic lesions. Blisters and superficial ulcers can occur and healing of these may produce scarring with ectropion and restriction of mouth opening. Keratoses and keratoacanthomas are common, and malignant tumors can develop from as early as 3 or 4 years: these include basal cell and squamous cell carcinoma, malignant melanoma, angiosarcoma and fibrosarcoma. Squamous cell carcinomas can occur also on the lips and the tip of the tongue.

Photophobia and conjunctivitis are common. Ectropion and destruction of the eyelids by carcinoma can lead to exposure keratitis and pigmented macules and malignancies can occur on the conjunctivae. Other abnormalities in XP patients include short stature, hypogonadism, microcephaly, mental retardation, deafness, choreoathetosis and ataxia. The diagnosis can be confirmed by studying the DNA repair process following UVR in cultured fibroblasts obtained from a skin biopsy.

Patients must be protected from exposure to UVR up to 320 nm (which includes emissions from some fluorescent lights) by all possible means including opaque sunscreens, covering clothing, hats and sunglasses. Observation for and early treatment of malignancies is mandatory.

Bloom's syndrome

This is an autosomal recessive disorder most common in the Ashkenazi Jewish race, with a photosensitive rash, growth retardation and an increased risk of malignancy.

The cutaneous lesions start between 1 and 2 years following sun exposure with a reticulate telangiectatic erythema occurring on the face, in a butterfly distribution resembling lupus, and also on the eyelids and ears and on the dorsa of the arms and hands. The condition worsens with continued sun exposure and scaling, and hemorrhagic crusting and blistering can occur. With stringent sun protection the rash improves and there is some spontaneous improvement after puberty. Over 50% of patients demonstrate multiple widespread café au lait spots. There is a severe proportionate dwarfism and patients often have a narrow pinched facies and a high arched palate. Testicular atrophy may occur. Patients are mentally normal.

Deficiency of one or more classes of immunoglobulins often occurs and these children suffer recurrent respiratory and gastrointestinal bacterial infections. Bloom's syndrome is one of the hereditary chromosomal breakage disorders and patients are at increased risk of malignancy, particularly leukemia but also lymphoma, squamous cell carcinoma, and nephroblastoma.

Cockayne's syndrome

In this rare autosomal recessive condition a photosensitive eruption occurs with erythema and scaling in light-exposed areas, particularly on the face after the first year of life. Later the photosensitivity decreases but hyperpigmentation and atrophy remain in the affected areas. Subcutaneous fat atrophy occurs on the face and the eyes are sunken due to loss of orbital fat. There is dwarfism with disproportionally long limbs and large hands and feet. Mental retardation is common and cerebellar and upper motor neuron dysfunctions occur. Other features are optic atrophy, retinal degeneration and progressive deafness.

The thymic hormone level is low and T cell function may be abnormal. Cultured fibroblasts are abnormally sensitive to killing by ultraviolet radiation and certain chemicals. Death is usual by 30 years, and at autopsy there is extensive demyelination of central and peripheral nervous systems.

Rothmund–Thomson syndrome

The syndromes described by Rothmund and Thomson may be genetically different but they are usually described together as the Rothmund–Thomson syndrome. Cases demonstrate both autosomal dominant and autosomal recessive inheritance, often with variable expressivity.

The skin is usually normal at birth and the first changes are seen between 3 and 24 months. The first sign is usually erythema, soon followed by a poikiloderma with atrophy, telangiectasia and patchy hyper- and hypopigmentation. The skin changes occur on the face, extremities and buttocks. Photosensitivity, sometimes severe, occurs in 30% of cases. In some patients verrucose lesions develop in late childhood on the dorsum and sides of hands and feet, on palms and soles, and occasionally elsewhere on the limbs. Once established, the cutaneous changes remain static throughout life. Squamous cell carcinoma may occur on both verrucose and atrophic lesions. There may be alopecia of scalp and secondary sexual hair, and nails may be dystrophic. Hypodontia may occur.

The patients are often of short stature with hypogonadism of variable degree. An increased incidence of hyperparathyroidism is reported. Ocular abnormalities, particularly juvenile cataracts, occur in over 50% of cases. A wide variety of skeletal abnormalities occur and there have been several reports of osteogenic sarcoma. Mental development and life expectancy are usually normal.

Erythropoietic porphyrias

The porphyrias are an important group of diseases which result from enzyme deficiencies in the heme synthesis pathway. Two important examples cause photosensitivity in childhood, and both are inherited.

Erythropoietic protoporphyria

This autosomal dominant condition is relatively common, and is associated with reduced ferrochelatase activity. It usually presents with photosensitivity which is relatively mild (cf. congenital erythropoietic porphyria). The child complains of burning of the skin either during or after exposure to sunlight, which may be followed by an erythematous rash in light-exposed areas. As the activating wavelengths are in the ultraviolet A and visible light spectra, the photosensitivity will also occur through window glass. Eventually small pock-like scars appear on the nose and cheeks, with thickening of the skin of the dorsum of the hands, which may give a clue as to the diagnosis. In due course, usually in adulthood, gallstones become a problem, and eventually hepatic cirrhosis may develop.

The diagnosis is confirmed by examination of the child's erythrocytes using a fluorescence lamp (400 nm radiation) when the red cells demonstrate a red fluorescent color. Erythrocyte protoporphyrin levels are markedly elevated, though the urinary and fecal porphyrins are normal.

The normal management of the child entails avoidance of the sun and the effective use of sunscreens (SPF 30+). In severe cases, treatment with β-carotene may be helpful at a dosage of 50–200 mg daily to maintain serum levels of 0.5 mg/100 ml.

Congenital erythropoietic porphyria (Gunther's disease)

This autosomal recessive type of porphyria is rare. It results from uroporphyrinogen III cosynthase deficiency.

The child presents with severe light sensitivity in infancy, with erythema, blistering (subepidermal blisters) and ulceration of the face, ears and the dorsum of the hands. This may also occur through window glass as the activating wavelengths are in the ultraviolet A and visible light spectra (320–450 nm). The child characteristically passes pink urine, and there may be a brown discoloration of the teeth, which fluoresce red under Wood's light. With the passage of time, very marked scarring may develop in the light-exposed areas, particularly of the face and ears, which may result in marked disfiguration. Hypertrichosis may be prominent on the face. Fingernails may be lost, as may the tips of the digits eventually. A fatal outcome is usual in the second or third decade due to anemia, hepatic or renal failure.

The diagnosis is made by estimation of the erythrocyte porphyrins (particularly coproporphyrin) which are very high, the finding of uroporphyrin and coproporphyrin in the urine, and coproporphyrin and protoporphyrin in the feces.

There is no satisfactory treatment at present. Management depends on avoidance of the sun and the use of the most powerful sunscreens (e.g. physical sunscreens such as zinc oxide and titanium dioxide).

INFECTIONS AND INFESTATIONS OF THE SKIN

VIRUS INFECTIONS

Herpes simplex (Plate 25.10)

Herpes simplex virus (HSV) infections are extremely common in children, and serological studies confirm that more than 90% of the population have been infected by adulthood. The commonest type is HSV1, though HSV2 is more important in adulthood, being the cause of genital herpes. Four distinct presentations are recognized in childhood.

Neonatal herpes simplex virus infection (Fig. 25.11)

This is a potentially devastating infection usually contracted during delivery from infected vaginal secretions (HSV2). However, intrauterine and postnatal infection may occur. Approximately 50% of infected infants have skin lesions which are manifested as grouped blisters localized initially on the presenting part, usually the head, with the onset usually between the fourth and eighth days of life. The eruption may become

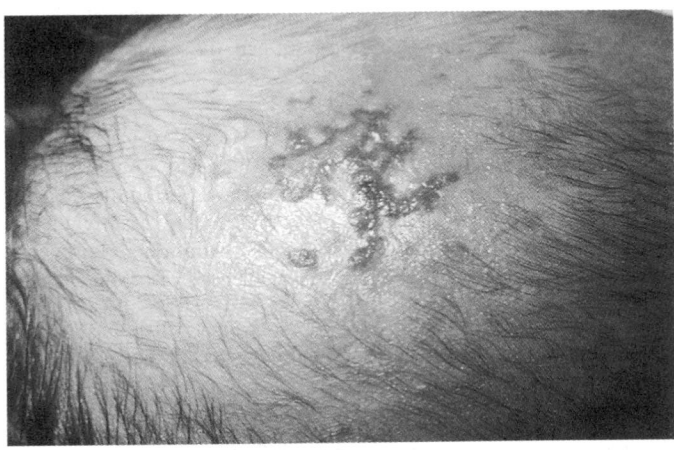

Fig. 25.11   Neonatal herpes on scalp.

widespread with individual lesions a few millimeters across coalescing to produce large erosions. A rapid immunofluorescence test on material from the blister base enables a diagnosis within a few hours. Culture of the virus takes several days. A rising titer of complement-fixing antibodies can be demonstrated comparing acute and convalescent sera.

The child with cutaneous neonatal herpes should be assessed urgently for the presence and extent of other organ involvement. Immediate treatment with intravenous acyclovir is indicated.

Primary herpetic gingivostomatitis (Fig. 25.12)

This is a common presentation of HSV infection in children. The child is systemically unwell with a high fever and there is severe swelling, erosion and bleeding of the gums and the anterior part of the buccal mucosa. Posterior spread is rare but anterior spread to the lips and the facial skin often occurs. There may be considerable soft tissue swelling and prominent lymphadenopathy. The condition is extremely painful and the child often refuses to eat or drink, necessitating parenteral fluids as the condition may take up to 2 weeks to resolve. Having the child suck ice blocks helps clean the mouth, or large cotton wool swabs soaked with water can be used. Oral antibiotics may be required

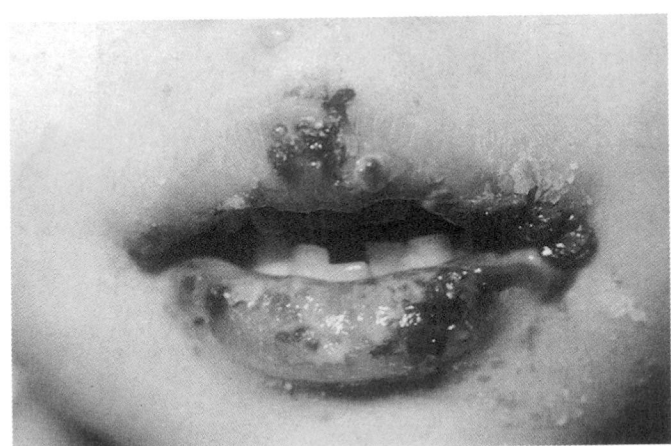

Fig. 25.12   Perioral herpes simplex.

for secondary bacterial infection. Unless the condition is very severe systemic antiviral therapy is not usually required.

Recurrent herpes simplex (herpes labialis)

Recurrent herpes simplex of the face, particularly around the lips (herpes labialis), is common in childhood. As in adults various factors, including fever and sun exposure, may reactivate the virus. Saline bathing of the lesions speeds resolution and prevents secondary infection. Topical antiviral agents are of limited value.

Disseminated herpes simplex (eczema herpeticum) (Fig. 25.13)

This occurs as a complication of atopic eczema and in immunosuppressed patients. It may originate from a primary or recurrent infection, or from external reinfection. Spread is both on the surface of the skin and also by hematogenous dissemination. The lesions are vesicles or pustules 2–4 mm across which may spread with alarming rapidity and have a tendency to coalescence to produce extensive and quite deep erosions. Topical agents should be avoided as their application may spread the virus. Secondary bacterial infection should be treated with oral antibiotics and saline or tap water packs relieve discomfort and dry out the lesions. In severe cases systemic acyclovir is indicated.

Herpes zoster (Fig. 25.14)

Herpes zoster (or shingles) is caused by the same herpes virus which produces chickenpox (the varicella zoster virus). It usually occurs when this virus, which has remained dormant in the cells of dorsal root or cranial nerve ganglia following an attack of

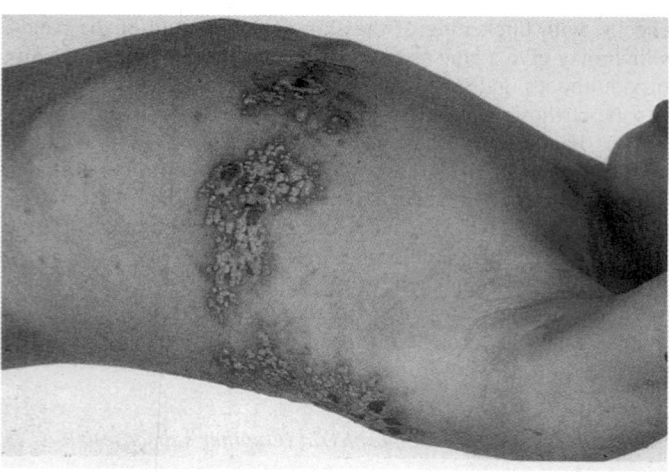

Fig. 25.14 Herpes zoster.

chickenpox, reactivates, replicates and spreads along the nerves from these ganglia to infect areas of skin supplied by them. Herpes zoster is much less common in children than adults but it may occur as early as the first year of life. In children who develop zoster in the first 2 years of life, there is rarely a history of previous chickenpox in the child but often a history of maternal chickenpox during pregnancy.

Herpes zoster presents as a segmental blistering eruption on an erythematous base. Crops of blisters erupt over 5–7 days spreading from a point nearest the central nervous system along the dermatome of skin supplied by the affected nerves to produce a solid or interrupted band of lesions, which may become pustular or hemorrhagic before drying and crusting over a further 1–2 weeks to leave normal skin or postinflammatory hypopigmentation. Scarring is rare in healthy patients and in the absence of severe secondary infection, although cicatricial alopecia may result from scalp lesions. Usually a single dermatome is affected but spread to one or two adjoining dermatomes may occur. The eruption is essentially unilateral though there may be minor spread to the opposite side on the trunk or brow. Up to 20 or 30 scattered lesions identical to chickenpox commonly occur. Infection involving the ophthalmic division of the 5th cranial (trigeminal) nerve may produce keratitis and uveitis, threatening vision. An important cutaneous sign of potentially dangerous herpes zoster ophthalmicus is blisters on the nose indicating involvement of the nasociliary branch. Blisters in the oral cavity occur with involvement of maxillary and mandibular divisions of the trigeminal nerve. Anogenital blistering and sometimes disorders of urination and defecation occur with involvement of sacral nerves.

Prolonged eruption of vesicles, severely necrotic lesions and postherpetic neuralgia are all very rare in children. Zoster in prepubertal children is usually a fairly mild condition with minimal morbidity and only moderate local pain while the blisters are erupting.

Management

This is directed at providing symptomatic treatment with wet compresses and appropriate analgesia, and dealing with any secondary bacterial infection. Early ophthalmological consultation is essential for ophthalmic zoster patients. Intravenous acyclovir is

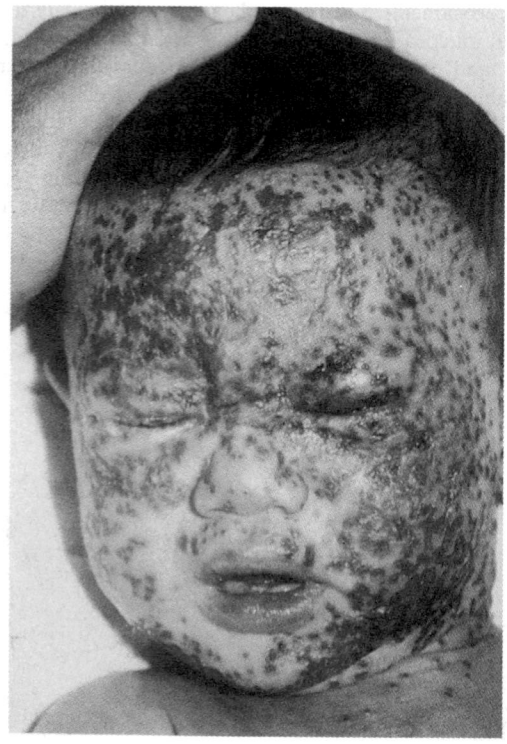

Fig. 25.13 Disseminated herpes simplex (eczema herpeticum).

indicated in very severe cases, particularly of ophthalmic zoster and for all immunosuppressed patients.

Most children with zoster are and remain in good general health: in an otherwise well child no immunological investigation or search for internal malignancy is indicated (Wurzel et al 1986).

Molluscum contagiosum (Plate 25.11)

This is a poxvirus infection, which is rare under 1 year of age, and occurs particularly in the 2–5 year age group. Outbreaks may occur among children who bath or swim together and in the adolescent age group sexual transmission becomes important. The typical lesion is spherical and pearly white with a central umbilication, but they may vary from tiny 1 mm papules to large nodules over 1 cm in diameter. They occur on any part of the skin surface with common sites being the axillae and sides of the trunk, the lower abdomen and anogenital area. Rarely they occur on the eyelids where they may cause conjunctivitis and punctate keratitis. A secondary eczema often occurs around lesions, particularly in atopics, and scratching of this spreads the mollusca. Hundreds of lesions may be present in an individual patient. Secondary bacterial infection may occur producing crusting, erythema and suppuration. However, these same changes may be seen during spontaneous resolution which occurs in most within several months leaving normal skin or small varicelliform scars.

Mollusca may clinically simulate warts or skin tags but they have a distinct histological appearance with lobulated downgrowths of epidermal cells containing intracytoplasmic inclusion bodies.

Management

Mollusca are surprisingly resistant to chemical therapies. The most definitive treatment is deroofing of the lesion with a large cutting-edged needle and wiping out the contents. The lesion itself is virtually anesthetic and this procedure can be performed almost painlessly with large lesions where the needle can be introduced into the molluscum without penetrating the surrounding or underlying skin. With multiple small lesions in a young child spontaneous resolution should be awaited, but if the lesions are troublesome due to site, surrounding eczema or frequent secondary infection removal under general anesthetic may rarely be considered.

Children should shower rather than bath and avoid heated swimming pools and spas; with these precautions the number of lesions spontaeously disappearing soon outweighs the number of new lesions appearing and the overall numbers drop off.

Warts

Warts are benign tumors caused by infection with a variety of papilloma viruses of the papova group.

The common wart (verruca vulgaris) occurs particularly on hands, knees and elbows. Plane or flat warts, 1–3 mm pink or brown barely raised papules, occur on the face and often spread along scratch marks or cuts. Plantar warts occur particularly over pressure points on the soles and can be differentiated from calluses by a loss of skin markings over the skin surface. Warts at mucocutaneous junctions often have a filiform or fronded appearance. Anogenital warts may be acquired from maternal

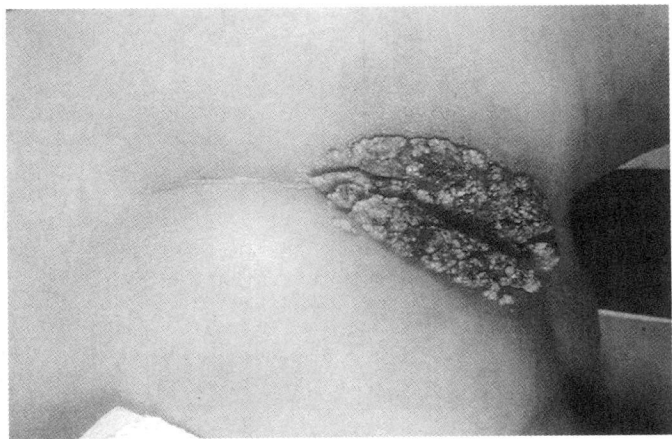

Fig. 25.15 Perianal warts.

infection during delivery, but their presence should always raise the suspicion of sexual abuse (Fig. 25.15).

Management

Various forms of treatment are available: they depend on the area, the type of wart and the age of the patient. Because spontaneous disappearance is common, aggressive treatment is usually inappropriate. Keratolytic wart paints (e.g. salicylic acid, lactic acid and collodion) are fairly effective provided they are applied diligently. These preparations are applied daily with or without plaster occlusion. For facial plane warts retinoic acid preparations are often effective. Podophyllin is useful for isolated anogenital warts but is extremely irritant and should be used with caution. Plantar warts can be treated with very strong keratolytics such as Upton's paste applied under plaster, or by a 20% formalin solution used daily to harden the surface, combined with serial paring. Cautery or diathermy are useful for lesions on the lips or anogenital area. Elsewhere recurrence is fairly frequent following their use and there is also a risk of producing a painful scar, particularly over the joints of digits or on palms or soles. Liquid nitrogen cryotherapy is a successful method of dealing with common warts and is useful for older children. Recently, oral cimetidine has been demonstrated to be a useful treatment in some cases of multiple refractory warts (Orlow & Paller 1993).

Papular acrodermatitis of childhood (Gianotti–Crosti syndrome) (Fig. 25.16)

Papular acrodermatitis of childhood was first described by Gianotti as an acrally distributed papular eruption occurring in young children with anicteric hepatitis subsequently shown to be due to the hepatitis B virus. However, a similar eruption may occur with a number of other viruses and the condition is best regarded as a reaction pattern with multiple etiologies (Taieb et al 1986). The viruses implicated include hepatitis B, hepatitis A, enteroviruses, adenoviruses, Epstein–Barr virus, cytomegalovirus, parainfluenza viruses, and rotavirus.

This pattern of exanthem occurs particularly in children between 1 and 4 years. The rash comprises discrete firm red papules 1–5 mm in diameter, sometimes surmounted by vesicles. Pruritus is variable and sometimes severe. The lesions involve the

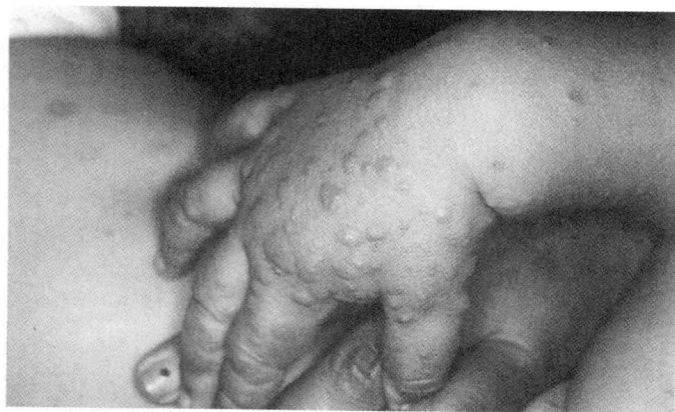

Fig. 25.16   Papular acrodermatitis of childhood.

limbs, particularly distally, and the face, with the trunk being essentially spared. The rash is persistent, lasting 3–12 weeks. Lymphadenopathy is usually present but the child is often otherwise remarkably well, leading to such misdiagnoses as insect bites and papular eczema.

Investigation should be aimed at excluding the more serious viral etiologies.

Pityriasis rosea (Fig. 25.17)

The etiology of this condition is unknown but epidemiological studies suggest a viral origin. It occurs in children and young adults and has no sexual or racial predilection.

The eruption commences with the appearance of the so-called herald patch, typically a single round or oval scaly lesion 1–5 cm

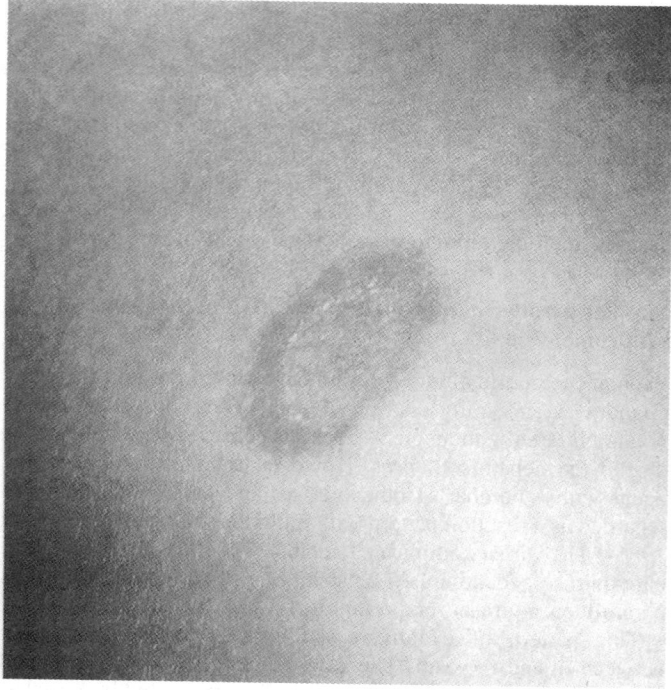

Fig. 25.17   Pityriasis rosea (herald patch).

in diameter, flat or slightly raised with a tendency to clear in the center. It usually occurs on the trunk, neck or proximal limbs. Some 5–15 days later the secondary eruption appears comprising multiple, variably pruritic, dull pink, oval macules with a peripheral collarette of scale. The typical distribution is on trunk and proximal limbs but may be very extensive. The long axis of the lesions on the trunk runs parallel with the ribs giving a 'fir tree' pattern. Rarer variants have lesions which are papular, urticarial, vesicular, purpuric or pustular but some of the typical lesions are usually intermingled. Lesions crop at 2–3 day intervals for 7–10 days and then spontaneous resolution occurs over several weeks. Sun exposure may speed this resolution and meanwhile symptomatic therapy can be used for the pruritus if this is troublesome.

BACTERIAL INFECTIONS

Staphylococcal and streptococcal infections of the skin are common in childhood. They take the following clinical forms:

Impetigo (Fig. 25.18)

This is a bacterial infection caused by *Staphylococcus aureus*, Group A streptococcus or a combination of these organisms. Recently there has been a worldwide increase in the predominance of staphylococci in the causation of impetigo (Coskey & Coskey 1987, Barton et al 1988).

Impetigo occurs in two forms, bullous and nonbullous (or crusted). Bullous impetigo is always due to staphylococci. Blisters arise on previously normal skin and increase rapidly in size and number, soon rupturing to produce superficial erosions with a peripheral brown crust. The erosions continue to expand, sometimes clearing centrally to produce annular lesions. The condition is usually neither itchy nor painful. Nonbullous impetigo may be due to either organism or to a combination. The lesions begin with a small transient vesicle on an erythematous base. The serum exuding from the ruptured vesicle produces a thick soft yellow crust, below which there is a moist superficial erosion. The lesions extend slowly and remain much smaller than those of bullous impetigo. Impetigo is often superimposed on other skin diseases such as insect bites, scabies, pediculosis and atopic eczema. As impetigo is an intraepidermal infection, the

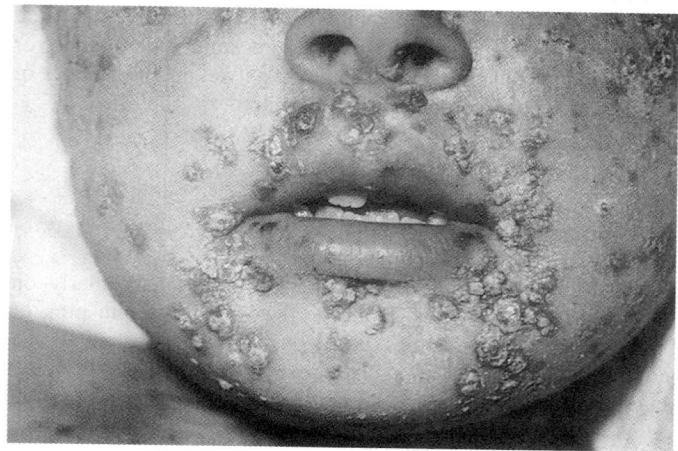

Fig. 25.18   Impetigo.

condition does not scar although postinflammatory pigmentation can occur, particularly in dark-skinned patients.

Management

Impetigo is very infectious and the patient should, if possible, be isolated. Saline bathing may be used to dry out the lesions and a swab for culture and sensitivity testing should always be taken. Topical mupirocin may be successful for localized early disease but in general oral antibiotics should be used. Because of the rarity in most areas of pure streptococcal impetigo, a penicillinase-resistant penicillin or erythromycin are the treatments of choice while awaiting culture results. In many areas of the world there is an emergence of erythromycin-resistant staphylococci (Rogers et al 1987, Coskey & Coskey 1987) and a knowledge of the local situation is important in selecting the antibiotic of first choice while awaiting sensitivity testing. Underlying diseases should be sought and treated appropriately if the pattern of impetigo suggests them. If a group A streptococcus is isolated the patient should be watched for 8 weeks for signs of glomerulonephritis.

Furunculosis

Furuncles or boils are cutaneous abscesses, centered around hair follicles, caused by a wide variety of types and strains of *Staphylococcus aureus* (*S. aureus*). When several furuncles are grouped they may become confluent, producing carbuncles with multiple draining points.

Furuncles are caused by the penetration of *S. aureus* through a hair follicle in an area of damaged, or more often clinically normal skin. Predisposing factors are friction, maceration and sweating, and so common sites are around the neck, axillae, groin and waistline. In the great majority of cases there is no impairment of host defenses but patients with diabetes, hypogammaglobulinemia, neutrophil function defects and general debility are at particular risk. Patients with recurrent attacks are often found to carry the virulent strains of *S. aureus* in their nose, axilla or perineum, or to be in close contact with another person who is a carrier. Boils commence as firm erythematous papules which evolve into fluctuant nodules which undergo central necrosis (pointing) and discharge their contained pus. Rarely they resorb and resolve without rupture.

Furunculosis should be treated with oral antistaphylococcal antibiotics after a swab has been taken for culture. Drainage of individual lesions is indicated only if they are mature and pointing and not discharging spontaneously: it should be avoided with lesions in the external auditory meatus and on the center of the face because of the remote risk of cavernous sinus thrombosis following spreading infection in these areas.

Chronic and recurrent furunculosis should be treated with a course of antibiotics of several weeks' duration and attempts to eliminate the carrier state with antibacterial soaps and washes and intranasal instillation of neomycin, bacitracin or fusidic acid. Other carriers who are in close contact should be identified and treated. Laundering in hot water is important to eliminate organisms from clothing and linen.

Cellulitis

This is an acute bacterial infection involving the subcutis as well as the dermis. The lesion is erythematous sometimes with a purple or blue hue. It is warm and tender and has a less well defined edge than erysipelas. Fever and malaise, leukocytosis and lymphadenopathy are usually present. When cellulitis follows a wound or other break in the skin, group A β-hemolytic streptococcus (GABHS) is the commonest cause. Other organisms involved in cellulitis include *Haemophilus influenzae*, *Streptococcus pneumoniae*, *Staphylococcus aureus* and *Pseudomonas aeruginosa*. Two special forms are discussed below.

Streptococcal perianal cellulitis (Plate 25.12)

This is a recently recognized entity occurring in children between 1 and 10 years. The child complains of painful defecation and bright blood is often found on the stool. There is a well-demarcated, very bright red erythema extending out several centimeters from the anus. The anal rim is often macerated and fissured. GABHS is grown from the skin and often also from the patient's throat. The condition may be surprisingly resistant to therapy, recurring after 5–10 days of oral penicillin therapy: an initial course of at least 14 days is advisable. The addition of topical mupurocin to the therapy further reduces the risk of recurrence. The newer term streptococcal perianal disease is preferred.

Facial cellulitis

Facial cellulitis in young children often occurs in the absence of any break in the skin and is due to *Haemophilus influenzae* or *Streptococcus pneumoniae* accompanying an upper respiratory tract infection or otitis media. Cellulitis due to these bacteria often has a lilac-blue color. The condition may be complicated by bacteremia, septicemia and meningitis. In all cases of facial cellulitis cultures should be taken from nasopharynx, ears, blood and, if indicated, cerebrospinal fluid. Needle aspiration from the lesion after saline injection may provide material from which the organism can be cultured.

Intravenous cefotaxime, a third generation cephalosporin, is the initial treatment of choice until an organism is identified and sensitivity tests performed.

Erysipelas

This is an acute bacterial infection of the dermal connective tissue and superficial lymphatics caused most often by group A β-hemolytic streptococcus but occasionally due to other streptococci, *Haemophilus influenzae* and *Staphylococcus aureus*. The lesion is brightly erythematous, hot, tender, and with a rapidly spreading distinct edge. Superimposed bullae may occur. There is accompanying fever and malaise and a leukocytosis. Predisposing factors include lymphatic obstruction and a break in the skin due, for example, to a wound, bite or tinea infection. The episode produces a lymphangitis which further damages the lymphatics, and chronic lymphedema may result from and further predispose to recurrent erysipelas. Treatment involves rest and high doses of the appropriate antibiotic, usually penicillin V, orally or intravenously depending on the severity.

Staphylococcal scalded skin syndrome (Figs 25.19 and 25.20)

Pathogenesis

The staphylococcal scalded skin syndrome (SSSS) is a widespread blistering disease caused by an epidermolytic toxin

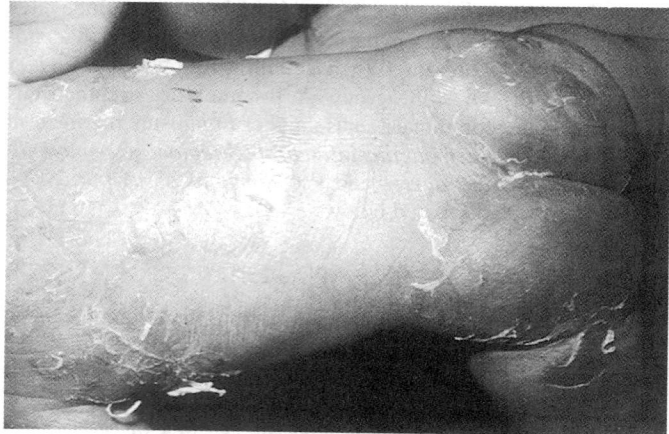

Fig. 25.19   Staphylococcal scalded skin syndrome.

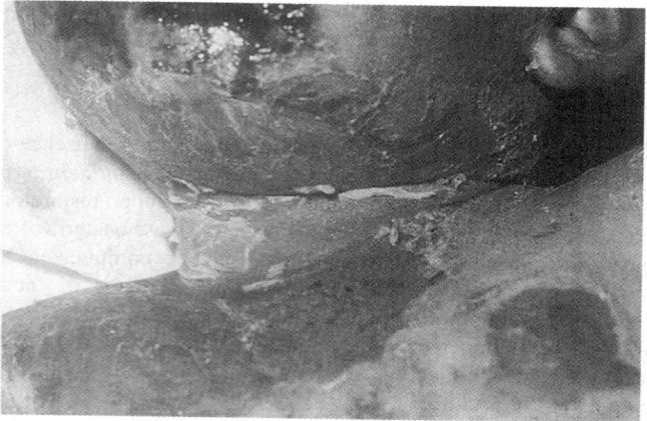

Fig. 25.20   Staphylococcal scalded skin syndrome.

produced by certain strains of *Staphylococcus aureus*, most often of phage group 2, types 70/71 or 51 but occasionally of phage group 1. This toxin produces a superficial splitting of the skin with the level of split being high in the epidermis. Clinical disease occurs when there is sufficient toxin load produced from an infection with these organisms. The commonest sites of infection are the umbilicus (in neonates), the nose, nasopharynx or throat, the conjunctiva and deep wounds.

Clinical features

The condition commences with a macular erythema initially on the face and in the major flexures and then becoming generalized. The skin is exquisitely tender and the child draws back from contact. After 2 days flaccid bullae develop and the skin wrinkles and shears off. The exfoliation is most marked in groin, neck fold and around the mouth and may involve the entire body surface but mucosa remain uninvolved. The child is usually febrile but because of the superficial level of the split fluid loss is rarely significant. The erosions crust and dry and heal with desquamation over the next 4–8 days leaving no sequelae.

Diagnosis

Cultures from skin and blister fluid are usually negative. Cultures should be obtained from any area of obvious infection but, if none is apparent, from nasopharynx and throat. The most important differential diagnosis is toxic epidermal necrolysis (TEN). In TEN the split is subepidermal and the blisters and erosions are usually hemorrhagic and mucosae are commonly involved. Microscopy of a Giemsa-stained section of the blister roof can detect the level of the split in the two conditions. Other conditions from which SSSS may be differentiated are scarlet fever, Kawasaki's syndrome and toxic shock syndrome, all of which show mucosal involvement and rarely demonstrate frank blistering.

Management

The child should be nursed naked on a nonstick material and handled as little as possible. No topical agents should be applied. A penicillinase-resistant penicillin is the treatment of choice and should be given orally if possible. Insertion and securing of an intravenous line is very painful in these patients and should be performed only if oral antibiotics are refused or if rehydration is required in a child refusing oral fluids. Analgesia is often necessary in the early stages. Emollients are useful once the skin dries and desquamation commences.

FUNGAL INFECTIONS

Tinea (Fig. 25.21)

This is an infection due to dermatophyte fungi: the source of the fungus is an animal (e.g. dog, cat, guinea pig, cattle), the soil or another human. Tinea occurs on any part of the skin surface and can involve hair and nails.

The classical features of tinea on the skin are itch, erythema studded with papules or pustules, annular or geographical lesions ('ringworm') with a tendency to central clearing and a superficial scale. On the palms and soles erythema and increased skin markings may be the only signs. Between the toes maceration with a thick white scale is the main finding and an annular lesion may extend onto the dorsum of the foot. On the soles there are deep seated blisters or pustules which dry to produce brown

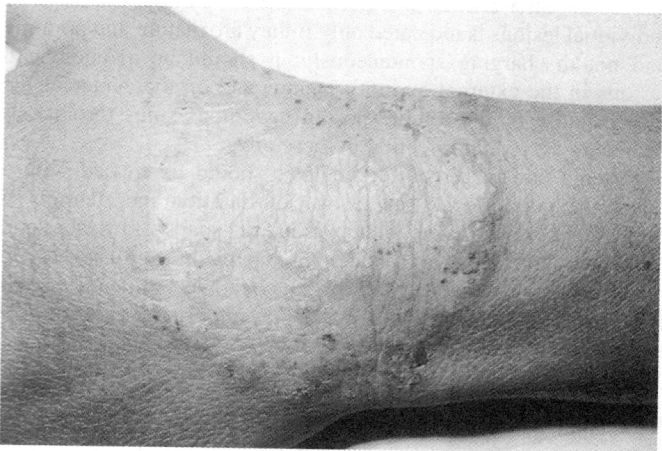

Fig. 25.21   Tinea.

crusts. Tinea is often unilateral and always asymmetrical, whereas eczema and psoriasis, which it may resemble, are often symmetrical in distribution. Nail tinea produces a white discoloration and crumbling of the nail plate with an accumulation of subungual debris.

On the scalp there is a characteristic combination of alopecia and inflammation with the hair loss being due to breaking of the hair shafts. Depending on the pattern of hair invasion by the fungus, the hairs are either broken off flush with the scalp or at lengths of up to 2–3 mm, but in an individual case all the hairs break at the same length. The inflammation varies from mild erythema and a fine dandruff-like scale to a pustular carbuncle-like lesion (kerion). Tinea causes a localized or patchy alopecia and the main conditions to be differentiated are trichotillomania and alopecia areata. In alopecia areata hairs are completely lost and there is no inflammation so the scalp is smooth and quite bald. In trichotillomania where hairs are plucked or twisted, breaks are seen at different lengths and inflammation is usually absent. Wood's light (an ultraviolet lamp) is useful in the diagnosis of some varieties of scalp tinea with the infected hairs fluorescing a bright green color. Other varieties of scalp tinea produce no typical fluorescence and the Wood's light has no place in the diagnosis of tinea on the skin surface. The diagnosis of tinea is confirmed by scraping hairs or scales onto a slide, adding 20% potassium hydroxide and examining the specimen microscopically. Septate branching hyphae are seen in skin scales and spores are found in hair. The fungus can be cultured on appropriate media.

Topical antifungals (Whitfield's ointment, imidazole creams) may be satisfactory for small localized patches of tinea on the skin. However, griseofulvin is the treatment of choice for longstanding or severe cutaneous tinea, and all hair and nail tinea: this fat-soluble drug is best taken after meals, preferably with a glass of milk. In general a 3-month course is used but nail tinea is treated until the nail grows out normally.

Candidiasis (moniliasis) (Fig. 25.22)

This is due to a nondermatophyte fungus, *Candida albicans*. It occurs on both skin and mucosal surfaces and certain factors predispose to its establishment. General predisposing factors include drug therapy with broad spectrum antibiotics, the oral

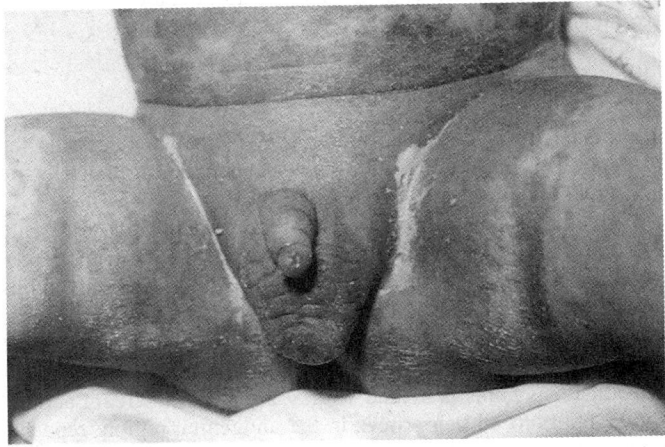

Fig. 25.22 Candidiasis.

contraceptive, corticosteroids and immunosuppressives, diabetes, pregnancy, general debility and any disease which interferes with immunological competence. Local predisposing factors are particularly those which create a warm moist environment. Flexural areas are susceptible, especially in the presence of sweating, obesity and other skin disease. The oral mucosa in infancy also has a particular susceptibility to this infection which is usually acquired during passage through an infected birth canal.

On the general body skin, where candidiasis rarely occurs except in the presence of immunodeficiency, the infection is manifested by small round erythematous lesions with a peripheral overhanging scale. Occasionally small papules or superficial pustules occur, especially in the neonate. In flexural areas the typical picture is of a cheesy white material deep in the folds and satellite lesions with the typical peripheral scale. On mucosae a curd-like white material is superimposed on a red base.

Chronic mucocutaneous candidiasis is a progressive candidal infection occurring in patients who have an inability to destroy candida due to a severe general immunodeficiency or due to a specific immunological defect. A variety of endocrinopathies may be associated with this syndrome. Initially, typical candida lesions become chronic and then become progressively hyperplastic, producing thick crusted plaques, even warty or horn-like lesions, occurring particularly around face and scalp, hands and feet. A nail dystrophy with thick crumbling nail plates and abundant subungual debris may occur and scalp hair may be lost. On the mucosae extensive thick white verrucose plaques occur.

The diagnosis is usually a clinical one which may be confirmed by microscopy and culture. Candida is frequently a secondary invader rather than a primary cause of skin disease and local and general predisposing factors should be eliminated. Once predisposing factors have been eliminated most localized infections respond well to topical agents including polyene antibiotics, nystatin and imidazole derivatives. Reduction of intestinal carriage with oral preparations is rarely necessary. Oral ketoconazole is useful in chronic mucocutaneous candidiasis and other candidal infections in the immunosuppressed.

Tinea versicolor (pityriasis versicolor)

This is an infection with *Pityrosporum* species which are part of the normal skin flora. It occurs mainly in tropical and temperate zones and usually affects adolescents and young adults. It presents as well-demarcated, asymptomatic or slightly itchy macules with a fine branny scale which is often only obvious on light scratching of the lesions. Primary macules 1–10 mm in diameter coalesce into larger patches. They occur in two colors, red-brown especially in the fair skinned and hypopigmented in darker skinned. In a partially tanned individual, lesions of both colors may he found. In young children it often presents with only facial lesions and almost invariably a parent or older relative will have tinea versicolor in the typical distribution.

Diagnosis is confirmed by microscopic examination of skin scrapings to which 20% potassium hydroxide has been added. Grape-like clusters of spores and short fragments of thick mycelia are seen. In its hypopigmented forms the condition must be distinguished from: (a) vitiligo, where the depigmentation is total and scale absent; (b) pityriasis alba where lesions are less well demarcated and some erythema may be seen; and (c) tuberculoid leprosy which is accompanied by anesthesia in the hypopigmented areas. The red-brown form has to be differentiated from seborrheic dermatitis, tinea and psoriasis, all of which lack the very fine branny type of scale.

Untreated the condition is persistent though some improvement may occur in winter. Various treatments are available. The treatment of choice is with topical imidazole creams. Alternatively two overnight applications of 2.5% selenium sulfide may be effective in the short term but relapse is frequent. With the depigmented form, whatever therapy is used sun exposure is required for full repigmentation.

ECTOPARASITIC INFESTATIONS

Scabies

This is due to *Sarcoptes scabei*, an eight-legged, oval-shaped mite less than 0.5 mm in length. The disease is transmitted by close physical contact: transmission by fomites is exceptional.

A small number of mites burrow into the skin in certain sites, particularly between the fingers, the ulnar border of the hand, around the wrists and elbows, the anterior axillary fold, nipples and penis and, in infants, the palms and soles. The pathognomonic primary lesion, a typical burrow, is rarely seen. It is a 2–3 mm long curved gray line with a vesicle at the anterior end. Other lesions which mark the sites of burrows are small blisters or papules, larger blisters on the palms and soles of infants, scratch marks, secondary eczema and secondary bacterial infection. Eczema or impetigo in the target areas for scabies should always raise suspicion of this disease as should blisters on the palms and soles of infants.

Often more prominent than the evidence of burrows is the so-called secondary eruption of scabies. This presents as multiple, very pruritic, urticarial papules which are soon excoriated. They occur particularly on the abdomen, thighs and buttocks. Young children may show a striking dermographism in the areas of scratch marks. When dermographism occurs in the first year of life scabies should always be suspected. Large inflammatory nodules may form part of the secondary eruption, occurring particularly on covered areas especially on axillae, scrotum, penis and buttocks. They may, however, be very widespread producing diagnostic difficulties. They may persist for months after effective scabies treatment.

The diagnosis of scabies is usually a clinical one but can be confirmed by demonstration of the mite, an art which can be mastered with practice. A burrow, which may be softened by the application of 20% potassium hydroxide, is scraped and the material smeared on a slide for microscopic examination. Burrows may be more easily identified by rubbing a thick black marking pen over suspicious areas and wiping with an alcohol swab leaving a burrow outlined with ink.

Management

The patient and all close contacts should be treated simultaneously. The treatment of choice is 5% permethrin cream: it should be applied to all body surfaces from the neck down and left on overnight. A repeat application should be administered after 1 week. Bedclothes and clothing should be washed in the normal way with no disinfection required. An irritant dermatitis may follow scabies treatment, particularly in atopics, and may require emollients and topical steroids once the miticide therapy is fully completed. Persistent nodules may respond to topical corticosteroids but a coal tar solution painted on is preferable for the very resistant ones.

Pediculosis (lice)

Human lice are ectoparasites dependent on man for survival. They are wingless six-legged insects, gray-white in color or red-brown when engorged with blood. The head louse (*Pediculus humanus capitis*) and the body louse (*Pediculus humanus humanus*) have a 2–4 mm long slim body and three similar pairs of legs. The pubic louse (*Pthirus pubis*, crab louse) has a wider, shorter body 1–2 mm long and the second and third pairs of legs are larger than the first, producing a crab-like appearance. The nits or ova are seen as oval gray-white 0.5 mm specks firmly attached by a chitinous ring to hairs or clothing.

Pediculosis capitis

This is a very common infection, occurring in epidemics amongst schoolchildren. The infestation is most severe in and may be confined to the occipital area. It is very itchy and excoriations are seen but secondary eczematization and bacterial infection may mask the condition. Nits may be differentiated from epidermal scales and hair casts by their firm attachment and by fluorescence with a Wood's light. Occasionally the head louse infects the eyelashes in children (Plate 25.13).

Pediculosis corporis

This is rare in children except in conditions of overcrowding and poor hygiene. The louse infects bedding and seams of clothing and nits are not found on the human. With body warmth the pediculi hatch and puncture the skin to produce small urticarial papules with hemorrhagic puncta. Pruritus is extreme and scratch marks are the main clinical sign.

Pediculosis pubis

The pubic hairs are the normal habitat of *Pthirus pubis* but it may also infect facial hair, eyelashes, general body hair and rarely the frontal margin of the scalp. Pubic infestation is usually sexually transmitted but bedding and towels may be responsible. Clinical signs may be minimal, even with severe itching, but excoriated papules and flat blue macules containing altered blood pigment may be seen as may evidence of secondary infection or eczematization. Eyelash infestation in children may occur from innocent close contact with an infected adult but the possibility of sexual abuse must always be considered.

Management of pediculosis

The management of pediculosis corporis involves removing the infestation from clothing with hot water laundering, hot electric drying, hot ironing or dry cleaning.

Permethrin shampoo is an effective pediculocide for scalp infestations but the efficacy as an ovicide is less certain and repeat application after a few days is recommended. Removal of nits with a fine comb can be facilitated by prior wrapping of the scalp for 1–2 hours in a towel soaked in vinegar which softens the chitin.

Pediculosis pubis is treated with 5% permethrin cream applied for 12 hours to all hairy areas in the anogenital region, repeated after 1 week. Sexual contacts should be treated simultaneously and all underclothing appropriately laundered.

Pediculosis of eyelashes is best treated with petroleum jelly applied thickly twice a day for a week.

Papular urticaria

This is a very common condition in children, and results from insect, flea or mite bites. In Britain dog, cat and bird fleas are the usual cause, but human fleas, bed bugs, mosquitoes and dog lice may be implicated. The child presents with papules and blisters on exposed skin such as the legs and arms. Each lasts for about 7–10 days before resolving.

It often takes the parents quite a lot of convincing of the cause of the condition. The family pet should be inspected and treated if necessary. In recurrent cases it is worth admitting the child to hospital upon which the child's rash will promptly disappear.

HYPERSENSITIVITY DISEASE (and those diseases clinically related)

TYPE I HYPERSENSITIVITY: ANAPHYLACTIC HYPERSENSITIVITY

Urticaria

This is a classical example of anaphylactic type hypersensitivity. It is induced by IgE-mediated allergy, as in atopic children with food allergy. Mast cells may degranulate by mechanisms which are apparently not immunologically mediated, e.g. urticaria due to aspirin and strawberries. It is convenient to discuss all types of urticaria under the heading of Type I hypersensitivity.

The most characteristic feature of urticaria is its transience. Erythematous swellings develop in the skin, which last for a few hours before disappearing; in chronic idiopathic urticaria, these swellings recur frequently. The urticarial wheals may be of variable size, and may have an obvious anular configuration. Angioedema (giant urticaria) is a variant of urticaria which affects the face and genital region and mainly involves the subcutaneous tissues with resultant gross swelling of the tissues.

Urticaria is common in all age groups, and is particularly so in children. It is due to increased permeability of capillaries or other small vessels, with resultant transudation of fluid. Several chemical mediators are involved, which are mainly released from mast cells: these include histamine, prostaglandins and leukotrienes. Mast cells are numerous in the skin, and are found in the dermis at a density of about $7000/mm^3$. Mast cell degranulation results from both immune (IgE, complement) and nonimmune mechanisms (Fig. 25.23).

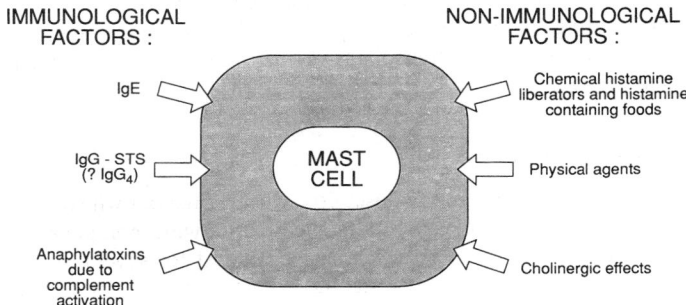

IMMUNOLOGICAL FACTORS :
- IgE
- IgG - STS (? IgG₄)
- Anaphylatoxins due to complement activation

NON-IMMUNOLOGICAL FACTORS :
- Chemical histamine liberators and histamine containing foods
- Physical agents
- Cholinergic effects

MAST CELL

Fig. 25.23 Pathogenesis of urticaria.

IgE-mediated urticaria and angioedema

Urticaria and angioedema following ingestion of food allergens is quite common in children with atopic eczema, and is often IgE mediated (confirmed by positive skin prick tests or radioallergosorbent tests). Swelling of the lips and tongue develops immediately after ingestion of the food, and contact urticaria may be seen if the food is in contact with the skin. If enough food allergen is ingested vomiting and diarrhea may occur, and the child may develop an asthmatic attack: generalized anaphylaxis may occur in a few children, especially with nuts. Widespread urticaria is common, usually occurring within 1 hour of ingestion of the food, which may last for a few hours. Common foods involved in such reactions include hens' eggs, cow's milk, fish, nuts and soya. Food allergy is commonly outgrown by the age of 5 years. IgE-mediated urticaria may also follow drug administration, particularly penicillin, and also insect stings, for example by bees or wasps.

Urticaria due to foods and drugs which is not apparently immunologically mediated

Certain foods such as strawberries, tomatoes and chocolate cause urticaria where no IgE-mediated mechanisms can be demonstrated. It seems likely that this is a direct effect on mast cells, and is similar to that caused by tartrazine (a common coloring in foods), benzoates and salicylates. Aspirin also commonly causes urticaria by a nonimmunological mechanism, but whether this is a direct effect on the mast cell or an effect on the cyclo-oxygenase pathway has yet to be determined.

Urticaria due to viral infections

In children, widespread urticaria is often the presenting feature of a number of viral infections, when it is accompanied by fever and malaise.

Chronic idiopathic urticaria

This type of urticaria is not very common in children. The urticaria recurs repeatedly for a period of years, with often daily exacerbations. By definition, no cause is found, but it is common for certain ingested chemicals in foods (e.g. salicylates, benzoates, food colorings) to make it worse.

Treatment of urticaria

The management of a child with urticaria depends on the cause. If a food is implicated, this is usually fairly obvious, except perhaps in infants where skin prick testing may be helpful. Any food implicated should be withdrawn from the diet, though it may be possible to reintroduce it when the child is older. In chronic idiopathic urticaria, treatment with an H1 antihistamine is indicated, such as terfenadine or astemizole.

TYPE II HYPERSENSITIVITY: CYTOTOXIC/CYTOLYTIC HYPERSENSITIVITY

This important group of conditions comprises the autoimmune diseases. By far the best understood of these diseases are pemphigoid and pemphigus, though both are rare in children.

Other conditions which have been ascribed to autoimmunity are chronic bullous disease of childhood, vitiligo and alopecia areata.

Juvenile pemphigoid

This is a rare blistering disease, which results from the formation of IgG antibodies to the basement membrane zone of the epidermis. The child presents with large and widespread blisters, which may (as in chronic bullous disease of childhood) be most marked on the face and around the genitalia. The diagnosis is confirmed by immunofluorescence of skin or serum (with appropriate substrate) to demonstrate antibasement membrane zone antibodies. Treatment is with oral steroids, which should be tapered off as the condition allows. In most the disease is self-limiting.

Pemphigus

Pemphigus is also rare in children, the most common type being pemphigus foliaceus. The blistering is less evident than in pemphigoid, though there may be widespread plaques and erosions. The diagnosis is confirmed by immunofluorescence studies of skin and serum, which demonstrate IgG antibodies to the intercellular substance of the keratinocytes in the epidermis. Treatment is with oral steroids, as in pemphigoid.

Chronic bullous disease of childhood (Plate 25.14)

This may well be a type of autoimmune disease, but the evidence for this is less strong than in pemphigoid or pemphigus. It is most commonly seen in young children, with blistering which is most marked around the neck and genital region. Immunofluorescence studies of skin show linear IgA deposition along the basement membrane zone of the epidermis with evidence of circulating IgA antibodies in some.

Treatment with dapsone or sulfapyridine usually clears the blisters very effectively. The disease is self-limiting, after months or years.

Vitiligo (Plate 25.15)

This is possibly an autoimmune disease. Though specific antimelanocyte antibodies cannot be demonstrated by immunofluorescence, complement-fixing antibody to melanocytes has been shown in some patients. It is well recognized that patients with vitiligo frequently have thyroid, gastric and adrenal autoantibodies: this is important because patients with autoimmunity often have more than one autoimmune disease. Vitiligo causes complete depigmentation of the skin (unlike tinea versicolor and pityriasis alba), and on histological examination there is an absence of melanocytes and melanin in the epidermis. Vitiligo is common in adults, and is not rare in children. The depigmentation is usually localized, but in some patients the condition is progressive to involve almost the whole body. Spontaneous repigmentation occurs more in children than in adults. In those that do not repigment photochemotherapy with topical 5-methoxypsoralen may be helpful. Otherwise stains may be applied to the depigmented skin to minimize disfiguration.

Alopecia areata (Plate 25.16)

It seems likely that at least in some patients with this condition the process is due to autoimmunity, though conclusive proof is lacking. As with vitiligo, there is an increased incidence of autoantibodies and autoimmune diseases. There is also an increased incidence of atopy, and atopic children are more likely to develop total alopecia. There may be a family history of alopecia areata.

Most children develop discoid areas of alopecia in the scalp with peripheral exclamation hairs, and these areas regrow hair normally in due course. In some children, however, particularly those with an ophiasifom distribution of hair loss (involving the temples and occipital region), the condition is progressive to become total and regrowth is much less likely. There are also nail changes, with fine pitting and horizontal depressions known as Beau's lines. Although alopecia areata is not a life threatening condition, it is obviously distressing for children and parents.

There is no effective treatment for alopecia areata at present. Intralesional steroids may cause some local hair growth but this has no permanent effect on the course of the alopecia. In older children, short contact dithranol treatment may induce hair growth but the result is rarely cosmetically acceptable. There is no evidence as yet that topical minoxidil is helpful.

TYPE III HYPERSENSITIVITY: IMMUNE COMPLEX-MEDIATED HYPERSENSITIVITY

This takes various forms, depending on the size of the vessel involved, the nature of the vessel, the size and solubility of the immune complexes and their antibody class, whether immune complexes are deposited from a distant site or formed locally, and the chronicity of immune complex formation. It follows then that immune complex-mediated reactions may take several different clinical forms. Examples include the following:

Allergic vasculitis (including Henoch–Schönlein purpura) (Plate 25.17)

This is relatively common, and is characterized by the development of purpura (often palpable) over the lower limbs, buttocks and forearms. Other organs involved in the vasculitis are the kidneys and intestinal vessels, resulting in proteinuria and hematuria, abdominal pain and gastrointestinal hemorrhage. In some children arthralgia is also prominent. In children it usually follows a virus or respiratory infection, the vasculitis resulting from deposition of immune complexes in the vessels of the skin, kidneys and intestines, with complement activation and resultant polymorph infiltration. In Henoch–Schönlein purpura the immunoglobulin deposited is IgA, whereas in other types of vasculitis it is IgG.

The prognosis is very variable. In most children the condition is self-limiting; others may develop renal failure (usually treatable with dialysis or renal transplant) or may die of gastrointestinal hemorrhage.

Urticarial vasculitis

This is a variant of allergic vasculitis, where urticarial wheals are prominent due to anaphylotoxin release following complement activation in vessels. The urticarial wheals last for several days, unlike those in 'classical' urticaria, where they last for a few hours. Urticarial vasculitis is often accompanied by arthralgia. A skin biopsy shows leukocytoclastic vasculitis, and complement studies reveal low CH50 and C3 levels. It may result from drug ingestion or infection, or may be a feature of lupus erythematosus.

Erythema nodosum

This is rare in young children. It is a type of vasculitis which occurs in the subcutaneous fat. Clinically, erythematous nodules develop, usually on the shins though sometimes on the thighs and forearms. They last for about 2–3 weeks and are characteristically tender. They resolve leaving bruising, but then tend to recur in crops. Causes include streptococcal infections, sarcoidosis, tuberculosis and sulfonamide ingestion: often it occurs without obvious reason. Treatment is of the underlying cause. Usually it resolves spontaneously, but occasionally treatment with oral steroids is indicated.

Erythema multiforme (Figs 25.24 and 25.25)

This is an uncommon condition in children which tends to follow herpes simplex infection, mycoplasma pneumonia and sulfonamide ingestion. Vasculitis which is predominantly lymphocytic is prominent on histological examination of the skin,

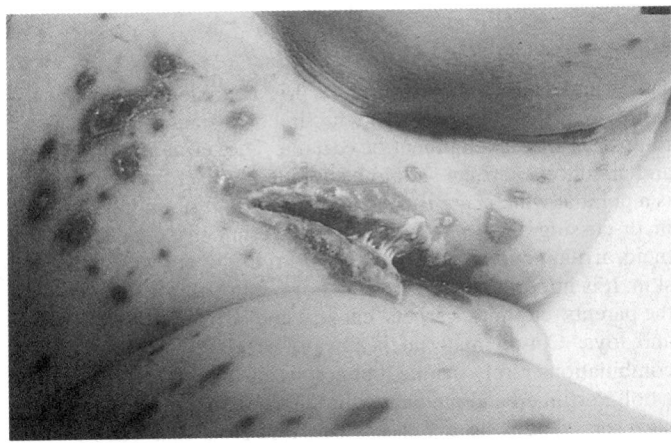

Fig. 25.24 Erythema multiforme, Stevens–Johnson: perineal.

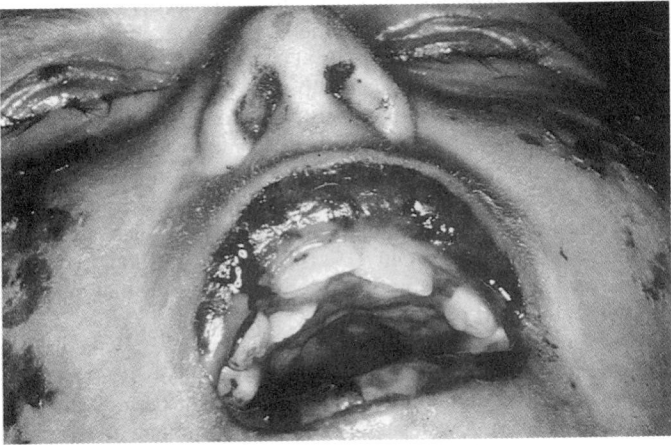

Fig. 25.25 Erythema multiforme, Stevens–Johnson: oral.

as is intraepidermal and subepidermal vesiculation. The role of immune complex deposition in this condition is still largely circumstantial, though intravascular IgM and C3 have been demonstrated to be associated with the vasculitis.

Clinically, it is characterized by the formation of circular target lesions on the limbs, with a red periphery and blue (often bullous) center. Stomatitis and genital involvement are common. The rash may be widespread, and the child is often toxic and ill ('Stevens–Johnson syndrome'). The rash usually fades within 10 days but may recur, particularly in the case of erythema multiforme following recurrent herpes simplex infection. In some children there is also marked eye involvement with purulent conjunctivitis, corneal ulceration, anterior uveitis or panophthalmitis. This usually resolves completely but occasionally may lead to blindness. In children with severe erythema multiforme treatment with oral steroids may be indicated.

Dermatitis herpetiformis

This may be a form of immune complex-mediated hypersensitivity, due to deposition of IgA in the dermal papillae of skin. It is a variant of celiac disease, and 80% have partial or subtotal villous atrophy of the small intestine, which returns to normal on a gluten-free diet.

It is more common in adults than in children, and is characterized clinically by the development of small intensely itchy blisters on the elbows, knees, shoulders and buttocks. These resolve with dapsone or sulfapyridine given orally, but recur when the drugs are stopped. The correct treatment is a gluten-free diet, when the blisters should resolve (permanently) within 2 years: the dapsone or sulfapyridine should be continued until this occurs.

TYPE IV HYPERSENSITIVITY: DELAYED TYPE HYPERSENSITIVITY

Allergic contact eczema

Allergic contact eczema is one of the main examples of delayed type hypersensitivity in the skin. It is much less common in children than in adults, probably due to lack of contact with sensitizing chemicals.

In the sensitized child, an epicutaneously applied chemical, which is usually a hapten, combines with epidermal proteins to form an antigen. It is then taken up by epidermal Langerhans cells which carry it via the lymphatics to the regional lymph nodes. It is thought that they present the antigen to T lymphocytes there (though it is possible that peripheral antigen presentation may also occur). Following interleukin 2 release clonal expansion of T cells follows, and specific T lymphocytes pass down the afferent lymphatics to the skin, where they recognize the antigen and set off a sequence of events that produces inflammation and eczema.

Clinically, allergic contact eczema is characterized by the development of erythema and small blisters (microvesication) at the site of contact with the allergen. The commonest allergen in children is nickel, which is contained in metal clips and studs (e.g. jeans studs) and in nongold earrings. It seems likely that a number of children are sensitized following piercing of the ears, and by wearing costume jewelry earrings. Other contact allergens in children include plants such as *Rhus* (particularly in the USA and Australia) (Plate 25.18), chemicals used in rubber production and topical medications such as neomycin and gentamicin.

Identification of the allergen is essential, and this is carried out by patch testing the child. The allergen is dissolved in a suitable vehicle (e.g. petrolatum) and applied in an aluminum chamber to the back of the child. This is removed at 48 hours, and note of erythema and microvesication is taken; a further reading is performed at 96 hours. Interpretation requires expertise, as not all reactions are necessarily specific delayed type hypersensitivity reactions.

ECZEMA AND DERMATITIS

Eczema and dermatitis are synonymous and are very often used interchangeably. The only type of eczema whose etiology is fully understood is allergic contact eczema. A number of other types of eczema are recognized which are not examples of delayed hypersensitivity.

ATOPIC ECZEMA (Figs 25.26 and 25.27)

Atopy is a genetically determined disorder with an increased tendency to form IgE antibody to inhalants and foods (see Ch. 28). There is increased susceptibility to asthma, allergic rhinitis and

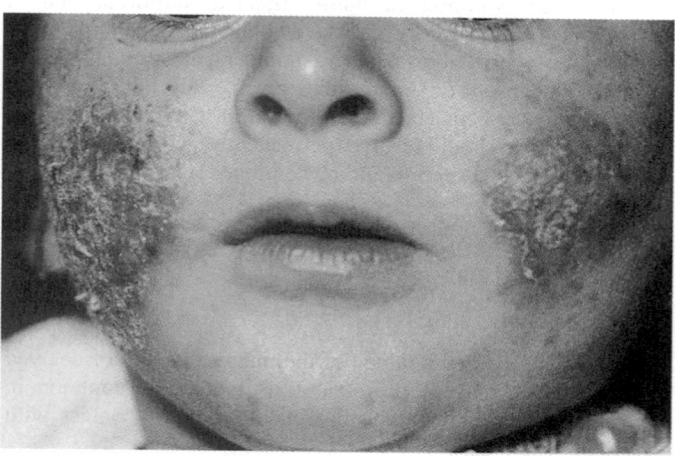

Fig. 25.26 Atopic eczema: facial in young infant.

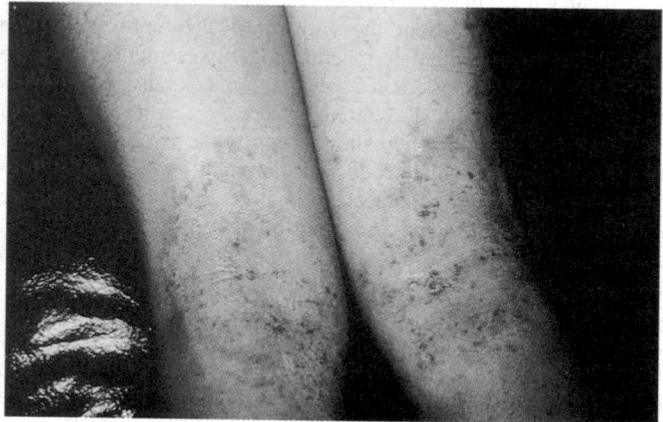

Fig. 25.27 Atopic eczema: flexural in older child.

atopic eczema. Although eczema may begin at any age, in 75% of patients first signs are present by 6 months.

Clinical features

The characteristic clinical features are a generalized dryness and a tendency to lichenification or thickening of the skin, pruritus and excoriations and patches of acute, subacute or chronic eczema. Involvement of the whole cutaneous surface may occur but the predominant areas are the face in infants, extensor aspects of the limbs as the child begins to crawl, and the limb flexures in older children. In severe cases the whole skin may be erythematous and in these patients white dermographism is often a prominent feature: this indicates that the condition is likely to be unstable and difficult.

Complications

Patients with atopic eczema may develop secondary bacterial infection which presents either as impetigo or folliculitis, or simply as worsening eczema. Mollusca contagiosa are common and atopic patients are at risk of developing severe widespread herpes simplex infections. The usual childhood immunizations are quite safe.

Management (see also Ch. 28)

These patients have an inherently dry, irritable skin. While the skin may become more stable with time, constant care is required to prevent the development of eczema. The terms infantile, baby and childhood eczema should be avoided as they imply that there is a point at which care is no longer needed. Time should be taken in discussing factors which act as external irritants. Wool is a major irritant and should never be worn in direct contact with the skin. It is important to warn that wool contact may also occur with the parents' clothing, carpets, car seat and stroller covers, blankets and toys. Cotton material is always safe and cotton polyester combinations rarely irritate, but acrylic may be as troublesome as wool. Perfumed and medicated products, disinfectants and strong cleansers should be avoided. Soap in excess and bubble baths overdry the skin, so soap substitutes should be used. Dealing with the basic dryness is essential and can be achieved with bath oils and the regular use of emollients, choosing one appropriate for the local climatic conditions. Urea-containing emollients sting broken skin and should be avoided. Emollients should be applied all over at least twice a day even when the skin is free of eczema.

Topical steroids are an essential part of the management and it should be emphasized to parents that as long as these are used only where and when there is active eczema overuse is unlikely, particularly if attention is paid to the general measures which prevent recurrences. The steroid preparation should be applied three times a day. In general, ointment bases, which are more emollient, are preferred. Only 1% hydrocortisone should be used on the face and in the groin but fluorinated steroids may be used elsewhere for short periods.

In severe cases failing to respond to routine therapy, the use of wet dressings is effective in achieving control. This is essentially an inpatient procedure but may be used for short periods at home on localized areas. A water-based emollient is applied all over and a steroid in a water miscible cream base is applied to the areas of eczema. Sheeting soaked in warmed tap water is applied and bandaged on with a crepe bandage held in place with a tubular gauze dressing. The procedure is repeated three times a day. These dressings increase the hydration of the skin, physically prevent scratching, immediately reduce itching and enhance the penetration of topical steroids. In infants only weak steroids should be used because of the risk of absorption and, in general, wet dressings should not be used for more than a few days at a time with topical steroids.

Obvious secondary bacterial infection should be treated with oral antibiotics. However, these are indicated in most patients with severe weeping eczema even in the absence of clinically obvious infection. Nocturnal sedation, usually with an antihistamine, is useful during acute flares. Oral steroids should be avoided because a severe rebound can occur on withdrawal and after several courses the eczema is rendered very unstable.

In children with a reported worsening of eczema after eating it is important first to take a careful history in order to exclude contact urticaria, a rapid development of redness and/or wheals at the site of contact with the food antigen. Foods which cause this reaction should be avoided. Otherwise no alteration to the child's diet should be considered unless the eczema has failed to respond to conventional topical therapy. Dietary manipulation in the management of refractory eczema is covered in Chapter 28. The role of the dust mite in these severe cases is covered in the same section.

Follow-up of patients with atopic eczema should be frequent and where possible with the same physician. As the child becomes older discussion about future careers is important as certain occupations are likely to aggravate the skin. It is important to develop a trusting and cooperative relationship with the patient and his parents as they will require much encouragement to help them cope with this distressing condition.

DISCOID ECZEMA (nummular eczema) (Fig. 25.28)

In children this is often a manifestation of the atopic state. Well-defined patches of acute eczema occur in a strikingly symmetrical distribution. In infants the commonest sites are the upper back and the tops of the shoulders; in older patients the extensor aspects of the limbs are particularly involved. The lesions may be very thick and exudative and they are very itchy. They have to be distinguished from tinea and impetigo which are less symmetrical

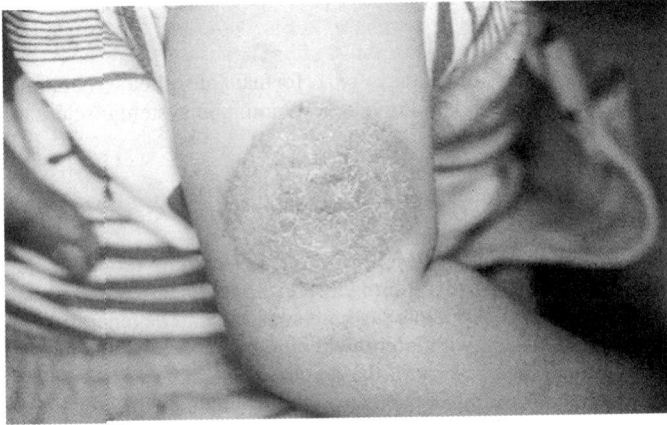

Fig. 25.28 Discoid eczema.

and psoriasis which is rarely moist. The management involves emollients and topical steroids as for atopic dermatitis, with the continued use of emollient helping to prevent recurrences.

PITYRIASIS ALBA

This condition appears as poorly defined, slightly scaly, hypopigmented patches occurring particularly on the face and the upper arms. It probably represents a very mild eczema which, however, produces a striking postinflammatory depigmentation. Occasionally some areas will show erythema and more definite eczematous changes. The condition is more common in atopics. The mild irritation and signs of mild eczema respond to emollients and weak topical corticosteroids but the hypopigmentation may be very persistent and require sun exposure over a prolonged period before repigmentation is complete. The condition should be differentiated from vitiligo where there is total depigmentation and no scale and from tinea versicolor which is rare on the face, has very well demarcated lesions and has a very fine branny scale.

SEBORRHEIC DERMATITIS

This is a condition of infancy and adult life; patients develop dermatitis in sites of greatest sebum production.

The rash has an erythematous background and a greasy yellow scale. In the flexures the scale may be absent and a glazed erythema the only sign. Scaling is particularly prominent on the scalp, producing the so-called 'cradle cap'. The main areas of involvement are scalp, glabella, behind and inside the ears, nasolabial folds, axillae and groin and in infants the neck and limb flexures. In the flexural areas candidiasis is commonly superimposed. The rash is usually asymptomatic.

Various conditions mimic seborrheic dermatitis including drug reactions (in children particularly due to phenytoin sodium), early psoriasis and Langerhans' cell histiocytosis. These should be considered when what appears to be a seborrheic dermatitis occurs at an unexpected age or fails to respond to therapy.

Seborrheic dermatitis usually responds quickly to weak topical corticosteroid preparations with the addition of an anticandidal agent for the flexural areas. On the scalp, sulfur and salicylic acid preparations left on overnight are usually more effective than corticosteroids. If the scale is very thick, warmed olive or paraffin oil can be used to soften it before the cream is applied. It should be emphasized that the disorder will tend to recur through infancy.

NAPKIN DERMATITIS

In all napkin dermatitis there is a combination of the elements of moisture, candidiasis and dermatitis, either seborrheic or primary irritant from the urine and feces. Miliaria or sweat duct occlusion is another common feature. Napkin dermatitis is only rarely due to laundering products. The newer superabsorbent disposable napkins are often preferable to cloth napkins.

Management

The napkin should be changed frequently. A combination cream of 1% hydrocortisone and antimonilial agent is usually effective and a silicone or zinc barrier cream may be added to protect the skin against moisture. There will usually be a quick response to therapy but recurrences are to be expected.

CONNECTIVE TISSUE DISEASES (Ch. 24)

LUPUS ERYTHEMATOSUS (LE)

This is rare in children but neonatal lupus erythematosus (also rare) is of considerable importance.

Neonatal lupus erythematosus (Plate 25.19)

This occurs due to the passage of maternal antibodies through the placenta, where the mother suffers from systemic LE, subacute cutaneous LE or the sicca syndrome. In 50% of cases the mother is asymptomatic but the vast majority have SS-A (anti-Ro) antibodies. The most important feature of neonatal LE is heart block of varying degrees. This is usually permanent, and without pacing there is a significant mortality (Ch. 13). Other features include autoimmune hemolytic anemia, thrombocytopenia, hepatitis, pneumonitis and splenomegaly.

The skin lesions resemble those of discoid LE in the adult, occurring on the face, neck and scalp, with erythematous macules or plaques with scaling, central atrophy and follicular plugging. They are often present at birth, and disappear within the first year of life. There may also be photosensitivity. A skin biopsy will usually show the features of adult discoid LE with liquefaction degeneration of the basal keratinocytes and a periappendageal lymphocytic infiltrate. Direct immunofluorescence is positive in 50% of infants, with a band-like deposition of IgG and complement at the dermoepidermal junction.

Treatment of the skin is with 1% hydrocortisone cream and protection from the sun.

Lupus erythematosus in the older child

This takes two main forms, systemic LE and discoid LE. It is thought that this is a spectrum of disease, as sometimes patients with discoid LE will progress to systemic LE and a proportion of those with discoid LE have circulating antinuclear antibodies, anemia, leukopenia and thrombocytopenia and other features such as Raynaud's phenomenon and arthralgia.

Discoid lupus erythematosus

This usually affects girls, who develop erythematous plaques on the face, the arms and dorsum of the hands. The most commonly affected parts of the face are the nose and the cheeks. Involvement of the scalp usually leads to scarring alopecia. Histological examination of the plaques shows characteristic liquefaction degeneration of the basal cell layer of the epidermis, and a periappendageal lymphocytic infiltrate in the dermis.

There may be mild anemia, leukopenia or thrombocytopenia and some children will have circulating antinuclear antibodies.

The prognosis is variable, as in some the plaques will resolve spontaneously whereas in others they tend to be persistent. Avoidance of sun exposure by the use of sunscreens and a hat is important.

Systemic lupus erythematosus

As in discoid LE this usually affects girls. It is a multisystem connective tissue disease which often carries a poor prognosis, due to renal involvement. This is discussed fully in Chapter 24.

The skin manifestations include a butterfly rash on the face, discoid plaques usually on the face, reticulate livedo most marked on the legs, panniculitis, vasculitic ulcers, cuticular hemorrhages at the fingernail folds, and alopecia.

DERMATOMYOSITIS

This is a rare connective tissue disease affecting the skin, muscle and blood vessels. Its etiology is unknown, though in some adults there is an association with carcinomas of internal viscera and lymphomas. The histological changes in the skin may resemble those of lupus erythematosus, though the dermal edema is more marked. In the later stages the dermis becomes sclerotic, and the picture may be similar to the changes in scleroderma.

The clinical manifestations are extremely variable. In some children the skin signs may be very prominent with minimal myositis, whereas in others there is polymyositis with little evidence of skin involvement. Myositis is manifested by a proximal muscular weakness with difficulty in climbing stairs and raising the arms above the shoulder girdle, and by a raised serum creatine phosphokinase. There may be concomitant fever and malaise.

The rash when present is very characteristic. A purplish–red heliotrope rash occurs on the face involving the eyelids, the forehead and upper cheeks. There may be marked edema of the hands and arms with an erythematous linear rash over the dorsum of the hands with nail fold telangiectasia. Erythema of the scalp may develop and there may be marked alopecia. Reticulate livedo is seen in some, and may lead to ulceration of the skin.

Calcification is common in children, affecting more than 50% of cases. It primarily involves the muscles, particularly around the pelvic and shoulder girdles, and may cause marked functional disability. It also occurs in the subcutaneous tissues, and there may be extrusion through the skin with ulceration.

The course of the disease is variable, but there is generally a good prognosis in children. Death may occur due to respiratory failure, difficulty in swallowing, or the side-effects of steroid therapy.

Treatment with oral corticosteroids is required with high doses of prednisone (1–2 mg/kg initially) tapering to a maintenance dose which should be carried on for months or years, till the serum creatine phosphokinase returns to normal and the signs of the disease have disappeared. Physiotherapy may be useful to prevent contractures.

SCLERODERMA

In children this may take two forms: morphea (localized scleroderma), which is relatively common, and systemic sclerosis which is very rare.

Morphea

This is a localized and benign form of scleroderma, though it can cause quite marked disfigurement. On histological examination, the dermis is at first edematous with swelling and degeneration of the collagen fibrils, with later thickening of the dermis and loss of appendages. The etiology of the condition is unknown.

The areas of morphea occur usually as either plaques or linear lesions of sclerosis in the skin, which are at first purplish in color, and later become white and waxy. Hairs are lost within the area, with loss of sweating. They occur on the trunk and limbs. When they involve a limb (usually linear lesions), they may involve muscles and bone leading to shortening of the limb.

A particular disfigurement which results from morphea is the so-called 'coup de sabre', which occurs in the frontoparietal area. This starts with contraction of the skin over the affected area with development of an ivory plaque with hyperpigmentation at the edge and telangiectatic vessels coursing over it. The resulting groove may extend downwards, affecting the mouth and mandible. The tongue may be atrophic on the affected side, and there may be marked alopecia. There is marked facial asymmetry with consequent disfigurement.

There is no effective treatment for morphea but intralesional triamcinolone may be helpful in some children.

Systemic sclerosis

This is very rare in children. The etiology is unknown, but as similar changes may be seen in graft versus host reactions, it may be some sort of rejection phenomenon.

In the majority of patients the condition starts with Raynaud's phenomenon which may continue for several years before other manifestations occur. These include: swelling of the hands; sclerodactyly with atrophy of the pulps of the fingers; calcinosis of the finger pulps which may be prominent; ulceration; and gangrene. In some, terminal phalangeal absorption also occurs.

Later, other features occur with beaking of the nose, radial furrowing around the mouth which becomes smaller, macroglossia, esophageal dilation and stricture, and abnormal colonic peristalsis.

The prognosis is variable, though most patients continue with the condition for many years with increasing deformity. There is no specific treatment, though oral corticosteroids may be helpful in some.

IDIOPATHIC PHOTOSENSITIVITY ERUPTIONS

Before considering a child to have an idiopathic photosensitivity eruption, it is important to exclude one of the hereditary diseases (q.v.), and photosensitive drug eruptions which are common and may be caused by a number of drugs (notably sulfonamides, tetracyclines and phenothiazines).

Polymorphic light eruption (PLE)

About 20% of patients with PLE present before the age of 10 years. A delayed reaction occurring several hours or the next day after exposure to the sun results in erythema, burning and itching, followed by papule and plaque formation. With avoidance of sun exposure this reaction will settle but will usually relapse when the child is exposed to the sun again. It usually presents during the summer, but in some children it is most marked in the spring and early summer, with remission of the symptoms in midsummer with 'hardening' of the skin.

Most children with PLE continue into adulthood with it. Action spectrum studies are usually normal, and are therefore unhelpful. Prevention of PLE depends on adequate topical photoprotection with sunscreens. In those children with severe PLE, photochemotherapy with oral psoralen and UVA light may be helpful.

Actinic prurigo

This condition is clinically similar to PLE but is now recognized to be a separate entity. It nearly always develops in early childhood and 80% of patients are female. There is usually progressive improvement in adolescence.

Clinically all exposed sites are affected, including face, lips, neck, ears, arms, dorsum of hands and lower legs. In the majority there is also involvement of covered skin, though to a lesser extent. It is worse during summer months but very often persists even in winter. In most cases there is a family history and there is also a strong association with atopy.

Action spectrum studies are abnormal in the majority with sensitivity to both UVA and UVB; however, in some children these studies are normal. Treatment is similar to that of PLE, but thalidomide has also been found to be particularly effective in this condition.

Hydroa vacciniforme

This is a very rare condition which invariably starts in childhood. On exposure to sunlight the child develops tingling and erythema followed by blistering and umbilicated papules on the face, ears, arms and dorsum of hands. These lead to crusting and varioliform scars.

Action spectrum studies are abnormal with sensitivity mainly involving UVA. Treatment is generally unsatisfactory, though broad spectrum topical sunscreens may be helpful.

SKIN DISEASES OF THE NEONATE

ERYTHEMA TOXICUM NEONATORUM

This is a benign self-limiting condition of unknown etiology occurring in up to 70% of neonates. The onset is from birth to 14 days but most cases start between 24 and 48 hours. The commonest lesions are erythematous macules and papules but in some cases pustules appear. Lesions occur anywhere on the body surface except palms and soles but with a predilection for face and trunk. In cases present at birth, lesions are more acrally distributed and are often pustular. A peripheral blood eosinophilia is present and smears from pustules demonstrate sheets of eosinophils. The condition usually resolves in a few days but, rarely, may persist for several weeks.

Its main importance is its simulation, especially when pustular, of serious neonatal infections.

ACROPUSTULOSIS OF INFANCY

This is a benign condition of unknown etiology occurring in otherwise healthy infants. The onset is usually in the neonatal period but may be delayed for some months. Recurrent crops of papules which quickly evolve into 2–4 mm vesicopustules occur, most commonly on the palms and soles and dorsa of hands and feet. Initially each crop takes 1–2 weeks to settle and new crops occur every 2–3 weeks. As time goes on the crops occur less frequently and the episodes are less severe and of shorter duration. Lesions are pruritic but are accompanied by no systemic symptoms. The condition finally resolves by 2–3 years.

The disease must be differentiated from other neonatal pustular conditions including herpes simplex, impetigo, scabies and candidiasis. Cultures of the lesions of infantile acropustulosis are sterile. A clinically identical condition can occur also as a postscabetic reaction in infants who have been successfully treated for scabies.

Topical therapy is usually ineffective. Oral antihistamines can be used if pruritus is severe.

TRANSIENT NEONATAL PUSTULAR DERMATOSIS

This is a benign condition in which superficial pustules are present at birth; it is rare for further lesions to develop postnatally. The pustules rupture within 24 hours, developing a brown crust which separates after a few days to leave normal skin or a hyperpigmented macule in dark-skinned individuals. Lesions occur mainly on chin, upper anterior trunk, lower back and buttocks. They are asymptomatic and the infant is otherwise well. Lesions are sterile on culture enabling differentiation from important neonatal infections. If hyperpigmented macules occur, they resolve over 3–4 months.

CUTIS MARMORATA (congenital livedo reticularis)

This term usually refers to a transient benign physiological vascular reaction occurring in both premature and full-term infants as a response to minor cooling. A blue or purple discoloration in a marbled or reticulate pattern occurs on trunk and limbs. It lasts minutes to hours but reverses quickly on warming the infant. The tendency to the condition lasts for weeks or months.

There are a number of important conditions which may be associated with more severe and persistent cutis marmorata. These include Down syndrome, trisomy 18, homocystinuria, de Lange syndrome, neonatal lupus and congenital hypothyroidism. A nevoid vascular disorder, cutis marmorata telangiectatica congenita, presents with reticulate purple lesions but the distribution is often segmental rather than generalized and atrophy and ulceration may occur in the affected areas.

MILIA

These represent retention cysts of the pilosebaceous follicles. They occur in approximately 50% of neonates as firm pearly white 1–2 mm papules particularly on the face. They usually disappear by 4 weeks of age. Persistent milia may be a marker for certain syndromes including Bazex's syndrome, orofaciodigital syndrome type I and Marie–Unna hypotrichosis.

MILIARIA (PRICKLY HEAT)

This is a sweat retention phenomenon common in young infants. Unlike the equivalent condition in older persons it can occur in the absence of fever or significant occlusive factors. An obstruction of unknown etiology occurs within the intraepidermal portion of the eccrine sweat duct with retention of sweat behind the block. Lesions commence as red macules on which are superimposed 2–3 mm papules, vesicles or pustules (Plate 25.20). Secondary infection can occur but most commonly these pustules are sterile. Characteristically the pattern and severity of the condition alter significantly from day to day enabling differentiation from infantile acne and infective conditions. Lesions occur most commonly on the face but scalp, neck and upper trunk are other common sites. The condition is also prone to occur under plastic napkins and napkin covers.

The management of miliaria involves keeping the child as cool as practicable, avoidance of contact with nonporous materials such as nylon and plastic, and of occlusive topical agents. The parents should be reassured that this is a transient condition and is uncommon after 6 months of age.

INFANTILE ACNE

This condition commences at about 3 months of age with lesions particularly on the cheeks. Open comedones predominate but closed comedones, papules, pustules and even cysts can occur. Deeper lesions may produce significant scarring. Untreated the condition usually lasts 2–3 years. In patients with a strong family history of acne the condition may be more severe and there may be difficult acne at puberty. Hormonal abnormalities are rarely found in these patients and investigation is indicated only in cases which are unusually severe, prolonged or unresponsive to therapy. Most patients respond well to topical retinoic acid used at nighttime. If pustules are present topical clindamycin can be added and intralesional steroid injection is indicated for the rare large cyst.

SUBCUTANEOUS FAT NECROSIS OF THE NEWBORN

This is a necrosis of subcutaneous fat in the newborn probably induced by ischemia. It occurs usually in healthy full-term infants. Often, however, there is a history of a difficult labor and delivery with such complications as prolonged labor, fetal distress, perinatal asphyxia due to meconium aspiration or other cause and forceps delivery. The condition has also been reported in an infant following hypothermic cardiac surgery.

The lesions appear between the second and third weeks of life as nontender, firm, skin-colored or red-purple nodules or plaques occurring particularly on buttocks, shoulders, upper back, proximal limbs and cheeks. New nodules may develop over several weeks. They usually disappear spontaneously without complication in several months leaving no trace. However, sometimes they become fluctuant, ulcerate or calcify. In patients with calcified lesions hypercalcemia may develop.

Fluctuant lesions should be aspirated, secondary infection should be dealt with if it complicates ulcerated lesions, and serum calcium levels should be monitored in the presence of calcified lesions. Otherwise management involves observation and reassurance.

HARLEQUIN COLOR CHANGE

This is a vascular phenomenon probably caused by an immature autonomic regulatory mechanism. When the neonate is lying on one side the lower half of the body is red and the upper half is pale with a clear midline separation. This color change is transient and can be reversed by altering the infant's position. It is a very transient phenomenon and is rare after the first few days of life. It does not indicate any significant neural or vascular abnormality.

NEOPLASTIC DISEASES

MASTOCYTOSIS

This refers to a group of conditions whose signs and symptoms are due to the infiltration of tissues by mast cells and to the release of the chemical mediators contained in these cells.

Mast cells are ubiquitous connective tissue cells containing granules which store mediators including histamine, prostaglandin D_2, heparin, proteases, leukotrienes and chemotactic factors. Mast cell degranulation with release of these substances may be triggered by immunological (IgE or complement-mediated) and nonimmunological stimuli, in particular a number of drugs. The effects of release of these chemicals may be local or general. Local effects include erythema and swelling ('urtication') of lesions on rubbing, dermographism, pruritus, hemorrhage and blistering. General effects include generalized pruritus, fever and flushing; tachycardia and hypotension; headache and irritability; vomiting, diarrhea, increased salivation and peptic ulceration; rhinorrhea and bronchospasm; increased lacrimation; and a generalized hemorrhagic diathesis.

Mastocytosis may present in childhood or adult life. The forms of the disease seen in childhood are mastocytomas, urticaria pigmentosa, diffuse cutaneous mastocytosis and rarely systemic mastocytosis.

Mastocytoma

This is a round to oval flesh-colored to yellowish nodule or plaque usually present at birth or appearing in the first months of life. Although usually solitary, some children develop a number of mastocytomas particularly on arms or trunk. They usually regress spontaneously over a few years but while present they urticate on rubbing, and blisters, which may be hemorrhagic, often occur in infancy. These children commonly have attacks of generalized flushing but other symptoms and signs of mediator release are rare.

Urticaria pigmentosa

Multiple macules, papules, nodules or plaques occur in a widespread distribution, particularly involving the trunk. The onset is usually between 1 and 9 months of age. The lesions erupt over several weeks, then become static and finally in most cases disappear over several years. The lesions are often significantly pigmented. They are usually pruritic and may blister. Urtication occurs and there may be dermographism in nearby clinically normal skin. Generalized pruritus and flushing may occur, and less frequently other signs of mediator release.

Diffuse cutaneous mastocytosis

This is a rare form of mastocytosis with the onset usually at birth. Massive mast cell infiltration into the skin produces a diffuse thickening with associated edema, erythema and blistering. The skin may have a leathergrain or peau d'orange appearance or be nodular or verrucose. The color is yellowish or red. Blistering is prominent and may be so severe that the presentation is that of a generalized bullous disease. The full spectrum of local and systemic symptoms and signs of mediator release may be seen and these are usually severe and disabling and may be life threatening. The cutaneous lesions tend to improve with time but some degree of infiltration usually remains.

Systemic mastocytosis

This implies the infiltration of mast cells into organs other than the skin, and not simply systemic features due to the release of mediators from cutaneous mast cell infiltrates. It is extremely rare in childhood and is almost always associated with diffuse cutaneous involvement in this age group. Hepatosplenomegaly and lymphadenopathy may occur; the cells may infiltrate renal parenchyma and gastrointestinal mucosa; skeletal involvement produces both osteoporotic and osteosclerotic lesions. Mast cell leukemia is a very rare complication.

Management

In general, mastocytosis is a self-limiting disease. If an isolated lesion is producing generalized flushing, excision can be considered. The patient should carry a list of agents (i.e. aspirin, morphine, codeine, d-tubocurarine, scopolamine, quinine, thiamin, procaine, polymixin B and radiographic contrast media) which stimulate mast cell degranulation and avoid these where possible. Physical trauma to the lesions should be avoided.

H1 antihistamines are rarely effective in controlling symptoms and signs of mediator release but combined with H2 blockers they may be more effective. In more severe cases oral disodium cromoglycate, ketotifen and nifedipine may be tried.

LANGERHANS CELL HISTIOCYTOSIS
(Histiocytosis X)

This condition is rare (Ch. 16), and the cells involved are Langerhans' cells (containing Birbeck granules, and with CD1 markers) and not true histiocytes. Three types are recognized:

Letterer–Siwe disease (Fig. 25.29)

This usually presents in the first year of life. Discrete yellow-brown papules develop on the scalp, face, upper trunk and flexures, with a distribution suggestive of seborrheic eczema. Purpura and crusting of the lesion may become evident. In some children mucous membranes are also involved, with gingivitis and oral and genital ulceration.

Signs of systemic involvement become manifest, with hepatosplenomegaly, lymphadenopathy and anemia. Chest X-ray shows miliary shadowing and bone scans may show osteolytic areas. The outcome has recently changed though the mortality is still high (50–60%) particularly for children under the age of 6

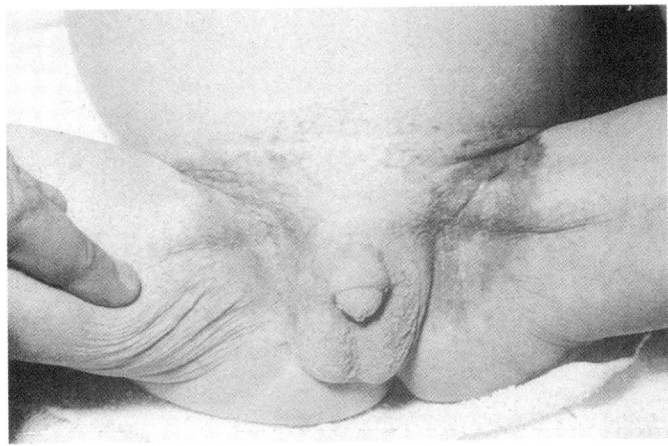

Fig. 25.29 Letterer–Siwe disease.

months due to fatal bacterial and viral infections. Treatment with steroids and cytotoxic drugs has reduced the mortality and slowed the progression.

Hand–Schüller–Christian disease

This is a more benign form of histiocytosis X, which follows a chronic nonfatal course. The usual manifestations are radiological bone defects, exophthalmos and diabetes insipidus. Skin lesions similar to those in Letterer–Siwe disease are present in 30%. The disease usually presents within the first 5 years of life, and treatment with vinblastine and prednisone may be indicated.

Eosinophilic granuloma

This is the most benign form of histiocytosis X. It commonly presents within the first 5 years of life, and skin involvement is rare. When it does occur, yellowish or brownish papules are found on the scalp and trunk in a distribution similar to the other forms of histiocytosis X. Spontaneous resolution usually occurs.

REFERENCES

Andersen S L C, Thomsen K 1971 Psoriasiform napkin dermatitis. British Journal of Dermatology 84: 316–319

Barton L L, Friedman A D, Portilla M G 1988 Impetigo contagiosa: a comparison of erythromycin and dicloxacillin therapy. Pediatric Dermatology 5: 88–91

Bell S D, MacDonald D M 1985 The prevalence of café-au-lait patches in tuberous sclerosis. Clinical and Experimental Dermatology 10: 562–565

Coskey R J, Coskey L A 1987 Diagnosis and treatment of impetigo. Journal of the American Academy of Dermatology 17: 62–63

Enjolras O, Mulliken J B 1993 The current management of vascular birthmarks. Pediatric Dermatology 10: 311–333

Enjolras O, Riche M C, Merland J J 1985 Facial port wine stains and Sturge Weber syndrome. Pediatrics 76: 48–51

Esterly N B, Margileth A M, Kahn G 1984 The management of disseminated eruptive haemangiomata in infants: special symposium. Pediatric Dermatology 1: 312–317

Freire-Maia N, Pinheiro M 1984 Ectodermal dysplasias: a clinical and genetic study. Alan R Liss, New York

Happle R 1991 How many epidermal nevus syndromes exist? Journal of the American Academy of Dermatology 25: 550–556

Illig W, Weidner F, Hundeeker M et al 1985 Congenital nevi <10 cms as precursors to melanoma. Archives of Dermatology 121: 1274–1281

Jacobs A H, Hurwitz S, Prose N et al 1984 The management of congenital nevocytic nevi: special symposium. Pediatric Dermatology 2: 143–156

Kaplan E N 1974 The risk of malignancy in large congenital nevi. Plastic and Reconstructive Surgery 53: 421–428

Lorentzen M, Pers M, Bretteville Jensen G 1977 The incidence of malignant transformation in giant pigmented nevi. Scandinavian Journal of Plastic and Reconstructive Surgery II: 163–167

Neville E A, Finn O A 1975 Psoriasiform napkin dermatitis – a follow up study. British Journal of Dermatology 92: 279–285

Orlow S J, Paller A 1993 Cimetidine therapy for multiple viral warts in children. Journal of the American Academy of Dermatology 28: 794–796

Pasyk K A 1987 Classification and histopathological features of haemangiomas and other vascular malformations. In: Ryan T J, Cherry G W (eds) Vascular birthmarks. Oxford University Press, Oxford, p 3

Rhodes A R, Sober A J, Calvin L et al 1982 The malignant potential of small congenital nevocellular nevi. Journal of the American Academy of Dermatology 6: 230–241

Rogers M 1992 Epidermal nevi and the epidermal nevus syndromes: a review of 233 cases. Pediatric Dermatology 9: 342–344

Rogers M, Dorman D C, Gapes M, Ly J 1987 A three year study of impetigo in Sydney. Medical Journal of Australia 147: 59–62

Rogers M, McCrossin I, Commens C 1989 Epidermal nevi and the epidermal nevus syndrome. Journal of the American Academy of Dermatology 20: 476–488

Solomon L M, Esterly N M 1975 Epidermal and other organoid nevi. Current Problems in Pediatrics 6: 1–56

Stevenson R F, Thompson H G, Marin J D 1974 Unrecognized ocular problems associated with port wine stain of the face in children. Canadian Medical Association Journal 11: 953–955

Taieb A, Plantin P, Du Pasquier P, Guillet G, Maleville J 1986 Gianotti Crosti syndrome: a study of 26 cases. British Journal of Dermatology 115: 49–59

Wurzel C L, Kahan J, Heitler M, Rubin L G 1986 Prognosis of herpes zoster in healthy children. American Journal of Diseases of Children 140: 477–478

26 Disorders of the eye

J. S. Cant

Examination of the eyes   1649
   Special methods of examination   1653
   Testing visual acuity   1656
The apparently blind baby   1657
   Amaurosis   1657
   Acute onset blindness   1658
   Transient blindness   1658
   Hysteria and malingering   1658
   The management of the blind or visually
      handicapped child   1658
Strabismus and amblyopia   1658
   Pseudo-squint   1659
   Heterophoria   1659
   Concomitant (non-paralytic) squint   1660
   Incomitant (paralytic) squint   1660
   Management of squint   1660
   Squint amblyopia   1660
External eye disease   1661
   The orbits   1661
   The eyelids   1661
   The conjunctiva   1663
   The cornea   1664
   The lacrimal apparatus   1664
Internal eye disease   1665
   Uveitis   1665

Cyclitis   1666
Degenerative diseases of the retina and choroid   1666
Disorders of the lens   1667
Tumors of the eye   1670
The optic nerve   1671
Papilledema   1671
Optic neuritis   1671
Pseudopapilledema   1671
Myelinated nerve fibers   1671
Optic atrophy   1671
Optic nerve glioma   1672
Orbital angioma and varices   1672
Buphthalmos (infantile glaucoma)   1672
Ocular signs of systemic disease   1673
   Disorders of metabolism   1673
   Endocrine disease   1674
   The collagen diseases   1674
   Diseases of the skin   1675
   Hypertension   1675
   Blood dyscrasia   1675
   Allergy   1675
   Connective tissue disorders   1676
   Systemic infective diseases   1676
   Nutritional disorders   1677
   Toxic disorders   1677

Ophthalmology is the study of the eyes and their adnexa together with all aspects of vision. Diseases of the eyes and disorders of vision cannot be considered in isolation from the rest of the body and ocular disease is commonly an extension or a reflection of general disease. Eye disease is closely related to systemic disease and ophthalmology should be considered in a medical context, just as diseases of the eye in children should, where possible, be treated in a children's hospital rather than in a segregated eye hospital.

This chapter deals with disorders of the eye in infancy and childhood. Where the condition is confined to the eye some detail is given but where it is an extension of systemic disease which is dealt with elsewhere, the etiology, course and treatment of the underlying condition are not discussed. Many investigative procedures and methods of treatment used in ophthalmology require sophisticated equipment and techniques which are not dealt with. Surgery, which is an important part of ophthalmology, although perhaps no longer the major part, is not detailed.

EXAMINATION OF THE EYES

Before examining the eyes a history should be taken concerning not only visual symptoms and ocular complaints but also concerning general health. Examination of the eyes should be preceded where possible by assessment of the visual acuity (taking each eye separately followed by the binocular acuity) as the acuity cannot be tested for some time after the use of an ophthalmoscope or other methods of illumination. The condition of the orbits and surrounding structures should be examined prior to the examination of the eyes themselves. Many congenital deformities involve the eyes, the eyelids, the bones of the orbit and face, and these are seldom isolated defects. Facial symmetry, the relative position of the eyes and the shape of the skull should be noted. The palpebral apertures are then inspected for size, shape and symmetry, followed by examination of the eyelid margins and eyelids. With the eyes in the primary position the lower eyelids should 'cut' the lower limbus of each eye (although this is a variable relationship) and the upper eyelid should 'cut' the cornea about 2 mm below the upper limbus with the margins of both upper eyelids on the same level. With a hand held firmly on the forehead to prevent action of the frontalis muscle there should be normal action of the levator palpebrae superioris. Ptosis is often accompanied by poor levator action. Minor degrees of ptosis may be indicated by the absence of the normal skin folds in the upper eyelid or by the presence of backward tilting of the head (an abnormal head posture).

The orbits are best examined by simple inspection followed by palpation. Inspection will reveal orbital asymmetry and orbital size differences and it will also show abnormalities in the position of the orbits, either in the face or relative to one another. Palpation of the orbital margins may reveal bony defects, soft swellings such as those caused by angioma or the hard firm swelling of a dermoid, all of which are often too small to be detected by inspection. The diagnosis of proptosis may be difficult, particularly as the eyes of an infant are large relative to the orbits. Bilateral proptosis in infants is generally due to symmetrical orbital deformities such as those associated with craniofacial dysostosis. Unilateral proptosis is more easily recognized because of the asymmetry produced (Fig. 26.1). The commonest causes of unilateral proptosis are traumatic orbital hemorrhage, meningocele or neoplasm. Under 2 years of age, orbital neoplasm is commonly metastatic due to neuroblastoma. Hemangioma, optic nerve glioma and rhabdomyosarcoma are found in children of all ages. In examining a child with apparent proptosis digital compression of the eye through the closed eyelid should be used as reduced compressibility indicates the presence of a space-occupying lesion. Where proptosis is obvious, displacement of the eye either directly forwards or obliquely gives an indication of the site of the lesion. When an eye is proptosed, a rim of sclera may be seen between the lower limbus and the lower eyelid margin and the amount of exposed sclera is a guide to the degree of proptosis. An exophthalmometer is a useful instrument to assess the rate of progression of proptosis although photography of the full face and profile is more helpful, particularly in follow-up. Scanning techniques have largely replaced photography and also radiology

in its various forms. When unilateral, it should be borne in mind that a common cause of apparent proptosis is enophthalmos or microphthalmos on the opposite side. Unilateral proptosis may be diagnosed in error in older children where the axial length of the eye is increased in unilateral high myopia. In all cases of proptosis or of orbital disease a stethoscope should be used to listen for a bruit in the orbital region.

In examining the globe of the eye the anterior segment should first be looked at using a focused light (not a diffuse light such as that of a simple pen-torch). The cornea should be clear with a smooth and regular surface reflex. The normal corneal diameter is 10 mm in the newborn baby and measures the adult size of approximately 12 mm by about 1 year of age. The cornea of the newborn infant is not optically clear for the first 2 weeks of life due to stromal opacity, particularly apparent in premature babies. Any pathological corneal opacity will be seen with a focused light although magnification is necessary should the opacity be very small.

The size and shape of the pupils should be compared, the direct and consensual light reactions examined and in infants over 6 months of age the pupillary reaction to accommodation studied. Large differences in pupil size must be investigated by ocular and neurological examination but small differences in pupil size are not uncommon in young children and have no effect on vision. These minor degrees of anisocoria (different size of pupil) seen in young babies become less marked over 2 years but may persist throughout life and are of no significance. Horner's syndrome (Fig. 26.2) is a relatively common cause of unequal pupils in infants and where present one drop of 2% cocaine should be instilled; if there is no pupillary dilation the lesion is in the peripheral sympathetic supply.

Congenital abnormalities of the iris are common and a particularly common defect is a sector coloboma (Fig. 26.3) of the lower part of the iris. A sector coloboma may be an isolated finding but it always justifies a full ocular examination, as other abnormalities are frequently associated. The irides should be compared for color differences. Heterochromia is generally of no significance and minor degrees are often found, but it may be associated with Horner's syndrome or a complication of uveitis. The presence of heterochromia always warrants a full eye examination. Sector heterochromia affecting part of the iris of one

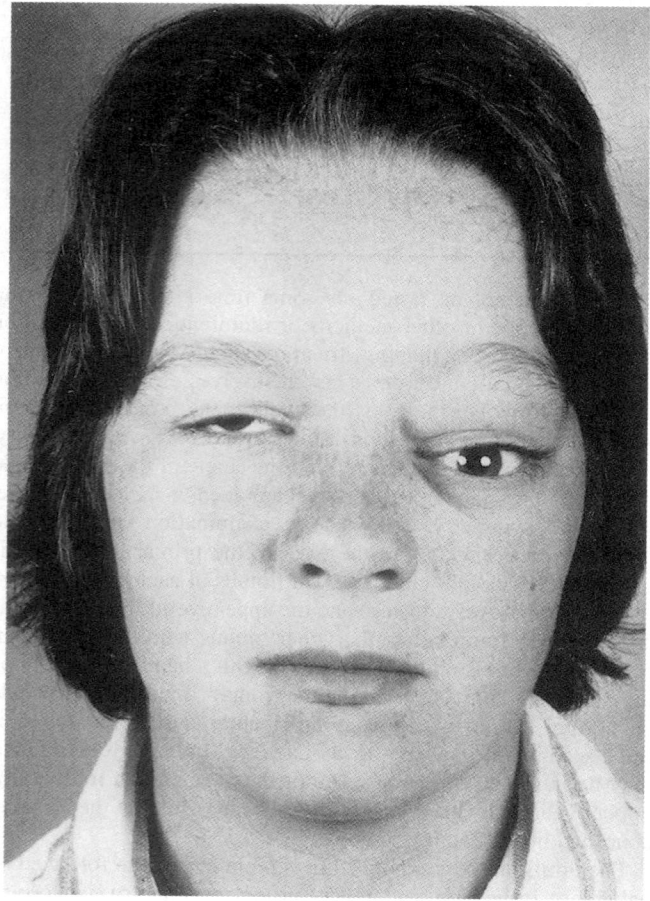

Fig. 26.1 Proptosis. Left-sided proptosis and facial asymmetry caused by an orbital tumor (hemangioma) which had been present since birth and had not resolved spontaneously. Eventually this tumor caused optic nerve compression and visual reduction but it was successfully removed intact.

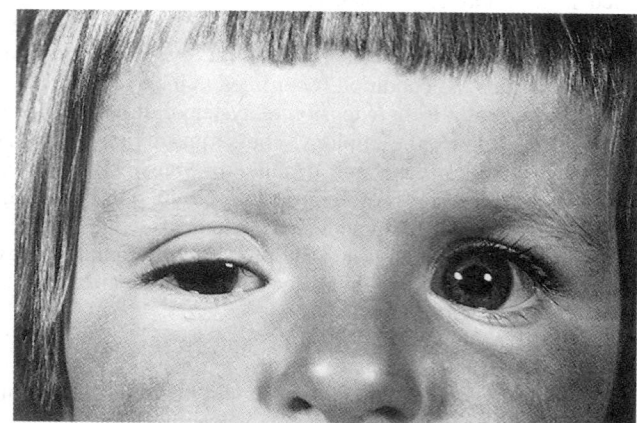

Fig. 26.2 Horner's syndrome. A child with right-sided Horner's syndrome showing ptosis and enopthalmos. The pupil of the right eye cannot be seen in this photograph but it is not occluded as the ptosis is only partial.

there should be a clear red reflex in the pupil (Plate 26.1). Any lens opacity will disturb the normally uniform red reflex (Plates 26.2 and 26.3). Opacities in the vitreous will become apparent on approaching the child's eye and putting increasingly strong 'plus' lenses in the ophthalmoscope. Indirect ophthalmoscopy (Fig. 26.4) is preferable for examination of the fundus as it gives a large field of view, overcomes the difficulties inherent in examining a constantly moving child's eye, and should be less alarming to the child than direct ophthalmoscopy. Indirect binocular ophthalmoscopy is an essential part of the detailed examination of the entire fundus, such as must be made in children with retinoblastoma. It is particularly useful in comparing the fundi as not only does it give a large field of view with a stereoscopic image, but also one can change rapidly from one eye to the other for comparison. Fine differences in color, vascularity and detail of the optic disks can be compared readily with the indirect ophthalmoscope (Plate 26.4).

In examining the fundus, the optic disk should first be sought, if necessary by tracing branching retinal vessels to their origin. The normal optic disk is pinkish in hue due to the presence of fine blood vessels and the disk margins are well defined. The detail of the lamina cribrosa can be discerned and the central area of the optic disk may be depressed (physiological cupping). Papilledema

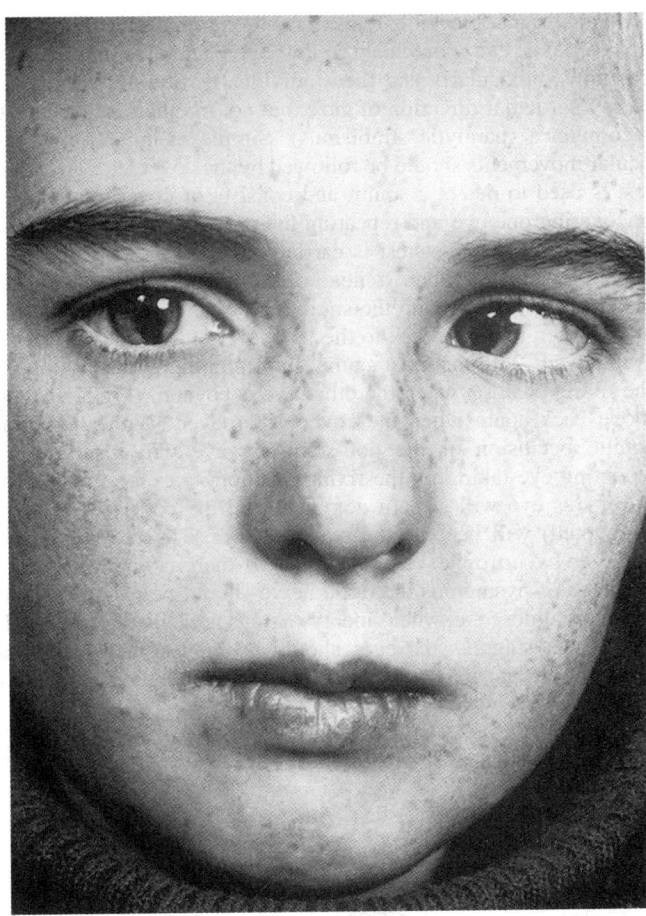

Fig. 26.3 Bilateral iris coloboma. This child has iris colobomata in the typical inferomedial position. The coloboma on the left side was associated with a coloboma of the fundus in a similar position with involvement of the macula and the resultant convergent squint.

eye only is of no significance. The eyes of a newborn infant are generally light blue in color but there should be color equality between the two irides and an equal distribution of color within each iris.

The undilated and dilated pupil should be black when seen in direct light; if the pupil or any part of it is other than black there may be a lens opacity or a mass in the vitreous. The commonest cause of a white or gray pupil is developmental cataract and the most serious cause of a loss of the normal pupillary appearance is retinoblastoma.

Ophthalmoscopy should only be carried out after examination of the anterior segment of the eye and of the pupil with a focused light. In the normal eye the fundus can be seen with the ophthalmoscope through the undilated pupil, but for full ophthalmoscopy the pupils must be dilated with a quick-acting mydriatic such as 1% cyclopentolate. Cycloplegics such as atropine or other belladonna alkaloids are seldom necessary. Direct ophthalmoscopy with the simple battery-operated ophthalmoscope is commonly used and gives a reasonable indication of the condition of the media and fundi, being most useful in examining the media, particularly the lens. When the pupil is fully dilated and the direct ophthalmoscope is held close to the observer's eye and at arm's length from the patient's eye,

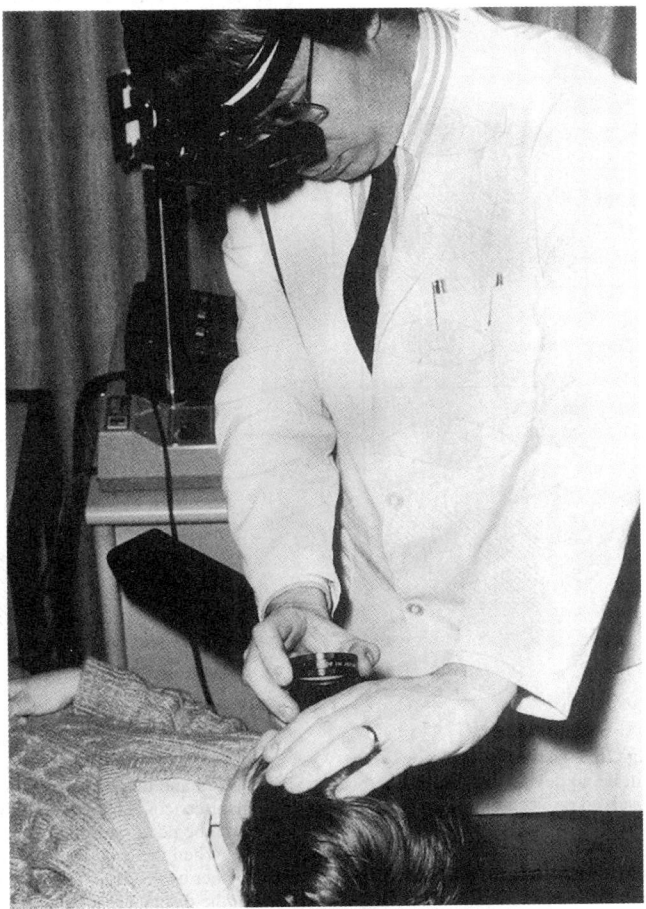

Fig. 26.4 The binocular indirect ophthalmoscope. The binocular indirect ophthalmoscope gives a stereoscopic view of a large area of the fundus. The instrument is worn on a headband and a condensing lens is held close to the patient's eye which has a fully dilated pupil.

is the disk abnormality on which the ophthalmologist is most often asked to give an opinion: in papilledema the optic disk first becomes a deeper pink color and its margins blurred; fine hemorrhages then develop on the disk and in the surrounding retina and there is elevation of the disk which can be made out readily using the indirect ophthalmoscope (Plates 26.5 and 26.6). The macula is two disk diameters to the temporal side of the optic disk on a slightly lower level and it should not be sought until the disk has been fully examined, as a bright light shining on the macula irritates the patient and causes the undilated pupil to constrict – it is for this reason that reduced illumination should be used when examining the macular area. The fovea appears as a bright red reflex in the center of the macula and it is studied by decreasing the intensity of illumination in the ophthalmoscope. The retina is next searched quadrant by quadrant, followed by examination of the retinal periphery, also quadrant by quadrant, and finally details of the retinal vessels are examined (Plate 26.4).

Detailed examination of the fundi may have unexpected results (Plates 26.7–26.9).

The ocular movements are examined superficially during the initial inspection of the eyes and face and detailed examination may be undertaken then or after full examination of the eyes but where the ocular movements are to be examined the pupils must be undilated. With the head in the erect position and the child fixing a distant object, the relative position of the eyes should first be noted. The eye should next follow an object to the nine cardinal positions, binocularly and then individually. Squint (strabismus) in any particular direction of gaze, but not in others, will indicate incomitance (paralytic strabismus). Simple examination of the ocular movements should be followed by the cover test. The cover test is used to detect a squint and consists of covering and then uncovering one eye and repeating the process with the other eye (Fig. 26.5). The cover test is carried out with the child fixing a distant object and then a near object. With latent squint the covered eye will take up the squinting position behind the cover and be seen to move back to the 'fixing' position when the cover is removed. With manifest squint, the squinting eye will move to the fixing position when the other eye is covered (Fig. 26.6) and move back again when the cover is removed. With alternating squint, occlusion of the non-squinting eye will result in the squinting eye taking up the fixing position, but on removing the cover this eye will remain dominant and the covered eye (now uncovered) will become the squinting eye. The cover test also analyzes hypertropia (vertical squint). If there is doubt about the presence of nystagmus the optic nerve should be examined with the ophthalmoscope, when fine nystagmus is easily discernible. In manifest nystagmus the eyes should be moved in the cardinal positions of gaze to determine if the nystagmus increases or decreases.

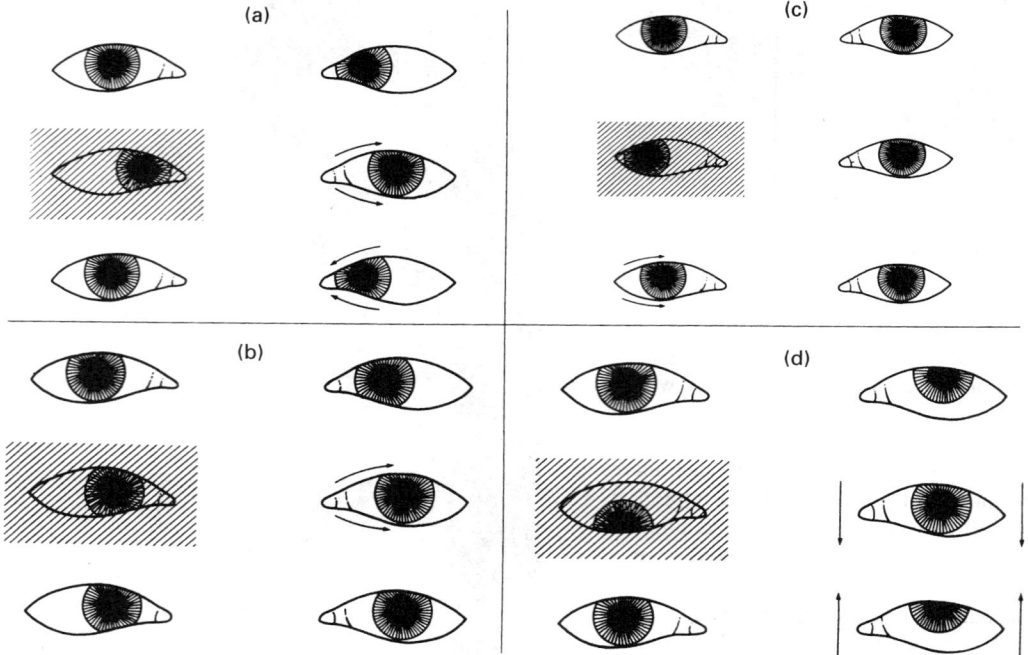

Fig. 26.5 The cover test for squint. Where there is no squint and there is normal binocular vision, both eyes maintain steady fixation on a distant object. There will be no deviation when one or other eye is covered and this is the basis of a cover test. When there is a latent or manifest squint some deviation will be observed on occluding one or other eye. (**a**) In manifest convergent squint the squinting eye is turned in and the non-squinting eye maintains fixation. If the squinting eye is occluded in the cover test there will be no variation in the angle of squint, but when the non-squinting eye ('fixing eye') is occluded it converges and the squinting eye takes up fixation. When the occluder is removed the original position of the eyes is resumed. (**b**) In alternating convergent squint either eye can maintain fixation while the other eye is turned in. If the squinting eye is occluded there is no alteration in the angle of deviation, but when the 'fixing eye' is occluded the opposite eye fixes the distant object and the previously straight eye converges. The former position is not resumed when the occluder is removed and the previously squinting eye maintains fixation (and the previously straight eye converges) until the occluder covers the originally squinting eye, when the originally fixing eye takes up position. (**c**) In latent squint both eyes will fix a distant object but when one eye is covered it deviates. When the cover is removed the eye with the latent squint resumes fixation. The other eye does not shift or lose fixation while the opposite eye is being covered or uncovered. (**d**) The cover test is used to diagnose vertical squint as in horizontal squint, e.g. in left hypertropia the left eye is elevated (or the right eye depressed) and when the fixing eye is covered the opposite eye moves vertically to take up fixation.

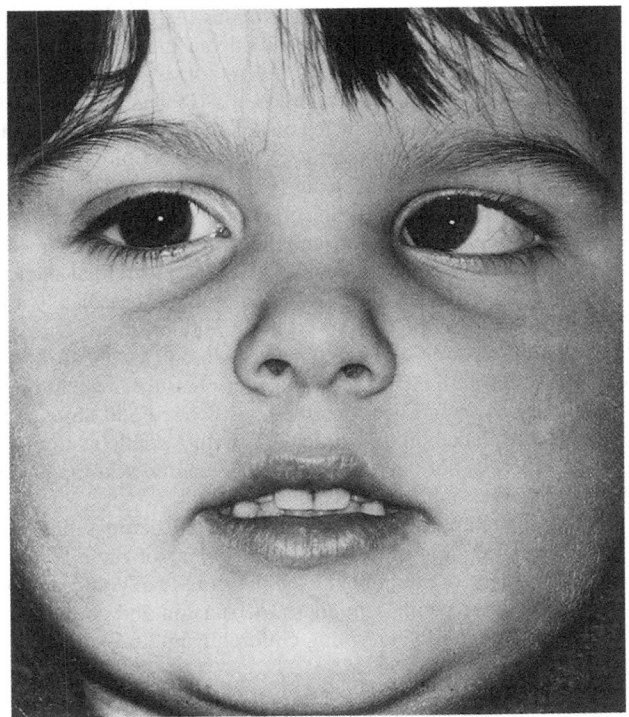

(a)

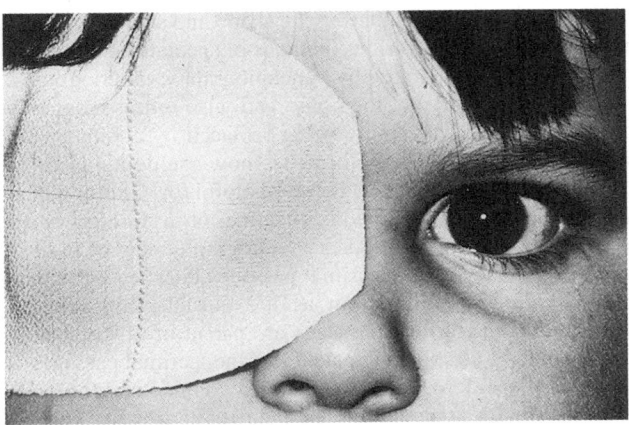

(b)

Fig. 26.6 (**a**) Convergent squint. A child with a left convergent squint and slight elevation on adduction of the left eye. The right eye has good vision but the left eye is intensely amblyopic. (**b**) Left convergent squint. The 'normal' right eye has now been totally occluded and the child is fixing with the left eye. The right eye will be converging behind the occluder.

SPECIAL METHODS OF EXAMINATION

The direct ophthalmoscope is the 'standard equipment' used in the examination of the eye.

The binocular indirect ophthalmoscope gives a stereoscopic image of the fundus (see above) and is preferred by the ophthalmologist.

Photography is used regularly to record details of examination and is invaluable for comparative purposes. The face, external eye, anterior segment (Fig. 26.7), lens and fundus can all be photographed without difficulty. Cine photography and video recording give useful records of the ocular movements including nystagmus. Fundus photography is used routinely in adults to record details of the retina, optic disk, etc. although examination

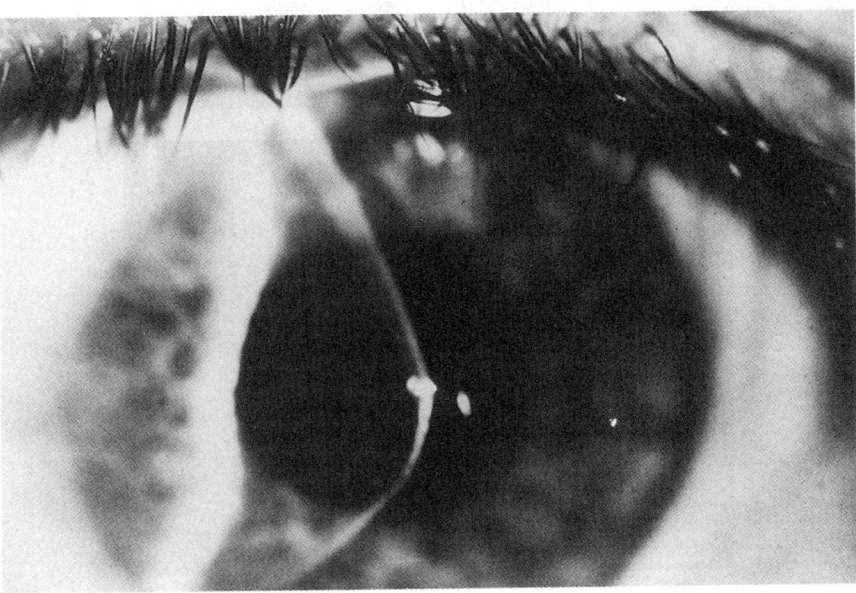

Fig. 26.7 Keratoconus. A slit lamp photograph of the cornea of an eye with conical cornea. Instead of the normal regular corneal curve a slit is cone shaped, and whereas the periphery of the cornea shows normal thickness, it is thinned at the apex of the cone.

of the color plates in this chapter will show that it is difficult to maintain equality of color (color temperature).

Radiology is useful in examining and measuring the shape and size of the orbits and in comparing the shape and size of the optic foramina. Until recently, various methods of specialized radiology including contrast orbitography, pneumography, arteriography, venography and dacryocystography and also ultrasonography were used but these are rapidly being replaced by computerized scanning techniques. Radiology is now seldom used in ophthalmology, although it may be very helpful for cases of ocular trauma and especially in the localization of a foreign body. Dacryocystography and macrodacryocystography may be used to examine the patency of the lacrimal passages but they contribute little useful clinical information as it is usually apparent on examination if the lacrimal passages are patent or obstructed. A simpler method of establishing patency of the lacrimal passages is to instil a drop of fluorescein into the lower conjunctival fornix. If fluorescein remains apparent in the conjunctival sac after about 5 minutes the lacrimal passage on that side is obstructed, or, alternatively, if fluorescein appears in the nostril or on blowing the nose the lacrimal passage is patent.

Fluorescein retinal angiography has become an established technique and is used to give details of the retinal and choroidal circulations and of lesions of the fundus. Angiography is valuable in assessing the presence of papilledema in doubtful cases, as it shows with certainty whether even minor degrees of papilledema are present. In established papilledema (Plates 26.5 and 26.6) the picture is characteristic when using the ophthalmoscope but in doubtful cases angiography is helpful. Fluorescein retinal angiography is useful in quantifying papilledema (Figs 26.8 and 26.9) and it is also helpful in following optic atrophy, in assessing vascular lesions of the retina and the retinopathies and in measuring the 'arm–retina circulation time'. Fluorescein retinal angiograms are taken by rapid serial fundus photography immediately after the intravenous injection of 10 ml of sodium fluorescein. This is now a routine ophthalmic investigative procedure.

The measurement of the intraocular pressure in a child presents difficulty as the cornea must be anesthetized and an applanation tonometer placed on the cornea, but with a gentle examiner and a child who has not been frightened this can be accomplished with accuracy even in the very young.

The slit-lamp binocular microscope ('slit lamp') must be used to examine details of the anterior segment of the eye. This is a standard piece of equipment used in virtually all eye examinations in the adult and with gentleness, persuasion and cooperation can be helpful even in very young children (Fig. 26.7).

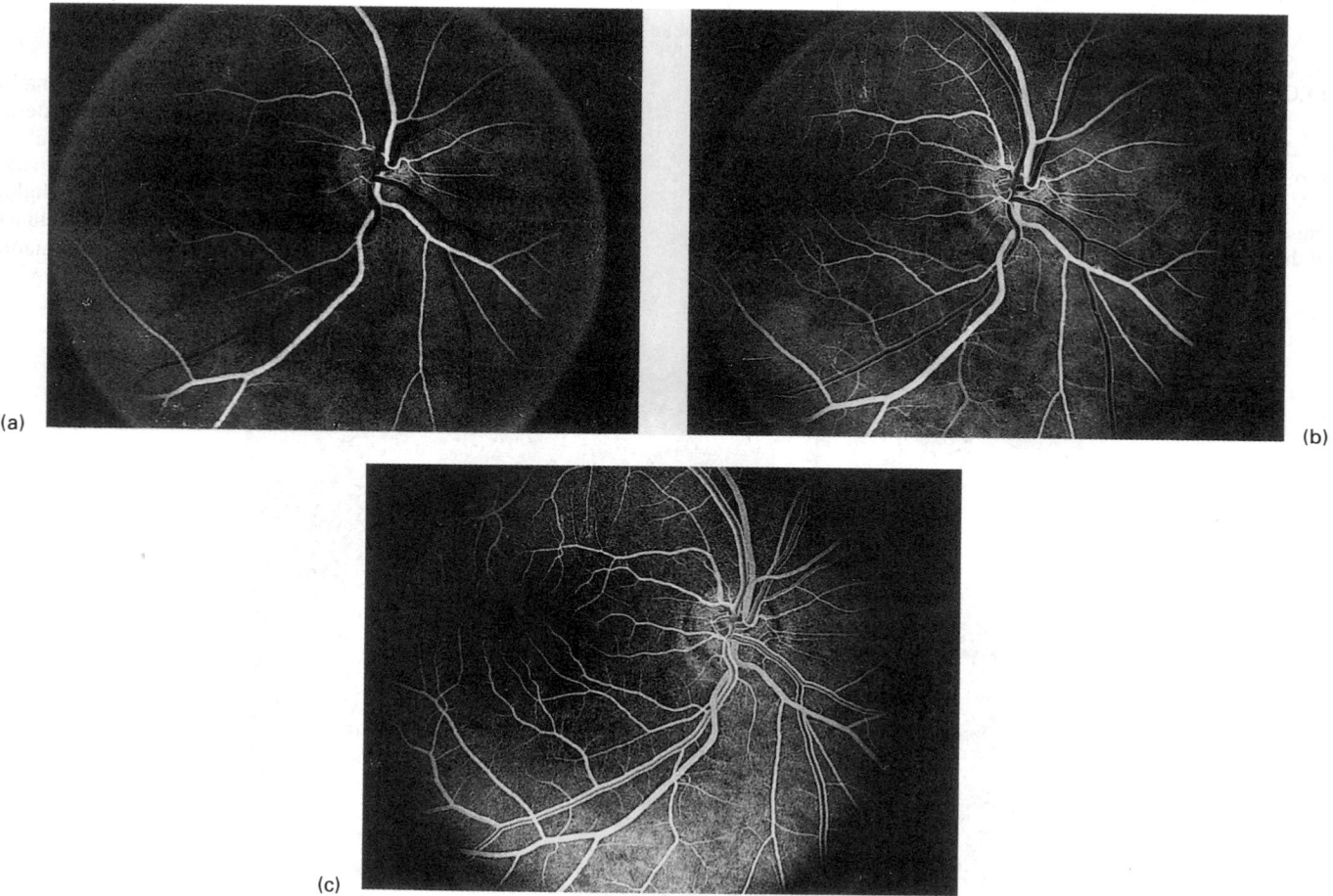

(a)

(b)

(c)

Fig. 26.8 Normal retinal fluorescein angiogram. A series of retinal photographs taken after the injection of sodium fluorescein intravenously: **(a)** (6 seconds after injection) shows fluorescein entering the normal retinal circulation; **(b)** (10 seconds after injection) shows filling of the normal arterial circulation; **(c)** (12 seconds after injection) shows the normal arterial circulation with developing venous filling with normal background fluorescence and a normal optic disk.

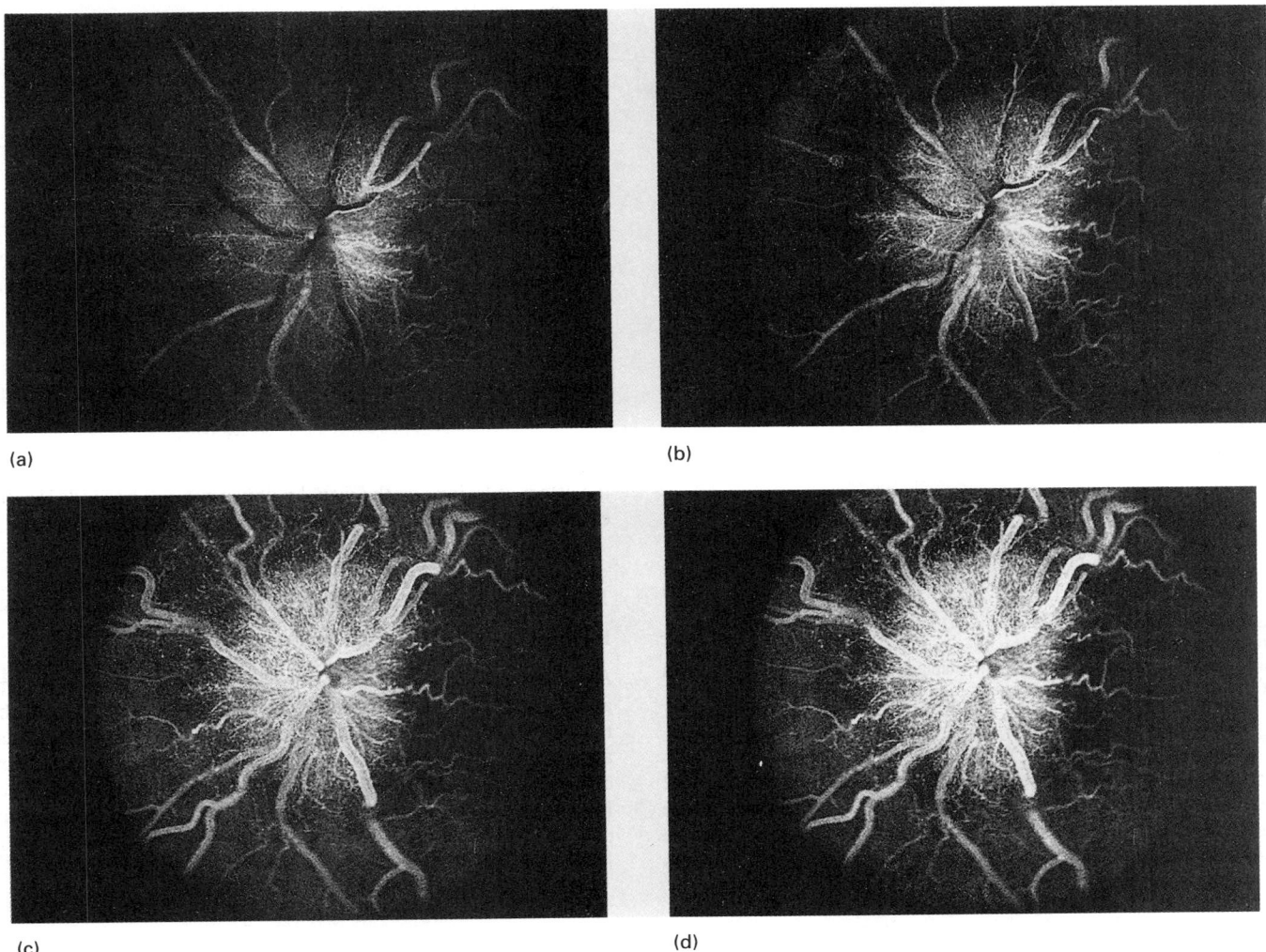

(a)

(b)

(c)

(d)

Fig. 26.9   Fluorescein angiograms of the optic disk in early papilledema: (**a**) (6 seconds) shows dye reaching the optic disk; (**b**) (8 seconds) shows established dye on the disk and early leakage; (**c**) (10 seconds) and (**d**) (12 seconds) show the typical appearance of a papilledematous disk with leakage of fluorescein from the optic disk, with irregular disk margins and dilated and tortuous retinal vessels.

Electrodiagnostic techniques have become available for routine use during the past two decades. These techniques include the electroretinogram (ERG), the electro-oculogram (EOG) and the visual evoked response (VER).

The electroretinogram depends upon the existence of a 'resting current' between the cornea and the posterior pole of the eye. It is useful in the diagnosis of circulatory diseases of the retina, detachment of the retina, retinal abiotrophies and choroidoretinal atrophy. The electroretinogram is made up of an early receptor potential, the 'a' wave, a 'b' wave and a 'c' wave (Fig. 26.10). There is also an 'off' effect whose position and nature is variable according to the type and timing of the initial stimulus flash. The electroretinogram is produced entirely by the retina and no other structures in or around the eye are involved in its production. The 'a' wave depends on the outer segments of the retinal receptors, the 'b' wave arises from the inner nuclear layer of the retina and the 'c' wave (which is variable and is not always present) probably arises from the pigment epithelium. These wave changes are very sensitive responses and can be modified or abolished by pathological conditions of the retina. The electroretinogram is reduced or abolished in the hereditary retinal degenerations apart from those conditions where the eye changes are strictly limited to the macula, such as Tay–Sachs disease (Plate 26.10). In recording the electroretinogram, a bright stimulus flash is used after placing a contact lens electrode on the eye. The tracing is recorded using a modified standard electronic bank.

The electro-oculogram depends on the modification of the 'resting current' when the eye moves. Two electrodes are attached to the skin near the inner and outer canthi and if the eye is adducted the nasal electrode will become positive relative to the temporal electrode; repeated eye movements are used to produce the electro-oculogram (Fig. 26.11). The electro-oculogram is reduced or abolished in abiotrophic lesions, in retinal degenerations such as those occurring in myopia, siderosis and chloroquin intoxication and in extensive inflammations of the retina and choroid. Electro-oculography is a simple technique using simple and portable equipment but it requires considerable cooperation from the patient and is difficult to perform in patients who cannot fix a target or who have very poor vision.

The visual evoked response uses scalp electrodes to record the

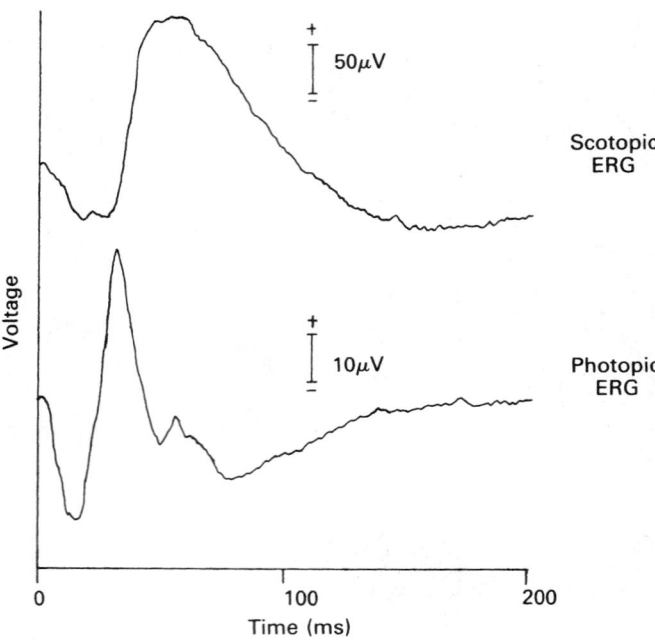

Fig. 26.10 A normal electroretinogram (ERG) showing the typical wave pattern and amplitude. The electroretinogram is taken under photopic (light adapted) conditions and scotopic (dark adapted) conditions. The wave pattern is reduced or abolished in various pathological conditions of the retina.

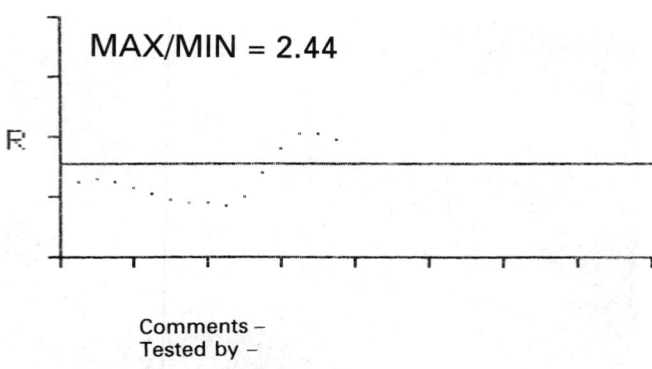

MAX/MIN = 2.44

Comments –
Tested by –

Fig. 26.11 This is a trace of a normal electro-oculogram (EOG). Each laboratory has its own baseline for carrying out these tests and for recording data and the traces are largely used for comparative purposes.

the effect of lesions on the visual pathways it will be modified, for example, by lesions within the eye, particularly at the macula.

TESTING VISUAL ACUITY (see Ch. 9)

Refractive errors

Emmetropia is the condition in which no refractive error is present and parallel rays of light are brought to a point focus upon the macula when the eye is at rest. Few normal adults eyes are absolutely emmetropic and minor degrees of refractive error are common. The refractive state of the eye depends upon a variety of factors including the length of the eye, the index of refraction of the media and the curvature of the cornea. There is a genetic influence upon the final refractive state.

electrical response to repeated light flashes to the eyes (Figs 26.12 and 26.13). The visual evoked response records essentially the function of the central visual pathways. It is useful in the diagnosis of, for example, optic neuritis but although it assesses

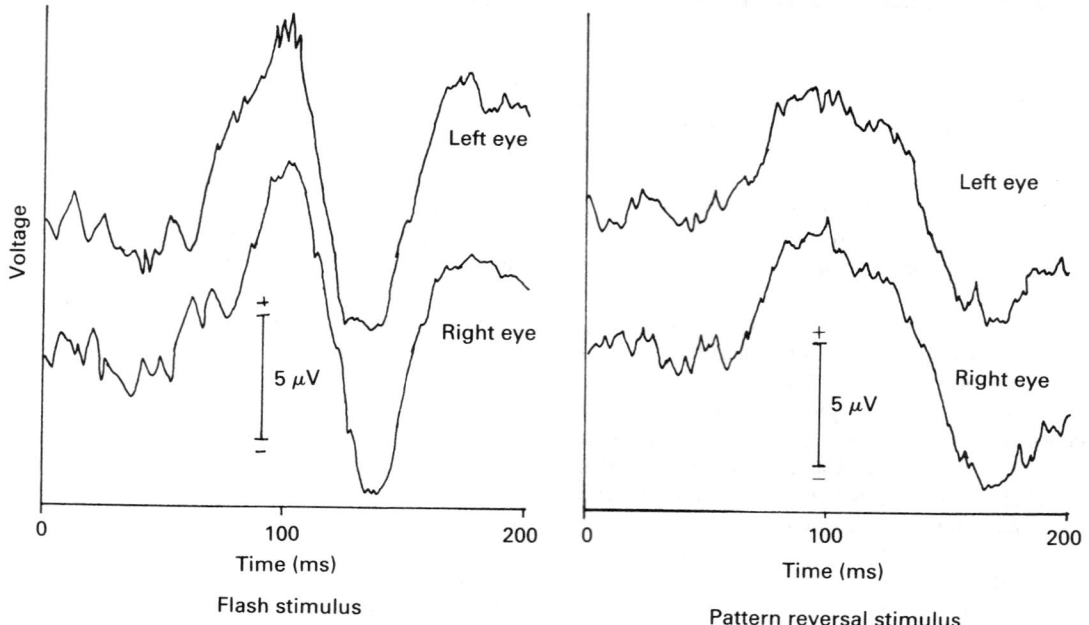

Flash stimulus

Pattern reversal stimulus

Fig. 26.12 Visual evoked response (VER). A visual evoked response uses repeated light flashes and records the function of the central pathways. Initially a simple light flash was used, but it was subsequently found that a checkerboard flash gave a better reaction and now pattern reversal is used for greater accuracy. The VER is useful in comparing an eye with even slightly reduced vision with the normal eye. Any major difference between the two sides indicates an abnormality in the visual pathway of the affected side.

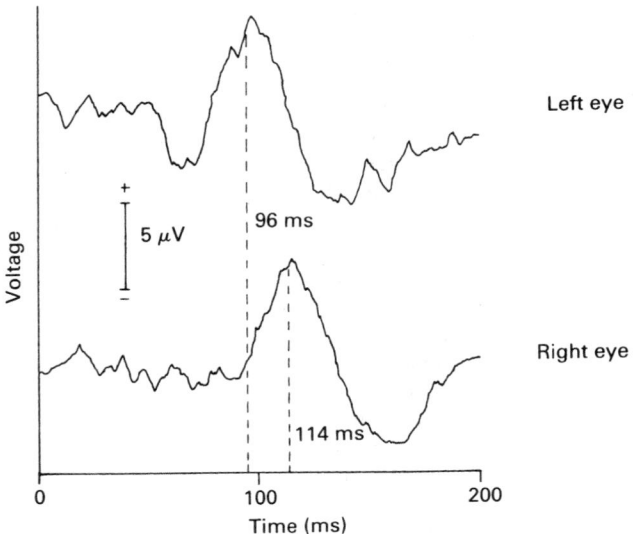

Fig. 26.13 Pattern reversal visual evoked response. The VER of two eyes where the left eye (upper trace) shows a normal pattern and there is a slight delay in the right eye (lower trace).

Hypermetropia (long sight) is the commonest refractive error and is due to the eye being relatively short in axial length. The eye at birth normally has about 3 diopters of hypermetropia and becomes emmetropic by about 3 years of age. When a child is hypermetropic he has good distance vision but difficulty with close vision and this may be accompanied by amblyopia or a squint. Aphakia (absence of the lens), whether congenital or surgical, is a special case of hypermetropia in that the eye is hypermetropic by about 12 diopters and has no accommodation. The same condition occurs if the lenses are completely dislocated.

Myopia (short sight) is caused by the eye being relatively long. Congenital myopia is rare and myopia usually develops between 7 and 14 years of age. After an eye becomes myopic there is usually some increase in the degree of myopia over several years until the final refractive stage is reached shortly after puberty. A myopic child should wear spectacles constantly. The wearing of spectacles does not 'cure' myopia but simply gives good corrected vision. Myopia is usually a genetically determined condition for which there is no cure apart from extremely rare cases of corneal or lenticular abnormality and although advertisements for treatment of myopia abound, the only safe help available is the use of spectacles or contact lenses which bring about good vision but do not have any therapeutic value.

Astigmatism is the condition in which parallel rays of light cannot be brought to a point focus upon the retina by any effort of accommodation or with the use of simple spherical spectacle lenses and images are always blurred for distant and near vision. Astigmatism must be corrected by a lens incorporating a cylinder.

Refractive errors are generally similar in the two eyes but occasionally there is inequality in the refraction or there may be a uniocular refractive error.

Anisometropia is the refractive state when there is a difference of more than 2 diopters in the refraction of the eyes and this may lead to amblyopia or a squint. In anisometropia the eye closest to emmetropia is generally used electively but occasionally a child will develop alternating vision using a hypermetropic eye for distance and the myopic eye for close vision.

Newborn children are almost always hypermetropic as the axial length of the eye is generally small at birth. As the axial length enlarges the eye progresses toward emmetropia or even, in some cases, after the age of about 7 years, to myopia. In newborn children there is often a very high degree of astigmatism which can vary in both magnitude and axis over the first year of life. The refractive error in the first few months of life changes rapidly and is seldom the same as the refractive error a few years after birth.

Testing for refractive errors

Children rarely complain of poor vision and even schoolchildren or young adults may accept poor vision produced by the onset of myopia without comment. For this reason it is essential that visual acuity should be tested regularly in schoolchildren and also in preschool children. No refractive error can be cured by spectacles but the use of spectacles allows the child to develop normal visual and binocular reflexes and enables him to have a normal acuity of vision. Children accept spectacles readily (where they are necessary) and, with the higher degrees of refractive error, contact lenses will be worn without difficulty.

If a refractive error is suspected the examination of refraction should be undertaken. Young children are unable to cooperate fully in subjective testing and older children are over-anxious to cooperate. For this reason refraction in children under about 8 years of age should be carried out objectively after using a weak cycloplegic. Where a refractive error is detected the refraction examination should be repeated in 6 months' time and then annually. Cycloplegia is not necessary on all occasions after the refractive error has become stabilized. A cycloplegic is used for its effect in paralyzing accommodation and not for the mydriasis which cycloplegics produce. Atropine drops (0.25%) may be used twice daily for 2 days prior to examination but care should be taken to occlude the lower lacrimal punctum when atropine drops are instilled in young children as there is a risk of toxicity should atropine be absorbed through lacrimal passages. Should atropine be used, the ointment (0.25%) is preferable to drops, being less readily absorbed, but this is rather more difficult to administer. The practice of 'atropinizing' the child before an ophthalmic examination without prior examination is to be deplored because of the risk of atropine toxicity. The routine use of atropine is now seldom necessary, as rapidly acting temporary cycloplegics such as tropicamide are useful in refraction. If no refractive error is found on refraction, or if the vision does not improve with the use of spectacles, a full ocular examination must be carried out.

Reading difficulties may be found in a schoolchild that are unrelated to any refractive error or ocular abnormality. Specific reading disability (dyslexia) occurs more commonly in boys than in girls and may initially be confused with a refractive error. Dyslexia may be associated with mixed lateral dominance, upsets in spatial orientation or visual agnosia. Children with dyslexia usually respond well to educational methods based initially on auditory rather than visual techniques.

THE APPARENTLY BLIND BABY (see Ch. 9)

AMAUROSIS

Amaurosis is commonly used to mean total or partial loss of vision in one or both eyes and implies total or partial blindness. Amaurosis should not be confused with amblyopia, which is the term commonly used to refer to a lazy eye (squint), although amblyopia is also used in cases where there is visual loss due to, for example, toxicity (e.g. toxic amblyopia).

The term amaurosis, meaning blind or partially blind, implies that an exact diagnosis has not been made. Amaurosis can be due to a congenital ocular or cerebral abnormality or a tumor in the eye or the orbit. It can also be due to degenerative lesions and infective processes. Where amaurosis is suggested in a child who has previously had good vision, full investigation is necessary.

ACUTE ONSET BLINDNESS

The acute onset of blindness in a child usually implies systemic or neurological disease rather than an ophthalmic condition. Acute onset total blindness is very rare. If the eyes are normal, neurological or systemic factors should be investigated. Where one eye shows blindness there should be pupillary signs of an afferent defect. In a totally blind eye due to an ocular or optic nerve lesion, on direct light stimulation neither the pupil of the apparently blind eye nor that of the other eye will respond but on shining a light into the normal eye both pupils will respond equally and fully.

TRANSIENT BLINDNESS

Transient blindness is unusual in children and is associated with papilledema. Where papilledema is present, episodes of transient blindness may last from a few seconds to a minute. The cause of such transient blindness (obscurations) is not understood but it is presumed to be related to raised intracranial pressure and changes in axoplasmic flow. Episodes of transient blindness can occur in late childhood due to migraine and although these may be associated with the usual phenomena connected with migraine they may be isolated and the diagnosis can be difficult. The sudden onset of diabetes mellitus in children is occasionally associated with wild swings in refraction and, should this cause a hypermetropic child to become temporarily myopic, it is occasionally interpreted as impending blindness.

HYSTERIA AND MALINGERING

'Hysterical amblyopia' and hysterical blindness are terms which are now seldom used. Teenage children very occasionally have psychological upsets which cause them to appear to be blind; these children are rather more commonly male than female. When such a patient presents it is usually evident that some psychiatric or neurological condition is present and, although the patient claims to be blind, he can usually navigate well. These patients usually have tubular visual fields or variable fields. As reproduction of their signs is always inconstant this in itself may be diagnostic. It is usually very difficult to establish a diagnosis from the ophthalmic aspect but the condition becomes apparent after a few days of observation. Hysterical amblyopia is often referred to as a visual conversion reaction but such a diagnosis should not be made until ophthalmic and neurological conditions have been excluded. Malingering is very occasionally met with in ophthalmology. A typical patient claims to have loss of vision or reduced vision in one eye only. Malingering was common in the days of conscription for national service (the army) but is now usually reserved for legal compensation cases. It is usually easy to diagnose by simple expedients.

THE MANAGEMENT OF THE BLIND OR VISUALLY HANDICAPPED CHILD

Where it is apparent that a child will become blind or almost totally blind, the diagnosis should be made after full examination and the position should be explained to the parents and also, most importantly, to the child. It causes great distress and psychological upset if false hope is given where no hope is possible and one always emphasizes that where blindness or almost total blindness is inevitable, this should be diagnosed as early as possible and the best available help should be offered. Blind children manage remarkably well where they are given help from the earliest possible moment. Many blind children, given minimal support, are able to pursue normal careers and normal lives. Unfortunately many blind children are sent to 'blind schools' where they meet and marry other blind children, which always adds to their difficulty and complicates the pedigree. In general, blind children should be encouraged to lead a perfectly normal life. Visually handicapped children are more difficult to recognize and diagnose as they come in between the area of what is normal and what is blind. As a general rule, where sight is impaired permanently and no treatment can be offered, a normal sighted education should be offered as far as possible and a normal background should be given, but it should be recognized and it should be explained fully to the child, parents and teachers that vision is reduced and that all available visual aids should be used in the furtherment of the best possible education and development.

STRABISMUS AND AMBLYOPIA

Strabismus is the condition in which the eyes deviate from normal. The visual axis of one eye (the squinting eye) is not directed at the object observed by the other eye (the fixing eye). The visual axis is the line joining the fovea to the fixation object. It is only during the past century that the understanding of strabismus has been put on a rational basis, with the result that treatment has become effective. Previous attempts at treatment of strabismus were based on surgery and were concerned solely with correcting the anatomical deviation but it is now realized that to correct strabismus good vision must be restored to each eye so that full binocularity eventually develops and maintains the eyes in the primary position associated with full stereoscopic vision.

The visual reflexes become established during the first few years of life and as full recovery of normal vision can only be brought about within a short time of the development of a squint, satisfactory treatment of strabismus depends upon an early diagnosis. The widespread belief that children may spontaneously 'grow out' of a squint is entirely fallacious and still results in many children being referred for treatment when it is too late. Although after delayed referral surgical cure may still be possible, the squinting eye usually remains amblyopic. The earliest possible diagnosis and treatment of a child with a squint is essential.

The commonest type of strabismus is of the concomitant convergent nature associated with a hypermetropic refractive error. No case of strabismus or pseudostrabismus should be treated lightly and the ocular fundus should always be examined in detail, bearing in mind that an inflammatory or neoplastic lesion involving the retina or visual pathways may cause strabismus through interference with afferent sensation. Although these cases are rare, strabismus can be an early diagnostic sign, and detailed examination of the eye may be helpful in preservation of vision or even of life.

The principal causes of squint are sensory and motor obstacles to the correct alignment of the eyes, together with refractive errors. Sensory obstacles include any defect in the afferent visual pathway, such as corneal scarring, cataract and disease of the retina or of the optic nerve. Any of these will reduce vision, disturb fusion of the two images and, in a child, may provoke a squint. An important cause in this group is occlusion of one eye by a pad or bandage during treatment of some other condition. If a child's eye is covered in the treatment of, for example, a corneal ulcer or facial injury, the eye may become amblyopic and very quickly a squint will develop. Motor obstacles causing squint include deformities of the orbit, congenital abnormalities of the extraocular muscles or disease of the muscles or their motor nerves.

Refractive errors are a common cause of strabismus and by far the commonest is hypermetropia which produces overconvergence resulting in convergent strabismus. Myopia results in underconvergence, leading to a divergent strabismus. Squint is not caused by anxiety, worry, fear, or by infectious disease, although a latent squint may become manifest during some intercurrent illness. Squint is frequently ascribed to the exanthematous infections, especially measles, but this has never been shown to be the direct cause, although there is the possibility that encephalitis following measles could cause an extraocular muscle palsy.

Almost 50% of all squinting children have a family history of squint or refractive error and when a child presents with a squint the other children in the family should be examined. Squint itself is not inherited but the factors producing a squint may be transmitted. These include facial or orbital anomalies and a particularly common hereditary factor is the presence of a refractive error.

PSEUDO-SQUINT

This implies the appearance of squint in a child when the visual axes are correctly aligned and no true squint is present. It is an appearance usually caused by marked epicanthal folds which may be bilateral (Fig. 26.14) or unilateral, a small or large interpupillary distance, a broad nasal bridge, or facial asymmetry. Most of these conditions give the false appearance of a convergent squint, less sclera being visible on the nasal side of the cornea than on the temporal side. These appearances tend to be exaggerated in photographs and when the child is looking upwards.

Pseudo-squint is a common condition among young children but with facial development it generally disappears. A child with a pseudo-squint should be examined carefully as there is always the possibility of a true squint also being present. A pseudo-squint can be diagnosed by alternately covering one eye and then the other while the child is fixing on a light (the cover test, p. 1652). If there is no movement of the eyes during this test only a pseudo-squint is present. No treatment is necessary for pseudo-squint nor is any treatment usually required for the cosmetic blemish responsible for the appearance. Facial asymmetry almost always lessens with growth of the child and even where the interpupillary distances are wide or narrow this generally becomes less obvious with growth. Epicanthal folds disappear or reduce spontaneously and should only be treated surgically in the rare condition where the skin folds are so gross as to be covering the iris or pupil of the eyes in the primary position.

HETEROPHORIA (LATENT SQUINT)

This is the condition in which there is extraocular muscle imbalance and although there is normally no deviation of the eyes, a potential deviation is present. In esophoria the eyes tend to turn

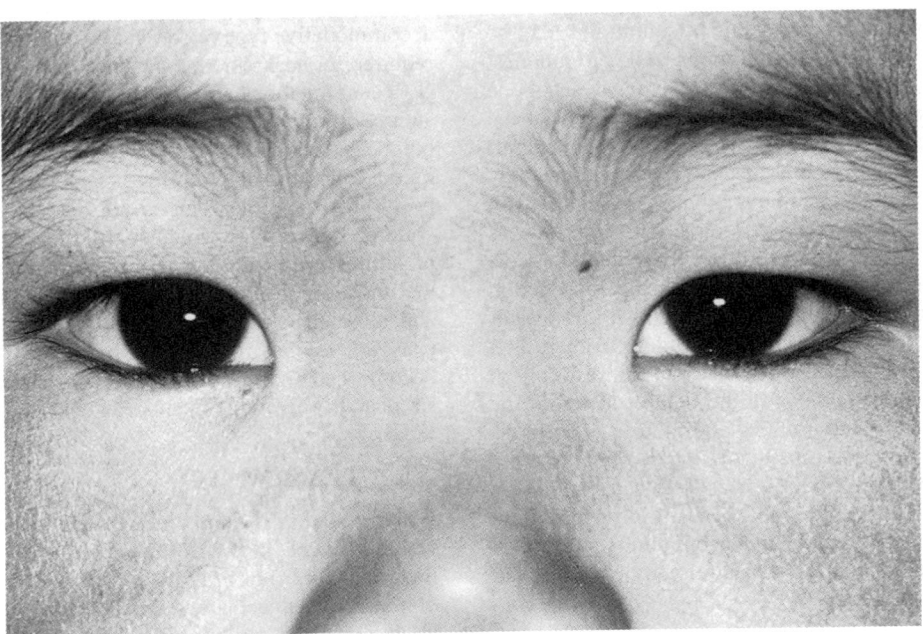

Fig. 26.14 Epicanthal folds. This child has a broad nasal bridge and also epicanthal folds. The skin folds cover the medial part of the sclera of each eye causing the eyes and the pupils to appear to be nearer to the inner canthi than normal, giving a pseudo-squint.

in, due to either convergence excess when the deviation is greatest for near vision, or divergence weakness when the deviation is greatest for distance vision. In exophoria the eyes tend to turn out, due to either divergence excess or convergence weakness. Hyperphoria and hypophoria refer to the tendency for an eye to turn upwards or downwards. The causes of latent squint are similar to the causes of manifest squint. In general, latent squint causes little trouble and does not develop into a true squint but a latent squint may break down into a true squint during illness or with a change in refractive error.

The treatment of latent squint may involve little more than the correction of a refractive error although sometimes orthoptic treatment or occasionally surgery is necessary.

Convergence insufficiency is a special form of latent squint in which the eyes cannot converge or sustain convergence on a close object causing a feeling of discomfort on attempting close vision which is interpreted as 'eye strain'. Convergence insufficiency is relatively common and is the only condition in which a squint or latent squint is associated with 'eye strain'. It responds rapidly to simple orthoptic treatment, together with the correction of any refractive error present.

CONCOMITANT (NON-PARALYTIC) SQUINT

In this condition the angle of deviation remains unchanged whatever the direction of the gaze. Concomitant squint may be convergent, divergent, hypertropic (where the squinting eye turns upwards) or hypotropic (where it turns downwards). The great majority of concomitant squints are horizontal but occasionally a squint has both a horizontal and a vertical element. A concomitant squint may be intermittent, being present only on fixation for certain distances or in certain direction of gaze, but it is generally manifest at all times.

INCOMITANT (PARALYTIC) SQUINT

This is much less common than concomitant squint and may be produced by a large number of conditions. The commonest squints in this group have a neurogenic cause due to paresis of one of the extraocular muscles (paralytic squint). Dysfunction of the sixth nerve is particularly prone to occur with external (lateral) rectus weakness. The extraocular muscles may also be affected by myogenic lesions, generally congenital anomalies associated with musculofascial abnormalities. Duane's retraction syndrome is typical of this group and in this condition the external rectus muscle becomes fibrosed and there may be associated enophthalmos and ptosis on eye movement. In the superior oblique tendon sheath syndrome (Brown's syndrome) there is a fascial anomaly involving the sheath of that muscle, resulting in loss of movement of the affected eye in the field of action of the inferior oblique muscle. Incomitant squint in a child is occasionally caused by severe trauma involving an orbital fracture with displacement of the eye, or it may be caused by a skull injury involving the third, fourth or most commonly the sixth intracranial nerves. The treatment of incomitant squint must include treatment of the underlying condition but extraocular muscle surgery is often necessary.

MANAGEMENT OF SQUINT

In the management of the squinting child the first essentials are

refraction and the assessment of visual acuity. Spectacles are prescribed to correct any refractive error. If vision in the squinting eye remains defective even after the constant wearing of spectacles, occlusion of the non-squinting eye for 1 or 2 weeks at a time is used to improve the central vision in the squinting eye. Occlusion may produce a rapid improvement in vision and this is greatest where amblyopia has been present for only a short time. If the squint is of long standing and amblyopia is intense it may be very difficult to obtain visual improvement by occlusion. Before occluding an eye it is necessary to be certain that fixation of the squinting eye is not eccentric, otherwise the covering of a non-squinting eye will cause any eccentric fixation to become established. The wearing of spectacles together with occlusion and orthoptic treatment may alone be sufficient to correct a squint and restore binocular vision and if this is the case no further treatment may be necessary, although continued orthoptic supervision is necessary until the child reaches the age of 7 or 8 to ensure that there is no breakdown in binocular function.

Surgical treatment may be necessary where the angle of deviation remains or is not fully corrected despite these other forms of treatment. Surgery is always carried out under general anesthesia and involves the shortening, lengthening or repositioning of the extraocular muscles. Where the squint has initially been of large angle, two operations are commonly necessary. Surgery is seldom carried out before orthoptic treatment, but in the very young child surgery is necessary at an early age if a satisfactory result is to be obtained. At whatever age surgery is performed, regular supervision is given until the surgeon is certain that full central vision and binocular vision are established.

Other methods used in the treatment of squint include the use of anticholinesterase drugs such as pilocarpine drops and diisopropylfluorophosphate (DFP) to cause a decrease in accommodation with a corresponding reduction in convergence. Pilocarpine and DFP are useful in the accommodative type of convergent squint where the initial angle is small and the squint is greatest for near vision. Bifocal spectacles are occasionally used in the accommodative type of squint to reduce the extra accommodation required for near vision, together with the associated convergence.

Recent methods of treatment include the use of adjustable sutures in which conventional strabismus surgery is carried out but the sutures are left tied in such a way that they may be adjusted on the following day to bring the eyes into as near to the primary position as possible. This is not difficult in adults and in older children but very few younger children will accept the adjustment of sutures even under local anesthesia. During the past few years the injection of botulinus toxin has been used to induce a partial and temporary paralysis of an extraocular muscle to allow the eyes to resume the primary position and binocular vision to become established. Should this technique find a place, many strabismus operations in children could be avoided.

SQUINT AMBLYOPIA

When a squint develops in an adult, double vision is produced which may be in the form of confusion (where two different images are seen) or of diplopia (in which a true and a false image of the same object are seen). When a child develops a squint double vision is rapidly followed by the suppression of vision in the squinting eye. This suppression may be temporary but generally leads to a permanent loss of central vision (amblyopia). In suppression, the image from the squinting eye is first ignored and is then positively suppressed by a central mechanism, and amblyopia is an extension of this process. A special type of suppression occurs in alternating squint when the suppression alternates from one eye to the other depending upon which eye is fixing.

Amblyopia is common in the concomitant squint of children but occasionally eccentric fixation develops in the squinting eye when a part of the retina other than the fovea is used for fixation. In some cases there is abnormal retinal correspondence in which the fovea of the non-squinting eye is used together with a non-foveal area of the retina of the squinting eye in an attempt to get some form of binocular function. Eccentric fixation and abnormal retinal correspondence are difficult to eliminate but they must be eradicated if normal foveal fixation is to be taught and established. Some children, particularly those with paralytic incomitant squints, develop abnormal head postures with tilting or turning of the head to one side or the other. This can be so marked as to simulate a torticollis and not uncommonly an incomitant squint in a child presents as an ocular torticollis.

The most important points concerning strabismus are that the diagnosis should be made as soon as possible and treatment given as early as possible while the binocular reflexes are still plastic. Where the possibility of squint is raised or where there is a family history of squint, the child should be referred for expert opinion as soon as possible.

EXTERNAL EYE DISEASE

THE ORBITS

A number of developmental abnormalities may arise due to premature closure of those orbital sutures which do not normally close until adult life; where closure is abnormal it is generally associated with defects in the closure of the sutures of the vault of the skull.

Craniostenosis

Oxycephaly (tower skull) is caused by premature closure of the coronal suture resulting in a high skull with a steep forehead. *Scaphocephaly* (boat-shaped skull) is caused by premature closure of the sagittal suture. *Plagiocephaly* is due to asymmetrical suture closure and *trigonocephaly* is caused by premature closure of the midline metopic suture of the frontal bone resulting in a triangularly shaped skull.

The craniostenoses are frequently of minor degree and cause only a cosmetic defect but where they are more advanced they may result in raised intracranial pressure, often indicated by papilledema. The presence of papilledema indicates prompt surgical decompression of the skull or optic foramina before optic atrophy develops. Shallow orbits may result in proptosis with corneal exposure and this may necessitate orbital decompression.

Cranial dysostosis

Craniofacial dysostosis (Crouzon's anomaly) is a hereditary association of oxycephaly, shallow orbits and aplasia of the maxilla with nasal and palatal defects. *Mandibulofacial dysostosis* (Treacher Collins' syndrome or Franceschetti's syndrome) includes malformations of the eyelids and ears with hypoplasia of the bones of the face and sometimes colobomas of the eyelids and

iris or fundus. *Hypertelorism* is a hereditary developmental anomaly in which the orbits are widely separated and other anomalies generally coexist together with mental retardation.

Infection

The most common inflammation of the orbit in childhood is acute cellulitis, usually pyogenic in origin due to spread of infection from a paranasal sinus. The origin is most often in the ethmoid sinuses in infants but in older children it may be from the ethmoid, frontal or maxillary sinuses. Orbital cellulitis develops rapidly and can lead to severe toxicity with a high fever. Complications include meningitis, cavernous sinus thrombosis and papilledema leading to optic atrophy and exposure keratitis. Orbital cellulitis settles rapidly with an appropriate systemic antibiotic. Acute orbital cellulitis may be mimicked by reactive edema of the eyelids, caused by inflammation in neighboring structures, but in this case there is no systemic toxicity, the eyelids are not acutely tender and when the eyelids are gently opened the eyes can be seen to be freely mobile.

Neoplasms

The most common tumor of the orbit in an infant is hemangioma. This is almost always benign and, if small, no treatment is necessary; if it is causing progressive proptosis, radiotherapy is the treatment of choice. If a hemangioma is neglected (Fig. 26.1) surgical excision may eventually be necessary. Orbital venous varices are not uncommon. Varices reduce in size spontaneously and treatment should not be attempted, as the rupture of a varix can lead to a massive orbital hemorrhage and the loss of sight through optic nerve compression or corneal exposure. Astrocytoma (glioma) of the optic nerve, a benign progressive tumor, causes exophthalmos and papilledema: it may be part of von Recklinghausen's disease. A dermoid cyst may occur as an isolated benign tumor or associated with a bony dehiscence and it should be excised surgically as there is the possibility of hemorrhage into the cyst, causing a rapid proptosis. Neuroblastoma is a malignant secondary tumor which occurs in the orbits of young children as a metastatic spread from a primary adrenal gland tumor. Of cases of proptosis in children, 2% are due to leukemia which occasionally presents in this way.

THE EYELIDS

Ptosis

Ptosis is the commonest developmental abnormality of the eyelids but it is not always congenital and may be considered under several headings.

Congenital ptosis is often an isolated finding but in many cases is associated with local ocular anomalies including marked epicanthal folds and squint, or with remote congenital defects including abnormalities of the fingers and toes, or as part of Turner's syndrome. Congenital ptosis is generally bilateral and often hereditary. It may be part of the Marcus Gunn jaw-winking syndrome in which there is elevation of the drooping eyelid on opening the mouth or lateral movement of the jaw.

Where congenital ptosis is slight in degree, surgery is best avoided. As a rule, surgery need not be undertaken unless there is interference with vision through occlusion of the pupil as happens most frequently in unilateral ptosis. In bilateral ptosis clear vision is obtained by a backward tilting of the head and in cases such as this surgery to both eyelids is required to correct the drooping eyelids and eliminate the abnormal head posture.

Sympathetic ptosis (Horner's syndrome; Fig. 26.2) results only in slight drooping of the eyelid, and surgery is not usually necessary.

Neurogenic ptosis is caused by involvement of the third nerve. It may be congenital in nature when there is often an associated paresis of the superior rectus muscle. The pupil may be fixed and dilated. The indications for treatment are the same as those in other congenital cases.

Mechanical ptosis results from drooping of an eyelid which has been thickened by traumatic or inflammatory scarring. Treatment is directed to the primary condition.

Coloboma

Coloboma of the eyelids (absence of a portion of the lid) may occur as an isolated defect, generally at the junction of the inner and middle thirds of the upper or lower eyelids, but it is more commonly associated with other developmental abnormalities in the orbital region (Plate 26.11).

Hemangioma

Hemangioma may involve the eyelid alone but often extends on to the skin of the face or scalp and sometimes includes the conjunctiva. The incidence of some degree of hemangioma of the skin in this region is just over 2%. A hemangioma may be present at the time of birth or appear within the first weeks of life (Fig. 26.15). It may grow rapidly during the first year but tends to disappear spontaneously over the course of a few years. The majority should be allowed to undergo spontaneous regression. Exposure to low dosage of radiation is effective in treating a hemangioma but is not advisable. If the hemangioma obscures the visual axis, treatment is necessary and intralesional injection of steroids is the treatment of choice. Sturge–Weber disease typically has a telangiectasis of the skin of one side of the face and there may be an associated hemangioma of the choroid, sometimes with buphthalmos.

Hordeolum

Hordeolum (stye) is an abscess of an eyelash follicle close to the eyelid margin (Fig. 26.16). The treatment of a simple stye is to

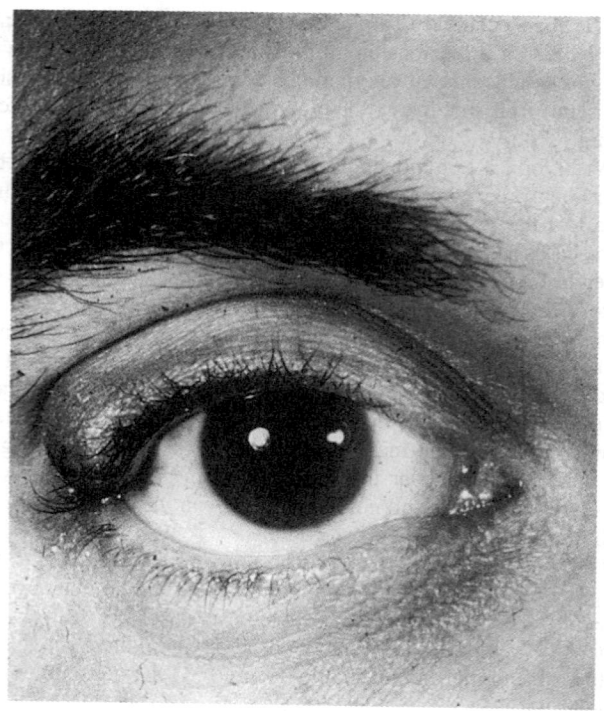

Fig. 26.16 Hordeolum (stye). This child has a stye at the outer end of the right upper eyelid. The swelling involves the eyelid margin and an eyelash and is tender.

allow it to point and if necessary to remove the eyelash at the tip of the follicle. Local antibiotics should not be used. Local heat may encourage a stye to point.

Meibomian cyst

Chronic granulation of a meibomian gland results in a small hard nodule in the eyelid unconnected with the eyelid margin, known as a meibomian cyst. The treatment is to excise it completely or to curette it (Fig. 26.17).

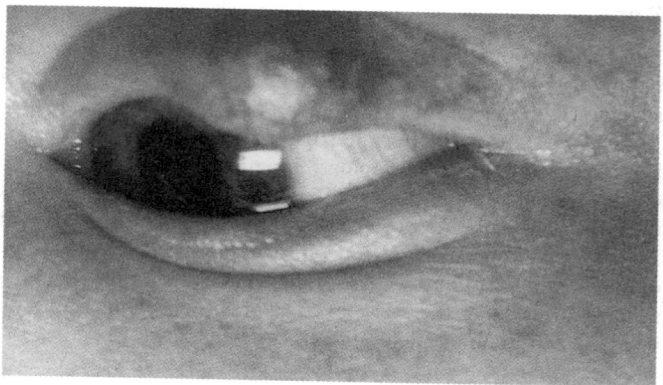

Fig. 26.15 Developmental hemangioma of the upper eyelid.

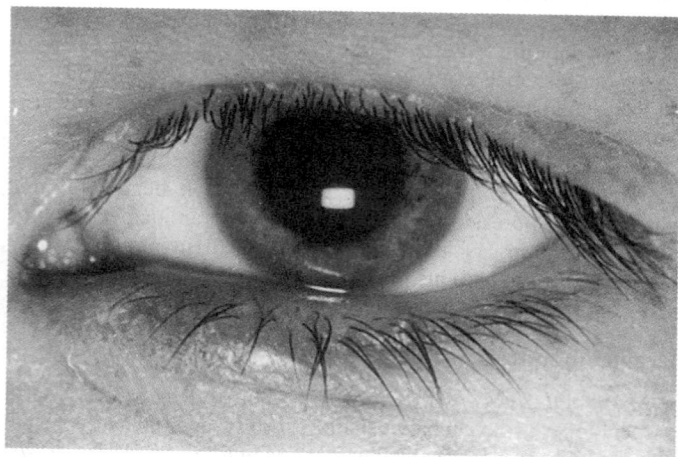

Fig. 26.17 Meibomian cyst (eyelid cyst). There is a small cyst situated inferomedially on the left lower eyelid but not involving the eyelid margin. The cyst will not be tender.

Blepharitis

Squamous blepharitis frequently occurs in young children, particularly those with seborrhea. There is reddening of the eyelid margins, crusting of the eyelashes and usually an associated mild conjunctivitis. Treatment should be directed to the seborrhea and to hygiene; the crusted eyelid margins should be bathed vigorously several times a day (a weak solution of sodium bicarbonate is helpful in softening crusts) and usually no further treatment is necessary. In resistant cases the application of corticosteroid ointment several times a day for a few days after removing the crusts may be beneficial.

Pediculosis blepharitis

Pediculosis blepharitis is occasionally associated with pediculosis infection (lice). Lice infestation is generally assumed to be associated with poor hygiene but this is not always the case. In persistent blepharitis, examination of the eyelids with magnification occasionally shows sign of pediculosis (Fig. 26.18). Both pubic and head lice may be involved and, where ova or adult lice are seen on the eyelash, the child should be examined thoroughly for signs of lice infestation and the appropriate treatment given should lice be found elsewhere. The lesions on the eyelid margins can be removed mechanically by vigorous bathing with moist cotton wool and this is helped by the application of pilocarpine drops or 0.5% eserine ointment, which cause paralysis of the organisms.

Molluscum contagiosum

This viral infection may involve the skin of the eyelids. In severe cases it causes a keratitis which will not respond until the molluscum lesions of the eyelids are treated and eradicated. Treatment is by expression of the individual lesions and if there is a recurrence in any lesion, chemical or electric cautery is effective.

Entropion

Inward turning of the eyelid margins occurs only rarely in children and is almost always spastic in nature, the most common cause being bandaging of the eye (see squint amblyopia). Where

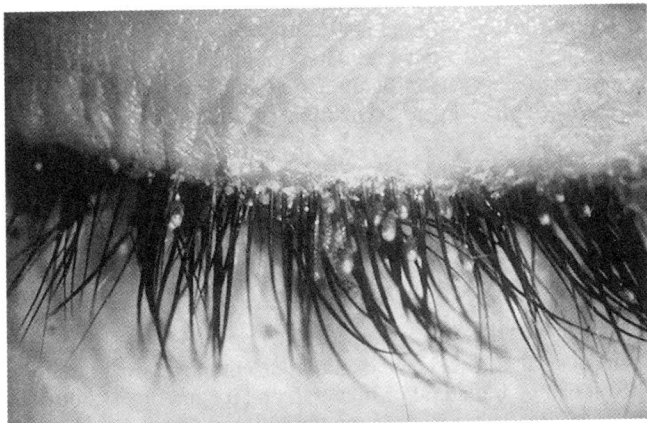

Fig. 26.18 Pediculosis (lice). This patient presented with apparently simple blepharitis but on magnification lice could be seen adherent to the eyelashes and were removed mechanically.

it occurs spontaneously it may be associated with multiple congenital orbital abnormalities and surgery may be necessary. Sometimes it occurs in babies with well-developed buccal pads of fat, when it is mechanical in nature and no treatment is necessary. Occasionally entropion is cicatricial, caused by scarring of the conjunctiva from inflammation, trauma, or a burn. Ectropion, outward turning of the eyelid, is usually cicatricial in children due to scarring of the skin below the lower eyelids and the majority of cases require treatment by surgery.

THE CONJUNCTIVA

Conjunctivitis

Conjunctivitis is an inflammation of the mucous membrane lining the eyelids and the globe of the eye. It is generally infective but it may have a chemical, traumatic or allergic origin. Where the cause is other than a primary infection a secondary infective element develops rapidly. The primary sign in conjunctivitis is hyperemia of the mucous membrane with production of mucus and sometimes of pus. There may be edema of the conjunctiva (chemosis) which can be associated with edema of the eyelids and orbit and in severe cases there may be small petechial conjunctival hemorrhages or larger subconjunctival hemorrhages.

In all cases of conjunctivitis the conjunctivae, eyelids and eyes should be examined carefully. It is particularly important to look for a foreign body on the bulbar conjunctiva, under the upper or lower eyelids or on the cornea, and the presence of conjunctival follicles should be sought. A culture should be taken from the conjunctival sac, the nose and the nasopharynx and it should be borne in mind that epidemics of conjunctivitis are common among school-children.

Acute purulent conjunctivitis results in a rapid inflammation of the conjunctiva with chemosis and edema of the eyelids. There is a copious discharge of mucus and pus and there is systemic toxicity. The causative organism is frequently a staphlycoccus but other pyogenic organisms may be responsible.

Ophthalmia neonatorum is an acute purulent conjunctivitis of newborn infants which may be due to the gonococcus (see Ch. 5). Severe untreated cases may cause ulceration of the cornea with possible rupture of the globe and blindness. An increasing number of mild cases of neonatal conjunctivitis are due to *Chlamydia trachomatis* (TRIC virus) (see below).

Membranous conjunctivitis is nowadays rare and is generally due to *Corynebacterium diphtheriae*. This is a rapidly developing inflammation with membrane formation and is associated with diphtheritic membranous lesions of the upper respiratory passages. Pseudomembranous conjunctivitis, also rare although it occurs more frequently than diphtheritic conjunctivitis, is caused by a number of organisms including the staphylococcus, pneumococcus and Koch–Weeks bacillus and is characterized by a fibrinous exudate on the conjunctiva which is not a true membrane.

Acute catarrhal conjunctivitis is a common condition in children in which there is hyperemia of the conjunctiva with a mucopurulent discharge. Complications are rare in this condition which persists for about 2 weeks. It may develop into chronic catarrhal conjunctivitis.

Exanthematous conjunctivitis often accompanies acute infective diseases and is generally part of the underlying disease but there may also be a secondary bacterial infection. It occurs particularly in measles, vaccinia (Plate 26.12) and varicella.

Phlyctenular conjunctivitis is less common than formerly. It is a localized inflammation on one part of the conjunctiva or occasionally the cornea where a small nodule develops which eventually ulcerates. The cause is probably a local allergy which, in the past, was generally due to tuberculin but there may be an allergy to other bacteria or toxins.

Simple allergic conjunctivitis produces a hyperemia of the conjunctiva with pronounced epiphora (Plate 26.13). This is frequently associated with asthma or hay fever but may occur alone. Vernal conjunctivitis occurs in children, is allergic in nature and occurs in spring and early summer, starting with hyperemic injection of the conjunctivae and mucoid discharge. There is always an intense itch in the region of the eyes. There is papillary hypertrophy of the conjunctivae which, together with conjunctival pallor, is striking.

Viral conjunctivitis is a large group due to many different organisms. A viral conjunctivitis in which the specific diagnosis can be made is inclusion blennorrhea caused by *Chlamydia* (the TRIC virus) which is pathogenic for the conjunctiva, cervix uteri and male urethra. This causes an apparently simple conjunctivitis in young children or 'swimming pool' conjunctivitis in older children. In these older children there is follicle formation (which does not occur in infants) and there is often corneal involvement. The diagnosis is made from examination of conjunctival scrapings for inclusion bodies. The chlamydial agent causes trachoma in tropical and subtropical countries. The treatment of inclusion blennorrhea is essentially prophylactic, avoiding contact with other cases of this type of conjunctivitis or with adults with urogenital infection. The condition responds to oral and to local sulfonamide or tetracycline therapy. Trachoma is still the greatest cause of preventable blindness in the world and has been identified since the earliest times in warm climates. Treatment can appear to be almost impossible because of appalling conditions of hygiene throughout a whole population and often the treatment of large groups of people is necessary, e.g. the topical administration of tetracycline twice daily to the population, and at the same time the general hygiene of the community should be improved and insects eliminated.

In temperate countries treatment is not such a problem but even in these situations the treatment of whole families may be necessary and the relationship of the disease to promiscuity explained.

Treatment of conjunctivitis

The essential in treating conjunctivitis is to bathe the eyes frequently to remove discharging mucus and pus. In mild cases, this together with hygiene is all that is required and antibiotics should be avoided. In more severe cases where pus is copious or there is edema of the eyelids, appropriate local antibiotics are indicated and should be used in the form of eyedrops. Local antibiotics should always be given frequently (e.g. 2 hourly) and pus should always be bathed from the eyelid margins before instilling an antibiotic drop, as local ocular antibiotics are ineffective in the presence of pus or mucus. Antibiotic and antiviral or antifungal agents are almost always given locally, but ophthalmia neonatorum is an exception in that antibiotics are given both locally and also systemically.

Allergic conjunctivitis is treated by identifying and treating the cause or, where this is impossible, avoiding the allergen. Systemic antihistaminics are useful in suppressing recurrences of allergic conjunctivitis but topical antihistaminics should be avoided.

Acute episodes of allergic conjunctivitis may be suppressed by the brief use of topical corticosteroids used in drop form for a very short period while the allergen is identified, but where prolonged local therapy is indicated sodium cromoglycate is the preferred therapeutic agent.

THE CORNEA

Inflammation of the cornea may be superficial or deep. Superficial keratitis may be associated with acute conjunctivitis when there are punctate discrete epithelial opacities. A true superficial corneal ulcer may be a primary response to infection, but frequently has its origin in minor trauma. Where a corneal ulcer is due to pneumococcal infection there is commonly an associated anterior uveitis with pus in the anterior chamber.

Viral keratitis is most commonly found to be due to herpes simplex virus and the initial inflammation usually develops as a herpetic keratoconjunctivitis. The primary infection in the majority of cases is unrecognized but some infants present with an acute follicular conjunctivitis. A typical dendritic figure may develop in the corneal epithelium in the primary stage but this generally appears during a recurrence of infection. Treatment of viral keratitis is usually unsatisfactory but herpes simplex keratitis responds to local treatment with 5-iodo-2-deoxyuridine (IDU) or to local aciclovir ointment which is more effective. It is important that viral infections of the cornea should not be treated with corticosteroids as this causes spread of the infection and has resulted in the loss of many eyes.

Interstitial keratitis is much less common than formerly. It is almost always due to syphilitic infection but very occasionally has been caused by other organisms. Interstitial keratitis develops as an acute anterior uveitis with corneal edema and infiltration with eventually a dense central corneal opacity which gradually clears to some extent. Treatment is directed to the underlying uveitis and to the systemic syphilitic infection. Where corneal scarring is permanent a corneal graft may be necessary.

Traumatic keratitis occurs and should always be considered where there is a red or painful eye. Corneal abrasion is not uncommon, often being caused by a scratch on the eye or an object coming into contact with the surface of the cornea. A corneal abrasion heals spontaneously and the pain can be relieved by the instillation of simple ointment and the use of a pad and bandage. Where corneal ulceration is present the cornea should be examined in detail with the possibility of a foreign body in mind. Traumatic keratitis (and traumatic conjunctivitis) in children is very occasionally self-inflicted and sometimes a disturbed child will scratch his cornea or instil a foreign substance into the conjunctival sac.

THE LACRIMAL APPARATUS

Disorders of the lacrimal gland are rare in children.

Acute dacryoadenitis

Acute dacryoadenitis may occur as a complication of mumps, when it can be unilateral or bilateral, and it sometimes follows an orbital injury. There is systemic toxicity with pain, swelling and tenderness in the region of the gland. No treatment is necessary unless orbital cellulitis develops, when antibiotics should be given systemically.

Congenital obstruction of the nasolacrimal duct

This occurs in about 2% of babies. Obstruction is usually due to a simple delay in canalization of the duct but a developed duct may be obstructed by mucus or debris or there may be a persistent membrane at the lower end of the duct. In a very few cases there is complete obstruction due to a failure in development of the duct or bony canal. Where the nasolacrimal duct is obstructed there is epiphora as soon as tear production develops and a mucoid conjunctival discharge. If the lacrimal sac becomes infected, pus can be expressed from the lacrimal puncta, appearing in the nose or welling back onto the eye.

Simple congenital obstruction of the tear passages tends to clear spontaneously. The eyelids should be bathed frequently with a moist sterile swab to remove mucus and debris and the skin over the lacrimal passages massaged. Where there is infection, mucopus should be expressed from the lacrimal sac several times daily, and the appropriate antimicrobial drop instilled. Unless there is infection, local antimicrobials should be avoided because of the likelihood of sensitivity. If an antimicrobial is given it should be used frequently in the form of an eyedrop and not as an ointment which would further obstruct the tear passages.

In the few cases which do not respond to these simple measures the tear passages may be probed under general anesthesia but this is a traumatizing procedure that is best avoided. Where there is a bony developmental anomaly surgery is necessary but should be postponed until after the age of 2 years.

Radiology is seldom useful in the diagnosis of tear passage lesions but it can occasionally detect a radiopaque obstruction within the tear passages or detect previously undiagnosed bony trauma. Radiology, including plain X-rays, and also dacryocystography, macrodacryocystography and lacrimal scintigraphy may help in localizing the site of an obstruction but are seldom required. The use of fluorescein drops in the conjunctival sac (see pp. 1653–1655) is the overall best and simplest technique in assessing the function of the lacrimal passages.

Acute dacryocystitis

This occasionally occurs in children but is unusual. It may arise spontaneously, possibly through pyogenic spread from the nasopharynx, or it may follow a congenitally obstructed tear passage. In some cases there has been trauma to the facial bones. There is a pyogenic infection with systemic toxicity, pain and tenderness over the tear sac with pain in the regional lymph nodes. There is a tendency for the abscess to point through the skin of the face in a few days' time and a fistula develops. The treatment of acute dacryocystitis is to give a systemic antimicrobial, together with local heat. When the condition subsides it is generally possible to irrigate through the tear passages but if it does not respond to simple irrigation and probing, dacryocystorhinostomy may be necessary after some months have elapsed.

INTERNAL EYE DISEASES

UVEITIS

The uveal tract is the vascular tunic of the eye and consists of the iris, the ciliary body and the choroid. Inflammation of the uvea is common and although it may present primarily as iritis, cyclitis or choroiditis it is rare for one part of the uveal tract alone to be inflamed. Even if an inflammatory process appears to be localized to one part of the uvea, adjacent areas are always involved. The term uveitis is used to describe inflammation of any part of the uveal tract with anterior uveitis referring to iritis and cyclitis and posterior uveitis referring to choroiditis. This clinical separation into anterior and posterior uveitis is a useful one.

Anterior uveitis

The etiology of anterior uveitis in children is unknown in the majority of cases. It is associated with rheumatoid arthritis in about 10% of cases, with sarcoidosis in about 8% and with tuberculosis in 4% of cases. Other much less common causes include syphilis, brucellosis and viral infections.

Typically there is a history of an abrupt onset of photophobia with lacrimation and a reduction in vision. The globe of the eye is intensely injected with the most obvious engorgement being round the limbus. The pupil is small and irregular and in advanced cases there is pus in the anterior chamber (hypopyon). Where there is no frank pus, inflammatory cells can be seen in the aqueous and on the back of the cornea with the binocular microscope or with a focused light and a lens. When uveitis is predominantly an iritis there is intense pain and rapid loss of vision; when predominantly a cyclitis, vision is blurred rather than lost and there are many 'floaters'.

Treatment is directed initially to full dilation of the pupil with topical atropine or, if necessary, subconjunctival injection of atropine. Local corticosteroids (e.g. 1% solution of hydrocortisone or 0.1% solution of betamethasone instilled every 2 hours) are used to suppress the inflammatory response. Where a specific etiology is found this must be treated.

Posterior uveitis

Choroiditis may occur alone but there is generally an element of associated cyclitis and the retina may also be involved to produce a choroidoretinitis. In contrast to anterior uveitis, a definite etiology can be found in about 65% of cases of posterior uveitis in children. Among the identifiable causes are tuberculosis, syphilis and brucellosis, the fungal infection histoplasmosis and the protozoal infection toxoplasmosis. Sarcoidosis, sympathetic ophthalmia and cytomegalic inclusion disease are responsible for a small proportion of cases. The nematode infections *Toxocara canis* and *Toxocara cati* have recently been shown to be responsible for a few cases.

Posterior uveitis is a painless condition and the only symptoms are visual. Where the site of infection is primarily at the posterior pole of the eye there is rapid blurring of vision with 'floaters' in the field of vision. When the macula is involved there is usually sudden and marked decrease in central vision. When the site is predominantly peripheral visual loss is variable depending on the site and extent of the inflammation. There may be only floaters with some slight blurring of vision. Even the adult may be slow to complain of the visual symptoms of uveitis and it is therefore particularly difficult to make an early diagnosis in children.

Ophthalmoscopically, the vitreous is seen to be hazy due to exudation and there may be discrete vitreous opacities. A recent focus of uveitis is seen as a whitish area in the fundus with indistinct borders and an older focus has a clear-cut white appearance with darkly pigmented borders. Many cases of posterior uveitis are self-limiting. Healed areas of choroiditis can be seen as atrophic areas of the retina and choroid through which the white sclera is easily seen. A focus of choroiditis causes a scotoma in the field of vision and, if at the macula, there is loss of central vision which in a child is likely to cause a squint.

The pupil should be fully dilated as in the treatment of anterior uveitis, and specific treatment given where indicated by the etiology. Systemic corticosteroids are effective in suppressing almost all forms of posterior uveitis.

CYCLITIS

Cyclitis, or pars planitis, is usually bilateral and presents as blurred vision associated with many spots. Before long the central visual acuity is obviously reduced. The eye is usually white and superficially quiet but there is vitreous involvement and before long edema of the macula develops. Cyclitis has a prolonged course and the etiology is seldom discovered.

DEGENERATIVE DISEASES OF THE RETINA AND CHOROID

These diseases can be divided broadly into the three groups discussed below. They are almost always hereditary although generally the appearance of the fundus is normal at birth. Both eyes are affected and although the rate of progression varies, the final clinical picture and the visual outcome are the same in both eyes. The term abiotrophy is used to describe disorders when there is a postnatal degeneration of tissues that have apparently developed normally. The term tapetoretinal degeneration is used to describe degenerations that involve the retina with its pigment epithelium and the choroid. Electrophysiology (q.v.) is becoming increasingly useful in making a precise diagnosis of these degenerative conditions and in monitoring their progression.

Central tapetoretinal degenerations

These conditions cause destruction of the central receptor cells of the retina which are predominantly cones and there is therefore a marked decrease in central vision with loss of color discrimination.

Infantile (Best's) macular degeneration

This is a rare condition which is not associated with degeneration elsewhere in the body.

Juvenile (Stargardt's) macular degeneration

This is the most common in this group. Its onset is generally between 5 and 15 years of age and both eyes are involved. The mode of inheritance is variable but the symptoms and clinical findings are alike in one pedigree. Initially, there is macular edema with mottled pigmentation and later the posterior pole of the retina takes on a yellowish appearance; central vision is reduced to 1/60 or less as there is a large central scotoma with poor color vision. The deterioration in vision generally takes place over a few years at the end of which time there is no further visual loss and no change in the final retinal picture (Plate 26.14).

Adolescent (Sorsby's) macular degeneration

This is similar to juvenile macular degeneration but occurs later in childhood and in young adult life. Clinical progression is slower with changes confined to the macula and although the visual deterioration is serious, it is not as great as in juvenile macular degeneration.

There are many variations in the picture seen in juvenile and adolescent macular degeneration and many cases do not fit clearly into either group. Some children develop hemorrhagic changes at the maculae, associated with macular edema, and after several years a disciform macular degeneration develops with clinically obvious exudation at the posterior pole of the eyes causing the maculae to be raised. Eventually, the picture seen in established juvenile or adolescent macular degeneration develops. These degenerations generally occur as isolated findings but may occur with other abnormalities.

Amaurotic family idiocy

This includes a group of conditions in which there is degeneration of the central nervous system and retina. The cardinal clinical findings are blindness and mental retardation with general deterioration. The infantile form with autosomal recessive inheritance is Tay–Sachs disease which occurs most commonly in Jews and is a lipid degeneration in the ganglion cells of the central nervous system. There is degeneration throughout the retina manifest as a gray appearance due to lipid degeneration, most pronounced at the macula. There is a cherry-red spot at the fovea caused by the exposed choriocapillaris (Plate 26.10). The affected child is normal at birth and signs of degeneration appear at about 6 months of age.

Juvenile amaurotic family idiocy (Batten–Mayou disease)

This develops at about 7 years of age. It is also autosomal recessive. The fundus picture is again similar to Tay–Sachs disease but without a cherry-red spot. Other forms of these degenerations have been described.

Niemann–Pick disease

This is similar to Tay–Sachs and has a similar ophthalmic picture.

Gaucher's disease

This gives a diffuse white appearance in the fundus but no cherry-red spot.

Peripheral tapetoretinal degenerations

Retinitis pigmentosa

The most common of the tapetoretinal degenerations is retinitis pigmentosa. Inheritance is variable but is generally recessive. There is degeneration of the receptor cells of the retina, principally the rods, and an associated degeneration of the pigment epithelium with migration of pigment from these cells into the stroma of the retina. The blood vessels of the retina become narrowed and eventually there is widespread retinal gliosis and optic atrophy. Clinically, in a developed case there are deposits of pigment occupying the mid-periphery of the fundus but not involving the area around the optic disk and macula or the extreme periphery. The clumps of pigment have a spidery appearance sometimes described as being like bone corpuscles. As the condition progresses pigment deposition becomes heavy, the optic disk atrophies and develops a waxy pallor and eventually posterior polar cataracts appear.

The first symptom is night blindness which generally begins in childhood and is followed by the development of ring scotomata in the fields of vision which are most obvious in poor lighting. The scotomata extend peripherally and then centrally to cause serious visual loss. The rate of visual deterioration varies but is usually very slow and serious visual loss may not develop until middle or late adult life. The patient is left with a very small area of central vision and because of the loss of peripheral vision is eventually severely handicapped. Retinitis pigmentosa may occur as an isolated defect or as part of the Laurence–Moon–Biedl syndrome. In this condition there is obesity, polydactyly, hypogenitalism and mental retardation. The fundus picture in retinitis pigmentosa varies very much but eventually there is dense peripheral pigmentation and attenuation of the retinal vessels (Plate 26.15).

No treatment is available for retinitis pigmentosa. Many forms of treatment have been suggested during the past 50 years varying from simple optical 'remedies' to the intraorbital injection of extract of placenta, the latter of which was in vogue in eastern Europe for a considerable time. No treatment has been shown to be effective where proper controls have been used.

Retinitis punctata albescens

This produces symptoms similar to retinitis pigmentosa but the onset is earlier. The ultimate visual loss is not as severe as in retinitis pigmentosa. The eventual clinical picture differs in that retinal pigmentation in the mid-periphery is not so marked and the pigment is interspersed with white spots.

Choroidal degenerations

Choroideremia is the most common condition in this group. Degeneration occurs primarily in the choroid with eventual destruction of the choroid and the outer part of the retina. Patches of degeneration appear in the mid-periphery of the fundus to leave discrete punched out areas, many of which coalesce and spread towards the anterior retina and the posterior pole to cause greatly reduced vision but never complete visual loss. Gyrate atrophy of the choroid is rare and produces a similar picture which is confined to the peripheral part of the retina.

Detachment of the retina

Detachment of the retina is essentially a disease of adult life and is unusual in children. There are two types of retinal detachment: primary or idiopathic detachment of the retina, and secondary detachment of the retina which is due to a condition not primarily retinal.

In primary retinal detachment there is a tear or hole in the retina with degeneration of the vitreous allowing fluid from the vitreous cavity to pass into the subretinal space. The primary retinal defect is generally in the peripheral part of the retina and there may be no obvious cause for it. In some children there is a strong family history of peripheral retinal degeneration; when this is the case the type of retinal degeneration and its position is similar within a pedigree. In some cases there is a history of trauma which has resulted in the development of a retinal hole. The symptoms of primary detachment of the retina are visual (these may not be commented on by the young child) and the treatment is surgical.

In secondary retinal detachment the subretinal fluid pushing the retina forward may arise from the vitreous or from the retinal or choroidal circulations. This subretinal fluid is a transudate and the primary causes embrace a wide variety of conditions including systemic hypertension, uveitis and primary and secondary tumors. Among the tumors are retinoblastoma (Fig. 26.19 and Plate 26.16) and the angiomata of von Hippel–Lindau disease and Sturge–Weber disease. In some cases the retina is pulled forward by the contraction of adherent fibrous bands which have developed in the vitreous following trauma or hemorrhage into the vitreous or following retinopathy of prematurity (see Ch. 5). The treatment of secondary detachment of the retina is directed to the primary condition and the course, prognosis and treatment of primary and secondary retinal detachment are so different that it is of paramount importance to make the diagnostic distinction between the two types.

DISORDERS OF THE LENS

Cataract is the term used to describe a lens which is partially or completely opaque and is also used to describe a discrete opacity within an otherwise clear lens. Five broad types of cataract are recognized in patients of all ages. These are developmental, secondary (to systemic disease), complicated (a complication of local ocular disease), traumatic and senile. The first four categories apply to children and in them there is considerable overlap between the first two categories which are here considered together. The disease to which the cataract is secondary is often a hereditary or developmental one.

Developmental cataract

Developmental cataract is present at birth or develops within the first few years of life. It was formerly called congenital cataract but this term is unsatisfactory as many opacities in this group develop after birth. Developmental cataract is not usually diagnosed until the child is several weeks or even several months old. The neonate sleeps a great deal and even when awake tends to keep his eyes closed and frequently does not appear to see. The pupils in the neonate are very small and for these reasons a cataract which may have been present at birth is frequently not detected until several months have passed and if it is so small as to interfere with vision slightly, or not at all, it may never be detected.

There are very many types of developmental cataract and they are best grouped into those where the cataract has a primary hereditary tendency and those where the cataract may be secondary to some underlying disease with a hereditary basis.

Hereditary cataracts

Where a cataract is hereditary it is commonly bilateral and the type of cataract is generally the same throughout a pedigree. These cataracts are frequently incomplete and in many cases do not interfere with vision. They are given morphological descriptions according to their shape and site in the lens, which depends upon the stage at which they develop. Not the least important of their implications to the ophthalmic surgeon is the

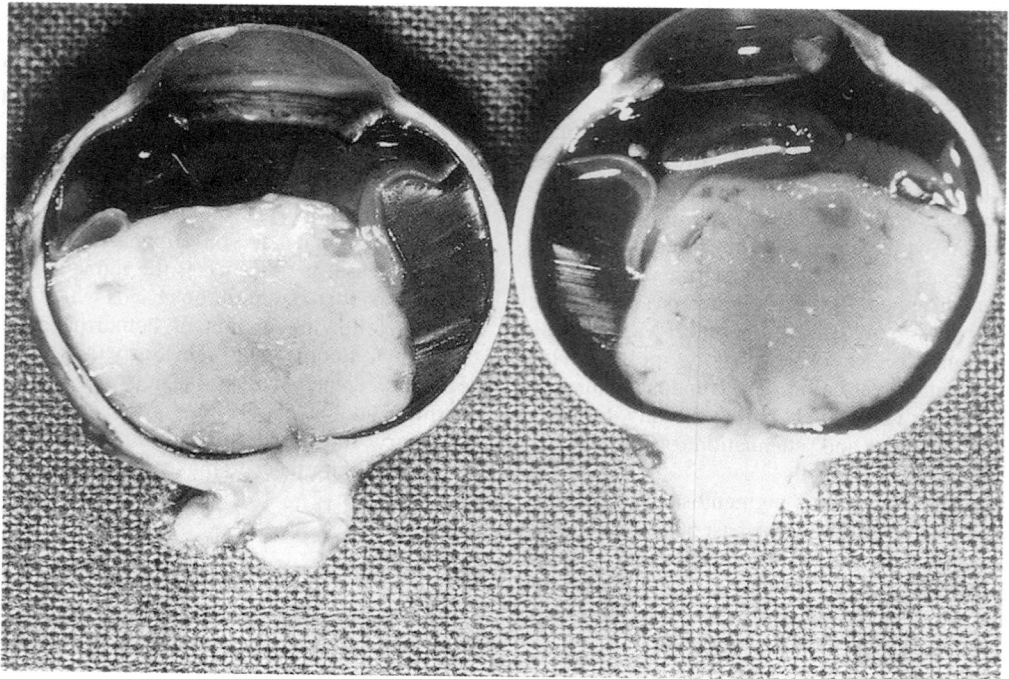

Fig. 26.19 An enucleated eye showing a large retinoblastoma causing detachment of the retina and almost filling the vitreous cavity.

ability to recognize them as developmental or inherited opacities since, if they are first noticed at a routine examination in adult life, they may be thought to be either senile or traumatic in nature. The commonest of these opacities is zonular (lamellar) cataract. This consists of lamellar opacity surrounding a clear or almost clear central zone in the lens. It occurs frequently and the extent of opacity and area of clear nucleus remaining depends upon the stage at which the cataract developed. Sutural cataract is an opacity involving only the anterior and posterior y-shaped sutures. Axial cataract involves the central axial region of the lens. Anterior polar cataract and posterior polar cataract are opacities in the axial area at the poles of the lens. Embryonic nuclear cataract is central in position. Coralliform cataract is centered on the lens nucleus and in configuration resembles coral. Total cataract occupies all the lens. The commonest mode of transmission in hereditary cataract is autosomal dominant but all patterns of transmission may be seen.

Secondary developmental cataracts

Where developmental cataract is not of the hereditary type there is frequently some coexisting systemic or ocular disease.

Rubella cataract may occur in an infant whose mother has had rubella during the first 3 months of pregnancy. The opacity is generally bilateral although the extent of opacity in the two eyes is usually unequal. The entire lens may be opaque or more commonly there is a dense central opacity with a clearer peripheral area. Sometimes the cataract is membranous in nature. Live rubella virus has been cultured from lens material removed from such eyes many months after birth. Where the lens is partially clear and the fundus can be seen there is pigment stippling at the posterior pole and it is not generally recognized

that children of mothers who have had rubella early in pregnancy but who have escaped cataract frequently have a fine pigmentary rubella retinopathy which is sufficient to cause a significant reduction in central vision which may be either undetected or whose nature may not be recognized.

Rubella cataract responds remarkably favorably to surgery, although the presence of rubella retinopathy prejudices the final visual result. It is becoming recognized that other viruses may produce a similar toxic developmental cataract. This has been seen in the children of mothers who have been affected during the first few months of pregnancy with viral diseases including measles, mumps, infectious mononucleosis, chickenpox, epidemic encephalitis and influenza.

Galactosemia cataract. This is a rare condition but it is among the few types of lens opacity which are reversible with treatment. All infants with developmental cataract should have the urine tested for galactose as a screening test. The earliest lens change in this disorder is in increase in refractivity of the fetal nucleus which then develops an appearance like an oil droplet. Up to this point the lens changes are reversible but if dietary treatment is not instituted the entire lens eventually becomes opaque. The cataract, which is bilateral, appears between the fourth and eighth weeks of life in untreated cases and increases rapidly until the lens is completely opaque by the tenth week. Where a complete lens opacity develops it is irreversible but the results of surgery are good.

Retinopathy of prematurity. Well-marked examples of this condition progress to develop lens opacity which is irreversible and surgery will only worsen an already disorganized eye.

Persistent hyperplastic primary vitreous is frequently associated with cataract. In this condition there is a failure in development of the definitive vitreous resulting in a mass of vascular tissue behind the lens.

Zonular cataract, which is exactly similar to the hereditary type of zonular cataract, may develop in early childhood, associated with vitamin D deficiency. The lens opacity is irreversible but does not progress when the diet is made good. Where the lamellae are thin this type of cataract is compatible with good vision, but should it progress to the point where surgery is required the ultimate vision is good.

Diabetic cataract. True diabetic cataract which occurs only in young and labile diabetics is rare. Initially, there is hydration of the lens with the development of discrete subcapsular opacities which increase rapidly in number and size. It is always bilateral and within a few days the entire lens in both eyes becomes opaque. In the early stages the lens opacities are reversible with correction of the metabolic state, but if the cataract becomes complete both eyes will be virtually blind and surgery is necessary. The results of surgery are very good.

Tetany cataract may develop in the first year of life where there is prolonged infantile tetany. There are discrete opacities situated centrally in the lens; similar opacities develop later in childhood or in adolescence where there is latent or manifest tetany. These lens opacities are not reversible but progression stops with systemic treatment.

Atopic cataract. Atopic dermatitis, which is often associated with cataract in the adult, is occasionally the cause of cataract in children. This is a bilateral lens opacity which appears initially in the anterior cortex and may progress steadily until the entire lens is opaque.

Coronary cataract occurs in the periphery of the lens and, although seldom present in infancy, develops during childhood or at puberty. The lens opacities fill the periphery of both lenses; they are club shaped and can be seen only when the pupil is fully dilated. These opacities are non-progressive and do not interfere with vision.

Down syndrome is commonly associated with cataract (about 75% of such children have lens opacities). The opacities are generally small and discrete and do not interfere with vision.

Complicated cataract

This is the type of cataract that develops as the result of some other ocular disease (e.g. retinoblastoma, uveitis, buphthalmos). It starts in the posterior part of the lens and progresses slowly. When this type of cataract appears the eye is usually seriously damaged by the underlying condition and the visual result of treatment depends upon the success of treatment of the primary condition.

Traumatic (and drug-induced) cataract

Lens opacities occur following any type of trauma to the eye. The most common trauma in a child is a penetrating injury which may result in a complete opacity but occasionally only part of the lens becomes opaque. If the eye is otherwise relatively undamaged, surgical treatment is successful. Other types of trauma which may cause cataract include blunt trauma electric shock and intense heat.

Corticosteroid-induced cataract may occur in children who have been treated with systemic corticosteroids for over a year. The cataract is bilateral and starts at the posterior pole of the lens. If corticosteroids are withdrawn the lens opacity is not progressive but if they are continued the opacity progresses with a rapid reduction in vision.

The diagnosis of cataract

Cataract can only be diagnosed when the pupil is fully dilated. Where the cataract is complete it will be seen as a white or gray area filling the dilated pupillary aperture, but where it is incomplete it may only be seen as a dark area against the red reflex visualized with the ophthalmoscope (Plate 26.2). Where a cataract is incomplete it is impossible to assess or even to guess at a child's vision by estimating the amount of opacity in the pupil but examination with the binocular microscope and slit lamp will give some indication of the visual prognosis as the further back in the lens the opacity is situated, the greater the interference with vision. It should always be remembered that many apparently large lens opacities, particularly those situated anteriorly in the lens, are compatible with almost normal vision.

Treatment of cataract

Apart from a few rare examples, such as diabetic cataract and galactosemia cataract where early treatment of an underlying condition may cause reversal of lens opacities, effective treatment is entirely surgical. Where vision is not reduced or only slightly reduced, treatment should not be offered. It is better for a child to accept some reduction in central vision with the retention of a full field of vision than to suffer aphakia with absolute dependence on spectacles (a pair for distance vision and a pair for reading) and a considerable reduction in the field of vision. There is the further consideration that lens extraction in a child has in the past been complicated by the development of retinal detachment even up to 20 years following surgery, although with modern surgical techniques this is no longer the hazard it once was.

Where a cataract is uniocular, lens extraction is probably best avoided as the only way of overcoming the resultant amblyopia due to uniocular aphakia is to fit the child with contact lenses together with spectacles to overcome the high hypermetropic refractive error in the aphakic eye and the aniseikonia (a difference in image size between the two eyes). Where developmental cataract is bilateral and advanced to the stage where vision is seriously reduced, surgery should be offered as soon as possible in the knowledge that the results of surgery may be excellent. In these cases, both eyes generally have surgery and the child wears spectacles. If a cataract is present from birth or appears within the first few weeks of life there may be failure in development of the fixation reflex with the onset of nystagmus. If there is a risk of nystagmus developing operation must be undertaken within the first 3 months of life. The visual result is particularly poor once nystagmus is established. Apart from the consideration of nystagmus, surgery should be offered as early as possible in suitable cases to allow the establishment of the fixation and binocular reflexes. Before offering surgery it must always be borne in mind that congenital cataract tends to be associated with other ocular or systemic disease which may seriously influence the visual result. For this reason, in all children with developmental cataract a detailed ocular examination is necessary, frequently involving preliminary ocular examination under general anesthesia to assess the state of the eyes, particularly the retinae and optic nerve. Unsuccessful cataract surgery is not only disappointing but can lead to an unsightly eye or the loss of an eye. Where a child has reduced vision which is not sufficiently bad to justify a lens extraction, or where because of systemic disease, mental retardation or other consideration, the major operation of lens extraction is best avoided, the minor procedure of optical iridectomy (the removal of a sector of the iris) may be employed to allow more light rays to enter the eye, with considerable improvement in vision (Plate 26.2). This procedure has been employed for many years but fell into disfavor with the advent of successful lens extraction.

Adult cataract surgery has changed dramatically in the past decade with the introduction of acrylic lens implants to replace the cataractous lens. These lens implants have been used since about 1950 but they have only been really successful in the last 10 years or so with improved materials and with the development of microsurgery. Lens implantation is now a routine procedure in adults but is not yet established in children, especially the very young. It is anticipated that before long lens implantation will be a practical procedure in young children and the approach to cataract surgery and its results should be greatly changed.

Dislocation of the lens

Lens dislocation in children is either congenital or occurs in infancy as an isolated hereditary defect or as part of Marfan's syndrome or homocystinuria (see p. 1108). Dislocation is usually bilateral but one lens may precede the other. Partial dislocation (subluxation) has the same origins as complete dislocation and often proceeds to complete dislocation (Plate 26.17). A dislocated lens may be cataractous but often remains clear for many years. Traumatic dislocation (unilateral) is rare in children and the lens becomes opaque.

TUMORS OF THE EYE

Retinoblastoma

Retinoblastoma is virtually the only malignant tumor that occurs in the eye in childhood. It was formerly described as a 'glioma' but since it is now known to be developed from retinoblasts, the term glioma is no longer used.

Clinical features

Retinoblastoma develops within the first few years of life, usually before the third year but is seldom congenital. A familial incidence is relatively common and in some instances the tumor is hereditary. Hereditary transmission, although well known, has been infrequent until recent times as patients with retinoblastoma rarely survived but nowadays, with adequate treatment, the proportion of hereditary cases of retinoblastoma is increasing and the absolute number of cases is also increasing. Retinoblastoma is unusual in having a hereditary and familial incidence and it is also unusual in being multifocal. About 25% of cases are bilateral and it is not uncommon to find more than one area of tumor in the same eye, although where this occurs the smaller area may have spread as a cell nest from the larger. Retinoblastoma starts as a small white area in the fundus or as multiple small elevations on the surface of the retina. The tumor may grow between the retina and choroid to cause a retinal detachment (a secondary detachment) or it may grow inward into the vitreous. Seedlings may spread throughout the eye and may develop as fresh areas of tumor on the retina or in the later stages they may be seen as white masses on the iris or forming a level in the anterior chamber. If the tumor is left untreated it grows to fill the eye and before long the

root of the iris is pressed forward by the tumor mass to cause secondary glaucoma with pain and enlargement of the eye. Eventually, the tumor ruptures through the choroid and sclera with relief of pain to form a fungating mass in the orbit. It fills the orbit rapidly with erosion of the orbital walls but before this stage is reached there has generally been direct spread down the optic nerve to the brain. Death is usually caused by direct spread to the brain and metastases are unusual except in the later stages. The rate of progression in retinoblastoma varies greatly and although spontaneous regression has occasionally been described the condition is usually rapidly fatal.

Retinoblastoma is usually advanced when detected and is often seen by the parents as a white mass in the pupil of the eye – the cat's eye reflex. It is occasionally seen in its earlier stages during the routine examination of the ocular fundus of a child who had presented with a squint, as when the primary site of the tumor is near the posterior pole of the eye, vision may fail rapidly and a squint may develop (Fig. 26.19 and Plate 26.16).

Treatment

Enucleation of the involved eye with the removal of as much of the optic nerve as possible is the accepted method of treatment. If the tumor is diagnosed early, radiation alone is completely successful. The excised optic nerve should be examined histologically and if there is any evidence of spread of tumor cells along the nerve toward the brain, enucleation should be followed by irradiation. Where there has been extension from the eye into the orbit, exenteration followed by irradiation is necessary but even this mutilating procedure is seldom successful in saving the child's life. Where there has been no extraocular spread, enucleation alone is frequently completely successful and, provided a second tumor does not develop in the other eye, the child will survive to a normal adult life with only the minor handicap of an ocular prosthesis and uniocular vision. In these cases it is most important that the second eye should be examined in detail at intervals of about 2 months until the child reaches the age of about 6 years. Retinoblastoma is unusual among tumors of neuroectodermal origin in that it is radiosensitive and, should a tumor develop in the second eye, it can be treated quite easily without loss of the eye and generally leaving almost full vision. Radiation is usually given by a cobalt-60 plaque sutured to the sclera or by deep X-ray therapy. Where radiation is used, photocoagulation and systemic antimetabolites may be used as adjuvant therapy.

In the past, treatment of retinoblastoma always involved enucleation of the first eye with observation of the second eye which would be enucleated should a tumor develop in it. The advent of radiotherapy in the past few decades has saved the lives and sight of many children with retinoblastoma as although the tumor in the presenting eye is usually too far advanced for conservative treatment, the second eye can almost always be treated by radiation provided there has been adequate supervision with consequent early diagnosis. The great tragedy in this condition is failure to ensure adequate follow-up or, more usually, failure of the family to comply with advice regarding the prognosis and follow-up. It is essential that the seriousness of the condition should be explained to parents. With the increased number of surviving children, more fresh cases are occurring and with really early diagnosis it is now practicable and safe to treat both eyes by conservative therapy. Some children with retinoblastoma treated by radiation develop sarcoma in or around the orbit in early adult life and all children with retinoblastoma treated by radiation should be kept under supervision indefinitely. Because of the genetic associations, families with this tumor require genetic counselling (see Ch. 3).

Other tumors of the eye include the phacomata and the very rare tumor astrocytoma of the retina and dictyoma and medulloepithelioma of the ciliary body, all of which are only locally invasive.

THE OPTIC NERVE

The optic nerve head (optic disk) is easily seen in the normal eye on ophthalmoscopy (Plate 26.4) and examination of the optic disk must be part of any routine ophthalmic or neurological examination. The abnormal conditions most frequently involving the optic disks are papilledema, papillitis (optic neuritis) and optic atrophy. The clinician should be familiar with the appearance of the normal optic disk and should be able to examine the disk through the undilated pupil. It is only through familiarity with the normal disk that unusual conditions such as optic nerve hypoplasia may be diagnosed, helping to explain reduced vision. The optic disks are best examined using the binocular indirect ophthalmoscope as the disks can then be compared. Fundus photography including the disk is very helpful for recording and comparative purposes. Fluorescein angiography is particularly helpful in confirming the diagnosis of optic disk lesions and although it is not used routinely in pediatric ophthalmology, fluorescein angiography is standard practice in adult ophthalmology. Angiograms can be taken in young children provided they cooperate in allowing drops to be instilled to dilate the pupils, in accepting an injection of sodium fluorescein into a vein (usually in the antecubital fossa) and in allowing photographs of the optic fundi to be taken.

PAPILLEDEMA

Optic disk edema refers to any swelling of the optic nerve head with the term papilledema being reserved for optic disk swelling caused by raised intracranial pressure. In fully developed papilledema the optic disk margins are blurred, the disk is elevated, the blood vessels are congested, there is loss of venous pulsation and there are hemorrhages and exudates surrounding the disk (Plate 26.6). The picture in established papilledema is easy to recognize but the earlier stages of papilledema (Plate 26.5) are difficult to identify and here angiography is particularly helpful. In papilledema the central vision is usually normal but there may be episodes of transient loss of vision involving only a few seconds and the blind spot may be enlarged.

The precise cause of papilledema is not understood but it is usually associated with a rise of intracranial pressure and stasis of axoplasmic flow.

Papilledema in young children is most frequently associated with tumors of the posterior fossa. The causes of papilledema in children are: intracranial lesions (raised intracranial pressure, e.g. tumor, meningitis, hemorrhage, thrombosis, hydrocephalus); orbital lesions (tumor, abscess, etc.); ocular lesions (uveitis, sudden reduction of intraocular pressure due to trauma, etc.); systemic conditions including hypotension, blood dyscrasias, cardiac failure, collagen disorders and renal disease.

Where the term papilledema is used, raised intracranial pressure is generally assumed to be present and should be excluded before any other diagnosis is reached.

OPTIC NEURITIS

Optic neuritis may give a clinical picture similar to papilledema. It is generally caused by inflammation or degeneration (demyelination) in the optic nerve but, unlike papilledema, there is commonly a profound loss of central vision. In optic neuritis, where the lesion is situated in the anterior part of the optic nerve, the appearance of the optic nerve head is that of early papilledema and the condition is termed papillitis, but where the lesion is behind the lamina cribrosa the optic nerve head may appear to be normal and the condition is then termed retrobulbar neuritis.

Optic neuritis is usually an acute condition beginning with a sudden and profound loss of vision. It is often part of generalized disease and a full neurological examination should be made. It may indicate the onset of, for example, Devic's disease or Schilder's disease, or it may be an early sign of multiple sclerosis. In older children it may indicate drug toxicity.

PSEUDOPAPILLEDEMA

The appearance of papilledema is occasionally caused by an elevated optic disk due to hyperplastic glial tissue on the optic nerve head or due to other developmental abnormalities of the optic disk. High hypermetropia can give the appearance of an elevated disk. Pseudopapilledema usually appears as an isolated finding and where it is present there is no other ocular abnormality, central vision is normal, the fields of vision are full and there is a normal blind spot and a normal fluorescein angiogram.

MYELINATED NERVE FIBERS

Myelinated nerve fibers (Plate 26.18) are occasionally seen close to the optic disk and are sometimes confused with papilledema or pseudopapilledema. Myelinated nerve fibers are due to myelin extending beyond the optic nerve head into the retina and are of no significance other than increasing the size of the normal blind spot.

OPTIC ATROPHY

When the optic nerve is damaged, optic atrophy results. The cause of optic atrophy may be congenital, degenerative, inflammatory, vascular or neoplastic and any of these conditions can result in permanent damage to the axons of the optic nerve. Optic atrophy is characterized by a pale optic disk with an associated loss of central and peripheral vision.

'Primary' optic atrophy is a degeneration of the optic nerve with no evidence of previous swelling or proliferation in the region of the optic nerve head on ophthalmoscopy (Plate 26.19). 'Secondary' optic atrophy is a reactive condition and generally follows an acute inflammation which leaves mesenchymal proliferation in the region of the optic nerve head.

In general, primary optic atrophy appears to be spontaneous and may present as an isolated finding. There are many causes including inheritance and toxicity. The appearance of a pale optic disk sharply outlined is characteristic. Secondary optic atrophy usually follows papilledema and has an irregular and pale disk with evidence of proliferation.

A specific cause of primary optic atrophy is Leber's hereditary optic atrophy which is an inherited degenerative disease of the optic nerve. Leber's optic atrophy is commonest in males in childhood and causes a serious loss of vision with a central scotoma. Leber's atrophy usually develops suddenly in one eye with blurring of vision, and the other eye follows rapidly. The cause is not understood but it is always inherited.

OPTIC NERVE GLIOMA

Glioma is a tumor of the optic nerve which occurs in children and can have a profound effect on vision. Histologically these tumors are similar to gliomata occurring elsewhere in the central nervous system. They cause proptosis, papilledema and a great reduction in central vision which may progress to blindness. The diagnosis of optic nerve glioma can be made clinically through reduction of vision, increase in hypermetropia due to raised intraorbital pressure and the presence of retinal folds and is easily confirmed by a scan of the orbit. The treatment of optic nerve glioma generally involves enucleation of the eye with the entire length of the optic nerve within the orbit and possibly a craniotomy to remove the optic nerve up to the optic chiasma. The recent tendency is to manage these tumors conservatively as they rarely spread and do not metastasize. In these circumstances, although the eye may be blind, the child only suffers the cosmetic blemish of proptosis with, possibly, strabismus.

ORBITAL ANGIOMA AND VARICES

Space-occupying lesions in the orbit may be of vascular origin consisting of angiomatous tissue. A hematoma may arise, especially in association with localized varices. Proptosis is likely to be the presenting sign and indentation of the orbit occurs.

BUPHTHALMOS (INFANTILE GLAUCOMA)

Buphthalmos is an uncommon disease of infancy in which the eye enlarges due to a rise in intraocular pressure.

Primary buphthalmos is caused by a congenital anatomical anomaly in the angle of the anterior chamber interfering with the drainage of aqueous humor. The precise anatomical defect is variable including absence or abnormality of the canal of Schlemm, a failure of mesodermal cleavage in the angle of the anterior chamber, or, most commonly, persistence of mesodermal tissue in the angle of the anterior chamber. When the eye is examined with the gonioscope, some anatomical abnormality in the angle of anterior chamber is usual but occasionally the angle appears to be normal. The anatomical defect in the angle of the anterior chamber is present at birth but enlargement of the eye sometimes does not appear until the child is a few months old or occasionally even 1 or 2 years old. Both eyes are generally involved in primary buphthalmos (Fig. 26.20) which is more common in boys than in girls.

Secondary buphthalmos can be due to a large variety of causes, many of which are similar to those producing secondary glaucoma in the adult. Any condition interfering with the drainage of aqueous humor from the eye causes a potential rise in intraocular pressure, leading to secondary glaucoma. Uveitis, ocular neoplasm, intraocular hemorrhage and trauma can all lead to this type of buphthalmos. The Sturge–Weber syndrome can cause buphthalmos through hemangioma of the choroid associated with

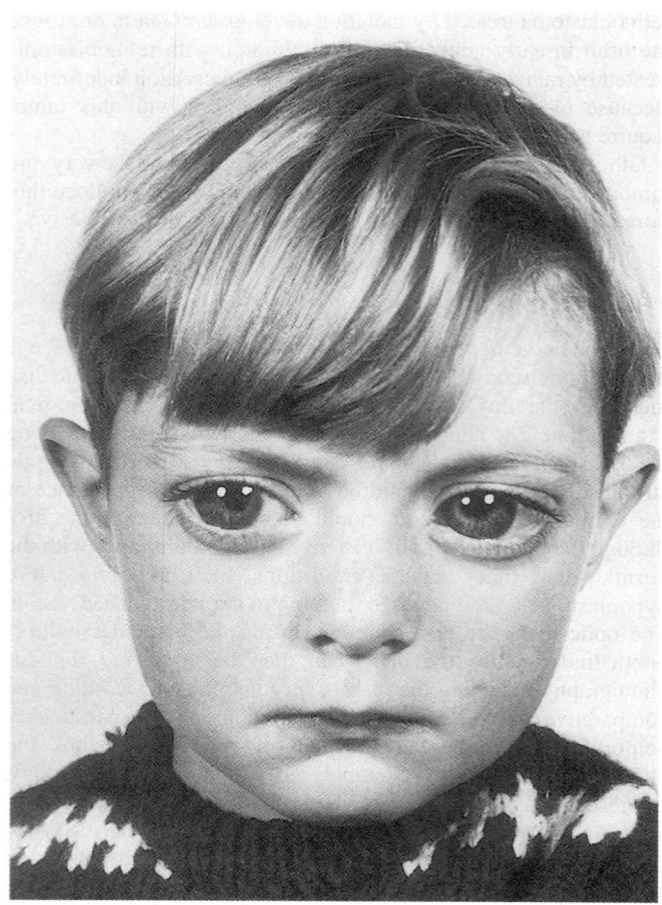

Fig. 26.20   Buphthalmos. A small boy with obviously large eyes due to buphthalmos (developmental glaucoma).

hemangioma in the face and sometimes of the cerebellum. In this case the buphthalmos is unilateral.

Clinical features of buphthalmos

In buphthalmos there is progressive enlargement of the eye as the coats of the immature eye of a young child cannot withstand an increased intraocular pressure. The anteroposterior diameter of the eye increases first and the corneal curvature then increases, with a resulting deepening of the anterior chamber. There is generally a progressive myopia. Eventually the cornea becomes hazy due to edema which follows ruptures in Descemet's membrane and with this edema there is reddening of the eye, photophobia and epiphora. The optic nerve head becomes atrophic and cupped due to raised intraocular pressure. When this stage is reached there is rapid and permanent reduction in vision. The presenting feature may be the enlarged eye which can be particularly striking in the unilateral case but an early and characteristic symptom is photophobia. The child with buphthalmos avoids light by lying face down in his cot burying his head in the pillow.

Buphthalmos is a serious condition and any child who appears to have enlarged eyes should be examined carefully with infantile glaucoma in mind. Megalocornea (anterior megalophthalmos) is a possible cause of enlargement of the eye in a baby but this is a rare condition which is bilateral and equal, causes no symptoms and is not associated with clouding of the cornea, cupping of the optic disk or raised intraocular pressure. A child suspected of having buphthalmos must be examined under general anesthesia when the corneal diameters can be measured, the tension of the eye assessed and the angle of the anterior chamber viewed through a gonioscope.

Treatment

Primary buphthalmos is treated surgically. Trabeculectomy is the treatment of choice in which the removal of a portion of the trabecular meshwork in the angle of the anterior chamber with a peripheral iridectomy increases drainage of aqueous from the eye and lowers the pressure in the eye. An alternative to trabeculectomy is goniotomy in which the tissues of the angle of the anterior chamber are divided with a small knife.

In secondary buphthalmos treatment must be directed to the underlying condition but a drainage operation may also be necessary.

Prognosis

The prognosis in primary buphthalmos is poor unless surgical treatment is instituted early. Even minimal enlargement of an infant's eye is associated with visual loss and many of these children are only diagnosed when one eye at least is obviously enlarged. If the condition is untreated complete blindness results, although in a very few cases spontaneous remission (in which there has been no further enlargement of the eye but no recovery of lost visual field) has been described. There is no place for medical therapy as definitive treatment in the form of topical substances or systemic agents to lower the intraocular pressure (although local or systemic therapy may be used for a few days while surgery is being arranged). Surgery must be performed as soon as buphthalmos has been diagnosed and as the condition is generally bilateral, the second eye should be examined and treated as necessary. It should be emphasized that all infants with apparently large eyes should be regarded as possibly having buphthalmos.

OCULAR SIGNS OF SYSTEMIC DISEASE

DISORDERS OF METABOLISM

Galactosemia (p. 1132)

This causes bilateral cataract which has already been described.

Albinism (p. 1107)

This, a disorder of tyrosine metabolism, almost always involves the eyes and vision. It is unusual to find complete ocular albinism but partial degrees of albinism, either associated with lack of pigmentation elsewhere in the body or confined to the eyes alone, are common. Where ocular albinism appears to be complete there is generally at least a trace of melanin present which increases slightly during infancy. In a true ocular albino there is deficiency of melanin throughout the eye which is most obvious in the iris and choroid. Extraneous scattered light is transmitted through the iris and the coats of the eye into the interior of the eye resulting in a red glow which is clearly discerned in the pupil and through the iris. The iris is hypoplastic and light gray in colour, not pink as in albino animals (Plate 26.20). The fundus is unpigmented (although blood pigment is normal) and there is, not uncommonly, absence of a defined macula. Pigment is lacking in the skin of the eyelids, and the cilia and eyebrows are white. Abnormal development of the fixation reflex results in a pendular nystagmus, and photophobia causes the child to develop a constant frown with hypertrophy of the orbicularis muscle and a leonine countenance. There is no treatment for ocular albinism but the child can be helped by correcting the refractive error which commonly accompanies the condition, and prescribing tinted lenses to reduce the photophobia. The provision of tinted contact lenses within the first 6 months of life will, in some cases, allow the child to develop normal fixation, refixation and binocular reflexes with the avoidance of nystagmus or strabismus. It is important to appreciate that if this type of lens is to be used to prevent nystagmus it should be fitted early in infancy.

Cystinosis (p. 1123)

This may result in a deposition of cystine crystals throughout the coats of the eye and in the iris. These very fine crystals are seen most readily in the cornea.

Homocystinuria (p. 1108)

This causes bilateral dislocation of the lenses, due to deficiency and eventual breakdown in the zonule. The dislocation may be congenital but the lenses are generally in the normal anatomical position at birth and tend to dislocate upwards within the first few years of life. The lenses usually remain clear. As the lens dislocates the eye becomes increasingly myopic due to increasing sphericity of the lens, but should the lens move out of the pupillary area there is a sudden change to aphakic hypermetropia, and at the point where the lens edge is in the center of the pupil there is a gross irregular astigmatism and vision is particularly poor (Plate 26.17). A sudden change from high myopia to high hypermetropia indicates complete dislocation of the lens. It is not uncommon for the lens to pass forward from its normal anatomical position behind the iris into the anterior chamber. As it passes through the pupil border it may be held in the pupil by contraction of the sphincter of the iris. Should this occur there is obstruction to the flow of aqueous humor with a resultant sudden rise in intraocular pressure causing a form of glaucoma which is accompanied by sharp pain in the eye with sudden reduction in vision. Unlike angle closure glaucoma, the treatment of this condition (inverse glaucoma) is to dilate the pupil with a mydriatic to free the lens. Dislocation of the lens in homocystinuria responds well to surgical lens extraction but as general anesthesia and surgery may be followed by the thrombotic episodes which are a feature of this disorder, and as children with homocystinuria are usually mentally retarded and difficult to nurse in the postoperative stage, lens extraction is best avoided unless the lens is completely dislocated and moving about freely or causing attacks of glaucoma.

The earliest clinical sign of subluxation of the lens is iridodonesis, a tremor of the iris seen on ocular movement, due to loss of the normal support given by the lens to the iris. As progressive dislocation occurs the lens edge becomes visible in the pupil. Peripheral retinal degeneration is commonly seen and there is a high incidence of retinal detachment. Subluxation of the lens can be prevented or its progression stopped by adequate dietary therapy, but medical treatment has no effect on an established dislocation.

Wilson's disease (hepatolenticular degeneration)

This causes the appearance of a Kayser–Fleischer ring in the cornea. This is a greenish-brown deposition of copper in Descemet's membrane. In developed cases there is a band of copper crystals about 2 mm wide extending round the periphery of the cornea. The ring is seldom complete and is not obvious at the upper and lower margins of the cornea. In early cases these rings can only be seen with the binocular microscope but in developed cases they can be seen readily at low magnification. With successful treatment of Wilson's disease the Kayser–Fleischer ring disappears but it tends to recur after a period of several years, even with successful maintenance therapy. Copper may be deposited on the lens capsule to cause a 'sunflower' cataract.

Lipidoses

These affect the eyes in several ways. Idiopathic hyperlipemia may cause lipemia retinalis in which there is pallor of the retinal vessels and fundus background due to the presence of lipids in the circulation. After several years arcus senilis, known in children as arcus juvenilis, appears at the periphery of the cornea. Arcus juvenilis generally differs from arcus senilis in that in the former the arcus is not separated from the sclera by a clear ring of cornea.

Tay–Sachs disease, Niemann–Pick disease and Gaucher's disease are considered in the appropriate sections.

ENDOCRINE DISEASES

Diabetes

Diabetes in a child may present with transient obscurations in vision due to an upset in refraction. When there is a rapid rise in blood sugar the aqueous humor becomes hypotonic relative to the lens with consequent hydration of the lens and an increase in its refractive power resulting in myopia. Rapid changes in refraction in a child should point to diabetes. With stabilization of the metabolic state the refraction is also stabilized but spectacles should not be prescribed or changed during a period of unstable control. Diabetic cataract is a rare complication of diabetes and when it does appear it is found only in adolescents and young adults. Retinopathy of diabetes is the best known of diabetic complications involving the eye but as it seldom appears in diabetes of less than 5 years' duration, it is rarely seen in a child. The earliest signs of retinopathy of diabetes are microaneurysms at the posterior pole of the eye followed by small retinal hemorrhages and accompanied by irregularity in venous caliber. Where retinopathy develops in a young diabetic it tends to progress to proliferative retinopathy and the prognosis for vision is poor. In the early stages of retinopathy the child (or adult) is not aware of any visual disturbance and routine testing of vision may not detect any central visual loss even when retinopathy is established. The earliest sign of visual disturbance is an upset in color vision which is sometimes present even in the preretinopathic stage. The development of microaneurysms can be shown by fluorescein retinal angiography before they can be seen with the ophthalmoscope. Oculomotor palsies due to diabetic peripheral neuropathy occur but are uncommon. Uveitis is rather commoner in diabetics than in non-diabetics.

Hyperthyroidism

Hyperthyroidism in a child causes bilateral upper lid retraction which gives the eye a staring appearance which can be confused with exophthalmos. True dysthyroid exophthalmos in a child is exceedingly rare.

Hypothyroidism

There is a high incidence of strabismus due to mental retardation with associated upset in the binocular reflexes. This strabismus responds to orthoptic and surgical treatment.

Hypoparathyroidism

Hypoparathyroid cataracts are bilateral, subcapsular opacities developing as lamellae in the lens, each of which corresponds to an attack of tetany. If the condition is untreated the lens opacity progresses towards maturity but with successful treatment there is no further opacification, although the isolated lamellae of opacity remain unchanged. Should the vision be depressed to the point where surgical interference is required, the response to a lens extraction is good.

Pheochromocytoma

Pheochromocytoma causes a rapidly progressive retinopathy of hypertension. Addison's disease does not affect the eye itself but causes pigmentation of the eyelids and conjunctivae.

THE COLLAGEN DISEASES

Disseminated lupus erythematosus

Disseminated lupus erythematosus causes a rapidly progressive retinopathy beginning with superficial hemorrhages and cytoid bodies at the posterior pole of the eye, progressing to extensive retinal hemorrhage, exudation and papilledema. The picture improves rapidly with systemic corticosteroid therapy.

Polyarteritis nodosa

Polyarteritis nodosa may cause a hypertensive retinopathy due to systemic vascular involvement and this retinopathy does not differ from classical hypertensive retinopathy. Where there is a specific lesion involving the central retinal artery or one of its branches there is the characteristic picture of arterial occlusion, but where a branch of the retinal artery alone is involved the classical fundus picture of a branch arterial occlusion is preceded by superficial retinal hemorrhage in the region of the occluded vessel.

Rheumatoid arthritis

Rheumatoid arthritis may be complicated by a bilateral anterior uveitis. In children this type of anterior uveitis may be painless and the accompanying deterioration in vision is insidious. Initially, there is exudation into the anterior chamber manifest by flare and cells and eventually the pupil becomes irregular with the iris atrophic and adherent to the lens. Secondary glaucoma may develop. In some cases a complicated cataract develops and longstanding cases show corneal opacities due to deposition of calcium in the interpalpebral strip of the cornea. Eventually there is atrophy of the eyeball. Anterior uveitis associated with rheumatoid arthritis responds in its early stages to simple local therapy including mydriatics and corticosteroids. In view of the painless and relatively quiet nature of the condition, all children with rheumatoid arthritis should have an eye examination, if necessary using sedation or even general anesthesia. Uveitis may be masked although not effectively treated by systemic corticosteroids. The condition almost always becomes binocular. It may present at any stage in the course of rheumatoid arthritis and both eyes should be examined regularly, even where previous examinations have shown them to be clear of inflammation.

Ankylosing spondylitis

Ankylosing spondylitis may be accompanied in children by episcleritis and scleritis. This starts as a mildly irritable eye with an injected area on the sclera where the sclera appears to be thin, although histological examination of a focus of episcleritis shows it to be infiltrated and thickened. There is always an accompanying uveitis which is frequently painful. The end result of scleritis is a perforated sclera and collapsed eye. Scleritis responds to systemic corticosteroids and local therapy similar to that for uveitis.

Dermatomyositis

Dermatomyositis can cause ptosis, proptosis or muscle palsy through orbital involvement, or uveitis and scleritis where the lesions involve the globe of the eye. In the acute stage there is commonly an acute retinopathy with venous distension and engorgement with retinal and preretinal hemorrhage and papilledema. All of these changes respond to systemic treatment.

DISEASES OF THE SKIN

Ulcerative blepharitis with its accompanying indolent conjunctivitis is commonly associated with seborrhea and will recur despite successful ocular therapy unless the seborrhea is also treated.

Molluscum contagiosum causes umbilicated vesicles on the eyelids and surrounding skin which should be expressed or cauterized. In marked cases of molluscum contagiosum there is a keratoconjunctivitis which clears completely when the skin lesions are treated.

Pediculosis (pubic or scalp)) may be accompanied by pediculosis of the eyelashes which can cause blepharitis and may result in chronic conjunctivitis. Ocular treatment is only successful if the cilia and the body are cleared of lice (see blepharitis; Fig. 26.18).

Stevens–Johnson syndrome (erythema multiforme) typically causes an acute conjunctivitis with membrane formation. There is a tendency to adhesion between the conjunctival surfaces and this may progress to symblepharon and obliteration of the fornices.

Although many other skin diseases of adult life involve the eye few of them do so in childhood. There is a group of conditions which may occur in late childhood or adolescence which, although not primarily diseases of the skin, all have skin lesions and may involve the eye. These include Reiter's syndrome, Behçet's syndrome, Vogt–Koyanagi syndrome and Harada's disease. All of these are uncommon and their ocular complication is uveitis.

HYPERTENSION

Hypertension of whatever origin tends to cause a characteristic retinopathy. The earliest sign in the fundus is narrowing and straightening of the arterioles due to constriction of the vessel walls. This is followed by 'cotton wool patches', the result of retinal infarcts, and then superficial and deep retinal hemorrhages appear with edema at the posterior pole. The characteristic signs in the fundus are the soft fluffy exudates with flame-shaped hemorrhages and a star figure at the macula which follows macular edema. Retinopathy of hypertension is bilateral and its rate of progression and extent depend upon the severity of the underlying condition. In the earliest stages where only the retinal vessels are involved the changes are completely reversible and although in the later stages the fundus picture may improve considerably with treatment, the background retinopathy is usually represented by macular scarring with pigmentation, and where there has been papilledema this is usually followed by secondary optic atrophy. Where hypertension has been of particularly rapid onset and is severe the retinopathy will progress steadily and is liable to cause massive exudation into and behind the retina, causing extensive retinal detachment and if this is bilateral, blindness can be the presenting symptom. In these cases effective lowering of the blood pressure results in resorption of the exudate with surprisingly good recovery of vision.

BLOOD DYSCRASIA

Severe anemia, whatever its origin, causes pallor of the retina and optic nerve head. The background retinopathy shows deep round hemorrhages and superficial linear hemorrhages with no exudation. Sickle-cell anemia produces a characteristic retinopathy in which there is a distinct tendency to massive vitreous hemorrhage; in this condition, whilst the central area of the retina may appear to be normal, the retinopathy starts in the periphery of the retina with venous dilation and new vessel formation which results in hemorrhage. Eventually there is fibrous tissue formation which may result in detachment of the retina and blindness but before this stage is reached sight may be lost by massive vitreous hemorrhage. This retinopathy responds in its early stages to treatment by photocoagulation.

Leukemia causes a retinopathy similar to that seen in anemia but generally with obvious venous distension and some superficial retinal exudation. Leukemic infiltration may occur in the orbit, resulting in orbital congestion or even proptosis.

ALLERGY

Allergic conjunctivitis is the most common ocular involvement in local or generalized allergy. This may present as an immediate conjunctivitis with rapidly developing conjunctival injection and chemosis, accompanied by extreme discomfort and copious lacrimation. The rather more common delayed conjunctivitis has a less rapid onset and produces less obvious local signs which, however, tend to persist, unlike the immediate type which disappears within a few days. Both of these types of allergic conjunctivitis respond to topical antihistaminics such as

Otrivine–Antistin (xylometazoline 0.05% w/v and antazoline 0.5% w/v) or corticosteroids (such as 0.1% solution of betamethasone given for not more than 1 week). Symptomatic relief is produced by topical vasoconstrictors (such as 1/100 000 adrenaline solution or 1% zinc sulfate solution) but these forms of treatment are only palliative and fundamental treatment involves diagnosis of the allergic nature of the conjunctivitis, finding the responsible allergen and giving treatment by desensitization. It is important to recognize the nature of allergic conjunctivitis as treatment of these children with local antibiotics, which frequently happens, eventually causes sensitivity to the antibiotic or its vehicle.

CONNECTIVE TISSUE DISORDERS

Marfan's syndrome characteristically has bilaterally dislocated lenses. Minor degrees of subluxation can only be diagnosed with a fully dilated pupil although the condition is generally indicated by an irregular refractive error. Marfan's syndrome is sometimes accompanied by high myopia and keratoconus.

Marchesani syndrome has multiple developmental defects in the anterior segment of the eye, the most typical of which is spherophakia, the increased sphericity of the lens causing myopia.

Osteogenesis imperfecta is accompanied by blue sclerae (blue sclerotics) due to scleral thinning with choroidal pigment showing through. There is a tendency to myopia and keratoconus. Children with osteogenesis imperfecta usually develop cataract in adult life. (Blue sclerae are seen in the normal infant up to about 6 months of age and in infantile glaucoma (buphthalmos) the sclerae also appear to be blue due to choroidal pigment showing through a stretched sclera.)

SYSTEMIC INFECTIVE DISEASES

Viral diseases

The viral diseases involving the eye include *measles*, which commonly causes an acute conjunctivitis or blepharoconjunctivitis with photophobia. Simple treatment is all that is required and local antibiotics should not be used unless there is a secondary infection. *Rubella* occasionally causes a mild conjunctivitis which does not require treatment. Rubella in a mother during the first trimester of pregnancy may cause a developmental cataract and rubella retinopathy in the baby. *Mumps* may cause a mild conjunctivitis. *Varicella* occasionally causes an acute conjunctivitis commencing with small pustules on the conjunctiva which rupture to produce minute ulcerated areas, and if there are multiple pustules on the conjunctiva there is liable to be corneal ulceration. *Herpes zoster* ophthalmicus involves the skin of the eyelids and is accompanied by an acute conjunctivitis with secondary bacterial infection. Where the nasociliary nerve is involved, indicated by vesicles at the tip of the nose, there will be anterior uveitis which develops with a sharp pain in the eye. It is important to examine the eye carefully in herpes zoster ophthalmicus, although this may be difficult due to inflammatory edema of the eyelids. *Epidemic keratoconjunctivitis* and *pharyngoconjunctival fever* both cause an acute conjunctivitis with extensive superficial keratitis shown by small spots of ulceration on the corneae. *Cytomegalic inclusion disease* may cause a choroidoretinitis.

Fungal diseases

Fungi are responsible for an increasing number of ocular and orbital inflammations. The increasing use of antibiotics and corticosteroids, both systemically and locally, is largely responsible for this increase. Fungal invasion causes the same signs of inflammation as other organisms, producing conjunctivitis, keratitis, uveitis, etc., depending upon the part of eye involved. Unilateral proptosis, ocular muscle paresis and obstruction of the tear passages all result from extraocular fungus invasion. Where any of these conditions appear to be indolent or unresponsive to treatment, fungus infection should always be borne in mind.

Protozoal diseases

Protozoal diseases, with the exception of toxoplasmosis, rarely involve the eye. *Congenital toxoplasmosis* causes a posterior uveitis, involving the region of the macula in one or both eyes. This is the commonest cause of posterior uveitis in infancy although by the time of birth the lesion may be healed. There is a punched out appearance of the fundus at the posterior pole of the eye giving a white area of approximately two optic disk diameters in size and surrounded by black pigment. Vision is always seriously reduced and a squint may be present. Acquired toxoplasmosis is uncommon in infancy but may be accompanied by a posterior uveitis.

The eye lesions of congenital toxoplasmosis generally remain quiet throughout life but there may be acute exacerbations due to the rupture of pseudocyst causing an acute inflammatory reaction. The result is a temporary further reduction in vision and a patch of fresh uveitis can be seen beside the original lesion accompanied by posterior vitreous haze. Treatment with sulfonamides and pyrimethamine is successful and should be accompanied by systemic corticosteroid therapy to suppress the inflammatory response.

Helminthic diseases

Toxocara canis (and rarely *Toxocara cati*) are the only helminthic diseases involving the eyes in temperate climates. *Toxocara canis* causes a posterior uveitis or choroidoretinitis giving an appearance similar to that seen in retinoblastoma. There is invasion of the posterior part of the eye by the *Toxocara* which causes a granuloma with persistent endophthalmitis which can result in loss of the eye. *Onchocerca* and *Loa loa* cause acute bilateral generalized uveitis due to helminthic invasion of the eyes in areas where these infections are common.

Onchocerciasis is responsible for much blindness in Africa where the sufferers are numbered in many millions. It also occurs in central America but does not occur in temperate climates. *Onchocerca volvulus* infects man through the black fly of the genus *Simulium* and the eye is invaded by the parasite to cause an extensive anterior and posterior uveitis. Treatment consists of excising infected skin nodules (onchocercomata) to eliminate dissemination of microfilariae and the use of piperazine derivatives such as diethylcarbamazine. At the same time communities should be removed from the source of infection which is always close to a river, but treatment of populations appears to be virtually impossible as although river areas are cleared and the river and its banks are sprayed to kill the fly, the population invariably return to the river and the infected fly also reappears.

Loa loa causes bilateral generalized uveitis due to helminthic invasion of the eyes. Loiasis is a much less serious ocular problem than other helminthic diseases as, although in some areas, for example in islands in the Pacific, almost 100% of the inhabitants are infected, there is seldom any evidence of invasion of the eye by filaria to set up a uveitis.

Bacterial infections

The eye can be involved in systemic bacterial infections of all types. The eye lesion depends upon direct organismal spread and varies from a simple acute conjunctivitis to metastatic uveitis with abscess formation. Where an infant develops a purulent uveitis or endophthalmitis, metastatic uveitis should be considered.

Diphtheria can cause a membranous conjunctivitis which generally accompanies or precedes the pharyngeal infection. The appearance and mechanism of production of the membrane are similar to that in the throat.

Tuberculosis which causes anterior or posterior uveitis with nodule formation was formerly considered to be an important cause of uveitis but its incidence is now reducing. There is an anterior uveitis with heavy exudation in the anterior chamber. The ocular lesions respond to systemic antituberculous treatment and local corticosteroids are generally also necessary. This type of tuberculous eye lesion can cause serious destruction or distortion of the ocular tissues. Where there is disseminated tuberculosis infection there may be multiple foci of posterior uveitis presenting as disseminated choroidoretinitis. This responds to systemic treatment and no local ocular therapy is necessary. Phlyctenular keratoconjunctivitis which causes lacrimation and photophobia and yellowish nodules on the conjunctiva was at one time common in young children. This is due to tuberculous bacterial allergy, and treatment must be given on general lines although relief of ocular symptoms can be produced with the use of local corticosteroids or vasoconstrictors.

Acquired *syphilis* causes granulomatous anterior and posterior uveitis but is rarely seen in children. Congenital syphilis is accompanied by interstitial keratitis in about 20% of cases. The keratitis may appear at any age in childhood and start as a violent inflammatory reaction with corneal swelling and epithelial edema accompanied by a sharp reduction in vision. It is generally bilateral, the second eye being involved 1 or 2 months following the first eye. When the corneal inflammation is established there is corneal vascularization and blood vessel invasion may be so heavy as to give the corneae a pink appearance. The condition tends to settle spontaneously with some improvement in vision although there is always evidence of keratitis having been present and ghost vessels can be seen in the corneal stroma. The primary lesion is always an anterior uveitis and is accompanied by a diffuse choroiditis. Systemic treatment must be given but there is a good response to local treatment of the uveitis.

Sarcoid, although not a bacterial infection, produces a picture similar to ocular tuberculosis. In systemic sarcoidosis nodules can be found in the skin of the eyelids, the conjunctiva, and in any of the tissues of the orbit. Conjunctival biopsy is occasionally used for diagnostic purposes. The commonest intraocular involvement is iridocyclitis in which there are large iris nodules. If left untreated, the sarcoidosis progresses as a chronic uveitis with eventual atrophy of the uvea leading to phthisis bulbae and collapse of the eye. In the early stages the response to systemic corticosteroid therapy is dramatic.

NUTRITIONAL DISORDERS

It is unusual for the eyes or vision to be involved in nutritional disorders unless the deficiency is gross. Vitamin deficiencies produce specific eye lesions.

Avitaminosis A, whether due to dietary defect or systemic disease, causes keratinization of the conjunctival and corneal epithelium which is called xerosis. This appears concurrently with changes in the gastrointestinal and respiratory epithelium. The conjunctiva loses its luster and becomes wrinkled whilst white foamy areas (Bitot's spots) are seen in the interpalpebral regions. As xerosis progresses the cornea becomes opaque with loss of its epithelium and there may be frank ulceration. This stage of corneal involvement (keratomalacia) leads to destruction of the cornea and loss of the eye. At any stage up to established keratomalacia there is a rapid improvement with massive doses of vitamin A given systemically. The earliest symptom of vitamin A deficiency is night blindness which is rarely commented upon by children. Even before night blindness is established there is delay in dark adaptation, and an assessment of the rate of dark adaptation gives an indication of the presence of vitamin A deficiency, but this is an unreliable test in children.

Avitaminosis B involves the eye should there be peripheral neuropathy or *Wernicke's encephalopathy* due to thiamin deficiency. Extraocular muscle palsies, ptosis and nystagmus may be produced. Riboflavin deficiency produces conjunctivitis with corneal vascularization in advanced cases. These eye changes probably only occur in extreme degrees of riboflavin deficiency and there is no justification for giving vitamin B to children with corneal vascularization.

Avitaminosis C can cause hemorrhage into the eye or the tissues surrounding the eye. There may be orbital hemorrhage with gross proptosis.

Avitaminosis D in early infancy produces bilateral lamellar cataracts (see pp. 301, 1194). Clear lens develops outside the areas of opacification when the deficiency is put right. Avitaminosis D in a mother produces corresponding lamellar cataracts in the fetus which appear as congenital cataracts.

TOXIC DISORDERS

Some drugs given systemically have serious effects on the eye or vision and are best considered at this stage. Systemic *corticosteroid* therapy may cause bilateral cataract when the drug has been given for a year or more. The cataract is situated in the posterior part of the lens and causes considerable reduction in vision. Systemic and local corticosteroid therapy given over a prolonged period may cause glaucoma of an insidious type which may only be detected when optic atrophy develops. Young children who have had systemic corticosteroid therapy for a prolonged period may develop papilledema when the steroid is withdrawn.

Chloroquine therapy causes corneal deposition of chloroquine crystals which disappear when the drug is withdrawn. Prolonged therapy causes a permanent bilateral pigmentary retinopathy with reduction in central vision. A similar retinopathy may be seen after prolonged antibiotic therapy, particularly with chloramphenicol.

The toxic effects of drugs on the eye can usually be detected by electrophysiology before there is any visual loss or any retinal ophthalmoscopic change.

Oxygen toxicity – retinopathy of prematurity (see Ch. 5).

Lead intoxication occasionally occurs in children when there may be optic neuritis with reduction in peripheral vision and the production of scotomata, together with extraocular muscle palsies and ptosis.

A number of drugs given systemically interfere with vision through pupillary dilation and reduction in accommodation. The most common of these drugs are the belladonna alkaloids of which atropine is the most commonly used. Antihistaminics which are commonly prescribed for motion sickness may cause visual disturbance.

Where drugs produce a teratogenic effect, the eye may be involved. Thalidomide taken in pregnancy caused microphthalmos and iris and retinal colobomata in about 25% of cases and there is the possibility that other congenital defects which have no obvious hereditary basis may be due to teratogenic agents.

Drug intoxication. An increasing number of teenage children are now becoming addicted to drugs by intravenous injection. Most of these drugs cause no more ocular abnormalities than blurred vision, double vision, dilated pupils and hallucinations, but where drugs are injected intravenously endophthalmitis can occur (usually due to *Candida albicans*) introduced by unsterilized needles and contaminated solutions used to dilute drug powders. *Candida albicans* causes endophthalmitis, pneumonitis and sternal chondritis. When the patient presents, the endophthalmitis is generally beyond the point where effective treatment is possible but fortunately only one eye is usually involved. Nowadays, when a youngster presents with an acutely inflamed eye and signs of endophthalmitis and in poor general health the question of drug abuse should be considered and urgent treatment given.

27 Disorders of the ear, nose and throat

D. L. Cowan   A. I. G. Kerr

THE EAR   1679
Congenital abnormalities   1679
Microtia/anotia/meatal atresia   1679
Meatal stenosis   1679
Ossicular abnormalities   1679
Injuries/foreign bodies   1680
Perforation of the tympanic membrane   1680
Wax   1680
Infections of the ears   1680
Otitis externa   1680
Furunculosis   1680
Acute otitis media   1680
Acute mastoiditis   1680
Chronic otitis media   1680
Referred otalgia   1681
Secretory otitis media   1681
Deafness   1682
Causes of sensorineural deafness   1682
Diagnosis of deafness   1683
Subjective audiometry   1683
Objective audiometry   1683
Treatment of deafness   1683
The phonic ear   1683
Cochlear implants   1683
D. L. Cowan

THE NOSE AND SINUSES   1683
The nose   1683
Foreign bodies   1684
Fracture of the nose   1684
Epistaxis   1684
Rhinitis   1684
Nasal septal deviation   1685
Disease of the paranasal sinuses   1685
Maxillary sinusitis   1685
Ethmoiditis   1685
Frontal sinusitis   1685
Nasal polyps   1685
Choanal atresia   1685
Diseases of the nasopharynx   1685
Adenoids (nasopharyngeal tonsil)   1685
Angiofibroma   1686
Pharyngitis   1686
Tonsils   1686
Disorders of phonation   1687
Dysphonia   1687
Aphonia   1688
A. I. G. Kerr
References   1688

THE EAR

CONGENITAL ABNORMALITIES

MICROTIA/ANOTIA/MEATAL ATRESIA

The auricle forms from six tubercles of His. Malformations include microtia, a misshapen auricle, or anotia, the absence of the auricle. Both may be associated with accessory auricles, which are small residual tubercles that may lie sometimes over the cheek without function. Either of these congenital abnormalities of the auricle may be associated with meatal atresia, the absence of the bony meatus. They are commonly associated together in a variety of congenital conditions and syndromes. They may present as a unilateral problem, e.g. first arch syndrome, or as a bilateral problem, e.g. craniofacial dysostosis. If the deformity is a unilateral one it is extremely important to investigate the normal ear to ensure that the hearing is normal on the unaffected side. Assuming the normal ear has normal hearing, then surgical or other intervention on the affected side becomes purely cosmetic. If the condition is bilateral, then the degree of conductive hearing loss should be established and, in the first instance, a bone-anchored hearing aid fixed by a head band should be fitted at an early age. In the past, attempts at surgical reconstruction of a pinna and/or fashioning of an external meatus have been unrewarding. They have been superseded by osseous integrated implants which can be fitted direct to the skull so that either a bone-anchored hearing aid can be attached to the implant or, alternatively, a prosthetic auricle. This surgery cannot be undertaken until the child is approximately 4 or 5 years old when the skull is thick enough to take a titanium implant screw.

MEATAL STENOSIS

Meatal stenosis may occur either as a congenital abnormality or as a result of chronic otitis externa. Down syndrome children have very narrow external auditory meati and they often have middle ear problems. This makes diagnosis of the middle ear problems more difficult.

OSSICULAR ABNORMALITIES

Congenital abnormalities of the ear ossicles are rarely seen in isolation and are usually associated with some other manifest congenital abnormality. Attempts at surgical repair of ossicles in children are not normally advisable and any bilateral hearing deficit should be treated by a hearing aid.

INJURIES/FOREIGN BODIES

Direct trauma to the auricle may produce a hematoma and is commonly seen in sporting injuries. The hematoma should be aspirated and a pressure bandage applied to avoid the cosmetic abnormality known as 'cauliflower ear'.

PERFORATION OF THE TYMPANIC MEMBRANE

This can be caused either by an object inserted into the ear or alternatively by pressure, e.g. in nonaccidental injury where a slap across the ear can cause a perforation of the drum due to the pressure of the air column in the narrow meatus. This form of injury is also seen in explosions or in diving accidents. Head injuries may be associated with perforation of the eardrum and also leakage of CSF.

Treatment of perforation of the eardrum is conservative; the ear is kept dry and in the great majority of traumatic perforations the eardrum will heal spontaneously. This healing may take several months but no attempt at surgical intervention should be considered for at least 6 months.

WAX

It is normal for wax to be present in ears and as a general rule this causes no problems unless the wax is impacted into the external auditory meatus by the use of cotton buds. The superficial squamous epithelial cells in the external meatus have a natural flow pattern outwards, so that wax will be naturally extruded from the ear and hence, if the wax is kept soft by the use of simple olive or almond oil drops, syringing of the ears should not be required. As a general rule it is preferable not to syringe children's ears as they will find it uncomfortable and it will interfere with the natural extrusion process.

INFECTIONS OF THE EARS

OTITIS EXTERNA

This condition does not occur as commonly in children. The basis of treatment is aural toilet and the application of topical antibiotic, with or without steroids, either on a small gauze dressing, which is preferable, or, alternatively, administered as eardrops. The skin of the meatus is often swollen and extremely tender and aural toilet may have to be carried out under a general anesthetic.

FURUNCULOSIS

A furuncle in the external meatus will produce an acutely painful ear which is tender to the touch. It is often associated with a tender lymph node over the mastoid tip and hence the combination is often mistaken as an acute mastoiditis. In acute mastoiditis, the maximum area of tenderness is rarely, if ever, over the mastoid tip. Treatment of furunculosis is oral antibiotics and local dressings.

ACUTE OTITIS MEDIA

This occurs commonly in infants and children as the eustachian tube is shorter, relatively wider and more horizontal than in the adult and also because children have adenoids which are close to the opening of the eustachian tube: hence, acute otitis media is a common accompaniment to upper respiratory tract infections and other infections. Clinically, the condition will present as an acutely painful ear, usually bilaterally, and the child will be fevered and may develop febrile convulsions.

The eardrum if inspected will appear either acutely inflamed or bulging, with obvious pus behind it, and the pain is due to the build-up of mucopurulent secretions in the middle ear. The first-aid treatment is analgesics/antipyretics, and antibiotics. If the eardrum perforates, the pain will subside. In the vast majority of patients the drum will heal once the infection has settled. The treatment of infants and children with recurrent attacks of acute otitis media is either by repeated use of antibiotics or by surgical intervention. In young children, whose adenoids have not developed, the insertion of ventilation tubes (grommets) in the tympanic membranes will prevent recurrent attacks of acute otitis media. In older children who have significant adenoids, their removal will reduce further attacks of otitis media.

ACUTE MASTOIDITIS

Acute mastoiditis still occurs but not nearly as frequently as it used to, due to the use of antibiotics for acute otitis media. Clinically, the child with acute mastoiditis will present with an acutely tender swelling in the postauricular region with the area of maximum tenderness being over the surface marking of the mastoid antrum which is at the level of the top of the tragus. If looked at from behind, the auricle will be seen to be projecting outwards from the skull due to the loss of the postauricular sulcus and this is most commonly due to the collection of subperiosteal pus. The ear may or may not be discharging. The child will usually be in considerable pain and will be febrile. Treatment is admission, administration of intravenous antibiotics and analgesics and careful monitoring of the pulse and temperature for 24–48 hours. If the postauricular swelling is increasing or if the temperature is not settling in that time, then surgical drainage of the subperiosteal pus and drilling away of the diseased cortical bone should be undertaken under general anesthesia. Acute mastoiditis rarely becomes a recurrent problem nor leads to chronic otitis media or cholesteatoma formation.

CHRONIC OTITIS MEDIA

Chronic otitis media is associated with a permanent perforation of the tympanic membrane. There are two quite distinct groups:

Tubotympanic disease

Usually such children have had recurrent attacks of otitis media which have either been inappropriately treated or which have resulted in a permanent residual anterior central perforation of the tympanic membrane. The clinical presentation is of intermittent quite profuse painless mucopurulent discharge from the ear. The profuse discharge occurs in association with an upper respiratory tract infection or following the child swimming or getting the ear wet. If treated with oral antibiotics, the discharge should cease. The hearing loss will be minimal. Effective antibiotic treatment of tubotympanic is required and the child should keep his ear dry. Closure of the perforation by myringoplasty using a temporalis fascia graft is not advisable until the child has gone at least 6 months without any discharge from the ear and this will rarely be before the age of 8 or 9.

Attico/antral disease

These children have a continuous painless moderate purulent or bloodstained discharge from the ear. There may be middle ear granulations. This discharge will often be foul-smelling as the commonest organism is *Pseudomonas pyocyaneas*. This form of chronic otitis media is more serious as it is usually associated with cholesteatoma in the mastoid antrum or mastoid cell system which may erode the ossicles and cause a significant hearing loss. If cholesteatoma is identified in the ear by suction clearance, under general anesthesia, then mastoid surgery is indicated as facial nerve palsy or cerebral complications will occur if the cholesteatoma is not cleared completely from the mastoid system.

REFERRED OTALGIA

Referred pain in the ear may be from the tonsils, sinuses or teeth, all of which must be considered in a child who has unexplained otalgia.

SECRETORY OTITIS MEDIA

This is a very common condition between 4 and 6 years and is commoner in boys. It is alternatively called nonsuppurative otitis media, seromucinous otitis media, exudative otitis media, or simply 'glue ear'. Children with secretory otitis media commonly present with a hearing loss due to the collection of fluid in their middle ears. Cytologically, the fluid contains polymorphonuclear leukocytes, macrophages and cell debris but no ciliated columnar cells or eosinophils. The fluid is invariably sterile and various searches for viruses have proved negative. Biochemically, the fluid contains glycoproteins and nucleoproteins and this gives the fluid its thick tenacious quality.

Natural history

Classically, a child with secretory otitis media will present with painless insidious bilateral conductive deafness, which if measured audiometrically, will not be greater than 40 decibels. Fluid will classically collect without prior middle ear infections and often the child does not remark on the loss of hearing. The problem may not be identified until routine audiometric testing is done at school. The fluid collects due to blockage of the eustachian tube. If children are left for up to 8 weeks, 20% of them will drain their fluid and their hearing will return to normal. Alternatively, a distinct group of children who have recurrent otitis media which has been treated appropriately by antibiotics develop a collection of sterile fluid in the middle ear which does not drain down the eustachian tube, presumably due to edema of the mucosa.

Prevalence

At any one time, 1 child in 100 will have secretory otitis media, and in a recent study from Riyadh, Saudi Arabia, 13.8% of 4214 children aged 1–8 were found to have secretory otitis media.

Diagnosis

Diagnosis is usually made by taking a careful history from the parents and/or the teachers, who are seeing the child on an everyday basis. Otoscopic examination will reveal an abnormal eardrum which may be retracted, bulging, dull, blue/yellow in color, or have air–fluid bubbles visible behind it. Puretone audiometry will reveal a conductive hearing loss which is usually bilateral and worse in the lower frequencies than the higher frequencies but never greater than 40 decibels. Impedance audiometry will give a flat tympanogram with a negative middle ear pressure and a greatly reduced tympanic membrane compliance.

Etiology

The underlying cause is believed to be some abnormality of eustachian tube function and, certainly, children with cleft palate, and hence impaired eustachian tube function, have a greatly increased risk of having secretory otitis media. Children with chronic secretory otitis media do have persistent negative middle ear pressure due to eustachian tube malfunction and this results in the loss of the elastic layer of the tympanic membrane with atelectasis or atrophy of the membrane. Adenoids blocking the eustachian tube orifice in the nasopharynx have long been associated with this condition and so their removal is often undertaken as a form of treatment. However, children without adenoids still get secretory otitis media and therefore there must be more complex factors involved. Attempts to associate nasal allergy with secretory otitis media have never been substantiated and apart from the already mentioned age and sex factors, the only other recently proven etiologic factor is passive smoking within the home environment (Maw et al 1992). Because the eustachian tube is situated so centrally, it is extremely difficult to investigate its function in these children, and hence the etiology remains obscure.

Treatment

The treatment of secretory otitis media remains controversial. Many suggest that surgical treatment should not be undertaken as the condition may resolve spontaneously with time. However, there is no doubt that some young toddlers who are slow to talk may turn out to have secretory otitis media, or that the school-child with secretory otitis media may well present with poor oral work in comparison to his written work. Parents of children with secretory otitis media are the first to notice when the hearing loss recurs and are always the quickest to demand treatment. Children tend to accept what is given to them and rarely complain when the condition recurs, although their behavior may alter. Another symptom not uncommonly seen in children with secretory otitis media, that of loss of balance, may also improve following treatment.

Attempts to treat the condition medically with long-term, low dose antibiotics and/or local or oral decongestants have never convincingly been proven to be effective and any positive results may well be due to the natural history of the condition and the spontaneous recovery in some children. If clearance of the fluid does not occur within 2 months then the only available treatment is surgical.

Surgery consists of myringotomy (drainage of the fluid), with adenoidectomy, or with grommet tube insertion, or with both. Attempts are still being made to draw up clearly defined identifiable clinical guidelines, but these are yet to be fully agreed. In my practice, I perform myringotomy and insertion of grommet tubes in children who have no significant adenoids, i.e. those under 2–2.5 years, or those who have already had their adenoids removed. In the group who do have significant adenoids (a history of chronic mouth breathing and snoring or with enlargement on a lateral X-ray of the nasopharynx) I will perform myringotomy and adenoidectomy. Of those children who have a simple myringotomy and adenoidectomy, 80% do not develop recurrent secretory otitis media and hence the grommet tubes can be reserved for the 20% who recur following the initial operation. Children with chronic secretory otitis media need grommet tubes to be inserted in an attempt to reduce the negative middle ear pressure, ventilate the middle ear and so prevent atelectasis of the tympanic membrane.

Children with grommet tubes are advised not to immerse their head under water, either in the bath or in the swimming pool. If children insist on diving deep in the swimming pool, then either a commercial earplug or cotton wool impregnated with petroleum jelly may be inserted into the ears to prevent water reaching the tympanic membrane. Classically, grommet tubes remain in place in the eardrums from 6 months to 1 year, but the range may be from 2 months to 2 years. Apart from infection, there are no long-term complications from the use of grommet tubes.

Outcomes

The number of children with chronic otitis media has fallen since treatment of secretory otitis media has been more active. As far as the final hearing goes, the long-term results appear to be reasonably good, although these have not been totally scientifically delineated.

DEAFNESS

Otitis media will produce a conductive deafness of approximately 40 decibels which can affect speech development.

A child with a hearing handicap should be identified as having a conductive deafness or sensorineural deafness (nerve deafness). In conductive deafness the disability is not so severe and often there may be a surgical or medical method of treating it. Sensorineural deafness in children is not uncommon. In developed countries, the incidence of bilateral significant sensorineural deafness is 1 in 1000 live births. 'Significant loss' is a loss of between 25 and 35 decibels in the better ear. It is the high frequency component of the loss that is usually important. If the loss in the better ear is at a level of 30 decibels when averaged over the four frequencies 500 Hz, 1 kHz, 2 kHz and 4 kHz, then the child will require some kind of amplification to attain normal speech and language.

CAUSES OF SENSORINEURAL DEAFNESS

Hereditary prenatal causes

There are large numbers of syndromes in which deafness is a recognized factor:

Waardenburg syndrome (p. 1560). This autosomal dominant condition with variable expression consists of some or all of the following characteristics: unilateral or bilateral perceptive deafness (20% of cases); hypertrichosis of the eyebrows which meet in the midline; heterochromia of the irises; or a white forelock.

Klippel–Feil syndrome (p. 1556). A short neck limits head movements, the hairline is low at the back, there may be paralysis of the external rectus muscle in one or both eyes and there is perceptive hearing loss which may be severe.

Alport's syndrome (p. 965) is X-linked dominant and affects boys more severely than girls. There is severe progressive glomerulonephritis and a progressive sensorineural loss which does not show itself until the boy is about 10 years old.

Pendred's syndrome (p. 1046) is autosomal recessive and causes simple goiter at about the age of 4–5 years. There is an associated deafness which is often severe.

Refsum's syndrome (pp. 787, 1173) consists of icthyosis, ataxia, retinitis pigmentosa, night blindness, mental retardation and a sensorineural deafness.

Usher's syndrome (p. 816) is autosomal recessive. There is retinitis pigmentosa with contraction of the visual fields and a severe sensorineural loss which may be progressive.

Jervell and Lange-Nielsen syndrome (p. 626) is autosomal recessive with a cardiac arrhythmia and a profound sensorineural deafness. These children may present with syncopal attacks and if untreated, these attacks can be fatal.

The inheritance of deafness is well recognized and in some children with recessive inheritance, the sensorineural hearing loss may be progressive. Nonhereditary prenatal deafness is due to maternal illness, especially in the first trimester of pregnancy. Cytomegalovirus infections, toxoplasmosis, glandular fever and rubella are the most common, while parental syphilis and the taking of certain ototoxic drugs by the mother may cause deafness in the baby.

Ototoxic drugs that should be specifically avoided during pregnancy are the aminoglycosides, quinine and to a lesser extent salicylates and alcohol.

Perinatal causes of deafness are basically related to prematurity and hypoxia. With the advances in neonatology, when extremely immature babies with complex neonatal problems are now surviving, the number of children with significant bilateral deafness sometimes associated with other abnormalities, and often related to hypoxia, is increasing. The cochlea is particularly sensitive to lack of oxygen. As neonatology improves further, the numbers of children with perinatal deafness will hopefully reduce.

Postnatal causes

Middle ear problems cause conductive deafness and the causes of these have already been discussed. Sensorineural loss may result from head injury, from the use of ototoxic drugs and as a result of specific infections. Parents whose children get repeated attacks of acute otitis media are often concerned that significant sensorineural loss may result, but this is extremely rare.

Measles and mumps. Measles and mumps remain the specific infections that can cause significant sensorineural hearing loss. Luckily, mumps, although it will cause a profound sensorineural loss, generally only produces a unilateral loss, while the increasing use of measles vaccine will reduce the incidence of deafness from this cause.

Meningitis. Meningococcal or pneumococcal meningitis may give severe bilateral sensorineural hearing loss which will be permanent and may progress in severity following recovery from the meningitis.

In summary, only about 50% of children with significant bilateral sensorineural loss have an identifiable cause.

DIAGNOSIS OF DEAFNESS

The first 2 years of life are absolutely vital for the acquisition of speech and language and hence the early detection of significant hearing loss in a baby is vital.

No child has no islands of hearing at all and with early detection and appropriate amplification the chances of the child learning to speak are greatly increased. The ideal would be to have a quick, simple, objective test that could be done on every child during the first 24 hours of life, but at present this is not available as a practical screening measure.

SUBJECTIVE AUDIOMETRY

Distraction audiometry

This is still a reliable, efficient method of testing which requires the minimum of equipment. The disadvantage is that it cannot be performed until the child is holding his head up unsupported. In the UK this is carried out by the health visitor as one of the routine screening tests at 7 or 8 months.

Conditioned audiometry

As the child gets older, he can be conditioned to perform a specific task in response to the input of sound.

Puretone audiometry

This is the main method of testing but cannot be done until the child will tolerate wearing headphones and can be relied upon to respond accurately to puretone sounds.

OBJECTIVE AUDIOMETRY

Brainstem evoked response audiometry

This is the most reliable form of objective audiometry and can be performed at any age. Disadvantages are that it takes a considerable time, it is not frequency specific, and the child will have to be lying quietly or else sedated for it to be performed satisfactorily. In some multiply-handicapped children it may have to be done under general anesthetic.

Otoacoustic emissions

This is a quick, efficient and very simple form of objective audiometry that is increasingly being suggested as the most useful test for screening children. Its disadvantage is that it does not distinguish between conductive deafness and sensorineural deafness and that any children who fail the otoacoustic emission test usually have to then progress to brainstem evoked response audiometry.

Impedance audiometry or tympanometry

This is a simple test that measures the compliance of the eardrum and the pressure of the air in the middle ear. It is ideally suited for identifying secretory otitis media patients and is useful in screening outpatients who have failed their routine school audiometric testing.

TREATMENT OF DEAFNESS

Treatment of conductive deafness has been discussed elsewhere in this chapter. There is no medical treatment for sensorineural deafness and treatment is based on prophylaxis. Genetic counseling and preventive measures such as immunization are important to avoid some causes of sensorineural hearing loss. As neonatology advances and hypoxia becomes less common, the incidence of deafness amongst ex-premature infants will be reduced. Sensorineural hearing loss is not normally progressive but in some congenital conditions it is, and so careful monitoring of the child's hearing is vital once the diagnosis has been made.

The mainstay of treatment remains amplification by some form of hearing aid. A large range of hearing aids is now available for children with sensorineural hearing loss and it is extremely important that the degree of handicap and the shape of the audiogram is known before the hearing aid is prescribed. Nowadays the hearing aid can be customized to the child's actual specific hearing loss.

THE PHONIC EAR

Teaching the deaf has been revolutionized by the advent of the phonic ear. This is a radio-aid type of hearing device where the mother or the teacher wears a microphone and a transmitter and the child wears the radio receiver. This means the child can sit anywhere in the class and be in direct radio contact with the teacher and hence the degree of amplification can be greatly enhanced. Many children with quite severe hearing handicap can therefore now be educated in their own local school rather than having to go to specific schools for the hearing impaired.

COCHLEAR IMPLANTS

This is the latest and most powerful form of hearing aid in which a small fenestration is made surgically in the basal turn of the cochlea and 22 electrodes on a very delicate wire are inserted into the cochlea itself. At present, these devices are extremely expensive and require considerable expertise and a huge amount of time for each individual electrode to be specifically tuned to the child's needs. This can only be done in highly specialized centers and children requiring these devices at present are only those who are deriving nothing whatsoever from the standardized hearing aids systems described above. The device is particularly of use in children who have become deaf after having learnt speech, for example those who have had meningitis with severe acquired hearing loss.

THE NOSE AND SINUSES

THE NOSE

The nose functions as an air conditioner for the lower respiratory tract. It achieves this by cleaning, warming and humidifying the inspired air. The turbinates (Fig. 27.1) project from the lateral wall, increasing the surface area and causing turbulence. This allows heat and fluid exchange and causes any particles to be deposited on the lining of the nose in the sticky mucus which then passes posteriorly and is swallowed. The function of the paranasal sinuses is unknown.

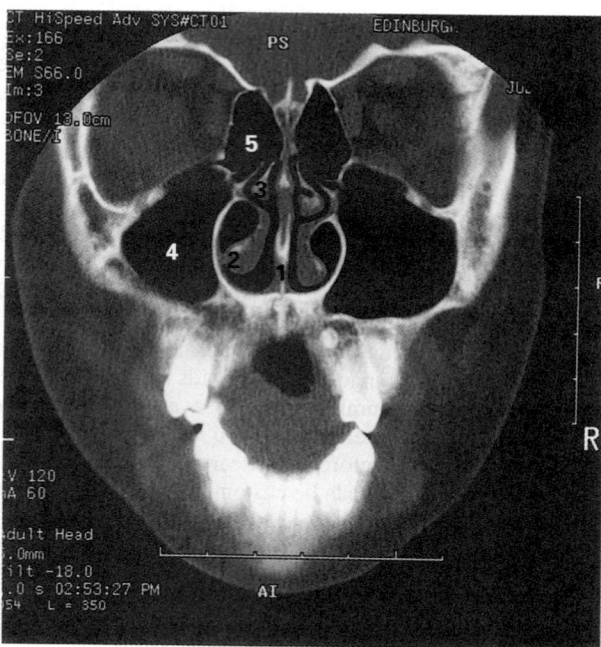

Fig. 27.1   Normal coronal CT scan of an 11-year-old boy showing: (1) nasal septum; (2) inferior turbinates; (3) middle turbinates; (4) maxillary sinuses; (5) ethmoid sinuses.

FOREIGN BODIES

These present as foul-smelling and sometimes bloodstained unilateral nasal discharge. They occur most often in children between the ages of 2 and 4 years, and are usually bits of foam rubber or toys which they have inserted themselves. It is rare for them to cause lower respiratory tract infections and the treatment is removal of the foreign body.

FRACTURE OF THE NOSE

The nose is the commonest bone in the body to be broken. In children nasal fractures are less common than in adults as the nasal bones are smaller and the tissues more pliant.

Nasal fractures result from direct trauma. Initially, there is swelling over the bridge of the nose and around the eyes which takes 5–7 days to subside. It is then possible to see whether the nasal bones are deviated, when manipulation under general anesthetic to straighten them is usually required. Manipulation must be carried out within 21 days of the injury otherwise the bones will become fixed.

Hematoma of the septum presents as severe blockage of the nose after an injury. This inevitably becomes infected and results in septal abscess and destruction of cartilage and requires surgical drainage and a broad spectrum antibiotic for 10 days.

EPISTAXIS

This is very common at any age. The bleeding can be spontaneous or secondary to mild trauma and usually arises in Little's area, in the anterior part of the nasal septum. Epistaxis can occur in patients with bleeding disorders (e.g. hemophilia or thrombocytopenia) but is rarely the presenting feature of these conditions.

After identifying the source of bleeding, local anesthetic (four parts 4% topical lignocaine to one part of 1 in 1000 adrenaline) is applied using cotton wool.

The area is then cauterized using a silver nitrate stick. In severe cases not responding to cautery, admission with nasal packing and intravenous fluid replacement may be required.

RHINITIS

This is extremely common and is characterized by swelling and inflammation of the nasal lining, often accompanied by clear or purulent rhinorrhea.

Viral rhinitis (the common cold or coryza)

This occurs very commonly with a pyrexial illness, runny nose, throat discomfort, sneezing and occasional earache. Treatment is symptomatic – analgesics and antipyretics as required. There is no proven place for decongestants in this condition. Viruses which have been identified as causing the common cold include rhinovirus, reovirus and adenovirus.

Viral rhinitis may be the precursor of laryngotracheobronchitis or pneumonia. A simple cold will normally last for 7–10 days and the child will not be unwell.

Bacterial rhinitis

This usually presents as purulent discharge following acute rhinitis. Antibiotics are rarely required unless the nasal blockage becomes worse or systemic symptoms such as fever and headaches occur when adenoiditis or sinusitis should be suspected. In some children there is a constant low grade bacterial rhinitis variable in severity, where no definitive underlying cause can be found. This can be associated with poor diet, damp housing and parental smoking. The underlying problem is thought to be lowered local nasal immunity. Most children with this condition will improve spontaneously from about the age of 8 years onwards. Immotile cilia syndrome is a rare cause and will often be associated with lower respiratory tract disease.

Allergic rhinitis

This usually occurs in children over 5 years old. It presents as sneezing, associated with clear rhinorrhea, nasal blockage and often conjunctivitis and sore throat. Seasonal rhinitis usually occurs in the summer and is caused by allergy to pollens. Perennial rhinitis can occur at any time of the year and can be associated with exposure to extrinsic allergens such as animals, e.g. cats or dogs or housedust mite.

The diagnosis is made from the history. On examination, the nasal lining will be slightly pale and swollen. Confirmation of the allergic basis can be made by carrying out skin testing or sending serum IgE assay.

Treatment is, if possible, by removal of the allergen but if this is not possible (e.g. seasonal rhinitis), a nonsedating antihistamine such as loratidine, supplemented by occasional use of a nasal steroid spray such as beclomethasone may be helpful. Allergy to housedust mite and housedust is increasingly recognized as a cause of rhinitis and allergic asthma. Treatment consists of cutting down the allergen in the bedroom by use of sprays or antiallergic sheeting. Nonsedating antihistamines and sometimes a short course of steroid sprays are also useful in combating this condition.

Nonallergic rhinitis (vasomotor rhinitis)

This presents as nasal blockage and catarrh and is differentiated from allergic rhinitis by negative allergy testing. Treatment is by antihistamine and decongestant combinations and occasionally by steroid sprays for 2 months. Where there is no response to medical treatment, surgical diathermy reduction of the inferior turbinate can be carried out.

NASAL SEPTAL DEVIATION

This can be traumatic but is more commonly developmental. Slight deviation is common and causes no symptoms, but more severe deviation will cause nasal obstruction, sometimes on both sides, occasionally with external nasal deformity. There may be associated allergic or vasomotor rhinitis. Surgery is only indicated for significant nasal blockage and is usually performed only in older children as surgery in young children can cause deformity which increases with age.

DISEASES OF THE PARANASAL SINUSES

The paranasal sinuses (maxillary, ethmoid, frontal and sphenoid; Fig. 27.1) are all derived from the nasal cavity and are lined by respiratory epithelium. The maxillary sinuses are small at birth and do not attain significant size until 4 or 5 years of age. The ethmoid sinuses are well developed at birth, but the frontal sinuses do not develop until 9 or 10 years old. The sphenoid sinuses rarely cause symptoms in childhood.

There is slight inflammation of the sinus mucosa in all forms of rhinitis and when the ostium to the sinus gets blocked, secretions are retained and purulent sinusitis develops. Treatment with antibiotics and local decongestants opens up the ostium and allows the sinuses to drain.

MAXILLARY SINUSITIS

This is rare under the age of 6 and it usually follows influenza or parainfluenza. The nose becomes very congested, there is copious purulent catarrh and there may be associated headache and fever. The commonest organisms found are pneumococcus and *Haemophilus influenzae*. Diagnosis is on suspicion and the finding of purulent catarrh in the nose and throat. Treatment is by ephedrine nosedrops, combined with a broad spectrum antibiotic such as amoxicillin or erythromycin for 1 week. X-rays are indicated when there is no response to the appropriate antibiotics, at which time surgical drainage may occasionally be required.

ETHMOIDITIS

This is a potentially serious condition which occurs in children from 3 years upwards. It usually follows an upper respiratory tract infection. The symptoms are of frontal headache and pain around the eye with fever and slight nasal blockage. Examination shows orbital cellulitis with swelling and tenderness and marked inflammation. If there is abscess formation it is usually periosteal and causes lateral displacement of the globe. The clinical diagnosis is now confirmed by a CT scan. Urgent treatment with parenteral broad spectrum antibiotic is required with surgical drainage if there is abscess formation (Arjmand et al 1993). If untreated, blindness or intracranial extension can occur.

FRONTAL SINUSITIS

This is less common than ethmoiditis and presents in children over 10. Like ethmoiditis, it is potentially serious with a risk of spread to involve the orbit or intracranial structures. It usually occurs after a cold or flu and causes severe frontal headache associated with inflammation and tenderness over the frontal sinus. Nasal symptoms are often minimal. Diagnosis and treatment similar to that for ethmoiditis. Spread can are occur inferiorly to involve the eye.

NASAL POLYPS

These present as unilateral or bilateral nasal blockage. Examination of the nose will show a pale, fleshy usually mobile structure. Most common is a unilateral *antrochoanal polyp* arising from the maxillary antra. These grow into the nose and down into the nasopharynx often causing total obstruction of one side with purulent catarrh. They are benign and treatment is removal.

Ethmoidal polyps are less common and cause nasal blockage and catarrh. Ethmoidal polyps occur in children with cystic fibrosis, when the histology is different from the usual 'allergic type'. Treatment is removal under local anesthetic.

CHOANAL ATRESIA

This rare anomaly is due to failure of breakdown of the nasobuccal membrane which normally occurs at 6 weeks fetal development. The incidence is 1 in 8000 and unilateral atresia is commoner than bilateral. 50% of cases are associated with the CHARGE syndrome – choanal atresia with ear, eye, heart and genital defects.

Bilateral choanal atresia is a neonatal emergency. The nose breathing neonate may gasp and make significant respiratory efforts but becomes hypoxic and requires airway support. Some cases may mouth breathe, but then have difficulty when feeding. The diagnosis is by suspicion and by inability to pass a catheter along the nose. The treatment consists of establishment of an airway, sometimes orotracheal, sometimes oral. A CT scan determines the extent of the atresia and defines whether it is bony or membranous. Corrective endoscopic surgery is carried out as soon as is practicable.

DISEASES OF THE NASOPHARYNX

ADENOIDS (NASOPHARYNGEAL TONSIL)

These are part of the Waldeyer's ring of lymphoid tissue which protects the upper airway. Adenoids are normally small at birth but enlarge from 18 months and regress normally at 8–9 years.

Adenoid hypertrophy

Since all children have adenoids, obstruction is a result of either a relatively small nasopharynx or large adenoids. Persistent enlargement causes snoring and often results in children having

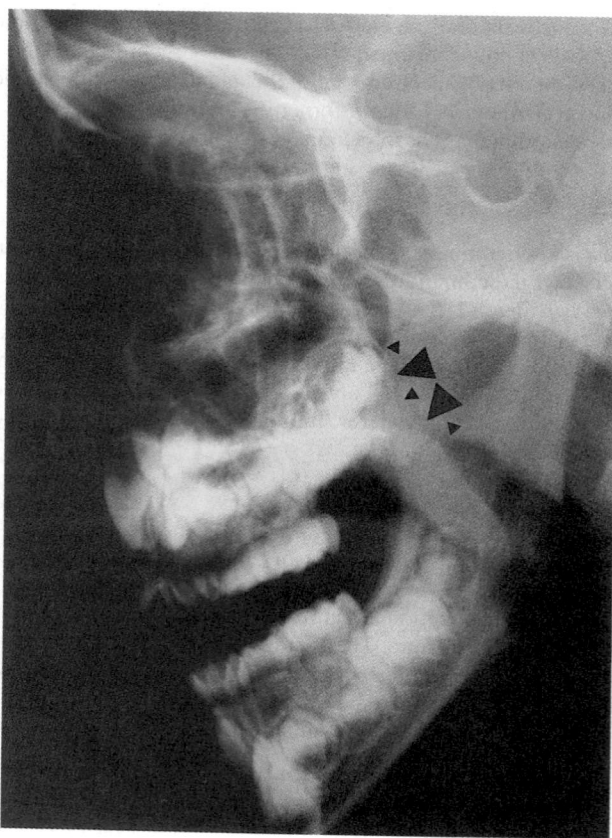

Fig. 27.2   Lateral soft tissue X-ray of a 4-year-old boy showing enlarged adenoids occluding the postnasal airway (arrowed).

upper respiratory tract infections which last for 3–4 weeks instead of for 7–10 days. Such children usually mouth breathe and have hyponasal speech. There is an association between enlarged or infected adenoids and middle ear disease.

Adenoid hypertrophy is suspected with the above history and on the finding of a patent anterior nasal airway. Confirmation of adenoid size can be carried out by a lateral soft tissue X-ray of the neck (Fig. 27.2). In mild or intermittent cases, treatment is reassurance that the adenoids will go away. Surgery should be reserved for more persistent problems.

Adenoiditis

Adenoiditis occurs with viral infections and exacerbates nasal blockage. It can be quite severe in a small child with fever and purulent nasal discharge. A broad spectrum antibiotic for 5 days is indicated in severe cases.

Adenoidectomy

Removal of the adenoids is indicated for:

1. airway obstruction in a small child (see airway obstruction, tonsillitis)
2. severe persistent nasal obstruction
3. otitis media.

Primary or secondary hemorrhage occurs in about 1 case in 200.

ANGIOFIBROMA

This is a benign tumor of the back of the nose and nasopharynx which presents in males in their early teens. Its symptoms are of nasal blockage with epistaxis. If expansion is rapid, cranial nerve compression can occur. The diagnosis is confirmed by endoscopy and a CT scan. Treatment is by surgery initially, radiotherapy being reserved for intracranial extension.

PHARYNGITIS

This is very common and usually of viral origin. It is a common presenting symptom of many upper respiratory tract infections, including the common cold, and may also precede the exanthemata of rubella or measles. There is generalized inflammation of the pharynx and often rhinitis. Treatment is supportive with antipyretics and analgesics as necessary.

TONSILS

The palatine tonsils, like the adenoids, are part of the body's defensive mechanism and serve to protect the upper airway from infection. Their removal, however, causes no subsequent immunological problems, nor is it associated with any deleterious long-term effect.

Acute tonsillitis

This is commonest between the ages of 3 and 8, but can occur at any age. 50% of cases are viral and 50% are bacterial with the β-hemolytic streptococcus commonest, although *Staph. aureus*, pneumococcus and *Haemophilus influenzae* are also implicated.

The onset is abrupt, with pain in the throat, associated shivering and a pyrexia up to 39°C. The pain may be severe and radiate to the ears. Swallowing is acutely sore and solid food is refused, although fluids may be accepted. The disease progresses over 48 hours, even with antibiotic therapy, and the swelling of the pillars and the tonsils may give dysphagia for fluids and even for saliva which may dribble from the mouth. Speech may become thick and muffled and there is often painful enlargement of cervical glands.

On examination, the mucosa of the pillars and soft palate are congested and as the disease progresses the tongue becomes coated and the breath become offensive. The tonsils are swollen and inflamed, with a purulent exudate. In severe cases, edema of the palate and the uvula may make the voice muffled and thick. Sometimes in streptococcal infections a scarlatiniform rash appears over the body.

Differential diagnosis

1. *Infectious mononucleosis.* This occurs in older children often accompanied by marked lymphadenopathy in the neck and other areas. The child is miserable with throat discomfort due to generalized congestion of the throat and swelling of the tonsils. Serological confirmation can resolve doubt and treatment is supportive with analgesia and fluids.
2. *Viral pharyngitis.* In this condition, the child is less ill and has other symptoms, e.g. blocked-up nose.
3. *Herpangina.* This self limiting condition due to Coxsackie virus has papular, vesicular and ulcerative lesions on the anterior pillars, the palate and the tonsils.

4. *Moniliasis*. White patches are present on the tongue and on the tonsils and pharynx. It is usually associated with immunodeficiency but can occur after antibiotic therapy.

Treatment

In mild tonsillitis, analgesia and adequate fluid intake is all that is required but in more severe cases penicillin V for 7–10 days is usually successful. Erythromycin may be used where there is penicillin sensitivity. Amoxicillin or co-amoxiclav is less suitable, and if given to a child with mononucleosis will result in an extensive skin rash. Parenteral penicillin may be required in persistent cases. Paracetamol is usually sufficient analgesia.

Complications of tonsillitis

1. *Peritonsillitis*. Inflammation spreads outwith the tonsillar area and the child develops increasing pain and fever, often with significant swelling of the soft palate. Parenteral penicillin for 3–4 days can be changed to oral medication as the fever and pain subside.

2. *Peritonsillar abscess (quinsy)*. When peritonsillitis localizes, an abscess can form. Although this condition is less common in children, it still presents as a serious and potentially lethal complication. It can occur during or just after an acute attack of tonsillitis presenting with increasing pain and swelling, usually on one side of the throat, with marked dysphagia and often otalgia. The child will have difficulty in opening his mouth. Examination is difficult but will show the affected tonsil to be very red, covered in pus and pushed medially. In addition, there will be gross swelling and redness of the palate and marked cervical lymphadenopathy on the ipsilateral side. If untreated, the abscess can spread to give rise to a parapharyngeal abscess with the risk of spread to the base of the skull or even into the superior mediastinum. The treatment is drainage under general anesthetic and can be a hazardous procedure. If it is not certain that pus is present, intravenous penicillin or erythromycin is given with fluids and analgesics.

3. *Airway obstruction*. This usually occurs in children aged 2–3 as a result of chronic hypertrophy of the adenoids and tonsils. The child breathes noisily at night and often during the day. Occasionally the parents will volunteer that the child stops breathing for short periods during the night and this can cause them some understandable alarm. At other times more direct questioning is required to elicit this symptom. If untreated, this relatively common complication of tonsillitis can lead to chronic hypoxia, pulmonary hypertension and, in severe cases, cor pulmonale. Where there is any suggestion of airway obstruction, the child should undergo a sleep study with monitoring of the oxygen saturation. If there are episodes of desaturation, indicative of sleep apnea, and there is no other cause for the airway obstruction, adenotonsillectomy usually cures the condition (Stradling et al 1990). Such children should be admitted to the high dependency unit on the night of surgery and their breathing pattern should be monitored. In some more severe cases the respiratory drive is depressed and they may need oxygen until the respiratory drive returns to normal.

5. *Rheumatic fever*. This is very rarely seen now as a complication of tonsillitis.

Indications for tonsillectomy

The following are indications for tonsillectomy (enlargement of the tonsils on their own is not an indication for their removal):

1. Airway obstruction is an absolute indication in small children with persistent noisy breathing and suspected or proven sleep apnea. The adenoids will also be removed.

2. Suspicion of other pathology, e.g. lymphoma, is also an absolute indication. There is usually a change in the architecture of the tonsil which would suggest lymphoma.

3. Recurrent acute tonsillitis. By this is meant six or seven attacks of definite tonsillitis in 1 year. Five attacks per year for 2 years or three to four attacks per year for 3 or more years are also indications for tonsillectomy.

4. Two or more attacks of peritonsillar abscess (Wolf et al 1995).

Complications of tonsillectomy

A primary hemorrhage occurs within the first 24 hours in 0.5–1.0% of children. Usually this is in the first 6 hours after surgery and the child will start coughing up blood or, if unrecognized, may vomit a variable quantity of blood. After fluid replacement the child is returned to the operating room where the bleeding vessels are identified and controlled by diathermy or ligature. A secondary hemorrhage occurs after 7–10 days. Often the child's throat will have started to become sore again and he then becomes aware of blood coming into his mouth. These children should be admitted, crossmatched and intravenous access obtained. A broad spectrum antibiotic such as amoxicillin is administered and local treatment consisting of hydrogen peroxide gargles and, occasionally, local adrenaline swabs can be carried out. If the bleeding persists, return to theater for ligature of the vessels or in rare cases packing of the tonsillar fossa.

DISORDERS OF PHONATION

DYSPHONIA

Dysphonia, or difficulty in producing sound, is usually associated with laryngeal disease (hoarseness). Some children have weakness or roughness of their voice in the course of an upper respiratory tract infection, this being a manifestation of laryngitis. Following recovery the voice usually returns to normal and no further investigation is required. Persistent hoarseness should be investigated and this can only be done by visualization of the larynx with a fiberoptic endoscope passed along the nose, into the nasopharynx. Where this is not possible, a direct laryngoscopy is indicated to define the pathology.

The causes of hoarseness in children are as follows:

1. *Vocal nodules*. These occur at the junction between the anterior third and posterior two-thirds of the vocal cords. They are usually secondary to voice abuse and in loud and noisy children are known as 'screamers' node. Small nodules can improve with speech therapy or if the nodules grow, surgery involving microscopic dissection is indicated. Histology shows hypertrophic squamous epithelium with underlying edema of the Reinke's space.

2. *Polyps of the larynx*. These occur spontaneously or following intubation and cause variable hoarseness. They are removed under general anesthetic.

3. *Laryngeal papillomas*. These are a rare cause of hoarseness associated with maternal genital warts (papilloma virus). They present as persistent hoarseness, sometimes with aphonia and occasionally airway obstruction. Treatment is by removal and multiple operations may be required. They do not become malignant but can spread into trachea and in rare cases, into bronchus.

4. *Unilateral vocal cord paralysis*. This can follow surgical or nonsurgical trauma to the neck, or occur following viral infections including mononucleosis. The voice may be breathy if the cord is abducted or well maintained if the cord is medialized. The diagnosis is usually made on fiberoptic endoscopy, and treatment consists of speech therapy.

APHONIA

Complete loss of voice can occasionally occur with laryngeal pathology, e.g. papillomas, and in most cases the larynx should be visualized. Complete aphonia in an otherwise healthy child should be viewed with suspicion. Functional or 'hysterical' aphonia occurs after emotional or physical trauma, e.g. tonsillectomy. It usually affects older children and in most cases is self-correcting. Occasionally a laryngoscopy may have to be carried out to establish the diagnosis, but usually explanation of the problem together with counseling will suffice.

REFERENCES

Arjmand E M, Lusk R P, Muntz H R 1993 Acute sinusitis, children and the eye. Otolaryngology – Head and Neck Surgery 109: 886–894

Maw A R, Parker A J, Lance G N, Dilkes M G 1992 The effects of parental smoking on outcome after treatment for glue ear in children. Clinics in Otolaryngology 17: 411–414

Strading J R, Thomas G, Warley A R H, Williams P, Freeland A 1990 Effect of adeno-tonsillectomy, on nocturnal hyponaemia, sleep disturbance and symptoms in snoring children. Lancet 335: 249–253

Wolf M, Euen-Chen I, Talmi Y P, Kronenberg J 1995 Tonsillectomy following per-tonsillar abscess. International Journal of Paediatric Otolaryngology 31: 43–46

28 Allergic disorders

T. J. David

Definitions and explanation of terms   **1689**
Timing of the allergic response   **1689**
Types of allergens   **1689**
Pollens   1689
Fungal (mold) spores   1690
House dust   1690
Insects   1691
Plants   1691
Foods   1691
Diagnosis of allergy – history   **1691**
Diagnostic testing for allergy   **1692**
Scratch, prick and intradermal skin tests   1693
Measurement of circulating IgE antibody   1693
Provocation challenge tests   1694
Allergic aspects of asthma   **1694**
Allergic aspects of atopic eczema   **1695**
Allergic aspects of urticaria   **1697**

Idiopathic urticaria   1697
Contact urticaria   1697
Food-provoked exercise-induced anaphylaxis   1697
Hay fever   **1697**
Perennial rhinitis   **1698**
Allergic conjunctivitis   **1698**
Behavior problems   **1698**
Food intolerance   **1698**
Cow's milk protein intolerance   1699
Egg intolerance   1700
Soya intolerance   1701
Intolerance to food additives   1701
Anaphylaxis   **1701**
Drug allergy   **1702**
Hyposensitization   **1702**
Prevention of atopic disease   **1703**
References   1704

DEFINITIONS AND EXPLANATION OF TERMS

The widespread misuse of the word allergy causes confusion. It is essential to have a definition or explanation of terms.

ALLERGY

Allergy is a reproducible adverse reaction to an extrinsic substance mediated by an immunological response, irrespective of the precise mechanism. The substance provoking the reaction may have been ingested, injected, inhaled or merely have come into contact with the skin or mucous membranes. The terms allergy and hypersensitivity have the same meaning and are interchangeable.

ATOPY

There is no good definition of atopy. The term was introduced to describe the 'asthma and hay fever group' of diseases. Subsequently atopy has been redefined as an hereditary predisposition to the production of IgE antibody, an unsatisfactory oversimplification. The atopic diseases comprise asthma, atopic eczema, allergic rhinitis, allergic conjunctivitis and some cases of urticaria.

FOOD INTOLERANCE

Food intolerance is a reproducible adverse reaction to a specific food or food ingredient, and it is not psychologically based. Food intolerance occurs even when the subject cannot identify the type of food which has been given. This definition does not take into account dosage. Clearly any food in vast excess will cause a reproducible adverse reaction. Such events are not generally covered by the term food intolerance.

TIMING OF THE ALLERGIC RESPONSE

When the airways, skin or conjunctivae are challenged by a single dose of allergen, a reaction can be classified as immediate, late, dual (that is both immediate and late), or delayed. The timing of these responses has been used to formulate hypotheses as to their immunopathogenesis (e.g. the Gell and Coombs types I to IV classification). However, these classifications mainly serve a didactic purpose, and may not relate to inflammation in disease. A single provocation with a large dose in the laboratory may differ greatly from the real life continuous or repeated exposure to smaller doses of allergens. In a study of patients with asthma who experienced only a late reaction after inhalation of low doses of allergen, the inhalation of a higher allergen dose resulted in a dual reaction (Ihre et al 1988). Most allergic reactions are not confined to a single Gell and Coombs type and usually involve a combination of mechanisms far more complex than such categorizations imply. A common error is to assume the presence of one type of reaction based on the timing of events. Thus immediate reactions (e.g. anaphylaxis) are often wrongly equated with a type I reaction. Another example is that most late bronchial reactions after allergen provocation are not type III reactions, but inflammatory consequences of a type I reaction. The pathogenesis and mechanisms of allergic disorders are reviewed elsewhere (Mygind 1986, Chapel & Haeney 1988, Holgate & Church 1993, Middleton et al 1993).

TYPES OF ALLERGENS

POLLENS

Grass pollen

There are hundreds of species of grass, but a relatively small number account for most cases of pollen allergy. These are timothy grass, red top grass, blue grass, orchard grass, sweet vernal grass, meadow grass, Bermuda grass, rye grass and cocksfoot. With the exception of Bermuda grass, skin prick testing demonstrates extensive cross-reactivity between these grass species (Middleton et al 1993). Pollen grains are only released during the day. Pollen counts are highest in the morning and early afternoon, and on hot, dry days. Wind can transport pollen many miles, and in cities the pollen count can remain high well into the evening. The timing of the peak pollen counts depends on the geographical location, the type of grass, and the weather conditions. In temperate regions in the northern hemisphere, a peak from mid-May to mid-July is usual.

Weed pollen

While grass pollens are the major trigger of allergic rhinitis and conjunctivitis in the UK, in North America the major cause are pollens of the various species of ragweed. Other weeds of importance in other places are mugwort, sagebrush, cocklebur, English plantain, Lamb's quarter, goosefoot, Russian thistle and burning bush. Peak levels of weed pollen occur in late summer and the autumn.

Tree pollen

Many deciduous trees produce pollen, usually in the spring. Birch pollen in Scandinavia, Japanese cedar pollen in Japan, and mountain cedar pollen in North America are all important causes of allergic rhinitis and conjunctivitis.

FUNGAL (MOLD) SPORES

Molds require a high relative humidity for growth, and reproduce by the production of spores. Yeasts are unicellular molds. Molds are ubiquitous. Exposure to molds is continuous rather than seasonal, and, as with house dust mites and in contrast to grass pollen, the extent to which a patient's symptoms can be attributed to mold allergy is often unclear. Occasionally the history may suggest mold allergy, e.g. symptoms occurring after being in a barn or raking leaves.

Outdoor molds

Cladosporium, Alternaria, Fusarium, smuts and rusts (and to a lesser degree *Aspergillus, Penicillium, Mucor, Didymella* and *Sporobolomyces*) are the most important outdoor causes of mold allergy. The major sources of exposure are rotting leaves, straw, hay, grass, grain and flour. Wet weather favors mold growth. Some spores (e.g. some species of *Cladosporium* and *Alternaria*) are released in sunny and windy conditions, but others (e.g. *Fusarium, Phoma, Basidiomycetes*) are released by processes that require free water, and high levels of these particles occur with rainfall, dew, fog and the relatively damp conditions which prevail during darkness. Light intensity and duration can also affect spore production in certain molds, and in *Cladosporium* species, for example, a dark interval appears necessary to ensure the formation of a single spore crop in each 24-h period. Thus circadian trends in humidity, temperature, air speed and light interact to produce a diurnal and nocturnal pattern of spore distribution. In addition, the type of vegetation affects the local air spora. Temperate grasslands and grain-growing areas are particular sources of the spores of *Alternaria* and *Cladosporium*. Forests abound with wood-rotting molds, and large orchards can raise levels of airborne yeasts.

Indoor molds

Aspergillus and *Penicillium* are the two molds most commonly cultured from houses, especially from basements, inaccessible crannies and bedding. These molds are often called storage fungi because they are common causes of rot in stored grain, fruits and vegetables. In contrast to most molds which require a relatively high moisture content (22–25%) in their substrate, *Aspergillus* can thrive on substrates with a lower moisture content (12–16%). *Penicillium* is the green mildew seen on articles stored in basements. Roquefort, Stilton and other blue cheeses owe their sharp aroma to veins of the bluish-green mold *Penicillium roquefortii* and Camembert and Brie are ripened from the outside by a coat of white *Penicillium camemberti* mold. The major sources of exposure to indoor molds are damp cellars, poorly ventilated bathrooms, wallpaper on cold walls, window frames (condensation), artificial humidifiers, damp textile materials, and stored food.

HOUSE DUST

House dust may contain a large number of antigens, including house dust mites, human and animal dander, fungi, algae, bacteria, food remnants and feathers (Middleton et al 1993). The composition of house dust varies from house to house, from region to region, and also changes with the season of the year.

House dust mites

The predominant house dust mite in Europe is *Dermatophagoides pteronyssinus*, but in the USA the dominant species is *Dermatophagoides farinae*. These mites feed from desquamated human skin scales, which are mainly shed in the bed and bedroom. The amount of skin shed by one person in a day provides enough food to supply thousands of mites for months, and the decisive factors which influence the number of mites are air humidity and temperature. The optimum conditions for mites are 70–80% relative humidity and an ambient temperature of 26°C. Mites cannot reproduce when the relative humidity falls below 60%, and cannot survive for more than a few days in a relative humidity of below 40% if the temperatures is above 25°C. The lack of mites at higher altitudes (e.g. alpine resorts) is due to the lower relative humidity. The mite antigen is predominantly found in mite fecal pellets which are of a similar size to pollen grains. It appears that the majority of house dust mite allergens are enzymes involved in digestion which become entrapped within the fecal pellet. Mites are found in bedding, mattresses, carpets, cuddly toys and upholstered furniture. They are also found in carpets and upholstered furniture in other parts of the house. Moisture from human skin causes particularly humid conditions in beds and bedding which creates favorable conditions for mite survival. The relationship between the season and mite density in houses is attributable to seasonal changes in the ambient indoor humidity. In temperate areas, the number of mites is lowest in the winter, when central heating dries the indoor air.

Storage mites

The most important species are *Glycophagus*, *Tyrophagus*, *Lepidoglyphus* and *Acarus*. They do not cross-react with the *Dermatophagoides* species. Storage mites are common in farm stores (e.g. stored hay), granaries, warehouses and places where food is stored. They are infrequent in houses unless the same room is used for cooking, eating and sleeping, as can happen with dwellings in the tropics.

Mammalian pets

The sources of allergens are dander (epidermal scales), hair, feathers, saliva and urine.

INSECTS

Stinging insects

The medically important Hymenoptera are bees, wasps, hornets, yellow jackets, fire ants and harvester ants (Middleton et al 1993). Hymenoptera venoms are complex mixtures of enzymes, peptides and other vasoactive substances. Thus reactions to insect stings can be immunological, pharmacological, or both.

Biting insects

Allergy to the salivary secretions of biting insects is common. Local immediate and delayed allergic reactions to bites from fleas (papular urticaria), mosquitoes, sandflies, deerflies and horseflies are common.

Inhalant allergens from insects

Inhalant allergies to moths, butterflies, bees and beetles have all been described in those exposed to them as a result of a hobby.

PLANTS

Plants are a cause of adverse reactions in the skin, but most reactions are not allergic. The major mechanisms of adverse reactions are allergic contact dermatitis (e.g. poison ivy, chrysanthemum, primula), irritant contact dermatitis (e.g. buttercup), pharmacological effects (e.g. stinging nettles), and phytophotodermatitis (e.g. giant hogweed).

FOODS

Foods as allergens are discussed in the section on food intolerance.

DIAGNOSIS OF ALLERGY – HISTORY

The lack of really useful laboratory tests for allergy (see below) means that there is no substitute for a careful history.

IMPORTANT QUESTIONS

The history should include questions about:

1. when symptoms occur
2. where symptoms occur
3. when or where the patient is free of symptoms
4. the presence of other allergic symptoms
5. family history of allergy or atopic disease.

OTHER CLUES FROM THE HISTORY

1. The symptoms are worse at night. Both asthma and eczema are often worse at night, but it is wrong to equate all nocturnal symptoms with house dust mite allergy, as there are other possible explanations. Circadian rhythms affecting airway caliber, bronchial reactivity (Sly & Landau 1986) and cortisol secretion account for some of the increase in symptoms at night in asthma. In eczema, heat, tiredness and low cortisol secretion may contribute to nocturnal symptoms. In theory a high concentration of house dust mite antigen found in some bedrooms could contribute to nocturnal symptoms in asthma, rhinitis or atopic eczema, but in one large study there was no association between worsening at night or on waking and the presence of house dust mite allergy (Murray et al 1983). Only improvement in the symptoms following the complete avoidance of house dust mites in the bedroom (very difficult to achieve – see below), and recurrence of symptoms on re-exposure, will prove the point. A study of the symptoms associated with house dust mite allergy showed that a history of symptoms being provoked during domestic activity that stirs up house dust (bedmaking, dusting, vacuuming, emptying a vacuum cleaner bag, sweeping, shaking out bedding) when house dust mite antigen becomes airborne, is probably the only reliable pointer to house dust mite allergy (Murray et al 1983).

2. The symptoms are worse at certain times of the year. The usual inference is that the symptoms are attributable to a seasonal allergen. Sometimes the history is convincing. For example, where sneezing and conjunctivitis occur each year in June and July on sunny days when the grass pollen count is high, it is highly probable that the symptoms are attributable to allergy to grass pollen. Often, the history is not so easy to interpret. For example, a worsening of asthma in August, September or October is often difficult to explain. Possibilities include allergy to inhaled molds, an increase in the number of house dust mites in the autumn, changes in the weather, or catching viral respiratory infections when returning to school after the summer holidays (Khot et al 1988, Storr & Lenney 1989).

3. The symptoms are worse in certain weather conditions. The reasons for attacks of asthma after a thunderstorm or heavy rainfall are not fully understood. Allergy to inhaled fungal spores, a fall in the barometric pressure, a sudden fall in air temperature, and release of allergenic starch granules from ruptured pollen grains are all possible explanations.

4. The symptoms improve when the patient is away from home (e.g. on holiday). Improvement in atopic eczema when the patient goes on holiday is frequently noted, but the reason is usually obscure. In one study (Turner et al 1991), there was a significant correlation between improvement in eczema and a more southerly holiday location; improvement was common in holidays taken in the Mediterranean or further south (63/92 – 69%), while holidays in northern Britain were more likely to be associated with deterioration (27/100 – 27%) than improvement (13/100 – 13%). The absence of pets or house dust mites may be the explanation in some cases, although the improvement which occurs on holidays (the disease often virtually disappears) is far greater than the modest improvement which can be seen after admission to hospital in the same patients. Exposure to sea water, sunlight or lack of stress are believed by some parents to be the explanation for such improvement, but there is no evidence to support these ideas. The improvement or complete disappearance of asthma at high altitude resorts, seen in some patients, is generally attributed to the absence of house dust mite and pet animal antigens.

5. *The presence or absence of a family history of atopic disease.* Patients with atopic disease often have a positive family history of atopic disease, though atopy is so common in the normal population (wheezing in 21%, eczema in 12% and hay fever in 4% of all children in the UK by the age of 5 years (Butler & Golding 1986)) that a positive family history is a rather nonspecific finding. In an apparently atopic child, the absence of a positive family history is more important, and should make the physician reconsider a diagnosis of atopic disease.

6. *Multiplicity of symptoms.* Allergic symptoms are usually multiple. It is important to inquire if the patient has other symptoms or signs that may be allergic in origin, in addition to the presenting complaint, and these features are: wheezing, sneezing, pruritus, urticaria, perioral erythema, eczema and conjunctivitis. Several symptoms may coexist. Unilateral symptoms, whether nasal, ocular or respiratory, suggest the presence of a nonallergic condition.

7. *Symptoms occurring after exposure to pets.* Several situations cause confusion:

a. The patient who is noted to have an immediate allergic reaction when stroking or being licked by, for example, a dog, but who is otherwise apparently able to live in the same house as the animal without obvious immediate allergic reactions; delayed reactions or enhanced bronchial reactivity may be overlooked.
b. The patient who apparently experiences an immediate allergic reaction to, for example, certain cats but not others; again, delayed reactions or enhanced bronchial reactivity may be overlooked.
c. The patient whose atopic disease predates the acquisition of a pet animal; the animal could still be an important trigger continuing to provoke the disease.
d. The patient who had a pet animal some years before the onset of symptoms; the animal could still be an important trigger.
e. The patient's symptoms did not improve when the pet was sent to live elsewhere for a few weeks; sufficient pet antigen to provoke disease may still be present in the household.

A major source of confusion is that parents equate allergy with immediate reactions, and are unaware that constant exposure to pet antigen in the home tends to cause chronic rather than acute symptoms. Many patients who are allergic to pets react to minute traces of the animal, for example a few hairs on someone's clothing, and this explains why the disease in question failed to improve after the pet was removed from the household. For therapeutic trials to be meaningful, extensive cleaning of carpets, upholstered furniture, clothing and bedding are necessary to remove the allergen.

8. *Food intolerance.* Food intolerance is generally associated with multiple symptoms, and it is rare for a single symptom (e.g. asthma, rhinitis, abdominal pain) to be caused by food intolerance. Parents commonly overvalue food intolerance as a cause of symptoms. In one study, double-blind food challenges provoked symptoms in only 27 of 81 (33%) of children whose parents had reported food intolerance (May & Bock 1978).

UNQUALIFIED REPORTS OF ALLERGY

It is unhelpful to write 'allergy' in a patient's notes without any description of the evidence for the diagnosis. Many untoward events are wrongly labeled as allergies. For example, there are several reasons why penicillin administration may be followed by an adverse event, but few justify a diagnosis of penicillin allergy. A rash during antibiotic therapy may be caused by an underlying infection, or by a coloring agent or preservative included in a liquid preparation of the antibiotic. Loose stools are likely to be due to an underlying viral infection or a disturbance of the gut flora, but it is common to find this described by parents as an allergy to the antibiotic. The incorrect and careless labeling of a child as having penicillin allergy may rob the patient of penicillin treatment for life. Common and similar examples are the patient said to be allergic to cow's milk, in whom inquiry reveals that this is based not on observation of the patient but on the fact that someone has placed the child on a cow's milk-free diet, or the patient said to be allergic to something solely on the basis of skin or blood tests.

SIMPLE CAUSE AND EFFECT

The interpretation of the observation that exposure to a single item (e.g. a cat) is followed within minutes by an obvious adverse event (e.g. sneezing and orbital edema) should be quite simple, but there are pitfalls. The history is more reliable if it is based on the parents' unprompted original observations. The parents' observations may be especially unreliable because:

1. There is a strong emotional underlay, e.g. strong attachment to a family pet, leading to underdiagnosis of allergy because the family do not want to part with the animal.
2. In the case of food intolerance, double-blind studies have repeatedly shown parental histories to be particularly unreliable (see below).
3. In the case of behavioral symptoms, there is a widespread but mistaken belief in the importance of adverse reactions to foods or food additives (David 1987).
4. A parent's report of alleged allergic reactions may have been fabricated (factitious illness).

In general, the quicker the onset of the allergic reaction, the more reliable is the history. A history of the same allergic symptoms after repeated exposure to an allergen is more reliable than a report of a single episode.

DIAGNOSTIC TESTING FOR ALLERGY

There is no ideal test which will predict with certainty whether avoidance of a specific allergen will improve or abolish symptoms in an individual patient. Some of the problems are due to difficulties intrinsic to the test, but some are inherent in the complex nature of atopic disease. Take, for example, a child with asthma who develops sneezing, conjunctivitis and angioedema of the orbit immediately after playing with a cat, and who has a positive skin prick test and positive RAST test to cat dander. Clearly it is logical that the child should avoid cats, but there is no guarantee that cat avoidance will help the patient's asthma. The reasons for the failure of allergen avoidance are discussed later, but can be summarized as:

1. the allergen was incompletely avoided

2. the allergen was only one of several factors provoking the patient's disease
3. the allergen was irrelevant to the patient's symptoms.

It is unrealistic to expect any clinical or laboratory test to cope with the first two of these problems. The best that can be hoped for is that a test will help establish the potential clinical relevance of a particular allergy. Regrettably, the currently available tests, described below, all suffer from serious limitations.

SCRATCH, PRICK AND INTRADERMAL SKIN TESTS

The principle of these skin tests is that the skin wheal and flare reaction to an allergen demonstrates the presence of mast-cell-fixed antibody. This is mainly IgE antibody, although in theory it could also be IgG_4 antibody. IgE is produced in plasma cells distributed primarily in lymphoid tissue in the respiratory and gastrointestinal tract, and is distributed in the circulation to all parts of the body, so that the sensitization is generalized and therefore can be demonstrated by skin testing. Age influences the reaction, and a child under 2 years of age produces much less reaction than an older child.

Short-acting antihistamines (H_1 receptor antagonists) must be discontinued at least 5 days prior to skin testing. However, astemizole and certain other nonsedating antihistamines are long acting, and suppression of the wheal and flare response has been noted as much as 5 months after discontinuation of astemizole. Because of the variability of cutaneous reactivity, it is necessary to include positive and negative controls whenever skin prick tests are performed. The negative control solution should consist of the diluent used to preserve the allergen extracts. The positive control solution usually consists of histamine, and is mainly used to detect suppression of reactivity, for example caused by H_1 antihistamine medication.

Scratch testing

A drop of allergen solution is placed on the skin which is then scratched so as to superficially penetrate the skin. The scratch test introduces an inconstant amount of allergen through the skin and is therefore poorly standardized and produces results which are too variable for routine clinical use (Lessof 1987, Bousquet & Michel 1993).

Prick testing

A drop of allergen solution is placed on the skin which is then pricked with a needle or lancet, and the result read after 15 min. The negative control should be negative, unless the patient has dermographism. The histamine control should be positive, unless the patient has recently received H_1 antihistamines, which would invalidate negative skin test results. The flare is ignored, and the diameter of the wheal is measured. Later reactions may occur, but their significance is unclear. Prick tests can also produce variable results, but the introduction of standardized precision needles for prick testing has made the method potentially more reproducible. Delegation of skin testing to untrained staff and the continued use of hypodermic needles lead to frequent errors and poor reproducibility.

The interpretation of skin prick tests is difficult. Skin test extracts vary in their potency and specificity. There is a lack of agreed definition about what constitutes a positive reaction (Lessof et al 1980). Most definitions of a positive reaction are based on the absolute diameter of the wheal, with arbitrary cutoff points for positivity at 1 mm, 2 mm or 3 mm. The problems with the interpretation of prick test results in an individual patient are:

1. Skin prick test reactivity may be present in subjects with no clinical evidence of allergy (Lessof 1987, Bousquet & Michel 1993).
2. Skin prick test reactivity may persist after clinical evidence of allergy has subsided (e.g. Ford & Taylor 1982).
3. Skin prick tests may be negative in some patients with allergies. For example, skin prick tests are negative in 13–17% of those with rhinitis provoked by pollen (Pepys 1975).
4. False negative results may occur in infants and toddlers. The whealing capacity of the skin is diminished in early infancy, and when wheals are produced they are smaller than in later life, so that the criteria for a positive wheal must be adjusted (Bousquet & Michel 1993). There are no age-related guidelines for what constitutes a positive reaction.
5. There is a poor correlation between the results of provocation tests and prick tests.
6. Skin prick tests for foods are especially unreliable (David 1993).

The results of skin tests cannot be taken alone, but need to account for the history and physical findings (Patterson 1985, Bousquet & Michel 1993). From a carefully taken history one might suspect a particular allergen, and the finding of a positive prick test would increase the likelihood that the allergen was causing symptoms. Few people, however, would be prepared to ignore a strong history of allergy in the face of a negative prick test, yet it is illogical to regard the prick test as significant when it confirms the history and to disregard it when it fails to do so. The contentious issues in clinical practice are whether a child with atopic disease will benefit from attempts to avoid household pets, house dust mites or certain foods, but skin prick tests are unreliable predictors of response to such measures.

Intradermal testing

Intradermal testing is painful, can cause fatal anaphylaxis, and is only performed for limited reasons and then only if a preliminary skin prick test is negative (Bernstein 1988). Intradermal tests are more sensitive than skin prick testing, and also produce more false positive reactions. As with skin prick testing, there is a lack of agreement as to what constitutes a positive reaction. The number of false positive reactions makes the interpretation of the results of intradermal testing even more difficult than skin prick testing.

Skin patch testing

Patch testing is used to identify causative allergens in suspected allergic contact dermatitis, and is discussed elsewhere (Wilkinson & Rycroft 1992).

MEASUREMENT OF CIRCULATING IgE ANTIBODY

In vitro tests for circulating allergen-specific IgE antibody (e.g. radioallergosorbent (RAST) tests) avoid possible confounding variables in skin testing, namely IgE affinity for mast cells, their tendency for degranulation, and skin reactivity to released mediators. Thus, in theory, the in vitro test should be more reliable than skin testing. However, the clinical interpretation of in vitro IgE antibody tests is subject to most of the same pitfalls as the interpretation of skin prick testing. Additional problems with IgE antibody tests are:

1. Cost.
2. The IgE antibody concentration in the plasma varies with allergen exposure. A few patients with allergic rhinitis are RAST negative before the pollen season, but become positive after the pollen season.
3. A very high level of total circulating IgE (e.g. in children with severe atopic eczema) may cause a false positive result.
4. A very high level of IgG antibody with the same allergen specificity as IgE antibody can cause a false negative result.
5. For each allergen, the test differs in the degree to which it is influenced by elevated total serum IgE.
6. In vitro IgE assays are slightly less sensitive than skin testing.

In vitro tests for IgE antibody are only preferable to skin testing where the patient has had a very severe reaction to the allergen in question (because of the small risk of anaphylaxis with skin testing), where the patient has widespread skin disease (e.g. atopic eczema), where the skin shows dermographism, or when H_1 antihistamines cannot be discontinued.

PROVOCATION CHALLENGE TESTS

With the exception of food challenges in patients with suspected food intolerance, provocation tests (bronchial, nasal, conjunctival) have little place in routine clinical practice but have been helpful in the study of the pathophysiology and pharmacology of atopic disease. The results suffer from the same major limitation as the results of skin or IgE antibody testing, which is that a positive result from an allergen challenge by no means proves that the allergen is contributing to the patient's disease.

Blinded oral food challenge

The test comprises the oral administration of a challenge substance, which is either the item under investigation or an indistinguishable inactive (placebo) substance. Neither the child, the parents nor the observers know the identity of the administered material at the time of the challenge. Food challenges are subject to a number of pitfalls:

1. There is a danger of producing anaphylactic shock, even if anaphylactic shock had not occurred on previous exposure to the food (Goldman et al 1963, David 1984).
2. Difficulties arise if a cooked food is used for testing and the patient is only sensitive to a raw food, or vice versa. Cooking reduces the sensitizing capacity of cow's milk, and intolerance to raw but not cooked egg, potato and fish are well described.
3. It is unclear what dosage of different foods is required to exclude food intolerance. The dosage used in studies employing encapsulated foods is inevitably limited. Larger quantities of food may cause an adverse reaction when smaller quantities do not. For example, Hill et al (1988) found that whereas 8–10 g of milk powder (corresponding to 60–70 ml of milk) was adequate to provoke a response in some patients with cow's milk protein intolerance, other patients (with late-onset symptoms) required up

to 10 times this volume of milk daily for more than 48 h before symptoms developed.

4. Failure to randomize the order of placebo with active substance or to employ a double-blind placebo-controlled methodology are errors common to many studies, especially those of food additives in chronic urticaria.
5. A food challenge performed during a quiescent phase of the disease may fail to provoke an adverse reaction. For example, in chronic urticaria intolerance to salicylates is confined to patients with active disease.
6. The regular administration of salicylates to patients with salicylate intolerance quickly leads to a state of tolerance to salicylate. It is possible, although unproven, that a similar phenomenon occurs with certain food additives. Thus a double-blind challenge performed while a patient is regularly consuming a foodstuff may fail to provoke an adverse reaction.
7. Where food intolerance exists in children with atopic dermatitis, it is common for the patient to be intolerant to several foods. The removal of only one offending item may fail to help the patient and reintroduction may not provoke deterioration.
8. In some situations, factors other than a food are necessary for positive challenges to occur. For example, in a subgroup of patients with exercise-induced anaphylaxis, symptoms only occur if exercise follows the ingestion of a particular food (Kidd et al 1983). Exercise or the food alone fail to provoke symptoms.

ALLERGIC ASPECTS OF ASTHMA

There is no doubt that exposure to various triggers can provoke or worsen asthma in certain patients. However, there is a lack of objective investigations to establish the qualitative importance of allergy. For example, it is impossible to state, for asthmatic children of any specific age, in what proportion exposure to an animal provokes an attack of asthma, or what proportion will benefit from removal of a household pet. The management of the allergic aspects of asthma is largely empirical. Some triggers are allergens, but others are not, so it is misleading to think of asthma solely as an allergic disease. Some triggers, in addition to causing airway smooth muscle contraction, also cause an increase in the nonspecific responsiveness of the airway smooth muscle. Nonallergic triggers are discussed in Chapter 12.

IMPORTANCE OF TRIGGERS

It is unknown whether the complete avoidance of all potential triggers, were this possible (which it plainly is not), would abolish asthma or merely cause improvement. The disappearance of asthma following the removal of household pets is a poorly documented but occasionally striking phenomenon. Observations of children with unusually severe asthma who are sent to alpine resorts, where the exposure to house dust mites and pets is greatly reduced or abolished, are that somewhere between one- and two-thirds become completely asymptomatic and can discontinue all therapy. Return home is followed by relapse in most patients. In the past it was believed that this improvement was due to separation from parents and 'family tension', but the current doctrine is that the benefit is due to the avoidance of inhaled allergens. A history may help identify intermittent triggers which provoke attacks, but may not identify allergens to which the patient is regularly exposed and which are responsible for maintaining the asthmatic state (e.g. house dust mites).

INVESTIGATIONS

Skin tests, RAST tests and provocation tests (see above) are unhelpful. A trial of specific allergen avoidance is the only logical approach.

ALLERGEN AVOIDANCE

It is impossible to avoid cold weather, exercise, laughing and crying. Viral infections, pollens and fungal spores are ubiquitous, and avoidance is impossible without unacceptable restrictions. The conventional half-hearted attempts to avoid house dust mites (daily mattress hoovering and bedroom dusting) usually fail to reduce the quantity of house dust mite antigen in the child's bedroom sufficiently to help the patient. The safety or clinical benefit of acaricides has not been established. Domestic air cleaning devices (mechanical filters, negative ion generators, electrostatic precipitators) fail to reduce the large reservoir of nonairborne household antigens and are unhelpful.

Since a large proportion of a child's life is spent in the bedroom, measures to reduce exposure to house dust mites must be focused on the bedroom, but it is unclear whether the implicit assumption that mites in other parts of the house are less important is true. Near complete avoidance of dust mites is theoretically possible in the bedroom but entails expense and an obsessional attention to detail:

1. Place the mattress and pillow in a plastic bag or vapor-permeable cover and seal.
2. Replace a divan bed base (which cannot be completely sealed in a cover) by a nonupholstered wooden or metal base.
3. Remove woolen blankets, eiderdowns, quilts and duvets, even if made of synthetic materials, and replace with cotton or acrylic blankets which are hot washed (at 130°F, 55°C) weekly.
4. If there is more than one bed in the bedroom, then the above precautions must be applied to all beds.
5. Remove floor carpet, and replace with flooring which can be wet mopped.
6. Remove upholstered furniture, teddy bears and similar furry creatures to another room.
7. Remove toys and clothing, other than items kept enclosed in a cupboard, to another room.
8. Remove all items on horizontal surfaces such as bedside tables, book shelves, window sills, tops of cupboards, so that these areas can be damp dusted daily.
9. Retain curtains, to be washed every 3 months. Do not replace with venetian blinds, which are more likely to accumulate dust.
10. Remove mobiles and lamp shades which cannot be wiped free of dust.

Measures for the rest of the house are lower priority. Ideally, the whole house is changed to minimize the sites in which mites can grow. This requires removal of all carpeting and replacement by polished flooring, removal of all upholstered furniture, and ensuring that all window blinds are washable (Platts-Mills et al 1995). In addition, humidity needs to be controlled by ventilation and measures to combat dampness, and extreme humidity by air conditioning. Acaricides such as tannic acid or benzyl benzoate only have short-lived effects (Woodfolk et al 1995) and are not substitutes for the measures described above.

Many parents and doctors would regard such measures as unacceptably restrictive, and such an extreme approach can only be justified in unusual cases where either there is a clear history that house dust mites play an important part or where conventional drug therapy has failed to control severe disease.

Avoidance of pets is possible but often unpopular or unacceptable to the family. Removal of the animal itself is insufficient, and if the level of pet antigen in the household is to be adequately reduced then also required are intensive carpet and furniture cleaning. Complete removal of cat antigen is especially difficult (if not impossible), and because of its adhesion to wall surfaces (Wood et al 1992), requires washing of the walls.

ROLE OF ANTIGEN AVOIDANCE IN THE MANAGEMENT OF ASTHMA

There are no objective data upon which to base clear recommendations, with the result that there are differences of opinion about the relevance of antigen avoidance. The cornerstone of the treatment of asthma is drug therapy, supplemented where possible or relevant by the avoidance of triggers. Even with the most enthusiastic approach to the identification and avoidance of triggers, it is rare for this alone to abolish symptoms. The major triggers which are at least potentially avoidable are house dust mites and pets. Since there is no clinical or laboratory test which can accurately identify those patients who will benefit from antigen avoidance, the only logical approach is to attempt a defined trial period of avoidance, including an assessment after an agreed period of time (e.g. 3 months) as to whether there has been any benefit.

ALLERGIC ASPECTS OF ATOPIC ECZEMA

We do not know what proportion of children with atopic eczema will benefit from antigen avoidance regimens. All advice in this area is empirical.

The management (see also Ch. 25) can be divided into first line approaches (e.g. use of emollients and topical steroids (David 1995), recognition and treatment of infection (David & Longson 1985, David & Cambridge 1986), use of sedating H_1 antihistamines at night), and if these are unsuccessful, possibly some form of antigen avoidance regimen.

The situations in which antigen avoidance should be considered are:

1. Severe disease. Exclusion diets are highly disruptive to family life, and are potentially nutritionally hazardous (David 1993), so it makes little sense to employ a diet when the condition is mild (under 10% of the skin surface area affected) and easily controlled with simple topical therapy. Such diets may be appropriate if 25% or more of the skin is affected.

2. History. A history of immediate urticarial or gastrointestinal reactions to foods is common. It is unproven whether the regular administration of a food which after a single exposure causes urticaria leads to the worsening of atopic eczema, but it seems reasonable to avoid foods for which there is a clear history of an immediate allergic reaction.

3. Multiple atopic disorders in infancy. The occurrence of more than one atopic disorder appears to increase the possibility of an important allergic element. This is especially true if atopic features such as eczema, asthma or rhinitis are accompanied by gastrointestinal symptoms such as persistent loose stools or vomiting.

4. Age. Elimination diets are simpler to administer and control in infancy and results are better at this age.

5. Severe eczema in exclusively breast-fed infants. In one study, in 6 of 37 breast-fed infants eczema improved when the mother avoided cow's milk protein and egg and relapsed when these were reintroduced (Cant et al 1986). It was impossible to predict which baby would respond to maternal dietary exclusion, and it is reasonable to try maternal avoidance of cow's milk and egg in an infant with eczema who is being exclusively breast-fed. Other foods can provoke eczema in this way, but their detection depends on parental suspicion followed by avoidance and challenge.

ANTIGEN AVOIDANCE IN ATOPIC ECZEMA

Diets

The important principles underlying any elimination diet are:

1. The diet should in the first instance be tried for a defined period of time (e.g. 6 weeks in patients with eczema) and not just imposed indefinitely.

2. At the end of this period the patient should be reassessed to see if the diet has been helpful. If it has not, then the diet should be discontinued. If the diet has helped, and the parents and doctor feel that the therapeutic benefit outweighs the inconvenience of the diet, then the items omitted should be reintroduced one by one (in eczema at the rate of about one new food every 5–7 days).

3. The help of a dietitian is important, to ensure that specific food items have been properly excluded from the diet, and to ensure the nutritional adequacy of the diet (David et al 1984, Devlin et al 1989, Mabin et al 1995a).

There are four varieties of dietary exclusion. All are empirical, and the details of which items are excluded may vary. Infants and toddlers are far more likely to benefit than teenagers.

Half-hearted attempts to 'have a go'

The very small quantity of food which can provoke an adverse reaction means that the 'try cutting down his milk' type of tinkering with the diet is most unlikely to succeed. The advantage of a carefully conducted diet is that even if it fails, at least the parents will be satisfied in the knowledge that it was tried properly.

Complete avoidance of known triggers

A trial of rigorous avoidance of known or suspected triggers is a logical first step. It is common to see a child with a clear history of intolerance to a food, but where the food is being incompletely avoided. An example would be a child with a history suggesting cow's milk protein intolerance who is avoiding cow's milk but consuming products which contain whey or casein, or who is receiving goat's milk.

Cow's milk and egg avoidance

The main place for this diet is in infancy. The chances of a useful clinical benefit are small.

Avoidance of 10 common food triggers

The patient avoids approximately 10 common food triggers, plus foods for which there is a history of intolerance. The foods usually chosen for exclusion are cow's milk, egg, wheat, fish, legumes (pea, bean, soya, lentil), tomato, nuts, berries and currants, citrus fruit and food additives (for a discussion of these see separate section below). The chances of a useful clinical benefit are small.

The few-food diet (oligoantigenic diet)

This consists of exclusion of all foods except for five or six items. These items should not include a food for which there is a history of intolerance. Such diets comprise a meat (usually lamb or turkey), three vegetables (e.g. potato, rice, and carrot or a brassica – cauliflower, cabbage, broccoli or sprouts), a fruit (usually pear) and possibly a breakfast cereal (e.g. Rice Crispies). There is scanty data on the outcome of few-food diets. In one study, a few-food diet was associated with marked improvement in 50% of patients (median age 2.9 years, range 0.4–14.8) with atopic eczema, but after 12 months' follow-up, the results were the same (marked improvement) in the group that improved, the group that failed to improve, and the group that tried a diet but were unable to cope (Devlin et al 1991a). In another study, 85 children (median age 2.3 years, range 0.3–13.3 years) with atopic eczema were randomly allocated to receive a few-foods diet supplemented with either a whey hydrolysate or a casein hydrolysate formula, or to remain on their usual diet and act as controls, for a 6-week period (Mabin et al 1995b). After 6 weeks, there was a significant reduction in all three groups in the percentage of surface area involved and skin severity score. 16 (73%) of the 22 controls and 15 (58%) of the 24 who received the diet showed a greater than 20% improvement in the skin severity score. This is the only controlled study of a few-food diet, and it failed to show benefit. However, the drawback to these two studies is the relatively high median age and the wide age range, which is important because it is general experience that the best results for elimination diets are in infants. Given the tendency for most children with food hypersensitivity to grow out of the problem by the age of 3 years, the inclusion of substantial numbers of older children in these studies biased the results against finding benefit from a diet.

Elemental diet

The application of an inpatient regimen of 4–6 weeks of a so-called elemental diet (e.g. Elemental 028, Tolerex) is the ultimate test of whether food intolerance is relevant or not, but until more data are available this approach must be regarded as experimental (Devlin et al 1991b). The drawbacks comprise the lack of a guarantee of success, family disruption associated with 2–3 months' hospitalization, loose stools (due to hyperosmolarity of the formula), weight loss and hypoalbuminemia.

House dust mites, pets

House dust mites and pets are of major importance as triggers in atopic eczema, and it is increasingly recognized that an important reason for a lack of therapeutic response to an elimination diet is failure to avoid them. However, the number of patients who experience benefit solely from the avoidance of pets or mites appears to be small. As with elimination diets, there is no test which predicts benefit from avoidance measures. Some patients with atopic eczema are worse during the pollen season or after grass has been cut, but avoidance is impossible.

ALLERGIC ASPECTS OF URTICARIA

Allergy or food intolerance is only relevant to idiopathic urticaria, contact urticaria, and food-provoked exercise-induced anaphylaxis. The general management of urticaria is described in Chapter 25.

IDIOPATHIC URTICARIA

Acute urticaria

Acute urticaria is the result of a variety of causes (often not identified) and mechanisms. The proportion of cases in which a cause is found varies; in childhood the most common cause of acute urticaria is a viral infection. Urticaria may develop during an illness or within 1–2 weeks after the illness, and remain a problem for a few days or weeks. Immediate allergic reactions to foods are the other major cause of acute urticaria. A parent notices, for example, that whenever a child eats fish his lips swell and he develops an urticarial rash. Fish is avoided, and the problem disappears. Occasional lapses of avoidance either demonstrate continued intolerance or, with time, loss of symptoms. Cases which come to medical attention are mostly severe (e.g. associated with laryngeal edema), atypical, or associated with other disorders notably atopic eczema. The common foods incriminated (egg, cow's milk, fish, nuts, tomatoes and fruit) are similar to those which cause allergic contact urticaria (see below), the difference being that children are in general more likely to touch raw foods than to eat them, and raw foods are on the whole more likely to trigger urticaria than cooked foods.

Chronic urticaria

In the majority of cases of chronic (i.e. lasting more than 2 months) urticaria, no cause is found and the disorder spontaneously improves over a period of 6–12 months. Most studies implicating food additives are seriously flawed (David 1993), but genuine cases of additive-provoked urticaria do exist, and this has been documented under double-blind placebo-controlled conditions for sodium benzoate, tartrazine, sunset yellow, amaranth, indigo carmine, monosodium glutamate and sodium metabisulfite (Supramaniam & Warner 1986). Aspirin has also been shown to provoke urticaria (Supramaniam & Warner 1986). In persistent and troublesome urticaria it is worth performing a trial of complete food additive avoidance for an arbitrary period of 4 weeks. If the urticaria disappears then it is simple to perform challenges with individual additives (Supramaniam & Warner 1986).

CONTACT URTICARIA

Irritant contact urticaria

Common causes are plants such as stinging nettles or creatures such as jellyfish, moths and caterpillars. Chemicals are a major cause of irritant contact urticaria, and this is important because the relevant chemicals are widely used in food, medicines and cosmetics.

Allergic contact urticaria

This is an immediate allergic reaction, and should not be confused with contact dermatitis which represents a delayed reaction. Although certain foods, such as raw egg, cow's milk, raw potatoes, raw fish, apples and nuts are particularly common causes of allergic contact urticaria, any food containing protein could in theory cause allergic contact urticaria. In addition to erythema and urticarial wheals, where the food is taken by mouth the symptoms often include itching or tingling of the lips. The tissues and secretions of pet mammals are also common causes of allergic contact urticaria in childhood. Chemicals can also cause allergic contact urticaria, and this includes a number of drugs applied topically, a few vehicles contained in topical medicaments and miscellaneous other chemicals (Fisher 1986).

FOOD-PROVOKED EXERCISE-INDUCED ANAPHYLAXIS

In simple exercise-induced anaphylaxis, exercise is followed by hypotension, accompanied by a varying combination of cholinergic urticaria (widespread tiny (1–3 mm) wheals with variable erythema which last 30–60 min and occur in association with sweating) and angioedema of the face and pharynx. In a curious but well-described variant of this disorder, attacks only occur when the exercise follows within a couple of hours of the ingestion of specific foods such as celery, shellfish, peaches or wheat (Kidd et al 1983). The mechanism of this rare food-dependent exercise-induced anaphylaxis is obscure but in these patients a simple double-blind food challenge performed without exercise will fail to validate a history of food intolerance.

HAY FEVER (Seasonal allergic rhinitis)

The incidence and peak months of hay fever depend upon the proportion of the population who are atopic and the type of pollen (e.g. grass, birch tree, ragweed, mugwort) which is prevalent (Mygind 1979).

The severity of the symptoms varies with the daily pollen count. The symptoms are multiple consecutive sneezes, rhinorrhea, nasal blockage, itching of the eyes, itching of the soft palate and referred itching in the ears (attributed to the common innervation (the glossopharyngeal nerve) of the ear and the pharyngeal mucosa). Asthmatic symptoms sometimes coexist with attacks of hay fever.

The diagnosis is based on the occurrence of the above symptoms each year during the pollen season. No investigations are required. Avoidance of pollen is impossible outdoors, and staying indoors during good weather is unjustifiable in view of the safe and effective therapy which is available. Nonsedating H_1 antihistamines are by far the simplest treatment for mild cases, given either at the onset of attacks or regularly during the pollen season. An advantage of H_1 antihistamines is that they also help eye symptoms, but they are less effective for nasal symptoms than prophylactic topical steroids. Prophylactic treatment comprises:

1. Sodium cromoglycate, but for greatest benefit this needs to be applied to the nasal mucosa at least four times a day, and is much less effective than steroids. The main use is as eyedrops, given 6-hourly.

2. Inhaled steroids: fluticasone (once daily), beclomethasone or budesonide (twice daily) are highly effective in most cases. A combination of steroids and nonsedating H_1 antihistamines is of greater benefit than steroids alone, and is logical in troublesome cases.

3. Oral decongestants (e.g. pseudoephedrine) cause central nervous system stimulation, or drowsiness if combined with a

sedating H_1 antihistamine, and are not very effective. Topical vasoconstrictors are unsatisfactory except for short-term use (e.g. air travel).

4. The short-term advantage of systemic steroids (short course of oral prednisolone or depot injection of a microcrystalline ester such as methylprednisolone acetate) may be offset by the small risk of fatal chickenpox resulting from temporary immunosuppression (Kasper et al 1990, Clogg 1992, Rice et al 1994).

PERENNIAL RHINITIS

Perennial rhinitis can be classified (Mygind 1979) as:

1. Perennial rhinitis (known allergic trigger). This accounts for most children with perennial rhinitis. If the patient has been exposed to the causative allergen in the last few days, then eosinophilia will be seen in a nasal smear in 80% of patients. Prophylactic topical sodium cromoglycate or steroids are effective. The important triggers are house dust mites or pets.

2. Perennial rhinitis (no identifiable allergic trigger, but nasal eosinophilia present). The cause is unknown, but the condition can sometimes be provoked by nonallergic mechanisms, e.g. alcoholic beverages. Prophylactic topical steroids are effective.

3. Perennial rhinitis (no identifiable allergic trigger, and no nasal eosinophilia). This mainly affects adults, and the etiology is unknown. The anticholinergic effect of sedating H_1 antihistamines (e.g. triprolidine) may be helpful.

ALLERGIC CONJUNCTIVITIS

Allergic conjunctivitis can be seasonal or perennial. The major symptom is itching. Rubbing gives immediate but only short-lasting relief, and this is followed by more itching and worsening inflammation of the conjunctivae. Sometimes this leads to a sensation that there is a foreign body present. In seasonal allergic conjunctivitis, allergen (pollen) avoidance is impossible. In perennial conjunctivitis, the identification and avoidance of allergens (e.g. house dust mites, pet animals) is as empirical as it is in asthma. The management of allergic conjunctivitis is mainly pharmacological.

SYMPTOMATIC TREATMENT

For immediate relief it is helpful to apply a crushed ice compress. This can be accompanied by either topical application of H_1 antihistamine with vasoconstrictor eyedrops (xylometazoline and antazoline eyedrops give effective symptomatic relief but cause quite marked transient stinging), or oral quick-acting, nonsedating H_1 antihistamines (e.g. terfenadine).

PROPHYLACTIC TREATMENT

This consists of either regular administration of oral H_1 antihistamines or 6-hourly sodium cromoglycate eyedrops. Topical steroids should only be used under the supervision of an ophthalmologist, for there is a danger of enhancement of herpes simplex corneal infection and a risk of producing glaucoma.

Vernal keratoconjunctivitis is a rare, severe chronic inflammation of the conjunctiva which may last 5 years or more. The characteristic feature is the presence of cobblestone-like papillae on the upper tarsal conjunctiva. The papillae do not themselves cause symptoms, and may be present when the disease is inactive. Exacerbations of conjunctivitis are often seasonal, during which keratitis may develop. The majority of patients have atopic eczema or asthma, but it is rare to find a trigger (allergic or otherwise). Approximately 85% of patients are boys, and the onset of the disorder is below the age of 10 years in about three-quarters of patients. The condition tends to start in the spring (this is the meaning of the word vernal), and the symptoms are itching, rubbing, a burning sensation, redness, a discharge and ptosis. During an exacerbation keratitis is common, causing photophobia and reduced visual acuity, and sometimes leading to an ulcer which may in turn cause permanent loss of vision. The management, which would always be supervised by an ophthalmologist, consists of topical steroids for exacerbations, topical antibiotics for secondary infection, and acetylcysteine eyedrops where there is a thick discharge. Topical sodium cromoglycate alone is only of benefit in the mildest cases.

BEHAVIOR PROBLEMS

Both hospital and community-based double-blind placebo-controlled studies have repeatedly failed to confirm any validity in the idea that food or food additives cause behavioral problems in otherwise healthy individuals (David 1987, David 1993). The avoidance of food additives seems to have only a very short-lived beneficial effect on hyperkinesis and other behavior problems, and any benefit from additive avoidance diets is likely to be a placebo response. One source of confusion has been the presence of atopic disease. If a food additive makes eczema or asthma worse, then the concentration span and behavior may also be expected to suffer, but there is no evidence that this is anything other than an indirect effect.

FOOD INTOLERANCE

The prevalence of food intolerance is unclear, although it is greater in infants than in adults, particularly atopic children. The difficulties in establishing the prevalence of food intolerance are the individual variation in tolerance of feelings and symptoms, the unreliability of unconfirmed parental observations, and the lack of definition of what constitutes a reaction to food. All eating causes reactions, for example satiety, the urge to defecate, a feeling of warmth, and weight gain. In the present context we are dealing with unwanted reactions, but families vary in their tolerance of events.

The prognosis for food intolerance is good. A prospective study showed that the offending food or fruit was back in the diet after only 9 months in half the cases, and virtually all the offending foods were back in the diet by the third birthday (Bock 1987). The mechanisms for food intolerance may be immunological (food allergy), metabolic (e.g. lactase deficiency), pharmacological (e.g. vasoactive amines), toxic (e.g. lectins in red kidney beans), irritant (e.g. curry) or unknown.

Intolerance to cow's milk protein, egg, soya and food additives are discussed below. Intolerance to other foods, such as fish, nuts, wheat, tomato, and fruits can occur, but these are mainly responsible for immediate allergic reactions. Skin and RAST tests are unhelpful, and where there is doubt about the diagnosis a challenge is required. The management consists of avoidance.

COW'S MILK PROTEIN INTOLERANCE

Cow's milk protein intolerance is a heterogeneous disorder. The most common antigens in cow's milk are β-lactoglobulin, casein, α-lactalbumin, bovine serum albumin and bovine γ-globulin. Digestion may result in the production of additional antigens. The marked antigenic similarity between cow's and goat's milk proteins (Crawford & Grogan 1961) explains why most children with cow's milk protein intolerance are intolerant to goat's milk. Intolerance to carbohydrates present in cow's milk and milk formulae is dealt with in Chapter 11.

The quantity of cow's milk required to produce an adverse reaction varies. Some patients develop anaphylaxis after ingestion of less than 1 mg of casein, β-lactoglobulin or α-lactalbumin. In contrast, Goldman et al (1963) showed that 29 out of 89 children (33%) with cow's milk intolerance did not react to 100 ml of milk but only to 200 ml or more. The median reaction onset time in those who reacted to 100 ml milk challenges was 2 h, but the median reaction onset time in those who required larger amounts of milk to elicit reactions was 24 h.

Most cow's milk formula-fed infants with cow's milk protein intolerance develop symptoms in the first 3 months of life. The age of onset of the first symptoms in breast-fed babies depends on the age at which cow's milk is first introduced. A few breast-fed infants develop symptoms during breast-feeding, because of the presence of cow's milk protein in the mother's breast milk (Gerrard 1979).

Symptoms

There is no single symptom or pattern of symptoms which is pathognomonic of cow's milk protein intolerance. Vomiting is a common immediate symptom. Frequent loose stools occur in 25–75% of patients. In an uncommon but florid picture, infants can present with heavily bloodstained loose stools, sometimes accompanied by mucus, giving rise to the clinical description of food-allergic colitis. Malabsorption may mimic celiac disease with bulky fatty stools, abdominal distention and poor weight gain, and protein-losing enteropathy may be an associated feature. In such cases a jejunal biopsy usually shows some degree of villous atrophy. Acute abdominal pain (often but not always accompanied by vomiting or loose stools) can be a striking symptom. The acute presentation of blood in the stools and abdominal pain may mimic intussusception.

Discomfort, crying or irritability are common and major features of cow's milk protein intolerance in infancy, but it is not clear whether this represents painful hyperperistalsis of the gut or discomfort associated with vomiting or other symptoms. They may occur in conjunction with other symptoms, particularly gastrointestinal symptoms, or they may occur alone. These symptoms usually commence within an hour of cow's milk protein ingestion, although this is not always noted by the parents, partly because irritability from one feed can merge into that caused by the next feed. Crying or screaming are nonspecific symptoms in infants, are often accompanied by drawing-up of the legs, and have a number of causes including hunger, tiredness, infection or pain. Many studies of colic as a possible symptom of cow's milk protein intolerance fail to define the term colic, to record associated symptoms that might suggest cow's milk protein intolerance, and to record any temporal relationship between symptoms and milk ingestion.

Wheezing, coughing or rhinitis are common symptoms of cow's milk protein intolerance, and are usually seen in combination with other symptoms such as atopic eczema or vomiting. The acute onset of stridor is occasionally seen within a few minutes of cow's milk ingestion, and indicates angioedema of the larynx or trachea. A persistent perioral erythematous rash, urticaria or eczema can be features of cow's milk protein intolerance. Anaphylactic shock is a rare but potentially fatal feature of cow's milk protein intolerance. The symptoms usually develop within minutes of ingestion of cow's milk protein, but anaphylaxis may be delayed for as much as 9 h after ingestion of cow's milk (David 1984).

Patients with cow's milk protein intolerance may be intolerant to other foods. In one hospital-based series of 100 children with cow's milk protein intolerance, over 50% exhibited intolerance to one or more other foods (Hill et al 1984).

Clues to the diagnosis in the history

1. Symptoms occur, or are made worse, soon after ingestion of cow's milk protein. Multiple affected systems (e.g. gut, chest and skin) make the diagnosis more likely; single symptoms make it most unlikely.
2. Symptoms date from the time, or soon after the time, that breast-feeding was stopped or cow's milk protein was first introduced into the diet. (NB Feeding changes often coincide with the onset of atopic disease, and do not prove a cause and effect relationship.)
3. A family history of cow's milk protein intolerance.
4. The presence of severe atopic disease in an infant under the age of 12 months.
5. The observation that spilling cow's milk onto noneczematous skin causes an urticarial rash.

Making the diagnosis of cow's milk protein intolerance

Most patients whose symptoms commence within an hour of cow's milk ingestion have a positive skin prick test, but most of those whose symptoms occur more slowly have negative skin prick tests. As is the case with most other examples of food intolerance, skin prick tests and RAST tests are unhelpful because of the high incidence of false positive and false negative results. A jejunal biopsy is unnecessary because it cannot replace the need for milk elimination and challenge, and the histological changes seen in the small intestine are not diagnostic for cow's milk protein intolerance.

The procedure required to diagnose cow's milk protein intolerance is:

1. A period of avoidance (2 days for those with symptoms occurring within an hour of milk ingestion; 14–28 days for those with delayed-onset symptoms) causing loss of symptoms.
2. Recurrence of symptoms on reintroduction of cow's milk protein.
3. Loss of symptoms after second withdrawal of cow's milk protein.
4. Continued abatement of symptoms with continued avoidance of cow's milk protein.

This strategy must be accompanied by regular attempts to reintroduce cow's milk protein, for example yearly, to see if the patient has grown out of the intolerance.

Failure of milk exclusion

The reasons why a trial period of cow's milk elimination may fail are:

1. The patient has an alternative cause for the reported symptoms.
2. The period of elimination was too short.
3. Foods containing cow's milk protein have not been fully excluded from the diet.
4. The patient is intolerant to the cow's milk substitute which has been given. This is common with goat's milk or sheep's milk. About 10% of patients with cow's milk protein intolerance are also intolerant to soya. A smaller proportion are intolerant to whey hydrolysate formulae (these vary in their antigenicity), and there are rare cases of intolerance to casein hydrolysate formulae (Pregestimil or Nutramigen).
5. Coexisting or intercurrent disease, e.g. gastroenteritis.
6. The patient is intolerant to other items which have not been withdrawn from the diet or the environment.
7. The patient's symptoms are trivial and have been exaggerated, or alternatively do not exist at all and have either been imagined or fabricated by the parents. Complete fabrication of symptoms by parents is rare, but the mistaken belief that a child's symptoms are attributable to food intolerance is common.

Milk challenge procedure

A challenge with cow's milk protein is done either to confirm the diagnosis or to see if the patient has grown out of the intolerance. If it is known that the child can tolerate small amounts of cow's milk at home then a formal challenge in hospital is not required, and the parents can continue to increase the quantity of cow's milk given at home.

During cow's milk protein challenge, symptoms may appear that had not been noted previously, the concern being anaphylactic shock. In Goldman's study (Goldman et al 1963), 3 of 89 patients developed anaphylactic shock as a new symptom during milk challenge (in a further 5, anaphylaxis had been noted prior to milk challenge). This means that in infancy milk challenges should be performed in hospital, the first dose should be minuscule (e.g. one drop of milk), and the child should be observed for approximately 12 h in case of delayed anaphylaxis (David 1984). If there are no symptoms, cow's milk should continue to be given to the child at home. Troublesome adverse reactions can still develop during the next few days. Cow's milk protein intolerance often lasts only a few months, and in many cases it has disappeared completely by the age of 12 months, hence the need for milk challenge at the age of 12 months in patients who were diagnosed in infancy. Most children become tolerant to cow's milk protein by the age of 3 years, although some degree of intolerance persists, occasionally into adult life, in a small number of patients.

Cow's milk-free diets

Cow's milk exclusion means the avoidance of all foods which contain cow's milk protein. A dietitian will be able to provide an appropriate diet sheet containing an up-to-date list of milk-free manufactured foods. Beef avoidance is unnecessary as the coexistence of intolerance to cow's milk and beef is unusual. Infants on a cow's milk-free diet require a cow's milk substitute.

The choice is between formulae based on soya, whey hydrolysate, casein hydrolysate (Pregestimil or Nutramigen) or amino acids (Neocate). Goat, sheep's and ass's milk are inadvisable because of the high incidence of cross-sensitivity, their high solute content, and the risk of serious gastrointestinal infections due to unhygienic methods of collection and distribution. Noninfant formulae soya-based milks are unsuitable because of their low calcium, vitamin and energy content (David 1993). If an infant is intolerant to both soya and casein hydrolysate, the options are donated human milk, a comminuted chicken-based formula, an elemental diet, or in exceptional circumstances intravenous feeding. After infancy, the rare cases of intolerance to all milk substitutes are dealt with by introducing milk-free solids with added calcium supplements (e.g. calcium and ergocalciferol tablets (which contain 97 mg calcium or 2.4 mmol of Ca)), effervescent calcium gluconate tablets (2.25 mmol elemental calcium per tablet) or calcium gluconate BPC tablets (1.35 mmol elemental calcium per tablet)). Even where a soya or casein hydrolysate infant milk formula is provided, the calcium intake may fall below the estimated requirements (Devlin et al 1989). The importance of such low intakes of calcium is unknown, but there may be special risks for patients with atopic eczema. In these children intestinal absorption may be impaired because of an associated enteropathy, the absence of lactose from the diet may impair calcium absorption, and there is a risk of vitamin D deficiency and consequently diminished gastrointestinal calcium absorption in children with atopic eczema who are kept out of sunlight (Devlin et al 1989).

EGG INTOLERANCE

The major allergens in egg white are ovalbumin, ovomucoid and ovotransferrin, and all three are also present in much smaller quantities in egg yolk. Cooking reduces the allergenicity of eggs by 70%. Almost all children with egg intolerance can tolerate cooked chicken. The eggs of turkeys, duck and goose contain similar allergens to hen's eggs.

Egg intolerance is most common in the first 6 months of life, and the most frequent presentation is the rapid onset of symptoms minutes after an infant is given egg for the first time. Reactions occurring within an hour of eating egg consist of an erythematous rash around the mouth, swelling and urticaria of the oral mucosa and angioedema of the face, sometimes with wheezing, stridor, conjunctivitis, rhinitis, vomiting, loose stools and in severe cases anaphylaxis. Those with immediate reactions also exhibit urticaria after skin contact with egg.

The diagnosis of egg intolerance is made from the history. Skin prick tests and RAST tests are unhelpful because of false positive and false negative results, and on the rare occasions when the diagnosis is in doubt it can only be confirmed by challenge. The management is to exclude egg from the diet. Egg intolerance is not a contraindication to measles or measles–mumps–rubella vaccination because modern measles vaccines are grown on fibroblasts and do not contain detectable quantities of egg protein. Studies have shown that measles–mumps–rubella vaccine can be safely given to children with egg allergy (Aickin et al 1994). The same may not apply to other vaccines such as influenza vaccine, which is grown in the allantoic cavity of chick eggs and which does contain traces of egg protein. In the majority of cases intolerance has disappeared by the age of 3 years. Where the presentation is after the age of 12 months, which is unusual, the duration of intolerance may be longer, and is occasionally lifelong.

SOYA INTOLERANCE

Soya protein is a common constituent of flour, and is widely distributed in manufactured foods including bread, pastry and sausages. Soya protein is also commonly employed as a meat extender and found in sausages, hamburgers and pie fillings. Soya and other beans can cause flatulence, abdominal pain and loose stools, which are due to the action of intestinal bacteria on poorly digestible oligosaccharides, mainly raffinose and stachyose.

Soya protein intolerance is less common than cow's milk protein intolerance. The clinical features and management of the two disorders are the same, but the widespread use of soya in manufactured foods means that soya protein avoidance is more difficult than cow's milk protein avoidance.

INTOLERANCE TO FOOD ADDITIVES

Food additives include coloring agents, preservatives, antioxidants, emulsifiers, stabilizers, sweeteners, other flavor modifiers and a large miscellaneous group of other agents. The scale of use of additives in food comes as a surprise to most people, and it is understandable that many should find these substances vaguely menacing. An obsession with food that is natural overlooks both the large number of toxic substances naturally occurring in food (Harris 1986) and the fact that most substances which provoke food intolerance are naturally occurring, such as eggs, cow's milk and nuts. There is an enormous discrepancy between the public's perception of food additive intolerance and objectively verified intolerance. In one study, 1372 of 18 582 people living in High Wycombe claimed to suffer from food additive intolerance, but double-blind challenges confirmed this in only two subjects, who were both shown to react adversely to the coloring agent annatto, which caused headache in one and abdominal pain in the other (Young et al 1987).

Tartrazine and benzoic acid

Tartrazine is a yellow coloring agent, and one of the group of azo dyes. It is used as a coloring agent in a wide range of foods and medicines. Benzoic acid and the related benzoates retard the growth of bacteria and yeasts, and are used as food preservatives. Small quantities occur naturally in certain foods such as cranberries and bilberries. Double-blind placebo-controlled studies have demonstrated that tartrazine can provoke urticaria, asthma or rhinitis in a small number of atopic subjects (David 1993). Similar studies have shown that benzoates can provoke urticaria. There is a lack of objective information about whether benzoates can provoke asthma. Tartrazine or benzoate intolerance can be identified by history (particularly unreliable in suspected food additive intolerance), elimination and challenge. It is possible that repeated administration of tartrazine or the benzoates leads to tolerance, and the severity of adverse reaction may not always be severe enough to warrant avoidance.

Sulfites

Sulfur dioxide and the sodium or potassium salts of sulfite or metabisulfite are widely used as food preservatives. Dried fruit is commonly treated with sulfur dioxide, and high levels of sulfite are sometimes found in wine, beer and salads in restaurants. Sulfites are sometimes used as preservatives in parenteral preparations of drugs, including several drugs used for the intravenous or inhalational treatment of asthma. Double-blind placebo-controlled studies have demonstrated that the oral administration of sulfite solutions can provoke bronchoconstriction in 35–70% of children with asthma.

A history of worsening of pre-existing asthma after consuming artificial drinks, eating in a restaurant or inhalation or injection of a drug containing sulfite raises the possibility of sulfite intolerance. Skin tests are unhelpful, and the diagnosis can only be confirmed by challenge, employing increasing doses of sulfite so as to establish the patient's threshold dose which can provoke asthma. Knowledge of the threshold enables the patient to avoid only those foods with a relatively high sulfite level, making a very restrictive diet unnecessary.

Other food additives

Evidence for harmful effects to children from other food additives does not exist, apart from those additives which can provoke urticaria (see above) and a single case of orofacial granulomatosis (Melkersson–Rosenthal syndrome) provoked by carmoisine, sunset yellow and monosodium glutamate (Sweatman et al 1986).

ANAPHYLAXIS

In this chapter, and in the clinical situation, the term anaphylaxis or anaphylactic shock is taken to mean a severe reaction of rapid onset, with circulatory collapse. In the past the term anaphylaxis was used to describe any immediate allergic reaction caused by IgE antibodies, however mild, but such usage fails to distinguish between, for example, trivial urticaria, and a life-threatening event. The mechanisms are believed to be IgE mediated (e.g. penicillin or insulin allergy), the generation of immune complexes (e.g. reactions to blood products), a direct (not involving antigens or antibodies) effect on mast cells or basophils causing inflammatory mediator release (e.g. reactions to radiocontrast media) and presumed abnormalities of arachidonic acid metabolism (e.g. anaphylactoid reactions to aspirin). It is possible to theoretically differentiate between anaphylaxis (immunologically mediated reactions) and anaphylactoid (nonimmunologically mediated) reactions. Previous sensitization is required for the former but not the latter.

The major causes of anaphylactic shock are drugs (e.g. penicillin, muscle relaxants), heterologous antisera (used for the prophylaxis and treatment of tetanus, diphtheria, rabies, snake bites and botulism), radiographic contrast media, the administration of blood products, hyposensitization injections, venoms from stinging insects (honeybee, wasp, hornet, yellow jacket) and foods (especially egg, cow's milk, nuts, fish and shellfish). Although delayed (12 h or more) anaphylactic reactions can occur, most cases of anaphylaxis produce symptoms within minutes after exposure to the causative agent. In general, the sooner the symptoms occur the more severe is the reaction. The first symptoms are feeling unwell, feeling warm, generalized pruritus, fear, faintness and sneezing. In severe cases these early symptoms are quickly (in seconds or minutes) followed by loss of consciousness, and death from severe bronchospasm, suffocation (edema of the larynx, epiglottis and pharynx) or shock and cardiac arrhythmia.

One cause of death in anaphylaxis is obstruction to the upper airway, and protection of the airway is vital, with endotracheal intubation or if this is impossible tracheostomy. Oxygen should be given early for airway obstruction and/or hypotension to prevent myocardial ischemia. Adrenaline 1 : 1000 solution, 0.01 ml/kg, is the most important drug. It should be given subcutaneously or intramuscularly, or if there is severe hypotension or imminent vascular collapse it should be diluted in 10 ml saline and given intravenously slowly over 3–5 min, remembering that this route carries the risk of ventricular arrhythmia. A second dose should be given at the site of the causative injection or sting to delay absorption. Adrenaline has a short half-life, and the injection can be repeated at 20-min intervals, as required and tolerated. Bronchoconstriction is treated with a nebulized β_2-agonist (e.g. salbutamol or terbutaline). Hypotension is treated with intravenous fluids. After injection of adrenaline, an H_1 antihistamine (e.g. chlorpheniramine) is administered by intramuscular or intravenous injection, and continued for 48 h to prevent recurrence of urticaria. Steroids take some hours to be effective and are unhelpful in the immediate treatment of anaphylaxis, but are of possible benefit in preventing a secondary relapse. Further management consists of avoidance of the cause, and in the case of insect venom stings consideration of hyposensitization.

For those who are at risk of a life-threatening anaphylactic reaction (the main risk factors are a previous life-threatening reaction, and asthma) there is a place for supplying syringes preloaded with adrenaline for use outside hospital. Parents and other responsible adults (e.g. teachers) must be trained when and how to administer the injection. Set against the possible therapeutic advantages are a lack of proven life-saving efficacy and a number of serious drawbacks which include the risks of overdosage, inadvertent intravenous injection and exclusion from school (Patel et al 1994). Alternatively, adrenaline is available as a metered-dose aerosol (Medihaler-Epi). About 10% of the drug reaches the lungs and is absorbed, the remainder being exhaled or deposited in the mouth and pharynx and swallowed. The aerosol can be fitted into the Volumatic spacer device. In healthy individuals, large doses (15–30 puffs) have to be given to achieve the same plasma levels as a 300 mg subcutaneous injection and the recommended dose for children is 10–15 puffs.

DRUG ALLERGY

The term drug allergy should be restricted to reactions proven to be the result of an immunological mechanism. Pseudoallergic reactions have similar clinical manifestations but are not the result of a reaction between the drug or a drug metabolite and specific antibodies. Although drugs may produce the spectrum of common allergic reactions discussed above, many manifestations attributed to drug allergy, such as a wide variety of skin rashes (e.g. exfoliative dermatitis, erythema multiforme or photosensitivity reactions), drug fever, serum sickness, and hematological (e.g. lupus erythematosus) reactions are rarely, if ever, produced by naturally encountered allergens. Only a few drugs such as large peptides (e.g. insulin), papain, streptokinase and foreign antisera are effective inducers of an immune response. The majority of drugs are simple chemicals of low molecular weight which are not immunogenic unless combined with serum or tissue proteins to form an immunogenic complex.

In general skin prick testing and in vitro tests (e.g. IgE antibodies) are unhelpful, and the main investigative tool is

readministration of the drug when the patient is asymptomatic, but the risk of inducing anaphylaxis restricts the use of this approach.

PENICILLIN ALLERGY

Degradation products of penicillin may bind with tissue or serum proteins to form an immunogenic complex which can elicit an immune response. Penicillin allergy is attributed either to the benzylpenicilloyl hapten (the so-called 'major' determinant because 95% of tissue-bound penicillin is in this form), or to a group of compounds collectively called the 'minor' determinants which are paradoxically responsible for many of the most severe allergic reactions. Adverse reactions to penicillin can be most simply classified by the timing of their occurrence. Immediate reactions occur within an hour of administration and are usually directed against the minor determinant antigens. The clinical features are urticaria, laryngeal edema, bronchospasm and anaphylactic shock. Accelerated reactions occur 1–72 h after penicillin administration, have the same clinical features as immediate reactions, and are usually directed against the major determinant. Late reactions, the mechanisms of which are generally less well understood, occur more than 72 h after drug administration. They comprise such disorders as a maculopapular (measles-like) rash, urticaria, serum sickness, erythema multiforme, hemolytic anemia, thrombocytopenia and neutropenia. Rarely, late reactions are due to the new development of an immediate or accelerated reaction.

Ampicillin can provoke the same allergic reactions as other penicillins, but in addition is associated with a particularly high incidence of a nonallergic maculopapular rash, beginning a week or more after starting therapy.

An inquiry about possible penicillin allergy is mandatory prior to an injection of penicillin. However, not all patients with penicillin allergy give a history of previous penicillin administration. In these patients either the history is incorrect and the patient has received penicillin therapy, or sensitization has occurred through inadvertent exposure to penicillin in other sources such as food, milk or even soft drinks. Where there is a history of penicillin allergy, the choice is either to withhold antibiotics or to avoid the use of penicillins, cephalosporins or imipenem, which like the penicillins contains a β-lactam ring and which shows extensive cross-reactivity with penicillin. Almost all deaths from anaphylaxis have resulted from injection of the drug, and the oral route has only been associated with a handful of fatal cases.

Skin prick testing and RAST testing are unhelpful, partly because mixtures of the minor determinants are unstable and not commercially available. On the very rare occasions in childhood (e.g. endocarditis) when treatment with penicillin is essential, then it is possible to hyposensitize the patient by oral and then continuous intravenous administration (Stark et al 1987), but this procedure carries a risk of fatal anaphylaxis. The protection from hyposensitization is short lived, although it is possible to maintain a state of hyposensitization by long-term administration of a low dose.

HYPOSENSITIZATION

Hyposensitization comprises the regular injection of allergen extracts with the object of reducing or abolishing the patient's reaction to the allergen. The mode of action of hyposensitization is poorly understood. The drawbacks to hyposensitization injections are:

1. lack of significant clinical benefit
2. the need for multiple injections
3. the need for prolonged (many years) treatment for benefit to be maintained
4. the risk of fatal anaphylaxis, particularly but not exclusively in subjects with asthma.

For these reasons, inhalant or other allergies in children with atopic disease are not indications for hyposensitization. The risk of death from anaphylaxis (26 deaths in the UK between 1967 and 1986) means that hyposensitization, which is only justified in patients with life-threatening allergy to bee or wasp venom (rare in childhood), can only be performed in hospitals with full facilities for cardiopulmonary resuscitation.

Intolerance to carbamazepine (skin rash) has been successfully treated by the oral administration of 0.1 mg daily and doubling the dose every 2 days, with a delay in increments if any skin rash appears. It is probable that intolerance to a number of other drugs could be approached in the same way (Battersby et al 1995), though there is a risk with some drugs (e.g. penicillin, see above) of provoking anaphylaxis. Oral hyposensitization has been achieved in a small number of children with food intolerance, but carries the risk of anaphylaxis and must be regarded as experimental.

PREVENTION OF ATOPIC DISEASE

Since it was reported that breast-feeding protects against atopic eczema, the notion that atopic disease can be prevented by breast-feeding has been surrounded by confusion. Not one study of this subject is without serious defect, and those from the greatest enthusiasts for breast-feeding are often the most flawed. Objections to previous studies include:

1. Observer bias. Doctors known to be protagonists of breast-feeding decided whether infants had eczema or not in the full knowledge of whether the baby was breast- or bottle-fed.

2. Nonblind ascertainment of history. Interviewers asking for feeding history are likely to be biased if they know of the child's outcome (i.e. atopic status). Knowledge of the outcome tends to create an association between exposure and outcome where none exists. Feeding histories must be taken by someone who knows nothing about the child, and should be taken before the outcome is known.

3. Reliance on prolonged maternal recall. A history taken years after the feeding period is prone to error regarding both the duration and exclusivity of breast-feeding. Prospective studies avoid this problem.

4. Adequate exclusivity of breast-feeding. If breast-feeding is protective it may be through exclusion of foreign proteins like egg or cow's milk, or protection may be due to protective substances in human milk. The consumption of other foods during breast-feeding may interfere with the protective effect of breast-feeding. Unless breast-feeding has been exclusive for a period of time, it is difficult to test the preventive effect of breast-feeding.

5. Definition of atopic diseases. The conditions being investigated must be carefully defined. There should be a close agreement between the observations of two observers and between the observations of the same observer at different times.

Skin rashes, wheezing and sneezing all have numerous causes. Not all are atopic.

6. Sufficient duration of breast-feeding. Brief exposure to human milk may not be expected to provide long-term protection against subsequent atopic disease. If breast-feeding is protective, then the longer the duration of breast-feeding the greater would be the expected protection against atopic disease.

7. Assessment of disease severity. Misleading information based on the failure to differentiate between minor and major forms of disease. Studies compared the total incidence of diseases such as eczema or asthma in babies fed different ways, but parents fear *severe* cases. The protective effect of breast-feeding is unlikely to be all or none, so that if there is a genuine protective effect there should be some dose–response relationship. The demonstration of a graded degree of outcome in response to varying duration of breast-feeding would strengthen the inference that breast-feeding prevented the outcome.

8. Controls are essential to exclude confounding variables such as family history of atopic disease, racial origin, social class, exposure to pets and so on. Atopic mothers may, for example, preferentially breast-feed in the hope of preventing atopic disease. This tends to bias the results against a protective effect of breast-feeding, because the breast-fed infant would then be at greater genetic risk of developing atopy.

9. Adequate follow-up is essential. Breast-feeding may simply delay the age of onset of disease. Thus a follow-up study lasting 12 months might show a protective effect, but a 24-month follow-up might show no protective effect. Delaying the age of onset might be beneficial or harmful.

Contrary to the current received wisdom that breast-feeding is protective, it is increasingly being recognized that ingested food antigens can pass into human milk (Gerrard 1979, Cant et al 1986, David 1993). Maternal avoidance of the food in question is followed by remission of atopic disease in the infant, and re-exposure followed by relapse. Some studies from Scandinavia have served to further undermine belief in the protective effect of breast-feeding, exclusive or otherwise. A prospective study from Finland showed a steadily *increasing* incidence of atopic disease the longer a mother exclusively breast-fed her infant (Savilahti et al 1987). A prospective study of breast-fed babies from Sweden showed that those who had been exclusively breast-fed in the first few days or life were *more likely* to develop atopic disease than those who were given supplementary cow's milk feeds for the first few days of life and then breast-fed (Lindfors & Enocksson 1988). Finally, a follow-up study of 69 preterm infants showed that the 38 infants fed exclusively with human milk to the age of 4 months had significantly more allergic symptoms than the 31 infants fed with adapted cow's milk formula from birth (Savilahti et al 1993).

Several studies have examined the effect of the inhalant environment in early infancy on the subsequent manifestations of allergic disease, by comparing the month of birth of patients with immediate skin reactions to specific allergens to the month of birth of a reference population (Zeiger 1993). A relationship between the month of birth and the subsequent development of an allergy has been claimed for birch tree pollen, grass pollen, ragweed pollen and house dust mites, but the evidence is far from clear. The inference has been made (but never substantiated) that allergy to these items could be avoided by ensuring that the birth of a child takes place shortly after the seasonal disappearance of the allergen, thereby avoiding sensitization in infancy.

REFERENCES

Aickin R, Hill D, Kemp A 1994 Measles immunisation in children with allergy to egg. British Medical Journal 309: 223–225

Battersby N C, Patel L, David T J 1995 Increasing dose regimen in children with reactions to ceftazidime. Clinical Experimental Allergy 25: 1211–1217

Bernstein I L 1988 Proceedings of the task force guidelines for standardizing old and new techniques used for the diagnosis and treatment of allergic diseases. Journal of Allergy and Clinical Immunology 82(suppl): 487–526

Bock S A 1987 Prospective appraisal of complaints of adverse reactions to foods in children during the first three years of life. Pediatrics 79: 683–688

Bousquet J, Michel F B 1993 In vivo methods for study of allergy. Skin tests, techniques, and interpretation. In: Middleton E, Reed C E, Ellis E F, Adkinson N F, Yunginger J W, Busse W W (eds) Allergy. Principles and practice. Mosby, St Louis, ch 22, pp 573–627

Butler N R, Golding J 1986 From birth to five. A Study of the health and behaviour of Britain's 5-year-olds. Pergamon, Oxford

Cant A J, Bailes J A, Marsden R A, Hewitt D 1986 Effect of maternal dietary exclusion on breast fed infants with eczema: two controlled studies. British Medical Journal 293: 231–233

Chapel H, Haeney M 1988 Essentials of clinical immunology, 2nd edn. Blackwell Science, Oxford

Clogg D K 1992 Varicella in children receiving steroids for asthma: Risks and management. Pediatric Infectious Disease Journal 11: 419–420

Crawford L, Grogan F 1961 Allergenicity of cow's milk proteins. Journal of Pediatrics 59: 347–350

David T J 1984 Anaphylactic shock during elimination diets for severe atopic eczema. Archives of Disease in Childhood 59: 983–986

David T J 1987 Reactions to dietary tartrazine. Archives of Disease in Childhood 62: 119–122

David T J 1993 Food and food additive intolerance in childhood. Blackwell Scientific Publications, Oxford

David T J 1995 Atopic eczema. Prescribers Journal 35: 199–205

David T J, Longson M 1985 Herpes simplex infections in atopic eczema. Archives of Disease in Childhood 60: 338–343

David T J, Cambridge G C 1986 Bacterial infection and atopic eczema. Archives of Disease in Childhood 61: 20–23

David T J, Waddington E, Stanton R H J 1984 Nutritional hazards of elimination diets in children with atopic eczema. Archives of Disease in Childhood 59: 323–325

Devlin J, Stanton R H J, David T J 1989 Calcium intake and cows' milk free diets. Archives of Disease in Childhood 64: 1183–1184

Devlin J, David T J, Stanton R H J 1991a Six food diet for childhood atopic dermatitis. Acta Dermatovenereologica 71: 20–24

Devlin J, David T J, Stanton R H J 1991b Elemental diet for refractory atopic eczema. Archives of Disease in Childhood 66: 93–99

Fisher A A 1986 Contact dermatitis, 3rd edn. Lea & Febiger, Philadelphia

Ford R P K, Taylor B 1982 Natural history of egg hypersensitivity. Archives of Disease in Childhood 57: 649–652

Gerrard J W 1979 Allergy in breast fed babies to ingredients in breast milk. Annals of Allergy 42: 69–72

Goldman A S, Anderson D W, Sellers W A, Saperstein S, Kniker W T, Halpern S R 1963 1. Oral challenge with milk and isolated milk proteins in allergic children. Pediatrics 32: 425–443

Harris J B 1986 Natural toxins. Animal, plant, and microbial. Clarendon Press, Oxford

Hill D J, Ford R P K, Shelton M J, Hosking C S 1984 A study of 100 infants and young children with cow's milk allergy. Clinical Reviews in Allergy 2: 125–142

Hill D J, Ball G, Hosking C S 1988 Clinical manifestations of cows' milk allergy in childhood. I. Associations with in-vitro cellular immune responses. Clinical Allergy 18: 469–479

Holgate S T, Church M K 1993 Allergy. Gower Medical, London

Ihre E, Axelsson I G K, Zetterstrom O 1988 Late asthmatic reactions and bronchial variability after challenge with low doses of allergen. Clinical Allergy 18: 557–567

Kasper W J, Howe P M 1990 Fatal varicella after a single course of corticosteroids. Pediatric Infectious Disease Journal 9: 729–732

Khot A, Burn R, Evans N, Lenney W, Storr J 1988 Biometeorological triggers in childhood asthma. Clinical Allergy 18: 351–358

Kidd J M, Cohen S H, Sosman A J, Fink J N 1983 Food-dependent exercise-induced anaphylaxis. Journal of Allergy and Clinical Immunology 71: 407–411

Lessof M H 1987 Skin tests. In: Lessof M H, Lee T H, Kemeny D M (eds) Allergy: an international textbook. John Wiley, Chichester, ch 16, pp 281–287

Lessof M H, Buisseret P D, Merrett J, Merrett T G, Wraith D G 1980 Assessing the value of skin tests. Clinical Allergy 10: 115–120

Lindfors A, Enocksson E 1988 Development of atopic disease after early administration of cow milk formula. Allergy 43: 11–16

Mabin D C, Sykes A E, David T J 1995a Nutritional content of few foods diet in atopic dermatitis. Archives of Disease in Childhood 73: 208–210

Mabin D C, Sykes A E, David T J 1995b Controlled trial of a few foods diet in severe atopic dermatitis. Archives of Disease in Childhood 73: 202–207

May C D, Bock S A 1978 A modern clinical approach to food hypersensitivity. Allergy 33: 166–188

Middleton E, Reed C E, Ellis E F, Adkinson N F, Yunginger J W, Busse W W 1993 Allergy. Principles and practice, 4th edn. Mosby, St Louis

Murray A B, Ferguson A C, Morrison B J 1983 Diagnosis of house dust mite allergy in asthmatic children: what constitutes a positive history? Journal of Allergy and Clinical Immunology 71: 21–28

Mygind N 1979 Nasal allergy, 2nd edn. Blackwell Scientific, Oxford

Mygind N 1986 Essential allergy. Blackwell Scientific, Oxford

Patel L, Radivan F S, David T J 1994 Management of anaphylactic reactions to food. Archives of Disease in Childhood 71: 370–375

Patterson R 1985 Allergic diseases. diagnosis and management, 3rd edn. Lippincott, Philadelphia

Pepys J 1975 Skin testing. British Journal of Hospital Medicine 14: 412–417

Platts-Mills T A E, Hayden M L, Woodfolk J A, Call R S, Sporik R 1995 House dust mite avoidance regimens for the treatment of asthma. In David T J (ed) Recent advances in paediatrics. Churchill Livingstone, Edinburgh, ch 4, pp 45–58

Rice P, Simmons K, Carr R, Banatvala J 1994 Near fatal chickenpox during prednisolone treatment. British Medical Journal 309: 1069–1070

Savilahti E, Tainio V M, Salmenpera L, Siimes M A, Perheentupa J 1987 Prolonged exclusive breast feeding and heredity as determinants in infantile atopy. Archives of Disease in Childhood 62: 269–273

Savilahti E, Tuomikoski-Jaakkola P, Jarvenpaa A L, Virtanen M 1993 Early feeding of preterm infants and allergic symptoms during childhood. Acta Paediatrica 82: 340–344

Sly P D, Landau L I 1986 Diurnal variation in bronchial responsiveness in asthmatic children. Pediatric Pulmonology 2: 344–352

Stark B J, Earl H S, Gross G N, Lumry W R, Goodman E L, Sullivan T J 1987 Acute and chronic desensitisation of penicillin-allergic patients using oral penicillin. Journal of Allergy and Clinical Immunology 79: 523–532

Storr J, Lenney W 1989 School holidays and admissions with asthma. Archives of Disease in Childhood 64: 103–107

Supramaniam G, Warner J O 1986 Artificial food additive intolerance in patients with angio-oedema and urticaria. Lancet 2: 907–909

Sweatman M C, Tasker R, Warner J O, Ferguson M M, Mitchell D N 1986 Oro-facial granulomatosis. Response to elemental diet and provocation by food additives. Clinical Allergy 16: 331–338

Turner M A, Devlin J, David T J 1991 Holidays and atopic eczema. Archives of Disease in Childhood 66: 212–215

Wilkinson J D, Rycroft R J G 1992 Contact dermatitis. In: Champion R H, Burton J L, Ebling F J G (eds), Rook/Wilkinson/Ebling textbook of dermatology. Blackwell Scientific, Oxford, ch 16, pp 611–715

Wood R A, Mudd K E, Eggleston P A 1992 The distribution of cat and dust mite allergens on wall surfaces. Journal of Allergy and Clinical Immunology 89: 126–130

Woodfolk J A, Hayden M L, Couture N, Platts-Mills T A E 1995 Chemical treatment of carpets to reduce allergen: comparison of the effects of tannic acid and other treatments on proteins derived from dust mites and cats. Journal of Allergy and Clinical Immunology 96: 325–333

Young E, Patel S, Stoneham M, Rona R, Wilkinson J D 1987 The prevalence of reaction to food additives in a survey population. Journal of the Royal College of Physicians of London 21: 241–247

Zeiger R S 1993 Development and prevention of allergic diseases in childhood. In: Middleton E, Reed C E, Ellis E F, Adkinson N F, Yunginger J W, Busse W W (eds) Allergy. Principles and practice. Mosby, St Louis, ch 44, pp 1137–1171

29 Poisoning, accidents and sudden infant death syndrome

J. Sibert   P. J. Fleming

Poisoning in childhood   1705
Accidental child poisoning   1705
Deliberate self-poisoning in older children   1706
Non-accidental poisoning   1706
Treatment of child poisoning   1706
Chronic poisoning   1708
Notes on poisoning with individual substances   1708
Accidents to children   1711
Mortality from accidents   1711
Morbidity from accidents   1712
Where to treat childhood accidents?   1712
General principles in treating childhood accidents   1712
Etiological factors in childhood accidents   1712
Prevention of childhood accidents   1712
Accidents to children at play and recreation   1713
Playground injuries   1713
Dog bites   1714

Horse accidents   1714
Burns and scalds in children   1714
Architectural accidents and falls   1715
Road traffic accidents   1715
Drowning and near-drowning in childhood   1716
J. Sibert
The sudden infant death syndrome   1719
Definition and historical perspective   1719
Incidence   1719
Epidemiology, risk factors and risk reduction campaigns   1719
Pathology and the medicolegal system   1720
Normal developmental physiology and possible pathophysiological processes   1721
Support for bereaved families   1722
Care of the next infant   1723
P. J. Fleming
References and Bibliography   1723

POISONING IN CHILDHOOD

Poisoning in children may be accidental, non-accidental, iatrogenic or, in older children, deliberate.

ACCIDENTAL CHILD POISONING

Epidemiology

Accidental poisoning is predominantly seen in children under the age of 5 years but older children may be involved if they are developmentally delayed. The peak age is between 1 and 4 years (Sibert 1975). More boys than girls take poisons accidentally.

Some children die from poisoning each year (Craft 1983), but the number of deaths has fallen over recent years, probably because of better treatment and because of the child-resistant container (CRC) regulations. Though the number of deaths are few, many more children are admitted to hospital for treatment and observation and even more present to hospital accident and emergency departments. Many of these are sent home directly because they have taken relatively non-toxic substances. In New Zealand 19% of children had at least one incident of poisoning or suspected poisoning by the age of 3 years. No medical help was sought in many of these incidents.

Substances taken

Children may take a variety of substances accidentally. These are conveniently divided into medicines (prescribed and non-prescribed), household products and plants. The majority of children who take poisons do not have serious symptoms (Wiseman et al 1987). Medicines may be of low toxicity, e.g. the oral contraceptive pill or antibiotics; intermediate toxicity, which may cause symptoms in young children; or potential high toxicity. Many of the household products children take may be relatively non-toxic, but a few such as caustic soda, soldering flux and paint stripper may cause serious harm (Craft et al 1984). The commonest household product that children take is white spirit and turpentine substitute. About 10% of these children have patchy chest X-ray changes. In developing countries paraffin (kerosene) poisoning is a particular problem as it is used as a cooking fuel and is often kept in open containers. These incidents are common in poor social circumstances and in summer and are probably largely related to thirst. Kerosene may cause serious aspiration pneumonitis and death.

A child may eat a poisonous plant accidentally or a group may sample a plant, such as laburnum, together. Most plants are relatively non-toxic, e.g. cotoneaster, rowan or sweet pea. However, some such as arum lily, deadly nightshade or yew can cause serious symptoms.

Etiology of accidental child poisoning

Perhaps surprisingly, the availability of poisons does not appear to be a major factor in accidental child poisoning. There is evidence that family psychosocial stress and behavioral problems, such as hyperactivity, predispose towards child poisoning (Sibert 1975, Bithoney et al 1986) and these family and personality findings have importance for the prevention of child poisoning.

Preventing child poisoning

Education

A campaign in Birmingham, UK, to publicize accidental child poisoning and to encourage the return of medicines concluded 'that publicity, storage and destruction of unwanted medicines have little preventive value'. A New Zealand study evaluated placing 'Mr Yuk' stickers on poisons together with a campaign to prevent child poisoning. No reduction in poisoning admissions was found. The link between accidental child poisoning and family psychosocial stress and hyperactivity make it unlikely on theoretical grounds that education will be effective. Families under stress will be unlikely to remember safety propaganda.

Child-resistant containers

Child-resistant containers (CRCs) were first suggested in 1959 by Dr Jay Arena in Durham, North Carolina. These containers were evaluated in a community in the United States by Scherz (1970) and found to be successful. They were then introduced into the United States for aspirin preparations, with successful results.

Following this work in the US, child-resistant closures were introduced by regulation in 1976 in the United Kingdom for junior aspirin and paracetamol preparations. This resulted in a fall in admissions of children under 5 years after salicylate poisoning (Sibert et al 1985, Jackson et al 1985). In 1978 CRCs were introduced by regulation for adult aspirin and paracetamol tablets. In 1982 a voluntary agreement was made between the government and the Royal Pharmaceutical Society where all prescribable solid dose medications would be placed in CRCs or safety packaging, with exceptions only for the elderly and infirm. Acceptance of CRCs by pharmacists after 1982 was not uniform but since January 1989 the Royal Pharmaceutical Society has made it a professional requirement. In 1985 the Department of Trade and Industry regulated for a number of household products (e.g. white spirit and turpentine substitute) to be sold in CRCs.

Other methods of preventing child poisoning

Lockable medicine cupboards have been suggested for the prevention of child poisoning. On theoretical grounds they are unlikely to be effective as parents under stress are less likely to remember to put their medicines away or lock the cabinets. Making household products unpalatable with bitter chemical agents (e.g. Bitrex – denatonium bromide; Sibert & Frude 1991) is a possible preventive measure to child poisoning but has not been evaluated. Serious accidental poisoning might also be prevented by a reduction in the prescribing of toxic drugs. This has been done for barbiturates and might also be done for quinine and vaporizing solutions.

DELIBERATE SELF-POISONING IN OLDER CHILDREN

A number of older children take poisons deliberately. They may take medications as a response to an emotional crisis (mainly adolescent girls) or ingest excess alcohol (predominantly adolescent boys). They form one end of an age spectrum of overdose in adults.

NON-ACCIDENTAL POISONING (see also Ch. 34)

The recognition of non-accidental poisoning as an extended syndrome of child abuse was made in 1976. These children are deliberately poisoned by their parents and may present with bizarre or unusual symptoms rather than poisoning directly. A number of medicines or household products may be given to children including salt in feeds to babies. These cases probably form part of the syndrome of factitious illness in childhood or the Munchausen syndrome by proxy (McClure et al 1996). The parents may or may not be psychiatrically disturbed and the children may also show other types of child abuse.

TREATMENT OF CHILD POISONING

Management of accidental poisoning in childhood

General

The majority of children who present to hospital after accidental poisoning do not have serious symptoms. There are nevertheless a few children who have taken a significant poison and who are potentially ill or are ill. We should clearly like to prevent unnecessary admissions to hospital whilst maintaining safety. A way round this dilemma is to classify the substance the child has taken into one of four categories: low toxicity, uncertain toxicity, intermediate toxicity or potential high toxicity. After classification children can be either sent home, observed in the accident and emergency department or admitted for observation or treatment. THE POISONS INFORMATION CENTER SHOULD BE CONTACTED IF THERE IS ANY DOUBT ABOUT THE TOXICITY OF A SUBSTANCE A CHILD HAS TAKEN OR THE TREATMENT THAT IS NEEDED. A list of some of the poisons commonly taken accidentally by children is shown in Table 29.1.

Older children who have taken poisons deliberately and cases of iatrogenic poisoning and non-accidental poisoning should all be admitted to hospital.

The parents of all children who present with accidental poisoning should be given advice regarding the storage of medicines and household products. The health visitor should be contacted in all cases, remembering that family psychosocial stress is often linked with accidental poisoning in childhood. There may be specific problems which need medical or social help.

Emptying the stomach

It used to be standard practice to empty the stomach in cases of accidental poisoning in childhood. This has recently come under review (Vale et al 1986, Wrenn et al 1993) and emesis using ipecacuanha pediatric mixture (ipecac) is now rarely used and activated charcoal should be used more frequently. Gastric lavage was largely abandoned some years ago. It is sometimes needed in certain cases, such as iron poisoning, for substances to be instilled into the stomach. The stomach should not be emptied in cases of hydrocarbon ingestion, such as paraffin or white spirit, or with corrosive substances such as caustic soda. In the United States it has been argued that ipecac should be kept in any home where there are young children. Ipecac is not recommended for home use in the UK.

Activated charcoal

Activated charcoal is being increasingly used in the management of childhood poisoning (Greensher et al 1987). Activated charcoal

Table 29.1 Guide to toxicity of substances taken in accidental child poisoning

Low toxicity

Medicines
Antibiotics (except ciprofloxacin, sulfasalazine and chloramphenicol)
Antacids
Calamine
Oral contraceptives
Vitamin preparations which do not contain iron
Zinc oxide creams

Household products
Chalks and crayons
Emulsion paints and water paints
Fabric softeners
Plant food and fertilizers
Silica gel
Toothpaste
Wallpaper paste
Washing powder (except dishwasher powder)

Plants
Begonia
Cacti
Cotoneaster
Cyclamen
Honeysuckle
Mahonia
Rowan
Spider plant
Sweet pea

Intermediate toxicity

Medicines
Cough medicines (most)
Fluoride
Ibuprofen
Laxatives
Lignocaine gel
Paracetamol elixir
Salbutamol

Household products
Alcohol-containing colognes, aftershaves and perfumes
Bleach
Detergents
Disinfectants (most)
Nail varnish remover
Paints (oil based)
Pyrethrins
Talc
Rat or mouse poison
Window cleaners

Plants
Berberis
Fuchsia
Holly
Pyracantha

Potentially toxic

Medicines
Benzodiazepines
Carbamazepine
Codeine-containing cough medicines
Clonidine
Digoxin
Diphenoxylate (Lomotil)
Iron
Mefenamic acid (Ponstan)
Metoclopramide
Mianserin (Bolvidon)
Paracetamol tablets
Phenytoin
Quinine
Salicylates
Hyoscine
Tricyclic antidepressants (including dothiepin and amitriptyline)
Theophyllines

Household products
Alcoholic beverages
Acids
Alkalis
Camphor and camphorated oil
Cetrimide
Disc batteries
Bottle-sterilizing tablets
Carbon monoxide
Essential oils (e.g. real turpentine, pine oil, citronella and eucalyptus)
Methylene chloride (paint stripper)
Organochloride insecticides
Organophosphorus insecticides
Paradichlorobenzene moth balls
Petroleum distillates (white spirit, paraffin, turpentine substitute)
Paraquat
Phenolic compounds
Slug pellets (metaldehyde)

Plants
Arum lily
Deadly nightshade
Philodendron
Laburnum
Yew

absorbs toxic materials in the gut by offering alternative binding sites. It is used either as an alternative to ipecac or more usually after ipecac-induced vomiting occurs. Its routine use is limited by its poor acceptance by children and in some cases it has to be instilled into the stomach by tube. Two preparations are available, Medicoal 5 g sachets and Carbomix 50 g. Activated charcoal is useful for a variety of drugs including aspirin, carbamazepine, digoxin, mefenamic acid, phenobarbitone, phenytoin, quinine and theophylline. It is particularly useful in tricyclic antidepressant poisoning.

Accidental poisoning with substances of low toxicity

Children who have taken substances of low toxicity can be allowed home after assessment. Their parents should be given advice regarding storage of medicines and the general practitioner should be contacted. If there is doubt over what substance has been taken, a child should be admitted for observation.

Accidental poisoning where there is uncertainty of toxicity

If there is any doubt about the toxicity of a substance a child may have taken, the Poison Information Center should be contacted day or night:

London – Guy's Hospital	Tel. 0171 407 7600 or 0171 635 9191
Edinburgh – Royal Infirmary	Tel. 0131 536 1000
Cardiff – Llandough Hospital	Tel. 01222 709901
Belfast – Royal Victoria Infirmary	Tel. 01232 240503

Some children arrive in hospital having taken unknown tablets or household products. Often research with the pharmacist will help. If there is doubt the child should be admitted for observation.

Intermediate toxicity

Children who have taken substances of intermediate toxicity accidentally should be observed for a period in hospital (usually up to 6 hours) until one can be confident that significant symptoms are not going to occur. This observation can be undertaken in many cases in an accident and emergency department which has a section for children or for short periods in the pediatric ward or day unit. If there are adverse factors, particularly social factors, children should be admitted to hospital for longer periods.

Accidental poisoning with potentially toxic substances

Children who have taken substances of potential toxicity should be admitted to hospital for observation and treatment

Treatment of individual poisons

Table 29.1 shows the toxicity of the substances which are most frequently taken accidentally by children under 5. The frequency of ingestion of substances has been assessed from data from Craft et al (1984).

Management of deliberate poisoning in older children

Deliberate poisoning in older children should be treated differently from accidental poisoning in younger children. These children form one end of the age spectrum of overdose in adults and such children are more likely to take significant amounts of poison. Substances that can be regarded as having intermediate toxicity when taken accidentally should be regarded as potentially toxic when taken deliberately.

Poisoning in older children should be recognized as a serious symptom and an indication of child and family disturbance. Children who deliberately take poisons show more disturbed family relationships than children referred for psychiatric help for other reasons. They have a high level of psychiatric symptoms, especially depression.

All children who take poisons deliberately should be admitted to hospital and should be assessed by a child or adolescent psychiatrist. Many will need educational, psychological and social work help as well as psychiatric assessment.

CHRONIC POISONING

Lead poisoning

Lead is a serious poison for children. Its toxic effects are due to its combination with sulfhydryl groups of essential enzymes resulting in disturbances in carbohydrate metabolism, cell membrane transport, renal tubular absorption and other body processes. The blood level at which toxic effects become evident varies from child to child but in general major symptoms are unlikely if the whole blood lead level is less than 2.5 μmol/l (52 μg/100 ml). It is probable that behavioral and learning difficulties may result from exposure to only moderately elevated lead levels between 1.4 and 2.9 μmol/l (Faust & Brown 1987). Low level fetal lead exposure at less than 1.4 μmol/l may also affect mental development (Dietrich et al 1987).

Children in the United Kingdom may be poisoned by sucking or chewing lead paint. Lead from burning batteries, lead shot for fishing and lead from old water pipes are other potential sources. Children from the Indian subcontinent may be poisoned by *surma*, the lead-containing eye make-up used even in young babies.

Clinical features

Children who are poisoned by lead are likely to present with pica (compulsive eating of substances other than food), anorexia, abdominal pain, irritability and failure to thrive. Severe lead poisoning may present with neurological symptoms including drowsiness, convulsions and coma from lead encephalopathy. Lead poisoning may also present as progressive intellectual deterioration.

The diagnosis is made by elevated blood lead levels and anemia with hypochromia and basophilic stippling. There may also be increased bone density with transverse bands at the ends of the long bones on radiological examination.

Treatment

The source of lead should be identified and removed. Chelating agents should be used to form non-toxic lead compounds. In mild cases D-penicillamine should be used orally in two daily doses of 10 mg/kg. In severe cases sodium calcium edetate (EDTA) should be used, 40 mg/kg by i.v. infusion over 1 hour twice daily for up to 5 days. Each gram of EDTA should be diluted in 100 ml normal saline. The effectiveness of EDTA can be enhanced by the deep i.m. injection of dimercaprol 2.5 mg/kg 4-hourly for 2 days, 2–4 times on the third day, then 1–2 times daily until recovery.

Mercury poisoning

This once common disorder was called 'pink disease' because of the color of the extremities or 'acrodynia' because of the accompanying pain. It was largely due to the use of mercury-containing teething powders which have now been withdrawn. There was anorexia, loss of weight and hypotonia as well as the characteristic painful red or pink extremities. A differential diagnosis of this condition is the red extremities of neglected children. Treatment of mercury poisoning is by the deep i.m. injection of dimercaprol 5 mg/kg 4-hourly for 2 days, 2.5 mg/kg twice daily for the third day and once daily for the next 10 days.

Chronic boric acid poisoning

Chronic boric acid poisoning was a major problem in the 1940s and 1950s. It was caused by ingestion of boric acid used either as a treatment for nappy rash or as a pacifier. It presented with convulsions, vomiting and diarrhea.

NOTES ON POISONING WITH INDIVIDUAL SUBSTANCES
(Craft et al 1984, Scherger et al 1988)

Intermediate toxicity

Medicines

Cough medicines. Most cough medicines do not cause serious symptoms in the doses available to children. Medicines based on antihistamines may cause drowsiness and anticholinergic effects. Drowsiness will usually not need treatment but if coma occurs resuscitative measures should be used. Medicines based on codeine should be regarded as potentially toxic.

Fluoride. Fluoride has a rapid action but is seldom toxic in the quantities taken by children. Symptoms include vomiting, nausea and abdominal pain.

Ibuprofen. Ibuprofen and other non-steroidal anti-inflammatory agents only seldom cause symptoms in children. Symptoms may include gastrointestinal irritation, kidney and liver damage. Oral fluids should be encouraged.

Laxatives. Serious symptoms after laxative ingestion are rare. If diarrhea occurs it occurs quickly. Occasional patients may need intravenous fluids. The child should be observed for serious symptoms for a short time.

Lignocaine gel. Local anesthetics such as lignocaine are toxic in overdose, causing convulsions and circulatory collapse. Significant amounts of lignocaine gel are seldom ingested accidentally by children.

Paracetamol elixir. Paracetamol elixirs such as Calpol are sweet and sickly in large doses and serious accidental poisoning is very rare. There is insufficient paracetamol in most small bottles of elixir to cause problems. Blood levels should be checked 4 hours after the ingestion if more than 150 mg/kg has been taken. Treatment (see potential toxicity section below) is only needed if the serum paracetamol level is above 200 mg/l at 4 hours (or in rare delayed cases in children above 50 mg/l at 12 hours). In most cases children can be discharged after a period of observation.

Salbutamol. There may be peripheral vasodilation, muscle tremors and agitation. Serious symptoms are rare although severe hypokalemia and arrhythmias have been seen.

Household products

Alcohol-containing perfumes, cologne and aftershave. Symptomatic cases are rare. Asymptomatic children can be allowed home after a short period of observation to make certain they do not become drowsy.

Bleach. Ingestion of household bleach causes fewer problems than would be expected (Craft et al 1984). Ipecac or lavage should not be used. Milk or antacids can be given orally. Local lesions in the mouth can be treated symptomatically and in the few cases where significant esophageal involvement is possible, endoscopy can be undertaken.

Detergents (anionic). Dishwashing liquid and shampoo are only toxic in large doses. Vomiting occurs in large doses. A period of observation may be needed.

Disinfectants. Serious cases are unusual.

Nail varnish remover (acetone). Observation for a period should be all that is needed but nausea and vomiting may occur, going on to coma if large amounts are taken.

Paints (oil based). Unless the paint has lead in it, the only problems that occur are caused by the petroleum distillate base. The stomach should not be emptied. In practice children do not seem to take significant amounts.

Pyrethrins. These insecticides are not usually a hazard if ingested or inhaled accidentally. The child should be observed for a short period.

Rat or mouse poison. The common ingredients of rat or mouse poison (warfarin or dichlorolose) are usually non-toxic in the doses taken by children. The exact type of poison should be identified using the poisons center and in most cases the child can be sent home after a short period of observation.

If large amounts of warfarin are ingested vitamin K can be used but this is not needed in most cases.

Talc. Talc is only toxic if inhaled. It may cause retching and choking due to pulmonary edema. Cases of ingestion only need a short period of observation to make certain inhalation did not occur.

Window cleaner. Most are non-toxic unless aspirated. The cleaner should be identified using the poisons center. In most cases the child can be sent home after a short period of observation.

Plants

Berberis. Very occasionally causes confusion, epistaxis or vomiting. The child should be observed for a short period.

Fuchsia. Unlikely to cause problems although potentially toxic. Observe for a short period.

Holly. Unlikely to cause problems although potentially toxic due to ilicin and theobromine.

Pyracantha. This causes nausea and vomiting but is unlikely to cause problems. The child should be observed for a short period.

Potential toxicity

Medicines

Barbiturates. May cause coma and hypotension. Cases are becoming less common, as they are less frequently prescribed. Activated charcoal can be used.

Benzodiazepines – tranquillizers and hypnotics such as diazepam (Valium) and nitrazepam (Mogadon). These can cause drowsiness and coma, but problems are unusual in accidental ingestion. In very young children respiratory depression may need treatment with artificial ventilation.

Carbamazepine. This drug has some anticholinergic activity. Paradoxically convulsions and violent reactions may occur as well as cardiac problems such as heart block. Activated charcoal is useful to adsorb carbamazepine.

Codeine-containing cough medicines. If significant amounts are taken there can be respiratory depression, for which the antagonist naloxone can be used (10 µg/kg i.v.)

Clonidine. Clonidine can cause bradycardia, hypotension, coma and gastrointestinal upset. The use of atropine and dopamine infusion for the hypotension is controversial and supportive treatment (including assisted ventilation) may be adequate for even the most severe cases (Yagupsky & Gorodischer 1983).

Digoxin. Digoxin can be a serious poison in children, with only a few tablets being fatal. Activated charcoal is useful. These children should be monitored very closely, probably in an intensive care unit, with careful ECG monitoring. Beta-blockers such as propranolol should be used in severe cases, with atropine if there is heart block. The serum potassium should not be allowed to go too low or too high. Digoxin-specific antibody fragments are now available for the reversal of life-threatening overdosage (Digibind, Wellcome).

Diphenoxylate (the active constituent in Lomotil, the antidiarrheal agent). This compound has an opiate-like action, which causes prolonged respiratory depression. Treatment is with the opiate antagonist naloxone (10 µg/kg as i.v. bolus). There may be a transient improvement followed by relapse and cases should be observed for at least 36 hours and repeated doses of naloxone given as necessary.

Hyoscine. Hyoscine may cause dilated pupils, dry mouth, tachycardia and delirium due to anticholinergic effects. Observation will be all that is needed with most patients.

Iron. Iron is a potentially very serious poison, initially causing vomiting and hematemesis, but going on to acute gastric ulceration and shock. Later convulsions and cardiac arrhythmias may occur. Iron tablets may be detected by X-ray of the abdomen. Further treatment should be aimed at preventing additional absorption of the iron, by the use of the chelating agent desferrioxamine methylate, instilled into the stomach (5–10 g in 50–100 ml of liquid). Desferrioxamine should also be used parenterally (15 mg/kg/hour to a maximum of 80 mg/kg) in all cases where a potentially toxic amount of iron may have been taken. The severity of a poisoning episode can be judged by the serum iron level. Levels above 16.1 mmol/l at 4 hours indicate significant poisoning.

Mefenamic acid (Ponstan). This drug rarely causes problems in young children. Activated charcoal is effective. Convulsions can be treated with diazepam.

Metoclopramide (Maxolon). In overdose this drug causes extrapyramidal signs, drowsiness and vomiting. If extrapyramidal signs develop antiparkinsonian drugs such as procyclidine can be used.

Mianserin (Bolvidon). Mianserin has milder anticholinergic effects than the tricyclic antidepressants. Serious problems are uncommon. Drowsiness is the most common symptom.

Paracetamol (acetaminophen). Serious accidental ingestion of paracetamol is rare in children because the tablets are bitter and difficult to swallow and the elixir is too sweet to take in toxic quantities. Serious paracetamol poisoning may cause hepatocellular necrosis. Patients at risk of liver damage can be identified by measurement of blood levels 4 hours after the ingestion. Treatment is needed if the serum paracetamol level is above 1.32 mmol/l (200 mg/l) at 4 hours (or in rare delayed cases in children, 0.33 mmol/l at 12 hours) (Rumack & Matthew 1975). Treatment is with oral methionine (at a dose of 1 g 4-hourly) for four doses. *N*-acetylcysteine intravenously is an alternative particularly in children who are vomiting or who present after 12–24 hours when methionine is ineffective.

Quinine. Quinine is a significant poison in children and has caused several deaths. It is used for night cramps. Quinidine and chloroquine are also toxic. Activated charcoal can be used.

Phenytoin. Phenytoin ingestion may cause ataxia and nystagmus. Activated charcoal can be used.

Salicylates. Severe poisoning is now rare as aspirin preparations are no longer used for children because of the dangers of Reye's syndrome. Hyperventilation is an early sign of significant salicylate poisoning due to stimulation of the respiratory center with resultant respiratory alkalosis. There may also be a metabolic acidosis. In severe cases there is disorientation and coma.

The severity of a poisoning episode can be judged by salicylate levels (Done 1960). Toxicity can occur at levels above 2.2 mmol/l (300 mg/l) in children. In asymptomatic and mild cases nothing more needs to be done apart from encouraging fluid and electrolyte replacement and giving vitamin K. Activated charcoal is useful. Forced alkaline diuresis can be used in moderate to severe cases but its use is controversial and alkalinization of the urine is the important thing rather than the induction of excessive urine flow. Peritoneal dialysis can also be effective.

Tricyclic antidepressants. Tricyclic antidepressants such as amitriptyline are serious poisons for young children. They may cause cardiac effects such as sinus tachycardia, hypotension and conduction disorders and death by their direct effect on the myocardium. There may be blurred vision and dry mouth from the anticholinergic effects. There may also be central effects of agitation, confusion, convulsions, drowsiness, coma and respiratory depression. Activated charcoal should also be used.

There is no specific antidote for tricyclic ingestion. The ECG should be monitored for cardiac arrhythmias. No treatment is indicated if there is adequate tissue perfusion and blood pressure. Metabolic acidosis should be corrected. Convulsions should be treated with diazepam. Life-threatening arrhythmias should be treated with propranolol. As tricyclics are protein bound active methods of elimination such as hemodialysis do not remove significant amounts of the drug.

Theophylline. Theophylline can cause restlessness, agitation, vomiting, convulsions, coma, hypotension, hypokalemia and ventricular tachycardia. Activated charcoal can be used. Convulsions can be treated with diazepam.

Household products

Alcoholic beverages. These may cause severe hypoglycemia. Blood alcohol levels are useful in management. Hypoglycemia should be detected by frequent blood glucose measurements, and prevented and treated by intravenous glucose infusions.

Acids. Acids tend to cause inflammation and ulceration at the pylorus rather than the esophagus. This may lead to stenosis (Rees et al 1986). Emesis or lavage should not be undertaken and chemical antidotes should not be given as the heat of the chemical reaction may increase injury. The extent of the injury should be assessed by endoscopy at an early stage. Steroids should be used to suppress the inflammation (prednisolone 2 mg/kg/day).

Alkalis. Alkalis such as caustic soda and dishwasher powder can cause burns to the mouth and esophageal ulceration, leading to stricture: review by esphagoscopy and treatment with steroids have improved the outlook for this condition. Emesis or lavage should not be undertaken, nor any chemical antidotes as the heat of the reaction may increase injury. The extent of the injury should be assessed by endoscopy at an early stage. Steroids should be used to suppress the inflammation (prednisolone 2 mg/kg/day).

Camphor and camphorated oil. These are dangerous poisons for children. They are absorbed quickly and because they are lipid soluble, enter the brain causing delirium, rigidity, coma and convulsions. Convulsions should be treated with diazepam.

Disk or button batteries. Mercury cell, alkaline manganese and silver cell batteries contain a strong alkali (usually potassium hydroxide) as a main ingredient. Mercury cell batteries contain toxic amounts of mercury. Silver cell batteries generally contain less toxic ingredients than the other types. Worn batteries are less toxic than new ones.

Disk batteries can cause problems if they lodge in the gut and become corroded and release their contents. They may cause ulceration or perforation from caustic injury if lodged in the esophagus or stomach (Votteler et al 1983) and should be removed endoscopically if they lodge there. If they go beyond the stomach they are usually passed without problem. Their progress should be monitored by abdominal X-ray. Mercury levels should be measured when appropriate. If the battery shows signs of leaking or breaking it should be removed surgically.

Bottle-sterilizing tablets. Bottle-sterilizing tablets contain a bleach-like substance (sodium dichloroisocyanurate). They effervesce with water to make a sterilizing solution. If this reaction takes place in the mouth considerable damage can take place with edema and ulceration. Cases need to be monitored for their airway patency and intravenous fluids may be needed. Monitoring for esophageal involvement by endoscopy may be needed in some cases. The use of steroids is logical in severe cases.

Cetrimide. Cetrimide is a cationic detergent and can be caustic when concentrated. Mucklow (1988) describes caustic burns in babies accidentally fed a dilute antiseptic solution containing cetrimide and chlorhexidine. The stomach should not be emptied. If problems with ulceration occur steroids should be used. Cetrimide may also have depolarizing muscle-relaxing effects leading to breathlessness.

Carbon monoxide. Hemoglobin has an affinity for carbon monoxide over 200 times greater than for oxygen. Carboxyhemoglobin will reduce the amount of hemoglobin available to carry oxygen and also hinders oxygen release. The incidence of carbon monoxide poisoning has fallen since house gas no longer contains this substance. Carbon monoxide poisoning should be treated with 100% oxygen over a period of several hours. Hyperbaric oxygen should be considered in severe cases if it is available.

Essential oils. Essential or volatile oils contain mixtures of cyclic hydrocarbons, ethers, alcohols and ketones. They include turpentine, pine oil, citronella and eucalyptus as well as such things as Karvol capsules. Their toxicity varies, with real turpentine (not to be confused with turpentine substitute) being very toxic. Symptoms of essential oils include vomiting, drowsiness and convulsions. Ipecac should not be used.

Methylene chloride (*paint stripper*). This is a very serious poison for children. It is caustic and may cause damage to skin, stomach, mucous membranes and pharynx. Vomiting, dizziness, confusion, toxic myocarditis and hemoglobinuria may occur. Methylene chloride is metabolized to carbon monoxide and carboxymethemoglobin concentrations may be elevated for several days. The stomach should not be emptied. Fluids should be given to dilute the methylene chloride. High-flow oxygen should be given if carboxyhemoglobin is present.

Organochloride insecticides. These include DDT, dieldrin and lindane. Symptoms include excitability, muscle twitching and convulsions. Activated charcoal is valuable.

Organophosphorus insecticides. A wide range of compounds which include malathion. They act by inhibiting cholinesterase in the blood. Symptoms include confusion, nausea, vomiting, wheezing and convulsions. If symptoms appear atropine (i.v.) 0.05 mg/kg and pralidoxime 20–60 mg/kg as required, depending on the severity of the poisoning, should be given by slow i.v. injection and repeated if needed.

Paradichlorobenzene mothballs. Most cases of accidental ingestion do not have serious symptoms. Ingestion may cause nausea and vomiting and cyanosis may develop due to methemoglobinemia. This should be treated with methylene blue.

Paraquat. Paraquat weedkiller is available in two forms: a concentrated form (Gramoxone) available only to farmers and horticulturists and a granular form (Weedol) which contains only 2.5% paraquat. Accidental ingestion of the concentrated form is rare and ingestion of the granular form rarely causes serious problems. Paraquat causes local ulceration and in severe cases a proliferative alveolitis. Treatment should be to prevent absorption by Fuller's earth or bentonite.

Petroleum distillates, *e.g. kerosene*, *turpentine*, *white spirit and turpentine substitute*. These substances may cause a pneumonitis from lung aspiration. Ipecac or lavage should not be used. Kerosene poisoning is a particular problem in the Third World. Rhonchi are the most common physical sign and X-ray changes are common. Treatment in mild cases is symptomatic, together with the use of prophylactic antibiotics. Corticosteroids are often used, but clear evidence of their effectiveness is lacking. Severe cases may need oxygen and intensive respiratory care.

Phenolic compounds. These include cresols, menthols, phenols and hexachlorophene. Coal tar vaporizing solution contains cresol. They may cause local corrosive damage and there may be cerebral symptoms. Activated charcoal can be used.

Slug pellets (*metaldehyde*). Slug pellets contain about 3% metaldehyde which is toxic in children and 4 g is said to be fatal for a child. Experience suggests that problems do not arise after accidental ingestion. The child should be observed for 4–6 hours to check for serious symptoms such as flushing, salivation and convulsions. Convulsions should be treated with diazepam.

Plants

Arum lily. Causes gastrointestinal side-effects and later CNS manifestations.

Deadly nightshade (*atropa*). This plant has an atropine effect causing photophobia, visual disturbance, dryness of mouth, flushed skin, etc. If there are symptoms a slow intravenous injection of physostigmine can be used.

Philodendron (*Swiss cheese plant*) *and Dieffenbachier*. This plant has a local caustic action due to oxalic acid and may cause a sore mouth and laryngeal edema. Steroids may be useful in severe cases.

Laburnum. Causes vomiting, diarrhea and nausea. Although quite commonly taken, serious problems are very rare (Bramley & Goulding 1981).

Yew. Causes gastrointestinal side-effects and later CNS manifestations. There may be severe hypotension.

ACCIDENTS TO CHILDREN

MORTALITY FROM ACCIDENTS

Accidents to children are important to the pediatrician. They are the most frequent cause of children dying over 1 year of age and thus are a challenge to any efforts to reduce mortality in childhood. In 1992, 559 children under 14 years died in England and Wales from injuries and poisoning (Table 29.2). Nearly twice as many children aged 5–14 years die from accidents as from malignant disease.

Road traffic accidents remain the most frequent cause of accidental death in children. Particularly important are deaths to child pedestrians but many children die on bicycles and in cars. Deaths from conflagrations and complications of burns and scalds have been highlighted with house fires due to foam furniture. They cause just under 100 deaths a year in England and Wales.

Table 29.2 Accidental deaths from injuries and poisoning England and Wales 1992 0–14 years

Cause	M	F	Total
Transport accidents	185	96	281
Accidental poisoning	6	4	10
Accidental falls	29	8	37
Medical misadventure	2	3	5
Fire and flames	47	35	82
Environmental	2	4	6
Accidental drowning	34	13	47
Inhalation	9	8	17
Mechanical suffocation	35	6	41
Others	22	11	33
Total	**371**	**188**	**559**

Nearly 50 children die each year from drowning (Table 29.2). There has been a reduction of the number of children dying from accidental causes over the years. For instance, the mortality rates for children aged 1–14 years have been reduced in England and Wales from over 200 children per million in 1931 to under 100 children per million in 1984 (Child Accident Prevention Trust 1989). This is probably due to improvements in the environment and the general care of children as well as better treatment.

MORBIDITY FROM ACCIDENTS

Accidents are a significant cause of handicap in children. Head injuries, which may follow pedestrian, cycle or passenger road traffic accidents, falls or child abuse are the major cause of handicap following injury. Children may be also brain damaged following near drowning or suffocation episodes. Cosmetic damage following burns, scalds and road traffic accidents may be psychologically damaging to the child. The child may be scarred by remembering the actual accident or from the effects of the subsequent hospital admission and treatment.

Childhood accidents are a frequent cause of attendance at accident and emergency departments. We recently found that one child in four attends our accident department in a year. On this basis it can be estimated that 2.33 million children attend an accident and emergency department annually. Although the majority of these injuries are relatively trivial, amongst them there are serious injuries. Twelve percent of children attending an accident and emergency department have fractures (Sibert et al 1981).

Childhood accidents are also a frequent cause of admission to hospital. Between 5% and 10% of the children who attend hospital require admission. In 1985 this proportion amounted to about 120 000 children in England and Wales (Department of Health and Social Security 1987).

WHERE TO TREAT CHILDHOOD ACCIDENTS?

Children should be treated in the best possible environment after an accident and if this is the accident and emergency department, it should not be hostile to the child. Children should not be managed in the same areas as seriously ill, violent or disturbed adults and this means separate waiting areas and accommodation. Such areas should have a bright, welcoming decor with toys. This can be provided at low cost in most accident and emergency departments (Richmond et al 1987).

GENERAL PRINCIPLES IN TREATING CHILDHOOD ACCIDENTS

Injured children may need the care of many separate medical specialties. After a road traffic accident, for instance, a child may need orthopedic surgeons, pediatric surgeons, plastic surgeons, neurosurgeons and anesthetists as well as the pediatrician. There should be a multidisciplinary co-ordinated approach between everyone looking after these children. In some cases, such as after head injuries in children, clear plans for patterns of care need to be discussed and agreed in advance.

The interests of the whole child and family after an accident should not be forgotten. Children can be emotionally scarred not only by the accident itself but by painful and insensitive treatment. Parents often feel guilty after an accident and may anyway have been under stress before the accident. Follow-up of children should pay attention not only to the injury itself but also to the psychological sequelae. Particular attention to reintegration into school may be required.

ETIOLOGICAL FACTORS IN CHILDHOOD ACCIDENTS

Social factors are important in childhood accidents. Road traffic accidents are five times more common in children whose fathers come from social class V compared to children from professional families and the death rate in boys aged 0–14 years from fires is 15 times higher in social class V than social class I (Office of Population Censuses and Surveys 1988). Similar social class gradients are seen in other accidents to children with disadvantaged children having more accidents. The reasons are complex. Poorer families usually live in more dangerous environments; for example, it is much easier for a child to have a road accident if his house opens straight onto a main road in the inner city than if he lives in a detached house with a garden. Pyschosocial stress factors are also involved in the etiology of many childhood accidents. Road traffic accidents are commoner in families under stress and accidental childhood poisoning was found to be strongly related to family stress factors. The children of mothers who are psychiatrically disturbed have an accident rate nearly four times higher than control children. In New Zealand accidents are twice as common in families with a life events score over 12 compared to those with a score under 4 (Beautrais et al 1982).

The question of personality in childhood accidents and whether children can be accident prone is difficult. It is much more likely that accident proneness is related to the environment, both physical and social, rather than to personality factors. It is probably more correct to speak of an accident-prone community than an accident-prone child.

PREVENTION OF CHILDHOOD ACCIDENTS

The prevention of accidents is an important public health issue. They are unlikely to be prevented by campaigns covering all accidents but well-researched multidisciplinary action on individual types of accidents may be successful. In preventing a particular type of accident a methodological approach is needed: looking first at the size and nature of the problem, then deciding what preventive solutions are possible, implementing them on a small scale and then introducing them more widely when they have proved to be effective.

There are three main strategies for accident prevention: education of children and parents, changing the environment and enforcing changes in the environment by law. Research suggests that whilst in some fields, such as teaching children to swim, education is important, most successes in accident prevention have followed environmental changes and that educational campaigns by themselves are only of limited value.

Environmental change in child accident prevention

Environmental change can prevent accidents. This has been shown in the use of child-resistant containers to prevent childhood poisoning, child safety seats to prevent injury in passenger car accidents, fencing private swimming pools to prevent drowning and by flameproofing of nightdresses to prevent burns. Sometimes an environmental measure, such as seat belts for cars, is effective but is not fully used by the population and has to be enforced by law.

Health education and childhood accidents

A number of studies have shown that education campaigns to prevent accidents to children by themselves are ineffective. A program directed at the parents of children to reduce home accidents (the Rockwood County study) made no difference in accident rates between control and target families. There was little evidence that the 'Play it Safe' television programs made any impact on accident rates in children (Sibert & Williams 1983). An education campaign with posters and literature in Cardiff only sensitized the population to trivial accidents (Minchom & Sibert 1984). There is evidence, however, that health visitors visiting the home giving specific attention to accident prevention can make a difference in the way that families behave, in particular with regard to the installation of safety equipment.

Health education therefore must be directed either on a one-to-one basis by people such as the health visitor or general practitioner or to educate public opinion to institute environmental change. For instance, parents can be educated that safe playground equipment is needed for their children. They can then press the local authority to act.

Action on childhood accidents

In 1977 Court and Jackson were instrumental in the formation of the Child Accident Prevention Trust (CAPT). The Trust brings many disciplines together to foster research and action on accidents to children: there are similar groups in other parts of the world.

As well as national action on accident prevention local action is needed. In Sweden, public health physicians led by Stangstrom from the Karolinska Institute in Stockholm developed the concept of local action through the concept of Safe Communities. Projects in Sweden using this approach reduced accidents by as much as 20% (Schelp 1987). The First World Injury Control Conference in 1989 approved a manifesto for Safe Communities: 'Safety – a universal concern for all' (WHO 1989). The Second World Conference in Atlanta confirmed this.

The basis of any program of injury control is surveillance. This needs close liaison between the community pediatrician and the accident department. Once an accident has happened it may happen again. For instance, a dangerous balcony which allowed a fall should be repaired straight away, together with others like it.

ACCIDENTS TO CHILDREN AT PLAY AND RECREATION

Playground injuries

Play is vital for children in their physical development and their ability to make social relationships. Although children do play at home and in organized groups, many play in playgrounds provided by local authorities and private organizations. Playgrounds provide an alternative to playing in dangerous places such as the road and need to be as safe as possible. However, there is evidence that playgrounds may be dangerous places for children. In Cardiff, about 1.5% of child hospital attendances are due to injuries sustained in a playground (Mott et al 1994). A few children die each year in playground accidents.

There has been much work in developing safer equipment and surfaces and in producing acceptable safety standards (BS 5696 and BS 7188). This work has been summarized by Heseltine et al (1989). Swings, slides, climbing frames and roundabouts are all commonly involved in playground accidents. They all can be designed for better safety. Impact-absorbing surfaces have been introduced to lessen the severity of a head injury from falling from equipment onto a hard surface (Chalmers et al 1996). These may be either bark, sand or special impact-absorbing rubberized tiles. However, recent criticisms of these surfaces include a lack of proven studies of their effectiveness and their high cost (Ball & King 1991).

Mott et al (1994) reviewed playground injuries in Cardiff. They found children injured on public playgrounds have a high hospital admission rate and fracture rate compared to other types of injury. Although taking injuries as a whole the bark-surfaced playgrounds were safer, significant numbers of children sustain fractures on bark surfaces from falls from equipment. There are many possible variables in playground injuries:

- type of equipment
- type of surface
- height of equipment
- numbers of children playing
- type of play of the children
- maintenance of the surface
- maintenance of the equipment
- weather
- supervision.

These factors are interlinked and the playground should be considered as a whole when preventive strategies are attempted. There is some evidence from Mott et al (1994) and from work in New Zealand that height of equipment may be one of the important variables as well as the surface.

Influencing playground design

The Consumers' Association (1988) found that in a sample of playgrounds in England and Wales there was evidence of bad design, poor maintenance, little safety surfacing and plentiful litter. Pediatricians will wish to influence playground safety in their districts by lobbying the local authority.

Sports and recreational injuries

All forms of sport and recreation have some risk. The whole ethos of preventing injuries to children during sport and recreation is a difficult one. Clearly, one cannot protect children from all risks in recreational activity, which is important in physical development and the development of personality. On the other hand, one does not want to expose children to unnecessary risk.

There has been little research on the risks of various sports, in particular whether rugby or soccer are dangerous for boys. A study in Wales (Hughes et al 1986) suggested that rugby may cause more injuries than soccer, in particular to the upper part of the body. There is also the danger of neck injuries and paraplegia with rugby.

There are few recreational activities that do not have some risk, but this risk can be reduced by sensible supervision and other safety measures. Hill and mountain climbing expeditions need careful supervision by experienced guides and teachers if disasters are to be prevented. Rugby teams should be of similar age and ability and referees should pay particular attention to collapsing the scrum.

DOG BITES

Dog bites to children are extremely common and as many as 1 in 100 children a year presents to an accident and emergency department with this problem (Sibert et al 1981). In an American study 20% of children (most under 5 years of age) were reported by their parents to have been bitten by a dog. German shepherds (Alsatians) were the commonest breed of dog involved. In America and Britain, many of the accidents occur in the home or with dogs well known to the children. However, a significant number of children are bitten in public areas, particularly play areas.

The majority of dog bites are minor, but severe lacerations, particularly facial lacerations, may occur. There are a few deaths, mainly children exposed to guard dogs. There has also been concern about potentially dangerous breeds of dog kept in the home.

Significant dog bites should be debrided and sutured. It is usual to give tetanus prophylaxis, but routine antibiotics are not needed. In many countries, particularly in India, the danger of rabies is present.

HORSE ACCIDENTS

Horse riding is a common leisure pursuit, particularly in girls around puberty. Horse-riding accidents are one of the few types of accident that are more common in girls than boys, with the peak incidence in 10–14-year-olds. The few deaths each year usually result from severe head injuries. They do not usually reach double figures in England and Wales.

Just under half of horse accidents arise from a fall leading to head injuries, limb fractures and occasionally spinal injuries. Some children get kicked and some are crushed by horses falling on them. Horses also sometimes bite and butt children and tread on their feet.

Many accidents to children on horses are caused by inexperience on the part of the rider, particularly when the horse is startled in traffic. Injury during competitions is rare. Good supervision and teaching are important in prevention and horse and rider should be matched. Good head protection is vital in preventing serious head injury. Many traditional riding hats offer little protection for the rider. In April 1984 a new British Standard, BS 6473, for protective hats was introduced. The importance of wearing such protection cannot be overemphasized.

BURNS AND SCALDS IN CHILDREN

Injuries from burns and scalds occur particularly in children under 5 years old from deprived backgrounds. They remain a significant cause of death in childhood, second only to road traffic accidents; 82 children died in England and Wales in 1992. The vast majority died in conflagrations in private dwellings. Many die from gas and smoke inhalation rather than by direct heat. There have been striking changes in the number of children who have died from burns and scalds in recent years. A major component of the reduction has been the fall in the number of deaths from the ignition of clothing following flameproofing regulations and the reduction of open fires.

As well as being an important cause of death in childhood, burns and scalds cause significant morbidity from long-term scarring and psychological damage. Over half the admissions to hospital from thermal injuries are caused by scalds, most of which are in children under 5. Children are scalded most commonly from a cup or a mug but significant numbers are scalded from teapots and kettles and from hot bath water. Bath scalds are usually caused by unsupervised children falling in the bath (Yeoh et al 1994) but the differentiation between accident and abuse can be difficult.

As well as in house fires, children are burnt from small igniting sources such as matches, outdoor fires, space heating and cooking equipment. Firework accidents have been reduced with the discontinuation of certain types of fireworks, the restriction in the minimum age of people to whom fireworks are sold and the limitation of time fireworks are available in the shops to a few weeks before 5 November.

Background factors to burn and scald accidents to children

There is little doubt that psychosocial factors are involved in burn and scald accidents to children. Mortality has been as much as 15 times higher in social class V boys than social class I boys. With house fires there is a strong relationship between non-owner occupation, population density and children in care. National cohort studies have also confirmed heavy social class gradients in morbidity from burn and scalds, with poorer families being more liable to these accidents. There is a strong correlation with lack of hot water and overcrowding in the housing.

Disadvantaged families live in environments where smoking is common, where there are open fires and where there is inflammable furniture, making them more liable to burns and scalds. These families are also under psychosocial stress, making supervision of young children difficult.

The prevention of burn and scald accidents to children

Burn accidents may be prevented by stopping the source of the fire and also by reducing the flammability of the child's environment. Many conflagrations are caused initially by smoking. Reducing smoking will also reduce house fires. The abolition of strike-anywhere matches would reduce the ability of young children to ignite a match. Accidents involving open fires have fallen with the introduction of central heating but they still remain a problem with poor families. Fireguards should be used with young families and should conform to BS 6539.

Injuries and deaths due to flammability of nightdresses have lessened with the Night-dress (Safety) Regulations in 1967. These injuries can be reduced still further by extending the regulations on night-dress safety (BS 5722) and by reducing the number of open fires.

Many children have died in house fires because of the flammability of upholstered furniture and from the toxic fumes produced when it burns. There is now legislation to ban the foam which causes dangerous fumes and replace it with a safety foam. The full effects of this legislation will take many years to come through because of the long life of furniture in homes. Smoke detectors are widely used in the United States and found to be effective (US Fire Administration 1980). They are becoming more established in Britain and their use should be encouraged both in public buildings and private housing.

The prevention of scalds in children is more difficult. A wider use of mugs and the elimination of unstable cups should be encouraged. A number of children injure themselves from spillage from kettles and these injuries can be avoided by the use of coil or short electric kettle flexes without large expense. Some children scald themselves by pulling saucepans down from cookers, incidents which could be prevented by reducing access to the cooker and by using cooker guards. Bath scalds could be prevented by reducing the temperature of the hot water in domestic systems so these accidents cannot occur (Yeoh et al 1994). This can be done in two ways: reducing the thermostat temperature in domestic hot water tanks and, more expensively, by thermostatically controlled mixer taps.

ARCHITECTURAL ACCIDENTS AND FALLS

There has been an increasing recognition that safety is an important consideration in the design of homes where children live. Many falls, glass accidents and burns can be prevented by good design. A dialog between architects and those treating accidents on safer design for children in new houses is needed. Practical design guidelines are now available (Child Accident Prevention Trust 1986).

Falls

Falls cause a significant number of deaths in childhood (37 in England and Wales in 1987) and are also the commonest cause of presentation to the accident and emergency department (Department of Trade 1987, Sibert et al 1981). They have a varied etiology. They may be on one level, such as falling on the pavement, at home or in the school playground. These may occur as a result of unruly behavior and better supervision of play is perhaps the only answer to prevent these injuries which are rarely fatal. Indeed, although such falls are a common presentation to a hospital (19%) there were no fatal falls on one level in an analysis of 253 fatal falls in children aged 0–14 years in England and Wales between 1975 and 1985 (Nixon et al 1987).

Falls can also be from one level to another. Younger children may be dropped (7.5% of fatal falls), fall from furniture (18% of fatal falls) or fall down the stairs (17% of fatal falls). The danger of falls from baby walkers has been highlighted and they can no longer be advised for children's use (Glendill et al 1987). Older children fall from trees, cliffs and mountains, play equipment and buildings. Poor window catches and design allow a number of accidents, particularly in high-rise flats. The introduction of safety catches or window guards will reduce these. In New York City a program providing free window guards (The Children Can't Fly Program) has been successful in preventing window falls in a poor area of New York.

Falls downstairs are a particular problem for toddlers (Nixon et al 1987). Much can be done to prevent them, by better stair design and stair gates. The use of stair gates can be encouraged by the health visitor, and a Safe Community program. Open stairs with wide gaps between balustrades may be esthetically beautiful, but are dangerous for young children. In 1985 building regulations were changed to make certain that a 100 mm sphere could not be passed through any opening or guard to a flight of stairs.

Glass injuries

Falls through glass may cause severe lacerations to hands, wrists and arms, and occasionally the face. Severe damage may result from injury to arteries, nerves and tendons, and internal injuries may also be found, with the bowel sometimes protruding from the abdominal wall. There are a few deaths each year, usually from uncontrolled arterial bleeding. There are also cases of scarring and permanent disability from nerve damage.

The child is usually injured by glass in doors or by low-level glazing. A typical story would be a child falling downstairs into a glass door. The sharp, jagged parts of the glass may cause severe lacerations to any parts of the body, particularly the upper limbs. First aid to severe bleeding from glass injuries is best done by pressure on the wound, using a pad after the glass has been removed. In some cases, quite extensive surgery is needed.

The whole problem of glass injuries in childhood could be prevented by the use of safety glass. There are a number of types of glass or plastic that can be used in building. Annealed flat glass breaks easily into shards and annealed wire glass cracks easily with exposed wires. Safety glass is either laminated, which absorbs impact and is resistant to penetration, or toughened tempered glass which shatters into small cuboid pieces. Other safe alternatives to annealed flat glass are polycarbonate sheet or plastic safety film. Laminated glass is only about 1.8 times more expensive than annealed flat glass. Safety glass is covered by the building regulations.

ROAD TRAFFIC ACCIDENTS

Road traffic accidents (RTAs) cause more deaths in children than any other type of accident. This presents a major challenge in prevention and treatment to all those who work in the field.

Pedestrian road traffic accidents

Pedestrian road traffic accidents are particularly common in the inner city and in children from socially deprived families. Fatality rates are correlated with the prosperity of the area. Psychosocial stress is an important factor in road traffic accidents and the interaction of a poor environment with stress is probably involved in many accidents.

Children under 10 years are particularly at risk from pedestrian RTAs. Boys between 5 and 8 years are at maximum risk. Parents may overestimate the ability of their children to handle traffic and let them go out on the road unsupervised. Children under the age of 8 are not able to estimate the speed or dangers of traffic. The behavior of children up to 9 years old is immature and marked by inability to foresee dangerous situations (Kohler & Ljungblom 1987). Sharples et al (1989), looking at deaths from head injuries in the northern region, found that 72% of these deaths occurred between 3 p.m. and 9 p.m. and mostly to boys playing after school.

Education and child pedestrian road traffic accidents

It is possible to teach some 6-year-old children elementary traffic rules in an artificial situation and when they know they are being observed but a large number of children do not learn them and it may be these children that have accidents. In Britain it was suggested that the Green Cross Code prevented accidents when it was introduced but analysis of the figures suggests this was not the case. Safety and traffic education are unlikely by themselves to prevent road traffic accidents (Roberts et al 1994).

Environmental change and child pedestrian road traffic accidents

The most important means of preventing pedestrian road traffic accidents is by modification of the environment. Residential areas can be redesigned to give priority to pedestrians and to separate them from traffic. The speed of traffic can be reduced by speed bumps and safe crossings can be provided. The 'Woonerf' schemes introduced in the Netherlands are good examples of what can be done. The provision of play areas will reduce the number of children on dangerous streets. The Safe Community approach is a way of introducing traffic calming.

Passenger accidents

The protection of children in cars from serious injury and death must be an important part of any child safety program whether on a national, local or individual level. A major part of such protection is the development of child-restraint systems and seat belts.

Much of the research on seat belts has been on adult passengers. There is good evidence that seat belts are effective in preventing death and serious injury but the educational campaigns used to persuade people to wear them were generally unsuccessful. Serious injuries fell by 20% following the 1983 legislation compelling the wearing of seat belts in front seats. There is evidence that child-restraint systems also prevent injury and death. The Transport and Road Research Laboratory (TRRL) found that no child died in a 2-year period when in a restraint whereas 264 non-restrained children were killed in that time. Serious injuries are much less common in restrained children. These differences are less pronounced in younger children. Child-restraint systems have the unexpected bonus of improving children's behavior and this probably improves driving standards.

Restraint systems in use

The best restraint depends very much on the age of the child. Carriers for babies less than 10 kg have been developed which are portable seats that can be fixed in the car with an adult safety belt. These have proved convenient and safe and restrain the baby directly. Their wider use can be encouraged by loan schemes.

Children between 10 and 18 kg should have a child car seat. These can be fixed directly to the car by two- or four-point anchorage or adult seat belts. Many good designs are now available. For children from 18 to 36 kg adult seat belts should be used with a booster cushion. These are as safe as child harnesses. A survey in Cardiff (Richmond et al 1989) has shown that only 47% of children under 9 months and 26% of older children are appropriately restrained in cars. There is legislation to insist that if cars are fitted with rear seat belts and children are carried, approved safety seats or belts have to be used.

Bicycle injuries

Bicycles play an important part in the life of most children, particularly boys between 3 and 12 years. Bicycle injuries are a significant cause of death and disability in children. In England and Wales in 1991 36 boys and 10 girls died from collisions of pedal cycles with motor vehicles (OPCS 1992). We showed in a study in Cardiff that 1 in 80 boys have a bicycle head injury severe enough to be admitted to hospital in childhood (Clarke & Sibert 1986). There are factors in bicycle design which are vital to safety; for example, the high-rise bicycle that was introduced into Britain in the late 1960s and early 1970s had features that made it more dangerous than standard models.

The prevention and reduction in severity of bicycle injuries may involve education and environmental change. Children's bicycle safety courses should include proper maintenance of chain, gear and brakes. Parents should be encouraged to give thought to the type of bicycle they buy for their child and to the use of protective clothing and helmets. The use of helmets is now accepted as a key part of preventing bicycle injuries. There are at least five case control studies that show the effectiveness of cycle helmets in preventing head injury:

- Thompson et al (1989) in Seattle. Cyclists had a 85% reduction in their risk of head injury by wearing helmets.
- Malmaris et al (1994) from Cambridge found there was a protective factor of 3.25 for wearing helmets.
- Thomas et al (1994) from Brisbane, Australia, showed a reduction of bicycle head injuries of 63% by the use of helmets.
- McDermott et al (1993) in Victoria, Australia, found head injury was reduced by 45% by approved helmets.
- Spaite et al (1991) from Tucson, Arizona, found the mean injury severity score much greater in those not wearing helmets.

DROWNING AND NEAR-DROWNING IN CHILDHOOD

Drowning is the third most common cause of accidental death in children in the UK. In 1988 and 1989 306 children had confirmed submersion incidents, 149 dying and 157 surviving after near-drowning (Kemp & Sibert 1992), 10 of whom sustained severe neurological deficit. The majority were less than 5 years of age. Many near-drowning cases admitted to hospital are seriously ill and have to be admitted to the intensive care unit.

The annual incidence in England and Wales of submersion accidents for children under 15 years of age was 1.5 per 100 000 with a mortality rate of 0.7 per 100 000. Many more boys drown than do girls which reflects the very different behavior patterns of boys. Boys under 5 had the highest incidence of submersion, 3.6 per 100 000. In Los Angeles County drowning death rates are as high as 1 : 8000 in boys aged 2–3 years (O'Carroll et al 1988). There are also very heavy social class gradients, with disadvantaged children more likely to drown. One mode of drowning that does not follow this pattern is death in private swimming pools.

Sites of drowning (Table 29.3)

Children can drown indoors and outdoors, and in deep or shallow water. Drowning and near-drowning in childhood can be divided by the site where the injury takes place, each site having a definite age range (Kemp & Sibert 1992, Nixon et al 1986) and corresponding to a stage in child development: babies who cannot protect themselves when they fall in bath water, toddlers who wander off and older children who die whilst swimming.

Bath drownings

Bath drownings occur in the babies. They can drown in quite shallow water and should not be left unattended. The possibility of non-accidental drowning should be remembered in young children (Kemp et al 1994a). Kemp and her colleagues found that accidental bath drownings were confined to children under 2.

Garden pond drownings

Garden pond drownings occur in toddlers. Children can drown in quite small shallow ponds. The commonest story is of an unsupervised toddler in a neighbor's garden or when visiting friends or relatives. Toddlers can also drown in pails, farm slurry pits, cattle troughs and puddles.

Domestic and private swimming pools

Toddlers and young children are also in danger when wandering off unsupervised into domestic swimming pools. Unsupervised children may either fall into the pool or crawl under the covers. These drownings are a particular problem in warm affluent countries. Children may also drown in private pools without supervision in hotels and holiday camps.

Public pools

Deaths from public pool drownings are a minor problem in the United Kingdom following health and safety regulations introduced in 1985 which insist that there is a high level of supervision of children in such pools (Health and Safety Commission 1988). Drownings in public pools are at a level of one per year in the UK, a tribute to the level of supervision (Kemp & Sibert 1992). Many of the children who are admitted to hospital

Table 29.3 Cases of drowning in children under 15 years of age in UK 1988–9 grouped according to site of incident (141 notified in 1988, 165 in 1989) (Kemp & Sibert 1992)

	Survivors near-drowning	Drowning deaths	Total	Mean age
Bath	19 (1)*	25	44	1 year 2 months
Garden pond	48 (4)*	11	59	1 year 10 months
Domestic pool	15 (2)*	18	33	2 years 4 months
Private pool	10	8	18	5 years 9 months
River, canal, lake	17 (2)*	56	73	6 years 10 months
Public pool	30 (1)*	2	32	7 years
Sea	9	20	29	7 years 10 months
Other	9	9	18	4 years 2 months
Total	157 (10)*	149	306	

* Survivors who sustained severe neurological handicap.

after nearly drowning in public baths have had effective poolside resuscitation.

Rivers, canal, lakes and sea

Drowning in rivers, canals and lakes is predominantly a problem of older boys who play unsupervised and get into trouble in deep water (Kemp & Sibert 1992). Many are non-swimmers. These boys correspond to the boys in Australia who drown in creeks. A few children drown at sea in England and Wales, some from falling into docks, some lost at sea in boating accidents and some drowned from the beach.

Pathophysiology of drowning and near-drowning

The excellent prognosis for some children rescued from apparent death has encouraged a better understanding of the pathophysiology of drowning. The majority of deaths from drowning, even amongst competent swimmers, occur within 10 meters of a safe refuge. This suggests that some physiological disturbance associated with the initial immersion is in many cases responsible for incapacitation. There may also be some pathological reason why a child drowns, such as epilepsy.

The survival of some children after a long period of immersion may be due to the vestigial diving reflex (active in diving mammals) where the peripheral circulation is shut down with a profound bradycardia and the brain receives the majority of the cardiac output. There is work to show, however, that the diving reflex is not active in humans (Ramey et al 1987). Harries (1986) has suggested that survival for prolonged periods under water is because the circulation fails as a secondary event sometime after the immersion and because of the protective effect of hypothermia. Orlowski (1988) has used the term 'ice water drowning' rather than 'cold water drowning' as a review of the world's medical literature revealed that all the cases with a good outcome after very prolonged immersion occurred in water with a temperature of 10°C or less. This suggests also that it may be the hypothermia that is protective.

Complications and sequelae of near-drowning

There is some controversy over how many children suffer severe brain damage after resuscitation following a near-drowning episode. Studies in the USA (Peterson 1977, Frates 1981) have shown that fixed dilated pupils and coma predicted those patients who would die or have neurological deficit after severe submersion incidents. These studies may have referred to children drowning in the relatively warm pools found there.

In contrast, in Britain some children do survive normally after severe submersion incidents despite being admitted to hospital unconscious with fixed dilated pupils (Kemp & Sibert 1991). Of 64 nearly drowned children unconscious on admission, 31 had normally reactive pupils and all but three (all of whom had severe pre-existing neurological disease and had secondary drowning complications) made a full recovery. Of the 33 patients with fixed dilated pupils on admission 10 children made a full recovery, 13 died and 10 sustained severe neurological deficit in the form of a spastic quadriplegia with profound learning difficulties. Spontaneous respiratory effort on admission was associated with normal survival. Pupils that remained dilated after 6 hours admission and fits continuing 24 hours after admission predicted a poor outcome. The prognosis for near-drowning episodes in warm water seem worse than for those occurring in cold or ice water (Orlowski 1988, Bolte et al 1988). Many children who have had a severe hypoxic episode following near-drowning will develop cerebral edema which may contribute to the ultimate brain damage suffered by these casualties.

Salt and fresh water drowning

There has been discussion about different mechanisms occurring in salt and fresh water drowning in children because of experimental animal data showing hemolytic crises following aspiration of fresh water in large volumes into the lungs. In practice, much smaller volumes are aspirated by humans and fears of hemolytic crises have proved to be unfounded. It may be that secondary drowning is more serious in salt water than in fresh water. The differences between salt and fresh water drowning in children are less important than those between warm and cold water drowning.

Aspiration pneumonia

A proportion of children who nearly drown aspirate water and develop a pneumonia with secondary infection. This is rarely a serious complication unless the child has developed brain damage.

Secondary drowning

Secondary drowning is a phenomenon in which respiratory deterioration occurs with pulmonary edema, between 1 and 72 hours after the original incident. Harries (1986) suggests that this complication occurs only in the first 24 hours and approximately 5% of near-drownings are affected. There may be a worse prognosis in salt water than in fresh water near-drownings. The alveolar membrane dysfunction is probably due to surfactant deficiency and should be treated by adequate intermittent positive pressure ventilation. The value of corticosteroid treatment is unproven, but they are often prescribed.

Treatment

The aims of treatment of a nearly drowned child are to restore adequate ventilation and circulation, prevent further heat loss and to correct acid–base status. Apart from correcting the acidosis directly these can usually all be achieved at the waterside. Simple first aid with mouth-to-mouth resuscitation, covering and warming are vital. Many children may vomit during resuscitation so it is important to insure a clear airway throughout the resuscitation procedure. As some apparently dead children may recover fully from near-drowning episodes, it is wise to attempt to resuscitate all apparently dead, drowned children. This is particularly the case in cold or ice water.

All children who may have inhaled water should be admitted to hospital. The presence of crepitations is helpful in deciding whether there has been aspiration. Children who have adequate ventilation and no apparent sequelae should be reviewed for 24 hours for signs of secondary drowning and supraventricular cardiac arrhythmias. They should have chest physiotherapy. Secondary drowning should be treated by positive end expiratory pressure and intermittent positive pressure ventilation.

Severely ill children who cannot maintain adequate oxygenation initially should be admitted to an intensive care unit where they can be mechanically ventilated. Those children who have neither respiration nor cardiac output should be ventilated, have external cardiac massage and have their acidosis corrected.

If the core temperature is below 28°C consideration should be given to slow rewarming although 'the optimal treatment of these children is unproven' (Orlowski 1988). The effect of hypothermia, barbiturate therapy and monitoring and regulating intracranial pressure in hypoxic/ischemic brain injury has been studied by Bohn et al (1986). They found that these measures provided little benefit and recommended that therapy should be directed at maintaining cerebral perfusion and adequate oxygenation.

Children who appear dead after exposure to drowning at very low temperatures should not be pronounced brain dead until they have been brought up to a near normal core temperature.

Prevention

Most drowning accidents occur with children too young to be able to swim. Preventing bath accidents in babies should be part of the health visitor's program of education with mothers. It should be emphasized that it is unsafe to leave young children unsupervised in the bath even for short periods. Mothers should also be told about the dangers of drowning in garden ponds and families with young children are well advised to fence or cover these. Much could be done to insist on protecting children from access to these ponds particularly in garden centers. There is evidence that fencing which prevents children from having access to domestic pools with self-shutting gates can prevent drowning. In Canberra, private swimming pools have to be fenced by law but there was no such legal sanction in Brisbane at the time of one study: only one child died in the Australian capital from a swimming pool accident over a 5-year period, compared with 55 in Brisbane. Fencing has now been introduced by regulation into Australia, South Africa, New Zealand and parts of the US. We still await such legislation in the UK.

To be unable to swim probably increases the risk of drowning. Teaching children to swim may reduce the number of deaths among 5–14-year-olds. Certainly, there has been an overall fall in the number of deaths of children from drowning which has coincided with better swimming training. A number of older children drown whilst swimming unsupervised in rivers, lakes and creeks: this unsupervised swimming should be discouraged but is impossible to prevent. The reduction in serious drowning in public swimming pools incidents with health and safety regulations has been most welcome (Kemp & Sibert 1992). This supervision at the waterside should remain a high priority for local authorities and should be extended to private pools and open water where swimming is common.

Life jackets and buoyancy aids are important in helping to prevent children who use boats and canoes from drowning if they fall overboard. Getting children to wear them is difficult but boat and canoe clubs can insist that their members wear them.

Accidental suffocation, choking and strangulation in childhood

Accidental mechanical asphyxia is a significant cause of death in children. Nixon and his colleagues (1995) reviewed deaths registered as choking, suffocation or strangulation in a total population study for the 2 years 1990–1991 in England and Wales. There is of course a differential diagnosis with deliberate suffocation.

Nixon et al found an overall annual incidence of 0.7 per 100 000 children at risk with two modal peaks at less than 1 year of age and in the early teenage years because of boys being found hanged. Twenty-one children died from choking, 12 on food, nine on non-food items. Thirty-nine children died from inhalation of vomit with 21 of these being associated with medical conditions. Twenty-eight children suffocated with a modal age for suffocation of 5 months. Nineteen occurred in beds or cots. Seven of these were in bed clothes or mattresses. Forty-eight children died from strangulation, of whom 35 children hanged. Younger children were strangled by ribbons and cords holding dummies (3), venetian blind cords (3), clothing and accessories (4) and in five cases by poorly maintained cots.

Some of these incidents are not true accidents and there may be problems of classification, with inhalation of vomit as an injury, non-accidental injury and the coexisting diagnosis of SIDS. The group of older boys found hanging are probably mainly not true suicide.

The numbers of children choking on food and dying emphasizes the importance of supervision whilst children eat. Few children now suffocate on a toy and that emphasizes the importance of European Standards for Toy Safety. Children may die by strangulation when in cots. Parents of young children should be discouraged from using poorly maintained cots, telephone wires or window cords near cots or necklaces or dummy cords when in cots.

THE SUDDEN INFANT DEATH SYNDROME (SIDS)

DEFINITION AND HISTORICAL PERSPECTIVE

Sudden unexpected deaths in infancy have been recognized since antiquity. Historically, many were attributed to overlaying, and in some countries legislation was enacted in an attempt to prevent babies being taken into bed with parents, particularly if they had been drinking alcohol (Norvenius 1995). In some societies parents were accused of infanticide. During the 20th century, as more babies in Western countries slept in cots, and overall infant mortality rates fell, it became clear that certain infant deaths, unexpected by history, remained unexpected after detailed post-mortem examination (Templeman 1892, Limerick 1992). Whilst a small proportion of such deaths were (and remain) a result of deliberate parental actions, in most there is no suspicion of such actions, and the consistent epidemiological features of the condition (e.g. age incidence, seasonality) make such a cause inherently very unlikely for the great majority (National Advisory Body for CESDI 1996).

In 1969, at a conference in Seattle, a definition was drawn up for the sudden infant death syndrome (SIDS):

The sudden death of an infant or young child, which is unexpected by history and in which a thorough post-mortem examination fails to demonstrate an adequate cause for death.

Many subsequent attempts have been made to improve upon this definition, particularly emphasizing the need for a review of the clinical history and the circumstances of death. At the 3rd SIDS International Meeting in Stavanger in 1994 a modified definition was proposed, which whilst retaining the inherent simplicity of the original definition, includes caveats to cover these concerns:

The sudden death of an infant, which is unexplained after review of the clinical history, examination of the circumstances of death, and post-mortem examination.

Whilst the cause or causes of such deaths remain unknown a more precise definition is unlikely to be achieved (Rognum & Willinger 1995).

The human definition, that of a family who put a loved and apparently healthy baby down to sleep only to find him or her a few minutes to a few hours later dead with no adequate explanation for the death even after detailed investigation, is the one with which the clinical pediatrician must struggle to cope and try to provide comfort and support to the family.

INCIDENCE

The reported incidence of SIDS varies widely between countries and over time. During the 1970s the incidence apparently rose in the United Kingdom and many other Western countries. This rise was attributed to diagnostic shift, in that the diagnosis of SIDS was not a registerable cause of death in the United Kingdom until 1971. Throughout the 1980s the incidence of SIDS in the United Kingdom remained between 1.6 and 2.2 per 1000 live births. In some countries (e.g. New Zealand) the rates were consistently higher, at 3–4 per 1000 live births, and in others (e.g. Hong Kong) much lower, at 0.2 per 1000 live births or less. The recognition in the late 1980s of the contributory role of prone sleeping position, and the implementation in many countries of campaigns to reduce the risk of SIDS (see below) has led to a remarkable fall in incidence, to 0.7 in the United Kingdom, and 1.4 in New Zealand. In the USA the rate, which had remained static between 1.2 and 1.4 per 1000 live births, has fallen after a risk reduction campaign to approximately 0.8 (provisional figure for 1995: National Institute of Child Health and Human Development, Washington DC).

EPIDEMIOLOGY, RISK FACTORS AND RISK REDUCTION CAMPAIGNS

Epidemiological features of SIDS

A number of characteristic and consistent features of SIDS have emerged from studies in various countries over the past 30 years, notably a characteristic age distribution, with very few deaths in the first 2 weeks after birth, a peak at 2–3 months and less than 10% of deaths occurring after 7 months; an excess of deaths in male babies and (until recently) a marked seasonality, with more deaths in the winter months, particularly in temperate or colder regions. This excess of deaths in the colder months, when the incidence of viral upper respiratory tract infections is highest, has led to an interest in the role of infection in the etiology of SIDS. Whilst most babies who die suddenly and unexpectedly have been apparently well in the preceding few days, an increased proportion compared to matched control infants have had signs or symptoms suggestive of minor viral infection (Gilbert et al 1990, Cole et al 1991). In a population-based case control study of the role of viral infection in SIDS, Gilbert et al (1992) did not find a significant excess of viral infections in the infants who died, but found that the combination of heavy wrapping and the presence of a viral infection was a major risk factor. A number of studies have found that recent immunization *reduced* the risk of SIDS (Mitchell et al 1995).

The association between infant mortality and socioeconomic deprivation has been recognized since the 19th century, and the marked excess of SIDS in the most deprived groups in society has been noted in several epidemiological studies, though this pattern is not significantly different from other causes of infant mortality (Taylor & Sanderson 1995, Spencer 1996). SIDS occurs within all socioeconomic groups, but certain factors have consistently been found to be associated with increased risk, notably young maternal age, high parity, maternal smoking or drug abuse, short gestation, low birthweight for gestation, multiple births and male sex. Such factors, whilst of value in identifying populations at increased risk of SIDS, and thus potentially suitable for inclusion in studies of possible pathophysiological processes, are not (with the exception of smoking and drug abuse) within the power of the parents to change, and are thus of limited value in any attempt to reduce the incidence of the condition. Certain other factors (e.g. breast or bottle-feeding, maternal alcohol intake) may act as markers of lifestyle or socioeconomic status, and have less consistently been found to have independent effects on the risk of SIDS (Fleming et al 1996). Whilst considerable attention has been focused on the subsequent siblings of SIDS victims as a group at increased risk of SIDS, large scale population-based studies have not confirmed a significantly increased risk for such infants independent of environmental or childcare factors (which are likely to remain constant within families, and may thus lead to an apparently increased risk for successive infants in the same family) (Irgens et al 1993).

A family history of a previous unexplained infant death or of recurrent apparent life-threatening episodes may be suggestive of an underlying abnormality of physiology or a metabolic disorder, but may also raise the question of imposed upper airway obstruction or other form of abuse (National Advisory Body for CESDI 1996) (see also Chapter 12, Apparent Life-Threatening events).

Potentially modifiable factors

Over the past decade attention has increasingly been given to a number of factors in the infant's pre- and postnatal environment which affect the risk of SIDS and *are* potentially amenable to change. Studies in Hong Kong, Holland, England, New Zealand and Australia have shown the strong association between the prone sleeping position and the risk of SIDS (Lee et al 1989, Jonge et al 1989, Fleming et al 1990, 1996, Beal & Finch 1991, Mitchell et al 1994). Heavy wrapping, a warm environment, soft bedding and covers which can slip over the baby's head have all been implicated as risk factors (Fleming et al 1990, 1996, Ponsonby et al 1993, Kemp et al 1994, Wilson et al 1994, Williams et al 1996). These studies have drawn attention to the importance of pre- and postnatal exposure to tobacco smoke as a risk factor for SIDS (Mitchell 1995, Blair et al 1996). In New Zealand, but not in the UK, breast-feeding had a protective effect independent of associated sociocultural factors (Ford et al 1993, Gilbert et al 1995, Fleming et al 1996). Bedsharing by parents with their baby was initially identified by the New Zealand cot death study group as a risk factor for SIDS, but more detailed analysis of their data showed that this was only the case for parents who smoked (Scragg et al 1993, 1995). These findings have subsequently been confirmed by studies in the United Kingdom and in the USA (Klonoff-Cohen et al 1995, Fleming et al 1996). The work of McKenna (McKenna et al 1993), an anthropologist who has studied the interactions between mothers and babies during bedsharing, raises the possibility that under certain circumstances these interactions may be protective, and reduce the risk of SIDS.

Risk reduction campaigns

The recognition of the apparent importance of the potentially modifiable risk factors led in the late 1980s and early 1990s to the introduction in several countries (e.g. New Zealand, the UK, Australia, Holland, Norway) of campaigns to change infant care practices in order to reduce the risk of SIDS (Stewart et al 1993a). Such campaigns have all included attempts to stop babies being placed in the prone position to sleep, and information on the adverse effects of exposure to tobacco smoke. Some have included advice on avoiding overheating, illness care, promotion of breast-feeding and avoidance of bedsharing. These campaigns have all been followed by a dramatic fall in the incidence of SIDS, which has been largely attributed to the avoidance of the prone sleeping position (Wigfield et al 1992, Mitchell et al 1994, Irgens et al 1995, Dwyer et al 1995, Wigfield & Fleming 1995). In the USA, the implementation of a concerted risk reduction campaign did not occur until 1994, but preliminary data show a significant fall in the SIDS rate by the end of 1995 (see above).

SIDS after a risk reduction campaign

Few studies have so far been published on the epidemiology of SIDS after risk reduction campaigns, but data from the Confidential Enquiry into Stillbirths and Deaths in Infancy (Fleming et al 1996, Blair et al 1996, National Advisory Body for CESDI 1996) show that in the UK, whilst some factors remain unchanged (e.g. male preponderance), others have changed significantly (e.g. there has been a marked reduction in the seasonal occurrence). The time that the death was discovered in this study was between 5 and 10 a.m. for almost 70% of the deaths. With the marked reduction in prevalence of prone sleeping, the overall incidence of SIDS has fallen (as noted above), but for those infants put down to sleep prone the risk of SIDS remains approximately eight times higher than for those who are supine. The side sleeping position, whilst safer than the prone position, carries approximately twice the risk of the supine position. The use of bedding (particularly duvets), which can slip over the baby's head was found to be a major risk factor. Exposure to tobacco smoke, either before or after birth, is now identified as the single largest potentially avoidable factor, with a population attributable risk estimated at 60% (i.e. it may be responsible for this proportion of the deaths).

The evidence linking some of the risk factors and SIDS is now very strong, amounting in the case of sleeping position and parental smoking to evidence of a *causal* relationship. This is not to say that all (or even a high proportion of) babies put to sleep prone or exposed to tobacco smoke will die as SIDS, but that these factors exert their effects somewhere in the pathway of causality, so that removing the factor will have a major influence on the incidence of SIDS. The ways in which risk factors are related to the process or processes which lead to death are largely unknown, though a number of hypotheses have been proposed.

PATHOLOGY AND THE MEDICOLEGAL SYSTEM

In England and Wales all sudden unexpected deaths must be reported to the coroner, who will order that certain basic information be collected (usually by the police or the coroner's officer) and that a post-mortem examination be carried out. The coroner's main responsibility is to ensure that deaths due to non-natural causes are identified. In Scotland the Procurator Fiscal has a similar role to that of the coroner. The quality of the post-mortem examination has varied widely in the past, but the adoption in 1993 by the Royal College of Pathologists of a recommended minimum standard for such examinations has led to increased consistency and quality of post-mortems in the United Kingdom (National Advisory Body for CESDI 1996). The CESDI report and the Allitt enquiry (Clothier 1994) both strongly recommend that most if not all such examinations be carried out by pathologists with particular expertise in pediatric pathology. The CESDI Report also emphasized the importance of obtaining a detailed clinical history (usually by a pediatrician) from the parents of all infants dying suddenly and unexpectedly. This history should be obtained if possible *prior* to the post-mortem, as it may be of importance in helping to direct the pathologist's attention to particular features.

Understanding and interpretation of the available information for the family is helped by holding a multidisciplinary case discussion meeting a few weeks after the death, which should usually be attended by the pathologist, the general practitioner, the health visitor and the pediatrician. The value of such meetings has been emphasized by the Report of the Confidential Enquiry into Stillbirths and Deaths in Infancy (National Advisory Body for CESDI 1996).

At post-mortem examination or the multidisciplinary case discussion meeting, a proportion of infant deaths which were sudden and apparently unexpected are found to have a complete explanation (e.g. overwhelming infection, inborn error of metabolism, non-accidental injury). Such deaths, which together comprise between 10% and 30% of all sudden deaths in infancy, should not therefore be classified as SIDS, but as deaths due to the identified cause. For comparative purposes information should be collected on all unexpected deaths, including both SIDS and those deaths which were fully explained (National Advisory Body for CESDI 1996).

Certain other findings are relatively common, and, whilst not giving an explanation for the death, do suggest that the infant may not have been completely well before death (e.g. viral upper respiratory tract infection, otitis media). Such deaths do come within the definition of SIDS, but should be separately identified for purposes of classification (Gilbert et al 1992, National Advisory Body for CESDI 1996). In the remaining cases, no evidence of pathological processes which may have contributed to the death is identified, but certain features are commonly seen which are characteristic of babies dying as SIDS. Such findings include liquid heart blood, the presence of bloodstained fluid at the nose or mouth and petechial hemorrhages on the serosal surfaces of intrathoracic organs. Post-mortem hypostatic staining may give information on the position in which the baby died if the baby lay in this position for a number of hours after death. It is important that skeletal X-rays are carried out to look for possible bony injuries, and that samples are taken for detailed microbiological and histological examination. Electrolyte determination of the vitreous humor may identify biochemical abnormalities present at the time of death.

NORMAL DEVELOPMENTAL PHYSIOLOGY AND POSSIBLE PATHOPHYSIOLOGICAL PROCESSES

The precise series of events which occurs during sudden infant death is unknown; nor is it known whether there is a single final common pathway or a number of possible pathophysiological pathways. The characteristic pathological findings outlined above have been interpreted as suggesting that respiratory failure is the final event in the majority of cases, perhaps preceded by one or more episodes of tissue hypoxia of variable severity (Naeye 1980).

Recent evidence from infants who died suddenly and unexpectedly whilst undergoing cardiorespiratory monitoring and recording (Meny et al 1994) showed that, in these cases at least, the first abnormal event was a sudden severe, prolonged bradycardia, followed by cessation of breathing.

The observation by Steinschneider (1972) that prolonged episodes of apnea were recorded from some infants who had presented with apparent life-threatening events, and that such episodes were also identified in infants whose siblings had died as SIDS, led to the 'apnea hypothesis' of SIDS. This postulated that the final event in most, if not all, SIDS victims was apnea, and that infants at risk of dying in this way were likely to have repeated apneic episodes prior to death. Several large studies have failed to find any evidence to support this hypothesis, and Southall et al (1983), in a large, population-based prospective study, found that none of those infants identified as having episodes of prolonged apnea in the first week or at 6 weeks subsequently died as SIDS. None of the infants in this study who died as SIDS had previously shown prolonged apnea. Despite this lack of supporting evidence, the use of 'pneumograms' to identify infants with prolonged or frequent apnea, who were then deemed to be at increased risk of SIDS, was widespread, particularly in the USA until recently. The use of apnea monitors or more complex monitoring and/or recording devices (including measures of oxygenation) for infants identified by any technique as being at high risk of SIDS has not to date been shown to be of value in reducing the death rates for such infants (Keens & Ward 1993) though a large study (the CHIME study) currently under way in the USA may go some way towards resolving this question. Similarly there is no evidence that the use of apnea or other monitors is of any direct value in the care of subsequent siblings of infants who have died as SIDS (p. 1723).

The absence of supporting evidence for the 'apnea hypothesis' does not rule out a defect of cardiac or respiratory control as an underlying part of the pathophysiology of SIDS. A number of studies have shown apparent differences in cardiac or respiratory pattern between normal control infants and those who subsequently died as SIDS, though such differences are relatively subtle, and of no value in identifying individual infants at particular risk (Schectman et al 1988, 1989). The very strong association between SIDS and sleep or presumed sleep has led to the suggestion, supported by some experimental evidence, that a part of the final common pathway to death may be a defect in the process of arousal (Hunt 1989).

During the first few months after birth complex developmental changes occur in a number of physiological systems, including the control of respiration, and thermoregulation. The effect of spontaneous and imposed disturbances on the pattern of respiration changes with age; prolonged and highly oscillatory responses to spontaneous deep breaths or brief exposure to increased CO_2 are most common at around 2–3 months of age. The presence of spontaneous oscillatory patterns of breathing (periodic breathing) is a normal feature of respiration in infants, particularly at this age (Fleming et al 1988).

There are characteristic changes in the organization of the sleep–wake cycle over the same time period, with a marked increase in the amount of time spent in quiet sleep at around 8–12 weeks of age, and evidence that some infants who die as SIDS may have immaturity of these processes. Many physiological control systems behave differently according to the infant's sleep state, e.g. control of respiration, heart rate, arousal and thermoregulation (Schectman et al 1992, Azaz et al 1992).

There is an increase in daytime and a decrease in night-time rectal temperature during early infancy. Rectal temperature changes little during night-time sleep in the newborn period but around the age of 8–16 weeks a characteristic pattern appears, with a relatively abrupt fall to below 36.5°C soon after sleep followed by a plateau and then a gradual rise in the early morning prior to waking. This pattern develops earlier in infants who are breast-fed, female, first-born and from more affluent families; infants gaining weight most rapidly mature later (Lodemore et al 1992).

The insulation provided by bedding and clothing, and room temperature have only a small effect upon infant rectal temperature during nocturnal sleep. Bottle-feeding or parental smoking individually did not affect rectal temperature but in combination, bottle-fed babies exposed to smoke had rectal temperatures 0.1°C higher for the entire night. In infants sleeping at home, the prone position is associated with an increased rectal temperature for some or all of the night (Tuffnell et al 1995).

Daytime metabolic rate increases rapidly during early infancy (Azaz et al 1992) but little is known about nocturnal maturation during this period. By 3 months of age the infant excretes approximately 50% more heat per unit surface area than in the first week after birth. The 3-month-old infant is thus better adapted to dealing with cold stress than the newborn, but may be more vulnerable to the effects of heat stress (Fleming et al 1993).

In a prospective study of normal infants, the metabolic rate during infection varied with age. In infants less than 3 months of age the metabolic rate commonly fell at the time of an infection, and fever was unusual, whilst in older infants the metabolic rate usually increased, and fever was more common (Fleming et al 1994). In infants of all ages developing viral infections, the fall in temperature during the night was reduced 3–7 days before clinical signs of illness appear. During this prodrome parents often reported that their infants were 'not right'. When clinical signs of infection appeared the fall in rectal temperature during the night returned to that expected for the infant's age, and few infants became pyrexial (Jackson et al 1994). These observations suggest that changes of body temperature (and possibly metabolic rate) occur in the absence of significant clinical signs of illness and may fit with the concept of SIDS occurring in the prodromal phase of infection. This would fit the observations of recent signs or symptoms suggestive of infection but the lack of objective post-mortem evidence of established infection in many infants (Gilbert et al 1990, 1992, Cole et al 1991). The concept of unrecognized illness preceding death and possibly leading to reduced weight gain prior to death has been the basis for the use of weighing scales as a means of monitoring infant well-being and perhaps allowing early identification of such illness. However, Brookes et al (1994) did not find any evidence of poor weight gain preceding SIDS in a large population-based study.

Blackwell et al (1995) have suggested a possible mechanism by which the prone sleeping position, heavy wrapping and the presence of a viral infection might predispose to the development of a secondary bacterial infection, with release of inflammatory mediators, particularly tumor necrosis factor, into the pharynx, leading to rapid and potentially lethal development of shock.

Exposure to tobacco smoke before or after birth may impair the development of autonomic function (as assessed by the infant's blood pressure response to changes in position from horizontal to a 60% head-up tilt) (White et al 1995), and may also contribute to deficient arousal in infants during hypoxia (Lewis & Bosque 1995).

Inborn errors of metabolism, particularly defects of fat oxidation (e.g. medium chain acyl-CoA dehydrogenase deficiency, p. 1129), have been reported in a small proportion of infants dying suddenly and unexpectedly, but probably account for only 1–3% of the total of apparent SIDS deaths (Holton et al 1991).

One current view of SIDS envisages a 'triple-risk' model of the pathophysiology. This suggests that infants compromised by the effects of antenatal or perinatal factors (e.g. poor fetal growth, maternal smoking, perinatal asphyxia) may go through a period during their development in which one or more physiological system (e.g. respiratory or cardiac control, arousal, thermoregulation) is vulnerable. The effect of a stressor (e.g. infection, thermal stress, hypoxemia) during this vulnerable period may be to cause failure of the vulnerable system. SIDS would thus be seen as the result of exposure to an exogenous stressor(s), during a critical developmental period, in vulnerable infants. Such a model may allow understanding of the ways in which many apparently unrelated factors may combine to contribute to the risk of death, particularly in infants predisposed by prenatal factors such as poor fetal growth, exposure to tobacco smoke, etc. Such a model does not imply that all such deaths occur as the result of the same insult or follow the same pathophysiological pathway, nor does it imply that all infants who die will necessarily have been identifiably compromised in utero or in the perinatal period (Filiano & Kinney 1994).

SUPPORT FOR BEREAVED FAMILIES

The death of a child is perhaps the worst tragedy that can befall any family. To lose a child suddenly, unexpectedly and with no subsequent explanation for what happened may impose unbearable stress on parents, surviving siblings and the extended family. Because of the circumstances of the death, and the inevitable involvement of the coroner and/or the police, many families bereaved in this way suffer the additional torture of the spoken or unspoken suspicion that they may have, deliberately or accidentally, contributed to the cause of their baby's death. Families bereaved by the sudden unexpected death of their babies have special needs, which healthcare professionals must recognize and provide for. Almost inevitably, parents feel guilty because of some perceived imperfection which they recall in the way in which they cared for their infant. In their anxiety to reassure parents, healthcare professionals may sometimes fail to listen effectively to what the parents are trying to say. There is no point in reassuring parents that they did all the right things in the care of their baby unless you have first listened in detail to exactly what they did and what happened.

Bereaved parents need and deserve a sensitive, compassionate, caring approach from professionals. They need to be given time to be together as a family, perhaps for the last time, but should not be made to feel isolated by being left alone for long periods in a strange place such as an accident and emergency department. If resuscitation attempts have been made in the A & E department, it is important that doctors and nurses realize that it is not necessary to leave the endotracheal tube in place after death, unless there has been a concern that it was not correctly placed and that this contributed to the death. If this is the case, the tube can be cut off at the lips, and then gently pushed further down the trachea, so that it is not visible from outside. The pathologist will easily be able to identify the placement of the tube, and the parents will be able to see their baby's face fully. Parents must be given clear, simple information (preferably written) on what will happen, and what will be required of them (e.g. registration of the death). They need to know that a post-mortem examination will be performed, and they need to know, in sensitive terms, what that will involve. They need to know exactly where their baby will be, and when and how they will be able to see him or her.

As soon as possible after the death, often whilst parents are still holding their baby, in their home or in the accident and emergency department, they should be given the opportunity to talk at length about what has happened. Experience in the Avon Infant Mortality Study and the CESDI study (Stewart & Fleming 1993, National Advisory Body for CESDI 1996) has shown the importance of this initial sensitive but detailed 'debriefing'. This interview should usually be carried out by an experienced senior doctor (pediatrician or general practitioner) or senior nurse, and careful notes recorded immediately afterwards. Information obtained at this interview may be of particular importance to the pathologist, in helping to direct specific investigations at the post-mortem examination. It may also be of particular value in helping the parents to start to come to terms with the death of their baby. The parents may have particular questions or concerns about what they believe may have happened, and eliciting this information early may allow the pathologist to give an answer. Unless the circumstances of the death or the post-mortem findings are unusual or suspicious, the great majority of SIDS deaths are not followed by an inquest. Usually the coroner will issue a death certificate very shortly after the pathologist gives an initial report, which should usually be within 48 hours of the death.

If the baby who died was a twin, consideration should be given to whether the family would be helped by admitting the surviving twin to hospital for a few days. Whilst the real risk of death of the second twin is probably small, the family are likely to be very worried about this, and may find it easier to express their grief if they feel that the surviving twin is safe. For other families keeping the surviving twin at home may be important.

Arrangements should be made for an experienced doctor (usually a consultant pediatrician) to see the family again, preferably at home, with their general practitioner or health visitor, within a few days, to talk through the preliminary results of the post-mortem examination, to give information on what is known about SIDS, and to try to answer their questions. This meeting will also give an opportunity to talk about the effects of grief on the members of the family (including siblings and grandparents), and their close friends. It may be the first opportunity which the members of the primary care team have had to talk in detail about what has happened with the parents and to establish their very important role in providing continuing support. For most families at least one further visit from the pediatrician will be appropriate, again usually with a member of the primary care team. A recent study (Dent et al 1996) showed the importance of this follow-up from both the primary care team and the pediatrician, but showed that for the majority of families this support was not made available. As noted above, a multidisciplinary case discussion and future care planning meeting a few weeks after the death, attended by the pediatrician and the primary care team, at which the clinical history, post-mortem findings and special needs of the family are discussed is of great value, and should be implemented as a routine (National Advisory Body for CESDI 1996).

Parents should be given information on national and local parents' support groups* and on parent befriending schemes run by volunteers from those groups.

CARE OF THE NEXT INFANT

A further value of a multidisciplinary case discussion meeting is in planning appropriate care for the family should they decide to have a further baby. Approximately 80% of bereaved families have another baby within 3 years, and parents will be very worried about the risk to the next baby. The real risk of SIDS for the next baby is approximately the same as if the baby who died were still alive. That is not to say that the risk is the same as for the rest of the population, since many risk factors (particularly those relating to socioeconomic factors) will still be present.

Bereaved families should be given the opportunity to discuss their concerns and have their questions answered during a subsequent pregnancy, and to be seen on one or more occasions after the baby's birth by a pediatrician with a particular interest in the care of such infants. In many areas of the United Kingdom the CONI (Care of Next Infant) program of the FSID may provide some additional help for such families. As noted above, there is no evidence that the use of any type of monitoring device is of direct value to the baby, but as part of a support package for the parents the use of a monitor may be of value for some families (Stewart & Fleming 1993, Stewart et al 1993b).

---

* For example, the Foundation for the Study of Infant Deaths, London; the Scottish Cot Death Trust, Glasgow; the Irish Sudden Infant Death Association, Dublin; Cot Death Research, Weston super Mare, Somerset.

REFERENCES AND BIBLIOGRAPHY

Arena J M 1959 Safety closure caps. Journal of the American Medical Association 169: 1187–1188

Azaz Y, Fleming P J, Levine M, McCabe R, Stewart A, Johnson P 1992 The relationship between environmental temperature, metabolic rate, sleep state and evaporative water loss in infants from birth to three months. Pediatric Research 32: 417–423

Backett E M, Johnston A M 1959 Social pattern of road accidents to childhood. Some characteristics of vulnerable families. British Medical Journal 1: 409–413

Bacon C J 1990 The thermal environment of sleeping babies and possible dangers of overheating. In: David T J (ed) Recent advances in paediatrics. Churchill Livingstone, Edinburgh, pp 123–136

Balarajan R, Raleigh V S, Botting B 1989 Sudden infant death syndrome and postneonatal mortality in immigrants in England and Wales. British Medical Journal 298: 716–720

Ball D, King K 1991 Playground injuries: a scientific appraisal of popular concerns. Journal of the Royal Society of Health August: 134–137

Beal S M, Finch C F 1991 An overview of retrospective case control studies investigating the relationship between prone sleeping position and SIDS. Journal of Pediatrics and Child Health 27: 334–339

Beautrais A L, Fergusson D M, Shannon F T 1982 Life events and childhood mortality: a prospective study. Pediatrics 70: 935–939

Bithoney W G, Snyder J, Michalek J, Newberger E H 1986 Childhood ingestions as symptoms of family distress. American Journal of Diseases of Children P 139: 456–459

Blackwell C C, Weir D M, Busuttil A et al 1995 Infection, inflammation and the developmental stage of infants: a new hypothesis for the aetiology of SIDS. In: Rognum T O (ed) Sudden infant death syndrome. New trends in the nineties. Scandinavian University Press, Oslo, pp 189–198

Blair P, Fleming P J, Bensley D et al 1996 Smoking and sudden infant death syndrome: results of the 1993–5 case-control study for the confidential enquiry into stillbirths and deaths in infancy. British Medical Journal 313: 195–198

Bohn D J, Biggar W D, Smith C R, Conn A W, Barker G A 1986 Influence of hypothermia, barbiturate therapy and intracranial monitoring on morbidity and mortality after near-drowning. Critical Care Medicine 14: 529–534

Bolte R G, Black P G, Bowers R S, Thorne J K, Cornelli H M 1988 The use of extracorporeal warming in a child submerged for 66 minutes. Journal of the American Medical Association 260: 377–379

Bramley A, Goulding R 1981 Laburnum 'poisoning'. British Medical Journal 283: 1220–1221

Brookes J G, Gilbert R E, Fleming P J et al 1994 Postnatal growth preceding sudden infant death syndrome. Pediatrics 94: 456–461

Brown G W, Davidson S 1978 Social class, psychiatric disorder of mother and accidents to children. Lancet 1: 378–381

Chalmers D J, Marshall S W, Langley J D, Evans M J, Brunton C R, Kelly A, Pickering A F 1996 Height and surfacing as risk factors in falls from playground equipment: a case-control study. Injury Prevention 2: 98–104

Child Accident Prevention Trust 1986 Child safety and housing. CAPT, London

Child Accident Prevention Trust 1989 Basic principles of child accident prevention. CAPT, London

Clarke A J, Sibert J R 1986 Why child cyclists should wear helmets. Practitioner 230: 513–514

Clarke A, Walton W W 1979 Effect of safety packaging on aspirin ingestion by children. Pediatrics 63: 687–693

Clothier C 1994 The Allitt Enquiry: independent enquiry relating to deaths and injuries on the children's ward at Grantham and Kesteven General Hospital during the period February to April 1991. HMSO, London

Cole T J, Gilbert R E, Fleming P J, Morley C J, Rudd P T, Berry P J 1991 Baby check and the Avon Infant Mortality Study. Archives of Disease in Childhood 66: 1077–1078

Consumers' Association (Which) April 1988 Playground safety. CA, London

Coombs R R A, Holgate S T 1990 Allergy and cot death: with special focus on allergic sensitivity to cow's milk and anaphylaxis. Clinical and Experimental Allergy 20: 359–366

Craft A W 1983 Circumstances surrounding deaths from accidental poisoning. Archives of Disease in Childhood 58: 544–546

Craft A W, Lawson G R, Williams H, Sibert J R 1984 Accidental childhood poisoning with household products. British Medical Journal 288: 682

Dent A, Condon L, Blair P, Fleming P J 1996 A study of bereavement care after a sudden and unexpected death. Archives of Disease in Childhood 74: 522–526

Department of Health and Social Security/Office of Population Censuses and Surveys 1987 Hospital in-patient enquiry main tables. Series MB4 No. 27. HMSO, London

Department of Trade 1987 Home accident surveillance system. DoT, London

Department of Trade and Industry 1988 HASS data, personal communication

Dietrich K N, Krafft K M, Bornschein R L et al 1987 Low level fetal lead exposure effect on neurobehavioural development in early infancy. Pediatrics 80: 721–730

Done A K 1960 Salicylate intoxication. Pediatrics 26: 800–807

Dwyer T, Ponsonby A L, Blizzard L, Newman N M, Cochrane J A 1995 The contribution of changes in the prevalence of prone sleeping position to the decline in sudden infant death syndrome in Tasmania. Journal of the American Medical Association 273: 783–789

Emery J L 1986 Families in which two or more cot deaths have occurred. Lancet i: 313–315

Emery J L, Chandra S, Gilbert-Barness E F 1988 Findings in child deaths registered as sudden infant death syndrome (SIDS) in Madison, Wisconsin. Pediatric Pathology 8: 171–178

Faust D, Brown J 1987 Moderately elevated blood lead levels: effects on neuropsychological functioning in children. Pediatrics 8: 623–629

Feldman K W, Schaller R J, Feldman J A, Mcmillon M 1978 Tap water scald burns in children. Pediatrics 62: 1–7

Filiano J J, Kinney H C 1994 A perspective on neuropathological findings in victims of sudden infant death syndrome: the triple-risk model. Biology of the Neonate 65: 194–197

Fleming P J, Blair P, Bacon C, Bensley D et al 1996 The environment of infants during sleep and the risk of the sudden infant death syndrome: results of the 1993–5 case-control study for the confidential enquiry into stillbirths and deaths in infancy. British Medical Journal 313: 191–195.

Fleming P J, Gilbert R, Azaz Y et al 1990 Interaction between bedding and sleeping position in the sudden infant death syndrome: a population based case control study. British Medical Journal 301: 85–89

Fleming P J, Howell T, Clements M, Lucas J 1994 Thermal balance and metabolic rate during upper respiratory tract infection in infants. Archives of Disease in Childhood 70: 187–191

Fleming P J, Levine M R, Azaz Y, Wigfield R 1993 The development of thermoregulation and interactions with the control of respiration in infants: possible relationship to sudden infant death. Acta Paediatrica Scandinavica 389 (suppl): 57–59

Fleming P J, Levine M R, Long A M, Cleave J P 1988 Postneonatal development of respiratory oscillations. Annals of the New York Academy of Sciences 533: 305–313

Ford R P, Taylor B J, Mitchell E A et al 1993 Breast feeding and the risk of sudden infant death syndrome. International Journal of Epidemiology 22: 885–890

Frates R C 1981 Analysis of predicative factors in the assessment of warm-water near-drowning in children. Americal Journal of Diseases of Children 135: 1006–1010

Froggatt P, Beckwith J B, Schwartz P J, Valdes-Dapena M, Southall D P 1988 Cardiac and respiratory mechanisms that might be responsible for sudden death infant syndrome. Ideas for future research. Annals of the New York Academy of Sciences 533: 421–426

Gilbert R E, Fleming P J, Azaz Y, Berry P J, White D G, Orreffu V, Rudd P T 1990 Signs of illness in babies preceding sudden unexpected infant death. British Medical Journal 300: 1237–1239

Gilbert R E, Rudd P T, Berry P J, Fleming P J, Hall E, White D G, Orreffu V, James P P 1992 Combined effect of infection and heavy wrapping on the risk of sudden infant death. Archives of Disease in Childhood 67: 272–277

Gilbert R E, Wigfield R E, Fleming P J, Berry P J, Rudd P T 1995 Bottle feeding and the sudden infant death syndrome. British Medical Journal 310: 88–90

Gilbert R, Rudd P, Fleming P J et al 1991 Infection and overwrapping in sudden infant death. Archives of Disease in Childhood 66

Glendill D N S, Robson W V, Cudmore R E, Tavistock R R 1987 Baby walkers – time to take a stand. Archives of Disease in Childhood 62: 491–494

Golding J, Limerick S, Macfarlane A 1985 Sudden infant death. Patterns, puzzles and problems. Open Books Publishing, Somerset

Greensher J, Mofenson H C, Caraccio T R 1987 Ascendancy of the black bottle. Pediatrics 80: 949–951

Guilleminault C, Heldt G, Powell N, Riley R 1986 Small upper airway in near-miss sudden infant death syndrome infants and their families. Lancet i: 402–407

Gunn T R, Tonkin S L 1989 Upper airway measurements during inspiration and expiration in infants. Pediatrics 84: 73–77

Guntheroth W G 1989 Crib death. The sudden infant death syndrome, 2nd edn. Futura, Mount Kisco, NY

Guntheroth W G, Lohmann R, Spiers P S 1990 Risk of sudden infant death syndrome in subsequent siblings. Journal of Pediatrics 116: 520–524

Harries M 1986 Drowning and near drowning. British Medical Journal 293: 123–124

Health and Safety Commission 1988 Safety in swimming pools. Sports Council, London

Heseltine P, Holborn J, Wenger J 1989 Playground management and safety. National Playing Fields Association, London

Hill C M, Brown B D, Morley C J, Davis J A, Barson A J 1988 Pulmonary surfactant. II. In sudden infant death syndrome. Early Human Development 16: 153–162

Hoffman H J, Damus K, Hillman L, Krongrad E 1988 Risk factors for SIDS. Results of the National Institute of Child Health and Human Development SIDS Cooperative Epidemiological Study. Annals of the New York Academy of Sciences 533: 13–30

Holton J B, Allen J T, Green C A et al 1991 Inherited metabolic disease in the sudden infant death syndrome. Archives of Disease in Childhood 66: 1315–1317

Hoppenbrouwers T 1987 Sleep in infants. In: Guilleminault C (ed) Sleep and its disorders in children. Raven Press, New York, pp 1–15

Hughes D R, Evans R C, Sibert J R 1986 Sports injuries to children. British Journal of Accident and Emergency Medicine 1: 4–13

Hunt C E 1989 Impaired arousal from sleep: relationship to sudden infant death syndrome. Journal of Perinatology 9: 184–187

Illingworth C W, Brennan P, Jay A, Al-Rawif E R, Collier M 1975 200 injuries caused by playground equipment. British Medical Journal 4: 332–334

Irgens L M, Markestadt T, Baste V, Shrevder P, Skjaerven R, Oyen N 1995 Sleeping position and sudden infant death syndrome in Norway 1967–91. Archives of Disease in Childhood 72: 478–482

Irgens L M, Oyen N, Skjaerven R 1993 Recurrence of sudden infant death syndrome among siblings. Acta Paediatrica 389 (suppl 82): 23–25

Irgens L M, Skjaerven R 1986 Sudden infant death syndrome and post perinatal mortality in Norwegian birth cohorts 1967–1980. Acta Paediatrica Scandinavica 75: 523–529

Irgens L M, Skjaerven R, Lie R T 1989 Secular trends of sudden infant death syndrome and other causes of post perinatal mortality in Norwegian birth cohorts 1967–1984. Acta Paediatrica Scandinavica 78: 228–232

Jackson J A, Petersen S A, Wailoo M P 1994 Body temperature changes before minor illness in infants. Archives of Disease in Childhood 71: 80–83

Jackson R H 1981 Laceration from glass in childhood. British Medical Journal 283: 1310–1312

Jackson R H, Craft A W, Lawson G R, Sibert J R 1985 Changing pattern of poisoning in children. British Medical Journal 287: 1468

Johnson P 1988 Airway reflexes and the control of breathing in post-natal life. Annals of the New York Academy of Sciences 533: 262–275

Jonge G A, Engleberts A C, Koomen-Liefting A J M, Kastense P J 1989 Cot death and prone sleeping position in The Netherlands. British Medical Journal 298: 722

Keens T G, Ward S L 1993 Apnea spells, sudden deaths and the role of the apnea monitor. Pediatric Clinics of North America 40: 897–911

Kemp A M, Mott A M, Sibert J R 1994a Accidents and child abuse in bathtub submersions. Archives of Disease in Childhood 70: 435–438

Kemp A M, Sibert J R 1991 Outcome for children who nearly drown: a British Isles study. British Medical Journal 302: 931–933

Kemp A M, Sibert J R 1992 Drowning and near drowning in children in the United Kingdom. Lessons for prevention. British Medical Journal 304: 1143–1146

Kemp J S, Nelson V E, Thach B T 1994b Physical properties of bedding that may increase the risk of sudden infant death syndrome in prone-sleeping infants. Pediatric Research 36: 7–11

Kinney H C, Filiano J J 1988 Brainstem research in sudden infant death syndrome. Pediatrician 15: 240–250

Klonoff-Cohen H S, Edelstein S L, Lefkowitz E S et al 1995 The effect of passive smoking and tobacco exposure through breast milk on sudden infant death syndrome. Journal of the American Medical Association 273: 795–798

Knowelden J, Keeling J, Nicholl J P 1985 Post neonatal mortality. A multicentre study undertaken by the Medical Care Research Unit, University of Sheffield. HMSO, London, pp 1–82

Kohler L, Ljungblom B-A 1987 Child development and traffic behaviour. Traffic and children's health. Nordic School of Public Health, Stockholm

Learmonth A 1979 Factors in child burn and scald accidents in Bradford 1969–73. Journal of Epidemiology and Community Medicine 33: 270–273

Lee N N Y, Chan Y F, Davies D P, Lau E, Yip D C P 1989 Sudden infant death syndrome in Hong Kong: confirmation of low incidence. British Medical Journal 298: 721

Lewis K W, Bosque E M 1995 Deficient hypoxia awakening response in infants of smoking mothers: possible relationship to sudden infant death syndrome. Journal of Pediatrics 127: 691–699

Limerick S A 1992 Sudden infant death in historical perspective. Journal of Clinical Pathology 45 (suppl): 3–6

Lodemore M R, Petersen S A, Wailoo M P 1992 Factors affecting the development of night time temperature rhythms. Archives of Disease in Childhood 67: 1259–1261

MacCleary L 1989 Playgrounds – Leisure accident surveillance system (LASS). Consumer Safety Unit, Department of Trade and Industry

McClure R J, Davis P M. Meadow S R, Sibert J R 1996 Epidemiology of Munchausen syndrome by proxy, non accidental poisoning and non accidental suffocation. Archives of Disease in Childhood 75: 57–61

Malmaris C, Summers C L, Browning C, Palmer C R 1994 Injury patterns in cyclists attending an accident and emergency department: a comparison of helmet wearers and non-wearers. British Medical Journal 308: 1537–1540

McDermott F T, Lane J C, Brazenor G A, Debney E A 1993 The effectiveness of bicycle helmets: a study of 1710 casualties. Journal of Trauma 34: 834–844

McKenna J J, Thoman E, Anders T, Sadeh A, Schectman V, Glotzbach S 1993 Infant-parent cosleeping in evolutionary perspective: implications for understanding infant sleep development and SIDS. Sleep 16: 263–282

Meny R G, Carroll J L, Carbone M T, Kelly D H 1994 Cardiorespiratory recordings from infants dying suddenly and unexpectedly at home. Pediatrics 93: 44–49

Minchom P, Sibert J R 1984 Does health education prevent childhood accidents? Postgraduate Medical Journal 60: 260–262

Mitchell E A 1995 Smoking: the next major and modifiable risk factor. In: Rognum T O (ed) Sudden infant death syndrome. New trends in the nineties. Scandinavian University Press, Oslo, pp 114–118

Mitchell E A, Brunt J M, Everard C 1994 Reduction in mortality from sudden infant death syndrome in New Zealand: 1986–92 Archives of Disease in Childhood 70: 291–294

Mitchell E A, Stewart A W, Clements M 1995 Immunisation and the sudden infant death syndrome. British Medical Journal 310: 88–90

Morris J A, Haran D, Smith A 1987 Hypothesis: common bacterial toxins are a possible cause of the sudden infant death syndrome. Medical Hypotheses 22: 211–222

Mott A, Evans R, Rolfe K, Potter D, Kemp K W, Sibert J R 1994 Patterns of injuries to children on public playgrounds. Archives of Disease in Childhood 71: 328–330

Mucklow E S 1988 Accidental feeding of a dilute antiseptic solution containing chlorhexidine 0.05% with cetrimide 1% to five babies. Human Toxicology 7: 567–569

Naeye R L 1980 Sudden infant death. Scientific American 242: 52–58

National Advisory Body for CESDI 1996 Annual Report for 1994. Department of Health, London

Nelson E A S, Taylor B J, Weatherall I L 1989 Sleeping position and infant bedding may predispose to hyperthermia and the sudden infant death syndrome. Lancet i: 199–201

Nicoll A, Gardner A 1988 Whooping cough and unrecognised postperinatal mortality. Archives of Disease in Childhood 63: 41–47

Nixon J W, Kemp A M, Levene S, Sibert J R 1995 Suffocation, choking and strangulation in childhood in England and Wales: epidemiology and prevention. Archives of Disease in Childhood 71: 7–14

Nixon J, Jackson H, Hayes M 1987 An analysis of childhood falls involving stairs and bannisters. Consumer Safety Unit, Department of Trade and Industry, London

Nixon J, Pearn J, Wilkey I, Corcoran A 1986 A fifteen year study of child drowning. Accident Analysis and Prevention 18: 199–203

Norvenius G 1995 Is SIDS a new phenomenon? In: Rognum T O (ed) Sudden infant death syndrome. New trends in the nineties. Scandinavian University Press, Oslo, pp 11–14

Norvenius S G 1987 Sudden infant death syndrome in Sweden in 1973–1977 and 1979. Acta Paediatrica Scandinavica (suppl) 333: 5–138

O'Carroll P W, Alkon E, Weiss B 1988 Drowning mortality in Los Angeles County 1976 to 1984. Journal of the American Medical Association 260: 380–383

Office of Population Censuses and Surveys 1988 Deaths by accidents and violence. Quarterly Monitors DH4 Series. OPCS, London

OPCS Bulletin DH6, No. 5. 1992 Office of Population, Censuses and Surveys. London 1992

Orlowski J P 1988 Drowning, near drowning and ice water drowning. Journal of the American Medical Association 260: 390–391

Pearn J H, Nixon J 1977 Are swimming pools becoming more dangerous? Medical Journal of Australia 1977: 702–704

Peterson B 1977 Morbidity of childhood after near-drowning. Pediatrics 59: 364–370

Peterson D R, Sabota E E, Daling J R 1986 Infant mortality among subsequent siblings of infants who died of sudden infant death syndrome. Journal of Pediatrics 108: 911–914

Ponsonby A L, Dwyer T, Gibbons L E, Cochrane J A, Wang Y G 1993 Factors potentiating the risks of sudden infant death syndrome associated with the prone position. New England Journal of Medicine 329: 377–382

Ramey C A, Ramey D N, Hayward J S 1987 Dive response of children in relation to cold water drowning. Journal of Applied Physiology 63: 665–668

Rees B I, Jenkins A R, Sibert J R 1986 Gastric stenosis caused by Everflux. British Journal of Clinical Practice 40: 303–304

Richmond P C W, Evans R C, Sibert J R 1987 Improving facilities for children in an accident and emergency department. Archives of Disease in Childhood 62: 299–301

Richmond P W, Skinner A, Kimche A 1989 Children's car restraints: use and parental attitudes. Archives of Emergency Medicine 6: 41–45

Roberts I, Ashton T, Dunn R, Lee-Joe T 1994 Preventing child pedestrian injury: pedestrian education or traffic calming? Australian Journal of Public Health 18: 209–212

Rognum T O, Willinger M 1995 The story of the 'Stavanger definition'. In: Rognum T O (ed) Sudden infant death syndrome. New trends in the nineties. Scandinavian University Press, Oslo, pp 21–25

Rognum T O, Saugstad O D, Oyasaeter S, Olaisen B 1988 Elevated levels of hypoxanthine in vitreous humor indicate prolonged cerebral hypoxia in victims of sudden infant death syndrome. Pediatrics 82: 615–618

ROSPA Firework Injuries Statistics 1987 Royal Society for Prevention of Accidents, Cannon Houses, The Priory Queensway, Birmingham B4 6BS

Rumack B, Matthew H 1975 Acetaminophen poisoning and toxicity. Pediatrics 55: 871–876

Sandels S 1977 Children in traffic. Elek, London

Schectman V L, Harper R M, Kluge K A et al 1988 Cardiac and respiratory patterns in normal infants and victims of the sudden infant death syndrome. Sleep 11: 413–424

Schectman V L, Harper R M, Kluge K A et al 1989 Heart rate variation in normal infants and victims of SIDS. Early Human Development 19: 167–181

Schectman V L, Harper R M, Wilson A J, Southall D P 1992 Sleep state organization in normal infants and victims of the sudden infant death syndrome. Pediatrics 89: 865–870

Schelp L 1987 Community intervention and changes in accident pattern in a rural Swedish municipality. Health Promotion 2: 109–125

Scherger D L, Wruk K M, Kulig K W, Rumack B 1988 Ethyl alcohol-containing cologne, perfume and after shave ingestions in children. Americal Journal of Diseases of Children 142: 630–632

Scherz R G 1970 Prevention of childhood poisoning. Pediatric Clinics of North America 17: 713

Schwartz P J 1988 The cardiac theory and sudden infant death syndrome. In: Culbertson J L, Krous H F, Bendell R D (eds) Sudden infant death syndrome. Medical aspects and psychological management. Edward Arnold, London, pp 121–138

Scragg R, Mitchell E A, Taylor B J et al 1993 Bed sharing, smoking and alcohol in the sudden infant death syndrome. British Medical Journal 307: 1312–1318

Scragg R, Stewart A W, Mitchell E A, Ford R P, Thompson J M 1995 Public health policy on bed sharing and smoking in the sudden infant death syndrome. New Zealand Medical Journal 108: 218–222

Sharples P M, Aynsley Green A, Eyre J A 1989 Annual Meeting of BPA

Sibert J R 1975 Stress in families of children who have ingested poisons. British Medical Journal ii: 87–89

Sibert J R, Clarke A J, Mitchell M P 1985 Improvements in child resistant containers. Archives of Disease in Childhood 60: 1155–1157

Sibert J R, Frude N 1991 Bittering agents in the prevention of accidental poisoning: children's reactions to denatonium benzoate. Archives of Emergency Medicine 8: 1–7

Sibert J R, Maddocks G B, Brown N 1981 Childhood accidents – an endemic of epidemic proportions. Archives of Disease in Childhood 56: 226–227

Sibert J R, Newcombe R G 1974 Bicycle injuries in childhood. British Medical Journal 1: 613–614

Sibert J R, Webb E, Cooper S 1987 Drowning and near drowning in children in Wales. Practitioner 232: 439–440

Sibert J R, Williams H 1983 Medicine and the media. British Medical Journal 286: 1893

Sidlak M Z, Gleeson M J, Weingraf C L 1985 Accidental ingestion of sterilizing tablets in children. British Medical Journal 290: 1707–1708

Southall D P 1988 Role of apnea in the sudden infant death syndrome: a personal view. Pediatrics 81: 73–84

Southall D P, Richards J M, de Swiet M et al 1983 Identification of infants destined to die unexpectedly during infancy: evaluation of predictive importance of prolonged apnoea and disorders of cardiac rhythm or conduction. British Medical Journal 286: 1092–1096

Spaite D W, Murphy M, Criss E A, Valenzuela T D, Meislin H W 1991 A prospective analysis of injury severity among helmeted and non helmeted bicyclists involved in collisions with motor vehicles. Journal of Trauma 31: 1510–1516

Spencer N 1996 Poverty and child health. Radcliffe Medical Press, Oxford

Steinschneider A S 1972 Prolonged apnea and the sudden infant death syndrome: clinical and laboratory observations. Pediatrics 50: 646–654

Sterman M B, Hodgman J 1988 The role of sleep and arousal in SIDS. Annals of the New York Academy of Sciences 533: 48–61

Stewart A J, Fleming P J 1993 Bereavement care for families. Health Visitor 66: 207–209

Stewart A J, Fleming P J, Howell T 1993b Follow-up support for families with subsequent children. Health Visitor 66: 244–247

Stewart A J, Mitchell E A, Tipene Leach D, Fleming P J 1993a Lessons from the New Zealand and United Kingdom Cot Death Campaigns. Acta Paediatrica Scandinavica 389 (suppl): 119–123

Taylor J A, Sanderson M 1995 A re-examination of the risk factors for the sudden infant death syndrome. Journal of Pediatrics 126: 887–891

Telford D R, Morris J A, Hughes P et al 1989 The nasopharyngeal bacterial flora in the sudden infant death syndrome. Journal of Infection 18: 125–130

Templeman C 1892 Two hundred and fifty eight cases of suffocation of infants. Edinburgh Medical Journal 38: 322–329

Thach B T 1988 The potential role of airway obstruction in sudden infant death syndrome. In: Culbertson J L, Krous H F, Bendell R D (eds) Sudden infant death syndrome. Medical aspects and psychological management. Edward Arnold, London, pp 62–93

Thomas S, Acton C, Nixon J, Battistutta D, Pitt W R, Clark R 1994 Effectiveness of bicycle helmets in preventing injury in children: a case control study. British Medical Journal 308: 173–176

Thompson R, Rivara F P, Thompson D C 1989 A case control study on the effectiveness of bicycle safety helmets. New England Journal of Medicine 320: 1361–1367

Tuffnell C, Petersen S, Wailoo M 1995 Prone sleeping infants have a reduced ability to lose heat. Early Human Development 43: 109–116

US Fire Administration (1980) An evaluation of residential smoke detectors under actual field conditions. Final Report EMW-C-002, Washington DC

Vale J A, Meredith T J, Proudfoot A T 1986 Syrup of ipecac – is it really useful? British Medical Journal 293: 1321–1322

Votteler T P, Nash J C, Rutledge J C 1983 The hazards of alkaline disc batteries. Journal of the American Medical Association 249: 2504–2506

Wennergren G, Milerad J, Lagercrantz H et al 1987 The epidemiology of sudden infant death syndrome and attacks of lifelessness in Sweden. Acta Paediatrica Scandinavica 76: 898–906

White M, Beckett M, O'Regan M, Matthew T 1995 The effect of maternal smoking in pregnancy on autonomic function in infants. In: Rognum T O (ed) Sudden infant death syndrome. New trends in the nineties. Scandinavian University Press, Oslo, pp 174–176

Wigfield R E, Fleming P J 1995 The prevalence of risk factors for SIDS: impact of an intervention campaign.. In: Rognum T O (ed) Sudden infant death syndrome: New trends in the nineties. Scandinavian University Press, Oslo, pp 124–128

Wigfield R, Fleming P J, Berry P J, Rudd P T, Golding J 1992 Can the fall in Avon's sudden infant death rate be explained by the observed sleeping position changes? British Medical Journal 304: 282–283

Wigglesworth J S, Keeling J W, Rushton D I, Berry P J 1987 Pathological investigations in cases of sudden infant death. Journal of Clinical Pathology 40: 1481–1483

Williams S M, Taylor B J, Mitchell E A et al 1996 Sudden infant death syndrome: insulation from bedding and clothing and its effect modifiers. International Journal of Epidemiology 25: 366–375

Wilson C A, Taylor B J, Laing R M, Williams S M, Mitchell E A 1994 Clothing and bedding and its relevance to sudden infant death syndrome: further results from the New Zealand Cot Death Study. Journal of Paediatrics and Child Health 30: 506–512

Wiseman H M, Guest K, Murray V S G, Volans G N 1987 Accidental poisoning in childhood: a multicentre study. Human Toxicology 6: 293–314

World Health Organization 1989 Manifesto for safe communities. 1st World Conference on Accident and Injury Prevention, Stockholm

Wrenn K, Rodewald L, Dockstader L 1993 Potential misuse of ipecac. Annals of Emergency Medicine 22: 1408–1412

Yagupsky P, Gorodischer R 1983 Massive clonidene ingestion in a 9 month old infant. Pediatrics 72: 500–501

Yeoh C, Nixon J W, Dickson W, Kemp A, Sibert J R 1994 Patterns of scald injuries to children in the bath. Archives of Disease in Childhood 71: 156–158

30 Psychiatric disorders

Peter Hoare   David Will   Robert Wrate

PSYCHIATRIC DISORDERS IN CHILDHOOD
   1727
Introduction   1727
Normal and abnormal psychological development
   1728
General features of psychiatric disturbance   1732
Assessment procedures   1734
Disorders in preschool children   1736
Psychiatric aspects of child abuse   1737
Childhood autism, schizophrenia and other
   psychoses   1737
Emotional disorders   1739
Mood disorders   1742
Conduct disorder   1742
Disorders of elimination   1743
Overactivity and hyperactivity   1744
Miscellaneous disorders   1744
Psychological effects of illness and handicap   1746
Treatment methods   1748
Peter Hoare

PSYCHIATRIC DISORDERS IN ADOLESCENCE   1749
Introduction   1749
Adolescent development   1750
How disorders develop   1750
Principles of assessment   1751
When to make a psychiatric referral   1752
Adolescent psychiatric services available   1753
Talking with adolescents   1753
Psychiatric syndromes   1754
Emotional disorders   1755
Eating disorders   1757
Sexual abuse and sexual offenders in adolescence   1759
Maladaptive responses to chronic physical disorders   1760
Brain-injured adolescents with behavioral disturbance   1761
Delinquency   1762
Substance abuse   1762
Principles of therapy   1763
David Will   Robert Wrate
References and Bibliography   1764

PSYCHIATRIC DISORDERS IN CHILDHOOD

INTRODUCTION

Child psychiatry is concerned with the assessment and treatment of children's emotional and behavioral problems. These problems are common, with prevalence rates of 10–20% in several community studies. The majority of disturbed children are not seen by specialist psychiatric services but by general practitioners, community health doctors and pediatricians, along with other professionals such as teachers and residential care staff. Consequently, knowledge about the range and variety of emotional and behavioral problems shown by children is important for all doctors involved in the care of children. The everyday work of the pediatrician provides clear evidence of the stressful effects of illness on the psychological well-being and adjustment of both the child* and the family.

Psychiatric disturbance in childhood is most usefully defined as an abnormality in at least one of the three areas: emotions, behavior or relationships. It is *not* helpful to regard these abnormalities as strictly defined disease entities with a precise etiology, treatment and prognosis. Rather, it is preferable to regard

them as deviations or departures from the norm which are distressing either to the child or to those involved with his welfare. Although child psychiatric disorders do not conform to a strict medical model of illness, it does not mean that these disorders are trivial or unimportant. Some disorders such as autism or conduct disorder have major implications for the child's development and adaptation in adult life.

In childhood, the distinction between disturbance and normality is sometimes imprecise or arbitrary. Isolated symptoms are common and not pathological. For example, many children will occasionally feel sad, unhappy or have temper tantrums. This does not mean that they are disturbed, as disturbance is characterized by the number, frequency, severity and duration of symptoms rather than by the form of symptomatology. In addition, disturbed children rarely have unequivocally pathological symptoms such as hallucinations or delusions. In clinical practice, it is often more important to establish why the child is the focus for concern rather than to adopt the more narrow perspective of whether the child is disturbed or not.

Another important feature of psychiatric disturbance in childhood is that several factors, rather than only a single factor, contribute to the development of disturbance. This makes assessment and treatment more difficult so that an essential prerequisite for successful treatment is the correct evaluation of the relative contribution of the different etiologic factors. Etiologic factors are usually categorized into two groups, constitutional and environmental. The former include heredity

---

* The male gender is used throughout this chapter wherever this could refer to either gender as the alternative wording is cumbersome and unwieldy.

factors, intelligence and temperament. The three major environmental influences are the family, schooling and the community. Another factor, physical illness or handicap, if present, can have a profound effect on the child's development and on his vulnerability to disturbance.

Three other considerations are of general importance in understanding children's behavior: the situation-specific nature of behavior; the impact of current stressful circumstances; and the role of the family. Children's behavior varies markedly in different situations, that is it is situation specific. For instance, a child may be a major problem at school but not at home, or vice versa. Consequently, there may well be an apparent discrepancy between accounts of the child's behavior from the parents and from the teachers. The most likely explanation for this discrepancy is that the demands and expectations upon the child in the two situations are different. It is therefore essential to obtain several independent accounts about the child's behavior wherever possible, in order to derive a more accurate and realistic assessment of the problem. This situation-specific nature of the behavior has implications for treatment, as it is important to explain to parents and to teachers the reasons for the discrepancy, thereby lessening the likelihood of misunderstanding.

Children are immature and developing individuals whose capacities and coping skills change markedly during childhood. Childhood is also a period of life characterized by change, challenge and the necessity for adaptation. Consequently it is not surprising that symptoms of disturbance may arise at times of stress when the demands on the child are excessive. Research in the past 15 years (Goodyer 1990) has shown that life events are associated with an increased psychiatric morbidity among children, a finding similar to that reported for adults. Some stresses such as the birth of a sibling or starting school are of course normal and inevitable, whereas others, such as marital break-up or life-threatening illness, are serious, with long-term implications for the child's well-being.

The child may, however, cope successfully with the stress, thereby enhancing the child's self-esteem and confidence. Alternatively, the child may be overwhelmed, responding with the development of symptomatic behavior. The latter may involve regressive behavior (i.e. behaving in a more immature, dependent fashion), or more specifically maladaptive behavior (e.g. aggression, excessive anxiety or withdrawal). A crucial feature of assessment is the identification of stressful factors that may be contributing to the problem, as this will influence treatment strategies and also the prognosis.

The family is the most potent force both for the promotion of health and for the development of disturbance in the child's life. Assessment of parenting qualities, the marital relationship and the quality of family interaction are essential components of child psychiatric practice. It is a frequent observation that it is the parents who are disturbed and not the child. One consequence of this observation is that in many cases the focus of treatment is likely to be the parents, or the whole family, rather than the child. Indeed, in many instances the main emphasis of treatment is the promotion of normal healthy family interaction as much as the specific treatment of the child's disturbed behavior.

Finally, many disturbed children do not complain about their distress or admit to problems, but rather it is their parents or other adults involved with their care who bring the child to the attention of professionals. Disturbed children more commonly manifest their distress or unhappiness indirectly through symptoms such as abdominal pain, aggression or withdrawal. Direct questioning of the child on first acquaintance is also unlikely to reveal the true extent of the child's feelings or the degree of his distress: sensitive observation during the interview and the use of indirect techniques such as play are necessary to elicit a more accurate view. This is only likely to be successful once a relationship of trust has been established between the child and the doctor.

NORMAL AND ABNORMAL PSYCHOLOGICAL DEVELOPMENT

Children are developing individuals. They are not small adults. A 2-year-old child is very different from a child of 12, whereas an adult of 25 may not differ that much from one of 35. During childhood, the child undergoes a remarkable transformation from a helpless, dependent infant to an independent self-sufficient individual with his own views and outlook, capable of embarking on a career and living separate from his family. Knowledge about the *mechanisms*, *processes* and *sequences* underlying these events is necessary in order to understand the nature of psychological disturbance in childhood. This knowledge also helps to define more clearly what is age-appropriate behavior and to distinguish the pathological from the normal. This section has three parts: developmental theories, developmental psychopathology and personality development.

DEVELOPMENTAL THEORIES (Table 30.1)

It is useful to define some terms at the outset as they are often used interchangeably. *Growth* refers to the incremental increase of a character, feature or attribute; *maturation* is that aspect(s) of development that is mainly due to innate or endogenous factors; *development* describes those changes in an organism's structure and behavior that are systematically related to age. Many behaviors (for example walking and talking) have a substantial maturational component, whereas others (for instance emotional and social development) are strongly influenced by environmental factors. The continuous interaction between maturational and environmental factors throughout childhood helps to mold the personality development of the child.

Developmental theories tend to focus on at least one of the following areas: cognitive, emotional and social. They differ widely in theoretical orientation, in supporting empirical evidence, and in the relative importance attributed to experience in influencing development. No single theory is satisfactory, so that most clinicians use some parts of the various theories to explain different aspects of development. The theories are usually described as stage theories, implying that they regard development as a series of recognizable phases of increasing complexity through which the child progresses (see Table 30.1).

Cognitive development

In 1929, the Swiss psychologist, Piaget elaborated the most comprehensive theory about cognitive development. Many of his conclusions were based on experiments conducted on his own children over a number of years. Piaget has had a tremendous impact on educational concepts and teaching, particularly in primary schools over the last 30 years. More recently, the theoretical basis and validity of Piaget's conclusions have been questioned by further empirical studies (Bee 1995). Despite these

Table 30.1 Summary of cognitive, emotional and social development

	Age in years				
	0	2	6	9	12 + upwards
Cognitive (Piaget)	*Sensorimotor* Differentiates self from objects Begins to act intentionally Achieves object permanence	*Preoperational* Learns to use language and to represent objects by image and words Thinking is egocentric (unable to see other viewpoint) and animistic (everything has feelings including inanimate objects)	*Concrete operational* Thinking is more logical and less egocentric Achieves conservation of number (age 6), volume (age 7) mass (age 8) Able to arrange objects in rank order		*Formal operational* Able to think in abstract manner about propositions and hypotheses
Emotional (Freud)	*Oral* Main concern is initially with satisfaction of basic needs such as hunger Later on, attachment to care giver	*Anal* Cooperative activity with caregiver Satisfaction with increased self-control and achievement	*Phallic* Learns to interact with peers, often leads to rivalry Aware of own sexuality causing Oedipal conflict, resolved by identification with the same sex parent Conscience begins to form	*Latency* Reduced sexual interest with main concerns about peer relationships and position within peer group	*Genital* Revival of earlier conflict, especially sexual conflict Four main tasks: separation from parents, sexual role, career choice, identity
Social and personality development	Social smiling (8 wks)	Attachment (6 mths) Stranger anxiety (10 mths)	Cooperative play (3 yrs)	Strong preference for same sex friends with stereotyped expectations (6–7 yrs)	Enduring relationships (8 yrs onwards)
	Erikson's stage of trust vs mistrust	*Erikson's stage of autonomy vs shame and doubt*	*Erikson's stage of initiative vs guilt*	*Erikson's stage of industry vs inferiority*	*Erikson's stage of identity vs role diffusion*

criticisms, Piaget's views remain the most useful account of cognitive development.

Piaget's theory is based within a biological framework. In order to survive, the individual must have the capacity to adapt to the demands of the environment. Cognitive development is the result of interaction between the individual and the environment. Four factors influence cognitive development: increased neurological maturation, enabling the child to appreciate new aspects of experience and to apply more complex reasoning as he gets older; the opportunity to practice newly acquired skills; the opportunity for social interaction and to benefit from schooling; and the emergence of internal psychological mechanisms or *structures* that allow the child to construct successively more complex cognitive models based on maturation and experience.

Piaget describes two types of intellectual structure, *schemas* and *operations*. The former are present at birth, the latter arise during childhood. *Schemas* are internal representations of some specific action, for instance sucking or grasping, whereas *operations* are internal rules of a higher order which have the distinctive feature that they are *reversible*, as, for example, multiplication is reversible by division. There are two ways whereby the child adapts his cognitive structure to the demands of the environment, *assimilation* and *accommodation*. The former refers to the incorporation of new objects, thoughts and behavior into existing structures, whereas the latter describes the change of existing structures in response to novel experiences. The child attends and learns most when his environment has a degree of novelty that challenges his curiosity but is not so strange that it becomes too confusing.

Piaget describes four main phases: *sensorimotor*, *preoperational*, *concrete operational* and *formal operational*. The

age range given for each stage is the average, though this can vary considerably depending upon intelligence, cultural background and social factors. However, the order is assumed to be the same for all children. Schemas predominate in the sensorimotor and preoperational stages, whereas operations predominate in the concrete operational and formal operational stages.

Sensorimotor (birth–2 years). Initially, behavior is dominated by innate reflexes such as feeding, sucking and following, hence the name for this period. Gradually, the infant realizes the distinction between *self* and *nonself*, namely where his body ends and the world outside begins. The infant also realizes that his behavior can influence the environment, so that intentional and purposeful behavior begins. Finally, the infant achieves *object permanence* whereby he recognizes that an object still exists even although it is no longer visible.

Preoperational period (2–7 years). Language development greatly facilitates cognition so that the individual begins to represent objects by symbols and words. Thinking is, however, *egocentric* and *animistic*. The former refers to the child's tendency to regard the world solely from his own position with the inability to see a situation from another viewpoint. Animistic thinking describes the child's tendency to regard everything in the world as endowed with feelings, thoughts and wishes. For instance, the moon is watching over you when you sleep, when the child bangs into the door he says 'naughty door'.

The child has problems with the principles of conservation for number, volume and mass. The essential principle underlying conservation is that the number, volume or mass of an object is not changed by any visual alteration in its display or appearance. For instance, the child readily believes that the more widely spaced of two rows of counters has more counters than the denser packed row, or that there is more water in a tall beaker when it is poured there from a shorter, more squat beaker.

The child also believes that every event has a preceding cause, rejecting the concept of chance or coincidence. Again, the child's moral sense is rigid and inflexible, so that punishment is invariable, irrespective of the circumstances. The child's concept of illness is radically different to that of the adult, with illness being a consequence for misdeeds, a punishment for a misdemeanor.

Concrete operational (7–12 years). Thinking becomes more logical and less dominated by immediate perceptual experience or by changes in appearance. Conservation of number, weight and mass are successively achieved during this period. The child becomes less egocentric, capable of seeing events from another person's standpoint. The child is able to appreciate and utilize reversibility, for example if 2 plus 2 equals 4, then 4 minus 2 must equal 2.

Formal operational (12 years and upwards). This stage represents the most complex mode of thinking. Its main characteristics are the ability to think in an abstract fashion, to formulate general rules and principles and to devise and test hypotheses, an approach similar to that used in mathematics or in scientific investigation. An example of such reasoning is the following: Joan is fairer than Susan; Joan is darker than Anne. Who is the darkest? (Answer: Susan). Prior to the formal operational stage, the child would require the aid of dolls to solve this problem. (It should be pointed out that not everyone achieves this stage of thinking, even as an adult!) The content of thinking also alters markedly with an emphasis on the hypothetical, the future and ideological issues.

Critical comment on Piaget

Recently, the Piagetian model has been criticized extensively for the lack of evidence to support the existence of the internal structures necessary for the concrete and formal operational stages as well as the elaboration of alternative explanations for the child's inability to carry out conservation tasks successfully before a certain age (Donaldson 1978, Matthews 1994). These criticisms are substantial, but they do not detract from the major conceptual contribution that Piaget has made to knowledge about cognitive development in children.

Recent developments in cognitive theory

Psychologists and psychiatrists have become increasingly interested in the development and application of cognitive theory to the understanding and treatment of psychiatric disorders (Beck et al 1979, Hawton et al 1995). The main principles underlying this theory are that an individual's beliefs about (a) himself, (b) the future, and (c) the world influence his mood and behavior, an idea similar in some ways to the Piagetian concept of schemas. When a person is depressed, his thoughts are self-defeating and he commits certain cognitive errors. Two common types of cognitive error are *personalization* and *dichotomous thinking*. The following two statements are examples of these two errors respectively: 'The reason my parents separated is all because of me', and 'I'm no good at tennis, so I'm bound to be useless at any other sport'.

A major extension of these ideas in childhood is the notion of the *self-concept*. By the age of 6 or 7 years, most children have very definite and clear ideas about themselves and their qualities. For example, they are able to compare themselves to other children with respect to popularity, attractiveness, scholastic ability, and so on. Self-concept is a construct similar to that of a schema in Piaget's theory. Another important facet of self-concept is the favorable or unfavorable evaluation that the child makes of himself, an aspect called *self-esteem*. Children with high self-esteem appear to do better in school, regard themselves as in control of their own destiny, have more friends and get along better with their families (Bee 1995).

Emotional and social development

Sigmund Freud (1953) elaborated the most comprehensive theory about emotional development, while Erikson (1965), also a psychoanalyst, applied psychoanalytic concepts within a social and cultural framework. Freudian theory emphasizes the biological and maturational components of development with an invariable sequence to development for everyone. Like Piaget's, it is a stage or phase theory with the individual progressing successively through each phase. A major criticism of Freudian theory is that its concepts do not lend themselves readily to scientific investigation, so that it is difficult to prove or disprove the validity of the theory.

Freud proposed that the individual goes through five stages prior to adulthood, namely *oral, anal, phallic, latency* and *genital*. These terms refer to the major developmental task or potential conflict that the individual has to achieve or resolve during this period. Table 30.1 describes the important features of the different stages, e.g. during the phallic stage, the Oedipal crisis arises. At this time (around age 3–4 years), the child becomes aware of his own sexual feelings and also that he is attracted in a sexual manner to the parent of the opposite sex. Moreover, the child is simultaneously aware that the parent of the same sex is a rival for the attention of the other parent. The conflict arises because the child is caught between the desire for one parent and the wrath of the other parent. The conflict is successfully resolved by the child identifying with the parent of the same sex, thereby eliminating the rivalrous feelings.

Erikson's major contribution has been to place psychoanalytic concepts in a social and cultural dimension (see Table 30.1). For Erikson, the most important task for the individual is to achieve a coherent sense of identity, a balanced and mature appraisal of one's abilities and limitations, with a recognition of the importance of previous experience and with realistic expectations for the future. Such a task occupies the individual throughout his lifetime. The individual passes through a series of developmental stages, all of which are polarized into two extremes, one successful and adaptive and the other unsuccessful and maladaptive. The two poles of the first stage are *trust* and *mistrust*. The former refers to the child's belief that the world is safe and predictable, and that he can influence events towards a favorable outcome, whereas a sense of mistrust implies a world that is cruel, erratic and unable to meet his needs. The role of the caregiver, usually the mother, is crucial to the achievement of a successful outcome. Erikson also believed that the individual carries forward the residues of earlier stages into the present, thereby giving the past an influence on contemporary behavior. Erikson's writings are a compelling and coherent account of development. A major weakness, however, is the lack of empirical evidence to support the conclusions.

Development of social relationships (Bee 1995)

A characteristic of human beings is their predilection for the establishment and maintenance of social relationships. Although Freud and Erikson refer to social relationships, it is only with the recent elaboration of *attachment theory* by Bowlby (1969) and by Ainsworth (1982) that a plausible theory for this phenomenon has been described. Attachment theory proposes that social relationships develop in response to the mutual biological and psychological needs of the mother and the infant. Mother–infant interaction promotes social relationships. Each member of the dyad has a repertoire of behavior that facilitates interaction: the infant by crying, smiling and vocalization; the mother by facial expression, vocalization and gaze. The mother can regulate the infant's state of alertness, for instance rocking and stroking to soothe the child, talking and facial expression to stimulate the child.

The term *attachment* describes the infant's predisposition to seek proximity to certain people and to be more secure in their presence. Bowlby maintains that there is a biological basis for this behavior, as it has been found extensively in other primates as well as in most human societies. It has considerable survival and adaptive value for the species, as it enables the dependent infant to explore from a secure base and also to use the base as a place of safety at times of distress. From the age of 6 months onwards, infants develop selective attachment to people, usually the mother initially, but not exclusively to her. This first relationship is regarded as the prototype of subsequent relationships, so that its success or failure may have long-term consequences. Clinicians distinguish between *secure attachment* and *anxious attachment*, with the former referring to healthy and the latter to potentially unsatisfactory relationships.

Bonding refers to the persistence of relationships over time, namely the child's capacity to retain the relationship despite the absence of the other individual. Much of the infant's behavior promotes the development of attachments by ensuring close proximity and interaction with the mother. These ideas have many implications for obstetric and pediatric practice, for the reduction of stress associated with hospitalization and for possibly explaining the origins of nonaccidental injury to children.

Other aspects of development

Gender and sex role concepts

Gender identity is part of self-concept, but the development of the child's understanding about 'boyness' or 'girlness' (the sex role concept) is a more elaborate process. Children usually acquire *gender identity* (correctly labeling themselves and others) by about age 2 or 3, followed by *gender stability* (permanence of gender identity) by about age 4. *Gender constancy* (gender identity unalterable by change in appearance) appears around 6 years, similar to other conservation-like concepts. Children show clear evidence of sex role stereotyping from an early age, with an excessively rigid concept for a brief period around age 6 or 7 years. Freudian theory explains these findings on the basis of identification whereby the child imitates the same sex parent, thus acquiring appropriate sex-typed behavior. Alternative explanations emphasize the importance of social reinforcement (Mischel 1970) or of cognition whereby the child acquires a schema about the respective roles and behavior of boys and girls (Kohlberg 1966).

Moral development

The acquisition of moral or ethical values is an important aspect of the socialization of children. Freud and Piaget both described how this process happens. Freudian theory maintains that the superego or conscience develops during the phallic stage, around age 4–5 years. At this time, the child is identifying strongly with the same sex parent in order to resolve the Oedipal conflict and, in consequence, acquires parental values and prohibitions. In contrast, Piaget hypothesizes a much more gradual or stage-like sequence to the acquisition of moral values. The child around 3 years old bases his judgment on the outcome rather than the intention of an act, with an emphasis on punishment following on from a misdemeanor. Subsequently, the child adopts a more conventional morality based upon conformity with family values. Finally, the adolescent derives a personal value system that combines his own idiosyncratic values with those of his family and of society with the intention of achieving the 'greatest good for the greatest number'.

DEVELOPMENTAL PSYCHOPATHOLOGY

This longwinded phrase refers to two important dimensions necessary to evaluate children's behavior: firstly, whether the behavior is age appropriate (the developmental aspect), and secondly, whether the behavior is abnormal (the psychopathological aspect). For example, separation anxiety is a normal phenomenon among children aged between 9 months and 4 years approximately, whereas it would be abnormal in a child aged 6 years.

The tripartite division of disturbance into abnormalities of behavior, emotions or relationships provides a useful way to analyze disturbance. Many behavioral problems can be conceptualized in terms of deficits or excesses. For instance, children with encopresis or enuresis can be regarded as having failed to acquire the skills necessary to use the toilet appropriately. Similarly, the aggressive child is showing excessive belligerent or assertive behavior at an inappropriate time. This approach also has implications for treatment, as the latter is often based on behavioral techniques designed to promote certain behaviors or, alternatively, eliminate others.

Anxiety is central to the understanding of emotional disturbance. It has physical manifestations such as palpitations and dry mouth as well as psychological manifestations such as fear and apprehension. Anxiety is a normal, indeed essential, part of growing up. Anxiety may occur in many situations: in response to external threat; in new or strange situations; or in response to the operation of conscience. Anna Freud (1936) developed the concept of *defense mechanisms* to explain how the individual dealt with excessive anxiety. This response is entirely healthy and appropriate in many situations, only becoming maladaptive when it is used exclusively or excessively, thus preventing the individual from learning how to cope with a normal amount of anxiety. Common defense mechanisms include *denial*, *rationalization*, *regression* and *displacement*. Denial is the child's reluctance or inability to accept the psychological impact of a particular event or situation. For instance, a child refuses to admit to stealing even though it is obvious that he is responsible, as the resultant loss of self-esteem and overwhelming guilt make admission impossible. Rationalization is the attempts to justify or minimize the psychological consequences of an event. 'I don't really like football, so that I am not bothered about playing for the team' is an example of the way in which the child may deal with a failure to gain selection for the school team. Regression occurs when a child behaves in a more developmentally immature manner, often at times of stress, for example becoming enuretic at the start of primary school. Displacement is the transfer of hostile or aggressive feelings from their original source onto another person, for instance getting angry with a sibling rather than with an adult.

Social relationships are often impaired among disturbed children. This may be a primary failure in some instances, such as autism, or more commonly a secondary phenomenon. Children with neurotic or conduct disorders are usually isolated and unpopular with their peer group as they either exclude themselves or are themselves excluded as a result of their deviant behavior. In addition, the behavior usually brings them into conflict with parents or other adults such as teachers.

PERSONALITY DEVELOPMENT

Childhood is the time during which personality is formed. Wordsworth's aphorism 'the child is father of the man' is substantially true. Personality is a broad concept referring to the enduring and uniquely individual constellation of attributes that distinguish one person from another. It comprises the cognitive, emotional, motivational and temperamental attributes that determine the individual's view about himself, his world and the future. Throughout childhood, the various elements interact with each other to mold the child's personality. Moreover, this process occurs in the context of the child's life experiences, particularly within the family but also subsequently in the world outside the family. Healthy personality formation is an important prerequisite for satisfactory adjustment during childhood and also during adult life.

Personality is influenced by two main groups of factors, constitutional and environmental, whilst a third, illness or handicap, if present, can have a profound effect on the child. Constitutional factors include hereditary factors, intelligence and temperament. Intelligence describes the individual's ability to think rationally about himself and his environment, while temperament refers to the individual's characteristic style or approach to new people or situations, his level of activity and prevailing mood. These temperamental traits influence the child's response to his environment and also shape the range and variety of his experiences.

The main environmental influences are the family, schooling and the community. The family is the most powerful force for promoting healthy development as well as for causing severe

disturbance in a child's life. Families fulfill many functions for children, including: the satisfaction of basic physical needs such as food and shelter; the provision of love and security; the development of social relationships with adults and peers; the promotion of cognitive and language skills; the experience of appropriate role models and socialization; and the acquisition of ethical and moral values.

Schooling has three main roles for children: the attainment of scholastic skills; the promotion of peer relationships; and the acceptance of adult authority other than the parents. The community, through the quality of housing and the availability of resources, also has a considerable influence on the child's development. Finally, physical handicap and illness, when present, exert a major effect on personality development. This effect arises not only from the direct restrictions or limitations that illness and handicap may impose on the child's abilities, but, more commonly and importantly, through their indirect effects on the child's self-esteem, through overprotectiveness by the parents and through the adverse effects on social relationships with siblings and peers.

Figure 30.1 is a diagrammatic representation of an interactive model of personality development which incorporates the ideas discussed in this section. As shown, constitutionally-determined temperamental traits have a direct effect on personality and behavior, with the environment also exerting a similar impact. Environmental and temperamental factors have direct effects on the self-concept, which in turn shapes and modifies the personality as well as the environment. These interactive processes continue throughout childhood in a dynamic manner to produce a final product, the individual.

GENERAL FEATURES OF PSYCHIATRIC DISTURBANCE

DIAGNOSTIC CLASSIFICATION

A single cause is rarely responsible for the development of disturbance. The usual pattern is for several factors to be involved, with a broad distinction into constitutional and environmental factors. The important constitutional factors are intelligence and temperament, whilst current life circumstances, the family, schooling and the community are the major environmental influences. One consequence of this multiple causation is that it is inappropriate to devise a diagnostic classification on the basis of etiology, as the relative contribution of each factor is often unclear.

Diagnostic practice is therefore descriptive or phenomenological, with three main categories of abnormality: *emotions*,

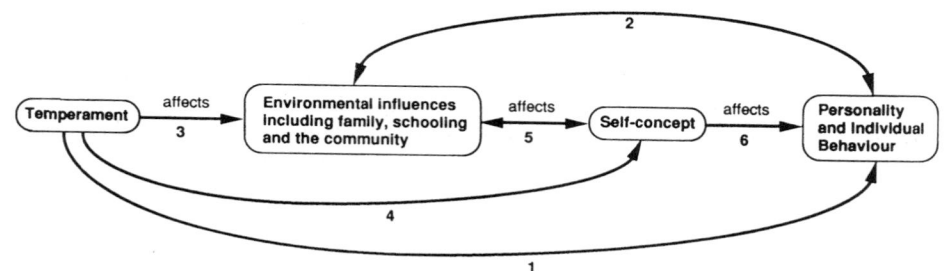

Fig. 30.1   Interactive model of personality development.

behavior and *relationships*. In addition, these abnormalities should be of sufficient severity that they impair the individual in his daily activities and/or cause stress to the individual or to those responsible for his well-being. A commonly used definition of disturbance is as follows: an abnormality of either emotions, behavior or relationships which is sufficiently severe and persistent to handicap the child in his social or personal functioning and/or to cause distress to the child, or to his parents, or to people in the community.

Another feature of contemporary diagnostic practice in child psychiatry is the adoption of a multiaxial framework to describe the various abnormalities or handicaps that are frequently present together in one child (Rutter et al 1975a). This is also a further recognition of the multifactorial nature of disturbance in childhood. The two commonest systems are the ICD-10 (WHO 1992) and DSM-IV (American Psychiatric Association 1994) (see Table 30.2). DSM-IV is used extensively in North America, whereas ICD-10 is popular in the UK. The two systems have similar underlying principles, with an emphasis on a clinical–descriptive approach to diagnosis and the categorization of children along several dimensions, with every child having a position on each dimension, even when there is no abnormality. ICD-10 uses a glossary, and DSM-IV uses operationally defined criteria to provide the basis for diagnosis. An important difference between ICD-10 and DSM-IV is that the latter allows for more than one diagnosis on the clinical syndrome axis, whereas ICD-10 prefers a single diagnosis, an approach more widely used.

DSM-IV places pervasive developmental disorders, including autism, and developmental disorders, such as specific reading disorder, on Axis I, whereas ICD-10 groups these conditions on a separate Axis 2, disorders of psychological development. The following list shows a convenient way to classify the important psychiatric syndromes in childhood:

1. conduct disorders
2. emotional disorders
3. mixed disorders of conduct and emotions
4. hyperkinetic disorders
5. disorders of social functioning
6. tic disorders
7. pervasive developmental disorders
8. miscellaneous disorders.

Table 30.2 DSM-IV and ICD-10 classification systems (modified for child psychiatry)

DSM-IV	ICD-10
Axis 1	*Axis 1*
Clinical syndrome	Clinical syndrome
Axis 2	*Axis 2*
Mental retardation	Disorders of psychological development
Personality disorders	
Axis 3	*Axis 3*
Physical disorders/illness	Mental retardation
Axis 4	*Axis 4*
Psychosocial and environmental problems	Medical illness
Axis 5	*Axis 5*
Global assessment of functioning	Abnormal psychosocial conditions
Axis 6	*Axis 6*
	Psychosocial disability

Conduct disorder is characterized by severe, persistent, socially disapproved of behavior such as aggression or stealing that often involves damage to, or destruction of property and is unresponsive to normal sanctions. The main feature of emotional disorder is a subjective sense of distress, often arising in response to stress. This group is further divided into phobic, anxiety, obsessional and conversion states together with severe reactions to stress. Many disturbed children show a mixture of emotional and behavioral symptoms, so that a mixed category is clinically useful. Hyperkinetic disorders cover a range of disorders characterized by overactivity, distractibility, impulsivity, aggression and short attention span. Large differences in the prevalence of this syndrome have been reported between the USA and the UK (see section on overactivity and hyperactivity). Disorders of social functioning comprise conditions such as elective mutism and attachment disorders. Pervasive developmental disorders include childhood autism, Rett's syndrome, childhood disintegrative disorder and Asperger's syndrome. The miscellaneous group contains a diverse group of problems such as encopresis, enuresis and developmental disorders. Other important but uncommon conditions such as schizophrenia and mood disorders are categorized in a similar fashion to that for adults, providing that the diagnostic criteria are fulfilled.

EPIDEMIOLOGY OF DISTURBANCE

Epidemiological research has provided accurate information about the frequency and distribution of disturbance throughout childhood and adolescence, the differences between urban and rural areas, and the effects of illness and handicap on vulnerability to disturbance, as well as providing clues about the relative importance of various etiologic factors (Rutter et al 1975b).

Most studies have shown prevalence rates of between 10 and 20%, depending on the criteria for deviance. The first and most influential study was the Isle of Wight study (IOW) carried out by Rutter et al (1970). Using strict definitions of disorder, they found rates of approximately 7% among 10- to 11-year-old children. Follow-up of these children into adolescence indicated a prevalence rate of around 7%, with more than 40% of the children with conduct disorder continuing with major problems. Disorders arising for the first time during adolescence were more adult-like in presentation, with a preponderance of females. Over 80% of the disorders were in the emotional, conduct or mixed categories. Emotional disorders were more common among girls, with anxiety as the commonest type. By contrast, conduct disorders, and to an important extent mixed disorders, were more common among boys, with an association with specific reading retardation. A comparative study of 10-year-olds living in London (Rutter et al 1975b) showed a rate of disturbance over twice that on the IOW. This study also showed that the difference in prevalence rate was entirely accounted for by the increased frequency of predisposing factors among children and their families in London compared with those on the IOW. These factors were family discord, parental psychiatric disorder, social disadvantage and inferior quality of schooling.

The IOW study also showed that children with chronic illness or handicap had much higher rates of disturbance than healthy children. For instance, children with central nervous disease such as epilepsy or cerebral palsy had a rate over 5 times that of the general population, while children with other illnesses such as asthma and diabetes were twice as likely to be disturbed as healthy children.

Studies of preschool children have found that about 20% of children have significant behavior problems, with 7% classified as severe. Follow-up studies of these children (Richman et al 1982) indicated that about 60% persisted, most commonly among overactive boys of low ability. An important association was found between language delay and disturbed behavior. Finally, problems were more likely to persist when there was marital discord, maternal psychiatric ill health and psychosocial disadvantage such as poor housing and large family size.

ASSESSMENT PROCEDURES

HISTORY TAKING AND EXAMINATION

Interview skills are essential to the elucidation, understanding and treatment of emotional and behavioral problems in children. Training in interview skills should be an important part of medical undergraduate and postgraduate training. Maguire & Rutter (1976) showed that doctors in training often lack these skills, but that it was possible to improve their skills with training. Points of general importance include: clarification about the nature of the problem and the reason for referral; obtaining adequate factual information; eliciting emotional responses and attitudes about past and current events; observing behavior during the interview; establishing trust and confidence of the child and family; providing the parents with a summary of problems and a provisional treatment plan at the end of the initial interview.

There are no absolute rules about interviewing, indeed flexibility is essential. However, the following guidelines are useful.

1. The interview room should be large enough to seat the family comfortably and also to allow the children to use the play material in a relaxed manner.

2. Avoid having a desk between the interviewer and the family, i.e. put the desk against the wall of the interview room.

3. Do not spend the interview writing down notes but rather encourage eye-to-eye contact, taking the minimum notes necessary.

4. The play material must be suitable for a wide age range and include crayons and paper, jigsaws, simple games, books (provides rough estimate of reading ability), doll's house, play telephones and miniature domestic and zoo animals.

5. The play material should be gradually introduced as appropriate and not left around in a haphazard manner.

6. Interview parents and young children together.

7. Older children and adolescents like to be seen separately from parents at some point during the interview.

8. Older children and adolescents are able to talk about problems openly once trust in the interviewer has been established.

9. Too direct questions usually elicit denial from the child, so open-ended questions are greatly preferable.

The interview should provide information about the following (bold type indicates essential facts):

1. **Presenting problem(s): frequency, severity, onset, course, exacerbating/ameliorating factors, effect on family. Help given so far**.
2. Other problems or complaints

   a. general health: eating, sleeping, elimination, physical complaints, fits or faints
   b. interests, activities and hobbies
   c. **relationship with parents and sibs**
   d. relationship with other children, special friends
   e. mood: happy, sad, anxious
   f. level of activity, attention span, concentration
   g. antisocial behavior
   h. **schooling: attainments, attendance, friendships, relationship with teachers**
     i. sexual knowledge, interests and behavior (when relevant).
3. **Any other problems not previously mentioned**.
4. Family structure
   a. **parents: ages**, occupations, **current physical and psychiatric state**, previous physical and psychiatric history
   b. sibs: ages, problems
   c. home circumstances.
5. Family function
   a. **quality of parenting, mutual support and help, level of communication and ability to resolve problems**
   b. **parent–child relationship: warmth, affection and acceptance, level of criticism, hostility and rejection**
   c. sibs' relationship
   d. pattern of family relationships.
6. Personal history
   a. pregnancy and delivery
   b. early mother–child relationship, postpartum depression, early feeding patterns
   c. temperamental characteristics: easy or difficult, irregular, restless baby and toddler
   d. developmental milestones
   e. **past illnesses and injuries, hospitalization**
   f. separations greater than 1 week
   g. previous schooling.
7. **Observation of child's behavior and emotional state**
   a. **appearance, nutritional state, signs of neglect or injury**
   b. activity level, involuntary movements, concentration
   c. mood: expressions or signs of sadness, misery, anxiety
   d. reaction to and relationship with the doctor, eye contact, spontaneous talk, inhibition and disinhibition
   e. relationship with parents: affection/resentment, ease of separation
   f. habits and mannerisms
   g. presence of delusions, hallucinations, thought disorder.
8. Observation of family relationships
   a. patterns of interaction
   b. clarity of boundaries between parents and child
   c. communication
   d. emotional atmosphere of family: mutual warmth/tension, criticisms.
9. Physical examination
   a. screening neurological examination
     (i) note any facial asymmetry
     (ii) eye movements: ask child to follow a moving finger and observe eye movement for jerkiness, uncoordination
     (iii) finger–thumb apposition: ask child to press the tip of each finger against the thumb in rapid succession, observe clumsiness, weakness
     (iv) copying pattern, drawing a man
     (v) observe grip and dexterity in drawing

(vi) observe visual competence when drawing
(vii) jumping up and down on the spot
(viii) hopping
(ix) hearing: capacity of child to repeat numbers whispered two meters behind him
b. Further medical examination (if relevant).

Formulation

At completion of the assessment, the clinician should be able to make a formulation. This is a succinct summary of the important features of the individual case. The formulation consists of the following: statement of main problems; diagnosis and differential diagnosis; relative contribution of constitutional and environmental factors to the etiology; probable short-term and long-term outcome; further information required (including special investigations); initial treatment plan. The formulation should be included in the case notes, thereby providing the clinician with a record of his views at referral.

PSYCHOLOGICAL ASSESSMENT

Psychological assessment, carried out by child psychologists, is an invaluable and integral part of the overall assessment of a child's problems in many situations. It can provide information about three aspects of development: general intelligence, educational attainments and special skills. Assessment is usually based upon the administration of standardized assessment procedures. These tests are either norm referenced or criterion referenced. The former compares the child's ability with other children of the same age, whereas the latter is on a pass/fail basis, for instance whether he can tie his shoelaces. Ideally, the test items should have good discriminatory value (distinguish between children of different ability), be reliable (give similar results when repeated) and valid (in agreement with other independent evidence). An important aspect of the assessment is that the tasks are carried out in a standardized fashion, thereby increasing their reliability and validity.

INTELLECTUAL ABILITY

Developmental assessment in infancy and early childhood

The commonly used tests are the Bayley scales of infant development, Griffiths mental development scale and the Denver developmental screening test (see Ch. 9).

Assessment of general intelligence amongst school-age children

The most popular test is the Wechsler intelligence scale for children – revised form (WISC-R) (Wechsler 1974). This covers an age range from 6 to 16 years. 10 subtests are usually used, measuring different aspects of the child's ability. Commonly, the tests are divided into 'verbal' and 'performance' categories, yielding a 'verbal IQ' and a 'performance IQ'. The verbal subtests commonly used are *information*, *comprehension*, *arithmetic*, *similarities* and *vocabulary*, whilst the performance subtests are *picture completion*, *picture arrangement*, *block design*, *object assembly* and *coding*. Each subtest has a mean score of 10 so that combining the 10 tests gives a 'full scale' IQ of 100 with a

standard deviation of 15. The 'normal' distribution of the test scores means that it is possible to state that 66% of children will be within the IQ range 85–115, 95% within IQ range 70–130, and 99% within IQ range 55–145. Other tests used include the Stanford–Binet (Form L-M) (Thorndike 1973) and the British ability scales (BAS) (Elliott et al 1983).

EDUCATIONAL ATTAINMENT

There are two commonly used reading tests, the Schonell graded word reading test and the Neale analysis of reading ability. The latter is more comprehensive, though taking longer to administer. It provides information about speed, accuracy and comprehension of reading. The scores are transformed into reading ages of so many years and months, for instance 6 years 11 months. Other attainment tests include the Schonell graded spelling test. There is no satisfactory standardized test of mathematical skills, although appropriate subtest scores of the WISC-R and the BAS can be used as a guide to mathematical ability.

Specific skills

Reynell development language scale, Bender motor gestalt test and the Vineland social maturity scales are examples of tests to assess the child's acquisition of certain abilities and skills. These are often helpful with some specific problems.

Limitations of assessment

Caution should always be exercised in the interpretation of test results. It is wrong to attribute undue significance to a single result, most often done with the IQ score. Many factors influence test results, including fatigue, poor testing conditions and the use of inappropriate tests. The results should be evaluated in the context of the overall assessment and the report from the child psychologist. A great deal of harm, upset and distress can happen to a child when he is incorrectly classified or labeled as either too able or too dull on the basis of an unreliable psychological assessment.

Additional information

A distinctive feature of child psychiatry practice is the importance attached to obtaining independent evidence about the child's behavior. This is for two reasons: firstly, a child's behavior varies from one situation to another, so that it is helpful to have information about the child's behavior in several contexts; secondly, parental accounts of the child's behavior are likely to be distorted in many cases, as it is the parents who are disturbed rather than the child. Consequently, an important part of assessment is to obtain reports from other professionals involved with the family, such as schools, health visitors or general practitioners. Another common practice is the use of questionnaires to supplement information provided by referrers and other more formal reports. Several questionnaires (e.g. Achenbach & Edelbrock 1983) have been devised to assess different age ranges and have satisfactory psychometric properties. The most commonly used questionnaires for school-age children in the UK are the Rutter parents' and teachers' scales, also known as Rutter A and Rutter B, respectively. These scales have established reliability and validity as well as classifying children into neurotic or emotional, conduct or antisocial and mixed categories.

DISORDERS IN PRESCHOOL CHILDREN

Except for rare but severe disorders such as childhood autism, psychiatric disorders in this age group are mostly deviations or delays from normality rather than psychiatric illness as such. Moreover, the child's behavior and development are so influenced by the immediate surroundings that it is often the environment which is responsible for the problems rather than the child.

ETIOLOGY

Four types of factors contribute to problems in varying degrees in the individual case: temperamental factors; physical illness or handicap; family psychopathology; and social disadvantage. The New York Longitudinal Study (Thomas & Chess 1982) showed clearly that children with certain types of temperamental characteristics, the so-called 'difficult child' and the 'slow to warm up child' profile, were more likely to develop problems. Again, physical illness or handicap can reduce activity, directly or indirectly affect developmental progress and increase parental anxiety, all of which potentiate the likelihood of behavioral disturbance. Parental psychiatric illness, marital disharmony and poor parenting skills are instances where disturbances in the parents adversely affect the child's behavior. There are high rates of depression among mothers with preschool children. Social disadvantages such as poor housing or inadequate recreational facilities increase the risk of disturbance among preschool children (Richman 1977).

FREQUENCY OF PROBLEMS

Table 30.3 shows the prevalence of common problems among 3- and 4-year-old children in the general population (Richman & Lansdown 1988).

Table 30.3 Problem behaviors in 3- and 4-year olds (Richman & Lansdown 1988)

Behavior	3-year-olds (%)	4-year-olds (%)
Poor appetite	19	20
Faddy eater	15	24
Difficulty settling at night	16	15
Waking at night	14	12
Overactive and restless	17	13
Poor concentration	9	6
Difficult to control	11	10
Temper	5	6
Unhappy mood	4	7
Worries	4	1
Fears	10	12
Poor relationships with siblings	10	15
Poor relationships with peers	4	6
Regular day wetting	26	8
Regular night wetting	33	19
Regular soiling	16	3

Problems are mainly about eating, sleeping and elimination, with a marked decrease in wetting and soiling over the 1-year period. Affective symptoms such as unhappiness and relationship problems are much less common, but probably more significant. Community studies indicate that 20% of children are regarded by their mothers as having problems, with 7% rated as severe.

COMMON PROBLEMS

Temper tantrums

They usually arise when the child is thwarted, angry or has hurt himself. They can occur in isolation or as part of a wider problem. They comprise a variety of behaviors, including screaming, crying, often with collapse to the floor and banging of feet. A child can be aggressive towards other people around him, but the child rarely injures himself. Most tantrums 'burn themselves out' so that specific intervention is not necessary. If it is, then the following points are useful: if necessary, restrain from behind by folding arms around child's body; minimize any additional attention to the child; only respond and praise when behavior is back to normal.

Feeding problems

They range in severity from a minor problem, such as the finicky child, to the severe disabling problem of nonorganic failure to thrive. Minor problems will usually respond to patient and attentive listening to the parents' concerns, counseling and specific advice. Severe nonorganic failure to thrive (prevalence 2%) is a complex problem requiring comprehensive assessment and a large amount of time and resources to remedy (Skuse et al 1992). Several factors are responsible in most cases, including poor mother–child relationship, often in the context of more widespread emotional and social deprivation, and factors in the child, including temperamental factors and aversion to feeding. *Pica*, the ingestion of inedible material such as dirt or rubbish, is a normal transitory phenomenon during the toddler period. Persistent ingestion is found amongst mentally retarded, psychotic and socially deprived children. Lead poisoning, though always mentioned, is a possible but uncommon danger from pica.

Sleep problems

These are common, with up to 20% of 2-year-olds waking at least five times per week (Richman 1981, Eaton-Evans & Dugdale 1988). The two most frequent problems are reluctance to settle at night and persistent waking up during the night. Several factors contribute to the problem, including adverse temperamental characteristics in the child, perinatal problems and maternal anxiety. It is also important to distinguish between those factors responsible for the onset of the problem and those responsible for maintaining the problem. Medication such as trimeprazine and promethazine are frequently prescribed but are usually ineffective. Their only genuine indication is to provide a brief respite for the parents as well as ensuring that the child has an uninterrupted night's sleep. The most successful management is a behavioral strategy (see treatment section). Douglas & Richman (1984) provide a useful summary of these techniques. Other sleep problems in older children are discussed in the miscellaneous section.

PSYCHIATRIC ASPECTS OF CHILD ABUSE

Originally this was restricted to the 'battered baby syndrome' (Kempe & Kempe 1978), but it has now been extended to include physical abuse, emotional abuse, sexual abuse and neglect. Several inquiries and controversies during the 1980s, particularly the Cleveland affair (Butler-Sloss 1988), have highlighted the importance of this topic for pediatricians. This section will concentrate on the psychiatric aspects: other sections discuss the diagnosis and the adolescent issues related to child abuse (see Chapter 34 and p. 1759). It is also important to remember that the different aspects of child abuse are frequently present in the same child and family and that many comments about the detection, management and treatment apply equally well to all aspects of child abuse. Several recently published books (Bentovim et al 1988, Cicchetti & Carlson 1989, Jones 1992, Monck et al 1995) provide very useful accounts of current practice about various aspects of child abuse, particularly in relation to sexual abuse.

PHYSICAL ABUSE

Diagnostic awareness and suspicion are the key elements in the detection and recognition of physical abuse. The following list summarizes the common characteristics of abused children and their families, although the most important factor to recognize is that child abuse can occur in any family, irrespective of class, color or creed.

Common characteristics of abused children and their families

Risk characteristics of the abused child:

1. product of unwanted pregnancy
2. unwanted child in family
3. low birthweight
4. separation from mother in neonatal period
5. mental or physical handicap
6. habitually restless, sleepless or incessantly crying
7. physically unattractive.

Risk characteristics of the parent(s):

1. single parent
2. young
3. were abused themselves as children
4. low self-esteem
5. unrealistic expectations of child and his development
6. inconsistent or punishment-orientated discipline.

Risk characteristics of social circumstances:

1. low income or unemployment
2. social isolation
3. current stress such as housing crisis, domestic friction, exhaustion or ill health
4. large family.

Management

Most cases of child abuse do not require the involvement of a child psychiatrist, as the principal concern is the protection of the child, practical support for the family and help with parenting skills. The child psychiatrist can make a useful contribution in two ways: firstly, to act as an outside consultant to other professionals and agencies working with the family on various aspects of detection, management and treatment; secondly, to provide individual and family therapy for the child, the parents or the family in particular instances, depending upon the assessment.

In addition to its immediate effects, child abuse may have medium-term and long-term sequelae. Many abused children continue to be exposed to emotional abuse and neglect throughout their childhood, so that they often show symptoms of disturbance such as unhappiness, wariness, untrusting, low self-esteem and poor peer relationships. This childhood experience in turn predisposes abused children to become abusing parents when adults (Kempe & Kempe 1978).

EMOTIONAL ABUSE

This term has been introduced to describe the severe impairment of social and emotional development resulting from repeated and persistent criticism, lack of affection, rejection, verbal abuse and other similar behavior by the parent(s) to the child. Affected children display a variety of symptoms: low self-esteem; limited capacity for enjoyment; severe aggression; impulsive behavior.

SEXUAL ABUSE

This became a topic of major public and pediatric concern in the late 1980s (Butler-Sloss 1988). The role of the child psychiatry team is more important here, as interviewing skills, psychotherapeutic expertise and the use of specialized equipment (anatomically accurate dolls) are often necessary at the detection and also the treatment stages of management. Detailed accounts of this work, including the use of the anatomical dolls, are described in the book by the Great Ormond Street child sex abuse team (Bentovim et al 1988, Monck et al 1995). The establishment of specialized assessment teams in every locality is another important recommendation of the Cleveland Enquiry (Butler-Sloss 1988).

NEGLECT

This varies markedly, ranging from relative inadequacy and incompetence in providing basic shelter, love and security for the child to severe failure in the provision of basic essentials, often combined with emotional and social deprivation.

MUNCHAUSEN SYNDROME BY PROXY (Meadow 1989)

This remarkable variant of physical abuse often occurs against the same background of parental psychopathology and social disadvantage as other forms of abuse. The role of the child psychiatrist is usually confined in most cases to offering counseling for the parents and/or family therapy when indicated.

CHILDHOOD AUTISM, SCHIZOPHRENIA AND OTHER PSYCHOSES

These conditions have been previously combined under the general term 'childhood psychosis', as they are severe and disabling, with clear-cut abnormalities. However, autistic children experience neither hallucinations nor delusions (the characteristics of psychosis), and, moreover, have had the abnormalities from early infancy. For these reasons, ICD-10 and DSM-IV have separated out childhood autism from other psychotic conditions in childhood into a new diagnostic category called pervasive developmental disorders. The latter category also includes Rett's syndrome, disintegrative disorder and Asperger's syndrome (Wing 1981).

CHILDHOOD AUTISM

Kanner's (1943) original description of 11 children with 'an extreme autistic aloneness' has not been improved upon, with its astute observation of 'inability to relate in an ordinary way to people and to situations' and 'an anxiously obsessive desire for the maintenance of sameness'. Most authorities now agree that three features are essential to the diagnosis: general and profound failure to develop social relationships; language retardation; ritualistic and compulsive behavior. Additionally, these abnormalities should be manifest before 30 months.

Prevalence

Epidemiological studies in childhood (Wing & Gould 1979) have found prevalence rates of 2/10 000 increasing to 20/10 000 when individuals with severe mental retardation and some autistic features are included. Boys are three times more affected than girls.

Clinical features

Impaired social relationships

Parental recollections of infancy often reveal that as an infant the child was slow to smile, unresponsive and passive with a dislike of physical contact and affection. Contemporary social deficits include the failure to use eye-to-eye gaze and facial expression for social interaction, rarely seeking others for comfort or affection, rarely initiating interaction with others, a lack of empathy (the ability to understand how others feel and think) and of cooperative play. The children are aloof and indifferent to people.

Language abnormalities

Language acquisition is delayed and deviant with many autistic children never developing language (approximately 50%). When present, language abnormalities are many and varied, including immediate and delayed echolalia (repetition of spoken word(s) or phrase(s)), poor comprehension and use of gesture, pronominal reversal (use of 'you' when 'I' is meant) and abnormalities in intonation, rhythm and pitch.

Ritualistic and compulsive behavior

Common abnormalities are rigid and restricted patterns of play, intense attachments to unusual objects such as stones, unusual preoccupations and interests (timetables, bus routes) to the exclusion of other pursuits and marked resistance to any change in the environment or daily routine. Tantrums and explosive outbursts often occur when any change is attempted.

Other features

Autistic children often exhibit a variety of stereotypies including rocking, finger twirling, spinning and tiptoe walking. They are often overactive with a short attention span. 70% of autistic children are in the retarded range of intelligence with only 5% having an IQ above 100. Occasionally, some have remarkable abilities in isolated areas, for instance computation, music and rote memory. About 20% will develop epilepsy during adolescence, though not usually severe.

Association with other conditions

Autistic behavior occurs in some patients with a diverse group of conditions including fragile X syndrome, rubella, phenylketonuria, tuberous sclerosis, neurolipoidoses and infantile spasms (Lord & Rutter 1994). More recently, Rett's syndrome, with its marked autistic features, has been described (Hagberg et al 1983) (see neurology section).

Etiology

Most people favor an organic basis as neurological abnormalities are common, and because of the association with epilepsy and various neurological syndromes, the increased rate of perinatal complications and higher concordance among monozygotic compared with dizygotic twins (Rutter & Schopler 1988, Lord & Rutter 1994). Application of new investigative techniques such as CAT scan, MRI and positron emission tomography have not revealed any consistent abnormality, though increased serotonin levels have been reported. The relationship between autism and the fragile X syndrome is also unclear, as the different rates in the various studies may be a reflection of the degree of mental handicap rather than of any etiologic significance. A most interesting psychological perspective on the autistic deficit is provided by the series of experiments described by Hobson (1993). Hobson concluded that the primary deficit in autism is a lack of empathy, namely the inability to perceive and interpret emotional cues.

Treatment

The explanation of the diagnosis is a vital first step in helping parents to accept the presence of handicap with the consequent lessening of the parental guilt about etiology. Counseling and advice are likely to be necessary throughout childhood. Lord & Rutter (1994) suggested that treatment aims should have four components: the promotion of normal development; the reduction of rigidity and stereotypies; the removal of maladaptive behavior; the alleviation of family stress. Behavioral methods, including operant conditioning and shaping (see behavioral treatment section), are the most likely ways to achieve some success with the first three aims, whilst counseling is important for the fourth. Special schooling, where the child's special social and educational needs are recognized, is very beneficial, sometimes on a residential basis. Drugs do not have an important part in management.

Outcome

Many autistic individuals are unable to live independently, with only 15% looking after and supporting themselves (Lockyer & Rutter 1969). Many are placed in institutions for the mentally handicapped, though government policy now favors community care. Autistic children with an IQ of at least 70, receiving proper education and coming from middle-class families do better than their counterparts.

OTHER PERVASIVE DEVELOPMENTAL DISORDERS

Disintegrative disorder (Lord & Rutter 1994)

This term refers to a group of conditions characterized by normal development until around 4 years of age, followed by profound regression and behavioral disintegration, with loss of language and other skills, impairment of social relationships and the development of stereotypies. It can follow on from a minor illness or from a more definite central nervous system disease such as measles encephalitis. The prognosis is poor, resulting from the underlying degenerative pathology.

SCHIZOPHRENIA (see adolescent section)

This is a rare disease during childhood. Even during adolescence, it has a frequency of less than 3 per 10 000. Symptomatology consists of delusions (fixed, false beliefs), hallucinations (perceptual experience in the absence of relevant sensory stimulus), distortions of thinking (thought insertion and withdrawal) and of movement, most commonly catatonia. It can present with acute disturbed behavior or insidiously with gradual withdrawal and failing schoolwork. There is good evidence of a genetic component, with approximately 10% of relatives having the disease. Diagnostically, it often can be difficult to distinguish from a major mood disturbance such as manic depressive psychosis or a drug-induced episode.

Treatment

Treatment must be comprehensive, including drug treatment with major tranquilizers such as chlorpromazine or haloperidol and antiparkinsonian drugs, individual and family therapy, as well as help with education. Favorable prognostic factors include high intelligence, acute onset, precipitating factors and normal premorbid personality.

DELIRIUM-LIKE CONDITIONS

Delirium-like conditions, with impairment of consciousness, hallucinations and illusions are common among children with acute infections. Rarely, a noninfective agent, for instance acute intermittent porphyria, is responsible.

EMOTIONAL DISORDERS

The primary abnormality is a subjective sense of distress due to anxiety which can be expressed overtly as in anxiety disorders or covertly as in somatization or conversion disorders. This group of disorders is similar in many respects to neurotic disorders in adults. They are further divided into the following categories: anxiety and phobic states; obsessional disorders; conversion disorders, dissociative states and somatization disorders; and reaction to severe stress and adjustment disorders. Many children often show a mixed pattern of symptoms, so that a clear-cut distinction into a single category is not possible. The IOW study found a prevalence rate of 2.5% with a female preponderance. Prognosis is generally favorable as many problems arise from an acute stress, so that the problems should resolve once the stressful effects lessen.

ANXIETY STATES

Clinical features

This is the commonest type of emotional disorder. Anxiety has physical and psychological components, with the former referring to palpitations and dry mouth, while the latter refers to the subjective sense of fear and apprehension. Somatic symptoms, particularly abdominal pain, are common. Again, many symptoms may represent the persistence and exaggeration of normal developmental fears, ranging in severity from an acute panic attack to a chronic anxiety state over several months. Predisposing factors include temperamental characteristics, over-involved and over-concerned parents and the 'special child syndrome'. The latter refers to children who are treated differently by their parents. This may arise in several circumstances, for instance the child is much wanted, previous ill health during pregnancy or infancy, resulting in 'anxious' attachment between the child and parents. In turn, 'anxious' attachment may lead to the parents inadvertently reinforcing normal fears and anxieties.

Treatment

Several approaches, including individual, behavioral and family therapy, are used, often in combination depending upon the assessment and formulation. Anxiolytic drugs such as diazepam do not have a major role except in certain situations and for a specified period.

PHOBIC STATES

Clinical features

Phobias are common and normal among children. For instance, toddlers are fearful of strangers, whereas adolescents are anxious about their appearance or weight. Pathological fears often arise from ordinary fears that are exacerbated by parental and/or social reinforcement. A phobia is defined as a special form of fear for specific objects or situations, for instance dogs or heights. Its characteristics are that it is out of proportion to the situation, is irrational, is beyond voluntary control and leads to avoidance of the feared situation. This avoidance behavior is the main reason the fear is maladaptive as it leads to increasing restriction and limitation of the child's activities.

Treatment

A behavioral approach, using graded exposure to the feared situation, is the most commonly used treatment. The rationale of this approach is that continued exposure to the feared stimulus reduces the anxiety associated with the stimulus, thereby decreasing avoidance behavior. The success of this method often depends on the ability of the therapist to devise a treatment program that combines gradual exposure without inducing too much anxiety. Occasionally, anxiolytic drugs are used in conjunction with this behavioral approach.

SCHOOL REFUSAL

This term, also known as school phobia, refers to the child's irrational fear about school attendance. It is also known as the masquerade syndrome (Waller & Eisenberg 1980) as it can present in a variety of disguises, including abdominal pain, headaches and viral infection. The child is reluctant to leave home in the morning to attend school, in contrast to the truant who leaves home but does not arrive at school. It occurs most commonly at the commencement of schooling, change of school, or the beginning of secondary school.

Most cases can be understood in terms of the following three mechanisms, often in combination: first, separation anxiety, whereby the child and/or the parent are fearful of separation, of which school is an example; second, specific phobia about some aspect associated with school attendance, such as traveling to school, mixing with other children, or some part of the school routine, for instance certain subjects, gym or assembly; third, an indication of a more general psychiatric disturbance such as depression or low self-esteem. The latter is more frequent among adolescents. Typically, most school refusers have good academic attainments, are conformist at school, but oppositional at home. School refusal can present either acutely or insidiously, often becoming a chronic problem in adolescence.

Treatment

The initial essential step is to recognize the condition itself, namely to avoid unnecessary and extensive investigations for minor somatic symptoms or to advise prolonged convalescence following minor illness. For the acute case, early return to school with firm support for the parents and liaison with the school is the most successful approach. For the more intractable cases, extensive work with the child and parents, along with a graded return to school is advisable. A specific behavioral program for the phobic elements may be necessary as well as the use of anxiolytic drugs in some instances. The chronic problem often requires a concerted approach, sometimes involving a period of assessment and treatment at a child psychiatric inpatient unit. Many clinicians also use family therapy to tackle the major relationship problems that exist in many cases. Two-thirds usually return to school regularly, whilst the remainder, usually adolescents from disturbed families, only achieve erratic attendance at school at best. Follow-up studies into adult life have found that approximately one-third continue with neurotic symptoms and social impairment.

OBSESSIVE–COMPULSIVE DISORDERS (see Fig. 30.2)

Definition

An obsession is a recurrent, intrusive thought that the individual recognizes is irrational but cannot ignore. A compulsion or ritual is the behavior(s) accompanying these ideas, the aim of which is to reduce the associated anxiety.

Clinical features

Most children display obsessional symptoms to a minor degree at some time, for instance avoiding cracks on paving stones or walking under ladders. They have no significance. It is when the behavior interferes with ordinary activities that it amounts to an illness. Common obsessive rituals are hand washing and dressing. Obsessional thoughts often have a foreboding quality, for instance that 'something could happen' to a parent or sibling, that he might die, or get run over. The rituals are maintained, though maladaptive, because they produce temporary reduction in

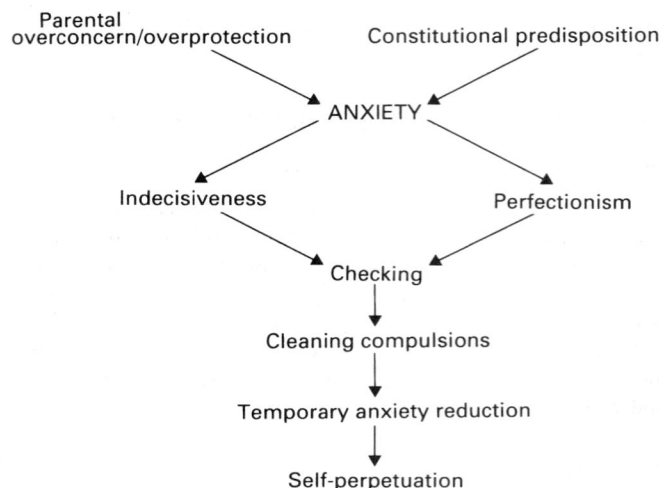

Fig. 30.2 Development of obsessional symptoms.

anxiety. Commonly, the child involves other members of the family in the performance of rituals, so that the child assumes a controlling role within the family.

The illness is rare (community prevalence 0.3%) but commoner among older children and adolescents with an acute or gradual onset. In addition to anxiety symptoms, many children exhibit depressive features.

Treatment

Behavioral methods, particularly response prevention, are successful in eliminating the obsessive–compulsive behavior. Response prevention consists of training the child to become aware of the cues that trigger the symptom and then using distraction techniques to make the performance of the ritual impossible. Medication, usually clomipramine, is helpful sometimes for anxiety and depressive symptoms. Involvement of other members of the family, whether specifically in family therapy or to assist the child in the elimination of rituals, is necessary. Some cases require inpatient admission. Two-thirds do well, with the remainder continuing to have problems, usually in a fluctuating fashion.

CONVERSION DISORDERS AND DISSOCIATIVE STATES

Clinical features

These are rare in childhood. Conversion disorder refers to the development of physical symptoms, usually of the special senses or limbs, without any pathological basis in the presence of identifiable stress and/or affective disturbance. The emotional conflict is said to be 'converted' into physical symptoms which are less threatening to the individual than the underlying psychological conflict. A dissociative state is the restriction or limitation of consciousness due to psychological causes; examples include amnesia and fugue. It is, however, extremely dangerous to diagnose the condition solely by the exclusion of organic disease as follow-up studies have found that a minority subsequently develop definite organic illness. There should always be positive psychological reasons to explain the development of the symptoms. Common reasons include major life events or stresses for the child, a similar illness among other family members/peers, or underlying depressive disorder.

Minor degrees of these disorders are extremely common and frequently occur as a transitory phenomenon during the course of many illnesses. A more general term 'abnormal illness behavior' has been coined to describe the situation when the individual persists with and exaggerates symptoms following on from an illness, akin to the physician's phrase 'functional overlay'.

Treatment

Successful treatment depends upon the recognition that the symptoms are 'real' for the child, psychic pain is as distressing as physical pain. Anger and confrontation are unhelpful. A firm sympathetic approach with little attention to the symptom per se as well as avoiding rewarding the symptom is probably best. Allow the child to give up his symptoms with good grace, preferably providing the child with some face-saving reason for improvement. The outcome is good for the individual episode, though other psychological problems may persist.

SOMATIZATION DISORDER (Lask & Fosson 1989)

Clinical features and management

Many children complain of somatic symptoms which do not have a pathological basis. Common symptoms are abdominal pain, headaches and limb pains with community prevalence rates of approximately 10% (Faull & Nicol 1986). Management involves the minimum necessary investigation to exclude any pathology, the identification of any stressful circumstances and a sensitive explanation of the basis for the symptoms. The prevention of restrictions and the active encouragement of normal activities are essential.

When somatic symptoms are persistent, chronic and involve several systems of the body, ICD and DSM use the term somatization disorder. In many cases, there is clear evidence of underlying anxiety or recent stressful events.

REACTION TO SEVERE STRESS AND ADJUSTMENT DISORDERS

This group of disorders arises in response to an exceptionally stressful event or a significantly adverse life change. The clinical features of the different syndromes vary considerably, with a preponderance of affective symptoms in most cases.

Adjustment disorder

Definition

This is a maladaptive response occurring within 3 months of an identifiable psychosocial stressor. The maladaptive response must be of sufficient severity to impair daily activities such as schooling, hamper social relationships and be greater than expected given the nature of the stressor. Finally, the reaction must not last longer than 6 months.

Clinical features

By definition, the symptoms vary with ICD and DSM recognizing more than 6 categories. Clinical practice shows that anxiety and depressive symptoms, often combined, are the most frequent categories. Common stressors include parental divorce, unemployment, family illness or family move.

Predisposing factors

Age has different effects, depending on the type of stressor. For instance, separation is more upsetting for the younger child than for the adolescent, whereas a loss or change of heterosexual relationship is far more important for an adolescent than for the younger child. Boys are also more vulnerable to the adverse effects of stress than girls. Temperamental characteristics such as 'difficult' or 'slow to warm up' style probably influence susceptibility as well. Again, the child's previous experience and repertoire of coping skills affect the response to the current stressor. For instance, if the child has successfully coped with adversity in the past, his resilience and ability to withstand the present situation are enhanced. Finally, the family, particularly the parents, can magnify or minimize the impact of a stressor, dependent on their resourcefulness and coping style.

Outcome

By definition, the disorder can only last for 6 months, after which time the diagnostic category must change. The more important clinical consideration is not the change in diagnostic category, but the adverse effect that chronic or repeated stresses can have on the child's long-term adjustment.

Post-traumatic stress disorder (Yule 1991)

The 'epidemic' of disasters which have involved British children over the past 10 years (the capsize of the *Herald of Free Enterprise*, the sinking of the cruise ship *Jupiter*, the Pan-Am Lockerbie air crash and the crushing disaster at the Hillsborough football stadium) have made clinicians acutely aware of this syndrome. Clinicians are now familiar with the wide symptomatology often found and have also become involved in treatment programs to reduce the distress in the immediate aftermath and also in the longer term. The events include accidents, or disasters as well as more personal trauma such as witnessing murder, rape or torture.

Clinical features

These include 'flashbacks' (the repeated reenactment of the event with intrusive memories, dreams or nightmares); a sense of detachment, 'numbness' and emotional blunting; irritability, poor concentration and memory problems. Following disasters, many survivors often experience an increased awareness of danger, a foreshortened view of the future ('only plan for today'), a feeling of 'survivor' guilt (self reproach about own survival, whilst companions died) and acute panic reactions.

Yule (1991) indicates that between 30 and 50% of children show significant psychological morbidity following disasters, with symptoms persisting for several months (Yule et al 1990).

Management

The available evidence (Yule 1991) suggests that postdisaster 'debriefing' sessions on an individual or group basis are helpful. Specific counseling sessions to help the child deal with phobic, anxiety or depressive symptoms are frequently necessary as well as helpful. Cognitive/behavioral approaches are particularly suitable for these types of problems.

MOOD DISORDERS

DEPRESSION (see p. 1754)

There is an important distinction between sadness and unhappiness on the one hand and a depressive disorder on the other. Transitory mood swings are a normal phenomenon affecting many children, particularly adolescents. Moreover, sadness and unhappiness are features found in several other psychiatric disorders including chronic anxiety and conduct disorder. By contrast, depressive disorder is characterized by a sustained lowered mood, anhedonia (inability to derive pleasure from life), low self-esteem, suicidal ideas and disturbances of eating and sleeping.

Until recently, it was thought that this syndrome did not occur in prepubertal children, except perhaps following certain illnesses such as infectious mononucleosis. However, the development of reliable interview schedules and questionnaires (Rutter 1988) has changed this view so that it is recognized that depressive illness does occur, though uncommonly (less than 1%). Bipolar or manic depressive illness is even more infrequent.

Assessment

A comprehensive assessment involving individual and family interview(s) is essential, along with information from the school. The interview(s) with the child has particular importance as it can involve the disclosure of suicidal ideas and also provide the opportunity for the child to unburden himself as well as establishing a trusting relationship with the therapist. The assessment of suicidal risk is important (see adolescent section). Detailed inquiry should be made about current stresses, particularly life events involving threat and loss of self-esteem and also about recent illnesses, particularly viral infections.

Treatment

Tricyclic antidepressants (imipramine or amitriptyline) are successful for some children with definite depressive disorder, though the problems with side-effects are common and occasionally disabling. The newer classes of antidepressants such as fluoxetine and paroxetine are now being used with some success, but controlled trials have not been carried out so far. Individual and family therapy are also used in most cases. Attempts should be made wherever possible to ameliorate any contributory stressful factors. Recently, some clinicians have also attempted to use cognitive–behavioral approaches in older children and adolescents (see adolescent section).

Outcome

Approximately two-thirds will respond to treatment with the remainder continuing either to show symptoms or to be vulnerable to further episodes.

CONDUCT DISORDER

Clinical features

This is usually defined as persistent antisocial or socially disapproved of behavior, that often involves damage to property and is unresponsive to normal sanctions. The IOW study found a prevalence rate of 4% when the mixed disorder category was included as well, with a marked male predominance (at least 3 : 1). There is no absolute criterion for deviance as societal and cultural values determine the seriousness or importance that is attached to antisocial behavior. Common symptoms include temper tantrums, oppositional behavior, overactivity, irritability, aggression, stealing, lying, truancy, bullying and wandering away from home/school. Delinquency (a legal term referring to a person committing an offense against the law) is a frequent feature among older children and adolescents. Stealing, vandalism, arson and firesetting are common forms of delinquency (male : female 10 : 1).

Traditionally, a distinction has been made between socialized and unsocialized antisocial behavior. The former describes behavior that is in accord with peer group values but contrary to those of society, for instance antisocial gang behavior such as stealing and vandalism. Unsocialized antisocial behavior implies more disturbed behavior as it is often done as a solitary activity with a background of parental rejection or neglect and poor peer relationships. Learning difficulties, especially specific reading retardation, occur more commonly among children with conduct disorders. This is a further reason why school is unpopular and a source of discouragement for these children. Additionally, many children with conduct disorder have affective symptoms such as anxiety or unhappiness, as well as low self-esteem and poor peer relationships. When these symptoms are prominent, it is often appropriate to classify the disorder as mixed, implying both emotional and behavioral symptomatology.

Etiology

Four factors, the family, the peer group, the neighborhood and constitutional, make some contribution in most cases, but the family is usually the most important. Families of children with conduct disorder are characterized by a lack of affection, rejection, marital disharmony, inconsistent and ineffective discipline, and parental violence and aggression. The families are often of large size, which aggravates the problems of supervision and care. Constitutional factors present in some cases include low intelligence and learning difficulties, along with adverse temperamental features such as overactivity and impulsiveness. Oppositional peer group values are an important feature in older children and adolescents. Many children with conduct disorder live in areas of urban deprivation with poor schooling. The intractable and chronic nature of these problems is a major reason for the continuation of conduct disorder into adolescence and adult life.

Treatment

Help for the family, by counseling for the parents or by family therapy, is often used. Again, a behavioral approach for some symptoms such as aggression is often successful. Educational support through remedial teaching or the provision of special education can be important in some cases. For many families, however, the role of psychiatric services is limited, with practical support with rehousing in order to alleviate social disadvantage the most important contribution.

Prognosis

Two-thirds continue to show problems into adult life. Bad prognostic features are many and varied symptoms, problems at home and in the community and antiauthority and aggressive attitudes (Robins 1966).

DISORDERS OF ELIMINATION

ENURESIS

This term refers to the involuntary passage of urine in the absence of physical abnormality after the age of 5 years. It may be nocturnal and/or diurnal. Bed wetting continuously, though not necessarily every night, since birth is termed primary enuresis, whereas when there has been a 6-month period of dry beds at some stage, recurrence of bed wetting is termed secondary or onset enuresis. Diurnal enuresis is much less common than nocturnal, but more common among girls and among children who are psychiatrically disturbed. Depending upon definition, approximately 10% of 5-year-olds, 5% of 10-year-olds and 1% of 15-year-olds will have nocturnal enuresis. The majority of children with nocturnal enuresis are not psychiatrically ill, though a substantial minority (approximately 25%) have signs of psychiatric disturbance.

Etiology

A combination of individual factors such as positive family history (approximately 70%), low intelligence, psychiatric disturbance and small bladder capacity, along with environmental factors such as recent stressful life events, large family size and social disadvantage are present in most cases.

Treatment

It is important to exclude any physical basis for the enuresis by history, examination and, if necessary, investigation of the renal tract. Assuming no physical pathology, the most important initial step is to minimize the handicap, namely to point out to the parents the very favorable natural outcome of the condition, and to relabel the child's enuresis as immaturity rather than laziness or willfulness. A star chart, the accurate recording of enuresis plus positive reinforcement for dry nights, provides an accurate

baseline as well as a successful treatment in its own right. An enuretic alarm is successful with older cooperative children. The success of this approach is probably because the child becomes more aware of the sensation of a full bladder along with the encouragement from parents for dry nights. The newer models of the buzzer are extremely compact and do not require a pad placed between the sheets, thereby increasing patient compliance considerably. It is useful to combine a buzzer with a star chart. Tricyclic antidepressants such as imipramine, 25–50 mg nocte, are very effective at stopping enuresis, though their major limitation is that the enuresis returns when they are stopped. Many pediatricians believe it is wrong to prescribe such drugs, as they may be lethal when taken in an overdose, either accidental or intentional.

SOILING AND ENCOPRESIS

Most children are continent of feces and clean by their fourth birthday. Encopresis is the inappropriate passage of formed feces, usually onto underclothes, in the absence of physical pathology after 4 years of age. Soiling (the passage of semisolid feces) is often used synonymously with encopresis. Symptoms vary widely in severity, ranging from slight staining of underclothes to encopresis with the smearing of feces onto the walls. It is uncommon, with a community prevalence among 8-year-olds of 1.8% for boys and 0.7% for girls. Psychiatric disturbance is common among children with encopresis. Enuresis may also be present.

Clinical features (Fig. 30.3)

Figure 30.3 shows a convenient way to classify encopresis with a broad distinction between children who retain feces with eventual overflow incontinence and those who deposit feces inappropriately on a regular basis. Some children have never achieved continence, a situation called continuous or primary encopresis, whilst others have had periods of cleanliness followed by relapse, the so-called discontinuous or secondary encopresis. Figure 30.3 also lists the common different patterns of interaction found among encopretic children and their parents. For instance, children with retentive encopresis have usually been subjected to coercive and obsessional toilet training practices, so that the encopresis is seen as a reaction, often of anger and aggression,

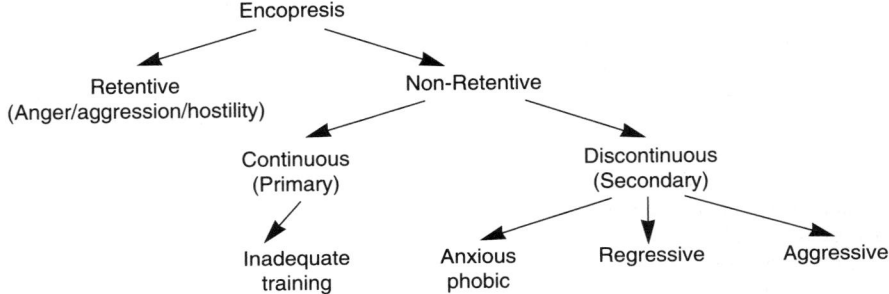

Three patterns are common:
- Child with primary encopresis
- Child with retentive encopresis
- Child with secondary encopresis

Fig. 30.3 Types of encopresis and their psychopathology.

towards this practice. Similarly, many children with continuous nonretentive encopresis come from disorganized chaotic families where regular training and toileting are not the norm. Again, encopresis can arise in some children as a response to a stressful situation. Finally, encopresis can reflect a poor parent–child relationship, often longstanding and usually associated with other aspects of psychiatric disturbance. The clinical picture is often, however, not as clear cut, with the different elements each making some contribution. There may be a previous history of constipation and occasionally anal fissure.

Treatment

A physical etiology such as Hirschsprung's disease must be considered before commencement of psychological treatment. The assessment must include an account of previous treatments and most importantly, the current attitude of the parents and the child to the problem. Treatment has two aims: the promotion of a normal bowel habit; and the improvement of the parent–child relationship. Initially, bowel washout and/or microenemata may be necessary to clear out the bowel. Judicious use of bowel smooth muscle stimulants (Senokot), stool softeners (Dioctyl) and bulk agents (Lactulose) is helpful for the child with retention. Again, suppositories are often useful from time to time. This should also be combined with parental and child education about the dietary importance of fiber. The psychological component includes behavioral (star chart) and individual psychotherapy to gain the cooperation and trust of the child along with parental counseling or family therapy, to modify attitudes and hostile interactions between the child and his parents. Encopresis usually resolves by adolescence, though other problems may persist. Occasional case reports of persistence into adult life have been published (Fraser & Taylor 1986).

OVERACTIVITY AND HYPERACTIVITY (Taylor 1994)

Clinical features

Terms such as overactivity or hyperactivity, hyperkinetic disorder and attention deficit disorder are used interchangeably, so that it is important to define the usage in each instance.

In the UK, hyperkinetic disorder is restricted to the small number of children (less than 0.1%) who show severe, pervasive (present in all situations) hyperactivity, are impulsive and distractible, with a short attention span. They are often aggressive with marked mood swings. Other associated features are male predominance (at least 3 : 1), low intelligence with learning difficulties and evidence on examination or investigation of neurological impairment. The hyperactivity is at its peak between the ages of 3 and 8 years.

Attention deficit disorder is a term mainly used in North America where it refers to a large group of children (approximately 5–10% of the population) whose principal abnormalities are a short attention span and distractibility. They are frequently hyperactive, aggressive and have learning difficulties.

Many disturbed children have overactive or hyperactive behavior as part of the clinical picture, but only in certain situations. Psychiatrists in the UK would probably classify these children as conduct disorder; North American clinicians would include them in the attention deficit disorder category.

Treatment

Medication, usually with stimulant drugs such as methylphenidate (up to 0.3 mg/kg/day) can be very valuable for children with severe hyperkinetic syndrome, but it should be restricted to this small group of children and not prescribed for every child with overactivity. Most importantly, treatment should be combined with behavioral approaches. Side-effects of methylphenidate include loss of appetite, insomnia, reduced growth rate and labile moods. Drug 'holidays', whereby the drug is stopped for periods of time are very useful, not only to minimize side-effects but also to show whether medication is still necessary. Behavioral techniques, parental counseling and the alteration and manipulation of the child's environment, particularly at school, to reduce and minimize distraction are the main components of treatment programs in most cases. An alternative approach adopted by some clinicians has been the use of exclusion diets on the basis that the child is allergic to certain substances, commonly tartrazine. Evidence for the efficacy of these exclusion diets other than as a placebo response is unconvincing, though Egger et al (1985), using a sophisticated methodological design, showed that children with severe hyperactivity and mental retardation did respond. It is, however, unclear whether these results would apply to children of normal intelligence with less severe problems, who make up the majority of overactive children.

Outcome

Hyperactivity and attention deficits lessen considerably by adolescence, though other major problems such as learning difficulties and behavior problems persist. A substantial minority continue to have problems in adult life, mainly of an antisocial nature.

MISCELLANEOUS DISORDERS

DEVELOPMENTAL DISORDERS

Language disorders (see developmental section)

Children with language disorders are more vulnerable to disturbance, mainly because of the associated anxiety and embarrassment caused by the disorder. Specific language delay (5–6/1000) is twice as common in boys than girls, with a strong association with large family size and lower social class. Approximately 25% of 3-year-olds with specific language delay have behavioral problems.

Stuttering, an abnormality of speech rhythm consisting of hesitations and repetitions at the beginning of syllables and words, is a normal, though transitory phenomenon, occurring at around 3–4 years of age. When it persists (approximately 3% of the general population), often due to inadvertent parental attention, it leads to anxiety and low self-esteem.

Elective mutism

This is not strictly a language disorder, as the main problem is the child's refusal to talk in certain situations, most commonly at school, rather than an inability to speak. Mild forms of the disorder are common but transitory, usually at the commencement of schooling, while the severe form occurs in about 1 per 1000 (Kolvin & Fundudis 1981). Other features include previous history of speech delay, excessively shy but stubborn temperament and parental overprotectiveness.

A combination of behavioral and family therapy techniques to promote communication and the use of speech is most commonly used, though some cases require inpatient assessment. Prognosis is good for approximately 50%, with failure to improve by the age of 10 years a poor prognostic sign.

Reading difficulties

Though mainly of educational concern, the pediatrician or child psychiatrist may get involved because of the associated behavioral or emotional problems. The two main types are first, general reading backwardness, when the retardation is a reflection of generalized intellectual delay, and second, specific reading retardation when the attainment in reading is significantly behind that expected on the basis of age and intelligence. The problem is usually 'significant' when the delay is at least 2 years. Dyslexia is a concept similar to that of specific reading retardation, implying a neuropsychological substrate for the specific reading difficulties. The use of this term is contentious, so that the more bland expression, specific reading retardation, is preferred by many clinical psychologists.

The etiology is multifactorial, involving genetic, social, perceptual and language deficits. A noteworthy feature is the strong association between specific reading retardation and conduct disorder, with the behavior problem most likely arising secondary to the frustration and disillusionment associated with the reading difficulty. Treatment involves detailed assessment of the precise nature of the problem by a psychologist, followed by an individualized remedial program carried out by a specialized teacher in collaboration with the psychologist. Help with the behavioral problem is also necessary in order to prevent more serious problems arising during adolescence.

TIC DISORDERS

Tics are rapid, involuntary, repetitive muscular movements, usually involving the face and neck, for instance blinks, grimaces and throat clearing. Simple tics occur as a transitory phenomenon in about 10% of the population, with boys outnumbering girls 3 to 1 and with a mean age of onset around 7 years. They range in severity from simple tics involving head and neck through to complex tics extending to the limbs and trunk and finally to Gilles de la Tourette's syndrome. The latter comprises complex tics accompanied by coprolalia (uttering obscene words and phrases) and echolalia (the repetition(s) of sounds or words). Like stammering, tics are made worse at times of stress and may be exacerbated by undue parental concern. The differential diagnosis of tics in childhood is principally from chorea, where the movements are less coordinated and predictable, are not stereotypic in form and cannot be suppressed. Other features of tics are positive family history and a previous history of neurodevelopmental delay. Many tics resolve spontaneously, but those that persist can be extremely disabling and difficult to treat.

Treatment

Several approaches are used singly or in combination, depending on assessment. Medication is effective but should be reserved for severe cases. Haloperidol (0.5–1.5 mg b.i.d.) is the drug of choice for the Tourette syndrome. If unsuccessful, alternative drugs are pimozide and clonidine. Many children with simple tics respond to explanation and reassurance along with advice for the parents. Individual and/or family therapy may be indicated when anxiety and tension are clearly making important contributions to the problem. Behavior therapy in the form of relaxation and or massed practice can also be helpful.

Prognosis

Simple tics have a good outcome with complete remission, whereas in the Tourette syndrome the condition fluctuates in a chronic manner with 50% continuing with symptoms even into adult life.

HABIT DISORDERS

Finger or thumb sucking and nail biting

These are extremely common and usually of no pathological significance. Excessive finger/thumb sucking can lead to deformity of teeth and fingers. Occasionally, they are signs of a more serious disturbance which itself requires treatment.

Rocking and head banging

Many normal otherwise healthy toddlers indulge in these habits when they are in their cot, causing much anxiety and distress to their parents who are also embarrassed by neighbors' complaints about the noise. Most children spontaneously cease these habits by around the fourth birthday so that reassurance and support for the parents is usually effective.

More serious self-injurious behavior occurs among some severely retarded children, some blind children and children with the Lesch–Nyhan syndrome.

Masturbation

This usually attracts attention and concern when it happens excessively. Most infants and toddlers engage in and enjoy touching their genitalia. During middle childhood, this appears less common and/or the child is more discreet. At adolescence, masturbation is probably universal among boys, though less common among girls. Excessive masturbation requires investigation and help. Causes include: local skin irritation, particularly among infants; sexual abuse among older children; and emotional deprivation, when the masturbation represents an attempt by the child to obtain some pleasure from an otherwise unloving environment. Some mentally retarded adolescents cause much embarrassment to their parents by masturbation in public. Clear guidance for the parents about what is acceptable and what is not, for instance masturbation in private is allowable, are the best way to help, along with encouragement for the parents to enforce these rules.

SLEEP DISORDERS (see also section on preschool children)

Night terrors

The usual pattern is for the child to wake up in a frightened, even terrified state, not to respond when spoken to, nor appear to see objects or people. Instead, the child appears to be hallucinating, talking to and looking at people/things not actually present. The child may be difficult to comfort, with the period of disturbed behavior and altered consciousness lasting up to 15 minutes, occasionally longer. Eventually the behavior settles, with or without comfort, and the child goes back to sleep, awakening in the morning with no recollection of the episode. The latter point is invaluable in helping to allay parental anxiety about the episodes. Night terrors arise from stage 4 or deep sleep. The peak incidence is between 4 and 7 years with a continuation of 1–3% into older children. It is also helpful to identify and ameliorate any identifiable stresses that may occasionally contribute to the problem. Lask (1988) described an apparently novel successful behavioral approach relying on waking the child 15 minutes prior to the expected time of the night terror.

Nightmares

These are frightening or unpleasant dreams, occurring during REM (rapid eye movement) sleep. The child may or may not wake up but there will be a clear recollection of the dream if he does wake up and also in the morning. There is no period of altered consciousness or inaccessibility as with night terrors.

Sleep walking (somnambulism)

The child, usually aged between 8 and 14 years, calmly arises from his bed with a blank facial expression, does not respond to attempts at communication and can only be awakened with difficulty. The child is in a state of altered consciousness at the deep level of sleep (stages 3 or 4). Any contributory anxiety should be treated, as well as giving the parents some advice about the safety and protection of the child during these episodes.

EATING DISORDERS (see also preschool and adolescent sections)

Obesity

This is a common problem affecting around 10% of children, depending upon definition. Psychological problems may be responsible for the onset of the obesity and/or may arise secondary to the obesity. The role of the psychiatrist or psychologist is to identify and treat these problems and more importantly, to enlist the cooperation of the child and family in adherence to a dietary regimen. Other treatment components include a behavioral program to modify eating patterns, for instance making the child more aware of the cues associated with excessive eating. A major problem with treatment programs is that they may not modify the eating habits sufficiently to ensure that the weight loss is maintained when the program is finished.

Anorexia nervosa

This condition, defined as a morbid fear of being fat accompanied by behavior designed to produce weight loss, does occur in prepubertal children, girls and boys, though much less frequently than among adolescents. Again bulimia, defined as periodic bouts of 'binge eating' or the consumption of high calorific food over a brief period often followed by self-induced vomiting, rarely occurs in children. The main features of these conditions are discussed in the adolescent section.

PSYCHOLOGICAL EFFECTS OF ILLNESS AND HANDICAP

Approximately 15% of children have some form of chronic illness or handicap. The IOW study of Rutter showed clearly that this group of children were much more at risk for disturbance, namely a rate of 33% among children with chronic illness affecting the central nervous system and of 12% among children with chronic illness not affecting the central nervous system compared with 7% among the general population. The IOW study also showed that children with chronic illness or handicap had the same range of disorders as other disturbed children, thereby implying that the mechanisms involved with this increased morbidity are probably indirect and nonspecific rather than direct and specific to each illness or handicap.

Effects on the child

Three aspects are important: the acquisition of skills and outside interests; the development of self-concept; and the development of adaptive coping behavior. Many illnesses or handicaps inevitably limit and restrict the child's ability or opportunity to acquire everyday skills and develop interests and hobbies: for example, the child with cerebral palsy by definition is motor handicapped, the dietary restrictions of diabetes, the exercise limitations of asthma and the avoidance by children with epilepsy of some activities such as cycling or swimming. Additionally, educational problems are common among this group of children for a variety of reasons, including increased absence from school, specific learning difficulties, especially among children with epilepsy, and low expectations of parents and teachers.

Illness and handicap can adversely affect the child's self-concept in several ways through the effects on the child's body image, his self-esteem and his ideas about the causation of the disability. Many children have a distorted view of their body, believing the handicap to be very prominent or disfiguring. These ideas can often be reinforced by comments from parents and peers. The other factor influencing the child's self-concept is his explanation for the cause of his disability. Young children below the age of 6 years often regard their disability as a punishment for some misdemeanor, whilst during middle childhood the child commonly thinks he has 'caught' the illness from someone or something. It is only from around 10 years onward that adult-like ideas of causation begin to appear.

Successful adaptation to a disability depends on the acquisition of a range of coping behaviors and defense mechanisms to lessen anxieties to an acceptable level. Effective coping strategies include rationing the amount of stress into containable amounts, obtaining information from several sources, rehearsing the possible outcomes of treatment and assessing the situation from several viewpoints. Parents, nursing staff and pediatricians have an important role in promoting this repertoire of skills among children with disability. Additionally, defense mechanisms such as denial, rationalization and displacement can be helpful for the child during the initial stages of adjustment to the illness or disability.

Effects on the parents

The parents can respond in various ways in the short term (see later section) and also in the long term. Most parents eventually achieve some degree of adaptation, though for a minority maladaptive behavior patterns emerge and are prominent. The common reaction is overprotection whereby the parent(s) is unable to allow the child to experience the normal disappointments and upsets inevitable during childhood, so that the child leads a 'cotton wool' existence. Less frequently, the parent(s) may be rejecting and indifferent to the child because the child's disability is so damaging to the parents' self-esteem or because the disability has exacerbated an already precarious parent–child relationship. Overprotection and rejection are sometimes combined together in the parental reaction to the child's disability.

The parents may also find it difficult to provide appropriate discipline and control as they irrationally fear that such control may aggravate the child's illness, e.g. induce a fit in an epileptic child.

Finally, the stress of coping with the child's illness may exacerbate parental marital disharmony, though in a minority it may paradoxically unite them as they face the adversity together.

Effects on siblings

This can manifest itself in several ways: the oldest sibling may be given excessive responsibility, such as looking after the handicapped sib; the sibs may lose friendships because they are reluctant to bring their friends home in case their handicapped sib is an embarrassment; finally, the sibling's own developmental needs may be neglected, with consequent resentment and frustration.

BREAKING BAD NEWS TO PARENTS

This distressing but inevitable aspect of pediatrics comes in various guises, such as the birth of a child with Down syndrome, or with the diagnosis of cystic fibrosis. Unfortunately, most undergraduate and postgraduate training includes very little teaching about this important subject. Though the details vary for each case, the following general principles are important:

1. Information should be given by the most senior and experienced doctor involved with the child's care.

2. Both parents must be seen together if at all possible, as this reduces misinformation and allows the parents to be mutually supportive from the outset.

3. Allow adequate time for the interview (*not* 10 minutes at the end of a ward round).

4. Privacy is essential, not only as a matter of courtesy and dignity but also because it allows parents to express emotions more freely.

5. Begin the interview by asking the parents to tell you what they know about the problems.

6. Tell parents frankly and honestly in simple and nontechnical language the nature of the problem, explaining the reasons for the investigations and the basis for the diagnosis.

7. Encourage the parents to ask questions (by asking them some open-ended questions).

8. Emphasize the positive as well as the negative aspects of the diagnosis, for instance the child will be able to have physiotherapy and special equipment, will be able to go to school and to receive effective control for pain.

9. Facilitate the expression of emotions by the parents, namely respond sympathetically and sensitively to the parent(s)' distress and crying.

10. Make a definite offer of a further appointment to talk things over again.

11. Many parents find it helpful to continue the discussion with a nurse or social worker after the interview.

REACTIONS TO HOSPITALIZATION

Admission to hospital is a common experience during childhood. While most parents and their children cope successfully with the admission, some, particularly those with repeated admissions for minor illnesses, show evidence of disturbance which may in turn have been the reason why the child was admitted in the first place (Quinton & Rutter 1976).

Admission to hospital can have adverse effects in the short term as well as in the long term. The contributory factors can be grouped under three headings: the child and family; the nature of the illness; and the attitudes and practices of the hospital and its staff. Important factors within the child and family include age, temperament of the child, previous experience of hospital, previous parent–child relationship and current family circumstances. Children between the ages of 1 and 4 years are particularly stressed by separation from familiar figures. Similarly, children with adverse temperamental characteristics, such as poor adaptability and irregularity of habits, are more vulnerable. If the child had a favorable experience when in hospital previously, this will ease the burden for any subsequent admission. If the parent–child relationship was poor prior to admission, hospitalization is likely to exacerbate this problem because of the additional stress. Adverse family circumstances, for instance financial, may also be aggravated by admission.

The nature of the illness, particularly the associated pain and the necessity for painful procedures, influences the child's response. Again, an acute admission is likely to be more stressful than an elective procedure.

The attitudes of the staff and hospital practices can minimize considerably the distress for the child. Helpful and favorable aspects include good rooming-in facilities, adequate preparation for painful or unpleasant procedures, nursing and medical staff trained to minimize distress and to offer comfort when required. The ward should be organized so that parents and sibs are encouraged to visit as well as ensuring the ready availability of play leaders and teachers. Medical and nursing staff should also have access to social work resources as well as to psychological and psychiatric services. Finally, joint liaison between the medical and psychiatric team and the establishment of a staff support group to enable staff to discuss their own anxieties about working in a stressful environment are likely to be beneficial.

CARE OF THE DYING CHILD (p. 927, Ch. 16)

Parents usually undergo two periods of grief response, firstly at the time of diagnosis ('initial phase') and then at the approach of death ('terminal phase'). These phases have the features of a grief response, namely shock and numbness, denial, development of somatic symptoms and/or affective features such as anger, anxiety or depression, followed by some degree of acceptance. Most concern is often expressed about what to tell the child. The latter is obviously influenced by the child's age and intelligence. Generally speaking, current hospital practice is to facilitate discussion with the child about his illness and its implications.

Parental wishes should, however, be respected, whilst indicating to the parents the advantages of a more open attitude. Consequently, there are no absolute rules but rather that a sensitive and flexible approach is most likely to be beneficial.

TREATMENT METHODS

Several factors are usually responsible for the development of disturbance so that it is unlikely that one treatment method will resolve the problem. All treatment approaches include active cooperation between the therapist and the child and family, agreement between them about the aims of treatment, and a mutual trust to enable these aims to be achieved. Careful analysis of the following elements is therefore necessary in order to devise an effective treatment program:

1. Individual
    a. physical illness or handicap
    b. intellectual ability
    c. type of symptomatology
2. Family
    a. developmental stage (for instance a family with preschool children or one with adolescents)
    b. psychiatric health of parents
    c. marital relationship
    d. parenting qualities
    e. communication pattern within the family
    f. ability to resolve conflict
    g. support network, for instance availability of extended family
3. School
    a. scholastic attainments
    b. attitude of child and parents to the authority of the school
    c. peer relationships
4. Community
    a. quality of peer relationships and of role models
    b. neighborhood and community resources.

The formulation of the problem along these four dimensions determines the suitability and likely success of treatment.

The three main types of treatment approach available are *drug treatment*, the *psychotherapies*, and *liaison* or *consultation work*. The latter refers to the common practice whereby the child psychiatrist or a member of the psychiatric team does not have direct contact with the referred child, but rather helps those involved with the child to understand and modify the child's behavior. Psychotherapies are those treatments that use a variety of psychological techniques to ameliorate disturbance. They include individual therapy, behavior therapy, family therapy and group therapy as well as counseling and advice for parents.

DRUG TREATMENT

This does not have a major treatment role in child psychiatry. Moreover, drugs should only be used to treat specific symptoms and only for a defined period of time. They are most likely to produce symptomatic relief rather than have a curative effect. Table 30.4 summarizes the important indications and side-effects of various drugs used in child psychiatry.

PSYCHOTHERAPIES

These are the commonest treatment approach in contemporary child psychiatric practice.

Table 30.4 Drug treatment in child psychiatry

Drug	Usage	Comment
Anxiolytics (e.g. diazepam)	Anxiety/phobic conditions	Short-term adjunct to behaviour treatment
Neuroleptics Phenothiazines (e.g. chlorpromazine)	Schizophrenia/ Hyperkinetic syndrome	Extrapyramidal side-effects common
Butyrophenones (e.g. haloperidol)	Complex tics/Tourette syndrome	Extrapyramidal side-effects common
Tricyclics Imipramine/amitriptyline	Enuresis	Effective, but high relapse rate
Clomipramine	Major affective disorder	Most useful with persistent and sustained mood disturbance
Stimulants Methylphenidate	Hyperkinetic syndrome	Effective short-term. Long-term side-effects on growth, sleep and appetite
Fenfluramine	Pervasive developmental disorder	Effectiveness not established. Side-effects include irritability, anorexia and weight loss
Hypnotics (e.g. trimeprazine/promethazine)	Persistent sleep disorder in preschool children	Only short-term
Lithium	Recurrent bipolar affective disorder	Close supervision of blood level for signs of toxicity
Laxatives (e.g. bulk-forming (methylcellulose) stimulants (senna), softener (dioctyl)	Encopresis with constipation	Facilitates formation and passage of feces
Central α-agonist (e.g. clonidine)	Unresponsive Tourette syndrome	Sedation and rebound hypertension

Individual psychotherapy

The therapist aims to: develop a trusting, nonjudgmental relationship with the child; enable the child to express his feelings and thoughts; understand the meaning of the child's symptoms, including his behavior during the therapeutic session; and provide the child with some understanding and explanation for his behavior. The indications for individual psychotherapy are not clearly established, though most usually it is for children with a neurotic or reactive disorder rather than for those with a constitutionally based disorder. For younger children the medium for communication is play, such as sand play or through drawing, whilst for older children verbal exchange and discussion are possible.

Behavioral psychotherapy (McAuley & McAuley 1977)

This approach is based upon the application of the findings from experimental psychology, particularly learning theory, to a wide range of problems such as enuresis, encopresis, tantrums and aggression. Its characteristics are as follows:

1. Define problem(s) objectively with reference to the antecedents, the behavior itself and the consequences (the ABC approach).
2. Emphasis on current behavior rather than on past events.
3. Set up hypotheses to account for the behavior.
4. Pretreatment baseline to determine the frequency and severity of the problem.
5. Devise behavioral programs on an individual basis to test the hypothesis.
6. Evaluate outcome of treatment programs.
7. Tackle one problem at a time.

As with other psychotherapies, success depends upon the establishment of a trusting relationship with the patient and the close supervision of the treatment program, together with the involvement of teachers and parents in many cases.

Family therapy (Barker 1992) (see adolescent section)

This is an extremely popular treatment approach now. The rationale underlying family therapy is that the child's disturbed behavior is symptomatic of the disturbance within the family as a group. There are many different theoretical approaches and techniques (see Barker 1992) but all usually involve interviewing the whole family on each occasion for about 1 hour. Most family work is short term, lasting about 6 months, with approximately monthly sessions. The emphasis is on current behavior, verbal and nonverbal, observed during the session rather than on past events. The main aim is to improve communication within the family so that dysfunctional patterns of behavior are replaced by more healthy and adaptive behavior.

Group therapy (see adolescent section)

Older children and adolescents often benefit from group therapy when the aim is to improve interpersonal relationships, particularly with the peer group, using a variety of theoretical models, for instance psychodynamic and social skills.

Supportive psychotherapy and counseling

The former is frequently used for the child with chronic illness or handicap, when the focus may be the child or the parents. It is especially beneficial at the time of diagnosis and also in the longer term when the implications of the disability become more evident. Parental counseling is also used to help the parents understand their child's behavior problems, the factors that may have led to them and that are responsible for their continuation, along with an emphasis on the parent–child relationship and the improvement of parenting skills. Counseling may therefore help parents to devise and implement a behavioral program to modify the child's behavior as well as to promote normal development.

LIAISON AND CONSULTATION PSYCHIATRY (Lask 1994)

This is a collaborative approach between the child psychiatry team and the professionals directly involved with the child, for instance hospital staff, teachers and residential care staff, in order to help these professionals to understand the child's disturbed behavior and their own possible contribution to the problem, and to suggest ways to improve the situation. Although the child psychiatrist may see the referred child in the first instance, subsequent contact is usually with the staff rather than with the child. This approach can also include the establishment and supervision of a staff support group whose aim is to look at the attitudes and emotional responses of the staff towards the behavior shown by the children under their care.

PSYCHIATRIC DISORDERS IN ADOLESCENCE

INTRODUCTION

PREVALENCE

The prevalence of emotional and behavioral disturbance is even greater in adolescence than in childhood. Depending upon the criteria employed and the sample population study, prevalence rates of up to 1 in 4 have been reported. In the original adolescent follow-up to the pioneering Isle of Wight Study a deviancy rate of 15% was found (Graham & Rutter 1973). However, as has already been pointed out, unlike most medical disorders a majority of these disorders represent the extreme end of normal distribution, and their causation is both multifactorial and rarely clear-cut.

PERSISTENCE OF CHILDHOOD DISORDERS

Many of the disorders present in adolescence arise during childhood, persisting with little modification. In the Isle of Wight follow-up, this was true for a majority of the adolescent conduct disorders and about a quarter of the emotional disorders.

Of the remainder that arise de novo during adolescence, clinical practice suggests that, in many cases, clear evidence of some preceding vulnerability can be found. For example, temperamental characteristics of persistent negative mood or unadaptability may have been prominent childhood characteristics of some adolescents with a behavior disorder. Likewise, childhood personality traits of obsessionality or perfectionism are often premorbid characteristics of adolescent anorexic patients. A childhood tendency towards anxious or depressive responses to stress often persists into adolescence. Similarly, although sexual disorders rarely arise before adolescence, some preceding disturbance or vulnerability is common (sometimes associated with, or secondary to, childhood sexual abuse).

NEW DISORDERS

Two psychiatric disorders typically arise during adolescence without any prominent childhood precursors: bipolar depressive illness and schizophrenia (Cawthron et al 1994). For this reason, even where there is a positive family history that ought to alert the clinician to their possible presence, symptoms of these two disorders may be misattributed to 'adolescence' as a developmental phase of notorious difficulty. The diagnosis may then only be made after the full clinical picture has developed. For example, an only daughter of a single parent became querulous and irritable in late childhood, and during adolescence battled with her mother, dropping out of school and experimenting with drugs. She was only recognized to have a manic–depressive illness when she was admitted from her bed-sit under a compulsory hospital order in a disheveled and deluded state.

Thus, adolescent psychiatry straddles both child psychiatry and general psychiatry, so to work effectively with adolescents it is necessary to have knowledge of both. It is also important to have knowledge of the developmental phases specific to adolescence, and some familiarity with the current social context of adolescents (e.g. youth culture, the effect of adverse family experience, socializing effects of school and workplace, unemployment, etc.).

ADOLESCENT DEVELOPMENT

THE TIMING AND DURATION OF DEVELOPMENT

There is no clear relationship between biological puberty and the onset of adolescence as a social phenomenon. The timing of biological puberty may affect adolescents' social experience. Early developers are held in higher esteem by their peers, but late developers achieve more at school, perhaps seeking compensatory satisfaction elsewhere, or less distracted by their emerging sexuality and the interest of others. There is no evidence firmly linking biological puberty with cognitive development; adolescents may have obtained their full height and have well-developed secondary sexual characteristics but cognitively may not have attained Piaget's stage of formal thinking, unable to reason in a fully abstract way.

Western perspectives on adolescence tend to emphasize the social aspects, and place developmental theories of adolescence within this context, but in other cultures the various 'rites de passage' of adolescence may have little or no link to biological puberty, occurring even as late as 28 or 30 years old (the Masai), whilst other cultures attach no particular significance to adolescence as a psychosocial stage. A simple definition of adolescence might be the period of significant dependence upon parents and other adults beyond biological puberty, which particular social circumstances might prolong. For example, even after gaining responsibility for young children of their own, the strong filial ties of young working class parents in some western communities may prevent them acquiring an adulthood status equal to that of their parents. An extended period of economic dependence upon parents (because of unemployment, continuing further education, chronic disability, etc.), or the necessity for frequent parental support because of single parent status, may also prolong this process. In Europe, the patterns of transition between adolescence and adulthood are probably becoming more pluralized and fragmented (Chisholm & Hurrlemann 1995).

SUBPHASES IN DEVELOPMENT

However long the period of prolonged dependence, in western cultures four subphases can generally be recognized. First, a *preadolescence* phase, which in girls does seem to immediately follow the onset of biological puberty, when youngsters begin to be intensely interested in youth culture and peer friendships become of much greater importance. *Early adolescence* (around 13–15 years) differs only in the development of a much more ambivalent, questioning attitude towards parents. Peer relationships, by contrast, are largely uncritical, since peers meet the early adolescent's intense dependency needs. These adolescents jointly examine and question aspects of the adult world they are now beginning to enter. In secondary school they have left the world of childhood behind, and have to deal with many teachers instead of the one or two to which they were previously accustomed. The first opportunities for part-time work occur at this time. In the *midadolescent* phase (14/15 to 16 years), the distinct maturational tasks of adolescence become more clearly apparent. First, acquiring a sexual identity, sexual feelings and drives now much stronger, enhancing adolescents' long-established gender role identity and promoting sexual role experimentation. Second, acquiring a social identity outwith their family. This occurs in two ways: a widening of their social network (to include a number of significant adults), and an altered relationship with their parents. The ambivalence within this relationship has started to diminish, so adolescents find they can once again begin to rely on parents, without immediately assuming that this will automatically lead to a loss of autonomy. This constitutes an important step in the third maturational task of adolescence: achieving emotional independence. Paradoxically, as Winnicott, the pioneering child psychoanalyst, pointed out (1965), it is only possible to develop a capacity for self-sufficiency if one is able to depend upon others at times of intimacy or stress, i.e. a capacity for mature dependence, whose full development often extends into the third or fourth decade of life. Establishing a satisfactory work identity is the fourth maturational stage of adolescence. The development of competency and sustained effort within the context of realistic goals permits achievement at work to become an important source of self-esteem. Such achievement is clearly affected by socioeconomic conditions such as high youth unemployment. By the last stage of adolescence, i.e. *late adolescence* (17/18 years of age onwards), a work and sexual identity should be well established, and whilst most still live within the parental home, their emotional and social emancipation will be apparent from their considerable emotional involvement with nonfamily members, evident within their regular nonoccupational shared activity with peers and other young adults.

HOW DISORDERS DEVELOP

CAUSAL FACTORS

Many different factors may be responsible for the development of a disorder in adolescence. In clinical practice it is often possible to develop clear hypotheses about why and how a disorder might have arisen. Three types of causal factor may be identified.

Precipitating factors

These are sudden stressful events facing the youngster or his family. They are usually closely linked in time to the onset of a disorder, such as the loss of a close relationship precipitating a depressive reaction, or parent(s)' or peers' persisting criticism of an adolescent girl's weight seeming to precipitate the onset of an anorexic illness. It is important to be aware that the stressful event may be an internal one, for example developmental anxieties associated with pubertal changes, or the overwhelming guilt which may follow a sudden feeling of jealousy or anger with a parent.

Predisposing factors

These factors either cause the adolescent or his family to be vulnerable to stressful events, or cause them to respond in a particular way, e.g. a tendency towards becoming intensely guilty about angry or jealous feelings, which in turn may be fostered by a family pattern of habitual conflict avoidance. In one family a predisposition towards emotional overinvolvement may be accentuated by the onset of chronic illness in one family member, whilst in another more disengaged family the same event may lead family members to further emotional withdrawal from one another.

Maintaining factors

These factors play a part in the maintenance of a disorder after its onset. They may be quite different from those responsible for its onset. For instance, once a pattern of deliberate weight loss has led to obvious food avoidance, an anorexic pattern of food refusal may develop and persist because it is the only way an adolescent girl feels she can maintain her autonomy in the face of intrusive parental concern. Similarly, deliberate exercise to reduce weight may eventually serve an additional function – the prevention of depressive feelings – which persists even after the wish to loose further weight has gone.

CAUSAL MECHANISMS

These concern how the various factors described above act to produce the symptoms characteristic of a particular disorder.

Various organic insults (or stressors) may produce a similar emotional response, the symptomatology largely determined by the type of personality involved. Anxiety, depression and anger are the basic emotional responses to stressful situations (Will & Wrate 1985), the manner of their expression as much determined by characteristics of the individual affected and his family as by the nature of the stressful event. For example, a major disappointment (as the precipitating event) might lead a shy, introverted adolescent (the predisposition) to become withdrawn (the symptom), whilst a rather omnipotent adolescent might respond by becoming even more overbearing.

Most psychiatric disorders of adolescence can be understood in these terms. However, this is not so true of the psychoses, even though family communication deviance and high levels of negative affect may precipitate the onset of psychotic illness in vulnerable adolescents (Goldstein 1985). Although there are no definitive biological markers for bipolar disorders or schizophrenia, there is strong circumstantial evidence that both illnesses are the result of biochemical abnormalities, probably involving serotonergic and dopaminergic neuron systems of the limbic system (Kendell 1988, Meltzer 1987). Although disorders sometimes appear to be precipitated by external stress (e.g. school

or university exam problems, or peer group difficulties), these 'stresses' may simply be early evidence of their insidious onset. Evidence for stress provoking a relapse has been established for schizophrenia (Kane 1987) but not for bipolar disorder. The primary defect in schizophrenia is probably cognitive, with secondary effects on emotion; in bipolar illness the reverse is likely.

SYMPTOMS AS MALADAPTIVE SOLUTIONS

Symptoms may arise in several ways. Some symptoms may develop as a response to others in the adjustment reaction (under the influence of predisposing or maintaining factors), whilst the remainder are often determined by the nature of the original stress (influenced by a combination of precipitating factors and factors responsible for the vulnerable predisposition). Take the previous example of the omnipotent adolescent who responded to disappointment by becoming overbearing. Firstly, his behavioral response might be characteristic of his emotional defense against many different kinds of stress. Secondly, this response is composed of a primary anxiety (which might be experienced by all subjects exposed to the same stress), and a secondary defense which many others might not share (attempting to control the disappointing environment so as to diminish his anxiety and prevent himself from becoming depressed). Amongst his behavioral response and vocal complaints might also be recognized elements of the disappointing event which precipitated his behavior. By this means many symptoms in adolescent psychiatry can be regarded as maladaptive solutions to stressful events facing the adolescent and his family.

Common experiences may become stressful life events because of the vulnerable predisposition of the adolescent and his family. For example, a mildly obsessional early-adolescent girl, who is a member of a family in which there is a taboo on anger, may respond to fears of her own anger by becoming obsessionally preoccupied with harm befalling others, especially her mother. As a consequence she may develop checking rituals and constantly seek reassurance. A similarly obsessional mid-adolescent boy, in a family where there is a taboo on sex, might respond to a sexually threatening experience or thought of his own by becoming obsessionally preoccupied with dirt; washing rituals may follow.

PRINCIPLES OF ASSESSMENT

A FRAMEWORK FOR ASSESSMENT

The psychiatric assessment of an adolescent has at least two main aims: diagnosis and formulation, and decision making:

1. to establish the nature of any psychiatric disorder present, and assess its duration and severity
2. to place the adolescent's disturbance within a developmental context and assess possible etiologic factors
3. to assess the positive features of the individual and family, e.g. the 'protective factors' described above
4. to form an opinion about prognosis and about what treatment is indicated, i.e. decision making.

A full assessment should therefore provide both a descriptive and an explanatory account of the adolescent's disturbance. This should include an assessment of how well the adolescent is accomplishing the maturational tasks described above and of the possible predisposing, precipitating and maintaining factors contributing to the disturbance.

To achieve this it is usually helpful to assess young people who are still living at home in a conjoint interview with their families, or if they are not living at home, to consult any other professionals involved in their current care, for example social workers or residential care staff. There may, for example, be 'maintaining' factors within the hostel or children's home that make it difficult to deal effectively with the adolescent's disturbance. An adequate assessment of the problems and their context may require consultation with all the professionals involved with a family. Indeed, since some adolescents generate considerable conflict between different professionals, such multiprofessional contact may be essential.

At the initial interview, the type of information that is described in the section on history taking above (p. 1734) is obtained. For effective communication with young people some additional skills, which are described below (p. 1753), are required. An assessment of the young person's mental state and of the functioning of his family are essential, often in the context of a family interview. On other occasions it is easier and indeed more appropriate to do a detailed assessment of the adolescent's mental state in a separate individual session (e.g. with adolescents with sexual problems and psychotically ill adolescents).

Case example

At the end of assessment, a *formulation* of the problems should be made, along the lines of this example:

Diagnosis. John, aged 15, is suffering from school refusal.

Maturational tasks. John is showing a marked delay in achieving emotional independence: he spends most of his time at home in the company of his mother. His social identity is highly restricted: he has no friends of his own age nor has he been involved in any age-appropriate social activities for at least 2 years. His sexual identity is immature: he has never had a girlfriend and denies all interest in girls or sex. He has no real work identity either: 18 months' schooling have been lost and he has no idea of what he would like to do after he leaves school.

Causal factors. Until he was 10 years old, John suffered severely from asthma and required numerous hospitalizations (*predisposing factors*). This resulted in his mother overprotecting him, which in turn led to conflict between mother and father about how to handle and discipline him (*early maintaining factors*). 2 years ago his maternal grandmother died and his mother, who had been very close to her mother, became depressed (*precipitating factors*). John's school refusal started from this time. Although mother is no longer depressed, the parents' inability to agree on whether or not John should be encouraged to return to school has resulted in John being allowed to remain at home (*additional maintaining factors*).

Summary. The same individual and family factors which have caused John to be overprotected by his mother (his asthma, and the marital conflict which has estranged the parents and reinforced John and mother's relationship) have contributed to John's school refusal and his lack of emotional independence. His school refusal, by impairing the development of a work and social identity, is interfering further with his adolescent maturation.

Prognosis. Guarded, in view of length of symptoms and length of familial disturbance.

Treatment. Initial interventions should be directed towards the

maintaining factors. A trial of family therapy is recommended, designed to foster a parental alliance in conjunction with a psychiatric recommendation that steps should be taken to return John to school as soon as possible.

WHEN TO MAKE A PSYCHIATRIC REFERRAL

The pediatrician is often in a dilemma about when to refer an adolescent to a psychiatrist. As has been mentioned, many *normal* adolescents may appear to be untrusting and reluctant to talk about their difficulties. So, unless the pediatrician has extensive experience of normal adolescent patients, or, indeed, has parental experience of normal adolescents, it may be difficult to distinguish what is normal adolescent *oppositionality* from something more sinister. This problem may be shared by the parents of some adolescents.

GUIDELINES FOR REFERRAL FOR A SPECIALIST PSYCHIATRIC OPINION

Mandatory

1. Any adolescent exhibiting signs suggestive of major *psychotic illness*. When any of the signs referred to in the sections below on schizophrenia (p. 1755) and depressive illness (p. 1754) are present.

2. Any adolescent who appears to be suffering from a major emotional illness, for example obsessional–compulsive disorder (p. 1756) or school refusal (p. 1756).

3. Adolescents suffering from *eating disorders* such as anorexia nervosa (p. 1757) or bulimia nervosa (p. 1759) should always be referred for psychiatric treatment if their symptoms have persisted for more than 3 months.

Strongly recommended

1. Any adolescent who has made any form of suicide attempt that is either inexplicable or where there may be an underlying depressive illness (see section on parasuicide, p. 1757).

2. Adolescents of either sex who disclose in their teenage years that they have experienced intrafamilial or extrafamilial sexual abuse (see p. 1759).

3. All adolescent perpetrators of sexually abusive activity, including exhibitionists, child molesters and rapists. There is a growing body of research which suggests that some of these adolescents become the adult child sexual abusers of tomorrow (see p. 1760).

Recommended

1. An opinion should be sought on adolescents who show evidence of conduct disorders where the influence of peer group and sociocultural pressures does not seem to account adequately for the behavioral difficulties.

2. Any adolescent living in a family whose poor functioning significantly impairs the adolescent's maturation and development.

3. Adolescents whose dependency upon such substances as alcohol, solvents and opiates (see p. 1762) appears to reflect individual or family problems rather than undesirable sociocultural patterns.

4. Any adolescent who is coping poorly with the psychological effects of chronic physical illness or handicap (see p. 1760).

HOW TO REFER

Few psychiatrically disturbed adolescents acknowledge from the outset that they are in need of help, perhaps because of their wish to emancipate themselves from dependence on adults. Accordingly, it is often difficult to persuade them that they need to see a psychiatrist. Where the youngster is under 16, the pediatrician should begin by helping the parents to see that a psychiatric opinion might be useful or even essential. The pediatrician should anticipate that, in many cases, the adolescent's psychiatrist will invite the parents *and* other family members to the first appointment. A family appointment may reduce the patient's feeling of stigmatization, but the request for all family members to attend may bewilder the parents and siblings. It is therefore important to orientate the parents and adolescent about what to expect (Will & Wrate 1985). This entails explaining the reason for the family appointment, i.e. it is often the best way to get to the bottom of the presenting problems and hence help them.

Many a taciturn adolescent has been enabled to 'open up' and talk about his problems when faced with both confirmatory and conflicting testimony from other family members. The oppositional adolescent may only reveal his particular perceptions of the family and its problems when disagreeing with the views of another family member. A neurotically inhibited young person may find the confirmation of his views by another family member (typically a sibling) a potent catalyst for self-expression. A family assessment meeting in a department of adolescent psychiatry is often a powerful forcing ground for the understanding and hence the resolution of adolescent problems.

ADOLESCENT PSYCHIATRIC SERVICES AVAILABLE

Most parts of Britain have an outpatient adolescent psychiatric service offering individual and family appointments. The age range for referrals is generally from 12 or 13 at the lower end to about 16 or so (i.e. school-leaving age) and some areas have an inpatient unit for young people. There is an enormous variation in available provision, which makes it imperative that the pediatrician is acquainted with the services available locally.

TALKING WITH ADOLESCENTS

There are some basic principles for successful communication with adolescent patients (Wrate 1989):

1. Ensure an adequate negotiation of expectations. For example, what they expect of the appointment, how the doctor sees its purpose and how it will proceed. It is vital to disabuse them of unnecessary anxieties about 'madness' or being seen as 'children'. This should include how much confidentiality can be assumed. The doctor might feel there are some matters it is essential to share with a youngster's parents or teacher. This can be negotiated, and *this is when to do it.*

2. Adolescents should feel that communication is taking place within a developing relationship. Relationship building is therefore important, for example by inquiring in an interested way about some of their personal circumstances and interests, career

intentions, previous contacts with hospitals and doctors, etc. A patronizing attitude on the part of the doctor or an opaque attitude, revealing little or nothing about himself as a person, are both equally unhelpful.

3. Effective communication is more than just talking. It involves a good capacity to listen, the ability to convey an attitude that the adolescent patient is in an expert position about himself and his concerns. Even if the adolescent cannot provide an answer to questions like 'Why do you think you get these headaches?', the doctor at least conveys an expectation of mutual problem solving. Empathic silence or uninterrupted listening may convey the same expectation.

4. The symmetry of communication: information-seeking questions tend to elicit information not affect, whilst affective data is most frequently elicited by specifically focusing on affect. Doctors tend to adopt a multiple-choice type questioning approach with unforthcoming patients, but as answers tend to mirror the questions, following up any slight lead the patient provides is important.

COMMON PROBLEMS

The most frequently voiced complaints of adolescents are:

1. not being listened to, or the adults only listening to what they want to hear
2. a talk turns into unsolicited advice or a mini-lecture
3. being patronized or the doctor being nosey (i.e. intrusive questioning against the adolescent's interests)
4. the doctor acting on behalf of particular adults rather than on the patient's behalf
5. the patient not understanding what is being asked of him, as simple straightforward language is not used
6. adults lacking humor or humanity, the patient feeling 'just a number'.

If the general principles described above prevail, these concerns should rarely be felt. Doctors, on the other hand, most often complain of adolescents being unforthcoming or sullen, even hostile. Sometimes the doctor's own attitude unwittingly contributes to this behavior, for example by failing to take time to build up a relationship, not being clear about the purposes of the appointment, or not taking the trouble to find out what the youngster feels would be a worthwhile outcome.

Persistently silent or sullen adolescents should not be allowed to feel their continued attitude will control the whole situation, as unchecked it will. Three steps to prevent this happening are possible:

1. By commenting on what is taking place in as uncritical a way as possible, assuming that the situation is no less difficult for the patient than for the doctor.

2. By indicating that the doctor can make time for the patient to talk about difficult feelings which may underlie their stuck position.

3. If no real progress ensues, by drawing the consultation to a close rather than prolonging it in an agonizing way. Where this situation arises, some patients are grateful if the doctor provides another opportunity for them to talk on their own whilst others are more relieved if any follow-up appointment includes the presence of some family members. Either way, the adolescent is being given a second opportunity to succeed.

MENTAL STATE EXAMINATION

In contrast to children, adolescents are generally able to give a good account of their feelings, of their habitual emotional responses to stressful situations, and their views about family relationships. Doctors should not be put off by their experience of a minority of adolescents who simply repeat 'dunno' to almost every question asked of them.

Except where there is suspicion of a psychotic illness, routine questions about the possible presence of psychotic symptomatology should not be asked, since they unnecessarily add to the patient's anxiety. On the other hand, questions about such affects as anger, sadness, and any specific worries they have are well tolerated since most adolescents are particularly interested in their emotional experiences, and these questions convey interest and concern. However, many adolescents tend to provide general answers to these questions, not relating their mood to any specific issues. It is therefore generally necessary to also ask how these feelings interfere with everyday functioning, for example concentration, maintaining interest and obtaining pleasure, affecting appetite and falling asleep, etc. In order to avoid increasing the patient's self-consciousness, it may be necessary to preface certain questions by such normalizing remarks as 'Young people sometimes feel...'.

Adolescents are generally intensely interested in how they are getting on in the world, including why misadventure befalls them, so they usually welcome an inquiry that attempts to determine precipitating, predisposing and maintaining factors associated with a particular mood, e.g. what leads up to a depressive mood swing or to their temper flaring up. A new intellectual understanding of an emotional state allows patients to feel more in control of themselves, less in the grip of their feelings.

PSYCHIATRIC SYNDROMES

As earlier stated, emotional and behavioral disturbance in adolescence may be largely unmodified extensions of disorders already present in childhood. Those characteristic of childhood have already been described. This section provides an account of those disorders more distinctive of adolescence, where much research and clinical development has taken place in the last 10 years.

DEPRESSION

There is a sudden increase in the prevalence of depressive symptomatology with adolescence. Recent studies suggest a community 1-year prevalence of about 10%, perhaps twice that rate for the whole adolescent period (Cooper & Goodyer 1993, Goodyer & Cooper 1993, Monck et al 1994), the risk rising for older adolescents. A continuum of severity can be identified from the majority who have mild or transient symptoms to the minority with a major depressive episode or some form of bipolar depressive illness.

Depressive reactions

A depressed mood, perhaps with tearfulness and feelings of hopelessness, occurring as an adjustment reaction to some external stress is a quite common cause of minor depression, for example precipitated by peer group difficulties, discordant family relationships, or bereavement. Sometimes the stress may be considered to have been exacerbated by factors within the internal world of the adolescent, for example low self-esteem, unfulfilled emotional needs, or frustrated adolescent emancipator strivings. In any of these reactive states the vegetative symptoms of clinical depression (e.g. impaired appetite with significant weight loss, impaired memory and concentration, motor restlessness and/or agitation) should not be present. Apart from the provision of general support, unless a major depression develops, no treatment except for brief counseling should be necessary.

Depressive syndromes

Many cases of so called 'neurotic' depression, attributed to life stressors or adolescent developmental problems, are now recognized to have arisen independent of these putative factors, and instead are assumed to have been at least partly determined by biological factors. Whatever the exact diagnosis, feelings of misery and anhedonia are invariably associated with these depressive syndromes, along with intermittent tearfulness, impaired concentration, loss of interest, irritability and sometimes loss of temper control. Sleep is usually disturbed (either an initial insomnia or sleeping excessively) and some preoccupation with suicidal thoughts is common. Although these may often be transient, such symptoms can follow a chronic or subchronic course, beginning in adolescence and producing considerable impairment of function. No longer described as 'neurotic', these 'dysthymic' disorders are considered as a subcategory of the depression spectrum, and a lifetime prevalence of at least 3–9% has been estimated. Without treatment there is increasing evidence of impaired social adjustment in adulthood (Kandel & Davies 1986), and of risk for a major depressive episode.

Major depression

Adolescents presenting with a depressive 'reaction' may actually be suffering from a major depressive episode, and those with dysthymia are at particular risk. Although the mean age for the onset of the syndrome of manic depressive disorder is mid to late twenties, many patients develop it earlier; there is a steady rate of increase in the onset of affective symptoms in adolescence (McGee et al 1992). Epidemiological studies in the UK (Cooper & Goodyer 1993) and the USA (e.g. Lewinsohn et al 1994) have shown that it is far more common than previously thought or currently diagnosed, and since many episodes last for months if untreated, adolescents can be left with psychosocial scars that time may not heal (Rhode et al 1994).

If the presence of a major depressive episode or the symptoms of a manic depressive disorder are suspected, referral to a psychiatrist should always follow. The marked vegetative symptoms and motor disturbance described above strongly suggest the presence of one of these two disorders. Motor retardation may be present, i.e. where gross motor movements are slow, speech is monotonous, thoughts seem slow, and there is a poverty of affect, but peer group social withdrawal is probably one of the most important indicators (Goodyer & Cooper 1993). Depressive thoughts might occasionally include delusional beliefs (e.g. of having cancer), or even hallucinatory experience (e.g. voices telling them they're bad or that they're going to die). This may make the diagnosis difficult to distinguish from schizophrenia, but the main clue lies in recognizing the presence of the prevailing depressive mood, so that the delusional thoughts and hallucinatory experience are recognized to arise from that mood. The first presentation of a manic depressive illness in adolescence is often a manic picture, i.e. elation, restlessness, grandiosity, a flight of ideas, insomnia, excitability, and often irritability.

The possibility of shared genetic vulnerability indicates that a family history of major depressive illness should always be sought on examining patients presenting with depression or psychotic elation.

Treatment

Treatment is always required for those with more serious psychiatric conditions – either medication or a psychological treatment. The choice of appropriate antidepressant remains uncertain, and even the efficacy of the tricyclic compounds, until recently the obvious first choice, remains unproven (Hazell et al 1995). These have usually been prescribed up to a daily dosage of 125–150 mg or up to 5 mg/kg bodyweight. Amitriptyline is generally prescribed where there is accompanying anxiety and/or sleep disturbance, imipramine where there is anergia or retardation, and clomipramine where obsessional or compulsive symptoms are present. All, to varying degree, present dangers of cardiac toxicity in overdose.

The advent of two new treatment methods has transformed the treatment of depression. Firstly, cognitive therapy, a highly structured form of psychotherapy which addresses an adolescent's negative dysfunctional beliefs (of himself, of the world, and of the future) which are assumed to underpin the depression (see Spence 1994). Secondly, the availability of selective serotonin reuptake inhibitors, because of their relative freedom from side-effects and emerging evidence of their effectiveness: fluoxetine and paroxetine (each 20–30 mg daily) and sertraline (100–150 mg daily) seem the most frequently chosen, taken as a single dose in the morning to prevent nighttime insomnia; the dosage is increased gradually to prevent nausea or diarrhea.

One of the neuroleptics (e.g. haloperidol or chlorpromazine) is the treatment of choice for manic states, and lithium carbonate as a maintenance treatment for the prevention for relapse in adolescents with a manic depressive illness (Allesi et al 1994). Carbamazepine and sodium valproate have both sometimes been used for mood stabilization but, as was once the case for lithium, their prescription remains controversial. Whatever the drug choice, effective chemotherapy depends upon good treatment compliance, so time and care is taken to acquaint the adolescent with all aspects of the treatment, including possible side-effects. Because of the seriousness of the diagnosis and the importance of the medication, similar time and care is taken with the adolescent's parents, most of whom need considerable support to accept the diagnosis and the necessity for quite long-term treatment.

SCHIZOPHRENIA

Onset and course during adolescence

Schizophrenia more often presents in adolescence with an insidious onset (Asarnow & Ben-Meir 1988). Delusions and hallucinations are often not present. Instead there is evidence of increasing social withdrawal and flattening of affect (Aarksog &

Motenson 1985), suspiciousness or hypersensitivity, feelings of vulnerability or depersonalization, eccentric or overvalued ideas, and sometimes hypochondriasis. Occasionally a more 'sociopathic' picture presents with temper outbursts and aggression (Aarksog & Motenson 1985). Childhood precursors of schizophrenia are few. Some studies suggest that in vulnerable adolescents the onset of the illness may be provoked by high levels of negative affect and poor family communication (Goldstein 1985).

Hallucinations, particularly auditory and visual, are more common in schizophrenia than in depressive psychosis, but in the early stages of the illness adolescents often conceal their presence. They may be suggested only by the patient appearing to respond to distracting stimuli or talking to himself when he believes he is not being observed. Likewise, disturbances of thought are generally concealed until the adolescent is frankly deluded. However, relatives are likely to report they feel the youngster has been behaving and thinking oddly for some time.

Differential diagnosis

Like manic depressive psychosis, schizophrenia is a rare condition in adolescence, but in at least 10% there is a positive family history. Against a diagnosis of schizophrenia is a history of drug misuse, good emotional contact maintained with the patient despite severe psychotic symptoms, and the rapid resolution of symptoms with neuroleptics.

Treatment

Where the presence of a schizophrenic illness is suspected, a referral should always be made to a psychiatrist. Treatment, which usually has to start on an inpatient psychiatric basis, has two key components. Firstly, adequate control of symptoms is established by the use of neuroleptic drugs. It is extremely important to avoid the adolescent experiencing unpleasant side-effects (particularly extrapyramidal ones), as experience of these invariably affects compliance. For this reason, newer neuroleptics such as sulpiride (Wagstaff et al 1994) and risperidone (Quintana & Keshavan 1995), which have lower extrapyramidal side-effects than older neuroleptics like the phenothiazines, are drugs of choice. In young people with refractory schizophrenia which has failed to respond to at least two neuroleptics, the use of clozapine is increasingly considered (Birmaher et al 1992).

Secondly, helping the adolescent to recover self-esteem and a competent identity after a psychotic episode is extremely important. Rebuilding adolescent's lives often involves modifying their aspirations and career intentions, limiting the expectations of both the youngsters and their families whilst ensuring some room for hope, activity and purpose to their lives, and avoiding the kind of levels of high emotion and critical comments which have found to be associated with relapse (Doane et al 1986).

EMOTIONAL DISORDERS

Some form of emotional 'turmoil' is present in about 40% of adolescents suffering from psychiatric disorder (Rutter et al 1976). In fact, anxiety, depression, preoccupation with health and body image and feelings of isolation, apathy and boredom are all relatively common during the adolescent period. Adverse social factors such as unemployment may further increase such feelings. Adolescents tend to present with emotional disorders that are less differentiated than neuroses in adults, with a wider and more fluid range of symptoms. The most distinct emotional disorders of adolescence include school refusal, obsessional neurosis and the depressive reactions described above.

SCHOOL REFUSAL IN ADOLESCENCE

Clinical picture

Although also common in children (see p. 1739), school refusal is an archetypal emotional disorder of early adolescence. The precursors of school refusal presenting in adolescence may include a past history of school refusal when starting primary school, other forms of separation problems (e.g. a reluctance to stay overnight with friends) and an excessive state of dependency between mother and child. School refusal is often precipitated by the move from primary to secondary school, the adolescent finding the usually stricter and more impersonal regimen of secondary school not to his liking. Often the most important predisposing factor is the position the youngster has come to occupy in his family. Not infrequently the panic-stricken youngster is an indulged martinet at home, supported by a coalition with one parent (Bryce & Baird 1986).

School refusers are often first referred to a pediatrician because they commonly present with a plethora of physical complaints – typically recurrent abdominal pain, headache and earache – which provide a rationale for their unwillingness to attend school. Prompt diagnosis and a cessation of the search for physical pathology is important since the prognosis is better if the problem is still acute and the adolescent still young (Steinberg 1983). Follow-up studies have shown that up to one-third of school refusers still have agoraphobic and other neurotic difficulties 3 years after treatment and that these persist in one-fifth at 10-year follow-up (Berg 1982).

Treatment

A range of treatments is used, including family therapy combined with a prompt return to school (Bryce & Baird 1986), and behavioral treatments (Yule 1985). The longer the patient is away from school, the more entrenched the problem is likely to become.

OBSESSIVE–COMPULSIVE DISORDER

At least 1 in 300 of an ordinary adolescent population experience obsessive–compulsive symptoms (see page 1740 for definition and description) that significantly interfere with their functioning.

Clinical picture

There are striking associations with other disorders, for example eating disorders (Whitaker et al 1990), Tourette syndrome, major depression and anxiety disorders (Swedo et al 1989). The commonest obsession shown by adolescents is a concern with dirt, germs or environmental toxins, while the commonest compulsions are excessive or ritualized handwashing, showering, bathing or grooming (Swedo et al 1989).

Treatment

Behavioral methods of treatment (Stern 1978) such as self-monitoring, thought stopping, modeling and response prevention (see p. 1764), have tended to replace psychotherapy in the treatment of adults and there is some reason to believe that such techniques are also appropriate with children (Wolff & Rappoport 1988). There is now considerable evidence that psychopharmacological treatment may help obsessive–compulsive symptoms. Clomipramine hydrochloride has been tested in at least six double-blind controlled trials with adults. In a similar trial (Flament et al 1985) significant improvement was found in a group of 19 adolescents with obseqssive–compulsive neurosis. Newer 5–HT uptake inhibitors (e.g. fluoxitene and fluvoxamine) may prove to have an even more potent effect (Flament et al 1987, Apter et al 1994). Despite vigorous treatment, however, it appears that the majority of adolescent patients will have persisting, if reduced, symptoms on follow-up at 2–7 years (Leonard et al 1993). It may be necessary to maintain such patients on long-term medication.

SUICIDE AND PARASUICIDE

Suicide

There is a recent increase in adolescent male suicides (McClure 1984). Under 14 years of age its incidence is rare: 1 in 100 000. There is often some forewarning, and evidence that some victims are very isolated or are facing a particularly painful loss (e.g. of a friendship, anticipated academic failure, etc.). Some are high achievers, as in Japan. Often an interpersonal conflict such as a 'disciplinary crisis' has preceded the suicide (perhaps as a last straw). Based on a review of the literature, Mack has suggested a set of eight factors which may all conspire to influence a child or adolescent towards suicide (Mack 1986):

1. The presence of constitutional factors producing a biological vulnerability towards depressive moods.
2. The presence of a profoundly depressed mood (a consequence of any one of the depressive disorders described above), presumably unrecognized or inadequately treated.
3. Early developmental influences, e.g. early loss of an important relationship, sensitizing the youngster to later losses.
4. Personality factors, in particular a combination of very vulnerable self-esteem and the presence of 'exalted and rigid' ego-ideals, i.e. wishful hopes of personal accomplishment and fulfillment incompatible with daily reality, leading the youngster to constantly feel not good enough, and thus unable to bounce back readily from disappointments and hurts.
5. To compensate for their deficient self-esteem, certain relationships with friends or significant adults may become overimportant, so that any loss of these may have a devastating effect.
6. In the weeks or months preceding the suicide, an increasing orientation towards death is sometimes evident.
7. The social context of the adolescent, for example normative anxieties about social injustice, or a possible world war, may adversely affect the youngster.
8. Finally, precipitating factors in the youngster's immediate social world (e.g. an impending house move, examination failure, a minor rejection or hurt, etc.) as the final straw.

Sometimes death or serious illness in the adolescent's immediate social environment may have been present, and suicide pacts or suicide affiliation may occur. The psychological trauma of adolescent suicides upon their surviving friends is now the subject of concern, specific targeting of these groups now replacing the ineffective schools campaigns set up in the 1980s (Shaffer et al 1988). Nonetheless, the majority of adolescents who kill themselves were not known to have been severely depressed at the time of their death, so it is generally difficult to argue that a professional intervention could have successfully forestalled a completed suicide. It is more easy retrospectively to identify missed opportunities to prevent one.

Parasuicide

This is a much more widespread phenomenon, which increases during the adolescent years, causing sufficient concern in the USA at least to have led to the development of school-based preventative programs (Shaffer et al 1988). Parasuicide is much more common amongst girls than boys, a reversal of the ratio for completed suicide (Allen 1987). This marked difference in sex ratio is the most striking individual characteristic of the adolescent parasuicide.

Over the last decade, certain other features of adolescent parasuicide have become well established. Social factors include youthful marriage, low social status, and long-term unemployment of the adolescent or within the family. The strong association between unemployment and parasuicide might be mediated through increasing the adolescent's vulnerability to stressful events through feelings of hopelessness and loss of self-esteem that long-term unemployment may engender. Even then other factors might exaggerate or diminish this effect of unemployment. As previously noted, environmental stress and adverse life events tend to cluster, and many of these have been found to be associated with parasuicide, for example family break-up or chronic family ill health, academic under-achievement, or other relationship difficulties and interpersonal conflict.

No psychiatric diagnosis has been found to be particularly predictive of adolescent parasuicide. The presence of depressive symptomatology is not necessarily evidence of a major depressive disorder; indeed, studies have repeatedly shown that conduct disorders are more highly correlated with adolescent parasuicide than major depressive disorders (Apter et al 1988). A parasuicidal act is most usually the outcome of maladaptive problem solving, impulsively carried out by a youngster disinhibited by anger or alcohol, where no other way out of a conflict is perceived.

Assessing adolescent parasuicides

Hawton (1986) offers a simple classification of adolescent parasuicides. A minority fall into one of two categories, both containing essentially normal youngsters facing stress who differ only in the duration of that stress: acute stress (less than 1 month); and chronic stress. The remainder are a group of youngsters under chronic stress who have also demonstrated considerable behavioral disturbance. On the basis of other studies, only this latter group is likely to be at risk of further parasuicide.

However, others (e.g. Shaffer et al 1988) argue against a categorical classification, suggesting instead that examining youngsters' typical emotional and intellectual responses to stress, their impulsivity and habitual coping styles, is the most effective means of assessing future risk.

Referral for a psychiatric opinion is only definitely indicated where it seems that individual factors are of at least equal importance to social ones, for example because no stressful precipitating event can be identified, or the adolescent appears depressed. Otherwise, reassurance and brief counseling may be all that is necessary, but consideration should always be given to involving the hospital social work department.

EATING DISORDERS

ANOREXIA NERVOSA

This condition consists of:

1. an intense fear of becoming obese, even when underweight
2. disturbance in body image, e.g. feeling fat or believing that one area of the body is 'too fat' even when emaciated
3. refusal to maintain a reasonable bodyweight (i.e. weight 15% or more below the expected percentile)
4. BMI <17.5 criterion only applies in older adolescents (>18 years)
5. amenorrhea in girls.

As weight falls, the patient begins to develop all the physical and psychological sequelae of starvation. These include psychological symptoms once considered etiologic: lowered mood, impaired concentration and short-term memory, narrowed interests and an excessive preoccupation with food. The condition occurs mainly in adolescent girls in western countries, where its incidence may be rising, and there is an overrepresentation of upper- and middle-class patients. Although there is accumulating evidence for a central biological control of eating responding to a 'set point' for body fat, perhaps mediated by glucagon-like peptide-1 in the hypothalamus (Turton et al 1996), social pressures on girls – for example to assume a fashionably slim body shape – are likely to be important precipitants, since it is known that amongst adolescents undereating and overeating concerns are widespread (Mueller et al 1995), present even before adolescence.

Psychological factors thought to be important in the development of the condition largely center around the patient's poor sense of personal autonomy, often linked in turn to perfectionistic strivings. An oversolicitous or intrusive relationship with their mother is not uncommonly observed. The marked cognitive distortions of anorexic patients (e.g. 'If I eat a full meal, I will immediately become fat') clearly play a potent role in perpetuating the illness, likewise the malnutrition-induced hypothalamic dysfunction. From a psychodynamic perspective, the anorexia seems to act at an unconscious level as both a means of avoiding maturation, for which the patient feels ill-equipped, and as a maladaptive act of autonomy. Many of these factors may be over-represented in adolescents with chronic physical illness, e.g. insulin-dependent diabetes, predisposing such patients to eating disorders (Neumark-Sztainer et al 1995).

Family factors long thought to be of etiologic importance for anorexia nervosa, including rigid, overly close family relationships and a poor capacity to resolve intrafamilial conflicts (Palazolli et al 1989), have not been readily supported by recent research (Grigg et al 1989, Blair et al 1995).

Apart from endocrine disturbances (e.g. thyroid suppression and hypocortisolemia), there are a number of well recognized medical complications:

1. lowered metabolic rate, with bradycardia, hypotension, peripheral cyanosis, cold intolerance, lanugo, and lassitude
2. amenorrhea, with evidence of early osteopenia (on DEXA bone studies) or of diminished growth
3. bone marrow suppression, i.e. anemia, leukopenia, and a thrombocytopenia, sometimes marked
4. reduced resistance to infections or bruising secondary to these problems
5. hypoalbuminemia, sometimes with evidence of ankle edema
6. constipation and raised serum urea and creatinine because of oral restriction of fluids
7. evidence of avitaminosis, including skin changes, hair loss, and a sensory peripheral neuropathy
8. hypoglycemic episodes
9. laxative-abuse-induced electrolyte disturbances, particularly hypokalemia
10. raised liver function tests.

Course

Anorexia usually starts relatively insidiously, with the patient gradually reducing her food intake, already influenced by a powerful fear of fatness (a significant proportion of patients may in fact have previously been overweight). At first carbohydrates and fats are selectively avoided but gradually the patient begins to avoid more and more types of food and even fluids. As weight is lost, symptoms such as depression, social withdrawal, poor concentration and sensitivity to the cold develop. In addition, as the disorder becomes chronic (i.e. extends into a second year), hidden maneuvers may be increasingly used to reduce weight including self-induced vomiting, purging with laxatives and copious physical exercise.

Treatment

Early or less severe adolescent patients can generally be successfully treated on an outpatient basis, using family therapy (Russell et al 1987) or other similar counseling approaches (Crisp et al 1991), reserving inpatient treatment for more severe cases where hospitalization becomes an essential component of a long-term treatment plan, indeed even life saving.

Figure 30.4 was drawn by a profoundly emaciated 15-year-old girl during a particularly depressed and treatment-resistant phase of a long admission. It was drawn on the front cover of a self-image questionnaire; part of the original line drawing printed on the questionnaire's cover is also shown to demonstrate how much she has altered it. Her weight was below the 3rd percentile whilst her height was above the 90th. The picture graphically conveys how despairing she was feeling, and confirms that, like most anorexic patients, the girl was fully aware of her state of emaciation.

Such severely emaciated patients require complete bed rest with increased exercise dependent on calorific intake. A behavioral reward program is commonly introduced but best avoided if a collaborative partnership with the patient is considered important. Intravenous or nasogastric feeding are rarely necessary, and require close monitoring to prevent complications (these can include a refeeding hypophosphatemia, fluid overload, misplaced NG tubes, and iatrogenic sepsis). Expert nursing is required throughout an anorexic's admission and it is on the quality of

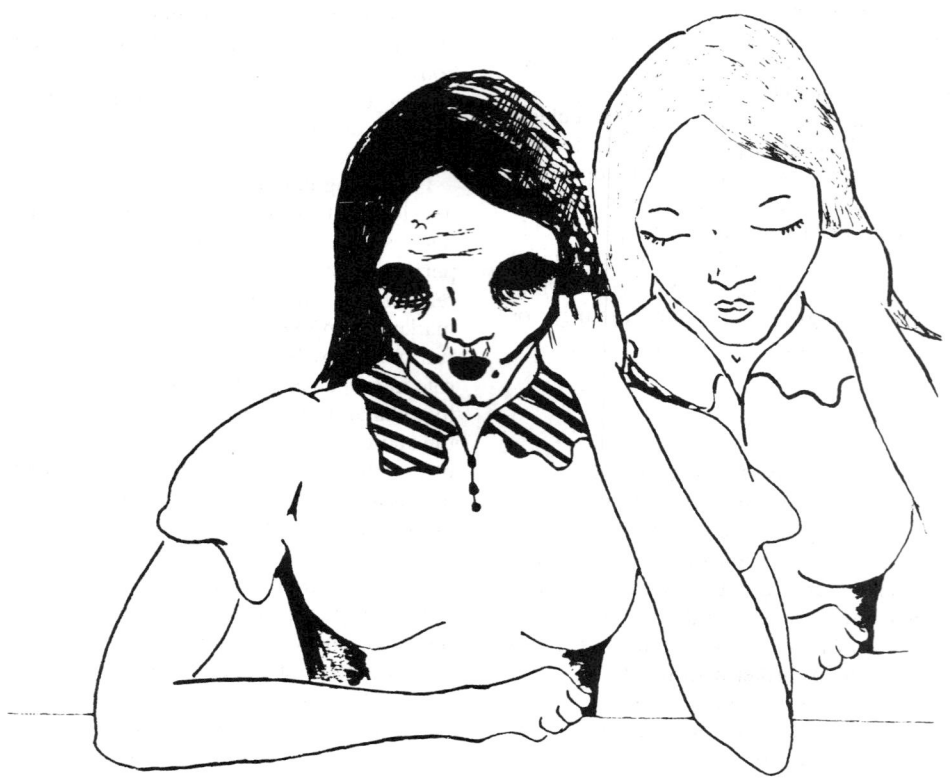

Fig. 30.4 See text for explanation.

nursing that the outcome of an admission will largely depend. Once the patient's weight has risen, individual psychotherapy or cognitive therapy is introduced in conjunction with family therapy. Except for the treatment of a co-morbid depression, which can sometimes develops during the course of the illness, drug treatment has little or no place.

Outcome

With treatment, follow-up studies show that about 50% make a full recovery and another 25% show considerable improvement but continue to have menstrual irregularities and minor eating problems; some 20–25% remain severely handicapped and their illnesses run a chronic course (see e.g. Ratnisuriya et al 1991). In Sweden, Gillberg and colleagues have convincingly demonstrated that poor adult outcome for adolescent anorexics is associated with particular personality problems, notably empathy deficits (Gillberg et al 1994), which may be important to address if chronicity is to be avoided. The mortality rate seems likely to be 10% or more, with death occurring most commonly from late-diagnosed infection, hypothermia, or irreversible hypoglycemia rather than from the direct effects of malnutrition (Russell 1986).

BULIMIA NERVOSA

This condition comprises:

1. preoccupation with food associated with episodes of gross overeating or 'bingeing'
2. a phobic fear of fatness, which, as in anorexia, must be avoided
3. the development of techniques to counteract the fattening effect of binges, particularly self-induced vomiting and the use of laxatives.

Like anorexia nervosa, bulimia is far more common in women. It is much more common in older adolescents, present in up to 1 in 20 18-year-olds. In some cases of bulimia there is evidence of a previous episode of anorexia (Russell 1986) but most often bulimia develops de novo as a syndrome in its own right. The disorder tends to persist. It is often kept secret from others and the repetitive eating binges can interfere with social relationships, the patient becoming guilty and depressed. The repeated vomiting and/or purging may lead to a variety of physical side-effects ranging from eroded dental enamel to hypokalemia and impaired renal function.

Treatment

The current treatment of choice is cognitive–behavioral therapy (Fairburn et al 1993). Work on the bulimic's distorted thinking may be combined with 'stimulus control' techniques to avoid or cope better with situations that typically elicit the bingeing behavior. Fluoxetine (which blunts appetite) has been recommended, but controlled trials have provided no convincing support for its use.

SEXUAL ABUSE AND SEXUAL OFFENDERS IN ADOLESCENCE

CHILD SEXUAL ABUSE AND THE ADOLESCENT

Sexual abuse is 'the involvement of dependent, developmentally immature children and adolescents in sexual activities they do not fully comprehend, to which they are unable to give informed consent, or that violate the social taboos of family roles'. This is a broad definition encompassing both intrafamilial and extrafamilial abuse and including not only abuse which involves physical contact but also 'noncontact' abuse such as exposing a child to pornographic books or videos. Using this definition, Baker & Duncan's (1985) community survey estimated that 10% of adults in the UK had been sexually abused as children. Intrafamilial sexual abuse most commonly begins when the child is prepubescent, between the ages of 8 and 10, although it is most commonly disclosed by the victim during adolescence (Peters et al 1986).

Precursors and precipitants

A number of high-risk factors in families which are associated with sexual abuse have been identified (Finkelhor & Baron 1986):

1. a poor mother–child relationship
2. a mother who is absent or unavailable, particularly as a result of illness
3. marital disharmony and violence
4. social isolation
5. alcoholism in the father figure
6. living in a stepfamily.

More girls than boys are subject to sexual abuse, although as the possibility of sexual abuse in boys is more widely recognized, more boy victims are being identified (Watkins & Bentovim 1992). The perpetrator is almost always male and usually known to the child: if not the father figure, a male trusted to look after the child or to babysit. The abuse often begins with fondling then becomes more intrusive with digital vaginal penetration, oral sex or sodomy and full vaginal intercourse.

The presentation of sexual abuse in adolescents

Adolescent sexual abuse victims may present in an overt way or more covertly. Overt presentations include actual disclosure of the abuse to a professional (e.g. a teacher), family friend or family member. The adolescent may first ask that the adult guarantees total confidentiality and promises not to report the disclosure. This guarantee must not be given since, if there are grounds for believing that the disclosure is true, then the relevant authorities – the police or social work department – must be informed.

Covert presentations of sexual abuse in adolescents may include pregnancy and venereal disease, particularly when the teenager appears distressed and vague about the identity of her partner. Other covert presentations include more general indices of distress such as depression, failing school performance, parasuicidal behavior and running away from home. Finally, sexual promiscuity may be a consequence of sexual abuse, since victims have often been trained from an early age to relate in a sexual way to others.

The treatment of adolescent victims of child sexual abuse

Two principles are central to successful treatment. Firstly, the victim must be protected from further abuse. This invariably requires ensuring that the perpetrator no longer lives under the same roof as the victim. Secondly, the victim should be provided with a supportive context in which to talk about the strong and sometimes conflicting feelings engendered by the abuse. This can be achieved in a number of ways.

Individual therapy is the mainstay of treatment, but group psychotherapy, composed exclusively of victims, is widely used (Bentovim et al 1991). Such groups can be very effective in a number of ways, including reducing the stigmatization victims feel by allowing them to meet other people who have been abused. Groups may be less effective at helping victims whose predominant experience is one of betrayal, who may find it very difficult to trust others, and their needs may be better met in individual psychotherapy (Morrison 1989).

ADOLESCENT SEXUAL OFFENDERS

There is a growing amount of evidence that adolescents may commit sexual offenses and perpetrate acts of sexually abusive behavior (Glasgow et al 1994). Most people who subsequently go on to sexually abuse children in their adult life appear to begin their pedophiliac 'careers' in adolescence (Vizard et al 1995). The assessment of adolescent sexual offenders should include obtaining a reliable account of their offenses, a systematic evaluation of their sexual knowledge and attitudes (Salter 1988) and an understanding of their social relationships. The most useful treatment programs are based on cognitive–behavioral principles (Becker & Kaplan 1993), which use a combination of social skills training, sex education, cognitive restructuring and covert sensitization (see also Will et al 1995).

MALADAPTIVE RESPONSES TO CHRONIC PHYSICAL DISORDERS

SOMATIZING DISORDERS

Vague or medically unexplained physical symptoms are common in adolescence. Fatigue/weakness, headaches, and recurrent abdominal pain are the most common, though a polysymptomatic presentation is also common, affecting up to 1 in 20 boys and twice as many girls. These syndromes are poorly understood (Campo & Fritsch 1994), and seem to be generally approached through any associated problem, e.g. undisclosed sexual abuse or other life stressors, or treating the comorbid condition, e.g. depression. Unwitting family reinforcement of an adolescent's symptomatology is a common clinical concern, but in a recent review Mrazek (1994) has warned against misattributing psychological explanations to symptoms simply because no physical explanation has been discovered.

CHRONIC FATIGUE SYNDROME

This must certainly be the most frequently referred somatic disorder in child and adolescent psychiatry (Garralda 1992). Often described as 'postviral', with a history of fever, headache, myalgia, tender 'swollen glands', and arthralgia, definitive laboratory findings are generally absent but a high degree of functional impairment is present because of unremitting or intermittently prolonged fatigue and exercise intolerance, leading to social restriction and repeatedly interrupted school attendance (Smith et al 1991, Carter et al 1995). Missed academic milestones, despite home tutoring, with peer group isolation, and regression into preadolescent type parental dependence are common sequelae. Both the etiology and the prognosis are uncertain. It is

important to obtain an understanding of the adolescent's premorbid personality and his psychosocial circumstances at the time of illness onset, but it is generally unhelpful to challenge the physical nature of the original illness episode. The frequent misunderstandings that can arise between patients' families and their doctors often seem to arise from the Cartesian trap of assuming the problem is either somatic or it is psychological, for example in relation to depression illness and the possible value of an antidepressant, since tearfulness and low mood are frequent, and a major depressive illness may be present in up to a third. Unlike depressive illness, the onset of chronic fatigue syndrome is generally sudden and even where depressive symptomatology is prominent there is usually little or no suicidal ideation. The possible role of antidepressants must still be considered, and the adolescent helped gradually to unlearn the 'learned helplessness' that so often develops over the long course of their illness. General support and reassurance about an eventual good outcome are also important; in other words, psychological interventions are an integral part of the treatment of chronic fatigue syndrome.

INDIVIDUAL ADAPTATION TO A CHRONIC PHYSICAL DISORDER

There is a general increase in susceptibility to emotional disturbance of all kinds with chronic physical disorder. This probably arises from multiple factors, which include:

1. The nature of the disorder: for example whether it is a chronic or relapsing condition, a progressive or a life-threatening course, and the degree and nature of any functional impairment. In addition, puberty may be associated with a change in the disorder, for example increased resistance to insulin upsetting previously satisfactory diabetic control.

2. The side-effects or complications of treatment procedures, for example feelings about dietary restriction or disfiguring effects of treatment (perhaps limb amputation or alopecia), cytotoxic effects on the CNS and IQ, or the necessity for repeated hospitalization and consequent disruption to schooling and peer group friendships.

3. The adolescent's developing self-image, in particular the discrepancy between social expectations and the youngster's own views of himself as different from his nonimpaired peers. Stigmatization, which adolescents feel acutely, has been shown to be particularly influenced by the visibility of the affliction and the degree to which it interferes with effective communication.

4. The adolescent's coping mechanisms.

The resilience and stoicism of chronically ill children and adolescents is well known. Three defense mechanisms can commonly be recognized: denial, sublimation, and intellectualization, of which denial is the most important. It produces an unconscious impairment in self-awareness, for example about how upset, demoralized, or frightened one really feels. Providing this denial is adaptive, and not, for example, blinding the diabetic adolescent to the necessity for reasonably strict dietary control, the adolescent's subjective sense of well-being remains surprisingly good. Sublimation is the defense mechanism whereby ambitions, drives, and interests that would otherwise be frustrated by the affliction are channeled into some genuinely satisfying outlet. Rationalization or intellectual self-justification, for example not liking football rather than not being able to play it as well as nonimpaired peers, can be a further means of maintaining self-esteem (Dunn-Geier et al 1986, Eiser 1990).

It is not clear why adaptive responses begin to fail, perhaps because for the most part they do not. In adolescence two developments occur that probably add to the vulnerability of youngsters with a chronic illness or disability. Firstly, their ego ideal, the adolescent's narcissistic concern for himself and his own expectations of himself in relation to social ideals, both of which are painfully confronted by his disability and the many real limitations it imposes. Depressive responses or a defense of anger and resentment are likely, and the eventual mastery of this phase can be likened to a bereavement process. Secondly, the adolescent's normal emancipatory drives are in conflict with his very real dependency needs (Johnson 1988). Where this is compounded by a lack of effective sublimation and a failure to realize unfulfilled potential, it may precipitate a diabetic youngster into reckless demonstrations of competency and independence that include rejecting the necessity for good treatment compliance, careless of the consequences, or denial that adverse consequences are possible.

FAMILY AND SOCIAL RESPONSES

Overprotection with chronic disorders, that is benevolent stigmatization, has become a source of contemporary concern. Anxiety has been concerned with different settings: the family; the social role of special schools and the atmosphere within them; and the way individuals with a particular disability may be lumped together by society as a distinctive subculture, obliterating the individuality of each.

The burden of care on families of patients with chronic psychiatric illness is considerable and has been discussed in the child psychiatry section. Much emphasis has been placed on the problems faced by parents and their disabled children, rather than approaching them through their resilience and problem solving. Beresford (1994) considers optimism, flexibility, a sense of personal control (e.g. recognizing controllable stressors), relying on active problem solving rather than palliative solutions to problems, and a capacity to galvanize effective social support as amongst the most important factors for parental coping (Beresford 1994), and provides a detailed review of the extensive research literature that has built up over the last 15 years.

DEPARTMENTAL RESPONSES

Given the opportunity, most chronically ill/disabled adolescents would be articulate spokesmen for their needs, and it is likely that a number of time-honored rituals on the pediatric wards and in outpatient clinics would come under criticism.

HELPING TO MODIFY MALADAPTIVE RESPONSES

There are four main ways of helping to modify maladaptive responses, which broadly address the need to help emotional coping and to increase practical coping:

1. normalization
2. ventilation
3. assist problem solving
4. psychodynamic working-through.

Normalization describes the process whereby adolescents and their families often benefit from learning that their experiences and feelings are shared by many others who are also facing the same situation. Feelings of inadequacy or unnecessary fears about being neurotic may be removed. A considerable amount of patient education may be necessary to make this effective. Opportunities to ventilate feelings are almost always welcome, particularly since the chronically ill and their carers often assume that their stoicism also meets an unspoken social expectation. Guilt, anger, despair, resentment, envy of those more fortunate than themselves, fears of the unknown, of relapse or of painful death may all need to be expressed before an adolescent or his family can assume more adaptive responses to his chronic illness. Counseling can provide a specific focus for examining conflicting needs or difficult decisions facing the adolescent and/or the family. It may help them to make difficult decisions or develop more effective coping styles. Psychotherapy, for the individual adolescent and/or the family, allows for the exploration and possible resolution of emotional or relationship conflicts, fears about separation and independence, feelings of guilt or a greater tolerance of depression and disappointments, any or all of which might be preventing a better adaptation to the adolescent's chronic illness (Landsdown & Goldman 1988). Often a sibling or a parent may be as much a beneficiary as the adolescent patient (Garber et al 1990).

These interventions can be provided in a variety of ways: the adolescents might be offered individual psychotherapy, parents might be provided with counseling, family therapy might be undertaken, or groups of families affected by chronic disability might meet together to permit a normalizing experience and the ventilation of feelings. All four intervention methods described above may coexist in psychotherapy groups specifically set up for adolescent patients with certain types of disorder like cystic fibrosis, diabetes, etc. The social groups/clubs arranged for these youngsters are rarely used to share and explore feelings; often there is a deliberate avoidance of doing so, demonstrating competency instead. There are also reports of special programs specifically directed towards promoting coping skills in particular patient groups, for example juvenile diabetics.

BRAIN-INJURED ADOLESCENTS WITH BEHAVIORAL DISTURBANCE

Significant cognitive improvement may occur for up to 2 years after a brain injury, and even after this computer-assisted learning can sometimes considerably help concentration. On the other hand, helping the youngster come to terms with his disability and reduced potential is a long and painful process. A first concern is to help the adolescent develop improved self-control techniques, often using a combination of cognitive–behavioral therapy and anxiety-management techniques. The brain-injured adolescent, usually a boy, is keen to be helped to reestablish a semblance of normal adolescence, and parents often need considerable help to enable them to establish effective but not over protective limit setting. Most reports of this work have largely been based on inpatient treatment (e.g. McCabe & Green 1987). For the best possible results these vulnerable youngsters need continuing support, with intermittently more active interventions, right until and often through early adulthood (Ylvisaker 1985). Contrary to what one might expect of brain-injured individuals, psycho-therapy can be an important treatment component (Prigatono 1986).

DELINQUENCY

Delinquency is a legal term, not a psychiatric diagnosis. A juvenile delinquent is conventionally defined as: a young person between the age of 10 (the age of 'criminal responsibility') and 17 years who has been prosecuted and found guilty of an offense that would be classified as a 'crime' if committed by an adult. In practice the term is now widely used to refer to criminal behavior committed by young people up to the age of about 20. Only a small minority of delinquent offenses consist of crimes of violence, drug or sex offenses. 90% of delinquent offenses in England are accounted for by the following kinds of behavior: theft, vehicle offenses, breaking and entry and vandalism.

PRECURSORS AND PRECIPITANTS

There appear to be at least four important influences: age, social environment, policing policy, and family characteristics.

Age. Delinquency reaches its peak for males at 15 and for females at 14, thereafter remaining high for the rest of adolescence before falling dramatically in early adulthood (Farrington 1995).

Social environment. The Cambridge Study in Delinquent Development, which began in south London in 1961, has thrown much light on the social origins of delinquency. Conduct disorder in childhood, particularly if associated with aggressive behavior, is especially associated with subsequent delinquency in adolescent boys and sociopathic personality disorder in adult life. Although enduring antisocial personality traits may seem to account for this persistence, the social effects of negative cycles between the youngster, the conduct disorder and the social environment should not be forgotten, nor should the impact of continuing social deprivation be underestimated.

Policing policy affects the rate of delinquency. The crime rate for adolescent boys increased threefold between 1957 and 1977, and that for girls increased by a factor of more than six (Rutter 1979). However, such statistics should be treated with caution, because delinquency is a legal term not a behavioral one. Changes in police practice may profoundly alter the number and nature of delinquents apprehended, and prevailing stereotypes about delinquency can become self-fulfilling prophecies because of their effect on policing policy.

Family influences have been shown to be related to delinquency. The Cambridge study found that both convicted and self-reported delinquents tended to come from large-sized low-income families with criminal parents or siblings, to have had unsatisfactory or inadequate rearing in childhood, and to be of below average intelligence.

It appears likely that these connections are mediated by environmental factors and social learning: the effects of growing up in a socially deprived area, in a deprived and highly stressed family where criminal behavior and violent acts are part of everyday life. Most delinquency is best explained in terms of sociological theory: as a natural reaction to environmental circumstances ... [rather than] suggesting that [delinquents] are weak or peculiar individuals in need of psychiatric attention. In a recent major review of findings from the Cambridge study, Farrington (1995) emphasized how offending was but one element of a larger syndrome of antisocial behavior, where preventative programs need to be directed to initiatives that foster social learning.

SUBSTANCE ABUSE

Substance abuse involves a wide range of drugs and other psychoactive substances. These range from the legally available caffeine, alcohol, tobacco and solvents, to opiates, hallucinogens, cannabis, amphetamines and barbiturates which are obtained illegally. Most adolescents in the UK never use illegal drugs. Of those who do, the majority take 'soft' drugs on an experimental or recreational basis, without developing dependence and, despite the media publicity about deaths following the use of Ecstasy, usually without adverse psychosocial sequelae.

EPIDEMIOLOGY

Teenage drinking

Alcohol is the substance most frequently used by young people in the UK and, in contrast to onset of smoking, there is evidence to suggest that the age at which it is first used decreased between the 1960s and 1980s, perhaps due to the halving of the real cost of alcohol. Underage drinking in pubs still seems widespread, although recent research indicates a higher proportion of non-drinking adolescents than 15 years ago (e.g. Foxcroft et al 1995 reporting on a large study in Humberside). This is a small comfort in otherwise bleak figures: in 1992, 38% of girls and 51% of boys reported having been drunk by the age of 13 years, their first drink most often obtained in their own home or in the house of a friend. Physical dependency before their 20th birthday is not unheard of.

Smoking

Tobacco is almost certainly the drug of abuse that causes the most damage to health. Despite the fact that it is illegal for anyone under the age of 16 to purchase cigarettes in the UK, many young adolescents smoke. The New Zealand birth cohort study found that over a third of nonsmokers at 14 years of age are smoking at 16 years; few of these subsequently stop smoking (Fergusson & Horwood 1995), perhaps influenced by their peer group affiliation, most of whose members also smoke (Fergusson et al 1995). Nonetheless, the single most important long-term predictor of daily smoking among young adults seems to be whether or not their mothers had smoked during their childhoods (Oygard et al 1995, Swan et al 1990).

Other substances

Marijuana is the most widely used illegal drug. It is usually smoked, providing a sense of mild euphoria. Its use in the UK has fluctuated over the years, probably in association with availability, which now seems widespread. Onset of use seems largely mediated by peer group influences and availability, though poor family cohesion may be important as an early vulnerability factor (Bauman & Ennett 1996). As with many of the other drugs used by adolescents, it seems likely that friendships may be increasingly determined by drug use, i.e. selecting their peers in relation to a drug culture. Use of amphetamines, barbiturates and LSD probably follow a similar pattern; where these are taken away from a rave or dance culture (the usual location for Ecstasy), polydrug use is probably far more common than reliance upon a single drug. Heroin and opiate use develops in older adolescents, e.g. in the UK the vast majority of registered addicts known to the

Home Office are aged over 19 years (Oppenheimer 1985), although where there has been a strong heroin subculture in some cities there are reports of a continuing epidemic of heroin abuse among younger adolescents.

Solvent abuse seems on the wane. It is predominantly an activity of the younger adolescent age group and indeed abuse may start as early as 8 or 9, predominantly as a peer group activity; only solitary use is indicative of psychological or psychiatric disturbance. A wide variety of substances containing toluene, acetone, naphtha, benzene and carbon tetrachloride have been inhaled by children and adolescents to produce effects of intoxication, e.g. glues and model-making cement, typing correction fluid, dry-cleaning fluid, petrol and propellant gases from aerosols. Watson (1986) provides an admirable summary of current knowledge about substance abuse which dispels many of the myths that have surrounded it.

RISK-TAKING BEHAVIOR

The proportion of early substance users who progress onto drugs with major immediate health risks is uncertain. Poor nutrition, susceptibility to infections, and accidental overdose are the main risks. The presence of unrecognized mental illness, including depression and early schizophrenia, probably accounts for some who develop major dependency problems, and in other instances a psychiatric illness episode may be precipitated or brought forward by drug misuse. In most instances, however, social factors are probably the most important influence: giving up drugs often means having to give up most friends and a whole way of life.

Adolescent risk-taking has been most frequently researched in relation to sexual behavior, and risk to HIV infection in particular. The *context* of the behavior seems most important (Donovan & McEwan 1995). For example, homelessness and the disinhibiting effects of alcohol place adolescents at social risk, where coercive or unprotected sex with multiple partners is much more likely. The risk of contracting AIDS through needle sharing has led to the development of a community drug service in Edinburgh aimed at harm reduction, prescribing oral methadone to drug users; a significant reduction in injecting drug use and a fall in HIV rates has been observed (Greenwood 1996).

PRIMARY PREVENTION

Health education schemes targeted at young people have been conspicuously unsuccessful; current efforts are now largely directed toward harm reduction. Otherwise, campaigns may best be directed toward indirect factors known to be strongly associated with adolescents' drug use, e.g. drug availability, the economic and employment status of their social circle, friends' norms and values (Bauman & Ennett 1996), adjusting the method to take account of the changing nature of peer group influences during adolescence.

PRINCIPLES OF THERAPY

INDIVIDUAL PSYCHOTHERAPY WITH ADOLESCENTS

Psychodynamic psychotherapy is designed to provide the patient with insight into the meaning, causes and significance of his symptoms and behavior, in the hope that such insight will lead to change. To achieve this, the adolescent psychotherapist makes interpretations which link current behavior and feelings with significant past experiences, demonstrating their impact on current realities.

Most adolescents are often extremely reluctant to acknowledge that they need help from an adult, since this contradicts their normal wish for independence. The adolescent psychotherapist therefore tends to use diminutives when describing his patients' feelings. He will say, 'So you were a bit sad when your mother died' rather than 'you were devastated when you mother died'. Adolescents often use their therapists as 'safe' adults with whom they can practice different modes of relating and different types of behavior. For these reasons, individual psychotherapy with adolescents is often an amalgam of psychodynamic psychotherapy, reality testing and cognitive therapy.

GROUP TREATMENT

Aims of group therapy

The section on maladaptive responses to chronic disorder referred to four types of treatment intervention which can all be met by group therapy: normalization, ventilation, counseling and psychotherapy. Group leaders may decide that their particular group should be especially concerned with only one of these, e.g. social skills counseling, but in practice these other aspects of work often occur as well. Within this general framework a number of different types of group may operate: for example, psychodynamic groups; social skills training using role play; focused discussion; and groups focusing on promoting particular coping skills in relation to a specific disorder (see previous section on chronic disorders).

Groups for relatives

In an adolescent department two types of useful groups might be present. First, groups for parents which allow them to ventilate feelings, share experience, and to also learn and gain support from one another. The second type of group is some form of family group, for example the multiple family group previously described (Gonzales et al 1987), in which, over eight sessions, patients and their families are helped in a structured way to share experience and develop better understanding of each other's difficulties and their common burdens. Mutual problem solving is then possible.

FAMILY THERAPY

Family therapy is the treatment of choice for many adolescent problems, because of the intimate relationship between adolescent behavior and family interaction. It is particularly indicated whenever an adolescent's emotional or behavioral difficulties seem to be underpinned by family dysfunction.

Family therapy only begins after an assessment of the adolescent's problems indicates that family dysfunction is an important predisposing or maintaining factor. A contract is made with the family to meet for a number of sessions to try and address these problems. Change is achieved first by experiential means such as setting tasks for the family, so that family members actually begin to behave differently with one another and hence begin to feel differently about one another (for example, asking the parents to draw up a rota of family chores to be performed by the children may have the effect of not only reestablishing the parents as a couple, but also of regrouping the children as a group of siblings).

The second main vehicle of change is interpretation. The family therapist interprets the meaning of characteristic family processes in order to effect change in the way the family functions. For example, one common dysfunctional process that occurs is for family members to start arguing or fighting with one another in response to a difficult and emotionally charged issue, such as a bereavement. The therapist will interpret this along the lines of: 'I am struck with what has just happened. We were beginning to talk about granny's death and all of a sudden an argument broke out. I wonder if its easier for you to fight with one another than to face the sad feelings you have when thinking about her death?'

COGNITIVE–BEHAVIOR THERAPY

Cognitive–behavior therapy (CBT) is a treatment approach that includes two related methods, cognitive therapy and behavior therapy. Behavior therapy is guided by two basic principles; first, that behavior is responsive to particular stimuli and to their consequences; second, that both aspects include social factors in the environment (that is the responses of other people). Behavior therapy techniques include systematic desensitization, flooding, response prevention and thought stopping.

Cognitive therapy is based on the idea that individuals are active interpreters of the world according to their own beliefs, expectations and attitudes. The way an individual interprets an event is held to significantly influence mood and behavior, so that idiosyncratic styles of cognition may, by themselves, lead to psychological disturbance (Blackburn & Davison 1995). Thus depression, for example, can be seen as the result of a number of cognitive errors such as personalization. This is incorrectly blaming oneself for someone else's behavior, e.g. 'The reason my parents separated is all because of me'. The cognitive therapist helps the individual explore then refute such 'automatic thoughts'. McAdam (1987) has argued that CBT is well suited to work with adolescents since it is a collaborative form of therapy in which the young person's own contribution is very important. It has an established efficacy in the treatment of depression in adults and its application to psychiatric problems in adolescence can be expected to grow substantially (Kendall 1989, Spence 1994).

RESIDENTIAL TREATMENT

Two types of residential inpatient treatment facilities for disturbed adolescents exist. First, admission facilities suitable for the treatment of acute psychiatric disorders, for example psychosis. In many parts of the UK this is provided by the general admission wards of the local mental health unit, rather than by a specialized adolescent inpatient unit. Most of these specialized units instead offer the second type of resource, i.e. medium-term admission (4 months to 1 year) for a small number of patients with chronic psychiatric disorders, for example adolescents with severe eating disorders (particularly anorexia nervosa) who fail to respond to outpatient treatment, those with chronic depression, and patients in the recovery stage of psychosis. Descriptive accounts of the work of these units are available elsewhere (Steinberg 1985, Singh 1987, Wrate et al 1994).

There are three main indications for inpatient treatment:

1. The provision of specialized and continuous care for suicidal adolescents.
2. The provision of specialized and continuous care of severely ill patients, e.g. those with severe anorexia nervosa or psychosis.
3. The need for detailed assessments, including the use of certain investigative procedures, and assessing the response to psychotropic medication.

Treatment methods

To carry out their aims most effectively, adolescent psychiatry inpatient units are increasingly involved in the community. For example, their inpatients are at home most weekends, they often attend a local school or are in part-time work throughout most of their admission, and inpatient staff work directly with the patients' families and liaise with other hospital departments, community agencies, etc. As this community integration increases, the structure and function of adolescent psychiatry inpatient units will undergo increasing change, focusing in particular on the most severely ill, for whom skilled psychiatric hospitalization may decisively alter the course of their disorder (Rothery et al 1995).

REFERENCES AND BIBLIOGRAPHY

Aarksog T, Motenson K V 1985 Schizophrenia in early adolescence – a study illustrated by long term cases. Acta Psychiatrica Scandinavica 72: 422–429

Achenbach T M, Edelbrock C S 1983 Manual for child behavior checklist and revised behavior profile. Achenbach, Burlington Vt

Ainsworth M D S 1982 Attachment: retrospect and prospect. In: Parkes C M, Stevenson-Hinde J (eds) The place of attachment in human behaviour. Basic Books, New York, p 3–30

Allen J P 1987 Youth suicide. Adolescence 22: 271–290

Allesi N, Naylor N W, Ghaziuddin M, Zubieta J K 1994 Update on lithium carbonate in children and adolescents. Journal of the American Academy of Child and Adolescent Psychiatry 33: 291–304

American Psychiatric Association 1994 Diagnostic and statistical manual of mental disorders, 4th edn. American Psychiatric Association, Washington DC

Apter A, Bleich A, Plutchik R, Mendelsohn S, Tyano S 1988 Suicidal behaviour, depression and conduct disorder in hospitalised adolescents. Journal of the American Academy of Child and Adolescent Psychiatry 27: 696–699

Apter A, Ratzoni G, King R, Weizman A, Iancu I, Binder M, Riddle M 1994 Fluvoxamine open label treatment of adolescent in-patients. Journal of the American Academy of Child and Adolescent Psychiatry 33: 342–348

Asarnow J R, Ben-Meir S 1988 Children with schizophrenic spectrum and depressive disorders: a comparative study of pre-morbid adjustment, onset pattern and severity of impairment. Journal of Child Psychology and Psychiatry 29: 477–488

Baker A W, Duncan S P 1985 The incidence and prevalence of intrafamilial and extrafamilial sexual abuse of female children. Child Abuse and Neglect 7: 133–146

Barker P 1992 Basic family therapy, 3rd edn. Collins, London

Bauman K E, Ennett S T 1996 On the importance of peer influence for adolescent drug use: commonly neglected considerations. Addiction 91: 185–198

Beck A T, Rush A J, Shaw B F, Emery G 1979 Cognitive therapy of depression. Wiley, New York

Becker J V, Kaplan M S 1993 Cognitive behavioral treatment of the juvenile sex offender. In: Barbaree H E, Marshall W L, Hudson S M (eds) The juvenile sex offender. Guildford Press, New York

Bee H 1995 The developing child, 7th edn. Harper, New York

Bentovim A, Elton A, Hildebrand J, Tranter M, Vizard E 1988 Child sexual abuse within the family: assessment and treatment. Wright, Bristol

Bentovim A, van Elburg A, Boston P 1991 In: Bentovim A, Elton A, Hildebrand J, Tranter M, Vizard E (eds) Child abuse within the family: assessment and treatment. John Wright, London

Beresford B A 1994 Resources and strategies: how parents cope with the care of a disabled child. Journal of Child Psychiatry and Psychology 35: 171–209

Berg I 1982 When truants and school refusers grow up. British Journal of Psychiatry 141: 208–210

Birmaher B, Baker R, Kapur S, Quintana H, Ganguli R 1992 Clozapine for the treatment of adolescents with schizophrenia. Journal of the American Academy of Child and Adolescent Psychiatry 31: 160–164

Blackburn I, Davison K 1995 Cognitive therapy for the treatment of depression and anxiety. Blackwell Scientific, Oxford

Blair C, Freeman C, Cull A 1995 The families of anorexia nervosa and cystic fibrosis patients. Psychological Medicine 25: 985–993

Bowlby J 1969 Attachment and loss. Vol 1. Attachment. Hogarth Press, London

Bryce G, Baird D 1986 Precipitating a crisis: family therapy and adolescent school refusers. Journal of Adolescence 9: 199–213

Butler-Sloss (Lord Justice) E 1988 Report of the inquiry into child abuse in Cleveland (1987). HMSO, London

Campo J V, Fritsch S L 1994 Somatisation in children and adolescents. Journal of the American Academy of Child and Adolescent Psychiatry 33: 1223–1235

Carter B D, Edwards J F, Kronenberger W G et al 1995 Case control study of chronic fatigue in pediatric patients. Pediatrics 95: 179–186

Cawthron P, James A, Dell J, Seagrott V 1994 Adolescent onset psychosis. A clinical and outcome study. Journal of Child Psychology and Psychiatry 35: 1321–1332

Chisholm L, Hurrlemann K E 1995 Adolescence in modern Europe. Pluralised transition patterns and their implications for personal and social risks. Journal of Adolescence 18: 129–158

Cicchetti D, Carlson V 1989 Child maltreatment. Theory and research on the causes and consequences of child abuse and neglect. Cambridge University Press, New York

Clark D B, Donovan J E 1994 The reliability and validity of the Hamilton anxiety rating scale in an adolescent sample. Journal of Child Psychology and Psychology 35: 354–360

Cooper P J, Goodyer I 1993 A community study of depression in adolescent girls. I. Estimates of symptom and syndrome prevalence. British Journal of Psychiatry 163: 369–374

Crisp A, Gowers S et al 1991 A controlled study of the effects of therapies aimed at adolescent and family psychopathologies in anorexia nervosa. British Journal of Psychiatry 159: 325–333

Doane J A, Goldstein M J, Miklowitz D J, Falloon I R M 1986 The impact of individual and family treatment on the affective climate of families of schizophrenics. British Journal of Psychiatry 148: 279–287

Donaldson M 1978 Children's minds. Fontana/Collins, Glasgow

Donovan C, McEwan R 1995 A review of the literature examining the relationship between alcohol use and HIV-related sexual risk-taking in young people. Addiction 90: 319–328

Douglas J, Richman N 1984 My child won't sleep. Penguin, Harmondsworth

Dunn-Geier B J, McGrath P J, Rourke B P et al 1986 Adolescent chronic pain: the ability to cope. Pain 26: 23–32

Eaton-Evans J, Dugdale A E 1988 Sleep patterns of infants in the first year of life. Archives of Disease in Childhood 63: 647–649

Egger J, Carter C, Graham P, Gumley D, Soothill J F 1985 A controlled trial of oligoantigenic treatment in the hyperkinetic syndrome. Lancet i: 540–545

Eiser C 1990 The psychological effects of chronic disease. Journal of Child Psychology and Psychiatry 31: 85–98

Elliott C, Murray D J, Pearson L 1983 The British abilities scales (new edition). National Foundation for Educational Research/Nelson, Windsor

Erikson E 1965 Childhood and society. Penguin, London

Fadden G B, Bebbington P, Kuipers L 1987 The burden of care: the impact of functional psychiatric illness in the patient's family. British Journal of Psychiatry 150: 285–292

Fairburn C G F, Marcus M D, Wilson G T 1993 Cognitive–behaviour therapy for binge eating and bulimia nervosa. In: Fairburn C G F, Wilson G T (eds) Binge eating: nature, assessment, and treatment. Guilford Press, New York

Farrington D P 1995 The twelfth Jack Tizard Memorial Lecture: The development of offending and antisocial behaviour from childhood: key findings from the Cambridge Study in Delinquency Development. Journal of Child Psychology and Psychiatry 36: 929–964

Faull C, Nicol R 1986 Abdominal pain in six year olds: an epidemiological study in a new town. Journal of Child Psychology and Psychiatry 27: 251–261

Fergusson D M, Horwood L J 1995 Transitions to cigarette smoking during adolescence. Addictive Behaviours 20: 627–647

Fergusson D M, Horwood L J, Lynskey M T 1995 Maternal depressive symptoms and depressive symptoms in adolescents. Journal of Child Psychiatry and Psychology 36: 1161–1178

Fergusson D M, Lynskey M T, Horwood L J 1995 The role of peer affiliations, social, family, and individual factors in continuities in cigarette smoking between childhood and adolescence. Addiction 90: 647–659

Finkelhor D, Baron L 1986 High-risk children. In: Finkelhor D (ed) A sourcebook on child sexual abuse. Sage, Beverley Hills

Flament M, Rappoport J, Berg C, Sceery W, Kitts C, Mellstromm B, Linnoila M 1985 Clomipramine treatment of childhood obsessive–compulsive disorder. Archives of General Psychiatry 42: 977–983

Flament M, Rappoport J, Murphy D S, Berg C J, Lake R 1987 Biochemical changes during clomipramine treatment of childhood obsessive–compulsive disorder. Archives of General Psychiatry 44: 219–225

Foxcroft D R, Lowe G, Lister-Sharp D J 1995 Teenage drinking: a 4-year comparative study. Alcohol and Alcoholism 30: 713–719

Fraser A M, Taylor D C 1986 Childhood encopresis extended into adult life. British Journal of Psychiatry 149: 370–371

Freud A 1936 The ego and the mechanisms of defence. Hogarth Press, London

Freud S 1953 Three essays on the theory of sexuality (1905). In: Collected Papers, vol. 7, standard edn. Hogarth Press, London

Garber J, Zeman J, Walker L S 1990 Recurrent abdominal pain in children: psychiatric diagnoses and parental pathology. Journal of the American Academy of Child and Adolescent Psychiatry 29: 648–656

Garmezy N, Masten A S 1994 Chronic adversities. In: Rutter M, Taylor E, Hersov L (eds) Child and adolescent psychiatry: modern approaches, 3rd edn. Blackwell, Oxford

Garralda M E 1992 A selective review of child psychiatric syndromes with a somatic presentation. British Journal of Psychiatry 161: 759–773

Gillberg I C, Rastam M, Gillberg C 1994 Anorexia nervosa outcome: a six-year controlled longitudinal study of 51 cases including a population cohort. Journal of the American Academy of Child and Adolescent Psychiatry 33: 729–739

Glasgow D, Horne L, Calam R, Cox A 1994 Evidence, incidence, gender and age in sexual abuse of children perpetrated by children: towards a developmental analysis of child sexual abuse. Child Abuse Review 3: 196–210

Goldstein M J 1985 Family factors that antedate the onset of schizophrenia and related disorders: the result of a fifteen year prospective longitudinal study. Acta Psychiatrica Scandinavica 71(suppl 139): 7–18

Gonzales S, Steinglass P, Reiss D 1987 Family-centred interventions for people with chronic disabilities: the eight-session multiple family discussion programme. George Washington University Medical Centre Publication

Goodyer I 1990 Life experiences, development and childhood psychopathology. Wiley, Chichester

Goodyer I, Cooper P J 1993 A community study of depression in adolescent girls. II. The clinical features of identified disorder. British Journal of Psychiatry 163: 374–380

Graham P, Rutter M 1973 Psychiatric disorder in the young adolescent: a follow up study. Proceedings of the Royal Society of Medicine 66: 1226–1229

Greenwood J 1996 Six years' experience of sharing the care of Edinburgh's drug users. Psychiatric Bulletin 20: 8–11

Grigg D N, Friesen J D, Sheppey M I 1989 Family patterns associated with anorexia nervosa. Journal of Marital and Family Therapy 15: 29–42

Hagberg B, Aicardi J, Dias K, Ramos O 1983 A progressive syndrome of autism, dementia, ataxia and loss of purposeful hand use in girls: Rett's syndrome. Archives of Neurology 14: 471–479

Hawton K 1986 Suicide and attempted suicide among children and adolescents. Developmental Psychology Series No.5, Sage, London

Hawton K, Salkovskis P, Kirk J, Clark D 1995 Cognitive behaviour therapy for psychiatric problems: a practical guide, 2nd edn. Oxford University Press, Oxford

Hazell P, O'Connell D, Heathcote D, Robertson J, Henry D 1995 Efficacy of tricyclic drugs in treating child and adolescent depression: a meta-analysis. British Medical Journal 310: 897–899

Hobson P 1993 Autism and the development of mind. Lawrence Erlbaum, Hove

Hospital Advisory Service, Child and Adolescent Mental Health Services 1995 Together we stand: the commissioning, role and management. HMSO, London

Johnson S B 1988 Psychological aspects of childhood diabetes. Journal of Child Psychology and Psychiatry 29: 729–738

Jones D 1992 Interviewing children who have been sexually abused, 4th edn. Royal College of Psychiatrists/Gaskell Press, London

Kandel D B, Davies M 1986 Adult sequelae of adolescent depressive symptoms. Archives of General Psychiatry 43: 255–263

Kane J M 1987 Treatment of schizophrenia. Schizophrenia Bulletin 16: 635–652

Kanner L 1943 Autistic disturbances of affective contact. The Nervous Child 2: 217–250

Kempe R S, Kempe C H 1978 Child abuse. Fontana, London

Kendell R E 1988 Schizophrenia (Ch 16) and affective disorders (Ch 17). In: Kendell R E, Zealley A K (eds) Companion to psychiatric studies, 4th edn. Churchill Livingstone, Edinburgh

Kohlberg L 1966 A cognitive developmental analysis of children's sex-role concepts and attitude. In: Maccoby E (ed) The development of sex differences. Stanford University, Stanford, CA

Kolvin I, Fundudis T 1981 Elective mute children: psychological development and background factors. Journal of Child Psychology and Psychiatry 22: 219–232

Landsdown R, Goldman A 1988 The psychological care of children with malignant disease. Journal of Child Psychology and Psychiatry 29: 555–567

Lask B 1988 Novel and non-toxic treatment for night terrors. British Medical Journal 297: 592

Lask B 1994 Paediatric liaison work. In: Rutter M, Taylor E, Hersov L (eds) Child and adolescent psychiatry: modern approaches, 3rd edn. Blackwell, Oxford, p 996–1005

Lask B, Fosson A 1989 Childhood illness: the psychosomatic approach. John Wiley, Chichester

Leonard H L, Swedo S, Lenane M, Rettew D C, Hamburger M S, Barko J J, Rappoport J L 1993 A two to seven year follow-up study of 54 obsessive compulsive children. Archives of General Psychiatry 50: 429–438

Lewinsohn P M, Clarke G N, Seeley J R, Rhode P 1994 Major depression in community adolescents: age of onset, episode duration, and time to reoccurrence. Journal of the American Academy of Child and Adolescent Psychiatry 33: 809–819

Lockyer L, Rutter M 1969 A five to fifteen year follow-up study of infantile psychosis. III. Psychological aspects. British Journal of Psychiatry 115: 865–882

Lord C, Rutter M 1994 Autism and other pervasive developmental disorders. In: Rutter M, Taylor E, Hersov L (eds) Child and adolescent psychiatry: modern approaches, 3rd edn. Blackwell, Oxford, p 569–593

McAdam 1987 Cognitive behavior therapy: a therapy for the troubled adolescent. In: Coleman J C (ed) Working with troubled adolescents – a handbook. Academic Press, London

McAuley R, McAuley P 1977 Child behavioural problems. An empirical approach to management. Macmillan, London

McCabe R J R, Green D 1987 Rehabilitating severely head-injured adolescents: three case reports. Journal of Child Psychology and Psychiatry 28: 118–126

McClure G M G 1984 Recent trends in suicide amongst the young. British Journal of Psychiatry 144: 134–138

McGee R, Feehan M, Williams S, Anderson J. 1992 DSM-III disorders from 11 to age 15 years. Journal of the American Academy of Child and Adolescent Psychiatry 31: 50–59

Mack J E 1986 Adolescent suicide: an architectural model. In: Klerman G L (ed) Suicide and depression among adolescents and young adults. American Psychiatric Press, Washington

Maguire G P, Rutter D R 1976 History taking for medical students. I. Deficiencies in performance. Lancet ii: 556–558

Matthews S 1994 Cognitive development. In: Bryant P, Colman A (eds) Developmental psychology. Longman, London

Meadow R 1989 Munchausen syndrome by proxy. ABC of child abuse. BMA, London, pp 37–39

Meltzer H Y 1987 Biological studies in schizophrenia. Schizophrenia Bulletin 13: 485–495

Mischel W 1970 Sex typing and socialisation. In: Mussen P H (ed) Carmichael's manual of child psychology, vol 2. Wiley, New York

Monck E, Graham P, Richman N, Dobbs R 1994 Adolescent girls. I. Self-reported mood disturbance in a community population. British Journal of Psychiatry 165: 760–769

Monck E, Bentovim A, Goodall G, Hyde C, Lwin R, Sharland E 1995 Child sexual abuse: a descriptive and treatment study. HMSO, London

Morrison J 1989 Working with sexual trauma: principles of individual therapy with adolescent victims of sexual abuse. Practice 2: 311–325

Mrazek D A 1994 Psychiatric aspects of somatic disease and disorders. In: Rutter M, Taylor E, Hersov L (eds) Child and adolescent psychiatry:

modern approaches, 3rd edn. Oxford, Blackwell

Mueller C, Field T, Yando R et al 1995 Undereating and over eating concerns among adolescents. Journal of Child Psychology and Psychiatry 36: 1019–1026

Neumark-Sztainer D, Story M, Resnick M D, Garwick A, Blum R W 1995 Body dissatisfaction and unhealthy weight-control practices among adolescents with and without chronic illness: a population-based study. Archives of Pediatrics and Adolescent Medicine 149: 1330–1335

Offord D R, Boyle M H, Szatmari P et al 1987 Ontario Child Health Study. II. Six month prevalence of disorders and service utilisation. Archives of General Psychiatry 44: 832–836

Oppenheimer E 1985 Drug taking. In: Rutter M, Hersov L (eds) Child and adolescent psychiatry: modern approaches. Blackwell, Oxford

Oygard L, Klepp K-I, Tell G S, Vellar O D 1995 Parental and peer influence on smoking among young adults: ten year followup of the Oslo youth study participants. Addiction 90: 561–569

Palazolli M S, Cirillos M, Sorrentino A M 1989 Family games: general models of psychotic processes in the family. Karnac Books, London

Peters S D, Wyatt E G, Finkelhor D 1986 Prevalence. In: Finkelhor D (ed) A sourcebook on child sexual abuse. Sage, Beverley Hills

Prigatono G P 1986 Neuropsychological rehabilitation after brain injury. Johns Hopkins University Press, Baltimore

Puig-Antich J, Orvashel H, Tabrizi M, Chambers W 1980 The assessment of affective disorder in children and adolescents by semi-structured interview. Archives of General Psychiatry 42: 696–702

Quintana H, Keshavan M 1995 Case study: risperidone in children and adolescents with schizophrenia. Journal of the American Academy of Child and Adolescent Psychiatry 34: 1292–1296

Quinton D, Rutter M 1976 Early hospital admission and later disturbances of behaviour: an attempted replication of Douglas's findings. Developmental Medicine and Child Neurology 18: 447–459

Ratnisuriya R H, Eisler I, Szmuckler G I, Russell G F M 1991 Anorexia nervosa outcome and outcome factors after 20 years. British Journal of Psychiatry 158: 495–512

Rhode P, Lewinsohn P M, Seeley J R 1994 Are adolescents changed by an episode of major depression? Journal of the American Academy of Child and Adolescent Psychiatry 33: 1289–1298

Richman N 1977 Behavioural problems in pre-school children. Family and social factors. British Journal of Psychiatry 131: 523–527

Richman N 1981 A community survey of characteristics of one-to-two-year-olds with sleep disruptions. Journal of the American Academy of Child Psychiatry 20: 281–291

Richman N, Lansdown R 1988 Problems of pre-school children. Wiley, Chichester

Richman N, Stevenson E J, Graham P 1982 Pre-school to school: a behavioural study. Academic Press, London

Robins L 1966 Deviant children grown up. Williams and Williams, Baltimore (reprinted 1973, Kriegen, Huntington, New York)

Rothery D J, Wrate R M, McCabe R, Aspin J, Bryce G 1995 Treatment goal planning: outcome findings of a prospective multi-centre study of adolescent inpatient units. European Journal of Child and Adolescent Psychiatry 4: 209–221

Russell G F M 1986 Anorexia and bulimia nervosa. In: Rutter M, Hersov L (eds) Child and adolescent psychiatry. Blackwell, Oxford

Russell G F M, Szmuckler G I, Dare C, Eisler I 1987 Evaluation of family therapy in anorexia nervosa and anorexia bulimia. Archives of General Psychiatry 44: 1047–1056

Rutter M 1979 Changing youth in a changing society. Nuffield Provincial Hospital Trust, London

Rutter M 1987 Psychosocial resilience and protective mechanisms. American Journal of Orthopsychiatry 57: 316–331

Rutter M 1988 Depressive disorders. In: Rutter M, Tuma A M, Lann I S (eds) Assessment and diagnosis in child psychopathology. Fulton, London p 347–376

Rutter M, Schopler E 1988 Autism and pervasive developmental disorders. In: Rutter M, Tuma A M, Lann I S (eds) Assessment and diagnosis in child psychopathology. Fulton, London, p 408–436

Rutter M, Tizard J, Whitmore K 1970 Education, health and behaviour. Longman, London

Rutter M, Shaffer D, Shepeherd M 1975a A multi-axial classification of child psychiatric disorders. WHO, Geneva

Rutter M, Yule B, Quinton D, Rowlands O, Yule W, Berger M 1975b Attainment and adjustment in two geographical areas. III. Some factors accounting for area differences. British Journal of Psychiatry 126: 520–533

Rutter M, Graham P, Chadwick O, Yule W 1976 Adolescent turmoil: fact or fiction? Journal of Child Psychology and Psychiatry 17: 35–56

Salter A 1988 Treating child sexual offenders and victims: a practical guide. Sage, Beverley Hills

Shaffer D 1994 Debate and argument: structured interviews for assessing children. Journal of Child Psychiatry and Psychology 35: 783–784

Shaffer D, Garland A, Gould M, Fisher P, Trantman P 1988 Preventing teenage suicide: a critical review. Journal of the American Academy of Child and Adolescent Psychiatry 27: 675–687

Singh N 1987 A perspective on therapeutic work with impatient adolescents. Journal of Adolescence 10: 119–132

Skuse D, Wolke D, Reilly S 1992 Failure to thrive. Clinical and developmental aspects. In: Remschmidt H, Schmidt M (eds) Child and youth psychiatry, European perspectives. Vol. II Developmental psychopathology. Hans Huber, Stuttgart

Smith M S, Mitchell J, Corey L et al 1991 Chronic fatigue in adolescents. Pediatrics 88: 195–202

Spence S H 1994 Practitioner review: cognitive therapy with children and adolescents: from theory to practice. Journal of Child Psychiatry and Psychology 35: 1191–1228

Steinberg D 1983 The clinical psychiatry of adolescence, Ch 10. Problems of feelings and behaviour. John Wiley, Chichester

Steinberg D 1985 The adolescent unit: work and teamwork in adolescent psychiatry. John Wiley, Chichester

Stern R S 1978 Obsessive thoughts: the problem of therapy. British Journal of Psychiatry 132: 200–205

Swan A V, Creeser R, Murray M 1990 When and why children first start to smoke. International Journal of Epidemiology 19: 323–330

Swedo S E, Rappoport J L, Leonard H L, Lenane M, Cheslow D 1989 Obsessive–compulsive disorder in children and adolescents: clinical phenomenology of 70 consecutive cases. Archives of General Psychiatry 46: 335–341

Taylor E 1994 Syndromes of attention deficit and overactivity. In: Rutter M, Taylor E, Hersov L (eds) Child and adolescent psychiatry: modern approaches, 3rd edn. Blackwell, Oxford p 285–307

Thomas A, Chess S 1982 Temperament and development. Brunner/Mazel, New York

Thorndike R L 1973 Stanford Binet intelligence scale, Form L-M, 1972 Norms tables. Houghton Mifflin, Boston

Turton M D, O'Shea D, Gunn I et al 1996 A role for glucagon-like peptide-1 in the central regulation of feeding. Nature 379: 69–72

Vizard E, Monck E, Misch P 1995 Child and adolescent sex abuse perpetrators: a review of the research literature. Journal of Child Psychology and Psychiatry 36: 731–756

Wagstaff A J, Fitton A, Benfield P 1994 Sulpiride. A review of its pharmacodynamic and pharmacokinetic properties and therapeutic efficacy in schizophrenia. CNS Drugs 2: 313–333

Waller D, Eisenberg L 1980 School refusal in childhood – a psychiatric–paediatric perspective. In: Hersoo L, Berg I (eds) Out of school – modern perspectives in school refusal and truancy. Wiley, Chichester

Watkins B, Bentovim A 1992 The sexual abuse of male children and adolescents: a review of current research. Journal of Child Psychology and Psychiatry 33: 197–248

Watson J 1986 Solvent abuse. Croom Helm, London

Wechsler D 1974 Manual for the Wechsler intelligence scale for children, revised. Psychological Corporation, New York

Werry J S, McLellan J M, Chard L 1991 Childhood and adolescent schizophrenic, bipolar and schizo-affective disorders: a clinical and outcome study. Journal of the American Academy of Child and Adolescent Psychiatry 30: 457–465

Whitaker A, Johnson J, Schaffer D et al 1990 Uncommon troubles in young people: prevalence estimates of selected psychiatric disorders in a non-referred adolescent population. Archives of General Psychiatry 47: 487–496

Will D, Wrate R 1985 Integrated family therapy. Tavistock, London

Will D, Douglas A, Wood C 1995 The evolution of a group treatment programme for adolescent perpetrators of sexually abusive behaviour. Journal of Sexual Aggression 1: 69–82

Williams B T R, Gilmour J D 1994 Annotation: sociometry and peer relations. Journal of Child Psychology and Psychology 35: 997–1013

Wing L 1981 Asperger's syndrome: a clinical account. Psychological Medicine 11: 115–129

Wing L, Gould J 1979 Severe impairments of social interaction and associated abnormalities in children: epidemiology and classification. Journal of Autism and Developmental Disorders 9: 11–30

Winnicott D 1965 The capacity to be alone. In: The maturational process and the facilitating environment. Hogarth Press, London

Wolff R A, Rappoport J L 1988 Behavioral treatment of childhood compulsive disorder. Behavior Modification 12: 252–266

Wood A, Moore A, Harrington R 1995 Properties of the mood and feelings questionnaire in adolescent psychiatric outpatients: a research note. Journal of Child Psychiatry and Psychology 36: 327–334

World Health Organization 1992 The ICD-10 classification of mental and behaviour disorders: clinical descriptions and diagnostic guidelines. WHO, Geneva

Wrate R M 1989 Talking to adolescents. In: Myerscough P (ed) Talking with patients. Oxford University Press, Oxford

Wrate R M, Rothery D J, McCabe R J R, Aspin J, Bryce G 1994 A prospective multi-centre study of admissions to adolescent psychiatry inpatient units. Journal of Adolescence 17: 221–237

Ylvisaker M 1985 Head injury rehabilitation. Taylor and Francis, London

Yule W 1985 Behavioural approaches. In: Rutter M, Hersov L (eds) Child and adolescent psychiatry: modern approaches. Blackwell, Oxford, pp 794–808

Yule W 1991 Work with children following disasters. In: Herbert M (ed) Clinical child psychology. Wiley, Chichester, p 349–363

Yule W, Udwin O, Murdoch K 1990 The 'Jupiter' sinking: effects on children's fears, depression and anxiety. Journal of Child Psychology and Psychiatry 71: 1051–1062

31 Surgical pediatrics

G. A. MacKinlay   A. C. H. Watson

Neonatal surgery   1768
Respiratory problems   1768
Causes of respiratory distress in the newborn   1768
Duodenal obstruction   1773
Small bowel obstruction   1774
Meconium plug syndrome/small left colon syndrome   1776
Hirschsprung's disease   1777
Urological problems in the neonate   1778
Exomphalos and gastroschisis   1779
Sacrococcygeal teratoma   1781
Anorectal anomalies   1781
Neonatal necrotizing enterocolitis (NEC)   1782
Biliary atresia   1782
Surgery of the infant and child   1783
Head and neck, face and mouth   1783
Pyloric stenosis   1784
Gastroesophageal reflux   1785
Intussusception   1786
Appendicitis   1786
Primary peritonitis   1787
Meckel's diverticulum   1787
Superior mesenteric artery syndrome   1787
Choledochal cyst   1788
Cholelithiasis   1788
Inguinal hernia and hydrocele   1788
Femoral hernia   1790

Umbilical hernia   1790
Epigastric hernia   1790
Surgical aspects of the genitourinary tract   1790
Anomalies of testicular descent   1790
The acute scrotum   1791
Circumcision   1792
Paraphimosis   1793
Hypospadias   1793
Epispadias   1794
Urinary tract infection – surgical aspects   1794
Labial adhesions   1795
Hydrocolpos   1795
Hematocolpos   1796
Vaginal agenesis and vaginal atresia – surgical aspects   1796
Ovarian cysts   1796
G. A. MacKinlay
Plastic surgery   1796
Cleft lip and palate   1796
Other craniofacial deformities   1797
Hemangiomas and vascular malformations   1797
Cystic hygroma: lymphangioma   1798
Melanocytic nevi   1798
Café-au-lait spots   1798
Burns   1798
A. C. H. Watson
References   1800

Pediatric surgery encompasses a wider range of surgery than any other surgical specialty. It is confined to an age group rather than an organ system. In the older child some commoner problems are often dealt with by adult surgeons.

Congenital problems presenting in the neonatal period or later, together with other conditions peculiar to childhood, should be treated in a specialist center by trained pediatric surgeons backed by pediatric anesthetists, pediatric radiologists, pediatric pathologists and experienced nursing staff specifically trained in the care of children. In a general hospital the child should be nursed on a children's ward and if there is no pediatric surgeon, care should be provided by the surgeon who is treating the child *together* with a pediatrician.

In the case of the neonate, a particular surgical challenge is encountered not only in the requirement for a meticulous surgical technique but also in careful pre- and postoperative management. The reward is the prospect of a full three score years and ten survival compared with the commonly sought 5-year survival in many aspects of adult surgery.

The presence of an anomaly requiring surgery is often detected antenatally by ultrasound, enabling discussion with the parents, obstetrician, pediatric surgeon and neonatologist. The parents can thus be prepared and reassured, where possible, that although an abnormality has been detected it can be treated. They can visit the surgical neonatal unit, meet the staff and, where appropriate, the timing of delivery may be planned to facilitate optimal transfer of the baby to the awaiting surgical unit or direct to the operating theater. Pregnancy is a time of potential parental stress and unless great care is taken in explaining the possible consequences of an antenatally diagnosed anomaly their anxiety will be increased.

NEONATAL SURGERY

RESPIRATORY PROBLEMS

Whilst respiratory distress in the newborn is primarily the domain of the neonatologist some causes may be surgical and early referral to a pediatric surgeon may be of lifesaving importance.

CAUSES OF RESPIRATORY DISTRESS IN THE NEWBORN

1. Upper airway
   a. choanal atresia
   b. nasal encephalocele
   c. tumors of the nasopharynx
   d. Pierre Robin syndrome

e. macroglossia
f. hemangio/lymphangiomata of oral cavity
g. laryngotracheoesophageal cleft
h. laryngeal web
i. laryngeal stenosis
j. hemangioma of larynx
k. laryngomalacia
l. tracheomalacia
m. tracheal stenosis
n. cystic hygroma
o. cervical teratoma
2. Intrathoracic
   a. congenital lobar emphysema
   b. cystic adenomatoid lung malformation
   c. bronchogenic and lung cysts
   d. enterogenous cysts
   e. pneumothorax
   f. sequestration of lung
   g. vascular ring
   h. congenital heart disease
   i. diaphragmatic hernia
   j. eventration of the diaphragm
   k. esophageal atresia and tracheoesophageal fistula.

Choanal atresia is obstruction of the posterior nares by a bony or occasionally membranous septum. If bilateral it is a neonatal emergency, as babies are obligate nasal breathers. An oral airway will overcome this problem until the obstruction is relieved.

An oral airway is also of benefit in *Pierre Robin syndrome* where there is a hypoplastic mandible, the tongue falling posteriorly to occlude the glottis. An airway can be maintained in position for several weeks, the baby being fed nasogastrically or via a gastrostomy. A tracheostomy may be easier to manage and is maintained until the mandible grows, keeping the tongue forward. It also facilitates repair of the cleft palate which is associated in the majority of cases.

A *laryngeal web*, if complete, leads to death in utero. If partial, the symptoms may merit emergency tracheostomy. *Laryngomalacia* leads to inspiratory stridor which usually resolves in the first 2.5 years of life. *Tracheomalacia* is commonly associated with esophageal atresia. It has been postulated that the hypertrophied upper pouch, containing swallowed liquor, compresses the developing trachea, preventing the normal growth of tracheal rings. The problem increases postoperatively sometimes making it impossible to extubate these babies. The diagnosis may be confirmed radiologically by lateral screening of the neck, observing the anteroposterior narrowing of the trachea with inspiration. Aortopexy, suturing the aorta to the back of the sternum, thus pulling the pretracheal fascia and hence the anterior tracheal wall forward, is sometimes of benefit. Prolonged intubation may allow time for the tracheal rings to become more supportive but may itself lead to subglottic stenosis. Tracheostomy is required in some cases.

Congenital lobar emphysema leads to overexpansion of a lung lobe with compromise of ventilation. Half the cases present within days of birth, the remainder usually in the first few months of life. The most common cause is bronchomalacia of the associated bronchus although some cases may be caused by external compression. The baby may present with feeding difficulties due to dyspnea. The diagnosis is made radiologically and the most commonly affected lobes are the left upper lobe or the right middle lobe. Treatment is lobectomy in severe cases but in many conservative management is appropriate.

Cystic adenomatoid lung and *congenital lung cysts* can present in much the same way as lobar emphysema. Their expansion produces respiratory distress. Congenital cysts tend to be unilocular and solitary. Cystic adenomatoid lung malformation is due to excessive overgrowth of bronchioles with multiple cysts lined by cuboidal and ciliated pseudostratified columnar epithelium. The left lower lobe is commonly affected and the appearance may antenatally or even postnatally be mistaken for a diaphragmatic hernia. Treatment is resection of the affected lobe.

Pulmonary sequestration is a mass of lung tissue not communicating with the bronchial tree and which receives its blood supply from an anomalous systemic vessel. It may be within the substance of the lung (intralobar sequestration) or completely separate (extralobar). Areas of sequestration are thought to arise from an extra bronchopulmonary bud of the foregut. They most commonly occur in the left lower lobe and the blood supply comes direct from the aorta, above or below the diaphragm. The anomalous blood supply may often be identified by ultrasound techniques avoiding the need for angiography. The condition usually presents with respiratory infections, more commonly after the neonatal period. The treatment is resection (Clements & Warner 1987).

Diaphragmatic hernia

Diaphragmatic hernia may be congenital or acquired, the latter usually being traumatic in origin. Congenital diaphragmatic hernia arises due to an abnormality in the formation of the diaphragm between the fourth and tenth weeks of fetal life.

The commonest herniation is the Bochdalek type, a posterolateral defect, possibly a failure of closure of the pleuroperitoneal canal. It has been postulated that the primary anomaly is in the developing lungs which fail to induce diaphragmatic closure and this may explain hypoplasia in the contralateral lung. A hernia through the foramen of Morgagni is less common in neonates. This defect is retrosternal, to the right or left of the midline. The third site for herniation is the esophageal hiatus – the so-called hiatus hernia.

The true incidence of congenital diaphragmatic hernia is difficult to ascertain as so many die at birth, others present as live births and others sometime after the neonatal period. This lesion represents 8% of major fatal congenital anomalies noted in a British perinatal mortality survey (present in 1 in 2200 of all births). It has a variable incidence in live births in different series from 1 in 4000 to 1 in 10 000. In Edinburgh the incidence is 1 in 7000 live births.

Some cases are now detected antenatally by ultrasound but the majority present with respiratory distress – cyanosis, dyspnea and tachypnea – either immediately after birth or within a few hours. Occasionally, particularly on the right side, the presentation may be later, the defect being present at birth but actual herniation of abdominal content occurring as a postnatal event. The later the onset of symptoms, the better the prognosis. Examination reveals a scaphoid abdomen, bowel sounds on auscultation of the affected side of the chest and a shift of the apex beat to the right in the case of a left-sided hernia. The right side is less common, perhaps due to plugging by the liver, but if a defect is present here it tends to be large with herniation of the liver as well as bowel.

Once air has been swallowed after birth a chest X-ray confirms the diagnosis, showing gas filled loops of bowel on the affected

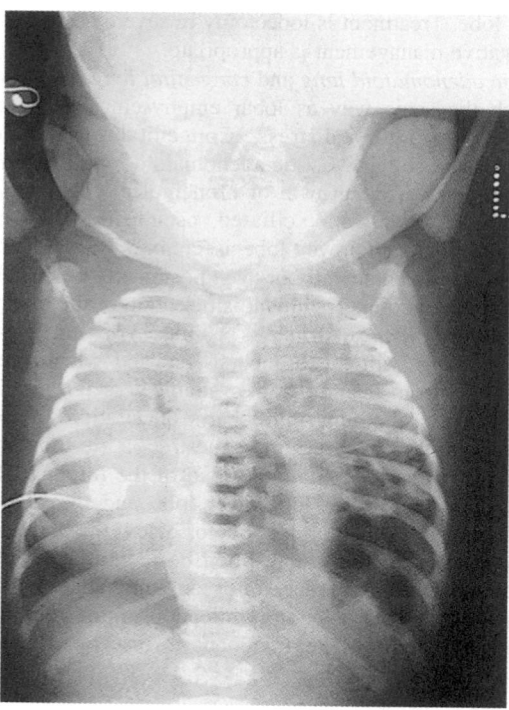

Fig. 31.1   Diaphragmatic hernia (left-sided Bochdalek defect).

side of the chest with displacement of the mediastinum to the opposite side (Fig. 31.1).

Treatment

A nasogastric tube is passed to reduce the gaseous distention of the bowel with air. In the past the surgical repair of the hernia was a true emergency, it being felt that the sooner the hernia was reduced the more easily the lungs could expand. Babies were operated on virtually regardless of condition and the survival rates in general were poor. It has been shown that respiratory mechanics, far from improving, frequently deteriorate as a result of repair of the hernia. The role of urgent surgery has thus been re-evaluated. It has always been known that the babies with the least hypoplastic lungs fared better. These also tend to be the cases that present after hours rather than immediately at birth. Now an initial, nonsurgical approach to diaphragmatic hernia has been adopted in many centers with the aim of improving pulmonary function and reducing pulmonary vascular resistance (Bohn et al 1987, Sakai et al 1987). After diagnosis the baby is intubated and hyperventilated and paralyzed. Metabolic acidosis is corrected with bicarbonate therapy and the respiratory rate and pressure are adjusted to reduce the $PaCO_2$ to <4.7 kPa (<35 mmHg). A chest X-ray is taken to verify the endotracheal tube position and exclude a pneumothorax. A preductal arterial line (radial) is sited for blood gas and pressure monitoring. The ventilatory index (mean airway pressure × respiratory rate) is calculated and this should be <1000 with a $PaCO_2$ <5.3 (<40 mmHg) prior to surgery. If the index is higher, high frequency oscillatory ventilation is instituted. Tolazoline may be administered to reduce pulmonary vascular resistance and prevent shunting through the ductus arteriosus. In some centers extracorporeal membrane oxygenation (ECMO) is

used for prolonged support with variable results. Whatever the method of stabilization preoperatively, it must be carried out in a surgical unit as it is the pediatric surgeon who must be in a position to determine the timing of surgery.

Operative treatment

An abdominal approach is usually preferred with a transverse upper abdominal incision on the side of the hernia. The bowel and other organs are reduced and the defect in the diaphragm examined. If the defect is large a patch of prosthetic material may be used. Approximating a defect under tension merely reduces lung compliance. An underwater seal drain is positioned prior to completion of the repair.

Postoperatively, support is maintained as before until the baby can be weaned from the ventilator. A few patients who require little or no ventilatory support preoperatively may be extubated immediately. Of the remainder the mortality rate still remains around 50%, although it is hoped that the change in preoperative management will improve the outlook.

Eventration of the diaphragm

This is due to a deficiency in the muscle of the diaphragm. The thin layer becomes attenuated and bulges up into the thorax. Extensive eventrations are similar to diaphragmatic hernia presenting in the neonatal period. Smaller eventrations present later and require localized plication.

Esophageal atresia

Atresia is absence or closure of a normal body orifice or passage (Greek *a* = negative, *tresis* = hole). A fistula is an abnormal communication between two epithelial surfaces.

Esophageal atresia is a congenital defect of unknown etiology, the great majority of cases being associated with a tracheoesophageal fistula. The incidence is approximately 1 per 3000 live births. Many babies with esophageal atresia are premature and of low birthweight. The lower the birthweight, the greater the mortality. More than half the babies presenting with esophageal atresia have associated congenital abnormalities. Commonly associated are vertebral, anorectal, cardiac, tracheoesophageal, renal and limb anomalies (VACTERL). This was formerly known as the VATER complex. The anatomical varieties of esophageal atresia and related disorders are illustrated in Figure 31.2.

Clinical features

Maternal hydramnios is so common that all babies born to a mother with hydramnios should have a tube passed to assess the patency of the esophagus. In cases with esophageal atresia the tube will be arrested about 10 cm from the lips. If the diagnosis is not made in this manner then the baby will be noted to froth at the mouth, choke, cough or become dyspneic and cyanosed. These symptoms will be exacerbated by attempts to feed the baby. The patency of the esophagus should then be tested by a firm tube of at least 10 or 12 FG, which should be passed orally. Acid secretions aspirated from the tube may have refluxed through the fistula so radiological confirmation of the position of the tube is necessary if suspicion is high.

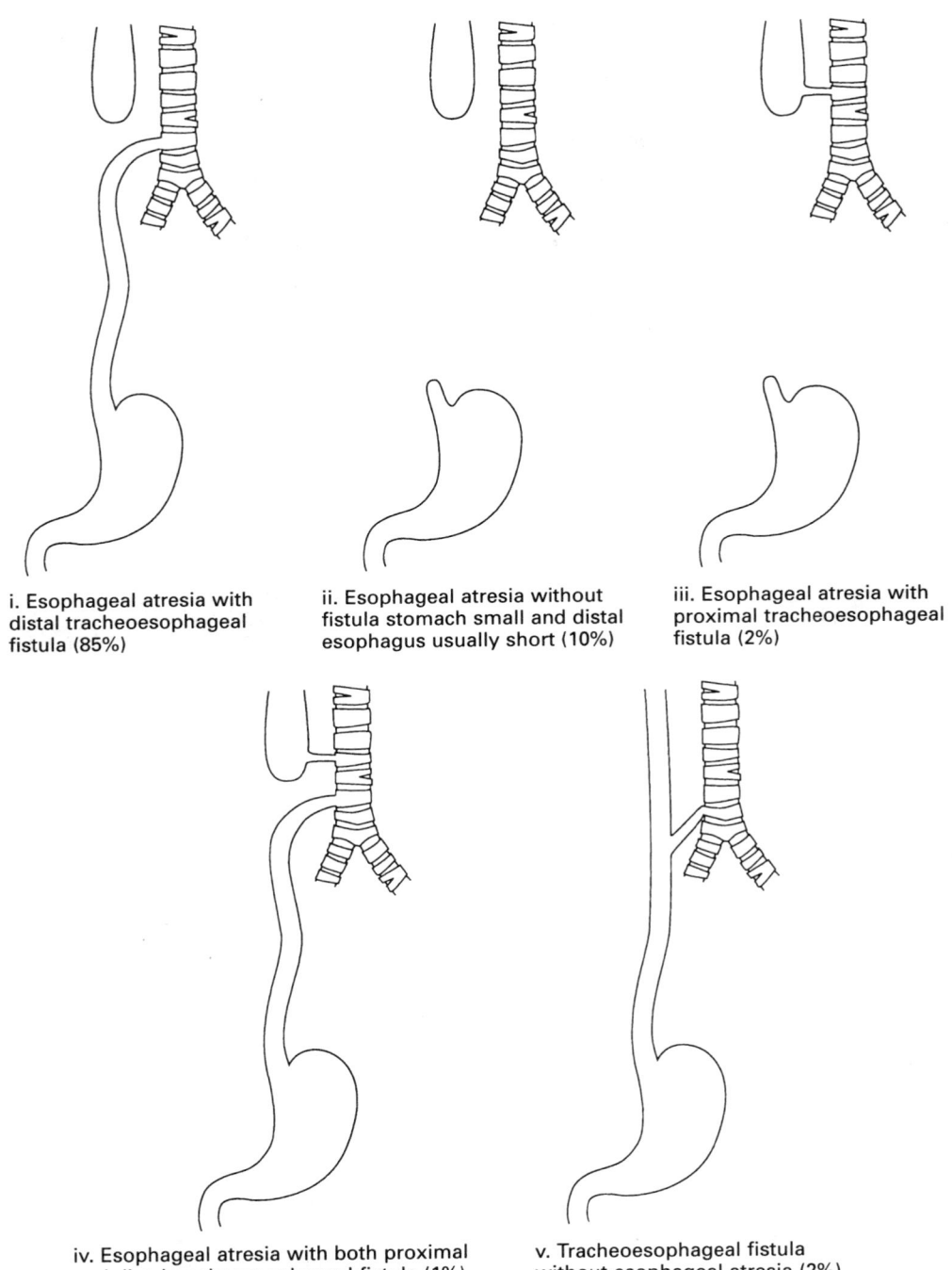

i. Esophageal atresia with distal tracheoesophageal fistula (85%)

ii. Esophageal atresia without fistula stomach small and distal esophagus usually short (10%)

iii. Esophageal atresia with proximal tracheoesophageal fistula (2%)

iv. Esophageal atresia with both proximal and distal tracheoesophageal fistula (1%)

v. Tracheoesophageal fistula without esophageal atresia (2%)

Fig. 31.2   Esophageal atresia and tracheoesophageal fistula.

A Replogle tube is a double lumen plastic catheter which can be passed via the nose into the upper esophageal pouch, enabling continuous suction to be applied without causing damage to the mucosa. Suction is applied to the end of the catheter, air passing along the finer of the two lumina as secretions are aspirated. If the latter are particularly thick, careful irrigation may be carried out via the finer lumen tube.

A plain chest X-ray with gentle pressure on the Replogle tube enables the distal extent of the pouch to be ascertained. The presence of air in the stomach and bowel confirms the presence of

a distal tracheoesophageal fistula (TEF) (Fig. 31.3). In the case of atresia without a fistula there is absence of air in the stomach (Fig. 31.4). Occasionally there may be associated duodenal atresia, but providing there is a TEF, then the gas pattern should suggest this (Fig. 31.5).

Some surgeons like to use 1–2 ml of contrast to define the upper pouch but there is great danger of spillage into the tracheobronchial tree and the procedure is unnecessary. Preoperatively, apart from adequate aspiration of the upper pouch, opinions differ as to the best position in which to nurse the baby. Some advocate the

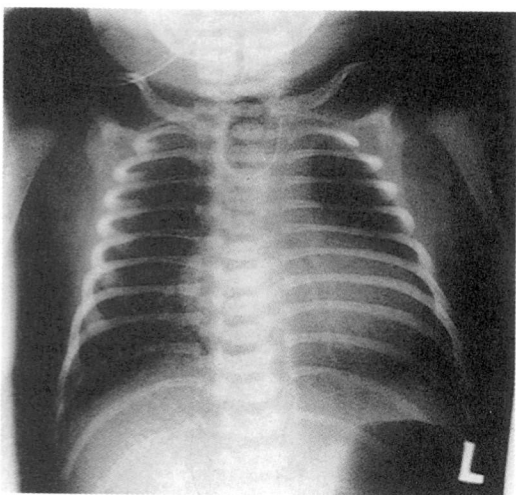

Fig. 31.3   Esophageal atresia with distal tracheoesophageal fistula.

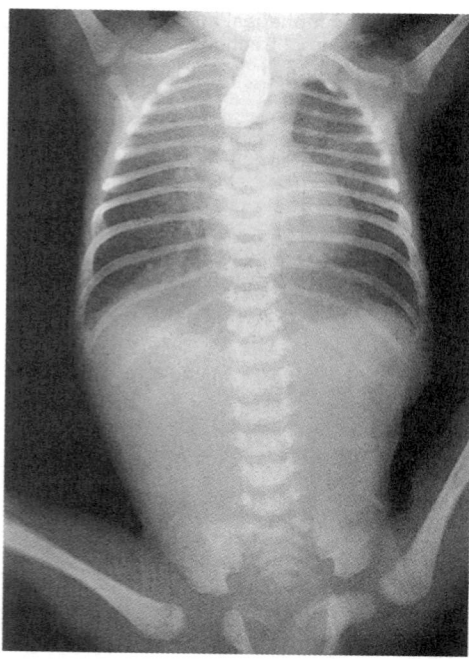

Fig. 31.4   Esophageal atresia without TEF.

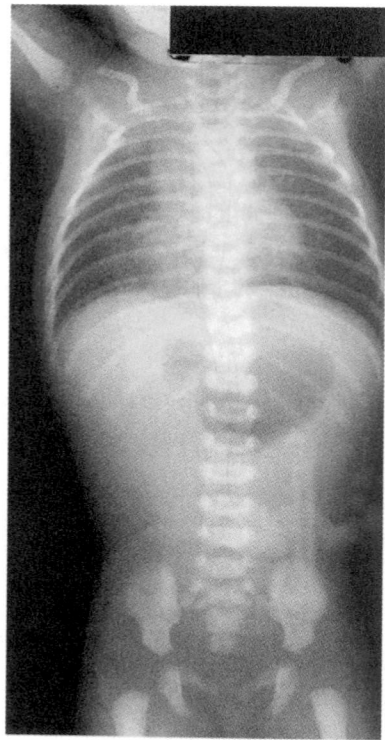

Fig. 31.5   Esophageal atresia with duodenal atresia.

Trendelenburg (head down) position to prevent aspiration of secretions but this may lead to reflux of gastric content via the fistula into the lungs (especially the right upper lobe). Others, to prevent this, advise a head up position. A horizontal and semiprone position reduces the incidence of right upper lobe collapse and seems satisfactory.

Treatment

In the commonest type of anomaly (with a distal TEF), surgery is carried out as an 'elective emergency'. It does not have to be performed immediately in the middle of the night but can be safely left until the following day. If pneumonitis is present, it is justifiable to delay treatment for 24 h or more to allow chest physiotherapy and appropriate antibiotics to be administered. A right posterolateral thoracotomy is made and, via an extrapleural approach, the fistula is divided and repaired and an end-to-end anastomosis between the proximal and distal esophagus is made in a single layer. A fine transanastomotic silastic tube is passed nasogastrically prior to completion of the anastomosis so that early nasogastric feeding can be instituted. Some surgeons prefer a gastrostomy but most find it unnecessary.

On the sixth or seventh postoperative day a contrast swallow is performed to confirm patency of the anastomosis and exclude leakage at this site. If leakage is present it can safely be managed conservatively if an extrapleural approach has been followed. Anastomotic stricture, if it occurs, is treated by esophagoscopy and bougienage or balloon dilation under X-ray control. Most children, following a successful repair, have a persistent brassy cough or 'seal bark' which may last for 1 or 2 years. This is probably due to a degree of tracheomalacia.

Dysphagia due to abnormal motility in the esophagus both above and below the anastomosis may be due to vagal nerve damage or, more probably, an intrinsic abnormality associated with the lesion. This, like the seal bark, usually resolves by the age of 2 years.

Cases of esophageal atresia without a fistula are best managed initially by gastrostomy and aspiration of the upper pouch via a replogle tube. In my experience, delayed primary anastomosis can be achieved after 3 months of regular stretching of the upper pouch by the nursing staff using a Nelaton catheter at feed times. Once there is radiological evidence of a gap of less than 3 cm, as visualized with a metal bougie in the lower pouch (passed per gastrostomy) and a radiopaque tube in the upper pouch, surgery can be carried out. Postoperatively, the infants are electively paralyzed and ventilated for up to 7 days to relieve the tension on the anastomosis, a technique also of value in tight anastomosis in the common type of atresia with a distal fistula (MacKinlay & Burtles 1987). Others favor construction of a cervical esophagostomy followed by colonic interposition or formation of a gastric tube to bridge the gap between the upper pouch and the stomach.

H-type tracheoesophageal fistula

These occasionally present in the first few weeks of life with coughing or cyanosis on feeding. More commonly they present much later with recurrent chest infections, a history of coughing on feeds, and sometimes abdominal distention. Because the fistula runs obliquely upwards from esophagus to trachea, the flow of esophageal content into the trachea is limited and intermittent. The diagnosis is made at a contrast swallow under screening. Treatment is surgical division of the fistula, usually via a cervical approach.

DUODENAL OBSTRUCTION

Duodenal obstruction may be intrinsic (atresia, membrane, stenosis or annular pancreas) or extrinsic (Ladd's bands with or without volvulus of the midgut).

Intrinsic duodenal obstructions (Fig. 31.6)

The etiology of duodenal atresias and other intrinsic duodenal obstructions differs from that of intrinsic obstructions in the remainder of the small intestine. It appears to be a failure of development due to an early insult and there are often associated abnormalities. Down syndrome is present in 30% of cases. In 10% there is esophageal atresia, and a further 10% have anorectal anomalies. Cardiac and renal anomalies may also be associated. Cardiac abnormalities are particularly common in those with Down syndrome.

Atresia or stenosis usually affects the second or occasionally the third part of the duodenum.

Complete obstructions present with vomiting within 24 h after birth. The vomitus may or may not be bile stained, depending on whether the obstruction is proximal or distal to the ampulla of Vater. In those with bile stained vomitus the meconium, if passed, may also be normally bile stained as there may be openings of the bile duct proximal and distal to the obstruction via Wirsung's and Santorini's ducts.

In maternity units where passage of a nasogastric tube is a routine soon after birth, aspiration of more than 20 ml of fluid may be indicative of a duodenal or small bowel obstruction.

Abdominal distention, if any, is confined to the upper abdomen due to obstruction of the stomach and duodenum.

The diagnosis is confirmed by a plain erect X-ray which demonstrates the characteristic 'double bubble' appearance of air fluid levels in the stomach and duodenum (Fig. 31.7). The double bubble may also be detected antenatally, ultrasound detecting fluid distention of the stomach and duodenum (Hancock & Wiseman 1989). An incomplete obstruction, stenosis, or membrane with a small hole in it may allow air to pass through to the rest of the bowel, thus masking the double bubble (Fig. 31.8), but a contrast study confirms the presence of obstruction (Fig. 31.9). Sometimes the diagnosis may be delayed several months or even a year or two if sufficient food can pass through.

Treatment

If there is any delay in diagnosis of a duodenal obstruction then any resulting metabolic disturbance must be corrected preoperatively. At laparotomy a duodenoduodenostomy is the procedure of choice (Fig. 31.10), or for a stenosis or membrane a duodenoplasty may be performed, opening the duodenum lengthways across the obstruction and closing it transversely. Resection of a diaphragm must be undertaken cautiously to avoid damage to the ampulla of Vater.

An annular pancreas (Fig. 31.10a) is caused by the failure of the normal migration of the ventral bud to join the dorsal one. It is rarely a true ring around the duodenum but more commonly associated with an intrinsic obstruction within the duodenum (membrane or stenosis). A duodenoduodenostomy is performed with no attempt to divide the pancreas for fear of fistula formation.

Extrinsic duodenal obstruction

Ladd's bands may obstruct the duodenum occasionally alone but more commonly in association with a midgut volvulus (volvulus neonatorum). Such a volvulus may present in the neonatal period or at any age and arises due to an incomplete, or malrotation of the bowel. By the sixth week of intrauterine life the gut tube elongates to a greater extent than can be accommodated in the developing abdominal cavity and thus herniation through the umbilical ring occurs. During the next month the bowel undergoes an anticlockwise rotation returning to the abdominal cavity by the tenth week. By the time the stomach has rotated to the left, the

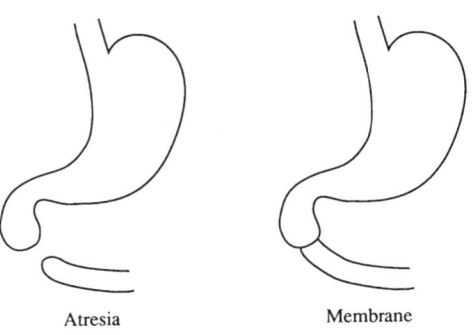
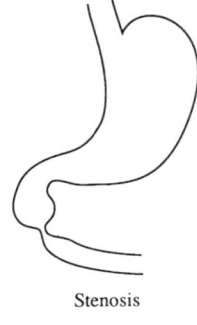
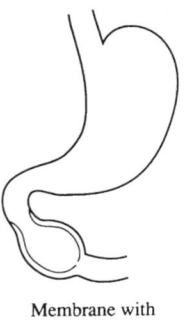

Atresia   Membrane   Stenosis   Membrane with windsock deformity

Fig. 31.6 Duodenal anomalies.

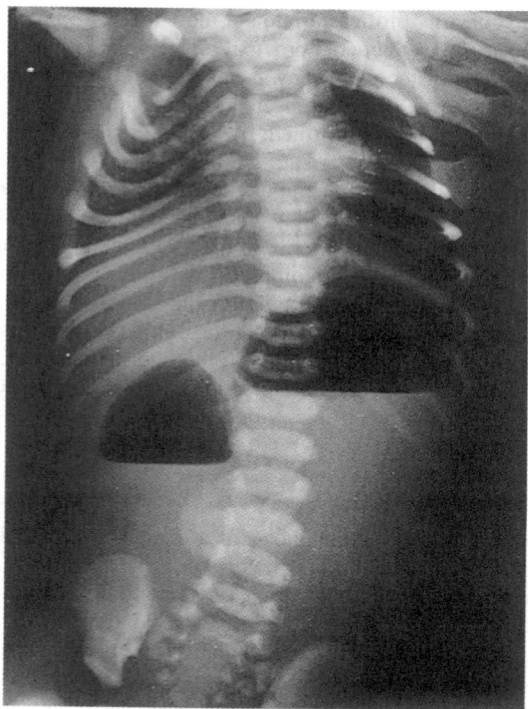

Fig. 31.7 'Double bubble' in duodenal atresia.

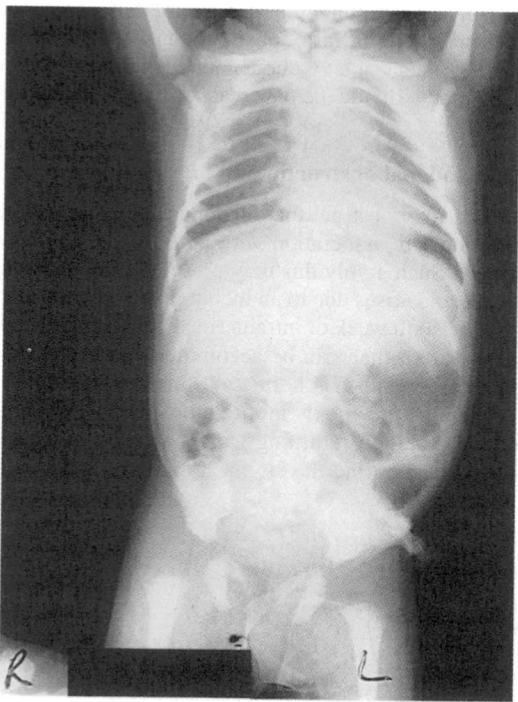

Fig. 31.8 Plain film of baby soon after birth.

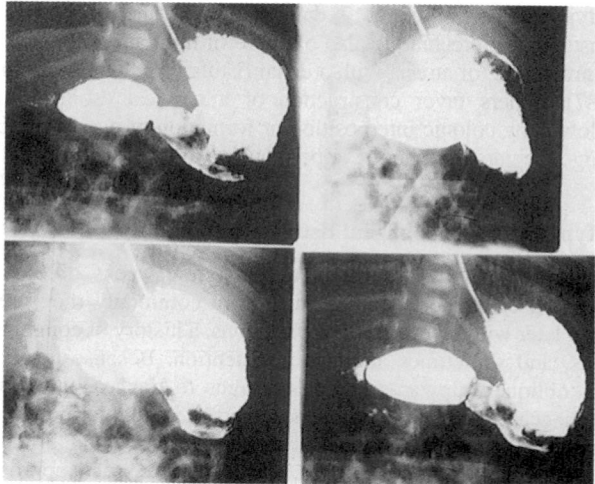

Fig. 31.9 Upper gastrointestinal contrast study on same baby as Figure 31.8.

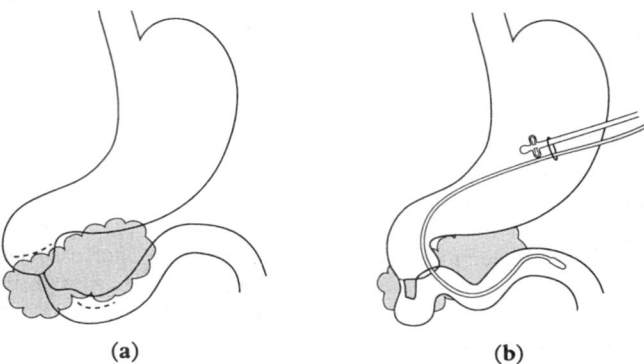

Fig. 31.10 (a) Annular pancreas with intrinsic duodenal membrane. (b) Duodenoduodenostomy with gastrostomy and transanastomotic silastic feeding tube.

the duodenojejunal flexure and the ileocecal region. Failure of the cecum and ascending colon to reach their normal position results in a short base to the midgut mesentery and peritoneal bands passing from the cecum (in the midline or to the left side) to the right posterior abdominal wall. These bands (Ladd's bands) obstruct the duodenum. In addition, the short base to the mesentery allows a midgut volvulus to arise, the bowel rotating in a clockwise direction, and resulting in duodenal obstruction. A plain X-ray will show a double bubble and usually a small amount of gas in the bowel more distally. Contrast studies may confirm the diagnosis. An upper gastrointestinal study may show a duodenal obstruction and a typical coiled spring sign. An enema may show an anomalous position of the cecum.

Once any electrolyte or acid–base disturbance is corrected, laparotomy must be performed without delay to avoid ischemia of the midgut.

SMALL BOWEL OBSTRUCTION

This may arise due to an abnormality directly associated with the bowel itself (intrinsic), pressure from without (extrinsic), or obstruction within the lumen (intraluminal).

duodenal C-loop has formed and the small bowel, followed by the large bowel, returns to the abdomen. The cecum and ascending colon pass to the right of the abdomen, the latter becoming retroperitoneal. The small bowel mesentery is then fixed between

Intrinsic anomalies

These are mainly atresias, membranes, stenoses and duplications of the bowel. Atresias may arise anywhere along the length of the bowel, being most common in the distal ileum and rarely seen in the colon. Their likely cause is an interruption of the mesenteric vessels in utero. These vary from membranous obstruction in continuity, those with or without an associated gap in the mesentery and multiple atresias, to the so-called apple peel type deformity with extensive loss of mesentery and bowel, the distal small bowel receiving its blood supply from the middle colic vessels through a precarious continuity between marginal arcades (Fig. 31.11).

The bowel proximal to the obstruction is distended and hypertrophied and distally the bowel is collapsed, often with a microcolon (unused) although babies with obstructions of this kind may pass meconium of normal appearance. The latter is dependent on the timing of the vascular accident in utero.

The diagnosis is confirmed by plain X-ray which will show a number of distended loops of small bowel with air–fluid levels in an erect view (Fig. 31.12). The level of obstruction can be estimated by the number of distended loops. There will be absence of air distal to a complete obstruction.

Contrast studies have a limited role in the diagnosis of such obstructions unless to exclude intraluminal or functional conditions.

Treatment

Preoperative treatment involves passage of a nasogastric tube and correction of electrolyte imbalance by appropriate administration of intravenous fluids. If the diagnosis is established early there is little or no requirement for intravenous resuscitation.

Operative treatment involves laparotomy, resection or tapering of grossly dilated bowel proximal to the atresia (to prevent problems of postoperative peristaltic inertia) and then anastomosis between the dilated proximal bowel and the collapsed distal bowel.

Duplications

Duplications of the alimentary tract can occur at any level from mouth to anus. A length of bowel may be duplicated, the two segments sharing a common blood supply and muscular wall yet having separate mucosal linings. They may or may not communicate, and it is the noncommunicating type that tends to

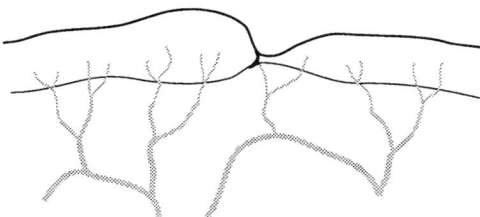

Intraluminal diaphragm

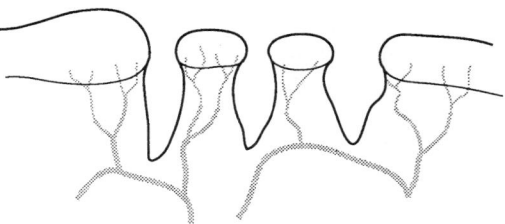

Multiple atresias

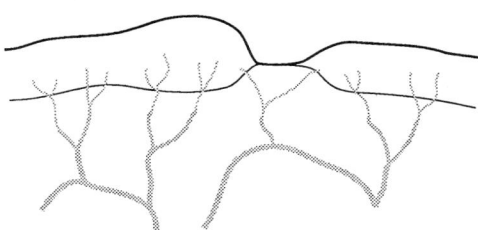

Atresia with cord like segment between ends of bowel

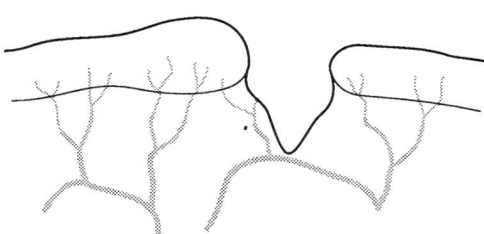

Complete separation of bowel ends with mesenteric defect

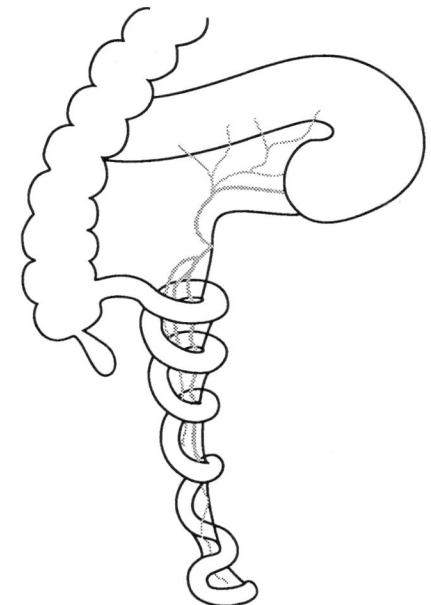

'Apple peel bowel' ~ Atresia with extensive mesenteric defect and tenuous blood supply to distal ileum

Fig. 31.11   Small bowel atresias.

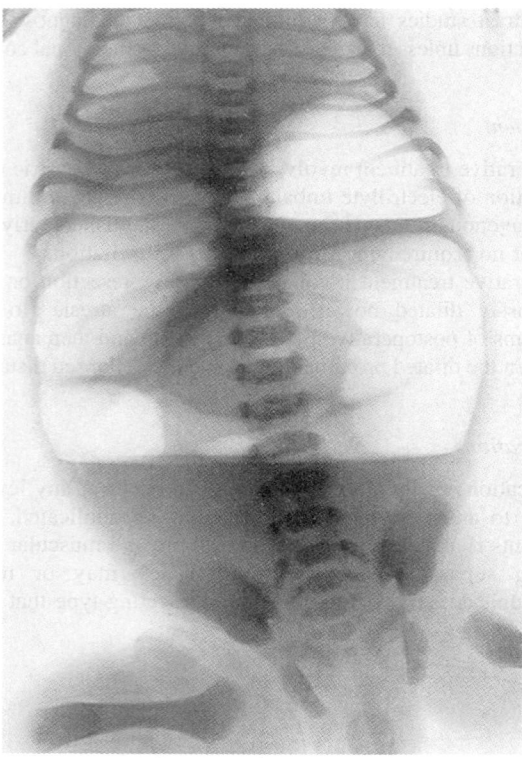

Fig. 31.12   Jejunal atresia.

form a short cystic segment which, by accumulation of secretions within it, leads to intestinal obstruction. Such duplications may be palpable as a cystic intra-abdominal mass which together with the signs of intestinal obstruction lead to the diagnosis. Ultrasound and contrast studies may be of value.

Treatment. The treatment usually involves a localized bowel resection but if the duplication is extensive in length or at a site such as the ileocecal junction, the mucosa of the duplicated segment should be dissected out, thus avoiding extensive resection or loss of the ileocecal valve.

Extrinsic anomalies

Extrinsic anomalies leading to intestinal obstruction include hernias (inguinal or internal), localized volvulus, bands, vitellointestinal remnants and mesenteric cysts.

An incarcerated inguinal hernia is the commonest cause of intestinal obstruction at any age. The inguinal region must thus be carefully examined when any patient, neonate or older, presents with intestinal obstruction. Internal hernias are rare and can only be identified at laparotomy.

Localized volvulus may arise in relation to bands, duplication cysts and vitellointestinal remnants. Treatment at laparotomy varies according to the causative factor and the condition of the affected bowel. Mesenteric cysts may lead to local volvulus or may present as a palpable cystic mass. They are treated by resection.

Intraluminal anomalies

Intraluminal causes of intestinal obstruction include meconium ileus, milk curd obstruction and meconium plug syndrome.

Around 10% of patients with cystic fibrosis present in the neonatal period with obstruction of the distal ileum (meconium ileus). The distal few centimeters of ileum contain pale gray 'rabbit pellets' of inspissated meconium proximal to which is a segment containing hard green-black meconium and, more proximally still, distended loops containing tarry fluid meconium and air. Distal to the obstruction is a microcolon and usually no meconium is passed, presenting signs being abdominal distention and bile stained vomiting within a few days of birth.

Plain abdominal films show gross abdominal distention with few fluid levels and often a ground glass appearance (of air bubbles in the viscid meconium) in the right iliac fossa. Sometimes there are signs of calcification from perforation and leakage of meconium antenatally.

Volvulus of the hypertrophied distended bowel may also lead to atresia, or perforation may occur after birth.

The presence of meconium ileus has no relationship to the subsequent 'severity' of the cystic fibrosis.

Conservative management

Treatment can be either conservative or operative. Conservative management involves the administration of a gastrografin enema under fluoroscopic control. Gastrografin with 0.1% Tween 80, a detergent, added as a wetting agent has a high osmolarity of 1900 mOsm/l and acts by drawing fluid into the bowel, thus freeing the inspissated meconium in the distal ileum. It is essential, therefore, that the baby is adequately hydrated and an intravenous infusion must be in progress. If necessary the procedure may be repeated after 24 h. If there is calcification the procedure is best avoided for fear of reperforation.

Surgical management

For cases in which there are complications such as perforation or signs of meconium peritonitis (calcification) or after failed gastrografin enema, operative treatment is required. Laparotomy is performed via an upper transverse abdominal incision. Intestinal resection is necessary for bowel that is grossly dilated or of doubtful viability. A Bishop Koop ileostomy is usually performed. This is a Roux-en-Y anastomosis between the end of the proximal limb of ileum and the side of the distal limb, bringing the end of the latter out of the abdomen as an end ileostomy in the right iliac fossa. This acts as a safety valve through which the distal ileum can be irrigated. In the case of continued obstruction the stoma will function. Once it is relieved, bowel contents pass the natural way.

Milk plug or mild curd obstruction also occurs in the distal ileum and may be due to the administration of inappropriately concentrated artificial milk feeds, or possibly a transient low bile acid excretion. The management is similar to that described above.

MECONIUM PLUG SYNDROME/SMALL LEFT COLON SYNDROME

Meconium plug syndrome must not be confused with meconium ileus. It is sometimes described as small left colon syndrome. The distal colon or rectum is plugged by sticky gray-white mucus distally with sticky meconium above it. The presentation is usually at about 2 days with a history of failure to pass meconium.

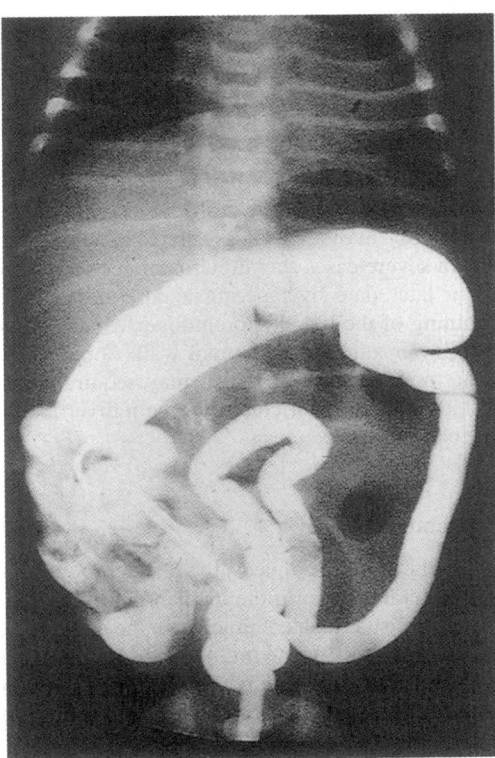

Fig. 31.13 Small left colon syndrome.

There is evidence of low intestinal obstruction with generalized abdominal distention, frequently with a history of bile stained vomiting and X-ray showing gaseous distention. There are multiple fluid levels present in the majority of cases.

The diagnosis is made by contrast enema. Initially barium is used to exclude Hirschsprung's disease, but then changed to water-soluble contrast when the appearance of a meconium plug is seen in a narrowed left colon. The colon is usually narrow up to the splenic flexure where it becomes dilated (Fig. 31.13). It has been postulated that there is a discrepancy in the activity of the parasympathetic supply from the vagus nerve (supplying the bowel to two-thirds of the way across the transverse colon to the splenic flexure) and the sacral parasympathetics which supply the remainder. Whatever the etiology, the enema invariably proves to be therapeutic with satisfactory evacuation of meconium. The abdomen in most cases decompresses over 24 h and feeds can then be introduced. If bowel evacuation is not normal then Hirschsprung's disease must be excluded.

HIRSCHSPRUNG'S DISEASE (Hirschsprung 1887)

Hirschsprung, a Danish pediatrician, described two patients who died at 7 and 11 months from constipation associated with gross abdominal distention and a highly dilated hypertrophied colon full of feces. There is absence of ganglion cells in the myenteric plexuses (both Auerbach's and Meissner's) of the most distal bowel and extending proximally for a variable distance. Aganglionosis involving only the rectum or rectosigmoid is often termed 'short segment' Hirschsprung's disease and affects males five times more commonly than females. 'Long segment' Hirschsprung's disease, extending above the sigmoid, has an

equal sex incidence and a greater likelihood of siblings being affected. In short segment disease there is a 1 in 20 risk that brothers will be affected and a 1 in 100 risk for sisters. In long segment disease the risk to all siblings is 1 in 10.

In a few cases there is total colonic aganglionosis with disease extending into the small bowel and in extremely rare cases involving the whole alimentary canal. At least 70% of cases are short segment, 25% long segment and about 5% total colonic.

Hirschsprung's disease differs from many other alimentary tract abnormalities in that the birthweight is usually within the normal range. It is uncommon in premature and low birthweight babies. Associated congenital anomalies are uncommon apart from Down syndrome which affects 1 in 20. The cause of the disease is unknown. It has been postulated that it is due to a failure of migration of ganglion cells from the neural crest which normally proceeds in a craniocaudal direction having entered the upper end of the alimentary tract (Bodian & Carter 1963). Differentiation of ganglion cells occurs in the wall of the gut between the seventh and eighth week of intrauterine life and proceeds in a craniocaudal direction.

Clinical features

Usually the symptoms of Hirschsprung's disease are manifest within the first few days of life. This is certainly the case in all long segment or total colonic cases but some short segment cases and especially 'ultrashort' segment cases may present later, even into old age.

Failure to pass meconium within the first 24 h, abdominal distention, bile stained vomiting and reluctance to feed are the main symptoms. Diarrhea may be the presenting feature of Hirschsprung's enterocolitis, a devastating complication of the condition which has a high mortality. The etiology of Hirschsprung's enterocolitis is unknown but apart from diarrhea it is associated with gross abdominal distention and circulatory collapse. A rectal examination results in the explosive passage of flatus and loose stool, deflating the abdomen.

Diagnosis

A plain abdominal X-ray shows distended small and large bowel, sometimes with multiple fluid levels on an erect film. A barium enema is best carried out without a previous rectal examination as then the narrow aganglionic bowel with dilation proximally is demonstrated. A delayed film at 24 h, again avoiding an invasive rectal examination, shows retained barium and often a clear indication of the level of disease with a cone-shaped transition zone between normal bowel above and the narrowed aganglionic distal segment.

Definitive diagnosis is by rectal biopsy. A suction biopsy is adequate to confirm the absence of ganglion cells in the submucosal plexus, specimens being taken at 1 and 3 cm above the dentate line. Histochemical staining will demonstrate excessive acetyl cholinesterase activity in abnormal nerve trunks and absence of ganglion cells.

Treatment

Once the diagnosis is made, a defunctioning colostomy, or ileostomy, is performed proximal to the diseased bowel. Frozen sections can be used if necessary to confirm that the stoma is sited in normal bowel. A definitive procedure is carried out when the infant is 3–12 months of age, depending on the surgeon's preference. It usually consists of excision of the aganglionic bowel and a 'pull through' procedure. Some, however, prefer an anorectal myectomy (Scobie & MacKinlay 1977) (a procedure also of use, alone, in very short segment disease combined with an anterior resection operation).

If enterocolitis supervenes (and it can even happen after a definitive procedure, especially if an aganglionic segment remains), then rapid replacement of lost fluid by a suitable electrolyte solution, often preceded by plasma, is required. This should be combined with saline bowel washouts using a two tube technique, one to run saline in, preferably above the aganglionic segment, the other at a slightly lower level to allow evacuation. Broad spectrum antibiotics are usually administered prophylactically although infection has not been shown to be the precipitating factor. Enterocolitis is certainly the most lethal complication of Hirschsprung's disease.

UROLOGICAL PROBLEMS IN THE NEONATE

Posterior urethral valves

The commonest obstructive uropathy in male children is valvular obstruction of the posterior urethra. Occasionally the diagnosis is made on antenatal ultrasound. A large proportion of cases present in the first 2 weeks of life, the majority in the first 6 months and the remainder, whilst usually becoming apparent in the first few years, may present as late as early adult life.

The neonate may present with retention of urine or dribbling and a palpably distended bladder with or without infection or uremia. Later presentation is usually with incontinence or infection.

The valves are classically folds of mucosa attached just below the verumontanum and attempts to void lead to apposition of the valves. The obstruction leads to dilation of the posterior urethra, the bladder, the ureter and renal pelvis.

As micturition commences in the fetus in the first trimester, the back pressure on the kidneys may lead antenatally to severe damage – renal dysplasia. Occasionally the bladder hypertrophy is such that reflux no longer occurs but the ureters remain dilated and tortuous.

Diagnosis

A micturating cystourethrogram (MCU) is diagnostic in this anomaly, demonstrating the gross dilation of the posterior urethra and usually the refluxing dilated ureters and bilateral hydronephrosis.

Treatment

Disruption of the valves is required. This may be affected by pulling the inflated balloon of a Fogarty catheter across the valves or by delicately disrupting them with a Whitaker hook. A resectoscope can be used transurethrally and the valves either fulgurated or, to avoid a deep destruction of tissue, cut with a cold knife. If renal function is particularly poor, temporary drainage via bilateral cutaneous ureterostomies (preferably ring ureterostomies) may be required.

Prune belly syndrome (triad syndrome)

This consists of deficiency of the anterior abdominal wall muscles, cryptorchidism and urinary tract deformities. The abdominal muscular deficiency is mainly in the lower abdomen, the whole abdominal wall taking on the wrinkled appearance of a prune (Fig. 31.14). The ribs may be flared outwards at the lower costal margin and respiratory infections are common.

Surgery is best avoided unless there is significant renal impairment. In severe cases ring ureterostomies may be required, followed at a later date by tapering and reimplantation of the ureters, trimming of the bladder, orchidopexies and excision and repair of the lower anterior abdominal wall. Some cases have a functional urethral obstruction which may require urethrotomy. Other cases show urethral stricture or even a diverticulum at the site of the prostatic utricle.

Urachal anomalies

The urachus in the embryo connects the bladder to the allantois. It is normally obliterated to form the median umbilical ligament. It may, however, persist as a patent urachus in the neonate, requiring repair. Occasionally the two extremities of the urachus close, leaving a cyst in the middle which becomes filled with secretions and may present as a mass or more commonly, when it becomes infected, as an abscess.

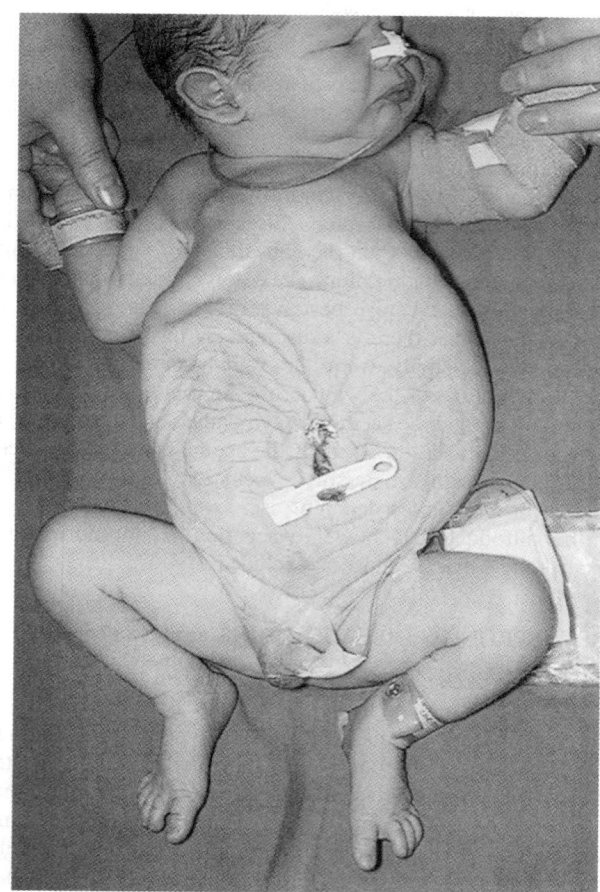

Fig. 31.14 Prune belly syndrome.

Bladder exstrophy (ectopia vesicae)

This is part of a range of lower abdominal wall defects, ranging from epispadias, through exstrophy of the bladder, to the even more catastrophic vesicointestinal fissure or cloacal exstrophy.

In bladder exstrophy there is a lower abdominal wall anomaly in which there is wide separation of the pubic bones, the bladder surface being flat and exposed with the two ureteric orifices clearly visible (Fig. 31.15). In the male there is complete epispadias with a strip of urethral mucosa on the dorsum of a short broadened flattened penis. In the female there is also an epispadiac urethra with a bifid clitoris and separation of the labia anteriorly at the level of the vaginal orifice.

The bladder is best repaired soon after birth. If necessary, bilateral iliac osteotomies enable the pubic bones to be better approximated thus facilitating the repair. Careful construction of the bladder neck is vital to achieve subsequent continence, and in the male later repair of the severe epispadiac deformity is required. If the bladder repair is unsuccessful it may be necessary to carry out a urinary diversion procedure.

EXOMPHALOS AND GASTROSCHISIS

These are two distinct conditions of different etiology. Although formerly exomphalos was believed to be more common, gastroschisis is now seen more frequently. Antenatal diagnosis of both conditions by ultrasound examination is now almost routine. Gastroschisis also gives rise to an elevated maternal serum α-fetoprotein and distinction from other anomalies such as neural tube defects is by ultrasonography. Gastroschisis is not an indication for termination of pregnancy whilst exomphalos major, with its high incidence (30–40%) of associated anomalies, may be.

Exomphalos

Exomphalos (omphalocele) is a herniation of intra-abdominal contents through the umbilical ring into the umbilical cord.

Defects less than 4 cm in diameter are classified as *exomphalos minor* (Fig. 31.16). There are rarely associated abnormalities in this group.

Exomphalos major (Fig. 31.17), on the other hand, commonly has coexisting abnormalities and a defect greater than 4 cm in diameter, presumably arising through failure of development of the anterior abdominal wall prior to herniation of the midgut loop. In a large defect, not only the intestines (small and large) herniate but also the liver, spleen, stomach, bladder and even ovaries and fallopian tubes in the female. Incomplete or malrotation of the bowel is common and the associated abnormalities often include cardiac defects; 20% of cases are anencephalic. In the *Beckwith–Wiedemann* syndrome there is exomphalos, macroglossia and gigantism. The baby is large for his gestational age with an exomphalos, a big tongue and large solid viscera. There is also a facial nevus flammeus in the center of the forehead and odd indentations in the ear lobe (Fig. 31.18). There may also be pancreatic hyperplasia leading to severe neonatal hypoglycemia.

An *omphalocele* is usually covered by a sac composed of the fused layers of amniotic membrane and peritoneum. The sac may rupture ante-, intra- or postpartum.

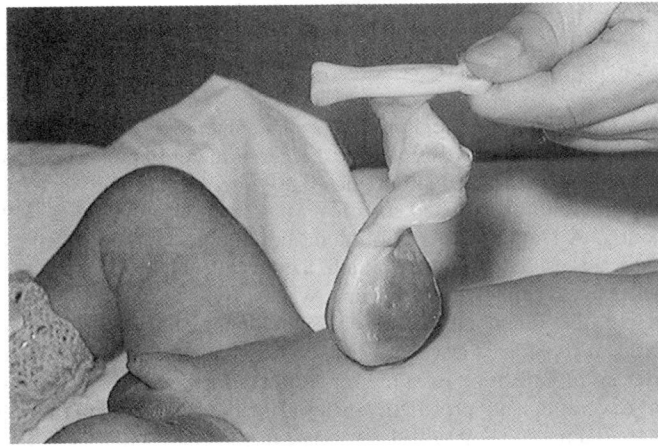

Fig. 31.16 Exomphalos minor.

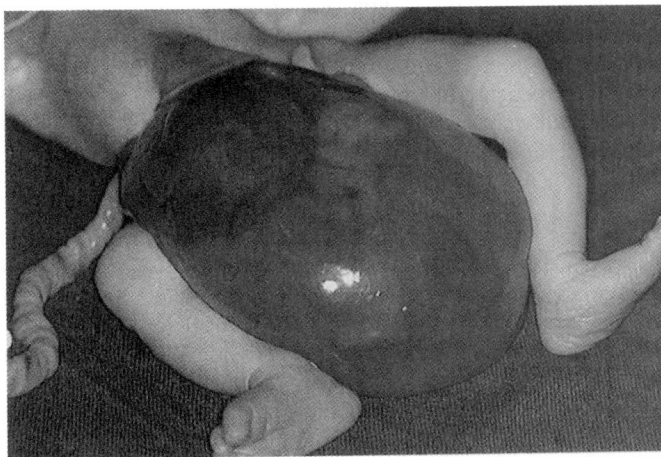

Fig. 31.17 Exomphalos major.

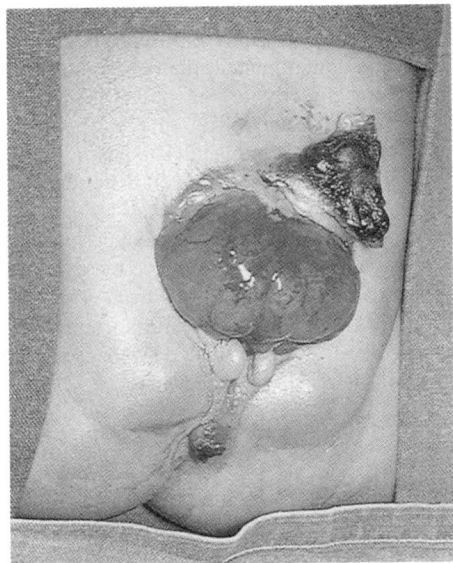

Fig. 31.15 Ectopic vesicae.

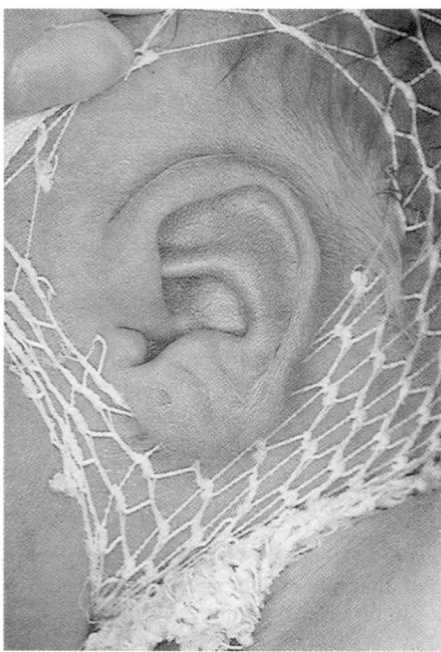

Fig. 31.18 Earlobe indentations in Beckwith–Wiedemann syndrome.

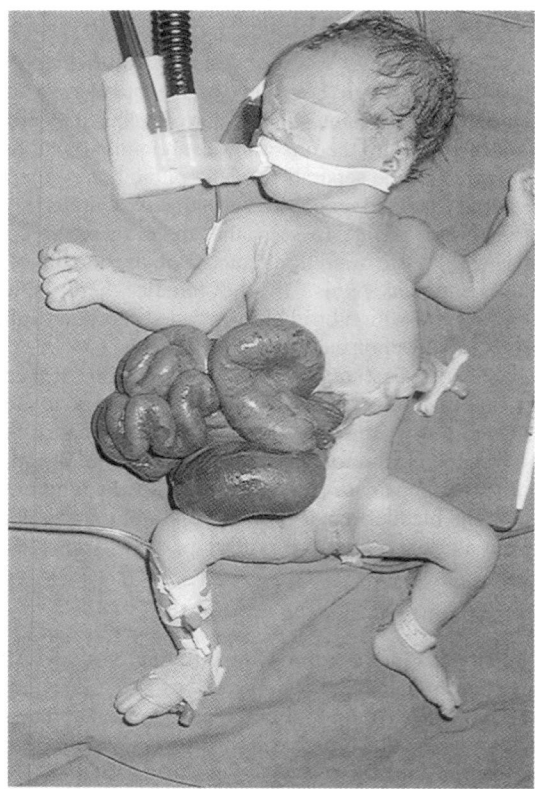

Fig. 31.19 Gastroschisis.

Treatment

In a large omphalocele, conservative management may be appropriate in the neonatal period. The danger of mercury poisoning has led to the recommendation that 0.5% mercurochrome in 65% alcohol solution be used for only 48 h, applying the solution 2 hourly. A simple alcohol solution should then be applied daily until an eschar forms. Epithelialization of the sac from the periphery results over the ensuing weeks. It may take 3–4 months before the infant can be discharged home, returning for later surgical repair of the ventral hernia. Other methods of treatment include mobilization of skin around the defect and skin coverage or coverage with prosthetic material such as Silastic, Dacron, human dura, etc., all with later repair of the ventral hernia. If the defect is small enough then with stretching of the anterior abdominal wall primary repair may be possible as in gastroschisis (see below). In cases with an apparently simple herniation through a small defect into the umbilical cord it is tempting to twist the cord to reduce the contained bowel into the abdominal cavity, then simply ligate the cord. Such a temptation must be strongly resisted as all too frequently there is a Meckel's diverticulum or another cause of adherence of the bowel to the sac and serious damage may result. Formal surgical repair is always indicated.

Gastroschisis

Gastroschisis is a complete defect through all layers of the anterior abdominal wall extending up to about 3 cm in length and usually lying to the right of a normally attached umbilical cord (Fig. 31.19). It is almost as though a short transverse incision had been made with a scalpel antenatally. The etiology is unknown. Almost all the small and large bowel are eviscerated through the small defect – in most instances from stomach to rectum inclusive. Other organs are rarely apparent. The eviscerated bowel is markedly thickened, apparently foreshortened, matted together and often covered with a confluent gelatinous layer, 'gut in aspic'.

If possible, delivery should be in a perinatal center close to the regional pediatric surgical center. The decision whether to deliver the baby with exomphalos or gastroschisis by cesarean section or vaginally is an obstetric one. The results of treatment of the baby are not significantly improved by cesarean delivery.

At delivery it is essential that the baby is placed in a plastic bag extending to above the level of the defect and leaving the head and, if necessary, the upper limbs exposed. The bowel must not be allowed to become contaminated, the baby being transferred in a transport incubator directly to the pediatric surgical operating table and the baby extracted from the bag aseptically, by the surgeon, once anesthesia is induced. The passage of a nasogastric tube prior to transfer reduces bowel distention and resulting ischemia if the anterior abdominal wall defect is very small. Transport in a polyethylene bag helps reduce hypothermia which would otherwise result from heat loss by evaporation. These babies rapidly drop their temperature from 37°C to 35°C when exposed for even a few minutes to site an intravenous infusion. The application of warm saline soaked swabs is not a good idea as they rapidly cool, increasing the heat loss.

Treatment

Providing the temperature has been adequately maintained and no fluid loss has occurred, direct transfer to the operating table for primary repair will achieve the best results. The anterior abdominal wall is slowly and gently, yet vigorously, stretched manually. Once the abdominal cavity has been sufficiently enlarged the bowel can be returned under minimal tension and the defect closed with an absorbable purse-string suture. It is essential that the baby is left with a reasonable umbilicus and this is achieved with a further purse-string suture to the skin. The defect is usually so small that the umbilicus is not eccentric in position.

Postoperatively, ventilatory support is often required for a few days. In addition a prolonged ileus necessitates intravenous nutrition for days or in some cases even weeks. The prognosis in gastroschisis cases treated in this manner is excellent.

On occasion the bowel wall is too thickened to allow complete reduction and in these cases a silastic 'silo' is constructed, the content being reduced gradually over succeeding days.

SACROCOCCYGEAL TERATOMA (p. 921)

A sacrococcygeal teratoma is the commonest teratoma presenting in the neonatal period. They tend to be large and protrude from the space between the anus and the coccyx (Fig. 31.20). The lesion is usually covered in skin but the most protuberant part may be necrotic due to vascular compromise. The tumor may also extend up into the pelvis and a large retrorectal component is palpable in all cases. In a presacral teratoma there is no protrusion behind the anus and the presentation may be later in the first year of life.

The tumor may be both solid and cystic in nature. A very large tumor may give rise to dystocia and if diagnosed antenatally is best delivered by cesarean section.

There is usually an elevated α-fetoprotein level in the baby at birth and this should decline appropriately following excision.

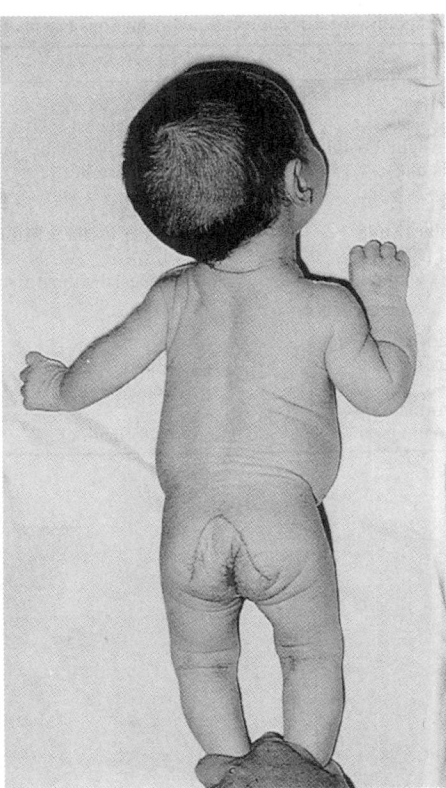

Fig. 31.21 Postoperative appearance of Figure 31.20.

Even benign tumors should be followed up into adulthood as recurrence of benign or malignant elements may occur.

Treatment is excision within the first few days of life. A double 'chevron' incision is made with the baby in a prone position and with careful excision and reconstruction of the pelvic floor which, despite its gross stretching, recovers normal function (Fig. 31.21).

ANORECTAL ANOMALIES

Congenital anomalies of the anus and rectum are reported to occur in 1 in 1800 to 1 in 10 000 live births. In Edinburgh the incidence is 1 in 3100. There is a wide spectrum of anomalies and many attempts have been made to classify them.

An anatomical approach simplifies matters (Table 31.1; Stephens 1984). The lesions are grouped according to whether the end of the rectum is above levator ani, *high* (supralevator), or below, *low* (translevator). There is also an *intermediate*, partially translevator group. The essential component of the levator ani in these malformations is the puborectalis sling which is the key to fecal continence.

In the male a high lesion commonly communicates with the urethra whereas in the female, with the genital tract intervening, the fistula is to the vagina. A low lesion may open onto the skin of the perineum, or in the male, track forwards along the median raphe of the scrotum (Fig. 31.22), or in the female, towards the vestibule. In addition, a severe cloacal anomaly may arise in girls with urethra, vagina and rectum opening into a common channel. Anal stenosis may arise in either sex and presents with the passage of toothpaste-like motions.

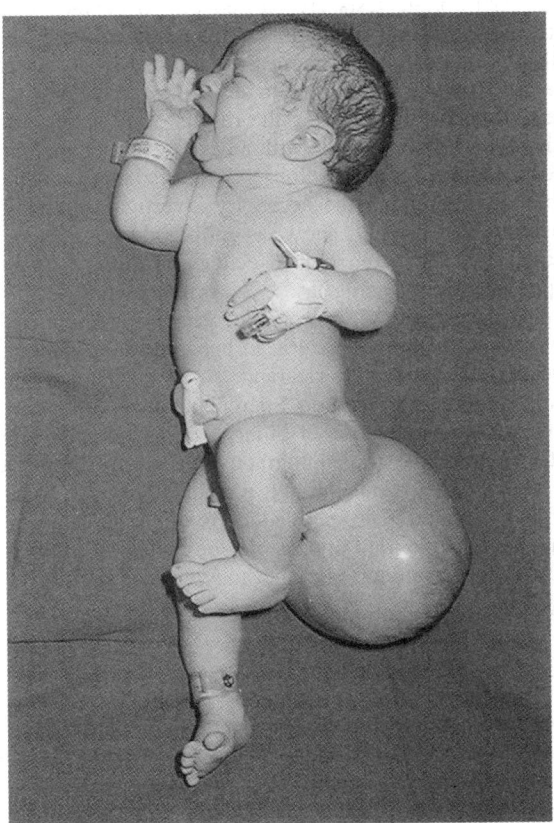

Fig. 31.20 Sacrococcygeal teratoma.

Table 31.1 Classification of anorectal malformations (Stephens 1984)

Female	Male
High	*High*
Anorectal agenesis:	Anorectal agenesis:
With rectovaginal fistula	With recto–prostatic–urethral fistula
Without fistula	Without fistula
Intermediate	*Intermediate*
Rectovestibular fistula	Rectobulbar urethral fistula
Rectovaginal fistula	
Anal agenesis without fistula	Anal agenesis without fistula
Low	*Low*
Anovestibular fistula	
Anocutaneous fistula	Anocutaneous fistula
Anal stenosis	Anal Stenosis
Cloacal malformations	
Rare malformations	Rare malformations

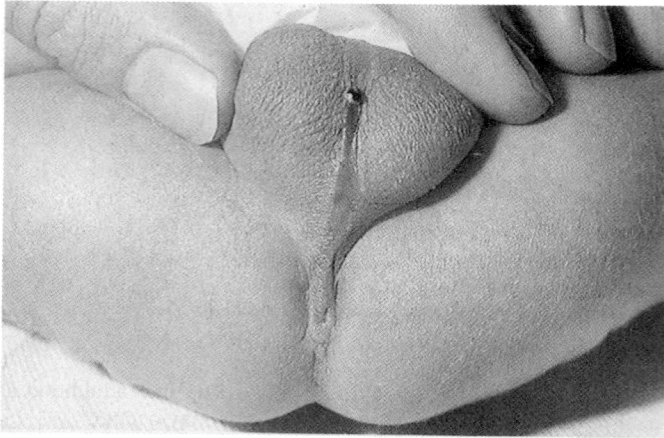

Fig. 31.22 Low anorectal anomaly.

Treatment

Anal stenosis is treated by graduated anal dilation with Hegar's dilators. A low lesion with a long subcutaneous tract should have the latter opened and an anoplasty performed. An anovestibular fistula can also be managed by a cutback procedure. This may result in rather close proximity of anal and vaginal openings (shotgun perineum) but the perineum develops as the child grows, separating the orifices. To avoid this appearance some prefer to transpose the anal opening to a more normal site.

High and intermediate lesions, and low lesions where the diagnosis is not at first obvious, require a defunctioning colostomy in the neonatal period. A sigmoid colostomy will enable subsequent adequate washouts of the distal loop, a procedure that is especially important in lesions communicating with the urinary tract. Prophylactic antibiotics are also required in such cases.

Once the colostomy is established, formal contrast studies via the distal loop (distal loopogram) define the level of the lesion accurately. Definitive repair is then deferred for a few weeks or months depending on the preference of the surgeon. The procedure of choice is the posterior sagittal anorectoplasty described by de Vries & Pena (1982), requiring meticulous technique and a thorough understanding of the anatomy.

NEONATAL NECROTIZING ENTEROCOLITIS (NEC)

This condition is described in detail on page 210. Presenting as it does with abdominal distention and bile stained vomiting, it is occasionally considered that the baby has intestinal obstruction but the presence of blood in the stool and pneumatosis intestinalis, often with portal venous gas, are pathognomonic of NEC. The management is conservative, i.e. nonoperative wherever possible with nasogastric decompression, intravenous feeding and broad spectrum antibiotics. The criteria for surgical management include pneumoperitoneum, persistent and increasing abdominal tenderness and continued clinical deterioration despite appropriate medical management. Operative management includes resection of necrotic bowel and stoma formation. Occasionally localized drainage under local anesthesia is of value in extremely ill babies, with appropriate intervention at a later date. Conservatively managed survivors often develop intestinal strictures requiring later resection. Asymptomatic strictures identified on contrast studies are best kept under review, reserving surgery for symptomatic cases.

BILIARY ATRESIA (see also p. 475)

Biliary atresia is a condition in which the extrahepatic bile ducts are grossly nonpatent. The condition is characterized by obstructive jaundice. There has traditionally been a division into 'correctable' biliary atresia, where only the distal ducts are occluded, and 'noncorrectable', in which the proximal ducts are occluded.

Presentation is with jaundice persisting beyond the first 2 weeks of life. Appropriate tests are carried out to exclude causes of hepatocellular disease (hepatitis A, hepatitis B, toxoplasmosis, rubella, cytomegalovirus, herpes, syphilis, listeriosis, galactosemia, fructosemia, α_1-antitrypsin deficiency, etc.) It is vital not to waste too much time awaiting the results of all tests as delay in treatment of biliary atresia will adversely affect the progress. Suspected cases must therefore be referred early to a center capable of undertaking the necessary investigation and surgery. Ultrasound will rarely show a gallbladder and may show increased hepatic parenchymal echoes in biliary atresia. An isotope liver scan using a ^{99m}Tc iminodiacetic acid (IDA) radiopharmaceutical will demonstrate good hepatic uptake but no excretion into the bowel at 24 h. In hepatocellular jaundice there is a decrease in hepatocyte clearance.

Some surgeons prefer to do a percutaneous liver biopsy which may be strongly indicative of biliary atresia, but others proceed directly to operative cholangiography if there is a positive IDA scan. This is carried out through a small transverse right upper abdominal incision. The gallbladder is often small and fibrotic making a cholangiogram impossible. Occasionally patency of the cystic duct and common bile duct may be identified and, rarely, biliary hypoplasia.

Treatment

The procedure of choice for extrahepatic biliary atresia is Kasai's hepatic portoenterostomy. This was first described in Japanese in 1959 and only in 1968 in English (Kasai et al 1968).

Kasai achieves a satisfactory bile drainage in 80% of cases. In other series this ranges from 35% to 75% (personal small series 75%). Many will develop portal hypertension and cholangitis (various modifications of Kasai's procedure are carried out to reduce this complication). Liver transplantation is of great value in cases who fail to achieve or maintain bile drainage following the Kasai procedure.

SURGERY OF THE INFANT AND CHILD

HEAD AND NECK, FACE AND MOUTH

Embryological

Branchial

Sinuses, fistulae, cysts and cartilaginous elements may be apparent at birth or may be noted in infancy or later in childhood. The first and second pharyngeal arches and clefts produce these anomalies. First cleft remnants are rare and include a tract from the external auditory canal to the upper lateral neck. They may present with recurrent abscesses in the neck, and treatment involves excision of the whole tract, which is usually a sinus being blind ending at the external auditory canal. Abnormal development of the first arch results in cleft lip and palate (pp. 1796–1797), abnormal shape of the pinna, and deafness due to malformation of the malleus and incus.

Second branchial remnants are more common. In theory sinuses should be more common than fistulae but the reverse is true and cysts are the least common, more often presenting in adult life. Fistulae have a skin opening over the anterior border of the lower third of the sternomastoid. This may be noted to discharge clear mucus. The tract passes upwards between the internal and external carotid arteries to open in the tonsillar fossa.

The length of this tract often necessitates two incisions to facilitate its removal, one being at the skin opening and the other parallel to it, at a higher level, to follow the tract through the carotid bifurcation.

Branchial cysts manifest themselves as they slowly enlarge with secretions, appearing in late childhood or young adulthood. They tend to lie deep to the anterior border of the upper third of the sternocleidomastoid muscle. They may become infected. The treatment is excision.

Cartilaginous branchial remnants may appear along the anterior border of sternocleidomastoid. They do not usually have an associated tract and are excised purely for cosmetic reasons.

Thyroglossal cysts

These are more common than branchial remnants. The thyroid develops as a diverticulum from the floor of the pharynx leaving it attached to the foramen cecum (at the junction of the anterior two-third, and posterior one-third of the tongue) by a stalk, the thyroglossal duct, which is normally completely reabsorbed. The track of a persistent thyroglossal duct should developmentally be ventral to the hyoid bone but differential growth results in part of the duct reaching its deep surface. A thyroglossal cyst arises typically in the midline of the neck anteriorly, or occasionally just to one or other side of the midline. By virtue of its attachment to the thyroglossal duct the cyst moves on swallowing or protrusion of the tongue (Fig. 31.23a, b and c). The cyst is usually at the level of or just below the hyoid bone but can be anywhere along the line of the duct. Surgery is best performed when the lesion is diagnosed, as infection may arise and lead to difficulty in complete excision. The operation involves not only removal of the cyst but the body of the hyoid and the tract must be followed up to the level of the foramen cecum. Failure to do this is likely to lead to recurrence.

Dermoid cysts

These usually occur at sites of embryological fusion. These may be in the midline. A dermoid cyst in the neck may be mistaken for a thyroglossal cyst although it will not move on swallowing or protrusion of the tongue. A common site is the external angular dermoid cyst in the eyebrow area at the outer angle of the eye.

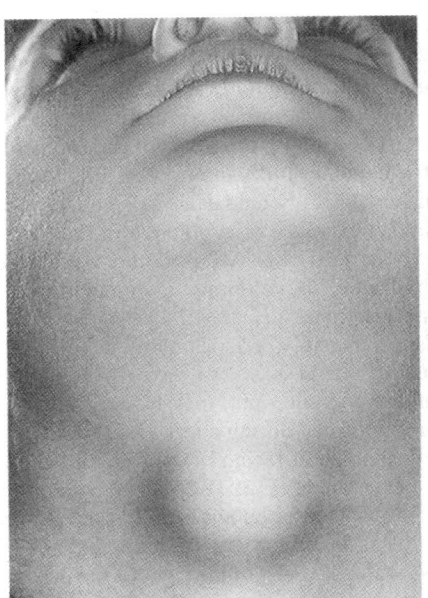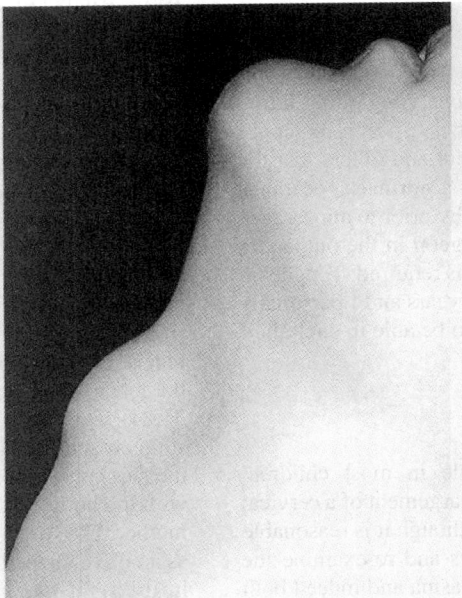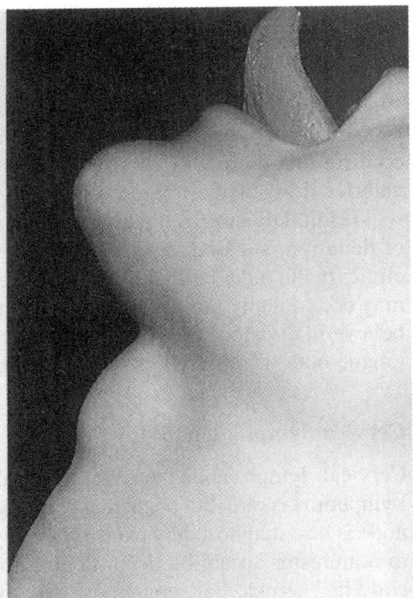

a   b   c

Fig. 31.23   (a) Thyroglossal cyst; (b) and (c) show elevation on tongue protrusion.

Occasionally there may be a dumbbell extension intracranially. They occur if ectodermal cells become buried beneath the skin surface during development. An inclusion dermoid cyst may similarly arise secondary to trauma.

Cystic hygroma

Commonly arising in the neck, these fluid filled lesions of lymphatic origin may be found elsewhere, including the axilla and groin or, rarely, on the trunk. They are either present at birth, sometimes being diagnosed on antenatal ultrasonography, or may appear within the first 2 years or sometimes later. Usually arising in the posterior triangle of the neck, they may sometimes be very large indeed extending into the floor of the mouth and tongue where complete excision may prove difficult, leading to disfigurement and occasionally to the need for a tracheostomy. Infection leads to difficulty with subsequent surgery which is thus best performed soon after diagnosis. Aspiration of the cysts and injection of a streptococcal derivative 'OK432' is a new treatment that is proving to be an effective alternative to surgery (Ogita 1996).

Salivary gland enlargement

This may arise secondary to a calculus in a duct (which may affect the submandibular duct in particular). Parotid duct calculi are rare but recurrent swelling of the gland may be due to sialectasis, seen on a sialogram as dilated duct radicles. The treatment is to advise the sucking of acid drop sweets to promote salivary flow and at the same time massaging the gland from back to front. If infection supervenes then antibiotics must be administered.

Ranula (Latin *rana* = frog)

This is a sublingual cyst which may be small or may fill the floor of the mouth. It may be related to a salivary or mucus gland. It is thin walled and contains clear viscid fluid. Care is required not to damage the submandibular duct during its excision and marsupialization is often safer.

Tongue tie

A short lingual frenum leads to maternal anxiety regarding future problems with speech and feeding difficulties. Speech therapists confirm that there will be no speech problem and others that the anterior third of the tongue will grow and a normal appearance will result. Division of the tongue tie in a baby prior to appearance of dentition is a simple procedure for a surgeon in the outpatient clinic. In the older child, general anesthesia is required. Tongue tie may occasionally present beyond the first 2 years and I personally believe in division, as all children deserve to be able to stick their tongue out – if only to lick an ice cream!

Cervical lymphadenopathy

Cervical lymph nodes are readily palpable in most children. Lymphoma is rare, but persistent painless enlargement of a cervical node is best diagnosed by excision biopsy although it is reasonable to administer an antibiotic in doubtful cases and re-examine the child in 2 weeks. Cat scratch disease, toxoplasma and indeed both tuberculosis and atypical mycobacterial infections may occur and usually affect jugulodigastric and submandibular nodes.

In mycobacterial infections nodes may feel fixed to deeper tissues and to skin, and may caseate and discharge. Sinus formation may result from abscess rupture or incomplete excision. Antituberculous chemotherapy is necessary once the diagnosis has become established.

Acute suppurative cervical lymphadenitis usually results from an upper respiratory tract infection. Early administration of antibiotics may lead to resolution without abscess formation but if an abscess does form it should be allowed to point before drainage. Kaolin poultices seem old fashioned but are still of value in this process.

Sternomastoid tumor

This is the commonest cause of torticollis in childhood (other causes include hemivertebrae, acute fasciitis, cervical adenitis and ocular muscle imbalance). The cause of this lesion is unknown. It is more common in babies born by breech presentation and was considered to be a result of trauma to the muscle during delivery. It seems likely, however, that it arises in utero, resulting in breech presentation. Within the muscle there is an area of endomysial fibrosis with atrophied muscle fibers surrounded by collagen and fibroblasts. The infant presents usually at 2–3 weeks of age with a hard swelling within the substance of sternocleidomastoid. The shortening of the muscle makes the infant look upwards and to the opposite side. It is important to commence physiotherapy as soon as the diagnosis is made. The parents are taught how to stretch the muscle by rotating the head towards the side of the tumor. These stretching exercises should be carried out twice daily and must continue for at least the first year, diminishing in frequency thereafter. Failure to treat adequately leads to shortening of deeper cervical structures and craniofacial asymmetry. Surgical division of the muscle and deeper strictures is necessary in cases that fail to respond or are missed in the neonatal period.

Thyroid swellings (see p. 1783)

PYLORIC STENOSIS

Though often called congenital, hypertrophic pyloric stenosis only very rarely has its onset of symptoms at birth and has never been described in a stillbirth. Vomiting normally commences around 2–3 weeks of age, becoming more frequent and projectile. The vomitus is of gastric content (milk) and is never bile stained. It may become brownish or visibly bloodstained due either to an accompanying gastritis or to rupture of capillaries in the gastric mucosa from frequent vomiting. The baby fails to thrive, becomes constipated and dehydrated, developing a hypochloremic alkalosis from the loss of gastric acid.

Examination reveals a hungry, worried looking baby and if recently fed, visible gastric peristalsis, with a wave traveling from the left hypochondrium towards the right, may be apparent (Fig. 31.24). The diagnosis is confirmed during a test feed. For this the surgeon and the nurse or mother sit facing in opposite directions, the surgeon to the left of the nurse (Fig. 31.25). The baby is fed with the bottle in the right hand or at the left breast of the nursing mother. The surgeon palpates the tumor with the left hand. It is felt as an olive-shaped mass which lies just to the right of the midline, in the right hypochondrium. Contraction of the tumor is noted with variation in palpability, thus confirming that one is not confusing it with a Riedel's lobe of liver, or similar anomaly. If

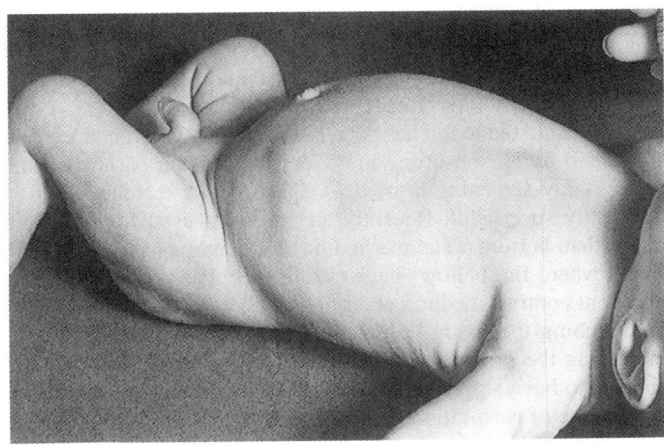

Fig. 31.24   Pyloric stenosis: visible peristalsis.

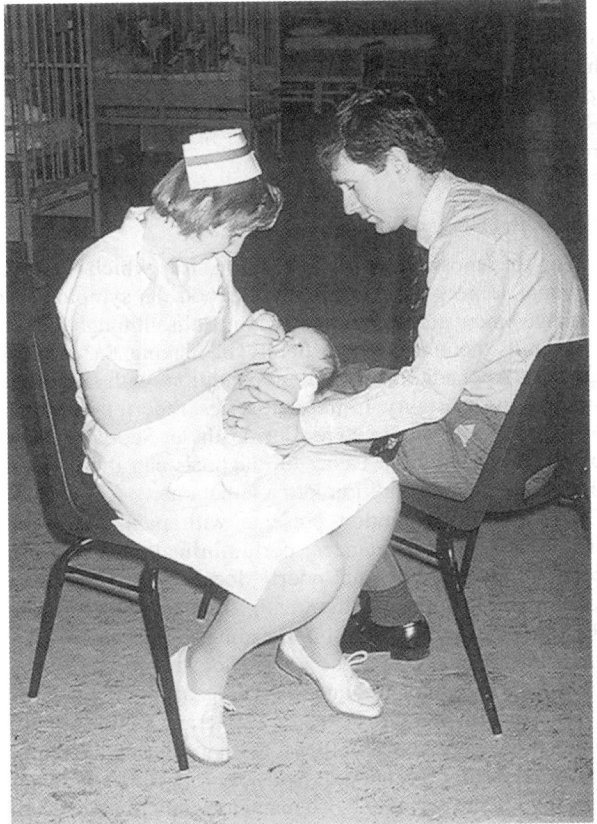

Fig. 31.25   Pyloric stenosis: test feed.

difficulty is encountered in palpating the tumor, the passage of a nasogastric tube to wash out the stomach may facilitate the procedure (it may be that the filled gastric antrum has previously obscured the pylorus). This seemingly ritual routine not only enhances the chance of palpating the tumor but avoids the calamity of the baby vomiting over the examiner's trousers!

Most surgeons will only operate if they can palpate the tumor but if difficulty is encountered in palpation, ultrasound examination is now the diagnostic investigation of choice.

Treatment

First the hypochloremic alkalosis together with any associated hypokalemia is corrected by administering 5% dextrose in 0.45% saline with added potassium chloride if required. Although the use of 0.45% saline takes twice as long to correct the deficit as normal saline would, it is safer to administer. Preoperative gastric lavage is also performed and the nasogastric tube left in situ.

Once the electrolyte and acid-base deficit is corrected, surgery is performed under general anesthesia. The universally accepted operation of choice is the pyloromyotomy attributed to Ramstedt. Actually the first recorded use of this procedure was by Sir Harold Stiles in the Royal Hospital for Sick Children, Edinburgh on 3 February 1910, a year prior to Ramstedt's operation performed on 28 July 1911 and published in 1912. Unfortunately Stiles' patient died on the fourth postoperative day, either from gastroenteritis or delayed chloroform poisoning!

The pylorus is delivered through a right transverse upper abdominal incision and an incision made from the pyloroduodenal junction well onto the antrum of the stomach. The incision extends down into the muscle which is then spread bluntly, all muscle fibers being ruptured, allowing the intact mucosa to bulge. The pylorus is returned to the abdomen and the wound closed.

Oral feeding can be commenced in 4 h. Some choose a graduated feeding regime of dextrose, half strength, then full strength milk introduced over 24–48 h. Others advise a more rapid return to normal feeds. Certainly breast-fed infants come to no harm from being returned to the breast initially for a short time, gradually increasing to normal feeding time.

Vomiting in the first 24 h postoperatively is not unusual and is presumably related to preoperative gastritis. If persistent it usually settles after gastric lavage. Most babies will be fit for discharge within 48–72 h after surgery.

GASTROESOPHAGEAL REFLUX

This is due to incompetence at the cardia and is another cause of vomiting which may commence as early as the neonatal period. The condition may or may not be associated with a hiatus hernia. The infant vomits effortlessly at any time, and usually appears unconcerned about the problem. The vomiting need not be related to feed times. The vomitus may be coffee ground or streaked with bright red blood if there is associated peptic esophagitis. The diagnosis is confirmed by barium studies and pH studies together with endoscopy if indicated. Most cases respond to conservative management of thickening the feeds, sitting the baby up at all times (although there is dispute about this) and the administration of an antacid such as Gaviscon. If, however, the infant fails to thrive, has persistent peptic esophagitis, recurrent aspiration pneumonitis or a proven large 'sliding' hiatus hernia, then a surgical antireflux procedure is required. If an esophageal stricture has already developed it will usually resolve after surgery but in some cases bouginage or balloon dilation is required. Various antireflux operations have been devised, the most popular being the Nissen fundoplication. The esophagus is mobilized, the right crus tightened and the gastric fundus mobilized and wrapped around the abdominal esophagus. This operation can now be performed laparoscopically, reducing postoperative discomfort and length of hospital stay.

Children with severe neurological handicap are especially prone to gastroesophageal reflux and hiatus hernia. Usually the surgical treatment of these children is welcomed by their parents, or carers, as their well-being is so obviously improved. Presumably they suffer a great deal of discomfort related to esophagitis and their frustration is increased by their inability to complain. The results of surgery in such cases is invariably rewarding.

INTUSSUSCEPTION

Intussusception is the invagination of part of the intestine into itself. An intussusception arising in the ileum may pass all the way round the large bowel to appear at the anus. The lead point is known as the intussusceptum, the sheath as the intussuscipiens and between these are the entering and returning layers of the bowel. Naturally, the mesentery with its vessels is drawn between the entering and returning layers, leading to engorgement of the vessels and diapedesis of red cells into the lumen of the bowel. Mucus is produced by the engorgement of the mucosal cells and, mixed with the red cells, produces the classical redcurrant jelly stool. Eventually a strangulating obstruction occurs and gangrene of the intussusceptum may result.

In infants the lead point is presumed to be an enlarged Peyer's patch, the lymphoid tissue presumably responding to a viral stimulant. This becomes the apex of the intussusception which then proceeds for a variable distance into the colon. The peak incidence is in infants 3–9 months of age. The timing has been attributed to a change in the bowel flora associated with weaning. In older children the lead point may be an invaginated Meckel's diverticulum, a polyp, an enteric cyst, or hemorrhage into the bowel wall in Henoch–Schönlein purpura or leukemia. It is more common in boys than in girls, some reporting a ratio as high as 5 : 1, but in Edinburgh the ratio is only 1.2 : 1. Some report seasonal variation, possibly related to infectious agents.

The presentation is with a painful cry, drawing up the knees and going pale, presumably in relation to colic (88% in our series). The colicky pain is intermittent and occurs with increasing frequency as the condition progresses, rather like labor pains. Vomiting is a common symptom (86%) and the passage of redcurrant jelly stools is frequent (56%).

On examination, between attacks of colic, an abdominal mass is usually palpable. This is typically sausage shaped and commonly palpable in the ascending or transverse colon. A small percentage of intussusceptions present at the anus.

Investigation

Plain abdominal X-ray will often show a filling defect corresponding to the intussusception and will demonstrate any obstruction by the presence of fluid levels within the bowel. Ultrasound can identify a 'target sign' corresponding to the layers of the intussusception. Occasionally a barium enema may be used diagnostically in frankly obstructed cases.

Treatment

First an intravenous infusion is set up. Some collapsed infants require blood or plasma for primary resuscitation, others only require isotonic fluids. A nasogastric tube may be passed, especially if vomiting has been a marked symptom at presentation. Preparation is as for a surgical reduction; the operating room is arranged in case it is required but in most cases

nonoperative reduction is first attempted. The only contraindications to nonoperative management are a seriously ill child with a prolonged history, marked intestinal obstruction or evidence of peritonitis (rare).

Hydrostatic reduction has been intermittently popular since first advocated by Hirschsprung in 1876. Nowadays a barium enema under X-ray screening is used as a therapeutic technique and is frequently successful. Recently air has been used for reduction rather than barium. (The method has for centuries found favor in China where fire bellows have traditionally been used.) Air is an excellent contrast medium and scientific control of the pressure is by attaching the rectal Foley catheter to a sphygmomanometer, increasing the pressure to 100 mmHg if necessary. This method appears to have a greater success rate than barium and in the rare occurrence of perforation, proves safer.

Surgical reduction is required for those in whom nonoperative reduction fails. The intussusception is reduced manually by stripping it back from the point the apex has reached. Pulling on the entering layer of bowel can lead to serosal splitting or rupture of the bowel. Once the intussusception is reduced appendectomy is usually performed. This may help to prevent recurrence by adherence of the cecum in the right iliac fossa. If reduction proves impossible then a limited bowel resection may be required.

Recurrence rates of 2–4% have been recorded and seem unrelated to the method of reduction.

APPENDICITIS

This is the most common condition for which emergency abdominal surgery is required in childhood. Its symptomatology and management are similar to those in adults although in the very young child there may be difficulty in making the appropriate diagnosis. Appendicitis is still a condition with a significant morbidity and mortality. In a recent series, reporting on the last 5 years of the 1970s, there were four deaths in Scotland related to appendicitis in children. Delay in diagnosis can thus convert an eminently treatable condition into a lethal one.

Classically the condition presents with pain, vomiting and fever. The pain commences periumbilically, the distended appendix causing dull and poorly localized midgut pain via visceral nerve fibers to the tenth thoracic nerve root. The pathology of appendicitis is of spreading inflammation from the mucosa through the wall to the serosa. Serosal inflammation leads to peritoneal inflammation and the pain is accurately localized to the right iliac fossa – classically at McBurney's point (two-thirds along a line from the umbilicus to the anterior superior iliac spine). Atypical presentation leads to difficulty in diagnosis, especially in the very young. Neonatal appendicitis is exceedingly rare and the mortality rate is high. In the preschool child the diagnosis is also difficult and a high perforation rate is encountered. The preschool child may present with anorexia, listlessness, fever, vomiting and diarrhea.

Care must be taken in the examination of the child with suspected appendicitis. The tongue may be coated and there is a classical 'fetor oris', a sweet smell on the breath perhaps partly related to ketones. The child is reluctant to climb onto the examination couch. The chest is examined to exclude a right lower lobe pneumonia which may easily lead to a mistaken diagnosis of appendicitis. Examination of the abdomen must be very gentle, starting in the left lower quadrant and gradually working round each quadrant to finish in the right iliac fossa.

Clumsy technique can lose a child's confidence and lead to voluntary guarding. Tenderness at McBurney's point remains the cardinal sign of appendicitis.

Involuntary guarding and rigidity are reliable signs of peritonism or peritonitis. There is no excuse in endeavoring to elicit rebound tenderness as, if present, the child's confidence is immediately lost, the pain being so severe, thus precluding subsequent examination. Likewise, rectal examination should be reserved for cases with negative or equivocal abdominal findings, where it may be the only means of diagnosis of a pelvic appendicitis. It may otherwise confirm a diagnosis of constipation or, in females, gynecological disease. It must be remembered that the appendix can adopt a variety of intra-abdominal positions circumferentially around the attachment to the cecum. A retrocecal appendix may have few abdominal signs initially, although psoas spasm may be apparent.

There are no investigations that can prove the presence of appendicitis. The white cell count need not be raised and an X-ray, whilst occasionally showing a fecolith, is generally unhelpful. Ultrasound is now of value in recognizing a thickened appendix with surrounding edema.

The differential diagnosis includes intestinal diseases such as gastroenteritis, Crohn's disease and other causes of terminal ileitis such as *Yersinia* infection, Meckel's diverticulitis and leukemic typhlitis, mesenteric adenitis and deep iliac adenitis. In addition, gynecological problems such as salpingitis and ovarian cysts must be considered. Urinary tract infection may also be confused with appendicitis, the situation being further complicated by the possible occurrence of pyuria when an inflamed appendix is adjacent to the bladder. Finally, medical disorders such as right basal pneumonia, diabetes mellitus, Henoch–Schönlein purpura and sickle-cell disease have all been misdiagnosed as appendicitis. In fact almost all causes of acute abdominal pain in childhood must be considered but appendicitis is the commonest surgical emergency.

Treatment

If necessary, preliminary resuscitation of the patient by administration of intravenous fluids should be considered. Once the patient has been adequately hydrated then appendectomy is carried out through a skin crease incision an inch or more below McBurney's point to leave a neat scar well below the 'bikini line'. At induction of anesthesia a single dose of broad spectrum antibiotics such as an aminoglycoside and metronidazole, to cover bowel flora including *E. coli* and *Bacteroides fragilis*, is administered to endeavor to prevent postoperative complications such as wound infections and intra-abdominal abscesses, especially pelvic and subphrenic. If an appendix mass is palpated some prefer conservative management with bed rest, intravenous fluids and antibiotics with an interval appendectomy at 3 months. Others proceed to appendectomy appropriately covered by antibiotic therapy.

PRIMARY PERITONITIS

This has a similar presentation to appendicitis but without a history of central pain moving to the right iliac fossa. The abdominal signs are those of peritonitis especially in the lower abdomen. At operation diffuse peritonitis is found with peritoneal exudate, yet no obvious focus of infection. The commonest causative organisms are pneumococci and streptococci. The source of infection has been thought to be the genital tract, the condition being commoner in girls, but the occasional occurrence in boys leads one to suspect blood-borne spread. There may be a preceding or coexisting upper respiratory tract infection. The management is appropriate antibiotic therapy (usually penicillin).

MECKEL'S DIVERTICULUM

Meckel's diverticulum arises from the vitellointestinal duct which leads from the primitive gut to the yolk sac. Persistence of the proximal end of the duct occurs in 2% of the population (the 2 foot from the ileocecal valve, 2 inch long story is erroneous: it may be a variable length and variable distance from the ileocecal valve).

The vitellointestinal duct can lead to a number of anomalies if it persists (Fig. 31.26). The duct itself may remain patent to the umbilicus and thus present as a fistula in neonates. Partial obliteration may give rise to cyst formation or a persistent fibrous cord from the umbilicus to the ileum may act as an axis for localized volvulus or lead to bowel obstruction.

A Meckel's diverticulum may become inflamed or lead to hemorrhage or invaginate into the ileum and cause intussusception. Meckel's diverticulitis has an identical presentation to acute appendicitis and must always be considered if a normal appendix is identified at surgery.

Bleeding in relation to a Meckel's diverticulum arises because the lining often contains heterotopic gastric mucosa (35–49%). This leads to peptic ulceration of the adjacent normal ileal mucosa (Fig. 31.27). Bleeding usually occurs in preschool children, especially toddlers. It may be intermittent passage of a small amount of altered blood in the stool, although massive hemorrhage with the passage of maroon or even bright red blood is more common. After adequate resuscitation, with blood replacement, a Meckel's scan should be performed. This is a ^{99m}Tc pertechnetate isotope scan which has an affinity for parietal cells. The stomach is visualized on the scan image, together with the bladder, as the isotope is excreted through the kidneys. A third 'blob' of isotope is likely to indicate ectopic gastric mucosa in a Meckel's diverticulum (or rarely in a duplicated segment of bowel). The scan image is enhanced by priming the patient with cimetidine for a few days.

The treatment is in all cases Meckel's diverticulectomy, the diverticulum being found on the antimesenteric aspect of the ileum 40–100 cm proximal to the ileocecal valve.

SUPERIOR MESENTERIC ARTERY SYNDROME

This syndrome, a cause of acute and chronic abdominal pain in childhood, is due to obstruction of the third part of the duodenum by the superior mesenteric artery. It has variously been called Cast syndrome, Wilkie's syndrome, chronic duodenal ileus and arteriomesenteric duodenal compression syndrome. It may be congenital or acquired, the latter being due to rapid growth without associated weight gain, rapid weight loss or from hyperextension of the vertebral column in a plastic cast. The presentation may be acute or chronic with acute obstructive symptoms or intermittent abdominal pain and vomiting. Contrast studies if performed between attacks may show little but if performed in an acute episode will demonstrate obstruction of the third part of the duodenum. The superior mesenteric artery

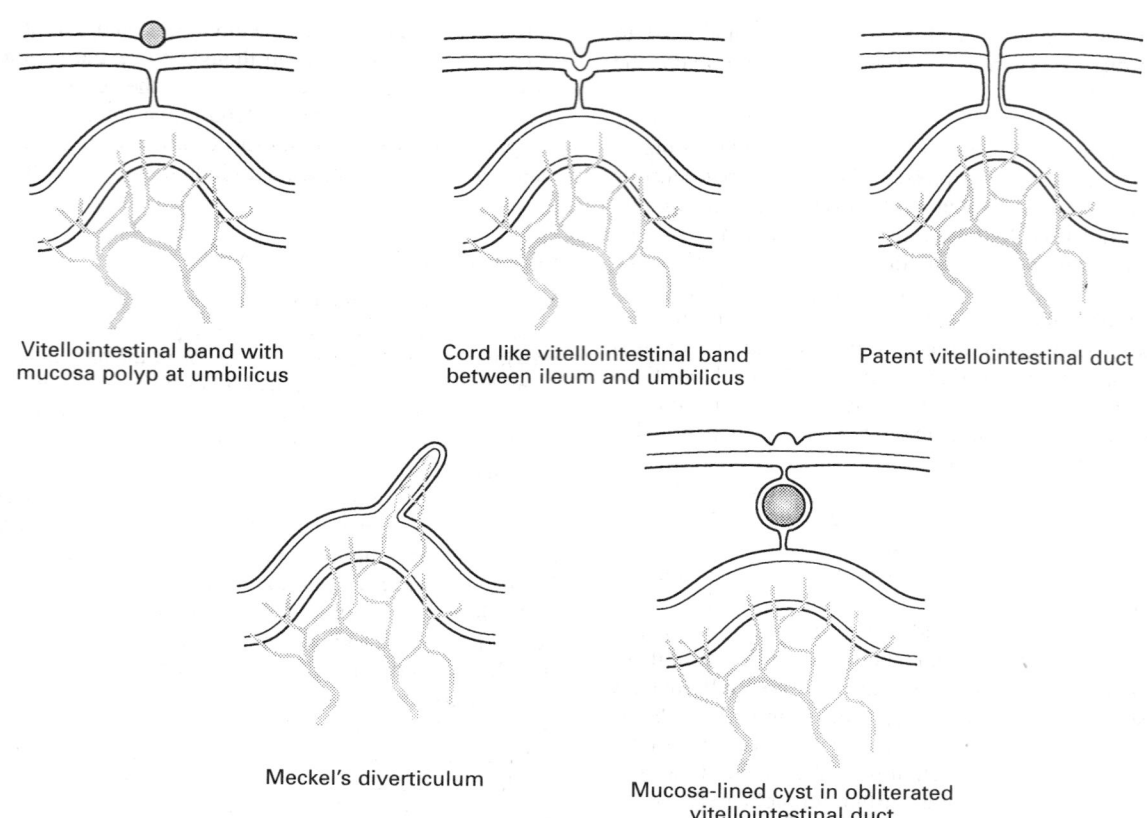

Vitellointestinal band with mucosa polyp at umbilicus

Cord like vitellointestinal band between ileum and umbilicus

Patent vitellointestinal duct

Meckel's diverticulum

Mucosa-lined cyst in obliterated vitellointestinal duct

Fig. 31.26 Vitellointestinal remnants.

normally subtends an angle of 45° with the aorta but under the conditions described above the angle may decrease to 15° thus occluding the underlying duodenum.

Management is conservative or surgical, the former being alteration of diet, nursing prone and removing or windowing a plaster cast if present. Surgical management entails division of the ligament of Treitz and transposition of the small bowel to the right side in a position of nonrotation (Wilson-Storey & MacKinlay 1986).

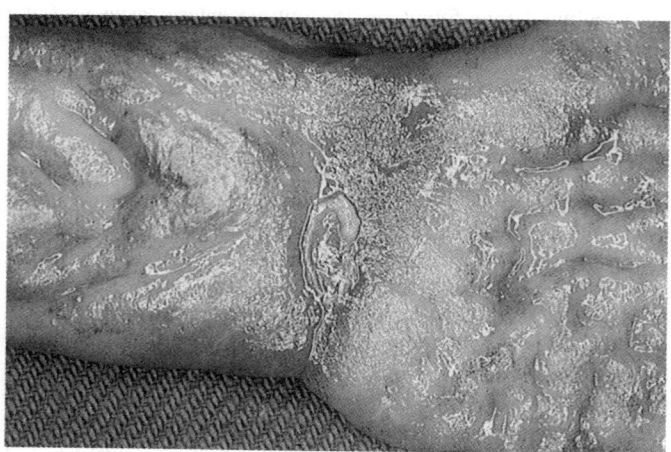

Fig. 31.27 Peptic ulcer at junction of gastric and ileal mucosa in Meckel's diverticulum.

CHOLEDOCHAL CYST

This is a cystic dilation of the choledochus (the common bile duct). The etiology is unknown but some believe it to be related to the reflux of pancreatic secretions into the common duct. The presentation may be in infancy with obstructive jaundice suggestive of biliary atresia, or in the older child with intermittent jaundice, abdominal pain and vomiting often associated with fever suggestive of ascending cholangitis. The diagnosis is by ultrasonography. Treatment consists of excision of the cyst and a Roux-en-Y choledochojejunostomy or hepaticojejunostomy. Failure to excise the entire cyst may result in carcinoma of the cyst wall in the long term.

CHOLELITHIASIS

Gallstones are uncommon in childhood but must be considered in children with hereditary spherocytosis. If metabolic stones develop then cholecystectomy is required, but in hemolytic disease the gallbladder is usually normal and simple cholecystotomy and removal of the stones is all that is required. This procedure should always be considered at the time of splenectomy in these children.

INGUINAL HERNIA AND HYDROCELE

These conditions have the same origin in childhood – the presence of a patent processus vaginalis. The only difference between them is the caliber of the processus (Fig. 31.28). If wide a hernia is

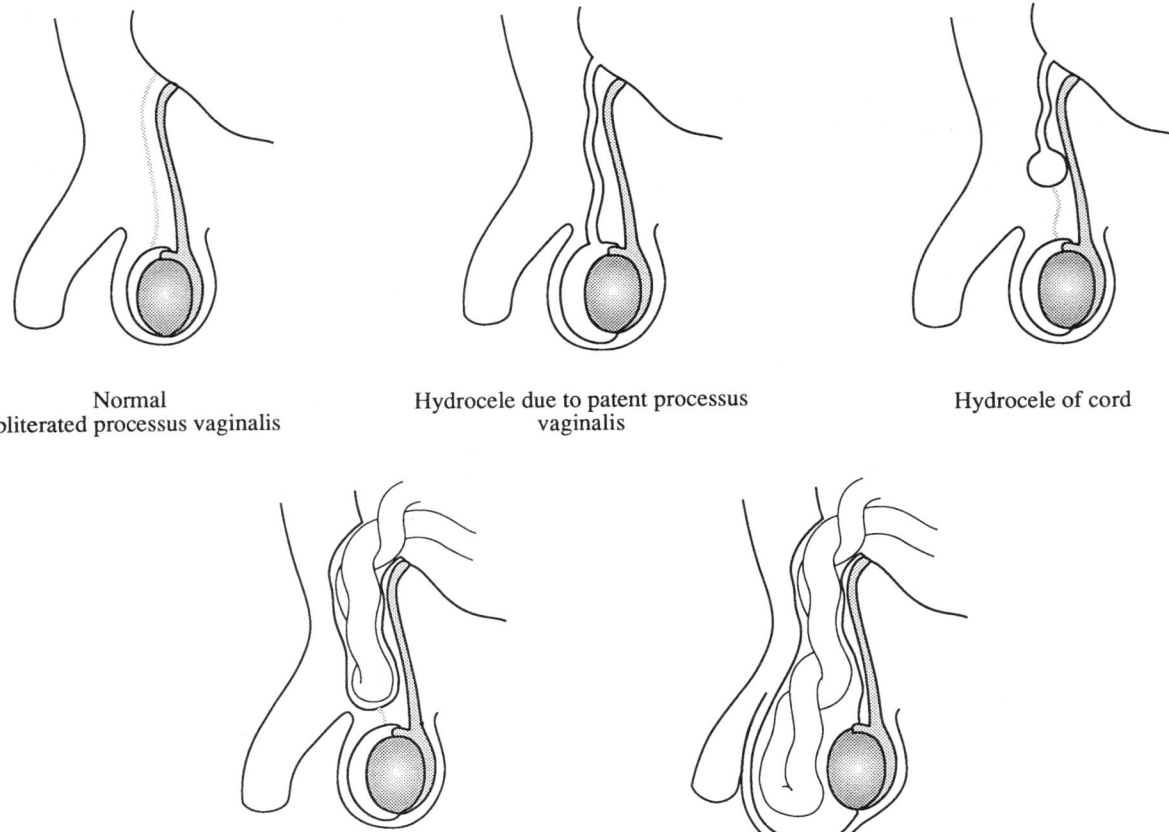

Normal
Obliterated processus vaginalis

Hydrocele due to patent processus vaginalis

Hydrocele of cord

Hernia of funicular type

Hernia of complete type

Fig. 31.28 Inguinal herniae and hydroceles.

produced, if narrow then peritoneal fluid may tract down to the tunica vaginalis. This explains the use of the term hydrocele from the Greek *hydro* = water, *kēlē* = hernia. (A similar derivation applies to encephalocele, omphalocele, ureterocele, etc.). Frequently hydrocele is spelt, erroneously, 'coele', even in textbooks: it is not derived from coelom (Greek *koilōma* = hollow).

The processus vaginalis is an outpouching of peritoneum drawn down by the descent of the testis. The distal portion persists as the tunica vaginalis but the intervening communication with the peritoneal cavity is normally obliterated. Persistence of a widely patent processus along its whole length results in a hernia of the 'complete' type – a scrotal hernia. Obliteration of the distal portion results in a 'funicular' hernial sac. Similarly, a hydrocele of the cord can arise, the distal portion being obliterated and the proximal communication narrowed.

These conditions are more common on the right side than the left, presumably related to the later descent of the right testis. They may also arise in girls, although hernias are less common. Occasionally an ovary may prolapse into a hernia – at surgery it must be inspected to confirm that it is indeed an ovary and not a testis in testicular feminization syndrome (Fig. 31.29). Chromosomal analysis may be of value in excluding this condition in girls with bilateral hernias but the incidence is extremely low. The hydrocele equivalent in a female is a hydrocele of the canal of Nuck – a small diverticulum of peritoneum accompanying the round ligament of the uterus through the inguinal canal.

In general, hydroceles are only treated surgically if they persist beyond the age of 1 year, the majority resolving spontaneously prior to that. In toddlers there is often a history of a hydrocele increasing in size towards the end of the day – the fluid slowly returns to the peritoneum through the narrow processus when the

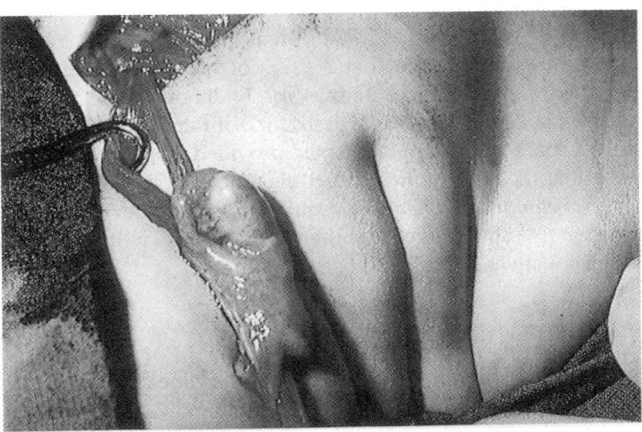

Fig. 31.29 External female genitalia and normal testis in testicular feminization syndrome.

child is recumbent at night. Surgery consists of ligation and division of the patent processus vaginalis through a small inguinal incision.

Inguinal hernias are treated with a similar operation. If the hernia is not obvious on examination, despite a typical history, tickling may increase the intra-abdominal pressure to demonstrate the hernia, but its presence can be confirmed by rolling the spermatic cord over the pubic bone with the index finger, thickening being apparent in the presence of a hernia.

If a scrotal swelling is present, a hydrocele can usually be distinguished from a hernia by the fact that one can get above it. Rarely does a hydrocele extend up into the inguinal canal. Transillumination may be misleading, as the thin bowel wall, with intraluminal fluid in a young infant, will also transilluminate.

The surgery is a semiurgent herniotomy. There is no requirement for herniorrhaphy (repair).

Incarceration of an inguinal hernia implies irreducibility which will lead to strangulation of the bowel if left untreated. Gentle reduction is attempted. Force must not be applied and unless reduction is easy the child should be sedated with i.m. morphine and tipped head down; occasionally gallows traction is of benefit. If reduction is unsuccessful, immediate surgical reduction and herniotomy are necessary. If it is successfully reduced then herniotomy must be performed before the infant is discharged.

Confirmation of the previous incarceration may be made by observing an increase in testicular size on the affected side (a positive Robarts' sign). This results from venous obstruction of the pampiniform plexus which can result in testicular infarction in cases where the hernia is not urgently reduced.

FEMORAL HERNIA

This is uncommon in children but, as in adults, is recognized by the swelling lying below the inguinal ligament and lateral to the pubic tubercle. Femoral herniorrhaphy is required.

UMBILICAL HERNIA

By the time the umbilical cord has separated in the newborn the umbilical ring has usually closed but in a proportion of children a defect is left, resulting in an umbilical hernia. There is a higher incidence of this condition in blacks than in whites. Umbilical hernia occurs in Beckwith's syndrome, Hurler's syndrome, trisomy 18, and trisomy 13.

The vast majority of umbilical hernias will resolve spontaneously within the first 2 years of life. Incarceration and strangulation in umbilical hernias in childhood are so rare that they need not cause concern. Persistence of the hernia beyond the age of 2 years merits surgical repair, provided that care is taken to ensure that the incision lies within the umbilical folds.

A *paraumbilical hernia* usually lies in the linea alba immediately above the umbilical ring. This will not close spontaneously and surgical repair is required.

EPIGASTRIC HERNIA

An epigastric hernia occurs through the linea alba, usually midway between the xiphisternum and the umbilicus. It presents as a pea-sized swelling occasionally associated with pain and results from herniation of extraperitoneal fat through the defect. It is best treated surgically although it can safely be left alone.

SURGICAL ASPECTS OF THE GENITOURINARY TRACT

ANOMALIES OF TESTICULAR DESCENT

It is best to consider the following distinct entities: the testis arrested in the normal line of descent (true undescended); ectopic testes; and retractile testes. In addition, testes may be atrophic or absent (anorchia).

Testes arrested along the normal line of descent

The term cryptorchidism (Greek *cryptos* = hidden, *orchis* = testis) should be reserved for impalpable, usually abdominal, testes. There is a higher incidence of undescended testis in premature than in full-term babies. Two-thirds of undescended testes in newborn infants will descend, usually by 6 weeks in term and 3 months in preterm babies. There is an increased incidence of cryptorchidism in anencephalics and other cerebral anomalies.

Ectopic testes

These have descended as far as the external inguinal ring and then become deviated into the superficial inguinal, perineal (Fig. 31.30), suprapubic or femoral ectopic sites. The commonest by far is the superficial inguinal pouch above and lateral to the external inguinal ring.

Retractile testes

The cremasteric reflex in young children will draw the testes into the region of the superficial inguinal pouch very readily but they can be manipulated back down to the bottom of the scrotum. The testis would normally reside in the scrotum if such a child is in a warm bath or relaxed in bed in a warm room with warm hands.

Anorchia

Anorchia may be on one or both sides. If on one side alone there may be ipsilateral renal agenesis. If the baby is fully masculinized but both testes are absent it must be assumed that they have atrophied subsequent to torsion or infarction during development. Absence of testicular tissue and therefore lack of müllerian

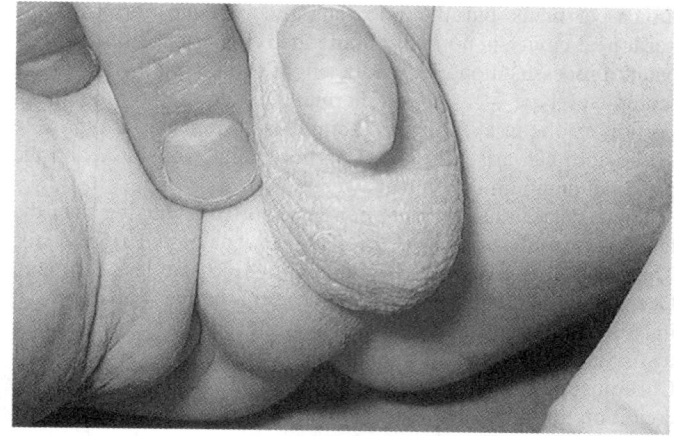

Fig. 31.30 Perineal ectopic testis.

inhibitory hormone during early gestation can lead to müllerian development along female lines. The lack of androgenic stimulation (testosterone) from the testes leads to failure of wolffian duct development.

'Ascending testis'

Some boys with recorded testicular descent at routine clinic checks in infancy may be found later at preschool or school medicals to have an undescended testis. This phenomenon of the 'ascending testis' has only been noted in recent years (Atwell 1985). It has been suggested that this is caused by failure of elongation of the spermatic cord during differential body growth, so that the testis is drawn up by absorption of the processus vaginalis. It may even be that in some cases the confines of a superficial inguinal pouch are sufficiently lax in some young boys that the testis can be manipulated well down into the scrotum. If the pouch remains static in size, differential growth will reveal that the testis is truly obstructed in its descent.

Treatment

It has been shown that adverse morphological changes occur in undescended testes from the second year of life onwards with a statistically significant reduction of spermatogonia and tubular growth. Most surgeons therefore choose to perform orchidopexies between 2 and 3 years of age. An associated hernia is an indication for earlier surgery. There is no place now for delaying surgery until 9 or 10 years of age. Any testis which has not descended in the first year of life will not appear later.

The treatment of the true undescended testis and the ectopic testis is orchidopexy, the testis and cord being mobilized via an inguinal approach and usually fixed in the scrotum in a subdartos pouch.

Malignancy in the undescended testis

Testicular malignancy occurs in 0.0021% of adult males. Undescended testes occur in 0.28% of the population and 12% of cases of testicular malignancy are reported to occur in testes known to have been undescended. There is thus a 40 times greater incidence of malignancy in cryptorchid patients than in the general population. Orchidopexy probably does not eradicate the problem but at least the testis is placed in a position where early malignancy may be detected. In unilateral undescended testes there is also an increased risk of malignancy in the contralateral testis.

Fertility

Only one-third of those following bilateral orchidopexy and two-thirds of those after unilateral orchidopexy appear to have a sperm count sufficient to be potentially fertile. It is hoped, however, that these figures will be improved by the change in policy over the past few years to operate on the majority of cases in the second year of life.

THE ACUTE SCROTUM

This may result from torsion of the testis, torsion of a testicular appendage, epididymo-orchitis or idiopathic scrotal edema or, rarely, a testicular tumor.

Torsion of the testis

Torsion of the testis most commonly occurs in the neonatal period or at puberty, with a few cases presenting in the intervening years. In the neonate the torsion occurs outside the tunica vaginalis. In the neonatal period there is a plane of mobility between the tunica vaginalis and the outer layer of the scrotum. Presentation is with a reddened hemiscrotum with a hard, swollen, often indurated testis. This is not infrequently noted 24 h after birth although the torsion may have occurred at delivery. On exploration the testis is often black and infarcted but usually it is 'given the benefit of the doubt', untwisted and replaced in the scrotum, although the majority will atrophy. The contralateral testis must be fixed at the same procedure to avoid undergoing torsion at a later date. After the newborn period torsion occurs secondary to an abnormally high investment of the tunica, the testis often being described as having bell-clapper fixation. Presentation is with pain which is usually testicular in position but theoretically, as testicular innervation is from T10, it should be felt centrally in the abdomen. Examination reveals a swollen hemiscrotum often with edema and erythema, depending on the length of history. There is exquisite tenderness on palpation. The treatment is emergency surgery as delay will affect the viability of the testis.

Preoperative isotope scanning or Doppler probing to confirm the diagnosis merely wastes time. The scrotum is explored, the testis derotated and, providing surgery is carried out within 6 h, the testis is likely to become pink under warm towels. It is then fixed in the scrotum. As the anomalous tunical attachment is likely to be bilateral, orchidopexy is also performed on the other side.

Torsion of testicular appendages

Embryological remnants are commonly attached to the testis. The hydatid of Morgagni is attached to the upper pole and is a müllerian duct remnant. It varies in size from a pinhead to a pea or may be absent. Other remnants include the appendix epididymis (a wolffian tubercle remnant), the paradidymis or organ of Giraldés (another mesonephric remnant) and the vas aberrans of Haller. The hydatid of Morgagni is the most common to undergo torsion which leads to less acute pain than testicular torsion, the pain being usually at the upper pole of the testis where occasionally a bluish nodule is seen through the scrotal skin. An infarcted hydatid can give rise to considerable swelling and inflammation and doubtful cases are best explored (Fig. 31.31) to exclude testicular torsion. In any case, the necrotic hydatid is best excised as an emergency, giving instant pain relief. If treated conservatively the pain lingers on for up to 2 weeks.

Epididymo-orchitis

This is rare in children unless there is an associated renal tract anomaly. If the latter has already been established then it is safe to treat with antibiotic therapy. If, however, the clinical picture cannot be distinguished from torsion of the testis, exploration is mandatory to establish the diagnosis.

Idiopathic scrotal edema

This is a fascinating entity presenting with erythema and edema of the scrotum suggestive of a possible underlying torsion. The erythema and edema spread beyond the scrotum however into the groin and perineum (Fig. 31.32). Usually the process is confined to one side of the scrotum and the adjacent groin and perineum.

The etiology is unknown. It may be an allergic phenomenon; it is occasionally associated with an eosinophilia and may respond to antihistamine therapy. Some suggest it may be caused by an insect bite. The testis is nontender and the condition settles within a few days.

CIRCUMCISION

Routine circumcision of the newborn as commonly practiced in the USA is to be condemned, the incidence of complications,

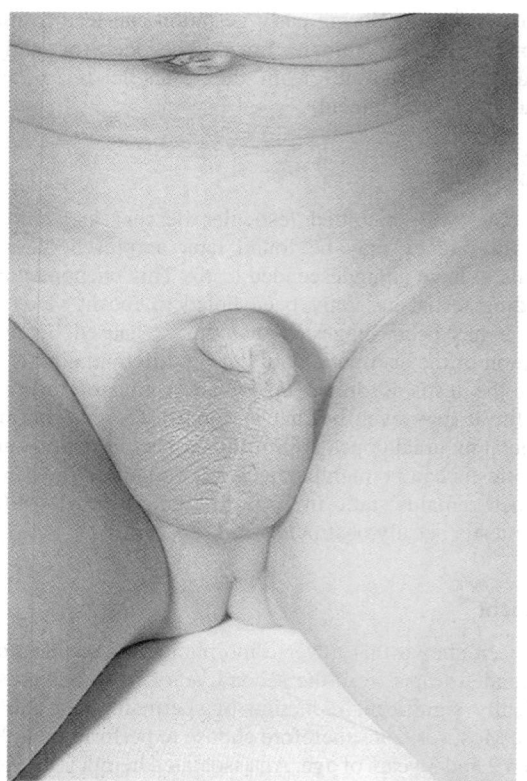

Fig. 31.32 Idiopathic scrotal edema.

including death, far outweighing the supposed advantage of avoiding such problems as carcinoma of the penis. The latter is virtually unknown in those who practice adequate hygiene. The fact that it is 'more hygienic' is often used as an excuse for circumcision but one does not chop off the ears to save washing them, or the feet because they may smell! It has been suggested that lack of carcinoma of the cervix in Jewish women is related to male circumcision but Aitken-Swan & Baird (1965) showed no

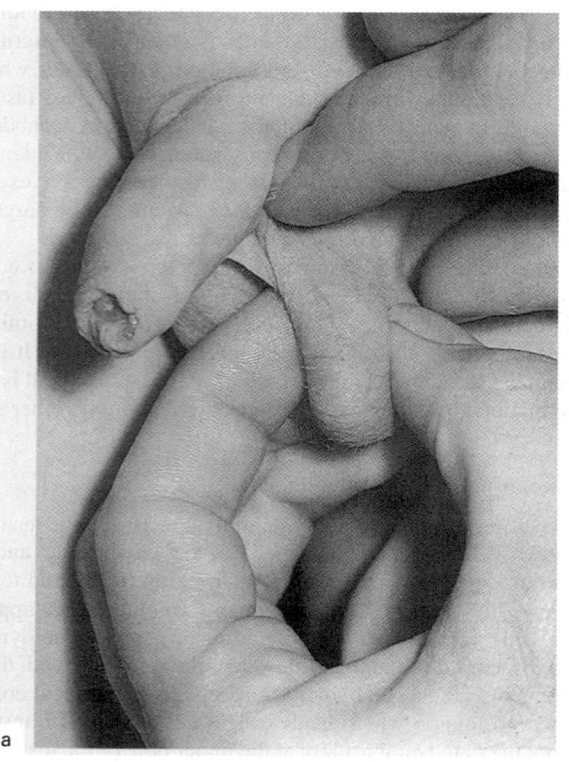

a

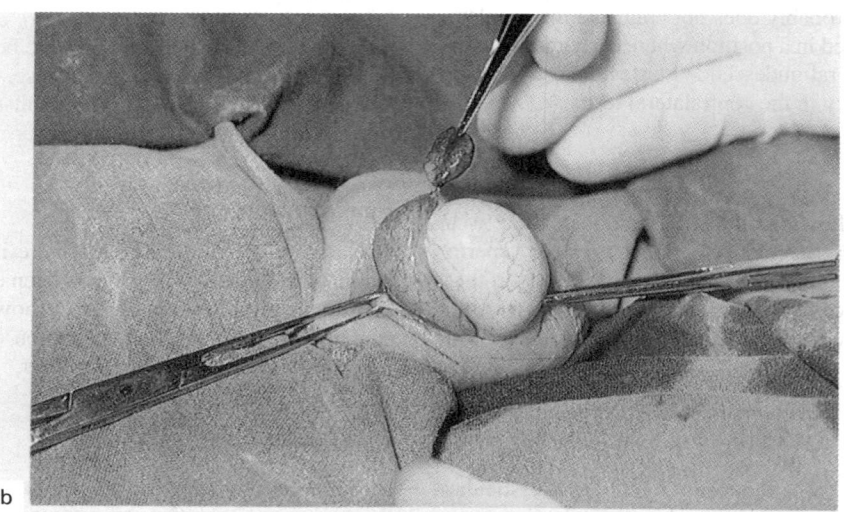

b

Fig. 31.31 Hydatid of Morgagni (a) clinical appearance (b) at operation.

difference in incidence in wives of circumcised and uncircumcised men. In 1975 a committee of the American Academy of Pediatrics stated: 'There is no absolute medical indication for the routine circumcision of the newborn. A program of good penile hygiene, simply retracting the foreskin to wash away accumulated smegma on a daily basis, would appear to offer all the advantages of circumcision without the attendant surgical risks or the increased risk of meatal stenosis' (Report of the Ad Hoc Task Force on Circumcision 1975).

Nonretractability of the prepuce, in childhood, should not be used as an excuse for 'lopping off an innocent and useful appendage'. Bokai in 1869 was the first to draw attention to the physiological adherence of the foreskin, there being fusion of the glans and the prepuce developmentally. Diebert, in 1933, showed that separation of the prepuce in the human penis is due to keratinization of the subpreputial epithelium, a process not complete at birth but accomplished during early childhood. Phimosis (a muzzling, from Greek *phimos* = muzzle) is thus physiological at birth.

Apart from religious or tribal reasons there are few indications for circumcision. The only valid one is a fibrous phimosis (Fig. 31.33). This may be due to inappropriate attempts at retraction at an early age, causing splitting and scarring of the preputial meatus, or perhaps is related to recurrent infections. In its most severe form it presents as balanitis xerotica obliterans with scarring of the underlying glans and urethral meatus. Meatal strictures also arise after neonatal circumcision secondary to meatitis which arises in the absence of the protective covering of the foreskin. Ballooning of the foreskin is often seen as an indication for circumcision but it will usually resolve in time.

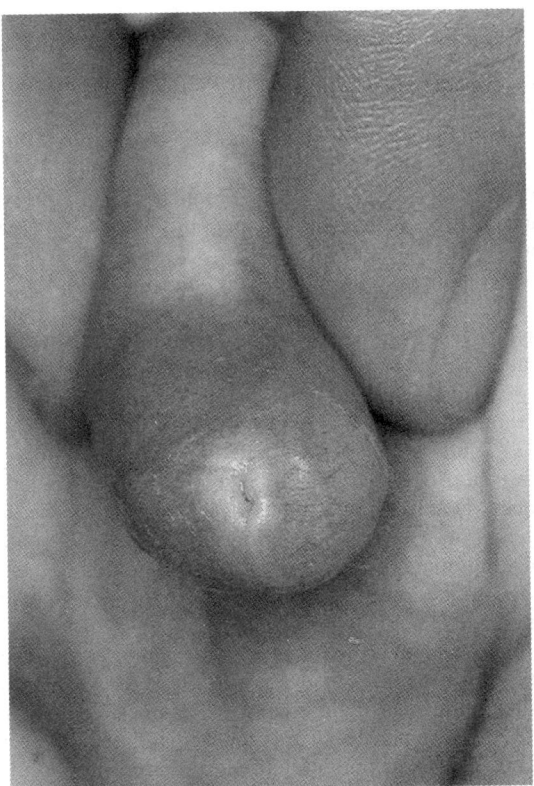

Fig. 31.33 Fibrous phimosis (balanitis xerotica obliterans).

Recurrent balanitis or balanoposthitis is possibly related to partial separation of preputial adhesion and infection of inadequately draining secretions. This can readily be resolved by separation of the adhesions. Previously this was normally carried out under general anesthesia but with the advent of EMLA cream (eutectic mixture of local anesthetics) the separation can readily be carried out painlessly and simply in the outpatient clinic or GP surgery (MacKinlay 1988). Daily retraction with application of petroleum jelly for a few days to prevent readherence followed subsequently by normal preputial hygiene is all that is required.

In examination of the foreskin in small boys it often appears tight on attempted retraction. The simple technique advocated in 1950 by Sir James Spence should be adopted: 'Retract the prepuce and you will see a pinpoint opening, but draw it forward and you will see a channel wide enough for all the purposes for which the infant needs the organ at that early age. What looks like a pinpoint opening at 7 months will become a wide channel of communication at 17 years.'

Operation

Circumcision is thus performed either for religious or tribal reasons, for fibrous phimosis or, perhaps most frequently, for remuneration! Hypospadias is a contraindication for neonatal circumcision, as is a buried penis. Neonatal circumcision is practiced, often without anesthesia using a plastibell or a Gomco clamp. In the former, a plastic ring is placed under the foreskin and a string tied round the foreskin in a groove in the plastic device. Redundant skin together with the device separates off within a few days leaving a very neat cosmetic result. A Gomco clamp has a similar action but rather than the string, a cutting device removes the prepuce and compresses the skin edges causing them to fuse and prevent hemorrhage. In older children a surgical cutting technique with absorbable sutures is used. In many cases of phimosis a foreskin preserving preputioplasty is sufficient.

PARAPHIMOSIS

This occurs when a narrowed foreskin is retracted behind the corona glandis penis and cannot be returned. The constriction leads to engorgement of the glans and of a cuff of foreskin distal to the tight band but behind the corona (Fig. 31.34). Firm manual compression with gauze and EMLA cream will usually reduce the edema and facilitate return of the foreskin. If this fails, injection of hyaluronidase into the swollen ring of prepuce, under general anesthesia, followed by compression, allows reduction (Fig. 31.35). Occasionally the tight constricting band needs to be incised. Circumcision is frequently advocated following paraphimosis but, surprisingly, the foreskin is usually easily retractable a fortnight after the event and recurrence is exceptional.

HYPOSPADIAS (Greek *hypo* = below, *spadon* = rent)

This is one of the commonest congenital anomalies, occurring in one in 400 live male births. The meatus lies in an abnormal position on the ventral aspect of the penile shaft or even scrotally or perineally. The foreskin tends to be deficient in its ventral

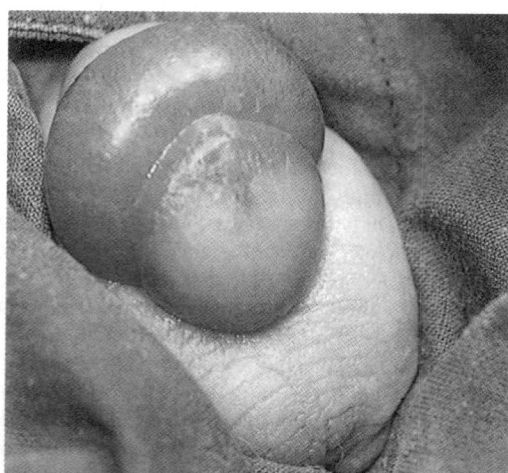

Fig. 31.34   Paraphimosis.

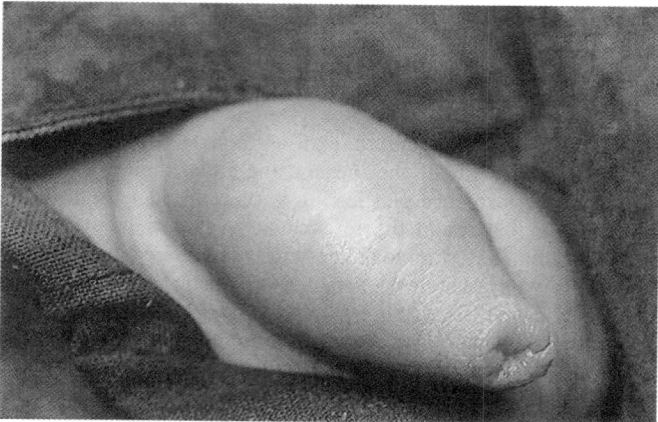

Fig. 31.35   Reduced paraphimosis.

aspect and thus is described as 'hooded'. Thirdly, there is chordee, a ventral flexion of the penis, the incidence and degree of which increases as the meatus is more proximally placed. The meatus itself may be narrowed leading to potential problems of back pressure. In the majority of cases the meatus is coronal in position, rarely it is glandular. Of the remainder, most are on the penile shaft but a few lie more proximally still in the scrotum or perineum. It is often thought that hypospadias is frequently associated with upper renal tract anomalies but in fact the incidence of these is much the same as in the general population, except perhaps in the most severe types of the deformity. In those penoscrotal and perineal types there may be associated undescended testes and the possibility of an intersex state must be investigated.

There are over 200 operations described in the literature for the correction of hypospadias. This gives some indication of the complication rate, each newly described repair aiming to be an improvement in this regard. The age for surgery is mainly the surgeon's preference. It has always been agreed that, where possible, correction should be complete by the time the boy starts school so that he may stand and pee like his peers! The more distally placed the meatus the easier it is to achieve a successful

result. For a coronal hypospadias the MAGPI repair (meatal advancement and glanduloplasty incorporated) has become very popular and is generally carried out at a few months of age. The essential components to the repair of the more severe varieties are release of the chordee and urethral reconstruction. The chordee is related to tight fibrous bands distal to the meatus and thought possibly to relate to atrophy of that portion of the corpus spongiosum. It is, however, possible to have chordee without hypospadias so the etiology is uncertain. Fistula formation is unfortunately common following hypospadias repair and a few unfortunate cases require multiple interventions to achieve successful closure. The aim of all modern repairs is to create a terminal meatus on a well-formed glans and a penile shaft which is straight on erection together with a good cosmetic result (a good 'body image').

EPISPADIAS

In its most extreme form this is associated with bladder exstrophy. Otherwise it may be balanic, penile or penopubic. It may also occur in girls. In epispadias the urethra is deficient dorsally. The penis is flattened with a splayed glans and shortened, the crura being attached to often separated pubic bones. The prepuce is deficient dorsally with a ventral hood prepuce and there is dorsal chordee. Occasionally the problem is not obvious, the foreskin being complete and phimotic and the penis buried, but once the prepuce is retractable the condition is revealed. In the female the clitoris is duplicated on either side of the wide open urethra, defective dorsally (Fig. 31.36). The treatment is likewise dependent on sex and severity and the degree of continence and the success rate is variable.

URINARY TRACT INFECTION – SURGICAL ASPECTS

Medical management of urinary tract infections in neonates is discussed on page 261 and in older children on page 949.

The commonest cause of infection is *vesicoureteric reflux*. There remains much controversy over the role of surgery in vesicoureteric reflux (White & O'Donnell 1990). Reflux in the presence of infection leads to pyelonephritis, the extension of the intrarenal reflux, if present, leading to scarring. If the child can be kept free of infection, the reflux may improve or resolve. Severe reflux should be treated surgically. This entails a transvesical operation to lengthen the submucosal tunnel of the ureter. It has a high rate of success but in a few cases leads to stenosis. More recently, a new technique involving the endoscopic injection of Teflon submucosally beneath the ureteric orifice has been devised (STING – subureteric Teflon injection). This has proved very successful but long-term results have yet to be evaluated. Other substances such as bioplastique or collagen may be used as concern has been raised that Teflon may migrate to the brain or elsewhere, although the original authors refute this concept.

Stenosis of the lower end of the ureter requires reimplantation, the stenotic segment being excised.

Duplex ureters may be an incidental finding without causing problems in the majority of cases. If detected in investigation of a urinary tract infection, there is usually an associated anomaly. The ureter from the upper pole tends to enter the bladder at a lower level. Thus the lower pole ureter has a shorter intramural course and a tendency to reflux. The upper pole ureter has a tendency to stenosis, an association with a ureterocele and a possible tendency

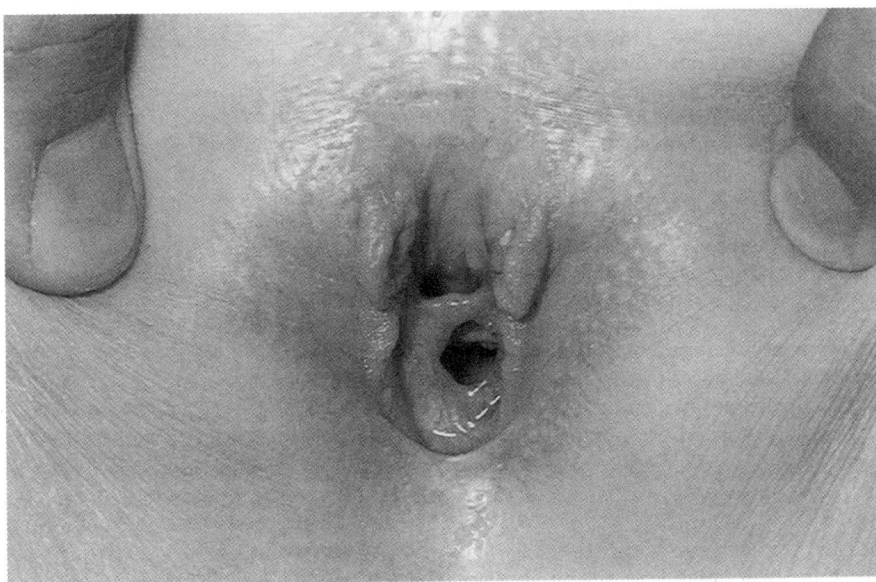

Fig. 31.36 Female epispadias.

to open below the bladder neck leading to incontinence. It may even open ectopically into the vagina.

If there is reflux of both ureters, reimplantation of both, in their common sheath, is usually the treatment of choice. Occasionally they join at a higher level leading to yo-yo reflux between the two and a predisposition to infection. This is treated either by heminephroureterectomy if one moiety is shown to have poor function on isotope studies, or else anastomosis at the level of the pelves may be advocated.

A *ureterocele* may arise in relation to the upper pole ureter. It represents herniation of the intramural portion of the ureter into the bladder. Its meatus may be stenosed, may open below the bladder neck or may even on occasion allow reflux. The ureterocele may obstruct the lower ureter or even lead to bladder outlet obstruction by prolapsing across the internal urethral meatus. The ureterocele may be incised endoscopically to relieve an acute problem, especially of value in the infant, or may be excised with ureteric reimplantation if appropriate. If an isotope scan shows minimal function in the affected moiety then partial nephroureterectomy may be the treatment of choice.

Hydronephrosis may be due to obstruction at the pelviureteric junction or, if the ureter is also dilated, to vesicoureteric obstruction or vesicoureteric reflux. Obstruction at the pelviureteric junction (PUJ) may be due to congenital narrowing, high insertion of the ureter, or aberrant renal vessels. The presentation is usually with investigation of a urinary tract infection. It may be diagnosed antenatally or in the older child may present with a Dietl's crisis, acute obstruction at the PUJ secondary to kinking after an abnormal fluid load. This may not present until the first beer drinking spree in a young adult! In the neonate, antenatally diagnosed hydronephrosis may be a stable condition which can be monitored with serial ultrasound examinations and isotope studies as some infants will acquire normal drainage across the PUJ as they grow. At any age an isotope study will indicate whether the kidney has already suffered major damage. If its contribution to total renal function is less than 10% then nephrectomy is the treatment of choice. If there is doubt in an acute presentation, a percutaneous nephrostomy tube may be inserted under ultrasound guidance and further isotope studies, after draining for 1–2 weeks, may show improvement. If there is reasonable function but a definite PUJ obstruction then the treatment of choice is a pyeloplasty. This involves excision of the redundant extra renal pelvis and pelviureteric junction with reanastomosis of the proximal ureter to the dependent portion of the repaired pelvis.

LABIAL ADHESIONS

It is surprising how often young girls are referred to the outpatient clinic with a diagnosis of vaginal agenesis when in fact the problem is a simple one of fusion of the labia minora. Unlike preputial adhesions in the male this is not a congenital problem but an acquired one, possibly a consequence of mild intertrigo. The adherence may lead to dysuria, there often being only a tiny orifice for the urine to escape. It may even lead to urinary tract infection or at least a positive culture on MSU. The labia are very delicate and adhere in the midline. They are readily separated, often merely by gently parting the labia with the thumbs or with a quick flick of a probe causing momentary discomfort. If the child is particularly apprehensive then the procedure may be performed under general anesthesia. Vaseline should be gently smeared across both edges in one maneuver and this must be repeated daily, for a week, by the mother. Some prefer the use of 0.01% dienestrol cream to keratinize the epithelium.

HYDROCOLPOS

This becomes apparent in the newborn with an imperforate hymen due to the stimulus of vaginal secretions under the influence of maternal estrogen. It may also be secondary to a vaginal septum. The back pressure may also lead to hydrometra, distention of the uterus and even hydrosalpinx, distention of the fallopian tubes. The obstruction is relieved surgically.

HEMATOCOLPOS

This arises at puberty for similar reasons, there presumably having been insufficient secretions in the neonatal period for the condition to become manifest. The uterus is often palpable as hydrometrocolpos develops. Displacement of the bladder lead to difficulty with micturition. The membrane is divided under anesthesia and antibiotic cover to prevent ascending infection.

VAGINAL AGENESIS AND VAGINAL ATRESIA – SURGICAL ASPECTS

In the case of agenesis, surgery is best deferred until well beyond the pediatric age group when the girl chooses to become sexually active. Atresia in the form of imperforate hymen or low vaginal septum is treated when it gives rise to hydrocolpos or hematocolpos as outlined above.

OVARIAN CYSTS

Benign and malignant cysts of the ovary may lead to a number of different problems for the surgeon. *Follicular* cysts may be very tiny or may enlarge, especially in the neonatal period and around puberty. Hemorrhage into them may cause sudden pain. Ovarian cysts are occasionally noted on pelvic ultrasound in the investigation of girls with abdominal pain. Whether or not they are the cause of the pain is often uncertain. They may induce torsion of the ovary with acute abdominal pain and necessitate oophorectomy. If possible, however, if cysts are causing problems, ovarian cystectomy is the treatment of choice. I have encountered torsion of such a degree as to lead to torsion of the uterus also with infarction of the contralateral ovary, necessitating hysterectomy and bilateral salpingo-oophorectomy. This must be exceedingly rare but does indicate the need for urgent exploration.

Other cystic changes in the ovary include teratoma, cystadenoma, yolk sac tumor, dysgerminoma and granulosa cell tumor (see Ch. 16, p. 922).

PLASTIC SURGERY

CLEFT LIP AND PALATE

Incidence

This group of congenital anomalies occurs in about 1.4 per 1000 births. About one-third of cases have a cleft palate only and two-thirds a cleft lip with or without a cleft palate. In about one-third of patients there is a definite history of a cleft defect in relatives. Where one sibling is affected, the risk of the same anomaly appearing in a subsequent sibling is about 1 : 25, or 1 : 8 if the parent also has a cleft. Where cleft palate forms part of a recognized syndrome, the inheritance follows differing patterns. Clefts are not infrequently associated with anomalies in other systems, e.g. cardiac, neurological, musculoskeletal and alimentary.

Etiology

In normal development, the lip, alveolus and a small portion of anterior hard palate are derived from fusion of the maxillary and medial nasal processes between the fifth and seventh weeks. The remainder of the palate fuses in the midline from anterior to posterior from the ninth to 12th weeks. Clefts result from failure

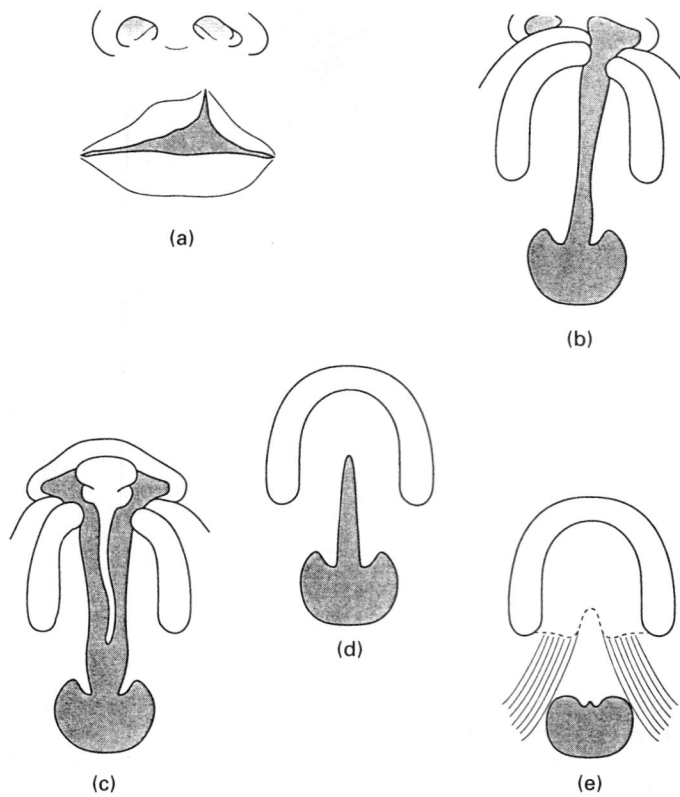

Fig. 31.37 (a) Incomplete unilateral cleft lip. (b) Complete unilateral cleft lip and palate. (c) Complete bilateral cleft lip and palate. (d) Isolated cleft of soft palate. (e) Submucous cleft palate.

of mesodermal penetration across any of these epithelial junctions and may range in severity from a notch in the free margin of the lip to a complete separation of the two halves of the maxilla. Clefts of the lip may be unilateral or bilateral. The most minor cleft of the palate is a bifid uvula which may indicate the presence of a submucous cleft, where there is no muscle union in the soft palate and a bony notch in the hard palate – a type often missed until the onset of defective speech. Figure 31.37 illustrates the major types of cleft lip and palate.

Cleft palate may be associated with underdevelopment of the mandible and neonatal respiratory embarrassment in the Pierre Robin sequence. Feeding may present problems. It improves spontaneously in the majority of cases.

Management

Clefts of lip and palate give rise to many problems other than deformity, including feeding, speech, facial growth, hearing, dentition and psychological development. Management is complex and involves specialists from many disciplines who must work closely together. The Royal College of Surgeons of England has recently recommended that units should only manage clefts if they see a minimum of 30 new clefts a year.

Feeding

The baby with a cleft lip whose palate is intact can breast feed successfully. Where the palate is cleft, breast-feeding is difficult but milk can be expressed and given from a bottle. Various special teats are available but a simple long teat with a larger hole in the tip is usually satisfactory. An orthodontic plate can sometimes help. The premature baby with a cleft may need to be tube fed initially.

Pierre Robin sequence

The infant should be nursed prone so that the force of gravity draws the tongue forward, clearing the airway. The face may be held off the bed by a frame, or a nasopharyngeal airway may be inserted. Operative tethering of the tongue or a tracheostomy are now rarely required.

Alveolar arch alignment; presurgical orthopedics

Where the cleft of lip and palate is complete, the two halves of the maxilla may be displaced but can be molded by serial orthodontic splints over several months, permitting a more precise operation.

Operation

The lip cleft can be closed in the neonatal period, but a better procedure is possible at 3–4 months. The nasal deformity and the alveolus may be repaired. The bilateral cleft lip may be closed in one or two stages. Primary closure of the palatal cleft is usually performed between 6 and 12 months to give the best chance of normal speech. Secondary surgery may be needed before the child goes to school.

Ear, nose and throat problems

Constant contamination of the nose with food can cause chronic irritation and infection. The eustachian tube is functionally impaired and 'glue ear' and acute otitis media are common. Infection must be vigorously treated with antibiotics. Long-term supervision is needed, including audiometry on each follow-up visit. Treatment may involve paracentesis of the eardrum and insertion of grommets. Adenoidectomy should be avoided if possible.

Orthodontic care

The orthodontist usually delays active treatment until secondary teeth are appearing. At 8 or 9 years, bone grafting may be needed to consolidate the alveolar arch. Good dental hygiene is fundamental to such work, and advice and supervision should continue throughout childhood.

Speech

A cleft palate may cause speech problems even after repair. Articulatory errors can be corrected by speech therapy, but if the soft palate (velum) does not close off the nasopharynx efficiently, or if there is a fistula causing air to escape down the nose, surgical correction is required.

When surgery is being considered, diagnostic methods include the ear of a skilled therapist, videofluoroscopy, nasopharyngoscopy and aerodynamic studies. Precise diagnosis permits an operation tailored to the individual patient.

Results of treatment of clefts have improved considerably in recent years. One of the most important reasons for this is the institution of multidisciplinary teams, bringing together at one time and place all those concerned with the child's care so that a coherent sequence of diagnosis and treatment can be followed.

OTHER CRANIOFACIAL DEFORMITIES

Cranial synostoses require urgent referral for release of the fused sutures to allow normal brain development. Craniofacial dysostosis (Crouzon's syndrome), acrocephalosyndactyly (Apert's syndrome), hypertelorism, craniofacial microsomia and mandibulofacial dysostosis (Treacher Collins' syndrome) and other major deformities are amenable to surgical correction in specialist centers. More common minor abnormalities include dermoid, branchial and thyroglossal cysts and fistulae which can be excised.

HEMANGIOMAS AND VASCULAR MALFORMATIONS

Hemangiomas are vascular tumors which enlarge by rapid cellular proliferation. Vascular malformations are structural anomalies which grow as the child grows but may expand with changes in vascular dynamics.

Hemangiomas

These may be in or under the skin or mucous membrane. They may be visible as a small red spot at birth but more commonly appear first at about 7 days of age. Rapid enlargement can continue for 3 months or more. In most instances, spontaneous regression by intravascular thrombosis starts at about a year but the process takes up to 7 years and may be incomplete. A central graying of the skin lesion and shrinkage in size are the visible stages of this process. Lesions liable to trauma, e.g. in the perineum, ulcerate easily, and healing thereafter always brings an obvious scar. Large lesions on the face are not only highly disfiguring but may destroy features if ulceration ensues.

The natural course of the disease must be discussed with parents so that they understand the timescale involved.

Treatment of hemangiomas

Cryotherapy and the injection of sclerosants have been used but may cause scarring. Babies with ulcerated perineal angiomas may need to be admitted to hospital. In some instances surgical removal can be performed with minimal scar but the only urgent indications are if vision or respiration are becoming obstructed. Most can be left to fibrose spontaneously. By the time the child goes to school, redundant remains of involuted hemangiomas can be reduced, if necessary, by a minor operation.

Complications of hemangiomas

Kasabach–Merritt syndrome. In the neonate, large or multiple hemangiomas are occasionally associated with a generalized bleeding disorder caused by the trapping of platelets within them which produces a profound thrombocytopenia. A course of prednisone, 2–4 mg/kg per 24 h can effect dramatic improvement, or, if this fails, embolization of the hemangioma can be considered.

Congestive cardiac failure. A combination of visceral and multiple cutaneous angiomas which can lead to cardiac failure is occasionally seen. Treatment with steroids is often effective; if it fails, embolic therapy is indicated.

Vascular malformations

The port-wine stain (nevus flammeus, nevus venosus)

It is present at birth. The skin is normal in all but color. The stain tends to darken and become nodular with age but varies between pale pink and a deep blue-red. It often picks out the cutaneous distribution of a sensory nerve, especially the trigeminal nerve in the face in part or whole.

Treatment is by laser, the best results at present being given by the pulsed tunable dye laser (Tan et al 1989).

Arteriovenous malformations

These may present with enlarged visible vessels, pain, trophic skin changes and progressive hypertrophy. They may lead to cardiac failure.

The Klippel–Trenaunay and Parks–Weber syndromes feature skin staining on a limb, congenital varicose veins and limb hypertrophy. The former is predominantly a venous malformation and remains fairly static; the latter is arteriovenous and tends to get worse.

CYSTIC HYGROMA: LYMPHANGIOMA

Lymphatic malformations

Multiple lymphatic cysts may present at birth in the neck and floor of the mouth (cystic hygroma) and cause obstruction to labor or respiratory embarrassment in the neonate. Urgent surgery may be required. They are also found elsewhere, often at the root of the limbs, sometimes with multiple vesicles in the skin or mucosa. They may be localized or diffuse. A proportion of those found in childhood resolve; those that do not can be very difficult to treat.

Primary lymphedema, caused by hypoplasia of the lymphatics, commonly appears at puberty but occasionally presents as a congenital condition (Milroy's disease). It is inherited as an autosomal dominant trait.

MELANOCYTIC NEVI

These are very common. Most are acquired after birth but some are congenital and may be very large. The question of their malignant potential is controversial and estimates vary between 5% and 40% for malignant change in giant congenital melanocytic nevi. They may cause severe disfigurement and psychological distress.

Treatment

Excision may be indicated for cosmetic reasons or because of worry about future malignant change. Tangential excision, dermabrasion or curettage in the first few weeks of life can be effective in some cases, but pigmentation may return. Hairs will not be removed by this technique and malignant potential may persist. In the older child full thickness skin excision is needed, with inevitable scarring. Skin grafts or flaps are needed for reconstruction of larger defects.

CAFÉ-AU-LAIT SPOTS

These may be associated with neurofibromatosis. They can be treated by laser.

BURNS

Thermal injury is a common childhood accident in all countries. Predisposing factors include primitive, poor or overcrowded housing, families under stress, flammable clothing, ignorance and lack of insight in parents. Nonaccidental injury may take this form, being suggested where the history and the physical findings are inconsistent or bizarre. The toddler, exploring his world on hands and knees or with unsteady gait, is a ready victim and boys are burned more often than girls.

Scalding with hot liquids is by far the commonest cause of injury in this age group. Flame burns are less common than they were, but house fires still claim victims with the added risk of smoke inhalation injury. Other causes include contact with hot objects, chemicals, friction and electric current.

Severity of injury

This depends on three main factors:

1. *Extent.* Heat damages the underlying capillaries, causing them to leak protein-rich fluid. The resulting loss from the circulation reaches a critical level when the extent of the burn exceeds about 10% of the body surface area, and the child will require intravenous resuscitation. Extent is measured by using a chart (Fig. 31.38) or by taking the area of the hand as about 1%. Erythema should be discounted when making this measurement.

2. *Depth.* Healing depends on whether epithelial elements survive in the dermis. Partial thickness burns will heal by outgrowth of epithelial cells from hair follicles and sweat glands; they can be subdivided into superficial, which heal in less than 3 weeks and do not cause scars, and deep dermal which take longer to heal and cause hypertrophic scars. Deep or full thickness burns can heal only from the margins. The depth of tissue destruction is determined by the temperature of the agent, the duration of its contact, the skin thickness and the victim's age.

3. *Site.* Burns of the face and hands are particularly serious, and those of the perineum cause problems in management. While the skin is the site of injury in most instances, the epithelial linings of the respiratory and upper alimentary tracts may be damaged separately or together with a skin burn.

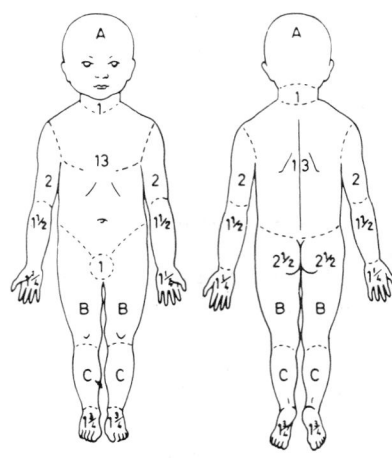

Fig. 31.38 Chart for calculating percentage area burned in childhood. A = $1/2$ of head; B = $1/2$ of one thigh; C = $1/2$ of one leg. The percentages of these areas varies with age.

Pathophysiology

Local

The fluid loss from the circulation is at its maximum immediately after the burn and decreases over the following 48 hours. A deep burn destroys significant numbers of red cells. The insulating and protective functions of skin are lost, and body heat, water and electrolytes pass from the body in much increased amounts. Nitrogen losses also rise.

General

There is a massive rise in the secretion of stress hormones (Smith et al 1995). Urinary water and sodium excretion fall and potassium and nitrogen losses increase. The larger the burn, the more profound the reaction tends to be. The catabolic phase lasts until the burn is healed.

Treatment

First aid

After separating the child from the source of the injury, clothing should be removed and the burn cooled by immersion in lukewarm water or by use of a wet cloth (the risk of hypothermia must be remembered). The burn can then be covered with a clean cloth or clingfilm until definitive local treatment is possible.

Pain

A partial thickness burn is very painful, while deeply burned skin is anesthetic. Potent analgesia by the intramuscular or intravenous route is essential. Throughout treatment, attention must be focused on the avoidance of pain during practical procedures; analgesic or anesthetic drugs should be selected and used with precision.

Shock

Where the area burned exceeds 10% of the body surface, an intravenous infusion will be required. The restoration and maintenance of an effective circulation can be achieved with plasma, purified protein solution, dextran or balanced salt solutions. The quantities to be given vary with the weight of the child and the extent of the burn. The rate of administration is rapid initially and usually lasts for 36–48 h. Close patient observation, hourly urinary output measurement by an indwelling urethral catheter, and serial hemoglobin and hematocrit estimations provide adequate control data. A central venous pressure line can be helpful in the severe case, but it has been indicted as a major source of infection if maintained for days in the burned patient.

System management

Respiratory system

Where a child has been rescued from a burning building or where clothing has burned over the face, airway problems can be anticipated. Arterial blood gases should be monitored and intubation and assisted ventilation may be necessary. Broncho-pneumonia is a frequent later complication of large burns.

Central nervous system

Toddlers with even minor scalds are liable to convulse in the first 2 days with serious or even fatal outcome. The cause is thought to lie with early fluid shifts and the lag that occurs within the brain and its meninges. Papilledema is not always present. Diazepam and mannitol (1 g/kg i.v. over 20 min) gain quick control of fits and brain swelling, and phenytoin sodium and dexamethasone prolong the effect. Focal neurological deficits may occur at any time, probably as a result of septic emboli.

Urinary system

In the first 2 days after injury increased levels of antidiuretic hormone limit urinary output. Infusion should be used circumspectly and a serum sodium level of not less than 130 mmol/l should be maintained.

In deep burns, thermal damage to red blood cells causes hemoglobinuria, which may lead to tubular necrosis and renal failure. If rapid restoration of circulating fluid volume does not clear the urine, a solute diuretic such as 20% mannitol should be given without delay. A catheter may be required to monitor urine output or avoid contamination of the burn. It should be removed as soon as possible.

Cardiovascular system

Electrical current injury may cause cardiac damage and an ECG examination is advisable after such an injury. General anesthesia is best avoided until the tracing has returned to normal.

Tachycardia persists throughout recovery from a large burn and is largely a product of a high metabolic rate to offset the high evaporative heat losses. Heat regulation is disturbed and the child must be kept warm to avoid hypothermia.

Hemopoietic system

Loss of red cells, destroyed by a deep burn, must be replaced by early transfusion. Further losses take place during surgery and erythropoiesis remains depressed until a large burn has healed. The red cell mass must be maintained by transfusion if the body is to achieve quick healing.

Alimentary system

Gastric stasis is common in the early hours after a large burn but oral intake should be started as soon as possible. Ranitidine has reduced the incidence of hemorrhagic gastritis and Curling's ulcer is now rarely seen.

Accurate naked weights, obtained twice weekly from admission, guide the clinician through the early weight gain of fluid retention, diuresis, the catabolic phase, and the anabolic phase that comes more quickly and strongly in the child.

Nutrition

Daily fluid intake must take account of increased losses through the burn wound. A high calorie intake is needed to balance heat loss and minimize lean tissue breakdown. A protein intake at the upper end of the normal range is adequate. Iron and vitamins C and B complex are supplemented to combat anemia and aid wound healing. The seriously burned child cannot take food in solid form and it is kinder and more effective to give most of this as a fortified liquid feed. A fine-bore nasogastric feeding tube for this purpose should be passed on all children with burns over 15%. The planned intake should be achieved stepwise over the first 1–2 weeks. Early forcing of high food intake may predispose to a post-stress diabetes which may be resistant to insulin. Neglect of food intake will result in a profound weight loss, hypoproteinemia, and failure of the burn to heal.

Musculoskeletal system

While immobilization may be unavoidable for practical reasons, its use will increase muscle wasting and delay the recovery of an effective musculature. Regular active exercises should be performed wherever possible. Joint positioning and joint movement require constant attention if severe, and possibly permanent, joint contracture is to be avoided.

Local care

Infection is the major complication of all but the smallest burn. It can destroy surviving epithelium and penetrate a deep burn, with a risk of invasive infection. The commonest organism is *Staphylococcus aureus* but the β-hemolytic streptococcus is feared for its destructive capabilities and *Pseudomonas aeruginosa* can be dangerous on extensive burns. Constant monitoring, scrupulous hygiene and prevention of overcrowding are essential to control infection. Large burns should be isolated. Where appropriate, early excision and grafting can lead to healing before infection can occur. Local antibacterial agents are valuable but systemic antibiotics must be used with care as they can easily lead to superinfection with resistant organisms or fungi.

A superficial burn will, if protected from infection and trauma, heal in less than 3 weeks and is usually dressed with a well-padded gauze and cotton wool dressing with a Vaseline gauze inner layer. Deeper burns need skin grafting, unless very small.

Toxic shock syndrome

This can follow even very minor burns in the child (Cole & Shakespeare 1990) and can have a mortality of 11% (de Saxe et al 1985). It is therefore essential to recognize and treat it on suspicion. Signs are of an unwell, irritable child, 3 or more days after a burn, with pyrexia and three or more of the following: rash, hypotension, diarrhea or vomiting, inflamed mucous membranes, *Staphylococcus aureus* on wound swabs and occlusive dressings.

Treatment is with i.v. fluids, gammaglobulins (0.4 g/kg) or fresh blood or fresh frozen plasma (10 ml/kg over 4 hours), exposure of the burn, topical antibacterial agent and i.v. antibiotics.

Scarring

A superficial burn should leave little physical trace; the healed skin will be dry and should be creamed several times a day. With deeper injuries, scarring is unavoidable. The hypertrophic scar reaction is most intense in childhood. On the face, it disfigures and distorts features. On the flexures, it limits joint movement. Unrelieved scar contracture impedes growth of that part and deforms the growing skeleton. Spontaneous resolution of the hypertrophic scar is slow, variable and incomplete. Its full development may be cut short and its regression accelerated by elastic compression, intralesional injection of steroid hormones, or application of silicone gel. Secondary surgical procedures are often required to replace the worst scars, their timing and scope being dictated by the physical, psychological and educational needs of the child.

Psychological support

A close rapport between child, nurse, parents and doctor is fundamental in such a taxing hospital stay, which can extend over months. The child deserves explanation, occupation, and freedom from recurring pain. The parents, whose guilt feelings should be appreciated, should be incorporated into the therapeutic effort. The help of an interested and experienced psychiatrist may be invaluable.

Prognosis

Intensive early therapy can resuscitate a child with the gravest of surface burns. However, long-term survival is rare where 70% or more of the skin is destroyed. A child who survives a burn with significant scarring faces the prospect of physical and psychological problems which will probably become worse during adolescence. Continued long-term support is needed for patient and family for many years.

REFERENCES

Aitken-Swan J, Baird D 1965 Circumcision and cancer of the cervix. British Journal of Cancer 19: 217–227

Atwell J D 1985 Ascent of the testis: fact or fiction. British Journal of Urology 57: 474–477

Bodian M, Carter C O 1963 A family study of Hirschsprung's disease. Annals of Human Genetics 26: 261–277

Bohn D, Tamura M, Perrin D, Barker G, Rabinovitch M 1987 Ventilatory predictors of pulmonary hypoplasia in congenital diaphragmatic hernia, confirmed by morphologic assessment. Journal of Pediatrics 111: 423–431

Bokai J 1869 A fitma (preputium) sejtes adatapadasa a makkoz gyermakelnel. Orvosi Hetil 4: 583–587

Clements B S, Warner J O 1987 Pulmonary sequestration and related broncho-pulmonary vascular malformations: nomenclature and classification based on anatomical and embryological considerations. Thorax 42: 401–408

Cole R P, Shakespeare P G 1990 Toxic shock syndrome in scalded children. Burns 16: 221–224

de Saxe M J, Hawtin P, Wieneke A A 1985 Toxic shock syndrome in Britain – epidemiology and microbiology. Postgraduate Medical Journal 61: 5–8

de Vries P A, Pena A 1982 Posterior sagittal anorectoplasty. Journal of Pediatric Surgery 17: 638–643

Diebert G A 1933 The separation of the prepuce in the human penis. Anatomical Records 54: 387–393

Hancock B J, Wiseman N E 1989 Congenital duodenal obstruction: the impact of an antenatal diagnosis. Journal of Pediatric Surgery 24: 1027–1031

Hirschsprung H 1887 Stuhlragheit Neugeborener in Fotge von Dilation und Hypertrophie des Colons. Jahreb Kinderheilk 27: 1–7

Kasai M, Kimura S, Asakura Y 1968 Surgical treatment of biliary atresia. Journal of Pediatric Surgery 3: 665–675

Kernahan D A, Rosenstein S W 1990 Cleft lip and palate. A system of management. Williams & Wilkins, Baltimore

MacKinlay G A 1988 Save the prepuce. Painless separation of preputial adhesions in the outpatient clinic. British Medical Journal 297: 590–591

MacKinlay G A, Burtles R 1987 Oesophageal atresia: paralysis and ventilation in management of the wide gap. Pediatric Surgery International 2: 10–12

Ogita S, Tsuto T, Nakamura K, Deguchi E, Tokiwa K, Iwai N 1996 OK-432 therapy for lymphangioma in children: why and how does it work? Journal of Pediatric Surgery 31: 477–480

Ramstedt C 1912 Zur Operation der angeborenen Pylorusstenose. Medizinische Klinik (Berlin) 8: 1702–1705

Report of the Ad Hoc Task Force on Circumcision 1975 Pediatrics 56: 610–611

Sakai H, Tamura M, Hosokawa Y, Bryan A C, Barker G, Bonn D 1987 Effect of surgical repair on respiratory mechanics in congenital diaphragmatic hernia. Journal of Pediatrics 111: 432–438

Scobie W G, MacKinlay G A 1977 Ano rectal myectomy in treatment of ultra-short Hirschsprung's disease. Archives of Disease in Childhood 52: 713–715

Smith A, McIntosh N, Thomson M et al 1995 The stress effect of thermal injury on the hormones controlling fluid balance. Baillière's Clinical Paediatrics. Baillière, London

Spence, Sir James (1950) 1964 Spence on circumcision. Lancet ii: 902

Stephens F D 1984 Wingspread Conference on Anorectal Malformations. Racine, Wisconsin

Stiles H J 1910 (original operation note 3 February 1910 – personal possession)

Tan O T, Sherwood K, Gilchrist B A 1989 Treatment of children with port-wine stains using the flashlamp-pulsed tuneable dye laser. New England Journal of Medicine 320: 416–421

White R H R, O'Donnell B 1990 Controversies in therapeutics. Management of urinary tract infection and vesico-ureteric reflux in children. 1. Operative treatment has no advantage over medical management (RHRW). 2. The case for surgery (BO'D) British Medical Journal 300: 1391–1394

Wilson-Storey D, MacKinlay G A 1986 The superior mesenteric artery syndrome. Journal of the Royal College of Surgeons of Edinburgh 31: 175–178

32 Emergency care

Tom Beattie   Louise E. Wilson

ACCIDENT AND EMERGENCY 1802
The home setting 1802
Community care 1804
Prehospital care 1804
The accident and emergency unit services 1805
Approach to the management of the severely ill or
    injured child in the accident and emergency
    department 1806
Approach to the severely injured child 1809
Management of the unstable child with underlying
    pathology 1813
Conclusion 1816
Tom Beattie

PEDIATRIC INTENSIVE CARE 1816
Transport services 1817
Initial assessment 1817
Respiratory support 1817
Cardiovascular support 1819
Postoperative care of the cardiac surgical patient 1822
Nitric oxide 1823
Acute renal replacement therapy 1823
Hepatic support 1824
Support of the neurological system 1825
Clinical applications – examples 1825
Support services 1826
Louise E. Wilson
References 1826

ACCIDENT AND EMERGENCY

In an ideal world there would never be a critically ill or injured child. We do not live, however, in an ideal world and consequently, for the forseeable future there will be a substantial requirement to provide for the treatment of critically ill and injured children.

The continuum of pediatric emergency care is summarized in Figure 32.1. Beginning in the home and community, care must be provided optimally in this setting and in a way appropriate to the problem and in a seamless fashion continued upstream by the emergency services to the pediatric accident and emergency unit, and, if necessary, onwards to the hospital with its intensive care facilities. Within this continuum there should be the desire to keep children out of hospital and, if possible, provide care within the home and community environment (Haller et al 1983).

THE HOME SETTING

For the first 5 years of life most children spend the bulk of their time within the home and immediate community. The majority of children coming into contact with emergency medical services do so as a result of infection or injury.

INFECTION

Most children will experience upper and lower respiratory tract infection with considerable frequency between the ages of 0 and 5 years. After this age it is much less frequent. Such illness can usually be managed within the home, providing parents have sufficient confidence and education to carry out the appropriate treatment. Much of the illness in this age group will be viral and will require little more than supportive measures such as antipyretic therapy and encouraging fluid intake. There is, however, an increasing demand for this type of treatment to be obtained from family doctors or emergency departments. The disintegration of the nuclear family is one factor increasing this demand on medical time, particularly in primary care. With education and confidence parents should be able to look after such minor illness themselves.

Bacterial infection will be present in a small number of cases and will require antibiotic therapy. In an even smaller number of cases significant infectious disease such as meningitis, septicemia or osteomyelitis will be present. Similarly, a small number of children with viral illness will develop further complications, e.g. febrile seizure, or bacterial infection may supervene. If parents are unprepared for these problems they will tend to lose confidence and this will undermine education for management of illness within the community.

An education program that teaches parents how to deal with febrile illness must also alert parents to the dangers of bacterial illness, which requires antibiotic treatment with or without a stay in hospital. Within this education program it is important to differentiate the needs of the infant under 3 months of age. The response of the younger child to infection is quite different from that of older children and adults and parents should be aware of how to get advice for these children should the need arise (Morley et al 1991).

INJURY

Despite the frequency of infections, injuries are the leading cause of morbidity and mortality for children between the ages of 1 and 15 years. Most of these accidents occur within the home setting,

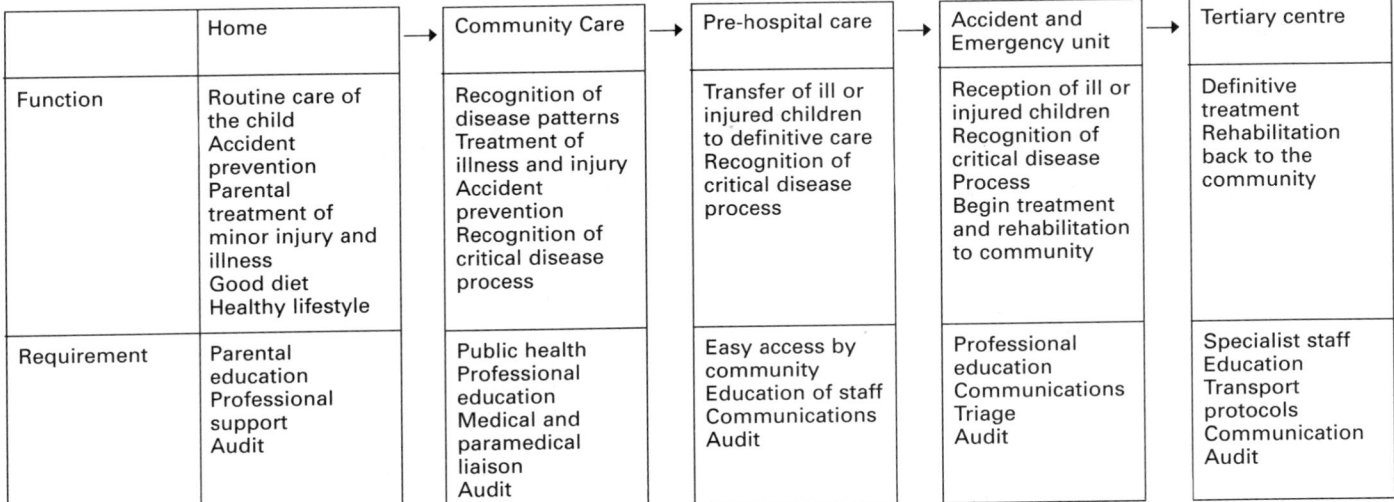

	Home	Community Care	Pre-hospital care	Accident and Emergency unit	Tertiary centre
Function	Routine care of the child Accident prevention Parental treatment of minor injury and illness Good diet Healthy lifestyle	Recognition of disease patterns Treatment of illness and injury Accident prevention Recognition of critical disease process	Transfer of ill or injured children to definitive care Recognition of critical disease process	Reception of ill or injured children Recognition of critical disease Process Begin treatment and rehabilitation to community	Definitive treatment Rehabilitation back to the community
Requirement	Parental education Professional support Audit	Public health Professional education Medical and paramedical liaison Audit	Easy access by community Education of staff Communications Audit	Professional education Communications Triage Audit	Specialist staff Education Transport protocols Communication Audit

Fig. 32.1 Components of a pediatric emergency medical system.

which includes the garden and its surroundings. Burns and scalds, poisonings, falls from a height, fingertip injuries and near drowning account for the vast majority of such injuries.

ACCIDENT PREVENTION PROGRAMS

One of the ways to tackle the toll wrought by injury in this age group is an integrated accident prevention program within an emergency medical system. The components of such an accident prevention system include:

1. accident surveillance
2. data analysis
3. identification of problems
4. development of strategies (based on 3)
5. implementation of strategies
6. continue surveillance (to assess effectiveness and begin again if necessary)

In many ways this is a completion of a typical audit cycle and relies on collaboration between emergency physicians, general practice, public health medicine, educationalists and health promotion agencies. These should bring their respective skills together in a coordinated fashion.

Accident surveillance

At present, injury surveillance is patchy, with much information being derived from inpatient databases. These are inaccurate and only reflect about 10% of the total number of accidents which occur. Without meaningful measures of injury severity this data is, at best, a reflection of current medical practice. A good example of this is the documentation of poisoning. Many children who are poisoned can be safely dealt with in the home without ever coming to hospital, provided adequate medical advice can be given with monitoring by telephone. If this advice is not available then many children will present to hospital. They will present to the emergency room, where their treatment will depend on the experience and confidence of the staff working in that department. Insecure, inexperienced junior staff will tend to admit because they are unsure of what to do. Senior staff who are experienced

and confident will be able to mange many of these children on an outpatient basis. The number of poisonings determined from an inpatient stay will vary with these units. This has nothing to do with the incidence of poisoning but all to do with medical practice. By changing medical practice one will demonstrate an apparent fall in the incidence of poisoning when in fact the incidence remains high. Failure to take cognizance of these matters when developing accident surveillance will lead to inappropriate preventive measures (Beattie 1996).

Effective data surveillance should start with a minimum data set (MDS). This MDS should aim to capture a small, important amount of information on every child who presents (Redmond et al 1992). If too much information is required, staff will tend not to collect it and parents will get irritated because they feel that their child should be treated rather than them answering questions. Typically, this MDS should include age, sex, postcode and proxies for social class and/or deprivation. Some idea of the causation should also be included. The international classification of disease E-codes (Ribbeck et al 1992) are universally accepted and usually adequate. Ideas on the most common diagnoses using a system such as the International Classification of Disease codes (ICD) could be included on discharge. If this information were to be collected on all children, one would rapidly develop a suitable accident surveillance system which could be expanded as the need arose.

Data analysis and problem identification

Once an accurate database that gathers details on a substantial proportion of injury occurring within the community is in place, then problem areas can be identified. This can be on the basis of: deprivation or need; clustering; type of accident, e.g. fall, poisoning; type of injury e.g. fracture, head injury. Once analyzed, this information can be available to health education agencies who can implement parts 4 and 5 of the audit cycle.

Devising a strategy

Before any strategy can be devised to protect against childhood accidents, three components have to be addressed:

1. the child
2. the family
3. the environment.

Tackling any of these areas on its own will fail: any strategy must concomitantly address the problems inherent in the other two areas. It is well recognized that some children are more accident prone than others. Is this because the family is poor or the environment is poor? Or is it that that child is inherently more prone to injury for reasons of clumsiness, poor eyesight/coordination/vision? To date many accident prevention programs have been simplistic, with individuals working in isolation without the complete umbrella of a pediatric emergency medical service (PEMS).

Implementing a strategy

Before a strategy can be successful, the lessons learnt from commercial advertisers have to be learned. Repeating the same message ad infinitum leads to message fatigue. The message must be appropriate to the target audience and must take note of all factors discussed above. In addition, the target audience must be identified and effectively targeted.

Re-audit

It is important to measure any effect of the prevention campaigns against the initial database. Failure to do so may lead to inappropriate and ineffective campaigning being continued indefinitely. If there has been no diminution in the levels of injury that one has targeted then the strategies need to be re-evaluated in the light of the data analysis and/or message.

Community education

In order for the child to be cared for within the home as effectively as possible, ideally without accessing emergency medical services, a substantial amount of effort must be paid to community education. The target audience must be defined. Does one tackle children in junior school or senior school in an effort to help future generations? Should one address the problem at antenatal classes, where there is a good chance that the message will reach an interested mother and perhaps the father? Is it appropriate to address the issue of safety in the postnatal period when the father is almost certainly not going to be present? These issues need to be urgently addressed if child accident prevention is to be taken forward in any meaningful manner.

COMMUNITY CARE

Within the context of a PEMS, community care should be directed at disease prevention. There will, however, still be a significant proportion of children who have transient episodes of acute illness requiring medical intervention. Interspersed with these will be children with chronic disability who may have more complicated needs for emergency care than their able-bodied peers.

For community care to work effectively there needs to be a network of experienced general practitioners and community pediatricians working alongside health visitors, district nurses, midwives and other paramedical staff. They will be aided and abetted by a public health system working alongside the medical fraternity. Good sanitation, maintenance of water supplies and attention to housing and overcrowding are all important issues in the prevention of disease and illness.

Disease surveillance by public health physicians and public health laboratories can identify trends in disease. Many infectious diseases, e.g. mycoplasma infection, occur in a cyclical fashion. Disease reporting can help identify when these infections are imminent and serological testing can help confirm that they have actually arrived. This will alert practitioners to the common types of disease that may be in the community setting at any given time. This may help direct treatment by the correct use of antibiotics and, if used efficiently, may avoid many unnecessary hospital admissions.

The health professionals within the community have several roles. The first is disease prevention, primarily in terms of immunization and accident prevention. Where immunization has been effective many diseases have almost been eradicated. Health professionals in the community should be able to give advice to parents on disease and accident prevention and they should also be able to recognize situations where family dynamics are breaking down, making accidents and child abuse more common. Sibert (1975) has identified many stress factors as a major cause of poisoning. Health visitors and family physicians should be able to recognize these family stresses and provide preemptive care.

Within the community it is vital to recognize the child who has a disease process which is not suitable for treatment in the community but needs further care within a hospital setting. A good example of this is bronchiolitis. Many cases of bronchiolitis can be cared for in the community, with children getting supportive care and advice. However, family practitioners should be in the position to identify the child at risk from significant airway distress, e.g. not feeding, a respiratory rate over 50, or apneic attacks (Isaacs 1995). In this situation the child needs hospital for further treatment which may include antiviral therapy and ventilation. Equally, the community services should be able to identify the child who may not be so ill but where the family circumstances are such that the child is not going to be adequately looked after at home. Situations where this may occur include poverty, a mother who is not coping because she has two or three other small children, single parents or families of drug abusers. In these situations, even though the child may not warrant admission for medical reasons, the social factors may indicate that the child needs to be transferred for inpatient care. Community practitioners are much better placed to identify these problems than hospital based-staff.

In order to facilitate adequate community care there needs to be a degree of professional education relevant to the needs of the community, with medical and paramedical liaison and an effective audit system.

PREHOSPITAL CARE

Prehospital care is a link between home and the community on one hand and the hospital based services of accident and emergency and tertiary level care on the other. The function of prehospital care is to transfer ill or injured children to places of either advanced or definitive care. Two issues are important within the prehospital care setting, namely access and education.

To be effective, prehospital care has to be easily accessed by all members of the community, e.g. in the UK, dialing '999' gains access to the ambulance service. This universal national access code, available to all and free of charge, is probably the most effective component in the prehospital setting.

Education is also vital. The role of general practitioners in prehospital care must be fully defined. It must be relevant to the

PEMS within which the prehospital care is practiced. For example, there will be differences between urban and rural areas in terms of decisions to 'stay and play' and 'scoop and run'. It must be remembered that the absolute numbers of true pediatric emergencies, be they illness or trauma, are relatively small, particularly compared to the adult population. The skills needed to carry out emergency care effectively require time to attain and practice to maintain. An integrated pediatric emergency medical system can best evaluate the needs of its catchment area and train the prehospital care staff accordingly. Where short distances are envisaged and transfer times are rapid, then training needs may be less demanding, with concentration on simple airway, breathing and circulation skills. In rural areas, where transport times may be prolonged, advanced life support skills may be necessary (Gallehr & Vukov 1993, Grossman et al 1995). Where land-based transport is adequate, training in driving skills may be all that is required. However, should air medical transport by helicopter or fixed-wing aircraft be necessary as a routine, then training in aviation medicine and associated problems will need to be included in the training package. Inner city areas with significant drugs problems may have a high incidence of penetrating trauma which will require an emphasis to be placed on treatment of such injuries within that setting.

The key to the prehospital care system is an integration between the community and the receiving units under the umbrella of a pediatric emergency medical system which can coordinate appropriate education and audit the interventions and outcomes.

THE ACCIDENT AND EMERGENCY UNIT SERVICES

Pediatric accident and emergency departments fall into three broad categories:

1. those attached to specialist pediatric hospitals which only treat children
2. those attached to large district or teaching hospitals which have combined pediatric and adult populations
3. those attached to small community or cottage hospitals, treating relatively small numbers of patients overall.

Within each of these three settings various problems exist.

The dedicated pediatric unit is usually situated in a large conurbation, often attached to a university or medical school. It will provide child and family centered care to an exceptionally high standard. However, experience of dealing with major injury and illness will often be much less than that in a comparable adult population. There will therefore have to be a greater emphasis paid to education regarding recognition and resuscitation skills to facilitate optimum care of ill and injured children when they present. Retention of these skills is also a major issue which needs to be addressed.

In a unit which combines pediatric and adult patients, general resuscitation skills and teamwork will be much more practiced but pediatric illness recognition and treatment skills may be comparatively deficient. The ability to provide a child and family centered approach is often more difficult than in the purely pediatric setting.

The cottage hospital may benefit from being able to provide care closer to the patient's home, but recognition of childhood illness and resuscitation skills may be significantly absent unless teaching programs are strong. Staff should rotate to busy units at regular intervals to update and recertify in pediatric skills.

In all settings the regular turnover of junior and nursing staff means that regular resuscitation updates are essential, e.g. pediatric advanced life support courses. Staffing and training in departments that have children attending should always build in adequate time for training and staff development to ensure that skills are maintained at an optimum level.

BASIC REQUIREMENTS

Within these settings certain basic concepts need to be addressed.

At the very least there should be *dedicated* facilities for the reception and treatment of children. Children are often already frightened and distressed by being in hospital and every effort should be made to keep them as calm and content as possible. An attractive environment which is child friendly facilitates this. Examination rooms should have sufficient toys and pictures to enable distraction therapy to be efficiently practiced. Play leaders are an invaluable resource to aid this process.

Resuscitation rooms should be fully equipped with all the various equipment that is required for pediatric resuscitation (see Table 32.1). Children change shape and size with age. It is almost impossible to recall accurately all the weights of children at various age groups. Drug and fluid therapy is usually done on a dose per weight basis. It is important to avoid calculations in 'the heat of the moment'. It is all too easy to place a decimal point in the wrong place and either over- or underdose children. For this reason charts should be available or tapes laid out on beds so that rapid determination of dosage depending on the weight/length of child can be established. These charts will also have details of the correct size of endotracheal tube, the length to which the tube should be cut and various other parameters necessary for effective pediatric resuscitation (Luten et al 1992, Oakley 1988).

Parents often arrive at the accident and emergency department with other siblings. The presence of play leaders will help entertain these children and enable the distressed relatives to be with the sick or injured child. Quiet rooms should be available so that bereaved or distressed relatives can be alone in their time of distress, though a staff member should always be available for this if required. Facilities should be available to enable nappy changing and breast-feeding to occur in private.

The function of staff within the accident and emergency unit will be to receive all ill and injured children and to institute treatment in a timely and appropriate fashion, depending on the urgency of the medically assessed need for treatment (triage).

Triage is usually performed by the nursing staff but it is equally valid for medical staff to perform this task. Objective triage is difficult in the pediatric population as there are very few objective pediatric scales which can be related to all types of problems presenting (medical, surgical, trauma or other). Much triage is subjective and will in part depend upon the volume of work. A well child presenting at a quiet time will very often get through the system more rapidly than an ill child presenting at a busy time.

Skills

Key within this setting are recognition skills. It is imperative that staff working within the accident and emergency unit are able to recognize the child who has a disease process which, if left untreated, will lead to serious incapacity or death. Key recognition skills are those of respiratory and circulatory compromise (see later).

Table 32.1 Equipment for the resuscitation room

Airway
Guedel airway – 0 → 5
Endotracheal tubes – 2.5 → 8 uncuffed and 7 → 10.5 cuffed
Introducers
Laryngoscope handles
Laryngoscope blades – straight and curved
Yankauer suction catheters
Argyle suction catheters
Suction device (with backup)
Cricothyroid puncture set (this may be commercial or 'homemade')
Jet insufflation system

Breathing
Round masks
Triangular masks
Bag–Valve–Mask device with reservoir bag
O_2 supply (with backup)
Ayres T-piece circuit (or equivalent)
Chest drains 10 → 32G
Drainage tubing and jars for underwater seal

Circulation
Intravenous cannulae 24 → 14F
Central venous cannulae and Seldinger introducer wire
Intraosseous cannulae 17F
Giving sets
Blood warmer
Infusion pumps
Defibrillator with facility for synchronized DC version capable of variable energy delivery

Disability
Cervical collars
Spinal boards
Arm and leg splints

Monitoring equipment
Pulse oximeter
Cardiac monitor
Blood glucose test machines
Blood gas analyzer

Other
Tapes for i.v. lines, ETT tubes, chest drains
Syringes 1 ml, 2 ml, 5 ml, 10 ml
3-way taps
Connection tubing

Other (contd)
Suture material
Suture packs
Chest drain packs
Urinary catheters
Nasogastric tubes
Clock
Warmth

Drugs
Adrenaline – 1 : 10 000 and 1 : 1000
Atropine
Lignocaine – 1%, 2%
Sodium bicarbonate – 1.84%, 4.2%, 8.4%
Morphine
Naloxone
Glucose – 50%, 25%, 10%
Glucagon
Diazepam – (as emulsion)
Phenytoin
Adenosine
Disopyramide
Beta-blocker
Propofol
Suxamethonium
Atracurium
Mannitol – 10%, 20%
β_2-agonists – nebulizer solution
Ipratropium – nebulizer solution
β_2-agonists – i.v. solution
Aminophylline
Hydrocortisone
Procyclidine

Fluids
Normal saline
Plasma

If neonates are expected the following equipment should also be available:
Resuscitaire
Heat source
Warm towels/wraps
Umbilical catheters

Allied to recognition skills are motor skills which enable appropriate therapies to be effectively carried out. These skills include:

1. the ability to definitively open and secure an airway
2. the ability to ensure that oxygenation is maintained
3. the ability to ensure that circulation is maintained.

The frequency with which these skills are practiced will depend on the population served and the effectiveness of the home, community and prehospital services. Communities which have poor home safety, poor community immunization rates and primitive public sanitation can expect to deal with large numbers of ill or injured children.

Where numbers are small, maintenance of recognition skills can only be maintained by appropriate teaching programs, e.g. PALS (pediatric advanced life support).

Transfer

Once a child has been received in the accident and emergency unit and the airway, breathing and circulation have been stabilized, the child needs to be transferred from the accident and emergency unit for definitive treatment. This will often be via an imaging facility to surgery, and from there to an intensive care setting. To complete the emergency medical system, safe transfer to and from each of these areas needs to be established. Even if the accident and emergency department is within the tertiary care center, transfer to the scanning suite or the intensive care unit can be fraught with danger if it is not performed expertly and efficiently.

A transport team should be a priority development in any pediatric emergency care system so that there can be safe transfer to the tertiary care center for definitive treatment.

Both within the accident and emergency setting and the tertiary care unit rehabilitation is important. This will enable the ill or injured child to regain their place as effectively as possible within the home/community setting.

APPROACH TO THE MANAGEMENT OF THE SEVERELY ILL OR INJURED CHILD IN THE ACCIDENT AND EMERGENCY DEPARTMENT

Most ill children will be brought to hospital by the prehospital services. In these situations airway care and circulatory support will have been instituted according to local training and policy guidelines. In addition there will be an element of warning so that the resuscitation team can be gathered and tasks allocated.

As it is very easy for parents or bystanders to pick up smaller children, children who are severely ill or injured will often be brought to hospital, unannounced and unexpected, in private transport. Consequently the components of the resuscitation team should be established in advance. It is important that one doctor is in charge to coordinate the resuscitation and decide on the priorities for care, with other staff in complementary roles.

INITIAL ASSESSMENT

Rapid assessment of the airway, breathing and circulation is mandatory (primary survey) (see also Ch. 12, Fig. 12.10).

Airway

The airway can be described as open, maintainable or unmaintainable. An open airway is defined as one with no obstruction present. This includes the absence of secretions, stridor, gurgling or other noises. An open airway needs no further management but should be kept under review.

A maintainable airway is defined as one which can be kept open with simple measures such as positioning, chin lift/head tilt, the use of an oropharyngeal airway, or the use of *gentle* suction.

An unmaintainable airway is one which is still at risk despite these simple measures, necessitating either intubation or the creation of a surgical airway (cricothyrotomy).

The airway should be maintained by the simplest measures available. Intubation, if required, must be done by experienced operators with skill and in a timely fashion. Any attempt taking longer than 30 seconds should be abandoned and the child oxygenated with a bag–valve–mask device pending a second attempt.

All sick or injured children require high flow oxygen. This should be administered using a face mask if the airway is open and maintainable. Otherwise, artificial ventilation should be established using a bag–valve–mask device (see below).

Breathing

The efficacy of breathing can be assessed only after the airway has been opened. The rate, volume and symmetry of respiration should be assessed by observation and auscultation.

Respiratory compromise can be characterized by either an increasing or decreasing work of breathing (Table 32.2).

If breathing is absent or diminished, ventilation using a bag–valve–mask device should be instituted as soon as possible. Absent breath sounds and hyperresonance to percussion on one side should lead one to consider a pneumothorax. This should be immediately drained using a needle thoracostomy. The needle should be inserted into the midclavicular line in the second intercostal space pending the insertion of a formal chest drain. Once inserted, the needle should be left in place until the chest drain is working properly. If signs of respiratory compromise (Table 32.2) are present, supplemental oxygen should be administered in the highest rate available.

Circulation

A central pulse should be palpated at this stage. The carotid pulse should be palpated lateral to the thyroid cartilage and medial to the sternocleidomastoid muscle in a child. In an infant the brachial pulse should be palpated in the upper arm.

If there is no pulse palpable (or pulse is less than 60 beats per minute in an infant less than 1 year of age) cardiac massage should be started at a rate of 80–100 beats per minute. If a pulse is palpable, other evidence of circulatory embarrassment should be sought (Table 32.3).

All children with circulatory embarrassment (indeed all children who are severely ill or injured) should have i.v. access established as soon as possible. Failure to establish peripheral i.v. access within a few minutes in children who are in circulatory distress should lead one to insert an intraosseous needle into the tibia or femur (p. 526). If signs of circulatory embarrassment or shock are present, fluid should be administered as a 20 ml/kg bolus. It does not matter at this stage whether the fluid is crystalloid or colloid but certainly electrolyte poor fluids should be avoided.

Blood pressure (BP) is an unreliable sign of circulatory compromise in children. Up to 40% of the circulating blood volume needs to be lost before the blood pressure will fall. A falling blood pressure is a late sign and indicates a failure of compensatory mechanisms to maintain perfusion to vital areas. Once BP falls, early and urgent treatment is indicated if permanent harm is to be avoided.

While the medical staff are assessing the airway, breathing and circulation, the nursing staff should help get the child undressed and should attach a cardiac monitor and a pulse oximeter.

With this initial assessment one should find oneself in one of the following situations:

1. a child in cardiac arrest
2. a traumatized child who requires further trauma-orientated resuscitation
3. an unstable child with continuing airway, breathing or circulatory compromise associated with underlying pathology
4. a stable child.

CARDIAC ARREST

Cardiac arrest is rare in the pediatric population but causes to consider include sudden infant death syndrome, trauma, drowning and asphyxia.

Table 32.2 Signs of respiratory compromise

Increased work of breathing	Decreased work of breathing
1. Increasing respiratory rate	1. Decreasing respiratory rate
2. Increasing heart rate	2. Poor respiratory effort
3. Use of accessory muscles in respiration	3. Poor lung expansion
4. Flared nostrils	4. Decreasing level of consciousness
5. Intercostal/sternal recession	
6. Decreasing level of consciousness	

Table 32.3 Physical signs of circulatory embarrassment

1. Rising pulse
2. Weakening peripheral pulses
3. Increasing capillary return (greater than 2 seconds)
4. Increasing peripheral core temperature difference
5. Decreased urine output
6. Altered level of consciousness

Cardiac arrest in children is primarily asystolic in nature. Occasionally, electromechanical dissociation ((EMD), also known as pulseless electrical activity (PEA)) or ventricular fibrillation (VF) is present. It is important to begin resuscitation but also consider definitive drug and fluid therapies as indicated by the underlying rhythm (Zideman et al 1994).

The outcome of cardiac arrest in children is dismal, particularly when it occurs in the community (Ronco et al 1995). Prolonged hypoxia, hypoglycemia and acidosis, in addition to the underlying disease process, all contribute to cell death, particularly in the myocardium and brain, making restoration of vital functions difficult. Even if cardiac function is restored, the prolonged insult to the brain usually leaves the child with permanent or profound neurological deficit.

Asystole

Asystole is characterized by a pulseless, apneic child associated with no complexes on the cardiac monitor. It is important to confirm that this is so by going through the following procedure:

1. turning up the gain on the cardiac monitor
2. ensuring that all the connections are made
3. checking that the monitor is not connected to 'paddles' of the cardioversion equipment.

The recommended sequence for dealing with asystole is found in Figure 32.2.

Electromechanical dissociation (EMD)

EMD is associated with a pulseless, apneic child and bizarre complexes on the cardiac monitor. Often this is associated with underlying pathology such as pneumothorax, cardiac tamponade, electrolyte imbalance, hypovolemia and hypothermia. Treatment should correct these underlying disorders. An algorithm for treating EMD can be seen in Figure 32.2.

Ventricular fibrillation

VF is much rarer in children than in adults, though recent reports have indicated that it might be more frequent than once suspected. An algorithm for treating ventricular fibrillation can be found in Figure 32.2.

STOPPING RESUSCITATION

The decision to terminate resuscitation will be a difficult one. Children who have been poisoned, drowned or who are hypothermic should have active resuscitation continued for a considerable time. This will usually occur within the intensive care setting with continuing resuscitation during transit. Post-traumatic cardiac arrest has a very poor prognosis and prolonged attempts at resuscitation should be avoided. Similarly, sudden infant death syndrome should not lead to unduly prolonged resuscitation attempts.

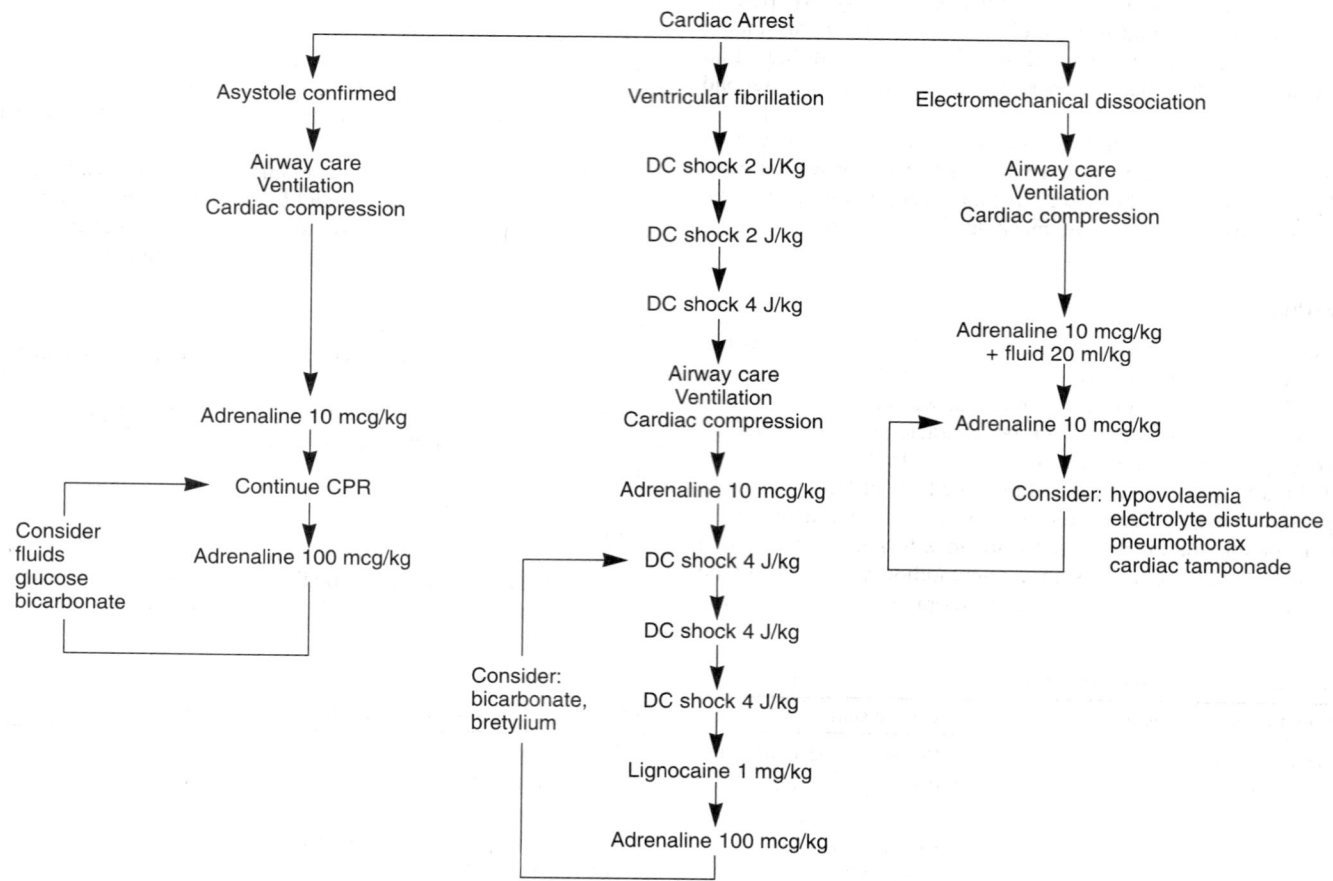

Fig. 32.2 Recommended sequences for cardiac arrest.

APPROACH TO THE SEVERELY INJURED CHILD

Major trauma is a relatively rare occurrence in the pediatric population compared to the adult population. 80% of children who die will be dead on arrival of the paramedical team at the scene, a fact which makes accident prevention all the more important. Care of the airway, breathing and circulation are of paramount importance. *One of the major differences, however, is that traumatized children are at risk of having damage to the spinal column, particularly the cervical spine.* In particular, this means that one has to be able to perform airway opening maneuvers without excessive movement in the cervical spine area. Measures such as chin lift without head tilt are important. Oropharyngeal airways are important adjuncts to the process.

SPINAL CORD INJURY WITHOUT RADIOLOGICAL ABNORMALITY (SCIWORA) (Ferguson & Beattie 1993)

This is a rare finding but has a potentially horrendous outcome.

Pathophysiology

Relative laxity of spinal ligaments associated with underdevelopment of the articular facets of the vertebrae in the spinal column allows excessive movement to take place during severe hyperflexion/extension injuries. This results in compression of the spinal cord. The column will return to its normal anatomy without any evidence of fracture or subluxation being present. Normal X-rays, therefore, in an unconscious child, should not lead one to assume that there is no possibility of spinal cord injury.

Implications for clinical practice

If the child is awake and is able to move all four limbs then SCIWORA is unlikely to be present. However, in those children who have an altered level of consciousness, SCIWORA must be suspected. In these children full spinal column immobilization measures must be implemented until the spine can be cleared either radiologically or clinically.

Simple measures to immobilize the spine will include: use of sandbags or other similar sized objects to immobilize the head; taping the head to a spinal board; and immobilizing the head on the shoulders using hands and arms.

The airway should be assessed and opened in the simplest way possible and this should be carried out without moving the cervical spine (see above).

BREATHING

Breathing abnormalities are reasonably common with trauma. Causes include pneumothorax, hemothorax, rib fractures and gastric dilation. All children with traumatic injuries should be given supplemental oxygen and any specific underlying disease treated. A pneumothorax should be decompressed by needle thoracotomy and gastric dilation should be decompressed via a gastric tube. If a basal skull fracture is suspected this tube should be passed via the mouth rather than the nose to avoid inadvertently siting it in the brain!

CIRCULATION

Problems with circulation may be due to hypovolemia, tension pneumothorax or cardiac tamponade. Hypovolemia is the most common and intra-abdominal injuries are a more common cause of hypovolemia than other injury. Small babies may become relatively hypovolemic due to intracerebral bleed but other causes must be sought. As a general rule hypovolemia should not be ascribed to a head injury: some other focus must be sought. The signs of hypovolemia will also be present following trauma, in particular an altered level of consciousness and poor peripheral pulses. A low blood pressure is a sign of great importance, indicating urgent fluid replacement.

Intravenous cannulae should be inserted into large veins, avoiding fractured limbs where possible. If the child is stable and blood is not required urgently, a simple 'group and save serum' is all that is required. Where the child is unstable, blood will be required urgently. Ideally this blood should be fully grouped and cross-matched, but occasionally O negative blood will be needed (Fig. 32.3).

DISABILITY

The relatively large head compared to the rest of the body makes the child more vulnerable to head injury than the adult. Most are minor, with the incidence of intracranial bleeding being less in the pediatric population than the adult population.

The first assessment does not need to calculate a complete coma score (e.g. the Glasgow Coma Scale); it is sufficient to document whether the child is Awake, responding to Verbal stimuli, responding to Painful stimuli, or Unresponsive (the AVPU scale). Pupillary reflexes may be documented but at this stage they will not alter management significantly.

While the medical team are assessing airway, breathing circulation and disability, the nursing team should undress the child, apply a cardiac monitor and a pulse oximeter and prepare to assist with airway and i.v. access procedures.

SECONDARY SURVEY

Once the airway, breathing and circulation have been addressed, a full secondary survey of the child should be carried out. Every part of the body will be examined both visually and by palpation. Judicious use of plain X-ray, ultrasound and computed tomography will aid the diagnostic process. Minor injuries which may have been missed on the first brief survey will be detected and will lead to further treatment and investigation. Injuries which are commonly detected during the secondary survey include bleeding from the ear and nose, small pneumothoraces, gastric dilation and minor fractures to the peripheries.

HEAD INJURY

Head injury is a significant cause of morbidity and mortality in the pediatric population. The relatively large head changes the center of gravity and the head is one of the most commonly injured parts of the body in the pediatric population.

The causes of significant head injury include falls from a height, motor vehicle accidents and nonaccidental injury.

While most children who sustain significant head injury will lose consciousness, it should be borne in mind that hypoxia,

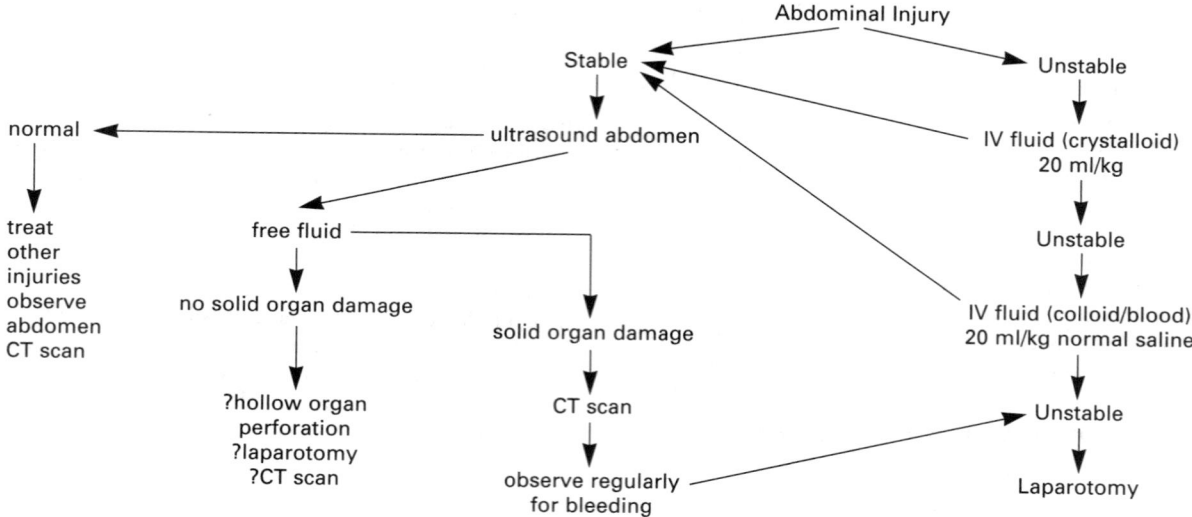

Fig. 32.3 Plan of action for abdominal injury.

hypovolemia or both are significant causes of altered level of consciousness. Sharples et al (1990) indicated that children transferred to a central neurosurgical unit with head injury are more likely to die as a result of associated hypoxia and/or hypovolemia due to respiratory or circulatory distress than to die from the head injury.

The role of the accident and emergency department in managing head injury is straightforward, but it is important to grasp the concept of primary and secondary brain injury.

Primary brain injury is that which occurs at the time of impact. Any damage done at this stage is usually irreversible. Secondary brain injury occurs due to an extra insult, commonly hypoxia, hypovolemia and brain edema. There is a complex relationship between the primary injury and these other secondary factors. The initial injury will cause swelling from a normal inflammatory response. Localized brain injury might occur if the child has been hit with a hard object such as a golf club or hammer. The inflammation will be localized and will not cause generalized brain edema. In contrast, the small baby who is exposed to vigorous shaking (nonaccidental injury) will have diffuse brain injury with a generalized inflammation throughout the brain. This malignant cerebral edema is almost impossible to treat and is usually the cause of significant morbidity and mortality associated with 'shaken baby syndrome'. Postmortem examination reveals multiple hemorrhages and diffuse brain edema. Most cases of head injury fall between these two extremes.

When an initial insult is associated with loss of consciousness, hypoxia will often ensue as a result of an obstructed airway. The hypoxia will cause cerebral anoxia with resultant cell damage and death and a generalized inflammatory response with a variable degree of cerebral edema being present. The same situation will occur if other causes of hypoxia ensue, e.g. pneumothorax, pulmonary contusion.

Similarly, a decrease in perfusion pressure to the brain secondary to hemorrhage or other cause of hypovolemia will result in failure to deliver glucose and oxygen to the brain and again generalized inflammation increases the intracranial pressure. Thus, unless there is adequate circulatory drive to perfuse the brain, a vicious cycle ensues.

ROLE OF THE ACCIDENT AND EMERGENCY DEPARTMENT

The role of the accident and emergency department is to ensure that the airway is open by whatever means possible, to ensure that ventilation is maximized, and that oxygen saturations are maintained between 95% and 100%. This helps to maintain circulation to enable cerebral perfusion to be normalized.

By the time the child gets to accident and emergency a degree of intracranial swelling may already have taken place. In the early stages this will often be from an intracranial hematoma. Children with head injury may have extradural, acute subdural or intracerebral bleeds and all of these can produce considerable pressure effects. Children may sustain extradural hematomas without fractures to the middle meningeal region (in contrast to the adult population). A normal skull X-ray therefore may be very misleading. Only when the airway, breathing and circulation are secure and any other life-threatening injury is identified and controlled can the child be transferred to the scanning suite for the formal diagnosis to be made. There may be a dilemma between obtaining surgical hemostasis (e.g. from a ruptured liver or spleen) and the management of significant intracranial hematoma. It is imperative in these situations to control the circulation and to ensure brain perfusion is maximized to reduce the effect of secondary brain injury from hypoxia and/or hypovolemia. This tension is not easy to resolve and it takes considerable experience to ensure that the correct sequence of events occurs.

Intracranial pressure

It is not uncommon for raised intracranial pressure to be present and the computed tomography scan to show no evidence of intracranial bleed. In this situation, cerebral edema is probable and it is important to try and reduce the pressure. Most of the measures to reduce cerebral edema will only work on a normal brain and are of dubious benefit: they include hyperventilation to ensure a $PaCO_2$ of about 4 kPa; use of mannitol or frusemide; and sedative techniques such as barbiturate anesthesia. Use of these agents should be discussed with the neurosurgeon.

There have been reports of experimental work suggesting that calcium blocking agents may be of some benefit. There is no evidence that steroids have any role to play in the management of post-traumatic cerebral edema.

Basal skull fractures

The accident and emergency department is responsible for identifying basal skull fractures by clinical examination. Physical signs that indicate that a basal skull fracture is present include: 'panda eyes' (racoon eyes); blood or CSF from the nose or ears; or Battle's sign (bruising over the mastoid process). If any of these are present, a basal skull fracture should be diagnosed clinically. Basal skull fractures are open fractures and there is a significant chance that infection will develop, usually during the first 12–24 hours though not uncommonly after this period. The use of antibiotics for the management of basal skull fractures is controversial. There is no clear evidence that antibiotics will reduce the subsequent chance of meningitis developing but this should be discussed with the local neurosurgical unit prior to definitive treatment being commenced.

Convulsions

Many children will convulse following a head injury. This can also result in hypoxia. After oxygen has been supplied and ventilation assisted, the fit should be stopped using diazepam 0.2 mg/kg. Assessment of the level of consciousness will then be difficult and such children should undergo CT scanning. Phenytoin 10–15 mg/kg may be used to reduce subsequent seizures after discussion with the neurosurgical unit.

Transfer

When the airway has been established, oxygenation maximized and circulation and perfusion restored to normal, the child should be transferred for definitive diagnosis to a computed tomography suite under stringent transfer conditions. Transfer from the safety of the resuscitation room should not be commenced until full transfer protocols have been instituted as transfer from the accident and emergency setting to the scanning suite may be as dangerous and perilous as traveling from one center to another.

THORACOABDOMINAL INJURIES

Thoracoabdominal injury is relatively rare in the pediatric population compared with the adolescent and adult population. Most injuries are blunt, although the increase in the use of firearms has meant that penetrating thoracoabdominal trauma in the pediatric population is rising. Many children with major thoracic injuries will die before reaching hospital although improvements in prehospital care mean an increasing number may survive. Injuries which fall into this category include traumatic dissection of the aorta and massive tension pneumothorax.

Traumatic dissection of the thoracic aorta

This is typically caused by rapid deceleration injury and most children will die in the prehospital phase. If they survive to reach hospital the diagnosis can be suspected by the presence of a widened mediastinum on a chest X-ray associated with fractures of the upper ribs. It is best confirmed by either arteriography or computed tomography. If suspected, the child should be transferred urgently to a thoracic surgical center.

Tension pneumothorax

Tension pneumothorax is treated by the insertion of a large-bore needle into the second intercostal space on the affected side. Signs of tension pneumothorax include signs of respiratory distress, and distended neck veins and absent breath sounds on the affected side. Once the pneumothorax is drained using the needle in the second intercostal space, a formal chest drain should be inserted and connected to an underwater seal. Drainage of a pneumothorax on one side may reveal the presence of a lesion on the other side and this should be treated appropriately.

Moderate chest injury

The greater use of seat belts and seat restraints has led to an increase in chest wall bruising from the physical restraint of the child. Children with seat belt abrasions to the chest or abdomen have been subjected to considerable deceleration forces. While the most likely thoracic injuries will be fractured clavicle with or without a fractured sternum, it should be borne in mind that underlying myocardial contusion is a possibility. This is extremely difficult to detect clinically. The presence of abnormal ECGs and raised cardiac enzymes are unreliable and if there is any doubt the child should be admitted for a period of observation with continuous cardiac monitoring.

Fractured ribs are rare in the pediatric population: if seen in the infant or toddler nonaccidental injury should be suspected. Relief of pain is all that is usually required but, occasionally, if there are more than three ribs fractured on one side, intercostal block may be needed. Bilateral rib fractures may lead to a flail chest though this is rare in the pediatric population.

Abdominal injury

As with thoracic injury, blunt trauma is the rule, with penetrating trauma increasing in frequency as children get older. Blunt trauma can result in hemorrhage and loss of perfusion from rupture of solid organs such as spleen, kidney and liver; or peritonitis from injury to the bowel and pancreas. A strong index of suspicion is always needed as the child can often have minimal abdominal signs at an early stage. This is particularly so in pancreatitis and bowel perforation where peritonitis can take between 6 and 12 hours to develop.

Any child who shows evidence of circulatory collapse following trauma should have intra-abdominal hemorrhage considered. Clinical diagnosis is unreliable and some form of imaging is indicated if the child is stable. Children who are unstable should always have intra-abdominal bleeding suspected. A plan of action is shown in Figure 32.3.

Ultrasound assessment should be done initially in the stable child. If there is any free fluid present in the abdomen a careful search should be made of the hepatic, splenic and renal areas. If these are considered normal, then bowel perforation should be suspected and a laparotomy performed. Computed tomography will help diagnose the problem.

Hepatic and splenic trauma should be treated conservatively provided the child remains stable. A full evaluation of the solid organs should be made using computed tomography once the initial injury is suspected on ultrasound examination.

Peritoneal lavage has been advocated in the diagnosis of intra-abdominal injury. The criteria for a positive test are subjective and the results are inferior to an ultrasound scan done by an expert. The ultrasound scan can also give a good indication as to the organ that is involved, particularly if solid organ injury is present, and can detect even small amounts of free fluid. Ultrasound cannot distinguish between blood and inflammatory exudate (e.g. from ruptured bowel), but it is much less invasive and does not cause the child any undue distress.

Seat belt injury

Chest injury is most usual from belts with three point fixation (e.g. a lap belt and harness fixation). If children are restrained using only a lap belt and they are involved in a high speed collision they will sustain a hyperflexion injury of the torso. This will usually result in intra-abdominal injury, often with significant hepatic or splenic component, and may be associated with a degree of spinal instability with fractures occurring in the L1, L2 region of the lumbar spine. Any child who has significant lap belt injury to the mid-abdominal region should have a spinal injury suspected and should have full spinal immobilization until the spine has been fully cleared both radiologically and clinically (see SCIWORA above).

ORTHOPEDIC INJURY

Orthopedic injury following trauma is common. Within the accident and emergency department there are three roles to be considered:

1. recognition of the fracture
2. identification of associated soft tissue injury which may cause compromise to the limb
3. splintage and analgesia.

Recognition of the fracture

A bent bone is obviously a broken bone. Of more concern is the occult undisplaced fracture as such fractures can bleed into tight fascia compartments with subsequent compartment syndrome. Particularly at risk of vascular compromise are fractures of the elbow, where the brachial artery may be involved, and the tibia. As a general rule, if there is any concern about the presence of an occult fracture, the area should be X-rayed to either confirm or deny its presence.

With all fractures the distal pulses should be palpated and distal neurological function should be checked. If the perfusion is adequate distal to the fracture site, then all that is needed is for the limb to be splinted until life-threatening conditions such hypoxia or hypovolemia are corrected. Nerve injuries need to be noted and examined further when the child is stable.

Identification of associated soft tissue injury

Soft tissue injuries associated with fractures include:

1. tissue loss
2. open wounds

3. vascular damage
4. nerve damage
5. tendon damage.

Tissue loss and open wounds associated with a fracture will lead to infection in the bone if not adequately treated and debrided. There is no place in the accident and emergency department to start this process but the wound should not be ignored. It is sufficient to assess the distal pulses and neurological function and, if these are intact, dress the wound with a disinfectant dressing leaving further management to the orthopedic department. Broad spectrum antibiotics effective against Gram-positive, Gram-negative and anaerobic organisms are important. Local policies determine which antibiotics are given. Tetanus prophylaxis is also important if the patient is not fully immunized.

Analgesia

Analgesia in children with long bone fracture is greatly under used. There is often a fear of masking intra-abdominal injury or of aggravating consciousness level if there has been coincident head injury. Both of these are inadequate reasons to withhold analgesia in a child who is in considerable pain. Two methods of analgesia exist in this situation:

1. local and peripheral nerve block
2. intravenous opiate.

Local and peripheral nerve block

The bone which is most amenable to this treatment is the femur. Successful blocking can be obtained by infiltrating a long-acting anesthetic such as bupivacaine around the femoral nerve where it passes under the inguinal ligament lateral to the artery. This will take 5–10 minutes to work and can be preceded by a more fast acting local anesthetic such as lignocaine or prilocaine. If adrenaline is used great care must be taken not to inject adrenaline into the femoral artery which is adjacent to the nerve. Some authors advocate the use of sciatic nerve block for tibial fractures.

Intravenous opiate

In trauma situations opiate analgesia should always be given intravenously. There is no place for the intramuscular route as it is unreliably absorbed and will not necessarily provide the effect required.

The weight of the child should be estimated by whatever means possible and the appropriate dose of opiate obtained. This should be further diluted to 10 ml. This can then be titrated 1 ml at a time over a period of 10 minutes to maximal effect. As soon as the child becomes settled the administration can be stopped and a further bolus given at intervals to maintain analgesia. Usually at this stage the pain drive will be sufficient to keep the child awake and to counteract any diminution of level of consciousness. If there is any concern subsequently about the ability to assess either the level of consciousness or abdomen then naloxone can be offered to reverse the opiate.

Once analgesia has been administered, the fractured limb should be splinted by whatever means possible until such time as the child can be brought to theater by the orthopedic surgeons.

It should be stressed that orthopedic injuries are a long way down the order of treatment. Priority should be given to airway, breathing and circulation prior to doing anything with orthopedic injuries.

BURN CARE (Ch. 31)

Burns are a common pediatric problem. Two issues need to be addressed:

1. the burn injury
2. complication such as smoke inhalation, hypothermia, toxic shock syndrome.

Although both the burn injury and an associated complication can occur together, usually either one or the other is the main problem on initial presentation to the accident and emergency department. There are many possible etiologies for burn injury (Table 32.4), but whatever the cause, the approach is the same: the airway, breathing and circulation should be assessed and looked after as in all previous circumstances. Once these have been addressed it is important to identify the size of the burn. Management of the burn will depend on the following factors:

1. area involved
2. depth of the burn
3. site of the burn.

Area of the burn

Small burns, i.e. less than 5% of total body surface area (TBSA), can be managed on an outpatient basis provided that the burn is superficial, does not involve an area such as the face, and there are no complications present. Treatment will consist of analgesia, usually oral, and dressings according to local policy. One method of dressing the burn is to use mupirocin-impregnated tulle gras which is an effective antistaphylococcal agent. If the burn is greater than 5% TBSA analgesia requirements will usually be greater than can be managed on an outpatient basis and the child should be admitted. Intravenous opiate will be required. Whether the wounds are dressed or left open is dependent on local practice. There is some evidence that leaving the burns open is more beneficial. If the burn is greater than 10% TBSA the child will need intravenous rehydration according to local formulae, e.g. Muir and Barclay formula. The child should be admitted for inpatient care.

Depth of the burn

Burns can be classified into superficial, partial thickness and full thickness. Superficial burns include those with erythema only or with small amounts of blistering. Partial thickness burns are those

Table 32.4   Causes of burn injury

1. Wet heat	Scald
2. Dry heat	Flame
	Hot surface
3. Radiation	Ultraviolet (sunburn)
	Iatrogenic (as radiation treatment in oncology)
4. Chemical	Acid
	Alkali
	Corrosive
5. Electrical	

which have a significant area of blistering, with either blisters intact or spontaneously burst. Full thickness burns present as white avascular areas which are insensitive to touch (it is not usually very kind to touch burns in children and inspection is usually all that is required for diagnosis).

In reality a mixture of superficial, partial thickness and full thickness is often present depending on the burning agent and the duration it has been in contact with the skin. All full thickness burns should be referred to a plastic surgeon for immediate assessment and treatment. Partial thickness burns may be suitable for outpatient care if they do not extend over a large surface area. Treatment is as discussed above.

Site of the burn

Burns to the face, airway, mouth, pharynx, buttock and perineum, hands and feet and any circumferential burn to either the trunk or a limb need to be treated with a great deal of caution. Burns in any of these areas need to be referred to a plastic surgeon for inpatient treatment. Burns to the face and airway in particular may require admission to an intensive care unit as the risk to the airway is quite considerable.

COMPLICATIONS OF BURNS

In the accident and emergency department it is important to identify those children with complications such as smoke inhalation or hypothermia, or which may be the result of nonaccidental injury.

Smoke inhalation

Smoke inhalation is a complex entity with several mechanisms for insult being present at one time. These include:

1. inhalation of toxic fumes such as carbon monoxide and/or cyanide
2. local action of soot and other organic particles
3. chemical burns from acids and other compounds.

Carbon monoxide poisoning and cyanide lead to asphyxia with red cells unable to release oxygen. It is the leading cause of death following house fires in children. Children who are suspected of having carbon monoxide poisoning should be resuscitated with 100% oxygen and consideration should be given to treatment with hyperbaric oxygen. If cyanide is suspected then treatment with standard cyanide kits is suggested, either with dicobalt edetate if the child is comatose and asystolic, or sodium nitrate and thiosulfate solutions if the child is comatose but still perfusing.

Bronchial lavage may be considered if particulate matter or acids are considered to be present in the airway.

The net result of the contamination is a fulminant inflammatory process leading to pulmonary edema. This can be of insidious onset, so all children who are suspected of having had smoke inhalation should be admitted for a period of observation until they are proved normal.

MANAGEMENT OF THE UNSTABLE CHILD WITH UNDERLYING PATHOLOGY

In this situation one will have secured the airway, breathing and circulation and probably have some idea as to the underlying pathology. It is easy, for instance, to identify a child who is in status epilepticus, with profound respiratory distress, or who is comatose. The real challenge is to identify the actual disease process and the etiologic factors so that the most appropriate therapy can be given.

In these situations the standard approach of taking history and then doing a physical examination should go by the wayside. Often a history will be available at this stage, but it may be scrappy and imprecise. Most information will be gained from a detailed physical examination. This is best done in a systematic fashion, excluding groups of illnesses in turn.

Patterns of illness include:

1. infection
2. seizure disorder and coma
3. metabolic abnormalities
4. cardiac lesions
5. respiratory disorders
6. surgical pathology
7. poisoning
8. life-threatening infection.

INFECTION

Life-threatening infection is relatively rare in the western world where vaccination and immunization are widespread. Diseases such as diphtheria and epiglottitis are more or less eradicated with effective vaccination but in areas where vaccination is less good or has waned these diseases continue to form important causes of mortality. Meningococcemia continues to be one of the most important life-threatening infections to appear acutely to the accident and emergency department.

When dealing with infection three broad age groups have to be considered:

1. those aged 0–3 months
2. those aged 3–36 months
3. those aged over 36 months.

Children aged 0–3 months

These children are either in or adjacent to the neonatal period and consequently have many of the problems associated with this time of life. The symptoms with which these children present are many and varied. They include going off feeds, failure to thrive, jitteriness and irritability. The origin of their symptoms may include congenital anomalies such as congenital heart disease or inborn errors of metabolism. Surgical causes such as intussusception and obstructed hernia may also present in this way.

Physical signs such as neck stiffness and bulging fontanels are imprecise in this age group. Blood parameters such as white cell count and preponderance of neutrophils to lymphocytes are also imprecise. Clinical suspicion therefore is the mainstay of diagnosis and if there is any doubt children should have blood cultures taken and antibiotic treatment started. These children are usually admitted until a diagnosis is reached.

Children aged 3 months to 3 years

The children at the lower end of this spectrum will still be prone to the problems in the younger age group. Viral illness is still more common than bacterial illness in this age group but underlying

bacterial illness or bacteremia should nevertheless be considered. Physical signs are more precise with these children often being pyrexial, tachycardiac and tachypneic. Signs such as neck stiffness may be more reliable in meningitis. Signs of chest infection, osteomyelitis and septic arthritis may also be easier to detect. There are still problems with the diagnosis of surgical causes such as acute abdomen (Baraff 1993, Baraff et al 1993).

Children aged 3 years and over

Significant bacterial disease is relatively rare in this age group but is a particular worry. Common causes include chest infection, septicemia, urinary tract infection and orthopedic infection. Meningitis and meningococcal septicemia are still relatively rare. Abdominal conditions are easier to diagnose in these children because they are better able to communicate symptoms.

Management of life-threatening infection

Children should be resuscitated and blood taken for full blood count, urea and electrolytes, blood glucose and culture. Chest X-ray, urine culture and lumbar puncture may also be indicated. Care should be taken not to perform lumbar puncture on children who are unconscious as this may produce herniation of the brain through the tentorium (coning) with resultant brain death.

Intravenous antibiotics should be administered according to local sensitivity patterns and protocols. Children should be admitted to a high dependency or intensive care unit where inotropic support may be needed.

SEIZURE DISORDER

Most seizure disorder presenting in this way will either be due to idiopathic epilepsy or febrile seizure disorder, or secondary to metabolic defects such as hypoglycemia or an electrolyte disorder. Trauma may also be considered. Treatment should be aimed at stopping the seizure and at the same time trying to identify underlying treatable causes such as hypoglycemia and electrolyte imbalance. If fever is present this should be reduced as rapidly as possible.

Management of seizure disorder in the emergency situation

First-line treatment is i.v. diazepam, 0.2 mg/kg to a maximum 0.6 mg/kg intravenously. This should be followed (if the seizure is not stopped) by a slow i.v. administration of phenytoin 10–15 mg/kg under ECG control. At this stage if the child is still fitting then consideration must be given to reducing intracranial pressure and it may be necessary to paralyze and ventilate the child for control of seizure. Airway and ventilation can also be better maintained and the child should be admitted to the intensive care/high dependency unit.

Blood sugar should always be tested by strip testing and in the laboratory. If the blood sugar is low this may reveal an underlying metabolic disorder. Further blood should be taken along with urine to help diagnose metabolic anomalies if present and the child should be given 25% glucose 1–2 ml/kg.

COMA

Comatose children are particularly at risk of airway problems so great care must be given to maintaining the airway and ventilation. Once this is secured, the underlying causes such as poisoning, epilepsy, head injury (or other trauma), hypoglycemia or intracranial infection should be suspected. Treatable causes should be identified and managed appropriately and the child transferred to a high dependency area. This may involve transfer via CT scanning if an intracranial lesion is suspected. If trauma is suspected (particularly NAI), the child should be treated as with any other trauma victim and resuscitated aggressively prior to transfer.

METABOLIC ABNORMALITIES

Diabetic abnormalities, either hypo- or hyperglycemia, are those most commonly presenting and should be managed as discussed in Chapter 20. Small babies may present critically ill as a result of an inborn error of metabolism and while these are rare, they should be suspected in any child who presents close to the neonatal period, particularly if an intercurrent infection is suspected. A strong clue may be hypoglycemia.

CARDIAC LESIONS

Children with cardiac lesions present either in heart failure or in cardiac arrest.

Heart failure

Heart failure is often due to progression of cardiac abnormalities, and underlying processes such as renal failure may also be present. Supraventricular tachycardia (SVT) is the commonest underlying cardiac dysrhythmia to cause heart failure, particularly in younger age groups. The treatment of heart failure should be aimed towards maximizing oxygenation and reducing the fluid load. Any underlying dysrhythmia should be treated appropriately according to local guidelines. The child should be transferred as soon as possible to a high dependency area, where future treatment can be monitored and inotropic support given if necessary.

Cardiac arrest

Cardiac arrest is considered earlier (p. 1807). The underlying causes may include hypertrophic cardiomyopathy or dysrhythmia.

RESPIRATORY DISORDERS

Common respiratory disorders presenting in accident and emergency departments include asthma, bronchiolitis, croup and foreign body in the airway. Recognition of respiratory distress/failure has been considered earlier (p. 522). All children with respiratory disease should have oxygen delivery maximized and then treatment directed specifically against the underlying cause.

If a foreign body is suspected wedged in the airway, the Heimlich maneuver or chest thrust maneuver may be necessary, depending on the level of consciousness of the child.

SURGICAL CAUSES

Surgical causes of collapse are often forgotten in the accident and emergency department, particularly in the younger age group. Intussusception and obstructed herniae commonly cause symptoms such as vomiting. This vomiting is not typical of that of gastroenteritis and may only consist of one or two vomits. After that the child becomes unduly collapsed. Intussusception in particular can present with a child who is deathly pale but without much else in the way of physical signs. The classic signs of redcurrent jelly stool and a palpable mass are often absent (MacDonald & Beattie 1995).

Pyloric stenosis may present with a dehydrated alkalotic child if the vomiting has been profuse.

As with all conditions, a strong index of suspicion is required. All of these conditions may require the child to be resuscitated according to standard guidelines and transferred for appropriate surgical opinion and intervention.

Of particular concern is the peripubertal girl presenting in a collapsed state. Two diagnoses should be considered: drug overdose (either intentional or accidental); and ectopic pregnancy. These may be related (i.e. the pregnancy may be the reason for the overdose). In both situations resuscitation is vital and should follow the lines as described above. Pregnancy may be the result of child sexual abuse and this should be managed, if suspected, along local guidelines.

POISONING (Ch. 29)

Poisoning in children is commonest between the second and third year of life. Children who are poisoned usually present with minimal signs or symptoms. The role of the accident and emergency department is to identify the child who is at risk of either airway or circulatory collapse and to deal with these problems accordingly. The detailed management of poisoning in this age group is beyond the scope of this section. Suffice to say that all doctors working in accident and emergency should have a good working knowledge of pharmacology of medications that are both prescribed and bought over the counter. The knowledge of the potential side-effects will help in determining which children can be discharged and which need to be admitted for further care. The local poison center phone number must be easily available in the unit.

The role of gastric decontamination in this age group is difficult. The current trend is to move away from gastric lavage, which is seen as a particularly unpleasant process to inflict on children. The role of syrup of ipecacuanha has also been challenged: there is evidence to suggest that it will only be effective (if at all) if administered within 1 hour of the ingestion (Bond et al 1993, Young & Bivins 1993). Current vogue for decontamination is to administer charcoal to the child. Most children will actually drink charcoal despite it looking unpleasant and this is probably the method of choice for all children who require gastric decontamination.

Specific antidotes are available for only a few poisons. Staff working within accident and emergency departments should be familiar with these and their usage.

MENINGOCOCCAL DISEASE (Ch. 23)

Infection with *Neisseria meningitidis* is probably one of the most significant causes of critical illness in children. Often starting as a vague nonspecific illness at any age, this infection can kill within hours. The florid purpuric rash is often not present initially, more often developing from a subtle finding in the early stages. In the community, treatment should consist of intramuscular benzylpenicillin and urgent transfer to hospital with supplemental oxygen by mask to raise the F_iO_2. In the accident and emergency department, i.v. access and fluid replacement will be added. Fluid volumes of 60 ml/kg may be needed (in 10–20 ml/kg bolus) to restore perfusion. A cephalosporin (e.g. cefuroxime or cefotaxime) will be added to penicillin to control infection. Prompt transfer to the intensive therapy unit should be arranged, when inotropic agents may be added.

SAFE TRANSFER

All categories of ill and injured children will require initial transfer to the accident and emergency department. Subsequent to this they will need to be transferred from the resuscitation room to facilitate further investigation and/or treatment. This may be in-house but some will require transport between hospitals. There should be careful liaison between the intensive care unit and the accident and emergency department to ensure that this transfer is as safe and expeditious as possible. Treatment and resuscitation may need to be continued during the transfer. In particular, care to the airway, breathing and circulation will be mandatory. The transport should be effected by people experienced in the care of all these areas and who are able to intervene en route if required.

Consideration should be given to the mode of transport to enable possible interventions en route.

STABLE CHILDREN

Stable children require work-up and disposal as appropriate but no active resuscitation. They should be regularly reviewed to ensure they remain stable.

CONCLUSION

In summary, the pediatric emergency medical system has many facets, all of which need to be coordinated to provide for the streamlined care of children. The aim should be prevention if at all possible. If prevention is not possible, then facilities must exist for the efficient care of all children within a seamless emergency medical structure capable of providing all aspects of emergency care and rehabilitation back to the community.

PEDIATRIC INTENSIVE CARE

Following initial resuscitation and treatment of the patient in the accident and emergency department, consideration must be given to the most appropriate location in which the child can receive ongoing medical and nursing care. This may be a general ward, a high dependency area, or an intensive care unit (ICU). The ICU is an area of the hospital which is staffed and equipped to a high standard specifically for the treatment of reversible acute or impending organ failure (Fig. 32.4). An appropriately trained member of the medical staff should always be present on the ICU, and the nurse to patient ratio is 1 : 1 or greater. On the ICU there should be the capacity to monitor a wide range of physiological

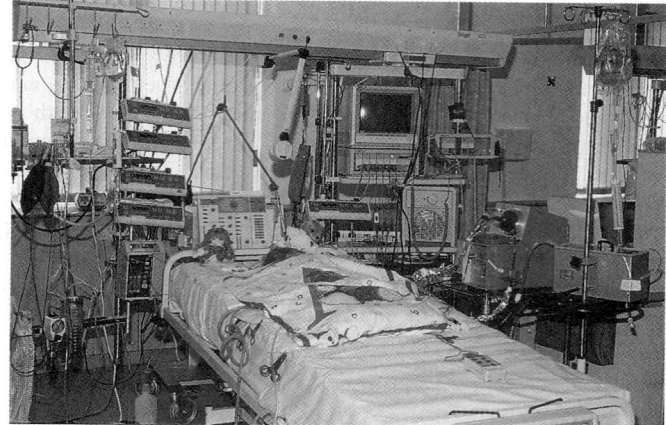

Fig. 32.4 Intensive care bed space with monitoring equipment.

variables, including: heart rate and rhythm; saturation by pulse oximetry; blood pressure (invasively and noninvasively); core temperature; central venous, atrial, or pulmonary artery pressure; intracranial pressure; and end-tidal carbon dioxide levels. There should be easy access to full laboratory services. There is a range of therapies which, irrespective of the child's underlying diagnosis, are most appropriately administered in the ICU setting (Table 32.5). In general these are interventions or techniques of life support which if suddenly withdrawn or accidentally interrupted would place the child's life at immediate risk.

Pediatric intensive care units usually admit children not only from the accident and emergency department but also from medical and surgical specialties. Admissions following surgery, trauma or as a result of infectious disease form the majority of admissions. This varied case mix means that the successful management of a child in the ICU will require a cooperative approach across the disciplines. Unfortunately, as highlighted by a recent report by the British Paediatric Association (British Paediatric Association 1993), intensive care services for children in the UK are highly fragmented, with only half the children requiring and receiving intensive care in 1991 treated in a pediatric intensive care unit. A lower mortality has been demonstrated in children who are treated in specialist intensive care units compared with children who are cared for in mixed adult and pediatric units in nontertiary hospitals (Pollack et al 1991). This, coupled with the effect of work volume (Farley & Ozminkowski 1992), and the impact of full time specialist appointments in pediatric intensive care (Pollack et al 1988), has led to the suggestion that pediatric intensive care may be most effectively delivered in the UK by large pediatric intensive care units (Shann 1993).

Table 32.5 Therapies and support administered in intensive care

Endotracheal intubation
Mechanical ventilatory support
Continuous invasive pressure measurement
Vasoactive drug infusion
Continuous antiarrhythmic infusions
Intra-aortic balloon counterpulsation
Extracorporeal life support
Nitric oxide administration

TRANSPORT SERVICES

The development of regional centers brings with it the need for the establishment of safe and efficient transport services for the critically ill child (Day 1993, Pon & Notterman 1993, Macrae 1994). The goal during transport should be to provide the same or better quality of care than the patient had before transport. A detailed log of transport requests should be kept. Information recorded should include the call time, demographic data, a brief history and diagnosis, a summary of interventions already undertaken and recommendations for further management tailored to the capabilities of the referring hospital. The transport team should be experienced in airway management, resuscitation and vascular access and should have specific training in transport medicine including aviation medicine. Equipment taken should enable continuous monitoring of physiological parameters during stabilization and transport of the patient (Table 32.6) as well as allow the team to perform any resuscitative measures that may be required. The child should be fully resuscitated and stabilized by the transport team prior to transfer.

INITIAL ASSESSMENT

Whether the patient has been transferred within or between hospitals, the initial assessment in the ICU is identical. The basic sequence of checking the airway, ensuring adequate ventilation and circulation is performed to ensure no ill effects of transport. After initial restabilization of the patient and review of the history and physical findings, management is usually directed at both specific and general support measures whilst investigations are performed to confirm the clinical diagnosis. Management of specific medical conditions is discussed in the relevant chapters elsewhere in this book. The rest of this chapter will adopt a more general approach and focus on major organ support. The support modalities used in any particular case will depend on the clinician's assessment of the condition of the child and the underlying disease process.

RESPIRATORY SUPPORT

Any critically ill child should receive oxygen in an attempt to restore and maintain oxygen delivery to the cells. The success of this treatment depends upon an adequately functioning respiratory system, satisfactory cardiac output and hemoglobin level. The child with respiratory distress may be cyanotic or pale, have tachypnea, dyspnea, tachycardia or agitation. A decreasing level of consciousness, falling respiratory rate and falling heart rate are preterminal signs. Simple techniques for maintenance of the airway have already been described (Ch. 12); however, endotracheal intubation may be required to guarantee an adequate airway. Intubation with spontaneous ventilation may be used in

the relief of upper airway obstruction, or in patients who have lost protective upper airway reflexes but have adequate ventilation.

Mechanical ventilation is one of the major support modalities used in pediatric intensive care. There are five major indications for assisted ventilation:

1. Respiratory failure caused by intrinsic pulmonary disease which includes alveolar and interstitial disorders as well as airway diseases.

2. Ventilatory failure due to neuromuscular disorders or respiratory muscle fatigue.

3. Circulatory problems with cardiovascular dysfunction such as shock syndrome or after cardiac arrest.

4. Central nervous system dysfunction, including head and spinal cord lesions, abnormalities in the control of breathing, status epilepticus or infectious encephalopathy.

5. Surgical indications, for example in the patient after cardiac surgery, prolonged and extensive abdominal surgery or after trauma.

VENTILATOR CHARACTERISTICS

In order to use ventilators effectively, a basic understanding of their functional characteristics and of lung mechanics is required (see pp. 159, 498). In practice, volume limited, time cycled ventilators are often used to ventilate older children and pressure limited, time cycled ventilators for infants. High frequency ventilation is considered separately.

In volume limited ventilation, the patient receives a specified tidal volume with each mechanical breath. The frequency of the breaths and the inspiratory time are specified. An adequate inspiratory flow rate must be provided through the ventilator so that the specified tidal volume can be delivered within the chosen inspiratory time. The maximum positive pressure reached during the respiratory cycle depends on the flow rate to the ventilator and the compliance and resistance of the circuit and patient's lungs. Thus the primary set parameter is the tidal volume, and the secondary or derived parameter is the peak pressure. With pressure limited ventilation, a peak pressure is specified and when that pressure is reached, excess flow to the ventilator is released through a pressure release valve. This ensures that the preset pressure is not exceeded. Time cycled pressure limited ventilation is a common mode used in neonatology in which an inspiratory flow rate, time and pressure limit are designated. The tidal volume delivered depends upon the compliance and resistance of the circuit and patient's lungs. The tidal volume delivered can be altered by changing the inspiratory flow rate, the inspiratory time or pressure limit. In this mode of ventilation the primary set parameter is the pressure whilst the secondary derived parameter is the volume of gas delivered.

Volume limited time cycled and pressure limited time cycled ventilators can be used in either an assist mode or control mode. In the assist mode, the patient initiates the ventilator cycle using a trigger system which detects altered flow or pressure in the circuit. When the ventilator senses the patient's breath, inspiratory flow is initiated and a preset volume or peak pressure is delivered to the patient. In control mode a preset tidal volume, or preset pressure and rate are set for the ventilator. The patient has no alternative but to breathe with the ventilator. There are some variants of the assist and control modes which allow patients to initiate inspiratory cycles on a background preset rate. This means that a minimum

Table 32.6 Monitoring capacity required during transport

ECG
Oxygen saturation
Blood pressure (by noninvasive and invasive means)
Temperature
Other invasive pressure, e.g. central venous pressure
End-tidal CO_2

level of mechanical ventilation is maintained should the patient become apneic or unable to trigger the ventilator. One such mode is intermittent mandatory ventilation. Here the patient can breath spontaneously between ventilator breaths. The ventilator breaths are time cycled and they may occur at any phase of the patient's own respiratory cycle. An improvement upon this is synchronized intermittent mandatory ventilation. Again the patient can breathe spontaneously and receives a fixed number of volume limited breaths at a set rate. This time the ventilator senses the patient's inspiratory effort and cycles so that the positive pressure breaths are synchronized with the patient's own breath. The application of positive end-expiratory pressure (PEEP) ensures that the airway pressure remains positive at the end of expiration. It can be applied in both pressure limited and volume limited ventilators and is used to increase functional residual capacity to improve gas exchange. Continuous positive airway pressure (CPAP) refers to the maintenance of positive airway pressure throughout the respiratory cycle when the patient is spontaneously breathing. Again the aim is to increase functional residual capacity. There are a variety of ways of delivering CPAP: via an endotracheal or nasopharyngeal tube; via nasal prongs or cannulae; or by a tight-fitting face mask. Excessive levels of CPAP or PEEP may cause problems with overdistension of the lung and impedance of systemic venous return and hence diminution of cardiac output.

CLINICAL APPLICATIONS

The exact nature of the ventilatory support chosen depends on the size of the child and the nature of the illness. When determining initial ventilator settings in the intubated patient the patient is often hand ventilated using a T-piece circuit with pressure monitor to gauge airway compliance. Clinical assessment should include the magnitude and symmetry of the chest movement. On a volume limited ventilator tidal breaths are usually set at 12–15 ml/kg and on a pressure limited ventilator a peak pressure is chosen that results in adequate chest expansion. A respiratory rate appropriate for the age of the child should be chosen.

Application of PEEP depends on the clinical circumstance, and further adjustments of the ventilator parameters are made following blood gas analysis. Children with upper airway obstruction may simply require an artificial airway to relieve this obstruction and may not necessarily need to be ventilated. Children with lower airway obstruction problems such as asthma are at risk of decreased cardiac output and hypotension during intubation and mechanical ventilation as positive pressure applied to already hyperinflated lungs may impede venous return, secondary to high intrathoracic pressure. When ventilating asthmatic children a prolonged expiratory phase is usually required. A volume limited ventilator is often used and a cuffed endotracheal tube may be required. In patients with acute respiratory distress syndrome, problems include a reduction in the functional residual capacity of the lung with an increase in the closing volume close to functional residual capacity, atelectasis and ventilation–perfusion mismatch. Maintenance of lung volume is therefore very important and this may be achieved with either CPAP or PEEP. In patients with severe acute respiratory distress syndrome, mild hypercapnia is often accepted, rather than induce barotrauma with aggressive ventilation (permissive hypercapnia). In children suffering from weakness of their respiratory muscles, a normal tidal volume and rate can be used with inspired oxygen concentration kept to a minimum. Wherever possible, an assist

mode is used to prevent disuse atrophy of the muscles. Ventilation in patients with heart failure may relieve alveolar collapse from edema and decrease oxygen demand by decreasing the work of breathing. Judicious use of PEEP or CPAP may relieve atelectasis. Manipulation of ventilation can often be used therapeutically in the treatment of disorders of pulmonary vascular resistance. Ventilation may be required in the postoperative cardiac surgical patient, depending on the age and preoperative status of the patient, the complexity and duration of the surgery. Controlled ventilation is normally used until hemodynamic stability is achieved. Following some surgical procedures such as the Fontan operation (p. 621), early extubation is the goal in order to avoid high intrathoracic pressures, which may impede passage of blood flow across the pulmonary vascular bed. In patients with raised intracranial pressure, ventilation may be used to manipulate pH and hence alter cerebral vascular resistance. Low PEEP pressures are used where possible as high intrathoracic pressures may impede cerebral venous return to heart.

Weaning starts when the pathology for which the patient was ventilated in the first place is resolving. The patient must be able to take over ventilation without excess energy expenditure, and there must be adequate respiratory muscle strength, hemodynamic stability and a good nutritional state. Extubation is performed when the patient is awake and alert with protective airway reflexes and is hemodynamically and metabolically stable with effective breathing.

Complications

Positive pressure ventilation is not without complications. Damage to the airway from the endotracheal tube can occur. This includes problems with nasal alar necrosis, development of palatal grooves, laryngeal edema, ulceration of the vocal cords and subglottic scarring and stenosis. Ventilation using high airway pressure can cause overdistension of alveoli and alveolar rupture, alterations in cardiac filling and output and altered mucociliary clearance. Problems can also occur with the equipment, with either mechanical failure of the ventilator or alarm failure, or problems with humidification of gases leading to endotracheal tube blockage.

High frequency ventilation

This is a term applied to a variety of ventilatory modes characterized by a supraphysiological ventilator rate and a low tidal volume which may be less than or equal to the physiological dead space during conventional ventilation. There is still marked debate as to how gas exchange actually occurs during high frequency ventilation (Wetzel & Gioia 1987). The three main modes are high frequency positive pressure ventilation, high frequency jet ventilation and high frequency oscillatory ventilation (HFPPV, HFJV, HFOV). In HFPPV the breath rate is set at 60–100 cycles per minute with a tidal volume of 3–4 ml/kg. A gas mix is intermittently delivered via a side arm of the main inspiratory limb. In HFJV a jet injects a gas mix at high velocity into the trachea with rates of 100–400 cycles per minute and tidal volume of 3–5 ml/kg (Wetzel & Gioia 1987, Smith et al 1993). In HFOV, which is used with a breath rate of 900–3600 cycles per minute, alternating positive and negative pressure is generated in the airway by a piston pump or diaphragm (Arnold et al 1993, Arnold et al 1994). Tidal volumes are in the range of 1–3 ml/kg. This is the only mode of high frequency ventilation with an active expiratory phase. High frequency ventilation is used clinically when it is important to minimize volutrauma to the lungs, in the treatment of bronchopleural fistula, and occasionally in patients with acute respiratory distress syndrome (Paulson et al 1995). The combination of high frequency ventilation with nitric oxide may prove useful in the treatment of persistent pulmonary hypertension of the newborn.

CARDIOVASCULAR SUPPORT

It is important to be able to recognize the child in need of cardiovascular support and to treat the circulatory dysfunction appropriately. A basic understanding of the principles that determine normal myocardial performance provides the background for formulating plans for appropriate therapy. The metabolic needs of the body for nutrients and adequate oxygen delivery are primarily met by changes in cardiac output. The cardiac output is determined by the heart rate and the stroke volume (the portion of blood that is ejected from the ventricle by a single heartbeat). The magnitude of this stroke volume is influenced by the myocardial end-diastolic fiber length (preload), the contractility of the myocardium and the ventricular afterload.

A decreased preload, and hence decreased cardiac output, occurs in a variety of conditions commonly encountered on the ICU. For example, decreased blood volume or plasma volume in hemorrhagic shock or sepsis may result in a decrease in diastolic volume. Supraventricular tachycardias can result in a markedly decreased diastolic filling time and hence decreased end-diastolic volume. Although heart rate is a determinant of cardiac output, at very fast rates the increase in heart rate cannot completely compensate for the decrease in end-diastolic volume and hence a low cardiac output state results. Atrial flutter or fibrillation may lower cardiac output due to the loss of the 'atrial kick' which augments late diastolic filling. Iatrogenic factors are also important causes of decreased venous return and low end-diastolic volume, for example high mean airway pressure in ventilated patients, excessive vasodilator therapy and aggressive diuresis. Clinically, right and left atrial pressures are used as indicators of ventricular end-diastolic pressure, the relationship between end-diastolic pressure and volume being determined by the compliance of the ventricle. Caution is needed when interpreting atrial pressure as a measure of ventricular preload. Factors which alter the distensibility of the myocardium may result in a decreased end-diastolic volume or a failure for the end-diastolic volume to increase normally in response to fluid challenge, whilst the end-diastolic pressure increases markedly. Hence, despite high systemic and pulmonary venous pressures there may be a normal or low end-diastolic volume. Major alterations in distensibility may occur in myocardium subjected to problems such as ischemia, hypoxia or acidosis. Rapid accumulation of a pericardial effusion can limit filling of the heart, resulting in a low end-diastolic volume and low cardiac output despite high measured filling pressures.

Depression of the contractile state of the myocardium can occur with a range of common disorders, for example sepsis, acidosis, hypoglycemia, hypoxia or hypocalcemia. In addition, a number of antiarrhythmic drugs used in the treatment of resistant rhythm disturbances, such as verapamil and procainamide, can also decrease the contractile state. Patients with cardiomyopathy and myocarditis may have an intrinsic decrease in the contractile state of their myocardium.

Alterations in afterload, the opposition to blood ejection from the ventricle, can have a marked effect on stroke volume. Systemic hypertension will lower the left ventricular stroke volume acutely, just as pulmonary hypertension will lower the right ventricular stroke volume. Coarctation of the aorta in the neonate can cause a sudden dramatic alteration in afterload when the duct constricts, resulting in a severe afterload increase on the left ventricle and reduction in cardiac output.

CLINICAL ASSESSMENT AND MANAGEMENT

The patient with severe cardiovascular dysfunction generally has decreased pulses, poor capillary refill, cool extremities, decreased urine output and altered sensorium. A low blood pressure is a preterminal sign, as blood pressure may be maintained by intense vasoconstriction even in the presence of a markedly reduced circulating volume. A chest X-ray gives basic information on heart size and lung fields, whilst an echocardiogram is useful for assessment of myocardial dysfunction as well as documenting the presence of any pericardial fluid. Management strategies can be divided in to those specifically aimed at altering the determinants of cardiac output discussed above, and more general measures.

As cardiac output is dependent on heart rate it is important to check that the patient's heart rate is appropriate for age. Supraventricular tachycardia can result in congestive heart failure and conversion to sinus rhythm by rapid overdrive pacing or cardioversion can dramatically relieve the problem. The postoperative cardiac surgical patient with a bradycardia may require pacing. The first step in the treatment for most ICU patients, however, will be to ensure an adequate preload has been achieved. Central venous lines are normally placed and central venous pressure increased by fluid therapy to levels of 8–10 mmHg. If perfusion, pulse, blood pressure and urine output are not normalized by the fluid challenge, manipulation of contractility or afterload reduction may be required. A range of inotropic drugs, discussed below, are used to manipulate the contractile state of the myocardium. If a decision is made to use vasodilators to reduce afterload, the placement of a Swan–Ganz catheter or Doppler determination of cardiac output may allow changes in cardiac output to be more readily followed.

Whilst trying to maximize cardiac output in infants and children, it is also vital to reduce cardiac work, in an attempt to allow the myocardium to recover. First among these more general therapies is mechanical ventilation with oxygen, coupled with appropriate sedation. Mechanical ventilation will alleviate the work of breathing which may be substantial if there is pulmonary edema or lung dysfunction present. Administration of oxygen, which is important in any ill child, will relieve arterial desaturation and adequate sedation and pain relief will limit endogenous catecholamine secretion and sympathetic vasoconstriction to pain. Anemia should be corrected. Prevention of fever will reduce the metabolic demand that must be met by the heart. It may also reduce heart rate and improve cardiac output by allowing adequate filling during diastole. Treatment of hypothermia will reduce systemic vascular resistance and hence afterload. Finally, a variety of mechanical devices may be used to support the failing heart when therapeutic manipulation of preload, afterload and contractility have failed. These include the intra-aortic balloon pump which reduces left ventricular afterload and improves coronary artery perfusion, and by a variety of extracorporeal life support devices, such as extracorporeal membrane oxygenation (ECMO) or ventricular assist devices which bypass one of the ventricles.

Vasoactive drugs

The three general categories of inotropic agents are the digitalis-like compounds, the phosphodiesterase inhibitors and catecholamines (Steinberg & Notterman 1994).

Digoxin related compounds inhibit the activity of the membrane bound sodium–potassium, adenosine triphosphatase. This results in a raised intracellular sodium which slows the rate of exchange of intracellular calcium for extracellular sodium. The resultant rise in intracellular calcium augments myocardial contractility. Due to its relatively long half life, potentiation by hypokalemia and predominantly renal clearance, digoxin is now less commonly used than continuous catecholamine infusions in the intensive care setting.

Bipyridines, such as amrinone, augment contractility by elevating intracellular cyclic AMP independent of the adrenergic receptor. Amrinone is an inhibitor of phosphodiesterase type III, an enzyme which degrades cyclic AMP. Amrinone is a positive inotrope and a systemic vasodilator, and this combination of inotrope and afterload reducer is useful in situations where myocardial workload should not be excessively increased.

Catecholamines act through stimulation of α and β adrenergic and dopaminergic receptors. A knowledge of the effect of stimulation of the receptors and the receptor profile of the individual catecholamines allows determination of their clinical effect: α-1 adrenergic receptors mediate vasoconstriction; stimulation of β-1 adrenergic receptors results in increased stroke work at a given preload and afterload, and chronotropy; β-2 adrenergic receptors mediate vasodilation and bronchodilation. Dopaminergic receptors are located primarily in the renal, visceral and coronary arteries and, when stimulated, cause blood flow to these organs to increase. The various catecholamines used to treat hemodynamic problems vary in the receptors at which they are active and this activity may also alter with the dose administered.

Dopamine is a neurotransmitter found in sympathetic nerve terminals and in the adrenal medulla. It is often employed to treat mild to moderate cardiogenic or distributive shock associated with moderate degrees of hypotension. At low infusion rates dopaminergic receptor effects predominate, whilst at intermediate rates β-1 and β-2 adrenergic receptor effects are more important, and at high rates α adrenergic receptor effects predominate (Notterman et al 1990, Seri 1995). To treat hypotension, therapy is usually initiated with an infusion rate of 5–10 μg/kg/min and increased until there is evidence of improved cardiac output (skin temperature, capillary refill and urine output) and restoration of appropriate blood pressure for age. Infusion rates greater than 20 μg/kg/min are not customary even if they maintain 'normal blood pressure'. Rates of this magnitude usually result in maintenance of blood pressure by an increase in systemic vascular resistance by α adrenergic activation, rather than improved cardiac output, and should prompt re-examination of the physiological diagnosis or selection of a different agent.

Dobutamine, a synthetic catecholamine is administered as a racemic mixture: (+) dobutamine is a strong β adrenergic receptor agonist and an α adrenergic receptor antagonist; (–) dobutamine is an α adrenergic receptor agonist and a weak β adrenergic receptor agonist (Perkin et al 1982). This results in a drug with significant inotropic activity and minimal chronotropic or vasopressor activity. The major indication for prescribing dobutamine in the pediatric age group is poor myocardial contractility with a normal to moderately decreased blood pressure. Therapy is started at an infusion rate of around 5 μg/kg/min, and the patient should be re-evaluated with a view to changing therapy if there is no substantial improvement with infusion rates of 20 μg/kg/min.

Noradrenaline is the principal neurotransmitter of the sympathetic nervous system. It is a moderately potent α adrenergic receptor agonist with some β-1 adrenergic receptor effect, but little or no β-2 adrenergic receptor activity. It is the agent of choice when the major hemodynamic disturbance involves hypotension with an abnormally low systemic vascular resistance and a normal or high cardiac output, such as may be seen in septic shock. The usual starting dosage is an infusion of 0.1 μg/kg/min up to a maximum of 1 μg/kg/min.

Adrenaline is the principal mediator of the stress response and produces widespread metabolic and hemodynamic effects. It activates adrenergic receptors of the α, β-1 and β-2 types. β adrenergic receptors are activated at low concentrations resulting in inotropy and chronotropy with peripheral β-2 adrenergic receptors promoting relaxation of resistance arteries. At intermediate infusion rates, α-1 adrenergic receptor activation also becomes important, and at very high infusion rates (greater than 1 μg/kg/min) α-1 adrenergic receptor mediated vasoconstriction predominates. Blood flow to individual organs may then be compromised and the associated increase in afterload may further impair myocardial function (Zaritsky & Chernow 1985). The principal use of adrenaline is in the treatment of shock associated with hypotension and myocardial dysfunction.

Intra-aortic balloon pump counterpulsation

The intra-aortic balloon pump is commonly used in adults as a temporary circulatory assist device after cardiac surgery, and is increasingly being used in pediatrics (Park et al 1993). The basic premise behind its development was that removal of blood from the arterial tree during ventricular systole and the rapid reinfusion of the same blood during diastole would increase coronary artery perfusion pressure and decrease the work of the left ventricle (Nanas & Moulopoulos 1994). A balloon catheter is positioned in the thoracic aorta and a gas source, usually helium, used to abruptly inflate and deflate the balloon. Inflation and deflation are triggered by an electrocardiogram in such a way that the balloon inflates in diastole with the closure of the aortic valve and deflates at the start of the systole. By raising diastolic pressure within the proximal aorta by balloon expansion during diastole, coronary perfusion pressure is increased and balloon deflation in systole leaves the aorta relatively empty, hence reducing left ventricular afterload. This decreases myocardial oxygen demand and increases cardiac output at any given level of filling pressure.

Clinical indications

Clinical indications for the insertion of an intra-aortic balloon pump include cardiogenic shock, postoperative low cardiac output syndrome and as an aid to weaning from cardiopulmonary bypass.

Complications

The device is usually inserted percutaneously through the femoral artery (Fig. 32.5), and in very small patients the caliber of the

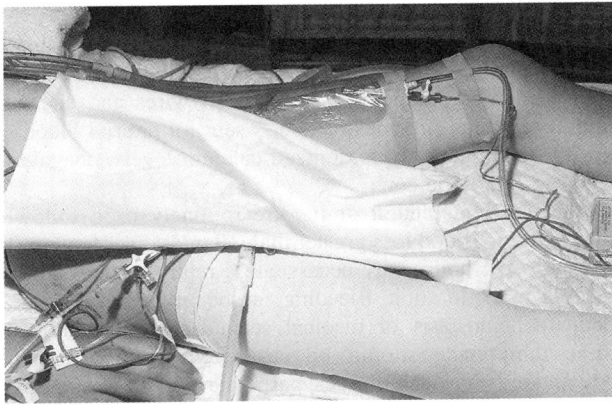

Fig. 32.5 Intra-aortic balloon pump inserted via left femoral artery.

femoral artery may limit the diameter of the gas channel of the device and this, in turn, may restrict balloon filling and emptying. In infants it may also become difficult to move a sufficient volume of gas in the brief time allowed by the short duration of the cardiac cycle. Tachycardia, at any age, has the same effect and arrhythmias may also interfere with the consistent timing of the balloon's cycle. Other problems associated with intra-aortic balloons include limb ischemia, balloon leak or rupture, trauma to the arterial wall incurred whilst inserting the balloon, dislodgment of thrombus during balloon removal and the risk of infection.

Extracorporeal life support

The term extracorporeal life support encompasses a range of techniques including extracorporeal membrane oxygenation (ECMO) and the use of ventricular assist devices. ECMO has been used to support the circulation in a variety of conditions (Table 32.7) (Meliones et al 1991, Butt et al 1992, Shanley et al 1994).

In venoarterial ECMO, blood is drained from the right internal jugular vein or right atrium, pumped through a membrane lung (oxygenator), warmed and returned back into the patient's internal carotid artery or aorta via an arterial catheter, thereby providing mechanical support for both the heart and the lungs (Fig. 32.6). It is sometimes necessary to drain the left atrium as well as the right atrium to the ECMO circuit if the left ventricle is too dysfunctional to pump out the scant amount of blood that enters it from the pulmonary circulation (via bronchial collateral vessels, ductus arteriosus or right ventricle) (Levy et al 1992). If the blood is returned to the right atrium (venovenous ECMO) (Cornish et al 1993), respiratory but no hemodynamic support is provided. ECMO is normally offered only when conventional mechanical

Table 32.7 Range of conditions which may require extracorporeal membrane oxygenation (ECMO)

Meconium aspiration

Congenital diaphragmatic hernia

Idiopathic persistent pulmonary hypertension of the newborn

Acute respiratory distress syndrome

Pneumonia

Following cardiac surgery

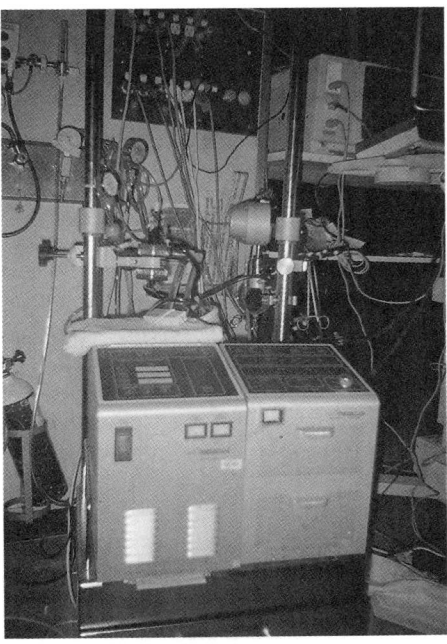

Fig. 32.6 Oxygenator, pump and warmer for ECMO.

ventilation and cardiovascular support fails, and the patient meets criteria for > 80% predicted mortality in the individual institution. The primary disease for which ECMO has been instituted must be reversible, and most centers prefer patients to have received less than 7 days of ventilatory support prior to institution of ECMO, because of the risk of ventilator induced barotrauma (Black et al, 1995, Green et al 1995). ECMO flow rates are adjusted based on blood gases and clinical perfusion of the child. When a patient has been placed on venoarterial ECMO, ventilator peak pressures are reduced and the rate reduced to 4–6 breaths per minute, thereby minimizing the risk of further barotrauma. Systemic heparinization is normally required with ECMO, leading to an increased risk of hemorrhage. Other complications include technical problems with the circuitry, an increased risk of infection, hemolysis and platelet consumption, risk of clot formation in the circuitry and embolization. ECMO is a labor intensive and costly treatment, the clinical benefits of which are difficult to evaluate in a controlled trial in the nonneonatal population because of the wide range in etiology of cardiorespiratory failure in this group (O'Rourke et al 1993).

Ventricular assist devices

Ventricular assist devices may be used in the support of the cardiovascular system after cardiac surgery (Karl et al 1991, Lee et al 1993). The circuitry is similar to, but simpler than that used for ECMO (Fig. 32.7). Blood is drained from the right atrium and pumped in to the pulmonary artery (right ventricular assist) or drained from the left atrium and returned to the aorta (left ventricular assist). A combination of right and left ventricular assist devices ('biVAD') is also possible. No oxygenator is used and a blood warmer is not usually required. Heat loss can be minimized by wrapping the circuitry in silver foil. As the blood is exposed to a foreign surface, anticoagulation is required and the complications are similar to those with ECMO.

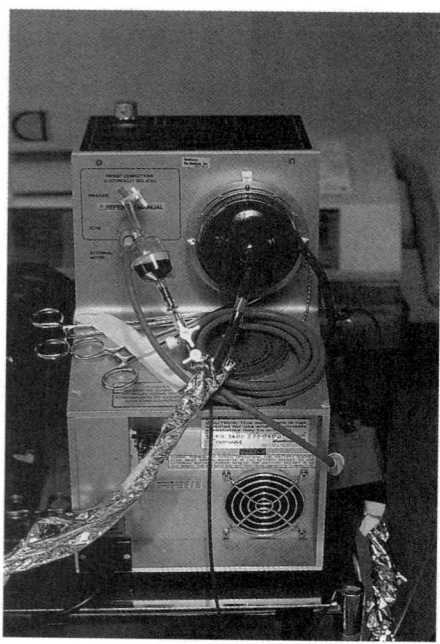

Fig. 32.7   Left ventricular assist device.

POSTOPERATIVE CARE OF THE CARDIAC SURGICAL PATIENT

Patients undergoing cardiac surgery form a special subset of intensive care patients. They may have preoperative organ system dysfunction, suffer transient myocardial ischemia with aortic cross-clamping, or have adverse systemic effects from cardiopulmonary bypass, and thus require skilled management of every major organ system in the immediate postoperative period. There are a number of well recognized postoperative consequences of prolonged cardiopulmonary bypass. These include decreased coagulation factors and platelets due to consumption, activation of the fibrinolytic system and the complement cascade and endothelial cell injury resulting in increased capillary permeability. Mechanical damage can occur to the cellular components of the blood resulting in hemolysis.

When the patient arrives in the ICU, they will have been subjected to a period of transport during which patient monitoring and control are at a minimum. Problems encountered during transport include hypotension due to cardiac dysfunction, volume shifts from moving the patient, or hypertension due to sympathetic stimulation or emergence from anesthesia. Any arrhythmia problem that can be encountered in the postoperative period can occur during the transport. There is also the risk of accidental extubation, or dislodgment of arterial or venous catheters, or drains.

On arrival in the ICU, ECG leads from the bedside monitor should be attached to the patient. If rhythm and blood pressure are stable, the arterial pressure transducer can be transferred to the bedside monitor and the patient placed on the ventilator and breath sounds auscultated. After this, central venous, pulmonary artery or atrial pressures should be transferred to the bedside monitor. A brief verbal account from the anesthetist and surgeon should then be obtained by the ICU team. This should include patient's preoperative history, the intraoperative course and current hemodynamic state including the use of any vasoactive or antiarrhythmic medicines. A full examination of the patient is performed and a chest X-ray is obtained. This is checked for endotracheal tube position, position of all wires and catheters, pneumothorax and effusions. Blood is sent for arterial blood gas analysis, serum electrolytes, ionized calcium levels, coagulation studies and full blood count.

Mediastinal and pleural drains are routinely used following cardiac surgery. Blood loss greater than 10 ml/kg in 1 hour or 3–5 ml/kg/h for 3–4 hours may necessitate a return to the operating theater for re-exploration. Bleeding can be either surgical due to inadequate hemostasis or medical secondary to coagulopathy. Cardiac tamponade should be suspected when a patient's postoperative course deteriorates, particularly if chest drain losses have suddenly diminished. A narrow pulse pressure, decreased blood pressure, rising right atrial pressure with jugular venous distention, tachycardia and poor peripheral perfusion may occur. Cardiac tamponade can be due to either global compression or regional compression of a low pressure chamber, e.g. the left atrium by hematoma. Prompt volume infusion is necessary to maintain cardiac output whilst the patient's chest is reopened.

POSTOPERATIVE COMPLICATIONS

Postoperative pulmonary hypertension may occur, for example after repair of ventricular septal defects, truncus arteriosus, or total anomalous pulmonary venous drainage. Initial therapy includes adequate sedation of the patient, optimization of lung volume, high alveolar oxygen tension and an alkaline blood pH. Thereafter consideration is given to treatment with specific vasodilators such as nitric oxide (see below). Dysrhythmias such as bundle branch block and complete heart block may develop in the postoperative period and be transient or permanent. Cardiac pacing may be an effective and reliable means of ensuring adequate heart rate and if postpericardotomy heart block is anticipated atrial and ventricular epicardial pacing wires are placed at the time of operation. Nodal tachycardias may require treatment with overdrive pacing, cooling or amiodarone. Postpericardotomy syndrome is an inflammation of the pericardium that can follow any surgical manipulation of the pericardium. It can present with signs of tamponade, or the patient can have a swinging fever and irritability. A pericardial friction rub may be present, with enlargement of the cardiac silhouette on chest X-ray because of pericardial fluid accumulation. The condition is generally self limiting but may require treatment with steroids or other anti-inflammatory agents.

The patient may develop acute renal failure, particularly if there is perioperative hypotension. Careful attention to fluid balance and electrolytes must be paid in all postoperative cardiac patients, with appropriate treatment of hypotension. Dialysis may be required in patients with an expanded extracellular volume, hyperkalemia, or acidosis, or to facilitate appropriate fluid management. Peritoneal dialysis is the usual first-line renal support, but continuous venovenous hemofiltration may be appropriate. Acute hepatic failure can also occur, particularly in those in whom an elevated venous pressure is required to maintain pulmonary blood flow. Bilirubin, serum transaminase levels, prothrombin and glucose levels should be followed, with appropriate treatment of hypoglycemia, coagulopathy or hyperammonemia.

Diaphragmatic paralysis can occur after cardiac surgery, as the phrenic nerve is susceptible to injury by transection, traction or cold injury. Phrenic nerve paralysis seen in the immediate postoperative period is not always irreversible, and recovery may occur after several days or weeks. Failure to wean from positive pressure ventilation may be the first clue to diaphragmatic paralysis, and the diagnosis can usually be made in the spontaneously breathing patient, where an elevated hemidiaphragm with paradoxical movement is noted. Positive pressure ventilation may be continued for several weeks to allow spontaneous recovery of the diaphragm to occur, otherwise plication of the diaphragm is required. In any patient who fails to wean from ventilation the possibility of a residual cardiac lesion must also be considered. Postoperative chylothorax results from injury to the thoracic duct or its intrathoracic tributaries. Pleural effusions develop which appear milky once feeds have been reinstituted. Management includes pleural drainage and a diet that is low in long chain fatty acids, but occasionally pleurodesis or ligation of the thoracic duct may be necessary.

NITRIC OXIDE

Treatment with inhaled nitric oxide is becoming a more common occurrence in the ICU. Nitric oxide (NO) is composed of a single atom of oxygen and a single atom of nitrogen. Recent research has revealed a major physiological role for NO in a variety of mammalian tissues. It is involved in the modulation of vascular tone in both the systemic and pulmonary circulation. It is a potent inhibitor of human platelet aggregation and may play a role in neurotransmission. In 1980, Furchgott and Zawadzki reported a relaxant effect of acetylcholine in vitro on arterial ring preparations with intact endothelium. They postulated the presence of an endothelium derived relaxing factor. Since then, two independent research groups have suggested that NO accounts for the action of endothelium derived relaxing factor (Ignarro et al 1987, Palmer et al 1987).

MECHANISM OF ACTION

NO activates soluble guanylate cyclase which stimulates the production of cyclic guanosine monophosphate which, in turn, promotes relaxation of smooth muscle cells (Moncada et al 1991). The mechanism of vasodilation of the commonly used drugs sodium nitroprusside and nitroglycerine is now attributed to the chemical conversion of these nitrovasodilators to NO by the endothelial cells of the blood vessels.

Endogenous NO is generated as a result of oxidation of L-arginine by nitric oxide synthase (NOS). There are two main forms of NOS, a constitutive form which is calcium and calmodulin dependent and an inducible form which is calcium independent. Vascular endothelial cells normally synthesize NO using the constitutive form of NOS and this enzyme is also responsible for the generation of NO by platelets. Inducible NOS, present in vascular endothelial cells, vascular smooth muscle and phagocytic cells, is activated by immunological stimuli. Stimulation of this enzyme in patients with septic shock may be responsible for overproduction of NO and profound vasodilation (Radomski et al 1987, Moncada et al 1991, Kilbourn & Griffith 1992).

Irrespective of its mode of production, NO has a short half life of 3–5 seconds and is quickly oxidized to yield nitrites and nitrates. Hemoglobin has a high binding affinity for nitric oxide inactivating it, resulting in the production of nitrosyl hemoglobin which, in the presence of oxygen, is oxidized to methemoglobin. When NO is inhaled, it diffuses from the alveoli through the walls of the nearby blood vessels causing vasodilation before reaching the bloodstream and being inactivated by hemoglobin. This restricts the vasodilatory effects of NO to the pulmonary vasculature and prevents widespread systemic vasodilation. Intravenously administered vasodilators may increase V/Q mismatch in the lung, whereas administration of inhaled nitric oxide should improve perfusion to ventilated areas of the lung. This has led to the introduction of inhaled NO as a therapeutic modality in the treatment of pulmonary hypertension.

CLINICAL USAGE

In adults with acute respiratory distress syndrome, low concentrations of inhaled NO can reduce pulmonary artery pressure without alteration in systemic mean arterial pressure, resulting in improved oxygenation (Rossaint et al 1993). Inhaled NO therapy is also used in the treatment of persistent pulmonary hypertension of the newborn (Kinsella et al 1992). Intravenously infused vasodilators may result in both pulmonary and systemic vascular dilation leading to increased intracardiac and intrapulmonary shunting. Inhalation of NO, however, can improve arterial oxygenation in these patients by decreasing pulmonary vascular resistance without systemic effect. NO may also have a role to play in the management of perioperative pulmonary hypertensive crisis in patients undergoing cardiac surgery (Tibballs 1993).

NO on exposure to oxygen is oxidized to nitrogen dioxide which is itself a strong oxidizing gas able to cause lung damage and induce pulmonary edema (Gaston et al 1994). When administering nitric oxide the concentration of nitric oxide and nitrogen dioxide to which the patient is exposed must be closely monitored. The length of contact time between nitric oxide and oxygen must be minimized and the minimum concentration of NO that produces the desired therapeutic effect is used (Tibballs et al 1993). Methemoglobin concentrations should also be regularly monitored in any patient receiving NO therapy.

Inhaled NO may diffuse from the alveoli not only to the vascular smooth muscle causing relaxation, but also to airway smooth muscle, resulting in bronchodilation. This opens up the possibility of using NO inhalation therapy as a treatment for bronchoconstriction. As mentioned earlier, inducible NOS may play an important role in the vasodilation seen in septic shock and research is concentrating on a possible therapeutic role of NOS inhibitors in patients with septic shock. However, because of the complexity of the physiological reactions in which nitric oxide is involved, the use of NOS inhibitors in humans may have deleterious side-effects.

ACUTE RENAL REPLACEMENT THERAPY

Acute renal failure occurs frequently in patients requiring intensive care, often secondary to a low cardiac output state, although hemolytic uremic syndrome, trauma, and drug toxicity are also important causes (Chesney et al 1975, Coulthard & Vernon 1995). Dialysis is indicated for patients who are volume overloaded and unresponsive to conservative medical therapy or who are developing complications of congestive heart failure or pulmonary edema. It is also used to treat those patients with severe electrolyte disturbances, symptomatic uremia or uncontrolled hypertension, or to enable parenteral nutrition to be employed. There are three main supportive therapies, peritoneal dialysis, hemodialysis and hemofiltration.

Peritoneal dialysis is simple to perform and is often sufficient therapy for the treatment of acute renal failure. Temporary dialysis catheters are simple to insert in the intensive care unit. However, there may be technical problems in performing peritoneal dialysis in children who have undergone recent abdominal surgery and large volumes of dialysate in the abdominal cavity may compromise respiratory function. Other problems include protein loss in the peritoneal dialysate, infection, and technical difficulties during fill and drainage (Reznik et al 1991). Hypertonic solutions used to increase fluid removal may result in high blood glucose levels, and in the intensive care setting peritoneal dialysis may not provide sufficiently fine control of fluid balance and electrolytes.

Hemodialysis can be used to remove any water soluble substance in the extracellular fluid that is not protein or tissue bound. It can be combined with charcoal hemoperfusion in the treatment of certain intoxications. It requires large bore vascular access, and the circuits and dialyzer must be carefully selected in relation to the child's circulating blood volume. The rate of removal and return of blood to the patient must balance so that hemodynamic instability does not occur. Anticoagulation is required as the blood is exposed to a foreign surface. Careful monitoring of cardiovascular status, temperature, electrolytes, hematocrit and clotting is required. Cardiovascular instability, hemolysis, temperature instability and air embolism are the major risks. Specialized equipment is required, and nurses specifically trained in hemodialysis to run the machine. Hemodialysis is infrequently used in the acute setting in intensive care.

In children for whom peritoneal dialysis is not appropriate, there is increasing use of continuous renal replacement therapy (Zobel et al 1991, Latta et al 1994, Fleming et al 1995). There are two main techniques of hemofiltration, continuous arteriovenous hemofiltration (CAVH) and continuous venovenous hemofiltration (CVVH). In CAVH two large bore cannulae, one arterial and one venous are required. The patient's own blood pressure provides the driving force to push the blood through the circuit. In continuous venovenous hemofiltration (CVVH) vascular access is obtained with a double lumen large bore venous catheter. The blood is then pumped at a preset flow rate, determined by the child's size, from the outlet lumen of the catheter through a filter returning to the venous circulation via the inlet lumen of the catheter. The flow through the circuit is independent of the patient's blood pressure. As many of the patients on ICU may be hemodynamically unstable, CVVH may allow better control of fluid balance than CAVH. In either technique, as the blood passes through the filter, ultrafiltrate is formed with an electrolytic composition equal to that of the patient's blood. Depending on the final fluid balance required, a proportion of the ultrafiltrate can be replaced intravenously by a replacement fluid which mimics the required electrolyte composition of serum. If electrolyte derangement is marked, a countercurrent flow dialysis circuit needs to be added, resulting in continuous venovenous hemodiafiltration (CVVHD; Bunchman et al 1995). In CVVHD the combination of a high blood flow, convective clearance and additional diffusion of solute clearance results in an increased clearance of urea and creatinine compared with CVVH. As blood is passed through an extracorporeal circulation, complications are similar to those seen with hemodialysis with the risk of air embolism, infection, accidental disconnection in the circuit and heat loss. Close supervision of fluid replacement therapy is also required, particularly if large volumes of ultrafiltrate are being removed as hypotension can readily occur. There is also a requirement for anticoagulation to prevent the rapid loss of ultrafiltration efficiency and clotting of the filter. The most widely used anticoagulant is heparin, although prostacyclin can be used if systemic coagulopathy or heparin-induced thrombocytopenia is a problem. Trials with heparin bonded membranes are currently underway.

HEPATIC SUPPORT

Liver failure occurs when the synthetic capacity of the liver is severely compromised, resulting in an array of symptoms, signs and biochemical abnormalities (discussed on p. 478). The major causes of liver failure in children are infectious, metabolic, toxic or due to biliary obstruction. Fulminant hepatic failure is a severe acute form of hepatic failure complicated by encephalopathy within 8 weeks of the start of symptoms, in a patient with no previous liver damage. Previously, treatment focused on meticulous medical treatment of these patients, enabling liver regeneration to occur and minimizing complications. Liver transplantation now offers an alternative treatment for some of these patients (Alonso et al 1992, Burdelski 1994).

Hepatic encephalopathy results in disordered consciousness and progressive deterioration of brain function. Clinical signs such as muscle tone, deep tendon reflexes and response to stimuli can be used to follow the course of the illness, but signs may become obscured in the intubated patient. Deteriorating conscious state with depression of cough reflex will lead to a compromised airway and the risk of aspiration. It is important to protect the airway and ensure adequate ventilation in these patients. Cerebral edema and intracranial hypertension may also occur and intracranial pressure monitoring may be useful. Conservative medical management of raised intracranial pressure by ensuring adequate airway and positioning with 30° head up tilt, avoidance of hypercapnia, hypoxemia and noxious stimuli, and maintenance of an adequate cerebral perfusion pressure remain the mainstays. Mannitol is considered if renal function is normal.

From a hemodynamic viewpoint, a high-flow low-resistance state with warm peripheries and bounding pulses may be seen. It is important to support the circulation appropriately, to maintain normovolemia and avoid decreased cerebral perfusion. Renal failure may occur as a consequence of hepatorenal syndrome. There will be a progressive rise in plasma creatinine with oliguria and a low urine sodium. Blood urea levels are an unreliable indicator of renal function due to impaired hepatic urea synthesis. Reduced levels of fibrinogen, prothrombin, and factors 5, 7, 9, 10 occur. Transplant criteria may be based in part upon clotting factor levels and levels must be interpreted in the knowledge of blood products given. Other general measures used in the treatment of hepatic failure include the use of dextrose 50% to maintain adequate glucose levels, and considering the use of branched chain amino acids rather than aromatic in nutritional support, along with vitamin supplementation. Lactulose may be administered to reduce the enteral contribution to the ammonia load, and H_2 receptor antagonists to decrease the risk of gastrointestinal bleeding.

All patients with hepatic failure should be frequently reassessed with a view to liver transplantation. In large liver transplant units children make up 30–50% of admissions (Scharschmidt 1984). Problems with pediatric liver transplants include the shortage of donors, technical problems related to vessel size, and previous surgery in children with biliary atresia. Transplantation should be considered in all children who have progressive chronic liver disease as well as those who have fulminant hepatic failure. The main contraindications are disseminated malignancy and systemic infection. Various techniques of size reduction of adult livers has increased the donor pool for children (Otte et al 1990), but there are still technical difficulties with the small size of the hepatic artery. The postoperative retransplantation rate is 18–27%, but higher in infants (Busuttil et al 1991, Salt et al 1992). The major complications are vascular, including hepatic artery thrombosis, biliary complications with obstruction or leakage of bile, and medical problems of hypertension, neurological or renal impairment. Overall 1-year survival is around 75%, with a large proportion of these children having normal liver function (Busuttil et al 1991, Otte et al 1989).

SUPPORT OF THE NEUROLOGICAL SYSTEM

The differential diagnosis of altered conscious state and investigations for determining etiology are discussed elsewhere (Ch. 14). Specific treatment for neurological disorders includes the treatment of infections, control of seizures, and drainage of hematomas, but the mainstay of treatment in the intensive care unit is supportive general medical management to minimize secondary hypoxic or ischemic damage (Pfenninger 1993).

Maintenance of an adequate airway, ventilation and circulation are paramount. In the treatment of raised intracranial pressure, therapy is directed at maintenance of adequate cerebral perfusion and substrate delivery. A variety of intracranial pressure monitoring devices are available; coupled with invasive arterial monitoring they can be used to monitor cerebral perfusion pressure. Simple measures to minimize raised intracranial pressure appropriate in all patients include attention to positioning, with the head in the midline, neck straight and bed head raised 30° to aid venous return. Adequate sedation is necessary in the intubated patient, decreasing sympathetic output, and noxious stimuli should be avoided. Patients should be maintained euvolemic with an adequate circulating volume, and crystalloid intake reduced, although hypoglycemia or hyperglycemia should be avoided. Hyperthermia increases cerebral metabolic requirements and should be avoided.

Neuromuscular blockade may be required to prevent Valsalva maneuvers in the intubated patient and to manipulate ventilation. Hyperventilation can be used to control episodic rises in intracranial pressure, although prolonged hyperventilation can lead to ischemic damage, and carbon dioxide reactivity of the vasculature may not be sustained. Mannitol may also be used to treat rises in intracranial pressure, providing renal function is adequate. Steroids may be useful in the treatment of raised intracranial pressure secondary to tumors where their use may reduce edema around the mass lesion, but have not proven useful in control of generalized edema, for example after trauma, in Reye's syndrome, or after hypoxic–ischemic damage. When control of the intracranial pressure is not achieved by these means, barbiturate coma may be used to reduce the cerebral metabolic rate. Central venous as well as intra-arterial monitoring should be used, as cardiovascular support may be required in these patients to maintain cerebral perfusion pressure.

CLINICAL APPLICATIONS – EXAMPLES

The application and interaction of the general support principles discussed above will now be illustrated in the management of a child admitted following near-drowning, and the child with meningococcal septic shock.

NEAR–DROWNING

Drowning has been defined as a submersion injury that causes death within 24 hours of the incident, whereas near-drowning is a submersion injury after which the patient survives for at least 24 hours. Many of these patients eventually die from organ damage caused by the initial injury (Fields 1992). The primary injury is the hypoxemia and ischemia which occur at the time of submersion and continue until adequate ventilation, oxygenation and perfusion are restored. The global ischemia affects all organs, but the primary morbidity and mortality are frequently due to brain ischemia.

Patients with altered mental status or respiratory dysfunction should be admitted to the ICU. Therapy concentrates on cardiopulmonary support and prevention of secondary central nervous system injury. Intrapulmonary shunting can result from aspiration, and mechanical ventilation with a positive end-expiratory pressure can improve ventilation perfusion match. Pulmonary edema that accompanies near-drowning can be controlled by titrating the level of positive end-expiratory pressure. Bronchospasm can be treated with bronchodilating agents. Currently the routine use of corticosteroids and prophylactic antibiotic therapy are not recommended. It is better to withhold antibiotics unless the fluid in which the drowning occurred was highly contaminated, or until there are definite clinical signs of infection. Acute respiratory distress syndrome (ARDS) may develop. A variety of mechanical ventilation strategies have been described for the treatment of ARDS. We follow a policy of permissive hypercapnia, aiming to provide adequate oxygenation with the lowest inspiratory pressures and oxygen concentrations possible. This strategy needs to be balanced against any need for manipulation of ventilation to control raised intracranial pressure. High frequency ventilation or extracorporeal life support for respiratory failure may be required.

Near-drowned children can present with a range of cardiovascular disturbances. They may be hypervolemic or hypovolemic, and myocardial ischemia may cause cardiogenic shock. Invasive monitoring, appropriate volume support, inotropic agents and afterload reduction may be required. Attention must be paid to normalizing body temperature and to the metabolic needs of the child, avoiding hyperglycemia or hypoglycemia. The insult may result in acute renal failure, and invasive support may be required.

The management of central nervous system injury is primarily directed at preventing further secondary injury. Adequate perfusion along with oxygenation, ventilation and cardiovascular support are required. Fluids may need to be restricted to limit cerebral edema. Hyperthermia and seizures should be aggressively managed. Intracranial pressure monitoring is less commonly used and steroids are not given (Bohn et al 1986). For the patient with suspected elevations in ICP, medical management with head elevation, hyperventilation, crystalloid fluid restriction, diuretic therapy and adequate sedation may be used. There are a variety of factors which are associated with a poor outcome from near-drowning. These include: a submersion time longer than 5 minutes; initial pH less than 7.1; continued requirement for cardiopulmonary resuscitation when the patient reaches hospital; persistence of coma; fixed, dilated pupils; elevated intracranial pressure. The chance of intact survival is extremely low for a near-drowned victim requiring cardiopulmonary resuscitation in the accident and emergency room (Nichter & Everett 1989, O'Rourke 1986). One exception to abnormal outcomes in asystolic patients involves ice water injuries (Biggart & Bohn 1990).

MENINGOCOCCAL SEPTIC SHOCK

The mortality rate for children presenting with meningococcal septic shock is around 50%. The child with meningococcal septicemia requires urgent initiation of treatment with antibiotics, and general support of all systems whilst concurrent diagnostic tests are carried out (Nadel et al 1995). Cardiac output and arterial oxygen content must be maximized, whilst oxygen requirements are minimized. Administration of oxygen is a simple basic treatment. Intubation and ventilation may be required for a variety of reasons, for example the child may have an altered mental status, decreased oxygenation secondary to ARDS, or pulmonary edema secondary to poor myocardial function. Elective mechanical ventilation should be considered as it will decrease the child's metabolic demands. The intubated child should be adequately sedated. Aggressive support of the cardiovascular system is required and maintenance of an adequate circulatory volume will require plasma expansion. Central venous access and the measurement of central venous pressure will enable preload of the heart to be more readily manipulated, although as these children have ongoing capillary leak there are no normal values for optimal central venous pressure. Children with sepsis can also have depressed myocardial contractility, and there should be early initiation of inotropic support. A mix of low dose dopamine with dobutamine may be used, with dobutamine substituted with adrenaline if there is poor response. Some children may require reduction of afterload to improve cardiac output, and low dose prostacyclin is most commonly used. Dialysis (peritoneal or hemofiltration) may be required in shocked patients who remain oliguric after restoration of adequate cardiac output. Neurological dysfunction may be due to a direct effect of the infection, hypoxia, decreased cerebral perfusion due to low cardiac output, or cerebral edema. Therapy is directed at the maintenance of an adequate cerebral perfusion pressure. The introduction of a scoring system for meningococcal septicemia (Sinclair et al 1987) has provided us with a useful means of assessing the severity of the disease and prognostic indicators are well known (Leclerc et al 1984). This means that children at high risk of death can be readily identified and benefit from early and aggressive treatment of their disease in the ICU, with the aim of reducing morbidity and mortality.

SUPPORT SERVICES

Although this section has focused on organ support in intensive care, in practice this physiological approach must be coupled with an awareness of the emotional needs of the child. Intensive care is a stressful environment for the child and family members, and adequate psychological and social support services must be readily accessible. Judicious use of analgesics and hypnotics should ensure that the child has minimal recall of a pain free admission to intensive care.

REFERENCES

Alonso E M, Gonzalez-Vallina R, Whitington P F 1992 Update of pediatric liver transplantation. European Journal of Pediatrics 151: S23–S31

Arnold J H, Truog R D, Thompson J E, Fackler J C, 1993 High-frequency oscillatory ventilation in pediatric respiratory failure. Critical Care Medicine 21: 272–278

Arnold J H, Hanson J H, Toro-Figuero L O, Gutierrez J, Berens R J, Anglin D L 1994 Prospective, randomized comparison of high-frequency oscillatory ventilation and conventional mechanical ventilation in pediatric respiratory failure. Critical Care Medicine 22: 1530–1539

Baraff L J 1993 Management of infants and children 3–36 months of age with fever without source. Pediatric Annals 28(8): 497–498, 501–504

Baraff L J, Bass J W, Fleischer G R et al 1993 Practice guidelines for the management of infants and children 0–36 months of age of fever without source. Annals of Emergency Medicine 22(7): 198–210

Beattie T F 1996 An accident and emergency based child accident surveillance system: is it possible? Journal Accident and Emergency Medicine 13(2): 116–118

Biggart M J, Bohn D J 1990 Effect of hypothermia and cardiac arrest on outcome of near-drowning accidents in children. Journal of Pediatrics 117: 179–183

Black M D, Coles J G, Williams W G et al 1995 Determinants of success in pediatric cardiac patients undergoing extracorporeal membrane oxygenation. Annals of Thoracic Surgery 60: 133–138

Bohn D J, Biggar W D, Smith C R, Conn A W, Barker G A 1986 Influence of hypothermia, barbiturate therapy and intracranial pressure monitoring on morbidity and mortality after near-drowning. Critical Care Medicine 14: 529–534

Bond G R, Requa R K, Krenzelok E P et al 1993 Influence of time until emesis on the efficacy of decontamination using acetaminophen as a marker in a paediatric population. Annals of Emergency Medicine 22(9): 1403–1407

British Paediatric Association 1993 Report of a multidisciplinary working party on paediatric intensive care. November 1993

Bunchman T E, Maxvold N J, Kershaw D B, Sedman A B, Custer J R 1995 Continuous venovenous hemodiafiltration in infants and children. American Journal of Kidney Diseases 25: 17–21

Burdelski M 1994 Liver transplantation in children. Acta Paediatrica Supplement 395: 27–30

Busuttil R W, Seu P, Millis J M et al 1991. Liver transplantation in children. Annals of Surgery 213: 48–57

Butt W, Karl T, Horton A, Shann F, Mullaly R 1992 Experience with extracorporeal membrane oxygenation in children more than one month old. Anaesthesia and Intensive Care 20: 308–310

Chesney R W, Kaplan B S, Freedom R M, Haller J A, Drummond K N 1975 Acute renal failure: an important complication of cardiac surgery in infants. Journal of Paediatrics 87: 381–388

Cornish J D, Heiss K F, Clark R H, Strieper M J, Boecler B, Kesser K 1993 Efficacy of venovenous extracorporeal membrane oxygenation for neonates with respiratory and circulatory compromise. Journal of Pediatrics 122: 105–109

Coulthard M G, Vernon B 1995 Managing acute renal failure in very low birthweight infants. Archives of Disease in Childhood 73: F187–F192

Day S E 1993 Intra-transport stabilization and management of the pediatric patient. Pediatric Clinics of North America 40: 263–274

Farley D E, Ozminkowski R J 1992 Volume-outcome relationships and inhospital mortality: the effect of changes in volume over time. Medical Care 30: 77–94

Ferguson F, Beattie T F 1993 Occult spinal cord injuries in traumatised children. Injury 24(2): 83–84

Fields A I 1992 Near-drowning in the pediatric population. Critical Care Clinics 8: 113–129

Fleming F, Bohn D, Edwards H et al 1995 Renal replacement therapy after repair of congenital heart disease in children. A comparison of hemofiltration and peritoneal dialysis. Journal of Thoracic and Cardiovascular Surgery 109: 322–331

Furchgott R F, Zawadzki J V 1980 The obligatory role of endothelial cells in the relaxation of arterial smooth muscle by acetylcholine. Nature 288: 373–376

Gallehr J E, Vukov L F 1993 Defining the benefits of rural emergency medical technician–defibrillation. Annals Emergency Medicine 22(1): 108–112

Gaston B, Drazen J M, Loscalzo J et al 1994 The biology of nitrogen oxides in the airways. American Journal of Respiratory and Critical Care Medicine 149(2 Pt 1): 538–551

Green T P, Noler F W, Goodman D M 1995 Probability of survival after prolonged extracorporeal membrane oxygenation in pediatric patients with acute respiratory failure. Critical Care Medicine 23: 1132–1139

Grossman D C, Hart L G, Rivara F P et al 1995 From roadside to bedside: the regionalisation of trauma care in a remote rural county. Journal of Trauma 38(1): 14–21

Haller J A, Shorter N, Miller D et al 1983 Organisation and function of a regional paediatric trauma centre: does a system of management improve outcome? Journal of Trauma 23: 691–696

Ignarro L J, Buga G M, Wood K S, Byrns R E, Chaudhuri G 1987 Endothelium derived relaxing factor produced and released from artery and vein is nitric oxide. Proceedings of The National Academy of Sciences of the USA 84: 9265–9269

Isaacs D 1995 Bronchiolitis. (Editorial.) British Medical Journal 310: 4–5

Karl T, Sano S, Horton S, Mee R B B 1991 Centrifugal pump left heart assist in pediatric cardiac operations. Indication, technique, and results. Journal of Thoracic and Cardiovascular Surgery 102: 624–630

Kilbourn R G, Griffith O W 1992 Overproduction of nitric oxide in cytokine-mediated and septic shock. Journal of the National Cancer Institute 84: 827–831

Kinsella J P, Neish S R, Shaffer E, Abman S H 1992 Low-dose inhalational nitric oxide in persistent pulmonary hypertension of the newborn. Lancet 340: 819–820

Latta K, Krull F, Wilken M, Burdelski M, Rodeck B, Offner G 1994 Continuous arteriovenous haemofiltration in critically ill children. Pediatric Nephrology 8: 334–337

Leclerc F, Beuscart R, Guillois B et al 1984 Prognostic factors of severe infectious purpura in children. Intensive Care Medicine 11: 140–143

Lee W A, Gillinov A M, Cameron D E et al 1993 Centrifugal ventricular assist device for support of the failing heart after cardiac surgery. Critical Care Medicine 21: 1186–1191

Levy F H, O'Rourke P P, Crone R K 1992 Extracorporeal membrane oxygenation. Anesthesia and Analgesia 75: 1053–1062

Luten R C, Wears R C, Broselow J et al 1992 Length-based endotracheal tube and emergency equipment in pediatrics. Annals Emergency Medicine 21(8): 900–904

MacDonald I A R, Beattie T F 1995 Intussusception presenting to a paediatric accident and emergency department. Journal of Accident and Emergency Medicine 12(3): 182–186

Macrae D J 1994 Paediatric intensive care transport. Archives of Disease in Childhood 71: 175–178

Meliones J N, Custer J R, Snedecor S, Moler F W, O'Rourke P P, Delius R E 1991 Extracorporeal life support for cardiac assist in pediatric patients. Review of ELSO Registry data. Circulation 84(SIII): 168–172

Moncada S, Palmer R M, Higgs E A 1991 Nitric oxide: physiology, pathophysiology and pharmacology. Pharmacological Reviews 43: 109–142

Morley C J, Thornton A J, Cole T J et al 1991 Baby check: a scoring system to grade the severity of acute systemic illness in babies under 6 months old. Archives of Disease in Childhood 66: 100–105

Nadel S, Habibi P, Levin M, 1995 Management of meningococcal septicaemia. Care of the Critically Ill 11: 33–38

Nanas J N, Moulopoulos S D 1994 Counterpulsation: historical background, technical improvements, hemodynamic and metabolic effects. Cardiology 84: 156–167

Nichter M A, Everett P B 1989 Childhood near-drowning: is cardiopulmonary resuscitation always indicated? Critical Care Medicine 17: 993–995

Notterman D A Greenwald B M, Moran F, DiMaio-Hunter A, Metakis L, Reidenberg M M 1990 Dopamine clearance in critically ill infants and children: effect of age and organ system dysfunction. Clinical Pharmacology and Therapeutics 48: 138–147

Oakley P A 1988 Inaccuracy and delay in decision making in paediatric resuscitation and a proposed reference chart to reduce error. British Medical Journal 297: 817–819

O'Rourke P P 1986 Outcome of children who are apnoeic and pulseless in the emergency room. Critical Care Medicine 14(5): 466–468

O'Rourke P P, Stolar C J, Zwischenberger J B, Snedecor S M, Bartlett R H 1993 Extracorporeal membrane oxygenation: support for overwhelming pulmonary failure in the pediatric population. Collective experience from the extracorporeal life support organisation. Journal of Pediatric Surgery 28: 523–528

Otte J B , de Ville de Goyet J, Alberti D et al 1989 Liver transplantation in children: University of Louvain Medical School (Brussels) experience with the first 139 patients. Clinical Transplants 4: 143–152

Otte J B, de Ville de Goyet J, Sokal E et al 1990. Size reduction of the donor liver is a safe way to alleviate the shortage of size-matched organs in pediatric liver transplantation. Annals of Surgery 211: 146–157

Palmer R M, Ferrige A G, Moncada S 1987 Nitric oxide release accounts for the biological activity of endothelium-derived relaxing factor. Nature 327: 524–526

Park J K, Hsu D T, Gersony W M 1993 Intraaortic balloon pump management of refractory congestive heart failure in children. Pediatric Cardiology 14: 19–22

Paulson T E, Spear R M Peterson B M 1995 New concepts in the treatment of children with acute respiratory distress syndrome. Journal of Pediatrics 127: 163–175

Perkin R M, Levin D L, Webb R, Aquino A, Reedy J 1982 Dobutamine: a hemodynamic evaluation in children with shock. Journal of Pediatrics 100: 977–983

Pfenninger J 1993 Neurological intensive care in children. Intensive Care Medicine 19: 243–250

Pollack M M, Katz R W, Ruttimann U E, Getson P R 1988 Improving the outcome and efficiency of intensive care: the impact of an intensivist. Critical Care Medicine 16: 11–17

Pollack M M, Alexander S R, Clarke N, Ruttimann U E, Tesselaar H M , Bachulis A C 1991 Improved outcomes form tertiary centre pediatric intensive care: a statewide comparison of tertiary and nontertiary care facilities. Critical Care Medicine 19: 150–159

Pon S, Notterman DA 1993 The organization of a pediatric critical care transport program. Pediatric Clinics of North America 40: 241–261

Radomski M W, Palmer R M, Moncada S 1987 The anti-aggregation properties of vascular endothelium: interactions between prostacyclin and nitric oxide. British Journal of Pharmacology 92: 639–646

Reznik K V M, Griswold W R, Peterson B M, Rodarte A, Ferris M E, Mendoza S A 1991 Peritoneal dialysis for acute renal failure in children. Pediatric Nephrology 5: 715–717

Ribbeck B M, Runge J W, Thomason M H, Baker J W 1992 Injury surveillance: a method for recording E-codes for injured emergency department patients. Annals Emergency Medicine 21(1): 37–40

Rodewald L E, Wrenn K D, Slovis C M 1992 A method for developing and maintaining a powerful but inexpensive computer database of clinical information about emergency department patients. Annals Emergency Medicine 21(1): 41–46

Ronco R, King W, Donley D K, Tilden S J 1995 Outcome and cost at a children's hospital following resuscitation for out-of-hospital cardiopulmonary arrest. Archives of Paediatrics and Adolescent Medicine 149(2): 210–214

Rossaint R, Falke K J, Lopez F, Slama K, Pison U, Zapol W M 1993 Inhaled nitric oxide for the adult respiratory distress syndrome. New England Journal of Medicine 328: 399–405

Salt A, Noble-Jamieson G, Barnes N D et al 1992 Liver transplantation in 100 children: Cambridge and King's College Hospital series. British Medical Journal 304: 416–421

Scharschmidt B F 1984 Human liver transplantation: analysis of data on 540 patients from four centres. Hepatology 4: 95S–101S

Seri I 1995 Cardiovascular, renal and endocrine actions of dopamine in neonates and children. Journal of Pediatrics 126: 333–344

Shanley C J, Hirschl R B, Schumacher R E et al 1994 Extracorporeal life support for neonatal respiratory failure. A 20-year experience. Annals of Surgery 220: 269–282

Shann F 1993 Australian view of paediatric intensive care in Britain. Lancet 342: 68

Sharples P M, Storey A, Aynsley-Green A, Eyre J 1990 Avoidable factors contributing to death of children with head injury. British Medical Journal 300: 87–91

Sibert R 1975 Stress in families of children who have ingested poisons. British Medical Journal (12 July): 87–89I

Sinclair J F, Skeogh C H, Hallworth D 1987 Prognosis of meningococcal septicaemia. Lancet 2: 38

Steinberg C, Notterman D A 1994 Pharmacokinetics of cardiovascular drugs in children. Inotropes and vasopressors. Clinical Pharmacokinetics 27: 345–367

Tibballs J 1993 Clinical applications of gaseous nitric oxide. Anaesthesia and Intensive Care 21: 866–871

Tibballs J, Hochmann M, Carter B, Osborne A 1993 An appraisal of techniques for administration of gaseous nitric oxide. Anaesthesia and Intensive Care 21: 844–847

Wetzel R C, Gioia F R 1987 High frequency ventilation. Pediatric Clinics of North America 34: 15–38

Young W F, Bivins H G 1993 Evaluation of gastric emptying using radionuclides: gastric lavage versus ipecac-induced emesis. Annals of Emergency Medicine 22(9): 1423–1427

Zaritsky A, Chernow B 1985 Use of catecholamines in paediatrics. Journal of Paediatrics 105: 341–350

Zideman D, Bingham R, Beattie T F et al 1994 Guidelines for paediatric life support. British Medical Journal 308: 1349–1355

Zobel G, Ring E, Kuttnig M, Grubbauer H M 1991 Five years experience with continuous extracorporeal renal support in paediatric intensive care. Intensive Care Medicine 17: 315–319

33 Practical procedures

Ian A. Laing   Edward Doyle

Introduction **1829**
Explanation 1829
Warmth, lighting and restraint 1829
Asepsis and antisepsis 1830
Cooling 1830
The treatment of pain 1830
Pain assessment 1830
Opioids 1831
Patient-controlled analgesia 1831
Non-steroidal anti-inflammatory drugs 1832
Regional anesthetic techniques 1832
Analgesia in the pediatric intensive care unit and
    neonatal unit 1832
Chronic and terminal pain 1833
Closure of wounds 1833
Blood pressure measurement 1833
Blood sampling 1834
Capillary 1834
Venous 1834
Arterial 1835
Arterial cannulation 1836
Venous cannulation 1836

Surgical venous cut down 1837
Percutaneous central venous cannulation 1837
Umbilical vessel catheterization 1838
Exchange transfusion 1838
Urine sampling 1839
Lumbar puncture 1840
Cisternal puncture 1840
Subdural tap 1841
Ventricular puncture 1841
Tracheal intubation 1841
Tracheostomy 1843
Joint aspiration 1843
Bone marrow 1844
Drainge of pneumothorax 1844
Paracentesis of the thorax 1845
Paracentesis of the abdomen 1845
Gastric lavage 1845
Liver aspiration 1845
Percutaneous renal biopsy 1845
Skin biopsy 1846
Muscle biopsy 1846
References 1846

INTRODUCTION

Practical procedures in pediatrics are best learnt in the treatment rooms and at the cot sides of children's hospitals. No chapter can substitute for close observation and repeated practice. Techniques for such procedures can, however, be written down. The authors offer suggestions, often based on personal experience, while recognizing that other clinicians may prefer methods which in their hands offer new advantages for the patient.

EXPLANATION

The aims of any procedure should first be explained to parents and a clear description of the method to be used should be given. There must be total frankness in discussing risks and in dealing with any questions the parents may ask. A bright 3-year-old also deserves to have a clear description of the forthcoming procedure. Being whenever possible at the same physical height as the child helps to allay the fears which multiply when a strange adult towers threateningly overhead. For some procedures it may be necessary to obtain consent in writing from the child's parents (or legal guardians) and especially if a general anesthetic is required. Parents who wish to be present may be allowed to observe minor procedures, provided that this does not impair the efficiency of the operators. A parent may be invaluable in reassuring a child during a stressful experience, but no parent should ever be responsible for restraining the child, nor for taking any active part in the work done. The child should if possible perceive the parent as being a protector rather than a treacherous collaborator.

WARMTH, LIGHTING AND RESTRAINT

A small infant is particularly vulnerable to cooling, and so all procedures which involve removing the child's clothing should only be done in warm surroundings. Room temperatures between 22°C and 28°C will probably protect the child, increase patient co-operation and improve the success rate of the practical procedure. Privacy is essential, partly for the dignity of the child and family, and partly to reduce the convection currents which follow the arrivals and departures of bustling personnel. For a partially clothed newborn infant the room temperature should always be above 25°C and serious consideration should be given to performing all the necessary work with the neonate in a prewarmed incubator at the child's neutral thermal environment. An open radiant heat warmer may be ideal for more major procedures requiring free access to the infant and skin servo-control may ensure that hypothermia does not contribute to the child's morbidity. A general anesthetic may inhibit the child's own thermoregulation, thus increasing the responsibility of the caring team to monitor the core temperature regularly.

Good lighting is essential and strip lighting in a treatment room should be supplemented if necessary by an angle-poise lamp, particularly during precision procedures such as insertion of a peripheral arterial cannula.

Physical restraint of the frightened child may be essential for the successful outcome of any practical procedure. Holding a wriggling toddler steady during lumbar puncture takes not only gentle firmness but also technical skill and some endurance! The skilled assistant should be able to guarantee immobilization of the operative site and a separate trained member of staff may be required to observe the patient during the procedure. The infant or young child may occasionally be restrained best by a blanket wrapping, but beware to protect the patient from inhalation of vomit or obstruction of the upper airway.

ASEPSIS AND ANTISEPSIS

All operative surfaces are cleaned beforehand with 0.5% chlorhexidine gluconate (Raymed) or an iodine-containing synthetic detergent such as Wescodyne (Amsco). For *minor procedures* the operator should scrub hands and forearms to the elbows with an effective cleaning agent such as 4% chlorhexidine (Hibiscrub, ICI) or hexachlorophene (EZ scrub, Parke Davis). The hands and forearms are then rinsed in warm running water, keeping the wrists above the elbows and finally meticulous drying is carried out prior to the procedure. The appropriate area of patient's skin is then cleaned with 70% isopropyl alcohol (Mediswab, Smith & Nephew) and the surface allowed to dry.

Major procedures require that the operator first put on protective cap and face mask, then carry out a 5-min scrub of hands and forearms using 7.5% povidone iodine (Betadine surgical scrub, Napp) or 4% chlorhexidine gluconate (Hibiscrub, ICI). Thereafter a careful rinse is followed by a thorough drying with sterile towels. The operator then puts on sterile gown and gloves. Three careful prolonged washes of the local area of the patient's skin are needed, using an agent such as 10% povidone iodine solution (Betadine antiseptic solution, Napp) or 0.5% chlorhexidine gluconate in 70% isopropyl alcohol (Hibitane tincture, Stuart Pharmaceuticals). The skin is then allowed to dry and sterile towel drapes are applied.

At the end of all procedures which involve iodine-containing solutions, particularly if the child is still in infancy, it is essential to remove the antiseptic solution completely in order to avoid skin burns and systemic effects including suppression of thyroid function.

COOLING

Hyperpyrexia may be defined as a core temperature above 40°C and is usually caused by exposure to extreme heat for several hours, but may occasionally occur in infective illnesses including malaria and pneumonia. Since the pyrexia itself can cause fits and irreversible harm to the child, rapid cooling is indicated in most cases. The child should be bathed or sprayed by cool water in a draught of cool air, thus increasing heat loss both by evaporation and by convection. In less extreme cases wet sponge cooling may be used regularly or wrapping the child intermittently in a wet sheet, followed by fanning the exposed body either by electric fan or manually with a blanket. An intramuscular injection of chlorpromazine (1 mg/kg) promotes vasodilation and may further cool the child by decreasing the amount of shivering. The patient's temperature should be measured at least every 10 min. Alternatively a continuous reading probe may be used. In anticipation of the hypothermia which may follow recovery from the previous pyrexia, therapy is stopped when the core temperature has dropped to 39°C.

THE TREATMENT OF PAIN

There is convincing evidence that until the mid-1980s postoperative pain in children was substantially undertreated compared with the practice in adults (Schechter 1989). It was thought that neonates and young infants did not feel pain and some clinicians feared the side-effects of analgesic drugs used perioperatively. There was also uncertainty about optimal doses and frequency of administration.

It is now clear that neonates and infants do feel pain. There is evidence that the complete central nervous system is active during fetal life (Flower 1985). The relevant neuroanatomical, neurophysiological and neurochemical mechanisms are mature enough in term and preterm neonates for them to experience pain. The density of cutaneous pain receptors is at least as rich in neonates as in adults (Anand & Hickey 1987). Neurological tracts in the spinal cord and brain involved in central transmission of pain are completely myelinated from the end of the third trimester (Pounder & Steward 1992). In neonates and infants undergoing surgical procedures with minimal anesthesia there is an increased release of catecholamines, glucagon, cortisol and growth hormone (Anand et al 1985, Milne et al 1986, Srinivasan et al 1986) in response to these procedures and this rise is attenuated when potent analgesia is provided (Anand et al 1985).

Analgesia and sedation should be provided both for acute and for chronic pain and careful consideration should also be given to providing combined analgesia and sedation whenever assisted ventilation is used.

Options for the treatment of pain in children include physical, psychological and pharmacological methods. Simple measures such as warmth, swaddling and feeding if appropriate may be useful. The presence of parents, reassurance and distraction are also important. Older children should be given a simple explanation of what is to happen and an assurance that any pain experienced will be treated as well as possible.

The main groups of drugs used for analgesia after surgery or trauma are opioids, local anesthetics and nonsteroidal anti-inflammatory drugs (NSAIDs), including paracetamol. It may be difficult to achieve adequate pain relief with opioids alone and multimodal or combined analgesic regimens may be superior. It is often desirable to use two or more analgesic drugs such as a local anesthetic block plus an opioid or a combination of opioid, regional technique and NSAID. These combinations may have synergistic effects. Analgesic regimens are most effective when given early and if possible in anticipation of the nociceptive stimulus. Reduced long-term pain after surgery (Tverskoy et al 1990) and a reduced incidence of phantom limb pain after amputation (Bach et al 1988) have been demonstrated when preemptive analgesia is used.

PAIN ASSESSMENT

A pain assessment tool should be able to detect the presence of pain, to estimate its severity and to determine the effectiveness of analgesic interventions. In children old enough to communicate, self-report numerical (Maunuksela et al 1987) or visual analog (Berde et al 1991) scales as used in adults have been shown to fulfill these requirements. In babies, infants and handicapped children subjective assessments are not possible and pain assessment is based upon indirect indicators, behavioral, physiological or biochemical (Grunau & Craig 1987, Hanallah et al 1987). In practice younger children should be observed by experienced pediatric nurses and scored using a simple five-point scale (Lloyd-Thomas & Howard 1994):

1 = pain free
2 = comfortable except on moving
3 = uncomfortable at rest
4 = distressed but can be comforted
5 = distressed and inconsolable.

The opinion of the parents can also be an excellent guide to the degree of a child's distress. The aim should be to have the child pain free at rest and with minimal discomfort during movement. During treatment for acute pain, assessments should be performed hourly to ensure efficacy.

OPIOIDS (Table 33.1)

Opioids are in widespread use for children undergoing intermediate and major surgery. They act both centrally and peripherally in the nervous system. They have a relatively narrow therapeutic range and marked variability in response between patients, particularly in children less than 3 months of age. In neonates and young infants there is an increased sensitivity to the depressant effects of opioids (Koren et al 1985, McNicol 1994). The concurrent use of other centrally acting sedative drugs with opioids puts the patient at considerable risk of oversedation and respiratory depression.

Intermittent intramuscular administration of opioids does not produce steady plasma levels and results in periods of inadequate pain relief (Berde 1989). This technique should therefore be avoided where possible. Intermittent intravenous administration of opioid when required is a useful method when the child is able to report pain and is particularly useful in the acute situation of emergency treatment of pain caused by trauma.

The technique of continuous infusion of opioid solution has become popular because of its efficacy, simplicity and wide range of indications. An infusion following a bolus dose has been demonstrated to provide better analgesia than intramuscular injections (Hendrickson et al 1990). An intravenous infusion of 10–40 µg/kg/hour of morphine following a bolus of 150 µg/kg provided equivalent analgesia to an epidural infusion of 0.1–0.4 ml/hour of 0.25% bupivacaine in infants undergoing abdominal surgery (Wolf & Hughes 1993). The effective use of intravenous infusions for pain relief requires close nursing supervision to ensure that the infusion rate is adequate and titrated against needs which will change with time and activity such as mobilization and physiotherapy.

An alternative method of delivery is to use subcutaneous routes. This technique has been shown to be effective in children (McNicol 1993), but is subject to the same potential dangers as the intravenous route.

PATIENT-CONTROLLED ANALGESIA (PCA)

PCA has the potential to provide good pain relief, flexible enough to respond to the changing needs of patients, their individuality and their current status. Patients who perceive pain are able to self-administer within their prescription limits without reference to medical or nursing staff. The staff can preset for the patient the bolus dosage, the obligatory delay between boluses (lockout interval), the presence or absence of a background infusion and the maximum dosage over a period of 4 h.

There is evidence that the optimal use of PCA after major surgery is associated with less postoperative morbidity and earlier discharge than with intermittent intramuscular analgesia (Wasylak et al 1990) and in pediatric practice the pain experienced is less with PCA (Berde et al 1991). A pediatric study comparing PCA using morphine with a continuous infusion of morphine demonstrated better pain relief with PCA (Bray et al 1995). PCA has also been used in children for chronic and terminal pain (Mowbray & Gaukroger 1990) and for terminal care (Doyle & Morton 1994). With explanation and postoperative supervision many children aged 8 years and older can use PCA appropriately, as can selected children as young as 5 years.

The risks of PCA are respiratory depression and oversedation. There is a danger of excessive drug administration because of incorrect drug dilutions, machine malfunction or incorrect programming of the infusion pump. If infusions are administered through the same intravenous cannula as intravenous fluids there is a danger that opioid will reflux into the intravenous fluids and a subsequent uncontrolled bolus may be administered. To prevent this, infusions should be delivered through a dedicated cannula or an antireflux valve.

Side-effects of opioids include respiratory depression, oversedation, nausea, vomiting, urinary retention and pruritus. It may be that pulse oximetry has a place in the monitoring of PCA (Hutton & Clutton-Brock 1993), given that mild hypoxemia may be an indicator of hypoventilation. A child who is asleep may provide a clinical problem in assessing whether the child is oversedated, but a child who is merely asleep will usually have a good color, unobstructed breathing, good perfusion and an oxygen saturation of above 95% in air. There should be regular checks on the infusion pump or PCA machine.

A variation on PCA which has been successfully used in children is nurse-controlled analgesia (Lloyd-Thomas & Howard 1994). With this technique a modest infusion of morphine (10–20 µg/kg/hour) is supplemented by boluses (10–20 µg/kg) given at

Table 33.1 Methods of morphine administration

Technique	Dilution	Dose
Bolus dose i.v.		100–200 µg/kg (precedes infusion)
Intravenous infusion	1 mg/kg in 50 ml saline (20 µg/kg/ml)	10–40 µg/kg/hour (0.5–2 ml/hour) 5–20 µg/kg/hour under 3 months
Subcutaneous infusion	1 mg/kg in 20 ml saline (50 µg/kg/ml)	10–40 µg/kg/hour (0.2–0.8 ml/hour)
Patient-controlled analgesia	1 mg/kg in 50 ml saline (20 µg/kg/ml)	Bolus dose 20 µg/kg (1 ml) lockout interval 5 min; background infusion 4 µg/kg/hour (0.2 ml/hour)
Nurse-controlled analgesia	1 mg/kg in 50 ml saline (20 µg/kg/ml)	Infusion 10 µg/kg/hour (0.5 ml/hour); bolus dose 20 µg/kg (1 ml); lockout 20–30 min
Oral		200–300 µg/kg 4-hourly

the discretion of the nurse caring for the child, and with a lockout interval of 15–30 min and a 4-hourly maximum dose. This offers the advantages of avoiding an overgenerous fixed infusion rate while offering a basal level of analgesia which can then be supplemented and titrated to the child's needs.

NONSTEROIDAL ANTI-INFLAMMATORY DRUGS

Tissue injury leads to nociception by direct mechanical and thermal damage to nerve endings, to inflammation by the release of chemicals and enzymes from nerves and damaged tissue and to hyperalgesia generated by algogenic substances and sprouting of damaged nerves into the injured tissue. After noxious stimuli to peripheral nerves, antidromic impulses in axons promote the release of substance P from nerve endings resulting in vasodilation and an increase in vascular permeability. This causes local edema and, in combination with the release of algogenic substances (prostaglandins, leukotrienes, bradykinin, serotonin and histamine), leads to inflammation and sensitization of nociceptors, resulting in hyperalgesia. The primary efferent neuron thus serves a dual function: transmission of neural stimuli and the peripheral release of mediators of inflammation at the site of injury.

Salicylates inhibit the biosynthesis of prostaglandins. Other NSAIDs probably act by several different mechanisms, including the increase of intracellular cyclic AMP which stabilizes cell membranes in polymorphonuclear leukocytes, thus reducing the enzymic component of the inflammatory response.

Subgroups of NSAIDs include salicylates (aspirin), indole derivatives (indomethacin and sulindac), propionic acid derivatives (ibuprofen and naproxen), oxicam derivatives (pyroxicam and tenoxicam), phenylacetic acid derivatives (diclofenac sodium) and the pyrrole derivative ketorolac trometamol. Their limitations are their relative lack of potency, and in major procedures they should be considered only as an adjunct to more powerful analgesics. Adverse side-effects of NSAIDs include peptic ulceration, impaired platelet function, bronchospasm, rhinitis and renal impairment. Where possible NSAIDs should be avoided in children with asthma. Apart from its use in chronic juvenile arthritis, aspirin is contraindicated in children less than 12 years old, because of an association with the development of Reye's syndrome.

Commonly used and effective NSAIDs are diclofenac sodium 1–3 mg/kg daily in two or three divided doses and ibuprofen 5 mg/kg 6-hourly. Diclofenac is available in water-soluble form and as suppositories and ibuprofen in a syrup form for children unable to swallow tablets. Ketorolac trometamol 1 mg/kg as a loading dose followed by 0.5 mg/kg 6-hourly (for a maximum of 48 h) is a potent NSAID regimen which is available for intravenous use. Paracetamol in a dose of 10–15 mg/kg 4–6-hourly is a useful analgesic during many forms of minor surgery or for non-specific pain. Its antipyretic effect may also be important. The rectal route has a bioavailability of about 80% of the oral route and therefore requires doses in the region of 20–30 mg/kg.

REGIONAL ANESTHETIC TECHNIQUES

The use of local anesthetics plays a major part in the provision of analgesia for children. Regional techniques include infiltration of a surgical wound, single nerve blockade, plexus blockade and central neuraxial block (epidural and spinal analgesia). Regional techniques are commonly combined with general anesthesia in order to decrease the dosage of general anesthetic used, and to provide analgesia lasting into the postoperative period.

Only those with proper training and experience should use regional anesthetic techniques. Resuscitation equipment and expert assistance should be at hand.

Common techniques include infiltration for suture of lacerations or invasive procedures such as lumbar puncture, digital nerve block, penile nerve block for circumcision, caudal epidural blockade for groin and lower limb surgery, and lumbar or thoracic epidural blockade for abdominal or thoracic surgery. The commonest regional technique used unsupplemented by general anesthesia is subarachnoid (spinal) anesthesia for inguinal hernia repair in premature neonates where this technique is associated with fewer respiratory complications than general anesthesia (Cote et al 1995). The most commonly used local anesthetic agents in children are lignocaine and bupivacaine. Bupivacaine is longer acting with a more pronounced sensory than motor block when used in dilute concentrations but it is more cardiotoxic than lignocaine. Lignocaine may be used at a dosage up to 3 mg/kg, whereas the maximum for bupivacaine is 2.5 mg/kg.

Potential complications include hematoma formation at the site of injection, intraneural injection during single nerve or plexus blockade, inadvertent subarachnoid injection during epidural blockade and systemic toxicity of local anesthetics from absolute overdose or inadvertent intravascular injection. Regional techniques produce a lack of sensation which may distress children if this has not been explained beforehand and presents the potential risk of injuries from incorrect positioning of a limb, plaster casts or compartment syndromes. More common effects are urinary retention and leg weakness following epidural blockade. The use of dilute solutions of local anesthetic for caudal epidural blockade has been shown to reduce the incidence of motor block without reducing the duration of analgesia. The manifestations of overdose or intravascular injection are convulsions and cardiovascular collapse. Treatment should be cessation of the injection, clearing the airway, artificial respiration with 100% oxygen, and closed cardiac massage if necessary. Anticonvulsants such as benzodiazepines or anesthetic induction agents should be titrated to effect. Fluids, pressor agents and antidysrhythmics are given as required.

The commonest regional anesthetic now used outside the operating theater is EMLA, the eutectic mixture of local anesthetics, which provides topical cutaneous anesthesia prior to venepuncture, venous cannulation and lumbar puncture. EMLA consists of a mixture of 2.5 mg/ml of lignocaine and 2.5 mg/ml of prilocaine. EMLA is available as a cream applied locally to the skin at least 1 h prior to the elective or semielective procedure as a pea-sized dollop covered by a tegaderm dressing.

ANALGESIA IN THE PEDIATRIC INTENSIVE CARE UNIT AND NEONATAL UNIT

Children receiving artificial ventilation in an intensive care unit or special care nursery are subject to a number of painful interventions. The provision of analgesia reduces the stress response, cardiovascular changes and rises in intracranial pressure associated with these interventions. While the need for analgesia may be obvious after surgery or trauma, it is less obvious but just as important in other patients in intensive care. The use of neuromuscular blockers to produce paralysis must always be accompanied by the administration of sedation and analgesia and the practice of inducing paralysis without these measures is now unacceptable. In most cases an infusion of an opioid such as morphine 20–40 µg/kg/hour or fentanyl 2–5 µg/kg/hour is useful, with the administration of boluses to deal with incident pain such as physiotherapy and tracheal suction. The use of NSAIDs and regional blocks is often inappropriate and opioids are the only analgesic used. In these circumstances the side-effects of respiratory depression and sedation may even be desirable, facilitating assisted ventilation and amnesia. By the time weaning is under way the requirements for opioid have usually been reduced to a point where respiratory depression is not a problem. Older children over 3 months may often require a sedative agent such as a benzodiazepine in addition to analgesia.

In premature neonates a bolus dose of 100–200 µg/kg of morphine over 1 or 2 hours followed by an infusion of 5–10 µg/kg/hour is usually effective. This regimen has been shown not only to provide analgesia but also to reduce the concentrations of circulating catecholamines in ventilated premature babies (Quinn et al 1993). The provision of analgesia and sedation may produce a favorable effect on outcome by moderating the uncontrolled catabolic response to stress in critically ill infants. Even when a continuous infusion of opioid is used to provide analgesia, invasive procedures such as chest drain insertion or lumbar puncture should be preceded by an additional bolus of opioid or by the infiltration of local anesthetic. Occasionally mild hypotension is seen after morphine administration, presumably as a consequence of histamine release and vasodilation (Quinn et al 1993), and tolerance appears to develop relatively quickly (Arnold et al 1990) although data on the pharmacokinetics of these doses are scarce in premature neonates. Other potential problems which cause concern include prolonged weaning from respiratory support, seizures and the development of a withdrawal syndrome.

CHRONIC AND TERMINAL PAIN (See Ch. 16)

Chronic pain occurs less commonly in children than in adults, but it may show as one of the chronic pain syndromes such as reflex sympathetic dystrophy or as part of a chronic or terminal illness. Reflex sympathetic dystrophy is characterized by recurrent limb pain associated with signs of sympathetic nervous system dysfunction in the affected limb such as cyanosis, mottling, dry skin, muscle atrophy and osteoporosis. This condition classically follows trauma to the limb. Treatment is based on a combination of counseling, physiotherapy, traditional analgesics and sympathetic blockade.

Neoplasms may cause pain either by direct tissue invasion or as a consequence of nerve or plexus invasion. Patients with neoplasms may undergo the pain of recurrent therapeutic procedures and investigations, and the use of general anesthetic for invasive events such as bone marrow aspiration can minimize this form of suffering for many children. Phantom limb pain may occur after amputation (Krane et al 1991). Ideally all such patients should be referred to a multidisciplinary pain service, where treatment is individualized. An 'analgesic ladder' may be used in which simple analgesics such as paracetamol or an NSAID followed by a weak opioid such as codeine may then progress to more potent opioids such as morphine. A wide range of dose requirements may be necessary in this group of children. Side-effects are common, including constipation, nausea and somnolence. Other measures, such as physiotherapy, tricyclic

antidepressants, steroids or specific nerve or plexus blocks, are employed on an individual basis.

Cystic fibrosis is commonly associated with chronic chest and abdominal pain, while sickle cell anemia, hemophilia and rheumatological conditions tend to cause severe acute exacerbations on a background of chronic pain. Acute episodes often require systemic opioids which should not be denied because of fears of addiction but should be weaned as quickly as possible. Long-term discomfort usually requires chronic NSAID and paracetamol use and possibly oral opioids such as codeine.

In summary it is almost always possible to provide satisfactory analgesia for children in pain. Appropriate and sensible use of the various analgesic drugs and techniques available combined with assessments of efficacy and side-effects will provide good quality analgesia with a wide margin of safety.

CLOSURE OF WOUNDS

The area is infiltrated with local anesthetic and 3 min is allowed to pass, remembering that an impatient operator can cause unnecessary discomfort to the patient by beginning before pain relief is maximal. The wound is then inspected and all foreign bodies and dirt removed by forceps and scrubbing brush. The wound edges and deeper layers of tissue are washed with sterile saline solution or 0.1% aqueous chlorhexidine. All non-viable tissue is excised to reduce the likelihood of future infection. Subcutaneous sutures for deep layers should be of an absorbable material, e.g. 3/0 plain catgut. The skin edges are apposed without tension and sutures are positioned 0.5–1 cm apart. The skin sutures are stitched with an atraumatic needle, ideally with silk suture affixed. For best cosmetic results only the finest silk suture should be used to repair face wounds.

In all but the cleanest wounds inquiry should be made about the patient's tetanus immunization status. Tetanus toxoid is given if indicated and consideration is given to further treatment with intramuscular injection of a long-acting penicillin (Triplopen). Subsequent infection in the wound should be treated by removal of selected sutures at the infected site to allow pus to drain to the surface. The extracted suture and a swab of pus are sent for bacteriological examination, and any cellulitis is treated with an appropriate antibiotic. Wound dehiscence can usually be managed by packing the gaping wound with an antiseptic (chlorhexidine) dressing.

BLOOD PRESSURE MEASUREMENT

The routine measurement of blood pressure at each thorough physical examination gives important information not only about the cardiovascular system, but may also provide a key physical sign in disease of renal, endocrine and central nervous systems. The cuff bladder must encircle the upper arm and its width should cover two-thirds of the distance from shoulder to elbow. Too small a cuff is a common reason for obtaining an inappropriately high reading. At a time when the child is as relaxed as possible, the cuff bladder is pumped up gently to 20 mmHg above the predicted systolic pressure, then the cuff is deflated slowly while the examiner auscultates carefully over the brachial artery in the antecubital fossa and records the systolic pressure when the first pulsation is heard. As the cuff deflates further the diastolic pressure is recorded when the pulsation changes from a distinct beat to a muffled sound.

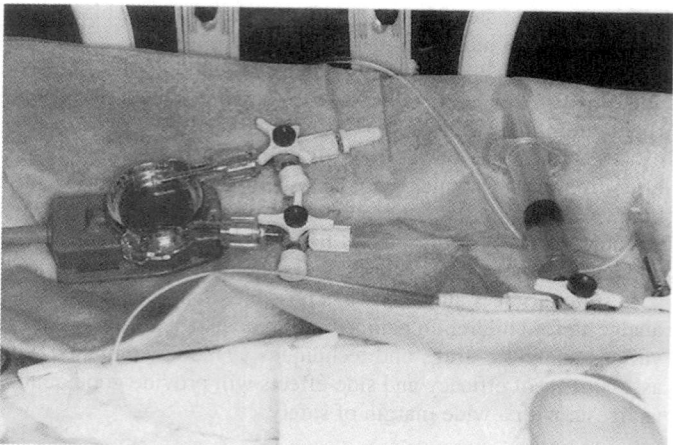

Fig. 33.1 Arterial pressure transducer with Luer lock connections.

Doppler ultrasound is useful for arterial blood pressure monitoring, particularly in vascular disease, but intra-arterial continuous pressure monitoring has revolutionized pediatric intensive care. An artery is cannulated as described below, and a pressure transducer (Hewlett Packard 1295 C) is connected via a three-way tap to the line under strict sterile precautions. Noncompliant tubing must be used and all connections should have Luer lock fittings (Fig. 33.1). Trends in the child's arterial pressure can be continuously observed on the monitor (Hewlett Packard 78834 A) even while the line is kept patent with a slow continuous flow of heparinized saline: accurate blood pressure measurements are taken by adjusting the three-way tap to connect the patient to the transducer alone, temporarily cutting off the flow of saline. Accidental introduction of air bubbles into the tubing may cause damping of the pressure signal.

BLOOD SAMPLING

CAPILLARY

If microtechniques are available in the local laboratory, a capillary blood sample may be adequate for blood gas tension and biochemical assessments. While satisfactory specimens for plasma glucose, bilirubin, sodium, chloride, urea, some drug concentrations and the Guthrie test are obtainable by this method, hemolysis may provide a falsely elevated plasma potassium concentration and a capillary hematocrit typically is misleadingly high compared to a venous sample. Capillary methods are contraindicated in shock and edema and also for blood culture. If blood is required for accurate gas tensions including PaO_2 (arterial oxygen tension) then an arterial sample is mandatory.

Capillary blood sampling in the neonate is best done on the plantar aspect of the foot, especially on the medial or lateral aspect of the posterior third (Fig. 33.2). In older children the side of the thumb or ventrolateral aspects of the fingers are suitable. The skin should be warmed beforehand and a check made to ensure good perfusion with rapid capillary return after blanching. The area is cleaned with a spirit swab, and some workers prefer to smear a thin film of Vaseline on the surrounding skin. The lancet tip should be no longer than 2.5 mm, and this should be pushed firmly through the epidermis – being unduly tentative with the lancet may cause a child the discomfort of a second or third stab or (worse still) the slow pain of prolonged squeezing. Only intermittent gentle coaxing is needed, and the blood will rise easily along a heparinized specimen tube by its own capillarity. A spring-loaded device (Autolet, Owen Mumford) may be used for older children, and those who require frequent sampling may prefer to carry out this procedure themselves.

If facilities for immediate analysis of capillary samples are not available, one end of the blood-filled capillary tube can be closed with sealing wax or plasticine, and then a fine iron mixing filament, a 'mouse', can be introduced. The other end is then sealed and finally the blood is agitated by moving the 'mouse' up and down the tube by means of a magnet. If there is to be much delay then the sample should be stored on ice.

VENOUS

In the newborn, blood will drip freely through a 21G needle from a vein on the dorsum of the hand. Older children are often remarkably co-operative if the antecubital fossa is chosen, a confident explanation is given, and the needle tip is kept out of sight until the last moment. The assigned helper encircles the

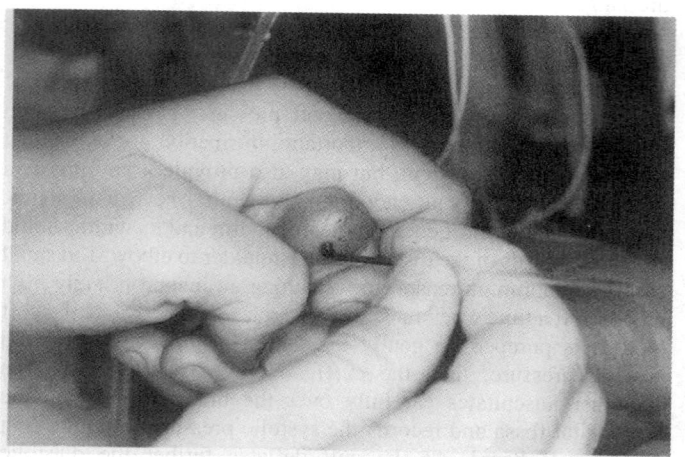
(a)

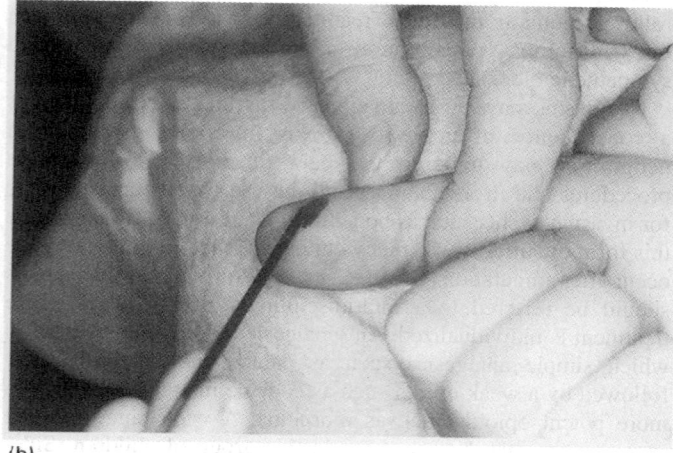
(b)

Fig. 33.2 Capillary blood sampling from (a) medial aspect of heel of a preterm infant and (b) lateral aspect of a child's thumb.

child's upper arm firmly to occlude venous return and to hold steady, while the other hand holds the child's forearm in firm supination (Fig. 33.3). The phlebotomist chooses a vein by touch and sight, anchoring it by gently stretching the overlying skin. After the needle has penetrated the skin a flashback of blood into the hub of the needle confirms that the needle tip is in the vein. Gentle negative pressure on the plunger of the syringe gathers the sample of blood required. Once the sample has been obtained, the assistant must release the venous occlusion in the upper arm before the needle is withdrawn. A sterile cotton wool ball will stop the bleeding, but pressure should not be applied until the needle is removed. Alcohol swabs should not be used at this stage as they will cause unnecessary discomfort to the child.

The child who presents in shock will urgently need a reliable intravenous cannula and in an intensive care unit blood sampling may well be best carried out using an indwelling arterial catheter. If blood is needed urgently from the poorly perfused infant it may be necessary to use the external jugular vein. The conscious, supine child is restrained by a blanket enveloping both arms and the head is held firmly below body level by an experienced assistant who must also observe the patient's breathing pattern and color. The head is then turned laterally to display the external jugular vein coursing over the sternomastoid muscle (Fig. 33.4).

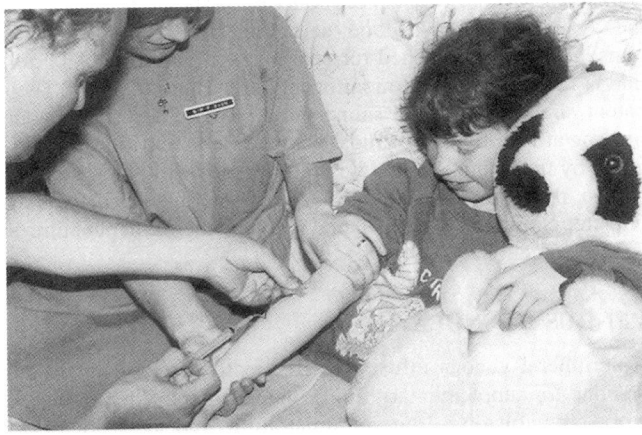

Fig. 33.3   Venous blood sampling from arm of a 9-year-old.

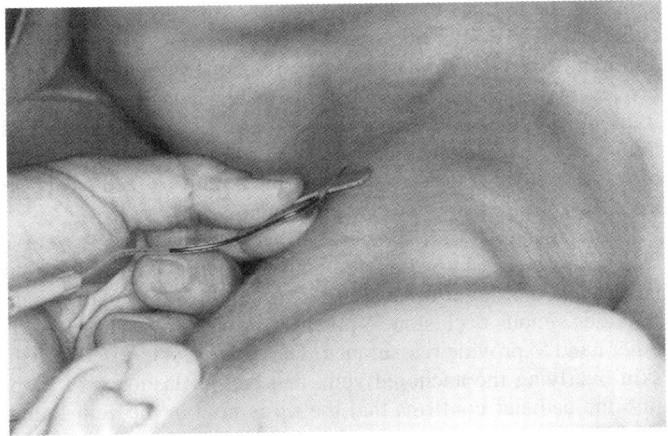

Fig. 33.4   Venous blood sampling from external jugular vein of a shocked 12-year-old.

Air embolus must be guarded against at all times, and many clinicians find that using a 21-G butterfly needle may simplify the technique provided that the needle remains attached to the syringe throughout the procedure. Taking the syringe off while the needle is still in the vein must never be done because it may result in air being sucked into the child's central veins. This procedure is very frightening to the child and is to be condemned as a regular method of blood sampling. Equally hazardous is the use of the femoral vein, where hemorrhage, thrombosis, inadvertent arterial sampling and infection (including septic arthritis) make this an unacceptable procedure except as a last resort. The vein lies medial to the artery in the femoral triangle. The leg should be immobilized in partial abduction and the skin is penetrated just medial to the femoral arterial pulse 0.5 cm distal to the inguinal crease. The needle is inserted only up to 0.5 cm deep in order to protect the hip joint against trauma. Particularly after jugular or femoral venous blood sampling, firm pressure is applied for 2 min to the venepuncture site and hemostasis is subsequently confirmed by close inspection.

When bacteriological culture of venous blood is required the clinician should wash hands and forearms meticulously, and clean the patient's skin locally with antiseptic as for a major procedure. A spirit swab removes excess antiseptic and the site is allowed to dry. A closed system of needle and syringe must always be used if bacteriological contamination is to be avoided. Venepuncture should be 'clean' with early entry into the vein. Once the sample is obtained the venepuncture needle is removed and replaced with another sterile needle which penetrates the sterile bung of the aerobic and anaerobic culture bottles. Blood cultures should be sent directly to the laboratory or, if delay is anticipated, they should be incubated at 37°C until transfer is convenient.

ARTERIAL

In the absence of an indwelling arterial catheter, arterial blood is best obtained by intermittent sampling from the radial artery, and in neonates the right radial artery (which is preductal) is generally selected. Puncturing the brachial artery should be avoided because ischemia of the forearm may occur. However, the dorsalis pedis and posterior tibial arteries offer satisfactory alternatives for safe sampling. Before embarking on radial arterial puncture it is advisable to check that the collateral blood supply is adequate. The modified Allen's test is done by passively clenching the child's hand, compressing both radial and ulnar arteries at the wrist, then after the hand has turned white, releasing the pressure over the ulnar artery. A good ulnar supply will allow flushing of the hand in less than 10 s. In all arterial sampling, it is important to check before the procedure that there is no clinical evidence of a coagulopathy. When a syringe is to be used for arterial blood gas sampling, 0.1 ml of heparin 5000 units/ml should be drawn up beforehand and then expelled, remembering that excess heparin in the syringe causes falsely low values of PCO_2 and pH. All air bubbles must also be removed since misleadingly high PO_2 and low PCO_2 values may be obtained. The blood-filled syringe should be sealed with a cap or a piece of plasticine and the sample stored on ice for the journey to the laboratory.

During radial arterial sampling the patient's wrist should be held in supination and extended by 30°. The radial artery is generally easy to palpate, although some clinicians prefer to visualize it by transilluminating the wrist with a fiberoptic light source. Anesthetic skin patches can be used to decrease the initial

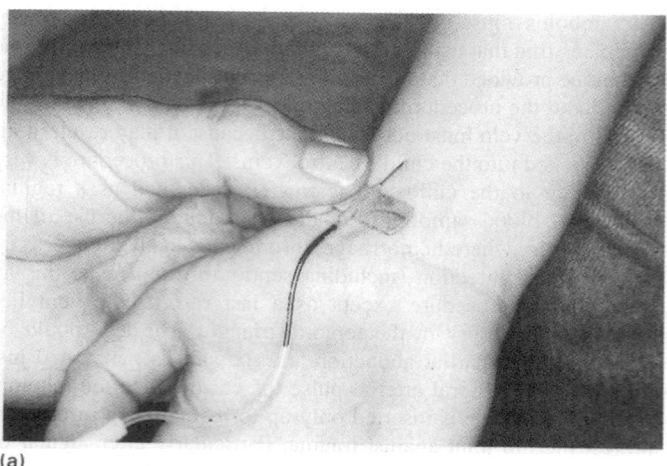
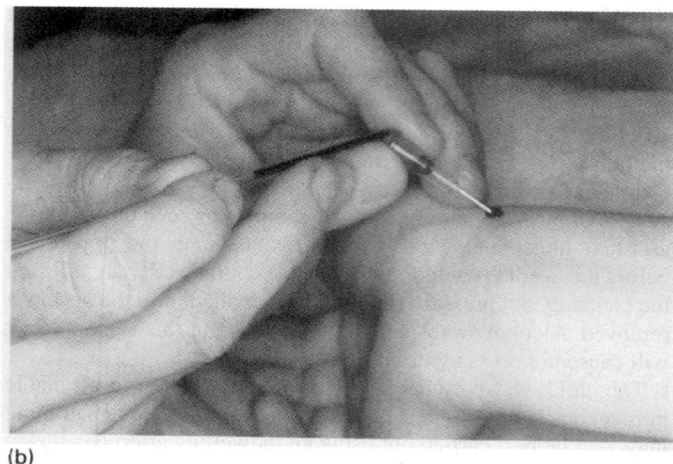

(a)   (b)

Fig. 33.5   Radial arterial blood sampling: (**a**) closed system; (**b**) collected by tube capillary.

discomfort but only by infiltrating the tissues around the artery with lignocaine *without adrenaline* can pain relief be complete. 3 minutes after infiltration of the local anesthetic, a 23G needle is inserted bevel upwards into the proximal flexion crease at 30° to the horizontal. Easier than using a butterfly needle connected to a syringe (Fig. 33.5a) is the collection of the sample in a preheparinized capillary tube (Fig. 33.5b). After the needle is withdrawn an assistant must press with a cotton wool ball on the puncture site for 5 min and then confirm hemostasis by 1 min observation. Both oxygen and carbon dioxide tensions fall rapidly as the child cries, and so rapidity of sampling is important for accurate results.

ARTERIAL CANNULATION

In the newborn period the first arterial line is usually an umbilical one, because of ease of insertion (see below). The radial arteries, posterior tibial and dorsalis pedis may also be used with a low complication rate. The femoral artery is increasingly used as the site of choice among anesthetists who are caring for children with cardiovascular surgical problems. Ischemia of the leg and foot can be a complication. Having carried out a modified Allen's test (see above) the clinician should splint the child's hand with a roll of gauze under the wrist to leave the hand in extension of 30°, and with the fingers still readily visible. The course of the artery can be marked on the skin, using palpation and a high intensity cold light source. An anesthetic skin patch is put on the skin and allowed to provide pain relief and then the deeper tissues are infiltrated with only 0.2 ml of 2% lignocaine *without adrenaline*: this small volume should give some deeper pain relief without distorting the course of the artery. While the local anesthetic is taking effect, a 10 ml syringe of normal saline is drawn up with 1 IU heparin/ml and this is flushed into extension tubing in preparation for connection to the catheter in situ.

A 22 or 24G cannula with stylet is selected and inserted bevel upwards into the skin immediately proximal to the wrist flexor creases and at 30° to the horizontal. The cannula and stylet are pushed quickly through the subcutaneous tissues to transfix the artery and then the stylet is removed. The cannula is then withdrawn very slowly until arterial backflow is established. The doctor's hand is then lowered so that the cannula is at 10° to the

horizontal and gentle rotation of the cannula tip may increase the ease with which the cannula is then threaded up the lumen of the artery. Firm pressure over the skin above the cannula tip will stem the flow of arterial blood until the anesthetic extension set is connected. A three-way tap or rubber bung should be inserted into the system for easy blood sampling and a blood pressure transducer can be attached for continuous monitoring. An arterial line is for sampling and monitoring only. The infusion to keep it patent should be normal saline with 1 IU of heparin/ml added, running at 1 ml/hour. No drugs (nor parenteral nutrition) should be given by this route. Minimizing interference with the system may reduce the complication rates. A transparent, sterile covering (Opsite, Smith & Nephew) may protect the skin puncture site against infection.

VENOUS CANNULATION

A peripheral venous infusion is frequently required in pediatric practice for supplementary fluids, management of hypoglycemia, blood transfusion, drug administration and occasionally for parenteral nutrition. Toddlers often have veins which are difficult to see, particularly if the child has a generous allocation of subcutaneous fat. The veins may, however, be coaxed into showing themselves by allowing the chosen arm to hang down, and particularly after prolonged local warming of the site. In children of races with marked skin pigmentation, palpation often proves more valuable than visualization. If an arm is to be immobilized, the child should first be asked (if appropriate) which thumb he/she prefers to suck, and also whether the child is right- or left-handed – social comfort and the ability to feed easily are important for the child's well-being and dignity.

Plastic cannulae 22, 24 or 26-G are satisfactory. A vein is selected as before by vision and palpation and the overlying skin is cleaned thoroughly. An assistant immobilizes the limb, and provides venous occlusion. A parent may wish to hold the child's other hand to provide reassurance. The cannula is inserted into the skin overlying the anchored vein, and then a flashback of blood into the catheter confirms that the tip is now in the vein lumen. With the cannula held steady, the central stylet is withdrawn and finally the cannula is threaded up the lumen of the vein. It is then attached to the T-extension and fixed securely so that during wakefulness or sleep the patient is unable to cause inadvertent disconnection of the system. While the antecubital fossa usually provides an easy site for cannulation and is therefore favored by the less experienced operator, a cannula in the forearm or dorsum of the hand allows the child greater freedom of movement. Fixation must not obscure subsequent observation of the skin, because full thickness chemical burns of the skin may occur due to subcutaneous infiltration of an infusate, and this is particularly common when calcium, phenytoin, hypertonic solutions or cytotoxic drugs are being administered.

In young infants scalp veins are numerous, superficial and accessible. Fixation of the cannula is easy because of the firmness of the skull, and the drip site can be kept under observation. The unwary may be tempted to try to cannulate a branch of the superficial temporal artery, but careful palpation of vessels coursing anterior to the ear should avoid this hazard. Injudicious placing of a cannula into an artery can be identified at the time of flushing with a syringe of heparinized saline, when the artery and other associated branches blanch rapidly in a manner never seen during successful venous cannulation. This error is important to identify because infiltration of infusate may cause serious focal ischemia and necrosis of local tissues. A small area of skin is shaved with a safety razor, and a cannula with wings is selected (Neoflon, Viggo). Taping of the cannula involves capturing the wings with a firm tape and ensuring that the position of the connecting tubing is out of reach of the infant's marauding hands.

SURGICAL VENOUS CUT DOWN

In shock, when no veins are available for percutaneous cannulation, it may be necessary to perform a surgical cut down, and this is most reliably done on the long saphenous vein. Full sterile technique is required for this major procedure, and equipment available beforehand in a sterile pack should include a scalpel, three pairs of curved artery forceps, mosquito forceps, small scissors, needle holder, bevelled Silastic catheter, fine catgut ties and also a 3/0 silk suture for the skin. The child's foot and ankle are immobilized in plantar flexion, and the area anterior and proximal to the medial malleolus anaesthetized. A small transverse incision is made, and the underlying vein is identified and dissected free using curved artery forceps. The saphenous nerve is separated from the vein, and the forceps are then passed underneath the vein to capture a double length of catgut which is then drawn through, cut into two, and then the distal half is tied off, occluding the vein, and left to provide traction. The proximal length is tied loosely and held with forceps to provide proximal traction and control of backflow of blood. A small 'v' is snipped in the vessel wall between the two ties, and the lumen is exposed with fine forceps. The Silastic catheter is inserted through the 'v' in a proximal direction, with momentary relaxation of the proximal restraining tie, and the tubing is passed up the vein to the desired distance. The suture is then firmly secured round the vein and indwelling catheter, the system is flushed with heparinized saline, and the skin wound is sutured with a 3/0 silk suture on an atraumatic needle.

Protection of the catheter site will be needed using sterile fixation (Steristrips), covered by a transparent sterile layer (Opsite) and firm splintage. If the outer borders of Opsite are sealed to the skin with tape (Dermiclear) it may be possible to avoid all interference with the wound site for as long as the intravenous line is required.

PERCUTANEOUS CENTRAL VENOUS CANNULATION

If a child is in shock or if central venous pressure monitoring is required or occasionally when parenteral nutrition is administered, a central venous line may be required. While it is possible to insert such a line by a surgical cut down, this technique leaves a cosmetic scar, whereas it is possible to carry out central venous cannulation by a percutaneous technique which leaves a preferable long-term cosmetic result.

The least hazardous technique uses the antecubital fossa, where the basilic vein (medially) and, less good, the laterally placed cephalic vein often show as sizable, easily palpable vessels into which a fine long catheter may be threaded. Full sterile technique is essential. The patient's elbow is splinted in extension and venous occlusion is provided by a simple elastic band for neonates or by a firm rubber cuff in older children. The operator first fills the chosen Silastic catheter with heparinized saline and measures on the patient the distance it is hoped to insert the catheter: the superior vena cava or right atrium may be suitable goals. The outer needle is then inserted into the large vein chosen, and when a rapid backflow is obtained the Silastic cannula is threaded by fine curved forceps upstream into the vein until the desired length of insertion has been achieved and then the outer steel needle is withdrawn, leaving the cannula in situ. Fixation of the inserted cannula is as before, using Steristrips, Opsite, Dermiclear and secure splintage.

The Seldinger technique is also of great value to the clinician who wishes to insert a reliable cannula into a large vein. The internal jugular and subclavian veins have been popular choices as sites for such a central line. It may be, however, that the femoral vein has been unjustly despised as a potential site for catheterization on the grounds that many bacteria proliferate in close proximity to the folds of the groin. If meticulous sterile technique is used, however, it is common to insert a central catheter into the femoral vein for long-term use and to have no further problems until the clinical need for intravenous feeding is past.

The leg is immobilized in partial abduction. Full sterile technique is used to clean the upper thigh, groin, genitals and suprapubic area, and the operative site is then carefully draped with sterile towels. Local anesthesia is administered and the femoral artery carefully palpated by the operator's gloved fingertips. The position of the femoral vein is easily established by needle and syringe immediately medial to the femoral artery pulse. The syringe is removed leaving the needle in the vessel, and the designated wire is threaded up the lumen of the needle into the femoral vein. The outer needle is then removed by a gentle rotating action leaving the wire in the femoral vein. Usually a gauze swab is required to staunch bleeding around the wire's exit from the skin. The definitive catheter is then threaded over the wire, until the operator can grasp the naked proximal end of the wire, allowing the cannula to be threaded easily up the inferior vena cava. The wire is then removed completely. The cannula is allowed to fill with venous blood and is then connected to an anesthetic extension set with heparinized saline. Except in times of great urgency, it is recommended practice to X-ray the child's abdomen and chest to establish the precise position of the catheter tip before beginning the infusion of fluids.

Similarly the internal jugular vein can be cannulated, although the recognized hazard of pneumothorax may increase the operator's anxiety level during this procedure. The child is immobilized supine and horizontally and then the bed is tilted head down by 15°. The child's head is then rotated laterally to the left. Under strict asepsis, the needle penetrates the skin over the anterior border of the sternomastoid muscle at the level of the thyroid cartilage and the needle tip points to the right nipple. The needle is advanced until blood flashback is obtained and then the Seldinger wire is threaded up the needle center as before. The technique is then completed as for the femoral venous catheterization described above.

It is only by practice that proficiency and a high success rate come to the operator's fingertips. The novice should not embark on the procedures unsupervised. Hematoma, pneumothorax, thrombosis, embolization (including air embolization) and sepsis may all have catastrophic effects on the child.

UMBILICAL VESSEL CATHETERIZATION

The umbilicus provides both venous and arterial access during the first week of life. Arterial catheterization is favored for monitoring blood pressure, gas tensions and by some authorities for exchange transfusions. A venous approach may be used for emergencies, exchange transfusion, central venous pressure monitoring, and rarely for access after failed arterial cannulation. The principles of the method of cannulation are the same for both, including warmth, restraint, full aseptic technique, careful monitoring and adequate oxygenation during the procedure.

Equipment includes small dissecting forceps, small toothed forceps, small scissors, scalpel, probe and a 3.5 or 5.0G catheter according to the size of vessel for cannulation. The catheter and a three-way tap are flushed with heparinized saline. The periumbilical skin of the anterior abdominal wall is washed with Betadine and the operative area is protected with sterile drapes. A gauze ribbon is tied loosely around the base of the umbilicus, and serves as a guard against subsequent hemorrhage. The scalpel is used to slice the umbilicus cleanly through, 0.5 cm from the anterior abdominal wall. It is a common error to begin with a stump which is too long, resulting in the creation of false passages bursting out of the vessels into the surrounding Wharton's jelly. The largest, thin-walled vessel is the vein and the two arteries (occasionally there is only one) often lie together as a pair, thick-walled and uninvitingly small. Two curved, self-retaining artery forceps should be clipped to the umbilical stump as close to the chosen vessel as possible. These are then laterally rotated so that the vessels stands proud from the cut surface of the umbilical stump (Fig. 33.6). The forceps are held steadily by the assistant who also is responsible for keeping the umbilical stump dry.

The operator then chooses the finest curved non-toothed forceps available and teases open the vessel so that the rim opens into the shape of a trumpet bell, and is then ready to receive the catheter. Touching the catheter only with sterile nontoothed forceps (Fig. 33.6), the operator passes the tip into the vessel and gently eases it along the lumen until blood flows back freely. For venous catheterization the aim is to coax the tip through the ductus venosus to the inferior vena cava: sites to avoid are hepatic vessels, portal vein and through the foramen ovale to the left atrium. The tip of an arterial catheter is ideally placed between the fifth and eighth thoracic vertebrae (T5–8) or inferior to the third lumbar vertebra (L3–L4). For a high arterial catheter satisfactory position is usually achieved by measuring the distance between the child's umbilicus and shoulder tip (x cm) and then inserting the catheter to a distance of $x + 1$ cm. The low arterial catheter

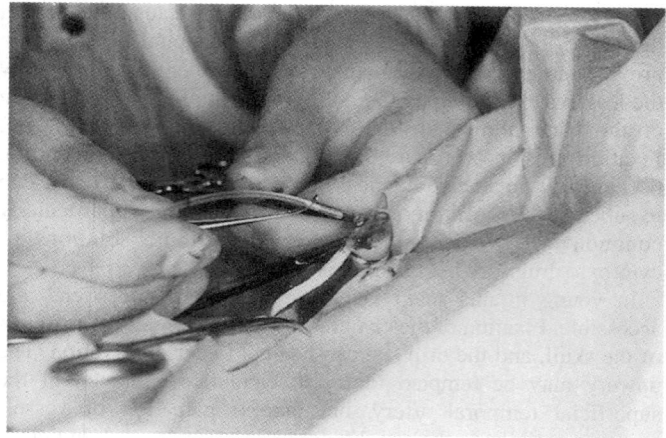

Fig. 33.6 Umbilical arterial catheterization: self-retaining forceps open the artery lumen for cannulation.

position is gained by passing the catheter into the vessel until arterial blood is obtained and then for a further 1–2 cm for a small or larger infant. The catheter should be secured very firmly by suturing to the strongest part of the base of the stump without stitching through the vessel just cannulated and avoiding the nearby skin which would cause the infant pain. Except in an emergency, the position of the catheter tip should be checked by X-ray or ultrasound.

Because of the risks of central infection umbilical catheters should be removed as soon as they are no longer essential. Thrombosis, embolism, hemorrhage and necrotizing enterocolitis may all be associated with central catheterization. Arterial catheters are associated with ischemia of buttocks and toes, and with hematuria. The catheter must therefore be removed as soon as vascular compromise is suspected. Prophylactic antibiotics are not indicated but many practitioners, having removed the catheter, may send the tip for bacteriological culture.

EXCHANGE TRANSFUSION

Full exchange transfusion is done most frequently for severe hyperbilirubinemia, but it may have a role in the management of profound anemia, resistant septicemia, coagulopathy and sclerema. The procedure can be carried out through a single umbilical vessel or else by a combined procedure, e.g. blood input through a large vein and output via the radial artery, although this is recommended only when umbilical access has proved impossible. It is essential to preserve the first blood samples for full investigation of the etiology of the hyperbilirubinemia, as the underlying diagnosis may be obscured by the exchange transfusion itself. If time allows, the blood used for exchange transfusion for rhesus incompatibility should be rhesus negative but otherwise crossmatched against the infant's own blood. If, however, it is anticipated antenatally that an exchange transfusion needs to be done soon after birth, the blood should be group O, rhesus negative red cells in AB serum compatible with maternal serum. The blood should be fresh, at most 48 h old, at room temperature and collected in citrate-phosphate-dextrose. It is then further warmed immediately prior to and during the procedure in a water bath with regulated heater coil. The blood transfusion laboratory may offer to remove some plasma, up to 25% of the total volume of whole blood, thus producing 'semipacked cells', which should maintain the infant's hematocrit close to 55%, although this is not appropriate if the exchange transfusion is to treat septicemia or coagulopathy.

Exchange transfusion is a life-threatening procedure which can take up to 4 h of continuous care from inserting catheter to completion of procedure. It should be carried out by an experienced clinician and assistant who can devote their full attention to the infant throughout the operation. It is unacceptable to have the operator providing cover for labor ward emergencies simultaneously and the assistant must be relieved of all other duties in the neonatal unit until the end of the exchange transfusion. Continuous electrocardiographic monitoring is important, and the environmental temperature should be in the neutral thermal range. Many clinicians prefer to have the infant nursed on an open radiant warmer with servo-control of skin temperature and this method has the advantage of providing ready access to the child throughout. Full sterile technique is employed. The assistant keeps 10-min records of pulse and respirations, half-hourly recordings of dextrostix and core temperature and must also document carefully a record of blood volume exchanged and drugs used. The assistant should also be a meticulous time-keeper who disciplines the operator to keep to schedule.

A timetable for the procedure is drawn up, planning to exchange 200 ml/kg bodyweight over a period of at least 1.5–2 h. This goal is achieved by exchanging 4 ml/kg bodyweight in 2-min cycles. The infant is given no fluids orally during the procedure and any very recent feed may be emptied from the stomach by gastric tube before the exchange begins. Umbilical catheterization is accomplished (see above) and the catheter connected to two three-way taps. A sterile, closed system is adopted (Fig. 33.7) whereby the infant's blood is aspirated in aliquots and then transferred to the disposable container. Meanwhile donor blood is drawn through the blood-warming bath and then directed gently into the infant's bloodstream. Some practitioners routinely give calcium gluconate (1 ml 10%) very slowly intravenously at hourly intervals, but many now regard this as unnecessary and potentially hazardous, reserving this therapy for infants who show lengthening of the QT interval on electrocardiography. Constant clinical observation is most important and at the end of the

procedure a final blood specimen should be taken for analysis of blood count, bilirubin, electrolytes, glucose, calcium and blood culture.

By a similar technique a partial plasma exchange transfusion can be carried out on a polycythemic infant. Concern about a hyperviscosity syndrome arises when the neonate's venous hematocrit is greater than 65–70%. Exchange of 20 ml/kg bodyweight is performed, using fresh frozen plasma, 5% albumin, or purified protein derivative as the donor medium. Advice should be sought from the blood transfusion service regarding the possibility of viral contamination and especially concerning which product is least likely to transmit non-A, non-B hepatitis or cytomegalovirus.

URINE SAMPLING

All samples require early transport to the bacteriology laboratory, if possible in less than 1 h from collection. Midstream urine and clean catch methods are similar techniques but the former requires the co-operation of the older child to control urine flow, such that the first urine passed is discarded, the next small volume is collected in a sterile container and the rest of the urine voided is again discarded. A clean catch collection is obtained in a sterile container by observing the infant or young child closely and patiently with equipment at the ready and opportunistically capturing a sample of urine in midflow. In both methods the perineum should first be thoroughly cleaned with sterile saline; boys should have the glans penis washed, no antiseptic should contact the urine to be collected and the penis or vulva should not touch the sterile container.

To obtain a sample of urine from neonates or infants, suprapubic aspiration (Fig. 33.8) is the most reliable method and it is also indicated in the ill child as part of an urgent screen before starting antibiotic treatment. The method is contraindicated if the child has a bleeding diathesis or if urine has been passed in the previous half hour – a 'dry tap' would almost certainly be the result. Prior to attempting aspiration of urine many neonatal units now use ultrasonography to demonstrate that the bladder contains a sufficient volume of urine; otherwise suprapubic dullness to percussion indicates a full bladder. With an assistant displacing the child's labia laterally or holding the penis gently to prevent premature passage of urine, the suprapubic region is cleaned with Betadine and allowed to dry. The child is held supine with legs abducted and a 23G needle connected to a syringe is introduced at the proximal transverse crease in the midline (Fig. 33.8). The needle should be angled 20° cranially, and negative pressure is gently applied to the syringe plunger as the needle is advanced. The recommended maximum depth is only 3 cm. Fresh urine is aspirated into the syringe and, after withdrawal of the needle, the assistant should press on the puncture site for 2 minutes while consoling the infant. With good technique, any bacterial growth in the urine obtained is interpreted as a urinary tract infection, although piercing the bowel is a recognized complication and may be misleading. Brief hematuria is occasionally noted after the procedure.

The fourth method of obtaining a reliable sample of urine for bacteriological culture is by perurethral catheterization of the bladder. This is indicated for definitive diagnosis of urinary tract infection if suprapubic puncture is contraindicated, to relieve urinary retention, to perform a micturating cystourethrogram or to measure the volume of bladder residue after passage of urine. The

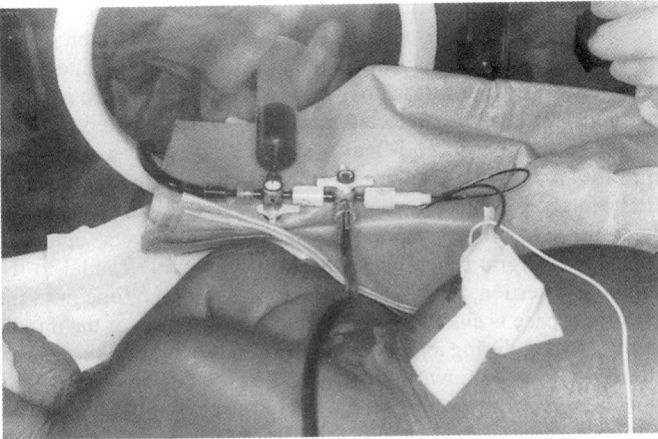

Fig. 33.7 Exchange transfusion for hyperbilirubinemia. Warmed rhesus-negative blood is drawn into the syringe from the left of picture; blood from the infant is disposed of via tubing, bottom center.

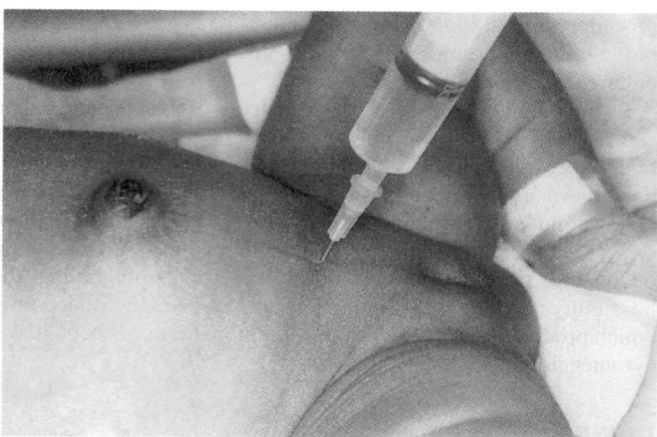

Fig. 33.8   Suprapubic aspiration of urine.

strictest asepsis is essential if the introduction of a new urinary tract infection is to be avoided. For the youngest children or for intermittent catheterization, Gibbons male and female catheters are available – 4, 6 and 8G in increasing size for infants – while older children can have up to size 14G inserted. Argyle feeding tubes (5 FG for a newborn, 6 FG for an infant and 8 FG for an older child) are also satisfactory for a brief procedure. If an indwelling catheter is required for an older child Foley catheters, which have balloon fixation, are preferable (8F–14F for 8–14-year-olds). The child is restrained supine and the perineum cleaned three times with aqueous chlorhexidine. The girl's labia are parted and washed with swabs held in forceps, wiping anterior to posterior. The catheter lubricated with sterile jelly is then inserted into the urethral orifice anterior to the vaginal introitus, until urine is obtained. The boy's penis is held in a swab in the clinician's left hand; the prepuce is retracted and the glans cleaned with chlorhexidine. The lubricated catheter is then inserted into the urethra using forceps held in the right hand. It is essential to remember that the operator's left hand is contaminated and must not contact the catheter during insertion. For indwelling catheters the balloon is inflated by gentle injection of sterile water into the catheter side arm. The tubing is taped to the patient's thigh and the prepuce replaced over the glans.

LUMBAR PUNCTURE

Lumbar puncture is needed to exclude the diagnosis of meningitis, to administer antibiotics intrathecally, and to instill contrast medium for myelography. If there is clinical evidence of raised intracranial pressure, and particularly if the child has a depressed conscious level, the advisability of performing the procedure should first be discussed with a neurosurgeon, so that help is readily at hand if the child should deteriorate due to 'coning' during or after the procedure. The decision to proceed with lumbar puncture when either coagulopathy or respiratory instability is present may be a difficult clinical judgment. One view is to delay the procedure for a few hours until the child is stable enough to withstand the investigation, but meanwhile to treat as though for meningitis, accepting that bacteriological cultures may be compromised on the basis of the presence of systemic antibiotics.

Lumbar puncture is usually done with the child in the left lateral decubitus position, although the sitting position is also appropriate, even in the neonate who can be supported throughout. The back should be well flexed, but no traction or flexion should be put on the neck. The patient's airway should never be compromised. Full aseptic technique is used and the space between lumbar vertebrae 3 and 4 is chosen – the third lumbar vertebra generally marks the junction of the line between the iliac crests and the vertebral column. It is traditional to use local anesthetic only for the older child, but local anesthetic patches or EMLA cream are appropriate for all children.

A lumbar puncture needle with stylet is required, otherwise an implantation dermoid may be a complication of the procedure. Appropriate sizes are, for a neonate, gauge 22 length 3.5 cm, and for an older child, gauge 20 length 5 cm. The needle and stylet are inserted gently in the midline into the intervertebral space, angling the needle 10° cranially, frequently withdrawing the stylet to see whether cerebrospinal fluid emerges. There is often a feeling of decreased resistance as the theca is entered. The stylet is then withdrawn and, if no clear fluid drips readily out, then the barrel of the needle is rotated without going deeper or withdrawing from the current position. If still no fluid emerges then the stylet is again inserted and the needle advanced less than a millimeter for the search to continue as before. The commonest complication, a traumatic tap, is usually due to the needle being inserted too far, with consequent rupture of a lumbar vein or venule. Samples of cerebrospinal fluid are collected for cell count, bacteriological and virological cultures and for protein and glucose concentrations, then the stylet is replaced and the whole system withdrawn. If frank blood, attributable to a traumatic tap, has been obtained, the offending needle should be withdrawn, replaced by a clean version and an adjacent intervertebral space selected for a further attempt. If, despite contamination with blood, cerebrospinal fluid has undoubtedly been obtained, this can be preserved for culture and a specimen sent for cell counting and comparison of the ratio of red to white cells. An unexpected predominance of white cells to red cells, particularly when compared to the ratio obtained in the patient's peripheral blood, may indicate meningitis.

CISTERNAL PUNCTURE

In the rare circumstance of a low spinal abscess or tumor, lumbar puncture may be contraindicated. Cisternal puncture, a potentially very hazardous procedure, may then be appropriate.

The sedated child is firmly restrained with the neck flexed. Full aseptic technique is required. All hair in the occipital and suboccipital areas is shaved and the area thoroughly cleaned with a prolonged series of Betadine washes. Sterile drapes are applied, and local anesthetic is injected into the skin immediately inferior to the occiput in the mid-line. A spinal needle is inserted in the midline and angled superiorly in order for the needle tip deliberately to contact the bone at the base of the skull. The needle is then withdrawn as far as the subcutaneous layers, and then reinserted several times, on each occasion slightly caudal to the previous insertion, and touching the skull base each time until the cisternal space is entered. The feeling of penetration of the dura is similar to that during a lumbar puncture. On each needle insertion, the stylet is withdrawn to check for flow of cerebrospinal fluid, which emerges when the needle tip has successfully entered the cisternal space. Subarachnoid fluid from the cisterna magna can then be collected for investigation.

Since faulty technique may cause paraplegia or death, cisternal puncture should always be carried out by (or under the direct supervision of) a clinician experienced in the procedure. Cisternal puncture is contraindicated in a child who has a myelomeningocele because the spinal needle could directly traumatize the herniated cerebellum.

SUBDURAL TAP

This procedure may be appropriate for the child less than 2 years of age whose coronal suture is still palpably patent, and where a subdural collection of fluid is to be diagnosed and drained. Older children will require a surgical burr hole to achieve these goals. The risks in a child with a bleeding diathesis should be carefully assessed.

The child is wrapped firmly in a blanket, and the clinical condition is kept under close surveillance during the tap. A generous area over and around the anterior fontanelle is shaved and washed thoroughly with Betadine. Full aseptic precautions are taken. The needle used may be 20G × 2.2 cm and must have a stylet and 'guard' which is fixed 5 mm from the tip, to prevent plunging inadvertently too deep into the tissues. A point is chosen on the coronal suture 3 cm from the mid-line and lateral to the anterior fontanelle. The firmness of the guard should be checked and the skin pierced. The skin is dragged laterally along the coronal suture by the needle tip which is then pushed firmly through the suture with rotating action. The stylet is removed and any subdural collection will show itself as straw-colored or blood-stained fluid welling up the spinal needle. Samples from the effusion should be collected for bacteriological and biochemical investigation. A maximum of 30 ml of fluid should be allowed to flow and then the needle is removed, the previous lateral drag on the skin providing a natural seal, which is supplemented with firm pressure for 5 minutes using a sterile dry swab. The other side may then be explored in the same way. The practitioner should not allow the needle tip to penetrate deeper than 5 mm. Complications of the procedure include infection, subgaleal fluid collection, trauma to the cerebral cortex and laceration of the superior sagittal sinus.

VENTRICULAR PUNCTURE

This invasive procedure is required where ventriculitis is suspected or where non-communicating hydrocephalus has occurred. Ultrasonography can demonstrate dilated ventricles and may provide a useful assessment of the thickness of cerebral cortex to be pierced. The need for restraint of the child and meticulous sterile technique are the same as for a subdural tap.

The lumbar puncture needle is inserted at the lateral angle of the anterior fontanel and the needle tip is directed towards the inner canthus of the contralateral eye. Ventricular fluid is usually very easy to obtain at the predicted depth. Pressure monitoring should be carried out, either by transducer or by simple manometry, normal values being less than 10 mmHg in older children and less than 5 mmHg in neonates at rest. Where pressure-measuring facilities are unavailable, rapid flow of ventricular fluid may be allowed until 20 ml have been collected and then the needle is withdrawn. If flow slows before 20 ml have drained, then the needle is withdrawn. A sterile dry dressing is applied to the skin at the site of entry. Porencephalic cysts can occur along the line of recurrent ventricular punctures. Because of the possibility that the ventricular tap may cause localized damage to brain tissue, it is customary to select the right ventricle for recurrent taps, so that

the left side (which is the side more likely to be the dominant hemisphere) is spared. Occasionally, however, the lateral ventricles do not communicate with one another and the left ventricle may require to be punctured in order to drain off loculated ventricular fluid under pressure.

TRACHEAL INTUBATION

This is a very important technique, best learnt by person-to-person instruction, demonstration and much personal practice on a model. Becoming accomplished at intubating neonates is essential for all pediatricians and the necessary skills are acquired in the delivery room. The technique of intubation of the older child is most rapidly mastered by attending pediatric surgical operating lists and caring for the child's airway under the guidance of the anesthetist. For the practitioner unskilled in endotracheal intubation it is safer to ventilate the apneic child by bag insufflation of oxygen through a mask tightly sealed against the patient's face, with the neck in partial extension and the mandible held forward (Fig. 33.9). The struggling child almost certainly does not need urgent intubation and can be managed by the delivery of 100% oxygen by face mask. Even the moderately experienced intubator, when confronted with a child who has Pierre Robin syndrome or suspected epiglottitis, should if possible delay until the arrival of the most experienced pediatric anesthetist available.

If time allows, all equipment should be checked beforehand, including the effectiveness of suction apparatus, all tubing connections, the maximum pressure escape valve (set to 25–30 cmH$_2$O for a neonate) and the laryngoscope battery and light bulb. An appropriate size of endotracheal tube is selected (Table 33.2), many practitioners preferring to choose one which has been stored in a refrigerator, giving it added firmness. The child lies supine with head partially extended. The laryngoscope is held lightly by the fingers of the left hand, the child's gums are parted by the clinician's right hand and then the laryngoscope blade is eased gently into the mouth (Fig. 33.10a), lifting the tongue forward. The blade tip advances until it enters the glossoepiglottic fold and the epiglottis is then raised by a lifting action of the left hand. Occasionally pressure is needed on the thyroid cartilage to bring the larynx into view. The endotracheal tube is then passed from the angle of the mouth on the right: if this technique is used then

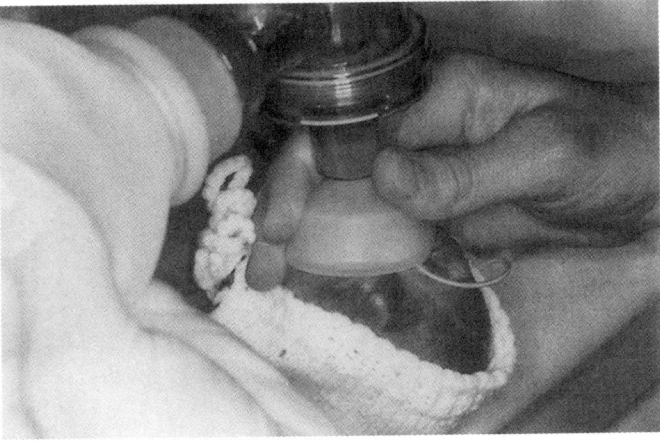

Fig. 33.9 Bag and mask insufflation of oxygen, demonstrating a tight seal of mask round infant's nose and mouth.

Table 33.2 Size of tube for endotracheal intubation

	Inside diameter (mm)
Weight of neonate	
Less than 1 kg	2
1 to 2 kg	2.5
2 to 3 kg	3
Age of child (years)	
1	3.5
2	4
5	5
7	6
10	7
14	8

the tube will not block the clinician's view of the vocal cords. In older children a cuff may then need to be inflated to minimize air escape. Air entry should be checked by observation of the movement of the chest wall and by auscultating bilaterally. Decreased air entry on the left side may mean that the endotracheal tube has been inserted too far and the tip is in the right main bronchus. Slowly easing the tube back while auscultating on the left side will allow an improved position with good breath sounds on both sides.

There is great variation in the methods used to fix an orotracheal tube firmly. The uncuffed Murphy endotracheal tube (Respiratory Support Products) is supplied with a convenient cross piece and slip lock, providing a system which is fairly reliable and cosmetically acceptable. An effective alternative is achieved by sliding a plastic flange and cylinder over the orotracheal tube and then suturing the tube to the surrounding cylinder wall (Fig. 33.10c). The flange is tied on either side by cotton ribbons to a nonstretch cap and then small dental rolls lift the plastic flange from the infant's cheeks to minimize frictional tauma (Fig. 33.10d).

Nasotracheal intubation is used in many centers for intensive care of neonates and older children, particularly if prolonged periods of artificial ventilation are anticipated. The sedated child should be supine and an anesthetic spray may be directed to the posterior nasopharynx if the child is conscious or likely to feel the discomfort of the procedure. The larger nostril is chosen for the procedure and an unshouldered tube for nasotracheal intubation is selected. The tip is lubricated with sterile jelly and passed into the nasopharynx. If there is resistance at the posterior nasopharynx,

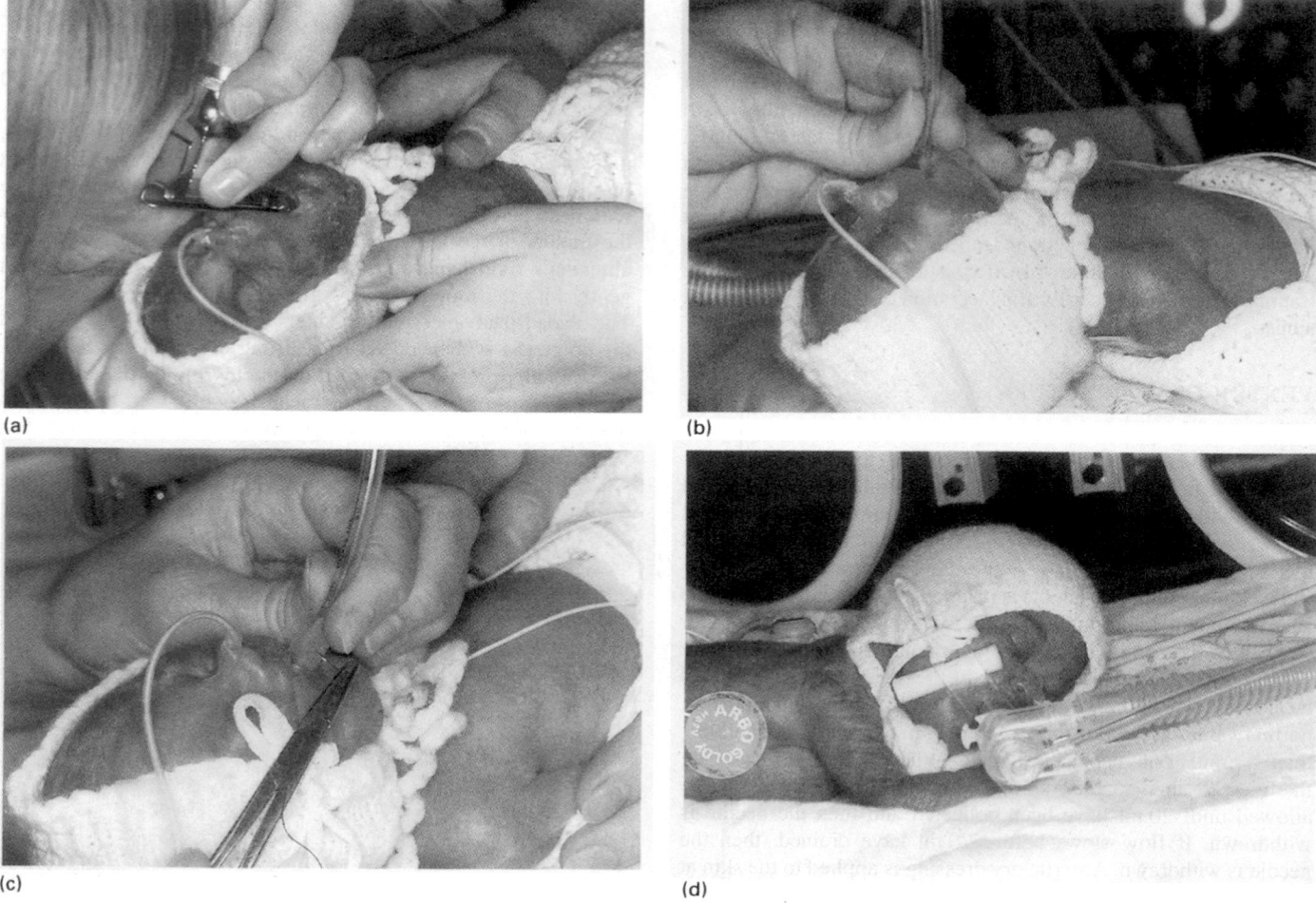

(a)   (b)

(c)   (d)

Fig. 33.10 Intubation of a preterm neonate. (**a**) Head held in partial extension. (**b**) Endotracheal tube gripped firmly using the infant's chin as a stabilizing platform. (**c**) Endotracheal tube is stitched to a flange and cuff, which ties firmly to a nonstretch cap. (**d**) Dental rolls protect infant's cheeks from frictional trauma.

then gentle but firm pressure is used directing the tube medially and posteriorly in the nostril. The tube must not be forced; better to try the opposite nostril or a smaller gauge of tube if the nasal route is strongly to be preferred. Once the tube is felt to pass into the posterior oropharynx, the laryngoscope is held in the left hand as before, and, lifting the tongue forward, the position of the tube tip is identified. A pair of Magill's forceps held in the right hand is used to coax the tip of the tube into the larynx above the vocal cords and then an assistant advances the tube tip by pushing the proximal end a little further into the nostril, while the clinician watches the tube tip advance deeper into the larynx. The correct length of tubing inserted is recorded by noting the marking on the side of the tube at the level of the nostril rim.

TRACHEOSTOMY

This procedure should usually be done electively by a skilled surgeon. However, on rare occasions the upper airway may obstruct acutely and there is failure to pass an endotracheal tube, e.g. in severe epiglottitis.

The child is placed supine with a small pillow under the shoulders to produce extension of the head. An assistant should

Table 33.3 Essential equipment for tracheostomy

Scalpel No. 15 blade

Five pairs curved self-retaining forceps

Two pairs straight self-retaining forceps

Small self-retaining retractor

Small toothed forceps

Curved (Metzenbaum's) scissors

Skin hook or tracheostomy hook

Tracheostomy spreader

Needle holder

Sterile swabs

Chromic catgut 3.0

Prolene or nylon sutures 4.0

Table 33.4 Shiley's tracheostomy tubes: size guidelines

Age of child (years)	Tube size
0	0
1	1
2	2
5	3
10	4
12	5
14	6

attempt to insufflate oxygen by bag and mask while emergency preparations are made and the neck is cleaned. Essential equipment for this procedure and recommended tube sizes are shown in Tables 33.3 and 33.4. If the child is comatose and near to death a transverse incision through the skin is made 1.5 cm above the sternal notch. Fascia is retracted laterally and the isthmus of thyroid is displaced superiorly. Stay sutures are put quickly into the trachea's lateral aspects and a longitudinal incision made in the trachea through the second and fourth tracheal rings in the mid-line. The stay sutures are retracted laterally and a tracheostomy tube is inserted, pointing downwards towards the carina. Artificial ventilation with 100% oxygen is carried out, auscultating bilaterally to insure equal air entry. The tracheal stay sutures are then removed and the ends of the skin incision are sutured. It normally takes a week for a tract to develop, during which time the tracheostomy tube should be supported in position by firm but atraumatic cotton ribbon (Fig. 33.11a). Complications include obstruction (particularly if inadequate humidity is provided – see Fig. 33.11b), infection, accidental extubation and chronic tracheal stenosis.

JOINT ASPIRATION

Aspiration of fluid from a joint may be required in the diagnosis of septic arthritis, hemarthrosis, crystal synovitis and occasionally for intra-articular steroid injection. A 19 or 21G needle should be used for large joints and 23 or 25G for the smallest. A small sandbag can be helpful for relaxed immobilization of the joint under investigation. The strictest aseptic technique should be used

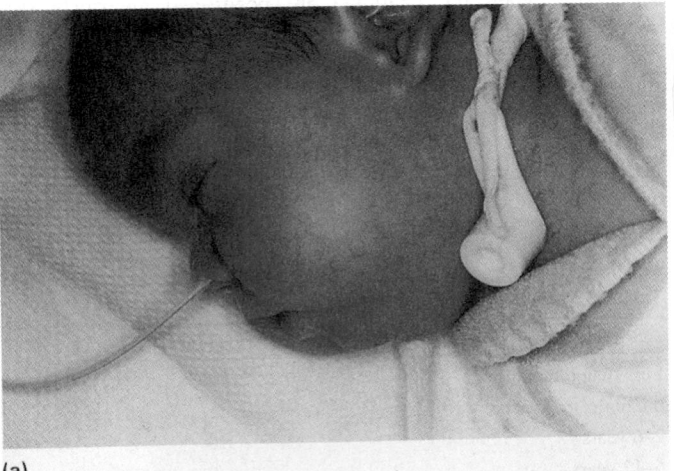

(a)

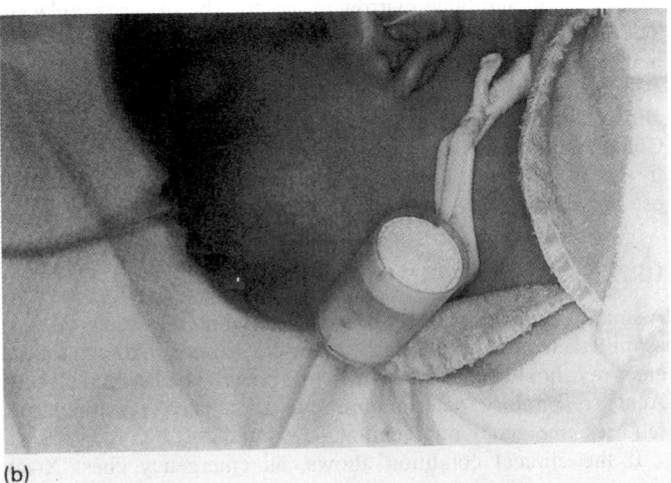

(b)

Fig. 33.11 Tracheostomy firmly fixed by cotton ribbon (**a**) and (**b**) with simple humidification system (Thermovent, Portex).

and local anesthetic without adrenaline injected into skin, subcutaneous tissues and down to the capsule of the joint. If the hip joint is the site of septic arthritis then open surgical drainage, with appropriate antibiotic cover, is usually required. Infection of metaphyses can cause sterile effusions in adjacent joints, hence needle tap over an area of metaphyseal erythema and tenderness may yield pus for culture.

BONE MARROW

Bone marrow examination may be required in anemia to rule out aplasia or leukemia, metastatic malignancy or a storage disease. It can also be used for rapid chromosomal analysis in the neonatal period and for marrow bacteriological culture in occult infection. It may be contraindicated in the bleeding diatheses, including hemophilia and Christmas disease, although the thrombocytopenic patient can be protected by a platelet transfusion before and during the procedure.

Analgesia and sedation are required for the procedure. General anesthetic may be best for the child who will need repeated bone marrow investigations. Where local anesthetic is used, plain lignocaine is infiltrated into the skin, subcutaneous tissues and periosteum: at the same time the depth of the periosteum is noted and this distance plus 2 mm is used as the length from marrow needle tip to the protective adjustable metal guard which will prevent the needle from penetrating too deeply. For the child under 3 months of age, the tibia is the preferred site: the medial subcutaneous surface is palpated and the needle inserted at the junction of the upper and middle third. The older infant or child should be placed in the lateral recumbent position: the site for marrow aspiration is on the posterior iliac crest 1 cm above the posterior superior iliac spine. The sternum is *never* used as the site of bone marrow aspiration in pediatric practice.

Strict aseptic technique is used. A 21G marrow needle is suitable for young infants and an 18G needle for older children – both needles must have a well-fitting trocar and a reliable adjustable metal guard. The needle and trocar are pushed through skin down to periosteum and the bone is penetrated by a rotating action. The needle becomes fixed in solid bone and then the trocar is withdrawn. A 20 ml syringe is connected to the needle and strong suction applied to draw up 0.2 ml of blood and marrow. If nothing appears the trocar is replaced, the needle advanced a further 1 mm and bone marrow aspirated. The trocar is replaced. The trocar and cannula are then withdrawn together and hemostasis obtained by 5 min of firm pressure. Meanwhile the aspirate is expelled onto several slides, smears are made and allowed to dry. A sterile dressing is placed over the puncture site. Complications of this procedure include bone fracture (especially if the tibia is the chosen site), subperiosteal hematoma and osteomyelitis.

DRAINAGE OF PNEUMOTHORAX

A small pneumothorax may produce no symptoms or may present as mild tachypnea with little systemic compromise. In such a child an X-ray should be taken and the child should be observed closely. Acute respiratory deterioration due to tension pneumothorax requires emergency intervention.

If the clinical condition allows, an emergency chest X-ray (ideally with a lateral view also) should be carried out to establish the site of intrapleural air. If the child is in extremis the diagnosis

can be made by percussion, auscultation, transillumination (by a torch or cold light source in a darkened room) and if necessary by intercostal needle aspiration. This last is done by connecting a 20 ml syringe to a butterfly needle (23-G for a neonate, 19G for an older child) via a three-way tap. Gas under tension is aspirated from the needle placed in the second intercostal space in the midclavicular line. There is no place for the emergency plunging of a definitive drain into a moribund child's chest. The tension pneumothorax can be accurately diagnosed and controlled by needle aspiration, while the appropriate equipment and sterile procedure pack are prepared. Analgesia and sedation are essential prior to the insertion of a chest drain and adequate time should be allowed to elapse for complete pain relief.

The choice of cannula size for formal drainage is shown in Table 33.5. Facial oxygen is given throughout. For the older child two commonly used sites of insertion are suitable: if the second intercostal space outside the midclavicular line is selected, the child lies back at 45°; if the fourth intercostal space in the midaxillary line is chosen the patient leans forward onto firm supporting pillows. Strict aseptic technique is used and local anesthetic is infiltrated into the skin, subcutaneous tissue and pleura. A transverse incision is then made in the skin just above the rib and the trocar and cannula inserted. During insertion it is essential to grip the trocar and cannula 1 cm from the tip, either between finger and thumb or with a sterile clamp, so that the vital organs deep to the intrapleural air do not get damaged during the procedure. The trocar is then withdrawn. The cannula is pushed in gently between 5 and 10 cm, clamped, connected to the underwater seal drainage (or a flutter valve) and the clamp is then released. The water level is checked for the presence of bubbling or a rhythmical swinging with respiration. A pursestring suture and adhesive tape ensure that the attachment is secure. A chest X-ray should then be arranged.

Twenty-four hours after the bubbling has stopped the cannula may be clamped. If a repeat X-ray confirms complete re-expansion of lung the chest drain may be removed, but only after the child has been given adequate analgesia and sedation. The pursestring is pulled tight and the wound covered with a sterile dressing. Bacteriological examination of the cannula tip is an important routine. Most clinicians order a further chest X-ray after the cannula has been removed.

Most babies are ventilated when supine and drainage is most successful when the cannulae are positioned anteriorly (the second intercostal space). The author, however, strongly favors the fifth intercostal space in the anterior axillary line, so that the internal mammary arteries are unlikely to be traumatized and for a superior cosmetic result in both boys and girls. Persuading the cannula tip to travel anteriorly in the chest can be reliably achieved by bending the trocar tip by 20° and inserting the trocar and cannula such that the tip is coaxed anterior to the collapsed lung. One of the commonest reasons for insertion of a second

Table 33.5   Tube size for chest drainage

Age	Argyle tube
Less than 6 months	12
6 months to 2 years	11
2–6 years	10
6–12 years	9
More than 12 years	8

drainage cannula is failure to maneuver the first cannula anteriorly.

PARACENTESIS OF THE THORAX

This procedure requires sedation, analgesia and strict aseptic technique. It can be used both diagnostically and therapeutically for removal of fluid, pus or blood. If well enough, the child sits up and is supported leaning forward on pillows. Chest X-rays, both anteroposterior and lateral, or ultrasonography assist with localization of chest fluid. Usually the eighth or ninth intercostal space in the posterior axillary line is chosen as the best site for paracentesis, but loculated fluid may need to be drained from an alternative position. When the local anesthetic has numbed the chosen area an 18G needle connected via a three-way tap to a 20 ml syringe is inserted just above bone. Fluid aspirated into the syringe is discharged via the three-way tap into a sterile outflow collecting system. Specimens are sent for bacteriological and pathological examination. Where large volumes of fluid are involved it may be decided to drain a proportion of the material at daily intervals, because pulmonary edema may result from rapid removal of too much fluid. Other complications are pneumothorax, hemothorax and the introduction of infection.

PARACENTESIS OF THE ABDOMEN

Aspiration of fluid from the abdomen may be used diagnostically (e.g. post-trauma and in malignant ascites) or therapeutically (e.g. in hepatic cirrhosis and the nephrotic syndrome). The child's bladder must be emptied prior to the procedure and consideration is given to deflating the intestines by a nasogastric tube on free drainage. The patient lies supine and the choice of paracentesis site is made – either in the midline half way between symphysis pubis and umbilicus or in the right or left iliac fossa lateral to the inferior epigastric artery. With full sterile precautions local anesthetic is infiltrated, a small scalpel incision made (avoiding previous scars) and a trocar and cannula inserted into the peritoneum. The trocar is then withdrawn and the cannula gently advanced further. A sterile drainage tube is attached to the cannula, which is then taped securely in position. Fluid is sent for estimation of electrolytes, glucose, protein, cell count, Gram stain and bacteriological culture.

Complications of paracentesis include hypovolemia (a spring clip will prevent too rapid flow of a large fluid volume), cannula blockage (correctable by manipulation of the tube or even injection of 5 ml of sterile saline) and bladder or bowel perforation. If air is aspirated as the cannula enters the peritoneal cavity, the bowel has probably been punctured and the cannula should be removed immediately. Appropriate antibiotic therapy is necessary, including therapy against anaerobic organisms. The puncture should seal spontaneously but peritonitis may ensue.

GASTRIC LAVAGE

This procedure has been largely abandoned in favor of inducing vomiting by ipecacuanha syrup, which is a safer and more effective technique. Neither gastric lavage nor ipecacuanha should be used if the child has swallowed paraffin, turpentine or related substances, nor if a corrosive has been consumed. The child must be fully conscious or, if unconscious, then a cuffed endotracheal tube must protect the airway.

Table 33.6 Choice of orogastric tube for gastric lavage

Age of child (years)	Gauge (FG)
0–2	28
2–4	30
Older than 4	34

An orogastric tube is selected as shown in Table 33.6. The distance between the child's chin and umbilicus is measured and marked on the tube, being the appropriate distance for insertion. The conscious child is then wrapped in a sheet and placed in the left semiprone position with head downwards over the edge of the bed. The orogastric tube is passed to the measured distance. If choking or cyanosis occurs the procedure must be stopped at least temporarily. If the child vomits during insertion, the tube must be removed fully to allow free emesis. Occasionally an oropharyngeal airway is required to keep the child from biting the orogastric tube during the procedure. Once the tube is in place, the stomach contents are aspirated with a large syringe. Rubber tubing and a funnel are connected to the orogastric tube and some tepid normal saline is poured in. The funnel end of the tubing is then lowered allowing the gastric contents to empty passively into the disposal bucket. Five cycles may be needed and then, if indicated, a drug may be instilled by the same route as the saline (e.g. desferrioxamine in treating iron poisoning) prior to removal of the orogastric tube.

LIVER ASPIRATION

Where large, chronic, amebic abscesses have not responded to treatment with amebicidal drugs, it may be necessary to aspirate pus. This procedure should not be attempted if the problem involves multiple small abscesses. The area of maximum pain and tenderness and a local mass are identified. Ultrasonography may assist the clinician in identifying the largest abscess or abscesses. Under aseptic conditions and opiate sedation or general anesthetic, an 18G needle is inserted into the mass and pus aspirated. If large amounts of pus are obtained the procedure may be repeated in 48 h with further benefit. It is essential that metronidazole and/or dehydroemetine are being administered at the same time to prevent further dissemination of disease.

PERCUTANEOUS RENAL BIOPSY

This procedure may provide important information in chronic nephritis but should be attempted only by an experienced operator. Renal biopsy is contraindicated in hydronephrosis, single kidney, a coagulopathy, systemic hypertension and uremia. A unit of blood must first be crossmatched and a preliminary X-ray or ultrasound scan done to localize the kidney relative to prepositioned radiopaque skin markers. The traditional method using a Vim–Silverman or Trucut needle is described here, but is now largely superseded by the renal biopsy gun as a day-case procedure.

The biopsy site is marked over the lower pole of the kidney, usually where the lateral edge of sacrospinalis muscle crosses the lowest rib. A combination of premedication and local anesthetic or light general anesthetic and muscle relaxant may be used. The child lies prone and a 10 cm No. 27 exploring needle is inserted first and as the lower pole of kidney is entered, the needle swings with respiration. The guard on the Vim–Silverman biopsy needle is adjusted to the same depth and the biopsy needle inserted in the same direction as the exploring needle. The kidney is entered while the child's breath is held in deep inspiration and then the needle is allowed to swing with respiration. The biopsy is taken while the patient's breath is again held – cutting blades are firmly inserted, then covered with the outer needle and the Vim–Silverman system removed. The wound is pressed firmly with a gauze swab, bandaged, then observed for bleeding for 24 h. The biopsy specimen is placed in 10% formalin solution immediately and in liquid nitrogen if immunofluorescent techniques are required.

Many believe that it is vital that the child be in bed and observed closely for 24 h with careful monitoring of blood pressure and pulse, although successful Trucut biopsies are described as a day-case procedure. Transient hematuria is an occasional complication. Some children have experienced postoperative hemorrhage requiring blood transfusion, surgical exploration and unilateral nephrectomy.

SKIN BIOPSY

Small skin lesions may be removed totally by excision biopsy. Pigmented nevi, if they require removal, should be excised by cutting down to, but not through, subcutaneous fascia. Sampling tissue of large lesions may be achieved by removing an elliptical specimen which includes the junction of normal and abnormal skin. The longitudinal axis of the ellipse should follow Langer's lines, which may be defined by wrinkling the skin and observing the lines on the epidermis which usually coincide with the direction of the growth of hairs.

After infiltration of local anesthetic, the incision is made with a No. 15 scalpel, held like a pen in one hand, while the other hand produces skin traction for hemostasis. Profusely bleeding vessels may be cauterized or ligatured with 4.0 or 5.0 absorbable suture, e.g. Vicryl or Dexon. The biopsy specimen is lifted with forceps while curved scissors free the skin by cutting subcutaneously. Most wounds can then be closed with a subcuticular 4.0 Vicryl suture, but if tension exists across the site then apposition is achieved with interrupted 4.0 prolene or nylon sutures.

Punches (2 mm and 5 mm) have been designed as an alternative skin biopsy technique. A punch is pushed through the skin by rotating clockwise and anticlockwise as far as the subcutaneous fat layer. The punch is then withdrawn and the circular specimen of skin is freed and removed as above. Hemostasis is achieved by suture or by pressure followed by the application of a small disc of Gelfoam.

MUSCLE BIOPSY

Most muscle biopsies are obtained from rectus femoris, gastrocnemius or deltoid muscles. After infiltration with local anesthetic, a linear incision is made with a No. 15 scalpel immediately over the muscle and parallel to Langer's lines (see Skin biopsy above). In the thigh a longitudinal incision is used. Bleeding blood vessels may be cauterized or ligatured and the muscle is exposed by sharp dissection through the deep fascia until the muscle belly protrudes. A small self-retaining retractor decreases local hemorrhage by traction. A muscle biopsy clamp is used to transfix and pick up the muscle section under constant tension and the specimen is then dissected free and transferred immediately, still under constant tension, into the laboratory medium, e.g. glutaraldehyde. Suturing of the muscle with 4.0 Dexon must include the investing fascia since muscle itself will not hold sutures. Subcutaneous and cutaneous layers are closed as for skin biopsy (see above).

REFERENCES

Anand K J S, Hickey P R 1987 Pain and its effects in the human neonate and fetus. New England Journal of Medicine 317: 1321–1329

Anand K J S, Brown M J, Bloom S R, Aynsley-Green A 1985 Studies on the hormonal regulation of fuel metabolism in the human newborn infant undergoing anaesthesia and surgery. Hormone Research 22: 115–128

Arnold J H, Truog R D, Orav E J, Scavone J M, Hershenson M B 1990 Tolerance and dependence in neonates sedated with fentanyl during extracorporeal membrane oxygenation. Anesthesiology 73: 1136–1140

Bach S, Noreng M F, Tjelldun N U 1988 Phantom limb pain in amputees during the first 12 months following limb amputation after preoperative lumbar epidural blockade. Pain 33: 297–301

Berde C B 1989 Pediatric postoperative pain management. Pediatric Clinics of North America 36: 921–940

Berde C B, Lehn B M, Yee J D, Sethna N F, Russo D 1991 Patient controlled analgesia in children: a randomized prospective comparison with intramuscular administration of morphine for postoperative analgesia. Journal of Pediatrics 118: 460–466

Bray R J, Woodhams A M, Vallis C J, Kelly P J, Ward Platt M 1995 A double-blind comparison of morphine infusion and PCA in children. Association of Paediatric Anaesthetists Annual Scientific Meeting

Cote C J, Zaslavsky A, Downes J J, Kurth D, Welborn L G, Warner L O, Malviya S V 1995 Postoperative apnea in former preterm infants after inguinal herniorrhaphy. Anesthesiology 82: 809–822

Doyle E, Morton N S 1994 Long term patient-controlled analgesia in terminal care. Paediatric Anaesthesia 4: 137–139

Flower M J 1985 Neuromaturation of the human fetus. Journal of Medical Philosophy 10: 237–251

Grunau R V E, Craig K D 1987 Pain expression in neonates; facial expression and cry. Pain 28: 395–410

Hanallah R S, Broadman L S, Belman A B, Abramowitz M D, Epstein B S 1987 Comparison of caudal and ilioinguinal nerve blocks for control of post-orchidopexy pain in pediatric ambulatory surgery. Anesthesiology 66: 832–834

Hendrickson M, Myre L, Johnson D G 1990 Postoperative analgesia in children: a prospective study of intermittent intramuscular injection vs continuous intravenous infusion of morphine. Journal of Pediatric Surgery 25: 185–191

Hutton P, Clutton-Brock T 1993 The benefits and pitfalls of pulse oximetry. British Medical Journal 307: 457–458

Koren G, Butt W, Chinyanga H, Soldin S, Tan Y K, Pape K 1985 Postoperative morphine infusion in newborn infants: assessment of disposition, characteristics and safety. Journal of Pediatrics 107: 963–967

Krane E J, Heller E B, Pomietto M L 1991 Incidence of phantom sensation and pain in pediatric amputees. Anesthesiology 75: A69

Lloyd-Thomas A R, Howard R F 1994 A pain service for children. Paediatric Anaesthesia 4: 3–15

Maunuksela E, Olkkola K T, Korpela R 1987 Measurement of pain in children with self-reporting and behavioural assessment. Clinical Pharmacology and Therapeutics 42: 137–141

McNicol L R 1993 Postoperative analgesia in children using continuous s.c. morphine. British Journal of Anaesthesia 71: 752–756

McNicol L R 1994 Paediatric analgesia. In: Nimmo W S, Rowbotham D J, Smith G (eds) Anaesthesia, 2nd edn. Blackwell Scientific Publications, Oxford

Milne E M G, Elliott M J, Pearson D T, Holden M P, Orskov H, Alberti K G M M 1986 The effect on intermediary metabolism of open-heart surgery with deep hypothermia and circulatory arrest in infants of less than 10kg body weight. Perfusion 1: 29–40

Mowbray M J, Gaukroger P B 1990 Long-term patient-controlled analgesia in children. Anaesthesia 45: 941–943

Pounder D R, Steward D J 1992 Postoperative analgesia: opioid infusions in infants and children. Canadian Journal of Anaesthesia 39: 969–974

Quinn M W, Wild J, Dean H G, Hartley R, Rushforth J A, Puntis J W L, Levene M I 1993 Randomised double-blind controlled trial of effect of morphine on catecholamine concentrations in ventilated pre-term babies. Lancet 342: 324–327

Schechter N L 1989 The undertreatment of pain in children: an overview. Pediatric Clinics of North America 36: 781–794

Srinivasan G, Jain R, Pildes R S, Kannan C R 1986 Glucose homeostasis during anesthesia and surgery in infants. Journal of Pediatric Surgery 21: 718–721

Tverskoy M, Cozacov C, Ayache M, Bradley E L, Kissin I 1990 Postoperative pain after inguinal herniorrhaphy with different types of anesthesia. Anesthesia and Analgesia 70: 29–35

Wasylak T J, Abbot F V, English M J M, Jeans M 1990 Reduction of postoperative morbidity following patient-controlled morphine. Canadian Journal of Anaesthesia 37: 726–731

Wolf A R, Hughes D G 1993 Pain relief for infants undergoing abdominal surgery: comparisons of infusions of i.v. morphine and extradural bupivacaine. British Journal of Anaesthesia 70: 10–16

34 Social and legal aspects of pediatrics

F. N. Bamford   David Lessels   A. G. M. Campbell

Vital statistics   1848
Special investigations of child health   1850
Organization of medical services for children   1852
Family influences on child health   1854
Deprivation   1857
Adoption   1858
Preschool and school health care   1860
The children of immigrants   1865
Child abuse   1866
F. N. Bamford

Legislation to protect children and to promote their welfare   1874
The Children Act 1989   1874
F. N. Bamford
The Children (Scotland) Act 1995   1876
David Lessels
The pediatrician and medical negligence   1877
A. G. M. Campbell
References and Bibliography   1880

Definition

Social pediatrics is the study of how children's health is affected by the circumstances in which they live and by their relationships to various members and groups of society. It is that part of pediatrics concerned with:

1. the organization and administration of public services providing health care for children
2. the application of measures to prevent disease and protect children from adverse social influences
3. the contribution of pediatric knowledge to the alleviation and solution of social and educational problems.

This chapter starts with an account of vital statistics and how they are collected because they are fundamentally important to the rational use of resources. It is followed by a brief outline of services in Britain. Prevention is dealt with elsewhere and will not be repeated here. An outline of relevant British law has been included because protection of children from adverse social influences often involves litigation requiring a pediatric contribution. The greatest part of the chapter is about the effect of various social influences on child health. For nearly all children, mothers are their first and most important contacts followed by families, nurseries and schools. Problems arising from these relationships are described successively and the chapter also includes an account of the effects of migration.

VITAL STATISTICS

Every country requires accurate information about its population for administrative and planning purposes including the efficient management of health services. In developed countries, national systems of vital statistics are based on data obtained by census and by registration of births, marriages and deaths.

Census

Populations have been enumerated from ancient times. The Doomsday Book of 1086 is the earliest known record in England. Most modern censuses developed during the 17th and 18th centuries and in Britain a decennial census has been taken since 1801 with the exception of 1941. Censuses are expensive and in most countries are carried out only every 10 years. They are compulsory and confidential. Attention to detail ensures that they are as accurate as possible and a great deal depends on the employment of conscientious enumerators and on the veracity of the respondents. Time precision is important and it is customary to count the number of residents of a household at midnight on the night of the census.

Since much of the value of vital statistics is derived from the study of changes over years, great care is necessary before the form of questions is changed, and additions or alterations are subject to parliamentary approval. Between censuses, estimates are made from figures obtained from the previous census, the Registrar of Births, Marriages and Deaths and migration records. Revised estimates are published following the next census.

The Office of Population Censuses and Surveys (OPCS) had the task of organizing censuses and of compiling and analyzing vital statistics from these and other sources. The OPCS was closely linked with the Central Statistical Office (CSO) which was responsible for the coordination of social statistics. In 1996, the two offices merged to become the Office of National Statistics (ONS).

Registration of births, marriages and deaths

Births, marriages and deaths have been recorded by the Church from early times and in Britain registration with the State became a statutory obligation in 1839.

Live births

Live birth is defined in the Births and Deaths Registration Act 1953 simply as the birth of a child born alive irrespective of the duration of the pregnancy. A definition recommended by the WHO is:

complete expulsion or extraction from its mother of a product of conception, irrespective of the duration of the pregnancy which, after such separation, breathes or shows any other evidence of life such as beating of the heart, pulsation of the umbilical cord, or definite movement of the voluntary muscles, whether or not the umbilical cord has been cut or the placenta is attached; each product of such a birth is considered live born.

It is not used by all countries and international differences in registration practice and definition should be taken into account when data are compared.

In Britain the local Registrar of Births and Deaths has to be informed within 42 days (21 days in Scotland) of every live birth and certain people have a legal responsibility to inform him. They are the mother; the father if married at the time of conception or birth; the occupier of the house or institution in which the birth occurred; a person present at the birth; or the person in charge of the child.

In the birth register is recorded the child's date and place of birth, name, surname and sex, the father's name, surname, place of birth and occupation, the mother's name, surname, place of birth, occupation and usual address, together with her maiden surname and the surname in which she contracted her latest marriage if different from her maiden surname, and the name, surname, address and qualification of the informant. The Population (Statistics) Act 1938 authorized the collection of particulars about fertility such as the ages, marital status and numbers of previous children of the parents but these are not entered in the register and are treated as confidential.

Either a short or full birth certificate is issued. The former is provided without charge and records only the name, date of birth and registration district of the child. Full certificates are provided for a small fee. Those issued in England and Wales differ slightly from those in Scotland but both record the name, sex, date and place of birth of the child, the names of both parents, the father's occupation and the mother's maiden surname. In Scotland the hour of the child's birth and the date and place of the parent's marriage (and their occupations) are included.

Stillbirths

A stillborn infant is defined as a child which has issued forth from its mother after the 24th week of pregnancy and which did not at any time after being completely expelled from its mother breathe or show any other signs of life: The Stillbirth (Definition) Act 1992. In England and Wales a stillbirth should be registered within 42 days (within 21 days in Scotland) and cannot be registered if more than 3 months have elapsed since the birth. Maternity Allowance is payable only for registered live and stillbirths.

The entry in the register includes the cause certified by a medical practitioner together with the date and place of stillbirth, the baby's name, if any, and the parent's full names, occupations, usual addresses and places of birth. If she does not wish the father to be identified in the register the mother's details are sufficient. Other confidential questions are asked for statistical purposes but are not included in the register.

Abortion

It is a statutory duty of any doctor who has performed an abortion to notify the event within 7 days. The data collected include the name, age and status of the mother and the place, date and method of abortion.

Deaths

When a child dies during an illness in which he has been attended by a registered medical practitioner, the practitioner is obliged by statute to send a certificate to the Registrar stating his opinion of the cause of death. He also supplies the parents or guardians with a certificate headed 'Notice to Informant' stating that he has signed a medical certificate of the cause of death and they must then register the death. They inform the Registrar of the full name, sex, address, date and place of birth and date and place of death of their child.

In the case of sudden, unexplained or postoperative deaths and deaths due to violence, the matter has to be referred to the Coroner in England and Wales, or to the Procurator Fiscal in Scotland. The Coroner usually orders a postmortem examination and conducts an inquiry including, in some cases, a formal inquest before issuing a certificate stating the cause of death. The Procurator Fiscal can order a postmortem and carry out an investigation and, depending upon the circumstances, may apply to the sheriff to hold a Fatal Accident Inquiry.

Annual tables can be compiled showing the effect of age, sex, occupational class, time of year and geographical situation on mortality. Most of the information is factual but causes of death are often opinions and known to be inaccurate. They should be considered critically during any inquiry or comparison.

An account of the secular changes in the child population, definitions of the indices used to measure mortality and tabulations of the principal causes of death in childhood can be found in Chapter 1.

Morbidity

As mortality has decreased information about illness has become more important. Unfortunately, it is not so well recorded as data about births and deaths but certain conditions and disabilities are notifiable by law. The most important sources of morbidity statistics are as follows:

Notification of infectious disease

This was introduced many years ago to facilitate the control of contagious infections by the isolation of affected persons and the protection of contacts. Underreporting is notorious but the Public Health (Control of Disease) Act 1984 requires any registered medical practitioner attending a person who he suspects may be suffering from a notifiable infectious disease to notify 'forthwith'

Table 34.1 Notification of infectious diseases in the UK

Anthrax	Puerperal fever
Cholera	Rabies
Diphtheria	Relapsing fever
Dysentery (amebic or bacillary)	Rubella
Erysipelas	Scarlet fever
Food poisoning	Smallpox
Legionellosis	Tetanus
Leptospirosis	Toxoplasmosis
Malaria	Tuberculosis
Measles	Typhoid fever
Meningococcal infection	Typhus
Mumps	Varicella (chickenpox)
Ophthalmia neonatorum	Viral hemorrhagic fevers (including yellow fever)
Plague	Viral hepatitis
Poliomyelitis	Whooping cough

the 'Proper Officer' of his district. The 'Proper Officer' is usually a designated consultant in public health medicine. There are official notification forms but telephone notification is requested for some conditions. Diseases which have to be notified are listed in Table 34.1. In some places notification of additional diseases may be required by local Acts of Parliament.

Genitourinary medicine clinics submit returns to the Department of Health which include some cases of congenital infection.

Hospital activity analysis

This is an administrative and planning instrument recording data on patients discharged from hospital. Information is obtained about the numbers of children hospitalized, their diagnostic categories and durations of stay.

Annual social surveys

These were published by the Office of Population Censuses and Surveys and, from 1996, will be published by the Office of National Statistics. They consist of the Family Expenditure Survey, a General Household Survey, a National Food Survey and various other surveys, some of them relevant to child health such as Day Care Services for Children and Children's Dental Health. The General Household Surveys contain information about self-reported acute and chronic sickness and consultations with general practitioners.

Notification of congenital malformations

In Britain a voluntary system of notification of congenital malformations recognizable at birth was introduced after the thalidomide epidemic of 1961. It was intended to give early warning of any further teratogenic disaster. Abnormalities are usually recorded by midwives on birth notification forms but the information is often incomplete and does not include malformations occurring in cases of fetal death. Population-based registers of children with specific conditions such as Down syndrome are usually more satisfactory.

Registers of handicapped children

In England and Wales (but not in Scotland) the Children Act 1989 (Sch. 2, pt. 1, s. 2) requires every local authority social services

department to maintain a register of disabled children and provide services minimizing the effect of their disabilities. For purposes of the Act a child is disabled if he is blind, deaf or dumb or suffers from mental disorder of any kind or is substantially *and* permanently handicapped by illness, injury or congenital deformity or such other disability as may be prescribed. Special Needs registers are often kept by health authorities but the information in them is often of poor quality. Similar registers are kept for purposes of educational administration.

Cancer registration

Children's Tumor registers have been established for many years. Information is supplied by oncologists and pediatricians voluntarily. They are diagnostic registers, based on geographically defined areas and as such provide more precise data than are available in other types of register.

British Paediatric Association Surveillance Unit

Several agencies collaborate in the surveillance of infections, infection-related conditions and epidemiological studies of uncommon disorders. It is a method of detection and monitoring based on the receipt of monthly postal returns from members of either the Royal College of Paediatrics and Child Health or the Faculty of Paediatrics of the Royal College of Physicians of Ireland. There is a high response rate (almost 95%) and important information about a variety of conditions has been obtained.

SPECIAL INVESTIGATIONS OF CHILD HEALTH

Special inquiries are necessary when questions cannot be answered by reference to existing data either because the information is not available or the form in which it exists is not sufficiently precise. There are three main types – descriptive, analytic and intervention studies.

Descriptive studies

These include accounts of incidence and distribution often dependent on retrospective data. Problems arise because of incomplete and inaccurate records, changing diagnostic criteria or population structures and difficulties in defining the timing of events.

Analytic studies

Such studies are used, for example, to evaluate the relative importance of different etiologic factors. There are three types:

1. Cross sectional studies – analysis of the characteristics of a group of children at a particular time.

2. Case-control studies – a group of children with a known disease or developmental characteristic is matched with an appropriately chosen control sample. Care has to be taken to avoid sampling bias and matched controls are usually selected from random number tables or case registers using either the next entry or entries at defined intervals. Birth, infant clinic and school registers can be used and in some studies hospital patients with diseases unrelated to the one being investigated serve as controls. Siblings are often good subjects because they have a matching home environment.

3. Cohort studies – a defined group of children is re-examined at intervals. Some of the best known and productive child health surveys have been of this type. They are prospective inquiries and are necessarily longer and usually more expensive than other types of inquiry. Care has to be taken to avoid errors due to changing techniques of examination during the study period and, especially in the case of larger studies, to minimize variation between different observers. Cohort studies in themselves may alter the behavior of parents and the health experience of their children because they are often educated and interested by the study.

Intervention studies

Clinical trials to determine the effectiveness of drugs or to evaluate different preventive and administrative measures are of this type. These studies are prospective and the choice of control groups is of critical importance. Great weight has to be given to ethical considerations in all child health investigations and intervention studies can be particularly difficult in this respect.

Child mortality and morbidity studies

The following are the most important postwar mortality and morbidity studies concerned with children in the UK.

Maternity Survey 1946

A Joint Committee of the Population Investigation Committee and the Royal College of Obstetricians and Gynaecologists undertook a survey into the operation and use of maternity services which had implications for child health. Through the staff of local authority health departments, data about nearly 14 000 confinements occurring throughout England, Scotland and Wales during one week in March 1946 were collected. The survey showed inequalities in the care received by women in different social classes and a clear relationship between social class and the incidence of low birth weight babies.

The National Survey of Health and Development

A sample of 5362 children from the Maternity Survey of 1946 were followed up and the data published in *Children under Five* (Douglas & Blomfield 1958) showed that children in rural areas were generally taller than those in towns and that children in Southern England were taller than those in Northern England, Scotland or Wales. The shortest children were in the lower social groups and class differences in height increased to the age of 5 years. It was inferred from the data that children of employed mothers were not disadvantaged. Families in the poorest homes were found to make the least use of the health services.

In *The Home and the School* (Douglas 1964), attainments of children in primary schools were described and it was shown that for middle-class children good maternal care and housing reinforced good performance at school. Observations of the children in secondary schools were the subject of a third report, *All Our Future* (Douglas et al 1968), in which it was reported that lower manual working-class children of high ability tended to leave school early. This was particularly marked when parental interest was lacking and school staffing and equipment deficient. In selective schools for the most intelligent there was a steady social class gradient in achievement and it was greatly influenced by the type of family from which the students came. Pupils in schools with lesser standards differed considerably in achievement according to social class. At all stages of school life the influence of home was an important determinant of the attainments of children.

1000 Family Study, 1947–62

In Newcastle upon Tyne from 1 May to 30 June 1947, 1142 newborn infants were enrolled into a special study group and their families visited regularly by nurses and doctors. Illnesses were recorded against known family and social backgrounds. The study continued for 15 years when most children left school. A great amount of data about child morbidity was collected (Spence et al 1954, Miller et al 1960).

Stillbirth and Infant Mortality Study

The influence of social class, maternal age, parity and geographical location on stillbirth, neonatal and postneonatal mortality was studied and 'vulnerable' or 'high risk' groups defined in biological and social terms (Morris & Heady 1955). It was shown that they exerted largely independent influences on stillbirth and neonatal mortality rates in England and Wales.

Mothers aged 35 years having a first baby and mothers of any parity over 40 years of age were found to be at high risk of producing stillborn children and postneonatal death occurred more frequently in the children of young mothers who had large families. Age and parity differences between the mothers in various social classes were insufficient to explain the separate mortality rates experienced by their children. Although mortality rates declined with remarkable uniformity between 1911 and 1949, rates of fall were not the same in each social class, improvement being least in the laboring classes. Three factors were thought to explain these findings: firstly, a time lag, different in each class, between social improvement and better health; secondly, changing composition of the social groups; and thirdly, cultural differences in lifestyles not directly related to economic factors (Morris & Heady 1955).

The Perinatal Mortality Survey, 1958

Information about 17 204 births in the week commencing the 3 March 1958 was collected and analysis confirmed the findings of the Stillbirth and Infant Mortality Study with respect to the influence of age, parity, geographic region and social class.

Perinatal mortality was highest for first infants and the babies of very young mothers and lowest for second infants and those born to mothers between 20 and 30 years. Rates escalated after the third child and with increasing maternal age. Standardization for age and parity left social class differences virtually unchanged and did not affect regional variation. Rates were lowest in Southeastern England and London and highest in Northeastern England and Scotland (Butler & Bonham 1963).

A second report addressed the effects on perinatal mortality of place of delivery and the availability of consultant services. Deaths due to causes amenable to good obstetric care were higher in rural than in urban areas. Inferior perinatal mortality rates in Northern England and Scotland were ascribed to differences in health, physique and reproductive habit rather than the quality of obstetric services (Butler & Alberman, 1969).

The National Child Development Study

Children enrolled into the Perinatal Mortality Survey were followed up and information collected on approximately 90% of the sample. All children had an educational assessment by their class teacher, a standardized examination by a community medical officer and a health visitor interviewed their parents. A great body of knowledge was assembled and published by the National Children's Bureau in a series of books. It was found, for example, that among 11 000 children at 7 years of age, girls were generally better readers than boys who in turn surpassed them at problem arithmetic. 5% of children had special educational help and teachers thought that 8% would have benefited from such help and that 2% should have attended a special school. The medical inquiry revealed the frequency of a number of problems such as stammer (1%), suboptimal vision in at least one eye (13%), impaired hearing (4.9%) and bedwetting after the age of 7 years (10%). Social class affected performance and adjustment at school and in general girls were found to be better adjusted than boys (Kellmer-Pringle et al 1966, Davie et al 1972).

Isle of Wight Survey

This was a study of children aged 9 to 12 years who were living in a clearly defined geographical area. In 1964 intellectual and educational retardation was surveyed and in 1965 psychiatric disorder and physical handicap. Children were selected by screening methods and they and controls were examined individually.

As expected, intellectual retardation with an IQ more than 2 SD below the mean was present in 2.5% of the children studied, but in 0.3% it was so severe as to prevent attendance at school. One-third of the severely retarded children had Down syndrome. Specific educational problems occurred in 4% of the children and 6.3% were backward at reading; the latter being more common in boys than girls. Few had received special help. Intellectually retarded children had much greater rates of neurological abnormality and emotional and behavioral disorder than controls.

The prevalence of psychiatric disorder in 10- and 11-year-old children was 6.8%. In all, 1 child in 54 was found to have a chronic or recurrent handicap at 9 to 11 years (Rutter et al 1970).

British Births Child Study

A cohort of 16 000 children born in the UK during a week in 1970

was studied, events during their first week of life recorded and detailed inquiries made about all deaths in the neonatal period. A random 10% sample was examined at 22 months and again at 3½ years.

As in earlier surveys of this type a great deal of information was produced. Half of the children had attended hospital on at least one occasion before 3½ years, a high proportion because of accidents, but many with head injuries were not taken to hospital. Children of working mothers had more accidents than those whose mothers did not go out to work.

Children from large families were more likely than only children to contract infectious diseases but less likely to be vaccinated. Among young children with lower respiratory tract infections the most significant associated factor was maternal smoking. The survey revealed a high proportion of errors in screening tests for hearing, vision, squint and congenital dislocation of the hips (Chamberlain & Simpson 1979).

A social index was devised, incorporating not only the Registrar General's classification by occupation but also education, housing and neighborhood of residence. Each of these was scored and the index produced was found to be a better discriminator of child development and the use of services than the Registrar General's classification alone.

ORGANIZATION OF MEDICAL SERVICES FOR CHILDREN

Children of economically privileged nations benefit from fairly sophisticated health services, contrasting starkly with the absence of provision for the majority in the rest of the world who live in poor rural areas. Patterns of health care vary from country to country because of accidents of historical development and economic and political difference but the UK child health services described below are similar in many respects to those in other parts of Northern Europe.

Public arrangements for child health care evolved gradually, usually starting as local voluntary efforts to meet perceived needs, followed by legislation to make them generally available; the present system is thus the latest point in a process of reform beginning with the Poor Law of the 16th century. Some statutory measures to protect the health of children were promulgated by individuals who influenced parliamentary opinion while other laws were enacted following royal commissions or government committees of inquiry. Not surprisingly, services developing in such diverse ways lacked coordination.

In the UK, a National Health Service was inaugurated in 1948 to provide free comprehensive care for the whole population. It used existing services. All children became eligible to receive advice and treatment without charge from a family practitioner of their parents' choice and hospital consultation and care when necessary. Hospital facilities and the number of pediatricians were expanded and this coincided with advances in therapeutics which greatly improved the treatment of common diseases. Local authorities retained responsibility for preventive health services including infant welfare, school health, immunization and health visiting.

Hospital, family practitioner and local authority services were administered separately leading to duplication of services and difficulties in planning. Discontent with the administrative structure led to a reorganization of the National Health Service in Scotland in 1973 and in England and Wales in 1974. The purposes of reorganization were to create a more integrated service, enable representation of consumer interests, define responsibility, facilitate professional contributions to decision making and reallocate resources according to need. A tier of administration was eliminated and responsibility for the preventive health services was transferred from the local authorities to the National Health Service.

The Committee on Child Health Services (Court Committee)

The Secretary of State for Social Services established an expert committee 'to review the provision made for the health services for children, up to and through school life; to study the use made of these services by children and their parents and to make recommendations.' The report, published in 1976, contains an unparalleled review of child health in England and Wales which should be consulted by all who are concerned with the welfare of children. It has influenced legislative and administrative change in the UK and several important recommendations have been implemented. The Committee asserted that 'We have found no better way to raise a child than to reinforce the ability of his parent(s) whether natural or substitute to do so', and they sought involvement of parents and the provision of services to support them.

In their opinion preventive and therapeutic services should not be separate and medical care for children should be based on family practice. They rejected the idea of total pediatric specialization in primary care as practiced in some developed countries but recommended limited specialization and involvement of family practitioners in preventive child health services. The term 'general practitioner pediatrician' was coined.

The Committee expressed concern that health visitors whose traditional work was to visit and advise mothers about infant health and nutrition had acquired many other duties and, as a consequence, young families received less attention. They proposed the formation of groups of children's nurses led by 'child health visitors' to undertake both preventive and therapeutic duties in the community.

Hospital treatment of sick children in children's departments of main hospitals was preferred to care in a multiplicity of small hospitals. They recommended the appointment of 'consultant community pediatricians' with special skills in developmental, educational and social pediatrics and with contractual duties in special schools and social service departments. This recommendation has now been implemented.

Multidisciplinary district handicap teams with responsibility for all handicapped children including the mentally handicapped were suggested and a right of direct access to them by parents was recommended. Such teams have been in place throughout the UK for several years.

The report discussed the nature and prevalence of psychiatric disorder and reaffirmed an accepted need for expansion of the child psychiatry services. It recommended the development of integrated child and adolescent psychiatry services capable of operating in a variety of settings.

The Committee was concerned to protect the interests of children both individually and collectively. It recommended that where there is suspicion of serious ill health for which treatment is not being sought, health visitors should initially seek access to the child by persuasion but in the event of failure should have the right to apply for a legally enforceable medical examination.

Likewise, it was recommended that head teachers having reasonable grounds to suspect parental neglect or abuse should have the right to request the examination of a child in their charge, if necessary without the consent of the parents. These recommendations were made more than a decade before legislation applying to England and Wales enabled courts to make 'Child Assessment Orders' requiring parents to make their children available for medical examination. Finally, the Committee advocated the formation of a statutory Joint Committee for Children to review and coordinate services, influence public opinion, disseminate advice on good practice and ensure the implementation of recommendations.

The Brotherston Report published in 1973 (Scottish Home and Health Department) made similar recommendations for Scotland.

Joint Working Party on Child Health Surveillance (Hall Committee)

This was set up in 1986 to review preventive health care of children. They reviewed the literature, examined various screening tests and recommended a core program of surveillance for preschool children. It was pointed out that, although surveillance and monitoring are almost universally regarded as good practice, there is lack of uniformity and a paucity of research on the effectiveness of its various components. There have been three editions of *Health for All Children* reporting their recommendations. The latest proposes fewer procedures, the need for targeting and flexibility and emphasizes the importance of primary prevention, preferring the term 'child health promotion' to surveillance (Hall 1996).

Financial problems and dissatisfaction with the quality and availability of hospital care led to a further review of health service administration in 1989. The following is a summary of the administrative arrangements at present.

Central government departments

The National Health Service in England is the responsibility of a cabinet minister, the Secretary of State for Health, who is answerable to Parliament. In Scotland there is a separate Health Department within the Scottish Office the responsibility of the Secretary of State for Scotland; and the Secretary of State for Wales is responsible for health services in Wales. Ministers helped by their departments decide about national policies and the allocation of resources. A Children's Division within the Department of Health deals with the administration of the services and there is a standing Children's Committee with an advisory role. From time to time expert committees of inquiry are appointed.

Health authorities

Responsibility for all services within geographically defined areas lies with Health Authorities (Health Boards in Scotland) directly funded by and accountable to central government. They determine priorities of expenditure on health and purchase services. There are no formal arrangements for pediatric advice to be given to them nor is there necessarily any pediatric representation. They must provide medical advice for local education authorities and those health authorities with university teaching hospitals. They also have an additional responsibility to provide training facilities.

National Health Service trusts

Health services other than general practitioner services are provided by trusts responsible for managing hospitals and community services within their districts. In some places hospital and community trusts are separate as in the early days of the National Health Service. The members of trusts are appointed by the Secretary of State for Health (or Secretaries of State for Scotland or Wales) and they compete with each other to provide services required by health authorities. Whether the arrangements will stifle innovative practice and the effect that they will have on the development of pediatric care, in particular expensive tertiary care, remains to be seen.

General practitioner services

The majority of consultations about children are provided by general practitioners who are not employees of the National Health Service. They are professionally independent but contract to provide services either directly for the health authorities or with funds allocated to their practice. A general practitioner contract, introduced in 1990, has had a substantial impact on child health services by increasing the uptake of immunization and involving many more practitioners in developmental surveillance of children.

FAMILY INFLUENCES ON CHILD HEALTH

Most children live with a mother and father in a separate household, and a married couple living together with children of their marriage is the traditional western concept of a normal family. Many now reject this but, although less than formerly, there are still considerable social pressures upon young people to get married and once married to have children. There was an expectation that families would contain more than one child because it was commonly believed that only children were at a disadvantage but this belief has been eroded by social and economic pressures and single-child families are now very common throughout Western Europe.

Most British parents are likely to think that child rearing within extended families is second best although in the world as a whole it is probably at least as common as parenting within nuclear families, and millions of children are brought up successfully in this way. Geographic dispersion of extended families in Britain during the past few generations has led to a number of problems because older members of families are no longer as easily available as they were to give advice, support and help in child care.

Children can be successfully raised in adoptive or other substitute families as well as in nuclear and extended families but lack of any family is usually disastrous. Deprivation or disruption of normal family care is a matter of considerable concern for the present and may have far-reaching consequences for the future because parents' knowledge of how to bring up children is derived substantially from their own childhood experiences. The well known adverse effects on child health of aberrant family care can, therefore, extend beyond one generation.

ONE-PARENT FAMILIES

A one-parent family is defined as a mother or a father living without a spouse with his or her never married, dependent child or children (and not cohabiting). The proportion of one-parent families in Britain increased from 8% (involving 1 million children) in 1971 to 19% (involving 2.2 million children) in 1991. Of lone mothers in 1991, approximately 37% were single, 36% divorced, 22% separated and 6% widowed. Lone fathers looked after 2% of one-parent families with dependent children.

Children in one-parent families differ from others because they have little or no contact with one of their parents, usually the father. The care that they receive varies, as with children in normal families and generalizations about disadvantage may be misleading in individual cases. Nevertheless, many children are adversely affected because of economic hardship, difficulties with housing or social isolation, loneliness and emotional debility of mothers arising from the unshared burden of bringing up young children.

Not surprisingly, therefore, many children in one-parent families differ from children in normal homes. There is, for example, a highly significant negative association between skeletal maturation and indices of socioeconomic status of which the best single predictor is the rate within an area of single-parent households. As well as physical health, behavior may also be adversely affected. According to the National Survey of Health and Development children of divorced or separated parents tended to be rough and troublesome and more likely than others to be delinquent. Family disruption is associated with antisocial behavior and absence of a father is thought to be of substantial importance in this respect. Studies have shown that among emotionally disturbed children, such as those attending special schools for behaviorally disordered children, children from one-parent families are over-represented. This does not mean that life in a single-parent household is necessarily damaging to all of them, nor that they cannot compensate for their circumstances, but simply that they are generally exposed to more social stress than other children.

Prolonged stress and insecurity from any cause has an adverse effect on school work and poor performance by children from one-parent families is common. However, the relationship is not straightforward.

Among children living in one-parent families, those born outside of marriage and continuing to live with their birth mothers appear to suffer most disadvantage, followed by children affected by parental separation or divorce, while those orphaned by death of a parent seem to do best. Some features of each of these groups are described in succeeding sections.

Children born outside marriage

A child was said to be illegitimate if his or her mother and father were not married to one another at the time of conception or at the time of the child's birth. It referred to a legal status but it was removed from legal use in England and Wales by the Family Law Reform Act 1987, and in Scotland by the Law Reform (Parent and Child) (Scotland) Act 1986.

The proportion of births outside marriage has changed substantially during the past 30 years in most western countries. In the UK the percentage of births outside marriage increased from 5.72% in 1961, through 8.94% in 1971, to 12.44% by 1981. During the next decade it more than doubled to 29.79% by 1991. Very similar rates were recorded in France but elsewhere in Europe, although the general trend was upwards, there were wide variations, e.g. in 1991 the rate was 2.4% in Greece and 46.5% in Denmark.

In the UK there has also been an increase in the proportion of births outside marriage registered by both parents – from 38% in 1961 to three-quarters by 1992. Many give the same address and it is probable that about a half of children born outside marriage are brought up by both parents living in nonmarital union.

Cohabitation, i.e. couples living together as husband and wife without legal marriage, has become more common. Rates are higher for divorced men and women many of whom have dependent children. The General Household Survey indicated that couples cohabiting before marriage have higher rates of divorce than those who do not cohabit before marriage.

When an unmarried mother becomes pregnant she has three alternatives. She may marry but this option has declined in popularity and a much greater proportion than in the past now take the second alternative of carrying the pregnancy to term and keeping the baby without getting married. The third choice, abortion, appears to have been made most often by those who formerly would have relinquished care of their children and, after the Abortion Act 1967, there was a sharp fall in the number of babies being offered for adoption by strangers.

Legal terminations of pregnancy increased gradually from 1971 when there were 133.1 thousand abortions to 1981 when there were 136.9 thousand. During the following decade there was a substantial increase to the 1991 figure of 181.9 thousand. Most but not all terminations are of pregnancies outside marriage.

The younger a mother the greater the probability that she will be unmarried. If she is unmarried her baby is much more likely than babies of married couples to be at a disadvantage because of late prenatal care or failure to book for confinement. She is more likely than a married mother to suffer social disadvantage and there is a marked tendency to downward social mobility among unmarried mothers who keep their children. These and other factors combine to lead to a greater than normal proportion of their pregnancies being associated with low birthweight. Children of mothers who are cohabiting suffer less detriment than those whose mothers are unsupported in pregnancy.

A relatively small but important group of unmarried mothers are those under 16 years of age. They are important not only because there is an increased risk of infant mortality and morbidity but also because maternity seriously prejudices the education and life opportunities of the mothers. In 1991 there were 7800 conceptions in girls under 16 years of age. The conception rate was 9.3/1000 girls aged 13–15 years. Although the conception rate was slightly higher than 20 years earlier the number of babies born to very young mothers fell because a greater proportion of their pregnancies were terminated. In 1971 the conception rate was 8.7/1000 with an abortion rate of 3.2/1000; in 1981 the conception rate was 7.2/1000 with an abortion rate of 4.1/1000; in 1991 the conception rate was 9.3/1000 with an abortion rate of 4.8/1000.

Babies born to unmarried mothers have higher mortality rates in all countries. Much of the increase in perinatal mortality can be accounted for by their smaller size at birth and, in countries with the lowest levels of perinatal mortality, higher rates among the babies of unmarried parents are due to an excess of late fetal death rather than greater early neonatal death. Differences in morbidity are not so clearly apparent although children living alone with their mothers were shown to be more accident prone and a higher proportion of them than children living with both parents had poor physical coordination or fidgety, restless behavior. In respect of growth and the attainment of developmental milestones, they were not significantly different.

The National Child Development Study found that by the age of 7 years illegitimate children, unless adopted in infancy, were below average for their age in general knowledge, oral ability, creativity, perceptual development, reading attainment and arithmetic skills. These disadvantages applied irrespective of whether the parents subsequently married and in all social classes. They had a higher incidence of behavioral and adjustment difficulties at school and maladjustment was more common especially among boys who were illegitimate at birth.

Mothers of children and, if they are married, their husbands have automatic 'parental responsibility' ('parental rights and responsibilities' in Scotland). The father of a child does not have 'parental responsibilities and rights' unless he is married to the mother. He may apply to a court for an order giving him 'parental responsibility' or, in Scotland, 'parental responsibilities or rights'. Alternatively, with the cooperation of the mother a formal parental responsibility agreement may be made which would confer on the father full parental rights and responsibilities. Others, e.g. grandparents, may apply for 'parental responsibility'. More than one person may have parental responsibility for the same child at the same time and each may act alone in discharging these responsibilities. They include decisions about religion, education, consent to adoption and marriage, medical treatment or overseas travel. Whether married or not the father of a child is liable for the payment of maintenance to the child and this is enforced through the Child Support Agency.

Parental separation and divorce

There is no doubt that persistent discord between parents is common, harmful to children and a relevant consideration in pediatric practice. In the UK divorce has increased but this may not reflect more marital disharmony so much as changes in the law which has made divorce easier. The UK has the highest divorce rate in the European Community and there are more lone-parent families due to divorce than to births outside marriage. In England the number of divorces doubled after the Divorce Reform Act 1969, and there was a record number in 1985 following the Matrimonial and Family Proceedings Act 1984 which permitted divorce petitions after 1 year of marriage. Recent changes in divorce law aim to reduce acrimony associated with the proceedings by removing the need of the applicant to prove fault. It is unlikely to reduce the number of divorce petitions. Recently the proportion of marriages ending in divorce has risen by about 1% per year although the total number of divorces has fallen because of the increase in people choosing to cohabit rather than marry.

Families disrupted by divorce have become so numerous that even assuming that many affected children are not significantly damaged the total morbidity arising from this event alone must be considerable. In 1991 the number of decrees absolute was 158 745 in England and Wales and 12 479 in Scotland. Of these 110 630 and 5552 respectively were of couples with one or more children, i.e. almost 70% of divorces in England and Wales involved children. In Scotland it was a smaller proportion (45%). Many of the children are very young – of those living in stepfamilies 72% started to do so before they were 10 years old.

Many different circumstances lead to divorce and it should be remembered that the situation is fluid. For many children there will be further separation arising from divorce. They are affected in various ways and there is marked variability in outcome. The reasons why some children do well and others do badly are not fully understood but multiple parenting changes are likely to be harmful.

It may be helpful to consider the various stages of the process separately. The reactions of children to them will vary with their personality, age and experience.

1. Preseparation

The period before parents separate may be very painful for children. They are often upset by parental argument and become especially frightened when faced with violent physical quarrels. During such altercations infants may be injured and older children may try to intervene. At this stage psychosomatic symptoms are common, e.g. asthma may become worse or enuresis recommence, or educational difficulties arise from loss of confidence. Separation of parents may be a relief to children but the concept of 'staying together for the good of the child' is supported by evidence suggestive of more behavior problems and poorer academic performance after divorce than before it.

2. Separation – loss of a parent

When parents separate, children may not be wholly relieved of the stress induced by acrimonious relationships because there is often contact between the parents prior to divorce. Nevertheless, it is inevitable that they have to begin to come to terms with the loss of a parent at this time. Children past toddler age may feel rejected and themselves reject the noncustodial parent but most wish to maintain contact with both parents. This is particularly the case when the mother is the noncustodial parent. Contact is a right of the child and it should be regular, reliable and take place in as natural circumstances as possible. Those who because of age or very prolonged separation have had no significant relationship with a parent may still need to meet him or her but very frequent contact under these circumstances may not be helpful and can be harmful if it threatens the security of existing relationships. In short, where contact is intended to maintain or develop relationships it needs to be fairly frequent, but where it is simply to enable children to know about their origins it need not be so frequent.

Older children may experience damaging conflicts of loyalty or may fear loss of the other parent. Their sense of self-worth may diminish and they may become prone to illness and accidents. They should be allowed to determine the frequency of contact when practicable and in legal proceedings in England under the Children Act 1989 (and the Children (Scotland) Act 1995 in Scotland) their wishes have to be ascertained and taken into account.

3. Litigation

In the UK, children do not have separate representation in divorce proceedings. Courts determine issues of where they are to reside and custody and the amount of contact they are to have with their parents on divorce. The Court has a positive duty to consider the welfare of children but their source of information about the children is usually a 'Statement of Arrangements' submitted by one of the parents. Unless there is parental disagreement judges are unlikely to be alerted to problems or bargains between parents that have little to do with child welfare. Occasionally they may call for welfare reports or, less commonly, for medical evidence and in a few cases they may interview children themselves. In England divorce courts have the power to commit children to the care of local authorities if they consider that neither parent is suitable.

4. After the divorce – disadvantage

Following divorce of their parents considerable numbers of children live in one-parent families. Downward social mobility and problems with housing and finance are common. Courts attempt to ensure that there is an equitable distribution of any resources and that a home is preserved for the children but there are sometimes changes of home, school, friends and surroundings to which children have to adapt. There are obvious difficulties and widespread and long-term poverty has been reported among families of broken marriages. Difficulties may arise because of children continuing to believe that their parents will be reconciled and using symptoms of illness to bring them together.

5. Stepfamilies

Some parents cohabit with a new partner before divorce and many remarry afterwards. If present trends continue 1 in 8 children under 16 years will live at some stage in a family in which one of their birth parents has either remarried or cohabited with somebody other than their birth parent. Children in these circumstances may be protected from poverty only to encounter problems associated with new relationships. Ambivalence or rejection by the new parent towards infants may lead to attachment problems and the risk of abuse. Older children may get on well with their stepparent but they are unlikely to regard his or her affection as an adequate substitute for that of their real father or mother. They are likely to be resentful of correction and particularly sensitive about criticism of their absent parent.

Better economic circumstances associated with life in a stepfamily do not protect children from the adverse effects of their parents' divorce. Stepchildren are at greater than normal risk of problems with social relationships, health, behavior and educational achievement. They tend to leave home earlier and receive less support than those growing up with both birth parents.

6. Long-term effects

Children who have lost a parent may feel insecure and anxious about further separation or loss. They may lack confidence to make new friends and there is an increased risk of emotional disturbance, poor educational attainment and delinquency. Divorced parents may be less inclined than others to seek assistance because of fear of criticism by their estranged spouse.

Prolonged lack of contact may give rise to problems in adolescence when a realistic knowledge of both parents is contributory to the development of personal identity. Later in life people tend to relate to their spouses much as their parents related to each other. Disadvantage may, therefore, be perpetuated in this respect.

Death of a parent

A relatively small but significant proportion of families have only one parent because of death. They may experience the same economic disadvantages and social isolation as other lone-parent families in addition to the emotional consequences of loss, but only in a minority is there prolonged disturbance.

Children need to mourn and reactions to death vary with age. Adverse effects on later personality were found to be greatest when parental death occurred during the child's third or fourth year, but loss of a parent at any age may be damaging. It depends partly upon the circumstances of death, partly upon the relationship that had existed between the parents prior to death, but above all upon the quality of care received by the child before and after bereavement. Most of these children suffer less adverse effect than those in other types of one-parent family.

In the National Survey of Health and Development it was shown that children who lost their fathers before they were 6 years old did better in a series of tests if their mothers had not remarried than if they were from families where remarriage or cohabitation had occurred. Children of fathers who had died after the child reached 11 years did not do so well and in secondary school children prolonged illness of the father before death appeared to be very disturbing. Delinquent behavior was not a particular problem in older boys who had lost a parent in contrast to those whose parents had separated or divorced.

Children of widows may be adversely affected by their mother's unresolved depression or by her fatigue if economic necessity causes her to go out to work. They are sometimes subjected to anxious, overprotective behavior with consequential immaturity of development, occasional psychosomatic symptoms or obesity.

DEPRIVATION

This term is used in respect of children who from loss of parents or from any other cause are deprived of a normal home life with their own parents or relatives. Most of them become the responsibility of local authority social service departments and many suffer substantial physical, intellectual and emotional morbidity. In the opinion of the author their management and, more importantly, prevention of the need for accommodation by local authorities are among the most vital problems confronting society.

In England and Wales there were, in 1991, 66 000 children or 5.5/1000 children under 18 years looked after by local authorities. This was substantially fewer than in 1981 when the figure was 99 000 or 7.6/1000 children under 18 years. This welcome downward trend has continued probably because of changes in practice arising from the introduction of the Children Act 1989.

Reasons for children being accommodated

Some children are looked after by or on behalf of local authorities for medical reasons, the commonest being short-term illness of their mothers, i.e. illness of less than 6 months' duration. There is no exact information about the illnesses but they are mostly psychiatric, gynecological or surgical illnesses in that order of frequency. A substantial number are accommodated because of confinement of their mothers, the implication being that their families are so isolated as to be without friends or relatives able or willing to help even in temporary difficulties. Long-term illness of mothers accounts for a smaller number of cases and fewer than

1000 children are accommodated each year because of death of one or both parents. About three-quarters of these children lose their mothers and either have no fathers or their fathers are unable to care for them.

The majority of the children are accommodated for more obviously social reasons although they too may have been influenced by medical conditions. Care Orders, housing difficulties and maternal desertion are the most frequent social reasons followed by abandonment and parental imprisonment. Children of imprisoned parents experience particular difficulties and have very limited opportunities for contact visits. There is accommodation in prisons for only 36 infants with their imprisoned mothers in England and Wales and none in Scotland or Northern Ireland.

Duration of accommodation

The length of time that children remain in local authority accommodation varies with individual circumstances but in the past many were continuously in care for 5 years or more. It is among older children who have been away from home for long periods that there is considerable emotional and intellectual morbidity.

Place of accommodation

There has been a trend towards accommodation in foster homes and away from admission to local authority children's homes. The proportion of accommodated children in foster homes increased from 38% in 1981 to 58% in 1991 and those in local authority children's homes fell from 28% in 1981 to 16% in 1991. Fewer children were looked after in the children's homes of voluntary charitable societies and in residential special schools in 1991 than in 1981.

Geographic variation

As might be expected, there are considerable differences between the proportions of children looked after by local authorities in urban and rural areas. There are also differences between regions, the highest rates being in London and the North West of England and the lowest in East Anglia. These variations are not simple reflections of differing social needs but vary with such factors as local policy, facilities for care and the efficiency of social service departments.

Medical examination on admission to care

In the UK there are statutory regulations requiring that children have a medical examination before or within 24 hours of being placed with fosterparents or in a children's home. The most striking feature of many of the children is their distress. Accommodation by the local authority is generally an upsetting and frightening event. There are a few children, particularly those who have been seriously deprived, who are happy to receive attention but there are many others, usually older children, who are withdrawn and resentful. This has two implications: firstly that unpleasant aspects of the examination should be omitted; and secondly, that satisfactory assessment is not practicable.

The usefulness of medical examinations is limited and they should be restricted to the attainment of the following objectives:

1. Safeguarding the child's medical welfare by initiating treatment when it is required or ensuring the continuity of existing treatment, e.g. anticonvulsant medicines in children who have epilepsy or insulin in the case of diabetic children.

2. Recording medical evidence which may subsequently be used in law to safeguard the welfare of children, by writing down the nature and extent of any injuries and describing in detail any evidence of neglect. In this context, early, accurate weighing and measuring is very important because of the known association between emotional deprivation and growth failure.

3. Preventing other children in foster homes or residential institutions from catching contagious diseases. This aspect has, in the past, been overemphasized.

4. Protecting fosterparents or the staff of children's homes from mischievous complaints by aggrieved parents, e.g. in respect of injuries, weight loss, etc. In rare instances examinations may also serve to protect children from harsh treatment by staff.

ADOPTION

Children whose birth parents are unable or unwilling to look after them need a substitute family. Adoption is one way of providing substitute care and has the advantage that it is permanent and legally secure. De facto adoption has occurred throughout history, but in the UK, unlike some other European countries, it was not recognized in law until the 20th century. For example the first Adoption Act in England and Wales was passed in 1926 (1930 in Scotland) and since that time the term 'adoption' has usually referred to the legal process.

Incidence

Adoption statistics are difficult to interpret but the number of orders made since the inception of legal adoption in England and Wales is shown in Figure 34.1. After reaching a peak in 1968, the year after the Abortion Act, there was a sharp fall, the greatest reduction being in the number of infants adopted by strangers. Less than a quarter of adopted children are under 1 year of age at the time of adoption. Before 1968 around a quarter of all illegitimate babies were adopted and of the remainder approximately a third stayed with their natural parents who subsequently married. After 1968, the proportion of illegitimate children being offered for adoption decreased and there was a concurrent increase in the number adopted by relatives. Orders granted to relatives or to a natural parent together with a stepparent accounted for about a half of all adoptions. The figures were then affected by great efforts that were made to place handicapped children and older children from institutions.

Mechanism

People wishing to adopt unrelated children must apply to an Adoption Agency – either a Local Authority Social Services Department or a charitable Adoption Society approved by the Secretary of State. Many of the latter have religious affiliations. It is not permissible for anybody (including doctors and nurses) to enter into agreements or facilitate placements of children with a view to adoption unless the proposed adopters are relatives of the child, and it is an offense to receive an unrelated child with a view

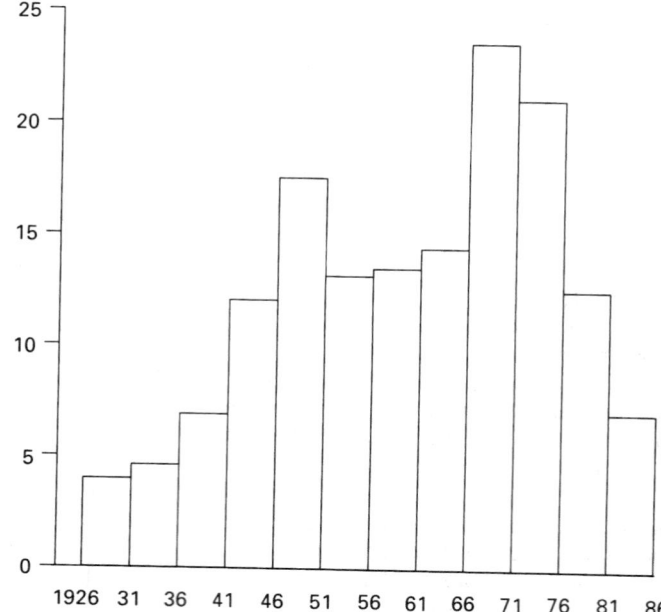

Fig. 34.1 Number of adoption orders made since the inception of legal adoption in England and Wales in 1926.

to adoption except through a local authority or approved Adoption Agency. Applicants must be at least 21 years old. They may be sole applicants of either sex if they are unmarried but if married, an order will be granted to a sole applicant only if his spouse cannot be found, is permanently separated or is incapable of applying because of ill health.

Applicants are interviewed by social workers to assess their suitability as parents and their homes are visited to determine whether they have satisfactory accommodation. Local authorities are approached to see if they know of anything against proposed placements. Couples beyond childbearing years are not usually considered for infant adoption although there is no legal bar to adoption at any age over 21 years. Unless one applicant is a natural parent or the child is over 16 years, the inquiry includes a medical examination, normally undertaken by the prospective adopter's family doctor. Its purpose is to make reasonably certain that applicants will be able to support and care for a child until the end of adolescence and that there are no conditions such as psychosexual problems that may jeopardize the stability of a placement. Previous illness, whether physical or psychiatric, does not preclude successful application provided that it is unlikely to affect the quality or continuity of care and affection received by the child.

Adoption agencies are required to establish at least one adoption panel. It has to have a medical adviser, usually a pediatrician or a senior clinical medical officer. Each application is considered by the adoption panel and, if it is agreed that the couple would make good parents, their names are entered onto a waiting list and they can expect to receive a child, sooner or later.

Registered agencies are allowed to advertise and to receive contributions towards their expenses and, conversely, may make payments to adopters in special circumstances. These include, for example, facilitating adoption of handicapped and long-term foster children and enabling large families of children to be kept together.

Consent and court procedure

After going to prospective adopters, the child has to have his home with them for at least 13 weeks before an Adoption Order can be made. The probationary period cannot start until 6 weeks of age although he or she may have been placed earlier. Placements are conditional upon free, informed and unconditional agreements by natural mothers and, in the case of legitimate children, fathers as well. Putative fathers' agreements are not required unless they have obtained a Parental Responsibility Order or Agreement.

An application for an Adoption Order can be made to a Magistrate's Court, a County Court, the High Court or in Scotland the Sheriff Court or Court of Session. The County Court or Sheriff Court deals with most adoption petitions. The application has to be accompanied by a witnessed, signed consent of the natural parent(s) and a form showing that the child has been medically examined. A date for the adoption hearing is then fixed.

When a court receives an application for an Adoption Order, it appoints a person called a 'guardian ad litem' (in Scotland 'curator ad litem') who is not associated with the Adoption Agency. His or her duty is to safeguard the welfare, especially the legal welfare, of the child. If children are old enough to understand the nature and effect of adoption courts are notified and have a duty to try to ascertain their wishes. In Scotland an Adoption Order can only be made in relation to a child aged 12 or under unless the child consents to the adoption. The guardian ad litem interviews anybody who has been interested in or involved with the adoption and makes sure that the agreement of the mother has been fully understood and freely and unconditionally given. Although birth parents cannot make their agreement conditional, e.g. with respect to religious upbringing, the Agency must have regard to their wishes.

Parental agreement can be given or dispensed with at an early stage by application to the courts for a 'freeing order'. An order can be given if at least one parent agrees to the adoption, or if the child is in the care of the local authority and there is an application to dispense with parental agreement. The effect of it is to transfer parental rights and duties to the Adoption Agency until an Adoption Order is made. Freeing orders reduce the period of uncertainty for all parties. They may be revoked on application by either parent after 12 months if placement for adoption has not occurred.

Applications are heard in private and natural parents do not have to attend court although they may do so if they wish. Unless there is a 'freeing order' consent may be withdrawn at any time until an Adoption Order is made. This happens in a small proportion of cases and is very distressing to prospective adopters who may have looked after the child for a considerable period.

In some cases adoption orders may be made without the agreement of the birth parents, either because they cannot be found or are unable to give their consent owing to mental or other incapacity. Furthermore, courts may grant orders against their wishes if they have persistently failed, without reasonable cause, to discharge the duties of a parent, have abandoned or neglected their child, have persistently ill-treated him or have seriously ill-treated him and there is no likelihood of rehabilitation. Parental consent can also be dispensed with if it is being withheld 'unreasonably' and in deciding this an English court must regard the child's welfare as the first but not the only consideration. In Scotland the child's welfare is the paramount consideration.

From the moment an order is made all parental rights and responsibilities are transferred to the adoptive parents and the child is treated as the legitimate child of their marriage. The rights of all other people are extinguished.

Access to birth records

Some adopted persons wish to know about their birth parents and in Scotland those over 17 (recently reduced to 16) always had a right of access to their original birth entry and court process record. In England and Wales access has been available only since 1975. Any adopted person over 18 years of age may apply to the Registrar General for a copy of his or her birth certificate. Those adopted before 1975 are obliged to be interviewed by a counselor before a certificate can be issued but for adoptions after 1975 counseling is optional. In 1992 the number of adopted people counseled was 3347 and approximately two-thirds of them expressed an intention to trace their natural parents.

Outcome

Infant adoption has proved to be remarkably successful and although there are well-known risks associated with illegitimacy, the very good care enjoyed by illegitimate children who are adopted enables them to develop normally despite their greater vulnerability at birth. Adopted children aged 7 years described in a report of the National Child Development Study did not differ from other children in respect of defects found at a physical examination including tests of vision, hearing and speech. Class teachers recorded that a greater proportion of adopted boys showed clumsiness, poor physical coordination and fidgety, restless behavior than other boys but the ability of adopted children in general knowledge, self-expression, creativity, reading and arithmetic was at least as good as their nonadopted peers and markedly better than illegitimate children in the care of their natural parents. Boys adopted into middle-class families experienced difficulties of adjustment more frequently than adopted girls or boys adopted into working-class homes.

Other studies have shown that these problems diminish with age except for children with markedly deviant parentage. Adoptees born to schizophrenic, alcoholic and criminal parents are at greater risk than other children. The IQs of adopted children correlate better with those of their birth parents than the IQs of their adopting families although some published studies of children adopted very early have reported average or above average intellectual ability. Children adopted in infancy before the 1970s were often screened by voluntary adoption agencies before placement and are a selected population as compared to those placed later. It is generally agreed that placement should be as early in the child's life as possible but late-adopted children, including those previously deprived, often show a remarkable capacity for recovery and adaptation. Institutional care does not inevitably lead to irreversible psychological disorder and studies have shown that neglected children can be adopted later in childhood with a good prospect of success. Children placed at around 2 years of age from a residential nursery showed a marked acceleration of intellectual ability and few behavioral problems. Older children from the same nursery did not improve as much in ability but their adoptions were, nevertheless, satisfying to their adoptive parents. The longer the period of adversity experienced by children before placement the longer are they likely to take to settle but their past is of less importance than their experience in their new home. There may be an initial need to control the behavior of older boys and the early stages of a placement are likely to be difficult but they make progress albeit slowly.

An investigation of adoptees reaching adult life has shown that 70% of them made a good or excellent life adjustment. The remainder were adjusting poorly or were at risk and 13% had been known to the police although most of their offenses were minor. A little more than a half of them were thought by their parents to have had emotional or behavioral problems while growing up but despite this 85% were satisfied with the adoption.

Trends in adoption

Until the 1970s the great majority of children who were placed for adoption were white infants, medically screened for normality, and placed soon after birth with infertile couples. Since the 1967 Abortion Act only a minority of children adopted have been healthy infants. Many have been older children with a history of neglect or with severe mental or physical disabilities. Children who in the past would have been considered unsuitable for adoption have been adopted. For many of them the consequences of nonadoption would have been continuing deprivation and this has been increasingly appreciated. Although some placements have broken down, the rate of breakdown, and the damage that arises from it, is less than a half of that experienced by children in long-term foster care.

Handicapped children need families as much, if not more, than those who are healthy but their care often imposes great strains on those who look after them. Parents proposing to adopt them need the fullest possible information and an opportunity to discuss with an expert the implications of their decision. This has become an increasing part of pediatric practice with respect to adoption. Adopting families also require continuing support and advice and the need for a postadoption service has been recognized.

During the 1980s attention was directed to the feelings of children adopted by families of different ethnic backgrounds to their own. Mixed race children adopted early generally do well but there can be problems of social acceptance, and current practice is to place them within their own group whenever possible.

Custodianship, which was intended for use when legal security but something less than adoption was needed, has now been displaced by subsequent statutory provisions in the Children Act 1989 and the children (Scotland) Act 1995. A review of adoption law has been undertaken but the likely legislative outcome and the implications for practice are not clear at present.

PRESCHOOL AND SCHOOL HEALTH CARE

Day care for children of working mothers

There are national and regional differences in the proportions of mothers of young children in paid employment. Some regions have had a tradition of female work but it is now general in the whole of the UK that many more mothers have jobs than in the past and there has been a corresponding increase in the need for day care facilities. The jobs undertaken by young mothers are often part time and low in skill, status and remuneration but women of all social classes are involved and those with professional qualifications are more likely than average to continue with their occupation during motherhood.

A majority of working mothers are employed outside school hours and during part of the school holidays. They must obtain either substitute care for their children at home or day care elsewhere. Nursery facilities fall far short of needs and the number of publicly funded nursery places in the UK is much lower than in other Western European countries. In 1990, only 2% of children under 3 years in the UK had a publicly funded nursery place compared to 20% in France and Belgium and 48% in Denmark. Fewer than 10% of working mothers used any kind of day nursery (Botting 1995).

The effect of maternal employment on children appears to depend partly on the quality of the alternative care that they receive. Children under 3 years of age are at greatest risk but maternal fatigue may be detrimental to children of any age if it impairs parent/child interaction. The National Child Development Study found that: 'in general, the children of working mothers do not show any marked ill-effects at the age of seven in terms of their attainments and adjustment at school' although, when they were examined at 11 years, children of mothers in full-time employment read less well than their peers. The latter finding was not consistent in all groups of children, illegitimate children and children of widows doing better when their mothers worked full time. Among middle-class children, educational attainment seems to be adversely affected by their mothers' work, whilst the reverse is true for working-class boys. In any individual case the effect is likely to depend on the mother's enjoyment of her work, whether it causes undue fatigue or anxiety, the age of her child and the quality and consistency of the care received.

Care at home

In the past, working mothers often relied on their families to look after children but the modern tendency to move from one area to another has reduced opportunities for this type of care. There are no legal restrictions or controls over the care of children in their own homes provided that they are not left unattended or in the charge of an unsuitable person. A few children receive inconsistent care from a succession of 'au pair' girls.

Child minders

When publicly funded day nurseries are not available, or are inconveniently located, or do not open for sufficient time, working mothers may use private nurseries but more commonly take their children to the homes of people who agree to mind them for a modest profit. They are called child minders and when they look after unrelated children of less than 8 years for more than 2 hours in any day they have to be registered with their local authority. Registration is not required by fosterparents, nannies or those with legal parental responsibility. Local authorities are required to keep a register of child minders and those who provide day care on domestic premises in their area. They must satisfy themselves about the fitness of those looking after children and the suitability of people likely to live or work on the premises. A certificate of registration is issued specifying conditions such as the number of children that may be looked after. The local authority must be informed of any change of persons caring for children or living on the premises. Inspections are obligatory at least once a year and there is a right of entry to the premises. Registration may be refused or canceled but there is an appeal mechanism.

Private nurseries

The same requirement to register with the local authority applies to private nurseries including nurseries and crèches attached to places of employment. Staff members and qualifications, the safety and suitability of the premises and arrangements for feeding and medical care are all considered in determining whether or not registration will be granted and how many children will be allowed. In 1991, there were 400 workplace nurseries in the UK.

Day nurseries

Nurseries for the day care of children developed separately from nursery schools and classes. They are the responsibility of social service departments and differ in that they may admit children under 2 years of age, open for longer hours and parents usually have to pay according to their means. Day nurseries are usually staffed by nursery nurses rather than teachers, although trained teachers may be employed to deal with older children.

Admission to day nurseries is generally restricted to children in certain priority groups: for example, when admission is part of a child protection 'Care Plan'; those whose mothers are ill or incapable of providing care; and those in circumstances where health, welfare or development are at risk.

Nursery education

Nursery schools differ from day nurseries in that they are closed during school holidays, mostly admit children part time and rarely before their third birthday. No charge is made. They are administered by local education authorities and have a head teacher and qualified teaching staff assisted by nursery nurses. Their primary function is educational.

The first nursery school in the UK was opened in 1816 by Robert Owen at his cotton mill in New Lanark. He emphasized the need for happy personal relationships, satisfaction of childish curiosity and exercise in the open air. Formal teaching and books played no part in the curriculum. The number of nursery schools greatly increased and by 1900, more than 40% of 3- and 4-year-old children were attending state schools. Unfortunately, rigid educational practices and herding of children into large unhygienic groups led to nursery classes being discredited and their numbers were reduced by governments concerned to save money.

The kindergarten movement developed concurrently with nursery schools during the latter part of the 19th century and served some middle-class children. It was influenced by the ideas of Froebel who attached great importance to play and self-expression. Educational thought was affected and there was an emphasis in schools on the provision of early experience to facilitate child development. The importance of physical well-being and environmental hygiene was also recognized.

Despite a prevalent view that the best place for children under 5 years is at home with their mothers, nursery education became more popular again. In 1960 use of nursery school places on a part-time basis in order to increase the number of children that could be admitted without increasing the cost was advocated officially. This practice was endorsed by the Central Advisory Council for Education (1967) who considered that separation of children from their homes for whole days was not desirable and that children under 3 years should not be admitted to schools. Their report (the Plowden Report) asserted the principle that nursery education should be available on demand for all children and is best remembered for introducing the concept of educational priority areas and the provision of services to offset the disadvantages of a poor environment. Urban aid schemes were subsequently developed and through them the number of nursery school places expanded.

There is little evidence that nursery education confers any permanent advantage on children other than the enjoyment of association with their peers. Teachers believe that children at nursery schools grow in self-control, self-confidence and independence but it is not clear whether their development in this respect is enhanced as compared to children who remain at home. Nevertheless some research studies suggest that nursery school children are happier and better able to adjust to primary school than other children. Many parents are now convinced that it confers an advantage and recent government policy has been directed towards trials of a voucher scheme to support admission to nursery schools.

A number of early intervention schemes aimed at offsetting social and economic disadvantage have been developed. The most notable were the 'Head-Start' programs in the US. They did not result in persisting rises of IQ although initial rises of between 5 and 15 points were shown. Similar programs have been tried elsewhere but their advantages tended to be lost unless they were continued into primary schools and the gap between children of different social classes was not reduced.

Structured language development programs in nursery schools have been advocated to help disadvantaged children because many of them do not have the opportunity to develop at home the more complex forms of language demanded at school. Improvements in language skills have been demonstrated but the methods used to stimulate language development remain controversial.

Play groups

Play groups originated in New Zealand but spread to Europe and in the 1960s their numbers in Britain expanded very rapidly. This occurred because parents appreciated the need of their children to play with others in a safe place. There is a great variety among play groups. Many cater for middle-class children and are organized and supervised by their mothers on a nonprofit basis. Others are run by charitable bodies and larger ones have trained staff. Children generally attend for a half day session each week although some play groups are open two or three times a week.

Child health clinics

The first infant consultation clinic was started in Paris by Budin and a similar clinic, called a 'goutte de lait', was opened in northern France. Like Budin's clinic its objective was to encourage breast-feeding but when it was impossible a substitute was recommended with advice as to the conditions necessary for success in artificial feeding. The first infant milk depot in the UK was set up in St Helens, Lancashire in 1899, and later in other industrial towns. Clinics had considerable success in ensuring safe artificial feeding and in preventing nutritional disease in infancy but they were less effective in encouraging breast-feeding.

The Maternity and Child Welfare Act 1918 gave local authorities power to make arrangements 'for safeguarding the health of expectant mothers and children less than 5 years of age not attending recognised schools'. Exchequer grants enabled the development of schemes intended to reduce infant mortality and morbidity. Mothers were invited to take well babies to clinics for weighing and consultation with a doctor. Infant foods were sold at discounted prices and this was a great incentive to attendance. The importance to children of their mother's health was recognized and in some clinics dinners were provided at minimal cost to improve their usual diet.

Immunization against infectious disease became an important part of clinic services and the range of prophylactic injections increased in the postwar years. Formerly, most children received immunoprophylaxis at child health clinics but following the introduction of a new contract encouraging general practitioners to undertake this service the proportion being immunized by general practitioners greatly increased as did the number of children receiving immunoprophylaxis.

Developmental screening examinations were introduced at clinics in the 1960s and gave them a renewed sense of purpose. An overwhelming majority of children in the UK were taken to child health clinics, the greatest proportion attending during the first year of life. There was social class variation in attendance at clinics, the highest proportion of attenders being children of skilled workers. Many children of the professional classes were not taken to clinics but of greater importance, many of the poorest children did not attend, especially if they were later born children of families.

Increased participation of general practitioners in child health activities was advocated in various reports including the report of a subcommittee on Child Welfare Centres (Central Health Services Council 1967; the Sheldon Committee) and the Committee on Child Health Services (1976; the Court Committee). The spirit of their recommendations was embodied in the 1990 general practitioner contract referred to above which introduced financial incentives for the first time. General practitioners now undertake the majority of child health surveillance and immunization in their own surgeries or health centers and there has been a rapid decline in the number of separate child health clinics. More than 80% of general practices now offer child health surveillance and except in urban conurbations where some continue, child health clinics have practically ceased to exist.

Child health surveillance

Child health surveillance involves:

1. oversight of the health and development of all children
2. measuring and recording growth
3. monitoring developmental progress
4. arranging treatment when it is needed
5. preventing disease and disability by immunization and health education.

It should be achieved by sympathetic consultations with parents, the principle purpose being to encourage them in the care of their children. Of great importance is the need to avoid causing unnecessary anxiety. Surveillance is not synonymous with screening and although good surveillance includes some screening tests the consultation should not consist simply of a series of obstacles to be overcome by the baby.

The benefits accruing from child health surveillance include the enhancement of relationships with parents and, arising from them, opportunities to advise on immunization, accident prevention and other child health topics and a chance to collect epidemiological data.

Screening tests

These are rapid examinations or tests enabling the recognition of unidentified disease (Cochrane & Holland 1971). The classical criteria of an ideal screening test are that it must be:

1. simple, quick and easy to interpret
2. acceptable to the public
3. accurate
4. repeatable
5. sensitive – positive when the disease is present
6. specific – negative when the disease is not present.

There are many screening tests and it is necessary to be selective. Programs should address important, treatable problems that are recognizable in their latent or early symptomatic stages and the tests used should be acceptable and lead to cost-effective treatments with favorable outcomes. Developmental screening does not fulfill the Cochrane & Holland criteria and it was concluded that routine developmental screening examinations using standardized screening tests were unnecessary for detecting serious disorder such as cerebral palsy or severe learning difficulty and of doubtful value in detecting less obvious disorders such as those of speech (Hall 1996). Such conditions would be more efficiently detected early if doctors undertaking surveillance knew about child development and considered it at each encounter with the child, took parents' concerns seriously and listened to teachers.

School Health Service

The purpose of a school health service is to help every child to derive full benefit from education. This entails the prevention of disease, making sure that ill children get appropriate treatment, caring for handicapped children and bringing medical expertise to bear on learning difficulties. Of these component parts the latter is the essentially unique function and may be called educational medicine.

The connection between the physical condition of children and their capacity to benefit from education has been appreciated for a long time and towards the end of the 19th century school health services were started in several European countries. In Britain education of blind and deaf children became compulsory in 1893 and local education authorities were permitted to provide services for mentally defective and epileptic children from 1899. It was in connection with this that doctors with statutory powers were first appointed, their purpose being to ascertain whether or not children were defective or epileptic. The impetus to mandatory medical examination came from public concern regarding the large number of army recruits for the Boer War who were physically unfit and in 1907 a law was passed requiring education authorities to arrange for medical inspection of children around the time of admission to public elementary schools. In some European countries, school doctors were at first preoccupied with the premises and conditions in which children were taught. Environmental hygiene continued to be a concern of school health personnel but in the UK the service from its inception was centered on medical examination. There was an emphasis on nutrition, hygiene and infectious disease and local authorities were obliged to ensure that pupils received any medical or dental treatment that was necessary. The School Health Service had a significant treatment role until the inception of the National Health Service in 1948, when, with the exception of dental treatment, the need declined.

As a consequence of the great reduction in prevalence of serious illness in children during the last 40 years, routine medical inspections have been criticized frequently and their content and timing reappraised. The majority of children are physically well but many have educational difficulties due to intellectual impairment, emotional illness, speech disorders or other conditions. There has been considerable interest in the early identification and care of these children and their management has been given greater emphasis in school medical work.

Administration and staff

In the UK and in most western countries except Germany and the US, authority over school health services lies with national parliaments. Before 1974 services in England and Wales were administered by local education authorities but they now operate as consultant-led services within the National Health Service.

Any registered medical practitioner may be employed in the British School Health Service without specific qualification. There are approved postgraduate training courses which are usually undertaken on an inservice basis shortly after appointment. The number of doctors engaged in school medical work in the UK has been greatly reduced in the past few years. Most have full-time appointments in community child health but some, including family practitioners, have part-time contracts. Staffing sometimes includes sessional commitments by ophthalmologists and other specialists. In addition to doctors, nurses, speech therapists, audiometricians, orthoptists, chiropodists, physiotherapists and occupational therapists are employed in school health work. It is costly in the use of trained personnel.

Senior and experienced staff may be required to give advice about children who are thought to have special educational needs and examinations may be undertaken to ascertain whether the health of children would be prejudiced by employment. School doctors have a statutory duty to provide information about pupils to the Employment Medical Advisory Service.

School medical inspection

Historically this has been by far the largest item of school health activity and continued for many years with relatively little modification. It has been undertaken wherever school health has been practiced and, although the recommended number of examinations has varied from country to country, universal examination of children at about the time of school entry has been regarded as an essential minimum. Despite recurrent criticisms of the examinations by professionals they have been generally appreciated by parents.

The provision of medical inspections for pupils is required by statute but parents are not obliged to allow their children to be examined. They have a right to be present at examinations. In many areas, routine medical examination on school entry has been

displaced by child health surveillance at $4\frac{1}{2}$ years, immediately before most children start school.

After the initial examination of all children at about the time of school entry there is, in most parts of the UK, a policy of selective examination. There is no general agreement about the method of selection and it may be on the basis of a screening examination by a school nurse, by head teacher referral, parental questionnaire or by selecting whole schools in deprived areas. The author favors selection based on annual measurements of height and weight and the use of growth charts. About 15% of children at routine medical inspections were found to have defects, many requiring follow-up to ensure effective management.

Screening of vision and hearing

This is undertaken in schools and is important because of the direct relevance of hearing and vision to learning. The tests are often carried out by school nurses although audiometricians and orthoptists are sometimes employed.

Vision. It has been recommended that visual acuity should be tested annually in all primary and secondary schools and in special schools but this frequency of testing is not always achieved. Tests are often done under less than ideal conditions but there is no doubt about their overall value because they lead to the initial detection of many visual defects.

Hearing. All children have their hearing tested in the first year of life by a health visitor using distraction methods, and children known to be at risk of deafness are tested by more sophisticated methods. By the time that they reach school most children with sensorineural deafness have been identified. The commonest remaining cause of hearing loss is middle ear infection which is especially prevalent in early childhood. Many children have only a single audiometric examination during their school life but this is not sufficient and it has been recommended that all children should have their hearing tested by a school nurse twice during primary education. There is also a strong case for ensuring that children who truant at a later age have their hearing tested.

Screening for other disorders

Screening has been advocated for a wide variety of disorders such as adolescent scoliosis, urinary tract infections, etc. Although some of them may fulfill the criteria for desirable screening tests it is arguable whether or not schools should be used to test for conditions that have no bearing on education.

Control of infection

School doctors have a role in immunoprophylaxis (see Ch. 7) and assist in the control of infectious disease in schools. School closure because of serious infection is now rare but many children, especially those at nursery schools, catch common childhood fevers or gastrointestinal infections and require exclusion from school. In the latter, normal practice is to exclude children until there is clinical recovery and three stool examinations have proved negative.

An occasional task of school doctors is the surveillance of children who have been exposed to tuberculosis through a member of staff or an older pupil. Contacts are tuberculin tested at school and arrangements are made for those with positive reactions to have a chest X-ray.

Hygiene inspections are carried out periodically by school nurses. Their purpose is to identify children with skin infections or ectoparasitic infestations especially pediculosis capitis. Treatment facilities may be provided. In some areas cleansing orders are issued to parents of verminous children and they are excluded from school. Unfortunately these children are often the ones who can least afford to miss school and some school doctors allow them to attend provided that they are assured that the child and family have been treated with an effective insecticidal shampoo.

Health education

The importance of health education has been recognized from the inception of the School Health Service but most school doctors do not have clearly defined responsibilities and much depends on their own enthusiasm. It is considered that teaching should be done by teachers but that school doctors and health visitors have a role in assisting them. They may help in discussions and seminars for older children and they should be more involved in teacher training. Important opportunities for health educational activity will be provided by the system of health interviews of senior pupils by school nurses that has been recommended.

Child guidance and the School Health Service

Child psychiatry provision in the UK developed in a very fragmented fashion and much of it was based on child guidance clinics initiated by local education authorities through their school health departments. There were, and still are, great regional variations in the availability and use of services. Local education authorities no longer employ psychiatrists but obtain psychiatric advice through cooperative arrangements with the National Health Service. Consulting psychiatrists occasionally undertake clinical sessions in schools or local authority premises and they make recommendations about the management and educational placement of children with maladaptive behavior.

Special educational need

Educational provision for handicapped children in the UK was greatly influenced by the recommendations of a Committee of Enquiry into the Education of Handicapped Children and Young People (1978; the Warnock Committee). They were incorporated into the Education Act 1981 and subsequent regulations. Their effect has been to shift the emphasis from provision for specific handicaps to meeting special educational need, i.e. focusing on need rather than disability.

Special educational need is defined as any learning difficulty calling for special educational provision. Learning difficulty means a significantly greater difficulty in learning than the majority of children of the same age and may or may not involve a disability preventing the child from taking full advantage of the education generally provided in schools. The definition also encompasses children under 5 years who have or will be likely to have special educational needs.

Those with severe or complex learning problems requiring either extra resources in ordinary schools or admission to special units or schools usually have a statutory assessment and a 'Statement of Educational Need' is made. Not every child with learning difficulty is formally assessed; it is estimated that up to

20% of children need special help at some time in their school lives but only 2% require 'Statements of Educational Need'. The majority are dealt with by arrangements such as remedial tuition within their own schools and are not subject to formal procedures. In England and Wales parents of children who have reached 2 years of age may be obliged to submit them for examination, or they may request an examination, if their child is thought to need special educational treatment. Education authorities in Scotland may examine children from birth and have a statutory duty to do so in the case of children over 5 years. Parents have a right to notice of examinations, to be present at them, to be informed of results and to appeal against decisions with which they disagree.

If a parent requests an assessment the local authority must comply. Statutory assessment may also be initiated following observations at school, recommendations by educational psychologists or information from other sources such as health authorities. The latter have a duty to inform education authorities whenever they think that a child under 5 years is likely to have special educational needs. They are also required to inform parents if they think that their child would be assisted by a voluntary body.

Assessments should be done either in the children's own homes or in familiar surroundings such as their schools and they should be part of a continuing process. Short periods of admission to special nurseries or schools may be valuable for assessment. Assessment in hospital may be required for those with severe or complex learning difficulties, those with medical conditions receiving treatment likely to impair future learning, children in psychiatric units and those admitted because of neglect or severe social problems.

Local education authorities are required by statute to seek written 'advice' on relevant matters affecting educational needs and how they may be met. It includes educational, psychological, medical and, when appropriate, social reports. Medical information is provided through a designated medical officer. Pediatricians and others who have provided medical care or opinion are usually invited to contribute to the assessment. Information from medical sources is coordinated and should include a description of what the child can do, a developmental prognosis and advice about any medical or paramedical treatment that may be required.

When the local authority has received all the advice requested it prepares a draft 'statement' incorporating the various reports. This is given to the parents and most agree with the recommendations. They have a right to ask for an interview with an officer of the local authority and if, having met him, they disagree with the draft statement they may require him to arrange a meeting with the person who provided the disputed advice.

Following agreement with the parents, or determination of an appeal, a final 'statement' is made. Local education authorities have a duty to ensure that provision is made for whatever is specified in 'Statements of Educational Need' and to allocate appropriate resources. It is intended that, when possible, children should be educated in normal schools and teachers may be designated to help and advise colleagues about those with special needs. Independent school placements may be paid for when authorities are unable to meet needs. Local education authorities are required to review 'statements' at least every year. In the event of significant changes of circumstance reassessment is undertaken. All children subject to 'Statements of Special Educational Need' are reassessed during the school year after they reach 13½ years to enable plans to be made and advice given about remaining education, transitional arrangements, further education, vocational training and employment. At the first annual review after the 14th birthday they must obtain an opinion from the Social Services Department about whether or not the child will be a 'Disabled Person' and entitled to statutory services under welfare acts.

THE CHILDREN OF IMMIGRANTS

Migrations have occurred throughout history and some, like the Arab occupation of North Africa and the European colonizations of Australia and the Americas, have produced profound and lasting changes. Significant alterations have taken place in the nature of British society because of the migrations from the Caribbean Islands, the Indian subcontinent and East Africa that occurred mostly between 1955 and 1965.

In England and Wales 8% of children under 16 years are now from ethnic minority communities. A number of special considerations apply to their health care.

Children born overseas. There are some diseases that are more common in immigrants irrespective of where they come from and occur with greater than normal frequency because of the social circumstances of migration. Another group of diseases are those prevalent in the migrant's country of origin.

Infections

Tuberculosis is the most important disease of migration. It is still common in developing countries. Many immigrant children with tuberculosis probably contract their disease in their host country as a consequence of social conditions under which they live at the time of arrival. For obvious financial reasons they often live in overcrowded houses in the period immediately after immigration. They are at risk of close contact with cases of tuberculosis. There is, therefore, a need to offer tuberculin testing and BCG vaccination to them as soon as possible after they arrive in the UK. Infants born to immigrant parents are at greater risk of tuberculous infection than others and BCG vaccine should be offered at birth.

Many children from underdeveloped countries arrive in the UK from rural communities which often lack water-borne sanitation. Not surprisingly infestations with soil-transmitted helminths are common. Prevalence varies considerably according to where the children have lived but microscopic examination of a single fecal smear revealed parasitic ova in the stools of about 20% of children of school age who had migrated to the UK from the Indian subcontinent. The majority of infested children do not have symptoms and it can be argued on the one hand that those with light infestations should not be treated. On the other hand, those with significant numbers of hookworms, roundworms or whipworms get abdominal symptoms and some, especially those with hookworms, become anemic. Their general health can be improved and it is advisable to arrange for examination of the stools of all children arriving from or returning from visits to rural areas of developing countries.

Relative to the total number of children involved a surprisingly small number are found to have enteric infections such as typhoid. It is always a possibility and any child who develops a pyrexial illness within a short time of arriving from the tropics should be strictly isolated and appropriate samples of blood, urine and feces sent to a laboratory. The investigation of pyrexia in children under these circumstances (and in children returning from exotic holidays) should always include the examination of a blood film for malaria parasites.

Perinatal problems

The fertility of West Indian and Asian immigrant women has been substantially greater than the average for the UK and this appears to have been a feature of immigration at other times in history. There are, therefore, increased obstetric risks associated with high multiparity and a tendency to short intervals between succeeding pregnancies.

Family planning is contrary to the religious beliefs of Muslims unless it is reliably determined that the mother's health will suffer greatly by frequent pregnancies. High fertility rates have continued in these immigrant groups, although not in others, and in the UK about 20 000 babies are born each year to Muslim mothers. Family planning and antenatal care may be difficult for some Asian mothers because of a reluctance to leave their homes, language problems and anxiety about being examined by male medical staff. The majority receive antenatal care although many do not present themselves until the third trimester. Unattended delivery is more common, presumably because of communication difficulties and the effects of multiparity.

The average birthweight of babies born to Asian immigrant mothers is less than that of babies born to European mothers and a difference of birthweight has been recorded between babies born to consanguineous and nonconsanguineous Asian immigrant parents. The offspring of consanguineous parents were reported to have a threefold increase in postneonatal deaths and serious chronic disease compared to others.

Children born to immigrant mothers before immigration are almost all breast-fed and breast-feeding is often prolonged. Infant feeding practices change shortly after the mothers arrive in the UK and in addition to the well-known general disadvantages of formula feeding there are hazards when mothers are unable to read or to understand instructions in English.

Genetic disease

There are higher rates of multiple congenital malformations and deafness in the children of Asian immigrant parents and there is a presumption that they are due to customary consanguinity. It is possible that socioeconomic factors and a greater number of pregnancies at high maternal age may play some part. In consanguineous pregnancies there is a 25-fold increase in autosomal recessive conditions and of affected offspring there is a 1 in 10 risk of death or mental retardation. Genetic counseling is a sensitive subject which presents particular difficulties in this group of patients.

Health in childhood

Children of Asian immigrant parents are more likely than others to live in large families and because of this and relatively greater socioeconomic deprivation, to share sleeping accommodation. Infant mortality rates for children of newly arrived immigrants were considerably higher than for children born to British mothers. The distribution of fatal conditions was not unusual and contrasted markedly with infant mortality patterns described in India.

Children of Asian immigrant mothers are brought to medical pediatric outpatient clinics only slightly more often than children of British mothers but are admitted to hospital much more frequently. Almost a half of children admitted have respiratory infections or asthma. Admission rates are probably influenced by adverse housing conditions and by difficulties in communication.

Metabolic bone disease has been a special problem in the children of Asian immigrants. In contrast to the children of other immigrants and the British urban poor it tends to occur throughout childhood and in all social groups. It is particularly common in adolescent girls and vitamin D deficiency continuing into pregnancy sometimes leads to the birth of infants with fetal rickets.

A number of explanations for these differences have been suggested but they are probably due to insufficient exposure of skin to ultraviolet light. For religious reasons most girls have clothing completely covering their limbs and from puberty onwards do not leave their homes as often as European children. Rickets in the children of Asian immigrants should be prevented by giving a dietary supplement of vitamin D.

Parental care

Illegitimacy is uncommon among the children of Asian mothers in the UK and very few are brought up in single-parent families. Their children receive a good deal of attention and security but young children tend to lack environmental stimulus as compared to their British counterparts. During infancy they often use their parents' native language and by school entry may have insufficient knowledge of English to progress. Diagnosis of a language disorder is twice as likely as in other children. Delays in reading have been recorded but the educational disadvantages are generally overcome by the time that they reach secondary school. The same is not true of children of Caribbean immigrants who experience a very different pattern of child rearing with a high incidence of maternal employment.

CHILD ABUSE

Children may be injured by acts or omissions of their caretakers and the likelihood of unnecessary suffering or avoidable impairment of health or development should lead to prompt and appropriate protective action. For the purposes of description, ill-treatment can be classified into:

1. physical abuse including burns and scalds
2. sexual abuse
3. Munchausen syndrome by proxy
4. neglect and failure to thrive
5. emotional abuse.

More than one form is commonly found in each case. They are all symptomatic of disordered parent–child relationships.

PHYSICAL ABUSE

The emotive term 'battered baby syndrome' was deliberately coined by C. H. Kempe to draw attention to the plight of physically abused children. He estimated that the incidence in the US was about 6 per 1000 live births. In Western Europe it is probably not very different but true prevalence is unknown

because many cases are concealed and there are problems of definition. Some children die and it is thought to be the cause of permanent disability in about 400 children in the UK each year. About a third of identified physical abuse occurs in children under 6 months of age, a third between 6 months and 3 years and a third over 3 years of age.

Prediction

In assessing whether children are likely to be abused it is useful to consider factors relating to the parents, the child and their social conditions separately. If parents have certain personality characteristics or have already demonstrated a capacity to assault children and their child is difficult or unrewarding, there is a strong possibility of injury being triggered by any social crisis. The following have been found to correlate with later ill-treatment.

1. The parents:

a. were abused or experienced family disruption in their childhood
b. lack family support and are unreasonably fearful of caring for their child
c. have unreasonable expectations of their baby and treat him as a much older child
d. have poor impulse control
e. may be generally rigid or authoritarian, e.g. the incidence of abuse is greater in some strict religious groups and in families of military personnel
f. one, usually the father, may be aggressively psychopathic and assault others within and without his family – about 5% of abusing parents fall into this category and a similar proportion are psychiatrically ill.

2. The child:

a. was unwanted and there may have been a denial of pregnancy, requests for abortion or talk of adoption
b. was separated from the mother at birth, e.g. because of prematurity, and initial attachment to him was prevented or interrupted
c. is disappointing either because of a defect or because a child of the opposite sex was wanted
d. is hyperactive by day and cries at night
e. is difficult because of illness
f. is different from the rest of the family.

3. Social factors:

a. crises relating to housing or the disconnection of services
b. loss of work – chronic unemployment increases the likelihood of abuse by fathers
c. poverty and crises relating to the use of money
d. loneliness or isolation of mothers when their partners have left or are working away from home
e. marital crises and new liaisons – stepchildren are at increased risk
f. unwanted pregnancy.

Diagnosis

Injuries to every part of the body have been recorded. Some are catastrophic, leading to death or permanent disability and prevention of them is vitally important. Most children who are killed or sustain lasting damage have been assaulted more than once. Recognition, followed by prompt reporting of significant minor injuries may be life saving because of a tendency for them to be repeated and to escalate in severity.

Physically abused children generally present in one of three ways. Those with very severe life-threatening injuries are often, but not always, taken to hospital without undue delay. Those with injuries obviously requiring treatment but not causing unconsciousness, collapse or convulsions may be taken either to hospital or to their family doctors but characteristically a delay of several days occurs between the injury and medical attention being sought. Most children with bruising or minor injuries are brought for opinion as a result of observations by teachers, nursery staff, other caretakers or members of the public. A small proportion are discovered at routine medical examinations.

The history

Only a small minority of parents bringing nonaccidentally injured children to hospital admit to having assaulted their child. They often conceal previous injuries and give a history that is clearly inconsistent with the clinical observations. Sometimes they deny any knowledge of the injuries or say that the child has injured himself. Such statements with respect to very young children are almost always untrue and lack of explanation for any injury should arouse suspicion. It is very important to write down the history at length, not only to enable it to be cross-checked at a later date but also because, in the event of criminal litigation, only contemporaneously written notes can be used in Court.

Children do not usually say much in a clinic setting but later, may make significant remarks that should be recorded verbatim. There is often a noticeable lack of warmth in the interaction between the parent and child. Parents often do not show appropriate concern about the injuries and fail to assist the child, e.g. with dressing, during the consultation. Collusion between parents is usual, but when they are in dispute one may give exaggerated accounts of assault by the other.

The injuries

Intracranial injury

This may be caused either by direct trauma or by violent shaking. Direct trauma may be caused by accident but children do not injure themselves until they become independently mobile. Rolling off a bed or climbing out of a cot does not commonly cause a skull fracture and the majority of simple parietal fractures require a free fall of at least 1 m, and at least twice as far is needed for complex fractures. Intracranial injury is uncommon even in children who fall downstairs. Severe head injury in infancy is, therefore, likely to be nonaccidental unless there has been a road traffic or similar accident.

Skull fractures usually involve a parietal bone. In abused children they tend to be multiple and irregular rather than single, narrow, uncomplicated, linear cracks. They are more frequently bilateral or multiple and nonparietal, i.e. the frontal and occipital bones are sometimes involved. Growing fractures, subdural hematomata and cerebral edema are all more common in nonaccidentally injured children than in others.

About one-half of children with subdural hematomata do not have fractures. They have been shaken by an enraged parent. It is believed that they are often thrown against walls or onto the floor at the end of the shaking episode so that the presence of a parietal fracture does not exclude the possibility of shaking injury. The children sometimes have small circular bruises on their upper arms or back corresponding to the position of their assailant's grip. Retinal hemorrhages are characteristically present and ophthalmologic examination is necessary in all cases of suspected nonaccidental injury.

Shaking causes shearing of vessels crossing the subdural space and in cases of nonaccidental injury subdural hemorrhage is seen characteristically in the posterior interhemispheric fissure. Cerebral edema is common and may arise either directly as a consequence of trauma or secondarily owing to anoxia. Neurological, intellectual and visual impairment occur in a significant proportion of severely shaken children.

Bone injuries

It has been estimated that 1 child in 8 who sustains a fracture before 18 months of age may have been nonaccidentally injured. In cases of suspected child abuse, especially in infants, it is almost always advisable to obtain skeletal X-rays because they may 'tell a story that the child is too young or too frightened to tell for himself'. Nonaccidental bone injuries are much more likely to be multiple and associated with bruising of the head and neck than accidental injuries. Classically, but not so commonly, they are located at the growing ends of bones. It is generally the case that transverse fractures are associated with direct blows, angulated fractures with leverage and spiral fractures with rotational forces. In nonaccidental injury the latter are the most common, especially spiral fractures of the humerus. They are often associated with marked periostial reaction because both are caused by gripping and twisting of the limb.

Rib fractures in healthy children, particularly those posteriorly at the costochondral junction, are almost always due to nonaccidental injury and are most commonly caused by severe chest compression. Substantial force is required because of the elasticity of young children's ribs. They are very unlikely to be broken during the course of vigorous resuscitation. Rib fractures are easily overlooked on radiographs taken before signs of healing are evident and they may be identified more easily by bone scintography.

Fractures at the growing ends of bones may be caused either by pulling and twisting of the limb or by the centrifugal force generated during shaking. A series of microfractures of the immature new bone are caused leading to detachment of all or part of the epiphysis and growth plate. It may appear on X-ray examination either as a translucent line, a corner fracture or a bucket handle fracture. A single metaphyseal fracture may be produced accidentally or in the course of rough play but multiple metaphyseal fractures are pathognomonic of abuse.

Multiple fractures are often in different stages of healing and are indicative of several episodes of trauma. Fractures without early callus or periosteal new bone formation, are usually less than 7–10 days old. The younger the child the earlier are signs of healing likely to be seen. Soft callus is visible after the first week and it gradually matures to a recognizably more dense appearance by the third or fourth week after the fracture. Thereafter there is remodeling of the bone and a previous fracture may be evident for as long as 1 year.

In infants, the periosteum is thicker and more vascular than in adults. Periosteal injuries, like posterior rib fractures, may not be immediately visible on radiographs and bone scintigraphy can be helpful. They are usually very painful. Irregularities in the outline of healing periosteum may denote that the child has sustained further trauma.

Superficial injuries

Bruises and abrasions are infrequent in healthy children during their first year but afterwards all children get them in the course of normal play and ill-treatment is inferred only if they are excessive in number or have a pattern characteristic of a particular form of punishment.

Abrasions. In many cases it is easy to tell what has happened. Children who have been hit with the buckle-end of a belt or with a chain have recognizable marks and, likewise, those who have been strapped with a stiff plastic belt may have J-shaped cuts on their limbs, back or buttocks. Blows to children wearing clothing of woven or cellular material often imprint a pattern. Linear abrasions around the ankles and wrists of children tied to their cots are easily identifiable as are the marks of ligatures tied to the penis of small boys to stop them wetting. Abraded skin heals within a few days but hyperpigmentation of affected parts often persists for several weeks.

Bruises. These may be flat or associated with swelling:

1. Those caused by finger pressure are usually flat and there is little associated swelling of the surrounding tissues. They are roughly circular, measure approximately 1 cm in diameter and occur, e.g. when a hand has been held firmly over a baby's mouth or when the limb of a child has been gripped very tightly.

2. Those caused by impact with a blunt object, such as a fist or hard surface, tend to be associated with swelling which persists for a few days.

Bruises are caused by extravasation of blood from broken capillaries under the skin. Initially they are red but quickly change to blue/purple. Pigment from disintegrating red cells gradually alters their color and after approximately 48–72 h they begin to have a brownish hue. After a further 2 or 3 days they turn green/yellow and usually fade within 7–10 days. The age of bruises cannot be stated precisely because times taken for absorption vary with the vascularity of the affected tissues. Slight variations in color are not, therefore, significant, but attempts should be made to state an approximate age because fresh and fading bruises on similar parts of the same child would be indicative or repeated trauma. The color of bruises on photographs is notoriously unreliable.

Account should be taken of the site of bruises because where subcutaneous tissues are lax as, e.g. on the face, they tend to spread from the site of injury. There may also be tracking of blood between tissue planes so that bruises may appear at sites distant from the point of trauma. In cases of trauma to relatively avascular areas, such as in bastinado when the soles of the feet have been severely beaten, there may be very few marks.

Some bruises are petechial in type, i.e. they consist of multiple pinpoints of bleeding. Bruises caused by negative pressure (love bites) are characteristically of this type and hard slaps across the face often leave a petechial type of bruise corresponding approximately to the size of the assailant's hand.

Pinches and bites. These also cause characteristic bruises.

Those due to pinches consist of two slightly curved parallel marks and there may be associated scratches from fingernails. They are most commonly found on arms or buttocks. Bites cause two hemispherical bruises with superimposed marks outlining the position of the teeth. They can be matched to dental impressions of possible assailants and salivary antibodies can be detected in samples taken from the unwashed skin of children who have been bitten. Specialist help from a forensic dental surgeon can be important and should be sought immediately.

Burns and scalds

Nonaccidental burns and scalds are often difficult to distinguish from those due to accidents and consistency of the history with the injury is particularly important. They may be inflicted in various ways but the following are worthy of mention:

Cigarette burns. If a child brushes against a lighted cigarette he experiences pain, withdraws immediately and no mark is left. A lighted cigarette stubbed out on the skin of an adult causes a circular area of erythema, usually without blistering, and it disappears after 24–48 h. Circular burns with blistering and secondary infection are caused by lighted cigarettes being held deliberately next to the skin for several seconds. Although the injuries may be trivial, they denote great callousness on the part of assailants. Nonaccidental cigarette burns are usually on parts that can be readily immobilized. Children of about 6 months sometimes grasp at cigarettes and the lighted end sticks in their palm. Accidental cigarette burns may also occur around the neck when lighted tobacco falls into the clothing of children.

Hotplate burns. Children are sometimes punished by sitting them on electric cookers or by holding them onto hot surfaces or electric appliances. A contact burn is produced, the severity depending on the temperature of the object and the duration of contact. Severe burns may be caused if a child is made to touch live electrical parts such as the bar of an electric fire.

Immersion burns. Children, especially those who are enuretic or encopretic, may be dipped into a bath of very hot water. If the temperature of the water exceeds 60°C (140°F) immersion will produce a full thickness scald in well under half a minute. The scald will be up to the level of immersion but the central parts of the buttocks may not be scalded where they are protected by contact with the bath. Children scalding themselves accidentally by turning on a hot tap jump about in the bath, usually sparing the soles of their feet and causing irregular splash marks on their legs.

Roasting. Some children are held over or very near to a fire or source of radiant heat as a form of punishment and sustain extensive erythema or blistering. When they have been held near flames their hair may be singed.

Hot feed scalds. Small trickle-mark scalds at the angle of the mouth occur when very hot milk has been carelessly given to children. Inflicted burns due to hot food tend to be around rather than within the mouth.

Chemical burns. Corrosive chemicals can produce very severe and disfiguring burns. They may be associated with staining of the skin.

Injuries to the mouth

Abused children often have injuries of their face and mouth. Older children may have teeth broken but infants tend to suffer tears of the frenulum of the upper lip. The latter are usually due to the flanges of feeding bottles being pushed hard into the mouth. Scars of the frenulum persist for many years and may give a clue to the quality of earlier care. Impatient feeding may also cause pharyngeal injuries when spoons are pushed far back into the mouth.

Visceral injuries

Although visceral injuries are less frequently recognized than head injuries, fractures and bruises, as a cause of death in nonaccidentally injured children they are surpassed only by central nervous system injuries. They may present considerable diagnostic difficulty because fist blows to the abdomen do not produce significant external marks and the nature of intra-abdominal injuries may not be recognized prior to surgical treatment.

The most common injuries are tears of mesentery and perforations of small intestine. Much force is required because the gut is mobile except at points of attachment in the epigastrium and right iliac fossa and severe blows may simply cause retroperitoneal hemorrhage. Perforations of the stomach or bladder are unusual as are tears of the liver or spleen but any of these injuries may be produced. Lung damage may occur in association with rib fractures but it is uncommon. When there have been kicks or blows to the back there may be frank or microscopic hematuria and urine should always be examined for red cells.

SEXUAL ABUSE

Sexually abused children are those who have been used in any way for the sexual gratification of adults. They may be of any age or either sex. A significant proportion have been physically as well as sexually abused and nonorganic failure to thrive has been recorded in between 5 and 10% of sexually abused children.

The abuse may include any form of sexual activity ranging from allowing the child to witness indecent acts, involvement in pornographic photography, inducing them to masturbate adults or lick their genitalia, being fondled, used for intercrural intercourse or oral sexual activity through to genital and/or anal penetration.

Abusers are usually known to the children and are commonly male relatives, household members or temporary carers. There are similarities to physical abuse in that offending parents have frequently been emotionally deprived or abused in their own childhood and have inappropriate expectations of their children. Mothers may know what is going on and collude by avoidance and there is often a gradual escalation in the nature of the abuse. Like physical abuse it can occur in all social groups but is said to be more common when living conditions are crowded and in geographically isolated areas. About a quarter of fathers convicted of incest have low intelligence.

Risk factors

Children are at particular risk if there is:

1. a family history of incest or sexual deviance
2. a member of the household with a record of sexual offenses
3. loss of maternal libido and sexual rejection of the father
4. alcohol misuse
5. a pedophile in the household – especially in relation to sex rings and pornography.

Presentation

Sexual abuse can be brought to attention by one or more of the following:

1. Statements made by children to parents, teachers or friends. They should be recorded verbatim and *exactly* what the child has said should be considered carefully. Unprompted explicit statements by young children are generally true. Less definite disclosure should lead to appropriate inquiry but interviews of children should be undertaken only by skilled personnel in carefully controlled circumstances. Repetitive questioning is potentially harmful and is likely to produce misleading and inaccurate answers.
2. Symptoms of local irritation or trauma such as urinary frequency, soreness, vaginal discharge or bleeding.
3. Symptoms due to the emotional effects of abuse such as secondary enuresis, encopresis, anorexia and failure to thrive.
4. Sexualized behavior or sexual knowledge inappropriate for the child's age. Both may be derived from video material or observation of their parents but when pain or the quality of semen is described physical interference is probable.

Examination

Genital examination requires the agreement of a parent or the direction of a court. Only in exceptional circumstances should mothers of preadolescent children not be present. Adolescent patients should be asked who they wish to be present. The examination should be undertaken as soon as is reasonably practicable after abuse is suspected but the cooperation of the child is required and if it cannot be obtained the examination should be deferred for a short time unless there is a pressing medical need. Repetitive genital examination should be avoided unless it is necessary for therapeutic purposes or there is a reasonable suspicion of continuing abuse. Colposcopic examination may be helpful in obtaining clearer definition of the clinical signs and photographs taken using a colposcope may be helpful in avoiding the need for second examinations for forensic purposes. Clinical findings rarely provide conclusive proof of abuse and many abused children do not have abnormal signs.

The weight to be given to any observed signs varies as follows:

1. Conclusive or very strong evidence

a. Semen, blood or hair foreign to the child within the vagina or anus.
b. Sexually transmitted diseases such as gonorrhea.

2. Presumption of sexual abuse if no alternative explanation

a. Significant damage of the hymen vaginalis, including posterior or lateral notches, transections and attenuation (loss of hymenal tissue).
b. Tears or other injury of the vaginal wall.
c. Marked enlargement of the hymenal opening. Most children have an opening of approximately 4 mm until they are approaching puberty. There are individual variations but an opening greater than 1 cm is not seen in normal prepubertal children. Hymenal size should not be used as a sole basis for diagnosis.

d. Tears or scars extending from the anal mucosa to perianal skin.

3. *Supportive but not diagnostic of abuse*

a. Patchy localized reddening on the inner sides of the labia.
b. Minor abrasions of the vulva.
c. Injury to or scarring of the posterior fourchette.
d. Perianal swelling, venous congestion or bruising without reasonable explanation.
e. Swelling or thickening of the anal verge skin.
f. Genital or anal warts.
g. Anal laxity or reduction of the power of the anal sphincter without other cause.
h. Reflex anal dilatation greater than 1.5–2 cm without stool in the ampulla.

Management

Good interprofessional communication is required. *The first duty is to children and there is no law of confidentiality which overrides their welfare.* Good pediatric care consists of:

1. safeguarding medical welfare by excluding sexually transmitted disease, treating injuries and obtaining help with psychological problems
2. assisting with the protection of children from further abuse by cooperating with responsible agencies
3. facilitating the collection of forensic evidence which may be important to the protection of children in the future.

In girls past puberty the possibility of pregnancy should be considered. An appreciable proportion of pregnancies arising from incest probably abort spontaneously and among those that survive to the 28th week, there is a high perinatal mortality rate – possibly as much as 15%. In addition to a markedly increased risk of recessively inherited traits, there is an incidence of nonspecific mental handicap among long-term survivors which may be as high as 60%. This has obvious implications for the management of pregnancy and for substitute care of liveborn children.

Psychological considerations

Victims of abuse often suffer from psychological malaise but some preadolescent children may be apparently undisturbed provided that the abuse was not aggressive. Some are threatened and may present with psychosomatic symptoms or behavioral disturbances. Although the cessation of abuse brings relief of anxiety it may be replaced by uncertainty about removal, separation and future care. Children are likely to be upset by family disruption and recrimination following detection and conviction.

During adolescence victims may become depressed, resentful and leave home early. They have a greater than normal chance of suffering psychosexual difficulties for many years afterwards. The effect of abuse on sexual orientation is uncertain.

Violent sexual assault by strangers is particularly frightening to children and they are not helped by the unexpected reactions of their parents and society. Despite their ordeal and suffering, anger rather than sympathy is often the initial response of parents when they learn about the assault. The anxiety of affected children may be increased by inevitable questioning by their parents and the police. They are likely to associate the latter with having done something wrong and a medical examination with having a disease or something wrong with them. Additional to their immediate distress, emotional and social adjustment can be seriously impaired and learning retarded. These children require careful and sympathetic handling and psychiatric advice should be sought in all cases.

Sexual exploitation

This may be either direct as in prostitution or indirect as in pornographic photography or entertainment.

The extent of child prostitution in the UK is uncertain but it includes homosexual prostitution by boys and the exchange of sex for money or accommodation by 'runaways' and delinquent teenage girls. Child sex rings have been described with young children recruited by older ones.

Laws have been enacted in both the UK and the US to protect children from exploitation by pornographic photography. There are longstanding legal restrictions on the employment of children in the entertainment industry. Children taking part in performances for which a charge is made have to be licensed by local authorities who before granting a license have to take into account 'health, comfort and moral protection'.

MUNCHAUSEN SYNDROME BY PROXY (Meadow 1982, 1993a)

This has been defined as the intentional production or feigning of physical or psychological signs or symptoms in another person who is under the individual's care. The motivation for the perpetrator's behavior is to assume the sick role by proxy (American Psychiatric Association 1994). It is not a discrete medical syndrome but a name given to a spectrum of events that may arise either from the invention of symptoms or the procurement of illness. They have in common that:

1. the illness is fabricated by a parent or someone who is in loco parentis
2. the child is taken for medical care, usually persistently, and often has multiple investigative procedures and/or inappropriate treatment
3. the parent denies causing the child's illness
4. the illness ceases on separation from the parent although, in some cases, there may be persistent disabilities arising from what has been done.

Excessive parental anxiety may have similar consequences for children because insistent demands for medical care are likely to lead to investigations that are sometimes invasive and treatment that is unnecessary. Exaggeration of symptoms, whether arising from anxiety or not, has the same effect. By seeking multiple consultations (doctor shopping) parents may cause the abuse to be compounded. The abusers are the doctors. Other consequences of excessive parental anxiety may be the encouragement of abnormal illness behavior and enforced invalidism in the case of children with relatively minor disabilities.

Whether or not excessive anxiety or exaggeration should be regarded as abusive depends entirely upon whether it has a significantly damaging effect on the child. It is not strictly Munchausen syndrome by proxy but is similar in several respects. In order to avoid confusion it is often best to state clearly what is thought to have happened rather than use a diagnostic umbrella.

A very wide range of symptoms or signs can be fabricated. It may involve simple, repetitive claims that events, such as convulsions, have occurred when there has not been a convulsion or it may consist of false reporting of apneic episodes to nursing staff who then incorporate them in the clinical records. Notes may be entered or erased by parents. Sometimes signs are also falsified, e.g. by the mother cutting her finger and putting blood into her child's nappy.

The key to the identification of invented illness is a detailed history of the time of each alleged event and who was present when an event commenced. An essential feature of the condition is dishonesty and it is necessary to cross-check the history with others who have had frequent contact with the child. When events occur in a young child and are infrequent it should not cause surprise if only the mother witnesses them but if they are frequent other household members see them if they are real.

A similarly detailed history is of critical importance in cases when illness has been procured by a parent. The two most important forms of procured illness are suffocation and poisoning.

Imposed upper airway obstruction (suffocation)

The victims are almost always infants. Pillows, towels or a hand are held across the face or the child's face is pressed into the mother's bosom. Occasionally plastic bags are used and, in older children, pressure over the trachea. The latter leaves characteristic bruising and often associated fingernail scratches but in most other cases there are few, if any external marks – perhaps a few petechiae, a subconjunctival hemorrhage or slight nose bleeding.

Suffocation may present as unexplained episodes of apnea or ill-defined seizures. Single or infrequent episodes may reflect intense hatred by the mother for the child or an impulsive action during stress but when it is due to Munchausen syndrome by proxy episodes are repetitive and very dangerous. Although the intention may be to procure an illness there is little time difference between suffocation producing transient unconsciousness and that causing neurological damage or death.

Recurrent apnea is not uncommon in preterm babies. In mature infants it is necessary to exclude seizures, cardiac and respiratory disorders, gastroesophageal reflux and electrolyte disturbances. An important feature of apnea due to suffocation is that it ceases when the child is separated from the mother. Covert video surveillance may be used to prove the diagnosis but it is not necessary in all cases.

A small proportion, thought to be between 2 and 10%, of cases of sudden infant death syndrome are attributable to suffocation – 'the gently battered baby.' Occasionally it is admitted by mothers who injure later-born children and it may come to light when there have been successive, unexplained, infant deaths.

Poisoning

Drugs may be prescribed because a false history of illness has been given or they may be used by parents to induce illness in their children. In the former type of case, anticonvulsants are particularly important because prescribed doses are sequentially increased in response to a history that adequate seizure control has not been achieved. Illness may be induced by many other substances. The most important are salt and purgatives (Meadow 1993b).

In salt poisoning children present with thirst, vomiting, drowsiness and/or convulsions. They are hypernatremic and have very high urinary sodium concentrations.

Those children given excessive purgatives or soap solutions over a period of time usually have diarrhea and/or vomiting, and there are negative findings to the usual investigations. They fail to thrive and the possibility should be considered when children failing to thrive feed avidly, have reasonably normal bowel function and put on weight when cared for in hospital by a nurse or when looked after for a period by family members other than their mothers.

In addition to being used in cases of Munchausen syndrome by proxy, drugs may play an important part in child abuse in other ways:

1. Nonprescribed drugs and drugs prescribed for others may be improperly administered to children. More than one type of drug may be given. Sedatives and tranquilizers are the most commonly used because of crying, wakefulness or hyperactive behavior. They may come to attention because nursery nurses or teachers notice repeated drowsiness or incoordination in the morning getting better later in the day. Other cases are recognized following the investigation of otherwise inexplicable symptoms in children taken to hospital. Whenever there is a suspicion of drug abuse, urine and blood samples should be obtained promptly and stored in the refrigerator for later analysis. The police should be informed early in the case so that the assistance of the forensic science laboratory can be obtained.

2. Prescribed drugs may have paradoxical effects making children unduly difficult to manage and, therefore, more likely to be physically abused. For example, phenobarbitone sometimes causes young children to be irritable and wakeful.

3. Drugs prescribed for parents, e.g. benzodiazepines, may affect control and make rage more likely.

4. Narcotics and alcohol both impair normal control and inhibition. They can lead to financial difficulties and child neglect. Children of heroin or cocaine addicts are at substantial risk because not only do their parents tend to be unpredictable but they may also administer dangerous drugs to them. They may present with drowsiness, pinpoint pupils and respiratory depression. Deaths from methadone overdosage have been recorded in children of addicts.

Munchausen syndrome by proxy is commonly associated with other forms of abuse. The type of illness fabricated in the same child can change with time. More than a third of children in one series had siblings with fabricated illness. Recurrence risks are high for children left with their mothers in unchanged circumstances and many have school problems, conduct and emotional disorders. Some learn to have Munchausen syndrome by proxy.

NEGLECT AND FAILURE TO THRIVE

Parents are required to provide food, warmth and shelter, protection from injury and necessary medical treatment or, if they are unable to provide them, to ensure that their child receives them from statutory or other sources.

Feeding is a basic function of parenting as is the provision of warmth and shelter. In western society it is unusual for children to be inadequately clothed for warmth although clothing may be dirty, torn or ill-fitting. Likewise inadequate shelter is uncommon because public authorities are required to provide housing for all except those who have intentionally made themselves homeless.

Children have a right to be protected against injury and in this respect there is a great deal of neglect. Those most at risk are children left alone or with siblings in locked houses. Every year lives are lost in house fires when parents have gone out for the evening. Children left unattended for longer periods often have a characteristically expressionless appearance when they are rescued and even at a young age the eldest children of these families have often assumed a parental role.

Failure to keep appointments for diagnostic or therapeutic purposes is common and, as a consequence, treatment of some conditions is too late. Important examples relate to vision and hearing; delayed treatment of squint sometimes leading to amblyopia. Some parents neglect to provide medical attention, common ailments such as otitis media, napkin rash, etc. going untreated, and in extreme cases the lives of children being put at risk. Failure to ensure necessary treatment should not be regarded as culpable if it conflicts with strongly held religious views of the parents although their children too may need protection.

Neglected children almost always suffer not one but many privations. They are often dirty, unkempt or verminous, with soiled clothing, poor growth and nutrition and chronic infections or sore napkin areas. Severe neglect occurs when children are unloved by parents who have low intelligence and inadequate resources.

Failure to thrive (see also Chs 11 and 21)

Failure to thrive is not simply poor weight gain. Thriving involves vigor, strength and developmental progress as well as growth. There is a problem of definition and, arising from it, difficulty in determining prevalence. Nevertheless, general pediatric experience is that among children admitted to hospitals failure to thrive is common and in the US figures of between 1 and 5% have been reported. Rates in nonhospital populations are unknown.

The ratio of children with organic disease to those with nonorganic failure to thrive varies in different reports but the proportions are, more or less, equally divided in hospital inpatients. The condition of those with organic disease is often made worse by social problems, particularly when prenatal or perinatal disorders make parenting difficult. The following classification therefore reflects the realities of pediatric practice more accurately:

1. nonorganic failure to thrive – one-half or more
2. failure to thrive due to organic disease alone – one-quarter or less
3. failure to thrive exacerbated by adverse social factors – one-quarter.

It follows from the inclusion of the latter group that a history of social adversity should not discourage a search for organic disease nor should an organic diagnosis deflect inquiry about social or emotional factors.

Presenting symptoms and diagnosis

Organic disease is usually associated with a characteristic history or findings on examination. Many of the children present with vomiting or symptoms of malabsorption and appropriate investigation of the gastrointestinal tract clinches the diagnosis.

There is a tendency, which should be resisted, to base the diagnosis of nonorganic failure to thrive on the exclusion of organic disease and many children are subjected to excessive investigation.

The presenting symptoms of nonorganic failure to thrive differ from those of organic disease. There is usually a complaint of persistent feeding difficulty, poor appetite or extreme selectivity in diet sometimes commencing soon after birth and continuing over a long period. Often parents describe adequate provision of food but say that their children will not eat it. Their primary concern is with eating rather than growth.

The most severely affected children are pale, lethargic and apathetic but most are simply small and look younger than their age. Their body proportions are immature with short limbs and relatively well preserved head growth. In nonorganic failure to thrive height and weight are usually in proportion, but more than 2 SD below the mean and head circumference is in the normal range. Growth velocity is consistently low but irregularities of growth occur with changes of circumstance. In some there is a failure to catch up weight lost during minor intercurrent illness.

Behavior and development in nonorganic failure to thrive

Nonorganic failure to thrive is usually due to a chronic failure to provide sufficient food but there is also an association with later psychosocial dwarfism.

In the latter group behavior similar to that described in deprived children is often exhibited. Infants sit with anxious watchfulness, rarely smiling or vocalizing and they may be restless or irritable if picked up. More severely affected infants are withdrawn and the less severely affected are difficult and demanding. Later they fail to show normal reserve with strangers and are not distressed by separation from their parents. Indiscriminate friendliness and aggressive egocentric behavior follow. They frequently have disorders of sleep and elimination. Affected children often underachieve in tests of language development and social adaptation. They are less task orientated, less persistent and achieve lower scores in mental development than controls.

Parenting in failure to thrive

Characteristically the children are later-born members of multiproblem families with a short interval between their birth and that of their older siblings. Mothers are often estranged from their own parents and may give a history of family disruption during their childhood. They receive little support from their husbands and health problems and feelings of anxiety, depression or isolation are common.

Interaction with their infant is impaired although in other respects behavior is normal. They may give little attention to the infant, ignoring approaches and look at him or her only infrequently. Inappropriate positions are adopted during feeding and there is less than normal physical contact. They may express negative feelings about infants and older children are frequently criticized, belittled or threatened. Others in the family may thrive despite similar circumstances and it is presumed that interaction with affected children has been influenced by adverse circumstances during pregnancy or delivery or by differences of infant personality or temperament. More simply the mother may have been worn out by the care of preceding children.

Prognosis and management

There is a close association between nonorganic failure to thrive and physical abuse. About 20% of battered children have had prior hospitalization for feeding problems or growth failure. Rigorous follow-up is necessary although parental cooperation is often poor. Accurate measurements of growth plotted on a centile chart provide a very sensitive and objective index of the quality of parenting, and young children should be weighed and measured whenever there is a change of circumstance and at intervals of no less than 3 months if they have been returned to the care of a previously abusing parent. Follow-up studies of children remaining with their parents have shown that almost a half remain more than 2 SD below the mean for height and/or weight.

There is a very wide spectrum of outcome and prognosis is difficult. It appears to depend upon whether the child was simply underfed by an overwhelmed mother or emotionally abused and suffering from true psychosocial failure to thrive. Serious emotional disorder is uncommon in the former group but a substantial number fail at school and there is a risk of some degree of intellectual deficit. In the latter group social adjustment is often impaired and persisting severe social pathology in some families provides a model for defiant antisocial behavior by their children.

Following admission to hospital the growth of most but not all of the children accelerates. The same occurs when transfer to a warm, nurturing fosterparent is arranged. Recovery occurs in other respects. Nocturnal secretion of growth hormone returns to normal within 3 weeks and developmental attainments improve over a longer period. The best that can be done within families is to provide encouragement, support and supervision. When improvement does not occur and in cases of true psychosocial dwarfism related to emotional abuse, serious consideration has to be given to permanent separation of children from their families.

Emotional abuse

Emotional abuse is difficult to define and, therefore, not surprisingly, underdiagnosed. It may be active or passive and there is an association with neglect and failure to thrive.

Victims of active emotional abuse may suffer in a wide variety of ways, for example:

1. repeated threats or intimidation
2. inappropriate restriction such as locking in dark cellars or cupboards
3. constant criticism, discouragement or ridicule undermining self-esteem
4. Cinderellas – regularly treated less well than siblings
5. restriction of normal peer relationships.

Passive emotional abuse may also be manifest in a number of ways. They are forms of neglect and deprivation including, for example, persistently:

1. leaving the child unattended for long periods
2. failing to provide warm, affectionate, parental contact
3. failing to assist or comfort after minor trauma or to visit when in hospital
4. failing to stimulate or encourage.

Anomalous child care practices such as extreme overprotectiveness may be just as damaging as emotional abuse but the former is distinguished by a concern and love for the child which is not shown by the abusing parent.

Management of child abuse

1. When children are thought to have been abused the overriding concern, in all cases, must be to ensure their safety. Often it is convenient to admit them to hospital even though their injuries or medical conditions do not in themselves necessitate hospitalization. Appropriate treatment should be given and skeletal X-rays, coagulation studies and any other investigations indicated by the child's condition should be arranged promptly.

2. If parents refuse to cooperate with investigation or attempt to remove their child from hospital or other safe accommodation legal steps should be taken to secure the child's safety (see p. 1874).

3. It is generally advisable to encourage parents to visit and in the case of children on Emergency Protection Orders there is an obligation to allow reasonable contact. Nursing staff need to be watchful but not critical and sometimes only supervised contact may be deemed reasonable. In very exceptional cases it may be necessary to exclude parents from hospitals to ensure the safety of other children.

4. As soon as a firm diagnosis has been made parents should be interviewed by a senior member of the pediatric staff accompanied by a witness. They should be told of the diagnosis but care should be taken to avoid making or being drawn into any personal accusation or assignment of blame. Parents should also be told of the pediatrician's duty to report the matter to the Social Services Department. In some countries, but not in the UK, reporting is required by law.

5. Inform the parents of the name of the social worker who will be visiting them and if possible introduce them. In cases of death or very serious injury communicate immediately with the police. Prompt involvement of the police is also advisable when poisoning is suspected.

6. A psychiatrist's opinion about the parents is often valuable and should be arranged if they need psychiatric help or are willing to be seen.

7. Within a few days of being informed a case conference should be convened by the Social Services Department under the child protection procedures for the locality.

8. Attend the child protection conference if at all possible but, in any event, provide a written report of the clinical findings and your opinion.

9. Arrange to examine any siblings.

10. *At every stage write very full notes*. In the event of criminal proceedings you will be allowed to refer only to contemporaneously written records. Ensure that they are kept in a secure place, especially in cases of suspected Munchausen syndrome by proxy.

11. In England, if a decision is taken to apply to the courts for a Care Order or a Supervision Order to be made in respect of a child, remember that proceedings under the Children Act 1989 are not adversarial. Continuing support and assistance for the parents should be offered although it may not always be accepted.

12. The Court will probably appoint a guardian ad litem. His or her function is to represent the interests of the child in the proceedings. Pediatricians have an obligation to assist the

guardian ad litem irrespective of who invited them to be involved in the proceedings.

13. Abused children should not be discharged from hospital without the knowledge of the Social Services Department.

14. After discharge progress should be monitored in the outpatient department. Many parents welcome medical follow-up.

LEGISLATION TO PROTECT CHILDREN AND TO PROMOTE THEIR WELFARE

150 years ago few people would have questioned the absolute power of fathers to determine what happened to their children. This is still the position today in many parts of the world. In the latter half of the 19th century various reforms were introduced in the UK to protect children from harmful occupations. They were included in, for example, the Factories Acts, the Coal Mines Acts and the Chimney Sweeps Acts. Several of them were consolidated in the first Children Act in 1908. Also in 1908, Juvenile Courts were introduced in England and Wales and the judiciary were no longer able to deal with children in the adult criminal justice system.

Various other measures concerning neglect and ill-treatment of children were incorporated in the law during the ensuing years, particularly in the Children and Young Persons Act 1933, the Children Act 1948, the Children and Young Persons Act 1963, the Social Work (Scotland) Act 1968 which set up the children's hearing system in Scotland, the Children Act 1975 and the Child Care Act 1980. Child care law became very complex.

The Children Act 1989 applies to England and Wales and there is comparable but by no means identical legislation in force in Scotland as a result of the Children (Scotland) Act 1995. Much of the previous English and Scots Law relating to children was consolidated in these Acts but they are not simply pieces of consolidating legislation. They both contain new principles regarding the care and upbringing of children and represent two of the most important statutes on child care law yet enacted.

THE CHILDREN ACT 1989

The principles to be followed by the courts are as follows:

1. The welfare of the child must be the paramount consideration.
2. Delay in reaching decisions is likely to be prejudicial to the child.
3. There is a presumption that it is best not to make a legal order.

Welfare of the child

Section 1 of the Children Act 1989 is quite unequivocal in making welfare of the child the Court's paramount consideration in any questions relating to children's upbringing or the disposition of their property.

Pediatric evidence is often essential when questions of welfare are being considered. Careful records of growth, development, nutrition, clothing, injuries and untreated illness may be vitally important. Records made at times when children change from one care giver to another may be especially important.

What would the child like to happen?

In deciding what to do a court has to have regard for the ascertainable wishes and feelings of the child, considered in the light of his age and understanding. This has the potential for absurdity because, theoretically, a lawyer instructed to represent the interests of a young child is obliged to present the child's requests. There is an escape from acceding to children's wishes if they are perceived to be damaging to their interests: although courts have to take them into account, they do not necessarily have to act on them. Opinions may be requested about the capacity of children to express their wishes reliably and it is, of course, important to recognize that they may be unduly influenced by parental pressure.

Parental responsibility

An underlying philosophy of the Children Act 1989, is that both parents should have responsibility for their children and that it should not be reduced either by family breakdown or illegitimacy. When parents are married at the time of a child's birth, each has parental responsibility for the child. If they are not married the father does not have parental responsibility but may acquire it either by a formal agreement with the mother or by application to a court or by marrying her. Other people with legitimate interests in the child (e.g. a grandparent) may also apply for a 'Parental Responsibility Order', so that more than one person may have parental responsibility for the same child at the same time.

Subject to some limitations, anyone with parental responsibility for a child can give valid consent to medical treatment. A person who does not have parental responsibility but has care of the child may not give consent but has a duty to do what is reasonable in the circumstances, such as taking him to the doctors if he is ill.

Orders with respect to children in family proceedings

These can have a bearing on pediatric practice. The orders available to courts are to define:

1. where and with whom the child will live – a Residence Order
2. who the child can go to see – a Contact Order
3. what medical treatment he may receive or where he may go to school or similar questions – a Specific Issue Order
4. what may not be done to the child, e.g. genital examinations or reference to a child psychiatrist – a Prohibited Steps Order.

Local authority support for children and families – children in need

The Act imposes certain duties on local authorities which they discharge through their social services departments. For example, they are required to regulate and inspect child minders and private day nurseries (see p. 1860). They are also required to provide for 'children in need'. The latter is an attempt to extend the law in relation to prevention.

'Children in need' are defined as those unlikely to achieve or maintain or have the opportunity of achieving or maintaining a reasonable standard of health without the provision of local authority services, or their health or development is likely to be significantly impaired or further impaired without the services, or they are disabled. There is a general duty placed on local authorities to safeguard and promote welfare and, insofar as it is consistent, to promote upbringing within families.

They have to take steps to identify needs, publish information about services and ensure that those who may benefit receive the relevant information. Unfortunately there are rather diverse interpretations of 'need' in different parts of England and Wales. Nevertheless, it is a useful concept because the family support provided can include, not only advice, guidance and counseling but also activities for children, e.g. crèches, home help services, including laundry, and assistance with travel and holidays.

If a 'child in need' is living away from his family, the local authority must take such steps as are practicable to promote contact with his family if it is consistent with his welfare. For the disabled, assistance can be given in kind and, exceptionally, in cash

Accommodation of children by local authorities

The Act has changed the emphasis on the way accommodation is provided for children. Formerly they could be received into the care of local authorities on a voluntary basis provided that certain criteria defined in the Children Act 1948 were fulfilled. Accommodation of a child is now viewed as a service providing support for families. Local authorities have a statutory duty to provide accommodation for 'children in need', e.g. in cases of parental illness or for respite care. Specifically, they have to provide accommodation when a child has no person with 'parental responsibility', when he is lost or abandoned and when his carers are prevented from providing suitable accommodation or care, e.g. during hospitalization or imprisonment. They have to provide accommodation for children in 'police protection' or in detention or on remand and they may, after ascertaining their wishes, provide for children between 16 and 21 years if it would safeguard their welfare.

Social services departments have to be informed if a child is kept in hospital for 3 consecutive months because they have a duty to decide whether his welfare is being adequately safeguarded. They are also required to provide aftercare services for those leaving health or educational accommodation.

Children for whom local authorities provide accommodation are now said to be 'looked after' by the authority rather than in their care. What is done for them must be for their welfare and they must be consulted. There has to be a 'care plan' and the principles guiding the plan are that placement should be near the child's home, siblings should be kept together and whenever possible accommodation should be arranged with relatives or friends. A review is required by statute 4 weeks, 3 months and 6 months after the child is accommodated.

Significant harm

The conditions necessary to obtain a Care Order for those children requiring protection have been changed by the Children Act 1989. In the past a retrospective test was applied. Now a court may make a Care Order or a Supervision Order only if it is satisfied that the child concerned *is* suffering or *is likely to* suffer significant harm and that the harm or likelihood of harm is attributable to the care being given to the child, or likely to be given to him, or that he is beyond parental control.

In determining whether or not the criteria are fulfilled, courts have interpreted 'is suffering' to mean at the time protective action was taken. Medical evidence of injuries that have already occurred and of the state of health and development of the child

will still be required. Welfare will be paramount and what will be best for the child will obviously involve not only the present but especially the future. It follows that prognosis will become critically important.

The Act defines 'harm' as 'ill-treatment or the impairment of health or development.' This is a very broad definition indeed. 'Development' means physical, intellectual, emotional, social or behavioral development, 'health' means physical or mental health and 'ill-treatment' includes sexual abuse and forms of ill-treatment that are not physical.

It remains to be seen whether courts will take the view that the significance of harm is in proportion to the severity of injuries. There is not a necessary relationship between the severity of an injury and the risk of recurrence. A child who has a minor injury can have a very poor prognosis for recurrent ill-treatment. It is not the abuse that is the principal problem because it is only a symptom of an underlying defect in the relationship between the parents and the child. Unless this can .be altered the outlook remains bad irrespective of whether actual assaults occur.

The effect of Care Orders and Supervision Orders

A *Care Order* requires a local authority to receive a child into its care and to keep him while the Order remains in force. During this period it has parental responsibility and may restrict the responsibility of parents or refuse to allow them reasonable contact with the child but only if it is necessary in order to safeguard or promote his or her welfare.

A *Supervision Order* requires the named supervisor to advise, assist and befriend the child, to do what is necessary to supervise effectively and to consider applying to the Court for discharge or variation of the Order when it is no longer being complied with or when it is considered to be no longer necessary. A supervisor may require the child to attend specified places or participate in particular activities. The child may be brought for medical examination but the underlying principle applies that the child's wishes have to be taken into account.

An *Education Supervision Order* may be made on an application by a local education authority in respect of a child of compulsory school age if he is not being properly educated, i.e. when a School Attendance Order is not being complied with or a pupil is not attending school regularly.

Child Assessment Orders

A local authority or an authorized person may apply to a court for a Child Assessment Order. It is appropriate when there is a reasonable suspicion of significant harm or the likelihood of significant harm, an assessment is required and the parents are obstructive. Child Assessment Orders are intended for use when there is insufficient information to justify an application for an Emergency Protection Order. When made, they may last for up to 7 days. Parents have to produce the child to a named person and comply with any directions specified in the Order. A child of sufficient understanding to make an informed decision may refuse to submit to examination or other forms of assessment.

Emergency Protection Order

A court may make an Emergency Protection Order if it is satisfied that, either (a) there is reasonable cause to believe that a child is suffering or is likely to suffer significant harm unless he is removed to or kept in a safe place or (b) there are reasonable grounds to suspect that the child is suffering significant harm or is likely to suffer significant harm and inquiries are being frustrated by access being unreasonably refused *and* that access is required as a matter of urgency. The Order may contain directions with respect to contact and medical and psychiatric examinations or other forms of assessment. A child of sufficient understanding may refuse to submit to examination or assessment.

The authority conferred by the Order is much the same as that conferred by Place of Safety Orders in the past but, consistent with the principle that delays in legal proceedings are generally harmful to children, the time scales have been compressed. Whereas Place of Safety Orders lasted for up to 28 days and subsequent Interim Care Orders for seemingly indefinite intervals thereafter, Emergency Protection Orders last for a period not exceeding 8 days and can be extended once only for a period of up to an additional 7 days. Furthermore the parents have a right to apply for an Emergency Protection Order to be discharged at any time after the expiry of 72 hours.

Interim Care Orders

These were abused in the past and are now also restricted in duration to 8 weeks for the first order and 4 weeks for second and subsequent orders. With the granting of Interim Care Orders, courts may give directions for medical and psychiatric examinations. Once again there is the proviso that if children are of sufficient age and understanding examinations or assessments can take place only with their agreement.

Police protection

This is intended for the short-term protection of children in emergency situations. A police constable can remove a child to suitable accommodation and keep him there if he has reasonable cause to believe that the child would be likely to suffer significant harm otherwise. He may also take reasonable steps to prevent the removal of a child from hospital or other accommodation. The local authority and the parents have to be informed as soon as practicable. No child may be kept in police protection for more than 72 hours.

THE CHILDREN (SCOTLAND) ACT 1995

This statute is underpinned by a number of important principles including the following:

1. Parents have legal responsibilities (listed in the Act) towards their children.
2. Parents have parental rights (again listed in the Act) only in order to allow them to discharge their parental responsibilities.
3. Parental responsibilities continue after divorce, subject to any orders the court may have made.
4. In coming to decisions over disputes regarding the exercise of parental rights and responsibilities, courts must regard the welfare of the child as the paramount consideration.
5. In reaching decisions courts should have regard to the wishes of the child.

6. In deciding disputes over the exercise of parental rights and responsibilities, the courts have a variety of orders available to them including:
   a. Residence orders (which are similar to what used to be called custody orders)
   b. Contact orders (formerly called access orders)
   c. Specific issue orders (e.g. an order relating to a specific matter such as whether consent should be given to a child's medical treatment)
   d. interdicts to prohibit a parent exercising a particular parental right.
7. Courts should not make an order (e.g. a residence or contact order) unless it would be better than making no order. This is to discourage parents from seeking unnecessary orders.
8. Parents are the best people to look after their children and the State should only interfere with the autonomy of the family if it is necessary for the protection of the child's welfare.

Duties of local authorities towards children in their area

Scottish local authorities, like their English counterparts, have obligations towards children, which they discharge through social work departments. In particular they must safeguard and promote the welfare of any child in their area who may be in need, and promote the upbringing of children by their families by providing an appropriate level of services. They must provide accommodation for a child where no-one has parental responsibility for him (e.g. because his parents are dead), or where he is lost or abandoned, or where the person who has been caring for him cannot do so (e.g. because of ill health or imprisonment). Under the law prior to the Children (Scotland) Act 1995 such children were described as being 'received into the care of a local authority', but now they are termed as being 'looked after' by the authority. Most such children are looked after on what might be called a 'voluntary' basis in that the parents have agreed that the local authority should take over caring for the child. However, in some circumstances it may be necessary when parents are failing to promote and safeguard the welfare of the child for the local authority to seek compulsory powers to protect the child's needs.

Child protection – compulsory measures

Children's hearings

Introduced by the Social Work (Scotland) Act 1968 but governed now by the Children (Scotland) Act 1995 (Part II), the children's hearing system is concerned with children who may require compulsory measures of supervision. The hearing is conducted before three trained lay persons, at least one of whom must be a woman and at least one of whom must be a man. Cases are brought before them by an individual who is designated the 'Reporter'. The children who are subject to the jurisdiction of the hearing must normally be under 16, but in certain circumstances the hearing's jurisdiction extends to children up to 18. There are 12 grounds on which the Reporter may refer a case to the hearing to consider whether the child concerned is in need of compulsory measures of supervision, including that he is likely to suffer unnecessarily due to lack of parental care; or has failed to attend school regularly without reasonable excuse; or has committed an offense. Should the child or parent accept the ground for referral, the hearing proceeds to dispose of the case, e.g. by imposing a supervision requirement placing the child in a residential establishment or a condition that the child be subject to a medical examination or treatment. It would be noted, however, that if the child is of sufficient maturity he or she can refuse to consent to the medical treatment/examination. If the ground for referral is not accepted the matter must be put before the sheriff who will decide if the ground is established. If it is, he will remit the case back to the hearing for disposal.

When a child is subject to a supervision requirement his or her parents retain, and can exercise, their parental rights and responsibilities, but only to the extent that they do not conflict with the orders made by the children's hearing.

Child Protection Order (CPO)

This court order was introduced by the 1995 Act to improve the procedure for removing a child in an emergency to a place of safety when the child was being seriously mistreated or neglected by his parents. The Act allows any person, e.g. a local authority or policeman, to apply to the sheriff court for a CPO which the sheriff can make if:

1. there are reasonable grounds to believe
   a. the child is suffering significant harm as a result of the way he is being mistreated or neglected, or
   b. the child will suffer such harm if not removed or kept in a place of safety (or does not remain in the place where he is currently being accommodated), and
2. a CPO is necessary to protect the child from significant harm.

The order authorizes the removal of the child to or his retention in a place of safety, and the sheriff can make directions, e.g. as to contact between the child and his parents, or to authorize medical treatment or assessment of the child. The Reporter can discharge the child from the place of safety but if he does not a children's hearing must be held on the second working day after the order is implemented. If the children's hearing is satisfied that the conditions for making the CPO are met, it can continue the order and a second children's hearing arranged to decide whether or not the child is in need of compulsory measures of supervision. The second hearing must take place on the eighth working day after the order is implemented.

A CPO can last for 8 days at the most although it may be recalled earlier by, for example, a children's hearing or the sheriff.

Emergency protection

There may be extreme emergencies involving mistreatment of children when it is crucial that they be removed immediately from dangerous situations, but it would take too long to get a child protection order from the sheriff authorizing the removal. In such a situation any person, e.g. a policeman, can apply to a justice of the peace (JP) for authority to remove the child to a place of safety. The JP can only give such authority if certain matters are satisfied including that the conditions for making a CPO are present. The maximum period for which the authorization endures under this provision is 24 hours but, depending on the circumstances, it may not extend beyond 12 hours if within that

period the child has not been taken to a place of safety or no application to the sheriff for a CPO has been made.

In certain emergency situations a police constable can remove a child to a place of safety without obtaining a JP's authorization. The power to keep the child in the place of safety does not extend beyond 24 hours from the time of removal.

The 1995 Act also introduced innovations to Scotland in the form of Child Assessment Orders (CAO) and Exclusion Orders (EO). The former are awarded by the sheriff where a local authority suspects that a child is suffering or is likely to suffer significant harm as a result of ill-treatment but the child's parents will not permit the child to be examined in order that the suspicions can be confirmed or not. In granting a CAO the sheriff will authorize a person, e.g. a doctor, to carry out the assessment. The assessment could normally take place without the child being removed from its home, but the Court can authorize the child to be taken and kept at a specified place for the purpose of the assessment. A CAO is only effective for 7 days at the most. The Exclusion Order allows the sheriff on the application of the local authority to exclude an abusing parent from the family home. At the latest an EO ceases to have effect 6 months after it was made, although the sheriff may order it to cease at an earlier date. An EO will only be made if: the child has suffered or is likely to suffer significant harm; it is necessary for his protection; and it would better safeguard the child's welfare than the removal of the child from the family home.

THE PEDIATRICIAN AND MEDICAL NEGLIGENCE

Compared with doctors in some other specialties, pediatricians are not frequent targets of litigation, but medical errors in the care of infants and children can result in particularly poignant tragedies for families and may have devastating consequences for the doctor or doctors concerned. As the child may be left with lifelong disability, negligence can also be very expensive and a considerable drain on the resources that might otherwise be made available elsewhere within the health service. In this section some areas of practice are indicated where pediatricians, by their attitude and approach, might avoid or minimize their vulnerability to legal action. Some underline the importance of good communication with colleagues and patients (and parents of the very young), but most simply represent the application of courtesy and common sense. All emphasize the importance of what is generally agreed to be 'good clinical practice'.

Over 50% in number (and about 85% of the costs) of negligence claims involving pediatricians result from problems that occur in the care of *newborn infants*. In about half of these the pediatrician may be involved as part of general allegations directed against the hospital and obstetric team that a baby was 'brain damaged' from intrapartum asphyxia. Allegations specifically made against the pediatric staff may include errors in the conduct of resuscitation in the delivery room or in the subsequent care needed in the nursery whether or not they are relevant to the unsatisfactory outcome. In *older children*, delays in diagnosis, and therefore delays in starting effective treatment, are common, notably in meningitis. Errors in management include failure to anticipate and prevent life-threatening crises like cardiorespiratory arrest, e.g. by elective ventilation; or failures in monitoring. At all ages, mistakes occur in the prescribing and administration of drugs (Campbell 1994).

Pointers to prevention

Attitude and communication

1. Always remain courteous and as calm as possible in dealing with a frightened child and anxious parents, even in circumstances of frustration and provocation. Listen carefully to the child (if appropriate) and to the parents and give them opportunities to express their feelings and ask questions. It is easy to become impatient and dismissive, particularly when exhausted after a difficult day or night on duty. Develop 'long antennae' that will be sensitive to misunderstandings and unspoken anxieties – many can be resolved immediately by taking a few minutes for explanation and reassurance. Inevitably you will have many other things to do but try not to appear rushed. If you cannot deal with the problem immediately because of an emergency elsewhere, say so, but find time to go back and see the parent(s) or relatives as soon as possible. To you as a pediatrician, it may be just one case among many; to the parents it is the only one that matters to them. If things go wrong, they will remember if the attitudes and actions of the doctor(s) concerned seemed uncaring or defensive.

2. Listen very carefully if a mother or experienced nurse expresses concern about a child's condition. They have more consistent contact with the child and are in a much better position to notice subtle but important changes. An experienced mother's concern about her infant being 'just not right' should always be taken seriously. Do not refuse to visit the ward to examine a sick child when requested by nurses or the parents. If you cannot attend immediately, explain why and make sure that you attend at the earliest opportunity. If necessary, ask a colleague to make the call on your behalf. Make a habit of reading the regular shift reports on the nursing Kardex and other nursing observation sheets. They will often provide important and helpful details about a child's condition and progress.

3. Hospital doctors sometimes become involved in legal actions that have been 'triggered' by a dismissive response to a diagnosis made by the referring general practitioner, e.g. 'Please see and advise. This may only be a viral illness but I am concerned that it could be meningitis'. Always take such a provisional diagnosis seriously until proved otherwise – the family doctor may be more experienced and will know the child and family better than you do. If admission is requested but you do not believe it is necessary, have good grounds for this decision and record them. If sending the child home, it is prudent to involve a more senior colleague and, if possible, to let the GP or practice receptionist know so that a follow-up visit may be arranged.

4. If a child is critically ill be as realistic as possible, but do not make exact predictions about the time of death or the chances of survival. Try to steer the difficult course between raising false hopes on the one hand and destroying all hope on the other. It is never possible to be absolutely sure about prognosis – the outcome may surprise you.

5. 'Medical accidents'. If a complication or error in treatment has occurred, deal with it immediately. Initiate corrective steps without delay. Obtain appropriate specialist consultations and tell the parents exactly what happened, as far as you know it, without admitting blame or blaming others. Maintain a caring and supportive attitude even in the face of parental hostility and threats of legal action. Like anyone else, doctors can make mistakes – parents recognize this but they will not readily forgive attempts to conceal the truth about what happened. Many a legal action has originated because parents believed it to be the only way of discovering the truth.

Consent

The standard consent form signed on admission is generally taken as sufficient for most routine investigations and procedures needed for initial diagnosis and treatment. However, with the exception of emergencies when a parent may not be available, be particularly careful about telling the parents and obtaining separate consent when complicated and potentially hazardous tests or treatments are planned. Give adequate explanations of the risks and benefits and give the parents opportunities to ask questions. Never refuse requests for a second opinion or specialist consultation but encourage them whenever appropriate. In carrying out investigations or treatments, stay within the limits of your own field of expertise, experience and training – otherwise, if something goes wrong, you may not have the support of your colleagues.

Note. While a signed consent form is *prima facie* evidence of consent to surgery or some other invasive procedure, in some circumstances the method or timing of obtaining the consent may be challenged. Ideally the standard consent form should be supported by some documentation in the medical record which verifies that the doctor discussed the planned procedure, its indication, risks and benefits, and that the patient/parents expressed understanding of what was involved.

Record keeping

1. A claim for negligence can succeed or fail on the quality of the clinical notes. As a doctor, your notes of what happened will be taken as a reflection of your style and standards of practice. Insisting that you did everything right will not help if there is nothing to support this in the record, particularly if the nursing reports give a different impression. Notes should be written contemporaneously, be legible, objective and as complete as possible. Get into the habit of making sure that they are always dated, timed and signed. The original entry must never be changed by 'doctoring' it with the benefit of hindsight. If it is necessary to add some clarifying details on a later occasion, these should be identified as such and also dated and timed. Altering the original record is always obvious, will raise suspicions of deceit and, should the matter ever come to court, will be catastrophic to your credibility. A doctor who changes the medical record in this way is also likely to get into difficulties with the General Medical Council.

A doctor who with intent to deceive, makes an entry in a patient's medical records, knowing it to be false or misleading, or amends an entry by adding or subtracting false information or by deleting genuine information, is deliberately falsifying the case notes. This is unethical and a doctor so doing will be liable, if the matter is reported to the council, to disciplinary proceedings.

2. The notes should include a *history* that reflects a comprehensive review of the child's background and current illness, and a description of the *examination* and *investigations* that contains sufficient detail to indicate a logical and thorough approach to solving the clinical problem. All important findings, including vital signs and important positive and negative findings should be recorded, rather than just 'ticked off'. The practice of

bracketing a large number of checks or tests with one 'tick' or 'NAD', while understandable, is to be discouraged. Each item should be considered (and recorded) separately. Scanty notes employing excessive use of shorthand imply haste and inattention to detail.

3. Make a point of writing regular *progress notes*, *at least* once a day if a child is seriously ill, but more frequently as changes in condition and treatment dictate. Progress notes can be the strongest or weakest elements in a doctor's defense. Deficiencies in the notes may be compared unfavorably with the regular and detailed shift notes completed by the nursing staff. In your notes include any important points discussed in conversations, including by telephone, with the parents. If handing over to colleagues, a brief note indicating the essential details of management and progress to date will not only be helpful to them but may prevent potentially harmful errors of omission and commission.

4. A doctor requesting *laboratory tests* should take responsibility for checking and recording the results. A system should be in place to ensure that laboratory report slips are properly reviewed before being filed in the case record. This is particularly important if the child has been discharged – many a doctor has ended up in court because a vital laboratory report has been filed without being seen by someone capable of recognizing its significance.

5. The accident and emergency department, where rapid clinical decisions are often needed, is a fruitful source of litigation. It is a hectic, noisy, high pressure and often understaffed part of the hospital where rapport with patients and parents may be more difficult to achieve. Families will be anxious and unhappy in such stressful surroundings and more likely to complain about an unsatisfactory outcome. It is also difficult to find the time for detailed note keeping, but try to make good notes, however brief, using a Dictaphone if necessary. Adequate notes make all the difference to mounting a successful defense of any claim for negligence.

6. Never write derogatory personal observations in the medical record, particularly those that are irrelevant to care of the patient.

Drugs

Be particularly careful with the prescribing and administration of drugs. Hospital drug errors are responsible for many medical accidents every year, some of them with tragic consequences.

All are preventable by adopting a few simple precautions; for example:

1. *Know the drug*. Become familiar with the drugs you prescribe and give. Inform the parents about the drugs prescribed for their child. They should know the name of the drug, the reason for using it, and any major adverse effects that could occur. (Consider preparing patient handouts with the basic information on frequently prescribed drugs.)

2. *Drug orders*. Make sure that your written drug instructions are clear. Print the drug name in capital letters. Avoid symbols and abbreviations, e.g. mcg should be written out fully as micrograms (see BNF). Be particularly careful with calculations involving the decimal point. Orders for potent drugs should not be given or accepted by telephone.

3. *Check it out*. If a nurse or pharmacist questions your drug order or dose, accept the query graciously and check it carefully.

You may be grateful to them for preventing a tragedy. To be absolutely sure, particularly about an unfamiliar drug, look it up in the BNF or one of the pediatric drug references. This point is particularly important if you are covering another ward or unit where the drugs used may not only be unfamiliar but highly toxic if used incorrectly. Doctors working temporarily on oncology wards are particularly vulnerable. Be especially careful with *intrathecal* drugs – only rarely are they necessary and only on specialized units. Check that the dose *and* preparation are appropriate for intrathecal use. No matter how much you trust the nurses or colleagues who work with you, always insist on personally checking any drug (including the diluent fluid) you inject or add to an infusion. Particularly potent or potentially dangerous preparations, e.g. potassium chloride, should always be stored separately from drugs or infusion fluids in regular use.

4. *Allergy*. Exclude a history of drug sensitivity or anaphylaxis before injecting penicillin or preparations derived from foreign protein. Ensure that an 'allergic history' is recorded prominently in the case record.

5. *Pediatric preparations*. As far as possible prescribe and use only *pediatric* formulations for children, and on mixed wards encourage their separate storage.

Delegation

Doctors in training learn through the gradual delegation of responsibility according to experience, competence and judgment. If delegation has been inappropriate, the senior doctor will be considered at least partly liable in any claim of negligence that may arise through the actions of his or her juniors. Doctors in training must be adequately supported and should not be asked to undertake tasks outwith their experience and competence without prior instruction or adequate supervision. In turn, junior doctors should only accept tasks they feel competent to carry out. When a junior doctor asks a senior doctor for advice, the time and substance of that advice should be recorded in the clinical notes. Senior doctors who are difficult to contact or who get irritated and upset when asked to help with difficult problems may have only themselves to blame if their juniors become involved in litigation.

Guidelines

The concept of guidelines is not new – textbooks and Department of Health circulars are guidelines. What is relatively new is agreement on what is 'good clinical practice' with colleagues and standardizing its application to patient care in an attempt to educate and improve overall performance in the management of recurring clinical problems, e.g. diabetic ketoacidosis, status asthmaticus, etc. For the guidance of junior doctors and nurses practice protocols may need to be more detailed and prescriptive; for more senior clinicians they can be statements of principle within which reasonable clinical judgment may be exercised but should be robust enough to withstand scrutiny as a competent standard. Doctors are expected to keep up to date and be familiar with the current procedures and treatments relevant to their sphere of practice. Clinical guidelines should be reviewed regularly in the light of experience and new knowledge. Doctors sometimes fear that guidelines could become misused medicolegally, but just as with textbooks they will not necessarily put a doctor on or take him off a legal hook. The test of negligence remains 'failure to act in accordance with a practice accepted as proper by a responsible body of medical men skilled in that particular art'. Where scientific uncertainty exists this should be made clear, but innovative treatments should not be used unless they are part of properly designed and authorized clinical trials.

Adolescents

Consent. The major part of a pediatrician's practice is with young children below the age of consent; hence most of the above remarks are relevant to the pediatrician/parent(s) relationship. Children over the age of 7 or 8 years will have an increasing understanding about the implications of their illness, treatment, etc. and it is right that, as they mature, they should be increasingly involved in discussions about their management but to an extent that should remain at the discretion of the doctor and parents. 16 years is the 'legal' age of consent, but some children of 14 years (and even younger) are mature enough to be capable of giving informed consent to treatment. The courts would probably support a pediatrician who honors an adolescent's informed consent to

treatment if the child demonstrated maturity and decision-making capacity. The underage adolescent, however, probably does not have the same right to *refuse* treatment, particularly in situations where refusal might have serious consequences such as death or disability. In these circumstances the views of the parents and responsible doctor(s) should probably prevail although seeking court approval might be the prudent course of action.

Confidentiality. The pediatrician should encourage adolescents to take part in collaborative decision making with their parents, but there will be circumstances where this is not possible or will be refused. Generally, a mature adolescent's wish for confidentiality must be observed and there must be good grounds, carefully recorded, for any breach of this to the parents or anyone else. Both the parents and the adolescent patient should be aware that information provided by the patient will be kept confidential unless (1) the adolescent requests parental involvement, or agrees to a parental request for information and (2) the pediatrician has good grounds to believe that the adolescent's behavior will lead to harm to him- or herself or to another person. The adolescent should understand these limits to confidentiality.

REFERENCES AND BIBLIOGRAPHY

American Psychiatric Association 1994 Daignostic and statistical manual of mental disorders, 4th edn. (DSM IV) American Psychiatric Association, Washington
Black D 1992 Children of parents in prison. Archives of Disease in Childhood 67: 967–970
Botting B (ed) 1995 The health of our children – a review in the mid 1990's. Decennial Supplement – OPCS (DS No 11). HMSO, London
British Paediatric Association 1987 The school health service. BPA, London
British Paediatric Association 1994 Evaluation of suspected imposed upper airway obstruction. BPA, London
Butler N R, Bonham D G 1963 Perinatal problems, first report 1958, British Perinatal Mortality Survey. Churchill Livingstone, Edinburgh
Butler N R, Alberman E D 1969 Perinatal problems, second report 1958, British Perinatal Mortality Survey. Churchill Livingstone, Edinburgh
Campbell A G M 1994 The paediatrician and medical negligence. In: Powers M J, Harris N H (eds) Medical negligence, 2nd edn. Butterworths, London, pp 688–743
Central Advisory Council for Education (England) 1967 Children and their primary schools (Plowden Report). HMSO, London
Central Health Services Council 1967 Report of a sub-committee of the Standing Medical Advisory Committee on Child Welfare Centres. (Chairman: Sir Wilfred Sheldon) HMSO, London
Chamberlain R N, Simpson R N 1979 The prevalence of illness in childhood. A report of the British Births Child Study into illness and hospital experiences of children during the first three and a half years of life. Pitman Medical, London
Chamberlain R N, Chamberlain G, Howlett B, Claiveaux A 1975 British births 1970. Vol 1: The first week of life. Heinemann Medical Books, London
Child adoption: a selection of articles on adoption theory and practice. Association of British Agencies for Adoption and Fostering, London
Children Act 1989 HMSO, London
Children (Scotland) Act 1995 HMSO, London
Cochrane A, Holland W 1971 Validation of screening procedures British Medical Bulletin 27: 3–8
Committee of Enquiry into the Education of Handicapped Children and Young People (Chairman: Warnock H M) 1978 Special educational needs. HMSO, London
Committee on Local Authority and Allied Personal Services (Chairman: Seebohm F) 1968 Report of the Committee on Local Authority and Allied Personal Services. HMSO, London
Committee on One Parent Families (Chairman: Finer Hon. Sir Morris) 1974 Report of the Committee on One Parent Families. HMSO, London
Committee on Child Health Services (Chairman: Court S D M) 1976 Fit for the Future. HMSO, London
Dale A, Marsh C 1992 Census users guide 1991. OPCS. HMSO, London
Davie R, Butler N R, Goldstein H 1972 National Child Development Study

second report: from birth to seven. Longman, London
Department of Health 1989 An introduction to the Children Act 1989. HMSO, London
Department of Health 1991 Child abuse: a study of enquiry reports 1980–89. HMSO, London
Department of Health and Social Security 1988 Diagnosis of child sexual abuse: guidance for doctors. HMSO, London
Douglas J W B 1964 The home and the school. MacGibbon & Kee, London
Douglas J W B, Blomfield J W 1958 Children under five. Allen & Unwin, London
Douglas J W B, Ross J M, Simpson H R 1968 All our future. Peter Davies, London
Education Act 1993 HMSO, London
Education (Handicapped Children) Act 1981 HMSO, London
Employment Medical Advisory Service Act 1972 HMSO, London
Forfar J O (ed) 1988 Child health in a changing society. Published for the British Paediatric Association by Oxford University Press, Oxford
Fratter J, Rowe J, Sapsford D, Thoburn J 1991 Permanent family placement: a decade of experience. British Agencies for Adoption and Fostering, London
Gatrad A R 1994 Attitudes and beliefs of Muslim mothers towards pregnancy and infancy. Archives of Disease in Childhood 71: 170–174
Hall D M B 1996 (ed) Health for all children. Report of the Third Joint Working Party on Child Health Surveillance. Oxford University Press, Oxford
HMSO 1988 Report of the Inquiry into Child Abuse in Cleveland 1987. HMSO, London
Hobbs C J, Wynne J M 1993 Child abuse: clinical paediatrics international practice and research. Baillière Tindall, London
Home Office, Department of Health, Department of Education and Science and Welsh Office 1991 Working together under the Children Act 1989: a guide to arrangements for inter-agency co-operation for the protection of children from abuse. HMSO, London
Johnson A 1995 Use of registers in child health. Archives of Disease in Childhood 72: 474–476
Kellmer-Pringle M L, Butler N R, Davie R 1966 National Child Development Study first report: 11,000 seven year olds. Longman, London
Knowlden J, Keeling J, Nichol J P 1985 Post neonatal mortality. A multicentre study undertaken by the Medical Research Unit, Sheffield University. Department of Health and Social Security, HMSO, London
Meadow S R 1982 Munchausen syndrome by proxy. Archives of Disease in Childhood: 57 92–98
Meadow S R (ed) 1993a ABC of child abuse, 2nd edn. British Medical Journal, London
Meadow S R 1993b Non-accidental salt poisoning. Archives of Disease in Childhood 68: 448–452
Meltzer H 1994 Day care services for children. OPCS (SS No 1296). HMSO, London

Miller F J W, Court S D M, Walton W S, Knox E G 1960 Growing up in Newcastle upon Tyne. Oxford University Press, London

Morris J N, Heady J A 1955 Social and biological factors in infant mortality. Lancet i: 343, 395, 445, 499, 554

Office of Population Censuses and Surveys (OPCS) 1993 Congenital malformation statistics notifications 1991. MB3 No 7. HMSO, London

Office of Population Censuses and Surveys (OPCS) 1994 Birth statistics 1992. FMI No 21. HMSO, London

Office of Population Censuses and Surveys (OPCS) 1994 Cancer statistics: registrations 1989. MBI No 22. HMSO, London

Office of Population Censuses and Surveys (OPCS) 1994 Communicable disease statistics 1992. MB2 No 19. HMSO, London

Office of Population Censuses and Surveys (OPCS) 1994 Marriage and divorce statistics 1992. FM2 No 20. HMSO, London

Office of Population Censuses and Surveys (OPCS) 1994 Mortality statistics: childhood 1992. DH6 No 6. HMSO, London

Office of Population Censuses and Surveys (OPCS) 1995 Abortion statistics 1992. AB No 19. HMSO, London

Office of Population Censuses and Surveys (OPCS) 1995 Census ethnic groups reports 1991. HMSO, London

Office of Population Censuses and Surveys (OPCS) 1995 Census topics report 1991 – children and young adults. HMSO, London

Office of Population Censuses and Surveys (OPCS) 1995 General household survey 1993. GHS No 24. HMSO, London

Office of Population Censuses and Surveys (OPCS) 1995 Mortality statistics: perinatal and infant 1992. DH3 No 26. HMSO, London

Office of Population Censuses and Surveys (OPCS) 1995 National diet and nutrition survey: children aged $1\frac{1}{2} - 4\frac{1}{2}$. HMSO, London

Rosenberg D A 1987 Web of deceit: a literature review of Munchausen syndrome by proxy. Child Abuse and Neglect 11: 547–563

Rowe J, Hundleby M, Garnett L 1989 Child care now: British Agencies for Adoption and Fostering, London

Royal College of Physicians 1997 Physical signs of sexual abuse in children: a report of the Royal College of Physicians. RCP, London

Rutter M, Graham P, Yules W 1970 A neuropsychiatric study in childhood. Clinics in Developmental Medicine 35–36. Heinemann, London

Scottish Home and Health Department 1973 Towards an integrated child health service (Brotherston Report). HMSO, Edinburgh

Spence J C, Walton W S, Miller F J W, Court S D M 1954 A thousand families in Newcastle upon Tyne. Oxford University Press, London

Staples B, Pharoah P O D 1994 Child health statistical review. Archives of Disease in Childhood 71: 548–554

Stewart-Brown S L, Haslum M 1988 Screening of vision in school: could we do better by doing less? British Medical Journal 297: 1111–1113

Thomson 1996 Family, law in Scotland, 3rd edn.

Wilson J M G, Jugner G 1968 Principles and practice of screening for disease. Public Health Papers No 34. WHO, Geneva

35 Child care in developing countries

W. A. M. Cutting   B. J. Brabin

Introduction   1882
Geographical regions and changes in the child
    health situation   1882
Measuring child well-being and its rate of change
    1883
The political factors and economic constraints on
    child health   1884
The socioethical situation and the health of children
    1885
    Cultural context of child health and the girl child
        1885
    Maternal education and child survival   1886
    Child exploitation   1887
        Types of exploitation   1887
        Street children   1887
    The rights of the child   1888

How the structure and fashions in health services affect children
    1888
The realities and the needs in the health care services for
    children   1889
Primary health care (PHC) and its implementation   1889
    PHC strategies   1889
    Problems facing PHC and the health services   1890
Special services   1890
    Perinatal care   1890
    Services for the disabled   1891
    Nutrition   1892
References   *1892*

INTRODUCTION

This chapter sets out some dimensions and trends in health problems affecting children in an international context. It also reviews the services attempting to tackle these problems at the end of the second millennium.

In the developing world there are differences of environment, inequalities of natural assets and maldistribution of resources. The result is many impoverished families and a large burden of morbidity and mortality on their children. The application of technology has reduced the mortality rate from some diseases more quickly than the birth rate. Consequently poverty and population growth mean that many families and countries have relatively little to spend on health care. The poorer countries of this world are underdeveloped or developing, but not necessarily tropical since many lie north of the tropic of Cancer or south of the tropic of Capricorn.

When planning to improve standards of health, essentials must come first. An adequate water supply in each community, satisfactory housing, agricultural aids, productive employment, stable markets, appropriate energy sources and improved female literacy. For the health of children the essentials also include sufficient and appropriate food, and a safe, stable and stimulating environment. A capable mother can compensate for many other deficiencies. Doctors and pediatricians should be aware that they can do little to influence many factors that limit the health of the world's children. Diagnosing and treating the sick child are important tasks, but the role of pediatricians includes informed advocacy, speaking out for children and supporting parents. Although the health of a child is dependent on many groups and individuals in general, ultimately it depends on one in particular – his or her mother.

GEOGRAPHICAL REGIONS AND CHANGES IN THE CHILD HEALTH SITUATION

Children of the world live in very varied environments and circumstances. The social, economic, demographic and environmental factors which affect their health and well-being are set out in a detailed set of tables at the end of each year's UNICEF report, *The State of the World's Children*. A few of the many facts from the 1996 report have been summarized in Table 35.1. Countries are grouped together by region and developmental status. The four types under consideration are industrialized countries, countries in transition, developing countries and the least developed countries (columns 6–9 in the Table 35.1). There are over 10 times as many children in developing and underdeveloped countries compared with industrial countries. Also in the developing and least developed countries children make up 37–50% of the total population. In contrast, in industrialized countries children constitute only about 20% of the population, but there is a higher proportion of people in the older age groups.

The under-5 mortality rate (U5MR) is an important measure of the development of countries and the well-being of their children. The U5MR is the number of children who die before completing 5 years of age per 1000 liveborn children in a country or community. In industrialized countries the U5MR has decreased from 37 in 1960 to 9 in 1994. The decrease in the least developed countries is from 282 to 170. Thus in 1960 a child born into the least developed countries had 7.7 times the chance of dying before age 5, compared with a child born in an industrial country. By the mid-1990s a child from the least developed countries had 19 times the chance of dying before its 5th birthday compared with one in an industrialized country. Many factors influence the U5MR, food

Table 35.1 International comparisons: children's health, mortality and associated factors

	Sub-Saharan Africa	Middle East & North Africa	South Asia	East Asia & Pacific	Latin America & Caribbean	Industrialized countries	Countries in transition	Developing countries	Least-developed countries
	[1]	[2]	[3]	[4]	[5]	[6]	[7]	[8]	[9]
Population under 16 years (millions)	262	154	482	540	170	169	105	1607	256
Percentage of total population	48	42	39	31	36	21	25	37	50
Under-5 mortality rates*									
1960	256	239	237	200	158	37	–	216	282
1980	204	142	179	80	87	15	–	138	222
1994	177	62	124	56	47	9	36	101	170
Under-5 mortality annual reduction rate (ARR) (%) 1980–94	1.0	5.9	2.6	2.5	4.4	3.8	–	2.2	1.9
Reduction rate required 1994–2000 (%)	15.9	4.1	9.6	6.9	4.5	4.8	–	10.2	14.8
Nutrition: percentage of children underweight, moderate to severe**	31	12	64	23	11	–	–	35	41
Adult literacy rate 1990									
Male (%)	63	70	59	88	86	–	99	76	56
Female (%)	42	46	32	72	83	–	97	57	34
Education: percentage reaching grade 5 primary	66	91	59	87	74	98	–	74	54
Percentage household consumption spent on food	38	39	51	45	34	14	–	41	–
Television sets per 1000 population	23	112	31	44	163	593	–	56	10
GNP† per capita ($US)	519	2129	309	871	2883	23 195	2000	987	238
GNP† per capita: annual growth rate 1980–1993 (%)	–0.3	0.6	2.9	6.8	–0.1	2.2	–0.6	2.9	0.7
Total fertility rate§									
1960	6.6	7.0	6.1	5.6	6.0	2.8	2.8	6.0	6.6
1994	6.2	4.4	4.0	2.3	3.0	1.9	1.7	3.5	5.7

Source: The State of the World's Children (UNICEF 1996)
* The number of deaths of children under 5 years of age per 1000 live births. More specifically this is the probability of dying between birth and exactly 5 years of age.
** Moderate and severe underweight means those that are below −2 standard deviations from the median weight for age of a reference population.
† Gross national product, expressed in current US dollars. GNP per capita growth rates are average annual growth rates that have been computed by fitting trend lines to the logarithmic values of GNP per capita at constant market prices for each year of the time period.
§ The number of children that would be born per woman according to the prevailing age-specific fertility rates.

availability, educational opportunity, etc., but the most striking differences are in the per capita income. In industrialized countries this is virtually 100 times that of the poorest countries. What is more, this maldistribution of wealth is increasing because the wealthier countries have been able to sustain in excess of a 2% per year growth rate, while in the poorest countries the growth rate is one-third of that, and in some situations inflation has undermined the financial stability. (The role of international borrowing and debt is referred to elsewhere.)

The large number of developing countries in the world have been divided by UNICEF into five groups (columns 1–5 in Table 35.1). These countries are characterized by having a high proportion of the population in the pediatric age group (31–48%) and a relatively low but variable GNP per capita, often with great contrasts of wealth and poverty within individual countries. In general these countries all had a high U5MR (158–256) 30 years

ago, and have been able to cut this figure in half by the mid-1990s. Some regions have done exceptionally well, for example North Africa and the Middle East and East Asia and the Pacific. In these regions the U5MR is approximately a quarter of what it was 35 years ago. The sub-Saharan Africa region has had a poor improvement of the U5MR. It has been hit by a series of catastrophes: droughts; political instability and coups; drop in world prices of its raw materials; and the epidemic of HIV infection, associated with other diseases and particularly tuberculosis.

MEASURING CHILD WELL-BEING AND ITS RATE OF CHANGE

The under-5 mortality rate (U5MR) is used as a principal indicator in the UNICEF's tabulations (UNICEF 1996) (Table 35.1, lines

3–5). Using this measurement has several advantages. First it relates to an end result of the development process rather than an 'input' such as school enrollment level, per capita calorie availability, or the number of doctors per 1000 population – all of which are means to an end. Second, the U5MR is the result of a wide variety of inputs: the nutritional health and the health knowledge of mothers; the level of immunization and use of oral rehydration; the availability of maternal and child health services including prenatal care; income and food accessibility in the family; clean water and sanitation; and the overall safety of the child's environment. Third, the U5MR is less susceptible than some measures, for example per capita GNP, to 'distortions of the average'. This is because the natural scale does not allow the children of the rich to be 1000 times as likely to survive, even if the man-made scale does permit them to have 1000 times as much money. In other words it is much more difficult for a wealthy minority to affect a nation's U5MR. It therefore presents a more accurate, if far from perfect, picture of the health status of the majority of children and the society they live in.

The speed of progress in reducing U5MR can be measured by calculating its average annual reduction rate (AARR) (line 6 in Table 35.1). Unlike the comparison of absolute changes, the AARR reflects the fact that the lower limits to the U5MR are approached only with increasing difficulty. This is because when the U5MR is low, a higher proportion of the deaths are due to the rarer and less easily preventable diseases like congenital malformations and malignancy. As the lower levels of under-5 mortality are reached, the same absolute reduction obviously represents a greater percentage of reduction. The AARR therefore shows a higher rate of progress for say a 10-point reduction if that reduction happens at the lower level of under-5 mortality. The gross national product (GNP) per person, expressed in US dollars is an index of wealth or poverty of a country. When the AARR is used in conjunction with GNP growth rates, the U5MR and its reduction rate gives a picture of the progress being made by any country or region, and over any period of time, towards achieving some of the most essential human needs.

The regional achievements of AARR, are shown in line 6 of Table 35.1. UNICEF has set a number of social and health goals to be achieved by the year 2000. Central among these is to achieve a U5MR rate in all countries of 70 per 1000 live births or of two-thirds of the 1990 rate, whichever is the lesser. The row in the table labeled 'Reduction rate required 1994–2000 (%)' (line 7 in Table 35.1) indicates the amount of progress required in the next few years to achieve that goal. It is striking that in some regions, for example the Middle East and North Africa, the reductions in mortality in the last 14 years suggests that the target is achievable. However, in other regions, for example sub-Saharan Africa and the least developed countries of the world, the required rate of reduction of mortality is 10–15 times what was achieved in recent years.

From Table 35.1 and the more comprehensive tables in *The State of the World's Children* (UNICEF 1996) there is no obvious relationship between the annual reduction of the U5MR and the annual growth in per capita GNP. The situation of individual countries is obscured in tables which collect the data from a variety of countries. On an individual national level the information indicates how policies, priorities and other factors determine the relationships between economic, social and health progress.

Since population pressure at the national or household level

affects child care, fertility rates are relevant. The national data shown in the UNICEF tables give the total fertility rate* for each country and its average annual rate of reduction. In Table 35.1 it can be seen that regions which have achieved substantial reductions in their U5MR have also achieved significant reductions in fertility.

THE POLITICAL FACTORS AND ECONOMIC CONSTRAINTS ON CHILD HEALTH

Development is a multifaceted process and child health is one essential component of that process. It has been said that child health reflects and determines the human condition, and measures of child health such as the infant mortality rate or percentage of stunted children are indicators of human development. The executive director of UNICEF, the late James P. Grant, stated: 'History may judge 1990 as the most momentous year ever for the world's children' because of the World Conference on Education for All, the Convention on the Rights of the Child, and the World Summit for Children, which resulted in 'unprecedented attention directed towards the most defenceless and needy among us' (Grant 1992). The decade of 1990 also marks UNICEF's 50th anniversary in 1996 and its 'State of the World's Children' report for that year outlines the international efforts made since 1946 to respond to children's needs (UNICEF 1996). The Declaration and Plan of Action of the 1990 World Summit for Children sets out future international goals – at the highest political level – to reduce rates of mortality and disease, malnutrition and illiteracy, and to reach specific targets by the year 2000. These goals, summarized in Table 35.2, are generally agreed health priorities; their attainment depends on political factors and economic

Table 35.2 Goals for the year 2000 (UNICEF 1996)

1. One-third reduction in 1990 under-5 death rates (or to 70 per 1000 live births, whichever is less)

2. A halving of 1990 maternal mortality rates

3. A halving of 1990 rates of malnutrition among the world's under-5s (to include the elimination of micronutrient deficiencies, support for breast-feeding by all maternity units, and a reduction in the incidence of low birthweight to less than 10%)

4. The achievement of 90% immunization among children under 1 year, the eradication of polio, the elimination of neonatal tetanus, a 90% reduction in measles cases, and a 95% reduction in measles deaths (compared with preimmunization levels)

5. A halving of child deaths caused by diarrheal diseases

6. A one-third reduction in child deaths from acute respiratory infections

7. Basic education for all children and completion of primary education by at least 80% – girls as well as boys

8. Safe water and sanitation for all communities

9. Acceptance by all countries of the Convention on the Rights of the Child, including improved protection for children in especially difficult circumstances

10. Universal access to high-quality family planning information and services in order to prevent pregnancies that are too early, too closely spaced, too late or too many

* The total fertility rate is the number of children that would be born per woman according to the prevailing age-specific fertility rates.

constraints affecting sustainable development. It will be very difficult for many countries to bring about these reductions in child mortality, disease rates and illiteracy. For some African countries it will be impossible because of political turmoil and economic crisis (Fig. 35.1). Currently about 70 of the poorest countries rely entirely on concessional lending and as a group they contain 80% of the world's population categorized as living in poverty. Roughly 45% of lending is to Africa and almost 50% of this targets poverty reduction activities such as nutrition, health, education and population efforts (Williams 1996). Total economic debts as a percentage of gross national product have increased in these countries over the period 1971–1993. Sub-Saharan Africa's debt, which has continued to soar, now surpasses its GNP. No single organization has an answer to the complex problems posed by this economic situation. Effective responses to problems of poverty are influenced by local realities shaped by culture, politics, wealth distribution, community values and household relations that cannot simply be altered by economic analysis or theoretical models. There needs to be a shift so that economic strategies focus on social conditions, and research should address the effects of economic policies at the household level.

The term 'adjustment' refers to a range of economic policies which have mostly been supported by loans from the World Bank and International Monetary Fund. These new loans broadly represent an attempt to strengthen the balance of payments by shifting towards a market-orientated system. The debt crisis and falling export prices reduced foreign exchange for most developing countries and the substantial loans available allowed countries to reduce these burdens and support the commodity process. This may be viewed as an unavoidable response to the debt crisis. Adjustment has potentially important effects on health and education, through its effects on market prices and employment. Households may have lower incomes which affect health-related activities, and reduced government spending may reduce health provision and educational opportunities. User-fees reduce access to clinic facilities and schools.

There has been little systematic evaluation of how structural adjustment policies and the terms of trade relate to child health and welfare. A recent analysis of adjustment and the health of mothers and children concludes that there is little evidence for the proposition that adjustment promotes sustainable economic growth in low income countries (Costello et al 1994). This view is pessimistic and partly reflects the difficulties which arise in trying to link health effects to economic policy in the short term. However, a recent analysis by Save the Children Fund (1996) also strongly questions whether this approach is wise. Using examples such as the cost of immunization and the new tuberculosis epidemic it illustrates that outside agencies may be getting it wrong – mainly by failing to support national structures in sustaining health care over the long term. Key aspects for the future may be based on adapting economic and health strategies to local circumstances and devolving decision making to communities.

Communities require social stability which is essential for economic growth. Civil breakdown results in major damage to the health infrastructure. Children have always been caught up in warfare and civil unrest, but recent situations have highlighted the dangers. Good governance and financial discipline of borrower countries are vital if governments are to provide services such as health and education effectively. UNICEF has adopted in 1996 an anti-war agenda which rests on the proposition that the tragedy befalling children is preventable. In the wars of the past decade, some 2 million children have been killed; 4–5 million disabled; 12 million left homeless; more than 1 million orphaned or separated from their parents and some 10 million psychologically traumatized (UNICEF 1996).

The task of those concerned with child health is to mitigate the effects of these circumstances, poverty and war, wherever and whenever possible. Political instability and the continuing economic stagnation of most of sub-Saharan Africa presents challenges to everyone as well as to the World Bank, governments, nongovernmental organizations and professional organizations. A continued emphasis on social stability should be embedded in any reforms, interventions or adjustment policies aimed at improving child health in less developed countries.

THE SOCIOETHICAL SITUATION AND THE HEALTH OF CHILDREN

CULTURAL CONTEXT OF CHILD HEALTH AND THE GIRL CHILD

The concept of childhood as a time free from gender is only true of children from wealthier families in the world. Gender has two components – biological and cultural. For girls, in many less developed countries the emphasis is on their reproduction role and this becomes established in childhood. The focus on the vulnerability of girls arises partly because of this but also because of discrimination against them in many societies due to male attitudes and a preference for sons over daughters. Parents favor sons because of the labor and old age security they provide and because they carry the family line. This discrimination limits access to food and medical facilities for girls which can have serious consequences for their health. Death rates for girls, after the neonatal period, are consistently higher than for boys of the same age in many less developed countries (Fig. 35.2).

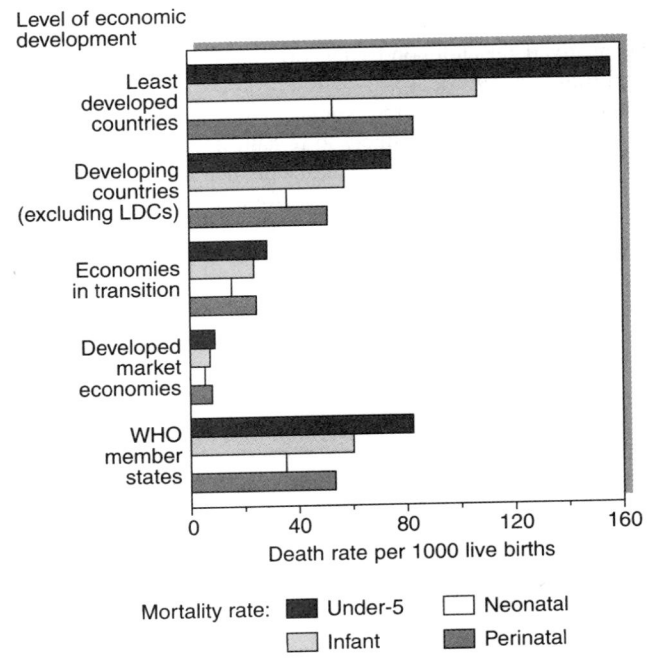

Level of economic development

Death rate per 1000 live births

Mortality rate: ■ Under-5   □ Neonatal
□ Infant   ■ Perinatal

Fig. 35.1 Economic development and deaths among children, 1995 (WHO 1996a).

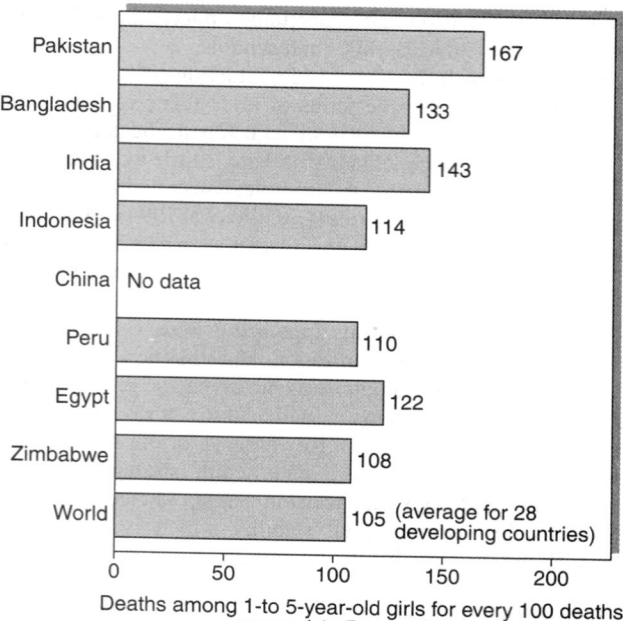

Fig. 35.2 Differences in female and male child mortality (modified from Rosen & Conley 1996).

Table 35.3 Strategies for improving female adolescent status (modified from Kurz et al 1994)

1. **Improve adolescents' food intake**
   - Increase household purchasing power
   - Educate adolescents about nutrition
   - Introduce meals at schools or work sites
   - Consider iron fortification or supplementation
   - Discourage gender differences in food intake

2. **Keep girls in school**
   - Ensure girls' safety and privacy at school
   - Establish schools close to home
   - Increase the proportion of female teachers
   - Make school hours more flexible
   - Introduce alternatives to formal education
   - Integrate food supplementation into school systems

3. **Postpone first births**
   - Postpone age at marriage
   - Offer appropriate family planning and reproductive health services for adolescents
   - Provide family life education and life options
   - Increase educational attainment for girls

4. **Reduce girls' workloads and improve work conditions**
   - Introduce mechanisms to reduce girls' workloads
   - Teach adolescents income-earning skills
   - Build partnerships with employers

5. **Improve adolescents' health**
   - Inform and educate adolescents about their health
   - Design and provide health services for adolescents
   - Develop effective communication strategies for adolescents

6. **Enhance girls' self-esteem**
   - Increase knowledge and skills
   - Provide opportunities for achievement
   - Increase girls' awareness of opportunities for the future
   - Establish means for communication

One measure of a child's position is the parental willingness to send him or her to school. In less developed countries deeply rooted traditional and religious attitudes often limit girls' educational and employment opportunities. For example in Pakistan, literacy rates are about 21% for women and 47% for men and only 35% of girls are enrolled in primary school, which is half the enrollment rates for boys, a ratio unchanged since 1970 (Rosen & Conley 1996). In contrast, the quality of family child health care is more often associated with maternal than paternal schooling, reflecting a cultural division of labor in which men are not involved in child care.

In some societies girls are considered an important asset to families (e.g. Cambodia) as, according to tradition, husbands come to live with their wives' family becoming an asset for income generation. For this reason girls are less likely to be abandoned. Girls also may have an economic value, fetching hundreds of dollars when sold into the sex trade as virgins (World Vision 1996).

The Declaration from the 1990 World Summit for Children does not mention girls as a special category, although it stresses the role of women in general and equal treatment opportunities for girls. Emphasis has been given to improving female reproductive capacity during childhood by improving the health of young adolescents, particularly their nutritional status (Table 35.3). Improving the reproductive capacity and health of adolescents is a key component for improved child survival, but it is also important that girls are enabled to reach their full intellectual and social potential in their own right. The aim should not be solely to produce reproductively efficient mothers.

MATERNAL EDUCATION AND CHILD SURVIVAL

There is a close relationship between child mortality and the length of formal schooling of the mother. Even after adjustment for economic factors 1–3 years' maternal education is associated with a fall of 20% in childhood mortality. This relationship exists in all major regions of the developing world and in countries with either well developed or poorly developed health care systems (Cleland & van Ginneken 1988). Literacy programs for adults who received no childhood education also show these benefits (Sandiford et al 1995).

When girls can assume some independence even when unmarried, they are more likely to remain in school. When older women are allowed to appear in public on their own initiative, then mothers are more likely to take action for a sick child and not wait to consult husband or brothers. With more autonomy women will be more likely to treat their daughters like their sons, providing better nutrition and health care. For these reasons a marked degree of female autonomy is probably essential for significant child mortality reduction in less developed countries (Caldwell 1986).

Several studies have demonstrated a close association between maternal education and infant and child mortality. The key analysis was by Caldwell (1979) who surveyed data from Ibadan, Nigeria, and demonstrated that the mother's education was a more decisive determinant of child survival than economic well-being. Although other studies have confirmed these initial findings the various mechanisms or intervening factors which lead to the lower mortality are not well understood. More equitable treatment of daughters and sons plays some role, but factors affecting water use, housing quality, and use of preventive and curative services are also important. Little is known about the intervening role of health beliefs and domestic practices, although these are probably very important.

The education advantage in survival is less pronounced during the neonatal period and higher male mortality rates during the first 4 weeks of life are reported. This is consistent with the overwhelming evidence that in childhood male biological risk, as opposed to cultural risk, of death is higher than female. Some understanding about the important causes of child mortality, such as diarrhea and pneumonia, is important for the successful introduction of key interventions, such as oral rehydration practices (Stapleton 1989) and community management strategies for early recognition and treatment of respiratory infection.

CHILD EXPLOITATION

Types of exploitation

There are a variety of damaging activities or omissions which endanger a child's health, well-being or safety. Children are exploited because they are vulnerable. Girls may be especially vulnerable because of the danger of physical abuse and sexual violation. Families in least favored circumstances will be those who are most likely to send their children out to work. Children from lower socioeconomic groups are those most likely to be sent to work and to be malnourished. Evidence for this comes from a study of childhood malnutrition and child labor in rural India (Satyanarayan et al 1986). Conversely, children kept at home to help with household duties and child care may not be able to attend school. Many children must combine domestic tasks in the home with waged labor outside; others are required to stay at home in order to free adults for labor outside the home.

Conceptions of exploitation are culturally related. Behaviors and attitudes acceptable in some areas and eras may be viewed as detrimental in others. In 18th and 19th century Europe employment of children as chimney sweeps was an acceptable practice. Crosscultural perspectives in child maltreatment depend on circumstances and should be considered in the context of:

1. cultural differences in child-rearing practices
2. departure from culturally acceptable behavior
3. societal harm of children which is beyond control of parents or care-takers (Tsitoura 1995).

Parents who exploit and abuse their children are themselves often under stress and a high proportion have a poor education. Premature, mentally retarded and physically disabled children may be at particular risk.

Children are generally the victims of violence rather than its perpetrators, yet one of the most deplorable developments in recent years has been the increasing use of children as soldiers. Recently in 25 countries, thousands of children under the age of 16 have fought in wars and in 1988 alone they numbered 200 000 (UNICEF 1996). In the Uganda conflict in 1986 approximately 25% of the forces were under 14 years of age. Such children have experienced the psychological trauma of violence, captivity, sexual abuse, undernutrition and torture and the effects of this on their psychological development is difficult to determine. In Uganda, trauma rehabilitation centers have been established to help abducted children rescued from areas of conflict. These provide counseling and nursing services and are facilitated by social workers to enable resettlement of children to their parents or next of kin. Similar initiatives have been developed in other war torn zones.

Street children

Most of the literature on street children concerns boys. There is no adequate information on the numbers of children who live on the streets or the comparative proportion of boys and girls who engage in specific street trade. It is estimated there are 50 000– 100 000 street children who manage to survive in Calcutta, India; and in Phnom Penh estimates vary between 5000 and 10 000. Such estimates do not account for the fluctuations of the street population, who may not live solely on the street but maintain links with the family. These numbers do not account for some of the most exploited children in Cambodia – girls sold into prostitution and hired labor – and they do not account for the full number of orphaned and abandoned children. In 1991 it was estimated that in Cambodia 1 in every 13 children had lost at least one parent and 45% of these have lost both parents (Paul 1995). Traditionally, such children are cared for by the extended family, but as this support is reduced by the effects of war or the HIV epidemic, then many children cater for their own needs. Not all these children are orphaned and many may be runaways who are escaping violence in the home. A recent survey by Paul (1995) showed that poverty, hunger, family disharmony and violence were the most common factors cited by children themselves as reasons they were on the street. She has classified the following groups of street children:

- slavery or bonded labor conditions after outright sale or adoption (including organized prostitution, military conscription and domestic service)
- semiorganized 'contractual' labor (market place labor and sifting for recyclables and food at main rubbish dumps)
- self-organized labor (begging, homosexual sex)
- daily or monthly hire situations (construction and coolie labor).

The problems and dangers faced by street children relate to their hazardous occupations, for example sifting rubbish with bare hands and feet. Some are sexually abused and become infected with sexually transmitted diseases. In Honduras 44% of street children were sexually active and almost all had been treated for sexually transmitted diseases (Wright et al 1993). They live in fear of bullying and losing their earnings as they have no safe place to keep them or their meager belongings. In a study of 30 child street hawkers in Port Harcourt, Nigeria, the children complained of adult abuse (13%), sexual harassment (42%, both boys and girls), education deprivation (17%), and disliking their work (27%). In traffic-polluted city centers such as Lagos, where a high number of street hawkers are children, air pollution resulting in respiratory morbidity is likely to be a significant hazard. A particular cause for concern are the Indian temple prostitutes, termed devadasis, who are low-caste girls estimated to be over 100 000 in number and who are given to temples of the goddess Yellema by their parents. These girls are sexually exploited from early puberty by devotees and have almost no option but to become prostitutes (Ennew 1994).

Seeking solutions to these problems involves a range of measures from immediate service provision to tackling the root causes. Many nongovernment agencies are involved in this work. One of the first initiatives in Calcutta was a drop-in center located on a busy railway station. Gradually the services were extended to include night shelter facilities. A city action plan has now been developed (Chaudhuri 1994). Fyfe (1989) presents five stages to assist working children which extend into tackling the 'root causes':

1. education and training (providing access to schooling)
2. welfare services (to disadvantaged children in the community as a whole, and not only to those in residential centers; rehabilitation of children leaving the sex industry)
3. protected work (placement schemes and sheltered workshops, community-based care at specific sites)
4. advocacy (emphasis on child rights, youth networks and local support groups)
5. regulation and enforcement (support for the training of police; child-specific provision within the court and prison systems).

These rights of children to be protected from violence and exploitation need to be highlighted so that appropriate funding for interventions and strategies for delivery can be ensured.

THE RIGHTS OF THE CHILD

Children's rights is a concept which is clearly related to the law. A child's rights approach to improving the situation for children in less developed countries establishes through recognition, but not necessarily legislation, the needs of children in health, education and security. The United Nations Convention on the Rights of the Child received universal ratification in 1993 from its member states. The Convention with its 52 articles provides a set of principles and standards for the planning and practice of pediatrics and child health for all children and young people up to the age of 18 years (HMSO 1991). The main article of the Convention concerned with the provision of health services is Article 24 which says that *all* children and young people under 18 years old have the right to 'the enjoyment of the highest attainable standard of health'. This includes such principles as:

- steps to reduce infant and child mortality
- providing primary health care
- providing pre- and postnatal care (UNICEF estimates that 500 000 women die annually in childbirth; the estimated maternal mortality rate for least developed countries is 603 per 100 000 births (UNICEF 1996))
- providing basic health promotion information
- developing preventive health care services.

Those providing services should also allow children to have their own views about their health and treatment and the services which affect them. This includes children with disabilities who have a right to appropriate services and support. Those from indigenous populations and ethnic, linguistic and religious minorities have the right to enjoy and practice their own cultures. Equal opportunities in education should be provided to children who are unable to attend school regularly.

Despite the importance of this milestone Convention, evidence suggests that inequalities in health between industrialized and developed countries are widening (see comments on under-5 mortality above). The main reason for their deaths is dire poverty preventing adequate nutrition and sanitation. Although a high percentage of children are now immunized against major diseases of infancy, extending vaccination to the remainder has slowed through lack of funding. Implementing the Convention in developing countries is restricted because of these realities. Nevertheless in daily work those responsible for child care may

look to the Convention as a source of authority in advocating children's rights. This is especially important for the most deprived and vulnerable children and those who are chronically sick, as it counterbalances complacent or defeatist views concerning the prospects for improving child life and health in poor countries.

HOW THE STRUCTURE AND FASHIONS IN HEALTH SERVICES AFFECT CHILDREN

Central planned health services were a feature in many countries after the Second World War. This was the case for both those which were newly achieving independence from the colonial system and the industrialized countries which were settling after the stresses of war. Even in poorer countries these services were moderately funded by local or international donor money. By the 1980s it appeared that the expectations and the costs of running increasingly expensive and comprehensive health services were beyond the capability of many national governments in wealthy as well as poor countries. Since then there has been a shift to a more capitalistic program with a range of services from simple indigenous care, which is generally cheap but not always effective, to sophisticated and often expensive 'fee for service programs'. This change has happened at a time of political and economic breakdown in a number of poorer countries where the government health provision has deteriorated. There is increasingly a contrast between the rich and the poor, both on an international scale and within countries. This is reflected by very varied health facilities and care provided for different groups.

Over the last 15 years there have also been changes in the fashion of provision of services and the emphases made by WHO, other UN agencies, bilateral aid and nongovernmental programs. In the 1950s and 1960s there were large centrally organized vertical programs against specific diseases; malaria and smallpox. Malaria control made dramatic advances in many countries in response to a military-like campaign and a unipurpose department. Ultimately resistance of the parasites to the cheaper antimalarial drugs, particularly chloroquine, and the resistance of the mosquito vectors to the most economic insecticides, particularly DDT, combined with inflation and social disruption in some areas to undermine the program. In contrast, a smallpox eradication program had identified a visible disease and vulnerable pathogen against which improved vaccine and delivery services were pushed home with appropriate financial backing, political will and a service which was flexible enough to deal with the epidemiological situation. This resulted in a major public health success and smallpox eradication has reduced mortality and disfigurement in a dramatic way. In the 1970s and 1980s the UN agencies and the government programs concentrated on specific themes for the improvement of health of children: under-5s clinics, charting growth to pre-empt malnutrition; child survival strategies which included appropriate rehydration for diarrheal disease; immunizations against the common childhood diseases; and the promotion of specific nutrients like vitamin A and iron. The WHO then focused its attention on primary health care 'for all by the year 2000'. This was to provide basic care with a minimum number of essential drugs and appropriate training for community-based health workers which would provide help at a local level in an economic way. In a wide variety of ways, grass-root services which used local personnel and simple methods had shown that it was possible, without great expense and advanced

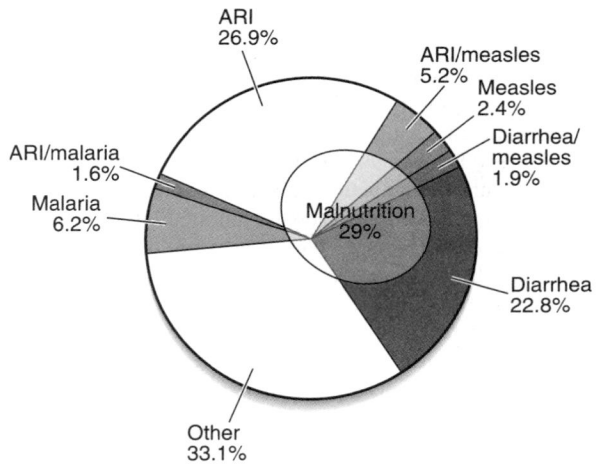

Percentages of deaths associated with:

Acute respiratory infections (ARI)	33.7%
Malnutrition	29.0%
Diarrhea	24.7%
Malaria	7.7%
Measles	9.5%
One or more of these conditions	71.0%

Fig. 35.3 Distribution of deaths among children less than 5 years old in developing countries, 1993 (WHO 1995b). For further information contact: The Director, Division of Diarrhoeal and Acute Respiratory Disease Control, World Health Organization, Avenue Appia, CH-1211 Geneva 27, Switzerland. Tel: +41 22 791 2632; Fax: +41 22 791 4853.

technology, to reduce mortality and morbidity rates (Newall 1975). There was inevitably some loss of focus from the specific disease emphasis of earlier decades.

The latest trend promoted by WHO and the UN agencies is 'integrated management of the sick child' which focuses on prompt and effective treatment (WHO 1995a). There is also a stress on major epidemiological threats from HIV infection and resurgent tuberculosis. In some ways the health emphases have come full circle, from disease-specific programs through special themes and the promotion of primary care back to the major killing diseases (Fig. 35.3). The services caring for children have a double problem. On the one hand they must provide day-to-day help for sick children and provide for groups with special needs. On the other hand they must utilize the funding and accept the emphases which the UN and national health services provide as 'flavor of the month'. The health of children should be more important than development fashions and political posturing.

THE REALITIES AND THE NEEDS IN THE HEALTH CARE SERVICES FOR CHILDREN

PRIMARY HEALTH CARE (PHC) AND ITS IMPLEMENTATION

PHC strategies

PHC has been a strategy for 'health for all' in developing countries which was promoted following the International Conference on Primary Health Care at Alma-Alta in 1978. Providing care for sick children along with interventions to keep them healthy are integral and essential components of PHC. This strategy is implemented through the promotion of community participation in planning, management, monitoring and through

the evaluation of the local health system. There should be integration and management strengthening at all levels of the health system. The term 'selective PHC' specifies interventions against morbidity and mortality from specific diseases implemented within the general health service. Key PHC interventions that have been implemented by governments and international organizations included: the Expanded Program on Immunization against the six key vaccine preventable diseases in children (tuberculosis, diphtheria, pertussis, tetanus, poliomyelitis, measles); the Diarrheal Disease Control Program promoting the correct use of oral rehydration fluids; the Acute Respiratory Infection Program promoting the early recognition of pneumonia in children through interpretation of common clinical signs and the appropriate use of antibiotics; and the Bamako Initiative, a controversial attempt to strengthen primary health care using community financing and participation. WHO and UNICEF are now developing 'integrated management of the sick child'. This focuses on symptomatic identification of illnesses in outpatient settings to ensure more appropriate and, where possible, combined treatment of all the major illnesses and to speed up referral of severely ill children. Health workers are trained in how to communicate key health messages to mothers. The approach gives attention to prevention of childhood disease as well as treatment.

The above concept acknowledges the coexistence of several illnesses in many children; for example those children living in malaria endemic areas may have clinical malaria together with diarrhea and/or pneumonia. Therefore the presence of respiratory or gastrointestinal symptoms does not exclude malaria. The prompt diagnosis and treatment of malaria, without microscopy, is a priority but is difficult because fever alone cannot be presumed to indicate malaria and presenting symptoms and signs vary according to the level of malaria transmission and hence acquired immunity. Therefore 'observation areas' for regular checking of diagnosis are necessary in health facilities in order to review management before outpatient discharge. Malaria microscopy remains the key element in malaria diagnosis.

When mothers arrive at a clinic, giving priority to very sick children is also essential. Introducing 'triage' (French: to sort) into first level health facilities is necessary for efficient screening for very sick children. Assigning children on simple clinical signs and symptoms into urgent or less urgent cases is required and the selection for earlier treatment needs to be explained to the parents.

Another crucial factor is whether health facilities are open for emergencies after normal working hours. Mothers should not be discouraged from bringing sick children outside 'normal' hours. The multipurpose nature of clinics needs emphasis or children with minor illnesses may be refused immunization unnecessarily or, conversely, sick children brought to immunization clinics may be refused treatment and asked to attend at a different time. Missed opportunities for immunization can reach figures as high as 30–40% in some under-5s clinics.

Integrated management of the sick child by health workers who are not doctors, although not a new concept (Morley 1973), is attractive because it addresses major health needs and could be cost effective. The algorithms developed for this program have not yet been fully evaluated in areas with varying endemicity of common childhood diseases. The approach addresses the sick child as a whole and not single diseases. Disease-specific control programs for diarrhea and pneumonia have been comprehensively evaluated and show good efficacy in reducing child mortality,

Table 35.4 Essential drugs for outpatient management of the sick child

- Oral rehydration salts
- Oral first and second line antibiotics
- Oral first and second line antimalarials
- Iron tablets
- Vitamin A capsules
- Paracetamol
- Mebendazole
- Tetracycline eye ointment
- Gentian violet for application to skin and mouth
- Quinine for intramuscular use
- Chloramphenicol for intramuscular use

particularly in research settings. Their implementation on a program basis requires good and regular health staff supervision and active health promotion. The supervisory aspects of these activities are easily neglected greatly reducing their impact and cost-effectiveness.

A minimum level of knowledge, skill and supplies is required to ensure health care of a reasonable quality. This includes availability of a short list of essential drugs for outpatient use. Health workers require a simple timing device for counting the respiratory rate, a liter measure for preparation of oral rehydration salts (ORS), a weight scale and a thermometer. A list of essential drugs for integrated outpatient management of the sick child proposed by WHO/UNICEF is shown in Table 35.4. In community settings simple delivery kits enabling hygienic cutting and tying of the umbilical cord are essential for use by traditional birth attendants in order to reduce the risk of hemorrhage and neonatal tetanus.

Perhaps the most widespread community primary intervention in the 1990s has been the introduction of vitamin A supplementation to mothers postnatally and to children generally over 6 months of age. The vitamin A administered to mothers enhances breast milk vitamin A content. Several large-scale epidemiological studies have demonstrated the benefits of this on mortality reduction, primarily due to reduced severity and complications from measles and severe diarrhea. These vitamin A supplementation programs take various forms and can operate both through the health services and with community involvement. There is some disagreement on this approach in terms of its sustainability. In the longer term more attention has to be given to improving the vitamin A intake from the general diet.

Problems facing PHC and the health services

As with the Expanded Program on Immunization these activities are often heavily donor supported and their sustainability is dependent on this. Competition between various initiatives is also dependent on resource allocations internally. There are difficult issues facing PHC, and the 1980s saw severe problems in financing these health initiatives, particularly in sub-Saharan Africa. If South Africa is excluded, external aid accounts for almost 20% of the total health expenditure in Africa compared to 0.6% in China and 1.6% in India. The demand for health services has also increased due to population growth, successful social mobilization and the AIDS pandemic with TB and other associated infections. In some countries this has led to an inadequate availability of medicines, equipment and a failure to pay health worker salaries. Two responses to this situation were firstly the Bamako Initiative and secondly Health Sector Reform. The objectives of the Bamako Initiative outlined by WHO related to universal accessibility to PHC. This would be attained through decentralization of health decision making to the district level, community level management of PHC, user-financing under community control, a realistic national drug policy and provision of essential drugs, leading to a self-sustaining PHC with emphasis on promoting the health of women and children. Initially the emphasis has been related to implementing user changes for essential drugs through a community-managed drug fund. This strategy has been subject to considerable criticism; nevertheless in five African countries the evidence suggests that most people manage to find the money needed to pay for health services through various community support mechanisms. It highlights the plight of those who cannot pay in time for children needing treatment for more acute illnesses (McPake et al 1993).

Although communities can provide to some extent for themselves they still require access to health services and these services should provide what people want. People do not accept poor quality services just because they are there and this leads to underutilization. Health Sector Reform has emerged as a priority for refining policies and reforming structures through which health improvements are implemented in developing countries. The main components emphasize decentralization in order to promote efficiency and public accountability. Governments of developing countries have to ensure that the appropriate share of public resources is allocated to health in a way that satisfies users who should also exercise some control over them. These initiatives have to be achieved in countries where per capita expenditure on health is about 2% of that in established market economies. In absolute terms, 36 countries, mostly in Africa, were each spending less than $20 per capita in 1990 (Cassels 1995). Can this be achieved in a health sector where staff are unmotivated and sometimes poorly trained, where patients face long clinic times at inconvenient hours and there are frequently inadequate supplies and drugs? In the private sector financial exploitation may occur with no safeguards against unnecessary or even dangerous treatments. Hospital management in most less-developed countries is a relatively neglected area, partly as a consequence of the international focus on PHC. Social, economic, demographic and epidemiological data are needed to guide reform procedures, although this alone cannot necessarily move governments into action.

Reform is likely to depend not only on the government services but also on other groups, such as nongovernmental organizations, user groups, university and research institutions, community organizations and private sector providers. International interest should take the form of a broader political approach to health services reform and policy, including support for such groups. In a recent realistic but pessimistic review Bergstrom & Mocumbi (1996) concluded: 'health for all is a distant dream, and, without concrete and credible actions to alleviate the pathology of poverty, we must expect it to remain a dream for many generations to come'.

SPECIAL SERVICES

Perinatal care

A high proportion of babies die in their first month of life, many in the first week. Perinatal and neonatal deaths are not always

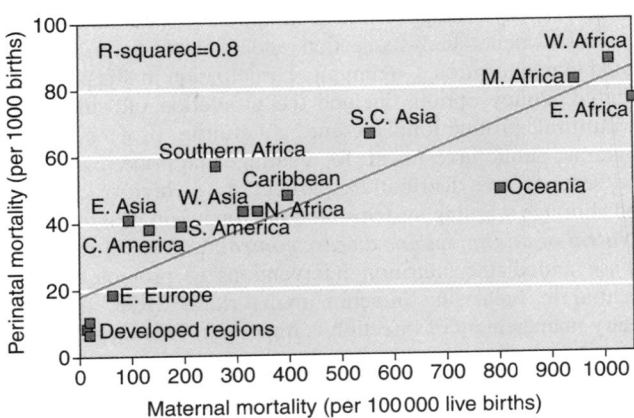

Fig. 35.4 Maternal and perinatal mortality by region (WHO 1996b).

Table 35.5 10 steps for successful breast-feeding

1. Have a written breast-feeding policy that is routinely communicated to all health care staff
2. Train all health care staff in skills necessary to implement this policy
3. Inform all pregnant women about the benefits and management of breast-feeding
4. Help mothers initiate breast-feeding within an hour of birth
5. Show mothers how to breast-feed, and how to maintain lactation even if they are separated from their infants
6. Give newborn infants no food or drink other than breast milk, unless medically indicated
7. Practice rooming-in – allow mothers and infants to remain together 24 hours a day
8. Encourage breast-feeding on demand
9. Give no artificial teats or pacifiers (also called dummies or soothers) to breast-feeding infants
10. Foster the establishment of breast-feeding support groups and refer mothers to them on discharge from the hospital or clinic

recognized as a real problem in many countries for cultural reasons and because they are so common. For this reason in some societies the baby is not given a name until it has survived a certain period. Some of the factors that lead to perinatal and neonatal death result from inadequate care of mothers and babies. In a typical sub-Saharan setting, about 1 out of every 20 families will be motherless because of pregnancy-related deaths. If each mother who dies has had on average, three or four children, 1 child in 6 will be in a motherless family. These are often orphans of poor perinatal care. In developing countries where 98% of perinatal deaths take place, the perinatal mortality rate is estimated to exceed 55 per 1000 live births, five time higher than in developed countries.

Most mortality and morbidity in the perinatal and neonatal periods is preventable. The causes are often classified as maternal, obstetric and fetal. They include factors such as poor maternal health and poor care during pregnancy, inappropriate management of maternal complications and delivery and lack of appropriate care for the newborn, especially the resuscitation of mildly asphyxiated babies. The significance of these factors will vary from place to place. A valuable summary of available information on perinatal mortality has been compiled by the Maternal Health and Safe Motherhood Programme of WHO (WHO, 1996b). Maternal and perinatal mortality rates by region (around 1995) are shown in Figure 35.4.

Lower perinatal mortality will result from interventions addressing the needs of the newborn – resuscitation when necessary (adequate provision of bag and masks), immediate breast-feeding (for example ensuring implementation of the baby-friendly initiative of UNICEF) (Table 35.5), warm, clean and hygienic delivery conditions and cord care, and early detection (or prevention) of perinatal infections or neonatal diseases. The prevention and management of anemia and control of malaria in pregnancy will reduce the low birthweight risk and improve survival. The mother–baby package (WHO 1994) introduced by WHO's Maternal Health and Safe Motherhood Programme in 1995 comprises a cluster of cost-effective interventions. The emphasis is on the birth attendant who can ensure carefully monitored deliveries and life-saving interventions, should complications occur. The mother–baby package offers a minimum list of essential interventions (Table 35.6). Low cost technologies for the newborn are especially important in developing countries.

One of the cheapest appropriate technologies for low birthweight newborn babies is close skin-to-skin contact with the mother. This is one of the ideas behind the kangaroo method which has been shown to be effective in reducing neonatal mortality. Research should be supported to evaluate these methods (Acolet & Harvey 1993).

Services for the disabled

Children in developing countries are more likely to suffer from one of the preventable causes of disability, like paralytic poliomyelitis, and are least likely to receive help and understanding. Disability is closely associated with poverty. Estimates of prevalence vary greatly because of varying definitions. WHO and UNICEF estimates are between 5 and 10%. The organization of services for these children depends on both community-based and institutional approaches to rehabilitation. Institutional approaches have the disadvantage that they are expensive, 'patient orientated', urban, can be difficult to integrate

Table 35.6 Mother–baby package: essential interventions

- Family planning to reduce incidence of unwanted and mistimed pregnancies
- Basic maternal care to all women
- Protection and support for early and exclusive breast-feeding
- Reduce anemia in pregnant women
- Reduce sexually transmitted diseases in pregnant women
- Reduce maternal deaths due to complications of abortions
- Reduce maternal deaths due to hemorrhage
- Reduce maternal deaths due to prolonged/obstructed labor
- Reduce maternal deaths due to puerperal sepsis
- Eliminate neonatal tetanus
- Reduce neonatal deaths due to birth asphyxia
- Reduce neonatal deaths associated with neonatal hypothermia
- Reduce ophthalmia neonatorum

into other activities and are usually run by well-trained professionals. Community-based rehabilitation (CBR) refers more to therapeutic measures applied by families to the disabled in their own homes. The focus is on the child in the community and the role of the professional is supportive. Local technologies and self-help become more important. Through this approach help can be given to many more children of all ages. The movement towards CBR has increased throughout the 1980s and important lessons have been learnt. These are reviewed in a recent report from the Netherlands (Schulpen & de Waal 1993). Regular newsletters (CBR News) are also published by the Appropriate Health Resource and Technologies Action Group (AHRTAG).

Nutrition

The Food Security Conference in Rome in 1974 declared that 'no child in the world will go to bed hungry by the year 2000'. There is a shortage of time and resolve to fulfill that hope. In the Convention on the Rights of the Child, two articles address the issue of nutrition. Article 24 says that 'Parties ... shall take appropriate measures to ... combat disease and malnutrition' through provision of adequate nutritious foods. Article 27 says that parties 'shall in case of need provide material assistance and support programmes, particularly with regard to nutrition, clothing and housing'.

Local, national, international and nongovernmental organizations have been working on the problem of malnutrition in many different ways for decades. There have been some changes in the profile of nutrition-related diseases during this time in several developing countries. In sub-Saharan Africa severe food shortages and, in places, near famine exists; while in Southeast Asia severe protein–energy malnutrition (PEM) has declined. Florid acute micronutrient deficiencies such as pellagra and keratomalacia have also declined, whereas chronic micronutrient deficiencies have become the major nutritional problems. These are iron and folate deficiency, goiter and other iodine deficiency disorders and the less severe forms of vitamin A deficiency. The possibility that zinc deficiency could have a bearing on PEM, vitamin A deficiency and anemia should be seriously considered. Zinc is a component of key enzymes and is involved in protein synthesis; its deficiency could therefore aggravate PEM.

Nutrition interventions to address these problems have been grouped into the following categories: household food security, nutrition and infectious disease control; caring capacity; controlling micronutrient deficiencies; and therapeutic nutrition through rehabilitation (United Nations Subcommittee on Nutrition 1991). These relate to the immediate causes at an individual level which are inadequate food intake and infectious disease incidence. Interventions normally require a judicious mix of policies with the priority given to a particular category varying from country to country.

Food security. The government should have state- and district-level assessment, analysis, action and evaluation of activities related to malnutrition. Community participation in this process is essential. Policy options include the promotion of: small-scale agricultural production; income generating projects; credit programs; public investment; food storage and price regulations; food security and distribution, particularly to high-risk groups; food shortage warning systems; and micronutrient programs.

Nutrition and infectious disease control. Control of infectious disease and dietary/nutrition interventions to promote this are essential to break the infection–malnutrition cycle. Improved dietary management of infection is important. This includes:

- continuation of breast-feeding (Table 35.6)
- maintenance of diet during infection, especially in persistent diarrhea
- administration of vitamin A in the management of measles and severe diarrhea
- the use of ORS in diarrhea
- dietary support in chronic infections
- use of low dose oral iron in anemia even if associated with malaria parasitemia
- treatment of intestinal parasites.

The dietary prevention of infection includes promoting exclusive breast-feeding for 4–6 months, and continued breast-feeding into the second year of life. Satisfactory weaning foods and supplemental vitamin A are valuable. Prevention of low birthweight by improving older girls' and women's nutritional status during pregnancy and lactation is a priority.

Caring capacity. Women's education and literacy affects almost all aspects of their caring capacity. In this context it determines much of their ability to cope with interventions. Investments in literacy, particularly of the girl child, could have large long-term benefits because of her future reproduction and caring role (Kurz et al 1994, Sandiford et al 1995).

Controlling micronutrient deficiencies. This can be achieved through supplementation programs with iodine, iron and vitamin A.

Therapeutic nutrition. Nutritional rehabilitation of individual undernourished children has a conventional sequence consisting of the resuscitation phase, first refeeding phase, rehabilitation itself and then preparation for returning home. The interventions in these phases are well described (Pelletier 1993). Nutritional rehabilitation is considered satisfactory when the child reaches 100% of reference weight for height. The child must be closely monitored throughout this 6- to 8-week period. This may not imply a lengthy stay in hospital as rehabilitation may continue in an appropriate center or preferably at home.

In summary, malnutrition is an extremely complex condition. A comprehensive understanding of its ecology is necessary to plan long-term solutions. The central role of women in interventions has been well demonstrated. There is no single way to eradicate malnutrition, but there are workable, sustainable strategies in which health workers and communities can cooperate.

REFERENCES

Acolet D, Harvey D 1993 Low cost technology for the newborn in developing countries. Archives of Disease in Childhood 69: 477–478

Bergstrom S, Mocumbi P 1996 Health for all by the year 2000? British Medical Journal 313: 316

Caldwell J C 1979 Education as a factor in mortality decline: an examination of Nigerian data. Population Study 33: 395–413

Caldwell J C 1986 Routes to low mortality in poor countries. Population and Development Review 12(2): 171–220

Cassels A 1995 Health sector reforms. Key issues in less developed countries. Journal of International Development 7: 329–347

Chaudhuri S 1994 Survival of street children in Calcutta. Child, Newsletter of the International Child Health Group, British Paediatric Association, November

Cleland J, Van Ginneken J K 1988 Maternal education and child survival in developing countries: the search for pathways of influence. Social Science and Medicine 27: 1357–1368

Community Based Rehabilitation News (CBR News) International newsletter on community based rehabilitation and the concerns of disabled people. AHRTAG, London

Costello A, Watson F, Woodward D 1994 Human face or human facade. Adjustment and the health of mothers and children. Centre for International Child Health, Institute of Child Health, London.

Ennew J 1994 Defining the girl child: sexuality, control and development. VENA Journal 6: 51–56

Fyfe A 1989 Child labour. Polity Press, Cambridge

Grant J P 1992 Children's needs climb towards top of world agenda. Forum for Applied Research and Public Policy 7(Spring): 66–72

Her Majesty's Stationery Office (HMSO) 1991 The UN Convention on the Rights of the Child. HMSO, London

Kurz K M, Peplinsky N L, Johnson-Welds C J 1994 Investigating the future: six principles for promoting the nutritional status of adolescent girls in developing countries. International Centre for Research on Women, Washington, DC

McPake B, Hanson K, Mills A 1993 Community financing of health care in Africa: an evaluation of the Bamako initiative. Social Science and Medicine 36: 1383–1395

Morley D C 1973 Paediatric priorities in the developing world. Butterworths, London

Newell K W 1975 Health by the people. WHO, Geneva

Paul D 1995 Street survival: children work and urban drift in Cambodia. World Vision Policy and Research Department, UK

Pelletier J G 1993 Severe malnutrition: a global approach. Children in the Tropics. International Children's Centre, Paris.

Rosen J E, Conly S R 1996 Pakistan's population programme: the challenge ahead. Population Action International, Washington, DC

Sandiford P, Cassel J, Montengro M, Sanchez G 1995 Impact of women's literacy on child health and its interaction with access to health services. Population Studies 49: 5–17

Satyanarayan K, Prasanna K T, Rao N B S 1986 Effect of early childhood undernutrition and child labour on growth and adult nutritional status of rural Indian boys around Hyderabad. Human Nutrition: Clinical Nutrition 400: 131–139

Save the Children Fund 1996 Poor in health. Save the Children Fund, London

Schulpen T W J, de Waal F C 1993 Crippling disorders in children, a global problem. Tropical and Geographical Medicine 45: 196–268

Stapleton M C 1989 Diarrhoeal diseases: perceptions and practices in Nepal. Social Science and Medicine 28: 593–604

Tsitoura S 1995 Child abuse and neglect. In: Lindstrom B, Spencer N (eds) Social paediatrics. Oxford University Press, Oxford, pp 310–330

UNICEF 1996 The state of the world's children. Oxford University Press, Oxford

United Nations Subcommittee on Nutrition 1991 Some options for improving nutrition in the 1990s. Supplement to SCN News No. 7. WHO, Geneva

Williams D 1996 Is the World Bank changing? In: Towards peace and justice. Discussion Paper, No. 3. World Vision, UK

World Health Organization 1994 Mother–baby package. Implementing safe motherhood in developing countries. (WHO/FHE/MSM/94.11) WHO, Geneva

World Health Organization 1995a Integrated management of the sick child. Bulletin of the World Health Organization 73(6): 735–740

World Health Organization 1995b The world health report 1995. Bridging the gaps. WHO, Geneva

World Health Organization 1996a The world health report 1996. WHO, Geneva

World Health Organization 1996b Perinatal mortality, a listing of available information. Maternal Health and Safe Motherhood Programme, Family and Reproductive Health. WHO, Geneva

World Vision 1996 The commercial sexual exploitation. World Vision Policy and Research Department, UK

Wright J D, Kaminsky D, Wittig M 1993 Health and social conditions of street children in Honduras. American Journal of Diseases of Children 147: 279–283

36 Practical aspects of diagnostic imaging

G. M. A. Hendry   A. G. Wilkinson

Introduction   1894
General discussion   1894
Equipment and imaging modalities   1894
Conventional X-rays   1895
Ultrasound   1896
Computerized tomography scanning   1896
Nuclear medicine   1897
Single photon emission tomography   1897
Positron emission tomography   1897
Magnetic resonance imaging   1898
Interventional procedures   1898

Body systems   1899
Respiratory system   1899
Alimentary tract   1901
Liver and biliary tract   1906
Pancreas and spleen   1907
Central nervous system   1907
Urinary tract   1909
Retroperitoneal abnormalities   1912
Genital system   1913
Skeletal system   1914
References   1919

INTRODUCTION

Imaging of the pediatric patient will be influenced by the availability of equipment and expertise.

Imaging has been revolutionized in recent years with the introduction of ultrasound (US), computerized tomography (CT), radioisotope scanning (RIS) and magnetic resonance imaging (MRI). However, the conventional techniques of plain X-rays and contrast studies are still of importance and, together with US, constitute the majority of investigations. The initial section of this chapter provides an insight into the various techniques available and the later sections discuss their applications to the various body systems.

GENERAL DISCUSSION

The child should be examined in a pleasant friendly environment. The X-ray rooms and waiting areas can be decorated with posters, paintings and a supply of friendly 'animals' and toys made available. In older children any procedure should be explained in understandable terms which often gains cooperation. Parents are encouraged to be present in the room to comfort their child. Sedation is very rarely necessary for conventional imaging techniques.

Trained personnel, be they radiologists, radiographers, nurses or anesthetists, are essential for a complete and successful pediatric imaging unit. In a general hospital at least two radiographers and one radiologist should be trained and have responsibility for the investigation and interpretation of pediatric problems.

Strict radiation protection is the rule in pediatric departments to avoid radiation damage to sensitive immature and developing structures and to avoid cumulative damage to the chromosomes of future generations. Radiation dose can be reduced by the correct choice of exposure factors, the use of rare earth screen and film combinations and carbon fiber backed X-ray cassettes and table tops which more easily transmit X-ray photons and hence lead to a reduction in exposure dose (Table 36.1). Variations in technique can result in up to 70-fold differences in entrance surface dose measurements for a given examination in the same size of child (Schneider et al 1995). Accurate coning of the X-ray beam to the area of the body to be examined, lead shielding of the gonads and avoidance of film retakes are important. These factors obviously require the presence of an experienced pediatric radiographer.

A close liaison between the clinician and radiologist will lead to the correct examination for the clinical problem, thus avoiding unnecessary and repeat investigations. Investigations should also begin with the least invasive procedure and proceed along recognized flow channels. (Royal College of Radiologists 1995).

EQUIPMENT AND IMAGING MODALITIES

Any hospital concerned with the investigation of children must have conventional X-rays and real-time US available (World Health Organization 1987a). It is preferable to have easy access to CT, nuclear medicine and MRI. In tertiary referral centers positron emission tomography (PET) and single photon emission computerized tomography (SPECT) are further specialist nuclear medicine investigations.

A department's standard X-ray generator should be of high performance allowing rapid exposure times of 1–2 ms (World Health Organization 1987a). This will reduce movement blur. Recording of the image by photographing the intensifier screen – indirect radiography – during screening will reduce the radiation dose by one-third to one-quarter.

Table 36.1 Estimates of radiation doses in children from various imaging methods

(a) Total dose in X-ray examination

Area of investigation	EDE (mSv) (total dose)	Absorbed skin doses (mSv)
Lumbar spine (anteroposterior + lateral)	2.7	5
Chest (anteriopositerior)	0.02	0.5
Skull (3 views)	0.15	7
Abdomen (anteroposterior)	1.8	1
Thoracic spine (anteroposterior + lateral)	0.9	9
Pelvis	1.6	1.5
Intravenous urogram	4.1	5
Barium meal	4.3	7
Barium enema	9.3	10
CT scans		
Chest	6	18
Abdomen	5	16
Head	7	26
Neonatal head	12	38

(b) Relative dose in isotope imaging

Isotope	EDE (mSv/MBq)	Administered dose (MBq) 1–12 years	Clinical indication
99mTc pertechnetate	0.0110	10–50	Meckel's diverticulum, duplication cyst, gastroesophageal reflux, thyroid imaging
99mTc MAG3	0.0063	5–10	Renography
99mTc DMSA	0.0160	25–40	Functioning renal mass
Disofenin	0.0200	6–60	Biliary imaging
99mTc diphosphonate	0.0060	60–300	Bone and soft tissue imaging
Gallium 67 citrate	0.3200	10–40	Infection, neoplasms
Indium 111-labelled white cells	0.6500	20–30	Abscess, infection
Xenon 133	0.00069	100–300	Pulmonary ventilation scanning

EDE = effective dose equivalent
MAG 3 = marcaploacetyl triglycerine

Digital imaging is the application of computers to radiography and allows a more flexible tissue analysis after a single exposure, eliminating retakes due to poor choice of exposure factors. Injection of contrast enhances vascular structures and increases the contrast differentiation between body tissues.

Careful positioning of the child for a radiological investigation is important. Immobilization may be necessary. The parent or helper in the department often will suffice by holding the child; bucky bands and foam pads may, however, be necessary. Pediatric screening units should have specialized cradles in which to secure the child. Radiographic views in different positions are thus possible without struggling, preventing excessive radiation exposure.

CONVENTIONAL X-RAYS

X-rays are high frequency electromagnetic waves. An image is produced by light exposure of the photographic film by fluorescent screens excited by the X-ray beam as it emerges from the patient. Plain films are almost universally used as the only or primary modality for investigation of suspected bony injury, pneumonia, mediastinal and lung masses and bowel obstruction or perforation. Healing of fractures is monitored by serial X-rays to confirm adequate union in a satisfactory position. Replacement of conventional 'hard copy' films with electronic images (digital radiographs) has been predicted for some years, but this technology is expensive and is confined to a few pilot sites at present. Fluoroscopy is a dynamic X-ray image produced when the emergent X-ray beam is directed onto a photomultiplier tube. The image can then be observed on a television monitor. The information from fluoroscopy can be digitized and the resultant data stored on hard disk with selected images transferred to hard

copy film. Barium meals, enemas, cystograms and interventional procedures are performed under fluoroscopic control.

The image on the X-ray film depends on the contrast produced by differential absorption of X-rays in different body tissues. Air, fat, bone and soft tissues are the natural contrasts. The contrast differences can be enhanced by giving artificial media, such as barium or iodine, as a water-soluble contrast. In pediatric practice nonionic water-soluble contrasts are now routinely used for intravenous, intra-arterial and intrathecal examinations.

The benefits of nonionic contrast are the low osmolality and diminished toxicity (Grainger 1984). Unfortunately nonionic contrasts are 4–5 times the cost of the previously used ionic media.

Flavored nonionic contrast media are used in the examination of swallowing mechanisms in suspected aspiration, tracheoesophageal fistula and in the diagnosis of bowel obstruction in the neonate. The contrast, being of low osmolality, is not diluted during passage through the gut. Traditionally sodium acetrizoate (Gastrografin), a hypertonic water-soluble contrast, has been used as a contrast medium in the diagnosis and treatment of meconium ileus, meconium plug syndrome and meconium ileus equivalent. As this contrast has 10 times the osmolality of plasma, it causes osmotic effects and dehydration, particularly in small children. Adequate fluid balance must therefore be maintained during the use of the contrast. This may require intravenous fluids. Nonionic water-soluble contrast only 2–3 times the osmolality of plasma has been shown to be equally effective in treatment of these conditions.

Barium sulfate is an inert, dense, safe contrast medium. It is exclusively used for gastrointestinal studies in selected densities. The contrast may be produced in liquid or powder form. Added flavoring is essential as children may be reluctant to drink the contrast.

Double contrast barium studies combine the use of high-density barium and air. The latter may be swallowed in sufficient volume by an apprehensive child but can be supplemented by bicarbonate contained in the barium suspension or by giving additional bicarbonate powders or tablets. These procedures provide an excellent thin barium coating of the gut mucosa enabling superficial ulcerations or polyps to be detected. Low-density barium mixtures are suitable for examination of the small bowel. The small bowel enema is a procedure where the contrast is injected directly through a nasojejunal tube followed by saline or methyl cellulose. This procedure may give more accurate assessment of mucosal detail.

ULTRASOUND

This noninvasive and inexpensive modality has revolutionized the imaging of pediatric diseases. A transducer produces high frequency sound waves of between 3.5 and 10 MHz which penetrate the tissues and are reflected from different tissue interfaces back to the transducer. Differing intensities of signal from varying interfaces in the tissue are then converted into a digital format, allowing a sectional image of the organ structure to be formed.

Several types of transducer are available. The sector scanner with a small head is useful when examining the brain through a small anterior fontanel or for an intercostal or subcostal approach to the chest and upper abdomen. Linear and curved linear array transducers have multiple crystals and are electronically controlled. In the former, the image produced is rectangular with excellent near-field detail which is useful for the examination of superficial structures. No known deleterious effects have been recorded in vivo (Wells 1987). Children rarely need sedation and feeding the baby before or while scanning leads to a quiet examination. Good transducer–skin contact using a coupling jelly is important. Reflection of ultrasound by gas can cause problems in the abdomen and chest and the lack of information behind bone makes it of limited value in intracranial investigation beyond infancy.

Real-time ultrasound is continuous sampling of the organs examined with a frame rate of 10–40 per second. Patient movement becomes therefore less significant. Ultrasound is a sectional technique and a mental image of the organ examined is formed during the procedure. Spot films can be made of any section.

Successful ultrasound is operator dependent and thus should only be performed by specialist trained sonographers.

Doppler ultrasound

Doppler ultrasound is a technique for assessing blood flow by measuring the frequency changes of sound reflected from flowing red blood cells. The information is presented as a spectrum of frequency versus time and, if the appropriate angle correction is made, velocity versus time. Duplex Doppler ultrasound refers to a simultaneous display of a two-dimensional ultrasound image together with the pulsed Doppler data. The Doppler signal can be sampled from any area of the cross-sectional image and this is facilitated if color Doppler is also available.

The main indications for Doppler ultrasound are:

1. the diagnosis of congenital heart disease (see section on cardiology, p. 592);
2. to demonstrate arterial and venous flow to confirm vessel patency;
3. to investigate hemodynamic disturbances in aneurysms and stenoses;
4. to detect physiological and pathological changes indicated by quantitative Doppler shifts;
5. to measure absolute blood flow (Winkler & Helmke 1989).

The parameters commonly used in quantifying Doppler changes are the pulsatility or the resistive index, peak systolic velocity, diastolic velocity and mean flow velocity.

For example, in examination of the brain decreased diastolic flow can be demonstrated in conditions such as hydrocephalus or cerebral edema where raised intracranial pressure is present. This is manifest by an increase in the resistance index or pulsatility index (Goh et al 1992).

Higher frequency shifts in systole indicating an increase in systolic velocity are noted at the site of arterial stenosis and this technique is useful in the investigation of renal and aortic vascular abnormalities in systemic hypertension and in demonstrating vascular thrombosis and stenosis following renal and hepatic transplantation.

It must always be remembered that associated physiological changes such as circulatory collapse and persistent ductus arteriosus can affect the Doppler spectrum and cause spurious abnormalities in the abovementioned parameters (Winkler & Helmke 1989).

Color Doppler

Color Doppler images both frequency shift and phase information. This allows red blood cell movement to be color encoded with hue dependent on the speed and direction of movement with respect to the transducer. Color imaging highlights blood flow against the gray background of the 2D image and has revolutionized the echocardiographic diagnosis of congenital heart disease, allowing small shunts to be detected accurately.

Power Doppler

A recent development in Doppler ultrasound is the so-called power Doppler. This technique measures the density rather than the velocity of the red blood cells in the sample area.

The amplitude of the signal is governed by the amount of blood within the sample volume. Large amplitude signals are portrayed as a bright hue and weak signals as a dim color on the monitor.

The technique is independent of the angle of insonation and the flow velocity of the red blood cells. The technique is also called ultrasound angiography as it gives a detailed road map of blood flow in an organ. The technique is three times more sensitive than conventional Doppler and shows smaller blood vessels at deeper depths. It also provides better edge enhancement of blood vessels. The disadvantage is the inability to provide functional information such as direction of flow (Babcock et al 1996) and flow velocity measurements.

Contrast agents are now being developed for ultrasound. These require the injection of microbubbles of air into the circulation which cause echo enhancement in blood vessels.

COMPUTERIZED TOMOGRAPHY SCANNING (CT)

In this technique an X-ray fan beam rotates around the body placed in the central aperture of the scanner and detectors record the emergent beam from every angle. The information from multiple interactions of the X-rays with the tissues is computerized and presented as a 2D image of a slice through the body. Conventional scanners perform one slice at a time with each slice taking 2 or 3 seconds. Modern scanners operate in a spiral fashion and can complete a scan of the abdomen or chest within half a minute, allowing this to be completed within a single breath hold and enabling much more efficient use of a rapid bolus of i.v. contrast. The section thickness can be collimated between 1 and 10 mm and sections may be contiguous or spaced (depending on the pitch of the spiral scanner). Thin sections allow more detailed imaging with high resolution (at the expense of a poorer signal-to-noise ratio) (White 1996). This fine section tomography is useful in the chest to assess bronchiectasis and interstitial lung disease or in the assessment of the petrous bone in suspected abnormalities of the middle and inner ears (Kuhn 1993).

Software packages can allow volume measurement (e.g. size of abdominal tumors) and 3D reconstructions are particularly useful for craniofacial abnormalities. The data can be reformatted in any plane.

The radiation dose can be reduced by tailoring the examination to the clinical problem. Technical advances with improving sensitivity of the detectors and a specific policy to reduce the kV and mA in children also contribute to a reduction in dose (Ambrosino et al 1994, Naidich 1994). Radiation doses are determined in relation to skin dose, bone marrow dose and gonadal dose.

CT scanners with fast scan times of between 1 and 2 seconds are of value in children, to minimize artifact due to child movement and gut motility. Rapid reconstruction of the image also shortens the examination. Children are not ideal subjects for CT as fat (the natural contrast to define certain organs) is lacking. Preparation of the child for the procedure is important. An explanation to the child and parents often overcomes anxiety and the presence of trained pediatric staff in the unit is a necessity. Triclofos in a dose of 80–100 mg/kg up to a maximum of 2 g is usually a satisfactory sedative in the under- 2-year-olds. Diazepam 0.2 mg/kg intravenously is appropriate for older children. In many centers general anesthesia is felt to be safer than sedation (Hubbard et al 1992). During sedation or anesthesia the child must be adequately monitored with oxygen saturation, blood pressure and respiration continuously recorded. A person trained in pediatric resuscitation should be available. The child should be fasted for 5 hours before sedation or general anesthesia (American Academy of Pediatrics 1988).

Contrast will allow differentiation of structures in the section. The gut is opacified with a 2–5% diluted solution of a nonionic contrast (300 mg/ml) in a dose of 100–500 ml, depending on the age of the child. Three-quarters of the dose is given 1 hour before the procedure, the remaining volume 15 minutes before. In pelvic examinations the rectum is opacified with a similar dilute contrast.

Intravenous nonionic water-soluble contrast will enhance vascular structures and visualize the renal tract. Rapid injection and immediate CT examination is termed dynamic scanning and provides additional information about vascular structures.

The indications for CT are numerous, including the assessment of retroperitoneal, pelvic, mediastinal, pleural, pulmonary and bony abnormalities (White 1996). CT is particularly useful in the investigation of head injuries, space-occupying lesions of the brain and imaging of the chest and abdomen in acute trauma

(Ruess et al 1995). However, MRI is increasingly being used as the primary imaging modality for the central nervous system. Orthopedic applications include the investigation of congenital abnormalities of the feet, Perthes disease of the hips, bone and soft tissue masses. With specialized software, assessment of the mineral content of bone is possible.

NUCLEAR MEDICINE

Nuclear medicine studies involve the administration, usually intravenous, of a radionuclide bound to a carrier molecule which is organ specific. The radionuclide emits radiation usually in the form of gamma rays and the technique can be used for both diagnostic and therapeutic purposes.

The most commonly used radionuclide is technetium 99m which has a physical half-life of 6 hours and emits gamma energy of 140keV. Iodine 123 (half-life 13 hours), iodine 131 (half-life 8.04 days), xenon 133 (half-life 5.3 days) and krypton 81m (half-life 13 seconds) are occasionally used. The child receives a weight/surface area-related dose of the radionuclide and the radiation dose from this technique is frequently less than that received from equivalent X-rays.

Recently specific monoclonal antibodies, e.g. UJ13A, 3F8, or metaiodobenzylguanidine (MIBG) have been labeled with large doses of [131]I (beta particle emitter) and used in the treatment of neuroblastoma. The use of radionuclides for therapeutic purposes is a potential growth area. Unlike other imaging modalities which provide anatomical images, radionuclide studies provide functional information and are of value in the diagnosis of renal disease, gastrointestinal disorders, lung disease, skeletal abnormalities and in tumor staging (Gordon 1993).

SINGLE PHOTON EMISSION TOMOGRAPHY (SPECT)

This is an allied technique which involves the use of the gamma camera rotating around the body during the examination, collecting data from multiple angles. Computer manipulation of this data produces a series of axial images allowing greater sensitivity in detecting smaller differences in activity and also more precise localization of abnormalities. This has multiple applications including more accurate detection of renal scars (^{99m}Tc DMSA), localizing a seizure focus in epileptic patients (^{99m}Tc HMPAO) and spinal abnormalities in patient with low back ache (^{99m}Tc MDP).

POSITRON EMISSION TOMOGRAPHY (PET)

This technique involves the use of a positron emitting radionuclide which is produced in a cyclotron. Positron emitters in use are carbon 11, fluorine 18, nitrogen 13 and oxygen 15. The compound is taken up in the body tissues following intravenous administration and is of particular value in studies of brain physiology where the regional chemistry of the compound at molecular level is portrayed in the scan. (Lancet 1989, Nunan et al 1995). Fluorodeoxyglucose (FDG) is proving of value in the staging of children with neuroblastoma and Ewing's sarcoma. The technique is extremely expensive and is dependent on the presence of a cyclotron. To date there are only five such facilities available in the United Kingdom and the technique must be regarded as a research tool.

MAGNETIC RESONANCE IMAGING (MRI)

This technique has imaging capabilities which are ideally suited to pediatrics and should become an essential feature of all pediatric centers. It depends on the ability of the nucleus of an atom to resonate under certain conditions in the presence of a magnetic field. The child is placed within a strong magnetic field and then exposed to a specific radiofrequency (RF) by means of a coil which fits the body part to be examined. This causes the nuclei in the subject to resonate about their equilibrium. When the RF pulse is terminated the nuclei continue to resonate with emission of RF detected as the MR signal, before returning to their original equilibrium position. The resonant frequency is proportional to the magnetic field strength.

The signal originates in protons within the body (largely from free water in the tissues). Differing RF pulse sequences and repetition times can be used to produce resonance from which an image can be constructed. Maximum contrast between tissues can be achieved by the correct choice of these variables.

Several different types of magnet are available. The low field strength magnets operate at 0.18–0.23 Tesla and usually have an open configuration rather than a tunnel so are less claustrophobic for children and are also quiet. The low field strength, however, results in a lower signal-to-noise ratio and hence reduced resolution and longer acquisition time for the image. Sequences have been developed to counteract these problems.

Mid-range magnets and high field strength magnets have magnetic field strengths of 0.3–0.5 and 1–2 Tesla. These systems are supercooled with helium, are more expensive and are noisier during data acquisition and require more shielding for the magnetic field. The systems are nearly all of tunnel configuration with corresponding problems of claustrophobia and access, particularly during anesthesia. The advantages of the high field strength systems are the ability to acquire the image data in a shorter time with generally better resolution from an improved signal-to-noise ratio. Spectroscopy and functional brain studies are possible with magnetic field strengths of 1.5 Tesla and above.

The time for acquisition of the data during the examination depends on the sequence chosen. This may vary from 1 to 9 minutes and usually three or more acquisitions are required to complete the examination. Modern echoplanar imaging (EPI) techniques will dramatically reduce the examination times (800 msec/slice) making the modality more suitable for restless children and enabling dynamic studies to be carried out. Other sequences include turbo spin, fat suppression techniques and MR angiography. At the present time, MRI is considered the examination of choice for central nervous system, intraspinal and musculoskeletal anatomy and pathology. Blood vessels, the heart and intraspinal contents can be well visualized without the need for administration of contrast medium. There is no artifact from adjacent bone and with brain and spinal cord accurate assessment of normal and abnormal myelination (Staudt et al 1994), intracranial hemorrhage and infarction, anoxic encephalopathy and the assessment of periventricular edema (Floodmark et al 1989, Byrd et al 1989a, b) is possible.

MRI also enables imaging of the heart and vascular system. In conventional spin echo images, flowing blood appears as a signal void which helps differentiate vessels from lymph nodes. Gradient echo images can be used to produce a high signal from flowing blood, allowing magnetic resonance angiography. With cardiac gating cine loop images of the heart can be obtained to give detailed information on cardiac function and congenital abnormalities such as coarctation of the aorta and intracardiac defects. Volume acquisition techniques allow the blood vessels in a given volume to be examined in any plane. Postprocessing using the maximum intensity projection technique (MIP) allows 3D reconstruction of vessels which can be rotated to permit visualization from any angle. Standard spin echo T1 images in coronal, sagittal and axial planes will outline vascular rings, including the double aortic arch and aberrant innominate artery. The relationship of the vessel with the trachea is clearly identified.

In the lung, metastases are less well demonstrated than with CT. In cystic fibrosis, mucus plugs produce a bright signal, as do areas of inflammation. It is not possible, however, to obtain the same parenchymal detail as achieved with high resolution CT.

MRI is a useful technique for imaging abdominal masses, particularly those arising in the liver, kidney or retroperitoneal areas. Fluid-filled structures are easily identified using the appropriate sequences and the relation of major blood vessels to the tumor is beautifully demonstrated. Being a multiplanar imaging technique, MRI is valuable in the assessment of presacral masses, the demonstration of the uterus and ovaries in intersex and endocrine abnormalities (Secaf et al 1994) and the assessment of the pelvic floor muscles in anorectal atresia.

As yet it is not possible to examine the gastrointestinal tract as gut movement causes multiple artifacts. In future, this may be possible with the use of contrast media and antispasmodics. MRI is also a recognized technique in the diagnosis of diseases involving the musculoskeletal system. Although cortical bone produces a signal void, it is the changes in marrow signal which identify the pathology of osteomyelitis, trauma, bleeding or edema.

It is important to remember that the signal from the pediatric bone marrow changes with the aging of the child. As more fat accumulates with increasing age, there is a corresponding increase in the marrow signal (Moore & Dawson 1990). MRI has been described as useful in the initial diagnosis of Perthes disease where a low signal is seen in the epiphysis of the femur on T1 and T2 images. Growth plate injuries, osteomyelitis and involvement of the bone marrow in metastatic disease may all be diagnosed with this technique (Jaramillo et al 1990, Darnman et al 1992).

INTERVENTIONAL PROCEDURES

These techniques have now been well integrated into pediatric practice (Towbin 1989). Percutaneous nephrostomy with catheterization and drainage of a hydronephrosis initially involves the ultrasonic guidance of a fine 22G needle into the renal pelvis. Following aspiration of urine, water-soluble contrast may be injected for fluoroscopic identification of the pelvicalyceal system. A guidewire is then inserted through the needle. The tract is dilated and finally a 5–8 French catheter is coiled in the renal pelvis. The procedure is best performed under general anesthetic. Balloon dilatation of pelviureteric junction obstruction and postoperative strictures can be performed, though insertion of a temporary ureteric stent is necessary to prevent occlusion of the ureter by inflammatory changes.

In the investigation of obstructive jaundice percutaneous transhepatic cholangiography (PTC) can be performed under ultrasound guidance. A 25G chiba needle is inserted into the dilated biliary system. Contrast injection followed by spot films delineates the level of obstruction.

Dilatation of esophageal strictures with a balloon catheter is now a well-described technique (Fig. 36.1). The procedure is performed under general anesthesia in conjunction with the surgical team. The stricture is initially outlined with contrast and the balloon catheter size selected (Sato et al 1988). A narrow feeding tube is then passed through the mouth and a guidewire fed through the feeding tube to cross the stricture. The preselected balloon catheter, varying in size from 6 mm to 20 mm, is passed over the guidewire and inflated with contrast under fluoroscopic control, until waisting at the stricture is abolished. Larger balloons of 30–35 mm have been used successfully in achalasia. Continuous ECG monitoring is essential as esophageal dilatation can cause bradycardia or apnea.

A similar technique has been described for small bowel and colonic strictures. A record of screening time and number of procedures is essential to monitor radiation exposure.

The hydrostatic reduction of intussusception and treatment of meconium ileus with water-soluble contrast will be discussed in the relevant sections.

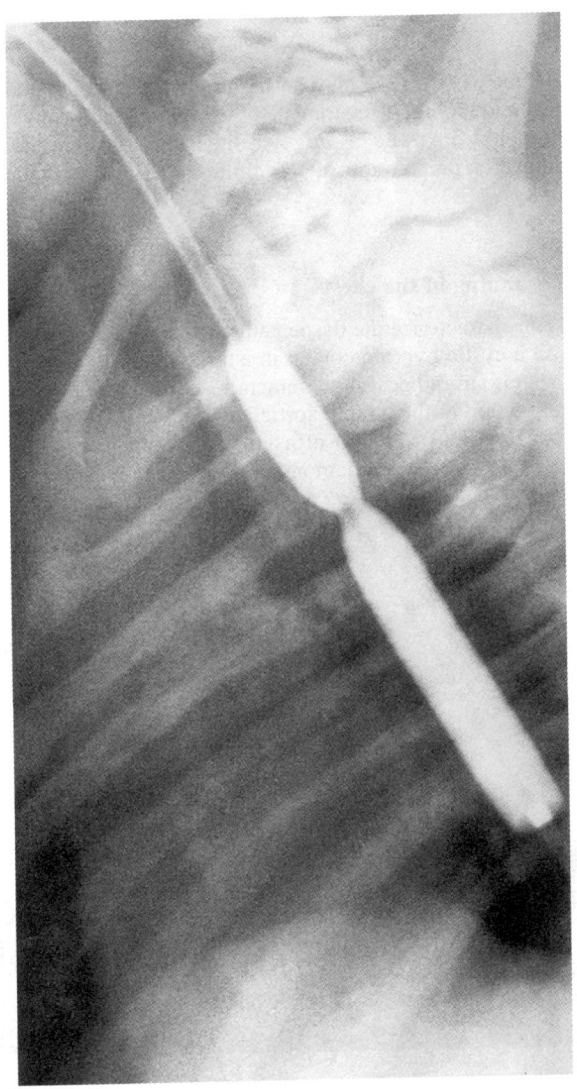

Fig. 36.1 Balloon dilatation of esophageal stricture. Note indentation on the contrast-filled balloon from the stricture.

Foreign bodies in the esophagus may be removed with a balloon catheter. The catheter is inserted through the mouth and the balloon inflated distal to the foreign body. In the prone head-down position the catheter is pulled cranially and the foreign body is removed from the mouth with forceps (McDermott et al 1995). Similarly magnetic material lying in the esophagus or stomach may be withdrawn using a magnet attached to a nasogastric tube. This is of particular value in withdrawing the small batteries now used in calculators and other devices. If left in situ these objects disintegrate, causing corrosive strictures and perforations of the esophagus and stomach (Volle et al 1989).

Recently the transjugular intrahepatic portosystemic shunt (TIPS) procedure has been used in children with portal hypertension caused by liver disease. A stent is inserted in the liver substance to connect the portal vein to the hepatic vein, reducing portal venous pressure and preventing complications such as bleeding varices.

Arteriovenous malformations can be embolized following selective catheterization of feeding vessels at angiography. Steel coils, acrylic glue or various types of particulate matter can be used to reduce flow through the abnormality.

BODY SYSTEMS

RESPIRATORY SYSTEM

Plain radiographs

Chest radiographs are the most frequently requested imaging procedure in children and there is opportunity for effective cost reduction and radiation protection by more careful vetting of requests (World Health Organization 1987b). Radiographic technique is important and an acceptable chest radiograph must include the whole chest from the thoracic inlet to diaphragm and be sufficiently penetrated to show major spinal abnormalities through the mediastinal shadow. Younger children are usually examined supine and older cooperative children can be examined erect. The routine use of lateral chest radiographs is unnecessary. Lung segments which are collapsed or consolidated can be located by their interference with normal mediastinal or diaphragmatic contours. Overinflation is assessed by the effects on rib configuration and the diaphragm level and shape. Pleural effusions previously detected by means of decubitus films should be confirmed with ultrasound. Obstructive emphysema, usually from foreign body obstruction, is demonstrated with films on inspiration and expiration exposed consecutively. This is important as a normal chest X-ray may be found in 20% of cases of inhaled foreign bodies.

When imaging children with stridor the standard radiographs are an anteroposterior chest radiograph, lateral neck radiograph and a high kV filter view of the trachea. Subglottic narrowing is seen in croup. A right-sided aortic knuckle usually deviates the trachea to the left. The presence of a vascular ring can be confirmed with a barium contrast swallow, the classic findings being a right-sided esophageal impression from a right aortic arch and an associated posterior impression on the esophagus from the double arch component or an aberrant left subclavian artery. The exact anatomy is clearly demonstrated with MRI.

The child with suspected epiglottitis should be admitted directly to the ward, the condition being diagnosed clinically or on direct laryngoscopy in theater. Fatalities have arisen secondary to airway obstruction during radiography of these children. Occasionally the diagnosis is confused clinically with croup, but the typical lateral neck radiographic appearance of a swollen epiglottis and aryepiglottic folds allows differentiation.

Contrast swallow

The contrast mainly used is barium sulfate. The indications are in the assessment of mediastinal masses and stridor when a vascular ring is suspected.

In children with swallowing problems, such as in cerebral palsy, where aspiration is suspected, iso-osmolar nonionic water-soluble contrast media should be used. This contrast does not provoke pulmonary edema if aspirated. Suspected 'H'-type tracheoesophageal fistulae are examined using video recording with the child in the prone or lateral position. A nasogastric tube is inserted into the esophagus. Contrast is injected to distend the esophagus during withdrawal of the tube from the cardia to the pharynx. Contrast is seen to cross from the esophagus forwards and upwards into the trachea. Video recording is necessary to avoid confusion with spillover of contrast from the larynx.

Fluoroscopy

Fluoroscopy of the chest is an infrequent examination but can be helpful in the assessment of diaphragmatic movements and obstructive airway disease, often from suspected foreign body aspiration.

Ultrasound

This noninvasive modality is the first-line investigation in congenital heart disease. The technique also provides a rapid method to determine the presence of a pericardial effusion. An opaque hemithorax, whether due to consolidation, pleural fluid or an underlying neoplasm, can be assessed. This avoids the need for further X-ray films. Ultrasound can differentiate between subpulmonary pleural fluid, subphrenic fluid and an elevated diaphragm and can assess diaphragmatic movement.

Pulmonary and mediastinal masses can be visualized with ultrasound if adjacent to the chest wall or heart. The consistency of the mass, whether cystic or solid, can be assessed. Sequestration of the lung is characterized by a solid or cystic mass in the lower zones and the supplying arterial vessel can often be visualized piercing the diaphragm. The characteristics of the blood flow in the vessel can be analyzed with a Doppler study. Angiographic confirmation of sequestration with anomalous arterial supply is now rarely required.

Computerized tomography scanning

This sectional technique is of value in the imaging of pulmonary and mediastinal masses. The technique will display any calcification, fat or bone destruction associated with the abnormality. The differentiation of primary pulmonary consolidation, abscess formation and empyema can be made with this technique. Contrast enhancement will outline the vascular pleura leaving the contents of an empyema unopacified. Primary pulmonary diseases including bronchiectasis (Fig. 36.2), interstitial fibrosis and emphysema can also be assessed using thin section high resolution technique (Kuhn 1993). Artifacts from areas of atelectasis are produced in the lung fields if a general

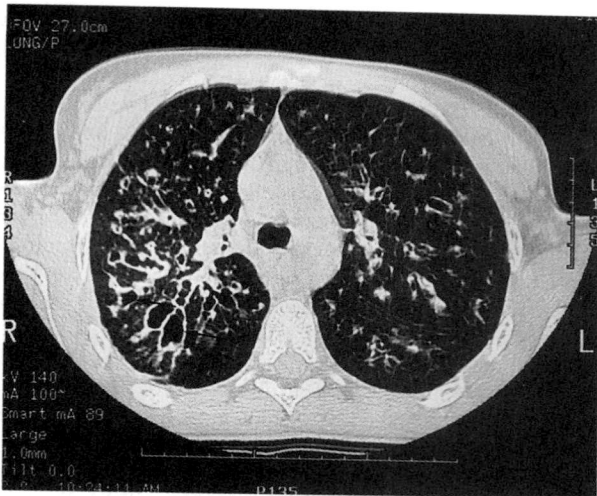

Fig. 36.2 High resolution computerized tomography scan of the lungs demonstrating diffuse bronchiectasis. Arrows highlight the dilated bronchi with thickened walls.

anesthetic is used. CT can also be used in the demonstration of tracheal and laryngeal anatomy. Bronchography and conventional tomography have been largely superseded by modern CT imaging. For preparation of the child for CT investigation, see page 1897.

MRI scanning of the chest

MRI can characterize the tissue nature of mediastinal masses, e.g. fluid in a cystic hygroma or fat in a teratoma. The technique can demonstrate intrathecal involvement of paravertebral masses and flowing blood in the double aortic arch in a child presenting with stridor (Fig. 36.3). Pleural effusions, thickening and pulmonary masses can also be well demonstrated.

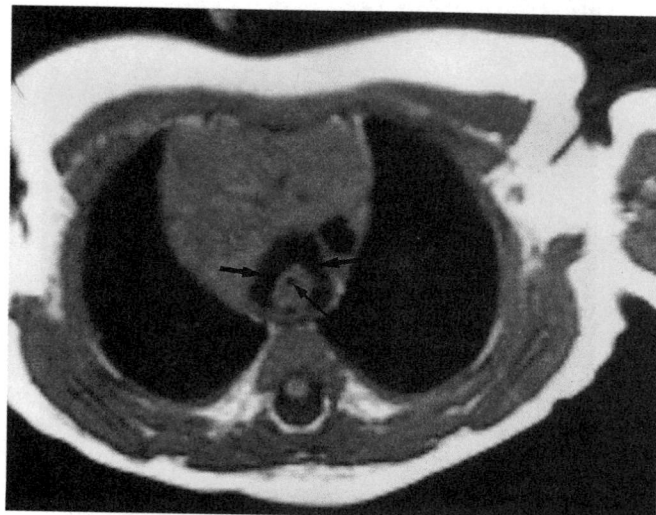

Fig. 36.3 Axial T1-weighted MRI scan of the chest demonstrating the double aortic arch which rings the trachea and esophagus (trachea – long arrow, vascular ring – short arrows).

The technique has the advantages of portraying the image in any plane (coronal, sagittal and axial) but does not as yet have the resolution of CT for the imaging of parenchymal lung disease. For the role of MRI in cardiac disease, see Chapter 13.

Radionuclide scanning

Radionuclide studies provide reliable information regarding lung perfusion and ventilation. Ventilation lung scans can be performed using xenon 133 or 127, with an aerosol ('Technegas') or krypton 81m. The use of xenon or an aerosol can be extremely difficult in a small, uncooperative child and, although difficult to obtain, krypton is particularly useful as it has a short half-life of 13 seconds, can be inhaled through a simple mask and provides better quality images. Perfusion scanning to assess the pulmonary blood flow to the lungs is usually carried out using technetium 99m macroaggregates of albumin (MAA), human albumin microspheres (HAM) or xenon 133 dissolved in saline. ^{99m}Tc MAA studies are currently favored with children. The pulmonary arterioles are temporarily occluded by the albumin particles. The number of arterioles and alveoli increase rapidly from about 4 months to 3 years before reaching the adult level at about 8 years. The number of particles injected should be reduced in proportion to the child's weight/surface area with a further 50% reduction if the child has a right to left shunt or pulmonary hypertension.

Lung scans are useful in the assessment of several congenital lung lesions, e.g. congenital lobar emphysema, sequestration, aplasia or hypoplasia. They also have a role in the preoperative and postoperative assessment of some forms of congenital heart disease, e.g. right to left shunts, pulmonary artery hyoplasia. They are valuable in the follow-up of children with foreign body aspiration, previous collapse and/or consolidation, bronchiectasis and cystic fibrosis. They can be used in the diagnosis of the occasional child with suspected pulmonary emboli.

ALIMENTARY TRACT

The radiographic investigations with the lowest positive yield are those referred for vague abdominal pain, encopresis and constipation (World Health Organization 1987a). Acute appendicitis is a clinical diagnosis which does not require the use of contrast studies although in young children more difficult diagnoses may be confirmed with ultrasound.

Cradles are useful devices for immobilizing infants for alimentary tract examinations, reducing handling and inducing reassurance analogous to wrapping an infant in a shawl. Infrared lamps attached to fluoroscopy units are invaluable in reducing heat loss in infants and are reassuring to older children (Gyll & Blake 1986).

Conventional radiography

Plain films are useful in assessing mechanical obstructions from esophagus to rectum, whether congenital or acquired, using air as the contrast medium (Gyll & Blake 1986). Supine films sometimes require supplementation with horizontal beam films which can be taken with the child erect, decubitus with right side raised or with a lateral shoot-through view with the child supine or prone. These views may demonstrate air fluid levels and evaluate any free intraperitoneal air following perforation. In children over 1 year of age the nature of dilated bowel loops can be recognized by the same criteria used in adults – jejunum with complete transverse folds, ileum featureless and colon with haustrations which do not extend across the whole lumen. However, in infancy the site and number of dilated loops is a better guide and in rectal atresia the rectum may not fill with swallowed air until 48 hours after birth, best demonstrated with the baby lying prone over a pillow or wedge.

Intussusceptions can be identified on plain films as a soft tissue density mass anywhere along the line of the colon. A degree of small bowel obstruction is often present. Ultrasound in expert hands can demonstrate the intussuscepting mass even when it is obscured on plain films due to dilated bowel loops.

In necrotizing enterocolitis the plain film findings include thickened bowel mucosa, immotile bowel loops, intramural gas which has a linear or bubble-like pattern and, rarely, portal venous gas seen as a branching lucent appearance within the liver (Fig. 36.4a & b). Positive contrast is not usually necessary for the diagnosis. Free intraperitoneal gas following perforation may be recognized on the supine film as a central lucency, the so-called

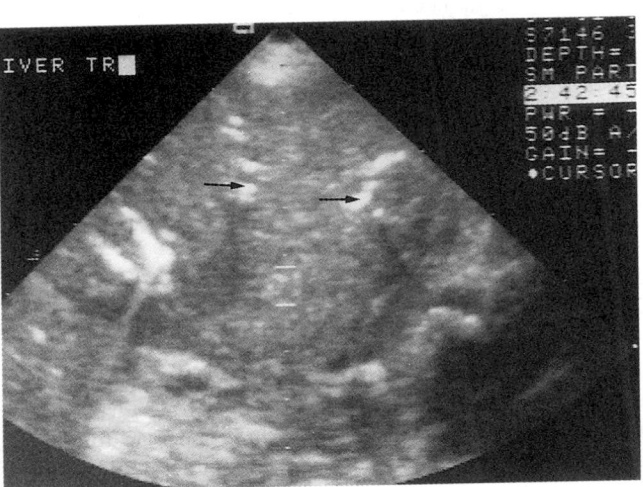

(a)

(b)

Fig. 36.4 Necrotizing enterocolitis in a neonate. (**a**) There is dilation of the small bowel. Intramural gas (small arrows) and gas in the biliary system (large arrows). (**b**) Sagittal ultrasound through the liver showing gas in the portal venous system as hyperechoic linear streaks (arrows).

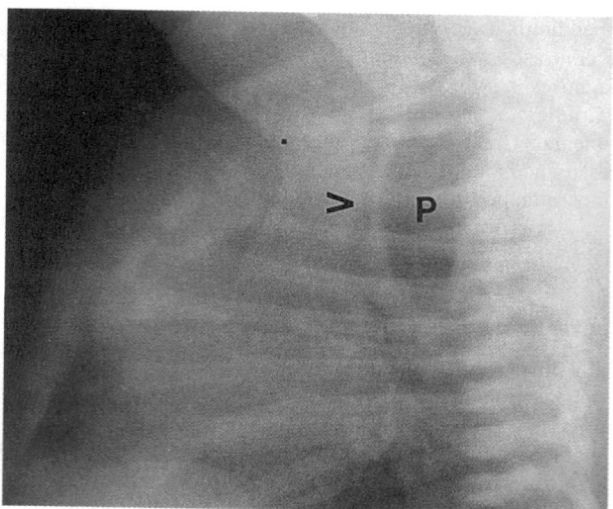

Fig. 36.5 Newborn with esophageal atresia. Note air filling the proximal esophageal pouch (P) indenting the trachea. Associated tracheal narrowing due to tracheomalacia (arrow head).

football sign, the central lace due to the outlined falciform ligament.

A gas-free abdomen is sinister in infancy – it may denote an infant so debilitated that the normal amount of air cannot be swallowed, a stomach filled with excess secretions in high obstruction or a high esophageal atresia without distal tracheoesophageal fistula. If there is clinical doubt a little air introduced through a nasogastric catheter will help to differentiate. A stiff opaque catheter held in the upper pouch during a plain film of the chest and upper abdomen is all that is required to confirm esophageal atresia (Fig. 36.5). The level of the atresia will be shown as well as any associated vertebral anomaly and the presence of a distal tracheoesophageal fistula will be confirmed by the presence of abdominal bowel gas.

Peritoneal calcification in the newborn denotes prenatal perforation (calcification can become visible within 4 days of perforation at this age) and is commonly secondary to obstructive bowel disease including atresia and meconium ileus. Apart from swallowed foreign bodies fecoliths are the commonest intra-abdominal opacities in the UK and can be extremely helpful in the diagnosis of appendicitis.

Loss of definition or displacement of the normal properitoneal fat and the psoas shadows in relation to inflammatory disease and neoplasm are useful in older children but are rarely seen in young infants.

Contrast studies

Barium sulfate is cheap and safe and is the most commonly used contrast in the alimentary tract. It is contraindicated in perforation as a leak may cause mediastinitis or peritonitis. It does not cause pulmonary edema if aspirated. When perforation is suspected low osmolality water-soluble contrast should be used. High osmolality water-soluble contrast should not be used in upper gastrointestinal studies in children due to the risk of pulmonary edema if aspirated.

Indications for barium studies in children include persistent vomiting, hematemesis, suspected peptic ulceration, aspiration

pneumonias and dysphagia. Milk isotope studies and pH monitoring have reduced the need for barium meals to detect gastroesophageal reflux and upper GI endoscopy may be preferred to detect peptic ulceration. Fasting for 4 hours is adequate preparation for barium meals and barium can be given from a bottle, feeder cup, beaker or straw. Barium is injected down a nasogastric tube when children cannot or will not swallow. High density barium (e.g. 250% weight for volume) should be used for double contrast technique studies to detect fine mucosal abnormalities in the esophagus, stomach and duodenum. Low density barium (50–100%) should be used for single contrast examinations to detect malrotation or for small bowel examinations. In a tiny premature neonate 5 ml of barium may suffice though an adolescent may require 500 ml to perform a small bowel examination.

The small bowel enema is a technique where contrast is injected directly into the jejunum through an appropriately placed nasogastric tube. This is followed by methyl cellulose, water, saline or air. Screening of the barium column as it passes through the gut improves visualization of individual bowel loops and is useful in the diagnosis of Crohn's disease and lymphoma.

Malabsorption is better investigated with biochemical techniques and biopsy studies. A symptomatic Meckel's diverticulum is rarely filled on barium follow-through investigation. In malrotation the position of the duodenojejunal flexure is low and to the right of the L1, L2 left-sided vertebral body pedicles. If volvulus has occurred partial duodenal obstruction may be present or the spiral shape of the twisted midgut noted (Fig. 36.6). If the diagnosis is in doubt then a follow-through study with screening of the ileocecal region is necessary. A barium enema is no longer regarded as the best investigation for the diagnosis of malrotation (Millar et al 1987).

Barium contrasts are also commonly used to examine the colon and rectum. The double contrast technique requires excellent cleansing of the large bowel. Preparation involves a low-residue diet for 24 hours, together with an orally effective laxative. This has largely superseded preparation enemas. High-density barium is used to fill the colon which is then drained to remove surplus contrast. Air is insufflated using a hand pump to distend the colon,

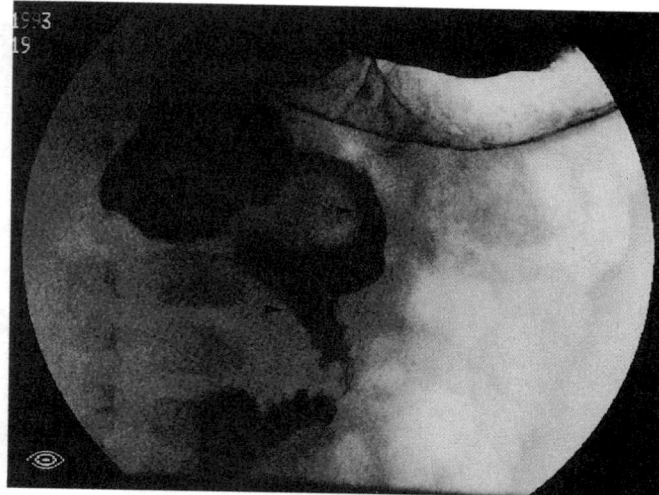

Fig. 36.6 Barium meal demonstrating spiral sign of the midgut volvulus (arrows). Twisted duodenojejunum.

leaving only a thin layer of barium coating the mucosa to demonstrate abnormalities such as ulceration or polyps (Fig. 36.7). Endoscopy may be preferred, particularly in situations where biopsy of the mucosa is required. Most information can be obtained with two decubitus views which should be inspected before other films are taken. The technique is best deferred for 7 days after full-thickness colonic biopsy. Unprepared single contrast enemas with low-density barium (50% w/v) may be performed in constipated children suspected of having Hirschsprung's disease to detect the zone of transition from the narrow aganglionic segment distally to the distended colon laden with feces proximally. Balloon catheters should not be used since this may obscure a transition zone in the rectum. A 24-hour film may show delayed colonic clearance of barium which may be diagnostic of Hirschsprung's disease. Rectal biopsy provides histological confirmation.

Reduction of an intussusception with contrast is a well-recognized procedure in the correct clinical setting. Contraindications are complete bowel obstruction, the presence of perforation or peritonitis and an extremely sick child. Conventionally, under fluoroscopic control dilute barium was run in from a height of 3 feet until retrograde filling of the terminal ileum indicated successful reduction. Recently the use of air pressure for reduction (Gu et al 1988) has become widely accepted. Air is pumped into the rectum with a hand pump, using a small valve (Kenny & Lutkin 1989) or a sphygmomanometer to limit the pressure to 120 mmHg. In some centers special pumps with flow rate and pressure controls have been devised. Air can be seen distending the distal colon and outlining the intussusception as a soft tissue mass that moves proximally. When the intussusception is reduced there is sudden loss of the soft tissue

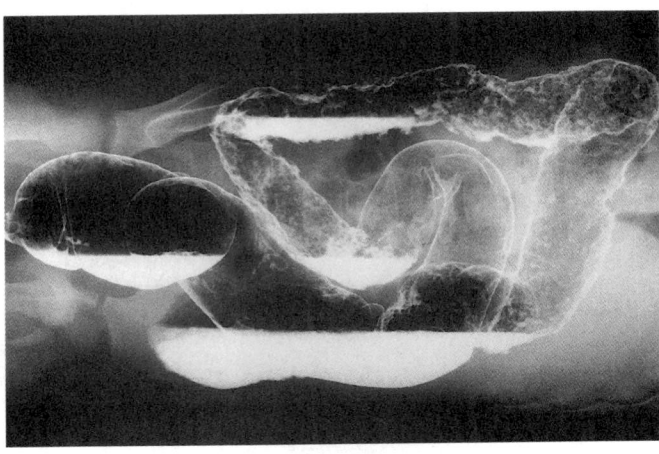

Fig. 36.7 Double contrast enema showing typical changes of ulcerative colitis with superficial and submucosal ulceration throughout the colon.

mass in the cecum and air distention of the terminal ileum (Fig. 36.8a & b). This endpoint of successful reduction can be more difficult to appreciate if there is gaseous distention of small bowel due to obstruction and a water-soluble contrast enema may then be helpful for confirmation. It is commonly observed that the child relaxes almost immediately following successful reduction.

The success rate of reduction is generally claimed to be higher for air than barium (over 90% for air). Perforation is rare and easily recognized by air outlining the liver. Perforation with air causes less peritoneal contamination and a smaller perforation defect as compared with barium (Shiels et al 1993). Respiratory

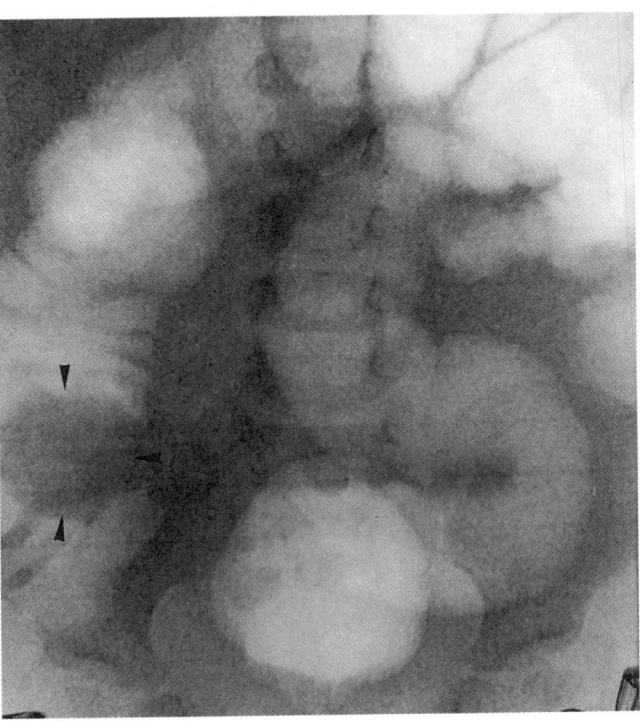

(a)

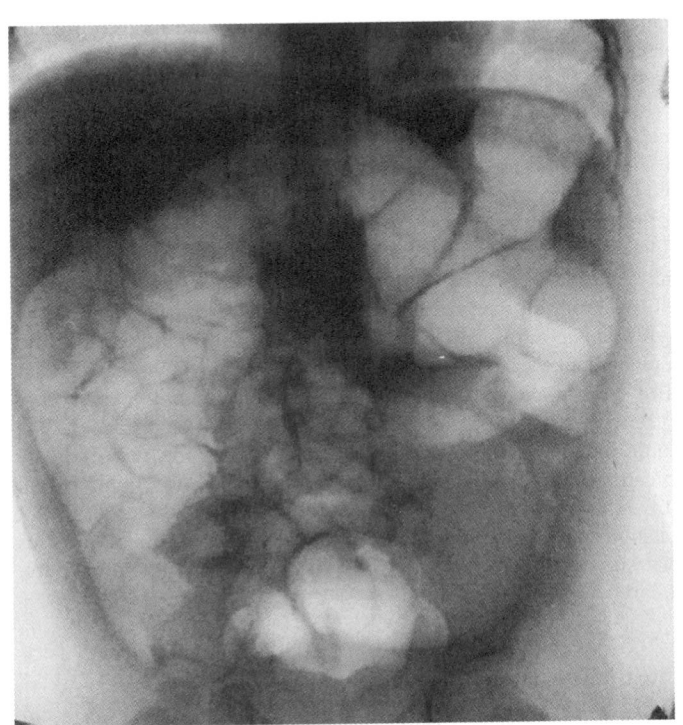

(b)

Fig. 36.8 Intussusception. (**a**) Air enema reduction of intussusception (arrow heads). (**b**) Final reduction showing free filling of the small bowel with gas and the disappearance of the soft tissue swelling of the intussusception.

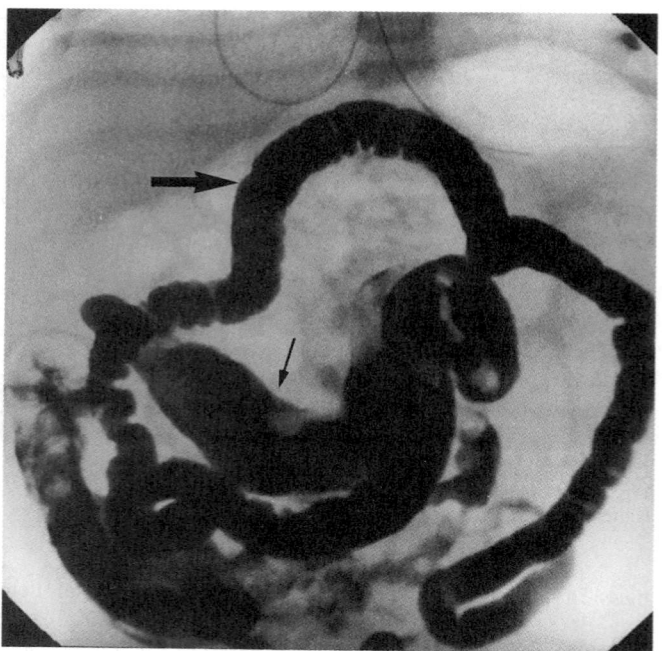

Fig. 36.9 Meconium ileus. Gastrografin enema demonstrates the presence of a microcolon. Contrast refluxes into the terminal ileum and proximally the dilated small bowel loops. (Colon thick arrow, small bowel thin arrow.)

distress from abdominal distention following perforation has been reported, though if air insufflation is stopped immediately, this will not occur. If air reduction is not complete on the first attempt, a further attempt performed a few hours later may be successful (Saxton et al 1995). Reduction of intussusception using saline as the hydrostatic medium together with ultrasound monitoring has recently been reported with a 91% success rate (Rohrschneider & Troger 1995).

In the diagnosis and treatment of meconium ileus and meconium plug syndrome hypertonic water-soluble contrast is used (Leonidas et al 1970). This contrast lubricates the obstructing plugs and, being hypertonic, draws fluid into the gut lumen, softening the plug (Fig. 36.9). Gastrografin, Hypaque 300 or Conray 280 are suitable contrast media. Undiluted Gastrografin may cause mucosal ulceration and in our practice the contrast is diluted from an osmolality of 2150 to 700 mosmol/l. The use of hypertonic contrast media requires simultaneous intravenous fluid replacement therapy to avoid dehydration in the small baby. Plain film evidence of perforation, either recent with free intraperitoneal air or old reflected by peritoneal calcification, is a contraindication to therapeutic enema. Perforation may indicate intestinal volvulus caused by meconium loading; small bowel atresia and a volvulus may be associated (Leonidas et al 1970). Liaison with the surgical team before therapeutic enema insures that should perforation occur as a complication of the procedure, it can be dealt with promptly.

Ultrasonic examination

The use of ultrasound examination in gastrointestinal problems is now well recognized. Ultrasound diagnosis of pyloric stenosis is 100% accurate in experienced hands and has replaced barium meal in most centers (Stunden et al 1986). The findings of the pyloric canal on ultrasound are of an elongated canal measuring over 14 mm in length, over 12 mm in diameter and with a muscle thickness of over 3.5 mm which fails to shorten and open in response to vigorous gastric peristalsis (Fig. 36.10). Ultrasound can also be used to diagnose intussusception and the typical appearances are of a target or doughnut shaped intra-abdominal mass (Fig. 36.11). The examination is particularly useful in those children presenting with obstruction where the mass is not seen on the plain film (Verschelden et al 1992). Ultrasound can demonstrate free intraperitoneal fluid indicating transudate caused by venous engorgement; air reduction can still be successful but should be undertaken with care since free fluid can also indicate necrosis of the bowel wall.

Recently color Doppler ultrasound has been used to indicate avascularity of the intussusception. This suggests ischemic change and is a contraindication for reduction (Lim et al 1994). The technique will also demonstrate duplication cysts of the bowel and dilated fluid-filled loops of gut in obstruction and evaluate mucosal thickening. Small amounts (more than 10 ml) of free intraperitoneal fluid can be clearly detected in the pelvis or subhepatic area.

Ultrasound is a sensitive and specific technique for the diagnosis of acute appendicitis. The criteria for diagnosis include noncompressibility of the appendix, a transverse diameter greater than 6 mm, mucosal edema and the presence of an appendicolith (Fig. 36.12) (Puylaert 1986, Vignault et al 1990, Siegel 1995).

In hemolytic uremic syndrome the clinical presentation of the child may be with abdominal pain and rectal bleeding. A target sign may be seen with ultrasound representing the hemorrhagic gut mucosa. This may be confused with an intussusception.

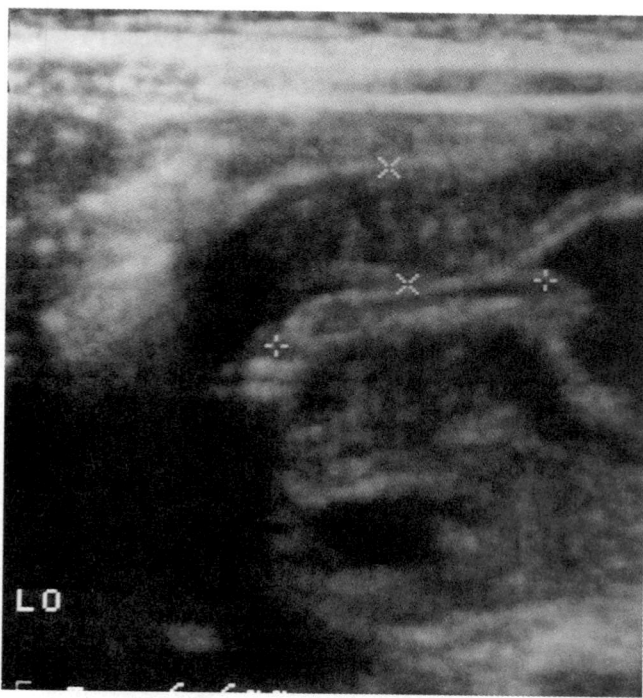

Fig. 36.10 Pyloric stenosis. Longitudinal ultrasound scan through the pylorus. The vertical crosses indicate the length of the canal, oblique crosses the thickness of muscle layer.

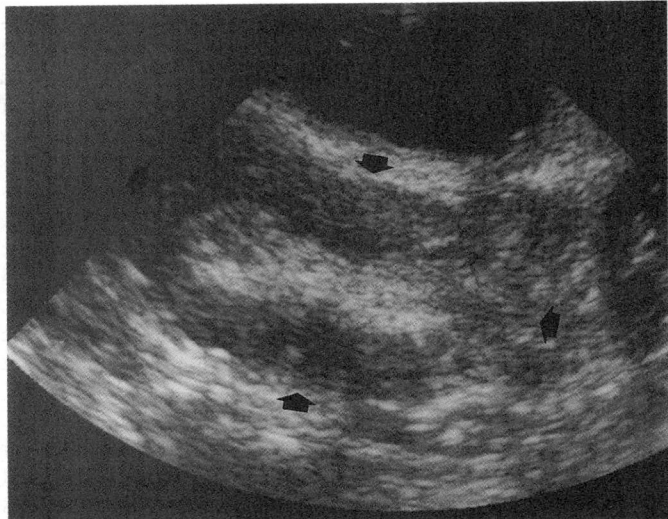

Fig. 36.11 Ultrasound scan of intussusception demonstrating doughnut sign (arrows).

Doppler ultrasound may reveal generalized avascularity of the gut (Friedland et al 1995) which is a manifestation of the ischemic vasculitis which occurs in this condition. It is worthy of note that the kidney parenchyma may be hyperechoic reflecting the glomerular vasculitis. It is to be noted that thickened mucosa can also be demonstrated on ultrasound in Crohn's disease (Fig. 36.13a & b) and ulcerative colitis.

The diagnosis of an intra-abdominal abscess is suggested by a thick-walled cystic lesion often sited in the pelvis. Ultrasound may also be used to assess upper gut obstruction and the injection of fluid into the stomach through a nasogastric tube allows visualization of a dilated fluid-filled duodenum secondary to

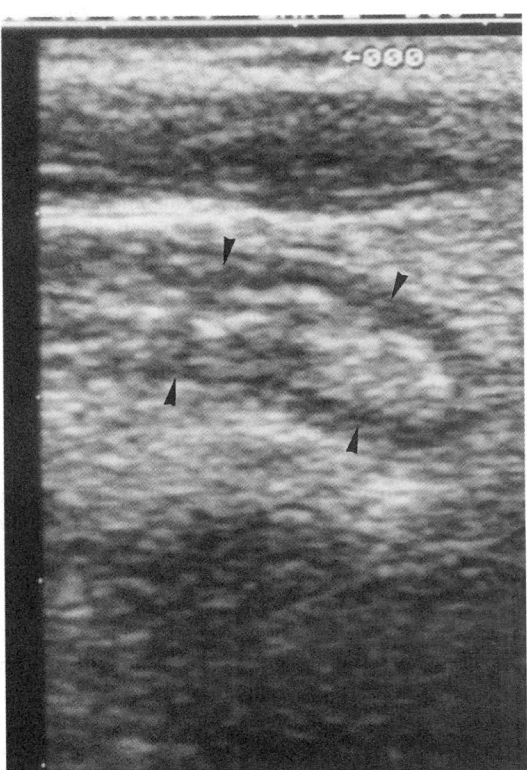

Fig. 36.12 Acute appendicitis. Ultrasound scan of the appendix in longitudinal section. The appendix was noncompressible with a width of 8 mm. The central echoes are thickened mucosa. The hypoechoic rim represents the edematous submucosa (arrow heads).

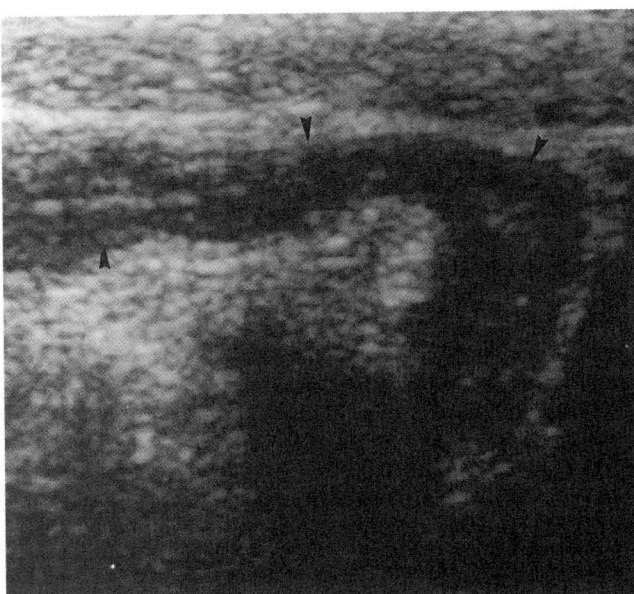

(a)

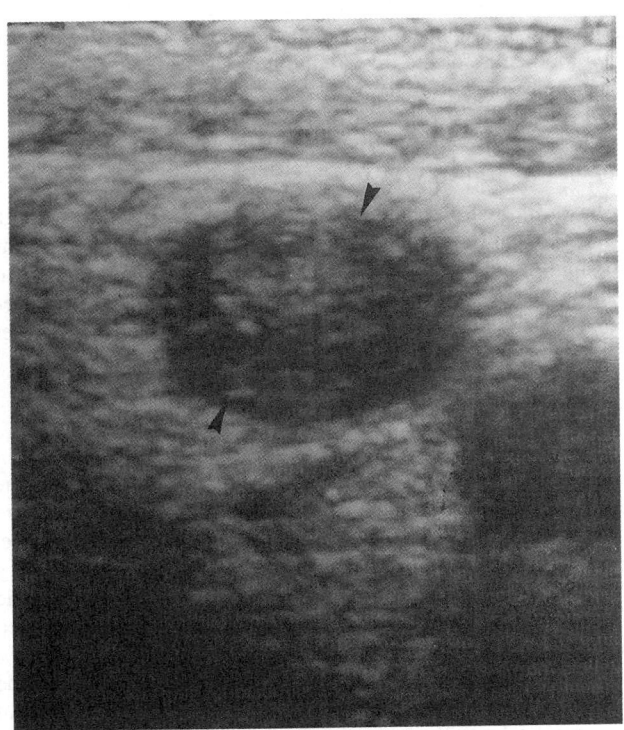

(b)

Fig. 36.13 Crohn's disease. Ultrasound scan through the terminal ileum showing hypoechoic edematous mucosa (arrow heads) representing the string sign: (a) longitudinal, (b) transverse sections.

duodenal obstruction. In malrotation the anatomical relationships of the superior mesenteric artery and vein are usually altered. Thus the transverse US section at the level of the uncinate lobe of the pancreas reveals the vein situated to the left of the artery compared with its normal right anterolateral position (Loyer & Dunne Eggli 1989). In anorectal atresia the fluid- or meconium-filled rectum can be identified as a transonic or mixed echoic structure. When scanning from the perineum the distance between the skin and the rectum can be measured directly. If this is less than 1 cm the atresia is unlikely to be complicated by the presence of a fistula and represents a so-called low lesion.

Nuclear medicine studies

Technetium 99m pertechnetate is taken up by the mucus secretory cells of gastric mucosa as well as by the thyroid gland and choroid plexus. Meckel's diverticulae or duplication cysts containing gastric mucosa will take up the radionuclide. The child should be fasted for 3–4 hours prior to the examination. Some centers have found the use of cimetidine in a dose of 20 mg per kg in three divided doses on the day before the examination with a double dose on the morning of the examination to be helpful, as it blocks secretion of pertechnetate from the gastric mucosa and improves the lesion-to-background ratio. An area of abnormal uptake of the radionuclide should appear at the same time as stomach activity and may be found anywhere in the abdomen.

Technetium sulfur colloid can be added to milk and used in the assessment of gastroesophageal reflux or gastric emptying. Technetium HMPAO (hexamethylpropyleneamine oxime) labeled white cells have recently been used in the diagnosis of inflammatory bowel disease such as ulcerative colitis and Crohn's disease. Increased activity in the small and large bowel occurs in areas involved with the disease (Charron et al 1994). The same radionuclide has replaced the use of indium 111 in the labeling of white blood cells for the investigation of suspected inflammatory lesions such as abdominal abscesses.

Computerized tomography

This has a limited place in gastrointestinal imaging, but is useful in the investigation of intraperitoneal abscesses and trauma to the abdominal organs (Ruess et al 1995). Contrast-enhanced CT has the ability to examine multiple organs as well as identifying free intraperitoneal air and coincidental damage to bony structures including the spine and pelvis.

LIVER AND BILIARY TRACT

The common clinical indications for radiological imaging of the liver are hepatomegaly, jaundice and portal hypertension. There are numerous causes of liver enlargement, including heart failure, hepatitis, septicemia, storage diseases, α1-antitrypsin deficiency and primary and secondary neoplasms. Plain X-rays are of little value but may demonstrate calcification in masses or increased radiolucency of the liver in fatty infiltration.

Ultrasound is the initial imaging method and will define the liver size, shape and consistency. Often only an enlarged organ but with normal echo pattern is seen. Decreased echoity generally or discrete hypoechoic masses are characteristic of leukemic and lymphomatous infiltration. Increased echoity is seen in fatty

infiltration, cirrhosis and hemochromatosis. Cysts and abscesses have a mainly transonic appearance with a rim of variable thickness. Fungal infection occurs in immunocompromised children and can appear as multiple areas of increased or decreased echogenicity, target lesions (concentric high and low echogenicity) or diffuse abnormality of echotexture; these lesions can be biopsied under ultrasound guidance. Primary liver tumors are usually hyperechoic (Pobiel & Bisset 1995). Areas of necrosis, however, impart a variable consistency with transonic and echoic features on ultrasound. Indeed, hemangioendotheliomas and mesenchymal hamartomas may have a large cystic component. Ultrasound can be used in the initial assessment of liver, splenic and renal trauma. Contusion or frank laceration may be seen but more commonly free intraperitoneal fluid is identified.

Ultrasound is also the mainstay in imaging of the biliary tract. The patient should be fasted from fatty foods and maintain a clear fluid intake for 6 hours before the examination. The bile-filled gall bladder is clearly demonstrated and the presence of gall stones and mucosal thickening assessed. An absent or small gall bladder is a feature of biliary atresia. Usually the findings in biliary atresia are nonspecific but it is now well recognized that the presence of a choledochal cyst in the intrahepatic portal region is suggestive of an underlying biliary atresia. In less than 5% of cases, dilatation of the intrahepatic biliary ducts is seen. The diameter of the common bile duct should be less than 4 mm. Obstructive biliary disease is rare in children but is described secondary to gall stones (seen in hemolytic disease, inflammatory bowel disease, therapy with certain drugs, especially cyclosporin, or prolonged parenteral nutrition), enlarged portal lymph nodes, lymphoma, retroperitoneal sarcomas or primitive pancreatic tumors.

Choledochal cysts are characterized by a transonic cystic mass separate from the gall bladder and in the line of the common bile duct (Fig. 36.14). A dilated gall bladder has been described in Kawasaki's disease, secondary to parenteral nutrition and in acalculus cholecystitis and is a nonspecific finding in many children who are sick from a variety of causes. Sludge and debris often layer along the gall bladder floor.

Analogs of iminodiacetic acid linked to technetium are excreted by hepatocytes and are used in the investigation of the biliary

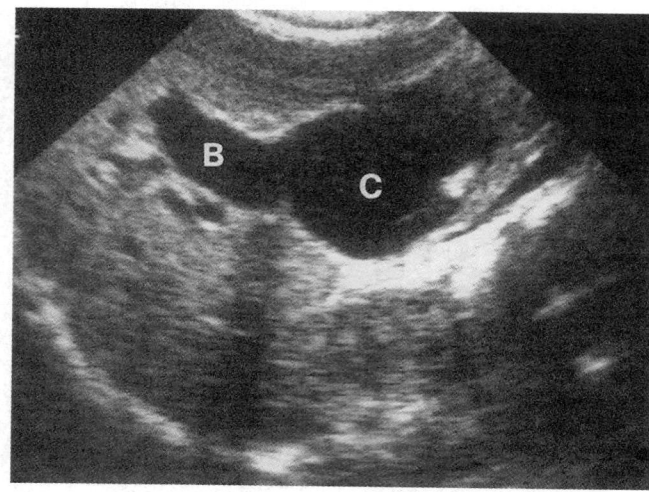

Fig. 36.14 Sagittal ultrasound section through the liver. Note transonic area representing the choledochal cyst (C) and associated dilatation of the common bile duct (B).

system. The third-generation derivative trimethyl bromoimino-diacetic acid (BROMIDA) is particularly useful in the jaundiced neonate suspected of having biliary atresia. The presence of radionuclide in the gut will exclude this diagnosis, though its absence does not confirm the diagnosis as severe hepatitis can cause a similar picture (Fig. 36.15). Uptake of the radionuclide is enhanced by giving the neonate a 5-day course of phenobarbitone 5 mg per kilogram per day in divided doses. BROMIDA scanning is also valuable in the follow-up of children with portoenterostomies for biliary atresia.

Doppler ultrasound is useful in the assessment of liver disease, particularly in biliary cirrhosis, portal hypertension and after liver transplantation. The hepatic arterial blood flow, portal venous and hepatic venous flow are assessed. Color Doppler enables the direction of flow to be more easily determined. In thrombosis of the vessels no flow is recorded. In portal vein thrombosis the normal portal vein is absent and replaced by peripheral collaterals. In stenosis of the portal vein frequency shifts at the level of the narrowing are noted. In progressive biliary cirrhosis reduced diastolic flow in the hepatic artery may be found. Thickening of the lesser omentum and varices can be visualized. The technique cannot measure portal venous pressure at present.

CT scanning can further evaluate the extent of the liver masses but in children appears to be less sensitive in detecting disease than ultrasonic investigation.

MRI scanning appears to be useful in outlining hepatic parenchyma and hepatic vessels and may well be the investigation of choice for detection of primary and secondary masses. MR is also useful for the detection of fatty infiltration.

Angiography may be indicated in the preoperative assessment of liver tumors and indirect portal venography is helpful if portosystemic shunting is being considered. Two-dimensional Doppler ultrasound is used, however, in the routine assessment of portal hypertension.

PANCREAS AND SPLEEN

These organs are best imaged with CT and ultrasound. The ultrasonic diagnosis of acute pancreatitis is characterized by a swollen pancreas of low echogenicity and ill-defined outline (Balthazar et al 1994). Chronic pancreatitis as seen in cystic fibrosis is characterized by a small hyperechoic organ. Pancreatic pseudocysts following trauma or inflammation are clearly defined as transonic areas. Splenic involvement with lymphoma or leukemia is characterized by discrete or diffuse areas of low echogenicity. Fungal abscesses may occur in immuno-compromised children and can have increased or decreased echogenicity or target appearance. Both ultrasound and CT are of value in assessing abdominal trauma (Fig. 36.16). Technetium 99m sulfur, tin or albumin colloid can be used to demonstrate the presence of functional splenic tissue following trauma. Care should be used with albumin colloid as there have been reports of anaphylactoid reactions with this material.

CENTRAL NERVOUS SYSTEM

The investigation of the central nervous system has been revolutionized with the introduction of ultrasound, CT and MR.

Plain radiographs

Plain skull X-rays may be considered obsolete if CT services are available, but are still useful in the initial assessment of suspected craniostenosis, intracranial calcification, long-standing raised

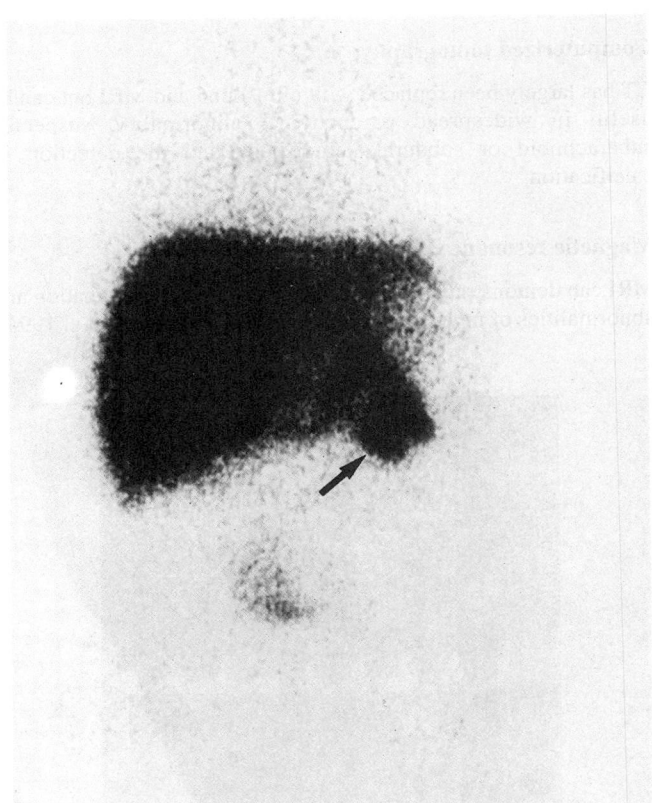

Fig. 36.15 Radioisotope liver scan using HIDA-derivative. This demonstrates isotope activity in the hepatocytes and within the small bowel on a 30-minute acquisition (arrow), thus indicating patency of the biliary tree.

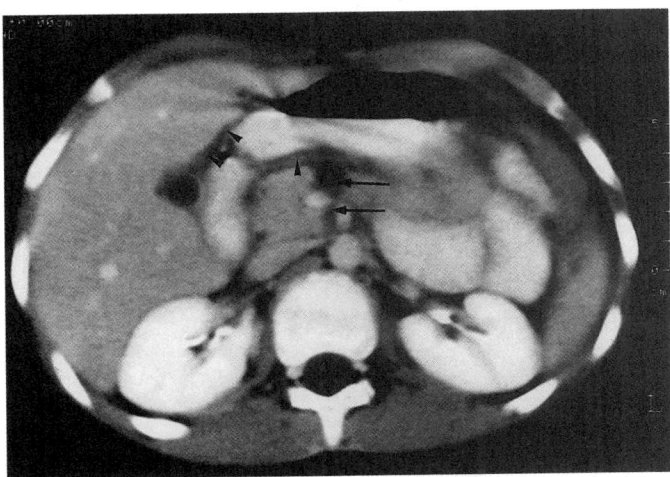

Fig. 36.16 Axial CT scans through the pancreas with contrast enhancement of the gut and kidney. Pancreatic laceration (long arrows), free fluid seen in the lesser sac and under the liver (arrow heads).

intracranial pressure, metastatic and metabolic bone disease and linear fractures of the skull. Conventional radiography is still the first investigation requested after trauma to the skull and spine but its place after skull trauma is the subject of ongoing acrimonious debate and probably the only universally acceptable statement is that it must never replace careful clinical assessment.

After suspected skull trauma two radiographs are taken with the child supine, an anteroposterior view and a shoot-through lateral with a horizontal X-ray beam to include the upper cervical spine. These views are supplemented by a tilted (Townes) anterior–posterior view to show the posterior fossa if occipital injury is suspected. A submentovertical (basal) view is indicated if there is bleeding from an ear.

Imaging of the spinal cord is now performed with MRI and myelography is rarely indicated. Plain films may be helpful in the immediate assessment of major spinal trauma, supplemented with CT if fractures and/or dislocation are suspected.

Ultrasound

A 7.5 MHz transducer is used in premature babies and neonates though a 5 MHz transducer is necessary to visualize the posterior fossa in older babies.

The indications for US are in the assessment of parenchymal changes following hypoxia in the neonate with detection and grading of intraventricular hemorrhage. Acute severe hypoxic injury can occur without visible changes on ultrasound and CT or preferably MRI should be performed if there is clinical doubt. Periventricular leukomalacia is characterized by initial periventricular echogenicity followed by developing cystic changes and enlarging ventricles (De Vries et al 1989) (Fig. 36.17). The position of drainage catheters can also be assessed. Inflammatory brain conditions may be represented by an overall increase in cortical echogenicity, secondary hydrocephalus and parenchymal echogenic areas representing complicating infarcts. Congenital brain abnormalities detectable on ultrasound include absence of the corpus callosum with a high midline 3rd ventricle and separation of the lateral ventricles, holoprosencephaly, midline brain cysts and the Arnold–Chiari malformations. Congenital brain tumors, papillomas and teratomas are rare.

Papillomas are of high echoity and usually present in the 3rd and lateral ventricles. Teratomas have a mixed echoity often with total disorganization of brain tissue. A widened subdural space is seen in children with macrocrania (Babcock et al 1988). This is often a benign appearance and in the absence of other clinical abnormalities, the appearance returns to normal with growth of the child. A wide space is also seen in the presence of pathological fluid collections following trauma or infection or associated with cerebral atrophy. With top quality techniques it is now possible to differentiate subdural from subarachnoid fluid collections (Veyrac et al 1989).

Doppler ultrasound is helpful in the physiological assessment of cerebral abnormalities, including anoxia and cerebral hemorrhage, and diastolic flow may be reduced or absent in raised intracranial pressure (Fig. 36.18) (Horgan et al 1989, Goh et al 1992). Doppler traces from the middle cerebral arteries can be obtained by scanning through the temporoparietal bones and the anterior cerebral arteries directly through the anterior fontanel. Assessment of AV malformations is possible (Fig. 36.19a & b) demonstrating feeding arteries, draining veins and turbulent flow within the malformation.

The spinal cord and brainstem can be visualized with ultrasonic imaging. The medullary pyramids and cerebellar vermis are assessed through either the anterior fontanel or foramen magnum. The position of the spinal cord, the conus and the cauda equina are assessed. In a child with obvious or occult spinal dysraphism, a tethered cord, the presence of a wide subarachnoid space or associated intraspinal lipoma may be recognized.

Computerized tomography

CT has largely been replaced with ultrasound and MRI but can be useful in widespread parenchymal abnormality, suspected subarachnoid or subdural hemorrhage and the detection of calcification.

Magnetic resonance imaging

MRI can demonstrate the normal development of myelination and abnormalities of myelination can be evaluated (Staudt et al 1994).

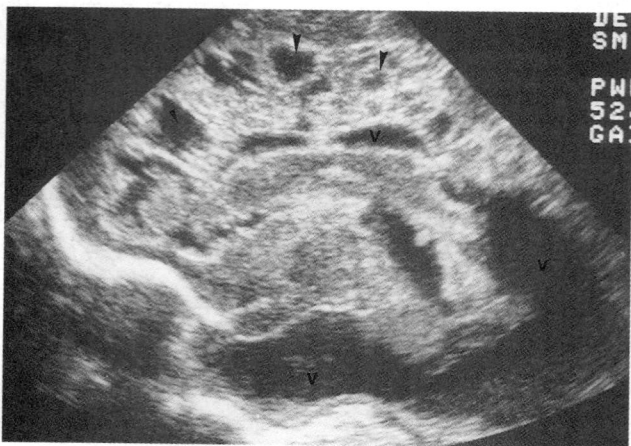

Fig. 36.17 Sagittal ultrasound scan through the brain reveals multiple cystic change in the periventricular area (arrow heads) (V – ventricles). Appearances compatible with the diagnosis of periventricular leukomalacia.

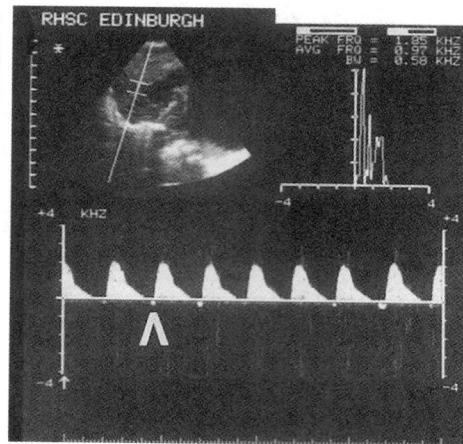

Fig. 36.18 Doppler examination of the anterior cerebral artery in a child with hydrocephalus. Note the reversal of diastolic flow (white arrow head). The intracranial pressure was raised at 30 mmHg.

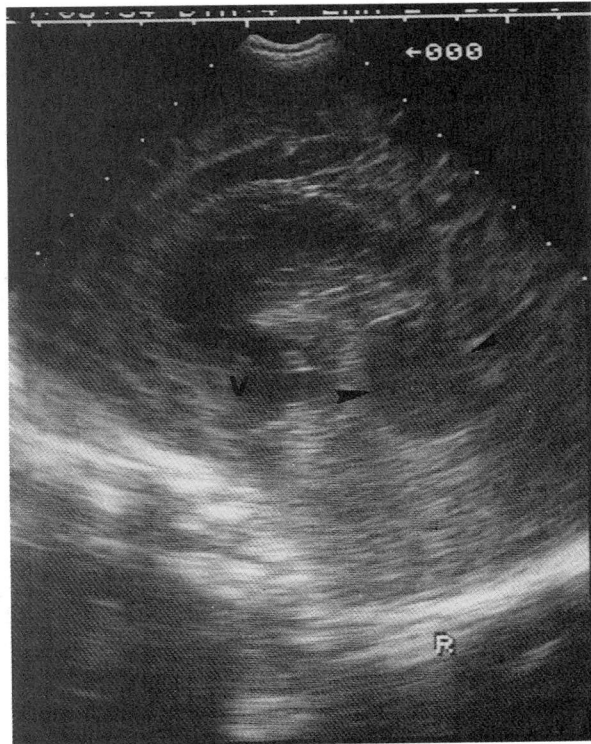

(a)

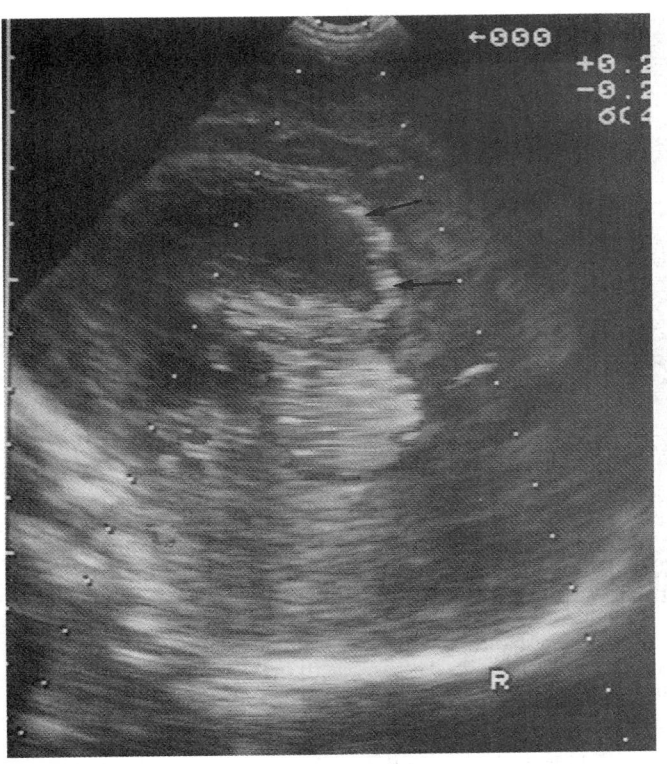

(b)

Fig. 36.19   Ultrasound of vein of Galen aneurysm. (**a**) Sagittal midline section of the brain demonstrating transonic appearance of a vein of Galen aneurysm (arrows) (V – 3rd ventricle). (**b**) Doppler ultrasound showing vascular flow in the posterior pericallosal artery supplying the AV malformation (arrows).

Migration anomalies such as schizencephaly and gray matter heteropia may only be appreciated on MRI (Fig. 36.20) (Byrd 1989a, b). Early ischemic changes may best be appreciated with specialized MRI sequences (Floodmark et al 1989, Barkovich & Truwit 1990, Christophe et al 1994). Special sequences can be used for demonstration of CSF flow in the evaluation of hydrocephalus. MR angiography can demonstrate anomalies such as arteriovenous malformations, aneurysms and vessel occlusions. MR can detect brain edema not visualized on CT and is invaluable in the assessment of patients with tumors, encephalitis, abscess formation and demyelination.

Angiography

Cerebral angiography may still be indicated in the investigation of vascular malformations, intracranial aneurysms and occlusive disease of the intracranial vessels, particularly if intervention is anticipated. Selective catheterization through the femoral route using the Seldinger technique is the safest and most usual method. Embolization of selected arteriovenous malformations and aneurysms may be possible.

SPECT scanning using 99m technetium HMPAO can be used in the assessment of regional cerebral blood flow. It is of particular value in localizing the focus of a seizure in children who fail to respond to medical therapy. There may be increased uptake of the radionuclide during an ictal scan with decreased uptake at the same site from an interictal study. It has been particularly useful in the assessment of children with temporal lobe epilepsy where surgery is contemplated.

URINARY TRACT

Ultrasound

This technique has revolutionized the imaging of the renal system. It is the initial modality used in children presenting with urinary tract infection (Whitaker & Sherwood 1984), hematuria, abdominal mass and enuresis. It is effective as a screen for congenital renal anomalies as part of chromosomal abnormalities and syndromes. The technique is also useful in assessing the natural history of fetal hydronephrosis and multicystic kidney (White 1989).

The examination is of value in the diagnosis of congenital malformations, be these horseshoe kidney, crossed renal ectopia or nonrotation. Duplex kidneys may be complicated by hydronephrosis, reflux and ureterocele. The dilated pelvicalyceal system, ureter and ureterocele can be directly visualized (Share & Lebowitz 1989) (Fig. 36.21a & b). Reflux nephropathy may produce a small kidney with an echogenic cortex. Localized renal scars are better demonstrated with ^{99m}Tc DMSA isotope scans.

Echogenic kidneys with or without loss of corticomedullary differentiation are seen in acute renal vein thrombosis, glomerular and interstitial disease, acute renal obstruction and autosomal recessive polycystic kidney disease. The kidneys are also enlarged in the acute stages of these diseases.

Echogenic but small kidneys are seen in chronic glomerular disease, the later stages of renal vein thrombosis and renal dysplasia. Autosomal dominant polycystic kidney disease is characterized by discrete cysts in the renal cortex. However, it may be difficult to distinguish from autosomal recessive

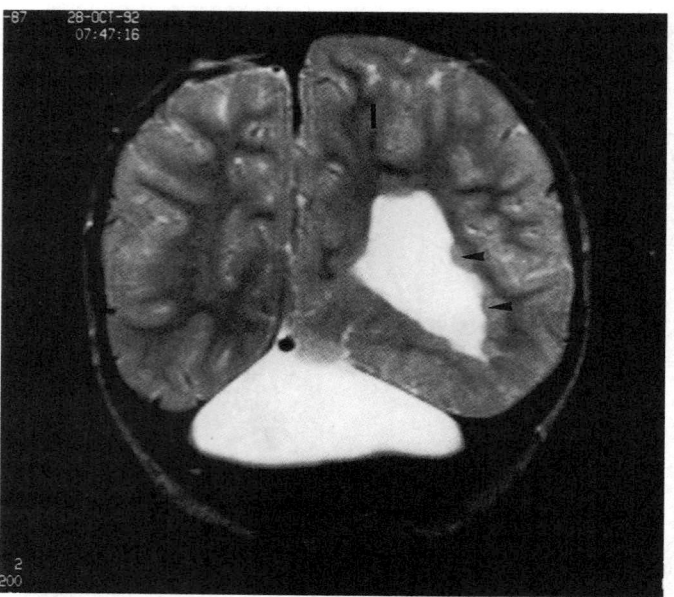

Fig. 36.20 Coronal MRI scan demonstrating hemimegalencephaly within enlargement of the left cerebral hemisphere (l) and the corresponding lateral ventricle. Gray matter heterotopia in the periventricular area (arrows).

polycystic kidney disease in the earlier stages when the kidneys may be enlarged with small cysts in both conditions. Multicystic kidney disease is unusually unilateral and characterized by multiple noncommunicating cysts.

Nephrocalcinosis is characterized by echogenic medullary pyramids. A similar appearance may be seen with deposition of proteins in the collecting tubules in acute tubular obstruction and in Tamm–Horsfall proteinuria of the newborn.

Ultrasonic examination is extremely sensitive in detecting minor widening of the pelvicalyceal system. This can lead to

difficulties in interpretation as it is a normal finding in well-hydrated children or secondary to ureteric distention from a full bladder. A false-positive diagnosis of early obstruction or vesicoureteric reflux may ensue. The AP diameter of the renal pelvis in the transverse scan should normally be less than 5–7 mm.

Renal calculi are easily seen in the cortex but may be overlooked when sited in the nondilated renal pelvis. Calculi lying in the focal plane of the transducer produce an acoustic shadow, allowing easier identification. The bladder should be assessed and the presence of a ureterocele, trabeculation, residual urine or calculus identified. In posterior urethral valves, a dilated posterior urethra may be detected and examination of this area via a perineal approach is of value (Cremin & Aaronson 1983). Primary renal tumors, the most common being a nephroblastoma, are initially assessed with ultrasound where the size, shape and staging of the tumor is possible. Extension into the inferior vena cava is well demonstrated with ultrasound.

Doppler ultrasound of the renal vessels is of value in the diagnosis of renal artery stenosis where changes in spectral tracings are seen at the site of stenosis and the poststenotic area. The technique is also of value in the assessment of post-transplant patients and in the estimation of renal vein patency in renal vein thrombosis. In hemolytic uremic syndrome, decreased flow in diastole is commonly seen in the active stages of the disease. Improvement in the RI usually precedes clinical recovery.

Intravenous urography

The requirement for this examination has decreased with the advances in US and radioisotope scanning. The indications are in the further evaluation of confusing results or for further imaging of an abnormality detected on ultrasound (Fig. 36.22). The technique may be required for further delineation of ureteric detail and assessment of minor congenital abnormalities.

In children under 2 years no preparation is required and in particular, dehydration is to be avoided. Nonionic contrast media

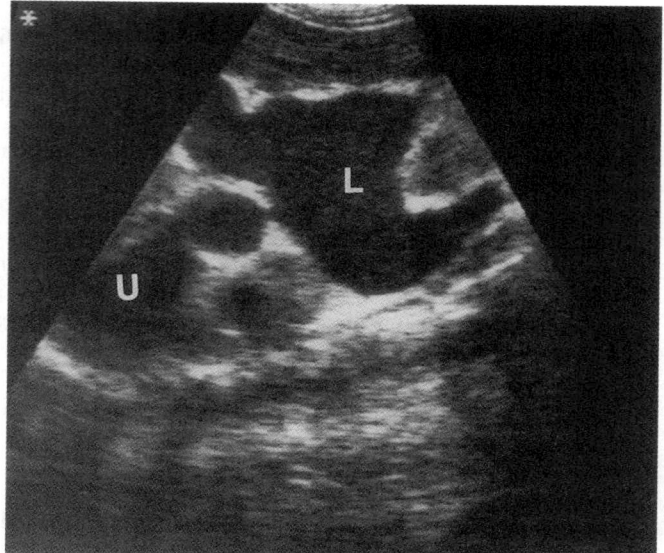

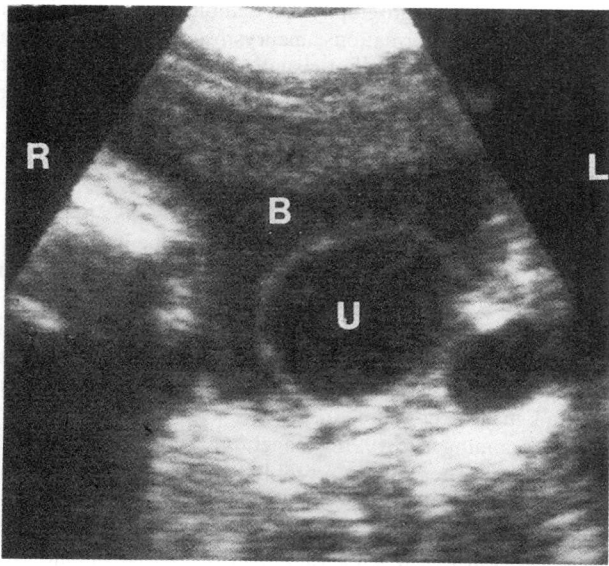

(a)

(b)

Fig. 36.21 Ultrasound examination of complicated duplex kidney. (**a**) Sagittal ultrasound section of duplex kidney. Dilated upper (U) and lower (L) pelves. Upper was associated with obstructing ureterocele demonstrated in Fig. 36.21(b). The lower moiety was dilated due to reflux. (**b**) Transverse ultrasound of the bladder demonstrating ureterocele (U – ureterocele, B – bladder, R – right, L – left).

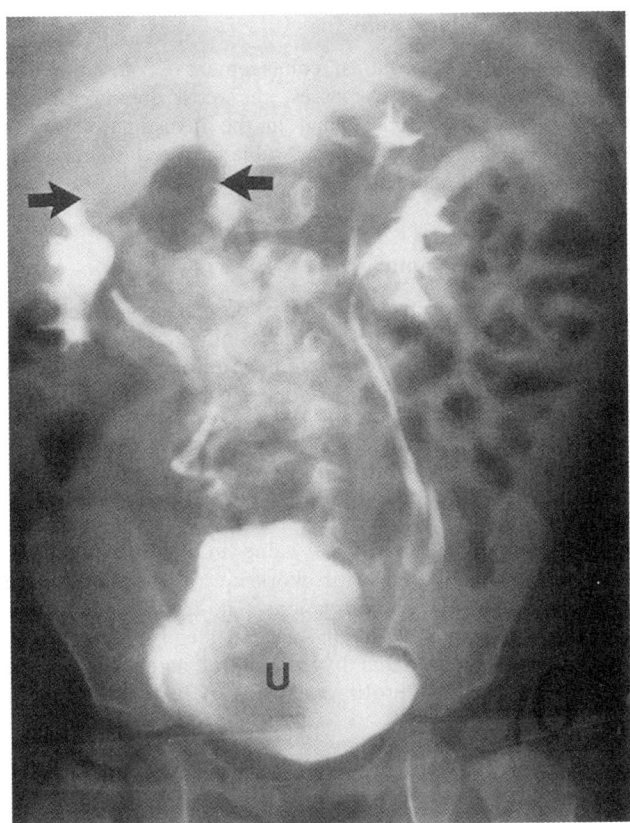

Fig. 36.22   Intravenous urogram in a child with bilateral duplex kidneys; note nonfunctioning right upper moiety causing lateral deviation of lower moiety pelvis (arrows). Filling defect noted in the bladder representing ureterocele (U) associated with the right upper moiety.

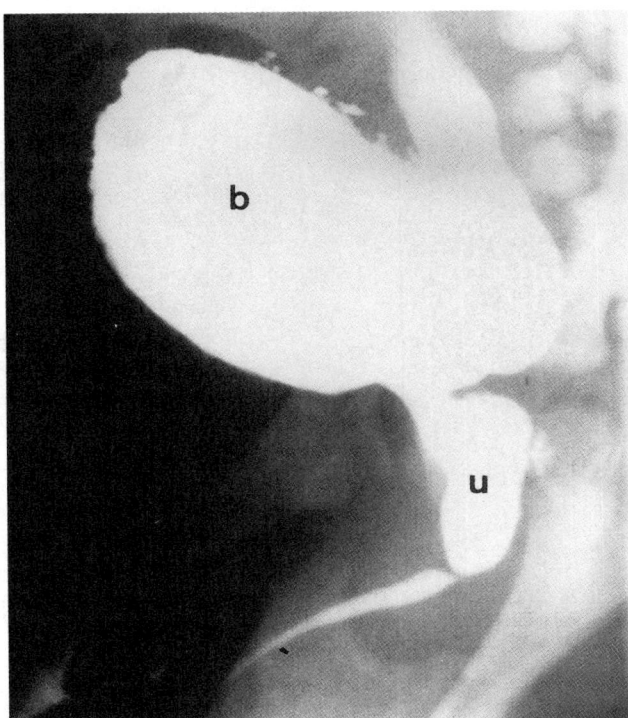

Fig. 36.23   MCU in a child with posterior urethral valves. Note trabeculated bladder (b) and dilated posterior urethra (u); associated vesicoureteric reflux is present.

should be used in a concentration of 300 mg iodine/ml. The standard dose is 2–3 ml/kg up to a maximum of 50 ml. Following an initial plain film a 15-minute full-length film of the renal tract often suffices for the examination. An early 5-minute film in the nephrogram phase may be helpful in determining the presence of renal scarring. Delayed prone films may be indicated in the presence of obstruction. Lateral or oblique films or spot films under fluoroscopic control may occasionally be helpful.

Micturating cystourethrography

The most common indication for MCU is usually in the investigation of urinary tract infection when reflux is suspected in a child less than 2 years of age. The examination is also indicated in those children found to have a dilated urinary tract on ultrasound. Vesicoureteric reflux is graded according to severity (Levitt 1981), significant reflux being that reaching the kidney. Other indications for cystography include a child with a poor urinary stream and where abnormalities of the urethra are suspected (Fig. 36.23).

Sedation is rarely required. Under sterile conditions a fine feeding tube is inserted into the bladder. If severe reflux is demonstrated during the procedure then the child should be started on antibiotics. The study is a dynamic process and a video recording of micturition with appropriate spot films is necessary. The configuration, shape and function of the bladder can be

assessed and the presence of urethral abnormalities, valves, diverticula or strictures noted in addition to vesicoureteric reflux. Girls may be examined supine but to demonstrate the urethra boys must be rotated into an oblique or lateral position.

Nuclear medicine studies

Technetium 99m DMSA (dimercaptosuccinic acid) is taken up by the proximal renal tubules and demonstrates the presence of functional renal tissue. It can be used to identify ectopic renal tissue and to assess horseshoe kidneys. It is particularly valuable in the work-up of the child with a urinary tract infection as it is the most sensitive method of detecting renal scarring (Fig. 36.24) (Gordon 1993). Areas of reduced uptake of the radionuclide will be found in over 20% of children with acute pyelonephritis and animal studies have demonstrated that these areas progress to scarring in the absence of adequate treatment. DMSA scanning can thus be used to highlight the 'at risk' kidney.

Technetium 99m DTPA (diethylenetriamine penta-acetic acid) is filtered by the glomeruli and time–activity renogram curves can be obtained which demonstrate abnormalities in uptake and excretion. Technetium 99m MAG3 (mercaptoacetyltriglycine) is primarily excreted by the proximal convoluted tubules although about 10% is filtered through the glomeruli. Its main advantage over DTPA is its superior image quality and its lower radiation dose. It is more difficult to prepare and is more expensive. These radionuclides are of value in the assessment of reflux in the cooperative toilet-trained child (indirect radionuclide cystogram). Reflux is identified by the presence of increased activity in the kidneys during micturition (Fig. 36.25). The technique is as

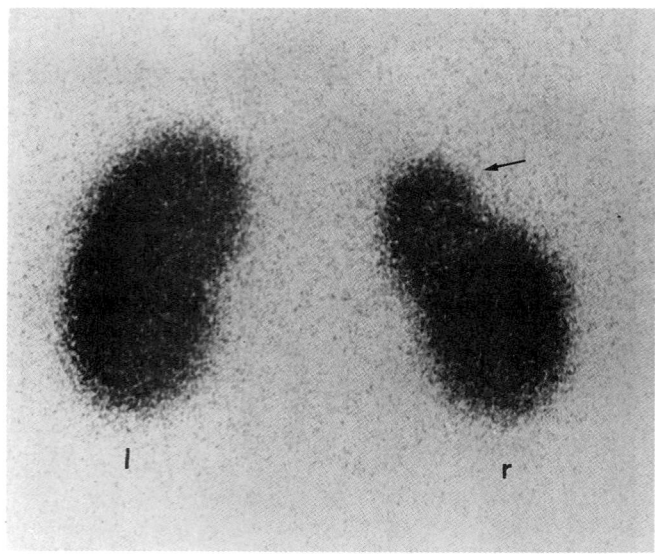

Fig. 36.24   Technetium 99m DMSA isotope scan of the kidney. This 2-hour scan reveals decreased uptake in the upper pole of the right kidney compatible with scarring (arrow).

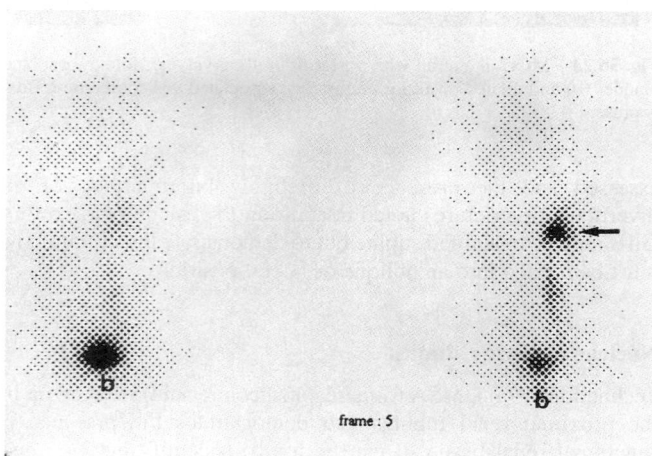

Fig. 36.25   Indirect study of vesicoureteric reflux using technetium 99m MAG3. On voiding isotope activity is seen to extend from the bladder (b) into the right kidney (arrow).

accurate as the micturating cystogram but involves significantly less radiation. In the younger child a direct isotope cystogram can be performed using technetium pertechnetate. The technique is extremely sensitive, involves a very low radiation dose but does not provide anatomical detail of the urethra.

Both DTPA and MAG3 can be used in the diagnosis of renal obstruction. A standard renogram study is performed initially and if the renogram curves are failing to fall by 20 minutes, intravenous frusemide is given to produce a diuresis. The renogram curve will fall rapidly with a time to half counts of less than 5 minutes in the presence of a dilated, nonobstructed system. The curve will be flat or continue to rise in the presence of obstruction. Unfortunately in a fairly large number of children there will be slow response to frusemide and here a retrograde or antegrade study may be helpful.

Computerized tomography

This technique with contrast enhancement is of value in the staging of primary renal masses, the most common being a Wilms' tumor (Fig. 36.26), and in the investigation of renal trauma. However, CT is of little value in the vast majority of urinary tract abnormalities.

Retrograde pyelography

This technique is useful in complex problems, particularly the anatomical demonstration of nonfunctioning duplex kidneys and the assessment of ureteric strictures. Retrograde or antegrade pyelography can be used to exclude mechanical obstruction in dilated systems where the use of renography is inconclusive.

Angiography

This technique is primarily of value in the investigation of hypertension following prior work-up of the patient with ultrasound and isotope investigations. The technique will reveal accurately the presence of renal arterial stenosis, segmental or main branch, fibromuscular hyperplasia or aortic abnormalities such as narrowing in neurofibromatosis and Takayasu's disease.

RETROPERITONEAL ABNORMALITIES

Investigation of the retroperitoneum will be required in primary adrenal gland masses, i.e. adenomas and carcinomas which commonly present with virilization. Other tumors include ganglioneuromas and neuroblastomas or cystic lesions, abscess or hemorrhage related to the gland. Storage diseases such as Wolman's disease are uncommon. Primary retroperitoneal tumors include neurogenic masses, teratomas, lymphomas and rhabdomyosarcomas. Masses may also arise secondary to vertebral abnormalities such as osteomyelitis and primary vertebral neoplasms.

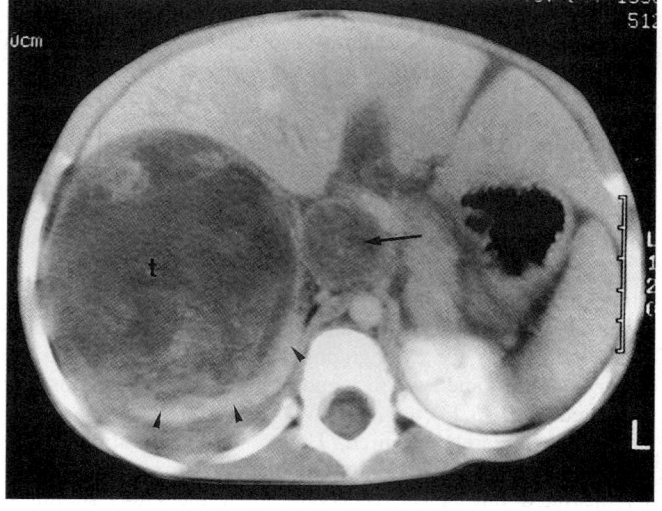

Fig. 36.26   Contrast-enhanced CT of the abdomen. Large Wilms' tumor (t) arising from and destroying the right kidney (arrow heads). Extension of the tumor into the IVC (long arrow).

Plain radiographs

The basic imaging methods include plain abdominal films to visualize any calcification in the mass and identify secondary erosions in the vertebral bodies or fat or bone content in a teratoma.

Ultrasonic imaging

Ultrasonic imaging will clearly demonstrate a mass greater than 1.5 cm, but often fails to depict spread into the retroperitoneal structures, particularly if the lesion is calcified or hidden by bowel gas. In adrenal hemorrhage the history, changing ultrasonic pattern from sonolucent to echogenic or vice versa associated with a decrease in size obviates the need for further radiological assessment (Fig. 36.27).

Computerized tomography scanning

CT scanning is useful for the deliniation of retroperitoneal masses if MRI is not available. Calcification within the mass and associated abnormalities of the vertebrae are well demonstrated. Hemorrhage into the psoas muscle in hemophilia is well demonstrated.

Magnetic resonance imaging

MRI is now the modality of choice for the demonstration of retroperitoneal and paraspinal abnormalities. Encroachment of infection or tumor into the spinal canal is demonstrated without the need for myelographic contrast. Tissue contrast is superior to that achieved with CT, increasing sensitivity in the detection of abnormalities and allowing accurate staging of tumors (Fig. 36.28). Follow-up scans can assess response to therapy. Marrow

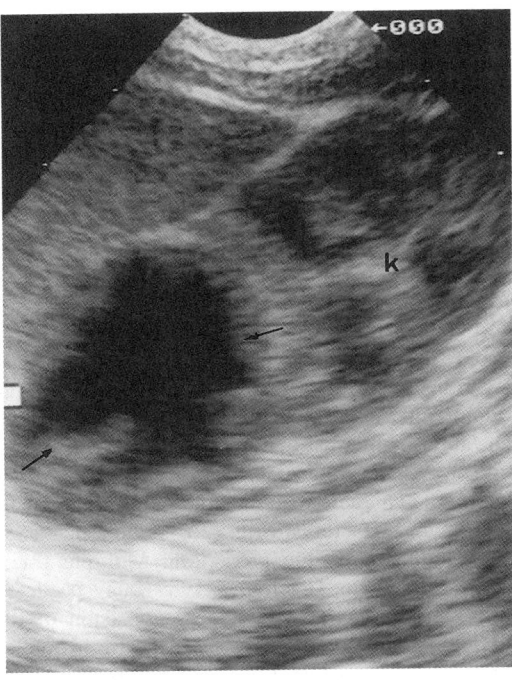

Fig. 36.27 Sagittal ultrasound scan through the right kidney showing a hypoechoic area in the right suprarenal gland. This represents an adrenal hemorrhage (arrows) (k – kidney).

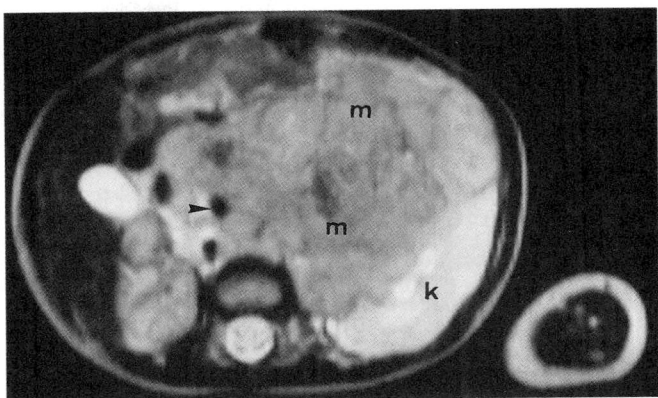

Fig. 36.28 T2-weighted axial MRI scan of the abdomen. This reveals a large medium signal mass invading the left kidney and extending across the midline and wrapping around the inferior vena cava and aorta. The appearances are of a neuroblastoma (m – mass, k – kidney, arrow – aorta).

abnormalities in the spine due to infection, tumor or abnormal hemopoiesis can be appreciated.

Nuclear medicine studies

Bone scintigraphy using 99m technetium methylene diphosphonate is more sensitive than conventional radiography in the detection of bony metastatic disease, the deposits usually being identified as areas of increased uptake of the radionuclide. Neuroblastoma and rhabdomyosarcoma frequently metastasize to bone. Two-thirds of children with neuroblastoma will show uptake of the bone scanning agent in the primary soft tissue tumor.

Meta-iodobenzylguanidine (MIBG) is a synthetic neurotransmitter analog with uptake and storage similar to that of noradrenaline. It can be linked to ^{131}I or ^{123}I and used in the detection of neural crest tumors such as neuroblastoma and pheochromocytoma. More than 90% of neuroblastomas are able to concentrate MIBG although this figure falls markedly if there is a delay in performing the initial scan. [123]I MIBG shows maximal tumor uptake at around 48 hours and can be used for therapeutic purposes, either following standard chemotherapy or at the time of the initial diagnosis.

The somatostatin analog octreotide gives similar uptake to MIBG in patients with neuroblastoma or pheochromocytoma but its uptake is superior in other neuroendocrine tumors.

Gallium scanning can be used in the initial staging and follow-up of children with Hodgkin's and non-Hodgkin's lymphoma. It has greater specificity than CT scanning in the diagnosis of residual disease.

GENITAL SYSTEM

The uterus, ovaries and vagina can be clearly assessed using ultrasound. This is dependent on visualization through a fluid-filled bladder. The developing ovary contains multiple follicles (Fig. 36.29). Charts are available for normal ovarian and uterine sizes in relation to age (Salardi et al 1985). The technique can thus be used to assess the internal organs in intersex states, precocious or delayed puberty and chromosomal abnormalities.

Uterine growth and vaginal mucosal thickness can be measured and related to hormone therapy. The presence of foreign bodies in

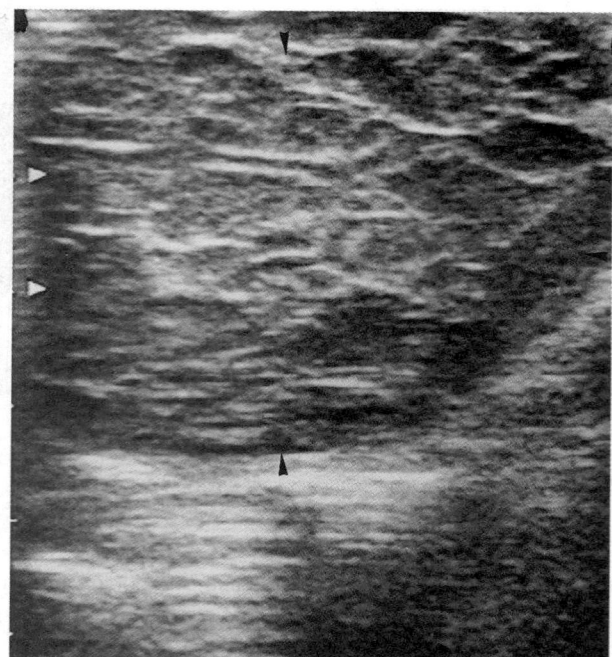

Fig. 36.29 Sagittal ultrasound section through the lower abdomen of a neonate showing a multiloculate cystic mass representing a torted ovary (arrow heads).

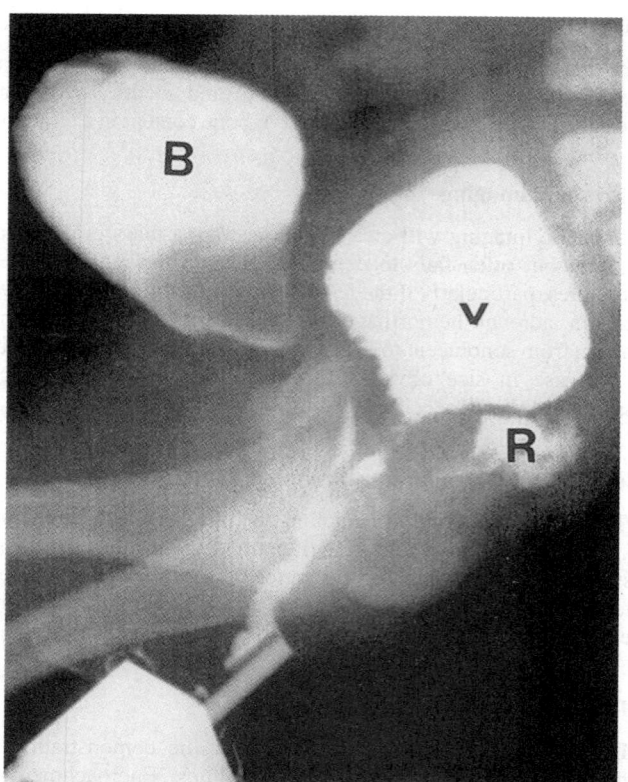

Fig. 36.30 Genitogram demonstrating persistent urogenital sinus with opening of the bladder (B), vagina (V) and rectum (R) into a common chamber.

the vagina as a cause of discharge can also be diagnosed. The imaging of ovarian and pelvic abnormalities may be improved by transvaginal ultrasound, but this is not normally performed in pediatric practice.

The imaging of cloacal and urogenital sinus abnormalities requires the technique of genitography where water-soluble contrast is injected into the perineal orifice followed by relevant radiographs (Fig. 36.30).

The scrotum and inguinal canal can be examined using a 7–10 MHz linear probe and abnormalities such as hydrocele, undescended testis, patent processus vaginalis, cyst of the spermatic cord and inguinal hernia demonstrated. When the clinical presentation is pain and swelling differentiation between epididymitis (swollen epididymis with increased color Doppler flow signals) and testicular torsion (swollen testis with absent Doppler flow signals) can be made reliably (Luker & Siegel 1994). Following trauma to the scrotum the testes can be examined for rupture. Torted appendix of Morgagni also causes pain and swelling and can usually be recognized as a cystic lesion with surrounding increased Doppler signals. Varicoceles occur rarely in children but can be recognized as multiple vascular channels with increased blood flow.

MRI is now being recognized as a multiplanar modality to image the uterus and ovaries. The technique can also be used to locate the position of undescended testis, most of which tend to be located high in the inguinal canal.

SKELETAL SYSTEM

Plain radiographs

The commonest indication for radiography is in the assessment of trauma. It is important to include the joints at both ends of the bone being examined and to have two views at right angles to each other. Greenstick fractures are common in childhood and can be recognized by kinks in the cortex with or without significant deformity. Undisplaced spiral fractures of the tibia are common in toddlers. The diagnosis may only be made on a follow-up film at least 7 days following the trauma. Periosteal reaction is present and the fracture line may be visible. Requests for radiography in trauma should be vetted to prevent inappropriate examinations in trivial trauma; this is particularly likely in minor skull, spine and chest injuries.

Views of the elbow with its six ossification centers are particularly difficult for inexperienced clinicians to interpret but a comparison view of the other elbow should rarely be necessary if the films are reviewed promptly by a pediatric radiologist. A range of normal films retained in the casualty department may be helpful. Plain films in osteomyelitis may be normal for several days after abnormalities are detectable by nuclear medicine, ultrasound or MRI. Nonaccidental injury to infants can be recognized by the characteristic metaphyseal fractures which can appear as 'corner' fractures (Fig. 36.31) or 'bucket handle' fractures depending upon the projection. Multiple fractures in various stages of healing (Kleinman 1987) may be detected on skeletal survey. Rib fractures due to compression of the chest characteristically occur posteriorly where the rib is bent over the tip of the transverse process or in the midaxillary line. Skull fractures and subdural collections may be found. MRI is proving to be the most valuable technique in that dating of subdural and extradural hemorrhages is possible (Fig. 36.32). A skeletal survey

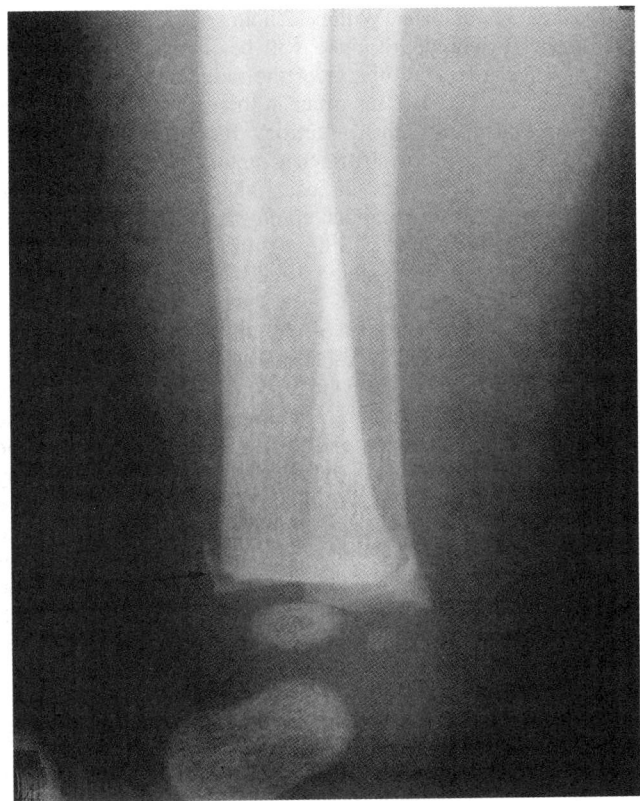

Fig. 36.31 Nonaccidental injury. Lateral view of the tibia and fibula demonstrating the typical corner fractures at the lower end of the tibia (arrow) and soft tissue swelling anterior to the tibia.

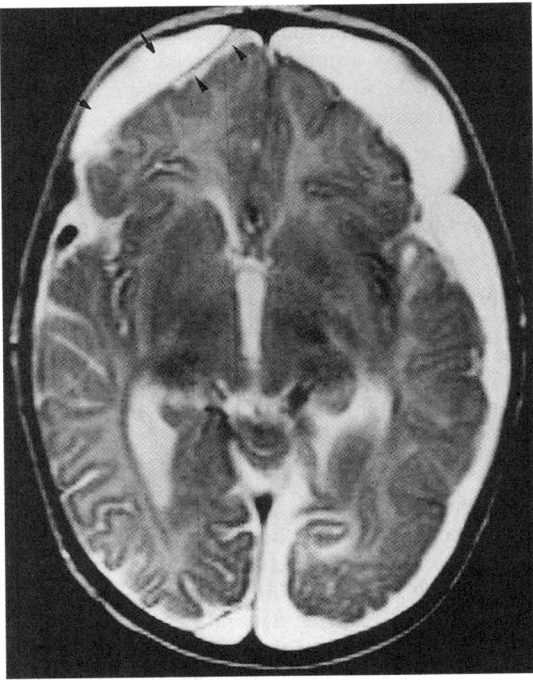

Fig. 36.32 Axial T2-weighted MRI scan of the brain of a child suffering nonaccidental injury. Increased signal in the subdural space (long arrows) and subarachnoid space (arrow heads) indicate areas of hemorrhage.

should include AP and lateral skull, lateral spine, chest, pelvis and AP limb X-rays. Coned views of the knee, ankle, elbow and wrist joints may be required to confirm minor metaphyseal fractures.

Skeletal survey is also performed in the assessment of bone dysplasias. The abnormality may be localized to the diaphyseal, metaphyseal or epiphyseal areas of the bones and may involve the spine. The survey for dysplasia need only include the limbs on one side of the body. Surveys for malignant disease are particularly useful in Langerhans' histiocytosis when the isotope scan may be unremarkable. In metabolic disease including rickets, hyperparathyroidism and lead poisoning a film of one wrist or knee is usually adequate for diagnosis and follow-up. Endocrine abnormalities may result in abnormal delay or advancement in bone age. This is usually assessed from a radiograph of the left hand and wrist by comparison with standards (Greulich & Pyle 1984) or by computation of a score using specific criteria (Tanner et al 1983).

Under 1 year of age the bone maturation may be assessed by counting the epiphyseal centers on one side of the body (Elgenmark 1946) or from assessment of the size and shape of the knee and foot epiphyses.

Plain films of the hip in Perthes disease may show flattening of the epiphysis, but in the early stages subarticular lucency is usually only demonstrated on the frog leg lateral film. The view is also invaluable in the diagnosis of slipped femoral capital epiphysis, particularly if the slip has been predominantly posterior.

Back pain in children is a significant symptom and should be taken seriously. Plain spinal radiographs are useful in the detection of trauma, congenital abnormalities including hemivertebrae, fused vertebrae and scoliosis. Discitis is represented by a narrow disc space with eventual destruction of the vertebral body end plates. Radioisotope scanning using ^{99m}Tc phosphate compounds is more sensitive in detecting the abnormality early when plain films may be normal. MRI will clearly depict changes in the disc space and vertebral body marrow (Fig. 36.33). The defects of spondylosis and spondylolisthesis may be detected on plain X-ray but are elegantly demonstrated on CT (Fig. 36.34). Secondary changes due to spinal canal masses or paraspinal masses, e.g. in neuroblastoma, may produce pedicle erosion. Many bone dysplasias, metabolic abnormalities and tumors have abnormalities revealed on plain radiographs. These include inferior beaking of the vertebral body in Hurler's syndrome, central and anterior beaking in spondyloepiphyseal dysplasia and vertebra plana in histiocytosis X. Multiple vertebral body collapse and generalized osteoporosis are found in neuroblastoma and leukemia.

Imaging of the spinal cord is now performed with MRI and myelography is rarely indicated. Plain films may be helpful in the immediate assessment of major spinal trauma, supplemented with CT if fractures and/or dislocation are suspected.

Nuclear medicine studies

Technetium 99m diphosphonate compounds (usually methylene diphosphonate – MDP) are used in the investigation of bone disorders including infection, trauma, tumors and avascular necrosis. Uptake of the radionuclide is dependent on blood flow and osteoblastic activity. A triple bone scan is usually performed when osteomyelitis is suspected and consists of a blood flow study followed immediately by a blood pool study with static

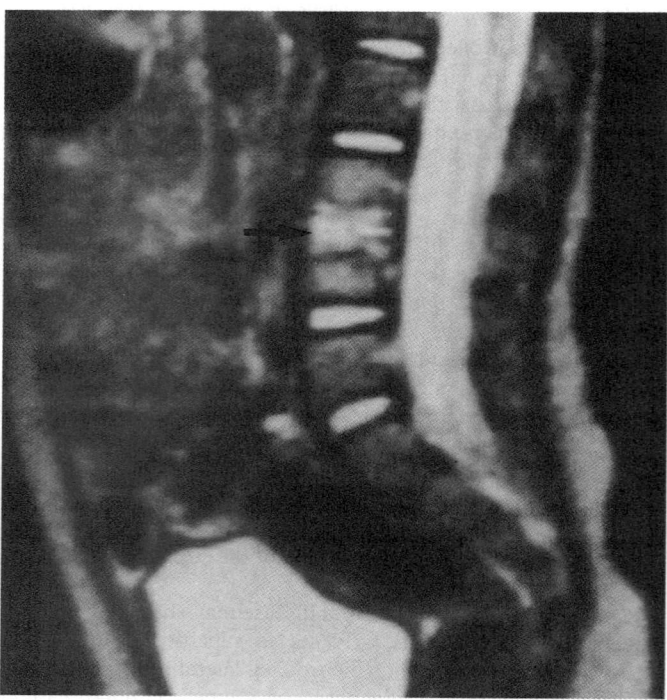

Fig. 36.33 Sagittal T2-weighted MRI scan of the spinal cord and vertebrae. This demonstrates increased signal in the L3–L4 vertebral bodies and a higher signal in the intervening disc space (arrow). Appearances are diagnostic of discitis.

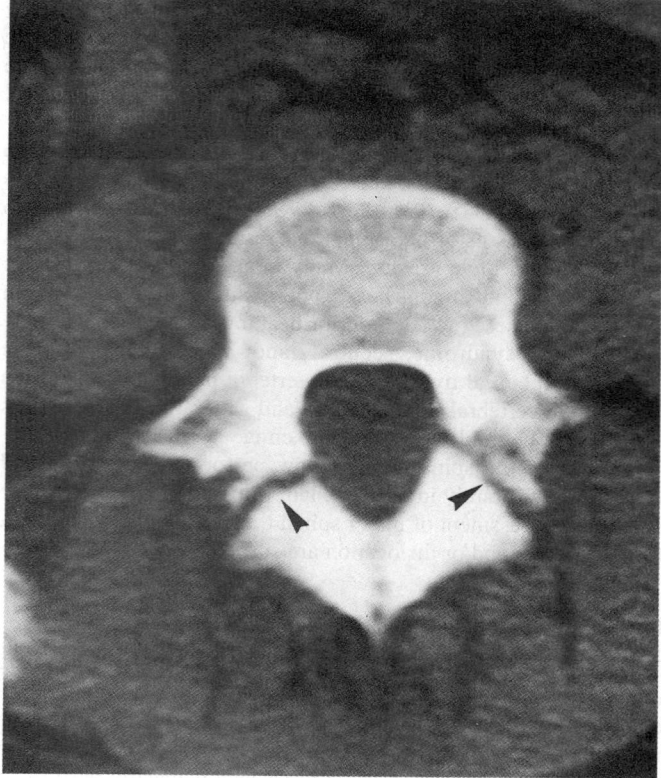

Fig. 36.34 Axial CT scan through the spine at the L5 level, bilateral spondylolisis defects in the pars interarticularis (arrows).

images some 3 hours later. Within 12 hours of the development of symptoms of osteomyelitis there will be increased blood flow, hyperemia and increased uptake of the radionuclide on the later pictures. False-negative scans occur in the neonate or when there is a particularly virulent infection. Increased blood flow, hyperemia, with a more diffuse late uptake may occur with a septic arthritis. In Perthes disease, where there is avascular necrosis of the femoral capital epiphysis, an area of reduced uptake of the radionuclide will be identified (cold area). A bone scan may detect unsuspected fractures in a child with nonaccidental injury.

Bone scintigraphy can be of value in the diagnosis and localization of benign lesions such as osteoid osteoma. It plays an important role in the assessment of bony metastatic disease in children with neuroblastoma, rhabdomyosarcoma, osteogenic sarcoma, Ewing's sarcoma and histiocytosis and should be routinely performed in the work-up of these children. Bony metastatic disease occurs less frequently with other tumors and a bone scan should only be performed in these children if they are experiencing bone pain, e.g. lymphoma, leukemia, or if the tumor has seeded into the spinal canal, e.g. medulloblastoma, ependymoma. Pulmonary metastatic deposits in a child with osteogenic sarcoma may show up as 'hot areas' in the lungs.

Magnetic resonance imaging

MRI scanning with its excellent contrast definition is the best modality to demonstrate the extent of intraosseous and extraosseous spread of primary bone tumors, though CT is used to detect lung metastases. A knowledge of the normal variations in T1 and T2 signals of marrow related to age is essential (Moore & Dawson 1990). Detailed information on marrow abnormalities is crucial when contemplating reconstructive surgery with prostheses. MRI will also assess marrow abnormalities in other tumors such as neuroblastoma and leukemia. The extent of osteomyelitis can be accurately assessed, usually showing a decreased T1 signal and high T2 signal in the acute stages. MRI demonstrates ischemic change in Perthes disease and sickle cell disease.

Computerized tomography scanning

The role of CT in tumor staging has been superseded by MRI. CT can be useful in trauma of the spine or pelvis to demonstrate small displaced fragments of bone. Limited CT can be used to investigate suspected rotatory subluxation of the atlantoaxial joint (Fig. 36.35). CT measurement of leg lengths and hip anteversion can be performed with low dose techniques (Fig. 36.36).

Ultrasound

Ultrasound examination of the infant hip is now well established as the method of choice in the investigation of developmental delay of the hip. It can be performed up to the age of 6 months after which ossification of the femoral head obscures acetabular detail. It allows assessment of the acetabular morphology which can be graded according to Graf (Graf 1984) or using the dynamic study of Harcke (1984). Stability can be assessed by stressing the hip during the ultrasound examination and observing the movement of the femoral head relative to the acetabulum (Fig.

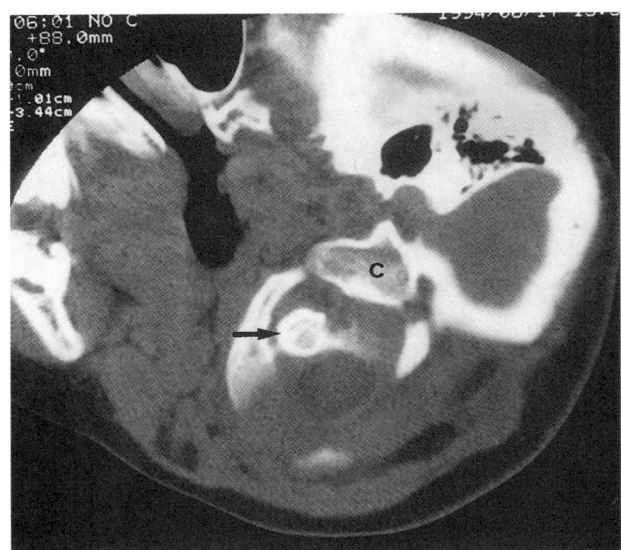

Fig. 36.35 Axial CT showing rotatory dislocation of C1 on CT following a road traffic accident. Note odontoid peg (arrow) and rotated C1 (c).

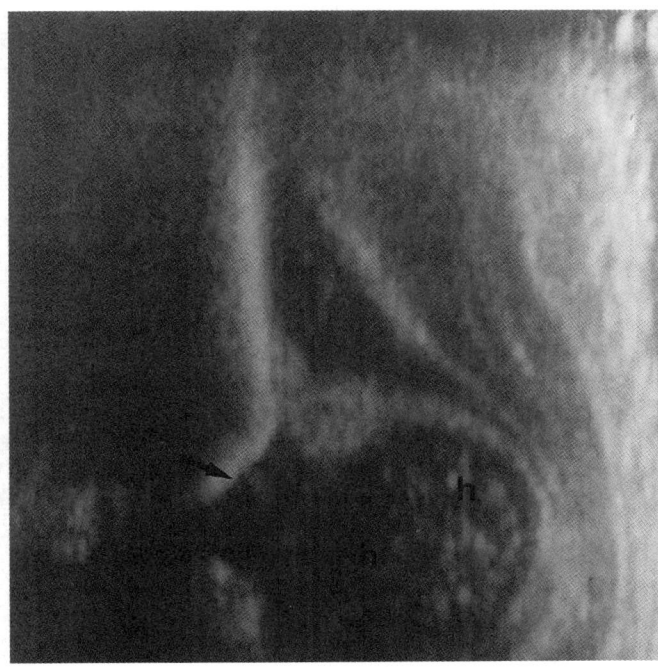

Fig. 36.37 Coronal ultrasound sections of a dislocated left hip. Note steep acetabular angle (short arrow) and displaced femoral head (h). Long arrows depict space between the femoral head and medial acetabular margin.

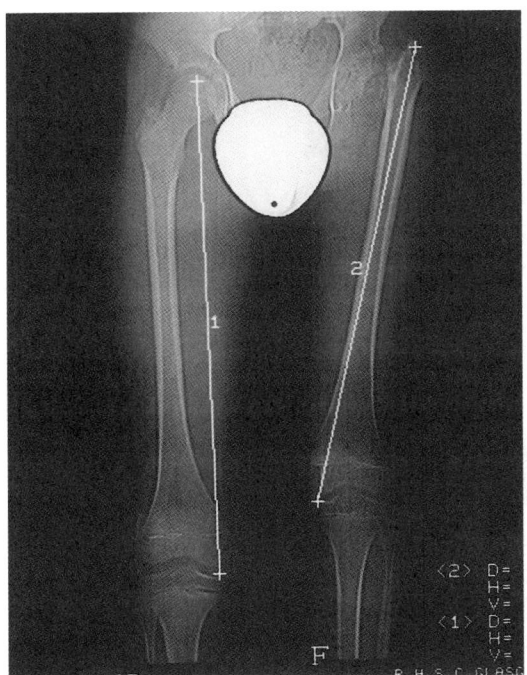

Fig. 36.36 The use of a CT scanogram in estimating leg length. Note destruction of the left femoral head. This was secondary to a septic arthritis.

36.37). Increasingly treatment is influenced by the ultrasound examination rather than dictated by clinical features alone.

Ultrasound can assess the presence and size of effusion in the painful hip and guide aspiration if clinically indicated (Miralles et al 1989) (Fig. 36.38). Soft tissue masses can be assessed using ultrasound which can identify lymph node enlargement, abscess formation, lipomata, cystic hygromas and popliteal cysts without the need for further investigation. Other soft tissue masses may require biopsy for identification and this can be guided by ultrasound. Early osteomyelitis can be diagnosed with ultrasound, demonstrating the presence of soft tissue edema and subperiosteal fluid (Fig. 36.39) before abnormalities can be demonstrated on plain radiographs.

Acknowledgments

We wish to thank Dr Ruth Mackenzie, Consultant Radiologist, Royal Hospital for Sick Children, Glasgow, for her contribution to the nuclear medicine sections.

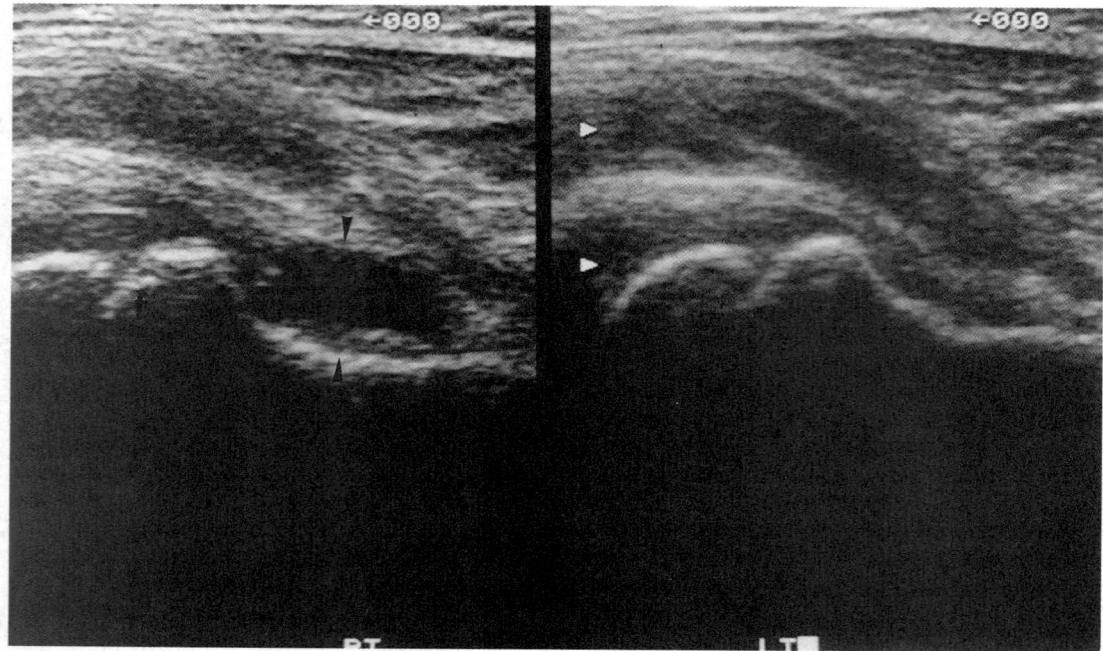

Fig. 36.38   Sagittal ultrasound scan of the right and left hips. Fluid distention of the right hip joint space (arrows) (f – femur).

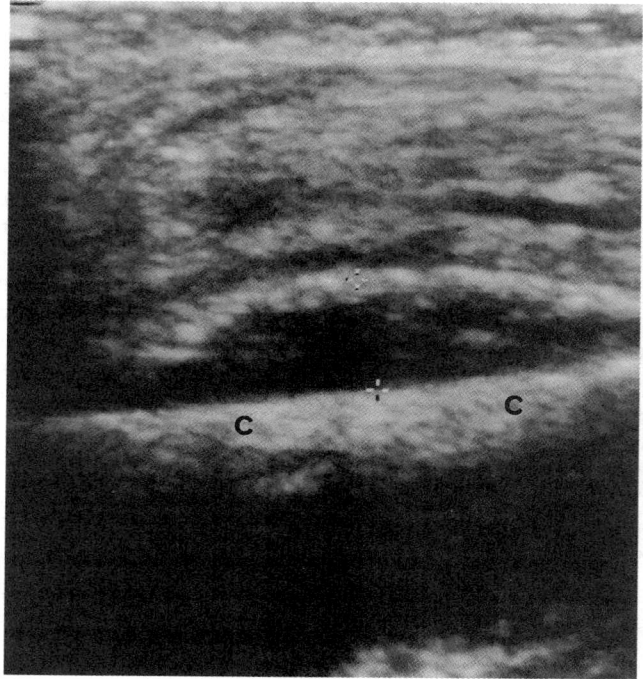

Fig. 36.39   Sagittal ultrasound of the distal tibia showing a subperiosteal edematous collection (crosses) (c – cortex of tibia).

REFERENCES

Ambrosino M M, Genieser K J, Roche A, Kaul A, Lawrence M 1994 Feasibility of high resolution low dose chest CT in evaluating the paediatric chest. Pediatric Radiology 24: 6–10

American Academy of Pediatrics, Committee on Drugs 1988 Guidelines for monitoring and management of pediatric patients during and after sedation for diagnostic and therapeutic procedures. Pediatrics 89: 1110–1115

Babcock D S, Han B K, Dine M S 1988 Sonographic findings in infants with macrocrania. American Journal of Roentgenology 150: 1359–1365

Babcock D S, Patriquin H, Lafortune M, Dauzat M 1996 Power Doppler sonography: basic principles and clinical applications in children. Pediatric Radiology 26: 109–115

Balthazar E J, Freeny P C, van Sonnenberg E 1994 Imaging and intervention in acute pancreatitis. Radiology 193: 297–306

Barkovich A J, Truwit C L 1990 Brain damage from perinatal asphyxia: correlation of MR findings with gestational age. American Journal of Neuroradiology 11: 1087–1096

Byrd S E, Osborn R E, Bohan T P, Naidich T P 1989a The CT and MR evaluation of migrational disorders of the brain. Part I. Lissencephaly and pachygyria. Pediatric Radiology 19: 151–156

Byrd S E, Osborn R E, Bohan T P, Naidich T P 1989b The CT and MR evaluation of migrational disorders of the brain. Part II. Schizencephaly heterotopia and polymicrogyria. Pediatric Radiology 19: 219–222

Charron M, Orenstein S R, Bhargava S 1994 Detection of inflammatory bowel disease in paediatric patients with Tc 99m HMPAO labelled leukocytes. Journal of Nuclear Medicine 35: 451–455

Christophe C, Clercx A, Blum D, Hasaert S D, Segebarth C, Perlmuter N 1994 Early MR detection of cortical and subcortical hypoxic ischaemic encephalopathy in full term infants. Pediatric Radiology 24: 581–584

Cremin B J, Aaronson I A 1983 Ultrasonic diagnosis of posterior urethral valves in neonates. British Journal of Radiology 56: 435–438

Darnman B C, Hoffer F A, Rand F F, O'Rourke E J 1992 Osteomyelitis in children. Gadolinium enhanced MR imaging. Radiology 182: 743–748

De Vries L S, Dubowitz L M S, Pennock J M, Bydder G M 1989 Extensive cystic leucomalacia: correlation of cranial ultrasound, magnetic resonance imaging and clinical findings in sequential studies. Clinical Radiology 40: 158–166

Elgenmark O 1946 The normal development of the ossific centres during infancy and childhood. Acta Paediatrica Scandinavica (suppl 1): 33

Floodmark O, Lupton B, Li D et al 1989 MR imaging of periventricular leukomalacia in childhood. American Journal of Roentgenology 152: 583–590

Friedland J A, Herman T, Siegel M J 1995 Escherichia: 0157–H7–associated haemolytic uraemic syndrome. Value of colonic colour doppler sonography. Pediatric Radiology 25: S65–S67

Goh D, Minns R A, Hendry G M A, Thambyayah M, Steers A J W 1992 Cerebrovascular resistive index assessed by duplex doppler sonography and its relationship to intra-cranial pressure in infantile hydrocephalus. Pediatric Radiology 22: 246–250

Gordon I 1993 Effect of nuclear medicine on paediatric imaging. British Journal of Radiology 66: 971–985

Graf R 1984 Fundamentals of sonographic diagnosis of the infant hip. Journal of Paediatric Orthopaedics 4: 735–741

Grainger R G 1984 Low osmolar contrast media. British Medical Journal 289: 144–145

Greulich W W, Pyle S I 1984 Radiographic atlas of skeletal development of the hand and wrist, 2nd edn. Stanford University Press, California

Gu L, Alton D J, Daneman A, Stringer D A, Liu P, Wilmot D M, Reilly B J 1988 Intussusception reduction in children with rectal insufflation of air. American Journal of Roentgenology 150: 1345–1348

Gyll C, Blake N S 1986 The neonatal abdomen. Paediatric diagnostic imaging. Heinemann, London, p 70

Harcke H T 1984 Examination of the infant hip with real time ultrasonography. Journal of Ultrasound Medicine 4: 131–137

Horgan J G, Rumack C M, Hay T, Manco-Johnson M L, Merenstein G B, Esola C 1989 Absolute intracranial blood flow velocities evaluated by duplex doppler sonography in symptomatic preterm and term neonates. American Journal of Roentgenology 152: 1059–1064

Hubbard A M, Marcovich R I, Kimmel B, Kroger M, Barkto M B 1992 Sedation for paediatric patients undergoing CT/MRI. Journal of Computerized Axial Tomography 16: 3–6

Jaramillo D, Hoffer F A, Shapiro F, Rand F 1990 MRI imaging of fractures of the growth plate. American Journal of Roentgenology 155: 1261–1265

Kenny I J, Lutkin J E 1989 A pressure valve for pneumonic reduction of intussusception. British Journal of Radiology 62: 497–498

Kleinman P K 1987 Diagnostic imaging of child abuse. Williams and Wilkins, Baltimore

Kuhn J P 1993 High resolution CT of paediatric pulmonary parenchymal disorders. Radiology Clinics of North America 31: 533–551

Lancet 1989 SPECT and PET in epilepsy. Lancet 1: 135

Leonidas J C, Berdon W E, Baker D H, Santulli T V 1970 Meconium ileus and its complications. American Journal of Roentgenology 130: 598–609

Levitt S B 1981 Medical versus surgical treatment of primary vesico-ureteric reflux. Report of the International Reflux Study Committee. Pediatrics 67: 392–400

Lim H K, Bae S H, Lee K H, Seo GS, Yoon GS 1994 Assessment of the reducibility of ileocoelic intussusception in children: usefulness of colour doppler sonography. Radiology 191: 781–785

Loyer E, Dunne Eggli K 1989 Sonographic evaluation of superior mesenteric vascular relationship in malrotation. Pediatric Radiology 19: 173–175

Luker G D, Siegel M J 1994 Colour doppler sonography of the scrotum in children (pictorial essay). American Journal of Roentgenology 163: 649–655

McDermott V G M, Taylor T, Wyatt J P, Mackenzie S, Hendry G M A 1995 Oro-gastric magnet removal of ingested disc batteries. Journal of Paediatric Sugery 31 29–33

Millar A J W, Rode H, Brown R A, Cywes S 1987 The deadly vomit: malrotation and mid gut volvulus. Paediatric Surgery International 2: 172–176

Miralles M, Gonzalez G, Pulpeiro J R 1989 Sonography of the painful hip in children. 500 consecutive cases. American Journal of Roentgenology 152: 579–582

Moore S G, Dawson K L 1990 Red and yellow marrow in the femur: age related changes in appearance at MR imaging. Radiology 175: 219–223

Naidich D P 1994 Helical CT of the thorax: clinical applications. Radiology Clinics of North America 32: 759–774

Nunan T, O'Doherty M, Croft D 1995 Clinical uses of positron emission tomography. Radiology Now 12: 19–22

Pobiel R S, Bisset J S III 1995 Imaging of liver tumours in the infant and child (pictorial essay). Pediatric Radiology 25: 495–506

Puylaert J B 1986 Acute appendicitis: ultrasound evaluation using graded compression. Radiology 158: 355–360

Rohrschneider W K, Troger T 1995 Hydrostatic reduction of intussusception under ultrasound guidance. Pediatric Radiology 25: 530–534

Royal College of Radiologists 1995 Making the best use of a department of clinical radiology. In: Guidlines for doctors, 3rd edn. RCR, London

Ruess L, Sivit C J, Eichelberger M R, Taylor G A, Bond S J 1995 Blunt hepatic and splenic trauma in children: correlation of a CT injury severity scale with clinical outcome. Pediatric Radiology 25: 321–325

Salardi S, Orsini L F, Cacciari E, Bovicelli L, Tassoni R, Reygiami A 1985 Pelvic ultrasound in premenarchal girls. Relation to puberty and sex hormone concentrations. Archives of Disease in Childhood 60: 120–125

Sato Y, Frey E E, Smith W L, Pringle K C, Soper R T, Franken E A 1988 Balloon dilatation of oesophageal stenosis in children. American Journal of Roentgenology 150: 639–641

Saxton V, Katz M, Phelan M, Beasley S 1995 Intussusception repeat delayed gas enema, increased reduction rate. European Society of Paediatric Radiology Abstracts, Utrecht, p 12

Schneider K, Koh M N, Ernst G, Endemann B, Panzer W, Padovani R, Wall B 1995 A closer look at the European wide survey of the variation in dose and image quality of common x-ray examinations of the 5 year old child. European Society of Paediatric Radiology Abstracts, Utrecht, p 46

Secaf E, Hricak H, Gooding CA et al 1994 Role of MRI in the evaluation of ambiguous genitalia. Pediatric Radiology 24: 231–235

Share J C, Lebowitz R L 1989 Ectopic ureterocele without ureteral and calyceal dilatation. American Journal of Roentgenology 152: 567–571

Shiels W E II, Kirks D R, Keller G L, Ryckman F, Daughery C, Speaker B, Summa D 1993 Colonic perforation by air and liquid enemas comparison study in young pigs. American Journal of Roentgenology 160: 931–935

Siegel M J 1995 Appendicitis in children: ultrasound and diagnosis. Pediatric Surgery International 10: 62–65

Staudt M, Schropp C, Staudt F, Obletter N, Bise K, Breit A, Weinmann H M 1994 MRI assessment of myelinization. An age standardisation. Paediatric Radiology 24: 122–127

Stunden R J, Le Quesne G W, Little K E J 1986 Improved diagnosis of infantile hypertrophic pyloric stenosis. Paediatric Radiology 16: 200–205

Tanner J M, Whitehouse R H, Cameron N, Marshall W A, Healey M J R, Golstein H 1983 Assessment of skeletal maturity and prediction of adult height (TW2 method). Academic Press, London

Towbin R B 1989 Paediatric interventional procedures in the 1980s. A period of development, growth and acceptance. Radiology 170(3): 1081–1091

Verschelden P, Filiatrault N, Garel L, Grignon A, Perreault G, Boisvert J, Dubois J 1992 Intussusception in children: reliability of ultrasound in diagnosis. A prospective study. Radiology 184: 741–744

Veyrac C, Baud C, Couture A 1989 Pericerebral effusion and ultrasound diagnosis. Follow up of 130 cases. Paediatric Radiology 19: 268 (abstract)

Vignault F, Filiatrault D, Brandt M L, Garel L, Grigson A, Ouiment A 1990 Acute appendicitis in children: evaluation with ultrasound. Radiology 176: 501–504

Volle E, Beyer P, Kaufmann H J 1989 Therapeutic approach to ingested button type batteries. Magnetic removal of ingested button type batteries. Paediatric Radiology 19: 114–118

Wells P N T 1987 The safety of diagnostic ultrasound. British Journal of Radiology (suppl 20)

Whitaker R H, Sherwood T 1984 Another look at diagnostic pathways in children with urinary tract infection. British Medical Journal 288: 839–841

White K S 1996 Helical/spiral CT scanning: a paediatric radiology perspective. Pediatric Radiology 26: 5–14

White R H R 1989 Fetal uropathy. British Medical Journal 298: 1408–1409

Winkler P, Helmke K 1989 Major pitfalls in Doppler examination of the cerebral vascular system. Pediatric Radiology 19: 267–268

World Health Organization 1987a Rational use of diagnostic imaging in paediatrics. Technical Report Series 757. HMSO, London

World Health Organization 1987b Unnecessary examinations. In: Rational use of diagnostic imaging in paediatrics. Technical Report Series 757. HMSO, London

37 Biochemical and physiological tables and reference ranges for laboratory tests

N. R. Belton

BIOCHEMICAL AND PHYSIOLOGICAL DATA

The *Système International d'Unités* or SI unit system has been widely adopted in basic sciences and medicine in many countries including the UK and, more recently, the US (American Academy of Pediatrics 1980, 1989). In this chapter reference values are generally given in SI units followed by traditional units. In Tables 37.1, 37.2 and 37.3 a *multiplication factor* has been given for each substance. This is the number by which the values in *traditional units* need to be *multiplied* in order to convert to *SI units* (thus also if the values in *SI units* are divided by this factor, the result will be given in traditional units).

The SI unit of quantity is the mole.

$$\text{Concentration in moles} = \frac{\text{weight in grams}}{\text{molecular weight}}$$

The unit of volume commonly used in clinical biochemistry is the liter. Hence moles/liter or mol/l is the standard unit used in these tables.

Similarly the smaller units are millimoles/l (mmol/l)
micromoles/l (μmol/l)
nanomoles/l (nmol/l)
and picomoles/l (pmol/l)

1 mole	=	10^3 millimoles
1 millimole	=	10^3 micromoles
1 micromole	=	10^3 nanomoles and
1 nanomole	=	10^3 picomoles

EXAMPLES OF CONVERSIONS

Urea has a molecular weight of 60

$$\therefore 180 \text{ mg/100 ml urea} = \frac{180 \times 10}{60} = 30 \text{ mmol/l}$$

(the factor 10 is used to convert from 100 ml to 1 liter).

Glucose has a molecular weight of 180

$$\therefore 90 \text{ mg/100 ml glucose} = \frac{90 \times 10}{180} = 5 \text{ mmol/l}$$

For *univalent* ions the units remain the same if the concentration was previously expressed in mEq/l

e.g. *sodium*   140 mEq/l = 140 mmol/l

For *divalent* ions, e.g. calcium, the old values are divided by two, the valency of calcium

$$\text{i.e.}\quad 5 \text{ mEq/l} = \frac{5}{2} = 2.5 \text{ mmol/l}$$

10 mg/100 ml calcium

$$= \frac{10 \times 10 \text{ (i.e. to convert from 100 ml to 1 liter)}}{40 \text{ (molecular weight of calcium)}} = 25 \text{ mmol/l}$$

Thus
10 mg/100 ml calcium = 5 mEq/l calcium = 2.5 mmol/l

ENZYMES

In serum and other tissues enzymes are always measured by their enzymatic activity alone, and never by absolute quantities of the enzyme. The units in which enzyme activity is expressed vary widely, in many cases depending primarily on the units used by the investigators who first estimated the enzyme clinically.

The International Union of Biochemistry recommended in 1964 that enzyme activities be expressed in international units (IU) where 1 IU is that amount of enzyme which will catalyze the transformation of 1 micromole of substrate per minute. A further unit of enzyme activity is the *Katal* which is that amount of an enzyme which will catalyze the transformation of 1 mole of substrate per second under defined conditions. The Katal is not in common usage.

However, despite this system of units, and because of the range of methods available – which may use different substrates to measure the same enzyme – the clinician should always be aware of the normal range of values relevant to the method used in his hospital. Units/liter or U/l is now in common use.

Table 37.1 Normal blood serum and plasma values

	Traditional units, normal ranges	Multiplication factor	SI units, normal ranges
Acetoacetate plus acetone (serum)	Up to 3.0 mg/100 ml	10	Up to 30 mg/l
Acid phosphatase (serum)	5.0–12.6 U/l 2.8–7.0 King–Armstrong units		
Adrenocorticotropic hormone (ACTH) (plasma)	10–80 g/l		<2–20 mU/l

Alanine aminotransferase (ALT) (glutamic-pyruvic transaminase) (serum)
  Infants
  Children
	
	10–80 U/l
	10–40 U/l
	10–35 spectrophotometric (Wroblewski) units		

Aldolase (serum)	2.6–13.5 U/l 3.5–18.3 Bruns units		

Aldosterone (plasma)
  Infants
  Children
	
	<108 ng/100 ml
	<36 ng/100 ml
		
		27.7
			
			<3000 pmol/l
			<1000 pmol/l

Alkaline phosphatase (ALP) (serum)
  Newborns and infants
  Children
	
	140–1100 U/l
	250–800 U/l
	8–27.5 King-Armstrong units		

Amino acids (serum) (all values are in nonfasting plasma, and may be up to two times higher in neonates; all other amino acid concentrations are normally less than 25 μmol/l)			
Alanine	1.6–4.3 mg/100 ml	112.4	180–480 μmol/l
α-aminobutyrate	0.1–0.4 mg/100 ml	97.1	10–40 μmol/l
Arginine	0.5–2.3 mg/100 ml	57.5	30–130 μmol/l
Asparagine	0.4–1.2 mg/100 ml	75.8	30–90 μmol/l
Aspartate	<2.3 mg/100 ml	75.2	<170 μmol/l
Citrulline	0.4–1.2 mg/100 ml	57.1	20–70 μmol/l
Cystine	0.5–2.6 mg/100 ml	41.7	20–110 μmol/l
Glutamate	<1.9 mg/100 ml	68	<130 μmol/l
Glutamine	7.9–12.3 mg/100 ml	68.4	540–840 μmol/l
Glycine	0.8–2.9 mg/100 ml	133.3	100–390 μmol/l
Histidine	<3.6 mg/100 ml	64.5	<230 μmol/l
Isoleucine	0.3–1.3 mg/100 ml	76.3	20–100 μmol/l
Leucine	0.8–3.0 mg/100 ml	76.3	60–230 μmol/l
Lysine	1.6–4.1 mg/100 ml	68.5	110–280 μmol/l
Methionine	<1.2 mg/100 ml	67.1	<80 μmol/l
Ornithine	0.4–1.3 mg/100 ml	75.8	30–100 μmol/l
Phenylalanine	0.3–2.1 mg/100 ml	60.6	20–130 μmol/l
Proline	1.0–3.2 mg/100 ml	87	90–280 μmol/l
Serine	0.8–3.0 mg/100 ml	95.2	80–290 μmol/l
Taurine	0.1–1.8 mg/100 ml	80	10–140 μmol/l
Threonine	1.0–2.6 mg/100 ml	84	80–220 μmol/l
Tryptophan	0.2–2.0 mg/100 ml	49	10–100 μmol/l
Tyrosine	0.5–1.8 mg/100 ml	55.2	30–100 μmol/l
Valine	1.2–3.9 mg/100 ml	85.5	100–330 μmol/l

α-amino nitrogen (plasma or serum)
  Newborns
  6 weeks–11 years
  (serum values are higher than those in plasma)
	
	3.7–11.7 mg/100 ml
	3.0–7.5 mg/100 ml
		
		0.714
			
			2.6–8.4 mmol/l
			2.1–5.4 mmol/l

Ammonia (blood)
  Newborns (higher in jaundiced and premature infants)
  Infants and older children
	
	90–150 μg/100 ml
	35–80 μg/100 ml
		
		0.587
			
			53–88 μmol/l
			21–47 μmol/l

Amylase (negligible at birth)
  Infants
  Children
	
	<50 U/l
	100–400 U/l
	60–200 Somogyi units		

α₁-antitrypsin (α₁-antiprotease) (serum)	1.8–4.0 g/l	1	1.8–4.0 g/l

Table 37.1 *Cont'd*

	Traditional units, normal ranges	Multiplication factor	SI units, normal ranges
Androstenedione (serum)			
Infants	<86 ng/100 ml	0.035	<3 nmol/l
Post-puberty			
Male	58–230 ng/100 ml		2–8 nmol/l
Female	58–315 ng/100 ml		2–11 nmol/l
Arginine vasopressin (AVP)			
Newborns	<10 pg/ml	1.0	<10 pmol/l
Thereafter	<5 pg/ml		<5 pmol/l
Ascorbic acid (plasma)	0.5–1.5 mg/100 ml	56.8	28–85 µmol/l
Aspartate aminotransferase (AST) (glutamic-oxaloacetic transaminase)			
Newborns	10–75 U/l		
Children	10–45 U/l		
	10–40 spectrophotometric (Karmen) units		
Atrial natriuretic peptide (ANP)			
Newborns	30–150 pg/ml	0.33	10–50 pmol/l
Thereafter	5–35 pg/ml		1.7–11.7 pmol/l
Base excess (blood) (usually below – 2.5 mmol/l in newborn)	+2.5 to –2.5 mEq/l	1.0	+2.5 to –2.5 mmol/l
Bicarbonate or total CO_2 (plasma)			
Newborns	18–23 mEq/l	1.0	18–23 mmol/l
Thereafter	20–26 mEq/l		20–26 mmol/l
Bilirubin, total (serum)			
Cord blood	Up to 2.9 mg/100 ml	17.1	Up to 50 µmol/l
Cord blood (premature infants)	Up to 3.4 mg/100 ml		Up to 58 µmol/l
First 24 h (higher in premature infants)	Up to 6.0 mg/100 ml		Up to 103 µmol/l
2–5 days (in the newborn period virtually all the bilirubin is present as free (unconjugated) bilirubin)	Up to 12 mg/100 ml		Up to 205 µmol/l
After 1 month (mainly unconjugated)	0.1–1.5 mg/100 ml		1.7–26 µmol/l
Blood volume			
At birth	61–100 (mean 78) ml/kg	1.0	61–100 (mean 78) ml/kg
Values increase slightly during 1st week			
Higher values are found in premature infants and when there is delayed clamping of the umbilical cord			
Thereafter values gradually fall towards adult values	53–87 (mean 71) ml/kg		53–87 (mean 71) ml/kg
Body water (expressed as a % of body weight – mean values)			
Total			
At birth	79%		79%
6 months	68%		68%
1 year and thereafter	60%		60%
Extracellular			
At birth	44%		44%
6 months	28%		28%
1 year	26%		26%
Falling gradually thereafter to	20%		20%
Intracellular			
At birth	35%		35%
6 months	38%		38%
1 year	34%		34%
Rising again by 2 years to	40%		40%
Ceruloplasmin (serum, plasma)			
Newborns	0.05–0.2 g/l	6.67	0.3–1.3 µmol/l
Thereafter	0.2–0.4 g/l		1.3–2.7 µmol/l
Calcium (serum)			
Cord blood	9.3–12.2 mg/100 ml	0.25	2.33–3.05 mmol/l
1st week			2.05–3.05 mmol/l
Breast-fed	8.2–12.2 mg/100 ml		1.85–2.75 mmol/l
Bottle-fed	7.4–11.0 mg/100 ml		2.20–2.75 mmol/l
Thereafter	8.8–11.0 mg/100 ml		
(About 40% of the calcium is protein bound, the remainder being ionized or ultrafiltrable. A slightly lower amount, 30–35%, is protein bound in the newborn period)			

Table 37.1 *Cont'd*

	Traditional units, normal ranges	Multiplication factor	SI units, normal ranges
Calcium, ionized (plasma)	4.0–5.2 mg/100 ml	0.25	1.00–1.30 mmol/l
Carotenes (serum)		0.0186	
Up to 1 year	70–340 μg/100 ml		1.3–6.3 μmol/l
1 year and older	100–150 μg/100 ml		1.9–2.8 μmol/l
Carbon dioxide, total (serum)		1.0	
Newborns	14–23 mmol/l		14–23 mmol/l
Increasing during first few hours of life to	18–27 mmol/l		18–27 mmol/l
PCO_2 – carbon dioxide, partial pressure (arterial blood) (higher values are found in newborn infants and in venous blood)	35–45 mmHg	0.133	4.7–6.0 kPa
Carboxyhemoglobin			
Newborns (higher in infants with Rh or ABO incompatibilities)	Up to 1.5% of total hemoglobin		Up to 1.5% total of hemoglobin
Older children	Up to 5% of total hemoglobin		Up to 5% of total hemoglobin
Catecholamines (plasma)			
Noradrenaline (norepinephrine)		5.911	
Supine	100–400 pg/ml		591–2364 pmol/l
Standing	300–900 pg/ml		1773–5320 pmol/l
Adrenaline (epinephrine)		5.458	
Supine	<70 pg/ml		<382 pmol/l
Standing	<100 pg/ml		<546 pmol/l
Dopamine		6.528	
Supine and standing	<30 pg/ml		<196 pmol/l
Chloride (serum)	95–106 mEq/l	1.0	95–106 mmol/l
Cholesterol (serum)		0.0259	
Cord blood	23–135 mg/100 ml		0.6–3.5 mmol/l
1–6 weeks	93–217 mg/100 ml		2.4–5.6 mmol/l
Increasing gradually until 1 year and older	119–263 mg/100 ml		3.1–6.8 mmol/l
Copper (serum)		0.157	
Cord blood	48–142 μg/100 ml		7.6–22.4 μmol/l
Older children	77–185 μg/100 ml		12.1–29.1 μmol/l
Copper oxidase (serum) Values are as for ceruloplasmin			
Cortisol (plasma) At birth (normally 1/5 to 1/2 of maternal plasma) lower values are seen in infants born by Cesarean section than by vaginal delivery)	3.4–22.1 μg/100 ml	27.6	94–610 nmol/l
12 h	16.0 (mean) μg/100 ml		440 (mean) nmol/l
24 h	7.0 (mean) μg/100 ml		193 (mean) nmol/l
Older children			
0800 h	8–26 μg/100 ml		200–720 nmol/l
2200 h (usually less than 50% of 0800 h value) (There is considerable diurnal variation such that the highest values are at about 0800 h and lowest around 2200–2400 h. This diurnal variation is absent in newborn infants up to about 5–6 weeks)	Below 7.4 μg/100 ml		Below 205 nmol/l
Creatine kinase (serum) (CK)			
Newborns	<300 units/l		
Children	<200 units/l		
Creatinine (plasma)		88.4	
Newborns (higher in preterm infants)	0.2–1.1 mg/100 ml		20–100 μmol/l
Thereafter	0.2–0.9 mg/100 ml		20–80 μmol/l
Dehydroepiandrosterone (DHA) (serum)			
Children 7–10 y	7–10 g		0.4–7 nmol/l
Children 11–14 y	11–14 g		1–20 nmol/l
Dehydroepiandrosterone sulfate (DHAS) (serum)			
Newborns			0.5–7 μmol/l
Thereafter			<1.4 μmol/l
1,25-dihydroxyvitamin (plasma)	25–45 pg/ml	2.4	60–108 nmol/l

Table 37.1 *Cont'd*

	Traditional units, normal ranges	Multiplication factor	SI units, normal ranges
2,3-diphosphoglycerate (blood)			
Newborn (1st day)	3.4–7.5 mmol/l red blood cells		3.4–7.5 mmol/l red blood cells
5th day	4.9–8.9 mmol/l red blood cells		4.9–8.9 mmol/l red blood cells
Decreasing thereafter until at 3 weeks and thereafter	3.9–6.8 mmol/l red blood cells		3.9–6.8 mmol/l red blood cells
Dopamine (plasma)			
Adrenaline (epinephrine) (plasma) } see Catecholamines			
Estradiol (serum)		36.7	
Newborns	27–52 ng/100 ml		1000–1900 pmol/l
Prepubertal	<1.9 ng/100 ml		<70 pmol/l
Adults			
Male	<4.1 ng/100 ml		<150 pmol/l
Female	>2.2 ng/100 ml		>80 pmol/l
Fats – see Lipids			
Fatty acids – see Lipids			
Ferritin			
Cord blood	70–200 ng/ml		
1 day–2 months	100–500 ng/ml		
Thereafter values fall to:			
4 months (mean)	100 ng/ml		
6 months (mean)	60 ng/ml		
1 year	16–100 ng/ml		
5–15 years	10–100 ng/ml		
α_1-fetoprotein (serum)			
Newborns	<55 000 units/ml (may be higher if premature)		
Infants at 8 weeks	<3100 units/ml		
Infants at 20 weeks	<40 units/ml		
Children	<15 units/ml		
Fibrinogen (plasma)		0.0294	
Newborns	150–350 mg/100 ml		4.4–10.3 μmol/l
Older children	200–400 mg/100 ml		5.8–11.6 μmol/l
Fibrin/fibrinogen degradation products (serum)	2.3–19.5 μg/ml	1.0	2.3–19.5 mg/l
Folic acid (serum) (higher values, up to 40 nmol/l are found in newborns and up to 50 nmol/l in preterm infants)	5–15 ng/ml	2.27	11–34 nmol/l
Follicle-stimulating hormone (FSH) (plasma)			
Children	<3.0 U/l		
Galactose (blood)		0.0556	
Newborns	0–20 mg/100 ml		0–1.1 mmol/l
Thereafter	<4.3 mg/100 ml		<240 μmol/l
Galactose-1-phosphate (blood)			
Children	<0.6 μmol/g Hb		
Galactose-1-phosphate uridyltransferase (erythrocytes)	>20 units/g Hb		
In galactosemia	<6 units/g Hb		
(Carriers)	(10–15 units/g Hb)		
Glucose (blood)		0.0556	
Fasting	60–100 mg/100 ml		3.3–5.5 mmol/l
Newborns	40–80 mg/100 ml		2.2–4.4 mmol/l
(Transiently low values below 2.2 mmol/l are commonly seen on the first day of life. Persistently low values should be investigated)			
Glutamic-oxaloacetic transaminase (serum) – see under Aspartate aminotransferase			
Glutamic-pyruvic transaminase (serum) – see under Alanine aminotransferase			
γ-glutamyltransferase (serum) (γGT)			
Newborns	<200 units/l		
Infants	<120 units/l		
Children	<35 units/l		

Table 37.1 *Cont'd*

	Traditional units, normal ranges	Multiplication factor	SI units, normal ranges
Glycogen (erythrocytes)			
Newborns	48–361 µg/g hemoglobin	1.0	48–361 µg/g hemoglobin
Older children	32–151 µg/g hemoglobin		32–151 µg/g hemoglobin
Growth hormone (serum)	<5 mU/l		
	Peak value should be above 15 mU/l		
	after appropriate stimulation		
Hemoglobin (blood) – see Table 37.9			
Hemoglobin, glycated (hemoglobin A$_1$)	4.7–7.9% of total Hb		
Haptoglobins (serum)	30–200 mg/100 ml	0.01	0.3–2.0 g/l
Hydrogen ion concentration (see also pH)	(pH 7.35–7.42)		38–45 nmol/l
17-α-hydroxyprogesterone (serum)			
Cord blood	<5000 ng/100 ml	0.03	<150 nmol/l
Newborns	<1000 ng/100 ml		<30 nmol/l
Children	<200 ng/100 ml		<6 nmol/l
25-hydroxyvitamin D (plasma) (there is a seasonal variation in values which are highest in summer and lowest in winter)	>10 ng/ml	2.5	>25 nmol/l
Immunoglobulins (see proteins)			
Insulin (serum)			
Fasting	5–40 µ units/ml	1.0	5–40 mU/l
Newborns (before first feed)	25–87 µ units/ml		25–87 mU/l
Iron (serum)			
Newborns	110–270 µg/100 ml	0.179	19.7–48.3 µmol/l
Falling in first 6 months, then rising by 3 years of age to (Higher values are found if determinations are done by atomic absorption spectrophotometry)	60–175 µg/100 ml		10.7–31.3 µmol/l
Iron-binding capacity (serum) – (TIBC)			
Newborns	59–175 µg/100 ml	0.179	11–31 µmol/l
Rising gradually during first 6 months to	250–400 µg/100 ml		45–72 µmol/l
Ketones	Up to 3 mg/100 ml	10	Up to 30 mg/l
Lactate (blood)			
Newborns	Up to 3.0 mEq/l	1.0	Up to 3.0 mmol/l
Thereafter	1.0–1.8 mEq/l		1.0–1.8 mmol/l
Lactate dehydrogenase (serum) (LDH)	58–230 units/l		
(Values may be twice as high in newborns)	or		
	120–480 spectrophotometric (Wroblewski) units		
Lactate dehydrogenase isoenzymes (serum)			
LDH$_1$ (heart)	24–34%		
LDH$_2$ (heart, red blood cells)	35–45%		
LDH$_3$ (muscle)	15–25%		
LDH$_4$ (liver, muscle)	4–10%		
LDH$_5$ (liver, muscle)	1–9%		
Lead (blood)	Up to 40 µg/100 ml	0.0483	Up to 1.9 µmol/l
Lipids (serum)			
Total			
Newborns	150–400 mg/100 ml	0.01	1.5–4.0 g/l
Thereafter	400–1000 mg/100 ml		4.0–10.0 g/l
Free (nonesterified) fatty acids			
Newborns	250–1000 µEq/l	1.0	250–1000 µmol/l
Older children	300–1450 µEq/l		300–1450 µmol/l
Phospholipids			
Cord blood	75–150 mg/100 ml	0.01	0.75–1.5 g/l
Newborns	170–250 mg/100 ml		1.7–2.5 g/l
Older children	150–300 mg/100 ml		1.5–3.0 g/l
Phospholipid phosphorus	5–10 mg/100 ml	0.323	1.6–3.2 mmol/l
Triglycerides (plasma) – fasting	100–1300 mg/100 ml	0.00133	0.6–1.7 mmol/l
Lipoproteins (serum)			
Newborns			
Alpha	71–176 mg/100 ml	0.01	0.71–1.76 g/l
Beta	51–158 mg/100 ml		0.51–1.58 g/l

Table 37.1 *Cont'd*

	Traditional units, normal ranges	Multiplication factor	SI units, normal ranges
Lipoproteins *Cont'd*			
Omega (chylomicrons)	48–106 mg/100 ml		0.48–1.06 g/l
Total	170–440 mg/100 ml		1.70–4.40 g/l
There is a fairly sharp rise in the first 10 days, then a further gradual rise until at 2 years and older			
Alpha	147–327 mg/100 ml	0.01	1.47–3.27 g/l
Beta	225–541 mg/100 ml		2.25–5.41 g/l
Omega (chylomicrons)	98–268 mg/100 ml		0.98–2.68 g/l
Total	490–1090 mg/100 ml		4.90–10.9 g/l
Luteinizing hormone (LH) (serum)			
Children	<1.9 U/l		
Magnesium (serum)			
Cord blood	1.50–2.50 mg/100 ml	0.41	0.62–1.03 mmol/l
Newborns	1.40–2.45 mg/100 ml		0.58–1.00 mmol/l
Older children	1.45–2.32 mg/100 ml		0.60–0.95 mmol/l
Methemoglobin (blood)	0–0.3 g/100 ml	10	0–3 g/l
In preterm infants	0–0.4 g/100 ml		0–4 g/l
Nonprotein nitrogen (serum)			
Cord blood	24–38 mg/100 ml	0.714	17–27 mmol/l
Newborns	20–33 mg/100 ml		14–24 mmol/l
Children	25–40 mg/100 ml		18–29 mmol/l
Noradrenaline (norepinephrine) (plasma) – see catecholamines			
Osmolality (serum)	275–295 mosmol/kg	1.0	275–295 mmol/kg
Oxygen capacity (blood)	1.335 ml oxygen/g hemoglobin	1.0	1.335 ml oxygen/g hemoglobin
Oxygen content (blood)			
Umbilical vein (umbilical artery values are usually 4–8 vol. % lower)	5.5–18.8 vol. %		
Children	13.7–17.5 vol. %		
Oxygen saturation (arterial blood)			
Umbilical artery	0–32%		
Umbilical vein	26–73% (mean 47%)		
Children	86–101%		
Oxygen saturation (venous blood)			
Newborns	30–80%		
Older children	60–85%		
Parathyroid hormone (plasma)	<0.2 U/l		
*P*CO$_2$ – see Carbon dioxide			
pH (arterial blood) (See also hydrogen ion) (Venous blood values are 0.03 lower)	7.35–7.42		
*P*O$_2$ – oxygen tension (arterial blood)			
Umbilical vein	12.8–32.0 mmHg	0.133	1.7–4.3 kPa
Newborns after first 24 h	77–100 mmHg		9.3–13.3 kPa
Older children	85–105 mmHg		11.3–14.0 kPa
Phenylalanine (plasma)			
Umbilical vein	0.4–2.0 mg/100 ml	60.5	25–119 μmol/l
Newborns (Transient values above 2.8 mg/100 ml may be found in the newborn period. Plasma concentrations are usually maintained at between 84 and 300 μmol/l in the treatment of phenylketonuria)	0.7–2.8 mg/100 ml		42–170 μmol/l
Phospholipids (serum) – see Lipids			
Phosphorus, inorganic (serum)			
Cord blood	3.2–7.6 mg/100 ml	0.323	1.03–2.45 mmol/l
Newborns, 1st week	5.8–9.0 mg/100 ml		1.87–2.91 mmol/l
Newborns, 2nd week	4.9–8.9 mg/100 ml		1.58–2.87 mmol/l
Up to 1 year	4.0–6.5 mg/100 ml		1.30–2.10 mmol/l
Thereafter	3.6–5.9 mg/100 ml		1.16–1.91 mmol/l
(Phosphorus values in the newborn period vary greatly depending very much on the type of milk feed; lower values are found in breast-fed infants)			

Table 37.1 *Cont'd*

	Traditional units, normal ranges	Multiplication factor	SI units, normal ranges
Plasma volume			
At birth	33.5–49.5 ml/kg	1.0	33.5–49.5 ml/kg
Rising until at 3–6 months of age the mean value is about	54 ml/kg		54 ml/kg
Thereafter it falls so that the range for older children is	31–54 ml/kg		31–54 ml/kg
Potassium (serum)			
Umbilical vein	3.3–6.8 mEq/l	1.0	3.3–6.8 mmol/l
Newborns	4.3–7.6 mEq/l		4.3–7.6 mmol/l
Older children	3.5–5.6 mEq/l		3.5–5.6 mmol/l
Progesterone (serum)			
Adults			
Male	<64 ng/100 ml	0.032	<2 nmol/l
Female	<2800 ng/100 ml		<90 nmol/l
Prolactin (serum)			
Newborns	<4000 mU/l		
Children	60–390 mU/l		

Proteins (serum)
Values in g/100 ml

	Total	Albumin	Globulins			
			α_1	α_2	β	γ
Newborns	4.6–7.7	2.5–5.0	0.1–0.3	0.4–0.6	0.3–0.6	0.8–1.2
1 year	5.6–7.3	3.5–5.0	0.2–0.4	0.4–1.0	0.5–1.0	0.5–1.3
4 years and over	6.0–8.0	3.7–5.0	0.2–0.4	0.4–1.0	0.6–1.1	0.5–1.8

Values in g/l (using multiplication factor of 10)

	Total	Albumin	α_1	α_2	β	γ
Newborns	46–77	25–50	1–3	4–6	3–6	6–14
1 year	56–73	35–50	2–4	4–10	5–9	4–12
4 years and over	60–80	37–50	2–4	4–10	6–10	5–12

(Low total protein and albumin values are found in immature infants)

Immunoglobulins (serum)

	IgG		IgA		IgM	
	mg/100 ml	g/l	mg/100 ml	g/l	mg/100 ml	g/l
Newborns	650–1450	6.5–14.5	0–10	0–0.1	0–30	0–0.3
1–3 months	200–650	2.0–6.5	5–40	0.05–0.4	10–100	0.1–1.0
4–6 months	150–800	1.5–8.0	10–60	0.1–0.6	10–100	0.1–1.0
1 year	300–1200	3.0–12.0	20–80	0.2–0.8	40–200	0.4–2.0
3 years and older	500–1500	5.0–15.0	30–300	0.3–3.0	40–200	0.4–2.0

(Immunoglobulin values vary widely in children, particularly in the first 6 months of life. Care should be taken therefore in interpreting marginal differences from the normal)

	Traditional units, normal ranges	Multiplication factor	SI units, normal ranges
Pyruvate (blood)	0.05–0.09 mEq/l	1000	50–80 µmol/l
Renin (plasma)	1.1–4.1 mg/ml/h		
Sodium (serum, plasma)			
Newborns	132–145 mEq/l	1.0	132–145 mmol/l
Thereafter	135–145 mEq/l		135–145 mmol/l
Standard bicarbonate (blood)			
Umbilical vein	12–21 mEq/l	1.0	12–21 mmol/l
Newborns	18–25		18–25 mmol/l
Thereafter	21–25		21–25 mmol/l
Sulfate (serum)	0.5–1.5 mg/100 ml	104.1	50–150 µmol/l
Testosterone (serum)			
Newborns (male)	Up to 200 mg/100 ml	0.0347	<7 nmol/l
Infants (male), 2–4 months	<375 mg/100 ml		<13 nmol/l
Boys			
Prepubertal	Up to 100 ng/100 ml	0.0347	Up to 3.5 nmol/l
Rising at puberty to	290–865 ng/100 ml		10–30 nmol/l
Girls	<100 ng/100 ml		<3.5 nmol/l
Thyrotropin or thyroid stimulating hormone – TSH (serum)			
Newborns	<25 mU/l		
Thereafter	0.3–5.0 mU/l		
Thyroxine – T_4 (serum)			
Cord blood and newborns	11–34 µg/100 ml	12.9	140–440 nmol/l
Infants	7–15 µg/100 ml		90–195 nmol/l
Children	5.4–14 µg/100 ml		70–180 nmol/l

Table 37.1   *Cont'd*

	Traditional units, normal ranges	Multiplication factor	SI units, normal ranges
Thyroxine, free (FT$_4$) (serum)	0.7–1.8 ng/100 ml	12.9	9–23 pmol/l
Triiodothyronine – T$_3$ (serum)		0.0154	
Cord blood (values are well below maternal serum values)	10–45 ng/100 ml		0.15–0.45 nmol/l
Newborns	50–400 ng/100 ml		0.8–6.2 nmol/l
Thereafter	100–250 ng/100 ml		1.5–3.8 nmol/l
Tyrosine (plasma)		0.0552	
Cord blood	0.7–2.0 mg/100 ml		39–110 µmol/l
Newborns (Transiently increased values may be found in the newborn, particularly in the immature infant. Markedly or persistently high values should be investigated)	0.7–5.6 mg/100 ml		39–309 µmol/l
Older children	0.7–1.1 mg/100 ml		39–61 µmol/l
Urea (blood) (Higher values are commonly seen during the first 6 months of life in infants fed on unmodified milks, i.e. those whose protein concentration is substantially above that of breast milk)	15–40 mg/100 ml	0.166	2.5–6.6 mmol/l
Urea nitrogen (blood) (See comment on protein intake under Urea as blood urea nitrogen also depends on protein intake as well as functional maturity of the kidneys)	7–19 mg/100 ml	0.357	2.5–6.8 mmol/l
Uric acid (serum)	2.0–7.0 mg/100 ml	0.0595	0.12–0.42 mmol/l
Vitamin A (serum)	20–100 µg/100 ml	0.0349	0.7–3.5 µmol/l
Vitamin C, ascorbic acid (plasma)	0.5–1.5 mg/100 ml	56.8	28–85 µmol/l
Vitamin E, α-tocopherol (plasma)		23.2	
Cord blood and newborn infants	0.2–0.6 mg/100 ml		5–14 µmol/l
Vitamin E concentrations increase slowly with age until at 2 years and older the normal range is	0.5–1.2 mg/100 ml		12–28 µmol/l
Newborn infants if artificially fed continue to have plasma concentrations similar to or slightly above the values quoted for cord blood. Breast-fed infants however have higher values similar to those of older children. Preterm infants have lower values than full-term infants			
Zinc (serum)		0.153	
Cord blood	72–212 µg/100 ml		11–32 µmol/l
Children	60–190 µg/100 ml		9–29 µmol/l

Table 37.2 Normal constituents of urine

	Traditional units, normal ranges	Multiplication factor	SI units, normal ranges
Acidity – see pH and Titratable activity			
Adrenaline	0.02–0.7 µg/kg/24 h	5.46	0.11–0.38 nmol/kg/24 h
Aldosterone – see Steroids			
Amino acids (these values may be up to two times higher in neonates)			
Alanine	232–717 mg/g creatinine	0.099	23–71 µmol/mmol creatinine
α-aminoadipate	18–145 mg/g creatinine	0.055	1–8 µmol/mmol creatinine
α-aminobutyrate	23–93 mg/g creatinine	0.086	2–8 µmol/mmol creatinine
β-aminoisobutyrate	23–581 mg/g creatinine	0.086	2–50 µmol/mmol creatinine
Arginine	59–216 mg/g creatinine	0.051	3–11 µmol/mmol creatinine
Asparagine	<90 mg/g creatinine	0.067	<6 µmol/mmol creatinine
Aspartate	106–455 mg/g creatinine	0.066	7–30 µmol/mmol creatinine
Citrulline	20–137 mg/g creatinine	0.051	1–7 µmol/mmol creatinine
Cystathionine			<20 µmol/mmol creatinine
Cystine	108–405 mg/g creatinine	0.037	4–15 µmol/mmol creatinine
Glutamate	<50 mg/g creatinine	0.060	<3 µmol/mmol creatinine
Glutamine	557–1459 mg/g creatinine	0.061	34–89 µmol/mmol creatinine
Glycine	958–4593 mg/g creatinine	0.118	113–542 µmol/mmol creatinine
Histidine	825–5754 mg/g creatinine	0.057	47–328 µmol/mmol creatinine
Isoleucine	15–90 mg/g creatinine	0.067	1–6 µmol/mmol creatinine
Leucine	30–164 mg/g creatinine	0.067	2–11 µmol/mmol creatinine
Lysine	115–475 mg/g creatinine	0.061	7–29 µmol/mmol creatinine
Methionine	34–153 mg/g creatinine	0.059	2–9 µmol/mmol creatinine
Ornithine	30–119 mg/g creatinine	0.067	2–8 µmol/mmol creatinine
Phenylalanine	74–315 mg/g creatinine	0.054	4–17 µmol/mmol creatinine
Phosphoethanolamine			2–25 µmol/mmol creatinine
Proline	<13 mg/g creatinine	0.077	<1 µmol/mmol creatinine
Serine	298–607 mg/g creatinine	0.084	25–51 µmol/mmol creatinine
Taurine	521–2281 mg/g creatinine	0.071	37–162 µmol/mmol creatinine
Threonine	149–338 mg/g creatinine	0.074	11–25 µmol/mmol creatinine
Tryptophan	23–186 mg/g creatinine	0.043	1–8 µmol/mmol creatinine
Tyrosine	102–306 mg/g creatinine	0.049	5–15 µmol/mmol creatinine
Valine	13–92 mg/g creatinine	0.076	1–7 µmol/mmol creatinine
α-amino nitrogen			
Premature infants	10.0–26.8 mg/kg/24 h	71.4	714–1910 µmol/kg/24 h
Newborns	6.8–20.7 mg/kg/24 h		485–1480 µmol/kg/24 h
Infants	3.4–8.5 mg/kg/24 h		243–607 µmol/kg/24 h
Children (values are lower in breast-milk-fed babies than in those fed on cow's milk)	0.9–2.9 mg/kg/24 h		64–207 µmol/kg/24 h
Using creatinine as an index the normal values in children are	0.14–0.78 mg α-amino nitrogen/µmol creatinine nitrogen	631	88–492 µmol α-amino nitrogen/µmol creatinine nitrogen
δ-aminolevulinic acid (high levels are found in lead poisoning and in some porphyrias)	Up to 0.5 mg/100 ml	7.63	Up to 38 µmol/l
Ammonia			
Newborns: 1st day	0.02–0.50 mEq/kg/24 h	1.0	0.02–0.50 mmol/kg/24 h
Newborns: 7th day	0.26–0.86 mEq/kg/24 h		0.26–0.86 mmol/kg/24 h
Children	0.52–1.08 mEq/kg/24 h		0.52–1.08 mmol/kg/24 h
	or 7–34 µEq/min/1.73 m^2		7–34 µmol/min/1.73 m^2
Ascorbic acid load test >5% of an oral dose of 20 mg/kg are excreted in 24 h			
Bicarbonate None when the pH is below 6.8			
Calcium			
Newborns (1st week of life)	0–0.7 mg/kg/24 h	25	0–17.5 µmol/kg/24 h
Infants	Up to 40 mg/24 h		Up to 1000 µmol/24 h
Older children	Up to 4 mg/kg/24 h		Up to 100 µmol/kg/24 h
	or 30–150 mg/24 h		or 750–3750 µmol/24 h
Calcium : creatinine ratio (estimated on the second morning urine, i.e. the first specimen voided after the overnight urine has been passed)	Up to 0.25 mg/mg	2.82	Up to 0.7 mmol/mmol
Catecholamines			
Total	0.4–2.0 µg/kg/24 h	5.91	2.4–11.8 µmol/kg/24 h – calculated as noradrenaline

Table 37.2 *Cont'd*

	Traditional units, normal ranges	Multiplication factor	SI units, normal ranges
Catecholamines *Cont'd*			
Adrenaline (epinephrine)	0.027–0.7 µg/kg/24 h	5.46	0.15–3.8 µmol/kg/24 h
Noradrenaline (norepinephrine)	0.4–1.6 µg/kg/24 h	5.91	2.4–9.5 µmol/kg/24 h
Cells			
Erythrocytes	0–2 mm^3	10^6	0–2 × 10^6/l
Leukocytes			
Males	0–4 mm^3		0–4 × 10^6/l
Females	0–20 mm^3		0–20 × 10^6/l
Chloride			
Newborn infant	Up to 3 g/l	28.2	Up to 85 mmol/l
Older children	Up to 4 mEq/kg/24 h		Up to 4 mmol/kg/24 h
	or 170–250 mEq/l		or 170–250 mmol/l
Concentrating capacity – see Osmolality			
Copper	Up to 40 µg/24 h	0.0157	Up to 0.6 µmol/24 h
	or <40 µg/100 ml		or <6.3 µmol/l
Coproporphyrin (increased excretion is found in lead poisoning, liver disease and some porphyrias)	Up to 0.1 µg/ml	1.53	Up to 0.15 µmol/l
Creatine			
Newborns	Up to 36 mg/kg/24 h	7.69	Up to 280 µmol/kg/24 h
Infants	Up to 15 mg/kg/24 h		Up to 115 µmol/kg/24 h
Values in girls are higher than those in boys			
There is a gradually decreasing creatine excretion with age to adult levels of	Up to 2 mg/kg/24 h		Up to 15 µmol/kg/24 h
Creatinine			
Newborns and infants	10–20 mg/kg/24 h	8.84	88–176 µmol/kg/24 h
Older children	5–40 mg/kg/24 h		44–354 µmol/kg/24 h
Creatinine clearance			
Newborns	40–65 ml/min/1.73 m^2		
Increasing gradually until at 1 year and older			
Males	98–150 ml/min/1.73 m^2		
Females	95–123 ml/min/1.73 m^2		
Galactose			
Infants on a milk diet may excrete up to	20–25 mg/100 ml	0.056	1.1–1.4 mmol/l
Much higher values are seen in galactosemia			
Glucose			
Newborns	Up to 20 mg/100 ml	0.056	Up to 1.1 mmol/l
Older children	Up to 5 mg/100 ml		Up to 0.28 mmol/l
Homovanillic acid (HVA)	3–16 µg/mg creatinine		
Increased in neuroblastoma			
5-hydroxyindole acetic acid	1.4–13.2 mg/24 h	5.26	7–70 µmol/24 h
4-hydroxy 3-methoxymandelate (HMMA) – see under Vanillylmandelic acid			
5-hydroxytryptamine (serotonin)	43–123 µg/24 h		
Lead	1.5–22 µg/24 h	4.83	7–106 nmol/24 h
Magnesium			
Newborns (1st week of life)	Up to 10 mg/24 h	41.1	Up to 411 µmol/24 h
Older children	1.24–4.4 mg/kg/24 h		51–181 µmol/kg/24 h
Magnesium/creatinine ratio	Up to 0.41 mg/mg	0.215	Up to 0.09 mmol/mmol
Metanephrine (high values, above 0.2, are found in pheochromocytoma)	0.02–0.16 µg/mg creatinine		
Mucopolysaccharides (expressed as hexuronic acid)	Increasing from 0.5 mg/24 h at age 2 years to 2–12 mg/24 h at 14 years		
Normetanephrine (increased in pheochromocytoma)	0.05–0.6 µg/mg creatinine		
Osmolality			
Newborns			
Delivery urine	79–118 mosmol/kg	1.0	79–118 mmol/kg
Maximum in neonatal period	600 mosmol/kg		600 mmol/kg

Table 37.2 *Cont'd*

	Traditional units, normal ranges	Multiplication factor	SI units, normal ranges
Osmolality (*cont'd*)			
After at least a 12-h thirst or in the 4 h after DDAVP the osmolality should be greater than 750 mosmol/kg (specific gravity 1.022)			>750 mmol/kg
Normal values of up to 1200 mosmol/kg may be observed but in newborns and young infants, until maturity of renal function is obtained, values of this order are not found			Up to 1200 mmol/kg
pH			
Newborns	5.0 or higher		
Older children	5.3–7.2		
Phosphorus			
Newborns (breast-fed) (values for cow's-milk-fed babies may be up to 10 times higher)	0–0.7 mg/24 h	0.0325	Up to 0.023 mg/kg/24 h
Infants	Up to 200 mg/24 h		Up to 6.5 mmol/24 h
Older children	15–20 mg/kg/24 h		0.49–0.65 mmol/kg/24 h
Porphobilinogen (no increase in lead poisoning)	Up to 0.2 mg/100 ml		
Potassium			
Newborns (breast-fed) (up to twice this value in infants fed on cow's milk formulae)	Up to 2.3 mEq/kg/24 h	1.0	Up to 2.3 mmol/kg/24 h
Older children (usually about half the sodium excretion)	Up to 2 mEq/kg/24 h		Up to 2 mmol/kg/24 h or 25–125 mmol/l
Protein			
Newborns	About 10 mg/24 h		
Older children	30–50 mg/24 h (about 25% albumin)		
Sodium			
Newborns (breast-fed)			
1st day	0.11–0.39 mEq/kg/24 h	1.0	0.11–0.39 mmol/kg/24 h
7th day	Up to 4.4 mEq/kg/24 h		Up to 4.4 mmol/kg/24 h or 1.5 mmol/h/1.73 m² (mean)
(Values are normally up to 50% above this level in infants fed on cow's milk formulae and in preterm infants)			
Older children	Up to 3.7 mEq/kg/24 h		Up to 3.7 mmol/kg/24 h or 40–225 mmol/24 h
Steroids			
Aldosterone	1–5 µg/24 h	2.774	2.7–14 nmol/24 h
17-hydroxycorticosteroids (17-oxogenic steroids)			
Newborns	Up to 1 mg/24 h	3.47	Up to 3.5 µmol/24 h
Up to 6 years	2–6 mg/24 h		7–21 µmol/24 h
6–9 years	6–8 mg/24 h		21–28 µmol/24 h
10–14 years	8–10 mg/24 h		28–35 µmol/24 h
17-ketosteroids (17-oxosteroids)			
Newborns (1st 2 weeks)	0.5–2.5 mg/24 h	3.47	1.7–8.7 µmol/24 h
2 weeks–2 years	0–0.5 mg/24 h		0–1.7 µmol/24 h
2–8 years	0–2.5 mg/24 h		0–8.7 µmol/24 h
8–10 years	0.7–4 mg/24 h		2.4–14 µmol/24 h
Thereafter there is a gradual increase during puberty to values of:			
Boys	2.5–13 mg/24 h		8.7–45 µmol/24 h
Girls	2.5–11 mg/24 h		8.7–38 µmol/24 h
Pregnanediol	0–1 mg/24 h	3.12	0.3–3 µmol/24 h
Pregnanetriol			
Newborns	0.2–0.3 mg/24 h	2.97	0.6–0.9 µmol/24 h
Older children	Up to 1.1 mg/24 h		Up to 3.3 µmol/24 h
Steroid ratio:			
$\dfrac{\text{11-deoxysteroids}}{\text{11-oxysteroids}}$	>0.5 (first week of life >0.8)		
This steroid 11-oxygenation index is a reflection of the efficiency of the last stage of cortisol biosynthesis High values are found in congenital adrenal hyperplasia			
Testosterone (before puberty)	Up to 5 µg/24 h	3.47	Up to 17 nmol/24 h

Table 37.2 *Cont'd*

	Traditional units, normal ranges	Multiplication factor	SI units, normal ranges
Titratable acidity Newborns Older children	45–110 µEq/min/1.73 m² or about 0.3 mEq/kg/24 h 35–70 µEq/min/1.73 m² or 1 mEq/kg/24 h	1.0	45–110 µmol/min/1.73 m² or about 0.3 mmol/kg/24 h 35–70 µmol/min/1.73 m² or 1 mmol/kg/24 h
Urea clearance (lower in newborns)	50–90 ml/min/1.73 m²		
Urobilinogen	Up to 3 mg/24 h		
Vanillylmandelic acid (VMA) or 4-hydroxy-3-methoxymandelate (HMMA) Newborns–6 months 6 months–15 years (Elevated levels are seen in children with neuroblastomas, gangliomas and pheochromocytomas)	Up to 200 µg/kg/24 h 60–150 µg/kg/24 h or <6 mg/24 h	5.05	Up to 1010 nmol/kg/24 h 300–760 nmol/kg/24 h or <30 µmol/24 h

Volume

1st and 2nd days:	15–60 ml	1–3 years:	500–600 ml
3–10 days:	50–300 ml	3–4 years:	600–700 ml
10 days–2 months:	250–450 ml	5–7 years:	650–1000 ml
2 months–1 year:	400–500 ml	8–14 years:	800–1400 ml

Many other substances which are either not normally present in the urine or which are present in small quantities may be estimated when appropriate. These include hemoglobin, homogentisic acid, phenylpyruvic acid, etc.

Table 37.3 Normal cerebrospinal fluid values

	Traditional units, normal ranges	Multiplication factor	SI units, normal ranges
β-n-acetylhexosaminidase	0–4 IU/l	1.0	0–4 IU/l
γ-aminobutyric acid (GABA)			83–383 pmol/l
α-amino nitrogen	1.0–1.5 mg/100 ml	0.714	0.7–1.1 mmol/l
Aspartate aminotransferase Newborns Older children (In the normal child the CSF level of this enzyme is about half that of the serum level. Increased CSF levels of the enzyme occur in infants and children with various intracranial pathological conditions such as acute bacterial meningitis)	1–10 Karmen spectrophotometric units (0.5–5.0 IU/l) 2–20 Karmen units (1–10 IU/l)		
Bicarbonate	21.3–25.9 mEq/l	1.0	21.3–25.9 mmol/l
Bilirubin Newborns (correlates with serum levels: most is unconjugated) Older children (CSF concentrations vary with changes in serum concentration. Free bilirubin can be identified if present in significant quantity on a spectrophotometric scan due to its characteristic flattened peak with a maximum at about 455 nm. Conjugated bilirubin (bilirubin glucuronides) has a maximum at 422 nm. Where bilirubin is present in increased amounts and there is spectrophotometric evidence of 'old' blood also, the most likely source of both is a CNS hemorrhage. Large amounts of bilirubin are seen in the CSF with no blood present in neonatal hyperbilirubinemia (Kjellin 1970, Hellstrom & Kjellin 1971)	0.04–0.44 mg/100 ml None	17.1	0.7–7.5 µmol/l None
Calcium Newborns Older children (Spinal fluid calcium concentration approximates to that of serum ionized calcium)	5.5–7.7 mg/100 ml 4.0–5.2 mg/100 ml	0.25	1.38–1.93 mmol/l 1.0–1.30 mmol/l

Table 37.3 *Cont'd*

	Traditional units, normal ranges	Multiplication factor	SI units, normal ranges
Cell count			
Erythrocytes			
During the first 14 days of life	Up to 675/mm³	10^6	Up to 675×10^6/l
Later	0–2/mm³		$0–2 \times 10^6$/l
Leukocytes: in newborns, particularly in premature infants	Up to 14/mm³		Up to 14×10^6/l
In the first year of life	Up to 10/mm³		Up to 10×10^6/l
After 1 year	Up to 5/mm³		Up to 5×10^6/l
Chloride	116–128 mEq/l	1.0	116–128 mmol/l
The range is slightly lower in newborn and young infants	109–123 mEq/l		109–123 mmol/l
Carbon dioxide			
Combining power (see also PCO_2)	22–28 mEq/l	1.0	22–28 mmol/l
Cholesterol	219–571 µg/100 ml	0.0259	5.7–14.8 µmol/l
Newborns	Up to 220 µg/100 ml		Up to 5.7 µmol/l
(approximately 35% is free cholesterol and 65% esterified)			
Creatine kinase			
Newborns	0.7–2.0 IU/l	1.0	0.7–2.0 IU/l
Older children	0.2–1.6 IU/l		0.2–1.6 IU/l
Glucose (The CSF level is less than, but varies with, changes in blood glucose. It is often low in newborn infants and pathologically low when the CSF is infected)	50–80 mg/100 ml	0.0556	2.8–4.4 mmol/l
β-glucuronidase	0–30 mIU/l	1.0	0–30 mIU/l
Glutamic-oxaloacetic transaminase – see Aspartate aminotransferase			
Homovanillic acid (HVA)	75–200 mg/ml		
5-hydroxyindole acetic acid			
Birth-1 year	90–150 ng/ml	5.24	470–785 nmol/l
1 year onwards	30–90 ng/ml		160–470 nmol/l
Lactate	7.2–22.0 mg/100 ml	0.112	0.8–2.4 mmol/l
(lactate : pyruvate ratio 14.3–17.6. Higher values are found in newborns following intrauterine or neonatal asphyxia)			
Lactic dehydrogenase			
Newborns	3–120 Wroblewski units (1.5–58 IU/l)	1.0	3–120 Wroblewski units (1.5–58 IU/l)
Older children	14–59 Wroblewski units (6.8–30 IU/l)		14–59 Wroblewski units (6.8–30 IU/l)
(Increased LDH activity in the CSF is observed in acute bacterial infections and in many cases of organic brain disease)			
Lipids			
Total	766–1740 µg/100 ml	0.01	7.7–17.4 mg/l
Free (nonesterified) fatty acids	42–98 µEq/l	1.0	42–98 µmol/l
Neutral fat (glycerides)	0–900 µg/100 ml	0.01	0–9 mg/l
Phospholipids	209–889 µg/100 ml	0.01	2.1–8.9 mg/100 ml
Magnesium			
Newborns	1.8–2.6 mEq/l	0.5	0.9–1.3 mmol/l
Older children	0.49–4.0 mEq/l		0.25–2.0 mmol/l
Nonprotein nitrogen	11–20 mg/100 ml	10	110–200 mg/l
Osmolality	273–304 mosmol/kg (mean 285)	1.0	273–304 mmol/kg (mean 285)
(It has been suggested that if the CSF osmolality is considerably greater than that of the serum, severe neurological disturbance may occur. This is particularly true in hyperosmolar hypernatremic dehydration (Habel & Simpson 1976)			
PCO_2			
Newborns	38–63 mmHg (mean 49)	0.133	5.1–8.4 kPa (mean 6.5)
Thereafter	40–51 mmHg		5.3–6.8 kPa
pH	7.32–7.37		

Table 37.3 *Cont'd*

	Traditional units, normal ranges	Multiplication factor	SI units, normal ranges
Potassium	2.1–3.9 mEq/l	1.0	2.1–3.9 mmol/l
(Levels in spinal fluid are largely independent of serum values. Infants may have lower values than the range quoted)			
Phosphorus, inorganic		0.323	
Newborns	0.7–3.1 mg/100 ml		0.23–1.00 mmol/l
Older children	1.4–2.2 mg/100 ml		0.45–0.71 mmol/l
Pressure			
Newborns	50–80 mm water		
Infants	40–150 mm water		
Children	70–200 mm water		
Protein			
Lumbar fluid	20–40 mg/100 ml	10	200–400 mg/l
Lumbar fluid contains more protein than fluid from the cisterna magna which in turn contains more protein than ventricular fluid. Thus the upper limit of normal			
for cisternal fluid is	25 mg/100 ml		250 mg/l
And that for ventricular fluid	15 mg/100 ml		150 mg/l
Newborns (lumbar fluid)	25–90 mg/100 ml		250–900 mg/l
Reducing to upper limits of normal at 1 month	70 mg/100 ml		700 mg/l
And at 6 months	40 mg/100 ml		400 mg/l
Even higher values up to	250 or 300 mg/100 ml		2500–3000 mg/l
may be found in premature infants and in some term infants			
Protein electrophoresis			
Newborns:			
Albumin (+ prealbumin)	50%		
α_1-globulins	7%		
α_2-globulins	9%		
β-globulins	14%		
γ-globulins	20%		
Gradually changing until in			
Older children:			
Albumin (+ prealbumin)	52%		
α_1-globulins	7%		
α_2-globulins	9%		
β-globulins	20%		
γ-globulins	12%		
Pyruvate	0.4–0.7 mg/100 ml	113	40–80 µmol/l
Newborns	0.6–1.2 mg/100 ml		70–140 µmol/l
Sodium	130–157 mEq/l	1	130–157 mmol/l
Urea nitrogen	7–18 mg/100 ml	0.166	1.2–3.0 mmol/l
Uric acid	0.5–2.6 mg/100 ml	0.0595	0.03–0.15 mmol/l
Volume			
Infants	40–60 ml		
Young children	60–100 ml		
Older children	80–120 ml		
Adults	100–160 ml		
Water content	98.3–99.6 g/100 ml		

Table 37.4   Normal constituents of stools

Amount
  Meconium: 70–90 g
  Newborns: Breast-milk-fed: 15–25 g/24 h
                 Cow's-milk-fed: 30–40 g/24 h
  2 months–6 years: 7–54 g/24 h
  Older children: 30–200 g/24 h
  (Amount is lower on a mainly meat diet, but may be higher than quoted values on a mainly vegetable diet)
Appearance
  69% of healthy newborns have their first stools within 12 h and 94% within 24 h
  Meconium: greenish-brown to black
  Infants: golden yellow (due to bilirubin), on breast milk, turning green (biliverdin) on standing, brown (stercobilin) on cow's milk
  Older children: brown (stercobilin, bilifuscin, mesobilifuscin) darkening on exposure to air; pitch black when hematin content is high due to stomach or upper intestinal tract hemorrhage; light gray when fat content is high, due to breakdown products of bile pigments
Bilirubin
  Meconium: 430–1750 µmol/kg (252–1020 mg/kg)
  The bilirubin content of stools falls as that of the plasma rises in the newborn period. This fall continues throughout the first year of life when adult values of 9–34 µg/kg (5–20 mg/24 h) are reached.
  Disturbances of intestinal flora by antibiotics can cause an increase in bilirubin content
Blood
  The Apt test for fetal hemoglobin may be performed on stool samples to show whether blood in the stool of a newborn infant is maternal in origin or from the infant (Apt & Downey 1955)
Calcium
  Meconium: 3.3–20 mmol/kg (130–800 mg/kg)
  Infants: 6.5–8.25 mmol/24 h (200–300 mg/24 h) increasing in childhood towards adult values of 7.5–32.5 mmol/24 h (300–1000 mg/24 h)
Copper
  Meconium: 157–393 µmol/kg (10–25 mg/kg) increasing to adult values of 0–79 µmol/24 h (0–5 mg/24 h)
Coproporphyrin
  See Porphyrins
Fat and fatty acids
  See Lipids
Iron
  Meconium: 215–484 µmol/kg (12–27 mg/kg) increasing to adult values of 102–120 µmol/24 h (5.7–6.7 mg/24 h)
Lactic acid
  Up to 0.44 mmol/24 h (40 mg/24 h)
  Increased in carbohydrate malabsorption
Lipids
  Total fats: in children greater than 90% of dietary fat should be absorbed where fat intake is normal. Although normal total fecal fat is usually less than 2 g/day, the upper limit of normal is usually set at about 4.5–5 g/day. In addition the proportion of fat is usually less than 50% of the fecal dry weight in young children up to 6 months and less than 25% in older children
  Free fatty acids: up to 1.4 g per 24 hours or about two-thirds of the total fat
Magnesium
  Meconium: 9–30 mmol/kg (219–729 mg/kg) increasing to adult value of 5–15 mmol/24 h (122–365 mg/24 h)
Nitrogen
  Meconium: 19 g/kg (mean value)
  Newborn infants: breast-milk-fed: 160 mg/24 h
  Cow's-milk-fed: 400 mg/24 h
  Adult: 1–2 g/24 h
Organic acids
  Up to 400 mmol/kg
pH
  Meconium: 5.7–6.4
  Newborns, breast-milk-fed: 4.6–5.2
  In general while infants on breast milk have acid stools, those on cow's milk have neutral or alkaline stools
  Older children: 5.0–8.8, but normally slightly alkaline (7.0–7.5)
  Stools with a pH of less than 5 should be further examined for reducing substances, etc.

Phosphorus
  Meconium: 2.4–7.9 mmol/kg (74–254 mg/kg)
  Infants: 4.9–6.0 mmol/24 h (157–193 mg/24 h) increasing in childhood towards adult values of 10–24 mmol/24 h (310–775 mg/24 h)
Porphyrins
  Coproporphyrin and protoporphyrin are found in stools in small quantities, usually less than 1–2 mg/24 h
  Coproporphyrin is related to the amount of meat in the diet. See also Bilirubin and Urobilinogen
Potassium
  Meconium: 12–51 mmol/kg
Protein
  Small amounts, mainly undigested nutrient protein and bacterial proteins are found
Sodium
  Meconium: 90–182 mmol/kg
Trypsin
  Meconium: None
  In a child of under 2 years of age, if a 1 in 50 dilution of fresh feces fails to digest gelatin, this finding is evidence of cystic fibrosis of the pancreas
Urobilinogen
  Rarely found in stools in the first week of life and only in small quantities up to 1 year of age. Later up to 240 nmol (200 mg) of urobilinogen/24 h may be found normally
Water
  Meconium: 68–82% of the total weight of stools
  Newborn–3 months: 65–85% of the total weight of stools (slightly higher in breast-fed babies)
  3 months–6 years: 82–86% of the total weight of stools

Table 37.5   Therapeutic ranges for commonly used drugs in children

Drug	Therapeutic range in blood (µmol/l unless stated otherwise)
Carbamazepine	12–50
Chloramphenicol	30–60
Diazepam	0.7–1.0
Digoxin	
Infants	Up to 5.1 nmol/l
Older children and adults	1.0–2.6 nmol/l
Ethosuximide	280–700
Gentamicin	7.5–9.0
Peak 15 min post i.v. or 60 min post i.m.	8.0–18.5
Trough-predose	<3.7
Paracetamol	
Toxic value at 4 h	>1300
Toxic value at 8 h	>650
Toxic value at 12 h	>300
Phenobarbitone	60–130
For febrile convulsions	>60
Phenytoin	30–70
Primidone	23–55
Theophylline	55–110
For preterm apnea	30–70
Tobramycin	11–21
Sodium valproate	300–600

Table 37.6 Normal amniotic fluid values

Acetone bodies
0.20 mg/l

Calcium
1.6–2.1 mmol/l (6.4–8.2 mg/100 ml). Values above this range may be found near to term

Chloride
113 mmol/l (113 mEq/l) is the mean value up to 30 weeks' gestation, decreasing to a mean value of 111 mmol/l (111 mEq/l) at term

Citrate
155–420 μmol/l (3.0–8.1 mg/100 ml)

Creatine kinase
4.5 ± 2.3 IU/l. No significant changes occur with increasing gestational age. Markedly elevated values (10–180 times normal) may be indicative of intrauterine death

Creatinine
Up to 28 weeks' gestation: <88 μmol/l (0.1 mg/100 ml) increasing gradually, 36 weeks–term, >141 μmol/l (1.6 mg/100 ml). Low values tend to be associated with stillborn infants or polyhydramnios. High values above 350 μmol/l (4.0 mg/100 ml) tend to be associated with toxemic and diabetic mothers. Creatinine concentration in amniotic fluid has been suggested as an index of fetal maturity as have several other substances such as uric acid, total protein, total hydroxyproline, and α-fetoprotein

Enzymes
Many enzymes have been detected and estimated in amniotic fluid. At present the measurement of enzymes in cultured amniotic fluid cells is mainly used for the detection of inborn errors of metabolism

α-fetoprotein
18 weeks: 2.4–23.8 mg/l (k units/ml)
25–42 weeks: 0–10.5 mg/l (k units/ml).
Values are high in spina bifida and anencephalus, but raised values have also been described in association with placental injury and fetal death, Turner's syndrome, congenital nephrosis, omphalocele and duodenal atresia

Glucose
See Sugar

5-hydroxyindole acetic acid
8–42 nmol/g protein in the 1st and 2nd trimester, increasing to 79–315 nmol/g protein (15–60 ng/mg protein) in the last trimester. Normal values occur in polyhydramnios but low values occur in association with anencephalus and spina bifida

α-ketoglutarate (2-oxoglutarate)
10–95 μmol/l (0.1–1.4 mg/100 ml)

Lactate
Generally higher levels are found in amniotic fluid than in peripheral venous blood. Two different ranges are available in the literature. They are 2.6–5.9 mmol/l (23–56 mg/100 ml) and 5.8–12 mmol/l (52–108 mg/100 ml). High levels appear to be associated with fetal distress or delay in onset of respiration. Lower values are found at Cesarean sections

Lecithin : sphingomyelin ratio
This ratio has been shown to be a good index of pulmonary surfactant in the fetus. Normally this ratio is between 0.8 and 1.9 up to 32 weeks and then increases rapidly up to values of 5 or 6 at term. When this ratio is below 1.5 just before birth, the possibility of respiratory distress syndrome occurring is high (about 80%). If the ratio is above 2.0 respiratory distress is unlikely even in a preterm infant. When the ratio is between 1.5 and 2.0, about 20% of newborns develop respiratory distress

Magnesium
18 weeks' gestation: 0.7–0.95 mmol/l (1.4–1.9 mEq/l)
Term: 0.25–0.7 mmol/l (0.5–1.4 mEq/l)

Nitrogen
0.6 g/l – about half is nonprotein nitrogen

Osmolality
About 280 mmol/kg (280 mosmol/kg) at 10 weeks' gestation gradually falling to 250–260 mmol/kg (250–260 mosmol/kg) at term

PCO_2
5.9–7.6 kPa (44–57 mmHg)

pH
7.04–7.20

Phosphorus, inorganic
0.42–0.81 (mean 0.65) mmol/l or 1.3–2.5 mg/100 ml (mean 2.0) at term

Potassium
3.3–5.2 mmol/l (3.3–5.2 mEq/l) – slight fall towards term

Protein, total
3–11 g/l (0.3–1.1 g/100 ml) mainly albumin (albumin : globulin ratio about 3.1)

Sodium
137 mmol/l (137 mEq/l) is the mean value up to 30 weeks' gestation decreasing to a mean value of 133 mmol/l (133 mEq/l) at term

Solids, total
0.9–1.7% at term. Probably similar throughout pregnancy

Standard bicarbonate
13.0–19.8 mmol/l (13.0–19.8 mEq/l)

Sugar, reducing
0–300 mg/l (0–30 mg/100 ml) with a mean value of 130 mg/l (13 mg/100 ml). Decreased in long pregnancy

Urea
2.1–6.2 mmol/l (12.7–37.1 mg/100 ml). Increases occur as pregnancy progresses but values are too widely scattered, particularly near term for this determination on its own to be a useful indicator of fetal maturity.

Uric acid
2nd trimester: 0.12–0.33 mmol/l (2.1–5.5 mg/100 ml)
Term: 0.33–0.65 mmol/l (5.5–11.0 mg/100 ml)
This increasing uric acid output later in pregnancy reflects the increasing urinary output of the maturing fetus and its increasing muscle mass

Volume (mean values)
10 weeks' gestation: 30 ml
20 weeks' gestation: 250 ml
30 weeks' gestation: 600 ml
36 weeks' gestation: 1000 ml
Term: 800 ml
Polyhydramnios (>2000 ml) is commonly associated with intestinal obstruction and an increased incidence of congenital malformations. Oligohydramnios (<300 ml) is found in association with renal agenesis

Table 37.7 Function tests

Alanine load test
250 mg L-alanine/kg bodyweight orally, in cold water, is given to fasted patient. In patients with unimpaired gluconeogenesis there is normally a significant increase in the blood glucose concentration with little or no increase in lactic acid. Alanine levels reach a peak by about 1 h, then rapidly return to normal

Calcium loading test
Calcium, 1 g/1.73 m^2 body surface area, is given as calcium gluconate (Sandocal), and the patient is given, after fasting, a standard breakfast containing approximately 300 calories, 25 mmol sodium, 100 mg calcium, and 100 mg phosphorus. Normal children have urinary calcium creatinine ratios below 0.8 before and in the 4 h after the calcium load

Creatinine clearance
Normal: 90–150 ml/min/1.73 m^2 (40–65 in newborns)

$$\text{Calculation:} \quad \frac{\text{urine creatinine (mmol/l)} \times \text{vol/min}}{\text{plasma creatinine (mmol/l)}} \times \frac{1.73}{\text{surface area}}$$

Dexamethasone suppression test (of adrenal corticosteroid secretion)
Low dose: 20 µg/kg/day in 4 equal doses at 6-hourly intervals for 2 days. Plasma cortisol < 1 nmol/l
Urine cortisol < 50 nmol/24 h
Most patients with Cushing's syndrome give greater levels than stated, irrespective of etiology
High dose: 80 µg/kg/day in 4 equal doses at 6-hourly intervals for 2 days. Suppression by this higher dose but not the low dose is most frequently seen in pituitary-dependent bilateral adrenal hyperplasia (Cushing's disease)

Glucose tolerance test
Dose – 1.75 g/kg, not to exceed 75 g. Diabetes should be diagnosed only when the fasting plasma glucose is 7.8 mmol/l or higher, the 2 h concentration is 11.1 mmol/l or higher, and a value taken between these times is also 11.1 mmol/l or higher. Impaired glucose tolerance is present in children with a normal fasting plasma glucose and a 2 h concentration above 7.8 mmol/l, even if the 2 h level and another taken between 0 and 2 h both exceed 11.1 mmol/l

Growth hormone stimulation tests
Response to insulin hypoglycemia, arginine, clonidine or Bovril – peak > 20 mU/l

Growth hormone releasing factor (GRF) test
Measurement of the plasma growth hormone response to biosynthetic GRF may be of value in assessing whether GH insufficiency, identified by the clonidine or insulin hypoglycemia tests is due to pituitary or hypothalamic dysfunction. After a baseline blood sample, 1 µg/kg bodyweight is given i.v. and blood samples collected at 15, 30, 45, 60, 75, 90 and 120 min. A normal response is a rise in GH greater than 30 mU/l, peaking at 15–30 min after GRF administration

Fat absorption
The normal daily fecal fat excretion in children is 14 mmol (4 g) or less when assessed in a 5-day collection

Renal functional capacity
GFR
Newborns: 40–65 ml/min/1.73 m^2 increasing steadily to 90–150 ml/min/1.73 m^2 in children aged 1 year or older

Maximum concentrating ability
Newborns: up to 600 mosm/kg
Infants after 6 months and children: 800–1200 mosm/kg
Minimum urinary pH: 5.3 (after acid load)

Synacthen screening test
Synacthen (Tetracosactrin BP) is given by intravenous injection (500 ng per 1.73 m^2) and blood samples collected at 30, 60, 90 and 120 min
Cortisol concentration at 30 min should reach at least 425 nmol/l, with an increase of at least 145 nmol/l above the basal concentration

Depot synacthen test
Dose 1 mg i.m. daily for 3 days. Plasma cortisol increases at least 3-fold over basal concentrations in normals. There is also a response in secondary adrenal insufficiency. An absent cortisol response is definitive evidence of primary adrenal insufficiency

Xylose absorption test
5 g dose xylose: normal urine excretion should be greater than 1 g/5-h period (> 20% of dose). Normal plasma xylose > 1.3 mmol/l, 1 h after 5 g xylose

(See Hindmarsh & Swift 1995 for a full assessment of growth hormone provocation tests)

Table 37.8 Conversion factors

Ionic concentration

$$\text{mmol/l} = \frac{\text{mg/100 ml} \times 10}{\text{molecular weight}}$$

$$\text{mEq/l} = \frac{\text{mg/100 ml} \times 10}{\text{equivalent weight}}$$

$$\left(\text{equivalent weight} = \frac{\text{atomic weight}}{\text{valency}}\right)$$

To convert mEq/l to mg/100 ml for the following ions:

Sodium	multiply by	2.30
Potassium	multiply by	3.91
Calcium	multiply by	2.00
Magnesium	multiply by	1.215
Phosphorus	multiply by	1.72 (at pH 7.4)
Chloride	multiply by	3.55
Bicarbonate	multiply by	6.1
Lactate	multiply by	9.0
Protein	multiply by	0.41

To convert mg/100 ml to mEq/l, divide by the conversion factors given in right-hand column

Temperature
To convert °Fahrenheit to °Centigrade subtract 32 and then multiply by 5/9
To convert °Centigrade to °Fahrenheit multiply by 9/5 and then add 32

Energy
To convert kilocalories (kcals) to kilojoules (kjoules) multiply by 4.18

Weight
To convert grams to pounds and ounces divide by 454 to obtain the complete number of pounds, divide the remainder by 28.4 to obtain number of ounces
To convert pounds and ounces to grams multiply pounds by 454, multiply ounces by 28.4 and add the two products together

Table 37.9 Normal hematological values (all values shown are means with the ranges in parentheses)

Age	Red blood cells (× 10^12/l)	Hemoglobin (g/dl)	Hematocrit (%)	White blood cells (× 10^9/l)	Neutrophils (%)	Lymphocytes (%)	Eosinophils (%)	Monocytes (%)	Reticulocytes (%)	Platelets (× 10^9/l)	MCV (fl)	MCH (pg)	MCHC (g/dl)
Birth	5.0–6.0	17 (14–20)	55 (45–65)	18 (9–30)	60 (40–80)	32	2	7–14	5 (3–7)	100–300	94–118	32–40	34–36
1 week	Values fall within 3 months to	17 (13–21)	54 (43–66)	12 (6–22)	39 (30–50)	46	3	7–14	2 (0–4)	150 to 450	88–108	32–40	34–36
2 weeks		16.5 (13–20)	50 (42–66)	12 (5–21)	40 (30–50)	48	3	6–12	1 (0–2)		86–106	32–40	34–36
6 months–6 years	3.5–5.6	12 (10.5–14)	38 (33–42)	10 (6–15)	42 (32–52)	51	2–3	4–8	1 (0–2)	150 to 450	76–88	24–30	30–36
Adult Female	3.9–5.6	14 (12–16)	42 (37–47)	7.5 (5–10)	60 (40–75)	30 (20–45)	1–6	2–10	0–2		76–98	27–32	30–35
Male	4.5–6.5	16 (14–18)	46 (42–52)								76–96	27–32	30–35

(See also Lilleyman & Hann 1992, Nathan & Oski 1993, Lanzkowsky 1995.)

In low birthweight infants (BW < 1500 g) the mean Hb value falls from 18 g% at birth to 10 g% at 6 weeks (rising slowly thereafter) and mean corpuscular volume falls from 115 fl to 95 fl over the same period. Up to 34–36 weeks of fetal life 90–95% of hemoglobin is fetal hemoglobin. Thereafter the proportion of fetal hemoglobin decreases at rate of 3–4% per week, until 40 weeks when mean is 75% and range 50–85%. Thereafter slow fall to <60% at 2 months after birth (range 40–60%).

Then more rapid fall to <30% at 3 months after birth
<15% at 4 months after birth
<5% at 6 months after birth
<2% at 3 years after birth.

Table 37.10   Systolic blood pressure (mmHg) in awake children by age and cuff size

Age	4 cm cuff			8 cm cuff			12 cm cuff		
	No. of children	Mean (SD) blood pressure	95th centile	No. of children	Mean (SD) blood pressure	95th centile	No. of children	Mean (SD) blood pressure	95th centile
4 days*	171	76.2 (9.9)	95						
6 weeks*	1129	95.7 (10.7)	113						
6 months	129	104.8 (10.7)	124	738	88.5 (12.3)	109			
1 year				1323	93.4 (11.1)	112			
2 years				1322	95.5 (10.6)	115			
3 years				1218	96.8 (9.7)	115			
4 years				1149	97.4 (9.3)	113			
5 years				777	96.2 (9.4)	114	218	89.1 (9.3)	107
6 years				449	95.8 (9.1)	112	626	90.0 (8.2)	104
7 years				187	97.3 (9.2)	114	881	90.0 (8.6)	104
8 years				55	96.2 (8.6)	110	1042	91.9 (8.4)	105
9 years							963	92.3 (8.7)	106
10 years							449	94.3 (8.8)	111

* Some of the babies were asleep at time of measurement.
(From de Swiet et al 1992.)

Table 37.11   Diastolic blood pressure (mmHg) in awake children by age and cuff size*

Age (years)	8 mm cuff			12 mm cuff		
	No. of children	Mean (SD) blood pressure	95th centile	No. of children	Mean (SD) blood pressure	95th centile
5	777	62.3 (9.5)	78	218	57.8 (9.5)	73
6	442	63.6 (9.4)	70	621	59.6 (9.5)	74
7	179	66.2 (7.6)	81	839	60.6 (8.2)	75
8	55	65.2 (7.8)	78	1016	60.7 (7.6)	74
9				954	60.2 (7.6)	73
10				442	61.8 (7.2)	75

* The numbers of children studied are less than in Table 37.10 because the diastolic blood pressure (Korotkoff V) could not be determined for every child.
(From de Swiet et al 1992.)

Table 37.12   Blood pressure levels for the 90th and 95th percentiles of blood pressure for boys aged 1 to 17 years by percentiles of height

Age (years)	Blood pressure percentile*	Systolic blood pressure by percentile of height† (mmHg)							Diastolic blood pressure by percentile of height† (mmHg)						
		5%	10%	25%	50%	75%	90%	95%	5%	10%	25%	50%	75%	90%	95%
1	90th	94	95	97	98	100	102	102	50	51	52	53	54	54	55
	95th	98	99	101	102	104	106	106	55	55	56	57	58	59	59
2	90th	98	99	100	102	104	105	106	55	55	56	57	58	59	59
	95th	101	102	104	106	108	109	110	59	59	60	61	62	63	63
3	90th	100	101	103	105	107	108	109	59	59	60	61	62	63	63
	95th	104	105	107	109	111	112	113	63	63	64	65	66	67	67
4	90th	102	103	105	107	109	110	111	62	62	63	64	65	66	66
	95th	106	107	109	111	113	114	115	66	67	67	68	69	70	71
5	90th	104	105	106	108	110	112	112	65	65	66	67	68	69	69
	95th	108	109	110	112	114	115	116	69	70	70	71	72	73	74
6	90th	105	106	108	110	111	113	114	67	68	69	70	70	71	72
	95th	109	110	112	114	115	117	117	72	72	73	74	75	76	76
7	90th	106	107	109	111	113	114	115	69	70	71	72	72	73	74
	95th	110	111	113	115	116	118	119	74	74	75	76	77	78	78
8	90th	107	108	110	112	114	115	116	71	71	72	73	74	75	75
	95th	111	112	114	116	118	119	120	75	76	76	77	78	79	80
9	90th	109	110	112	113	115	117	117	72	73	73	74	75	76	77
	95th	113	114	116	117	119	121	121	76	77	78	79	80	80	81
10	90th	110	112	113	115	117	118	119	73	74	74	75	76	77	78
	95th	114	115	117	119	121	122	123	77	78	79	80	80	81	82

Table 37.12 *Cont'd*

Age (years)	Blood pressure percentile*	Systolic blood pressure by percentile of height† (mmHg)							Diastolic blood pressure by percentile of height† (mmHg)						
		5%	10%	25%	50%	75%	90%	95%	5%	10%	25%	50%	75%	90%	95%
11	90th	112	113	115	117	119	120	121	74	74	75	76	77	78	78
	95th	116	117	119	121	123	124	125	78	79	79	80	81	82	83
12	90th	115	116	117	119	121	123	123	75	75	76	77	78	78	79
	95th	119	120	121	123	125	126	127	79	79	80	81	82	83	83
13	90th	117	118	120	122	124	125	126	75	76	76	77	78	79	80
	95th	121	122	124	126	128	129	130	79	80	81	82	83	83	84
14	90th	120	121	123	125	126	128	128	76	76	77	78	79	80	80
	95th	124	125	127	128	130	132	132	80	81	81	82	83	84	85
15	90th	123	124	125	127	129	131	131	77	77	78	79	80	81	81
	95th	127	128	129	131	133	134	135	81	82	83	83	84	85	86
16	90th	125	126	128	130	132	133	134	79	79	80	81	82	82	83
	95th	129	130	132	134	136	137	138	83	83	84	85	86	87	87
17	90th	128	129	131	133	134	136	136	81	81	82	83	84	85	85
	95th	132	133	135	136	138	140	140	85	85	86	87	88	89	89

* Blood pressure percentile was determined by a single measurement.
† Height percentile was determined by standard growth curves.
(Reproduced by permission of Pediatrics 98: 653–654; 1996)

Table 37.13 Blood pressure levels for the 90th and 95th percentiles of blood pressure for girls aged 1 to 17 years by percentiles of height

Age (years)	Blood pressure percentile*	Systolic blood pressure by percentile of height† (mmHg)							Diastolic blood pressure by percentile of height† (mmHg)						
		5%	10%	25%	50%	75%	90%	95%	5%	10%	25%	50%	75%	90%	95%
1	90th	97	98	99	100	102	103	104	53	53	53	54	55	56	56
	95th	101	102	103	104	105	107	107	57	57	57	58	59	60	60
2	90th	99	99	100	102	103	104	105	57	57	58	58	59	60	61
	95th	102	103	104	105	107	108	109	61	61	62	62	63	64	65
3	90th	100	100	102	103	104	105	106	61	61	61	62	63	63	64
	95th	104	104	105	107	108	109	110	65	65	65	66	67	67	68
4	90th	101	102	103	104	106	107	108	63	63	64	65	65	66	67
	95th	105	106	107	108	109	111	111	67	67	68	69	69	70	71
5	90th	103	103	104	106	107	108	109	65	66	66	67	68	68	69
	95th	107	107	108	110	111	112	113	69	70	70	71	72	72	73
6	90th	104	105	106	107	109	110	111	67	67	68	69	69	70	71
	95th	108	109	110	111	112	114	114	71	71	72	73	73	74	75
7	90th	106	107	108	109	110	112	112	69	69	69	70	71	72	72
	95th	110	110	112	113	114	115	116	73	73	73	74	75	76	76
8	90th	108	109	110	111	112	113	114	70	70	71	71	72	73	74
	95th	112	112	113	115	116	117	118	74	74	75	75	76	77	78
9	90th	110	110	112	113	114	115	116	71	72	72	73	74	74	75
	95th	114	114	115	117	118	119	120	75	76	76	77	78	78	79
10	90th	112	112	114	115	116	117	118	73	73	73	74	75	76	76
	95th	116	116	117	119	120	121	122	77	77	77	78	79	80	80
11	90th	114	114	116	117	118	119	120	74	74	75	75	76	77	77
	95th	118	118	119	121	122	123	124	78	78	79	79	80	81	81
12	90th	116	116	118	119	120	121	122	75	75	76	76	77	78	78
	95th	120	120	121	123	124	125	126	79	79	80	80	81	82	82
13	90th	118	118	119	121	122	123	124	76	76	77	78	78	79	80
	95th	121	122	123	125	126	127	128	80	80	81	82	82	83	84
14	90th	119	120	121	122	124	125	126	77	77	78	79	79	80	81
	95th	123	124	125	126	128	129	130	81	81	82	83	83	84	85
15	90th	121	121	122	124	125	126	127	78	78	79	79	80	81	82
	95th	124	125	126	128	129	130	131	82	82	83	83	84	85	86
16	90th	122	122	123	125	126	127	128	79	79	79	80	81	82	82
	95th	125	126	127	128	130	131	132	83	83	83	84	85	86	86
17	90th	122	123	124	125	126	128	128	79	79	79	80	81	82	82
	95th	126	126	127	129	130	131	132	83	83	83	84	85	86	86

* Blood pressure percentile was determined by a single reading.
† Height percentile was determined by standard growth curves.
(Reproduced by permission of Pediatrics 98: 653–654; 1996)

Table 37.14   Composition of infant milk and formula feeds (all values refer to the concentration per 100 ml of normally reconstituted feeds)

Milk or formula (manufacturer)	Energy		Protein			Fat				Carbohydrate				Minerals					
	kJ	kcal	Total (g)	Casein (%)	Whey (%)	Total (g)	Saturated (%)	Unsaturated (%)	Type	Total (g)	Lactose (g)	Maltodextrin (g)	Other (g)	Na (mg)	K (mg)	Ca (mg)	P (mg)	Mg (mg)	Fe (µg)
Human (breast) milk (mature) (average values)	293	70	1.1	32	68	4.2	51	49		7.0	7.0			15	60	35	15	2.8	76
Cow's milk (average values)	267	64	3.1	77	23	3.8	63	37		4.7	4.7			53	136	112	89	11	58
Modified milks																			
Aptamil (Milupa)	281	67	1.5	40	60	3.6	50	50	Veg. oils, milk fat	7.2	7.2			23	82	66	42	5.2	700
Boots Formula 1	280	67	1.5	40	60	3.48	48	52	Veg. oils	7.41	7.41			19	46	39	25	6.3	800
Boots Formula 2	283	68	1.61	80	20	3.63	48	52	Veg. oils	7.15	7.15			22	73	59	45	5.2	800
Farley's First	284	68	1.45	39	61	3.82	41.5	58.5	Veg. oils, fish oils	7.0	7.0			19	57	35	29	5.2	650
Farley's Second	277	66	1.7	77	23	2.9	35.9	64.1	Veg. oils	8.3	2.8		5.5	25	86	61	48	6	660
Milumil (Milupa)	283	67	1.9	80	20	3.1	53	47	Veg. oils	8.0	6.1	1.9		27	98	88	57	7	700
Plus (Cow and Gate)	277	66	1.7	80	20	3.4	41	56	Veg. oils	7.2	7.16			25	90	80	47	5.4	500
Premium (Cow and Gate)	277	66	1.41	40	60	3.6	41	56	Veg. oils	7.1	7.0			18	67	53	27	5.1	510
SMA White	280	67	1.6	80	20	3.6	43	57	Veg. oils	7.0	7.0			22	80	56	44	5.3	800
SMA Gold Cap (Wyeth)	280	67	1.5	40	60	3.6	43	57	Veg. oils	7.2	7.2			16	65	46	33	6.7	800
Preterm milks (for low birthweight babies)																			
Neutriprem (Cow and Gate)	336	80	2.2	40	60	4.4	41	59	Veg. oils, marine oil	8.0	4.0	4.0		32	71	108	54	8	900
Neutriprem 2 (Cow and Gate)	310	74	1.8	40	60	4.1	42	58	Veg. oils	7.5	6.0	1.5		24.8	73	80	40	6	1100
Osterprem (Farley's)	334	80	2.0	39	61	4.6	41.6	58.4	Veg. oils, milk fat	7.65	6.0	1.65		42	72	110	63	5	40
Prematil (Milupa)	335	80	2.4	40	60	4.4	43	57	Veg. oils	7.9	6.2	1.7		41	80	100	50	10	900
Prem Care (Farley's)	301	72	1.85	39	61	3.96	42	58	Milk fat, veg. oils, fish oil	7.24	6.2	1.04		22	78	70	35	5.2	650
SMA Low Birth Weight	343	82	2.0	40	60	4.4	50	50	Veg. oils, MCT	8.6	4.3	4.3		35	85	80	42.5	8	800
Soya milks																			
Infasoy (Cow and Gate)	277	66	1.8			3.6	41	59	Veg. oils	6.7		6.7		18	65	54	27	5	800
Isomil (Abbott)	286	68	1.8			3.7	43	57	Corn oil, coconut oil	6.9		4.2	2.7	32	77	70	50	5	1200
Farley's Soya	293	70	1.95			3.8	37	53	Veg. oils	7.0		7.0		25	75	56	37	5.7	700
Prosobee (Mead Johnson)	283	67	2.0			3.6	43	57	Veg. oils	6.6		6.6		24	81	64	51	7.4	1200
Wysoy (Wyeth)	274	65	1.8			3.6	43	57	Veg. oils	6.9		6.5	1.4	18	70	60	42	6.7	670
Follow-on milks																			
Boots Milk Drink powder	272	65	2.15	62	38	3.41	47	53	Milk Fat, veg. oils	6.43	6.04	0.39		29	97	69	58	8.5	1260
ready-to-feed	301	72	2.52	80	20	3.19	47	53	Veg. oils	8.29	6.34	1.95		29	132	91	80	9	1400
Farley's Follow-on	285	68	2.1	64	36	3.1	41	59	Veg. oils, milk fat	8.0	5.3	2.7		31	91	72	55	7.8	1200
Forward (Milupa)	311	74	2.1	80	20	3.3	48	52	Veg. fat	9.0	7.0	2.0		30	115	87	62	8.5	1200
Progress (SMA)	281	67	2.2			3.0	46	54	Veg. oils	7.8	7.8			33	107	90	62	8	1300
Step-Up (Cow and Gate)	293	70	1.8	80	20	3.8	36	64	Veg. oils	7.2	7.2			23	86	88	50	6	1300

For powdered preparations, reconstitution is normally made by diluting 1 levelled scoop of powder in 30 ml of water. Only the scoop provided by the manufacturer for that powder should be used. (For further information on the composition of infant milks and foods see Department of Health and Social Security (1977, 1980, 1988), Department of Health (1994), ESPGAN (1977, 1981, 1982, 1987, 1990) and Tsang et al (1993).

Minerals					Vitamins													Choline (mg)	Carnitine (mg)	Inositol (mg)	Taurine (mg)
Cu (μg)	Zn (μg)	Mn (μg)	Cl (mg)	I (μg)	A (μg)	B_1 (μg)	B_2 (μg)	Pantothenic acid (μg)	B_6 (μg)	B_{12} (μg)	Biotin (μg)	Folic acid (μg)	Niacin (μg)	C (mg)	D (μg)	E (mg)	K (μg)				
39	295		43	7	60	16	31	260	5.9	0.01	0.76	5.2	230	3.8	0.01	0.35					
21	400	3	97	26	50	30	165	350	60	0.4	1.9	6	80	1.0	0.03	0.09					
40	500	10	53	10	60	40	120	400	40	0.2	1.0	10	700	8	1.0	0.6	3.0				7.0
39	390	3.9	39	5.2	84	65	78	260	65	0.22	1.3	3.9	800	9.8	1.0	1.0	3.9				
35	500	3.5	45	10	70	50	60	300	60	0.18	1.03	7.0	900	8.0	1.0	0.7	6.0				
42	340	3.4	45	4.5	100	42	55	230	35	0.14	1.0	3.4	690	6.9	1.0	0.48	2.7				
40	330	3.3	55	10	97	39	53	220	33	0.13	1.0	3.3	660	6.6	1.0	0.46	2.6				6.0
30	500	8	59	9.1	63	40	60	400	40	0.2	1.0	11	800	8	1.1	0.6	3.2				4.6
40	400	7	56	9.9	80	40	100	300	40	0.2	1.5	10	800	8	1.1	0.81	5.0	7			4.6
41	380	7	40	9.9	76	38	110	250	38	0.2	1.5	10	750	7.6	1.1	0.81	5.1	7			4.6
33	600	10	55	10	75	100	150	300	60	0.2	2.0	8	900	9	1.1	0.74	6.7	6.7	0.6		3.8
33	600	10	43	10	75	100	150	300	60	0.2	2.0	8	900	9	1.1	0.74	6.7	10	1.3		3.8
80	700	14	45	20	100	100	160	500	80	0.2	3.0	48	1550	28	2.4	0.96	9	6	1.5	3	5.5
60	600	7	45	15	107	80	120	600	70	0.2	3.0	20	1600	18	1.58	1.2	7.0				
96	880	3	60	8	100	95	180	500	100	0.2	2.0	50	1000	28	2.4	10.0	7	5.6	1.0	3.2	5.1
80	700	5	48	14	108	140	200	1000	120	0.2	3.0	48	3000	16	2.4	3	6.6	10	2	30	5.5
57	600	5.0	45	4.5	100	95	100	400	80	0.2	1.1	25	400	15	1.3	1.5	6.0				
82.5	800	10	60	10	90	120	200	450	72	0.3	2.4	48	1320	11	1.5	1.2	8	15	2.7	4.5	7
40	600	25	40	13	80	40	100	300	40	0.2	1.5	10	800	8.0	1.1	1.3	5	7	1.5	3.5	4.6
50	500	20	59	10	60	40	60	500	40	0.3	3.0	10	900	5.5	1.0	1.7	10		1.2		4.5
42	540	34	50	8.4	100	42	56	240	36	0.15	1.1	3.5	700	9	1.1	0.50	2.8	4.9	0.85	4.0	5.1
51	810	17	54	10	61	54	61	340	41	0.2	2.0	11	680	8.1	1.0	1.4	5.4	8.1	0.85	11.5	
47	500	20	40	6	60	67	100	300	42	0.2	3.5	5	500	5.5	1.0	0.64	10	8.5	1	10	3.8
380	410	5.1	72	6.5	110	42	63	250	33	0.16	1.2	3.9	770	10	2.0	0.85	3.7				
	500	2	76	4	63	45	150	450	60	0.3	2.2	10.5	520	7	1.08	0.78	7.2				
41	400	4.0	68	11	80	40	150	360	40	0.2	3.0	7	650	10	1.1	0.48	2.7				
70	600	10	71	12.4	62	40	150	400	40	0.2	1.0	11	730	9.0	1.0	0.6	3.0				
40	600	10	62	12	75	100	150	300	60	0.2	2.0	8	900	9	1.2	0.74	6.7	9	0.8		0.5
49	700	11	51	11	60	40	100	300	40	0.2	1.6	11	800	8.0	1.8	0.81	5.6	7			

Table 37.15 Composition of special formula infant feeds and supplements (all values refer to the concentration per 100 ml of normally reconstituted feeds except where otherwise stated

Feed (manufacturer)	Type/clinical indications	Energy		Protein		Fat		Carbohydrate	
		kJ	kcal	g	Type	g	Type	g	Type
AL 110 (Nestlé)	Lactose free	280	67	1.9	Casein	3.3	Milk fat, corn oil	7.4	Maltodextrin from corn starch
Alfaré (Nestlé)	Hypoallergenic	301	72	2.5	Whey, amino acids	7.0	MCT, milk fat, corn oil	7.8	Maltodextrin, starch
Caprilon (Cow and Gate)	For fat malabsorption	275	66	1.5	Whey, casein	3.6	MCT oil, Soy oil	7.0	Glucose syrup, lactose
Enfamil AR (Mead Johnson)	Pre-thickened, for posseting and reflux	287	69	1.7	Casein, whey	3.5	Veg. oils	7.55	Glucose polymer, lactose, rice starch
Galactomin 17 (Cow and Gate)	Low lactose, for galactosemia	280	67	1.9	Sodium + calcium caseinates	3.4	Palm, Canola, coconut and sunflower oils	7.4	Glucose syrup
Galactomin 19 (Cow and Gate)	Low lactose, for glucose-galactose intolerance	288	69	1.9	Casein	4.0		6.4	Fructose, trace of lactose
Locasol (Cow and Gate)	Low calcium for hypercalcemia	278	67	1.9	Casein, demineralized whey	3.4	Vegetable oils, milk fat	7.0	Lactose
MCT Pepdite (0–2) (SHS)	Free from lactose, gluten, fructose, sucrose	286	68	2.1	Hydrolyzed non-milk protein, amino acids	2.7	Coconut oil, sunflower oil	8.9	Glucose syrup
HN 25 (Milupa)	Low lactose, for treatment of diarrhea	242	57	2.6	Milk protein	1.2	Vegetable fat	9.1	Maltodextrin, starch
Monogen (SHS)	For lipid and lymphatic disorders	312	74	2.0	Whey, aminoacids	2.0	MCT (93%)	12	Glucose syrup
Neocate (Scientific Hospital Supplies)	Free of protein, lactose and sucrose Hypoallergenic	300	72	1.95	Amino acids	3.45	Safflower, coconut and soya oils	8.1	Glucose syrup
Nutramigen (Mead Johnson)	Free of protein, lactose and sucrose	284	68	1.9	Enzymatically hydrolyzed casein	3.4	Palm, soy, coconut and sunflower oils	7.4	Glucose polymers corn starch
Pepdite (0–2) (SHS)	Free from lactose, gluten, fructose, sucrose	297	71	2.1	Hydrolyzed non-milk protein, amino acids	3.5	Coconut oil, peanut oil, animal fat	7.8	Glucose syrup
Pepti-Junior (Cow and Gate)	Hypoallergenic	276	66	1.78	Whey hydrolysate	3.62	Corn oil, MCT oil	6.6	Glucose syrup, lactose
Pregestimil (Mead Johnson)	Free of protein, lactose and sucrose	284	68	1.9	Enzymatically hydrolyzed casein	3.8	Corn, soy, safflower and MCT oils	6.9	Glucose polymers corn starch
Prejomin (Milupa)	Hypoallergenic	313	75	2.0	Hydrolysate	3.6	Vegetable fats	8.6	Maltodextrins, starch
XP Analog (SHS)	Phenylalanine free, for PKU	300	72	1.95	Amino acids	3.5	Safflower, coconut and soya bean oils	8.1	Glucose syrup
Components used in special feeds									
Calogen (SHS)*	High calorie fat emulsion	1850	450	–		50	Arachis oil, peanut oil	–	Glucose polymer
Comminuted chicken meat (Cow and Gate)	Carbohydrate free	212–266	51–64	7.0–8.0	Chicken meat	2.5–3.5		–	None
Duocal (SHS) (liquid) (1 to 3 dilution)	High energy supplement	661	158	–		7.4	Maize oil, coconut oil	24.2	Glucose syrup
Instant carobel (Cow and Gate)	Instant feed thickener	Does not add energy to feed (contains carob bean gum flour, calcium lactate)							
Liquigen (SHS)	Fat (MCT) supplement, for malabsorption	1850	450	–		50	MCT	–	
Maxijul (SHS)	Carbohydrate source	†1615	380					95	Maltodextrin
Maxipro (SHS) (1 to 5 dilution)	Protein supplement, free from gluten fructose, sucrose	332	79	16.0	Whey protein, amino acids	1.2		<1.0	Lactose
MCT Duocal (SHS)	Energy supplement, free of protein, lactose, gluten, sucrose	†2116	505	–		23.2	MCT, LCT	74	Glucose syrup
MCT oil (Cow and Gate)	Medium chain triglycerides	3515	855			95	Medium chain triglycerides		
Nestargel (Nestlé)	Feed thickener	Does not add energy to feed							
Polycal (Cow and Gate)	Carohydrate source	†1610	380	–		–		94.5	Maltodextrin, maltose, glucose
Scandishake (SHS)	High energy supplement	†2153	514	4.7		24.7		68.2	
Seravit, paediatric (SHS)	Vitamin, trace element and mineral mixture								
Super Soluble Duocal (SHS)	Free from gluten, protein, lactose	†2061	492	–		22.3		72.7	
Super Soluble Maxijul (SHS)	Carbohydrate source	†1615	380	–		–		95	

* SHS = Scientific Hospital Supplies.
† Concentrations per 100 g.
‡ Concentrations per 17 g (recommended daily intake from 6 months).
All values refer to the normal dilution as recommended by the manufacturer.

	Minerals							Vitamins													
Na (mg)	K (mg)	Ca (mg)	P (mg)	Mg (mg)	Fe (µg)	Cu (µg)	Zn (µg)	A (µg)	B_1 (µg)	B_2 (µg)	Pantothenic acid (µg)	B_6 (µg)	B_{12} (µg)	Biotin (µg)	Folic acid (µg)	Niacin (µg)	C (mg)	D (µg)	E (mg)	K (µg)	Osmolality (mOsm/kg H_2O)
23	80	60	40	6.7	800	40	500	60	40	90	300	50	0.15	1.5	6	500	5.4	1.0	0.8	5.5	5
44	90	60	38	9	900	40	540	72	40	100	320	50	0.16	1.6	10	760	7.6	2	0.9	5.9	
18	65	54	27	5	500	40	400	80	40	100	300	40	0.2	1.5	10	760	7.6	2	0.8	5.1	233
24	85	55	44	5.4	800	44	700	61	54	61	340	41	0.2	2.0	10.8	670	8.1	1.0	1.35	5.4	
27	97	83	55	6.6	500	80	400	79	40	100	300	40	0.2	1.6	10	900	8	1.1	0.9	5.2	210
20	66	55	27	8.0	500	79	400	81	40	100	300	40	0.2	1.5	10	900	8.1	1.3	1.0	5.3	487
27	97	≤7	55	6.6	500	40	400	80	40	100	300	40	0.2	1.6	10.5	900	8	<0.004	0.8	5.2	310
35	58	45	35	5.1	825	60	585	80	60	90	255	52	0.45	3.9	5.8	675	6.2	1.1	0.7	6.8	9.8
39	109	66	48	8	1000	30	200	56	40	100	400	30	0.2	1	10	400	9	1.1	0.7	2	
35	58	45	35	5.1	800	60	600	80	60	90	250	52	0.15	3.9	5.8	680	6.1	1.1	0.7	6.7	280
18	63	49	34	5.1	1050	68	750	80	59	90	400	78	0.19	3.9	5.7	675	6.0	1.3	0.7	3.2	353
32	74	64	43	7.4	1200	51	700	61	54	61	338	41	0.2	2	10.8	680	8.1	1.0	1.35	5.4	320
35	58	45	35	5.1	825	60	585	80	60	90	255	52	0.15	3.9	5.8	675	6.2	1.1	0.7	6.8	9.8
30	100	81	41	12	800	58	600	116	60	160	390	60	0.3	2.3	16	1300	12	2	1.8	7.8	210
32	74	63	42	7.5	1200	66	470	78	66	60	320	40	0.37	2	11	850	7.5	1.1	1.6	11	320
42	92	57	29	11	1800	60	600	71	50	60	500	40	0.2	2.0	12	1100	7.5	1.2	0.8	4.7	225
18	63	49	34	5.1	1050	70	750	79	60	90	400	80	0.19	3.9	5.7	680	6	1.3	0.7	3.1	353
10	50	9	45	8	400	50	200														131
≤1.7	≤1.7	≤1.7	≤1.7																		310
28																					
<20	<5		<5																		to 284 (1 to 4 dilution)
26	94	100	66																		
30	3.7																				
(MCT oil should always be diluted before use)																					
50	50	50	100																		
106	306	118	235	9.4																	
‡<2	Trace	43.7	291	60.7	11700	780		7800	710	540	2890	580	1.46	36	52	5950	68		4.9	28.2	
<5	<5	<5	<5																		
<20	<5		<5																		

Table 37.16 Examples of pediatric enteral feeds

Feed	Protein	Composition per 100 ml					Special features	Manufacturer
		Protein g	Energy kcal	kJ	Fat g	Carbohydrate g		
Nutrison Paediatric (Standard)	Caseinates	2.75	100	420	4.5	12.2		Cow & Gate
Nutrison Paediatric (Energy Plus)	Caseinates	3.4	150	630	6.8	18.8		Cow & Gate
Paediasure	Whey and caseinate	3.0	100	420	5.0	11.0		Abbott Laboratories
Elemental 028	Essential and nonessential amino acids	2.0	76	322	1.3	14.1	Severe GI tract impairment	Scientific Hospital Supplies
Elemental 028 Extra	Essential and nonessential amino acids	2.5	85	358	3.5	11.0	Severe GI tract impairment	Scientific Hospital Supplies
Generaid Plus	Whey and branched chain amino acids	2.42	102	428	4.2	13.6	Hepatic disorders. Fat: 35% MCT : 65% LCT	Scientific Hospital Supplies
Kindergen P.R.O.D.	Whey and essential amino acids	1.5	101	424	5.2	12.1	Chronic renal failure	Scientific Hospital Supplies
Peptide 2+	Soya and beef peptides	2.8	88	369	3.5	11.4	GI tract impairment	Scientific Hospital Supplies
MCT Peptide 2+	Soya and beef peptides	2.8	91	381	3.6	11.8	GI tract impairment + fat malabsorption. Fat: 83% MCT : 17% LCT	Scientific Hospital Supplies

Table 37.19 Reference nutrient intakes for vitamins and minerals

Age	Thiamin (mg/d)	Riboflavin (mg/d)	Niacin (nicotinic acid equivalent) (mg/d)	Vitamin B_6 (mg/d)§	Vitamin B_{12} (µg/d)	Folate (µg/d)	Vitamin C (mg/d)	Vitamin A (µg/d)	Vitamin D (µg/d)
0–3 months	0.2	0.4	3	0.2	0.3	50	25	350	8.5
4–6 months	0.2	0.4	3	0.2	0.3	50	25	350	8.5
7–9 months	0.2	0.4	4	0.3	0.4	50	25	350	7
10–12 months	0.3	0.4	5	0.4	0.4	50	25	350	7
1–3 years	0.5	0.6	8	0.7	0.5	70	30	400	7
4–6 years	0.7	0.8	11	0.9	0.8	100	30	500	–
7–10 years	0.7	1.0	12	1.0	1.0	150	30	500	–
Males									
11–14 years	0.9	1.2	15	1.2	1.2	200	35	600	–
15–18 years	1.1	1.3	18	1.5	1.5	200	40	700	–
19–50 years	1.0	1.3	17	1.4	1.5	200	40	700	–
50+ years	0.9	1.3	16	1.4	1.5	200	40	700	†
Females									
11–14 years	0.7	1.1	12	1.0	1.2	200	35	600	–
15–18 years	0.8	1.1	14	1.2	1.5	200	40	600	–
19–50 years	0.8	1.1	13	1.2	1.5	200	40	600	–
50+ years	0.8	1.1	12	1.2	1.5	200	40	600	†
Pregnancy	+0.1‡	+0.3	*	*	*	+100	+10	+100	10
Lactation:									
0–4 months	+0.2	+0.5	+2	*	+0.5	+60	+30	+350	10
4+ months	+0.2	+0.5	+2	*	+0.5	+60	+30	+350	10

* No increment.   † After age 65 the RNI is 10 µg/d for men and women.   ‡ For last trimester only.
§ Based on protein providing 14.7% of EAR for energy.   ** Phosphorus RNI is set equal to calcium in molar terms.
†† 1 mmol sodium = 23 mg.   ‡‡ 1 mmol potassium = 39 mg.   §§ Corresponds to sodium 1 mmol = 35.5 mg.
*** Insufficient for women with high menstrual losses where the most practical way of meeting iron requirements is to take iron supplements.
(From Department of Health 1991).

Table 37.17 Estimated average requirements (EARs)† for energy

Age	EARs MJ/d (kcal/d) Males	EARs MJ/d (kcal/d) Females
0–3 months	2.28 (545)	2.16 (515)
4–6 months	2.89 (690)	2.69 (645)
7–9 months	3.44 (825)	3.20 (765)
10–12 months	3.85 (920)	3.61 (865)
1–3 years	5.15 (1230)	4.86 (1165)
4–6 years	7.16 (1715)	6.46 (1545)
7–10 years	8.24 (1970)	7.28 (1740)
11–14 years	9.27 (2220)	7.92 (1845)
15–18 years	11.51 (2755)	8.83 (2110)
19–50 years	10.60 (2550)	8.10 (1940)
51–59 years	10.60 (2550)	8.00 (1900)
60–64 years	9.93 (2380)	7.99 (1900)
65–74 years	9.71 (2330)	7.96 (1900)
75+ years	8.77 (2100)	7.61 (1810)
Pregnancy		+0.80*(200)
Lactation:		
1 month		+1.90 (450)
2 months		+2.20 (530)
3 months		+2.40 (570)
4–6 months (group 1)		+2.00 (480)
4–6 months (group 2)		+2.40 (570)
>6 months (group 1)		+1.00 (240)
>6 months (group 2)		+2.30 (550)

*Last trimester only.

Group 1 mothers: those breast-feeding for up to 6 months.
Group 2 mothers: those breast-feeding for more than 6 months.
† EAR Estimated average requirement of a group of people for energy or protein or a vitamin or mineral. About half will usually need more than the EAR, and half less.
(From Department of Health 1991.)

Table 37.18 Reference nutrient intakes* for protein

Age	Reference nutrient intake** (g/d)
0–3 months	12.5†
4–6 months	12.7
7–9 months	13.7
10–12 months	14.9
1–3 years	14.5
4–6 years	19.7
7–10 years	28.3
Males:	
11–14 years	42.1
15–18 years	55.2
19–50 years	55.5
50+ years	53.3
Females:	
11–14 years	41.2
15–18 years	45.0
19–50 years	45.0
50+ years	46.5
Pregnancy‡	+6
Lactation:‡	
0–4 months	+11
4+ months	+8

* These figures, based on egg and milk protein, assume complete digestibility.
† No values for infants 0–3 months are given by WHO. The RNI is calculated from the recommendations of COMA.
‡ To be added to adult requirement through all stages of pregnancy and lactation.
** RNI Reference nutrient intake for protein or a vitamin or mineral. An amount of the nutrient that is enough, or more than enough, for about 97% of people in a group. If average intake of a group is at RNI, then the risk of deficiency in the group is very small.
(From Department of Health 1991.)

Calcium (mg/d)	Phosphorus** (mg/d)	Magnesium (mg/d)	Sodium (mg/d)††	Potassium (mg/d)‡‡	Chloride (mg/d)§§	Iron (mg/d)	Zinc (mg/d)	Copper (mg/d)	Selenium (µg/d)	Iodine (µg/d)
525	400	55	210	800	320	1.7	4.0	0.2	10	50
525	400	60	280	850	400	4.3	4.0	0.3	13	60
525	400	75	320	700	500	7.8	5.0	0.3	10	60
525	400	80	350	700	500	7.8	5.0	0.3	10	60
350	270	85	500	800	800	6.9	5.0	0.4	15	70
450	350	120	700	1100	1100	6.1	6.5	0.6	20	100
550	450	200	1200	2000	1800	8.7	7.0	0.7	30	110
1000	775	280	1600	3100	2500	11.3	9.0	0.8	45	130
1000	775	300	1600	3500	2500	11.3	9.5	1.0	70	140
700	550	300	1600	3500	2500	8.7	9.5	1.2	75	140
700	550	300	1600	3500	2500	8.7	9.5	1.2	75	140
800	625	280	1600	3100	2500	14.8***	9.0	0.8	45	130
800	625	300	1600	3500	2500	14.8***	7.0	1.0	60	140
700	550	270	1600	3500	2500	14.8***	7.0	1.2	60	140
700	550	270	1600	3500	2500	8.7	7.0	1.2	60	140
*	*	*	*	*	*	*	*	*	*	*
+550	+440	+50	*	*	*	*	+6.0	+0.3	+15	*
+550	+440	+50	*	*	*	*	+2.5	+0.3	+15	*

Table 37.20 Safe intakes

Nutrient	Safe intake*
Vitamins:	
Pantothenic acid	
adults	3–7 mg/d
infants	1.7 mg/d
Biotin	10–200 µg/d
Vitamin E	
men	Above 4 mg/d
women	Above 3 mg/d
infants	0.4 mg/g polyunsaturated fatty acid
Vitamin K	
adults	1 µg/kg/d
infants	10 µg/d
Minerals:	
Manganese	
adults	1.4 mg (26 µmol)/d
infants and children	16 µg (0.3 µmol)/d
Molybdenum	
adults	50–400 µg/d
infants, children and adolescents	0.5–1.5 µg/kg/d
Chromium	
adults	25 µg (0.5 µmol)/d
children and adolescents	0.1–1.0 µg (2–20 µmol)/kg/d
Fluoride (for infants only)	0.05 mg (3 µmol)/kg/d

* Safe intakes have been set for some nutrients for which there are insufficient reliable data on human requirements to set any dietary reference values. However, these safe intakes were set particularly for infants and children. The safe intake was judged to be a level or range of intake at which there is no risk of deficiency, and below a level where there is a risk of undesirable effects.
(From Department of Health 1991.)

Table 37.21 Food and Nutrition Board, National Academy of Sciences–National Research Council recommended dietary allowances* revised 1989. 'Designed for the maintenance of good nutrition of practically all healthy people in the United States'

Category	Age (years) or condition	Weight†		Height†		Protein (g)	Fat-soluble vitamins			
		kg	lb	cm	in		Vitamin A (µg RE)††	Vitamin D (µg)**	Vitamin E (mg α-TE)§	Vitamin K (µg)
Infants	0.0–0.5	6	13	60	24	13	375	7.5	3	5
	0.5–1.0	9	20	71	28	14	375	10	4	10
Children	1–3	13	29	90	35	16	400	10	6	15
	4–6	20	44	112	44	24	500	10	7	20
	7–10	28	62	132	52	28	700	10	7	30
Males	11–14	45	99	157	62	45	1000	10	10	45
	15–18	66	145	176	69	59	1000	10	10	65
	19–24	72	160	177	70	58	1000	10	10	70
	25–50	79	174	176	70	63	1000	5	10	80
	51+	77	170	173	68	63	1000	5	10	80
Females	11–14	46	101	157	62	46	800	10	8	45
	15–18	55	120	163	64	44	800	10	8	55
	19–24	58	128	164	65	46	800	10	8	60
	25–50	63	138	163	64	50	800	5	8	65
	51+	65	143	160	63	50	800	5	8	65
Pregnant						60	800	10	10	65
Lactating	1st 6 months					65	1300	10	12	65
	2nd 6 months					62	1200	10	11	65

* The allowances, expressed as average daily intakes over time, are intended to provide for individual variations among most normal persons as they live in the US under usual environmental stresses. Diets should be based on a variety of common foods in order to provide other nutrients for which human requirements have been less well defined.
† Weights and heights of reference adults are actual medians for the US population of the designated age, as reported by NHANES II (NHANES II = National Health and Nutrition Examination Survey (1976–1980)). The median weights and heights of those under 19 years of age were taken from Hamill et al (1979) The use of these figures does not imply that the height-to-weight ratios are ideal.
†† Retinol equivalent. 1 retinol equivalent = 1 µg retinol or 6 µg β-carotene. See text for calculation of vitamin A activity of diets as retinol equivalents.
** As cholecalciferol. 10 µg cholecalciferol = 400 IU of vitamin D.
§ α-tocopherol equivalents. 1 mg d-α-tocopherol = 1 α-TE. See text for variation in allowances and calculation of vitamin E activity of the diet as α-tocopherol equivalents.
‡ 1 NE (niacin equivalent) is equal to 1 mg of niacin or 60 mg of dietary tryptophan.
(From National Research Council 1989.)

Table 37.22 Estimated safe and adequate daily dietary intakes of selected vitamins and minerals*

Category	Age (years)	Vitamins		Trace elements†				
		Biotin (µg)	Pantothenic acid (mg)	Copper (mg)	Manganese (mg)	Fluoride (mg)	Chromium (µg)	Molybdenum (µg)
Infants	0–0.5	10	2	0.4–0.6	0.3–0.6	0.1–0.5	10–40	15–30
	0.5–1	15	3	0.6–0.7	0.6–1.0	0.2–1.0	20–60	20–40
Children and adolescents	1–3	20	3	0.7–1.0	1.0–1.5	0.5–1.5	20–80	25–50
	4–6	25	3–4	1.0–1.5	1.5–2.0	1.0–2.5	30–120	30–75
	7–10	30	4–5	1.0–2.0	2.0–3.0	1.5–2.5	50–200	50–150
	11+	30–100	4–7	1.5–2.5	2.0–5.0	1.5–2.5	50–200	75–250
Adults		30–100	4–7	1.5–3.0	2.0–5.0	1.5–4.0	50–200	75–250

* Because there is less information on which to base allowances, these figures are not given in Table 37.19 and are provided here in the form of ranges of recommended intakes.
† Since the toxic levels for many trace elements may be only several times usual intakes, the upper levels for the trace elements given in this table should not be habitually exceeded. (From National Research Council 1989).

Water-soluble vitamins							Minerals						
Vitamin C (mg)	Thiamin (mg)	Riboflavin (mg)	Niacin (mg NE)‡	Vitamin B_6 (mg)	Folate (µg)	Vitamin B_{12} (µg)	Calcium (mg)	Phosphorus (mg)	Magnesium (mg)	Iron (mg)	Zinc (mg)	Iodine (µg)	Selenium (µg)
30	0.3	0.4	5	0.3	25	0.3	400	300	40	6	5	40	10
35	0.4	0.5	6	0.6	35	0.5	600	500	60	10	5	50	15
40	0.7	0.8	9	1.0	50	0.7	800	800	80	10	10	70	20
45	0.9	1.1	12	1.1	75	1.0	800	800	120	10	10	90	20
45	1.0	1.2	13	1.4	100	1.4	800	800	170	10	10	120	30
50	1.3	1.5	17	1.7	150	2.0	1200	1200	270	12	15	150	40
60	1.5	1.8	20	2.0	200	2.0	1200	1200	400	12	15	150	50
60	1.5	1.7	19	2.0	200	2.0	1200	1200	350	10	15	150	70
60	1.5	1.7	19	2.0	200	2.0	800	800	350	10	15	150	70
60	1.2	1.4	15	2.0	200	2.0	800	800	350	10	15	150	70
50	1.1	1.3	15	1.4	150	2.0	1200	1200	280	15	12	150	45
60	1.1	1.3	15	1.5	180	2.0	1200	1200	300	15	12	150	50
60	1.1	1.3	15	1.6	180	2.0	800	800	280	15	12	150	55
60	1.0	1.2	13	1.6	180	2.0	800	800	280	10	12	150	55
70	1.5	1.6	17	2.2	400	2.2	1200	1200	320	30	15	175	65
95	1.6	1.8	20	2.1	280	2.6	1200	1200	355	15	19	200	75
90	1.6	1.7	20	2.1	260	2.6	1200	1200	340	15	16	200	75

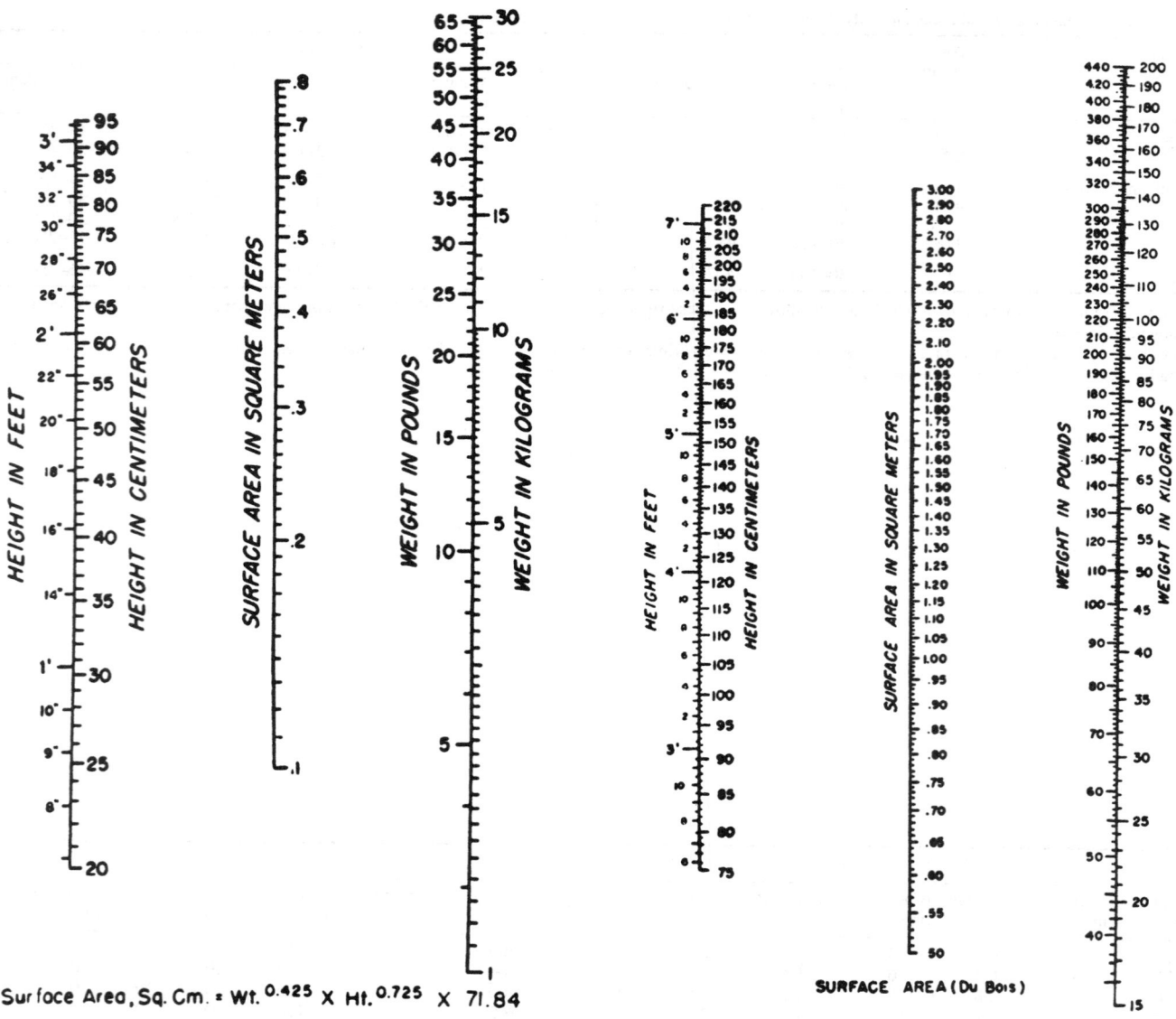

Surface Area, Sq. Cm. = Wt.$^{0.425}$ X Ht.$^{0.725}$ X 71.84

SURFACE AREA (Du Bois)

Fig. 37.1 Nomograms for body surface area (after du Bois & du Bois (1916) and Crawford et al (1950)). A rapid rough method for estimating surface area from weight alone is: suface area m^2 = $\dfrac{4W + 7}{W + 90}$ (where W = weight in kilograms) (Costeff 1966). (See also Fig. 37.2.)

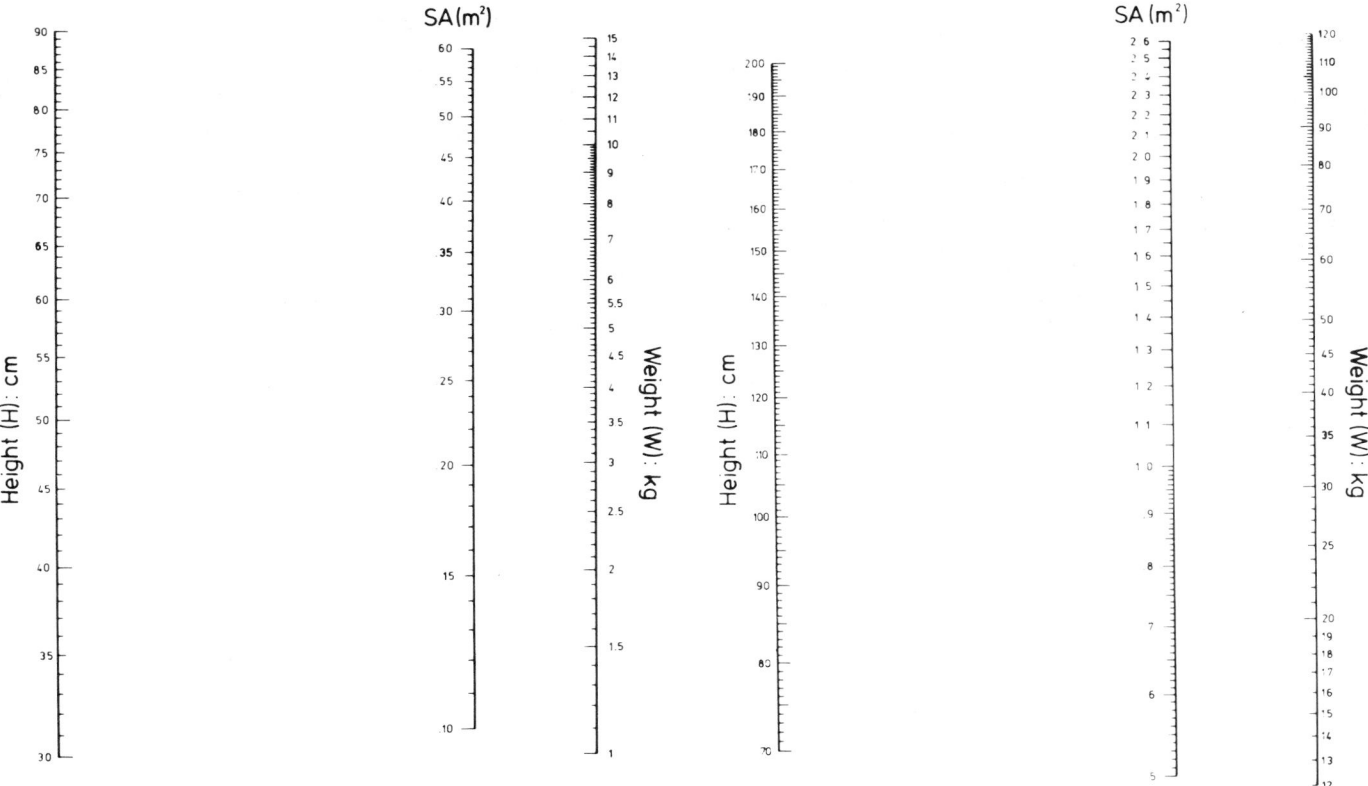

Fig. 37.2 Nomograms for body surface area (Haycock et al 1978). Surface area was calculated geometrically from 34 body measurements and the following formula derived: surface area (m^2) = weight (kg)$^{0.5378}$ × height (cm)$^{0.3964}$ × 0.024265.
Haycock et al state that as the du Bois formula (see Fig. 37.1) increasingly underestimates surface area as values fall below 0.7 m^2, their nomograms are more accurate in this lower range and particularly so for newborn infants.

REFERENCES AND BIBLIOGRAPHY

Apt L, Downey W S 1955 Melena neonatorum. The swallowed blood syndrome. A simple test for the differentiation of adult and foetal haemoglobin in bloody stools. Journal of Pediatrics 47: 6–12

American Academy of Pediatrics 1980 Committee on Hospital Care: metrication and SI units. Pediatrics 65: 659–664

American Academy of Pediatrics 1989 Committee on Drugs: S.I. units. Pediatrics 83: 129–131

Chantler C, Barratt T M 1972 Estimation of glomerular filtration rate from plasma clearance of 51-chromium edetic acid. Archives of Disease in Childhood 47: 613–617

Costeff H 1966 A simple empirical formula for calculating approximate surface area in children. Archives of Disease in Childhood 41: 681–683

Crawford J D, Terry M E, Rourke G M 1950 Simplification of drug dosage calculation by application of the surface area principle. Pediatrics 5: 783–790

Department of Health 1991 Dietary values for food, energy and nutrients for the United Kingdom. Report on Health and Social Subjects No. 41. HMSO, London

Department of Health 1994 Weaning and the weaning diet. Report on Health and Social Subjects No. 45. HMSO, London

Department of Health and Social Security 1977 The composition of human milk. Report on Health and Social Subjects No. 12. HMSO, London

Department of Health and Social Security 1980 Artifical feeds for the young infant. Report on Health and Social Subjects No. 18. HMSO, London

Department of Health and Social Security 1988 Present day practice in infant feeding: third report. Report on Health and Social Subjects No. 32. HMSO, London

de Swiet M, Fayers P, Shinebourne E A 1992 Blood pressure in the first 10 years of life; the Brompton study. British Medical Journal 304: 23–26

Du Bois D, Du Bois E F 1916 Clinical calorimetry. Tenth paper. A formula to estimate the approximate surface area if height and weight be known. Archives of Internal Medicine 17: 863

ESPGAN Committee on Nutrition 1977 Guidelines on infant nutrition I. Recommendations for the composition of an adapted formula. Acta Paediatrica Scandinavica Supplement 262: 1–20

ESPGAN Committee on Nutrition 1981 Guidelines on infant nutrition II. Recommendations for the composition of follow-up formula and beikost. Acta Paediatrica Scandinavica Supplement 287: 1–25

ESPGAN 1982 European Society for Pediatric Gastroenterology and Nutrition 1982 recommendations for infant feeding. Acta Paediatrica Scandinavica Supplement 302: 1–27

ESPGAN 1987 Nutrition and feeding of preterm infants. Acta Paediatrica Scandinavica Supplement 336: 1–14 and Blackwell, Oxford, pp 1–248

ESPGAN Committee on Nutrition 1990. Comments on the composition of cow's milk based follow-up formulas. Acta Paediatrica Scandinavica 79: 250–254

Habel A H, Simpson H 1976 Osmolar relation between cerebrospinal fluid and serum in hypersomolar hypernatraemic dehydration. Archives of Disease in Childhood 51: 660–666

Haggerty R J, Moroney M W, Nadas A S 1956 Essential hyperetension in infancy and childhood. American Journal of Diseases of Children 92: 535–549

Hamill P V V, Drizd T A, Johnson C L, Reed R B, Roche A F, Moore W M 1979 Physical growth: National Center for Health Statistics percentiles. American Journal of Clinical Nutrition 32: 607–629

Haycock G B, Schwartz G J, Wisotsky D H 1978 Geometric method for measuring body surface area: A height–weight formula validated in infants, children and adults. Journal of Pediatrics 93: 62–66

Hellstrom B, Kjellin K G 1971 The diagnostic value of spectrophotometry in the newborn period. Developmental Medicine and Child Neurology 13: 789–797

Hindmarsh P C, Swift P G F 1995 An assessment of growth hormone provocation tests. Archives of Disease in Childhood 72: 362–368

Hughes I A 1986 Handbook of endocrine investigations in children. Wright, Bristol

Insley J (ed) 1996 A paediatric vade-mecun, 13th edn. Edward Arnold, London

Kjellin K G 1970 Bilirubin compounds in the CSF. Journal of the Neurological Sciences 13: 161–173

Lanzkowsky P 1995 Manual of pediatric hematology and oncology, 2nd edn. Churchill Livingstone, New York

Lilleyman J S, Hann I M 1992 Paediatric haematology. Churchill Livingstone, Edinburgh

McLaren D S, Burman D, Belton N R, Williams A F (eds) 1991 Textbook of paediatric nutrition, 3rd edn. Churchill Livingstone, Edinburgh

Nathan D G, Oski F A 1993 Hematology of infancy and childhood. 4th edn. Saunders, Philadelphia

National High Blood Pressure Education Program Working Group on Hypertension Control in Children and Adolescents 1996 Update on the 1987 Task Force Report on High Blood Pressure in Children and Adolescents: a working group report from the National High Blood Pressure Education Program. Pediatrics 88: 649–658

National Research Council 1989 Recommended dietary allowances, 10th edn. National Academy Press, Washington

Soldin S J, Hicks J M 1995 Pediatric reference ranges. AACC Press, Washington DC

Soldin S J, Rifai N, Hicks J M B 1992 Biochemical basisi of pediatric disease. AAAC Press, Washington DC

Task Force on Blood Pressure Control in Children 1987 Report of the Task Force on Blood Pressure Control in Children – 1987. Pediatrics 79: 1–25

Tsang R C, Lucas A, Uauy R, Zlotkin S 1993 Nutritional needs of the preterm infant. Williams & Wilkins, Baltimore

38 Pediatric prescribing

R. E. Olver   D. Haddad   A. M. MacConnachie

Physiological variables   1953
Body size and composition   1953
Renal and hepatic function   1953
Routes of administration   1953
Oral   1953
Rectal   1954
Inhalation   1954
Intramuscular and intravenous   1954
Skin   1954
Dose size and frequency   1954

Therapeutic drug monitoring   1954
Use of the drug dosage tables   1954
Product license and liability   1955
Neonatal prescribing   1955
Antibiotics, antiviral and antifungal drugs   1955
Drugs other than antimicrobials   1956
Prescribing for children beyond the neonatal period   1958
References and Bibliography   1980

Rational pediatric prescribing requires a clear understanding of the normal variability of drug handling and response, particularly in the neonate and young child. Important factors include increasing size, changing body composition and maturation of hepatic and renal function. In addition, certain disease states may alter drug metabolism and excretion.

PHYSIOLOGICAL VARIABLES

BODY SIZE AND COMPOSITION

In the progression from full-term newborn to adult, bodyweight increases by a factor of about 20 and surface area by a factor of 8 (see Table 38.4). Increase in size necessitates increase in drug dosage because of greater volume of distribution, metabolic rate and speed of elimination (see below).

Drug distribution is influenced by changes in body water and body fat. Both total body water (TBW) and extracellular fluid volume (ECF) as a proportion of total bodyweight are highest in the newborn and fall thereafter (TBW as a percentage of bodyweight: newborn 80%, 3 months 70%, 1 year 60%, adult 55%; ECF as a percentage of bodyweight: newborn 45%, 3 months 33%, 1 year 28%, adult 20%). Thus water-soluble drugs, which are mainly distributed in the extracellular fluid, have their largest volumes of distribution in the neonatal period and early infancy. Body fat is low in the newborn, rises to a maximum in the first 3 months and then decreases until the age of 6 years. The larger the body fat depots, the more will fat-soluble drugs be sequestered in such depots.

Although there are changes in protein binding of drugs, this property being lowest in the newborn period and early infancy, the differences are small and clinically insignificant.

RENAL AND HEPATIC FUNCTION

Most drugs are excreted through the kidneys and hence developmental changes in glomerular filtration and tubular secretion are the most important factors determining the rate of excretion. Glomerular filtration rate per unit surface area in the newborn is approximately a third of that in the adult and tubular secretion is similarly reduced. On a basis of comparative surface area, both properties reach adult levels by 3–6 months of age and thereafter tend to be higher than in the adult. This has clear implications for the use of drugs eliminated by glomerular filtration (e.g. aminoglycosides) or by tubular secretion (e.g. penicillins).

By rendering drugs more water soluble, hepatic microsomal enzyme systems enhance their efficient excretion. On a bodyweight basis, oxidation and glucuronidation are reduced in the neonate whereas demethylation and sulfation are little different from in the adult. Thus drugs which are oxidized (e.g. lignocaine, phenobarbitone, phenytoin and diazepam) and those which are glucuronidated (e.g. chloramphenicol) show prolonged half-lives and tend to accumulate in neonates. Microsomal oxidation of drugs such as anticonvulsants and theophylline is more rapid than in adults, gradually decreasing towards adolescence.

ROUTES OF ADMINISTRATION

ORAL

For most children and most conditions this is the preferred route. However, vomiting and lack of cooperation may each reduce efficacy. Liquid preparations are often appropriate for infants and young children. Potential disadvantages include sucrose base and shortened shelf life (particularly if diluted).

Crushed tablets administered in a suitable drink or mixed with food should be considered as a possible alternative to liquid preparations. The majority of children aged 4 years or more can swallow an average sized whole tablet.

RECTAL

This route of drug administration is unpleasant and unreliable. It may, however, be useful for administration of diazepam rectal solution, antiemetic suppositories, paracetamol suppositories (where the oral route is precluded), and for metronidazole suppositories prior to bowel surgery.

INHALATION

Apart from the administration of antibiotics and Dornase alfa in cystic fibrosis, the main indication for inhalation is the treatment of asthma. β-adrenoceptor agonists, muscarinic antagonists, steroids and sodium cromoglycate may be given by this route. Choice of appliance appropriate for the age of child is all important. Irrespective of age, the use of a pressurized nebulizer and mask is indicated for all severe episodes of asthma unresponsive to other forms of therapy and is the only well-established method of delivering drugs to the airways of children under the age of about 3 years. From 3 years onwards a pressurized aerosol used in conjunction with a spacer incorporating a one-way valve near the mouthpiece may be satisfactory. Powder preparations can successfully be administered from the age of about 5. Few children under the age of about 9 years can coordinate their breathing sufficiently well to be able to use a pressurized aerosol satisfactorily without a spacer.

INTRAMUSCULAR AND INTRAVENOUS

Intramuscular injections are painful and drugs administered in this way may be erratically absorbed (e.g. chloramphenicol and phenytoin). The intramuscular route may be appropriate for the administration of phenothiazines to stop vomiting. Intramuscular drug therapy may sometimes be appropriate in the treatment of epilepsy in the child with an intercurrent illness and vomiting who requires prophylaxis. Intramuscular injections must be avoided in hemophilia and other bleeding disorders. The intravenous route is preferred for systemic administration of drugs for which there is no appropriate oral formulation and in the treatment of serious illness in which both certainty of administration and high blood levels are necessary.

SKIN

Significant absorption of topically applied drugs may occur in infants because of their large surface/volume ratio and especially in the presence of broken or inflamed skin. Absorption may be further increased by the occlusive effect of plastic pants. Thus, hexachlorophene and boric acid applied to the nappy area may give rise to toxicity, and the use of steroids over a large area may have significant systemic effects. Prolonged use of potent steroids may cause skin atrophy.

DOSE SIZE AND FREQUENCY

Detailed pharmacokinetic and pharmacodynamic data relating to drugs used in children are frequently lacking. Hence, the calculation of a pediatric dose may be derived from the adult dose, reduced on the basis of bodyweight or surface area. Beyond the newborn period, drug doses per unit surface area are similar throughout childhood and this is generally the most satisfactory basis for deriving pediatric doses from adult doses (see Table 38.4).

For most drugs, the younger the child the larger will be the weight-related single dose of the drug. For drugs primarily excreted by the kidneys (e.g. aminoglycosides, penicillins) the daily doses expressed per unit bodyweight are similar at most ages beyond 6 months. In the newborn period, however, renal and hepatic immaturity dictate that daily doses per unit bodyweight are relatively low. Furthermore, the appropriate daily dose of most antibiotics varies both with gestational and postnatal age (Table 38.1); this is generally achieved by varying dose frequency.

Frequency of administration is inversely related to the elimination half-life of the drug. Where no relationship between plasma concentration and effect is known, the drug should be given once or twice a day in order to maximize compliance.

Drug steady-state plasma concentrations are generally not achieved until about five elimination half-lives have elapsed. A loading dose is advisable for emergency therapy, particularly for drugs with a long half-life (e.g. digoxin, phenobarbitone).

THERAPEUTIC DRUG MONITORING

The measurement of drugs in body fluids is only worthwhile if it can be demonstrated that there is a correlation between concentration and therapeutic or toxic effects. The major indications for monitoring blood levels of drugs are:

1. where a drug has a narrow therapeutic index, i.e. where potentially toxic levels are not greatly in excess of therapeutic levels
2. where a conventional dose has either failed to produce the desired therapeutic effect or has induced toxicity
3. in patients whose normal elimination pathways are functionally impaired.

USE OF THE DRUG DOSAGE TABLES

TABLES 38.1 and 38.2

Because of the need for accuracy of dose calculation in the newborn, only weight-related doses are given. Changing renal and hepatic function in the preterm infant, with corresponding changes in elimination half-lives, is reflected by variations in dose frequency.

TABLE 38.3

Depending on the data source, dosages are given on the basis of bodyweight or age (or both). Very occasionally doses are expressed per unit surface area. Because of the age-related changes in drug handling mentioned above, the appropriate dose expressed per unit weight tends to decline with increasing age beyond early infancy (particularly for those drugs requiring microsomal metabolism in the liver prior to elimination). For this reason, where a range of weight-related doses is given, doses towards the higher end of the range will often be most appropriate in late infancy and early childhood. In the obese child, calculation of the correct dose per kg is dependent upon the use of ideal bodyweight derived from height and age. Where a single dose is given for an age range it refers to the mid-age point and some extrapolation may be necessary at the extremes.

Where new or potentially toxic drugs are used, the manufacturer's data sheet should be consulted. Daily doses may need to be reduced in the presence of hepatic or renal disease. Drugs for which caution needs to be exercised even in the presence of mild renal impairment (GFR: 20–50 1/min per 1.73 m², creatinine 150–300 μmol/l) are marked with an asterisk.

The complexity and toxicity of chemotherapy regimes used for the treatment of malignant disease are such that it is not appropriate to include them in this section. The reader is referred to Chapters 15 and 16.

PRODUCT LICENSE AND LIABILITY

All medicines, with the possible exception of those under development, e.g. used in clinical trials, must receive a product license (PL) which is issued by the appropriate licensing authority – The Medicines Control Agency in the UK or Federal Drugs Authority in the USA. The PL specifies, amongst other things, the licensed indications for the drug together with its recognized dosage range. Not infrequently, however, pediatric use of a drug is not recognized in the PL, usually because there was insufficient clinical experience at the time of licensing for it to be promoted in younger age groups. Nevertheless, children may benefit from treatment with unlicensed medicines and use of a medicine outwith its product license may be justified. Doctors should remember, however, that they are largely responsible for the safety of the medicines which they prescribe and that their liability may increase when prescribing unlicensed medicines or unlicensed dosages.

Drugs listed in the following text are as far as possible licensed in the UK for use in children in the stated dosage range. If in doubt, prescribers should first check with their local pharmacy.

Table 38.1 Neonatal prescribing: antibiotics, antiviral and antifungal drugs

Drug	Route	Single dose	Gestation or birthweight	Frequency of administration per 24 h with corresponding postnatal age			Notes
				<7 days	7–14 days	>14 days	
Acyclovir*	i.v.	10 mg/kg	All gestations	3	3	3	Infuse over 1 h
Amoxicillin	i.m., i.v., oral	30 mg/kg	<37 weeks	2	3	4	
			≥37 weeks	4	4	4	
Amoxicillin and clavulanic acid	i.m., i.v., oral	30 mg/kg	<37	2	3	4	Dose given in terms of amoxicillin
			≥37 weeks	4	4	4	
Amphotericin	i.v.	0.25 mg/kg	All gestations	1	1	1	Infuse over 6 h Increase dose as tolerated to max. of 1.0 mg/kg daily Nephrotoxic Electrolyte disturbances
Ampicillin	i.m., i.v., oral	30 mg/kg	<37 weeks	2	3	4	Double dose for meningitis
			≥37 weeks	4	4	4	
Augmentin – see amoxicillin and clavulanic acid							
Azlocillin	i.m., i.v.	50 mg/kg	<37 weeks	2	2	2	
		100 mg/kg	≥37 weeks	2	3	3	
Aztreonam	i.v.	30 mg/kg	All gestations	2	3	3–4	Increase to 50 mg/kg in severe infection
Benzyl penicillin	i.m., i.v.	50 mg/kg	<37 weeks	2	3	4	Double dose for meningitis
			≥37 weeks	4	4	4	
Cefotaxime	i.m., i.v.	50 mg/kg	All gestations	2	3	3	
Ceftazidime	i.v.	25 mg/kg	All gestations	2	3	3	
Cefuroxime	i.m., i.v.	30 mg/kg	<37 weeks	2	3	3	
			≥37 weeks	2†	3	3	
Chloramphenicol	i.v. not i.m.	12.5 mg/kg	<37 weeks	2	2	2‡	
			≥37 weeks	2	2	3	
Flucloxacillin	i.m., i.v., oral	30 mg/kg	<37 weeks	2	3	4	
			≥37 weeks	4	4	4	
Flucytosine*	i.v. infusion, oral	50 mg/kg	All gestations	2	2	2	
Gentamicin*	i.m., i.v. (slow)	2.5 mg/kg	≤28 weeks	1	2	2	Monitor blood levels and adjust dose/frequency. Therapeutic range: peak 8–10 mg/l, trough <2 mg/l
		2.5 mg/kg	29–35 weeks	1–2	2	2	
		2.5 mg/kg	≥36 weeks	2	2	2	

Table 38.1   *Cont'd*

Drug	Route	Single dose	Gestation or birthweight	Frequency of administration per 24 h with corresponding postnatal age			Notes
				<7 days	7–14 days	>14 days	
Metronidazole	i.v.	7.5 mg/kg	All gestations	3	3	3	
Miconazole	oral	62.5 mg	Term	2	2	2	Oral gel 125 mg/5 ml
Netilmicin*	i.m., i.v. (slow)	As for gentamicin		As for gentamicin			As for gentamicin
Nystatin	Oral	100 000 units	All gestations	3	3	3	
Piperacillin	i.m., i.v.	100 mg/kg	<37 weeks	2	2	3	
			≥37 weeks	2	3	3	
Teicoplanin							
Loading dose	i.v.	16 mg/kg	All gestations	Single dose			Administer as i.v. bolus
Maintenance	i.v.	8 mg/kg		1	1	1	or 30 min infusion
Vancomycin*	i.v. infusion	15 mg/kg	All gestations	2	2	2	Infuse over 60 min. Dose may be increased for septicemia. Therapeutic range: peak 18–26 mg/l, trough 5–10 mg/l

* Indicates that caution is required even in the presence of mild renal impairment   (GFR: 20–50 ml/min per 1.73 m², plasma creatinine: 150–300 µmol/l
† Age ≥4 days: dose frequency 3/24 h;
‡ Age ≥4 weeks: dose frequency 3/24 h. Avoid oral route preterm.

Table 38.2   Neonatal prescribing: drugs other than antimicrobials

Drug	Route	Dose schedule	Frequency per 24 h	Notes
Adrenaline	i.v. or intracardiac i.v.	For cardiac arrest: 0.1–0.3 ml/kg (1/10 000) For severe hypotension: 0.5 µg/kg per min increasing until effect achieved	Single dose	May be repeated
Alprostadil – see prostaglandin E₁				
Aminophylline – see theophylline				
Atropine	i.v., s.c., i.m.	10 µg/kg	Single dose	i.v. for bradycardia, s.c. or i.m. for premedication
Bendrofluazide	Oral	0.4 mg/kg	1	
Caffeine citrate	Oral, i.v.	Loading dose: 20 mg/kg Maintenance: 5 mg/kg	1 1	Caffeine citrate contains approx 50% caffeine. Therapeutic range 8–20 mg/l (expressed as caffeine)
Calciferol	Oral	Prophylaxis: 400 units Treatment: 1000–2000 units	1 1	
Calcium chloride (dihydrate)	Oral	30 mg/kg	4	
Calcium gluconate	Oral i.v.	100 mg/kg 0.2 ml/kg of 10% solution in 4.8 ml/kg of 0.9% saline	4 Single dose	Infuse over 10 min. Watch for bradycardia
Calcium resonium	Oral, rectal	0.5 g/kg	Single dose	Repeat 4-hourly as required
Carbamazepine	Oral	5–10 mg/kg	1–2	Therapeutic range 4–12 mg/l
Carbimazole	Oral	0.25 mg/kg	3	
Chloral hydrate	Oral	30–50 mg/kg	Single dose	Repeat up to 3 × per 24 h
Chlorothiazide	i.v., oral	10 mg/kg	2	

Table 38.2 *Cont'd*

Drug	Route	Dose schedule	Frequency per 24 h	Notes
Chlorpromazine	i.m. (deep), i.v., oral	0.5 mg/kg	4	For i.v.: dilute ×5
Cimetidine	Oral, i.v. (slow)	2.5–5 mg/kg	4	Increases serum levels of theophylline and phenytoin
Clonazepam	i.v.	Loading dose: 250 µg, maintenance: 10 µg/h	Single dose	Therapeutic range 25–85 µg/l
Dexamethasone	i.m., i.v., oral	0.2 mg/kg	3	
Diamorphine	i.m., i.v. / Oral	25–50 µg/kg / 75 µg/kg	4–6	For i.v. start with 12.5 µg/kg and inject very slowly
Diazepam	i.v., rectal	0.3 mg/kg	Single dose	Repeat as necessary, watch for respiratory depression
Digoxin*	i.v. (slow) / Oral	10 µg/kg } digitalization / 15 µg/kg	Total of 3 doses	
	i.v. (slow) / Oral	8 µg/kg } maintenance / 10 µg/kg	1–2	Individualize dosage to achieve blood levels of 1–2.6 nmol (0.8–2 µg)/l
Disopyramide*	i.v. (slow) / Oral	Starting dose: 1 mg/kg / Maintenance: 5–10 mg	3	Repeat i.v. doses of up to 4 mg/kg
Dobutamine	i.v.	5 µg/kg per min		Infuse in 5% dextrose, increase dose for effect
Dopamine	i.v.	5 µg/kg per min		Infuse in 5% dextrose, increase dose for effect
Edrophonium	i.v. (slow)	0.2 mg/kg	Single dose	
Ethamsylate	i.m., i.v.	12.5 mg/kg	4	Watch for transient hypotension
Folic acid	Oral	0.25 mg/kg	1	
Frusemide	i.v., oral	1–3 mg/kg	Single dose	Start with low dose. Repeat 12-hourly as necessary. Caution with aminoglycosides
Glucagon	i.v.	0.3 mg/kg / 10 µg/kg per h	Single dose / Infusion	May be repeated after 20 min
Hepatitis B vaccine H-B Vax / Engerix	i.m. / i.m.	10 µg (0.5 ml) / 20 µg (1.0 ml)	{ At birth, 1 and 6 months	Antihepatitis B virus immunoglobulin also given at birth
Hydrocortisone	i.m., i.v.	10 mg/kg	Single dose	Increase ×4 for laryngeal edema
Immunoglobulin Anti-hep B	i.m.	200 units	At birth	Repeat at 1 month if not vaccinated within 48 h of birth
Anti-varicella-zoster	i.m.	250 mg		For infants born to mothers who develop varicella up to 6 days before birth or within 1st postnatal week
Indomethacin	i.v., oral	0.2–0.3 mg/kg	Up to 2	Max. total dose 0.6 mg/kg
Isoprenaline	i.v.	0.2 µg/kg per min in 5% glucose		Increase at 10-min intervals for effect. Maximum 2 µg/kg per min
Lignocaine	i.v.	Loading dose: 1 mg/kg, maintenance: 20–50 µg/kg per min	Single dose	Repeat after 5–10 min if necessary to a maximum total loading dose of 5 mg/kg
Magnesium chloride	Oral	30 mg/kg	3	
Magnesium sulfate	i.m. / i.v.	0.1 ml/kg (50% soln) / 2.5–5 ml/kg (1% soln)	Single dose / Single dose	Infuse over 1 h with ECG monitoring
Mannitol	i.v.	0.5–1 g/kg	Single dose	20% solution. Infuse over 30 min. Can be repeated
Morphine	i.m., i.v. / Oral	50–100 µg/kg / 100–200 µg/kg	4–6	For i.v. start with 25 µg/kg and inject very slowly or infuse at 25–50 µg/kg per h

Table 38.2 *Cont'd*

Drug	Route	Dose schedule		Frequency per 24 h	Notes
Naloxone	i.v., s.c. i.m.	10 µg/kg 60 µg/kg		Single dose Single dose	May be repeated at 2- to 3-min intervals Onset slower than i.v.
Neostigmine	i.v.	80 µg/kg		Single dose	To reverse pancuronium
Pancuronium	i.v.	30–60 µg/kg		Single dose	Repeat 1- to 4-hourly as necessary
Paraldehyde	Deep i.m.	0.1 ml/kg		Single dose	Repeat 4- to 6-hourly as necessary
Phenobarbitone	i.m., i.v. Oral	Loading dose: 20 mg/kg Maintenance: 2.5 mg/kg		Single dose 2	Therapeutic range 15–40 mg/l
Phenytoin	i.v.	20 mg/kg: loading dose			Loading: 2 doses of 10 mg/kg 1 h apart. Inject slowly. May cause myocardial depression
	i.v. Oral	2 mg/kg 5–7 mg/kg	} maintenance	2	Therapeutic range 10–20 mg/l
Phytomenadione	Oral, i.v., i.m.	Prophylaxis	<1 kg: 0.5 mg single dose >1 kg: 1.0 mg single dose		
Prostaglandin E₁	i.v. infusion	0.05–0.4 µg/kg per min			May cause apnea. Start with lowest dose
Pyridoxine	i.v.	100 mg/kg		Single dose	Inject over 1 min with EEG monitoring
Sodium iron edetate (Sytron)	Oral	5 ml of 50% solution		1	
Sodium valproate	Oral	Loading dose: 10 mg/kg Maintenance: 10 mg/kg		Single dose 2	Up to 3 loading doses in first 24 hours if fits continue
Theophylline	Oral, i.v.	Loading dose: 5 mg/kg Maintenance: 2 mg/kg		Single dose 2–3	Inject over 20–30 min. Aminophylline is 80% theophylline. Therapeutic range 28–56 µmol/l
Tolazoline	i.v.	Starting dose: 2 mg/kg Maintenance: 1–2 mg/kg per h		Single dose	Infuse over 10 min
Vitamin D₂ – see calciferol Vitamin K – see phytomenadione					

* Indicates that caution is required even in the presence of mild renal impairment (GFR: 20–50 ml/min per 1.73 m², plasma creatinine: 150–300 µmol/l)

Table 38.3 Precribing for children beyond the neonatal period

Drug	Route	Single dose/kg	Single dose for different age groups (unless stated otherwise)				Times daily	Comments
			>1 month <1 year	1–4 years	5–12 years	>12 years		
Acetaminophen – see paracetamol								
Acetazolamide	Oral, i.v.	2–6 mg/kg	Dose based on bodyweight at all ages				3–4	Adjust dose to achieve ketosis in treatment of epilepsy
Acetylcysteine	i.v. (slow)		Initial dose 150 mg/kg in 5% glucose over 15 min followed by 50 mg/kg over 4 h then 100 mg/kg over next 16 h (total dose 300 mg/kg in 20 h)					Much less effective if given later than 15 h after paracetamol overdose
Acetylsalicylic acid – see aspirin								
ACTH – see corticotropin								
Acyclovir* For herpes simplex	Oral		100 mg	<2 years 100 mg >2 years 200 mg	200 mg	200 mg	5	Double dose in the immunocompromised

Table 38.3   *Cont'd*

Drug	Route	Single dose/kg	Single dose for different age groups (unless stated otherwise)				Times daily	Comments
			>1 month <1 year	1–4 years	5–12 years	>12 years		
Acyclovir* (continued) For herpes simplex or varicella-zoster	i.v.		250 mg/m²	250 mg/m²	250 mg/m²	5 mg/kg	3	i.v. infusion over 1 h. Double dose in the immunocompromised
5% cream	Topical (skin)						5	
3% ointment	Topical (eye)						5	
Adrenaline 1 in 1000 (1 mg/ml)	i.m.		0.05–0.1 ml	0.1–0.25 ml	0.25–0.5 ml	0.5 ml	Single dose	Repeat for anaphylaxis every 10–15 min until improvement occurs
0.5% + 1% drops	Topical (eye)						1–2	
Alfacalcidol	Oral		<20 kg: 0.05 µg/kg per day		>20 kg: 1 µg/day		1	Adjust dose to avoid hypercalcemia
Allopurinol*	Oral	10–20 mg/kg	100 mg	100–200 mg	200–300 mg	300 mg	1	Reduce doses of concurrent azathioprine and 6-mercaptopurine
Alprostadil – see Prostaglandin E₁								
Amethocaine 0.5% drops	Topical (eye)							
Amikacin*	i.m., i.v.	7.5 mg/kg	Dose based on bodyweight at all ages				2–3	Maintain plasma concentrations at 25 mg/l (peak), 2–4 mg/l (trough)
Aminophylline	i.v.		Initially: 5 mg/kg by slow i.v. injection over 20 min Maintenance: 0.8–1 mg/kg per h by slow i.v. infusion (max. 20 mg/kg per 24 h)					Omit loading dose if patient already receiving xanthines. Maintain plasma concentrations of theophylline at 55–110 µmol/l for all routes
	Oral		–	–	100–225 mg	225–450 mg	2	Start at low dose (approx. 5 mg/kg) and increase slowly. Doses for sustained-release preparations given
Amitriptyline	Oral		–	–	>7 years 10–20 mg	25–50 mg	1	Max. treatment period of 3 months for enuresis
Amoxicillin	Oral		62.5 mg	125 mg	250 mg	250–500 mg	3	
	i.v., i.m.	12.5–25 mg/kg	62.5–250 mg	125–400 mg	250 mg–1 g	500 mg–1 g	4–6	No advantage over ampicillin when given parenterally
Amoxicillin and clavulanic acid	Oral		31.3–125 mg	62.5–250 mg	125–500 mg	500 mg	3	All doses given in terms of amoxicillin
	i.v.	25 mg/kg	75–250 mg	250–400 mg	400 mg–1 g	1 g	3–4	
Amphotericin	i.v.		0.25 mg/kg initially, increasing to 1 mg/kg depending on individual response and tolerance				1	i.v. infusion over 6 h Nephrotoxic Electrolyte disturbances
Oral candidiasis	Oral		100 mg suspension	100 mg suspension	10 mg lozenge	10 mg lozenge	4	Negligible absorption from oral administration
Intestinal candidiasis	Oral		100 mg	100 mg	100 mg	100–200 mg	4	
Amphotericin liposomal and colloid complex	i.v.		1 mg/kg initially, increasing to 4 mg/kg depending on individual response and tolerance				1	Better tolerated than conventional amphotericin if high dose required. Infuse over 1 h
Ampicillin	Oral		62.5–125 mg	125–250 mg	250–500 mg	500 mg	4	
	i.v., i.m.	12.5–25 mg/kg	62.5–250 mg	125–400 mg	250 mg–1 g	500 mg–1 g	4–6	Up to 400 mg/kg per day given for meningitis
Ascorbic acid	Oral		25–50 mg at all ages				1	
Aspirin	Oral	10–20 mg/kg	Risk of Reye's syndrome. Avoid in children <12 years unless specifically indicated, e.g. juvenile chronic arthritis			300–900 mg	4–6	Take after food. Optimum anti-inflammatory plasma salicylate concentration 250–300 mg/l

Table 38.3 *Cont'd*

Drug	Route	Single dose/kg	Single dose for different age groups (unless stated otherwise)				Times daily	Comments
			>1 month <1 year	1–4 years	5–12 years	>12 years		
Astemizole	Oral		–	–	5 mg	10 mg	1	
Atenolol	Oral i.v. (slow)	1 mg/kg initially, rising to maximum of 2 mg/kg depending on response and tolerance					1	
Atropine sulfate 1% drops	i.v., i.m., s.c. Topical (eye)	10–20 µg/kg	Dose based on bodyweight up to 12 years			300–600 µg		Premedication dose
Augmentin – see amoxicillin and clavulanic acid								
Azathioprine	Oral, i.v.	1–4 mg/kg	Dose based on bodyweight at all ages				1	Reduce dose to one-quarter if used with allopurinol
Azithromycin	Oral		50–100 mg	200 mg	300 mg	500 mg		Pediatric suspension 200 mg/5 ml available
Azlocillin	i.v.	75–100 mg/kg	100 mg/kg	1–1.5 g	1.5–3 g	2–5 g	3	
Aztreonam	i.v.	30–50 mg/kg	Dose based on bodyweight at all ages				3–4	Maximum dose 8 g/day i.v. bolus or 30 min infusion for high doses
Baclofen	Oral	Initially 2.5 mg 2–4 times daily increased gradually over 2 weeks to a maximum total daily dose of 40 mg (<8 years) or 60 mg (>8 years)					3–4	Withdraw gradually
Beclomethasone dipropionate	Inhalation		50 µg	50–100 µg	100–300 µg	200–400 µg	2–4	Lung penetration enhanced by prior inhalation of a bronchodilator
	Intranasal		–	50 µg	50–100 µg	100 µg	2–4	
Bendrofluazide	Oral	0.1–0.2 mg/kg	1.25 mg	1.25–2.5 mg	2.5 mg	2.5–5 mg	1	
Benorylate	Oral	25 mg/kg	–	250 mg	500 mg	1–2 g	4	Contains aspirin. Under 12 years indicated for treatment of juvenile chronic arthritis only. Adjust dose to maintain a plasma salicylate concentration of 250–300 mg/l
Benzoic acid – see Whitfield's ointment								
Benzoyl peroxide 2.5%, 5% and 10% topical preparations	Topical (skin)						1–2	
Benztropine	i.v., oral	Can be used with caution in children >3 years. Adult dose for acute dystonic drug reactions: 1–2 mg i.v., then 1–2 mg orally twice daily						
Benzyl benzoate 25%	Topical (skin)	Scabies: apply over whole body omitting head and neck. Repeat without bathing the following day and wash off 24 h later. In severe cases repeat 2–3 times						Dilute to 12.5% for children and 6.25% for infants
Benzyl penicillin	i.m.		15 mg/kg	150–300 mg	300–600 mg	600 mg–1.2 g	4	
	i.v.	25–50 mg/kg	Dose based on bodyweight at all ages				4–6	Use highest dose and frequency for meningitis
Bephenium	Oral		2.5 g	<2 years: 2.5 g >2 years: 5 g	5 g	5 g	Single dose	Dose may be repeated after 2–3 days
Betamethasone	Oral	5–50 µg/kg	Dose based on bodyweight at all ages				2	Adjust dose according to response
	i.v.		1 mg	2 mg	4 mg	5 mg	3–4	
0.1% and 0.025%	Topical (skin)							
0.1% drops	Topical (ear, eye or nose)							
0.1% eye ointment								

Table 38.3 *Cont'd*

Drug	Route	Single dose/kg	Single dose for different age groups (unless stated otherwise)				Times daily	Comments
			>1 month <1 year	1–4 years	5–12 years	>12 years		
Bisacodyl	Oral		2.5 mg	5 mg	5–10 mg	10 mg	1	Night
	Rectal		2.5 mg	5 mg	5–10 mg	10 mg	1	Morning
Brompheniramine			0.1–0.25 mg/kg	1–2 mg	2–4 mg	4–8 mg	3–4	
Budesonide	Inhalation (aerosol)		50–100 µg	50–200 µg	100–400 µg	200–600 µg	2	Lung penetration enhanced by prior inhalation of a bronchodilator
Buprenorphine	Sublingual Oral	100 µg 100–200 µg 200–300 µg	Patients 15–25 kg bodyweight Patients 25–40 kg bodyweight Patients >40 kg bodyweight					
	i.v., i.m.	3–6 µg/kg	Dose based on bodyweight over 15 kg				3–4	
Caffeine – see Table 38.2 Calciferol Prophylaxis	Oral		400 units	400 units	400 units	400 units	1	
Treatment	Oral		1500 units	1500 units	1500–3000 units	3000–6000 units	1	Adjust dose according to response. Doses 5–10 times higher required in resistant rickets
Calcitonin	s.c., i.m.	4–8 units/kg	Dose based on bodyweight at all ages				1	Adjust dose according to response. Doses 5–10 times higher required in resistant rickets
Calcitriol	Oral	0.01–0.05 µg/kg	Dose based on bodyweight at all ages				1	Adjust dose to avoid hypercalcemia
Calcium gluconate 10% Hypocalcemia	Oral, i.v.	100 mg/kg	Dose based on bodyweight at all ages				4	Adjust dose according to response. For i.v. dilute to 2.5% solution (1 ml/kg plus 3 ml 0.9% saline/kg) and infuse over 10 min with cardiac monitoring
Cardiac resuscitation	i.v.	100 mg/kg	Repeat every 10 min					
Calcium polystyrene sulfonate	Oral, rectal	0.25 g/kg	1–2.5 g	2.5–5 g	5–10 g	15 g	3–4	Dose may be halved for maintenance therapy
Captopril*	Oral		<12 years: initial dose 0.5 mg/kg then 1–2 mg/kg 1 h before meals			25–50 mg	3	Start with the lower dose for maintenance
Carbamazepine	Oral	5–10 mg/kg	25–100 mg	50–200 mg	100–400 mg	200–600 mg	2	Start with the lower dose and increase gradually. Optimum therapeutic plasma concentration 5–10 mg/l
Carbimazole	Oral	0.25 mg/kg	0.25 mg/kg	2.5 mg	5 mg	10 mg	3	Reduce dose when symptoms controlled
Carfecillin	Oral	10–20 mg/kg	50–200 mg	100–300 mg	250–500 mg	500 mg – 1 g	3	Only for *Pseudomonas* UTI
Cefaclor	Oral	7 mg/kg	62.5 mg	125 mg	250 mg	500 mg	3	Double dose in severe infection
Cefadroxil	Oral	12.5 mg/kg	62.5–125 mg	250 mg	500 mg	500 mg–1 g	2	
Cefixime	Oral	4 mg/kg	Dose based on bodyweight at all ages				2	
Cefotaxime	i.v., i.m.	50 mg/kg	250–500 mg	500–750 mg	750 mg–1 g	1–2 g	2–4	Maximum 200 mg/kg daily in severe infection
Ceftazidime	i.v., i.m.	25–50 mg/kg	Dose based on bodyweight at all ages				3–4	Use the higher dose in cystic fibrosis and severe acute infection
Ceftriaxone	i.v.	50 mg/kg	Dose based on bodyweight at all ages				1	Infuse over 30 min to 1 h. Up to 100 mg/kg in life-threatening infection

Table 38.3 *Cont'd*

Drug	Route	Single dose/kg	Single dose for different age groups (unless stated otherwise)				Times daily	Comments
			>1 month <1 year	1–4 years	5–12 years	>12 years		
Cefuroxime	i.v., i.m.	20–30 mg/kg	30 mg/kg	250–500 mg	0.5–1 g	0.75–1.5 g	3–4	Up to 240 mg/kg daily in meningitis reduced to 120 mg/kg after 3 days or on clinical improvement
	Oral		–	–	125 mg	250 mg	2	Double dose in otitis media
Cephalexin	Oral		62.5 mg	125 mg	250 mg	250–500 mg	3–4	
Cephradine	i.v., i.m.	12.5–50 mg/kg	Dose based on bodyweight at all ages				4	
	Oral	6.3–12.5 mg/kg	62.5 mg	125 mg	250 mg	500 mg	4	
Charcoal, activated	Oral		Give 5–10 times the dose of drug or poison up to a maximum of 50 g; 5–10 g in water repeated every 15–20 min until the appropriate total dose has been given					
Chloral hydrate								Take well diluted with water
Sedative dose	Oral	6–12 mg/kg	Dose based on bodyweight at all ages				4	
Hypnotic dose	Oral	30–50 mg/kg	200 mg	250–500 mg	500 mg–1 g	500 mg–2 g	1	Use hypnotic dose for procedures up to 5 years
Chloramphenicol	i.v., oral	12.5–25 mg/kg	Dose based on bodyweight at all ages				4	Start with the higher dose. Recommended peak plasma concentrations 15–25 mg/l
0.5% drops, 1% ointment	Topical (eye)							
5% and 10% drops	Topical (ear)							
Chlormethiazole edisylate 0.8%	i.v.		Initially 80 µg/kg min increased every 2–4 h until seizures abolished					Watch for respiratory depression or hypotension Accumulation may occur
Chloroquine*								
Malaria prophylaxis	Oral	5–6 mg/kg <6 weeks: 37.5 mg	75 mg	150 mg	225 mg	300 mg	Weekly	Start 1 week before and continue 4 weeks after leaving endemic area. Doses given in terms of chloroquine base. 150 mg chloroquine base = 200 mg chloroquine sulfate = 250 mg chloroquine phosphate (approx.)
Malaria treatment	Oral		12 mg/kg initially followed by a single dose of 6 mg/kg after 6–8 h, and on each of the following 2 days					
	i.v.	5–20 mg/kg	Dose based on bodyweight at all ages				2	Danger of arrhythmias. Infuse over 4 h and change to oral regime when possible
Chlorothiazide	Oral	5–20 mg/kg	Dose based on bodyweight at all ages				2	
Chlorpheniramine	Oral		0.1 mg/kg	1–2 mg	2–4 mg	4 mg	3	
	s.c., i.m., i.v.		0.25 mg/kg	2.5–5 mg	5–10 mg	10 mg	Single	For i.v. dilute in syringe with blood and give slowly
Chlorpromazine	Oral i.m. (deep)	0.5 mg/kg	–	0.5 mg/kg	10–25 mg	25 mg	3–4	
	Rectal	1 mg/kg	–	12.5–25 mg	25–50 mg	50–100 mg	3–4	
Chlortetracycline*	Oral		–	–	–	250–500 mg	4	Contraindicated under 12 years
3% cream and ointment	Topical (skin)						3	
1% ointment	Topical (eye)							
Chlorthalidone	Oral		2.5 mg/kg	25 mg	25–50 mg	50 mg	1	May be given on alternate days (double dose)
Cholera vaccine	s.c., i.m.		1st dose: Subsequent doses: 0.3 ml	0.1 ml 0.3 ml	0.3–0.5 ml 0.5 ml	0.5 ml 1 ml		Primary course consists of 2 vaccinations, preferably 1 month apart. Booster every 6 months where required

Table 38.3 *Cont'd*

Drug	Route	Single dose/kg	Single dose for different age groups (unless stated otherwise)				Times daily	Comments
			>1 month <1 year	1–4 years	5–12 years	>12 years		
Cholestyramine Hyper-cholesterolemia	Oral		0.17 g/kg	1.5–2.5 g	2.5–8 g	8–12 g	1–3	Other drugs should be given at least 1 h before or 4 h later. Fat-soluble vitamin supplements may be required
Pruritus	Oral		0.05–0.1 g/kg	0.5–1.5 g	1–4 g	4–8 g	1	
Choline salicylate 8.7% dental gel	Topical (oral)							
Cimetidine	Oral, i.m., i.v. (slow)	5–10 mg/kg	5–10 mg/kg	100 mg	100–200 mg	200 mg	4	Increases serum levels of theophylline and phenytoin
Ciprofloxacin	Oral		–	125 mg	250 mg	500 mg	3	For treatment of pseudomonas infection in CF. May cause arthropathy. May increase serum levels of theophylline
	i.v.	2.5–5 mg/kg	Dose based on bodyweight at all ages				2	
Cisapride	Oral	0.2 mg/kg	Dose based on bodyweight at all ages				3–4	
Clarithromycin	Oral	7.5 mg/kg	50–75 mg	125 mg	125–250 mg	250 mg	2	Pediatric suspension available
Clindamycin	Oral	4–5 mg/kg	37.5 mg	75 mg	75–150 mg	150–450 mg	3–4	Reserve for serious infections and discontinue in the event of diarrbea
	i.v., i.m.	5–10 mg/kg	Dose based on bodyweight up to 12 years			300–600 mg	4	Infuse over 30 min
Clobazam	Oral	0.2–1 mg/kg	Dose based on bodyweight at all ages				2	Start with the lower dose
Clobetasol propionate 0.05% preparations	Topical (skin)						1–2	
Clobetasone butyrate 0.05% cream and ointment	Topical (skin)						1–4	
Clofazimine	Oral		Weekly:	100 mg plus	150 mg plus	150 mg plus		Part of a multidrug regime as recommended by WHO. Monthly dose given under supervision
			Monthly:	100 mg	150 mg	200 mg		
Clonazepam	Oral	Initially:	0.25 mg	0.25 mg	0.5 mg	1 mg	Night	Start with a low dose and increase every 4 days according to response
		Maintenance:	0.5 mg	0.5–1.5 mg	1.5–3 mg	2–4 mg	2	
	i.v. (slow)		50 µg/kg	50 µg/kg	30–40 µg/kg	25 µg/kg	Single	Maximum dose <5 years: 0.5 mg; >5 years: 1 mg
Clotrimazole 1% cream, solution, spray and dusting powder	Topical (skin)						2–3	
Cloxacillin	Oral, i.v. (slow)		62.5–125 mg	125–250 mg	250 mg	500 mg	4	Double dose for serious infections
Coal tar Ointment, paint and paste in various strengths	Topical (skin)						1–3	
Co-amoxiclav – see amoxicillin and clavulanic acid								
Cocaine 4% drops	Topical (eye)							
Colistin	Oral		0.25 mega units	0.25–0.5 mega units	0.75–1.5 mega units	1.5–3 mega units	3	Not absorbed when given by mouth. Used for bowel sterilization
	Inhalation		–	0.5 mega units	1.0 mega units	1.0 mega units	2	For treatment of CF

Table 38.3 *Cont'd*

Drug	Route	Single dose/kg	Single dose for different age groups (unless stated otherwise)				Times daily	Comments
			>1 month <1 year	1–4 years	5–12 years	>12 years		
Corticotropin Infantile spasms	s.c., i.m.		Initially 40 units/day reducing to 20 units/day				1	Reduce dose according to response. May be given on alternate days
Asthma, rheumatoid arthritis			1 unit/kg	1 unit/kg	1 unit/kg	40 units	1	
Co-trimoxazole	Oral, i.v. infusion		120–240 mg	240 mg	480 mg	960 mg	2	480 mg co-trimoxazole contains 80 mg trimethoprim and 400 mg sulfamethoxazole. Increase dose by 50% in severe infections
Pneumocystis carinii	Oral i.v. infusion	30 mg/kg	Dose based on bodyweight at all ages				4	
Cyclizine	Oral i.v., i.m.		– –	25 mg –	25 mg –	50 mg 50 mg	3 3	
Cyclopentolate 0.5% and 1% drops	Topical (eye)							
Cycloserine*	Oral	5 mg/kg	Dose based on bodyweight at all ages				2	Adjust dose to maintain plasma concentration below 30 mg/l
Cyclosporine*								See Chapter 16
Danazol	Oral		Precocious puberty: 100–400 mg daily according to age and weight					
Dapsone	Oral		–	25 mg	50–100 mg	100 mg	1	Given as part of a multidrug regime as recommended by WHO
Dehydroemetine	i.m.	0.5–0.7 mg/kg	Dose based on bodyweight at all ages				2	Maximum single dose: 45 mg
Demeclocycline*	Oral		–	–	–	150 mg	4	Contraindicated under 12 years
Desferrioxamine* Iron poisoning	Oral, i.m., i.v.		Initially 0.5–1 g i.m. and 5 g in 50–100 ml water by mouth after lavage then 1–2 g i.m. every 12 h or (if patient collapsed) 15 mg/kg/h i.v. to a max. of 80 mg/kg in 24 h					
Iron overload	s.c. infusion		0.5–4 g over 12 h on 5–7 nights/week					
Desmopressin (DDAVP) Diabetes insipidus	Intranasal Oral		– –	5–10 µg 100 µg	5–10 µg 100–200 µg	10–20 µg 200 µg	1 or 2 3	Titrate dose to obtain optimum control
	i.m., i.v.		–	0.4 µg	0.4 µg	1–4 µg	Single	
Nocturnal enuresis	Intranasal Oral		– –	– –	>7 years 200–400 µg	200–400 µg	Bedtime Single Bedtime	Long-term use not recommended
Dexamethasone Cerebral edema	Oral, i.v.	50 µg/kg	0.25–0.5 mg	0.5–0.75 mg	0.75–2 mg	2–4 mg	4	Doses shown are for maintenance. First dose may be doubled
0.1% drops	Topical (eye)							
Dexamphetamine	Oral		Initially:	2.5 mg (3–5 years)	5–10 mg (>6 years)		Morning	Increase dose by 2.5–5 mg/week up to 10–20 mg twice daily
Diamorphine	s.c., i.m.	50–100 µg/kg	Dose based on bodyweight at all ages				6	Increased according to requirement in severe pain
Diazepam Cerebral spasticity	Oral		0.25 mg/kg	2.5 mg	5 mg	10 mg	2	
Convulsions	i.v. (slow)	0.2–0.3 mg/kg	Dose based on bodyweight under 12 years		10–20 mg		Single dose	Beware of transient respiratory depression
	Rectal		–	5 mg	5–10 mg	10 mg	Single dose	Use solution not suppository

Table 38.3 *Cont'd*

Drug	Route	Single dose/kg	Single dose for different age groups (unless stated otherwise)				Times daily	Comments
			>1 month <1 year	1–4 years	5–12 years	>12 years		
Diazoxide Hypoglycemia Hypertension	Oral i.v.	 5 mg/kg	Initially 5 mg/kg per day – increase as required Dose based on bodyweight at all ages				2–3 Single dose	May be repeated after 30 min. Usual maximum single dose 150 mg
Diclofenac	Oral	0.5–1 mg/kg	–	5–15 mg	7.5–40 mg	25–50 mg	2–3	
Dicyclomine	Oral		0.5 mg/kg	5–10 mg	10 mg	10–20 mg	3	Avoid use <6 months because of possible apnea
Dienestrol 0.025% and 0.01% cream	Topical							Potential systemic estrogen effects
Diethylcarbamazine	Oral		1 mg/kg initially, increasing over 3 days to 2 mg/kg. Treat for 21 days				3	
Digoxin* Digitalization	Oral i.v. (slow)		<2 years 60–80 µg/kg in 24 h, >2 years 40–60 µg/kg in 24 h. 50% of 24 h dose initially then 25% at 8 and 16 h					Lower dose for parenteral route
Maintenance			12.5% of total digitalizing dose based on bodyweight at all ages				2	Therapeutic plasma range 1–2.6 nmol (0.8–2 µg)/l
Digoxin-specific antibody fragments	i.v. infusion							Approximately 60 mg binds 1 mg digoxin
Dihydrocodeine	Oral		–	–	10–30 mg	30 mg	4–6	
Dihydrotachysterol	Oral		0.05–0.1 mg	0.1–0.5 mg	0.5–1 mg	0.5–1 mg	1	Adust dose to avoid hypercalcemia
Diiodohydroxy quinoline	Oral	10 mg/kg	50–100 mg	100–200 mg	150–600 mg	600 mg	3	Usual course 20 days
Diloxanide furoate	Oral		–	–	125–250 mg	250–500 mg	3	Usual course 10 days in chronic amebiasis. Double dose for 5–10 days in acute infection
Dimenhydrinate	Oral		–	12.5–25 mg	25–50 mg	50–100 mg	2–3	
Dimercaprol	i.m.		2.5–3 mg/kg 4-hourly for 2 days; 2–4 times on the third day then 1–2 times daily					
Dioctyl sodium sulfosuccinate – see docusate								
Diphenoxylate	Oral		–	–	2.5 mg	2.5–5 mg	3	Not recommended under 4 years
Diphenylpyraline	Oral		–	–	2.5–5 mg	5–10 mg	2	Slow-release preparation
Diphtheria antitoxin	i.m., i.v.		10 000–30 000 units increased to 40 000–100 000 units in severe cases					Doses up to 30 000 units should be given i.m. For doses over 40 000 units the bulk should be given i.v.
Diphtheria vaccine adsorbed	i.m., s.c.		0.5 ml × 3 at monthly intervals during 1st year of life. Reinforcing dose at school entry					Combined vaccines – diphtheria and tetanus and diphtheria, tetanus and pertussis available
Dipyridamole	Oral	1.25 mg/kg	5–12.5 mg	12.5–25 mg	25–50 mg	50–100 mg	4	
Disopyramide	Oral		2.5–7.5 mg/kg	25–75 mg	50–150 mg	50–150 mg	4	
Dithranol 0.1%–2% preparations	Topical (skin)							
Dobutamine	i.v. (infusion)		2.5 µg/kg per min rising to maximum of 15 µg/kg per min according to effect					Monitor ECG and blood pressure
Docusate	Oral		12.5 mg	12.5–25 mg	25–50 mg	100 mg	3	Not recommended under 6 months
Domperidone	Oral Rectal	0.2–0.4 mg/kg 1 mg/kg	1–4 mg Dose based on bodyweight at all ages	2–5 mg	5–10 mg	10–20 mg	3–4 4	
Dopamine	i.v. (infusion)		2 µg/kg per min rising to maximum of 15 µg/kg per min according to effect					Rarely doses up to 50 µg/kg per min may be used. Monitor heart rate

Table 38.3 *Cont'd*

Drug	Route	Single dose/kg	Single dose for different age groups (unless stated otherwise)				Times daily	Comments
			>1 month <1 year	1–4 years	5–12 years	>12 years		
Dornase alfa	Inhalation	2.5 mg	–	–	2.5 mg	2.5 mg	1	Administer via jet nebulizer. Twice daily admin. may be warranted
Doxycycline	Oral		–	–	–	100 mg	1	Double dose given on 1st day. Contraindicated under 12 years
Droperidol Premedication	Oral, i.m.	0.3 mg/kg	Dose based on bodyweight at all ages				Single dose	Usual maximum dose for premedication: 5 mg
Antiemetic	i.m., i.v.	0.02–0.075 mg/kg	Dose based on bodyweight at all ages				Single dose	Repeated 1- to 4-hourly as required
Edrophonium	i.v.	0.1 mg/kg	Give 1/5 of the dose initially; if tolerated give remainder				Single dose	
Ephedrine 0.5% and 1% drops	Oral Topical (nose)		7.5 mg	15 mg	30 mg	30–60 mg	3	
Erythromycin	Oral		62.5–125 mg	125–250 mg	250–500 mg	500 mg	4	Double oral and i.v. doses in severe infection
	i.v. infusion	6 mg/kg	Give as a 0.1–0.5% solution over 20–60 min				4	
Ethambutol*	Oral	25 mg/kg for 60 days thereafter reduced to 15 mg/kg					1	May cause visual impairment. Avoid in young children
Ethamsylate – see neonatal section								
Ethinylestradiol	Oral			Starting dose:	1–2 µg		1	Increase as appropriate for stage of puberty
Ethosuximide	Oral		–	125–250 mg	250–750 mg	250 mg–1 g	2	Start with low dose and increase gradually. Therapeutic range 40–100 mg/l
Fenoterol	Inhalation (aerosol)		–	–	200 µg	200–400 µg	3–4	
	Inhalation (nebulizer)		–	–	0.5–1 mg	1 mg	3	
Ferrous fumarate	Oral		70 mg	140 mg	210 mg	200–400 mg	2	Ferrous fumarate 200 mg = 65 mg iron
Ferrous gluconate	Oral		–	–	300 mg	300–600 mg	3	Ferrous gluconate 300 mg = 35 mg iron
Ferrous succinate (106 mg/5 ml elixir)	Oral		1 ml	2.5 ml	5 ml	–	3	Ferrous succinate 106 mg = 37 mg iron
Ferrous sulfate	Oral		60 mg	120 mg	180 mg	200 mg	3	Ferrous sulfate 200 mg = 60 mg iron
Flucloxacillin	Oral		62.5 mg	125 mg	250 mg	250–500 mg	4	
	i.m., i.v. (slow)	12.5 mg/kg	Dose based on bodyweight at all ages				4	Use i.v. and double dose in severe infection
Fluconazole Superficial infection	i.v. infusion	1–2 mg/kg	Dose based on bodyweight at all ages				1	
Systemic infection	i.v. infusion	3–6 mg/kg	Dose based on bodyweight at all ages				1	
Flucytosine*	Oral, i.v.	25–50 mg/kg	Dose based on bodyweight at all ages				4	Infuse over 30 min
Fludrocortisone	Oral	5 µg/kg	5 µg/kg	50–100 µg	100 µg	200 µg	1	
Flumazenil	i.v. (slow)		Adult dose: 0.2 mg over 15 s, then 0.1 mg at 1 min intervals if required. Usual dose range 0.3–0.6 mg. Max. total dose 1 mg (2 mg in intensive care unit)					
Fluocinolone acetonide 0.0025–0.025% preparations	Topical (skin)						1–3	Potent topical corticosteroid

Table 38.3 *Cont'd*

Drug	Route	Single dose/kg	Single dose for different age groups (unless stated otherwise)				Times daily	Comments
			>1 month <1 year	1–4 years	5–12 years	>12 years		
Fluticasone	Inhalation (aerosol) (dry powder)		One or two inhalations (50–100 µg) for all ages over 4 years				2	Establish on minimum effective maintenance dose
	Intranasal		One spray (50 µg) to each nostril for all ages over 4 years				2	
Folic acid	Oral		0.5 mg/kg	5 mg	5 mg	5 mg	1	Larger doses may be required in malabsorption
Folinic acid	Oral, i.v., i.m.							See Chapter 16
Framycetin 0.5% cream	Topical (skin)						3	
0.5% drops and ointment	Topical (ear/eye)						3	
Frusemide	Oral	1–2 mg/kg	Dose based on bodyweight up to 12 years			20–40 mg	1–3	Avoid concurrent use of aminoglycosides
	i.m., i.v. (slow)	0.5–1.5 mg/kg	Dose based on bodyweight up to 12 years			20–50 mg	1	
Furazolidone	Oral	1.25 mg/kg	Dose based on bodyweight at all ages				4	
Fusidic acid	Oral		12.5 mg/kg	250 mg	250–500 mg	500–750 mg	3	
	i.v.		6–7 mg/kg as diethanolamine fusidate. Dose based on bodyweight at all ages				3	Give well diluted over at least 6 h. Dose may be doubled for severe infection
2% preparations	Topical (skin)						3	
1% gel	Topical (eye)						2	
Gamma globulin – see immunoglobulin								
Gentamicin*	i.m, i.v.		2.5 mg/kg	2.5 mg/kg	2.5 mg/kg	2 mg/kg	3	Maintain plasma concentrations at 6–10 mg/l (peak) and <2 mg/l (trough)
0.3% preparations	Topical (skin/ear/eye)						3–6	
Glucagon	s.c., i.m., i.v.	0.025 mg/kg	0.025 mg/kg	0.5 mg	0.5–1 mg	1 mg	Single dose	If not effective in 10 min, intravenous glucose should be given
Gonadorelin	s.c., i.v.		100 µg	100µg	100 µg	100 µg	Single dose	
Granisetron	i.v.	40 µg/kg	Single dose based on bodyweight at all ages. Maximum 3 mg					Rapid infusion over 5 min just before chemotherapy
Griseofulvin	Oral	10 mg/kg	10 mg/kg	100–150 mg	150–500 mg	500 mg–1 g	1	
Growth hormone – see somatropin								
Haloperidol	Oral, i.m., i.v.	25 µg/kg	25 µg/kg	0.25–0.4 mg	0.4–1 mg	1.5 mg	2	Dose may be increased gradually to maximum of 10 mg daily (12 years or under) or 30 mg (>12 years). Exceptionally these doses may be exceeded
Heparin	i.v. infusion	25 units/kg per h	25 units/kg per h	250–400 units per h	400–1000 units per h	1000–1500 units per h	–	Adjust dose to maintain clotting time or thrombin time at 2–3 times normal
Hepatitis B vaccine H-B-Vax	i.m.		<10 years: 0.5 ml repeated at 1 and 6 months; >10 years: 1.0 ml repeated at 1 and 6 months					Double dose in immunocompromised.
Engerix B	i.m.		1.0 ml at all ages, repeated at 1 and 6 months					Hepatitis B immunoglobulin may also be given to those contaminated with virus

Table 38.3 *Cont'd*

Drug	Route	Single dose/kg	Single dose for different age groups (unless stated otherwise)				Times daily	Comments
			>1 month <1 year	1–4 years	5–12 years	>12 years		
Homatropine 1% and 2% drops	Topical (eye)							
Hyaluronidase	i.m., s.c.		1 500 units in total					
Hydralazine Hypertensive crisis	i.m., i.v. (slow)	0.2 mg/kg	Dose based on bodyweight at all ages				Single	May be repeated after 30 min or given as infusion
Maintenance	Oral	0.25–0.5 mg/kg	0.25–0.5 mg/kg	2.5–8 mg	4–12.5 mg	12.5 mg	4	Initial doses stated. Maximum daily dose 8 mg/kg
Hydro-chlorothiazide	Oral	1 mg/kg	1 mg/kg	12.5 mg	12.5–25 mg	25–50 mg	2	
Hydrocortisone Replacement	Oral		20 mg/m² per day. Dose based on surface area at all ages					2/3 dose in morning, remainder in evening. Dose increased in periods of stress
Therapeutic	i.m., i.v. (slow)		50 mg	50 mg	100 mg	100 mg	4	Increase dose fourfold for infantile laryngeal edema
0.5%, 1%, 2.5% preparations	Topical (skin)							
Hydroflumethiazide	Oral	1 mg/kg	1 mg/kg	10–15 mg	15–40 mg	25–50 mg	1	
Hydroxocobalamin	i.m.		Initially 1 mg repeated 5 times at intervals of 2–3 days. Maintenance dose 1 mg every 3 months					
Hydroxyzine	Oral		–	5–10 mg	10–25 mg	25–50 mg	4	
Hyoscine hydrobromide Motion sickness	Oral		–	–	75–150 µg	150–300 µg		First dose to be taken 30 min before journey; 6-hourly thereafter
Premedication	s.c., i.m.	10–15 µg/kg	–	100–200 µg	150–400 µg	400–600 µg	Single dose	
Hypromellose 0.3%, 0.5%, 1% drops	Topical (eye)							
Ibuprofen	Oral	5 mg/kg	–	50–75 mg	75–200 mg	200–400 mg	3–4	Maximum dose of 500 mg/day in children under 30 kg
Ichthammol 5%, 10% preparations	Topical (skin)							
Idoxuridine 5%, 40% solutions	Topical (skin)							Made up in dimethyl sulfoxide
0.1% drops 0.5% ointment	Topical (eye)							
Imipenem–cilastatin*	i.v. infusion	15 mg/kg	50–150 mg	150–250 mg	200–500 mg	500 mg	3–4	Dose given in terms of imipenem. Not recommended under 3 months
Imipramine Enuresis	Oral		–	–	25–50 mg	50–75 mg	Bedtime	Max. treatment period 3 months. Not recommended under 7 years
Depression	Oral				10 mg	25 mg	3	
Immunoglobulin Normal	i.m.		Usual prophylactic dose: 0.02–0.04 ml/kg. For prolonged exposure or in areas of high endemicity: 0.06–0.12 ml/kg and repeat every 4–6 months on continued exposure				Single dose	Gives protection for 3 months
								Specific preparations available for hepatitis B, rabies, tetanus and varicella-zoster

Table 38.3   *Cont'd*

Drug	Route	Single dose/kg	Single dose for different age groups (unless stated otherwise)				Times daily	Comments
			>1 month <1 year	1–4 years	5–12 years	>12 years		
Indomethacin Anti-inflammatory	Oral		–	–	25 mg	25–50 mg	2–3	
Closure of ductus arteriosus	See neonatal section							
Influenza vaccine	i.m., s.c. (deep)		–	–	0.5 ml	0.5 ml	Single dose	Repeated once after 4–6 weeks for primary vaccination
Insulin Short acting	i.m., s.c., i.v.		Soluble Insulin Inj					All preparations 100 units/ml
Intermediate acting	s.c.		Isophane Insulin Inj; Biphasic Insulin Inj; Insulin Zinc Susp. (amorphous); Insulin Zinc Susp. (crystalline); Insulin Zinc Susp. (30% amorphous, 70% crystalline)					
Long acting	s.c.		Protamine Zinc Insulin Inj					
Ipecacuanha 0.14% elixir	Oral		5–10 ml	15 ml	15 ml	20–30 ml	Single dose	Follow dose with 100–200 ml water. Repeat dose after 20 min if necessary
Ipratropium	Inhalation (aerosol)		–	18 μg	18–36 μg	18–36 μg	3	18 μg/metered dose
	Inhalation (nebulizer)		12.5 μg/kg	125 μg	250 μg	500 μg	3	250 μg/ml
Iron sorbitol 50 mg Fe/ml	i.m. (deep)	1.5 mg/kg	Given once daily or on alternate days. Max. single dose: 100 mg					Total dose 10–24 injections according to initial hemoglobin level. Not recommended in infants under 3 kg
Isoniazid	Oral, i.m., i.v.		10–15 mg/kg	10 mg/kg	10 mg/kg	300 mg	1	Monitor hepatic function; consider concurrent pyridoxine therapy to prevent peripheral neuropathy
Isoprenaline	i.v. infusion	0.1–4 μg/kg per min.	Dose based on bodyweight at all ages					
Ivermectin	Oral	150 μg/kg					Single dose	
Ketoconazole	Oral	3 mg/kg	–	50 mg	100 mg	200 mg	1	Monitor liver function carefully
Ketamine Anesthesia	i.v. (slow)	2 mg/kg	Dose based on bodyweight at all ages				Single dose	May be repeated
	i.m.	10 mg/kg	Dose based on bodyweight at all ages				Single dose	
Subanesthesia	i.m.	5–7 mg/kg	Dose based on bodyweight at all ages					Dose for procedures
Ketotifen	Oral		–	1 mg	1 mg	1–2 mg	2	
Labetalol	Oral		–	–	–	Initially: 100 mg	2	Increase as necessary by 200 mg daily every 2–3 days to usual maintenance of 400–800 mg daily (max. 2400 mg daily)
	i.v.		–	–	–	Initially: 20 mg	Single dose	Then 40–80 mg at 10-min intervals
Lactulose 3.35 g/5 ml	Oral	Starting dose:	2.5 ml	5 ml	10 ml	15 ml	2	
Lamotrigine Combination with sodium valproate	Oral	200 μg/kg/day 500 μg/kg/day 5 mg 1–5 mg/kg/day	Starting dose: all patients >25 kg First incremental dose: all patients >25 kg Alternate days starting dose if <25 kg Maintenance dose for all patients				1–2	Add-on therapy only First 14 days Next 14 days Monitor liver/kidney function. Also clotting studies

Table 38.3   *Cont'd*

Drug	Route	Single dose/kg	Single dose for different age groups (unless stated otherwise)				Times daily	Comments
			>1 month <1 year	1–4 years	5–12 years	>12 years		
With anticonvulsants other than sodium valproate		1 mg/kg 2.5 mg/kg 2.5–7.5 mg/kg	Starting dose: all ages First incremental dose: all ages Maintenance dose: all ages				2	First 14 days Next 14 days Discontinue if rash develops
Levamisole	Oral	3 mg/kg	10–30 mg	30–45 mg	45–120 mg	120–150 mg	Single dose	
Lignocaine	i.v. (slow)	0.5–1 mg/kg	Dose based on bodyweight at all ages					Dose may be repeated twice, then infuse 20–50 µg/kg per min
0.5% and 1% solutions	s.c.							
2–5% preparations	Topical							
Liothyronine sodium	Oral	Maintenance:	2.5–10 µg	10–15 µg	10–25 µg	10–25 µg	2–3	Initial dose 5 µg daily increased gradually to maintenance dose
Loperamide	Oral		–	0.5 mg	1–2 mg	2 mg	4	Not recommended for acute diarrhea in infants
Lorazepam Premedication	Oral	0.05 mg/kg	–	–	0.5–2.5 mg	2–3 mg	Single dose	
Lypressin 2.5 units/squeeze	Intranasal		–	2.5–5 units	2.5–5 units	2.5–5 units	3–7	Adjust dose and frequency according to response
Magnesium hydroxide 550 mg/10 ml	Oral	0.5 ml/kg	–	5–10 ml	5–15 ml	10–20 ml	Single dose	Osmotic laxative
Malathion 0.5% alcoholic lotion	Topical (skin)							
Mannitol	i.v. infusion	0.5–2 g/kg	For oliguria 0.1–0.2 g/kg as test dose; give remainder only if diuresis induced				Single dose	Administer over 30–60 min. Dose may be repeated
Mebendazole Threadworm	Oral		–	100 mg	100 mg	100 mg	Single dose	Not recommended under 2 years
Whipworm, roundworm and hookworm	Oral		–	100 mg	100 mg	100 mg	2	Treat for 3 days
Mecillinam	i.v., i.m.	5–15 mg/kg	25–150 mg	50–240 mg	75–600 mg	200–600 mg	3–4	Use the lower dose and frequency for urinary tract infection
Mefenamic acid	Oral	8 mg/kg	50 mg	100 mg	150–200 mg	250 mg	3	Not to exceed 7 days' treatment except in juvenile chronic arthritis. Not recommended under 6 months
Menadiol sodium phosphate	Oral	0.5 mg/kg	–	5 mg	5–20 mg	10–40 mg	1	Use phytomenadione in neonates
Mepacrine Giardiasis	Oral	2 mg/kg	5–20 mg	20–30 mg	30–100 mg	100 mg	3	Treat for 5–7 days
Meropenem	i.v.	20–40 mg/kg	Dose based on bodyweight at all ages				3	Highest dose in treatment of meningitis. 12-hourly dosing in moderate renal failure
Methicillin	i.v. (slow) i.m.	25–100 mg/kg	0.1–1 g	0.25–1.5 g	0.4–4 g	1–4 g	4–6	Use the higher doses and frequency for severe infection
Methionine	Oral	50 mg/kg	50 mg/kg	500–750 mg	750–2000 mg	2500 mg	6	
Methylcellulose	Oral		50 mg/kg	0.45–0.9 g	0.5–1.5 g	0.5–2 g	2–3	
Methyldopa	Oral	3 mg/kg	3 mg/kg	25–50 mg	50–125 mg	125–250 mg	3	May be increased to 65 mg/kg per day but not to exceed daily dose of 3 g
	i.v.	5–10 mg/kg	Dose based on bodyweight at all ages				4	

Table 38.3 *Cont'd*

Drug	Route	Single dose/kg	Single dose for different age groups (unless stated otherwise)				Times daily	Comments
			>1 month <1 year	1–4 years	5–12 years	>12 years		
Methylphenidate	Oral		–	–	5 mg	5 mg	2	Give before breakfast and lunch
Methylprednisolone	i.v.	15–30 mg/kg	Dose for treatment of shock (not septicemic)				1	May be repeated twice. Maximum daily dose 1 g
Methyltestosterone	i.m.		50 mg monthly for 6 months then 100 mg monthly					Absorption by mouth unreliable
Metoclopramide	Oral, i.m., i.v.		0.1 mg/kg	1–2 mg	2.5–5 mg	5–10 mg	2–3	Maximum daily dose 0.5 mg/kg. Risk of dystonic reactions
Metoprolol	Oral	2.5 mg/kg	–	25–40 mg	40–100 mg	50–100 mg	2	
Metriphonate	Oral	7.5 mg/kg	Dose based on bodyweight at all ages				Single dose	Give 3 doses at intervals of 2 weeks
Metronidazole	Oral, i.v. infusion	7.5 mg/kg	7.5 mg/kg	75-100 mg	100–300 mg	200–500 mg	3	
	Rectal		125 mg	250 mg	500 mg	1 g	3	
Metyrapone	Oral		In the differential diagnosis of Cushing's syndrome 15 mg/kg (minimum dose 250 mg) is given 4-hourly for 6 doses					
Mexiletine	Oral	2.5–4 mg/kg	Dose based on bodyweight at all ages				3–4	
	i.v. (slow)	2–4 mg/kg	Dose based on bodyweight at all ages				Single dose	After initial dose an infusion of 2–4 mg/kg/h may be given
Miconazole	i.v. infusion	10–15 mg/kg	40–150 mg	100–250 mg	150–600 mg	600 mg	3	Infuse over at least 30 min
2% gel	Topical (oral)						2–4	
2% cream and powder	Topical (skin)						2	For napkin rash apply at each nappy change
Minocycline	Oral		–	–	–	50–100 mg	2	Contraindicated under 12 years
Minoxidil	Oral		0.1 mg/kg per dose initially, increasing to a maximum daily dose of 2 mg/kg according to response and tolerance				1–2	
Monosulfiram	Topical (skin)		25% solution (dilute with 2–3 parts of water before use)				Single dose	Apply diluted solution over whole body except head and neck. Repeat if necessary for 2–3 nights
Morphine	s.c., i.m.	0.1–0.2 mg/kg	0.2 mg/kg	2.5–5 mg	5–10 mg	10 mg	6	
	Oral		0.2–0.4 mg/kg increased according to requirement in severe pain				6	
Mupirocin 2% ointment	Topical (skin)						3	
2% ointment	Topical (nose)						2–3	
Nalidixic acid	Oral	12.5 mg/kg	12.5 mg/kg	150–250 mg	250–500 mg	500 mg–1 g	4	Not recommended under 3 months
Naloxone – see also neonatal section	i.v., i.m.	5–10 µg/kg	Dose based on bodyweight at all ages					i.v. preferred. Repeat according to response. Consider infusion for severe narcosis
Naproxen*	Oral	5 mg/kg	–	–	75–250 mg	250–500 mg	2	
Natamycin 1% suspension	Topical (oral)		4 drops	10 drops	10 drops	10 drops	After meals	
Neomycin	Oral	15 mg/kg	50–200 mg	200–300 mg	250–500 mg	1 g	6	Little or no oral absorption but exercise caution in renal failure
0.5% cream, ointment	Topical (skin)						3	
0.5% drops, ointment	Topical (eye)						3–4	

Table 38.3 *Cont'd*

Drug	Route	Single dose/kg	Single dose for different age groups (unless stated otherwise)				Times daily	Comments
			>1 month <1 year	1–4 years	5–12 years	>12 years		
Neostigmine	Oral	0.5–1 mg/kg	1–7.5 mg	7.5 mg	15 mg	15–30 mg	4–6	Initial dose given. Concurrent anticholinergic may be required
	i.v.	50 µg/kg	0.15–0.5 mg	0.5–0.75 mg	0.75–2 mg	2–2.5 mg	Single dose	For reversal of nondepolarizing muscle relaxants. Give with atropine
Netilmicin*	i.v., i.m.	2–2.5 mg/kg	Dose based on bodyweight at all ages				3	Maintain plasma concentrations at 6–10 mg/l (peak) and <2 mg/l (trough)
Niclosamide T. saginata T. solium D. latum	Oral		<2 years: 500 mg	2–6 years: 1 g	>6 years: 2 g		Single dose	Tablets should be taken (chewed or crushed) after a light breakfast and followed by a purgative 2 hours later
H. nana	Oral		<2 years: 250 mg	2–6 years: 500 mg	>6 years: 1 g		1	Give double dose on first day. Treat for 7 days
Nicotinamide Prophylaxis	Oral		5–10 mg	10 mg	15 mg	15–20 mg	1	
Nifedipine	Oral	125–250 µg/kg	Dose based on bodyweight at all ages				2–3	Dose may be increased to maximum of 1 mg/kg daily
Nitrazepam	Oral	0.25 mg/kg	1–2.5 mg	2.5–4 mg	2.5–5 mg	5–10 mg	2	Anticonvulsant dose given
Nitrofurantoin*	Oral	2.5 mg/kg	2.5 mg/kg	25 mg	50 mg	100 mg	4	For prophylaxis give single dose every night. Contraindicated in neonates
Noradrenaline acid tartrate	i.v. infusion		Initially 0.2 µg/kg per min, then 0.1–0.2 µg/kg per min					Give as a 8 µg/ml solution in 5% dextrose/water
	Intracardiac		25–150 µg (undiluted) according to age					
Nystatin	Topical (oral)		100 000 units at all ages				4	Not absorbed after oral administration
100 000 units/g	Topical (skin)		Various preparations available				2–4	
Ondansetron	i.v. infusion		–	–	5 mg/m²	5 mg/m²	Single dose	Infuse over 15 min immed. prior to chemotherapy and follow with oral ondansetron for up to 5 days
	Oral		–	–	4 mg	4–8 mg	3	
Orciprenaline hydrochloride	Oral	0.5–1 mg/kg	5–10 mg	5–10 mg	10–20 mg	20 mg	3–4	
	Inhalation (aerosol)		–	0.75 mg	0.75–1.5 mg	0.75–1.5 mg	2–4	
Orphenadrine	Oral		Adults and children: 150 mg daily in divided doses gradually increased					Maximum 400 mg daily
Oxamniquine	Oral	10–15 mg/kg	Dose based on bodyweight at all ages				2	Treat for 1–3 days
Oxprenolol	Oral	1 mg/kg	3–10 mg	10–15 mg	15–40 mg	40 mg	3	
Oxymetholone	Oral	1 mg/kg	3–10 mg	10–15 mg	15–40 mg	40–50 mg	2–3	Monitor skeletal maturation
Oxytetracycline	Oral		–	–	–	250–500 mg	4	Contraindicated under 12 years
Pancreatin	Oral		Individualize dose according to stool number and consistency. <2 years open capsule(s) and mix contents with feeds					Various preparations available containing protease, amylase and lipase: Cotazym, Creon, Nutrizym, Pancrease, Pancrex and Pancrex V. High doses associated with colonic strictures
Pancuronium – see also Table 38.2	i.v.		60–100 µg/kg initially, then 10–20 µg/kg every 30–60 min as necessary				Single dose	
Paracetamol	Oral, rectal	12 mg/kg	60–120 mg	120–250 mg	250–500 mg	0.5–1 g	4	Suppositories generally not used >4 years

Table 38.3 *Cont'd*

Drug	Route	Single dose/kg	Single dose for different age groups (unless stated otherwise)				Times daily	Comments
			>1 month <1 year	1–4 years	5–12 years	>12 years		
Paraldehyde	i.m. (deep), rectal		0.1 ml/kg	1–4 ml	5–6 ml	5–10 ml	Single dose	Administer rectal dose as a 10% enema in 0.9% saline or as a 50% enema in arachis or olive oil
Paromomycin	Oral	10 mg/kg	Dose based on bodyweight at all ages				3	
Pemoline	Oral		–	–	>6 years: 20–40 mg each morning			Dose may be increased at weekly intervals to maximum of 100 mg daily
Penicillamine*	Oral	5 mg/kg	–	50–75 mg	75–200 mg	125–250 mg	3–4	For rheumatoid arthritis start with 50 mg/day before food increasing at 4-weekly intervals. Monitor for blood dyscrasias and proteinuria
Penicillin V	Oral		62.5 mg	125 mg	250 mg	250–500 mg	4	Take at least 1/2 hour before food. For prophylaxis give twice daily up to maximum of 500 mg/day
Pentagastrin	s.c. i.v. infusion	6 μg/kg 0.6 μg/kg per h	Dose based on bodyweight at all ages Dose based on bodyweight at all ages				Single dose	
Pentamidine isethionate* *P. carinii*	i.v. infusion	4 mg/kg	Dose based on bodyweight at all ages				1	Treat for at least 14 days
Leishmaniasis Visceral	i.m. (deep)	3–4 mg/kg	Dose based on bodyweight at all ages				Alternate days	Maximum 10 injections
Cutaneous	i.m. (deep)	3–4 mg/kg	Dose based on bodyweight at all ages				Once or twice weekly	Treat until condition resolves
Pentazocine	Oral		–	–	25 mg	25 mg	4–8	
	s.c., i.m.	1 mg/kg	–	10–15 mg	15–30 mg	30 mg	4–8	
	i.v.	0.5 mg/kg	–	5–7.5 mg	7.5–15 mg	15 mg	4–8	
Pethidine	Oral, i.m.	0.5–2 mg/kg	1 mg/kg	10–15 mg	15–50 mg	50–100 mg	4–6	
Phenindione	Oral	1–3 mg/kg	Dose based on bodyweight up to 12 years			50–150 mg	1	Warfarin preferred. Adjust dose according to prothrombin time
Phenobarbitone Maintenance	Oral, i.m.	4–6 mg/kg	4–6 mg/kg	30–60 mg	60–90 mg	90 mg	1	Maintain plasma concentrations of 15–40 mg/l
Loading dose	i.v., i.m.	12–20 mg/kg	Dose based on bodyweight at all ages				Single	Give i.v. over 5 min
Phenoxybenzamine	Oral	0.5–1 mg/kg	Dose based on bodyweight at all ages				2	
Phenoxymethyl penicillin – see penicillin V								
Phentolamine	i.v., i.m.		1–5 mg according to age				Single dose	
Phenylephrine 0.25% drops	Topical (nose)							3- to 4-hourly. Use with caution under 3 months
2.5%, 10% drops	Topical (eye)							
Phenytoin Maintenance	Oral	2.5–5 mg/kg	Dose based on bodyweight at all ages				2	Can be given as a single daily dose. Maintain plasma concentrations between 10 and 20 mg/l
Status epilepticus	i.v. (slow)	10–15 mg/kg	Dose based on bodyweight at all ages				Single dose	Inject slowly at a rate not exceeding 1 mg/kg per min, preferably under ECG control
Pholcodine	Oral		100 μg/kg	1–2.5 mg	5 mg	10 mg	3–4	

Table 38.3 *Cont'd*

Drug	Route	Single dose/kg	Single dose for different age groups (unless stated otherwise)				Times daily	Comments
			>1 month <1 year	1–4 years	5–12 years	>12 years		
Phytomenadione (vitamin K₁) – see also Table 38.2	Oral, i.m., i.v. (slow)	0.3 mg/kg	1–3 mg	5 mg	5–10 mg	10 mg	Single dose	May be repeated
Pilocarpine 0.5%, 1% drops	Topical (eye)							
Piperacillin	i.v.	25–75 mg/kg	Dose based on bodyweight at all ages				4	Use high dose in severe infection and in CF
Piperazine *E. vermicularis*	Oral	50–75 mg/kg	50–75 mg/kg	750 mg	1.5 g	2 g	1	Treat for 7 days
Ascariasis	Oral	100 mg/kg	100 mg/kg	1.5 g	3 g	4 g	Single dose	
Piroxicam	Oral	0.3–0.6 mg/kg	–	–	5–15 mg	15–20 mg	1	Contraindicated under 6 years
Pivampicillin	Oral		20 mg/kg	175–250 mg	250–500 mg	500 mg	2–3	
Pivmecillinam	Oral	5–10 mg/kg	25–100 mg	50–150 mg	75–200 mg	200–400 mg	4	Use dose 50% above the highest shown here for treatment of salmonellosis
Pizotifen	Oral		–	–	500 µg	500 µg	3	May be given as a single daily dose of 1 mg at night
Pneumococcal vaccine	s.c., i.m.		–	0.5 ml	0.5 ml	0.5 ml	Single dose	Contraindicated under 2 years
Podophyllum 15% paint	Topical (skin)						1	
Polysaccharide iron complex	Oral	2 mg/kg	2 mg/kg	25 mg	50 mg	100 mg	2	Dose given in terms of elemental iron
Polystyrene sulfonate resin	Oral, rectal	0.25 g/kg	1–2.5 g	2.5–5 g	5–10 g	15 g	3–4	
Potassium chloride	Oral i.v. infusion	Daily dose: 2.5–3.5 mmol/kg			2–2.5 mmol/kg	1.5–2 mmol/kg	1.5 mmol/kg		Oral: give in divided (3) doses. i.v.: maximum concentration 40 mmol/l. 75 mg potassium chloride contains 1 mmol K⁺
Potassium permanganate 0.01% solution	Topical (skin)							
Pralidoxime	i.v. (slow)	20–60 mg/kg	Dose based on bodyweight at all ages				Single dose	Dose can be repeated
Praziquantel	Oral	20–25 mg/kg	Dose based on bodyweight at all ages				3–4	
Prazosin	Oral	0.05 mg/kg per dose initially, increasing to maximum daily dose of 0.4 mg/kg according to response and tolerance					2–3	Start with twice daily dosage
Prednisolone	Oral, i.m., i.v.	125–500 µg/kg	Dose based on bodyweight at all ages				1–4	Dose and frequency depend on condition being treated
0.5% drops	Topical (eye, ear)							
Primaquine	Oral	0.25 mg/kg	1–2.5 mg	2.5–5 mg	5–10 mg	10–15 mg	1	Treat for 14–21 days. Reduce dose in G6PD deficiency
Primidone	Oral	10–15 mg/kg for maintenance	Dose based on bodyweight at all ages				2	Start with a low dose at bedtime. Metabolized to phenobarbitone. Optimum plasma concentration of phenobarbitone 15–40 mg/l
Probenecid	Oral	10 mg/kg	–	10 mg/kg	150–250 mg	250–500 mg	4	Initially 25 mg/kg as a single dose. Not recommended under 2 years
Procainamide*	Oral	8 mg/kg	25–80 mg	80–125 mg	125–250 mg	250–500 mg	4–6	
	i.v. (slow)	2 mg/kg initially, repeated every 10–30 min (max. 100 mg) then 0.5 mg/kg per h						

Table 38.3 *Cont'd*

Drug	Route	Single dose/kg	Single dose for different age groups (unless stated otherwise)				Times daily	Comments
			>1 month <1 year	1–4 years	5–12 years	>12 years		
Procaine penicillin	i.m.	10 mg/kg	10 mg/kg	100–150 mg	150–300 mg	300–600 mg	1	
Prochlorperazine	Oral	125–250 µg/kg	–	1.25–2.5 mg	2.5–5 mg	5–10 mg	2–3	Possible dystonic reactions; caution indicated under 10 kg bodyweight
	i.m. (deep)	125–250 µg/kg	–	1.25–2.5 mg	2.5–6.25 mg	6.25–12.5 mg	2–3	
	Rectal	250 µg/kg	–	2.5 mg	5–12.5 mg	12.5–25 mg	2–3	
Procyclidine	i.m., i.v. (slow)		2.5 mg	2.5 mg	5 mg	5–10 mg	Single	May be repeated after 20 min
Proguanil	Oral		25 mg	50 mg	100 mg	150 mg	1	Malaria prophylaxis
Promethazine Antihistaminic	Oral		2.5–5 mg	5–10 mg	10–15 mg	15–20 mg	2–3	
Sedative	Oral		5–10 mg	15–20 mg	20–25 mg	25–50 mg	Single dose	
Propranolol	Oral	0.25–0.5 mg/kg	0.25–0.5 mg/kg	2.5–7.5 mg	5–20 mg	10–40 mg	3–4	Initial dose stated; adjust according to response
	i.v. (slow)	25–50 µg/kg	Dose based on bodyweight at all ages				3–4	Give i.v. injection under ECG control
Propylthiouracil*	Oral		–	–	15–50 mg	50–100 mg	3	Initial dose stated; reduce when hyperthyroidism is controlled
Prostaglandin E₁ – see Table 38.2								
Protamine sulfate	i.v. (slow)		Maximum rate 5 mg/min (1 mg neutralizes 100 units heparin given in the previous 4 h)					Maximum dose 50 mg
Protirelin (TRH)	i.v.		200 µg	200 µg	200 µg	200 µg	Single dose	
Proxymetacaine 0.5% drops	Topical (eye)							
Pseudoephedrine	Oral		5–15 mg	15 mg	30 mg	60 mg	3	
Pyrantel	Oral	10 mg/kg	10 mg/kg	125 mg	250–500 mg	500–750 mg	Single dose	Maximum daily dose 1 g
Pyrazinamide	Oral	5 mg/kg	Dose based on bodyweight at all ages				4	Only used in children if no alternative
Pyridostigmine	Oral		5–30 mg	30 mg	60 mg	60 mg	4–6	Initial doses given; adjust according to response
Pyridoxine – see also Table 38.2	Oral	0.5–1 mg/kg	5–10 mg	10–20 mg	20–50 mg	50 mg	2–3	
Pyrimethamine Toxoplasmosis	Oral	0.5 mg/kg	–	6.25 mg	12.5 mg	25 mg	1	Double dose for first 3 days. Use with sulfadimidine and calcium folinate
Pyrvinium	Oral	5 mg/kg	Dose based on bodyweight at all ages				Single dose	
Quinine sulfate	Oral	10 mg/kg	10 mg/kg	100–150 mg	150–600 mg	400–600 mg	3	Treat for 7 days. Dose valid for quinine hydrochloride and dihydrochloride
Quinine dihydrochloride	i.v. infusion	10 mg/kg	10 mg/kg	100–150 mg	150–600 mg	400–600 mg	3	Infuse over 4 h. A loading dose of 20 mg/kg can be given. Reduce i.v. dose to 6.7 mg/kg after 3 days
Ranitidine	Oral i.v. (slow)	2 mg/kg 0.3–0.7 mg/kg	2 mg/kg	20–30 mg	30–100 mg	100–150 mg	2 3	
Reproterol	Inhalation (aerosol)		–	–	0.5 mg	1 mg	3	
Ribavarin – see tribavarin								
Riboflavin Therapeutic	Oral	1 mg/kg	5–10 mg	10–15 mg	15–30 mg	30 mg	1	Physiological requirement 0.4–1.8 mg/day according to age

Table 38.3 *Cont'd*

Drug	Route	Single dose/kg	Single dose for different age groups (unless stated otherwise)				Times daily	Comments
			>1 month <1 year	1–4 years	5–12 years	>12 years		
Rifampicin Tuberculosis	Oral, i.v.	10–20 mg/kg	10–20 mg/kg	100–300 mg	150–450 mg	450–600 mg	1	Maximum dose of 8 mg/kg in impaired liver function. Maximum daily dose 600 mg
Meningococcal carriers	Oral	5–10 mg/kg	5–10 mg/kg	10 mg/kg	10 mg/kg	600 mg	2	Treat for 2 days. Use the lower dose/kg, <3 months
Salbutamol	Inhalation (aerosol)		–	100–200 μg	100–200 μg	200 μg	3–4	
	Inhalation (powder)		–	200 μg	200 μg	200–400 μg	3–4	
	Inhalation (nebulizer)		1.25 mg	2.5 mg	2.5–5 mg	5–10 mg	4	
	Oral		1 mg	1–2 mg	2–4 mg	4 mg	3–4	
	Oral (slow release)		–	4 mg	4 mg	8 mg	2	Preparation not recommended under 3 years
	i.v.	5 μg/kg injected over 15 min followed by 5 μg/kg per h						Monitor heart rate. Infusion rate may be increased according to response (max. 20 μg/kg per h)
Salicylic 2% ointment	Topical (skin)						2–3	
Salmeterol	Inhalation (aerosol) (powder)		–	–	50 μg	50–100 μg	2	Long acting
Senna	Oral	–	–	3.75–7.5 mg	7.5–15 mg	15–30 mg	Once (bedtime)	Dose given in terms of total sennosides
Sodium aurothiomalate*	i.m. (deep)	1 mg/kg	Dose based on bodyweight (max. 50 mg total)				Once weekly	Give test dose of 100–200 μg/kg for 2–3 weeks
Sodium bicarbonate	i.v. (slow)	1–2 mg/kg	Dose based on bodyweight and calculated deficit				Single	May be repeated
Sodium calciumedetate	i.v. infusion	40 mg/kg	40 mg/kg	400–600 mg	600 mg–1.5 g	1.5–3 g	2	Treat for up to 5 days
Sodium cellulose phosphate	Oral		3 g	3 g	3–4 g	5 g	3	
Sodium chloride – see Chapter 10								
Sodium cromoglycate	Inhalation (aerosol)		–	5–10 mg	5–10 mg	5–10 mg	4–8	
	Inhalation (powder)		–	20 mg	20 mg	20 mg	4–8	
	Inhalation (nebulizer)		–	20 mg	20 mg	20 mg	4–6	
2% drops and spray	Topical (nose)						4–6	
2% drops, 4% ointment	Topical (eye)						2–4	
Sodium fusidate – see fusidic acid								
Sodium hypochlorite 0.1–0.5% solutions	Topical (skin)							
Sodium ironedetate	Oral		95 mg	95 mg	190 mg	190–380 mg	3	Twice daily <1 year. Sodium ironedetate 190 mg = 27.5 mg iron
Sodium nitrite	i.v. (slow)	10 mg/kg	Give as 3% solution over 3 min					Follow by 250 mg/kg sodium thiosulfate over 10 min

Table 38.3 *Cont'd*

Drug	Route	Single dose/kg	Single dose for different age groups (unless stated otherwise)				Times daily	Comments
			>1 month <1 year	1–4 years	5–12 years	>12 years		
Sodium picosulfate	Oral	–		2.5 mg	2.5–5 mg	5–10 mg	1	Night-time dose. Active in 10–14 h
Sodium salicylate	Oral	12.5–17.5 mg/kg	Risk of Reye's syndrome; avoid in children <12 years unless specifically indicated, e.g. juvenile chronic arthritis			500 mg–2 g	3–4	Take with food; therapeutic plasma concentration 125–300 mg/l
Sodium stibogluconate	i.m., i.v.	10 mg/kg	10 mg/kg	100–150 mg	150–400 mg	400–600 mg	1	Treat visceral leishmaniasis for 30 days and cutaneous leishmaniasis for 10 days
Sodium thiosulfate	i.v. (slow)	250 mg/kg	Dose based on bodyweight at all ages					Given over 10 min
Sodium valproate	Oral i.v. (slow)	6–12.5 mg/kg	6–12 mg/kg	60–200 mg	100–400 mg	200–700 mg	3	Start with 6–7 mg/kg and increase as necessary
Somatropin	i.m., s.c.	0.5–0.7 unit/kg weekly divided into 2 or 3 doses (i.m.) or 6–7 doses (s.c.)						Dose may need to be increased at puberty
Spironolactone	Oral	1–1.5 mg/kg	1–1.5 mg/kg	12.5–25 mg	12.5–50 mg	50–100 mg	2	Dose may be doubled and given once a day. Carcinogenic in rodents
Stanozolol	Oral		–	2.5 mg	2.5–5 mg	2.5–10 mg	1	Hereditary angioedema. Reduce to lowest effective maintenance dose
Streptokinase	i.v.	Loading dose: 2500–4000 µ/kg by infusion over 25 min Maintenance: 500–1000 µ/kg/h by continuous infusion						Strict observation essential. Monitor fibrinogen levels frequently
Streptomycin*	i.m.	15 mg/kg	50–150 mg	150–250 mg	250–500 mg	500 mg	2	Maximum total daily dose 1 g
Sulfadiazine	i.v. (slow)	25 mg/kg	75–250 mg	250–400 mg	400 mg–1 g	1 g	4	Initial dose = 50 mg/kg. For i.v. injection or infusion dilute to 5% or less. After 2 days change to oral route
	Oral	37.5 mg/kg	Dose based on bodyweight at all ages				4	
Sulfadimidine	Oral i.v. (slow) i.m. (deep)	25 mg/kg	25 mg/kg	0.25–0.5 g	0.75–1 g	1–1.5 g	4	Initial dose = 50 mg/kg
Sulfasalazine	Oral	10–15 mg/kg for acute attack; maintenance: 5–7.5 mg/kg					4	
Suxamethonium	i.v.	1–1.5 mg/kg initially then 1/3 of initial dose						
Synacthen – see tetracosactrin								
Talampicillin	Oral	7 mg/kg	7 mg/kg	62.5–125 mg	125–250 mg	250 mg	3	Dose may be doubled in severe infections
Teicoplanin*	i.v., i.m.	10 mg/kg loading doses given 12-hourly × 3 6–10 mg/kg maintenance at all ages					1	Higher doses used in cystic fibrosis
Temazepam	Oral	0.5–1 mg/kg	Premedication dose for all ages					Administer 1 h preoperatively. Controlled drug in UK
Terbutaline	Inhalation (aerosol)	–	–	250 µg	250–500 µg	250–500 µg	4	
	Inhalation (powder)	–	–	500 µg	500 µg	500 µg	4	
	Inhalation (nebulizer)	–	–	2–3 mg	3–5 mg	5–10 mg	2–6	
	Oral	–	–	0.75 mg	0.75–2.5 mg	2.5–5 mg	3	
	s.c., i.m. i.v. (slow)	0.01 mg/kg	–	0.1–0.15 mg	0.15–0.3 mg	0.25–0.5 mg	4	
Terfenadine	Oral	–	–	–	30 mg	60 mg	2	Risk of cardiac arrhythmias if prescribed with erythromycin, clarithromycin and some oral antifungals. Also, avoid combination with other arrhythmogenic drugs, e.g. phenothiazines, antidepressants

Table 38.3 *Cont'd*

Drug	Route	Single dose/kg	Single dose for different age groups (unless stated otherwise)				Times daily	Comments
			>1 month <1 year	1–4 years	5–12 years	>12 years		
Tetrachlorethylene	Oral	0.1 ml/kg	–	–	1.5–5 ml	2.5–5 ml	Single dose	Maximum dose 5 ml. Avoid in young children
Tetracosactrin	i.m., i.v.		36 µg/kg	250 µg	250 µg	250 µg	Single dose	Dose for short ACTH stimulation test
Tetracosactrin zinc	i.m.		0.25 mg	0.25–0.5 mg	0.25–1 mg	0.5–1 mg		Initially given daily then every 2–8 days
Tetracycline*	Oral		–	–	–	250–500 mg	4	Contraindicated under 12 years
	i.v. infusion		–	–	–	250–500 mg	2	Maximum concentration for i.v. infusion 0.5%
1% drops	Topical (eye)							
1% ointment	Topical (eye, ear)							
Theophylline Sustained release	Oral	10–12 mg/kg	–	100–180 mg	125–250 mg	250–500 mg	2	Maintain plasma concentration of 10–20 mg/l
Conventional preps (tabs or liquid)	Oral	3–5 mg/kg	3–4 mg/kg	5 mg/kg	4–5 mg/kg	4 mg/kg	3–4	Give three times a day up to 6 months and above 16 years
Thiabendazole	Oral	25 mg/kg	25 mg/kg	250–500 mg	500 mg–1 g	1–1.5 g	2	Take with food. Tablets should be chewed before swallowing
Thiamin	Oral, i.m.		5 mg	10 mg	20 mg	25 mg	1	Dose increased 10-fold in severe deficiency
Thiopentone	i.v.	2–7 mg/kg	Dose based on bodyweight at all ages				Single dose	
Thioridazine	Oral	0.5–2 mg/kg	0.5 mg/kg	5–12.5 mg	25–75 mg	75–150 mg	2	
Thyroxine	Oral	–	6–8 µg/kg	5 µg/kg	4 µg/kg	3 µg/kg	1	Adjust dose according to response
Ticarcillin	i.m., i.v.	50–75 mg/kg	0.25–0.75 g	0.5–1 g	0.75–3 g	2–4 g	4	Use the higher dose in CF
Ticarcillin and clavulanic acid	i.v. infusion	75 mg/kg	0.25–0.75 g	0.75–1 g	1–3 g	3 g	4	Dose given in terms of ticarcillin
Tinidazole	Oral	50–75 mg/kg	0.2–0.75 g	0.5–1 g	0.75–2 g	1–2 g	1	Intestinal amebiasis: treat for 3 days. Hepatic amebiasis: treat for 5 days
Tioconazole 28% solution	Topical (nails)						2	Treat for up to 6–12 months
Tobramycin*	i.v., i.m.	2–2.5 mg/kg	Dose based on bodyweight at all ages				3	Maintain plasma concentrations at 6–10 mg/l (peak) and <2 mg/l (trough)
Tocopheryl acetate	Oral	1–5 mg/kg	25 mg	50 mg	50–100 mg	100 mg	1	Dose used in cystic fibrosis
Tolmetin	Oral	5–10 mg/kg	–	50–150 mg	75–400 mg	400 mg	3	Not recommended under 2 years
Tolnaftate 1% cream	Topical (skin)						2	
Tramadol*	Oral i.v. i.m.		Not yet licensed in the UK for children <12 years but single doses 1–2.5 mg/kg have been used				Repeated 4- to 8 hourly as required	
Tranexamic acid	Oral	25 mg/kg	0.1–0.25 g	0.25–0.5 g	0.25–1 g	1–1.5 g	2–3	
	i.v. (slow)	10 mg/kg	10 mg/kg	0.1–0.15 g	0.15–0.5 g	0.5–1 g	3	
Triamcinolone acetonide 0.1% cream and ointment	Topical (skin)	Apply sparingly for short periods					2–4	Potent topical corticosteroid
Triamterene	Oral	1–2 mg/kg	5–20 mg	10–30 mg	25–75 mg	50–100 mg	2	

Table 38.3   *Cont'd*

Drug	Route	Single dose/kg	Single dose for different age groups (unless stated otherwise)				Times daily	Comments
			>1 month <1 year	1–4 years	5–12 years	>12 years		
Tribavirin	Inhalation	A solution containing 20 mg/ml is administered by aerosol inhalation or nebulization for 12–18 h per day for 3–7 days						
Triclofos	Oral	–	0.1–0.25 g	0.25–0.5 g	0.5–1 g	1 g	Single dose	Hypnotic dose stated
Trifluoperazine	Oral	20–50 μg/kg	–	0.25 mg	0.25–1 mg	1–2 mg	4	
	i.m.	25 μg/kg	Dose based on bodyweight at all ages					
Triiodothyronine – see liothyronine								
Trimeprazine Pruritus	Oral	0.25 mg/kg	0.25 mg/kg	2.5 mg	5 mg	10 mg	3	
Premedication	Oral	2–4 mg/kg	Dose based on bodyweight at all ages				Single dose	
Trimethoprim	Oral	4 mg/kg	25–50 mg	50 mg	100–150 mg	200 mg	2	
	i.v. (slow)	3 mg/kg	Dose based on bodyweight < 12 years			150–250 mg	2–3	
Triprolidine	Oral	–	1 mg	2 mg	2–3 mg	2.5–5 mg	3	
Trisodium edetate	i.v. infusion	Up to 60 mg/kg	Dose based on bodyweight at all ages				Single dose	
Tropicamide 0.5% and 1% drops	Topical (eye)							
Tubocurarine	i.v.	0.3–0.5 mg/kg	Dose based on bodyweight at all ages					Initial dose stated. Supplementary doses of 0.06–0.1 mg/kg may be administered
Undecenoates	Topical (skin)	Creams, ointments and dusting powders available						
Vancomycin*	i.v. infusion	15 mg/kg	15 mg/kg	150–250 mg	250–600 mg	600 mg	3	Infuse over 60 min. Maintain plasma concentrations at 18–26 mg/l (peak) and 5–10 mg/l (trough)
	Oral	5 mg/kg	5 mg/kg	50–75 mg	75–200 mg	250 mg	4	Not absorbed following oral administrations
Verapamil	Oral	2–3 mg/kg	10–20 mg	20–40 mg	40–80 mg	80–120 mg	2–3	
	i.v.	0.1–0.2 mg/kg	0.75–2 mg	2–3 mg	2.5–5 mg	5 mg	Single dose	
Vigabatrin*	Oral	20–50 mg/kg	–	0.25–0.5 g	0.5–1 g	1–2 g	2	Add-on therapy. Low initial dose, then titrate. Monitor neurological function
Vitamin A	Oral							Physiological requirement 1500–5000 units according to age
Vitamin B group		See thiamin (B$_1$), Riboflavin (B$_2$), pryridoxine (B$_6$) and hydroxocobalamin (B$_{12}$)						
Vitamin C – see ascorbic acid								
Vitamin D – see calciferol								
Vitamin E – see tocopheryl acetate								
Vitamin K – see phytomenadione								
Warfarin	Oral	0.1–0.2 mg/kg for maintenance. Loading dose 0.2–0.6 mg/kg					1	Adjust dose according to prothrombin time
Whitfield's ointment	Topical (skin)						2	Contains 6% benzoic acid and 3% salicylic acid
Xylometazoline 0.05% and 0.1% drops	Topical (nose)						1–2	
Zidovudine*	Oral	150–180 mg/m^2. Dose based on surface area at all ages					4	
Zinc sulfate 0.25% drops	Topical (eye)							

This table should be used in conjunction with the section on pp. 1953–1955, 1980.
* Indicates that caution is required even in the presence of mild renal impairment (GFR: 20–50 ml/min per 1.73 m^2, plasma creatinine: 150–300 μmol/l). Drug dosage may need to be reduced in the presence of hepatic disease and in the critically ill patient in whom hepatic and renal function may be impaired.

Table 38.4

Age	Ideal bodyweight		Height		Body surface (m²)	Percentage of adult dose
	kg	lb	cm	in		
Newborn*	3.4	7.5	50	20	0.23	12.5
1 month*	4.2	9	55	22	0.26	14.5
3 months*	5.6	12	59	23	0.32	18
6 months	7.7	17	67	26	0.40	22
1 year	10	22	76	30	0.47	25
3 years	14	31	94	37	0.62	33
5 years	18	40	108	42	0.73	40
7 years	23	51	120	47	0.88	50
12 years	37	81	148	58	1.25	75
Adult						
Male	68	150	173	68	1.8	100
Female	56	123	163	64	1.6	100

* The figures relate to full-term and not preterm infants.

REFERENCES AND BIBLIOGRAPHY

British National Formulary September 1996 British Medical Association and Royal Pharmaceutical Society of Great Britain, London

Data Sheet Compendium 1996–1997 Association of the British Pharmaceutical Industry, London

McCracken G H, Nelson J D 1983 Antimicrobial therapy for newborns, 2nd edn. Grune & Stratton, New York

Roberton N R C 1992 Textbook of neonatology. Churchill Livingstone, Edinburgh

Rylance G 1987 Drugs for for children. World Health Organization, Geneva

Yaffe S J 1992 Pediatric pharmacology. Grune & Stratton, New York

Index

A985G mutation, medium chain acyl-CoA dehydrogenase deficiency, 1129
'ABC' approaches
 behavioral psychotherapy, 1749
 resuscitation, **522–524**
Abdomen
 actinomycosis, 1473
 birth trauma, 121
 circumference, fetus, 82, 115
 computed tomography, 1906
 diagnostic radiation doses, 1895 (Table)
 distension
  history taking, 17
  neonate, 211 (Table)
 examination, **32–33**
 germ cell tumors, 922
 injuries, **1811–1812**
 imaging, 1907
 masses, leukemias, 871
 neuroblastoma, 910, 911
 non-accidental injury, 1869
 paracentesis, **1845**
 shaking injury, 701
 small noncleaved lymphomas, 907
 tuberculosis, **1345**
 X-rays
  erect and supine, 433–434
  intestinal obstruction, 210
  necrotizing enterocolitis, **211,** 282
  teratoma, 291 (Table)
  with ultrasonography, urinary tract infections, 952
Abdominal aorta, fetal blood flow, 115
Abdominal epilepsy, 685
Abdominal migraine, 461, 717, 718
Abdominal pain
 Henoch–Schönlein purpura, 1609
 histoplasmosis, 1476
 history taking, 17
 Kawasaki disease, 1479
 measles, 1354
 nephroblastoma, 913
 nephrotic syndrome, 969
 recurrent, **460–461**
Abdominal reflexes, 35, 36 (Table)
Abdominal thrusts, resuscitation, 522
Abdominal wall, anomalies, 1778–1781
Abduction contracture of hip, congenital, **1552**
Aberrant innominate artery, 573
Abetalipoproteinemia, **446,** 1150 (Table), **1152–1153**
 dietary management, 1214 (Table)
 vs Friedreich's ataxia, 765
 hemolysis, 864
 neurology, **767,** 790 (Table)
 vitamin E deficiency, 1197–1198
Abidec, preterm supplements, 154
Abiotrophy, 1666
Abnormal illness behavior, 1741
ABO blood groups

codominance, 66
 hemolytic disease of the newborn, 216–217, 231, **233–234**
 protection against rhesus disease, 232
Abortion, *see also* Termination of pregnancy
 definition, 94
 threatened, 80, 88
 toxoplasmosis, 1464
Abortive poliomyelitis, 1379
Abrasions, non-accidental injury, 1868
Abscesses, *see also* Cold abscesses; *specific sites*
 amebic, 1468
  aspiration, 1469, 1845
 Bartholin's, 1425, 1428
 BCG vaccination, 1339
 Brodie's, 1590
 cerebellum, 762
 cervical lymphadenitis, **1784**
 cystic fibrosis, 556
 environmental mycobacteria, 1349
 ethmoiditis, 1685
 hyperIgE syndrome, 1261
 liver, *see* Liver, abscesses
 lungs, 569
 vs mumps, 1372
 pelvis, FUO investigations, 1283 (Table)
 peritonsillar, 1687
 retropharyngeal, 563
  tuberculosis, 1592
 ultrasonography, 1905
Absence seizures, 675, *see also* Childhood absence epilepsy
Absent atrioventricular connection, 597
Absent pulmonary valve, pulmonary regurgitation, 609
Absorbents, diarrheal diseases, 1296
Absorption, *see also* Intestinal absorption
 colon, 455
 steroids, napkin area, 1066
Absorptive hypercalciuria, 1056
ABVD regimen, Hodgkin's disease, 910
Acanthamoeba culbertsoni, 1467, **1469–1470**
Acanthamoeba keratitis, 1470
Acanthocephala, **1513**
Acanthocytosis, abetalipoproteinemia, 1152
Acardiac twins, umbilical cord ligation, 115
Acatalasia, 1174
Accelerated allergic reactions, penicillin, 1702
Accelerated BCG reaction, 1339
Accelerated starvation, 1083
Acceleration injuries, 705
Accessory auricles, 1679
Accessory muscles of respiration, 512
Accidental hemorrhage, *see* Placenta, abruption
Accidental hypothermia, 149–150
Accidental poisoning, **1705–1708**
Accident and emergency departments, **1805–1808**

attendance rates, 1712
 injuries treated, 11 (Table)
 major trauma, 1810–1811
 and negligence, 1879
 referral rates from general practice, 9
 sudden infant death syndrome, 1722–1723
Accident proneness, 1712
Accidents, **1711–1719**
 age-specific mortality, 7
 head injuries, **704–709**
 medical, 1878
 mortality trends, 8
 prevention, 339–340, **1803–1804**
Accommodation, intellectual, 1729
Accommodation of children, **1857–1858,** **1875,** 1876
Acellular vaccine, pertussis, **345,** 1318
Aceruloplasminemia, 1146
Acetaminophen, *see* Paracetamol
Acetazolamide
 administration, 1958 (Table)
 benign intracranial hypertension, 665
 familial paroxysmal ataxias, 764
 hydrocephalus, 665
  posthemorrhagic, 252
Acetoacetyl-CoA thiolase deficiencies, 1130
Acetone poisoning, 1709
N-Acetyl aspartate, proton magnetic resonance spectroscopy, birth asphyxia, 128
Acetyl-CoA, glucose-6-phosphatase deficiency, 1137
Acetyl-CoA:*N*-acetyl-glucosaminide *N*-acetyl transferase deficiency, 1160
N-Acetylcysteine, 1710
 administration, 1958 (Table)
Acetylcysteine, bronchoalveolar lavage, alveolar proteinosis, 578
N-Acetyl-galactosamine-6-sulfatase deficiency, 1160
N-Acetyl-galactosaminidase, absence, 1168
α-*N*-Acetylgalactosaminidase deficiency, 780 (Table)
N-Acetylglucoaminyltransferase II deficiency, 1175
N-Acetyl-glucosamine-1-phosphotransferase deficiency, 1169
N-Acetyl-glucosamine-6-Sulfate sulfatase deficiency, 1160
N-Acetyl-D-glucosaminidase deficiency, 1160
N-Acetylglutamate synthetase deficiency, 1110
β-n-Acetylhexosaminidase, cerebrospinal fluid, normal values, 1933 (Table)
Achalasia, **429**
Achlorhydria, vitamin B$_{12}$ deficiency, 853 (Table)
Achondrogenesis, 1570–1571
 type II, inheritance, 1566 (Table)
Achondroplasia, 370–371, **1572–1575**

airway obstruction in sleep, 531
 homozygous, 1571
 inheritance, 1566 (Table)
Achromatopsia, 271
Acid–base disturbances, **415–422**
 clinical judgement, 421–422
 respiratory disorders, **504–505**
Acid esterase deficiency, *see* Wolman's disease
Acid hydrolases, lysosomes, 1156
Acid infusion, esophagus, asthma, 542
Acidity, urine
 neonate, 257
 normal values, 1933 (Table)
Acid lipase deficiency, *see* Wolman's disease
Acid maltase deficiency, *see* Pompe's disease
Acidosis, *see also* Metabolic acidosis
 acute diarrhea, 453, 1293–1294, 1296
 acute renal failure, 259, 975
 fetus, 116, 125, 133
 ionized calcium, 299
 malaria, 1452–1453
 neonatal jaundice, 218
 neonatal kidney function, 108
 osteomyelitis, 283
 potassium levels, 411
 respiratory distress syndrome, 177
  correction, 179
 rewarming, 150
 ventilation, 161
 vomiting, 212
Acid phosphatase
 and Gaucher disease, 1166
 normal values, 1922 (Table)
Acids, 415, *see also* Gastric acid
 household, poisoning, 1710
Acini
 liver, 470
 lung, 494–495
Ackee fruit, 1117
Acne, infantile, 1646
Aconitase deficiency, with succinate dehydrogenase deficiency, 1126
Acoustic blink reflex, 36 (Table)
Acquired central deafness, *see* Auditory agnosia
Acquired hypogammaglobulinemia, 1256
Acquired pneumonia, neonate, 280
Acridine orange, central venous line sepsis, 1224
Acrocentric chromosomes, 53
Acrocephalopolysyndactyly, 1561
Acrocephalosyndactyly, **1560–1561**
Acrocephaly, 1560
Acrodermatitis chronica atrophicans, 1313
Acrodermatitis enteropathica, 444, 447, 1147, 1201, **1627**
 candidiasis, 1470–1471
Acrodynia, *see* Mercury poisoning
Acromelia, 76 (Table)
Acropustulosis, 1628, 1629
 of infancy, **1645–1646**
Acrylic, atopic eczema, 1642

ACTH, **1038**, *see also* Synacthen screening test
Addison's disease, tests, 1068
administration, 1964 (Table)
growth, 1068
on adrenal cortex, **1038**, 1059–1060
at birth, 109
blood sampling, 297
congenital adrenal hyperplasia, 986
deficiency, 1041
excess, 1041
feedback on, 1059
fetus, 1003
hereditary unresponsiveness, 1068
for infantile spasms, 687
normal values, 1922 (Table)
Actin
Duchenne muscular dystrophy, 729
small round cell tumors, 912 (Table)
Actinic prurigo, 1645
Actinobacillus muris, **1322**
Actinomycin, toxic effects, 894 (Table), 897
Actinomycosis, 570, 1471 (Table), **1473**
Action spectrum studies, idiopathic photosensitivity eruptions, 1645
Activated charcoal, **1706–1707**, 1815
administration, 1962 (Table)
Activated protein C resistance, 882
Activator deficiency (AB variant GM₂-gangliosidosis), 1163–1164
Active hydrocephalus, 658
clinical features, 659–660
very low birth weight, outcome, 171–172
Active immunity, 341
Active surveillance, African trypanosomiasis, 1457
Activin, 1024
Actual bicarbonate, 419
Acuity card procedure, 269–270
Acute bronchitis, postneonatal mortality, 5 (Table)
Acute carditis, **628–629, 1597–1598**
Acute catarrhal conjunctivitis, 1663
Acute disseminated encephalomyelitis, 1361
Acute febrile pharyngitis, 1370
Acute glomerulonephritis, **961–962**
Acute hemorrhagic conjunctivitis, **1385**
Acute herpetic gingivostomatitis, 1363, 1364–1365, **1438**
Acute herpetic keratoconjunctivitis, 1364
Acute infantile hemiplegia, cystathione synthase deficiency, 1108
Acute infective diarrhea, **451–454**
Acute intermittent porphyria, 790 (Table), 1100, **1143**
Acute leukemias, 868
Acute lymphoblastic leukemia, 868
immune deficiency, 889
obesity, 1190
prognostic factors, 872
relapse management, 873–874
survival rates, 898 (Table)
treatment, **872–874**
trisomy 21, 887
tumor markers, 912 (Table)
Acute metabolic disorders, neonate, 304–307
Acute monocytic leukemia, 927
Acute myeloblastic leukemia, 868–869
management, **874**
Acute myeloid leukemia, secondary, epipodophyllotoxins, 898
Acute myocarditis, Coxsackie B viruses, 1382
Acute nephritic syndrome, 961
Acute nonlymphoblastic leukemia, survival rates, 887 (Table)
Acute onset blindness, **1658**
Acute otitis media, **1680**
Acute parainfectious polyneuritis, 725–726
Acute phase reactants, 1234

neonatal sepsis, 277
Acute porphyrias, **1143**
Acute purulent conjunctivitis, 1663
Acute pyelonephritis, 950
Acute renal failure, **973–979**
bee stings, 1524
after cardiac surgery, 1822
management, **1823–1824**
neonate, **257–259**, 974
snake bite, 1523
urinary tract infections, 950
Acute respiratory disease (ARD), 1370
Acute respiratory illness programs, 1889
World Health Organization, 490, 493, 567
Acute retinopathy of prematurity, 266
Acute rheumatic fever, *see* Rheumatic fever
Acute severe asthma, **547–549**
falciparum malaria, 1453
neonate, 258
Acute tubular obstruction, ultrasonography, 1910
Acyanotic congenital heart disease
with arteriovenous shunt, **599–613**
without arteriovenous shunt, **606–613**
Acyclovir
administration, 1955 (Table), 1958–1959 (Table)
bone marrow transplant recipients, 875
CNS infections, 696
drug resistance, 1530
herpes simplex, 287, 1365, **1440**
pregnancy, 1441–1442
varicella in cancer treatment, 895
viral pneumonia, 535
Acylcarnitines, 1129
fatty acid disorders, 1129
plasma, 297
Acyl-CoA dehydrogenases, 1128
deficiency, 297
Acyl-CoA derivatives, N-acetylglutamate synthetase deficiency, 1110
Acyl-CoA oxidase deficient adrenoleukodystrophy, 786 (Table), 1174
ADA, *see* Adenosine deaminase deficiency
Adaptive development, *see* Cognitive development
Added sounds, respiratory, 512
Adder bites, **1520–1521**
Addiction, fear of, 928
Addiphos, 1222 (Table), 1223 (Table)
Addisonian crisis, 1068
treatment, 415
Addison's disease, **1067**
adrenoleukodystrophy, 786 (Table), 1174
anemia, 865
vs anorexia nervosa, 1023
eye, 1674
mucocutaneous candidiasis, 1251
Addition, drug combinations, 1528
Additrace, 1221
Adelaide coma scale, 695
Adenine phosphoribosyl transferase deficiency, 1141
Adenohypophysis, *see also* Anterior pituitary hormones
diseases, **1041–1043**
Adenoidectomy, 1686
deafness, 817
secretory otitis media, 1682
Adenoiditis, 1686
Adenoids
hypertrophy, 1685–1686
noisy breathing, 508–509
obstructive sleep apnea, 531
secretory otitis media, 1681
speech, 810
Adenomas, thyroid gland, 1052
Adenoma sebaceum, *see also* Angiofibromas

tuberous sclerosis, 801
Adenomatous polyposis, familial, 448
liver tumors, 924
Adenomatous polyps, colon, 448
Adenosine, for paroxysmal supraventricular tachycardia, 627
Adenosine deaminase deficiency, 1141, 1242 (Table), **1250–1251**
enzyme replacement, 1270
gene therapy, 1270
Adenosine diphosphate, *see* ADP
Adenosine monophosphate, *see* Cyclic adenosine monophosphate
Adenosine triphosphate, *see* ATP
Adenoviruses, **1370–1371**
bronchiolitis, 564, 576
eye, **1384–1385**
pharyngitis, 560
pneumonia, 568, 1370
viral diarrhea of infancy, 1384
Adenylate cyclase, steroidogenesis, 1059
Adenylate kinase deficiency, 1141
Adenylosuccinase deficiency, 1141
Adhesins, *Haemophilus influenzae*, 1307
Adhesion molecules, 1234–1235
neonate, 275
sepsis, 276 (Table)
Adhesive tape method, *see* Cellulose tape method
Adipose tissue, *see* Body fat
Adjustable sutures, squint, 1660
Adjustment, third world economics, 1885
Adjustment disorder, **1741**
Adjuvants, vaccines, 341, 342
Adolescence
age range for, 17
asthma, 540–541, 550
cancer, 897
Chlamydia trachomatis, 1430, **1432**
contraception, 994–995
death, 928
diabetes mellitus, 1080
disease incidence, 13
epilepsy, 691
essential hypertension, 636
girls, improving status, 1886 (Table)
goiter, 1048
gonorrhea, **1425**
growth, 352, **357–362**
gynecology, **991–993**
and medical negligence, **1880**
neural tube defect, 657
nutrition, 1189
diabetes mellitus, 1210
preventive medicine, 340–341
psychiatric disorder, **1749–1764**, *see also* Residential treatment
assessment, **1751–1752**
psychiatric referral, **1752–1753**
recurrent patellar dislocation, 1553
scoliosis, 1558
sexual abuse, 1752, **1759–1760**, 1870
smoking, 493, 1762
social development, 385
Adolescent coxa vara, **1596**
Adolescent macular degeneration, 1666
Adoption, **1858–1860**
Adoption Agencies, 1858
Adoption Orders, 1859
Adoptive lactation, 328
ADP, platelet aggregation, 227
ADP storage pool disease, 229
Adrenal cortex, **1059–1069**
ACTH on, **1038**, 1059–1060
androgens, 1024
and corticosteroid therapy, 546
hypofunction, **1067–1069**
precocious pseudopuberty, 1027
Adrenal gland, **1059–1069**, *see also* Adrenal medulla
carcinoma, 1065
control of labor, 1005
death from asthma, 537
dexamethasone suppression test,

1938 (Table)
fetus, 1003
hemorrhage
birth trauma, 121
neonate, 224
imaging, 1912
neuroblastoma, 911
Adrenal hypercorticism, **1065–1067**
Adrenaline (epinephrine), 1069
administration, 1959 (Table)
neonate, 1956 (Table)
aerosol, 1524
for anaphylaxis, 1702
antivenom treatment, 1523
cardiac stimulation, 135
emergency supply, 134 (Table)
hypersensitivity reactions, 1306
intensive care, 1820
on lung maturation, 176
nebulized, croup, 563
normal values, 1924 (Table)
urine, 1930 (Table)
resuscitation, **525–526**
doses, 527 (Fig.)
Adrenal medulla, **1069**
function in SGA baby, 137
neural crest cells, 641
Adrenarche, 377, 1003, **1060–1061**
α-Adrenergic agonists, 1748 (Table)
neurogenic bladder, 657
β-Adrenergic agonists
on lung maturation, 176
tocolysis, 116
transient hyperinsulinemia, 295
β2-Adrenergic agonists, *see* Bronchodilators
Adrenergic receptors
asthma, 538
bronchi, 497
types, 1820
Adrenocorticotrophic hormone, *see* ACTH
Adrenoleukodystrophy, 72 (Table), 786 (Table), **1068, 1174**
neonatal, 308, 785 (Table), 1173
Adrenomedullary unresponsiveness, 1069
Adrenomyeloneuropathy, 1174
Adriamycin, toxic effects, 894 (Table)
Adult developmental disability, **842**
Adult GM₁-gangliosidosis, 1163
Adult height
achondroplasia, 1575
prediction, 362–363
Adult hemoglobin, 849
Adult polycystic kidney disease, *see* Autosomal dominant polycystic kidney disease
Adult respiratory distress syndrome, **578–579**
Adults, *vs* children, cholera, 1304
Adversive seizures, 673
Advisory committees, infant research, 103
Adynamic ileus, potassium depletion, 412
AEC syndrome, 1626 (Table)
Aedes aegypti, arboviruses, 1389
Aerosol dispensers, 1954
adrenaline, 1702
Affective disorders, **1742**
Afibrinogenemia, 230, 881, *see also* Fibrinogen, deficiency
Afipia spp., 1520
Africa
demography, 2 (Table)
HIV vertical transmission, 288
sub-Saharan, 1883
yaws, 1417, 1419
African green monkeys, Marburg virus disease, 1388, 1389
African trypanosomiasis, **1453–1458**
control, 1457–1458
Afterload, cardiac, 1819
Agammaglobulinemia, *see also* Bruton's agammaglobulinemia; X-linked agammaglobulinemia
gastrointestinal disease, 444

Aganglionosis, Hirschsprung's disease, 1777
Age groups
    disease incidence, **9–13**
    drug dosages, 1980 (Table)
    mortality rates, 3, **5–7**
Age standards, pubertal development, 360–361
Aggressive psychopathy, physical abuse risk, 1866
Agnosia
    auditory, 807, 815
    finger agnosia, 669
    verbal, 807
    visual, 822
Agonadism, 1010
Agranulocytosis, antithyroid drugs, 1051
Aicardi-Goutieres syndrome, 797 (Table)
Aicardi's syndrome, 245, 284 (Table), **647,** 830 (Table)
AIDS, **1392–1398,** see also HIV infection
    gastrointestinal tract, 444, 1394
    risk-taking behavior, 1763
Air
    neonatal resuscitation, 133
    passage to bowel, 108
Airborne infections, 1281
Air bronchogram, respiratory distress syndrome, 178
Air embolism (pneumatosis arterialis), neonate, 190
Air enema, intussusception, 1786, 1903–1904
Air entry, endotracheal intubation, 1842
Air leaks, see also Surgical emphysema
    pulmonary, see also Pneumothorax
    neonate, **187–190, 576–577**
Air mode, incubators, 148
Air pollution, **492–493,** 542, see also Smoke
Air pressure reduction, intussusception, 1786, 1903–1904
Air temperature, incubator settings, 148
Air transport, medical, 1805
Airway (Guedel), 524
Airways
    cervical spine injuries, **1809**
    closure, 501, see also Dynamic airway narrowing
    conductance, 498
    diameter vs age, 496 (Table)
    function, **498–501**
    obstruction, **499–501,** 522, see also Epiglottitis; Upper airway obstruction
        anaphylaxis, 1702
        congenital abnormalities, 1769
        imposed, **1871,** see also Suffocation
        tonsillitis, 1687
    resistance, 496–497, **498**
    responsiveness, 499, see also Bronchi, provocation tests
        allergens, 542
        asthma, 536–537, **537–538,** 543–544
        cystic fibrosis, 554
        resuscitation, **522, 524, 1807,** 1810
Akathisia, 772
ALA dehydratase porphyria, 1142 (Table)
ALA (δ-aminolevulinic acid), 1142
Alae nasi, 76 (Table)
Alagille syndrome, 221, **474,** 1145
Aland Island disease, 1108
Alanine
    elevation, 1125
    fasting plasma levels, 1103
    gluconeogenesis, SGA baby, 137
    load test, 1938 (Table)
β-Alanine, 1115
Alanine aminotransferase, 472 (Table)
    inborn errors of metabolism, 306
    normal values, 1922 (Table)
ALA synthetase, 1142
Albendazole
    ascariasis, 1485

enterobiasis, 1488
helminthoma, 1494
hookworm, 1490
hydatid disease, 1506
onchocerciasis, 1497
Albers–Schönberg disease, see Osteopetrosis
Albinism, 1106–1107
    delayed visual maturation, 272
    Griscelli syndrome, 1254
    Hermansky–Pudlack syndrome, 879
    oculocutaneous, 72 (Table), **1107, 1629, 1673**
        frequency, 47 (Table)
    with sensorineural deafness, 1107–1108
Albright's hereditary osteodystrophy, 1057
Albright's solution, 415
Albumin
    bilirubin binding, 214
    chronic liver disease, 480
    congenital analbuminemia, 1175
    cystic fibrosis, 1208
    failure to thrive, 467
    fetus, 471
    levels
        liver disease, 472 (Table)
        nutrition, 1188
        preterm infant, 142
    for neonatal jaundice, 219
    nephrotic syndrome, infusions, 970
    osmotic pressure, 407
    protein-losing enteropathy, 443
    urine, 966
Albumin colloid, scintigraphy, 1907
Alcohol
    abuse, 1762
        adolescents, 341
    congenital heart disease, 596
    consumption, 15 (Table)
    epilepsy, 690
    on fetus and neonate, 91 (Table)
    hypoglycemia, 1082, 1710
    muscle injection, 759
    neoplasms, 890
    preconceptual care, 80
    pregnancy, 338, 641, 642
    solution, central venous line occlusion, 1225
    thiamin deficiency, 1198
Aldolase A defect, 1135
Aldolases, see also Fructose-1-phosphate aldolase deficiency
    normal values, 1922 (Table)
Aldosterone, 410
    heart failure, 599
    isolated biosynthesis defects, 1068–1069
    neonates, 143
    normal values, 1922 (Table)
        urine, 1932 (Table)
    plasma, 1051
    salt wasting, 1006
    renal action, 942
    zona glomerulosa, 1059
Alertness, neonate, 238 (Fig.)
Alexander's leukodystrophy and spongiform degeneration, 797 (Table)
Alexia, 821
Alfacalcidol
    administration, 1959 (Table)
    for familial hypophosphatemia, 948
Alginate-producing Pseudomonas aeruginosa, cystic fibrosis, 555
Alimentary tract, see also Gastrointestinal tract
    congenital disorders, severely handicapped children affected, 14 (Table)
Alkaline phosphatase, see also Bone alkaline phosphatase
    Crohn's disease, 457
    inborn errors, **1176–1177**
    levels, 472 (Table)

osteopenia of prematurity, 302–303
    normal values, 1922 (Table)
    nutrition, 1188
    osteosarcoma, 917
    syphilis, 1408
    vitamin D deficiency, 1195–1196
Alkalinization, see Urine, alkalinization
Alkalis, poisoning, 1710
Alkalosis
    hypochloremic, 1785
    hypokalemic, **946–947**
    ionized calcium, 299
    potassium levels, 411
    respiratory, 307, 419, 420, 504
    vomiting, 212
Alkaptonuria, 1107
Alkylating agents
    avoiding, 910
    leukemia from, 890
    and radiotherapy, 893
    toxic effects, 894 (Table)
Alkyl DHAP synthase deficiency, 1174
Alleles, 64
Allelic mutations, 1100
Allen's test, modified, 1835
Allergens
    asthma, **541**
        early exposure, 540
    avoidance, **1695–1696**
        time of birth, 1703
    respiratory disorders, 493
    types, **1689–1691**
Allergic bronchopulmonary aspergillosis, **550, 556**
Allergic colitis, 456
Allergic conjunctivitis, **1698–1699**
    antihistamines, 1664, 1675–1676
    simple, 1664
Allergic contact eczema, 1641–1642
Allergic contact urticaria, 1697
Allergic disorders, **1689–1705,** see also Hypersensitivity reactions
    and immunodeficiency, 1248
Allergic keratoconjunctivitis, **1698–1699**
Allergic reactions, 1689, 1703
    reporting, 1692–1693, 1879
Allergic rhinitis, 1684–1685
    vs common cold, 560
Allergic vasculitis, 1640
Allergy, 1689
    and breast-feeding, 327
    IgA deficiency, 1258
Allogeneic bone marrow transplantation, 875
Alloimmune neonatal thrombocytopenic purpura, 228–229, see also Isoimmune thrombocytopenia
Allopurinol
    administration, 1959 (Table)
    for chemotherapy, 897
    on free radical production, 131
    leukemias, 871
    test for ornithine transcarbamylase deficiency, 1110–1111
All-trans retinoic acid, for acute promyelocytic leukemia, 874
Almitrine, 531
Alopecia
    AIDS, 1395
    syphilis, 1406
    tinea, 1637
Alopecia areata, 1640
    vs tinea, 1637
Alper's disease, 736, 797 (Table), 1125, 1127
α1-antitrypsin
    deficiency, **577,** 1100, **1175–1176**
    liver, 473
    fecal protein measurement, 448
α-adrenergic receptor antagonists, neurogenic bladder, 657
α-aminolevulinic acid, normal values, urine, 1930 (Table)

α-fetoprotein
    amniotic fluid, 1937 (Table)
    antenatal care, 80
    causes of elevation, 81 (Table)
    congenital nephrotic syndrome, 972
    Down syndrome, 56
    germ cell tumors, 921, 922
    liver tumors, 924
    normal values, 1925 (Table)
    sacrococcygeal teratoma, 1781
    serum levels, 472 (Table)
α-glucosidases, preterm infant, 151
α-hemolytic streptococci (S. viridans), **1333**
    infective endocarditis, 630
Alphalipoprotein deficiency, familial, 724, 790 (Table), 1150 (Table), 1153
α thalassemia, 72 (Table)
    maternal, 89 (Table)
α-o thalassemia, 226
Alport's syndrome (hereditary nephritis), **965–966,** 1113
    deafness, 1682
    mechanisms, 1567
Alternate-day corticosteroid therapy, 1069
    asthma, 546
    regimes, 1016
Alternating hemiplegia syndrome, 713
Alternating squint, 1652
Alternative therapies, respiratory disorders, 494
Aluminium, parenteral nutrition, 1221 (Table)
Aluminium hydroxide
    and chronic renal failure, 980
    phosphorus deficiency, 1200
Alveolar air equation, 504
Alveolar arch alignment, cleft palate surgery, 1797
Alveolar–arterial oxygen difference, 163, **504**
Alveolar cells, maturation, 176
Alveolar cysts, hydatid disease, 1505
Alveolar hypoventilation, **503–504**
Alveolar macrophages, 532
Alveolar proteinosis, **578**
Alveolar rhabdomyosarcoma, 916
Alveolar ventilation, 160
Alveoli, pulmonary
    development, 175, **495**
    diameter vs age, 496 (Table)
    postnatal lung growth, 177
    rupture, 187
Alzheimer's disease, 797 (Table)
    apoE gene mutations, 1152
    Down syndrome, 55
Amantadine, influenza, 1369, 1530
Amastigotes, 1454 (Fig.)
    Leishmania spp., 1460
    T. cruzi, 1458
Amaurosis, **1657–1658**
Amaurotic family idiocy, 1666
Ambiguous atrioventricular connections, 597
Ambiguous genitalia, **986–987,** 998, 1006
    21-hydroxylase deficiency, 1062
    3β-hydroxysteroid dehydrogenase deficiency, 1064
Ambisome (liposomal amphotericin B), 1463, 1472, 1478
Amblyopia, 1657–1659, **1660–1661**
    hemangiomas, 1619
    testing visual acuity, 395
Ambroxol, 179
Ambulances
    neonates, 156–157
    policy, 1805
Ambulatory electrocardiography, 624
Ambulatory electroencephalography, 677
Ambulatory monitoring, suffocation vs fits, 700
Ambulatory peritoneal dialysis, continuous, 981

Ambulatory pH measurement, esophagus, 427, 429–430
Amebiasis, **1467–1469**
  hepatic, **478**
    abscess aspiration, 1469, 1845
  meningitis, CSF white cells, 1290
Amebic dysentery, 1468
  antibiotic, 454 (Table)
Amegakaryocytic thrombocytopenia, 856
Amelia, 1545
Amenorrhea, 1035
  exercise, 1026
  primary, **989–991**
  secondary, **992–993**
American Academy of Pediatrics, calcium and phosphorus supplements, 304
American cutaneous leishmaniasis, 1461 (Table)
American football sign, 210
American mucocutaneous leishmaniasis, 1461 (Table)
American Society for Clinical Nutrition, recommendations for parenteral nutrition, 1221
American Task Force on Blood Pressure Control in Children, 636, 637
American trypanosomiasis, **1458–1460**
Americas, demography, 2 (Table)
Amidopyrine, neutropenia from, 867
Amiel-Tison system, trunk tone, 240 (Fig.)
Amies' medium, 1423
Amikacin
  administration, 1959 (Table)
  environmental mycobacteria, 1350
  neonate, 279 (Table)
Amiloride
  cystic fibrosis, 558
  for hypokalemic alkalosis syndromes, 947
Amino acid restricted diet, **1119–1120**
Amino acids, see also Branched chain amino acids
  absorption, 207, 446
  brain development, 643
  breast milk, score, 332
  deprivation on insulin-like growth factors, 1023
  excretion promotion, 307
  intestinal absorption, 438
  metabolism disorders, 248, 297, 305 (Table), **1102–1118**
    not causing mental retardation, 1102
  normal values, 1922 (Table)
    urine, 1930 (Table)
  parenteral nutrition, 1220, 1222 (Table)
  plasma levels
    formula feeding, 332
    nutrition, 1188
  requirements, 1120, **1181**
    preterm infant, 157–158
  transport disorders, **1120–1123**
  tubular reabsorption, 943, 1122
  urine, 1103
    testing, 306
ω-Amino acids, metabolism disorders, 1115–1116
Aminoacidurias, 1103, 1121
  generalized, 1122
α-Aminoadipic aciduria, 1113
p-Aminobenzoic acid, urine, cystic fibrosis, 553
γ-Aminobutyric acid, see Gamma-aminobutyric acid
Aminoglycosides
  deafness, 1127
  dosage considerations, 1527
  mechanism, 1527
  not in myasthenia, 728
  Pseudomonas aeruginosa, cystic fibrosis, 557
β-Aminoisobutyric acid, 1115
α-Aminolevulinic acid, normal values, urine, 1930 (Table)
δ-Aminolevulinic acid, 1142

Aminolevulinic dehydratase porphyria, 1143
α-Amino nitrogen, normal values, 1922 (Table)
  cerebrospinal fluid, 1933 (Table)
  urine, 1930 (Table)
Aminophylline, 548
  administration, 1959 (Table)
  apnea attacks, 198 (Table)
  danger of seizures, 547
  hypokalemia, 145
5-Aminosalicylic acid, Crohn's disease, 457
Aminosidine, **1463**
Amiodarone, 626–627
  hypertrophic cardiomyopathy, 634
Amish, Ellis–van Creveld syndrome, 47
Amitriptyline, 1755
  administration, 1959 (Table)
  migraine, 717 (Table)
Ammonia, 472 (Table), see also Hyperammonemia
  normal values, 1922 (Table)
    urine, 1930 (Table)
  Proteus mirabilis, 1320
  renal secretion, 944
Ammoniacal dermatitis, vs monilial napkin rash, 1472
Ammonium chloride, 420 (Table)
  for alkalosis, 421
  renal tubular acidosis test, 944
Amniocentesis, **80–81**
  on airway development, 494
  chromosome preparations from, 50
  cystic fibrosis, 552
  Down syndrome, 56
  hexosaminidases, 1164
  21-hydroxylase deficiency, 1061–1063
  mental retardation prevention, 841
  sialic acid storage diseases, 1169
Amnionitis, prolonged rupture of membranes, pneumonia, 183
Amniotic debris
  aspiration, 186
  swallowing, 210
Amniotic fluid, 253
  normal values, 1937 (Table)
  volumes, 115
    normal, 1937 (Table)
    postterm pregnancy, 83
Amniotomy, 84, 87
Amocarzine, onchocerciasis, 1497
Amodiaquine
  adverse effects, 1448
  malaria treatment, 1452 (Table)
Amoxicillin
  administration, 1955 (Table), 1959 (Table)
  and clavulanic acid, see Clavulanic acid, with amoxicillin
  gonorrhea, 1427 (Table)
  prophylaxis, infective endocarditis, 632 (Table)
  and scarlatiniform rashes, 1332
  Streptococcus pyogenes pharyngitis, 560
  urinary tract infections, 952 (Table)
Amphetamine
  extrapyramidal effects, 771, 772
  overactivity, 841
  tics, 768
Amphotericin B, 1434, 1472, **1477–1478**
  administration, 1955 (Table), 1959 (Table)
  aspergillosis, 536, 1474
  coccidioidomycosis, 1475
  cryptococcosis, 1476
  liposomal, 1463, 1472, 1478, 1959 (Table)
  mechanism, 1530
  neonate, 289
  nephrotoxicity, 1478, 1530
Ampicillin
  administration, 1955 (Table), 1959 (Table)

allergy, 1702
  bacterial meningitis, 1291
  deafness, congenital syphilis, 1415
  Escherichia coli resistance, 951
  gonorrhea, 1427 (Table)
  Listeria monocytogenes, 284
  neonatal pneumonia prevention, 184
  neonate, 279 (Table)
  pyogenic osteitis, 1590
  rashes
    chickenpox, 1361
    infectious mononucleosis, 1366
    scarlatiniform, 1332
Amplified auditory input, see Hearing aids
Amputations (congenital), 1545
Amputations (surgical), osteosarcoma, 919
Amrinone, intensive care, 1820
Amygdala, growth hormone regulation, 1012–1014
Amygdalohippocampectomy, 686
Amylase, 436
  serum measurement, 461
Amyl nitrite, migraine, 716
Amyloid, kidneys, cystic fibrosis, 556
Amyloid A, 1177
Amyloidosis, 966, **1177**
  central nervous system, 794 (Table)
  juvenile chronic arthritis, 1603
  leprosy, 1310
Amyloid precursor gene, Alzheimer's disease, 55
Amylopectin, 436
Amylose, 436
Amyoplasia congenita, 1587
Amyotrophic lateral sclerosis, 721, 726
  dysarthria, 812
Anabolic steroids, see also Androgenic steroids
  for growth disorders, 1020
  for hyperammonemia, 1111
  liver tumors, 890, 924
Anal fissure, 17, 462
  syphilis, 1406
Analgesia, 1830
  fractures in major trauma, **1812**
Analgesic ladder, 1833
Analgesics
  dysmenorrhea, 992
  sickle cell crises, 863
Anal period, 1729 (Table)
Anal reflex, 36 (Table)
Analytic studies, child health, 1851
Anaphase, 47
Anaphylactoid purpura, see Henoch–Schönlein purpura
Anaphylactoid reactions, 1701
Anaphylatoxins, septicemia, 1287
Anaphylaxis, **1701–1702**
  cow's milk protein intolerance, 1699, 1700
  food-provoked exercise-induced, 1697
  insect stings, 1524
Anaplastic astrocytomas, 903
Anaplastic nephroblastoma, 914
Anatomical dead space, 498
Anchovy sauce pus, 1469
Ancylostoma spp., **1488–1490**
  larval disease, 1484 (Table)
Anderson's disease, 789 (Table)
Androgenic steroids, see also Anabolic steroids
  for Addison's disease, 1068
  adrenal, 1059
  adrenal cortex, 1024
  adrenarche, 1060–1061
  for Fanconi's anemia, 854
  on fetus and neonate, 91 (Table)
  genital development, 986
  hereditary angioedema, 1263
  liver tumors, 890
  peripheral metabolism disorders, 1009
  reticularis cells, 1059
Androgen insensitivity syndrome, complete, 991
Androgen receptor defects, 1009

Androstenedione
  normal values, 1923 (Table)
  ovaries, 1024
Anemia, **850–867**
  acute renal failure, 976
  African trypanosomiasis, 1455
  and cerebral microcirculation, 714–715
  chronic renal failure, 865–866, 979, 980
  congenital syphilis, 1412
  copper deficiency, 1201
  epidermolysis bullosa, 1622
  inborn errors of metabolism, 306
  leishmaniasis, 1462
  leukemia, 870
  malaria, 1447–1448, 1449, **1451**
    cerebral, 1450–1451
    management, 1453
  neonate, **223–226**
    organisms, 285 (Table)
  parvovirus B19, 1359
  progressive systemic sclerosis, 1608
  retinopathy, 1675
  schistosomiasis, 1510
  secondary, **865–867**
  toxocariasis, 1485
  typhoid fever, 1325
Anencephalic congenital adrenal hypoplasia, 1067
Anencephaly, 648, 1558
  exomphalos, 1779
  fetal zone, adrenal cortex, 1003
  gestation length, 1005
  growth, 1003
  recurrence risks, 74
Anerobic metabolism, brain, 694, 754
Aneuploidies, 46
  cytogenetic nomenclature, 53
Aneurysms
  cardiac
    Chagas' disease, 1458
    ventricular septum, 600
  cerebral, 709, **710**
    mortality, 711
  Kawasaki disease, 1479
  sinus of Valsalva, 608
  vein of Galen, ultrasonography, 1909 (Fig.)
Angelman syndrome, 59, 60 (Table), 830 (Table), 1022
Angina, anomalous origin of left coronary artery from pulmonary artery, 612
Anginose glandular fever, 1366
Angioblastic tissue, 847
Angioedema, 1639
Angiofibromas, 1686, see also Adenoma sebaceum
  tuberous sclerosis, 1625
Angiography
  atrial septal defect, 602
  atrioventricular septal defect, 604
  cardiac, 593–594
  cerebral, **1909**
    aneurysms, 710
  gastrointestinal hemorrhage, 460
  liver, 1907
  pulmonary, 514
  renal, 972, 973, 1912
  retina, with fluorescein, 1654, 1671
  small intestine, 447
Angiokeratoma corporis diffusum, see Fabry disease
Angiokeratomata, 1164
Angiomatosis, encephalotrigeminal, see Sturge–Weber syndrome
Angioneurotic edema, hereditary, **1175,** 1262–1263
Angiostrongyliasis, **1493–1494**
Angiostrongylus caninum, larval disease, 1484 (Table)
Angiostrongylus constaricensis, 1494
Angiotensin converting enzyme inhibitors
  heart failure, 599
    neonatal, 205
  preconceptual care, 79
  renal hypertension, 973

Angiotensin II
  heart failure, 599
  respiratory distress syndrome, 142
Angular stomatitis, 424
Anhedonia, 1742
Anhidrosis, 34
Anhidrotic ectodermal dysplasia, 150
Anicteric hepatitis, 477
Animistic thinking, 1729
Anion gap, 1118 (footnote)
Aniridia, 290
Aniridia–Wilms' tumor syndrome, 59, 60
    (Table), 913
Anisakiasis, **1494**
Anisakis marina, larval disease, 1484
    (Table)
Aniseikonia, 1669
Anisocoria, 1650
Anisometropia, 1657
Ankle clonus, 38 (Table)
Ankle–foot arthroses, 757
Ankle jerk, 35, 38 (Table)
Ankyloblepharon ectodermal dysplasia
    and clefting, 1626 (Table)
Ankylosing spondylitis, **1605**
  eye, 1675
Ankylostomiasis, diarrhea, 1295
Ann Arbor staging system, 910 (Table)
Annual social surveys, 1850
Annular pancreas, 1773, 1774 (Fig.)
Anogenital warts, 1442, 1443, **1444**
Anomalads, 75
Anomalous origin of left coronary artery
    from pulmonary artery, 612
Anomalous pulmonary venous drainage,
    vs persistent fetal circulation, 182
Anopheles spp., 1445
Anorchia, 1790–1791
Anorectal manometry, 464–465
Anorexia, 467
  juvenile chronic arthritis, 1210
Anorexia nervosa, 371–372, 1746,
    1757–1759
  endocrine effects, 1014–1024
  puberty, 1023
Anoxic seizures, 672
  reflex, 672
Anserine, 1114, 1115
Antacids, and esophagitis, 429
Antagonism, drug combinations, 1528
Antecubital fossa, central venous
    cannulation, 1837
Antenatal care, **80–83**, *see also*
    Ultrasonography, pregnancy
  at-risk groups, 113–114
  immigrants, 1865
  syphilis, 1410
  twin pregnancies, 90
Antenatal diagnosis, *see* Prenatal
    diagnosis
Antenatal screening, congenital syphilis,
    1403
Antenatal therapy, 21-hydroxylase
    deficiency, 1062
Antenatal transfer, 157
Antepartum hemorrhage, **88–90**
Anterior cleavage syndrome, *see* Anterior
    segment cleavage syndrome
Anterior fontanel bones, 1558
Anterior horn cells, **719–721**
Anterior pituitary hormones, **1038–1039**,
    see also Adenohypophysis
Anterior segment cleavage syndrome, 264,
    265 (Fig.), 270
Anterior temporal lobectomy, 686
Anterior uveitis (iridocyclitis), **1665**
  neonate, organisms, 284 (Table)
  rheumatoid arthritis, 1674
Anterior visual pathway disorders,
    270–271
Anthracycline toxicity, 634, 894 (Table),
    896, 897
Anthrax, **1300**
Anthropometry, 76, **1186–1187**
  liver disease, 1209

Anti-A isoagglutinins, toxocariasis, 1485
Antiarrhythmic drugs, **626–627**
Antibiotics, **1526–1530**, *see also named
    diseases and organisms*
  AIDS, 1396
  appendicitis, 1787
  asplenia, 613
  atopic eczema, 1643
  bacteremia, 1287
  bone marrow transplant recipients, 875
  candidiasis, 1470
  cat-scratch disease, 1520
  cerebrospinal fluid, 696
  combinations, **1528**
  conjunctivitis, 1664
  Crohn's disease, 457–458
  cystic fibrosis, **557–558**
  for diarrhea, 454, 1296
  dosages, **1527–1528, 1955–1956**
    (Table)
  eye toxicity, 1677
  fulminating colitis, 459
  Helicobacter pylori, 432
  for immunodeficiency, 1267
  immunosuppression by, 1265
  impetigo, 1635
  infective endocarditis, 631, 632 (Table)
  interstitial pneumonitis, 534
  intrathecal, *see* Intrathecal route
  laboratory monitoring, 1300
  leukemia, 870
  meningitis
    bacterial, **1291**
    neonatal, 247, 282
  meningococcal disease, 1816
  necrotizing enterocolitis, 211
  neonate, **278–279**
  in nephrotic syndrome, 969
  in neutropenia, 894–895
  open fractures, 1812
  pneumonia, 568
  and preterm labor, 116
  prophylaxis, **1528–1529**
    chronic granulomatous disease, 1260
    gonorrhea, 1429
    Haemophilus influenzae, 1309
    immunodeficiency, 533, 1529
    meningitis, 1292
    Neisseria meningitidis, 1315
    neonatal pneumonia, 184
    vesicoureteric reflux, 956–957
  pyogenic osteitis, 1590–1591
  reactions, 1692–1693
  resistance, **1529**
    Neisseria gonorrhoeae, 1421–1422
  rheumatic fever, 1599–1600
  septic arthritis, 1592
  septicemia, 1288
  serum levels, 1530
  sickle cell disease, 863
  skull fractures, basal, 1811
  after splenectomy, 857
  on sputum bacteriology, 1298
  superinfections, 1295
  syphilis, 1401
  tonsillitis, 1687
  treponematoses, endemic, 1419–1420
  urinary tract infections, 951
    neonate, 261
Antibiotic susceptibility tests, *Neisseria
    gonorrhoeae,* 1424
Anti-B isoagglutinins, toxocariasis, 1485
Antibodies, **1236–1237**
  anticandidal, neonate, 1470
  deficiency
    with complement deficiencies, 1263
    with normal immunoglobulins, 1259
  detection, 1300
    pneumonia, 567
  functional tests, 1245
  herpes simplex virus, 1437
  HIV infection, 1264
  to lymphocytes, therapeutic, 1265
  malaria, 1447
  neonate, 275

  passive immunity, 341
  production defects, **1255–1259**
  syphilis, 1402–1403
  systemic lupus erythematosus, 1605
  toxoplasmosis, 1465–1466
Antibody-dependent cellular cytotoxicity,
    1235
Anticholinergic drugs
  asthma, 547
  for extrapyramidal syndromes, 769, 772
  neurogenic bladder, 657
  tall stature, 1020
Anticholinesterases, *see* Cholinesterase
    inhibitors
Anticipation, myotonic dystrophy, 66
Anticipatory vomiting, chemotherapy, 896
Anticoagulants
  and cerebrovascular disease, 715
  maternal therapy, 230
Anticonvulsants
  ataxia, 762
  birth asphyxia, 130
  calcitonin, 1057
  child abuse, 1871
  vs degeneration, 796 (Table)
  encephalopathies, 697
  on learning, 690
  maternal therapy, 230
  neonate, 246–247
  pregnancy, 114, 691
Anti-D immunoglobulin, pregnancy, 338
Antidiuretic hormone, 409, **1039**, *see also*
    Vasopressin
  acceptor blockade, 948
  deficiency, 1039
  effect, cytotoxic drugs, 896
  inappropriate secretion, *see also*
      Syndrome of inappropriate ADH
      secretion
    birth asphyxia, 129
    diabetic ketoacidosis, 1076
    preterm infant, 142
  neonates, 143
  normal values (arginine vasopressin),
      1923 (Table)
  respiratory distress syndrome, 142
Antiemetics, migraine, 717 (Table), 718
Antifungal chemotherapy, **1477–1478,
    1530**
Antigenic drift, shift, 1368
Antigen-presenting cells, 1235, *see also*
    Dendritic cells
Antigen-processing cells, *see* Phagocytes
Antigen recognition activation motifs,
    1239–1240
Antigens
  immune system, 1231–1232
  pneumonia, 567
  presentation, 1233 (Fig.), **1235–1236**
  response testing, 1246
Antihistamines
  allergic conjunctivitis, 1664, 1675–1676
  and allergy skin tests, 1693
  anaphylaxis, 1702
  antivenom treatment, 1523
  mastocytosis, 1647
  seasonal asthma, 549
  seasonal rhinitis, 1697
Anti-IgA, 1258, 1268
Anti-Kell, anti-Fya antibodies,
    isoimmunization, 234
Antilymphocyte globulin, 1265
Antimalarials, and glucose-6-phosphate
    dehydrogenase deficiency, 859
    (Table)
Antimetabolites, toxic effects, 894 (Table)
Antimitotic drugs, and breast-feeding,
    329–330
Antimony (pentavalent antimony
    compounds), **1462–1463**
Antimotility drugs, 453–454
Antimuscarinic drugs, *see* Anticholinergic
    drugs
Antinuclear antibodies, juvenile chronic
    arthritis, 1601, 1602

Antinuclear factor, Hashimoto's
    thyroiditis, 1048
Antiphospholipid antibody syndrome,
    prenatal care, 114
Antipyrine test, total body water, 403
Antiretroviral therapy, **1397–1398**
Anti-Ro
  heart block, 635
  lupus erythematosus, 1606
Antisecretory drugs, 453–454
Antisepsis, for procedures, **1830**
Antiseptic baths, epidemic methicillin-
    resistant *S. aureus,* 1329
Antiseptics
  Burkholderia cepacia, 1321
  poisoning, 1711
Antisocial behavior, socialized, 1742
Antistreptolysin O titers, 628, 962,
    1330
  infectious mononucleosis, 1367
  rheumatic fever, 1599
Antithrombin III, 227, 231, 882
  α_1-antitrypsin deficiency, 1176
  disseminated intravascular coagulation,
      231
Antithyroid antibodies, 1048
Antithyroid drugs, 1051
Antitoxins
  botulism, 1302
  diphtheria, **1306–1307**
  tetanus, 1333, 1334
  equine, 285
α_1-Antitrypsin
  deficiency, **577, 1100, 1175–1176**
    liver, 473
  fecal protein measurement, 448
Antivenoms
  adder, 1521
  Chironex fleckeri, 1526
  Latrodectus, 1524–1525
  scorpion stings, 1526
  snake bite, 1522–1523
Antiviral drugs, **1530**
  immunodeficiency, 1267
Antrochoanal polyp, 1685
Antrum, stomach, 430
Anuria, neonate, 258
Anus, *see also* Rectal atresia; *entries
    starting* 'Anal'
  anomalies, **1781–1782**
  carcinoma, 1445
  enterobiasis, 1486, 1487
  examination, 33
  gonorrhea, 1425
  herpes simplex, 1438–1439
  internal sphincter spasm, *see* Short
      segment Hirschsprung's disease
  neural tube defect, 657
  sexual abuse, 1870
  stenosis, 462
Anxiety, 1731
  learning disorder, 824–825
Anxiety states, **1739**
Anxiolytics, 1748 (Table), *see also*
    Tranquilizers
  chemotherapy, 896
Anxious attachment, 1731, 1739
Aorta
  Marfan's syndrome, 1589
  poststenotic dilation, 607
  right-sided, imaging, 1899
  thoracic, traumatic dissection, **1811**
Aortic arch, *see also* Double aortic arch
  ultrasonography, 591
Aortic regurgitation
  congenital, 608
  rheumatic, 629
  ventricular septal defect, 600, 601
Aortic sinus, aneurysm, 608
Aortic stenosis, 32, **606–607**
  vs carotid bruit, 594
  signs, 587 (Table)
  Turner's syndrome, 370
Aortic valve stenosis, neonate, 203
Aortopexy, tracheomalacia, 1769

Aortopulmonary septal defect, 605
Aparalytic hemisyndrome, 741
Apert's syndrome, 830 (Table), 1560
    inheritance, 1566 (Table)
Apex beat, 586
    position, 31, 32
Apgar scores, 111, **125**, 126, 134
    vs fetal blood sampling, 119
    prognostic value, 131–132
Aphakia, 1657, 1669
Aphonia, 809, 1688
Apical murmur, 594
Apical trabecular region hypoplasia, right
    ventricle, 611
Apical tuberculosis, 1336
Aplasia cutis congenita, **1620**
Aplastic anemias, **854–856**
Aplastic crises, 852, 856
    erythema infectiosum, 1359
    sickle cell disease, 862
Apnea, **509**, **528–530**, *see also*
        Respiration, delay at birth
    Duchenne muscular dystrophy, 732
    gastroesophageal reflux, 212
    neonates, **196–198**
    recurrence, 198
    sudden infant death syndrome, 1721
    suffocation, 1871
    tracheoesophageal fistula, 573
Apnea monitors, 197, **530**
Apnea test, brain death, 709
apoE gene mutations, Alzheimer's
    disease, 1152
Apoferritin : ferritin ratio, 1146
Apollo 11 disease, **1385**
Apoprotein B, absence, 446
Apoproteins, 1149
Apoptosis, neurons, birth asphyxia, 127
Apparent life-threatening events, **528–
    530**
Apparent mineralocorticoid excess
    hypokalemic alkalosis, 946
    syndrome, 1065–1067
Appendicitis, **1786–1787**
    chickenpox, 1361
    histoplasmosis, 1476
    maternal, 89 (Table)
    measles, 1354
    strongyloidiasis, 1492
    ultrasonography, 1904
Appendix
    ascariasis, 1483
    beef tapeworm, 1500
    Enterobius vermicularis, 1487
    schistosomiasis, 1509
Appendix of Morgagni, torsion, 1914
Appetite, 17
    cystic fibrosis, 553
Apple peel deformity, small bowel
    obstruction, 1775
Appropriate for gestation (AGA), size,
    definition, 94
Aprotinin, 228
Aptamil, 112 (Table)
Apt test, 224, 230, 1936 (Table)
APUD cells, 642
Aquaporins, 942
Aqueduct of Sylvius, obstruction, 658
Arachidonic acid, 333, 1182
Arachnodactyly, 39, **1588**
    congenital contractural, **1589**
Arachnoid cysts, **651**
Arachnoiditis, tuberculosis, 1345
Arboviruses, **1389–1390**
    liver, 1388
Arc 5 test, hydatid disease, 1506 (Fig.)
Archicerebellum, 749
Architectural accidents, **1715**
Arcuate fiber damage, transcortical
    aphasias, 815
Arcus juvenilis, 1674
Arginine
    supplements, 307, 1111, 1112
    urea cycle disorders, 1110, 1111

L-Arginine, for hyperammonemia, 1112
Argininemia, 1111
Arginine vasopressin, *see also* Antidiuretic
        hormone; Vasopressin
    response, neonate, 257
Argininosuccinic aciduria, 1103, **1111**
    ataxia, 762
Argyle feeding tubes, urethral
        catheterization, 1840
Argyll Robertson pupils, 1413
Arias syndrome, 218
Arithmetic, *see also* Dyscalculia
    development, 825 (Fig.)
Arm, measurement, 20
Armadillo, *Mycobacterium leprae*, 1309
Arm muscle area, 1186
Arm recoil, neonate, 44, **237**
    gestation age, 41 (Fig.)
Arm release, prone neonate, 238 (Fig.)
Arm traction, neonate, 237 (Fig.)
Arnold–Chiari malformation, 645, **647**,
    657
    ataxia, 753
L-Aromatic amino acid decarboxylase
    defect, 1107
Arrested hydrocephalus, *see* Compensated
        hydrocephalus
Arrhythmias, **623–628**, *see also*
        Dysrhythmias
    amphotericin B, 1478
    after cardiac surgery, 1822
    carditis, 1598
    Chagas' disease, 1459
    faints, 672
    mitral valve prolapse, 610
    neonate, 203
    toxoplasmosis, 1465
Arsenic, 1185 (Table)
Arterial blood
    oxygen saturation, 593
    oxygen tension, 194–195
        respiratory distress syndrome, 179
    pH, 416, 505
    sampling, **505**, **1835–1836**
        osteomyelitis, 283
    vs venous blood, acid—base indices,
        419
Arterial cannulation, **1836**
    inadvertent, 1837
Arterial jugular venous oxygen difference,
    708
Arterial switch operation, transposition of
        great arteries, 615
Arterioles, infantile cortical hyperostosis,
    1583
Arteriomesenteric duodenal compression
        syndrome, **1787–1788**
Arteriosclerosis, 712
Arteriovenous fistulae, 605
    intracranial, 711
Arteriovenous malformations, 1798
    cerebral, *see* Vein of Galen aneurysm
    embolization, 1899
    intracranial, 709, **710–711**
    ultrasonography, 1908
Arteriovenous shunt, acyanotic heart
        disease with, **599–613**
Arteritides
    renal involvement, 966
    stroke, 711–712
Arthralgia, syphilis, 1408
Arthritis, *see also* Polyarthritis; Septic
        arthritis
    chickenpox, 1361
    Chlamydia trachomatis, 1430
    cystic fibrosis, 556
    erythema infectiosum, 1358–1359
    gonococcal, 1426, 1428
    Kawasaki disease, 1479
    Lyme disease, 1313, **1611–1612**
    rubella, 1357
    salmonellosis, 1324
    syphilis, congenital, 1413
    tuberculosis, **1345–1346**

X-linked agammaglobulinemia, 1255
Arthrogryposis, myopathic, 728
Arthrogryposis multiplex congenita, 29
    (Fig.), **1586–1587**
Articulatory dyspraxia, **807**, 818
    acquired, 814
Arum lily poisoning, 1711
Arylsulfatase C deficiency (steroid
        sulfatase deficiency), 1164, 1165
Arylsulfatases, 1164
    Maroteaux–Lamy syndrome, 1161
    mucolipidoses, 1171
Asbestos, and neoplasms, 891
Ascariasis, **1481–1485**
    larval disease, 1484 (Table)
    liver, 478
Ascending aorta, poststenotic dilation,
    607
Ascending infection, neonatal pneumonia,
    183–184
Ascending testis, 1791
Ascites, 28 (Fig.)
    examination, 33
    management, 482
    tuberculosis, 1345
Asepsis, **1830**
Aseptic meningitis, *see* Viral infections,
        meningitis
Aseptic necrosis, osteochondroses, 1594
Ashkenazi Jews, 1100
    Tay–Sachs disease, 1164
Ash leaf macules, 1625
Asia, demography, 2 (Table)
Asian immigrants, 1865–1866
Askin tumor, tumor markers, 912 (Table)
Ask-Upmark kidney, 253–254
Asparaginase, toxicity, 894 (Table), 896
Aspartame, 1105
Aspartate aminotransferase, 472 (Table)
    inborn errors of metabolism, 306
    normal values, 1923 (Table)
        cerebrospinal fluid, 1933 (Table)
    Wilson's disease prognosis, 481
        (Table)
Aspartylglucosaminuria, 780 (Table), 1157
    (Table), **1167**
Asperger's syndrome, 807, 824
Aspergilloma, 1474
Aspergillosis, 570, 1471 (Table),
    1473–1474
    allergens, 1690
    allergic bronchopulmonary, 550, 556
    bone marrow transplant recipients, 874
    immunocompromised patient, **536**
Asphyxia, 123, 124
    hypophosphatasia, 1176
    meconium passage, 185
    neonate
        cardiovascular aspects, 205
        mortality, 4 (Table), 7
        physiological, 107
        vomiting, 212
Asphyxiating thoracic dystrophy, *see*
        Jeune's asphyxiating thoracic
        dystrophy
Aspiration
    amebic abscesses, 1469, 1845
    cerebral palsy, 428
Aspiration pneumonias
    drowning, 1718
    neonates, **185–187**, 280
    respiratory distress syndrome, 182
Aspirin, 1832
    administration, 1959 (Table)
    for cerebrovascular disease, 715
    Kawasaki disease, 633, 1480
    migraine, 717 (Table), 718
    platelets, 229, **879**
    poisoning, 1710
    pregnancy, 81
    prenatal therapy, 114
    rheumatic diseases, 1603
    rheumatic fever, 628, 1599
    toddler diarrhea, 464

Asplenia, 613
    septicemia, 1288, 1292
    Streptococcus pneumoniae, 1319, 1320
Assimilation, intellectual, 1729
Assist mode ventilation, 1817, *see also*
        Patient triggered ventilation
Associations, congenital, 75
Ass's milk, 1700
Astemizole
    administration, 1960 (Table)
    and allergy skin tests, 1693
Astereognosis, 35
Asthma, 491, **536–550**
    acute severe, **547–549**
    air pollution, 492–493
    allergic aspects, **1694–1695**
    auscultation, 30
    breathing exercises, 521, 545
    bronchial provocation tests, 501
    cystic fibrosis, 555
    diagnosis, **542–544**
    functional residual capacity, 501
    meconium aspiration syndrome, 186
    mortality, 490 (Table), 536
    natural history, 539–541
    patterns for drug therapy, 545
    pets, 493, 545
    prognosis, 541
    pruritus, 510
    psychological factors, 493–494, 542,
        545
    recurrence risks, 74
    severely handicapped children affected,
        14 (Table)
    sputum, 507
    sulfites, 1701
    triggers, **541–542**
    vs tuberculous emphysema, 1342
    ventilation, 1818
Astigmatism, 1657
Astrocytomas, **902–903**
    optic nerve, *see* Optic gliomas
    relative incidence, 900 (Table)
    spinal cord, 906
Astroviruses, gastrointestinal tract, 1384
Asymmetric growth retardation, 744, 1191
Asymmetric muscle tone (hemisyndrome),
    741
Asymmetric tonic neck reflex, 37 (Table),
    382
    neonatal gestation age, 40 (Table)
Asymptomatic virus shedding, herpes
        simplex, 1436, 1437
Asystole, resuscitation, **525–526**, **1808**
Ataxias, **762–765**, *see also* Friedreich's
        ataxia
    acute, **762–764**
    cerebral palsies, 738–739, **749–753**
    dyspraxia, 669
    gait, 34, 35
    heredodegenerative, 764
    Lennox–Gastaut syndrome, 674
    physiological truncal, 668
    progressive, 764, 792 (Table)
    speech, 809
Ataxia telangiectasia, 290, **766–767**, 792
        (Table), 799 (Table), 1142, 1242
        (Table), **1253**
    germ cell tumors, 920
    liver tumors, 924
    neoplasms, 888 (Table), 889–890,
        1248
Ataxic diplegia, hydrocephalus, 745
Ataxic dysarthria, 813
Atelectasis, *see* Collapse (pulmonary
        lobe); Recurrent segmental
        collapse
Atenolol, 637 (Table), 973 (Table), 1960
        (Table)
Athetosis, 770
Atlantoaxial joint, computed tomography,
    1916
ATM gene, 1253
Atomic bombs, neoplasms, 890

Atopic asthma, 540
  cystic fibrosis, 555
Atopic cataract, 1669
Atopic eczema, **1642–1643**
  allergic aspects, **1695–1696**
Atopy, 1689
  asthma, 536–537, **540**, 541
  breast milk protection, 152
  bronchiolitis, 564, 565
  environment, 492
  eosinophilic gastroenteritis, 442
  family history, 1692
  preventive measures, **1703**
  transient food intolerance, 441
Atosiban, 116
ATP
  hypoxia, 127
  magnetic resonance spectroscopy, birth asphyxia, 128
Atransferrinemia, 1146
Atrax robustus, 1525
Atresia, definition, 1770
Atria, situs, 597
Atrial fibrillation, 625
Atrial flutter, 625
Atrial hypertrophy, electrocardiography, 589
Atrial natriuretic peptide
  neonates, 143
  normal values, 1923 (Table)
Atrial redirection, transposition of great arteries, 615
Atrial septal defect, **601–602**
  M mode echocardiography, 590 (Fig.), 591 (Fig.), 602
  signs, 587 (Table)
Atrial septostomy, 598
  Rashkind balloon, 205
    transposition of great arteries, 614–615
Atrial tachycardia, 625
Atrioventricular connection, congenital heart disease, 597
Atrioventricular septal defect, 198, **603–605**
At-risk groups, *see* High-risk pregnancy, fetus and infant
Atropine
  administration, 1960 (Table)
    neonate, 1956 (Table)
  for bradycardia, 627
  cardiac stimulation, 135
  emergency supply, 134 (Table)
  organophosphorus poisoning, 1711
  refractive error testing, 1657
  resuscitation, doses, 526 (Table), 527 (Fig.)
Attachment, anxious, 1731, 1739
Attachment theory, 1731
Attention, 819–820
Attention deficit disorder, **1744**
  epilepsy, 690
  ex-preterm infants, 171
Attenuated severe combined immunodeficiency, 1249
Attenuated vaccines, *see* Live attenuated vaccines
Attico/antral disease, 1681
Attitude of doctor, 1878
Atypical nevi (dysplastic nevi), 1618
Atypical pneumonia
  Chlamydia pneumoniae, **1432–1433**
    primary, 1374
Atypical verrucose endocarditis, 635
Auchmeromyia luteola, 1514
Audiometry, **816–817, 1683**
  secretory otitis media, 1681
  syphilis
    congenital, 1414
    secondary, 1408
Auditory agnosia, 807, 815
Auditory comprehension of language, Test of (TACC), 400
Auditory evoked potentials,

hypoglycemia, 137
Auditory nerve
  examination, 34
  neonatal damage, organisms, 284 (Table)
Auditory orientation, neonate, 238 (Fig.)
Auditory pathway, investigation, 243–244
Auditory response cradle, 244
Augmentative communication, 814
Augmentin, 1955 (Table), 1959 (Table)
Aura, 673
  migraine, 717
Auramine–rhodamine staining, *Mycobacterium tuberculosis,* 1335
Auranofin, 1604
Auricle, **1679–1680**
Auriscopic examination, 21, 511
  otitis media, 561
Aurothiomalate, sodium, administration, 1976 (Table)
Auscultation
  chest, 30
  heart, **32, 586–587**
  intermittent, fetal monitoring, 117
  neonatal heart, 199
Auscultatory method, blood pressure, 20
Austin Flint murmur, 629
Australia
  breast-feeding rates, 326 (Table)
  marine animal stings, 1526
  snake bite, 1523, 1524
Australia antigen, *see* Hepatitis B surface antigen
Australian tiger snake venom, 1521
Autism, 818, **1737–1739**
  fragile X mental retardation, 63
  nomenclature, 834–836
  semantic-pragmatic disorder, 807
  severely handicapped children affected, 14 (Table)
  vs speech disorder, 808
  succinylpurinemic, 790 (Table)
  tuberous sclerosis, 801
Autistic behavior, epilepsy, 690
Autoantibodies
  systemic lupus erythematosus, 1605
  tissue (test), 472 (Table)
Autografts, and cryopreservation, ovaries, 1033
Autoimmune diseases
  adrenal gland, 1067
  chronic active hepatitis, **480**
  complement deficiency disorders, 1262, 1263
  endocrine, 998
  enteropathy, 443
  gastritis, 430
  hemolytic anemias, **863–864**
  and hypoparathyroidism, 1057
  IgA deficiency, 1258
  and immunodeficiency, 1248
  myasthenia gravis, 727
  neonatal thrombocytopenia, 229
  neutropenia, 867
  skin, **1639–1640**
  thyroiditis, *see* Hashimoto's thyroiditis
Autoimmunity
  Chagas' disease, 1459
  diabetes mellitus, 1074
Autoinfection, strongyloidiasis, 1492
Autologous marrow rescue, high dose chemotherapy, 874
Automatic resuscitators, 524–525
Autonomic discharge, fits, 673
Autonomic dysfunction, sacral, herpes simplex, 1439
Autonomic nervous system, *see also* Riley–Day syndrome
  cerebrospinal fluid production, 658
Autonomous functioning nodules, hyperthyroidism, 1052
Autopsy
  brain injury dating, 703
  coroner's, 1720–1721

inborn errors of metabolism, 307
neonatal death, **173–174**, 175
sudden infant death syndrome, 1720–1721, 1723
virology, 1352
Autoregulation, cerebral blood flow, 699
Autosomal dominant polycystic kidney disease, 72 (Table), 89 (Table), **254, 940–941,** 959
  ultrasonography, 1909–1910
Autosomal inheritance, **65–66**
Autosomal recessive chronic granulomatous disease, 1242 (Table)
Autosomal recessive hyperIgM syndrome, 1242 (Table)
Autosomal recessive hypohidrotic ectodermal dysplasia, 1625 (Table)
Autosomal recessive limb girdle dystrophy, 733
Autosomal recessive polycystic kidney disease, 254, 940
  ultrasonography, 1909–1910
Auxotyping, *Neisseria gonorrhoeae,* 1422
Available oxygen, 225
Avascular necrosis, femoral head, 1594–1595
  from splinting, 1551
Average annual reduction rates, under-5 mortality rates, 1884
Avermectins, *see also* Ivermectin
  hookworm, 1490
AV node, conduction defects, **626**
Axial cataract, 1668
Axillae, neurofibromatosis, 1628
Axillary hair, puberty, 357
Axillary lymph nodes, examination, 30
Axillary temperature, 147
Axonal transport, herpes simplex virus, 1436
Axons, degeneration, 722
Ayerza's syndrome, 1510
Ayre's T-piece, Jackson–Rees modification, 524
Azathioprine
  administration, 1960 (Table)
  autoimmune chronic active hepatitis, 480
  immunosuppression, 1265
  systemic lupus erythematosus, 1606
Azithromycin
  administration, 1960 (Table)
  environmental mycobacteria, 1350
  nongonococcal urethritis, 1432
Azlocillin
  administration, 1955 (Table), 1960 (Table)
  Pseudomonas aeruginosa, cystic fibrosis, 558 (Table)
AZT, *see* Zidovudine
Aztreonam
  administration, 1955 (Table), 1960 (Table)
  Pseudomonas aeruginosa, cystic fibrosis, 558 (Table)
Azul, see Pinta

B19, *see* Parvoviruses, B19
Babinski reflex, 37 (Table), 239–240
'Baby Doe' case, 102–103
Baby Friendly Hospital Initiative, 339
Baby walkers, 1715
Bacille Calmette-Guerin, *see* BCG vaccination
Back slaps, resuscitation, 522
Backwash ileitis, 458
Baclofen
  administration, 1960 (Table)
  cerebral palsy, 758–759
Bacteremia, **1286–1287**
  gonococcal, 1426

salmonellosis, 1324
  schistosomiasis, 1509
  Staphylococcus aureus, **1329**
  urinary tract infections, neonate, 261
Bacteria
  evolution, 1279 (Table)
  overgrowth, protracted diarrhea, 454
Bacterial index, leprosy, 1310
Bacterial infections, **1297–1351,** *see also* Bacterial meningitis
  cystic fibrosis, **554–555**
  diarrhea, 452
  eye involvement, **1677**
  HIV infection, 1393–1394, 1396
  home care, 1802
  hypothermia, 149
  leishmaniasis, 1462
  malaria, 1453
  neonatal jaundice, 218
  neonate, 1282
  peritonitis, spontaneous, **483**
  postulated, and sudden infant death syndrome, 1722
  respiratory, 491, 569
    community-acquired pneumonia, **565–568**
  on influenza, 1368, 1369
  respiratory distress syndrome, 181–182
  rhinitis, 1684
  skin, **1634–1636**
  snake bites, 1521
  tracheitis, 563 (Table), 564
  United Kingdom, mortality, 1276 (Table)
  vaginosis, 116, **1435**
  varicella, 1361, 1362
  vs viral infections, pneumonia, 567 (Table)
Bacterial killing disorders, 1259–1262
Bacterial killing tests, neutrophils, 1247
Bacterial meningitis
  acute, **1288–1292**
    bacteriology, 1298
    vs gastroenteritis, 1294–1295
    Haemophilus influenzae, 1307, **1308**
    prevention, **1292**
  deafness, 816
Bacterial polysaccharide immune globulin, 1309
Bacteriology
  cancer treatment, 895
  laboratory methods, **1297–1300**
    antibiotic sensitivity and resistance, **1529**
  diphtheria, 1306
Bacteriophage *N*X174, antibody tests, 1245
Bacteriuria
  and preterm labor, 116
  significant, 950
Bag and mask ventilation
  apnea attacks, 197
  neonatal resuscitation, 133–134
Bag-valve–mask systems, 524
BAIB (β-aminoisobutyric acid), 1115
Bairnsdale ulcer, 1349–1350
Balance, development, 382
Balanced polymorphism, sickle cell gene, 860
Balanced reciprocal translocations, chromosomal, 52 (Fig.), 53
Balancing movements, 38, 39 (Fig.)
Balanitis, 1793
  neonate, organisms, 284 (Table)
Balantidiasis, 1470
'Ball and socket' deformity, achondroplasia, 1574
Ballerina syndrome (toe walking), 668, 760
Balloon atrial septostomy, *see* Atrial septostomy
Balloon dilation
  coarctation of aorta, 205, **594,** 611–612
  esophagus, 1899

Balloon valvuloplasty, 593, 594
  pulmonary stenosis, 609
Ball playing, development, 382
Baltic myoclonic epilepsy, 795 (Table)
Bamako Initiative, 1889, **1890**
Banding, chromosomes, cytogenetic
    nomenclature, 54
Banked human milk, 152
Bantu, hemosiderosis, 1146–1147
Baptism, neonatal death, 173
Barbiturates
  for acute-onset stroke, 715
  neoplasms, 890
  poisoning, 1709
  for raised intracranial pressure, 699
    coma therapy, 1825
  trigonocephaly, 1560
  withdrawal effects, 772
Bare lymphocyte syndromes, 1242
    (Table), 1250
Baringer's syndrome, 752
Barium enema reduction, intussusception,
    1903
Barium studies, **1902–1904**, *see also*
    Contrast swallow
  colon, 464
  Crohn's disease, 457
  diagnostic radiation doses, 1895 (Table)
  double contrast, 464, 1896, 1902–1903
  esophagus, 429
  Hirschsprung's disease, 1777
  respiratory disorders, **514–517**
  small intestine, 447
  stomach, 435
  Trichuris trichiuria, 1491, 1492 (Fig.)
  ulcerative colitis, 459
  vascular ring, 573, 612, 1899
Barium sulfate, 1895
Barlow maneuver, 41
Barotrauma, 160–161
  air embolism, 190
  bronchopulmonary dysplasia, 194
Barrier nursing, 1281
Bartholinitis, gonococcal, 1425
  treatment, 1428
Barth syndrome, 1128, **1156**
Bartonellosis, **1300–1301**
  cat-scratch disease, 1520
  emergence, 1279 (Table)
  hemolysis, 864
Bart's hydrops, 860, 862
Bartter's syndrome, 260, **946**
  vs congenital chloridorrhea, 446
Basal cell nevus syndrome, corpus
    callosum, absence, 647
Basal ganglia, 767–768
  astrocytomas, 903
  calcification, **774**
  classification of diseases, 770–774
  kernicterus, 754
  postasphyxial dyskinesia, 755
  syndromes, 738
Basal metabolic rate, 1181
Baseline rate, fetal heart, 117 (Table)
Basement membrane nephropathy, 966
Bases, 415
  deficit, normal fetal blood, 119 (Table)
  excess, 419, 504
  normal values, 1923 (Table)
Basic life support, **522–524**
Basilar impression, 1559
Basilar migraine, 717
Basket weave appearance, hereditary
    nephritis, 965
Bejel, see Endemic syphilis
Belgium, hypothyroidism, preterm infant,
    1046
Bell-shaped chest, 720
Bell's nerve palsy, 725
Bell's palsy, 725
Bender Gestalt test, 400
Bendrofluazide, administration, 1960
    (Table)
  neonate, 1956 (Table)
Bengal strain, *Vibrio cholerae,* 1303

Bats, rabies from, 1377
Batten disease, 796–797 (Table), 1171
Batten–Mayou disease (juvenile amaurotic
    family idiocy), 1666
Batteries
  poisoning, 1710–1711
  swallowed, 435
    removal, 1899
Battle's sign, 1811
Bayley and Griffith scales of infant
    development, 167
Bayley scales of infant development, 400,
    827
B cell leukemias, 868
B cell lymphomas
  chemotherapy, 909
  gene rearrangements, 906
B cells, *see* B lymphocytes
BCG vaccination, 341, **1338–1340**
  AIDS, 1396
  contraindications, 342 (Table)
  failure, 1339
  foreign travel, 345
  for leprosy, 1311
  neonate, 286, 1339, 1340, 1346
  WHO on, 346 (Table)
Beaking, vertebral bodies, 1915
Beans, flatulence, 1183
Beau's lines, 1640
Becker muscular dystrophy, 732
Beckwith syndrome, 830 (Table)
Beckwith–Wiedemann syndrome, *see also*
    Sotos syndrome
  hepatoblastoma, 924
Beclomethasone, administration, 1960
    (Table)
Bed rest
  juvenile chronic arthritis, 1603
  rheumatic fever, 1599
Bedrooms, allergen avoidance, 1695
Bedsharing, sudden infant death
    syndrome, 1720
Bed wetting, history taking, 18
Beef, and cow's milk protein intolerance,
    1700
Beef tapeworm (*Taenia saginata*),
    1499–1500
Beer odor, methionine malabsorption,
    1122
Beetles, toxins, **1525**
Bee venom, 1524
Behavior
  cerebral palsy, 761
  epilepsy, 690–691
  history taking, 18
  mental retardation, 834, 841
  respiratory disorders, 510
Behavioral program, chronic constipation,
    462–463
Behavioral psychotherapy, 1749, *see also*
    Cognitive–behavior therapy
Behavioral tests of vision, 269–270
Behavior disorders
  adoptees, 1860
  foods and additives, 1698
  Sanfilippo's syndrome, 1160
  severely handicapped children affected,
    14 (Table)
Behavior scales, 400
Behçet's syndrome, 424, 1611
  eye, 1675
Behr's autosomal recessive optic atrophy,
    271

Benign familial neonatal seizures, 245,
    247, 680 (Table)
Benign intracranial hypertension, **665,**
    715, 718
Benign myoclonic epilepsy of infancy,
    680 (Table)
Benign neonatal sleep myoclonus, 245
Benign occipital epilepsy with occipital
    spike-waves, 681 (Table)
Benign partial epileptic syndromes, 684
Benign recurrent cholestasis, 1145
Benign rolandic epilepsy, 681 (Table),
    684
Benorylate, 1960 (Table)
Bentiromide, pancreatic function tests,
    451
Benzathine benzyl penicillin, endemic
    treponematoses, 1419–1420
Benzathine penicillin
  rheumatic fever, 629, 1600
  syphilis, 1409
Benzhexol, with haloperidol, 841
Benzidazole, 1460
Benzodiazepines
  and child abuse, 1871
  encephalopathies, 697
  for extrapyramidal rigidity, 769
  poisoning, 1709
Benzoic acid, in food, 1701
Benzoyl peroxide, 1960 (Table)
N-Benzoyl-1-tyrosyl *p*-aminobenzoic acid
    test, cystic fibrosis, 553
Benztropine, administration, 1960 (Table)
Benzyl benzoate, scabies, 1517, 1960
    (Table)
Benzyl penicillin
  actinomycosis, 1473
  administration, 1955 (Table), 1960
    (Table)
    bacterial meningitis, 1291
    β-hemolytic streptococci, 1332 (Table)
    gonorrhea, 1427, 1428
    Lyme disease, 1314 (Table)
    ophthalmia neonatorum, 1429
    pyogenic osteitis, 1590–1591
    rheumatic fever, 1599–1600
    syphilis, 1410
      congenital, 1415
Benzylpenicilloyl hapten, 1702
Bephenium, 1490, 1960 (Table)
Berberis, poisoning, 1709
Bereavement, 928–929
  sudden infant death syndrome,
    1722–1723
Bereavement counseling, 174–175
Bereavement folders, 173
Bereavement response, mental retardation,
    839
Bereavement services, 928
Bergstrom & Mocumbi, on health care in
    developing countries, 1890
Beri beri, *see* Thiamin, deficiency
Bernard–Soulier syndrome, 229, 877,
    879
Berry aneurysms, 710
'Best buy' interventions, infectious
    diseases, 1279
'Best interests' principle, 101
Best's macular degeneration, 1666
β-adrenergic receptor antagonists, 626
  and Chagas' disease, 1460
  on fetus and neonate, 91 (Table)
  hypertrophic cardiomyopathy, 634
  Marfan's syndrome, 1589
  renal hypertension, 972–973
β-aminoisobutyric acid, 1115
Beta-blockers, *see* β-adrenergic receptor
    antagonists
β cells, pancreas, 1071
  hypoglycemia, 1083
β-fetoprotein
  cholestatic jaundice, 220
  serum levels, 471
β-glucuronidase, breast milk, 219

β-hemolytic streptococci (*S. pyogenes*),
    1330–1332
  group A
    impetigo, 1635
    pharyngitis, heart disease
      prophylaxis, 628
    throat swabs, 1298
  group B
    maternal immunization, 1267
    neonatal meningitis, 247
    neonatal sepsis, 278, **280–281,** 1240
    vs persistent fetal circulation, 182
    pneumonia, 184
    rheumatic fever, 1597
  neonatal meningitis, 247 (Table)
  perianal cellulitis, 1635
  pharyngitis, 560
  pneumonia, 569
Beta-human chorionic gonadotropin
  liver tumors, 924
  tumor marker, 921, 922
Betaine, for cystathione synthase
    deficiency, 1109
Betamethasone
  administration, 1960 (Table)
  eyedrops, interstitial keratitis, 1415
β thalassemia, 72 (Table)
  maternal, 89 (Table)
  mutations, 69
Bezoars, 435
Bicarbonate, *see also* Carbonic
    acid/bicarbonate buffer system;
    Sodium bicarbonate
  for air contrast, 1896
  alimentary secretions, 411 (Table)
  cholera, loss, 1303
  colonic secretion, 455
  concentrations, 404, 406 (Table)
  fractional excretion, 260
  gastroenteritis
    loss, 1293
    replacement, 1296
  intestinal absorption, 438
  and mixed acidosis, 504
  normal values, 1923 (Table), 1928
    (Table)
    amniotic fluid, 1937 (Table)
    cerebrospinal fluid, 1933 (Table)
  pancreas, cystic fibrosis, 551
  reabsorption, 257, 941, 944
    failure, 945
  renal threshold, neonate, 108
  resuscitation, doses, 526 (Table), 527
    (Fig.)
  urine, 1930 (Table)
Biceps jerk, 35, 38 (Table)
  neonate, 239
Bicuspid aortic valve, **607**
Bicycles
  epilepsy, 691
  injuries, **1716**
Bifid ureters, 255
Bifocal spectacles, squint, 1660
Bifunctional protein deficiency,
    adrenoleukodystrophy, 786
    (Table), 1174
'Big bang' theory, reflux nephropathy, 262
Bilateral renal agenesis, 253
Bile
  bilirubin excretion, 215–216
  electrolytes, 411 (Table)
  neonate, 471
Bile acids
  metabolism disorders, **1145**
  peroxisomal disorders, 1172 (Table)
Bile salts
  cystic fibrosis, 449
  lipid digestion, 437
  neonate, 471
  preterm infant, 207
  serum levels, 472 (Table)
  short gut syndrome, 445
  vitamin D absorption, 301
Bile-stained vomiting, neonate, 210

Bilharziasis, see Schistosomiasis
Bilharziomas, 1509
Biliary atresia, 1782–1783
  extrahepatic, 475
  hepatitis syndrome in infancy, 473
  I-131 rose bengal fecal excretion test, 221
  intrahepatic, lipoprotein X, 1153–1154
  vs intrahepatic cholestasis, 474
Biliary calculi, 856, 1788
  cystic fibrosis, 484
  ultrasonography, 472
Biliary cirrhosis
  causes, 482 (Table)
  extrahepatic biliary atresia, 475
Biliary hypoplasia, 221, 472 (Table)
  intrahepatic, 474
Biliary tract
  cystic fibrosis, 556
  embryology, 206–207
  imaging, 1906–1907
  obstruction
    ascariasis, 1483
    coagulation disorder, 882
    rhabdomyosarcoma, 916
  spontaneous perforation, 472 (Table), 475–476
  typhoid fever, 1325
Bilirubin
  cerebrospinal fluid, 1933 (Table)
  encephalopathy, 232
  metabolism
    disorders, 1144–1145
    neonate, 214–216
  normal values, 1923 (Table)
    stools, 1936 (Table)
  parenteral lipids, 1220
  serum levels, 472 (Table)
    exchange transfusion indication, 219, 233
    phototherapy indication, 218
  Wilson's disease prognosis, 481 (Table)
Binding proteins, see also High-affinity human growth hormone-binding protein (hGHBP); named substances bound
  insulin-like growth factors, 351, 365–366, 374, 1019
Binet, Alfred, see Stanford–Binet intelligence scale
Binocular indirect ophthalmoscopy, 1651, 1671
Biochemical nutritional assessment, 1187–1188
Bioethical committees, 101
Biofeedback, migraine, 719
Biological false positive reaction, cardiolipin antigen tests, 1402
Biophysical profile, fetus, 115
Biopsy, 891, see also Renal biopsy
  amyloidosis, 1177
  bronchial, 520
  celiac disease, 440, 441
  Ewing's sarcoma, 919
  liver, 221, 472–473
    tumors, 925
  lymphomas, 908
  metabolic myopathies, 1132
  muscle
    Duchenne muscular dystrophy, 730, 732
    technique, 1846
  osteosarcoma, 917
  pleural, 521
  polymyositis, 1607
  rectum, 464
  Reye's syndrome, 479
  skin, 1846
  small intestine, 447–448
  syphilis, 1402
Biosynthetic growth hormone, 1019
Biotin, 1184 (Table)
  deficiency, 1199
  estimated safe and adequate daily

intakes, 1949 (Table)
for hereditary lactic acidosis, 1125
metabolism disorders, 1148
for 3-methylcrotonylglycinuria, 1117
multiple carboxylase deficiency, 1254
for organic acidurias, 1119
parenteral nutrition, 1221 (Table)
for propionic acidemia, 1117
safe intakes, 1948 (Table)
Biotinidase deficiency, 790 (Table), 1148
Biparietal diameter, 80, 82
Biphasic renal failure, bee stings, 1524
Bipolar depressive illness, adolescence, 1750, 1751, 1755
Bipyridines, intensive care, 1820
Birbeck granules, 925
Bird-fancier's lung, 577
Birth, see also Delivery; Intrapartum care; Marriage, births outside
  disease incidence at, 13
  rates, 1
    per female, 15 (Table)
  registration, 1849
Birth asphyxia, 123–132, see also Postasphyxial dyskinesia
  and acute renal failure, 259, 974
  ataxia, 752
  and cerebral palsy, 119, 738, 741
  deafness, 1682
  failure to thrive, 465–466
  hyperglycemia, 298
  hypoglycemia, 294–295, 1006
  management, 129–131
  meconium passage, 185
  prognosis, 131–132
  pseudobulbar palsy, 812
  stillbirth rates, 4 (Table)
Birth history, 18, 41
Birth records, adopted persons' access, 1859
Births and Deaths Registration Act 1953, live births definition, 1849
Birth trauma, 120–123
  cerebral palsy, 741
  eyes, 264, 267
  growth hormone deficiency, 372
  head injuries, 121–122, 699
  intracranial, 121–122
  large for gestational age infant, 138
  neonatal mortality, 4 (Table)
  nonprogressive ataxia, 752
  skull fractures, 121 (Table), 707
  stillbirth rates, 4 (Table)
  trends, 7
Birthweight, see also Low birthweight
  on childhood mortalities, 3 (Table)
  definitions, 94
  immigrants, 1865
  outcome, 167, 170–171
  subsequent growth, 356, 1023
Birthweight ratio, 167
Bisacodyl, administration, 1961 (Table)
Bishop Koop ileostomy, 1776
Bismuth poisoning, mouth, 424
Bismuth subcitrate, Helicobacter pylori, 432
Bites
  bruises, 1868
  and stings, 1520–1526
    allergy, 1691
Bithionol, liver and lung flukes, 1513
Bitot's spots, 1194, 1677
Blackfan–Diamond syndrome, 856
Blackheads, demodicidosis, 1514–1515
Black locks albinism and sensorineural deafness syndrome, 1107
Black widow spider bites, 1524
Bladder, see also Neuropathic bladder
  abdominal examination, 32, 33
  carcinoma
    cyclophosphamide, 890
    schistosomiasis, 1509
  development, 934
  exstrophy, 256, 1779

innervation, 656
micturating cystourethrography, 1911
rhabdomyosarcoma, 915
schistosomiasis, 1508, 1509
ultrasonography, 1910
Bladderworm larva, see Cysticercus bovis
Blalock–Hanlon procedure, transposition of great arteries, 615
Blalock–Taussig operation, 617
Blaschko, lines of, 1618
Blastomycosis, 570, 1471 (Table), 1474–1475
Bleach, poisoning, 1709
Bleeding disorders, see Coagulation disorders
Bleeding time, 228
Bleomycin, toxic effects, 894 (Table)
Blepharitis, 1663
  ulcerative, 1675
Blepharophimosis, 76 (Table)
Blindness, 1657–1658, see also Visual impairment
  cerebral palsy, 761
  cortical, 273
  genetic, 46
  hydrocephalus, 666
  hypertensive retinopathy, 1675
  menarche, 1043
  neonate, investigation, 273
  prediction by visual evoked potentials, 243
  severely handicapped children affected, 14 (Table)
  very low birthweight, 171
Blinking, neonate, 241
Bliss symbolic system, 814
Blister beetles, toxins, 1525
Blisters, epidermolysis bullosa, 1622–1623
Blocks, developmental examination, 392, 393
Blood, 847–884, see also Hemopoiesis
  acid–base status, 419, see also Blood gases
  buffers, 417–418
  feces, 1936 (Table)
  neonate, 108
  storage temperature, 851 (Table)
Blood cultures, 1297–1298
  central venous line sepsis, 1224
  infective endocarditis, 631
  neonatal meningitis, 282
  neonatal sepsis, 276
  pneumonia, 567
  pyogenic osteitis, 1590
  salmonellosis, 1324
  technique, 1835
  typhoid fever, 1325–1326
Blood films
  African trypanosomiasis, 1456
  Chagas' disease, 1459
  malaria, 1452
  neonate, 223
Blood flow
  cerebral, 661, 698–699, 708
    fetal hypoxia response, 124
    fits, 673
    resistance index, 661, 707
    status epilepticus, 692
    ventilation, 1818
  Doppler ultrasonography, 1896
  fetal
    abdominal aorta, 115
    hypoxia response, 123–124
    middle cerebral artery, 115
  lung fields, 200
  regional cerebral, single photon emission computed tomography, 1909
  skin, preterm infant, 147
  uterine artery, 81
Blood fluke infection, see Schistosomiasis
Blood gases, 505, see also Blood, acid–base status

acute severe asthma, 548
fetus, cerebral circulation, 82
hypoglycemia, 297
neonatal care, 159, 160
respiratory distress syndrome, 178, 179
Blood group antigens, development, 223
Blood group incompatibility
  hemolytic disease of the newborn, 216–217
  neonate, 231–234
Blood islands, 221, 847
Blood loss
  acute, neonate, 224
  hookworm, 1489
Blood pressure
  cerebral blood flow, 699
  measurement, 20, 636–637, 1833–1834
  neonate, 199–200
  neonatal meningitis, 282
  normal values, 1940–1941 (Table)
  resuscitation, 1807, 1809
Blood product infusions, immunodeficiency, 1267
Blood sampling, 1834–1836
  calcium metabolism, 1053
  coagulation disorders, 227
  fetal scalp, 86, 119
  hemoglobin, 223
  leukemia, 871
  methemoglobinemia, 864
  preterm infant, anemia from, 225
  virology, 1351
Blood transfusion, see also Blood product infusions; Exchange transfusion
  acute renal failure, 976
  amounts, 851 (Table)
  bronchopulmonary dysplasia prevention, 195
  Chagas' disease, 1458
  congenital erythropoietic porphyria, 1144
  cytomegalovirus, 1366
  gastrointestinal hemorrhage, 433
  gentian violet, 1458, 1460
  hepatitis C virus, 1387
  intravascular fetal, 114
  malaria, 1453
  neonate, 224
    for sepsis, 1267, see also Exchange transfusion
    for respiratory distress syndrome, 179
  siderosis, 1201
  syphilis from, 1401
  terminal care, 928
  for thalassemia, 863
  trauma, 1809
Blood urea nitrogen, hypernatremia, 414
Blood vessels
  development, 847
    brain, 642
  neck, strokes, 711
Blood volume, 851 (Table)
  neonate, 222–223
  normal values, 1923 (Table)
  umbilical cord, clamping, 108, 222
Bloody tap, CSF white cells, 1290
Bloom's syndrome, 289, 1142, 1253, 1631
  neoplasms, 888 (Table), 1248 (Table)
Blount's disease, 1554
Blow-off valve, resuscitation equipment, 133
Blueberry muffin baby, 248
Blue bottle jellyfish, 1526
Blue diaper syndrome, 1122
Blush, cranial ultrasonography, very low birth weight, 172, 251
B lymphocytes
  activation, 1240
  antibody production, 1237
  fetus, 1240
  measurement, 1246
  neonate, 275
Bobble-headed doll, 651, 658, 771

Bochdalek foraminal hernia, 575, 1769, 1770 (Fig.)
  pulmonary hypoplasia, 191
Body fat, 1953
  adolescent body changes, 361–362
  marbling, growth hormone deficiency, 1016 (Fig.)
Body image, 382
Body length, fetal growth, 350
Body louse, 1518
Body mass index, 364, **1021, 1186**
Body proportions, 20
  abnormal, 999
Body surface area
  and drug dosage, 1954, 1980 (Table)
  GFR measurement, 942
  nomograms, 1950 (Fig.), 1951 (Fig.)
Body temperature, *see* Temperature
Body water, **402–403**
  normal values, 1923 (Table)
Bogalusa Heart Study, lipid levels, 1149
Boils, *see* Furunculosis
Bolus feeding, enteral nutrition, 1217–1218
Bonding, 1731
Bone age, **362,** 1012, 1915
  growth hormone deficiency, 373–374
  hypothyroidism, 1050
Bone alkaline phosphatase
  growth marker, 1012
  neonate, 302
Bone diseases, skull foramina, 811
Bone marrow
  aspiration, 850
    neonatal infection, 277
  chromosome preparations from, 49
  failure, 854–856
  hemopoiesis, 847
  Hodgkin's disease, 910
  immunodeficiency, 1245
  magnetic resonance imaging, 1898
  malaria, 1447–1448, 1451
  neonatal thrombocytopenia, 229
  neuroblastoma, 911
  sampling, **1844**
  suppression by cytotoxic drugs, 894 (Table)
  tumor diagnosis, 891
  typhoid fever, 1326
Bone marrow transplantation, 874–875, **1268–1270**
  acute leukemias, **874**
  adrenoleukodystrophy, 1174
  aplastic anemias, 856
  Fanconi's anemia, 854
  Hurler's syndrome, 1159
  immunosuppression, 1265
  infections, 533–534
  lysosomal disorders, 1102, 1158
  osteopetrosis, 1582
  thalassemia major, 863
Bone mass, peak, 1053
Bones
  calcitonin on, 1055
  congenital syphilis, 1412, 1413
  copper deficiency, 1202
  dysplasias, *see* Skeletal dysplasias
  Gaucher disease, 1166
  hemoglobinopathies, 862
  hydatid disease, 1505
  imaging, **1914–1917**
  infarction, sickle cell disease, 862
  leukemia, 868
  magnetic resonance imaging, 1898, 1916
  Menkes' kinky hair syndrome, 1146
  mineral content, measurement, 302
  nephroblastoma metastases, 913
  neuroblastoma, 911
  neurofibromatosis, 800
  oxalosis, 947
  pain, mefenamic acid, 928
  sarcomas, second primary tumors, 898 (Table)

scintigraphy, 1913, **1915–1916**
sodium, 408 (Table)
syphilis, 1407–1408
  congenital, 1412, 1413
tuberculosis, 1336, **1345–1346,** 1592
tumor incidence, 886 (Table)
Bonnevie-Ulrich syndrome, 830 (Table)
Booking, antenatal care, 80–81
Boomslangs, bites, 1522, 1523
Booster phenomenon, tuberculin test, 1338
Borderline leprosy, 1310
Bordetella pertussis, 1315
  specimens, 1298
Boric acid
  poisoning, 1708
  urine specimen bottles, 951
Bornholm disease, **1382**
  chest pain, 509
Boron, 1185 (Table)
Borrelia afzelli, 1313
Borrelia burgdorferi, emergence, 1279 (Table), *see also* Lyme disease
Borrelia garinii, 1313
Borrelia specific antibody, 1612
Borrelia spp., relapsing fever, 1322
Bot fly, 1514
Botryoid rhabdomyosarcoma, 916, 993–994
Bottle caries, 1189
Bottle feeding, *see also* Formula feeding
  cleft lip and palate, 1797
  developing countries, respiratory tract infections, 559
Bottle-sterilizing tablets, poisoning, 1711
Bottom shufflers, 667
Botulinum toxin
  cerebral palsy, 759–760
  floppy baby syndrome, 726
  squint, 1660
Botulism, **1301–1302**
'Bouafle' group, trypanosomes, 1454
Bounding pulses, 32, 586
Bovine pro-opiomelanocortin, 1038
Bovine serum albumin, antibodies to, 327
Bovine surfactant (Survanta), 179
Bowel movements
  history taking, 17
  normal frequencies, 461
Bowel sounds, 33
Bowlby, J., attachment theory, 1731
Bow legs (genu varum), 38, **1553**
Box jellyfish, 1526
Brachial plexus, birth trauma, 123, 721–722
Brachycephaly, 21 (Fig.), 1560
Brachydactyly, 39, 76 (Table), 1546 (Table), **1548**
Bradycardia
  at birth, 135, 139
  carditis, 1598
  fetus, 86, 133
  neonate
    apnea, 197
    management, 205
  respiratory disorders, 511
  resuscitation, 523
  sinus, 624
  treatment, 627–628
Bradykinesia, 769
Brain, *see also* Central nervous system
  abscess
    neonatal meningitis, 282
    specimens, 1298
  biopsy
    encephalitis, 1352
    viral infections, 1376
  development, 107, **641–645**
    environmental factors, **667,** 827–828
    growth, 363, 644, 645
    stimulation, 828
  herniations, 698, 708, 812
  second primary tumors, 898 (Table)
  shaking injury, 701–702

shrinkage, hypernatremia, 414
swelling
  birth asphyxia, 130–131
  trauma, 1810
Brain damage, **1810,** *see also* Cerebral palsy
  alexia, 821
  behavioral disturbance from, adolescents, **1761**
  and development, 386
  hypernatremia, 415
  learning disorder, 820
  mental retardation, 828–829
  near-drowning, 1717–1718
  neonate, **249–252**
  non-accidental injury, 704
  nonketotic hyperglycinemia, 305
  preterm infant, 102
  syntactic dysgraphia, 824
  vaccination, 343
Brain death, 709
Brainstem
  akinetic mutism, 815
  coning, 698
    upward, 663
  failure, 703
  flaccid bulbar palsy, 811–812
  gliomas, **903–904**
  neural tube defects, 657
  shaking injury, 701
  tumors, signs, 900
Brainstem auditory evoked potentials, 244, 817
  audiometry, 1683
Braking, expiration, 505
Branched chain amino acids
  hyperinsulinemia, 296
  metabolism disorders, **1116–1118**
Branchial arches, 206
Branchial remnants, 1783
Branching enzyme deficiency, 1138–1139
Brazelton, states of alertness, 235 (Table)
Brazilian purpuric fever, 1307
Breakbone fever (dengue fever), **1389**
Breaking bad news to parents, **1747**
Break point, cerebral blood flow autoregulation, 699
Breast
  carcinoma
    and breast-feeding, 327
    Klinefelter's syndrome, 62
    oral contraceptive pill, 995
    second primary, 898 (Table)
    soft tissue sarcomas, 889, 915
  development, 359, 360, 989, 1000
    premature, 1027–1028
  disorders, feeding difficulties, 209
  neonatal gestation age, 42 (Fig.)
  neurofibromatosis, 800
  puberty, 357
Breast-feeding, 111, **113, 326–331,** 1188
  acute diarrhea, 453
  atopic disease, flawed studies, **1703**
  atopic eczema, 1696
  bilirubin, normal range, 218
  bronchiolitis, 564
  cleft lip and palate, 1796–1797
  contraindications, 329–330
  cystic fibrosis, 1207
  developing countries, 1892
  failure to thrive, 331
  HIV infection, 288, 329
  management, 328–329
  pneumonia, 568
  preterm infant, 153
  prevalence, 326
  promotion, 339
  SGA baby, 137
  social class, 15 (Table), 326
  and sudden infant death syndrome, 327, 1720
  test weighing, 111
  and urinary tract infections, 950
  vitamin K, 230

Breast milk, **112,** 326, 327 (Table), 1188, *see also* Lactation
  amino acids, 1119, 1120 (Table)
  calcium absorption from, 301
  calcium and phosphorus, 304
  composition, 330 (Table), 332–333, 1942–1943 (Table)
  cow's milk proteins, 1699
  fat absorption from, 207–208
  fortification, 152
  lactoferrin, 1234
  vs necrotizing enterocolitis, 210
  potassium, 145
  preterm infant, 152
  selenium, 1202
  sodium, 143, 332
  solute load, 333
  yield, 328
Breast milk jaundice, **219–220**
Breast milk substitutes, *see* Formula milks
Breast nodule diameter, neonatal gestation age, 40 (Table)
Breath, history taking, 17
Breath-holding attacks, **672**
Breathing, **505–506**
  control, **196–198**
  examination, 19
  fetus, 495, 496
  noisy, **507–509**
  resuscitation, **522–523, 524–525,** 1807
  sleep, *see* Sleep, breathing
  trauma, **1809**
Breathing exercises, 521
  asthma, 521, 545
Breathing movements, lung development, 175, 191 (Table)
Breathlessness, history taking, 17, **509**
Breath sounds, 30, **512**
  cystic fibrosis, 554
Breath tests
  carbon-13 urea, *Helicobacter pylori,* 431
  hydrogen, 448
Breech delivery, **87–88**
  internal hemorrhage, 224
Breech presentation, 83
  preterm delivery, 120
  sternomastoid tumor, 1784
Bretylium, 526
Bricks, developmental examination, 392, 393
Bright thalamus, 251
Brill–Zinsser disease, 1390 (Table), **1391**
British ability scales, 400
British Births Child Study, 1852
British Institute of Funeral Directors, 175
British language development scales, 400
British Paediatric Association Surveillance Unit, 1281, **1850**
British picture vocabulary tests, 400
Brodie's abscess, 1590
BROMIDA scintigraphy, biliary tract, 1907
Bromide, 1185 (Table)
Bromocriptine
  growth hormone secretion, 1012
  tall stature, 1020
Brompheniramine, administration, 1961 (Table)
Bromsulfthalein secretion, hyperbilirubinemias, 1145
Bronchi, *see also* Airways, responsiveness
  biopsy, 520
  ciliated epithelium, 532
  congenital abnormalities, **573**
  development, 175, **494,** 495, 496
  provocation tests, 500 (Fig.), **501**
  selective intubation, pulmonary interstitial emphysema, 189
  smooth muscle
    asthma, **538**
    development, 497
  stenosis, 573–574
  tuberculosis, 1341

Bronchial breathing, 30, 512
Bronchial casts, 507
Bronchiectasis, 532, **576**
  causes, 575
  Chagas' disease, 1458
  computed tomography, 1900 (Fig.)
Bronchioles, diameter *vs* age, 496 (Table)
Bronchiolitis, 489, 559, **564–565**
  chest movement, 512
  community *vs* hospital care, 1804
  measles, 1354
  mortality, 490 (Table)
  obliterative, 565, **576**
  predisposing factors, 498
  respiratory syncytial virus, 564, 1370
Bronchitis, 489, **565**
  measles, 1354
  postneonatal mortality, 5 (Table)
Bronchoalveolar lavage, 520
  alveolar proteinosis, 578
  asthma, 537
  pneumonia in immunocompromised
    patient 534
Bronchoconstriction, anaphylaxis, 1702
Bronchodilator responsiveness
  asthma, 543
  cystic fibrosis, 554
Bronchodilators, 545–546
  acute severe asthma, 547–548
  cystic fibrosis, 558
  and episodic wheeze, 549
  repeat prescription monitoring, 544
Bronchogenic cysts, 192, 574
Bronchography, 514
Bronchomalacia, 495, 512, **574–575**
Bronchopulmonary aspergilloma, 1474
Bronchopulmonary aspergillosis, allergic,
    550, 556
Bronchopulmonary dysplasia, **193–195**
  definitions, 194
  vs gastroesophageal reflux, 212
  metabolic bone disease, 302
  respiratory distress syndrome, 181
  water balance, 142, 143
Bronchopulmonary schistosomiasis, 1510
Bronchopulmonary-vascular
    malformations, **573–574**
Bronchoscopy, 519–520
  pulmonary tuberculosis, 1342
Bronchovesicular breath sounds, 30
Brønsted–Lowry terminology, acids and
    bases, 415
Bronzed diabetes, 1147
Broselow tape measure, 526
Brotherston Report, 1853
Brown adipose tissue, 146
Brown's syndrome, 1660
Brown widow spider bites, 1524
Brucellosis, **1302–1303**
  FUO investigations, 1283 (Table)
Brudzinski's sign, 38
Brugia malayi, 1496 (Table), 1498
Brugia timori, 1498
Bruises
  birth trauma, 120–121
  non-accidental injury, 1868
    head injury, 700
Bruits
  arteriovenous fistulae, 605
  arteriovenous malformation, 711
  carotid, 594
  liver, 471
Brush border, carbohydrate digestion, 437
Brush border oligopeptidase, neonate, 207
Brushfield's spots, Down syndrome, 23,
    27 (Fig.), 55
Bruton's agammaglobulinemia
  neoplasms, 889 (Table)
  respiratory tract infections, 533
Bruton tyrosine kinase gene defect, 1255
B scan, *see* Cross-sectional
    echocardiography
Bubonic plague, 1318
Buccal mucosa, 424–425

'Bucket handle' fractures, 1914
Buckler–Tanner growth standards, 1014
Budesonide, administration, 1961 (Table)
Budin, 'goutte de lait,' 1861
Budin, Pierre, neonatal unit (1895), 96
Buffer base, 419, 420
Buffers, **416–418**
  bicarbonate, 504
  renal tubular acidosis, 944
Buffy coat smear, neonatal sepsis, 276
Bulbar palsy, flaccid, 810–812
Bulbar poliomyelitis, 1380
Bulbourethral glands, gonorrhea, 1425
Bulimia nervosa, **1759**
Bullae, 577
  incontinentia pigmenti, 803
Bull ant bites and stings, 1524
Bullneck appearance, diphtheria, 1306
Bullous disease of childhood, chronic,
    1640
Bullous ichthyosis, 1620, 1621 (Table)
Bullous impetigo, 1634
Bullous varicella, 1361
Bundle branch block, 626
Bundle of His, conduction defects, **626**
Bung eye, 1499
Buphthalmos (infantile glaucoma), 23, 27
    (Fig.), 43, 264, **1672–1673**
Bupivacaine, 1832
Buprenorphine, administration, 1961
    (Table)
Burden of disease, developing countries,
    1276, 1280 (Table)
Burkholderia cepacia, 1321
  cystic fibrosis, 555
Burkitt's lymphoma, 891, 906
  incidence, 886 (Table)
  presentation, 907
Burns, **1714–1715, 1798–1800**
  accident and emergency care, **1813**
  hemolysis, 864
  lungs, **571–572**
  non-accidental injury, 700, **1868**
Burrows, scabies, 1638
Buruli ulcer, 1349–1350
'Busoga' group, trypanosomes, 1454
Busulfan, on fetus and neonate, 91 (Table)
Butterfly rash, 1605
Button batteries, poisoning, 1710
Button kidney, small, 254
Butyrophenones, 1748 (Table)
Buzzers, enuresis, 1743
Byler disease, 1145

C1-esterase inhibitor deficiency, **1175,**
    1262
C3b (complement), 1232
C3 nephritic factor, 1263
C3 receptor deficiency, 1263
Cadaverinuria, 1121
Café au lait macules, neurofibromatosis,
    798, **800,** 1628, 1798
Café au lait patches, and tuberous
    sclerosis, 1625
Café au lait pigmentation, congenital
    syphilis, 1412
Cafergot suppositories, migraine, 717
    (Table)
Caffeine
  administration, neonate, 1956 (Table)
  for apnea attacks, 198
  migraine, 718
Caffey's disease, **1583–1585**
Cairn's syndrome, 737
Calabar swelling, 1497
Calcaneonavicular joint, fusion, 1555
Calcaneum, osteochondrosis, **1595**
Calciferol, *see* Vitamin D
Calcification
  basal ganglia, **774**
  cysticercosis, 1501
  dermatomyositis, 1644

dermatomyositis-polymyositis, 1608
liver tumors, 924
peritoneum, 1902
  meconium ileus, 1776
pineal gland, 1044
  tumors, 904
schistosomiasis, 1509 (Fig.)
Sturge–Weber syndrome, 802
toxoplasmosis, 1465
tuberculosis, 1335, 1341
tuberous sclerosis, 801
Calciopenic rickets, **1056, 1057, 1058**
  hypoparathyroidism, 1057
Calcitonin, **1055**
  administration, 1961 (Table)
  disorders, 1057
  fetus, 298, 1004
  medullary carcinoma of thyroid, 1052
  neonate, 299
Calcitriol
  administration, 1961 (Table)
  osteopetrosis, 1583
Calcium, 1185 (Table)
  abnormal excretion, 1058
  absorption, cows milk-free diets, 1700
  cell death, birth asphyxia, 127
  concentrations, 404 (Table), 406 (Table)
  concentration units, 1921
  deficiency, **1200**
  fetus, 1004
  gastroenteritis, 1294, 1297
  for hyperkalemia, 145
  loading test, 1938 (Table)
  metabolism, **1053–1059**
  neonate
    absorption, 301–302
    late neonatal tetany, 300
    metabolism disorders, **298–300**
    serum levels, 1053
  normal values, 1923–1924 (Table)
    amniotic fluid, 1937 (Table)
    cerebrospinal fluid, 1933 (Table)
    stools, 1936 (Table)
    urine, 1930 (Table)
  osteopenia of prematurity, plasma
    levels, 302
  parenteral nutrition, 1221, 1222 (Table),
    1223 (Table)
  preterm supplements, 154–155
  Recommended Dietary Allowances,
    1949 (Table)
  reference nutrient intakes, 1947 (Table)
  requirements, 1181 (Table)
    preterm infant, 152 (Table), 301–302
  restriction, osteopetrosis, 1582
  serum, forms, 1053
  sources, 1185 (Table)
  supplements
    cow's milk-free diets, 1700
    neonate, 299, 304
  tubular reabsorption, 943
  in utero accretion, 301
Calcium carbonate, chronic renal failure,
    980
Calcium channel blockers, **131,** 627
  cerebral edema, 1811
  mdr-1 partial reversal, 893
  migraine, 717 (Table)
  for preterm labor, 116
Calcium chloride
  neonate, administration, 1956 (Table)
  osmolality, 405
  resuscitation, doses, 526 (Table), 527
    (Fig.)
Calcium : creatinine ratio, urine, 943, 959
  normal values, 1930 (Table)
Calcium gluconate
  acute renal failure, 975
  administration, 1057, 1961 (Table)
    neonate, 1956 (Table)
  exchange transfusion, 1839
  hyperkalemia, 259, 415, 975
  hypocalcemia, 299, 300, 975, 1961
    (Table)

Latrodectus bites, 1524
  resuscitation, 135, 527 (Fig.)
Calcium glycerophosphate, 1221
Calcium losing tubulopathy, *see* Bartter's
    syndrome
Calcium polystyrene sulfonate,
    administration, 1961 (Table)
Calcium resonium
  administration, 259
    neonate, 1956 (Table)
  hyperkalemia
    acute renal failure, 975
    enema, 145 (Table)
Calculi, *see also* Biliary calculi;
    Nephrolithiasis; Urolithiasis
  calcium hyperabsorption, 1200
  cystinuria, 1121
  hyperoxaluria, 1112, 1113
  oxalosis, 1112
  salivary, 1784
Calcutta, street children, 1887–1888
Calipers, cerebral palsy, 757
Callus, 1867
  time of appearance, 703
Calories, *see also* Energy, requirements;
    Protein–energy malnutrition
  bronchopulmonary dysplasia
    prevention, 195
  deficiency, neonatal jaundice, 218
  fluid intake relationship, 403
  inborn errors of metabolism,
    management, 307
  preterm infant
    milk formulae, 152
    requirements, 151 (Table)
    supplements, 154
Calorie to nitrogen ratio, preterm
    requirements, 157
Calpol preparations, migraine, 717 (Table)
Calvé's disease, 1594–1595
cAMP, *see* Cyclic adenosine
    monophosphate
Camphor, poisoning, 1710
Camptodactyly, 76 (Table), 1546 (Table),
    1549
Camptomelic dysplasia, **1572,** 1573 (Fig.)
  inheritance, 1566 (Table)
Campylobacter spp.
  antibiotic, 454 (Table)
  emergence, 1279 (Table)
  encephalopathy, 683, 693
  Guillain–Barré syndrome, 726
  United Kingdom, 1277 (Fig.)
Camurati-Engelmann disease, 1582
    (Table)
Canada, breast-feeding rates, 326 (Table)
Canal of Nuck, hydrocele, 1789
Canavan's disease, 791 (Table), 1116
Cancrum oris, **1354**
Candidiasis, **1433–1434, 1470–1472**
  AIDS, 1395, 1397
  antifungal drug resistance, 1530
  diarrhea, 1294, 1295
  endophthalmitis, 1678
  and hypoparathyroidism, 1057, 1470
  and inhaled corticosteroids, 546
  mouth, 425
  mucocutaneous, chronic, 1243 (Table),
    1251, 1637
  myeloperoxidase deficiency, 1260
  neonate, 276, 277, **289,** 1433, 1470
  parenteral nutrition, 1590
  respiratory tract, **535–536**
  sexually transmitted, detection or
    exclusion, 1399
  skin, **1637**
  vs tonsillitis, 1687
  upper respiratory tract, specimens,
    1298
  vulvovaginitis, 988
Canthal index, 22
Cantharidin, 1525
Capillariasis, **1495**
  larval disease, 1484 (Table)

Capillary blood, **1834**
  diabetes mellitus monitoring, 1079
  gases measurement, 160
  hematological assessment, 849
  hemoglobin, 223
Capillary hemangioma, intracranial, 710
Capillary malformation (port-wine stain), 1620, 1798
Capsular antigens, *Haemophilus influenzae*, 1307–1308
Captia Syphilis M (commercial IgM test), 1404, 1405
Captopril
  administration, 1961 (Table)
  cyanotic heart disease, dosage, 202 (Table)
  for cystinuria, 1121
  glomerular disease in scleroderma, 966
  heart failure, 599
  hypertension, 637 (Table), 638
    renal, 973
Caput succedaneum, 21 (Fig.), 121
Carate, see Pinta
Carbamazepine, 686
  administration, 1961 (Table)
    neonate, 1956 (Table)
  hyposensitization, 1703
  mania, 1755
  migraine, 719
  poisoning, 1709
  therapeutic ranges, 1936 (Table)
Carbamino compounds, carbon dioxide as, 417
Carbamylglutamate, for urea cycle disorders, 1110
Carbamyl phosphate synthetases, 1110, 1141
Carbaryl
  head lice, 1518
  pubic lice, 1519
Carbidopa
  dihydropteridine reductase deficiency, 1106
  tyrosine hydroxylase deficiency, 1107
Carbimazole, 1051
  administration, 1961 (Table)
    neonate, 1956 (Table)
  neonatal hyperthyroidism, 1051
  transplacental, 1005
Carbohydrate-deficient glycoprotein syndrome, 1156, **1175**
Carbohydrate exchange system, 1077
Carbohydrates
  absorption, 207
    preterm infant, 151
  dietary, **1182–1183**
    acute porphyrias, 1143
    diabetes mellitus, 1209–1210
    enteropathies, 1214–1215
    sources, 1182 (Table)
  digestion, 423
    small intestine, 436–437
  feces, 448
  malabsorption, **445–446**, 448
  metabolism, **1071–1084**
    disorders, **1131–1135**
    neonate, 471
    progressive ataxias, 765
  parenteral nutrition, 1220, 1222 (Table)
  preterm requirements, 158
  proportion in energy intake, 1180
  puberty, 1028
  requirements, preterm infant, 151 (Table)
Carbohydrate utilization tests, *Neisseria gonorrhoeae*, 1423
Carbomix, 1707
Carbon-13 urea breath test, *Helicobacter pylori*, 431
Carbon dioxide, *see also* $PaCO_2$; PCO_2
  combining power, cerebrospinal fluid, 1934 (Table)
  gas exchange, 160
  measurement, 505

normal values, 1924 (Table)
  plasma content, 417
  production rate, 417
  transport, 502
Carbonic acid/bicarbonate buffer system, 416, **417**
Carbonic anhydrase, erythrocytes and renal tubules, 417–418
Carbonic anhydrase II deficiency, **1177**
Carbonic anhydrase II gene, osteopetrosis, 1582
Carbon monoxide
  diffusing capacity, 505
  poisoning, 572, 1711, 1813
    dyskinesia, 754
Carboxyhemoglobin, normal values, 1924 (Table)
Carbuncles, 1635
Carcinogenesis, 340
  transplacental, 289
Carcinoid syndrome, pellagra-like symptoms, 1114
Card agglutination test for trypanosomiasis, 1456
Cardiac arrest, **1807–1808**, 1815, *see also* Resuscitation
  hyperkalemia, 412
Cardiac catheterization, **593–594**
  atrial septal defect, 602
  atrioventricular septal defect, 604
  vs Doppler ultrasonography, pulmonary stenosis, 608
  neonate, 201
    interventional, 205–206
  pulmonary angiography, 514
  ventricular septal defect, 601
Cardiac failure, *see* Heart failure
Cardiac output, 1819
  acute renal failure, 974
  neonate, management, 205
  reduced at birth, **135**, 139
  ventilation, 1818
Cardiac position, 598, **612–613**
Cardiac prostheses, antibiotic prophylaxis, 631
Cardiac stimulation
  at birth, 135
  catecholamines, 1069
Cardiac surgery, *see* Heart surgery
Cardiac tamponade
  after cardiac surgery, 1822
  pneumopericardium, 189
Cardiolipin antigen tests, syphilis, **1402**
  monitoring, 1404, 1410
Cardiomegaly, 31, 587
Cardiomyopathy, **633–634**
  angiotensin converting enzyme inhibitors, 599
  Chagas' disease, 1458
  Friedreich's ataxia, 765
  hemolytic uremic syndrome, 977, 978
  neonate, 205
Cardiomyotomy, Heller's, 429
Cardiopulmonary bypass, 164–165
  hypothermia, 149
  postoperative care, 1822
Cardiopulmonary resuscitation, *see* Resuscitation
Cardiothoracic ratio, 587–588
Cardiotocography, 86–87, 115, **117–119, 124–125**, 129
Cardiotoxicity
  cytotoxic drugs, 894 (Table), **896**, 900
  potassium, 259
  sodium stibogluconate, 1462–1463
Cardiovascular support, **1819–1821**
Cardiovascular system
  disorders, **584–640**
    with apnea, 197 (Table)
    and birthweight, 369
    Marfan's syndrome, 1589
  Doppler ultrasonography, 1896
  examination, **30–32**, 585–587
    neonate, **199–200**

fetal-neonatal transition, **107**
  magnetic resonance imaging, 1898
  neonatal disease, **198–206**
    management, 205–206
Cardioversion, 527 (Fig.)
  paroxysmal supraventricular tachycardia, 627
Carditis, acute, **628–629, 1597–1598**
Care of Next Infant program, 1723
Care Orders, 1875
Care (statutory), **1857–1858, 1875**, 1876
  children in, 15 (Table)
Carfecillin, administration, 1961 (Table)
Caribbean immigrants, 1866
Caries, *see also* Bottle caries
  fluoride, 1202
Carnitine, *see also* L-carnitine
  deficiency, **736**, 1188
  depletion in organic acidurias, 1119
  for Fanconi's syndrome, 1122
  and parenteral nutrition, 1220
  supplements, 297, 1112
  transport defects, 735–736, 1129
Carnitine/acylcarnitine translocase deficiency, 1129
Carnitine cycle, defects, 1129
Carnitine palmitoyl transferases, 1128
  deficiencies, 736, **1129**, 1132
Carnosine, 1114, 1115
β-Carotene, erythropoietic protoporphyria, 1631
Carotenemia, familial, 1148
Carotenes, normal values, 1924 (Table)
Carotid arteries, stroke, 711
Carotid body, neural crest cells, 642
Carotid bruit, 594
Carpenter syndrome, 1561
Carriers
  amebiasis, 1467
  β-hemolytic streptococci, 1330
  cystic fibrosis, 552
  diphtheria, 1307
  Duchenne muscular dystrophy, 732
  hemophilia A, 880
  hepatitis B virus, 1386, 1387
  herpes simplex virus, 1436, 1437
  inborn errors of metabolism, 1101
  maple syrup urine disease, 1101
  salmonellosis, 1323
  Staphylococcus aureus, 1328–1329
  Streptococcus pneumoniae, 1319
  Streptococcus pyogenes, 560
  typhoid fever, 1324, 1326
  viral hepatitis type B, 476, **477**
Cartilage, **1567**
Cartilage–hair hypoplasia, 856, 1242 (Table), 1254, 1578
Carukia barnesi, 1526
Carybdeid jellyfish, 1526
Casals necklace, 1198
Caseation, tuberculosis, 1335, 1336, 1341
Case-control studies, 1851
Caseins, *vs* whey proteins, infant formula, 332, 1188
Case notes, *see* Record keeping
Casoni test, 1506
Casts, hematuria, 958
Cast syndrome (superior mesenteric artery syndrome), **1787–1788**
Catalase, peroxisomal disorders, 1172 (Table)
Cataract, 472 (Table), **1667–1670**
  cerebellar ataxias, 753
  from corticosteroids, 1669, 1677
  diabetes mellitus, 1669, 1674
  galactitol, 1133, 1134
  hypoparathyroidism, 1674
  inborn errors of metabolism, 305
  mental retardation, 835 (Table)
  organisms, neonate, 284 (Table)
  rubella, 24 (Fig.), 1668
  severely handicapped children affected, 14 (Table)

sunflower, 1674
Catarrhal conjunctivitis, acute, 1663
Catarrhal jaundice (hepatitis A virus), **476, 1386**
Catarrhal phase, pertussis, 1315
CATCH 22 syndrome, 596
Catch-up growth, 364, 1014
  low birthweight, 368
Catecholamines, **1069**
  as hormones, 997 (Table)
  intensive care, 1820
  on lung maturation, 176
  neuroblastoma, 911–912
  normal values, 1930 (Table)
  urine, 1930–1931 (Table)
Caterpillars, 1526
Cat eye syndrome, 830 (Table)
Catheterization, *see also* Cardiac catheterization; Central venous lines; Urethra, catheterization
  transtracheal, 507
Catheters
  enema continence, 463
  peritoneal dialysis, 259
  umbilical vessels, 231, **1838**
Catheter specimen of urine, 950, 1299
Cats, 1519 (Table)
  allergens, 1695
  Toxoplasma gondii, 1464
Cat-scratch disease, **1519–1520**
Cat urine odor, 1117
Cauda equina, ependymomas, 902
Caudal regression syndrome, 641
Caudate nucleus, necrosis, 773
Caustic soda, poisoning, 1710
Cautery, epistaxis, 1684
Cavernous hemangiomas
  disseminated intravascular coagulation, 231
  intracranial, 710–711
C-banding, 49
CD3 deficiencies, 1242 (Table), 1250
CD4 : CD8 ratio, T lymphocytes, 1246
  HIV infection, 1264
CD4 lymphocytopenia, idiopathic, 1252
CD4 receptor, AIDS, 1393
CD5 surface marker, B lymphocytes, 1237
CD7 deficiency, 1250
CD40 ligand deficiency (hyperIgM syndromes), 1242 (Table), 1256
CD antibodies, 1231–1232
  for graft-*versus*-host disease, 1269
CD surface markers
  defects, 1250
  T lymphocytes, 1238–1239
    neonate, 1240–1241
Cebocephaly, 649
Cefaclor, 1961 (Table)
Cefadroxil, 1961 (Table)
Cefixime, 1961 (Table)
  gonorrhea, 1427 (Table)
Cefotaxime, 1955 (Table), 1961 (Table)
  bacterial meningitis, 1291
  CNS infections, 696
  facial cellulitis, 1635
  gonorrhea, 1428 (Table)
  Lyme disease, 1314 (Table)
  neonate, 279 (Table)
  meningitis, 247, 282
  osteomyelitis, 283
  urinary tract infections, 952 (Table)
Cefoxitin, environmental mycobacteria, 1350
Ceftazidime
  administration, 1955 (Table), 1961 (Table)
  bacterial meningitis, 1291
  cystic fibrosis, 558 (Table)
  neonate, 279 (Table)
  pseudomonas pneumonia, 185
  urinary tract infections, 261
Ceftizoxime, gonorrhea, 1428 (Table)

Ceftriaxone
  administration, 1961 (Table)
  bacterial meningitis, 1291
  gonorrhea, 1427 (Table), 1428
  Lyme disease, 1314 (Table)
  neonate, 279 (Table)
  ophthalmia neonatorum, 1429
  typhoid fever, 1326
Cefuroxime
  administration, 1955 (Table), 1962
    (Table)
  bacterial meningitis, 1291
  gonorrhea, 1427
  neonatal meningitis, 247
  urinary tract infections, 952 (Table)
CELF (clinical evaluation of language
    function), 400
Celiac axis angiography, 447
Celiac disease, **439–441**
  abnormal gait, 753
  vs cystic fibrosis, 554
  dermatitis herpetiformis, 1641
  dietary management, 1214 (Table)
  ESPGAN protocol, 441
  iron deficiency, 1201
  severely handicapped children affected,
    14 (Table)
  water secretion, 436
Cell division, genetics, 47–48
Cell-mediated immunity, 273–275
  disorders, 1248–1254, *see also named
    disorders*
  HIV infection, 1393
  leprosy, 1309–1310
  neonate, 1240–1241
  nonspecific, **1234–1235**
  specific, 1237–1239
  tests, 1246–1248
  tuberculosis, 1336
Cell membranes, 405
Cellulitis, 1329, **1635**
  vs erysipelas, 1332
  orbit, 1661
Cellulose tape method, enterobiasis, 1488
Censuses, 1848, *see also* Office of
    Population, Censuses and Surveys
Centers for Disease Control
  HIV infection classification, 1393, **1395
    (Table)**
  Sexually Transmitted Disease Treatment
    Guidelines, maternal herpes
    simplex, 1441–1442
Centile charts
  blood pressure, 636
  growth, 353, 465, 1014–1015
CentiMorgans (map units), 72
Centipedes, 1526
Central Advisory Council for Education,
    nursery schools, 1861
Central apnea, 197 (Table)
Central core disease, 734, 735 (Table)
Central deafness, acquired, *see* Auditory
    agnosia
Central hypoventilation syndrome
  congenital, **530–531**
  drug-induced, 772
Centralization of care, neoplasms, 885
Central nervous system, *see also* Brain;
    Radiotherapy, central nervous
    system
  acute lymphoblastic leukemia, 872–873
  acute myeloblastic leukemia therapy,
    874
  African trypanosomiasis, 1455
  AIDS, 1394, 1397
  breathing, 505–506
  burns, 1799
  Chagas' disease, 1459
  congenital malformations, 15 (Table),
    645–657
    diabetes insipidus, 1040 (Table)
    postneonatal mortality, 5 (Table)
  cryptococcosis, 1476
  cytotoxic drugs, 896–897, 899

development, 107, 381, **641–645**
  and breast milk, 152, 327
  chronic renal failure, 981
  malnutrition, 1193
  outcome of apneic attacks, 198
  outcome of prematurity, **165–172**
  outcome of respiratory distress
    syndrome, 182
  thyroid hormones, 1003
developmental disorders, **666–670**
disorders, **641–846**
  with apnea, 197 (Table)
  growth failure, 1017
  hypothyroidism from, 1049
  precocious puberty, 1029
  and vaccination, 342 (Table)
Duchenne muscular dystrophy, 729
and endocrine system, 997
Gaucher disease, 1166
glucose transport defects, 1123
glycolysis defects, 1131–1132
growth failure, causes, 1017
growth hormone regulation, 1012
hemolytic uremic syndrome, 977–978
hereditary lactic acidosis, 1125
hydatid disease, 1505
hypoglycemia
  damage, 293
  SGA baby, 137
imaging, **1907–1909**
incontinentia pigmenti, 1626
intracranial teratomas, 922
leukemia, 871
lymphomas, 908
  chemotherapy, 909
magnetic resonance imaging, 1898,
  1908
neoplasms, **900–907**
  ataxia, 763
  cerebrospinal fluid, 1290
  headache, 715
  hemorrhage into, 709–710
  incidence, 886 (Table)
  neonate, 292 (Table)
    incidence, 290 (Table)
  strokes, 714
phenylketonuria, 1103
puberty, 1026–1027
racemose cyst, 1501
schistosomiasis, 1510
shigellosis, 1328
syphilis, *see also* Neurosyphilis
  congenital, 1412
tuberculosis, **1344–1345**
viral infections, 694, **1375–1378**
Wilson's disease, 1146
Central pontine myelinosis, 797 (Table)
Central precocious puberty, 1029–1030
Central progressive cerebellar ataxias,
  766–767
Central retinal artery occlusion,
  polyarteritis nodosa, 1674
Central Statistical Office, 1848
Central tapetoretinal degenerations, **1666**
Central venous lines
  cancer treatment, infection avoidance,
    894
  fracture of, 1225
  occlusion, 1225
  parenteral nutrition, 159, **1223–1225**
  sepsis, 1224–1225
  technique, **1837–1838**
Central venous pressure, 1819
  acute blood loss, 224
Centric fusions, *see* Robertsonian
  translocations
Centrifugal lipodystrophy, 1156
Centromeres, 53
  staining, 49
Centronuclear myopathy, 734, 735 (Table)
Cephalexin, administration, 1962 (Table)
Cephalhematoma, 21 (Fig.), 121
Cephalhydrocele (growing skull fracture),
  700, 707

Cephalosporins, 568
  dosage considerations, 1527
  neonatal meningitis, 282
  site of action, 1527
Cephradine
  administration, 1962 (Table)
  urinary tract infections, 952 (Table)
Ceramidase deficiency, Farber syndrome,
  1167
Ceramide, 1162
Cercariae, schistosomiasis, 1508
Cerebellum
  abscesses, 762
  agenesis, 753
  astrocytomas, **902–903**
  ataxias, **749–753**
    acute, 762
  congenital malformations, **645–647**
  degeneration, GM2 gangliosidosis,
    765–766
  developmental disorders, 669
  fits, 674
  hemorrhage, 251
  primitive neuroectodermal tumors, *see*
    Medulloblastomas
  surgery, 760
  tumors, signs, 900
  vermis, ultrasonography, 1908
Cerebral abnormalities, **647–651,** *see also*
  Cortical dysplasias
  high body temperature, 150
Cerebral angiography, **1909**
  aneurysms, 710
Cerebral arteries, fetus, Doppler
  ultrasonography, 82
Cerebral arteriovenous malformation, *see*
  Vein of Galen aneurysm
Cerebral atrophy
  cerebral palsy, 171
  periventricular hemorrhage, 664
Cerebral blood flow, **661, 698–699,** 708,
  see also Cerebral hemodynamics
  fetal hypoxia response, 124
  fits, 673
  status epilepticus, 692
  ventilation, 1818
Cerebral cortex, *see* Cortical dysplasias
Cerebral cysticercosis, 1501, 1502
Cerebral dominance, 645
  delay, 820–821
Cerebral dysrhythmia, **673–676**
Cerebral edema
  birth asphyxia, 126
  diabetic ketoacidosis, 1076
  hypernatremia, 414
  infarction, 714
  magnetic resonance imaging, 1909
  non-accidental injury, 701–702
  trauma, 703, 1810
Cerebral function monitoring, prognosis in
  birth asphyxia, 132
Cerebral function monitors, 243
Cerebral gigantism (Sotos syndrome), 832
  (Table), 833, 1043
Cerebral hemodynamics, *see also* Cerebral
  blood flow; Cerebral perfusion
  pressure
  birth asphyxia, 128–129
Cerebral infarction, 709
  germinal matrix hemorrhage, 250
  neonatal seizures, 245
Cerebral injury, *see* Brain damage
Cerebral lesions, vomiting, 212
Cerebral malaria, **1450–1451**
Cerebral metabolism
  hypoxic ischemia, 694
  neonatal seizures, 244–245
  status epilepticus, 692
Cerebral necrosis, hemorrhagic, 281
Cerebral palsy, 43 (Fig.), 165, 166, 167,
  738–762
  aspiration, 428
  constipation management, 463
  cranial ultrasonography, 171

definition, 738
early stages, 833
epidemiology, 738–739
and epilepsy, **685,** 738, 761
esophageal peristalsis, 426
etiology, classification, 739, 740 (Table)
and fetal monitoring, 119
hypocapnia, 161
management, 755–761
obesity, 1190
pseudobulbar palsy, 812
severely handicapped children affected,
  14 (Table)
Cerebral perfusion pressure, 659, **661,
  698,** 707–708
  neonate, 243
Cerebral protection, 708, 715
Cerebral venous thrombosis,
  gastroenteritis, 1294
Cerebral vesicles, development, **642–644**
Cerebral vessels, *see also* Cerebral arteries
  Doppler ultrasonography, 1908
  magnetic resonance imaging, 1909
Cerebrohepatorenal syndrome, *see*
  Zellweger syndrome
Cerebromacular degeneration, 1115
Cerebrospinal fluid
  acanthamebic disease, 1469
  African trypanosomiasis, 1456
  antibiotic penetration, 1527
  antibody levels, 1245
  bacterial meningitis, 1289, **1290**
  bacteriology specimens, **1298**
  bicarbonate on, 504
  birth asphyxia, 128
  drugs on production, 664
  head injuries, sampling, 708
  herpes simplex meningitis, 1439
  immunoglobulin infusion, 1267
  infection investigation, 696
  kinetics, **658**
  lactate, 1125
    meningitis, 1290
  leptospirosis, 1312
  leukemia, 871–872
  mumps meningitis, 1371
  neonatal meningitis, 281–282
  neonatal sepsis, 276
  neonate, **242**
  neurosyphilis, 1405
  non-accidental head injury, 703
  normal pressure, 1935 (Table)
  normal values, 1933–1935 (Table)
  normal volume, 1935 (Table)
  obstruction, 658
  opening pressure, cerebral malaria,
    1451
  pleocytosis, 663
  protein
    Dejerine–Sottas disease, 723
    Guillain-Barré syndrome, 726
    subarachnoid hemorrhage, 710
  therapeutic removal, 699
  tuberculous meningitis, 1344
  ventriculitis, 663
  viral infections, 1376
  viral meningitis, 1375
  virology, **1352**
Cerebrotendinous xanthomatosis, 789–790
  (Table), 1145, **1156**
Cerebrovascular accidents, *see*
  Hemiplegia; Strokes
Cerebrovascular disease, **709–715**
Ceredase, Gaucher disease, 1166
Ceroid, Hermansky–Pudlak syndrome,
  1107
Ceroid lipofuscinosis, 1171
  neuronal, 796–797 (Table), 1171
Certificates of disposal, cremations, 174
Certification, neonatal death, 174
Ceruloplasmin
  vs age, infants, 471
  normal values, 1923 (Table)
  Wilson's disease, 481

Cervical intraepithelial neoplasia, 994
Cervical lymphadenitis, environmental
  mycobacteria, **134**
Cervical lymphadenopathy, 511, **1784**
  diphtheria, 1306
  Kawasaki disease, 1479
  mycobacteria, 1343
  roseola infantum, 1359
Cervical ribs, 1557
Cervical spine, shaking injury, 701
Cervical suture, 116
Cervix
  Chlamydia trachomatis, 1432
  gonorrhea, 1420, 1425
  labor, 84
    induction, 87
  tumors, 993–994
  warts, 1443
Cesarean section, 116
  autoimmune neonatal
    thrombocytopenia, 229
  breech presentation, 87–88
  herpes simplex, 288, 1441
  placenta previa, 90
  preterm delivery, **119–120**
  resuscitation, 133
  transient tachypnea of the newborn,
    182
  wet lungs, 107
CESDI report, coroner's post-mortems,
  1721
Cestodes, **1499–1506**
Cetrimide, poisoning, 1711
Cetyltrimethyl ammonium bromide test,
  837
C-fos gene, osteopetrosis, 1582
CH50 (total hemolytic complement test),
  1245
Chagas' disease, **1458–1460**
Chagoma, 1458, **1459**
Challenge tests (provocation tests), **1694,**
  see also named substances
Chanarin–Dorfman syndrome, ichthyosis,
  1622 (Table)
Chancres, **1405–1406**
  trypanosomal, 1455
Charcoal, activated, **1706–1707,** 1815
  administration, 1962 (Table)
Charcot–Marie–Tooth atrophy, 72 (Table),
  721, 722–723, 765
Chediak–Higashi syndrome, 1107, 1242
  (Table), 1245, **1261,** 1629 (Table)
  vs Griscelli syndrome, 1254
  neoplasms, 889 (Table)
Cheeses, molds, 1690
Chelating agents, dermatomyositis-
  polymyositis, 1608
Chemical burns, 1868
Chemical conjunctivitis, neonate, 263
Chemical potential, 405
Chemicals
  aplastic anemia, 856 (Table)
  neoplasms, 890–891
Chemiluminescence, phagocytosis assay,
  1247
Chemoprophylaxis, *see also* Antibiotics,
  prophylaxis
  malaria, **1448–1449**
  tuberculosis, **1340**
Chemoreceptor control, respiration,
  disorders, 530–531
Chemoreceptor reflex, laryngeal, 528
Chemosis, 1663
Chemotaxis, 274, 1235
  assessment, 1247
  neutrophil disorders, 1260–1262
Chemotherapy (antifungal), **1477–1478,**
  1530
Chemotherapy (oncological), **892–893,**
  see also named tumors
  brain tumors, 901
  drug toxicity effects, **894 (Table)**
  Hodgkin's disease, 910
  infections, 533

leukemias, 872–874
lymphomas, 908–909
neonate, 290
Chemotherapy (tuberculosis), **1347–1348,**
  see also named drugs
Cherry red spot, **270,** 1163, 1164, 1666
  type I sialic acid storage disease, 1169
Cherubism (familial fibrous dysplasia of
  the jaws), 1565
Chest, *see also* Rib recession
  cancer therapy, late effects, 900
  cardiac surgery, scars, 586
  circumference, 30
  compressions, resuscitation, 523–524
  deformity, **512**
    cystic fibrosis, 554
  drainage, **521, 1845,** *see also* Pleural
    tap
    pneumothorax, 1807, **1844–1845**
    sedation, 521
  Ewing's sarcoma, 917, 918
  examination, 30
  expansion, 30, 512
  injuries, **1811,** 1812
  leads, *see* Precordial leads
  neonate, 43
  neuroblastoma, 911
  osteosarcoma metastases, 917, 918
  pain, **509**
  physiotherapy, neonatal intensive care,
    97
  rhabdomyosarcoma, 916
  structural defects, **1556–1558**
Chester porphyria, 1143
Chest leads, electrocardiography, 588
  (Fig.)
Chest X-rays, **513–514, 1899–1900**
  aortic stenosis, 607
  asthma, 544
  atrioventricular septal defect, 604
  bronchiolitis, 564
  bronchopulmonary aspergilloma, 1474
  coarctation of aorta, 611
  congenital heart disease, 598
  congenital lung cysts, 574
  cystic fibrosis, **554**
  diaphragmatic hernia, 575
  dysphagia, 426
  heart disease, **587–588**
  heart failure, 599
  hydatid disease, 1506 (Fig.)
  hyperlucency, 576
  idiopathic dilation of pulmonary artery,
    609
  immunodeficiency, 1244
  left ventricular inflow obstructions, 609
  mitral stenosis, 629
  neonatal cardiovascular system, 200
  nephroblastoma, 913
  persistent ductus arteriosus, 603
  pneumonia, 567
  pneumothorax, 187–188
  pulmonary hypertension, 606
  radiation doses, 1895 (Table)
  total anomalous pulmonary venous
    connection, 623
  toxocariasis, 1486
  tuberculosis, 1336
  ventricular septal defect, 601
Chewing movements, neonate, 236
Chiari malformations, **646–647**
Chiasm, optic gliomas, 904
Chickenpox, **1360–1362,** *see also*
  Varicella-zoster virus
  AIDS, 1396
  ataxia, 762
  eye, 1676
  intracranial hemorrhage, 713
  mouth, 424
  neurological complications, 1376
Chicleros, cutaneous leishmaniasis, 1463
Chief cells, stomach, 430
Chignon, 121
Chigoe flea, **1514**

Chikungunya virus, 1389
Child abuse, 18, **1866–1874,** *see also*
  Non-accidental injury
  Children Act 1989, 1875
  failure to thrive, 469
  growth failure, 1017
  management, **703–704**
  vs Menkes' kinky hair syndrome, 1146
  pancreatitis, 450
  precocious pseudopuberty, 1028
  prevention, 340
  psychiatric aspects, **1737**
Child Accident Prevention Trust, 1713
Child Assessment Orders, 1853, **1875**
Child Assessment Orders (Scotland), 1877
Childbirth, *see* Birth; Intrapartum care
Child development centers, 399–400
Child exploitation, **1887–1888**
Child guidance, 1864
Child health clinics, **1861–1862**
Child health promotion, 340
Child health surveillance, **1862**
  Joint Working Party on, 1853
Child health visitors, 1853
Childhood
  age range for, 17
  demographic definition, 3
Childhood absence epilepsy, 680 (Table),
  684
  learning, 690
Childhood phase, growth, 352, 364
Child labor, 1887
Child minders, 1860
Child population, **1,** 2
Child pregnancy, 15 (Table), 341
Child Protection Orders (Scotland), **1877**
Childrearing, restrictive, 828
Children Act 1989, 1873, **1874–1876**
Children in need, Children Act 1989,
  1874–1875
Children's Coma Scale, 704 (Table)
Children (Scotland) Act 1995, **1876–1877**
Children's hearings (Scotland),
  1876–1877
Children's homes, of local authorities,
  1857
Children's Liver Disease Foundation, 485
Children under Five (National Survey of
  Health and Development), 1851
Child-resistant containers, 1706
Child-restraint systems, passenger
  accident prevention, 1716
CHIME study, sudden infant death
  syndrome, 1721
Chimpanzee, adrenarche, 1061
China
  demography, 2 (Table)
  intussusception, fire bellows, 1786
Chinese food, migraine, 716
Chinese restaurant syndrome, 1115–1116
Chingleput trial, BCG vaccination, 1339
Chironex spp., 1526
Chix, enteral feeding, short gut syndrome,
  445
Chlamydia pneumoniae, 569, **1373–1374,**
  1432–1433
Chlamydia psittaci, see Psittacosis
Chlamydia spp., **1429–1433**
  eye, 1384
  pneumonitis, 196, 564
  sexually transmitted diseases, 994
    detection or exclusion, 1399, 1400
  United Kingdom, 1277
Chlamydia trachomatis, **1374,** 1385,
  1429–1432
  epididymo-orchitis, doxycycline, 1432
  inclusion blennorrhea, 1664
  ophthalmia neonatorum, **263–264,** 283
  pertussis-like illness, 561–562
  pneumonia, 566, **569, 1431–1432**
    cough, 280, 1374
    radiology, 567
  pneumonitis, 564
  vertical transmission, 1400

Chloral hydrate, administration, 1962
  (Table)
  neonate, 1956 (Table)
Chlorambucil, nephrotic syndrome, 971
Chloramphenicol
  administration, 1955 (Table), 1962
    (Table)
  cerebrospinal fluid, 1527
  eye toxicity, 1677
  'gray baby' syndrome, 108
  mechanism, 1527
  meningitis, 1292
    bacterial, 1291
    neonatal, 282
    plague, 1318
  neonate, 279 (Table)
  therapeutic ranges, 1936 (Table)
  typhoid fever, 1326
  typhus, 1391
Chloride, 1185 (Table)
  alimentary secretions, 411 (Table)
  colonic absorption, 455
  concentrations, 404, 406 (Table)
  feces
    cholera, 1303 (Table)
    gastroenteritis, 1293
  intestinal absorption, 438
  movement across membranes, 406
  normal values, 1924 (Table)
    amniotic fluid, 1937 (Table)
    cerebrospinal fluid, 1934 (Table)
    urine, 1931 (Table)
  reference nutrient intakes, 1947
    (Table)
  requirements, preterm infant, 152
    (Table)
Chloride channels, cystic fibrosis, 551
'Chloride shunt' syndrome (Gordon's
  syndrome), 947
Chloridorrhea, congenital, 446–447
Chlormethiazole
  administration, 1962 (Table)
  on phenytoin treatment, 697
Chloroquine, 289
  amebiasis, 1469
  eye toxicity, 1677
  malaria
    administration, 1962 (Table)
    prophylaxis, 1448–1449
    resistance, 1448
    treatment, 1452
  poisoning, 1710
Chlorothiazide
  administration, 1962 (Table)
  neonate, 1956 (Table)
  for hypertension, 637 (Table)
Chlorpheniramine, administration, 1962
  (Table)
Chlorpromazine
  administration, 1962 (Table)
  neonate, 1957 (Table)
  for hyperpyrexia, 1830
Chlorpropamide, transient
  hyperinsulinemia, 295
Chlortetracycline, administration, 1962
  (Table)
Chlorthalidone, administration, 1962
  (Table)
Choanal atresia, **193, 1685,** 1769
  vs common cold, 560
Choking, **1718–1719,** 1815
Cholangiocarcinoma, *Opisthorchis
  viverrini,* 1512
Cholangiography, *see also* Endoscopic
  retrograde
    cholangiopancreatography
  biliary atresia, 1782
  endoscopic retrograde, 451, 472
  percutaneous transhepatic, 472, 1898
Cholangitis, extrahepatic biliary atresia,
  475
Cholecalciferol, 1053
Cholecystokinin, pancreatic function tests,
  451

Choledochal cysts, **475, 1788**
  ultrasonography, 1906
Cholelithiasis, *see* Biliary calculi
Cholera, **1303–1305**
  enterotoxins, 452, 1303, 1304
  vaccination, 1962 (Table)
Cholestanol, cerebrotendinous
  xanthomatosis, 1156
Cholestasis, 473, *see also* Intrahepatic
  cholestasis
  benign recurrent, 1145
  neonate, 219, **220–221**
    α_1-antitrypsin deficiency, 1176
    scintigraphy, 472
  parenteral nutrition, **159,** 1225–1226
  phototherapy, 219
Cholesteatoma, 1681
Cholesterol
  familial hypercholesterolemia type II,
    1151
  marasmus, 1192
  normal values, 1924 (Table)
    cerebrospinal fluid, 1934 (Table)
  plasma levels, 1149, 1150
  steroidogenesis, 1059
  synthesis disorders, **1156**
Cholesterol desmolase deficiency, 1008,
  1064
Cholesterol esters, digestion, 437
Cholestyramine
  administration, 1963 (Table)
  hypercholesterolemia, 1152
  short bowel syndrome, 1212
Choline
  administration (salicylate), 1963 (Table)
  for cystathione synthase deficiency,
    1109
Cholinergic drugs
  extrapyramidal effects, 768
  growth hormone secretion, 1012
  neurogenic bladder, 657
Cholinesterase inhibitors
  myasthenia gravis, 727–728
  squint, 1660
Chondrodysplasia punctata (Conradi's
  disease), 830 (Table), 1173–1174,
  1571–1572
  ichthyosis, 1622 (Table)
Chondrodysplasias, *see* Skeletal
  dysplasias
Chondrodystrophies, 1017
Chondroectodermal dysplasia, *see*
  Ellis–van Creveld syndrome
Chondromas, multiple enchondromatosis,
  1585–1586
Chondrosarcoma, *vs* osteosarcoma, 918
Chordee, 256, 1794
Chorea, **772**
  rheumatic, 1597, **1598–1599**
  vs tics, 772, 1745
Choreiform disorders, **767–774**
Choreiform movements, 769
Choreoathetosis, 770
  paroxysmal, 772–773
  posticteric, 753–754
Chorioamnionitis
  pneumonia, 183
  sepsis, 277
Choriocarcinoma, 921
Chorionepithelioma, ovaries, ectopic
  gonadotropin secretion, 1029
Chorionic villus sampling, 80–81
  chromosome preparations from, 50
  cystic fibrosis, 552
  21-hydroxylase deficiency, 1062
Chorioretinitis, toxoplasmosis, 1465, 1466
Choroid, *see also* Gyrate atrophy of
  choroid and retina
  degenerative diseases, **1666–1667**
Choroid cyst of third ventricle,
  hydrocephalus, 658
Choroideremia, 1667
Choroiditis, 1665–1666
Choroidoretinitis

neonate, 284 (Table)
  syphilis, 1408
  congenital, 1412, 1414
Choroid plexectomy, 664
Choroid plexus, 1043
  cerebrospinal fluid production, 658
  neoplasms, **905–906**
Christmas disease, 230, **881**
Christmas eye, 1525
Christ Siemens Touraine syndrome, 1625
  (Table)
Chromatography, feces, 448, 454–455
Chromium, 1185 (Table)
  deficiency, 1202
  estimated safe and adequate daily
    intakes, 1949 (Table)
  parenteral nutrition, 1221
  safe intakes, 1948 (Table)
  sources, 1185 (Table)
Chromium-51 albumin, fecal protein
  measurement, 448
Chromium-51-EDTA-labeled target cells,
  cytotoxicity assays, 1247
Chromosomally mediated resistant
  Neisseria gonorrhoeae, 1421, 1427
Chromosomal syndromes, **54–67**
Chromosome atlases, 60
Chromosome breakage syndromes,
  immunodeficiency disorders,
  1253–1254
Chromosome disorders, **48–67**
  central nervous system, 645
  congenital heart disease, 596
  growth failure, 1017
  immunodeficiency disorders,
    1241–1242
  leukemias, 869, 872
  malignant neoplasms, **887–889**
  speech disorder, 808
Chromosome karyotypes, preparation,
  48–50
Chromosome 'paints,' 50
Chromosome rearrangements, 73
  neuroblastoma, 911
  rhabdomyosarcoma, 915
Chromosomes, **48–54**
  Fanconi's anemia, 854
Chromosome studies, indications, 50–51
Chronic aggressive hepatitis, HBV
  infection, 477
Chronic benign neutropenia, 867
Chronic bullous disease of childhood,
  1640
Chronic disease, *see also* Disability;
  Handicap
  growth, 368, 372, **1017–1018,** 1031
  maladaptive responses, **1760–1761**
  psychological effects, **1746–1748**
Chronic fatigue syndrome, 1760
  Epstein–Barr virus, 1367
Chronic granulocytic leukemia, 872
Chronic granulomatous disease, 533, 1243
  (Table), **1259–1260**
  nitroblue tetrazolium test, 533, 1247
Chronic idiopathic urticaria, 1639
Chronic leukemias, 868
Chronic liver disease, 471, **480–484**
Chronic lung diseases, 576, *see also*
  named diseases
  breathing in sleep, 506
  neonatal, **193–196**
    cardiovascular aspects, 206
  obstruction after asthma, 539
  and oxygen therapy, 504
  prematurity, 491
Chronic mucocutaneous candidiasis, 1243
  (Table), **1251,** 1637
Chronic otitis media, **1680–1681**
Chronic pain, **1833**
Chronic persistent hepatitis, HBV
  infection, 477
Chronic poisoning, **1708**
Chronic progressive external
  ophthalmoplegia, 1127

Chronic pulmonary insufficiency of
  prematurity, **196**
Chronic pyelonephritis, *see* Reflux
  nephropathy
Chronic refractory diarrhea, 1295
Chronic renal failure, **978–982**
  anemia, 865–866, 979, 980
  neonate, **259–260**
  nephroblastoma, 914
Chrysotherapy, 1603–1604
Chvostek's sign, 300
Chylomicronemia with
  prebetalipoproteinemia, 1150
  (Table)
Chylomicron retention disease, 1153
Chylomicrons, 1148 (Table), 1149
  secondary disorders, 1154 (Table)
Chylothorax, **193**
  after cardiac surgery, 1823
Chymotrypsins, 437
  feces, cystic fibrosis, 553
Cigarette burns, 1868
Cilia, 532
Ciliary dyskinesia, 495, 520, **532, 577,** *see*
  also Mucociliary escalator
Ciliated epithelium, bronchi, 532
Cimetidine
  administration, 1963 (Table)
  neonate, 1957 (Table)
  scintigraphy for Meckel's diverticulum,
    1906
  warts, 1633
Cingulate gyrus, herniation, 698
Ciprofloxacin
  actinomycosis, 1473
  administration, 1963 (Table)
  cat-scratch disease, 1520
  environmental mycobacteria, 1350
  gonorrhea, 1427, 1428
  mechanism, 1527
  Pseudomonas aeruginosa, cystic
    fibrosis, 557
  Pseudomonas urinary tract infections,
    951
  resistance, *Neisseria gonorrhoeae,* 1421
  typhoid fever, 1326
Circadian rhythms, *see also* Diurnal
  variation
  ACTH secretion, 1038
  breast milk, 332
  congenital adrenal hyperplasia
    treatment, 1064
  cortisol, 1059
  glomerular filtration rate, 941
  neonatal intensive care, 98
  parathyroid hormone secretion, 1054
  temperature, 1282
  urine, Ondine's curse, 530
Circinate erythema, African
  trypanosomiasis, 1455
Circulation, *see also* Cardiovascular
  support
  resuscitation, **523–524, 525–526, 1807**
  trauma, **1809**
Circumcision, **1792–1793**
  and urinary tract infections, 261,
    949–950
Circumoral pallor, scarlet fever, 1285
Cirrhosis, **481–484**
  hepatitis B virus, 477
  hepatitis C virus, 478
  hepatocellular carcinoma, 924
Cisapride
  administration, 1963 (Table)
  gastroesophageal reflux, 155, 571
Cisplatinum, toxicity, 894 (Table), 896
Cisternal puncture, **1840–1841**
Citrate, and chemotherapy, 897
Citric acid, for hyperammonemia, 1112
Citric acid cycle, disorders, 1126
Citrulline, for lysinuric protein
  intolerance, 1121
L-Citrulline, for ornithine
  transcarbamylase deficiency, 1110

Citrullinemia, 1111
Cladosporium spp., spores, 1690
Clarithromycin
  administration, 1963 (Table)
  environmental mycobacteria, 1350
  leprosy, 1311
Clasp knife hypertonia, 35
Classical hemorrhagic disease of the
  newborn, 230
Classification
  accidental poisoning, 1706
  basal ganglia diseases, 770–774
  central nervous system tumors,
    899–900
  diabetes mellitus, 1072
  epilepsy, **674–676**
  failure to thrive, 465
  infections, **1274–1275 (Table)**
  leukemias, 868–869
  lipoprotein disorders, **1150–1151**
  non-Hodgkin's lymphoma, 907–908
  psychiatric disorder, **1732–1733**
  psychosis, 835–836
  retinopathy of prematurity, 266
  snakes, 1521 (Table)
  speech and language disorders, 805
    (Table)
  unexpected deaths, 1721
Clathrin, 1156
Clavicle
  birth trauma, 121 (Table)
  congenital pseudarthrosis, 1556
  pyknodysostosis, 1583
Clavulanic acid
  with amoxicillin, 1959 (Table)
    gonorrhea, 1427 (Table)
    neonate, 1955 (Table)
    urinary tract infections, 261, 952
    (Table)
  with ticarcillin, 1978 (Table)
Claw hand deformity, mucolipidosis III,
  1170
Clean-catch midstream urine specimens,
  950, 1299
Cleansing orders, 1864
Clear-cell adenocarcinoma, cervix and
  vagina, 994
Clear-cell sarcoma, kidney, 914
Cleft lip, 76, 424, **1796–1797**
  recurrence risks, 74
Cleft of anterior mitral leaflet, 604
Cleft palate, 810, **1796–1797**
  recurrence risks, 74
  Wolf-Hirschhorn syndrome, 58
Cleidocranial dysplasia, **1562**
Clindamycin
  administration, 1963 (Table)
  bacterial vaginosis, 1435
  infective endocarditis, prophylaxis, 632
    (Table)
  pyogenic osteitis, 1590
Clinical evaluation of language function,
  400
Clinical nutritional assessment, 1188
Clinodactyly, 55, 76 (Table), **1548–1549**
Clitoral reduction, 1065
Clitoromegaly, 1008
Cloaca, 206
  anomaly, 1781
    imaging, 1914
  common, 987
  exstrophy, 256
Clobazam, administration, 1963 (Table)
Clobetasol, administration, 1963 (Table)
Clobetasone, administration, 1963 (Table)
Clofazimine
  administration, 1963 (Table)
  environmental mycobacteria, 1350
  leprosy, 1311
Clomipramine, 1755
  obsessive–compulsive disorders, 1756
Clonazepam
  administration, 1963 (Table)
  neonate, 1957 (Table)

Clonazepam (Contd)
  birth asphyxia, 130
  neonatal seizures, 246 (Table)
Clonic seizures, neonate, 244 (Table)
Clonidine
  growth hormone secretion, 1012
  migraine, 717 (Table), 719
  poisoning, 1709
Clonorchiasis, 1512
  life cycle, 1511 (Table)
  liver, 478
Clonus, neonate, 239
Clostridium botulinum, 1301–1302
Clostridium tetani, 285, 1333
CLO test, see Rapid urease test
Clothing, protective, infection prevention, 1282
Clotrimazole, 1434, 1474, 1963 (Table)
Cloxacillin
  administration, 1963 (Table)
  Staphylococcus aureus, 1329 (Table)
Clozapine, 1755
Clubbing, 511, 543, 585
  cystic fibrosis, 554
  Trichuris trichiuria, 1491
Club foot, see Equinus deformity; Talipes equinovarus
Clue cells, bacterial vaginosis, 1435
Clumsiness, 668
Cluster headache, 716
Clustering, leukemia, 868, 889, 890
Cluttering of speech, 806
Clutton's joints, 1413
CLVPP regimen, Hodgkin's disease, 910
C-myc proto-oncogene, Burkitt's lymphoma, 906
Coagulation disorders, 879–882
  neonate, 227–231
Coagulation factor VII, deficiency, 881
Coagulation factor VIII, 227, see also Factor VIII-related antigen; Hemophilia A; Von Willebrand's disease
  dosage, 35, 851 (Table)
Coagulation factor IX, see also Christmas disease
  deficiency, 881
  dosage, 851 (Table)
Coagulation factor X, deficiency, 230, 881
Coagulation factor XIII, deficiency, 230, 881
Coagulation factors
  deficiencies, neonate, 229–231
  normal values, 228 (Table)
Coagulation therapy, dosage, 851 (Table)
Coal tar ointment, 1963 (Table)
Coal tar vaporizing solution, poisoning, 1711
Co-amoxiclav, see Clavulanic acid, with amoxicillin
Coarctation of aorta, 32, 200, 611–612
  balloon dilation, 205, 594, 611–612
  cardiac afterload, 1819
  pulses, 585, 598, 611
  signs, 587 (Table)
  Turner's syndrome, 370, 596, 611
Coat's retinopathy, 732
Cobalamin
  lysosomal storage disorder, 1157 (Table)
  metabolism disorders, 1147–1148
Cobalt, 1202
Cobras, bites, 1522
'Coca-Cola' urine, 859
Cocaine
  on brain development, 642
  crack, 248
Coccidioidin test, 1475
Coccidioidomycosis, 570, 1471 (Table), 1475
Cochlear implants, 818, 1683
Cockayne's syndrome, 1630
  type A, 1142
Cocktail party chatter, 804, 818

Codeine
  cough medicines, poisoning, 1709
  migraine, 717 (Table)
Codman's triangle, 917
Codominance, 66
Codons, 68–69
Coeliac Society, 485
Coe virus, 1372, 1382
Cognitive–behavior therapy, 1764
Cognitive development, 383–384, 667, 1728–1730
  epilepsy, 690
Cognitive learning, 819
Cognitive status epilepticus, 676, see also Status epilepticus, nonconvulsive
Cognitive therapy, depression, 1755
Cohabitation, 1855
Cohen technique, ureteric reimplantation, 956
Cohort studies, 1851
COL1A1 allele mutations, 1568
COL1A2 allele mutations, 1569
COL2A1 gene mutations, 1571, 1577, 1580
Cold, common, 492, 559–560, 1372–1373, 1684
Cold abscesses
  bones, 1345–1346
  lymph nodes, 1343
  spine, 1592
Cold autoimmune hemolytic anemia, 864
Cold climate, respiratory disorders, 492
Cold hemolysins, congenital syphilis, 1414
Colestipol, hypercholesterolemia, 1152
Colic
  vs cow's milk protein intolerance, 1699
  infantile, 461
Colistin, administration, 1963 (Table)
Colitis
  cow's milk protein intolerance, 1699
  hemolytic uremic syndrome, 977
  salmonellosis, 1324
Collagen, 1565–1567
  metabolism, markers, 1012, 1567
Collagenase, on uterine cervix, 84
Collagen vascular diseases, see Connective tissue disorders
Collapse, neonatal heart disease, 203
Collapse (lung), tuberculosis, 1341
Collapse (pulmonary lobe), 514, see also Recurrent segmental collapse
  cystic fibrosis, 556
  pertussis, 1316
Collapsing pulse, 32
Collateral ventilation, 497
Collecting ducts, renal, 259
Collectins, 1234
Colligative properties, 405
Collodion baby, 1621
Colloid, thyroid, 1044
Colloid osmotic pressure, 407
  preterm infant, 142
Coloboma
  eyelid, 1662
  iris, 1650
  Wolf-Hirschhorn syndrome, 58
Colomycin, Pseudomonas aeruginosa, cystic fibrosis, 558 (Table)
Colon, 455–460, see also Colorectal carcinoma
  amebiasis, 1468
  Chagas' disease, 1458, 1459
  Crohn's disease, 457
  cystic fibrosis, 554
  helminthoma, 1494
  investigation, 464–465
  motility, 451
    investigations, 464–465
  polyps, 448
  schistosomiasis, 1509
  temperature, 147
  X-ray appearance, 1901

Colonoscopy, 464
  rectal bleeding, 460
Color blindness, red–green, inheritance, 67
Color Doppler ultrasonography, 1896
  flow mapping, heart disease, 593
  intussusception, 1904
Colorectal carcinoma
  Crohn's disease, 458
  ulcerative colitis, 459
Colostrum, 112, 332
Colposcopy, sexual abuse, 1869
Colubridae, 1521
Colubrid venoms, 1521, 1522
Columella, 76 (Table)
Coma
  cerebral malaria, 1450
  cholera, 1304
  emergency care, 1815
  investigation, 695
  neonate, 236
  postasphyxial encephalopathy, 127
Coma scales, 695
Combative behavior, transient, 1520
Combination analgesia, 1830
Combination vaccines, 342
Combined hyperlipidemia, 1150 (Table), 1152
Combined immunodeficiencies, 1248–1254
  replacement therapy, 1268–1270
Combined modality therapy, Hodgkin's disease, 910
Combined sulfite oxidase and xanthine oxidase deficiency, 791 (Table)
Combined ventricular hypertrophy, electrocardiography, 589
Comminuted chicken, 1208
Committee on Child Health Services, 1853
Common bile duct
  ascariasis, 1483
  ultrasonography, 1906
Common cold, 492, 559–560, 1372–1373, 1684
Common variable immunodeficiency, 1242 (Table), 1243, 1256–1257
  gastrointestinal disease, 444
  neoplasms, 1248 (Table), 1256
  vs X-linked agammaglobulinemia, 1255
Communicable disease centers, guidelines, 1281
Communicable diseases, see Infectious diseases; Notifiable diseases
Communicable Disease Surveillance Centre, 1281
Communicating hydrocephalus, 659
Communication, 1878, see also Speech, disorders
  with adolescents, 1753–1754
  alternative media, 814
  cancer, 897–898
  cerebral palsy, 761
  with mentally handicapped children, 836–837
  on mental retardation, 839
  nonverbal, 818
  normal development, 384–385
  with parents, 99–100
Communication systems, kernicterus, 754
Community-acquired pneumonia, 565–568
Community-based rehabilitation, developing countries, 1891
Community care, 1804
  mental retardation, 842
Community pediatricians, consultant, 1853
Companion in labor, 84
Compartment injury, 1812
Compensated hydrocephalus, 659
  clinical features, 659
Complement deficiency disorders, 1262–1263

Complement factor 4, sclerosing cholangitis vs autoimmune chronic active hepatitis, 481
Complement receptors, 1234
  CR3, neonate, 274
Complement system, 1232–1234
  endotoxins on, 1287
  fetus, 1240
  hyposplenia, 1266
  measurements, 1245
  neonate, 275, 1240–1241
Complete androgen insensitivity syndrome, 991
Complete heart block, neonate, 203
Complete regression, neoplasms, 893
Complete testicular feminization, 1010
Complex carbohydrates, 1183
Complex partial seizures, 675
  prognosis, 687
Compliance
  chemotherapy (tuberculosis), 1347
  gonorrhea treatment, 1427
Compliance (respiratory), 496, 501
Complicated cataract, 1669
Component vaccines, 341
Compound fractures, skull, 707
Compound nevi, 1618
Compression head injuries, 699
  birth trauma, 122
Compressive head wrapping, 664
Compulsions, 1740
Compulsive water drinking, 1039
Computed tomography, 1896–1897
  abdomen, 1906
  birth asphyxia, 128
  brain tumors, 901
  central nervous system, 1908
  chest, 519, 1900
  cysticercosis, 1502
  epilepsy, 678
  head injuries, 706
  hydrocephalus, 661
  liver, 472
  neonate, cranial, 242
  obliterative bronchiolitis, 576
  radiation doses, 1895 (Table)
  retroperitoneum, 1913
  subarachnoid hemorrhage, 710
  subdural hemorrhage, 703
  trauma, 1916
  tuberculosis, 1342
  urinary tract, 1912
Computer games, epilepsy, 691
Computers
  learning disorders, 825
  parenteral nutrition, 1221–1223
  speech disorders, 814
Concomitant immunity, schistosomiasis, 1508
Concomitant squint, 1660
Concordant atrioventricular connections, 597
Concordant ventriculoarterial connections, 597
Concrete operational period, development, 1729 (Table), 1730
Conditioned audiometry, 1683
Conditioned reflex learning, 819, 838
Conditioning therapy, nocturnal enuresis, 957
Condoms, 994
Conduct disorder, 1733, 1742–1743
Conduction aphasia, 815
Conduction defects, 626–628
  atrial septal defect, 602
Conduction heat loss, 146
Conductive deafness, 816, 817, 1682
Condyloma acuminatum, 1442, 1443
  treatment, 1444
Condylomata lata, 1407
Confidentiality
  adolescents, 1753, 1880
  and sexual abuse, 1759
Confusion, double vision, 1661

Congenital abnormalities, *see also* Congenital malformations; Dysmorphic syndromes
  aspiration pneumonia, 186
  central nervous system, *see* Central nervous system, congenital malformations
  delayed visual maturation, 272–273
  eye examination, 268
  genitalia, 986
  immigrants, 1865
  inborn errors of metabolism, 305
  kidney, 253–256
  leukemia risk, 868
  limbs, **1545–1556**
  malformation syndromes, **75–76**
    neoplasms, 290
  neonatal care, **110–111**
  neonatal mortality, 4 (Table)
  neonatal seizures, 245 (Table)
  neoplasms, 887–888
  notification, 1850
  postneonatal mortality, 5 (Table)
  respiratory tract, **572–576**
  screening, 339 (Table)
  SGA baby, 137–138
  spinal cord, 651–657
  stillbirth rates, 4 (Table)
  surgery, 1768
  trends, 7–8
  urinary tract, **253–256**, 935
Congenital adrenal hyperplasia, 72 (Table), 109, 999, **1061–1065**
  ambiguous genitalia, 1006
  fetus, 985, **986**
  frequency, 47 (Table)
  gestation length, 1006
  hypertension, 1006, 1065, 1070
  management, 1064
  precocious pseudopuberty, 1027
  vomiting, 212
Congenital adrenal hypoplasia, **1067**
  puberty, 1061
Congenital aortic regurgitation, 608
Congenital aplasia cutis, **1620**
Congenital Chagas' disease, 1458, 1459
Congenital chloridorrhea, 446–447
Congenital contractural arachnodactyly, **1589**
Congenital deformations, **75–76**
  definition, 645
Congenital dislocation of hip, 39 (Fig.), 40–41, **1549–1551**
  recurrence risks, 74
  severely handicapped children affected, 14 (Table)
Congenital enteropathies, 442–443
Congenital erythropoietic porphyria, **865,** 1142 (Table), 1144, **1631**
Congenital familial telangiectasia, tongue, 425
Congenital fiber type disproportion, myopathy, 735 (Table)
Congenital folate malabsorption, 1147
Congenital glaucoma, 23, 27 (Fig.), 43, **1672–1673**
Congenital glucagon deficiency, 297
Congenital heart disease, **595–623**
  congenital rubella, 286, 596
  Down syndrome, 55, 596
  duct-dependent, 198–199
  etiology, 596
  hypoglycemia, 295
  incidence, 95 (Fig.), **595–596**
  magnetic resonance imaging, 1898
  maternal, 89 (Table)
  maternal hyperphenylalaninemia, 1104 (Table)
  mental retardation, 835 (Table)
  mortality trends, 8
  nomenclature, 597–598
  nutrition, **1210**
  vs persistent fetal circulation, 182
  Pierre Robin syndrome, 1562

  postneonatal mortality, 5 (Table)
  pulmonary lymphangiectasis, 193
  recurrence risks, 74, 597
  severely handicapped children affected, 14 (Table)
  signs, 587 (Table)
  symptoms, 584
Congenital hemiplegia, 740–741
Congenital hemolytic anemia, 217–218
Congenital hepatic fibrosis, **483–484**
Congenital hypoaldosteronism, 260
Congenital hypopituitarism, 297, 999
Congenital hypothyroidism, *see* Cretinism
Congenital ichthyosiform erythroderma, 1621
Congenital livedo reticularis, 1646
Congenital lobar emphysema, **192, 574,** 1769
Congenital lung cysts, **574,** 1769
Congenitally corrected transposition of great arteries, **616**
Congenital lymphedema, 1798
  chromosome studies, 51
Congenital malaria, 1450
Congenital malformations, *see also* Central nervous system, congenital malformations; Congenital abnormalities
  cerebellar ataxia, 752–753
  developing countries disease burden, 1280 (Table)
Congenital mesoblastic nephroma, 255, 292 (Table)
Congenital muscular dystrophy, 728–729, 735 (Table)
  Fukuyama type, 650, 729
Congenital myasthenia, 727
Congenital nephrogenic diabetes insipidus, 260
Congenital nephrotic syndrome, 971–972
  Finnish type, neonate, 261
Congenital nonhemolytic hyperbilirubinemias, 218
Congenital nystagmus, *see* Infantile nystagmus
Congenital panhypopituitarism, adrenal insufficiency, 1041
Congenital ptosis, 1661–1662
Congenital pulmonary regurgitation, 609
Congenital sensorineural deafness, 816
Congenital spherocytosis, maternal, 89 (Table)
Congenital syphilis, 248, **284, 1404–1405, 1411–1415**
  diagnosis, 1414–1415
  stigmata, 1414
  treatment, 1415
Congenital tuberculosis, **1346**
Congenital type 1 fiber dominance, myopathy, 735 (Table)
Congenital word blindness, 821
Congo red test, amyloidosis, 1177
Coning
  brainstem, 698
    upward, 663
  stroke, 714
Conjugate bases, 415
Conjugated bilirubin
  cerebrospinal fluid, 1933 (Table)
  estimation, 219
Conjugated hyperbilirubinemia, prolonged, **220–221**
Conjunctiva
  bilharzial granuloma, 1509
  telangiectasia, 766
Conjunctivitis, **1663–1664,** *see also* Allergic keratoconjunctivitis; Ophthalmia neonatorum
  acute hemorrhagic, **1385**
  Chlamydia trachomatis, **1430–1431**
  erythema multiforme, 1675
  follicular, 1370, 1385
  gonococcal, *see* Ophthalmia neonatorum

Kawasaki disease, 1479
  measles, **1354,** 1355
  pederin, 1525
  respiratory disorders, 510
  staphylococcal, 281
Connective tissue disorders, **1596–1613**
  anemia, 865
  complete heart block, 203
  eye, **1674–1675**
  fibrosing alveolitis, 578
  heart, **635–636**
  heart block, 203, 626
  skin, **1644–1645**
Conn's syndrome, 1066
Conradi–Hunermann chondrodysplasia punctata, 1173, **1572**
Conradi's disease, *see* Chondrodysplasia punctata
Consanguinity, 1865
Consciousness, 820, *see also* Coma
  cholera, 1304
  examination, 34
  history taking, 17
  respiratory disorders, 510
Consent, *see* Informed consent
Conservation, perception, 1729
Consolability, neonate, 236, 238 (Fig.)
Consolidation, 565
  breath sounds, 512
  radiology, 513–514
Consonance, loss of, puberty, 1027–1029, 1034–1035, 1069
Constipation
  chronic, **461–463**
  cystic fibrosis, 554
  dietary management, **1211**
  mental retardation, 841
  neonate, **213–214**
  neural tube defect, 657
  presacral tumors, 921
  rectal bleeding, 460
  terminal care, 928
  urinary tract infections, 950
  vinca alkaloids, 896
Constitutional delay of growth and puberty, **372,** 990, **1031**
  management, 1035
Constitutional factors, psychiatric disorder, 1727
Constitutional short stature, 371
Constitutional tall stature, 375–376
Constriction bands, congenital, **1547**
Constructional dyspraxia, 669
Consultant community pediatricians, 1853
Consultation psychiatry (liaison psychiatry), 1749
Consumption coagulopathy, *see* Disseminated intravascular coagulation
Contact eczema, 1641–1642
Contact infections, 1281
Contact lenses, albinism, 1673
Contact Orders, 1874, 1876
Contacts (infectious diseases)
  diphtheria, 1307
  genital warts, 1445
  gonorrhea, treatment, 1429
  syphilis, treatment, 1410
  tuberculosis, **1340**
Contact urticaria, **1697**
  atopic eczema, 1643
Continuation phase, chemotherapy, acute lymphoblastic leukemia, 873
Continuous ambulatory electrocardiography, arrhythmias, 624
Continuous ambulatory peritoneal dialysis, 981
Continuous arteriovenous hemofiltration, 976, 1824
Continuous cerebral dysrhythmias, **691–693,** *see also* Status epilepticus

Continuous cycling peritoneal dialysis, 981
Continuous feeding, *vs* intermittent feeding, preterm infant, 153
Continuous hemodialfiltration, 976–977, 1824
Continuous infusion, enteral nutrition, 1217, 1218 (Table)
Continuous murmurs, 586–587, 603
Continuous negative extrathoracic pressure, 162
Continuous positive airways pressure, **161–162,** 1818
  apnea attacks, 197
  obstructive sleep apnea, 531
  pneumothorax, 187
  respiratory distress syndrome, 180
Continuous renal replacement therapy, 1824
Continuous venovenous hemodialfiltration, 1824
Continuous venovenous hemofiltration, 976, 1824
Contraception, *see also* Oral contraceptive pill
  adolescence, 994–995
  Islam, 1865
Contractions, uterine, 84
  fetal heart rate, 86
Contractural arachnodactyly, congenital, **1589**
Contractures
  arthrogryposis multiplex congenita, 1587
  congenital hemiplegia, 744
  flexion, congenital, **1549**
  prevention, 757
Contrast media, 1895
  computed tomography, 1897
  hypertonic, meconium ileus, 1904
  transplacental, 1005
  ultrasonography, 1896
Contrast swallow, 571, **1900**
Control groups, birthweight outcome, 167
Control mode ventilation, 1817
Control of breathing, 196–198
Controls, case-control studies, 1851
Convalesced patient plasma, for Lassa fever, **1388**
Convalescent serum samples, lymphocytic choriomeningitis, 1376
Convective heat loss, 146
Conventional osteosarcoma, 917–918
Convention on the Rights of the Child, United Nations, **1888,** 1891
Convergence insufficiency, 1660
Convergent strabismus, 265
Conversion disorders, **1740–1741**
Conversion factors, units, 1921, 1938 (Table)
Convulsions, *see* Seizures
Cooking, scald prevention, 1715
Cooling, **1830**
Coombs' test, hemolytic disease of the newborn, 216–217, 232
Coordination, 749, 823
  examination, 35
  history taking, 17
Coordination disorders, developmental, 668
Copper, 1185 (Table)
  breast milk, 332
  deficiency, **1201–1202**
    metabolic bone disease, 301–302
    preterm infant, 225
  estimated safe and adequate daily intakes, 1949 (Table)
  Indian childhood cirrhosis, 484
  metabolism disorders, **1145–1146**
  normal values, 1924 (Table)
    stools, 1936 (Table)
    urine, 1931 (Table)
  parenteral nutrition, 1221 (Table)
  reference nutrient intakes, 1947 (Table)

Copper, 1185 (Table) (Contd)
  requirements, preterm infant, 152
    (Table)
  sources, 1185 (Table)
  therapy, Menkes' kinky hair syndrome,
    1146
  Wilson's disease, 481
Copper oxidase, see Ceruloplasmin
Coprolalia, 1745
Coproporphyria, hereditary, 1142 (Table),
    1143
Coproporphyrin, normal values
  stools, 1936 (Table)
  urine, 1931 (Table)
Coproporphyrinogens, 1142, 1144
  hyperbilirubinemias, 1145
Coproporphyrin oxidase, red cells, 1143
Coralliform cataract, 1668
Coral snakebites, 1522
Cord blood hemoglobin, 223
Cordocentesis, for thrombocytopenia, 229
Cordylobia anthropophaga (tumbu fly),
    1514
Core temperature, 1282
Cori's disease, 789 (Table)
Cornea, 1664–1665, see also Keratitis
  disorders, 270
  examination, 1650
  Fabry disease, 1164
  Hurler's syndrome, 1159
  neonate, 264
    examination, 268
  ophthalmia neonatorum, 263
  ulcers, 1664
  xerosis, 1194
'Corner' fractures, 1914
Cornstarch, glucose-6-phosphatase
    deficiency, 1137
Coronary arteries
  disease and birthweight, 369
  fistula, 605
  malformations, 612
Coronary cataract, 1669
Coronary sinus, total anomalous
    pulmonary venous connection, 623
Coronary sinus atrial septal defect, 601
    (Fig.)
Corona veneris, 1406
Coronaviruses, 1373
Coroners, 1720–1721, 1849
Cor pulmonale, 502
  bronchopulmonary dysplasia, 194
  cystic fibrosis, 556
Corpus callosum
  absence, 647
  division, 686–687
Corpus striatum, 767
Corrected plasma calcium, neonate,
    298–299
Corrected QT interval, ionized calcium,
    298–299
Cortical dysplasias, 642, 649–651
  epilepsy, 685
Cortical hyperostosis, infantile, 1583–1585
Cortical layers, 642
Cortical thickness, bone development, 302
Cortical visual impairment, 273
Corticosteroid-binding globulin, 1059
Corticosteroids
  allergic conjunctivitis, 1664, 1676, 1698
  anterior uveitis, 1665
  antivenom treatment, 1523
  asthma, 546
    acute severe, 548–549
  atopic eczema, 1642–1643
  autoimmune chronic active hepatitis,
    480
  benign intracranial hypertension, 665
  biosynthesis, inborn errors, 1009
  birth asphyxia, contraindicated, 131
  on brain, 699
  bronchopulmonary dysplasia, 195
  cancer therapy, toxic effects, 894
    (Table)

Candida albicans, 289
  candidiasis, 1470
  cataract from, 1669, 1677
  congenital syphilis, 1415
  Crohn's disease, 457
  Cushing's syndrome from, 1065
    cyclical, Duchenne muscular dystrophy,
      731
  cysticercosis, 1502
  cystic fibrosis, 558
  dermatomyositis, 1644
  dermatomyositis-polymyositis, 1608
  excess administration, hypertension,
    1070
  eye toxicity, 1677
  geniculate herpes, 725
  growth failure, 1016
  hemangiomas, 1619
  as hormones, 997(Table)
  household products poisoning, 1710
  idiopathic fibrosing alveolitis, 578
  idiopathic thrombocytopenic purpura,
    879
  immunosuppression, 1265
  infantile cortical hyperostosis, 1585
  infectious mononucleosis, 1368
  juvenile chronic arthritis, 1604
    local injections, 1605
  Kawasaki disease, 1481
  leprosy, 1311
  myocarditis, infective, 630
  myopathy from, 736
  nebulized, croup, 563
  nephrotic syndrome, 969, 970–971
    response and dependency, 971
  normal values, urine, 1932 (Table)
  osteopetrosis, 1582
  Pneumocystis carinii pneumonia, 535
  poliomyelitis, 1379
  polymyositis, 737
  postinfectious encephalitis, chickenpox,
    1362
  preterm labor, 116
  raised intracranial pressure, 714, 1825
  respiratory distress syndrome, 104, 114,
    161, 178–179, 338
  rheumatic fever, 628, 1599–1600
  seasonal rhinitis, 1697, 1698
  systemic lupus erythematosus, 1606
  for thrombocytopenia, 229
  toxoplasmosis, 288–289
  trichinosis, 1494–1495
  tuberculosis, 1347
    meningitis, 1345
    miliary, 1343
    pericarditis, 1343
    pulmonary, 1342
  typhoid fever, 1326
  ulcerative colitis, 459
  viral keratitis, contraindicated, 1664
  for vitamin D intoxication, 1055
  withdrawal, adrenal crisis, 1068
Corticosterone methyloxidase deficiency,
    1068
Corticotropin, see ACTH
Corticotropin releasing hormone,
    molecule, 1037 (Table)
Cortisol
  ACTH secretion, 1038
  at birth, 109
  deficiency, hypoglycemia, 297
  fasciculata cells, 1059
  fetal hypoxia response, 124
  normal values, 1924 (Table)
  plasma, 1059
  secretion pattern, 1059
  secretion tests, 1938 (Table)
Cortisol : cortisone ratio, 11β-
    hydroxysteroid dehydrogenase
    deficiency, 1066
Cor triatriatum, 609
Corymbose syphilide, 1407
Corynebacterium diphtheriae, 1305
Coryza, see Common cold

Cosmetics
  India, lead, 1708
  poisoning, 1709
Cosmetic surgery, craniosynostosis,
    1561–1562
Costal margin recession, 30, see also
    Intercostal indrawing; Rib
    recession
Cost-benefit analysis, 105
Cost-effectiveness analysis, 105
Costochondral junctions, 30
  rickets, 1195, 1196
  scurvy, 30, 1199
Costs
  consideration for antibiotics, 1528
  genetic disorders, 46
Cost utility analysis, 105
Cot death, see Sudden infant death
    syndrome
Cotransporters, see Sodium/glucose
    cotransporters
Co-trimoxazole
  administration, 1964 (Table)
  bone marrow transplant recipients, 875
  cat-scratch disease, 1520
  environmental mycobacteria, 1350
  for immunodeficiency, 1266
  Pneumocystis carinii, 535, 577
    cancer treatment, 895
    HIV infection, 1397
  pneumonia, 568
  prophylactic, 533
    cancer treatment, 894
Cottage hospitals, accident and emergency
    departments, 1805
Cough, 506–507
  Chlamydia trachomatis, 280, 1374
  cystic fibrosis, 554
  history taking, 17
  pertussis, 1315
  toxocariasis, 1485
  tracheoesophageal fistula, 1772
  tuberculosis, 1342
Cough medicines
  bronchitis, 565
  poisoning, 1708–1709
Cough reflex, 36 (Table)
Coumarins, 230
Couney, Martin, neonatal care, 96
Counseling, see also Genetic counseling
  bereavement, 174–175
  mental retardation, 838
  parents, psychiatry, 1749
Countercurrent immunoelectrophoresis,
    meningitis, 1290
  neonatal, 282
Counterimmunoelectrophoresis, 277
Coup de sabre, 1645
Court Committee (Committee on Child
    Health Services), 1853
Courts, neonatal intensive care decisions,
    101, 102–103
Cover test, 395, 1652
  pseudo-squint, 1659
Cowdry type A inclusions, herpes simplex,
    1437
Cowper's glands, gonorrhea, 1425
Cow's milk, 112 (Table), 153, 331
  amino acids, 1119, 1120 (Table)
  composition, 331 (Table), 1942–1943
    (Table)
  formula milk manufacture, 333
  intolerance, 212
    careless reporting, 1692
    challenge testing, 1694, 1700
    diarrhea, 1293
    dietary management, 1214 (Table)
    and postgastroenteritis lactose
      intolerance, 333
    proteins, 155, 213, 441–442, 1201,
      1215, 1699–1701
  iron, 333
  for malnutrition, 1193
  metabolic effects, 108

  molybdenum, 1202
  neonatal tetany, 299–300
  proteins, in formula milks, 332
  sensitivity, 327
  solute load, 333
    after weaning, 334
Cow's milk colitis, 213
Coxa magna, 1595
Coxa vara
  adolescent, 1596
  congenital, 1551–1552
Coxiella burnetii (Rickettsia burnetii),
    1374, 1375
Coxsackie viruses, 1381–1383
  congenital infection, 286 (Table)
  group A, 1381–1382, see also Coe virus
  group B, 1382–1383
  group B4, diabetes mellitus, 1074
  group B5, myositis, 724
  myelitis, neuropathy, 724, 725–726
  respiratory infections, 1372
C peptide, 1071
CR3, see Complement receptors, CR3
Crab louse (Pthirus pubis), 1518–1519,
    1638
Crabs, Paragonimus spp., 1513
Crab yaws, 1417
Crack cocaine, 248
Cracked pot sign, intracranial pressure, 20,
    1290
Crackles, respiratory, 512
Cradle cap, 1643
Cramps, vs myotonic syndromes, 733
Cranial nerves
  examination, 34
  flaccid bulbar palsy, 810–812
  neonate, 264, 265
  osteopetrosis, 1582
  palsies
    meningitis, 1289
    tumors, 900
  primitive reflexes, 36 (Table)
  raised intracranial pressure, 708
Cranial sutures, see Sutures (cranial)
Cranial ultrasonography, 242, 678
  intracranial hemorrhage, 249–250
  prematurity outcome studies, 167
  ventricular index, 252
  very low birthweight, outcome, 171
Craniodiaphyseal dysplasia, 1581 (Table)
Craniofacial deformities, surgery, 1797
Craniofacial dysostosis (Crouzon's
    syndrome), 1561, 1661
  inheritance, 1566 (Table)
Craniomeningoceles, 648
Craniometaphyseal dysplasias, 1581
    (Table)
Craniopharyngioma, 373, 794 (Table),
    905, 1000, 1042
  diabetes insipidus, 1040 (Table)
  obesity, 1022
Craniostenosis, 1558–1560, 1661
Craniosynostosis, 242, 1797
  genetic analysis, 76
  premature, 1559–1560
Craniotabes, 20, 1195
Craniotomy, craniosynostosis, 1561
Craniotubular dysplasias, hyperostoses,
    1581
Cranium, examination, 20
Cranium bifidum, 647–648
Crawling, motor development, 667
Crawling reflex, 38 (Table)
C-reactive protein, 1234
  cerebrospinal fluid, meningitis, 1290
  neonatal sepsis, 276 (Table), 277
Creams, 1617
Creatine
  for gyrate atrophy of choroid and retina,
    1111
  normal values, urine, 1931 (Table)
  synthesis disorder, 1116
Creatine kinase
  normal values, 1924 (Table)

Creatine kinase (Contd)
  amniotic fluid, 1937 (Table)
  cerebrospinal fluid, 1934 (Table)
  polymyositis, 1607
Creatine phosphokinase
  Duchenne muscular dystrophy, 730
  neonate, 729
Creatinine
  amniotic fluid, 1937 (Table)
  clearance, 1931 (Table), 1938 (Table)
  GFR measurement, 942
  normal values, 1924 (Table)
    urine, 1931 (Table)
  plasma levels
    neonate, 257 (Table), 258, 259
    preterm infant, 142
  urine
    neonates, 142 (Table)
    renal failure, 974
  vs urine flow rate, very low birth
    weight, 142
Creeping, motor development, 667
Creeping eruption, see Cutaneous larva
  migrans
Cremasteric reflex, 35, 37 (Table), 1790
Cremations, certificates of disposal, 174
Crepitations, see Crackles
Crescentic glomerulonephritis, 962–963,
  965
Cresols, poisoning, 1711
CREST syndrome, 1608
Cretinism, 22 (Fig.), 248, 1046–1048
  Kocher–Debré–Sémélaigne syndrome,
    737
Creutzfeldt–Jakob disease, 1378
Crib-O-Gram, 244
Cricoid cartilage split, for subglottic
  stenosis, 196
Cricothyroid muscle, 808
Cri du chat syndrome, 58, 830 (Table)
Crigler–Najjar syndrome, 218, 219, 1144
Criterion referenced tests, psychological,
  1735
Crocodile tears, 725
Crohn's disease, 456–458
  FUO investigations, 1283 (Table)
  mouth, 424
  nutrition, 457, 458, 1206–1207
  self-help groups, 485
  ultrasonography, 1905
  water secretion, 436
Crohn's in Childhood Research Appeal,
  485
Cromoglycate, see Sodium cromoglycate
Crossed ectopic kidney, 939
Crossed extension reflex, 37 (Table), 240
  neonatal gestation age, 40 (Table)
Cross-reacting antigens, Haemophilus
  influenzae, 1308
Cross-sectional echocardiography,
  591–592
Cross-sectional studies
  disease, 1851
  growth, 352
Cross syndrome, 1107, 1629 (Table)
Crotamiton, scabies, 1517
Crotonic acidemia, 1113
Croup, 563, see also Diphtheria
  imaging, 1899
  spasmodic, 508
Crouzon's syndrome, see Craniofacial
  dysostosis
Crown–heel length, fetal growth, 350
Crown–rump length, 19–20, 80
  fetal growth, 350
  sitting height, 363–364
Crude birth rate, 1
Crude protein content, breast milk, 332
Cry, 34
  neonate, 238 (Fig.)
Crying
  asthma, 542
  on blood gases, 505
  neonate, 236

Cryoprecipitate, 230, 881
  dosage, 851 (Table)
Cryopreservation, and autografts, ovaries,
  1033
Cryosurgery, for subglottic stenosis, 196
Cryotherapy
  genital warts, 1445
  retinopathy of prematurity, 267
  warts, 1633
Cryptococcosis, 1471 (Table), 1475–1476
Cryptogenic tuberculosis, 1336,
  1343–1344
Cryptorchidism, 290, 1007, 1037, 1790
  tumors, 922, 1791
Cryptosporidiosis
  AIDS, 1397
  emergence, 1279 (Table)
  United Kingdom, 1277 (Fig.)
Cryptothyroidism, 1049
Crypts of Lieberkühn, 435
c-src gene, osteopetrosis, 1582
CTAB test (cetyltrimethyl ammonium
  bromide test), 837
Ctenocephalides spp., 1503 (Fig.)
C-terminal fragments, parathyroid
  hormone, 1054
CT scan, see Computed tomography
Cubes, developmental examination, 392,
  393
Cubitus valgus, Turner's syndrome, 61
Cuffed catheters, central venous lines,
  1224, 1225
Cultures, see also Blood cultures; Urine,
  cultures
  candidiasis, 1434
  Chlamydia spp., 1430
  Neisseria gonorrhoeae, 1423
  ophthalmia neonatorum, 263
  shell viral cultures, 1366
Curare, ventilation for RDS, 181
Curators ad litem, 1859, 1873–1874
Curosurf (porcine surfactant), 179
Curved linear array transducers,
  ultrasonography, 1896
Cushing reflex, 706
  neonate, 243
Cushing's disease, 1041
Cushing's syndrome, 1000, 1065–1066
  hypertension, 1065, 1070
  maternal, 89 (Table)
  obesity, 1190
  short stature, 375
Custodianship, 1860
Cutaneous anthrax, 1300
Cutaneous larva migrans, 1490–1491
  organisms, 1484 (Table)
Cutaneous leishmaniasis, 1461 (Table),
  1463–1464
Cutaneous nerve segments, see
  Dermatomes
Cutaneous polyarteritis, 1610
Cutaneous reflexes, 36–37 (Table)
Cut down, surgical venous, 1837
Cutis marmorata, 1646
Cutis marmorata telangiectatica congenita,
  1646
Cyanide-nitroprusside test, 837, 1109
Cyanide poisoning, 1813
Cyanosis, 511, 585
  diagnostic algorithm, 613 (Table)
  episodes of sudden onset (Southall),
    528
  history taking, 17, 584
  neonate, 110, 201–202
    and heart failure, 203
  nitrogen washout test, 200–201
  normal children, episodes, 585
  respiratory distress syndrome, 177
Cyanotic breath-holding attacks, 672
Cyanotic congenital heart disease,
  613–623
  stroke, 713
Cycle specific cytotoxic drugs, 892
Cyclic adenosine monophosphate (cAMP)

adrenal cortex, 1059
cardiac function, 1820
cholera, 1303
growth endocrinology, 364
hypoparathyroidism, 1059
parathyroid hormone release, 1054
Cyclical corticosteroids, Duchenne
  muscular dystrophy, 731
Cyclical neutropenia, 867, 1259
Cyclical parenteral nutrition, 1226
Cyclical vomiting, 717
Cycling, see Bicycles
Cycling peritoneal dialysis, continuous,
  981
Cyclitis, 1666, see also Anterior uveitis
Cyclizine, administration, 1964 (Table)
Cyclooxygenase inhibition, 229
Cyclopentolate, administration, 1964
  (Table)
Cyclophosphamide
  on fetus and neonate, 91 (Table)
  focal segmental glomerulosclerosis, 971
  hemorrhagic cystitis, 959
  immunosuppression, 1265
  leukemia from, 890
  nephrotic syndrome, 970 (Fig.), 971
  systemic lupus erythematosus, 1606
  toxic effects, 894 (Table), 896, 897
Cyclopia, 58, 649
Cycloplegics, refractive error testing, 1657
Cycloserine, administration, 1964 (Table)
Cyclosporine, 1265
  administration, 1964 (Table)
  liver transplantation, 484–485
  mdr-1 partial reversal, 893
  nephrotic syndrome, 970 (Fig.)
CYP21 genes, 21-hydroxylase deficiency,
  1062
Cyproheptadine, migraine, 717 (Table),
  719
Cyproterone
  polycystic ovarian disease, 993
  precocious puberty, 1030, 1031
Cystathione, neuroblastoma, 911–912
Cystathione synthase deficiency, 1100
Cystathionine, metabolism disorders, 1109
Cystathionine synthase deficiency,
  1108–1109
Cysteamine
  for cystinosis, 1123
  therapy, 945
Cysteine, 1108
  preterm requirements, 157
Cystic adenomatoid malformation, 192,
  1769
Cystic astrocytomas, 903
Cystic disease, renal, 254–255, 940–941
Cysticercoids, Hymenolepis spp., 1502
Cysticercosis, 1501–1502
Cysticercus bovis, 1500
Cystic fibrosis, 72 (Table), 491, 550–559,
  see also Meconium ileus
  analgesia, 1833
  arthropathy, 1611
  and bronchiolitis, 564
  bronchoscopy, 520
  clinical diagnosis, 552–553
  cost, 46
  diabetes mellitus, 556, 1082
  ethmoidal polyps, 1685
  frequency, 47 (Table)
  genetic diagnosis, 73
  giardiasis, 1466
  liver, 484, 556
  malabsorption, 445, 449, 553
  mortality, 490 (Table)
  neonatal jaundice, 220
  nutrition, 450, 1207–1209
  pancreas and intestine, 449–450
  physiotherapy, 521, 557
  Pseudomonas aeruginosa, 555, 557,
    558 (Table), 1320
  screening, 339 (Table), 552
    antenatal care, 80

severely handicapped children affected,
  14 (Table)
specialist care, 559
treatment, 557–559
vitamin E deficiency, 1198
Cystic Fibrosis Research Trust, 485
Cystic fibrosis transmembrane
  conductance regulator gene, 550,
  551
Cystic hygroma, 22 (Fig.), 1784, 1798
Cystine, 1108
Cystin-lysinuria, 1121
Cystinosis, 945, 1123, 1157 (Table)
  eye, 1673
Cystinuria, 446, 947–948, 1121
Cystitis, 950
  cytotoxic drugs, 894 (Table), 896, 959
  hematuria, 958, 959
Cystography, radionuclide, 1911–1912
Cystometrography, 656
Cystoscopy, hematuria, 960
Cysts, see also Lung cysts
  cerebral palsy, 171
  periventricular leukomalacia,
    ultrasonography, 242, 251
Cytocentrifugation, cerebrospinal fluid,
  696
Cytochrome b₅ reductase deficiency,
  1131–1132
Cytochrome reductase deficiency, stroke,
  713
Cytogenetics
  Duchenne muscular dystrophy, 729, 732
  dystrophia myotonica, 734
  Huntington's chorea, 773
  leukemias, 869
  neoplasms, 891
  tuberous sclerosis, 802
Cytokeratins, small round cell tumors, 912
  (Table)
Cytokine receptors, 365, 1232
Cytokines, 1232, 1233 (Table)
  hemopoiesis, 849
  for immunodeficiency, 1270
  juvenile chronic arthritis, 1210
  and macrophages, 1235
  for neonatal infections, 1267
  neonate, 273, 275, 1241
  neoplasm treatment, 893
  production defects, 1250
Cytology, tracheal aspirate,
  bronchopulmonary dysplasia, 194
Cytomegalic congenital adrenal
  hypoplasia, 1067
Cytomegalic inclusion disease, 1365–1366
  eye, 1676
  FUO investigations, 1283 (Table)
Cytomegalovirus, 1365–1366
  AIDS, 1396
  bone marrow transplant recipients,
    874–875
  cancer treatment, 895
  congenital infection, 286 (Table), 287,
    1284
  detection, 817
  hepatitis, 1388
  immunosuppression, 1264
  neonates, 196, 248
  nephrotic syndrome, 972
  pneumonitis, immunocompromised
    patient, 535
Cytoplasmic immunoglobulin, small
  round cell tumors, 912 (Table)
Cytoplasm modifying test, toxoplasmosis,
  1465
Cytosine, toxic effects, 894 (Table)
Cytosolic acetoacetyl-CoA thiolase
  deficiency, 1130
Cytotoxic drugs, 892, see also
  Antimetabolites; Antimitotic drugs
  gonadal function, 899
  immunosuppression, 1265
  toxicity effects, 894 (Table)
Cytotoxic edema, birth asphyxia, 126

Cytotoxic hypersensitivity, skin, **1639–1640**
Cytotoxicity assays, lymphocyte function, 1247
Cytotoxic snake venoms, 1521
Cytotoxic T cells, tuberculosis, 1336
Cytotoxins
  bacterial diarrhea, 452
  Shigella spp., 1327

D1-pyrroline-5-carboxylic acid, excretion, 1114
Dacarbazine, toxic effects, 894 (Table)
Dacryoadenitis, acute, 1664
Dacryocystitis, acute, 1665
Dacryocystography, 1654
Dactylitis
  sickle cell disease, 862 (Fig.)
  syphilis, 1412
  tuberculous, **1593**
Daily record cards, asthma, 543
Daily rhythms, *see* Circadian rhythms
Dampness, respiratory disorders, 492
Danazol
  administration, 1964 (Table)
  fetal masculinization, 986
  for hereditary angioneurotic edema, 1175
Dancing eye syndrome, 752
  neuroblastoma, 763
Dandy–Walker cyst (syndrome), **645**, 658, 753
Dane particles, 1386
Dantrolene
  cerebral palsy, 759
  scoline myotonia, 733
Dapsone, 1311, *see also* Maloprim
  administration, 1964 (Table)
  methemoglobinemia, 864
Dark adaptation, vitamin A deficiency, 1677
Dark ground microscopy
  cholera, 1304
  syphilis, 1402
Darrow's solution, 1296
Daunomycin, toxic effects, 894 (Table)
Day care, **1860–1861**
Day nurseries, 1861
DDAVP, *see* Desmopressin
DDT, poisoning, 1711
Deadly nightshade poisoning, 1711
Dead space, 498
  V/Q mismatch, 502
Deafness, **1682–1683**
  acquired central, *see* Auditory agnosia
  Alport's syndrome, 966
  conductive, 816, 817, 1682
  DIDMOAD syndrome, 1081
  genetic, 46
  kernicterus, 248–249, 816
  meningitis, 1291, 1292, 1682
  profound childhood, recurrence risks, 74
  secretory otitis media, 1681
  sensorineural, **816–818, 1682**
    screening, 243–244
  severely handicapped children affected, 14 (Table)
  syphilis
    congenital, 1413, 1414, 1415
    secondary, 1408
  very low birthweight, 171
Deamidated human growth hormone, 365
Death, 927–928, *see also* Sudden death; Sudden infant death syndrome
  of parent, **1857**
  unexpected, 1720–1721
Death certificates, **1849**, *see also* Certification, neonatal death
Debranching enzyme deficiency (limit dextrinosis), 735, **1138**
Debriefing, sudden infant death syndrome, 1723

Debt, developing countries, 1885
Deceleration injuries, 705
Decelerations, fetal heart rate, 86, 117
Decerebrate rigidity, 747 (Fig.)
Deciduous teeth, eruption times, 27
Decongestants
  common cold, 560
  seasonal rhinitis, 1697–1698
Decosohexenoic acid, brain development, 643
Deep electrode EEG studies, 678
  mesial temporal sclerosis, 686
  for temporal lobectomy, 686
Deep flexor tendons, congenital shortness, 1549
Deep mycoses, 1470
Defecation, normal frequencies, 461
Defective apoprotein B-100, 1150 (Table), 1152
Defense mechanisms
  psychological, 1731–1732, 1760–1761
  respiratory, 497, **531–532**
Deferiprone, for thalassemia, 863
Defibrillation, **526**, 527 (Fig.), *see also* Cardioversion
Deficiency anemias, **850–853**
Deformations, *see* Congenital deformations
Deformities, musculoskeletal, **38–39**
Degenerate code, 68–69
Degenerative brain diseases, **774–798**
  investigations, 798 (Table)
  pseudobulbar palsy, 812
Deglutition, *see* Swallowing
Dehiscence, wounds, 1833
Dehydration, **409–411**, *see also* Hypernatremia
  acute diarrhea, 413, **452–453, 1293–1294**
  acute renal failure, 974
  cholera, management, 1304
  diabetic ketoacidosis, 1075
  examination, 1286, **1287 (Table)**
  fluid therapy, **413–415, 453, 1295–1296**
  neonate, 144
    jaundice, 218
    phototherapy, 218
  preterm infant, 141
  treatment, **413**
Dehydration fever, 1282
Dehydroemetine, administration, 1964 (Table)
Dehydroepiandrosterone, 1059
  fetus, 1003
  normal values, 1924 (Table)
Dejerine–Sottas disease, 723
De Lange syndrome, 23 (Fig.), 830 (Table)
  heart, 596
Delayed type hypersensitivity, 1689
  skin, **1641–1642**
  skin tests, 1247
  syphilis, 1401
  tuberculosis, 1336
Delayed visual maturation, 272–273
Delegation, and negligence, 1879
Deletions, 69
  chromosomal, 51, 52 (Fig.)
    aniridia–Wilms' tumor syndrome, 913
    neoplasms, 887–889
    neuroblastoma, 911
  chromosome 13, **59**
Deliberate poisoning, *see* Non-accidental poisoning; Self-poisoning
Delinquency, 1742, **1762**
Delirium-like conditions, 1739
Delivery
  herpes simplex virus transmission, **1441–1442**
  high-risk, 116–120
  place of, 83–84
  preterm infant, **138–139**
  room temperature, 147

squatting position, 107
Delta agent, hepatitis, 477, **1387**
δ-aminolevulinic acid, 1142
Delta brush pattern, electroencephalography, preterm infant, 243
δ cells, pancreas, 1071
ΔF508 deletion, cystic fibrosis, 73, 551
Delta virus, hepatitis, 477, **1387**
Demand feeding, 328
Demeclocycline, administration, 1964 (Table)
Dementia
  epilepsy, 687
  vs mental retardation, 826
  presenile, Down syndrome, 55
  tuberous sclerosis, 801
Demethylchlortetracycline, 1041
Demodicidosis, **1514–1515**
Demography, **1–15**
De Montbeillard, Count P., growth charts, 352
Demyelination, peripheral nerves, 722, 723
Dendrites, development, 643
Dendritic cells, 1242
Dengue fever, **1389**
Dengue hemorrhagic shock syndrome, 1389
Denial, 1731, 1760
  terminal care, 929
Denmark, *vs* Sweden, celiac disease, 440
Dental care
  δ-hemolytic streptococcal infection, 1333
  antibiotic prophylaxis, infective endocarditis, 631, 632 (Table)
  tuberculosis, 1336, 1340
Dental caries
  mental retardation, 841
  rates, 15 (Table)
Dental health, infants, 334
Dentatorubral atrophy, 792 (Table), *see also* Ramsay Hunt syndrome
Dentatorubral-pallidoluysian atrophy, 766
Dentinogenesis imperfecta, 1568
Denver screening test, 400
Deoxycorticosterone, 11-β hydroxylase deficiency, 1064
Deoxyguanosine triphosphate, 1250
Deoxypyridinoline, urine, 1567, 1612
11-Deoxysteroids, normal values, urine, 1932 (Table)
Depigmented macules, tuberous sclerosis, 802
Depot synacthen test, 1938 (Table)
Depressed fractures, 700, 702
Depression, **1742**
  adolescence, **1754–1755**
  vs chronic fatigue syndrome, 1760
Derived indices, anthropometric nutritional assessment, 1186
Dermatitis, *see also* Eczema
  ammoniacal, 1472
  beetle toxins, 1525
  napkin rash, 1643
  Paederus, 1525
  Physalia, 1526
  seborrheic, 1643
  vs tinea versicolor, 1637
Dermatitis herpetiformis, 1285, **1641**
Dermatobia hominis, 1514
Dermatobia spp., larval disease, 1484 (Table)
Dermatomes, 35
  definition, 1436
Dermatome-to-myotome stimulation, myelomeningocele, 653
Dermatomyositis, **737, 1606–1608, 1644**
  eye, 1675
Dermatophagoides spp., 1690
Dermis, 1616
Dermographism
  atopic eczema, 1642
  scabies, 1638

Dermoid cysts, 1783–1784
  orbit, 1661
  ovaries, 993
Dermolytic epidermolysis bullosa, 1622, 1624 (Table)
δ-6 Desaturase, 1206
Descemet's membrane, 264
Descriptive studies, child health, 1850
Desensitization, Hymenoptera stings, 1524
Desferrioxamine
  administration, 1964 (Table)
  iron poisoning, 1710
  for thalassemia, 863
Desmin, small round cell tumors, 912 (Table)
17,20-Desmolase deficiency, 1009
Desmopressin, 1040
  administration, 1964 (Table)
  hemophilia A, 880
  nocturnal enuresis, 957
  screening for diabetes insipidus, 943
  Von Willebrand's disease, 881
Desquamation, Kawasaki disease, 1285, 1479
Desquamative interstitial pneumonitis, 578
Detection bias, 327
Detergents, poisoning, 1709
Detoxification, cytotoxic drugs, 893
Detrusor, neurogenic bladder, 656
Detrusor instability, **957**
  vs enuresis, 957 (Table)
Deuterium dilution studies, 403
Developing countries, **1882–1893**
  bottle feeding, respiratory tract infections, 559
  disease burdens, 1276, 1280 (Table)
  formula feeding, 327
  gastroenteritis, mortality, 1293
  gonorrhea, 1421
  immunization schedules, 343–345
  mortality, **7**
    infections, 1274
  pneumonia diagnosis, 566
  respiratory disorders, **493**
  salmonellosis, 1323
  Shigella spp., 1327
  short stature, 1019
  tuberculosis, 1335
    HIV infection, 1346
Developing true hemiplegia, 741–742
Development, **349–380**
  adolescence, **1750**
  arithmetic, 825 (Fig.)
  assessment, **386–400**
    failure to thrive, 469
    interpretation, **396–399**
  Children Act 1989, 1875
  chronic renal failure on, 981
  ear, 816
  electrocardiography changes, 589
  immune system, **1240–1241**
  liver function, 471
  malnutrition, 1193
  psychological, **1728–1732**
  psychomotor, **381–400**
  puberty, ratings, 357–360
  sleep changes, 530
  speech, **804–805**
Developmental cataracts, **1667–1669**
Developmental disorders
  central nervous system, **666–670**
  pervasive, **834–836**, 1733, **1737–1739**
  speech, **670, 805–807**
Developmental history, 18
Developmental psychopathology, **1731–1732**
Developmental screening examinations, 1862
Developmental support, 98
Developmental test of visual perception, Frostig, 400
Developmental tic, simple, 771
Devic's disease, 793 (Table)

Dexamethasone
  administration, 1964 (Table)
    neonate, 1957 (Table)
  antiemetic, 896
  bronchopulmonary dysplasia, 195
  congenital adrenal hyperplasia, 1064
    antenatal management, 985
  croup, 563
  growth plate experiment, 1014
  Haemophilus influenzae meningitis, 1291, 1309
  21-hydroxylase deficiency, antenatal therapy, 1062
  tuberculosis, meningitis, 1345
  typhoid fever, 1326
Dexamethasone-suppressible hyperaldosteronism, 1066
Dexamethasone suppression test, 1066, 1938 (Table)
Dexamphetamine, administration, 1964 (Table)
5'-Dexoxyadenosyl-cobalamin, deficient synthesis, 1117
Dextrocardia, 598, 612
Dextrose
  for dehydration, 413
  for hyperammonemia, 1111
  hyperglycemia, 298
  for hypoglycemia, 294–295, 296
    pyruvate dehydrogenase deficiency, 306
  with insulin, for hyperkalemia, 145 (Table), 259, 415, 975
  parenteral nutrition, 158
  resuscitation, doses, 526 (Table), 527 (Fig.)
  for Reye's syndrome, 479
  strengths in fluid therapy, 1296
  treatment of hypernatremia, 414
DFMO (difluoromethyl-ornithine), 1457
D-glycerate dehydrogenase deficiency, 1112
D-glycericacidemia, 1113
Diabetes insipidus, **1039**
  congenital nephrogenic, 260
  DIDMOAD syndrome, 1081
  FUO investigations, 1283 (Table)
  head injuries, 709
  investigation, 943
  nephrogenic, **948–949,** 1039
Diabetes mellitus, **1072–1081,** *see also* Ketosis
  acid–base balance, 419, 421
  adrenarche, 1061
  and breast-feeding, 327
  calcium metabolism, 299
  candidiasis, 1470
  cataract, 1669, 1674
  caudal regression syndrome, 641
  celiac disease, 440
  chromium deficiency, 1202
  clinics, 1077
  congenital heart disease, 596
  control problems, 1080–1081
  cystic fibrosis, 556, 1082
  vs enuresis, 957 (Table)
  eye, **1674**
  fetus, 1005
    hemopoiesis, 225
  hyperlipoproteinemia, 1153, 1154 (Table)
  hypertrophic cardiomyopathy, neonate, 205
  hyperviscosity, 713, 715
  immune system, 1266
  incidence, 1072–1074
  inheritance, 998
  insulin-like growth factors, 351
  intracellular water loss, 406
  after intrauterine growth retardation, 1005
  large for gestational age infant, 138
  long-term management, 1076–1082
  maternal, 89 (Table), 295

mucocutaneous candidiasis, 1251, 1637
nephropathy, 966
neuropathy, 724
nutrition, **1209–1210**
obesity, risk, 1022
post-pancreatectomy, 1084
preconceptual care, 79
pregnancy, 114, 116
preventive strategies, 1081
recurrence risks, 74
refraction, 1658
screening, 339 (Table)
severely handicapped children affected, 14 (Table)
sodium levels, 404
thyroid disease, 1048
transient neonatal, 298
type II, with or without deafness, 1127
Diabetic foods, 1210
Diagnosis coding, 1803
Diagnostic imaging, *see* Imaging
Dialysis, *see also* Hemodialysis; Peritoneal dialysis
  acute renal failure, 976–977
  after cardiac surgery, 1822
  dietary management, 1211 (Table)
  for hyperammonemia, 1112
  inborn errors of metabolism, 307
  intensive care, 1823–1824
  neonate, 258, 259
  for organic acidurias, 1119
Diamorphine, 928
  administration, 1964 (Table)
    neonate, 1957 (Table)
Diapers, *see* Napkins
Diaphragm, 505, *see also* Phrenic nerve, paralysis
  breathing in sleep, 530
  congenital abnormalities, **575–576**
  diphtheria, 1306
  eventration, **575–576,** 1770
  examination, 512
  neonate, 495
  neuroblastoma, 911
  plication, phrenic nerve trauma, 122
Diaphragmatic hernia, 43, **575,** **1769–1770**
  intrauterine surgery, 115
  pulmonary hypoplasia, 191
Diaphragm contraceptives, 995
Diaphyseal aclasis, **1585**
Diaries
  asthma, 543
  dietary nutritional assessment, 1187
Diarrhea, 424, 467–468, *see also* Gastroenteritis; Toddler diarrhea; Z-lumirubin, loose stools
  acute infective, **451–454**
  AIDS, 1397
  bacteriology, 1299
  cancer treatment, 896
  Capillaria philippinensis, 1495
  causes, **1286**
  cow's milk protein intolerance, 1699
  dehydration, treatment, 413
  developing countries disease burden, 1276 (Table), 1280 (Table)
  giardiasis, 1466
  hemolytic uremic syndrome, 974, 977
  Hirschsprung's enterocolitis, 1777
  hyponatremia, 411
  metabolic disorders, 305
  necrotizing enterocolitis, 210, 212
  neonate, **212–213**
  neuroblastoma, 911
  nutrition, 1215
  protracted, in early infancy, **454–455**
  salmonellosis, 1324
  short bowel syndrome, 1212
Diarrheal Disease Control Program, 1889
Diary cards, asthma, 543
Diastematomyelia, **652,** 1557
Diastolic murmurs, 586

Diastolic velocity, Doppler ultrasonography, 1896
Diastrophic dwarfism, hitchhiker thumb, 76
Diastrophic dysplasia, **1577**
  inheritance, 1566 (Table)
Diazepam
  administration, 1964 (Table)
    neonate, 1957 (Table)
  computed tomography, 1897
  encephalopathies, 697
  febrile convulsions, 683
  on fetus and neonate, 91 (Table)
  resuscitation, doses, 527 (Fig.)
  seizures
    acute renal failure, 975
    emergency care, 1814
    head injuries, 1811
    neonatal, 246 (Table)
  status epilepticus, 692
  tetanus, 285, 1334
  therapeutic ranges, 1936 (Table)
Diazoxide
  administration, 1965 (Table)
  for hyperinsulinism, 296
  for hypertension, 637 (Table), 1965 (Table)
  neonate, acute renal failure, 259
  nesidioblastosis, 1085
Dibasic aminoaciduria, isolated, 1121
Dicarboxylic acids
  excretion, 1119
  fasting, 1128
Dicarboxylic aminoaciduria, 1121
Dichotomous thinking, 1730
Diclofenac, 1832
  administration, 1965 (Table)
Dicyclomine, administration, 1965 (Table)
DIDMOAD syndrome, 1084
diduchwa, see Endemic syphilis
Dieffenbachier, poisoning, 1711
Dieldrin, poisoning, 1711
Diencephalic astrocytomas, 903
Diencephalic epilepsy, 684
Diencephalic syndrome, 1043
Diencephalon, 642
Dienestrol cream
  administration, 1965 (Table)
  labial adhesions, 1795
Dientameba fragilis, enterobiasis, 1487
Diet(s), *see also* Exclusion diets; *named diseases*
  adolescents, 341
  amino acid restricted, **1119–1120**
  carbohydrates, acute porphyrias, 1143
  for celiac disease, 441, 442
  celiac disease incidence, 440
  chronic renal failure, 980
  cirrhosis, 482
  cystic fibrosis, **557**
  debranching enzyme deficiency, 1138
  diabetes mellitus management, 1077–1080
  diarrhea from, 1293
  failure to thrive, 466
  familial hyperchylomicronemia type I, 1151
  fructose-1-phosphate aldolase deficiency, 1135
  galactose-1-phosphate uridyltransferase deficiency, 1133
  gastrointestinal disorders, 469–470
  glucose-6-phosphatase deficiency, 1137
  and health, 340
  hepatic encephalopathy, 483
  history, 17, 1187
  hypercholesterolemia, 1152
  hyperphenylalaninemia, 1104, 1105
  inborn errors of metabolism, 307
  for intestinal lymphangiectasia, 444
  iron deficiency, 850
  low-methionine, 1109
  for malnutrition, 1193

maple syrup urine disease, 1116–1117, 1119
maternal, breast milk composition, 332
for migraine, 718
nephrotic syndrome, 970
normal, **1188–1189**
obesity, 1190
organic acidurias, 1119
oxalosis, 1113
protein, for hyperammonemia, 1112
for protracted diarrhea, 455
social class, 15 (Table)
sodium, 408
for toddler diarrhea, 464
Dietary intolerance, *see* Food intolerance
Dietary nutritional assessment, **1187**
Dietary reference values (definition), 1180
Diethylcarbamazine
  cutaneous larva migrans, 1491
  filariasis, 1498
  loiasis, 1497
  onchocerciasis, 1497
  toxocariasis, 1486
Diethylstilbestrol
  on fetus and neonate, 91 (Table)
  genital abnormalities from, 994
  neoplasms in offspring, 890
Dietl's crisis, 1795
Difetarsone, *Trichuris trichiura,* 1491
Differential tone, postasphyxial encephalopathy, 127
Diffuse cutaneous leishmaniasis, 1463
Diffuse cutaneous mastocytosis, 1647
Diffuse infantile hemangiomatosis, 1619
Diffuse mesangial sclerosis, 972
Diffusible nonionized calcium, 299
Diffusing capacity for carbon monoxide, 505
Difluoromethyl-ornithine, 1457
DiGeorge syndrome, 59, 60 (Table), 300, 444, 1242 (Table), **1252,** 1470
  congenital heart disease, 596
  incidence, 1243 (Table)
Digestion, 423
  small intestine, **436–437**
  stomach, 430
Digital imaging, 1895
Digitalis, and Chagas' disease, 1460
Digital subtraction angiography
  liver, 472
  lung vessels, 514
Digoxin, 627 (Table)
  administration, 1965 (Table)
    neonate, 1957 (Table)
  Coxsackie B myocarditis, 1382
  heart failure, 599
  infective myocarditis, 630
  intensive care, 1820
  neonate, 205
  paroxysmal supraventricular tachycardia, 627
  poisoning, 1709
  therapeutic ranges, 1936 (Table)
Digoxin-specific antibody fragments, 1709, 1965 (Table)
Dihydrocodeine, administration, 1965 (Table)
Dihydroemetine, amebiasis, 1469
Dihydrofolate reductase
  deficiency, 852
  overproduction, 892
Dihydropteridine reductase, 1106
  deficiency, 1106, 1114
  tetrahydrobiopterin test, 1105
Dihydropyrimidinase deficiency, 1142
Dihydropyrimidine dehydrogenase deficiency, 1142
Dihydrotachysterol, administration, 1965 (Table)
Dihydrotestosterone, 1004, 1024
  deficiency, 1009
  genital development, 986
2,8-Dihydroxyadenine, 1141

1,25-Dihydroxycholecalciferol, 304
  fetus, 1004
  neonate, 301
1,25-Dihydroxy vitamin D, 1054, 1058
  disorders, 1056
  fetus, 1053
  neonate, 1053
24,25-Dihydroxy vitamin D, 1054
Diiodohydroxyquinoline, administration,
  1965 (Table)
Diiodotyrosine, 1044
Diisopropylfluorophosphate, squint, 1660
Dilanoxide furoate, 1469, 1965 (Table)
Dilated cardiomyopathy, **633–634**
  neonate, 205
Dimenhydrinate, administration, 1965
  (Table)
Dimercaprol, 1708
  administration, 1965 (Table)
Dimercaptosuccinic acid scan, urinary
  tract infections, 953
Dimerization, growth hormone receptor,
  1013–1014
Dimers, human growth hormone, 365
Dimorphous leprosy, 1300
Dinner fork deformity, chorea, 1598
Dioralyte, 413, 453 (Table)
Dipetalogaster maximus, xenodiagnosis,
  1459
Diphenoxylate
  administration, 1965 (Table)
  poisoning, 1709–1710
Diphenylpyraline, administration, 1965
  (Table)
2,3-Diphosphoglycerate
  neonate, 108, 177
  normal values, 1925 (Table)
Diphtheria, 560, **561, 1305–1307**
  antibiotic prophylaxis, 1529
  ataxia, 762
  conjunctivitis, 1677
  myocarditis, 630, 1305, 1306
  neuropathy, **724**
  pharyngeal membrane, 511
  prevalence, 490
  re-emergence, 1278
  trends, 7
  United Kingdom, 1277, 1278 (Fig.)
  vaccination, 1965 (Table)
Diphtheria antitoxin, 561, **1306–1307**
  administration, 1965 (Table)
Diphtheria toxoid, linked *Haemophilus
  influenzae* antigen, 341
Diphyllobothrium latum, **1503–1504**
  vitamin B$_{12}$ deficiency, 853, 1199,
    1503–1504
Diplegia, 35, 43 (Fig.), **744–748**
  walking, 758
Diploid number, 47
Diploidy, 51
Diplomyelia, 652
Diplopia, 1661
Dip slides, urine bacteriology, 951, 1299
Dipsticks
  hematuria, 958
  proteinuria, 967
  urine bacteriology, 951, 1299
Dipylidium caninum, **1502–1503**
Dipyridamole
  administration, 1965 (Table)
  Kawasaki disease, 1480–1481
Direct antiglobulin test, malaria, 1448
Direct Coombs' test, idiopathic
  thrombocytopenic purpura, 878
Direct isotope cystography, 953
Direct radionuclide cystography, 1912
Dirofilaria immitis, **1499**
Dirofilaria spp., larval disease, 1484
  (Table)
Disability, *see also* Handicap
  definition, 167
  developing countries, **1891**
  incidence, **13**
  neural tube defects, 655

registers of, 1850
  responses, **1760–1761**
  trauma, 1809
Disability adjusted life years, 1276
Disaccharidases, 207
  defects, 445
  enteropathies, 1214–1215
Disaccharides, *see also* Lactose,
    intolerance
  diarrhea, 445
  digestion, 437
Disc batteries, poisoning, 1710
Discitis, imaging, 1915
Discoid eczema, **1643**
Discoid lupus erythematosus, 1644
Discordant atrioventricular connections,
  597
Discordant ventriculoarterial connections,
  597
Disease-specific control programs,
  primary health care, 1889–1890
Disease surveillance, 1804
Dishwasher powder, poisoning, 1710
Disinfectants
  Burkholderia cepacia, 1321
  poisoning, 1709
  cetrimide, 1711
Disintegrative psychosis, 796 (Table), 836,
  1739
Disomy, uniparental, 1017
Disopyramide, 627 (Table)
  administration, 1965 (Table)
  neonate, 1957 (Table)
Dispermy, 51
Displacement, defense mechanism, 1732
Disproportionate short stature, 1017
Disseminated adenovirus infection, 1371
Disseminated gonococcal infection,
  1420–1421, **1425–1426**
  tests, 1423
  treatment, 1428
Disseminated herpes simplex (eczema
  herpeticum), 1284, 1439, **1632**
  pregnancy, 1438
Disseminated histoplasmosis, 1477
Disseminated intravascular coagulation,
  882
  African trypanosomiasis, 1455
  birth asphyxia, 129
  leukemia, 870
  maternal, 89 (Table)
  Neisseria meningitidis, 1314
  neonate, 42, 231
    jaundice, 218
    organisms, 285 (Table)
  Plasmodium falciparum, 1448
  polycythemia, SGA baby, 137
  septicemia, 1287, 1288
  stroke, 713
Disseminated lupus erythematosus, *see*
  Lupus nephritis; Systemic lupus
  erythematosus
Disseminated monilial infection, 1472
Disseminated sclerosis in childhood, 793
  (Table)
Disseminated tuberculosis, 1336,
  1343–1344
Dissociation, ionic, 405
Dissociative states, **1740–1741**
Distal intestinal obstruction syndrome,
  449
  cystic fibrosis, 554
Distal nephron, 942
Distal renal tubular acidosis, 260
  permanent, 945
Distal renal tubule, 259
  function, **944**
Distal spinal muscular atrophy, 721
Distance chart
  fetal growth, 350
  postnatal growth, 352
Distraction audiometry, **816–817,** 1683
Distraction testing, deafness screening,
  244

Distraction therapy, accident and
  emergency departments, 1805
District handicap teams, 400, 1853
District hospitals, maternity services, 156
Disturbance, psychiatric, 1727–1728,
  1732–1734
Dithranol, 1629
Diuresis, postnatal, 257
Diuretic phase, respiratory distress
  syndrome, 180
Diuretics
  acidosis from, 420 (Table)
  ascites, 482
  on fetus and neonate, 91 (Table)
  heart failure, 599
    neonatal, 205
  hypertension, 638
    renal, 973 (Table)
  nephrotic syndrome, 970
  patent ductus arteriosus, 143
Diurnal enuresis, 1743
Diurnal rhythms, *see* Circadian rhythms
Diurnal variation
  dystonias, 774, 793 (Table)
  muscle tone, 756
Diving, grommet tubes, 1682
Diving reflex, 123, 627, 1717
Divorce, **1855–1856**
Dizygotic twins, 90
DMSA scan, urinary tract infections, 953
DNA, **68–70**
  analysis, limitations, 1100
  antibodies, systemic lupus
    erythematosus, 1606
  extraction, 70
  fingerprinting, *see* Restriction
    endonuclease fingerprinting
  mitochondrial, 1126
  Neisseria gonorrhoeae, detection, 1424
  neuroblastoma, content, 911
  repair, 69–70
  repair syndromes, **1142**
    Fanconi's anemia, 854
    neoplasms, 888 (Table)
Dobutamine
  administration, 1965 (Table)
    neonate, 1957 (Table)
  cyanotic heart disease, dosage, 202
    (Table)
  intensive care, 1820
Docosahexanoic acid, 332, 1182
Docusate, administration, 1965 (Table)
Dog bites, 1714
Dog hookworms, 1490
Dogs, 1519 (Table)
  Dirofilaria immitis, 1499
  hydatid disease, 1504
    praziquantel, 1506
  leishmaniasis control, 1464
  rabies from, 1377
  Taenia solium, 1501
  Toxocara canis, 1485, 1486
Dolichocephaly, 1560
Dolichols, urine, 1171
Doll's eye reflex, 36 (Table), 241
Dominance, *see* Cerebral dominance
Dominant inheritance, 64, **65–66**
  central nervous system malformations,
    645
  X-linked, **67**
'Domino' scheme, 84
Domperidone, administration, 1965
  (Table)
Donath–Landsteiner test, 1414
Donnan membrane equilibrium, 407
Dopamine
  administration, 1965 (Table)
    neonate, 1957 (Table)
  basal ganglia, 768
  cyanotic heart disease, dosage, 202
    (Table)
  heart failure, 599
  intensive care, 1820
  multiple tics, 771

  normal values, 1924 (Table)
  volume depletion, acute renal failure,
    974
Dopamine β-hydroxylase deficiency, 1107
Dopamine hydroxylase deficiency, 1069
Dopaminergic receptors, 1820
Doppler equation, 592
Doppler ultrasonography, **1896,** *see also*
  Echocardiography
  vs cardiac catheterization, pulmonary
    stenosis, 608
  cerebral blood flow, 661
  cerebral hemodynamics, birth asphyxia,
    128–129
  flow velocity waveform, umbilical
    artery, 82–83, 115
  gastrointestinal tract, 1904, 1905
  heart, 592–593
  innocent murmurs, 595
  intracranial lesions, 1908
  liver, 1907
  prognosis in birth asphyxia, 132
  renal vessels, 1910
  umbilical artery, flow velocity
    waveform, 82–83, 115
  urinary tract infections, neonate, 262
  uterine artery blood flow, 81, **82**
Dornase alfa, administration, 1966 (Table)
Dosage, **1954–1955**
  adult dose percentages, 1980 (Table)
  antibiotics, **1527–1528, 1955–1956
    (Table)**
  tables, **1954–1980**
Dot blotting, 70, 71 (Fig.)
Double aortic arch, 573, 612
  magnetic resonance imaging, 1900
Double bubble appearance, duodenal
  atresia, 1773, 1774 (Fig.)
Double compartment hydrocephalus, 659
Double contrast barium studies, 464,
  1896, 1902–1903
Double diffusion Arc 5 test, hydatid
  disease, 1506 (Fig.)
Double Dutch method, contraception, 995
Double heterozygotes,
  hemoglobinopathies, 66
Double inlet left ventricle, 620
Double inlet ventricle, 203 (Table), 597,
  620–621
Double outlet right ventricle, **622**
Double outlet ventricle, 597
Double ring sign, optic nerve hypoplasia,
  271
Double vision, 1661
Dounreay, neoplasms, 890
Down syndrome, **54–57,** 830 (Table),
  1190
  airway obstruction in sleep, 531
  atrioventricular septal defect, 604
  Brushfield's spots, 23, 27 (Fig.), 55
  cataract, 1669
  celiac disease, 440
  chromosome studies, 50
  congenital heart disease, 55, 596
  cytogenetic nomenclature, 53
  duodenal atresia, 55, 1773
  dysphonia, 809
  ear, 1679
  5-hydroxytryptamine, 841
  5-hydroxytryptophan, 768
  growth charts, 1017
  and Hashimoto's thyroiditis, 1049
  immunodeficiency, 1254
  intelligence, 829
  leukemia, 55, 289, 291 (Table), 887
  polycythemia, 226
  pulmonary vessels, 495
  screening, 339 (Table)
    antenatal care, 80
  severely handicapped children affected,
    14 (Table)
  and thyroid dysgenesis, 1049
  tongue, 425
  translocations, 53, **55–56**

Doxapram
  apnea attacks, 198
  Ondine's curse, 531
Doxorubicin, cardiotoxicity, 896
Doxycycline
  administration, 1966 (Table)
  Chlamydia trachomatis, epididymo-
    orchitis, 1432
  malaria prophylaxis, 1449
  oral absorption, 1527
  pelvic inflammatory disease, 1432
  syphilis, 1409 (Table), 1410 (Table)
D-penicillamine, Wilson's disease, 1146
DPT vaccine, 1305, 1317
  adverse effects, 343
  linked *Haemophilus influenzae* antigen,
    341
  mortality, 343 (Table)
  WHO on, 346 (Table)
DR3/DR4 heterozygosity, diabetes
    mellitus, 1073–1074
Dracunculosis, **1495–1496**
Drainage, *see also* Chest, drainage
  septic arthritis, 1592
  tracheoesophageal fistula, 210
Drash syndrome, 913, 914, 972
Dravet, severe myoclonic epilepsy, 688
    (Table)
Drawing
  development, 383–384, 670
    examination, 391 (Table), 393
  Goodenough–Harris drawing test, 400,
    670
  tremor, 396
Dried milks, for malnutrition, 1193
Drinking, 1762
Drinks, infants, 334
Drip breast milk, *see* Foremilk
Drooling, cerebral palsy, 761–762
Drop attacks, division of corpus callosum,
    687
Droperidol, administration, 1966 (Table)
Drowning, **571, 1716–1718,** *see also*
    Near-drowning
  mortality, 1712
  neurofibromatosis, 800
Drowsiness, respiratory disorders, 510
Drug abuse, **1762–1763**
  candidiasis and endophthalmitis, 1678
  child abuse, 1871
  neonatal hyperalertness, 236
  neonatal seizures, 245
  tremor, 770–771
Drug allergy, **1702–1703**
Drug rashes
  ampicillin, chickenpox, 1361
  vs scarlet fever, 1332
  vs seborrheic dermatitis, 1643
Drug resistance, *see also* Antibiotics,
    resistance
  Escherichia coli, 951
  gonorrhea, 1421–1422, 1427
  malaria, 1448
  neoplasms, 892–893
  Staphylococcus aureus, 1329
  tuberculosis, 1347–1348
Drugs, *see also* Medicines
  aplastic anemia, 856 (Table)
  Cushing's syndrome from, 1066
  developing countries, primary health
    care, 1890
  emergency departments, dosage charts,
    1805
  excretion, acute renal failure, 976
  extrapyramidal effects, 768, 772
  eye toxicity, **1677–1678**
  fibrosing alveolitis, 577
  folate deficiency, 852–853
  and glucose-6-phosphate dehydrogenase
    deficiency, 859 (Table)
  goitrogenic, 1049
  hematuria, 959
  immunosuppression, 1265
  improper administration, 1871

lupus, 1605
mastocytosis, 1647
maternal, on fetus and neonate, **90–91,**
    772
  medical negligence, **1879**
  metabolism, neonate, 471
  neoplasms from, 890
  neutropenia from, **866–867**
  overdose, 1815, *see also* Self-poisoning
    and porphyrias, 1143
  prophylaxis, 340
  psychiatry, 1748
  sideroblastic anemia, 867
  skin reactions, *see* Drug rashes
  therapeutic ranges, 1936 (Table)
  thrombocytopenia, 878, 879
  toxic encephalopathy, 694 (Table)
  transplacental, 772, 1005
  urticaria, 1639
Drug withdrawal, 772
  neonate, 771
Drunkenness, *see* Alcohol, abuse
D-serine-6 GnRH analogue, for
    precocious puberty, 1030
DSM
  pervasive developmental disorders,
    834–836
  psychiatric diagnosis, 1733
DTPA, *see* Renography
DTP vaccine, *see* DPT vaccine
D-tryptophan-6 GnRH analogue, for
    precocious puberty, 1030
Dual allergic reactions, 1689
Dual energy radiographic densitometry,
    302
Dual energy systems, parenteral nutrition,
    1220
Duane's retraction syndrome, 1660
Duarte variant, galactose-1-phosphate
    uridyltransferase deficiency, 1133
Dubin–Johnson syndrome, 218, **1145**
Dubowitz & Dubowitz, neonatal
    neurological examination, 237–
    239
Dubowitz score, gestation age, 41–42
Duchenne muscular dystrophy, 72,
    729–732
  assessment scale, 731
  genetic diagnosis, 73
  inheritance, 67
  mutations, 69
  screening, 339 (Table)
Ductus arteriosus, **198–199,** *see also*
    Persistent ductus arteriosus
  closure, 107, 203, 205
    nitrogen washout test, 200
  interventional radiology, 206
  murmur, 203 (Table)
Ductus venosus, **199**
Duffy blood group antigens, malaria, 1447
Dumb rabies, 1377
Dummies (nonnutritive sucking), 154
Duncan's syndrome, 1366
Duocal, for cystic fibrosis, 1208
Duodenal capsule, parasite diagnosis,
    1492–1493
Duodenum, 435
  atresia, 210, 1771, **1773–1774**
    Down syndrome, 55, 1773
  duplication cysts, thoracic involvement,
    192
  ileus, **1787–1788**
  intubation, 448
    pancreatic function tests, 451
  obstruction, **1773–1774**
  ulcer, 431
  ultrasonography, 1906
Duplex collecting systems, 937–938
Duplex Doppler ultrasonography, 1896
Duplex kidneys, 937
  ultrasonography, 1910 (Fig.)
Duplex ureters, 255–256, 1794–1795
Duplication cysts, duodenum, thoracic
    involvement, 192

Duplications, gastrointestinal tract,
    1775–1776
Duration of treatment, antibiotics, **1528**
Dusts, fibrosing alveolitis, 577
Dwarfism, *see also* named types; Short
    stature
  mental retardation, 834
  severely handicapped children affected,
    14 (Table)
Dwarf tapeworm, 1502
Dydrogesterone, 992
Dye test, toxoplasmosis, 1465–1466
Dying child, *see* Terminal care
Dynamic airway narrowing, **498–499,** 513
  asthma, 539
Dynamic deformities, cerebral palsy, 760
Dysanaptic growth, 496
Dysarthria, 810–814
Dysautonomia, *see* Familial dysautonomia
Dyscalculia, 824
Dyschondrosteosis, 1581
Dysdiadochokinesis, 35, 752
Dysentery, *see also Shigella* spp.
  amebic, 1468
  antibiotics, 454 (Table)
  schistosomiasis, 1509
Dysequilibrium syndrome, 646
Dysfibrinogenemia, 230
Dysfunctional uterine bleeding, 991–992
Dysgerminomas, *see also* Germinomas
  ovaries, 920, 993
Dysgraphia, 821–824
Dyshormonogenesis, congenital
    hypothyroidism, 1046
Dyskeratosis congenita, **854–855,** 1625
    (Table)
Dyskinesias, **767–774**
  cerebral palsy, 738
  dysgraphia, 822–823
Dyskinetic bulbar palsies, 813
Dyskinetic cerebral palsy, 753–755
Dyslexia, **820–821,** 1657, 1745
Dysmenorrhea, 992
Dysmorphic stigmata, mental retardation,
    834, 835 (Table)
Dysmorphic syndromes, *see also*
    Congenital abnormalities;
    Malformation syndromes
  hyperphagic, obesity, 1190
  short stature, 369–370
Dysosteosclerosis, 1581 (Table)
Dysostosis multiplex, 1158
Dysphagia, **426–427**
  tracheoesophageal fistula, 1772
Dysphasia, 814–815
  congenital, 807
Dysphonia, **808–809, 1687–1688**
  and inhaled corticosteroids, 546
Dysplasia, 76 (Table)
Dysplastic nevi, 1618
Dyspnea, *see* Breathlessness
Dyspraxia, *see also* Articulatory
    dyspraxia
  developmental, 670
  established true hemiplegia, 742
Dyspraxic dysgraphia, 823
Dysrhythmias, *see also* Arrhythmias
  cerebral, **673–676**
  speech, **805–806,** 809
Dysthymia, 1754
Dystonia
  drug reactions, 772
  kernicterus, 754
  neck, Sandifer syndrome, 428
  Niemann–Pick disease type C, 1167
Dystonia musculorum deformans,
    773–774, 793 (Table)
Dystonic phase, diplegia, 744, **746–747**
Dystonic syndrome of low birthweight,
    745
Dystrophia myotonica, 733–734
  congenital, 811
  maternal, 89 (Table)
Dystrophic epidermolysis bullosa, 1622

    (Table), 1624 (Table)
  mechanisms, 1567
Dystrophin, 729–730, 732
Dystrophin gene, 72, 73
Dysuria syndromes, 949

e antigen, hepatitis B virus, 1386
Ear
  development, 816
  disorders, **1679–1683**
    congenital syphilis, 1413–1414
  examination, 20–21
  neonatal gestation age, 42 (Fig.)
Ear lobes
  Beckwith–Wiedemann syndrome, 1780
    (Fig.)
  fragile X mental retardation, 63
  neonatal gestation age, 40 (Table)
Early childhood hyperkalemia, 947
Early congenital syphilis, **1411–1412**
  treatment, 1415
Early hemorrhagic disease of the newborn,
    230
Early infancy, disease incidence, 13
Early infantile epileptic encephalopathy,
    245
Early morning urine specimens, 1299
Early neonatal hypocalcemia, 299
Early neonatal mortality, 3, **4**
Early neonatal period, definition, 94
Early-onset pneumonia, neonate, 183–184
Eastern equine encephalitis, 1389
East Germany, *vs* West Germany, atopy,
    492
Eating disorders, **1746, 1757–1759,** *see
    also* Feeding problems
Eaton–Lambert syndrome, 728
Eaton's agent, 1374
Ebola virus disease, 1389
  emergence, 1279 (Table)
Ebstein's anomaly, **618–619**
Ecchymosis, eyelids, 1607
Echinococcosis, *see* Hydatid disease
Echocardiography, **590–592**
  atrial septal defect, 602
  cardiomyopathy, 634
  color Doppler, 1896
  infective endocarditis, 631
  mitral stenosis, 629
  mitral valve prolapse, 610
  neonate, 201
  total anomalous pulmonary venous
    connection, 623
  ventricular septal defect, 601
Echogenic kidneys, 1909
Echolalia, 1745
Echoplanar imaging, magnetic resonance
    imaging, 1898
ECHO viruses, 1381, **1383**
  congenital infection, 286 (Table)
  fits, 682
  respiratory infections, 1372
  X-linked agammaglobulinemia, 1255
ECM (erythema chronicum migrans),
    1312, **1313**
Econazole, 1434, **1478**
Economics, *see also* Cost-benefit analysis;
    Costs
  developing countries, 1885
  gross national products, 1883 (Table),
    1884
  neonatal care, **104–106**
Ecthyma gangrenosum, 1321
  Pseudomonas spp., 1287
Ectodermal defects, spine, 651
Ectodermal dysplasias, **1624–1625**
  teeth, 425
Ectopia cordis, 1556
Ectopia vesicae, 256, **1779**
Ectopic beats
  supraventricular, 624
    neonate, 203
  ventricular, 625

Ectopic gastric mucosa, 1787
  scintigraphy, 447, 460
Ectopic kidney, 254, 939
Ectopic pregnancy, 1815
Ectopic testes, 1790
Ectopic ureter, 937, 939, 1794–1795
  vs enuresis, 957 (Table)
Ectopic ureterocele, 256
Ectrodactyly, 76 (Table)
Ectrodactyly ectodermal dysplasia and
  clefting, 1626 (Table)
Ectropion, 1663
Eczema, 1642–1643
  and breast-feeding, 327
  early weaning, 333
Eczema herpeticum, see Disseminated
  herpes simplex; Kaposi's
  varicelliform eruption
Edema, 30 (Fig.)
  acute glomerulonephritis, 962
  African trypanosomiasis, 1455
  diuretic-resistant, 412
  heart failure, 585
  neonate, 43
    gestation age, 42 (Fig.)
  nephrotic syndrome, 968–969
  preterm infant, 141
  rhesus incompatibility, 233
  Turner's syndrome, 61 (Fig.)
Edinburgh articulation test, 400
Edrophonium
  administration, 1966 (Table)
    neonate, 1957 (Table)
  testing myasthenia, 727
EDTA, see Sodium calcium edetate
Education, see also Schooling
  asthma, 544–545, 549
  cancer survivors, 899
  cerebral palsy, 761
  chronic renal failure, 981
  on epilepsy, 691
  mental retardation, 840
  sexually transmitted diseases,
    1398–1399
  special needs, 340, 1864–1865
  Streptococcus pneumoniae, 1319–
    1320
Educational attainment, assessment,
  1735–1736
Education campaigns
  accident prevention, 1713
    pedestrian road accidents, 1716
    poisoning, 1706
  home care, 1804
  sudden infant death syndrome, 1720
Education Supervision Orders, 1875
Edwards' syndrome, see Trisomy 18
EEC syndrome, 1626 (Table)
Efflux resistance, antibiotics, 1529
Eflornithine (difluoromethyl-ornithine),
  1457
Egg counts, hookworm, 1490
Egg laying stages, schistosomiasis,
  1508–1509
Egg protein
  intolerance, 442, 1700–1701
  reference, parenteral nutrition, 1220
Eggs, see also Operculate eggs
  flukes, 1511 (Fig.), 1512 (Fig.)
  head louse, 1518, 1638
  Salmonella spp., 1323
  schistosomiasis, finding, 1510
Egocentric thinking, 1729
Egypt, zinc deficiency, 1201
Egyptian splenomegaly, 1510
Ehlers–Danlos syndrome, 875, 1612, see
  also Occipital horn syndrome
  mechanisms, 1567
  type VI, 1113
Ehrlichia chaffeensis, emergence, 1279
  (Table)
Ehrlich's aldehyde test, 837
18q-syndrome, 58
Einhorn's staging, carcinoma of testis, 922

Eisenmenger's syndrome, 606
Ejection click, 32, 586, 607
  coarctation of aorta, 611
Ekbom, restless leg syndrome, 769
Elapidae, 1521
Elapid venoms, 1521, 1522
Elastase, 437
  hemolytic uremic syndrome, 978
Elbow, radiography, 1914
Elective mutism, 1744–1745
Electrical axis, heart, 589
Electrical burns, heart, 1799
Electricity, and neoplasms, 890
Electrocardiography, 588–589
  acute carditis, 628
  anomalous origin of left coronary artery
    from pulmonary artery, 612
  aortic stenosis, 607
  after apparent life-threatening events,
    529
  arrhythmias, 623, 624
  atrial septal defect, 602
  atrioventricular septal defect, 604
  carditis, 1598, 1599
  congenitally corrected transposition of
    great arteries, 616
  dextrocardia, 613
  diphtheria, 1306
  Duchenne muscular dystrophy, 730
  Ebstein's anomaly, 619
  endocardial fibroelastosis, 610
  hyperkalemia, 145, 412
  hypokalemia, 145
  innocent murmurs, 595
  ionized calcium, 298–299
  lysosomal a-1,4-glucosidase deficiency,
    1138
  neonate, 200, 598
  persistent ductus arteriosus, 603
  pulmonary hypertension, 606
  pulmonary stenosis, 608
  transposition of great arteries, 614
  tricuspid atresia, 620
  ventricular septal defect, 601
Electrocautery, genital warts, 1445
Electroclinical dissociation, status
  epilepticus, 693
Electroencephalography, 676–678, see
  also Deep electrode EEG studies
  birth asphyxia, 129
  febrile convulsions, 683
  fits, 673
  mesial temporal sclerosis, 686
  neonate, 243
    seizures, 244, 246
  prognosis in birth asphyxia, 132
  status epilepticus, 693
  viral infections, 683
Electrolytes, 403–404, see also Feces,
    electrolytes
  disturbance, 409–415
  intestinal absorption, 438
  disorders, 446–447
  movement across membranes, 406–
    407
Electrolyte solutions, for dehydration,
  413, 452, 453, 1296, 1304
Electromagnetic fields, and neoplasms,
  890
Electromechanical dissociation, 1808
Electromyography
  Duchenne muscular dystrophy, 730
  dystrophia myotonica, 734
  muscle phosphorylase deficiency, 735
  myasthenia gravis, 727
  polymyositis, 737, 1607
  spasticity, 756
  spinal muscular atrophies, 720
Electronic fetal monitoring, see
  Cardiotocography
Electron transfer flavoprotein, 1128
Electron transport chain, disorders,
  1126–1128
Electro-oculogram, 1655

Electrophysiology
  hearing, 817
  intracardiac, 624
  vision tests, 270
Electroretinogram, 273, 1655
Elemental diets, 1213–1214
  atopic eczema, 1696
  Crohn's disease, 1206–1207
Elemental medical foods, 470, 1119
  hyperphenylalaninemia, 1105
Elephantiasis, neurofibromatosis, 800
Elimination diets, see Exclusion diets
Elliptocytosis, hereditary, 226, 858
Ellis–van Creveld syndrome, 831 (Table),
  1573 (Fig.), 1575–1576
  vs asphyxiating thoracic dystrophy,
    1577
  frequency, 47 (Table)
El Tor cholera, 1304
Embden–Meyerhof pathway, 859 (Fig.)
  glucose-6-phosphatase deficiency,
    1137
  methemoglobin reductase sideshoot
    process, 864
Embolism, see also Thromboembolic
    disease
  cerebral, 713
Embolization (therapeutic), arteriovenous
  malformations, 1899
Embryo
  definition, 94
  gut development, 1773
Embryology
  gastrointestinal tract, 206–207
  respiratory tract, 494–496
Embryonal carcinoma, 920–921
Embryonal rhabdomyosarcoma, 916
Embryonal tumors, central nervous
  system, 899
Embryonic nuclear cataract, 1668
Emergencies, 1802–1828
  Addisonian crisis, 1068
  diabetes mellitus, 1075
Emergency drugs, 134
Emergency protection, Children
  (Scotland) Act 1995, 1877
Emergency Protection Orders, 1873,
  1875–1876, see also Child
  Protection Orders (Scotland)
Emerging infections, 1278
Emery–Dreifuss muscular dystrophy, 72
  (Table), 732
Emetine, amebiasis, 1469
EMG syndrome, see
  Beckwith–Wiedemann syndrome
EMLA cream, 1832
Emmetropia, 1656
Emollients, atopic eczema, 1642–1643
Emotional abuse, 1737, 1873
Emotional deprivation, on brain growth,
  828
Emotional development, 1729 (Table)
Emotional disorders, 1733, 1739–1742
  adolescence, 1755–1757
Emphysema, 30, see also Lobar
    emphysema
  α1-antitrypsin deficiency, 1175
  functional residual capacity, 501
  obstructive, imaging, 1899
Empirical antimicrobial therapy, 1527
Employment
  cancer survivors, 899
  mental retardation, 840
Empty sella syndrome, 1043
Empyema, 568–569
  tuberculosis, 1341
  ultrasonography, 517
Enalapril, renal hypertension, 973 (Table)
Enamel defect, primary teeth, 28 (Fig.)
Enamel hypoplasia, neonate, 299
Enanthem, chickenpox, 1360
Encephalitis, see also Postinfectious
    encephalitis
  brain biopsy, 1352

dysarthria, 812
  ECHO viruses, 1383
  infectious, vs medulloblastoma, 901
  parvovirus B19, 1359
  poliomyelitis, 1379
  rabies vaccination, 1377
  roseola infantum, 1359
  stroke, 713–714
Encephaloceles, 646 (Fig.), 647 (Fig.),
  648
  occipital, 642, 752
Encephalocraniocutaneous lipomatosis,
  799 (Table), 803–804
Encephalomyelitis, measles, 1354
Encephalopathy, see also Hemorrhagic
  shock and encephalopathy
  syndrome; Reye's syndrome
  acute, 693–699
  AIDS, 795 (Table), 1394, 1397
  cat-scratch disease, 1520
  hemolytic uremic syndrome, 977–
    978
  hepatic, 478–479, 482, 483, 1824
    nutrition, 1209
  low birthweight, see Little's disease
  management, 695–699
  metabolic disorders, 305
  reactive arsenical, 1457
  shigellosis, 1328
  trauma, 695, 700
  vaccination, 343
  vincristine toxicity, 896
Encephalotrigeminal angiomatosis, see
  Sturge–Weber syndrome
Enchondromas, multiple
  enchondromatosis, 1585–1586
Encopresis, 17, 1743–1744
  vs constipation, 461
End-diastolic volume and pressure,
  1819
Endemic flea-borne typhus fever, 1390
  (Table), 1392
Endemic goiter, 1048
Endemicity
  giardiasis, 1466
  malaria, 1447
Endemic syphilis, 1418–1419
  organism, 1401
Endemic treponematoses, 1398,
  1415–1420
  control, 1419–1420
Endocardial cushion defect, see
  Atrioventricular septal defect
Endocardial fibroelastosis, 610
  Coxsackie B viruses, 1383
Endocarditis, see also Infective
    endocarditis
  atypical verrucose, 635
  gonococcal, 1426
    treatment, 1428
  monilial, 1472
  Q fever, 1374–1375
Endocrine disorders, 996–1098
  cancer survivors, 898–899
  eye, 1674
  hepatitis syndrome in infancy, 474
    (Table)
  neonate, 248–249
  tests, 1000–1002
Endocrine function, gastrointestinal tract,
  424
Endocrine myopathies, 736–737
Endodermal sinus tumor, 921
  testis, 922
Endodyogeny, Toxoplasma gondii, 1464
Endometriosis, 992
Endomyocardial fibrosis, 631–632
Endophthalmitis
  candidiasis, 1678
  neonate, organisms, 284 (Table)
Endoprostheses, osteosarcoma surgery,
  918
Endorphins, growth hormone secretion,
  1013

Endoscopic retrograde
    cholangiopancreatography, 451,
    472
Endoscopy
    colon, 464
    Crohn's disease, 457
    peptic ulcers, 432
    rectal bleeding, 460
    small bowel biopsy, 447
    stomach, 435
    ulcerative colitis, 459
    upper gastrointestinal hemorrhage, 433
    varices, 483
Endotoxins, 273, 1287
Endotracheal intubation, **524**, 1807,
    1841–1843
    bacteriology, 1298
    bronchoscopy, 520
    complications, 1818
    drugs via, 526
    emergency equipment, 1805
    epiglottitis, 562–563
    fluid aspiration, 186
    meconium aspiration syndrome, 186
    neonatal pneumonia, 183
    neonatal resuscitation, 134, 179
        preterm infant, 139
    respiratory support, 162
    subglottic stenosis, 196
    sudden infant death syndrome,
        1722–1723
    tracheomalacia, 1769
    tube sizes, 524 (Table), 527 (Fig.)
Endotracheal suction, neonate, 97, 104,
    163
End-stage renal failure, 979
End-tidal CO_2 sampling, 505
Enema continence catheter, 463
Enemas
    gastrografin, meconium ileus, 1776
    intussusception, 1786
    meconium plug syndrome, 1777
Energy, see also Calories; Protein–energy
        malnutrition
    obesity, 1190
    requirements, 466, **1180–1181**, 1947
        (Table)
        congenital heart disease, 1210
        cystic fibrosis, 1208
        liver disease, 1209
    parenteral nutrition, 1220
    unit conversion factors, 1938 (Table)
Energy generation, mitochondria,
        disorders, **1123–1130**, see also
        Mitochondrial myopathies
England, regional genetic services, 76
Enophthalmos, 23
Entamoeba histolytica, 1467
Entamoeba spp., 1467
Enteral feed reservoirs, 1219
Enteral nutrition, 467, 470, **1217–1219**,
        see also Tube feeding
    cystic fibrosis, 557
    formulae, 1219, 1946 (Table)
    preterm infant, **150–155**
    self-help groups, 485
    short bowel syndrome, 445, 1212
    tubes, 1218
Enteric-coated formulations, antibiotics,
        1527
Enteric-coated pancreatic enzyme
        supplements, 557, 1208
Enteric fever, definition, 1323
Enteric non-A, non-B hepatitis, **478, 1387**
Enteritis, see also Gastroenteritis;
        Necrotizing enterocolitis
    neonate, organisms, 284 (Table)
    nephroblastoma radiotherapy, 914
    salmonellosis, 1324
Enterobius vermicularis, see Pinworms
Enterococci, 1333
Enterocolitis, 1293
    Hirschsprung's, 1295, 1777, 1778
Enterocytes, 436, 437–438

congenital disorders, diarrhea, 213
Enteroglucagon, deficiency in short gut
        syndrome, 445
Enterokinase, 437
Enteropathies, **1214–1215**
Enteropathogenic *Escherichia coli*
        disease, see *Escherichia coli*,
        gastroenteritis
Enterostomies, 1218
Enterotoxins, 452
    cholera, 452, 1303, 1304
    Staphylococcus aureus, 1330
Enteroviruses, **1378–1383**
    apnea, 528
    vs measles, 1355
    meningitis, 1375, 1376
    vs rubella, 1357
    X-linked agammaglobulinemia, 1255
Entropion, 1663
Enuresis, **957, 1743**
    diabetes mellitus, 1075
Environmental change
    accident prevention, 1713, 1716
    infections, 1279 (Table)
Environmental factors
    asthma, 536
    on brain development, **667**, 827–828
    on child health, **13–14**, 15 (Table)
    leukemia, 868
    neoplasms, **890–891**
    neural tube defects, 651
    respiratory disorders, 492–493
Environmental history, 18
Environmental mycobacteria, **1348–1350**
Environment of care
    neonates, **96–103**
    procedures, 1829
Enzootic trypanosomiasis, 1454
Enzyme immunoassay
    filariasis, 1498
    syphilis, **1403, 1404**
Enzyme-linked immunoassay, β-hemolytic
        Lancefield group A streptococci,
        1298
Enzyme-linked immunosorbent assays
    giardiasis, 1467
    Lyme disease, 1313
    toxocariasis, 1486
Enzymes
    alleles and activity, 1100
    deficiencies, metabolic effects,
        1100–1101
    inactivation, antibiotic resistance, 1529
    measurement, 1921–1922
    replacement, immunodeficiency, 1270
Eosinophilia, **868**
    anisakiasis, 1494
    ascariasis, 1482, 1484
    enterobiasis, 1488
    hookworm, 1490
    pulmonary, **570**, 1484
    toxocariasis, 1486
Eosinophilic gastroenteritis, 442
Eosinophilic granuloma, 1648, see also
        Langerhans cell histiocytosis
Eosinophilic meningitis,
        angiostrongyliasis, 1494
Eosinophils
    fetus, 222, 848
    neonate, 848
        counts, 223
    normal counts, 1939 (Table)
Ependymomas, **902–903**
    relative incidence, 900 (Table)
    spinal cord, 902, 906
Ephedrine
    administration, 1966 (Table)
    nose drops, common cold, 560
Epibulbar dermoid, oculoauriculovertebral
        dysplasia, 1564 (Fig.)
Epicanthal folds, pseudo-squint, 1659
Epicutaneo-cava catheter, Vygon, 1224
Epidemic jaundice (hepatitis A virus), **476,
        1386**

Epidemic keratoconjunctivitis, 1370,
        1385, 1676
Epidemic louse-borne typhus, see Typhus
Epidemic methicillin-resistant *S. aureus*,
        1329
Epidemic pleurodynia, see Bornholm
        disease
Epidemics
    giardiasis, 1466
    measles, United Kingdom, 1276
    pertussis, 1315
    sleeping sickness, 1454
'Epidemiologic' treatment
    gonorrhea, 1429
    syphilis, 1410
Epidemiology
    genetic disorders, **45–47**
    gonorrhea, 1421
    malaria, **1446–1447**
    Neisseria gonorrhoeae, typing, 1422
    neonates, **94–95**
        sepsis, 275–276
    neoplasms, 289, **886–887**
    psychiatric disorder, **1733–1734**
    statistics collection, **1848–1852**
Epidermal growth factor, fetus, 1005
Epidermal nevi (and syndrome), **1618**
Epidermis, 1616
Epidermolysis bullosa, **1621–1623**
    dystrophic, 1622 (Table), 1624 (Table)
    mechanisms, 1567
    epidermolytic, 1622
Epidermolytic hyperkeratosis, see Bullous
        ichthyosis
Epididymitis
    gonococcal, 1425
        treatment, 1428
    vs torsion of testis, ultrasonography,
        1914
    tuberculosis, 1346
Epididymo-orchitis, 1791
    Chlamydia trachomatis, doxycycline,
        1432
Epidural analgesia, 1832
    fetal bradycardia, 86
    vs intravenous morphine, 1831
    preterm labor, 119
    twin pregnancy, 90
Epigastric hernia, 1790
Epiglottitis, 561, **562–563**
    bacteriology, 1298
    Haemophilus influenzae, 1308
    and imaging, 1899–1900
    mortality, 490 (Table)
    posture, 511
Epilepsy, **671–693**
    autism, 1738
    cerebral palsy, **685**, 738, 761
    classification, **674–676**
    congenital hemiplegia, 744
    degenerative diseases, 795 (Table)
    diplegia, 748
    vs dyskinesia, 768
    with electrical status in slow sleep, 689
        (Table)
    after febrile convulsions, 683
    in head injuries, **709**
    hydrocephalus, 666
    lesional syndromes, **684–686**
    malignant syndromes, **687**
    maternal, 89 (Table)
    and migraine, 717
    with myoclonic absences, 680 (Table)
    neurofibromatosis, 800
    after neonatal seizures, 247
    paroxysmal choreoathetosis, 773
    preconceptual care, 79
    pregnancy, 114
    prognosis, **687–691**
    recurrence risks, 74
    reflex 'reading,' 821
    restrictions, 691
    severely handicapped children affected,
        14 (Table)

single photon emission computed
        tomography, 679, 1897, **1909**
    Sturge–Weber syndrome, 803
    temporal lobe, 819
    vs tetanus, 1334
    tuberous sclerosis, **679**, 801, 802, 1625
    and vaccination, 342 (Table)
Epimastigotes, 1454
    T. cruzi, 1458
Epimerase deficiency, 1134
Epinephrine, see Adrenaline
Epiphyses
    maturation, 362
    separation, birth trauma, 121 (Table)
Epiphysiodesis, 1022
Epipodophyllotoxins
    secondary acute myeloid leukemia, 898
    toxic effects, 894 (Table)
Episodic arthritis, cystic fibrosis, 1611
Episodic wheeze, 539–540, 541, 543,
        549–550
Epispadias, 256, **1794**
Epistaxis, 1684
    idiopathic thrombocytopenic purpura,
        878
    Von Willebrand's disease, 881
Epithelioid cells, tuberculosis, 1335
Epithelium, small intestine, **435–436**, 437
Epsilonaminocaproic acid, 228
Epstein–Barr virus, **1366–1368**
    aplastic anemia, 856
    Burkitt's lymphoma, 868
    fits, 682
    Hodgkin's disease, 909
    immunosuppression, 1264
    infection-associated hemophagocytic
        syndrome IAHS, 926
    liver transplantation, 484
    lymphocyte function testing, 1245,
        1246
    neoplasms, 891, 1366, 1367
    receptor, 1234
    X-linked lymphoproliferative
        syndrome, 1251
Epstein's pearls, 43
Equine tetanus antitoxin, 285
Equinus deformity, see also Talipes
        equinovarus
    treatments, 758 (Table)
Equipment
    neonatal care
        requirements, 96
        transport, 157
    phototherapy, 218
Equivalent weight, 405
Erb palsy, birth trauma, 122
Erect and supine abdominal X-rays,
        433–434
Ergocalciferol, 1053
Ergotamine, migraine, 717 (Table), 718
Erikson, psychological development, 1729
        (Table), 1730–1731
Erlenmeyer flask deformity, 1166
Erysipelas, **1332, 1635**
Erythema chronicum migrans, 1312,
        1313
Erythema infectiosum, **1358–1359**
    rash, 1285
Erythema marginatum, 1598
Erythema multiforme, **1641**
    conjunctivitis, 1675
Erythema nodosum, 1336, 1641
    coccidioidomycosis, 1475
    tuberculosis, 510
Erythema nodosum leprosum, **1310**, 1311
Erythema toxicum neonatorum, 1284,
        1645
Erythroblastosis fetalis, 234–235, see also
        Hemolytic disease of the newborn
    hypoglycemia, 295
Erythrocyte carbonic anhydrase buffer
        system, 417–418
Erythrocyte porphobilinogen deaminase,
        1143

Erythrocytes, see Red cells
Erythrocyte sedimentation rate
  neonatal sepsis, 276 (Table), 277
  rheumatic fever, 1599
Erythromycin
  administration, 1966 (Table)
  β-hemolytic streptococci, 1332 (Table)
  chlamydial infection
    conjunctivitis, 1431
    pregnancy, 1432
  diphtheria, 1306
  gonorrhea, pregnancy, 1428
  Lyme disease, 1314 (Table)
  mechanism, 1527
  neonate, 279 (Table)
    chlamydial conjunctivitis, 283
    inclusion conjunctivitis, 1385
    pneumonia, 280
  ophthalmia neonatorum prophylaxis,
    ointment, 263, 1429
  pertussis, 1317
  rheumatic fever, 629
  syphilis, 1409 (Table), 1410 (Table)
  yaws control, 1420
Erythrophagocytosis, 925, 927
Erythropoiesis
  developmental, 222
  malaria, 1447–1448
Erythropoietic protoporphyria, 1142
  (Table), 1144, 1630–1631
Erythropoietin, 222
  neonate, 223, 849
  preterm infant, 225
  recombinant, 980
    chronic renal failure, 865–866
Escalator, see Mucociliary escalator
Escherichia coli
  antibiotic, 454 (Table)
  diarrhea, 452
  encephalopathy, 683, 693
  food poisoning, emergence, 1278
  gastroenteritis, 1293, 1294
  hemolytic uremic syndrome, 977
  neonatal meningitis, 247
  neonatal sepsis, 278
  urinary tract infections, 951–952
Eserine, pediculosis blepharitis, 1663
Esophageal speech, 809
Esophagitis
  herpes simplex, 1439
  reflux, 428
Esophagogram, 517
Esophagoscopy, 429 (Table), 430
Esophagus, 425–430, see also Varices
  acid infusion, asthma, 542
  atresia, 1770–1773
    radiology, 1902
    risk calculation, 75
  causes of recurrent inhalation, 570
  Chagas' disease, 1458, 1459
  embryology, 206
  foreign body removal, 1899
  investigations, 429–430
  preterm infant, 150
  progressive systemic sclerosis, 1608
  reflux, see Gastroesophageal reflux
  respiratory disorders, 513
  radiology, 514–517
  stricture, balloon dilatation, 1899
Esophoria, 1659
Esotropia, infantile, 265
ESPGAN Committee on Nutrition,
    calcium and phosphorus
    supplements, 304
ESPGAN protocol, celiac disease, 441
Espundia, 1463
Essential hypertension, 636
Essential oils, poisoning, 1711
Essential tremor, 770
Estimated average requirements (EAR),
    1180, 1181 (Table)
  energy, 1181, 1947 (Table)
  vitamins, 1184 (Table)
Estradiol

normal values, 1925 (Table)
  ovaries, 1023
Estriol, Down syndrome, 56
Estrogen cream, 988
Estrogens
  childhood, 987
  for constitutional tall stature, 376
  exogenous, precocious pseudopuberty,
    1028
  puberty, 1024
    induction, 1035
    precocious, 989
  for tall stature, 1020
  testis, 1024
  for Turner's syndrome, 1033–1034
Estrone, ovaries, 1023
E subunits, pyruvate dehydrogenase
    deficiency, 1126
ETF: CoQ oxidoreductase, 1128
Ethambutol
  administration, 1966 (Table)
  environmental mycobacteria, 1350
  tuberculosis, 1347, 1348
    meningitis, 1345
Ethamsylate
  administration, neonate, 1957 (Table)
  dysfunctional uterine bleeding, 992
Ethical development (moral development),
    1731
Ethics
  genetic screening, 77
  long-term parenteral nutrition, 1226
  neonatal care, 99–103
  quadriplegia, 749
  stopping resuscitation, 135
Ethinylestradiol
  administration, 1966 (Table)
  polycystic ovarian disease, 993
  primary amenorrhea, 990
  puberty induction, 1035
Ethionamide, tuberculosis, 1348
  meningitis, 1345
Ethmocephaly, 649
Ethmoidal polyps, 1685
Ethmoiditis, 1685
Ethnic factors, see also Immigrants,
    children of
  adoption, 1860
  birth rates, 1
  childrearing, 828
  genetic disorders, 47
  glucose-6-phosphate dehydrogenase
    deficiency, 859
  growth, 367–368
  21-hydroxylase deficiency, 1062
  lactase, 445
  leprosy, 1309
  motor development, 668
  respiratory disorders, 493
  risk calculation in multifactorial
    inheritance, 75
Ethnic groups, 15 (Table)
  antenatal screening, 80
  tuberculosis, 1335
  weaning, 334
Ethosuximide
  administration, 1966 (Table)
  therapeutic ranges, 1936 (Table)
Ethyl chloride spraying, 1490
Ethylene glycol poisoning, oxaluria, 1113
Etoposide
  infection-associated hemophagocytic
    syndrome IAHS, 926
  toxic effects, 894 (Table)
Euploidy, 51
Europe
  chronic renal failure incidence, 978
  demography, 2 (Table)
  HIV vertical transmission, 288
European Community, travel, epilepsy,
    691
European Court of Human Rights, sex
    education, 1399
Eustachian tube

cleft palate, 1797
  secretory otitis media, 1681
Evans' syndrome, 864
Evaporative heat loss, 146, 149
Eventration of diaphragm, 575–576,
    1770
Event recorders, arrhythmias, 624
Ewing's sarcoma, 918–920
  incidence, 885, 886 (Table)
  vs osteosarcoma, 917
  peripheral, tumor markers, 912
    (Table)
  survival rates, 887 (Table)
Examination, 19–44, see also
    Cardiovascular system,
    examination; Eye, examination
  admission to care, 1857–1858
  adoptive parents, 1858
  compulsory, 1853
  dehydration, 1286, 1287 (Table)
  developmental, 387–393, 393–396
  endocrinology, 998–1000
  epiglottitis, 562
  immunodeficiency, 1244
  liver disease, 471
  mental retardation, 833–834
  non-accidental injury, 703
  psychiatric disorder, 1734–1735
    adolescents, 1754
  respiratory disorders, 510–513
  school health services, 1863
  sexual abuse, 1869–1870
    sexually transmitted diseases, 1400
  skin disorders, 1617
  speech disorder, 808
  unstable child with underlying
    pathology, 1814
Exanthems, 1353–1365
  conjunctivitis, 1663
  and squint, 1659
Exanthem subitum, see Roseola infantum
Exchange transfusion, 219, 1838–1839
  for ABO incompatibility, 234
  amounts, 851 (Table)
  for hyperkalemia, 145
  inborn errors of metabolism, 307
  malaria, 1453
  for neonatal sepsis, 279, 1267
  neonatal thrombocytopenia, 229
  partial, polycythemia, 227
  prenatal blood loss, 224
  for rhesus incompatibility, 232, 233
  sickle cell disease, 863
  syphilis transmission, 1401
Exclusion diets, 1213, 1695–1696
  cow's milk protein, 1700–1701
  hyperactivity, 1744
  for migraine, 718
  special formula feeds, 1944 (Table)
Exclusion Orders (Scotland), 1877
Exercise, 15 (Table), 341
  aortic stenosis, 607
  asthma, 501, 541–542, 545, 549
  cerebral palsy, 758
  diabetes mellitus, 1078
  Duchenne muscular dystrophy, 731
  energy expenditure, 1181
  food intolerance, 1694
  hematuria, 959
  migraine, 716, 717 (Table)
  poliomyelitis, 1379
  proteinuria, 967
  puberty, 1026
Exercise-induced anaphylaxis, food-
    provoked, 1697
Exercise tests
  arrhythmias, 623
  semi-ischemic, 1139
Exoerythrocytic phase, Plasmodium spp.,
    1445
Exomphalos, 1779–1780
  Edwards' syndrome, 57
Exons, 69
Exophoria, 1660

Exophthalmos, 23
Exostoses, multiple, 1585
Exosurf, 179
Exotoxins, 273
  diphtheria, 1305
Expanded Program of Immunization,
    1280, 1889, 1890
Expiration, 505
Expiration films, chest X-rays, 513
Expiratory flow volume curve, 499 (Fig.),
    500
Expiratory grunting, respiratory distress
    syndrome, 177
Expiratory time constant, 500
  prolongation, 496
Expired air ventilation, 522, 523–524
Exploitation of children, 1887–1888
Expressed milk, 329
  vs drip milk, 152
Expressive dysphasia, 814
Expressivity, 65
Exstrophy
  bladder, 256
  cloaca, 256
Extended families, 1854
Extended Moebius' syndrome, 719
Extensor dystonia, 769–770
Extensor hypertonus, 44
  diplegia, 745, 746
  paroxysmal, causes, 671 (Table)
Extensor reflexes, 37 (Table)
External cardiac massage
  at birth, 135
  chest compressions, 523–524
External cephalic version, 83
External hydrocephalus, 659
External jugular vein, blood sampling,
    1835
Extracellular fluids, 403
  vs bodyweight, 1953
  electrolytes, 403–404
    normal values, 1923 (Table)
  potassium, 408 (Table), 411
  preterm infant, 139
  sodium, 408 (Table)
  volume regulation, 410
Extracorporeal hemofiltration, see
    Hemofiltration
Extracorporeal life support, 1821
Extracorporeal membrane oxygenation,
    164–165, 1821
  diaphragmatic hernia, 1770
  persistent pulmonary hypertension of
    the newborn, 204–205
  pulmonary hypoplasia, 192
Extradural hematoma, 702
  skull fracture, 707
Extramedullary hemopoiesis, 222
Extrapyramidal bulbar palsies, 813
Extrapyramidal disorders, 767–774
Extravasation, parenteral nutrition, 159
Extrinsic primary resistance, tumor cells,
    892
Exudative otitis media (secretory otitis
    media), 816, 1681–1682
Eye, 1649–1678
  acute lymphoblastic leukemia, 874
  acyclovir ointment, 1440
  Alport's syndrome, 965
  cerebellar ataxias, 753
  Chlamydia trachomatis, 1430, see also
    Trachoma
  congenital rubella, 286
  cysticercosis, 1501
  distance apart, 21–22
  erythema multiforme, 1641
  examination, 21–27, 1649–1657
    neonate, 241, 267–268, 273
  hemorrhage, birth trauma, 264
  herpes zoster, 1632, 1676
  incontinentia pigmenti, 1626
  leprosy, 1310, 1311
  Lyme disease, 1313
  measles, 1354, 1676

Eye, **1649–1678** (Contd)
  mental retardation, defects, 835 (Table)
  movements
    disorders, see also Ophthalmoplegia
      diphtheria, 1306
      oculocraniosomatic syndrome, 735
        (Table), 736
      preterm infant, 267
    examination, 1652
  myasthenia gravis, 727
  neonate, 43, **262–273**
    examination, 241, **267–268**, 273
    general appearance, 238 (Fig.)
    infections, organisms, 284 (Table)
  neurofibromatosis, 800
  osteogenesis imperfecta, 1568, 1676
  respiratory disorders, 510
  river blindness, 1527
  sheep nasal bot fly, 1514
  spitting cobra envenomation, 1522,
    1523
  Sturge–Weber syndrome, 802–803
  toxocariasis, 1486
  toxoplasmosis, 289, 1676
  viruses, **1384–1385**
Eyelashes
  pediculosis, 1639
  Pthirus pubis, 1519
Eyelids, **1661–1663**
  dermatomyositis, 1607
  ecchymosis, 264
  hemangiomas, 1619, 1662
  normal, 1649

Fabry disease, 776 (Table), 1157 (Table),
  1164
  replacement enzyme infusion, 1102
  stroke, 711
Face, see also Facies
  actinomycosis, 1473
  acute glomerulonephritis, 962
  cellulitis, 1635
  DiGeorge syndrome, 1252
  innate recognition, 107
  mental retardation, 835 (Table)
  Sturge–Weber syndrome, 802, 803
Facemasks, resuscitation, 524
Facial hair, puberty, 357
Facial nerve
  Bell's palsy, 725
  birth trauma, 122
  examination, 34
  lesions, 811
  palsy, 25 (Fig.), 43
    geniculate herpes, 1363
    Moebius' syndrome, 209
    poliomyelitis, 1380
Facial nevus, with vermis aplasia, 646
Facial syndromes, 1560–1565
Facies, 19, see also Face
Facile hyperketosis, 1130
Facioscapulohumeral muscular dystrophy,
  72 (Table), 732, 811
FACS analysis, phagocytosis, 1247
Factitious fever, 1283 (Table)
Factitious hematuria, 959
Factitious vaginal bleeding, 1028
Factor VIII-related antigen, hemolytic
  uremic syndrome, 978
Factors, see Coagulation factors
Fahr's syndrome, 797 (Table)
Failure to thrive, **465–469, 1191**, see also
  Growth, retardation
  breast-feeding, 331
  chromosome studies, 51
  congenital heart disease, 1210
  Munchausen syndrome by proxy, 1871
  neglect, 1871–1873
  nonorganic, **468–469**, 1736, **1872–1873**
  sexual abuse, 1869
Faints, 672
  definition, 671
Fallopian tubes, tuberculosis, 1346

Fallot's tetralogy, **616–618**
Fallout, nuclear tests, neoplasms, 890
Falls, 1715
Famciclovir, **1440–1441**
Familial adenomatous polyposis, 448
  liver tumors, 924
Familial alphalipoprotein deficiency, 724,
  790 (Table), 1150 (Table), 1153
Familial dysautonomia (Riley–Day
  syndrome), 209, 724, 832 (Table),
  1069, 1107
  tongue, 425
Familial dysbetalipoproteinemia type III,
  1150 (Table), 1152
Familial erythrophagocytic
  lymphohistiocytosis, 925, **927**
Familial fibrous dysplasia of the jaws,
  1565
Familial glucocorticoid deficiency, 1067
Familial hyperbetalipoproteinemia, see
  Familial hypercholesterolemias,
  type II
Familial hypercholesterolemias
  type II, 1151–1152
  type II A, 1150 (Table)
Familial hyperchylomicronemia type I,
  1150 (Table), 1151
Familial hyperphosphatasia, 1177
Familial hypobetalipoproteinemia, 1150
  (Table)
Familial hypocalciuric 'benign'
  hypercalcemia, 1058
Familial hypophosphatemia, 260, **948**
  inheritance, 67
Familial isolated growth hormone
  deficiency type IA, 367
Familial juvenile nephronophthisis, 941,
  see also Medullary cystic disease
Familial lecithin-cholesterol
  acyltransferase deficiency, 1150
  (Table), 1153
Familial marrow dysfunction, **855**
Familial nonsyndromic deafness, 1127
Familial paroxysmal ataxias, 764
Familial polyposis coli, 888 (Table), 889
Familial recurrent hematuria syndrome,
  966
Familial short stature, 371
Familial spastic-ataxic syndrome, 792
  (Table)
Familial spastic paraplegia, 792 (Table)
Familial striatal necrosis, 773
Families
  breakdown, 1804
  on child health, **1854–1857**
    immigrants, 1866
  chronic illnesses, responses, 1761
  dysfunction, failure to thrive, 468–469
  mental retardation, 839
  personality development, 1732
  psychiatric disorder, 1728
  psychiatric referral, 1753
  tuberculosis, 1340
Family history, 18
  atopy, 1692
  development, 387
  endocrinology, 998
  failure to thrive, 466
  Graves' disease, 1051
  neonates, 41
    eyes, 268
Family planning, Islam, 1865
Family studies, regional genetic services,
  76
Family support
  acute renal failure, 976–977
  cancer, 897
  chronic renal failure, 982
  congenital adrenal hyperplasia
    treatment, 1065
  diabetes mellitus, 1075
  thin child, 1023
Family therapy, 1749, **1763–1764**
Fanconi–Bickel syndrome, 1134

Fanconi's anemia, 289, **854**, 1254
  liver tumors, 890, 924
  neoplasms, 854, 888 (Table)
Fanconi's syndrome, 831 (Table), 941,
  944–945, 1122
  cystinosis, 1123
  hypophosphatemia, 944, 1058
  potassium citrate mixture, 415
  proteinuria, 967
  rickets, 1058
  tyrosinemia type I, 1106
Fansidar
  adverse reactions, 1448
  malaria treatment, 1452
Farber syndrome, 779 (Table), 1157
  (Table), **1167**
Farmer's lung, 577
Fasciculata cells, cortisol, 1059
Fascioliasis, 478, **1512–1513**
  fluke life cycle, 1511 (Table)
Fasciolopsiasis, 1513
  fluke life cycle, 1511 (Table)
Fas deficiency, lymphocytes, 1250
Fasting, see also Starvation
  dicarboxylic acids, 1128
  on growth factors, 1023
  hormone tests, 1000
  hypoglycemia, 1082–1083
  plasma amino acids, 1102–1103
  stress tests, inborn errors of
    metabolism, 1131
Fasting glucagon test, debranching
  enzyme deficiency, 1138
Fasting migrating motor complex, 208
Fat embolism, parenteral nutrition, 159
Fathers, one-parent families, 1854
Fatigue, see also Chronic fatigue
  syndrome
  myasthenia gravis, 727
Fat necrosis, subcutaneous
  birth trauma, 121
  neonate, 43, 1646
Fats, see also Body fat; Lipids
  absorption, 207–208
    preterm infant, 151
  breast milk, 332–333
  dietary, **1182**
    enteropathies, 1214
    for liver disease, 1209
    sources, 1182 (Table)
  digestion, 423
    small intestine, 437
    stomach, 430
  feces, see Feces, fats
  intravenous solutions, neonatal
    platelets, 229
  malabsorption, **446**
  metabolism, 1149
  milks, 332–333
  parenteral nutrition, 1220, 1222
    (Table)
  preterm requirements, 151 (Table), 158
  proportion in energy intake, 1180,
    1189
  and toddler diarrhea, 463, 464
Fat-soluble vitamins, 1182
  absorption, 437
Fatty acids, see also Free fatty acids;
  Polyunsaturated fatty acids; Short
  chain fatty acids; Very long chain
  fatty acids
  brain development, 643
  cystic fibrosis, 1208
  dietary sources, 1182 (Table)
  on ionized calcium, 299
  metabolism disorders, **1128–1130**
  oxidation defects, 1083
    dietary management, **1205 (Table)**
    mitochondrial, 297
Fauces
  gonorrhea, 1420
  vesicles, 560
Favism, 859
F cells, pancreas, 1071

Febrile convulsions, **682–684**
  inheritance studies, 682
  measles, 1354
  phenobarbitone, therapeutic ranges,
    1936 (Table)
  roseola infantum, 1359
  status epilepticus, 683, 692
  stroke, 713–714
Fecal impaction, neural tube defect, 657
Fecal water loss, preterm infant, 140
Feces
  amebiasis, **1468–1469**
  bacteriology, **1299**
  Candida spp., 1472
  carbohydrates, 448
  cholestatic jaundice, 220
  chromatography, **448, 454–455**
  cystic fibrosis, 553
  electrolytes
    cholera, 1303–1304
    gastroenteritis, 1293
  examination, 33
  fats, 448
    cystic fibrosis, 553, 1207, 1208
    measurement, 1938
    normal values, 1936 (Table)
  giardiasis, 1466–1467
  hepatitis A virus, 476, 1386
  hepatitis syndrome in infancy, samples,
    474
  history taking, 17
  neonate, 111
  normal amounts, 1936 (Table)
  normal properties, 1936 (Table)
  polioviruses, 1379
  protein, 443, 448
  protracted diarrhea, 454–455
  salmonellosis, 1324
  typhoid fever, 1326
  virology, 1384
  viruses, **1352**
  water output, 403 (Table)
Feedback, tubuloglomerular, 942
Feeding
  bronchiolitis, 564
  common cold, 560
  gastroesophageal reflux, 571
  quadriplegia, 748, 749
  speech therapy, 813
Feeding plates, see Palatal appliance
Feeding problems, 208–209, see also
  Eating disorders; Overfeeding
  failure to thrive, 466–467, 469
  preschool children, 1736
  vomiting, 209
Feeding pumps, 1218–1219
Feed reservoirs, 1219
Feed scalds, hot, 1868
Feet, see Foot
Felty's syndrome, 865
Female pseudohermaphroditism, 1007
Femoral artery, disadvantages as sampling
  site, 505
Femoral head
  avascular necrosis, 1594–1595
    from splinting, 1551
  slipped epiphysis, 1596
Femoral hernia, 1790
Femoral nerve block, 1812
Femoral pulses, 585–586
Femoral torsion, **1552–1553**
Femoral vein
  blood sampling, 1835
  central venous cannulation, 1837
Femur, see also Femoral head
  birth trauma, 121 (Table)
  hemopoiesis, 848 (Fig.)
  osteosarcoma distribution, 917
Fenfluramine, 1748 (Table)
Fenoterol, administration, 1966 (Table)
Fentanyl
  dystonia, 672
  transdermal patches, 928
  with ventilation, 1833

Ferritin, 1146
  neuroblastoma, 912
  normal values, 1925 (Table)
  serum levels, 1188
Ferrochelatase, 1142
Ferrous iron
  administration, 1966 (Table)
  dosages, 851–852
Ferrous sulfate, 851–852
Fertility index, 1
Fertility rates, world figures, 1883 (Table),
  1884
Fetal alcohol syndrome, 642, 753
  cortical dysplasia, 685
Fetal circulation, 106, 107, see also
  Persistent fetal circulation
  hypoxia response, 123–124
  necrotizing enterocolitis, 210
Fetal distress, 124
  resuscitation, 132
Fetal heart rate, 86, 116, 117
  preterm labor, 119
Fetal hemoglobin, 108, 214, 222, 225, 860
  cyanosis, 585
  normal ratios, 1939 (Table)
  synthesis, 849
Fetal hemopoiesis, juvenile chronic
  myeloid leukemia, 872
Fetal intestinal alkaline phosphatase, 302
Fetal motor complex, 208
Fetal-neonatal transition, 42, 106–109, 110
Fetal sclerosis, kidney, 934
Fetal surveillance, 115
Fetal transfusion, irradiated platelets, for
  thrombocytopenia, 229
Fetal zone, adrenal cortex, 1003, 1060
Fetofetal transfusion, see Twin–twin
  transfusion
Fetomaternal hemorrhage, 224
Fetomaternal transfusion, blood group
  incompatibilities, 231, 232
Fetoproteins, see α-fetoprotein;
  β-fetoprotein
Fetor oris, 1786
Fetoscopy, operative, 115
Fetus, see also Prenatal growth
  auditory response, 243
  breathing, 495, 496
  calcium homeostasis, 298
  calcium regulation, 1053
  congenital adrenal hyperplasia, 985,
    986
  definition, 94
  disease incidence, 11
  endocrinology, 1002–1005
  gonadotropins, 1003, 1023
  gynecology, 985
  hemopoiesis, 221–222, 848
  hydrocephalus, 665
  immune system, 1240
  lead poisoning, 1708
  long chain 3-hydroxyacyl-CoA
    dehydrogenase deficiency, 1130
  lung development, 175–176
  maternal drugs, 90–91
  monitoring, labor, 86–87
  nutrition, 151
  pre-eclampsia/pregnancy-induced
    hypertension, 90
  swallowing reflex, 426
  toxoplasmosis, 1465
  ultrasound measurements, 82
Feuerstein–Mims syndrome, 804
Fever, 20, see also Hyperpyrexia; named
    diseases
  Ewing's sarcoma, 919
  febrile convulsions, 683
  fluid replacement, acute renal failure,
    975
  head injuries, 708
  Hodgkin's disease, 909
  infections, 1282–1284
  Kawasaki disease, 1479
  management, 684

melarsoprol reaction, 1457
neonate, 150, 1282
nephroblastoma, 913
pneumonia, 566
respiratory disorders, 510
typhoid fever, 1325
Fever of unknown origin, 1282–1283
  blood cultures, 1297
Few foods diet, 1213, 1696
Fiber, dietary, 1183, 1211
  diabetes mellitus, 1078–1079
  sources, 1182 (Table)
Fibrillary astrocytoma, 903
Fibrillin, congenital contractural
  arachnodactyly, 1589
Fibrillin 1, Marfan's syndrome, 1587
Fibrin degradation products, 228
  disseminated intravascular coagulation,
    231, 882
Fibrin, fibrinogen degradation products,
  normal values, 1925 (Table)
Fibrin glue pleurodesis, 188
Fibrinogen
  deficiency, 881
  inherited disorders, 230
  neonatal sepsis, 277
  normal values, 228, 1925 (Table)
  plasma levels, disseminated
    intravascular coagulation, 231
Fibrinolysis, 228
Fibrin stabilizing factor, see Coagulation
  factor XIII
Fibroblast fusion experiments, ataxia
  telangiectasia, 1253
Fibroblast growth factor receptor genes
  mutations, 370, 1567, 1572, 1575
  thanatophoric dysplasia, 1570
Fibroblast growth factor receptors, 1567
Fibroblast growth factors, 351, 1567
Fibroblast pneumocyte factor, 176
Fibroblasts, chromosome preparations
  from, 49–50
Fibrodysplasia ossificans congenita, 1586
Fibrohistiocytoma, malignant, 918
Fibrolamellar hepatocellular carcinoma,
  925
Fibromas, neurofibromatosis, 800
Fibromuscular hyperplasia, stroke,
  711–712
Fibronectin
  fetal, vagina, 116
  for neonatal infections, 1267
  neonate, 275
Fibrosarcoma, vs osteosarcoma, 917
Fibrosing alveolitis, 577–578
  vs obliterative bronchiolitis, 576
Fibrous dysplasia, see also Polyostotic
    fibrous dysplasia
  localized, 1589
  tibia, 1549
Fibrous phimosis, 1793
Fiévre boutonneuse, 1392
Fifth day fits, 245
Fifth disease, see Erythema infectiosum
Fight and flight responses, epilepsy, 690
Filariasis, 1496–1499
Filariform larvae, hookworm, 1489
Filigree pattern, Ewing's sarcoma, 919
Filters, parenteral nutrition, 1223
Filter views, chest radiography, 514
Fine section computed tomography, 1897
Finger agnosia, 669
Fingers, see also Dactylitis
  length, 39
  movements
    neonate, 236
    normal development, 382
Finger sucking, 1745
Finished consultant episodes, 9
Finland, Chlamydia pneumoniae,
  1373–1374
Finnish type congenital nephrotic
  syndrome, 971–972
Fireguards, 1714

Fires, 15 (Table), 1714
  mortality, 1711
Fireworks, 1714
First aid, burns, 1799
First breath, 107
Fish, anisakiasis, 1494
Fisher's syndrome, 726, 762
Fish eye disease, 1150 (Table), 1153
Fish tank granuloma, 1349
Fish tapeworm, see Diphyllobothrium
    latum
Fistula, definition, 1770
Fits, 673–674, see also Seizures
  definition, 671
  first aid, 691
  history taking, 17
  non-accidental head injury, 700
Fitz-Hugh and Curtis syndrome, 1430
5-HT₃ antagonists, 896
5-hydroxytryptamine
  Down syndrome, 841
  normal values, urine, 1931 (Table)
5-hydroxytryptamine uptake inhibitors,
    obsessive–compulsive disorders,
    1756
5-hydroxytryptophan
  dihydropteridine reductase deficiency,
    1106
  Lesch–Nyhan syndrome, 768
5P-syndrome (cri du chat syndrome), 58,
    830 (Table)
Fixing eye, strabismus, 1658
Flaccid bulbar palsy, 810–812
Flapping tremor, 771
Flare, cranial ultrasonography, very low
    birth weight, 172, 251
Flash visually evoked potentials, 270
Flat foot, 1555
Flatulence, beans, 1183
Flavine adenine nucleotide, 1198
Flaviviruses, hepatitis, 477–478
Flea-borne typhus fever, endemic, 1390
    (Table), 1392
Fleas, see also Jigger flea
  Dipylidium caninum, 1502–1503
  typhus, 1391
Flecainide, 627 (Table)
Flexion contractures, congenital, 1549
Flexor dystonia, 769
Flies, 1513–1514
  larvae, 1484 (Table), 1513
Floppy baby syndrome, botulinum toxin,
    726
Flow limitation, airways, 499
Flow velocity waveform, Doppler
    ultrasonography, umbilical artery,
    82–83, 115
Flow volume curve, expiratory, 499 (Fig.),
    500
Flubendazole
  ascariasis, 1485
  hookworm, 1490
Flucloxacillin
  administration, 1955 (Table), 1966
    (Table)
  immunosuppression, 1265
  neonatal pneumonia, 280
  osteomyelitis, 283
  pyogenic osteitis, 1590
  Staphylococcus aureus, 1329 (Table)
Fluconazole, 1478
  administration, 1966 (Table)
  candidiasis, 536, 1434
Flucytosine, 1472, 1478, 1530
  administration, 1955 (Table), 1966
    (Table)
5-Flucytosine, neonatal candidiasis, 289
Fludrocortisone, see 9α-Fluorocortisol
Fluid balance, see also Water, balance
  charts, preterm infant, 141
  pneumothorax, 188
  preterm infant, 139–143
  restoration, 413–415
Fluid intake, phototherapy, 218

Fluid management
  acute renal failure, 974–975
  intracranial birth trauma, 122
  raised intracranial pressure, 714
  respiratory distress syndrome, 180
Fluid restriction
  birth asphyxia, 131
  metabolic bone disease, 302
  neonatal meningitis, 282
  nephrotic syndrome, 970
  raised intracranial pressure, 714
  syndrome of inappropriate ADH
    secretion, 1040
Fluid therapy
  acute diarrhea, 453, 1295–1296
  acute renal failure, 258
  congenital nephrogenic diabetes
    insipidus, 260
  dehydration, 413–415, 453, 1295–1296
  diabetic ketoacidosis, 1075
  hypernatremia, 453
  malaria, 1453
  meningococcal disease, 1816
  neonate, sodium, 143
  potassium, 411
  preterm infant, 140
  resuscitation, 526, 527 (Fig.)
  salmonellosis, 1324
Flukes (trematodes), 1506–1513
Flumazenil, administration, 1966 (Table)
Flunarizine, 131
  migraine, 717 (Table)
Fluocinolone, administration, 1966 (Table)
Fluorescein, eye examination, 1654, 1665,
    1671
Fluorescein angiography, 1671
  diabetic retinopathy, 1080
Fluorescein dilaurate, pancreatic function
    tests, 451
Fluorescence microscopy
  Mycobacterium tuberculosis,
    1334–1335
  syphilis, 1402
Fluorescent in situ hybridization, 50
Fluorescent Treponemal Antibody
    Absorbed Test, 1403
  congenital and neurosyphilis, 1405
Fluoride, 1202
  estimated safe and adequate daily
    intakes, 1949 (Table)
  poisoning, 1709
  safe intakes, 1948 (Table)
  supplements, 334
Fluorine, 1185 (Table)
9α-Fluorocortisol
  Addison's disease, 1068
  administration, 1966 (Table)
  congenital adrenal hyperplasia
    treatment, 1065
  for sweat tests, 553
Fluorodeoxyglucose, positron emission
    tomography, 1897
Fluoroquinolones
  joint pain, 556
  resistance, Neisseria gonorrhoeae, 1421
  salmonellosis, 1324
  typhoid fever, 1326
Fluoroscopy, 1895
  chest, 514, 1900
  dysphagia, 426
  foreign bodies, inhalation, 571
Fluorosis, 1202
5-Fluorouracil, dihydropyrimidine
    dehydrogenase deficiency, 1142
Fluoxetine, 1755
  bulimia nervosa, 1759
Flush method, blood pressure, 20
Fluticasone, administration, 1967 (Table)
Flynn–Aird syndrome, 753
FMR 1 gene, fragile X mental retardation,
    63
Foam furniture, 1715
Focal segmental glomerulosclerosis,
    971–972

Focal seizures, 684
Foerster's sign, 667
Fog test, 668
Folate/folic acid, 1184 (Table)
  administration, 1967 (Table)
    neonate, 1957 (Table)
  deficiency, 852–853, 1198
    DNA synthesis, 852 (Fig.)
  fragile X mental retardation, 63
  hereditary spherocytosis, 226
  for homocystinuria, 1109
  with ion exchange resins, 1152
  for malnutrition, 1193
  metabolism disorders, 1147
  with methotrexate, 1604
  neural tube defects, 652
  normal values, 1925 (Table)
  organic acidurias, 1119
  parenteral nutrition, 1221 (Table)
  preconceptual care, 80
  pregnancy, 114, 338
  Recommended Dietary Allowances,
    1949 (Table)
  requirements, preterm infant, 152
    (Table), 225
Foley catheters, 1840
Folinic acid
  administration, 1967 (Table)
  dihydropteridine reductase deficiency,
    1106
  folic acid deficiency, 1198
Folinic acid-responsive seizures, 1147
Follicle stimulating hormone, 1038
  childhood, 987
  fetus, 1003
  normal values, 1925 (Table)
  pulses, 1026
    hypothyroidism, 1028
  spermatogenesis, 1024
Follicular conjunctivitis, 1370, 1385
Follicular cysts, ovary, 1796
Follicular epithelium, thyroid neoplasms,
    1052
Folliculitis, Pseudomonas aeruginosa,
    1321
Follow-on formula, 331
Follow-up, sudden infant death syndrome,
    1723
Fontanels, 20, 242
  bulging, neonatal meningitis, 281
Fontan procedure, 621
  hypoplastic left heart syndrome, 620
  ventilation, 1818
Food additives
  intolerance, 1701
  urticaria, 1697
Food allergy, 1213–1214, 1639
  atopic eczema, 1695–1696
  contact urticaria, 1643
  urticaria, 1697
Food challenges, 1214, 1694, see also
    Cow's milk, intolerance, challenge
    testing
Food frequency questionnaires, 1187
Food intolerance, 212, 1213–1214, 1689,
    1698–1701
  asthma, 542, 545
    infantile, 550
  chronic constipation, 462
  diets for, 470, 1213
  history taking, 1692
  from infections, 454
  kwashiorkor, 1193
  multiple, 442
  toddler diarrhea, 463, 464
  transient, 441–442
Food manufacturing, infections, 1278
Food poisoning, 1278
  salmonellosis, 1323
  Staphylococcus aureus, 1329–1330
  typhoid fever, 1324–1325
  United Kingdom, 1276–1277
Food-provoked exercise-induced
    anaphylaxis, 1697

Foods, see also Milks
  goitrogens, 1049
  history taking, 17
  migraine, 716, 717 (Table)
Food security, 1892
Foot
  congenital abnormalities, 1554–1556
  dorsiflexion, neonate, 44
    gestation age, 40 (Table), 41 (Fig.)
  Duchenne muscular dystrophy, 730
  Edwards' syndrome, 57
  Friedreich's ataxia, 765
  writing with, 822
Football sign, 1902
Foot drop, vincristine, 896
Foramen cecum, 1043
Foramen magnum, see also Coning
  impaction syndrome, 647
  neoplasm, vs degenerative disease, 796
    (Table)
Foramen of Monro
  obstruction, 658
  tumors, tuberous sclerosis, 802
Foramen ovale, 199
  closure, 107
Forced alkaline diuresis, salicylate
    poisoning, 1710
Forced-choice technique, 269
Forced expiratory flow, 497
Forced expiratory volume, 499–500
  cystic fibrosis, 554
Forced vital capacity, 500
Forceps delivery
  preterm, 119, 120
  resuscitation, 133
Foregut, 206
Foreign bodies
  airway, 522, see also Choking
    vs common cold, 560
  inhalation, 571
  nose, 1684
  removal from esophagus, 1899
  swallowed, 435
  vagina, 987
Foreign material, inhalation, 570–572
Foreign travel, see Travel, international
Foremilk (drip milk), vs expressed milk,
    152
Foreskin, nonretractability, 1793
Formalin, plantar warts, 1633
Formal operational period, 1730
  development, 1729 (Table)
Form boards, 383
Formoterol, 546
Formula feeding, 113, 331–332, 1188, see
    also Formula milks
  acute diarrhea, 453
  vs breast-feeding, growth, 330
  preterm infant, 153
  SGA baby, 137
  Third World, 327
Formula milks, 112–113, 1188, see also
    Bottle feeding
  bilirubin, normal range, 218
  calcium absorption from, 301
  calcium and phosphorus from, 303
  calcium deficiency, 1200
  composition, 331 (Table), 1942–1943
    (Table)
    special formulae, 1944–1945 (Table)
  and hypernatremia, 414, 415
  hypomagnesemia, 300
  intolerance, 212
  manufacture from cow's milk, 333
  for maple syrup urine disease, 1120
  for marasmus, 1192
  medium chain triglycerides, 208
  neonatal tetany, 299
  preterm infant, 152–153
  sucrase-isomaltase deficiency, 446
Formulations, psychiatric, 1735, 1752
Forsius–Eriksson syndrome, 1108
Fortification, breast milk, 152
48XXXXY, 62

49XXXXY, 62
47XXX (triple X), 62
Foscarnet, cytomegalovirus, 1366
Foster homes, 1857
Four chamber view, echocardiography,
    591
4-syndrome, 58
Fourth nerve, see Trochlear nerve
Fourth ventricle
  entrapment, 659
  outflow obstruction, 658
Fractional excretion, 943
  bicarbonate, 260
  sodium (FE^{Na}), 256–257
    intrinsic renal failure, 258
Fractionation, radiotherapy, 893
Fractures, 38
  accident & emergency attendance rates,
    1712
  arthrogryposis multiplex congenita,
    1587
  birth trauma, 121
  dating, 703
  major trauma, 1812–1813
  non-accidental injury, 1867–1868
    head injury, 700
  nose, 1684
  osteogenesis imperfecta, 1570
    radiography, 1914–1915
  ribs, 1811, 1867, 1914
    shaking injury, 701
  tibia, congenital, 1549
Fragile X syndrome, 46, 62–64, 72
    (Table), 398
  articulatory dyspraxia, 818
  autism, 1738
  genetic diagnosis, 73
    (Renpenning), 831 (Table)
Framboesia, see Yaws
Frameshift mutations, 69
Framycetin, administration, 1967 (Table)
France, toxoplasmosis, 1465
Franceschetti's syndrome
    (mandibulofacial dysostosis), 25
    (Fig.), 1563–1564, 1661
Francisella tularensis, 1350
Free bilirubin, cerebrospinal fluid, 1933
    (Table)
Free erythrocyte protoporphyrin, 1188
Free fatty acids, 1148
  marasmus, plasma levels, 1192
  normal values, 1926 (Table)
    cerebrospinal fluid, 1934 (Table)
    stools, 1936 (Table)
  and parenteral nutrition, 1220
Free hormone levels, thyroid function
    tests, 1045, 1046
Freeing orders, adoption, 1859
Free radicals, asphyxia, 127
Free radical scavengers, 131
Free water clearance, 409–410
Freezing of meat, Taenia saginata
    prevention, 1500
Freiberg's disease, 1595
French–American–British classification,
    leukemias, 868
French sizes, enteral feeding tubes, 1218
Frequency syndromes, 949
Fresh frozen plasma, 230
  for birth trauma, 121
  disseminated intravascular coagulation,
    231
  dosage, 851 (Table)
Fresh water drowning, 1718
Freud, S., emotional development, 1729
    (Table), 1730–1731
Friction rub, pericardial, 32
Friedreich's ataxia, 28 (Fig.), 34, 72
    (Table), 764–765 (Fig.), 792 (Table)
  dysarthria, 813
  heart, 596
  hypertrophic cardiomyopathy, 634
Frog leg lateral radiography, hip, 1915
Frog position, scurvy, 1199

Frogs, sparganosis from, 1504
Fröhlich's syndrome, 1022
Frontal lobe glioma, 794 (Table)
Frontal sinusitis, 1685
Frontal vector loop, electrocardiography,
    588 (Fig.)
Frontometaphyseal dysplasia, 1581 (Table)
Frostig developmental test of visual
    perception, 400
'Frozen watchfulness,' 1018 (Fig.)
Fructokinase deficiency, 1135
Fructosamine, glycemic control, 1079
Fructose
  cholestasis, 220
  intestinal absorption, 438
  metabolism disorders, 1134–1135
Fructose-1,6-diphosphatase deficiency,
    296, 1135
Fructose-1-phosphate aldolase deficiency,
    1134–1135
Fructose tolerance test, 1134–1135
Fruit juices, toddler diarrhea, 463, 464
Frusemide
  acute renal failure, 975
  administration, 1967 (Table)
    neonate, 1957 (Table)
  on CSF production, 664
  heart failure, 599
  for hypertension, 637 (Table)
  intracranial pressure, 708
  Irukandji sting, 1526
  nephrotic syndrome, 970
  renal hypertension, 973 (Table)
  respiratory distress syndrome, 142
  resuscitation, doses, 526 (Table)
  syndrome of inappropriate ADH
    secretion, 1040
  for vitamin D intoxication, 1055
FTA-ABS, see Fluorescent Treponemal
    Antibody Absorbed Test
Fuchsia, poisoning, 1790
Fucosidosis, 780 (Table), 1157 (Table),
    1167–1168
Fugitive swelling, 1497
Fukuyama type congenital muscular
    dystrophy, 650, 729
Full term gestation, definitions, 94
Fulminant liver failure, 478–479, 1824
Fulminating colitis, 459
Fumarase deficiency, 788 (Table), 1126
Fumarylacetoacetate hydrolase deficiency,
    1106
Functional antibody deficiency, 1259
Functional antibody tests, 1245
Functional assessment of nutrition, 1186
Functional mapping, epilepsy, 679
Functional murmurs, 594
Functional residual capacity, 159, 501
  neonate, 496
Fundal height (uterus), 81, 115
Fundoplication, 429, 1785
Fundoscopy, see Ophthalmoscopy
Funerals, neonatal death, 174
Fungal infections, 1470–1478
  AIDS, 1397
  bone marrow transplant recipients, 875
  cancer treatment, 895
  eye, 1676
  immunocompromised patient, 535–536
  liver, ultrasonography, 1906
  respiratory tract, 570
  skin, 1636–1637
  spleen, ultrasonography, 1907
  systemic, 1471 (Table)
Fungal meningitis, 248
Fungal spores, allergens, 1690
Funicular hernia, 1789
Funnel chest, 1556
Funnel web spider, 1525
Funny turns, 671, 672–673
Furazolidone
  administration, 1967 (Table)
  giardiasis, 1467
Furious rabies, 1377

Furosemide, see Frusemide
Furunculosis, **1635**
    ear, **1680**
Fusidic acid
    administration, 1967 (Table)
    mechanism, 1527
    pyogenic osteitis, 1590
    Staphylococcus aureus, 1329 (Table)
Fusion, kidneys, 939

GABA, see Gamma-aminobutyric acid
Gaboon vipers, envenomation, 1522
Gag reflex, 36 (Table)
    neonate, 241
Gait
    examination, 34
    hemiplegia, 34, 35, 743–744
    history taking, 17
    running, 35
    truncal ataxia, 751
Galactitol, cataract, 1133, 1134
Galactokinase deficiency, 1134
Galactorrhea, 1039
Galactose
    absorption, 207, 438
    cholestasis, 220
    metabolism disorders, **1132–1134**
    normal values, 1925 (Table)
        urine, 1931 (Table)
    tolerance test, debranching enzyme
        deficiency, 1138
Galactosemia, 72 (Table), 329
    cataract, 1668
    dietary management, **1203 (Table)**
    neonate, 297
    vomiting, 212
Galactose-1-phosphate, normal values,
    1925 (Table)
Galactose-1-phosphate uridyltransferase
    deficiency, 1132–1133
    red cells, normal values, 1925 (Table)
Galactosialidosis, 781 (Table), 1157
    (Table), 1169
α-Galactosidase deficiency, 1164
β-Galactosidase deficiency, 1160
    GM₁-gangliosidosis, 1163
Galactosylceramide β-galactosidase
    deficiency, 1165
Galant reflex, see Trunk, incurvation
    reflex
Gallbladder
    Kawasaki disease, 1479
    ultrasonography, 1906
Gallium scintigraphy, lymphomas, 1913
Gallop rhythm (triple rhythm), 32, 598
Gallstones, see Biliary calculi
Gambian sleeping sickness, 1453, 1454
Gametocytes, *Plasmodium* spp., 1446
Gamma-aminobutyric acid
    metabolism disorders, 1115
    normal values, cerebrospinal fluid, 1933
        (Table)
    prolactin secretion, 1039
Gamma-aminobutyric acid receptors,
    infantile spasms, 687
Gamma-benzene hexachloride
    head lice, 1518
    pubic lice, 1519
    scabies, 1517
γ chain deficiency, interleukin-2 receptor,
    see X-linked severe combined
    immunodeficiency syndrome
Gammaglobulin, see also Immunoglobulin
    for mucocutaneous lymph node
        syndrome, 633, 1480
Gamma-interferon, malaria immunity,
    1447
Ganciclovir
    bone marrow transplant recipients, 875
    cytomegalovirus, 1366
        pneumonitis, 535
    drug resistance, 1530

Ganglion cells, rectum, chronic
    constipation, 463
Ganglioneuroma, dancing eye syndrome,
    763
Gangliosides, 1162
    development, 643
    injection, Guillain–Barré syndrome
        from, 726
Gangliosidoses, **775–776 (Table)**, 1159,
    see also GM₁ gangliosidoses; GM₂
    gangliosidoses
Gangosa, 1417
Ganthostoma spp., larval disease, 1484
    (Table)
Gap junctions, myometrium, 84
Garden pond drownings, 1717
Gardner's syndrome, 448, 888 (Table)
Gargoylism, see Hurler's syndrome
Garré's diffuse sclerosing osteitis, 1590
Gas chromatography, organic acidurias,
    1119
Gas chromatography–mass spectrometry,
    urine, 306
Gas contrast, abdominal X-rays,
    1901–1902
Gases, medical, neonatal resuscitation,
    133
Gas exchange, **502–505**, see also Blood
    gases
    asthma, 539
    development, **497**
    lungs, 160
    ventilator settings, 162–163
Gas gangrene, antibiotic prophylaxis,
    1529
Gas–liquid chromatography, urine, 306
Gasterophilus spp.
    larval disease, 1484 (Table)
    myiasis, 1514
Gas transport, **502–505**, see also Blood
    gases
Gastric acid
    preterm infant, 150, 207
    production, 430
Gastric aspirates, see also Gastric suction
    pneumonia diagnosis, 184
    preterm infant, 208
    tuberculosis, 1342
Gastric carcinoma, ataxia telangiectasia,
    290
Gastric distension, respiratory
    embarrassment, 155
Gastric juice
    cholera, protective effect, 1304
    electrolytes, 411 (Table)
Gastric lavage
    accidental poisoning, 1706, 1815
    technique, **1845**
Gastric lipase, 207, 437
Gastric mucosa, ectopic, 1787
    scintigraphy, 447, 460
Gastric suction, **430**, 435, see also Gastric
    aspirates
    accidental poisoning, 1706
    infants, 104
    neonate, 208
    preterm infant, 150
    trauma, 1809
Gastrin, 430
    short gut syndrome, 445
Gastritis
    autoimmune, 430
    Helicobacter pylori, 431
    neonatal, 210
Gastroenteritis
    acute infective diarrhea, **451–454**
    adenoviruses, 1371
    dehydration, **452–453**
        treatment, 413
    ECHO viruses, 1383
    fits, 683
    infantile, 327, **1292–1297**
        recovery, 1297
    and malnutrition, 1193

measles, 1354
    neonate, 282
        viral, 212–213
    nutrition, 1215
    viruses, **1384**, see also Rotaviruses,
        gastroenteritis
Gastroesophageal junction, 426
Gastroesophageal reflux, 212, **427–429**,
    466, **1785–1786**
    apparent life-threatening events, 528
    asthma, **542**, 547
    cystic fibrosis, 1209
    milk scans, 212, **519**
    positional deformity, 749
    preterm infant, 150
    respiratory disorders, 570, 571
        aspiration pneumonia, 187
    respiratory distress syndrome, 182
    scintigraphy, 1906
    ventilation, 155
Gastrogenic cysts, thoracic, 192
Gastrografin, 1895
    meconium ileus, 553, 1776, 1904
Gastrointestinal hemorrhage, see also
    Hematemesis; Rectal bleeding
    cirrhosis, management, **482–483**
    extrahepatic biliary atresia, 475
    hemorrhagic disease of the newborn,
        230
    Meckel's diverticulum, 1787
    upper, **433**
Gastrointestinal tract, **423–470**
    acute intermittent porphyria, 1143
    AIDS, 444, 1394
    amino acid transport systems, 1121
        (Table)
    anthrax, 1300
    blood loss, 1201
    burns, 1799
    calcitonin on, 1056
    chronic symptoms, **460–464**
    contrast media, 1895
        computed tomography, 1897
    defenses, **438–439**
    development, 107–108
        function, **150–151**
    disorders
        feeding problems, 469
        growth failure, 1018
    electrolytes and volume of secretions,
        411 (Table)
    failure to thrive, 466, **466–467**, 469
    function, **423–424**
    Henoch–Schönlein purpura, 1609
    IgA deficiency, 1258
    imaging, **1901–1906**
    infections, see also Gastroenteritis;
        named diseases
        iron supplements, 155
        United Kingdom, mortality, 1276
            (Table)
    kwashiorkor, 1192, 1193, 1194
    neonate, **206–214**
        mortality, 4 (Table)
    neoplasms, **448–449**
    polioviruses, 1379
    viruses, **1383–1384**
Gastroschisis, 1779, **1780–1781**
Gastroscopy, see Endoscopy
Gastrostomies, 1218, 1219 (Table)
Gastrostomy buttons, 1218
Gaucher disease, **778 (Table)**, 1157
    (Table), 1162, **1165–1166**
    human β glucosidase, 1102
    neonate, 308
    retina, 1666
    treatment, 1158
GB agents, 478
G-banding, 48
Gel cysts, vs hydatid disease, 1506
Geliophysic dwarfism, 1157 (Table)
Gels, skin treatment, 1617
Gender, see also Sex ratios
    low birthweight and outcome, 167–168

Gender identity, intersex disorders, 1010
Gender issues, developing countries,
    1885–1886
Gender reassignment, 1011
Gender role, 1731
Gene mapping, **72–73**
Gene probes, **70**
General acyl CoA dehydrogenase
    deficiency, 297
General anesthesia
    computed tomography, 1897
        chest, 1900
    examination of visual system, 273
    syndrome of inappropriate ADH
        secretion, 1040
General Household Surveys, 1850
Generalized herpetic infection, 1364
Generalized lipodystrophy, 1155
Generalized seizures, 675
General Medical Council, on record
    keeping, 1878
General paralysis of the insane, juvenile,
    1413
General practice
    child health activities, 1862
    consultation rates, 10 (Table)
    contract, 1854
    infectious diseases data, 1277–1278,
        1280 (Table)
    morbidity rates, **8–9**
    National Health Service, 1854
General practitioner pediatricians, 1853
Genes, **68–70**
Gene sequencing, 72
Gene therapy, adenosine deaminase
    deficiency, 1270
Genetic counseling, **76–77**, 114, 338
    congenital adrenal hyperplasia, 986
    congenital heart disease, 597
    Down syndrome, 56
    limb malformations, 1545
    mental retardation, 840
    retinoblastoma, 923
Genetic epilepsies, **679–684**
Genetic instability syndromes, neoplasms,
    888 (Table), 889–890
Genetics, **45–78**, see also Cytogenetics
    antibiotic resistance, 1529
    febrile convulsions, 683
    growth control, **366–367**
    21-hydroxylase deficiency, 1062
    immunodeficiency disorders,
        1241–1243
    inborn errors of metabolism, 1099–1101
    of mitochondria, 1126
Genetic screening, 338, 339 (Table)
    Down syndrome, 56–57
    ethics, 77
Geniculate herpes, 725, 1363
Genitalia, see also Ambiguous genitalia
    baby care, 112
    candidiasis, 1433
    Chlamydia trachomatis, 1430
    examination, 34
    female, embryology, 1004
    growth, 363
    imaging, **1913–1914**
    neonatal gestation age, 42 (Fig.)
    puberty, 357
    schistosomiasis, 1509
    syphilis, secondary, 1407
Genital period, emotional development,
    1729 (Table)
Genital tubercle, 986
Genitography, 1914
Genline, Internet URL, 1099
Genomic imprinting
    Prader–Willi syndrome, 1022
    Turner's syndrome, 1032
Gentamicin
    administration, 1955 (Table), 1967
        (Table)
    brainstem auditory evoked potentials,
        244

Gentamicin (*Contd*)
cat-scratch disease, 1520
Listeria monocytogenes, 284
neonate, 279 (Table)
meningitis, 247
pneumonia, 184
ophthalmia neonatorum, eye ointment, 1429
prophylaxis, infective endocarditis, 632 (Table)
Pseudomonas aeruginosa, cystic fibrosis, 558 (Table)
pyogenic osteitis, 1590
therapeutic ranges, 1936 (Table)
tularemia, 1351
urinary tract infections, 952 (Table)
Gentian violet
blood transfusions, 1458, 1460
for oral moniliasis, 1472
Genu recurvatum, **1553**
Genu valgum, 38, **1553**
Genu varum (bow legs), 38, **1553**
Geographic tongue, 27 (Fig.), 425
Geography
celiac disease, 440
diabetes mellitus, 1073
endemic treponematoses, 1416 (Fig.), 1417
hemoglobinopathies, 860
neoplasms, 885
schistosomiasis, 1507 (Table)
Gerbils, leishmaniasis control, 1464
German measles, *see* Rubella
Germ cells, ontogeny, 1002
Germ cell tumors, **920–923**
incidence, 886 (Table)
pineal, 904
Germinal cell mutations, 69
Germinal matrix hemorrhage, 249, 250
outcome, 171
Germinal plate, telencephalon, 642
Germinomas, 920
diabetes insipidus, 1040 (Table)
pineal gland, 1043
Germ tubes, *Candida albicans,* 1433, 1434
Gestation, WHO definitions, 94
Gestation age
fetus, 80
neonate, 40 (Table), **41**
outcome, 167, **168–170**
respiratory distress syndrome, 177
Ghana, yaws, 1417
Ghon focus, 1336
Ghost vessels, syphilitic keratitis, 1413
Gianotti–Crosti syndrome, **1633–1634**
Giant axonal neuropathy, 793 (Table)
Giant cell arteritis, 1611
Giant cell pneumonia, measles, 510, **535, 1354**
Giant cells, tuberous sclerosis, 801
Giant pigmented hairy nevus, 804
Giardia lamblia, **1466–1467**
AIDS, 1397
United Kingdom, 1277 (Fig.)
Gibbons catheters, 1840
Gigantism, 1021
cerebral (Sotos syndrome), 832 (Table), 833, 1043
pituitary, 376
Gilbert's syndrome, 218, **1144–1145**
Gilles de la Tourette's syndrome, 768, **771,** 824, 836, 1745
Gingivostomatitis, herpetic, 1363, 1364–1365, **1438, 1631–1632**
vs hand, foot and mouth disease, 1382
Girls, developing countries, 1885–1886
Gitelman's syndrome, 946
Glabella reflex, 36 (Table)
neonatal gestation age, 40 (Table)
Glanders, 1321
Glandular fever, *see* Infectious mononucleosis
Glandular tularemia, 1351

Glanzmann's disease, 229, 879
Glasgow coma scales, 695, 704 (Table)
Glass injuries, **1715**
Glaucoma
from corticosteroids, 1677
homocystinuria, 1673
infantile, 23, 27 (Fig.), 43, 264, **1672–1673**
Glia, cerebral, development, 642
β-Gliadin, intolerance, 439, 440
Glial-specific protein, 643
Gliding contusions, 701
Glioblastoma multiforme, 903
Gliomas, 899
frontal lobe, 794 (Table)
hypothalamus, 1042
vs neurofibromatosis, 801
optic, **904,** 1661, **1672**
stroke, 714
Globe dislocation, orbits, 264
Globins, hemoglobinopathies, 860
Globoid cell leukodystrophy, 777 (Table), 1157 (Table), **1165**
Glomerular basement membrane, *see* Basement membrane nephropathy
Glomerular filtration rate, 941, 1938 (Table)
measurement, **942–943**
neonate, 108, 934
postnatal development, 256, 1953
preterm infant, 140
Glomerular proteinuria, 968
Glomeruli
bleeding, 958
fetal sclerosis, 934
focal segmental glomerulosclerosis, 971
proteinuria, 967
Glomerulonephritis, **960–966**
hematuria, 958–959, 960
nephroblastoma, 914
Plasmodium falciparum, 1448
proteinuria, 961–962, 968
scabies, 1516
syphilis, 1408
tuberculosis, 1346
Glomerulotubular imbalance, neonates, 143
Glossina spp., *see* Tsetse flies
Glossopharyngeal nerve, 811
examination, 34
Gloves, infection prevention, 1282
Glucagon, **1072**
amino acid plasma levels, 1102
congenital deficiency, 297
fetus, 1004
for hypoglycemia, 1080
therapy, 1967 (Table)
neonate, 295, 296, 1957 (Table)
Glucagon test, debranching enzyme deficiency, 1138
Glucoamylase, 437 (Table)
Glucocorticoids
growth hormone gene transcription, 367
on lung maturation, 176
Gluconeogenesis
alanine load test, 1938 (Table)
disorders, 1126
liver, SGA baby, 137
neonate, 290–293
Glucose, 1182, *see also* Dextrose
absorption, 207, 438
blood levels
acute-onset stroke, 715
vs cerebrospinal fluid, 242
emergency care, 1814
hypoglycemia definition, 1080
neonate, 1005
nocturnal, 1072
chromium deficiency, 1202
concentration units, 1921
emergency supply, 134 (Table)
fetus and neonate, 290–293
hydrogen breath test, 448
intrapartum infusions, 296

neonatal resuscitation, 135–136
normal values, 1925 (Table)
cerebrospinal fluid, 1934 (Table)
urine, 1931 (Table)
parenteral nutrition, 1220, 1223 (Table)
regulation, fetus, 1004
renal reabsorption, 257
tolerance, disorders and birthweight, 369
tolerance test, 1938 (Table)
glucose-6-phosphatase deficiency, 1137
not in pyruvate dehydrogenase deficiency, 1125
transporters, defects, **1123**
Glucose CSF/blood ratio, meningitis, 1290
Glucose–galactose malabsorption, 446, 448, 1123, 1214 (Table), 1215
Glucose-6-phosphatase deficiency, 788 (Table), **1136–1137**
neutrophils, 1199, 1242 (Table), 1260
Glucose-6-phosphate dehydrogenase deficiency, 217, 218, **226, 858–859,** 1100
and drugs, 859 (Table)
maternal, 89 (Table)
primaquine, 1453
and sulfonamides, 859 (Table), 1528
Glucose-6-phosphate translocase deficiencies, 1137
Glucose polymers, for cystic fibrosis, 1208
α-Glucosidases, preterm infant, 151
β-Glucosidases, Gaucher disease, 1166
Glucosylceramide, 1162
β-Glucuronidase
breast milk, 219
cerebrospinal fluid, normal values, 1934 (Table)
deficiency, Sly syndrome, 1161
Glucuronidation, drugs, 1953
Glucuronyltransferase, 214–215
inhibition, breast milk jaundice, 219–220
Glue ear (secretory otitis media), 816, **1681–1682**
Glutamate, neurotransmission, 127
Glutamate dehydrogenase deficiency, 1115–1116
Glutamate formiminotransferase deficiency, 852, 1147
Glutamine
plasma levels, nutrition, 1188
short bowel syndrome, 1212
urine, 1103
γ-Glutamyl cycle, **1115**
γ-Glutamylcysteine synthetase deficiency, 1115
γ-Glutamyltransferase
deficiency, 1115
normal values, 1925 (Table)
γ-Glutamyltranspeptidase
deficiency, 1115
serum levels, 472 (Table)
prognosis, 473
Glutaric acidemia, 773, 1113
type II, **308,** 1130
Glutaric aciduria type II (MAD:S), 1130
α-Glutaryl-CoA oxidase deficiency, 1174
Glutathione
cytotoxic drug resistance, 893
synthesis, 1115
Glutathione instability, neonatal red cells, 849
Glutathione peroxidase, red cells, 1188
Glutathione reductase
deficiency, 1131
red cells, riboflavin deficiency, 1198
Glutathione synthetase deficiency, 1115, 1260
Gluten challenge, 441
Gluten intolerance, 439
GLUTs, defects, 1123
Glycated hemoglobin, normal values,

1926 (Table)
d-Glyceric acidemia, 773
Glycerin suppositories, 213
Glycerol
fructose-1,6-diphosphatase deficiency, 1135
intolerance, 1130
Glycerol kinase deficiency, 1130
Glyceryl trinitrate
for adrenoleukodystrophy, 1174
thrombophlebitis prevention, 1223
Glyceryl trioleate, for adrenoleukodystrophy, 1174
Glycine
for isovaleric acidemia, 1117
metabolism disorders, **1112–1113**
plasma levels, organic acidurias, 1119
urine, 1103
Glycinuria, with glycosuria, 1122
Glycoasparagines, aspartylglucosaminuria, 1167
Glycogen, 1135–1136
muscle biopsy, 1132
red cells, normal values, 1926 (Table)
Glycogenolysis, fetus and neonate, 290
Glycogen storage diseases, 296–297, 308, **1135–1140**
central nervous system, **788–789 (Table)**
dietary management, **1205 (Table)**
liver, hyperlipoproteinemia, 1153, 1154 (Table)
myopathy, 735
Glycogen synthase deficiency, 1140
Glycollate, excretion, 1113
Glycolysis
defects, **1131–1134**
fetal hypoxia response, 124
Glycoprotein 91 phagocytic oxidase gene defect, 1259
Glycoproteinoses, 1157 (Table), **1167–1169**
Glycosuria
false positive, 1131
with glycinuria, 1122
preterm infant, 257
proximal tubular function, 943
Glycosylated hemoglobin, 1079
Glyoxylate excretion, 1113
GM₁ gangliosidoses, 775 (Table), 1157 (Table), **1162–1163**
type I, neonate, 308
GM₂ gangliosidoses, 775 (Table), 1157 (Table), **1163–1164**
cerebellar degeneration, 765–766
GMH, *see* Germinal matrix hemorrhage
GMH-IVH, 249
Goat's milk, 153, **333,** 1700
intolerance, 1699
Goiter, 1045–1050
Goitrogens, 1049
Gold, *see* Chrysotherapy
Goldenhar's syndrome, 1557, 1563 (Table), 1564
Goldie–Goldman model, chemotherapy, 893, 910
Gold therapy, 1603–1604
Golgi apparatus, pH, effect of CFTR, 552
Gonadal dysgenesis, 990, 1008–1011, **1031–1035**
gonadoblastoma, 921
Gonadoblastoma, 921
Turner's syndrome, 62, 370
Gonadorelin, administration, 1967 (Table)
Gonadotropin-independent precocious puberty, 1030
Gonadotropin releasing hormone, 1039
childhood, 987, 1024–1026
delayed puberty investigation, 1031
low-dose test, precocious puberty, 1030
molecule, 1038 (Table)
Gonadotropin releasing hormone analogues, for precocious puberty, 1031

Gonadotropins, **1038**
  deficiency, 1031, 1041
  delayed puberty investigation, 1034
  fetus, 1002
  Turner's syndrome, 370
Gonads
  abnormal differentiation, 1010–1011
  fetus, 1003–1004
  one only, 1010
Goniotomy, buphthalmos, 1673
Gonorrhea, **1420–1429**
  detection or exclusion, 1399, 1400
  tests of cure, 1429
  treatment, **1426–1429**
  vertical transmission, 1400
Goodenough–Harris drawing test, 400, 670
Goodpasture's syndrome, 965
Gordon's syndrome, 947
Gorlin's syndrome, 888 (Table)
Goundou, 1417
Gout, 1140
'Goutte de lait' (Budin), 1861
Gower's sign, 730
Gp91 phox defect, 1259
Gp120, HIV, 1393
G-protein coupled receptors, 364
G proteins, 1057–1058
Graded balls test, see STYCAR graded balls test
Grading, radiological, respiratory distress syndrome, 178
Graft survival, renal transplantation, 981
Graft-versus-host disease
  bone marrow transplantation, 534, 874, 1269
  severe combined immunodeficiency syndrome, 1249
Grammar, normal development, 385
Gram-negative bacteria
  lysis, 273
  meningitis, 1290
    neonatal, 247 (Table), 248
Gram-negative septicemia, 1287
  complement deficiency, 1263
  disseminated intravascular coagulation, 231
  epidemiology, 276
  neonatal thrombocytopenia, 229
Gramoxone, poisoning, 1711
Gram-positive bacteria
  lysis, 273
  sepsis epidemiology, 276
Granisetron, administration, 1967 (Table)
Granulocyte colony stimulating factor, 849, 1233 (Table)
  for neonatal infections, 1267
  for neutropenias, 867, 1259
Granulocyte-macrophage colony stimulating factor, 1233 (Table)
  for neonatal sepsis, 279
Granulocytes
  fetus and neonate, 848
  transfusion, 279
Granulomas, tuberculosis, 1335
Granulomatous amebic encephalitis, 1469
Granulomatous diseases, see also Chronic granulomatous disease
  gastrointestinal, 444
  hypercalcemia, 1056
Granulosa cells, 1004
Granulosa cell tumors, ovary, 921, 989
Granulosa-theca cell tumors, ovary, 1028
Gräsbeck, syndrome of proteinuria with vitamin B$_{12}$ malabsorption, 853
Grasp
  examination, 388 (Table), 389 (Table)
  normal development, 382–383
Grasp reflexes, 36 (Table)
  neonatal gestation age, 40 (Table)
Grass pollens, allergy, 1689–1690
Gratings, vision test, 269
Graves, neonatal death, 174
Graves' disease, **1051–1052**

neonatal hyperthyroidism, 998
'Gray baby' syndrome, 108
Gray matter heterotopia, magnetic resonance imaging, 1910 (Fig.)
Greek helmet, Wolf-Hirschhorn syndrome, 58
Green Cross Code, 1716
Green monkey disease (Marburg virus disease), **1388–1389**
Greenstick fractures, 1914
Greig's syndrome (hypertelorism), 22, 24 (Fig.), 76 (Table), 647, 1562, 1661
Greulich and Pyle system, bone age, 362
Grief, 928–929, 1747
  for parent, 1857
  of parents, neonatal deaths, 172
Griffiths test, 398, 400
Griscelli syndrome, 1254
Griseofulvin, **1637**
  administration, 1967 (Table)
  mechanism, 1530
Grommets, tympanic membrane, 1680, 1681, 1682
Gross national products, 1883 (Table), 1884
Ground glass appearance
  Pneumocystis carinii pneumonia, 534 (Fig.)
  respiratory distress syndrome, 178
Ground itch, 1489
Group amino acid transport systems, 1121 (Table)
Group aminoacidurias, 1121
Group psychotherapy, 1749, **1763**
  sexual abuse, 1760
Growing pains, **1612–1613**
Growing skull fracture, 700, 707
Growth, 349–380, 1011–1023, see also Brain, growth; Hypothalamopituitary–somatotroph axis
  ACTH therapy, 1069
  assessment, **1011–1012**
    admission to care, 1858
  asthma, 540–541
  biochemical markers, 1012
  calcium and phosphate metabolism, 1053
  cancer on, 898
  chronic renal failure, 979
  constitutional delay, **372**, 1015
  and corticosteroid therapy, 546
  Cushing's syndrome, 1065
  disorders, 1015–1018
  energy expenditure, 1181
  hemiplegia, 744
  hypercortisolism, 1041
  mental retardation, 833–834
  normal, **349–364**
  overeating, 1022
  postnatal, 352–364
  psychological, 1728
  rapid, **1021**
  rates, total plasma alkaline phosphatase, 302
  regulation, 1014
  respiratory disorders, 510
  of respiratory tract, **496**
  retardation, 465, **1013–1019**, see also Failure to thrive
    asymmetric, 744, 1191
    bronchopulmonary dysplasia, 195
    Crohn's disease, 457
    diets causing, 1183
    neglect, 1873
    symmetric, 1191
    ulcerative colitis, 459
  spurts, 352, 360, **361**
  Turner's syndrome, 1032
Growth charts, **352–353**, 465, 1014–1015
Growth curve, 352
  breast-feeding, 330
  referral criteria for short stature, 368

Growth factors, see also named growth factors
  on bone and cartilage, 1567
  fetus, 1005
  prenatal growth, 351
  retinopathy of prematurity, 265
Growth hormone, 364–365, **1012–1014**
  anorexia nervosa, 1023
  deficiency, 372–374, 1015–1016
    growth pattern, 356
    with hypogammaglobulinemia, 1257
    hypothalamopituitary hypothyroidism, 1049
    short stature, 1014–1018
  delayed puberty investigation, 1034
  environmental factors, 371, 372
  exogenous, 1014
  fetus, 1003
  genes, **366–367**
  inherited deficiencies, 367
  and insulin-like growth factors, 366
  investigation, 374, 1018
  isoforms, 365, 366–367
  normal values, 1926 (Table)
  and nutrition, 1022–1023
  obesity, 1022
  pituitary gigantism, 376
  placental, 1005
  provocation tests, 374
  pseudohypoparathyroidism, 1057
  stimulation test response, 1938 (Table)
  therapy, 374, **1019–1020**
    cancer survivors, 898
    chronic renal failure, 980
    cranial radiotherapy, 1042
    and hormone replacement therapy, 990
    hypochondroplasia, 1575
    low birthweight children, 368–369
    precocious puberty, 1030
    skeletal dysplasias, 371
  Turner's syndrome, 370, 1019, 1033
Growth hormone antibodies, 1020
Growth hormone-binding protein, 1012–1014
  Laron-type dwarfism, 1017
Growth hormone insensitivity syndrome (Laron-type dwarfism), 365, 367, 374–375, 1012, 1013, **1017**
Growth hormone receptor, **365**, **1013–1014**
Growth hormone receptor-associated tyrosine kinase, 1013
Growth hormone receptor gene, **367**
Growth hormone-releasing hormone, **364**, 1012–1013
  abnormality of release, 1015–1016
  growth hormone response, insulin tolerance test, 1019
  molecule, 1038 (Table)
  test, 1938 (Table)
  therapy, 1019
Growth hormone-releasing hormone receptor, gene mutations, 366
Growth hormone-releasing peptides, 1020
  synthetic, 1013
Growth plates, 'catch-up' growth, 1014
Gruinard, anthrax spores, 1300
Grunting, expiratory, respiratory distress syndrome, 177
Gs subunit gene, McCune–Albright syndrome, 1028
GTP cyclohydrolase defect, 1106
Guanarito virus, emergence, 1279 (Table)
Guanylate cyclase activation, 1823
Guardians ad litem, 1859, 1873–1874
Guarding, 33
Guedel oropharyngeal airway, 524
Guidelines, medical practice, **1879–1880**
Guillain–Barré syndrome, 725–726
Guilt, terminal care, 929
Guinea pig kidney, heterophile antibody test, 1367
Guinea worm (dracunculosis), **1495–1496**
Gummata, 1401, 1413

Gums, 425, see also Gingivostomatitis
  hypertrophy, leukemias, 871
Gunther's disease, see Congenital erythropoietic porphyria
Guthrie test, 841
Guttate psoriasis, 1628
Gynecology, **985–995**
Gynecomastia, **1036–1037**
Gyrate atrophy of choroid, 1667
Gyrate atrophy of choroid and retina, 1111
Gyri, development, 642

H$_2$-antagonists, see Histamine H$_2$-receptor antagonists
Habenula, inhibition of puberty, 671
Habit disorders, **1745**
Habit spasms, vs rheumatic chorea, 1598
Habituation, neonate, 237 (Fig.)
Haem, see Heme
Haemophilus influenzae, **1307–1309**
  cystic fibrosis, 555, 557
  meningitis, 1289 (Table), **1292**
    chemoprophylaxis, 1292
    deafness, 816
    dexamethasone, 1291, 1309
    hemiplegia, 713
  otitis media, 561, 1307
  pneumonia, 566, 568
  septic arthritis, 1592
  upper airway obstruction, 562
Haemophilus influenzae antigen, in vaccines, 341, see also Hib immunization
Haemophilus influenzae type b
  epiglottitis, bacteriology, 1298
  United Kingdom, 1277 (Fig.)
    mortality, 1276
  young children, 1241
Haemophilus spp., neonatal meningitis, 247 (Table)
Hair
  cartilage–hair hypoplasia, 1254
  fragility, arginosuccinic aciduria, 305
  head lice, 1518
  hypothyroidism, 1050
  Pthirus pubis, 1519
  scalp, neonatal gestation age, 40 (Table)
  tinea, 1637
Hair follicle mite, **1514–1515**
'Hair-on-end' appearance, hemoglobinopathy, 863 (Fig.)
Half-lives, radionuclides, 1897
Half-PINNT, 1226
Hall Committee (Joint Working Party on Child Health Surveillance), 1853
Hallermann–Streiff syndrome, **1562**
Hallervorden–Spatz syndrome, 773, 794 (Table), 1147
Hallucinations
  bereavement, 929
  schizophrenia, 1755
Hallux, short, myositis ossificans, 1586
Hallux valgus, and metatarsus varus, **1555–1556**
Halo nevi, 1618
Haloperidol
  administration, 1967 (Table)
  extrapyramidal syndromes, 772
  for rage reactions, 841
  Tourette syndrome, 1745
Halzoun, 1512
Hamartomas
  intracranial, precocious puberty, 1028
  tuberous sclerosis, 802
Hamburgers, hemolytic uremic syndrome, 1278
Hamstring myoclonus, 673
Hand
  Edwards' syndrome, 57
  function, congenital hemiplegia, 740, 742
  malformations, 1545
    classification, 1546 (Table)

Hand (*Contd*)
skills, 382–383
development, **668–669**
history-taking, 18
Hand, foot and mouth syndrome, 1284,
1381–1382
Hand–foot syndrome, sickle cell disease,
862
Handicap, **399–400**, *see also* Cerebral
palsy; Disability; Neurological
handicap
adoption, 1860
definition, 167
head injuries, 709
incidence, **13**
on personality development, 1732
psychiatric disorder, 1733–1734
psychological effects, **1746–1748**
registers of, 1850
Handicap teams, district, 400, 1853
Handling, neonatal intensive care, 97–98,
99
Hand opening reflex, 37 (Table)
Hand–Schüller–Christian disease, 1648
central nervous system, 794 (Table)
Handwashing, 276, 1282
Hanging, 1719
H₂-antagonists, *see* Histamine H₂-receptor
antagonists
H antibodies, typhoid fever, 1326
Haploidentical bone marrow
transplantation, 1268
Haploid number, 47
Haptoglobins
deficiencies, 1175
malaria, 1451
neonatal sepsis, 277
normal values, 1926 (Table)
Harada's disease, eye, 1675
Harderoporphyria, 1142 (Table), 1143
HARDE syndrome, 753
Harlequin color change, 42, 1646
Harlequin fetus, 1621
Harm (Children Act 1989), 1875
Harpenden stadiometer, 353, 356 (Fig.)
Harrison's sulci, 30, 512
Hartnup disease, 446, 799 (Table), 1122
Harvest procedure, bone marrow
transplantation, 874
Hashimoto's thyroiditis, **1048–1049**
diabetes mellitus, 1080
growth delay, 1016
hyperthyroidism, 1051
treatment, 1050
Hatching behavior, 667
Haverhill fever, **1322**
Hawkinsinuria, 1107
Hay fever, 1684, **1697–1698**
Hay–Wells syndrome, 1626 (Table)
HBcAb IgM, 476 (Table)
HBeAb, HBeAg, HBsAb, 476 (Table)
HBsAg, *see* Hepatitis B surface antigen
HBV DNA, 476 (Table)
HBV specific DNA polymerase, 476
(Table)
HCV (coronaviruses), 1373
Head
examination, **20–29**
growth, 363
prematurity, 43
rhabdomyosarcoma, 915
Headaches, **715–719**, 900
boomslang bites, 1522
history taking, 17–18
psychogenic vomiting, 434
Head banging, 1745
Head circumference, **20**, 363–364
mental retardation, 834
neonate, 242
Head control, 382
examination, 389 (Table)
neonate, 237 (Fig.)
Head injuries, **699–709, 1809–1811**, *see
also* Non-accidental injury

ataxia, 764
birth trauma, **121–122, 699**
dysarthria, 812
management, 703
prevention
cycling, 1716
horse-riding, 1714
prognosis, **709**
strokes from, 714
tympanic membrane perforation, 1680
Head lag, neonate, 237 (Fig.)
gestation age, 40 (Table), 41 (Fig.)
Head louse, **1517–1518**
Head raising, prone neonate, 237 (Fig.)
Head rotation, neonatal gestation age, 40
(Table)
Head's reflex, 107, 196, 496
Head-Start programs, 1861
Head turning reflexes, neonatal gestation
age, 40 (Table)
Head turn to light (primitive reflex), 36
(Table)
Head wrapping, compressive, 664
Heaf gun, BCG vaccination, 1339
Heaf test, **1338**
Health, Children Act 1989, 1875
Health Authorities, 1853
Health education, school health services,
1864
Health for all children (Hall Committee),
1853
Health Sector Reform, **1890**
Health services
central, 1888
National Health Service, 1852–1853,
1853–1854
mental retardation, 838
staff, BCG vaccination, 1338
Health visitors, 1853
accident prevention, 1713
child development centers, 399
Health workers, developing countries,
1889–1890
Hearing
examination, 394–395
school health services, 1863
neonate, 241
Hearing aids, 817–818, 1683
congenital abnormalities, 1679
Hearing impairment, developmental tests,
400
Hearing loss, *see also* Deafness
congenital rubella, 286
history taking, 18
peripheral, 816–818
Heart, *see also* Valves
birth asphyxia, 129
diphtheria, 1305, 1306
diseases, **584–640**, *see also*
Cardiovascular system, disorders
growth failure, 1017
electrical axis, 589
electrical burns, 1799
enlargement, 31, 587
fetal-neonatal transition, **107**
hemolytic uremic syndrome, 977
hypertrophy, heart sounds, 32
Lyme disease, 1313
poliomyelitis, 1380
position, 598, **612–613**
thiamin deficiency, 1198
Heart block, **626**
anti-Ro, 635
neonate, 203
Heart failure
congenital heart disease, 598, **599**
congestive
angiomas, 1797–1798
doxorubicin, 896
emergency care, 1815
history taking, 584
neonate, 202–203, 205
hypoglycemia, 295
physical signs, 585

rheumatic heart disease, 1598
Heart-lung transplantation
cystic fibrosis, 556, **558–559**
obliterative bronchiolitis, 576
Heart muscle disease, *see*
Cardiomyopathy
Heart rate, *see also* Fetal heart rate
cardiac output, 1819
heart failure, 585
normal ranges, **32**
normal variations, 624
Heart sounds, 32, **586**
aortic stenosis, 607
atrial septal defect, 602
congenital heart disease, 598
congenitally corrected transposition of
great arteries, 616
Ebstein's anomaly, 619
pulmonary stenosis, 608
Heart surgery
chest scars, 586
dyskinesia, 754
hypothermia, 149
neonate, 206
postoperative care, **1822–1823**
ventilation, 1818
Heart transplantation, brain death, 709
Heartworm, *see Dirofilaria immitis*
Heat, *see* Warmth, excessive
Heat balance, preterm infant, 146
Heated cot, preterm infant temperature
control, 147–148
Heat loss, neonate, 111
Heat rash (miliaria), 1646
Heatstroke, hemorrhagic shock and
encephalopathy syndrome, 1288
Heave, right ventricular, 586
Heavy metal poisoning
basal ganglia, 768
neuropathy, 724
Heel to ear maneuver, neonatal gestation
age, 40 (Table), 41 (Fig.)
Height, *see also* Adult height
charts, **352–353**, 1014–1015
referral criteria for short stature, 368
mental retardation, 833–834
overeating, 1021
prognosis, puberty onset, 1029
social differences, 1851
velocity, 352–353
charts, 352–353
delayed puberty, 1031
hypothyroidism treatment, 1050
measurement, 355–356
precocious puberty treatment, 1030
tall stature, 375
Turner's syndrome, 1032
Height-for-age, 1186
Height-velocity, 1186
Heinz bodies, neonate, 849
Helicobacter pylori, **431–432**
emergence, 1279 (Table)
Helium equilibration, lung volume, 501
HELIX, DNA-based diagnoses register,
1099
Heller's cardiomyotomy, 429
Helmets, bicycle injury prevention, 1716
Helminthic diseases, **1481–1513**
control, 1481
developing countries disease burden,
1276 (Table)
and interventions, 1280 (Table)
eye, **1676–1677**
immigrants, 1865
laboratory methods, 1299
Helminthoma, **1494**
Helplessness, learned, 834
Hemangioblastomas, von Hippel–Lindau
syndrome, 803
Hemangiomas, 472 (Table), **1619–1620,
1797–1798**
eyelid, 1619, 1662
intestinal, 449
orbit, 1661, 1672
Sturge–Weber syndrome, 802–803

subglottic, **572**
tuberous sclerosis, 802
Hemarthroses, hemophilia A, 880, 881
Hematemesis
Apt test, 224
neonate, 111–112, 210
positional deformity, 749
Hematin, for acute porphyrias, 1143
Hematocolpos, 990 (Fig.), 991, 1796
Hematocrit
head injuries, 708
neonate, 223
polycythemia, 226, 227
normal values, 1939 (Table)
red cell volume from, 403
tetralogy of Fallot, 617
Hematocrit method, African
trypanosomiasis, 1456
Hematology
assessment, **849–850**
neonate, problems, **221–235**
normal values, 1939 (Table)
Hematoma
auricle, 1680
nasal septum, 1684
Hematophagous trophozoites, amebiasis,
1467
Hematopoiesis, *see* Hemopoiesis
Hematuria, **958–961**
hemophilia A, 880, 881
infective endocarditis, 630
neonate, **260–261**
nephroblastoma, 913
Heme
metabolism, 214
synthesis defects, **865–866, 1142–1144**
Hemianopia, congenital hemiplegia, 744
Hemiatrophy, congenital, **1545–1547**
Hemiballismus, 768
Hemichorea, 1598
Hemiconvulsion, hemiplegia, epilepsy
syndrome, 683
Hemifacial microsomia, 1563 (Table),
1564
Hemihypertrophy, 913
congenital, **1545, 1547** (Fig.)
hepatoblastoma, 924
syndrome, 290
Hemimegalencephaly, magnetic resonance
imaging, 1910 (Fig.)
Hemimelia, 1545
Hemiplegia, *see also* Cerebrovascular
disease
acute infantile, cystathione synthase
deficiency, 1108
acute-onset, management, 714–715
cerebral palsy, 739–744
epilepsy, 685
febrile convulsions, 683
gait, 34, 35, 743–744
head circumference, 20
hydrocephalus, 665–666
status epilepticus, 693
Sturge–Weber syndrome, 803
Hemiplegic dystonia, 770
Hemiplegic migraine, 716, 717
Hemispherectomy, 686
Hemisyndromes, 44, **741**
birth trauma, 122
Hemivertebrae, 651
congenital, 1557
Hemizygosity, 66
Hemochromatosis, **1147,** 1201
Hemodialfiltration, continuous
venovenous, 1824
Hemodialysis
acute renal failure, 976
chronic renal failure, 981
dietary management, 1211 (Table)
intensive care, 1824
water movement, 406
Hemofiltration
acute renal failure, **976–977,** 1824
neonate, 259

Hemoglobin, 860
  as buffer, 416, 417–418
  glycated, normal values, 1926 (Table)
  glycosylated, 1079
  levels
    vs age, 848
    neonate, 223
    normal, 1939 (Table)
    pyruvate kinase deficiency, 860
    rhesus incompatibility, 232, 233
  neonate, 214
  nitric oxide on, 1823
  transcutaneous saturation monitoring,
    see Transcutaneous oxygen
    monitoring
  types, fetus, 222
Hemoglobin F, see Fetal hemoglobin
Hemoglobin Gower, 849
Hemoglobinopathies, 226, 860–863
  double heterozygotes, 66
  genetic counseling, 114
  growth failure, 1017
  methemoglobinemia, 861, 862,
    864–865
  screening, 339 (Table)
Hemoglobin Portland, 849
Hemoglobin SC disease, 861
  immunodeficiency, 1266
Hemoglobinuria, 856
Hemolymphatic stage, African
  trypanosomiasis, 1455
Hemolysis
  African trypanosomiasis, 1455
  bee stings, 1524
  hemolytic uremic syndrome, 977
  malaria, 864, 1447–1448
  vitamin E deficiency, 1197
Hemolytic anemias, 220, 857–865
  folate deficiency, 852
  glutathione synthetase deficiency, 1115
  glycolysis defects, 1131
  purine nucleotide phosphorylase
    deficiency, 1250
  pyrimidine 5-nucleotidase deficiency,
    1142
Hemolytic crisis, glucose-6-phosphate
  dehydrogenase deficiency, 859
Hemolytic disease of the newborn,
  216–218, 225–226, 231
  rhesus incompatibility, 232
Hemolytic uremic syndrome, 974,
  977–979, 1327
  Doppler ultrasonography, 1910
  hamburgers, 1278
  rectal bleeding, 460
  ultrasonography, 1905
Hemophilia, 66–67, 72 (Table)
  analgesia, 1833
  computed tomography, 1913
  severely handicapped children affected,
    14 (Table)
Hemophilia A, 230, 880–882
Hemopoiesis, 847–849
  developmental, 221–222
  fetal, juvenile chronic myeloid
    leukemia, 872
Hemoptysis, 507
  cystic fibrosis, 554, 556
  Goodpasture's syndrome, 965
Hemorrhage, see also Blood loss; specific
    sites
  abdominal injury, 1811
  abdominal organs, birth trauma, 121
  accidental, see Placenta, abruption
  antepartum, 88–90
  cancer treatment, 895
  after cardiac surgery, 1822
  delayed, 881
  fetomaternal, 224
  gums, 425
  head injuries, 706
  hemophilia A, 880, 881
  internal, breech delivery, 224
  iron deficiency blood picture, 851

leukemia, 870
  neonatal mortality, 4 (Table)
  postpartum, labor induction, 87
  snake bites, 1522
  tonsillectomy, 1687
Hemorrhagic anemia, 224
Hemorrhagic cerebral necrosis, 281
Hemorrhagic chickenpox, 1360–1361
Hemorrhagic conjunctivitis, acute, 1385
Hemorrhagic disease, secondary, see
  Disseminated intravascular
  coagulation
Hemorrhagic disease of the newborn, 108,
  229–230, 1197
Hemorrhagic fevers, 1389–1390
  with renal syndrome, 1390
Hemorrhagic measles, 1354
Hemorrhagic pulmonary edema,
  hypothermia, 150
Hemorrhagic shock and encephalopathy
  syndrome, 1288
Hemosiderinuria, 856
Hemosiderosis, 1146–1147, see also
  Siderosis
  pulmonary, 578
Hemostasis, see also Coagulation factors
  disorders, 875–882
  neonate, 227–228
Hemotoxic snake venoms, 1521, 1522
Hemozoin, 1448
Hemsath fracture, 707
Henderson–Hasselbalch equation, 416,
  417, 504
Henoch–Schönlein purpura, 875, 961,
  1609–1610, 1640
  and mesangial IgA nephropathy, 963
  nephritis, 964, 1609–1610
  rash, 1285, 1609–1610
  rectal bleeding, 460
Heparan N-sulfatase deficiency, 1160
Heparan sulfate, 1160
Heparin
  administration, 1967 (Table)
  arterial blood sampling, 1835
  bronchoalveolar lavage, alveolar
    proteinosis, 578
  and disseminated intravascular
    coagulation, 231
  for hemofiltration, 1824
  for hemorrhagic skin purpura, 876
  major vessel thrombosis, 231
  parenteral nutrition, 158
  resistance, 882
  therapy
    disseminated intravascular
      coagulation, 882
    dosages, 851 (Table)
Hepatic cholesterol ester storage disease,
  1155
Hepatic fibrosis
  autosomal recessive polycystic kidney
    disease, 254
  congenital, 483–484
Hepatic gluconeogenic enzyme
  deficiencies, 296–297
Hepatic vein thrombosis, 28 (Fig.)
Hepatitis, see also Neonatal hepatitis
  FUO investigations, 1283 (Table)
  gonococcal, 1426
  infancy, 473–474
    cystic fibrosis, 484
  Kawasaki disease, 1479
  nephroblastoma radiotherapy, 914
  screening, antenatal care, 80
  toxoplasmosis, 1465
  vs tyrosinemia, 1106
Hepatitis A virus infection, 476, 1386
Hepatitis B surface antigen, 476 (Table),
  1386
  polyarteritis with, 1610
Hepatitis B virus
  hepatocellular carcinoma, 924
  infection, 476–477, 1386–1387
    congenital, 286 (Table), 288

polyarteritis, 1610
  vaccination, 1967 (Table)
    neonate, 1957 (Table)
  vertical transmission, 1386, 1400
Hepatitis C virus
  hepatocellular carcinoma, 478, 924
  IgA deficiency, 1264
  from immunoglobulin therapy, 1268
  infection, 477–478, 1387
    congenital, 288
    emergence, 1279 (Table)
Hepatitis D, 477, 1387
Hepatitis E virus, 478, 1387
Hepatitis F virus, 1388
Hepatitis immunoglobulin, 288
Hepatitis vaccine, 288
Hepatobiliary recirculation, 470
Hepatoblastoma, 924, 925
  ectopic gonatropin secretion, 1029
  malformation syndromes, 290
  neonate, 292 (Table)
    incidence, 290 (Table)
Hepatocellular carcinoma, 924, 924–925
  HBV infection, 477
  hepatitis C virus, 478, 924
Hepatocyte plates, 470–471
Hepatocytes, Dubin–Johnson syndrome,
  1145
Hepatoerythropoietic porphyria, 1142
  (Table), 1144
Hepatolenticular degeneration, see
  Wilson's disease
Hepatomegaly, 471
  cystic fibrosis, 556
  glucose-6-phosphatase deficiency, 1136
  heart failure, 585, 599
  inborn errors of metabolism, 305
  mental retardation, 835 (Table)
  toxocariasis, 1485
  typhoid fever, 1325
Hepatorenal failure, 483
Hepatosplenomegaly, neonate, organisms,
  284 (Table)
Hepatotoxicity
  aspirin, 1603
  cytotoxic drugs, 894 (Table), 897
  isoniazid, 1347
  valproate, 684
Herald patch, pityriasis rosea, 1634
Herd immunity, 341
Hereditary amyloidosis, 1177
Hereditary angioedema, 1262–1263, see
  also C1-esterase inhibitor
  deficiency
Hereditary cataracts, 1667–1668
Hereditary coproporphyria, 1142 (Table),
  1143
Hereditary elliptocytosis, 226, 858
Hereditary fructose intolerance,
  1134–1135
Hereditary hemolytic anemias, 857–864
Hereditary hemorrhagic telangiectasia,
  875
Hereditary hypophosphatemia, 260, 948
Hereditary lactic acidosis, 1124–1125
Hereditary motor and sensory
  neuropathies, 722–723
  Roussy–Levy type, 723, 764
Hereditary nephritis, see Alport's
  syndrome
Hereditary sensory neuropathies, 723–724
Hereditary spherocytosis, 226, 857–858
Hereditary stomatocytosis, 858
Hereditary thyroglobulin deficiency, 1044
Hereditary unresponsiveness to ACTH,
  1068
Heredodegenerative ataxias, 764
Heredopathia atactica polyneuritiformis,
  see Refsum's disease
Hering–Breuer reflexes, 196, 496
Hermansky–Pudlak syndrome, 879, 1107,
  1108, 1629 (Table)
Hermaphroditism, true, 986–987, 1010,
  see also Pseudohermaphroditism

Hernias, 1788–1790, see also
  Diaphragmatic hernia
  intestinal obstruction, 1776
  strangulated, 33, 1815
Herniations, brain, 698, 708, 812
Heroin, abuse, 1762–1763
Herpangina, 560, 1381
  vs acute herpetic gingivostomatitis,
    1364–1365
  vs hand, foot and mouth disease, 1382
  vs tonsillitis, 1686
Herpes genitalis, primary, 1438–1439
Herpes simplex virus, 1363, 1435–1436
  distribution of types, 1437
  infection, 1363–1365, 1435–1442,
    1631–1632
    AIDS, 1395
    congenital, 248, 286 (Table), 287,
      1284
    diagnosis, 1439–1440
    geniculate ganglion, 725, 1363
    immunocompromised patient, 535
    keratitis, 1664–1665
    meningitis, 713
    treatment, 1440–1441
    type 1, rash, 1284
  neonate, 1400
  ophthalmia neonatorum, 263
  virology, 1400
Herpes stomatitis, 424–425
Herpesviruses, 1360–1365, see also
  Human herpesviruses
Herpes zoster, 1284, 1362–1363,
  1632–1633
  chest pain, 509
  eye, 1632, 1676
Herpetiform epidermolysis bullosa, 1622
  (Table)
Heterochromia, 1650–1651
Heterogeneity, genetic disorders, 77
Heterophile antibody test, 1367
Heterophoria (latent squint), 1652,
  1659–1660
Heterophyes heterophyes, 1513
Heteroplasmy, mitochondrial DNA, 1126
Heterotopias, 685
  cerebral, 642, 650
  neurofibromatosis, 800
Heterozygosity, 64, 1101
Hetol, liver flukes, 1513
Heubner's artery, 249
Hexachlorobenzene, toxic porphyria, 1144
Hexachlorophene, poisoning, 1711
Hexanoylglycine, 1129
Hexarelin, 1012
Hexosaminidase A deficiency, 721
Hexosaminidases, 1163, 1164
  mucolipidoses, 1171
Hexose monophosphate shunt, 859 (Fig.)
HHH syndrome, 1111
Hib immunization, United Kingdom, 344
HIDA cholescintigraphy, technetium-99m,
  221
Hidrotic ectodermal dysplasia, 1625
  (Table)
High-affinity human growth hormone-
  binding protein (hGHBP), 365
High-density lipoprotein, 1148 (Table),
  1149
  secondary disorders, 1154 (Table)
High-dose chemotherapy, 875, 893
  astrocytomas, 903
  neuroblastoma, 913
High-dose phenobarbitone, birth asphyxia,
  130
High-frequency ventilation, 164, 188,
  1818–1819
  pneumothorax prevention, 188
  pulmonary interstitial emphysema, 189
High-pitched crying, 236
High-risk delivery, 116–120
High-risk pregnancy, fetus and infant,
  113–116
Hindgut, 206

Hip joints
 congenital abnormalities, 1549–1553
 imaging, 1916–1917, 1918 (Fig.), *see also* Perthes disease
 lysosomal storage disorders, 1158
 tuberculosis, **1593**
Hippocampus
 growth hormone regulation, 1012
 mesial temporal sclerosis, 685
Hiroshima atomic bomb, neoplasms, 890
Hirschsprung's disease, 33, 210, 462, **1777–1778**, *see also* Short segment Hirschsprung's disease
 barium enema, 1903
 diarrhea, 1293
 enterocolitis, 1295, 1777, 1778
 exclusion, 213
 vs gastroenteritis, 1295
 recurrence risks, 74
Hirsutism, 1000
 polycystic ovarian disease, 993
His, bundle of, conduction defects, **626**
Hiskey Nebraska test, 400
Histamine H_2-receptor antagonists
 gastroesophageal reflux, 429
 peptic ulcer, 432
 short bowel syndrome, 1212
Histidine
 metabolism disorders, **1114–1115**
 urine, 1103
Histidinemia, 1114
Histidinuria, 1115, 1122
Histiocytes, development, 925
Histiocytic lymphoma, 927–928
Histiocytoses, **925–927**, 1262
 fibrosing alveolitis, 578
 incidence, 886 (Table)
Histiocytosis X, *see* Langerhans' cell histiocytosis
Histoplasmin test, 1477
Histoplasmosis, 570, 1471 (Table), **1476–1477**
Historical aspects
 cystic fibrosis, 550
 diabetes mellitus, 1072–1073
 preterm neonate, 96–97
History of present illness, **17–18**
History-taking, **16–18**
 allergy, **1691–1693**
 apparent life-threatening events, 529
 cow's milk protein intolerance, 1699
 development, 387
 endocrinology, 998
 heart disease, 584
 immunodeficiency, 1243–1244
 mental retardation, 833
 neonate, 109
 physical abuse, 1867
 psychiatric disorder, **1734–1735**
 respiratory disorders, **506**
 skin disorders, 1616–1617
Hitchhiker thumb, diastrophic dwarfism, 76
HIV, 1393
 risk-taking behavior, 1763
HIV antigen testing, 1393
HIV infection, **1392–1398**, *see also* AIDS; Lymphoid interstitial pneumonitis
 antibody testing, 1399
 BCG vaccination, 1339
 and breast-feeding, 288, 329
 candidiasis, 1433, 1434
 congenital infection, 288
 dementia, 795 (Table)
 donated milk, prevention, 152
 emergence, 1278, 1279 (Table)
 environmental mycobacteria, 1350
 FUO investigations, 1283 (Table)
 hemophilia A, 881
 immunosuppression, 1264–1265
 neonate, 248, 286 (Table)
 neoplasms, 891
 papulonodular demodicidosis, 1515

poliomyelitis vaccination, 1381
 prevention, 1398
 respiratory tract infections, 533
 syphilis, 1401
  treatment, 1410
 toxoplasmosis, 1397, 1465
 tuberculosis, **1346–1347**
 visceral leishmaniasis, 1462
HLA antigens, 1235–1236
 autoimmune adrenal disease, 1069
 celiac disease, 440
 defects, 1250
 diabetes mellitus, 1073
 Graves' disease, 1051
 21-hydroxylase deficiency, 1062
 juvenile chronic arthritis, 1602
 Lyme disease, 1313
 myasthenia gravis, 727
 psoriatic arthritis, 1611
HMG-CoA lyase deficiency, 297
HMG-CoA reductase inhibitors, 1152
Hoarseness, *see* Dysphonia
Hodgkin's disease, **909–911**
 ataxia, 766
 incidence, 886 (Table)
 second primary, 898
 survival rates, 887 (Table), 898 (Table)
 therapy on gonadal function, 899
Holding dead infant, 173
Holidays, allergic symptoms, 1691–1692
Holland, *vs* United States, neurodevelopmental outcome of prematurity, 166
Holly, poisoning, 1709
Holocarboxylase synthetase deficiency, 1148
Holophrastic speech, 805
Holoprosencephaly, 57–58, **649**
Holt–Oram syndrome, heart, 596
Home and the School, The (National Survey of Health and Development), 1851
Home care, working mothers, 1860
Home management
 diabetes mellitus, 1075, **1076–1080**
 emergencies, **1802–1803**
 enteral feeding, 1219
 parenteral nutrition, 470, **1226**
Home monitoring, arrhythmias, 624
Home nebulizers, 547
Homeobox genes, growth hormone expression, **367**
Home uterine monitoring, tocography, 116
Homocarnosine, 1114
Homocitrulline, 1111
Homocysteine, 1108
Homocysteine methyltransferase deficiency, 852
Homocystine, 1108
 cobalamin disorders, 1148
Homocystinuria, 376, 790 (Table), 1100, 1108–1109
 5'-dexoyadenosyl-cobalamin defects, 1117
 dietary management, **1205 (Table)**
 eye, 1673
 vs Marfan's syndrome, 77
 with methylmalonic aciduria, 853, 1109
 stroke, 711
Homogentisic acid, alkaptonuria, 1107
Homoplasmy, mitochondrial DNA, 1126
Homosexuality, congenital adrenal hyperplasia, 1065
Homovanillic acid
 familial dysautonomia, 1069
 neuroblastoma, 911
 normal values
  cerebrospinal fluid, 1934 (Table)
  urine, 1931 (Table)
Homozygosity, 64
Homozygous achondroplasia, 1571
Honey, botulism, 1302
'Honeymoon' period, diabetes mellitus, 1077

Hong Kong, demography, 2 (Table)
Honking (psychogenic cough), 507
Hookworm, **1488–1491**
 blood loss rate, 1201
Hopi Indians, oculocutaneous albinism, 47
Hordeolum, 1662, 1663 (Fig.)
Horizontal beam radiography, chest, 514
Horizontal vector loop, electrocardiography, 588 (Fig.)
Hormone replacement therapy, primary amenorrhea, 990
Hormones
 activity *vs* concentration, 1002
 mechanisms, **996–998**
Horner's syndrome, 24 (Fig.), 34, 1662
 examination, 1650
Horse accidents, 1714
Horse erythrocytes, agglutinins, infectious mononucleosis, 1367
Horse serum
 diphtheria, 1306
 tetanus, 1334
Horseshoe kidney, 254
Hospital activity analysis, 1850
Hospital admission, *see also* Residential treatment, adolescent psychiatry
 acute severe asthma, **548–549**
 bronchiolitis, 1804
 child abuse, 1873
 head injuries, criteria, 706
 local authority notification, 1875
 rates, 9
  accidents, 1712
  immigrants, 1866
  reactions, 1747
Hospital costs, neonatal care, 105–106
Hospital discharge data, infectious diseases, 1280 (Table)
Hospitals
 delivery in, 84
 infection control, **1281–1282**
 nutrition support, 1215–1216
Hospital services
 Court Committee, 1853
 usage rates, 9, 11–12 (Table), 12 (Fig.)
Host defense boosting, neonatal sepsis, 279, 280 (Table)
Hot feed scalds, 1868
Hotplate burns, 1868
House dust (allergy), 1684–1685, **1690–1691**
House dust mites, 493, **1690**
 asthma patterns, 541
 atopic eczema, 1696
 exposure reduction, 545, 1694, **1695**
Household products, poisoning, 1705, **1709, 1710–1711**
Housing, respiratory disorders, 489, 492
5-HT_3 antagonists, 896
H-type tracheoesophageal fistula, 573, 1773
Human African trypanosomiasis, *see* African trypanosomiasis
Human alphaherpesvirus, *see* Herpes simplex virus
Human β glucosidase, Gaucher disease, 1102
Human chorionic gonadotropin, *see also* Beta-human chorionic gonadotropin
 antenatal care, 80
 Down syndrome, 56
 fetus, 1004, 1005
 placental, 1024
 puberty induction, 1035
 testes, development, 1004
Human coronaviruses, 1373
Human Genome Organization, 1099
Human growth hormone, *see* Growth hormone
Human growth hormone/placental lactogen gene cluster, 366–367
Human growth hormone receptor gene, **367**

Human herpesviruses, *see also* Herpes simplex virus; Varicella-zoster virus
 emergence, 1279 (Table)
 roseola infantum, 1285, 1359
Human immunoglobulin, *see also* Gammaglobulin; Immunoglobulin
 measles prevention, cancer treatment, 895
Human insulins, 1076, 1079
Human milk, *see* Breast milk
Human pancreatic polypeptide, fetus, 1004
Human papilloma viruses, 1400
 cervical intraepithelial neoplasia, 994
 infection, **1442–1445**
Human placental lactogen (HPL), 327, 1005
Human rabies immunoglobulin, 1377–1378
Human rights, *see* United Nations, Declaration of the Rights of the Child
Human T-cell leukemia virus, 868, 891
Human T-cell lymphotropic viruses, 906
 emergence, 1279 (Table)
Human tetanus immune globulin, 285, 1334
Humerus
 birth trauma, 121 (Table)
 fracture, shaking injury, 701
 osteosarcoma distribution, 917
Humidity
 incubators, 148
 ventilation, 163
Humoral immunity, 275
 nonspecific, **1232–1234**
 tests, 1245
Hunter's syndrome, 783–784 (Table), 1102, 1157 (Table), 1158, **1159–1160**
Huntington's chorea, 773, 793 (Table)
 vs rheumatic chorea, 1598
Hunt's cerebellar degeneration, 752
Hurler/Scheie syndrome (MPS I-H/S), 783 (Table), 1157 (Table), 1159
Hurler's syndrome, 23 (Fig.), 1102, 1157, **1158–1159**
 spine, 1915
Hutchinson's incisors, 1414
Huttenlocher's disease (Alper's disease), 736, 797 (Table)
Hyaline membrane disease, *see* Respiratory distress syndrome
Hyaloid vascular complex, 262–263
Hyaluronidase, administration, 1968 (Table)
Hycanthone, schistosomiasis, 1510–1511
Hydatid disease, **1504–1506**
 liver, **478**, 1505
Hydatid of Morgagni, torsion, 1791
Hydralazine
 acute renal failure, 974
 administration, 1968 (Table)
 on fetus and neonate, 91 (Table)
 heart failure, 599
 hypertension, 637 (Table), 638
  renal, 973 (Table)
 pyridoxine deficiency, 1198
Hydramnios
 esophageal atresia, 1770
 laryngeal clefts, 572
Hydranencephaly, 648–649
Hydration, for organic acidurias, 1119
Hydroa vacciniforme, 1645
Hydrocele, 34, **1788–1790**
Hydrocephalus, 21 (Fig.), **657–666**
 achondroplasia, 371, 1574
 assessment, 660–661
 ataxia, 753
 ataxic diplegia, 745
 causes, 660 (Table)
 clinical features, 659–660
 Dandy–Walker syndrome, 645

Hydrocephalus, 21 (Fig.), **657–666** (Contd)
  vs hydranencephaly, 649
  in utero shunting, 115
  magnetic resonance imaging, 1909
  from meningitis, 1289, 1291–1292
  neonatal meningitis, 282
  vs neonatal meningitis, 247
  neonate, **252**
  posthemorrhagic, see Posthemorrhagic
    hydrocephalus
  prenatal diagnosis, 252–253
  prognosis, 666
  progressive, see Active hydrocephalus
  severely handicapped children affected,
    14 (Table)
  shunted, 167, see also Shunting,
    hydrocephalus
  treatment, **662–666**
  tuberculosis, meningitis, 1345
  without head enlargement, 834
Hydrochloric acid
  central venous line occlusion, 1225
  defense role, 438
  production, 430
Hydrochlorothiazide, administration, 1968
  (Table)
Hydrocolpos, 987, 1795
Hydrocortisone, 1628
  Addison's disease, 1068
  administration, 1968 (Table)
    neonate, 1957 (Table)
  for congenital adrenal hyperplasia, 1064
  fulminating colitis, 459
  hypersensitivity reactions, 1306
  for infantile spasms, 689
  for transient hyperinsulinemia, 295
  for vitamin D intoxication, 1055
Hydroflumethiazide, administration, 1968
  (Table)
Hydrogen breath tests, 448
Hydrogen ion activity, 416
Hydrogen ions
  concentrations, 416–417
  gastric juice, 411 (Table)
  normal values, 1926 (Table)
  output, 417
Hydromyelia, 657
Hydronephrosis, 1795
  congenital, 936
  hematuria, 959
  neonate, 255
  neurogenic bladder, 656
Hydrophiid venoms, 1521
Hydrops, nonimmune fetal, lysosomal
  storage disorders, 1156
Hydrops fetalis, 232, **234–235**
  cystic adenomatoid malformation, 192
  parvovirus B19, 1359
Hydrostatic osmotic pressure, 407
Hydrostatic reduction, intussusception,
  1786
Hydrotherapy, juvenile chronic arthritis,
  1604
Hydroxocobalamin, dosage, 854, 1968
  (Table)
Hydroxychloroquine, juvenile chronic
  arthritis, 1604
1α-Hydroxycholecalciferol, 304
  for chronic renal failure, 980
25-Hydroxycholecalciferol
  liver disease, 1209
  neonate, 301
17-Hydroxycorticosteroids, normal values,
  urine, 1932 (Table)
D-2-,L-2-Hydroxyglutaric aciduria, 1118
5-Hydroxyindole acetic acid
  amniotic fluid, 1937 (Table)
  normal values
    cerebrospinal fluid, 1934 (Table)
    urine, 1931 (Table)
3-Hydroxyisobutyryl-CoA deacylase
  deficiency, 1117–1118
Hydroxykynureninuria, 1114
11β-Hydroxylase deficiency, 1008, 1062

(Table), **1064**
  virilization, 1008
17α-Hydroxylase deficiency, 1009, **1064**
18-Hydroxylase deficiency, 1064
21-Hydroxylase deficiency, 986, 1011,
  1027, **1062–1064**
  heterozygote detection, 1062
  screening, 1007
Hydroxylation, vitamin D, 1054
Hydroxylysinemia, 1113
4-Hydroxy-3-methoxymandelate, normal
  values, urine, 1933 (Table)
3-Hydroxy-3-methylglutaryl-CoA lyase
  deficiency, 297, 1130
β-Hydroxymethyl glutaryl-CoA synthase
  deficiency, 1130
4-Hydroxyphenylpyruvate dioxygenase
  reaction, 1107
17-Hydroxyprogesterone
  21-hydroxylase deficiency screening,
    1007
  normal values, 1926 (Table)
17α-Hydroxyprogesterone (17OHP),
  congenital adrenal hyperplasia,
  986, 1064
Hydroxyproline
  metabolism disorders, 1113, **1114**
  urine, 1567
    marasmus, 1192
3β-Hydroxysteroid dehydrogenase
  deficiency, 1008, 1009, 1028, 1062
  (Table), **1064**
  fetus, 1005
11β-Hydroxysteroid dehydrogenase
  deficiency, 946, 1066–1067
17β-Hydroxysteroid dehydrogenase
  deficiency, 1009
3β-Hydroxy-C27-steroid
  dehydrogenase/isomerase
  deficiency, 1145
3-Hydroxysteroid-Δ5-oxidoreductase
  deficiency, 1145
5-Hydroxytryptamine uptake inhibitors,
  obsessive–compulsive disorders,
  1756
5-Hydroxytryptophan
  dihydropteridine reductase deficiency,
    1106
  Lesch–Nyhan syndrome, 768
Hydroxyurea, sickle cell disease, 863
25-Hydroxy vitamin D, 1054, 1058, 1196
Hydroxyzine, dosage, 1968 (Table)
Hygiene inspections, school nurses, 1864
Hymen
  imperforate, 1796
  sexual abuse, 1869
Hymenolepis spp., **1502**
Hymenoptera, stings, **1524**
Hyoscine
  administration, 1968 (Table)
  poisoning, 1710
Hyperactivity, 819, **1744,** see also
  Hyperkinetic disorder
  ex-preterm infants, 171
  severely handicapped children affected,
    14 (Table)
Hyperadrenocorticism, **1065–1067**
Hyperalaninemia, 1115
Hyperaldosteronism, **1065–1067**
  chloridorrhea, 446
  screening, 637
Hyperalertness
  neonate, 236
  postasphyxial encephalopathy, 127
Hyperammonemia, 307
  birth asphyxia, 129
  disorders with, **1110–1112**
  inborn errors of metabolism, 305–306
  lysinuric protein intolerance, 446, 1121
  neonate, 248
  secondary causes, 1111
  SGA baby, 138
Hyperbilirubinemia, 248–249, see also
  Jaundice

inborn errors of metabolism, 306,
  1144–1145
  neonatal unconjugated, teeth, 425
  urinary tract infections, 261
Hypercalcemia, 1056, see also Idiopathic
  hypercalcemia
  chemotherapy, 897
  differential diagnosis, 1058
  hyperlipoproteinemia, 1154 (Table)
  hypophosphatasia, 1176
  infantile (Lightwood's syndrome), 831
    (Table)
  multiple endocrine neoplasia
    syndromes, 1056
  neonate, 300
  vitamin D toxicity, 1197
Hypercalciuria, 943, 1058
  absorptive, 1056
  idiopathic, 959
Hypercapnia, 161, **503–504**
  inadvertent PEEP, 163
  permissive, 1818, 1825
  respiratory response, 196
Hypercholesterolemia
  dietary management, 1206 (Table)
  hypothyroidism, 1153
  secondary, 1154 (Table)
Hypercoagulable states, stroke, 713
Hypercyanotic attacks, tetralogy of Fallot,
  617
Hyperendemic trachoma, 1430
Hyperextension, respiratory disorders, 511
Hyperflexion injury, seat belt injuries,
  1812
Hypergammaglobulinemia, HIV infection,
  1393, 1396
Hyperglycemia, neonate, 297–298
Hyperglycinemia, non-ketotic, 1103, **1112**
HyperIgE syndromes, 1242 (Table), 1245,
  1261
HyperIgM syndromes, 1242 (Table), 1255
Hyperimmune immunoglobulin
  in AIDS, 1396
  immunodeficiency, 1267
  viral hepatitis B, 477
Hyperinfection syndrome,
  strongyloidiasis, 1492
Hyperinflation, 499, 512
  asthma, 539
  cystic fibrosis, 554
  diaphragm, 505
Hyperinsulinemia, transient, 295–296
Hyperinsulinism, 1083, 1084
  neonate, 295–296
  obesity, 1022
Hyperkalemia, 145, 412
  acute renal failure, 975
    neonate, 258–259
  renal tubular, 947
  treatment, **415**
Hyperkeratosis, genital warts, 1442
Hyperketosis, facile, 1130
Hyperkinetic bulbar palsies, 813
Hyperkinetic disorder, 819, 1733, **1744**
  mental retardation, 841
Hyperleucine-isoleucinemia, 1116
Hyperlipemia
  diabetic ketoacidosis, 1074
  idiopathic, 1674
  plasma sodium, 404
Hyperlipoproteinemias, 1150 (Table),
  1151–1152
  secondary, 1153–1154
Hyperlucency, chest X-rays, 576
Hyperlymphoproliferative syndrome,
  neoplasms, 890
Hyperlysinemia, 1113
Hypermetabolic myopathy, 735 (Table)
Hypermetropia, 1657
  pseudopapilledema, 1672
Hypermobility syndrome, **1612**
Hypernatremia, 453, 1039
  cerebrospinal fluid, 1934 (Table)
  diabetic ketoacidosis, 1075

  gastroenteritis, 1294
  intracranial hemorrhage, 414, 713
  neonates, 144
  treatment, **414–415**
Hypernephroma
  metastases, cerebellum, 753
  von Hippel–Lindau syndrome, 803
Hyperornithinemia, 1111
Hyperoxaluria, calculi, 1112, 1113
Hyperoxia, see also Nitrogen washout,
  test
  retinopathy, 161, **265**
Hyperoxic test, 598
Hyperparathyroidism
  maternal, 89 (Table), 299, 300
  primary, **1056–1057**
  secondary, 980
Hyperphagic dysmorphic syndromes,
  obesity, 1190
Hyperphenylalaninemia, 1103–1106
Hyperphoria, 1660
Hyperphosphatasia, **1176–1177**
  congenital, 1582 (Table)
Hyperphosphatemia
  chemotherapy, 897
  chronic renal failure, 980
  hemolysis, 864
  neonate, 299
Hyperpipecolic acidemia, 308, 1173
Hyperplastic osteoperiostitis, congenital
  syphilis, 1413, 1414
Hyperprolactinemia, 1044
Hyperprostaglandin E syndrome, see
  Bartter's syndrome
Hyperpyrexia, 150, **1830**
  hereditary sensory neuropathy type 2,
    724
  malaria, 1453
  muscle relaxants, 733
Hyperreactive malarial splenomegaly,
  1451
Hypersensitivity
  African trypanosomiasis, 1455
  chemotherapy (tuberculosis), 1347
  diphtheria antitoxin, 1306
Hypersensitivity reactions, see also
  Allergic disorders
  lips, 424
  skin, **1639–1642**
  transient food intolerance, 441
Hypersplenism, 864, 877, 882
  cystic fibrosis, 556
  liver disease, 865
Hypertelorism (telecanthus), 22, 24 (Fig.),
  76 (Table), 647, 1562, 1661
Hypertension, **636–638**
  acute glomerulonephritis, 962
  acute renal failure, 975
  adrenal steroidogenesis, 1061
  birthweight, 369
  chronic renal failure, 979
  congenital adrenal hyperplasia, 1006,
    1064, 1069
  Cushing's syndrome, 1065, 1070
  diazoxide, 637 (Table), 1965 (Table)
  endocrine, **1069–1071**
  fetal adrenal gland, 1003
  after hemolytic uremic syndrome, 978
  11β-hydroxylase deficiency, 1008, 1064
  hypokalemic alkalosis, 946
  after intrauterine growth retardation,
    1005
  neonate, 203–204, 258
    acute renal failure, 259
    seizures, 245 (Table)
  nephroblastoma, 913
  neuroblastoma, 911
  pregnancy, **90,** 114
    risk assessment, 81
  recombinant erythropoietin therapy, 980
  renal, 636, 637, **972–973,** 1069
  retinopathy, **1675**
  Turner's syndrome, 61
  and vesicoureteric reflux, 949

Hypertensive crisis, drugs for, 973 (Table)
Hyperthermia, *see* Hyperpyrexia
Hyperthreoninemia, 1118
Hyperthyroidism, **1050–1052**
  eyelid retraction, 1674
  maternal, 89 (Table), 1005
  neonate, 998, 1005, 1050
  tall stature, 377
Hypertonicity, 35, 44
  neonate, 236
Hypertonic saline, sputum stimulation, 534
Hypertrophic cardiomyopathy, 72 (Table), **634**
  diabetes mellitus, neonate, 205
Hypertrophic peripheral neuropathy, 723
Hypertrophic pulmonary osteoarthropathy, cystic fibrosis, 1611
Hypertrophic pyloric stenosis, *see* Pyloric stenosis
Hyperuricemia, **1140–1141**
  acute renal failure, 975
  glucose-6-phosphatase deficiency, 1136, 1137
  muscle phosphorylase deficiency, 1139
  organic acidurias, 1119
Hypervalinemia, 1116
Hyperventilation
  diabetic ketoacidosis, 1075
  electroencephalography, 677
  intracranial pressure, 1825
  Joubert's syndrome, 646
  neuropathology from, 131
  psychogenic, 509
  therapeutic, 165, 698, **699,** 708
Hyperviscosity, 713, 715
Hyperviscosity syndrome, partial plasma exchange transfusion, 1839
Hyphae, candidiasis, 1433
Hyphema, birth trauma, 264
Hypnogogic myoclonus, 673
Hypnotics, 1748 (Table)
Hypnozoites, *Plasmodium* spp., 1446
Hypoalbuminemia
  acute renal failure, 974
  Crohn's disease, 457
  nephrotic syndrome, 969
Hypoaldosteronism, congenital, 260
Hypoallergenic feeds, 455
Hypobetalipoproteinemia, 1153
Hypocalcemia, 1058
  acute-onset stroke, 715
  acute renal failure, 975
  candidiasis, 1470
  differential diagnosis, 1056–1058
  encephalopathy, 682
  gastroenteritis, 1294, 1297
  maternal factors, 1005
  neonate, 28 (Fig.), **298–300**
    late, **299–300,** 1200
    seizures, 245, 247
  SGA baby, 137
Hypocapnia, 161
Hypochloremic alkalosis, 1785
Hypochondrogenesis, 1570–1571
  inheritance, 1566 (Table)
Hypochondroplasia, 370, 371, 1573 (Fig.), **1575**
  inheritance, 1566 (Table)
Hypoderma spp., larval disease, 1484 (Table)
Hypofibrinogenemia, 230
Hypogammaglobulinemia, **1255–1259**
  HIV infection, 1393
Hypoglossal nerve, 811
  examination, 34
Hypoglycemia, **1082–1084**
  acute-onset stroke, 715
  Addison's disease, 1067
  alcohol, 1080, 1710
  breast-feeding, 328
  cholera, 1304
  diabetes mellitus, **1080–1081,** 1210
  diazoxide, 1965 (Table)

encephalopathy, 682
falciparum malaria, 1450, 1451, 1452
glucose-6-phosphatase deficiency, 1136
hypoketotic, 1131
inborn errors of metabolism, 296–297, 306, **1130–1131**
induction, 1075
with lactic acidosis, 1135
large for gestational age infant, 138
leucine-induced, 1117
neonate, 135–136, 139, 249, **290–298, 1006,** 1081, 1083
  seizures, 245 (Table), 247
pentamidine, 1456
recurrent, 998
rewarming, 150
SGA baby, **137**
Hypoglycin, 1117
Hypogonadism
  galactose-1-phosphate uridyltransferase deficiency, 1133
  hypogonadotropic, 372, 1031, 1034
Hypohidrotic ectodermal dysplasia, 1625 (Table)
Hypokalemia, **145,** 411, 412
  cholera, 1304
  Fanconi's syndrome, 944, **944**
  myopathy, 736–737
  treatment, **415**
Hypokalemic alkalosis, **946–947**
Hypoketotic hypoglycemia, 1131
Hypokinetic bulbar palsies, 813
Hypolipoproteinemias, 1150 (Table)
  secondary, 1154 (Table)
Hypomagnesemia, 1201
  acute renal failure, 975
  diabetes mellitus, 299
  encephalopathy, 682
  hypoparathyroidism, 1057, 1058
  neonate, 300–301
    seizures, 245
  primary, 447
Hypomelanosis of Ito, 799 (Table), 804
Hyponatremia
  acute renal failure, 975
  Addison's disease, 1068
  asthma treatment, 549
  causes, 412
  diabetic ketoacidosis, 1075
  diarrhea, 411
  kwashiorkor, 1193
  neonates, 143–144
Hypoparathyroidism, **1056**
  candidiasis, 1057, 1470
    mucocutaneous, 1251
  cataract, 1674
  neonate, 300
  vs pseudohypoparathyroidism, 1058
Hypophoria, 1660
Hypophosphatasia, **1176**
  primary dentition, 425
Hypophosphatemia, 260, **948,** 1058
  familial, 260, **948**
  Fanconi's syndrome, 944, 1058
Hypophosphatemic rickets, 1123
Hypopigmentation, 1107
Hypopituitarism
  anemia, 865
  congenital, 297, 998
Hypoplastic left heart syndrome, 203 (Table), **619–620**
  pulses, 598, 619
Hypoproteinemia
  celiac disease, 441
  epidermolysis bullosa, 1622
  erythroblastosis fetalis, 235
Hypoprothrombinemia, 230
Hypopyon, 1665
Hyposensitization, **1702–1703**
  immunotherapy, 545
  and seasonal asthma, 549
Hypospadias, 256, **1793–1794**
Hyposplenia, 1266
  Streptococcus pneumoniae, 1319, 1320

Hyposthenuria, sickle cell disease, 862–863
Hypostop gel, 1080
Hypotelorism, 58, 76 (Table), 1562
Hypotension
  anaphylaxis, 1702
  inborn errors of metabolism, 307
  neonate, management, 205
  oxygenation, 160
  rewarming, 149
  status epilepticus, 693
Hypothalamic syndrome, leukemia, 871
Hypothalamopituitary congenital hypothyroidism, 1046
Hypothalamopituitary-dependent hypothyroidism, 1049
Hypothalamopituitary–somatotroph axis, **362–366**
Hypothalamopituitary unit, **1037–1043**
Hypothalamus, 997, 1037
  astrocytomas, 903
  delayed puberty, 1031
  glioma, 1043
  hypothyroidism, 1006–1007
  obesity, 1022, 1190
  primary amenorrhea, 990
  puberty, 670–671
  secondary amenorrhea, 993
  thyroid function tests, 1045
  tumors, diabetes insipidus, 1040 (Table)
Hypothermia, 20
  for birth asphyxia, 131, 149
  from brainstem failure, 703
  drowning, 571, 1717
  endocrine disorders, 1007
  gastroschisis, 1780
  neonate, **149–150,** 295
  preterm infant, 147
  SGA baby, 137
Hypothyroidism, 242, **1046–1050**
  anemia, 865
  ataxia, 752
  calcitonin, 1057
  growth delay, 1016
  on growth hormone expression, 367, **375**
  hypercholesterolemia, 1153
  hypothermia, 149
  maternal, 89 (Table)
  mucocutaneous candidiasis, 1251
  myopathy, 737
  neonatal jaundice, 220, 999, 1006
  obesity, 1190
  puberty, 1028, 1050
  radioactive iodine, 1052
  screening, 339 (Table), 1007
  short stature, 375
  strabismus, 1674
  transient, preterm infant, 1045
  transplacental drugs, 1005
Hypotonia, 29 (Fig.), 34, 35, 44
  vs botulism, 1302
  kernicterus, 754
  neonate, 236
  shuffling, 667
Hypotonic dehydration, 413
Hypouricemia, 1123
Hypoventilation, nocturnal, **509**
Hypovolemia
  brain damage, 1810
  nephrotic syndrome, 970
  trauma, **1809**
Hypoxanthine-guanine phosphoribosyltransferase deficiency, 1140
Hypoxemia, **502–503**
  apnea, 197 (Table)
  asthma, 539
  cirrhosis, 483
  cystic fibrosis, 554
  respiratory response, 196
  V/Q mismatch, 502
Hypoxia, *see also* Anoxic seizures
  basal ganglia, 768

disseminated intravascular coagulation, 231
fetus, 82
  labor, 86
  response, **123–125**
head injury, 1809–1810
ischemia, encephalopathy, 694
on lung development, 495
mesial temporal sclerosis, 686
in neoplasms, 892
respiratory distress syndrome, 177
retinopathy of prematurity, 265–266
tetralogy of Fallot, 617
Hypoxic-ischemic encephalopathy, **125–128,** *see also* Postasphyxial dyskinesia
  grade and prognosis, 132
  management, 130–131
  seizures, 245, 247
  strokes, 714
Hypsarrhythmia, infantile spasms, 687
Hysteresis, joint angle *vs* torque, 756
Hysterical amblyopia, blindness, **1658**

Iatrogenic transplacental virilization, 1008
Ibuprofen
  administration, 1968 (Table)
  cystic fibrosis, 558
  juvenile chronic arthritis, 1603
  migraine, 717
  persistent ductus arteriosus, respiratory distress syndrome, 204
  poisoning, 1709
ICD-10, psychiatric diagnosis, 1733
Ice, typhoid fever, 1324–1325
I-cell disease, 782 (Table), **1170–1171**
  neonate, 308
Ice packs, stings, 1524
Ice water drowning, 1717, 1826
ICF syndrome, 1253
Ichthyoses, 1621
  with diplegia, 799 (Table)
Ichthyosis vulgaris, 1620, 1621 (Table)
ICRF 187, iron chelation, cardioprotection in chemotherapy, 896
Ictal behavior, 690
Ictal SPECT, 679
Icterus gravis neonatorum, 232
Ictus, 674
Idiopathic CD4 lymphocytopenia, 1252
Idiopathic dilation of pulmonary artery, **609**
Idiopathic fibrosing alveolitis, **578**
Idiopathic hypercalcemia, 212, 1200
  of infancy, 1056
Idiopathic hypercalciuria, 959
Idiopathic hyperlipemia, 1674
Idiopathic neonatal hepatitis, 221
Idiopathic nephrotic syndrome, **968–971**
Idiopathic partial epilepsy of infancy, 680 (Table)
Idiopathic photosensitivity eruptions, **1645**
Idiopathic rapidly progressive glomerulonephritis, 965
Idiopathic scrotal edema, 1791–1792
Idiopathic thrombocytopenic purpura, **877–878**
  maternal, 89 (Table)
  neonatal thrombocytopenia from, 229
  rash, 1285
  vs rubella, 1357
Idiopathic torsion dystonia, 773–774, 793 (Table)
Idiopathic transient neonatal hyperinsulinism, 296
Idiopathic urticaria, **1697**
  chronic, 1639
Idoxuridine preparations, 1968 (Table)
α-L-Iduronidase, 1157
IFAT, African trypanosomiasis, 1456
Ifosfamide
  encephalopathy, 897
  nephrotoxicity, 896
  toxic effects, 894 (Table)

IgA, 1236 (Table), 1237
  ataxia telangiectasia, 766
  breast milk, 332
  deficiency, 1243, **1257–1258**
    gastrointestinal disease, 444
    hepatitis C, 1264
    respiratory disorders, 533
    true, neoplasms, 889 (Table)
  detection, 1300
  fetus and neonate, 275
  gastrointestinal immune response, 439
  low, transient food intolerance, 441
  measurements, 1245
IgA nephropathy, mesangial, 962–963
IgD, 1236 (Table), 1237
IgE, 1236 (Table), 1237
  asthma, investigation, 541
  circulating, **1693–1694**
  measurement, 1245
  skin tests, 1693
IgE-mediated urticaria, 1640
IGFBP3 (IGF binding protein), 366
IgG, 1236 (Table), 1237
  deficiencies, **532–533**
  development, 1241
  fetus and neonate, 275
  idiopathic thrombocytopenic purpura,
    877
  Lyme disease, 1314
  subclass deficiency, 1258
    with IgA deficiency, 1258
  subclass estimations, 1245
  syphilis, 1402
IgM, 1236 (Table), 1237
  congenital rubella, 1358
  detection, 1300
  fetus and neonate, 275
  syphilis, 1402, **1404**
    congenital, 1405
Ileal brake, 438
Ileocecal valve, 445
Ileostomy Association, 485
Ileum, 435
  congenital stenosis, 553
  resection, 1212
  salmonellosis, 1323
  X-ray appearance, 1901
Ileus, 208
  adynamic, potassium depletion, 412
  hypothermia, 150
  vinca alkaloids, 895
Ilia, lysosomal storage disorders, 1158
Iliac horn, *see* Nail–patella syndrome
Illegitimacy, *see* Marriage, births outside
Ill-treatment, Children Act 1989, 1875
Image intensifiers, 1894
Imaging, **1894–1920**
  cystic fibrosis, lungs, **554**
  epilepsy, **678–679**
  head injuries, 706–707
  neoplasms, 891
  renal hypertension, 972
  respiratory disorders, **513–519**
  urinary tract infections, 952–954
Imerslund, syndrome of proteinuria with
    vitamin B$_{12}$ malabsorption, 853
Imerslund–Grasbeck syndrome, 1199
Imidazoles, 1434, **1478**
  mechanism, 1530
Imino acids, disorders, **1113–1114**, 1121
Iminodiacetic acid derivatives, liver
    scintigraphy, 472, 474
  biliary atresia, 1782
Iminodipeptiduria, 1114
Iminoglycinuria, 446, 1121–1122
Imipenem, 1703
  administration, 1968 (Table)
  environmental mycobacteria, 1350
  Pseudomonas aeruginosa, cystic
    fibrosis, 558 (Table)
Imipramine, 1755
  administration, 1968 (Table)
  enuresis, 1743
  nocturnal enuresis, 957

Immature teratomas, 920
  management, 923
Immature/total neutrophil ratio, neonatal
    sepsis, 276 (Table), 277
Immediate allergic reactions, 1689
  penicillin, 1702
Immersion burns, 1868
Immigrants, children of, **1865–1866**
Immobility in utero, 654
Immobilization
  for bites and stings, 1523
  radiography, 1895
Immotile cilia syndrome, 1684
Immune competence, evaluation in HIV
    infection, 1393
Immune complex-mediated
    hypersensitivity, skin, **1640–1641**
Immune deficiency, *see*
    Immunodeficiency
Immune response
  celiac disease, 439–44
  Chagas' disease, 1459
  hepatitis B virus, 476
  neonate, 109, **273–280**
  neoplasms, 892
  respiratory tract, 532
Immune system, 906, **1231–1241**
  ataxia telangiectasia, 766
  development, **1240–1241**
  gastrointestinal tract, 439
  Kawasaki disease, 1480
Immunity, 1231
  Haemophilus influenzae, 1308
  malaria, **1447**
  schistosomiasis, 1508
Immunization in practice (WHO), 346
Immunization (vaccination), 340,
    341–346, *see also named diseases*
  adverse reactions, 342–343
  in AIDS, **1396**
  contraindications, **342,** 343
  developing countries, 1889
  diphtheria, 1305
  failure in Wiskott–Aldrich syndrome,
    1254
  failure of programs, 1278, 1279 (Table)
  hemophilia A, 881
  hepatitis A virus, 476
  hepatitis B virus, 477, **1387**
  historical aspects, 1862
  immunodeficiency, 1267
  improving uptake, 345–346
  leishmaniasis, 1464
  measles, 895, **1356**
    United Kingdom, 1276
  of mothers, 1267
  myths, 1318
  nephrotic syndrome, 969, 970
  pertussis, **1317–1318**
    vs incidence, 1315–1316
  rates, 15 (Table)
  respiratory disorders, effect on
    prevalence, 489–490
  rubella, 287, **1357**
  schedules, **343–345**
  for splenectomy, 857
  Streptococcus pneumoniae, 1319
  success, 1280
  and sudden infant death syndrome,
    1719
  tetanus, 1333
  tuberculosis, *see* BCG vaccination
Immunocompromised patient
  bacteremia, 1287
  cytomegalovirus, 1365
  fibrosing alveolitis, 577
  FUO investigations, 1284
  herpes simplex virus, 1441
Immunodeficiency, **1241–1270**
  AIDS, differential diagnosis, 1396
  antibiotic prophylaxis, 533, 1529
  BCG vaccination, 1339
  carcinoma, 1248
  diarrhea, 213

environmental mycobacteria, 1350
  and gastrointestinal disease, 444
  glucose-6-phosphate translocase
    deficiencies, 1137
  herpes simplex, 1439
  management, **1266–1270**
  measles vaccination, 1356
  neoplasms, 889, 1248
  parenteral lipids, 1220
  pneumonia, 568
  purine disorders, 1141
  respiratory disorders, **532–536**
  secondary, **1263–1266**
Immunofluorescence, *Bordetella pertussis*,
    1317
Immunofluorometric assays, 1001
Immunoglobulin gene deletions, 1242
    (Table)
Immunoglobulins, **1236–1237,** *see also*
    IgA; IgD; IgE; IgG; IgM
  deficiencies, 1102, **1255–1259**
  development, 1241
  fetus and neonate, 275, 1240
  functional tests, 1245
  gastrointestinal immune response, 439
  normal values, 1928 (Table)
  serum levels, 472 (Table), 1245
    HIV infection, 1264–1265
  transplacental, 343
  viral infections, 1351
  Wiskott–Aldrich syndrome, 1254
Immunoglobulin therapy, *see also*
    Hyperimmune immunoglobulin
  administration, 1968 (Table)
  in AIDS, 1396, 1397
  Guillain–Barré syndrome, 726
  Haemophilus influenzae, 1309
  hepatitis A virus, 1386
  hepatitis B virus, 1387
    neonate, 1957 (Table)
  for humoral immune defects,
    1267–1268
  idiopathic thrombocytopenic purpura,
    878
  IgA deficiency, 1258
  immunodeficiency, 533
  for infantile spasms, 687
  measles, 1355
    prevention, cancer treatment, 895
  neonatal sepsis, 279–280, **1267**
  neonatal thrombocytopenia, 229
  rubella, 1357
  tetanus, 1333, 1334
  varicella-zoster, neonate, 1957
    (Table)
Immunological reconstitution, AIDS,
    1398
Immunologic assays, enzymes, 1100
Immunology
  African trypanosomiasis, 1456
  techniques, 1300
Immunophenotyping, tumor diagnosis,
    891
Immunoradiometric assays, 1001–1002
  TSH, 1045
Immunoreactive trypsin, cystic fibrosis
    screening, 552
Immunosuppression, 1265
  for aplastic anemias, 856
  bronchoalveolar lavage, 520
  cancer treatment, 895
  Crohn's disease, 457
  cystic fibrosis, 558
  dermatomyositis-polymyositis, 1608
  diabetes mellitus, 1081
  infection-associated hemophagocytic
    syndrome IAHS, 926
  for juvenile chronic arthritis, 1604
  neoplasms, 890
  for polymyositis, 737
  renal transplantation, side-effects, 981
  systemic lupus erythematosus, 965,
    1606

Immunotherapy
  hyposensitization, 545
  for neonatal sepsis, 279–280
  neoplasms, 893
Impact-absorbing surfaces, playgrounds,
    1713
Impact injuries, 701, **705**
Impairment
  definition, 167
  incidence, **13**
Impedance audiometry, 817, 1683
  secretory otitis media, 1681
Imperforate hymen, 1796
Imperforate vagina, 990–991
Impetigo, 1284, 1329, **1634–1635**
  vs perineal herpes, 1365
  streptococcal, **1332**
Implantable devices, central venous lines,
    1224
Impression cytology, conjunctiva, 263
Imprinting, genetic disorders, 59
Impulse sound pressures, incubators, 97
Inactivated vaccine, 341
  poliomyelitis, 345
INAH, *see* Isoniazid
Inappropriate ADH secretion, *see also*
    Syndrome of inappropriate ADH
    secretion
  asthma treatment, 549
Inborn errors of digestion and absorption,
    445–447
Inborn errors of metabolism, **1099–**
    1178
  formula milks for, manufacturers, 1120
    (Table)
  heterozygotes, 66
  hypoglycemia, 296–297, 306,
    1130–1131
  incidence, 1101
  neonate, **304–309**
  seizures, 245
  not affecting fetus, 1105
  nutrition, 1203
  sudden infant death syndrome, 1722
  viral infections, 694
Inborn errors of testosterone biosynthesis,
    1008
Incarceration of inguinal hernia, 1790
Incest, 1101
  pregnancy, 1870
Incision, snake bite, 1523
Inclusion blennorrhea, 1385, 1664
Inclusion cell disease, *see* I-cell disease
Inclusion conjunctivitis, **1385**
Inclusions
  chlamydial infection, 1429–1430
  herpes simplex, 1437
Incomes, world figures, 1883
Incomitant squint, **1660**, 1661
Incontinence, 957
  history taking, 18
Incontinentia pigmenti, 799 (Table), 803,
    831 (Table), **1626–1627**
  eosinophil counts, 223
  inheritance, 67
Incubation period, *see also named*
    diseases
  vs prepatent period, malaria, 1446
Incubators, **148**
  noise levels, 97
  procedures, 1829
  transport, 157
Independence
  adolescence, 1750
  cerebral palsy, 762
Indeterminate colitis, 456
India
  BCG vaccination, 1339
  cosmetics, lead, 1708
  temple prostitutes, 1887
Indian childhood cirrhosis, 484, 1145
Indian tick typhus, 1392
Indican, urine, 1114, 1122
Indirect challenge procedure, 542

Indirect fluorescent antibody test, toxocariasis, 1486
Indirect micturition cystourethrography, urinary tract infections, 954, 955 (Fig.)
Indirect ophthalmoscopy, 1651–1652
Indirect radiography, 1894
Indirect radionuclide cystography, 1911–1912
Individualized prognostic strategy, 102
Individual psychotherapy, 1749, **1763**
sexual abuse, 1760
Indoles, urine, 1122
Indomethacin
administration, 1969 (Table)
neonate, 1957 (Table)
cyanotic heart disease, dosage, 202 (Table)
juvenile chronic arthritis, 1603
nephrogenic diabetes insipidus, 949
persistent ductus arteriosus, 205, 603
respiratory distress syndrome, 204
on platelets, 229
Inducible nitric oxide synthase, 1823
Induction of labor, **87**
postterm pregnancy, 83
rhesus incompatibility, 233
Industrial chemicals, parental exposure, neoplasms, 890–891
Industrialized countries, infections, mortality, 1275–1276
Inermicapsifer madagascarensis, 1506
Infancy, 98
AIDS, 1393
blood pressure, 20
Coxsackie B myocarditis, 1382
definition, 16, 94
dietary nutritional assessment, 1187
disease incidence, 13
fever, **1282–1283**
infections, emergency care, 1814
normal diet, **1188–1189**
pain, 1830
parenteral nutrition, regimens, 1223 (Table)
Infancy–childhood–puberty growth model, 1013
Infancy phase, growth, 352, 356, 364
Infant, newborn, *see* Neonate; Preterm infant
Infant feeding, *see also* Bottle feeding; Breast-feeding
intake levels, 333
Infant formula, *see* Formula milks
Infantile acne, 1646
Infantile colic, **461**
Infantile cortical hyperostosis, **1583–1585**
Infantile genetic agranulocytosis (Kostmann syndrome), **867,** 1259
Infantile glaucoma, 23, 27 (Fig.), 43, 264, **1672–1673**
Infantile GM$_1$-gangliosidosis, 1162, 1163
Infantile hypercalcemia (Lightwood's syndrome), 831 (Table)
Infantile hypertrophic pyloric stenosis, *see* Pyloric stenosis
Infantile macular degeneration, 1666
Infantile Marfan's syndrome, 1588
Infantile neuroaxonal dystrophy, 793 (Table)
Infantile nystagmus, 272
severely handicapped children affected, 14 (Table)
Infantile polyarteritis, 1610
heart, 636
Infantile Refsum's disease, 308, 785 (Table), 1173
Infantile scoliosis, 1557–1558
Infantile sialic acid storage disease, 1157 (Table), 1169
Infantile spasms, 673, *see also* West's syndrome
positron emission tomography, 679
Infantile tibia vara, **1554**

Infant milk depots, 1861
Infant mortality, **5**
rates, 3, 94
Infarction, *see also* Cerebral infarction
bones, sickle cell disease, 862
Infection-associated hemophagocytic syndrome IAHS, 926
Infection control
AIDS, 1396
hospitals, **1281–1282**
teams, 1282
Infections, **1273–1543,** *see also* Skin, infections
apnea, 197 (Table)
ataxia, 762
bone marrow transplant recipients, 874–875
and breast-feeding, 327
breast milk protection, 152
burns, 1800
cancer treatment, **894–895**
central nervous system, 794–795 (Table)
cerebrospinal fluid shunts, 662
chronic, secondary anemia, 865
complement deficiency disorders, 1262, 1263
diabetes mellitus, nutrition, 1210
emergency care, **1814**
encephalopathy, 693–694, 696
head injuries, **708**
hemolytic uremic syndrome, 977 (Table)
hepatitis syndrome in infancy, 474 (Table)
HIV infection complications, **1393–1394**
home care, 1802
from immunodeficiency, 1243
immunodeficiency from, 1263–1265
kwashiorkor, 1193
leukemia, 870
leukemia from, 868
liver transplantation, 484–485
maternal, 11
myelomeningocele, 653
neonate, **273–289**
chronic pulmonary, **196**
emergency care, 1814
mortality, 4 (Table)
seizures, 245
thrombocytopenia, 229
nephrotic syndrome, 969, 1288
neutropenia, 867
persistent pulmonary hypertension of the newborn, 205
postneonatal mortality, 5 (Table)
purpura, 876
sickle cell disease, 862
spina bifida occulta, 652
stillbirth rates, 4 (Table)
strokes, 713–714
thrombocytopenia, 878
Infectious diseases, *see also* Notifiable diseases
home care, 1802
nutrition and control, 1892
reporting, 1804
schools, **1863–1864**
Infectious encephalitis, *vs* medulloblastoma, 901
Infectious hepatitis (hepatitis A virus), **476, 1386**
Infectious mononucleosis, 560, **1366–1368**
vs cytomegalovirus disease, 1365
vs diphtheria, 1306
FUO investigations, 1283 (Table)
immunosuppression, 1264
liver, 1388
vs measles, 1355
vs mumps, 1372
pharyngeal membrane, 511
vs scarlet fever, 1331
vs tonsillitis, 1686, 1687

Infectious units, *Neisseria gonorrhoeae*, 142
Infective diarrhea, acute, **451–454**
Infective endocarditis, **630–631,** 1333
antibiotic prophylaxis, 1528
aortic stenosis, 607
duration of therapy, 1528
FUO investigations, 1283 (Table)
mitral valve prolapse, 610
pulmonary stenosis, 609
Infective myocarditis, **630**
Inferior vena cava
computed tomography, 1912 (Fig.)
ultrasonography, 1910
Infertile male syndrome, 1009
Infertility
anticonvulsants, 691
cancer survivors, 899
congenital adrenal hyperplasia, 1065
cyclophosphamide in nephrotic syndrome, 971
cystic fibrosis, 551
Down syndrome, 55
galactose-1-phosphate uridyltransferase deficiency, 1133
testicular descent anomalies, 1791
Inflammation
chronic, secondary anemia, 865
mediators, 273
muscle, **737–738**
phagocytosis, 1235
syphilis, 1401
Inflammatory bowel disease, **456–459**
arthropathy, **1611**
glucose-6-phosphate translocase deficiencies, 1137
nutrition, **1206–1207**
scintigraphy, 1906
self-help groups, 485
ultrasonography, 1905
Influenza, 286 (Table), **1368–1369**
immunosuppression, 1264
vs measles, 1355
vaccine
administration, 1969 (Table)
egg intolerance, 1700
viruses, 1368
type A, 566
Information sheets/booklets
nephrotic syndrome, 971
urinary tract infection prevention, 952
Informed consent, **1878**
adolescents, **1880**
adoption, 1859
procedures, 1829
research, parents, 103, 166
Infrared lamps, fluoroscopy, 1901
Infratentorial tumors, 900
Infundibular obstruction, *see* Right ventricle, outflow obstruction
Infusion pumps, insulin, 1081
Infusion sets, parenteral nutrition, 1225
Inguinal canal, ultrasonography, 1914
Inguinal hernia, **1788–1790**
intestinal obstruction, 1776
INH, *see* Isoniazid
Inhalation of foreign material, **570–572**
Inhalers, 545, **1954**
Inherited disorders, *see also entries starting* Hereditary
causing cirrhosis, 482 (Table)
fetus, 11
hepatitis syndrome in infancy, 473 (Table)
Inhibins, **1024,** 1027
Initial infection, herpes simplex virus, 1436
Injections, epiglottitis, 562
Injection sclerotherapy, varices, 483
Inlet ventricular septal defect, 600
Innate developmental behaviors, **667**
Innocent murmurs, **594–595**
neonatal, 203 (Table)
Innominate artery, aberrant, 573

Inotropic drugs, neonate, management, 205
INR, *see* Prothrombin time
Insecticides
aplastic anemia, 856 (Table)
poisoning, 1711
typhus control, 1391
Insects
allergens, **1691**
repellents, 1448
stings, 1524
Insensible water loss
fluid replacement, 975
neonate, 258
preterm infant, 140
Inside out rule, telencephalon, 642
In situ hybridization, 73
Inspiratory and expiratory times, ventilation for RDS, 163, 181
Institutional care, outcome, 1859
Insulin, **1071,** *see also* Hyperinsulinism
administration, 1969 (Table)
amino acid plasma levels, 1102
blood sampling, 297
with dextrose, for hyperkalemia, 145 (Table), 259, 415, 975
for diabetic ketoacidosis, 1075
fetus, 1004
for inborn errors of metabolism, 307
normal values, 1926 (Table)
parenteral nutrition, 298, 1220
puberty, 1026
regimens, 1072–1081
response, SGA baby, 137
tolerance test, 1018
growth hormone secretion, 1018
for transient neonatal diabetes mellitus, 298
Insulin dependent diabetes mellitus, 1072–1081
Insulin hypoglycemia test, growth hormone secretion, 1018
Insulin-like growth factor binding proteins, 351, 365–366, 374, 1018
Insulin-like growth factor receptors, 351
Insulin-like growth factors, 351, **365–366,** 1013
environmental factors, 371, 372
fetus, 1004
on growth hormone gene transcription, 367
and nutrition, 1022
paracrine, 1013
pituitary gigantism, 376
serum levels, measurement, 1018
testing, 374
Turner's syndrome, 370
Integrins, b$_2$, 1235
Intelligence, 820, **826–827,** 1732, *see also* IQ
adopted children, 1859
assessment, **1735**
autism, 1738
and breast-feeding, 327, 339
cerebral palsy, 761
congenital hemiplegia, 744
development, **381–400**
diplegia, 748
effect of epilepsy, 690
hydrocephalus, 666
Isle of Wight studies, 1852
skills in tests, 669, 670
Intensification therapy, acute lymphoblastic leukemia, 873
Intensive care, **1816–1826**
analgesia, **1832–1833**
head injuries, 708
neonates, 95, 96, **155–175**
environment, **97–99**
services, **155–157**
post-resuscitation, **526–528**
Intensive care units, infections, 1281
Intention myotonia, 733
Intention tremor, 752

Intercostal drainage, *see* Chest, drainage
Intercostal indrawing, recession, 30, *see also* Costal margin recession; Rib recession
Intercostal muscles, 505
Intercostal needle aspiration, 1844
Interference phenomena, 820–821
Interferon-α
  hepatitis B virus, 1387
  neonate, 275
  neoplasms, 893
Interferon-γ, 1233 (Table)
  for chronic granulomatous disease, 1260
  for immunodeficiency, 1270
  for neonatal infections, 1267
  receptor defect, 1250, 1262
Interferons, 1234, 1530
  cytomegalovirus, immunocompromised patient, 1366
  viral hepatitis B, 477, 1387
Intergroup rhabdomyosarcoma study, 916
Interhemispheric cysts, 651
Interictal behavior, 691
Interictal EEG, neonatal seizures, 247
Interictal SPECT, 679
Interim Care Orders, **1876**
Interleukin-2
  for common variable immunodeficiency, 1257
  for neonatal infections, 1267
Interleukin-2 receptor, γ chain deficiency, *see* X-linked severe combined immunodeficiency syndrome
Interleukins, 1233 (Table)
  tuberculosis, 1336
Interlobular bile ducts, paucity, **474**
Intermediate density lipoprotein, 1149
  secondary disorders, 1154 (Table)
Intermediate filament proteins, small round cell tumors, 912 (Table)
Intermediate fragments, parathyroid hormone, 1054
Intermediate leprosy, 1300
Intermittent auscultation, fetal monitoring, 117
Intermittent continuous infusion, enteral nutrition, 1218
Intermittent feeding, *vs* continuous feeding, preterm infant, 153
Intermittent mandatory ventilation, 1818
  respiratory distress syndrome, 181
Intermittent photic stimulation, 677
Intermittent positive pressure ventilation, 162
  respiratory distress syndrome, 180
Intermittent proteinuria, 967–968
Internal hydrocephalus, 659
Internal jugular vein
  central venous cannulation, 1837–1838
  central venous lines, 1224
International League Against Epilepsy, classification, 674
International Liaison Committee on Resuscitation, 522
International Society of Pediatric Oncology, MMT 95 Study, rhabdomyosarcoma management, 916
International travel, *see* Travel, international
International units, enzymes, 1921–1922
Internet
  inborn errors of metabolism, 1099
  phenylketonuria, 1103
Interphase, 47
Interpretation, family therapy, 1764
Intersex, *see also* Ambiguous genitalia; Sexual differentiation disorders
  chromosome studies, 50–51
Interstitial emphysema, pulmonary, neonate, **188–189**
Interstitial fluid, 403 (Table), 404 (Table)
  preterm infant, 141

Interstitial keratitis, 1664
  syphilis, 1677
    late congenital, **1413**, 1414, 1415
Interstitial pneumonitis, 534, 578, *see also* Lymphoid interstitial pneumonitis
  lymphocytic, 533
  neonates, 196
Interventional cardiac catheterization, 593, 594
  neonate, 205–206
Interventional radiology, **1898–1899**
  persistent ductus arteriosus, 593, 594, 603
  renal hypertension, 973
Intervention studies, 1851
Interviews
  parents of mentally handicapped children, 839
  psychiatric disorder, **1734–1735**
Intestinal absorption, 207–208, **437–438**
  colonic, 455
  preterm infant, 151
Intestinal alkaline phosphatase, fetal, 302
Intestinal juices
  loss, 411
  potassium, 409 (Table)
  sodium, 408 (Table)
Intestinal lymphangiectasia, **443–444**
  dietary management, 1214 (Table)
  immunodeficiency, 1259
Intestinal obstruction, 433–434
  ascariasis, 1483
  chronic granulomatous disease, 1259
  cystic fibrosis, 554
  neonate, 210
  ultrasonography, 1906
Intestinal pseudo-obstruction, 210, **451**
Intestinal stasis, neonatal jaundice, 220
Intestines
  amebiasis, 1468
  candidiasis, 1471
  fluke infection, **1513**
  motility, *see* Motility
  permeability, preterm infant, 151
  schistosomiasis, 1509
  traumatic perforation, 1811
  tuberculosis, 1345
Intra-aortic balloon pump, 1819, **1820–1821**
Intra-arterial continuous pressure monitoring, **1834**
Intracardiac electrophysiological studies, 624
Intracardiac injection, 135
  calcium gluconate contraindicated, 135
Intracarotid amylobarbital procedure, 679
Intracellular fluids, 403, **404**
  normal values, 1923 (Table)
  potassium, 408 (Table)
  sodium, 408 (Table)
Intracerebral hemorrhage, **709–710**, 713
Intracranial birth trauma, **121–122**
Intracranial hemorrhage, 224, **709–711**
  alloimmune neonatal thrombocytopenic purpura, 229
  birth trauma, 126
  cerebrospinal fluid, 703
  disseminated intravascular coagulation, 231
  encephalopathy, 695
  head injuries, management, 706
  hypernatremia, 414, 713
  idiopathic thrombocytopenic purpura, 878
  magnetic resonance imaging, 1914, 1915 (Fig.)
  neonate, **249–250**, 709
    mortality, 4 (Table)
    seizures, 245
  outcome, 171, 172
  trauma, 1810
Intracranial injury, *see* Head injuries; Intracranial birth trauma

Intracranial lesions, precocious puberty, 1029
Intracranial pressure
  ataxia, 763
  benign intracranial hypertension, 665
  birth asphyxia, 130–131
    monitoring, 128
  cracked pot sign, 20, 1290
  craniosynostosis, 1561
  decompression effects, 664
  headache, 715
  hepatic encephalopathy, 1824
  hydranencephaly, 649
  hydrocephalus, 658–659
  infarction, 714
  intensive care, 1825
  vs lacunar skull, 1559
  monitoring, 661, 663, **697–698**
  near-drowning, 1825–1826
  neonate, 243, 661
  status epilepticus, 693
  trauma, 703–704, **707–708**, 1810–1811
  tumors, 900
Intradermal testing, allergic disorders, 1693
Intrahepatic biliary atresia, lipoprotein X, 1153–1154
Intrahepatic biliary hypoplasia, **474**
Intrahepatic cholestasis
  vs biliary atresia, 474
  maternal, 89 (Table)
Intralipid, 158, 1220, 1223 (Table)
Intralobar nephroblastomatosis, 913
Intramuscular injections, **1954**
  opiates, 1831
  poliomyelitis, 1379
Intraocular pressure, measurement, 1654
Intraosseous osteosarcoma, 918
Intraosseous venous access, 526
Intrapartum care, **83–88**
Intrapartum complications, *see* Birth asphyxia; Birth trauma
Intrapartum glucose infusions, 295–296
Intrapartum infection, pneumonia, 183
Intraperitoneal fluid therapy, 413
Intrathecal route
  amphotericin B, doses, 1478
  antibiotics, 663
  baclofen, 759
  penicillin overdose, 676
  prescriptions, 1879
Intrauterine accretion, calcium, phosphorus, 301
Intrauterine amputation, 1545
Intrauterine contraceptive devices, 995
Intrauterine death, creatine kinase, 1937 (Table)
Intrauterine growth retardation, **82–83**, 465, 1005
  cell-mediated immunity, 1241
  gut perfusion, 151
  insulin-like growth factors, 351
  organisms, 284 (Table)
  short stature, 1014
    growth hormone therapy, 1019
Intrauterine hypoxia, stillbirth rates, 4 (Table)
Intrauterine positional deformity, 719
Intravascular fetal blood transfusion, 114
Intravenous access, *see also* Venous cannulation
  parenteral nutrition, 1223–1224
  resuscitation, **526**, 1807, 1809
Intravenous fluids
  for dehydration, 413
  preterm infant, 140
  sodium, neonates, 143
Intravenous immunoglobulin preparations, 1267–1268
Intravenous infusion, opiates, 1831–1832
Intravenous route, **1954**
  acyclovir, 1440
  benzyl penicillin, 1427, 1428 (Table)
  gonorrhea treatment, 1428

Intravenous urography, **1910–1911**
  diagnostic radiation doses, 1895 (Table)
  urinary tract infections, 952–953
Intraventricular hemorrhage, 122
  cerebrospinal fluid, 1290
  eye movements, 265
  and noise, 97
  pneumothorax, 188
  respiratory distress syndrome, 181
Intrinsic factor, 430
  deficiency, 853
  Schilling test, 1199
Intrinsic factor antibodies, 853 (Table)
Intrinsic primary resistance, tumor cells, 892
Intrinsic renal failure, neonate, 258
Introns, 69
Introtalker (Reybus), 814
Intubation, *see* Endotracheal intubation
Intussusception, 460, **1786**
  adenoviruses, 1384
  collapse from, 1815
  vs cow's milk protein intolerance, 1699
  vs gastroenteritis, 1294
  Henoch–Schönlein purpura, 1609
  imaging, 1901
    barium enema reduction, 1903
    ultrasonography, 1904
  palpation, 33
  pressure reduction, 1786, 1903–1904
Inulin, GFR measurement, 942
In utero accretion, calcium, phosphorus, 301
Invasive treatment, reducing, 99
Inverse glaucoma, 1673
Inversions, chromosomal, **51**, 52 (Fig.)
Involucrum, osteitis, 1590
Involuntary movements, history taking, 17
Iodide, *see also* Potassium iodide
  expectorants, 1045
  tissues absorbing, 1044
Iodination, salt, 1048
Iodine, 1185 (Table)
  antiseptics, 1830
  compounds, transplacental, 1005
  deficiency, 1045, **1048**
    developing countries disease burden, 1280 (Table)
  excess intake, 1202
  Recommended Dietary Allowances, 1949 (Table)
  reference nutrient intakes, 1947 (Table)
  requirements, 1181 (Table)
  sources, 1185 (Table)
Iodine-123, 1897
  thyroid scintigraphy, 1047
Iodine-131, 1897
Iodine-131 iodide, *see* Radioactive iodine
Iodine-131 metaiodobenzylguanine scan, neuroblastoma, 911
Iodine-131 rose bengal fecal excretion test, biliary atresia, 221
5-Iodo-2-deoxyuridine, herpes simplex, 1365
Iodothyronine hormones, 998 (Table)
Ion exchange resins, hypercholesterolemia, 1152
Ionized calcium, plasma levels, neonate, 298–299
Ions, concentration units, 1921
  conversion factors, 1938 (Table)
Ipecac, 1706, 1815, 1969 (Table)
Ipratropium bromide, 547, 549
  administration, 1969 (Table)
  episodic wheeze, 550
IQ, **827**, 1735
  cerebral palsy, 761
  congenital hemiplegia, 744
  congenital hypothyroidism, treatment delay, 1047
  effect of epilepsy, 690
  meningitis, 1292
  terminology, 826
  Turner's syndrome, 1032

Iran
  anthrax case, 1300
  zinc deficiency, 1201
Ireland, celiac disease incidence, 440
Iridocyclitis
  juvenile chronic arthritis, 1602
  leprosy, 1311
  syphilis, 1408
Iridodonesis, 1673
Iris
  albinism, 1673
  examination, 1650
Iritis, see Anterior uveitis
Iron, 1185 (Table)
  absorption, 430
  breast milk, 332
  chelation
    ICRF 187, cardioprotection in chemotherapy, 896
    thalassemia, 863
  deficiency, 850–852, 1201
    diagnosis, 1188
    with folate deficiency, 853
    hookworm, 1489
    on immune system, 1266
    mucocutaneous candidiasis, 1251
    prevention, 340, 341
      infants, 334
  distribution, 1146
  Hallervorden–Spatz syndrome, 773
  metabolism disorders, 1146–1147
  milks, 333
  normal values, 1926 (Table)
    stools, 1936 (Table)
  overload, 1201
  parenteral nutrition, 1222 (Table), 1223 (Table)
  poisoning, 1710
  preterm supplements, 155
  Recommended Dietary Allowances, 1949 (Table)
  reference nutrient intakes, 1947 (Table)
  replacement therapy, 851–852
  requirements, 1181 (Table)
    preterm infant, 152 (Table), 225
  serum levels, 1188
  sources, 1185 (Table)
  supplements, 331, 850
    polysaccharide complex, 1974
    vitamin E deficiency, 1197
  therapy, teeth, 425
Iron-binding capacity, 1146
  normal values, 1926 (Table)
Iron-binding proteins, 1234
Iron sorbitol, administration, 1969 (Table)
Irradiated platelets, fetal transfusion for thrombocytopenia, 229
Irregularly irregular rhythm, 32
Irritability, neonate, 238 (Fig.)
Irritable bowel syndrome, 461
Irritant contact urticaria, 1697
Irukandji sting, 1526
Ischemia
  hypoxia, encephalopathy, 694
  mesial temporal sclerosis, 686
  status epilepticus treatment, 693
Ischemic heart disease
  familial hypercholesterolemia type II, 1151
  genetic factors, 74
Islam, family planning, 1865
Isle of Wight studies, 1852
  psychiatric disorder, 1733–1734
    chronic illness, 1746
Islet cell antibodies, 1074
Islets of Langerhans, 1071
Isochromosomes, 51, 52 (Fig.)
  cytogenetic nomenclature, 54
Isoenzymes, 1100
Isohemagglutinins, 1245
Isoimmune neonatal thrombocytopenic purpura, 228–229
Isoimmune thrombocytopenia, 878, see also Alloimmune neonatal

thrombocytopenic purpura
Isolation
  bone marrow transplantation, 1269
  hospital care, 1281
  immunodeficiency, 1266
Isoleucine, degradation pathway, 1116 (Fig.)
Isomaltase, 437
  sucrase–isomaltase deficiency, 445–446, 448
Isomerism, atrial level, 597
Isoniazid (INH)
  administration, 1969 (Table)
  pellagra, 1198
  pyridoxine deficiency, 1198
  sideroblastic anemia, 867
  tuberculosis, 285, 1347, 1348
    chemoprophylaxis, 1340
    meningitis, 1345
    pregnancy, 1346
    pulmonary, 1342
Isoprenaline
  administration, 1969 (Table)
    neonate, 1957 (Table)
  for bradycardia, 627
  cardiac stimulation, 135
Isosmotic solutions, 405
Isosorbide, on CSF production, 664
Isospora belli, AIDS, 1397
Isotonic dehydration, 413
Isotonic solutions, 405
Isotopic dilution method, sodium, 408
Isotretinoin, congenital heart disease, 596
Isovaleric acidemia, 1117
ISPAD declaration, diabetes management, 1076
Itching, terminal care, 928
Ito, hypomelanosis, 799 (Table), 804
Itraconazole, 1478
  aspergillosis, 536
  oral absorption, 1527
Ivermectin
  administration, 1969 (Table)
  filariasis, 1498
  mites, 1517
  onchocerciasis, 1497
Ixodid ticks, Lyme disease, 1312

Jackson–Rees modification, Ayre's T-piece, 524
Jackson–Weiss syndrome, 1561
  inheritance, 1566 (Table)
JAK-3 defect, 1250
Jamaica, breast-feeding rates, 326 (Table)
Jamaican vomiting sickness, 1117
Jansen type metaphyseal chondrodysplasia, 1578, 1579 (Table)
  inheritance, 1566 (Table)
Jansky–Bielschowski disease, 1171
Janus kinase, defect, 1250
Janus kinase 2, 1013
Japan
  cystinuria, 947
  demography, 2 (Table)
  Kawasaki disease, 1480
Jargon aphasia, 814
Jarisch–Herxheimer reaction, 1323, 1411
Jaundice, see also Neonatal jaundice
  biliary atresia, 475
  brainstem auditory evoked potentials, 244
  cytomegalovirus, 1366
  history taking, 17
  liver tumors, 924
Jaw, Burkitt's lymphoma, 907
Jaw jerk, 35, 38 (Table)
Jaw-winking syndrome, 1661
JC virus, 1378
JEB protocol, germ cell tumors, 923
Jejunal biopsy, 447–448, 468
  celiac disease, 440, 441
  cystic fibrosis, 1209

Jejunostomies, 1219 (Table)
Jejunum, 435
  resection, 1212
  X-ray appearance, 1901
Jellyfish stings, 1526
Jervell syndrome, 626
  deafness, 1682
  heart, 596
Jet ventilation, 164, 1818
Jeune's asphyxiating thoracic dystrophy, 1576–1577
  vs hypophosphatasia, 1176
  renal involvement, 254
Jews, see also Ashkenazi Jews
  lysosomal diseases, 1164
Jigger flea, 1514
Jitteriness, 236–237, 673
  neonatal tetany, 300
Job's syndrome, 1261
Jo'burg virus disease, 1388–1389
Johns Hopkins University Genome Data Base, 1099
Joint Committee for Children, 1853
Joints
  aspiration, 1843–1844
    septic arthritis, 1592
  disorders, 1596–1613
  examination, 39–41
  excess mobility, 39
  hemophilia A, 880
  Henoch–Schönlein purpura, 1609
  leukemia, 870
  progressive systemic sclerosis, 1608
Joint Working Party on Child Health Surveillance, 1853
Jones criteria, rheumatic fever, 1597
Joubert's syndrome, 646, 831 (Table)
Judges, neonatal intensive care decisions, 101, 102–103
Jugular venous oxygen content, 708
Jugular venous pressure, 31
Jugular venous pulse, 585
Jumper ant bites and stings, 1524
Junctional epidermolysis bullosa, 1622, 1623 (Table)
Junctional nevi, 1618
Junior doctors, and negligence, 1879
Juvenile absence epilepsy, 681 (Table)
Juvenile amaurotic family idiocy, 1666
Juvenile chronic arthritis, 1600–1605
  nutrition, 1210–1211
  vs psoriatic arthritis, 1611
Juvenile chronic myeloid leukemia, 872
Juvenile general paralysis of the insane, 1413
Juvenile GM₁-gangliosidosis, 1163
Juvenile laryngeal papillomatosis, 1443–1444
Juvenile macular degeneration, 1666
Juvenile mass treatment, yaws, 1420
Juvenile myoclonic epilepsy, 681 (Table)
  inheritance studies, 682
Juvenile pemphigoid, 1640
Juvenile polyps, 448
Juvenile rheumatoid arthritis
  amyloidosis, 966
  FUO investigations, 1283 (Table)
  heart, 635
  IgA deficiency, 1258
Juvenile spinal muscular atrophy type 3, 721, 722 (Fig.)
Juvenile tabes dorsalis, 1413

Kabure itch, 1508
Kala azar, 1461–1463
Kallmann's syndrome, 1025, 1031
Kanamycin
  neonate, 279 (Table)
  ophthalmia neonatorum, 1429
Kangarooing, 97–98
Kangaroo method, perinatal care, 1891
Kaposi's sarcoma, 1396

Kaposi's varicelliform eruption, 1364, 1439, see also Disseminated herpes simplex
Kartagener's syndrome, 577, 612
Karyotypes, preparation, 48–50
Kasabach–Merritt syndrome, 1619, 1797, see also Cavernous hemangiomas, disseminated intravascular coagulation
Kasai operation (portoenterostomy), 475, 1782–1783
Kashin–Bek disease, 1146–1147, 1202
Katal (unit), 1922
Katayama syndrome, 1508
Kaufman Assessment Battery for Children, 827
Kawasaki disease (mucocutaneous lymph node syndrome), 633, 710, 1478–1481
  FUO investigations, 1283 (Table)
  gall bladder, 1906
  vs measles, 1355
  rash, 1285
  vs scarlet fever, 1331
Kay-Cee-L (potassium chloride syrup), 415
Kay Picture Test, 396
Kayser–Fleischer ring, 481, 1145, 1674
Kearns–Sayre syndrome, 787 (Table), 1127
Keloid scars, BCG vaccination, 1339
Kenya, breast-feeding rates, 326 (Table)
Kenyan tick typhus, 1392
Keratinocytes, 1616
Keratitis, 1664–1665
  acanthamoeba, 1470
  Pseudomonas aeruginosa, 1320
Keratoconjunctivitis
  acute herpetic, 1364
  allergic, 1698–1699
  epidemic, 1370, 1385, 1676
Keratoconus, 1653 (Fig.)
Keratolytics
  ichthyoses, 1620
  warts, 1633
Keratomalacia, 1194, 1677
Kernicterus, 232, 248–249, 754
  Crigler–Najjar syndrome, 1144
  deafness, 248–249, 816
  hyperkinetic bulbar palsy, 813
Kernig's sign, 38, 1289
Kerosene poisoning, 1705, 1711
Keshan disease, 1202
Ketamine, administration, 1969 (Table)
Ketoconazole, 1478
  administration, 1969 (Table)
  for precocious puberty, 1030
α-Ketoglutarate, amniotic fluid, 1937 (Table)
α-Ketoglutarate dehydrogenase deficiency, 1126
Ketones
  metabolism disorders, 1130
  methylmalonic acidemia, 1117
  normal values, 1922 (Table), 1926 (Table)
    amniotic fluid, 1937 (Table)
Ketorolac, 1832
Ketosis, 420 (Table)
  diabetes mellitus, 1075–1076
  hypertonicity, 415
  dicarboxylic acids, 1128
  facile hyperketosis, 1130
  hypoglycemia, 1082, 1131
  17-Ketosteroids, normal values, urine, 1932 (Table)
3-Ketothiolase enzymes, 1130
'Ketotic hyperglycinemia,' 1119
Ketotic hypoglycemia, 1083, 1131
Ketotifen, administration, 1969 (Table)
Kettles, scalds, 1715
Keyboards, dysgraphia, 825
Ki-1 antigen expression, large cell lymphoma classification, 907

Kidneys, *see also* Nephrogenic diabetes insipidus; Nephrotoxicity; *entries starting* Renal
  acid/base balance, **418–419**
  amino acid transport systems, 1121 (Table)
  amyloid, cystic fibrosis, 556
  birth asphyxia, 129
  calcitonin on, 1055
  and cerebellar syndromes, 753
  development, 934–935
  diseases
    nutrition, **1211**
    pregnancy, 114
    severely handicapped children affected, 14 (Table)
  enlargement, 471
  examination, 33
  function, **941–944**
    assessment, **942–944**, 1938 (Table)
    after hemolytic uremic syndrome, 978–979
    hyperkalemia, 145
    neonate, **108**, 143, 934–935
    postnatal development, **256–257**, 1953
    rickets, 1058
  galactose-1-phosphate uridyltransferase deficiency, 1133
  hemopoiesis, 222
  hemorrhage, neonate, 224
  Henoch–Schönlein purpura, 1609–1610
  malaria, 1448
  neonate, 108, **253–262**
    infection, organisms, 284 (Table)
  neoplasms, 913–915
    incidence, 886 (Table)
  non-accidental injury, 1869
  oxalosis, 1112
  potassium excretion, 409
  reduced mass, proteinuria, 968
  single photon emission computed tomography, 1897
  size *vs* GFR, 943
  sodium excretion, 408
  systemic lupus erythematosus, 1605–1606
  tuberculosis, 1346
  tumors, tuberous sclerosis, 802
  ultrasonography, 1909–1910
Killed vaccine, *see* Inactivated vaccine
Killian–Pallister syndrome, 59–60
Killing, cellular, 274
Kindergarten movement, 1861
Kinesiogenic dystonia, paroxysmal, 673, 773
Kinesthetic memory, 669, 822
Kinky hair syndrome, Menkes', 711, 791 (Table), 1146, 1202
Klebsiella spp., urinary tract infections, neonate, 283
Kleihauer test, 224, 231
Klinefelter's syndrome, **62**, 376, 1010, **1036**, 1037 (Fig.), 1190
  cytogenetic nomenclature, 53
  germ cell tumors, 920
  and Hashimoto's thyroiditis, 1049
  lexical deficit, 807
  neoplasms, 289
Klippel–Feil syndrome, 651, **1556–1557**
  deafness, 1682
Klippel–Trelaunay syndrome, 1620, 1798
Kloref (potassium chloride syrup), 415
Klumpke palsy, 122
Knee-elbow position, for breech presentation, 83
Knee jerk, 35, 38 (Table)
  chorea, 1598
  neonate, 239
Knee joint
  congenital abnormalities, 1553
  rickets, 1195

synovial effusion, 39–40
Knemometry, 1012
Kniest syndrome, 1157 (Table), **1577**
  inheritance, 1566 (Table)
Kniest-type dysplasia, 1577
Knock-knee, 38, **1553**
Knockout mouse studies, growth factors, 351
Knudson, 'two-hit' hypothesis, 868
Köbner's phenomenon, 1600
Kocher–Debré–Séméliegne syndrome, 737
Koch-type reaction, tuberculin test, 1337
Köhler's disease, **1595**
Koplik's spots, 1353
Korean hemorrhagic fever, 1390
Korsakoff's psychosis, 819
Korsakoff's syndrome, posttraumatic, 709
Kostmann syndrome (infantile genetic agranulocytosis), **867**, 1259
Kozlowski type metaphyseal chondrodysplasia, 1579 (Table)
Krabbe disease, 777 (Table), 1157 (Table), **1165**
Krait snakebites, 1522
Krebs cycle, disorders, 1126
Krypton-81m, 517, 1897, 1901
  scan radiation dose, 513
Kufs disease, 1171
Kugelberg–Welander disease (juvenile spinal muscular atrophy type 3), **721**, 722 (Fig.)
Kuru, 1378
Kwashiorkor, 371, **1192–1194**
  vs beri beri, 1198
  pellagra, 1198
Kyasanur Forest fever, 1390
Kynureninase deficiency, 1114
Kyphoscoliosis, 1558
  metatropic dysplasia, 1577
Kyphosis, 38, 1558

Labeling neonates, 111
Labetalol
  acute renal failure, 975
    neonate, 259
  administration, 1969 (Table)
  hypertension, 637
    renal, 973 (Table)
Labial adhesions, 988, **1795**
Labor, **84–87**, *see also* Induction of labor
  control of onset, 1005
  monitoring, 116–119
  twin pregnancies, 90
Laboratory methods, *see also* Bacteriology, laboratory methods
  endocrinology, 1000–1001
  gonorrhea, **1422–1424**
  liver disease, **471–472**
  syphilis, **1402–1404**
  tularemia, infection danger, 1351
  virology, **1351–1353**
Laboratory reports, and negligence, 1879
Labor ward routines, **111**
Laburnum poisoning, 1711
Labyrinthine reflexes, 36 (Table), 39 (Fig.)
Lacrimal apparatus, **1665–1666**
Lacrimal passages, investigation, 1654, 1665
β-Lactamase blocking agents, 1528
β-Lactamases
  antibiotic resistance, 1529
  Neisseria gonorrhoeae, 1422, 1427, 1428
  Staphylococcus aureus, 1328
Lactase, 207, 437
  deficiency, 445, 1214, *see also* Lactose, intolerance
  preterm infant, 151
Lactate
  amniotic fluid, 1937 (Table)
  blood levels

glucose tolerance test, glucose-6-phosphatase deficiency, 1137
  normal fetus, 119 (Table)
  sampling, 297
  cerebrospinal fluid, 1125
    meningitis, 1290
  hypoxic ischemia, 694
  metabolism disorders, **1124–1126**
  normal values, cerebrospinal fluid, 1934 (Table)
  proton magnetic resonance spectroscopy, birth asphyxia, 128
Lactate dehydrogenase, 1124
  Ewing's sarcoma, 919
  isoenzyme 1, 921
  normal values, 1926 (Table)
    cerebrospinal fluid, 1934 (Table)
  osteosarcoma, 917
Lactation, 327–328
Lactic acid
  excretion, 1119
  normal values, stools, 1936 (Table)
D-Lactic acidemia, 1125
Lactic acidosis, 307, 420 (Table), 1119, 1124–1125
  with hypoglycemia, 1135
  multiple carboxylase deficiency, 1254
Lactoferrin, 1234
Lactogenic receptors, growth hormone, 365
Lacto-ovo-vegetarian diet, 1189 (Table)
Lactose
  breast milk, 332
  intolerance, 155, 212–213
    postgastroenteritis, 333, 454, 1215
Lacto-vegetarian diet, 1189 (Table)
Lactulose
  administration, 1969 (Table)
  hydrogen breath test, 448
  liver failure, 1824
Lacunar skull, 1559
Ladder pattern, abdomen, 32
Ladd monitor, 243
Ladd's bands, 1773–1774
Laerdal bag, neonatal resuscitation, 133–134
Lafora body disease, 795 (Table)
Lamellar bodies, surfactant, 176
Lamellar cataract (zonular cataract), 1668, 1669
Lamellar exfoliation of newborn, 1621
Lamellar ichthyosis, 1620, 1621 (Table)
Lamina propria, small intestine, 435
Laminated glass, 1715
Lamotrigine, 686
  administration, 1969–1970 (Table)
Lampona cylindrata, bites, 1525
Lamprene, *see* Clofazimine
Lancefield groups, β-hemolytic streptococci, 1330
Lancets, 1834
Landau–Kleffner syndrome, 676, 689 (Table), 815
Landry's paralysis, 726
Lange-Nielsen syndrome, 626
  deafness, 1682
  heart, 596
Langer–Giedion syndrome, 60 (Table)
Langerhans' cell histiocytosis (histiocytosis X), 373, 925–926, **1647–1648**, 1915
  diabetes insipidus, 1040 (Table)
  gums, 425
  neonate, 293 (Table)
  severe combined immunodeficiency syndrome features, 1249
Langerhans' cells, 925, 1616
Langer's dwarfism, 1581
Langer's lines, 1846
Language, 804
  development, 392, 393
    autism, 1738
    delay, 398–399, 1744
    disorders, **1744–1745**

    examination, 388–391 (Table)
    normal, **384–385**
    social factors, 818, 828
  disorders, 807, **814–815**
    classification, 805 (Table)
    IQ, 827
  mental retardation, **836–837**
Language development programs, nursery schools, 1861
Language units, schools, 808
Lanugo, neonatal gestation age, 42 (Fig.)
Laparotomy
  ambiguous genitalia, 986, 987
  and hydrocolpos, 987
Lap belt injury, 1812
Large cell lymphomas, 907
Large for gestational age infant, **138**
  definition, 94
Large multicystic kidney, 254
L-arginine, for hyperammonemia, 1112
L-aromatic amino acid decarboxylase defect, 1107
Laron-type dwarfism, 365, 367, 374–375, 1012, 1013, **1017**
larva currens, 1492
Larval disease
  cestodes, 1499
  organisms, 1484 (Table)
Larval pneumonitis, ascariasis, 1482, 1484
Laryngeal dysfunction syndrome, 539
Laryngomalacia, **193, 572**, 1769
Laryngoscopes, resuscitation, 524
  neonatal, 134
Laryngotracheobronchitis, acute, 1369
Larynx
  chemoreceptor reflex, 528
  clefts, **572–573**
  cysts, 573
  diphtheria, 1306
  dysphonia, 809, 1687–1688
  Farber syndrome, 1167
  hemangiomas, 1619
  papillomas, **1443–1444**, 1688
  stenosis, **572**
  webs, 572, 1769
Laser therapy
  port-wine stain, 1798
  retinopathy of prematurity, 267
L-asparaginase, toxicity, 896
Lassa fever, **1388**
Late allergic reactions, 1689
  penicillin, 1702
Late bronchial reaction, asthma, 537
Late congenital syphilis, **1412–1414**
  treatment, 1415
Late fetal mortality, *see* Stillbirth
Late infancy, disease incidence, 13
Latency, herpes simplex virus, 1436
Latency period, emotional development, 1729 (Table)
Late neonatal hypocalcemia, **299–300**, 1200
Late neonatal mortality rate (LNMR), 3, **4**
Late neonatal period, definition, 94
Latent squint, 1652, **1659–1660**
Latent syphilis, 1401
  early, 1408
Late-onset hemorrhagic disease of the newborn, 230
Late-onset hypogammaglobulinemia, 1256
Late-onset liver failure, 478
Late-onset pneumonia, neonatal, 185
Lateral chest radiograph, 514
Lateral geniculate nucleus, development, 263
Lateralization, cerebral cortex, 644–645, 669, 821
Lateral popliteal palsy, 725
Late skin reaction, asthma, 541
Latex agglutination tests
  β-hemolytic Lancefield group A streptococci, 1298
  meningitis, 1290, 1298

Latex agglutination tests (*Contd*)
  neonatal, 282
  neonatal sepsis, 277
  toxoplasmosis, 1466
Latin America, demography, 2 (Table)
Latrodectus spp., bites, 1524
Lattice work appearance, hereditary
    nephritis, 965
Laughter, asthma, 542
Laurence–Moon–Biedl syndrome, 831
    (Table), 1190, 1667
  obesity, 1022
Lavage, *see also* Bronchoalveolar lavage;
    Gastric lavage
  peritoneal, diagnostic, 1812
  tracheal, 163
Lavatory seats, *Shigella* spp., 1327
Laxatives, 462, 1748 (Table)
  abuse, 1759
  child abuse, 1871
  poisoning, 1709
  urinary tract infection prevention,
    954–956
'Lazy leukocyte' syndrome, 1261
L-carnitine, 1128, *see also* Carnitine
  for fatty acid disorders, 1129
  for glutaric acidemia, 1113
  for hereditary lactic acidosis, 1125
  for hyperammonemia, 1112
  for isovaleric acidemia, 1117
  for organic acidurias, 1119
L-citrulline, *see also* Citrulline
  for ornithine transcarbamylase
    deficiency, 1110
L-dopa
  cerebral palsy, 759
  dihydropteridine reductase deficiency,
    1106
  extrapyramidal syndromes, 772, 774
  parkinsonism, 768
  tics, 771
  tyrosine hydroxylase deficiency, 1107
Lead
  expected values, 1926 (Table)
    urine, 1931 (Table)
  poisoning, 724, **1708**
    blood, 865
    eye, 1678
    mouth, 424
    pyrimidine 5-nucleotidase inhibition,
      1142
    toxocariasis, 1486
Leadbetter Politano technique, ureteric
    reimplantation, 956
Leaky severe combined
    immunodeficiency, 1249–1250
Lean body mass, 361, 1190
Learned helplessness, 834
Learning, 667, **819–820**
  biological factors, 386
Learning disorders, **819–842**, 1864
  central nervous system, radiotherapy,
    875, 899
  congenital hemiplegia, 744
  diplegia, 748
  epilepsy, 690
  headaches, 716, 718, 719
  and helminthic infections, 1481
  management, 824–826
  mental retardation, **826–842**
  motor skills, 752
  neonatal intensive care environment,
    97, **98**
  severely handicapped children affected,
    14 (Table)
Leber's optic atrophy (amaurosis), 68,
    271, 1127, 1672
Lecithin-cholesterol acyltransferase
    deficiency, familial, 1150 (Table),
    1153
Lecithin:sphingomyelin ratio, amniotic
    fluid, 1937 (Table)
Left atrial hypertrophy,
    electrocardiography, 589

Left atrial myxoma, 636
Left-to-right shunt
  airway obstruction, 573
  atrioventricular septal defect, 604
  foramen ovale, 199
  necrotizing enterocolitis, 210
  oxygen saturation measurements, 593
  pulmonary hypertension, 606
  ventricular septal defect, 600
Left ventricle
  enlargement, 31
  hypertrophy, 32
    electrocardiography, 589
  inflow obstructions, **609–610**
  outflow tract obstruction
    cardiomyopathy, 634
    transposition of great arteries, 614
Left ventricle to right atrium defect,
    605–606
Left ventricular failure, late cord
    clamping, 182
Legal issues, *see also* Medicolegal aspects
  medical negligence, **1877–1880**
  neonatal intensive care decisions, 101,
    102–103
Legionnaire's disease, **569**
  emergence, 1279 (Table)
Legislation, **1874–1877**
Leg recoil, neonate, 237 (Fig.)
  gestation age, 41 (Fig.)
Legs
  deformities, 38–39
  length
    computed tomography, 1916, 1917
      (Fig.)
    subischial, 363–364
    measurement, 20
    traction, neonate, 237 (Fig.)
Leigh's encephalopathy, 788 (Table),
    1125, 1127, *see also* Familial
    striatal necrosis
  ataxia, 762
Leishman–Donovan bodies, 1460
Leishmania recidivans, 1463
Leishmaniasis, **1460–1464**
  pentamidine, 1973
Leishmanin skin test, 1462, 1464
Length, **19–20**
Length–tension measurements, 756
Lennox–Gastaut syndrome, 688 (Table),
    795 (Table)
  ataxia, 674
  intelligence, 690
Lens, **1667–1670**
  dislocation, 1670
    homocystinuria, 1673
    inborn errors of metabolism, 305
    Marfan's syndrome, 1676
  dystrophia myotonica, 734
  extraction for cataract, 1669
  implantation, 1670
  neonate, 264
Lepidopterism, 1526
Leprechaunism, 298
Lepromatous leprosy, 1310
Leprosy, **1309–1311**
  neuropathy, 724
  tuberculoid, 1310
  vs tinea versicolor, 1637
Leptospirosis, **1311–1312**
  FUO investigations, 1283 (Table)
Leri–Weill disease (dyschondrosteosis),
    1581
Lesch–Nyhan syndrome, 773, 790 (Table),
    1102, **1140–1141**
  heterogeneity, 1100
  5-hydroxytryptophan, 768
Lesional epileptic syndromes, **684–686**
Lesionectomy
  for epilepsy, 686
  infantile spasms, 687
Let-down reflex, 112
Letterer–Siwe disease, 1647–1648, *see
    also* Langerhans cell histiocytosis

Letter tests, *see* Snellen test; STYCAR
    letter test
Leucine
  degradation pathway, 1116 (Fig.)
  maple syrup urine disease, 1117
Leucine-induced hypoglycemia, 1117
Leucine-sensitive hypoglycemia, 296
leucoderma colli, 1407
Leukemias, **867–875**
  from antitumor therapy, 890
  chromosome abnormalities, 289–290,
    889
  chromosome studies, 51
  clustering, 868, 890
  Down syndrome, 55, 289, 291 (Table),
    887
  and growth hormone deficiency, 1020
  incidence, 886 (Table)
  intracranial hemorrhage, 714
  lung function, 899
  vs lymphomas, 907
  myelogenous, glucose-6-phosphate
    translocase deficiencies, 1137
  neonate, 291 (Table)
    incidence, 290 (Table)
  pharyngitis, 560
  proptosis, 1662
  rash, 1285
  retinopathy, 1675
  second primary tumors, 898 (Table)
  severely handicapped children affected,
    14 (Table)
  spine, 1915
  vitamin K safety, 339
Leukemoid reactions
  Down syndrome, 289, 887
  myelocytic, plague, 1318
  neonate, 291 (Table)
Leukocoria, 268
Leukocyte adhesion deficiencies, 1242
    (Table), 1260–1261
  mismatched BMT, 1270
Leukocyte differentiation antigens,
    1231–1232
Leukocyte elastase, pulmonary interstitial
    emphysema, 188
Leukocytes, 866–875
  vs age, 849 (Table)
  cerebrospinal fluid
    neonate, 242
    normal values, 1934 (Table)
  examination, neonatal sepsis, 276
    (Table)
  immunodeficiency, 1244–1245
  inborn errors of metabolism affecting,
    1137
  infectious mononucleosis, 1367
  neonate, 223 (Table)
    sepsis, 277
  normal values, 1939 (Table)
    urine, 1931 (Table)
  technetium-99m-labelled, colon, 464
  urine, 950–951, 1299
Leukodystrophy, Krabbe disease, 1165
Leukoencephalopathy, CNS
    chemotherapy, 896
Leukoerythroblastosis, 856
Leukomalacia, birth asphyxia, 126
Leukopoiesis, developmental, 222
Leukostasis, 870, 871
Levamisole
  administration, 1970 (Table)
  ascariasis, 1485
  nephrotic syndrome, 970 (Fig.)
Levator palpebrae superioris, examination,
    1649
Level of consciousness, *see also* Coma,
    investigation
  febrile convulsions, 683
  trauma, 1809
Levene grading, intracranial hemorrhage,
    249
Levocardia, 598, 612, 613
Lewis antigens, fucosidosis, 1167–1168

Lexical deficit, 807
Leydig cell hypoplasia, 1008
Leydig cells, 1004
  puberty, 357
Leydig cell tumors, testis, 921
Lhermitte's sign, 901
Liability, multifactorial inherited
    disorders, 74
Liaison diabetes nurses, 1077
Liaison psychiatry, 1749
Libman–Sacks endocarditis, 635
Lice, **1517–1519**, *see also* Pediculosis
  relapsing fever, 1322
  typhus, 1391
Licenses, *see* Product licenses
Lichen sclerosis et atrophicus, 989
Liddle syndrome, 946
Lie, obstetric, 83
Life cycle, *Plasmodium* spp., **1445–1446**
Life events, mental retardation, 839
    (Table)
Life expectancy, 2
Life support, basic, **522–524**
Li–Fraumeni syndrome, 888 (Table), 889
  germ cell tumors, 920
Ligandin, 214
Ligands, malaria red cell invasion, 1446
Ligase chain reaction
  Chlamydia spp., 1430
  Neisseria gonorrhoeae, 1424
Light exposure, neonatal intensive care,
    97, 99
Light habituation, neonate, 237 (Fig.)
Lighting, for procedures, 1829
Lightwood's syndrome, 831 (Table)
Lignocaine, 1832
  administration, 1970 (Table)
    neonate, 1957 (Table)
  for arrhythmias, 627 (Table)
  for neonatal seizures, 246
  resuscitation, doses, 526 (Table)
  ventricular tachycardia, 627
Lignocaine gel, poisoning, 1709
Limb girdle dystrophy, autosomal
    recessive, 733
Limb leads, electrocardiography, 588
    (Fig.)
Limb pains with no organic disease,
    1612–1613
Limbs
  congenital abnormalities, **1545–1556**
  hypertrophy, vascular malformations
    with, 1620
  lengthening procedures, 1017
  rhabdomyosarcoma, 916
  tone and power, neonate, 237–239
Limit dextrinosis (debranching enzyme
    deficiency), 735, **1138**
Limit dextrins, 436
Lincomycin, mechanism, 1527
Linctus, bronchitis, 565
Lindane, poisoning, 1711
Linear array transducers, ultrasonography,
    1896
Linear scleroderma, 1608
Linear sebaceous nevus, 799 (Table),
    804
Lines of Blaschko, 1618
Lingraine, 717 (Table)
Lingual lipase, 207, 437
Lingual thyroid gland, 425
Linkages, genetic, 72, 73
Linkage studies, genetic epilepsies, 682
Linoleic acid
  requirements, 1182
  vitamin E deficiency, 1197
Linolenic acid, 332
α-Linolenic acid, requirements, 1182
Liothyronine, administration, 1970
    (Table)
Lipases, 207–208, 437
  for cystic fibrosis, 557
Lipemia retinalis, 1674
Lipid myopathies, 735–736

Lipids, see also Fats
  muscle biopsy, 1132
  normal values, 1926 (Table)
    cerebrospinal fluid, 1934 (Table)
    stools, 1936 (Table), 1938 (Table)
    plasma, disorders, **1148–1158**, 1674
Lipid storage disorders, **1154–1155**
  eye, 1674
Lipoamide dehydrogenase, ataxia, 765
Lipoatrophic diabetes, 1155
Lipodystrophy, 26 (Fig.), **1155–1156**, see
    also Partial lipodystrophy
Lipofundin, 1220
Lipofuscin, 1171
Lipohypertrophy, insulin injection, 1077,
    1079 (Fig.)
Lipoic acid, for pyruvate dehydrogenase
    deficiency, 1126
Lipoid adrenal hyperplasia, see
    Cholesterol desmolase deficiency
Lipolysis, SGA baby, 137
Lipomas
  encephalocraniocutaneous lipomatosis,
    804
  intraspinal, 652
Lipophilic antibiotics, 1527
α-Lipoprotein, see High-density lipoprotein
β-Lipoprotein, see also Low-density
    lipoprotein
  deficiency, 767
Lipoprotein(a), 1152
Lipoproteins
  normal values, 1926–1927 (Table)
  plasma, disorders, **1148–1158**
Liposomal amphotericin B, 1463, 1472,
    1478, 1959 (Table)
Lipoteichoic acid, β-hemolytic
    streptococci, 1330
β-Lipotropin, 1038
Lips, 424
Lipschutz inclusions, herpes simplex,
    1437
Liquid ventilation, 165
Liquor picis carbonis, 1628
Lisch spots, 800
Lissencephaly, 642, **650**
Listeria-type reaction, tuberculin test,
    1337
Listeriosis
  FUO investigations, 1283 (Table)
  meconium staining, 185
  meningitis, 1290
    neonate, 284
    meningitis, 247
Literacy
  mothers, 1886
  rates, 1883 (Table)
Lithium, 1041, 1185 (Table), 1748
    (Table), 1755
  Ebstein's anomaly, 596
Litigation, divorce, 1856
Little mouse, 366
Little's area, 1684
Little's disease, 35, **745**
Live attenuated vaccines, 341
  contraindications, 342 (Table)
Live births, 1849
  definition, 1
Liveborn baby, definition, 94
Livedo reticularis, congenital, 1646
Liver, **470–471**, see also Biopsy, liver;
    Viral hepatitis
  abscesses, **478**
    aspiration, **1845**
  amebiasis, 1468
  bronchiolitis, 564
  congenital syphilis, 1412
  cystic fibrosis, **484**, 556
  debranching enzyme deficiency, 1138
  disease
    amino acids, plasma levels, 1103
    anemia, 865
    Children's Liver Disease Foundation,
      485

cholestatic jaundice, 220–221
    vs Christmas disease, 881
    chronic, 471, **480–484**
    coagulation disorder, 882
    hyperlipoproteinemia, 1153–1154
    nutrition, **1209**
  drug metabolism, 1953
  embryology, 206
  examination, 33
  fetus, growth hormone on, 1002
  fructose-1-phosphate aldolase
    deficiency, 1134
  galactose-1-phosphate uridyltransferase
    deficiency, 1133
  gluconeogenesis, SGA baby, 137
  gluconeogenic enzyme deficiencies,
    297
  glucose-6-phosphatase deficiency, 1137
  glycogen storage diseases, 1136
  hemopoiesis, 221, 222, 847
  hydatid disease, **478**, 1505
  imaging, **1906–1907**
  malaria, 1448, 1449
  mitochondrial DNA depletion, 1127
  neonate, 108
    mass, 292 (Table)
    rupture, 224
  neoplasms, 484, **924–925**
    incidence, 886 (Table)
    ultrasonography, 1906
    neuroblastoma, 911
    radiotherapy, 912
  parenteral nutrition, 1226
  rhabdomyosarcoma, 916
  schistosomiasis, 478, 1509–1510
  transaminases, inborn errors of
    metabolism, 306
  transplantation, **484–485**, 1825
    α₁-antitrypsin deficiency, 1176
    for hyperammonemia, 1112
    inborn errors of metabolism, 1102
    with thymus grafts, 1268
    tyrosinemia, 1106
    Wilson's disease, 481
  trauma, 1812
  tyrosinemia, 1106
Liver alkaline phosphatase, neonate, 302
Liver failure
  acute, **478–479**
    after cardiac surgery, 1822
    intensive care, **1824–1825**
Liver fluke infection, **1512–1513**
Liver function tests, 472 (Table)
  infectious mononucleosis, 1367
Liver–kidney transplantation, for oxalosis,
    947
Liver phosphorylase and liver
    phosphorylase b kinase
    deficiencies, 1139
Liver span, 33
Living standards, respiratory disorders,
    489, 559
Lizard skin, onchocerciasis, 1497
LMB group, B cell lymphoma
    chemotherapy, 909
Loa loa, 1496, 1497, **1497**
  eye, 1676, 1677
  specimens, 1299
Lobar emphysema
  congenital, **192, 574**, 1769
  tuberculosis, 1341, 1342
Lobar sequestration, **574**
Lobectomy, cystic adenomatoid
    malformation, 192
Local anesthesia, arterial blood sampling,
    505
Local anesthetic agents, 1832
Local authorities
  care (statutory), **1857–1858, 1875**, 1876
  childhood accidents, 1713
  and child minders, 1860
  Children Act 1989, 1874–1875
  Children (Scotland) Act 1995, 1876
  special educational need, 1864

swimming pools, 1718
Lockable medicine cupboards, 1706
'Locked in' children, 813
Locomotor system, examination, 38–39
Locus, single gene, 64
Lod scores, 73
Löffler's syndrome, **570, 1484**
Logarithms, hormone values, 1001
Loin pain–hematuria syndrome, 959
Lomidine, 1456
Lomotil, diphenoxylate poisoning,
    1709–1710
London, vs Isle of Wight, psychiatric
    disorder, 813
Lone parent families, 15 (Table)
Long-chain acyl CoA dehydrogenase
    deficiency, 297
Long-chain fatty acids, 1148
  polyunsaturated, breast milk, 152
Long-chain glucose polymers,
    bronchopulmonary dysplasia
    prevention, 195
Long-chain 3-hydroxyacyl-CoA
    dehydrogenase deficiency,
    1129–1130
Long-chain lipid emulsions, for cystic
    fibrosis, 1208
Long-chain/very-long-chain acyl-CoA
    dehydrogenase deficiency, 1130
Longitudinal data, growth, 352
Long QT interval syndromes, 626
Long-stay care, mental retardation,
    839–840
Long-term outcomes, information lack,
    104
Long-term parenteral nutrition, 1226
Long-term sequelae, survival, neoplasms,
    897–899, 914
Loop diuretics
  hypokalemia, 145
  nephrotic syndrome, 970
Loop of Henle, 259
Loperamide
  administration, 1970 (Table)
  short bowel syndrome, 1212
  toddler diarrhea, 464
Lorazepam
  premedication, 1970 (Table)
  status epilepticus, 693
Lordosis, 38
Lorenzo's oil, for adrenoleukodystrophy,
    1174
Loss of your baby, The, 175
Lotions, 1617
Louping ill, 1390
Louse-borne relapsing fever, 1322
Louse-borne typhus, epidemic, see Typhus
Low birthweight, 350, **368–369**, see also
    Small for gestational age infant
    (SGA)
  brain damage, 745
  hypoglycemia, 293
  infection, 276
  late effects, 367
Low-density lipoprotein, 1148 (Table),
    1149
  secondary disorders, 1154 (Table)
Lowe and Costello, symbolic play test,
    400
Lower esophageal sphincter, 426
Lower motor neurone lesions, facial
    nerve, 34
Lower reference nutrient intake, 1180
Lower respiratory tract infections,
    564–570, see also named
    conditions
  from common cold, 560
  Haemophilus influenzae, 1307
  mortality, 490 (Table)
  specimens, **1298–1299**
  United Kingdom, mortality, 1276
    (Table)
Lower segment Cesarean section, preterm
    delivery, 120

Lowe's syndrome (oculocerebrorenal
    syndrome), 831 (Table), 948,
    1122–1123
Loxosceles, bites, 1525
L-penicillamine, for cystinuria, 1121
L-thyroxine, see also Sodium-l-thyroxine
  with antithyroid drugs, 1051
L-transposition (congenitally corrected
    transposition of great arteries),
    616
Lucidolytic epidermolysis bullosa, 1622,
    1623 (Table)
Lucey Driscoll syndrome, 219–220
Luft's syndrome, 1127
Lugol's iodine, neonatal hyperthyroidism,
    1051
Lumbar abscess, tuberculosis, 1592
Lumbar puncture, **1840**
  bacteremia, 1287
  bacterial meningitis, **1290**
  cancer treatment, 895
  emergency care, 1814
  and head injuries, 708
  mumps meningitis, 1372
  neonatal meningitis, 281, 282
  neonate, 242
  status epilepticus, 692–693
  subarachnoid hemorrhage, 710
  and tuberculous meningitis, 665
Lumbar spine, diagnostic radiation doses,
    1895 (Table)
Lumboperitoneal shunts, 662
Lumps, see Swellings
Lung:bodyweight ratio, pulmonary
    hypoplasia, 191
Lung compliance, respiratory distress
    syndrome, 177
Lung cysts, 192, 577
  congenital, **574**, 1769
Lung fields, blood flow, 200
Lung function tests, see Respiratory
    function tests
Lungs
  abscesses, 569
  absence, 575
  actinomycosis, 1473
  birth asphyxia, 129
  burns, **571–572**
  cancer survivors, 899
  cirrhosis of liver, 483
  congenital abnormalities, **573**
  congenital syphilis, 1412
  cystic fibrosis, pathophysiology,
    551–552
  cytotoxic drugs, 894 (Table)
  development, **175–177**
    anomalies, **191–193**
    role of kidney, 256
  environmental mycobacteria, **1350**
  examination, 30, **511–513**
  fetal-neonatal transition, **106–107**
  fluke infection, **1513**
  hookworm, 1489
  hydatid disease, 1505, 1506
  hypoplasia, 575
  imaging, **1899–1901**
  magnetic resonance imaging, 1898
  neonate, disorders, **175–198**
  nephroblastoma radiotherapy, 914
  osteosarcoma metastases, 917, 918,
    1916
  scintigraphy, **1901**
  segments, 494 (Fig.)
  tropical eosinophilia syndrome, **1498**
  tuberous sclerosis, 802
  ventilation mechanics, 159
  ventilation trauma, 160–161
  water output, 403 (Table)
Lung volume, testing, **501**
Lupus, see Neonatal lupus erythematosus;
    Systemic lupus erythematosus
Lupus erythematosus, 1644
Lupus nephritis, 964–965
  vs mesangial IgA nephropathy, 963

Luque procedure, 731
Luteinizing hormone, **1038**
  delayed puberty investigation, 1034
  fetus, 1003
  gonadotropin releasing hormone
      modulation, 1024–1026
  levels, 987
  normal values, 1927 (Table)
  spermatogenesis, 1024
Luteinizing hormone:follicle stimulating
      hormone, polycystic ovarian
      disease, 993
Lutzomyia spp., leishmaniasis, 1460
Lyme disease, **1312–1314**
  arthritis, 1313, **1611–1612**
  central nervous system, 795 (Table)
  Fluorescent Treponemal Antibody
      Absorbed Test, 1403
  myeloradiculitis, 725–726
  neonate, 248
Lymphadenitis, *see also* Mesenteric
      adenitis
  BCG vaccination, 1339
  cervical, environmental mycobacteria,
      1349
Lymphadenopathy, *see also* Cervical
      lymphadenopathy
  African trypanosomiasis, 1455
  HIV infection, **1395**
  infectious mononucleosis, 1366
  leishmaniasis, 1462
  leukemias, 871
  neonate, organisms, 284 (Table)
  rubella, 1356
  syphilis
      congenital, 1412
      primary, 1406
      secondary, 1407
  toxoplasmosis, 1465
  tuberculosis, **1343**
      intrathoracic, 1340–1341
Lymphadenosis benigna cutis, 1313
Lymphangiectasia, 193
  intestinal, **443–444**
Lymphangiography, Hodgkin's disease,
      910
Lymphangitis, streptococcal, 1332
Lymphatic filariasis, **1498**
Lymphedema, *see also* Congenital
      lymphedema
  Turner's syndrome, 61 (Fig.), 370
Lymph nodes
  axillary, examination, 30
  head and neck, 30
  immunodeficiency, 1244
Lymphoblastic lymphomas, 907
  chemotherapy, 908–909
  presentation, 907
Lymphocyte depletion, Hodgkin's disease,
      909
Lymphocyte-predominant Hodgkin's
      disease, 909
Lymphocytes
  blood
      fetus and neonate, 848
      normal counts, 1939 (Table)
  cerebrospinal fluid, 696
      mumps meningitis, 1371
      neurosurgery, 664
  gastrointestinal, 439
  HIV infection, 1393
  meningitis, 1290
  metabolism defects, **1250–1251**
  neonate, 223
  pokeweed mitogen test, 1245, 1246
  respiratory tract, 532
  tests, 1245–1247
  tuberculosis, 1335–1336
Lymphocytic choriomeningitis, **1376**
Lymphocytic interstitial pneumonitis, 533
Lymphocytic meningitis, **1375–1376**
Lymphocytosis, pertussis, 1317
Lymphogranuloma venereum, 1432
Lymphoid hyperplasia syndrome, **1395**

Lymphoid interstitial pneumonitis, HIV
      infection, **1395**, 1397
  congenital, 1264
  Epstein–Barr virus, 1366–1367
Lymphoid tissue
  gastrointestinal, 439
  growth curve, 363 (Fig.)
  respiratory, 495, 532
Lymphokines, Langerhans cell
      histiocytosis, 925
Lymphomas
  ataxia telangiectasia, 290
  gallium scintigraphy, 1913
  histiocytic, 927–928
  immune deficiency, 1248
  incidence, 886 (Table)
Lymphopoietic system, neonate, 274–275
Lyonization
  Duchenne muscular dystrophy, 729
  X chromosomes, 67, 948
Lypressin, administration, 1970 (Table)
Lysine, metabolism disorders, **1113**
Lysine dehydrogenase deficiency, 1113
Lysinuria, 1121
Lysinuric protein intolerance, 446, 1121
Lysosomal enzymes, infusion, 1102
Lysosomal a-1,4-glucosidase deficiency,
      see Pompe's disease
Lysosomal storage disorders, **1156–1157**
  central nervous system, **775–779**
      (Table)
Lysosomal transport defects, **1123**
Lysosomes, 1156
Lysozyme, 1234
Lytta, cantharidin, 1525

M2 receptor, asthma, 538
Macleod's syndrome, 576
Macroaggregates, perfusion lung scans,
      517, 1901
Macrocephaly, *see* Megaloencephaly
MACRODUCT sweat test, 552
Macrogametocytes, *Plasmodium* spp., 1446
Macroglossia, 425
Macrolides, pneumonia, 568
Macroorchidism, fragile X mental
      retardation, 63
Macrophage colony stimulating factor,
      1233 (Table)
Macrophage colony stimulating factor 1
      gene, osteopetrosis, 1582
Macrophages, 273–274
  cerebrospinal fluid, 696
  neurosurgery, 664
  HIV infection, 1264
  malaria immunity, 1447
  phagocytic function, 1235
Macrophthalmos, 268
Macula, 1652
Maculae cerulae, pthiriasis, 1519
Macular degenerations, 1666
Macular syphilide (roseola), 1406
Maculopapular rashes, **1285**
MAD deficiency (multiple acyl-CoA
      dehydrogenase deficiencies), 308,
      1130
Madelung's deformity, **1548**
MAD:M (riboflavin-responsive
      dicarboxylic aciduria), 1130
MAD:S (glutaric aciduria type II), 1130
Madura foot, 1477
Maffucci's syndrome, 1586
MAG 3, *see* Renography
Maggots, wounds, 1514
Magnesium, **409**, 1185 (Table)
  concentrations, 404 (Table), 406 (Table)
  deficiency, 1188, **1200–1201**
      NMDA calcium channels, 127
  normal values, 1927 (Table)
      amniotic fluid, 1937 (Table)
      cerebrospinal fluid, 1934 (Table)
      stools, 1936 (Table)
      urine, 1931 (Table)

oral dosage
  chloride, neonate, 1957 (Table)
  hydroxide, 1970 (Table)
  parenteral nutrition, 1222 (Table), 1223
      (Table)
  Recommended Dietary Allowances,
      1949 (Table)
  reference nutrient intakes, 1947 (Table)
  requirements, 1181 (Table)
      preterm infant, 152 (Table)
  sources, 1185 (Table)
  supplements, 302
Magnesium/creatinine ratio, normal
      values, 1931 (Table)
Magnesium hydroxide
  administration, 1970 (Table)
  phosphorus deficiency, 1200
Magnesium sulfate
  administration, neonate, 1957 (Table)
  for birth asphyxia, 131
  on fetus and neonate, 91 (Table)
  for hypomagnesemia, 300–301, 975
  for neonatal tetany, 300
  persistent pulmonary hypertension of
      the newborn, 204
Magnetic resonance imaging, 800–801,
      1898
  birth asphyxia, 128
  bones, 1898, 1916
  brain tumors, 901
  central nervous system, 1898, **1908**
  cerebral palsy, 171
  chest, **1900–1901**
  cranial, neonate, 242
  epilepsy, 678–679
  genital system, 1914
  headache, indications, 715
  head injuries, 707
  Hodgkin's disease, 910
  intracranial hemorrhage, 1914, 1915
      (Fig.)
  liver, 1907
  mesial temporal sclerosis, 686
  myelination failure, 642
  retroperitoneum, **1913**
  thorax, **519**
Magnetic resonance spectroscopy, birth
      asphyxia, 128
'Magoo head', birth trauma, 699
MAGPI procedure, 256, 1794
Maintainable airway, 1807
Maintaining factors, adolescent disorders,
      1751
Maintenance fluid, 1295–1296
Maize, pellagra, 1198
Majewski syndrome, 1571
Major histocompatibility complex
      molecules, 1235, *see also* HLA
      antigens
  common variable immunodeficiency
      and IgA deficiency, 1243
  defects, 1250
Major illness, poliomyelitis, 1379
Major vessel thrombosis, 231
Makaton, 837
Make-believe play, 383
Malabsorption, **439–445**, 467, 1902
  ascariasis, 1482
  cow's milk protein intolerance, 1699
  cystic fibrosis, 445, 449, 553
  diarrhea, 1293
  extrahepatic biliary atresia, 475
  folate deficiency, 852
  giardiasis, 1466
  hypolipoproteinemia, 1154 (Table)
  short gut syndrome, 444–445
  tyrosyluria, 1106
  vitamin B₁₂, 853, 1199
  vitamin D deficiency, 1196
Maladaptive solutions, adolescent
      psychiatric disorder, 1751
Maladie de tics, 768, 771
Malaria, **1445–1453**, 1865
  Burkitt's lymphoma, 891

chloroquine, *see* Chloroquine, malaria
clinical features, **1449–1451**
control, **1453**, 1888
developing countries disease burden,
      1276 (Table), 1280 (Table)
diagnosis, **1451–1452**
  FUO investigations, 1283 (Table)
hemolysis, 864, 1447–1448
immunosuppression by, 1263
neonate, 289
nephrotic syndrome, 968, 1448, 1451
primary health care, 1889
and sickle cell disease, 47
and sickle cell trait, 860
treatment, **1452–1453**
vs visceral leishmaniasis, 1462
Malaria antibodies, 1447
Malassezia spp., 289
Malathion
  head lice, 1518
  pubic lice, 1519
Mal de pinto, *see* Pinta
Male fetus, inadequate masculinization,
      986
Male pseudohermaphroditism, **1008–**
      1010
Malformation syndromes, **75–76**
  neoplasms, 290
Malignancy, *see* Neoplasms
Malignant diarrhea, *see* Refractory
      diarrhea
Malignant epileptic syndromes, **687**
Malignant fibrohistiocytoma, 918
Malignant histiocytosis, 927, **927**
Malignant hyperphenylalaninemia,
      1105–1106
Malignant hyperpyrexia, 150
Malignant teratomas, 920
Malingering, 1658
Malinosculation, 573
Malmö splint, congenital dislocation of
      hip, 1551
Malnutrition, *see also* Protein–energy
      malnutrition
  accelerated BCG reaction, 1339
  acute infective diarrhea, 451–452
  ascariasis, 1482
  chronic disease, 1215–1216
  delayed puberty, 1031
  developed countries, 1186
  developing countries, **1892**
  on growth, 367, 371–372
  growth failure, 1017
  hypothermia, 149
  immunodeficiency, 444, 1265–1266
  mental retardation, 829, 834
  neoplasms, 891
  respiratory disorders, 493, 533
  respiratory tract infections, 559
  thinness, 1023
  tuberculin test, 1337, 1338
  world figures, 1883 (Table)
Malonyl-CoA decarboxylase deficiency,
      1130
Maloprim
  adverse reactions, 1448
  malaria, prophylaxis, 1449
Malpresentations, 83
Malrotation, 210, 1773–1774
  barium studies, 1902
  ultrasonography, 1906
Maltese crosses, Fabry's disease, 1164
Mamba bites, 1522
Mammals, *see* Pets
Mandibulofacial dysostosis
      (Treacher–Collins syndrome),
      25 (Fig.), **1563–1564**, 1661
  speech, 810
Manganese, 1185 (Table), 1202
  estimated safe and adequate daily
      intakes, 1949 (Table)
  parenteral nutrition, 1221 (Table)
  neurological impairment, 1226
  safe intakes, 1948 (Table)

Manic depression, *see* Bipolar depressive
   illness
Manifest squint, 1652
Manipulative skills, 382–383
   development of, **668–669**
   history taking, 18
Mannan-binding lectin (MBL), 1234
   deficiency, 1263
   measurement, 1245
Mannerisms, 771
   mental retardation, 834
Mannitol
   administration, 1970 (Table)
    neonate, 1957 (Table)
   birth asphyxia, 131
   on brain, 699
   brain swelling, 708, 1799
   and cerebral microcirculation, 715
   on CSF production, 664
   status epilepticus, 693
Mannose-binding lectin, *see* Mannan-
   binding lectin
Mannosidoses, 780 (Table), 1157 (Table),
   1159, **1168**
Manometry
   anorectal, 464–465
   esophageal, 429
Mansonella spp., 1496 (Table),
   1498–1499
M antigen, β-hemolytic streptococci, 1330
Mantoux reaction, 286, 1337–1338
Manufacturers, formula milks for inborn
   errors of metabolism, 1120 (Table)
Maple syrup urine disease, 297,
   1116–1117
   carriers, 1101
   diet, 1116–1117, 1119, **1203 (Table)**
   formula milk for, 1120 (Table)
Map units, 72
Marasmus, 371, 1192
Marble bones disease, *see* Osteopetrosis
Marbling, fat, growth hormone deficiency,
   1016 (Fig.)
Marburg virus disease, **1388–1389**
Marchesani syndrome, eye, 1676
Marcus Gunn jaw-winking syndrome,
   1661
Marfan's syndrome, 72 (Table), 376, 596,
   875, **1587–1589**
   eye, 1676
   vs homocystinuria, 77
   inheritance, 1566 (Table)
Margins, economic, 105
Marijuana, 1762
Marine animals, stings, 1526
Marinesco–Sjögren syndrome, 646, 753,
   831 (Table)
Marker proteins, antiviral therapy, 1530
Maroteaux–Lamy disease, 784 (Table),
   1157 (Table), **1161,** 1164
Maroteaux type metaphyseal
   chondrodysplasia, 1579 (Table)
Marriage, births outside, 1854–1855
   adoption, 1858
   school performance, 1859
Masculinization, congenital, 986
Masquerade syndrome, *see* School refusal
Mass chemoprophylaxis, malaria, 1449
Mass immunization campaigns, 345
   BCG vaccination, 1338
Massive pulmonary hemorrhage, *see*
   Pulmonary hemorrhage
Mass spectrometry, organic acidurias,
   1119
Mast cells, 1647
Masticatory nucleus, 811
Mastocytoma, 1647
Mastocytosis, **1646–1647**
Mastoiditis
   acute, 1680
   environmental mycobacteria, 1349
   measles, 1355
   Pseudomonas aeruginosa, 1320
Masturbation, 1745

Matched related donor bone marrow
   transplantation, 1269
Matched unrelated donor bone marrow
   transplantation, 874, 1270
Matches, 1714
Maternal age
   on childhood mortalities, 3 (Table)
   Down syndrome, 56
   Klinefelter's syndrome, 62
   trisomy 18, 57
Maternal anticoagulant therapy, 230
Maternal anticonvulsant therapy, 230
Maternal anxiety, feeding difficulties,
   209
Maternal breast milk membrane, 219
Maternal diabetes mellitus, 89 (Table),
   295
   hypoglycemia, 1083
Maternal disease, stillbirth rates, 4
   (Table)
Maternal drugs, on fetus and neonate,
   90–91, 772
Maternal factors
   composition of breast milk, 332
   endocrine diseases, 998, **1005**
   neoplasms, 889
Maternal Health and Safe Motherhood
   Program (World Health
   Organization), 1891
Maternal hyperparathyroidism, 89 (Table),
   299, 300
Maternal hyperphenylalaninemia,
   1104–1105
Maternal immunization, group B
   streptococcus, 1267
Maternal immunoglobulins, 1240
Maternal infections, 11
Maternal medullary carcinoma of thyroid,
   300
Maternal serum α-fetoprotein, Down
   syndrome, 56
Maternal specific IgG platelet antibody,
   228
Maternal vitamin B_{12} deficiency, 853
Maternity and Child Welfare Act 1918,
   1862
Maternity services, district hospitals, 156
Maternity Survey 1946, 1851
Maternofetal transfusion, 227
Mathematics, *see* Dyscalculia
Mattresses, heated water-filled, 147–148
Maturation, psychological, 1728
Mature dependence, adolescence, 1750
Mature teratomas, 920
   management, 922
Maturity-onset diabetes in the young
   (MODY), 1072, 1081
Mauriac's syndrome, 1079
Maxilla
   cleft palate surgery, 1797
   osteomyelitis, 22 (Fig.)
Maxillary sinusitis, 1685
Maximal mid-expiratory flow, cystic
   fibrosis, 554
Maximum concentrating ability, kidney,
   1938 (Table)
Maximum expiratory flow volume,
   499–500
Maximum intensity projection, magnetic
   resonance imaging, 1898
Maxolon, *see* Metoclopramide
May–Hegglin anomaly, 876, 879
Mazzoti test, 1497
MBL associated protein (MASP), 1234
McArdle syndrome (muscle
   phosphorylase deficiency), 735,
   789 (Table), 1139
McBurney's point, 1786
McCarthy Scales of Children's Abilities,
   827
McCoy cell culture, *Chlamydia* spp., 1430
McCune–Albright syndrome (polyostotic
   fibrous dysplasia), 1028–1029
   1589

M cells, gastrointestinal immune response,
   439
McKusick's gene catalogs, 77
Mdr-1 gene, cytotoxic drug resistance,
   893
Mean airway pressure
   vs oxygenation, 163
   ventilation for RDS, 181
Mean corpuscular hemoglobin
   concentration
   vs age, 849 (Table)
   neonate, 223 (Table)
   normal values, 1939 (Table)
Mean corpuscular volume
   vs age, 849 (Table)
   neonate, 223 (Table)
   normal values, 1939 (Table)
Mean transit times, cerebral blood flow,
   661
Measles, 286 (Table), 510, **1353–1356**
   AIDS, 1396
   cancer treatment, 895
   deafness, 1682
   electroencephalography, 683
   eye, **1354,** 1676
   giant cell pneumonia, 510, **535, 1354**
   immunosuppression, 1264
   mouth, 424, **1354**
   neurological complications, 1376
   prevalence, 490
   rash, 1285
   vs scarlet fever, 1331, 1354
   strabismus, 1659
   trends, 7
   United Kingdom, 1276, 1277 (Fig.)
   vaccination
    contraindications, 342 (Table)
    early, 344
    egg intolerance, 1700
    foreign travel, 345
    mass, 345
    mortality, 343 (Table)
    UK, 345
   vaccine, 1356
    and subacute sclerosing
    panencephalitis, 343
Measles–mumps–rubella vaccine, *see*
   MMR vaccine
Measles virus, inflammatory bowel
   disease, 456
'Measly' meat, 1500
Meatal atresia, ear, 1679
Meatal stenosis, 1679
Meat tenderizer, insect stings, 1524
Mebendazole
   Acanthocephala, 1513
   administration, 1970 (Table)
   ascariasis, 1485
   enterobiasis, 1488
   helminthoma, 1494
   hookworm, 1490
   Trichuris trichiuria, 1491
Mechanical ptosis, 1662
Mecillinam, administration, 1970 (Table)
Meckel–Gruber syndrome, **646,** 752, 753
Meckel's diverticulum, **1787,** 1902
   ascariasis, 1483
   scintigraphy, 447, 460, 1787, **1906**
Meconium
   amniotic fluid staining, 116–117, 124,
    132–133, 185
   first passage, 108, 110, 111
   normal values, 1936 (Table)
Meconium aspiration syndrome, 129, 165,
   185–186
   pneumothorax, 185, 187
Meconium ileus, 210, **449,** 551, 553, 1776
   contrast enema, 1904
Meconium plug syndrome, **1776–1777**
Median facial cleft syndrome, 647
Mediastinal shift, pulmonary interstitial
   emphysema, 188
Mediastinum
   Hodgkin's disease, 909

   treatment, 910
   masses, 575
   non-Hodgkin's lymphoma, 909
   teratomas, 922
Medical evidence, admission to care, 1858
Medical gases, neonatal resuscitation, 133
Medical inspection, school health services,
   1863
Medical negligence, **1877–1880**
Medical records, *see* Record keeping
Medical services, pediatric, **1852–1853**
Medical staff, neonatal care, 96
Medicine cupboards, lockable, 1706
Medicines, *see also* Drugs
   poisoning by, 1705, **1708–1709**
Medicoal, 1707
Medicolegal aspects, *see also* Legal issues
   non-accidental injury, head injuries, **703**
   prescribing, 1955
   sudden infant death syndrome,
    1720–1721
Medilog system (Oxford), 243
Mediterranean fever (fiévre boutonneuse),
   1392
Medium chain acyl CoA dehydrogenase
   deficiency, 297, 1083, **1129**
Medium chain fatty acids, 1148
Medium chain triglycerides
   breast milk substitutes, 208
   restriction, hepatic encephalopathy, 483
Medroxyprogesterone, Ondine's curse,
   531
Medulla
   neural tube defects, 657
   ultrasonography, 1908
Medullary carcinoma of thyroid, 1052
   maternal, 300
Medullary cystic disease, kidney, 255, 941
Medullary sponge kidneys, 941
Medulloblastomas, 899, 900, **901–902,**
   906
Mefenamic acid, 928
   administration, 1970 (Table)
   dysfunctional uterine bleeding, 992
   dysmenorrhea, 992
   poisoning, 1710
Mefloquine, 1449, 1452 (Table)
Megacolon, 642
   chronic constipation, 462
   neurofibromatosis, 800
   toxic, 458, 464
Megacystis–megaureter, 255
Megakaryoblastic leukemia, 869
Megakaryocytes, fetus, 222
   and neonate, 848
Megalencephaly, 834
Megaloblastic anemia, **852–854**
   Diphyllobothrium latum, 1503–1504
Megaloblastic erythrocytes, primitive, 848
Megalocornea, 1672–1673
Megaloencephaly, 1558
Megalopyge spp., shock syndrome, 1526
Megavoltage radiotherapy, neoplasms, 893
Meibomian cyst, 1662
Meige's syndrome, 772
Meiosis, **47–48**
Melanocytes, 641, 1616
   neurofibromatosis, 800
Melanocyte stimulating hormones,
   1037–1038
Melanocytic nevi, **1617–1618, 1798**
Melanoma
   from nevi, 1618
    risk, 1617
   second primary, 898 (Table)
Melarsoprol, **1457**
MELAS syndrome, 682, 711, **736,** 1127
Melatonin, 1043
Melena, 459
   Apt test, 224
Melioidosis, 1321
Meloidae, *see* Blister beetles
Melorheostosis, **1585**
Melphalan, neuroblastoma, 913

Membrane
  diphtheria, 561, 1305, 1306
  pharynx, 511, 560
Membrane defects, hereditary hemolytic
    anemias, 857–860
Membrane potential, 404, 405, **406–407**
Membranes, permeability, **405**
Membranoproliferative
    glomerulonephritis, **963–964**
  complement deficiency, 1263
Membranous conjunctivitis, 1663
Membranous glomerulonephritis, 964
Memorials, neonatal death, 174
Memory, 820
  kinesthetic, 669, 822
Menadiol, 1209, 1970 (Table)
Menarche, 357, 1026
  twins, 366
Meninges
  leukemia, 870, **871**
  rhabdomyosarcoma, 915
Meningitis, 1814, see also Bacterial
    meningitis; Viral infections,
    meningitis
  borreliosis, 1313
  Coxsackie A viruses, 1381
  Coxsackie B viruses, 1382
  deafness, 1291, 1292, 1682
  duplication cysts of duodenum, 192
  ECHO viruses, 1383
  eosinophilic, angiostrongyliasis, 1494
  febrile convulsions, 683
  gonococcal, 1426
    treatment, 1428
  head injuries, **708**
  herpes simplex, 1439, 1442
  leptospirosis, 1312
  mental retardation, 842
  mortality, trends, 7
  mumps, 1371, 1372
  neonate, **247–248**, 281–282, 284
    (Table)
    antibiotic therapy, 279
    bacterial, 1289
    mortality, 4 (Table)
    seizures, 245 (Table), 247
  plague, 1318
  Pseudomonas aeruginosa, 1320
  Streptococcus pneumoniae, see
    Streptococcus pneumoniae,
    meningitis stroke, 713
  vs subarachnoid hemorrhage, 707
  vs tetanus, 1334
  tuberculosis, see Tuberculosis,
    meningitis
  United Kingdom, mortality, 1276
    (Table)
  vomiting, 212
Meningoceles, 653
  craniomeningoceles, 648
Meningococcus, see Neisseria
    meningitidis
Meningoencephalitis
  African trypanosomiasis, 1455–1456
  cryptococcosis, 1476
  neonate, 284 (Table)
  primary amebic, **1469**
  primary herpetic, 1364, 1365
  Q fever, 1374
  toxoplasmosis, 1465
Menkes' kinky hair syndrome, 711, 791
    (Table), 1146, 1202
Menstruation
  estimation of excess, 991–992
  migraine, 717
Mental Health (Scotland) Act, mental
    retardation, 840
Mental retardation, **826–842**
  chromosome studies, 50
  congenital rubella, 286
  Dandy–Walker syndrome, 645
  Duchenne muscular dystrophy, 729,
    730
  dystrophia myotonica, 734

genetic disorders, 46
gonadotropin deficiency, 1031
Hurler's syndrome, 1158
from incest, 1870
language disorder, 818
management, **837–841**
maternal hyperphenylalaninemia, 1104
    (Table)
medical ascertainment, **829–834**
metabolic screening, 1102
neuroleptic drugs, 772
obesity, 1022
Pierre Robin syndrome, 1562
preventive measures, **841–842**
profound, 839–840
recurrence risks, 74
Sanfilippo's syndrome, 1160
screening, **837**, 840
severely handicapped children affected,
    14 (Table)
stereotypies, 673
tuberous sclerosis, 1625
Mental state examination, see
    Examination, psychiatric disorder
Menthols, poisoning, 1711
Mepacrine, giardiasis, 1467, 1970 (Table)
Meptazinol, 1323
β-Mercaptolactate-cysteine disulfiduria,
    1109
Mercaptopropionylglycine, for cystinuria,
    1121
6-Mercaptopurine
  acute lymphoblastic leukemia, 873
  immunosuppression, 1265
  toxic effects, 894 (Table)
Mercurochrome, omphalocele, 1780
Mercury poisoning, 1708
  mouth, 424
  nephrotic syndrome, 972
  primary dentition, 425
Merkel cells, 1616
Meropenem, administration, 1970 (Table)
Merosin, congenital muscular dystrophies,
    729
Merozoites, Plasmodium spp., 1445–1446
MERRF syndrome, 682, 736, 787 (Table),
    1127
Merrill Palmer Scales of Mental
    Development, 827
Mesangial IgA nephropathy, 962–963
Mesencephalon, 642
Mesenteric adenitis, adenoviruses, 1384
Mesentery, 435
Mesial temporal lobe structures, epilepsy
    and learning, 690
Mesial temporal sclerosis, 685–686
Mesna, 896
Mesoblastic hemopoiesis, 221
Mesoblastic nephroma, **915**
  congenital, 255, 292 (Table)
  incidence, 290 (Table)
Mesocardia, 598, 612, 613
Mesodermal defects, spine, 651
Mesomelia, 76 (Table)
Mesomelic dysplasia, **1580–1581**
Messenger RNA, 68, 69
Metabolic acidosis, 419, 420, 504
  correction, 307
  glutathione synthetase deficiency, 1115
  inborn errors of metabolism, 305
  and organic acidurias, **1118–1119**
Metabolic alkalosis, 419, 420, 504
Metabolic bone disease
  preterm infant, **301–304**, see also
    Osteopenia
  radiography, 1915
Metabolic disorders, see also Inborn errors
    of metabolism
  acute, neonate, 304–307
  apnea, 197 (Table)
  ataxia, 762, 765
  causing acute cerebral dysrhythmias,
    675 (Table)
  complications of parenteral nutrition,

1225–1226
  with dysmorphic features, 308
  emergency care, 1814, 1815
  eye signs, **1673–1674**
  myopathies, 735–736, **1132**
  neonate, 248–249, **290–309**
  neutrophil chemotactic defects, 1261
  screening, 1101–1102
    heart muscle disease, 635 (Table)
  storage disorders, 307–308, see also
    Lysosomal storage disorders;
    substance names
  vomiting, 212
Metabolic rates
  under radiant warmer, 149
  and sudden infant death syndrome,
    1722
Metacentric chromosomes, 53
Metachromatic leukodystrophies, **776–777**
    (Table), 1157 (Table), **1164–1165**
Metacyclic trypomastigotes, 1454
Metagonimus yokogawai, 1513
Meta-iodobenzylguanidine (MIBG), 1913
Metaldehyde poisoning, 1711
Metanephrine, normal values, urine, 1931
    (Table)
Metanephros, 253, 934
Metaphase, 47
Metaphyseal chondrodysplasias,
    1578–1579
  inheritance, 1566 (Table)
Metaphyseal fractures, non-accidental
    injury, 1867
Metaphyses, shaking injury, 701
Metastases
  bone scintigraphy, 1916
  Ewing's sarcoma, 919
  nephroblastoma, 913
  osteosarcoma, 917, 918
  rhabdomyosarcoma, management, 917
  transplacental, 289
Metastatic uveitis, 1677
Metatarsus varus and hallux valgus,
    1555–1556
Metatropic dysplasia, **1577**
Metencephalin, 1038
Methadone withdrawal, neonatal seizures,
    245
Methemalbumin, 856
Methemoglobin, expected values, 1927
    (Table)
Methemoglobinemia, 202 (Table), **864–865**
  hemoglobinopathies, 861, 862, **864–865**
  neonate, 849
Methemoglobin reductase, 864
Methicillin
  administration, 1970 (Table)
  neonate, 279 (Table)
Methicillin-resistant S. aureus, 1329
Methionine, 1108
  administration, 1970 (Table)
  cobalamin disorders, 1148
  malabsorption of, 1122
  for paracetamol poisoning, 1710
  plasma levels
    homocystinuria, 1109
    neonate, 1109
Methionine adenosyl transferase
    deficiency, 1109
Methotrexate
  acute lymphoblastic leukemia
    central nervous system, 873
    continuation therapy, 873
  on fetus and neonate, 91 (Table)
  immunosuppression, 1265
  juvenile chronic arthritis, 1604
  resistance, 892
  toxic effects, 894 (Table), 896, 897
2-Methylacetoacetyl-CoA thiolase
    deficiency, 1130
Methyl B₁₂ synthesis, cobalamin
    disorders, 1148
Methylcellulose, administration, 1970
    (Table)

3-Methylcrotonylglycinuria, 1117
Methyldopa, administration, 1970
    (Table)
Methylene blue, for methemoglobinemia,
    864–865
Methylene chloride, poisoning, 1711
N⁵,¹⁰-Methylenetetrahydrofolate reductase
    deficiency, 1109
3-Methylglutaconyl-CoA hydratase defect,
    1117
Methylhistidine, 1114, 1115
Methylmalonic acidemias, 297, 1100,
    1117
Methylmalonic acidosis, 420 (Table)
Methylmalonic aciduria, with
    homocystinuria, 853, 1109
Methylmalonic semialdehyde
    dehydrogenase defect, 1117–1118
Methylmalonyl-CoA, catabolism,
    cobalamin disorders, 1148
Methylphenidate, 1744, 1748 (Table)
  administration, 1971 (Table)
  extrapyramidal effects, 771, 772
  overactivity, 841
  tics, 768
Methylprednisolone
  administration, 1971 (Table)
  nephrotic syndrome, 970
  Pneumocystis carinii pneumonia, 535
  systemic lupus erythematosus, 1606
Methyltestosterone, administration, 1971
    (Table)
N⁵-Methyltetrahydrofolate cyclohydrase
    deficiency, 852
α-Methyltransferase, 641
Metoclopramide
  administration, 1971 (Table)
  antiemetic, 896
  poisoning, 1710
  vs tetanus, 1334
Metolazone, nephrotic syndrome, 970
Metoprolol, administration, 1971 (Table)
Metriphonate
  administration, 1971 (Table)
  schistosomiasis, 1511
Metronidazole
  administration, 1956 (Table)
  amebiasis, 1469
    hepatic, 478
  bacterial vaginosis, 1435
  Crohn's disease, 457–458
  dracunculosis, 1496
  giardiasis, 1467
  mechanism, 1527
  neonate, 279 (Table)
    pneumonia prevention, 184
  pelvic inflammatory disease, 1432
  trichomoniasis, **1435**
Metronomic myoclonus, 769
Metyrapone, administration, 1971 (Table)
Mevalonic aciduria, 1156
Mexiletine, administration, 1971 (Table)
Mianserin, poisoning, 1710
Micelles, 437
Miconazole, 289, 1434, 1472, **1478**
  administration, 1956 (Table), 1971
    (Table)
Microalbuminuria
  diabetes mellitus, 966, 1080
  after hemolytic uremic syndrome, 978
Microaneurysms, diabetic retinopathy,
    1674
Microangiopathic hemolytic anemia, 864
Microbiology, see also Bacteriology
  neonate, 276–277
Microcephaly, 21 (Fig.), 642, 650, 1558
  IQ, 834
  maternal hyperphenylalaninemia, 1104
    (Table)
  severely handicapped children affected,
    14 (Table)
Microcystic disease
  congenital nephrotic syndrome, 971
  kidney, 255

Microdysgenesis, cerebral cortex, 685
Microencephaly, **649–650**
Micro-ESR, 276 (Table), 277
Microfibrils, Marfan's syndrome, 1587
Microgallbladder, cystic fibrosis, 484
Microgametocytes, *Plasmodium* spp., 1446
Micrognathia, 25 (Fig.), 43
Micro-IF test, *Chlamydia pneumoniae*, 1433
Microlithiasis, alveolar, 578
Micromoles, 1921
Micronutrient deficiencies, *see also specific nutrients*
  developing countries, 1892
Micropapular psoriasis, 1628
Micropenis, 1006–1007
Micropolygyria, 642
Microscopy
  African trypanosomiasis, 1456
  candidiasis, 1434
  cholera, 1304
  syphilis, 1402
  trichomoniasis, 1434–1435
  urine, 950–951, 958, 959, 1299
Microsomal enzyme systems, drug metabolism, 1953
Microsphere pancreatic enzyme supplements, enteric-coated, 557
Microspherocytes, 857
Microspherocytosis, 217
Microtia, 1679
Microvillous atrophy, congenital, 442–443
Micturating cystourethrography, **1911**
  neonate, 262
  urinary tract infections, 953
  vesicoureteric reflux, 956, **1911**
Micturition, *see also* Wetting problems
  history taking, 18
  neonate, 110, 111
  neural tube defect, 656
'Midcavity' forceps delivery, preterm, 120
Middle cerebral artery
  aneurysms, 710
  fetal blood flow, 115
  infarction, seizures, 245
Middle finger length, *vs* total hand length, 39
Midgut, 206
Midline defects, growth hormone deficiency, 372, 1016
Midline shift, intracranial, 698
Mid-pregnancy, antenatal care, 81
Midstream urine specimens, 950
  clean-catch, 950, 1299
Mid upper arm circumference, 1186
Midwife units, delivery in, 84
Migraine, **716–719**
  abdominal, 461, 717, 718
  ischemic episodes, 671
  management, 717–719
  psychogenic vomiting, 434
  transient blindness, 1658
  vascular spasm, 712–713
Migraleve, 717 (Table), 718
Migrating motor complexes, 438
Migril, 717 (Table)
Milia, 1646
  epidermolysis bullosa, 1622
Miliaria, 1646
Miliary tuberculosis, 1336, **1343–1344**
Milk curd obstruction, 1776
Milk feeds
  small-volume, preterm infant, 151
  technetium-99m sulfur colloid scintigraphy, 1906
Milks, **112–113,** *see also* Breast milk; Formula milks
  absorption, 207
  Actinobacillus muris, 1322
  amino acids, 1119, 1120 (Table)
  aspiration, 186
    preterm infant, 155
  brain lipid formation, 643

composition, 1942–1943 (Table)
  special formulae, 1944–1945 (Table)
cystic fibrosis, 1207–1208
folate content, effect of heating, 852
intake levels, 333
for malnutrition, 1193
for necrotizing enterocolitis, 212
preterm infant, **152–153**
toddlers, 1189
vitamin D fortification, 1196–1197
vitamin K, 230
Milk scans, gastroesophageal reflux, 212, **519**
Miller Diekker syndrome, 59, 60 (Table), 650
Millimetres of mercury, 698
Millimoles, 1921
Millipore filters
  cerebrospinal fluid cell collection, 696
  parenteral nutrition, 159
Milroy's disease, *see* Congenital lymphedema
Mineralocorticoid excess, *see also* Apparent mineralocorticoid excess
  hypokalemic alkalosis, 946
Minerals
  deficiencies, **1200–1203**
  dietary, 1183, 1185 (Table)
  parenteral nutrition, 1221
  preterm milk formulae, 152
  Recommended Dietary Allowances, 1949 (Table)
  safe intakes, 1948 (Table)
Miniature anion exchange centrifugation technique, African trypanosomiasis, 1456
Miniature congenital adrenal hypoplasia, 1067
Minicore disease, 735 (Table)
Minimal change disease, nephrotic syndrome, 968–969
  congenital, 972
Minimal hemiparesis, 744
Minimal inhibitory concentrations, antibiotics, **1529**
Minimal inhibitory dilutions, 1530
Minimal residual disease, leukemia, 869
Minimum data sets, accident surveillance, 1803
Mini-pill, 995
Minocycline
  administration, 1971 (Table)
  leprosy, 1311
Minor illness, poliomyelitis, 1379
Minoxidil
  administration, 1971 (Table)
  hypertension, 637 (Table)
  renal, 973 (Table)
Minute ventilation, 160, 163
Miscarriages
  genetic disorders, 46
  previous history, 18
Miscarriage, stillbirth and neonatal death, 175
Mismatched bone marrow transplantation, 1269–1270, *see also* Parent-to-child bone marrow transplantation
Missile injuries, 705
Mist, bronchiolitis, 564–565
Mistrust *vs* trust (Erikson), 1730
Mites, 1517, *see also* Demodicidosis; Scabies
  scrub typhus, 1392
Mitochondria, *see also* DNA, mitochondrial
  energy generation, disorders, **1123–1130**
  genetics, 1126
Mitochondrial acetoacetyl-CoA thiolase deficiency, 1130
Mitochondrial cytopathy, 68, 209
Mitochondrial DNA, depletion, 1127
Mitochondrial encephalopathy with lactic acidosis and stroke-like episodes

(MELAS), 682, 711, 736, 787 (Table), 1127
Mitochondrial inheritance, **68**
Mitochondrial myopathies, 736
  with multiple deletions of mtDNA, 1127
Mitochondrial neurogastrointestinal encephalopathy (MNGIE), 1127
Mitochondrial oxidation defects, fatty acids, 297
Mitogen responses, lymphocytes, 1246
Mitogens, 48
Mitosis, **47**
Mitral atresia, 620
Mitral regurgitation
  acute carditis, 628
  atrioventricular septal defect, 604
  rheumatic, 629
Mitral stenosis
  congenital, 609
  rheumatic, 629
Mitral valve
  cleft of anterior leaflet, 604
  prolapse, **610**
    atrial septal defect, 602
Mixed acidosis, 504
Mixed apnea, 197 (Table)
Mixed cellularity Hodgkin's disease, 909
Mixed connective tissue disease, **1609**
Mixed gonadal dysgenesis, 1009–1010
Mixed micellar vitamin K, 230
MK-801 (NMDA receptor antagonist), 131
M mode echocardiography, 590
  atrial septal defect, 590 (Fig.), 591 (Fig.), 602
  mitral stenosis, 629
MMR vaccine, 287, 1356
  delay after gammaglobulin therapy, 1480
  egg intolerance, 1700
Modified Allen's test, 1835
Modular feeds, cystic fibrosis, 1208
Modules, cerebral cortex, 644–645
Moebius' syndrome, 209, 719, 811
Mohr's syndrome, 1564, 1565 (Table)
Molality, 405
Molarity, 405
Molar sodium bicarbonate, respiratory distress syndrome, 179
Molding of muscle, 756
Molds, spores, 1690
Molecular biology, vaccine development, 342
Molecular genetics
  Duchenne muscular dystrophy, 729
  neoplasms, 891
  techniques, **70–72**
Molecular heterogeneity, 69
Mole (unit), 405, 1921
Molluscicides, 1511
Molluscum contagiosum, **1388, 1633**
  AIDS, 1395
  vs anogenital warts, 1444
  eyelids, 1663
  eye region, 1675
Molluscum fibrosum, 1628
Molybdenum, 1185 (Table), 1202
  estimated safe and adequate daily intakes, 1949 (Table)
  parenteral nutrition, 1221 (Table)
  safe intakes, 1948 (Table)
Molybdenum cofactor deficiency, **1147**
Monetary units, cost comparisons, 104, 105
Mongolian blue spots, 42
Moniliasis, *see* Candidiasis
Monitoring
  antimicrobial therapy, **1529–1530**
  after apparent life-threatening events, 529
  asthma, **544**
  birth asphyxia, **128–129**
  blood gases, 160

epilepsy, 691
fetus, labor, 86–87
head injuries, 708
intracranial pressure, 661, 663, **697–698**
  preterm infant, 197
  therapeutic ranges, **1954**
Monkeys, Marburg virus disease, 1388, 1389
Monoblastic leukemia, 869
Monoclonal antibodies
  lymphocyte tests, 1246
  lymphoma classification, 907
  therapeutic radionuclides, 1897
Monocytes, 925
  CD14, 1232 (Table)
  count
    neonate, 223 (Table)
    normal, 1939 (Table)
  fetus, 222
    and neonate, 848
  HIV infection, 1264
  phagocytic function, 1235
    defects, 1262
  tissue factor, 231
Monoiodotyrosine, 1044
Monosodium glutamate, 1115–1116
  migraine, 716
Monospot test, infectious mononucleosis, 1367
Monosulfiram, scabies, 1517, 1971 (Table)
Monounsaturated fatty acids, 1182
Monozygotic twins, 90
Mood
  disorders, **1742**
  history taking, 18
Moon's molar, 1414
MOPP regimen, Hodgkin's disease, 910
Moral development, 1731
Morbidity, **8–9**
  accidents, **1712**
  asthma, 536
  infections, 1276
  neonates, 95
  statistics, **1849–1850**
  status epilepticus, 692
  studies, **1851–1852**
Morbus errorum, 1518
Morgagni foraminal hernia, 1769
Morganella spp., 1320
Morning dip, asthma, 549
Moro reflex, 37 (Table), 238 (Fig.), 240
  gestation age, 40 (Table)
Morphea, 1644–1645
Morphine, 928
  administration, 1971 (Table)
    neonate, 1957 (Table)
  intravenous, *vs* epidural analgesia, 1831
  preterm infant, 1833
  with ventilation, 1833
Morphological index, leprosy, 1310
Morquio syndrome, 784 (Table), 1159, **1160–1161,** 1573 (Fig.), 1580
  vs GM$_1$-gangliosidosis, 1163
'Morsitans' group tsetse flies, 1454
Mortality, **2–8,** 1849
  accidents, **1711–1712**
  anorexia nervosa, 1759
  apneic attacks, 198
  appendicitis, 1786
  asthma, 490 (Table), 536
  bronchopulmonary dysplasia, 195
  cerebral malaria, 1451
  congenital heart disease, 595–596
  diphtheria, 1305
  Down syndrome, 55
  epilepsy, 687
  genetic disorders, 46
  HIV vertical transmission, 288
  hypernatremia, 415
  infections, **1275–1281**
  Kawasaki disease, 1480
  malnutrition, 1193
  measles, 1353

Mortality (*Contd*)
neonate
definitions, 94
hyperthyroidism, 1051
sepsis, 277, 278
from parenteral nutrition, 1226
pneumopericardium, 189
pneumothorax, 188
pulmonary interstitial emphysema, 189
respiratory disorders, **489–490**
schooling of mothers, **1886–1887**
status epilepticus, 692
studies, **1851–1852**
trends, **7–8**
under-5, **1882–1884**
vaccination, 343 (Table)
vitamin A deficiency, 1194
Morular cells, African trypanosomiasis, 1455
Mosaicism, 51, 53
cytogenetic nomenclature, 54
Down syndrome, 56
Killian–Pallister syndrome, 60
Klinefelter's syndrome, 62
Turner's syndrome, 62, 370, 1032
Mosquitoes, avoiding, 1448, 1453
Mothballs, paradichlorobenzene, poisoning, 1711
Mother–baby package (WHO), 1891
Mothering, 112
Mothers, *see also* Working mothers; *entries starting* Maternal age, 15 (Table)
antenatal transfer, 157
attachment to, 1731
care of neonate, 110–111
death in childbirth, 1891
developing countries, 1882
fetomaternal transfusion, 224
neonatal thrombocytopenia from, 229
one-parent families, 1854
and phototherapy, 218–219
psychiatric illness, 1712
schooling of, **1886–1887**, 1892
syphilis treatment, 284
unmarried, 1855
as widows, 1857
Motility
colon, 451
investigations, 464–465
intestinal, 424, **451**
preterm infant, 208
small intestine, 208, **438**
stomach, 430
Motion sickness, migraine, 717
Motivation, learning, 819
Motor development, examination, 388–391 (Table), 393
Motor disability, chronic, management, 755–761
Motor dysgraphia, 821–823
Motor retardation, 1754
Motor skills, *see also* Articulatory dyspraxia; Dyspraxia
ataxia, 752
normal development, **381–383**
Mott cells, African trypanosomiasis, 1455
Mourning, *see* Grief
'Mouse', capillary blood sample, 1834
Mouse inoculation, rabies, 1377
Mouse poison, 1709
Mouth, **424–425**, *see also* Oral hygiene; Oral moniliasis
examination, **27–29**, 511
Kawasaki disease, 1479
measles, 1354
neonate, 43
non-accidental injury, 1868–1869
Mouth to cecal transit time, 438
Movement assessment battery, 400
Movement disorders, **738–774**
on development, 386
dysgraphia, 822–823
examination, 34

infancy in terms of, 741
Movements, *see also* Motor development
developmental disorders, **667–668**
involuntary, history taking, 17
neonate, 236
spontaneous
fetus, 115
neonate, 44
Moxalactam, neonate, 279 (Table)
Moya moya, 711
Mucociliary escalator, 497, **532**
scintigraphy, 517
Mucocutaneous candidiasis, chronic, 1243 (Table), **1251**, 1637
Mucocutaneous leishmaniasis, 1463
metastasis prevention, 1464
Mucocutaneous lymph node syndrome, *see* Kawasaki disease
Mucolipidoses, 1157 (Table), 1159, **1169–1171**
type I, *see* Sialic acid storage diseases
type II, *see* I-cell disease
type III, 782 (Table)
type IV, 782 (Table), 1169
Mucolytic agents, bronchial instillation, 520
Mucopolysaccharides, normal values, urine, 1931 (Table)
Mucopolysaccharidoses, 783–784 (Table), 1157, **1158–1162**
neonate, 307
urine tests, 837
Mucormycosis, 1471 (Table)
Mucosa
oral, 424–425
small intestine, 435
Mucositis, cytotoxic drugs, 896
Mucous patches
endemic syphilis, 1419
syphilis, 1407
Mucus
bronchi, 532
stomach, 430–431
Müllerian duct system
failure syndromes, 991
persistent structures, 1008
Müllerian inhibiting hormone, 1004
Multiaxial systems, psychiatric diagnosis, 1733
Multicore disease, 735 (Table)
Multicystic kidney disease, 254, 936–937
ultrasonography, 1910
Multicystic ovaries, anorexia nervosa, 1023
Multidisciplinary district handicap teams, 400, 1853
Multidisciplinary meetings, sudden infant death syndrome, 1721, 1723
Multidrug resistance protein, Dubin–Johnson syndrome, 1145
Multifactorial inheritance, **74–75**
risk calculation, 75
Multinucleate giant cells, tuberculosis, 1335
Multiple acyl-CoA dehydrogenase deficiencies, 308, 1130
Multiple birth, *see also* Multiple pregnancy
on childhood mortalities, 3 (Table)
Multiple carboxylase deficiency, 1117, 1148, 1254
Multiple co-carboxylase deficiency, 1242 (Table)
Multiple congenital abnormalities, chromosome studies, 50–51
Multiple drug resistance gene, 893
Multiple enchondromatosis, **1585–1586**
Multiple endocrine deficiency disease, Hashimoto's thyroiditis, 1048
Multiple endocrine neoplasia syndromes, 1056
type II, 1052
Multiple epiphyseal dysplasia, 370, 371, 1579–1580

inheritance, 1566 (Table)
Multiple exostoses, **1585**
Multiple food intolerances, 442
Multiple myeloma
amyloid, 1177
proteinuria, 967
Multiple pregnancy, **90**, *see also* Multiple birth
Multiple puncture tuberculin tests, **1338**
Multiple sulfatase deficiency, 784 (Table), 1157 (Table), 1164, 1165
Multiple tics, 771–772
Multivitamins
for inborn errors of metabolism, 307
preterm supplements, 154
Mumps, **1371–1372**
deafness, 1682
eye, 1676
Munchausen syndrome by proxy, 1737, **1870–1871**
factitious epilepsy, 700
factitious hematuria, 959
FUO investigations, 1283 (Table)
growth failure, 1017
precocious pseudopuberty, 1028
Mupirocin, *S. aureus*, 1329
Murder rates, 700
Murine typhus, 1390 (Table), **1392**
Murmurs
aortic regurgitation, 629
atrial septal defect, 602
carditis, 628, 1597–1598
coronary artery fistula, 605
Ebstein's anomaly, 619
examination, 32, **586–587**
neonate, 43
innocent, **594–595**
iron deficiency, 851
mitral regurgitation, 629
mitral stenosis, 629
neonate, 203
persistent ductus arteriosus, 107, 603
pulmonary stenosis, 608
ventricular septal defect, 600
Murphy endotracheal tube, 1842
Muscle adenylate kinase deficiency, 1141
Muscle–eye–brain disease, 650
Muscle imbalance, myelomeningocele, 654
Muscle paralysis, *see* Paralysis
Muscle phosphofructokinase deficiency, 735, **1139–1140**
Muscle phosphorylase deficiency, 735, 789 (Table), 1139
Muscle relaxants, *see also* Pancuronium
myotonia, 733
pneumothorax prevention, 188
Muscles, **726–738**, *see also* Biopsy, muscle; Tone
examination, 39
glycogen storage diseases, 1136
inflammation, **737–738**
potassium, 411
stiffness, 756
toxoplasmosis, 1465
trichinosis, 1494
Muscles of mastication, 811
Muscular dystrophies, **728–729**
severely handicapped children affected, 14 (Table)
Muscularis, small intestine, 436
Muscular ventricular septal defect, 600
Mustard procedure, transposition of great arteries, 615
Mutase apoenzyme defects, methylmalonic acidemia, 1117
Mutations, **69–70**
Hunter's syndrome, 1160
inborn errors of metabolism, 1100
mitochondrial DNA, 1126, 1127
Mutism
elective, 1744–1745
receptive dysphasia, 815
MVPP regimen, Hodgkin's disease, 910

Myadenylate deaminase deficiency, 1141
Myalgic encephalopathy, Epstein–Barr virus, 1367
Myasthenia gravis, 23 (Fig.), **727–728**
dysarthria, 811
maternal, 89 (Table)
Myasthenic crisis, 728
Mycobacterium africanum, 1334
Mycobacterium bovis, 1334, 1335
Mycobacterium leprae, 1309–1310
Mycobacterium spp., 570, **1334–1348**
AIDS, 1396
cystic fibrosis, 555
environmental mycobacteria, **1348–1350**
immunosuppression by, 1263
Mycobacterium tuberculosis, **1334–1335**, *see also* Tuberculosis
vs Nocardia spp., 1477
Mycobacterium vaccae, 1340
Mycoplasmal infection, otitis media, 511
Mycoplasma pneumoniae, **1374**
pertussis-like illness, 561–562
pneumonia, 566, **569**
radiology, 567
Mydriatics, 1651
Myelinated nerve fibers, retina, **1671**
Myelination
central nervous system, 643–644
failure, 642
fatty acids, intake requirements, 332
postasphyxial dyskinesia, 755
Myelitis, postinfectious, **1376**
Myelocytic leukemoid reaction, plague, 1318
Myelodysplasias, 651, **652**, 868, 869
Myelogenous leukemia, glucose-6-phosphate translocase deficiencies, 1137
Myeloid hemopoiesis, 221, 222
Myelokathexis, *vs* infantile genetic agranulocytosis, 867
Myelomeningocele, **653–657**, *see also* Spina bifida
cisternal puncture contraindicated, 1841
neuropathic bladder, 957
severely handicapped children affected, 14 (Table)
Myelomonocytic syndrome, 872
Myeloperoxidase deficiency, 1242 (Table), 1260
Myiasis, **1513–1514**
Myoadenylate deaminase deficiency, 736
Myocarditis
African trypanosomiasis, 1455
Coxsackie B viruses, **1382–1383**
diphtheria, 630, 1305, 1306
infective, **630**
neonate, 205
organisms, 284 (Table)
rheumatic, 628
Myocardium
birth asphyxia, 129
Chagas' disease, 1458, 1459
contractile state, 1819
contusion, 1811
Duchenne muscular dystrophy, 730
ischemia
brain effects, 694
neonatal asphyxia, 205
Myoclonic astatic epilepsy, *see* Lennox–Gastaut syndrome
Myoclonic epilepsy
'salaam' attacks, 34
severely handicapped children affected, 14 (Table)
Myoclonic epilepsy with ragged red fiber myopathy (MERRF), 682, 736, 1127
Myoclonic seizures, neonate, 244 (Table)
Myoclonus
funny turns, 673
metronomic, 769

Myoglobinuria, metabolic myopathies, 1132
Myometrium, 84
Myopathies, **734–737**
    with cytochrome oxidase deficiency, 1127–1128
    debranching enzyme deficiency, 1138
    feeding difficulties, 209
    metabolic, **735–736, 1132**
Myophosphorylase deficiency, 735, 789 (Table), 1139
Myopia, 267, 1657
    vs proptosis, 1650
    very low birthweight, 171
Myosin
    muscular dystrophies, 729
    small round cell tumors, 912 (Table)
Myosis, 34
Myositis, see also Polymyositis
    Coxsackie virus, group B5, 724
    influenza, 1369
Myositis ossificans, **1586**
Myotomy, see Heller's cardiomyotomy
Myotonia congenita, 733
Myotonic dystrophy, 72 (Table)
    anticipation, 66
    genetic diagnosis, 73
    IgG, 1259
Myotonic syndromes, 733–734
Myotoxic snake venoms, 1521, 1522
Myotubular myopathies, 734, 735 (Table)
Myringotomy, secretory otitis media, 1681–1682
Myrmecia spp., bites and stings, 1524
Myths, immunization, 1318
Myxedema, 1049 (Fig.), 1050
    myotonia, 733
    voice, 809
Myxoma, left atrial, 636

NADPH oxidase defects, 1259
Naegleria fowleri, 1467, 1469
Nagasaki atomic bomb, neoplasms, 890
Nail–patella syndrome, **1553**
Nails
    alopecia areata, 1640
    chronic mucocutaneous candidiasis, 1637
    examination, 19
    syphilis, 1407, 1414
    tinea, 1637
Nail varnish remover, poisoning, 1709
Nairobi eye, 1525
Nalidixic acid
    administration, 1971 (Table)
    mechanism, 1527
    urinary tract infections, 952 (Table)
Naloxone
    administration, 1971 (Table)
        neonate, 1958 (Table)
    birth apnea, 134
    diphenoxylate poisoning, 1709–1710
    emergency supply, 134 (Table)
    resuscitation, doses, 527 (Fig.)
Napkin area, topical steroid absorption, 1067
Napkin dermatitis, 1643
Napkin psoriasis, 1628, 1629
Napkin rash, 988–989
    monilial, 1472
Napkins, blue staining, 1122
Naproxen
    administration, 1971 (Table)
    juvenile chronic arthritis, 1603
Nasal bridge, 76 (Table)
Nasal epithelial potential difference, cystic fibrosis, 553
Nasal escape, 810
Nasal fracture, birth trauma, 121 (Table)
Nasal meningoceles, 648
Nasal polyps, 1685
    cystic fibrosis, 555
Nasal route, insulin, 1081

Nasal septum
    deviation, 1685
        vs common cold, 560
    hematoma, 1684
Nasal specula, specimens for sexually transmitted diseases, 1400, 1423
Nasogastric tubes
    bronchiolitis, 564
    enteral nutrition, 1218
    neonate, 111
    vs oral tubes, preterm infant feeding, 153
Nasojejunal feeding, loose stools, 212
Nasolacrimal duct, congenital obstruction, 1665
Nasopharyngeal reflux, 425, 426
Nasopharyngeal tube, oxygen therapy, 568
Nasopharynx, **1685–1687**
    carcinoma, Epstein–Barr virus, 891
    Chlamydia trachomatis, 1432
    sampling
        bacteriology, 1298
        bronchiolitis, 564
        pertussis, 1317
        pneumonia, 567
        virology, 1351, 1352
    tumors, speech, 809, 810, 811
Nasotracheal intubation, 1842–1843
Natamycin, 1474, 1971 (Table)
National Association for Colitis and Crohn's disease, 485
National Child Development Study, 1852
National Health Service, 1852–1853, **1853–1854**
National Organization for Rare Diseases, 1099
National Survey of Health and Development, 1851
'Natural' antibodies, 1236
Natural killer cells, 1235
    CD subsets, 1232 (Table)
Nausea, 433
    cytotoxic drugs, 894 (Table), 895–896
    migraine, 717
Navajo Indians, glucuronyltransferase inhibition, 220
Navicular bone, osteochondrosis, **1595**
N-benzoyl-1-tyrosyl p-aminobenzoic acid test, cystic fibrosis, 553
Near-drowning, 571, **1716–1718**
    intensive care, **1825–1826**
Nebulized adrenaline, croup, 563
Nebulizers, 545, 1954
    acute severe asthma, 547–548
    home, 547
Necator americanus, 1488
    larval disease, 1484 (Table)
    tetrachlorethylene, 1490
Neck
    blood vessels, strokes, 711
    dystonia, Sandifer syndrome, 428
    examination, 29–30, 511
    neuroblastoma, 911, 912
    radiography, 513
    rhabdomyosarcoma, 915
    stiffness
        meningitis, 1289, 1814
        neonatal meningitis, 281
    tone, neonate, 239
    tonic reflexes, 240
Neck-righting reflex, neonatal gestation age, 40 (Table)
Necrotizing enterocolitis, 151, **210–212**, 282, 1782
    birth asphyxia, 129
    breast milk protection, 152
    diarrhea, 210, 212
    disseminated intravascular coagulation, 231
    enteral feeding, 155
    hypothermia, 150
    radiology, 1901
    water balance, 143
Neglect, 1737

failure to thrive, 469, **1871–1873**
Negligence, **1877–1880**
Negri bodies, 1377
Neisseria cinerea, 1423
Neisseria gonorrhoeae, 1420
    complement deficiency disorders, 1262, 1266
    laboratory methods, 1422–1424
    ophthalmia neonatorum, 263, 264, 283
Neisseria meningitidis
    carriers, rifampicin, 1976 (Table)
    complement deficiency disorders, 1262, 1266
    emergency care, **1815–1816**
    meningitis, 1289 (Table), 1290, **1292**
        deafness, 816
        neonatal, 247 (Table)
        prophylaxis, 1292, 1528
    rashes, **1285**, 1314, 1315, 1816
    septicemia, **1314–1315**
    septic shock, **1826**
    United Kingdom, 1277 (Fig.)
        mortality, 1276
    vaccine, 341
Nematocyst dermatitis, Physalia, 1526
Nematodes, **1481–1485**
Neocerebellum, 750
Neomycin
    administration, 1971 (Table)
    chlamydial conjunctivitis, 1431
Neonatal adrenoleukodystrophy, 308, 785 (Table), 1173
Neonatal death, **172–175**
    preterm delivery, 170
Neonatal hemochromatosis, 1147
Neonatal hepatitis, 221
    α_1-antitrypsin deficiency, 1176
    cystic fibrosis, 556
Neonatal intensive care
    analgesia, 1833
    withdrawing, **100–103**, 173
Neonatal jaundice, 110, 216–221, see also Posticteric choreoathetosis
    glucose-6-phosphate dehydrogenase deficiency, 859
    hypothyroidism, 220, 999, 1007
    rhesus incompatibility, 232
    urinary tract infections, 950
Neonatal lupus erythematosus, **1606, 1644**
Neonatal mortality, 3, **4**, 94
Neonatal myasthenia, 727
Neonatal rickets, see Osteopenia
Neonatal unconjugated hyperbilirubinemia, teeth, 425
Neonate, **93–325**
    acute renal failure, **257–259**, 974
    antimicrobial therapy monitoring, 1529
    BCG vaccination, 286, 1339, 1340, 1346
    blood changes, 848–849
    blood pressure, 20
    calcium, see Calcium, neonate
    candidiasis, 276, 277, **289**, 1433, 1470
    cerebral palsy, 741
    Chlamydia trachomatis, 1374, **1430–1432**
    congenital heart disease, management, 598–599
    Coxsackie B myocarditis, 1382
    deafness, 1682
    definitions, 16, 94
    diabetes mellitus, 1081
    dietary nutritional assessment, 1187
    disease incidence, 13
    drug withdrawal, 771
    dystrophia myotonica, 734
    ECHO viruses, 1383
    endocrinology, **1006–1011**
    examination, **41–44, 109–110**
    fever, **150, 1282**
    functional residual capacity, 496
    gas exchange, 497

gestation age, 40 (Table), **41**
    hemodialysis, 976
    herpes simplex, 1364, **1441–1442, 1631**
        liver, 1388
    hypermethioninemia, 1109
    hyperphenylalaninemia, 1104
    hyperthyroidism, 998, 1005, 1050
    hypertyrosinemia, 1106
    hypocalcemia, 28 (Fig.), **298–300**
        late, **299–300**, 1200
        seizures, 245, 247
    hypoglycemia, 135–136, 139, 249, **290–298, 1006**, 1081–1082
        seizures, 245 (Table), 247
    immune system, 1240–1241
        intervention, **1267**
    infections, see Infections, neonate
    intracranial hemorrhage, see Intracranial hemorrhage, neonate
    intracranial pressure, 243, 661
    lipid levels, 1149
    liver function, 471
    maternal drugs, **90–91**
    maternal sex hormones, 987
    medical negligence, 1877
    meningitis, see Meningitis, neonate
    mitochondrial disorders, 1127
    mortality rates, male, 1887
    neural tube defect management, 655
    neuroblasts, 911
    ovarian cysts, 985
    pain, **98**, 1830
    parenteral nutrition
        formulae, 1220
        regimens, 1222 (Table)
    phenylalanine, normal values, 1927 (Table)
    prescribing, 1956–1958 (Table)
    preventive pediatrics, **338–339**
    rashes, 1284
    reflexes, 36–38 (Table), 238 (Fig.), **239–240**
    refractive errors, 1657
    renal electrolyte reabsorption, 942
    respiratory tract, 496
    resuscitation, **132–136**
    routine examination, **42–43, 109–110**
    salivary amylase, 436
    screening, see Screening, neonate
    sepsis, see Sepsis, neonate
    sexually transmitted diseases, 1400
    skin diseases, **1645–1646**
    tetanus, **285**, 1333, 1334
    tetany (late neonatal hypocalcemia), **299–300**, 1200
    thrombocytopenia, **228–229**, 878–879
    thyroid function, 1044–1045
    tuberculosis, 285–286, **1346**
    urea cycle defects, 1110
    urine screening, amino acids, 1103
    urology, **1778–1779**
    varicella neonatorum, 1360, **1361**
Neoplasms, see also Central nervous system, neoplasms; Oncology; Second tumors
    adrenal cortex, 1069
    anemia, 865
    chromosome studies, 51
    common variable immunodeficiency, 1248 (Table), 1256
    dyskeratosis congenita, 855
    endocrine dysfunction, 1043
    epilepsy, 686
    Epstein–Barr virus, 891, 1366, 1367
    etiology, 887–892
    eye, **1670–1671**
    Fanconi's anemia, 854, 888 (Table)
    FUO investigations, 1283 (Table)
    growth mechanisms, 892
    gynecological, **993–994**
    heart, **636**
    hypercalcemia, 1056
    immunodeficiency, 889, 1248

Neoplasms, (Contd)
  incidence, 885
  intersex disorders, 1011
  intestine, 448–449
  liver, see Liver, neoplasms
  mortality trends, 8
  neonate, 289–290
  neurofibromatosis, 800
  pain, **1833**
  from papillomavirus lesions, 1445
  registers, 1850
  response standards, 893
  skin, **1646–1648**
  spine, imaging, 1912–1913
  thyroid gland, **1052–1053**
    from irradiation, 890
  and vitamin K, 230
  vitamin K safety, 339
  xeroderma pigmentosum, 888 (Table),
    1630
Neostigmine, 1972 (Table)
  myasthenic crisis, 728
  neonate, 727, 1958 (Table)
Nephrectomy, renal hypertension, 973
Nephritis, acute, complement deficiency,
  1263
Nephroblastoma, survival rates, 887
  (Table)
Nephroblastoma (Wilms' tumor), 888
  (Table), **913–914, 959**
  computed tomography, 1912 (Fig.)
  hepatoblastoma, 924
  incidence, 886 (Table)
  malformation syndromes, 290
  neonate, 292
  survival rates, 898 (Table)
Nephrocalcinosis, 1197 (Fig.)
  distal renal tubular acidosis, 260
  hematuria, 959
  permanent distal renal tubular acidosis,
    945
  ultrasonography, 1910
Nephrogenic diabetes insipidus, **948–949,**
  1039
  congenital, 260
  vs pituitary diabetes insipidus, 943
Nephrolithiasis, purine disorders, 1140,
  1141
Nephrons
  development, 253, 934
  hyperfiltration, 968
Nephropathica epidemica, 1390
Nephrosis, facial edema, 26 (Fig.)
Nephrostomy, see Percutaneous
  nephrostomy
Nephrotic syndrome, 961, **968–972**
  hyperlipoproteinemia, 1153, 1154
    (Table)
  infections, 969, 1288
  malaria, 968, 1448, 1451
  membranous glomerulonephritis, 964
  neonate, **261**
  syphilis, 972, 1408
    congenital, 1412
Nephrotoxicity
  acyclovir, 1440
  amphotericin B, 1478, 1530
  cytotoxic drugs, 894 (Table), 896
Nephrotoxic snake venoms, 1521
Nerve blocks, 1832
  fractures in major trauma, 1812
Nerve growth factor
  fetus, 1005
  neurofibromatosis, 798
Nervous system, see also Autonomic
  nervous system; Central nervous
  system; Peripheral nervous system;
  Riley–Day syndrome
  examination, 34–38
    neonate, **43–44, 235–244**
    psychiatric disorder, 1734–1735
  glycolysis defects, 1131–1132
Nesidioblastosis, 296, **1085**
  pancreas, 249

Netherton's syndrome, ichthyosis, 1622
  (Table)
Netilmicin, see also Gentamicin,
  administration
  administration, 1972 (Table)
  neonate, 279 (Table)
  pneumonia, 184
Nettleship–Falls syndrome, 1107–1108
Neural crest
  formation, **641–642**
  malformations, ocular anterior segment,
    270
Neural crest tumors, neurofibromatosis,
  800
Neuralgia, postherpetic, 1363
Neuralgic amyotrophy, 725
Neural tube
  closure, **641–642**
  defects, 641, **651–657**
    family recurrence rates, 74
    folate supplements, 114, 1198
    frequency, 47 (Table)
    management, **655–657**
    prevention, 338
    screening, 339 (Table)
      antenatal care, 80
Neuraminidase, hemolytic uremic
  syndrome, 978
α-Neuraminidase deficiency, sialidoses,
  1169
Neurenteric cysts, thoracic, 192
Neuroaxonal dystrophy, infantile, 793
  (Table)
Neuroblastoma, **910–913**
  ataxia, 766
  cystathionine excretion, 1109
  dancing eye syndrome, 763
  vs Ewing's sarcoma, 919
  incidence, 886 (Table)
  neonate, 291 (Table)
    incidence, 290 (Table)
  orbit, 911, 1661
  radiotherapy, iodine-131, 1897
  scintigraphy, 911, 1913
  spine, 911, 1915
  survival rates, 887 (Table), 898
    (Table)
Neuroblasts, neonate, 911
Neurodermatomes, definition, 1436
Neurodermatoses, **774–804**
Neurodevelopment, see Central nervous
  system, development
Neuroenteric cyst, 1557
Neurofibromatosis, 72 (Table), 77, 642,
  798–801, 888 (Table)
  astrocytomas, 903
  expressivity, 65
  liver tumors, 924
  optic gliomas, 904
  pseudarthrosis of tibia, 1549
  skin, **1628**
Neurofilament, small round cell tumors,
  912 (Table)
Neurogenic bladder, see Neuropathic
  bladder
Neurogenic ptosis, 1662
Neuroleptic drugs, 1755
  tardive dyskinesia, 772
Neurological disorders
  constipation management, 463
  intensive care, **1825**
  Lyme disease, 1313
  pertussis, 1316
  severely handicapped children affected,
    14 (Table)
  sleeping sickness, 1455–1456
  syphilis, see also Neurosyphilis
    secondary, 1408
Neurological handicap
  gastroesophageal reflux, 1785–1786
  meningitis, 1292
Neurology, neonate, **235–248**
  assessment, **43–44**
Neuromuscular junctions, **726–728**

Neuromyelitis optica, 793 (Table)
Neuronal apoptosis-inhibitor protein gene,
  719
Neuronal death, birth asphyxia, 126–127
Neuronopathic types, Gaucher disease,
  1166
Neurons
  cerebral, development, 642
  computer analogy, 644
  herpes simplex, 1436
  hypoxia, 694
Neuron-specific enolase
  cerebrospinal fluid, birth asphyxia, 128
  neuroblastoma, 912
  nonconvulsive epilepsy, 690
  small round cell tumors, 912 (Table)
Neuropathic bladder (neurogenic bladder),
  656–657, 957
  vs enuresis, 957 (Table)
  investigation, 954–956
Neuropathies, see also Peripheral
  neuropathies
  arthrogryposis multiplex congenita,
    1587
  cytotoxic drugs, 894 (Table), 896
  feeding difficulties, 209
Neuropathy, ataxia with retinitis
  pigmentosa (NARP), 1127
Neuroplasty, birth trauma, 123
Neurosurgery, cerebrospinal fluid
  pleocytosis, 664
Neurosyphilis, 795 (Table), **1413**
  diagnosis, **1405**
  treatment, 1410
Neurotensin, growth hormone secretion,
  1013
Neurotoxic snake venoms, 1521, 1522
Neurotransmitters
  ACTH secretion, 1038–1039
  and endocrine system, 997
  hypothalamus, 1039
Neurotripsy, 760
Neutral fat, see also Triglycerides
  cerebrospinal fluid, normal values, 1934
    (Table)
Neutral maltase, lysosomal a-1,4-
  glucosidase deficiency, 1138
Neutral phosphates, for familial
  hypophosphatemia, 948
Neutropenia, **866–867, 1259**
  antithyroid drugs, 1051
  cancer treatment, **894–895**
  inborn errors of metabolism, 306
  leukemia, 870
  Schwachman's syndrome, 450
  SGA baby, 137
Neutrophils
  count
    neonate, 223
    normal values, 1939 (Table)
  fetus, 1240
    and neonate, 848
  function tests, 1247–1248
  glucose-6-phosphate deficiency, 1199,
    1242 (Table), 1260
  hemolytic uremic syndrome, 977–978
  neonate, 261
  phagocytic function, 1235
  vitamin B$_{12}$ deficiency, 1199
Neutrophil secondary granules deficiency,
  1260
Nevi, **1617–1620**
  facial, with vermis aplasia, 646
Nevoid basal cell carcinoma, 888
  (Table)
Newborn baby, see Neonate
New South Wales, adult developmental
  disability, **842**
Nezelof syndrome, 1252
Niacin, 1184 (Table), see also Nicotinic
  acid
  conditions responding to, 1148
  parenteral nutrition, 1221 (Table)
  Recommended Dietary Allowances,

  1949 (Table)
  reference nutrient intakes, 1946
    (Table)
Nicardipine, 131
Nickel, 1185 (Table)
  contact eczema, 1641
Niclosamide
  administration, 1972 (Table)
  Inermicapsifer madagascarensis, 1506
  intestinal flukes, 1513
  Taenia saginata, 1500
Nicolle–Novy–MacNeal medium,
  1459
Nicotinamide
  for hereditary lactic acidosis, 1125
  for organic acidurias, 1119
  prophylaxis, 1972 (Table)
  therapy, 1198
Nicotinic acid
  deficiency, 1198
    tryptophan metabolism disorders,
      1114
  for Hartnup disease, 1122
Niemann–Pick diseases, **778–779 (Table),**
  1157 (Table), **1166–1167**
  eye, 1666
  neonate, 308
Nievergelt's mesomelic syndrome, 1581
Nifedipine
  acute renal failure, 975
  administration, 1972 (Table)
  hypertension, 637 (Table), 638
    renal, 973 (Table)
  hypertrophic cardiomyopathy, 634
  migraine, 717 (Table)
Nifurtimox, 1457, 1460
Night, see also entries starting
  'Nocturnal'
  epilepsy, 691
  neonatal intensive care, 98
Night-dresses, flammability, 1714
Nightmares, 1746
Night splints, 757
Night sweats, Hodgkin's disease, 909
Night terrors, 1745–1746
Nijmegen breakage syndrome, 1253–
  1254
Nipple confusion, 328, 329
Nipples, neonatal gestation age, 42 (Fig.)
Nipple stimulation, 112
Niridazole, dracunculosis, 1496
Nissen fundoplication, 429, 1785
Nitrate, urine dipsticks, 951
Nitrazepam
  administration, 1972 (Table)
  for extrapyramidal rigidity, 769
  for infantile spasms, 687
Nitric oxide, 127, **1823**
  inhalation, 165, **1823**
    persistent pulmonary hypertension of
      the newborn, 204, 1823
    pulmonary hypoplasia, 192
Nitric oxide synthase, 1823
  inhibitors, 131, 1823
Nitroblue tetrazolium test, 1247
  chronic granulomatous disease, 533,
    1247
  neonatal sepsis, 277
Nitrofurans, and glucose-6-phosphate
  dehydrogenase deficiency, 859
    (Table)
Nitrofurantoin
  administration, 1972 (Table)
  urinary tract infections, 952 (Table)
Nitrogen, see also Amino acids;
    Nonprotein nitrogen; Proteins;
    Urea nitrogen
  normal values
    amniotic fluid, 1937 (Table)
    stools, 1936 (Table)
Nitrogen dioxide, 1823
Nitrogen washout
  pneumothorax, 188
  test, 200–201

Nitroprusside
acute renal failure, 975
heart failure, 599
for hypertension, 637 (Table)
renal hypertension, 973 (Table)
Nitroprusside test, 837, 1109
Nitrosoureas
gonadal function, 899
toxic effects, 894 (Table)
Nits, 1518, 1638
Njovera, see Endemic syphilis
NK cells, *see* Natural killer cells
NMDA calcium channels, 127
NMDA receptor antagonists, 131
N-myc amplification, neuroblastoma, 911
Nociception, neonates, 98
Nocturnal asthma, 549
Nocturnal blood glucose levels, 1072
Nocturnal enuresis, **957**, 1743
Nocturnal hypoventilation, **509**
Nocturnal pulsatile growth hormone
release, testing, 1019
Nocturnal symptoms, allergy, 1691–1692
Nodular sclerosis, Hodgkin's disease, 909
Nodules, thyroid gland, 1052
Noise pollution, neonatal intensive care,
97, 99
Noisy breathing, **507–509**
Nomenclature, Paris Conference on
Standardization in Human
Cytogenetics, 53, 54 (Table)
Non-accidental injury, **1737, 1866–
1869**
bath drowning, 1717
brain injury, 1810
dating, 703
encephalopathy, 695
head injury, **700–704,** 1867, 1914, 1915
(Fig.)
vs hemophilia A, 880
imaging, 1914–1915, 1916
nonorganic failure to thrive, 1873
tympanic membrane perforation, 1680
Non-accidental poisoning, 1706
Nonacute porphyrias, **1144**
Nonadrenergic noncholinergic inhibitory
system, asthma, 538
Non-A, non-B hepatitis
enteric, **478, 1387**
transfusion-associated, *see* Hepatitis C
virus
Noncavitating transient parenchymal
echodensity, very low birth weight,
outcome, 172
Noncleaved cell lymphomas, 907
Noncommunicating hydrocephalus, *see*
Internal hydrocephalus
Nondisjunction, 51
retinoblastoma, 888
Nonesterified fatty acids, *see* Free fatty
acids
Nongonococcal urethritis, 1432
Nonhemolytic hyperbilirubinemias,
congenital, 218
Nonhemolytic streptococci, **1333**
Non-Hodgkin's lymphoma, **906–909**
vs Hodgkin's disease, 909–910
incidence, 886 (Table)
second primary tumors, 898 (Table)
small intestine, 449
survival rates, 887 (Table), 898 (Table)
tumor markers, 912 (Table)
Nonimmune fetal hydrops, lysosomal
storage disorders, 1156
Non-insulin-dependent diabetes mellitus,
1072
Nonionic contrast media, 1895
intravenous urography, 1910–1911
swallowing studies, 1900
Nonionized calcium, diffusible, 298–299
Nonketotic hyperglycinemia, 790 (Table),
1103
brain damage, 305

Non-NMDA calcium channels, 127
Non-nucleoside reverse transcriptase
inhibitors, 1397
Nonnutritive sucking, 154
Non-paralytic squint, **1660**
Nonprogressive cerebellar ataxia, *see*
Ataxia, cerebral palsies
Nonprotein nitrogen
breast milk, 332
normal values, 1927 (Table)
amniotic fluid, 1937 (Table)
Nonrapid eye movement sleep, *see also*
Quiet sleep
breathing, 196
Nonshivering thermogenesis, 146–147
Nonspecific immune mechanisms,
1232–1234
neonate, 1241
Nonspecific urethritis, 1429
Non-steroidal anti-inflammatory drugs,
1832
migraine, 718
peptic ulcers, 432
poisoning, 1709
rheumatic diseases, **1603**
thrombophlebitis prevention, 1223
Nonstressed testing, cardiotocography, 115
Nonsuppurative otitis media (secretory
otitis media), 816, **1681–1682**
Nonthrombocytopenic purpuras, **875–876**
Nonverbal communication, 818
Noonan's syndrome, 72 (Table), 370, 596,
1035
and Hashimoto's thyroiditis, 1049
Noradrenaline, 1069
administration, 1972 (Table)
intensive care, 1820
normal values, 1924 (Table)
Noradrenergic receptors, multiple tics,
771–772
NORD (National Organization for Rare
Diseases), 1099
Norethisterone
dysfunctional uterine bleeding, 992
dysmenorrhea, 992
fetal masculinization, 986
and puberty induction, 1035
Normal care, neonates, 95
Normal development, psychological,
381–385
Normalization
maladaptive response to chronic illness,
1761
mental retardation, 837, 838
Normal ranges, *see also named substances*
cautions, 1001
Normetanephrine, normal values, urine,
1931 (Table)
Norm referenced tests, psychological,
1735
Norrbottnian type, Gaucher disease, 1166
North American blastomycosis, 1471
(Table), **1474–1475**
Northern blot, 70
Northway grading, bronchopulmonary
dysplasia, 194
Norwalk virus, gastroenteritis, 1384
'Norwegian scabies,' 1516
Nose, **1683–1686,** *see also* Nasal polyps;
Postnasal drip
cytology, 577
development, 496
diphtheria, 1306
examination, **511**
filtration, 497
Nosocomial infections, **1281–1282**
AIDS prevention, 1396
diarrhea, 1295
neonatal intensive care units, 183, 276
Pseudomonas spp., 1321
Notes, *see* Record keeping
Notifiable diseases, 1280, **1849–1850**
rates, **9,** 10 (Table)
pertussis, 1315

Notochord, endodermal separation failure,
206
'Not tolerating feeds', 208
N protein, *see* G proteins
NTBC (pHPPA hydroxylase inhibitor),
1106
N-terminal fragments, parathyroid
hormone, 1054
Nuclear families, 1854
Nuclear fuel reprocessing plants,
neoplasms, 890
Nuclear magnetic resonance spectroscopy,
phosphorus-31, metabolic
myopathies, 1132
Nuclear medicine, *see* Scintigraphy
Nuclear messengers, signal transduction,
1240
Nuclear test fallout, neoplasms, 890
Nucleated red cell count, neonate, 223
(Table)
Nucleic acid tests, *Neisseria gonorrhoeae,*
1424
Nucleotides, 68
Nucleus ambiguus, 809
Nummular eczema, **1643**
Nurse-controlled analgesia, 1831–1832
Nursery care
mental retardation, 840
private, 1861
publicly funded, 1860
Nursery education, **1861**
Nurses
child development centers, 399
neonatal care, 96, 156
Nursing, preterm infant temperature
control, 147
Nutrition, **1179–1230**
acute renal failure, 975
AIDS, 1397
assessment, **1186–1188**
preterm infant, 155
bronchopulmonary dysplasia
prevention, 195
burns, 1799–1800
chronic renal failure, 980
Crohn's disease, 457, 458, **1206–1207**
cystic fibrosis, 450, **1207–1209**
developing countries, **1891–1892**
gastrointestinal disorders, **469–470**
on growth, 367
hypoglycemia, 295
requirements, 466, **1179–1183,** *see also*
Energy, requirements; *named
nutrients*
preterm infant, **151–152,** 157–158
supplements
chronic renal failure, 980
preterm infant, **154–155**
ulcerative colitis, 459, 1206
Nutritional imprinting, 1005
Nutritional rehabilitation, 1892
Nutrition nurse specialists, 1226
Nutrition support, **1215–1226**
teams, **1215–1217**
Nystagmus
albinism, 1673
anterior visual pathway disorders, 270
cataract, 1669
congenital, *see* Infantile nystagmus
delayed visual maturation, 272
examination, 1652
neonate, 43, 265, **271**
optic gliomas, 904
Nystatin, 289, **1434,** 1472, 1477–1478
administration, 1956 (Table), 1972
(Table)
mechanism, 1530
neonate, 279 (Table)
site of action, 1527
thrush diarrhea, 1295

O antibody, typhoid fever, 1326
Oast house syndrome, 1122

Obesity, 999, **1021–1023, 1190–1191**
Duchenne muscular dystrophy, 731
on growth, 367
hypertension, 1069
measurements, 364
plasma amino acids, 1102
psychological factors, 1746
and tallness, 1020
tall stature, 375
Objective audiometry, **1683**
Object permanence, sensorimotor
development, 1729
Obliterative bronchiolitis, 565, **576**
Obscurations (transient blindness), 1658
Obsessive–compulsive disorders, **1740**
adolescence, **1756**
Obstetric history, 18
neonates, 41
syphilis, 1411
Obstetrics
cerebral palsy, 738, 741
complications, **88–91**
developing countries, 1891
Obstructive apnea, 530 (Table)
Obstructive emphysema, imaging, 1899
Obstructive jaundice,
hyperlipoproteinemia, 1153–1154
Obstructive nephropathy, 255–256
Obstructive sleep apnea, 530, **531**
Obstructive uropathies, 950, *see also*
Postrenal failure
in utero shunting, 115, 935
management, 954–956
Obturator neurectomy, 760
Occipital horn syndrome, 1146
Occipital lobectomy, Sturge–Weber
syndrome, 803
Occipital subluxation, birth trauma, 121
(Table)
Occipitofrontal head circumference, *see*
Head circumference
Occlusion, for squint, 1660
Occult fecal blood tests, 459
Occult filariasis, 1498
Occupational health, pregnancy, 80
Occupational therapists, child
development centers, 399
Occupational therapy, juvenile chronic
arthritis, 1604
Oceania, demography, 2 (Table)
Ochronosis, 1107
Octanoic acid, 682
Octanoylglycine, 1129
Octasacchariduria, GM$_1$-gangliosidosis,
1163
Octreotide
neuroendocrine tumor scintigraphy,
1913
tall stature, 1020
Ocular albinism, 1107–1108
Ocular hemorrhage, birth trauma, 264
Ocular movements, *see* Eye, movements
'Ocular promiscuity', 1430
Oculoauriculovertebral dysplasia, 1557,
1563 (Table), 1564
Oculocerebrorenal syndrome (Lowe's
syndrome), 831 (Table), 948,
1122–1123
Oculocraniosomatic syndrome, 735
(Table), 736
Oculocutaneous albinism, *see* Albinism
Oculodentodigital syndrome, 1564
Oculomandibulodyscephaly with
hypotrichosis, **1562**
Oculomotor nerve (third nerve)
examination, 34
neurogenic ptosis, 1662
palsy, 265
raised intracranial pressure, 708
Oculopharyngeal muscular dystrophy, 811
Odontoid hypoplasia, Morquio–Brailsford
syndrome, 1160
Odor, examination, 19
Oedipal crisis, 1730

Oesophagostomum genera, 1494
Oestrus ovis, 1514
OFD syndrome (orofacial dysostosis), **1564**, 1565 (Table)
Office of Population, Censuses and Surveys, United Kingdom, 1281, 1848
  respiratory disorders, 489–490
Ofloxacin, gonorrhea, 1427 (Table)
Ohtahara syndrome, 688 (Table)
Ointments, 1617
OJEC regimen, neuroblastoma, 912, 913
'OK432' (streptococcal derivative), cystic hygroma, 1784
OKT4 deficiency, 1250
Old tuberculin, 1337
Old World cutaneous leishmaniasis, 1461 (Table)
Olfactory nerve, examination, 34
Oligemia, lung fields, 200 (Table)
Oligohydramnios, 115, 1937 (Table)
  deformations, 76
  pulmonary hypoplasia, 191, 192
Oligomeganephronia, 254, 938
Oligosaccharides, 1182–1183
Oligosacchariduria, GM₁-gangliosidosis, 1163
Oliguria
  acute renal failure, 258
  postnatal, 257
  preterm infant, 142
  respiratory distress syndrome, 180
Olivopontocerebellar atrophy, 792 (Table)
Ollier's disease, **1585–1586**
ω3:ω6 fatty acid ratio, breast milk, 332, 333
ω-3 polyunsaturated fatty acids, ulcerative colitis, 1206
OMIM catalog numbers, 1099, 1101
Ommen's syndrome, 1250, **1252**
Omphalocele, 1779
Omsk hemorrhagic fever, 1390
Onchocerciasis, **1496–1497**
  eye, 1676–1677
Onchocercomata, 1497
Oncogenes, 889
  rhabdomyosarcoma, 915
Oncology, **884–933**
Oncotic pressure, 407
Ondansetron, administration, 1972 (Table)
Ondine's curse, *see* Central hypoventilation syndrome
One parent families, 15 (Table), **1854–1857**
Onion bulb formation, 723
On-line Mendelian Inheritance of Man, *see* OMIM catalog numbers
Oocysts, *Plasmodium* spp., 1446
Oogenesis, 48
Oogonia, 1004
Ookinetes, *Plasmodium* spp., 1446
OPEC regimen, neuroblastoma, 912, 913
Open airway, 1807
Operating theaters, temperature control, 149
Operations, intellectual, 1729
Operative fetoscopy, 115
Operculate eggs
  Diphyllobothrium latum, 1504 (Fig.)
  flukes, 1511 (Fig.), 1512
Ophthalmia neonatorum (conjunctivitis), **263–264**, 283, 1663
  Chlamydia trachomatis, **263–264**, 283
  gonorrhea, 1420, 1421, **1424**, 1426
  prophylaxis, **1429**
  treatment, **1429**
  organisms, 284 (Table)
Ophthalmic zoster, *see* Supraophthalmic zoster
Ophthalmoplegia, 43, *see also* Eye, movements, disorders
  Niemann–Pick disease type C, 1167
Ophthalmoscopy, 25–27, 1000, **1651–1652**

diabetes mellitus, 1080
  tuberculous meningitis, 1344
Opiates, **1831**
  abuse, 1762–1763
  diarrheal diseases, 1296
  major trauma, 1812
  preterm labor, 119
  terminal care, 928–929
Opisthorchiasis, 1512
  fluke life cycle, 1511 (Table)
  liver, 478
Opisthotonus, 239
  cerebral malaria, 1450 (Fig.)
  diplegia, 746
Opitz syndrome, 831 (Table)
Opportunistic infections
  cancer treatment, **894**
  HIV infection, 1393–1394
  liver transplantation, 484–485
Opportunity costs, 104
Op-Site (plastic film), transcutaneous oxygen tension measurement, 160
Opsoclonus, 265
Opsoclonus/myoclonus, neuroblastoma, 911
Opsonization, 1232, 1234, 1235
  neonate, 274
Optical iridectomy, 1670
Optic atrophy, 271, **1671–1672**
  DIDMOAD syndrome, 1081
  Friedreich's ataxia, 765
  neonate, organisms, 284 (Table)
Optic blink reflex, 36 (Table)
Optic disc, 1651–1652, 1671
  septo-optic dysplasia, 647
Optic gliomas, **904**, 1661, **1672**
Optic nerve, **1671**
  examination, 34
  hypoplasia, 271
Optic neuritis, 725, **1671**
  ethambutol, 1347
Optokinetic nystagmus
  neonate, 241
  testing, 396
Oral contraceptive pill, **995**
  accidental ingestion, 1028
  anticonvulsants, 691
  for dysfunctional uterine bleeding, 992
  migraine, 717
  for polycystic ovarian disease, 993
Oral hygiene, cancer treatment, 894, 896
Oral moniliasis, 1470–1471, 1472
Oral mucosa, 424–425
Oral period, 1729 (Table)
Oral polio vaccine, 345
  WHO on, 346 (Table)
Oral rehydration solutions, **413**, 452, **453**, **1296**, 1304
Oral route, **1953–1954**
  antibiotics, absorption, 1527
  morphine dosage, 1831 (Table)
Oral tubes, *vs* nasal tubes, preterm infant feeding, 153
Oralytes, cholera, 1304
Orbit, **1661–1662**
  cellulitis, 1661
  examination, 1649–1650
  globe dislocation, 264
  neuroblastoma, 911, 1661
  rhabdomyosarcoma, 915
  tuberculosis, 1343
Orchidopexy, 1791
Orchitis, mumps, 1372
Orciprenaline, administration, 1972 (Table)
Orf, **1388**
Organic acidurias
  dietary management, **1204 (Table)**
  and metabolic acidosis, **1118–1119**
Organochloride, organophosphorus insecticides, poisoning, 1711
Organ transplantation
  brain death, 709
  cytomegalovirus disease, 1365

Ornidyl (difluoromethyl-ornithine), 1457
Ornithine transcarbamylase deficiency, **1110–1111**, 1113
  ataxia, 762
  valproate on liver, 684
Orofacial digital syndrome, 646
Orofacial dyskinesia, 768–769, 772, 813
Orofacial dysostosis, **1564**, 1565 (Table)
Orofacial granulomatosis, food additives, 1701
Orogastric tubes, sizes, 1845 (Table)
Oropharyngeal airway (Guedel), 524
Oropharyngeal infection, gonorrhea, 1425
  treatment, 1428
Orosomucoid, neonatal sepsis, 277
Orotic acid, ornithine transcarbamylase deficiency, 1110–1111
Orotic aciduria, 1141–1142
Orphans, accommodation, 1857
Orphenadrine, administration, 1972 (Table)
Orthodontics, cleft palate, 1797
Orthomyxoviruses, 1368
Orthopedic injury, **1812–1813**
Orthopedics
  cerebral palsy, 760
  limb malformations, 1545
  neural tube defects, 655
Orthostatic proteinuria, 967–968
Orthotics
  cerebral palsy, 757–758
  Duchenne muscular dystrophy, 731
  neural tube defects, 655
Ortolani's test, 41
Os calcis, osteochondrosis, **1595**
Osgood–Schlatter disease, **1595**
Osler–Weber–Rendu disease, 875
Osmolal clearance, 409
Osmolality, 405–406, 409
  normal values
    amniotic fluid, 1937 (Table)
    cerebrospinal fluid, 1934 (Table)
    plasma, 1039, 1040
    regulation, 410
    serum, normal values, 1927 (Table)
    urine, *see* Urine, osmolality
Osmolarity, 405
Osmometers, 405–406
Osmotic diarrhea, 455, 467, 468
  stool, 454 (Table)
Osmotic equilibrium, ECF *vs* ICF, 404
Osmotic fragility curve, hereditary spherocytosis, 857
Osmotic pressure, **405–406**, 407
Ossicles, congenital abnormalities, 1679
Osteitis, BCG vaccination, 1339
Osteoblasts, parathyroid hormone receptors, 1054
Osteochondritis dissecans, **1595–1596**
Osteochondrodysplasias, *see* Skeletal dysplasias
Osteochondromas, 917
Osteochondroses, **1593–1595**
Osteochondrosis tibiae, **1554**
Osteoclast development genes, osteopetrosis, 1582
Osteogenesis imperfecta, 72 (Table), **1567–1570**
  eye, 1568, 1676
Osteogenic sarcoma, *see* Osteosarcoma
Osteomyelitis (osteitis)
  environmental mycobacteria, 1350
  FUO investigations, 1283 (Table)
  imaging, 1914, 1916, 1917, 1918 (Fig.)
  maxilla, 22 (Fig.)
  neonate, 282–283
    antibiotic therapy, 279

  organisms, 284 (Table)
  osteosarcoma from, 917
  Pseudomonas aeruginosa, 1320–1321
  sickle cell disease, 862
    salmonella, 1323–1324, 1590
  staphylococcal, 281
  triple bone scan, 1915–1916
Osteopenia
  of prematurity, 301–304
  preterm infant, 154
Osteoperiostitis, hyperplastic, congenital syphilis, 1413, 1414
Osteopetrosis, 1177, 1200, **1581–1583**
  inheritance, 1566 (Table)
Osteoporosis, 301, 1053, 1200
  glucose-6-phosphatase deficiency, 1137
  Turner's syndrome, 61
Osteosarcoma, **917–918**
  chromosome deletion, 889
  survival rates, 887 (Table)
Osteosclerosis, leukemias, 870
Ostermilk, 112 (Table)
Ostium primum atrial septal defect, 601–602
Ostium secundum atrial septal defect, 601
Otitis externa, **1680**
Otitis media, 561, 1283, **1680–1682**
  Chlamydia trachomatis, 1374, 1432
  cleft palate, 1797
  from common cold, 560
  eardrum, 511
  environmental mycobacteria, 1349
  Haemophilus influenzae, 561, 1307
  measles, 1354
  neonate, 283–284
  Pseudomonas aeruginosa, 1320
  tympanocentesis, 1298
Otoacoustic emissions, 244
  audiometry, 1683
Otomandibular dysostosis (hemifacial microsomia), 1563 (Table), **1564**
Ototoxicity
  cytotoxic drugs, 894 (Table), 897
  drugs in pregnancy, 1682
Otrivine–Antistin, 1676
Outcomes, information lack, 104, 105
Outcome studies, prematurity, research, 165–172
'Outlet' forceps delivery, preterm, 120
Outlet ventricular septal defect, 600
Outpatient referrals, **9**
Outwardly rectifying chloride channel, cystic fibrosis, 551
Ovaries
  chorionepithelioma, ectopic gonatropin secretion, 1029
  cryopreservation and autografts, 1033
  cysts, 993, **1796**
    fetus, 985
    neonate, 985
    puberty, 1028
  delayed puberty, 1031–1035
  dysgenesis, Turner's syndrome, 370
  dysgerminomas, 920, 993
  embryology, 1004
  function, cancer survivors, 899
  germ cell tumors, 922
  premature failure, 992
  puberty, 1023
  teratomas, 993
  tumors
    precocious pseudopuberty, 1027
    precocious puberty, 989
  Turner's syndrome, 1032–1033
  ultrasonography, 1913
Overactivity, *see* Hyperactivity; Hyperkinetic disorder
Overdose, *see* Self-poisoning
Overeating, 1021–1024
Overfeeding, constipation, 213–214
Overheating, neonate, **150**
Overlearning, 669
Overprotection, 1747, 1761, 1873

Owen, Robert, nursery school, 1861
Oxalosis, 947, 1112–1113
Oxamniquine
    administration, 1972 (Table)
    schistosomiasis, 1511
Oxandrolone
    for CDGP, 372
    for Turner's syndrome, 1033
Oxantel, *Trichuris trichiuria*, 1491–1492
Ox erythrocytes, heterophile antibody test, 1367
Oxford Medilog system, 243
Oxidation
    drugs, 1953
    water production, 410
β-Oxidation
    fatty acids, 1128
        defects, 1083, *see also* Riboflavin
            responsive multiple acyl-CoA
            dehydrogenase deficiencies
        sudden infant death syndrome, 1722
    peroxisomal enzymes, 1171
Oxitropium bromide, 547
Oxoprolinase deficiency, 1115
3-Oxo-Δ4-steroid-5β-reductase deficiency, 1145
Oxprenolol, administration, 1972 (Table)
Oxybutynin, bladder dysfunction, 957
Oxycephaly, 21 (Fig.), 1560, 1661
Oxygen
    affinity of fetal hemoglobin, 225
    consumption rate, 417
    dissociation curve, 502, 503
        pyruvate kinase deficiency, 860
    gas exchange, 160
    lung toxicity, 161, 194, 195
    neonatal resuscitation, 133, 134, 135
    on nitric oxide, 1823
    normal values, 1927 (Table)
    retinopathy of prematurity, 265
    saturation, *see also* PaO_2; PO_2
        cardiac chambers, 593
    therapy, 521–522
        bronchiolitis, 564
        for bronchopulmonary dysplasia, 195
        carbon monoxide poisoning, 1711
        cardiovascular support, 1819
        and chronic lung disease, 504
        pneumonia, 568
        preterm infants, 104
        pulmonary hypertension, 606
        respiratory distress syndrome, 177–178, **179**
        respiratory response, 196
        resuscitation, 1807
    transport, 502–503
Oxygenation
    vs mean airway pressure, 163
    ventilator settings, 162
Oxymetholone,
    administration, 1972 (Table)
    for Fanconi's anemia, 854
Oxyphenbutazone, 1603
Oxypurinol, on free radical production, 131
11-Oxysteroids, normal values, urine, 1932 (Table)
Oxytetracycline
    administration, 1972 (Table)
    nongonococcal urethritis, 1432
    syphilis, 1409 (Table), 1410 (Table)
Oxytocin, 1039
    fetus, 1003
    labor, 84, 87
    release, milk production, 112
Oxytocin antagonists, 116
Oxyuriasis, *see* Pinworms

P53 gene, 888
    and drug resistance, 892
P-450$_{c17}$ enzyme deficiencies, 1009
P-450$_{scc}$ gene, cholesterol desmolase deficiency, 1009
Pacemakers, 627–628

hypertrophic cardiomyopathy, 634
Pachyonychia congenita, 1626 (Table)
Pacing, after cardiac surgery, 1822
Packed cells
    exchange transfusion, 233
    transfusion amounts, 851 (Table)
Packed cell volume, neonate, 142, 223 (Table)
    and fetus, 848
$PaCO_2$
    asthma, 539
        acute severe, 548
    birth asphyxia, 131
    cerebral blood flow, 699
    head injuries, 708
    hypercapnia, 503–504
    normal values, 1924 (Table)
    recommended values, 161
    ventilator settings, 162
Paederus, rove beetle dermatitis, 1525
Pain
    assessment, **1830–1831**
    burns, 1799
    chronic, **1833**
    history taking, 17
    insensitivity, 723
    neonates, **98,** 1830
    pancreatitis, 450
    preterm infant, 241
    referred to ear, 1681
    relief, **1830–1833**
        cardiovascular support, 1819
        preterm labor, 119
    terminal care, 928–929
Paints, poisoning, 1709
Paint stripper (methylene chloride), poisoning, 1711
Palatal appliance, preterm infant tube feeding, 153–154
Palate
    disorders, 810
    disproportion syndrome, 810
    palsy, diphtheria, 1306
Paleocerebellum, 750
Pallidal syndrome, 769
Pallid breath-holding attacks, 672
Pallor, history taking, 17
Palmar crease, Down syndrome, 55
Palmar grasp reflex, neonate, 238 (Fig.), 241
Palmar syphilide, 1406–1407
Palmitic acid, 207
Palmitoyl protein thioesterase defect, 1171
'Palpalis' group tsetse flies, 1454
Palpatory method, blood pressure, 20
Palpebral fissures, Down syndrome, 55
p-aminobenzoic acid, urine, cystic fibrosis, 553
Pancreas, **449–451, 1071**
    adenoma *vs* nesidioblastosis, 296
    cells, 1071
    annular, 1773, 1774 (Fig.)
    cystic fibrosis, 551, 553
        exocrine function testing, 553
    embryology, 207
    enzymes, preterm infant, 150–151
    enzyme supplements, 450, 1208
        administration, 1972 (Table)
        enteric-coated microspheres, 557
    fetus, 1004
    function tests, 451
    hypoglycemia causes, 1082 (Table), 1083
    imaging, **1907**
    islet cells, 1071
        fetus, growth hormone on, 1003
    kwashiorkor, 1193
    nesidioblastosis, 249
Pancreatectomy, nesidioblastosis, 1085
Pancreatic juice, electrolytes, 411 (Table)
Pancreatic lipase, 207, 437
Pancreatic polypeptide, 1071
Pancreatitis, **450–451**
    calcitonin, 1057

congenital syphilis, 1412
    cystin-lysinuria, 1121
    mumps, 1372
    viruses, 1384
Pancuronium
    administration, 1972 (Table)
    neonate, 1958 (Table)
    ventilation, 164
        for RDS, 181
    water balance, 142
Pancytopenia, 854–856
Panda eyes, 1811
Pandemics
    influenza, 1368
    scabies, 1515
Panhypopituitarism, congenital, adrenal insufficiency, 1041
Panstrongylus megistus, 1458
Pantothenic acid, 1184 (Table), 1199
    estimated safe and adequate daily intakes, 1949 (Table)
    parenteral nutrition, 1221 (Table)
    safe intakes, 1948 (Table)
Panventricular hydrocephalus, 659
PaO_2, 160, 195
    asthma, 539
    cyanosis, 585
    hypoxemia, 503–504
    neonate, 497
    recommended values, 161
Papile grading, intracranial hemorrhage, 249
Papilledema, 27, 1651–1652, **1671**
    craniostenosis, 1661
    fluorescein retinal angiography, 1654
    meningitis, 1290
    respiratory disorders, 510
    transient blindness, 1658
Papillitis, 1671
Papillomas
    choroid plexus, 905
        ultrasonography, 1908
    larynx, **1443–1444,** 1688
    yaws, 1417
Papillomavirus, *see* Human papillomaviruses
Papillon Lefevre syndrome, 1242 (Table), 1261
Pappataci fever (sandfly fever), **1390**
Papua New Guinea, swollen belly syndrome, 1492
Papular acrodermatitis of childhood, **1633–1634**
Papular acrolocated syndrome, 1383
Papular, papulosquamous syphilide, 1406–1407
Papular urticaria, **1639**
Papulonodular demodicidosis, 1515
Paracentesis, **1845,** *see also* Chest, drainage; Pleural tap
Paracentric inversions, chromosomal, 51
Paracetamol, 1832
    administration, 1972 (Table)
    migraine, 717 (Table)
    poisoning, 1709, **1710**
    therapeutic ranges, 1936 (Table)
Parachute responses, 382
Paradichlorobenzene mothballs, poisoning, 1711
Paradoxical embolism, 713
Paraffin poisoning, 1705, 1711
Parafollicular cells, medullary carcinoma of thyroid, 1053
Parafrenal glands, gonorrhea, 1425
Paragonimiasis, **1513**
    fluke life cycle, 1511 (Table)
Parainfectious neuropathies, 724–726
Parainfluenza virus infections, **1369**
Paraldehyde
    administration, 1973 (Table)
        neonate, 1958 (Table)
    encephalopathies, 697
    neonatal seizures, 246
    status epilepticus, 693

Paralysis, 1380
    for lactic acidosis, 307
    spinal muscular atrophy type 1, 720
    ventilation, 164
    writing, 822
Paralytic hemisyndrome, 44
Paralytic ileus, pelvic inflammatory disease, 1426
Paralytic poliomyelitis, 1379–1380
Paralytic squint, **1660,** 1661
Paramax sachet, migraine, 717 (Table)
Parameningeal rhabdomyosarcoma, 915
Paramyotonia, 733
Paranasal sinuses, **1685,** *see also* Sinusitis
    development, 496
    radiography, 513
Paraphimosis, **1793**
Paraphrasias, 814
Paraplegia, *vs* diplegia, 744–745
Paraquat poisoning, 577, 1711
Parasites, neonate, **288–289**
Parasuicide, **1757**
Parasympathetic nerve supply, meconium plug syndrome, 1777
Parathyroid gland, 1053
    fetal suppression, 298
    fetus, 1004
Parathyroid hormone, **1054–1055**
    disorders, **1056–1058**
    neonate, 299
    normal values, 1927 (Table)
    primary hyperparathyroidism, 1056
    serum levels
        hypercalcemia, 1058
        rickets diagnosis, 1057
        vitamin D deficiency, 1195
Paratyphoid fever, 1326–1327
Paraumbilical hernia, 1790
Paraurethral glands, gonorrhea, 1425
Parenchymal brain lesions, neonate, 249–250
Parenchymal intracranial cysts, echodensity, very low birth weight, outcome, 172
Parenchymatous egg capsules, *Inermicapsifer madagascariensis,* 1506
Parental responsibility, 1855
    Children Act 1989, 1874
Parenteral antibiotics, urinary tract infections, 951
Parenteral infections, diarrhea, 1293
Parenteral nutrition, 470, **1219–1226**
    anorexia nervosa, 1758
    candidiasis, 1590
    Crohn's disease, 1207
    hyperglycemia, 298
    liver disease from, **474–475**
    for malignant diarrhea, 1297
    metabolic bone disease, 302, 304
    necrotizing enterocolitis, 212
    neonates, **157–159**
        for hypoglycemia, 294
    persistent diarrhea, 1215
    protracted diarrhea, 455
    regimens, 1221–1223
    self-help groups, 485
    short bowel syndrome, 1212
    small intestine, 436
    vitamin K, 230, 1221 (Table)
    withdrawing, 102
Parenting classes, 80
Parents, *see also* Parental responsibility
    acrimony, 1856
    breaking bad news to, **1747**
    counseling, psychiatry, 1749
    death of, **1857**
    and development, 385–386
    and disabilities, 386, 1746–1747
    and epilepsy, 691
    excessive anxiety, 1870
    grief, neonatal deaths, 172
    group psychotherapy, 1763
    and height, 1015

Parents, (Contd)
  informed consent to research, 103, 166
  mental retardation, 839
  neonatal intensive care, 96–98, **99–100**
  and phototherapy, 218–219
  physical abuse risk, 1866
  and practical procedures, 1829
  preterm infant, 139
  psychiatric disorder, 1728
  smoking, 493
    asthma, 545
    sudden infant death syndrome, 1722–1723
  tall stature, 375
Parent-to-child bone marrow transplantation, 1268
Parietal cell antibodies, vitamin B$_{12}$ deficiency, 853 (Table)
Parietal cells, stomach, 430
Parietal foramina, 1558–1559
Paris Conference on Standardization in Human Cytogenetics, nomenclature, 53, 54 (Table)
Parity, on childhood mortalities, 3 (Table)
Parkes–Weber syndrome, 1620, 1798
Parkinsonism, 768, 769, 770
  drug-induced, 772
  juvenile, 793 (Table)
Paromomycin, administration, 1973 (Table)
Parosteal osteosarcoma, 918
Parotid gland
  enlargement, 1784
  mumps, 1371
Parotitis, 425
  lymphoid interstitial pneumonitis, 1395
  recurrent, 1372
  secondary syphilis, 1408
Paroxetine, 1755
Paroxysmal ataxias, familial, 764
Paroxysmal choreoathetosis, 772–773
Paroxysmal cold hemoglobinuria, 864
  congenital syphilis, 1414
Paroxysmal dystonia, 774
  kinesiogenic, 673, 773
Paroxysmal extensor hypertonus (tonic seizures)
  causes, 671 (Table)
  neonate, 244 (Table)
Paroxysmal nocturnal hemoglobinuria, 856
Paroxysmal phase, pertussis, 1315
Paroxysmal supraventricular tachycardia, **627**
Parrot's nodes, 1412
Parrot's pseudoparalysis, 1412
Partial albinism, Griscelli syndrome, 1254
Partial exchange transfusion, polycythemia, 227
Partial lipodystrophy, 1155–1156
  C3 nephritic factor, 1263
  membranoproliferative glomerulonephritis, 963–964
Partial liquid ventilation, 165
Partially-digested starches, 1193
Partial plasma exchange transfusion, 1839
Partial prothrombin time, 879 (Fig.)
Partial regression, neoplasms, 893
Partial seizures, 675
Partial thromboplastin time, 228
Partograms, 84, 85 (Fig.)
Parturition, see Birth; Intrapartum care
Parvoviruses
  aplastic anemia, 856
  B19, 1358
    congenital infection, 288
    emergence, 1279 (Table)
    and pyruvate kinase deficiency, 859
    rash, 1285
    and sickle cell disease, 862
Passenger accidents, **1716**

Passive emotional abuse, 1873
Passive immunity, 341
  diphtheria, 1305
  Haemophilus influenzae, 1308
  herpes simplex virus, 1437
Passive immunization, see Immunoglobulin therapy
Passive movements, neonate, 237–239
Passive smoking, secretory otitis media, 1681
Passmore classification, leukemias, 868
Pastes, 1617
Pasteurized cow's milk, after weaning, 334
Pastia's sign, 1331
Patau's syndrome, see Trisomy 13
Patch testing
  allergic disorders, 1693
  contact eczema, 1642
Patellar instability, **1553**
Patellar tap, 40
Patent ductus arteriosus, see Persistent ductus arteriosus
Patient-controlled analgesia, **1831**
Patient-triggered ventilation, 164
Pattern reversal visual evoked response, 1657 (Fig.)
Pattern visually evoked potentials, 270
Pauciarticular onset juvenile chronic arthritis, 1602
Paucity of interlobular bile ducts, **474**
Paul–Bunnell reaction, **1367**
Pavlik harness, congenital dislocation of hip, 1551
PC$_{20}$, bronchial provocation tests, 501
PCO_2, 419
  normal values
    amniotic fluid, 1937 (Table)
    cerebrospinal fluid, 1934 (Table)
Peabody picture vocabulary tests, 400, 827
Peak bone mass, 1053
Peak expiratory end pressure, ventilation for RDS, 181
Peak expiratory flow, 499–500
  asthma, 543, 544
Peak height velocity, adolescence, 361
Peak inspiratory pressure, respiratory distress syndrome, ventilation, 163
Peanuts
  in foods, 1213
  inhaled, 571
Pearson's marrow/pancreas syndrome, 1127
Pea soup meconium staining, 186
Peau d'orange
  Hunter's syndrome, 1159
  necrotizing enterocolitis, 211
Pectin, short bowel syndrome, 1212
Pectus carinatum, 30, 512, 1556
Pectus excavatum, 28 (Fig.), 512, 574, 1556
Pederin, rove beetle dermatitis, 1525
Pedestrian road traffic accidents, 1715–1716
Pediatric emergency medical systems, 1802, 1803 (Table)
Pediatric hospitals, accident and emergency departments, 1805
Pediatricians
  community, 1853
  indications for calling to birth, 132–133, 138
  infectious diseases data, 1280 (Table)
  mental retardation, 842
Pediatric medical services, **1852–1853**
Pedicle erosion, 1915
Pediculosis, **1517–1518, 1638–1639**
  blepharitis, 1663
  eye involvement, 1675
  schoolchildren, 1864
Pedigrees, **65–67**
  gene mapping, 72–73
Peditrace, 158, 1221, 1222 (Table), 1223 (Table)

Pelican itch, 1508
Pelizaeus Merzbacher syndrome, 797 (Table)
Pellagra, 1198
  Hartnup disease, 446, 1122
  tryptophan metabolism disorders, 1114
Pelvicalyceal system, ultrasonography, 1910
Pelvic floor, dyssynergia, 957
Pelvic inflammatory disease, **1426**
  Chlamydia trachomatis, 1430, 1432
  gonorrhea, 1420–1421, 1425
Pelvis
  abscess, FUO investigations, 1283 (Table)
  achondroplasia, 1575
  diagnostic radiation doses, 1895 (Table)
  neuroblastoma, 911
  osteosarcoma distribution, 917
  rickets, 1195
Pelviureteric junction obstruction, 255, 936, 1795
Pemoline, administration, 1973 (Table)
Pemphigoid, juvenile, 1640
Pemphigus, 1640
  vs incontinentia pigmenti, 803
  syphilitic, 1411
Pena–Shokier syndrome, 57
Penciclovir, 1440–1441
Pendlebury catheter, 259
Pendred's syndrome, 1046
  deafness, 1682
Penetrance, 67
Penetrating injuries, 705
Penicillamine, 481
  administration, 1973 (Table)
  Indian childhood cirrhosis, 484
  juvenile chronic arthritis, 1603, 1604
  for lead poisoning, 1708
  pyridoxine deficiency, 1198
D-Penicillamine, Wilson's disease, 1146
L-Penicillamine, cystinuria, 1121
Penicillin
  acute glomerulonephritis, 962
  allergy, **1702**
    careless reporting, 1692–1693
  bacterial meningitis, 1291
  congenital syphilis, 285, 1415
  diphtheria, 561, 1306
  endemic treponematoses control, 1419–1420
  gonococcal conjunctivitis, 264, 283
  hyposensitization, 1702
  intrathecal, overdose, 676
  Lyme disease, 1314 (Table)
  Neisseria gonorrhoeae, susceptibility tests, 1424
  neonate, 279 (Table)
    meningitis, 247
    pneumonia, 184
  pneumonia, 568
  resistance, *Neisseria gonorrhoeae,* 1421–1422
  rheumatic fever, 628, 629
  scarlet fever, 1332
  Streptococcus pyogenes pharyngitis, 560
  syphilis, **1408–1410**
    congenital, 285, 1415
  tetanus, 285
Penicillins
  cerebrospinal fluid, 1527
  dosage considerations, 1527
  site of action, 1527
Penicillin V, see Phenoxymethyl penicillin
Penicillium spp., allergens, 1690
Pen injectors, insulin, 1077, 1080
Penis
  candidiasis, 1433
  congenital abnormalities, 255, 256
  development, 358, 360
  examination, 34
  herpes simplex, 1438
  median raphe, gonorrhea, 1425

Penmanship, 821–823
Pentagastrin
  administration, 1973 (Table)
  stimulation test, medullary carcinoma of thyroid, 1052, 1055
Pentamidine
  leishmaniasis, 1973
  Pneumocystis carinii pneumonia, 535, 1973 (Table)
    AIDS, 1397
    cancer treatment, 895
  sleeping sickness, **1456**
Pentavalent antimony compounds, **1462–1463**
Pentazocine, administration, 1973 (Table)
Pentosuria, 1131
Pepper and salt fundus, see Salt and pepper fundus
Pepsinogen, 430
Pepsins, 430, 437
  neonate, 207
  preterm infant, 150
Peptic stricture, esophagus, 428
Peptic ulceration, **432**
Peptides
  absorption, 207
  digestion, 437
  hormones, 998 (Table), 999
  intestinal absorption, 438
Percentile charts, see Centile charts
Perception
  developmental examination, 388–391 (Table)
  preoperational period, 1729–1730
  for writing, 822
Percussion
  abdomen, 33
  chest, 30
  heart, 32
  respiratory disorders, 512
Percutaneous central venous cannulation, **1837–1838**
Percutaneous endoscopic gastrostomy, 1218
Percutaneous liver biopsy, **472–473**
Percutaneous nephrostomy, 1898
  renal failure, 974
Percutaneous oxygenation, 162 (Table), 165
Percutaneous transhepatic cholangiography, 472, 1898
Perennial rhinitis, 1684, **1698**
Perez reflex, 37 (Table), 770
Perfluorocarbon associated gas exchange (PAGE), 165
Perforation
  intestinal, 210
    intussusception reduction, 1904
    meconium ileus, 1904
    radiology, 1901–1902
    typhoid fever, 1325, 1326
  tympanic membrane, 21, **1680**
Performance IQ, 1735
Performance testing, audiometry, 817
Perfusion, see Ventilation and perfusion
Perfusion lung scans, 517–519, 1901
Perianal region
  enterobiasis, 1487, 1488
  streptococcal cellulitis, 1635
  thrush diarrhea, 1295
  warts, 988
Peribiliary capillary plexus, 470
Pericardial effusion, 635
  amebiasis, 1468
  Neisseria meningitidis, 1315
  tuberculosis, 1342–1343
Pericardial friction rub, 32
Pericarditis, 628, **634–635**
  Coxsackie B viruses, 1383
  gonococcal, 1426
  neonate, organisms, 284 (Table)
  tuberculosis, **1342–1343**
Pericentric inversions, chromosomal, 51
Perihepatitis, 1426, 1430

Perimembranous ventricular septal defect, 600
Perinatal asphyxia, *see* Birth asphyxia; Postasphyxial dyskinesia
Perinatal care, developing countries, **1890–1891**
Perinatal intensive care units, 156
  neonatal deaths, 172–173
Perinatal mortality, 3, 94
  developing countries, 1891
  Scotland, 841
  twin pregnancies, 90
  unmarried mothers, 1855
Perinatal Mortality Survey 1958, 1851–1852
Perinatal period
  definition, 94
  developing countries disease burden and interventions, 1280 (Table)
  dyskinetic cerebral palsy, causes, 753
  immigrants, 1865
  nonprogressive ataxia, causes, 752
  respiratory tract infections, 559
  tuberculosis, **1346**
  typhoid fever, 1325
Perinatal strokes, 740
Perineum
  amebiasis, 1468
  examination, **33–34**
  herpes, 1363–1364
  rhabdomyosarcoma, 916
Periodic breathing, 196, 1721
Periodic syndrome, 434
Periosteal osteosarcoma, 917, 918
Periosteal sarcoma, 917, 918
Periosteum
  infantile cortical hyperostosis, 1583
  non-accidental injury, 1867, 1868
  scurvy, 1200
Periostitis
  neonate, organisms, 284 (Table)
  syphilis, 1407–1408, 1412
Peripheral blood stem cell harvesting, 874
Peripheral hearing loss, 816–818
Peripheral infusions, parenteral nutrition, 159
  venous access, 1223
Peripheral nerves, **721–726**
  birth trauma, **122–123**
  diphtheria, 1305, 1306
  leprosy, 1310
  metachromatic dystrophy, 1165
  neurofibromatosis, 800
  surgery for cerebral palsy, 760
Peripheral nervous system, 719–738
Peripheral neuropathies, **722–726**
  acute intermittent porphyria, 1143
  borreliosis, 1313
  isoniazid, 1347
  pentamidine, 1456
  progressive ataxia, 766
Peripheral stem cell harvest, 1270
Peripheral tapetoretinal degenerations, **1666–1667**
Peripheral temperature, 1282
Peripheral venous access, *see* Peripheral infusions; Venepuncture
peripylaria forms, *Leishmania* spp., 1460
Peristalsis
  esophagus, 426
  preterm infant, 150
  visible, 32
Peritoneal dialysis
  acute renal failure, 976
  continuous, 981
  dietary management, 1211 (Table)
  for hypernatremia, 414
  intensive care, 1824
  neonate, 259
Peritoneal lavage, diagnostic, 1812
Peritoneum
  calcification, 1902
    meconium ileus, 1776
  CSF shunts to, 662

Peritonitis
  abdominal injury, 1811
  necrotizing enterocolitis, 211
  nephrotic syndrome, 969
  primary, **1787**
  Pseudomonas aeruginosa, 1320
  spontaneous bacterial, **483**
  tuberculosis, 1345
Peritonsillitis, 1687
Periventricular hemorrhage, 161, **249–250**
  hydrocephalus, 664
  vs Little's disease, 745
  ocular deviation, 241
Periventricular leukomalacia, 161, **250–251**
  birth asphyxia, 126
  outcome, 171, 172
  strabismus, 267
  ultrasonography, 242, 1908
Perléche, 1198
Permanent distal renal tubular acidosis, 945
Permeability, membranes, **405**
Permethrin
  head lice, 1518
  scabies, 1638
Pernasal swab, pertussis, 1317
Pernicious anemia, 853, 1199
  mucocutaneous candidiasis, 1251
Peroneal muscular atrophy (Charcot–Marie–Tooth atrophy), 72 (Table), 721, 722–723, 765
Peroxidase deficiency
  congenital hypothyroidism, 1046
  thyroid scintigraphy, 1047
Peroxisomal alanine glyoxylate aminotransferase defect, 1112
Peroxisomal 3-oxoacyl-CoA thiolase deficiency, 786 (Table), 1174
Peroxisomes, disorders, **785–787 (Table), 1171–1174**
Persistent asymptomatic proteinuria, 968
Persistent diarrhea, 1215
Persistent ductus arteriosus, 198–199, **602–603**
  Doppler ultrasonography, 1896
  interventional radiology, 593, 594, 603
  respiratory distress syndrome, 181, **204**
  signs, 587 (Table)
  water balance, 142–143
Persistent fetal circulation, 160, 165
  transient tachypnea of the newborn, 182
Persistent hyperplastic primary vitreous, 1668
Persistent hypoglycemia, 296
Persistent parenchymal echodensity, very low birth weight, outcome, 172
Persistent proteinuria, 968
Persistent pulmonary hypertension in the newborn, 202
  nitric oxide inhalation, 204, 1823
  respiratory distress syndrome, 204–205
Persistent vegetative state, 709
Personal independence, 762
Personality development, 1729 (Table), **1732**
Personalization, 1730, 1764
Perthes disease, **1594–1595**
  magnetic resonance imaging, 1898
  vs multiple epiphyseal dysplasia, 1580
  radiography, 1915
  scintigraphy, 1916
Pertussis, **561–562, 1315–1318**
  antibiotic prophylaxis, 1529
  apnea, 528
  intracranial hemorrhage, 713
  mortality, 490
  re-emergence, 1278
  trends, 7
  vaccination, 345
    adverse effects, 343
    contraindications, 342 (Table), 343
    early, 343–344
  vaccines, 341, 1317, 1318

Pervasive developmental disorders, **834–836**, 1733, **1737–1739**
Pes cavus, **1556**
Pes planus, **1555**
Petechiae
  birth trauma, 121
  infective endocarditis, 630
  neonate, organisms, 285 (Table)
  non-accidental injury, 1868
Petechial rashes, **1285**
  neonate, 1284
Pethidine, administration, 1973 (Table)
Petit mal, severely handicapped children affected, 14 (Table)
Petroleum distillates, poisoning, 1711
Pets
  allergy, 1691, **1692**, 1695, 1696
  asthma, 493, 545
  deworming, 1486
Peutz–Jeghers syndrome, 424, **448**
Peyer's patches, typhoid fever, 1325
Pfeiffer's syndrome, 1561
  bulbar palsy, 813
  inheritance, 1566 (Table)
pH, 416, 419, 420
  alimentary secretions, 411 (Table)
  amniotic fluid, 1937 (Table)
  esophagus
    ambulatory measurement, 427, 429–430
    asthma, 542
    neonatal reflux studies, 212
  fetal blood
    labor, 86
    normal, 119 (Table)
  Golgi apparatus, effect of CFTR, 552
  in nanomoles, 417
  normal values, 1926 (Table), 1927 (Table)
  urine, 1932 (Table)
  regulation, **417–419**
  respiratory distress syndrome, 179
  stomach, 430
  stools, 1936 (Table)
  urine
    minimum, 1938 (Table)
    proteinuria diagnosis, 967
  ventilation, 161
Phadebact Monoclonal GC test, 1423
Phagocytes, 274, 925, 1235
  disorders, **1259–1262**
Phagocytic assays, 1247
Phakomatoses, 245
Phallic period, 1729 (Table), 1730
Phantom limb pain, 1833
Pharmacokinetics, antimicrobials, **1527**
Pharyngitis, **560**, 1686
  acute febrile, 1370
  β-hemolytic streptococci, 1330
  diphtheria, 1306
Pharyngoconjunctival fever, 1370, **1385, 1676**
Pharynx
  aspirates, cystic fibrosis, 555
  Chlamydia trachomatis, 1432
  examination, 29, 511
  Fasciola hepatica, 1512
  gonorrhea, 1425
    management, 1423, 1428
    sexual abuse, 1421
  lymphomas, 908
  non-accidental injury, 1869
  suction, neonates, 104, 111
Phase specific cytotoxic drugs, 892
Phasic spasticity, 747
Phenindione, administration, 1973 (Table)
Phenobarbitone
  administration, 1973 (Table)
    neonate, 1958 (Table)
  birth asphyxia, 130
  BROMIDA scintigraphy, 1907
  and child abuse, 1871
  febrile convulsions prophylaxis, 684
  on fetus and neonate, 91 (Table)

  intracranial birth trauma, 122
  for neonatal jaundice, 219
  neonatal seizures, 246
  scintigraphy for neonatal cholestasis, 472
  status epilepticus, 693
  therapeutic ranges, 1936 (Table)
  vitamin K deficiency, 230
Phenolic compounds, poisoning, 1711
Phenothiazines, 1748 (Table)
  antiemetic, 895–896
  extrapyramidal syndromes, 772
Phenotypes, diverse genotypes for, 77
Phenoxybenzamine, 637 (Table), 1973 (Table)
Phenoxymethyl penicillin
  administration, 1973 (Table)
  β-hemolytic streptococci, 1332 (Table)
  Lyme disease, 1314 (Table)
  rheumatic fever, 629, 1599
Phentolamine
  administration, 1973 (Table)
  renal hypertension, 973 (Table)
Phenylacetylglutamine, degradation, 1103
Phenylalanine
  brain development, 643
  deficiency, 1105
  metabolism disorders, **1103–1106**
    bulbar palsy, 811
  normal values, 1927 (Table)
  tolerance test, 1105
Phenylalanine:tyrosine ratio, 1105
Phenylbutazone, 1603
Phenylbutyrate, amino acid excretion, 307
Phenylene diisothiocyanate, *Ancylostoma* spp., 1490
Phenylephrine, administration, 1973 (Table)
Phenylketonuria, 19, 72 (Table), 790 (Table), 1100–1101, **1103**
  diagnosis, 1105
  dietary management, **1204 (Table)**
  maternal, congenital heart disease, 596
  plasma amino acids, 1103
  screening, 339 (Table)
  severely handicapped children affected, 14 (Table)
Phenylpropionic acid test, medium-chain acyl CoA dehydrogenase deficiency, 1083
Phenylpropionylglycine, 1129
Phenytoin, 686
  administration, 1973 (Table)
    neonate, 1958 (Table)
  birth asphyxia, 130
  cerebellar atrophy, 762
  congenital heart disease, 596
  dystonia, 673
  emergency care, 1814
  encephalopathies, 697
  on fetus and neonate, 91 (Table)
  gums, 425
  head injuries, 709, 1811
  and myasthenia, 728
  neonatal seizures, 246
  neoplasms, 890
  poisoning, 1710
  pregnancy, 691
  seizures caused by, 697
  status epilepticus, 693
  therapeutic ranges, 1936 (Table)
  vitamin K deficiency, 230
Pheochromocytoma, 642, **1072**
  retinopathy, 1674
  scintigraphy, 1913
Philadelphia chromosome, 869, 872
Philodendron poisoning, 1711
Philtrum, 76 (Table)
Phimosis, 1793
Phlebotomus pappatasi, 1390
Phlebotomus spp., leishmaniasis, 1460
Phlebotomy, hereditary sideroblastic anemia, 866
Phlyctenulae, 510

Phlyctenular conjunctivitis, 1336, 1337, **1664,** 1677
Phobic states, **1739**
Phocomelia, 76 (Table), 1545
  writing, 822
Pholcodine, administration, 1973 (Table)
Phonation, 808, **1687–1688**
Phone numbers, *see* Telephone numbers
Phonic ear, 1683
Phonology, 804
Phosphate diabetes, 260, **948**
Phosphate (phosphorus), 1185 (Table)
  abnormal excretion, **1058**
  absorption, neonate, 301–302
  buffer, 416, **418**
    renal tubular acidosis, 944
  concentrations, 404, 406 (Table), 1053
    hypocalcemia, 1058–1059
    late neonatal tetany, 300
    osteopenia of prematurity, 302
  deficiency, **1200**
    neonate, 302
  intake, hypomagnesemia, 300
  neutral, for familial hypophosphatemia, 948
  normal values, 1927 (Table)
    amniotic fluid, 1937 (Table)
    cerebrospinal fluid, 1935 (Table)
    stools, 1936 (Table)
    urine, 1932 (Table)
  parenteral nutrition, 1221, 1222 (Table)
  reabsorption
    calculation, 1054
    renal, 257, 943
  Recommended Dietary Allowances, 1949 (Table)
  reference nutrient intakes, 1947 (Table)
  requirements, preterm infant, 152 (Table), 301–302
  restriction, chronic renal failure, 980
  sources, 1185 (Table)
  supplements
    neonate, 304
    preterm, 154–155
  in utero accretion, 301
Phosphatidylcholine, lamellar bodies, 176
Phosphocellulose, for trimethylaminuria, 1113
Phosphocreatine:inorganic phosphorus, magnetic resonance spectroscopy, 128
Phosphocysteamine, for cystinosis, 1123
Phosphodiesterase inhibition, 546
Phosphoenolpyruvate carboxykinase deficiency, 296–297, 1126
Phosphoethanolamine, hypophosphatasia, 1176
Phosphofructokinase deficiency, muscle, 735, **1139–1140**
Phosphoglycerate kinase deficiency, 1131
Phospholipase A2 inhibition, 546
Phospholipids, 1182
  digestion, 437
  normal values, 1926 (Table)
    cerebrospinal fluid, 1934 (Table)
Phosphomannomutase deficiency, 1175
Phosphopenic rickets, 1056, 1058
Phosphorus, *see* Phosphate
Phosphorus-31 nuclear magnetic resonance spectroscopy, metabolic myopathies, 1132
Phosphorus-32, cerebellar astrocytomas, 903
Phosphorylase b kinase deficiency, *see* Liver phosphorylase and liver phosphorylase b kinase deficiencies
Phosphorylases, glycogen metabolism, 1136
Photic stimulation, intermittent, 677
Photoconvulsive response, 677
Photography
  eye examination, **1653–1654,** 1671
  neonatal death, 173
Photon absorptiometry, 302

Photophobia, albinism, 1673
Photosensitive disorders, hereditary, **1629–1631**
Photosensitive epilepsy, 680 (Table)
  television, 691
Photosensitivity
  idiopathic eruptions, **1645**
  nonacute porphyrias, 1144
Phototherapy, 215–216, **218–219,** 233
  loose stools, 212
pHPPA hydroxylase inhibitors, NTBC, 1106
Phrenic nerve
  birth trauma, 122
  pacing, 531
  paralysis, 576
    after cardiac surgery, 1823
Phycomycosis, 1471 (Table)
Physalia, 1526
Physical abuse, *see* Non-accidental injury
Physical environment, neonatal care, 97
Physical examination, *see* Examination
Physiological anemia, 223
Physiological asphyxia, 107
Physiological dead space, 498
Physiological developmental ataxia, 752
'Physiological' immunodeficiency, 1240
Physiological jaundice of the newborn, 216, 218
Physiological nystagmus, 272
Physiological truncal ataxia, 668
Physiotherapists, child development centers, 399
Physiotherapy
  and bronchiolitis, 565
  cerebral palsy, 757
  chest, neonatal intensive care, 97
  cystic fibrosis, 521, 557
  genetic diplegia, 746
  juvenile chronic arthritis, 1604
  mental retardation, 838
  respiratory disorders, **521**
Phytanic acid
  peroxisomal disorders, 1172 (Table)
  storage disease, *see* Refsum's disease
Phytates, 334
Phytomenadione, administration, 1974 (Table)
  neonate, 1958 (Table)
Phytosterolemia, 1156
Phytosterols, parenteral nutrition, 1226
Phytosterols, *see* Phytosterols
PIA1, isoimmune thrombocytopenia, 878
Piaget, cognitive development, 1728–1729
Pia mater, subpial heterotopia, 685
Pica, 1201, 1736
  toxocariasis, 1485
Picornaviruses, 1381
Picture vocabulary tests, 400
Piebald syndromes, 1107
Pierre Robin syndrome, 110 (Table), 831 (Table), **1562–1563,** 1769, 1796, 1797
  airway obstruction in sleep, 531
Pigeon chest, 30, 512, 1556
Pigmentary retinopathies, 271
Pigmentation
  Addison's disease, 1068
  mouth, 424
  reduced, 1629 (Table), *see also* Albinism; Vitiligo
Pigs
  Taenia solium, 1501
  trichinosis, 1494
Pilocarpine
  pediculosis blepharitis, 1663
  squint, 1660
  sweat test, 552
Pilocytic astrocytomas, 902, 903
Pi (protease inhibitor) MM α₁-antitrypsin deficiency, 1175
Pinches, bruises, 1868
Pineal gland, **1043**
  tumors, **904–905,** 1043
Pineal tumors, retinoblastoma gene, 888

Pink disease, *see* Mercury poisoning
PINNT (Patients on Intravenous and Nasogastric Nutrition Therapy), 1226
Pinta, **1415–1417**
  organism, 1401
Pinworms, **1486–1488**
  vulvovaginitis, 987
Pipecolic acid, 308, 1173
L-Pipecolic acid, peroxisomal disorders, 1172 (Table)
Piperacillin, administration, 1956 (Table), 1974 (Table)
Piperazine
  administration, 1974 (Table)
  ascariasis, 1485
  ataxia, 762
  and enterobiasis, 1488
Pi (protease inhibitor) MM α₁-antitrypsin deficiency, 1175
Pirenzipine, tall stature, 1020
Piroxicam, administration, 1974 (Table)
PIT-1 gene, 367
Pituitary-derived growth hormone preparations, 1019
Pituitary diabetes insipidus, *vs* nephrogenic diabetes insipidus, 943
Pituitary fossa, *see* Empty sella syndrome
Pituitary gigantism, 376
Pituitary gland, 1037
  delayed puberty, 1031
  embryology, 1003
  hyperplasia, hypothyroidism, 1028
  hypoplasia, growth hormone deficiency, 372
  hypothyroidism, 1007
  neonatal disorders, 109
  neural crest cells, 641
  obesity, 1190
  primary amenorrhea, 990
  secondary amenorrhea, 993
  thyroid function tests, 1045
Pituitary hormone deficiencies, craniopharyngioma, 905
Pityriasis alba, 1643
  vs tinea versicolor, 1637
Pityriasis rosea, **1634**
  vs rubella, 1357
Pityriasis versicolor, **1637–1638**
Pivampicillin, 1974 (Table)
Pivmecillinam, 1974 (Table)
Pizotifen, 1974 (Table)
  migraine, 717, 717 (Table), 719
Placebo effect, growth hormone therapy, 1019
Placenta, *see also* entries starting Transplacental
  abruption, **88,** 89 (Table)
  cerebral palsy, 741
  congenital nephrotic syndrome, 972
    Finnish type, 261
  hormone secretion, 1005–1006
  insufficiency, 136–137
  skin, 42
  long-term cardiovascular disease and diabetes mellitus, 1066
  nostrum for retinitis pigmentosa, 1667
Placental lactogen, genes, 366
Placental transfusion, preterm infant, 222
Placenta previa, **88–90**
Place of Safety Orders, 1876, *see also* Child Protection Orders (Scotland)
Placing reflex, 37 (Table)
  neonate, 240
Plagiocephaly, 21 (Fig.), 1559–1560, 1661
Plague, **1318**
Plantar creases
  Down syndrome, 55
  neonatal gestation age, 42 (Fig.)
Plantar grasp reflex, neonate, 241
Plantar reflex, 37 (Table), 239–240
Plantar response, 35
Plantar syphilide, 1406–1407

Plantar warts, 1633
Plant lectin mitogen tests, lymphocytes, 1246
Plants
  adverse reactions, 1691
  poisoning, 1705, 1709, 1711
Plant sterols, *see* Phytosterols
Plasma
  buffers, 417–418
  convalesced patient, for Lassa fever, **1388**
  electrolytes, 403–404
  infusion
    for dehydration, 413
    hemolytic uremic syndrome, 978
    for immunodeficiency, 1268
  osmotic particles, 406 (Table)
  pH, 416
  postprandial, parenteral nutrition, 1297
  potassium, 411
  volume, 403
    normal values, 1928 (Table)
  water, 404
Plasma cells, gastrointestinal immune response, 439
Plasma exchange, hemolytic uremic syndrome, 978
Plasma exchange transfusion, partial, 1839
Plasmalogens, peroxisomal disorders, 1172 (Table)
Plasmapheresis
  Guillain–Barré syndrome, 726
  myasthenia gravis, 727, 728
Plasma proteins
  glycemic control, 1080
  inborn errors, **1175–1177**
Plasmid-mediated resistance, *Neisseria gonorrhoeae,* 1421–1422
Plasmids, antibiotic resistance, 1529
Plasmin, 228
Plasmodium falciparum, 1445, 1446, 1447, 1448
  clinical features, **1449–1450**
  treatment, 1452
Plasmodium spp., 1445–1446
Plastering, serial, 757
Plastezote jackets, 757–758
Plastic bag, gastroschisis, 1780
Plastic film (Op-Site), transcutaneous oxygen tension measurement, 160
Plastic properties of muscle, 756
Plastic surgery, **1796–1800**
  cleft palate, 810
Platelet activating factor, septicemia, 1287
Platelet antigens, 228
Platelets, 227
  aggregation
    Kawasaki disease, 1480
    ristocetin-induced, Von Willebrand's disease, 881
  counts, 228 (Table), *see also* Thrombocytopenic purpuras
    normal, 1939 (Table)
    percutaneous liver biopsy, 472
  fetus, 222
    and neonate, 848
  function disorders, **879**
    neonate, 229–230
  infantile cortical hyperostosis, 1583
  irradiated, fetal transfusion, 229
  neonatal sepsis, 276 (Table), 277
  polycythemia, SGA baby, 137
  storage pool diseases, 879
Platelet transfusions
  cancer treatment, 895
  disseminated intravascular coagulation, 231
  Wiskott–Aldrich syndrome, 1254
Platybasia, 1559
Play, and development, 386
Playground injuries, 1713
Play groups, 1861
Play leaders, accident and emergency departments, 1805

Pleotrophic cytotoxic drug resistance, 893
Pleroceroids, 1503, 1504
Plethora, lung fields, 200 (Table)
Plethysmography
    cystic fibrosis, 554
    lung function, **500**, 501
Pleural aspiration, *see* Chest, drainage;
        Pleural tap
Pleural biopsy, 521
Pleural effusions
    drainage, 1845
    imaging, 1899
    neonate, 193
        organisms, 284 (Table)
    pneumonia, **568–569**
    tuberculosis, 1341, 1342
    ultrasonography, 517
Pleural friction, 30
Pleural rub, 513
Pleural tap, **520–521**, *see also* Chest,
        drainage
    emergency, 1807
    for pneumothorax, 188, **1844–1845**
Pleurodesis, 556
    fibrin glue, 188
Pleurodynia, *see* Bornholm disease
Plexiform neurofibroma, 800
Plexiform neuromas, 1628
Ploidy, neuroblastoma, 911
Plowden Report, nursery schools, 1861
Pluripotent stem cells, hemopoiesis, 221
'Plus' disease, retinopathy of prematurity,
        266
Pneumatosis arterialis, *see* Air embolism
Pneumococcus, *see* Streptococcus
        pneumoniae
Pneumocystis carinii pneumonia,
        534–535, *see also* Co-trimoxazole,
        Pneumocystis carinii
    cancer treatment, 895
    HIV infection, 533, 1397
    preterm infant, 196
Pneumograms, after apparent life-
        threatening events, 529
Pneumomediastinum, neonate, 187, **189**
Pneumonia, *see also under named
        organisms*
    adenoviruses, 568, 1370
    vs appendicitis, 1786
    asthma patients, 547
    bacterial, measles, 1354, 1355
    bacteriology, 1298–1299
    chest pain, 509
    community-acquired, **565–568**
    crackles, 512
    immunocompromised patient, **534–536**
    mortality, 490 (Table)
        postneonatal, 5 (Table)
        trends, 7
    neonate, **183–185**, 280
        mortality, 4 (Table)
        organisms, 284 (Table)
        staphylococcal, 281
    primary atypical, 1374
    respiratory distress syndrome, 181–182
'Pneumonia season,' 1319
Pneumonic plague, 1318
Pneumonic tularemia, 1351
Pneumonitis, *see also* Interstitial
        pneumonitis
    Chlamydia spp., 196, 564
    cytomegalovirus, immunocompromised
        patient, 535
    larval, ascariasis, 1482, 1484
    varicella, 1361
Pneumopericardium, neonate, **189**
Pneumoperitoneum, neonate, 187,
        189–190
Pneumothorax, 577
    chest drainage, 1807, **1844–1845**
    chest pain, 509
    cystic fibrosis, 555–556
    meconium aspiration syndrome, 185,
        187

neonate, **187–188**
    respiratory distress syndrome, 181, 187
    resuscitation, 1807, 1811
    tension pneumothorax, 187, 188, **1811,
        1844**
PO₂, 419
    normal values, 1927 (Table)
Podophyllin, 988, **1444–1445**, 1633
Podophyllotoxin preparation, 1445
POEMS (otoacoustic emissions detection),
        244
Point mutations, 69
Poisoning, **1705–1711**, 1815
    child abuse, **1871**
    hemolysis, 864
    medical practice on incidence figures,
        1803
Poisonous animal bites and stings,
        1520–1526
Poisons Information Centers, 1706
    telephone numbers, **1707**
Pokeweed mitogen test, lymphocytes,
        1245, 1246
Poland's anomaly, 512
Polar bear liver, 1194
Polar bodies, 48
Police
    child abuse, 1873
    Children (Scotland) Act 1995, 1877
Police protection, 1876
Policing policy, delinquency, 1762
Poliomyelitis, 286 (Table), **1378–1381**
    immunization, world performance,
        1280, 1380
    trends, 7
    United Kingdom, 1277, 1278 (Fig.)
    vaccination, 345, 1381
        AIDS, 1396
        diarrhea and vomiting, 342 (Table)
        mass programmes, 345
        risks, 343
    virology, differential diagnosis, 1351
Poliomyelitis-like illness, ECHO viruses,
        1383
Polioviruses, **1379**, 1380
Political action, 337–338
Political instability, developing countries,
        1885
Pollens, 1689–1690
Polyarteritis, **1610–1611**
Polyarteritis nodosa, 1479
    heart, 636
    renal involvement, 966
    retinopathy, 1674
Polyarthritis, rheumatic fever, 1597
Polyarticular onset juvenile chronic
        arthritis, 1601–1602
Polycystic kidney disease, 254, **940–941**,
        see also Autosomal dominant
        polycystic kidney disease
    tuberous sclerosis, 801
    ultrasonography, 1909–1910
Polycystic ovaries, 993, **1034**, 1061
    21-hydroxylase deficiency, 1064
    puberty, 1028
Polycythemia, 713
    and hypoglycemia, 294
    liver tumors, 924
    neonate, **226–227**
    partial plasma exchange transfusion,
        1839
    SGA baby, 137
Polydactyly, 76, 1546 (Table), **1548**
Polydipsia, 1039
Polyembryoma, 921
Polyenes, *see* Amphotericin B; Nystatin
Polyethylene glycol conjugated ADA, 1270
Polyethylene glycol conjugated interleukin
        2, for common variable
        immunodeficiency, 1257
Polygenic inheritance, congenital heart
        disease, 596
Polyglandular autoimmune disease type 1,
        1057

Polyglandular enlargement, HIV infection,
        1395
Polyhydramnios, 1937 (Table)
    cystic adenomatoid malformation, 192
    mesoblastic nephroma, 915
Polyionic solution, for hypernatremia,
        414
Polymerase chain reaction, **70–71**
    cerebrospinal fluid, 1298
    HIV, 1393
    Mycobacterium tuberculosis, 1335
    rubella, 287
Polymorphic light eruption, 1645
Polymorphonuclear leukocytes, neonate,
        274
Polymyositis, **737–738, 1606–1608**, 1644
Polymyxins, site of action, 1527
Polyneuropathies, *see* Peripheral
        neuropathies
Polyostotic fibrous dysplasia
        (McCune–Albright syndrome),
        1028, 1029, **1589**
Polyploidy, 51
Polyposis, familial adenomatous, 448
    liver tumors, 924
Polyposis coli, 72 (Table)
    familial, 888 (Table), 889
Polyps
    gastrointestinal tract, **448,** 460
    larynx, 1687
    nasal, 1685
        cystic fibrosis, 555
Polyribosyl-ribitol phosphate (PRP),
        Haemophilus influenzae, 1308,
        1309
Polysaccharide-based oral rehydration
        solutions, 1304
Polysaccharide iron complex,
        administration, 1974 (Table)
Polysaccharides, antibody response
        deficiency, 1258
Polysaccharide vaccines, 341
Polysplenia, 613
Polystyrene sulfonate resin,
        administration, 1974 (Table)
Polyunsaturated fatty acids, 1148, 1182
    dietary sources, 1182 (Table)
    juvenile chronic arthritis, 1210
    long-chain, breast milk, 152
    milks, 332–333
    vitamin D absorption, 301
    and vitamin E requirement, 225
ω-3 Polyunsaturated fatty acids, ulcerative
        colitis, 1206
Polyurethane, enteral feeding tubes, 1218
Polyuria, 1039
Polyvinylchloride, enteral feeding tubes,
        1218
Pompe's disease, 596, 788–789 (Table),
        1138, 1157 (Table)
    neonate, 307
Pond fracture, birth trauma, 707
Pons, gliomas, 903
Ponstan, *see* Mefenamic acid
Popliteal angle, neonate, 44, 237, 239
    gestation age, 40 (Table), 41 (Fig.)
Popliteal pterygium syndrome, **1554**
Population density, **2 (Table)**
Populations, 1, 2, 1883 (Table)
Population (Statistics) Act 1938, birth
        registration, 1849
Porcine surfactant (Curosurf), 179
Porencephaly, 650
    very low birth weight, outcome, 172
Pores of Kohn, 177
Porins, and antibiotic resistance, 1529
Pork
    Taenia solium, 1501
    trichinosis, 1494
Pornography, 1870
Porphobilinogen, 1142
    normal values, urine, 1932 (Table)
Porphobilinogen deaminase, erythrocytes,
        1143

Porphyria cutanea tarda, 1142 (Table),
        1144
Porphyrias, **1142–1144, 1630–1631**
    congenital erythropoietic, **865**
    teeth, 425
Porphyrins, normal values, stools, 1936
        (Table)
Portal fibrosis, 221
Portal hypertension
    extrahepatic biliary atresia, 475
    management, **482–483**
    portal vein obstruction, **483**
Portal systemic shunting, schistosomiasis,
        1510
Portal tract, necrotizing enterocolitis, 282
Portal vein
    Doppler ultrasonography, 1907
    obstruction, portal hypertension, **483**
Portoenterostomy, 475, 1782–1783
Portuguese man-of-war, 1526
Port-wine stain, 1620, 1798
Position, obstetric, 83
Positional deformities, cerebral palsy,
        748–749
Positional sense, examination, 35
Positive end-expiratory pressure
        ventilation, 163, 1818
    near-drowning, 1825
    for pulmonary hemorrhage, 191
Positron emission tomography, **1897**
    brain tumors, 901
    epilepsy, 679
Posseting, 209
Postasphyxial dyskinesia, 753, **754–755**
Postasphyxial encephalopathy, **125–128**
    grade and prognosis, 132
Postaxial polydactyly, 76 (Table)
Posterior fossa
    hemorrhage, birth trauma, 122
    radiography, 1908
    tumor, gastroesophageal reflux, 428
Posterior pituitary hormones, **1039**
Posterior urethral valves, 255, 935, **937,**
        950, **1778**
    vs enuresis, 957 (Table)
    ultrasonography, 1908
Posterior uveitis, 1665–1666
Posterior visual pathway disorders,
        272–273
Postgastroenteritis lactose intolerance,
        333, 454, 1215
Postgonococcal urethritis, 1425
Posthemorrhagic hydrocephalus, 664–665
    preterm infant, 252–253
Postherpetic neuralgia, 1363
Postictal behavior, 690
Postictal period, 674
Posticteric choreoathetosis, 753–754
Postinfectious encephalitis
    chickenpox, 1361, 1362
    mumps, 1371–1372
Postinfectious encephalomyelitis, measles,
        1354
Postinfectious myelitis, **1376**
Post-kala azar dermal leishmaniasis, 1463
Postmaturity, *see also* Postterm pregnancy
    definitions, 94
Post-mortems, *see* Autopsy
Postnasal drip, 506
Postnatal development, renal function,
        256–257, 1953
Postnatal growth, **352–364**
Postnatal hemorrhage, 224
Postnatal investigation, urinary tract
        abnormalities, 936–937
Postnatal lung growth, 177
Postnatal ward routines, **111–112**
Postnecrotic cirrhosis, causes, 482 (Table)
Postneonatal mortality, 3, **5**
    Stillbirth and Infant Mortality Study,
        1851
Postoperative pain, 1830
Postpartum care, 88

Postpericardotomy syndrome, 1822
Post-polio syndrome, 1380
Postprandial motility, 208
Postprandial plasma, parenteral nutrition, 1297
Postprimary coccidioidomycosis, 1475
Postprimary tuberculosis, **1336**
pulmonary, 1342
Postrenal failure, 258
Poststenotic dilation of ascending aorta, 607
Poststreptococcal glomerulonephritis, 961
vs membranoproliferative glomerulonephritis, 963
vs mesangial IgA nephropathy, 963
Postterm pregnancy, 83
Post-traumatic stress disorder, **1741–1742**
Postural control, 382
Postural drainage, 521
Postural proteinuria, 967–968
Postural scoliosis, 1557
Posture, *see also* Ataxias; Prone sleeping
asymmetric skull, 1559
development of skills, 668 (Table)
Duchenne muscular dystrophy, 730
examination, 388 (Table), 389 (Table)
gastroesophageal reflux, 429, 571
history taking, 17
neonate, 44, 236–239
gestation age, 40 (Table), 41 (Fig.)
regional ventilation, 502
respiratory disorders, 511
tracheoesophageal fistula, 1771
Potassium, 408–409, 1185 (Table), 1223 (Table), *see also* Hyperkalemia
alimentary secretions, 411 (Table)
colonic secretion, 455
concentrations, 404 (Table), 406 (Table)
depletion, 421, 946–947
congenital chloridorrhea, 446–447
for diabetic ketoacidosis, 1076
disorders, **411–412**
renal pH control, **418–419**
feces
cholera, 1303 (Table)
gastroenteritis, 1293
fluid therapy for dehydration, 413
gastroenteritis, replacement, 1296
intestinal absorption, 438
movement across membranes, 405, 406
neonates, **144–145**
intravenous supplements, 145
urine, 142 (Table)
normal values, 1928 (Table)
amniotic fluid, 1937 (Table)
cerebrospinal fluid, 1935 (Table)
meconium, 1936 (Table)
urine, 1932 (Table)
parenteral nutrition, 1222 (Table)
per gram of noncollagen nitrogen, 411
reference nutrient intakes, 1947 (Table)
requirements, 413 (Table)
preterm infant, 152 (Table)
sources, 1185 (Table)
Potassium chloride
administration, 1974 (Table)
for alkalosis, 421
preparations, 415
Potassium citrate mixture, 415
Potassium iodide, sporotrichosis, 1473
Potatoes, fructose-1-phosphate aldolase deficiency, 1135
Potter's sequence, 108, 110, 253
Pott's disease, *see* Spine, tuberculosis
Pourcelot resistance index, birth asphyxia, 128–129, 132
Poverty
developing countries, 1883
divorce, 1856
Povidone iodine, ophthalmia neonatorum prophylaxis, 263, 1429
Powders
for inhalation, 1954
skin treatment, 1617

Power, limbs, neonate, 237–239
Power Doppler ultrasonography, **1896**
Poxviruses, specimens, 1352
PPNG, *see* β-lactamases, *Neisseria gonorrhoeae*
Prader orchidometer, 358
Prader–Willi syndrome, 831 (Table), 1006, 1022, 1190
bulbar palsy, 811
deletion, 59, 60 (Table)
depigmentation, 1107
obesity, 1022
Pralidoxime
administration, 1974 (Table)
organophosphorus poisoning, 1711
Praziquantel
administration, 1974 (Table)
cysticercosis, 1502
hydatid disease, dogs, 1506
Hymenolepsis spp., 1502
intestinal flukes, 1513
liver flukes, 1513
schistosomiasis, 1510
Taenia saginata, 1500
Prazosin
administration, 1974 (Table)
hypertension, 637 (Table)
renal, 973 (Table)
Preaxial polydactyly, 76 (Table)
Prebetalipoproteinemia type IV, 1150 (Table), 1152
Prechtl & Bientema, states of alertness, 235 (Table)
Precipitating factors, adolescent disorders, 1750–1751
Precocious puberty, 377, **1027–1031**
acute lymphoblastic leukemia treatment, 875, 1024
female, 989
hepatoblastoma, 924
21-hydroxylase deficiency, 1063
hypothyroidism, 1050
pineal gland, 1043
rapid growth, 1020
Preconceptual care (prepregnancy care), **79–80, 114**
folate, 652
Preconceptual prevention, 338
Precordial examination, 586
Precordial leads, electrocardiography, 588 (Fig.)
Precordial pulsation, 32
Prediction of adult height, 362–363
Predisposing factors, adolescent disorders, 1751
Prednisolone
acute severe asthma, 549
administration, 1974 (Table)
asthma, 546
autoimmune chronic active hepatitis, 480
Crohn's disease, 457
hemangiomas, 1619
idiopathic thrombocytopenic purpura, 878
infantile cortical hyperostosis, 1585
juvenile chronic arthritis, 1604
nephrotic syndrome, 970–971
polymyositis, 737
tuberculosis, 1347
ulcerative colitis, 459
Prednisone
ascariasis pneumonitis, 1484
Duchenne muscular dystrophy, 731
Pre-eclampsia, 90
uterine artery blood flow, 81
Preemptive analgesia, 1830
Pre-exposure prophylaxis, rabies, 1378
Preferential looking, 269
Pregnancy, *see also* Antenatal care; Maternal factors
anticonvulsants, 114, 691
bacterial vaginosis, **1435**
calcium metabolism, effect of fetus, 1053

cerebral palsy, 741
Chlamydia trachomatis, 1432
gonorrhea, treatment, 1428
herpes simplex, **1441–1442**
homocystinuria, 1108
incest, 1870
Plasmodium falciparum, 1448
preventive measures in, 338
rubella, 1357–1358
sexually transmitted diseases, **1400**
syphilis, 1410
systemic herpes simplex virus infection, 1438
teenage, 994, 1815, 1855
toxoplasmosis, 1464–1465
tuberculosis, **1346**
Pregnancy-induced hypertension, 90
Pregnanediol, normal values, urine, 1932 (Table)
Pregnanetriol
congenital adrenal hyperplasia, 986
normal values, urine, 1932 (Table)
Pregnenolone, 1060 (Fig.), 1064
Prehospital care, **1804–1805**
Preictal behavior, 690
Preimplantation diagnosis, in vitro fertilized embryos, cystic fibrosis, 552
Prekallikrein, 228
Pre-lipoprotein, *see* Very low density lipoprotein
Preload, cardiac, 1819
Premature craniosynostosis, **1559–1560**
Prematurity, *see* Preterm gestation; Preterm infant
Premutation, fragile X mental retardation, 63
Prenatal causes of deafness, 1682
Prenatal diagnosis, 338
cardiovascular disorders, 201
central nervous system malformations, 645
chest disorders, 517
chromosome preparations, 50
congenital heart disease, 597
congenital nephrotic syndrome, 972
cystic fibrosis, **552**
cystinosis, 945
Duchenne muscular dystrophy, 732
gynecology, 985
hemoglobinopathies, 863
hemophilia A, 880
Hunter's syndrome, 1160
21-hydroxylase deficiency, 1062–1063
immunodeficiency, **1248**
mental retardation, 841
red cell enzyme defects, 858
renal tumors, 915
urinary tract abnormalities, 256, **935–941**
ventriculomegaly, 252
Prenatal growth, **349–352,** 1002–1003
Prenatal infections, 284 (Table)
Prenatal radiation, neoplasms, 889–890
Prenatal therapy, **114–115**
galactose restriction, 1133
Preoperative period, development, 1729–1730
Prepatent period, malaria, 1446
Prepregnancy care, *see* Preconceptual care
Preprogrammed behaviors, **667**
Prepuce, nonretractability, 1793
Prerenal failure, 974
neonate, 258
Presacral tumors, 921
Preschool children
blood pressure, 20
definition, 17
disease incidence, 13
psychiatric disorder, 1734, **1736**
Preschool health care, **1860–1865**
Prescribing, 1953–1980
Prescriptions, 1879
Presenile dementia, Down syndrome, 55

Presentation, obstetric, 83
Pressure gradients
cardiac catheterization, 593
spectral Doppler ultrasonography, 592–593
Pressure immobilization, for bites and stings, 1523
Pressure limited ventilation, 1817
Pressure measurements, *see also* Manometry
cardiac catheterization, 593
Pressure–volume curve, lungs, 159
Pressure–volume index, response, intracranial, 698
Preterm delivery
breast milk composition, 332
twin pregnancies, 90
Preterm gestation, 11
chronic lung disease, 491
definition, 94
neonatal mortality, 4 (Table)
skin, 42
stillbirth rates, 4 (Table)
temperature, 20
Preterm infant
alkaline phosphatase, 302
anemias, **224–226**
Apgar score, **125,** 126
birth apnea, 135
theophylline therapeutic range, 1936 (Table)
birth asphyxia, 131
body composition, 151 (Table)
bone mineral deficit, 304
calcium requirements, 152 (Table), 301–302
care, **138–155**
cerebral palsy, 738–739
cough absence, 506
deafness, 1682
dyskinetic cerebral palsy, 753, 754
electroencephalography, 243
failure to thrive, 465–466
folate deficiency, 852
heart disease, 206
hyperglycemia, 298
hypoglycemia, 293, 294
immunity, 1240
infection, 276
metabolic bone disease, 301–304
morphine, 1833
'not tolerating feeds', 208
ophthalmic sequelae, 267
parenteral nutrition, 1220
persistent ductus arteriosus, 603
phosphorus requirements, 301–302
pneumonia, 183
posthemorrhagic hydrocephalus, 252–253
renal function, 257
respiratory tract, 496
resuscitation, 132
retinopathy, 1668
seizures, 245
sepsis, 277
thyroid function, 1045
umbilical cord clamping, 108, 139, 222, 225
vision, 738
Preterm labor, **115–116**
breech presentation, 87–88
management, 119
manual work, 80
Prevalence
cerebral palsy, **738,** 739
diabetes mellitus, 1073–1074
mental retardation, 826
and screening, 1001
Preventive measures, *see also* Immunization; *named diseases*
accidents, 705, **1712–1713**
burns and scalds, 1714–1715
diabetes mellitus, 1081
drowning, 1718

Preventive measures (*Contd*)
mental retardation, **841–842**
poisoning, 1706
sexually transmitted diseases, **1398–1399**
tuberculosis, **1340**
Preventive pediatrics, **337–348**
Hall Committee, 1853
malnutrition, 1194
urinary tract infections, **952,** 954–956
Previous history, 18
Prickly heat (miliaria), 1646
Prick testing, allergic disorders, 1693
Primaquine, 1453, 1974 (Table)
Primary atypical pneumonia, 1374
Primary biliary cirrhosis, 1145
Doppler ultrasonography, 1907
Primary brain injury, *vs* secondary brain injury, **1810**
Primary health care, *see also* General practice
developing countries, **1889–1890**
Primary hemochromatosis, 1147
Primary herpetic meningoencephalitis, 1364, 1365
Primary hyperoxaluria type I, 948
Primary hyperparathyroidism, **1056–1057,** 1058
Primary hypertension, 636
Primary infection, herpes simplex virus, 1436–1437, 1438–1439
pregnancy, 1441
Primary oocytes, 1004
Primary peritonitis, **1787**
Primary prevention, 338
Primary pseudohypoaldosteronism, 947
Primary resistance, tumor cells, 892
Primary syphilis, **1405–1406**
Primary tuberculosis, **1336**
progressive, **1341–1342**
pulmonary, **1340–1342**
Primene R, 157, 158 (Table)
Primidone
administration, 1974 (Table)
therapeutic ranges, 1936 (Table)
Primitive neuroectodermal tumors, 900, **901–902**
peripheral, tumor markers, 912 (Table)
pineal, 904
supratentorial, **906**
Primitive reflexes, 35, 36 (Table), 240, 382
Primordial follicle, 1004
PR interval, 589
carditis, 1598, 1599
Prisons, accommodation of children, 1857
Probenecid
administration, 1974 (Table)
gonorrhea, 1427 (Table)
syphilis, 1410
Procainamide, administration, 1974 (Table)
Procaine penicillin
administration, 1975 (Table)
syphilis, 1409, 1410
congenital, 1415
Procarbazine, gonadal function, 899
Procedures, practical, **1829–1847**
Processus vaginalis, 1788–1789
Prochlorperazine, administration, 1975 (Table)
Procoagulant inhibitors, 227
Procollagen peptides, osteogenesis imperfecta, 1568, 1569
Procollagen type I C-terminal propeptide, 1012
Procollagen type III N-terminal propeptide, 1012
Proctoscopy, 464
rectal bleeding, 459
Procurator Fiscal, 1849
Procured illness, 1871

Procyclidine, administration, 1975 (Table)
Pro-drugs, antibiotics, 1527
Product licenses, **1955**
Proenzymes, small intestine, 437
Progenitor stem cells, 221–222
Progeria, 26 (Fig.)
Progesterone, normal values, 1928 (Table)
Progestogen-like drugs, for precocious puberty, 1030
Progestogen-only pill, 995
Progestogens
and puberty induction, 1035
transplacental virilization, 1008
Proglottids, tapeworms, 1500, 1501
Prognosis
remarks on, 1878
respiratory disorders, 492
Prognostic scores, Wilson's disease, 481
Prognostic strategy, individualized, 102
Progressive ataxias, 764, 792 (Table)
Progressive coccidioidomycosis, 1475
Progressive disease, neoplasms, 893
Progressive hydrocephalus, *see* Active hydrocephalus
Progressive multifocal leukoencephalopathy, 795 (Table), **1378**
Progressive myoclonic epilepsy syndrome, 689 (Table), 795 (Table)
Progressive primary tuberculosis, **1341–1342**
Progressive systemic sclerosis, **1608–1609,** *see also* Scleroderma
glomerular disease, 966
heart, 636
renal crisis, 966
Progress notes, 1879
Proguanil, malaria, prophylaxis, 1448–1449, 1975 (Table)
Prohibited Steps Orders, 1874
Proinsulin, 1071 (Fig.)
Projectile vomiting, 434
Prokinetic drugs, gastroesophageal reflux, 429
Prolactin, 327–328, **1039,** *see also* Hyperprolactinemia
delayed puberty, 1031
levels, 1034
fetus, 1003
hyperprolactinemia, 1041
normal values, 1928 (Table)
respiratory distress syndrome, 176
secretion, 112
secondary amenorrhea, 993
Prolactin receptor, 1012
Prolidase deficiency, 1114
Proline, metabolism disorders, **1113–1114**
Prolonged jaundice, neonate, **219–221**
Prolonged rupture of membranes
pneumonia, 183
sepsis, 277
Promastigotes, 1454 (Fig.)
Leishmania spp., 1460
Promethazine, administration, 1975 (Table)
Promyelocytic leukemia, 869
Pronated foot, **1555**
Prone sleeping
apparent life-threatening events, 528
sudden infant death syndrome, 1720
Pro-opiomelanocortin, 1038
Properdin, 1232
'Proper Officers,' infectious disease notification, 1850
Prophase, 47
Prophylaxis, *see also* Antibiotics, prophylaxis
antifungal, 1530
co-trimoxazole, cancer treatment, 894
drugs, 340
febrile convulsions, 683–684
malaria, **1448–1449**
ophthalmia neonatorum, 1429
rabies, 1378

rheumatic fever, 1600
Propionic acidemia, 1117
Propofol, dystonia, 673
Propranolol, 627 (Table)
administration, 1975 (Table)
growth hormone secretion, 1013
hypertension, 637 (Table), 638
renal, 973 (Table)
hyperthyroidism, 1051
long QT interval syndromes, 627
migraine, 717 (Table), **718**
neonatal hyperthyroidism, 1051
tetralogy of Fallot, 617
Proprioception, writing, 822
Proptosis, 1650
craniostenosis, 1661
neuroblastoma, 911
neurofibromatosis, 800
orbital neoplasms, 1661
Prosencephalon, 642
Prospective studies, respiratory disorders, 492
Prostacyclin, 227
cyanotic heart disease, dosage, 202 (Table)
for hemofiltration, 1824
hemolytic uremic syndrome, 978
persistent pulmonary hypertension of the newborn, 204
Prostaglandin inhibitors, for preterm labor, 116
Prostaglandins
for congenital heart disease, 598–599
cyanotic heart disease, 202
E_1, neonate, 1958 (Table)
E_2
sodium balance, 142–143
urinary potassium loss, 144–145
for hematemesis, 210
labor, 84
induction, 87
role of adrenal gland, 1005
Prostaglandin synthetase inhibitors
dysfunctional uterine bleeding, 992
nephrogenic diabetes insipidus, 949
Prostate, rhabdomyosarcoma, 916
Prostheses
ear abnormalities, 1679
juvenile chronic arthritis, 1605
limb malformations, 1545
osteosarcoma surgery, 918
Prostitution, 1870, 1887
gonorrhea, 1421
Protamine, administration, 1975 (Table)
Protease inhibitors, 1397
Proteases, on uterine cervix, 84
Protective clothing, infection prevention, 1282
Protein binding, drugs, 1953
Protein bound calcium, 298–299, 1053
Protein C, 227, 231, 882
stroke, 713
Protein:creatinine ratio
after hemolytic uremic syndrome, 978
nephrotic syndrome, 969
urine, 967
Protein electrophoresis, cerebrospinal fluid, normal values, 1935 (Table)
Protein–energy malnutrition, **1191–1194**
developing countries, 1892
disease burden, 1280 (Table)
growth failure, 1017
immunodeficiency, 1265
juvenile chronic arthritis, 1210
Protein hydrolysate milks, 1215
for cystic fibrosis, 1208
Protein-losing enteropathy, **443**
Protein malnutrition, in insulin-like growth factors, 1023
Protein S, 228, 231, 882
disorder, stroke, 713
Proteins
absorption, 207

breast milk, quality, 332
as buffers, 416
concentrations, 404 (Table), 406
diet
enteropathies, 1214
for hepatic encephalopathy, 1209
for hyperammonemia, 1112
for inborn errors of metabolism, 307
dietary sources, 1182 (Table)
digestion, 423
preterm infant, 150
small intestine, 437
feces, 443, 448
inborn errors of metabolism, replacement, 1102
intolerance, *see also* Cow's milk, intolerance
lysinuric, 446, 1121
kwashiorkor, plasma levels, 1193
loss
cystic fibrosis, 1208
progressive systemic sclerosis, 1608
secondary immunoglobulin deficiency, 1259
malabsorption, **446**
metabolism, neonate, 471
milks, 332
normal values
amniotic fluid, 1937 (Table)
cerebrospinal fluid, 1935 (Table)
serum, 1928 (Table)
urine, 1932 (Table)
preterm milk formulae, 152
preterm supplements, 154
proportion in energy intake, 1180
Recommended Dietary Allowances, 1948 (Table)
reference nutrient intakes, 1947 (Table)
requirements, 1181–1182
parenteral nutrition, 1220
preterm, 151 (Table), 157–158
restriction
chronic renal failure, 980
hepatic encephalopathy, 483
stools, 1936 (Table)
transport into cells, 1123
urine, 967
Protein selectivity index, 967
Proteinuria, **966–972,** *see also* Nephrotic syndrome
glomerulonephritis, 961–962, 968
neonate, **261**
penicillamine, 1604
with vitamin B_{12} malabsorption, 853
Proteus spp., **1320**
Weil–Felix test, 1391
Prothrombin, deficiency, 881–882
Prothrombin time, 228, 879 (Fig.), 1188
acute liver failure, 479
liver disease, 472 (Table)
chronic, 480
percutaneous liver biopsy, 472
Wilson's disease prognosis, 481 (Table)
Protirelin, administration, 1975 (Table)
Proton magnetic resonance spectroscopy, birth asphyxia, 128
Proton pump inhibitors
gastroesophageal reflux, 429
Helicobacter pylori, 432
peptic ulcer, 432
short bowel syndrome, 1212
Proto-oncogenes, 889
Protoporphyrins, 1142
erythropoietic protoporphyria, 1144
Protozoa
infections, **1445–1470**
laboratory methods, 1299
Protracted diarrhea in early infancy, **454–455**
Providencia stuartii, 1320
Provocation tests, **1694,** *see also named substances*
Proximal renal tubular acidosis, 260, 944, **945–946**

Proximal tubules, 259
  function, 941, **943**, 944–945
Prozone phenomenon, cardiolipin antigen
  tests, 1402
PRP (polyribosyl-ribitol phosphate),
  Haemophilus influenzae, 1308,
  1309
PRPP-synthetase excess, 1141
Prune belly syndrome (triad syndrome),
  75, 255, **1778**
Pruritus
  asthma, 510
  enterobiasis, 1487
Pseudarthrosis, congenital, **1549**
  clavicle, 1556
Pseudoachondroplasia, 1580
  inheritance, 1566 (Table)
Pseudoallergic reactions, drugs, 1702
Pseudobulbar palsy, 812–813
Pseudocysts, pulmonary interstitial
  emphysema, 188
Pseudodeficiency, metachromatic
  dystrophy, 1165
Pseudoephedrine, administration, 1975
  (Table)
Pseudohermaphroditism, 1007, **1008–1010**
Pseudo-Hurler polydystrophy, 782 (Table)
Pseudohypertrophic muscular dystrophy,
  29 (Fig.), 39
Pseudohypoaldosteronism, 946, 1006,
  1067, 1068
  primary, 947
  type II (Gordon's syndrome), 947
Pseudohypoparathyroidism, 999 (Fig.),
  1000 (Fig.), **1057–1059**
  vs hypoparathyroidism, 1058
Pseudohypophosphatasia, 1176
Pseudomembranous conjunctivitis, 263,
  1663
Pseudomembranous enterocolitis, 1293
  antibiotic, 454 (Table)
Pseudomonas aeruginosa, **1320–1321**
  blue napkin staining, 1122
  cystic fibrosis, 555, 557, 558 (Table),
  1320
  pneumonia, 1320
Pseudomonas mallei, 1321
Pseudomonas pseudomallei, 1321
Pseudomonas pyocyanea, otitis media,
  1681
Pseudomonas spp., **1320–1321**
  ecthyma gangrenosum, 1287
  neonatal meningitis, 247 (Table)
  neonatal pneumonia, ceftazidime, 185
  urinary tract infections, ciprofloxacin,
  951
Pseudomonic acid, *S. aureus,* 1329
Pseudoneonatal adrenoleukodystrophy, *see*
  Acyl-CoA oxidase deficient
  adrenoleukodystrophy
Pseudo-obstruction, intestinal, 210, **451**
Pseudo-osteochondroses, 1594
Pseudopapilledema, **1671–1672**
Pseudoparalysis, 1380
Pseudopolyps, 449
Pseudoprecocious puberty, *see*
  Consonance, loss of
Pseudopseudohypoparathyroidism, 1057
Pseudopuberty, *see* Consonance, loss of
Pseudosepticemia, 1321
Pseudo-squint, **1659**
Pseudotrisomy 18, 57
Pseudotubercles, schistosomiasis, 1508
Pseudoxanthoma elasticum, 710, 875
Pseudo-Zellweger syndrome (peroxisomal
  3-oxoacyl-CoA thiolase
  deficiency), 786 (Table), 1174
Psittacosis, **569, 1373,** 1432
  FUO investigations, 1283 (Table)
Psoas abscess, 1592
Psoas hemorrhage, computed tomography,
  1913
Psoriasis, **1628–1629**

arthritis, **1611**
  vs tinea versicolor, 1638
Psychiatric disorders, **1727–1767**
  attendance rates, 9
  mental retardation, 834, 835 (Table)
  physical abuse risk, 1866
Psychiatric symptoms, acute intermittent
  porphyria, 1143
Psychiatry services
  Court Committee, 1853
  school health services, 1864
Psychogenesis, 644–645
Psychogenic breathlessness, 509
Psychogenic cough, 507
Psychogenic headache, 715–716
Psychogenic vomiting, **434–435**
Psychological assessment, **1735**
Psychological development, **1728–1732,**
  see also Development,
  adolescence; Psychomotor
  development
  congenital hypothyroidism, 1048
  Turner's syndrome, 1033
Psychological effects
  growth hormone therapy, 1020
  sexual abuse, 1870
Psychological factors
  accidents and management, 1712
  asthma, 493–494, 542, 545
  burns, 1800
  cancer survivors, 899–900
  chemotherapy, 897
  cystic fibrosis, 559
  diabetes management, 1077
  Duchenne muscular dystrophy, 731–732
  precocious puberty, 1031
  recurrent abdominal pain, 460
  respiratory disorders, **493–494**
Psychological support
  inflammatory bowel disease, 456
  parents and neonatal care, 100
  short stature, 1020
Psychologists, child development centers,
  399
Psychometric tests, **400**
Psychomotor development, **381–400**
Psychosine, 777 (Table)
Psychosis
  classification, 835–836
  speech, 818–819
Psychosocial deprivation, 1017
  growth, 368, 372
Psychotherapies, **1748–1749, 1763–1764**
  maladaptive response to chronic illness,
  1761
  sexual abuse, 1760
5-syndrome (cri du chat syndrome), **58,**
  830 (Table)
Pterins, 1105
Pterygium, 76 (Table)
Pthirus pubis, **1518–1519,** 1638
Ptosis, 23, **1661–1662**
  examination, 1649
Pubertal phase, growth, 352
Puberty, *see also* Precocious puberty
  assessment, 998, **1026–1027**
  asthma, 540–541
  cancer survivors, 898
  central nervous system development,
  670
  delay, 998, **1031–1036**
  constitutional, 372
  Crohn's disease, 457
  disorders, **1026–1035**
  endocrinology, **1024–1035**
  epilepsy, 691
  gynecology, **989–993**
  headache, 718
  height velocity, 356
  hypothyroidism, 1028, 1050
  induction, 1035
  Turner's syndrome, 370
  melatonin, 1043
  migraine, 717

physical changes, 357–361
  psychosocial aspects, 1750
  sex education, 1398
Pubic hair
  female, 989
  precocious pseudopuberty, 1027
  premature, 1060
Pubic hair stages, 358–359, 360
Pubic louse (*Pthirus pubis*), **1518–1519,**
  1638
Public Health (Control of Disease) Act
  1984, 1849–1850
Puff adders, envenomation, 1522, 1523
Pulmonary air leaks, neonate, **187–190,**
  576–577
Pulmonary angiography, 514
Pulmonary arteries, *see also*
  Bronchopulmonary-vascular
  malformations
  aberrant, 516 (Fig.), 573
  banding, ventricular septal defect, 601
  idiopathic dilation, **609**
  murmur, 203 (Table)
Pulmonary arterioles, fetal, 107
Pulmonary artery pressure
  fetal-neonatal transition, 107
  systolic, spectral Doppler
  ultrasonography, 592–593
Pulmonary artery sling, 612
Pulmonary aspergillosis, 1474
Pulmonary atresia, 613, **618**
  with ventricular septal defect, **617–618**
Pulmonary capillary hemangiomatosis, 575
Pulmonary disorders, neonate, **175–198**
Pulmonary edema
  chest X-ray, 588
  crackles, 512
  drowning, 1718
  hemorrhagic, hypothermia, 150
  pulmonary hemorrhage, 190
  rhesus incompatibility, 233
  sympathomimetic drugs, 116
Pulmonary eosinophilia, **570,** 1484
Pulmonary fibrosis, functional residual
  capacity, 501
Pulmonary flow murmur, 594
Pulmonary hemorrhage
  Goodpasture's syndrome, 965
  neonate, **190–191,** 224
  SGA baby, 138
Pulmonary hemosiderosis, **578**
Pulmonary histoplasmosis, 1476
Pulmonary hypertension, **606,** *see also*
  Persistent pulmonary hypertension
  in the newborn
  bronchopulmonary dysplasia, 194
  after cardiac surgery, 1822
  meconium aspiration, 185
  neonate, **198**
  persistent ductus arteriosus, 603
  pulmonary hypoplasia, 192
  ventricular septal defect, 600–601
Pulmonary hypoplasia, 175–176,
  191–192, 495, **575**
Pulmonary interstitial emphysema,
  neonate, **188–189**
Pulmonary lymphangiectasis, **193**
Pulmonary moniliasis, 1471, 1472
Pulmonary outflow tract
  distal narrowing, interventional
  radiology, 594
  double inlet ventricle, 620
Pulmonary regurgitation, congenital, 609
Pulmonary schistosomiasis, 1510
Pulmonary sequestration, **193,** 515 (Fig.),
  573, **574,** 1769
  ultrasonography, 1900
Pulmonary sling, 573
Pulmonary stenosis, 32, **608–609**
  signs, 587 (Table)
  tetralogy of Fallot, 616
  transposition of great arteries, 614
Pulmonary systemic flow ratio, 593
Pulmonary tuberculosis

mortality, 490 (Table)
  postprimary, 1342
  primary, **1340–1342**
Pulmonary valve stenosis, neonate, 203
Pulmonary vascular disease, histological
  grading, 606 (Table)
Pulmonary vascular resistance, 160
  calculation, 606
  neonate, **198**
Pulmonary vasodilators, 165
Pulmonary vessels
  development, 495
  heart disease, chest X-ray, 588, 601
  ventilation, 160
Pulsatile gonadotropin releasing hormone
  release, 1024, 1025
Pulsatile growth hormone release,
  nocturnal, testing, 1019
Pulsatility index
  Doppler ultrasonography, 1896
  intrauterine growth retardation, 82
Pulseless disease (Takayasu's disease),
  1610–1611
Pulseless electrical activity
  (electromechanical dissociation),
  1808
Pulse oximetry, 160, 505, 521
  acute severe asthma, 547
  fetal, 119
  patient-controlled analgesia, 1831
Pulses, 32, 585–586, *see also* Heart rate
  coarctation of aorta, 585, 598, 611
  congenital heart disease, 598
  hypoplastic left heart syndrome, 598,
  619
  neonate, 199
  persistent ductus arteriosus, 603
  resuscitation, 1807
Pulsus paradoxicus, **511**
Punch biopsy
  cutaneous leishmaniasis, 1464
  skin, 1846
Punishment, illness seen as, 1730
Pupillary reflexes, 36 (Table)
  neonatal gestation age, 36 (Table), 40
  (Table)
Pupils
  examination, 23–25, **1650**
  neurosyphilis, 1413
Pure gonadal dysgenesis, 1010
Puretone audiometry, 1683
Purgatives, *see* Laxatives
Purified protein derivative, tuberculin test,
  1337
Purine nucleotide cycle, 1141
Purine nucleotide phosphorylase
  deficiency, 1141, **1251**
Purines, metabolism disorders, **1140–1141**
Purpura fulminans, hemorrhagic
  chickenpox, 1361
Purpuras
  neonate, organisms, 284 (Table)
  nonthrombocytopenic, **875–876**
  thrombocytopenic, **876–879**
Purpuric rashes, **1285**
  Neisseria meningitidis, 1314, 1315
  neonate, 1284
Purtilo syndrome, neoplasms, 889 (Table)
Purtscher's retinopathy, 702
Purulent conjunctivitis, acute, 1663
Purulent pericarditis, 634, 635
Pus, amebiasis, 1469
Pustular dermatosis, transient neonatal,
  1646
Pustular psoriasis, 1628, 1629
Pustular syphilide, 1407
Putamen, necrosis, 773
Putsi fly (tumbu fly), 1514
P wave, 589
Pyelonephritis
  acute, 950
  chronic, *see* Reflux nephropathy
  FUO investigations, 1283 (Table)
  hematuria, 958

Pyeloplasty, 1795
Pygmies, yaws, 1417
Pyknocytes, 225
Pyknodysostosis, **1583**
  calcitonin, 1057
Pyle's disease, 1581 (Table)
Pyloric stenosis, 28 (Fig.), 33, 420
    (Table), **434, 1784–1785,** 1815
  recurrence risks, 74 (Table)
  risk calculation, 75
  ultrasonography, 1904
Pyloric tumor, 33
Pyloromyotomy (Ramstedt), 434, 1785
Pylorus, 430
Pyocyanin, 1320
Pyoderma, *see* Impetigo
Pyogenic osteitis, 1276, 1590
Pyracantha, poisoning, 1709
Pyrantel
  administration, 1975 (Table)
  Ancylostoma spp., 1490
  ascariasis, 1485
  enterobiasis, 1488
Pyrazinamide
  administration, 1975 (Table)
  tuberculosis, 1347, 1348
    meningitis, 1345
    pregnancy, 1346
    pulmonary, 1342
Pyrethrins, poisoning, 1709
Pyrethroids
  head lice, 1518
  scabies, 1517
Pyrexia, *see* Fever; Hyperpyrexia
Pyridinole, urine, 1612
Pyridinoline, urine, 1567
Pyridostigmine
  administration, 1975 (Table)
  myasthenia gravis, 728
Pyridoxal-5'-phosphate,
    hypophosphatasia, 1176
Pyridoxine
  administration, 1975 (Table)
    neonate, 1958 (Table)
  deficiency, 1113, 1198
  for gyrate atrophy of choroid and retina,
    1111
  for hereditary lactic acidosis, 1125
  for homocystinuria, 1108, **1109**
  for infantile spasms, 687
  with isoniazid, 1347
  for organic acidurias, 1119
  for oxalosis, 948, 1113
  parenteral nutrition, 1221 (Table)
  pregnancy, tuberculosis, 1346
Pyridoxine-dependent conditions, 1148
Pyridoxine-dependent convulsions, 245,
    1115
Pyrimethamine, *see also* Fansidar;
    Maloprim
  toxoplasmosis, 288, 1464, **1466,** 1975
    (Table)
Pyrimidine 5-nucleotidase deficiency,
    1142
Pyrimidines, metabolism disorders,
    1141–1142
Pyroglutamic aciduria, 1115
Pyruvate
  metabolism disorders, **1124–1126**
  normal values, 1928 (Table)
    cerebrospinal fluid, 1935 (Table)
Pyruvate carboxylase deficiency, 297,
    1126
Pyruvate dehydrogenase deficiency,
    1125–1126
  ataxia, 765–766
Pyruvate kinase deficiency, 226, **859–860,**
    1260
Pyrvinium pamoate
  administration, 1975 (Table)
  enterobiasis, 1488
Pyuria, 1299

Q-banding, 49

Q fever, 569, **1374–1375,** 1390 (Table),
    1392
QRS complex, 589
18Q-syndrome, **58**
QT interval, 589, *see also* Long QT
    interval syndromes
  corrected, ionized calcium, 299
Quadriplegia, cerebral palsy, 748
  epilepsy, 685
Quality adjusted life years (QALY), 105
Quality of life, 101
Quantitative buffy coat technique, African
    trypanosomiasis, 1456
Quarantine, measles, 1355
Quartan malaria, 1446, 1449
Queensland tick typhus, 1392
Questionnaires, educational attainment,
    1735–1736
Quiet sleep, *see also* Nonrapid eye
    movement sleep
  breathing, 530
Quinidine, poisoning, 1710
Quinine, 1452
  administration, 1975 (Table)
  poisoning, 1710
Quinolones
  dosage considerations, 1527
  mechanism, 1527
Quinsy, 1687

Rabies, **1376–1378**
  vs tetanus, 1334
Rabitidine, administration, 1975 (Table)
Raccoon eyes, 1811
Racemose cyst, central nervous system,
    1501
Rachischisis, 641
Rachitic rosary, 1195
Racial prejudice, 94
Radesyge, see Endemic syphilis
Radial artery, puncture, 505, 1835–1836
Radial defects, 1545
  hand, 1546 (Table)
Radial nerve
  acute palsy, 725
  birth trauma, 122–123
Radiant warmers, **148–149**
  acute renal failure, fluid replacement,
    975
  procedures, 1829
Radiation
  ataxia telangiectasia, 766–767
  leukemia, 868
  neoplasms, **889–890**
  sensitivity, 890
Radiation doses, diagnostic imaging, 1895
    (Table)
Radiation heat loss, 146
Radiation protection, 340, 1894
Radiculopathy, borreliosis, 1313
Radioactive iodine, 1051
  neoplasms, 1052
Radioallergosorbent test, 541
Radiofrequency surgery, pulmonary
    atresia, 618
Radiographic densitometry, dual energy,
    302
Radioimmunoassays, *vs*
    immunoradiometric assays, 1001
Radioisotopes, *see also* Radionuclides;
    Scintigraphy
  sodium, 408
Radiological grading, respiratory distress
    syndrome, 178
Radiology, **1895–1896,** *see also* Skeletal
    surveys
  colon, 464
  congenital dislocation of hip, 41,
    1550
  craniopharyngioma, 905
  cysticercosis, 1501
  eye, 1617
  gastrointestinal tract, **1901–1904**
  neuroblastoma, 911

osteitis, 1590
osteochondroses, 1594
osteopetrosis, 1582
osteosarcoma, 917
  recurrent abdominal pain, 461
rickets, 1196
  of prematurity, 302
scurvy, 1199–1200
small intestine, 447
*Radiology of syndromes, metabolic
    disorders and skeletal dysplasias*
    (Taybi and Lachman), 1099
Radionuclides, 1897, *see also*
    Scintigraphy
  radiotherapy, 1897
Radiopharmaceuticals, radiation doses,
    1895 (Table)
Radiotherapy
  central nervous system, 899, 901, *see
    also named tumors*
    acute lymphoblastic leukemia, 873
    effects on growth, 898
    endocrine aspects, long-term effects,
    1042–1043
    learning difficulties, 875, 899
    growth hormone deficiency, 373, 1016
  Hodgkin's disease, 910
  immunosuppression, 1265
  neonate, 290
  for neoplasms, 893, *see also named
    tumors*
    neoplasms from, 890
    osteosarcoma from, 917
    radionuclides, 1897
    retinoblastoma, 1670–1671
    second primary tumors, 898
    strokes, 714
Radio transmission aids, 817
Radioulnar synostosis, 62, **1548**
Radius, *see* Thrombocytopenia with
    absent radii
Rage reactions
  epilepsy, 690
  mental retardation, 841
Ragged-red fiber myopathy
  diagnosis, 1128
  myoclonic epilepsy with (MERRF),
    682, **736,** 1127
  oculocraniosomatic disease, 736
Ragged-red fibers, 1127
Rain, allergic symptoms, 1691
Ramp stretching, 756
Ramsay Hunt syndrome, 1363, *see also*
    Dentatorubral atrophy
Ramstedt's pyloromyotomy, 434, 1785
Randomized controlled trials, 104
Ranula, 1784
Rape, 1870
Rapid carbohydrate utilization test,
    Neisseria gonorrhoeae, 1423
Rapid eye movement sleep
  breathing, 196, 506, **530**
  cerebral blood flow, 661
  muscle tone, 756
  neonatal intensive care, 97
Rapidly progressive glomerulonephritis,
    962–963, **965**
Rapid Plasma Reagin test, **1402**
Rapid rate ventilation, *see* High frequency
    ventilation
Rapid urease test, *Helicobacter pylori,*
    431
Rapp Hodgkins syndrome, 1626 (Table)
Rashes, **1284–1285,** *see also named
    diseases*
  African trypanosomiasis, 1455
  AIDS, 1395
  antithyroid drugs, 1051
  cow's milk protein intolerance, 1699
  cystic fibrosis, 556
  dermatomyositis, 737, 1644
  ECHO viruses, 1383
  examination, 19, 1617
  Henoch–Schönlein purpura, 1285,
    1609–1610

history taking, 17
juvenile chronic arthritis, 1600
Neisseria meningitidis, **1285,** 1314,
    1315, 1816
respiratory disorders, 510
scabies, 1516
scarlet fever, 1285, 1331
syphilis
  congenital, 1411–1412
  secondary, 1406–1407
systemic lupus erythematosus, 1605
typhus, 1391
Rashkind balloon, *see* Atrial septostomy
Rasmussen's syndrome, 686
ras proto-oncogene signaling pathway,
    351
Rastelli procedure, transposition of great
    arteries, 615
RAST (radioallergosorbent test), 541
Rat-bite fevers, **1321–1322**
Rathke's pouch, 1002
Rationalization, 1731–1732, 1760–1761
Rat poison, 1709
Rats, murine typhus, 1392
Rat tapeworm, 1502
Rattle habituation, neonate, 237 (Fig.)
Rattle (toy), developmental examination,
    387
Rattly breathing, 509
Raven's Progressive Matrices, 400, 827
Reabsorption
  amino acids, 1122
  renal function, 941–942
Reactivation, herpes simplex virus, 1436
Reactive arsenical encephalopathy, 1457
Reading, tests, 1735
Reading difficulties, 1657, 1745
Reading retardation, **820–821,** 1657,
    1745
Real-time ultrasonography, 1896
Rebound phenomenon, rheumatic fever,
    1600
Rebound tenderness, 32–33, 1787
Rebuck skin window test, 1247
Receptive dysphasia, 814–815
Receptor-operated calcium channels,
    127
Receptors, endocrine disorders, 1002
Recessive inheritance, 64, **66**
  central nervous system malformations,
    645
  X-linked, **66–67**
Recessive X-linked ichthyosis, 1620, 1621
    (Table)
Reciprocal inhibition, cerebral palsy
    treatment, 757
Reciprocating gait orthoses, neural tube
    defect, 655
Reciprocating tachycardia, *see*
    Supraventricular tachycardia
Recognition skills, accident and
    emergency departments, 1805
Recombinant factor VIII, 881
Recombinant growth hormone treatment,
    374, 375
Recombinant human DNase 1, cystic
    fibrosis, 558
Recombinant human erythropoietin,
    refractory early anemia of
    prematurity 225
Recombination activating genes, Swiss
    type SCID, 1250
Recombination fraction, 73
Recommended Daily Amount, 1180
    (Table)
Recommended Dietary Allowance, 1180
    (Table), 1948–1949 (Table)
Recommended Nutrient Intakes (RNI),
    1180 (Table), 1181 (Table)
  cystic fibrosis, 1208
Record cards, asthma, 543
Record keeping
  antenatal care, 80
  child abuse, 1873
  and negligence, 1878–1879

Record systems, immunization, 346
Recreational injuries, 1713–1714
Recrudescent typhus, see Brill–Zinsser disease
Rectal atresia
 radiology, 1901
 ultrasonography, 1906
Rectal biopsy, immunodeficiency, 1245
Rectal bleeding, **459–460**
Rectal examination, **33**
 appendicitis, 1787
 cancer treatment, avoidance, 894
Rectal prolapse
 recurrent, cystic fibrosis, 553
 Trichuris trichiura, 1491
Rectal route, **1954**
 diazepam
  febrile convulsions, 683
  status epilepticus, 693
 paracetamol, 1832
 paraldehyde, encephalopathies, 697
Rectal snip, schistosomiasis, 1510
Rectal swabs, 1299
 virology, 1352
Rectal temperature, 111, 147, 149
Rectum, see also Rectal examination
 anomalies, **1781–1782**
 Crohn's disease, 457
 embryology, 206
 gonorrhea, 1420, **1425**
  treatment, 1428
 herpes simplex, 1438–1439
 suction biopsy, 464
Recurrence, herpes simplex virus, **1364,** 1436, **1439,** 1632
 pregnancy, 1441
Recurrence risk, congenital heart disease, 74, 597
Recurrent abdominal pain, **460–461**
Recurrent inhalation, **570–571**
Recurrent laryngeal nerve, 809
Recurrent parotitis, 1372
Recurrent segmental collapse, 550
Red blood cells, see Red cells
Red cell enzyme defects, 858–860
Red cell mass, neonate, 223
Red cells, see also Erythrocyte sedimentation rate
 burns, 1799
 erythema infectiosum, 1359
 fetus, 225
 galactose-1-phosphate uridyltransferase, normal values, 1925 (Table)
 glutathione peroxidase, 1188
 glutathione reductase, riboflavin deficiency, 1198
 glycogen, normal values, 1926 (Table)
 glycolysis defects, 1131
 malaria invasion, ligands, 1446
 malaria sensitization, 1448
 neonate
  cerebrospinal fluid, 242
  counts, 223 (Table)
  normal values
   cerebrospinal fluid, 1934 (Table)
   counts, 1939 (Table)
   urine, 1931 (Table)
 primitive megaloblastic, 848
 transfusion, preterm infant, 225–226
Red cell transketolase, 1188
Red cell volume, 403
 fetus and neonate, 848
Redcurrant jelly stool, 1786
'Red ears', 561
Red–green color blindness, inheritance, 67
Red reflex
 absence, 268
 ophthalmoscopy, 1651
Reduced vision, see Visual impairment
Reducing substances, urine, neonate, 220
5α-Reductase, 1004
 deficiency, **1009,** 1010
Reed–Sternberg cells, 909–910
Re-emerging infections, **1278**

Re-entry circuit, supraventricular tachycardia, 624
Reference nutrient intakes, 1180
 minerals, 1947 (Table)
 vitamins, 1184 (Table), 1946 (Table)
Referred pain, to ear, 1681
Reflex anoxic seizures, 672
Reflexes, 35–38
 extensor dystonia, 770
 hand, 668–669
 hypoxia response, 123
 myelomeningocele, 653–654
 neonate, 36–38 (Table), 238 (Fig.), **239–240**
  gestation age, 40 (Table)
 respiratory tract, 496
Reflex excitability, 756
Reflex hemisyndrome, 44, 741
Reflex 'reading' epilepsy, 821
Reflex rhinorrhea, 492
Reflex sympathetic dystrophy, **1833**
Reflux nephropathy, **262,** 949–950
 hypertension, 972
Refractive errors, **1656–1657**
 diabetes mellitus, 1674
 homocystinuria, 1673
 strabismus from, 1658
Refractory anemias, 869
Refractory diarrhea, 1297
 chronic, 1295
Refractory early anemia of prematurity, 225–226
Refrigerant spraying, 1490
Refrigeration
 bacteriology specimens, 1297
 virology specimens, 1352
Refsum's disease, 724, 787 (Table), 799 (Table), 1174
 deafness, 1682
 ichthyosis, 1622 (Table)
 infantile, 308, 785 (Table), 1173
Regional anesthesia, **1832**
Regional breast-feeding rates, UK, 326
Regional genetic services, England, 76
Registration
 births, marriages and deaths, **1849**
 neonatal death, 174
Regressed retinopathy of prematurity, 266
Regression, 1732
 development, 387
Regurgitation, 427–428
Rehabilitation, nutritional, 1892
Rehidrat, 413, 453 (Table)
Reifenstein's syndrome, 1010
Reiter's syndrome, 1432, **1611**
 eye, 1675
Rejection
 liver transplantation, 484
 parental, 1747
Relactation, 328
Relapsing fever, **1322–1323**
Release
 developmental examination, 389 (Table)
 motor development, 382
Religious care, neonatal death, 173
Religious diets, 1189
Remedial programs
 learning disorders, 826
 mental retardation, 838
Remission induction, acute lymphoblastic leukemia, 873 (Fig.)
REM sleep, see Rapid eye movement sleep
Renal agenesis, 253, 937–938
 facies, 22 (Fig.)
 pulmonary hypoplasia, 495
 recurrence risks, 74
Renal arterial thrombosis, neonate, 258
Renal biopsy, 960–961
 acute poststreptococcal glomerulonephritis, 962
 mesangial IgA nephropathy, 963
 nephrotic syndrome, 969, 970
 technique, **1845–1846**
Renal cortical necrosis, neonate, 258, 259

Renal diabetes insipidus, see Nephrogenic diabetes insipidus
Renal dysplasia, 254, 938
Renal failure
 acyclovir dosage, 1440
 birth asphyxia, 129
 calcitonin, 1057
 cirrhosis, 483
 dehydration, 1293–1294
 dietary management, 1211 (Table)
 drug dosage, 1955
 glucose-6-phosphatase deficiency, 1137
 hemorrhagic fever with renal syndrome, 1390
 hyperkalemia, 412
 liver failure, 1824
 neonate, **257–260**
Renal Fanconi syndrome, 1122
Renal feeds, 975
Renal hypertension, 636, 637, **972–973,** 1069
Renal hypoplasia, 253–254, 938
Renal osteodystrophy, 979–980, 1058
'Renal solute load', infant feeding, 333
Renal threshold, glucose, preterm infant, 298
Renal transplantation, **981–982**
 acceptance rates, 979
 cystinosis, 945, 1123
 hexosaminidases, 1164
 oxalosis, 1113
Renal tubular acidosis, 259–260, **945–946**
 hypophosphatemia, 1058
 tests, 944
Renal tubular function
 disorders, 259–260, **944–949**
 postnatal development, 256–257
Renal tubular hyperkalemia, 947
Renal tubules, cystic fibrosis transmembrane conductance regulator, 552
Renal vein thrombosis, 231
 gastroenteritis, 1294
 hematuria, 959
 hypernatremia, 414
 neonate, 258
Renin, normal values, 1928 (Table)
Renin–angiotensin–aldosterone system
 heart failure, 599
 neonates, 143, 257
Renography, 1912
 urinary tract infections, 953–954
Renutrition, therapeutic, 1892
Reoviruses, **1373**
Replacement fluid, 1295
Replicative segregation, mitochondrial DNA, 1126
Replogle tube, 1770–1771
Reporters (Scotland), 1876, 1877
Reprocessing plants, nuclear fuels, neoplasms, 890
Reproterol, administration, 1975 (Table)
Reptilase time, 228
Request forms, bacteriology, 1297
Research
 economic, 105–106
 ethics, **103**
 outcome studies, prematurity, 165–172
Research Trust for Metabolic Diseases in Children, 1099
Reservoirs, ventricular, 663
 intracranial pressure measurement, 697
 tuberculous meningitis, 666
Residence Orders, 1874, 1876
Residential treatment, adolescent psychiatry, **1764**
Residual volume, 501
Resistance index
 cerebral blood flow, 661, 707
 Doppler ultrasonography, 1896
Resistant starches, 1183
Resolution, vs visibility, 268
Resonant frequency, muscle, 756
Resonium A, 415

Resources
 measurement, 104
 neonatal care requirements, 96
Respiration, see also Control of breathing
 control of CO_2 tension, **418**
 delay at birth, 125, **134–136**
 development and SIDS, 1721
Respiratory acidosis, 419, 420, 504
 inborn errors of metabolism, correction, 307
 treatment, 421
Respiratory alkalosis, 307, 419, 420, 504
Respiratory compromise, 1807
Respiratory depression, prostaglandin therapy, 599
Respiratory disorders, **489–583**
 emergency care, 1815
Respiratory distress, **1768–1773**
 anemia, malaria, 1451
 inspection, 43
 parenteral lipids, 1220
 vascular ring, 612
Respiratory distress syndrome, **177–182**
 acid–base balance, 419–420
 adult, **578–579**
 cardiovascular aspects, 204–205
 chest movement, 511–512
 corticosteroids, 104, **114,** 161, 178–179, 338
 disseminated intravascular coagulation, 231
 effectiveness of treatments, 104
 lecithin:sphingomyelin ratio, amniotic fluid, 1937 (Table)
 near-drowning, 1825
 vs neonatal meningitis, 247
 neonatal mortality, 4 (Table)
 nitric oxide inhalation, 1823
 vs pneumonia, 183
 pneumothorax, 181, 187
 prevention, 179
 pulmonary hemorrhage, 190
 renal function, 257
 ventilation, 162–164, **180–181,** 1818
 water balance, 142
Respiratory embarrassment, see also Respiratory compromise
 gastric distension, 155
Respiratory epithelial surface, 497
Respiratory failure
 alveolar air equation, 504
 cystic fibrosis, 556
 definition, 502
 Duchenne muscular dystrophy, 730
 poliomyelitis, 1379
Respiratory function tests, **497–498**
 airway obstruction, **499–501**
 asthma, 538, 544
 cystic fibrosis, **554**
Respiratory inversion, 30
Respiratory muscles
 poliomyelitis, 1379
 sleep, 530
 strength measurement, 506
Respiratory paralysis
 neurotoxic snake venoms, 1522
 poliomyelitis, 1379, 1380
Respiratory rates, 510, 511
 vs age, **30**
 Joubert's syndrome, 646
 pneumonia, 566
 respiratory distress syndrome, 177
Respiratory reflexes, 196
Respiratory support, see Ventilation
Respiratory symptoms, cystic fibrosis, **554**
Respiratory syncytial virus, 492, **1370**
 apnea, 528
 bronchiolitis, 564, 1370
 bronchopulmonary dysplasia, 195
 hypothermia, 149
 immunoglobulin therapy, 1267
 prevention of transmission, 565
 virology, 1352
Respiratory time constant, 502

Respiratory tract, *see also* Lower respiratory tract infections; Upper respiratory tract
  burns, 1799
  development, **494–497**
  disorders, postneonatal mortality, 5 (Table)
  early weaning, 333
  examination, 30
  imaging, **1899–1901**
  infections, **559–570**, 1802
    AIDS, 1397
    developing countries disease burden, 1276 (Table), 1280 (Table)
    general practice, consultation rates, 1277–1278
    immunodeficiency, 1267
    viral, **1368–1373**, 1802
  neonatal examination, 110
  physiology, **497–506**
Respiratory transition period, birth, 42, **106–109**, 110
Respiratory water loss, preterm infant, 139
Respite care, mental retardation, 838
Resting cells, neoplasms, 892
Resting metabolic rate, 1180–1181
Restless leg syndrome of Ekbom, 769
Restraint
  for procedures, 1830
  radiography, 1895
Restraint systems, passenger accident prevention, 1716
Restriction endonuclease fingerprinting, herpes simplex virus, 1437, 1439
Restriction enzymes, 70
Restriction fragment length polymorphism analysis, 70
  prenatal diagnosis of immunodeficiency, 1248
Restrictive childrearing, 828
Resuscitation, **522–528, 1806–1809**
  chart, 527 (Fig.)
  head injuries, 706
  neonate, **132–136**
    failure to respond, **135**
    service provision, 156
  stopping, **1808**
Resuscitation rooms, 1805
  equipment, 1806 (Table)
Resuscitation trolley, 133
Resuscitators, automatic, 524–525
Retardation, motor, 1754
Retention of urine
  birth asphyxia, 129
  terminal care, 928
Reticular dysgenesis, 855, 1242 (Table), 1250
  vs infantile genetic agranulocytosis, 867
Reticularis cells, androgens, 1059
Reticulocytes
  vs age, 849 (Table)
  counts
    neonate, 223 (Table)
    normal, 1939 (Table)
    rhesus incompatibility, 233
  Plasmodium vivax, 1446
Retina, *see also* Gyrate atrophy of choroid and retina; Retinopathy
  albinism, 1673
  connective tissue disorders, 1674–1675
  degenerative diseases, **1666–1667**
  detachment, 1667
    retinopathy of prematurity, 267
  disorders, 270–271
  dysplasia, 271
    Walker–Warburg syndrome, 646
  examination, *see* Ophthalmoscopy
  hemangioma, von Hippel–Lindau syndrome, 803
  hemorrhage
    birth trauma, 264
    leukemia, 870
    trauma, 702
  homocystinuria, 1673

incontinentia pigmenti, 803
vascular development, 263
Retinal angiography, with fluorescein, 1654, 1671
Retinitis pigmentosa, 76, 268, **1666–1667**
Retinitis punctata albescens, 1667
Retinoblastoma, **923–924, 1670–1671**
  13q14 deletion, 59, 73, 289
  gene, 923
  incidence, 886 (Table)
  mutations, 887–888
  neonate, 293 (Table)
    incidence, 290 (Table)
  and osteosarcoma, 917
  retinal detachment, 1667
  second primary, 898
  survival rates, 898 (Table)
  vs toxocariasis, 1486
Retinoids
  for epidermal nevi, 1618
  ichthyoses, 1620
Retinol-binding protein defect, 1148
Retinopathy
  anemias, 1675
  diabetes mellitus, 1674
    examination, 1080
  hyperoxia, 161, **265**
  hypertension, **1675**
  leukemia, 1675
  lysosomal disorders, 1171
  mental retardation, 835 (Table)
  neonatal intensive care, light exposure, 97
  non-accidental injury, 702
  of prematurity, *see* Retrolental fibroplasia
  rubella, 1668
  very low birthweight, 171
Retractile testes, 1790
Retrobulbar neuritis, 1671
Retrocecal appendix, 1787
Retrograde pyelography, 1912
Retroinfection, enterobiasis, 1486
Retrolental fibroplasia, **265–267**
  severely handicapped children affected, 14 (Table)
Retroperitoneum
  germ cell tumors, 922
  imaging, **1912–1913**
Retropharyngeal abscess, 563
  tuberculosis, 1592
Retroviruses, neoplasms, 891
Rett's syndrome, 796 (Table)
Reversal reaction, leprosy, **1310**, 1311
Reversed barrier nursing, 1281
Reverse genetics, 72
Reverse transcriptase inhibitors, 1397
Reverse triiodothyronine, fetus, 1003
Reversibility, perception of, 1730
Rewarming, hypothermia, 149–150
Reye's syndrome, **479–480**, 1113
  amino acids, 1103
  chickenpox, 1361
  vs hemorrhagic shock and encephalopathy syndrome, 1288
  influenza, 1369
  vs ornithine transcarbamylase deficiency, 1110
Reynell developmental language scale, 400
Reynell Zinkin scales, 400
Rhabditiform larvae
  hookworm, 1489, 1490
  Strongyloides stercoralis, 1492, 1493 (Fig.)
Rhabdoid nephroblastoma, 914
Rhabdomyoma
  heart, 636
  tuberous sclerosis, 801, 802
Rhabdomyosarcoma, **915–917**, 1913
  botryoid, 916, 993–994
  vs Ewing's sarcoma, 919
  survival rates, 887 (Table)
  tumor markers, 912 (Table)

Rhagades, 1411, 1414
rhDNase, *see* Recombinant human DNase 1
Rhesus disease, 216, **232–233**
  disseminated intravascular coagulation, 231
  intravascular fetal blood transfusion, 114
  maternal incompatibility, 89 (Table)
  prevention, 338
  screening, 81, 339 (Table)
Rheumatic fever, **628–629, 1596–1600,** 1687
  antibiotic prophylaxis, 1529
Rheumatic heart disease, **628–630**
  history taking, 584
Rheumatism, acute, trends, 7
Rheumatoid arthritis, *see also* Juvenile chronic arthritis
  analgesia, 1833
  anterior uveitis, 1674
  fibrosing alveolitis, 578
  secondary anemia, 865
Rheumatoid factor, juvenile chronic arthritis, 1601–1602
Rhinitis, **1684–1685**
  congenital syphilis, 1411, **1412**
  perennial (seasonal), 1684, **1698**
Rhinopharyngitis mutilans, 1417
Rhinosporidiosis, 1471 (Table)
Rhinoviruses, **1372–1373**
Rhizomelia, 76 (Table)
Rhizomelic chondrodysplasia punctata, 308, 786 (Table), 1173–1174, 1571–1572
Rhizotomy, selective dorsal, cerebral palsy, 759
Rhodesian sleeping sickness, 1453, 1454
Rhodnius prolixus, 1458
Rhombencephalitis, 762
Rhus, contact eczema, 1641
Ribavirin
  bronchiolitis, 565
  bronchopulmonary dysplasia, 195
Riboflavin, 1184 (Table)
  administration, 1975 (Table)
  conditions responding to, 1148
  deficiency, 1198
    eye, 1677
  for glutaric acidemia, 1113
  for hereditary lactic acidosis, 1125
  for mitochondrial bioenergetic defects, 1128
  for organic acidurias, 1119
  parenteral nutrition, 1221 (Table)
  Recommended Dietary Allowances, 1949 (Table)
  reference nutrient intakes, 1946 (Table)
Riboflavin-responsive dicarboxylic aciduria (MAD:M), 1130
Riboflavin-responsive multiple acyl-CoA dehydrogenase deficiencies, 308
Ribonucleoprotein antigen, antibody, 1609
Rib recession, 505, 510, 511–512, *see also* Costal margin recession; Intercostal indrawing
  pneumonia, 566
  respiratory distress syndrome, 177
Ribs
  Ewing's sarcoma, 919
  fractures, 1811, 1867, 1914
    shaking injury, 701
  hemopoiesis, 848 (Fig.)
Rice-based oral rehydration solutions, 1296
Rich focus, 1344
Richner–Hanhart syndrome, 1106–1107
Rickets, 331, 1056 (Table), **1194–1196,** *see also* Calciopenic rickets; Familial hypophosphatemia; Osteopenia
  differential diagnosis, 1058
  hypophosphatemic, 1123
  immigrants, 1866
  phosphopenic, 1056, 1058

of prematurity, 301–304
Rickettsia burnetii, 1374, 1375
Rickettsial pox, 1390 (Table), **1392**
Rickettsia spp., infections, **1390–1392**
Rickety rosary, 30
Riding accidents, 1714
Rifabutin, environmental mycobacteria, 1350
Rifampicin
  cat-scratch disease, 1520
  environmental mycobacteria, 1350
  Haemophilus influenzae type b prophylaxis, 1309
  leprosy, 1311
  mechanism, 1527
  meningitis prophylaxis, 1292
  Neisseria meningitidis, carriers, 1976 (Table)
  tuberculosis, 1347, 1348, 1976 (Table)
    chemoprophylaxis, 1340
    meningitis, 1345
    pregnancy, 1346
    pulmonary, 1342
Right atrial hypertrophy, electrocardiography, 589
Rights, **1888**, *see also* United Nations, Declaration of the Rights of the Child
Right-sided aorta, imaging, 1899
Right-to-left shunts, **160**, 502–503, *see also* Eisenmenger's syndrome
  foramen ovale, 199
  pulmonary stenosis, 608
  respiratory distress syndrome, 177
Right ventricle
  dysplasias, 610–611
  endomyocardial fibrosis, 633
  enlargement, 31
  hypertrophy, 32
    electrocardiography, 589
  outflow obstruction, **608–609**
    tetralogy of Fallot, 616, 617
    ventricular septal defect, 600, 601
  pulmonary atresia, 618
Right ventricular heave, 586
Rigidities, 769–770
Rigid/spastic phase, diplegia, 747
Rigid spine syndrome, 732
Riley–Day syndrome (familial dysautonomia), 209, 724, 832 (Table), 1069, 1107
  tongue, 425
Rimantadine, 1530
  influenza, 1369
Ring chromosomes, 51, 52 (Fig.)
  cytogenetic nomenclature, 54
Ringworm, 1636
Risk assessment, pregnancy, **113–114**
Risk factors, sudden infant death syndrome, 1719–1720
Risk-taking behavior, **1763**
Risperidone, 1755
Ristocetin-induced platelet aggregation, Von Willebrand's disease, 881
Risus sardonicus, tetanus, 25 (Fig.)
Ritodrine, on fetus and neonate, 91 (Table)
Ritter's disease, *see* Scalded skin syndrome
Rituals, obsessive–compulsive disorders, 1740
River blindness, 1497
Riyadh (Saudi Arabia), secretory otitis media, 1681
RNA, 68
  Neisseria gonorrhoeae, detection, 1424
Road traffic accidents, **1715–1716**, *see also* Seat belts, injuries
  head injuries, 705 (Fig.)
  mortality, 1711
Roasting, 1868
Robarts' sign, 1790
Robertsonian translocations, 52 (Fig.), 53
  Down syndrome, 55, 56

Robin anomalad, 75, *see also* Pierre Robin syndrome
Robinow's syndrome, 1581
Rocker-bottom feet, 1555
    Edwards' syndrome, 57
Rocking (habit disorder), 1745
Rocky Mountain spotted fever, 1390 (Table), **1392**
Rokitansky–Kuster–Hauser syndrome, 991
Rolling, motor development, 667
Romana's sign, 1459
Rombergism, 35
Rooming-in, 329
Rooting reflex, 36 (Table)
    neonate, 238 (Fig.), 240–241
    gestation age, 40 (Table)
Rosary, rachitic, 1195
Roseola infantum, 1285, **1359**
    vs measles, 1355
Roseola (macular syphilide), 1406
Rose spots, 1325
Rotation-plasty, osteosarcoma surgery, 918
Rotaviruses, 1373
    emergence, 1279 (Table)
    gastroenteritis, 452, 1293, **1384**
        water secretion, 436
    United Kingdom, 1277 (Fig.)
    vaccines, 1295
Rothmund–Thomson syndrome, **1631**
Rotor's syndrome, 218, 219, **1145**
Roundworms (nematodes), **1481–1485**
Roussy–Lévy syndrome, 723, 764
Rove beetles, toxins, 1525
Royal College of Physicians, neonatal care cot numbers, 156
RSR pattern, atrial septal defect, 602
RTMDC (Research Trust for Metabolic Diseases in Children), 1099
Rubella, 136, 286–287, 832 (Table), **1356–1358**
    cataract, 24 (Fig.), 1668
    congenital heart disease, 286, 596
    vs erythema infectiosum, 1359
    eye, 1676
    hearing loss, 816, 817
    immunosuppression, 1264
    maternal, 89 (Table), **1357–1358**
    vs measles, 1355
    mouth, 424
    neonate, 248, **286–287**, 1284
    neurological complications, 1376
    panencephalitis, 795 (Table), **1378**
    rash, 1285
    vs scarlet fever, 1331, 1357
    severely handicapped children affected, 14 (Table)
    vaccination, 1357
    UK, 345
Rubenstein–Taybi syndrome, 60 (Table), 832 (Table)
Rud's syndrome, 803
Rugby, injuries, 1714
Rumination, 209, 428
    history taking, 17
Running, gait, 35
Rupture of membranes, *see* Prolonged rupture of membranes
Rural cutaneous leishmaniasis, 1463
Russell's viper bites, 1522, 1523
Russian spring–summer encephalitis, 1390
RUS system, bone age, 362
Rutter scales, educational attainment, 1735–1736
Ruvalcaba–Myhre–Smith syndrome, 1129
R wave, 589
Rye classification, Hodgkin's disease, 909

S100 protein, small round cell tumors, 912 (Table)
Saber tibia, 1413, 1414

Sabiá virus, emergence, 1279 (Table)
Sabin vaccines, 1381
Saccharopinuria, 1113
Saccular aneurysms, 710
Sacral agenesis, 641, 1557
Sacral autonomic dysfunction, herpes simplex, 1439
Sacral pit, 110
Sacrococcygeal tumors, **921**
    teratomas, 920, **1781**
Sacrum, Ewing's sarcoma, 919
Saddle nose, 1412
Safe bladder, 657
Safe Communities, 1713
Safe intakes, nutrients, 1180, 1948 (Table)
Safety glass, 1715
Sagittal sinus entrapment syndrome, 699
Sail sign, pneumomediastinum, 188 (Fig.)
'Salaam' attacks, myoclonic epilepsy, 34
Salbutamol
    administration, 1976 (Table)
    hyperkalemia, acute renal failure, 975
    pertussis, 562
    poisoning, 1709
    resuscitation, doses, 527 (Fig.)
Saldino–Noonan syndrome, 1571
Salicylates, 1832
    administration, 1977 (Table)
    and glucose-6-phosphate dehydrogenase deficiency, 859 (Table)
    neonatal platelets, 229
    poisoning, 1710
        acid–base balance, 420
        vs diabetic ketoacidosis, 1075
    rheumatic fever, 628, 1599
Salicylic acid, 1628
    skin treatment, 1976
Saline
    hypertonic, sputum stimulation, 534
    intravenous infusion, acid–base balance, 420 (Table)
    intussusception reduction, 1904
    strengths for fluid therapy, 1296
Saliva
    amylase, 436
    electrolytes, 411 (Table)
    hormone tests, 1001
    virology, 1351
Salivary glands, 425
    enlargement, **1784**
    mumps, 1371
Salk vaccines, 1381
Salla disease, 1157 (Table), 1169
Salmeterol, 546, 1976 (Table)
Salmonella spp., **1323–1327**
    antibiotic, 454 (Table)
    bacteremia, 1324
        schistosomiasis, 1509
    and Oroya fever, 1301
    sickle-cell disease, 1323–1324, 1590
Salmonella typhimurium, United Kingdom, 1277
Salt
    absorption, 208
    child abuse, 1871
    deficiency
        chronic renal failure, 979–980
        cystic fibrosis, 553
    iodination, 1048
    osmolality, 405
Salt and pepper fundus, 1412
Salt baths, vulvovaginitis, 988
Salt-losing crisis, congenital adrenal hyperplasia, 1064
Salt wasting, 1007
    adrenocortical hypofunction, 1067–1069
    21-hydroxylase deficiency, 1061, 1063
Salt water drowning, 1718
Salvage functions, colon, 455, 456
Sanctity of life, 101
Sanctuaries, pharmacological, 892
Sandflies, leishmaniasis, 1460
Sandfly fever, **1390**

Sandhoff disease, 775 (Table), 1157 (Table), **1163**, 1164
Sandifer syndrome, 428
Sand worm, *see* Cutaneous larva migrans
Sandy patches, schistosomiasis, 1509
Sanfilippo's syndrome, 784 (Table), 1158, **1160**
San Joaquin Valley fever, *see* Coccidioidomycosis
Saposin B defect, 1165
Sarcoidosis
    central nervous system, 763
    eye, 1677
    fibrosing alveolitis, 578
    hypercalcemia, 1056
Sarcomas
    neonate, 292 (Table)
        incidence, 290 (Table)
    post-radiation, 57
Sarcoptes scabiei, 1515–1517, 1638
Sarcosinemia, 1113, 1147
Saturated fatty acids, 1182
Saw-scaled viper bites, 1522
Saying goodbye to your baby, 175
Scabies, **1515–1517, 1638**
    postscabetic eruption, 1646
Scalded skin syndrome, 281
    staphylococcal, 1288, 1328, **1635–1636**
Scalds, **1715, 1798**
    non-accidental injury, 1868
Scalp
    blood sampling, fetus, 86, 119
    lacerations, 706
    psoriasis, 1629
    seborrheic dermatitis, 1643
    tinea, 1637
Scalp hair, neonatal gestation age, 40 (Table)
Scalp veins, 1837
    parenteral nutrition for malignant diarrhea, 1297
Scanogram, computed tomography, 1917 (Fig.)
Scaphocephaly, 21 (Fig.), 1560, 1661
Scapula, Sprengel's shoulder, **1548**, 1549 (Fig.)
Scarf sign, neonatal gestation age, 40 (Table), 41 (Fig.)
Scarlatina, 1285
Scarlet fever, **1331–1332**
    vs erythema infectiosum, 1359
    vs measles, 1331, 1354
    rash, 1285, 1331
    vs rubella, 1331, 1357
    tongue, 425, 1285
Scarring
    burns, 1800
    Ehlers–Danlos syndrome, 1612
    epidermolysis bullosa, 1622
    hemangiomas, 1619
Schedule of growing skills, 400
Scheie syndrome, 1157 (Table), 1158, **1159**
Schemas, intellectual, 1729
Scheuermann's disease, 1594–1595
Schilder's disease, *see* Adrenoleukodystrophy
Schilling test, 853 (Table), 1199
Schindler disease, 1157 (Table), 1164, **1168–1169**
Schistosomiasis, **1507–1511**
    hematuria, 958
    larval disease, 1484 (Table)
    liver, 478, 1509–1510
    nephrotic syndrome, 968
    salmonellosis, 1324
Schizogony, *Plasmodium* spp., 1445, 1446
Schizophrenia, 818–819, 836, 1739
    adolescence, 1750, 1751, **1755**
    vs depression, 1754–1755
    recurrence risks, 74
Schmidt's syndrome, 1048
Schmid type metaphyseal

chondrodysplasia, 1578, 1579 (Table)
    inheritance, 1566 (Table)
Schmorl's nodes, 1594
School children
    blood pressure, 20
    definition, 17
    disease incidence, 13
    normal diet, 1189
School failure, ex-preterm infants, 171
School health care, **1860–1865**
    services, **1862–1865**
Schooling, *see also* Education; Nursery education
    adopted children, 1859
    BCG Programme, 1340
    cerebral palsy, 761
    congenital hemiplegia, 744
    developing countries, 1885–1886
    Duchenne muscular dystrophy, 732
    immigrant children, 1866
    of mothers, **1886–1887**, 1892
    National Child Development Study, 1852
    National Survey of Health and Development, 1851
    personality development, 1732
    speech and language disorder, 808
    world figures, 1883 (Table)
School refusal, **1739–1740**
    adolescence, **1756**
Schultz–Charlton sign, 1331 (Fig.)
Schwachman syndrome, **450**, 1242 (Table), 1244, 1261
    vs infantile genetic agranulocytosis, 867
Schwartzmann reaction, 1318
Sciatic nerve, umbilical artery injection, 722
Scimitar sign, 193
Scimitar syndrome, 574
Scintigraphy, **1897**
    biliary atresia, 1782
    biliary tract, 1907
    bones, 1913, **1915–1916**
    cerebral blood flow, 661
    colon, 464
    congenital hypothyroidism, 1047
    esophagus, 429
    gastrointestinal tract, **1906**
    hepatitis syndrome in infancy, 474
    hydronephrosis, 936
    liver, 472
        chronic disease, 480
    lungs, **1901**
    Meckel's diverticulum, 447, 460, 1787, **1906**
    neuroblastoma, 911, 1913
    osteitis, 1590
    osteomyelitis, 283
    radiation doses, 1895 (Table)
    rectal bleeding, 460
    respiratory disorders, **517–519**
    retroperitoneum, **1913**
    small intestine, 447
    urinary tract, **1911–1912**
        infections, 953–954, 955 (Fig.)
Scissor excision, genital warts, 1445
SCIWORA (spinal cord injury without radiological abnormality), **1809**
Sclerae
    blue, 1676
    osteogenesis imperfecta, 1568
Sclerema neonatorum, 43
Scleritis, ankylosing spondylitis, 1675
Scleroderma, **1644–1645**, *see also* Progressive systemic sclerosis
Sclerosing cholangitis, **480–481**
    hepatitis syndrome in infancy, 473
Sclerosteosis, 1582 (Table)
Sclerotherapy, varices, 483
Scoline, myotonia, 733
Scoliosis, 38, **1557–1558**
    abduction contracture of hip, 1552
    breathing, 505

Scoliosis (Contd)
  Duchenne muscular dystrophy, 730, 731
  Friedreich's ataxia, 765
  idiopathic adolescent, recurrence risks, 74
  neural tube defect, 657
  neurofibromatosis, 800
  respiratory function tests, 498
  severely handicapped children affected, 14 (Table)
Scoring, pain, 1831
Scorpion stings, **1525–1526**
Scotland, see also Children (Scotland) Act 1995
  birth certificates, 1849
  infectious diseases surveillance, 1281
  National Health Service, 1853
Scratch testing, allergic disorders, 1693
Screamers node, 1687
Screening, **1862**, see also Genetic screening; Growth, assessment
  abnormal metabolites, 1119
  antenatal, **80**, 338
  celiac disease, 440–441
  cystic fibrosis, 339 (Table), **552**
  deafness, 816, 1683
  and development, 386
  endocrinology, 1007
  familial adenomatous polyposis, 448
  hemostasis, 228
  21-hydroxylase deficiency, 1008, 1062
  hypercholesterolemia, 1152
  mental retardation, **837**, 840
  metabolic disorders, 1101–1102
    heart muscle disease, 635 (Table)
  neonate, 339
    cystic fibrosis, **552**
  neuroblastoma, 913–914
  nutritional anthropometry, 1187
  peroxisomal dysfunction, 1172
  porphyrias, 1143
  and prevalence, 1001
  retinopathy of prematurity, 267
  school health services, **1863**
  sensorineural deafness, 243–244
  siblings, Wilson's disease, 481
  syphilis, 1403
  thyroid disease, congenital, 1003, 1046
Scriver et al., Metabolic and molecular bases of inherited disease (1995), 1099
Scrotum
  acute, **1791–1792**
  examination, 34
  Henoch–Schönlein purpura, 1610
  hernia, 1789
  idiopathic edema, 1791–1792
  neonatal gestation age, 40 (Table)
  ultrasonography, 1914
Scrubbing up, 1830
Scrub typhus, 1390 (Table), **1392**
Scurvy, 875, **1199–1200**
  costochondral junctions, 30, 1199
  eye, 1677
  tyrosyluria, 1106
Sea-blue histiocyte syndrome, 1157 (Table)
Seal bark, 1772
Sea snakes, bites, 1522
Seasonal asthma, 549
Seasonal rhinitis, 1684, **1697–1698**
Seasonal variations
  allergic symptoms, 1691
  growth, 368
  sudden infant death syndrome, 1719
Seat belts, 1716
  injuries, 1811, **1812**
Seatworms, **1486–1488**
Sea wasp, 1526
Sebopsoriasis, see Napkin psoriasis
Seborrheic dermatitis, 1643
  vs tinea versicolor, 1638
Seckel syndrome, 832 (Table), 1254
Secondary biliary hypoplasia, 221

Secondary brain injury, vs primary brain injury, **1810**
Secondary diabetes mellitus, 1081
Secondary drowning, 1718
Secondary granule deficiency, 1242 (Table)
Secondary hemorrhagic disease, see Disseminated intravascular coagulation
Secondary hyperaldosteronism, 1067
Secondary oocytes, 1004
Secondary prevention, 338
Secondary proximal renal tubular acidosis, 260
Secondary resistance, tumor cells, 892–893
Secondary survey, trauma, 1809
Secondary syphilis, **1406–1408**
  vs anogenital warts, 1444
Second Task Force on Blood Pressure Control in Children, 636
Second tumors, 890, **898**
  nephroblastoma radiotherapy, 914
Secretin, pancreatic function tests, 451
Secretory diarrhea, 455, 468
  stool, 454 (Table)
Secretory otitis media, 816, **1681–1682**
Secretory piece deficiency, IgA, 1245, 1257
Secretory response, antibodies, 439
Sector coloboma, 1650
Sector scanners, ultrasonography, 1896
Secure attachment, 1731
Sedation, 1830
  bronchoscopy, 519
  colonoscopy, 464
  computed tomography, 1897
  pleural drainage, 521
  ventilation, **1832–1833**
Sedatives
  hypothermia, 149
  improper administration, 1871
Segawa's disease, 1106, 1107
Segawa type dystonia, 673, 759
SEH, see Subependymal hemorrhage
Seizures, 671, see also Fits
  acute renal failure, 975
  apnea, 528
  arteriovenous fistulae, 711
  bacterial meningitis, 1291
  birth asphyxia, 130
  burns, 1799
  cholera, 1304
  definitions, 671
  emergency care, **1814–1815**
  first aid, 691
  folinic acid-responsive, 1147
  head injuries, **1811**
  history taking, 17
  hypernatremia, 414
  infarction, 714
  intracranial birth trauma, 122
  lactic acidosis, 307
  malaria, 1452
  neonatal tetany, 300
  neonate, 236, **244–247**
  non-accidental head injury, 700
  from phenytoin, 697
  pyridoxine-dependent, 245, 1115
  shigellosis, 1328
  from vaccination, 343
Seldinger technique, central venous cannulation, 1837
Selectins, 1234
Selective bronchial intubation, pulmonary interstitial emphysema, 189
Selective dorsal rhizotomy, cerebral palsy, 759
Selective IgA deficiency, 1242 (Table)
  incidence, 1243 (Table)
  neoplasms, 1248 (Table)
Selective IgM deficiency, 1258
Selective primary health care, developing countries, 1889

Selective serotonin reuptake inhibitors, 1755
Selenium, 1185 (Table), 1202–1203
  parenteral nutrition, 1221
  Recommended Dietary Allowances, 1949 (Table)
  reference nutrient intakes, 1947 (Table)
  requirements, 1181 (Table)
  sources, 1185 (Table)
Self-concept, 1730
Self-esteem, 1730
Self-help groups
  gastrointestinal and liver disease, 485
  sudden infant death syndrome, 1723
Self-management, asthma, 547
Self-mutilation, 771, 834, 841
Self-poisoning, 1706, **1708**, 1815
Self vs non-self, 1729
Sellafield, neoplasms, 890
Semantic dysgraphia, 824
Semantic-pragmatic disorder, 807
Semantics, 804
Semi-ischemic exercise test, 1139
Seminomas, see Germinomas
Semipacked cells, exchange transfusion, 1839
Semiskimmed milk, 334
Semi-vegetarian diet, 1189 (Table)
Semon's law, 809
Senna, administration, 1976 (Table)
Senning procedure, transposition of great arteries, 615
Sensation
  congenital hemiplegia, 744
  examination, 35
    neonate, 241–242
Sensorimotor experiences, 98
Sensorimotor period, development, 1729
Sensorineural deafness, **816–818, 1682**
  screening, 243–244
Sensory handicap
  cerebral palsy, 761
  neural tube defect, 656
  very low birthweight, 171
Sensory nerve segments, see Dermatomes
Sensory neurons, herpes simplex, 1436
Separation, marital, **1855–1856**
Sepsis
  central venous lines, **1224–1225**
  disseminated intravascular coagulation, 231
  and galactose-1-phosphate uridyltransferase deficiency, 1132–1133
  neonatal jaundice, 217
  neonate, 273, **277–278**
    complement deficiency, 1263
    hypoglycemia, 294
    inborn errors of metabolism, 305
    temperature, 1282
  parenteral nutrition, 159
  vomiting, 210, 212
Septic arthritis, 1589, **1591–1592**
  FUO investigations, 1283 (Table)
  gonococcal, 1426
  vs Lyme arthritis, 1612
  neonate, 282–283
  organisms, 284 (Table)
Septicemia, **1287–1288**, see also Gram-negative septicemia
  cancer treatment, 894
  epiglottitis, 562–563
  hemolysis, 864
  Neisseria meningitidis, **1314–1315**
  neonate, 205
  Pseudomonas aeruginosa, 1320
  salmonellosis, 1323, 1324
  Staphylococcus aureus, **1329**
  United Kingdom, mortality, 1276 (Table)
Septic shock, 1287
  Neisseria meningitidis, **1826**
  neonate, 205
Septo-optic dysplasia, 109, 472 (Table), 647, 1043

growth hormone deficiency, 372–373, 1016
Sequences, congenital, 75
Sequential segmental analysis, congenital heart disease, 597
Sequestra, osteitis, 1590, 1592
Sequestration, see also Pulmonary sequestration
  Plasmodium falciparum, 1446, 1448
Sequestration crisis, sickle cell disease, 862
Serial plastering, 757
Serological markers, viral hepatitis type B, 476 (Table)
Serology, **1300**
  chlamydial infection, 1430
  Lyme disease, 1313–1314
  malaria, 1452
    epidemiology, 1447
  pneumonia, 567
  syphilis, **1402–1404**
  viruses, **1351**
Seromucinous otitis media (secretory otitis media), 816, **1681–1682**
Serotonin, production block, 1114
Serous meningitis, 1344
Serovars, Neisseria gonorrhoeae, 1422
Sertoli cells, 1004
Sertoli cell tumors, testis, 921
Sertraline, 1755
Serum
  electrolytes, 403–404
  water, 404
Serum carnosinase deficiency, 1114
Serum hepatitis, see Hepatitis B virus
Serum sickness, heterophile antibody test, 1367
Servo mode, incubators, 148
Sessile warts, genitalia, 1443
Severe combined immunodeficiency syndrome, 1141, **1248–1250**
  bone marrow transplantation, 1268–1270
  diarrhea, 213
  genetics, 1241
  incidence, 1243 (Table)
  neoplasms, 889 (Table)
  respiratory tract infections, 533
Severe myoclonic epilepsy of Dravet, 688 (Table)
Severe X-linked myotubular myopathy, 735 (Table)
Sever's disease, **1595**
Sex, see also Gender
  low birthweight and outcome, 167–168
Sex chromosome abnormalities, **60–63**
Sex determination, intersex disorders, 1011
Sex-determining region of Y chromosome, 1004
Sex education, 1398–1399
Sex hormones
  accidental ingestion, 1028
  congenital dislocation of hip, 1550
  for constitutional tall stature, 376
  diabetes mellitus complications, 1080
  growth hormone tests, delayed puberty investigation, 1034
  and porphyrias, 1143
Sex-influenced inheritance, 65, **66–67**
Sex ratios
  cystic fibrosis, 551
  general, 15 (Table)
  infection, 276
Sex role, see Gender role
Sex steroid priming, 372
Sexual abuse, 949, **1737, 1869–1870**
  adolescents, 1752, **1759–1760**, 1870
  gonorrhea, 1420, 1421
  microbiology, 1299
  precocious pseudopuberty, 1027
  sexually transmitted diseases, investigation, 1400
  warts, 988

Sexual assault, 1870
Sexual behavior, risk-taking behavior, 1763
Sexual development (*Plasmodium* spp.), 1446
Sexual differentiation disorders, **1007–1011**, *see also* Ambiguous genitalia
  camptomelic dysplasia, 1572
Sexual exploitation, 1870, 1887
Sexual function, neural tube defect, 657
Sexually transmitted diseases, 994, **1398–1415, 1420–1445**
  congenital, developing countries disease burden, 1276 (Table)
  detection or exclusion, 1399
  emergence, 1278
  microbiology, **1299**
  United Kingdom, 1277
Sexual promiscuity, and sexual abuse, 1759
Sexual transmission, pediculosis, 1638
Shagreen patches, 1625
Shake lotions, 1617
Shaken baby syndrome, 1810, 1867
Shaking injury, *see* Whiplash shaking injury
Shapes, matching, 383
Shared care hospitals, 873
Sharps disposal, 1282
Sheath contraception, 994
Sheep
  bot fly, 1514
  hydatid disease, 1504
  milk, 333, 1700
  orf, 1388
Sheep red cell agglutinins, infectious mononucleosis, 1367
Shellfish, toxic paralysis, 727
Shell viral cultures, 1366
Sheridan, tests of vision, 395, 396
Shifting dullness, 33
Shigella sonnei, United Kingdom, 1277 (Fig.)
Shigella spp., **1327–1328**
  antibiotic, 454 (Table)
  dysentery, 452
  encephalopathy, 683, 693
Shiley's tracheostomy tubes, sizes, 1843 (Table)
Shingles, *see* Herpes zoster
Shock, *see also* Hypovolemia; Septic shock
  blood sampling, 1835
  burns, 1799
  Neisseria meningitidis, 1315
  neonate, blood loss, 224
  resuscitation, 1807
  treatment, 433
Short bowel syndrome, **444–445, 1211–1212**
Short chain acyl-CoA dehydrogenase deficiency, 1130
Short chain fatty acids, 1148, 1182
  colon, 455–456
  short bowel syndrome, 1212
Short chain 3-hydroxyacyl-CoA dehydrogenase deficiency, 1130
Short gut syndrome, **444–445, 1211–1212**
Short-limbed dwarfism, immunodeficiency, 1254
Short rib–polydactyly syndromes, **1571**
Short segment Hirschsprung's disease, 463, 465, 1777
Short stature, **368–375**, 998, **1014–1020**, *see also* Dwarfism
  chronic renal failure, 979, 980
  cultural advantages, 1019
Shoulder dystocia, 138
Shouldering, fetal heart rate, 86
Showers, epilepsy, 691
Shprintzen syndrome, 1252
Shuffling, 667

Shunt bilirubin, 214
Shunting
  hydrocephalus, **662–664**
    blindness, 666
    blockage, 663, 796 (Table)
    clinical features, 660
    epilepsy, 666
    neural tube defects, 655
    tuberculous meningitis, 665
  malfunction monitoring, 661
Shwachman–Diamond syndrome, **855,** 1578, 1579 (Table)
Sialectasis, 1784
Sialic acid storage diseases, 781 (Table), 1157 (Table), **1169**
Sialidoses, 781 (Table), 1157 (Table)
Sialogogues, 1001
Sialuria, 1169
Sialyl lewis X, 1234, 1261
Sibbens, *see* Endemic syphilis
Siberian tick typhus, 1392
Siblings
  diabetes mellitus, 1073
  disability on, 1747
  genetic epilepsies, 679–682
  HIV vertical transmission, 288
  Kawasaki disease, 1480
  screening, Wilson's disease, 481
  vs twins, menarche, 366
  vesicoureteric reflux, 956
Sickle cell disease, 72 (Table), 226, 861–863, 1100
  analgesia, 1833
  double heterozygotes, 66
  frequency, 47 (Table)
  genetic diagnosis, 73
  hematuria, 959
  and hookworm, 1489
  immunodeficiency, 1266
  and malaria, 47
  maternal, 89 (Table)
  mutation, 69
  osteitis, 862
    salmonella, 1323–1324, 1590
  parvovirus B19, 1359
  retinopathy, 1675
  screening, 339 (Table)
  stroke, 713
Sickle cell trait, 860
  maternal, 89 (Table)
  screening, antenatal care, 80
Sick sinus syndrome, 624
Sideroblastic anemias, 866, *see also* Myelodysplasias
Siderosis, blood transfusions, 1201
Sigmoidoscopy, 464
Signal transduction, immune system, 1239–1240
  defects, 1250
Significant bacteriuria, 950
Sign languages, 814, 837
Silicon, 1185 (Table)
Silicone, enteral feeding tubes, 1218
Silver nitrate, ophthalmia neonatorum prophylaxis, 263, 283, 1429
Silver–Russell syndrome, **369–370**, 1007, 1015, 1017, 1545
  precocious puberty, 1030
Silver syndrome, 832 (Table)
Simian crease, 55
Simian virus 40, 1378
Simon focus, 1336
Simple allergic conjunctivitis, 1664
Simple developmental tic, 771
Simple partial seizures, 675
Simvastatin, 1152
Singer's nodules, 809
Single contrast barium enema, 1903
Single dose therapy, gonorrhea, 1427
Single gene disorders, **64–68**
  congenital heart disease, 596
  neoplasms, 888 (Table)
Single outlet ventriculoarterial connections, 597

Single photon emission computed tomography, **1897**
  epilepsy, 679, 1897, **1909**
  language disorder, 808
  regional cerebral blood flow, **1909**
Single rooms, hospital care, 1281, 1282
Single ventricle (double inlet ventricle), 203 (Table), 597, **620–621**
Sinoatrial block, 624
Sinus arrest, 624
Sinus arrhythmia, 32, 624
Sinus bradycardia, 624
Sinus histiocytosis and massive lymphadenopathy, 926
Sinusitis, **1685**
  cystic fibrosis, 555
Sinus of Valsalva, aneurysm, 608
Sinusoidal stretching, 756
Sinusoids, liver, 470
Sinus tachycardia, 624, 628
Sinus venosus atrial septal defects, 601 (Fig.), 602
Sitting, 668
  development, 382
  examination, 389 (Table)
  femoral torsion, 1552
Sitting height, 363–364, 1017
Situation-specific behavior, 1728
Situs, 612–613
  atria, 597
  chest X-ray, 588
Situs inversus, 472 (Table), 612
SI unit system, 1921
Sixth disease, *see* Roseola infantum
Sixth nerve, *see* Abducens nerve
Size for gestation, definitions, 94
'Sizostat' (Tanner), 1014
Sjögren–Larsson syndrome, 791 (Table), 799 (Table), 803, 832 (Table)
  ichthyosis, 1622 (Table)
Sjögren's syndrome, 1606
Skeletal age, *see* Bone age
Skeletal dysplasias (osteochondrodysplasias), 370–371, 1017, **1565–1586**
  short stature, 1017
  management, 1019
  Turner's syndrome, 1032
Skeletal surveys, 1914–1915
  non-accidental injury, 700, 703
Skene's glands, gonorrhea, 1425
Skerljevo, *see* Endemic syphilis
Skills, accident and emergency departments, 1805–1806
Skin, **1616–1648**, *see also* Rashes
  absorption of drugs, **1954**
  acyclovir cream, 1440
  AIDS, **1395–1396**
  amebiasis, 1468
  asepsis for procedures, 1830
  ataxia telangiectasia, 1253
  biopsy, **1846**
  blood flow, preterm infant, 147
  Candida spp., 1472
  color, vitamin B$_{12}$ deficiency, 853
  dehydration, preterm infant, 141
  diphtheria, 561
  discoloration, phototherapy, 219
  disseminated gonococcal infection, 1426
  examination, 19
  eye, **1675**
  hemorrhage in, 876
  history taking, 17
  infections, **1631–1639**
    neonate, organisms, 285 (Table)
  leprosy, 1310
  leukemias, 871
  neonatal lupus erythematosus, 1606
  neonates, 42
    gestation age, 42 (Fig.)
  nonacute porphyrias, 1144
  North American blastomycosis, 1474
  onchocerciasis, 1497

progressive systemic sclerosis, 1608
Pseudomonas aeruginosa, 1321
second primary tumors, 898 (Table)
SGA baby, 138
spina bifida occulta, 652
staphylococcal infection, **1329**
  neonate, 281
syphilis
  congenital, 1411–1412
  secondary, 1406–1407
systemic lupus erythematosus, 1605, 1644
tuberculosis, 1343
virology, **1352**
vitamin D synthesis, 1053–1054
water output, 403 (Table)
Skinfold calipers, 999 (Fig.), 1011, 1021
Skinfold thicknesses, 364, 1186
Skin temperature, 147
  incubator settings, 148
Skin tests
  allergic disorders, **1693**
  asthma, 541
  toxoplasmosis, 1466
Skin window test (Rebuck), 1247
Skull
  achondroplasia, 1573, 1574
  basal fractures, 707, **1811**
    diabetes insipidus, 709
    gastric decompression, 1809
    X-rays, 1908
  foramina, obstruction, 811
  fractures, **707**
    birth trauma, 121 (Table), 707
    non-accidental injury, **700**, 1867
  hemoglobinopathy, 863 (Fig.)
  hydrocephalus, 660
  hypophosphatasia, 1176
  leukemia, 870
  lysosomal storage disorders, 1158
  Marfan's syndrome, 1588
  prematurity, 43
  structural defects, **1558–1565**
  X-rays, **1907–1908**
    epilepsy, 678
    radiation doses, 1895 (Table)
Skye, asthma, 493, 542
Slapped cheek appearance, 1285
Slapped cheek disease, *see* Erythema infectiosum
Sleep
  breathing, 196, 506, **528–531**
    muscular dystrophies, 732
  cerebral blood flow, 661
  developmental changes, 530
  electroencephalography, 677
  epilepsy, 691
  funny turns, 673
  growth hormone secretion, 1012
  heart rate, 624
  LH and FSH secretion, 1025
  muscle tone, 756
  neonatal intensive care, 97
  neonate, 236
  sudden infant death syndrome, 1721–1722
Sleep deprivation, epilepsy, 691
Sleep disorders, **1745–1746**
  African trypanosomiasis, 1455–1456
  preschool children, 1736
Sleeping arrangements, sudden infant death syndrome, 1720
Sleeping posture, neonate, 112
Sleeping sickness, *see* African trypanosomiasis
Sleep myoclonus, benign neonatal, 245
Sleep studies, airway obstruction, tonsillitis, 1687
Sleep walking, 1746
Slipped upper femoral epiphysis, **1596**
Slit-lamp binocular microscope, 1654
Slit ventricles, 659
Slit ventricle syndrome, 659, **664**

Slope clearance methods, GFR measurement, 942
Slow acetylators, isoniazid, 1347
Slow K, 415
Slow virus diseases, **1378**
Slug pellets, poisoning, 1711
Sly syndrome, 784 (Table), 1157 (Table), **1161–1162**
Small bowel, see Small intestine
Small bowel meal (enema), 1896, 1902
  Crohn's disease, 457
Small button kidney, 254
Small for gestational age infant (SGA), **136–138,** 465, **1005, 1007,** see also Low birthweight
  antenatal care, 81–82
  definition, 94
  diabetes mellitus, 1081
  feeding, 151
  hypoglycemia, 1082
  incidence, 15 (Table)
  long-term cardiovascular disease and diabetes mellitus, 1066
  maternal hyperphenylalaninemia, 1104 (Table)
  symphysis–fundal height, 81
Small intestine, **435–436,** see also Small bowel meal
  causes of failure to thrive, 468
  cystic fibrosis, 551
  investigations, **447–448**
  kwashiorkor, 1192, 1193, 1194
  motility, 208, **438**
  obstruction, **1774–1776**
  progressive systemic sclerosis, 1608
  resection, 1211–1212
Small left colon syndrome (meconium plug syndrome), **1776–1777**
Small noncleaved lymphomas, 907
Smallpox, eradication, 1888
Small round cell tumors, tumor markers, 912 (Table)
Smiling, development, 388 (Table)
Smith–Lemli–Opitz syndrome, 832 (Table), 1156
  neonatal seizures, 245
Smith–Magenis syndrome, 60 (Table)
Smoke
  inhalation, **571–572, 1813**
  respiratory disorders, developing countries, 493
  respiratory epithelial surface, 497
Smoke detectors, 1715
Smoking, 15 (Table), 340–341, see also Passive smoking
  adolescents, 493, 1762
  α1-antitrypsin deficiency, 1175
  parents, 493
    asthma, 545
  preconceptual care, 80
  pregnancy, 338, 495
  respiratory disorders, **493**
  sudden infant death syndrome, 340, 1720, 1722
Snails
  angiostrongyliasis, 1494
  control, 1511
  trematodes, 1507 (Table)
Snail-track ulcers, 1407
Snake bites, **1520–1524**
Snellen test, 268, 395
Snoring, 509
Snout reflex, 770
Soap solutions, child abuse, 1871
Soccer, injuries, 1714
Social behavior
  autism, 1738
  disorder, 1733
  examination, 388–391 (Table)
Social class
  accidents, 1712
  breast-feeding, 15 (Table), 326
  burns and scalds, 1714
  on childhood mortalities, 3 (Table)

diet, 15 (Table)
  height, 1014
  IQ, 827
  language development, 818
  Maternity Survey 1946, 1851
  mental retardation, 828–829
  sudden infant death syndrome, 1719–1720
Social contacts, neonatal care, 97–98
Social development, 1729 (Table), **1731**
Social factors
  AIDS, 1396
  cancer survivors, 899
  child abuse, 1866
  on child health, **13–14,** 15 (Table)
  cystic fibrosis, 559
  failure to thrive, 466, 468–469
  infectious disease emergence, 1279 (Table)
  IQ, 827
  language development, 818, 828
  learning, 819
  respiratory disorders, **492**
Social function of weaning, 333–334
Social history, 18
Social independence, 762
Social index, British Births Child Study, 1852
Social interaction, normal development, 385
Socialized antisocial behavior, 1742
Social pediatrics, **1848–1881**
Social services, mental retardation, 838
Social workers, child development centers, 399
Socioeconomic factors, growth, 368
Sociology, delinquency, 1762
Sodium, 407–408, 1185 (Table)
  abnormal steady state value, 413
  absorption, 208, 438
  alimentary secretions, 411 (Table)
  amniotic fluid, 253
  breast milk, 143, 332
  chloridorrhea, loss, 446
  colonic absorption, 455
  concentrations, 404, 406 (Table)
    units, 1921
  depletion, 409, **410–411**
    neonates, 144
  excretion, 410
    preterm infant, 142
  feces
    cholera, 1303 (Table)
    gastroenteritis, 1293
  movement across membranes, 405, 406–407
  normal values, 1928 (Table)
    amniotic fluid, 1937 (Table)
    cerebrospinal fluid, 1935 (Table)
    meconium, 1936 (Table)
    urine, 1932 (Table)
  oral rehydration solutions, 453
  parenteral nutrition, 1222 (Table)
  preterm infant, **143–144**
  preterm supplements, 154
  reabsorption, 941
    neonatal kidney, 108
  reference nutrient intakes, 1947 (Table)
  requirements, 413 (Table)
    preterm infant, 152 (Table)
  tubular reabsorption, postnatal development, 256–257
  urine, 408
    neonates, 142 (Table), 143
    renal failure, 974
Sodium benzoate
  amino acid excretion, 307
  for hyperammonemia, 1111
  for hyperglycinemia, 1112
Sodium bicarbonate, 104, see also Bicarbonate
  for acidosis, 259, 306–307, **421**
    acute renal failure, 975
    in hypernatremia, 414, 421

administration, 1976 (Table)
  diabetic ketoacidosis, 1076
  emergency supply, 134 (Table)
  glutathione synthetase deficiency, 1115
  for hyperkalemia, 145 (Table), 259, 415
    acute renal failure, 975
  neonatal resuscitation, 135
  for organic acidurias, 1119
  for renal tubular acidosis, 260
  respiratory distress syndrome, 179
Sodium calcium edetate
  administration, 1976 (Table)
  for lead poisoning, 1708
Sodium cellulose phosphate, administration, 1976 (Table)
Sodium cromoglycate
  administration, 1976 (Table)
  allergic conjunctivitis, 1664
  asthma, 546
  seasonal rhinitis, 1697
Sodium dantrolene, see Dantrolene
Sodium deficit, calculation, 975
Sodium-dependent carbohydrate absorption, 207
Sodium/glucose cotransporters, 1123
  glucose–galactose malabsorption, 446
  oral rehydration, 452
Sodium glycerophosphate, 1222 (Table)
Sodium hydroxide, Apt test, 224
Sodium iron edetate, 852
  administration, 1976 (Table)
    neonate, 1958 (Table)
Sodium lactate, for acidosis, 421
Sodium-l-thyroxine, 1047, 1050 see also L-thyroxine
Sodium nitrite, administration, 1976 (Table)
Sodium nitroprusside, see Nitroprusside
Sodium phenylacetate, phenylbutyrate, for hyperammonemia, 1111
Sodium picosulfate, administration, 1977 (Table)
Sodium polystyrene sulfonate resin, 415
Sodium-potassium-ATPase system
  gastrointestinal tract, 424, 438
  kidneys, 941
Sodium stibogluconate, **1462–1463,** 1977 (Table)
Sodium thiosulfate, administration, 1977 (Table)
Sodium valproate, see Valproate
Sodoku, **1321–1322**
Soft tissue
  Ewing's sarcoma, 919
  injuries
    birth trauma, **120–121**
    with fractures, 1812
  ultrasonography, 1917
Soft tissue sarcomas, 886 (Table), **915–917**
  breast cancer in mother, 889
  second primary tumors, 898 (Table)
Soiling, **1743–1744**
Sokosha, **1321–1322**
Soldiers, children as, 1887
Sole creases, neonatal gestation age, 40 (Table)
Solids, normal values, amniotic fluid, 1937 (Table)
Solivito, 158
Solivito N, 1222 (Table)
Solute load, see 'renal solute load'
Solvent abuse, 1763
  neuropathy, 724
Solvents, aplastic anemia, 856 (Table)
Somatic cell hybridization, 73
Somatic cell mutations, 69
Somatizing disorders, **1741,** 1760
Somatostatin, **364, 1012–1014,** 1071
  analogs
    nesidioblastosis, 1083
    short bowel syndrome, 1212

for hyperinsulinism, 296
    molecule, 1037 (Table)
Somatostatin-secreting cells, pancreas, 1005
Somatropin, administration, 1977 (Table)
Somnambulism, 673
'Somnolence syndrome', 901
Somogyi effect, 1079
Sorbitol, 1210
Sore throat, history taking, 17
Sorsby's macular degeneration, 1666
Sotalol, 626–627
Sotos syndrome, 376, 832 (Table), 1043
South American blastomycosis, 1471 (Table), **1474–1475**
South American trypanosomiasis, **1458–1460**
Southern blotting, **70**
  fragile X, 64 (Fig.)
Soviet Union (former), demography, 2 (Table)
SOX9 gene, camptomelic dysplasia, 1572
Soya, enteropathy, dietary management, 1214 (Table)
Soya milks (protein), 153, **333,** 1700
  celiac disease, 442
  composition, 1942–1943 (Table)
  and cystic fibrosis, 553
  galactose-1-phosphate uridyltransferase deficiency, 1133
  infant formula, 332, 1188
Space-occupying lesions
  endocrine aspects, 1042–1043
  hydrocephalus, 658
Spahr type metaphyseal chondrodysplasia, 1579 (Table)
Spanish fly, cantharidin, 1525
Sparganosis, 1504
Spasmus nutans, 272
Spastic diplegia, 35, 398
Spastic dysarthria, 812–813
Spasticity, 393, 742–744, 755, **756**
  gait, 34
  upper limb, 35
Spastic phase, diplegia, 747–748
Spatial learning, disorders, **670**
Special care, neonates, 95–96
  analgesia, 1833
  preterm, **139–155**
Special care units, neonates, 156
Special child syndrome, 1739
Special educational needs, 340, **1864–1865**
Special inquiries, child health, **1850–1852**
Special Needs registers, 1850
Special senses, defects on development, 386
Specific heart muscle disease, **634,** 635 (Table)
Specific immune mechanisms, 1232, **1235–1239**
Specific Issue Orders, 1874, 1876
Specimens
  bacteriology, 1297
    Neisseria gonorrhoeae, 1422–1423
  inborn errors of metabolism, at death, 307
  ophthalmia neonatorum, 263
  sexually transmitted diseases, 1399, 1400
Spectacles, 1657
Spectral analysis, crying, 236
Spectral Doppler ultrasonography, 592
  mitral stenosis, 629
Spectrin defect, hereditary spherocytosis, 226
Spectrophotometry, cerebrospinal fluid, 710
Speech, 34
  cleft palate, 1797
  development, **804–805**

Speech (Contd)
  developmental disorders, **670, 805–807**
  disorders, **804–819**
    severely handicapped children
      affected, 14 (Table)
  dyspraxia, 669
  history taking, 17
  phonation, 808, **1687–1688**
  retardation, 806
    congenital hemiplegia, 744
    dyslexia, 820
Speech therapists, child development
  centers, 399
Speech therapy, 807–808
  cerebral palsy, 761–762
  stammer, 806
Spelling dysgraphia, 823–824
Spence, Sir James, on foreskin, 1793
Spermatic cord, inguinal hernia, 1790
Spermatogenesis, 48, 1024
  puberty, 357
Sperm banking, cancer survivors, 899
SPf66 vaccine, 1449
Spherocytosis, hereditary, 226, **857–858**
Sphingolipidoses, 1157 (Table),
  1162–1167
Sphingomyelinase deficiency, 1166
Sphingosines, 1162
Spider bites, **1524–1525**
Spielmeyer–Vogt disease, 1171
Spina bifida, 1557, see also
  Myelomeningocele
  empiric risks, 74
Spina bifida complex, see Neural tube,
  defects
Spina bifida cystica, **652–657**
Spina bifida occulta, **652**
Spinal accessory nerve, examination, 34
Spinal analgesia, 1832
Spinal cord
  achondroplasia, 371
  adrenoleukodystrophy, 1174
  birth trauma, **123**
  congenital abnormalities, **651–657**
  constipation management, 463
  vs diplegia, 745
  ependymomas, 902, 906
  vs Guillain–Barré syndrome, 726
  isolated segment, 653–654
  myelomeningocele, lesion types,
    653–654
  poliomyelitis, 1379
  subacute combined degeneration, 1199
  tumors, **906–907**
  ultrasonography, 1908
  von Hippel–Lindau syndrome, 803
Spinal cord injury without radiological
  abnormality (SCIWORA), **1809**
Spinal muscular atrophies, 719–721
Spinal paralysis, poliomyelitis, 1379, 1380
Spine
  achondroplasia, 1573, 1574–1575
  deformities, 38
  diagnostic radiation doses, 1895 (Table)
  imaging, 1908, 1915
  immobilization, 1809
  lap belt injury, 1812
  lysosomal storage disorders, 1157, 1158
  magnetic resonance imaging, 1913
  Morquio–Brailsford syndrome, 1160
  neoplasms, imaging, 1912–1913
  neuroblastoma, 911, 1915
  neurofibromatosis, 800
  osteitis, 1592
  osteochondroses, 1594–1595
  radiotherapy, 901
    endocrine effects, 1042
  single photon emission computed
    tomography, 1897
  tuberculosis, 1344, 1346, **1592–1593**
Spin echo T1 images, magnetic resonance
  imaging, 1898
Spinnaker sign, pneumomediastinum, 188
  (Fig.)

Spinocerebellar ataxia type 1, 766
Spinocerebellar degenerations, 766
Spinoepiphyseal dysplasia, 1157 (Table)
Spiral fractures, tibia, 1914
Spiramycin, toxoplasmosis, 1466
Spirillum minus, **1321–1322**
Spirograms, 500
Spirometra genus, 1504
Spironolactone, 145
  administration, 1977 (Table)
  heart failure, 599
  nephrotic syndrome, 970
  renal hypertension, 973 (Table)
Spitting cobras, 1522, 1523
Spleen
  aspiration, leishmaniasis, 1462
  congenital syphilis, 1412
  examination, 33
  hemopoiesis, 222, 847–848
  imaging, **1907**
  rupture, neonate, 224
  trauma, 1812
Splenectomy
  hereditary spherocytosis, 857–858
  and Hodgkin's disease, 910
  idiopathic thrombocytopenic purpura,
    878
  osteopetrosis, 1582
  thalassemia, 863
Splenectomy Trust, address, 1320
Splenomegaly, 471
  idiopathic thrombocytopenic purpura,
    878
  leishmaniasis, 1462
  leukemias, 870–871
  malaria, 1448, 1449
    endemicity, 1447
    hyperreactive, 1451
  measles, 1354
  mental retardation, 835 (Table)
  schistosomiasis, 1510
  sickle cell disease, 862
  toxocariasis, 1485
  typhoid fever, 1325
Splintering, skull, birth trauma, 707
Splints
  cerebral palsy, 757–758
  congenital dislocation of hip, 1551
  juvenile chronic arthritis, 1604
Split hand and foot defects, 1546 (Table)
Split sternum, 1556
Spondyloepiphyseal dysplasia congenita,
  1580
  inheritance, 1566 (Table)
Spondyloepiphyseal dysplasias, 370, 371,
  1579–1580
  vs Morquio–Brailsford syndrome,
    1161
  spine, 1915
Spondylolisthesis, 1557
  imaging, 1915
Spondylolysis, 1557
Spondylosis, imaging, 1915
Spongiform encephalopathies, subacute,
  1378
Spontaneous abortion,
  hyperphenylalaninemia, 1104
  (Table)
Spontaneous bacterial peritonitis, **483**
Spontaneous perforation, bile ducts, 472
  (Table), **475–476**
Sporotrichosis, 1470, 1471 (Table),
  1472–1473
Sporozoites, *Plasmodium* spp., 1445
Sports
  asthma, 545
  epilepsy, 691
  injuries, 1713–1714
  mental retardation, 838
Spotted fevers, 1390 (Table), 1392
SP proteins, lamellar bodies, 176
Sprengel's shoulder, **1548**, 1549 (Fig.)
Spring-loaded lancets, 1834
Sputum, **507**

bacteriology, 1298
cystic fibrosis, 554
hydatid disease, 1506
stimulation, 534
tuberculosis, 1342
viruses, 1352
Squamous blepharitis, 1662
Square window test, neonatal gestation
  age, 41 (Fig.)
Squint amblyopia, **1660–1661**
Squint baby syndrome, 30, 749
SRY gene, XX males, 62
Stable disease, neoplasms, 893
Stable malaria, 1447
Stadiometer, 999 (Fig.)
Staff
  child development centers, 399–400
  neonatal deaths, 172, 175
  support, neonatal care, 100
Staffing, neonatal care, 96, 156
Stage theories, psychological
  development, 1728
Staging
  Hodgkin's disease, 909–910
  lymphomas, 908–909
  nephroblastoma, 914
  neuroblastoma, 912
  retinopathy of prematurity, 266
  tuberculous meningitis, 1345
Stairs, falls from, 1715
Stammering, **806**, 1744
Standard bicarbonate, 419
Standard deviation, weight, 19
Standard deviation scores
  nutritional assessment, 1187
  obesity, 1190
Standard errors, hormone values, 1001
Standardized birth rate, 1
Standard Precautions, hospital infection
  prevention, 1281
Standards of living, and respiratory
  disorders, 489, 559
Standing height, 353–354
Stanford–Binet intelligence scale, 400,
  826–827
Stanozol, administration, 1977 (Table)
Staphylinidae (rove beetles), toxins, 1525
Staphylococcus aureus, **1328–1330**
  cystic fibrosis, 555, 557–558
  furunculosis, 1635
  infective endocarditis, 630
  pneumonia, 566, 568
    radiology, 567
  vs scarlet fever, 1331–1332
  toxic shock syndrome, 1329
    emergence, 1279 (Table)
Staphylococcus epidermidis, 276, 278,
  281, **1330**
  meningitis, **1292**
Staphylococcus spp., **1328–1330**
  erythromycin-resistant, 1635
  neonate
    meningitis, 247
    rash, 1284
    sepsis, 281
  pneumonia, measles, 1355
  scalded skin syndrome, 1288, 1328,
    1635–1636
Star charts, enuresis, 1743
Starches, 1183
  digestion, 436
  glucose-6-phosphatase deficiency, 1137
  sources, 1182 (Table)
Stargardt's macular degeneration, 1666
Startles, neonate, 238 (Fig.)
Starvation, 1072, 1082–1083, see also
  Fasting
  accelerated, 1083
  growth hormone secretion, 365
  on intestine, 445
  plasma amino acids, 1102–1103
  small intestine, 436
  stress tests, inborn errors of
    metabolism, 113

Statements of Educational Need, 1864
State of the world's children (UNICEF),
  1882
States of alertness, 235–236
Station, obstetric, 83
Statistics, vital, see Epidemiology
Status epilepticus, **676, 691–693**
  cerebral palsy, 685
  febrile convulsions, 683, 692
  mental retardation, 842
  nonconvulsive, infantile spasms, 687
Status migrainosus, 717
Steady states, abnormal electrolyte values,
  413
Steatocrit, 448
  cystic fibrosis, 553
Steatorrhea
  cystic fibrosis, 553
  liver disease, nutrition, 1209
Steinberg thumb sign, 1588
Stemetil, migraine, 717 (Table)
Stenocephaly, **1559–1560**
Stepfamilies, 1856
Stepping reflex, neonate, 240
Stereotactic surgery, cerebral palsy, 760
Stereotypes, 771
  mental retardation, 673
Sterile pyuria, 1299
Sterilizing tablets, poisoning, 1711
Sternal recession, respiratory distress
  syndrome, 177
Sternomastoid tumor, 29, **1784**
  birth trauma, 121
Sternum
  hemopoiesis, 848 (Fig.)
  malformations, 1556
Steroidogenesis, adrenal cortex,
  1059–1060
  disorders, 1061–1069
Steroid ratio, normal values, urine, 1932
  (Table)
Steroid sulfatase deficiency, 1164, 1165
Sterols, see Phytosterols
Stethoscope, neonatal resuscitation, 134
Stevens–Johnson syndrome, 424, 1641
  conjunctivitis, 1675
Stibogluconate, **1462–1463**, 1977 (Table)
Stickler syndromes, 75, 810, 1580
  inheritance, 1566 (Table)
Stiff baby syndrome, 732, 733
Stiffness, muscle, 756
Stiles, Sir Harold, pyloromyotomy, 1785
Stillbirth
  causes, rates, 4 (Table)
  definition, 94
  grief, 172
  preterm delivery, 170
  previous history, 18
  rates, definitions, 3, 94
  registration, 1849
Stillbirth and Infant Mortality Study, 1851
Stillbirth and Neonatal Death Society, 175
Still's disease, 1600
  IgA deficiency, 1258
Still's murmur, 203 (Table), 594
Stimulants (psychiatry), 1748 (Table)
Stimulation
  apnea prevention, 197
  brain development, 828
  neonatal intensive care, 99
Stinging insects, 1691
'Stingose', 1524
STING procedure, 956–957, 1794
Stings and bites, **1520–1526**
Stippled epiphyses, see Chondrodysplasia
  punctata
St Jude modified lymphoma staging
  system, 908 (Table)
Stokes–Adams attacks, 626
Stomach, **430–435**, see also entries
  starting Gastric
Stomatitis, ulcerative, 1363, 1364–1365,
  1438
Stomatocytosis, hereditary, 858

Stools, *see* Defecation; Feces
Storage disorders, metabolic, 307–308, *see also* Lysosomal storage disorders; *substance names*
Storage mites, 1691
Stoss therapy, 1055
Strabismus, **1658–1661**
  cerebral palsy, 761
  convergent, 265
  examination, 395, 1652
  hypothyroidism, 1674
  isolated sixth nerve weakness, 725
  neonate, 265
  preterm infant, 267
  severely handicapped children affected, 14 (Table)
Straight leg raising, 38
Strangulated hernia, 33, 1815
Strangulation (asphyxia), 1718–1719, 1871
Strawberry tongue, 425, 1285, 1331, 1479
Street children, **1887–1888**
  gonorrhea, 1421
Streptococcal derivative 'OK432,' cystic hygroma, 1784
Streptococcus agalactiae, 1332
Streptococcus faecalis, 1333
Streptococcus pneumoniae, **1318–1320**
  antibiotic prophylaxis, 1529
  febrile convulsions, 683
  meningitis, 1289 (Table), 1290, **1292,** 1319
    deafness, 816
    neonatal, 247 (Table)
  pneumonia, 566, 568
  vaccination, 341, 1974 (Table)
    in nephrotic syndrome, 970
Streptococcus pyogenes, see β-hemolytic streptococci
Streptococcus spp., **1330–1333,** *see also* Poststreptococcal glomerulonephritis
Streptococcus viridans, see α-hemolytic streptococci
Streptokinase, 228, 231, 1977 (Table)
Streptolysins, 1330
Streptomycin
  administration, 1977 (Table)
  plague, 1318
  pregnancy, contraindication, 1346
  tuberculosis, 1347, 1348
    contraindication in HIV infection, 1347
    meningitis, 1345
Stress
  accident rates, 1712
  adolescent psychiatric disorder, 1751
  congenital adrenal hyperplasia treatment, 1064
  disorders, **1741–1742**
  fetal response, 124
  on hormone levels, 1000
  and porphyrias, 1143
  psychiatric disorder, 1728
  thermal, 146–147
Stress ulcers, 432
  neonate, 210
Stretch relaxation, 756
Strictures
  epidermolysis bullosa, 1622
  peptic, esophagus, 428
Stridor, **508, 509 (Table),** 513, 563
  cow's milk protein intolerance, 1699
  diphtheria, 1306
  imaging, 1899, 1900
  laryngomalacia, 572
  neonate, 193
  neurogenic, 659
  ultrasonography, 517
Strobe lights, epilepsy, 691
Strokes, **711–715,** *see also* Hemiplegia
  migraine, 717
  perinatal, 740
  tetralogy of Fallot, 617

Stroke volume, 1819
Strongyloides fülleborni, 1492, 1493
Strongyloides spp., larvae, *vs* rhabditiform larvae, 1490
Strongyloides stercoralis, **1492–1493**
  larval disease, 1484 (Table)
Structural genes, 69
Structural scoliosis, 1557–1558
Structures, intellectual, 1729
Sturge–Weber syndrome, 710, 799 (Table), **802–803,** 1620, 1662
  buphthalmos, 1672
Stuttering, **806,** 1744
St Vincent declaration, diabetes management, 1076
STYCAR graded balls test, 395
STYCAR letter test, 395
Stye (hordeolum), 1662, 1663 (Fig.)
Subacute combined degeneration of spinal cord, 1199
Subacute sclerosing panencephalitis, 794 (Table), **1355, 1378**
  dyskinesia, 769
  and measles vaccine, 343
  multiple tics, 772
Subacute spongiform encephalopathies, **1378**
Subaponeurotic hemorrhage, 121, 224
Subarachnoid hemorrhage, **710**
  birth trauma, 126
  neonate, 252
  perinatal, 122
Subcapsular hematoma, 224
Subclavian artery, aberrant, 200
Subclavian vein, central venous lines, 1224
Subconjunctival hemorrhage
  birth trauma, 121
  respiratory disorders, 510
Subcortical leukomalacia, birth asphyxia, 126
Subcostal recession, *see* Rib recession
Subcultural mental retardation, **827–829**
Subcutaneous emphysema, *see* Surgical emphysema
Subcutaneous fat necrosis
  birth trauma, 121
  neonate, 43, 1646
Subcutaneous immunoglobulin therapy, 1268
Subcutaneous layer, 1616
Subcutaneous nodules
  neuroblastoma, 911
  rheumatic heart disease, 1598
Subcutaneous route
  fluid therapy, 413
  insulin, 1077
    analogues, 1081
  opiates, 1831
Subdural effusions, meningitis, 1289, 1291
Subdural hemorrhage, **702–703**
  birth trauma, 126, 128, 699
  computed tomography, 703
  neonate, 251
  perinatal, 122
  retinopathy, 702
  stroke, 714
Subdural tap, **1841**
Subdural ultrasonography, 1908
Subependymal hemorrhage
  neonate, 249
  outcome, 171
Subependymal layer, 642
Subependymomas, 902
Suberylglycine, 1129
Subglottic hemangiomas, **572**
Subglottic stenosis, **196,** 572
Subischial leg length, 363–364
Subjective audiometry, **1683**
Sublimation, 1760
Sublingual glands, mumps, 1371
Submandibular glands
  enlargement, 1784

mumps, 1371
'Submerged tenth', 827
Submetacentric chromosomes, 53
Submucosal injection, vesicoureteric reflux, 956–957, 1794
Subperiosteal hemorrhage, 121
  scurvy, 1200
Subpial heterotopia, 685
Subregional centers, neonatal care, 156
Subscapular skinfold, 1187 (Table)
Substance abuse, **1762–1763,** *see also* Drug abuse
Substance P, 1832
  growth hormone secretion, 1013
Substrate competition, antibiotic resistance, 1529
Subtalar joint, fusion, 1555
Subtertian malaria, 1449
Subtle seizures, neonate, 244
Subtotal pancreatectomy, 1084
Subtotal thyroidectomy, 1052
Subtotal villous atrophy, 440, 441
Subureteric Teflon injection, 956–957, 1794
Subvalvar aortic stenosis, 607
Succinate dehydrogenase deficiency, with aconitase deficiency, 1126
Succinic acid dehydrogenase, brain development, 643
Succinylacetone, tyrosinemia, 1106
Succinyl-CoA:3-ketoacid-CoA transferase, 1130
Succinylpurinemic autism, 790 (Table)
Succus entericus, electrolytes, 411 (Table)
Sucking, 111, 112
  development, 107–108
  disorders, 209
  lactation, 327
  mechanism, 328
  nonnutritive, 154
  preterm infant, 150
Sucking reflex, 36 (Table), 238 (Fig.), 240–241
  gestation age, 40 (Table)
Sucrase, 437
Sucrase–isomaltase deficiency, **445–446,** 448
Sucrose, maximum intake, 334
Sucrose-based oral rehydration solutions, 1304
Suction
  endotracheal, neonate, 97, 104, 163
  neonatal resuscitation, 133
  pharynx, neonates, 104, 111
  snake bite, 1523
Sudden death, 927
  aortic stenosis, 607
  cancer survivors, 899
  Haemophilus influenzae, 1308
  hypertrophic cardiomyopathy, 634
  laryngeal stridor, 572
  medium chain acyl CoA dehydrogenase deficiency, 297, 1129
  mitral valve prolapse, 610
  notification, 1849
  overheating, 150
Sudden infant death syndrome, 491, **1719–1723**
  and apparent life-threatening events, 528, 530
  botulism, 1302
  and breast-feeding, 327, 1720
  mortality, 489, 490 (Table)
    neonatal, 4 (Table)
    postneonatal, 5 (Table)
    United Kingdom, 1276
  prevention, 340
  suffocation, 1871
Sudden unexpected death syndrome, epilepsy, 687
Suffocation, 700, 1718–1719, *see also* Airways, obstruction, imposed
Sugars, 1182–1183, *see also* Reducing substances

normal values, amniotic fluid, 1937 (Table)
Suicide, **1756–1757**
Sulfadiazine
  administration, 1977 (Table)
  rheumatic fever, 629
  toxoplasmosis, 288, 1466
Sulfadimidine
  administration, 1977 (Table)
  toxoplasmosis, 288
Sulfadoxine, *see* Fansidar
Sulfamethoxazole, *see also* Co-trimoxazole
  Pneumocystis carinii, cancer treatment, 895
Sulfasalazine
  administration, 1977 (Table)
  Crohn's disease, 457
  juvenile chronic arthritis, 1604
  ulcerative colitis, 459
Sulfatase deficiencies, **1164–1165**
Sulfate
  intracellular fluids, 404 (Table)
  normal values, 1928 (Table)
Sulfhemoglobinemia, 864
Sulfite oxidase deficiency, 773, 1109, *see also* Combined sulfite oxidase and xanthine oxidase deficiency
Sulfites, in food, 1701
Sulfonamides
  and glucose-6-phosphate dehydrogenase deficiency, 859 (Table), 1528
  immunosuppression, 1265
  mechanism, 1527
  nocardiosis, 1477
  toxoplasmosis, 1464
Sulfosalicylic acid, proteinuria diagnosis, 967
Sulfur-containing amino acids, metabolism disorders, 1108–1109
'Sulfur' granules, actinomycosis, 1473
Sulpiride, 1755
Sumatriptan, 716
  migraine, 717 (Table), **718**
Sunflower cataract, 1674
Sunlight
  idiopathic photosensitivity eruptions, 1645
  neoplasms, 890
  vitamin D, 1194
Sunscreen preparations
  albinism, 1108
  porphyrias, 1144, 1631
Sunsetting, 241, 659
Superantigens, 1236
Superficial temporal artery
  avoidance, 1837
  migraine, 716
Superior laryngeal nerve, 808
Superior mesenteric artery syndrome, **1787–1788**
Superior oblique tendon sheath syndrome, 1660
Superoxide dismutase defect, 721, 726
Supervision Orders, 1875
Supervision requirements (Scotland), 1877
Supinator jerk, 35
Supine length measurement, 353
Supplementary feeding, 328
Supplements, breast-feeding, 330–331, *see also specific nutrients*
Supporter (companion in labor), 84
Support groups, *see* Self-help groups
Supportive psychotherapy, 1749
Support therapy, birth asphyxia, 130
Suprabulbar palsy, 209
Supraophthalmic zoster, 1363
Suprapubic aspiration, 950, 1299, 1839
Suprapubic puncture, cystometrography, 656
Suprapylaria forms, *Leishmania* spp., 1460
Suprasellar arachnoid cysts, 651
Suprasternal thrills, 586

Supratentorial hemorrhage, birth trauma, 122
Supratentorial tumors, 900–901
  astrocytomas, **903**
  primitive neuroectodermal tumors, **906**
Supravalvar aortic stenosis, 607
Supravalvar pulmonary stenosis, 608
Supravalvar ring, left ventricular inflow obstruction, 609
Supraventricular ectopic beats, 624
  neonate, 203
Supraventricular tachycardia, **624–625,** 1815, 1819
  neonate, 203
  paroxysmal, **627**
  vs sinus tachycardia, 624
Sural nerve, 722
Suramin, **1456**
  onchocerciasis, 1497
Surface antigens, *see* Leukocyte differentiation antigens
Surface area, *see* Body surface area
Surfactant, 176
  activity measurements, 178
  administration
    intracranial hemorrhage prevention, 250
    meconium aspiration syndrome, 186
    Pneumocystis carinii pneumonia, 535
    pulmonary hemorrhage, 190, 191
    respiratory distress syndrome, 104, 162, 179, 188
  deficiency, 159, 177
  development, 496
  synthetic, 179
Surgery, **1768–1801**
  acute-onset stroke, 715
  for ambiguous genitalia, 1065
  antibiotic prophylaxis, 1528
  brain tumors, 901, *see also named tumors*
  cataract, 1669–1670
  cerebral palsy, 760
  choanal atresia, 193
  congenital adrenal hyperplasia, 986
  Crohn's disease, 458
  Cushing's syndrome, 375
  for epilepsy, 686–687
  Ewing's sarcoma, 919–920
  gastroesophageal reflux, 429
  hepatoblastoma, 925
  for intracranial hemorrhage, 711
  intrauterine, 115
  juvenile chronic arthritis, 1604–1605
  neonate, **1768–1782**
    abdominal, 210
    cardiac, 206
    neoplasms, 893
    nephroblastoma, 914
    neural tube defects, 655
    osteosarcoma, 918
    parenteral nutrition, 1220
    preterm infant, thermoregulation, 149
    primary hyperparathyroidism, 1056
    pyogenic osteitis, 1591
    sacrococcygeal tumors, 921, 922–923
    for short bowel syndrome, 1212–1213
    squint, 1660
    Sturge–Weber syndrome, 803
    tall stature, 1020
    ulcerative colitis, 459
Surgical emphysema, 43, 190
  neonate, 187
Surgical venous cut down, **1837**
Survanta (bovine surfactant), 179
Surveillance, *see also* Child health surveillance
  accident prevention, 1803
  infections, **1280–1281**
Surveillance case definitions, congenital syphilis, 1404–1405
Survival, neoplasms, 885, 887 (Table), 897–898
Survival motor neuron gene, 719

Sustanon, puberty induction, 1035
Sutural cataract, 1668
Sutures (cranial), 20
  diastasis, choroid plexus neoplasms, 905
  examination, 242
  leukemias, 870
Sutures (surgical)
  adjustable, squint, 1660
  skin biopsy, 1846
  wound closure, **1833**
Suxamethonium
  administration, 1977 (Table)
  and metrifonate, 1511
SV40 (simian virus 40), 1378
Sverdlovsk, anthrax outbreak, 1300
Swabs, bacteriology, 1297
Swallowing, 425–426
  development, 107
  diphtheria, 1306
  disorders, 570, 571
    neonate, 209
  history taking, 17
Swallowing reflex, 36 (Table)
  neonate, 240–241
Sweat
  electrolytes, causes of increase, 553
  tests, cystic fibrosis, 449–450, **552–553**
  water output, 403 (Table)
Sweat glands, 1616
  cystic fibrosis, 551
Sweating
  preterm infant, 140, 147
  respiratory disorders, 510
Sweaty feet odor, 1117
  MAD-S deficiency, 308
Sweden
  breast-feeding rates, 326 (Table)
  vs Denmark, celiac disease, 440
Sweep visually evoked potentials, 270
Sweets, vision test, 395
Swellings, history taking, 17
Swimmer's itch, 1508
Swimming
  asthma, 542
  epilepsy, 691
  grommet tubes, 1682
Swimming pool conjunctivitis, 1664
Swimming pool granuloma, 1349
Swimming pools, drowning, 1717, 1718
Swiss type severe combined immunodeficiency syndrome, 1242 (Table), 1250
Swollen belly syndrome, Papua New Guinea, 1492
Sydenham's chorea, 1597, **1598–1599**
  tics, 772
Sydney funnel web spider, 1525
Symbolic play test of Lowe and Costello, 400
Symmers' liver, 1509
Symmetric growth retardation, 1191
Sympathetic nervous system
  Horner's syndrome, 34
  neoplasms, incidence, 886 (Table)
Sympathetic stimulation, heart failure, 599
Sympathomimetic drugs
  for attention disorder, 819
  for preterm labor, 116
Symphalangism, 76, 1546 (Table), **1547**
Symphysis–fundal height, 81, 115
Synacthen screening test, 1938 (Table)
Synapsis, meiosis, 47
Synchronized ventilation, 164
  intermittent mandatory, 1818
Syncope, *see* Faints; Stokes–Adams attacks
Syndactyly, 76, 1546 (Table), **1547–1548**
  Apert's syndrome, 1560
Syndrome of inappropriate ADH secretion, 412, **1040–1041**
  neonate, 257
Syndromes, 75

Syndromic cystic disease, renal, 254–255
Synergy, drug combinations, 1528
Syngeneic bone marrow transplantation, 874
Synophyris, 76 (Table)
Synovectomy, juvenile chronic arthritis, 1604
Syntax, 804, **805,** 821
  dysgraphia, 824
Syphilis, **1401–1415,** *see also* Congenital syphilis; Endemic syphilis; Neurosyphilis
  acquired, clinical features, **1405–1408**
  vs anogenital warts, 1444
  detection or exclusion, 1399, 1400
  eye, **1677**
  laboratory methods, **1402–1404**
  nephrotic syndrome, 972, 1408
  retreatment, 1410
  teeth, 425
  treatment, **1408–1411**
  vertical transmission, 1400, **1411**
Systemic arterial pressure, fetal-neonatal transition, 107
Systemic carnitine deficiency, 736
Systemic lupus erythematosus, 964–965, **1605–1606,** *see also* Lupus nephritis
  complement deficiency, 1262, 1263
  complete heart block, 203
  fetal bradycardia, 86
  heart, 635
  IgA deficiency, 1258
  maternal, 89 (Table)
  neonatal thrombocytopenia from, 229
  pregnancy, 114
  retinopathy, 1674
  skin, 1605, 1644
Systemic mastocytosis, 1647
Systemic sclerosis, 1645, *see also* Progressive systemic sclerosis
Systolic velocity, Doppler ultrasonography, 1896
Sytron, *see* Sodium iron edetate

Tabes dorsalis, juvenile, 1413
Tache noir, 1392
Tachyarrhythmias, neonate, 203
Tachycardia, *see also* Ventricular tachycardia
  carditis, 1598
  fetus, 86, 117 (Table)
  heart failure, 585
  respiratory disorders, 511
  sinus, 624, 628
Tachyphylaxis
  and β2-adrenergic agonists, 546
  desmopressin, 880
  opioids, 928
Tachypnea, 511
  fluid replacement, acute renal failure, 975
  heart failure, 585
  inborn errors of metabolism, 305
  Joubert's syndrome, 646
Tacrolimus, 1265
Taenia asiatica, 1499
Taenia saginata, **1499–1500**
Taenia solium, 1499, **1500–1502**
Taiwan, hepatocellular carcinoma, 477
Takayasu's disease, **1610–1611**
Talampicillin, administration, 1977 (Table)
Talc, inhalation, 1709
Talipes, severely handicapped children affected, 14 (Table)
Talipes calcaneovalgus, **1555**
Talipes equinovarus (club foot), **1554–1555,** *see also* Equinus deformity
  recurrence risks, 74
Tall stature, **375–377, 1020**
  referral criteria, 375

Talus, congenital vertical, 1555
Tamm–Horsfall protein, 942, 967
Tamm–Horsfall proteinuria, ultrasonography, 1910
Tamponade, *see* Cardiac tamponade
Tangier disease (familial alphalipoprotein deficiency), 724, 790 (Table), 1150 (Table), 1153
Tanner–Whitehouse bone age, 362–363
Tanner–Whitehouse growth charts, **352–353,** 1014
T antigens, β-hemolytic streptococci, 1330
Tape measures, resuscitation, 526
Tapetoretinal degenerations, 271, **1666–1667**
Tapeworms, **1499–1506**
Tardive dyskinesia, 768, **772,** 813
Target heights, 353
Tars, psoriasis, 1628
Tartrazine, 1701
Tarur's disease, 735
Taurine, 1108
  deficiency, parenteral nutrition, 1226
  preterm requirements, 157
  urine, 1103
Taussig–Bing malformation, 622
Taybi and Lachman, *Radiology of syndromes, metabolic disorders and skeletal dysplasias,* 1099
Tay–Sachs disease, 775 (Table), 1157 (Table), **1163,** 1164, 1666
  frequency, 47 (Table)
  vs Sandhoff disease, 1163
T cell lymphomas, gene rearrangements, 906
T cell receptor, 1237–1238
  antigen presentation, 1235–1236
  signal transduction, 1239–1240
T cells, *see* T lymphocytes
T-cryptantigen, 978
Tea, 334
Teats, preterm infant, 154
Technetium-99m, 1897
  bone scan
    neuroblastoma, 911
    osteosarcoma, 917
  diphosphonate compounds, 1915
  DMSA, DTPA, urinary tract, 1911
  HIDA cholescintigraphy, 221
  HMPAO scanning, abdominal inflammation, 1906
  MAG3, urinary tract, 1911–1912
Technology, infectious disease emergence, 1279 (Table)
Teeth, 425
  congenital syphilis, 1414
  eruption times, **27–29**
  hypophosphatasia, 1176
  incontinentia pigmenti, 1626
Teflon injection, subureteric, 956–957, 1794
Teicoplanin
  administration, 1956 (Table), 1977 (Table)
  neonatal staphylococcal infection, 281
  prophylaxis, infective endocarditis, 632 (Table)
Telangiectasia
  ataxia telangiectasia, 766, 1253
  capillary hemangioma, 710
  congenital familial, tongue, 425
  hereditary hemorrhagic, 875
Telangiectatic osteosarcoma, 918
Telecanthus (hypertelorism), 22, 24 (Fig.), 76 (Table), 647, 1562, 1661
Telencephalon, development, **642–644**
Telephone numbers, Poisons Information Centers, **1707**
Television
  photosensitive epilepsy, 691
  set ownership, world figures, 1883 (Table) ·

Telogen effluvium, 1406
Telomeres, 53
Telophase, 47
Temazepam, administration, 1977 (Table)
Temperament, 1732
Temperature, **20, 1282**
  measurement
    preterm infant, **147**
    rectal, 111
    for procedures, 1829
    and sudden infant death syndrome, 1722
    unit conversion factors, 1938 (Table)
Temperature regulation, *see also*
      Hypothermia
  disorders
    with apnea, 197 (Table)
    ectodermal dysplasias, 1624
    neonates, mortality, 4 (Table), 149–150
  neonate, 112, 139
  preterm infant, **145–150**
  skin, 1616
Temper tantrums, 1736
Temple prostitutes, India, 1887
Temporal lobe, *see also* Mesial temporal
    sclerosis
  arachnoid cysts, 651
  basilar migraine, 717
  epilepsy, 819
  mesial structures, epilepsy and learning, 690
Temporal lobectomy, anterior, 686
Temporal vein, central venous lines, 1224
Tenckhoff catheter, 259
Tenderness, abdomen, 32–33
Tendo Achillis
  Duchenne muscular dystrophy, 730
  Emery–Dreifuss muscular dystrophy, 732
  surgery, 749, 760
Tendon reflexes
  neonatal, 38 (Table)
  tone measurement, 756
Tendon transplant, birth trauma, 123
Teniasis, **1499–1506**
Tenotomy, 760
Tension headache, 715–716
Tension pneumothorax, 187, 188, **1811, 1844**
Tentorial herniation, 698
  pseudobulbar palsy, 812
Teratogenesis, **90–91**, 114
  congenital heart disease, 596
  diabetes mellitus, 114
  DiGeorge syndrome, 300
  drugs causing, 338
  eye, 1678
Teratologic dislocation of hip, 1549–1550, 1551
Teratomas, 920
  ectopic gonatropin secretion, 1029
  intracranial, 922
    ultrasonography, 1908
    management, 922–923
    neonate, 291 (Table)
      incidence, 290 (Table)
    ovaries, 993
    pineal, 904, 922
Terbutaline
  acute severe asthma, 548
  administration, 1977 (Table)
Terfenadine, administration, 1977 (Table)
Terminal bronchioles, diameter *vs* age, 496 (Table)
Terminal care, **927–929, 1747–1748**
  analgesia, **1833**
Terminal deoxynucleotidyl transferase, 1238
  lymphomas, 907
  small round cell tumors, 912 (Table)
Terminal ileum, 445
Terminal trace, cardiotocography, 125
Terminal transverse defects, hand, 1546 (Table)

Termination mutations, 69
Termination of pregnancy, 94, 338, 1855
  adolescence, 994
  central nervous system malformations, 645
  mental retardation prevention, 841
  notification, 1849
  rubella, 1358
Ternidens deminutus, 1494
  eggs, 1490
Tertian malaria, 1446, 1449
Tertiary prevention, 338
Testes, *see also* Orchitis; Torsion, testes
  anomalies of descent, **1790–1791**, *see also* Cryptorchidism
  complete androgen insensitivity syndrome, 991
  delayed puberty, 1033
  embryology, 1003–1004
  examination, 34
  fragile X mental retardation, 63
  function, cancer survivors, 899
  Henoch–Schönlein purpura, 1610
  hypothyroidism, 1028
  incarceration of inguinal hernia, 1790
  leukemias, 871, 873
  lymphomas, 908
  neonatal gestation age, 40 (Table)
  puberty, 357, 1024
  radiotherapy, 899
  rhabdomyosarcoma adjacent, 916
  seminomas, 920
  tumors, 922, 1791
    gonadal dysgenesis, 1011
    precocious pseudopuberty, 1027
  volume measurement, 358, 360
Test feed, infantile hypertrophic pyloric stenosis, 1784–1785
Testicular feminization, 1010
  vs inguinal hernia, 1789
Test of auditory comprehension of language (TACC), 400
Testosterone, 1003–1004, 1024
  congenital adrenal hyperplasia, 986
  deficient fetal biosynthesis, 1008
  depot, phallus growth prediction, 1010
  genital development, 986
  for hyperammonemia, 1111
  normal values, 1928 (Table)
    urine, 1932 (Table)
  for organic acidurias, 1119
  ovaries, 1023
  puberty induction, 1035
  5-reductase deficiency, 1009
Testotoxicosis, 1030
Test-weighing, breast-feeding, 331
Tetanospasmin, 1333
Tetanus, **1333–1334**, *see also* Stiff baby syndrome
  antibiotic prophylaxis, 1529
  neonate, **285, 1333, 1334**
  prophylaxis, 1833
  snake bite, 1522
  risus sardonicus, 25 (Fig.)
Tetany, 1057
  gastroenteritis, 1294, 1297
  neonate (late neonatal hypocalcemia), **299–300, 1200**
Tetany cataract, 1669
Tethering, spinal cord, 652
*tet*M gene, tetracycline resistance, *Neisseria gonorrhoeae*, 1422
Tetmosol soap, scabies, 1517
Tetrabromophenol blue, proteinuria diagnosis, 967
Tetrachlorethylene, 1483
  administration, 1978 (Table)
  intestinal flukes, 1513
  Necator americanus, 1490
Tetracosactrin, administration, 1978 (Table)
Tetracycline
  administration, 1978 (Table)
  cholera, 1304

  on fetus and neonate, 91 (Table)
  Lyme disease, 1314 (Table)
  malaria, 1452
  mechanism, 1527
  plasmid-mediated resistance, *Neisseria gonorrhoeae*, 1422, 1427
  syphilis, 1409 (Table), 1410 (Table)
  teeth, 425
  typhus, 1391
  yaws control, 1420
Tetracycline ointment, ophthalmia neonatorum prophylaxis, 263, 1429
Tetracyclines, leptospirosis, 1312
Tetrahydrobiopterin, 1106
  pterin synthetic defects, 1105
Tetralogy of Fallot, **616–618**
Tetraploidy, 51
T_{H1} and T_{H2} responses, 1238
Thailand, thalassemia, 47
Thalamus
  hemorrhage, neonate, 251
  lesions, and epilepsy, 684
Thalassemia intermedia, 862, 863
Thalassemias, 72 (Table), 860, 862, 863
  frequency, 47 (Table)
  maternal, 89 (Table)
  mutations, 69
  neonate, 226
  screening, antenatal care, 80
Thalidomide syndrome, 91 (Table), 1545, *see also* Phocomelia
  eye, 1678
THAM-E perfusion, for cystine stones, 1121
THAM (tris-hydroxyaminomethane), 715
Thanatophoric dysplasia, **1570**
  inheritance, 1566 (Table)
Theca cells, ovary, 1004
Theca cell tumors, ovary, 921, 989
Thecoperitoneal shunts, 662
Thelarche, isolated premature, 1027
Thelarche variant, 1027
T helper cells, 1238
  tuberculosis, 1335–1336
Theophylline, 195
  acute severe asthma, 547
  administration, 1978 (Table)
    neonate, 1958 (Table)
  for apnea attacks, 197–198
  asthma, 546–547
  respiratory distress syndrome, ventilator weaning, 181
  therapeutic ranges, 1936 (Table)
Therapeutic index, 1528
Therapeutic ranges, 1936 (Table)
  monitoring, **1954**
Therapeutic renutrition, 1892
Thermal stress, 146–147
Thermogenesis, energy expenditure, 1181
Thermometers, 1282
Thermoregulation, *see* Hypothermia; Temperature regulation
Thiabendazole, 1485
  administration, 1978 (Table)
  capillariasis, 1495
  cutaneous larva migrans, 1491
  dracunculosis, 1496
  and enterobiasis, 1488
  toxocariasis, 1486
  trichinosis, 1494
Thiacetazone, tuberculosis, 1347, 1348
Thiamin, 1184 (Table)
  administration, 1978 (Table)
  deficiency, 1198
    assessment, 1188
    eye, 1677
    neuropathy, 724
  for hereditary lactic acidosis, 1125
  for maple syrup urine disease, 1117
  for organic acidurias, 1119
  parenteral nutrition, 1221 (Table)
  for pyruvate dehydrogenase deficiency, 1126

Recommended Dietary Allowances, 1949 (Table)
  reference nutrient intakes, 1946 (Table)
  therapy, 1198
Thiamin-dependent maple syrup urine disease, 1116
Thiamin-responsive conditions, 1148
Thiazides
  for hyperinsulinism, 295
  neonate
    hypoglycemia, 296
    platelets, 229
  nephrogenic diabetes insipidus, 948
Thin layer chromatography, urine, 306
Thinness, 1023, **1021–1022**
Thin section computed tomography, 1897
Thiobendazole, strongyloidiasis, 1493
Thiopentone
  administration, 1978 (Table)
  on phenytoin treatment, 697
  status epilepticus, 693
  and stroke management, 715
Thiopentone coma, neonatal seizures, 246
Thioridazine, administration, 1978 (Table)
Thiouracil, transplacental, 1006
Third heart sound, 32
Third nerve, *see* Oculomotor nerve
Third ventricle, cysts, 658
Third ventriculostomy, 664
Third World, *see* Developing countries
Thirst, 410, 411
  history taking, 17
  neonate, 143, 213, 214
Thomsen–Friedenreich antigen, 978
Thomsen's disease, *see* Myotonia congenita
Thoracic aorta, traumatic dissection, **1811**
Thoracic dystrophy, hypophosphatasia, 1176
Thoracic spine, diagnostic radiation doses, 1895 (Table)
Thoracoscopy, 569
Thoracotomy, osteosarcoma metastases, 918
Thorax, *see* Chest
Thorny-headed worms (Acanthocephala), **1513**
1000 Family Study 1947, 1851
Threadworms, **1486–1488**, *see also* Pinworms
Threatened abortion, 80, 88
Three day fever, *see* Roseola infantum
Threonine-induced acidosis, 1118
Threshold retinopathy of prematurity, 267
Thrills, precordial examination, 586
Thrive index, 1191
Throat swabs
  bacteriology, 1298
  virology, 1351
Thrombasthenia, 229, 878
Thrombin time, 228
Thrombocytopenia
  African trypanosomiasis, 1455
  alloimmune, intravascular fetal blood transfusion, 114
  amegakaryocytic, 855
  cancer treatment, 895
  congenital syphilis, 1412
  hemorrhagic chickenpox, 1361
  HIV infection, 1393, **1397**
  inborn errors of metabolism, 306
  indomethacin contraindicated, 204
  Kasabach–Merritt syndrome, 1619
  leishmaniasis, 1462
  neonate, **228–229**, 878–879
  Plasmodium falciparum, 1448
  polycythemia, 227
  rhesus incompatibility, 232
  Schwachman's syndrome, 450
  SGA baby, 137
  Wiskott–Aldrich syndrome, 1254
Thrombocytopenia with absent radii, 879
Thrombocytopenic purpuras, **876–879**

Thrombocytosis
    Crohn's disease, 457
    Kawasaki disease, 1480
    liver tumors, 924
Thromboembolic disease
    cystathione synthase deficiency, 1108,
        1109
    stroke, 713
Thromboembolism, parenteral nutrition,
    1226
Thrombolytic agents, neonates, 231
Thrombophlebitis, parenteral nutrition,
    1223
Thrombopoiesis, 222
Thrombosis, **882**
    intracranial, **713,** 715
    major vessels, 231
    nephrotic syndrome, 969
    parenteral nutrition, 159
    venous, gastroenteritis, 1294
Thrombotest, 228
Thrush, see Candidiasis
Thumb movements, neonate, 236
Thumb sucking, 1745
Thunderstorms, allergic symptoms, 1691
Thymectomy, myasthenia gravis, 728
Thymidine kinases, on acyclovir, 1440
Thymoma, aplastic anemia, 856
Thymus, **1044**
    ataxia telangiectasia, 766
    immunodeficiency, 1245
    replacement therapy, 1268
Thyrocerebrorenal syndrome, 753
Thyroglobulin, 1044
    hereditary deficiency, 1046
Thyroglossal cysts, 1044, 1049, **1783**
Thyroid antibodies, myasthenia gravis,
    727
Thyroid-binding globulin, congenital
    deficiency, 1175
Thyroidectomy, subtotal, 1052
Thyroid function tests, **1045–1046**
Thyroid gland, **1044–1053**
    cancer survivors, 898–899
    disorders, severely handicapped
        children affected, 14 (Table)
    dysgenesis, 1046, 1049–1050
    fetus, 1003
    lingual, 425
    neoplasms, **1052–1053**
        from irradiation, 890
    neural crest cells, 642
    precocious pseudopuberty, 1028
    second primary tumors, 898 (Table)
Thyroid hormones
    biosynthesis, 1045 (Fig.)
        at birth, 109
    brain development, 643
    on lung maturation, 176
    neonate, 248
    unresponsiveness, 1050
Thyroid stimulating hormone, see
    Thyrotropin
Thyroid stimulating hormone receptor,
    1051
Thyroid stimulating immunoglobulins,
    1051
Thyrotoxicosis, see Hyperthyroidism
Thyrotropin-releasing hormone
    molecule, 1037 (Table)
    prenatal, 114, 179
    prolactin secretion, 1039
    sex hormone secretion, 1050
    tests, 1045
Thyrotropin (TSH), **1039**
    deficiency, 1041–1042
    hypersecretion, 1052
    hypothyroidism, 1049
        screening, 1007, 1046
    normal values, 1928 (Table)
    serum levels, 1045
Thyroxine, 1044
    administration, 1978 (Table)
    fetus, 1003

on growth hormone expression, 367
    hypothyroidism screening, 1007, 1046
    normal values, 1928–1929 (Table)
    therapy, adrenal insufficiency, 1040
l-Thyroxine, see also Sodium-l-thyroxine
    with antithyroid drugs, 1051
Tibia
    bone marrow sampling, 1844
    bowing, congenital, **1549**
    hemopoiesis, 848 (Fig.)
    osteosarcoma distribution, 917
    spiral fractures, 1914
    torsion, **1554**
Tibial tubercle, osteochondrosis, **1595**
Tibia vara, infantile, **1554**
Ticarcillin, administration, 1978 (Table)
Tic disorders, **1745**
Tick-borne arbovirus infections, **1390**
Tick-borne spotted fevers, **1392**
Ticks
    bites, paralysis, **1525**
    Lyme disease, 1312
    relapsing fever, 1322
Tics, 673, 768–769, **771–772**
    drugs causing, 768
Tidal volume, ventilation, 1817
Time constant, respiratory, 502
Time cycled pressure limited ventilation,
    1817
Tinea, **1636–1637**
Tinea versicolor, **1637–1638**
Tinidazole
    administration, 1978 (Table)
    amebiasis, 1469
    giardiasis, 1467
Tioconazole, administration, 1978 (Table)
Tissue factor, monocytes, 231
Tissue factor III, 227
Tissue nonspecific alkaline phosphatase,
    1176
Tissue pH monitoring, fetal, 119
Tissue toxicity, cytotoxic drugs, 894
    (Table), 895
Titratable acidity, normal values, urine,
    1933 (Table)
T lymphocytes, 439, 1044, **1237–1239,**
    see also T cell receptor
    activation, 1239–1240
    bone marrow grafts, removal, 1270
    CD subsets, 1231–1232
    combined immunodeficiencies,
        1248–1249
    deficiency, candidiasis, 1470
    development, 1240–1241
    functions, 1240
    hyperIgE syndrome, 1261
    malaria immunity, 1447
    neonate, 274–275
    tests, 1245–1247
    tuberculosis, 1335–1336
Tobramycin
    administration, 1978 (Table)
    neonate, 279 (Table)
    Pseudomonas aeruginosa, cystic
        fibrosis, 558 (Table)
    therapeutic ranges, 1936 (Table)
Tocography, home uterine monitoring, 116
Tocopherol succinate, preterm infant, 225
Tocopheryl acetate, administration, 1978
    (Table)
Toddler diarrhea, **463–464**
Toddlers
    normal diet, 1189
    nutrition, diabetes mellitus, 1210
Todd's paresis, 741
Toes, webbing, 110
Toe walking, 668, 760
Togaviruses, see Arboviruses
Toilet training, neural tube defect, 656,
    657
Tolazoline
    administration, neonate, 1958 (Table)
    cyanotic heart disease, dosage, 202
        (Table)

diaphragmatic hernia, 1770
    persistent pulmonary hypertension of
        the newborn, 204
    pulmonary vasodilation, 165
    ventilation for RDS, 181
Tolbutamide, neonatal thrombocytopenia,
    229
Tolmetin
    administration, 1978 (Table)
    juvenile chronic arthritis, 1603
Toluidine blue test, 837
Tomography, chest, 514
Tone
    examination, 35
    history taking, 17
    measurement, 755–756
    neonate, 236–239
        gestation age, 40 (Table)
    rigidities, 769–770
Tongue, 425
    movement, 34
    nerve supply, 811
    scarlet fever, 425, 1285
    and speech disorder, 810
Tongue thrusting, neonate, 236
Tongue tie, 1784
Tonic hemisyndrome, 44
Tonic neck reflexes, 240
Tonic seizures, see Paroxysmal extensor
    hypertonus
Tonic spasticity, 747
Tonsillectomy, **1687**
    poliomyelitis, 1379, 1380
Tonsillitis, **1686–1687**
    β-hemolytic streptococci, 1330, 1331
    stroke after, 711
Tonsils, **1686–1687**
    examination, 29
    familial alphalipoprotein deficiency,
        1153
    infectious mononucleosis, 1366
    noisy breathing, 508–509
    obstructive sleep apnea, 531
Topical anesthesia, bronchoscopy, 519
Topical steroids, Cushing's syndrome
    from, 1065
TORCH, 817
    neonate, 248
Torkildsen shunt, 664
Torsion
    appendix of Morgagni, 1914
    ovarian cysts, 1796
    testes, **1791**
        vs epididymitis, ultrasonography,
            1914
Torsion dystonia, idiopathic, 773–774, 793
    (Table)
Torticollis, 25 (Fig.), 38, 1784
    incomitant squint, 1661
Torulopsis glabrata, vaginitis, 1433
Torulosis (cryptococcosis), 1471 (Table),
    1475–1476
Total anomalous pulmonary venous
    connection, **622–623**
Total anomalous pulmonary venous
    drainage, 203 (Table)
    ductus venosus closure, 199
Total body irradiation
    gonadal function, 899
    on growth, 373, 898
    late sequelae, 874
Total body water, **402–403**
    vs bodyweight, 1953
Total cataract, 1668
Total cavopulmonary connection, 621
Total CO$_2$ content, 419
Total energy expenditure, 1181
Total hemolytic complement test, 1245
Total hormone levels, thyroid function
    tests, 1045–1046
Total iron binding capacity, 1188
Total lung capacity, 501
Total mass treatment, yaws, 1420
Total mobility packages, 758

Total plasma alkaline phosphatase,
    neonate, 302–303
Total respiratory system resistance, 500
Tourette syndrome, 768, **771,** 824, 836,
    1745
Tourists, see also Travel, international
    sleeping sickness, 1455
Tourniquets, and snake bites, 1523
Toxascaris leonina, 1486
Toxic encephalopathy, 694–695
Toxic epidermal necrolysis, vs
    staphylococcal scalded skin
    syndrome, 1636
Toxic megacolon, 458, 464
Toxic neuropathies, 724
Toxic paralysis, 726–727
Toxic porphyria, 1144
Toxic shock syndrome, **1288**
    burns, 1800
    Staphylococcus aureus, 1329
    emergence, 1279 (Table)
Toxigenic Corynebacterium diphtheriae,
    1305
Toxins, see also named types e.g.
    Endotoxins, Cytotoxins
    neuromuscular junctions, 726–727
Toxocara canis, **1485–1486**
Toxocara cati, 1486
Toxoplasma gondii, 1464
Toxocara spp.
    eye involvement, 1676
    larval disease, 1484 (Table)
Toxoids, 341
Toxoplasmosis, **1464–1466**
    congenital infection, 248, 287 (Table),
        288–289, **1464–1465**
    eye, 289, 1676
    fits, 682
    FUO investigations, 1283 (Table)
    hearing loss, 816, 817
    HIV infection, 1397, 1465
    immunosuppression, 1264
    nephrotic syndrome, 972
    stroke, 713
Toy discrimination, audiometry, 817
Toys, vision test, 396
TPHA (Treponema pallidum
    Hemagglutination Assay),
    1403–1404
    index, cerebrospinal fluid, 1405
Trabeculectomy, buphthalmos, 1673
Trace alternant pattern,
    electroencephalography, preterm
    infant, 243
Trace elements, see also Minerals
    estimated safe and adequate daily
        intakes, 1949 (Table)
Trachea, see also Endotracheal intubation
    aspiration
        cytology, bronchopulmonary
            dysplasia, 194
        meconium aspiration syndrome, 186
        pneumonia diagnosis, 184
    cysts, 574
    diameter vs age, 496 (Table)
    lavage, 163
    neonate, 496
    pulmonary artery sling, 612
    stenosis, 573–574
Tracheitis, bacterial, 563 (Table), 564
Tracheoesophageal fistula, 209, **573,**
    1771–1773
    contrast studies, 1900
    drainage, 210
    laryngeal clefts, 572
    radiology, 514–517
Tracheomalacia, 574, 575, **1769**
    tracheoesophageal fistula, 573
Tracheostomy, **1843**
    aphonia, 809
    bacteriology, 1298
    bulbar poliomyelitis, 1380
    Pierre Robin syndrome, 1769
    for subglottic stenosis, 196

Trachoma, **1385**, 1430, 1664
Tracking
  lipid levels, 1150
  neonate, 241
  obesity, 1190
Training
  accident and emergency departments, 1805
  neonatal care, 157
Tramadol, administration, 1978 (Table)
Tramline appearance, Sturge–Weber syndrome, 802
Tranexamic acid
  administration, 1978 (Table)
  dysfunctional uterine bleeding, 992
  hemophilia A, 881
Tranquilizers, see also Anxiolytics
  improper administration, 1871
Transaminases, liver, inborn errors of metabolism, 306
Transbronchial biopsy, 520
Transcellular fluids, 403
Transcobalamin deficiencies, 1147
Transcobalamin II deficiency, 853, 854, 1242 (Table), 1257
  neutrophil killing defect, 1260
Transcortical aphasias, 815
Transcortin, 1059
Transcription factors
  growth hormone, 367
  immune system, 1240
Transcutaneous oxygen monitoring, 160, **161**, 195, 505, 521
  nitrogen washout test, 200
Transdermal patches
  fentanyl, 928
  thrombophlebitis prevention, 1223
Transepidermal water loss, 146
  preterm infant, 140
Transesophageal echocardiography
  atrial septal defect, 602
  infective endocarditis, 631
Transfatty acids, requirements, 1182
Transfer, within hospital, 1806, 1811, 1816, **1817**
Transferrin, 1146
  carbohydrate-deficient glycoprotein syndrome, 1175
Transforming growth factors, 351
  α, fetus, 1005
  β, 1233 (Table)
Transfusion-associated non-A, non-B hepatitis, see Hepatitis C virus
Transient blindness, **1658**
Transient combative behavior, 1520
Transient diabetes mellitus, neonate, 1081
Transient food intolerance, **441–442**
Transient hyperinsulinemia, 295–296
Transient hyperphosphatasemia, 1177
Transient hypogammaglobulinemia of infancy, 1259
Transient hypothyroidism, preterm infant, 1046
Transient ischemic attacks, **672**
Transient neonatal diabetes mellitus, 298
Transient neonatal hyperammonemia, 1110
Transient neonatal hyperinsulinism, idiopathic, 296
Transient neonatal hypoglycemia, 294–295
Transient neonatal pustular dermatosis, 1646
Transient tachypnea of the newborn, 106, **182–183**
  pneumothorax, 187
Transient vascular systems, eye development, 262–263
Transillumination
  pneumothorax, 188
  scrotum, 34
Transit eggs
  Capillaria hepatica, 1495
  Fasciola spp, 1513

Transitional milk (colostrum), 112, 332
Transition period, respiratory, birth, 42, **106–109**, 110
Transit times, mean, cerebral blood flow, 661
Transjugular intrahepatic portosystemic shunts, 1899
Transketolase, red cells, 1188
Translocations, 52 (Fig.), **53**
  Burkitt's lymphoma, 906
  cytogenetic nomenclature, 54
  Down syndrome, 53, **55–56**
  Ewing's sarcoma, 919
  leukemias, 869, 872
  trisomy 13, 58
Transmission, enterobiasis, 1486
Transmission-based precautions, hospital infection prevention, 1281
Transplacental carcinogenesis, 289
Transplacental drugs, 772, 1005
Transplacental immunoglobulins, 343
Transplacental infection, 276
  neonatal jaundice, 218
  pneumonia, 183, 280
Transplacental metastases, 289
Transplacental thyroid hormone analogues, 176
Transplacental virilization, 1008
Transplantation, for short bowel syndrome, 1213
Transport, 1816, **1817**, see also Transfer, within hospital
  after cardiac surgery, 1822
  gastrointestinal tract, 424
  neonate, **156–157**
  prehospital care, 1805
  preterm infant, 149
Transport disorders, metabolites, **1120–1123**
Transport media, Neisseria gonorrhoeae, 1423
Transport proteins, inborn errors, 1175
Transport resistance, cytotoxic drugs, 892–893
Transposition of great arteries
  complete, **613–616**
  congenitally corrected, **616**
Transposition of great vessels, 203 (Table)
Transpyloric feeding, preterm infant, 153
Transtracheal aspiration, 507, 1298
Trapezius, 34
Trapped fourth ventricle, 659
Trauma
  auricle, 1680
  cataract, 1669
  developing countries disease burden, 1276 (Table)
  diabetes insipidus, 1040 (Table)
  encephalopathy, 695, 700
  incomitant squint, 1660
  keratitis, 1664
  major, **1809–1813**
  migraine, 716
  pancreatitis, 450
  peripheral nerves, 721–722
  stroke, 711, **714**
Trauma rehabilitation centers, Uganda, 1887
Traumatic dissection of thoracic aorta, **1811**
Traumatic herpetic infection, 1364
Traumatic pneumothorax, neonate, 187
Traumatic tap, lumbar puncture, 1840
  vs subarachnoid hemorrhage, 710
Travel, international
  epilepsy, 691
  infectious disease emergence, 1279 (Table)
  malaria prophylaxis, 1448–1449
  vaccination, 345, 346 (Table)
Treacher–Collins syndrome, see Mandibulofacial dysostosis
Tree pollens, 1690
Trematodes, **1506–1513**

Tremors, 770–771
  drawing, 396
  neonate, 238 (Fig.)
Trendelenburg position, tracheoesophageal fistula, 1771
Trendelenburg test, 1550 (Fig.)
Treponema carateum, 1415, 1417
Treponema pallidum, see also TPHA
  subspecies, **1400–1401**
Treponematoses, **1400–1420**
  endemic, 1398, **1415–1420**
    control, **1419–1420**
Triad syndrome (prune belly syndrome), 75, 255, **1778**
Triage, 1805
  developing countries, primary health care, 1889
Trial of feeding, failure to thrive, 466–467, 469
'Trial of life', 102
Trials, randomized controlled, 104
Triamcinolone
  juvenile chronic arthritis, local injections, 1605
  skin, 1978 (Table)
Triamterene, administration, 1978 (Table)
Triatoma infestans, 1458
Triatomine bugs, 1458
  control, 1460
Triazoles, mechanism, 1530
Tribavain, administration, 1979 (Table)
Triceps jerk, 35
Triceps skinfold, 1187 (Table)
Trichinosis, **1494–1495**
Trichlorophone, Mansonella spp., 1499
Trichomonas vaginalis, detection or exclusion, 1399, 1400
Trichomoniasis, **1434–1435**
Trichorrhexis nodosa, 1111
Trichostrongylus spp., eggs, 1490
Trichotillomania, vs tinea, 1637
Trichuris trichiuira, **1491–1492**
Trichuris vulpis, 1491
Triclofos, 1897, 1979 (Table)
Tricuspid atresia, 203 (Table), 620
  echocardiography, 591 (Fig.)
Tricuspid regurgitation, neonate
  asphyxia, 205
  murmur, 203
Tricuspid valve, Ebstein's anomaly, 618
TRIC virus, see Chlamydia trachomatis
Tricyclic antidepressants, 1748 (Table), 1755
  enuresis, 1743
  poisoning, 1710
Trident hand deformity, achondroplasia, 1573
Triethylene tetramine, Wilson's disease, 1146
Trifluoperazine, administration, 1979 (Table)
Trigeminal nerve, examination, 34
Trigger finger, congenital, **1549**
Triggers, see also Allergens
  asthma, **541–542**
Triglycerides, 1149, see also Medium chain triglycerides
  digestion, stomach, 430
  normal values, 1926 (Table)
  parenteral nutrition, 1220
  plasma levels, 1149
    marasmus, 1192
  secondary disorders, 1154 (Table)
Trigonocephaly, 1560, 1661
Triiodothyronine, 1045
  fetus, 1003
  normal values, 1929 (Table)
  therapy, 1047–1048
Trimeprazine, administration, 1979 (Table)
Trimethoprim, see also Co-trimoxazole
  administration, 1979 (Table)
  Escherichia coli resistance, 951
  mechanism, 1527

Pneumocystis carinii, cancer treatment, 895
  urinary tract infections, 952 (Table)
Trimethylaminuria, 1113
Triose phosphate isomerase deficiency, 1131
Triple bone scan, osteomyelitis, 1915–1916
Triple rhythm (gallop rhythm), 32, 598
Triplet repeats, 69
Triple vaccine, see DPT vaccine
Triple X, **62**
Triploidy, 51
Triprolidine, administration, 1979 (Table)
Tris-hydroxyaminomethane, 715
Trisodium edetate, administration, 1979 (Table)
Trisomies
  congenital heart disease, 596
  polycythemia, 227
Trisomy 13, **57–58**, 832 (Table)
  congenital heart disease, 596
Trisomy 18, **57**, 832 (Table)
  congenital heart disease, 596
Trisomy 21, 55
  acute lymphoblastic leukemia, 887
Tristan da Cunha islanders, asthma, 493
Trizoles, **1478**
TRNG (tetracycline, plasmid-mediated resistance, N. gonorrhoeae), 1422, 1427
Trochlear nerve
  examination, 34
  palsy, 265
Trombicula spp., 1392
Trophic feeding, 151, 208
Trophozoites, hematophagous, amebiasis, 1467
Tropical eosinophilia syndrome, **1498**
Trousseau's sign, 300
True hermaphroditism, 986–987, 1010, see also Pseudohermaphroditism
True IgA deficiency, neoplasms, 889 (Table)
Truncal ataxia, 750–752
  physiological, 668
Truncus arteriosus, 203 (Table), **621–622**
Trunk
  incurvation reflex, 37 (Table), 770
    neonatal gestation age, 40 (Table)
  rhabdomyosarcoma, 915
  tone
    Amiel-Tison system, 240 (Fig.)
    neonate, 239
Trusts, National Health Service, 1854
Trust vs mistrust (Erikson), 1730
Trypanosoma brucei 'subspecies', 1453
Trypanosoma cruzi, 1458
Trypanosomiasis, **1453–1460**
Trypomastigotes, 1454
  T. cruzi, 1458
Trypsins, 437
  neonate, 207
  stools, 1936 (Table)
Tryptophan
  Hartnup disease, 1122
  metabolism disorders, **1114**
Tryptophanemia, 1114
Tsetse flies, 1454
  control, 1458
Tsutsugamushi fever (scrub typhus), 1390 (Table), **1392**
Tube feeding, 470, see also Enteral nutrition
  anorexia nervosa, 1758
  burns, 1800
  debranching enzyme deficiency, 1138
  elemental diets, 1207
  glucose-6-phosphatase deficiency, 1137
  heart failure, 599
  liver disease, 1209
  for malnutrition, 1193
  preterm infant, **153–154**, 208

Tuberculin positivity, **1336–1338**
  after BCG vaccination, **1340**
  BCG vaccination (need for), 1339
  environmental mycobacteria, 1349
  measles on, 1355
  vs tuberculosis, 1335
Tuberculoid leprosy, 1310
  vs tinea versicolor, 1637
Tuberculoma, **1344, 1345**
Tuberculosis, **1334–1348,** *see also*
  Pulmonary tuberculosis
  Addison's disease, 1068
  bones, 1336, **1345–1346,** 1592
    and joints, **1592–1594**
  bronchial biopsy, 520
  cervical lymphadenopathy, 1784
  chemotherapy, **1347–1348**
    return to school, 1348
  children of immigrants, 1865
  developing countries disease burden,
    1276 (Table)
  drug resistance, 1347–1348
  duration of therapy, 1528
  erythema nodosum, 510
  eye, **1677**
  FUO investigations, 1283 (Table)
  hematuria, 958
  hypercalcemia, 1056
  measles, 1355
  meningitis, 693, 1336, **1344–1345**
    CSF, 1290
    isoniazid, 1347
    management, 696
    stroke, 713
    ventricular dilation, 665
  mortality, 489–490
  neonate, 285–286, **1346**
  phlyctenulae, 510
  school doctors, 1863
  trends, 7
  United Kingdom, 1277, 1278 (Fig.),
    1335
  urine specimens, 1299
Tuberous sclerosis, 72 (Table), 799
    (Table), **801–802, 1625**
  on brain development, 642
  cortical dysplasia, 685
  epilepsy, **679,** 801, 802, 1625
  infantile spasms, 687
  lesionectomy, 686
  renal involvement, 254
  rhabdomyomas of heart, 636
Tubocurarine, administration, 1979
    (Table)
Tubotympanic disease, 1680
Tubular function, development, 1953
Tubular proteinuria, 967, 968
Tubular reabsorption, amino acids, 943,
    1122
Tubuloglomerular feedback, 942
Tuftsin deficiency, 1266
Tularemia, **1350–1351**
Tumbu fly, 1514
Tumor calcinosis, 1058
Tumor cell resistance, **892–893**
Tumor lysis syndrome, 871, 897
  acute renal failure, 975
  non-Hodgkin's lymphoma, 907
Tumor markers, 291–293 (Table), 891
  central nervous system tumors, 899
  germ cell tumors, 921
  small round cell tumors, 912 (Table)
Tumor necrosis factor, malaria immunity,
    1447
Tumor necrosis factor-α, neonate, 275
Tumors, *see* Neoplasms
Tumor suppressor genes, 888
Tunga penetrans, 1515 (Fig.)
Tungiasis, **1514**
Tunica vasculosa lentis, 263
Tunneling, central venous lines, 1224
Turbinates, 1683
Turner's syndrome, 26 (Fig.), 38, **60–62,**
    370, 833 (Table), 990, 1007

coarctation of aorta, 370, 596, 611
congenital heart disease, 596
cytogenetic nomenclature, 53
delayed puberty, 1032–1034
growth failure, 1017
growth hormone, 370, 1019, 1033
  and Hashimoto's thyroiditis, 1049
inheritance, 67
Turpentine poisoning, 1711
Turpentine substitute poisoning, 1705,
    1711
Turricephaly, 21 (Fig.), **1560, 1661**
TWAR strain, *Chlamydia psittaci,* 569,
    see also Chlamydia pneumoniae
T wave, 589
Tween 80
  gastrografin enema, 1776
  tuberculin test, 1337
Twins
  acardiac, umbilical cord ligation, 115
  cerebral palsy incidence, 167
  diabetes mellitus, 1073
  fetal growth, 350
  HIV vertical transmission, 288
  hospital admission, 116
  pregnancy with, 90
  vs siblings, menarche, 366
  sudden infant death syndrome, 1723
Twin studies, genetic epilepsies, 679
Twin–twin transfusion, 90, **224,** 227
  operative fetoscopy, 115
Two glass test, 1425
'Two-hit' hypothesis, Knudson, 868
Two-point discrimination, 35
2SP transport medium, *Chlamydia
    trachomatis,* 1431
Ty 21a vaccine, typhoid fever, 1326
Tympanic membrane
  examination, 21
  perforation, 21, **1680,** *see also* Chronic
    otitis media
Tympanocentesis, otitis media, 1298
Tympanometry, 817
Typhoidal tularemia, 1351
Typhoid fever, **1324–1326,** 1865
  antibiotic, 454 (Table)
  FUO investigations, 1283 (Table)
Typhus, 1390 (Table), **1391**
Tyrosinase-negative albinism, 1107, 1629
    (Table)
Tyrosinase-positive albinism, 1629 (Table)
Tyrosine
  catecholamines from, 1069
  metabolism, 1104 (Fig.)
    disorders, **1106–1108**
    normal values, 1929 (Table)
  thyroid hormone biosynthesis, 1045
Tyrosine hydroxylase defect, 1107
Tyrosine kinases
  growth-hormone-receptor-associated,
    1013
  immune system, 1239
  phosphorylation, 351
Tyrosinemia, 1106–1107
Tyrosinosis, 1107
Tyrosyluria, 1106
Tyson's glands, *see* Parafrenal glands

Ubiquinone
  for hereditary lactic acidosis, 1125
  for mitochondrial bioenergetic defects,
    1128
Uganda, trauma rehabilitation centers,
    1887
Uhl's disease, 610–611
UK8501 protocol, lymphoma
  chemotherapy, 908
UKCCSG 9004 protocol, lymphoma
  chemotherapy, 909
Ulcerative blepharitis, 1675
Ulcerative colitis, **458–459**
  nutrition, 459, 1206
  self-help groups, 485

Ulcerative stomatitis, 1363, 1364–1365,
    1438
Ulceroglandular syndrome, 1351
Ulcers
  amebic, 1469
  BCG vaccination, 1339
  hemangiomas, 1619
  oral mucosa, 424
  peptic, **432**
Ulegyria, 642
Ulnar defects, hand, 1546 (Table)
Ultrasonography, **1896,** *see also* Cranial
    ultrasonography;
    Echocardiography
  abdominal injury, 1811, 1812
  antenatal care, measurements, 81–82
  biliary atresia, 1782
  biliary tract, 1906
  birth asphyxia, 128
  brain, **1908**
  chest, **517, 1900**
  chronic liver disease, 480
  congenital dislocation of hip, 1551
  congenital nephrotic syndrome, Finnish
    type, 261
  double inlet ventricle, 620
  Down syndrome screening, 56–57
  fetal growth, 350
  gastrointestinal tract, **1904–1906**
  genitalia, 1913–1914
  head injuries, 706–707
  heart disease, **589–593**
    stroke, 713
  hydrocephalus, 660
  intussusception, 1786
  liver, 472, 1906
  neonatal meningitis, 247
  neonatal neurology, 242
  nephroblastoma, 913
  pancreas, 451
  pneumothorax, 188
  pregnancy, 80, 350
    hydrocephalus, 661
    screening, 81
    urinary tract abnormalities, 256,
      935–936
  renal failure, 974–975
  retroperitoneum, 1913
  skeletal system, **1916–1917**
  total anomalous pulmonary venous
    connection, 623
  twin pregnancies, 90
  urinary tract, **1909–1910**
    infections, 952
    neonate, 262
  ventricular septal defect, 601
Ultraviolet radiation
  neoplasms, 890
  xeroderma pigmentosum, 1630
Umbilical artery
  blood gases monitoring, 160
  Doppler ultrasonography, flow velocity
    waveform, 82–83, 115
  single, 42
Umbilical artery injection, sciatic nerve,
    722
Umbilical catheters, major vessel
    thrombosis, 231
Umbilical cord, 42
  acardiac twins, ligation, 115
  antiseptic dressings, 104
  clamping, 107, 111
    blood volume, 108, 222
    preterm infant, 108, 139, 222, 225
    transient tachypnea of the newborn,
      182
  compression in childbirth, 86
  delayed separation, 1261
  developing countries, 1890
  postnatal care, 112
Umbilical hernia, 1790
  neonate, 1106
Umbilical vessel catheterization, **1838**
Uncinaria stenocephala, 1488–1489

Unconjugated hyperbilirubinemia,
    1144–1145
  neonatal, teeth, 425
  prolonged, **219–220**
Under-5 mortality rates, **1882–1884**
  causes, 1889 (Fig.)
Undulant fever, *see* Brucellosis
Unemployment
  parasuicide, 1757
  respiratory disorders, 492
UNICEF
  health goals, 1884–1885
  State of the world's children, 1882
Unidentified bright objects, magnetic
    resonance imaging, 801
Unilateral facial agenesis (hemifacial
    microsomia), 1563 (Table), **1564**
Unilateral hydrocephalus, 659
Unilateral renal agenesis, 253
Uniparental disomy, 1017
United Kingdom
  breast-feeding rates, 326 (Table)
  celiac disease incidence, 440
  cystinuria, 947
  deafness screening, 244
  demography, 2 (Table)
  gonorrhea in children, 1421
  growth standards, 352–353
  immunization schedules, 344
  infections
    data sources, 1280 (Table)
    statistics, **1276–1278**
  neonatal death, 173–174
  Office of Population Censuses and
    Surveys, 1281, 1848
  perinatal mortality, **3**
  pertussis, 1315–1316
  respiratory disorders, 489–490
  stillbirth rates (SBR), **3**
  tuberculosis, 1277, 1278 (Fig.), **1335**
  vs United States, costing neonatal care,
    105
United Nations
  Convention on the Rights of the Child,
    1888, 1891
  Declaration of the Rights of the Child, 1
  health initiatives, **1888,** 1889
United States
  breast-feeding rates, 326 (Table)
  gastroenteritis, mortality, 1293
  gonorrhea in children, 1421
  HIV vertical transmission, 288
  vs Holland, neurodevelopmental
    outcome of prematurity, 166
  immunization schedules, 344 (Table)
  pertussis, 1315
  poliomyelitis vaccination, 345
  vs United Kingdom, costing neonatal
    care, 105
Units
  conversion factors, 1921, 1938 (Table)
  hormone values, 1000
  pressure, intracranial pressure, 698
Unmaintainable airway, 1807
Unmarried mothers, 1855
Unrelated donor bone marrow
    transplantation, 873
Unsafe bladder, 657
Unstable child with underlying pathology,
    1813–1816
Unstable malaria, 1447
Unverricht's disease, 795 (Table)
Upper airway obstruction, *see also*
    Epiglottitis
  burns, 572
  diphtheria, 1306
  infections, **562–564**
  mortality, 490 (Table)
Upper motor neurone lesions, facial nerve,
    34
Upper respiratory tract
  examination, **511**
  hemangiomas, 1619
  infections, **559–561,** 1282–1283

Upper respiratory tract (*Contd*)
  bacteriology specimens, **1298**
  ECHO viruses, 1383
  meningococcemia, 1314
  minimal change nephrotic syndrome, 969
  noisy breathing, 508–509
  virology specimens, **1351–1352**
  radiography, 513
Urachus, anomalies, 1778
Urates, urine color, 958
Urban cutaneous leishmaniasis, 1463
Urea
  amniotic fluid, 1937 (Table)
  concentration units, 1921
  normal values, 1929 (Table)
  plasma levels, 406 (Table), *see also* Blood urea nitrogen
  nutrition, 1188
  urine
    neonates, 142 (Table)
    renal failure, 974
Urea clearance, normal values, 1933 (Table)
Urea cycle, 1110
  defects, 248, 305 (Table), 306, 307, 1110–1111
  ataxia, 762
  dietary management, **1204 (Table)**
  protein tolerance, 1120
Urea nitrogen, normal values, 1929 (Table)
  cerebrospinal fluid, 1935 (Table)
Ureaplasma pneumonia, 196
Urease
  Helicobacter pylori, 431
  Proteus mirabilis, 1320
Uremia
  immune system, 1266
  infant, 935
  neuropathy, 724
  plasma sodium, 404
  SGA baby, 138
Ureteric bud, 934
Ureterocele, 256, 937, 1795
Ureters
  anomalies, 1794–1795
  congenital abnormalities, 255–256
  percutaneous nephrostomy, 1898
  reimplantation, 262, 956, **956–957**
  schistosomiasis, 1509
Urethra
  catheterization, 1839–1840
    infections, 1320
    neuropathic bladder, 657, 957
    urine specimens, 950, 1299
  congenital abnormalities, 255
  gonorrhea, 1425
  micturating cystourethrography, 1911
Urethral valves, *see* Posterior urethral valves
Urethritis
  gonorrhea, 1420
  nongonococcal, **1432**
Uric acid
  amniotic fluid, 1937 (Table)
  excretion, 1140
  normal values, 1929 (Table)
    cerebrospinal fluid, 1935 (Table)
Uric acidemia, SGA baby, 138
Uridine, for orotic aciduria, 1142
Uridine diphosphate galactose, 1134
Uridine diphosphate galactose-4-epimerase deficiency, 1134
Uridine diphosphoglucuronic acid, 218
Uridine diphosphoglucuronyltransferase, Crigler–Najjar syndrome, 218
Uridine triphosphate, cystic fibrosis, 558
Urinary tract, **934–984**
  burns, 1799
  imaging, **1909–1912**
  infections, **949–956**
    antibiotic prophylaxis, 1529
    vs appendicitis, 1787

vs enuresis, 957 (Table)
    hematuria, 958
    investigations, **952–956**
    maternal, 89 (Table)
    neonate, **261–262**, 283
      organisms, 284 (Table)
    Proteus mirabilis, 1320
    Pseudomonas aeruginosa, 1320
    surgical aspects, **1794–1795**
    tuberculosis, 1346
    vomiting, 212
  neonate, **253–262**
  obstruction
    acute renal failure, 974
    neurogenic bladder, 656
    renography, 1912
Urine
  acid excretion, 417, 418
  alkalinization
    cystinuria, 947
    salicylate poisoning, 1710
  amino acids, 1103
    testing, 306
  blue-green, 1122
  calcium:creatinine ratio, 943, 959
    normal values, 1930 (Table)
  Candida spp., 1472
  chemotherapy, 896
  circadian rhythm, Ondine's curse, 530
  color, 958
    blue-green, 1122
    infant, 471
  concentration, 942, 943
  cultures, 951
    neonatal sepsis, 276–277
    vesicoureteric reflux, 956
  diabetes mellitus monitoring, 1079
  dilution, 942
  dilution and concentration, postnatal development, 257
  fetus, 253
  flow rate
    vs creatinine, very low birth weight, 142
    preterm infant, 140, 141–142
  gonorrhea, 1425
  growth hormone measurements, 1019
  history taking, 18
  hormone tests, 1000
  hypoglycemia, investigations, 297–298
  mental retardation, 837
  neonate, 108, 110, 111
  neuroblastoma, 911–912, 913–914
  normal constituents, **1930–1933 (Table)**
  obligatory output, 973
  odors in inborn errors of metabolism, 305
  osmolality, 943, 1040
    neonatal, 108
    vs plasma osmolality, 1040
    preterm infant, 140
    renal failure, 974
  protein, 967
  reducing substances, neonate, 220
  renal failure, 974 (Table)
  retention, *see* Retention of urine
  sampling, **1839–1840**
    bacteriology, **1299**
    urinary tract infections, 950–951
    virology, 1352
  specific gravity, preterm infant, 141–142
  steroids, 1060
  typhoid fever, 1326
  volume, normal values, 1933 (Table)
  water output, 403 (Table)
Urobilinogen, normal values
  stools, 1936 (Table)
  urine, 1933 (Table)
Urocanic aciduria, 1115
Urogenital ridge, teratomas, 922
Urokinase, 228, 231
  central venous line occlusion, 1225

Urolithiasis
  cystinuria, 947
  hematuria, 959
  Proteus mirabilis, 1320
  ultrasonography, 1910
Urology, neonate, **1778–1779**
Uromucoid protein, *see* Tamm–Horsfall protein
Uroporphyrinogens, 1142, 1144
Urticaria, **1639**
  allergic aspects, **1697–1698**
  neonate, 1284
Urticarial vasculitis, 1640–1641
Urticaria pigmentosa, 1647
User charges, Bamako Initiative, 1890
Usher's syndrome, 816, 817, 1172
  deafness, 1682
USSR (former), demography, 2 (Table)
Usual interstitial pneumonitis, 578
Uterine artery blood flow, Doppler ultrasonography, 81, **82**
Uterine branches
  Taenia saginata, 1500
  Taenia solium, 1501
Uteroplacental insufficiency, 1005
Uterus
  absence, 991
  fetal growth restriction, 350
  parturition, 84
  rhabdomyosarcoma, 916
  tuberculosis, 1346
  ultrasonography, 1913
Utstein templates, 522
Uveitis, **1665–1666**, *see also* Anterior uveitis
  metastatic, 1677
  sarcoidosis, 1677
  syphilis, 1408
  tuberculosis, 1677

Vaccination, *see* Immunization
Vaccine-preventable diseases, developing countries disease burden, 1276 (Table), 1280 (Table)
Vaccines, **341–342**, *see also* Acellular vaccine; DPT vaccine; *named diseases and organisms*
  antibody tests, 1245
  cancer treatment, 895
  egg intolerance, 1700
  Haemophilus influenzae type b, 1292, **1309**, *see also* Hib immunization
  hepatitis B virus, 477, **1387**
  immunodeficiency, 1267
  malaria, 1449
  pertussis, 341, 1317, 1318
  rabies, 1377
  rotavirus, 1295
  and severe combined immunodeficiency syndrome, 1249
  Streptococcus pneumoniae, 341, 970, **1319**, 1974
  viral, immunosuppression by, 1264
Vaccinia, 286 (Table)
Vaccinology, 342
VAC regimen, Ewing's sarcoma, 920
VACTERL complex, 1770
Vacuum extraction, 120, 121
Vagabond's disease, 1518
Vagal maneuvers, paroxysmal supraventricular tachycardia, 627
Vagina
  agenesis, atresia, 1796
  bleeding
    factitious, 1028
    neonate, 110
  congenital absence, 988
  discharge, 1425
    enterobiasis, 1487
  fetal fibronectin, 116
  germ cell tumors, 922
  imperforate, 990–991

organisms, neonatal infection, 276
  reconstruction, 1065
  rhabdomyosarcoma, 916
  tumors, 993–994
  ultrasonography, 1913–1914
Vaginal caps, 995
Vaginitis, *see also* Vulvovaginitis
  candidiasis, 1433
Vaginosis, bacterial, 116, **1435**
Vagus nerve
  dysphonia, 809
  efferents, asthma, 538
  examination, 34
  to lungs, development, 495–496
  maneuvers, paroxysmal supraventricular tachycardia, 627
Valaciclovir, 1441
Valency, concentration units, 1921
Valgus foot, **1555**
Valine
  degradation pathway, 1116 (Fig.)
  hyperglycinemia, 1112
Valproate, 682
  administration, 1977 (Table)
    neonate, 1958 (Table)
  febrile convulsions prophylaxis, 684
  on fetus and neonate, 91 (Table)
  for infantile spasms, 687
  mania, 1755
  neonatal seizures, 246
  pregnancy, 691
  teratogenesis, 114
  therapeutic ranges, 1936 (Table)
Valsalva maneuver, neonatal cry, 107
Valuing of resources, 104–105
Valve prostheses, antibiotic prophylaxis, 631
Valves, CSF shunts, 662
Valvotomy, aortic stenosis, 607
Valvuloplasty, neonate, 205
Vamin, parenteral nutrition, 1220
Vamin 9, 1223 (Table)
Vamin-9-glucose, 158 (Table)
Vamin Infant (amino acid solution), 158 (Table)
Vaminolact, 1223 (Table)
Vanadium, 1185 (Table)
Van Buchem craniotubular hyperostosis, 1582 (Table)
Vancomycin
  administration, 1956 (Table), 1978 (Table)
  necrotizing enterocolitis, 211
  neonate, 279 (Table), 281
    pneumonia, 280
  prophylaxis, infective endocarditis, 632 (Table)
  site of action, 1527
  Staphylococcus aureus, 1329 (Table)
Vanillylmandelic acid, 1069
  neuroblastoma, 911
  normal values, urine, 1933 (Table)
Variability, fetal heart rate, 86, 117 (Table)
Variant surface glycoprotein, *Trypanosoma brucei*, 1455
Varicella, congenital syndrome, 1361
Varicella bullosa, 1361
Varicella gangrenosa, 1361
Varicella neonatorum, 1360, **1361**
Varicella-zoster virus
  AIDS, 1395
  cancer treatment, 895
  immunization, 345, 969
  immunocompromised patient, 535
  infection, 1360–1363, **1632–1633**
    congenital, 248, 286 (Table), 287, 1284
  rash, 1284
Varices
  extrahepatic biliary atresia, 475
  management, 483
  orbit, 1661, 1672
  upper gastrointestinal hemorrhage, 433
Varicoceles, 1914

Variegate porphyria, 1142 (Table), 1143
Variola, 286 (Table)
Vascular disease
   cystathione synthase deficiency, 1108
   syphilis, 1401
Vascular endothelial growth factor,
   retinopathy of prematurity, 265
Vascular factors, hemostasis, 227
Vascular headache, 715
Vascular malformations, **1619–1620,**
   1797, **1798,** *see also* Arteriovenous
   malformations;
   Bronchopulmonary-vascular
   malformations
   anencephaly, 642
   congenital stridor, **573**
Vascular nevi, **1618–1620**
Vascular ring, **573, 612**
   imaging, 1899
Vascular spasm, intracranial, 712–713
Vascular systems, transient, eye
   development, 262–263
Vasculitic syndromes, **1609–1610**
   skin, **1640–1641**
Vasculitis
   abdomen, Doppler ultrasonography,
      1905
   renal involvement, 966
Vas deferens, congenital bilateral absence,
   551
Vasoactive intestinal peptide
   growth hormone secretion, 1013
   neuroblastoma, 911
   prolactin secretion, 1039
Vasoconstriction, catecholamines, 1069
Vasoconstrictors, topical, allergic
   conjunctivitis, 1676
Vasodilators
   neonatal heart failure, 205
   renal hypertension, 973
Vasogenic edema, birth asphyxia, 126
Vasomotor change, hemiplegia, 744
Vasomotor rhinitis, 1685
Vasopressin, *see also* Antidiuretic
   hormone
   ACTH secretion, 1038
   fetus, 1003
   renal function, 942
VATER complex, 75, 1770
VATERL, heart, 596
Vaughan Williams classes, antiarrhythmic
   drugs, 626–627
VDRL, *see* Venereal Disease Research
   Laboratory carbon antigen test
Vector loops, electrocardiography, 588
   (Fig.)
Vegan diets, 1189
   carnitine deficiency, 1188
Vegetarian diets, **1189**
   weaning, 334
Vein of Galen aneurysm, 203 (Table),
   710–711
   ultrasonography, 1909 (Fig.)
Velocity (charts), 1011, *see also* Height,
   velocity
   fetal growth, 350
   postnatal growth, 352
Velofaciocardiac syndrome, 1252
Venepuncture
   blood cultures, 1298
   blood sampling, **1834–1835**
   osteomyelitis, 283
Venereal Disease Research Laboratory
   carbon antigen test, **1402**
   congenital and neurosyphilis, 1405
Venesection, porphyrias, 1144
Venoms, snakes, 1521
Veno-occlusive syndrome,
   nephroblastoma radiotherapy, 914
Venous arteriovenous malformation, 711
Venous blood
   vs arterial blood, acid–base indices, 419
   sampling, **1834–1835**
Venous cannulation, **1836–1837**

percutaneous central, **1837–1838**
Venous congestion
   cirrhosis, 482 (Table)
   lung fields, 200 (Table)
Venous cut down, surgical, **1837**
Venous hum, 32, 594
Venous thrombosis, gastroenteritis, 1294
Ventilation, **1817–1819,** *see also* Bag and
   mask ventilation; Endotracheal
   intubation
   air embolism, 190
   alkalosis, 299
   apnea attacks, 198
   bronchiolitis, 565
   bronchopulmonary dysplasia, 193, 194,
      195
   cardiovascular support, 1819
   complications, 1818
   diaphragmatic hernia, 1770
   expired air, **522,** 523–524
   lung trauma from, 160–161
   meconium aspiration syndrome, 186
   near-drowning, 1825
   neonatal care, **159–165**
      subglottic stenosis, 572
   Ondine's curse, 531
   pertussis, 562
   pneumothorax, 187
   poliomyelitis, 1380
   respiratory distress syndrome, 162–164,
      180–181, 1818
   resuscitation, 1807
   Reye's syndrome, 479
   rhesus incompatibility, 233
   sedation and analgesia, **1832–1833**
   water balance, 142
Ventilation and perfusion, **501–502,** 503
   asthma, 539
   mismatch, 160
Ventilation lung scans, **517–519,** 1901
   foreign body inhalation, 571
   radiation dose, 513
Ventilation of feelings, maladaptive
   response to chronic illness, 1761
Ventilation trauma, lungs, 160–161
Ventilatory index, diaphragmatic hernia,
   1770
Ventral hernia, 1780
Ventral suspension, 388 (Table)
   neonate, 44, 237 (Fig.)
   gestation age, 41 (Fig.)
Ventricles (brain)
   access, *see also* Reservoirs
      hydrocephalus monitoring, 661
      stroke from, 714
   dilation, *see also* Hydrocephalus
      very low birth weight, outcome,
         171–172
   measurement, fetus, 661
   raised pressure, 659–660
Ventricles (cardiac)
   enlargement, 31
      neonate, outcome, 252–253
   hypertrophy, 32
      electrocardiography, 589
      precordial examination, 586
Ventricular amniotic shunt, fetal
   hydrocephalus, 665
Ventricular assist devices, **1821**
Ventricular ectopic beats, 625
Ventricular fibrillation, resuscitation, **526,**
   1808
Ventricular index, cranial ultrasonography,
   252
Ventricular inversion, 616
Ventricular puncture, 664, **1841**
Ventricular septal aneurysm, 600
Ventricular septal defect, 198, **599–601**
   angiotensin converting enzyme
      inhibitors, 599
   double outlet right ventricle, 622
   neonate, murmur, 203
   with pulmonary atresia, **617–618**
   signs, 587 (Table)

tetralogy of Fallot, 616
   transposition of great arteries, 614
Ventricular tachycardia, 625–626
   neonate, 203
   treatment, 627
Ventriculitis, **663,** 1289
   neonate, 281
Ventriculoarterial connections, congenital
   heart disease, 597
Ventriculoatrial shunts, 252, 662
Ventriculocisternotomy, 664
Ventriculoperitoneal shunts, 662
   brain tumors, 901
   posthemorrhagic hydrocephalus, 252
Verapamil, 627 (Table)
   administration, 1978 (Table)
   hypertrophic cardiomyopathy, 634
   migraine, 717 (Table)
Verbal agnosia, 807
Verbal IQ, 1735
Vermis, aplasias, **645–647**
Vernal conjunctivitis, 510
Vernal keratoconjunctivitis, 1664,
   1698–1699
Verocytotoxin, hemolytic uremic
   syndrome, 977–978
Verrucose endocarditis, atypical, 635
Verrucous lesions, bartonellosis, 1301
Vertebrae
   beaking, 1915
   congenital abnormalities, 651
   hemopoiesis, 848 (Fig.)
Vertebral column, *see* Spine
Vertebra plana, 1594
Vertical talus, congenital, 1555
Vertical transmission
   hepatitis B virus, 1386, 1400
   herpes simplex, **1441–1442**
   HIV infection, 288, 329, 1392, 1398
   human papillomavirus, 1444
   sexually transmitted diseases, 1400
   sleeping sickness, 1454
   syphilis, 1400, **1411**
   toxocariasis, 1486
Veruga peruana, 1301
Vervet monkey disease, *see* Marburg virus
   disease
Very long chain fatty acids
   adrenoleukodystrophy, 1174
   peroxisomal disorders, 1172 (Table)
Very low birth weight
   Candida albicans, 289
   cerebral palsy, 738–739
   creatinine, *vs* urine flow rate, 142
   hyperkalemia, 146
   intracranial hemorrhage, 249
      serial ultrasonography, 250
   magnesium balance, 1201
   necrotizing enterocolitis, 210
   neurodevelopmental outcome, 166
   potassium loss, 145
   seizures
      incidence, 245
      prognosis, 247
   Wilson–Mikity syndrome, 195
Very low density lipoprotein, 1148
   (Table), 1149
   secondary disorders, 1154 (Table)
Vesicles, fauces, 560
Vesicoamniotic shunting, 935
Vesicoureteric junction obstruction, 255,
   936
Vesicoureteric reflux, 255, 256, **262,** 937,
   949–950, **956–957**
   indirect radionuclide cystography,
      1911–1912
   surgery, 1794
Vesicular rashes, **1284–1285**
Viability
   definition, 94
   preterm labor, 119
Vi antibodies, typhoid fever, 1326
Vi antigen, *Salmonella* spp., 1323
Vibration sense, 35

Vibrio cholerae, 1303
Vibrio cholerae 0139, emergence, 1279
   (Table)
Video/EEG studies, 677
Video games, epilepsy, 691
Videotaping, trial of feeding, 469
Vigabatrin
   administration, 1978 (Table)
   for infantile spasms, 687
Villi, small intestine, 435
Villous atrophy, *see also* Microvillous
   atrophy
   subtotal, 440, 441
Vimentin, small round cell tumors, 912
   (Table)
Vim-Silverman needle renal biopsy, 1846
Vinca alkaloids
   constipation, 896
   toxic effects, 894 (Table)
Vincristine
   continuation therapy, acute
      lymphoblastic leukemia, 873
   neuropathy, 896
Vinegar, *Chironex* stings, 1526
Viper berus, bites, **1520–1521**
Viperidae, 1521
Viper venoms, 1521
Viral coinfection (delta virus), 477, **1387**
Viral gastroenteritis, neonate, 212–213
Viral hepatitis, **476–478,** 1386–1388, *see
   also* Delta virus
   hemophilia A, 880
   maternal, 89 (Table)
   vs Weil's syndrome, 1312
Viral inactivation, intravenous
   immunoglobulin preparations,
   1268
Viral infections, **1351–1390,** *see also*
   Croup; HIV infection
   in AIDS, 1395, 1396
   anterior horn cells, 719
   arthritis, 1612
   vs bacterial infections, pneumonia, 567
      (Table)
   cancer treatment, 895
   central nervous system, 694, **1375–1378**
   cerebellitis, 762
   conjunctivitis, 1663, 1664
   developmental cataract, 1668
   diabetes mellitus, 1074
   diarrhea, 452
   eye involvement, **1676**
   febrile convulsions, 683
   gastroenteritis, 1293
   hemorrhagic cystitis, 958
   immunosuppression by, 1264–1265
   keratitis, **1664–1665**
   meningitis, **1375–1376**
      neonate, 248
   myocarditis, **630**
   neonate, **286–288,** 1282
   neoplasms, 891
   neutropenia, 866
   pneumonia, 566
      immunocompromised patient, **535**
   respiratory tract, **1368–1373,** 1802
   skin, **1631–1634**
   sudden infant death syndrome, 1719,
      1722
   United Kingdom, mortality, 1276
      (Table)
   urticaria, 1697
   wheeze, 540, 541, 565
Viral liposomes, vaccines, 342
Virilization, *see also* Sexual differentiation
   disorders
   21-hydroxylase deficiency, 1063–1064
Viruses
   antibody tests, 1245
   leukemia, 868
Visceral larva migrans, *see also Toxocara
   canis*
   organisms, 1484 (Table)
Visceral leishmaniasis, **1461–1463**

Visibility, *vs* resolution, 268
Visible peristalsis, 32
Vision
  cerebral palsy, 738, 761
  craniopharyngioma, 905
  development, **268–270**, 382
  examination, 25, **395–396**
  migraine, 717
  neonate, **262–273**
    examination, 241
  optic gliomas, 904
Visual acuity, **268**, 395
  neonate, 241
  testing, 1649, **1656–1657**
    school health services, 1863
Visual agnosia, 822
Visual fields, examination, 27
Visual impairment, **270–273**, *see also*
      Blindness
  developmental test, 400
  examination, 396
  history taking, 17
  nystagmus, 272
  severely handicapped children affected,
      14 (Table)
Visually evoked potentials, 270, 273,
      1655–1656, 1656 (Fig.), 1657
      (Fig.)
  neonate, 243
Visual orientation, neonate, 238 (Fig.)
Visual pathway, development, 263
Visuospatial developmental disorders, **670**
Visuospatial motor dysgraphia, 822
Vital capacity, 500 (Fig.), 501
Vital statistics, *see* Epidemiology
Vitamin A, 1184 (Table)
  for abetalipoproteinemia, 1153
  cystic fibrosis, 1208
  deficiency, 1188, **1194**
    developing countries disease burden,
      1280 (Table)
    eye, 1677
    immunodeficiency, 1266
  liver disease, 1209
  for malnutrition, 1193
  normal values, 1929 (Table)
  parenteral nutrition, 1221 (Table)
  Recommended Dietary Allowances,
      1948 (Table)
  reference nutrient intakes, 1946 (Table)
  sources, 1184 (Table)
  supplements
    cystic fibrosis, 557
    developing countries, 1890
  therapy, 1194
  toxicity, 1194
Vitamin B₁, *see* Thiamin
Vitamin B₂, *see* Riboflavin
Vitamin B₆, 1184 (Table), *see also*
      Pyridoxine
  deficiency, 1198
    sideroblastic anemia, 866
  Recommended Dietary Allowances,
      1949 (Table)
  reference nutrient intakes, 1946 (Table)
Vitamin B₁₂, 1184 (Table)
  deficiency, **853–854**, 1188, **1199**
    Diphyllobothrium latum, 853, 1199,
      1503–1504
    neuropathy, 724
  DNA synthesis, 853 (Fig.)
  metabolism disorders, **1147–1148**
  for methylmalonic acidemia, 1117
  normal levels, 1199
  for organic acidurias, 1119
  parenteral nutrition, 1221 (Table)
  preterm infant, 225
  Recommended Dietary Allowances,
      1949 (Table)
  reference nutrient intakes, 1946 (Table)
  serum levels, 854
  therapy, 1199
Vitamin C, 1184 (Table)
  administration, 1959 (Table)

deficiency, eye, 1677
  for hereditary lactic acidosis, 1125
  load test, 1930 (Table)
  for methemoglobinemia, 865
  for mitochondrial bioenergetic defects,
      1128
  normal values, 1923 (Table), 1929
      (Table)
  oxalosis, 1113
  parenteral nutrition, 1221 (Table)
  Recommended Dietary Allowances,
      1949 (Table)
  reference nutrient intakes, 1946 (Table)
Vitamin D, 299, **1053–1055**, 1184
      (Table), *see also* 1,25-Dihydroxy
      vitamin D
  analogues for hypoparathyroidism,
      1057
  deficiency, **1194–1196**
    cow's milk intolerance, 1700
    immigrants, 1866
    zonular cataract, 1669, 1677
  dosage as calciferol, 1961 (Table)
    neonate, 1956 (Table)
  for late neonatal tetany, 300
  liver disease, 1209
  maternal deficiency, 299
  neonate, 301
    supplements, 303
  normal values, 1924 (Table), 1926
      (Table)
  and nutritional assessment, 1188
  parenteral nutrition, 1221 (Table)
  Recommended Dietary Allowances,
      1948 (Table)
  reference nutrient intakes, 1946 (Table)
  sources, 1184 (Table)
  supplements, 331
    cystic fibrosis, 1208
  therapy, 1196, 1197
  toxicity, 1196–1197
Vitamin D-resistant rickets, 260, **948**
  treatment, 1197
Vitamin E, 1184 (Table)
  abetalipoproteinemia, 767, 1153
  absorption defect, 1148
  cystic fibrosis, 1208
  deficiency, 446, 1188, **1197–1198**
  liver disease, 1209
  normal values, 1929 (Table)
  parenteral nutrition, 1221 (Table)
  preterm infant, 225
    deficiency, 225
  Recommended Dietary Allowances,
      1948 (Table)
  safe intakes, 1948 (Table)
  sources, 1184 (Table)
Vitamin E-deficient hemolysis, 155
Vitamin K, 220, 229–230, 1184 (Table)
  for abetalipoproteinemia, 1153
  administration, 1974 (Table)
  deficiency, 882, **1196**
  for hereditary lactic acidosis, 1125
  infants, 154
  liver disease, 1209
  for mitochondrial bioenergetic defects,
      1128
  neonate, 111, 121
  parenteral nutrition, 230, 1221 (Table)
  prophylaxis, 230, 339
  Recommended Dietary Allowances,
      1948 (Table)
  safe intakes, 1948 (Table)
  sources, 1184 (Table)
  supplements, **330–331**, 1197
Vitamins, **1182**
  cystic fibrosis, 553–554, 1208
  deficiencies, **1194–1200**
    assessment, 1188
  Estimated average requirements (EAR),
      1184 (Table)
  estimated safe and adequate daily
      intakes, 1949 (Table)
  fat-soluble, 1182

absorption, 437
  for hereditary lactic acidosis, 1125
  for inborn errors of metabolism, 307
  infant supplements, 334
  liver disease, 1209
  metabolism disorders, **1147–1148**
  for organic acidurias, 1119
  parenteral nutrition, 1221
  preterm milk formulae, 152
  preterm requirements, 152 (Table), 158
  preterm supplements, 154
  Recommended Dietary Allowances,
      1948–1949 (Table)
  safe intakes, 1948 (Table)
Vitellointestinal duct
  anomalies, 1787
  regression failure, 206
Vitiligo, 1640
  vs pityriasis alba, 1644
  vs tinea versicolor, 1637
Vitlipid N Infant, 158, 1222 (Table)
Vitrectomy, retinopathy of prematurity,
      267
Vitreous humor
  opacities, 1651
  sudden infant death syndrome
      investigation, 1721
Vi vaccine, typhoid fever, 1326
Vocal cords, 808, 809
  paralysis, **572**
    unilateral, 1688
Vocal nodules, 1687
Vocal resonance, 30
Vogt cephalodactyly, 1560
Vogt–Koyanagi syndrome, eye, 1675
Voice breaking, 357
Volatile substance abuse, 15 (Table)
Volitional ataxia, 752
Voltage-dependent calcium channels, 127
Volume depletion, acute renal failure, 974
Volume expansion
  burns, 1799
  upper gastrointestinal hemorrhage, 433
Volume limited ventilation, 1817
Volume overload, acute renal failure, 975
Volumetric flow, spectral Doppler
      ultrasonography, 593
Volutrauma, 160–161
Volvulus, 210, 1776
  barium studies, 1902
  with Ladd's bands, 1773–1774
Vomiting, **433–435**, 467
  acid–base balance, 420
  adder bite, 1520
  bulimia, 1759
  causes, **1285–1286**
  cyclical, 717
  cytotoxic drugs, 894 (Table), 895–896
  duodenal atresia, 1773
  gastroesophageal reflux, 1785
  history taking, 17
  infantile hypertrophic pyloric stenosis,
      1784
  mental retardation, 841
  neonate, 111–112, **209–212**
    after first week, 212
  opioids, 928
  potassium chloride for alkalosis, 421
Von Gierke's disease, *see* Glucose-6-
      phosphatase deficiency
Von Hippel–Lindau syndrome, 72 (Table),
      753, 799 (Table), 803
Von Recklinghausen disease, *see*
      Neurofibromatosis
Von Willebrand factor, hemolytic uremic
      syndrome, 978
Von Willebrand's disease, 230, 881
V/P ratio, hydrocephalus, 660
Vulva
  candidiasis, 1433
  enterobiasis, 1487
Vulvovaginitis, **987–988**, 1421,
      1424–1425
  herpetic, 1363–1364, 1438

neonate, organisms, 284 (Table)
Vygon Epicutaneo-cava catheter, 1224

Waardenburg syndrome, 816, 1560–1561
  deafness, 1682
  genetic studies, 76
WADA test (intracarotid amylobarbital
      procedure), 679
Waiter's tip position, 122
Walker–Warburg syndrome, 646, 650
Walking
  cerebral palsy, 758
  delay, 397–398
  development, 382
  Duchenne muscular dystrophy, 730
  neural tube defects, 655
  slow development, 667–668
Walking reflex, 37 (Table)
  neonate, 238 (Fig.)
  gestation age, 40 (Table)
War, 1885
Warble fly, 1514
Warfarin
  dosages, 1979 (Table)
  maternal, 89 (Table), 91 (Table), 230
  poisoning, 1709
Warm autoimmune hemolytic anemia, 864
Warmth, excessive, apparent life-
      threatening events, 528
Warm-up exercises, asthma, 542, 549
Warnock Committee, 1864
Warts, **1633**
  genital, **1442–1445**
  perianal, 988
  vulvar, 988
Wassermann reaction, infectious
      mononucleosis, 1367
Wasting, spinal muscular atrophy type 2,
      720
Water
  absorption, 208
    small intestine, 436
  balance, 403
    acute renal failure, 258
    antidiuretic hormone, 1039
    preterm infant, **139–140**
      assessment, 141–142
  body, **402–403**
    normal values, 1923 (Table)
  for breast-fed babies, 331
  colonic absorption, 455
  depletion, 409, **410**
  deprivation tests, **943**, 948, 1039
  dracunculosis, 1496
  drinking, infants, 334
  environmental mycobacteria, 1349
  fluoridation, 1202
  for growth, 139
  hepatitis A virus, 1386
  intestinal absorption, 437
  intoxication, **412**
    desmopressin therapy, 1040
    dystonia, 673
  movement across membranes, 405,
      406–407
  normal values
    body, 1923 (Table)
    cerebrospinal fluid, 1935 (Table)
    stools, 1936 (Table)
  output, *vs* calories expended, 403
      (Table)
  reabsorption, 941
  requirements, 413 (Table)
    preterm infant, 140–141, 151 (Table)
  restriction, syndrome of inappropriate
      ADH secretion, 1040
  schistosomiasis control, 1511
Water-filled mattresses, heated, 147–148
Water-hammer pulse, 32
Waterhouse–Friderichsen syndrome, 1068,
      1314
Watershed zones, 714
Waterston anastomosis, 617

Wave forms, intracranial pressure, 698
Wave of Leao, migraine, 716
Wax, ears, 1680
Weaning, weaning foods, 330, **333–334,** 426, 1189
  amino acid restricted diets, 1119
  celiac disease, 440
  cystic fibrosis, 1208
  and failure to thrive, 466
  kwashiorkor, 1192
Weanling's dilemma, 1192, 1193 (Fig.)
Weather, allergic symptoms, 1691
Wechsler intelligence scales, 400, 827, 1735
  adult, 827
Weedol, poisoning, 1711
Weed pollens, 1690
Wegener's granulomatosis, 1610
Weight, 1022–1024
  calculating surface area, 1950 (Fig.)
  charting, 364
  dehydration, fluid therapy, 1295
  and drug dosage, 1954, 1980 (Table)
  expected, calculation, **19**
  fetus, 350
  history taking, 17
  neonate, 111
  and prescribing, 1953
  preterm infant, 141
  for puberty, 1026
  unit conversion factors, 1938 (Table)
Weight for height, 1186
  obesity, 1190
Weight for length, 20
Weight gain
  sex hormone treatment, 992
  and sudden infant death syndrome, 1722
Weight loss
  Hodgkin's disease, 909
  large for gestational age infant, 138
  for polycystic ovarian disease, 993
  postnatal, preterm infant, 139
Weil–Felix test, 1391
Weil's syndrome, 1312
Weintraub's syndrome, 824
Wenckebach phenomenon, 626
Werdnig–Hoffman disease, 72 (Table), 720, 753
Wernicke's area, 814
Western blot, 70
Western equine encephalitis, 1389
West Germany, vs East Germany, atopy, 492
West's syndrome, 676, 688 (Table), see also Infantile spasms
  treatment, **687**
Wet dressings, atopic eczema, 1642–1643
Wetting problems, **957**
  urinary tract infection prevention, 956
Wheelchairs
  cerebral palsy, 758
  Duchenne muscular dystrophy, 731
Wheeze, 491, **508, 512–513**
  and asthma, 536
  gastroesophageal reflux, 571
  history taking, 17
  physiology, 499
  pneumonia, 566
  toxocariasis, 1485
  viral infections, 540, 541, 565
Wheezy baby syndrome, 539–540
Whey proteins, vs caseins, infant formula, 332, 1188
Whiff test, bacterial vaginosis, 1435
Whiplash shaking injury, **700–701,** 705
  encephalopathy, 695
  stroke, 714
Whipworm (Trichuris trichiuria), **1491–1492**
Whispering pectoriloquy, 30

Whistling face syndrome, 811
White cell counts
  bacteremia, 1286–1287
  cerebrospinal fluid, 1290
  differential, pertussis, 562
White pupil (leukocoria), 268
White spirit, poisoning, 1705, 1711
White-tailed spider, bites, 1525
Whitfield's ointment, 1979 (Table)
Whitlow, herpetic, 1364
Whole cell vaccine, pertussis, 345
Whoop, pertussis, 1315
Widal test, 1326
Wilkie's syndrome (superior mesenteric artery syndrome), **1787–1788**
Williams–Campbell syndrome, 576
Williams syndrome, 59, 818, 833 (Table), 1197
  calcitonin, 1058
  heart, 596
Wilms' tumor, see Nephroblastoma
Wilson–Mikity syndrome, **195**
Wilson's disease, **481,** 791 (Table), 1145–1146, 1202
  eye, 1674
  hemolysis, 864
Wimberger's sign, 1412
Winchester syndrome, 1157 (Table)
Window cleaner, poisoning, 1709
Windows, falls from, 1715
Windswept deformity, 749
Wing & Gould's classification, psychosis, 835–836
Wiskott–Aldrich syndrome, 444, 878, 1242 (Table), 1245, **1253–1254**
  neoplasms, 889 (Table), 1248 (Table)
  and vaccines, 1267
Witch's milk, 110, 1039
Withdrawal, see Drug withdrawal
Withdrawal reflex, 37 (Table), 241–242
Withdrawing neonatal intensive care, **100–103,** 173
Wolffian ducts, 253, 1004
Wolff–Parkinson–White syndrome, **625**
  congenitally corrected transposition of great arteries, 616
Wolf–Hirschhorn syndrome, **58**
Wolfram syndrome (DIDMOAD syndrome), 1081
Wolman's disease, 776 (Table), 1154–1155
  neonate, 308
Wood's light, tinea diagnosis, 1637
Wool, atopic eczema, 1642
Woolsorter's disease, 1300
Word blindness, congenital, 821
Word deafness, 807
Word processors, dysgraphia, 825
Working mothers, 15 (Table), **1860–1861**
Work of stretch, 756
World, see also Geography
  infections, **1275–1276**
World Health Organization
  accident prevention, 1713
  acute respiratory illness program, 490, 493, 567
  AIDS definition, 1393, **1395**
  central nervous system tumor classification, 900 (Table)
  contact address, 1889 (Fig.)
  electrolyte solution, 413
  emerging infections, 1278
  endemic treponematoses, policies, 1420
  filariasis, 1496
  health initiatives, 1888–1889
  immunization
    guidelines, 346 (Table)
    schedules, 344
  immunodeficiency classification, 1241–1242
  live births definition, 1849

  lower respiratory tract infections, 565–566
  Maternal Health and Safe Motherhood Program, 1891
  neonates, definitions, 94
  oral rehydration solutions, **453,** 1296
  pertussis diagnosis, 1316–1317
World population, 1, **2**
World Summit for Children 1990, 1884–1885, 1886
Worm load
  ascariasis, 1482–1483
  enterobiasis, 1487
  hookworm, 1489
  Trichuris trichiuria, 1491
Worster Drought syndrome, 813
Wounds
  antibiotic prophylaxis, 1529
  cleansing, rabies, 1377
  closure, **1833**
  maggots, 1514
Wrapping, compressive, head, 664
Wrist drop, vincristine, 896
Writing disorders, 821–824
Wuchereria bancrofti, 1496 (Table), **1498**
  specimens, 1299

Xanthine oxidase, 127
  deficiency, see Combined sulfite oxidase and xanthine oxidase deficiency
Xanthine oxidase inhibitors, 131
Xanthinuria, 1141
Xanthochromia, 703, 710
  cerebrospinal fluid, neonate, 242
Xanthurenic aciduria, 1114
X chromosome inactivation studies, 1248
X chromosomes
  extra, 62
  hereditary hypophosphatemia, 948
  lyonization, 67, 948
Xenodiagnosis, 1459
Xenon-133, 517, 1897
Xeroderma pigmentosa, 70, 1142, 1254, **1630**
  neoplasms, 888 (Table), 1630
Xerophthalmia, 1194
X-linked agammaglobulinemia, 1242 (Table), 1255
  incidence, 1243 (Table)
  neoplasms, 1248 (Table)
X-linked chronic granulomatous disease, 1242 (Table)
X-linked dominant inheritance, **67**
X-linked hyperIgM syndrome, 1242 (Table)
X-linked hypogammaglobulinemia, bacteriophage X174 antibody test, 1245
X-linked hypophosphatemia, 260, **948**
X-linked lymphoproliferative syndrome, 1242 (Table), 1251, see also Duncan's syndrome
  neoplasms, 1248 (Table)
X-linked myotubular myopathy, 735 (Table)
X-linked recessive inheritance, **66–67**
  Fabry disease, 1164
  Hunter's syndrome, 1160
X-linked severe combined immunodeficiency syndrome, 1242 (Table), 1250
X-ray departments, 1894
X-rays, 1895
  generators, 1894
XX males, 62, 1010
47XXX (triple X), **62**
49XXXXY, **62**
48XXXY, **62**
Xylometazoline, 1979 (Table)

Xylose absorption test, 1938 (Table)
Xylulose, urine, 1131
XYY syndrome, **62**

Yaws, **1417–1418**
  and congenital syphilis, 1411
  control, 1419
  organism, 1401
Y chromosome
  Q-banding, 49
  sex-determining region, 1004
  Turner's syndrome, 1032
Yeast cells, feces, 1472
Yeast HBs vaccines, 1387
Yeast opsonization defect, 1263
Yellow fever, **1389**
Yellow mutant albinism, 1629 (Table)
Yersinia pestis, 1318
Yew, poisoning, 1711
Yolk sac, 206
  hemopoiesis, 847
Yolk sac tumor, see Endodermal sinus tumor
Yom Kippur, fasting, 1083
Y protein (ligandin), 214
Yupik Eskimos, congenital adrenal hyperplasia, 47

'Zambezi' group, trypanosomes, 1454
ZAP 70, 1239
  deficiency, 1242 (Table), 1250
Zellweger-like phenotype with structurally intact peroxisomes, 308
Zellweger-like syndrome, 785 (Table), 1174
Zellweger syndrome, 785 (Table), 1171 (Fig.), **1172–1173**
  on brain development, 642
  cerebellum, 753
  hemosiderosis, 1147
  neonate, 308
    seizures, 245
  retinal dystrophy, 271
Zidovudine, 1397
  administration, 1979 (Table)
  drug resistance, 1530
Zimbabwe, anthrax epidemic, 1300
Zinc, 1185 (Table)
  breast milk, 332
  Crohn's disease, 457
  deficiency, 444, 447, 1188, **1201, 1627,** 1892
    immunodeficiency, 1266
    on insulin-like growth factor, 1023
  for malnutrition, 1193
  metabolism disorders, **1147**
  normal values, 1929 (Table)
  parenteral nutrition, 1221
  Recommended Dietary Allowances, 1949 (Table)
  reference nutrient intakes, 1947 (Table)
  requirements, 1181 (Table)
    preterm infant, 152 (Table)
  sources, 1185 (Table)
Zinc acetate, for Wilson's disease, 1146
Zinc sulfate, for Wilson's disease, 481
Z-lumirubin, 216
  loose stools, 218
Zollinger–Ellison syndrome, 432
  multiple endocrine neoplasia syndrome, 1056
Zones, adrenal cortex, 1059
Zonular cataract, 1668, 1669
Zoster, see Herpes zoster
Zoster immune globulin, 1361, 1362
Zoster varicellosa, 1362
Zovirax, see Acyclovir
Zymogens, blood coagulation, 227

DEPT. OF PGMDE